W0331674

PEDIATRIA
di
NELSON

Dello stesso editore

Bartolozzi G., Guglielmi M. et al – Pediatria – III edizione (con CD-Rom)
Cattorini P. – Bioetica – III edizione
Fabrizi G. – Dermatologia pediatrica
Fabrizi G., Massi G. – Nevi e melanomi nel bambino
Graziella Fava Vizziello (a cura di) – Paternità in cerca d'autore
Italian Resuscitation Council, Società Italiana di Medicina d'Emergenza e Urgenza Pediatrica – PALS – Pediatric Advanced Life Support – Supporto delle funzioni vitali in pediatria
Lorini R., Di Pietro P., Romano C. (a cura di) – Pediatria d'urgenza
Marcelli D. – Psicopatologia del bambino – VI edizione
Moroni M., Esposito R., De Lalla F. – Malattie infettive – VII edizione (con CD-Rom)
Netter F.H. – Atlante di anatomia umana – III edizione (con CD-Rom)
Parigi G.B. – Chirurgia pediatrica
Pavone L., Ruggieri M. – Neurologia pediatrica – II edizione
Rapoport J.L., Ismond D.R. – DSM-IV. Guida alla diagnosi dei disturbi dell'infanzia e dell'adolescenza
Sadler T.W. – Embriologia medica di Langman – IV edizione
Ugazio A.G., Cavagni G. – Il bambino con infezioni ricorrenti
Villani A., Serafini G. – Anestesia neonatale e pediatrica

Per una consultazione dell'intero catalogo, visitate il sito Internet **www.elsevier.it**

PEDIATRIA di NELSON

Robert M. Kliegman, MD
Professor and Chair
Department of Pediatrics
Medical College of Wisconsin
Pediatrician-in-Chief
Pamela and Leslie Muma Chair in Pediatrics
Children's Hospital of Wisconsin
Executive Vice President
Children's Research Institute
Milwaukee, Wisconsin

Richard E. Behrman, MD
Clinical Professor, Department of Pediatrics
University of California, San Francisco
San Francisco, California
George Washington University
Washington, DC

Hal B. Jenson, MD
Chief Academic Officer
Baystate Health
Dean of the Western Campus of Tufts University
School of Medicine
Springfield, Massachusetts

Bonita F. Stanton, MD
Professor and Schotanus Family Endowed Chair
Carman and Ann Adams Department
of Pediatrics
Wayne State University
Pediatrician-in-Chief
Children's Hospital of Michigan
Detroit Medical Center
Detroit, Michigan

18ª EDIZIONE

VOLUME 2

Presentazione dell'edizione italiana di
Pasquale Di Pietro
Presidente della Società Italiana di Pediatria

ELSEVIER

MASSON

Titolo originale: Nelson Textbook of Pediatrics, 18/E
Copyright © 2007 by Saunders, an imprint of Elsevier Inc.

Books Publishing Director: Tiziano Strambini
Developmental Editor: Paola Leschiera

Production Director: Cristian Bertilaccio
Books Production Manager: Ornella Ceresa

Realizzazione editoriale: ART Servizi Editoriali S.p.A. - Bologna
Traduzione dalla lingua inglese: Ada Lisa Badocco, Alessandro Ballestrazzi, Silvia Bianchi, Luca Boccaccio, Laura Fenati, Elena Gentilcore, Gabriele Guerini Rocco, Silvia Adelina Mainardi, Alessandra Meneghel, Alda Maria Olivero, Gloria Anna Maria Rossi, Barbara Sambo, Calogero Trapani, Elisa Trevisan, Ornella Trunfio

Revisione scientifica della traduzione: Stefano Alboresi, Medico chirurgo con specializzazione in Pediatria Preventiva e Puericultura; Alessandro Ballestrazzi, Medico chirurgo con specializzazione in Pediatria e Fisioterapia; Luigi Nespoli, Professore ordinario di Pediatria, Direttore Clinica Pediatrica, Università degli Studi dell'Insubria, Varese

© 2009 Elsevier Srl - Tutti i diritti riservati
Printed in China

ISBN 978-88-214-3070-1

I diritti di traduzione, di memorizzazione elettronica, di riproduzione e adattamento totale o parziale, con qualsiasi mezzo (compresi i microfilm e le copie fotostatiche), sono riservati per tutti i Paesi. Tuttavia il lettore potrà effettuare fotocopie per uso personale nei limiti del 15% del presente volume dietro pagamento alla SIAE del compenso previsto dall'art. 68, comma 4, della legge 22 aprile 1941 n. 633 ovvero dall'accordo stipulato tra SIAE, AIE, SNS e CNA, CONFARTIGIANATO, CASA, CLAAI, CONFCOMMERCIO, CONFESERCENTI il 18 dicembre 2000.

Le riproduzioni ad uso differente da quello personale potranno avvenire, per un numero di pagine non superiore al 15% del presente volume, solo a seguito di specifica autorizzazione rilasciata da: AIDRO, via delle Erbe 2, 20121 Milano, telefax 02 809506, e-mail: aidro@iol.it.

La medicina è una scienza in continua evoluzione. La ricerca e l'esperienza clinica ampliano costantemente le nostre conoscenze, soprattutto in relazione alle modalità terapeutiche e alla farmacologia. Qualora il testo faccia riferimento al dosaggio o alla posologia di farmaci, il lettore può essere certo che autori, curatori ed editore hanno fatto il possibile per garantire che tali riferimenti siano conformi allo stato delle conoscenze al momento della pubblicazione del libro. Tuttavia, si consiglia il lettore di leggere attentamente i foglietti illustrativi dei farmaci per verificare personalmente se i dosaggi raccomandati o le controindicazioni specificate differiscano da quanto indicato nel testo. Ciò è particolarmente importante nel caso di farmaci usati raramente o immessi di recente sul mercato.

ELSEVIER

Elsevier Srl
Via Paleocapa 7, 20121 Milano – Tel. 02.88.184.1
Sito Internet: www.elsevier.it

Finito di stampare nel mese di Gennaio 2009 presso "China Translation & Printing Services" Ltd, Hong Kong

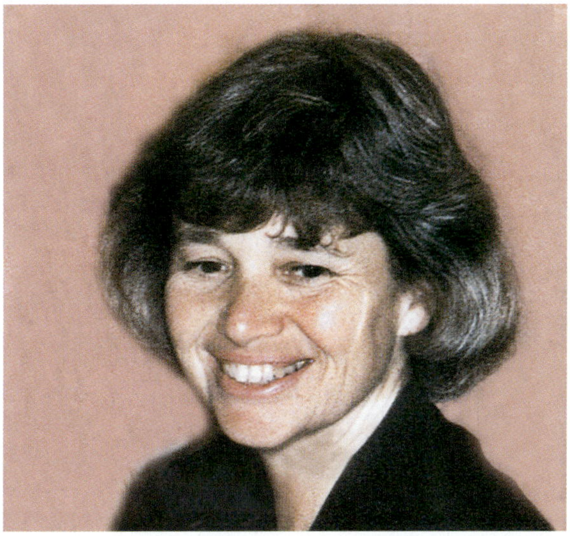

Questa edizione è dedicata ad Ann Nelson Behrman, che vivrà per sempre nei nostri cuori come moglie, madre, nonna, educatrice e amica amorevole e devota. Ann è strettamente legata a molte delle edizioni del Nelson Textbook of Pediatrics e sarà ricordata per il suo insaziabile amore per la vita, la curiosità intellettuale, lo stile aggraziato e il sincero impegno per tutti i bambini. La sua gentilezza e il suo calore hanno illuminato non solo la sua famiglia ma anche i numerosi studenti, medici e professori che ha accolto nella sua casa. A noi tutti manca profondamente.

Presentazione dell'edizione italiana

Con grande piacere ho accettato l'invito di Elsevier a presentare l'edizione italiana della diciottesima edizione del *Nelson Textbook of Pediatrics* che, ancora una volta, rispetta le aspettative della comunità pediatrica che ha sempre visto in questo trattato la "bibbia" della Pediatria. È un testo completo, aggiornato, facile da consultare, nonostante la grande massa di informazioni contenute, e complemento indispensabile per tutti i pediatri.

Pur rimanendo nella sua struttura generale uguale alle altre edizioni, il volume propone molte novità e parecchi capitoli sono stati rivoluzionati, modificati e aggiornati alla luce delle più recenti ricerche.

La caratteristica più importante di questo testo è la maniera organica con cui vengono descritte le varie problematiche; nella sua sintesi c'è tutto e chi lo consulta riesce ad inquadrare il problema. È un testo che il pediatra, sia ospedaliero sia di famiglia, non può non avere vicino e consultare quando nella pratica assistenziale lo assalgano i dubbi diagnostici.

È molto interessante sfogliare le edizioni precedenti e constatare il progressivo modificarsi dei concetti e lo sforzo di proporre gli aggiornamenti con saggezza, in accordo con il progredire della ricerca medica.

Un'importante novità di questa edizione è uno spazio molto più ampio dedicato alla pediatria generale, con i contributi del nuovo Editor Bonita F. Stanton. Tutti i pediatri trarranno vantaggio dalle novità descritte in relazione alle differenti terapie: antibiotica, antivirale, antiparassitaria, antimicotica e altre. La farmacoterapia è stata aggiornata senza tralasciare indicazioni precise sui dosaggi da utilizzare.

Il "Nelson" rimane a tutt'oggi il testo più consultato dai pediatri e basta visitare uno studio medico per constatare come sia il libro più "consumato".

Una domanda sorge spontanea: nell'era di Internet è ancora utile un testo dove si descrive sistematicamente la quasi totalità delle patologie pediatriche? La risposta è sì perché proprio la moltitudine di informazioni che si possono trarre consultando Internet pone al pediatra il problema di saper scegliere tra le informazioni che servono e quelle che si devono scartare. Internet non "filtra" ciò che ha evidenza scientifica da ciò che non ne ha.

Il grande pregio di questo testo è di permettere al pediatra un aggiornamento facile, veloce, preciso e sicuro su tutti i temi della Pediatria moderna al fine di fornirgli informazioni che possano aiutarlo sempre a fare scelte corrette per il proprio paziente.

Pasquale Di Pietro

AVVERTENZA PER IL LETTORE
I dati forniti si riferiscono agli Stati Uniti. Il lettore deve quindi tenere presente, soprattutto per quanto riguarda ad esempio il calendario delle vaccinazioni o le terapie proposte, che i farmaci e i relativi dosaggi si riferiscono alla pratica clinica statunitense.

Prefazione

La 18ª edizione del *Nelson Textbook of Pediatrics* unisce un'importante sintesi della pediatria clinica con le ultime acquisizioni nel campo della genomica, della diagnostica, delle tecniche di imaging e della terapeutica. La 18ª edizione continua a rappresentare lo "stato dell'arte" della cura del neonato, del bambino e dell'adolescente, in buona salute e malato, fornendo sia il quadro della medicina basata su evidenze sia le più significative esperienze cliniche di Autori di fama internazionale.

La promessa che la medicina traslazionale migliorerà la vita di tutti i bambini è più grande che mai. La conoscenza dello sviluppo, del comportamento e delle malattie umane, dal livello molecolare a quello sociologico, sta avanzando a una velocità eccezionale. Questo ha portato a una più profonda comprensione delle condizioni di salute e di malattia del bambino, così come a un sostanziale miglioramento della qualità dell'assistenza sanitaria per coloro che hanno accesso alle cure mediche. Questi straordinari progressi scientifici fanno inoltre sperare di poter combattere in modo efficiente le nuove malattie che minacciano i bambini e le loro famiglie.

Purtroppo molti bambini di tutto il mondo non beneficiano dei significativi passi avanti compiuti nella prevenzione e nel trattamento dei problemi sanitari, innanzitutto per mancanza di volontà politica e per un'errata valutazione delle priorità. Inoltre, molti bambini sono esposti ai rischi sostanziali derivanti dagli effetti avversi della povertà, della guerra e del bioterrorismo. Per far sì che le nostre crescenti conoscenze rechino vantaggio a tutti i bambini e a tutti i ragazzi, è necessario che i progressi medici e una buona pratica clinica si sposino con una legislazione efficace.

Questa nuova edizione del *Nelson Textbook of Pediatrics* si propone di fornire i contenuti essenziali che medici, staff infermieristico, studenti di medicina e altri care provider impegnati nell'assistenza pediatrica sono tenuti a conoscere per gestire in modo efficace l'enorme gamma di problemi biologici, psicologici e sociali che i nostri bambini e i nostri ragazzi possono incontrare. È nostro scopo fornire un testo esaustivo e allo stesso tempo conciso e di facile lettura, abbracciando sia le ultime novità scientifiche sia l'arte della pratica pediatrica più consacrata dal tempo.

La 18ª edizione è frutto di una riorganizzazione e revisione sostanziale della precedente edizione. Nuovi capitoli sono stati aggiunti, con la trattazione di nuove malattie, e altri sono stati notevolmente ampliati o modificati. Sono state inoltre inserite numerose tabelle, fotografie, immagini diagnostiche ed esplicative, oltre a riferimenti bibliografici aggiornati. Ogni argomento è stato analizzato allo scopo di aggiornarne e migliorarne l'esposizione, per la massima utilità di coloro che si occupano di fornire assistenza sanitaria in ambito pediatrico.

Anche la patologia più rara è di importanza centrale per un bambino che ne è affetto e per la sua famiglia, così come per il medico che lo ha in cura; tuttavia, non è stato possibile affrontare tutti i problemi sanitari con lo stesso grado di approfondimento in un unico testo generale di Pediatria come il presente. Perciò, sono inclusi nella bibliografia articoli generali e testi specialistici, che devono essere consultati ogniqualvolta si rendono necessarie ulteriori informazioni.

L'indiscutibile valore della 18ª edizione del testo si deve ai suoi esperti e autorevoli Autori. Noi tutti siamo debitori nei loro confronti per il duro lavoro svolto, per la competenza, la capacità di analisi e il buon senso. Un sincero apprezzamento va inoltre a Judy Fletcher e a Jennifer Shreiner della Elsevier e a Carolyn Redman del Pediatric Department of the Medical College of Wisconsin. Abbiamo tutti lavorato sodo per pubblicare un'edizione che potesse essere d'aiuto a coloro che forniscono assistenza a neonati e bambini e a coloro che desiderano sapere di più della salute infantile a tutto campo.

Per questa edizione abbiamo potuto contare sul contributo informale di molti medici e membri del personale del Medical College of Wisconsin e della Wayne State University School of Medicine. L'aiuto di queste persone e di numerosi pediatri di tutto il mondo, che hanno speso tempo per offrire il loro ponderato feedback e i loro suggerimenti, è sempre molto gradito e di grande utilità.

In ultimo, ma non certo per importanza, desideriamo ringraziare le nostre famiglie per la pazienza e la comprensione, senza le quali realizzare questo libro non sarebbe stato possibile.

Robert M. Kliegman, MD
Richard E. Behrman, MD
Hal B. Jenson, MD
Bonita F. Stanton, MD

Autori

Amy C. Abraham, PhD
Volunteer Clinical Faculty, Department of Psychiatry, Tulane University Health Sciences Center, School of Medicine; Clinical Psychologist, Lafayette Psychotherapy Group, New Orleans, Louisiana

Jon S. Abramson, MD
Professor and Chair of Pediatrics, Wake Forest University School of Medicine, Winston-Salem, North Carolina

Mark J. Abzug, MD
Professor of Pediatrics (Pediatric Infectious Diseases), University of Colorado School of Medicine; The Children's Hospital, Denver, Colorado

James D. Acton, MD
Assistant Professor, Department of Pediatrics, University of Cincinnati College of Medicine; Director, Cystic Fibrosis Center, Division of Pulmonary Medicine, Cincinnati Children's Hospital Medical Center, Cincinnati, Ohio

Ira Adams-Chapman, MD
Assistant Professor of Pediatrics, Department of Pediatrics, Division of Nematology, Emory University School of Medicine; Medical Director, Developmental Progress Clinic, Emory University School of Medicine, Atlanta, Georgia

Hoover Adger, Jr., MD, MPH
Professor of Pediatrics, Johns Hopkins University School of Medicine; Professor of Pediatrics, Johns Hopkins Hospital, Baltimore, Maryland

John Aiken, MD
Associate Professor of Surgery, Medical College of Wisconsin, Milwaukee, Wisconsin

Hassan H. A-Kader, MD
Associate Professor of Pediatrics; Chief, Division of Gastroenterology, Hepatology, and Nutrition, University of Arizona, Tucson, Arizona

Ramin Alemzadeh, MD
Associate Professor of Pediatrics, Section of Endocrinology and Diabetes, Medical College of Wisconsin; Director, Diabetes Program, Children's Hospital of Wisconsin, Milwaukee, Wisconsin

Karl E. Anderson, MD
Professor, Department of Preventive Medicine and Community Health, Internal Medicine, and Pharmacology and Toxicology; Staff, University of Texas Medical Branch, Galveston, Texas

Alia Antoon, MD
Assistant Clinical Professor, Harvard Medical School; Chief of Pediatrics, Shriners Hospital for Children, Shriners Burns Hospital, Boston, Massachusetts

Jacob V. Aranda, MD, PhD, FRCPC, FAAP
Professor, Department of Pediatrics, Pharmacology and Pharmaceutical Sciences, Wayne State University School of Medicine and College of Pharmacy and Allied Health; Director, Clinical Pharmacology and Toxicology and the Pediatric Pharmacology Research Unit Network (PPRU), Children's Hospital of Michigan, Detroit, Michigan

Carola A.S. Arndt, MD
Associate Professor of Pediatric and Adolescent Medicine, Chair, Division of Pediatric Hematology/Oncology, Mayo Clinic, Rochester, Minnesota

Stephen S. Arnon, MD
Founder and Chief, Infant Botulism Treatment and Prevention Program, California Department of Health Services, Richmond, California

Stephen C. Aronoff, MD, MBA
Professor and Chairman of Pediatrics, Temple University School of Medicine; Temple University Children's Medical Center, Philadelphia, Pennsylvania

David M. Asher, MD
Chief, Laboratory of Bacterial, Parasitic and Unconventional Agents, Division of Emerging and Transfusion-Transmitted Diseases, Office of Blood Research and Review, Center for Biologics Evaluation and Research, U.S. Food and Drug Administration, Kensington, Maryland

Joann L. Ater, MD
Professor of Pediatrics, University of Texas M.D. Anderson Cancer Center; Professor of Pediatrics, Children's Cancer Hospital, University of Texas M.D. Anderson Cancer Center, Houston, Texas

Dan Atkins, MD
Assistant Professor of Pediatrics, University of Colorado Health Sciences Center; Professor of Pediatrics, Director, Ambulatory Pediatrics, National Jewish Medical and Research Center, Denver, Colorado

Marilyn Augustyn, MD
Associate Professor, Boston University; Assistant Director, Division of Developmental and Behavioral Pediatrics, Boston Medical Center, Boston, Massachusetts

Ellis D. Avner, MD
Associate Dean for Research and Professor of Pediatrics (Nephrology), Medical College of Wisconsin; Director, Children's Research Institute, Children's Hospital Health System of Wisconsin, Milwaukee, Wisconsin

Parvin H. Azimi, MD
Clinical Professor of Pediatrics, University of California, San Francisco, San Francisco, California; Director of Children's Hospital and Research Center at Oakland, Oakland, California

Thomas Bahk, MD
Assistant Professor, Department of Pediatrics, Loma Linda University Medical Center, Loma Linda, California

William F. Balistreri, MD
Medical Director, Pediatric Liver Care Center; Associate Chair for Subspecialty Training, Department of Pediatrics, Cincinnati Children's Hospital Medical Center, Cincinnati, Ohio

Robert S. Baltimore, MD, FAAP
Professor of Pediatrics and Epidemiology, Departments of Pediatrics and of Epidemiology and Public Health, Yale University School of Medicine; Attending Physician, Pediatrics, Yale-New Haven Children's Hospital, New Haven, Connecticut

Shahida Baqar, PhD
Infectious Diseases Directorate, Enteric Diseases Department, Naval Medical Research Center, Silver Spring, Maryland

Fred F. Barrett, MD
Professor of Pediatrics (Retired), University of Tennessee Health Science Center; Medical Director, LeBonheur Children's Medical Center, Memphis, Tennessee

Christine E. Barron, MD
Assistant Professor of Pediatrics, Brown Medical School; Clinical Director, Child Protection Program, Hasbro Children's Hospital, Providence, Rhode Island

Dorsey M. Bass, MD
Associate Professor of Pediatrics, Stanford University; Attending Physician, Gastroenterology, Lucile Salter Packard Children's Hospital, Stanford, California

Michael D. Bates, MD, PhD
Assistant Professor, Department of Pediatrics, University of Cincinnati College of Medicine; Division of Gastroenterology, Hepatology and Nutrition; Division of Developmental Biology, Cincinnati Children's Hospital Medical Center, Cincinnati, Ohio

Mark Batshaw, MD
Professor and Chair of Pediatrics, George Washington University; Chief Academic Officer, Children's Hospital National Medical Center, Washington, District of Columbia

Howard Bauchner, MD
Boston University School of Medicine; Boston Medical Center, Boston, Massachusetts

Richard E. Behrman, MD
Clinical Professor of Pediatrics, University of California, San Francisco, San Francisco, California; George Washington University, Washington, District of Columbia; Stanford University, Stanford, California; Lucile Salter Packard Children's Hospital, Palo Alto, California; Executive Chair, Federation of Pediatric Organizations, Pediatric Education Steering Committee, Menlo Park, California

Michael J. Bennett, PhD
Professor of Pathology and Laboratory Medicine, University of Pennsylvania; Director, Metabolic Disease Laboratory, Children's Hospital of Philadelphia, Philadelphia, Pennsylvania

Daniel Bernstein, MD
Alfred Woodley Salter and Mabel G. Salter Endowed Professor, Chief, Division of Pediatric Cardiology, Stanford University; Co-Director Children's Heart Center, Lucile Salter Packard Children's Hospital, Palo Alto, California

Michelle Bestic, PharmD
Instructor of Pediatrics, Case Western Reserve University; Division of Pediatric Clinical Pharmacology and Toxicology, Rainbow Babies and Children's Hospital, Cleveland, Ohio

Zulfiqar Ahmed Bhutta, MB, FRCP, FRCPCH, FCPS, PhD
Husein Lalji Dewraj Professor and Chairman of Pediatrics and Child Health, Aga Khan University, Karachi, Pakistan

Leslie G. Biesecker, MD
Adjunct Associate Professor, Johns Hopkins University School of Public Health; Chief, Genetic Disease Research Branch, National Human Genome Research Institute, National Institutes of Health; NIH Clinical Center, National Institutes of Health, Bethesda, Maryland

Ari Bitnum, MD, MSc, FRCPC
Assistant Professor of Pediatrics, University of Toronto; Staff Physician, Pediatrics (Division of Infectious Diseases) Hospital for Sick Children, Toronto, Ontario, Canada

Samra S. Blanchard, MD
Associate Professor of Pediatrics, Division of Pediatric Gastroenterology, University of Maryland School of Medicine, Baltimore, Maryland

Ronald Blanton, MD, MSc
Center for Global Health and Disease, Case Western Reserve Institute; Attending Physician, Wade Park Veterans' Administration Hospital, Cleveland, Ohio

Archie Bleyer, MD
Professor and Mosbacher Chair of Pediatrics, University of Texas; Director, Community Clinical Oncology Program, University of Texas M.D. Anderson Cancer Center, Houston, Texas

Lynell Boamah, MD
Fellow, Pediatric Gastroenterology, Hepatology, and Nutrition, Cincinnati Children's Hospital Medical Center, Cincinnati, Ohio

Steven R. Boas, MD
Associate Professor of Pediatrics, Northwestern University, Feinberg School of Medicine; Pediatric Pulmonologist, Evanston Hospital, Evanston, Illinois, Children's Memorial Hospital, Chicago, Illinois

Thomas F. Boat, MD
Professor and Chair, Department of Pediatrics, University of Cincinnati College of Medicine; Chair, Department of Pediatrics, Director, Cincinnati Children's Research Foundation, Cincinnati Children's Hospital Medical Center, Cincinnati, Ohio

Mark Boguniewicz, MD
Professor, Division of Pediatric Allergy-Immunology, Department of Pediatrics, National Jewish Medical and Research Center and University of Colorado School of Medicine, Denver, Colorado

Robert A. Bonomo, MD
Associate Professor of Medicine, Pharmacology, and Molecular Biology and Microbiology, Case Western Reserve School of Medicine; Section Chief, Infectious Diseases, Louis Stokes Cleveland Veterans' Affairs Medical Center, Cleveland, Ohio

Neil W. Boris, MD
Associate Professor, Community Health Sciences, Tulane University School of Public Health and Tropical Medicine; Associate Professor of Psychiatry and Neurology, Tulane University Health Sciences Center, New Orleans, Louisiana

Christopher M. Borrillo, MD
Assistant Professor of Child and Adolescent Psychiatry, Tulane University School of Medicine; Southeast Louisiana Hospital, Youth Services, Mandeville, Louisiana, Jefferson Parish Human Services Authority, Division of Child and Family Services, Metairie, Louisiana

Laurence A. Boxer, MD
Professor and Director, Division of Pediatric Hematology/Oncology, Vice-Chair, Department of Pediatrics, Henry and Mala Dorfman Family Professor in Pediatric Hematology/Oncology, University of Michigan; Director, Pediatric Hematology/Oncology, C.S. Mott Children's Hospital, Ann Arbor, Michigan

Mary Brigid Bradley, MD
Associate Professor of Clinic Pediatrics, Columbia University; Assistant Attending Pediatrician, Morgan Stanley Children's Hospital of New York Presbyterian, New York, New York

David Branski, MD
Professor of Pediatrics, Hebrew University Medical School; Professor and Chair of Pediatric Departments, Hadassah University Hospitals, Jerusalem, Israel

David T. Breault, MD, PhD
Instructor in Pediatrics, Harvard Medical School; Assistant in Medicine, Division of Endocrinology, Children's Hospital Boston, Boston, Massachusetts

W. Ted Brown, MD, PhD
Chair, Department of Human Genetics, Director, George A. Jervis Clinic; Director, New York State Institute for Basic Research in Developmental Disabilities, Staten Island, New York

Rebecca H. Buckley, MD
J. Buren Sidbury Professor of Pediatrics, Professor of Immunology, Duke University Medical Center, Durham, North Carolina

Cynthia Budek, MS
Pediatric Nurse Practitioner, Children's Memorial Hospital, Chicago, Illinois

E. Stephen Buescher, MD
Professor of Pediatrics, Eastern Virginia Medical School, Norfolk, Virginia

Karen Burns, MD, MS
Assistant Professor of Clinical Pediatrics, Department of Hematology and Oncology, Cincinnati Children's Hospital Medical Center, Cincinnati, Ohio

Mitchell S. Cairo
Professor of Pediatric Medicine and Pathology, Columbia University; Division Head, Pediatrics, Morgan Stanley Children's Hospital of New York Presbyterian, New York, New York

Bruce M. Camitta, MD
Rebecca Jean Slye Professor of Pediatrics, Medical College of Wisconsin; Director, Midwest Children's Cancer Center, Pediatrics (Hematology and Oncology), Children's Hospital of Wisconsin, Milwaukee, Wisconsin

Rebecca G. Carey, MD
Fellow, Pediatric Gastroenterology, Hepatology and Nutrition, University of Cincinnati; Fellow, Pediatric Gastroenterology, Hepatology and Nutrition, Cincinnati Children's Hospital Medical Center, Cincinnati, Ohio

Andrew J. Carroll, III, PhD
Professor of Genetics, University of Alabama at Birmingham, Birmingham, Alabama

James T. Cassidy, MD
Professor Emeritus, Child Health-Pediatric Rheumatology, University of Missouri Health Care, Columbia, Missouri

Ellen Gould Chadwick, MD
Professor of Pediatrics, Northwestern University, Feinberg School of Medicine; Associate Director, Section of Pediatric, Adolescent, and Maternal HIV Infection, Division of Infectious Diseases, Children's Memorial Hospital, Chicago, Illinois

Sharon F. Chen, MD, MS
Department of Pediatric Infectious Diseases, Stanford University; Attending Physician, Department of Pediatric Infectious Diseases, Lucile Packard Children's Hospital, Stanford University Medical Center, Stanford, California

Yuan-Tsong Chen, MD, PhD
Professor of Pediatrics and Genetics, Duke University; Duke University Medical Center, Durham, North Carolina

Wanda L. Chenoweth, PhD, RD
Professor Emeritus, Department of Food Science and Human Nutrition, Michigan State University, East Lansing, Michigan

Russell W. Chesney, MD
Le Bonheur Professor and Chair, Department of Pediatrics, University of Tennessee Health Science Center; Vice President for Academic Affairs, Le Bonheur Children's Medical Center, Memphis, Tennessee

Robert D. Christensen, MD
Director of Research, Department of Neonatology, Intermountain Healthcare, Inc.; Medical Director, Department of Neonatology, Urban North Area, Intermountain Healthcare, Inc., Ogden, Utah

Theodore J. Cieslak, MD
Clinical Professor of Pediatrics, University of Texas Health Science Center at San Antonio, San Antonio, Texas; Clinical Associate Professor of Pediatrics, Uniformed Services University of the Health Sciences, Bethesda, Maryland; Chairman, San Antonio Military Pediatric Center, Fort Sam Houston, Texas

Thomas G. Cleary, MD
Professor of Pediatrics, University of Texas Medical School, Houston, Houston, Texas

Pinchas Cohen, MD
Professor of Pediatrics, David Geffen School of Medicine at University of California, Los Angeles; Chief, Endocrinology, Mattel Children's Hospital at University of California, Los Angeles

F. Sessions Cole, MD
Park J. White, MD, Professor of Pediatrics, Assistant Vice Chancellor for Children's Health, Washington University School of Medicine; Director, Division of Newborn Medicine, Chief Medical Officer Pediatrics, St. Louis Children's Hospital, St. Louis, Missouri

John L. Colombo, MD
Professor of Pediatrics, University of Nebraska College of Medicine; Chief, Pediatric Pulmonology, University of Nebraska, Omaha, Nebraska

Anne Comi, MD
Assistant Professor, Neurology and Pediatrics, Kennedy Krieger Institute, Johns Hopkins University School of Medicine; Faculty, Neurology and Developmental Medicine, Kennedy Krieger Institute, Baltimore, Maryland

Tania Condurache, MD
Resident in Pediatrics, University of Louisville School of Medicine, Louisville, Kentucky

Arnold Coran, MD
Professor of Surgery, Section of Pediatric Surgery, University of Michigan, Ann Arbor, Michigan

Roger Cornwall, MD
Assistant Professor of Orthopaedic Surgery, University of Pennsylvania School of Medicine; Attending Pediatric Hand and Upper Extremity Surgeon, Children's Hospital of Philadelphia, Philadelphia, Pennsylvania

Ronina A. Covar, MD
Assistant Professor of Pediatrics, University of Colorado Health Sciences Center; Assistant Professor of Pediatrics, National Jewish Medical and Research Center, Denver, Colorado

Kenneth L. Cox, MD
Professor, Pediatrics; Division Chief, Division of Pediatric Gastroenterology, Hepatology, and Nutrition, Lucile Salter Packard Children's Hospital, Palo Alto, California

Susan E. Crawford, MD
Research Associate, Pediatric Infectious Diseases, University of Chicago; Clinical Instructor, General Academic Pediatrics, Children's Memorial Hospital, Chicago, Illinois

James E. Crowe, Jr., MD
Ingraham Professor of Pediatrics, Microbiology, and Immunology, Vanderbilt University Medical Center, Nashville, Tennessee

Steven J. Czinn, MD
Professor and Chair of Pediatrics, University of Maryland School of Medicine; Chief of Pediatrics, University of Maryland Hospital for Children, Baltimore, Maryland

Richard Dalton, MD
Professor of Child/Adolescent Psychiatry, Tulane University Health Sciences Center; Clinical Professor of Pediatrics, Tulane University Health Sciences Center, New Orleans, Louisiana

Jorge H. Daruna, PhD
LA-YES-Louisiana Youth Enhanced Services, Office of Mental Health, State of Louisiana

Toni Darville, MD
Professor of Pediatrics and Microbiology/Immunology, University of Arkansas for Medical Sciences, Little Rock, Arkansas

Robert S. Daum, MD
Professor of Pediatrics, University of Chicago, Chicago, Illinois

Richard S. Davidson, MD
Associate Professor of Orthopaedic Surgery, University of Pennsylvania School of Medicine; Associate Professor of Orthopaedic Surgery, Children's Hospital of Philadelphia, Philadelphia, Pennsylvania

Ira D. Davis, MD, MS
Associate Professor of Pediatrics, Case Western Reserve University School of Medicine; Chief, Division of Pediatric Nephrology, Rainbow Babies and Children's Hospital, Cleveland Ohio

Peter S. Dayan, MD
Associate Professor of Clinical Pediatrics, Columbia University College of Physicians and Surgeons; Associate Director, Division of Pediatric Emergency Medicine, The Children's Hospital of New York Presbyterian, New York, New York

Michael R. DeBaun, MD, MPH
Associate Professor of Pediatrics, Biostatistics, and Neurology, Washington University School of Medicine; Pediatrics, St. Louis Children's Hospital, St. Louis, Missouri

Jacqueline L. Deen, MD, MSc
Research Scientist, International Vaccine Institute, Seoul, Korea

Katherine MacRae Dell, MD
Assistant Professor of Pediatrics, Case Western Reserve University School of Medicine; Attending Pediatric Nephrologist, Rainbow Babies and Children's Hospital, Cleveland, Ohio

Arlene E. Dent
Instructor, Center for Global Health and Diseases, Case Western Reserve University; Instructor, Department of Pediatrics, Pediatric Infectious Diseases and Rheumatology Division, Rainbow Babies and Children's Hospital, Cleveland, Ohio

Marie Descartes, MD
Associate Professor of Pediatrics and Genetics, University of Alabama, at Birmingham, Birmingham, Alabama

Robert Desnick, MD, PhD
Professor and Chairman of Human Genetics, Mount Sinai School of Medicine; Attending Physician, Pediatrics, Mount Sinai Hospital, New York, New York

Joseph DiCarlo, MD
Assistant Professor, Department of Pediatrics, Stanford University, Palo Alto, California

Angelo M. DiGeorge, MD
Emeritus Professor of Pediatrics, Temple University School of Medicine, Philadelphia, Pennsylvania

Mary K. Donovan, RN, MS, PNP
Manager of Nurse Practitioners, Care Coordination, and Outpatient Department, Shriners Burns Hospital, Boston, Massachusetts

John P. Dormans, MD, FACS
Professor of Orthopaedic Surgery, University of Pennsylvania School of Medicine; Chief, Division of Orthopaedic Surgery, Children's Hospital of Philadelphia, Philadelphia, Pennsylvania

M. Denise Dowd, MD, MPH
Professor, Department of Pediatrics, University of Missouri-Kansas City; Chief, Section of Injury Prevention, The Children's Mercy Hospital, Kansas City, Missouri

Daniel A. Doyle, MD
Assistant Professor of Pediatrics, Thomas Jefferson University, Philadelphia, Pennsylvania; Staff, Endocrinology Division, A.I. Dupont Hospital for Children, Wilmington, Delaware

Stephen Dreskin, MD, PhD
Professor of Medicine, Division of Allergy and Immunology, University of Colorado Health Sciences Center, Denver, Colorado; Director, Allergy, Immunology, and Rheumatology Practices, University of Colorado Hospital, Aurora, Colorado

Denis S. Drummond, MD
Professor Emeritus, University of Pennsylvania School of Medicine; Emeritus Chief of Pediatric Orthopaedic Surgery, Children's Hospital of Philadelphia, Philadelphia, Pennsylvania

Anne M. Dubin, MD
Associate Professor of Pediatrics, Stanford University, Stanford, California; Director of Pediatric Electrophysiology Laboratory, Pediatrics Cardiology, Lucile Salter Packard Children's Hospital, Palo Alto, California

Golde Dudell, MD
Associate Professor of Pediatrics, Emory University; Attending Physician, Children's Healthcare at Atlanta, Emory Cranford Long, Grady Memorial Hospital, Atlanta, Georgia

J. Stephen Dumler, MD
Professor, Department of Pathology, Division of Medical Microbiology, Johns Hopkins University School of Medicine, Professor, Department of Molecular Microbiology and Immunology, Johns Hopkins University Bloomberg School of Public Health; Associate Director, Division of Medical Microbiology, Director, Parasitology Laboratory, Department of Pathology, Division of Medical Microbiology, Johns Hopkins Hospital, Baltimore, Maryland

Paula M. Duncan, MD
Professor of Pediatrics, University of Vermont College of Medicine, Burlington, Vermont

Peter F. Ehrlich, MD
Associate Professor of Surgery, Section of Pediatric Surgery, University of Michigan, Ann Arbor, Michigan

Jack S. Elder, MD
Carter Kissell Professor of Urology, Professor of Pediatrics, Vice Chairman, Department of Urology, Case Western Reserve University School of Medicine; Director of Pediatric Urology, Rainbow Babies and Children's Hospital, Cleveland, Ohio

Dianne S. Elfenbein, MD
Associate Professor of Pediatrics, Division of Adolescent Medicine, University of Massachusetts Medical School; Medical Director, Teen-Tot Program, University of Massachusetts Memorial Health Care, Worcester, Massachusetts

Maria Enrione, MD
Assistant Professor, Neoucom; Pediatric Intensivist, Children's Hospital Medical Center of Akron, Akron, Ohio

Susan Feigelman, MD
Associate Professor of Pediatrics, University of Maryland School of Medicine, Baltimore, Maryland

Marianne E. Felice, MD
Professor and Chair, Department of Pediatrics, University of Massachusetts Medical School; Physician-in-Chief, University of Massachusetts Memorial Children's Medical Center, Worcester, Massachusetts

Eric I. Felner, MD
Assistant Professor of Pediatrics, Department of Pediatrics, Division of Endocrindogy, Emory University School of Medicine, Atlanta, Georgia

Patricia Ferrieri, MD
Chairman's Fund Endowed Chair in Laboratory Medicine and Pathology; Professor, Department of Pediatrics, Division of Infectious Diseases, University of Minnesota Medical School; Director, Clinical Microbiology Laboratory, University of Minnesota Medical Center, Fairview, Minneapolis, Minnesota

Jonathan D. Finder, MD
Associate Professor of Pediatrics, University of Pittsburgh School of Medicine; Attending Pulmonologist, Children's Hospital of Pittsburgh, Pittsburgh, Pennsylvania

Margaret C. Fisher, MD
Professor of Pediatrics, Drexel University College of Medicine, Philadelphia, Pennsylvania; Medical Director, The Children's Hospital at Monmouth Medical Center, Long Branch, New Jersey

Emily Fitzpatrick, MD
Pediatric Resident, Department of Pediatrics, Eastern Virginia Medical School; Pediatric Resident, Department of Pediatrics, Children's Hospital of the Kings Daughters, Norfolk, Virginia

David M. Fleece, MD
Assistant Professor of Pediatrics, Temple University School of Medicine, Philadelphia, Pennsylvania

Robert G. Flood, MD
Director, Pediatric Emergency Medicine; Assistant Professor, Department of Pediatrics, Temple University School of Medicine/Temple University Children's Medical Center, Philadelphia, Pennsylvania

Patricia M. Flynn, MD
Professor of Pediatrics and Preventive Medicine, University of Tennessee Health Science Center; Member, Department of Infectious Diseases, St. Jude Children's Research Hospital, Memphis, Tennessee

Joel A. Forman, MD
Associate Professor of Pediatrics, Mount Sinai School of Medicine; Vice Chair for Medical Education, Department of Pediatrics, Mount Sinai Hospital, New York, New York

Norman Fost MD, MPH
Professor, Director, Program in Bioethics, Department of Pediatrics, Medical History and Bioethics, University of Wisconsin Medical School; Pediatrician, University of Wisconsin Hospital and Clinics, Madison, Wisconsin

Lorry R. Frankel, MD, MBA
Associate Professor, Pediatrics, Stanford University School of Medicine; Director, Critical Care Services, Lucile Salter Packard Children's Hospital, Palo Alto, California

Melvin H. Freedman, MD, FRCPC, FAAP
Professor Emeritus of Pediatrics, University of Toronto Faculty of Medicine; Senior Scientist Emeritus, Research Institute, Hospital for Sick Children, Toronto, Ontario, Canada

Madelyn Freundlich, MSW, MPH, JD, LL.M
Excal Consulting Partners LLC, New York, New York

Jared E. Friedman, BA
Clinical Research Coordinator, Division of Orthopaedic Surgery, The Children's Hospital of Philadelphia, Philadelphia, Pennsylvania

Peter Gal, PharmD, BCPS, FCCP, FASHP
Clinical Professor, Division of Pharmacotherapy and Experimental Therapeutics, School of Pharmacy, University of North Carolina, Chapel Hill, Chapel Hill, North Carolina; Neonatal Pharmacotherapy Specialist, Department of Neonatology, Women's Hospital, Moses Cone Health System, Greensboro, North Carolina; Director, Graduate Pharmacy Education, Greensboro Area Health Education Center, Greensboro, North Carolina

Paula Gardiner, MD, MPH
Clinical Research Fellow, Division for Research and Education in Complementary and Integrative Medical Therapies, Osher Institute, Harvard Medical School, Boston Massachusetts

Luigi Garibaldi, MD
Professor of Pediatrics, Division of Pediatric Endocrinology, University of Pittsburgh School of Medicine; Clinical Director, Division of Pediatric Endocrinology, Children's Hospital of Pediatric Endocrinology, Children's Hospital of Pittsburgh, Pittsburgh, Pennsylvania

Abraham Gedalia, MD
Professor of Pediatrics and Head, Division of Pediatric Rheumatology, Louisiana State University Health Sciences Center; Head, Department of Rheumatology, Children's Hospital, New Orleans, Louisiana

Michael A. Gerber, MD
Professor of Pediatrics, University of Cincinnati College of Medicine; Attending Physician, Division of Infectious Disease, Cincinnati Children's Hospital Medical Center, Cincinnati, Ohio

Fayez K. Ghishan, MD
Horace W. Steele Endowed Chair in Pediatric Research, Head, Department of Pediatrics, Director, Steele Children's Research Center, University of Arizona College of Medicine; Faculty Member, Department of Pediatrics, The University of Arizona College of Medicine, Tucson, Arizona

Purushottam A. Gholve, MD, MBMS, MRCS
Research Fellow, The Children's Hospital of Philadelphia, Philadelphia, Pennsylvania

Francis Gigliotti, MD
Professor of Pediatrics, Microbiology, and Immunology, Chief, Pediatric Infectious Diseases, Associate Chair for Academic Affairs, Department of Pediatrics, University of Rochester School of Medicine and Dentistry; Attending Physician, Pediatrics, Golisano Children's Hospital at Strong, Rochester, New York

William S. Gilliam, PhD
Assistant Professor of Child Psychiatry and Psychology, Child Study Center, Yale University School of Medicine, Director, Edward Zigler Center in Child Development and Social Policy, Yale University; Yale-New Haven Children's Hospital, New Haven, Connecticut

Charles M. Ginsburg, MD
Marilyn R. Corrigan Distinguished Chair of Pediatric Research, Associate Dean for Academic Affairs, University of Texas Southwestern Medical Center at Dallas, Dallas, Texas

Bertil Glader, MD, PhD
Professor of Pediatrics and Pathology, Stanford University School of Medicine, Palo Alto, California; Division of Hematology-Oncology, Lucile Salter Packard Children's Hospital, Palo Alto, California

Frances Page Glascoe, PhD
Adjunct Professor of Pediatrics, Vanderbilt University, Nashville, Tennessee

Mary Margaret Gleason, MD
Clinical Assistant Professor, Brown Medical School, Providence Rhode Island; Clinical Assistant Professor, Tulane University School of Medicine, New Orleans, Louisiana

Donald Goldman, MD
Professor of Pediatrics, Children's Hospital, Harvard Medical School; Senior Associate in Infectious Diseases, Children's Hospital Boston, Boston, Massachusetts

Denise M. Goodman, MD
Associate Professor, Pediatric Critical Care Medicine, Northwestern University, Feinberg School of Medicine; Attending Physician, Pediatric Intensive Care Unit, Children's Memorial Hospital, Chicago, Illinois

David Gozal, MD
Children's Foundation Chair of Pediatric Research, Professor of Pediatrics, Pharmacology and Toxicology, Psychology and Brain Sciences, University of Louisville; Director, Rosair Children's Hospital Sleep Medicine and Apnea Center, Louisville, Kentucky

Michael Green, MD, MPH
Professor of Pediatrics and Surgery, University of Pittsburgh School of Medicine; Division of Infectious Diseases, Children's Hospital of Pittsburgh, Pittsburgh, Pennsylvania

Thomas P. Green, MD
Professor and Chairman of Pediatrics, Northwestern University, Feinberg School of Medicine; Children's Memorial Hospital, Chicago, Illinois

Larry A. Greenbaum, MD, PhD
Director, Division of Pediatric Nephrology, Emory University School of Medicine; Medical Director of Dialysis, Children's Healthcare of Atlanta, Atlanta, Georgia

David Grossman, MD, MPH
Professor of Pediatrics, University of Washington; Director, Harborview Injury Prevention and Research Center, Seattle, Washington

Gabriel G. Haddad, MD
Professor of Pediatrics and Neuroscience, Chairman, Department of Pediatrics, University of California, San Diego; Physician-in-Chief, Rady Children's Hospital of San Diego, San Diego, California

Joseph Haddad, Jr., MD
Professor and Vice Chairman, Otolaryngology/Head and Neck Surgery, Columbia University College of Physicians and Surgeons; Lawrence Savetsky Chair and Director, Pediatric Otolaryngology/Head and Neck Surgery, Morgan Stanley Children's Hospital of New York, New York

Joseph F. Hagan, Jr., MD, FAAP
Clinical Professor of Pediatrics, University of Vermont College of Medicine; Attending Physician in Pediatrics, Fletcher Allen Health Care, Burlington, Vermont

Scott B. Halstead, MD
Adjunct Professor, Preventive Medicine and Biometrics, Uniformed Services University of the Health Sciences, Bethesda, Maryland; Director, Research Department, Pediatric Dengue Vaccine Initiative, International Vaccine Institute, Seoul, Korea

Margaret R. Hammerschlag, MD
Professor of Pediatrics and Medicine; Director, Division of Pediatric Infectious Diseases, State University of New York Downstate Medical Center, Brooklyn, New York

Aaron Hamvas, MD
Professor of Pediatrics, Washington University School of Medicine; Medical Director, Neonatal Intensive Care Unit, St. Louis Children's Hospital, St. Louis, Missouri

James C. Harris, MD
Professor of Psychiatry and Behavioral Sciences, Pediatrics, and Mental Hygiene, Johns Hopkins University School of Medicine; Director, Developmental Neuropsychiatry, Johns Hopkins Hospital, Baltimore, Maryland

David B. Haslam, MD
Associate Professor, Pediatrics and Molecular Microbiology, Washington University School of Medicine; Attending Physician, Pediatric Infectious Diseases, St. Louis Children's Hospital, St. Louis, Missouri

Robert H.A. Haslam, MD, FAAP, FRCP(C)
Emeritus Professor and Chairman, Department of Pediatrics and Professor of Medicine (Neurology), University of Toronto; Emeritus Pediatrician-in-Chief, Hospital for Sick Children, Toronto, Canada

Fern R. Hauck, MD, MS
Associate Professor of Family Medicine and Public Health Sciences, University of Virginia School of Medicine; Attending Physician, Family Medicine, University of Virginia Health System, Charlottesville, Virginia

Gregory F. Hayden, MD
Professor of Pediatrics, University of Virginia School of Medicine; Attending Pediatrician, University of Virginia Children's Hospital, Charlottesville, Virginia

Jacqueline T. Hecht, PhD
Professor of Pediatrics, Vice-Chair for Research, Department of Pediatrics, University of Texas-Houston; Active Scientific Staff, Clinical Genetics Consultant, Houston Unit, Shriners Hospital for Children, Houston, Texas

Sabrina M. Heidemann, MD
Associate Professor, Pediatrics, Wayne State University School of Medicine; Pediatric Intensivist, Children's Hospital of Michigan, Detroit, Michigan

William C. Heird, MD
Professor of Pediatrics, Baylor College of Medicine, Houston, Texas

J. Owen Hendley, MD
Professor of Pediatrics, University of Virginia School of Medicine, Charlottesville, Virginia

Fred M. Henretig, MD
Professor of Pediatrics and Emergency Medicine, University of Pennsylvania School of Medicine; Director, Section of Clinical Toxicology, Division of Emergency Medicine, The Children's Hospital of Philadelphia, Philadelphia, Pennsylvania

Gloria P. Heresi, MD
Associate Professor of Pediatrics, Pediatric Infectious Diseases Division, University of Texas Health Science Center at Houston; Pediatrics, Memorial Herrmann Children's Hospital, Houston, Texas

Cynthia E. Herzog, MD
Associate Professor of Pediatrics, University of Texas M.D. Anderson Cancer Center, Houston, Texas

Lauren D. Holinger, MD
Professor, Otolaryngology – Head and Neck Surgery, Northwestern University Feinberg School of Medicine; Head, Division of Pediatric Otolaryngology, Children's Memorial Hospital, Chicago, Illinois

Steve Holve, MD
Clinical Instructor, Johns Hopkins University School of Medicine, Baltimore, Maryland; Chief of Pediatrics, Tuba City Regional Healthcare Corporation, Tuba City, Arizona

Jeffrey D. Hord, MD
Associate Professor of Pediatrics, Northeastern Ohio Universities College of Medicine, Rootstown, Ohio; Director, Pediatric Hematology/Oncology, Children's Hospital Medical Center of Akron, Akron, Ohio

B. David Horn, MD
Assistant Professor, Orthopaedic Surgery, University of Pennsylvania; Division of Orthopaedic Surgery, The Children's Hospital of Philadelphia, Philadelphia, Pennsylvania

William A. Horton, MD
Professor of Molecular and Medical Genetics, Oregon Health and Science University; Director of Research, Shriners Hospitals for Children, Portland, Oregon

Harish S. Hosalkar, MD, MBMS(Orth), FCPS(Orth), DNB(Orth)
Clinical Instructor, Department of Orthopaedic Surgery, University of Pennsylvania School of Medicine; Editor-in-Chief, University of Pennsylvania Orthopedic Journal, University of Pennsylvania School of Medicine, Philadelphia, Pennsylvania

Peter J. Hotez, MD, PhD, FAAP
Walter G. Ross Professor and Chair, Department of Microbiology, Immunology and Tropical Medicine, The George Washington University; President, The Sabin Vaccine Institute, Washington, District of Columbia

Michele S. Howenstine, MD
Professor of Clinical Pediatrics, Indiana University School of Medicine; Pediatric Pulmonologist, Section of Pediatric Pulmonology, James Whitcomb Riley Hospital for Children, Indiana University, Indianapolis, Indiana

Vicki Huff, PhD
Associate Professor, Department of Cancer Genetics, University of Texas M.D. Anderson Cancer Center, Houston, Texas

Denise Hug, MD
Assistant Professor, Departments of Ophthalmology and Pediatrics, University of Missouri – Kansas City School of Medicine; Children's Mercy Hospitals and Clinics, Kansas City, Missouri

Carl E. Hunt, MD
Adjunct Professor of Pediatrics, Uniformed Services University of the Health Sciences; National Heart, Lung, and Blood Institute, National Institutes of Health, Bethesda, Maryland

Melissa Hurwitz, MD
Assistant Professor of Pediatrics; Attending Physician, Division of Pediatric Gastroenterology, Hepatology, and Nutrition, Lucile Salter Packard Children's Hospital, Palo Alto, California

Sunny Zaheed Hussain, MD, MRCP
Director, Division of Pediatric Gastroenterology and Nutrition, Christus-Schumpert Sutton Children's Hospital, Shreveport, Louisiana

Elias S. Hyams, MD
Resident in Urology, New York University School of Medicine, New York, New York

Jeffrey S. Hyams, MD
Professor of Pediatrics, University of Connecticut School of Medicine, Farmington, Connecticut; Head, Division of Digestive Diseases, Hepatology, and Nutrition, Connecticut Children's Medial Center, Hartford, Connecticut

Richard F. Jacobs, MD, FAAP
Horace C. Cabe Professor, Department of Pediatrics, University of Arkansas for Medical Sciences; President, Arkansas Children's Hospital Research Institute, Little Rock, Arkansas

Norman Jaffe, MD, DipPaed, DSc
Professor of Pediatrics, University of Texas; Pediatric Oncologist, University of Texas M.D. Anderson Cancer Center, Houston, Texas

Renée R. Jenkins, MD
Professor and Chair, Department of Pediatrics and Child Health, Howard University; Adjunct Professor, Department of Pediatrics, George Washington University; Chair, Department of Pediatrics and Child Health, Howard University Hospital, Washington, District of Columbia

Peter S. Jensen, MD
Ruane Professor of Child Psychiatry and Director, Center for the Advancement of Children's Mental Health, Department of Psychiatry, Columbia University, New York, New York

Hal B. Jenson, MD
Professor of Pediatrics and Dean of the Western Campus of Tufts University School of Medicine; Chief Academic Officer, Baystate Health, Springfield, Massachusetts

Chandy C. John, MD
Associate Professor of Pediatrics and Medicine, Director, Global Pediatrics Program, University of Minnesota Medical School; Attending Physician, University of Minnesota Children's Hospital, Fairview, Minneapolis, Minnesota

Charles F. Johnson, MD
Emeritus Professor of Pediatrics, The Ohio State University College of Medicine and Public Health, Columbus, Ohio

Michael V. Johnson, MD
Departments of Neurology, Pediatrics, and Physical Medicine and Rehabilitation, Johns Hopkins University School of Medicine, Baltimore, Maryland; Chief Medical Officer, Kennedy Krieger Institute, Baltimore, Maryland

Richard B. Johnston, Jr., MD
Professor of Pediatrics, University of Colorado School of Medicine; Associate Dean for Research Development, University of Colorado School of Medicine; Executive Vice President for Academic Affairs, National Jewish Medical and Research Center, Denver, Colorado

James F. Jones, MD
Research Medical Officer, Chronic Viral Diseases Branch, Division of Viral and Rickettsial Diseases, National Center for Zoonotic, Vectorborne, and Enteric Diseases, Coordinating Center for Infectious Diseases, Centers for Disease Control and Prevention, Atlanta, Georgia

Saraswati Kache, MD
Clinical Assistant Professor of Pediatrics, Stanford University School of Medicine; Attending Physician, Pediatric Intensive Care Unit, Lucile Salter Packard Children's Hospital, Palo Alto, California

Nina S. Kaddan-Lottick, MD, MSPH
Assistant Professor of Pediatrics, Yale University School of Medicine; Medical Director, HERO's Clinic for Survivors of Childhood Cancer, Yale–New Haven Hospital, New Haven, Connecticut

Harry J. Kallas, MD
Associate Clinical Professor, Department of Pediatrics, University of California, San Francisco at Fresno, Fresno; Chair, Pharmacy, Therapeutics, and Utilization Committee, Department of Anesthesia and Critical Care, Children's Hospital, Central California, Madera, California

Michael Kashgarian, MD
Professor of Pathology and Molecular, Cellular, and Developmental Biology, Yale University School of Medicine; Attending Pathologist, Yale-New Haven Hospital; Director, Diagnostic Electron Microscopy, Yale-New Haven Hospital, New Haven, Connecticut

Alessandra N. Kazura, MD
Assistant Professor, Department of Psychiatry and Human Behavior, Brown Medical School; Assistant Professor, Hasbro Children's Research Center, Rhode Island Hospital, Providence, Rhode Island

James Kazura, MD
Professor, Center for Global Health and disease, Case Western Reserve University School of Medicine; Professor, Medicine and Pathology Departments, University Hospitals of Cleveland, Cleveland, Ohio

Virginia Keane, MD
Associate Professor of Pediatrics, University of Maryland School of Medicine

Desmond P. Kelly, MB, Ch.B
GHS Professor of Clinical Pediatrics, University of South Carolina School of Medicine; Medical Director, Division of Developmental-Behavioral Pediatrics, Donald A. Gardner Center for Developing Minds; Children's Hospital, Greenville Hospital System, Greenville, South Carolina

Kathi J. Kemper, MD, MPH
Caryl J. Guth Chair for Holistic and Integrative Medicine, Professor of Pediatrics and Public Health Sciences, Wake Forest University Baptist Medical Center; Staff, Department of Pediatrics, North Carolina Baptist Hospital, Winston-Salem, North Carolina

Eitan Kerem, MD
Professor, Department of Pediatrics, Hebrew University; Director, Department of Pediatrics, Mount Scopus Campus, Hadassah University Hospital, Jerusalem, Israel

Joseph E. Kershner, MD, FACS, FAAP
Chief, Pediatric Otolaryngology and Academic Vice Chairman, Department of Otolaryngology and Communication Sciences, Senior Associate Dean of Clinical Affairs, Medical College of Wisconsin; Medical Director, Pediatric Otolaryngology, Children's Hospital of Wisconsin, CEO, Children's Specialty Group, Children's Hospital of Wisconsin and Medical College of Wisconsin, Milwaukee, Wisconsin

Seema Khan, MBBS
Associate Professor, Department of Pediatrics, Thomas Jefferson University Medical College, Philadelphia, Pennsylvania; Department of Pediatric Gastroenterology, Alfred I. du Pont Hospital for Children, Wilmington, Delaware

Leila Kheirandish, MD
Assistant Professor of Pediatrics, Division of Pediatric Sleep Medicine, University of Louisville, Kentucky

Charles H. King, MD
Center for Global Health and Diseases, Case Western Reserve University School of Medicine, Cleveland, Ohio

Stephen L. Kinsman, MD
Associate Professor of Pediatrics and Neurology, University of Maryland School of Medicine; Pediatric Neurologist, University of Maryland Hospital for Children; Consulting Neurologist, Kennedy Krieger Institute, Baltimore, Maryland

Priya S. Kishnani, MD
Associate Professor of Pediatrics, Division of Medical Genetics, Duke University; Associate Professor of Pediatrics, Interim Division Chief, Division of Medical Genetics, Duke University Medical Center, Durham, North Carolina

Bruce L. Klein, MD
Associate Professor, Pediatrics and Emergency Medicine, The George Washington University School of Medicine and Health Sciences; Chief, Division of Transport Medicine, Children's National Medical Center, Washington, District of Columbia

Michael D. Klein, MD
Arvin I. Philippart III, MD Chair and Professor of Surgery, Wayne State University School of Medicine; Surgeon-in-Chief at Children's Hospital of Michigan, Detroit, Michigan

Marisa S. Klein-Gitelman, MD, MPH
Associate Professor, Northwestern University, Feinberg School of Medicine; Children's Memorial Hospital, Chicago, Illinois

Robert M. Kliegman, MD
Professor and Chair, Department of Pediatrics, Medical College of Wisconsin; Pediatrician-in-Chief, Pamela and Leslie Muma Chair in Pediatrics, Children's Hospital of Wisconsin; Executive Vice President, Children's Research Institute, Milwaukee, Wisconsin

William C. Koch, MD
Associate Professor of Pediatrics, Division of Infectious Diseases, Virginia Commonwealth University School of Medicine; Attending Physician, Pediatrics, Division of Infectious Diseases, Medical College of Virginia Hospitals, Richmond, Virginia

Gideon Koren, MD, FRCPC
Professor, Department of Pediatrics, Pharmacology, Pharmacy, Medical Genetics, University of Toronto, University of Western Ontario; Department of Pediatrics, The Hospital for Sick Children, Toronto, Ontario, Canada

Bruce R. Korf, MD, PhD
Wayne H. and Sara Crews Finley Professor and Chair, Department of Genetics, University of Alabama at Birmingham, Birmingham, Alabama

Peter J. Krause, MD
Professor of Pediatrics, University of Connecticut School of Medicine, Farmington, Connecticut; Director of Infectious Diseases, Department of Pediatrics, Connecticut Children's Medical Center, Hartford, Connecticut

Heather Krell, MD, MPH
Voluntary Clinical Associate Professor, Department of Psychiatry and Biobehavioral Sciences, Los Angeles, California

John Kuttesch, Jr., MD, PhD
Ingraham Associate Professor of Cancer Research, Department of Pediatrics, Vanderbilt University; Director, Brain Tumor Program, Associate Professor, Hematology and Oncology, Monroe Carell Jr. Children's Hospital at Vanderbilt; Ingraham Associate Professor of Cancer Research, Pediatric Hematology and Oncology, Vanderbilt-Ingraham Cancer Center, Nashville, Tennessee

Catherine S. Lachenauer, MD
Assistant Professor of Pediatrics, Harvard Medical School; Attending Physician, Division of Infectious Diseases, Children's Hospital, Boston, Massachusetts

Stephan Ladisch, MD
Professor and Vice Chairman of Pediatrics, George Washington University; Director, Center for Cancer and Immunology Research, Children's Research Institute, Children's National Medical Center, Washington, District of Columbia

Stephen LaFranchi, MD
Professor of Pediatrics, Oregon Health and Science University; Staff Physician, Doernbecher Children's Hospital, Portland, Oregon

Richard Lampe, MD
Professor and Chairman, Department of Pediatrics, Texas Tech University Health Sciences Center, Lubbock, Texas

Philip J. Landrigan, MD, MSc
Professor and Chairman, Department of Community and Preventive Medicine; Professor of Pediatrics, Mount Sinai School of Medicine, New York, New York

Gregory L. Landry, MD
Professor of Pediatrics, University of Wisconsin School of Medicine and Public Health; Team Physician, University of Wisconsin-Madison Athletic Teams, Madison, Wisconsin

Carole Lannon, MD, MPH
Professor, Department of Pediatrics, University of Cincinnati; Co-Director, Center for Health Care Quality, Cincinnati Children's Hospital Medical Center, Cincinnati, Chio

Philip LaRussa, MD
Professor of Clinical Pediatrics, Columbia University, New York, New York

Oren Lakser
Assistant Professor of Pediatrics, University of Chicago; Director, Fellowship Program in Pediatric Pulmonary; Director, Pediatric Flexible Fiberoptic Bronchoscopy Services, Section of Pediatric Pulmonary Medicine, University of Chicago, Chicago, Illinois

Charles T. Leach, MD
Professor of Pediatrics, University of Texas Health Science Center at San Antonio; Staff, University Hospital; Staff, Christus Santa Rosa Children's Hospital, San Antonio, Texas

Chul Lee, PhD
Associate Professor, University of Texas Medical Branch, Galveston, Texas

J. Steven Leeder, PharmD, PhD
Professor of Pediatrics and Pharmacology, Schools of Medicine and Pharmacy, University of Missouri-Kansas City; Marion Merrell Dow Chair in Pediatric Pharmacogenomics, Section of Developmental Pharmacology and Experimental Therapeutics, Children's Mercy Hospitals and Clinics, Kansas City, Missouri

Margaret W. Leigh, MD
Professor of Pediatrics, University of North Carolina, Chapel Hill; Attending Physician, North Carolina Children's Hospital, Chapel Hill, North Carolina

Steven Lestrud, MD
Instructor of Pediatrics, Northwestern University, Feinberg School of Medicine; Attending Physician, Children's Memorial Hospital, Chicago, Illinois

Donald Y.M. Leung, MD, PhD
Professor of Pediatrics, University of Colorado Medical School; Head of Pediatric Allergy-Immunology Division, National Jewish Medical and Research Center, Denver, Colorado

Stephen Liben, MD
Associate Professor of Pediatrics, McGill University; Director, Palliative Care Program, Department of Pediatrics, The Montreal Children's Hospital of the McGill University Health Center, Montreal, Québec, Canada

Andrew H. Liu, MD
Associate Professor, Division of Allergy and Clinical Immunology, Department of Pediatrics, National Jewish Medical and Research Center; Associate Professor of Pediatrics, University of Colorado Health Sciences Center, Denver, Colorado

Franco Locatelli, MD
Associate Professor of Pediatrics, Pavia University School of Medicine, Pavia, Italy; Head of Pediatric Hematology/Oncology Division, IRCCS Policlinico San Matteo, Pavia, Italy

Kelsey Logan, MD
Assistant Professor, Connecticut Children's Medical Center; Staff Physician, Elite Sports Medicine, Hartford, Connecticut

Sarah S. Long, MD
Section of Infectious Diseases, St. Christopher's Hospital for Children, Philadelphia, Pennsylvania

Daniel J. Lovell, MD, MPH
Joseph E. Levinson Professor of Pediatrics, University of Cincinnati Medical Center; Associate Director, Division of Rheumatology, Cincinnati Children's Hospital Medical Center, Cincinnati, Ohio

G. Reid Lyon, PhD
Senior Research Professor, Whitney International University and the American College of Education, Dallas, Texas

Helen N. Lyon, MD, SM
Instructor, Department of Pediatrics, Harvard Medical School; Staff Physician, Division of Genetics/Program in Genomics, Children's Hospital Boston, Boston, Massachusetts

Prashant V. Mahajan, MD, MPH, MBA
Associate Professor of Pediatrics and Emergency Medicine, Vice-Chief and Research Director of Pediatric Emergency Medicine, Carman and Ann Adams Department of Pediatrics, Wayne State University; Children's Hospital of Michigan, Detroit, Michigan

Joseph A. Majzoub, MD
Thomas Morgan Rotch Professor of Pediatrics, Harvard Medical School; Chief, Division of Endocrinology, Department of Medicine, Children's Hospital Boston, Boston, Massachusetts

Arik V. Marcell, MD, MPH
Assistant Professor of Pediatrics, University of Maryland, School of Medicine, Baltimore, Maryland

Joan C. Marini, MD, PhD
Branch Chief, Bone and Extracellular Matrix Branch, National Institute of Child Health, National Institutes of Health, Bethesda, Maryland

Morri Markowitz, MD
Professor of Pediatrics, Albert Einstein College of Medicine; Interim Chief, Division of Pediatric Endocrinology and Member, Division of Pediatric Environmental Sciences, Children's Hospital at Montefiore Hospital, Bronx, New York

Stacene R. Maroushek, MD, PhD
Pediatric Infectious Diseases and General Pediatrics, Division of Pediatrics Infectious Diseases, University of Minnesota and Hannepin County Medical Center, Minneapolis, Minnesota

Wilbert Mason, MD, MPH
Professor of Clinical Pediatrics, Keck School of Medicine of the University of Southern California; Head, Division of Infectious Disease, Department of Pediatrics, Children's Hospital Los Angeles, Los Angeles, California

Reuben Matalon, MD, PhD
Professor of Pediatrics, University of Texas Medical Branch, Children's Hospital, Galveston, Texas

Lawrence H. Mathers, Jr., MD, PhD
Associate Professor of Pediatrics and Surgery, Stanford University School of Medicine; Attending Physician, Pediatric Intensive Care Unit, Lucile Salter Packard Children's Hospital, Palo Alto California

Robert Mazor, MD
Assistant Professor of Pediatrics, University of Washington; Attending Pediatric Cardiac Intensivist, Pediatric Critical Care Medicine, Children's Hospital and Regional Medical Care, Seattle, Washington

Paul L. McCarthy, MD
Professor of Pediatrics, Yale School of Medicine; Head, Division of General Pediatrics and Director of Patient Services, Children's Hospital at Yale-New Haven, New Haven, Connecticut

Susannah A. McColley, MD
Associate Professor of Pediatrics, Northwestern University, Feinberg School of Medicine; Division Head, Pulmonary Medicine, Director, Cystic Fibrosis Center, Children's Memorial Hospital, Chicago, Illinois

Andrea C.S. McCoy, MD
Associate Professor of Pediatrics, Temple University School of Medicine; Associate Professor of Pediatrics, Temple University Children's Medical Center, Philadelphia, Pennsylvania

Margaret M. McGovern, MD, PhD
Professor of Human Genetics and Pediatrics, Mount Sinai School of Medicine; Attending Physician, Mount Sinai Hospital, New York, New York

Kenneth McIntosh, MD
Professor of Pediatrics, Harvard Medical School; Emeritus Chief, Division of Infectious Diseases, Children's Hospital Boston, Boston, Massachusetts

Rima McLeod, MD
Professor, Ophthalmology and Visual Sciences, Pedriatrics (Infectious Diseases) and the Committees on Molecular Medicine, Immunology, and Genetics and The College, The University of Chicago; Attending Physician, Department of Medicine and Pediatrics, Hospitals of the University of Chicago, Michael Reese Hospital and Medical Center, Chicago, Illinois

Peter C. Melby, MD
Professor, Department of Medicine, Division of Infectious Diseases, University of Texas Health Science Center at San Antonio; Associate Chief of Staff for Research and Development, Research Service, South Texas Veterans' Health Care System, San Antonio, Texas

Marian G. Michaels, MD, MPH
Professor of Pediatrics and Surgery, University of Pittsburgh School of Medicine; Division of Infectious Disease, Children's Hospital of Pittsburgh, Pittsburgh, Pennsylvania

Peter H. Michelson, MD
Assistant Professor of Pediatrics, Duke University School of Medicine, Durham, North Carolina

Henry Milgrom, MD
Professor of Pediatrics and Professor of Clinical Science, University of Colorado Health Sciences Center; Professor of Pediatrics, National Jewish Medical and Research Center, Denver Colorado

Michael L. Miller, MD
Associate Professor of Pediatrics, Northwestern University, Feinberg School of Medicine; Attending Physician, Children's Memorial Hospital, Chicago, Illinois

Grant A. Mitchell, MD
Professor of Pediatrics, Division of Medical Genetics, Department of Pediatrics, Centre Hospitalier Universitaire Sainte-Justine, Montreal, Quebec, Canada

Robert R. Montgomery, MD
Professor of Pediatric Hematology, Medical College of Wisconsin; Attending Physician, Pediatric Hematology, Oncology and Transplant, Children's Hospital of Wisconsin; Senior Investigator, Blood Research Institute, Blood Center of Wisconsin, Milwaukee, Wisconsin

Joseph G. Morelli, MD
Professor of Dermatology and Pediatrics, University of Colorado School of Medicine; Section Head, Pediatric Dermatology, The Children's Hospital, Denver, Colorado

Anna-Barbara Moscicki, MD
Professor of Pediatrics, University of California, San Francisco, San Francisco, California

Hugo W. Moser, MD
Professor of Neurology and Pediatrics, Johns Hopkins University; Director of Neurogenetics Research, Kennedy Krieger Institute, Johns Hopkins University School of Medicine, Baltimore, Maryland

Flor M. Munoz, MD
Assistant Professor of Pediatrics and Molecular Virology and Microbiology, Baylor School of Medicine; Attending Physician for Pediatric (Infectious Diseases), Texas Children's Hospital, Houston, Texas

Daniel J. Murphy, Jr., MD
Associate Professor of Pediatrics (Cardiology), Stanford University; Associate Chief, Pediatric Cardiology, Lucile Salter Packard Children's Hospital, Director, Adult Congenital Heart Clinic, Stanford University Hospital, Palo Alto, California

James R. Murphy, PhD
Research Professor in Pediatrics, University of Texas Medical School, Houston, Houston, Texas

Martin G. Myers, MD
Professor of Pediatrics and Preventive Medicine, University of Texas Medical Branch; Executive Director, National Network for Immunization Information, Galveston, Texas

William A. Neal, MD
Professor of Pediatrics, West Virginia University; Director, Preventive Cardiology, West Virginia University Children's Hospital, Morgantown, West Virginia

Robert M. Nelson, MD, PhD
Associate Professor of Anesthesiology, Critical, Care, and Pediatrics, University of Pennsylvania School of Medicine; Director, Center for Research Integrity, The Children's Hospital of Philadelphia, Philadelphia, Pennsylvania

Mary A. Nevin, MD, FAAP
Assistant Professor of Pediatrics, Northwestern University Feinberg School of Medicine; Attending Physician, Pulmonary Medicine, Children's Memorial Hospital, Chicago, Illinois

Zehava Noah, MD
Associate Professor of Pediatrics, Northwestern University, Feinberg School of Medicine; Attending Physician, Pediatric Critical Care, Children's Memorial Hospital, Chicago, Illinois

Lawrence M. Nogee, MD
Associate Professor of Pediatrics, Division of Neonatalogy, Johns Hopkins University School of Medicine; Attending Neonatalogist, Johns Hopkins Hospital, Baltimore, Maryland

Theresa J. Ochoa, MD
Assistant Professor, Center for Infectious Diseases, University of Texas-Houston Health Science Center, Houston, Texas

Robin K. Ohls, MD
Professor of Pediatrics, University of New Mexico; Director, Neonatal-Perinatal Fellowship Program, Department of Pediatrics, University of New Mexico, Albuquerque, New Mexico

Keith T. Oldham, MD
Professor and Chief, Department of Pediatric Surgery, Medical College of Wisconsin; Marie Z. Uihlein Chair and Surgeon-in-Chief, Children's Hospital of Wisconsin, Milwaukee, Wisconsin

Scott Olitsky, MD
Professor of Ophthalmology and Pediatrics, University of Missouri, Kansas City School of Missouri; Children's Mercy Hospitals and Clinics, Kansas City, Missouri

John Olsson, MD
Associate Professor, East Carolina University, Brody School of Medicine; Staff, Pitt County Memorial Hospital, Greenville, North Carolina

Susan Orenstein, MD
Professor of Pediatric Gastroenterology, University of Pittsburgh School of Medicine, Pittsburgh, Pennsylvania

Walter A. Orenstein, MD
Professor of Medicine and Pediatrics, Emory University School of Medicine; Associate Director, Emory Vaccine Center, Atlanta, Georgia

Gary D. Overturf, MD
Professor of Pediatrics and Pathology, University of New Mexico School of Medicine; Director, Pediatric Infectious Diseases, Department of Pediatrics, Children's Hospital of New Mexico; Medical Director, Infectious Diseases Section, TriCore Reference Laboratories, Albuquerque, New Mexico

Judith A. Owens, MD, MPH
Associate Professor of Pediatrics, Brown University Medical School; Director, Pediatric Sleep Disorders Clinic, Director, Learning, Attention, and Behavior Clinic, Hasbro Children's Hospital, Providence, Rhode Island

Lauren M. Pachman, MD
Professor of Pediatrics, Northwestern University Feinberg School of Medicine; Director, Molecular and Cellular Pathobiology, Children's Memorial Institute of Education and Research (CMIER); Professor, Department of Rheumatology, The Children's Memorial Hospital, Chicago, Illinois

Demosthenes Pappagianis, MD, PhD
Professor of Medical Microbiology and Immunology, University of California School of Medicine, Davis, Davis, California

John S. Parks, MD, PhD
Professor of Pediatrics, Director of Pediatric Endocrinology, Emory University School of Medicine; Attending Physician, Pediatrics Department, Children's Healthcare of Atlanta, Atlanta, Georgia

Diane E. Pappas, MD
Associate Professor of Pediatrics, University of Virginia School of Medicine, Charlottesville, Virginia

Ligia Peralta, MD, FAAP
Associate Professor, Department of Pediatrics and Epidemiology, University of Maryland Medical School; Chief, Division of Adolescent and Young Adult Medicine, Department of Pediatrics, University of Maryland Medical School, Baltimore, Maryland

Norma Pérez, DO
Pediatric Infectious Disease Fellow, University of Texas Health Science Center at Houston, Houston, Texas

Michael A. Pesce, Phd
Clinical Professor of Pathology, Columbia University, College of Physicians and Surgeons; Director of the Specialty Laboratory, New York Presbyterian Hospital, Columbia University Medical Center, New York, New York

John Peters, DO
Director, Division of Pediatric Gastroenterology, Janet Weis Children's Hospital, Geisinger Medical Center, Danville, Pennsylvania

Ross E. Petty, MD, PhD
Professor Emeritus, Department of Pediatrics, University of British Columbia and British Columbia's Children's Hospital, Vancouver, British Columbia, Canada

Anthony J. Piazza, MD
Assistant Professor of Pediatrics, Emory University School of Medicine, Division of Neonatal-Perinatal Medicine, Atlanta, Georgia

Larry K. Pickering, MD, FAAP
Professor of Pediatrics, Emory University School of Medicine; Senior Advisor to the Director, National Center for Immunization and Respiratory Diseases, Atlanta, Georgia

Dwight A. Powell, MD
Professor of Pediatrics, Ohio State University College of Medicine; Chief, Section of Infectious Diseases, Pediatrics Department, Children's Hospital, Columbus, Ohio

Keith R. Powell, MD
Professor and Chair, Department of Pediatrics, Northeastern Ohio Universities College of Medicine; Vice President and Dr. Noah Miller Chair of Medicine, Akron Children's Hospital, Akron, Ohio

Charles G. Prober, MD
Professor of Pediatrics, Medicine, Microbiology, and Immunology; Senior Associate Dean of Education, Stanford University School of Medicine, Stanford, California

Natoshia Raishevich
Research Associate, Department of Psychiatry, Columbia University College of Physicians and Surgeons, New York, New York

Robert Rapaport, MD
Professor of Pediatrics, Director of Division of Pediatric Endocrinology and Diabetes, Mount Sinai Medical Center, New York, New York

Stanley E. Read, MD, PhD, FRCPC, FAAP
Professor of Pediatrics, University of Toronto; Professor of Pediatrics, Infectious Disease Consultant, Hospital for Sick Children, Toronto, Ontario, Canada

Michael Reed, PharmD, FCCP, FCP
Professor of Pediatrics, Case Western Reserve University School of Medicine; Director, Pediatric Clinical Pharmacology and Toxicology, Pediatrics Department, Rainbow Babies and Children's Hospital, Cleveland, Ohio

Gary Remafedi, MD, MPH
Professor, University of Minnesota, Minneapolis, Minnesota; Executive Director, University of Minnesota Youth and AIDS Projects, Minneapolis, Minnesota

Jack S. Remington, MD
Professor Emeritus, Department of Medicine, Division of Infectious Diseases and Geographic Medicine, Stanford University School of Medicine, Stanford, California; Marcus A. Krupp Research Chair and Chairman, Department of Immunology and Infectious Diseases, Research Institute, Palo Alto Medical Foundation, Palo Alto, California

Jorge Reyes, MD
Professor of Surgery, University of Washington School of Medicine; Division Chief, Transplant Surgery, University of Washington Medical Center, Seattle, Washington

Iraj Rezvani, MD
Emeritus Professor of Pediatrics, Temple University; Chief, Section for Endocrine, Diabetes, and Metabolic Disorders, Temple University Children's Medical Center, Philadelphia, Pennsylvania

Frederick P. Rivara, MD, MPH
George Adkins Professor of Pediatrics, University of Washington, Seattle, Washington

Nathaniel H. Robin, MD
Associate Professor of Genetics, University of Alabama at Birmingham; University Hospital, University of Alabama at Birmingham, Children's Hospital, Birmingham, Alabama

Luther K. Robinson, MD, AB
Associate Professor of Pediatrics, State University of New York at Buffalo School of Medicine and Biomedical Sciences; Director, Dysmorphology and Clinical Genetics, Women and Children's Hospital of Buffalo, Buffalo, New York

George C. Rodgers, Jr., MD, PhD
Professor of Pediatrics and Pharmacology/Toxicology, Department of Pediatrics, University of Louisville; Associate Medical Director, Kentucky Regional Poison Center, Koasir Childrens Hospital, Louisville, Kentucky

Genie E. Roosevelt, MD, MPH
Assistant Professor of Pediatrics, University of Colorado School of Medicine; Attending Physician, The Children's Hospital, Denver, Colorado

David S. Rosenblatt, MD
Professor and Chairman, Department of Human Genetics, McGill University; Director, Division of Medical Genetics, Department of Medicine, McGill University Health Centre; Chief, Department of Medical Genetics, Sir Mortimer B. Davis Jewish General Hospital, Montreal, Quebec, Canada

Anne H. Rowley, MD
Professor of Pediatrics and of Microbiology/Immunology, Northwestern University, Feinberg School of Medicine; Attending Physician, Division of Infectious Diseases, Children's Memorial Hospital, Chicago, Illinois

Ranna Rozenfeld, MD
Associate Professor of Pediatrics, Northwestern University, Feinberg School of Medicine; Attending Physician, Pediatric Critical Care Medicine, Children's Memorial Hospital, Chicago, Illinois

Colin D. Rudolph, MD, PhD
Professor and Chief, Pediatric Gastroenterology and Nutrition, Medical College of Wisconsin; Children's Hospital of Wisconsin, Milwaukee, Wisconsin

Robert A. Salata, MD
Professor of Medicine, Epidemiology/Biostatistics, and International Health, Case Western Reserve University School of Medicine; Attending Physician, Chief, Division of Infectious Diseases and HIV Medicine, University Hospitals Case Medical Center, Cleveland, Ohio

Denise A. Salerno, MD
Associate Professor of Pediatrics, Temple University School of Medicine; Associate Professor of Pediatrics, Temple University Children's Medical Center, Philadelphia, Pennsylvania

Hugh Sampson, MD
Professor of Pediatrics and Immunobiology, Mount Sinai School of Medicine; Attending Physician, Mount Sinai Hospital, New York, New York

Joseph M. Sanfilippo, MD, MBA
Professor of Obstetrics, Gynecology, and Reproductive Sciences, University of Pittsburgh School of Medicine; Staff, Magee-Women's Hospital, Pittsburgh, Pennsylvania

Ashok P. Sarnaik, MD
Professor of Pediatrics, Wayne State University School of Medicine; Division Chief, Pediatric Critical Care Medicine, Children's Hospital of Michigan, Detroit, Michigan

Harvey B. Sarnat, MD, FRCPC
Professor of Paediatrics, Pathology (Neuropathology), and Clinical Neuroscience, University of Calgary Faculty of Medicine; Head, Division of Paediatric Neurology, Alberta Children's Hospital, Calgary, Alberta, Canada

Mark R. Schleiss, MD
Professor, Director of Pediatric Infectious Diseases, American Legion Chair of Pediatrics, Co-Director for the Center for Infectious Diseases and Microbiology Translational Research, and Associate Chair for Research, Pediatrics, University of Minnesota; Attending Physician, Pediatrics Department, University of Minnesota Medical Center, Fairview; Attending Physician, Pediatrics Department, University of Minnesota Children's Hospital, Fairview, Minneapolis, Minnesota; Consulting Physician, Pediatrics Department, Children's Hospitals and Clinics of Minnesota, Minneapolis and St. Paul, Minnesota

Robert L. Schum, PhD
Associate Professor of Pediatrics, Medical College of Wisconsin; Clinical Psychologist, Child Development Center, Children's Hospital of Wisconsin, Milwaukee, Wisconsin

Gordon G. Schutze, MD
Professor of Pediatrics and Pathology, University of Arkansas for Medical Sciences, College of Medicine; Arkansas Children's Hospital, Little Rock, Arkansas

J. Paul Scott, MD
Professor of Pediatrics, Medical College of Wisconsin; Attending Hematologist/Director, Wisconsin Sickle Cell Center, Department of Pediatrics, Hematology, Oncology, and Transplant, Children's Hospital of Wisconsin; Investigator, Hemostasis Research Section, Blood Research Institute, Blood Center of Wisconsin, Milwaukee, Wisconsin

Theodore C. Sectish, MD
Associate Professor, Stanford University School of Medicine; Director, Residency Training Program, Lucile Salter Packard Children's Hospital, Palo Alto, California

George B. Segel, MD
Professor of Pediatrics and Medicine, University of Rochester School of Medicine; Golisano Children's Hospital, Rochester, New York

Janet R. Serwint, MD
Professor of Pediatrics, Johns Hopkins University School of Medicine; Professor of Pediatrics, Director, Pediatric Resident Education, Johns Hopkins Hospital, Baltimore, Maryland

Jane Seward, MBBS, MPH
Acting Deputy Director, Division of Viral Diseases, National Center for Immunizations and Respiratory Diseases, Centers for Disease Control and Prevention, Atlanta, Georgia

Prachi E. Shah, MD
Associate Professor of Pediatrics, Baylor College of Medicine; Developmental and Behavioral Pediatrician: Meyer Center for Developmental Pediatrics, Texas Children's Hospital, Houston Texas

Bruce K. Shapiro, MD
Associate Professor of Pediatrics and Arnold Cepute, MD, MPH Chair in Neurodevelopmental Disabilities, Johns Hopkins University School of Medicine; Vice President, Training, Kennedy Krieger Institute, Johns Hopkins University School of Medicine, Baltimore, Maryland

Eugene D. Shapiro, MD
Professor, Department of Pediatrics, Epidemiology and Public Health, and Investigative Medicine, Yale University; Attending Physician, Pediatrics Department, Children's Hospital of Yale-New Haven

Bennett A. Shaywitz, MD
Professor of Pediatrics and Neurology; Co-Director, Yale Center for the Study of Learning, Reading, and Attention, Department of Pediatrics, New Haven, Connecticut

Sally E. Shaywitz, MD
Professor of Pediatrics; Co-Director, Yale Center for the Study of Learning, Reading, and Attention, Department of Pediatrics, New Haven, Connecticut

Joel Shilyanski, MD, FACS, FAAP
Associate Professor, Department of Surgery, University of Iowa; Director of Pediatric Surgery, University of Iowa Hospitals and Clinics, Iowa City, Iowa

Melanie Shim, MD
Adjunct Assistant Professor, Department of Pediatric Endocrinology, University of California at Los Angeles; Adjunct Assistant Professor, Department of Pediatric Endocrinology, University of California at Los Angeles, Los Angeles, California; Partner Physician, Department of Pediatric Endocrinology, Kaiser Permanente, Harbor City, California

Benjamin L. Shneider, MD
Professor of Pediatrics, Mount Sinai School of Medicine; Attending Physician, Mount Sinai Medical Center, New York, New York

Stanford T. Shulman, MD
Professor of Pediatrics, Northwestern University, Feinberg School of Medicine; Chief, Division of Infectious Diseases, Children's Memorial Hospital, Chicago, Illinois

George K. Siberry, MD, MPH
Assistant Professor, Department of Pediatrics, Johns Hopkins University School of Medicine; Medical Director, Harriet Lane Clinic, Department of Pediatrics, Johns Hopkins Hospital, Baltimore, Maryland

Scott H. Sicherer, MD
Associate Professor of Pediatrics, Jaffe Food Allergy Institute, Division of Pediatric Allergy and Immunology, Mount Sinai School of Medicine, New York, New York

Mark D. Simms, MD, MPH
Professor of Pediatrics and Chief, Section of Developmental Pediatrics, Medical College of Wisconsin; Medical Director, Child Development Center, Children's Hospital of Wisconsin, Milwaukee, Wisconsin

Eric F. Simoes, MD, DCH
Professor of Pediatrics, Section of Infectious Diseases, University of Colorado at Denver and Health Sciences Center; Professor of Pediatrics, Section of Infectious Diseases, The Children's Hospital, Denver, Colorado

Joseph A. Skelton, MD
Assistant Professor of Pediatrics, Medical College of Wisconsin; Director, NEW (Nutrition, Exercise, and Weight management) Kids Program™, Children's Hospital of Wisconsin, Milwaukee, Wisconsin

Thomas I. Slovis, MD
Professor of Radiology and Pediatrics, Wayne State University School of Medicine; Professor of Radiology and Pediatrics, Staff Radiologist, Children's Hospital of Michigan, Detroit, Michigan

Laura P. Smith, MD
Associate Professor of Ophthalmology and Pediatrics, University of Missouri, Kansas City School of Medicine; Staff, Children's Mercy Hospitals and Clinics, Kansas City, Missouri

Manu Sood, MD, MRCP, MBBS
Associate Professor, Medical College of Wisconsin; Director of Gastrointestinal Motility, Children's Hospital of Wisconsin, Milwaukee, Wisconsin

Joseph D. Spahn, MD
Associate Professor of Pediatrics, Division of Allergy, Immunology, and Rheumatology; Director, Immunopharmacology Lab, Division of Clinical Pharmacology; Director, Pediatric Allergy Immunology Fellowship Program, National Jewish Medical and Research Center, Denver, Colorado

Mark A. Sperling, MD
Professor, Department of Pediatrics, University of Pittsburgh; Professor, Division of Pediatric Endocrinology, Diabetes, and Metabolism, Children's Hospital of Pittsburgh, Pittsburgh, Pennsylvania

David A. Spiegel, MD
Assistant Professor of Orthopaedic Surgery, University of Pennsylvania School of Medicine; Orthopaedic Surgeon, The Children's Hospital of Philadelphia, Philadelphia, Pennsylvania

Jürgen Spranger, MD
Professor Emeritus of Pediatrics, University of Mainz, Germany; Formerly Head of Children's Hospital, Mainz, Germany

Brian Stafford, MD, MPH
Assistant Professor of Psychiatry and Pediatrics, University of Colorado Health Sciences Center; Consult-Liaison Psychiatrist, Department of Psychiatry/Behavioral Sciences, The Children's Hospital; Medical Director, Post-partum Depression Intervention Program, Kempe Center, Denver, Colorado

Sergio Stagno, MD
Professor and Chairman, Department of Pediatrics, The University of Alabama at Birmingham; Physician-in-Chief, Children's Hospital of Alabama, Birmingham, Alabama

Lawrence R. Stanberry, MD, PhD
John Sealy Distinguished Chair and Professor, Department of Pediatrics, University of Texas Medical Branch; Director, Sealy Center for Vaccine Development, University of Texas Medical Branch, Galveston, Texas

Charles A. Stanley, MD
Professor of Pediatrics, University of Pennsylvania School of Medicine; Chief, Division of Endocrinology, The Children's Hospital of Philadelphia, Philadelphia, Pennsylvania

Bonita F. Stanton, MD
Schotanus Professor and Chair, Department of Pediatrics, Wayne State University School of Medicine; Pediatrician-in-Chief, Carman and Ann Adams Department of Pediatrics, Children's Hospital of Michigan, Detroit, Michigan

Jeffrey R. Starke, MD
Professor and Vice Chairman, Department of Pediatrics, Baylor College of Medicine; Chief of Pediatrics, Ben Taub General Hospital; Infection Control Officer, Texas Children's Hospital, Houston, Texas

Barbara W. Stechenberg, MD
Professor of Pediatrics, Tufts University School of Medicine; Director, Pediatric Infectious Diseases, Vice Chairman, Pediatrics Department, Baystate Children's Hospital, Springfield, Massachusetts

Barbara J. Stoll, MD
George W. Brumley, Jr., Professor and Chair, Department of Pediatrics, Emory University School of Medicine, Atlanta, Georgia

Laura Stout Sosinsky, PhD
Postdoctoral Associate, Yale Child Study Center, Yale University School of Medicine, New Haven, Connecticut

Ronald G. Strauss, MD
Professor of Pathology and Pediatrics, University of Iowa College of Medicine; DeGowin Blood Center Faculty, Department of Pathology, University of Iowa Hospitals and Clinics, Iowa City, Iowa

Frederick J. Suchy, MD
Professor and Chair of Pediatrics, Mount Sinai School of Medicine; Pediatrician-in-Chief, Mount Sinai Hospital, New York, New York

Stuart C. Sweet, MD, PhD
Associate Professor, Department of Pediatrics, Washington University in St. Louis, St. Louis, Missouri

Robert P. Thomas, MD
Clinical Assistant Professor, University of Texas Health Science Center; Methodists Children's Hospital and Christus Santa Rosa Children's Hospital, San Antonio, Texas

Norman Tinanoff, DDS, MS
Professor and Chair, Department of Health Promotion and Policy, University of Maryland Dental School, Baltimore, Maryland

James K. Todd, MD
Professor of Pediatrics, Microbiology, and Preventive Medicine/Biometrics, University of Colorado School of Medicine; Director of Epidemiology, Clinical Microbiology and Clinical Outcomes, Department of Epidemiology and Community Pediatrics, The Children's Hospital, Denver, Colorado

Philip Toltzis, MD
Associate Professor of Pediatrics, Case Western Reserve University School of Medicine; Attending Physician, Division of Pharmacology and Critical Care, Rainbow Babies and Children's Hospital, Cleveland, Ohio

Lucy Tompkins, MD
Lucy Becker Professor of Medicine, Professor of Microbiology and Immunology, Chief, Division of Infectious Diseases and Geographic Medicine, Stanford University School of Medicine; Medical Director, Hospital Epidemiology and Infection Control, Stanford Hospitals and Clinics, Stanford, California

David G. Tubergen, MD
Medical Director, M.D. Anderson Physicians Network, University of Texas M.D. Anderson Cancer Center, Houston, Texas

Ronald B. Turner, MD
Professor of Pediatrics, University of Virginia School of Medicine, Charlottesville, Virginia

MacDara Tynan, MD, FAAP
Adjunct Clinical Associate Professor, Department of Pediatrics, University of North Carolina, Chapel Hill, North Carolina; Director of Hospitalist Group, Department of Pediatrics, Levine Children's Hospital, Charlotte, North Carolina

Rodrigo E. Urizar, MD (Retired)
Professor of Pediatrics, Nephrology, Director of Pediatric Dialysis Services, Albany Medical College, Union University; Attending Pediatric Nephrologist, Children's Hospital, Albany Medical Center, Albany, New York

Douglas Vanderbilt, MD
Assistant Professor of Pediatrics, Boston University School of Medicine; Staff, Division of Developmental and Behavioral Pediatrics, Boston Medical Center, Boston, Massachusetts

Andrea Velardi, MD
Professor of Hematology, Perugia University School of Medicine, Perugia, Italy

Elliott Vichinsky, MD
Medical Director, Hematology/Oncology, Children's Hospital and Research Center, Oakland, California

Beth A. Vogt, MD
Associate Professor, Case Western Reserve University; Staff Physician, Rainbow Babies and Children's Hospital, Cleveland, Ohio

Linda A. Waggoner-Fountain, MD
Associate Professor of Pediatrics, University of Virginia School of Medicine, Charlottesville, Virginia

Kimberly Danieli Watts, MD
Fellow, Pediatric Pulmonary Medicine, Northwestern University, Feinberg School of Medicine; Children's Memorial Hospital, Chicago, Illinois

Martin E. Weisse, MD
Professor of Pediatrics, West Virginia University School of Medicine; Chief, Department of Infectious Diseases, Director, Pediatric Residency Program, West Virginia University School of Medicine, Morgantown, West Virginia

Lawrence Wells, MD
Assistant Professor, Orthopaedic Surgery, University of Pennsylvania School of Medicine; Attending Surgeon, The Children's Hospital of Philadelphia, Philadelphia, Pennsylvania

Steven L. Werlin, MD
Professor of Pediatrics, Medical College of Wisconsin; Children's Hospital of Wisconsin, Milwaukee, Wisconsin

Michael Wessels, MD
Professor of Pediatrics and Medicine (Microbiology and Molecular Genetics), Harvard Medical School; Chief, Division of Infectious Diseases, Children's Hospital, Boston, Massachusetts

Ralph Wetmore, MD
Professor of Otorhinolaryngology, University of Pennsylvania School of Medicine; Senior Surgeon, Division of Pediatric Otolaryngology, Children's Hospital of Philadelphia, Philadelphia, Pennsylvania

Randall Wetzel, MD
Professor of Pediatrics and Anesthesiology, Keck School of Medicine; Chairman, Anesthesiology Critical Care Medicine, The Children's Hospital, Los Angeles, California

Isaiah D. Wexler, MD, PhD
Attending Pediatrician, Department of Pediatrics, Mount Scopus Campus, Hadassah University Hospital, Jerusalem, Israel

Perrin C. White, MD
Professor of Pediatrics, University of Texas Southwestern Medical Center; Chief, Endocrinology, Children's Medical Center, Dallas, Texas

Michael Wilschanski, MBBS
Director, Pediatric Gastroenterology Unit, Hadassah University Hospitals; Senior Lecturer, Division of Pediatrics, Hebrew University, Jerusalem, Israel

Glenna B. Winnie, MD
Associate Professor of Pediatrics, George Washington University; Chief, Division of Allergy, Pulmonary, and Sleep Medicine, Children's National Medical Center, Washington, District of Columbia

Paul H. Wise, MD, MPH
Professor of Pediatrics, Richard E. Behrman Professor of Child Health and Society, Stanford University School of Medicine; Director, Center for Policy, Outcomes and Prevention, Department of Pediatrics, Lucile Salter Packard Children's Hospital, Palo Alto, California

Charles R. Woods, MD
Associate Professor of Pediatrics, Wake Forest University School of Medicine; Brenner Children's Hospital, Winston-Salem, North Carolina

Laura Worth, MD, PhD
Associate Professor of Pediatrics, Medical Director, Cell Therapy, University of Texas M.D. Anderson Cancer Center; Assistant Professor, University of Texas Health Science Center, Memorial Hermann Hospital, Houston, Texas

Peter Wright, MD
Shedd Chair in Pediatric Infectious Diseases; Professor of Pediatrics, Pathology and Microbiology & Immunology; Chief, Division of Pediatric Infectious Diseases, Vanderbilt University School of Medicine, Nashville, Tennessee

Terry W. Wright, PhD
Associate Professor of Pediatrics and Microbiology & Immunology, University of Rochester School of Medicine, Rochester, New York

David T. Wyatt, MD
Professor of Pediatrics, Section of Endocrinology and Diabetes, Medical College of Wisconsin; Chief, Pediatric Endocrinology, Children's Hospital of Wisconsin, Milwaukee, Wisconsin

Robert Wyllie, MD
Chairman, Division of Pediatrics; Physician-in-Chief, Cleveland Clinic Children's Hospital, Cleveland, Ohio

Anthony Wynshaw-Boris, MD
Professor of Pediatrics and Medicine Department, Director, Center for Human Genetics and Genomics, Chief, Division of Genetics, Department of Pediatrics, University of California, San Diego School of Medicine; Rady Children's Hospital, San Diego, California

Stavra A. Xanthakos, MD, MS
Assistant Professor of Pediatrics, Department of Pediatrics, Division of Gastroenterology, Hepatology, and Nutrition, Cincinnati Children's Hospital Medical Center, Cincinnati, Ohio

Nada Yazigi, MD
Assistant Professor of Clinical Pediatrics, University of Cincinnati Medical School; Assistant Professor of Clinical Pediatrics, Division of Gastroenterology, Hepatology, and Nutrition, Cincinnati Children's Hospital Medical Center, Cincinnati, Ohio

Ram Yogev, MD
Professor of Pediatrics, Northwestern University; Director, Section of Pediatric, Addescent, and Maternal HIV Infection, Department of Pediatrics, Children's Memorial Hospital, Chicago, Illinois

Nader Youssef, MD, MBA
Assistant Professor of Pediatrics, University of Medicine & Dentistry of New Jersey – The New Jersey Medical School; Director, Center for Pediatric Irritable Bowel & Motility Disorders, Goryeb Children's Hospital at Atlantic Health, Morristown, New Jersey

Anita K.M. Zaidi, MBBS, SM
Associate Professor of Pediatrics and Microbiology, Aga Khan University; Pediatric Infectious Diseases Consultant, Aga Khan University Hospital, Karachi, Pakistan

Lonnie K. Zeltzer, MD
Professor of Pediatrics, Anesthesiology, Psychiatry, and Biobehavioral Sciences, David Geffen School of Medicine; Director, Pediatric Pain Program; Mattel Children's Hospital at University of California, Los Angeles, California

Maija H. Zile, PhD
Professor of Food Science and Human Nutrition, Michigan State University, East Lansing, Michigan

Barry S. Zuckerman, MD
The Joel and Barbara Alpert Professor and Chair of Pediatrics, Boston University School of Medicine, Professor of Public Health, Boston University School of Public Health; Chief, Pediatrics, Boston Medical Center, Boston, Massachusetts

Indice

VOLUME 1

VOLUME 2

Parte XVIII ■ Apparato respiratorio 1769

Parte XX ■ Malattie del sangue 2053

Parte XVII ■ Apparato digerente

Sezione 1 — Manifestazioni cliniche delle malattie gastrointestinali — Robert Wyllie

Capitolo 302 ■ Normali fenomeni del tratto digerente

La funzione gastrointestinale va incontro a cambiamenti a seconda del grado di maturità; un evento che è fisiologico in un neonato o in un lattante può essere sintomo di una patologia in un'età successiva. Il feto è in grado di deglutire liquido amniotico già alla 12ª settimana di gestazione, ma la suzione a scopo nutritivo nei neonati inizia a svilupparsi verso la 34ª settimana. I movimenti orali e faringei coordinati necessari per la deglutizione dei solidi si sviluppano nei primissimi mesi di vita; prima di questo periodo, la lingua spinge verso l'alto e verso l'esterno per spremere il latte dal capezzolo, anziché muoversi all'indietro per sospingere i solidi verso l'apertura dell'esofago. Dal primo mese di vita il bambino sembra mostrare una certa preferenza per i cibi dolci e salati. Il suo interesse per i solidi aumenta intorno all'età di 4 mesi; di conseguenza, la raccomandazione di introdurre questi alimenti all'età di 6 mesi si basa su considerazioni di carattere nutrizionale e culturale più che sulla maturazione del processo della deglutizione (vedi Capitolo 42). Durante l'alimentazione i lattanti inghiottono aria ed è quindi importante stimolare l'eruttazione per prevenire la distensione gassosa dello stomaco.

Nel cavo orale si possono osservare numerose varianti anatomiche che non hanno alcun significato patologico. Un **frenulo linguale breve** ("lingua legata") può destare preoccupazione nei genitori, ma è raro che interferisca con l'alimentazione o con l'articolazione del linguaggio e in genere non necessita di alcun trattamento. La presenza di **solchi sulla lingua** (lingua a carta geografica o scrotale) è di solito un reperto normale. L'**ugola bifida** può essere normale o associata a schisi sottomucosa del palato molle.

Il **rigurgito**, dovuto al reflusso gastroesofageo, è un evento comune nel primo anno di vita. Il cibo rigurgitato può fuoriuscire dalla bocca sotto forma di sbavamento oppure in modo vigoroso. In un bambino altrimenti sano che presenta rigurgito, il volume dell'emesi è in genere di circa 15-30 mL, ma talvolta superiore. Dopo un episodio di rigurgito di solito il bambino non dà segni di malessere, anche se può comparire fame. Gli episodi possono non verificarsi affatto oppure ripetersi diverse volte al giorno. Il rigurgito si risolve gradualmente nell'80% dei soggetti entro i 6 mesi di vita e nel 90% entro i 12 mesi. Se il problema persiste o insorgono complicanze, il reflusso gastroesofageo viene considerato non più un fenomeno normale connesso allo sviluppo, bensì un evento patologico e come tale richiede un'ulteriore valutazione e il trattamento. Tra le sue complicanze vi sono il deficit di crescita staturoponderale, le malattie polmonari (apnea o polmonite ab ingestis) e l'esofagite con relative sequele (vedi Capitoli 320 e 321).

I lattanti e i bambini piccoli talvolta mangiano in modo irregolare e ciò può essere fonte di ansia per i genitori. Un bambino ai primi passi può mangiare in modo insaziabile o rifiutare un pasto; è inoltre diffusa la tendenza ad accettare una limitata varietà di cibi. Bisognerebbe quindi invitare i genitori a considerare l'apporto alimentare nell'arco di più giorni e a non preoccuparsi troppo riguardo ai singoli pasti. L'infanzia e l'adolescenza sono periodi di rapida crescita, in cui le elevate esigenze nutrizionali possono associarsi a fame vorace. L'inappetenza del bambino ai primi passi o in età prescolare spesso preoccupa i genitori, che sono abituati a un apporto dietetico relativamente più elevato durante l'infanzia; per rassicurarli occorre dimostrare loro che la curva della crescita presenta un andamento appropriato per l'età.

Il numero, il colore e la consistenza delle feci possono variare moltissimo nello stesso soggetto e tra bambini della medesima età, senza un motivo apparente. Le prime feci emesse dopo la nascita sono costituite dal meconio, una sostanza viscosa, scura, che normalmente viene evacuata nelle prime 48 ore di vita. Con l'inizio dell'alimentazione, il meconio viene sostituito dalle feci di transizione, di colore verde-marrone, spesso contenenti latte cagliato e, dopo 4-5 giorni, dalle feci da latte, giallo-marrone. La **frequenza dell'alvo** è estremamente variabile nei bambini normali, potendo andare da 0 a 7 scariche al giorno. I neonati allattati al seno possono dapprima evacuare quantità piccole ma frequenti di feci poco formate (dette di transizione) per poi emettere, dopo 2-3 settimane, feci morbide molto raramente. Alcuni lattanti possono non evacuare per 1-2 settimane e poi avere una normale evacuazione intestinale morbida. Il colore delle feci ha scarso significato, a meno che non sia presente sangue o non si riscontri l'assenza dei prodotti della bilirubina (in tal caso il colore sarà bianco grigiastro anziché giallo-marrone). La presenza di materia vegetale, come piselli o cereali, nelle feci di un lattante più grande o di un bambino ai primi passi che ingerisce cibi solidi è normale e deve far pensare a una masticazione insufficiente, non a malassorbimento. Da 1 a 3 anni di vita è di comune riscontro la cosiddetta **diarrea del bambino ai primi passi**, con emissione intermittente di feci poco formate. Questi soggetti, che per il resto crescono in buona salute, spesso consumano quantità eccessive di bevande contenenti carboidrati. In genere le scariche alvine si verificano durante le ore diurne e non di notte. Il volume di liquidi ingeriti è spesso eccessivo; limitando l'assunzione delle bevande contenenti zuccheri e aumentando l'apporto di grassi con la dieta spesso si ottiene la risoluzione del quadro.

Spesso nei bambini piccoli e in quelli ai primi passi si osserva un addome globoso, soprattutto dopo pasti abbondanti. Tale fenomeno può essere dovuto a una combinazione di fattori: muscolatura addominale debole, organi addominali relativamente grandi e atteggiamento in lordosi. Nel primo anno di vita, è comune palpare il fegato 1-2 cm al di sotto del margine costale destro. Il fegato normale è di consistenza soffice e alla percussione risulta di dimensioni normali per l'età. Il lobo di Riedel è una sottile proiezione del lobo epatico destro che può essere palpata nella parte inferiore dell'addome, sul lato destro. Anche un apice della milza palpabile, di consistenza soffice, rappresenta un reperto normale. Nei bambini piccoli magri, la colonna vertebrale è facilmente palpabile e una struttura sovrastante può essere scambiata per una massa. È possibile apprezzare le pulsazioni dell'aorta. Spesso si riscontrano feci normali nel quadrante inferiore sinistro del colon discendente o del sigma.

L'**emissione di sangue** dal tratto gastrointestinale non è mai normale, ma il sangue deglutito può essere scambiato per un'emorragia gastrointestinale. Il sangue materno può essere ingerito al momento del parto o in seguito, durante l'allattamento, in caso di sanguinamento dal capezzolo. Talvolta il sanguinamento nasale o orofaringeo viene confuso con un'emorragia gastrointestinale (vedi Capitolo 103.4). I coloranti rossi contenuti nei cibi e nelle bevande possono tingere le feci, ma non producono positività al test per il sangue occulto nelle feci.

L'**ittero** è comune nei neonati, specialmente nei prematuri, e di solito è dovuto all'incapacità del fegato immaturo di coniugare la bilirubina, con conseguente aumento della frazione indiretta (vedi Capitolo 102.3). La persistenza di livelli di bilirubina indiretta troppo elevati, nei bambini allattati al seno, può essere secondaria all'ittero da latte materno, che di solito è un'entità benigna nei neonati a pieno termine. Elevati livelli di bilirubina diretta non sono normali e suggeriscono un'epatopatia, sebbene nei neonati possano essere secondari a infezione extraepatica (infezione delle vie urinarie) o ad accumulo di sangue con un eccessivo carico di bilirubina che viene rilasciato in circolo (emorragia endocranica). La frazione di bilirubina diretta non dovrebbe rappresentare più del 15-20% della bilirubina sierica totale; un suo aumento può essere secondario a iperbilirubinemia indiretta, poiché il fegato converte l'eccesso di bilirubina indiretta in bilirubina diretta e la fase *rate-limiting* dell'escrezione della bilirubina passa dalla glucuronazione della bilirubina all'escrezione della bilirubina diretta nel canalicolo biliare. L'iperbilirubinemia indiretta, che è comune nei neonati normali, tende a colorare le sclere e la cute di giallo oro, mentre quella diretta produce una tinta giallo-verdastra.

Capitolo 303 ■ Principali sintomi e segni delle malattie del tratto digerente

Le malattie a carico di organi che non fanno parte dell'apparato gastrointestinale possono produrre sintomi e segni che simulano le patologie del tubo digerente e che quindi dovrebbero essere prese in considerazione nella diagnosi differenziale (Tab. 303-1). La conoscenza della possibile patogenesi dei sintomi consentirà di prendere decisioni diagnostiche e terapeutiche razionali. Nei bambini con crescita e sviluppo normali, il trattamento può essere stabilito alla luce di una diagnosi presuntiva basata sull'anamnesi e sull'esame obiettivo, senza indagini diagnostiche formali. Lo scarso aumento di peso o il calo ponderale sono spesso associati a un processo patologico significativo e di solito necessitano di test diagnostici più formali.

TABELLA 303-1. Cause non digestive di sintomi gastrointestinali nei bambini

ANORESSIA
Malattie sistemiche (infiammatorie, neoplastiche)
Compromissione cardiorespiratoria
Iatrogena: terapia farmacologica, diete terapeutiche sgradevoli
Depressione
Anoressia nervosa
VOMITO
Errori congeniti del metabolismo
Farmaci (eritromicina, chemioterapia)
Ipertensione endocranica
Tumori cerebrali
Infezioni (vie urinarie)
Labirintite
Insufficienza surrenalica
Gravidanza
Psicogena
Emicrania addominale
Tossine
DIARREA
Infezioni (otite media, urinarie)
Uremia
Farmaci (antibiotici, cisapride)
Tumori (neuroblastoma)
Pericardite
STIPSI
Ipotiroidismo
Spina bifida
Ritardo psicomotorio
Disidratazione (diabete insipido, lesioni tubulari renali)
Farmaci (narcotici)
Intossicazione da piombo
Botulismo infantile
DOLORE ADDOMINALE
Pielonefrite, idronefrosi, colica renale
Polmonite
Malattia infiammatoria pelvica
Porfiria
Angioedema
Endocardite
Emicrania addominale
Febbre mediterranea familiare
Abuso fisico o sessuale
Lupus eritematoso sistemico
Fobia della scuola
Crisi falcemica
Infiammazione del disco vertebrale
Farmaci (FANS)
Osteomielite pelvica
DISTENSIONE O MASSA ADDOMINALE
Ascite (sindrome nefrosica, neoplasia, insufficienza cardiaca)
Massa distinta (tumore di Wilms, idronefrosi, neuroblastoma, cisti mesenterica, epatoblastoma, linfoma)
Gravidanza
ITTERO
Malattia emolitica
Infezione delle vie urinarie
Sepsi
Ipotiroidismo
Panipopituitarismo

FANS, farmaci antinfiammatori non steroidei.

DISFAGIA. La disfagia, o difficoltà di deglutizione, può essere causata da un difetto strutturale o da un disturbo della motilità. I difetti strutturali che causano un impedimento fisso al passaggio del bolo alimentare sono dovuti a restringimenti all'interno dell'esofago oppure a stenosi, membrane o tumori. L'ostruzione estrinseca è per lo più imputabile a un anello vascolare (vedi Capitolo 432). In genere i difetti strutturali causano più problemi di deglutizione dei solidi che dei liquidi. La maggior parte delle cause non strutturali di disfagia è dovuta ad anomalie della motilità dell'orofaringe o dell'esofago. La deglutizione è un processo complesso, che inizia già nel cavo orale: qui la masticazione e la lubrificazione del cibo portano alla formazione del bolo, che viene poi sospinto nella faringe dalla lingua. La fase faringea della deglutizione è rapida e comprende meccanismi protettivi per evitare che il cibo entri nelle vie aeree. L'epiglottide si abbassa sopra la laringe mentre il palato molle si solleva contro la parete nasofaringea; vi è un temporaneo arresto della respirazione mentre lo sfintere esofageo superiore si apre per consentire al bolo di entrare nell'esofago. Nell'esofago, contrazioni muscolari peristaltiche coordinate spingono il bolo alimentare verso lo stomaco. Dato che lo sfintere esofageo inferiore si rilassa subito dopo lo sfintere esofageo superiore, i liquidi che attraversano rapidamente l'esofago fanno il loro ingresso nello stomaco senza incontrare alcun impedimento.

La disfagia durante la fase orofaringea della deglutizione viene denominata **disfagia di trasferimento** ed è solitamente associata a malattie neuromuscolari (paralisi cerebrale). Il **globo** (in passato denominato *globo isterico*), ossia la sensazione che qualcosa si sia arrestato nell'esofago superiore, è tipicamente associato a reflusso gastroesofageo.

Quando la disfagia è associata a un ritardo nel passaggio del bolo attraverso l'esofago, il bambino può essere in grado di indicare il livello del torace in cui avverte un rallentamento; i sintomi esofagei possono irradiarsi all'incisura soprasternale. Quando il bambino indica questo punto, il blocco può trovarsi a qualsiasi livello dell'esofago.

Disfagia di trasferimento. Il passaggio del cibo nell'esofago superiore dipende da una complessa sequenza di eventi neuromuscolari. Perché avvenga l'allattamento è necessario che le labbra si chiudano attorno al capezzolo aderendo a esso mentre la lingua si sposta posteriormente. Quando la glottide si chiude per proteggere le vie aeree, il palato molle si solleva a chiudere il rinofaringe, i muscoli cricofaringei si rilassano e il cibo entra nella parte posteriore della faringe. Anche l'ingestione dei solidi richiede una serie di azioni coordinate; le grosse porzioni di cibo vengono triturate grazie al movimento delle mandibole e dei denti. Le secrezioni salivari, stimolate dall'anticipazione e dall'atto dell'ingestione, lubrificano i cibi quando passano attraverso la bocca. Le anomalie relative all'innervazione, alla forza o alla coordinazione dei muscoli coinvolti nel processo dell'ingestione sono associate a tale forma di disfagia nei bambini. In questi casi, un problema orofaringeo quasi sempre fa parte di un disturbo neurologico o muscolare più generalizzato (botulismo, difterite, malattia neuromuscolare). Lesioni orali dolorose, come quelle causate dalla stomatite virale acuta o di origine traumatica, interferiscono talvolta con l'ingestione. Se il passaggio dell'aria attraverso il naso è quasi completamente ostruito, la difficoltà di respirare provoca gravi disturbi durante la suzione. Sebbene ci si aspetti che gravi anomalie strutturali, dentali e salivari possano interferire con l'alimentazione, quest'ultima procede relativamente bene nella maggior parte dei bambini affetti, se sono affamati.

Disfagia non di trasferimento. I disturbi primari della motilità che causano compromissione della funzione peristaltica e disfagia sono rari nei bambini. La motilità dell'esofago distale risulta compromessa dopo la riparazione della fistola tracheoesofagea. Le discinesie possono accompagnare le collagenopatie vascolari. L'**acalasia** si verifica raramente nei bambini. Le membrane esofagee, i residui tracheobronchiali o gli anelli vascolari possono causare disfagia in età pediatrica. Un **restringimento** esofageo secondario a reflusso gastroesofageo cronico ed esofagite talvolta si manifesta con disfagia come sintomo di esordio. L'anello di Schatzki, un sottile anello di tessuto in prossimità dello sfintere esofageo inferiore, è un'altra causa meccanica di disfagia ricorrente che si presenta dopo l'infanzia. La disfagia può essere causata anche da un **corpo estraneo** esofageo o da un restringimento secondario all'ingestione di caustici.

RIGURGITO. Il rigurgito è la risalita spontanea del contenuto dello stomaco nell'esofago e nella bocca. Non solo non è mai associato a malessere, ma il bambino è spesso affamato subito dopo l'episodio. Lo sfintere esofageo inferiore impedisce il reflusso del contenuto gastrico nell'esofago (vedi Capitolo 320); il rigurgito o "spitting" è quindi secondario al reflusso gastroesofageo che avviene attraverso uno sfintere esofageo inferiore incompetente e, nei bambini, immaturo. Spesso si tratta di un fenomeno legato allo sviluppo, che si risolve con la maturazione. È importante distinguerlo dal vomito, termine che sta a indicare un riflesso attivo con un'ampia diagnosi differenziale (Tab. 303-2).

ANORESSIA. I centri della fame e della sazietà sono localizzati nell'ipotalamo; è probabile che i nervi afferenti dal tratto gastrointestinale a questi centri cerebrali siano importanti fattori coinvolti nell'anoressia tipica di molte malattie dello stomaco e dell'intestino. Il segnale di sazietà, stimolato dalla distensione dello stomaco o del tratto superiore dell'intestino tenue, viene trasmesso da fibre sensitive afferenti, la cui densità è particolarmente elevata nell'intestino prossimale. Anche i chemiorecettori presenti nell'intestino, stimolati dall'assimilazione delle sostanze nutritizie, influenzano il flusso afferente ai centri della fame. Alcuni impulsi raggiungono l'ipotalamo partendo dai centri superiori, probabilmente sotto l'influsso del dolore o del turbamento emotivo che una malattia intestinale comporta. Tra gli altri fattori di regolazione vi sono gli ormoni, la grelina, la leptina e il glucosio plasmatico, che a loro volta riflettono le funzioni intestinali.

TABELLA 303-2. Diagnosi differenziale dell'emesi durante l'infanzia

LATTANTE	BAMBINO	ADOLESCENTE
COMUNI		
Gastroenterite	Gastroenterite	Gastroenterite
Reflusso gastroesofageo	Infezione sistemica	GERD
Iperalimentazione	Gastrite	Infezione sistemica
Ostruzione anatomica	Ingestione di sostanze tossiche	Ingestione di sostanze tossiche
Infezione sistemica	Sindrome della pertosse	Gastrite
Sindrome della pertosse	Farmaci	Sinusite
Otite media	Reflusso (GERD)	Malattia infiammatoria intestinale
	Sinusite	Appendicite
	Otite media	Emicrania
		Gravidanza
		Farmaci
		Abuso di ipecacuana/bulimia
RARE		
Sindrome adrenogenitale	Sindrome di Reye	Sindrome di Reye
Errori congeniti del metabolismo	Epatite	Epatite
Tumore cerebrale (ipertensione endocranica)	Ulcera peptica	Ulcera peptica
Emorragia subdurale	Pancreatite	Pancreatite
Intossicazione alimentare	Tumore cerebrale	Tumore cerebrale
Ruminazione	Ipertensione endocranica	Ipertensione endocranica
Acidosi tubulare renale	Malattia dell'orecchio medio	Malattia dell'orecchio medio
	Chemioterapia	Chemioterapia
	Acalasia	Vomito ciclico (emicrania)
	Vomito ciclico (emicrania)	Colica biliare
	Restringimento esofageo	Colica renale
	Ematoma duodenale	
	Errori congeniti del metabolismo	

GERD (*GastroEsophageal Reflux Disease*), malattia da reflusso gastroesofageo.

VOMITO. Il vomito è un processo riflesso estremamente coordinato che può essere preceduto da aumentata salivazione e inizia con conati involontari. Il violento abbassamento del diaframma e la contrazione dei muscoli addominali, con rilassamento del cardias, spingono attivamente il contenuto gastrico in senso retrogrado verso l'esofago. Questo processo è coordinato dal centro midollare del vomito, che è influenzato direttamente dall'innervazione afferente e indirettamente dalla zona trigger chemiorecettoriale e dai centri superiori del sistema nervoso centrale (SNC). Sono molti i processi acuti o cronici che possono provocare il vomito (Tabb. 303-1 e 303-3).

Il vomito causato dall'ostruzione del tratto gastrointestinale è probabilmente mediato dai nervi afferenti viscerali intestinali che stimolano il centro del vomito (vedi Tab. 303-1). Se l'ostruzione è distale alla seconda porzione del duodeno, il vomito è di solito tinto di bile. La presenza di bile si riscontra anche in caso di vomito ripetuto in assenza di ostruzione, quando il contenuto duodenale refluisce nello stomaco. Anche le lesioni non ostruttive del tubo digerente possono provocare il vomito, in particolare le malattie dell'intestino prossimale, del pancreas, del fegato o dell'albero biliare. Alterazioni del SNC o metaboliche possono portare a emesi grave e persistente.

Il **vomito ciclico** è una sindrome caratterizzata da numerosi episodi di vomito intervallati da periodi di benessere. L'esordio avviene di solito tra i 2 e i 5 anni di vita; la frequenza degli episodi è variabile (in media 12 all'anno) e ciascuno di essi dura tipicamente 2-3 giorni, con quattro o più attacchi di emesi all'ora. I pazienti possono presentare prodromi come pallore, intolleranza al rumore o alla luce, nausea, letargia e cefalea o febbre. Tra i fattori precipitanti vi sono le infezioni, lo stress e l'eccitamento. Il vomito ciclico idiopatico può essere un equivalente emicranico (**emicrania addominale**) oppure essere dovuto ad alterazioni della motilità intestinale o a mutazioni del DNA mitocondriale. La **diagnosi differenziale** comprende anomalie gastrointestinali (malrotazione, cisti da duplicazione, cisti coledociche), malattie

TABELLA 303-3. Cause di ostruzione gastrointestinale

ESOFAGO	Malrotazione/bande di Ladd
Congenite	Atresia ileale
Atresia esofagea	Ileo da meconio
Anelli vascolari	Diverticolo di Meckel con volvolo o intussuscezione
Anello di Schatzki	Ernia inguinale
Residuo tracheobronchiale	Duplicazione intestinale
Acquisite	**Acquisite**
Stenosi esofagea	Aderenze postchirurgiche
Corpo estraneo	Morbo di Crohn
Acalasia	Intussuscezione
Malattia di Chagas	Sindrome da ostruzione ileale distale (fibrosi cistica)
Collagenopatia vascolare	Ematoma duodenale
STOMACO	Sindrome dell'arteria mesenterica superiore
Congenite	**COLON**
Membrane antrali	**Congenite**
Stenosi pilorica	Tappo di meconio
Acquisite	Malattia di Hirschsprung
Bezoar/corpi estranei	Atresia del colon, stenosi
Stenosi pilorica (ulcera)	Ano imperforato
Malattia granulomatosa cronica dell'infanzia	Stenosi rettale
Gastroenterite eosinofila	Pseudo-ostruzione
Morbo di Crohn	Volvolo
Epidermolisi bollosa	Duplicazione del colon
INTESTINO TENUE	**Acquisite**
Congenite	Colite ulcerosa (megacolon tossico)
Atresia duodenale	Malattia di Chagas
Pancreas anulare	Morbo di Crohn
Malrotazione/volvolo	Colonpatia fibrosante (fibrosi cistica)

del SNC (neoplasie, epilessia, patologia vestibolare), nefrolitiasi, colelitiasi, idrocefalo, patologie metaboliche-endocrine (ciclo dell'urea, metabolismo degli acidi grassi, malattia di Addison, porfiria, angioedema ereditario, febbre mediterranea familiare), appendicite cronica e malattia infiammatoria intestinale. Gli **esami strumentali**, che si basano su un'anamnesi e un esame obiettivo scrupolosi, possono comprendere, se indicate, l'endoscopia, la radiografia gastrointestinale con mezzo di contrasto, la RM cerebrale e le indagini metaboliche (lattato, acidi organici, ammoniaca). Il trattamento consiste nell'idratazione e nella somministrazione di ondansetron. La prevenzione è possibile grazie agli agenti antiemicranici (amitriptilina o ciproeptadina).

La possibili complicanze dell'emesi sono elencate nella Tabella 303-4. Le strategie di trattamento del vomito in generale e delle sue cause specifiche sono indicate a grandi linee nelle Tabelle 303-5 e 303-6.

DIARREA. La definizione più corretta è quella che considera la diarrea come l'eccessiva perdita di liquidi ed elettroliti con le feci. Normalmente, un bambino in tenera età evacua circa 5 g/kg di feci al giorno; nell'adulto il loro volume aumenta a 200 g/24 h. La maggiore quantità di acqua viene assorbita nell'intestino tenue; il colon concentra il contenuto intestinale contro un elevato gradiente osmotico. L'intestino tenue di un adulto può assorbire 10-11 L/die di una combinazione di liquidi ingeriti e secreti, mentre il colon ne assorbe circa 0,5 L. Le malattie che interferiscono con l'assorbimento nell'intestino tenue tendono a produrre diarrea abbondante, mentre quelle che compromettono l'assorbimento a livello del colon producono diarrea di volume inferiore. La **dissenteria** (feci ematiche, frequenti, di volume ridotto e miste a muco, con tenesmo e urgenza) è il sintomo predominante della colite.

All'origine di tutti i tipi di diarrea vi è un'alterazione del trasporto intestinale di soluti; il passaggio dell'acqua attraverso le membrane intestinali è passivo e determinato dal flusso tanto attivo quanto passivo di soluti, in particolare di sodio, cloro e glucosio. La patogenesi della maggior parte degli episodi di diarrea è attribuibile ad anomalie secretorie, osmotiche o della motilità oppure a una combinazione di queste (Tab. 303-7).

La **diarrea secretoria** è spesso causata da un secretagogo, come la tossina colerica, che si lega a un recettore sulla superficie dell'epitelio intestinale stimolando l'accumulo intracellulare di adenosina monofosfato ciclico o guanosina monofosfato ciclico. Alcuni acidi grassi e sali biliari intraluminali inducono la secrezione da parte della mucosa del colon attraverso questo stesso meccanismo. Anche la diarrea non associata a un secretagogo esogeno può avere una componente secretoria (malattia da inclusione dei microvilli). La diarrea secretoria tende a essere acquosa e a elevato volume; l'osmolarità delle feci può essere spiegata dalla presenza di elettroliti. Questa forma di diarrea in genere persiste anche quando non si somministra alcun alimento per bocca.

La **diarrea osmotica** si verifica dopo l'ingestione di un soluto che viene scarsamente assorbito, o in conseguenza della sua stessa natura (magnesio, fosfato, lattulosio o sorbitolo) o per effetto di una malattia dell'intestino tenue (lattosio in caso di deficit di lattasi o glucosio in caso di diarrea da rotavirus). Il carboidrato responsabile va incontro a fermentazione nel colon, ove si producono acidi grassi a catena corta (SCFA, *Short-Chain Fatty Acids*). Sebbene gli SCFA possano essere assorbiti nel colon e utilizzati come fonte di energia, l'effetto netto è un aumento del carico di soluto osmotico. Di solito questa forma di diarrea è di volume minore rispetto a quella secretoria e cessa con il digiuno.

TABELLA 303-4. Complicanze del vomito

COMPLICANZA	FISIOPATOLOGIA	ANAMNESI, ESAME OBIETTIVO ED ESAMI DI LABORATORIO
Metabolica	Perdita di liquidi nell'emesi	Disidratazione
	Perdita di HCl nell'emesi	Alcalosi; ipocalcemia
	Perdita di Na e K nell'emesi	Ipernatriemia; ipocalcemia
	Alcalosi →	
	Na nelle cellule	
	Perdita di HCO_3 nelle urine	pH urine 7-8
	Perdita di Na e K nelle urine	Na urinario ↑, K urinario ↑
	Ipocloremia → Cl conservato dai reni	Cl urinario ↓
Nutrizionale	Emesi di calorie e nutrienti	Malnutrizione; deficit di crescita
	Anoressia per calorie e nutrienti	
Lacerazione di Mallory-Weiss	Conati di vomito → lacerazione in corrispondenza della piccola curvatura della giunzione gastroesofagea	Emesi vigorosa → ematemesi
Esofagite	Vomito cronico → esposizione cronica all'acido	Pirosi; positività del test per il sangue occulto nelle feci
Aspirazione	Aspirazione di vomito, specialmente in caso di ottundimento del sensorio	Polmonite; disfunzione neurologica
Shock	Grave perdita di liquidi nell'emesi o nella diarrea associata	Disidratazione (la diarrea associata può spiegare l'acidosi?)
	Grave perdita di sangue nell'ematemesi	Deplezione del volume ematico

Cl, cloro; HCl, acido cloridrico; HCO_3, bicarbonato; K, potassio; Na, sodio.
Da Kliegman RM, Greenbaum LA, Lye PS (ed): *Practical Strategies in Pediatric Diagnosis and Therapy*, 2nd ed. Philadelphia, Elsevier, 2004, p 318.

TABELLA 303-5. Terapie farmacologiche per gli episodi di vomito

MALATTIA/CONDIZIONE	CLASSE TERAPEUTICA DEL FARMACO: AGENTE SPECIFICO (DOSE)
Reflusso	Antagonista dopaminergico: metoclopramide (0,1-0,2 mg/kg qid per os/ev)
	Antagonista dopaminergico periferico: domperidone (0,2-0,6 mg/kg tid-qid per os)
Gastroparesi	Metoclopramide, domperidone; vedi sopra
	Agonista della motilina: eritromicina (2-4 mg/kg tid-qid per os/ev)
Pseudo-ostruzione intestinale	Stimolazione dei complessi mioelettrici migranti intestinali:
	Octreotide (1 μg/kg bid-tid sc)
Chemioterapia	Metoclopramide; vedi sopra (0,5-1,0 mg/kg qid ev, con profilassi antistaminica degli effetti collaterali extrapiramidali)
	Antagonisti serotoninergici 5-HT_3: ondansetron (0,15-0,3 mg/kg tid ev/per os)
	Fenotiazine (effetti collaterali extrapiramidali, ematologici):
	Proclorperazina (≈0,3 mg/kg bid-tid per os)
	Clorpromazina (>6 mesi di vita: 0,5 mg/kg tid-qid per os/ev)
	Steroidi: desametasone (0,1 mg/kg tid per os)
	Cannabinoidi: nabilone (tetraidrocannabinolo) (0,05-0,1 mg/kg bid-tid per os)
Postoperatorio	Ondansetron, fenotiazine; vedi sopra
Chinetosi; malattie vestibolari	Antistaminici: dimenidrinato (1 mg/kg tid-qid per os)
	Anticolinergici: scopolamina (adulti: 1 cerotto/3 giorni)
Crisi adrenergica	Steroidi: cortisolo (2 mg/kg bolo ev seguito da 0,2-0,4 mg/kg/h ev [±1 mg/kg im])
Sindrome del vomito ciclico	Terapia di supporto:
	Analgesici: meperidina (1-2 mg/kg ogni 4-6 h ev/im)
	Ansiolitici, sedativi: lorazepam (0,05-0,1 mg/kg ogni 6 h ev)
	Antistaminici, sedativi: difenidramina (1,25 mg/kg ogni 6 h ev)
	Terapia abortiva:
	Antagonisti serotoninergici 5-HT_3:
	Ondansetron: vedi sopra
	Granisetron (10 μg/kg ogni 4-6 h ev)
	Farmaci antinfiammatori non steroidei (ulcera gastrica come effetto collaterale):
	Ketorolac (0,5-1,0 mg/kg ogni 6-8 h ev)
	Antagonisti serotoninergici 5-HT_{1D}: sumatriptan (>40 kg; 20 mg per via intranasale/25 mg per os, in monosomministrazione giornaliera)
	Profilassi (se >1 attacco al mese di sindrome da vomito ciclico; assunto quotidianamente)
	β-bloccante adrenergico, antiemicranico: propranololo (0,5-2,0 mg/kg bid per os)
	Antistaminico, antiemicranico: ciproeptadina (0,25-0,5 mg/kg/die ÷ bid-tid per os)
	Antidepressivo triciclico, antiemicranico: amitriptilina (0,33-0,5 mg/kg tid per os e aumentare gradualmente fino a un massimo di 3,0 mg/kg/die, al bisogno; effettuare un ECG di base all'inizio della terapia e prendere in considerazione il monitoraggio dei livelli del farmaco)
	Antiepilettico, antiemicranico: fenobarbital (2-3 mg/kg prima di coricarsi alla sera)
	Eritromicina: vedi sopra
	Contraccettivi orali a basso contenuto di estrogeni: prendere in considerazione episodi di sindrome da vomito ciclico catameniale

bid, due volte al giorno; ECG, elettrocardiogramma; im, per via intramuscolare; ev, per via endovenosa, sc, per via sottocutanea; tid, tre volte al giorno; qid, quattro volte al giorno.
Da Kliegman RM, Greenbaum LA, Lye PS (ed): *Practical Strategies in Pediatric Diagnosis and Therapy*, 2nd ed. Philadelphia, Elsevier, 2004, p 317.

Il contenuto di elettroliti da solo non è sufficiente a spiegare l'osmolarità delle feci, in quanto bisogna tener conto anche di un'altra componente osmotica: la differenza tra il contenuto di elettroliti (somma di [Na^+], [K^+] e anioni associati) e l'osmolarità fecale è >50 mOsm (vedi Capitolo 337). I disturbi della motilità possono essere associati a transito rapido o ritardato e in genere non comportano una diarrea di elevato volume. La motilità rallentata può essere correlata a iperproliferazione batterica come causa di diarrea. La diagnosi differenziale delle cause comuni di diarrea acuta e cronica è presentata nella Tabella 303-8.

STIPSI. Ogni definizione di stipsi è relativa e dipende dalla consistenza delle feci, dalla frequenza e dalla difficoltà delle evacuazioni. Il bambino normale può evacuare feci morbide anche ogni 2-3 giorni, senza alcuna difficoltà: in questo caso non si tratta di stipsi. L'evacuazione difficoltosa di feci dure ogni 3 giorni dovrebbe essere considerata come stipsi. Il disturbo può originare da un difetto tanto del riempimento quanto dello svuotamento del retto (Tab. 303-9).

Il lattante può presentare evacuazioni molto infrequenti di feci di consistenza normale, ma questo di solito è un reperto normale. La stipsi vera e propria nel periodo neonatale è più probabilmente secondaria a malattia di Hirschsprung, pseudo-ostruzione intestinale o ipotiroidismo.

Il difetto del riempimento rettale si verifica quando la peristalsi del colon è inefficace (in caso di ipotiroidismo o uso di oppiacei, oppure quando l'ostruzione intestinale è causata da un'anomalia strutturale o dalla malattia di Hirschsprung). La conseguente stasi del colon favorisce la perdita d'acqua delle feci e inibisce i riflessi rettali che normalmente scatenano l'evacuazione. Lo svuotamento del retto per evacuazione spontanea dipende dal riflesso della defecazione avviato dai recettori di pressione localizzati nel muscolo rettale. La ritenzione fecale, pertanto, può essere secondaria a lesioni che interessano tali muscoli, le fibre afferenti ed efferenti del midollo spinale sacrale o i muscoli dell'addome e del pavimento pelvico; anche un alterato rilassamento dello sfintere anale vi contribuisce.

La stipsi tende ad autoperpetuarsi, a prescindere dalla sua causa. Grandi quantità di feci dure accumulatesi nel retto rendono l'evacuazione non solo difficile, ma anche dolorosa; di conseguenza, la ritenzione aumenta e si instaura un circolo vizioso. La distensione del retto e del colon influisce negativamente sulla sensibilità al riflesso della defecazione e sull'efficacia della peristalsi. Alla fine, il contenuto acquoso dal colon prossimale può percolare attorno alle feci ritenute e passare attraverso il retto senza che il bambino se ne accorga. Questa **encopresi** involontaria può essere confusa con la diarrea. La stipsi di per sé non ha effetti sistemici deleteri, ma nei casi gravi, di vecchia data, si può sviluppare stasi delle vie urinarie e la stipsi può ingenerare ansia, con importanti ripercussioni emotive sul paziente e sulla famiglia.

TABELLA 303-6. Terapie di supporto e non farmacologiche per gli episodi di vomito

MALATTIA	TERAPIA
Tutte	Trattare la causa: ostruzione ⟶ operare; allergia ⟶ modificare la dieta (±steroidi); errori del metabolismo ⟶ difetto all'Rx; malattia da acido peptico ⟶ H_2RA, PPI ecc. (dubbio del traduttore)
Complicanze	
Disidratazione	Liquidi ev; elettroliti
Ematemesi	Trasfusione, correggere la coagulopatia
Esofagite	H_2RA, PPI
Malnutrizione	Alimentazione mediante gocciolamento NG o ND utile per molte condizioni croniche
Ileo da meconio	Clistere con Gastrografin®
DIOS	Clistere con Gastrografin®; soluzione di lavaggio del colon bilanciata
Intussuscezione	Clistere con bario; riduzione non chirurgica mediante clisma con aria
Ematemesi	Endoscopica: scleroterapia di iniezione o legatura delle varici esofagee; terapia iniettiva, applicazione di fibrina sigillante oppure elettrocauterizzazione con sonda di calore per lesioni selettive del tratto gastrointestinale superiore
Volvolo del sigma	Decompressione del colon
Reflusso	Posizione adeguata; misure dietetiche (bambini piccoli: fiocchi di riso, 1 cucchiaio ogni 30 g di latte artificiale)
Componenti psicogene	Psicoterapia; antidepressivi triciclici; ansiolitici (per es. diazepam 0,1 mg/kg/tid-qid per os)

DIOS (*Distal Intestinal Obstruction Syndrome*), sindrome da ostruzione intestinale distale; H_2RA (*Histamine₂-Receptor Antagonists*), antagonisti del recettore H_2 dell'istamina; NG, nasogastrico; ND, nasodigiunale; PPI (*Proton Pump Inhibitors*), inibitori della pompa protonica; qid, quattro volte al giorno; tid, tre volte al giorno.
Da Kliegman RM, Greenbaum LA, Lye PS (ed): *Practical Strategies in Pediatric Diagnosis and Therapy*, 2nd ed. Philadelphia, Elsevier, 2004, p 319.

DOLORE ADDOMINALE. Notevoli sono le differenze che si riscontrano da un bambino all'altro per quanto riguarda la percezione e la tolleranza del dolore addominale. Questo è uno dei motivi per cui la valutazione del dolore addominale cronico è difficile. Il dolore addominale funzionale (in assenza di cause organiche identificabili) può essere sgradevole per il bambino quanto quello dovuto a cause organiche. Tale distinzione è un elemento estremamente importante nella valutazione medica, che guida le strategie di work-up e terapeutiche. Più il dolore è specifico e suggestivo di una diagnosi in particolare, maggiori saranno le probabilità che esso abbia una base organica. Una crescita e un esame obiettivo (comprendente l'esplorazione rettale) normali sono rassicuranti nel bambino in cui si sospetta un dolore funzionale.

Per quanto la causa specifica possa essere difficile da identificare, di solito è possibile determinare la natura e la localizzazione di una lesione che provoca dolore basandosi sulla descrizione clinica. A trasmettere gli stimoli dolorosi nell'addome sono due tipi di fibre nervose: le fibre A, nella cute e nei muscoli, mediano il dolore trafittivo localizzato, mentre le fibre C, che si irradiano dai visceri, dal peritoneo e dai muscoli, trasmettono il dolore sordo, scarsamente localizzato. I corpi cellulari di tali fibre afferenti sono situati nei gangli delle radici dorsali e alcuni assoni attraversano la linea mediana per poi risalire al midollo, al tronco cerebrale e al talamo. Il dolore viene percepito nella corteccia del giro postcentrale, che riceve gli impulsi provenienti da entrambi i lati del corpo.

Il **dolore viscerale** tende a essere avvertito nel dermatomero da cui l'organo afferente riceve innervazione. Gli stimoli dolorosi che hanno origine dal fegato, dal pancreas, dall'albero biliare, dallo stomaco o dall'intestino tenue superiore sono riferiti all'epigastrio, mentre quelli che derivano dall'intestino tenue distale, dal cieco, dall'appendice o dal colon prossimale vengono percepiti nella regione ombelicale; infine, il dolore proveniente dall'intestino crasso distale, dalle vie urinarie o dagli organi pelvici è solitamente sovrapubico. Quando il dolore si irradia ad aree lontane innervate dallo stesso neuromero dell'organo ammalato, tale fenomeno di solito indica un aumento di intensità degli stimoli causali. Il **dolore parietale**, i cui impulsi sono trasmessi dalle fibre C dei nervi corrispondenti ai dermatomeri T6-L1, tende a essere più localizzato e intenso del dolore viscerale.

Nell'intestino, lo stimolo che solitamente provoca dolore è la tensione o lo stiramento. Le lesioni infiammatorie possono abbassare la soglia del dolore, ma i meccanismi responsabili del dolore o dell'infiammazione non sono chiari. I metaboliti tissutali rilasciati in prossimità delle terminazioni nervose probabilmente servono a spiegare il dolore causato dall'ischemia. La percezione di tali stimoli dolorosi può essere modulata dagli input provenienti dai centri cerebrali o dalla periferia. I fattori psicologici sono particolarmente importanti. Le caratteristiche del dolore addominale sono descritte nelle Tabelle 303-10 e 303-11.

EMORRAGIA GASTROINTESTINALE. Il sanguinamento può verificarsi in qualunque punto dell'apparato gastrointestinale e l'identificazione della sua sede può essere difficoltosa (Tab. 303-12). Per rendere più agevole la valutazione dell'intestino tenue si ricorre alla videocapsula endoscopica: il dispositivo di visualizzazione, delle dimensioni di una capsula, viene deglutito dai bambini più grandi o introdotto endoscopicamente in quelli più piccoli.

TABELLA 303-7. Meccanismi della diarrea

MECCANISMO PRIMARIO	DIFETTO	ESAME DELLE FECI	ESEMPI	COMMENTO
Secretorio	Ridotto assorbimento, aumentata secrezione, trasporto elettrolitico	Feci acquose, osmolarità normale; osmoli = 2 × (Na^+ + K^+)	Colera, *E. coli* enterotossigena; carcinoide, VIP, neuroblastoma, cloridorrea congenita, *Clostridium difficile*, criptosporidiosi (AIDS)	Persiste durante il digiuno; il malassorbimento di sali biliari può aumentare la secrezione intestinale di acqua; assenza di leucociti nelle feci
Osmotico	Maldigestione, difetti di trasporto, ingestione di soluti non assorbibili	Feci acquose, acide e positive per sostanze riducenti; aumento dell'osmolarità; osmoli >(Na^+ + K^+)	Deficit di lattasi, malassorbimento di glucosio-galattosio, lattulosio, abuso di lassativi	Cessa con il digiuno; aumento dell'idrogeno nell'aria espirata in caso di malassorbimento dei carboidrati; assenza di leucociti nelle feci
Aumento della motilità	Tempo di transito ridotto	Emissione di feci poco formate o normali, stimolata dal riflesso gastrocolico	Sindrome dell'intestino irritabile, tireotossicosi, sindrome da svuotamento postvagotomia	Anche le infezioni possono contribuire all'aumento della motilità
Riduzione della motilità	Difetti delle unità neuromuscolari Stasi (iperproliferazione batterica)	Feci poco formate o normali	Pseudo-ostruzione, ansa cieca	Possibile iperproliferazione batterica
Diminuzione dell'area di superficie (osmotica, motilità)	Ridotta capacità funzionale	Feci acquose	Sindrome dell'intestino corto, celiachia, enterite da rotavirus	Può richiedere una dieta elementare, oltre alla nutrizione parenterale
Invasione della mucosa	Infiammazione, diminuzione del riassorbimento del colon, aumento della motilità	Sangue e aumento dei leucociti nelle feci	Infezione da *Salmonella*, *Shigella*; amebiasi; infezione da *Yersinia*, *Campylobacter*	Dissenteria evidente nel sangue, nel muco e nei leucociti

K^+, potassio; Na^+, sodio; VIP (*Vasoactive Intestinal Peptide*), peptide intestinale vasoattivo.
Da Kliegman RM, Greenbaum LA, Lye PS (ed): *Practical Strategies in Pediatric Diagnosis and Therapy*, 2nd ed. Philadelphia, Elsevier, 2004, p 274.

TABELLA 303-8. Diagnosi differenziale della diarrea

	LATTANTE	BAMBINO	ADOLESCENTE
ACUTA			
Comune	Gastroenterite Infezione sistemica Associata ad antibiotici Iperalimentazione	Gastroenterite Intossicazione alimentare Infezione sistemica Associata ad antibiotici	Gastroenterite Intossicazione alimentare Associata ad antibiotici
Rara	Deficit primario di disaccaridasi Colite tossica di Hirschsprung Sindrome adrenogenitale Astinenza neonatale da oppiacei	Ingestione di sostanze tossiche	Ipertiroidismo
CRONICA			
Comune	Postinfettiva secondaria a deficit di lattasi Intolleranza al latte vaccino/latte di soia Diarrea cronica aspecifica dell'infanzia Eccessiva ingestione di succhi di frutta (sorbitolo) Celiachia Fibrosi cistica Enteropatia da AIDS	Postinfettiva secondaria a deficit di lattasi Sindrome dell'intestino irritabile Celiachia Intolleranza al lattosio Ingestione di succhi di frutta (sorbitolo) in quantità eccessiva Giardiasi Malattia infiammatoria intestinale Enteropatia da AIDS	Sindrome dell'intestino irritabile Malattia infiammatoria intestinale Intolleranza al lattosio Giardiasi Abuso di lassativi (anoressia nervosa) Stipsi con encopresi
Rara	Deficit immunitari primitivi Malassorbimento di glucosio-galattosio Malattia da inclusione del microvillo (atrofia del microvillo) Deficit di trasporto congeniti (cloro, sodio) Malassorbimento primario degli acidi biliari Sindrome di Munchausen per procura Malattia di Hirschsprung Sindrome di Shwachman Tumori secernenti Acrodermatite enteropatica Linfangectasia Abetalipoproteinemia Gastroenterite eosinofila Sindrome dell'intestino corto Sindrome della diarrea intrattabile Enteropatia autoimmune	Deficit immunitari acquisiti Tumore secernente Pseudo-ostruzione Deficit di saccarasi-isomaltasi Gastroenterite eosinofila	Tumore secernente Tumore intestinale primario Infezioni parassitarie e malattie veneree Ascesso appendicolare Malattia di Addison

Da Kliegman RM, Greenbaum LA, Lye PS (ed): *Practical Strategies in Pediatric Diagnosis and Therapy*, 2nd ed. Philadelphia, Elsevier, 2004, p 272.

TABELLA 303-9. Cause di stipsi

NON ORGANICA (FUNZIONALE) - RITENTIVA

ORGANICA

Anatomica
Stenosi anale
Ano imperforato
Ano dislocato anteriormente
Stenosi intestinale (postenterocolite necrotizzante)

Muscolatura anormale
Prune-belly syndrome
Gastroschisi
Sindrome di Down

Anomalie dei nervi o dei muscoli intestinali
Malattia di Hirschsprung
Pseudo-ostruzione (miopatia o neuropatia viscerale)
Displasia neuronale intestinale

Difetti del midollo spinale
Midollo ancorato
Traumi midollari spinali
Spina bifida

Farmaci
Anticolinergici
Narcotici

Farmaci
Antidepressivi
Agenti chemioterapici (vincristina)
Enzimi pancreatici (colonpatia fibrosante)
Piombo
Intossicazione da vitamina D

Malattie metaboliche
Ipocalcemia
Ipercalcemia
Ipotiroidismo
Diabete mellito

Malattie intestinali
Celiachia
Intolleranza alle proteine del latte vaccino
Fibrosi cistica (equivalente dell'ileo da meconio)
Malattia infiammatoria intestinale (stenosi)
Tumore

Malattie del tessuto connettivo
Lupus eritematoso sistemico
Sclerodermia

Diagnosi psichiatrica
Anoressia nervosa

L'erosione della mucosa del tratto gastrointestinale è la causa più comune di emorragia, sebbene il sanguinamento da varici secondario a ipertensione portale si verifichi abbastanza frequentemente da dover essere preso in considerazione. La **gastropatia da prolasso** (**traumatica**) produce emorragie subepiteliali con prolasso dello stomaco nell'esofago durante l'emesi vigorosa. Tale fenomeno può essere più comune delle lesioni di Mallory-Weiss secondarie a lacerazioni mucose associate a emesi. Le malformazioni vascolari di rado causano emorragie gastrointestinali nei bambini e sono difficili da identificare.

L'emorragia che ha origine dall'esofago, dallo stomaco o dal duodeno può causare **ematemesi.** Il sangue a contatto con i succhi gastrici o intestinali si scurisce rapidamente fino ad assomigliare al fondo di caffè, mentre è probabile che l'emorragia massiva sia di colore rosso. La presenza di sangue rosso o bordeaux nelle feci, o **ematochezia,** indica un'emorragia distale o un'emorragia massiva prossimale all'ileo distale. Un sanguinamento da moderato a lieve proveniente da sedi prossimali all'ileo distale tende a causare feci nere di consistenza catramosa (**melena**); anche emorragie di notevole entità nel duodeno o superiori possono provocare melena.

I bambini possono sviluppare **anemia sideropenica,** secondaria a emorragia enterica cronica, anche quando l'apposito test effettuato alla cieca non rileva sangue occulto nelle feci. L'emorragia gastrointestinale può produrre ipotensione e tachicardia, ma raramente provoca sintomi gastrointestinali; l'emorragia duodenale o gastrica attiva può determinare nausea, vomito o diarrea. I prodotti di degradazione del sangue intraluminale favoriscono il coma epatico, se la funzione del fegato è già compromessa, e portano a un aumento della bilirubina sierica.

TABELLA 303-10. Dolore addominale ricorrente o cronico nei bambini

MALATTIA	CARATTERISTICHE	INDAGINI CHIAVE
NON ORGANICA		
Sindrome del dolore addominale ricorrente (dolore addominale funzionale)	Dolore aspecifico, spesso periombelicale	Anamnesi ed esame obiettivo; altri test come indicato
Sindrome dell'intestino irritabile	Crampi intermittenti; diarrea e stipsi	Anamnesi ed esame obiettivo
Dispepsia non ulcerosa	Sintomi similulcerosi senza anomalie alla valutazione del tratto gastrointestinale superiore	Anamnesi; esofagogastroduodenoscopia
TRATTO GASTROINTESTINALE		
Stipsi cronica	Storia di ritenzione fecale, segni di stipsi all'esame obiettivo	Anamnesi ed esame obiettivo; radiografia diretta dell'addome
Intolleranza al lattosio	I sintomi possono essere associati a ingestione di lattosio; gonfiore, gas, crampi e diarrea	Ciclo di dieta priva di lattosio; breath test al lattosio
Infezione parassitaria (specialmente da *Giardia*)	Gonfiore, gas, crampi e diarrea	Valutazione delle feci per uova e parassiti; immunoassay specifici per *Giardia*
Eccessiva ingestione di fruttosio o sorbitolo	Dolore addominale aspecifico, gonfiore, flatulenza e diarrea	Abbondante consumo di mele, succhi di frutta o caramelle/chewing gum dolcificati con sorbitolo
Morbo di Crohn	Vedi Capitolo 333	
Ulcera peptica	Dolore epigastrico urente o tormentoso, che peggiora al risveglio o prima dei pasti ed è alleviato dagli antiacidi	Esofagogastroduodenoscopia o radiografie del tratto gastrointestinale superiore con mezzo di contrasto
Esofagite	Dolore epigastrico con pirosi retrosternale	Esofagogastroduodenoscopia
Diverticolo di Meckel	Dolore addominale periombelicale o inferiore; può esserci sangue nelle feci	Ecografia del diverticolo di Meckel o enteroclisi
Intussuscezione ricorrente	Grave dolore addominale crampiforme parossistico; può essere presente sangue nelle feci con l'episodio	Identificare l'intussuscezione durante l'episodio o il punto principale nell'intestino tra gli episodi mediante studi con mezzo di contrasto del tratto gastrointestinale
Ernia intestinale, inguinale o della parete addominale	Dolore addominale sordo o dolore della parete addominale	Esame obiettivo, TC della parete addominale
Appendicite cronica o mucocele appendicolare	Dolore ricorrente al quadrante inferiore destro; spesso fonte di diagnosi sbagliate, può essere una rara causa di dolore addominale	Clistere con bario, TC
Colecisti e pancreas		
Colelitiasi	Dolore al quadrante superiore destro, che può peggiorare con i pasti	Ecografia della colecisti
Cisti coledocica	Dolore al quadrante superiore destro, massa ± aumento della bilirubina	Ecografia o TC del quadrante superiore destro
Pancreatite ricorrente	Dolore fastidioso persistente, che può irradiarsi alla schiena, vomito	Amilasi e lipasi sieriche ± tripsinogeno sierico; ecografia o TC del pancreas
TRATTO GENITOURINARIO		
Infezione delle vie urinarie	Dolore sovrapubico sordo, dolore al fianco	Esame delle urine e urinocoltura, ecografia renale
Idronefrosi	Dolore addominale monolaterale o dolore al fianco	Ecografia dei reni
Urolitiasi	Dolore grave, progressivo; dal fianco alla regione inguinale e al testicolo	Esame delle urine, ecografia, pielografia endovenosa, TC
Altre malattie genitourinarie	Dolore sovrapubico o all'addome inferiore; sintomi genitourinari	Ecografia dei reni e della pelvi; valutazione ginecologica e uroandrologica
ALTRE CAUSE		
Emicrania addominale	Vedi testo; nausea, storia familiare di emicrania	Anamnesi
Epilessia addominale	Può avere prodromi convulsivi	EEG (può essere necessario più di uno studio, incluso l'EEG da privazione del sonno)
Sindrome di Gilbert	Dolore addominale lieve (causale o coincidente?); bilirubina non coniugata leggermente aumentata	Bilirubina sierica
Febbre mediterranea familiare	Episodi parossistici di febbre, dolore addominale grave e dolorabilità con altri segni di polisierosite	Anamnesi ed esame obiettivo durante un episodio, diagnosi DNA
Crisi falcemica	Anemia	Valutazione ematologica
Intossicazione da piombo	Dolore addominale vago ± stipsi	Livello sierico del piombo
Porpora di Schönlein-Henoch	Dolore addominale crampiforme, grave, ricorrente, sangue occulto nelle feci, rash caratteristico, artrite	Anamnesi, esame obiettivo, esame delle urine
Edema angioneurotico	Edema del volto o delle vie aeree, dolore crampiforme	Anamnesi, esame obiettivo, radiografie gastrointestinali con mezzo di contrasto, inibitore della C1 esterasi sierica
Porfiria intermittente acuta	Dolore grave precipitato da farmaci, digiuno o infezioni	Esame estemporaneo delle urine per le porfirine

TABELLA 303-11. Caratteristiche distintive del dolore gastrointestinale acuto nei bambini

MALATTIA	ESORDIO	LOCALIZZAZIONE	IRRADIAZIONE	QUALITÀ	COMMENTI
Pancreatite	Acuto	Epigastrio, quadrante superiore sinistro	Schiena	Costante, penetrante, fastidioso	Nausea, emesi, dolorabilità
Ostruzione intestinale	Acuto o graduale	Periombelicale, addome inferiore	Schiena	Alternanza di crampi (colica) e periodi di benessere	Distensione, stipsi, emesi, aumento dei rumori intestinali
Appendicite	Acuto	Periombelicale, quindi localizzato al quadrante inferiore destro; generalizzato in caso di peritonite	Schiena o pelvi, se retrocecale	Penetrante, costante	Anoressia, nausea, emesi, dolorabilità locale, febbre in caso di peritonite
Intussuscezione	Acuto	Periombelicale, addome inferiore	Nessuna	Crampiforme, con periodi senza dolore	Ematochezia, ginocchia portate verso il grembo
Urolitiasi	Acuto, improvviso	Posteriore (monolaterale)	Inguine	Netto, intermittente, crampiforme	Ematuria
Infezione delle vie urinarie	Acuto, improvviso	Posteriore	Vescica	Profondo o netto	Febbre, dolorabilità costocondrale, disuria, pollachiuria

TABELLA 303-12. Diagnosi differenziali dell'emorragia gastrointestinale nell'infanzia

LATTANTE	BAMBINO	ADOLESCENTE
COMUNI		
Enterite batterica	Enterite batterica	Enterite batterica
Allergia alle proteine del latte	Fissurazione anale	Malattia infiammatoria intestinale
Intussuscezione	Polipi del colon	Ulcera peptica/gastrite
Ingestione di sangue materno	Intussuscezione	Gastropatia da prolasso (traumatica) secondaria a emesi
Fissurazione anale	Ulcera peptica/gastrite	Sindrome di Mallory-Weiss
Iperplasia linfonodale	Epistassi deglutita	Polipi del colon
	Gastropatia da prolasso (traumatica) secondaria a emesi	
	Sindrome di Mallory-Weiss	
RARE		
Volvolo	Varici esofagee	Emorroidi
Enterocolite necrotizzante	Esofagite	Varici esofagee
Diverticolo di Meckel	Diverticolo di Meckel	Esofagite
Ulcera gastrica da stress	Iperplasia linfonodale	Teleangiectasia-angiodisplasia
Coagulopatia (malattia emorragica del neonato)	Porpora di Schönlein-Henoch	Malattia intestinale di Gay
	Corpo estraneo	Graft versus host disease
	Emangioma, malformazione arterovenosa	
	Abuso sessuale	
	Sindrome emolitico-uremica	
	Malattia infiammatoria intestinale	
	Coagulopatia	

DISTENSIONE ADDOMINALE E MASSE ADDOMINALI. La dilatazione dell'addome può essere dovuta a una diminuzione del tono della muscolatura della parete o all'aumento del contenuto in liquidi, gas o solidi. L'**ascite**, ossia l'accumulo di liquido nella cavità peritoneale, distende l'addome sia lateralmente sia anteriormente, quando è di grandi dimensioni. Questo liquido si sposta con i movimenti del paziente e trasmette un'onda di percussione.

Di solito il liquido ascitico è un trasudato con una bassa concentrazione di proteine, dovuta alla diminuzione della pressione colloido-osmotica plasmatica dell'ipoalbuminemia e/o all'aumento della pressione venosa portale. In caso di ipertensione portale, la perdita di liquido probabilmente si verifica dai vasi linfatici sulla superficie del fegato e dai capillari peritoneali viscerali, ma di solito l'ascite non compare finché i livelli di albumina sierica non si riducono. L'escrezione di sodio nelle urine subisce una notevole diminuzione via via che il liquido ascitico si accumula e, pertanto, l'ulteriore sodio introdotto con la dieta si trasferisce direttamente nello spazio peritoneale, portando con sé più acqua. Un liquido ascitico contenente un'elevata concentrazione di proteine di solito è un essudato prodotto da una lesione infiammatoria o neoplastica.

Quando il liquido distende l'intestino, si dovrebbe sospettare l'ostruzione o uno squilibrio tra assorbimento e secrezione. I fattori che causano accumulo di liquido nel lume intestinale spesso provocano anche accumulo di gas, che può manifestarsi con gorgoglii udibili. Nonostante il meteorismo sia di solito dovuto all'aria ingerita, la flora endogena può aumentare notevolmente negli stati di malassorbimento e produrre eccessive quantità di gas quando il substrato raggiunge l'intestino distale. La presenza di gas nella cavità peritoneale (pneumoperitoneo), forse segnalata dal tono timpanico alla percussione anche al di sopra di organi solidi come il fegato, indica la perforazione di un viscere.

Un organo addominale può ingrandirsi in modo uniforme oppure essere interessato da una massa ben definita. Nel tubo digerente, tali masse possono svilupparsi nel lume, nella parete o nel mesentere. Nel bambino con stipsi, si riscontrano spesso masse fecali mobili non dolenti. La parete intestinale può essere interessata da anomalie, cisti o malattie infiammatorie; le neoplasie a sua carico sono estremamente rare nei bambini. Il fegato può aumentare uniformemente di volume in risposta a varie patologie. Le masse epatiche distinte possono essere isole di tessuto epatico in via di rigenerazione in un fegato cirrotico oppure avere origine infiammatoria o neoplastica.

ITTERO. Vedi Capitoli 102.3 e 353.

American Academy of Pediatrics Subcommittee on Chronic Abdominal Pain: Chronic abdominal pain in children. *Pediatrics* 2005;115:812–815.

Armon K, Stephenson T, MacFaul R, et al: An evidence and consensus based guideline for acute diarrhoea management. *Arch Dis Child* 2001;85:132–142.

Boey CC, Goh KL: Psychosocial factors and childhood recurrent abdominal pain. *J Gastroenterol Hepatol* 2002;17:1250–1253.

Carty HM: Paediatric emergencies: Non-traumatic abdominal emergencies. *Eur Radiol* 2002;12:2835–2848.

Chong SK: Gastrointestinal problems in the handicapped child. *Curr Opin Pediatr* 2001;13:441–446.

Eccleston C, Morley S, Williams A, et al: Systematic review of randomised controlled trials of psychological therapy for chronic pain in children and adolescents, with a subset meta-analysis of pain relief. *Pain* 2002;99:157–165.

Golden CB, Feusner JH: Malignant abdominal masses in children: Quick guide to evaluation and diagnosis. *Pediatr Clin North Am* 2002;49:1369–1392.

Heuschkel RB, Fletcher K, Hill A, et al: Isolated neonatal swallowing dysfunction: A case series and review of the literature. *Dig Dis Sci* 2003;48:30–35.

Khan S, Di Lorenzo C: Chronic vomiting in children: New insights into diagnosis. *Curr Gastroenterol Rep* 2001;3:248–256.

Li BU, Misiewicz L: Cyclic vomiting syndrome: A brain-gut disorder. *Gastroenterol Clin North Am* 2003;32:997–1019.

Mulvaney S, Lombert EW, Garber J, Walker LS: Trajectories of symptoms and impairment for pediatric patients with functional abdominal pain. *J Am Acad Child Adolesc Psychiatry* 2006;45:737–744.

Rubin G: Constipation in children. *Clin Evid* 2003;10:369–374.

Russell G, Abu-Arafeh I, Symon DN: Abdominal migraine: Evidence for existence and treatment options. *Paediatr Drugs* 2002;4:1–8.

Sezione 2 — Il cavo orale — Norman Tinanoff

Capitolo 304 ■ Sviluppo e anomalie di sviluppo dei denti

INIZIO

I denti decidui, detti anche primari o da latte, si sviluppano nelle cripte dentarie che originano da una banda di cellule epiteliali presenti in ciascun mascellare in via di sviluppo. A partire dalla 12ª settimana di vita intrauterina, ciascuna di queste bande epiteliali (**lamine dentarie**) presenta cinque aree di rapida crescita su ciascun lato dei mascellari superiore (mascella) e inferiore (mandibola), osservabili come ingrossamenti rotondi simili a gemme. Con l'organizzazione del mesenchima adiacente in ciascuna area di crescita epiteliale, i due elementi assieme costituiscono l'abbozzo del dente.

Una volta che si sono costituite queste cripte per i 20 denti decidui, si forma un'altra generazione di germi dentari lingualmente (in direzione della lingua), i quali si svilupperanno nei successivi incisivi, canini e premolari permanenti, destinati a sostituire i denti decidui. Questo processo si svolge all'incirca dal 5° mese di gestazione per gli incisivi centrali e fino al 10° mese di vita per i secondi premolari. I primi, secondi e terzi molari, invece, si sviluppano dall'estensione delle lamine dentarie distalmente ai secondi molari decidui e le gemme per questi denti si formano, rispettivamente, all'incirca al 4° mese di gestazione, a 1 e a 4-5 anni di età.

ISTODIFFERENZIAZIONE-MORFODIFFERENZIAZIONE. A mano a mano che la gemma epiteliale prolifera, la superficie più profonda s'invagina comportando l'inclusione parziale di una massa di mesenchima. Le cellule epiteliali si differenziano in ameloblasti, che depongono una matrice organica destinata a formare lo smalto, mentre il mesenchima forma la dentina e la polpa dentaria.

CALCIFICAZIONE. Una volta formatasi la matrice organica, da diversi siti di calcificazione ha inizio la deposizione di cristalli minerali inorganici che in seguito si fondono. Le caratteristiche delle parti inorganiche di un dente possono essere alterate da (1) disturbi nella formazione della matrice, (2) una minore disponibilità di minerali o (3) inclusione di materiali estranei. Tali fenomeni talvolta influiscono su colore, struttura o spessore della superficie del dente. La calcificazione dei denti decidui inizia al 3-4° mese di vita intrauterina e termina circa 12 mesi dopo la nascita con la mineralizzazione dei secondi molari decidui (Tab. 304-1).

ERUZIONE. Al momento della formazione del germe dentario, ogni dente inizia un movimento continuo verso il cavo orale. I tempi di eruzione dei denti decidui e permanenti sono riportati nella Tabella 304-1.

TABELLA 304-1. Calcificazione, completamento della corona ed eruzione

DENTE	PRIMA EVIDENZA DI CALCIFICAZIONE	CORONA COMPLETATA	ERUZIONE
DENTIZIONE DECIDUA			
Mascellare superiore			
Incisivo centrale	3-4 mesi in utero	4 mesi	7½ mesi
Incisivo laterale	4½ mesi in utero	5 mesi	8 mesi
Canino	5½ mesi in utero	9 mesi	16-20 mesi
Primo molare	5 mesi in utero	6 mesi	12-16 mesi
Secondo molare	6 mesi in utero	10-12 mesi	20-30 mesi
Mascellare inferiore			
Incisivo centrale	4½ mesi in utero	4 mesi	6½ mesi
Incisivo laterale	4½ mesi in utero	4¼ mesi	
Canino		5 mesi in utero	9 mesi
Primo molare	5 mesi in utero	6 mesi	12-16 mesi
Secondo molare	6 mesi in utero	10-12 mesi	20-30 mesi
DENTIZIONE PERMANENTE			
Mascellare superiore			
Incisivo centrale	3-4 mesi	4-5 anni	7-8 anni
Incisivo laterale	10 mesi	4-5 anni	8-9 anni
Canino		4-5 mesi	6-7 anni
Primo premolare	1½-1¾ anni	5-6 anni	10-11 anni
Secondo premolare	2-2¼ anni	6-7 anni	10-12 anni
Primo molare	Alla nascita	2½-3 anni	6-7 anni
Secondo molare	2½-3 anni	7-8 anni	12-13 anni
Terzo molare	7-9 anni	12-16 anni	17-21 anni
Mascellare inferiore			
Incisivo centrale	3-4 mesi	4-5 anni	6-7 anni
Incisivo laterale	3-4 mesi	4-5 anni	7-8 anni
Canino	4-5 mesi	6-7 anni	9-10 anni
Primo premolare	1¾-2 anni	5-6 anni	10-12 anni
Secondo premolare	2¼-2½ anni	6-7 anni	11-12 anni
Primo molare	Alla nascita	2½-3 anni	6-7 anni
Secondo molare	2½-3 anni	7-8 anni	11-13 anni
Terzo molare	8-10 anni	12-16 anni	17-21 anni

Modificata da Logan WHG, Kronfeld R: Development of the human jaws and surrounding structures from birth to age 15 years. *J Am Dent Assoc* 1993;20:379.

ANOMALIE ASSOCIATE ALLO SVILUPPO DEI DENTI

Durante lo sviluppo dei denti si possono osservare sia carenze sia eccessi del numero dei denti. Il mancato sviluppo dei denti può essere dovuto a un trauma ambientale, un difetto genetico che coinvolge solo i denti, oppure essere la manifestazione di una sindrome. L'**anodonzia**, o assenza di denti, può essere dovuta a mancata formazione dei germi dentari (displasia ectodermica o assenza familiare di denti) o a un disturbo del normale sito d'inizio (l'area di una palatoschisi). I denti più comunemente assenti sono i terzi molari, gli incisivi laterali superiori e i secondi premolari inferiori.

La produzione di un numero di germi dentari superiori alla norma da parte della lamina dentaria comporta la formazione di denti sovrannumerari, molto spesso nell'area tra gli incisivi centrali superiori. Poiché essi tendono a influire negativamente sulla posizione e sull'eruzione dei denti adiacenti normali, è importante identificarli mediante radiografia. I denti sovrannumerari si osservano anche in presenza di displasia cleidocranica (vedi Capitolo 308) e nell'area di una palatoschisi.

Il **twinning**, cioè l'unione di due denti, si osserva molto spesso negli incisivi inferiori della dentizione decidua. Può essere distinto in geminazione, fusione e concrescenza. La **geminazione** consiste nello sdoppiamento di un unico germe dentario a formare una corona bifida su una radice singola con un canale pulpare comune: nell'arcata dentaria sembra essere presente un dente in più. La **fusione** è l'unione di denti con sviluppo incompleto che, a causa di pressione, trauma o affollamento, continuano a svilupparsi come un unico elemento. I denti fusi sono talora uniti per tutta la loro lunghezza, mentre in altri casi si osserva un'unica ampia corona sostenuta da due radici. La **concrescenza** è l'unione di due o più radici di denti adiacenti prossimali in seguito a un'eccessiva deposizione di cemento. Questo tipo di twinning, a differenza degli altri, si osserva molto spesso nella regione dei molari superiori.

Le anomalie della differenziazione possono comportare alterazioni della morfologia dentaria, quali **macrodonzia** (denti grandi) o **microdonzia** (denti piccoli). Gli incisivi laterali superiori possono assumere una forma troncoconica affusolata (**incisivi laterali conoidi**).

L'**amelogenesi imperfetta** rappresenta un gruppo di condizioni ereditarie che danno luogo a difetti dello smalto dei denti sia decidui sia permanenti, senza evidenza di disturbi sistemici (Fig. 304-1). I denti sono rivestiti da un sottile strato di smalto sviluppatosi in maniera anomala, attraverso cui si intravede la sottostante dentina gialla. I denti decidui sono generalmente più colpiti rispetto ai permanenti. La sensibilità alla carie è bassa, ma lo smalto va soggetto a distruzione da abrasione. Talvolta è indicato ricoprire completamente la corona per proteggere la dentina, ridurre la sensibilità dentaria e migliorare l'aspetto estetico.

La **dentinogenesi imperfetta**, o dentina opalescente ereditaria, è una condizione analoga all'amelogenesi imperfetta in cui gli odontoblasti non riescono a compiere una differenziazione normale, comportando la formazione di dentina scarsamente calcificata (Fig. 304-2). Questo disturbo autosomico dominante può anche presentarsi in pazienti con **osteogenesi imperfetta**. La giunzione amelodentinale subisce alterazioni che provocano il distacco dello smalto. La dentina esposta risulta quindi predisposta all'abrasione; in alcuni casi, l'usura arriva fino alla gengiva. I denti sono opachi e perlacei e le camere pulpari sono generalmente obliterate dalla calcificazione. Di norma sono interessati i denti sia decidui sia permanenti.

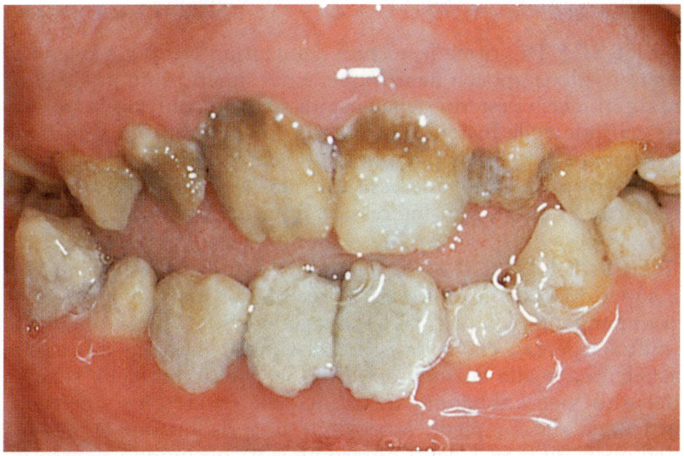

Figura 304-1. Amelogenesi imperfetta, tipo ipocalcificato. I difetti dello smalto consistono in discromia ed erosione, causate da errori durante la fase di mineralizzazione dello sviluppo dentario e da colorazione secondaria. (Da Nazif MM, Martin BS, McKibben DH, et al: Oral disorders. In Zitelli BJ, Davis HW [editors]: *Atlas of Pediatric Physical Diagnosis*, 4th ed. Philadelphia, Mosby, 2002, p 703.)

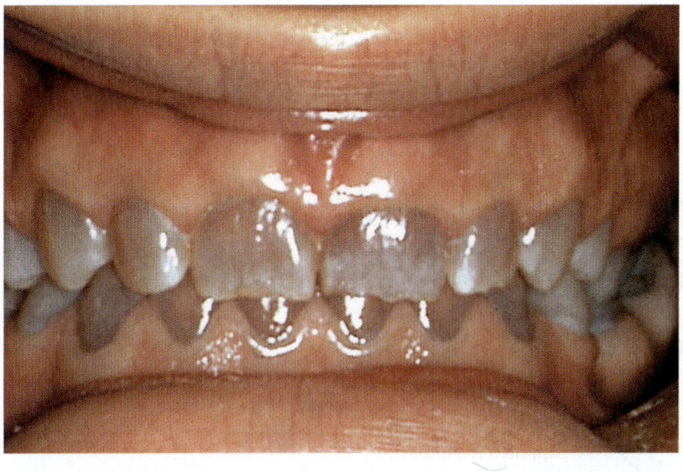

Figura 304-2. Dentinogenesi imperfetta. La lucentezza opalescente bluastra osservabile in molti di questi denti deriva da una dentina geneticamente difettiva. Questa condizione può essere associata a osteogenesi imperfetta. (Da Nazif MM, Martin BS, McKibben DH, et al: Oral disorders. In Zitelli BJ, Davis HW [editors]: *Atlas of Pediatric Physical Diagnosis*, 4th ed. Philadelphia, Mosby, 2002, p 703.)

I disturbi localizzati della calcificazione che si correlano a periodi di malattia, malnutrizione, nascita prematura o trauma durante il parto sono comuni. L'**ipocalcificazione** si presenta sotto forma di linee orizzontali o chiazze bianche opache sul dente; l'**ipoplasia**, più grave, consiste nella formazione di pozzetti o aree prive di smalto. Ai difetti della smalto sono associate condizioni sistemiche quali insufficienza renale o fibrosi cistica. Il trauma locale a carico degli incisivi decidui può influire anche sulla calcificazione degli incisivi permanenti.

La **fluorosi** (macchie sullo smalto) può dipendere da un assorbimento sistemico di fluoro >0,05 mg/kg/die durante la formazione dello smalto. Questo elevato assorbimento può essere dovuto al fatto di risiedere in una zona con acqua potabile a elevato contenuto di fluoro (>2 ppm), all'uso eccessivo di dentifricio con fluoro o a scorrette prescrizioni di fluoro e derivati. Durante lo sviluppo dello smalto, tale fenomeno influisce sulla funzione ameloblastica, comportando la comparsa di difetti di varia entità, che vanno da poche chiazze bianche sparse fino a gravi discromie (discolorazioni) brunastre e ipoplasia. Queste ultime alterazioni si osservano con concentrazioni di fluoro nell'acqua potabile >5 ppm.

La discromia dei denti può essere dovuta all'assorbimento da parte dello smalto di sostanze estranee durante lo sviluppo. L'iperbilirubinemia neonatale può determinare una discromia bluastra o nerastra nella dentizione decidua, mentre la porfiria produce una colorazione rosso-marrone. Le tetracicline, che vengono assorbite in maniera estesa dalle strutture ossee e dentarie, se somministrate durante il periodo di formazione dello smalto possono comportare una discromia giallo-marrone e ipoplasia. Tali elementi dentari si presentano fluorescenti alla luce ultravioletta. Il periodo a rischio va dal 4° mese di gestazione al 7° anno di vita. Una terapia ripetuta o prolungata con tetracicline aumenta il rischio.

L'eruzione ritardata dei 20 denti decidui può essere una caratteristica ereditaria o indicare la presenza di disturbi di natura sistemica o nutrizionale quali ipopituitarismo, ipotiroidismo, displasia cleidocranica, trisomia 21, progeria, osteodistrofia ereditaria di Albright, incontinentia pigmenti, rachitismo e sindromi multiple. La mancata eruzione di uno o più denti può derivare da cause locali come denti malposizionati o sovrannumerari, cisti, denti decidui ritenuti. Molto spesso la perdita prematura dei denti decidui è causata dall'eruzione prematura di quelli permanenti. Se l'intera dentizione è avanzata per l'età e per il sesso, occorre considerare una pubertà precoce o ipertiroidismo.

La presenza di **denti natali** si osserva in circa 1/2000 neonati; solitamente ve ne sono due nella posizione degli incisivi centrali inferiori. I denti natali sono presenti alla nascita, mentre quelli **neonatali** erompono nel primo mese di vita. I denti natali/neonatali, la cui inserzione è generalmente limitata al margine gengivale, con scarsa formazione di radice o sostegno osseo, possono essere costituiti da un dente sovrannumerario o da uno deciduo prematuramente erotto. Per distinguere queste due condizioni è sufficiente una radiografia. I denti natali sono associati a palatoschisi, sindrome di Pierre Robin, sindrome di Ellis-Van Creveld, sindrome di Hallermann-Streiff, pachionichia congenita e altre anomalie. Nel 15-20% dei bambini affetti è presente un'anamnesi di denti natali o eruzione prematura.

Talvolta i denti natali/neonatali, oltre a esitare in dolore e rifiuto dell'alimentazione, possono provocare disagio nella madre a causa dell'abrasione del capezzolo durante l'allattamento. Vi è il remoto pericolo di un distacco, con conseguente aspirazione, del dente. Per la sua posizione tra i processi alveolari durante la nascita, la lingua può subire lacerazioni e, talvolta, amputazione della punta (**malattia di Riga-Fede**). Occorre valutare caso per caso se sia o meno opportuno estrarre i denti decidui erotti prematuramente.

Si parla di mancata caduta di un dente deciduo quando esso non cade prima dell'eruzione del suo successore permanente. Molto spesso il dente deciduo alla fine cade spontaneamente, ma in certi casi può richiedere l'estrazione. Questo avviene per lo più nella regione degli incisivi inferiori.

Capitolo 305 ■ Disturbi del cavo orale associati ad altre condizioni

I disturbi dei denti e delle strutture adiacenti possono verificarsi in forma isolata o in associazione con altre affezioni sistemiche (Tab. 305-1). Molto spesso le condizioni mediche che si verificano durante lo sviluppo dei denti possono influire sulla formazione o sull'aspetto estetico dei denti stessi. Il danno subito dai denti durante il loro sviluppo è permanente.

TABELLA 305-1. Problemi dentali associati a specifiche condizioni mediche

CONDIZIONE MEDICA	REPERTI DENTALI O ORALI COMUNI ASSOCIATI
Labioschisi e palatoschisi	Denti mancanti, denti sovrannumerari, spostamento di segmenti dell'arco palatale, difficoltà di alimentazione, problemi di fonazione
Insufficienza renale	Chiazze nello smalto (denti permanenti), dismorfia facciale
Fibrosi cistica	Denti pigmentati per esteso uso di farmaci, chiazze nello smalto
Immunosoppressione	Candidosi orale con rischio di candidosi sistemica, iperplasia gengivale indotta da ciclosporine
Basso peso alla nascita con prolungata intubazione orale	Solco palatale, arco palatale stretto
Difetti cardiaci con predisposizione all'endocardite batterica	Batteriemia da procedure o traumi dentali
Deficit chemiotattico dei neutrofili	Parodontite giovanile (perdita dell'osso di sostegno)
Diabete giovanile (incontrollato)	Parodontite giovanile
Disfunzione neuromotoria	Trauma orale da caduta; malocclusione (*open bite*); gengivite da mancanza di igiene
Prolungata malattia (generalizzata) durante la formazione dei denti	Ipoplasia dello smalto nelle porzioni coronali formatesi durante la malattia
Convulsioni	Ingrossamento gengivale legato all'uso di fenitoina
Infezioni materne	Sifilide-denti di forma anomala
Rachitismo vitamina D-dipendente	Ipoplasia dello smalto

Capitolo 306 ■ Malocclusione

Il cavo orale è essenzialmente uno strumento masticatorio. I denti anteriori sono deputati a staccare con un morso porzioni di ampie quantità di cibo, mentre i posteriori hanno il compito di ridurre il boccone in un bolo tenero e umido. Le guance e la lingua spingono il bolo alimentare sulle aree di contatto fra i denti. Per ragioni fisiologiche ed estetiche è importante stabilire una corretta relazione tra denti superiori e inferiori.

VARIAZIONI DEI MODELLI DI CRESCITA. I modelli di crescita sono classificati in tre principali tipi di occlusione, determinati con i mascellari chiusi e i denti in occlusione (Fig. 306-1). Secondo la Classificazione della Malocclusione di Angle, nell'**occlusione di classe I** (normale) le cuspidi dei denti posteroinferiori intercuspidano in avanti e dentro le corrispondenti cuspidi dei denti superiori antagonisti, dando luogo un profilo facciale normale. Nella **malocclusione di classe II** ("denti di cavallo") le cuspidi dei denti posteroinferiori si trovano dietro e all'interno delle corrispondenti cuspidi dei denti superiori. Questa frequente disarmonia occlusale, che si osserva in circa il 45% della popolazione, si traduce in un profilo facciale con "mento sfuggente" (retrognazia) o denti anteriori protrusi. Il maggiore spazio tra i denti anteriori superoinferiori che si viene così a formare incoraggia le cattive abitudini di suzione del dito e spinta della lingua in avanti. Inoltre, i bambini con pronunciata malocclusione di classe II sono a maggior rischio di danni traumatici agli incisivi. Nella **malocclusione di classe III** (*under bite*) le cuspidi dei denti inferoposteriori intercuspidano a un dente o più in avanti rispetto ai loro antagonisti superiori. I denti anteriori si presentano in *cross bite* (morso inverso), con gli incisivi inferiori che protrudono oltre gli incisivi superiori. Il profilo facciale è caratterizzato dal "mento protruso" (**prognazia**).

CROSS BITE. Di norma le cuspidi dei denti inferiori si trovano in una posizione appena dentro quelle dei superiori, in modo che i margini incisivi esterni delle cuspidi stesse incontrino la porzione centrale delle fosse degli antagonisti superiori. La situazione contraria è detta *cross bite* (morso inverso). Il cross bite, distinto in anteriore quando interessa gli incisivi e posteriore quando riguarda i molari, può interessare uno o più denti.

OPEN BITE E CLOSED BITE. Quando i denti posteriori inferiori e superiori entrano in contatto reciproco, ma i denti anteriori rimangono separati, si ha una condizione detta *open bite* (morso aperto), che può essere dovuta al modello di crescita scheletrica o alla suzione del dito. Se l'abitudine della suzione del dito viene abbandonata prima che la crescita scheletrica e dentale sia completa, è possibile una risoluzione spontanea dell'open bite. Se i denti anteroinferiori occludono dentro gli anterosuperiori in una posizione di sovraocclusione, si configura il quadro del *closed bite* (morso chiuso) o *deep bite* (morso profondo). Il trattamento dell'open e del closed bite si basa sulla correzione ortodontica, eseguita generalmente in età prepubere e adolescenziale. Alcuni casi richiedono la chirurgia ortognatica al fine di posizionare i mascellari in maniera ottimale in una direzione verticale (per ottenere un corretto allineamento delle arcate dentarie).

AFFOLLAMENTO DENTALE. In presenza di mascellari troppo piccoli o di denti troppo grandi per un loro adeguato allineamento si può avere una sovrapposizione (*overlap*) degli incisivi. La crescita dell'osso avviene per lo più a livello delle regioni poste-

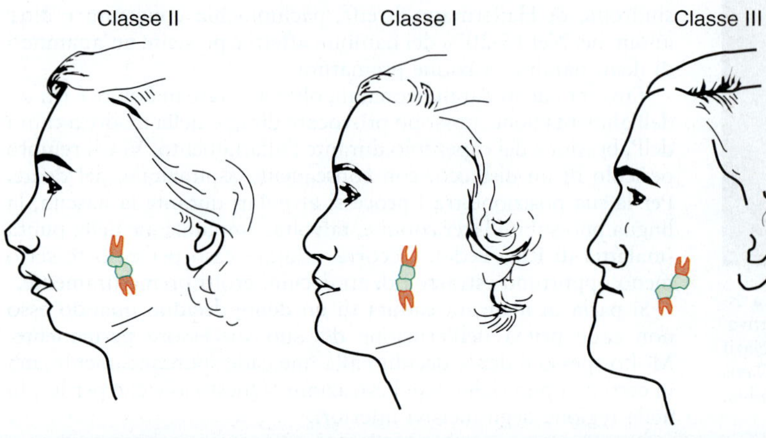

Figura 306-1. Classificazione della malocclusione di Angle. È illustrata la tipica corrispondenza tra il profilo facciale e il rapporto tra molari.

riori della mandibola e della mascella e, pertanto, se lo spazio anteriore risulta insufficiente all'età di 7-8 anni, questa situazione non si risolverà con la crescita dei mascellari. La presenza di diastemi della dentizione decidua non solo è normale, ma favorisce un adeguato allineamento dei denti successivi.

SUZIONE DEL DITO. Riguardo alla cattiva abitudine dei bambini di succhiarsi il dito sono state avanzate varie teorie eziologiche e proposte di correzione, anche in contrasto tra loro. La prolungata suzione del dito può causare l'allargamento a ventaglio (**flaring**) degli incisivi superiori, un open bite e un cross bite posteriore. I bambini cominciano a perdere questo vizio a partire dai 2 anni di età e il 10% circa lo perde entro i 5 anni. Se tale abitudine viene abbandonata poco dopo l'eruzione degli incisivi superiori permanenti (7-8 anni di età), ci sono buone probabilità che non influisca negativamente sulla dentizione. Sono stati suggeriti vari trattamenti, dalla modifica del comportamento all'applicazione di un apparecchio con estensioni che impedisca di introdurre il dito in bocca. La maggiore probabilità di successo si ha nei casi in cui il bambino smette di succhiarsi il dito di sua spontanea volontà. Tuttavia, questa interruzione non correggerà una malocclusione causata da un precedente modello di crescita deviante.

Capitolo 307 ■ Labioschisi e palatoschisi

Le schisi del labbro e del palato sono entità distinte ma strettamente collegate dal punto di vista embriologico, funzionale e genetico. Nonostante siano state formulate varie teorie al riguardo, si ritiene comunemente che la schisi labiale (labioschisi o labbro leporino) si verifichi a seguito dell'ipoplasia dello strato di cellule mesenchimali, con conseguente mancata saldatura delle due porzioni del labbro superiore. La schisi del palato (palatoschisi) sembra riconducibile alla mancata approssimazione o fusione dei due lati del palato.

INCIDENZA ED EPIDEMIOLOGIA. Nei neonati bianchi l'incidenza della labioschisi con o senza palatoschisi è di circa 1/750, mentre l'incidenza della sola palatoschisi è di circa 1/2500. Le schisi labiali sono più frequenti nei maschi. Le possibili cause comprendono l'esposizione materna ai farmaci, un complesso sindrome-malformazione o fattori genetici. Quantunque possa sembrare che le due condizioni si verifichino sporadicamente, la presenza di geni sensibili sembra importante. Vi sono famiglie in cui labioschisi o palatoschisi, o entrambe, sono ereditate in maniera dominante (*sindrome di Van der Woude*) ed è importante un accurato esame dei genitori per distinguere questo tipo di patologia dagli altri poiché il rischio di ricorrenza è del 50%. L'incidenza della schisi labiopalatale è influenzata anche da fattori etnici; l'incidenza è più elevata negli asiatici e negli indiani d'America, e più bassa nei neri. L'incidenza di malformazioni congenite associate (corredo cromosomico aneuploide, oloprosencefalia) e la compromissione dello sviluppo è maggiore nei bambini affetti da schisi, in particolare in quelli con sola palatoschisi. I rischi di ricorrenza delle schisi nell'ambito di una stessa famiglia sono trattati nei Capitoli 80 e 83.

MANIFESTAZIONI CLINICHE. La labioschisi può essere di vario grado, da una piccola incisione nel bordo vermiglio a una completa separazione a carico di cute, muscolo, mucosa, denti e struttura ossea. Le schisi, unilaterali (per lo più sul lato sinistro) o bilaterali, possono interessare la cresta alveolare. Reperti associati sono denti deformi, sovrannumerari o assenti. La sola palatoschisi si osserva alla linea mediana e può interessare solo l'ugola o estendersi dentro o attraverso il palato molle e il palato duro fino al forame incisivo. Quando è associata a labioschisi, la lesione può interessare la linea mediana del palato molle ed estendersi fino al palato duro su uno o entrambi i lati, esponendo una o entrambe le fosse nasali come nel caso di una palatoschisi uni- o bilaterale. Il palato può anche presentare una schisi sottomucosa, indicata dalla presenza di un'ugola bifida, una separazione parziale del muscolo con mucosa intatta o un'incisione palpabile nella regione posteriore del palato.

TRATTAMENTO. Un programma completo di riabilitazione per il bambino con schisi labiale o palatale può richiedere anni di trattamento da parte di un'équipe composta da pediatra, chirurgo plastico, otorinolaringoiatra, chirurgo orale e maxillofacciale, pedodontista, protesista dentale, logopedista, genetista, sociologo, psicologo e assistente sanitario. Spetta al pediatra la responsabilità di coordinare i vari specialisti e rappresentare un punto di riferimento per i genitori.

In un bambino con schisi labiale o palatale congenita, il primo problema da affrontare è l'alimentazione. Anche se alcuni studiosi sostengono l'opportunità di costruire otturatori in resina, la maggior parte ritiene che sia sufficiente usare tettarelle morbide e con ampi fori, una bottiglietta deformabile (biberon in materiale morbido) e fornire corrette istruzioni ai genitori per risolvere il problema in modo relativamente facile ed efficace.

La chiusura chirurgica di una labioschisi viene normalmente eseguita entro il 3° mese di vita, se il bambino ha raggiunto un peso soddisfacente e non è affetto da eventuali infezioni orali, respiratorie o sistemiche. L'intervento più comune si basa su una modifica della tecnica di rotazione-avanzamento secondo Millard; una linea di sutura a zig-zag riduce al minimo le indententature del labbro dovute a retrazione del tessuto cicatriziale. La riparazione può essere rivista a 4-5 anni di età. La chirurgia correttiva del naso può essere rimandata fino all'adolescenza o venire eseguita al momento della riparazione del labbro. I risultati estetici dipendono dall'ampiezza del difetto originale, dal potenziale di guarigione del soggetto, dall'assenza di infezione e dall'abilità del chirurgo.

Poiché le palatoschisi possono presentare dimensioni, forma e grado di deformità molto diversi, è opportuno scegliere il momento della correzione chirurgica caso per caso. Sulla decisione influiranno criteri quali l'ampiezza della schisi, l'adeguatezza dei segmenti palatali esistenti, la morfologia delle aree adiacenti (ampiezza dell'orofaringe) e dalla funzione neuromuscolare del palato molle e delle pareti faringee. Gli obiettivi della chirurgia sono: saldare i segmenti separati, conseguire una fonazione comprensibile e gradevole, ridurre il rigurgito nasale ed evitare che la lesione interessi la mascella in crescita.

In un bambino esente da altre patologie, la chiusura del palato di solito viene eseguita entro il primo anno di vita al fine di promuovere il conseguimento di una fonazione normale. Quando la correzione chirurgica è rimandata oltre il terzo anno di età, nella regione posteriore di una protesi dentaria superiore si può applicare un bulbo opportunamente modellato (*speech bulb*) per favorire l'articolazione del linguaggio. Tale accorgimento fa sì che la contrazione dei muscoli faringei e velofaringei porti i tessuti in contatto con il bulbo stesso in modo da ottenere l'occlusione del rinofaringe e aiutare il bambino a sviluppare un linguaggio intelligibile.

La palatoschisi di solito attraversa la cresta alveolare e interferisce con l'eruzione dei denti nella regione superoanteriore. I denti nell'area di schisi possono presentarsi spostati, malformati o mancanti. Questi ultimi, come pure eventuali denti non funzionali, possono essere sostituiti da dispositivi protesici.

CURA POSTOPERATORIA. Durante l'immediato periodo postoperatorio, è indispensabile un'assistenza infermieristica particolare. La delicata aspirazione del rinofaringe riduce al minimo le possibilità d'insorgenza di complicanze comuni quali atelettasia e polmonite. I principali obiettivi durante la cura postoperatoria sono mantenere pulita la linea di sutura ed evitare tensione lungo i punti di sutura. Il bambino viene nutrito con il biberon della Mead Johnson, immobilizzando le braccia con manicotti per gomiti. La dieta deve essere liquida o semiliquida per 3 settimane; l'alimentazione viene continuata con il biberon della Mead Johnson o una tazza. Bisogna evitare che il sito chirurgico venga in contatto con le mani del paziente, come pure con eventuali giocattoli e altri oggetti estranei.

POSTUMI DELLA LABIOSCHISI E DELLA PALATOSCHISI. In presenza di palatoschisi sono frequenti otite media ricorrente e perdita dell'udito. Lo spostamento delle arcate mascellari e la malposizione dei denti richiedono di norma la correzione ortodontica.

I difetti di fonazione, spesso associati a labioschisi e palatoschisi, possono essere presenti e persistere a causa di una scorretta chiusura del palato. La fonazione in questi casi è caratterizzata dall'emissione di aria dal naso e dal timbro fortemente nasale di certi suoni. La disfonia, presente prima e talvolta anche dopo la chirurgia palatale, è causata da inadeguatezza funzionale dei muscoli palatini e faringei. I muscoli del palato molle e delle pareti laterali e posteriori del rinofaringe costituiscono un diaframma che separa il rinofaringe dall'orofaringe durante la deglutizione e la produzione di alcuni suoni. Se tale diaframma non funziona adeguatamente è difficile che nella bocca si formi una pressione sufficiente a produrre le esplosive *p*, *b*, *d*, *t*, *i* o le sibilanti *s*, *sc*, *ch*: le parole contenenti tali suoni risultano perciò poco comprensibili. Dopo l'intervento chirurgico o l'inserimento di un apparecchio per la fonazione, è necessario affidare il paziente alle cure di un logopedista.

INCOMPETENZA VELOFARINGEA. La disfonia caratteristica del bambino con palatoschisi può essere dovuta anche ad altre anomalie ossee o neuromuscolari laddove non si venga a formare un'adesione sigillante efficace tra orofaringe e rinofaringe durante la deglutizione o la fonazione. L'anomalia può essere nella struttura del palato o della faringe o nei muscoli che vi si inseriscono. In un bambino a rischio di anomalie del linguaggio l'adenoidectomia può aggravare l'ipernasalità. Anche una palatoschisi sottomucosa può favorire questo problema. In tali casi, la massa adenoidea può aver facilitato la chiusura velofaringea al contatto con il palato molle in elevazione. Se la funzione neuromuscolare è adeguata, si può avere una compensazione nel movimento velofaringeo con conseguente miglioramento della disfonia, pur essendo necessario l'intervento di un logopedista. In altri casi, una lenta involuzione delle adenoidi può consentire una graduale compensazione della funzione dei muscoli palatali e faringei. Può essere questo il motivo per cui un difetto fonatorio risulta quasi impercettibile in alcuni bambini con palatoschisi sottomucosa o un'anomalia analoga che predispone all'incompetenza velofaringea. L'incompetenza velofaringea (VPI, *VeloPharingeal Incompetence*) si può riscontrare anche in soggetti con intrinseca anomalia palatale (sindrome velocardiofacciale). È opportuno che la VPI sia valutata da un'équipe composta da esperti in disturbi craniofacciali e da un genetista.

Manifestazioni cliniche. Sebbene i segni clinici siano diversi, i sintomi della VPI sono simili a quelli della palatoschisi. Vi possono essere: (1) fonazione ipernasale (che si nota in particolare nell'articolazione di consonanti la cui produzione richiede pressione, quali *p*, *b*, *d*, *t*, *v*, *f*, e *s*); (2) vistosi movimenti di contrazione delle narici durante la fonazione, (3) incapacità di fischiare, fare gargarismi, spegnere una candela o gonfiare un palloncino; (4) perdita di liquido dal naso quando il bambino beve con la testa reclinata verso il basso; (5) otite media; (6) ipoacusia. L'esame orale può evidenziare: (1) una palatoschisi o un palato relativamente corto con un ampio orofaringe; (2) un'attività muscolare assente, estremamente asimmetrica o minima del palato molle e della faringe durante la fonazione o il gagging; (3) una schisi sottomucosa. Quest'ultima è suggerita dalla presenza di (1) un'ugola bifida, (2) una membrana traslucida lungo la linea mediana del palato molle (indicativa di una soluzione di continuità dei muscoli) e (3) un'incisione palpabile lungo il margine posteriore del palato duro, anziché un processo spinoso della spina nasale nell'area posteriore oppure (4) uno spostamento o una scanalatura in avanti o a forma di V sul palato molle durante la fonazione o il gagging.

La VPI è evidenziabile anche radiograficamente. La testa va posizionata accuratamente in modo da ottenere una vera proiezione laterale. Si esegue una lastra con il paziente a riposo e un'altra durante l'emissione continua della vocale *u*, come nella parola "boom". Il palato molle entra in contatto con la parete faringea posteriore se la funzione è normale, mentre tale contatto è assente in caso di VPI. Per una valutazione più accurata della VPI si ricorre alla rinoscopia.

In casi selezionati, il palato può essere retroposizionato o si può eseguire la faringoplastica con un lembo tissutale prelevato dalla parete faringea posteriore. Anche i dispositivi dentali per il miglioramento della fonazione sono stati usati con successo. I reperti della rinoscopia permettono di scegliere il tipo di intervento chirurgico in base alle esigenze individuali.

Capitolo 308 ■ Sindromi con manifestazioni orali

Molte sindromi presentano manifestazioni specifiche o di accompagnamento di tipo orale, dentale o facciale (sindrome di Apert, Capitolo 592; sindrome di Crouzon, Capitolo 592; sindrome di Down, Capitolo 81).

L'osteogenesi imperfetta è spesso accompagnata da una serie di conseguenze sui denti, la cosiddetta **dentinogenesi imperfetta** (vedi Capitolo 304, Fig. 304-2). In base alla gravità della presentazione, il trattamento della dentizione va dal monitoraggio preventivo e conservativo di routine alla ricopertura dei denti posteriori affetti con corone in acciaio inossidabile al fine di ridurre l'abrasione da masticazione. La dentinogenesi imperfetta può manifestarsi anche in forma isolata, senza effetti sulle strutture ossee.

Un'altra sindrome, la **displasia cleidocranica**, è caratterizzata da variazioni orofacciali come bozze frontali prominenti, prognatismo mandibolare e un'ampia base nasale. L'eruzione dentaria è spesso in ritardo. Si osservano una ritenzione anomala dei denti decidui e la mancata eruzione di quelli permanenti. I denti sovrannumerari sono frequenti, specie nell'area dei premolari. I denti, pur essendo di norma esenti da ipoplasia, presentano spesso variazioni di dimensioni e forma. In caso di lesioni cariose è opportuno eseguire il restauro dei denti decidui e permanenti erotti. Talvolta è necessaria un'intesa terapia di riabilitazione dentale per mantenere una masticazione efficace.

Le **displasie ectodermiche** (vedi Capitolo 648) sono un gruppo eterogeneo di condizioni caratterizzato da manifestazioni orali che vanno da un interessamento scarso o nullo (la dentizione è completamente normale) a casi in cui i denti possono essere totalmente o parzialmente assenti o malformati. Poiché in mancanza dei denti l'osso alveolare non si sviluppa, i processi alveolari possono essere totalmente o parzialmente assenti e la risultante sovraocclusione della mandibola provoca la protrusione delle labbra. Lo sviluppo facciale non presenta altre anomalie. I denti, quando presenti, possono avere dimensioni normali o ridotte e forma conoide. In caso di aplasia delle ghiandole mucose labiali e vestibolari possono osservarsi secchezza e irritazione della mucosa orale. I soggetti con displasia ectodermica possono avere bisogno di protesi totali o parziali, anche in età molto giovane. In tal modo si ripristina l'altezza dei mascellari, migliorando la posizione delle labbra e il profilo facciale. Anche la funzione masticatoria migliora, con effetti positivi sulle abitudini alimentari.

La **sindrome di Pierre Robin** consiste in una micrognazia accompagnata da una palato molto arcuato o da una palatoschisi (Fig. 308-1). La lingua è solitamente di dimensioni normali, ma il pavimento della bocca è ridotto. L'ostruzione delle vie aeree,

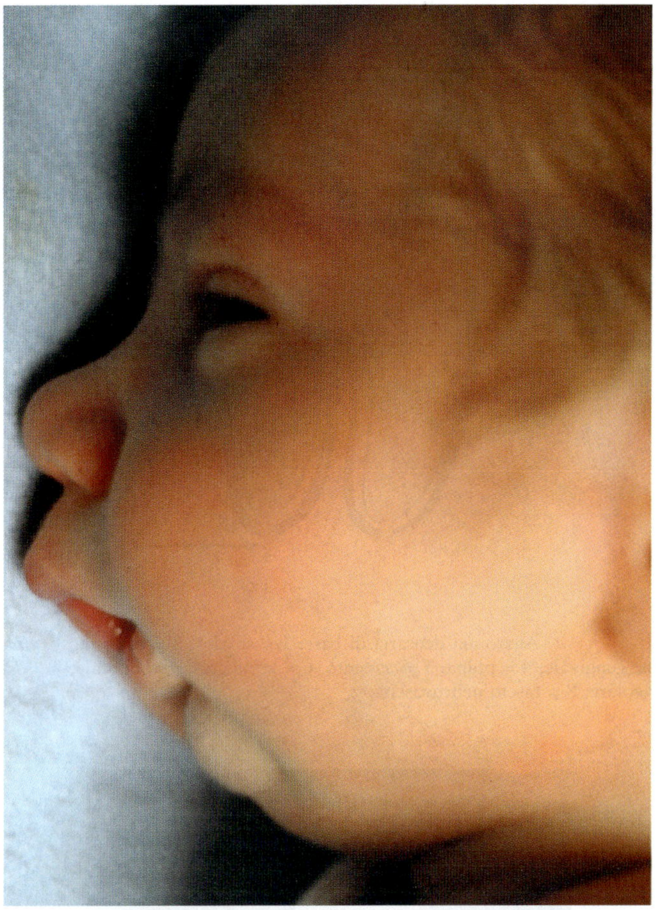

Figura 308-1. Sindrome di Pierre Robin. (Da Clark DA: *Atlas of Neonatology*, 7th ed. Philadelphia, WB Saunders, 2000, p 144.)

che può verificarsi soprattutto durante l'inspirazione, richiede di norma il trattamento per prevenire l'asfissia. Il bambino va mantenuto in posizione prona o parzialmente prona in modo che la lingua cada in avanti per alleviare l'ostruzione respiratoria. Alcuni soggetti possono richiedere l'intubazione endotracheale o, raramente, la tracheotomia. Interventi di spostamento della mandibola nel neonato possono migliorare le dimensioni mandibolari e la respirazione e rendere più agevole l'alimentazione orale. In presenza di ostruzione mandibolare, questa metodica è un'alternativa importante alla tracheotomia.

Talvolta è possibile che nel giro di pochi mesi si verifichi una crescita mandibolare spontanea sufficiente ad alleviare l'ostruzione delle vie aeree. Spesso la crescita della mandibola raggiunge un profilo normale in 4-6 anni. L'alimentazione dei neonati affetti da ipoplasia mandibolare, pur richiedendo grande attenzione e pazienza, di norma può essere ottenuta senza dover ricorrere al *gavage*. Le anomalie dentarie richiedono di solito un trattamento individualizzato. Una percentuale compresa tra il 30 e il 50% dei bambini con sindrome di Pierre Robin presenta la sindrome di Stickler, una condizione autosomica dominante che comprende altri reperti quali artrite e problemi oculari precoci.

Nella **disostosi mandibolofacciale** (sindrome di Treacher Collins o di Franceschetti), la facies è caratterizzata da rime palpebrali inclinate verso il basso, coloboma delle palpebre inferiori, ossa mascellari infossate, fistole cieche che si aprono tra gli angoli della bocca e le orecchie, pinne nasali deformi, crescita atipica dei capelli in estensione verso le guance, mento sfuggente e bocca grande. Sono comuni schisi facciali, anomalie delle orecchie e sordità. Il disturbo è autosomico dominante, spesso con penetranza incompleta. La mandibola è di norma ipoplasica; il ramo può mancare e i processi coronoide e condilare sono piatti o addirittura aplasici. La volta palatina può essere alta o con una schisi. Seppur di rado, si possono osservare macrostomia uni- o bilaterale o insufficienza della fusione embrionale dei processi intermascellari. Le malocclusioni dentarie sono frequenti. I denti possono presentare ampi diastemi, essere ipoplasici, spostati o presentare open bite. Sono indicati la terapia ortodontica e il trattamento dentario di routine.

La **microsomia emifacciale**, di norma caratterizzata da ipoplasia unilaterale della mandibola, può essere associata a paralisi parziale del nervo facciale, macrostomia, fistole cieche tra gli angoli della bocca e le orecchie e malformazioni a carico dell'orecchio esterno. Talvolta si sviluppano grave asimmetria facciale e malocclusione per l'assenza o l'ipoplasia del condilo mandibolare sul lato affetto. La deformità condilare congenita tende a peggiorare con l'età. Per minimizzare l'anomalia può essere indicata la chirurgia craniofacciale precoce. Il disturbo può essere associato ad anomalie vertebrali e oculari (spettro oculo-auricolo-vertebrale, compresa la sindrome di Goldenhar); pertanto, bisogna fare riferimento alle radiografie delle vertebre e delle coste per determinare l'entità dell'interessamento scheletrico.

Capitolo 309 ■ Carie dentaria

EZIOLOGIA. Lo sviluppo della carie dentaria dipende dall'interazione che si viene a creare tra superficie dei denti, carboidrati introdotti con la dieta e batteri orali specifici. Gli acidi organici prodotti dalla fermentazione batterica dei carboidrati riducono il pH della placca fino a provocare la demineralizzazione del dente. La lesione cariosa iniziale si presenta come un punto bianco opaco sullo smalto; con la progressiva perdita di minerale dentario si sviluppa una cavitazione.

All'insorgenza della carie è associato lo ***Streptococcus mutans***. I microrganismi di questa specie hanno la capacità di aderire allo smalto, produrre abbondante acido e sopravvivere in presenza di un basso pH. Una volta formatasi una cavitazione nella superficie dello smalto, altri microrganismi orali (lattobacilli) colonizzano il dente, producendo acido e favorendo la demineralizzazione della struttura dentaria. L'entità di tale demineralizzazione conseguente alla produzione di acido da parte dei batteri dipenderà dalla frequenza del consumo e dal tipo di carboidrati assunti. Il saccarosio è lo zucchero più cariogeno perché uno dei suoi sottoprodotti durante il metabolismo batterico è il glucano, un polimero che favorisce l'adesione dei batteri alla struttura dentaria. Il potenziale cariogeno di un biberon contenente una bevanda edulcorata consumata durante la notte o durante il riposo pomeridiano è molto più elevato rispetto a quello della stessa quantità di bevanda ingerita in un solo pasto. Analogamente, il saccarosio contenuto nei dolciumi gommosi, che rimangono a lungo in bocca, è più cariogeno dello zucchero dei prodotti alimentari che vengono a contatto con i denti per breve tempo.

EPIDEMIOLOGIA. Anche se l'incidenza della carie dentaria è diminuita nei Paesi sviluppati negli ultimi 30 anni, la sua prevalenza si mantiene elevata nei bambini provenienti da famiglie a basso reddito e in quelli originari di Paesi in via di sviluppo. Il calo è dovuto ai progressi compiuti nel campo della prevenzione, e in particolare all'uso del fluoro. Più della metà dei bambini statunitensi è affetto da carie dentaria, localizzata soprattutto nei pozzetti e nelle fessure delle superfici occlusali (masticatorie) dei molari.

MANIFESTAZIONI CLINICHE. Nella dentizione decidua la carie inizia a svilupparsi di norma nei pozzetti e nelle fessure. Le lesioni piccole possono essere difficili da diagnosticare, mentre quelle più estese si presentano come cavitazioni della superficie occlusale. La seconda localizzazione più frequente della carie è nelle aree dentarie interprossimali (le superfici di contatto tra i denti); in

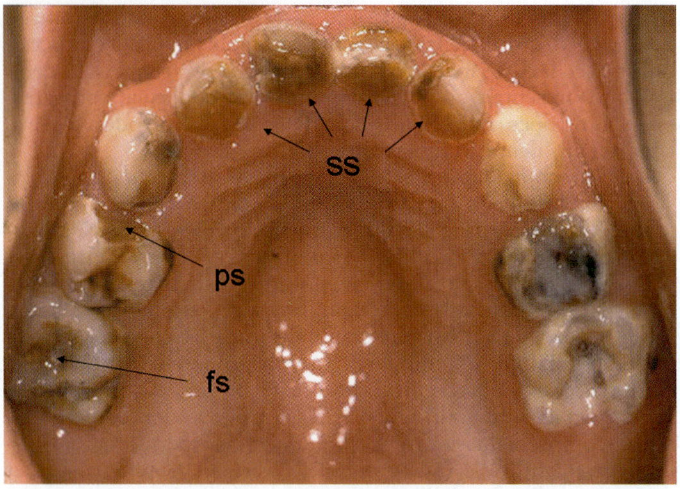

Figura 309-1. Carie florida o destruente (carie infantile precoce) in un bambino di 3 anni. Si notino le carie sulle superfici lisce degli incisivi (ss), sulla superficie interprossimale del primo molare deciduo (ps) e la fessura del secondo molare deciduo (fs).

molti casi, queste lesioni possono essere individuate soltanto mediante radiografie intraorali. Le lesioni cariose delle superfici lisce esposte (vestibolari e linguali) generalmente si osservano solo nei bambini con carie florida o destruente (Fig. 309-1).

La carie florida o destruente nei neonati e nei bambini fino al secondo anno di vita, detta **carie infantile precoce** o carie da biberon, viene attribuita a una scorretta alimentazione con il biberon. Pur essendo critica l'associazione di infezioni da batteri cariogeni nel bambino e frequente consumo di zucchero, nel biberon o in cibi solidi, non è escluso che al fenomeno carioso possano contribuire anche altri fattori, tra cui l'ipoplasia dello smalto dei denti decidui legata a carenze nutrizionali durante la gravidanza o la nascita prematura. Gli studi hanno inoltre stabilito una correlazione tra carie infantile precoce e allattamento al seno "a volontà" nei bambini più grandi. È interessante osservare che il latte vaccino è meno associato alla carie, probabilmente per il suo maggior contenuto di calcio e fosforo rispetto al latte materno.

La carie infantile precoce è frequente, con una prevalenza documentata del 30-50% nei bambini di stato socioeconomico basso, arrivando al 70% in alcuni gruppi di indiani d'America. Può presentarsi sin dal 12° mese di vita, molto prima che il bambino giunga all'attenzione del dentista. Spetta ai pediatri esaminare i denti del piccolo sia alla ricerca di eventuali carie, sia per stabilire un opportuno contatto paziente-dentista prima che il bambino a rischio di carie infantile precoce compia un anno di vita. I fattori di rischio comprendono elevato consumo di zucchero (assunto con le bevande o gli alimenti), appartenenza a famiglie di basse condizioni socioeconomiche, bambini immigrati, genitori o fratelli con elevati indici di carie ed evidenza di lesioni sui denti.

Coloro che presentano carie in tenera età sono considerati ad alto rischio di svilupparne altre con la crescita. Pertanto, una corretta prevenzione della carie infantile precoce può eliminare i principali problemi dentali nei bambini al secondo anno di vita e comportare minori rischi di carie negli anni a seguire.

COMPLICANZE. Se non è curata, la carie di norma distrugge la maggior parte del dente e invade la camera pulpare (Fig. 309-2), provocando un'infiammazione della polpa (**pulpite**) e dolore intenso. La pulpite può progredire in necrosi, con un'invasione dell'osso alveolare che causa un ascesso dentario (Fig. 309-3). L'infezione di un dente deciduo può compromettere il normale sviluppo del dente permanente successivo. In una piccola percentuale di casi, questo processo conduce a sepsi e a infezione della regione facciale.

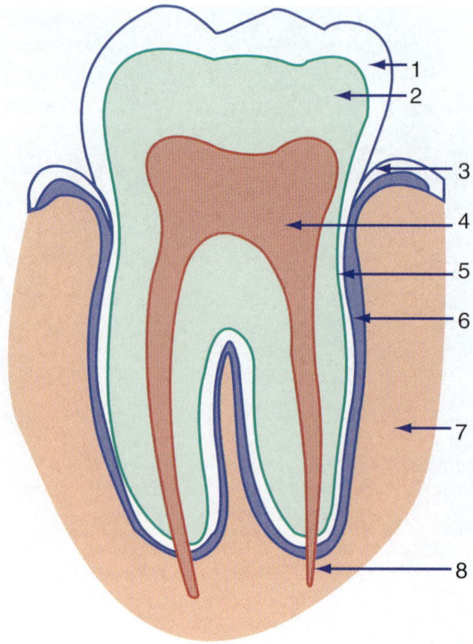

Figura 309-2. Anatomia dentaria di base: 1 = smalto; 2 = dentina; 3 = margine gengivale; 4 = polpa; 5 = cemento; 6 = legamento parodontale; 7 = osso alveolare; 8 = fascio neurovascolare.

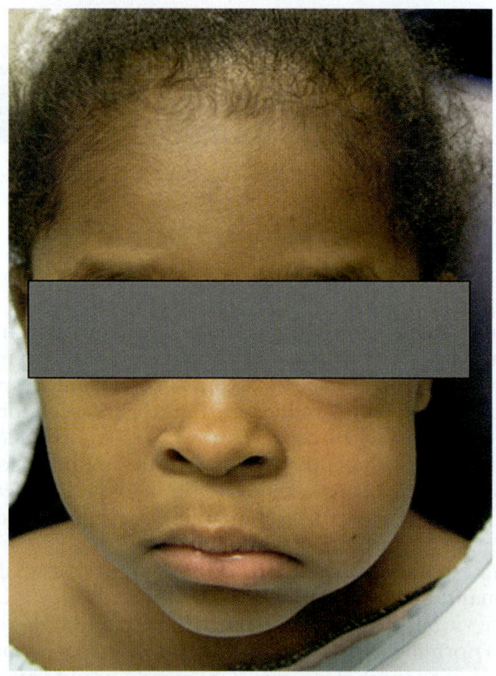

Figura 309-3. Edema facciale causato da ascesso in un molare deciduo. La risoluzione dell'infiammazione può essere ottenuta con una terapia antibiotica seguita dall'estrazione o dalla terapia endocanalare del dente interessato.

TRATTAMENTO. L'età alla quale si verifica la carie è importante nel trattamento odontoiatrico. I soggetti di età inferiore ai 3 anni, non essendo ancora in grado di collaborare con il dentista, spesso richiedono immobilizzazione, sedazione o anestesia generale. Dopo i 4 anni, i bambini sono generalmente in grado di affrontare il trattamento odontoiatrico in anestesia locale.

Il trattamento odontoiatrico, che si basa sull'uso di amalgama d'argento, resine composite o corone in acciaio inossidabile, può restaurare la maggior parte dei denti affetti da carie. Se la carie interessa la polpa, può rendersi necessario il ricorso a una rimozione parziale (pulpotomia) o totale (pulpectomia) della polpa. In caso di estrazione di un dente, può essere indicato l'uso di un mantenitore di spazio per prevenire la migrazione dei denti, responsabile di una scorretta posizione dei denti permanenti successivi.

Il trattamento clinico del dolore e dell'infezione associati a carie dentaria non curata varia in base all'entità dell'interessamento e alle condizioni mediche generali. L'infezione dentaria circoscritta all'unità dentoalveolare può essere trattata con misure locali (estrazione, pulpectomia). Gli antibiotici orali sono indicati per le infezioni dentarie associate a cellulite, edema facciale o difficoltà di anestetizzare il dente in presenza di infiammazione. La penicillina è l'antibiotico di scelta, tranne che nei soggetti con anamnesi di allergia a tale farmaco; clindamicina ed eritromicina sono le possibili alternative. Gli analgesici orali, come l'ibuprofene, sono di norma efficaci per il controllo del dolore. Se l'infezione interessa un'area vitale (cioè lo spazio sottomandibolare, che può causare l'angina di Ludwig, il triangolo facciale, che può condurre a trombosi del seno cavernoso, o lo spazio periorbitario, che può portare, anche se raramente, a interessamento della regione orbitaria), è opportuno somministrare gli antibiotici per via parenterale.

PREVENZIONE.

Fluoro. La misura preventiva più efficace contro la carie dentaria consiste nell'ottimizzare il contenuto di fluoro della rete idrica comunale portandolo a 1 ppm. I bambini che risiedono in aree con acque potabili non fluorurate e che sono a rischio di carie trarranno beneficio da una dieta arricchita con integratori a base di fluoro (Tab. 309-1). Di norma è possibile conoscere il livello di fluoro contenuto nell'acqua potabile telefonando all'apposito ente. È molto importante conoscere tale livello prima di prescrivere integratori fluorati. Per evitare una potenziale overdose non si devono prescrivere più di 120 mg di fluoro in totale. Una significativa overdose acuta di fluoro (>5 mg/kg) necessita di immediata attenzione medica. L'uso di agenti topici fluorati, applicati in ambulatorio o a casa, è benefico per i bambini a rischio di carie.

Igiene orale. Per prevenire la carie può essere utile spazzolare i denti ogni giorno, specie con un dentifricio con fluoro. Siccome la maggior parte dei bambini di età inferiore agli 8 anni non ha la coordinazione richiesta per eseguire adeguatamente questa operazione, dovrebbero essere i genitori a farsene carico. Per i bambini piccoli, che non sono in grado di espettorare, è bene applicare sullo spazzolino una quantità piccolissima di dentifricio fluorurato, della grandezza di un pisello o anche meno.

Dieta. Ridurre la frequenza di assunzione di zucchero previene la carie dentaria. Pertanto, l'uso prolungato e frequente di biberon contenenti bevande edulcorate va scoraggiato e i bambini a rischio di carie dovrebbero consumare meno merendine contenenti zucchero. Il frequente consumo di succo di frutta dal biberon o dalla tazzina ha un alto potenziale cariogeno, che però spesso non viene riconosciuto. È quindi importante spiegare ai genitori che il loro bambino dovrebbe consumare i succhi di frutta solo durante i pasti e per una quantità complessiva non superiore a circa 180 mL/die.

Sigillante dentale. I sigillanti dentali (*sealant*) si sono rivelati efficaci nella prevenzione della carie se applicati sui pozzetti e nelle fessure dei molari decidui e permanenti. L'efficacia massima si ottiene applicando i sigillanti subito dopo l'eruzione dei denti (di norma entro 1-2 anni) e facendone uso in soggetti che presentano solchi e fessure nei molari.

TABELLA 309-1. Programma di dosaggio degli integratori fluorati

	FLUORO NELL'ACQUA POTABILE DI USO DOMESTICO (PPM)		
ETÀ	< 0,3	0,3-0,6	> 0,6
6 mesi-3 anni	0,25*	0	0
3-6 anni	0,50	0,25	0
6-16 anni	1,00	0,50	0

*Milligrammi di fluoro/die.

Capitolo 310 ■ Malattie parodontali

Il parodonto comprende la gengiva, l'osso alveolare, il cemento e il legamento parodontale (vedi Fig. 309-2).

GENGIVITE. La scarsa igiene orale comporta l'accumulo di placca dentaria all'interfaccia dente-gengiva; la placca a sua volta scatena una risposta infiammatoria, che si manifesta sotto forma di arrossamento e gonfiore della gengiva, localizzato o diffuso. Oltre la metà dei bambini statunitensi in età scolare ha sofferto di gengivite nel corso della sua vita. Nei casi gravi, si osservano sanguinamento spontaneo della gengiva e alitosi. Il trattamento consiste in una corretta igiene orale (accurato spazzolamento dei denti e uso del filo interdentale), sufficiente per determinare una completa guarigione. Le fluttuazioni dei livelli ormonali che si verificano all'inizio della pubertà possono aumentare la risposta infiammatoria alla placca. Nei bambini sani è improbabile che la gengivite evolva in parodontite (infiammazione del legamento parodontale che porta a perdita dell'osso alveolare).

PARODONTITE AGGRESSIVA NEI BAMBINI (PARODONTITE PREPUBERALE). La parodontite nei bambini in età prepubere è una malattia rara, che inizia spesso durante il periodo di eruzione dei denti decidui e all'età di 4-5 anni. La malattia si presenta in forma localizzata o generalizzata. Si osserva una rapida perdita ossea, che spesso porta alla perdita prematura dei denti decidui. Spesso è associata a patologie sistemiche, tra cui neutropenia, difetti dell'aderenza o della migrazione leucocitaria, ipofosfatasia, sindrome di Papillon-Lefèvre, leucemia e istiocitosi X. In molti casi, tuttavia, non si ha evidenza alcuna di un sottostante problema medico. Nondimeno, sono necessarie indagini diagnostiche per escludere un'eventuale sottostante malattia sistemica.

Il trattamento comprende un'aggressiva pulizia dentaria professionale, l'estrazione strategica dei denti affetti e la terapia antibiotica. Si dispone di pochi studi che documentino il successo del trattamento a lungo termine nella regressione della perdita ossea dei denti decidui circostanti.

PARODONTITE AGGRESSIVA NEGLI ADOLESCENTI (PARODONTITE GIOVANILE LOCALIZZATA). La parodontite aggressiva negli adolescenti è caratterizzata da un rapido riassorbimento dell'osso alveolare, in particolare attorno agli incisivi e ai primi molari permanenti. La prevalenza complessiva negli USA è >1%, ma la prevalenza tra gli afroamericani è del 2,50%. Questa forma di parodontite è associata al ceppo batterico *Actinobacillus*. Inoltre, nei soggetti con parodontite aggressiva i neutrofili possono avere difetti chemiotattici o fagocitici. Se non è curata, i denti affetti perderanno il proprio apparato d'attacco e potranno cadere. Il trattamento varia a seconda del grado di interessamento. I pazienti diagnosticati all'insorgenza della malattia sono di norma trattati con curettage chirurgico o non chirurgico in associazione a terapia antibiotica. La prognosi dipende del grado di interessamento iniziale e dalla compliance con la terapia.

ERUZIONE DENTARIA. La dentizione può essere accompagnata da un intermittente fastidio localizzato nell'area interessata dall'eruzione dei denti decidui, irritabilità, febbricola e salivazione eccessiva; comunque, molti bambini non hanno fastidi evidenti. *Il trattamento dei sintomi comprende analgesici orali e anelli di gomma raffreddati per alleviare il fastidio.* Manifestazioni analoghe possono verificarsi anche in concomitanza con l'eruzione dei primi molari permanenti, intorno ai 6 anni di età.

IPERTROFIA GENGIVALE INDOTTA DA CICLOSPORINA O FENITOINA. L'uso della ciclosporina per sopprimere le reazioni di rigetto d'organo o della fenitoina nella terapia anticonvulsivante e, in alcuni casi, dei calcioantagonisti è associato a ipertrofia generalizzata della gengiva. La fenitoina e i suoi metaboliti hanno una diretta azione stimolatoria sui fibroblasti gengivali, comportando un'accelerazione della sintesi del collagene. Questo farmaco provoca minore iperplasia gengivale nei soggetti che seguono una meticolosa igiene orale.

L'ipertrofia gengivale si presenta nel 10-30% dei pazienti trattati con fenitoina. Le manifestazioni gravi possono comprendere: (1) vistosa ipertrofia della gengiva, che talvolta arriva a coprire i denti; (2) edema ed eritema della gengiva; (3) infezione secondaria, che porta a formazione ascessuale; (4) migrazione dei denti; (5) inibizione dell'esfoliazione dei denti decidui e successiva inclusione dei denti permanenti. Il trattamento consiste nella prevenzione e, se possibile, nella sospensione della ciclosporina o della fenitoina. I pazienti in trattamento a lungo termine con questi farmaci dovrebbero essere sottoposti a frequenti esami dentali e accurata igiene orale. Le forme gravi di iperplasia gengivale sono trattate con la gengivectomia, ma la lesione recidiva se si continua l'uso di farmaci.

PERICORONITE ACUTA. L'infiammazione acuta del lembo di gengiva che ricopre parzialmente la corona di un dente con eruzione incompleta è frequente nei molari permanenti inferiori. L'accumulo di detriti alimentari e batteri tra il lembo gengivale e il dente accelera la risposta infiammatoria. Una variante di questa condizione è l'ascesso gengivale dovuto all'intrappolamento dei batteri per l'uso di bande ortodontiche o corone artificiali. Trisma e dolore severo possono essere associati a infiammazione. I casi non curati possono esitare in infezioni della regione facciale e cellulite facciale.

Il trattamento comprende la pulizia locale e l'irrigazione dell'area interessata, risciacqui con soluzione salina tiepida e una terapia antibiotica. Con la regressione della fase acuta, l'estrazione del dente o la resezione del lembo gengivale prevengono la recidiva. L'individuazione precoce dell'inclusione parziale dei terzi molari inferiori e la loro successiva estrazione impediscono lo sviluppo di pericoronite in queste aree.

MALATTIA PARODONTALE NECROTIZZANTE (GENGIVITE ULCERONECROTICA ACUTA). La malattia parodontale necrotizzante, in passato denominata anche "bocca da trincea", è una particolare parodontopatia, associata a spirochete orali e fusobatteri. Non è chiaro, tuttavia, se i batteri provochino la malattia o siano secondari a essa. Si sviluppa raramente nei bambini sani dei Paesi sviluppati, con una prevalenza negli USA <1%, ma si osserva più spesso in bambini e adolescenti provenienti da aree in via di sviluppo dell'Africa, dell'Asia e del Sudamerica. In alcuni Paesi africani, dove i bambini affetti in genere soffrono di malnutrizione proteica, la lesione può estendersi nei tessuti adiacenti, causando necrosi delle strutture facciali (*cancrum oris* o noma).

Le manifestazioni cliniche della malattia parodontale necrotizzante comprendono: (1) necrosi e ulcerazione della gengiva interdentale, (2) una pseudomembrana grigiastra aderente sulla gengiva affetta, (3) alitosi, (4) linfoadenopatia cervicale, (5) malessere e (6) febbre. La condizione può essere scambiata per gengivostomatite erpetica acuta. La microscopia in campo scuro dei frustoli prelevati dalle lesioni necrotizzanti rivelerà la presenza di dense colonie di spirochete.

La terapia della malattia parodontale necrotizzante consiste nel trattamento acuto con pulizia locale, agenti ossigenanti (applicazione diretta di perossido di urea al 10% in glicerolo anidro quattro volte al giorno) e nella somministrazione di analgesici. In genere si osserva una regressione notevole entro 48 ore. Se il paziente è febbrile, può essere indicato potenziare la terapia con antibiotici (penicillina o metronidazolo). Una seconda fase del trattamento può rendersi necessaria se la fase acuta della malattia ha causato un danno morfologico irreversibile al parodonto. Si tratta di una forma non contagiosa.

Capitolo 311 ■ Trauma dentario

Le lesioni traumatiche del cavo orale possono essere suddivise in tre gruppi: (1) lesioni ai denti, (2) lesioni ai tessuti molli (ecchimosi, abrasioni, lacerazioni, punture, avulsioni e ustioni) e (3) lesioni ai mascellari (fratture del mascellare inferiore o superiore o di entrambi).

TRAUMI DEI DENTI. Circa il 10% dei soggetti di età compresa tra i 18 mesi e i 18 anni di età subisce un trauma dentario importante. Le fasce di età in cui questo evento si manifesta con maggiore frequenza sembrano essere tre: (1) bambini piccoli (1-3 anni), di norma a causa di cadute o maltrattamenti subiti; (2) soggetti in età scolare (7-10 anni), di solito per cadute dalla bicicletta o incidenti di gioco durante la ricreazione; (3) adolescenti (16-18 anni), spesso in conseguenza di colluttazioni, scontri atletici e incidenti automobilistici. Le lesioni a carico dei denti sono più frequenti nei bambini con denti anteriori protrusi. Anche i bambini con anomalie craniofacciali o deficit neuromuscolari sono a rischio di traumi dentari, che possono interessare i tessuti dentari duri, la polpa (nervo) e le strutture parodontali (attorno all'osso e all'apparato d'attacco) (Fig. 311-1 e Tab. 311-1).

Le fratture dei denti possono essere non complicate (confinate ai tessuti dentari duri) o complicate (quando interessano la polpa). L'esposizione della polpa, con conseguente contaminazione batterica, che può condurre a infezione e necrosi pulpare, complica la terapia e può ridurre le probabilità di un esito favorevole.

I denti più esposti ai traumi sono gli incisivi superiori. Il trattamento delle fratture coronali non complicate consiste nel coprire la dentina esposta e nell'applicare un restauro estetico. Le fratture coronali complicate di norma richiedono la *terapia endodontica* (terapia del canale radicolare). Le fratture coronoradicolari e quelle radicolari di solito richiedono un'estesa terapia odontoiatrica. Tali lesioni a carico dei denti decidui possono interferire con il normale sviluppo della dentizione permanente; pertanto gli incisivi decidui che hanno subito un trauma di notevole entità sono di norma trattati con l'estrazione.

Le lesioni traumatiche orali vanno segnalate quanto prima al dentista, che dovrebbe esaminare subito il paziente anche qualora i denti apparissero integri. I reperti di base (radiografie, modelli di mobilità, risposte a stimoli specifici) gli consentono di valutare la probabilità che insorgano complicanze in futuro.

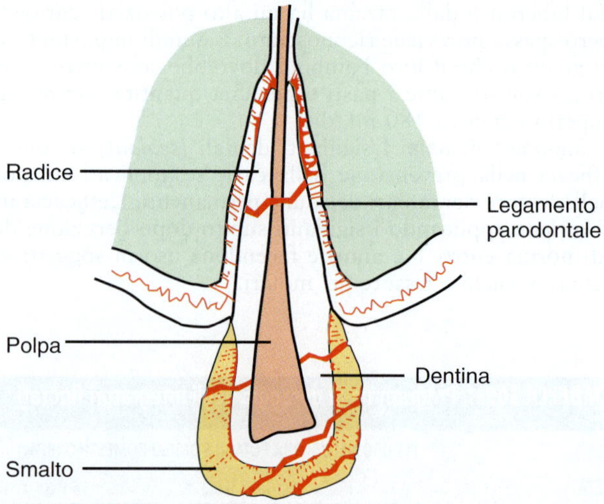

Figura 311-1. Le fratture dentarie possono coinvolgere lo smalto, la dentina o la polpa e verificarsi nella corona o nella radice di un dente. (Da Pinkham JR: Pediatric Dentistry: *Infancy Through Adolescence.* Philadelphia, WB Saunders, 1988, p 172.)

TABELLA 311-1. Lesioni a carico della corona del dente

TIPO DI TRAUMA	DESCRIZIONE	TRATTAMENTO E VISITA
Infrazione dello smalto (screpolatura)	Frattura incompleta dello smalto senza perdita di struttura dentaria.	All'inizio può non richiedere la terapia, ma dovrebbe essere valutata periodicamente dal dentista.
Fratture dello smalto	Frattura del solo smalto dentario.	Il dente può essere sottoposto a levigatura o trattato al fine di sostituire il frammento perso.
Frattura dello smalto e della dentina	Frattura dello smalto e dello strato dentinale del dente, che può essere sensibile al freddo o all'aria. La polpa può necrotizzare e portare ad ascesso periapicale.	Inviare il paziente dal dentista il prima possibile. È opportuno trattare l'area al fine di mantenere l'integrità della polpa sottostante.
Frattura dello smalto e della dentina con interessamento pulpare	La contaminazione batterica può condurre a necrosi pulpare e ascesso periapicale. Il dente può presentare sanguinamento o una piccola macchia rossa.	Inviare immediatamente il paziente dal dentista. La terapia dentale elettiva dipende dall'entità della lesione, dalle condizioni della polpa, dallo sviluppo del dente, dal tempo trascorso dalla lesione e da eventuali altre lesioni a carico delle strutture di sostegno. La terapia è diretta a ridurre al minimo la contaminazione nel tentativo di migliorare la prognosi.

Da Josell SD, Abrams RG: Managing common dental problems and emergencies. *Pediatr Clin North Am* 1991;38:1325-1342.

LESIONI ALLE STRUTTURE PARODONTALI. Il trauma dentario con associata lesione alle strutture parodontali di sostegno è in genere caratterizzato da elementi dentari mobili o spostati. Tali lesioni sono più frequenti nella dentizione decidua che in quella permanente. I tipi di trauma al parodonto comprendono: (1) concussione, (2) sublussazione, (3) lussazione intrusiva, (4) lussazione estrusiva e (5) avulsione.

Concussione. Le lesioni che provocano minor danno al legamento parodontale sono denominate concussioni. I denti interessati non sono mobili o spostati, ma reagiscono chiaramente alla percussione (applicazione delicata di colpi sul dente con uno strumento). Questo tipo di lesione di norma non richiede alcuna terapia e si risolve senza complicanze. A seguito di concussione, gli incisivi decidui possono cambiare colore, indicando così una degenerazione pulpare, e dovrebbero pertanto essere sottoposti all'attenzione del dentista.

Sublussazione. I denti sublussati presentano mobilità orizzontale da lieve a media, mobilità verticale o entrambe. Di solito si osserva emorragia lungo il colletto del dente, al margine gengivale, mentre non si registra alcuno spostamento del dente. Molti denti sublussati richiedono l'immobilizzazione con un tutore per garantire un'adeguata riparazione del legamento parodontale; alcuni di essi sviluppano necrosi pulpare.

Intrusione. I denti intrusi si affossano nel loro alveolo, a volte al punto da risultare clinicamente invisibili. Gli incisivi decidui possono dare la falsa impressione di essere avulsi; per accertarsi che si tratti di vera avulsione si consiglia di eseguire una radiografia (Figg. 311-2 e 311-3).

Estrusione. Questo tipo di lesione è caratterizzato dallo spostamento del dente dal proprio alveolo verso l'esterno, di solito in direzione linguale, con frattura della parete dell'alveolo osseo. Questi casi necessitano di un trattamento immediato; più si tarda a intervenire, maggiori saranno le probabilità che il dente rimanga fissato nella posizione ectopica. La terapia mira alla riduzione dell'estrusione (riposizionamento) e alla fissazione del dente (*splinting*). Inoltre, poiché va spesso incontro a necrosi, la polpa di tali denti richiede la terapia endodontica. La lussazione estrusiva nella dentizione decidua di solito viene trattata con l'estrazione in quanto le complicanze delle procedure di riduzione e fissazione possono comportare problemi per lo sviluppo della dentizione permanente.

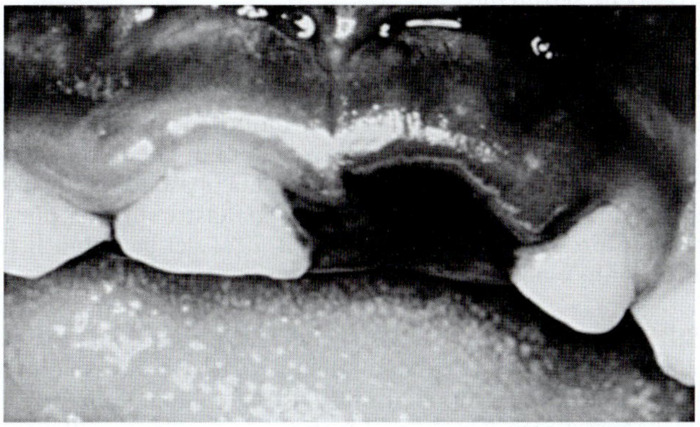

Figura 311-2. Incisivo deciduo intruso che si presenta come avulso.

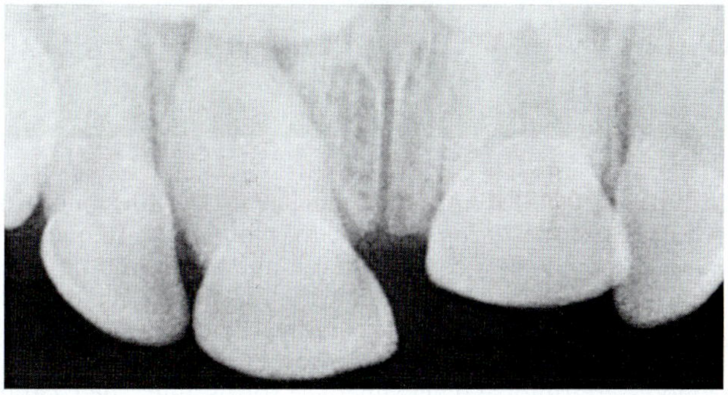

Figura 311-3. La radiografia occlusale documenta l'intrusione del "dente mancante" presentato nella Figura 311-2.

Avulsione. Se i denti permanenti avulsi vengono reimpiantati nel giro di 20 minuti dopo la lesione, è possibile ottenere un buon risultato; al contrario, se il ritardo supera le 2 ore, gli insuccessi (riassorbimento radicolare, anchilosi) sono frequenti. La probabilità che al reimpianto del dente segua il suo normale riattacco dipende dalla vitalità del legamento parodontale. I genitori che si trovano ad affrontare questa situazione d'emergenza devono essere istruiti a:

1. **Trovare il dente.**
2. **Risciacquarlo senza strofinare, stando ben attenti a non toccare la radice. Dopo aver tappato lo scarico del lavandino, tenere il dente per la corona e risciacquarlo sotto l'acqua corrente.**
3. **Inserire il dente nel suo alveolo. (Rimetterlo delicatamente nella sua posizione normale. Non preoccuparsi se estrude leggermente. Se questa manovra suscita eccessiva apprensione nel genitore o nel bambino, è meglio immergere il dente nel latte di mucca freddo o in altra soluzione isotonica fredda.)**
4. **Rivolgersi subito al dentista. (Durante il viaggio, il bambino dovrebbe tenere il dente nell'alveolo con un dito. Il genitore dovrebbe assicurare il bambino nel suo seggiolino con la cintura di sicurezza e guidare con prudenza.)**

È necessario immobilizzare il dente reimpiantato per facilitarne il riattacco; la terapia endodontica è sempre richiesta. I segni iniziali di complicanze associate al reimpianto possono presentarsi subito (una settimana dopo il trauma) o più tardi (anche a diversi anni di distanza). È indicato un attento follow-up dentale per almeno un anno.

PREVENZIONE. Per ridurre al minimo la probabilità di lesioni dentarie è opportuno attenersi alle seguenti regole:

1. **Ogni bambino o adolescente che pratichi sport di contatto dovrebbe indossare un paradenti, costruito dal dentista o acquistato in un negozio di articoli sportivi.**
2. **I bambini o gli adolescenti con problemi neuromuscolari o disturbi convulsivi dovrebbero indossare caschi con protezioni per il viso per salvaguardare la testa e il viso in caso di cadute.**
3. **È necessario indossare tali caschi anche quando si va in bici, si pattina o si fa skateboarding.**
4. **Tutti i bambini o gli adolescenti con incisivi protrusi dovrebbero essere valutati da un ortodontista o un dentista pediatrico.**

ULTERIORI CONSIDERAZIONI. I bambini con trauma dentario potrebbero aver subito anche un trauma cranico o cervicale e, pertanto, vanno sottoposti a una valutazione neurologica. È opportuno prendere in considerazione la profilassi antitetanica in qualsiasi caso di lesione che abbia compromesso l'integrità dei tessuti orali. Bisogna inoltre tenere presente la possibilità che il bambino sia stato vittima di maltrattamenti.

Capitolo 312 ■ Lesioni comuni dei tessuti molli orali

CANDIDOSI OROFARINGEA (vedi Capitolo 231.1). L'infezione orofaringea da *Candida albicans* (mughetto, moniliasi) è frequente nei neonati, che vengono a contatto con il microrganismo nel canale della nascita o durante l'allattamento. Le lesioni da candidosi orofaringea (COF) si presentano come macchie bianche che coprono totalmente o in parte la mucosa orofaringea. Queste placche possono essere rimosse dalla superficie sottostante, che è caratterizzata da infiammazione con emorragie petecchiali. La conferma della diagnosi si ottiene mediante l'esame microscopico diretto su striscio al potassio idrossido e la messa a coltura di frammenti prelevati per raschiamento da tali lesioni. Anche se nel neonato sano la COF segue di norma un decorso indipendente da influenze esterne, il trattamento con nistatina accelererà la guarigione e ridurrà il rischio di diffondere l'infezione ad altri bambini. Le infezioni persistenti dovrebbero essere trattate con fluconazolo.

La COF inoltre rappresenta un problema rilevante durante la terapia mielosoppressiva. La **candidosi sistemica** (CS), una causa maggiore di morbilità e mortalità durante la terapia mielosoppressiva, si sviluppa quasi esclusivamente in soggetti che hanno avuto in precedenza candidosi orofaringea, esofagea o intestinale. Questa osservazione implica che la prevenzione della COF dovrebbe ridurre l'incidenza di CS. L'uso di un regime multiplo, basato sull'impiego di una soluzione al 0,2% di clorexidina e fluconazolo, per la profilassi della COF nei bambini sottoposti a trapianto di midollo osseo può essere efficace nella prevenzione di COF, CS o esofagite da candida.

ULCERE AFTOSE. L'ulcera aftosa è un tipo particolare di lesione orale, tendente alla recidiva. La diagnosi differenziale è illustrata nella Tabella 312-1. Come riportato, le ulcere aftose si sviluppano nel 20% della popolazione. La loro eziologia non è chiara, ma sono state implicate cause infettive, come l'*Helicobacter pylori*, il virus dell'herpes simplex e anche il morbillo. Clinicamente queste ulcere sono caratterizzate da lesioni ulcerose ben circoscritte con una base necrotica bianca circondata da un alone rosso. Le lesioni durano 10-14 giorni e guariscono senza cicatrizzazione. I farmaci costosi acquistabili dietro presentazione di ricetta medica sembrano offrire scarsi vantaggi rispetto ai farmaci palliativi da banco disponibili.

TABELLA 312-1. Diagnosi differenziale dell'ulcerazione orale

CONDIZIONE	COMMENTO
COMUNE	
Ulcera aftosa	Lesioni dolorose circoscritte
Trauma	Incidenti, abitudine cronica di mordersi la guancia o anestesia dentale locale
Sindrome mani, piedi, bocca	Dolore, lesioni su lingua, regione anteriore del cavo orale, mani e piedi
Angina erpetica	Dolore, lesioni limitate al palato molle e all'orofaringe
Gengivostomatite erpetica	Vescicole lungo i bordi mucocutanei; dolore, febbre
Herpes labiale recidivante	Vescicole sulle labbra; dolore
Ustioni chimiche	Alcali, acidi, acido acetilsalicilico; dolore
Ustioni da calore	Cibo bollente, elettricità
NON COMUNE	
Deficit dei neutrofili	Agranulocitosi, leucemia, neutropenia ciclica; dolore
Lupus eritematoso sistemico	Recidivante, può essere asintomatico
Sindrome di Behçet	Assomiglia alle lesioni aftose; associata a ulcere genitali, uveite
Gengivostomatite ulcerosa necrotizzante	Stomatite di Vincent; dolore
Sifilide	Ulcere veneree o gomme; indolore
Morbo di Crohn del cavo orale	Simile all'afta; dolore
Istoplasmosi	Linguale
Sindromi con febbre ricorrente	Vedi Capitolo 162

GENGIVOSTOMATITE ERPETICA (vedi Capitolo 249). Dopo un periodo di incubazione di circa una settimana, l'infezione da virus dell'herpes simplex si manifesta con febbre e malessere generale. Il cavo orale può presentare diversi aspetti, tra cui eritema gengivale e grappoli di piccole vescicole in eruzione in tutta la bocca. Di norma, i sintomi scompaiono nel giro di 2 settimane senza lasciare cicatrici. È opportuno raccomandare un'abbondante assunzione di liquidi perché il bambino può andare incontro a disidratazione. Analgesici e risciacqui anestetici possono alleviare il disagio del paziente. L'aciclovir per via orale è utile per abbreviare la durata dei sintomi. È importante evitare l'autoinoculazione o la trasmissione dell'infezione agli occhi.

HERPES LABIALE RICORRENTE. Circa il 90% della popolazione sviluppa anticorpi contro il virus dell'herpes simplex. In periodi di quiescenza, si suppone che tale virus rimanga latente nei neuroni sensitivi. A differenza della gengivostomatite erpetica primaria, che si manifesta con vescicole multiple dolorose su labbra, lingua, palato, gengiva e mucosa, l'herpes recidivante è generalmente limitato alle labbra. Si tratta di un'affezione fastidiosa, in quanto causa dolore e un aspetto poco attraente, ma che in genere non dà sintomi sistemici. Si ritiene che la riattivazione del virus sia una conseguenza dell'esposizione ai raggi ultravioletti, di un trauma tissutale, dello stress o di un rialzo febbrile. In un soggetto affetto da herpes recidivante ma per altri aspetti sano la terapia antivirale risulta di scarso vantaggio rispetto alle cure palliative.

NODULI DI BOHN. Si tratta di piccole anomalie dello sviluppo situate lungo i versanti vestibolari e linguali delle creste mandibolare e mascellare e nel palato duro del neonato. Queste lesioni derivano dai residui di tessuto ghiandolare mucoso. Non richiedono il trattamento, in quanto scompaiono dopo poche settimane.

CISTI DELLA LAMINA DENTARIA. Sono piccole lesioni cistiche osservabili nel neonato, situate lungo la sommità delle creste mandibolare e mascellare, derivanti dai residui epiteliali della lamina dentaria. Il trattamento non è necessario in quanto scompaiono entro poche settimane.

GRANULI DI FORDYCE. Quasi l'80% degli adulti presenta multipli granuli bianco-giallastri riuniti in grappoli o in aree simili a placche, situati sulla mucosa orale, molto spesso sulla mucosa vestibolare o sulle labbra. Si tratta in realtà di ghiandole sebacee aberranti che sono presenti alla nascita, ma possono ipertrofizzarsi e presentarsi sotto forma di papule giallastre distinte durante il periodo preadolescenziale in circa il 50% dei bambini. Il trattamento non è necessario.

PARULIDE. La parulide, o ascesso gengivale, è una papula rossastra molle adiacente alla radice di un dente affetto da ascesso cronico. Insorge nel punto terminale di una fistola dentale drenante. Una volta diagnosticato l'ascesso, il trattamento consiste nell'estrarre il dente colpito oppure nel sottoporlo a terapia endocanalare.

CHEILITE. Questa secchezza delle labbra, seguita da desquamazione e screpolature e accompagnata da una caratteristica sensazione di bruciore, è comune nei bambini. Causata in genere da ipersensibilità al contatto con determinate sostanze (dai giocattoli agli alimenti) e all'azione della luce solare, è aggravata dall'abitudine di umettarsi le labbra con la lingua e dall'azione disseccante del vento, soprattutto nella stagione fredda. La cheilite si presenta spesso in associazione con la febbre. La frequente applicazione di vaselina, oltre ad accelerare la guarigione, ha funzione preventiva.

ANCHILOGLOSSIA. Causa dell'anchiloglossia, o "lingua legata", è un frenulo linguale anormalmente corto che può ostacolare il movimento della lingua, ma raramente interferisce con l'allattamento o l'articolazione dei suoni. Il frenulo può allungarsi spontaneamente con la crescita del bambino. Un'anchiloglossia grave può influire negativamente sulla fonazione e richiedere l'intervento chirurgico correttivo.

LINGUA A CARTA GEOGRAFICA. Detta anche glossite migrante, è una lesione benigna e asintomatica, caratterizzata da una o più chiazze lisce di colore rosso fuoco, che spesso presentano un margine membranoso giallo, grigio o bianco sul dorso di una lingua ruvida, ma per altri aspetti normale. Di eziologia ignota, non richiede alcun trattamento (vedi Capitolo 663).

LINGUA FISSURATA. Detta anche lingua scrotale, è una malformazione che si manifesta clinicamente con la comparsa di numerosi piccoli solchi o scanalature sulla superficie dorsale (vedi Capitolo 663). Se la lingua è dolente, è possibile ridurre la proliferazione batterica nelle fessure spazzolandola o irrigandola con acqua.

Capitolo 313 ■ Malattie delle ghiandole salivari e dei mascellari

Con l'eccezione della parotite epidemica acuta (vedi Capitolo 245), le malattie delle ghiandole salivari sono rare nei bambini. La tumefazione bilaterale delle ghiandole sottomascellari può insorgere in presenza di AIDS, fibrosi cistica, infezione da virus di Epstein-Barr e malnutrizione e, in modo transitorio, durante gli attacchi acuti di asma. Il vomito cronico può essere accompagnato da un ingrossamento delle parotidi. L'ipertrofia benigna delle ghiandole salivari è stata associata a endocrinopatie: malattia tiroidea, diabete e disturbi dell'asse ipofisosurrenalico.

PAROTITE RICORRENTE. In bambini altrimenti sani è possibile l'insorgenza di edema idiopatico delle parotidi recidivante. La tumefazione è in genere unilaterale, ma entrambe le ghiandole possono essere coinvolte, contemporaneamente o in successione. Il dolore è di lieve entità; la tumefazione è limitata alla ghiandola e di solito dura 2-3 settimane. L'incidenza sembra essere più alta in primavera.

PAROTITE SUPPURATIVA. Questa condizione, di norma dovuta a *Staphylococcus aureus*, può essere primaria o insorgere come complicanza di una parotite di eziologia diversa. Solitamente unilaterale, può essere accompagnata da febbre. La ghiandola è tumefatta, sensibile e dolente. La parotide suppurativa risponde a un'adeguata terapia antibatterica basata sulla coltura di materiale prelevato dal dotto di Stenone o al drenaggio chirurgico, che tuttavia di rado è necessario.

RANULA. Si tratta di una cisti associata a una ghiandola salivare maggiore sita nella zona sublinguale. Si manifesta con una tumefazione estesa, di consistenza molle e contenente muco, osservabile nel pavimento della bocca. Si verifica a qualsiasi età, compresa l'infanzia. In questi casi è opportuno asportare la cisti ed esteriorizzare il dotto reciso.

MUCOCELE. È una lesione della ghiandola salivare provocata dall'ostruzione del dotto di una ghiandola salivare. Molto comune sul labbro inferiore, ha l'aspetto di una vescicola piena di liquido o di un nodulo fluttuante ricoperto da una mucosa di colore normale. Il trattamento consiste nell'asportazione chirurgica, con la rimozione della ghiandola salivare accessoria interessata.

FOSSETTE LABIALI CONGENITE. Sono depressioni causate da fistole che conducono alle ghiandole mucose incluse nel labbro inferiore. Secernono saliva, in particolare a seguito di stimolazione salivare. Possono presentarsi come anomalie isolate o essere osservabili in pazienti con schisi labiale o palatale. Il trattamento è l'asportazione chirurgica del tessuto ghiandolare.

CISTI ERUTTIVA. È una tumefazione molliccia e indolore che compare sopra il dente in eruzione. In caso di sanguinamento nell'area cistica, può assumere un colore blu o nero bluastro. Nella maggior parte dei casi non è indicato alcun trattamento e la cisti si risolve con la completa eruzione del dente.

XEROSTOMIA. Nota anche come "secchezza della bocca", può essere associata a febbre, disidratazione, farmaci anticolinergici, GVHD (*Graft Versus Host Disease*), malattia di Mikulicz (infiltrati leucemici), sindrome di Sjögren o dosi tumoricide di radiazioni quando le ghiandole salivari si trovano nel campo di irradiazione. La xerostomia a lungo termine è un elevato fattore di rischio per la carie dentaria.

NEOPLASIE DELLE GHIANDOLE SALIVARI. Vedi Capitolo 500.

ISTIOCITOSI X (vedi Capitolo 507). L'eziologia e la patogenesi dell'istiocitosi restano oscure. Nella forma grave si osservano lesioni orali caratterizzate da dolore, edema, necrosi gengivale e distruzione dell'osso alveolare, con conseguente esfoliazione prematura dei denti. Il trattamento varia in base all'entità della patologia; in caso di malattia focale si ricorre al curettage chirurgico o alla terapia radiante. Per il trattamento della forma disseminata in vari organi possono rendersi necessari la chemioterapia con agenti multipli e il trapianto di midollo osseo.

TUMORI DEI MASCELLARI. Il **fibroma ossificante**, un comune tumore benigno dei mascellari, è spesso asintomatico e viene individuato con esami radiografici di routine. Il trattamento consiste nell'enucleazione o nel curettage. Il **granuloma gigantocellulare centrale** è un'altra lesione comune, considerata reattiva più che neoplastica. Sebbene generalmente asintomatica, questa condizione può espandersi, con o senza divergenza dei denti. Il trattamento consiste nel curettage completo o nell'escissione chirurgica. Le **cisti dentigere** sono lesioni comuni a carico della corona di un dente incluso o non erotto. Sebbene generalmente asintomatiche, possono ingrandirsi e diventare distruttive. Il trattamento è la rimozione chirurgica.

I tumori maligni primari dei mascellari nei bambini comprendono linfoma di Burkitt, sarcoma osteogenico, linfosarcoma, ameloblastoma e, più raramente, fibrosarcoma.

Capitolo 314 ■ Radiologia diagnostica nella valutazione dentale

La **radiografia panoramica** fornisce un'unica immagine tomografica dei mascellari superiore e inferiore, comprendente tutti i denti e le strutture di sostegno. Il tubo a raggi X ruota attorno alla testa del paziente con un movimento reciproco della lastra durante l'esposizione. Le immagini panoramiche, grazie alle quali è possibile visualizzare corpi, rami e condili mandibolari, i seni mascellari e molti contrafforti facciali, sono utilizzate per evidenziare anomalie del numero dei denti, del pattern di eruzione e sviluppo e lesioni cistiche o neoplastiche, infezioni ossee e fratture, oltre alle carie e alla malattia parodontale (Fig. 314-1).

Le **radiografie cefalometriche** sono immagini radiografiche posteroanteriori e laterali del cranio, ottenute utilizzando un **cefalostato** (posizionatore della testa) e tecniche in grado di visualizzare chiaramente lo scheletro e i tessuti molli della faccia. In ambito pediatrico si utilizzano protocolli analoghi in tutto il mondo. Basandosi su queste immagini, è possibile individuare i punti e i piani craniofacciali e confrontarli con gli standard ottenuti da migliaia di lastre radiografiche. La crescita facciale di un bambino può essere valutata serialmente grazie alle radiografie cefalometriche in sequenza. I rapporti tra i mascellari e tra base cranica e scheletro facciale possono essere determinati in maniera quantitativa. Inoltre, l'allineamento dei denti e il loro rapporto rispetto all'osso di sostegno sono misurabili serialmente.

Le radiografie dentali intraorali forniscono immagini dirette e molto dettagliate che mostrano le sezioni dei denti e delle strutture ossee di sostegno nel bambino. La lastra è posta lingualmente ai denti, mentre il fascio di raggi X è diretto attraverso i denti e le loro strutture di sostegno. Le immagini risultanti permettono non solo di rilevare la presenza di carie dentaria, perdita di osso alveolare (malattia parodontale), ascessi radicolari e traumi a carico di denti e osso alveolare, ma anche di analizzare il grado di sviluppo dei denti permanenti all'interno del tessuto osseo.

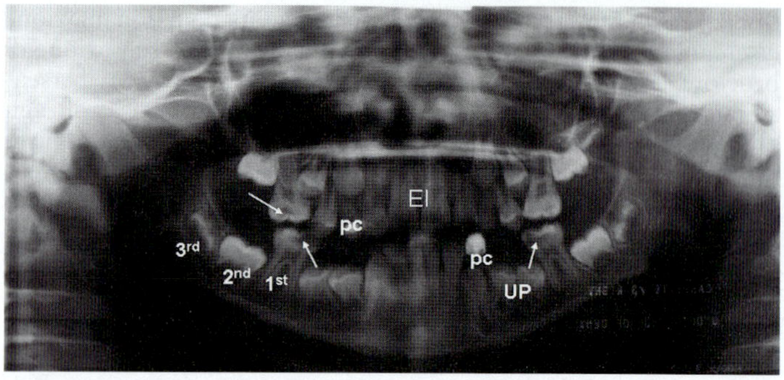

Figura 314-1. Radiografia panoramica di un bambino di 10 anni che mostra estesa carie dentaria dei primi molari permanenti (frecce), come pure strutture normali: primo molare permanente erotto, secondo molare permanente non erotto e terzo molare permanente non erotto; incisivi erotti (EI, *Erupted Incisors*), premolari non erotti (UP, *Unerupted Premolars*) e canini decidui erotti (pc, *primary canines*).

Andreasen JO, Andreasen FM: *Essentials of Traumatic Injuries to the Teeth*. Copenhagen, Munksgaard, 1990.

Bellinger DC, Trachtenberg F, Barregard L, et al: Neuropsychological and renal effects of dental amalgam in children. *JAMA* 2006;295:1775–1782.

Califano JV; American Academy of Periodontology Research, Science and Therapy Committee: Position paper: Periodontal diseases of children and adolescents. *J Periodontol* 2003;74:1696–1704.

Davidkin I, Jokinen S, Paananen A, et al: Etiology of mumps-like illnesses in children and adolescents vaccinated for measles, mumps, and rubella. *J Infect Dis* 2005;191:719–723.

Denny AD, Amm C: New techniques for airway correction in neonates with severe Pierre Robin sequence. *J Pediatr* 2005;147:97–101.

De Rouen TA, Martin MD, Leroux BG, et al: Neurobehavioral effects of dental amalgam in children. *JAMA* 2006;295:1784–1792.

Flaitz CM: Oral pathologic conditions and soft tissue anomalies. In Pinkham JR (editor): *Pediatric Dentistry: Infancy Through Adolescence*, 3rd ed. Philadelphia, WB Saunders, 1999, p 12.

Griffen AL (editor): Pediatric oral health. *Pediatr Clin North Am* 2000; 47.

Hale KJ; American Academy of Pediatrics Section on Pediatric Dentistry: Oral health risk assessment timing and establishment of the dental home. *Pediatrics* 2003;111:1113–1116.

Lin YTJ, Lu PW: Retrospective study of pediatric facial cellulitis of odontogenic origin. *Pediatr Infect Dis J* 2006;25:339–342.

Nelson LP, Shusterman S: Emergency management of oral trauma in children. *Curr Opin Pediatr* 1997;9:242–245.

Scully C: Aphthous ulceration. *N Engl J Med* 2006;355:165–172.

Selwitz RH, Ismail AI, Pitts NB: Dental caries. *Lancet* 2007;369:51–58.

Sonis A, Zaragoza S: Dental health for the pediatrician. *Curr Opin Pediatr* 2001;13:289–295.

Tinanoff N, Kanellis MJ, Vargas CM: Current understanding of epidemiology, mechanisms, and prevention of dental caries in preschool children. *Pediatr Dent* 2002;24:543–551.

Sezione 3 — Esofago

Capitolo 315 ■ Embriologia, anatomia e funzione dell'esofago

Susan Orenstein, John Peters, Seema Khan, Nader Youssef e Sunny Zaheed Hussain

L'esofago è un organo muscolare cavo, separato dalla faringe cranialmente e dallo stomaco caudalmente attraverso due sfinteri tonicamente chiusi. La sua funzione principale è di trasportare il materiale ingerito dalla bocca allo stomaco. In gran parte privo di ghiandole ed enzimi digestivi ed esposto soltanto brevemente alle sostanze nutritive, esso non svolge alcun ruolo attivo nella digestione.

EMBRIOLOGIA. L'esofago si sviluppa dall'intestino anteriore retrofaringeo e può essere distinto dallo stomaco nell'embrione di 4 settimane. Alla stessa epoca, la trachea inizia a gemmare appena anteriormente all'esofago in via di sviluppo; il solco laringotracheale che ne deriva si estende dando luogo ai polmoni. Alterazioni di questa fase possono portare ad anomalie congenite come la **fistola tracheoesofagea**. La lunghezza dell'esofago è di 8-10 cm alla nascita e raddoppia nelle prime 2-3 settimane di vita, raggiungendo i 25 cm circa nell'adulto. La sua porzione addominale è grande quanto lo stomaco nel feto di 8 settimane ma gradualmente si accorcia fino a misurare pochi millimetri alla nascita, raggiungendo una lunghezza finale di 3 cm circa dopo pochi anni di vita. Questa localizzazione intraddominale dell'esofago distale e dello sfintere esofageo inferiore (LES, *Lower Esophageal Sphincter*) è un importante meccanismo antireflusso, poiché gli aumenti della pressione intraddominale sono trasmessi anche allo sfintere, aumentando la sua azione protettiva. La deglutizione, osservabile in utero già a 16-20 settimane di gestazione, favorisce la circolazione del liquido amniotico; pertanto, il **polidramnios** è tipico dell'assenza di una deglutizione normale oppure di un'ostruzione dell'esofago o del tratto gastrointestinale superiore. Suzione e deglutizione raggiungono la completa coordinazione solo nella 34ª settimana di gestazione e ciò rappresenta un fattore che contribuisce alle difficoltà di alimentazione nei neonati prematuri.

ANATOMIA. Il lume dell'esofago è rivestito da epitelio squamoso stratificato non cheratinizzato, protettivo, spesso, che improvvisamente si trasforma in epitelio colonnare semplice a livello del margine superiore dello stomaco, in corrispondenza della **giunzione gastroesofagea** (**GEJ**, *GastroEsophageal Junction*). Tale epitelio squamoso è relativamente resistente al danneggiamento da parte delle secrezioni gastriche (a differenza dell'epitelio colonnare ciliato del tratto respiratorio), ma l'irritazione cronica da parte del contenuto gastrico può provocare alterazioni morfometriche e conseguente metaplasia delle cellule da squamose a colonnari che rivestono l'esofago inferiore. Gli strati più profondi della parete esofagea sono costituite in successione dalla lamina propria, dalla muscolaris mucosae, dalla sottomucosa e da due strati di tonaca muscolare propria (uno circolare circondato da uno strato longitudinale). I due sfinteri delimitanti dell'esofago, lo **sfintere esofageo superiore** (**UES**, *Upper Esophageal Sphincter*) a livello del muscolo cricofaringeo e il **LES** in corrispondenza della **GEJ**, costringono il lume esofageo a livello dei suoi limiti prossimale e distale. La muscolare propria del terzo superiore dell'esofago è prevalentemente striata, mentre quella dei due terzi inferiori è costituita da muscolo liscio. Le condizioni cliniche che interessano il muscolo striato (disfunzione cricofaringea, paralisi cerebrale) colpiscono l'esofago superiore, mentre quelle che interessano il muscolo liscio (acalasia, esofagite da reflusso) colpiscono l'esofago inferiore. Tra il LES muscolare è la "linea Z" mucosa della GEJ ci può essere una differenza di diversi centimetri.

FUNZIONE. L'esofago può essere suddiviso in tre aree: lo UES, il corpo esofageo e il LES. A riposo, la pressione del LES tonico è normalmente di 20 mmHg circa; valori <10 mmHg sono solitamente considerati anormali, anche se pare che la competenza nei confronti del flusso retrogrado di materiale gastrico sia mantenuta se la pressione del LES è >5 mmHg. La pressione del LES aumenta durante le amplificazioni della pressione intragastrica, causate da contrazioni dello stomaco e dei muscoli della parete addominale (straining) o dalla pressione esterna applicata alla parete addominale. Essa aumenta anche in risposta a stimoli colinergici, gastrina, alcalinizzazione gastrica e alcuni farmaci (betanecolo, metoclopramide, cisapride). La pressione dello UES, più variabile, è spesso superiore a quella del LES; essa si riduce quasi a zero durante il sonno profondo ma aumenta enormemente durante lo stress e lo straining.

La **deglutizione** inizia con il sollevamento della lingua, che sospinge il bolo nella faringe. La laringe si solleva e si sposta anteriormente, aprendo lo UES rilassato, mentre le pieghe ariepiglottiche opposte si chiudono. L'epiglottide ricade all'indietro ricoprendo la laringe per dirigere il bolo sopra la laringe e nello UES. Il palato molle occlude il nasofaringe. La peristalsi primaria così avviata è una contrazione che origina nell'orofaringe e attraversa l'esofago in senso aborale (Fig. 315-1). Il LES, tonicamente contratto per opporre una barriera al reflusso gastroesofageo, si rilassa quando ha inizio la deglutizione, quasi contemporaneamente al rilassamento dello UES. Il rilassamento del LES dura molto più a lungo, finché l'onda peristaltica lo attraversa e lo chiude. La normale velocità peristaltica esofagea è di circa 3 cm/s; l'onda impiega almeno 4 s per attraversare i 12 cm di esofago nel bambino piccolo e un tempo significativamente più lungo in quello più grande. La stimolazione del volto con un soffio d'aria può indurre la deglutizione e la peristalsi esofagea nei bambini piccoli sani, fenomeno detto **riflesso di Santmyer**.

Oltre che per permettere la progressione del materiale deglutito oltre la GEJ e il suo ingresso nello stomaco, il LES normalmente si rilassa per consentire il passaggio dell'aria deglutita o l'espulsione retrograda di materiale dallo stomaco. Forse come estensione di tali funzioni, il LES normale permette anche episodi fisiologici di reflusso, che sono di breve durata e si verificano circa cinque volte nella prima ora postprandiale, in particolare nello stato di veglia, ma altrimenti sono rari. Il suo **rilassamento transitorio**, non associato a deglutizione, costituisce il principale meccanismo alla base del **reflusso patologico** (vedi Fig. 315-1).

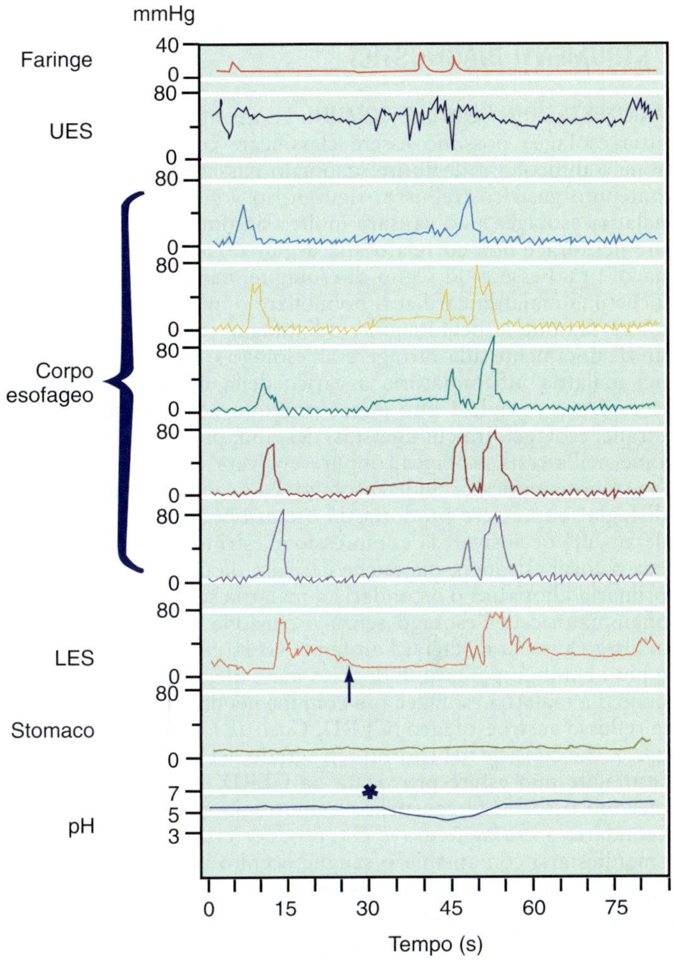

Figura 315-1. Un tracciato continuo della motilità esofagea che mostra due deglutizioni, come indicato dalla contrazione faringea associata al rilassamento dello sfintere esofageo superiore (UES, *Upper Esophageal Sphincter*) e seguita dalla peristalsi nel corpo dell'esofago. Anche lo sfintere esofageo inferiore (LES, *Lower Esophageal Sphincter*) mostra un rilassamento transitorio (*freccia*) non associato a una deglutizione. Vi è un episodio di reflusso gastroesofageo (*) registrato da un sondino per il pH al momento del rilassamento transitorio del LES. (Per gentile concessione di John Dent e Geoffrey Davidson.)

I complicati meccanismi di protezione funzionale del tratto respiratorio durante il movimento retrogrado del contenuto gastrico e la deglutizione si spiegano considerando lo stretto legame tra l'anatomia dell'apparato digerente superiore e quella dell'albero respiratorio superiore. Le funzioni protettive comprendono il tono del LES, il suo rafforzamento da parte delle crura diaframmatiche circostanti e la "protezione di supporto" del tono dello UES. Anche la peristalsi secondaria, simile alla peristalsi primaria ma priva di una componente orale, fa procedere dall'esofago il contenuto gastrico refluito. Un altro riflesso protettivo è la "deglutizione faringea" (che inizia cranialmente all'esofago, ma senza partecipazione della lingua). Tra i molteplici livelli di protezione nei confronti dell'aspirazione vi sono la coordinazione ritmica tra deglutizione e respirazione e tutta una serie di riflessi protettivi con afferenze ed efferenze esofago-faringee che chiudono lo UES o la laringe. Questi riflessi comprendono il riflesso contrattile esofago-UES, il riflesso contrattile faringe-UES, il riflesso di chiusura esofagoglottico e due riflessi di adduzione faringoglottica. Questi ultimi due riflessi sono stimolati da appositi chemiorecettori siti sulla superficie laringea dell'epiglottide e meccanorecettori sulle pieghe ariepiglottiche. È probabile che le interazioni tra l'esofago e il tratto respiratorio, responsabili delle manifestazioni extraesofagee della malattia da reflusso gastroesofageo, saranno spiegate da sottili anomalie in questi riflessi protettivi.

315.1 • Manifestazioni cliniche comuni e strumenti diagnostici

MANIFESTAZIONI CLINICHE COMUNI. Le manifestazioni della malattia esofagea possono essere classificate come dolore, ostruzione o difficoltà a deglutire, anomalo passaggio retrogrado del contenuto gastrico (reflusso, rigurgito o vomito), emorragia; la malattia esofagea può causare inoltre sintomi respiratori. Il dolore nel torace non correlato alla deglutizione (**"bruciore di stomaco"**) può essere un segno di esofagite, ma può rappresentare anche una malattia cardiaca, polmonare o muscoloscheletrica. Il dolore durante la deglutizione (**odinofagia**) localizza la malattia più distintamente alla faringe e all'esofago e spesso rappresenta una malattia infiammatoria a carico della mucosa. L'ostruzione esofagea completa può essere prodotta acutamente da corpi estranei esofagei, tra cui una stasi del cibo; può essere congenita, come nell'atresia esofagea; oppure evolvere nel tempo, quando una stenosi peptica occlude l'esofago. La deglutizione difficoltosa (**disfagia**) può essere prodotta da ostruzione esofagea non completamente occlusiva (da compressione estrinseca, stenosi intrinseca o corpi estranei), ma anche derivare da dismotilità esofagea (primaria/idiopatica o secondaria a malattia sistemica). Le lesioni infiammatorie dell'esofago senza ostruzione o dismotilità sono un'altra causa di disfagia; l'esofagite eosinofila, che colpisce per lo più i bambini più grandi di sesso maschile, è relativamente comune. La malattia esofagea più comune nei bambini è la **malattia da reflusso gastroesofageo** (**GERD**, *GastroEsophageal Reflux Disease*), che consiste nel ritorno retrogrado del contenuto gastrico. L'esofagite può essere provocata da GERD, malattia eosinofila, infezioni o sostanze caustiche. L'**emorragia** esofagea può essere secondaria a esofagite grave che produce erosioni o ulcerazioni e manifestarsi con anemia o sangue occulto nelle feci. Un'emorragia più acuta o grave può essere dovuta alla rottura di **varici esofagee**. L'ematemesi che ne consegue deve essere distinta dalle emorragie più prossimali (epistassi o emottisi). I sintomi respiratori della malattia esofagea possono essere dovuti all'ingresso del contenuto luminale nel tratto respiratorio oppure a risposte respiratorie riflesse in seguito a stimoli esofagei.

STRUMENTI DIAGNOSTICI. L'esofago viene valutato mediante radiografia, endoscopia, istologia, scintigrafia, manometria, pH-metria (associata come indicato ad altra polisonnografia) e impedenza intraluminale. Lo studio radiografico con mezzo di contrasto (solitamente bario) solitamente comprende lo studio fluoroscopico temporale in modo da potere valutare la motilità e l'anatomia. Sebbene sia richiesto per lo più per la valutazione della GERD, esso non è sensibile né specifico per questo scopo; tuttavia, può identificare le sue complicanze (stenosi o ernia iatale) o condizioni che la simulano (stenosi pilorica o malrotazione con volvolo intermittente). La fluoroscopia con bario è ottimale per la valutazione delle anomalie strutturali, come duplicazioni, stenosi o compressione esofagea esterna da parte di un vaso sanguigno aberrante, oppure per lo studio delle cause di dismotilità, come l'acalasia. Varianti dello studio fluoroscopico di routine con bario vengono utilizzate in situazioni particolari. Quando si sospetta una fistola tracheoesofagea "tipo H", il test è più sensibile se il radiologo, con il paziente prono, distende l'esofago introducendo il bario attraverso un sondino nasogastrico. La valutazione videofluoroscopica della deglutizione effettuata con bario di varie consistenze ("deglutizione con bario modificato," videoesofagogramma orofaringeo o *cookie swallow*) valuta in modo ottimale i bambini con disfagia dimostrando l'incoordinazione delle fasi faringea ed esofagea della deglutizione e l'eventuale aspirazione associata. In alcuni centri, la valutazione della deglutizione mediante endoscopia a fibre ottiche (FEES, *Fiberoptic Endoscopic Evaluation of Swallowing*) utilizza l'endoscopia nasofaringea per visualizzare la faringe e la laringe durante la deglutizione di pasti colorati quando si sospettano disfagia, penetrazione laringea o aspirazione. Questa è spesso associata al *sensory testing* (ST) del riflesso degli adduttori laringei in risposta a un puff di aria calibrato attraverso l'endoscopio alle aritenoidi: si esegue così la FEESST composita, che esamina i meccanismi dell'eventuale aspirazione presente. L'endoscopia consente la visualizzazione diretta della mucosa esofagea, ha valore terapeutico in quanto permette di rimuovere i corpi estranei e trattare le varici esofagee e rende inoltre possibile il prelievo bioptico di campioni, migliorando così la diagnosi della GERD "endoscopia-negativa", differenziandola dall'esofagite eosinofila e identificando le cause virali o fungine dell'esofagite. Le scansioni scintigrafiche sono utili nella valutazione dell'efficienza della peristalsi e nella dimostrazione degli episodi di reflusso. Esse possono essere specifiche, sebbene non molto sensibili, per l'aspirazione e permettono di quantificare lo svuotamento gastrico, suggerendo così la causa della GERD. Il salivagramma radionuclidico correlato può dimostrare l'aspirazione anche di piccole quantità di saliva. La manometria esofagea valuta la dismotilità dalla faringe allo stomaco; mediante misurazioni quantitative sincronizzate della pressione lungo l'esofago, essa individua e caratterizza le disfunzioni che talvolta sfuggono alla radiografia. La manometria è spesso di difficile realizzazione nei bambini piccoli; il modo migliore per valutare gli sfinteri è utilizzare speciali cateteri di Dent, anziché port semplici disponibili per il corpo esofageo. Il monitoraggio esteso del pH dell'esofago distale è un test sensibile per gli episodi di GER acido che permette di quantificare la durata e il grado di acidità, ma non il volume degli episodi di reflusso. Esso è collegato alla polisonnografia (uno "pneumogramma") quando si sospetta che il GER provochi apnea o sintomi simili. L'impedenza elettrica transluminale è un metodo per l'identificazione pH-indipendente dei movimenti del bolo nell'esofago; con una sonda pH incorporata, essa può distinguere tra reflusso liquido acido e non acido e reflusso gassoso.

Shaker R, Hogan WJ: Reflex-mediated enhancement of airway protective mechanisms. *Am J Med* 2000;108:8S–14S.

Capitolo 316 ■ Anomalie congenite: atresia esofagea e fistola tracheoesofagea

Susan Orenstein, John Peters, Seema Khan, Nader Youssef e Sunny Zaheed Hussain

L'atresia esofagea (EA, *Esophageal Atresia*) è la più frequente anomalia congenita dell'esofago, che colpisce circa 1/4000 neonati; di questi, più del 90% presenta una fistola tracheoesofagea associata (TEF, *TracheoEsophageal Fistula*). Nella forma più comune di EA, l'esofago superiore termina in una sacca a fondo cieco e la TEF comunica con l'esofago distale. I tipi di EA e di TEF e le loro frequenze relative sono illustrati nella Figura 316-1. Tale difetto presenta tassi di sopravvivenza >90%, grazie soprattutto al miglioramento della terapia intensiva neonatale, all'identificazione più precoce e alla correttezza degli interventi. I neonati che pesano <1500 g alla nascita presentano il rischio di mortalità più elevato. Il 50% dei neonati è non sindromico senza altre anomalie, mentre il restante 50% presenta anomalie associate, per lo più nel contesto della sindrome VATER/VACTERL (*Vertebral, Anorectal, [cardiac], Tracheal, Esophageal, Renal, radial, [limb]*, vertebrale, anorettale, [cardiaca], tracheale, esofagea, renale, radio, [arti]); queste sindromi dovrebbero essere associate a intelligenza normale. Nonostante la scarsa concordanza tra gemelli e la bassa incidenza di casi familiari, in alcuni pazienti i fattori genetici concorrono alla patogenesi della TEF, come

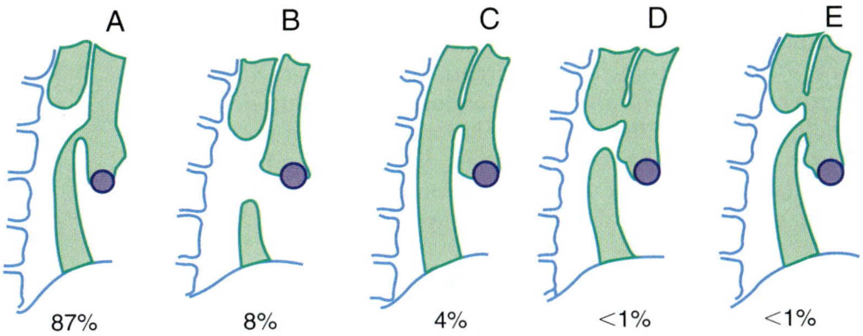

Figura 316-1. Rappresentazione schematica delle cinque forme più comuni di atresia esofagea e fistola tracheoesofagea, presentate in ordine di frequenza.

suggerito da distinte mutazioni nei casi sindromici: sindrome di Feingold (*N-MYC*), sindrome CHARGE (*CHD7*) e sindrome anoftalmia-esofagea-genitale (*SOX2*).

PRESENTAZIONE. Il neonato con EA in genere presenta aria schiumosa e gorgogliante nella bocca e nel naso dopo il parto, oltre a episodi di tosse, cianosi e distress respiratorio. L'alimentazione esacerba questi sintomi, provoca rigurgito e può precipitare l'aspirazione. L'aspirazione del contenuto gastrico attraverso una fistola distale causa una polmonite più dannosa rispetto a quella delle secrezioni faringee dalla sacca superiore a fondo cieco. Il bambino con una TEF isolata in assenza di EA (fistola "a H") può giungere all'attenzione medica più tardi per problemi respiratori cronici, tra cui broncospasmo refrattario e polmoniti ricorrenti.

DIAGNOSI. Nel caso del distress respiratorio a esordio precoce, l'impossibilità di introdurre un sondino nasogastrico o orogastrico nel neonato è suggestivo di atresia esofagea. Il polidramnios materno può indurre il medico a sospettare l'EA. La radiografia diretta nella valutazione del distress respiratorio può evidenziare un tubo di nutrizione attorcigliato nella tasca esofagea e/o nello stomaco disteso dall'aria, che indica la compresenza di una TEF (Fig. 316-2). Al contrario, l'EA pura può presentarsi sotto forma di un addome scafoide, privo di aria. Nella TEF isolata, un esofagogramma con mezzo di contrasto iniettato sotto pressione può dimostrare il difetto. In alternativa, l'orifizio è identificabile alla broncoscopia o quando il blu di metilene, iniettato nel tubo endotracheale durante l'endoscopia, viene osservato nell'esofago durante l'inspirazione forzata.

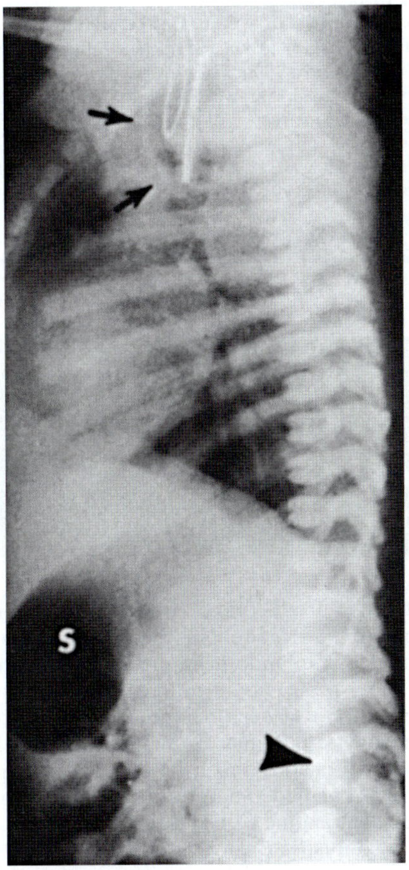

Figura 316-2. Fistola tracheoesofagea. Radiografia laterale che dimostra un sondino nasogastrico attorcigliato (*frecce*) nel segmento prossimale dell'esofago atresico. La fistola distale è suggerita dalla dilatazione gassosa dello stomaco (*S*) e dell'intestino tenue. La *punta* indica una fusione vertebrale, mentre un soffio cardiaco e la cardiomegalia fanno supporre la presenza di un difetto del setto ventricolare. Questo paziente presenta elementi dell'anomalia VATER (*Vertebral, Anorectal, Tracheal, Esophageal, Renal, radial*, vertebrale, anorettale, tracheale, esofagea, renale, del radio). (Da Balfe D, Ling D, Siegel M: The esophagus. In Putman CE, Ravin CE [ed]: *Textbook of Diagnostic Imaging*. Philadelphia, WB Saunders, 1988.)

TRATTAMENTO. Inizialmente, è fondamentale mantenere la pervietà delle vie aeree e prevenire l'aspirazione delle secrezioni. La posizione prona riduce al minimo il passaggio delle secrezioni gastriche in una fistola distale e l'aspirazione esofagea fa sì che una minor quantità di secrezioni si sposti dalla sacca cieca alle vie aeree. L'intubazione endotracheale con ventilazione meccanica deve essere evitata, se possibile, poiché può peggiorare la distensione dei visceri addominali. Quando possibile, si effettuano la legatura chirurgica della TEF e l'anastomosi primaria terminoterminale dell'esofago. Nel bambino prematuro o con altre complicanze, si può ritardare la chiusura primaria, prendendo tempo mediante legatura della fistola e posizionamento del tubo di gastrostomia. Se lo spazio tra le estremità atresiche dell'esofago è >3-4 cm, non è possibile procedere alla riparazione primaria; tra le possibili alternative vi è l'utilizzo di segmenti gastrici, digiunali o colici interposti a costituire un neoesofago. Si devono ricercare con attenzione le comuni anomalie associate, di natura cardiaca e di altro tipo.

PROGNOSI. La maggior parte dei bambini crescendo arriva a condurre una vita normale, ma le complicanze sono spesso impegnative, in particolare durante l'infanzia. Tra le complicanze della chirurgia vi sono fessure anastomotiche, rifistolizzazione e stenosi anastomotica. In molti casi a complicare il trattamento interviene anche la malattia da reflusso gastroesofageo (GERD, *GastroEsophageal Reflux Disease*), imputabile ad anomalie intrinseche della funzione esofagea, spesso combinata al ritardato svuotamento gastrico. La GERD contribuisce significativamente alla patologia respiratoria (**malattia respiratoria reattiva**) che spesso complica l'EA e la TEF, oltre a peggiorare le frequenti stenosi anastomotiche dopo la riparazione dell'EA.

316.1 • Anomalie congenite: difetti laringotracheoesofagei

Queste rare anomalie compaiono quando il setto tra l'esofago e la trachea non si sviluppa in modo completo, portando alla comparsa di un canale comune tra il lume faringoesofageo e quello laringotracheale, che rende incompetente la chiusura laringea durante la deglutizione o il reflusso. Nei primi mesi di vita il bambino presenta stridor, soffocamento, cianosi, aspirazione del cibo e infezioni toraciche ricorrenti. La diagnosi è difficile e di solito richiede la visualizzazione endoscopica diretta della laringe e dell'esofago. Quando si esegue la radiografia con mezzo di contrasto, spesso si osserva il materiale nell'esofago e nella trachea. Il trattamento consiste nella riparazione chirurgica, che però può essere complessa se i difetti sono lunghi.

Adzick NS, Nance ML: Pediatric surgery: I. *N Engl J Med* 2000;342:1651–1657.

Carr MM, Clark KD, Webber E, et al: Congenital laryngotracheoesophageal cleft. *J Otolaryngol* 1999;28:112–117.

Romeo C, Bonanno N, Baldari S, et al: Gastric motility disorders in patients operated on for esophageal atresia and tracheoesophageal fistula: Long-term evaluation. *J Pediatr Surg* 2000;35:740–744.

Sharma AK, Shekhawat NS, Agrawal LD, et al: Esophageal atresia and tracheoesophageal fistula: A review of 25 years' experience. *Pediatr Surg Int* 2000;16:478–482.

Shaw-Smith C: Oesophageal atresia, tracheo-oesophageal fistula and the VACTERL association: review of genetics and epidemiology. *J Med Genet* 2006;43:545–554.

Capitolo 317 ■ Malattie ostruttive e discinesie esofagee

Susan Orenstein, John Peters, Seema Khan, Nader Youssef e Sunny Zaheed Hussain

Le lesioni ostruttive producono classicamente **disfagia** per i **solidi** più precocemente e in modo più evidente rispetto ai liquidi e possono manifestarsi quando nella dieta del bambino si iniziano a introdurre cibi solidi; ciò le differenzia dalla **disfagia** dovuta a **discinesia,** in cui la deglutizione di liquidi è compromessa contemporaneamente o prima di quella dei solidi. In molti casi di disfagia, la valutazione inizia con la fluoroscopia, che può comprendere l'esame videofluoroscopico della deglutizione, in particolare se l'aspirazione è un sintomo primario. Le indagini di secondo livello sono spesso endoscopiche se si sospetta un'ostruzione intrinseca, manometriche se si sospetta una discinesia e di altro tipo nei casi particolari. Per le lesioni congenite può essere necessario l'intervento chirurgico, mentre le membrane e le stenosi peptiche possono rispondere in modo adeguato alla dilatazione endoscopica mediante palloncino (o *bougie*). In caso di stenosi peptiche, dopo la dilatazione, si dovrebbe prendere in considerazione la fundoplicatio per la profilassi continua.

ESTRINSECHE. Le **cisti esofagee da duplicazione** comprendono le duplicazioni dell'intestino anteriore di più frequente riscontro. Tali cisti sono delimitate da epitelio intestinale, possiedono una parete muscolare liscia ben sviluppata e sono collegate al tratto gastrointestinale normale; due terzi di esse si verificano sul lato destro dell'esofago. La presentazione più comune è il distress respiratorio, causato da compressione delle vie aeree adiacenti. La disfagia è un sintomo frequente nei bambini più grandi. L'emorragia gastrointestinale superiore può essere riconducibile alla presenza di mucosa gastrica secernente acido nella parete di duplicazione. Le **cisti neuroenteriche** possono contenere elementi gliali e sono associate ad **anomalie vertebrali.** La diagnosi viene posta grazie allo studio con bario o alla TC del torace. Il trattamento è chirurgico; è possibile anche l'approccio laparoscopico all'excisione.

Linfonodi mediastinici o sottocarenali ingranditi, causati da infezioni (tubercolosi, istoplasmosi) o neoplasie (linfoma), sono le masse esterne più comuni che comprimono l'esofago e provocano sintomi ostruttivi. Anche le **anomalie vascolari** possono esercitare una compressione sull'esofago; si definisce *disfagia lusoria* la disfagia prodotta da un'arteria succlavia destra aberrante o da un arco aortico collocato a destra o doppio (vedi Capitolo 432.1).

INTRINSECHE. La stenosi intrinseca del lume esofageo può essere congenita o acquisita. L'eziologia è suggerita dalla localizzazione e dal carattere della lesione, oltre che dalla situazione clinica. L'esofago inferiore è la sede più comune delle stenosi peptiche, che in genere sono piuttosto irregolari e misurano diversi centimetri di lunghezza. Anche gli anelli membranosi sottili, tra cui l'anello di Schatzki a livello della giunzione squamocolonnare, possono occludere quest'area. Nell'esofago medio, la stenosi congenita si associa talvolta ad atresia esofagea/fistola tracheoesofagea complessa, in cui alcune lesioni, incorporando cartilagine, non possono essere dilatate in tutta sicurezza; in alternativa, l'esofagite da reflusso può provocare una stenosi irregolare ed estesa che appare più prossimale della stenosi peptica consueta, spesso a causa di un'ernia iatale associata. A restringere l'esofago superiore possono essere membrane o anelli congeniti, come pure una stenosi infiammatoria che si verifica in seguito a ingestione di caustici o epidermolisi bollosa. L'acalasia cricofaringea può manifestarsi radiograficamente con una "barra" cricofaringea, nella parte posteriore dell'esofago superiore.

Enterline H, Thompson J: *Pathology of the Esophagus.* New York, Springer-Verlag, 1984.

Janssen M, Baggen MG, Veen HF, et al: Dysphagia lusoria: Clinical aspects, manometric findings, diagnosis, and therapy. *Am J Gastroenterol* 2000;95:1411–1416.

Capitolo 318 ■ Discinesia

Susan Orenstein, John Peters, Seema Khan, Nader Youssef e Sunny Zaheed Hussain

DISCINESIA (MUSCOLO STRIATO) DELL'ESOFAGO SUPERIORE E DELLO SFINTERE ESOFAGEO SUPERIORE. L'**acalasia** cricofaringea comporta il mancato rilassamento dello sfintere esofageo superiore (UES, *Upper Esophageal Sphincter*), mentre l'**incoordinazione** cricofaringea implica il completo rilassamento dell'UES, ma con mancata coordinazione tra il rilassamento e la contrazione faringea. Queste entità sono solitamente identificate alla valutazione videofluoroscopica della deglutizione (che talvolta evidenzia una sporgenza cricofaringea, denominata *barra*, ma spesso per una definizione più precisa della disfunzione bisogna ricorrere alla manometria. Una forma autolimitata di incoordinazione cricofaringea si verifica nell'infanzia e si risolve spontaneamente nel primo anno di vita se l'alimentazione orale viene proseguita nonostante la disfagia. Nei bambini più grandi, lo **spasmo** cricofaringeo idiopatico è solitamente trattato mediante la miotomia dell'UES. Tuttavia, è importante valutare tali bambini in modo completo, includendo la RM dell'encefalo per identificare le **malformazioni di Arnold-Chiari,** che possono presentarsi in questo modo ma sono trattate mediante decompressione craniale, anziché con la chirurgia esofagea. Lo spasmo cricofaringeo può essere così grave da produrre un **diverticolo** faringeo posteriore (di Zenker) al di sopra dello sfintere ostruttivo, entità che peraltro si verifica raramente nei bambini.

Tra le **cause sistemiche** di disfunzione della deglutizione che possono colpire l'orofaringe, l'UES e l'esofago superiore vi sono la paralisi cerebrale, le malformazioni di Arnold-Chiari, la siringomielia, la paralisi bulbare o i deficit dei nervi cranici (sindrome di Möbius, paralisi infantile transitoria del nervo laringeo superiore), la disfunzione muscolare faringea transitoria, l'atrofia muscolare spinale (tra cui la malattia di Werdnig-Hoffmann), la distrofia muscolare, le infezioni (botulismo, tetano, poliomielite, difterite), le malattie infiammatorie e del tessuto connettivo (dermatomiosite, miastenia gravis, polinevrite, sclerodermia) e la disautonomia familiare. Tutte queste condizioni possono produrre disfagia. I farmaci (nitrazepam, benzodiazepine) e la tracheostomia possono compromettere la funzione dell'UES e quindi provocare disfagia.

DISFUNZIONE (MUSCOLO LISCIO) DELL'ESOFAGO INFERIORE E DELLO SFINTERE ESOFAGEO INFERIORE. Tra le cause di disfagia dovute a discinesia esofagea primaria più distale sono incluse l'acalasia, lo spasmo esofageo diffuso, l'esofago a schiaccianoci e lo sfintere esofageo inferiore (LES, *Lower Esophageal Sphincter*) ipertensivo; tutte queste condizioni, tranne l'acalasia, sono rare nel bambino.

L'**acalasia** è una malattia motoria primitiva dell'esofago a eziologia sconosciuta, caratterizzata da perdita del rilassamento del LES e della peristalsi esofagea, che a sua volta contribuisce a un'ostruzione funzionale dell'esofago distale. Possibili cause sono fattori degenerativi, autoimmuni (anticorpi diretti contro il plesso di Auerbach) e infettivi (malattia di Chagas). In rari casi, la patologia è familiare o fa parte della sindrome acalasia, alacrimia e insensibilità alla corticotropina. Dal punto di vista anatomopatologico, l'infiammazione circonda le cellule gangliari, che sono di numero ridotto. Si verifica una perdita selettiva dei neuroni inibitori postgangliari che normalmente determinano il rilassamento dello sfintere, mentre i neuroni colinergici postgangliari rimangono indenni. Questo squilibrio produce elevate pressioni basali del LES e suo insufficiente rilassamento. La perdita della peristalsi esofagea può essere un fenomeno secondario. L'acalasia si presenta con disfagia per i solidi e i liquidi e può essere accompagnata da iponutrizione o sintomi respiratori; il cibo ritenuto in esofago può provocare esofagite. L'età media nei bambini è di 8,8 anni, con una durata media dei sintomi prima della diagnosi di 23 mesi; la patologia è rara prima dell'età scolare. La radiografia del torace mostra un livello idroaereo in un esofago dilatato. La **fluoroscopia con bario** evidenzia un affusolamento regolare dell'esofago inferiore fino al LES, con un aspetto "a becco di uccello" (Fig. 318-1). Spesso si osserva perdita della peristalsi primaria nell'esofago distale con ritenzione di cibo e scarso svuotamento. La **manometria** conferma la diagnosi ed evidenzia l'incompleto rilassamento di un LES a elevata pressione durante la deglutizione, spesso accompagnato da contrazioni simultanee non propulsive nell'esofago distale. Le due **opzioni di trattamento** più efficaci sono la dilatazione pneumatica e la miotomia chirurgica (di Heller). Spesso i chirurghi completano la miotomia con una procedura antireflusso per prevenire la malattia da reflusso gastroesofageo, che altrimenti fa spesso la sua comparsa quando lo sfintere è reso meno competente. I calcioantagonisti (nifedipina) e gli inibitori della fosfodiesterasi alleviano temporaneamente la disfagia. L'iniezione endoscopica di **tossina botulinica** nel LES contrasta la perdita selettiva dei neurotrasmettitori inibitori attraverso l'inibizione del rilascio di acetilcolina dalle terminazioni nervose e può essere una terapia efficace. La tossina botulinica è costosa; nella metà dei pazienti può essere necessaria la reiniezione entro un anno.

Lo **spasmo esofageo diffuso**, che colpisce adulti e adolescenti, provoca dolore toracico e disfagia. Esso viene diagnosticato mediante **manometria** e può essere trattato con nitrati o calcioantagonisti.

La **malattia da reflusso gastroesofageo** rappresenta la causa più comune di anomalie aspecifiche della funzione motoria esofagea, probabilmente attraverso l'effetto dell'infiammazione esofagea sulla muscolatura.

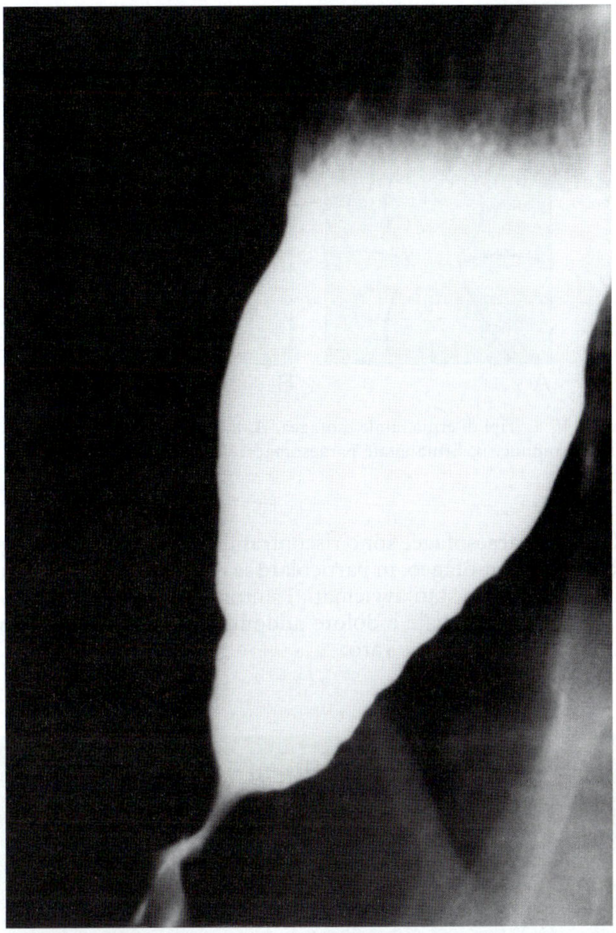

Figura 318-1. Esofagogramma con pasto baritato in un paziente con acalasia, che dimostra dilatazione dell'esofago e restringimento in corrispondenza dello sfintere esofageo inferiore. Si notino le secrezione ritenute che si stratificano al di sopra del bario, nell'esofago.

Orenstein SR: Oral, pharyngeal and esophageal motor disorders in infants and children. In Goyal R, Shaker R (editors): *GI Motility Online*. New York, Nature Publishing Group 2006. doi: 10.1038/gimo 38. View at www.nature.com/gimo/index.html

Capitolo 319 ■ Ernia iatale

Susan Orenstein, John Peters, Seema Khan, Nader Youssef e Sunny Zaheed Hussain

L'erniazione dello stomaco attraverso lo iato esofageo può verificarsi sotto forma di una comune ernia da scivolamento, in cui la giunzione gastroesofagea risale nel torace, oppure può essere paraesofagea, in cui una porzione dello stomaco (di solito il fondo) si insinua accanto all'esofago, all'interno della giunzione gastroesofagea, nello iato (Fig. 319-1). Le ernie da scivolamento sono spesso associate a reflusso gastroesofageo, specialmente nei bambini con ritardo dello sviluppo. La relazione con l'ernia iatale degli adulti non è chiara. Il trattamento medico non è rivolto all'ernia, ma al reflusso gastroesofageo.

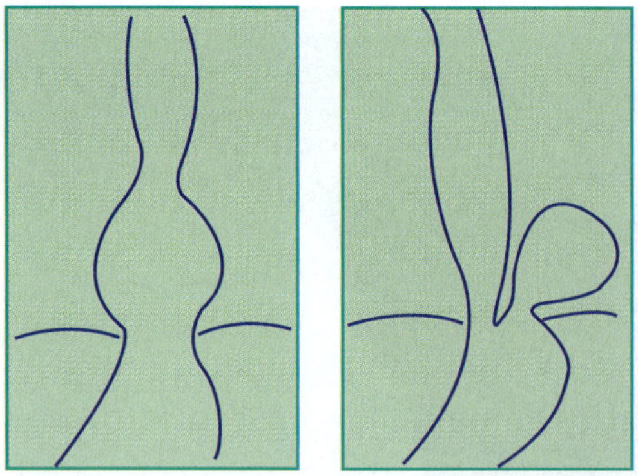

Figura 319-1. Tipi di ernia iatale esofagea. *A*, Ernia iatale da scivolamento, il tipo più comune. *B*, Ernia iatale paraesofagea.

Le ernie paraesofagee sono riscontrabili dopo fundoplicatio per reflusso gastroesofageo, in particolare se i bordi dello iato esofago dilatato non sono stati avvicinati. I sintomi abituali sono senso di pienezza postprandiale e dolore addominale superiore. L'infarto dello stomaco erniato è raro.

Capitolo 320 ■ Malattia da reflusso gastroesofageo

Susan Orenstein, John Peters, Seema Khan, Nader Youssef e Sunny Zaheed Hussain

La malattia da reflusso gastroesofageo (GERD, *GastroEsophageal Reflux Disease*) è la patologia esofagea più comune nei bambini di tutte le età. Il reflusso gastroesofageo consiste nel passaggio retrogrado di contenuto gastrico nell'esofago attraverso lo sfintere esofageo inferiore (LES, *Lower Esophageal Sphincter*). Sebbene forme occasionali di reflusso siano fisiologiche (per es. rigurgito che si osserva nei bambini normali), il fenomeno diventa patologico (GERD) in presenza di episodi più frequenti o persistenti, che quindi provocano esofagite o sintomi esofagei, oppure nei pazienti con sequele respiratorie.

FISIOPATOLOGIA. Tra i fattori che determinano le manifestazioni esofagee del reflusso vi sono la durata dell'esposizione esofagea (un prodotto della frequenza e della durata degli episodi di reflusso), la causticità del materiale refluito e la suscettibilità dell'esofago alle lesioni. Il LES, supportato dalle crura del diaframma in corrispondenza della giunzione gastroesofagea, oltre a espletare le funzioni similvalvolari proprie dell'anatomia della giunzione esofagogastrica, costituisce una barriera antireflusso. Nel contesto anche dei normali aumenti della pressione intraddominale che si verificano durante la vita quotidiana, la frequenza degli episodi di reflusso aumenta se il LES non presenta un tono insufficiente, se va incontro a rilassamenti con una frequenza anomala e se è presente un'ernia iatale, che impedisce il proporzionale aumento della pressione del LES durante lo straining (eccessivo impegno muscolare) addominale. I normali aumenti della pressione intraddominale possono essere ulteriormente accentuati dallo straining o dagli sforzi respiratori. A prolungare la durata degli episodi di reflusso sono l'assenza della deglutizione (durante il sonno) e i difetti della peristalsi esofagea. Si instaura quindi un circolo vizioso poiché l'esofagite produce disfunzione della peristalsi esofagea (onde di scarsa ampiezza, disturbi di propagazione), riduzione del tono del LES e accorciamento infiammatorio dell'esofago che porta a ernia iatale, tutti fattori che peggiorano il reflusso.

Il **rilassamento transitorio del LES** (TLESR, *Transient LES Relaxation*) è il meccanismo primario che consente l'insorgenza del reflusso. I TLESR si verificano indipendentemente dalla deglutizione, riducendo la pressione a 0-2 mmHg (al di sopra dello stomaco), e durano >10 s; essi compaiono a partire dalla 26ª settimana di gestazione. Sono regolati da un riflesso vasovagale, composto da meccanocettori afferenti nello stomaco prossimale, un pattern generatore di ritmo del tronco cerebrale e vie efferenti nel LES. La distensione gastrica (postprandiale o dovuta ad anomalo svuotamento gastrico o ingestione di aria) è il principale stimolo per i TLESR. Si discute se la GERD sia causata da una maggiore frequenza di TLESR o da una maggiore incidenza di reflusso durante i TLESR; entrambe le spiegazioni sono plausibili, in individui differenti. Lo straining durante un TLESR e le posture che abbassano la giunzione gastroesofagea al di sotto dell'interfaccia aria-liquido, nello stomaco, rendono più probabile il reflusso. Altri fattori che influenzano le dinamiche pressione-volume dello stomaco, come l'aumento delle evacuazioni, lo straining, l'obesità, i pasti copiosi o iperosmolari e un lavoro respiratorio aumentato (tosse, respiro affannoso), possono avere lo stesso effetto.

EPIDEMIOLOGIA E STORIA NATURALE. Il **reflusso nel bambino piccolo** diventa evidente nei primissimi mesi di vita, raggiunge un picco a circa 4 mesi per poi risolversi nella maggior parte dei casi entro i 12 mesi e quasi sempre entro i 24 mesi. I sintomi nei bambini più grandi tendono a essere cronici, crescenti o decrescenti, ma si risolvono completamente in non più della metà dei casi, che assomigliano a pattern adulti. È probabile che nella GERD entrino in gioco fattori predisponenti di carattere genetico; è stato identificato un raggruppamento familiare per i sintomi della GERD, l'esofagite endoscopica, l'ernia iatale, l'esofago di Barrett e l'adenocarcinoma. Essendo una malattia continuamente variabile e comune, è probabile un'ereditarietà complessa che interessa più geni e fattori ambientali. È stata proposta sul cromosoma 13q14 una forma pediatrica autosomica dominante con manifestazioni otolaringoiatriche e respiratorie.

MANIFESTAZIONI CLINICHE. La maggior parte delle manifestazioni cliniche di malattia esofagea può indicare la presenza di GERD. Il **reflusso nel bambino piccolo** si manifesta per lo più con rigurgito (soprattutto postprandiale), segni di esofagite (irritabilità, inarcamento della schiena, soffocamento, conati di vomito, avversione al cibo) e conseguente deficit di crescita staturoponderale; nella maggior parte dei casi, i sintomi si risolvono spontaneamente entro i primi 12-24 mesi. I **bambini più grandi**, al contrario, possono avere rigurgito in età prescolare; sintomi di dolore addominale e toracico sopraggiungono nella tarda infanzia e nell'adolescenza. Alcuni si presentano con contorsioni del collo (inarcamento della schiena, rotazione della testa da un lato) che configurano la cosiddetta **sindrome di Sandifer**. Le presentazioni respiratorie dipendono anche dall'età: nei pazienti più piccoli la GERD può manifestarsi sotto forma di apnea ostruttiva oppure stridor o malattia delle basse vie aeree, in cui il reflusso complica la patologia respiratoria primaria come la laringomalacia o la displasia broncopolmonare. L'otite media, la sinusite, l'iperplasia linfoide, la raucedine, i noduli delle corde vocali e l'edema laringeo sono stati tutti associati a GERD. Al contrario, le manifestazioni respiratorie nei bambini più grandi sono correlate con maggiore frequenza all'asma e a malattie otolaringoiatriche come la laringite e la sinusite.

DIAGNOSI. Nella maggior parte delle presentazioni tipiche di GERD, un'anamnesi e un esame obiettivo esaustivi sono sufficienti per porre la diagnosi inizialmente. Tale prima valutazione ha lo scopo di identificare i positivi pertinenti a supporto della GERD e le complicanze di questa, oltre ai negativi che rendono improbabili altre diagnosi. L'anamnesi può essere facilitata e standardizzata mediante questionari (I-GERQ [*Infant Gastroesophageal Reflux Questionnaire*] e derivati, I-GERQ-R), che permettono anche di utilizzare i punteggi quantitativi per la discriminazione diagnostica e la valutazione del miglioramento o aggravamento dei sintomi. Altre importanti **diagnosi** da prendere in considerazione nella valutazione di un bambino con vomito cronico sono l'allergia al latte o ad altri alimenti, la stenosi pilorica, l'ostruzione intestinale (soprattutto la malrotazione con volvolo intermittente), le malattie infiammatorie non esofagee, le infezioni, gli errori congeniti del metabolismo, l'idronefrosi, l'aumento della pressione endocranica, la ruminazione e la bulimia. In seguito, la valutazione iniziale può essere integrata da esami diagnostici mirati, a seconda della presentazione e della diagnosi differenziale.

La maggior parte dei test esofagei è piuttosto utile in particolari pazienti con sospetta GERD. Lo **studio radiografico con mezzo di contrasto** (di solito **bario**) dell'esofago e del tratto gastrointestinale superiore viene realizzato nei bambini con vomito e disfagia per escludere l'acalasia, i restringimenti o le stenosi esofagee, l'ernia iatale e l'ostruzione dello sbocco gastrico o l'ostruzione intestinale (Fig. 320-1). Il **monitoraggio prolungato del pH** dell'esofago distale, pur non essendo più considerato la *condicio sine qua non* della diagnosi di GERD, fornisce una documentazione quantitativa e sensibile degli episodi di reflusso acido, il più importante tipo di episodi di reflusso patologico. La sonda che rileva il pH dell'esofago distale viene collocata a un livello corrispondente all'87% della distanza narici-LES, calcolata con equazioni di regressione basate sull'altezza del paziente, oppure mediante visualizzazione fluoroscopica o identificazione manometrica del LES. I valori normali dell'esposizione dell'esofago distale all'acido (pH <4) sono generalmente stabiliti come <5-8% del tempo monitorato totale, anche se questi parametri di riferimento quantitativi non sono sufficienti per stabilire o escludere una diagnosi di GERD patologica. Le indicazioni più importanti al monitoraggio del pH esofageo sono la valutazione dell'efficacia della soppressione acida in corso di trattamento, la valutazione degli episodi di apnea in congiunzione con uno pneumogramma e forse l'impedenza (vedi oltre) e la valutazione delle presentazioni atipiche di GERD come la tosse cronica, lo stridor e l'asma. Nella diagnosi della GERD extraesofagea vengono utilizzate le sonde doppie per il pH, con l'aggiunta di una sonda esofagea prossimale alla sonda standard distale, identificando come valori soglia di anormalità i tempi di esposizione acida dell'esofago superiore pari a circa l'1% del tempo totale. L'**endoscopia** consente la diagnosi di esofagite erosiva (Fig. 320-2) e di complicanze come le stenosi o l'esofago di Barrett; le biopsie esofagee possono diagnosticare l'esofagite istologica da reflusso in assenza di erosioni, escludendo simultaneamente le cause allergiche e infettive. L'endoscopia trova impiego anche in campo terapeutico per dilatare le stenosi indotte dal reflusso. La scintigrafia radionuclidica con tecnezio può mostrare l'aspirazione e il ritardato svuotamento gastrico quando queste condizioni sono sospettate. Il test dell'**impedenza intraluminale** è una metodica impegnativa, raramente utilizzata in ambito clinico; ciononostante, la sua documentazione del reflusso non acido ha rivelato l'importanza del reflusso neutro nei bambini, in particolare in quelli con sintomi respiratori.

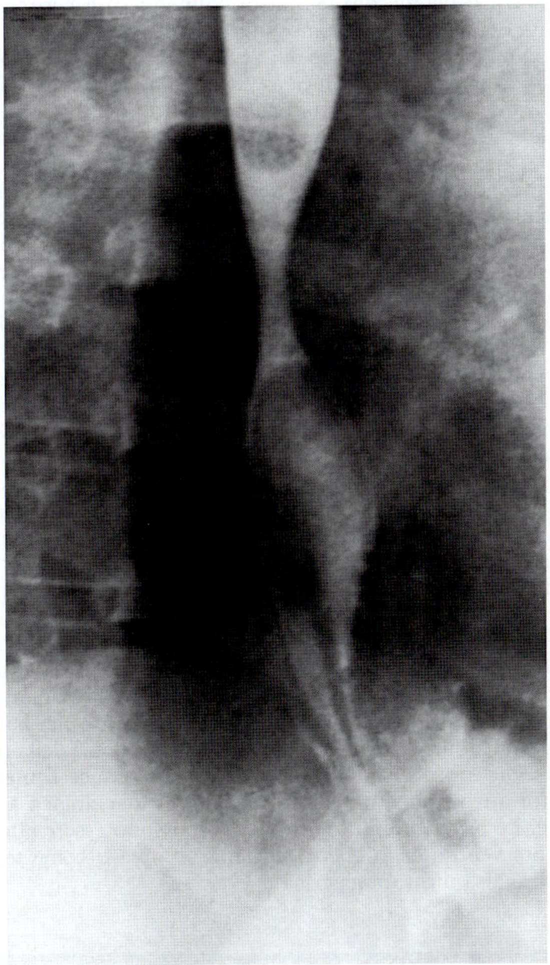

Figura 320-1. Esofagogramma con bario che dimostra reflusso gastroesofageo libero. Si noti la stenosi causata da esofagite peptica. Le pieghe gastriche longitudinali al di sopra del diaframma indicano l'insolita presenza di un'ernia iatale associata.

La **laringotracheobroncoscopia** valuta i segni delle vie aeree visibili che sono associati a GERD extraesofagea, come l'infiammazione laringea posteriore e i noduli delle corde vocali; questo esame può consentire la diagnosi di aspirazione silente (durante la deglutizione o il reflusso) mediante lavaggio broncoalveolare, con successiva quantificazione dei macrofagi carichi di lipidi nelle secrezione respiratorie. La manometria esofagea permette di valutare la discinesia, specialmente in preparazione alla chirurgia antireflusso.

La **terapia empirica antireflusso**, consistente in un breve ciclo con un inibitore della pompa protonica (PPI, *Proton Pump Inhibitor*) ad alte dosi, si è dimostrata una strategia con un buon rapporto costo-beneficio per la diagnosi negli adulti; sebbene non ufficialmente valutata nei bambini più grandi, essa è stata applicata anche a tale gruppo di età. La mancata risposta a tale trattamento empirico, o la necessità di proseguire il trattamento per periodi prolungati, rende obbligatoria la valutazione diagnostica formale.

TRATTAMENTO. La terapia conservativa e le modificazioni dello stile di vita costituiscono le basi del trattamento della GERD. Tra le misure dietetiche previste per i bambini vi sono la normalizzazione delle tecniche di alimentazione, dei volumi e della frequenza, se alterati. L'ispessimento del latte in formula con un cucchiaio di fiocchi di riso per 30 g circa di formula riduce la frequenza degli episodi di rigurgito, aumenta la densità calorica (1 kcal/g) e riduce la durata del pianto, sebbene possa non modificare il numero di episodi di reflusso non rigurgitante. Si può effettuare un breve ciclo con una dieta ipoallergenica per escludere l'allergia al latte o alle proteine della soia prima della farmacoterapia. Ai bambini più grandi e agli adulti si dovrebbe consigliare di evitare i cibi (pomodori, cioccolato, menta) e le bevande (succhi di frutta, bevande gassate e contenenti caffeina, alcol) acidi o che inducono reflusso. La riduzione del peso per i pazienti obesi e la sospensione dell'esposizione al fumo sono altre misure fondamentali a tutte le età.

Le **misure posturali** sono particolarmente importanti per i bambini piccoli, che non sono in grado di controllare la posizione del corpo in modo autonomo. La posizione seduta peggiora il reflusso nel bambino piccolo e andrebbe sempre evitata nei pazienti pediatrici con GERD. Nonostante dal monitoraggio del pH esofageo sia emerso un numero significativamente maggiore di episodi di reflusso nei bambini in posizione supina e distesi su un fianco rispetto a quelli proni, l'American Academy of Pediatrics e la North American Society of Pediatric Gastroenterology and

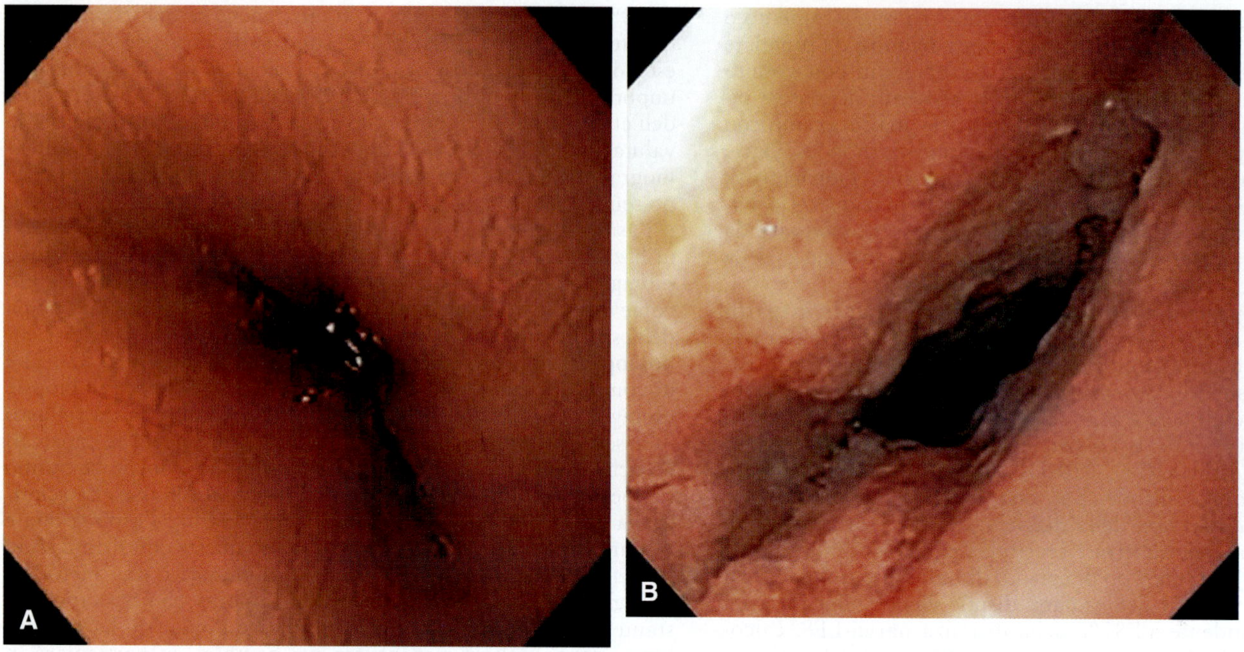

Figura 320-2. Immagine endoscopica di un esofago normale (*A*) ed esofagite peptica erosiva (*B*).

Nutrition raccomandano la posizione supina durante il sonno da quando si è scoperto che riduce il rischio di sindrome della morte improvvisa del lattante. Quando il bambino è sveglio e sotto osservazione, è possibile tenerlo in posizione prona o diritta in braccio al fine di ridurre al minimo il reflusso. Non si sa fino a che punto la postura influisca su questo disturbo nei bambini più grandi, ma alcuni dati suggeriscono un vantaggio della posizione laterale sinistra e del sollevamento della testa durante il sonno. Per tenere il capo del paziente in posizione elevata si consiglia di sollevare la testata del letto, invece di utilizzare molti cuscini, per evitare la flessione e la compressione dell'addome che potrebbero peggiorare il reflusso.

La **terapia farmacologica** ha lo scopo di migliorare l'acidità del contenuto gastrico o di favorirne il movimento aborale. Gli **antiacidi**, facilmente reperibili come farmaci da banco, sono la terapia antireflusso di più comune impiego. Essi determinano un rapido ma transitorio sollievo dai sintomi attraverso la neutralizzazione dell'acido. Tuttavia, il loro uso regolare a lungo termine non è raccomandabile, a causa degli effetti collaterali come diarrea (magnesio) e stipsi (alluminio) e dei rari casi riportati di conseguenze più gravi dovute all'uso cronico.

Gli **antagonisti del recettore H2 dell'istamina** (H2RA, *Histamine-2 Receptor Antagonists*: cimetidina, famotidina, nizatidina e ranitidina) sono farmaci antisecretori ampiamente utilizzati, che agiscono attraverso l'inibizione selettiva dei recettori dell'istamina sulle cellule parietali gastriche. La loro efficacia nel trattamento dell'esofagite da reflusso lieve o moderata è ben dimostrata. Gli H2RA sono stati raccomandati come terapia di prima linea grazie al loro eccellente profilo di sicurezza complessivo, ma stanno per essere soppiantati dagli inibitori della pompa protonica, grazie all'acquisizione di un'esperienza e di una sicurezza di utilizzo maggiori in ambito pediatrico, all'approvazione della Food and Drug Administration e alla disponibilità di formulazioni e posologie pediatriche.

Gli **inibitori della pompa protonica** (**PPI**, *Proton Pump Inhibitors*: omeprazolo, lansoprazolo, pantoprazolo, rabeprazolo ed esomeprazolo) esplicano l'effetto antireflusso più potente, bloccando i canali dell'ATPasi ione idrogeno-potassio della via finale comune nella secrezione di acido gastrico. Gli PPI sono superiori agli H2RA nel trattamento dell'esofagite grave ed erosiva. Le dosi di omeprazolo efficaci nei bambini sono state identificate (0,7-3,3 mg/kg/die) e sono superiori a quelle utilizzate negli adulti per quanto riguarda la dose in base al peso corporeo.

I **farmaci procinetici** disponibili negli Stati Uniti comprendono la metoclopramide (antagonista del recettore 2 della dopamina e del 5HT-3), il betanecolo (agonista colinergico) e l'eritromicina (agonista del recettore della motilina). La maggior parte di questi farmaci aumenta la pressione del LES; alcuni migliorano lo svuotamento gastrico o la clearance esofagea, ma nessuno modifica la frequenza dei TLESR. Gli studi clinici controllati condotti finora non hanno dimostrato grande efficacia nella GERD. Diversi nuovi farmaci procinetici che potrebbero rivelarsi utili non sono stati ancora adeguatamente studiati per tale indicazione nei bambini.

La **chirurgia**, solitamente la **fundoplicatio**, è una terapia efficace per la GERD intrattabile nei bambini, in particolare in quelli con esofagite o stenosi refrattarie e in quelli a rischio di morbilità significativa da malattia polmonare cronica. Essa può essere associata a una gastrostomia per la nutrizione o per lo svuotamento. La disponibilità di potenti farmaci acidosoppressori rende obbligatoria un'analisi più rigorosa dei rischi relativi (o costi) e dei benefici di tale trattamento relativamente irreversibile rispetto alla famacoterapia a lungo termine. Alcuni rischi della fundoplicatio sono una plicatura "troppo tesa" (con conseguente disfagia o dilatazione gassosa) o "troppo lassa" (e quindi incompetente). In base alla loro esperienza e alla malattia del paziente, i chirurghi possono scegliere se effettuare una plicatura "tesa" (a 360°, secondo Nissen) o "lassa" (<360°, secondo Thal ecc.) o se aggiungere una procedura di drenaggio gastrico (piloroplastica) per migliorare lo svuotamento gastrico. L'accuratezza preoperatoria della diagnosi di GERD e l'abilità del chirurgo sono i due più importanti fattori predittivi di una prognosi favorevole. Dagli studi a lungo termine risulta che le fundoplicatio diventano spesso incompetenti tanto nei bambini, quanto negli adulti; tale riscontro, unito alla potenza della terapia con PPI che è ora disponibile, in molti casi induce il medico a cambiare atteggiamento verso la terapia farmacologica a lungo termine. Le procedure di fundoplicatio possono essere effettuate come interventi a cielo aperto, in laparoscopia o come tecniche endoluminali (plicatura gastrica).

Benhamou PH, Francoual C, Glangeaud MC, et al: Risk factors for severe esophageal and gastric lesions in term neonates: A case-control study. Groupe Francophone d'Hepato-Gastroenterologie et Nutrition Pediatrique. *J Pediatr Gastroenterol Nutr* 2000;31:377–380.

Davidson G, Omari TI: Pathophysiological mechanisms of gastroesophageal reflux disease in children. *Curr Gastroenterol Rep* 2001;3:257–262.
Fonkalsrud EW, Ashcraft KW, Coran AG, et al: Surgical treatment of gastroesophageal reflux in children: A combined hospital study of 7,467 patients. *Pediatrics* 1998;101:419–422.
Lehman GA: Endoscopic and endoluminal techniques for the control of gastroesophageal reflux: Are they ready for widespread clinical application? *Gastrointest Endosc* 2000;52:808–811.
Lidums I, Lehmann A, Checklin H, et al: Control of transient lower esophageal sphincter relaxations and reflux by the $GABA_B$ agonist baclofen in normal subjects. *Gastroenterology* 2000;118:7–13.
Orenstein SR: Pediatric gastroesophageal reflux disease. In Orland RC (editor): *Gastroesophageal Reflux Disease.* New York, Marcel Dekker, 2000.
Orenstein SR, Di Lorenzo C: Postfundoplication complications in children. *Curr Treat Options Gastroenterol* 2001;4:441–449.
Orenstein SR, Peters JM: Vomiting and regurgitation. In Kliegman RM (editor): *Practical Strategies in Pediatric Diagnosis and Therapy,* 2nd ed. Philadelphia, Elsevier. 2004, pp 291–321.
Orenstein SR, Shalaby TM, Barmada MM, et al: Genetics of gastroesophageal reflux disease: A review. *J Pediatr Gastroenterol Nutr* 2002;34:506–510.
Orenstein SR, Shalaby TM, Cohn JF: Reflux symptoms in 100 normal infants: Diagnostic validity of the infant gastroesophageal reflux questionnaire. *Clin Pediatr* 1996;35:607–614.
Rothman M, Orenstein SR, Kleinman L, et al: Development of a revised infant gastroesophageal reflux questionnaire. *Acta Gastroenterol Belgica* 2003:73 (presented at the Second European Pediatric Gastrointestinal Motility meeting, Bruges, Belgium, April 23–26, 2003).
Rudolph CD, Mazur LJ, Liptak GS, et al: Pediatric gastroesophageal reflux clinical practice guidelines: Guidelines for evaluation and treatment of gastroesophageal reflux in infants and children. *J Pediatr Gastroenterol Nutr* 2001;32:S1–S31.
Salvia G, De Vizia B, Manguso F, et al: Effect of intragastric volume and osmolality on mechanisms of gastroesophageal reflux in children with gastroesophageal reflux disease. *Am J Gastroenterol* 2001;96:1725–1732.
Thompson M, Fritscher-Ravens A, Hall S, et al: Endoluminal gastroplication in children with significant gastro-oesophageal reflux in disease. *Gut* 2004;53:1745–1750.
Willging JP, Thompson D: Pediatric FEESST: Fiberoptic endoscopic evaluation of swallowing with sensory testing. *Curr Gastroenterol Rep* 2005;7: 240–243.

320.1 • Complicanze della GERD

ESOFAGEE: ESOFAGITE E STENOSI, ESOFAGO DI BARRETT, ADENOCARCINOMA. L'esofagite si può manifestare con irritabilità, inarcamento della schiena e avversione al cibo nei bambini piccoli; dolore toracico o epigastrico nei bambini più grandi; e (raramente) ematemesi, anemia o sindrome di Sandifer a qualunque età. L'esofagite grave e prolungata porta alla formazione di stenosi, in genere localizzate nell'esofago distale, che a loro volta causano disfagia, richiedendo dilatazioni esofagee ripetute e spesso la fundoplicatio. L'esofagite a lungo termine predispone alla trasformazione metaplastica del normale epitelio squamoso esofageo in epitelio cilindrico intestinale, denominata **esofago di Barrett**, un precursore dell'adenocarcinoma esofageo. L'esofago di Barrett e l'adenocarcinoma colpiscono con maggiore frequenza i maschi bianchi e i soggetti che presentano sintomi da reflusso di maggiore durata, frequenza e gravità. Tale trasformazione aumenta con l'età fino a raggiungere un plateau nella quinta decade di vita; l'adenocarcinoma è quindi raro nell'infanzia. L'esofago di Barrett, raro nei bambini, deve essere sottoposto a biopsie periodiche di sorveglianza, terapia farmacologica aggressiva e fundoplicatio per le lesioni progressive.

NUTRIZIONALI. L'esofagite e il rigurgito possono essere così gravi da determinare deficit di crescita staturoponderale a causa dello scarso apporto calorico. Talvolta per il trattamento di tali carenze si rende necessaria la nutrizione enterale (nasogastrica o nasodigiunale, oppure percutanea gastrica o digiunale) o parenterale.

EXTRAESOFAGEE: PRESENTAZIONI RESPIRATORIE ("ATIPICHE"). La GERD dovrebbe essere compresa nella diagnosi differenziale dei bambini con sintomi otolaringoiatrici o respiratori inspiegati o refrattari. Essa può produrre sintomi respiratori per contatto diretto del contenuto gastrico refluito con il tratto respiratorio (aspirazione, penetrazione laringea o microaspirazione) oppure per interazioni riflesse tra l'esofago e il tratto respiratorio (che inducono chiusura della laringe o broncospasmo). Spesso avviene che la GERD e una malattia respiratoria primaria, come l'asma, interagiscano instaurando un circolo vizioso da cui entrambe risultano aggravate. Molti bambini con queste presentazioni extraesofagee non presentano i sintomi tipici della GERD, rendendo difficile la diagnosi. Queste presentazioni atipiche richiedono un approccio scrupoloso alla diagnosi differenziale che prenda in considerazione tutta una serie di malattie primitive otorinolaringoiatriche (infezioni, allergie, gocciolamento postnasale, eccessivo utilizzo della voce) e polmonari (asma, fibrosi cistica). La terapia per la GERD deve essere più intensa (solitamente includendo un PPI) e prolungata (di solito almeno 3-6 mesi). L'assistenza specialistica dal punto di vista della malattia respiratoria (otorinolaringoiatra, pneumologo) e della malattia da reflusso (gastroenterologo) è spesso necessaria per gli esami diagnostici specialistici e per l'ottimizzazione della terapia intensiva.

APNEA E STRIDOR. Tali presentazioni delle vie respiratorie superiori sono state collegate alla GERD in alcuni case report e studi epidemiologici; il nesso temporale tra questi sintomi e gli episodi di reflusso è stato dimostrato in alcuni pazienti mediante il monitoraggio del pH esofageo; una risposta positiva alla terapia per la GERD è di ulteriore aiuto in numerose casistiche. Uno studio condotto su 1400 bambini piccoli con apnea attribuiva alla GERD il 50% dei casi, ma altri studi non sono riusciti a dimostrare tale associazione. L'apnea dovuta a reflusso è in genere ostruttiva, a causa del laringospasmo, che può essere considerato un riflesso protettivo patologicamente intenso. I bambini piccoli con questo tipo di apnea vengono spesso posizionati in modo provocativo (supini o seduti in flessione), hanno appena mangiato e presentano segni di apnea ostruttiva con sforzi respiratori improduttivi. Lo stridor scatenato dal reflusso in genere si verifica in bambini anatomicamente predisposti (laringomalacia, micrognazia). Il croup spasmodico, una spaventosa ostruzione episodica delle vie aeree superiori, può essere una condizione analoga nei bambini più grandi. Lo studio del pH esofageo può non riuscire a stabilire una relazione tra queste manifestazioni e il reflusso, a causa del tamponamento del contenuto gastrico da parte del latte in formula e della natura episodica delle condizioni. Gli pneumogrammi possono non identificare l'apnea ostruttiva, se non sono appositamente concepiti per rilevare tale fenomeno mediante misurazione del flusso aereo nasale.

La **laringite da reflusso** e altre manifestazioni otorinolaringoiatriche possono essere attribuite alla GERD. Tra i sintomi citati vi sono **raucedine**, affaticamento della voce, schiarimento della gola, tosse cronica, faringite, sinusite, otite media e una sensazione di nodo. La scarsità di valutazioni ben controllate al riguardo contribuisce a far sì che tali associazioni vengano considerate con un certo scetticismo. Altri fattori di rischio che irritano i condotti respiratori superiori possono predisporre alcuni pazienti con GERD a presentarsi prevalentemente con questi sintomi.

Nel 50% circa dei bambini con **asma**, quest'ultima patologia risulta associata alla GERD, riscontro che contrasta con la prevalenza di ciascuna condizione a sé stante, osservabile nel 10% circa dei bambini. I pazienti pediatrici con asma in cui è più probabile che il fattore scatenante sia la GERD sono quelli con sintomi di malattia da reflusso, con asma refrattario o steroide-dipendente e con aggravamento notturno dell'asma. La valutazione endoscopica che evidenzia le sequele esofagee della GERD rappresenta uno stimolo a intraprendere la terapia aggressiva (alte dosi e durata di molti mesi) della GERD.

Le erosioni dentali costituiscono la lesione orale più comune della GERD, distinguendosi per la loro localizzazione sulla superficie linguale.

Bauman NM, Bishop WP, Sandler AD, et al: Value of pH probe testing in pediatric patients with extraesophageal manifestations of gastroesophageal reflux disease: A retrospective review. *Ann Otol Rhinol Laryngol* 2000; 109:18–24.

El-Serag HB, Gilger MA, Kuebeler M, et al: Extraesophageal associations of gastroesophageal reflux disease in children without neurologic defects. *Gastroenterology* 2001;121:1294–1299.

Fuloria M, Hiatt D, Dillard RG, et al: Gastroesophageal reflux in very low birth weight infants: Association with chronic lung disease and outcomes through 1 year of age. *J Perinatol* 2000;4:235–239.

Goldenhersh MJ, Ament M: Asthma and gastroesophageal reflux in infants and children. *Immunol Allergy Clin North Am* 2001;21:439–448.

Harding SM, Sontag SJ: Asthma and gastroesophageal reflux. *Am J Gastroenterol* 2000;95:S23–S32.

Irwin RS, Madison JM: Anatomical diagnostic protocol in evaluating chronic cough with specific reference to gastroesophageal reflux disease. *Am J Med* 2000;108:126S–130S.

Kimball AL, Carlton DP: Gastroesophageal reflux medications in the treatment of apnea in premature infants. *J Pediatr* 2001;138:355–360.

Linnett V, Seow WK: Dental erosion in children: A literature review. *Pediatr Dent* 2001;23:37–43.

Nostrant TT: Gastroesophageal reflux and laryngitis: A skeptic's view. *Am J Med* 2000;108:149S–152S.

Orenstein SR: Update on gastroesophageal reflux and respiratory disease in children: A review. *Can J Gastroenterol* 2000;14:131–135.

Rosbe KW, Kenna MA, Auerbach AD: Extraesophageal reflux in pediatric patients with upper respiratory symptoms. *Arch Otolaryngol Head Neck Surg* 2003;129:1213–1220.

Sacco O, Fregonese B, Silvestri M, et al: Bronchoalveolar lavage and esophageal pH monitoring data in children with "difficult to treat" respiratory symptoms. *Pediatr Pulmonol* 2000;30:313–319.

Suskind DL, Zeringue GP III, Kluka EA, et al: Gastroesophageal reflux and pediatric otolaryngologic disease: The role of anti-reflux surgery. *Arch Otolaryngol Head Neck Surg* 2001;127:511–514.

Capitolo 321 ■ Esofagite eosinofila ed esofagite non GERD

Susan Orenstein, John Peters, Seema Khan, Nader Youssef e Sunny Zaheed Hussain

ESOFAGITE EOSINOFILA. L'epitelio esofageo è infiltrato da eosinofili, tipicamente a una densità >15 per campo ad alto ingrandimento. I sintomi di presentazione comprendono vomito, dolore toracico o epigastrico e disfagia con occasionale arresto del cibo o stenosi. La maggior parte dei pazienti è di sesso maschile. L'età media alla diagnosi è di 7 anni (intervallo 1-17 anni) e la durata dei sintomi è di 3 anni. Spesso sono presenti atopia, associata ad allergie alimentari, eosinofilia periferica (≈50% dei pazienti) ed elevati livelli di immunoglobuline E (IgE). Dal punto di vista endoscopico, l'esofago ha un aspetto granulare, con solchi o configurazione ad anello (Fig. 321-1); l'istologia esofagea rivela eosinofilia. L'esofagite eosinofila si differenzia dalla malattia da reflusso gastroesofageo (GERD, *GastroEsophageal Reflux Disease*) per la generale assenza di esofagite erosiva, per la maggiore densità eosinofila e per la refrattarietà alle terapie antireflusso. Il **trattamento** si basa sulle diete di esclusione per i soggetti con allergie dimostrate, mentre i corticosteroidi inalati e sistemici sono stati utilizzati con successo per i soggetti non responder e per l'esofagite eosinofila non allergica ("primaria"). Tra le terapie allo studio vi sono gli inibitori del leucotrieni (montelukast) e l'anticorpo anti-interleuchina 5 (anti-IL5, mepolizumab). Poco si sa della storia naturale della malattia, ma sembra che, in assenza di trattamento, l'esofagite eosinofila possa portare alla formazione di stenosi.

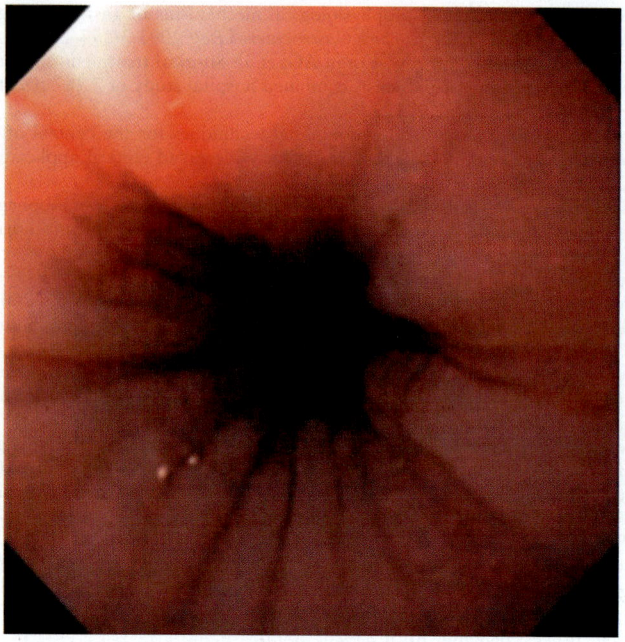

Figura 321-1. Immagine endoscopica dell'esofagite eosinofila.

ESOFAGITE INFETTIVA. L'esofagite infettiva, peraltro rara, colpisce con maggiore frequenza i bambini immunocompromessi; è causata da funghi come la *Candida* e la *Torulopsis glabrata*, da virus come l'herpes simplex e (raramente) da malattie batteriche, tra cui la difterite e la tubercolosi. I segni e i sintomi di presentazione tipica sono odinofagia, disfagia e dolore retrosternale, cui possono aggiungersi febbre, nausea e vomito. La candidosi esofagea, che comunemente (ma non sempre) si presenta sotto forma di infezione orofaringea concomitante, può colpire i pazienti pediatrici immunocompetenti e immunodepressi. Anche le infezioni virali esofagee possono presentarsi in ospiti immunocompetenti sotto forma di una malattia acuta febbrile. L'esofagite infettiva, come altre forme di esofagite infiammatoria, occasionalmente progredisce verso la stenosi esofagea. La diagnosi di esofagite infettiva viene posta mediante endoscopia ed esame istopatologico; l'aggiunta della reazione a catena della polimerasi (PCR, *Polymerase Chain Reaction*), della coltura tessuto-virus e dell'immunoistochimica aumenta la sensibilità diagnostica. Il trattamento si basa sull'uso di appropriati agenti antimicrobici, analgesici e antiacidi.

ESOFAGITE DA "PILLOLA". Si tratta di una lesione acuta causata dal contatto con un agente lesivo. Nello sviluppo di questa patologia sono stati implicati tetraciclina, cloruro di potassio, solfato ferroso e farmaci antinfiammatori, soprattutto se assunti sotto forma di compresse all'ora di andare a letto e con una quantità inadeguata di acqua. Tale prassi di frequente provoca un fastidio acuto, seguito da dolore retrosternale, odinofagia e disfagia; l'endoscopia mostra una lesione focale, comunemente localizzata in una delle regioni anatomiche stenotiche dell'esofago o a livello di un restringimento patologico non sospetto. La terapia è di supporto; anche se mancano dati che ne avvalorino l'efficacia, spesso si utilizzano antiacidi, anestetici topici e diete leggere o liquide.

Arora AS, Murray JA: Iatrogenic esophagitis. *Curr Gastroenterol Rep* 2000;2:224–229.

Diaz M, Leal N, Olivares P, et al: Infectious strictures requiring esophageal replacement in children. *J Pediatr Gastroenterol Nutr* 2001;32:611–613.

Khan S, Orenstein SR: Eosinophilic disorders of the gastrointestinal tract. In Feldman M, Friedman LS, Brandt LJ (editors): *Sleisinger & Fordtran's Gastrointestinal & Liver Disease,* 8th ed (in press).

Orenstein SR, Shalaby TM, Di Lorenzo C, et al: The spectrum of pediatric eosinophilic esophagitis beyond infancy: A clinical series of 30 children. *Am J Gastroenterol* 2000;95:1422–1430.

Ramanathan J, Rammouni M, Baran J Jr, et al: Herpes simplex virus esophagitis in the immunocompetent host: An overview. *Am J Gastroenterol* 2000;95:2171–2176.

Sant'Anna AM, Rolland S, Fournet JC, et al: Eosinophilic esophagitis in children: Symptoms, histology and pH probe results. *J Pediatr Gastroenterol Nutr* 2004;39:373–377.

Vodovnik A, Cerar A: Synchronous herpes simplex virus and cytomegalovirus esophagitis. *Z Gastroenterol* 2000;38:491–494.

Capitolo 322 ■ Perforazione esofagea

Susan Orenstein, John Peters, Seema Khan, Nader Youssef e Sunny Zaheed Hussain

La maggior parte delle perforazioni esofagee nei bambini è dovuta a trauma contusivo (incidenti automobilistici, ferite da arma da fuoco, abuso di minore) o è iatrogena. Il massaggio cardiaco, la manovra di Heimlich, il posizionamento del sondino nasogastrico, la laringoscopia traumatica o l'intubazione endotracheale, l'aspirazione postpartum troppo vigorosa delle vie aeree durante la rianimazione neonatale, la difficile endoscopia superiore, la scleroterapia delle varici esofagee e la dilatazione pneumatica per la terapia dell'acalasia sono stati tutti implicati. La rottura esofagea ha inoltre fatto seguito a vomito forzato nei pazienti con anoressia o ingestione di caustici.

La rottura spontanea dell'esofago (**sindrome di Boerhaave**), meno frequente, è associata ad aumenti improvvisi della pressione intraesofagea provocati da situazioni come vomito, tosse o sforzo durante la defecazione. Nei bambini e negli adulti la lacerazione interessa la parete esofagea laterale sinistra, poiché è a questo livello che si trova lo strato muscolare liscio; nei neonati (sindrome di Boerhaave neonatale) la rottura spontanea è a destra.

Tra i sintomi da perforazione esofagea vi sono dolore, dolorabilità al collo, disfagia, crepitio sottocutaneo, febbre e tachicardia; diversi pazienti con perforazioni cervicali hanno presentato polidipsia da acqua fredda, nel tentativo di alleviare il dolore alla gola. Le perforazioni a carico dell'esofago toracico prossimale tendono a creare segni (pneumotorace, versamenti) nel torace sinistro, mentre i segni delle lacerazioni distali sono più spesso a destra. Le radiografie del rachide cervicale e del torace, che mostrano ingrandimento mediastinico o aria libera paracervicale, sono spesso diagnostiche. Se le lastre radiografiche risultassero normali, si dovrebbe effettuare un esofagogramma con mezzo di contrasto idrosolubile, nonostante meno del 30% delle perforazioni cervicali sfugga a questa indagine. Pertanto, un esofagogramma con mezzo di contrasto idrosolubile negativo dovrebbe essere seguito da uno studio con bario; la maggiore densità del mezzo di contrasto permette di visualizzare meglio un difetto di piccole dimensioni, seppure con un maggiore rischio di mediastinite infiammatoria. L'endoscopia, che può anch'essa rivelarsi utile, porta con sé un tasso di falsi negativi del 30%. Nei casi difficili si può ricorrere alla TC del torace.

Il trattamento deve essere personalizzato. Se le piccole lacerazioni e la minima contaminazione mediastinica possono essere trattate in modo conservativo, con antibiotici ad ampio spettro, intervento chirurgico, "nulla per bocca", drenaggio gastrico e nutrizione parenterale, per la maggior parte delle perforazioni esofagee pediatriche si rende necessario il trattamento chirurgico.

Capitolo 323 ■ Varici esofagee

Susan Orenstein

L'ipertensione portale viene definita come un aumento della pressione venosa portale superiore a 10-12 mmHg rispetto alle pressioni normalmente presenti nella vena cava inferiore (vedi Capitolo 364). La decompressione di questa ipertensione attraverso la circolazione collaterale portosistemica mediante la vena coronaria, in associazione alla vena gastrica sinistra, dà origine alle varici esofagee. Queste ultime nella maggior parte dei casi sono "varici ascendenti"; quelle che originano in assenza di ipertensione portale e in caso di ostruzione della vena cava superiore, meno comuni, sono invece denominate "varici discendenti". Il loro trattamento è rivolto alla causa sottostante dell'anomalia della vena cava superiore. L'emorragia da varici esofagee è la principale causa di morbilità e mortalità da ipertensione portale. La presentazione è con ematemesi e melena significative; anche se la maggior parte dei pazienti presenta epatopatia, è possibile che alcuni bambini con patologie come la trombosi venosa portale extraepatica siano stati precedentemente asintomatici. Di fronte a ogni bambino con ematemesi e splenomegalia si dovrebbe supporre un'emorragia da varici esofagee fino a prova contraria.

Occasionalmente è possibile visualizzare le varici tramite esame fluoroscopico con mezzo di contrasto, anche se si preferisce ricorrere all'endoscopia superiore in quanto consente sia la diagnosi definitiva sia la terapia per gli episodi acuti di sanguinamento mediante la scleroterapia o la legatura a banda.

Il trattamento dei bambini con varici mediante scleroterapia profilattica, allo scopo di prevenire una prima emorragia, può ridurre l'incidenza dell'emorragia esofagea. I pazienti trattati possono sanguinare per gastropatia congestizia e non è riscontrabile alcun miglioramento nel tasso di sopravvivenza. Anche i β-bloccanti non selettivi, come propranololo, sono stati utilizzati per prevenire il sanguinamento da varici. La legatura endoscopica delle varici negli adulti riduce il rischio di un primo sanguinamento rispetto ai controlli non trattati e ai pazienti trattati con β-bloccanti; la diminuzione della mortalità si nota solo rispetto al gruppo di controllo (vedi Capitolo 364).

Goncalves ME, Cardoso SR, Maksoud JG: Prophylactic sclerotherapy in children with esophageal varices: Long-term results of a controlled prospective randomized trial. *J Pediatr Surg* 2000;35:401–405.

Imperiale TF, Chalasani N: A meta-analysis of endoscopic variceal ligation for primary prophylaxis of esophageal variceal bleeding. *Hepatology* 2001; 33:1003–1004.

Capitolo 324 ■ Ingestione di sostanze

Susan Orenstein

324.1 • Corpi estranei nell'esofago

La maggior parte (80%) dei casi di ingestione di corpi estranei si verifica nei bambini, per lo più di età compresa fra 3 mesi e 6 anni. Particolarmente a rischio sono anche i ragazzi con ritardi dello sviluppo e quelli con malattie psichiatriche. Le monete e le piccole componenti dei giocattoli sono i corpi estranei più comunemente ingeriti. Gli arresti di cibo sono meno comuni nei bambini che negli adulti e di solito si verificano nei soggetti con un'anomalia strutturale sottostante o un disturbo della motilità, come dopo riparazione dell'atresia esofagea o in presenza di esofagite eosinofila. La maggior parte dei corpi estranei esofagei si ferma a livello del cricofaringe (sfintere esofageo superiore), dell'arco aortico o appena al di sopra del diaframma, in corrispondenza della giunzione gastroesofagea (sfintere esofageo inferiore).

Almeno il 30% dei bambini con corpi estranei esofagei può essere totalmente asintomatico, per cui ogni storia di ingestione di corpi estranei dovrebbe essere presa in seria considerazione e indagata. Un primo attacco di soffocamento, con conati di vomito e tosse, può essere seguito da eccessiva salivazione, disfagia, rifiuto del cibo, emesi o dolore al collo, alla gola o alle regioni dell'incisura sternale. Se il corpo estraneo urta contro la laringe o la parete tracheale posteriore, membranosa, si possono riscontrare sintomi respiratori come stridor, respiro affannoso, cianosi o dispnea. Edema, eritema o crepitii sottocutanei a livello cervicale suggeriscono la perforazione dell'orofaringe o dell'esofago prossimale.

La valutazione del bambino con una storia di ingestione di corpi estranei inizia con le radiografie dirette anteroposteriori del collo, del torace e dell'addome, assieme alle proiezioni laterali del collo e del torace. La superficie piana di una moneta nell'esofago viene osservata in proiezione anteroposteriore, mentre il bordo è visualizzabile in proiezione laterale (Fig. 324-1). Il contrario vale per le monete conficcate nella trachea: a questo livello il bordo viene osservato in proiezione anteroposteriore e il lato piano in proiezione laterale. I materiali come la plastica, il legno, il vetro, l'alluminio e le ossa possono essere radiotrasparenti; la mancata visualizzazione dell'oggetto alle radiografie dirette in un paziente sintomatico giustifica l'endoscopia d'urgenza. Sebbene gli studi con mezzo di contrasto baritato possano essere utili nel paziente asintomatico occasionale con radiografie dirette negative, il loro utilizzo deve essere scoraggiato per la possibilità di aspirazione e per il rischio di rendere più difficoltosa la successiva visualizzazione e rimozione dell'oggetto.

Di solito il **trattamento** si basa sulla visualizzazione endoscopica dell'oggetto e della mucosa sottostante, con successiva rimozione del corpo estraneo; l'endoscopia terapeutica viene realizzata più conservativamente con un tubo endotracheale che protegge le vie aeree. Oggetti appuntiti nell'esofago, batterie a disco o corpi estranei associati a sintomi respiratori rendono obbligatoria la rimozione d'urgenza. Le batterie a disco, in particolare, devono essere rimosse con particolare tempestività, in quanto possono danneggiare la mucosa nel giro di un'ora e tutti gli strati esofagei entro 4 ore. Oggetti smussi e monete localizzati nell'esofago, in assenza di sintomi, si possono osservare fino a 24 ore prima del loro passaggio nello stomaco. Se non vi sono problemi di gestione delle secrezioni, si osserva un arresto del bolo carneo per un lasso di tempo che può raggiungere le 12 ore. Nei pazienti che non sono stati sottoposti in precedenza a interventi chirurgici esofagei, talvolta il glucagone (0,05 mg/kg ev) può essere utile per facilitare la progressione dei boli alimentari dell'esofago distale riducendo la pressione dello sfintere esofageo inferiore. L'uso di agenti che rendono tenera la carne o che formano gas può portare a perforazione e non è quindi raccomandato. Una tecnica alternativa per la rimozione delle monete conficcate nell'esofago da meno di 24 ore, che per maggiore sicurezza deve essere affidata a radiologi esperti, consiste nell'introdurre un catetere di Foley oltre la moneta sotto fluoroscopia, gonfiare il palloncino e quindi tirare indietro simultaneamente il catetere e la moneta, con il paziente in posizione prona obliqua. Preoccupazioni relative all'impossibilità di visualizzare direttamente la mucosa e, quando non si usa l'intubazione endotracheale, l'assenza di protezione delle vie aeree suggeriscono cautela nell'uso di questa tecnica.

Kay M, Wyllie R: Pediatric foreign bodies and their management. *Curr Gastroenterol Rep* 2005;7:212–218.

324.2 • Ingestione di caustici

L'ingestione di sostanze caustiche porta a esofagite, necrosi, perforazione e formazione di stenosi (vedi Capitolo 58). La maggior parte dei casi (70%) è costituita da ingestioni accidentali di alcali

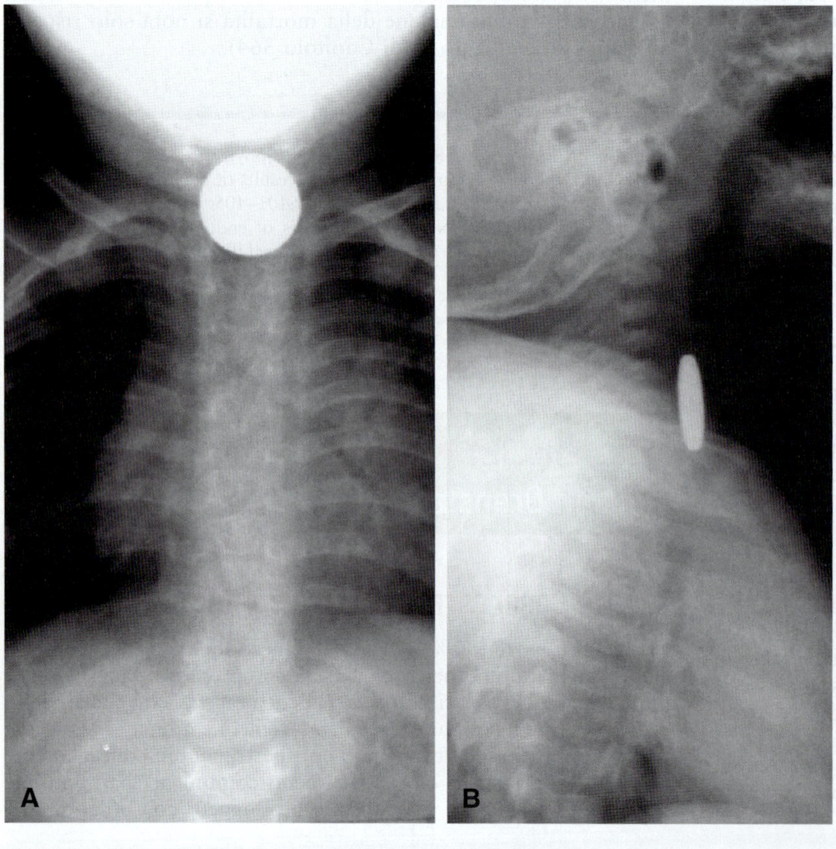

Figura 324-1. Radiografie di una moneta nell'esofago. Quando i corpi estranei si fermano a questo livello, la superficie piatta dell'oggetto viene osservata in proiezione anteroposteriore (*A*), mentre il bordo è visibile in proiezione laterale (*B*). Per gli oggetti che si fermano nella trachea si verifica il contrario. (Per gentile concessione di Beverley Newman.)

liquidi che producono necrosi liquefattiva grave, profonda; i disgorganti dei tubi di scarico sono i più comuni; essendo insapori, vengono ingeriti in grandi quantità. Le **sostanze acide** (20% dei casi) invece, essendo più amare, vengono ingerite in quantità inferiore; oltre a produrre necrosi coagulativa e un'escara spessa, alquanto protettiva, esse possono provocare gastrite grave, mentre gli acidi volatili possono determinare sintomi respiratori. L'ingestione di caustici produce segni e sintomi come vomito, scialorrea, rifiuto dei liquidi, ustioni orali, disfagia, dolore addominale e stridor. Il 20% dei pazienti sviluppa stenosi esofagee. L'assenza di lesioni orofaringee non esclude la possibilità di significative lesioni esofagogastriche, che possono portare a perforazione o stenosi. La mancanza di sintomi solitamente è associata a lesioni minime o assenti; al contrario, l'ematemesi, il distress respiratorio e la presenza di almeno tre sintomi sono predittivi di lesioni gravi. L'endoscopia superiore, raccomandata come il metodo più efficace per la rapida valutazione del danno tissutale, deve essere effettuata in tutti i bambini sintomatici. Come trattamento acuto si raccomanda la diluizione con acqua o latte, mentre la neutralizzazione, l'emesi indotta e il lavaggio gastrico sono controindicati. Il trattamento dipende dalla gravità e dall'estensione della lesione. Il rischio di stenosi è aumentato in caso di ulcerazioni circonferenziali, con placche e perdita della mucosa; tali lesioni possono rendere necessario il trattamento con dilatazione, mentre in alcuni gravi casi occorre procedere alla resezione chirurgica e all'interposizione del colon o dell'intestino tenue. Gli stent di silicone (autoespandenti), posizionati endoscopicamente dopo una procedura di dilatazione, possono essere un approccio alternativo e conservativo al trattamento delle stenosi. Sono stati riportati rari casi tardivi di carcinoma esofageo sovrapposto.

Gupta SK, Croffie JM, Fitzgerald JF: Is esophagogastroduodenoscopy necessary in all caustic ingestions? *J Pediatr Gastroenterol Nutr* 2001;32:50–53.

Broto J, Asensio M, Vernet JMG: Results of a new technique in the treatment of severe esophageal stenosis in children: Poliflex stents. *J Pediatr Gastroenterol Nutr* 2003;37:203–206.

de Jong AL, Macdonald R, Ein S, et al: Corrosive esophagitis in children: A 30-year review. *Int J Pediatr Otorhinolaryngol* 2001;57:203–211.

Sezione 4 — Stomaco e intestino

Capitolo 325 ■ Sviluppo, struttura e funzioni normali Robert Wyllie

SVILUPPO. L'intestino primitivo, che diventa riconoscibile a partire dalla 4ª settimana di gestazione, risulta composto dall'intestino anteriore, dall'intestino medio e dall'intestino posteriore. L'**intestino anteriore** dà origine al tratto gastrointestinale superiore, che comprende l'esofago, lo stomaco e il duodeno fino all'inserzione del dotto epatico comune. L'**intestino medio** dà origine alla restante parte dell'intestino tenue e del crasso fino alla prima metà del colon traverso. A partire dall'**intestino posteriore** si formano la parte rimanente del colon e il canale anale prossimale. Nel corso dello sviluppo fetale, la rapida crescita dell'intestino medio ne provoca la protrusione al di fuori della cavità addominale attraverso l'anello ombelicale. Successivamente esso ritorna nella cavità peritoneale e ruota in senso antiorario finché il cieco non si localizza nel quadrante addominale inferiore destro. Questo processo di norma risulta completato entro l'8ª settimana di gestazione. Il fegato origina dal diverticolo epatico, dal quale si sviluppano le cellule parenchimali, i dotti biliari, le strutture vascolari e le cellule ematopoietiche e di Kupffer. I dotti biliari extraepatici e la colecisti iniziano a svilupparsi come cordoni solidi, che poi si canalizzano entro il 3° mese di gestazione. Gli abbozzi pancreatici dorsale e ventrale si sviluppano a partire dall'intestino anteriore entro la 4ª settimana di gestazione e si fondono entro la 6ª. La funzione secretoria esocrina è presente a partire dal 5° mese. Sequenze genomiche *cis*-regolatorie controllano l'espressione genica durante lo sviluppo. I moduli di queste sequenze *cis* sono collegati tra loro e realizzano una cascata di regolazione genica che controlla lo sviluppo funzionale. Anche alcuni fattori estrinseci sono in grado di influenzare l'espressione genica. A livello dell'intestino l'espressione genica è condizionata da numerosi fattori di crescita, tra cui il fattore β, il fattore simil-insulinico e quelli presenti nel colostro umano (fattore di crescita umano ed epidermico).

La propulsione del cibo lungo il tratto gastrointestinale avviene grazie all'azione coordinata dei muscoli della parete intestinale. Le contrazioni sono regolate dal sistema nervoso enterico sotto l'influsso di vari peptidi e ormoni. Il sistema nervoso enterico deriva dalle cellule della cresta neurale che migrano in senso craniocaudale; tale migrazione del tessuto della cresta neurale risulta completata entro la 24ª settimana di gestazione; la sua interruzione causa la **malattia di Hirschsprung**. I pattern motori intestinali del neonato sono diversi da quelli dell'adulto. La motilità gastrointestinale alta a digiuno è normalmente caratterizzata da un pattern trifasico, noto come complesso motorio migrante. Quest'ultimo è di riscontro meno frequente nei neonati, che presentano un'attività fasica non migrante, responsabile di una propulsione inefficace, soprattutto nei prematuri. La motilità post-prandiale consiste di una serie di contrazioni anulari che si propagano caudalmente per distanze variabili.

DIGESTIONE E ASSORBIMENTO. La parete dello stomaco, dell'intestino tenue e del colon è costituita da quattro strati: mucosa, sottomucosa, strato muscolare e sierosa. L'85% della mucosa gastrica è rivestito da ghiandole ossintiche, che contengono cellule secernenti acido cloridrico, pepsinogeno e fattore intrinseco, e cellule mucose ed endocrine, che secernono peptidi con funzioni paracrine ed endocrine. Il pepsinogeno è il precursore dell'enzima proteolitico pepsina e il fattore intrinseco è necessario per l'assorbimento della vitamina B_{12}. Le ghiandole piloriche, localizzate nell'antro, contengono cellule secernenti gastrina. La produzione di acido e i livelli di gastrina sono inversamente correlati tra loro, tranne che negli stati secretori patologici. La secrezione di acido è bassa alla nascita, ma aumenta notevolmente nell'arco di 24 ore. La secrezione di acido e pepsina raggiunge un picco nei primi 10 giorni, per poi diminuire tra i 10 e i 30 giorni dopo la nascita. La secrezione di fattore intrinseco aumenta lentamente nelle prime due settimane di vita.

L'intestino tenue, che nel neonato a termine misura circa 270 cm, raggiunge la lunghezza di 450-550 cm, propria dell'adulto, entro il quarto anno di età. La sua mucosa è costituita da villi, protrusioni digitiformi della mucosa nel lume intestinale che espandono significativamente la superficie di assorbimento. La superficie mucosa risulta ulteriormente espansa da un orletto a spazzola che contiene enzimi digestivi e meccanismi di trasporto per i monosaccaridi, gli aminoacidi, i dipeptidi, i tripeptidi e i grassi. Le cellule dei villi originano da cripte adiacenti a essi e diventano funzionali quando migrano da queste ai villi. La mucosa dell'intestino tenue si rinnova nel giro di 4-5 giorni, grazie a un meccanismo di riparazione rapida di eventuali danni; nei bambini molto piccoli o malnutriti, tuttavia, questo processo può essere ritardato. Inoltre, le cellule delle cripte secernono fluidi ed elettroliti. I villi si sviluppano nel duodeno entro l'8ª settimana di gestazione e nell'ileo entro l'11ª. L'attività della disaccaridasi risulta misurabile a partire dalla 12ª settimana, ma quella della lattasi non raggiunge i suoi livelli massimi prima della 36ª. In genere, tuttavia, anche i neonati prematuri tollerano il latte artificiale contenente lattosio grazie al recupero dei carboidrati da parte dei batteri colici. Nelle popolazioni asiatiche e africane i livelli di lattasi possono cominciare a scendere dopo il quarto anno di età, provocando un'intolleranza al latte dei mammiferi. I meccanismi di digestione e assorbimento delle proteine, compresi gli enzimi pancreatici e i meccanismi di trasporto degli aminoacidi, dei dipeptidi e dei tripeptidi attraverso la mucosa, sono attivi entro la 20ª settimana di gestazione. I carboidrati, le proteine e i grassi vengono normalmente assorbiti nella metà superiore dell'intestino tenue, mentre i segmenti più distali rappresentano un'ampia riserva di capacità assorbitiva. La maggior parte del sodio, del potassio, del cloro e dell'acqua viene assorbita nell'intestino tenue. L'assorbimento selettivo dei sali biliari e della vitamina B_{12} avviene nell'ileo distale, mentre quello del ferro si verifica nel duodeno e nel digiuno prossimale. La digestione intraluminale dipende dal pancreas esocrino. Secretina e colecistochinina stimolano la sintesi e la secrezione di bicarbonato ed enzimi digestivi, che vengono rilasciati dalla mucosa dell'intestino prossimale in risposta a vari stimoli intraluminali, tra i quali i componenti della dieta.

La **digestione dei carboidrati** rappresenta solitamente un processo molto efficiente, che viene completato nel duodeno distale. Gli amidi vengono scissi in glucosio, oligosaccaridi e disaccaridi dall'amilasi pancreatica. I polimeri di glucosio residui subiscono un'ulteriore scissione a livello della mucosa a opera della glucoamilasi. Il lattosio viene scisso a livello dell'orletto a spazzola dalla lattasi, dando luogo al glucosio e al galattosio, mentre il saccarosio viene scisso dalla saccarasi isomaltasi in fruttosio e glucosio. Il trasporto all'interno della cellula di galattosio e il glucosio avviene principalmente tramite un processo sodio- ed energia-dipendente, mentre quello del fruttosio si verifica per diffusione facilitata.

Le **proteine** vengono idrolizzate dagli enzimi pancreatici, tra cui tripsina, chimotripsina, elastasi e carbossipeptidasi, ad aminoacidi singoli e oligopeptidi. Gli enzimi pancreatici vengono secreti come proenzimi, destinati a essere attivati tramite il rilascio di un enzima della mucosa detto enterochinasi. Gli oligopeptidi vengono ulteriormente scissi in dipeptidi, tripeptidi e aminoacidi a livello dell'orletto a spazzola da parte delle peptidasi. Le proteine possono entrare nella cellula grazie a trasportatori non competitivi specifici, che possono veicolare aminoacidi singoli o dipeptidi e tripeptidi, analoghi a quelli del tubulo renale. L'intestino umano nelle prima settimana di vita può assorbire proteine antigeniche intatte a causa della "lassità" delle giunzioni tra gli enterociti. L'ingresso di potenziali antigeni proteici attraverso la barriera mucosa potrebbe avere un ruolo nel successivo sviluppo dei disturbi indotti da alimenti o microrganismi.

L'**assorbimento dei grassi** avviene in due fasi. I trigliceridi della dieta vengono scissi dalla lipasi e dalla colipasi pancreatiche in monogliceridi e acidi grassi liberi; questi ultimi, una volta emulsionati dai sali biliari, a formare micelle di fosfolipidi e altre sostanze liposolubili, vengono trasportati fino alla membrana cellulare, dove avviene l'assorbimento. I grassi vengono riesterificati negli enterociti formando i chilomicroni, che giungono al dotto toracico attraverso i vasi linfatici intestinali. Più efficiente è l'assorbimento dei grassi a catena media, che possono entrare direttamente nella cellula. Essi vengono successivamente trasportati al fegato attraverso il sistema portale. L'assorbimento dei grassi può subire alterazioni in qualunque fase della digestione e del processo assorbitivo: nella fibrosi cistica si può verificare una riduzione degli enzimi pancreatici, le epatopatie colestatiche riducono la produzione di sali biliari e la formazione di micelle, la malattia celiaca può alterare la superficie mucosa, una formazione anomala di chilomicroni si verifica nell'abetalipoproteinemia e la linfangectasia intestinale altera il trasporto dei chilomicroni.

L'assorbimento dei grassi è meno efficiente nel neonato rispetto all'adulto. I neonati prematuri possono perdere fino al 20% delle calorie fornite dai grassi, rispetto a ≤6% dell'adulto. A ciò contribuiscono fattori come la ridotta sintesi di acidi biliari e lipasi pancreatica e la minore efficienza dell'assorbimento ileale. Nei neonati la digestione dei grassi è facilitata dalle lipasi linguali e gastriche. La lipasi del latte umano, che viene stimolata dai sali biliari, aumenta l'azione della lipasi pancreatica. Per alimentare i neonati con malassorbimento dei grassi solitamente si ricorre a latti artificiali con una percentuale più alta di trigliceridi a catena media, che vengono assorbiti indipendentemente dai sali biliari.

Il colon è un tubo di 75-100 cm con aspetto sacculato per via di tre strie di muscolatura longitudinale denominate *taeniae coli*, che ne percorrono l'intera lunghezza dividendo la mucosa in austrature. Austrature e tenie compaiono entro la 12ª settimana di gestazione. L'attività motoria più comune nel colon è la segmentazione ritmica non propulsiva, che serve a mescolare il chimo e a esporre il contenuto luminale alla mucosa colica. Tipicamente si verificano dei movimenti di massa all'interno del colon dopo il pasto. Il colon assorbe altra acqua ed elettroliti dal contenuto luminale per rendere le feci parzialmente o completamente solide. oltre a eliminare i sottoprodotti della degradazione batterica dei carboidrati. Le feci ristagnano nel retto finché la sua distensione stimola il riflesso della defecazione che, se accompagnato dal rilasciamento volontario dello sfintere esterno, consente l'evacuazione.

Capitolo 326 ■ Stenosi pilorica e anomalie congenite dello stomaco

Robert Wyllie

Il segno distintivo dell'ostruzione gastrica è il vomito non biliare; tra gli altri sintomi figurano il dolore addominale e la nausea. I segni dell'ostruzione dello svuotamento gastrico comprendono la distensione addominale e il sanguinamento da infiammazioni secondarie della mucosa gastrica o esofagea.

La causa più comune di vomito non biliare è la stenosi ipertrofica del piloro tipica dei neonati. Sintomi analoghi possono essere associati a varie altre malformazioni gastriche, tra cui l'atresia pilorica, le membrane antrali, le duplicazioni e i volvoli gastrici. La diagnosi differenziale comprende inoltre il reflusso gastroesofageo, l'ulcera peptica, la sindrome adrenogenitale con perdita di sali, la gastroenterite eosinofila, i bezoari e diverse altre anomalie del metabolismo e della motilità.

326.1 • Stenosi ipertrofica del piloro

La stenosi ipertrofica del piloro colpisce 1-3 neonati su 1000 negli Stati Uniti. È più comune tra i bianchi con antenati provenienti dal Nord Europa, meno comune negli afroamericani e rara negli asiatici. I maschi (specialmente i primogeniti) vengono colpiti quattro volte più delle femmine. I figli di madri, e in misura minore di padri, con una stenosi pilorica presentano un rischio elevato di sviluppare questa patologia. Essa infatti si sviluppa nel 20% circa dei figli maschi e nel 10% delle figlie femmine di madri affette. L'incidenza di stenosi pilorica risulta aumentata nei neonati con gruppo sanguigno B e 0. La stenosi pilorica è associata con altri difetti congeniti, tra cui la fistola tracheoesofagea e l'ipoplasia o l'agenesia del frenulo labiale inferiore.

EZIOLOGIA. La causa della stenosi pilorica non è conosciuta, ma sono stati implicati numerosi fattori. La condizione non è solitamente presente alla nascita e presenta una concordanza maggiore tra i gemelli monozigoti rispetto a quelli dizigoti. Rara nei feti nati morti, probabilmente si sviluppa dopo la nascita. È stata associata con la gastroenterite eosinofila, le sindromi di Apert e di Zellweger, la trisomia 18, le sindromi di Smith-Lemli-Opitz e di Cornelia de Lange. Inoltre, è stata evidenziata un'associazione variabile con l'eritromicina somministrata nei neonati per la profilassi della pertosse dopo esposizione. Sono stati implicati un'innervazione muscolare anomala, livelli sierici elevati di prostaglandine e l'ipergastrinemia nel neonato. Sono stati evidenziati dei livelli ridotti di nitrossido sintetasi pilorica con un'alterata espressione della regione regolatoria 1c dell'esone della nitrossidosintetasi neuronale (*neuronal Nitric Oxide Synthase*, nNOS), che influenza l'espressione del gene nNOS. La riduzione dell'ossido nitrico potrebbe contribuire alla patogenesi della stenosi pilorica.

MANIFESTAZIONI CLINICHE. Il vomito non biliare, che rappresenta il sintomo di esordio della stenosi pilorica, all'inizio può essere o meno proiettivo, ma di solito è progressivo e si verifica immediatamente dopo il pasto. Può far seguito a ogni pasto oppure essere intermittente. In genere compare dopo la 3ª settimana di vita, ma i sintomi possono manifestarsi anche nella 1ª e fino al 5° mese. Dopo il vomito, il neonato è affamato e desidera mangiare di nuovo. Se il disturbo persiste, la perdita progressiva di fluidi, idrogenioni e cloro provoca un'alcalosi metabolica ipocloremica. I livelli sierici di potassio vengono solitamente mantenuti, ma può verificarsi anche un deficit del potassio corporeo totale. Grazie a una maggiore attenzione verso i sintomi della stenosi pilorica, ora è possibile l'identificazione precoce dei pazienti con gradi più lievi di malnutrizione cronica o disidratazione severa.

L'ittero, associato alla riduzione dei livelli di glucuroniltransferasi, si osserva nel 5% circa dei neonati affetti. L'iperbilirubinemia indiretta in genere si risolve in breve tempo, una volta eliminata l'ostruzione.

Tradizionalmente, la **diagnosi** si effettua palpando la massa pilorica, che risulta solida, mobile, della lunghezza di circa 2 cm, a forma di oliva, dura, meglio palpabile dal fianco sinistro e localizzata al di sopra e a destra dell'ombelico, nell'epigastrio medio, al di sotto del margine epatico. Nei neonati sani la somministrazione del pasto può essere d'aiuto per la diagnosi, perché permette di osservare un'onda peristaltica gastrica che attraversa l'addome (Fig. 326-1). Dopo il vomito la muscolatura addominale è più rilassata e l'"oliva" più facile da palpare. Per agevolare la visita si può ricorrere alla sedazione, che tuttavia non è di solito necessaria. Un esaminatore esperto è in grado di porre diagnosi clinicamente nel 60-80% dei casi.

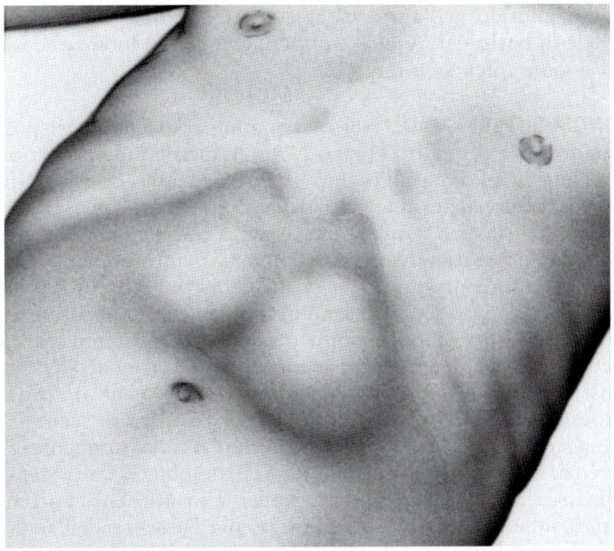

Figura 326-1. Onda peristaltica gastrica in un neonato con stenosi pilorica.

L'esame ecografico funge da conferma nella maggior parte dei casi e consente una diagnosi precoce nei neonati sospetti, ma che non presentano una massa pilorica all'esame obiettivo. I criteri diagnostici comprendono uno spessore del piloro >4 mm o una lunghezza complessiva >14 mm (Fig. 326-2). L'ecografia presenta una sensibilità del 95% circa. L'esame con mezzo di contrasto evidenzia un canale pilorico allungato, una protuberanza del

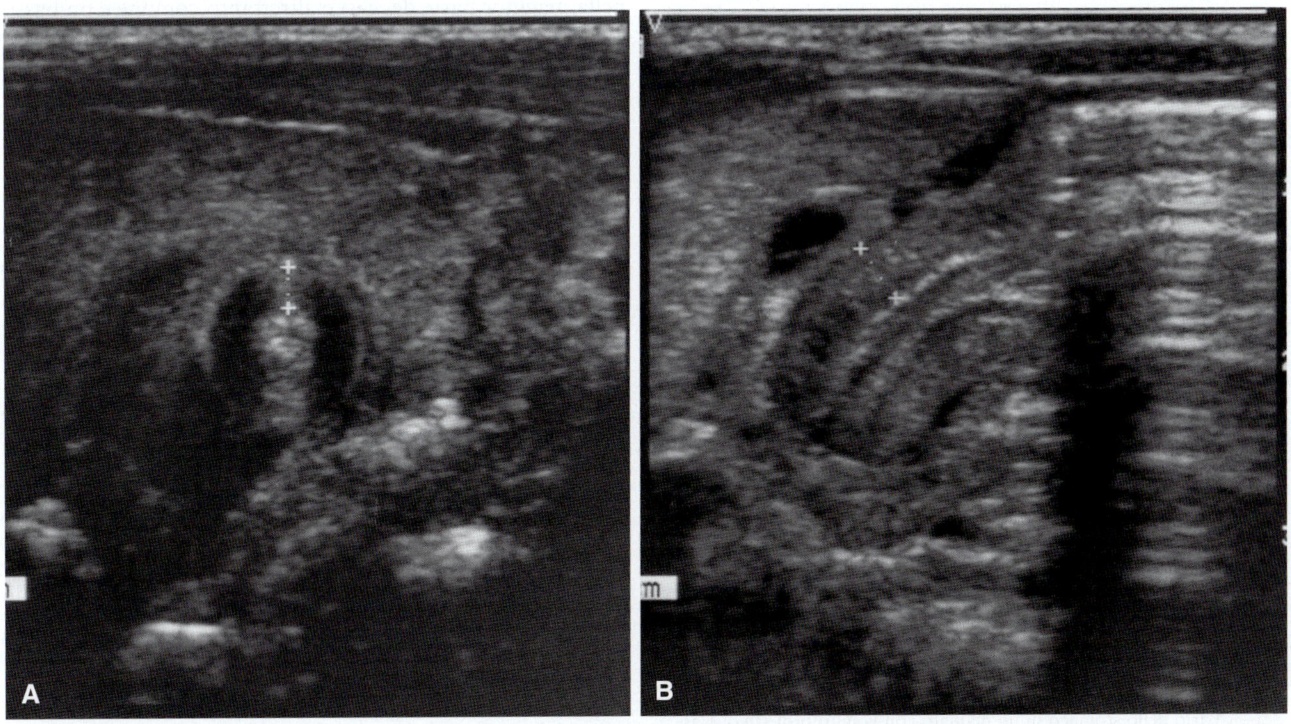

Figura 326-2. *A*, Scansione ecografica trasversale che mostra una parete muscolare pilorica spessa >4 mm (distanza tra le due crocette). *B*, Immagine orizzontale che mostra un canale pilorico lungo >14 mm (spessore della parete evidenziato dalle due crocette) in un neonato con stenosi pilorica.

muscolo pilorico nell'antro (il cosiddetto *shoulder sign*) e strie parallele di bario nel canale stenotico, che danno luogo al cosiddetto *double track sign* (Fig. 326-3).

DIAGNOSI DIFFERENZIALE. Nei casi comuni possono essere poste la diagnosi per il quadro clinico caratteristico e l'identificazione di una massa pilorica all'esame obiettivo o all'ecografia. I neonati eccezionalmente reattivi agli stimoli esterni, quelli nutriti da persone ansiose o con poca esperienza o quelli che non hanno stabilito un adeguato rapporto con la madre possono avere frequenti episodi di vomito nelle prime settimane di vita. Tali soggetti possono presentare caratteristiche che fanno pensare alla stenosi pilorica, poiché il vomito può essere persistente e anche proiettivo. Occasionalmente nei neonati piccoli ed emaciati, senza stenosi pilorica, sono visibili onde gastriche. Anche il reflusso gastroesofageo, con o senza ernia iatale, può venire scambiato per una stenosi pilorica, nonostante questo accada raramente. Per differenziare la malattia da reflusso gastroesofageo dalla stenosi pilorica si ricorre agli studi radiografici. L'insufficienza surrenalica può simulare una stenosi pilorica, ma l'assenza dell'acidosi metabolica e delle elevate concentrazioni sieriche di potassio e urinarie di sodio, tipiche della prima, sono d'aiuto nella diagnosi differenziale. Le alterazioni congenite del metabolismo possono provocare un'emesi ricorrente con alcalosi (ciclo dell'urea) o acidosi (acidemia organica) e letargia, coma o convulsioni. Il vomito con diarrea è suggestivo di gastroenterite, ma anche i pazienti con stenosi pilorica occasionalmente presentano diarrea. È raro che una membrana o una duplicazione pilorica determinino un vomito proiettivo, una peristalsi visibile e, nel caso della duplicazione, una massa palpabile. La stenosi duodenale prossimale all'ampolla di Vater può presentare le caratteristiche cliniche della stenosi pilorica, dalla quale tuttavia si differenzia per la presenza della massa pilorica all'esame obiettivo o all'ecografia.

TRATTAMENTO. Il trattamento preoperatorio è finalizzato a correggere le perdite di liquidi ed elettroliti e a ripristinare l'equilibrio acido-base. La somministrazione endovenosa di liquidi viene iniziata con una soluzione salina allo 0,45-0,9%, in 5-10% di destrosio, con l'aggiunta di cloruro di potassio alla concentrazione di 30-50 mEq/l. La somministrazione di liquidi dovrebbe essere continuata fino a ottenere la reidratazione del neonato e una concentrazione di bicarbonato è <30 mEq/l, segno che l'alcalosi è stata corretta. La correzione dell'alcalosi è essenziale per prevenire l'apnea postoperatoria che può essere associata con l'anestesia. La maggior parte dei neonati può essere efficacemente reidratata entro 24 ore. Il vomito in genere si interrompe quando lo stomaco è vuoto, e solo in rari casi è necessaria l'aspirazione nasogastrica.

La **procedura chirurgica di scelta** è la pilorotomia. Il tradizionale intervento di Ramstedt comporta una breve incisione cutanea trasversale; la sottostante massa pilorica viene sezionata senza incidere la mucosa e l'incisione viene richiusa. La tecnica laparoscopica è altrettanto efficace. Un vomito postoperatorio, che si verifica nella metà dei neonati, viene ritenuto secondario all'edema del piloro nella sede dell'incisione. Nella maggior parte dei neonati, tuttavia, l'alimentazione può essere iniziata entro le prime 12-24 ore dall'intervento chirurgico e continuata con il mantenimento per via orale entro le 36-48 ore. La persistenza del vomito suggerisce una pilorotomia incompleta, una gastrite, un reflusso gastroesofageo oppure una diversa causa di ostruzione.

Il trattamento chirurgico della stenosi pilorica è curativo, con una mortalità operatoria dello 0-0,5%. La terapia medica conservativa, che consiste in pasti piccoli e frequenti e nella somministrazione di atropina, si è rivelata efficace in un piccolo gruppo di pazienti. La dilatazione endoscopica con palloncino è risultata efficace nei neonati con vomito persistente dovuto a una pilorotomia incompleta.

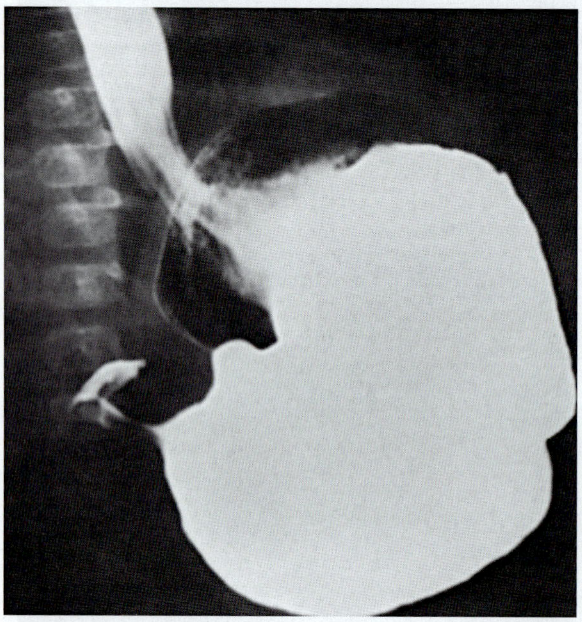

Figura 326-3. Bario nello stomaco di un neonato con vomito proiettivo. L'assottigliamento del canale pilorico è tipico della stenosi ipertrofica congenita del piloro.

326.2 • OSTRUZIONE CONGENITA DELLO SVUOTAMENTO GASTRICO

L'ostruzione dello svuotamento gastrico derivante dall'atresia del piloro o da membrane antrali è rara ed è responsabile di <1% di tutte le atresie e diaframmi del tratto alimentare. La causa di questo difetto è sconosciuta. L'atresia del piloro è stata associata con l'**epidermolisi bollosa** e solitamente si manifesta nella prima infanzia (vedi Capitolo 653). La sua distribuzione nei due sessi è sovrapponibile.

MANIFESTAZIONI CLINICHE. I neonati con atresia del piloro presentano vomito non biliare, difficoltà di alimentazione e distensione addominale nel primo giorno di vita. Il **polidramnios** si verifica nella maggior parte dei casi e altrettanto comune è un basso peso alla nascita. L'aspirato gastrico alla nascita è abbondante (>20 mL di liquido) e dovrebbe essere eliminato per prevenire l'aspirazione. Nelle prime 12 ore di vita può verificarsi la rottura dello stomaco. I pazienti con membrane antrali possono presentare sintomi meno drammatici, a seconda del grado di ostruzione. I bambini più grandi con membrane antrali presentano nausea, vomito, dolore addominale e calo ponderale.

DIAGNOSI. La diagnosi di ostruzione congenita dello svuotamento gastrico è suggerita dal riscontro di uno stomaco ingrandito e dilatato alla radiografia diretta dell'addome o all'ecografia prenatale. Gli studi gastrointestinali seriati con mezzo di contrasto in genere sono diagnostici e rivelano una retrazione pilorica. Una membrana antrale può presentarsi come un sottile setto in prossimità del canale pilorico. Nei bambini più grandi l'endoscopia si è rivelata utile per identificare queste strutture.

TRATTAMENTO. Il trattamento dell'ostruzione dello svuotamento gastrico nei neonati inizia con la correzione della disidratazione e dell'alcalosi ipocloremica. Occorre cercare di attenuare il vomito persistente con la decompressione nasogastrica. Il trattamento endoscopico o chirurgico dovrebbe essere intrapreso quando il paziente è stabile.

326.3 • DUPLICAZIONE GASTRICA

Le duplicazioni gastriche sono rare strutture cistiche o tubulari, in genere localizzate all'interno della parete dello stomaco. La maggior parte di esse ha un diametro <12 cm e di solito non comunica con il lume gastrico. Anomalie associate sono presenti almeno nel 35% dei pazienti. Le duplicazioni sono state poste in relazione con un difetto della ricanalizzazione dopo la fase solida dello sviluppo intestinale.

Le manifestazioni cliniche più comuni dipendono da un'ostruzione dello svuotamento gastrico parziale o completa. La cisti è palpabile nel 33% dei pazienti. Le duplicazioni comunicanti possono causare ulcerazioni gastriche ed essere associate a ematemesi o melena.

Le duplicazioni gastriche vengono visualizzate negli studi seriati del tratto gastrointestinale superiore come difetti estrinseci, solitamente localizzati lungo la piccola curvatura gastrica. La tomografia computerizzata (TC) o l'ecografia possono essere d'aiuto per definire la struttura cistica. Il trattamento delle duplicazioni gastriche sintomatiche consiste nell'escissione chirurgica.

326.4 • Volvolo gastrico

Il volvolo gastrico si presenta con una **triade** di sintomi a esordio improvviso: epigastralgia severa, conati incoercibili con emesi e impossibilità di introdurre un tubo nello stomaco. Lo stomaco è ancorato longitudinalmente dai legamenti gastroepatico, gastrosplenico e gastrocolico, mentre il suo asse traverso viene mantenuto in sede dal legamento gastrofrenico e dall'adesione retroperitoneale del duodeno. Si verifica un volvolo quando uno di questi legamenti è mancante oppure allungato, il che consente allo stomaco di ruotare su se stesso. Nella maggior parte dei bambini sono presenti altri difetti associati, tra i quali la malrotazione intestinale, i difetti diaframmatici o l'asplenia. Un volvolo può verificarsi lungo l'asse longitudinale (volvolo organoassiale) oppure lungo quello trasversale (volvolo mesenteroassiale).

MANIFESTAZIONI CLINICHE. La presentazione clinica del volvolo gastrico è aspecifica e suggerisce un'ostruzione intestinale alta. Il volvolo gastrico dell'età infantile è solitamente associato con il vomito non biliare. Un volvolo acuto può progredire rapidamente fino allo strozzamento e alla perforazione. La forma cronica è più comune nei bambini più grandi; in tal caso il paziente presenta un'anamnesi positiva per emesi, dolore addominale e sazietà precoce.

La **diagnosi** è suggerita dalla presenza di una dilatazione gastrica alle radiografie in bianco dell'addome. Le radiografie addominali in posizione eretta mostrano un doppio livello fluido con un caratteristico "becco" (per il quale si usa in genere la denominazione inglese "beak", NdR) in prossimità della giunzione esofagea inferiore nel volvolo mesenteroassiale. Nel volvolo organoassiale si può osservare invece un singolo livello gas-liquido senza il caratteristico becco. Il trattamento del volvolo gastrico acuto consiste nell'intervento chirurgico in emergenza, dopo che il paziente è stato stabilizzato. In casi selezionati di volvolo cronico in pazienti più grandi si è rivelata efficace la correzione endoscopica.

326.5 • Gastropatia ipertrofica

La gastropatia ipertrofica è rara nei bambini e, contrariamente a quanto accade nell'adulto (malattia di Ménétrier), costituisce in genere una condizione transitoria, benigna e autolimitante. Nella maggior parte dei casi risulta secondaria a un'infezione da Cytomegalovirus, ma sono stati implicati anche altri microrganismi, tra i quali i virus dell'herpes simplex, la ***Giardia*** e l'***Helicobacter pylori***. Le manifestazioni cliniche comprendono vomito, anoressia, dolore addominale alto, diarrea, edemi (da enteropatia protidodisperdente ipoproteinemica), ascite e, raramente, ematemesi in caso di ulcerazioni. L'esame endoscopico con biopsie conferma la diagnosi. L'età media alla diagnosi è di 5 anni (range 2 giorni-17 anni); la malattia in genere dura 2-4 settimane ed è sempre seguita dalla risoluzione completa. La **diagnosi differenziale** comprende la gastroenterite eosinofila, il linfoma o il carcinoma gastrico, il morbo di Crohn e lo pseudotumore infiammatorio.

Hoffer V, Finkelstein Y, Balter J, et al: Ganciclovir treatment in Ménétrier's disease. *Acta Paediatr* 2003;92:983–985.

Kawahara H, Imura K, Nishikawa M, et al: Intravenous atropine treatment in infantile hypertrophic pyloric stenosis. *Arch Dis Child* 2002;87:71–74.

Parrini S, Di Maggio G, Latini G, et al: Abnormal oral mucosal light reflectance in infantile hypertrophic pyloric stenosis. *J Pediatr Gastroenterol Nutr* 2004;39:53–55.

Saur D, Vanderwinden JM, Seidler B, et al. Single-nucleotide promoter polymorphism alters transcription of neuronal nitric oxide synthase exon 1c in infantile hypertrophic pyloric stenosis. *Proc Natl Acad Sci U S A* 2004;101:1662–1667.

To T, Wajja A, Wales PW, Langer JC: Population demographic indicators associated with incidence of pyloric stenosis. *Arch Pediatr Adolesc Med* 2005;159:520–525.

Yagmurlu A, Barnhart DC, Vernon A, et al. Comparison of the incidence of complications in open and laparoscopic pyloromyotomy: A concurrent single institution series. *J Pediatr Surg* 2004;39;292–296.

Capitolo 327 ■ Atresia, stenosi e malrotazione intestinale

Robert Wyllie

CONSIDERAZIONI GENERALI. L'ostruzione intestinale si verifica in circa 1/1500 neonati. Può essere parziale o completa, riconducibile ad anomalie intrinseche o estrinseche dell'intestino. È inoltre classificabile come semplice o strozzata: la prima è caratterizzata dalla mancata progressione in senso aborale del contenuto luminale; nella seconda si verifica inoltre una riduzione del flusso ematico all'intestino. Se l'ostruzione strozzata non viene risolta al più presto, può portare all'infarto e alla perforazione intestinale.

Tipicamente si verifica un accumulo di alimenti ingeriti, gas e secrezioni prossimalmente al livello dell'ostruzione, che provoca la distensione dell'intestino, la quale a sua volta determina una riduzione dell'assorbimento intestinale e un aumento della secrezione di liquidi ed elettroliti. Questa migrazione di liquidi ed elettroliti induce una deplezione di liquidi intravascolare isotonica, solitamente associata a ipokaliemia. L'attività contrattile dell'intestino prossimale all'ostruzione, dopo un iniziale aumento, va incontro a una spiccata diminuzione con riduzione dei borborigmi. La combinazione di accumulo di liquidi (distensione) e ipomotilità è associata con nausea e vomito.

Le lesioni ostruttive congenite dell'intestino possono essere suddivise in intrinseche (atresia, stenosi, ileo da meconio, megacolon agangliare) ed estrinseche (malrotazione, briglie costrittive, ernie intraddominali, duplicazioni). Prima di procedere all'intervento chirurgico si dovrebbe tentare di localizzare la lesione. Quando l'ostruzione è completa non ci dovrebbero essere grosse difficoltà nel riconoscimento del quadro clinico, ma quando essa è incompleta o intermittente la diagnosi può presentare notevoli difficoltà. Nel caso si riscontrasse **polidramnios**, che accompagna frequentemente le ostruzioni intestinali alte, sarebbe indispensabile aspirare il contenuto gastrico del paziente immediatamente dopo la nascita. L'aspirazione di 15-20 mL o più di liquidi gastrici, in particolare se tinti da bile, è suggestiva di un'ostruzione intestinale alta.

Inizialmente può essere osservato il transito del meconio se l'ostruzione è localizzata nella parte alta dell'intestino tenue o se si sviluppa tardivamente nel corso della vita intrauterina.

Quando l'ostruzione è incompleta (come in caso di stenosi intestinali, briglie costrittive, duplicazioni, volvoli incompleti), i segni (vomito, distensione addominale, stipsi ostinata) possono apparire rapidamente dopo la nascita oppure essere ritardati per un tempo indefinito. Questi segni possono raggiungere la severità dell'ostruzione completa oppure essere così lievi e sporadici da passare inosservati, finché un episodio acuto o l'esecuzione di accertamenti diagnostici non mettono in evidenza la lesione.

Con il termine “atresia” si indica un’ostruzione completa del lume intestinale, mentre parlando di stenosi si intende un blocco parziale del contenuto luminale. La prima, comune nel duodeno, nel digiuno e nell’ileo, rara nel colon, è responsabile del 33% circa di tutti i casi di ostruzione intestinale neonatale e colpisce con la stessa frequenza maschi e femmine. Essa altera inoltre lo sviluppo del plesso mienterico al di sotto del livello dell’atresia stessa, comportando i disordini della motilità osservati dopo l’intervento di correzione chirurgica.

Per effetto della dilatazione il flusso sanguigno all’intestino ostruito diminuisce e si allontana dalla mucosa, che perde quindi la sua integrità. Nell’intestino ostruito si assiste a una rapida proliferazione di batteri (in prevalenza coliformi e anaerobi) che, insieme alla perdita d’integrità della mucosa, attraversano la parete dell’organo, potendo provocare endotossiemia, batteriemia e sepsi.

La presentazione clinica dell’ostruzione intestinale varia a seconda della causa, del livello colpito e del tempo trascorso tra l’evento ostruttivo e la valutazione del paziente. I **sintomi classici** comprendono nausea e vomito, distensione addominale e stipsi ostinata. Un’ostruzione localizzata nella parte alta del tratto intestinale fino a interessare il duodeno o il digiuno prossimale provoca frequenti episodi di abbondante vomito biliare. Il dolore, intermittente e solitamente alleviato dal vomito, si localizza nell’epigastrio o nella regione ombelicale e la distensione addominale è di lieve entità. Un’ostruzione nella parte distale dell’intestino tenue determina invece una distensione addominale moderata o severa, con vomito progressivamente fecaloide. Il dolore è generalmente diffuso a tutto l’addome.

Non esistono esami di laboratorio che consentano di porre la diagnosi di ostruzione o di differenziare l’ostruzione semplice da quella associata a infarto intestinale. Un’ostruzione nel tratto gastrointestinale superiore è spesso associata a un’alcalosi metabolica ipocloremica. Una marcata leucocitosi, con o senza trombocitopenia, acidosi metabolica ed ematochezia, in un paziente con un quadro ostruttivo, suggerisce un infarto intestinale. Si dovrebbe sempre procedere alla determinazione dell’amilasi e della lipasi sieriche per escludere una pancreatite.

La diagnosi di ostruzione intestinale viene in genere suggerita dall’anamnesi clinica (comprendente l’ecografia prenatale) e dall’esame obiettivo. Le metodiche di imaging vengono utilizzate per confermarla e per localizzare la sede dell’ostruzione. Gli accertamenti iniziali consistono nelle radiografie dell’addome in posizione supina, eretta e in decubiti particolari.

Spesso radiografie dirette in posizione distesa ed eretta forniscono informazioni preziose sulla localizzazione delle lesioni ostruttive congenite dell’intestino. In caso di lesioni completamente ostruenti, si osserva una distensione intestinale al di sopra del livello dell’ostruzione ed è possibile rilevare una serie di livelli idroaerei nelle anse distese, nella posizione eretta o laterale obliqua. In caso di **perforazione** si può osservare uno **pneumoperitoneo**, con aria libera nelle regioni subfreniche o al di sopra del fegato, in decubito laterale sinistro. La presenza di una **calcificazione** all’interno della cavità peritoneale indica in genere un **ileo da meconio**. Raramente un’ostruzione con una calcificazione intraluminale risulta associata con una fistola rettourinaria, con l’agangliosi colica o con l’atresia intestinale. Nei pazienti con ileo da meconio si può osservare un caratteristico aspetto a vetro smerigliato nel quadrante inferiore destro, con bolle d’aria intrappolate all’interno del meconio ostruente. Nello stomaco di un lattante normale, subito dopo la nascita, di solito è possibile evidenziare radiograficamente la presenza di aria, la quale entro un’ora può raggiungere la porzioni prossimali dell’intestino tenue e i segmenti colici e dalle 3 alle 18 ore dopo può rendersi visibile nella parte distale del colon. Nei bambini di età <2 anni talvolta è difficile stabilire con certezza se l’ostruzione riguarda l’intestino tenue o il crasso.

L’ecografia è d’aiuto per identificare la stenosi pilorica, la malrotazione e il volvolo o l’intussuscezione e per differenziare la stenosi pilorica da altre cause di ostruzione prossimale. Le indagini con mezzo di contrasto o la TC sono indicate quando le radiografie dirette o l’ecografia non riescono a identificare l’origine dell’ostruzione. Le metodiche con mezzo di contrasto idrosolubile evitano il rischio di contaminazione del peritoneo con il bario, nei casi in cui vi sia una significativa possibilità di perforazione non evidenziata dalla presenza di pneumoperitoneo alla radiografia diretta. I clismi con mezzo di contrasto idrosolubile sono utili nella diagnosi di malrotazione, ileo da meconio, tappo da meconio e intussuscezione. In questi ultimi tre casi il clisma può essere sia diagnostico sia terapeutico, eliminando l’ostruzione. Per identificare le lesioni ostruttive dell’intestino prossimale (atresia, volvolo, malrotazione) il mezzo di contrasto viene introdotto per via orale o tramite sondino nasogastrico. Anche in questo caso si ricorre a mezzi di contrasto idrosolubili qualora si sospetti una perforazione. La TC dell’addome è sensibile e specifica anche per la diagnosi delle piccole ostruzioni intestinali, soprattutto nei bambini di età >2 anni.

TRATTAMENTO. I lattanti e i bambini con ostruzione intestinale presentano sia un blocco del transito intestinale, sia una perdita di liquidi ed elettroliti. I pazienti con strozzamento vascolare possono sviluppare anche un’ischemia intestinale con sepsi e shock. Il trattamento iniziale deve essere volto al **ripristino dei liquidi** e alla stabilizzazione del paziente. La **decompressione nasogastrica** in genere allevia il dolore e il vomito. Dopo appropriate colture, nei lattanti di aspetto sano con ostruzione intestinale o con sospetto infarto da strozzamento si instaura una copertura antibiotica ad ampio spettro. Quelli che presentano uno strozzamento devono essere trattati immediatamente con un intervento chirurgico, prima che l’intestino vada incontro a un infarto, che provocherebbe gangrena e perforazione intestinale. Una necrosi intestinale estesa determina una sindrome dell’intestino corto (vedi Capitolo 335.7). Il trattamento conservativo non chirurgico in genere viene limitato ai casi con sospette aderenze o stenosi infiammatorie, che possono essere risolte con la decompressione nasogastrica e farmaci antinfiammatori. Se non si ottengono segni clinici di miglioramento entro 12-24 ore, in genere è indicato l’intervento chirurgico.

327.1 • OSTRUZIONE DUODENALE

Si ritiene che l’atresia duodenale derivi da un difetto della ricanalizzazione del lume dopo la fase solida dello sviluppo intestinale nella 4ª-5ª settimana di gestazione. L’incidenza dell’atresia duodenale è di 1/10 000 neonati e corrisponde al 25-40% di tutte le atresie intestinali. In metà dei casi si tratta di soggetti prematuri. L’atresia duodenale può assumere diverse forme, tra le quali una membrana integra che ostruisce il lume, un breve cordone di tessuto fibroso che congiunge due tasche duodenali cieche o un’interruzione tra estremità non connesse del duodeno. Un raro tipo di ostruzione consiste in una membrana a forma di “manica a vento”, che rappresenta un lembo di tessuto dilatabile, associata ad anomalie del sistema biliare. Quella membranosa è la forma di atresia più comune e in questo caso l’ostruzione si verifica, nella maggior parte dei pazienti, distalmente all’ampolla di Vater. L’ostruzione duodenale può rappresentare anche la conseguenza di una compressione estrinseca, come nel caso del pancreas anulare oppure delle briglie di Ladd nei pazienti con malrotazione. La sindrome di Down è presente nel 20-30% dei pazienti con atresia duodenale. Altre anomalie congenite che si associano ad atresia duodenale comprendono la malrotazione (20%), l’atresia esofagea (10-20%), le cardiopatie congenite (10-15%) e le anomalie anorettali e renali (5%).

MANIFESTAZIONI CLINICHE. Il segno caratteristico dell’ostruzione duodenale è il **vomito biliare** senza distensione addominale, che si manifesta in genere già nel primo giorno di vita. Fin dalla fase precoce della malattia è possibile visualizzare onde peristaltiche. La metà delle gravidanze è caratterizzata da una storia di **polidramnios**, dovuto a un difettoso assorbimento del liquido amniotico da parte dell’intestino distale. L’ittero è presente in un terzo dei neonati. La diagnosi è suggerita dalla presenza del "**segno della doppia bolla**" alla radiografia diretta dell'addome (Fig. 327-1). Quest'ultimo quadro è determinato dalla distensione dello stomaco e del duodeno, che risultano pieni d'aria. Gli studi con mezzo di contrasto, pur non essendo di solito necessari e comportando un rischio di aspirazione, possono occasionalmente rivelarsi utili per escludere una malrotazione o un volvolo, poiché se quest'ultimo non viene eliminato entro 6-12 ore si può verificare un infarto intestinale. La diagnosi prenatale di atresia duodenale può essere effettuata tramite l'ecografia fetale.

TRATTAMENTO. Il trattamento iniziale dei neonati con atresia intestinale comprende la decompressione naso- o orogastrica e il ripristino dei liquidi per via endovenosa. Occorre poi effettuare un ecocardiogramma e una radiografia del torace e della colonna vertebrale per escludere eventuali anomalie associate. Il 30% circa dei neonati con atresia duodenale presenta anomalie congenite associate, che possono compromettere la sopravvivenza. La correzione definitiva dell'atresia viene in genere posticipata per valutare e trattare queste anomalie, che possono mettere a repentaglio la vita del paziente.

L'intervento chirurgico standard per la correzione dell'atresia consiste nella duodeno-duodenostomia, con eventuale riduzione del tratto dilatato di intestino prossimale per migliorare la peristalsi. È possibile posizionare un sondino gastrostomico per drenare lo stomaco e proteggere le vie aeree. Sono necessari un supporto nutrizionale per via endovenosa o tramite sondino digiunale transanastomotico finché il neonato non inizia ad alimentarsi per via orale. La prognosi dipende soprattutto dalla presenza di anomalie associate.

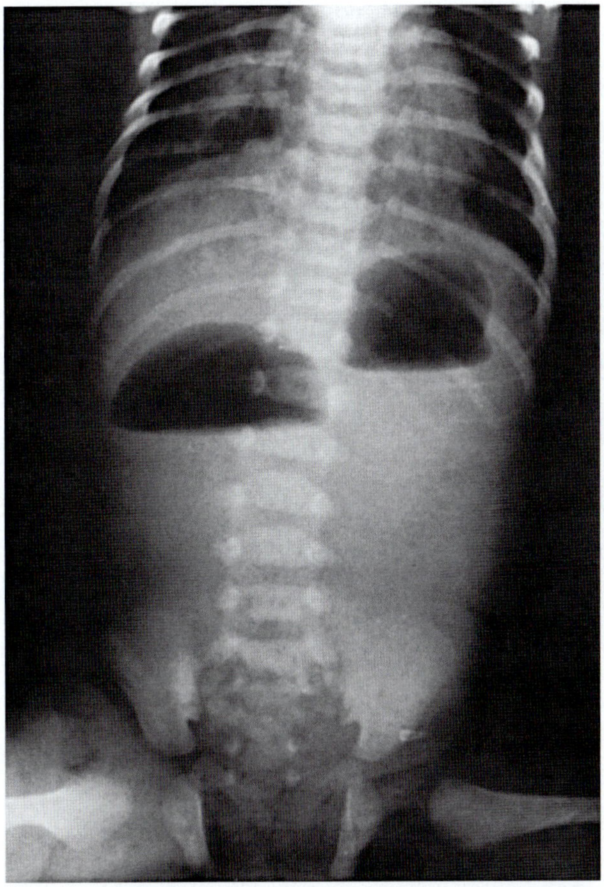

Figura 327-1. Radiografia addominale di un neonato affetto da atresia duodenale congenita, tenuto in posizione eretta. Si osservino le due aree scure in alto dovute al gas, con un'immagine di "doppia bolla", e l'assenza di gas nell'intestino distale.

Se l'ostruzione è dovuta alle briglie di Ladd con malrotazione, si rende necessario un intervento chirurgico immediato. Dopo la separazione delle pliche peritoneali anomale o delle briglie, tutto l'intestino crasso, una volta asportata l'appendice, viene posizionato nella parte sinistra dell'addome, con il tenue a destra (posizione che corrisponde a quella fetale in assenza di rotazione). L'appendicectomia viene effettuata per evitare una successiva diagnosi errata di appendicite. La malrotazione può coesistere anche con un'ostruzione duodenale intrinseca, come una membrana o una stenosi, identificabili facendo passare un catetere con punta a palloncino nel digiuno a valle dell'ostruzione, gonfiando il palloncino e infine ritirando lentamente il catetere stesso. L'intervento di scelta per il pancreas anulare è la duodeno-duodenostomia senza divisione del pancreas, in modo da lasciare un'ansa non funzionante più breve possibile. L'ostruzione duodenale diaframmatica viene trattata con una duodenoplastica.

327.2 • ATRESIA E OSTRUZIONE DIGIUNALE E ILEALE

Si ritiene che le atresie digiunoileali dipendano da danni vascolari intrauterini, che portano alla necrosi ischemica dell'intestino sterile e al riassorbimento dei segmenti colpiti. Vengono distinti quattro diversi tipi di atresia digiunale e ileale (Fig. 327-2). Il tipo I corrisponde al 20% delle atresie ed è caratterizzato da un diaframma intraluminale che ostruisce il lume, la cui continuità tra l'intestino prossimale e distale viene tuttavia mantenuta. Nel tipo II, che rende conto del 35% circa dei difetti, un cordone solido di piccolo diametro congiunge l'intestino prossimale a quello distale. Il tipo III viene suddiviso in due sottotipi. Il tipo IIIa corrisponde al 35% circa delle atresie e si verifica quando entrambe le estremità intestinali terminano con un'ansa cieca e sono accompagnate da un piccolo difetto mesenteriale. Il tipo IIIb è associato con un esteso difetto mesenteriale e con la perdita del normale apporto ematico all'intestino distale. L'ileo distale si avvolge attorno all'arteria ileocolica, dalla quale deriva il suo intero apporto ematico, dando luogo a un aspetto "a buccia di

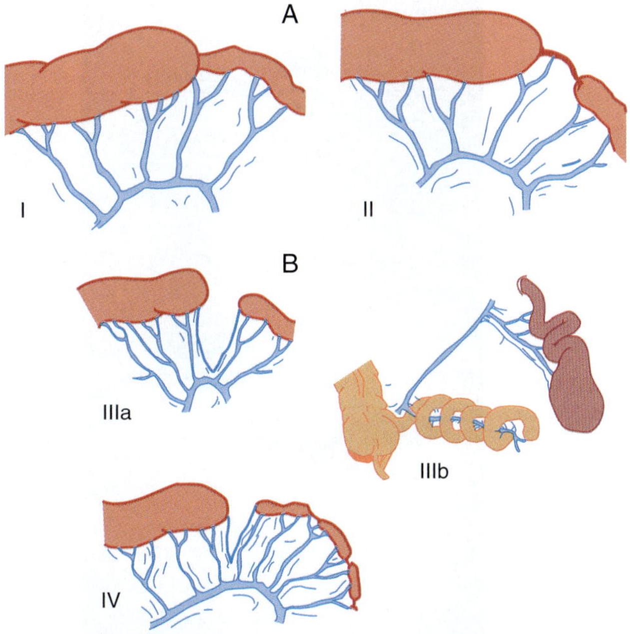

Figura 327-2. *A* e *B*, Classificazione dell'atresia intestinale. Tipo I: Ostruzione mucosa causata da una membrana intraluminale con integrità della parete intestinale e del mesentere. Tipo II: Estremità cieche separate da un cordone fibroso. Tipo IIIa: Estremità cieche separate da un difetto mesenteriale a forma di V. Tipo IIIb: Aspetto "a buccia di mela". Tipo IV: Atresie multiple. (Da Grosfeld J: Jejunoileal atresia and stenosis. In Welch KJ, Randolph JG, Ravitch MM [editors]: *Pediatric Surgery*, 4th ed. Chicago, Year Book Medical publishers, 1986.)

mela". Quest'anomalia è associata alla prematurità e in genere a un accorciamento dell'ileo distale e dell'intero intestino. Il tipo IV, che rappresenta il 5% circa di tutti i casi, consiste in multipli segmenti di atresia intestinale. Le atresie del colon presentano analogie con quelle digiunoileali, ma sono molto meno comuni.

L'**ileo da meconio** interessa principalmente i neonati con fibrosi cistica, il 10% dei quali lo sviluppa; per contro, l'80-90% dei neonati che presentano un ileo da meconio è affetto da fibrosi cistica. Nell'ileo da meconio semplice, gli ultimi 20-30 cm di ileo sono collassati e riempiti da pallottole di feci ipocromiche, mentre a monte di questo tratto un'ansa dilatata di lunghezza variabile risulta ostruita da meconio avente la consistenza di un denso sciroppo di glucosio. La peristalsi non riesce a sospingere in avanti questo materiale molto viscido, che rimane quindi impattato nell'ileo. Volvoli, atresia o perforazioni intestinali accompagnano l'ileo da meconio complicato. La perforazione in utero provoca una **peritonite da meconio**. A livello intraperitoneale il meconio può causare spesse aderenze, che dopo la nascita danno luogo a ostruzioni intestinali, e **calcificare** rapidamente.

Nel 5% dei pazienti con **malattia di Hirschsprung**, il segmento agangliare non comprende solo l'intero colon ma anche l'ileo terminale. Questa condizione determina una dilatazione anche dell'intestino tenue che possiede pareti provviste di gangli, ma per certi versi ipertrofiche, una zona di transizione ipogangliare a forma di imbuto e un tratto di intestino distale agangliare collassato.

MANIFESTAZIONI CLINICHE. Le anomalie extragastrointestinali sono meno comuni nell'atresia dell'intestino distale che nelle atresie duodenali. La diagnosi di atresia digiunoileale è possibile grazie all'ecografia prenatale. Il polidramnios si verifica nel 25% dei pazienti affetti. I gemelli monozigoti sono a maggior rischio di atresia rispetto a quelli dizigoti o ai figli unici. La nascita prematura avviene nel 30% dei casi. L'atresia è stata inoltre associata con un basso peso alla nascita, con parti multipli e con il consumo di cocaina o il fumo di sigaretta da parte della madre.

La maggior parte dei soggetti diventa sintomatica nel primo giorno di vita, con distensione addominale e vomito o aspirato gastrico tinto di bile. Nel 60-75% dei neonati non avviene il transito del meconio. L'ittero è stato rilevato nel 20-30% dei casi. La radiografia diretta visualizza numerosi livelli idroaerei (Fig. 327-3) o calcificazioni peritoneali associate alla peritonite da meconio. Gli esami con mezzo di contrasto dell'intestino superiore e inferiore possono individuare il livello dell'ostruzione e differenziare l'atresia dall'ileo, dai tappi da meconio e dalla malattia di Hirschsprung. L'ecografia addominale può distinguere l'ileo da meconio dall'atresia dell'ileo e identificare una malrotazione intestinale.

Nell'ileo da meconio la radiografia in bianco dell'addome mostra un tipico aspetto nebbioso o a vetro smerigliato nel quadrante inferiore destro. In questa sede sono disperse piccole bolle di gas intrappolate nel meconio (vedi Capitolo 102.1). A causa del loro contenuto vischioso, le anse intestinali, che risultano moderatamente dilatate, non presentano i livelli idroaerei solitamente presenti nelle radiografie in proiezione eretta. In caso di peritonite da meconio si possono osservare calcificazioni a placche, in genere in corrispondenza dei fianchi. Lo **pneumoperitoneo** è identificabile senza difficoltà per la presenza di aria libera tra il fegato e il diaframma in una radiografia addominale in posizione eretta; l'aria libera esercita una distensione dell'intero addome che può assumere l'aspetto di un pallone; talvolta il legamento rotondo è chiaramente visibile sulla linea mediana.

Nei neonati in molti casi non è possibile distinguere l'intestino tenue dal crasso alla radiografia diretta dell'addome. Se le radiografie dirette non sono specifiche, può essere necessario un esame del colon con mezzo di contrasto idrosolubile (Gastrografin, Hypaque) per distinguere le ostruzioni dell'intestino tenue e del crasso. Un colon piccolo, il cosiddetto "microcolon", ne suggerisce un utilizzo ridotto e la presenza di un'ostruzione prossimale alla valvola ileocecale. Si raccomanda cautela nell'utilizzo di clismi idrosolubili per la diagnosi e la terapia dell'ileo da meconio, poiché la loro iperosmolalità può richiamare liquidi nel colon e

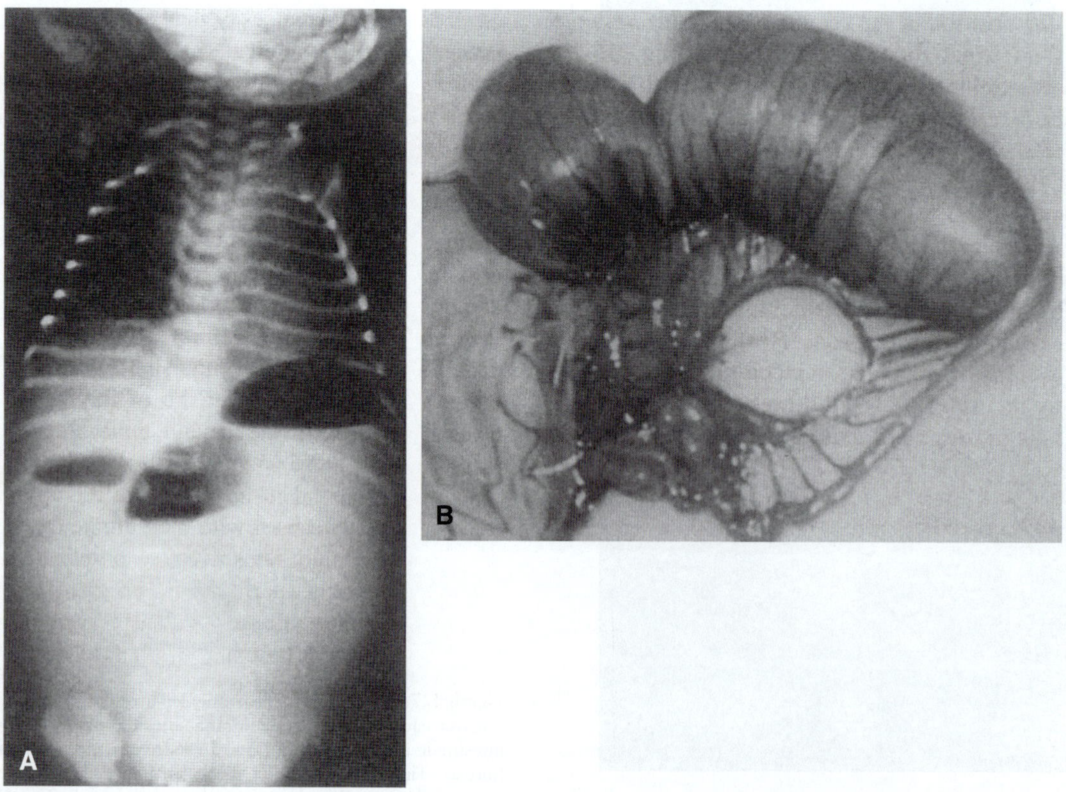

Figura 327-3. *A*, Radiografia addominale in un neonato con vomito biliare, che mostra alcune anse intestinali dilatate con livelli idroaerei. *B*, Alla laparotomia si è potuta osservare un'atresia digiunale di tipo I (mucosa). (Da O'Neill JA Jr, Grosfeld JL, Fonkalsrud EW, et al [editors]: *Principles of Pediatric Surgery*, 2nd ed. St. Louis, Mosby, 2003, p 493.)

causare disidratazione; inoltre, la pressione del clisma può richiamare liquidi nel colon e provocare una perforazione.

TRATTAMENTO. Prima di eseguire l'intervento chirurgico o di effettuare tentativi radiologici di disostruzione, occorre accertarsi che i pazienti con ostruzione dell'intestino tenue siano stabili e presentino un adeguato bilancio idroelettrolitico, a meno che non si sospetti un volvolo. Le infezioni dovrebbero essere trattate con antibiotici appropriati. Prima dell'intervento chirurgico in genere si somministra una profilassi antibiotica.

In caso di atresia ileale o digiunale è necessaria la resezione della porzione prossimale dilatata dell'intestino, seguita da un'anastomosi terminoterminale. Se è presente un semplice diaframma mucoso, una digiuno- o ileoplastica con escissione parziale della membrana rappresenta un'alternativa accettabile alla resezione. Nell'ileo da meconio non complicato, i clismi con Gastrografin consentono di porre la diagnosi di ostruzione e rimuovere il materiale denso. Il Gastrografin è ipertonico e deve essere utilizzato con attenzione per evitare la disidratazione, lo shock e la perforazione intestinale. Può essere necessario ripetere il clisma dopo 8-12 ore. Non è necessaria la resezione dopo riduzione, a meno che non si siano verificate complicanze ischemiche.

Il 50% circa dei pazienti con ileo da meconio semplice non risponde adeguatamente ai clismi idrosolubili e necessita di una laparotomia. Il trattamento chirurgico è indicato quando non è possibile eliminare l'ostruzione nonostante ripetuti tentativi terapeutici non chirurgici, oltre che nei neonati con ileo da meconio complicato. L'estensione dell'intervento chirurgico dipende dal grado di patologia. Nell'ileo da meconio semplice, il tappo può essere rimosso con la manipolazione o per irrigazione enterale diretta con *N*-acetilcisteina, dopo enterotomia. I casi complicati possono richiedere la resezione intestinale, il lavaggio peritoneale, il drenaggio addominale e il confezionamento di una stomia. Talvolta si rende necessaria la nutrizione parenterale totale.

327.3 • Malrotazione

La malrotazione consiste nella rotazione incompleta dell'intestino durante lo sviluppo fetale. L'intestino si forma come una struttura tubulare lineare che unisce lo stomaco al retto. L'intestino medio (dal duodeno distale al mesocolon trasverso) inizia ad allungarsi e progressivamente protrude all'interno del cordone ombelicale, fino a localizzarsi completamente al di fuori della cavità addominale. Nella rotazione dell'intestino in via di sviluppo all'interno e all'esterno della cavità addominale, l'arteria mesenterica superiore, che è responsabile dell'apporto ematico, funge da asse. Il duodeno, quando rientra nella cavità addominale, si sposta fino alla regione del legamento di Treitz e il colon che segue viene indirizzato verso il quadrante superiore sinistro. Successivamente il cieco ruota in senso antiorario all'interno della cavità addominale e raggiunge il quadrante inferiore destro. Il duodeno si fissa alla parete addominale posteriore prima che il colon abbia compiuto una rotazione completa. Dopo la rotazione, anche il colon destro e sinistro e la radice mesenterica si fissano all'addome posteriore. Questi punti di attacco forniscono un'ampia base di sostegno per il mesentere e l'arteria mesenterica superiore, prevenendo così la torsione della radice mesenterica e l'attorcigliamento delle strutture vascolari. La rotazione e l'ancoraggio addominale risultano completati entro il terzo mese di gestazione.

Una mancata rotazione si verifica quando l'intestino perde la sua capacità di ruotare dopo essere rientrato nella cavità addominale. La prima e la seconda porzione duodenale si trovano già nella loro posizione normale, ma il resto del duodeno, il digiuno e l'ileo occupano la parte destra dell'addome finché il colon è localizzato a sinistra. La malrotazione e la mancata rotazione si associano a eterotassia addominale e sindrome asplenia-polisplenia, con malformazioni cardiache congenite che tendono ad accumularsi una dopo l'altra (vedi Capitolo 431.11).

Il tipo più comune di malrotazione consiste nell'impossibilità del cieco di migrare fino al quadrante inferiore destro (Fig. 327-4).

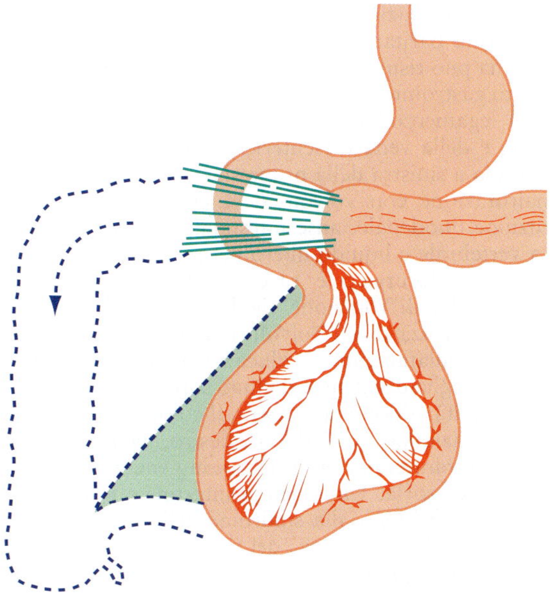

Figura 327-4. Meccanismo dell'ostruzione intestinale con rotazione incompleta dell'intestino medio (malrotazione). Le *linee punteggiate* indicano il percorso che avrebbe dovuto compiere il cieco. La mancata rotazione ha portato alla formazione di briglie ostruttive, che incrociano il duodeno, e di uno stretto peduncolo per l'ansa dell'intestino medio, che lo pone a rischio di formare un volvolo. (Da Nixon HH, O'Donnell B: *The Essentials of Pediatric Surgery*. Philadelphia, JB Lippincott, 1961.)

La localizzazione normale del cieco è nell'area sottoepatica. Il cieco, non compiendo la rotazione corretta, non può formare la normale aderenza ad ampia base alla parete addominale posteriore. Il mesentere, arteria mesenterica superiore compresa, è ancorato da uno stretto peduncolo, che può avvolgersi su se stesso e dare luogo a un volvolo dell'intestino medio. Inoltre delle briglie di tessuto (le cosiddette **briglie di Ladd**) possono estendersi dal cieco al quadrante superiore destro, attraversando e talvolta ostruendo il duodeno.

MANIFESTAZIONI CLINICHE. La maggior parte dei pazienti manifesta sintomi di ostruzione acuta o cronica durante il primo anno di vita. I lattanti spesso presentano **vomito biliare** e ostruzione intestinale acuta nella prima settimana di vita, mentre i bambini più grandi vanno incontro a episodi di dolore addominale acuto simili a coliche. In questi soggetti la malrotazione si può presentare con episodi ricorrenti di vomito, dolore addominale o entrambi. Occasionalmente i pazienti presentano **malassorbimento** o **enteropatia protidodisperdente**, associati con una proliferazione batterica. La causa dei sintomi è da ricercare in un volvolo intermittente o nella compressione del duodeno esercitata da briglie di Ladd o da aderenze che interessano l'intestino tenue o crasso. Il 25-50% degli adolescenti con malrotazione è asintomatico. Quelli che diventano sintomatici presentano un'ostruzione intestinale acuta o un'anamnesi con episodi ricorrenti di dolore addominale e (con minore frequenza) di vomito e diarrea. I pazienti di ogni età con un'anomalia della rotazione possono sviluppare un volvolo intestinale acuto, che pone a rischio la sopravvivenza, anche senza sintomi preesistenti.

La presentazione acuta di un'ostruzione del tenue in un paziente non sottoposto in precedenza a interventi intestinali rappresenta in genere la conseguenza di un **volvolo** associato a malrotazione. Questa è una complicanza della malrotazione che pone a rischio la sopravvivenza, assomiglia a un addome acuto o a una sepsi acuta e costituisce la principale ragione per la quale bisognerebbe sempre approfondire le indagini in presenza di sintomi suggestivi di malrotazione. La diagnosi viene posta tramite l'ecografia o metodiche radiografiche con mezzo di contrasto. La radiografia diretta dell'addome, pur non essendo in genere specifica, può evidenziare un'ostruzione intestinale con il segno della doppia bolla. Il clisma baritato in genere mostra il malposizionamento del cieco, ma può risultare normale nel 10% dei pazienti. Gli studi del tratto gastrointestinale superiore evidenziano una posizione errata del legamento di Treitz. L'ecografia rivela un'inversione dell'arteria e della vena mesenterica superiore; la localizzazione della seconda a sinistra della prima suggerisce una malrotazione. Una malrotazione con volvolo deve essere sospettata in caso di ostruzione duodenale, anse intestinali ispessite a destra della colonna vertebrale e liquido libero nel peritoneo.

L'intervento chirurgico è raccomandato per ogni paziente con un'anomalia di rotazione significativa, indipendentemente dall'età. In presenza di un volvolo l'intervento chirurgico viene effettuato immediatamente: si riduce il volvolo e si procede a liberare da ogni briglia duodeno e digiuno superiore, che vengono lasciati nella cavità addominale destra. Il colon viene liberato dalla aderenze e posizionato nell'addome destro, mentre il cieco viene posto nel quadrante inferiore sinistro, in genere dopo un'appendicectomia accessoria. Un'ischemia intestinale estesa provocata da un volvolo dà luogo alla sindrome dell'intestino corto (vedi Capitolo 335.7). La persistenza dei sintomi dopo la correzione di una malrotazione dovrebbe suggerire un disturbo della motilità simile a una pseudo-ostruzione.

Basu R, Burge DM: The effect of antenatal diagnosis on the management of small bowel atresia. *Pediatr Surg Int* 2004;20:177–179.
Escobar MA, Ladd AP, Grosfeld JL, et al: Duodenal atresia and stenosis: Long-term follow-up over 30 years. *J Pediatr Surg* 2004;39:867–871.
Forrester MB, Merz RD: Population-based study of small intestinal atresia and stenosis, Hawaii, 1986–2000. *Public Health* 2004;118:434–438.
Karnak I, Ciftci AO, Senocak ME, et al: Colonic atresia: Surgical management and outcome. *Pediatr Surg Int* 2001;17:631–635.
Khen N, Jaubert F, Sauvat F, et al: Fetal intestinal obstruction induces alteration of enteric nervous system development in human intestinal atresia. *Pediatr Res* 2004;56:975–980.
Kumaran N, Shankar KR, Lloyd DA, Losty PD: Trends in the management and outcome of jejuno-ileal atresia. *Eur J Pediatr Surg* 2002;12:163–167.
Mehall JR, Chandler JC, Mehall RL, et al: Management of typical and atypical intestinal malrotation. *J Pediatr Surg* 2002;37:1169–1172.
Millar AJ, Rode H, Cywes S: Malrotation and volvulus in infancy and childhood. *Semin Pediatr Surg* 2003;12:229–236.
Pickhardt PJ, Bhalla S: Intestinal malrotation in adolescents and adults: Spectrum of clinical and imaging features. *AJR Am J Roentgenol* 2002;179:1429–1435.
Werler MM, Sheehan JE, Mitchell AA: Association of vasoconstrictive exposures with risks of gastroschisis and small intestinal atresia. *Epidemiology* 2003;14:349–354.

Capitolo 328 ■ Duplicazioni intestinali, diverticolo di Meckel e altri residui del dotto onfalomesenterico

Robert Wyllie

328.1 • Duplicazioni intestinali

Le duplicazioni del tratto gastrointestinale sono anomalie rare, che consistono in strutture tubulari o sferiche completamente formate, adese all'intestino, con il quale condividono l'apporto ematico. Il rivestimento delle duplicazioni assomiglia a quello del tratto gastrointestinale. Le duplicazioni sono localizzate sul margine del mesentere e possono comunicare con il lume intestinale. Esse sono classificabili in tre categorie: duplicazioni localizzate, duplicazioni associate con difetti del midollo spinale e malformazioni vertebrali e duplicazioni del colon. Le duplicazioni multiple sono di riscontro occasionale (nel 10-15% dei casi).

Le **duplicazioni localizzate** possono verificarsi in qualunque segmento del tratto gastrointestinale, ma sono più comuni nell'ileo e nel digiuno. Si tratta solitamente di strutture cistiche o tubulari poste all'interno della parete intestinale. La loro causa non è nota, ma il loro sviluppo è stato attribuito a difetti della ricanalizzazione del lume intestinale dopo la fase solida dello sviluppo embrionale. Le duplicazioni intestinali che si verificano in associazione con **anomalie delle vertebre e del midollo spinale** (emivertebre, spina bifida anteriore, stria legamentosa tra la lesione e la colonna cervicale o toracica) potrebbero derivare da un'interruzione della notocorda nell'embrione in via di sviluppo. La **duplicazione del colon** è in genere associata con anomalie del tratto urinario e dei genitali. Si può verificare anche una duplicazione dell'intero colon, del retto, dell'ano e dell'ileo terminale. Si ritiene che questi difetti siano secondari a un accoppiamento caudale, con duplicazione dell'intestino posteriore, dei genitali e del tratto urinario inferiore.

MANIFESTAZIONI CLINICHE. I sintomi dipendono dalle dimensioni, dalla localizzazione e dal rivestimento mucoso. Le duplicazioni possono provocare un'ostruzione intestinale comprimendo il lume intestinale adiacente oppure rappresentare il punto di partenza di un'intussuscezione o costituire la sede di un volvolo. Se sono rivestite da mucosa acidosecernente, provocano ulcerazioni, perforazioni ed emorragie nell'intestino adiacente. I pazienti possono presentare dolore addominale, vomito, una massa palpabile oppure un'emorragia gastrointestinale acuta. Le duplicazioni intestinali a livello toracico (cisti neuroenteriche) si possono manifestare con distress respiratorio, mentre quelle dell'intestino inferiore possono causare stipsi o diarrea oppure essere associate al prolasso ricorrente del retto.

La diagnosi viene sospettata sulla base dell'anamnesi e dell'esame obiettivo. Le indagini radiologiche, come gli esami con bario, l'ecografia, la TC e la risonanza magnetica (RM), sono utili ma spesso aspecifiche, mettendo in evidenza una struttura cistica o un effetto massa. La scintigrafia con il radioisotopo tecnezio può localizzare una mucosa gastrica ectopica. La terapia delle duplicazioni consiste nella resezione chirurgica e nel trattamento dei difetti associati.

328.2 • Diverticolo di Meckel e altri residui del dotto onfalomesenterico

Il diverticolo di Meckel è un residuo del sacco vitellino embrionario, che viene denominato anche dotto onfalomesenterico o vitellino. Il dotto onfalomesenterico congiunge il sacco vitellino all'intestino nell'embrione in via di sviluppo, al quale fornisce il nutrimento fino alla formazione della placenta. Tra la 5ª e la 7ª settimana di gestazione questo dotto si riduce e si separa dall'intestino. Subito prima della sua involuzione, l'epitelio del sacco vitellino sviluppa un rivestimento simile a quello dello stomaco. Una mancata involuzione parziale o completa del dotto onfalomesenterico determina la formazione di varie strutture residue. Il diverticolo di Meckel è la più comune e costituisce la più frequente anomalia gastrointestinale congenita, potendosi riscontrare nel 2-3% di tutti i lattanti. Il diverticolo di Meckel tipico consiste in un'estroflessione di 3-6 cm dell'ileo lungo il bordo antimesentrico a 50-75 cm dalla valvola ileocecale (Fig. 328-1). La distanza dalla valvola ileocecale dipende dall'età del paziente. Di più raro riscontro sono altri residui del dotto onfalomesenterico, tra cui un dotto pervio, un cordone solido o con una cisti centrale oppure un diverticolo associato con la persistenza di un cordone tra il diverticolo e l'ombelico.

MANIFESTAZIONI CLINICHE. I sintomi del diverticolo di Meckel solitamente insorgono nei primi due anni di vita (in media a 2,5 anni), ma i sintomi iniziali possono manifestarsi fino ai dieci anni di età. La maggior parte dei diverticoli di Meckel sintomatici è rivestita da mucosa ectopica, compresa la mucosa acidosecernente che provoca un sanguinamento rettale non doloroso in-

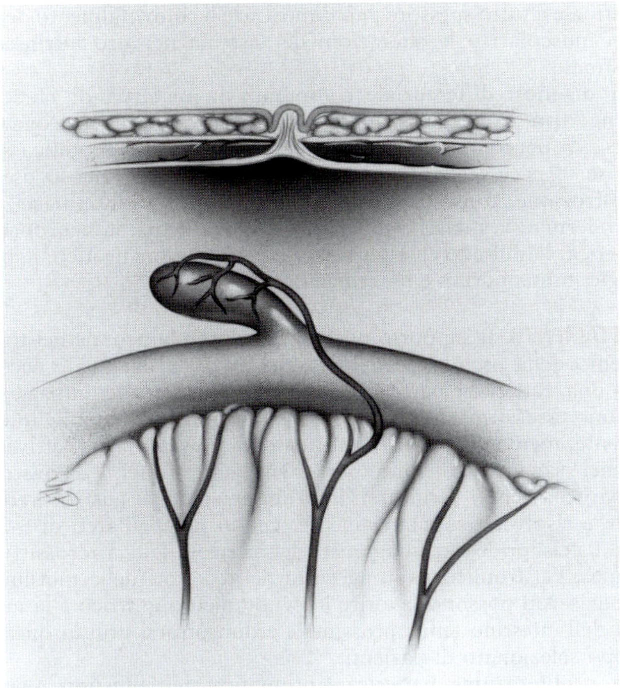

Figura 328-1. Un tipico diverticolo di Meckel localizzato sul margine antimesenterico.

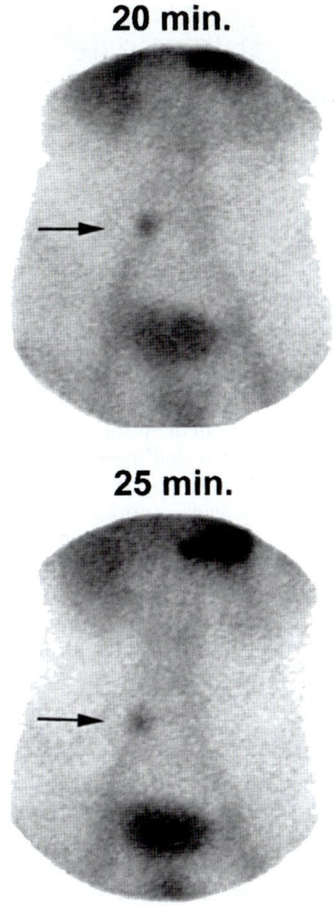

Figura 328-2. Scintigrafia per la ricerca del un diverticolo di Meckel, che mostra un accumulo di Tecnezio nello stomaco (sopra), nella vescica (sotto) e a livello della mucosa acidosecernente del diverticolo.

termittente per ulcerazione dell'adiacente mucosa ileale normale. Contrariamente a quanto accade a livello della mucosa duodenale superiore, l'acido in questo caso non viene neutralizzato dal bicarbonato pancreatico.

Le feci vengono tipicamente descritte come di color mattone oppure a gelatina di ribes. Il sanguinamento può determinare un'anemia significativa, ma è in genere autolimitante per la contrazione dei vasi splancnici, che si verifica quando il paziente diventa ipovolemico. Il sanguinamento da un diverticolo di Meckel può essere anche meno eclatante, con feci melaniche.

È meno frequente che il diverticolo di Meckel sia associato con un'ostruzione intestinale parziale o completa. Il meccanismo più comune di ostruzione è quello in cui il diverticolo costituisce il punto di partenza di un'intussuscezione. L'età media di insorgenza dell'ostruzione è inferiore a quella dei pazienti che presentano il sanguinamento come sintomo di esordio. L'ostruzione può derivare anche da briglie intraperitoneali che uniscono residui del dotto onfalomesenterico all'ileo o all'ombelico. Queste briglie causano l'ostruzione per erniazione interna oppure per la formazione di un volvolo dell'intestino tenue attorno a esse. Un diverticolo di Meckel può occasionalmente infiammarsi (diverticolite) e configurare un quadro simile a quello dell'appendicite acuta. In questi casi il bambino è più grande, con un'età media di 8 anni. La diverticolite può evolvere in perforazione e peritonite.

DIAGNOSI. La diagnosi dei residui del dotto onfalomesenterico dipende dalla loro presentazione clinica. Se un lattante o un bambino presentano un sanguinamento rettale significativo senza dolore, si dovrebbe sospettare un diverticolo di Meckel. La sua conferma può esser difficile: le radiografie dirette dell'addome non sono di alcun aiuto e negli esami baritati di routine raramente il diverticolo si riempie. La metodica più sensibile è una specifica scintigrafia con radionuclidi, effettuata previa infusione endovenosa di tecnezio-99m pertecnetato. Le cellule mucosecernenti della mucosa gastrica ectopica assumono il pertecnetato, consentendo la visualizzazione del diverticolo di Meckel (Fig. 328-2). Tale assorbimento può essere amplificato con vari agenti, tra cui la cimetidina, il glucagone e la gastrina. La sensibilità della scintigrafia con amplificazione è pari a circa l'85%, con una specificità del 95%. Altre metodiche per l'identificazione di questo diverticolo comprendono l'ecografia addominale, l'angiografia della mesenterica superiore, la TC addominale e la laparoscopia esplorativa. Nei pazienti che presentano un'ostruzione intestinale o un quadro di appendicite con un residuo del dotto onfalomesenterico, è raro che la diagnosi venga formulata prima dell'intervento chirurgico. La terapia del diverticolo di Meckel sintomatico consiste nell'escissione chirurgica.

Baldisserotto M, Maffazzoni DR, Dora MD: Sonographic findings of Meckel's diverticulitis in children. *AJR Am J Roentgenol* 2003;80:425–428.

Emamian SA, Shalaby-Rana E, Majd M: The spectrum of heterotopic gastric mucosa in children detected by Tc-99m pertechnetate scintigraphy. *Clin Nucl Med* 2001;26:529–535.

Fenton LZ, Buonomo C, Share JC, Chung T: Small intestinal obstruction by remnants of the omphalomesenteric duct: Findings on contrast enema. *Pediatr Radiol* 2000;30:165–167.

Lee KH, Yeung CK, Tam YH, et al: Laparascopy for definitive diagnosis and treatment of gastrointestinal bleeding of obscure origin in children. *J Pediatr Surg* 2000;35:1291–1293.

Swaniker F, Soldes O, Hirschl RB: The utility of technetium-99m pertechnetate scintigraphy in the evaluation of patients with Meckel's diverticulum. *J Pediatr Surg* 1999;34:760–764, discussion 765.

Capitolo 329 ■ Patologie della motilità e malattia di Hirschsprung Robert Wyllie

329.1 • Pseudo-ostruzione intestinale cronica

La pseudo-ostruzione intestinale cronica comprende un gruppo di patologie caratterizzate da segni e sintomi di ostruzione intestinale, in assenza di lesioni anatomiche. Essa si può verificare come patologia primitiva oppure essere secondaria a un gran numero di condizioni che alterano la motilità intestinale in maniera transitoria o permanente. La pseudo-ostruzione rappresenta un ampio spettro di patologie, da un'attività mioelettrica anomala alle alterazioni nervose (**neuropatia intestinale**) o muscolari (**miopatia intestinale**) a carico dell'intestino, che possono colpire l'intero tratto gastrointestinale oppure solo alcuni organi, come lo stomaco o il colon. Le varie anomalie patologiche verranno trattate insieme per via delle loro somiglianze cliniche.

La maggior parte delle forme di pseudo-ostruzione si verifica sporadicamente. All'interno di alcuni gruppi di individui autosomici dominanti o recessivi sono stati segnalati casi associati ad anomalie nervose o muscolari dell'intestino. I pazienti affetti da forme autosomiche dominanti di pseudo-ostruzione presentano espressioni variabili della malattia. Le forme acquisite possono manifestarsi dopo episodi di gastroenterite acuta, che si suppone abbiano danneggiato il plesso mioenterico.

Nella maggior parte delle pseudo-ostruzioni congenite è possibile dimostrare alterazioni nervose o muscolari. Nelle malattie muscolari lo strato muscolare esterno longitudinale viene sostituito da materiale fibrotico. Nelle malattie neuronali si può osservare una disorganizzazione dei gangli oppure un'ipo- o un'iperganglionosi. In alcuni bambini sono state rilevate anomalie delle cellule interstiziali di Cajal, in altri, invece, difetti mitocondriali.

MANIFESTAZIONI CLINICHE. Più della metà dei bambini con pseudo-ostruzione congenita manifesta sintomi già nei primi mesi di vita. Due terzi dei neonati con sintomi nei primi giorni di vita sono prematuri e il 40% circa presenta una malrotazione dell'intestino. Nel 75% di questi pazienti i sintomi insorgono già nel primo anno di vita, mentre gli altri diventano sintomatici in seguito. I **sintomi più comuni** sono la distensione addominale e il vomito, presenti nel 75% dei bambini affetti. La stipsi, il ritardo di crescita e il dolore addominale si riscontrano nel 60% circa dei pazienti, mentre la diarrea si verifica nel 30-40%. La sintomatologia si aggrava e si attenua spontaneamente nella maggior parte dei casi; la malnutrizione e le patologie intercorrenti tendono a esacerbare i sintomi. Nel 40% dei bambini con miopatia si osserva un **interessamento del tratto urinario**, che può presentarsi con infezioni urinarie ricorrenti, megacisti o sintomi ostruttivi. Le anomalie del tratto urinario sono meno comuni in caso di patologia neuronale.

La diagnosi di pseudo-ostruzione si basa sulla presenza di sintomi compatibili, in assenza di ostruzione anatomica. Alle radiografie dirette dell'addome si apprezzano livelli idroaerei nell'intestino tenue. I neonati con evidenza di ostruzione alla nascita presentano un microcolon. Dal momento che le metodiche di indagine con mezzo di contrasto evidenziano un transito rallentato del bario, bisognerebbe prendere in considerazione l'impiego di agenti idrosolubili.

Altre indagini possono fornire informazioni sulla fisiopatologia sottostante. La motilità esofagea è alterata nella metà circa dei pazienti. Gli studi della motilità antroduodenale e dello svuotamento gastrico producono risultati anormali in caso di interessamento dell'intestino tenue. L'evidenza di un complesso motorio migrante e di un'attività postprandiale normali alla manometria dovrebbe reindirizzare la valutazione diagnostica. La motilità anorettale risulta normale, reperto che permette di differenziare la pseudo-ostruzione dalla malattia di Hirschsprung. La biopsia intestinale a tutto spessore può dimostrare il coinvolgimento degli strati muscolari o le alterazioni del sistema nervoso intrinseco intestinale.

La **diagnosi differenziale** comprende la malattia di Hirschsprung, altre cause di ostruzione meccanica, la stipsi psicogena, la vescica neurologica e la sindrome dell'arteria mesenterica superiore. È necessario escludere cause secondarie di ileo o pseudo-ostruzione, come l'ipotiroidismo, l'assunzione di oppiacei, la sclerodermia, la malattia di Chagas, l'ipokaliemia, la neuropatia diabetica, l'amiloidosi, la porfiria, l'edema angioneurotico, le patologie mitocondriali e da radiazioni.

TRATTAMENTO. Il supporto nutrizionale è fondamentale nel trattamento della pseudo-ostruzione. Nel 30-50% dei casi è necessaria una nutrizione parenterale parziale o totale. Alcuni pazienti possono essere trattati con una supplementazione enterale intermittente, mentre per altri è sufficiente una dieta orale selettiva. I farmaci procinetici di solito non si rivelano efficaci. Una gastroparesi isolata può verificarsi dopo un episodio di gastroenterite virale e risolversi spontaneamente, per lo più nell'arco di 6-24 mesi. La cisapride (un antagonista dei recettori della 5-idrossitriptamina), l'eritromicina (un agonista dei recettori della motilina) e il tegaserod possono favorire lo svuotamento gastrico e la motilità dell'intestino tenue prossimale e dimostrarsi utili in questo gruppo selezionato di pazienti.

La **proliferazione batterica** sintomatica nell'intestino tenue, che può essere associata a steatorrea e malassorbimento, viene solitamente trattata con antibiotici per via orale; gli antibiotici, tuttavia, dovrebbero essere utilizzati con giudizio poiché possono portare alla selezione di batteri farmacoresistenti. Il trattamento dei pazienti con sintomi peptici consiste nella somministrazione di inibitori della secrezione acida (vedi Capitolo 332). Alcuni bambini traggono beneficio da un'ileostomia o colostomia decompressiva. La colectomia con anastomosi ileorettale è efficace quando la sede principale delle anomalie motorie è l'intestino crasso. Il trapianto di intestino può essere utile in pazienti selezionati (vedi Capitolo 336).

Haftel LT, Lev D, Barash V, et al: Familial mitochondrial intestinal pseudo-obstruction and neurogenic bladder. *J Child Neurol* 2000;15:386–389.
Iyer K, Kaufman S, Sudan D, et al: Long-term results of intestinal transplantation for pseudo-obstruction in children. *J Pediatr Surg* 2001;36:174–177.

329.2 • Stipsi funzionale

La stipsi viene definita come un ritardo o una difficoltà nella defecazione che persiste per almeno 2 settimane. In genere è possibile distinguere la stipsi funzionale (nota anche come stipsi idiopatica o ritenzione fecale) da quella secondaria a cause organiche sulla base dell'anamnesi e dell'esame obiettivo. Diversamente dalle malformazioni anorettali e dalla malattia di Hirschsprung, la stipsi funzionale tende a manifestarsi dopo il periodo neonatale, di solito in seguito a un transito fecale con evacuazione dolorosa, che induce alla ritenzione volontaria delle feci per evitare il dolore. A scatenare lo stimolo doloroso può essere un'infiammazione perianale imputabile a un'allergia alle proteine del latte. Il bambino che presenta lo stimolo alla defecazione adotta alcuni atteggiamenti tipici: in particolare, contrae i muscoli glutei irrigidendo le gambe quando è disteso oppure aggrappandosi a un mobile quando si trova in posizione eretta. Alcuni bambini si accovacciano o si nascondono durante il transito delle feci. Coloro che si occupano del bambino possono interpretare erroneamente queste attività come sforzi. Nella stipsi funzionale è comune l'encopresi diurna e alcuni pazienti presenteranno in anamnesi perdite ematiche con le feci, osservate durante un transito intestinale con movimenti dell'intestino crasso. I reperti suggestivi di una patologia sottostante comprendono difficoltà di crescita, calo ponderale, dolore addominale, vomito oppure ragadi o fistole anali persistenti.

L'**esame obiettivo** evidenzia spesso una grossa massa fecale palpabile nella regione sovrapubica; all'esplorazione rettale la cavità rettale si rivela dilatata, piena di feci negative al test al guaiaco. La presenza di un ciuffo di peli sulla colonna vertebrale o di una depressione spinale oppure la difficoltà a suscitare il riflesso cremasterico o il riflesso anale sono suggestive di una patologia spinale. Una compressione midollare in atto è suggerita dalla riduzione o dall'assenza dei riflessi degli arti inferiori. Si possono verificare lesioni del midollo spinale con alterazioni della cute sovrastante. I sintomi a carico del tratto urinario comprendono le infezioni ricorrenti; talvolta si evidenzia un'ostruzione nei bambini con stipsi e patologie del midollo spinale. I bambini senza evidenza di alterazioni all'esame obiettivo necessitano raramente di una valutazione con esami radiologici. Nei pazienti refrattari (con stipsi intrattabile), bisognerebbe prendere in esame l'opportunità di prescrivere esami specialistici per escludere condizioni come l'ipotiroidismo, l'ipocalcemia, la tossicità da piombo e la malattia celiaca. In alcuni bambini selezionati possono essere utili una RM della colonna vertebrale per identificare i processi intraspinali, una serie di accertamenti volti a individuare eventuali miopatie o neuropatie intestinali sottostanti oppure un clisma con bario per visualizzare anomalie strutturali. Gli studi della motilità rettale possono evidenziare un quadro di contrazioni paradosse dello sfintere anale esterno durante la defecazione, trattabile con modificazioni comportamentali. La valutazione della motilità colica può guidare la terapia nei casi refrattari, mostrando alterazioni segmentarie risolvibili con un intervento chirurgico.

La terapia della stipsi funzionale consiste nell'educare il paziente, nel favorire l'eliminazione del fecaloma e nel rendere più morbide le feci. I genitori dovrebbero comprendere che le perdite di feci associate all'incontinenza da sovrariempimento dipendono da un difetto della normale sensibilità e non da un atto volontario. Un programma regolare di educazione intestinale, che includa il restare seduti in bagno per 5-10 minuti dopo il pasto e l'annotare la frequenza delle evacuazioni, spesso è d'aiuto per ristabilire la regolarità intestinale. Se è presente un fecaloma all'esame obiettivo iniziale, di solito è necessario un clistere per eliminarlo, mentre viene iniziata una terapia di mantenimento con preparati che ammorbidiscano le feci. Gli schemi terapeutici classici comprendono l'utilizzo di preparati a base di **polietilenglicole**, lattulosio o olio minerale. Si sconsiglia l'uso prolungato di stimolanti come la senna o il bisacodil. I bambini con problemi comportamentali che interferiscono con l'efficacia del trattamento possono trarre beneficio da un appoggio psicoterapico. La terapia di mantenimento in genere viene continuata fino al ripristino della regolarità intestinale; è inoltre importante che il paziente impari a non considerare il transito fecale come un'esperienza dolorosa. I bambini con patologie spinali possono essere trattati efficacemente con la somministrazione di piccole quantità di liquidi attraverso una ciecostomia o un sondino sigmoideo.

Brooks RC, Copen RM, Cox DJ, et al: Review of the treatment literature for encopresis, functional constipation, and stool-toileting refusal. *Ann Behav Med* 2000;22:260–267.

Corazziari E, Badiali D, Bazzocchi G, et al: Long-term efficacy, safety, and tolerability of low daily doses of isosmotic polyethylene glycol electrolyte balanced solution (PMF-100) in the treatment of functional chronic constipation. *Gut* 2000;46:522–526.

Emmanuel AV, Kamm MA: Response to a behavioral treatment, biofeedback, in constipated patients is associated with improved gut transit and autonomic innervation. *Gut* 2001;49:214–219.

Kim HL, Gow KW, Penner JG, et al: Presentation of low anorectal malformations beyond the neonatal period. *Pediatrics* 2000;105:E68.

Rosen R, Buonomo C, Andrade R, Nurko: Incidence of spinal cord lesions in patients with intractable constipation. *J Pediatr* 2004;145:409–411.

Youssef NN, Di Lorenzo C: Childhood constipation: Evaluation and treatment. *J Clin Gastroenterol* 2001;33:199–205.

329.3 • Megacolon agangliare congenito (malattia di Hirschsprung)

La malattia di Hirschsprung, o megacolon agangliare congenito, è causata da un'anomala innervazione dell'intestino, che inizia a livello dello sfintere anale interno e si estende in senso prossimale coinvolgendo l'intestino per una lunghezza variabile. Questa patologia rappresenta la più comune causa di ostruzione intestinale nei neonati, con un'incidenza complessiva di 1/5000 nati vivi. I maschi ne sono affetti più delle femmine (4:1); la prematurità è rara. È emersa un'incidenza familiare aumentata nella malattia del segmento lungo. La malattia di Hirschsprung può essere associata con altri difetti congeniti, tra cui le sindromi di Down, Smith-Lemli-Opitz, Waardenburg, l'ipoplasia cartilagine-capelli e la sindrome da ipoventilazione congenita ("maledizione di Ondina"), oltre che con anomalie urogenitali e cardiovascolari. La malattia di Hirschsprung è stata osservata in associazione con la microcefalia, il ritardo mentale e anomalie faciali, con l'autismo oppure con la palatoschisi, l'idrocefalo e la micrognazia.

ANATOMIA PATOLOGICA. La causa della malattia di Hirschsprung è l'assenza delle cellule gangliari nella parete intestinale, che si estende a partire dall'ano in maniera continua e in senso prossimale per un tratto di lunghezza variabile. L'assenza dell'innervazione neurale è una conseguenza dell'arresto della migrazione dei neuroblasti dall'intestino prossimale a quello distale. Si tratta in genere di una patologia sporadica; in alcuni nuclei familiari sono emersi pattern di ereditarietà sia dominanti sia recessivi. Sono stati identificati difetti in vari geni che codificano per proteine della via di segnale RET (*RET*, *GDNF* e *NTN*), coinvolte nella via del recettore di tipo B dell'endotelina (EDN) (*EDNRB*, *EDN3* ed *EVE-1*). Le forme sindromiche della malattia di Hirschsprung sono state associate con i geni *LICAM*, *SOX10* e *SIP1*.

Il segmento agangliare è limitato al rettosigma nel 75% dei pazienti; nel 10% dei casi tutto il colon è privo di cellule gangliari. L'agangliosi intestinale totale è rara. Da un punto di vista istologico si osservano l'assenza dei plessi mioenterico e di Auerbach e fibre nervose ipertrofiche con un'elevata concentrazione di acetilcolinesterasi tra gli strati muscolari e nella sottomucosa.

MANIFESTAZIONI CLINICHE. La sintomatologia della malattia di Hirschsprung di solito si manifesta alla nascita, con un transito del meconio ritardato. Il 99% dei neonati a termine elimina il meconio nel giro di 48 ore dalla nascita. La malattia di Hirschsprung dovrebbe essere sospettata in tutti i neonati a termine (dal momento che la patologia è rara nei prematuri) che presentino un transito rallentato delle feci. Anche soggetti con un transito del meconio normale possono sviluppare in seguito un quadro di stipsi cronica. Un ritardo di crescita con ipoproteinemia da enteropatia protidodisperdente costituisce una presentazione meno comune, poiché in genere la malattia di Hirschsprung viene riconosciuta precocemente. I neonati allattati al seno possono presentare una forma meno severa rispetto a quelli nutriti con latte artificiale.

Il transito delle feci difficoltoso provoca la dilatazione dell'intestino prossimale e la distensione addominale. La dilatazione dell'intestino determina un aumento della pressione intraluminale, causando una riduzione del flusso ematico e il deterioramento della barriera mucosa. La stasi favorisce la proliferazione batterica, che può causare un'enterocolite (da *Clostridium difficile*, *Staphylococcus aureus*, anaerobi, coliformi) associata a sepsi e segni di ostruzione intestinale. La diagnosi tempestiva della malattia di Hirschsprung, prima dell'insorgenza dell'enterocolite, è fondamentale per ridurre morbilità e mortalità.

Nei bambini più grandi questa patologia deve essere distinta dalle altre cause di distensione addominale e dalla stipsi cronica (Tab. 329-1 e Fig. 329-1). L'anamnesi spesso rivela una progressiva difficoltà nel transito delle feci, che inizia nelle primissime settimane di vita. Una grossa massa fecale è palpabile nel quadrante addominale inferiore sinistro; il retto è solitamente vuoto. Le feci evacuate possono consistere in piccole pallottole, essere

TABELLA 329-1. Caratteristiche che permettono di distinguere la malattia di Hirschsprung dalla stipsi funzionale

VARIABILE	FUNZIONALE (ACQUISITA)	MALATTIA DI HIRSCHSPRUNG
ANAMNESI		
Esordio della stipsi	Dopo i due anni di età	Alla nascita
Encopresi	Comune	Molto rara
Ritardo di crescita	Infrequente	Possibile
Enterocolite	Assente	Possibile
Educazione intestinale coercitiva	Frequente	Assente
ESAME OBIETTIVO		
Distensione addominale	Infrequente	Comune
Scarso aumento ponderale	Raro	Comune
Tono anale	Normale	Normale
Esplorazione rettale	Feci in ampolla	Ampolla vuota
Malnutrizione	Assente	Possibile
INDAGINI STRUMENTALI		
Manometria anorettale	La distensione del retto causa il rilasciamento dello sfintere interno	Mancato rilasciamento dello sfintere o aumento paradosso della pressione
Biopsia rettale	Normale	Assenza delle cellule gangliari, aumentata colorazione per l'acetilcolinesterasi
Clisma baritato	Quantità massive di feci, zona di transizione assente	Zona di transizione, evacuazione ritardata (>24 ore)

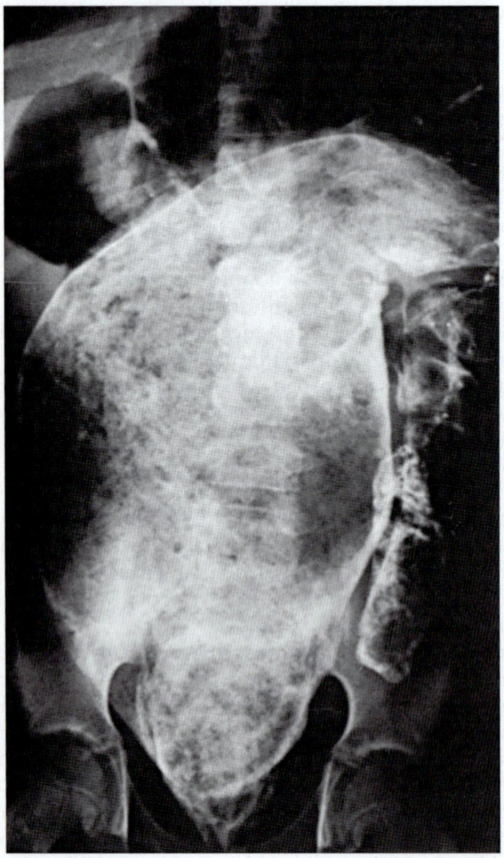

Figura 329-1. Clisma baritato in un paziente di 14 anni con stipsi severa. La notevole dilatazione del retto e del colon distale è tipica del megacolon funzionale acquisito.

nastriformi oppure avere una consistenza fluida; sono assenti le voluminose masse fecali e l'incontinenza tipici dei pazienti con stipsi funzionale. Nei neonati la malattia di Hirschsprung deve essere differenziata dalla sindrome da tappo di meconio, dall'ileo da meconio e dall'atresia intestinale; nei pazienti più grandi occorre prendere in considerazione la **triade di Currarino** (**malformazioni anorettali** come l'ano ectopico e la stenosi anorettale, **anomalie dell'osso sacro** come l'ipoplasia o la ridotta segmentazione oppure **masse presacrali** come il meningocele anteriore, il teratoma o la cisti).

L'esplorazione rettale evidenzia un tono anale normale ed è solitamente seguita dall'emissione esplosiva di feci e gas maleodoranti. Gli attacchi intermittenti di ostruzione intestinale da ritenzione fecale possono essere associati a dolore e febbre.

DIAGNOSI. La manometria rettale e la biopsia rettale tramite aspirazione rappresentano le metodiche più semplici e affidabili per la diagnosi della malattia di Hirschsprung.

Le biopsie rettali con aspirazione costituiscono la **procedura di scelta** e dovrebbero essere effettuate a più di 2 cm dalla linea dentata per evitare la normale area di ipoganglionosi della rima anale. Il materiale bioptico, che dovrebbe comprendere un adeguato campione di sottomucosa per valutare la presenza delle cellule gangliari, può essere colorato per la ricerca dell'acetilcolinesterasi, al fine di facilitare l'interpretazione. I pazienti con aganglionosi presentano un gran numero di fibre nervose ipertrofiche che si colorano positivamente per l'acetilcolinesterasi e l'assenza di cellule gangliari.

La manometria anorettale misura la pressione dello sfintere anale interno mediante un palloncino gonfiato nel retto. Negli individui normali la distensione rettale determina una riduzione riflessa della pressione dello sfintere interno. Nei pazienti con malattia di Hirschsprung la pressione non diminuisce oppure subisce un aumento paradosso con la distensione rettale. Questo test diagnostico, la cui accuratezza è >90%, è tuttavia di difficile esecuzione nei lattanti per motivi tecnici. Una risposta normale durante la valutazione manometrica esclude la diagnosi di malattia di Hirschsprung; una risposta ambigua o paradossa rende necessario ripetere lo studio di motilità o procedere alla biopsia rettale.

La diagnosi radiologica di malattia di Hirschsprung si basa sulla presenza di una zona di transizione tra il colon prossimale, normale, dilatato, e il colon distale, ostruito e di piccolo calibro, causata dal mancato rilasciamento dell'intestino agangliare. Questa zona di transizione, che non è solitamente presente prima delle due settimane di vita, sulla radiografia consiste in una porzione di intestino a forma di imbuto tra il colon prossimale dilatato e l'intestino distale ristretto. La valutazione radiologica dovrebbe essere effettuata senza preparazione onde evitare la dilatazione transitoria del segmento agangliare. Sono d'aiuto anche le lastre effettuate 24 ore dopo (Fig. 329-2). Se nel colon è ancora presente una quantità significativa di bario, questo reperto aumenta il sospetto di malattia di Hirschsprung, anche se non viene identificata la zona di transizione. Lo studio con clisma baritato è utile per determinare l'estensione dell'agangliosi prima dell'intervento chirurgico e per valutare le altre malattie che comportano un'ostruzione intestinale bassa nel neonato. Una biopsia rettale a tutto spessore può essere effettuata durante l'intervento chirurgico per confermare la diagnosi e l'estensione.

TRATTAMENTO. Una volta stabilita la diagnosi, il trattamento definitivo consiste nell'intervento chirurgico. Occorre decidere se eseguire una procedura definitiva appena posta la diagnosi oppure una colostomia temporanea, attendendo che il bambino raggiunga i 6-12 mesi di vita per effettuare la correzione definitiva. Tre sono le opzioni chirurgiche principali. La prima procedura chirurgica di successo descritta da Swenson consisteva nel resecare il segmento agangliare e nell'anastomizzare l'intestino prossimale normale al retto, 1-2 cm sopra la linea dentata. Dal momento che questo intervento è tecnicamente difficile, sono state messe a punto altre due procedure. Duhamel ha descritto una procedura per creare un neoretto, portando in basso l'intestino normalmente innervato, dietro il retto agangliare. Il neoretto così ottenuto presenta una metà anteriore agangliare dotata della nor-

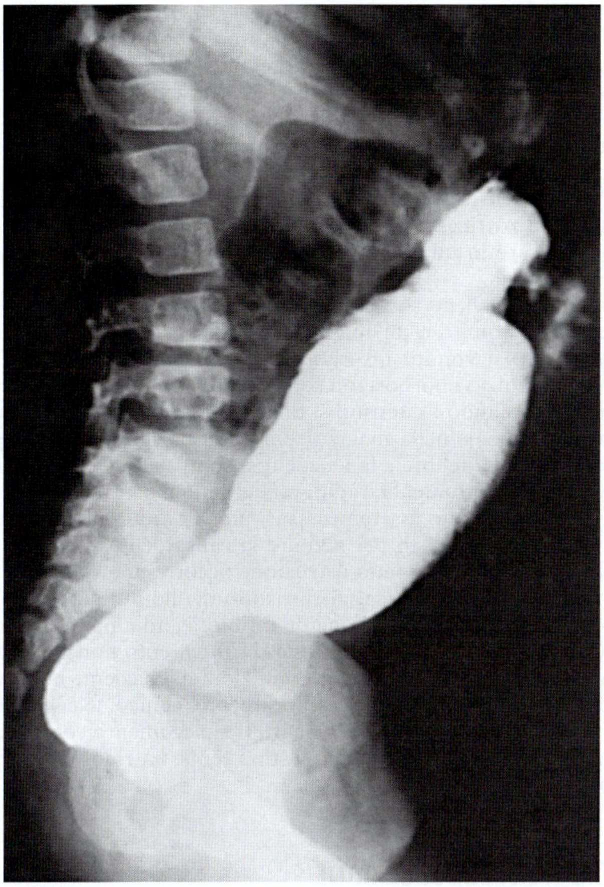

Figura 329-2. Proiezione laterale di un clisma baritato in una bambina di 3 anni con malattia di Hirschsprung. Il segmento distale agangliare è ristretto, con un intestino normale disteso a monte di esso.

male sensibilità e una metà posteriore gangliare con una propulsione normale. La procedura endorettale *pull-through* descritta da Boley prevede la resezione della mucosa dal retto agangliare e il passaggio del colon normalmente innervato attraverso il manicotto muscolare residuo, superando così l'intestino anomalo dall'interno. I progressi compiuti in queste tecniche hanno reso possibile sviluppare procedure endorettali *pull-through* laparoscopiche, che rappresentano il **trattamento di scelta**.

Nella malattia di Hirschsprung **segmentaria ultracorta** o acalasia dello sfintere interno, il tratto agangliare è limitato allo sfintere interno. I sintomi clinici sono simili a quelli che si osservano nei bambini con stipsi funzionale. Alla biopsia rettale tramite aspirazione sono presenti le cellule gangliari, ma la motilità rettale è anormale. L'asportazione di una striscia di muscolatura rettale determina solitamente un pattern intestinale più regolare.

La malattia di Hirschsprung **a segmento lungo**, che interessa tutto il colon e parte dell'intestino tenue, rappresenta un problema complesso. Gli studi di motilità rettale e la biopsia del retto mediante aspirazione mostrano un quadro di malattia di Hirschsprung, ma gli studi radiologici sono difficili da interpretare in quanto non è possibile identificare una zona di transizione colica. L'estensione dell'agangliosi può essere determinata accuratamente tramite biopsia al momento della laparotomia. Quando l'intero colon è agangliare, spesso con il parziale coinvolgimento dell'ileo terminale, l'anastomosi ileo-anale rappresenta il trattamento di scelta, conservando parte del colon agangliare per favorire l'assorbimento dell'acqua e produrre feci formate.

La prognosi della malattia di Hirschsprung trattata chirurgicamente è in genere soddisfacente; gran parte dei pazienti raggiunge la continenza fecale. I problemi postoperatori comprendono le enterocoliti ricorrenti, le stenosi, i prolassi, gli ascessi perianali e l'incontinenza fecale. In alcuni bambini è necessaria la miectomia o una nuova procedura *pull-through*.

329.4 • Displasia neuronale intestinale

Questa patologia può assomigliare alla malattia di Hirschsprung, ma invece dell'assenza delle cellule gangliari intestinali essa presenta nel **tipo A** l'assenza o l'ipoplasia dell'innervazione simpatica dei plessi mienterico e sottomucoso con un aumento delle fibre nervose parasimpatiche, un'iperplasia del plesso mienterico e un'infiammazione della mucosa colica e nel **tipo B** un plesso sottomucoso displastico con gangli giganti e fibre nervose ispessite, aumentata colorazione per l'acetilcolinesterasi e cellule gangliari isolate nella lamina propria.

Le **manifestazioni cliniche** comprendono distensione addominale, stipsi ed enterocoliti. Il tratto di intestino colpito può avere una lunghezza variabile (da un segmento all'intero tratto intestinale). Alcuni pazienti hanno una malattia di Hirschsprung associata, mentre altri presentano prematurità, sindrome del colon sinistro piccolo e sindrome da tappo di meconio.

Il **trattamento** è lo stesso previsto per la stipsi funzionale; se si rivela inefficace, è indicato l'intervento chirurgico.

Benailly HK, Lapierre JM, Laudier B, et al: *PMX2B*, a new candidate gene for Hirschsprung's disease. *Clin Genet* 2003;64:204–209.

Cucchiara S, Borrelli O, Salvia G, et al: A normal gastrointestinal motility excludes chronic intestinal pseudoobstruction in children. *Dig Dis Sci* 2000;45:258–264.

DeLorijn F, Reitsma JB, Voskuijl WP, et al: Diagnosis of Hirschsprung's disease: A prospective comparative accuracy study of common tests. *J Pediatr* 2005;146:787–792.

Hackam DJ, Reblock K, Barksdale EM, et al: The influence of Down's syndrome on the management and outcome of children with Hirschsprung's disease. *J Pediatr Surg* 2003;38:946–949.

Haftel LT, Lev D, Barash V, et al: Familial mitochondrial intestinal pseudo-obstruction and neurogenic bladder. *J Child Neurol* 2000;15: 386–389.

Keshtgar AS, Ward HC, Clayden GS, de Sousa NM: Investigations for incontinence and constipation after surgery for Hirschsprung's disease in children. *Pediatr Surg Int* 2003;19:4–8.

Langer JC, Durrant AC, de la Torre L, et al: One-stage transanal Soave pullthrough for Hirschsprung disease: A multicenter experience with 141 children. *Ann Surg* 2003;238:569–583, discussion 583–585.

Lapointe SP, Rivet C, Goulet O, et al: Urological manifestations associated with chronic intestinal pseudo-obstructions in children. *J Urol* 2002;168: 1768–1770.

Mousa H, Hyman PE, Cocjin J, et al: Long-term outcome of congenital intestinal pseudoobstruction. *Dig Dis Sci* 2002;47:2298–2305.

Pensabene L, Youssef NN, Griffiths JM, Di Lorenzo C: Colonic manometry in children with defecatory disorders. Role in diagnosis and management. *Am J Gastroenterol* 2003;98:1052–1057.

Teitelbaum DH, Coran AG: Reoperative surgery for Hirschsprung's disease. *Semin Pediatr Surg* 2003;12:124–131.

329.5 • Sindrome dell'arteria mesenterica superiore (sindrome di Wilkie, sindrome da ingessatura, sindrome da compressione duodenale arteriomesenterica)

La sindrome dell'arteria mesenterica superiore consiste in una compressione estrinseca del duodeno che si verifica nei bambini dopo un rapido calo ponderale e in posizione supina. Si ritiene che la compressione sia dovuta alla perdita di grasso del mesentere che porta l'arteria mesenterica superiore a collassare sul duodeno, comprimendolo tra l'arteria mesenterica superiore anteriormente e l'aorta posteriormente. In alternativa, la causa potrebbe essere la perdita del grasso di supporto nella seconda e terza porzione duodenale, in conseguenza della quale il duodeno collassa contro la colonna vertebrale.

L'**esempio classico** è rappresentato da un adolescente che inizia a vomitare dopo un intervento di chirurgia ortopedica con l'applicazione di un'ingessatura. Altri fattori associati comprendono l'anoressia, l'allettamento prolungato, il calo ponderale, la chirurgia addominale e una lordosi lombare eccessiva. La diagnosi viene stabilita radiologicamente con la dimostrazione di un'interruzione del duodeno appena a destra della linea mediana. L'ostruzione duodenale può essere accompagnata dalla dilatazione gastrica e duodenale prossimale.

Il **trattamento** della sindrome acuta consiste nella risoluzione dell'ostruzione e nel miglioramento della nutrizione per modificare i rapporti anatomici tra il duodeno e le strutture circostanti. Quando i pazienti adottano il decubito laterale o la posizione prona si ha l'allontanamento del duodeno dalle strutture potenzialmente ostruttive, che talora consente la ripresa dell'alimentazione. Possono essere d'aiuto farmaci procinetici come la metoclopramide e la cisapride. Se riposizionare il paziente non permette di alleviare i sintomi, è possibile inserire un sondino nasodigiunale oltre il punto dell'ostruzione per riprendere la nutrizione. In alcuni pazienti bisogna ricorrere alla nutrizione parenterale totale per ricostituire il grasso corporeo perduto e talvolta si rende necessario l'intervento chirurgico.

Capitolo 330 ■ Ileo, aderenze, intussuscezioni e occlusioni ad ansa chiusa Robert Wyllie

330.1 • Ileo

L'ileo consiste in un'insufficienza della peristalsi intestinale senza evidenza di ostruzione meccanica. L'assenza della normale attività motoria dell'intestino interferisce con il movimento in senso aborale del contenuto intestinale e nei bambini è associata, nella maggior parte dei casi, a interventi o infezioni addominali (polmonite, gastroenterite, peritonite). L'ileo, oltre ad accompagnare alcune alterazioni metaboliche, come l'uremia, l'ipokaliemia, l'ipercalcemia, l'ipermagnesiemia o l'acidosi, si verifica con la somministrazione di alcuni farmaci, come gli oppioidi e la vincristina, e può insorgere anche in seguito all'utilizzo di agenti che bloccano la motilità, come la loperamide, nel corso di episodi di gastroenterite.

L'ileo si presenta con distensione addominale ingravescente e vomito; il dolore, che, inizialmente è molto lieve, aumenta con il progredire della distensione. I borborigmi sono minimi o assenti, a differenza di quanto avviene nell'ostruzione meccanica precoce, nella quale sono iperattivi. Le radiografie dirette dell'addome mostrano livelli idroaerei multipli in tutto l'addome. Le radiografie in serie in genere non rivelano una distensione progressiva, come avviene invece nel caso dell'ostruzione meccanica. Le radiografie con mezzo di contrasto, se effettuate, mostrano un lento movimento del bario attraverso un lume pervio.

Il **trattamento** implica la correzione dell'anomalia sottostante. Si ricorre alla decompressione nasogastrica se la distensione addominale è associata a dolore o per alleviare il vomito ricorrente. L'ileo che si sviluppa dopo procedure chirurgiche addominali di solito si risolve con un ritorno alla normale motilità intestinale nel giro di 24-72 ore. Farmaci procinetici come la metoclopramide o l'eritromicina possono favorire il ripristino della normale motilità intestinale ed essere d'aiuto nei bambini con ileo prolungato. La somministrazione orale di farmaci che bloccano i recettori gastrointestinali degli oppiacei, ma non l'azione degli oppiacei stessi sul sistema nervoso centrale, può ridurre l'ileo nei pazienti che ricevono narcotici dopo un intervento chirurgico.

330.2 • Aderenze

Le aderenze sono bande fibrose di tessuto che rappresentano una causa comune di ostruzione postoperatoria dell'intestino tenue dopo chirurgia addominale. Il rischio che si formi un'aderenza in grado di determinare sintomi ostruttivi non è stato ben studiato nell'infanzia, anche se questa evenienza pare verificarsi nel 2-3% dei pazienti sottoposti a chirurgia addominale. La maggior parte delle ostruzioni è associata con un'aderenza singola e si può verificare in qualsiasi momento dopo la seconda settimana postoperatoria.

La **diagnosi** viene sospettata nei pazienti con dolore addominale, stipsi, vomito e un'anamnesi di chirurgia intraperitoneale. La nausea e il vomito insorgono subito dopo la comparsa del dolore. All'inizio i borborigmi sono iperattivi e l'addome è piatto; in seguito, quando l'intestino si dilata dando luogo a una distensione addominale nella maggior parte dei pazienti, i borborigmi scompaiono. La febbre e la leucocitosi sono suggestive di necrosi intestinale e peritonite. Le radiografie dirette mostrano un quadro ostruttivo e possono essere necessari una TC addominale o studi con mezzo di contrasto per definire la causa dell'ostruzione.

Nei pazienti con sospetta ostruzione occorre procedere alla decompressione nasogastrica, al ripristino dei liquidi per via endovenosa e alla somministrazione di antibiotici ad ampio spettro in previsione dell'intervento chirurgico. L'intervento non chirurgico è controindicato, a meno che le condizioni del paziente non siano stabili, con chiari segni di miglioramento clinico. Nei bambini con aderenze o ostruzioni ricorrenti, il ripiegamento con colla di fibrina delle anse adiacenti di intestino tenue ha ridotto il rischio di problemi ricorrenti.

330.3 • Intussuscezione

L'intussuscezione si verifica quando una porzione del tratto digerente si invagina telescopicamente all'interno di un segmento adiacente; essa rappresenta la causa più comune di occlusione intestinale tra il 3° mese e il 6° anno di età. Il 60% dei pazienti è di età inferiore a 1 anno e l'80% dei casi si verifica prima dei 24 mesi; si tratta tuttavia di un fenomeno raro nei neonati. L'incidenza varia da 1 a 4/1000 nati vivi; il rapporto maschi:femmine è di 4:1. Anche se una piccola percentuale delle intussuscezioni si riduce spontaneamente, la maggior parte di esse, se non trattata, porta a infarto intestinale, perforazione, peritonite e morte.

EZIOLOGIA ED EPIDEMIOLOGIA. Nella maggior parte dei casi, la causa non è nota. L'incidenza stagionale presenta dei picchi in primavera e autunno. L'intussuscezione, oltre a essere stata osservata in correlazione con una pregressa o concomitante infezione respiratoria da adenovirus (di tipo C), può complicare un'otite media, una gastroenterite, una **porpora di Schönlein-Henoch** o le infezioni del tratto respiratorio superiore. Il rischio è risultato aumentato nei bambini di età inferiore all'anno cui era stato somministrato un vaccino tetravalente rhesus-umano per il rotavirus, oggi non più disponibile, nelle prime due settimane di immunizzazione; in particolare, esso risulta molto maggiore dopo la prima dose di vaccino rispetto alle dosi successive alla seconda. L'Advisory Committee on Immunization Practice non raccomanda più questo vaccino. Sebbene il rotavirus produca un'enterotossina, non c'è alcuna associazione tra il rotavirus umano di tipo selvaggio e l'intussuscezione. I vaccini per rotavirus attualmente approvati potrebbero non essere associati con un rischio aumentato di intussuscezione (vedi Capitolo 262).

Si ipotizza che un'infezione gastrointestinale o l'introduzione di nuovi alimenti contenenti proteine provochino il rigonfiamento delle placche di Peyer nell'ileo terminale. L'iperplasia nodulare linfoide è un altro fattore di rischio correlato. I mammelloni prominenti di tessuto linfatico provocano il prolasso della mucosa ileale nel colon, causando così un'intussuscezione. Nel 2-8% dei pazienti si identificano **cause riconoscibili** per questa condizione, come un diverticolo di Meckel, un polipo intestinale, un neurofibroma, una duplicazione intestinale, un emangioma o neoplasie maligne come il linfoma. L'intussuscezione può complicare un'emorragia mucosa, come nella porpora di Schönlein-Henoch o nell'emofilia. La fibrosi cistica rappresenta un ulteriore fattore di rischio. Le intussuscezioni postoperatorie sono ileoileali e solitamente si verificano entro 5 giorni dall'intervento addominale. Le cause riconoscibili sono più comuni nei bambini di età >2 anni. L'intussuscezione intrauterina può essere associata con lo sviluppo di atresia intestinale. Il fenomeno è raro nei neonati prematuri.

ANATOMIA PATOLOGICA. Le intussuscezioni sono per lo più ileocoliche; quelle ciecocoliche sono meno comuni e quelle esclusivamente ileali sono piuttosto rare. Molto raramente l'appendice costituisce l'apice di un'intussuscezione. Il segmento prossimale dell'intestino, **invaginato** (intussusceptum), si introflette in quello distale, **invaginante** (intussuscipiens), spingendo anche il proprio mesentere dentro l'ansa che l'avvolge. La costrizione subita dal mesentere ostacola il ritorno venoso dando luogo alla congestione dell'intussusceptum con edema e al sanguinamento della mucosa, con conseguente comparsa di feci ematiche, talvolta contenenti muco. L'apice dell'intussuscezione si può estendere nel colon traverso, discendente o sigmoideo, fino a raggiungere e attraversare l'ano nei casi trascurati. Questa presentazione deve essere distinta dal prolasso rettale. La maggior parte delle intussuscezioni non strozza l'intestino nelle prime 24 ore, ma può esitare successivamente in gangrena e shock.

MANIFESTAZIONI CLINICHE. Nei casi tipici si assiste all'esordio improvviso, in un bambino precedentemente in stato di benessere, di un dolore colico intenso, parossistico, che si ripresenta a intervalli frequenti, accompagnato da notevoli sforzi con le ginocchia flesse e da forte pianto. Il bambino, che all'inizio, tra i parossismi del dolore, può sentirsi bene e riprendere a giocare come al solito, diventa sempre più debole e letargico se l'intussuscezione non viene ridotta. Talvolta la **letargia** è sproporzionata rispetto ai segni addominali. Nelle forme più gravi si può sviluppare uno stato simile allo shock, con febbre. Il polso diventa debole e sottile, la respirazione si fa superficiale e rumorosa e il dolore può essere espresso solo con gemiti. Il vomito, presente nella maggior parte dei casi, di solito è più frequente nella fase precoce; nella fase più avanzata appare tinto di bile. Nelle prime ore dopo la comparsa dei sintomi si può verificare l'evacuazione di feci di aspetto normale; in seguito però le escrezioni fecali diventano più scarse o, più spesso, cessano del tutto e il transito di gas intestinali è minimo o assente. Il transito del sangue si osserva in genere nelle prime 12 ore, ma talvolta non avviene per 1-2 giorni e in rari casi non si verifica affatto; nel 60% dei bambini si assiste all'evacuazione di feci contenenti sangue di colore rosso vivo e muco, le cosiddette feci a gelatina di ribes. Alcuni pazienti presentano solo irritabilità con una letargia alternante o progressiva.

La palpazione dell'addome solitamente evidenzia una massa a forma di salsicciotto, moderatamente dolente, dai margini talvolta non ben definiti, che può aumentare di dimensioni e fissità durante un parossismo doloroso ed è più spesso localizzata nel quadrante addominale superiore destro, con l'asse maggiore in direzione cefalocaudale. Se questa massa viene percepita in epigastrio, il suo asse maggiore è trasversale. Il 30% circa dei pazienti non presenta una massa palpabile. La presenza di muco ematico sul dito dell'esaminatore, dopo l'esplorazione rettale, avvalora la diagnosi di intussuscezione. La distensione e la tensione addominale si sviluppano quando l'ostruzione intestinale si fa più acuta. In rare occasioni l'intestino in avanzamento prolassa attraverso l'ano. Questo prolasso si differenzia da quello rettale perché è caratterizzato dalla comparsa di un solco tra l'intestino protrudente e la parete del retto, che invece non si osserva nel prolasso rettale.

L'intussuscezione ileoileale può essere caratterizzata da un quadro clinico meno tipico, con segni e sintomi analoghi a quelli dell'occlusione dell'intestino tenue. Un'**intussuscezione ricorrente** viene osservata nel 5-8% dei casi ed è più comune dopo una riduzione idrostatica che chirurgica. L'intussuscezione cronica, nella quale i sintomi si manifestano in forma lieve e a intervalli ricorrenti, si verifica per lo più durante o dopo un'enterite acuta e può insorgere sia nei bambini più grandi sia nei lattanti.

DIAGNOSI. Quando l'anamnesi e il reperto obiettivo sono suggestivi di intussuscezione, viene tipicamente effettuata un'ecografia. Se si opta per una radiografa diretta dell'addome, essa può mostrare una densità anomala nell'area colpita. Le ecografie di screening per sospetta intussuscezione aumentano la resa dei clismi diagnostici/terapeutici e riducono l'esposizione non necessaria alle radiazioni nei bambini con esame ecografico negativo. I reperti diagnostici all'ecografia comprendono una massa tubulare nelle scansioni longitudinali e un aspetto ad anelli concentrici o a bersaglio nelle scansioni trasversali (Fig. 330-1). I clismi con contrasto ad aria, idrostatico (soluzione fisiologica) e, meno frequentemente, idrosolubile hanno sostituito gli studi con bario. I clismi con contrasto evidenziano un difetto di riempimento o un'immagine a coppa in cima al mezzo di contrasto dove la sua progressione è impedita dall'invaginazione (Fig. 330-2). Possono risultare visibili una colonna centrale lineare di mezzo di contrasto nel lume ristretto del tratto invaginato e un sottile margine di bario intrappolato attorno all'intestino invaginato nelle pliche della mucosa all'interno dell'invaginante (segno della molla elicoidale), soprattutto dopo l'evacuazione. La regressione dell'intussuscezione sotto pressione, visualizzata radiograficamente o ecograficamente, documenta una riduzione efficace. Rispetto alle tecniche con contrasto idrostatiche tradizionali, la riduzione con aria è associata a un minor numero di complicanze e a una minore esposizione alle radiazioni.

DIAGNOSI DIFFERENZIALE. Può essere particolarmente difficile diagnosticare un'intussuscezione in un bambino che presenta già una gastroenterite; a mettere in allarme il medico dovrebbe essere qualunque cambiamento nel quadro della malattia, nelle caratteristiche del dolore o nella natura del vomito, oppure l'insorgenza di un sanguinamento rettale. In genere le feci ematiche e i crampi addominali che accompagnano l'enterocolite possono essere differenziati dall'intussuscezione poiché nell'enterocolite il dolore è meno severo e meno regolare, è presente diarrea e il bambino è visibilmente sofferente anche negli intervalli tra un parossismo doloroso e l'altro. Il sanguinamento di un diverticolo di Meckel in genere non è accompagnato da dolore. I sintomi articolari oppure la porpora accompagnano solitamente, ma non invariabilmen-

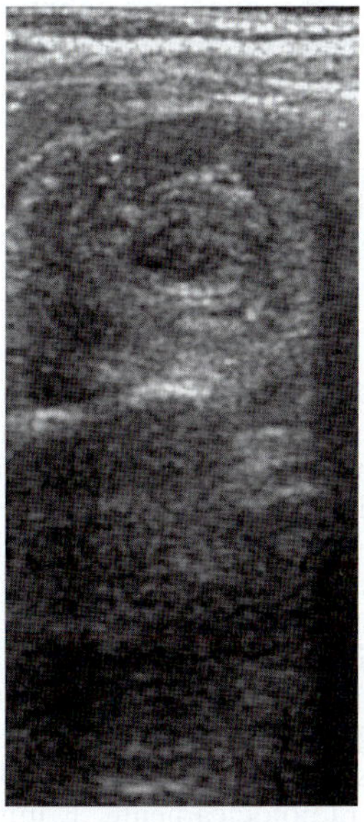

Figura 330-1. Scansione trasversale di un'intussuscezione ileocolica. Si osservino gli anelli all'interno delle anse intestinali.

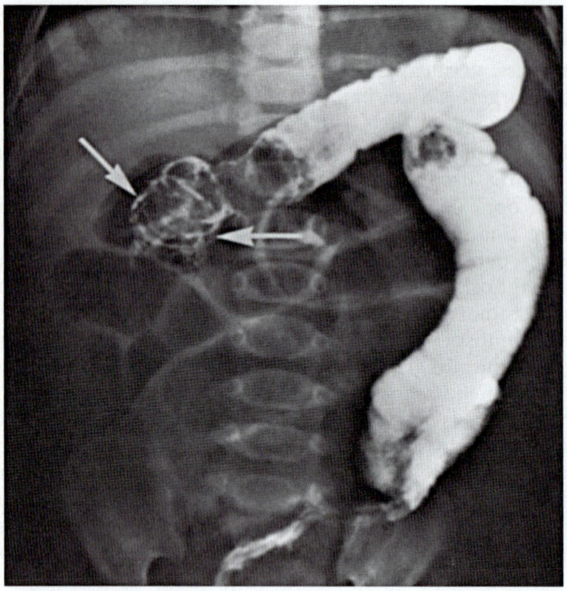

Figura 330-2. Intussuscezione in un neonato. È evidente l'ostruzione nel colon traverso prossimale. Il mezzo di contrasto tra l'invaginato e l'invaginante è responsabile dell'aspetto a molla elicoidale.

te, l'emorragia intestinale nella porpora di Schönlein-Henoch. Poiché l'intussuscezione rappresenta una complicanza di questa patologia, può essere necessaria un'ecografia per distinguere le due condizioni.

TRATTAMENTO. La riduzione di un'intussuscezione acuta costituisce una procedura di emergenza, da effettuarsi immediatamente dopo la diagnosi, in preparazione a un eventuale intervento chirurgico. Tuttavia, essa non va tentata in caso di intussuscezione prolungata con segni di shock, irritazione peritoneale, perforazione intestinale o pneumatosi intestinale.

La percentuale di successo della riduzione idrostatica radiologica sotto guida fluoroscopica o ecografica è ≈50% se i sintomi sono presenti da più di 48 ore e del 70-90% se la procedura viene effettuata nelle prime 48 ore. Le perforazioni intestinali si verificano nello 0,5-2,5% dei tentativi di riduzione con bario o idrostatica (con soluzione fisiologica). La percentuale di perforazione con la riduzione ad aria è pari allo 0,1-0,2%.

Il metodo migliore per individuare un'**intussuscezione ileoileale** è l'ecografia addominale. La riduzione per instillazione di mezzi di contrasto, soluzione fisiologica o aria potrebbe non essere possibile. Queste intussuscezioni possono svilupparsi insidiosamente dopo la chirurgia intestinale e richiedere un reintervento se non si riducono spontaneamente. Se è impossibile procedere a una riduzione manuale o se l'intestino non è vitale, si rende necessaria la resezione dell'intussuscezione, con un'anastomosi terminoterminale.

PROGNOSI. Nei lattanti le intussuscezioni non trattate risultano solitamente fatali; le possibilità di guarigione sono direttamente correlate alla durata dell'intussuscezione prima della riduzione. La maggior parte dei lattanti guarisce se viene effettuata una riduzione nelle prime 24 ore, dopodiché il tasso di mortalità aumenta rapidamente, soprattutto dopo il secondo giorno. Non è rara la riduzione spontanea durante la preparazione per l'intervento.

La **percentuale di recidiva** dopo riduzione è ≈10% e dopo riduzione chirurgica è del 2-5%; non si verificano recidive dopo la resezione chirurgica. I corticosteroidi possono diminuire la frequenza delle intussuscezioni recidivanti, che di solito non possono venire ridotte radiologicamente. È improbabile che un'intussuscezione causata da una lesione come un linfosarcoma, un polipo o un diverticolo di Meckel venga ridotta con successo con una manovra radiologica. Con un'adeguata gestione chirurgica, la riduzione operatoria presenta una percentuale di mortalità molto bassa nei casi diagnosticati precocemente.

330.4 • Occlusioni ad ansa chiusa

L'occlusione intestinale può essere causata da difetti del mesentere ("**ernie interne**") nei quali si introducono e rimangono intrappolate anse dell'intestino tenue. La congestione vascolare dell'intestino intrappolato, se non viene prontamente eliminata, provoca ischemia e gangrena intestinale. I sintomi consistono in vomito biliare, distensione e dolore addominale. I segni peritoneali suggeriscono un'ischemia intestinale. Alla radiografia diretta si apprezzano segni di ostruzione dell'intestino tenue oppure aria libera, in caso di perforazione intestinale. La terapia di supporto comprende liquidi per via endovenosa, antibiotici e decompressione nasogastrica. Al fine di prevenire la gangrena intestinale è indicata la pronta eliminazione chirurgica dell'occlusione. Talvolta i sintomi possono essere transitori, cronici o ricorrenti se l'intestino erniato scivola fuori dal difetto mesenterico, risolvendo spontaneamente l'ostruzione.

Bajaj L, Roback MG: Postreduction management of intussusception in a children's hospital emergency department. *Pediatrics* 2003;112:1302–1307.

Bines JE, Liem NT, Justice FA, et al: Risk factors for intussusception in infants in Vietnam and Australia: Adenovirus implicated, but not rotavirus. *J Pediatr* 2006;149:452–460.

Burke MS, Ragi JM, Karamanoukian HL, et al: New strategies in nonoperative management of meconium ileus. *J Pediatr Surg* 2002;37:760–764.

Centers for Disease Control and Prevention: Postmarketing monitoring of intussusception after Rota Teg vaccination—United States, February 1, 2006–February 15, 2007. *MMWR* 2007;56:218–222.

Crystal P, Hertzanu Y, Farber B, et al: Sonographically guided hydrostatic reduction of intussusception in children. *J Clin Ultrasound* 2002;30: 343–348.

Fischer TK, Bihrmann K, Perch M, et al: Intussusception in early childhood: A cohort study of 1.7 million children. *Pediatrics* 2004;114:782–785.

Henrikson S, Blane CE, Koujok K, et al: The effect of screening sonography on the positive rate of enemas for intussusception. *Pediatr Radiol* 2003;33:190–193.

Henry MCW, Brever CK, Tashjian DB, et al: The appendix sign: a radiographic marker for irreducible intussusception. *J Pediatr Surg* 2006;41:487–489.

Koumanidou C, Vakaki M, Pitsoulakis G, et al: Sonographic detection of lymph nodes in the intussusception of infants and young children: Clinical evaluation and hydrostatic reduction. *AJR Am J Roentgenol* 2002;178: 445–450.

Kubota A, Imura K, Yagi M, et al: Functional ileus in neonates: Hirschsprung's disease-allied disorders versus meconium-related ileus. *Eur J Pediatr Surg* 1999;9:392–395.

O'Ryan M, Lucero Y, Pena A, Valenzuela MT: Two year review of intestinal intussusception in six large public hospitals of Santiago, Chile. *Pediatr Infect Dis J* 2003;22:717–721.

Shteyer E, Koplewitz BZ, Gross E, Granot E: Medical treatment of recurrent intussusception associated with intestinal lymphoid hyperplasia. *Pediatrics* 2003;111:682–685.

Capitolo 331 ■ Corpi estranei e bezoar

Robert Wyllie

331.1 • Corpi estranei nello stomaco e nell'intestino

Una volta nello stomaco, il 97% degli oggetti ingeriti transita senza difficoltà attraverso il resto del tratto gastrointestinale. Si calcola che meno dell'1% di tutti i corpi estranei ingeriti dia luogo a perforazione; quest'ultima tende ad avere luogo in corrispondenza degli sfinteri fisiologici (piloro, valvola ileocecale), all'altezza di angolazioni acute (C duodenale), nelle zone caratterizzate da malformazioni intestinali congenite (membrane, diaframmi, diverticoli) o nelle aree sottoposte in precedenza a chirurgia intestinale.

I pazienti con corpi estranei non alimentari spesso presentano un'anamnesi di ingestioni accidentali; nel caso dei bambini piccoli un testimone può avere assistito all'evento. Il 90% circa dei corpi estranei è radiopaco. L'esame radiologico viene effettuato di routine per determinare il tipo, il numero e la localizzazione degli oggetti sospetti. Per visualizzare alcuni di essi, per esempio parti in plastica o giocattoli, possono essere necessarie radiografie con mezzo di contrasto.

È indicato un trattamento conservativo per la maggior parte dei corpi estranei transitati attraverso l'esofago ed entrati nello stomaco. La maggior parte degli oggetti transita attraverso l'intestino in 4-6 giorni, sebbene alcuni possano impiegare anche 3-4 settimane. Nel frattempo, si consiglia ai genitori di continuare a somministrare al paziente la dieta consueta e di esaminare le feci alla ricerca dell'oggetto ingerito. Si raccomanda di evitare i lassativi troppo drastici. Gli oggetti eccezionalmente lunghi o acuminati di solito vengono monitorati radiologicamente. Si dovrebbero istruire il paziente e i suoi genitori a segnalare immediatamente al medico la comparsa di dolore addominale, vomito, febbre persistente, ematemesi e melena. La mancata progressione dell'oggetto entro 3-4 settimane implica raramente una perforazione imminente, ma può essere associata con una malformazione congenita o con un'anomalia intestinale acquisita.

Alcuni oggetti sono più pericolosi di altri. I piccoli magneti utilizzati per fissare gli orecchini sono stati associati con la perforazione intestinale. Quando i magneti si mescolano al cibo, dopo l'ingestione, possono attrarsi l'uno l'altro attraverso la parete intestinale, provocando necrosi e perforazione da pressione. Le parti metalliche dei giocattoli economici contenenti piombo possono provocare **tossicità da piombo.** Nonostante sia raro che l'ingestione delle pile provochi problemi, la loro degradazione nel tratto gastrointestinale può causare sintomi dovuti alla fuoriuscita di sostanze alcaline o metalli pesanti (mercurio). È stata riportata anche una tossicità da litio. Le monete più recenti, inoltre, possono andare incontro a corrosione quando vengono sottoposte all'azione degli acidi gastrici per un tempo prolungato; tuttavia, a meno che non vengano ingerite numerose monete, è improbabile che i metalli pongano rischi clinici.

Nei bambini più grandi e negli adulti gli oggetti ovali con diametro >5 cm o spessore >2 cm tendono a posizionarsi nello stomaco, dal quale andrebbero recuperati endoscopicamente. Vanno rimossi anche gli oggetti sottili con lunghezza >10 cm, che non riescono a superare la C duodenale e, nei neonati e nei bambini che iniziano a camminare, gli oggetti lunghi più di 3 cm o di diametro >20 mm, che di solito non passano attraverso il piloro. Si raccomanda di recuperare endoscopicamente anche le spille di sicurezza aperte, mentre altri oggetti acuminati possono essere gestiti in maniera conservativa. Se il bambino ha ingerito farmaci o droga (pillole aggregate di ferro, bustine di cocaina) può essere necessario procedere alla rimozione chirurgica; come il primo intervento è possibile effettuare un lavaggio intestinale con polietilenglicole.

Talvolta capita che i bambini si introducano oggetti nel retto: quelli piccoli e smussati in genere fuoriescono spontaneamente, mentre quelli di grandi dimensioni o acuminati tipicamente devono essere rimossi. È essenziale somministrare una sedazione adeguata per rilassare lo sfintere anale prima di tentare la rimozione endoscopica o tramite speculum. Se l'oggetto è localizzato prossimalmente al retto, l'osservazione per 12-24 ore ne permetterà la discesa.

331.2 • Bezoar

Con il termine "bezoar" si indica un accumulo di materiale esogeno nello stomaco o nell'intestino. La maggior parte dei casi è stata riscontrata nelle donne con disturbi della personalità o negli individui con alterazioni neurologiche. I pazienti che sono stati sottoposti a chirurgia addominale presentano un rischio aumentato di sviluppo di bezoar. Il picco dell'esordio dei sintomi coincide con la seconda decade di vita. Questi accumuli vengono classificati in base alla loro composizione. I **tricobezoar** sono costituiti dai capelli del paziente stesso, mentre i **fitobezoar** sono composti da una combinazione di materiale vegetale e animale. I **lactobezoar**, che in passato venivano riscontrati per lo più nei neonati prematuri, sono attribuibili all'elevato contenuto di caseina o calcio di alcune formule artificiali per prematuri. Le gomme da masticare ingerite possono occasionalmente portare alla formazione di bezoar.

Talvolta i tricobezoar raggiungono notevoli dimensioni formando masse che dallo stomaco possono passare nel duodeno prossimale: ne conseguono i sintomi dell'ostruzione intestinale parziale o dell'impedimento allo svuotamento gastrico, che comprendono vomito, anoressia e calo ponderale. I pazienti possono lamentare dolore addominale, distensione e severa alitosi. L'esame obiettivo può evidenziare chiazze alopeciche e una massa solida nel quadrante superiore sinistro. I pazienti occasionalmente presentano anemia sideropenica, ipoproteinemia o steatorrea, causate da gastrite cronica associata. I fitobezoar si manifestano in maniera analoga.

Una radiografia diretta dell'addome può suggerire la presenza di un bezoar, che può essere confermata con l'ecografia o la TC. In genere i bezoar dello stomaco possono essere rimossi endoscopicamente. Se l'endoscopia non è efficace, può essere necessario un intervento chirurgico. I lactobezoar solitamente si risolvono con la sospensione dei pasti per 24-48 ore.

Aktay AN, Werlin SL: Penetration of the stomach by an accidentally ingested straight pin. *J Pediatr Gastroenterol Nutr* 2002;34:81–82.

Centers for Disease Control and Prevention: Gastrointestinal injuries from magnet ingestion in children—United States, 2003–2006. *MMWR* 2006;55: 1296–1300.

Cerri RW, Liacouras CA: Evaluation and management of foreign bodies in the upper gastrointestinal tract. *Pediatr Case Rev* 2003;3:150–156.

Kaneko H, Tomomasa T, Kubota Y, et al: Pharmacobezoar complicating treatment with sodium alginate. *J Gastroenterol* 2004;39:69–71.

Karjoo M, Kader H: A novel technique for closing and removing an open safety pin from the stomach. *Gastrointest Endosc* 2003;57:627–629.

Mallon PT, White JS, Thompson RL: Systemic absorption of lithium following ingestion of a lithium button battery. *Hum Exp Toxicol* 2004;23: 193–195.

Puig S, Scharitzer M, Cengiz K, et al: Effects of gastric acid on euro coins: Chemical reaction and radiographic appearance after ingestion by infants and children. *Emerg Med J* 2004;21:553–556.

Schalamon J, Haxhija EQ, Ainoedhofer H, et al: The use of a hand-held metal detector for localisation of ingested metallic foreign bodies—a critical investigation. *Eur J Pediatr* 2004; 163:257–259.

VanArsdale JL, Leiker RD, Kohn M, et al: Lead poisoning from a toy necklace. *Pediatrics* 2004; 114:1096–1099.

Capitolo 332 ■ Malattia ulcerosa peptica nei bambini Samra S. Blanchard e Steven J. Czinn

La malattia ulcerosa peptica, che costituisce il risultato finale dell'infiammazione dovuta a uno squilibrio tra i fattori citolitici e citoprotettivi nello stomaco e nel duodeno, si presenta con vari gradi di gastrite o franca ulcerazione. La sua patogenesi è multifattoriale, ma la via finale comune per lo sviluppo delle ulcere è l'azione dei contenuti acidi e ricchi di pepsina dello stomaco sulla mucosa gastrica e duodenale e l'incapacità dei meccanismi di difesa della mucosa di mitigarli. L'endoscopia permette di visualizzare le anomalie della mucosa gastrica e duodenale, con o senza alterazioni istologiche. Le lesioni profonde a carico della muscularis mucosa della parete gastrica o duodenale vengono definite **ulcere peptiche**. Le ulcere gastriche sono in genere localizzate sulla piccola curvatura dello stomaco mentre le ulcere duodenali vengono per lo più riscontrate nel bulbo (90% dei casi). Malgrado la mancanza di studi pediatrici basati su una grossa popolazione, la frequenza di malattia ulcerosa peptica nell'infanzia sembra essere bassa. Grandi centri pediatrici riportano aneddoticamente un'incidenza annuale di 5-7 bambini con ulcere gastriche o duodenali ogni 2500 accessi ospedalieri.

Le ulcere nei bambini possono essere classificate come **primarie** (croniche e più spesso duodenali) o **secondarie** (caratterizzate in genere da un esordio più acuto e più spesso gastriche). Sebbene le ulcere primarie siano per lo più associate con l'infezione da *Helicobacter pylori*, le forme idiopatiche rendono conto anche del 20% delle ulcere duodenali nei bambini. Le ulcere peptiche secondarie possono essere conseguenza di stress dovuti sepsi, shock o lesioni intracraniche (ulcere di Cushing) oppure di un severo danno da ustione (ulcere di Curling). Le ulcere secondarie possono essere attribuite all'uso di acido acetilsalicilico o farmaci antinfiammatori non steroidei (FANS), agli stati ipersecretivi come la sindrome di Zollinger-Ellison (vedi Capitolo 332.1), alla sindrome dell'intestino corto e alla mastocitosi sistemica.

PATOGENESI

SECREZIONE ACIDA. Entro i 3-4 anni di età la secrezione acida gastrica si avvicina ai valori tipici dell'adulto. L'acido inizialmente secreto dalle cellule ossintiche dello stomaco ha un pH intorno allo 0,8, mentre il pH del contenuto gastrico è 1-2. Un'eccessiva secrezione acida è associata con una grande massa di cellule parietali, con l'ipersecrezione da parte delle cellule G antrali e con un aumento del tono vagale, che dà luogo a una secrezione acida aumentata o sostenuta in risposta al pasto e a una secrezione aumentata durante la notte. Il controllo della secrezione acida viene ottenuto attraverso molteplici meccanismi di feedback, che coinvolgono vie endocrine, paracrine e neurali. I secretagoghi che stimolano la produzione acida gastrica comprendono l'acetilcolina rilasciata dal nervo vago, l'istamina secreta dalle cellule enterocromaffini e la gastrina rilasciata dalle cellule G dell'antro. I mediatori che riducono la secrezione acida gastrica e aumentano la produzione di mucina protettiva comprendono le prostaglandine.

DIFESA DELLA MUCOSA. La mucosa gastrointestinale è rivestita da uno strato continuo di muco, di consistenza gelatinosa, che funge da barriera di diffusione per gli ioni idrogeno e per altre sostanze chimiche. La produzione e la secrezione di muco sono stimolate dalla prostaglandina E_2. L'epitelio, al di sotto del rivestimento mucoso, forma una barriera di seconda linea, le cui caratteristiche sono determinate dalla biologia delle cellule epiteliali e dalle loro giunzioni serrate. Un'altra importante funzione delle cellule epiteliali è quella di secernere chemiochine a ogni minaccia di attacco da parte di microrganismi. La secrezione di bicarbonato all'interno del rivestimento mucoso, che viene regolata dalle prostaglandine, è importante per la neutralizzazione degli ioni idrogeno. Se si verifica una lesione mucosa, l'*epithelial growth factor*, il *transforming growth factor*-α, l'*insulin-like growth factor*, la gastrina e la bombesina scatenano rapidamente un'attiva proliferazione e migrazione delle cellule mucose, che vanno a ricoprire l'area in cui l'epitelio è danneggiato.

MANIFESTAZIONI CLINICHE

I sintomi di presentazione della malattia ulcerosa peptica variano a seconda dell'età del paziente. Ematemesi e melena sono riportate nella metà dei pazienti con malattia ulcerosa peptica. È più comune che i bambini in età scolare e gli adolescenti lamentino dolore epigastrico e nausea, come avviene generalmente negli adulti, mentre i neonati e i bambini piccoli di solito presentano difficoltà nell'alimentazione, vomito, episodi di pianto, ematemesi o melena. Nel periodo neonatale la perforazione gastrica può costituire la presentazione iniziale.

Il sintomo classico dell'ulcera peptica, ossia il dolore epigastrico alleviato dall'ingestione di cibo, è presente solo in una minoranza di bambini. Molti pazienti pediatrici presentano un dolore addominale poco localizzato, che può essere periombelicale. La stragrande maggioranza dei pazienti con dolore o fastidio periombelicale o epigastrico non ha un'ulcera peptica, bensì un disturbo gastrointestinale funzionale, come la sindrome del colon irritabile o la dispepsia funzionale. I pazienti con ulcera peptica raramente si presentano con un dolore addominale acuto da perforazione oppure con i segni e sintomi di pancreatite da ulcera penetrante posteriore. Occasionalmente può essere osservata l'emissione di sangue rosso vivo dal retto, se la velocità del sanguinamento è elevata e il tempo di transito intestinale è breve. Il vomito può essere un segno di impedimento allo svuotamento gastrico.

Il dolore viene spesso descritto come sordo o persistente, anziché penetrante o urente come nell'adulto. Esso può durare da pochi minuti ad alcune ore; i pazienti vanno incontro a frequenti esacerbazioni e remissioni, che durano per settimane o mesi. Il dolore notturno è comune nei bambini più grandi. Un'anamnesi di dolore ulceroso tipico con pronto sollievo dopo l'assunzione di antiacidi è rilevabile in $<30\%$ dei bambini. Nei pazienti con perdita ematica acuta o cronica, la penetrazione dell'ulcera nella cavità addominale o in organi adiacenti può provocare (per quanto raramente) shock, anemia, peritonite o pancreatite. Se l'infiammazione e l'edema sono estesi, si può verificare un'ostruzione acuta o cronica allo svuotamento gastrico.

DIAGNOSI

L'esofagogastroduodenoscopia rappresenta la metodica di scelta per stabilire la diagnosi di malattia ulcerosa peptica. Questa indagine, se affidata a gastroenterologi pediatrici esperti, può essere effettuata senza rischi a tutte le età. L'endoscopia, tramite la diretta visualizzazione dell'esofago, dello stomaco e del duodeno, consente di identificare le lesioni specifiche a carico di questi organi. È necessario effettuare prelievi bioptici dall'esofago, dallo stomaco e dal duodeno, non solo ai fini della valutazione istologica, ma anche per lo screening dell'infezione da *H. pylori*. L'endoscopia offre inoltre l'opportunità di effettuare una terapia emostatica iniettiva o tramite *heater probe* o elettrocoagulazione, se necessario.

ULCERE PRIMITIVE

GASTRITE DA *HELICOBACTER PYLORI*. Quella da *H. pylori* rappresenta una delle più comuni infezioni batteriche negli esseri umani. L'*H. pylori* è un bacillo Gram-negativo a forma di S, produttore di ureasi, catalasi e ossidasi, che può giocare un ruolo nella patogenesi della malattia ulcerosa peptica. Il meccanismo di acquisizione e trasmissione di questo microrganismo non è chiaro, sebbene la più probabile via di trasmissione sia orofecale o oro-orale. Questa ipotesi è supportata da alcuni studi dai quali risulta che l'organismo vitale di *H. pylori* può essere posto in coltura a partire dalle feci o dal vomito dei pazienti infetti. Sulla prevalenza dell'infezione incidono anche altri fattori di rischio, come il basso livello socioeconomico dei bambini o dei familiari affetti. I bambini infettati da *H. pilori* sviluppano tutti una gastrite cronica attiva, ma sono spesso asintomatici. Nei pazienti pediatrici l'infezione si può presentare con dolore addominale o vomito e, meno frequentemente, con un'anemia sideropenica refrattaria o un ritardo di crescita. L'*H. pylori* può essere associato, sebbene raramente, con una trombocitemia autoimmune cronica. La colonizzazione cronica da questo microrganismo predispone i bambini a un rischio significativamente aumentato di sviluppare un'ulcera duodenale, un cancro gastrico come l'adenocarcinoma o un linfoma MALT (*Mucosa-Associated Lymphoid Tissue*, tessuto linfatico associato alla mucosa). Il rischio relativo di carcinoma gastrico è di 2,3-8,7 volte superiore negli adulti infetti rispetto ai soggetti non infetti. L'*H. pylori* è stato classificato dall'Organizzazione Mondiale della Sanità come un cancerogeno di gruppo I.

La diagnosi di infezione da *H. pylori* viene effettuata istologicamente, evidenziando il microrganismo nei campioni bioptici (Fig. 332-1). I test sierologici, sebbene possano essere d'aiuto nello screening dei bambini per la presenza di questo microrganismo, utilizzando la ricerca validata degli anticorpi tipo immunoglobuline G (IgG), non aiutano a predire l'infezione attiva per determinare il successo dell'antibioticoterapia. Anche il breath test con ^{13}C-urea e il test per l'antigene fecale sono metodi non invasivi disponibili per rilevare l'infezione da *H. pylori*; malgrado ciò, nei bambini con sospetta infezione da *H. pylori*, si raccomanda di eseguire innanzitutto l'endoscopia superiore per confermare la diagnosi. Lo spettro di reperti endoscopici nei bambini con infezione da *H. pylori* varia da un aspetto macroscopicamente normale alla presenza di una gastrite aspecifica con pliche prominenti, nodularità (Fig. 332-2) o ulcere. Poiché la mucosa antrale sembra macroscopicamente normale in un numero significativo di bambini con gastrite primaria da *H. pylori*, è necessario effettuare biopsie del corpo e dell'antro gastrici indipendentemente dall'aspetto endoscopico. Una volta identificato l'*H. pylori*, bisognerebbe proporre la terapia eradicante anche nei bambini asintomatici (Tabb. 332-1 e 332-2).

ULCERE IDIOPATICHE. Le ulcere duodenali negative per *H. pylori* nei bambini che non presentano un'anamnesi di assunzione di FANS rappresentano il 15-20% delle ulcere duodenali di competenza pediatrica. Questi pazienti non presentano nodularità nell'antro gastrico né evidenza istologica di gastrite. Nelle ulcere idiopatiche la sola soppressione acida rappresenta il trattamento efficace di scelta. Si possono utilizzare sia gli inibitori della pompa protonica sia gli antagonisti dei recettori H_2. Le ulcere idiopatiche presentano un'elevata frequenza di recidiva dopo l'interruzione della terapia antisecretiva. Si raccomanda di seguire strettamente questi bambini e di riprendere la terapia antisecretiva in caso di ricomparsa dei sintomi. Se il bambino ha più di un anno, per la terapia di mantenimento si preferiscono gli inibitori della pompa protonica, dimostratisi superiori agli antagonisti dei recettori H_2 nella prevenzione delle ulcere ricorrenti.

ULCERE SECONDARIE

ACIDO ACETILSALICILICO E ALTRI FANS. I FANS provocano lesioni della mucosa per irritazione locale diretta e per inibizione della formazione di ciclo-ossigenasi e prostaglandine. Poiché le prostaglandine aumentano la resistenza della mucosa al danno, una loro produzione ridotta aumenta il rischio di lesioni mucose. La gastropatia erosiva severa provocata dai FANS può esitare in ulcere sanguinanti o perforazioni gastriche, localizzate più spesso a livello dello stomaco (soprattutto nell'antro) che del duodeno.

ULCERE "DA STRESS". Si verificano solitamente entro 24 ore dall'inizio di una malattia molto grave, che comporta uno stress fisiologico. In molti casi il sanguinamento proviene da erosioni più che da ulcere gastriche. Circa il 25% dei bambini con malattie molto gravi, ricoverati in un reparto di terapia intensiva pediatrica, avrà un'evidenza macroscopica di sanguinamento gastrico. Anche i neonati pretermine e a termine nelle unità di terapia intensiva neonatale sviluppano lesioni della mucosa gastrica e possono presentare emorragie gastrointestinali alte o ulcere perforate. Sebbene le misure profilattiche per prevenire le ulcere da stress nei bambini non siano standardizzate, nei reparti di terapia intensiva pediatrica vengono spesso utilizzati i farmaci che inibiscono la produzione acida gastrica (vedi oltre) per ridurre la frequenza di erosioni o ulcere gastriche.

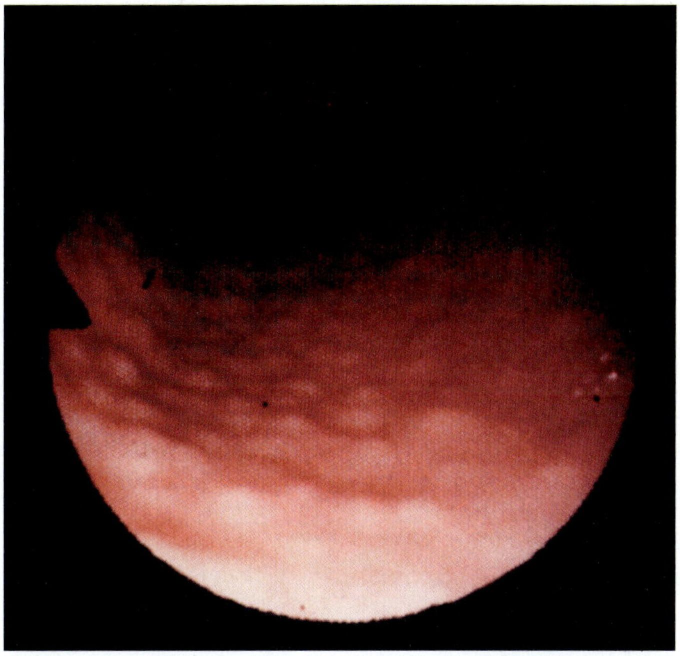

Figura 332-2. Aspetto endoscopico dell'iperplasia nodulare linfoide dell'antro gastrico. (Da Campbell GI, Thomas JE: Helicobacter pylori infection in paediatric practice. *Arch Dis Child Edu Pract Ed* 2005;90:ep25-ep30.)

TABELLA 332-1. Terapie eradicanti raccomandate per la malattia associata a *H. pylori* nei bambini

FARMACI	POSOLOGIA	DURATA DEL TRATTAMENTO
Amoxicillina	50 mg/kg/die ÷ bid	14 giorni
Claritromicina	15 mg/kg/die ÷ bid	14 giorni
Inibitore della pompa protonica	1 mg/kg/die ÷ bid	1 mese
Amoxicillina	50 mg/kg/die ÷ bid	14 giorni
Metronidazolo	20 mg/kg/die ÷ bid	14 giorni
Inibitore della pompa protonica	1 mg/kg/die ÷ bid	1 mese
Claritromicina	15 mg/kg/die ÷ bid	14 giorni
Metronidazolo	20 mg/kg/die ÷ bid	14 giorni
Inibitore della pompa protonica	1 mg/kg/die ÷ bid	1 mese

Adattata da Gold BD et al: Medical position statement: The North American Society for Pediatric Gastroenterology and Nutrition. Helicobacter pylori infectious children: Recommendations for diagnosis and treatment. *J Pediatr Gastroenterol Nutr* 2000;31:490-497.

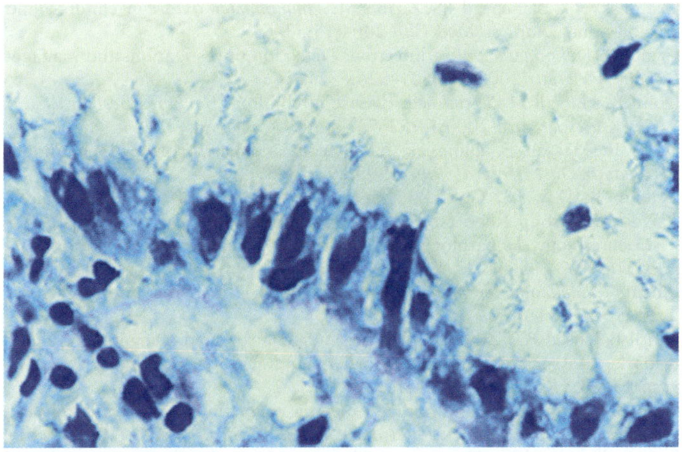

Figura 332-1. Aspetto dell'*Helicobacter pylori* sulla superficie della mucosa gastrica alla colorazione di Giemsa (alto ingrandimento). (Da Campbell GI, Thomas JE: Helicobacter pylori infection in paediatric practice. *Arch Dis Child Edu Pract Ed* 2005;90:ep25-ep30.)

TABELLA 332-2. Terapia antisecretiva con dosaggi pediatrici

FARMACO	DOSAGGIO PEDIATRICO	FORME DI SOMMINISTRAZIONE
ANTAGONISTI DEI RECETTORI H_2		
Cimetidina	20-40 mg/kg/die suddivisi in 2-4 somministrazioni/die	Sciroppo: 300 mg/mL Compresse: 200, 300, 400, 800 mg
Ranitidina	4-10 mg/kg/die suddivisi in 2-3 somministrazioni/die	Sciroppo: 75 mg/5 mL Compresse: 75, 150, 300 mg
Famotidina	1-2 mg/kg/die suddivisi in 2 somministrazioni/die	Sciroppo: 40 mg/5 mL Compresse: 20, 40 mg
Nizatidina	10 mg/kg/die suddivisi in 2 somministrazioni/die	
INIBITORI DI POMPA PROTONICA		
Omeprazolo	1,0-3,3 mg/kg/die <20 kg: 10 mg/die >20 kg: 20 mg/die Approvato per l'utilizzo nei bambini con età >2 anni	Capsule: 10, 20, 40 mg
Lansoprazolo	0,8-4 mg/kg/die <30 kg: 15 mg/die >30 kg: 30 mg/die Approvato per l'utilizzo nei bambini con età >1 anno	Capsule 15, 30 mg Bustine: 15, 30 mg Compresse solubili: 15, 30 mg
Rabeprazolo	Dosaggio nell'adulto: 20 mg/die	Compresse: 20 mg
Pantoprazolo	Dosaggio nell'adulto: 40 mg/die	Compresse: 40 mg
AGENTI CITOPROTETTIVI		
Sucralfato	40-80 mg/kg/die	Sospensione: 1000 mg/5 mL Compresse: 1000 mg

TRATTAMENTO DELLA MALATTIA ULCEROSA PEPTICA

La terapia dell'ulcera ha due obiettivi: la cicatrizzazione dell'ulcera e l'eliminazione della causa primaria. Altri aspetti importanti sono l'attenuazione dei sintomi e la prevenzione delle complicanze. I **farmaci di prima linea** per il trattamento della gastrite e della malattia ulcerosa peptica nei bambini sono gli antagonisti dei recettori H_2 e gli inibitori della pompa protonica (vedi Tab. 332-2); questi ultimi, più potenti nella cicatrizzazione dell'ulcera, possono essere utilizzati in aggiunta agli agenti citoprotettori se sono presenti lesioni mucose. Per il trattamento delle ulcere associate a *H. pylori* si devono utilizzare gli antibiotici in combinazione con un inibitore della pompa protonica (vedi Tab. 332-1).

Gli antagonisti dei recettori H_2 (cimetidina, ranitidina, famotidina, nizatidina) inibiscono competitivamente il legame dell'istamina con i recettori H_2 delle cellule della parete gastrica. Gli inibitori della pompa protonica bloccano la pompa H^+/K^+ ATPasi delle cellule della parete gastrica in maniera dose-dipendente, riducendo la secrezione acida gastrica basale e stimolata. Negli Stati Uniti sono disponibili almeno cinque inibitori della pompa protonica: omeprazolo, lansoprazolo, pantoprazolo, esomeprazolo, rabeprazolo. Sebbene non tutti siano approvati per l'impiego nei bambini, essi sono ben tollerati con effetti collaterali di scarsa entità, come diarrea (1-4%), cefalea (1-3%) e nausea (1%). Dal punto di vista dell'efficacia terapeutica, l'evidenza suggerisce che tutti gli inibitori della pompa protonica hanno un'efficacia sovrapponibile nel trattamento della malattia ulcerosa peptica, se utilizzati a dosaggi standard, e che sono superiori agli antagonisti dei recettori H_2; in particolare, questi farmaci esplicano il massimo effetto se assunti prima dei pasti.

TRATTAMENTO DELLA MALATTIA ULCEROSA PEPTICA CORRELATA A *H. PYLORI*. In pediatria gli antibiotici e i sali di bismuto sono stati utilizzati in combinazione con gli inibitori della pompa protonica per trattare l'infezione da *H. pylori* (vedi Tab. 332-1). La percentuale di eradicazione nei bambini varia dal 68 al 92%, quando viene utilizzata una terapia duplice o triplice per 4-6 settimane. La percentuale di cicatrizzazione dell'ulcera varia dal 91 al 100%. La triplice terapia consente di ottenere una percentuale di guarigione più elevata rispetto alla duplice. Il regime ottimale per l'eradicazione dell'infezione da *H. pylori* nei bambini deve ancora essere stabilito, ma l'impiego di un inibitore della pompa protonica in combinazione con claritromicina e amoxicillina o metronidazolo per 2 settimane rappresenta una soluzione ben tollerata e quindi raccomandata (vedi Tab. 332-1). Sebbene i bambini di età <5 anni possano andare incontro a una reinfezione, le ragioni più comuni del fallimento della terapia sono la scarsa *compliance* o la resistenza agli antibiotici.

TERAPIA CHIRURGICA. Da quando è stato scoperto l'*H. pylori* e si sono rese disponibili le moderne terapie mediche contro questo microrganismo, è estremamente raro che la malattia ulcerosa peptica necessiti di un trattamento chirurgico. Le indicazioni alla chirurgia rimangono il sanguinamento incontrollato, la perforazione e l'ostruzione. Grazie all'introduzione degli antagonisti dei recettori H_2, al riconoscimento e al trattamento dell'*H. pylori* e all'impiego degli inibitori della pompa protonica, l'incidenza della chirurgia per sanguinamento e perforazione si è ridotta notevolmente.

332.1 • SINDROME DI ZOLLINGER-ELLISON

Questa rara sindrome è caratterizzata da una malattia ulcerosa peptica severa e refrattaria, causata da un'ipersecrezione gastrica imputabile alla secrezione autonoma di gastrina da parte di un tumore neuroendocrino, il gastrinoma. La presentazione clinica è simile a quella della malattia ulcerosa peptica, con l'aggiunta della diarrea. La diagnosi viene sospettata per la presenza di ulcere ricorrenti, multiple o con localizzazione atipica. Più del 98% dei pazienti presenta elevati livelli di gastrina a digiuno. La sindrome di Zollinger-Ellison costituisce un'evenienza frequente nei pazienti con **neoplasie endocrine multiple** (*Multiple Endocrine Neoplasia*, **MEN1**), mentre è di raro riscontro in caso di **neurofibromatosi** e **sclerosi tuberosa**. Nella terapia è essenziale il trattamento immediato ed efficace dell'ipersecrezione acida gastrica. Gli inibitori della pompa protonica rappresentano i farmaci di scelta per via della loro efficacia e durata d'azione prolungata. Anche gli antagonisti dei recettori H_2 sono efficaci, ma sono necessarie dosi più elevate di quelle utilizzate per la malattia ulcerosa peptica.

Blecker U, Gold BD: Gastritis and peptic ulcer disease in childhood. *Eur J Pediatr* 1999;158:541–546.

Campbell DI, Thomas JE: *Heliobacter pylori* infection in paediatric practice. *Arch Dis Child Edu Pract Ed* 2005;90:ep25–ep30.

Chelimsky G, Blanchard SS, Czinn SJ: *Helicobacter pylori* in children and adolescents. *Adolesc Med Clin* 2004;15:53–66.

Czinn SJ: *Heliobacter pylori* infection: Detection, investigation, and management. *J Pediatr* 2005;146:S21–S26.

Dohil R, Hassall E: Peptic ulcer disease in children. *Baillieres Best Pract Res Clin Gastroenterol* 2000;14:53–73.

Dohil R, Hassall E, Dimmick J: Gastritis and gastropathy of childhood. *J Pediatr Gastroenterol Nutr* 1999;29:378–394.

Drumm B, Day AS, Gold B, et al: *Helicobacter pylori* and peptic ulcer: Working Group Report of the Second World Congress of Pediatric Gastroenterology, Hepatology, and Nutrition. *J Pediatr Gastroenterol Nutr* 2004;39:S626–S631.

Elitsur Y: *Helicobacter pylori* diagnostic tools: Is it in the stool? *J Pediatr* 2005;146:164–167.

Gibril F, Jensen RT: Zollinger-Ellison syndrome revisited: Diagnosis, biologic markers, associated inherited disorders, and acid hypersecretion. *Curr Gastroenterol Rep* 2004;6:454–463.

Gold BD: Current therapy for *Helicobacter pylori* infection in children and adolescents. *Can J Gastroenterol* 1999;13:571–579.

Kato S, Sherman PM: What is new related to *Heliocobacter pylori* infection in children and teenagers? *Arch Pediatr Adolesc Med* 2005;159:415–421.

Mulberg A, Linz C, Bern E, et al: Identification of non-steroidal anti-inflammatory drug-induced gastroduodenal injury in children with juvenile rheumatoid arthritis. *J Pediatr* 1993;122:647–649.

Sabbi T, De Angelis P, Colistro F, et al: Efficacy of noninvasive tests in the diagnosis of *Helicobacter pylori* infection in pediatric patients. *Arch Pediatr Adolesc Med* 2005;159:238–241.
Shah R: Dyspepsia and helicobacter pylori. *BMJ* 2007;334:41–43.

Capitolo 333 ■ Malattie infiammatorie intestinali croniche Jeffrey S. Hyams

Si definiscono *malattie infiammatorie intestinali croniche* (IBD, *Inflammatory Bowel Disease*) due diverse patologie con infiammazione intestinale cronica idiopatica: il morbo di Crohn e la rettocolite ulcerosa. Entrambe le patologie, le cui eziologie non sono ancora chiare, sono caratterizzate da riacutizzazioni e remissioni imprevedibili. Il momento di esordio più comune delle IBD è nell'epoca prepubere e nella prima età adulta. È stata dimostrata una distribuzione bimodale, con un inizio precoce a 10-20 anni di età e un secondo picco, meno accentuato, a 50-80 anni di età. Il 25% dei pazienti presenta la patologia prima dei 20 anni. Malgrado ciò, le IBD possono iniziare anche nel primo anno di vita e nell'ultimo decennio si è registrata un'aumentata incidenza tra i bambini piccoli. I bambini con un esordio precoce di IBD hanno una probabilità maggiore di presentare un interessamento colico. Nei Paesi industrializzati, queste patologie costituiscono la causa principale di infiammazione intestinale cronica tra i bambini nei primi anni di vita. Una terza categoria meno comune, quella delle coliti indeterminate, rappresenta il 10% circa dei pazienti pediatrici.

Nella patogenesi delle IBD sono coinvolti fattori sia genetici sia ambientali. La loro incidenza nei bianchi e non bianchi è sovrapponibile negli Stati Uniti ed è bassa nei neri in Africa. La prevalenza di morbo di Crohn negli Stati Uniti è molto più bassa tra gli ispanici e gli asiatici rispetto ai bianchi e ai neri. Tra i membri della famiglia di un individuo affetto è stato riportato un rischio di IBD compreso tra il 7 e il 30%; un bambino i cui genitori sono entrambi affetti da IBD presenta un rischio >35% di acquisire la malattia. I parenti di un individuo con rettocolite ulcerosa presentano un rischio superiore di acquisire la rettocolite ulcerosa rispetto al morbo di Crohn, mentre quelli di un individuo con il morbo di Crohn presentano un rischio aumentato di sviluppare questa patologia; nella stessa famiglia possono verificarsi entrambe le malattie. Il rischio che si verifichi una IBD tra i parenti di individui con il morbo di Crohn è per certi versi superiore che per gli individui con rettocolite ulcerosa.

L'importanza dei fattori genetici nello sviluppo delle IBD viene evidenziato dalla maggiore probabilità che entrambi i gemelli siano affetti se sono monozigoti anziché dizigoti. La concordanza tra i gemelli è più alta per il morbo di Crohn (36%) che per la rettocolite ulcerosa (16%). Le patologie genetiche che sono state associate con le IBD comprendono la sindrome di Turner, la sindrome di Hermansky-Pudlak, la glicogenosi di tipo Ib e varie immunodeficienze. Le analisi di associazione genetica, tramite lo studio del genoma completo, hanno identificato numerosi loci di suscettibilità, designati con le sigle da IBD1 a IBD6, rispettivamente sui cromosomi 16, 12, 6, 14, 5 e 19. Il locus IBD1, che ha mostrato la maggiore associazione, viene denominato *NOD2/CARD15*. Sono stati descritti tre polimorfismi principali (*R702W*, *G908R*, *1007fs*). Ulteriori alleli comprendono *SNP5*, *JW1* e *3020insC*. Mentre il possesso di una copia dell'allele a rischio determina un piccolo aumento del rischio di sviluppare il morbo di Crohn (da 2 a 4 volte), il possesso di 2 copie (in omozigosi o eterozigosi composta) aumenta il rischio di 20-40 volte. Queste varianti genetiche alterano l'attivazione del fattore nucleare κB (NF-κB, *Nuclear Factor κB*) intestinale in risposta ai lipopolisaccaridi e ai peptidoglicani batterici. Altri loci IBD possono codificare per il gene della resistenza multifarmaco e per i geni nel cluster dei geni trasportatori di cationi organici. Solo il 20% dei pazienti con morbo di Crohn è omozigote per le varianti di *NOD2*. Il possesso degli alleli a rischio *NOD2/CARD15* è associato con i fenotipi ileale e stenosante. Questi geni sono rari nei pazienti afroamericani, mentre sono presenti nel 40-50% dei pazienti bianchi.

Gli anticorpi anti-citoplasma neutrofilo di tipo perinucleare (p-ANCA, *Perinuclear Antineutrophil Antibody*), evidenziati nel 70% circa degli individui con rettocolite ulcerosa e in meno del 20% di quelli con morbo di Crohn, si pensa rappresentino un marcatore di disturbi immunoregolatori controllati geneticamente. Il 55% circa degli individui con morbo di Crohn risulta positivo per gli anticorpi anti-*Saccharomyces cerevisiae* (ASCA, *Anti-Saccharomyces Cerevisiae Antibody*).

Importanti sono inoltre i fattori ambientali, che presumibilmente spiegano la discordanza tra i gemelli e le variazioni del rischio all'interno della stessa razza nelle diverse regioni geografiche; i precisi fattori di rischio restano sconosciuti. Gli individui che emigrano nei Paesi industrializzati sembrano spesso acquisire la maggiore frequenza di IBD associata con queste regioni. Il fumo di sigaretta costituisce un fattore di rischio per il morbo di Crohn, ma paradossalmente protegge dalla rettocolite ulcerosa. Nessun agente infettivo specifico è stato associato in maniera riproducibile con le IBD.

Un'alterazione dell'immunoregolazione della mucosa intestinale potrebbe essere di primaria importanza nella patogenesi delle IBD. L'intestino è sottoposto a una costante stimolazione immunologica da parte degli agenti microbici e degli antigeni alimentari. In risposta a ciò, la mucosa normalmente sviluppa un'infiammazione "fisiologica". Nelle IBD il meccanismo che mantiene sotto controllo questa reazione non funziona e ne deriva un'infiammazione patologica. Non è chiaro se essa rappresenti una risposta abnorme agli abituali antigeni enterici oppure una risposta normale contro un microrganismo non ancora identificato. Vengono coinvolti i mediatori dell'infiammazione (citochine, metaboliti dell'acido arachidonico, metaboliti reattivi dell'ossigeno, fattori di crescita), che portano alla distruzione dei tessuti e a un rimodellamento con fibrosi. La maggior parte delle terapie ha lo scopo di interferire con l'attività di questi mediatori.

Solitamente è possibile distinguere la rettocolite ulcerosa dal morbo di Crohn sulla base della presentazione clinica e dei reperti radiologici, endoscopici e istopatologici (Tab. 333-1). Nel 10%

TABELLA 333-1. Confronto tra morbo di Crohn e rettocolite ulcerosa

CARATTERISTICA	MORBO DI CROHN	RETTOCOLITE ULCEROSA
Sanguinamento rettale	Occasionale	Comune
Diarrea	Variabile	Comune
Dolore addominale	Comune	Variabile
Massa addominale	Comune	Assente
Difetto nella crescita	Comune	Variabile
Malattia perianale	Comune	Insolita
Malattia rettale	Occasionale	Universale
Pioderma gangrenoso	Raro	Presente
Eritema nodoso	Comune	Meno comune
Ulcere orali	Comuni	Rare
Trombosi	Meno comune	Presente
Malattia colica	50-75%	100%
Malattia ileale	Comune	Assente, eccetto ileite da reflusso
Malattia gastroesofagea	Rara	Assente
Stenosi	Comuni	Insolite
Ragadi	Comuni	Assenti
Fistole	Comuni	Insolite
Megacolon tossico	Assente	Presente
Colangite sclerosante	Meno comune	Presente
Rischio di neoplasia	Aumentato	Molto aumentato
Lesioni discontinue (skip/segmentarie)	Comuni	Assenti
Interessamento transmurale	Comune	Insolito
Ascessi criptici	Meno comuni	Comuni
Granulomi	Comuni	Insoliti
Ulcere lineari	Rare	Comuni
Anticorpi anticitoplasma dei neutrofili con pattern perinucleare	Rari	Comuni citoplasmatici (pANCA)
Anticorpi anti-*Saccharomyces cerevisiae*	Comuni	Rari

circa degli individui con colite cronica non si giunge a stabilire una diagnosi definitiva (cosiddetta *colite indeterminata*). Talvolta, in un bambino che inizialmente si pensava fosse affetto da rettocolite ulcerosa sulla base del quadro clinico, in seguito viene posta diagnosi di morbo di Crohn. Il trattamento del morbo di Crohn e della rettocolite ulcerosa è sovrapponibile.

Le manifestazioni extraintestinali si verificano un po' più spesso nel morbo di Crohn che nella rettocolite ulcerosa (Tab. 333-2). Un ritardo di crescita viene osservato alla diagnosi nel 15-35% degli individui con morbo di Crohn. Delle manifestazioni extraintestinali che si verificano nelle IBD, l'interessamento articolare, cutaneo, oculare, orale ed epatobiliare tende a essere associato con la colite, sia ulcerosa sia di Crohn. Per alcune manifestazioni, tra cui l'artrite periferica, l'eritema nodoso e l'anemia, l'attività correla con quella della malattia intestinale. L'attività del pioderma gangrenoso correla meno bene con quella della malattia intestinale, mentre l'attività della colangite sclerosante, della spondilite anchilosante e della sacroileite non correla con la malattia intestinale. L'artrite si presenta con tre quadri: artrite periferica migrante che interessa soprattutto le grandi articolazioni, spondilite anchilosante e sacroileite. L'artrite periferica delle IBD tende a non essere distruttiva. La spondilite anchilosante inizia nella terza decade di vita ed è più comune negli individui con rettocolite ulcerosa che presentano il fenotipo dell'antigene leucocitario umano B27. I sintomi consistono nel dolore lombosacrale e nella rigidità mattutina; vengono tipicamente colpite la

TABELLA 333-2. Complicanze extraintestinali delle malattie infiammatorie intestinali croniche

MUSCOLOSCHELETRICHE
- Artrite periferica
- Monoartrite granulomatosa
- Sinovite granulomatosa
- Artrite reumatoide
- Sacroileite
- Spondilite anchilosante
- Ippocratismo digitale e osteoartropatia ipertrofica
- Periostiti
- Osteoporosi, osteomalacia
- Rabdomiolisi
- Osteomielite pelvica
- Osteomielite multifocale ricorrente
- Policondrite recidivante

CUTE E MEMBRANE MUCOSE
- Lesioni orali
- Cheilite
- Stomatite afosa, glossite
- Morbo di Crohn orale granulomatoso
- Ragadi iperplastiche infiammatorie e mucosa ad acciottolato
- Peristomatite vegetante

DERMATOLOGICHE
- Eritema nodoso
- Pioderma gangrenoso
- Sindrome dolce (*sweet syndrome*)
- Morbo di Crohn metastatico
- Psoriasi
- Epidermolisi bollosa acquisita
- Segni cutanei perianali
- Poliarterite nodosa

OCULARI
- Congiuntiviti
- Uveiti/iriti
- Episcleriti
- Scleriti
- Neurite retrobulbare
- Corioretinite con distacco di retina
- Cheratopatia del morbo di Crohn
- Alterazioni del segmento posteriore
- Vasculopatia retinica

BRONCOPOLMONARI
- Bronchite cronica con bronchiectasie
- Bronchite cronica con infiltrati neutrofilici
- Alveolite fibrosante
- Vasculite polmonare
- Malattia delle piccole vie aeree e bronchiolite obliterante
- Pneumopatia eosinofila
- Pneumopatia granulomatosa
- Ostruzione tracheale

CARDIACHE
- Pleuropericardite
- Miocardiopatia
- Endocardite
- Miocardite

MALNUTRIZIONE
- Ridotto introito alimentare: IBD, restrizioni dietetiche
- Malassorbimento: IBD, resezioni ileali, deplezione di sali biliari, eccessiva proliferazione batterica
- Perdite intestinali: elettroliti, minerali, nutrienti
- Aumentate necessità caloriche: infiammazione, febbre

EMATOLOGICHE
- Anemia: carenza di ferro (perdite ematiche)
- Vitamina B_{12} (malattia o resezione ileale, eccessiva proliferazione batterica, deficit di folati)
- Anemia da infiammazione cronica
- Porpora anafilattoide (morbo di Crohn)
- Iposplenismo
- Anemia emolitica autoimmune
- Alterazioni della coagulazione
  - Aumentata attivazione dei fattori della coagulazione
  - Attivazione della fibrinolisi
  - Anticorpi anticardiolipina
  - Rischio aumentato di trombosi arteriose o venose con stroke cerebrovascolare, infarto miocardico, occlusioni periferiche arteriose e venose

RENALI E GENITOURINARIE
- Metaboliche: formazione di cristalli urinari (nefrolitiasi, acido urico, ossalati)
- Nefropatia ipokaliemica
- Infiammazione: ascessi retroperitoneali, fibrosi con ulcerazioni ureterali, formazione di fistole
- Glomeruliti
- Membranonefriti
- Amiloidosi renale, sindrome nefrosica

PANCREATITE
- Secondaria ai farmaci (sulfasalazina, 6-mercaptopurina, azatioprina, nutrizione parenterale)
- Morbo di Crohn ampollare
- Pancreatite granulomatosa
- Riduzione della funzione esocrina pancreatica
- Colangite sclerosante con pancreatite

EPATOBILIARI
- PSC
- PSC dei piccoli dotti (pericolangite)
- Carcinoma dei dotti biliari
- Infiltrazione grassa del fegato
- Colelitiasi
- Epatite autoimmune

ENDOCRINE E METABOLICHE
- Ritardo di crescita, sviluppo sessuale ritardato
- Tiroidite
- Osteoporosi, osteomalacia

NEUROLOGICHE
- Neuropatia periferica
- Meningiti
- Disfunzione vestibolare
- Pseudotumor cerebri

IBD (*Inflammatory Bowel Disease*), malattia infiammatoria cronica intestinale; PSC (*Primary Sclerosing Cholagitis*), colangite sclerosante primitiva.
Modificata da Kugathasan S: Diarrhea. In Kliegman RM, Greenbaum IA, Lye PS (ed): *Practical Strategies in Pediatric Diagnosis and Therapy*, 2nd ed. Philadelphia, Elsevier/Saunders, 2004, p. 285.

schiena, le anche, le spalle e le articolazioni sacroiliache. La sacroileite isolata di solito è asintomatica, ma a un'indagine attenta risulta frequente. Tra le manifestazioni cutanee, la più comune è l'eritema nodoso. Anche gli individui con eritema nodoso o pioderma gangrenoso presentano un'elevata probabilità di sviluppare un'artrite. La glomerulonefrite e uno stato ipercoagulativo sono altre rare manifestazioni che si verificano nell'infanzia. Nei bambini con IBD è stata descritta una malattia tromboembolica cerebrale. L'uveite colpisce il 5% circa dei bambini con IBD ed è solitamente asintomatica e transitoria; la sua comparsa non ha alcun rapporto con l'attività della malattia intestinale. Esiste una scarsa correlazione tra fenotipo e genotipo per i sintomi e le complicanze.

333.1 • Rettocolite ulcerosa cronica

La rettocolite ulcerosa, una patologia infiammatoria cronica idiopatica, colpisce il colon risparmiando il tratto gastrointestinale superiore. La malattia di solito inizia a livello del retto per poi estendersi prossimalmente per una distanza variabile. Quando è localizzata nel retto, viene denominata proctite ulcerosa, mentre se interessa l'intero colon prende il nome di pancolite. Quest'ultima si osserva nella maggior parte dei bambini. La proctite ulcerosa si associa meno facilmente con manifestazioni sistemiche, sebbene possa rispondere al trattamento meno della malattia diffusa. Nel 30% circa dei bambini che presentano una proctite ulcerosa si verifica una diffusione prossimale della malattia. Raramente si è osservata una presentazione della rettocolite ulcerosa nella prima infanzia. È facile che l'intolleranza alle proteine assunte con la dieta venga diagnosticata erroneamente come rettocolite ulcerosa in questo gruppo di età. L'intolleranza alle proteine della dieta (proteine del latte vaccino) è una patologia transitoria, i cui sintomi sono associati direttamente con l'assunzione dell'antigene lesivo.

L'incidenza di rettocolite ulcerosa è rimasta relativamente costante, in antitesi con l'aumento osservato nel morbo di Crohn, ma varia a seconda del Paese d'origine. È più elevata nei Paesi dell'Europa settentrionale e negli Stati Uniti (15/100 000), più bassa in Giappone e Sudafrica (1/100 000). L'incidenza di rettocolite ulcerosa in Israele varia a seconda dell'area d'origine; i bambini nati in Asia o in Africa presentano il rischio minore. La prevalenza di rettocolite ulcerosa nei Paesi dell'Europa settentrionale e negli Stati Uniti varia da 100 a 200/100 000 abitanti. Gli uomini presentano un rischio leggermente più elevato delle donne di acquisire la rettocolite ulcerosa, mentre per il morbo di Crohn è vero l'opposto.

MANIFESTAZIONI CLINICHE. Il sangue nelle feci e la diarrea costituiscono la presentazione tipica della rettocolite ulcerosa. Si può osservare stipsi nei pazienti con proctite. Sono comuni sintomi come il tenesmo, l'urgenza, il dolore addominale crampiforme (soprattutto in concomitanza con la defecazione) e le evacuazioni notturne. Per quanto riguarda la modalità di insorgenza, la malattia può presentarsi sia in forma insidiosa, con una progressione graduale dei sintomi, sia in forma acuta e fulminante. La colite fulminante è caratterizzata dalla presenza di febbre, anemia severa, ipoalbuminemia, leucocitosi e più di 5 evacuazioni ematiche al giorno per 5 giorni. La cronicità costituisce un aspetto importante ai fini della diagnosi; quando un bambino presenta i sintomi da 1-2 settimane, è difficile stabilire se sia affetto da una colite infettiva transitoria subfulminante o da una rettocolite ulcerosa. La presenza di sintomi oltre questo periodo spesso risulta essere secondaria a una IBD. Possono essere presenti anoressia, calo ponderale e un deficit di crescita, sebbene queste complicanze siano più tipiche del morbo di Crohn.

Le manifestazioni extraintestinali che tendono a verificarsi più comunemente in caso di rettocolite ulcerosa che di morbo di Crohn comprendono il pioderma gangrenoso, la colangite sclerosante, l'epatite cronica attiva e la spondilite anchilosante. La carenza di ferro può derivare tanto dalle perdite ematiche croniche quanto dal ridotto assorbimento. L'infiammazione cronica e la produzione di svariate citochine infiammatorie possono interferire con l'eritropoiesi e provocare un'anemia da malattia cronica. Nelle ragazzine è comune un'amenorrea secondaria durante i periodi di attività della malattia.

Il decorso clinico della rettocolite ulcerosa è caratterizzato da riacutizzazioni e remissioni, spesso senza un'apparente spiegazione. Dopo il trattamento dei sintomi iniziali, il 5% circa dei pazienti pediatrici con rettocolite ulcerosa presenta una remissione prolungata (>3 anni). Il 25% dei bambini che si presentano con una rettocolite ulcerosa severa necessita della colectomia entro 5 anni dalla diagnosi, contro il 5% di quelli che si presentano con una malattia lieve. È importante considerare la possibilità di un'infezione intestinale con sintomi ricorrenti; queste infezioni possono simulare una riacutizzazione oppure effettivamente provocare una recidiva. C'è chi ritiene che l'impiego di farmaci antinfiammatori non steroidei predisponga alle esacerbazioni.

In generale è diffusa l'opinione che il rischio di cancro del colon inizi ad aumentare dopo 8-10 anni di malattia, trascorsi i quali potrebbe aumentare dello 0,5-1% all'anno. Il rischio insorge circa 10 anni più tardi negli individui con colite limitata al colon discendente. La proctite isolata non è virtualmente associata ad alcun aumento del rischio rispetto alla popolazione generale. Poiché il cancro del colon è solitamente preceduto dalle alterazioni tipiche della displasia mucosa, si raccomanda di sottoporre i pazienti affetti da rettocolite ulcerosa da >10 anni a uno screening con colonscopia più biopsie ogni 1-2 anni. Sebbene questo rappresenti lo standard attuale della pratica clinica, non è chiaro se questo approccio modifichi la morbilità e la mortalità. Due aspetti contrastanti a proposito di questo programma di gestione restano irrisolti: (1) gli studi originali possono aver sovrastimato il rischio di cancro del colon e, pertanto, la necessità di sorveglianza è stata amplificata esageratamente; (2) lo screening per la displasia potrebbe non essere adeguato per la prevenzione del cancro del colon nella rettocolite ulcerosa qualora alcuni tumori maligni non fossero preceduti dalla displasia.

DIAGNOSI DIFFERENZIALE. Le principali patologie da escludere sono la colite infettiva, quella allergica e quella di Crohn. In ogni bambino con rettocolite ulcerosa di nuova diagnosi si dovrebbe effettuare una coprocoltura per i patogeni intestinali, un esame delle feci alla ricerca di uova e parassiti ed eventualmente degli studi sierologici per l'ameba (Tab. 333-3). In caso di assunzione di antibiotici, si dovrebbe valutare la possibilità di una colite pseudomembranosa secondaria al *Clostridium difficile*. L'infezione da Cytomegalovirus può mimare la rettocolite ulcerosa oppure essere associata a un'esacerbazione della malattia già esistente. La distinzione più difficile è quella dal morbo di Crohn, poiché in questa patologia l'infiammazione del colon inizialmente può apparire identica a quella della rettocolite ulcerosa. L'aspetto macroscopico della colite o lo sviluppo di una malattia dell'intestino tenue alla fine portano alla diagnosi corretta, ma ciò può avvenire anni dopo la presentazione iniziale.

All'esordio la colite della sindrome emolitico-uremica può essere identica a quella della rettocolite ulcerosa precoce. Negli stadi più avanzati, i segni di emolisi microangiopatica (la presenza di schistociti sullo striscio di sangue periferico), la trombocitopenia e la successiva insufficienza renale dovrebbero confermare la diagnosi di sindrome emolitico-uremica. La porpora di Schönlein-Henoch, pur potendo presentarsi con dolore addominale e feci ematiche, non è solitamente associata a colite. La malattia di Behçet è riconoscibile per le sue caratteristiche peculiari (vedi Capitoli 160 e 333.3). Altre patologie da considerare sono la proctite attinica, la colite virale negli individui immunocompromessi e la colite ischemica (Tab. 333-4). Nella prima infanzia l'intolleranza alle proteine alimentari può essere confusa con la rettocolite ulcerosa, sebbene la prima rappresenti un problema transitorio che si risolve eliminando la proteina dannosa. La malattia di Hirschsprung può dare luogo a un'enterocolite prima della correzione chirurgica o anche qualche mese dopo; è improbabile che essa venga confusa con una rettocolite ulcerosa.

TABELLA 333-3. Agenti infettivi che simulano le malattie infiammatorie intestinali croniche

AGENTE	MANIFESTAZIONI	DIAGNOSI	COMMENTI
BATTERICI			
Campylobacter jejuni	Diarrea acuta, febbre, feci ematiche e leucocitosi	Coprocoltura	Comune negli adolescenti, può recidivare
Yersinia enterocolitica	Diarrea acuta ⟶ cronica, dolore al quadrante inferiore destro, adenite mesenterica-pseudoappendicite, feci ematiche e leucocitosi	Coprocoltura	Comune negli adolescenti come febbre di origine sconosciuta, calo ponderale, dolore addominale
Clostridium difficile	Esordio dopo terapia antibiotica, diarrea acquosa ⟶ ematica, pseudomembrane alla sigmoidoscopia	Ricerca delle citotossine	Può essere nosocomiale Possibile il megacolon tossico
Escherichia coli 0157 : H7	Colite, feci ematiche, dolore addominale	Coprocoltura e tipizzazione	Sindrome emolitico-uremica
Salmonella	Diarrea acquosa ⟶ ematica, food borne, leucociti fecali, febbre, dolore, crampi	Coprocoltura	Solitamente acuta
Shigella	Diarrea acquosa ⟶ ematica, leucociti fecali, febbre, dolore, crampi	Coprocoltura	Sintomi da dissenteria
Edwardsiella tarda	Diarrea ematica, crampi	Coprocoltura	Ulcerazioni all'endoscopia
Aeromonas hydrophila	Crampi, diarrea, feci ematiche	Coprocoltura	Può essere cronica Acqua potabile contaminata
Plesiomonas	Diarrea, crampi	Coprocoltura	Da frutti di mare
Tubercolosi	Raramente bovina, ora da *Mycobacterium tuberculosis* Regione ileocecale, formazione di fistole	Coprocoltura, PPD, biopsie	Può simulare il morbo di Crohn
PARASSITI			
Entamoeba histolytica	Diarrea ematica acuta e ascessi epatici, colica	Trofozoiti nelle feci, ulcerazioni "a fiasco" nella mucosa colica, test sierologici	Viaggi in aree endemiche
Giardia lamblia	Diarrea acquosa maleodorante, crampi, flatulenza, calo ponderale; non interessamento colico	Trofozoiti "a civetta" e cisti nelle feci; raramente intubazione duodenale	Può essere cronica
ENTEROPATIA AIDS-CORRELATA			
Cryptosporidium	Diarrea cronica, calo ponderale	Esame microscopico delle feci	Reperti mucosi diversi dalle IBD Localizzazione tropicale
Isospora belli	Come per il *Cryptosporidium*		
Cytomegalovirus	Ulcerazioni coliche, dolore, diarrea ematica	Coprocoltura, biopsie	

IBD (*Inflammatory Bowel Disease*), malattie infiammatorie intestinali croniche; PPD (*Purified Protein Derivative*), derivato proteico purificato.

TABELLA 333-4. Patologie intestinali simili alle malattie infiammatorie croniche

INFEZIONI (VEDI TAB. 333-3)
Batteriche
Parassitarie

AIDS-CORRELATE
Tossine

IMMUNOINFIAMMATORIE
Immunodeficienze congenite
Immunodeficienze acquisite
Enterocolite da proteine alimentari
Malattia di Behçet
Iperplasia nodulare linfoide
Gastroenterite eosinofila
Graft versus host disease

PATOLOGIE VASCOLARI-ISCHEMICHE
Vasculiti sistemiche (LES, dermatomiosite)
Porpora di Schönlein-Henoch
Sindrome emolitico-uremica

ALTRE
Colite prestenotica
Colite da diversione
Colite attinica
Enterocolite necrotizzante neonatale
Tiflite
Colite di Hirschsprung
Linfoma intestinale
Abuso di lassativi

LES, lupus eritematoso sistemico.

DIAGNOSI. La diagnosi di rettocolite o proctite ulcerosa necessita della presentazione tipica, in assenza di una causa specifica identificabile (vedi Tabb. 333-3 e 333-4) e dei tipici reperti endoscopici e istologici (vedi Tab. 333-1). Bisognerebbe essere cauti a diagnosticare una rettocolite ulcerosa in un bambino che ha presentato i sintomi per meno di 2-3 settimane, almeno finché non è stata esclusa un'infezione. Se si sospetta questa patologia in un bambino con sintomi subacuti, il medico dovrebbe porre la diagnosi definitiva solo quando vi sia evidenza di cronicità alle biopsie del colon. Gli esami di laboratorio possono evidenziare anemia (da carenza di ferro o malattia cronica) o ipoalbuminemia. Sebbene la velocità di eritrosedimentazione sia spesso elevata, essa può risultare normale anche in caso di colite fulminante. Un aumento dei leucociti viene osservato in genere solo nei casi di colite più severa. Il clisma baritato è suggestivo ma non diagnostico di malattia acuta (Fig. 333-1) o cronica spenta (Fig. 333-2).

La diagnosi di rettocolite ulcerosa deve essere confermata dall'esame endoscopico e istologico del colon. Classicamente la malattia comincia nel retto, con un aspetto macroscopico caratterizzato da eritema, edema, perdita del reticolo vascolare, granulosità e friabilità. Ci può essere un "confine" che demarca il margine tra l'infiammazione e il colon normale, oppure può essere coinvolto l'intero colon. Talvolta l'intensità dell'infiammazione risulta variabile anche nelle aree colpite. La sigmoidoscopia con endoscopio flessibile può confermare la diagnosi; la colonscopia permette di valutare l'estensione della malattia ed escludere una colite di Crohn. Non bisognerebbe effettuare la colonscopia quando si sospetta una colite fulminante, per il rischio di provocare un *megacolon tossico* o causare una perforazione durante la procedura. Il grado della colite può essere valutato dall'aspetto macroscopico della mucosa. Generalmente non si osservano ulcere separate, che sarebbero più suggestive di colite di Crohn. I reperti endoscopici della rettocolite ulcerosa derivano dalle microulcere, che conferiscono un aspetto di anormalità diffusa. In caso di colite cronica molto severa si possono osservare degli pseudopolipi. Le biopsie del colon interessato evidenziano un'infiammazione acuta e cronica della mucosa. I reperti tipici sono la criptite, gli ascessi criptici, la separazione delle cripte da parte delle cellule infiammatorie, i foci di cellule infiammatorie acute, l'edema, la deplezione mucosa e la ramificazione delle cripte. Quest'ultimo reperto non viene osservato nelle coliti infettive. I granulomi, le ragadi o il coinvolgimento a tutto spessore della parete intestinale (solitamente più nelle biopsie chirurgiche che in quelle endoscopiche) suggeriscono un morbo di Crohn. Anche le biopsie rettali possono distinguere un'IBD cronica da una colite acuta autolimitante.

La malattia perianale, con l'eccezione di una lieve irritazione locale o delle ragadi anali associate alla diarrea, dovrebbe

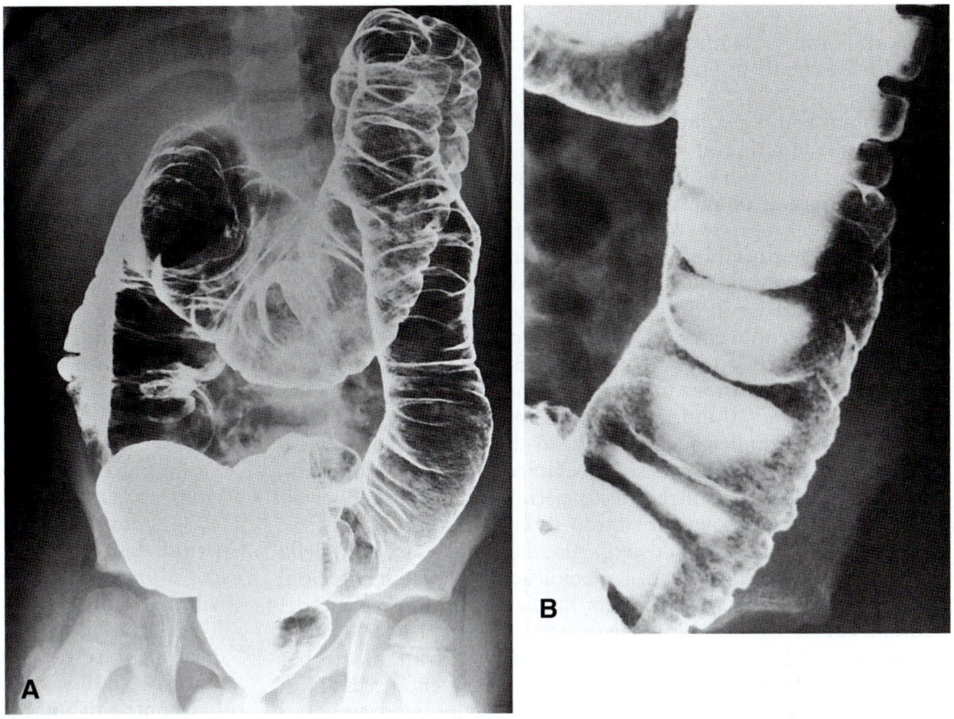

Figura 333-1. Rettocolite ulcerosa: clisma baritato a doppio contrasto in un bambino di 5 anni che aveva presentato sintomi intestinali ed extraintestinali dall'età di 3 anni. *A*, Piccole ulcere sono distribuite uniformemente sulla circonferenza colica e in maniera continua dal retto al colon traverso prossimale. Questo tipo di interessamento è tipico della rettocolite ulcerosa. *B*, In questa immagine conica del sigma nello stesso paziente, le piccole ulcerazioni sono rappresentate da minute spicole sulla superficie colica nella visione tangenziale e dalla fine punteggiatura della superficie colica frontalmente. (Da Hoffman AD, Hilton SW, Edwards DK [ed]: The child with diarrhea. In *Practical Pediatric Radiology*, 2nd ed. Philadelphia, WB Saunders, 1994, p 260.)

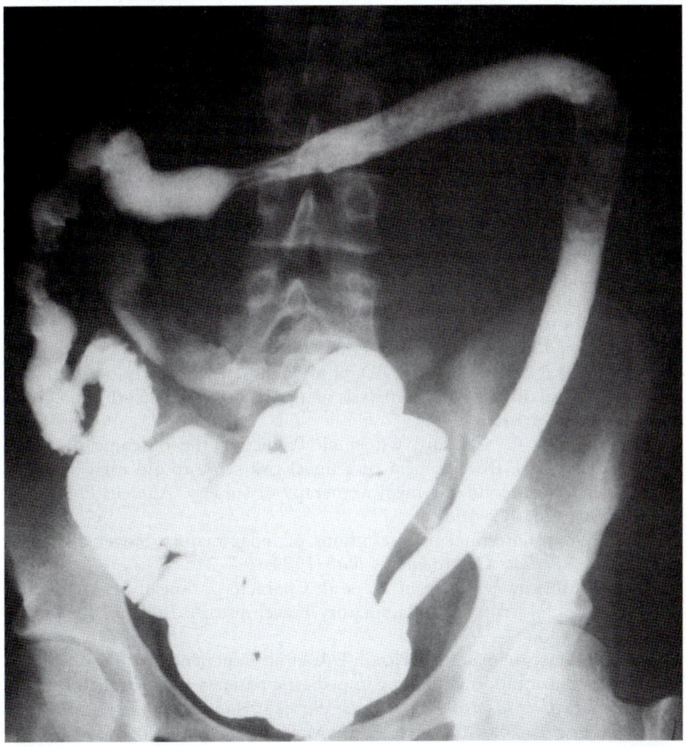

Figura 333-2. Rettocolite ulcerosa: alterazioni tardive. Questo clisma baritato a contrasto singolo mostra le alterazioni tardive della rettocolite ulcerosa in una ragazzina di 15 anni. Il colon è appiattito, di calibro ridotto e accorciato. È presente dilatazione dell'ileo terminale (ileite da reflusso). (Da Hoffman AD, Hilton SW, Edwards DK [ed]: The child with diarrhea. In *Practical Pediatric Radiology*, 2nd ed. Philadelphia, WB Saunders, 1994, p 262.)

indurre il medico a pensare al morbo di Crohn. Le radiografie dirette dell'addome possono mostrare la perdita dei segni delle austrature nel colon disteso dall'aria o una marcata dilatazione nel megacolon tossico. In caso di colite severa il colon può apparire dilatato; un diametro >6 cm, misurato radiologicamente in un adulto, suggerisce un megacolon tossico. Se è necessario esaminare radiologicamente il colon di un bambino con colite severa (per valutare l'estensione dell'interessamento o per cercare di escludere il morbo di Crohn), talvolta è d'aiuto effettuare un Rx transito o clisma del tenue con contrasto del tratto gastrointestinale superiore e poi osservare le scansioni tardive sul colon. Il clisma baritato è controindicato nel contesto di un potenziale megacolon tossico.

TRATTAMENTO. Non esiste una terapia medica curativa per la rettocolite ulcerosa; il trattamento ha lo scopo di controllare i sintomi e ridurre il rischio di recidiva. L'intensità del trattamento dipende dalla severità dei sintomi. Il 20-30% degli individui con rettocolite ulcerosa presenta un miglioramento spontaneo dei sintomi. I primi farmaci da utilizzare in caso di colite lieve sono gli aminosalicilati. La sulfasalazina è costituita da una componente sulfurea legata alla molecola attiva 5-aminosalicilato; questo legame impedisce un assorbimento precoce del farmaco nel tratto gastrointestinale superiore, consentendo al principio attivo di giungere nel colon, dove le due componenti vengono separate dal clivaggio batterico. La dose di sulfasalazina è di 50-75 mg/kg/24 ore (divisi in 2-4 dosi); generalmente non si superano i 2-3 g/24 ore. Si raccomanda di aumentare il dosaggio gradualmente fino alla dose piena nella prima settimana di terapia per evitare i sintomi gastrointestinali (nausea, dolore addominale) e la cefalea e per identificare un'eventuale ipersensibilità alla componente sulfurea. Possono passare diverse settimane prima che il farmaco cominci a fare effetto. La sulfasalazina tratta la colite ed è in grado di prevenire le recidive. Si raccomanda di continuarne l'assunzione anche quando la malattia è in remissione. L'ipersensibilità alla componente sulfurea rappresenta l'effetto collaterale principale, che si verifica nel 10-20% degli individui. In tal caso sono utili altre preparazioni meno allergeniche di 5-aminosalicilato (mesalazina, 50-70 mg/kg/die), la cui efficacia nel trattare la rettocolite ulcerosa e prevenire le recidive è pari a quella della sulfasalazina.

Forse il 10-20% degli individui che presenta una reazione allergica alla sulfasalazina presenterà una reazione simile con un altro 5-aminosalicilato. In rare occasioni questi farmaci causano un'esacerbazione della colite. Gli aminosalicilati possono essere somministrati anche in forma di clismi, che si rivelano utili soprattutto per le proctiti, per trattare le quali vengono utilizzati anche i clismi di idrocortisone (100 mg). Entrambe le forme di clisma possono essere somministrate ai bambini più grandi una volta al giorno (solitamente prima di coricarsi) per 2-3 settimane. Molti pazienti in età pediatrica preferiscono i farmaci orali ai clismi.

I bambini con pancolite o colite da moderata a severa non responsiva alla terapia con 5-aminosalicilati dovrebbero essere trattati con corticosterodi orali, più comunemente prednisone. La dose iniziale abituale di questo farmaco è di 1-2 mg/kg/24 ore (dose massima 40-60 mg). Se i sintomi non sono severi, il prednisone può essere assunto in un'unica somministrazione al mattino per ridurre la soppressione surrenalica. In caso di colite severa la dose può essere suddivisa in due somministrazioni al giorno ed essere assunta per via endovenosa. L'obiettivo è di scalare gradualmente a una dose a giorni alterni nel giro di 1-3 mesi e poi sospendere il farmaco. La persistenza di sintomi malgrado il trattamento con steroidi per 7-10 giorni o l'impossibilità di ridurre la dose costituiscono un'indicazione all'utilizzo di altri principi attivi o al trattamento chirurgico. Bisogna evitare l'impiego quotidiano prolungato di steroidi oltre questo periodo per i molteplici effetti collaterali, tra i quali il ritardo di crescita, la soppressione surrenalica, la cataratta, l'osteopenia, la necrosi asettica della testa del femore, l'intolleranza glucidica, il rischio di infezioni e gli effetti estetici. Con la terapia medica la maggior parte dei bambini raggiunge la remissione entro 3 mesi; il 10-15% tuttavia continua ad avere sintomi non responsivi al trattamento per oltre 6 mesi. A molti bambini con una malattia che necessita di frequenti trattamenti con corticosteroidi vengono somministrati immunomodulatori come l'azatioprina (1,5-2,5 mg/kg/die) o la 6-mercaptopurina (1-1,5 mg/kg/die). Alcuni dati non controllati suggeriscono un effetto di risparmio sui corticosteroidi in molti individui trattati. La ciclosporina, dimostratasi associata con un miglioramento in molti bambini con sintomi severi, non sembra influire sulla storia naturale della malattia. L'infliximab, un anticorpo monoclonale chimerico per il fattore di necrosi tumorale α (TNF-α, *Tumor Necrosis Factor* α), è stato utilizzato in alcuni casi di colite fulminante. Negli adulti con malattia moderata o severa la terapia di induzione e di mantenimento è risultata efficace nel determinare una risposta clinica positiva. Gli agenti probiotici possono avere un ruolo nel mantenere la remissione ed essere altrettanto efficaci della mesalazina nel prevenire le ricadute.

La colectomia viene effettuata in caso di malattia intrattabile, di complicanze della terapia e di malattia fulminante non responsiva alla terapia medica. Non è stato osservato un chiaro beneficio derivante dall'impiego della nutrizione parenterale totale o della dieta elementare continua per via entrale nel trattamento della rettocolite ulcerosa severa. Malgrado ciò, la nutrizione parenterale viene spesso utilizzata se l'introito orale è insufficiente, in modo che il paziente possa essere pronto da un punto di vista nutrizionale per la chirurgia, qualora la terapia medica si rivelasse inefficace. Con ogni terapia medica per la rettocolite ulcerosa occorre sempre soppesare i rischi del farmaco o del trattamento, tenendo conto del fatto che la colite può essere trattata con successo chirurgicamente.

La terapia chirurgica della colite intrattabile o fulminante è la colectomia totale. L'approccio ottimale consiste nel combinare la colectomia con un pull-through endorettale in cui si effettuano una resezione del retto e della sottomucosa rettale. L'ileo distale viene tirato in basso e suturato all'ano interno con una pouch a J creata con l'ileo immediatamente al di sopra del moncone rettale. Grazie a questa procedura, il bambino mantiene la continenza. Spesso viene confezionata un'ileostomia temporanea per proteggere la delicata anastomosi tra il manicotto della pouch e il retto. Di solito l'ileostomia viene chiusa dopo qualche mese, ricostituendo la continuità intestinale. In quel momento la frequenza delle evacuazioni è solitamente aumentata, ma il quadro può essere migliorato con la loperamide. La principale complicanza di questo intervento è la *pouchite*, una reazione infiammatoria cronica della pouch, che provoca diarrea ematica, dolore addominale e, occasionalmente, febbricola. La causa di questa complicanza è sconosciuta, sebbene sia più frequente quando la pouch ileale è stata confezionata per la rettocolite ulcerosa che per altre indicazioni (poliposi familiare del colon). La pouchite, osservabile nel 30-40% dei pazienti in precedenza affetti da rettocolite ulcerosa, di norma risponde al trattamento con metronidazolo o ciprofloxacina per via orale.

Il supporto psicosociale costituisce un aspetto importante del trattamento. Esso può comprendere un'adeguata discussione delle manifestazioni e del trattamento della malattia tra paziente e medico, un counseling psicologico per il bambino, se necessario, e un sostegno per il nucleo familiare fornito da un assistente sociale. I gruppi di sostegno si sono rivelati d'aiuto per alcune famiglie. I bambini con rettocolite ulcerosa dovrebbero essere incoraggiati a partecipare pienamente alle attività adatte alla loro età; tuttavia, potrebbe rendersi necessaria una riduzione delle attività durante i periodi di riacutizzazione della malattia.

PROGNOSI. Il decorso della rettocolite ulcerosa è segnato da remissioni e riacutizzazioni. Nella maggior parte dei bambini con questa patologia la terapia medica inizialmente si rivela efficace. Molti pazienti con manifestazioni lievi continuano a rispondere bene ai farmaci e possono persistere in remissione per lunghi periodi grazie a preparati di 5-aminosalicilati somministrati a scopo profilattico. Talvolta però un bambino con esordio lieve sviluppa più tardi dei sintomi intrattabili. Oltre la prima decade di malattia il rischio di sviluppare un cancro del colon inizia ad aumentare rapidamente. Tale rischio può essere ridotto con colonscopie di sorveglianza a partire dagli 8-10 anni di malattia. Il riscontro di una displasia significativa alla biopsia costituisce un'indicazione alla colectomia.

Arts J, D'Haens G, et al: Long-term outcome of treatment with intravenous cyclosporine in patients with severe ulcerative colitis. *Inflamm Bowel Dis* 2004;10:73–78.

Beattie RM, Croft NM, Fell JM, et al: Inflammatory bowel disease. *Arch Dis Child* 2006;91:426–432.

de Saussure P, Lavergne-Slove A, Mazeron MC, et al: A prospective assessment of cytomegalovirus infection in active inflammatory bowel disease. *Aliment Pharmacol Ther* 2004;20:1323–1327.

Dobson G, Hickey C, Trinder J: *Clostridium difficile* colitis causing toxic megacolon, severe sepsis and multiple organ dysfunction syndrome. *Intensive Care Med* 2003;29:1030.

Dolgin SE, Shlasko E, Gorfine S, et al: Restorative proctocolectomy in children with ulcerative colitis utilizing rectal mucosectomy with or without diverting ileostomy. *J Pediatr Surg* 1999;34:837–839.

Heyman M, Kirschner BS, Gold BD, et al: Children with early onset inflammatory bowel disease (IBD): Analysis of a pediatric IBD consortium registry. *J Pediatr* 2004;146:35–40.

Ho GT, Mowat C, Goddard CJ, et al: Predicting the outcome of severe ulcerative colitis: Development of a novel risk score to aid early selection of patients for second-line medical therapy or surgery. *Aliment Pharmacol Ther* 2004;19:1079–1087.

Hyams JS: Extraintestinal manifestations of inflammatory bowel disease in children. *J Pediatr Gastroenterol Nutr* 1994;19:7–21.

Hyams JS, Markowitz J, Treem W, et al: Characterization of hepatic abnormalities in children with inflammatory bowel disease. *Inflamm Bowel Dis* 1995;1:27–33.

Kader HA, Mascarehnas MR, Piccoli DA, et al: Experience with 6-mercaptopurine and azathioprine therapy in pediatric patients with severe ulcerative colitis. *J Pediatr Gastroenterol Nutr* 1999;28:54–58.

Kruis W, Fric P, Pokrotnieks J, et al: Maintaining remission of ulcerative colitis with the probiotic *Escherichia coli* Nissle 1917 is as effective as with standard mesalazine. *Gut* 2004;53:1617–1623.

Kugathasan S, Judd RH, Hoffmann RG, et al: Epidemiologic and clinical characteristics of children with newly diagnosed inflammatory bowel disease in Wisconsin: A statewide population-based study. *J Pediatr* 2003;143: 525–531.

Mamula P, Markowitz JE, Baldassano RN: Inflammatory bowel disease in early childhood and adolescence: Special considerations. *Gastroenterol Clin North Am* 2003;32:967–995.

Mamula P, Markowitz JE, Cohen LJ, et al: Infliximab in pediatric ulcerative colitis: Two-year follow-up. *J Pediatr Gastroenterol Nutr* 2004;38:298–301.

Rutgeerts P, Sandborn WJ, Feagan BG, et al: Infliximab for induction and maintenance therapy for ulcerative colitis. *N Engl J Med* 2005;353: 2462–2476.

333.2 • Morbo di Crohn (enterite regionale, ileite regionale, colite granulomatosa)

Il morbo di Crohn, una patologia infiammatoria cronica idiopatica dell'intestino, colpisce qualunque segmento del tratto alimentare, dal cavo orale all'ano. Anche se molte sono le analogie con la rettocolite ulcerosa, occorre sottolineare anche importanti differenze nel decorso clinico e nella distribuzione della malattia nel tratto gastrointestinale (vedi Tab. 333-1). Il processo infiammatorio tende a essere eccentrico e segmentarlo, spesso con zone di risparmio (tratti normali di intestino tra aree infiammate). Mentre nella rettocolite ulcerosa l'infiammazione è limitata alla mucosa (tranne che nel megacolon tossico), nel morbo di Crohn l'interessamento gastrointestinale è spesso transmurale. Nei bambini con morbo di Crohn, la presentazione iniziale nella maggior parte dei casi interessa l'ileo e il colon (ileocolite), ma riguarda solo l'intestino tenue nel 30% circa dei casi (il 70% di questi pazienti presenta solo un'ileite terminale) o solo il colon nel 10-15%. Pure l'interessamento gastrointestinale superiore (esofago, stomaco, duodeno) viene osservato nel 30% dei bambini. La malattia colica isolata è comune nei soggetti di età <8 anni. Il morbo di Crohn tende ad avere una distribuzione per età bimodale, con il primo picco a partire dall'adolescenza. Una diagnosi prima dei 20 anni di età è associata con una maggiore probabilità di malattia dell'intestino tenue, con lo sviluppo di stenosi e quindi con la necessità di intervenire chirurgicamente rispetto a una diagnosi effettuata dopo i 40 anni di età.

L'incidenza del morbo di Crohn è risultata in aumento, mentre quella della rettocolite ulcerosa è stabile. L'incidenza riportata di morbo di Crohn è di circa 3-4/100 000 e la prevalenza è di circa 30-100/100 000. La prevalenza di morbo di Crohn tra i bianchi e i neri sembra essere pari a 3-10 volte quella degli ispanici e degli asiatici che vivono negli Stati Uniti.

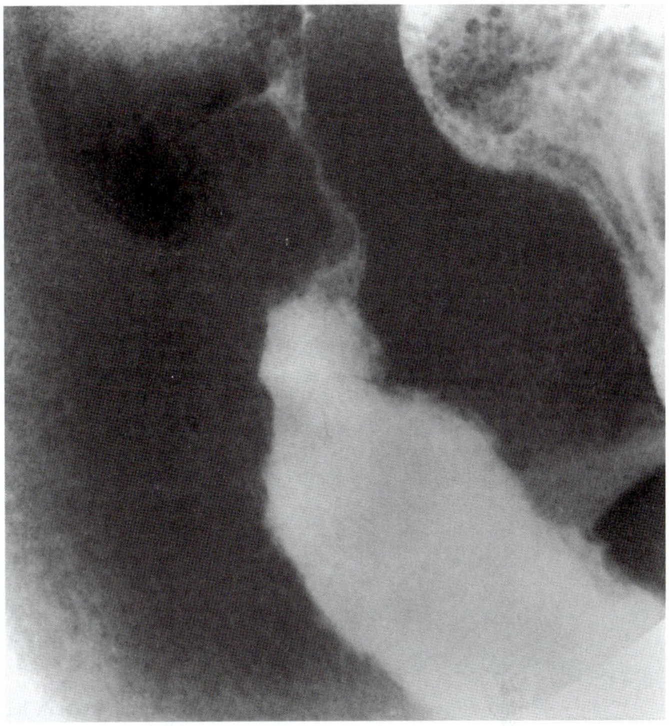

Figura 333-3. Morbo di Crohn stenotico. In questo ragazzino di 16 anni è presente una stenosi severa dell'ileo terminale. Il segmento non stenotico prossimale è caratterizzato dalla scomparsa di origine infiammatoria delle pliche mucose e da piccole ulcerazioni. (Da Hoffman AD, Hilton SW, Edwards DK [ed]: The child with diarrhea. In *Practical Pediatric Radiology*, 2nd ed. Philadelphia, WB Saunders, 1994, p 267.)

MANIFESTAZIONI CLINICHE. La classificazione di Vienna dei sottotipi di morbo di Crohn (le cui variabili comprendono l'età, la localizzazione e il comportamento della malattia, che può essere di tipo infiammatorio [non stenosante o fistolizzante], stenosante o fibrostenosante oppure fistolizzante) è stata proposta, ma non convalidata come strumento prognostico, sia negli adulti sia nei bambini. I pazienti con malattia dell'intestino tenue hanno maggiori probabilità di presentare un quadro di tipo ostruttivo (più spesso con dolore nel quadrante inferiore destro), caratterizzato da fibrostenosi, mentre quelli con malattia colica tendono a presentare sintomi derivanti dall'infiammazione (diarrea, sanguinamento, crampi). I fenotipi di malattia spesso variano mano a mano che si prolunga la durata della malattia (la malattia infiammatoria diventa stenosante). I segni e sintomi sistemici sono più comuni nel morbo di Crohn che nella rettocolite ulcerosa. Sono frequenti febbre, malessere e facile affaticabilità. Un deficit di crescita con ritardata maturazione ossea e ritardato sviluppo sessuale possono precedere gli altri sintomi di 1-2 anni e si verificano almeno due volte più facilmente nel morbo di Crohn che nella rettocolite ulcerosa. I bambini possono presentare come unica manifestazione del morbo di Crohn un deficit di crescita, le cui cause comprendono un introito calorico inadeguato, un assorbimento subottimale o un'eccessiva perdita di nutrienti, gli effetti dell'infiammazione cronica sul metabolismo osseo e l'impiego dei corticosteroidi nella terapia. È comune l'amenorrea, primaria o secondaria. Al contrario di quanto avviene nella rettocolite ulcerosa, è comune la malattia perianale (*skin tags* o marische [pliche cutanee], fistole, ascessi). L'interessamento gastrico o duodenale può essere associato a vomito ricorrente e dolore epigastrico. Un'ostruzione parziale dell'intestino tenue, spesso secondaria a un restringimento del lume intestinale dovuto all'infiammazione o a una stenosi, può provocare sintomi di dolore addominale crampiforme (specialmente con i pasti), borborigmi e distensione addominale intermittente (Fig. 333-3). Dovrebbe essere sospettata una stenosi se il bambino rileva un miglioramento dei sintomi in associazione con un'improvvisa sensazione di gorgoglio del contenuto intestinale in una regione ben localizzata dell'addome. Una rara complicanza del morbo di Crohn è l'ostruzione ureterale (solitamente dal lato destro), secondaria all'estensione del processo infiammatorio.

Per la diagnosi di **malattia fistolizzante** è necessario rilevare la formazione di una fistola. Le fistole enteroenteriche o enterocoliche (tra segmenti intestinali) sono spesso asintomatiche, ma possono contribuire al malassorbimento sono ad alta portata o provocano un'eccessiva proliferazione batterica (Fig. 333-4). Le fistole enterovescicali (tra intestino e vescica urinaria) originano dall'ileo o dal sigma e si presentano con segni di infezione urinaria, pneumaturia o fecaluria. Le fistole enterovaginali originano dal retto, provocano secrezioni fecaloidi dalla vagina e sono difficili da trattare. Le fistole enterocutanee (tra intestino e cute addominale) sono spesso causate da pregresse anastomosi chirurgiche con deiscenza. Gli ascessi intraddominali possono essere associati a febbre e dolore, ma provocare relativamente pochi sintomi. Gli ascessi epatici o splenici si verificano con o senza una fistola locale. Gli ascessi anorettali spesso originano immediatamente sopra l'ano a livello delle cripte di Morgani. La struttura delle fistole perianali è complessa per via dei diversi strati di tessuto. Mentre gli ascessi perianali sono in genere molto dolorosi, le fistole tendono a produrre meno sintomi del previsto. Alle esse è spesso associato un drenaggio purulento. Un *ascesso dello psoas* secondario a una fistola perianale si può presentare con dolore all'anca, riduzione dell'estensione dell'anca (segno dello psoas) e febbre.

Le manifestazioni extraintestinali sono più comuni nel morbo di Crohn che nella rettocolite ulcerosa; quelli particolarmente associati al morbo di Crohn comprendono le ulcere afose orali, l'artrite periferica, l'eritema nodoso, l'ippocratismo digitale, l'episclerite, i calcoli renali (acido urico, ossalato) e i calcoli biliari. Ognuna delle affezioni extraintestinali descritte nel paragrafo sulle IBD si può verificare con questa patologia (vedi Tab. 333-2). L'artrite periferica non è deformante. La comparsa di manifestazioni extraintestinali di solito è correlata alla presenza di colite. Durante i periodi di attività della malattia è comune l'amenorrea secondaria.

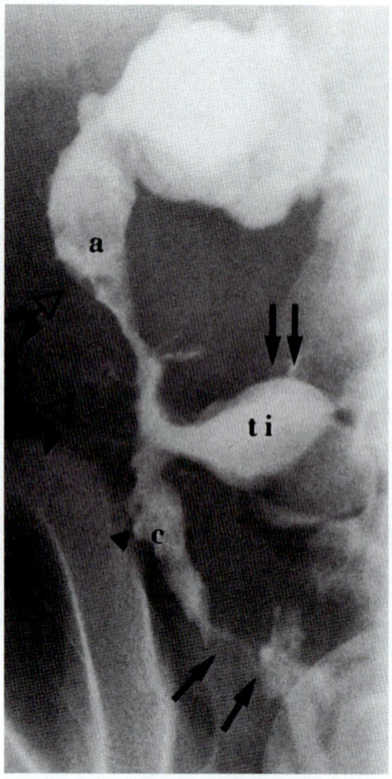

Figura 333-4. Morbo di Crohn: dilatazioni e fistole. Un'ileocolite severa ha provocato una fistola ileocecale (*frecce singole*, *in basso*) e la formazione di una dilatazione nel colon ascendente (a) [*frecce grandi*]. c, cieco (*punta di freccia*); ti, ileo terminale (*frecce accoppiate*). (Da Hoffman AD, Hilton SW, Edwards DK [ed]: The child with diarrhea. In *Practical Pediatric Radiology*, 2nd ed. Philadelphia, WB Saunders, 1994, p 268.)

Un interessamento esteso dell'intestino tenue, soprattutto in associazione con una resezione chirurgica, può dare luogo alla sindrome dell'intestino corto, che è rara nei bambini. Le complicanze della disfunzione o della resezione dell'ileo terminale comprendono il malassorbimento degli acidi biliari con diarrea secondaria e quello della vitamina B_{12}. La steatorrea cronica può provocare ossaluria con calcoli renali secondari. Anche il rischio di colelitiasi è aumentato, secondariamente alla deplezione di acidi biliari.

Una patologia con questa varietà di manifestazioni può avere un impatto notevole sullo stile di vita del paziente. Fortunatamente la maggior parte dei bambini con morbo di Crohn è in grado di proseguire le sue normali attività, dovendole limitare solamente nei periodi di esacerbazione dei sintomi.

DIAGNOSI DIFFERENZIALE. Le diagnosi che più comunemente devono essere distinte dal morbo di Crohn sono le enteropatie infettive (nel caso del morbo di Crohn: ileite terminale acuta, colite infettiva, parassiti enterici e ascesso periappendicolare) (vedi Tabb. 333-3, 333-4 e 333-5). La *Yersinia* può determinare molti dei reperti radiologici ed endoscopici dell'intestino tenue distale che vengono osservati nel morbo di Crohn. I sintomi della dissenteria batterica possono essere più facilmente confusi con la rettocolite ulcerosa che con il morbo di Crohn. È stato osservato che la malattia celiaca o l'infezione da *Giardia* danno luogo a una presentazione simile a quella del morbo di Crohn, comprendente diarrea, calo ponderale ed enteropatia protidodisperdente. La tubercolosi gastrointestinale è rara, ma può simulare il morbo di Crohn. La perforazione dell'intestino tenue da parte di corpi estranei (stuzzicadenti) può simulare un morbo di Crohn in una regione localizzata. Il linfoma dell'intestino tenue, pur potendo a sua volta simulare questa patologia, tende a essere associato con difetti di riempimento nodulari dell'intestino senza ulcerazioni o restringimenti del lume. Il linfoma intestinale è molto meno comune nei bambini rispetto al morbo di Crohn. Il dolore addominale funzionale ricorrente può simulare il dolore del morbo di Crohn dell'intestino tenue. L'*iperplasia nodulare linfoide* dell'ileo terminale (un reperto normale) può essere confusa con l'ileite di Crohn. Il dolore o una massa accompagnata da ipertermia nel quadrante addominale inferiore destro possono essere la conseguenza di un ascesso periappendicolare. Questa entità è occasionalmente associata anche con la diarrea. La digiunite necrotizzante è una rara condizione di infiammazione acuta e transitoria del digiuno (o, meno comunemente, dell'ileo o del colon), che può essere ricorrente.

Il difetto di crescita può rappresentare l'unica manifestazione del morbo di Crohn; devono essere prese in considerazione altre patologie come il deficit di ormone della crescita, l'enteropatia glutine-dipendente (celiachia) o l'anoressia nervosa. Se l'artrite precede le manifestazioni intestinali, può essere posta una prima diagnosi di artrite reumatoide giovanile. L'anemia refrattaria può costituire la caratteristica di presentazione ed essere confusa con una patologia ematologica primitiva. La leucemia si può presentare con dolore addominale acuto in associazione con un'alterazione dell'emocromo e venire inizialmente scambiata per morbo di Crohn. La malattia granulomatosa cronica dell'infanzia può provocare alterazioni infiammatorie nell'intestino con granulomi alla biopsia. Il restringimento antrale in questa patologia talora viene confuso con una stenosi secondaria al morbo di Crohn.

DIAGNOSI. Il morbo di Crohn si può presentare con svariate combinazioni di sintomi, che all'esordio possono essere subdoli (ritardo di crescita, dolore addominale isolati); ciò spiega perché non è possibile porre la diagnosi prima che siano trascorsi 1-2 anni dall'inizio dei sintomi. La diagnosi di morbo di Crohn dipende dal riscontro delle caratteristiche cliniche tipiche della patologia (anamnesi, esame obiettivo, esami di laboratorio e reperti endoscopici o radiologici), escludendo entità specifiche che possono avere analoghe manifestazioni e dimostrando la cronicità. L'anamnesi può comprendere qualunque combinazione di dolore addominale (specie nel quadrante inferiore destro), diarrea, vomito, anoressia, calo ponderale, ritardo di crescita e manifestazioni extraintestinali. Solo il 25% presenta inizialmente

TABELLA 333-5. Diagnosi differenziale dei sintomi di presentazione del morbo di Crohn

PRINCIPALE SINTOMO DI PRESENTAZIONE	DIAGNOSI DA CONSIDERARE
Dolore addominale nel quadrante inferiore destro, con o senza massa	Appendicite, infezione (per es. da *Campylobacter*, *Yersinia* spp.), linfoma, intussuscezione, adenite mesenterica, diverticolo di Meckel, cisti ovarica
Dolore addominale cronico periombelicale o epigastrico	Sindrome del colon irritabile, stipsi, intolleranza al lattosio, malattia peptica
Sanguinamento rettale senza diarrea	Ragade, polipo, diverticolo di Meckel, sindrome ulcerosa del retto
Diarrea ematica	Infezione, sindrome emolitico-uremica, porpora di Schönlein-Henoch, ischemia intestinale, colite attinica
Diarrea acquosa	Sindrome del colon irritabile, intolleranza al lattosio, giardiasi, infezione da *Cryptosporidium*, sorbitolo, lassativi
Malattia perirettale	Ragade, emorroide (rara), infezione streptococcica, condiloma (raro)
Ritardo nella crescita	Endocrinopatia
Anoressia, calo poderale	Anoressia nervosa
Artrite	Patologia vascolare del collagene, infezione
Alterazioni epatiche	Epatite cronica

Da Kugathasan S: Diarrhea. In Kliegman RM, Greenbaum LA, Lye P (ed): *Practical Strategies in Pediatric Diagnosis and Therapy*, 2nd ed. Philadelphia, Elsevier/Saunders, 204, p. 287.

la triade con diarrea, calo ponderale e dolore addominale; la maggior parte non ha diarrea e solo il 25% va soggetto a sanguinamento gastrointestinale.

I bambini con morbo di Crohn spesso appaiono in condizioni di sofferenza cronica: presentano comunemente una perdita di peso e sono spesso malnutriti. È frequente che un ritardo lineare della crescita preceda la presentazione clinica anche di 1-2 anni; questa manifestazione potrebbe non venire apprezzata finché non è stata stabilita la diagnosi. I pazienti in età pediatrica appaiono spesso pallidi, con livelli ridotti di energia e scarso appetito; quest'ultimo reperto talvolta deriva da un'associazione tra i pasti e il dolore addominale oppure la diarrea. Può essere presente tensione addominale, sia diffusa sia localizzata al quadrante inferiore destro. Talvolta è palpabile una massa dolente o una "pastosità" (pseudomassa) nel quadrante inferiore destro. La malattia perianale, quando presente, può essere caratteristica. Marische sulla cute anale (del diametro di 1-3 cm) o fistole perianali con drenaggio purulento sono suggestivi di morbo di Crohn. Possono essere presenti ippocratismo digitale, reperti dell'artrite e manifestazioni cutanee. L'emocromo completo evidenzia comunemente un'anemia, spesso con una componente sideropenica. La velocità di eritrosedimentazione, pur essendo spesso elevata, può anche essere normale; è comune un'elevata conta piastrinica ($>600\,000/mm^3$). Il numero dei leucociti può essere normale o lievemente aumentato. Il livello sierico dell'albumina può essere basso e il livello fecale di α_1-antitrispina elevato, reperto compatibile con l'enteropatia protidodisperdente. La calprotectina o la lattoferritina fecali sono solitamente elevate. Nel 55% dei bambini con morbo di Crohn, ma solo nel 5% di quelli con rettocolite ulcerosa, vengono identificati anticorpi anti-*Saccharomyces cerevisiae*.

Nei bambini con sospetto morbo di Crohn occorre studiare tanto l'intestino tenue quanto il crasso. La scelta iniziale della colonscopia o di un esame radiologico dipende in parte dalla presunta localizzazione della malattia. In caso di interessamento dell'intestino tenue, la prima indagine da effettuarsi dovrebbe essere un esame con contrasto del tratto gastrointestinale superiore con clisma del tenue. Gli studi radiologici permettono di evidenziare svariati reperti. Le radiografie dirette dell'addome possono essere normali oppure mostrare i reperti dell'ostruzione parziale dell'intestino tenue o l'impronta della parete colica. Uno studio con contrasto del tratto gastrointestinale superiore con clisma del tenue può evidenziare ulcerazioni aftose e pliche ispessite e nodulari, così come restringimenti del lume a qualunque livello del tratto gastrointestinale. Le ulcere lineari conferiscono alla superficie mucosa un aspetto ad acciottolato. Le anse intestinali sono spesso separate per effetto dell'ispessimento della parete intestinale e del mesentere. L'ileo terminale è il più comunemente interessato. Le aree malate tendono a essere eccentriche ed è possibile evidenziare aree normali tra i segmenti malati (aree di risparmio). L'endoscopia con videocapsula ha rivelato lesioni mucose a carico dell'intestino tenue in alcuni pazienti con valutazione radiologica normale.

Altri reperti radiologici che suggeriscono un morbo di Crohn più severo sono le fistole tra anse intestinali (enteroenteriche o enterocoliche), tratti tortuosi e le stenosi (vedi Figg. 333-3 e 333-4). Seguendo il flusso anterogrado del bario nel colon può essere evidenziata una malattia colica nel lato destro. L'ecografia e la TC con mezzo di contrasto sono gli esami più utili per individuare gli ascessi intraddominali. Alla TC è rilevabile una parete intestinale ispessita. La RM può localizzare aree di malattia intestinale attiva, sebbene questo esame non sia probabilmente migliore per identificare un ascesso. La RM è utile anche per valutare il morbo di Crohn in gravidanza poiché non comporta l'impiego di radiazioni ionizzanti. La scintigrafia con radionuclidi utilizzando globuli bianchi marcati con Indio può essere d'aiuto per localizzare le aree affette.

La colonscopia con biopsie può essere più utile degli studi radiologici o con radionuclidi per valutare la malattia colica e per stabilire la diagnosi. L'incannulamento ileale in corso di colonscopia risulta talvolta prezioso per chiarire una diagnosi dubbia di morbo di Crohn ileale. Tra i reperti alla colonscopia vi sono alterazioni infiammatorie aspecifiche irregolari (eritema, friabilità, perdita del reticolo vascolare), ulcere afose, ulcere lineari, nodularità e stenosi. I reperti alla biopsia possono consistere anche solo in alterazioni infiammatorie aspecifiche. I granulomi non caseosi, simili a quelli della sarcoidosi, costituiscono il reperto istologico più caratteristico, sebbene spesso non siano presenti. Anche l'infiammazione transmurale è caratteristica, ma identificabile solo sui campioni chirurgici.

TRATTAMENTO. Il morbo di Crohn non può essere guarito né con la terapia medica né con quella chirurgica. Lo scopo del trattamento è di alleviare i sintomi, prevenire le complicanze dell'infiammazione cronica (anemia, ritardo nella crescita), evitare le riacutizzazioni e, se possibile, far cicatrizzare la mucosa. Le specifiche modalità terapeutiche impiegate dipendono dalla localizzazione geografica, dalla severità dell'infiammazione, dall'età del paziente e dalla presenza di complicanze (ascessi). Per un morbo di Crohn lieve dell'ileo terminale o del colon si può fare un primo tentativo con la mesalazina (50-70 mg/kg/die). Sono state formulate preparazioni farmaceutiche specifiche che rilasciano il principio attivo 5-ASA nell'ileo e nel colon. La sulfasalazina può essere efficace per la colite di Crohn lieve, ma non è utile nella malattia dell'intestino tenue. Anche la budesonide, un corticosteroide con attività antinfiammatoria locale sulla mucosa intestinale e con un elevato metabolismo di primo passaggio epatico, viene impiegata per la malattia lieve ileale o ileocecale (dose nell'adulto: 9 mg/die). In caso di malattia del tenue o del colon più estesa o severa, la maggior parte dei medici inizia una terapia con corticosteroidi (prednisone, 1-2 mg/kg/die, massimo 40-60 mg). L'obiettivo è scalare gradualmente a una singola somministrazione al mattino a giorni alterni appena la malattia diventa quiescente. Tipicamente lo scalare può cominciare entro 3-4 settimane e continuare per alcuni mesi. I clinici variano i loro schemi di riduzione, ma la maggior parte diminuisce la dose giornaliera di 2,5-5,0 mg ogni 6-8 giorni, fino a portarla a 0,5 mg/kg, dopodiché una riduzione analoga viene effettuata a giorni alterni in cicli di 6-8 giorni (25 mg alternati a 20 mg per 8 giorni, seguiti da 25 mg alternati a 15 mg per 8 giorni e così via). Alla fine il prednisone viene somministrato solo a giorni alterni e poi questa dose viene scalata secondo la tolleranza. Si tratta di un approccio ben tollerato, anche se nel frattempo la patologia può riacutizzarsi. Non si è dimostrata efficace la prosecuzione quotidiana o a giorni alterni del prednisone come terapia di mantenimento per prevenire le ricadute.

La crescita del bambino viene ritardata sia dalla malattia attiva sia dalla terapia quotidiana con corticosteroidi, ma non dal trattamento a giorni alterni. Gli effetti collaterali degli steroidi somministrati ogni giorno tendono a verificarsi più rapidamente e a essere più severi quando il livello sierico di albumina è ridotto. Per la malattia colica distale sono stati impiegati sotto forma di clismi. La budesonide, spesso utilizzata per attenuare gli effetti collaterali dei corticosteroidi, pare essere efficace quanto la mesalazina nella malattia lieve e moderata dell'ileo e del colon destro, ma meno del prednisone. Ancora non si è appurato se essa abbia un minore effetto di soppressione della crescita rispetto al prednisone.

Purtroppo fino al 50% dei bambini con morbo di Crohn diventerà refrattario alla terapia con corticosteroidi oppure dipendente dalla somministrazione quotidiana, andando rapidamente incontro a riacutizzazioni della malattia quando il dosaggio viene ridotto. Gli immunomodulatori come l'azatioprina (1,5-2,5 mg/kg/die) o la 6-mercaptopurina (1,0-1,5 mg/kg/die) possono risultare efficaci in alcuni individui che presentano una scarsa risposta al prednisone o che sono steroidodipendenti. Poiché l'effetto benefico di questi farmaci può comparire anche 3-6 mesi dopo l'inizio della terapia, essi non risultano efficaci acutamente. Il loro impiego precoce può ridurre la dose cumulativa di prednisone per i primi 1-2 anni di terapia. Alcune varianti genetiche nei sistemi enzimatici responsabili del metabolismo di questi farmaci (tiopurina S-metiltransferasi o TPMT) possono condizionare la risposta e la potenziale tossicità. Se si riscontra una resistenza all'azatioprina oppure si verifica una tossicità, si utilizza il metotrexato (25 mg/1,73 m^2 alla settimana).

Per i pazienti con morbo di Crohn si ricorre alla terapia con anticorpi diretti contro i mediatori dell'infiammazione. L'infliximab (5 mg/kg somministrati per via endovenosa), un anticorpo monoclonale chimerico contro il TNF-α, è stato approvato per il trattamento iniziale e la successiva terapia di mantenimento degli adulti con morbo di Crohn. Esso viene comunemente utilizzato nei bambini, e delle serie non controllate pubblicate suggeriscono un notevole miglioramento dei sintomi nel 50-70% dei pazienti. Ha un inizio d'azione abbastanza rapido e viene somministrato inizialmente in tre infusioni per un periodo di 6 settimane (settimana 0, 2 e 6). La durata della risposta all'infliximab è variabile e può essere di sole 4-8 settimane, rendendo necessaria una terapia di mantenimento. Gli effetti collaterali comprendono le reazioni all'infusione, un'aumentata incidenza di infezioni (in particolare la riattivazione di una tubercolosi latente), una malattia demielinizzante, talvolta una neoplasia e lo sviluppo di autoanticorpi. Lo sviluppo di anticorpi contro l'infliximab è associato a un'aumentata incidenza di reazioni infusionali e a una ridotta durata della risposta. L'impiego concomitante di immunomodulatori come l'azatioprina è associato a livelli ridotti di anticorpi contro l'infliximab. La sicurezza a lungo termine di questa terapia biologica sembra buona, ma è necessaria un'osservazione a lungo termine per valutare i potenziali effetti collaterali tardivi come il linfoma. Prima di iniziare l'infliximab si dovrebbe effettuare un test per la tubercolosi con il derivato proteico purificato (PPD, *Purified Protein Derivative*). Un'infezione addominale (ascesso) attiva o latente costituisce una controindicazione a questo trattamento. Sono in fase di valutazione degli anticorpi umanizzati contro il TNF-α, l'interleuchina 12 e le molecole di adesione leucocitaria (natalizumab contro l'α-integrina).

Per le fistole perirettali sono disponibili molte opzioni terapeutiche. Il metronidazolo (10-20 mg/dL/die) risulta spesso efficace, ma se somministrato a lungo termine può causare una neuropatia con parestesie, che richiede la sospensione del trattamento. In questa situazione si sono rivelate efficaci l'azatioprina e la 6-mercaptopurina. Anche l'infliximab è utile, sebbene siano comuni le recidive.

La terapia nutrizionale è efficace sia come trattamento primario sia come trattamento complementare. L'approccio nutrizionale enterale (con diete elementari o polimeriche) risulta altrettanto rapido nell'inizio della risposta e altrettanto efficace rispetto ad altre terapie. In altri studi il prednisone è risultato più efficace per il controllo acuto della malattia. Poiché le diete elementari sono relativamente non palatabili, vengono somministrate tramite infusione nasogastrica o gastrostomica. In caso di malattia severa e acuta, si può optare per un'infusione continuativa nelle 24 ore; il trattamento può poi essere effettuato a cicli con infusioni notturne a casa. Si dovrebbe pianificare la sazietà in base al peso ideale per consentire un aumento del peso.

La maggior parte dei bambini non accetta facilmente l'infusione nasogastrica, ma dopo averla sperimentata cambia atteggiamento. I vantaggi sono che (1) è relativamente priva di effetti collaterali, (2) evita i problemi associati alla terapia con corticosteroidi ed (3) è contemporaneamente volta alla riabilitazione nutrizionale. I pazienti possono condurre una vita normale durante il giorno. Questo approccio comporta però un importante svantaggio, che peraltro è comune ad altre terapie: la ricaduta precoce alla sospensione del trattamento. Inoltre, la malattia anale e colica non rispondono bene. Ciononostante, l'infusione nasogastrica è l'ideale per i bambini con difetto della crescita.

I supplementi orali ipercalorici, sebbene efficaci, spesso non vengono tollerati per la sazietà precoce o l'esacerbazione dei sintomi (dolore addominale, vomito o diarrea). Malgrado ciò, dovrebbero essere proposti ai bambini con aumento di peso subottimale. La somministrazione notturna continua di nutrienti per via nasogastrica è risultata efficace in caso di malnutrizione cronica e ritardo nella crescita, con un rischio di complicanze molto inferiore rispetto all'iperalimetazione parenterale. Di notte è possibile somministrare una formulazione complessa di 5000-1000 kcal; c'è chi considera altrettanto efficace il trattamento con 50-80 kcal/kg ogni notte per un mese, ogni 4 mesi.

L'esordio iniziale o una riacutizzazione del morbo di Crohn possono essere acuti, con dolore severo, anoressia, febbre, tensione addominale e leucocitosi. Di fronte a un quadro simile è difficile escludere un processo infettivo che interessa la parete intestinale (microperforazione). Oltre a somministrare i corticosteroidi per via endovenosa, si dovrebbe subito instaurare una copertura antibiotica endovenosa ad ampio spettro per la flora intestinale (batteri Gram-negativi e anaerobi), da sospendere solo qualora non sembri esservi un processo infettivo. È necessaria una valutazione mediante ecografia o TC con mezzo di contrasto dell'addome per escludere un ascesso intraddominale. La formazione di una fistola enteroenterica o colica può essere evidenziata alla TC, sebbene venga meglio individuata con uno studio convenzionale con contrasto dell'intestino tenue.

Il trattamento chirurgico andrebbe riservato a indicazioni molto precise. La percentuale di recidiva dopo una resezione intestinale è elevata (>50% a 5 anni); il rischio che la chirurgia si renda nuovamente necessaria aumenta con ogni intervento. Le potenziali complicanze comprendono la formazione di una fistola o di una stenosi, la deiscenza anastomotica, l'ostruzione parziale postoperatoria dell'intestino tenue secondaria alle aderenze e la sindrome dell'intestino corto. La chirurgia rappresenta il trattamento di scelta per la malattia localizzata del tenue o del colon che non risponde alla terapia medica, per la perforazione intestinale, per le stenosi fibrotiche con ostruzione parziale sintomatica dell'intestino tenue e per il sanguinamento intrattabile. Gli ascessi intraddominali o epatici talvolta vengono trattati con successo mediante drenaggio tramite catetere sotto guida ecografica o TC e una concomitante terapia antibiotica per via endovenosa. Se questo approccio non risulta efficace, si rende necessario il drenaggio aperto chirurgico. Gli ascessi perianali spesso richiedono un drenaggio, a meno che non drenino spontaneamente. In generale le fistole perianali dovrebbero essere trattate con la terapia medica, anche se in caso di sintomatologia severa può rendersi necessaria la fistulectomia; questa procedura dovrebbe essere presa in considerazione solo se la localizzazione consente di non danneggiare lo sfintere. In passato il ritardo di crescita veniva considerato un'indicazione alla resezione; oggi però è stato dimostrato che questo approccio, in assenza di altre indicazioni, non è vantaggioso e vengono preferite la terapia medica, quella nutrizionale oppure entrambe.

L'approccio chirurgico in caso di morbo di Crohn consiste nell'asportare un tratto di intestino, il più breve possibile. Non vi sono evidenze che la resezione intestinale fino ai margini istologicamente liberi da malattia abbia un esito migliore della resezione delle sole aree colpite macroscopicamente; quest'ultima procedura inoltre riduce il rischio di sindrome dell'intestino corto. Un approccio alle stenosi sintomatiche dell'intestino tenue consiste nell'effettuare una stritturoplastica anziché una resezione. Il chirurgo effettua un'incisione longitudinale attraverso la stenosi, ma poi richiude l'incisione con punti di sutura in senso trasversale. Questa è la scelta ideale per le stenosi brevi senza malattia attiva. Le percentuali di reintervento con tale approccio non sono superiori a quelle della resezione, mentre viene preservata la lunghezza dell'intestino. Spesso viene somministrato un trattamento medico postoperatorio con farmaci come l'azatioprina per ridurre la probabilità di recidive postoperatorie.

La malattia perianale severa può essere invalidante e difficile da trattare qualora non risponda alla terapia medica. La diversione colica può consentire di ridurre l'attività in questa regione; la patologia solitamente si riattiva, tuttavia, alla ricanalizzazione del colon. Pertanto il trattamento chirurgico delle forme severe può richiedere la colectomia. Generalmente nel morbo di Crohn vengono sconsigliate le procedure che consentono di creare un'ileostomia continente o un *pull-through* endorettale, per il rischio di recidive nell'intestino rimanente. In caso di colectomia si effettua un'ileostomia convenzionale.

Le problematiche psicosociali per i bambini con morbo di Crohn comprendono una sensazione di diversità, la preoccupazione per l'immagine corporea, la consapevolezza di non poter prendere parte a tutte attività adatte alla propria età e il conflitto familiare provocato dallo stress che questa malattia comporta. Per questo il sostegno sociale rappresenta un'importante componente del trattamento del morbo di Crohn. I genitori sono spesso interessati a conoscere altri bambini con problemi simili, ma i diretti interessati possono essere restii a partecipare. Il supporto sociale e il counseling psicologico individuale sono importanti per consentire al paziente di affrontare un problema gravoso, in un'età che spesso comporta di per sé difficoltà di adattamento. I pazienti con forti legami sociali sono avvantaggiati. La progressiva educazione sulla malattia costituisce un aspetto importante del trattamento perché i bambini in generale affrontano meglio la situazione se capiscono i problemi e sono preparati ad affrontarli. La Crohn and Colitis Foundation of America ha sedi in tutti gli Stati Uniti (in Italia esiste la Federazione Nazionale AMICI [Associazione Malattie Infiammatorie Croniche dell'Intestino], *N.d.C.*).

PROGNOSI. Il morbo di Crohn è una patologia cronica associata con un'elevata morbilità, ma con una bassa mortalità. I sintomi tendono a recidivare malgrado il trattamento e spesso senza ragioni apparenti. Un'eccezione è che i sintomi di ostruzione parziale dell'intestino tenue possono verificarsi dopo un pasto ricco di fibre, in presenza di una stenosi dell'intestino tenue. Il calo ponderale e il deficit di crescita di solito migliorano con la terapia e l'attenzione alle esigenze nutrizionali del paziente. Fino al 15% degli individui con un precoce ritardo di crescita secondario al morbo di Crohn presenta una riduzione permanente della crescita lineare. L'osteopenia è particolarmente diffusa tra quelli con scarsa nutrizione cronica e con frequente esposizione a dosi elevate di corticosteroidi. Alcune delle manifestazioni extraintestinali (per es. la colangite sclerosante, l'epatite cronica attiva, il pioderma gangrenoso e la spondilite anchilosante) possono costituire di per sé cause importanti di morbilità.

Con il tempo la malattia può interessare tratti di intestino sempre più estesi, sebbene tipicamente alla progressione rapida che si osserva nelle fasi iniziali faccia seguito un rallentamento. Le complicanze del processo infiammatorio, tra cui stenosi intestinali, fistole, malattia perianale e ascessi intraddominali o retroperitoneali, tendono ad aumentare con il passare del tempo. Quasi tutti i soggetti con morbo di Crohn alla fine devono sottoporsi a intervento chirurgico per una di queste numerose complicanze; la percentuale di reintervento è elevata. Il lasso di tempo che intercorre tra l'esordio dei sintomi e la necessità della chirurgia sembra essere più breve nei bambini che negli adulti. La chirurgia difficilmente è curativa e dovrebbe essere evitata, eccetto che per le indicazioni specifiche precedentemente riportate. Le resezioni ripetute dell'intestino tenue, talvolta inevitabili, possono provocare un malassorbimento secondario alla sindrome dell'intestino corto (vedi Capitolo 335.7). La resezione dell'ileo terminale può dare luogo a un malassorbimento degli acidi biliari con diarrea e malassorbimento di vitamina B_{12}. Il rischio di cancro del colon negli individui con colite di Crohn di lunga durata si avvicina a quello associato con la rettocolite ulcerosa; è quindi indicata una colonscopia di screening dopo 10 anni di malattia colica.

Malgrado queste complicanze, la maggior parte dei bambini con morbo di Crohn conduce una vita piena e attiva con riacutizzazioni intermittenti dei sintomi.

Ardizzone S, Maconi G, Sampietro GM, et al: Azathioprine and mesalamine for prevention of relapse after conservative surgery for Crohn disease. *Gastroenterology* 2004;127:730–740.

Baert F, Noman M, Vermeire S, et al: Influence of immunogenicity on the long-term efficacy of infliximab in Crohn's disease. *N Engl J Med* 2003;348:601–608.

Baldassano RN, Han PD, Jeshion WC, et al: Pediatric Crohn's disease: Risk factors for postoperative recurrence. *Am J Gastroenterol* 2001;196: 2169–2176.

Brown SL, Greene MH, Gershon SK, et al: Tumor necrosis factor antagonist therapy and lymphoma development: Twenty-six cases reported to the Food and Drug Administration. *Arthritis Rheum* 2002;46:3151–3158.

Canani RB, de Horatio LT, Terrin G, et al: Combined use of noninvasive tests is useful in the initial diagnostic approach to a child with suspected inflammatory bowel disease. *J Pediatr Gastro Nutr* 2006;42:9–15.

Cosnes J, Cattan S, Blain A, et al: Long-term evolution of disease behavior of Crohn's disease. *Inflamm Bowel Dis* 2002;8:244–250.

Dietz DW, Laureti S, Strong SA, et al: Safety and long-term efficacy of stricture plasty in 314 patients with obstructing small bowel Crohn's disease. *J Am Coll Surg* 2001;192:330–337.

Dubinsky MC, Yang H, Hassard P: 6-MP metabolite profiles provide a biochemical explanation for 6-MP resistance in patients with inflammatory bowel disease. *Gastroenterology* 2002;122:904–915.

Gaya DR, Russell RK, Nimmo ER, Satsangi J: New genes in inflammatory bowel disease: lessons for complex disease? *Lancet* 2006;367: 1271–1284.

Hampe J, Franke A, Rosensteil P, et al: A genome-wide association scan of nonsynonymous SNPs identifies a susceptibility variant for Crohn disease in ATG16 L1. *Nat Genet* 2007;39:207–211.

Hanauer SB, Feagan BG, Lichtenstein GR, et al: Maintenance infliximab for Crohn's disease: The ACCENT I randomised trial. *Lancet* 2002;359: 1541–1549.

Hanauer SB, Korelitz BI, Rutgeerts P, et al: Postoperative maintenance of Crohn's disease remission with 6-mercaptopurine, mesalamine, or placebo: A 2 year trial. *Gastroenterology* 2004;127:723–729.

Heuschkel RB, Menache CC, Megerian JT, et al: Enteral nutrition and corticosteroids in the treatment of acute Crohn's disease in children. *J Pediatr Gastroenterol Nutr* 2000;31:8–15.

Keane J, Gershon S, Wise RP, et al: Tuberculosis associated with infliximab, a tumor necrosis factor α–neutralizing agent. *N Engl J Med* 2001;345:1098–1104.

Kobayashi KS, Chamaillard M, Ogura Y, et al: *NOD2*-dependent regulation of innate and adaptive immunity in the intestinal tract. *Science* 2005; 307:731–738.

Kugathasan S, Collins N, Maresso K, et al: *CARD15* gene mutations confers an increased risk for early surgery in pediatric-onset Crohn's disease. *Clin Gastroenterol Hepatol* 2004;2:1003–1009.

Levine A, Weizman Z, Broide E, et al: A comparison of budesonide and prednisone for the treatment of active pediatric Crohn disease. *J Pediatr Gastroenterol Nutr* 2003;36:248–252.

Mannon PJ, Fuss IJ, Mayer L, et al: Anti–interleukin-12 antibody for active Crohn's disease. *N Engl J Med* 2004;351:2069–2078.

Markowitz J, Grancher K, Kohn N, et al: A multicenter trial of 6-mercaptopurine and prednisone in children with newly diagnosed Crohn's disease. *Gastroenterology* 2000;119:895–902.

Miele E, Markowitz JE, Mamula P, et al: Human antichimeric antibody in children and young adults with inflammatory bowel disease receiving infliximab. *J Pediatr Gastroenterol Nutr* 2004;38:502–508.

Neurath MF: IL-23: a master regulator in Crohn disease. *Nat Med* 2007;13: 26–28.

Peltekova VD, Wintle RF, Rubin LA, et al: Functional variants of OCTN cation transporter genes are associated with Crohn disease. *Nat Genet* 2005;36:471–475.

Russell RK, Drummond HE, Nimmo ER, et al: The contribution of the DLGS 113A variant in early-onset inflammatory bowel disease. *J Pediatr* 2007;150:268–273.

Sandborn WJ, Hanauer S, Loftus EV Jr, et al: An open-label study of the human anti-TNF monoclonal antibody adalimumab in subjects with prior loss of response or intolerance to infliximab for Crohn's disease. *Am J Gastroenterol* 2004;99:1984–1989.

Sands BE, Anderson FH, Bernstein CN, et al: Infliximab maintenance therapy for fistulizing Crohn's disease. *N Engl J Med* 2004;350:876–885.

Selby WS: Mycobacterium avium subspecies paratuberculosis bacteriemia in patients with inflammatory bowel disease. *Lancet* 2004;364:1013–1014.

Sentongo TA, Semeao EJ, Piccoli DA, et al: Growth, body composition, and nutritional status in children and adolescents with Crohn's disease. *J Pediatr Gastroenterol Nutr* 2002;31:33–40.

Stephens MC, Shepanski MA, Mamula P, et al: Safety and steroid-sparing experience using infliximab for Crohn's disease at a pediatric inflammatory bowel disease center. *Am J Gastroenterol* 2003;98:104–111.

Weiss B, Shamir R, Bujanover Y, et al: *NOD2/CARD15* mutation analysis and genotype-phenotype correlation in Jewish pediatric patients compared with adults with Crohn's disease. *J Pediatr* 2004;145:208–212.

333.3 • Malattia di Behçet

La malattia di Behçet è una vasculite sistemica rara nei bambini (vedi Capitolo 160). Sebbene la patogenesi precisa rimanga sconosciuta, si osservano un'elevata prevalenza dell'antigene leucocitario umano (HLA, *Human Leucocyte Antigen*) B51, un'espressione aumentata della *heat shock protein* 60 e delle risposte immunitarie Th1-dominanti. Pare esservi una significativa aggregazione familiare. Stomatite afosa, eritema nodoso e artrite sono tra le manifestazioni più comuni. Le ulcere, che hanno un diametro di 2-10 mm, si sviluppano ovunque nella bocca e nella faringe posteriore; quelle intestinali possono simulare il morbo di Crohn. Esse sono ricoperte da membrane bianco-giallastre, hanno i bordi arrossati e sono dolorose. Altri segni sono le ulcere genitali, l'interessamento del sistema nervoso centrale (SNC) e la miosite. I reperti oculari (iridocicliti) sono meno comuni nei bambini che negli adulti. Il trattamento iniziale consiste solitamente nella somministrazione di farmaci antinfiammatori non steroidei, corticosteroidi, immunossoppressori e colchicina. Le terapie comprendono anche l'interferone-α/β, gli anticorpi anti-TNF e la talidomide. In caso di interessamento del SNC si è fatto ricorso alla somministrazione settimanale di metotrexato a basso dosaggio.

Kone-Paut I, Geisler I, Wechsler B, et al: Familial aggregation in Behçet's disease: High frequency in siblings and parents of pediatric probands. *J Pediatr* 1999;135:89–93.

Kone-Paut I, Yurdakul S, Bahabri AS, et al: Clinical features of Behçet's disease in children: An international collaborative study of 86 cases. *J Pediatr* 1998;132:721–725.

Suzuki Kurokowa M, Suzuki N: Behcet's disease. *Clin Exp Med* 2004;4:10–20.

Wechsler B, Sable-Fourtassou R, Bodaghi B, et al: Infliximab in refractory uveitis due to Behçet's disease. *Clin Exp Rheumatol* 2004;22:S14–S16.

Capitolo 334 ■ Allergie alimentari (ipersensibilità alimentare)

Jeffrey S. Hyams

Le allergie alimentari sono un gruppo di patologie nelle quali i sintomi derivano da risposte immunologiche a specifici antigeni alimentari (vedi Capitolo 150). Le allergie alimentari si verificano almeno nel 6% dei bambini fino ai 3 anni di vita, di cui il 2-3% è rappresentato da lattanti e bambini ai primi passi allergici al latte vaccino. Le reazioni vengono classificate come IgE-mediate e non IgE-mediate. Le reazioni IgE-mediate, caratterizzate da un rapido sviluppo dei sintomi, sono causate da mediatori dell'infiammazione che vengono rilasciati quando gli antigeni alimentari si legano a specifici anticorpi IgE sui mastociti e sui basofili. Le reazioni non IgE-mediate vengono mediate da cellule e si sviluppano nell'arco di ore o giorni. Per alcune condizioni cliniche sembrano essere coinvolti molteplici meccanismi.

MANIFESTAZIONI CLINICHE. Gli antigeni alimentari possono determinare sintomi respiratori, cutanei o gastrointestinali. Le manifestazioni gastrointestinali possono verificarsi in qualunque punto del tratto alimentare e spesso sono predominanti. Sono state descritte manifestazioni comportamentali, che però sono oggetto di dibattito.

IPERSENSIBILITÀ ALIMENTARE IgE-MEDIATA.

Sindrome da allergia orale. Il contatto dell'allergene con l'orofaringe provoca prurito o bruciore e angioedema delle labbra, della lingua, del palato e della gola. I sintomi possono precedere altre manifestazioni IgE-mediate di allergia alimentare. Anche l'allergia ai pollini (febbre da fieno) è comune in questi pazienti. L'eritema facciale da contatto con prodotti a base di agrumi o pomodoro non viene considerata una risposta immunitaria.

Anafilassi gastrointestinale. Dopo ingestione di un allergene si verifica la rapida insorgenza di nausea, dolori addominali crampiformi, vomito o diarrea o la combinazione di questi disturbi. Le proteine più comunemente implicate sono quelle del latte, delle uova, delle arachidi, della soia, dei cereali e del pesce.

Altre manifestazioni non gastrointestinali. Comprendono quelle cutanee, come orticaria, angioedema e dermatite atopica (eczema), quelle respiratorie, come asma e rinocongiuntivite, e l'anafilassi sistemica. Le reazioni pericolose per la vita sono tipicamente associate all'ingestione di arachidi, nocciole, pesce e molluschi. Questi soggetti presentano spesso una concomitante storia di asma.

IPERSENSIBILITÀ ALIMENTARE MISTA (IgE- E NON IgE-MEDIATA).

Queste patologie sono caratterizzate da un'intensa infiltrazione eosinofila degli specifici organi interessati. L'infiltrato infiammatorio può colpire la mucosa, la muscolare oppure la sierosa dello stomaco o dell'intestino tenue. L'infiltrazione eosinofila della muscolare provoca ispessimento e nodularità, determinando sintomi da ostruzione (dolore e vomito), mentre l'infiltrazione della sierosa provoca l'ascite eosinofila. Molti pazienti con queste patologie rispondono all'eliminazione di alcuni antigeni alimentari dalla dieta (latte), mentre altri necessitano di una restrizione più drastica di tutte le proteine, con l'impiego concomitante di proteine idrolizzate o di latte in polvere a base di aminoacidi. Occasionalmente alcuni pazienti richiedono una terapia con corticosteroidi.

Esofagite eosinofila allergica. Questa patologia è caratterizzata da un'intensa infiltrazione eosinofila della mucosa esofagea. Tra i lattanti e i bambini piccoli il vomito rappresenta il sintomo più comune, mentre nei bambini più grandi sono più comuni la disfagia e il dolore addominale oppure la pirosi (vedi Capitolo 321). Raramente sono presenti stenosi esofagee nei bambini più grandi e negli adolescenti: il medico diagnostica erroneamente un reflusso gastroesofageo in questi pazienti, che però non rispondono alle terapie consuete; inoltre, il test per il pH con sonda intraesofagea risulta normale. Il trattamento di solito comporta modificazioni dell'alimentazione nei pazienti più giovani, talora con la necessità temporanea di una dieta a base di aminoacidi; i pazienti più grandi vengono solitamente trattati con i corticosteroidi.

Gastrite eosinofila allergica. Questa patologia, più comune nell'infanzia e nell'adolescenza, si presenta con dolore addominale, vomito, anoressia, ematemesi, scarso aumento ponderale e, raramente, ostruzione allo svuotamento gastrico. Essa può simulare la stenosi del piloro nei bambini più piccoli. Nel 50% dei pazienti si osservano caratteristiche atopiche, come elevati livelli sierici di IgE ed eosinofilia periferica. Le biopsie gastriche evidenziano un'intensa infiltrazione eosinofila della mucosa e della sottomucosa, in particolare nell'antro.

Gastroenterocolite eosinofila allergica. Questi pazienti presentano sintomi simili a quelli descritti per l'esofagite e la gastrite eosinofila. È comune un difetto di crescita e la maggior parte degli individui affetti presenta sintomi atopici. Una marcata enteropatia protidodisperdente si può presentare con edema generalizzato e ipogammaglobulinemia.

PATOLOGIE NON IgE-MEDIATE.

Proctocolite allergica. I lattanti possono presentare tra il primo giorno e i 3 mesi di vita macchie o striature di sangue e muco nelle feci e occasionalmente una lieve diarrea. Possono verificarsi un aumento dei leucociti nelle feci e un'eosinofilia periferica. Tipicamente è presente una colite lieve a chiazze; l'iperplasia nodulare linfoide insorge nel 25% circa dei pazienti. Nella maggior parte dei casi la proctocolite deriva da un'ipersensibilità al latte vaccino. Questa patologia si verifica anche in paziente allattati esclusivamente al seno e talvolta per alleviarla è sufficiente modificare la dieta materna eliminando dei latticini. I bambini non allattati al seno possono essere trattati con latte artificiale con idrolisati di proteine. Talvolta si rende necessario un latte artificiale a base di aminoacidi.

Enterocolite indotta dagli alimenti. Vomito a diarrea protratti insorgono tra 1 settimana e 3 mesi di età. Reazioni meno severe possono verificarsi nei bambini più grandi e negli adulti. Le feci contengono sangue occulto, neutrofili ed eosinofili. Le biopsie digiunali evidenziano villi appiattiti, edema e cellule infiammatorie. I sintomi si risolvono entro 72 ore dall'eliminazione dell'alimento lesivo e recidivano entro 1-6 ore dalla sua reintroduzione. Il numero di neutrofili nel sangue aumenta di almeno $3,5 \times 10^9$/L 4-6 ore dopo la stimolazione alimentare. I bambini più grandi, nel passaggio dal latte materno o artificiale al comune latte vaccino, possono sviluppare una sindrome poco caratterizzata con anemia, ipoproteinemia e difetto di crescita. È comune l'eosinofilia. Nella maggior parte dei pazienti si rivela efficace un trattamento con latte artificiale contenente idrolisato di caseina o a base di aminoacidi.

Enteropatia indotta dagli alimenti. Malassorbimento, diarrea protratta, vomito e deficit di crescita causati da un'ipersensibilità alimentare si verificano nella maggior parte dei casi nel primo mese di vita. Le biopsie dell'intestino tenue evidenziano un'atrofia dei villi a chiazze con una risposta di cellule infiammatorie mononucleate. La reazione alla stimolazione alimentare e la risoluzione dei sintomi dopo l'eliminazione dell'alimento lesivo possono richiedere molti giorni o settimane.

Celiachia (enteropatia glutine-sensibile) e dermatite erpetiforme. Entrambe queste entità, che si possono verificare contemporaneamente, rappresentano una risposta immunologica all'ingestione di glutine. Vedi Capitolo 335.2.

Emosiderosi polmonare (sindrome di Heiner). Consiste in una combinazione di infiltrati polmonari da emorragie polmonari, sanguinamento gastrointestinale, anemia sideropenica, eosinofilia periferica e deficit di crescita secondari a un'intolleranza alimentare (spesso alle proteine del latte vaccino), che si risolve con l'eliminazione dell'alimento lesivo dalla dieta.

DIAGNOSI. Si sospetta un'allergia alimentare quando l'introduzione di determinati alimenti è seguita da sintomi tipici. Vanno esclusi altri meccanismi non allergici di intolleranza alimentare (compromissione dei processi digestivi o assorbitivi, contaminazione con microbi o tossine, attività farmacologica degli alimenti). Quando si sospetta un'allergia al latte vaccino bisognerebbe prendere in considerazione l'intolleranza al lattosio. La dieta di eliminazione e la successiva stimolazione controllata con placebo in doppio cieco (DBPCFC, *Double-Blind Placebo-Controlled Food Challenge*) rappresentano il *gold standard* per la diagnosi delle allergie alimentari. Nella DBPCFC gli alimenti sospetti vengono somministrati in capsule a dosi progressivamente crescenti, alternandoli con un placebo, e le reazioni vengono valutate in cieco. Le stimolazioni alimentari aperti, sebbene comunemente effettuati, sono meno affidabili (tranne che nei lattanti di pochi mesi). I sintomi possono essere riprodotti dalla DBPCFC solo nel 40% dei bambini con sospetta allergia alimentare. La stimolazione non va effettuata quando l'ingestione di un alimento è stata seguita da anafilassi: in tal caso, il bambino deve essere valutato da un allergologo.

L'impiego giudizioso di un prick test cutaneo o di un *RadioAllergoSorbent Test* (RAST) può essere molto utile per determinare se la causa dell'allergia alimentare è una reazione allergica IgE. I bambini possono essere valutati per le reazioni IgE agli alimenti a qualunque età poiché le IgE vengono prodotte entro le 24 settimane di gestazione. Un test per le IgE negativo, soprattutto se il paziente ha un'età >1 anno, indica con notevole accuratezza che la reazione non è IgE-mediata. Il significato di un test per le IgE positivo deve essere determinato in base all'anamnesi e all'età del paziente. Il test cutaneo risulta positivo pressoché nel 100% dei bambini di età ≥ 3 anni con DBPCFC positivo. Le IgE sieriche totali non sono affidabili nella diagnosi di un'allergia alimentare.

Nell'infanzia l'ipersensibilità è associata nella maggior parte dei casi con l'ingestione di latte vaccino o proteine della soia. Sebbene l'allattamento in genere le prevenga, si possono verificare comunque manifestazioni di allergia alimentare, soprattutto la proctocolite. Il latte vaccino nella dieta materna rappresenta la causa più comunemente identificabile di reazioni allergiche alimentari nei bambini allattati al seno; le reazioni ad arachidi, soia o uova nella dieta della madre sono meno frequenti.

Nei lattanti e bambini con allergie alimentari, il 90% delle reazioni è causato da uova, latte, arachidi, soia o frumento. Il 75% dei bambini con allergia alimentare comprovata reagisce a un unico alimento. Rappresentano un'eccezione i pazienti con gastroenterite eosinofila allergica, che spesso reagiscono a più di un alimento.

TRATTAMENTO E PROGNOSI. Il solo trattamento rivelatosi efficace per le allergie alimentari è una dieta di eliminazione. La maggior parte delle manifestazioni gastrointestinali si risolve nell'arco di alcuni giorni, sebbene alcune possano richiedere settimane (enteropatia indotta da alimenti). Un bambino a rischio di sviluppare una reazione IgE-mediata severa minacciosa per la sopravvivenza dovrebbe ricevere adrenalina iniettabile e un antistaminico. I progressi compiuti di recente nello sviluppo di una terapia anti-IgE potrebbero rivelarsi utili per i bambini con malattia severa. I bambini ad alto rischio di sviluppare un'allergia alimentare possono trarre beneficio dall'allattamento al seno e dall'eliminazione degli alimenti solidi e delle proteine del latte vaccino dalla loro dieta per i primi 6 mesi di vita.

Almeno il 30% dei neonati con allergia al latte vaccino presenta una sensibilità anche alle proteine della soia. Generalmente questi pazienti migliorano grazie alla somministrazione di latte artificiale con idrolisati proteici; nei soggetti (meno del 5%) che continuano a presentare sintomi il problema si risolve con il latte artificiale a base di aminoacidi. La ripresa dell'allattamento costituisce un'alternativa quando l'allergia al latte vaccino si presenta precocemente. Il 50% circa dei neonati colpiti da proctocolite durante l'allattamento migliora con l'eliminazione del latte vaccino dalla dieta materna. Negli altri bisogna decidere se i sintomi sono abbastanza severi (anemia e ipoproteinemia) da giustificare il passaggio al latte artificiale con idrolisatii proteici.

L'85% dei bambini con ipersensibilità alimentare non IgE-mediata alle proteine del latte non presenta più sintomi alla stimolazione alimentare entro i 3 anni di età. È comune la risoluzione dei sintomi da ipersensibilità alle proteine del latte vaccino o della soia entro il primo anno di vita. Al momento di reintrodurre il latte nella dieta, si dovrebbe cominciare offrendo un cucchiaino da tè o meno, per poi aumentare progressivamente la dose nell'arco di alcuni giorni, se l'alimento viene tollerato. Anche i bambini più grandi e gli adulti possono perdere la loro sensibilità a un alimento lesivo se quest'ultimo viene eliminato dalla dieta per 1-2 anni. I sintomi di un'allergia IgE-mediata alle arachidi, alle nocciole, al pesce o ai molluschi costituiscono un'eccezione e non si risolvono.

Brownell J, Casale TB: Anti-IgE therapy. *Immunol Allergy Clin North Am* 2004;24:551–568.

Hill DJ, Heine RG, Hosking CS: The diagnostic value of skin prick testing in children with food allergy. *Pediatr Allergy Immunol* 2004;15:435–441.

Liacouras CA, Ruchelli E: Eosinophilic esophagitis. *Curr Opin Pediatr* 2004;16:560–566.

Muraro A, Dreborg S, Halken S, et al: Dietary prevention of allergic diseases in infants and small children. Part III: Critical review of published peer-reviewed observational and interventional studies and final recommendations. *Pediatr Allergy Immunol* 2004;15:291–307.

Sampson HA: Update on food allergy. *J Allergy Clin Immunol* 2004; 113:805–819.

Sampson HA, Anderson JA: Summary and recommendations: Classification of gastrointestinal manifestations due to immunologic reactions to foods in infants and young children. *J Pediatr Gastroenterol Nutr* 2000;30: S87–S94.

Scurlock AM, Burks AW: Peanut allergenicity. *Ann Allergy Asthma Immunol* 2004;93:S12–S18.

Sicherer SH, Teuber S: Current approach to the diagnosis and management of adverse reactions to foods. *J Allergy Clin Immunol* 2004;114:1146–1150.

Snyder JD, Rosenblum N, Wershil B, et al: Pyloric stenosis and eosinophilic gastroenteritis in infants. *J Pediatr Gastroenterol Nutr* 1987;6:543–547.

334.1 • Gastroenterite eosinofila

Questa entità è costituita da un gruppo di patologie rare e ancora poco conosciute che hanno in comune l'infiltrazione dello stomaco e dell'intestino tenue da parte degli eosinofili e l'eosinofilia periferica. Anche l'esofago e l'intestino crasso possono essere colpiti. L'infiltrazione eosinofila dei tessuti può essere osservata nella mucosa, nella muscolare o nella sierosa. L'interessamento mucoso determina nausea, vomito, diarrea, dolore addominale, sanguinamento gastrointestinale, enteropatia protidodisperdente o malassorbimento. L'interessamento della muscolare può causare ostruzione (soprattutto del piloro), mentre l'attività sierosa dà luogo all'ascite eosinofila.

Questa condizione clinicamente si sovrappone all'ipersensibilità alle proteine della dieta dell'intestino tenue e del colon (vedi Capitolo 334). Sono di frequente riscontro allergie a molteplici alimenti e le IgE sieriche risultano comunemente elevate. Un'eosinofilia periferica è presente in più del 50% degli individui con questa patologia. La forma mucosa è la più frequente e viene diagnosticata identificando numerosissimi eosinofili sui campioni bioptici dell'antro gastrico o dell'intestino tenue.

In genere la patologia assume un andamento cronico e debilitante, con sporadiche esacerbazioni severe. Pochi pazienti traggono beneficio dalla dieta di eliminazione o dall'impiego di disodiocromoglicato, mentre la maggior parte richiede la somministrazione di steroidi sistemici. L'esofagite eosinofila isolata, non responsiva al trattamento del reflusso gastroesofageo, può migliorare con una dieta di eliminazione; in assenza di interessamento dello stomaco o dell'intestino tenue, essa può rappresentare un'entità a sé stante.

Heine RG: Pathophysiology, diagnosis and treatment of food protein induced gastrointestinal disease. *Curr Opin Allergy Clin Immunol* 2004;4:221.

Ngo P, Furuta G, Burks W: The pathobiology of esoinophilic gastroenteritis of childhood: Is it really the eosinophil, allergic mediated, or something else? *Curr Gastroenterol Rep* 2004;6:436–440.

Rothenberg ME: Eosinophilic gastrointestinal disorders (EGID). *J Allergy Clin Immunol* 2004;113:11–28.

TABELLA 335-1. Malattie da malassorbimento associate a difetto generalizzato della mucosa intestinale

ENTEROPATIA INDOTTA DA ALIMENTI
Enteropatia sensibile al glutine (celiachia)
Enteropatie sensibili al latte vaccino e ad altre proteine
Enteropatia eosinofila
DIFETTI CONGENITI DELLA MUCOSA INTESTINALE
Malattia da inclusione dei microvilli
Enteropatia a ciuffi (*tufting enteropathy*)
Sindrome da difetto della glicolisazione delle glicoproteine
Carenza di eparansolfato negli enterociti
Anendocrinosi enterica (mutazione NEUROG 3)
ENTEROPATIA PROTEINODISPERDENTE
Linfangiectasia (congenita e acquisita)
Patologie che provocano infiammazioni della mucosa intestinale
INFEZIONI INDOTTE
Infezioni da parassiti (per es. *Giardia* e *Cryptosporidium*)
Eccessiva proliferazione batterica
Sprue tropicale
Enteropatia postinfettiva
MALATTIE DA IMMUNODEFICIENZA
Malattie da immunodeficienza congenita
Carenza di IgA selettiva (può essere associata a celiachia)
Immunodeficienza combinata grave
Agammaglobulinemia
Ipogammaglobulinemia legata al cromosoma X
Sindrome di Wiskott-Aldrich
Malattia da immunodeficienza variabile comune
Malattia granulomatosa cronica
Immunodeficienza acquisita
Infezione da HIV
Terapia immunosoppressiva e post-trapianto di midollo osseo
ENTEROPATIA AUTOIMMUNE
VARIE
Malattia immunoproliferativa da intestino corto
Sindrome dell'intestino corto
Malnutrizione cronica
Enterite da radiazioni

Capitolo 335 ■ Malattie da malassorbimento

Manu Sood

Le malattie da malassorbimento costituiscono un ampio spettro di patologie a eziologia multipla e con manifestazioni cliniche varie. Sono tutte associate a un ridotto assorbimento intestinale di una o più sostanze nutritive presenti nella dieta. Il malassorbimento può dipendere sia da un difetto di **digestione** di quel determinato nutriente a livello del lume intestinale, sia da un cattivo **assorbimento** da parte della mucosa. Queste patologie si possono suddividere in anomalie generalizzate della mucosa, che di solito derivano dal malassorbimento di più sostanze nutritive (Tab. 335-1), e fenomeni di malassorbimento di un nutriente specifico (carboidrati, grassi, proteine, vitamine, minerali) (Tab. 335-2).

APPROCCIO CLINICO IN CASO DI SOSPETTO MALASSORBIMENTO IN ETÀ PEDIATRICA

Le caratteristiche cliniche dipendono dalla quantità e dal tipo di sostanza che non viene assorbita, ma le più comuni, specialmente se il malassorbimento interessa bambini da 1 a 3 anni, sono diarrea, distensione addominale, mancato incremento ponderale e quindi una caduta del percentile di crescita. I dati fisici comprendono scomparsa del grasso sottocutaneo, deperimento o ipotrofia muscolare e cute eccessivamente lassa per l'età pediatrica (Fig. 335-1). Nei bambini molto piccoli le conseguenze nutrizionali del malassorbimento sono più drammatiche, a causa delle limitate riserve d'energia e dell'aumentato fabbisogno calorico richiesto per l'aumento ponderale e per la crescita. Nei bambini più grandi la malnutrizione può provocare un ritardo della crescita, come nei pazienti in età pediatrica con diagnosi tardiva di celiachia. Se la malattia non viene curata, la crescita lineare rallenta e, in caso di malnutrizione prolungata, può sopravvenire anche la morte (vedi Capitolo 43), sebbene questo esito estremo di solito sia limitato ai bambini che vivono nei Paesi in via di sviluppo, dove le possibilità di ricorrere alla nutrizione enterale o parenterale possono essere limitate. Riscontri specifici nel corso della visita medica possono essere indicativi del tipo di alterazione; generalmente si verifica un edema, associato a enteropatia proteino-disperdente, ippocratismo digitale con la fibrosi cistica e la celiachia, escoriazione perianale e distensione addominale gassosa con il malassorbimento dei carboidrati, rash perianale e periorale con l'acrodermatite enteropatica, anomalie dei capelli con la sindrome di Menkes e le caratteristiche facciali tipiche della sindrome di Johannson-Blizzard.

Molti bambini affetti da problemi di malassorbimento hanno un ottimo appetito e tentano di compensare le perdite fecali di energia e di proteine. Nell'insufficienza pancreatica esogena perdite fecali contenenti fino al 40% delle proteine e delle sostanze energetiche ingerite non provocano malnutrizione, fino a che le perdite sono compensate da un aumento dell'appetito. Nelle patologie associate ad atrofia villosa o a infiammazione (celiachia, enteropatia postinfettiva), le perdite fecali di proteine e carboidrati sono solitamente modeste, ma possono comunque portare a malnutrizione, qualora siano associate ad anoressia o a ridotto assorbimento dei cibi.

TABELLA 335-2. Classificazione delle malattie da malassorbimento in base al principale nutriente non assorbito

MALASSORBIMENTO DEI CARBOIDRATI
Malassorbimento del lattosio
Carenza congenita di lattasi
Ipolattasia (tipo adulto)
Carenza di lattasi secondaria
Carenza congenita di saccarasi-isomaltasi
Malassorbimento di glucosio e galattosio
MALASSORBIMENTO DEI LIPIDI
Insufficienza pancreatica esocrina
Fibrosi cistica
Sindrome di Shwachman-Diamond
Pancreatite cronica
Sindrome di Pearson
Malnutrizione calorico-proteica
Patologie epatiche e biliari
Epatopatia colestatica
Difetti della sintesi degli acidi biliari
Malassorbimento degli acidi biliari (malattia ileale terminale)
Cause che interessano la mucosa intestinale
Abetalipoproteinemia
Ipobetalipoproteinemia omozigote
Malattia da ritenzione di chilomicroni (malattia di Anderson)
MALASSORBIMENTO DEGLI AMINOACIDI
Intolleranza lisinurica alle proteine (difetto del trasporto di aminoacidi dibasici, vedi Capitolo 74.3)
Malattia di Hartnup (difetto degli aminoacidi liberi neutri)
Sindrome del pannolino blu (malassorbimento del triptofano isolato)
Malattia delle urine dall'odore di luppolo (difetto dell'assorbimento di metionina)
Sindrome di Lowe (malassorbimento di lisina e arginina)
MALASSORBIMENTO DEI MINERALI E DELLE VITAMINE
Diarrea da cloro congenita
Difetto congenito dell'assorbimento del sodio
Acrodermatite enteropatica (malassorbimento dello zinco)
Malattia di Menkes (malassorbimento del rame)
Rachitismo vitamina D-dipendente
Malassorbimento dei folati
Congenito
Secondario a danneggiamento della mucosa intestinale (celiachia)
Malassorbimento della vitamina B_{12}
Anemia perniciosa autoimmune
Riduzione degli acidi gastrici (H_2-bloccanti o inibitori della pompa protonica)
Malattia ileale terminale (per es. morbo di Crohn) o resezione
Errori congeniti del trasporto e del metabolismo della vitamina B_{12}
Ipomagnesiemia primitiva
INDOTTO DA FARMACI
Sulfasalazina: malassorbimento dell'acido folico
Colestiramina: malassorbimento di calcio e lipidi
Fenitoina: malassorbimento del calcio

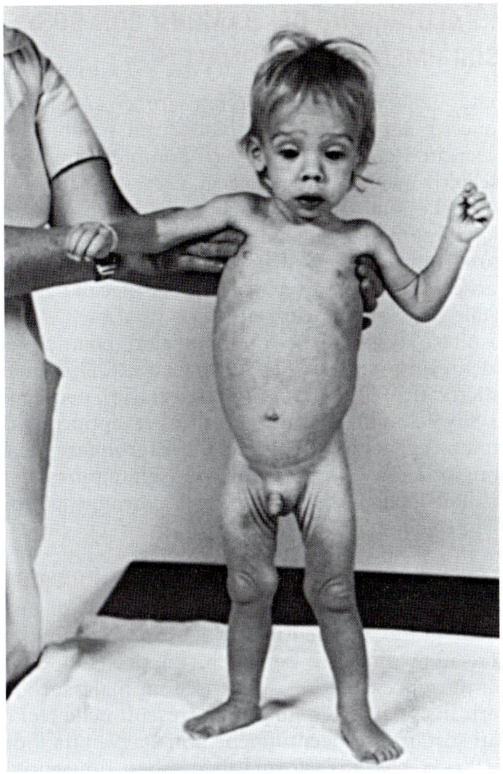

Figura 335-1. Maschio di 18 mesi affetto da celiachia attiva. Si notino le pliche cutanee lasse, il marcato deperimento muscolare prossimale e l'addome globoso. Il bambino ha un aspetto sofferente.

La valutazione nutrizionale è parte integrante dell'esame clinico dei bambini affetti da malattie dovute a malassorbimento (vedi Capitolo 43). A lungo termine il malassorbimento di calcio e vitamina D può provocare una riduzione della densità minerale ossea e una malattia del metabolismo osseo con aumentato rischio di fratture. Il malassorbimento della vitamina K può provocare coagulopatia, a prescindere dal meccanismo sottostante (malassorbimento dei grassi, atrofia delle mucose). L'enteropatia grave proteino-disperdente, spesso associata a sindromi da malassorbimento (celiachia, linfangiectasia intestinale), provoca ipoalbuminemia ed edema. Altre carenze di nutrienti comprendono il malassorbimento del ferro, che provoca anemia microcitica e una ridotta conta reticolocitaria, ridotti livelli sierici dei folati in patologie associate ad atrofia delle mucose e inoltre, nel malassorbimento dei grassi, una ridotta concentrazione sierica delle vitamine A ed E.

L'anamnesi da sola può non essere sufficiente a ottenere una diagnosi specifica, ma può guidare il pediatra a un approccio investigativo più strutturato e razionale. La diarrea è la principale espressione clinica del malassorbimento; la sua comparsa nella primissima infanzia suggerisce un difetto congenito (Tab. 335-3). Nella cloridorrea congenita e nella malattia da inclusione dei microvilli, le feci sono acquose e possono essere scambiate per urine. L'insorgenza di sintomi in seguito a introduzione di un particolare alimento nella dieta del bambino può fornire alcuni indizi diagnostici, come quelli legati all'assunzione di saccarosio nella carenza di saccarasi-isomaltasi. Un dato utile può essere costituito dalla natura della diarrea: scariche acquose ed esplosive fanno pensare a malassorbimento di carboidrati; feci sciolte e voluminose sono associate alla celiachia; feci pastose, giallastre e fetide sono indicative di insufficienza pancreatica esocrina. Di solito il colore delle feci non aiuta; se sono verdastre con "piselli e carote" indigeriti possono far pensare a un transito intestinale rapido nella diarrea del lattante, una malattia autolimitante che non impedisce la crescita.

TABELLA 335-3. Malattie diarroiche che si manifestano in età neonatale

PATOLOGIA	CARATTERISTICHE CLINICHE
Atrofia congenita dei microvilli	Diarrea acquosa intrattabile
Enteropatia a ciuffi (*tufting enteropathy*)	Diarrea acquosa intrattabile
Malassorbimento congenito del glucosio-galattosio	Diarrea acida
Carenza di lattasi congenita	Diarrea acida
Diarrea da cloro congenita	Idramnios, diarrea acquosa intrattabile
Scambio Na^+/H^+ difettoso nel digiuno, congenito	Idramnios, diarrea acquosa intrattabile
Malassorbimento congenito degli acidi biliari	Steatorrea
Carenza congenita di enterochinasi	Mancato accrescimento, edema
Anendocrinosi enterica (mutazione NEUROG 3)	Acidosi ipercloremica, mancato accrescimento

Adattata da Schmitz J: Maldigestion and malabsorption. In Walker WA, Durie PR, Hamilton JR et al (ed): *Pediatric Gastrointestinal Disease*, 3rd ed. Hamilton, Ontario, BC Decker, 2000, p 55.

335.1 • VALUTAZIONE DEI BAMBINI CON SOSPETTO MALASSORBIMENTO INTESTINALE

Nella scelta delle indagini da effettuare ci si basa in genere sull'anamnesi e sull'esame obiettivo. Se un bambino manifesta diarrea, le prime analisi dovrebbero comprendere la ricerca di sangue occulto e leucociti nelle feci per escludere malattie infiammatorie, l'esame microscopico delle feci e test anticorpali alla ricerca di parassiti come la *Giardia*, il pH fecale e la ricerca di sostanze riducenti per identificare un malassorbimento dei carboidrati e l'esame quantitativo dei grassi fecali per identificare un eventuale malassorbimento lipidico.

Può risultare utile anche un conteggio ematico completo, comprendente uno striscio periferico che evidenzi un'eventuale anemia microcitica, linfopenia (linfangiectasia), neutropenia (sindrome di Shwachman) e acantocitosi (abetalipoproteinemia). Se si sospetta una celiachia, si dovrebbero determinare i livelli sierici di immunoglobulina A (IgA) e della transglutaminasi tissutale. In base ai risultati delle indagini iniziali, si potranno poi pianificare esami più specifici.

INDAGINI PER IL MALASSORBIMENTO DEI CARBOIDRATI. La valutazione dei carboidrati nelle feci, con utilizzo di un reagente Clinitest® in grado di identificare le sostanze riducenti, è un test di screening piuttosto semplice. La presenza di feci acide con sostanze riducenti >2/+ suggerisce un malassorbimento dei carboidrati. Il saccarosio o gli amidi presenti nelle feci non sono considerati sostanze riducenti finché non è avvenuta l'idrolisi con acido cloridrico, che li trasforma in zuccheri riducenti.

Il **breath test all'idrogeno** si usa per scoprire quali carboidrati siano malassorbiti. Al paziente, a digiuno dalla mezzanotte, si somministra lo zucchero sospetto (lattosio o saccarosio) in soluzione orale (carico di carboidrati 1-2 g/kg, massimo 50 g). Nel malassorbimento, lo zucchero non è digerito né assorbito a livello del tenue, ma passa nel colon, dove viene metabolizzato dalla normale flora batterica. Uno dei prodotti di questo processo è l'idrogeno, che viene assorbito dalla mucosa del colon ed escreto nel respiro. Elevate concentrazioni di questo gas in campioni di respiro possono quindi essere indicative di un malassorbimento dei carboidrati. Un suo aumento nel respiro pari a 20 parti per milione (ppm) oltre la *baseline* è considerato un test positivo. Il bambino non dovrebbe essere sottoposto a terapia antibiotica, perché la flora presente nel colon è essenziale per la fermentazione degli zuccheri.

Tramite una **biopsia della mucosa dell'intestino tenue** si può ottenere una misurazione diretta della concentrazione di disaccaridasi nella mucosa (lattasi, saccarasi, maltasi, palatinasi). Nelle carenze enzimatiche primitive, i livelli enzimatici nelle mucose sono bassi, mentre la morfologia della mucosa intestinale è normale. L'atrofia totale o parziale dei villi può provocare una carenza di disaccaridasi secondaria e un'intolleranza transitoria al lattosio in presenza di celiachia o successiva gastroenterite da rotavirus. Una volta guarita la mucosa, i livelli di disaccaridasi ritornano nella norma.

INDAGINI PER IL MALASSORBIMENTO DEI LIPIDI. La presenza di globuli di grasso nelle feci suggerisce un malassorbimento dei lipidi. La capacità di assimilare i grassi varia con l'età; un neonato prematuro può assorbire solo il 65-75% dei grassi presenti nella dieta, mentre un neonato a termine ne assorbe quasi il 90% e un bambino più grande >95% di quelli contenuti in una dieta tipica. Pertanto, può essere normale trovare globuli lipidici nelle feci di un neonato o di un lattante nato prematuro, mentre questo reperto è piuttosto insolito in un bambino più grande. Per poter effettuare una diagnosi definitiva di malassorbimento lipidico le feci andranno raccolte per 3 giorni, in modo da valutare l'escrezione quantitativa dei lipidi e determinare il coefficiente di assorbimento lipidico (coefficiente di assorbimento lipidico [%] = [assunzione lipidi (g) − perdite lipidiche nelle feci (g) / assunzione di grassi (g)] × 100). Poiché le indagini sul bilancio fecale dei lipidi sono pesanti, costose e spiacevoli, di solito si preferiscono analisi più semplici. Di questi test fecali il più affidabile è lo steatocrito acido. Anche l'aspirato duodenale può essere utile per valutare i livelli di acidi biliari nei rari casi in cui il malassorbimento lipidico è causato da una carenza di acidi biliari.

Il malassorbimento lipidico e l'insufficienza pancreatica esocrina sono generalmente associati a carenze delle vitamine liposolubili A, D, E e K. Le concentrazioni sieriche delle vitamine A, D ed E sono misurabili. Un tempo di protrombina prolungato è un test indiretto per la valutazione di un'eventuale carenza di vitamina K.

INDAGINI PER LA PERDITA DI PROTEINE NEL TRATTO GASTROINTESTINALE. Le proteine alimentari ed endogene secrete nel tratto gastrointestinale vengono assorbite completamente; <1 g di proteine provenienti da queste fonti passa nel colon. La maggior parte dell'azoto fecale deriva da proteine batteriche presenti nell'intestino. Un'eccessiva perdita di proteine intestinali si manifesta generalmente sotto forma di **ipoalbuminemia**. Le nefropatie sono la causa più comune di ipoalbuminemia nei bambini; pertanto, sarà utile determinare l'escrezione di proteine nelle urine. Altre potenziali cause includono le epatopatie (produzione ridotta) e un'assunzione di proteine inadeguata. La concentrazione di **α_1-antitripsina** nelle feci è uno screening dell'enteropatia proteinodisperdente. Questa proteina sierica ha un peso molecolare simile all'albumina ma, al contrario dell'albumina, resiste alla digestione nel tratto intestinale. Un'eccessiva escrezione di α_1-antitripsina nelle feci dovrebbe indurre a eseguire ulteriori indagini per identificare la causa specifica di questa perdita proteica intestinale.

INDAGINI PER LA FUNZIONE PANCREATICA ESOCRINA (FIG. 335-2). La fibrosi cistica è la causa più comune d'insufficienza pancreatica esocrina nei bambini; perciò, per valutare un'eventuale insufficienza esocrina, prima di intraprendere test invasivi deve essere eseguito il test del sudore. Molti casi di fibrosi cistica vengono individuati tramite programmi di screening neonatale comprendenti test genetici; le rare mutazioni occasionali non vengono individuate. La valutazione dell'**elastasi-1 fecale** è un test sensibile atto ad analizzare la funzione pancreatica esocrina nella pancreatite cronica e nella fibrosi cistica. L'elastasi-1 è un'endoproteasi specifica sia dell'organismo umano in generale sia del pancreas in particolare. È stabile nelle patologie da transito intestinale anomalo e non si altera con la supplementazione di enzimi pancreatici. L'unico svantaggio del test dell'elastasi-1 nelle feci è l'impossibilità di differenziare completamente l'insufficienza pancreatica esocrina primitiva dalla disfunzione pancreatica esocrina secondaria ad atrofia dei villi intestinali. Questo test può inoltre dare un falso positivo negli episodi di diarrea acuta. Anche la concentrazione di **tripsinogeno sierico** può essere usata come screening dell'insufficienza pancreatica. Nella fibrosi cistica, i livelli sono molto elevati nelle prime fasi della vita per poi calare gradualmente, cosicché a 5-7 anni la maggior parte dei pazienti affetti da fibrosi cistica e da insufficienza pancreatica presenta livelli inferiori alla norma. Per monitorare la funzione pancreatica esocrina di questi pazienti può essere utile osservare il trend del tripsinogeno sierico seriale. Nella sindrome di Shwachman, un'altra patologia associata a insufficienza pancreatica esocrina, il livello di tripsinogeno sierico è basso. Altre analisi per individuare un'insufficienza pancreatica (test NBT-PABA e test al dilaurato di fluorescina [Pancreolauril test®]) misurano la concentrazione nelle urine o nel respiro di sostanze rilasciate e assorbite attraverso la superficie della mucosa in seguito alla digestione pancreatica. Questi test mancano di specificità e raramente si usano nella pratica clinica. Il gold standard della funzionalità pancreatica esocrina è l'analisi diretta dell'**aspirato duodenale** per il bicarbonato, il tripsinogeno e la lipasi in seguito a stimolazione con secretina e colecistochinina. Questo test richiede l'intubazione duodenale: negli Stati Uniti i centri in grado di effettuarlo sono pochi (per i particolari, vedi Capitolo 345).

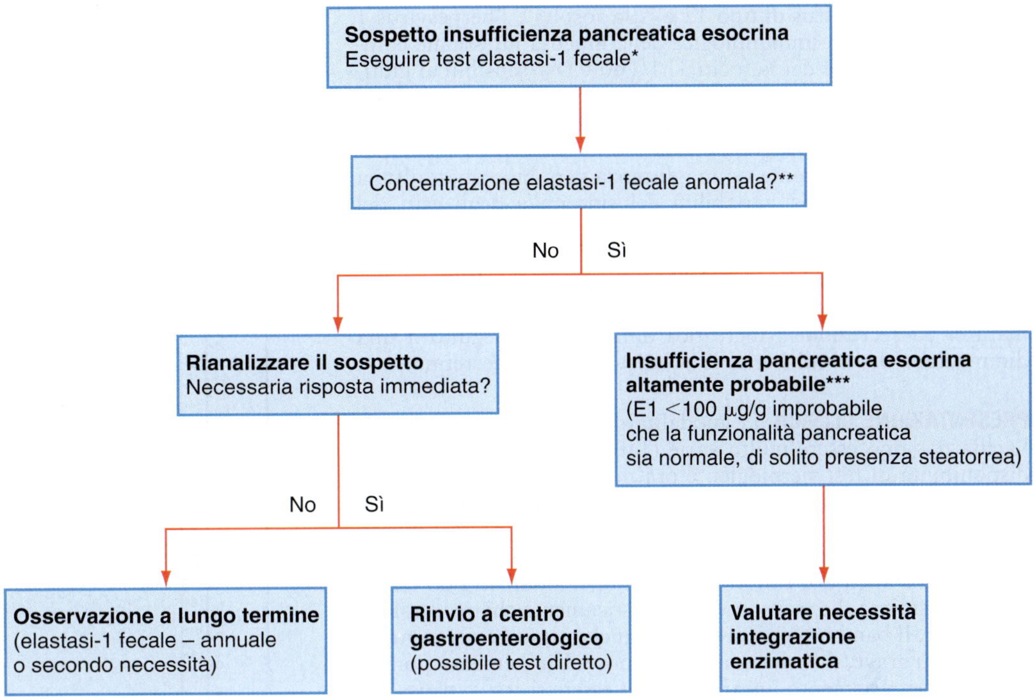

Figura 335-2. Algoritmo di valutazione della funzionalità pancreatica esocrina. *Se non disponibile, ricorrere a un altro tipo di test. Eseguire appropriati studi di imaging del pancreas. **In caso di valori borderline, prendere in esame la ripetizione del test con tre campioni indipendenti. ***Considerare la diagnosi differenziale (in particolare l'atrofia villosa e l'effetto di diluizione da parte delle feci acquose). (Adattata da Walkowiak J, Nousia-Arvanitakis S, Henker J, et al: Indirect pancreatic function tests in children. *J Pediatr Gastroenterol Nutr* 2005;40:107-114.)

INDAGINI PER LE PATOLOGIE DELLA MUCOSA INTESTINALE. La formulazione di una diagnosi specifica del malassorbimento richiede spesso un esame istologico della biopsia della mucosa dell'intestino tenue. I campioni si ottengono tramite endoscopia, che permette un prelievo multiplo, in quanto la mucosa può essere interessata in modo irregolare, soprattutto nella celiachia. Le lesioni della mucosa intestinale possono anche essere segmentali, in caso di linfangiectasia intestinale. In queste situazioni una sequenza di radiografie dell'intestino tenue può identificare una regione ispessita responsabile di una perdita proteica. Nel corso dell'endoscopia, si possono prelevare campioni bioptici della mucosa anche per misurare l'attività dei disaccaridi nella mucosa stessa ed eseguire aspirati duodenali per misurare la concentrazione degli enzimi pancreatici e per effettuare culture batteriche quantitative. Possono essere utili anche degli aspirati che valutino infezioni diverse, per esempio quella da *Giardia*.

PROCEDURE DI IMAGING. Tramite radiografie e il contrasto con bario si possono individuare il sito e la causa di una stasi intestinale. Sebbene la flocculazione del bario e la dilatazione dell'intestino con ispessimento delle pliche mucose siano state attribuite a lesioni diffuse da malassorbimento, come nel caso della celiachia, queste anomalie sono aspecifiche.

335.2 • ENTEROPATIA DA SENSIBILITÀ AL GLUTINE (CELIACHIA)

La celiachia è un'enteropatia immunomediata provocata da sensibilità permanente al glutine in individui geneticamente predisposti. Sebbene gli studi epidemiologici condotti in Europa e negli Stati Uniti suggeriscano che si tratti di un'affezione comune che può interessare lo 0,5-1,0% della popolazione generale, spesso tra l'inizio dei sintomi e la diagnosi intercorre un intervallo di tempo piuttosto lungo. Sulla scorta di un gran numero di studi effettuati negli Stati Uniti e in Europa, si stima che la prevalenza della celiachia in età pediatrica, tra i 2,5 e i 15 anni nella popolazione generale, vada da 3 a 13/1000 bambini, ovvero da ≈1/300 a 1/80 bambini. Pertanto, su 1500 bambini seguiti da un pediatra, è probabile che da 5 a 20 siano affetti da celiachia, che sia stata o meno diagnosticata. Negli Stati Uniti si stima che per ogni paziente celiaco ci siano 53 soggetti non diagnosticati, a causa del quadro clinico multiforme.

PATOGENESI. La celiachia esordisce solo dopo l'introduzione nella dieta del glutine, una proteina presente nel frumento, nella segale e nell'orzo. L'attività del glutine risiede nella frazione gliadinica, che contiene determinate sequenze ripetute di aminoacidi (motif), i quali causano sensibilizzazione dei linfociti della lamina propria. Il principale elemento scatenante della risposta infiammatoria in individui suscettibili può essere un peptide 33-mer, che reagisce con la transglutaminasi ed è un potente induttore delle linee T-linfocitiche derivate dall'intestino. Si può pensare a una predisposizione genetica quando, in gemelli omozigoti, esiste una concordanza prossima al 100%. Dal 2 al 5% dei parenti di primo grado manifesta un'enteropatia sintomatica da sensibilità al glutine e fino al 10% dei parenti di primo grado presenta un danno asintomatico alla mucosa dell'intestino tenue compatibile con questa patologia. Questa malattia è associata a un aumento degli alleli DQA1*0501 e DQB1*0201 del complesso maggiore di istocompatibilità (MHC, *Major Histocompatibility Complex*) di classe II. Questa combinazione allelica HLA-DQ2 si riscontra nel 98% dei celiaci del Nord Europa. Nel Sud dell'Europa il DQ2 è presente nel 92% dei pazienti con celiachia conclamata. La celiachia è associata a determinati tipi (B8, DR7, DR3, e DQw2) dell'antigene leucocitario umano (HLA, *Human Leucocyte Antigen*). Perché la malattia si sviluppi, possono essere necessarie altre influenze genetiche, non legate all'HLA, dato che, secondo le stime, il tasso di discordanza in fratelli HLA-identici è pari al 30-50%. Si stima che quasi il 30% della popolazione generale del Nord America sia positivo per il DQ2. Sono stati riferiti altri loci genici che possono essere associati alla celiachia. Anche se lo sviluppo di questa patologia è multigenico, il DQ2 e il DQ8 sono i componenti essenziali. Nel diabete di tipo 1, un test sierologico positivo per la celiachia si riscontra per lo più nei soggetti con genotipo HLA DQ2 o DQ8. Negli individui affetti da sindrome di Down la celiachia è per lo più legata all'eterodimero HLA DQ2, con una percentuale di *carriage* di circa il 100%. Un ulteriore allele è risultato implicato nel 20% dei pazienti affetti da sindrome di Down. La celiachia si verifica con maggiore frequenza nei bambini affetti da diabete di tipo 1 ed è 50 volte più comune in quelli affetti da sindrome di Down. Un aumento della frequenza si riscontra anche nei bambini con sindrome di Turner, sindrome di William, tiroidite e carenza selettiva di IgA.

Anche i fattori ambientali come i virus possono svolgere un ruolo nell'espressione di questa predisposizione genetica. Un alto grado di omologia nelle sequenze di aminoacidi si riscontra tra la gliadina e l'adenovirus di tipo 12 e 7, la rosolia e l'herpesvirus 1 umano. La risposta immunologica della mucosa intestinale comprende l'attivazione dei linfociti Th1/Th0 CD4⁺ sensibili al glutine. La risposta infiammatoria provoca atrofia dei villi e iperplasia delle cripte e danneggia l'epitelio superficiale dell'intestino tenue. Le alterazioni sono maggiori nell'intestino tenue prossimale per poi estendersi distalmente su una distanza variabile; quest'ultima osservazione spiega la variabilità dei sintomi e degli esiti del malassorbimento tra i soggetti affetti da enteropatia sensibile al glutine. L'enteropatia indotta dal glutine riduce la capacità di digestione e di assorbimento dell'area superficiale dell'intestino tenue e produce un relativo aumento delle cellule epiteliali immature. La secrezione pancreatica diminuisce in seguito a una diminuzione dei livelli sierici di colecistochinina e secretina.

PRESENTAZIONE CLINICA. Le modalità di presentazione della celiachia possono essere molto varie (Tab. 335-4), ma, grazie alla disponibilità di test sierologici, è ora possibile diagnosticare anche pazienti con sintomi addominali lievi. La **presentazione tipica** con diarrea, distensione addominale e mancato accrescimento sta diventando sempre meno comune nei bambini molto piccoli. La diarrea è ancora il sintomo più comune; all'inizio può essere acuta o insidiosa. Le feci sono caratteristicamente chiare, sciolte e sgradevoli. Il bambino può presentare anche attacchi ricorrenti di diarrea più grave, talvolta con feci acquose. L'incremento ponderale e/o l'accrescimento lineare possono essere scarsi, a causa del malassorbimento o di una diminuzione dell'appetito (Fig. 335-3). Sono presenti anche sintomi neurologici; molti bambini sono introversi, irritabili e stizzosi. Altre manifestazioni e associazioni non gastrointestinali della celiachia sono riportate nella Tabella 335-5. Spesso si ha un'anamnesi di distensione addominale e alcuni bambini lamentano dolori addominali, che tuttavia di solito non sono severi. Possono essere presenti deperimento e perdita di forza muscolare con ipotonia e il bambino può acquisire tardivamente le attività motorie più importanti.

Molti adolescenti e giovani adulti sono affetti da celiachia in forma latente e non presentano perdite né diarrea. In questi pazienti le manifestazioni includono affaticamento, dolori addominali, meteorismo e anemia.

SCREENING E DIAGNOSI. Lo screening della celiachia viene raccomandato per i fattori di rischio specifici (Fig. 335-4). I test per gli anticorpi IgA antiendomisio e per gli anticorpi IgA anti-transglutaminasi tissutale sono molto sensibili e specifici nell'identificare i soggetti affetti da questa malattia. Il test per l'anticorpo IgA antiendomisio è una tecnica d'immunofluorescenza relativamente costosa; l'interpretazione dipende dall'operatore ed è passibile d'errore, per cui questo esame è stato ampiamente sostituito dai test per gli anticorpi IgA anti-transglutaminasi tissutale, che sono di più semplice esecuzione pur avendo sensibilità e specificità analoghe. I test per gli anticorpi IgA e IgG antigliadina e per gli anticorpi IgA antireticolina non sono più raccomandati, in quanto privi di specificità. I test

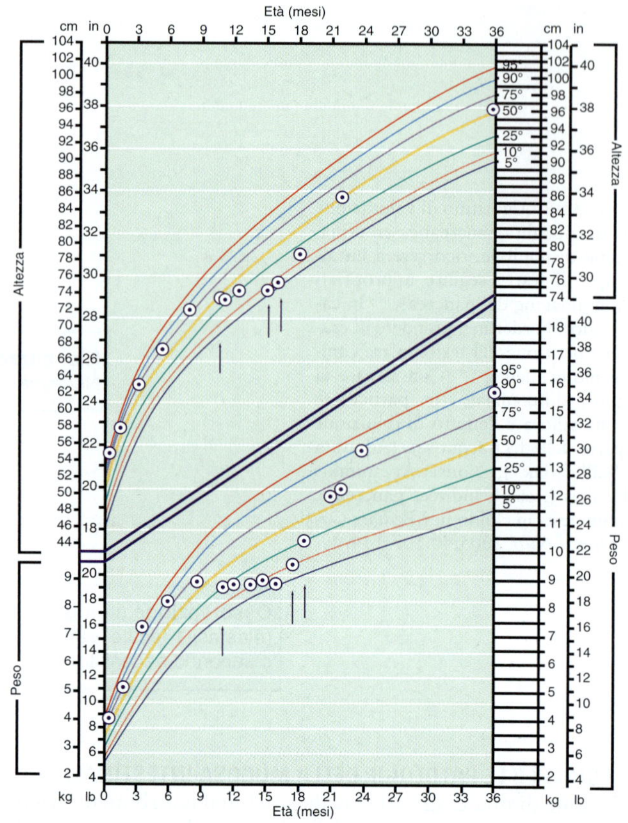

Figura 335-3. Enteropatia sensibile al glutine. La curva di crescita mostra una crescita inizialmente normale, da 0 a 9 mesi, seguita da scarso appetito con vomito e diarrea intermittenti, con l'avvio di una dieta contenente glutine (*freccia singola*). Una volta ottenuta la conferma della diagnosi mediante biopsia, il trattamento con dieta priva di glutine (*freccia doppia*) migliora la crescita.

TABELLA 335-4. Celiachia attiva dell'infanzia: 42 casi

SINTOMI	N. DI PAZIENTI
Mancato accrescimento	36
Diarrea	30
Irritabilità	30
Vomito	24
Anoressia	24
Feci maleodoranti	21
Dolore addominale	8
Eccesso di appetito	6
Prolasso rettale	3
SEGNI	
Altezza <25° percentile	30
Peso corporeo <25° percentile	37
Wasting muscolare	40
Distensione addominale	33
Edema	14
Ippocratismo digitale	11

TABELLA 335-5. Manifestazioni non intestinali e associazione con la celiachia

Ipoplasia dello smalto dei denti permanenti
Osteopenia/osteoporosi
Bassa statura
Pubertà ritardata
Anemia da carenza di ferro che non risponde alla somministrazione orale di ferro
Epatite (enzimi epatici elevati)
Artrite
Epilessia con calcificazione occipitale
Cefalea
Depressione
Atassia
Mielopatia
Autoimmunità
- Diabete mellito di tipo 1
- Tiroidite
- Cirrosi biliare primitiva
- Malattia di Addison
- Dermatite erpetiforme

Sindromi
- Turner
- Down
- William

Tumori maligni

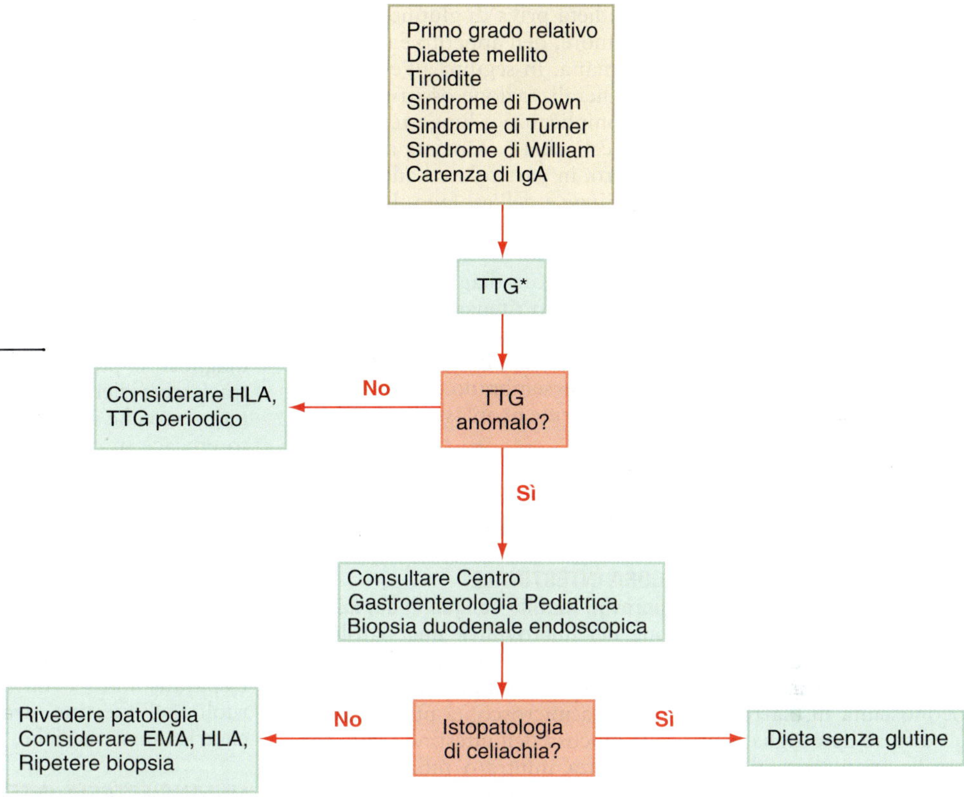

*TTG IgG raccomandata per individui con carenza IgA nota.

Figura 335-4. Test sierologici come il test anticorpale IgA antiendomisio (EMA), il test anticorpale IgA antitransglutaminasi tissutale (TTG) e il test dei genotipi HLA DQ2 o DQ8 sono utili per valutare i soggetti asintomatici affetti da diabete mellito, tiroidite, sindrome di Down, sindrome di Turner, sindrome di William o carenza di IgA, patologie che presentano un'alta incidenza di celiachia, e per esaminare anche i parenti di primo grado dei pazienti affetti da celiachia. (Adattata da Hill ID, Dirks MH, Liptak GS, et al: Guideline for the diagnosis and treatment of celiac disease in children: Recommendation of the North American Society for Pediatric Gastroenterology, Hepatology e Nutrition. *J Pediatr Gastroenterol Nutr* 2005;40:1-19.)

per gli anticorpi IgA antiendomisio e per gli anticorpi IgA antitransglutaminasi tissutale possono dare falsi negativi in presenza di carenza di IgA, che è associata a un aumento dell'incidenza della celiachia. La misurazione della concentrazione sierica di IgA è necessaria per poter escludere con sicurezza i falsi negativi negli individui con carenza di IgA. Se si sospetta una celiachia in pazienti affetti da carenza di IgA, può essere necessaria una biopsia intestinale. Poiché uno screening degli anticorpi può identificare pazienti senza celiachia documentata alla biopsia, è importante stabilire un limite inferiore dei titoli anticorpali abbastanza alto da evitare falsi positivi.

Biopsia dell'intestino tenue. La **diagnosi definitiva** di celiachia richiede una biopsia dell'intestino tenue, poiché nessuno dei test sierologici disponibili è affidabile al 100%. I cambiamenti istologici caratteristici comprendono atrofia totale o parziale dei villi, allungamento delle cripte e riduzione del rapporto villi/cripte, aumento del numero di linfociti intraepiteliali, indice mitotico dei linfociti intraepiteliali >0,2%, riduzione dell'altezza delle cellule epiteliali e perdita della polarità nucleare. Poiché la mucosa può essere interessata in modo discontinuo, è necessario effettuare più di una biopsia. I criteri per la diagnosi di celiachia basati sulla biopsia intestinale sono stati pubblicati dall'European Society of Pediatric Gastroenterology, Hepatology e Nutrition e rivisti nel 1990. In base ai criteri revisionati, nei bambini che presentano caratteristiche istologiche tipiche e una risposta clinica inequivocabile alla sospensione del glutine si può prendere in considerazione una diagnosi definitiva di celiachia. La normalizzazione dei test sierologici positivi in seguito alla sospensione del glutine è considerato una prova di conferma. Nei bambini di età <2 anni, l'enteropatia da sensibilità alle proteine del latte può produrre mutamenti simili a quelli dati dalla celiachia; talvolta può essere necessario confermare la diagnosi con un test di challenge per il glutine. Ciò richiede tre biopsie: una iniziale, alla presentazione, la seconda per documentare la guarigione in seguito a sospensione del glutine e la terza per evidenziare un danno ricorrente dopo reintroduzione del glutine.

TRATTAMENTO. *L'unico trattamento della celiachia è l'esclusione del glutine per tutta la vita, ovvero l'adozione di una dieta priva di frumento, orzo e segale.* In passato anche l'avena era considerata responsabile dell'enteropatia indotta da glutine; nonostante si abbiano le prove che questo cereale non dà problemi nei celiaci, rimane la preoccupazione che si possa verificare una sua contaminazione con il glutine durante la mietitura o la macinazione. A meno di non poter garantirne l'assoluta purezza, la sicurezza dell'avena rimane opinabile. In seguito a sospensione del glutine si ha una rapida remissione dei sintomi, un miglioramento della mineralizzazione ossea e l'inversione dell'insufficienza di crescita e delle carenze nutrizionali. Nei pazienti asintomatici diagnosticati in seguito ai test di screening, dopo la sospensione del glutine migliora il benessere tanto fisico quanto psicologico. Ci sono prove che anche una piccola quantità di glutine ingerita a intervalli regolari possa provocare danni alla mucosa. In passato, i prodotti contenenti <200 ppm erano considerati privi di glutine, ma attualmente le linee guida del Codex Alimentarius definiscono "privo di glutine" un valore <20 ppm e la National Food Authority ha ridefinito le diciture "privo di glutine" e "a basso tenore di glutine" indicando nel primo caso l'assenza di glutine e nel secondo livelli <200 ppm. È importante che un dietologo esperto con competenze specifiche nel campo della celiachia educhi la famiglia e il bambino stesso sulle restrizioni alla dieta alle quali occorre attenersi. Adottare un'alimentazione priva di glutine può essere difficile, specialmente per i bambini più grandi. Si raccomanda di seguire i bambini affetti da celiachia con visite periodiche, in modo da poter valutare i sintomi e la crescita, effettuare un esame fisico e controllare l'aderenza alla dieta priva di glutine: è stata riferita la totale mancanza di compliance nel 6-37% dei pazienti. Misurare i livelli di transglutaminasi tissutale 6 mesi dopo la sospensione del glutine, in modo da documentare la riduzione dei titoli anticorpali, può risultare utile come prova indiretta dell'aderenza a una dieta priva di glutine. Nei pazienti asintomatici si controllano annualmente gli anticorpi; la loro ricomparsa fa ipotizzare una mancata compliance, che può non essere intenzionale, ma dovuta a errori nella dieta.

PROGNOSI. La risposta clinica alla dieta priva di glutine di solito comporta un miglioramento dell'umore, dell'appetito e una riduzione della diarrea entro una settimana. In seguito all'esclusione del glutine, di solito anche la demineralizzazione ossea si riduce. Non è stata riconosciuta alcuna complicanza a lungo termine legata a questo regime dietetico. La celiachia è associata a linfoma intestinale e ad altre forme di cancro, in particolare l'adenocarcinoma dell'intestino tenue, della faringe e dell'esofago. Il linfoma T-linfocitico associato a enteropatia è una forma rara di linfoma linfocitico non Hodgkin di alto grado, che insorge in pazienti a cui in precedenza o in concomitanza è stata diagnosticata anche la celiachia. Vari studi di follow-up fanno ritenere che una dieta priva di glutine protegga dallo sviluppo del cancro, in particolare se viene iniziata nei primi anni di vita. Pertanto, una diagnosi precoce e strette restrizioni dietetiche sembrano essere l'unica possibilità per prevenire il rischio di forme neoplastiche associate alla celiachia, rare ma aggressive.

335.3 • Altre sindromi da malassorbimento

DIFETTI CONGENITI DELLA MUCOSA INTESTINALE

Malattia da inclusione dei microvilli (atrofia congenita dei microvilli). La malattia da inclusione dei microvilli è una patologia autosomica recessiva che si manifesta alla nascita con **diarrea secretiva acquosa profusa**. Si tratta della causa più comunemente riconosciuta di diarrea congenita. La microscopia ottica mostra un diffuso assottigliamento della mucosa dell'intestino tenue con atrofia ipoplastica dei villi, ma senza infiltrato infiammatorio. La microscopia elettronica rivela la presenza di enterociti con microvilli sparsi o assenti. Il citoplasma apicale degli enterociti contiene granuli secretori elettrondensi; un reperto caratteristico è la presenza di microvilli all'interno delle involuzioni della membrana apicale. Di solito le ecografie prenatali evidenziano la presenza di molte anse intestinali dilatate e ripiene di liquido e polidramnios. I neonati di solito presentano disidratazione e insufficienza della crescita. Nonostante il ricorso all'alimentazione parenterale, la diarrea prosegue e inizialmente è difficile gestire i liquidi. In assenza di alimentazione parenterale a lungo termine, la patologia è letale e comunque la maggior parte dei bambini muore nei primi mesi di vita o nella primissima infanzia. Come **trattamento** è stato utilizzato l'octreotide, un analogo della somatostatina che, in alcuni lattanti, è in grado di ridurre il volume delle feci. Il trapianto intestinale è l'unica terapia definitiva di questa rara patologia (vedi Capitolo 336).

Displasia epiteliale intestinale. L'enteropatia epiteliale intestinale o enteropatia *tufting* insorge nelle prime settimane di vita con **diarrea acquosa persistente** e interessa una piccola percentuale di lattanti affetti da diarrea. Tipicamente i sintomi non si manifestano subito dopo la nascita, bensì nella primissima infanzia. La caratteristica distintiva che si evidenzia all'esame bioptico della mucosa dell'intestino tenue è la presenza di "ciuffi" epiteliali focali (gruppi "a forma di lacrima" di enterociti strettamente associati tra loro con arrotondamento apicale della membrana plasmatica), che si presentano nell'80-90% della superficie epiteliale. In altre enteropatie note, questi "ciuffi" interessano <15% della superficie epiteliale. L'epitelio del colon risulta normale. Al microscopio elettronico si evidenzia un accorciamento ma non l'assenza dei microvilli. Non si conosce la patogenesi della malattia, che potrebbe essere dovuta a un'alterazione delle interazioni tra cellula e cellula e della matrice cellulare, a causa di una distribuzione anomala di α_2-β_1-integrina lungo l'asse villo-cripta, un'aumentata espressione di desmogleina e mutamenti ultrastrutturali dei desmosomi. Al momento nessun **trattamento** si è dimostrato efficace e di conseguenza gli unici interventi possibili rimangono l'alimentazione parenterale permanente ed eventualmente il trapianto dell'intestino (vedi Capitolo 336).

Anendocrinosi enterica. Mutazioni del gene *NEUROG3* producono un malassorbimento generalizzato della mucosa, vomito, diarrea, insufficienza della crescita, disidratazione e acidosi metabolica ipercloremica. L'alimentazione orale con qualunque alimento che non sia acqua provoca diarrea. Il trattamento quindi può essere rappresentato soltanto dall'alimentazione parenterale totale e dal trapianto dell'intestino tenue, oppure sia del fegato sia dell'intestino tenue.

SINDROME DA DIFETTO DELLA GLICOSILAZIONE DELLE GLICOPROTEINE E DEFICIT DI EPARANSOLFATO NEGLI ENTEROCITI. Il **disordine congenito della glicosilazione** (CDG, *Congenital Disorder of Glycosylation*) è un'alterazione genetica dell'assemblaggio degli N-glicani nel reticolo citosolico ed endoplasmatico che provoca una serie di manifestazioni (vedi Capitolo 87.6). Tutti i sottotipi di CDG I sono associati a **enteropatia proteino-disperdente**. La **diagnosi** si può determinare tramite focusing isoelettrico della trasferrina sierica, analisi enzimatica e/o analisi del DNA. Dal momento che il mannosio orale può rappresentare un **trattamento** efficace in caso di CDG Ib, si dimostra utile l'identificazione precoce dei bambini che presentano ipoglicemia, ipotiroidismo e/o carenza di globulina legante gli ormoni tiroidei.

La **carenza congenita di eparansolfato negli enterociti** è una causa rara di diarrea non trattabile associata a enteropatia proteino-disperdente e che può essere una manifestazione insolita della sindrome da difetto della glicosilazione delle glicoproteine (CDGS, *Carbohydrate-Deficient Glycoprotein Syndrome*) di tipo 1 (nota anche come sindrome di Jaeken) (vedi Capitolo 87.6). L'eparansolfato è un glicosaminoglicano che svolge molteplici ruoli nell'intestino, tra cui la restrizione delle macromolecole elettricamente cariche, quali l'albumina, nel lume vascolare.

LINFANGIECTASIA INTESTINALE. L'ostruzione del drenaggio linfatico dell'intestino può essere dovuta a difetti congeniti della formazione del dotto linfatico oppure a cause secondarie (Tab. 335-6). La forma **congenita** è spesso associata ad anomalie linfatiche in altri distretti del corpo, come avviene nelle sindromi di Turner, Noonan e Klippel-Trenaunay-Weber. Le cause della linfangiectasia **secondaria** includono pericardite ostruttiva, insufficienza cardiaca, fibrosi retroperitoneale, tubercolosi addominale e tumori maligni retroperitoneali. La linfa, ricca di proteine e

TABELLA 335-6. Cause dell'enteropatia proteino-disperdente

Linfangiectasia intestinale primitiva
Linfangiectasia intestinale secondaria
Pericardite costrittiva
Insufficienza cardiaca congestizia
Successiva a procedura di Fontan
Malrotazione
Linfoma
Sarcoidosi
Radioterapia
Infiammazioni della mucosa intestinale
Infezioni
Cytomegalovirus (CMV)
Eccessiva proliferazione batterica
Infezioni batteriche invasive
Infiammazioni gastriche
Malattia di Menetrier
Gastroenterite eosinofilica
Infiammazioni intestinali
Celiachia
Morbo di Crohn
Enteropatia proteinosensibile
Sprue tropicale
Enterite da radiazioni
Infiammazioni del colon
Malattie infiammatorie dell'intestino
Enterocolite necrotizzante
Malattie congenite della glicosilazione

linfociti, passa nel lume intestinale provocando enteropatia proteino-disperdente e deplezione linfocitaria. Spesso si verificano ipoalbuminemia, ipogammaglobulinemia, edema, lifocitopenia, malassorbimento dei lipidi e delle vitamine liposolubili e ascite chiloso. Anche la linfangiectasia intestinale si può presentare con ascite, edema periferico e ridotti livelli di albumina sierica.

La **diagnosi** è suggerita dai riscontri tipici in associazione con elevati livelli fecali di α_1-antitripsina. Un reperto caratteristico all'esame radiologico è l'ispessimento simmetrico e uniforme delle pliche mucose. La biopsia della mucosa intestinale mostra vasi chiliferi dilatati con distorsione dei villi in assenza di infiltrato infiammatorio. Il **trattamento** della linfangiectasia prevede una restrizione della quantità di grassi a catena lunga ingeriti tramite somministrazione di un latte artificiale contenente proteine e trigliceridi a catena media (MCT, *Medium-Chain Triglycerides*). L'integrazione di una dieta povera di grassi con olio di MCT, da utilizzarsi per cuocere, si applica nel trattamento dei bambini più grandi affetti da linfangiectasia. Raramente è necessario ricorrere all'alimentazione parenterale. Se è interessata soltanto una parte dell'intestino si può prendere in considerazione la resezione chirurgica.

ENTEROPATIA AUTOIMMUNE. I sintomi dell'enteropatia autoimmune si manifestano solitamente dopo i primi 6 mesi di vita. Spesso la prima diagnosi è quella di celiachia, ma la mancata risposta a una dieta priva di glutine porta a un'ulteriore valutazione. I reperti istologici nell'intestino tenue includono atrofia parziale o totale dei villi, iperplasia delle cripte e aumento delle cellule infiammatorie croniche nella lamina propria. Specifici anticorpi sierici antienterociti si possono individuare in ≥50% dei pazienti tramite colorazione all'immunofluorescenza indiretta delle mucose normali dell'intestino tenue e del rene. Può essere interessato anche il colon. Frequenti sono le **malattie autoimmuni extraintestinali** tra cui artrite, glomerulonefrite membranosa, diabete insulinodipendente, trombocitopenia, epatite autoimmune, ipotiroidismo e anemia emolitica. Il **trattamento** consiste nella somministrazione di prednisone, azatioprina, ciclofosfamide, ciclosporina o tacrolimus, oltre che nel trapianto di midollo osseo.

MALASSORBIMENTO DEGLI ACIDI BILIARI. Nel malassorbimento primitivo degli acidi biliari, la mutazione del gene cotrasportatore degli acidi biliari/Na1/bile nell'ileo, l'*SLC10A2*, provoca diarrea congenita, steatorrea, interruzione della circolazione enteroepatica degli acidi biliari e ridotti livelli plasmatici di colesterolo. Gli acidi biliari sono sintetizzati nel fegato a partire dal colesterolo e poi secreti nell'intestino tenue, dove facilitano l'assorbimento dei grassi, delle vitamine liposolubili e del colesterolo. Gli acidi biliari, una volta riassorbiti dall'intestino, ritornano al fegato tramite la circolazione portale e vengono di nuovo secreti nella bile. Normalmente, la circolazione enteroepatica degli acidi biliari è un processo quanto mai efficiente; il 10% degli acidi biliari intestinali sfugge al riassorbimento ed è eliminato tramite le feci. La secrezione di acidi biliari è ampiamente autoregolata, ma esiste soltanto una capacità limitata di aumentare la secrezione di acidi biliari. La riduzione della quantità di acidi biliari a causa del loro malassorbimento provoca steatorrea, che richiede una dieta povera di grassi. Gli acidi biliari non assorbiti stimolano l'escrezione di cloruro nel colon, con conseguente diarrea, la quale risponde alla colestiramina, una resina legante gli anioni. Il malassorbimento degli acidi biliari secondario può dipendere da un'affezione a carico dell'ileo, come il morbo di Crohn, oppure da una resezione ileale.

ABETALIPOPROTEINEMIA (VEDI CAPITOLO 86). Questa rara malattia autosomica recessiva del metabolismo delle lipoproteine è associata a grave malassorbimento lipidico a partire dalla nascita. In tutto il primo anno di vita i lattanti vanno incontro a un arresto di accrescimento, mentre le feci sono chiare, maleodoranti e voluminose. L'addome è disteso e i riflessi tendinei profondi sono assenti in seguito a neuropatia periferica, secondaria a carenza di vitamina E. Lo sviluppo intellettivo tende a essere lento. Dopo i 10 anni, i sintomi intestinali sono meno gravi, si sviluppa atassia e vi è una perdita della sensibilità di posizione e vibrazione con esordi di tremore intenzionale. Questi ultimi sintomi riflettono il coinvolgimento delle colonne posteriori, del cervelletto e dei gangli basali. Nell'adolescenza si sviluppa retinite pigmentosa atipica.

La **diagnosi** si basa sulla presenza di acantociti nel sangue periferico e su livelli di colesterolo plasmatico estremamente bassi (<50 mg/dL); i trigliceridi sono estremamente ridotti (<20 mg/dL). Non si riscontrano chilomicroni né lipoproteine a bassissima densità e la frazione delle lipoproteine a bassa densità (LDL, *Low Density Lipoproteins*) è praticamente assente dal circolo sanguigno; nella mucosa duodenale a digiuno si forma un marcato accumulo di trigliceridi negli enterociti dei villi. Nei pazienti più piccoli si manifesta steatorrea, ma permangono gli altri processi di assimilazione. Il rachitismo può essere un'insolita manifestazione iniziale dell'abetalipoproteinemia e dell'ipobetalipoproteinemia. Il rachitismo è provocato da perdite di calcio indotte dalla steatorrea. I pazienti presentano mutazioni del gene della proteina microsomiale di trasporto dei trigliceridi (MTP, *Microsomal Triglyceride transfer Protein*), con conseguente mancata funzionalità dell'MTP nel tenue. Questa proteina è necessaria per un normale assemblaggio e una normale secrezione delle lipoproteine a bassissima densità e dei chilomicroni. Non è disponibile alcun **trattamento** specifico. Occorre somministrare dosi elevate di vitamine liposolubili A, D, E e K. Le vitamine E (100-200 mg/kg/24 h) e A (10 000-25 000 UI/die) possono arrestare la degenerazione neurologica e retinica. Per alleviare i sintomi intestinali si può limitare l'assunzione di grassi a catena lunga, mentre i trigliceridi a catena media possono servire a integrare l'apporto di grassi.

IPOBETALIPOPROTEINEMIA OMOZIGOTE (VEDI CAPITOLO 86). Questa malattia si trasmette come carattere autosomico dominante. La forma omozigote è indistinguibile dall'abetalipoproteinemia. I genitori di questi pazienti, in quanto eterozigoti, presentano concentrazioni ridotte di LDL e di apoproteina β nel sangue, mentre quelli dei pazienti con abetalipoproteinemia presentano livelli normali. Esaminando al microscopio elettronico le biopsie dell'intestino tenue, si nota che nelle due forme (abetalipoproteinemia e ipobetalipoproteinemia) i vacuoli lipidici hanno dimensioni diverse: nell'ipobetalipoproteinemia sono molti e piccoli, mentre nell'abetalipoproteinemia sono di grandi dimensioni.

MALATTIA DA RITENZIONE DI CHILOMICRONI (MALATTIA DI ANDERSON). In questa rara malattia recessiva si ha un difetto dell'esocitosi dei chilomicroni da parte degli enterociti. La Sar1-GTP promuove la formazione di reticolo endoplasmatico per l'apparato del Golgi; nella malattia di Anderson la Sar1-b risulta carente. Questi pazienti presentano sintomi intestinali gravi con steatorrea, diarrea cronica e arresto della crescita. L'acantocitosi è rara e le sue manifestazioni neurologiche sono meno gravi di quelle osservate nell'abetalipoproteinemia. I livelli di colesterolo plasmatico sono moderatamente ridotti (<75 mg/dL); i trigliceridi a digiuno sono normali, ma i livelli di vitamine liposolubili, in particolare la A e la E, sono molto ridotti. Il trattamento consiste in una terapia aggressiva precoce con vitamine liposolubili e nella modifica dell'assunzione di grassi tramite la dieta, come nell'abetalipoproteinemia.

MALATTIA DI WOLMAN. Questa rara malattia dell'immagazzinamento dei grassi porta ad accumulo di lipidi in molti organi, tra cui l'intestino tenue. Oltre a vomito, diarrea grave ed epatosplenomegalia, i pazienti possono presentare steatorrea da ostruzione linfatica. Questa malattia è causata da una carenza di lipasi lisosomiale acida (vedi Capitolo 86). Il successo a lungo termine dei trapianti di midollo osseo ha portato alla normalizzazione dell'attività della lipasi lisosomiale acida nei leucociti periferici, con conseguente risoluzione della diarrea e ripresa delle tappe fondamentali dello sviluppo.

335.4 • Infezioni intestinali associate al malassorbimento

Il malassorbimento, pur manifestandosi raramente nei bambini immunocompetenti in seguito a infezioni intestinali primitive, si può verificare in conseguenza di infezioni da *Giardia*, rotavirus, *Campylobacter*, *Shigella*, *Salmonella* e coccidioidosi. Queste cause infettive sono più comuni nei bambini immunocompromessi.

ECCESSIVA PROLIFERAZIONE BATTERICA. I batteri sono normalmente presenti in gran numero nel colon e hanno un rapporto simbiotico con l'ospite, a cui forniscono sostanze nutritive e che proteggono dai microrganismi patogeni. Tuttavia, una loro eccessiva quantità nell'intestino tenue o nello stomaco è dannosa. Di solito, essi sono presenti soltanto in numero ridotto sia nello stomaco sia nell'intestino tenue. Il pH degli acidi gastrici impedisce ai microrganismi ingeriti di colonizzare il tenue, che grazie alla motilità di cui è dotato e al complesso motorio migrante viene ripulito tra un pasto e l'altro e durante la notte; la valvola ileocecale impedisce ai batteri di passare dal colon all'ileo; le difese delle mucose, quali le mucine e le immunoglobuline, prevengono l'eccessiva proliferazione batterica nell'intestino tenue. Tuttavia tale proliferazione può dipendere da determinate condizioni cliniche in grado di alterare il pH gastrico o la motilità dell'intestino tenue, tra cui alterazioni come ostruzione parziale dell'intestino, presenza di diverticoli, ridotte dimensioni intestinali, duplicazioni intestinali, diabete mellito e sclerodermia. Nascita prematura, immunodeficienza e malnutrizione sono altri fattori associati a eccessiva proliferazione batterica dell'intestino tenue.

La **diagnosi** si può effettuare tramite colture di aspirato dell'intestino tenue o il breath test al lattulosio; quest'ultimo è un disaccaride sintetico che non viene digerito dagli enzimi dell'orletto a spazzola mucoso, ma può essere fermentato dai batteri. Alti livelli basali di idrogeno e un rapido aumento di questo gas nei campioni di aria espirata vanno a sostegno di tale diagnosi, anche se i falsi positivi sono comuni.

L'eccessiva proliferazione batterica comporta un'inefficiente trasformazione intraluminale dei grassi introdotti con la dieta e conseguente steatorrea, provocata da deconiugazione batterica dei sali biliari, malassorbimento della vitamina B_{12} e danneggiamento dell'orletto a spazzola dei microvilli che presentano malassorbimento. L'eccessiva produzione di D-lattato (l'enantiomero dell'L-lattato) può causare intontimento, disfunzione neurologica e shock dovuto ad acidosi D-lattica. Si dovrebbe sospettare una diagnosi di acidosi lattica nei bambini a rischio di eccessiva proliferazione batterica con deterioramento neurologico e acidosi metabolica con alto gap anionico non spiegabile con gli acidi misurabili, come l'L-lattato. È necessario misurare l'enantiomero del D-lattato poiché l'analisi standard del lattato misura solo l'L-enantiomero.

Il **trattamento** è incentrato sulla correzione delle cause sottostanti, come per esempio l'ostruzione parziale. La somministrazione orale di antibiotici è la terapia d'elezione. Un ciclo iniziale di metronidazolo, assunto per 2-4 settimane, può dare sollievo per molti mesi. Sono necessari cicli ripetuti di antibiotici, tra cui azitromicina, trimetoprim/sulfametoxazolo, ciprofloxacina e metronidazolo. In alternativa si possono somministrare antibiotici non assorbibili, come gli aminoglicosidi. Occasionalmente può essere necessario ricorrere a una terapia antifungina, per controllare l'eccessiva proliferazione fungina nell'intestino.

SPRUE TROPICALE. I nativi di alcune regioni tropicali, anche se risiedono all'estero, possono presentare lesioni diffuse alla mucosa del tenue, dovute a sprue tropicale, anche molto tempo dopo essersi trasferiti. Le regioni endemiche sono L'India meridionale, le Filippine e alcune isole dei Caraibi; la malattia è invece poco comune in Africa, Giamaica e nel Sudest asiatico. L'eziologia non è chiara; si sospetta un'origine infettiva perché la sprue compare in seguito ad attacchi diarroici acuti e migliora con la terapia antibiotica. L'incidenza sembra in diminuzione, forse grazie all'uso frequente di antibiotici per curare le gastroenteriti nei Paesi in via di sviluppo.

I sintomi clinici includono febbre e malessere, seguiti da diarrea acquosa. Dopo circa una settimana le caratteristiche acute diminuiscono; in compenso, il malassorbimento, la diarrea intermittente e l'anoressia provocano una grave malnutrizione caratterizzata da glossite, stomatite, cheilosi, cecità notturna, iperpigmentazione ed edema. Spesso il deperimento o ipotrofia muscolare (wasting) è marcato e l'addome disteso. L'anemia megaloblastica è dovuta alle carenze di folati e di vitamina B_{12}. La **diagnosi** si ottiene tramite una biopsia dell'intestino tenue che evidenzi appiattimento dei villi, iperplasia delle cripte e un infiltrato cellulare infiammatorio cronico della lamina propria, con adiacente accumulo lipidico nell'epitelio superficiale.

Il **trattamento** consiste nell'integrazione delle sostanze nutritive carenti, come i folati e la vitamina B_{12}. Per prevenire la ricomparsa periodica, si raccomanda di somministrare acido folico orale (5 mg) e tetraciclina o sulfamidici per 6 mesi. Il 10-20% dei pazienti che ancora risiedono nella regione tropicale endemica è soggetto a recidive; possono essere necessari ulteriori cicli di antibiotici.

335.5 • Disordini da immunodeficienza

Il malassorbimento si può manifestare anche in caso di malattie da **immunodeficienza congenita**, tra cui carenza selettiva di IgA, grave immunodeficienza combinata, agammaglobulinemia, sindrome di Wiskott-Aldrich, malattia da immunodeficienza variabile comune e malattia granulomatosa cronica. Anche se di norma la carenza selettiva di IgA è asintomatica, si possono verificare malassorbimento causato da giardiasi, enteropatia aspecifica con eccessiva proliferazione batterica e carenza di disaccaridasi. Si dovrebbe innanzitutto escludere la celiachia, in quanto questa patologia è molto comune nei pazienti affetti da carenza di IgA. L'infezione cronica da rotavirus, la giardiasi, la proliferazione batterica e l'enteropatia proteinodipendente sono complicanze facilmente riconoscibili dell'agammaglobulinemia legata all'X che provocano malassorbimento. Il malassorbimento si verifica nel 10% circa dei pazienti affetti da ipogammaglobulinemia comune variabile a insorgenza tardiva, spesso secondaria a giardiasi. Nella malattia granulomatosa cronica, la funzionalità fagocitica è spesso compromessa, per cui in tutto il tratto gastrointestinale si sviluppano granulomi, che mimano il morbo di Crohn. Sono stati riferiti anche diarrea, steatorrea e malassorbimento della vitamina B_{12}.

Malnutrizione, diarrea e arresto dell'accrescimento sono comuni nei bambini affetti da **infezione da HIV** non trattata. Il rischio d'infezione gastrointestinale è legato alla riduzione del conteggio di CD4. Le infezioni opportunistiche includono *Cryptosporidium parvum*, Cytomegalovirus, *Mycobacterium avium-intracellulare*, *Isospora belli*, *Enterocytozoon bieneusi*, *Candida albicans*, astrovirus, calicivirus, adenovirus e i normali enteropatogeni batterici. In questi pazienti il *Cryptosporidium* può provocare una diarrea secretoria cronica.

La **chemioterapia antineoplastica** può causare un danno alla mucosa intestinale con conseguente malassorbimento secondario del lattosio. In seguito a trapianto di midollo osseo, il danneggiamento della mucosa dovuto a GvHD (**Graft vs Host Disease,** reazione del trapianto contro l'ospite) può provocare diarrea e malassorbimento. L'esame bioptico dell'intestino tenue mostra una lieve atrofia aspecifica dei villi, infiltrato cellulare infiammatorio misto e apoptosi. La chemioterapia antineoplastica e il trapianto di midollo osseo sono stati entrambi associati a danno pancreatico con conseguente insufficienza pancreatica.

335.6 • Malattia immunoproliferativa dell'intestino tenue

La malattia immunoproliferativa dell'intestino tenue (**linfoma mediterraneo**) colpisce soprattutto bambini tra i 10 e i 13 anni d'età che vivono nel bacino del Mediterraneo, nel Medio e nell'Estremo Oriente e in Africa. È una patologia linfoproliferativa da IgA che può esitare in un linfoma dei linfociti B.

La povertà ed episodi frequenti di gastroenterite nella prima infanzia costituiscono fattori di rischio antecedenti. In alcune aree l'incidenza di questa malattia è diminuita grazie al miglioramento delle condizioni socioeconomiche. Casi sporadici sono stati riferiti in Europa e in America, per lo più in immigrati provenienti da Paesi in via di sviluppo. Una patologia simile è stata descritta in pazienti affetti da AIDS. Inizialmente la malattia si presenta con diarrea intermittente e dolori addominali; in seguito subentrano diarrea cronica persistente, malassorbimento, enteropatia proteinodisperdente, calo ponderale, ippocratismo digitale e arresto dell'accrescimento. La **diagnosi** richiede biopsie multiple della mucosa del duodeno e del digiuno, volte a dimostrare la presenza di linfomi del tessuto linfoide associati alle mucose. Nella maggior parte dei casi si riscontra la presenza di un marker sierico dell'IgA (α-paraproteina a catena pesante). In alcuni pazienti con malattia precoce, un **trattamento** prolungato (circa 6 mesi) con tetracicline o metronidazolo può alleviare i sintomi. Lo stadio prelinfomatoso e i linfomi necessitano di chemioterapia.

335.7 • SINDROME DELL'INTESTINO CORTO

La sindrome dell'intestino corto deriva da malformazioni congenite o dalla resezione dell'intestino tenue. Le cause di questa sindrome sono elencate nella Tabella 335-7. La perdita di >50% dell'intestino tenue, con o senza una porzione del colon, può provocare i sintomi di una patologia da malassorbimento generalizzato o la carenza di una sostanza nutritiva specifica, a seconda della regione dell'intestino resecata. Alla nascita, l'intestino tenue è lungo da 200 a 250 cm; in età adulta esso raggiunge i 300-800 cm. La resezione dell'intestino ha una prognosi migliore nel lattante che nell'adulto, a causa del potenziale di crescita dell'intestino stesso. Un lattante a cui sia rimasta una porzione di tenue di non meno di 15 cm in presenza di valvola ileocecale, oppure una porzione di non meno di 20 cm in assenza della valvola, può sopravvivere ed essere portato allo svezzamento tramite nutrizione parenterale totale (TPN, *Total Parenteral Nutrition*).

TABELLA 335-7. Cause della sindrome dell'intestino corto

Congenite
Sindrome dell'intestino corto congenita
Atresie multiple
Gastroschisi
Resezione dell'intestino
Enterocolite necrotizzante
Volvolo con o senza malrotazione
Malattia di Hirschsprung a segmento lungo
Peritonite da meconio
Morbo di Crohn
Trauma

Oltre alla lunghezza dell'intestino, è importante anche la collocazione anatomica della resezione. Il digiuno ha un numero maggiore di pliche circolari e villi più lunghi. Il tratto prossimale del digiuno (100-200 cm) costituisce il sito principale di assorbimento di carboidrati, proteine, ferro e vitamine liposolubili, mentre l'assorbimento dei grassi avviene su un tratto di tenue più lungo. A seconda della regione intestinale resecata, si può verificare il malassorbimento di una sostanza nutritiva specifica. La vitamina B_{12} e i sali biliari vengono assorbiti soltanto nell'ileo distale (Fig. 335-5). Le resezioni del digiuno sono generalmente meglio tollerate della resezione dell'ileo, perché quest'ultimo può subire adattamenti al fine di assorbire nutrienti e liquidi. L'assorbimento netto di sodio e acqua è relativamente molto più alto a livello ileale. Di conseguenza, la resezione dell'ileo ha un effetto profondo sull'assorbimento dei liquidi e degli elettroliti a causa del malassorbimento di sodio e acqua nella porzione ileale residua; il malassorbimento ileale dei sali biliari stimola l'aumento della secrezione di liquidi ed elettroliti in corrispondenza del colon.

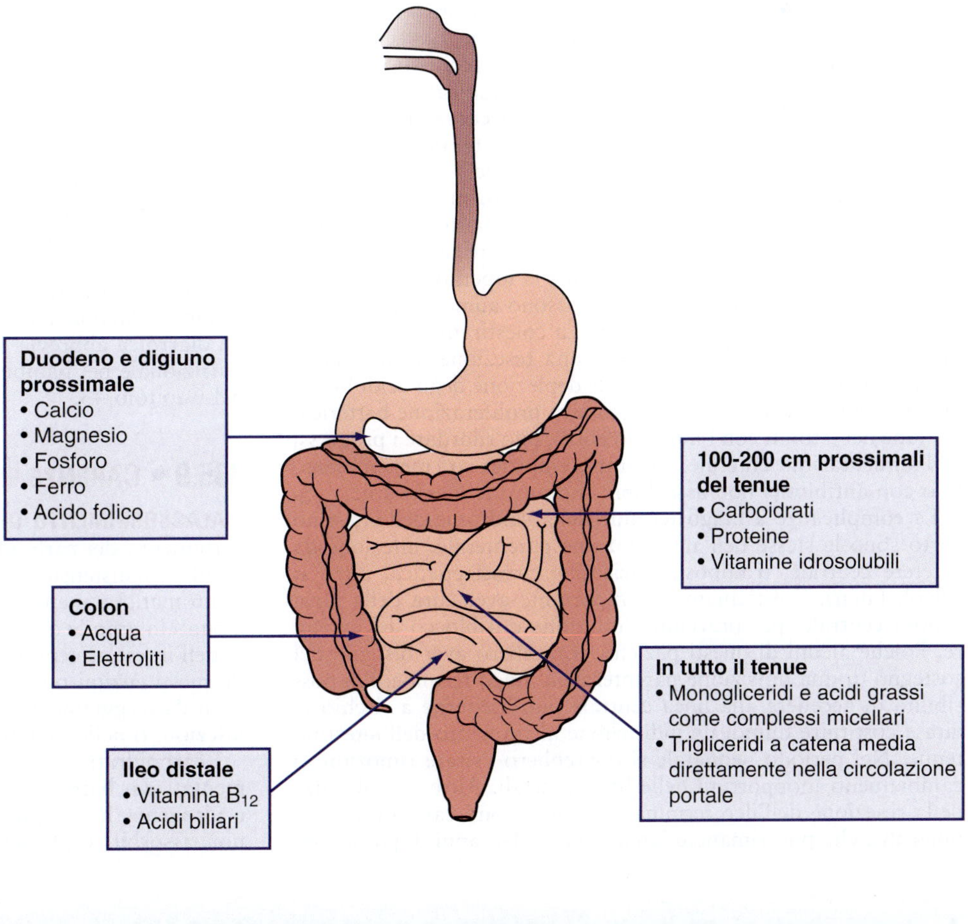

Figura 335-5. L'assorbimento delle sostanze nutritive nell'intestino tenue varia a seconda della regione interessata.

TRATTAMENTO. Dopo la resezione dell'intestino, la terapia della sindrome dell'intestino corto si concentra inizialmente sulla sostituzione delle massicce perdite di liquidi e di elettroliti, man mano che l'intestino si adatta ad assorbire queste perdite. Di norma l'alimentazione è fornita per via parenterale; a tal fine, si dovrebbe inserire un catetere venoso centrale. Si raccomanda di misurare la stomia addominale e valutare la produzione di feci in modo da fornire un'adeguata compensazione delle perdite di liquidi ed elettroliti. La misurazione dell'Na^+ nelle urine, che consente di valutare le sue riserve nell'organismo, è utile per impedirne la deplezione. Per assicurarsi un adeguato apporto di Na^+ bisogna assicurarsi che i suoi livelli urinari si mantengano più alti di quelli del K^+. L'uso di soluzioni gluco-elettrolitiche orali migliora il riassorbimento del sodio, in particolare in pazienti a cui è stato resecato il colon. Dopo le prime settimane post-resezione, le perdite di liquidi ed elettroliti si stabilizzano e la terapia si accentra sulla riabilitazione dell'intestino con reintroduzione graduale della nutrizione enterale. Al momento di iniziare la reintroduzione continuativa di piccoli volumi di sostanze nutritive enterali trofiche, si dovrebbero utilizzare un idrolisato proteico e un latte formulato arricchito con trigliceridi a catena media, per stimolare gli ormoni intestinali e promuovere la crescita della mucosa. L'alimentazione enterale aumenta anche il flusso pancreobiliare e riduce l'epatotossicità indotta dall'alimentazione parenterale. Appena possibile, si dovrebbe somministrare al lattante una piccola quantità d'acqua, poi latte formulato per os in modo da mantenere l'interesse per l'alimentazione orale e ridurre al minimo o evitare lo sviluppo di **avversione orale**. Gli acidi grassi essenziali devono essere somministrati per via parenterale o enterale. Man mano che prosegue l'adattamento dell'intestino, l'alimentazione enterale aumenta e l'integrazione parenterale diminuisce. Con la crescita, la mucosa intestinale prolifera e l'intestino stesso si allunga. Una volta raggiunta la massima capacità di assorbimento dell'intestino, bisognerà provvedere al trattamento delle carenze di un micronutriente o una vitamina specifici e curare i problemi transitori dovuti a malassorbimento della mucosa imputabile a infezione. Le infezioni gastrointestinali come quella da rotavirus o l'eccessiva proliferazione batterica nell'intestino tenue possono provocare difficoltà al raggiungimento dell'alimentazione enterale completa in pazienti con funzionalità assorbitiva marginale. In caso di marcato aumento della produzione di feci oppure evidenze di malassorbimento dei carboidrati (feci con pH $<5,5$ e presenza di sostanze riducenti) è controindicato aumentare ulteriormente l'alimentazione enterale. Si raccomanda invece di aumentare lentamente i tassi di nutrizione enterale continua fino a riuscire a somministrare per via enterale tutte le sostanze nutritive, dopodiché si potrà cambiare l'alimentazione aumentandone gradualmente i volumi per os o per bolo. Se il paziente ha un'abbondante emissione di feci, può essere utile aggiungere fibre solubili e agenti antidiarroici come la loperamide e gli anticolinergici, anche se questi farmaci possono aumentare il rischio di eccessiva proliferazione batterica. La colestiramina può essere utile nei pazienti che hanno subito una resezione ileale distale, anche se in questo caso la potenziale deplezione degli acidi biliari può aumentare la steatorrea. L'eccessiva proliferazione batterica, comune nei lattanti con l'intestino corto, può ritardare i progressi dell'alimentazione enterale. La terapia empirica con metronidazolo o con antibiotici non assorbibili si dimostra spesso utile.

Le **complicanze a lungo termine** della sindrome dell'intestino corto sono le stesse dell'alimentazione parenterale: infezione da catetere centrale, trombosi, colestasi e cirrosi epatica, oltre ai calcoli biliari. È estremamente importante aver cura della linea venosa centrale, per prevenire l'infezione e il blocco del catetere. Poiché alcuni di questi pazienti potrebbero aver bisogno del sostegno di una nutrizione parenterale a lungo termine, l'impossibilità di accedere alla linea centrale può metterne a rischio la vita e costituire quindi un'indicazione al trapianto dell'intestino tenue. Nel periodo neonatale si dovrebbero evitare rimozioni o cambiamenti inopportuni delle linee centrali. Altre complicanze della resezione dell'ileo terminale comprendono carenza di vitamina B_{12}, che può rimanere latente fino a 1-2 anni dopo la conclusione della nutrizione parenterale. È importante effettuare un monitoraggio a lungo termine per individuare eventuali carenze di vitamina B_{12}, folati, ferro, vitamine liposolubili e oligoelementi come zinco e rame. I **calcoli renali** si possono manifestare in conseguenza dell'iperossaluria secondaria a steatorrea (il calcio si lega ai grassi in eccesso ma non agli ossalati, che quindi vengono riassorbiti ed eliminati con le urine in quantità maggiore). La trombosi venosa e la carenza di vitamine sono state associate a iperomocistinemia nella sindrome dell'intestino corto. Con il progredire dell'alimentazione enterale si può manifestare diarrea sanguinolenta, secondaria a una lieve colite con disposizione a chiazze. Questa "colite da alimentazione", la cui patogenesi è ignota, di solito è benigna e può migliorare con una dieta ipoallergenica o somministrando sulfasalazina.

Nei pazienti che non sono in grado di raggiungere l'alimentazione enterale completa dopo vari anni di riabilitazione nutrizionale, si può prendere in considerazione un intervento chirurgico di allungamento dell'intestino. In alcuni bambini che mostrano complicanze o che hanno un accesso venoso marginale a causa dell'alimentazione parenterale continua, si può prendere in esame il trapianto d'intestino tenue (vedi Capitolo 336).

335.8 • Malnutrizione cronica

Nei Paesi avanzati la malnutrizione primitiva è rara. La maggior parte dei bambini affetti da malnutrizione presenta anche una malattia digestiva cronica sottostante. Se il piccolo è trascurato o se non si rispettano le corrette modalità di preparazione del latte artificiale si possono manifestare problemi di malnutrizione anche grave. La malnutrizione primitiva rimane comune nei paesi in via di sviluppo ed è una causa frequente di mortalità (vedi Capitolo 43). A essere danneggiati dalla malnutrizione proteico-energetica sono la struttura intestinale, la digestione e l'assorbimento dei nutrienti, come pure la funzionalità della barriera immunologica e della mucosa intestinale. In età pediatrica ne consegue un ciclo di diarrea protratta, probabilmente imputabile a un'eccessiva proliferazione batterica nel tenue. Nel kwashiorkor può essere presente una grave atrofia dei villi, simile a quella che si riscontra nella celiachia. L'attività di disaccaridasi della mucosa è ridotta, anche se tipicamente non si osserva intolleranza grave al lattosio. Nel marasma la struttura dei villi è relativamente ben conservata, nonostante al microscopio elettronico si apprezzino cambiamenti dei microvilli e anomalie intracellulari. Anche la funzionalità pancreatica esocrina è compromessa e ciò contribuisce a peggiorare il malassorbimento dei grassi e delle vitamine liposolubili.

Le carenze cliniche e subcliniche di micronutrienti hanno un notevole impatto sulla risposta del tratto intestinale ai patogeni intestinali. La riabilitazione nutrizionale corregge le anomalie dell'assorbimento gastrointestinale. L'integrazione di vitamina A riduce la mortalità e la gravità della diarrea nei Paesi in via di sviluppo. Analogamente, l'integrazione di zinco in corso di malattia diarroica abbrevia la durata della patologia. La riabilitazione nutrizionale nei bambini affetti da malnutrizione è stata trattata nel Capitolo 43.

335.9 • Carenze enzimatiche

MALASSORBIMENTO DEI CARBOIDRATI. I sintomi di un malassorbimento dei carboidrati includono diarrea sciolta e acquosa, flatulenza, distensione addominale e dolore. Alcuni bambini sono asintomatici a meno che i carboidrati malassorbiti non vengano assunti in grande quantità. Sulla membrana con orletto a spazzola dell'intestino tenue sono presenti le disaccaridasi: una carenza di questi enzimi può essere dovuta a un difetto genetico oppure a un danneggiamento dell'epitelio del tenue, come avviene nelle infezioni o nelle malattie infiammatorie.

I carboidrati non assorbiti penetrano nel colon e vengono fermentati dai batteri intestinali, con produzione di acidi organici e idrogeno. Il gas può provocare disagio, mentre i carboidrati non assorbiti e gli acidi organici provocano diarrea osmotica, caratterizzata da pH acido e da presenza di zuccheri (riducenti o non riducenti) nelle feci.

CARENZA DI LATTASI. La **carenza di lattasi congenita** è rara ed è associata agli stessi sintomi che si manifestano in seguito a esposizione al lattosio del latte. In tutto il mondo sono stati riferiti meno di 50 casi. L'**ipolattasia primitiva dell'adulto** è provocata da una diminuzione fisiologica della lattasi che si verifica con l'età nella maggior parte dei mammiferi. A livello dell'orletto a spazzola la lattasi è ridotta per tutta la vita fetale; la sua attività aumenta alla fine del periodo fetale e presenta un picco dalla nascita a termine fino ai 3 anni d'età, dopodiché i livelli cominciano a calare gradualmente. Questa riduzione dei livelli di lattasi varia a seconda del gruppo etnico di appartenenza, cosicché nella popolazione adulta degli Stati Uniti la carenza di questo enzima si manifesta in circa il 15% dei bianchi, nel 40% degli asiatici e nell'85% dei neri. La lattasi è codificata da un solo gene (*LCT*) di circa 50 kb situato sul cromosoma 2q21. La *down-regulation* del gene della lattasi è identificabile in età pediatrica fin dal 2° anno di vita. La persistenza della lattasi nelle popolazioni bianche discendenti da ceppi dell'Europa settentrionale e centrale e in alcune tribù nomadi dell'Africa è probabilmente dovuta al fatto che la presenza di questo enzima costituiva un vantaggio per quelle popolazioni, la cui dieta si basava principalmente su latte e prodotti caseari. L'**intolleranza al lattosio secondaria** deriva da un danneggiamento della mucosa del tenue (celiachia, infezione da rotavirus) e di solito è transitoria, in quanto si supera con la guarigione della mucosa.

Per la **diagnosi** ci si avvale del breath test all'idrogeno oppure si misura la concentrazione di lattasi nella mucosa previa biopsia dell'intestino tenue. Questi test diagnostici non sono però d'obbligo e spesso, per ottenere il sollievo dei sintomi, è sufficiente apportare piccoli cambiamenti dietetici che riducano o eliminino il lattosio dalla dieta.

Il **trattamento** per la carenza di lattasi consiste in una dieta priva di latte. Nei lattanti si può ricorrere a un latte artificiale privo di lattosio (a base di soia o di latte vaccino). I bambini più grandi possono bere latte con lattosio predigerito con lattasi, il che permette loro di assumere modeste quantità di latte. Inoltre è possibile somministrare durante i pasti una compressa che favorisca l'attività della lattasi. Sul mercato è disponibile un latte preconfezionato con un preparato a base di lattasi e con lattosio predigerito al 100%. Lo yogurt con fermenti vivi contiene batteri produttori di lattasi e di conseguenza è tollerato anche dai pazienti affetti da carenza di questo enzima. I formaggi duri, che contengono una percentuale ridotta di lattosio, sono in genere ben tollerati.

SINDROME DA INGESTIONE DI SUCCHI. I bambini che consumano grandi quantità di succhi contenenti sciroppo di amido ricco di fruttosio possono manifestare diarrea, distensione addominale e basso incremento ponderale; questi sintomi talvolta mimano le alterazioni da malassorbimento dei carboidrati. Ridurre la quantità di succo ingerito con la dieta è sufficiente a risolvere i sintomi e permette di evitare indagini non necessarie.

CARENZA DI SACCARASI-ISOMALTASI. Si tratta di una rara malattia autosomica recessiva, caratterizzata da carenza totale di saccarasi e ridotta attività digestiva della maltasi. Il complesso saccarasi-isomaltasi è composto da 1927 aminoacidi, codificati da un mRNA di 3364 bp. Il locus genico sul cromosoma 3 ha 30 esoni intorno a 106,6 kb. La maggior parte delle mutazioni della saccarasi-isomaltasi impedisce la sintesi della proteina enzimatica (mutazione null). Sono stati identificati anche difetti di elaborazione post-traslazionale. Circa il 2% degli americani di origine europea è eterozigote mutante. La carenza di saccarasi è particolarmente comune negli abitanti della Groenlandia (circa il 5%), in cui questo problema è spesso associato a carenza di lattasi.

I sintomi della carenza di saccarasi-isomaltasi si manifestano in genere quando il lattante viene sottoposto a una dieta contenente saccarosio o polimeri di glucosio; ciò si può verificare con l'ingestione di latte artificiale per neonati privo di lattosio oppure in seguito all'introduzione di alimenti in purea, in particolare la frutta e le sostanze dolci. Si osservano diarrea, dolore addominale e rallentamento della crescita. Alcuni pazienti possono giungere all'attenzione del medico durante la tarda adolescenza o addirittura in età adulta, ma un'anamnesi accurata appurerà che in realtà questi sintomi si erano già manifestati in precedenza. La **diagnosi** richiede l'idrolisi acida delle feci per le sostanze riducenti, in quanto la saccarasi è uno zucchero non riducente. In alternativa, si può procedere al breath test all'idrogeno o alla valutazione enzimatica di un campione bioptico del tenue.

Il fulcro del **trattamento** è una dieta di restrizione che escluda in via definitiva tutti gli alimenti contenenti saccarosio. La sostituzione enzimatica con un enzima di lievito purificato, la saccarosidasi, costituisce un'integrazione molto utile.

MALASSORBIMENTO DI GLUCOSIO-GALATTOSIO. Sono state identificate più di 30 mutazioni differenti del gene cotrasportatore del sodio/glucosio (*SGLT1*). Queste mutazioni causano una rara malattia autosomica recessiva del sistema di cotrasporto intestinale del glucosio e galattosio/Na^+, che provoca diarrea osmotica. Poiché la maggior parte degli zuccheri presenti nella dieta è polisaccaride o disaccaride con frazioni di glucosio o galattosio, la diarrea deriva dall'ingestione di glucosio, latte materno o anche latti formulati tradizionali. La disidratazione e l'acidosi possono essere gravi e addirittura letali. Le feci sono acide e contengono zuccheri. I soggetti che presentano questo difetto hanno un assorbimento del fruttosio normale e anche la struttura e la funzionalità dell'intestino tenue sono normali sotto tutti gli altri aspetti. La glicosuria intermittente o permanente dopo un digiuno o in seguito a un carico di glucosio è un dato frequente, causato dalla presenza di un difetto del trasporto anche a livello renale. Il reperto di sostanze riducenti positive nelle feci acquose e di una leggera glicosuria, nonostante i livelli degli zuccheri ematici siano bassi, è un indice fortemente indicativo di un malassorbimento di glucosio-galattosio. Quest'ultimo può essere identificato facilmente per mezzo del breath test all'idrogeno. È opportuno effettuare il primo test con una dose di 0,5 g/kg di glucosio; se necessario, si potrà eseguire un secondo test somministrandone 2 g/kg. L'idrogeno nel respiro aumenterà di più di 20 ppm. Una biopsia dell'intestino tenue può essere utile per appurare se l'architettura dei villi e le attività della disaccaridasi sono normali. L'identificazione di mutazioni dell'*SGLT1* rende possibile l'esecuzione di uno screening prenatale nelle famiglie a rischio di questa malattia.

Il **trattamento** consiste in una rigorosa restrizione del glucosio e del galattosio. Il fruttosio, l'unico carboidrato che si può assumere in sicurezza, andrebbe aggiunto al latte formulato privo di carboidrati a una concentrazione del 6-8%. L'assunzione di questo tipo di latte fa sì che la diarrea cessi immediatamente. Sebbene il difetto sia permanente, in un periodo successivo della vita il paziente riuscirà a tollerare quantità limitate di glucosio (negli amidi) o di saccarosio.

INSUFFICIENZA PANCREATICA ESOCRINA. Le patologie associate a insufficienza pancreatica esocrina saranno discusse nel Capitolo 346. La fibrosi cistica è la più comune malattia congenita associata all'insufficienza pancreatica esocrina. La seconda causa di insufficienza pancreatica in età pediatrica è la sindrome di Shwachman, peraltro rara. Altre malattie rare che provocano insufficienza pancreatica esocrina sono la sindrome di Johannson-Blizzard (steatorrea grave, aplasia delle pinne nasali, sordità, ipotiroidismo, difetti del cuoio capelluto), la sindrome di Pearson, che colpisce il midollo osseo (anemia sideroblastica, neutropenia di grado variabile, trombocitopenia), e la carenza di enzimi pancreatici isolati (lipasi, colipasi, tripsinogeno, amilasi, lipasi-colipasi).

L'APECED (*Autoimmune PolyEndocrinopathy-Candidiasis-Ectodermal Dystrophy*, poliendocrinopatia autoimmune-candidosi-distrofia ectodermica) è una rara malattia autosomica recessiva. La candidosi mucocutanea cronica è associata a insufficienza delle paratiroidi, della corteccia surrenale, delle cellule β pancreatiche, delle gonadi, delle cellule parietali gastriche e della tiroide. A questa patologia sono state associate anche insufficienza pancreatica e steatorrea.

335.10 • Patologie epatiche e biliari che provocano malassorbimento

Nell'epatopatia colestatica il malassorbimento lipidico deriva da una ridotta concentrazione di acidi biliari nel duodeno a cui può essere associata una disfunzione pancreatica esocrina. Oltre a presentare steatorrea, i pazienti affetti da queste malattie presentano carenze di vitamine liposolubili (A, D, E e K). Nella maggior parte dei casi i bambini affetti da epatopatia cronica hanno un aumentato fabbisogno energetico cui non possono tuttavia far fronte a causa dell'anoressia associata alla malattia. Scopo del trattamento nutrizionale di questi piccoli pazienti è fornire un adeguato apporto di calorie e azoto tramite l'integrazione di sostanze liposolubili. Può inoltre essere necessario somministrare integratori anche per via enterale o mediante PEG (*Percutaneous Endoscopic Gastrostomy*, gastrostomia endoscopica percutanea).

La **carenza di vitamina E** in pazienti affetti da colestasi epatica cronica è associata a sindrome neurologica progressiva con neuropatia periferica (sotto forma di perdita dei riflessi tendinei profondi e oftalmoplegia), atassia cerebellare e disfunzione posteriore della colonna. Se si interviene precocemente la patologia è almeno in parte reversibile, mentre può risultare irreversibile in caso di intervento tardivo. Può essere difficile identificare la carenza di vitamina E perché la presenza di elevati livelli ematici di lipidi, nell'epatopatia colestatica, può tradursi in livelli falsamente elevati di vitamina E sierica. Di conseguenza, è importante misurare il rapporto tra vitamina E sierica e lipidi sierici totali; i valori normali per i pazienti di età <12 anni sono >0,6, e per i pazienti di età ≥12 anni, <0,8. La malattia neurologica si può prevenire somministrando per os un preparato di vitamina E idrosolubile ([TPGS, *d-α-Tocopherol Polyethylene Glycol 1000 Succinate*, D-α tocoferil polietilenglicole 1000 succinato) in dosi da 25-50 UI/die nei neonati e 1 UI/kg/die nei bambini.

La **malattia ossea metabolica** si può sviluppare in seguito a carenza di vitamina D. La somministrazione contemporanea di vitamina D e un preparato di vitamina E idrosolubile (TPGS) potenzia l'assorbimento di vitamina D. Nella prima infanzia si somministra vitamina D_3 per os alla dose di 1000 UI/kg/24 h. Dopo un mese, se i livelli sierici di 25-idrossivitamina D dovessero risultare bassi, si mescola la stessa dose di vitamina D per via orale con TPGS. In seguito bisognerà monitorare la 25-idrossivitamina D ogni 3 mesi, adattando le dosi al bisogno.

La **carenza di vitamina K** si può verificare in conseguenza di colestasi epatica e scarso assorbimento dei grassi. Il primo segno può essere costituito da facilità alle ecchimosi. Nella colestasi epatica del neonato si può manifestare coagulopatia dovuta a carenza di vitamina K. Sarà quindi opportuno determinare di routine il tempo di protrombina (un test più sensibile) e il tempo di tromboplastina parziale, in modo da monitorare la carenza di vitamina K. La somministrazione di integratori di vitamina K dovrebbe essere una terapia di routine in tutti i casi di colestasi epatica in età pediatrica.

La **carenza di vitamina A** è associata a cecità notturna, xeroftalmia e aumentata mortalità in caso di morbillo. Occorre monitorare i livelli sierici di vitamina A e valutare se ricorrere o meno a una supplementazione.

335.11 • Difetti di assorbimento o di trasporto

DIFETTI DEL TRASPORTO DI AMINOACIDI. In molte alterazioni congenite specifiche del trasporto di aminoacidi si può manifestare un difetto del trasporto intestinale di queste sostanze. Almeno tre vettori specifici dell'intestino tenue sembrano essere coinvolti nel trasporto attivo di aminoacidi. L'assorbimento degli aminoacidi nella mucosa intestinale risulta difettoso nella **cistinuria**, anche se questi pazienti non presentano sintomi gastrointestinali. Nella **malattia di Hartnup**, il malassorbimento degli aminoacidi neutri, tra cui il triptofano, provoca atassia, deterioramento cellulare, un'eruzione simile alla pellagra e talvolta diarrea. Le manifestazioni cliniche sono dovute al malassorbimento del triptofano con conseguente carenza di nicotinamide. La somministrazione orale di nicotinamide produce un notevole miglioramento clinico. Il **malassorbimento della metionina** è associato a episodi diarroici nei bambini ritardati di carnagione chiara che presentino urine di odore dolciastro e contenenti un eccesso di acido β-idrossibutirrico. Nella **sindrome del pannolino blu** è invece difettoso l'assorbimento del triptofano.

MALATTIE DELL'ASSORBIMENTO DI VITAMINE E MINERALI.

Malassorbimento di vitamina B_{12}. La carenza di vitamina B_{12} può dipendere da diminuita assunzione (lattanti allattati al seno da madri con carenza non diagnosticata di vitamina B_{12} a causa di diete vegetariane strette), anomalie dell'assorbimento (resezione gastrica, anemia perniciosa autoimmune con diminuzione del fattore intrinseco), competizione per la vitamina B_{12} nell'intestino (eccessiva proliferazione batterica), disturbo dell'assorbimento in tutta la superficie ileale (morbo di Crohn, sprue tropicale), oppure da errori innati del trasporto e del metabolismo della vitamina B_{12}.

Diversi difetti congeniti rari possono influire sull'assimilazione della vitamina B_{12}. Queste patologie sono molto meno comuni della carenza di vitamina B_{12} nella dieta o del malassorbimento secondario a resezione ileale terminale o dovuto a una disfunzione. Nell'**anemia perniciosa giovanile**, la produzione di fattore intrinseco nello stomaco è carente: ne consegue un malassorbimento di vitamina B_{12}, che a sua volta provoca un'anemia megaloblastica e insufficienza di crescita. La struttura e la funzionalità gastrica sono per altri versi normali. La **carenza di transcobalamina II** è un difetto ereditario di una proteina necessaria per il trasporto intestinale di vitamina B_{12}, che dà luogo ad anemia megaloblastica grave, diarrea e vomito. La **sindrome di Imerslund** si verifica in pazienti con assorbimento ileale di vitamina B_{12} difettoso; per altri versi la struttura e la funzionalità ileali sono normali. L'anemia megaloblastica, che si sviluppa verso la fine del primo anno, di norma è associata a proteinuria.

Il **trattamento** di queste malattie consiste nella somministrazione di vitamina B_{12} tramite iniezione: 1000 μg due volte alla settimana per le carenze di transcobalamina II e 100 μg al mese per le altre. Quando i pazienti sono in remissione ematologica in seguito a terapia intramuscolare con vitamina B_{12}, si può passare alla vitamina B_{12} **intranasale** (500 μg a dosi fisse una volta alla settimana).

Malassorbimento congenito dell'acido folico. Il malassorbimento congenito isolato dei folati è stato descritto in meno di 20 pazienti. Può essere conseguenza di un difetto selettivo del vettore dei folati nella barriera intestinale ed ematoencefalica. Gli studi sull'ereditarietà fanno pensare a malattia autosomica recessiva. L'anemia megaloblastica grave si osserva a partire dal 3° mese. I sintomi neurologici comprendono atassia, convulsioni, ritardo mentale e calcificazioni intracraniche, mentre quelli gastrointestinali, che si possono presentare nella prima settimana di vita, includono ulcerazioni orali, diarrea e mancato accrescimento. La diagnosi si desume da un mancato aumento dei folati nel liquido cerebrospinale o nel siero in seguito a test da carico con acido folico orale (5 mg). Un **trattamento** precoce e aggressivo con acido folinico parenterale è fondamentale e dovrebbe essere guidato da una documentazione di miglioramento dei livelli di folati nel liquor. La terapia successiva, volta a mantenere stabili i livelli di folati nel siero, negli eritrociti nel liquido cerebrospinale, richiede la somministrazione di forti dosi orali (fino a 100 mg/die) di acido folico, folinico o metiltetraidrofolico.

Rachitismo dipendente dalla vitamina D. In questa malattia autosomica recessiva, un difetto specifico del metabolismo della vitamina D causa malassorbimento di calcio. La funzionalità intestinale è per altri versi normale (vedi Capitolo 48).

Diarrea clorodisperdente. Si tratta di una rara malattia ereditaria recessiva, provocata da mutazioni di un gene posto sul cromosoma 7, principalmente nota come adenoma *DRA* (*DownRegulated in Adenoma*). Il meccanismo del trasporto del cloruro/bicarbonato nell'ileo distale e nel colon è difettoso, il che provoca grave diarrea acquosa, a partire dalla nascita. È normale riscontrare un polidramnios materno. La diarrea acquosa porta a disidratazione e a gravi squilibri elettrolitici consistente in ipokaliemia, ipocloremia e alcalosi, un quadro quanto mai insolito nei bambini affetti da diarrea cronica. Gli altri aspetti dell'assorbimento intestinale sono normali. Le feci hanno un contenuto di cloruro superiore alla somma di sodio/potassio (125-150 mEq/L). Il **trattamento** non ha effetto sulla diarrea, ma riduce le complicanze. La modalità migliore per compensare tutte le perdite di elettroliti e acqua è per via endovenosa, mentre le soluzioni orali sono tollerate in genere dopo il primo mese di vita. Se si effettua una diagnosi precoce nel periodo neonatale e si inizia immediatamente una terapia adeguata il bambino affetto da questa patologia avrà una crescita e uno sviluppo perfetti.

Diarrea da sodio congenita. La base evidente di questa rara sindrome è un difetto dello scambio sodio-idrogeno nell'intestino tenue e nel colon. Come avviene nella diarrea da cloro congenita, il paziente fin dalla nascita presenta una diarrea secretiva acquosa profusa e un'anamnesi di polidramnios materno. Al contrario della diarrea da cloro congenita, tuttavia, questa patologia è caratterizzata da acidosi e una concentrazione di cloro nelle feci inferiore rispetto a quella di sodio (addirittura 145 mEq/L). Il **trattamento** con soluzione da idratazione orale è efficace per garantire una crescita normale.

Ipomagnesiemia primitiva. Questo difetto specifico del trasporto intestinale del magnesio provoca grave ipomagnesiemia e tetano ipocalcemico secondario nel periodo neonatale. Gli altri aspetti della funzionalità intestinale sono normali. Questi esiti si compensano con forti integrazioni di magnesio, che dovranno proseguire indefinitamente.

ACRODERMATITE ENTEROPATICA (VEDI CAPITOLO 670). Nei primi mesi di vita questa forma si presenta con eruzioni attorno alle giunzioni mucocutanee e alle estremità, alopecia, diarrea cronica e talvolta steatorrea. La concentrazione sierica di zinco e l'attività della fosfatasi alcalina sono basse. La carenza di zinco acquisita si presenta in modo analogo. I campioni bioptici della mucosa intestinale mostrano inclusioni di cellule di Paneth che scompaiono con la terapia. L'analisi delle concentrazioni di zinco nel latte materno può contribuire a differenziare l'acrodermatite enteropatica dalla carenza di zinco acquisita, in cui tali valori sono bassi. Il **trattamento** con solfato di zinco orale, 1-2 mg di zinco elementare/kg/24 h, porta a una rapida guarigione delle lesioni cutanee e a miglioramento della diarrea nell'acrodermatite enteropatica.

SINDROME DI MENKES (CAPELLI TORTI) (VEDI CAPITOLO 661). La malattia di Menkes è una patologia del metabolismo del rame, letale, multisistemica, legata al cromosoma X, dominata da sintomi neurodegenerativi e problemi del tessuto connettivo. Il gene di Menkes si trova sul braccio lungo del cromosoma X in Xq13.3 e il suo prodotto è un'adenosintrifosfatasi alcalina tipo P (ATPasi). È presente un diffuso difetto del trasporto cellulare del rame a carico sia dell'intestino sia di altri tessuti. Il rame ingerito si accumula nell'intestino e il suo assorbimento è difettoso. La malattia di Menkes è caratterizzata da ritardo di crescita, anomalie dei capelli, degenerazione cerebellare, grave vasculopatia, fratture e morte precoce. I livelli sierici di rame e ceruloplasmina sono bassi, mentre aumenta il contenuto di rame nelle cellule. Il **trattamento** attualmente accettato consiste nella somministrazione di rame parenterale; sono pochi i pazienti privi di complicanze neurologiche.

DIFETTI DELL'ASSORBIMENTO INDOTTI DA FARMACI. Alcuni farmaci hanno un impatto diffuso sull'epitelio del tenue. Il **metotrexato** può provocare un arresto della mitosi degli enterociti e di conseguenza lesioni della mucosa; anche forti dosi di neomicina influiscono sulla struttura della mucosa. La **sulfasalazina** interferisce con l'assorbimento dell'acido folico. La **colestiramina** si lega ai sali biliari e al calcio nel lume intestinale causando ipocalcemia e steatorrea. La **fenitoina** interferisce con l'assorbimento del calcio e può causare rachitismo.

Sindromi da malassorbimento

Branski D, Lerner A, Lebenthal E: Chronic diarrhea and malabsorption. *Pediatr Clin North Am* 1996;43:307–331.
Couper R, Oliver M: Pancreatic function tests. In Walker WA, Goulet O, Kleinman RE. et al (editors): *Pediatric Gastrointestinal Disease,* 4th ed. Hamilton, Ontario, BC, Decker, 2004, pp 1816–1829.
Khouri M, Huang G, Shiau Y: Sudan stain of fecal fat: New insight into an old test. *Gastroenterology* 1989;96:421–427.
Kleinman RE, Klish W, Lebenthal E, et al: Role of juice carbohydrate malabsorption in chronic nonspecific diarrhea in children. *J Pediatr* 1992; 120:825–829.
Riby JE, Fujisawa T, Kretchmer N: Fructose absorption. *Am J Clin Nutr* 1993;58:748S–753S.
Riddlesberger MM: Evaluation of the gastrointestinal tract in the child: CT, MRI, and isotopic studies. *Pediatr Clin North Am* 1988;35:281–310.
Tabrez S, Roberts IM: Malabsorption and malnutrition. *Prim Care* 2001; 28:505–522.
Wang J, Cortina G, Wu SV, et al: Mutant neurogenin-3 in congenital malabsorptive diarrhea. *N Engl J Med* 2006;355:270–280.
Weaver LT, Amarri S, Swart GR: 13C mixed triglyceride breath test. *Gut* 1998;43:S13–S19.

Celiachia

Barker CC, Mitton C, Jevon G, Mock T: Can tissue transglutaminase antibody titers replace small-bowel biopsy to diagnose celiac disease in select pediatric populations? *Pediatrics* 2005;115:1341–1346.
Bibgley PJ, Williams AJK, Norcross AJ, et al: Undiagnosed coeliac disease at age seven: Population based prospective birth cohort study. *Br Med J* 2004;328:322–324.
Bostwick H, Berezin S, Halata M, et al: Celiac disease presenting with microcephaly. *J Pediatr* 2001;138:589–592.
Branski D, Fasano A, Troncone R: Latest developments in the pathogenesis and treatment of celiac disease. *J Pediatr* 2006;149:295–300.
Catassi C, Bearzi I, Holmes GK: Association of celiac disease and intestinal lymphomas and other cancers. *Gastroenterology* 2005;128:S79–S86.
Ciclitira PJ, King AL, Fraser JS: AGA technical review on celiac sprue. American Gastroenterological Association. *Gastroenterology* 2001;120:1526–1540.
Farrell R, Kelly C: Current concepts: Celiac sprue. *N Engl J Med* 2002; 346:180–188.
Green PHR, Fleischauer AT, Bhagat G, et al: Risk of malignancy in patients with celiac disease. *Am J Med* 2003;115:191–195.
Hill ID, Dirks MH, Liptak GS, et al: Guideline for the diagnosis and treatment of celiac disease in children: Recommendation of the North American Society for Pediatric Gastroenterology, Hepatology and Nutrition. *J Pediatr Gastroenterol Nutr* 2005;40:1–19.
Hoffenberg E, Haas J, Drescher A, et al: A trial of oats in children with newly diagnosed celiac disease. *J Pediatr* 2000;137:361–366.
Labate A, Gambardella A, Messina D, et al: Silent celiac disease in patients with childhood localization-related epilepsies. *Epilepsia* 2001;42:1153–1155.
Larizza D, Calcaterra V, De Giacomo C, et al: Celiac disease in children with autoimmune thyroid disease. *J Pediatr* 2001;139:738–740.
Liu E, Li M, Bao F, et al: Need for quantitative assessment of transglutaminase autoantibodies for celiac disease in screening-identified children. *J Pediatr* 2005;146:494–499.
[No authors listed]: Revised criteria for diagnosis of coeliac disease. Report of Working Group of European Society of Paediatric Gastroenterology and Nutrition. *Arch Dis Child* 1990;65:909–911.
Norris JM, Barriga K, Hoffenberg EJ, et al: Risk of celiac disease autoimmunity and timing of gluten introduction in the diet of infants at increased risk of disease. *JAMA* 2005;293:2342–2351.
Pellechia M: Idiopathic cerebellar ataxia associated with celiac disease: Lack of distinctive neurological features. *J Neurol Neurosurg Psychiatry* 1999; 66:32–35.

Pueschel S, Romano C, Failla P, et al: A prevalence study of celiac disease in persons with Down's syndrome residing in the United States of America. *Acta Paediatr* 1999;88:953–956.
Swigonski NL, Kuhlenschmidt HL, Bull MJ, et al: Screening for celiac disease in asymptomatic children with Down syndrome: cost-effectiveness of preventing lymphoma. *Pediatrics* 2006;118:594–602.
Van Rijn JCW, Grate FK, Oostdijk W, et al: Short stature and the probability of coeliac disease, in the absence of gastrointestinal symptoms. *Arch Dis Child* 2004;9:882–883.
Watson PGP: Diagnosis of coeliac disease. *Br Med J* 2005;330:739–740.
Zachor DA, Mroczek-Musulman E, Brown P: Prevalence of celiac disease in Down syndrome in the United States. *J Pediatr Gastroenterol Nutr* 2000;31:275–279.
Zelnick N, Pacht A, Obeid R, Lerner A: Range of neurologic disorders in patients with celiac disease. *Pediatrics* 2004;113:1672–1676.

Difetti congeniti della mucosa intestinale

Damen G, de Klerk H, Huijmans J, et al: Gastrointestinal and other clinical manifestations in 17 children with congenital disorders of glycosylation type Ia, Ib, and Ic. *J Pediatr Gastroenterol Nutr* 2004;38:282–287.
Kennea N, Norbury R, Anderson G, Tekay A: Congenital microvillous inclusion disease presenting as antenatal bowel obstruction. *Ultrasound Obstet Gynecol* 2001;17:172–174.
Murch SH, Winyard PJ, Koletko S, et al: Congenital enterocyte heparan sulphate deficiency with massive albumin loss, secretory diarrhea, and malnutrition. *Lancet* 1996;347:1299–1301.
Patey N, Scoazec JY, Cuenod-Jabri B, et al: Distribution of cell adhesion molecules in infants with intestinal epithelial dysplasia (tufting enteropathy). *Gastroenterology* 1997;113:833–843.
Reifen RM, Cutz E, Griffiths AM, et al: Tufting enteropathy: A newly recognized clinicopathological entity associated with refractory diarrhea in infants. *J Pediatr Gastroenterol Nutr* 1994;18:379–385.
Walker-Smith J, Murch S: Miscellaneous disorders of the small intestine. In Walker-Smith J and Murch S (editors): *Diseases of the Small Intestine in Childhood,* 4th ed. Oxford, Isis Medical Media, 1999, pp 380–381.

Enteropatia proteinodisperdente

Cheong JL, Cowan FM, Modi N. Gastrointestinal manifestations of postnatal cytomegalovirus infection in infants admitted to a neonatal intensive care unit over a five-year period. *Arch Dis Child Fetal Neonatal Ed* 2004; 89:F367–F369.
Salvia G, Cascioli C, Ciccimarra F, et al: A case of protein losing enteropathy caused by intestinal lymphangiectasia in a preterm infant. *Pediatrics* 2001;107:416–417.
Schmider A, Henrich W, Reles A, et al: Isolated fetal ascites caused by primary lymphangiectasia: A case report. *Am J Obstet Gynecol* 2001;184: 227–228.
Vardy PA, Lebenthal E, Shwachman H: Intestinal lymphangiectasis: A reappraisal. *Pediatrics* 1975;55:842–851.

Infezioni che provocano malassorbimento

Farthing MJG: The molecular pathogenesis of giardiasis. *J Pediatr Gastroenterol Nutr* 1997;24:79–88.
Liebman WM, Thaler MM, Dehorimier A, et al: Intractable diarrhea of infancy due to intestinal coccidiosis. *Gastroenterology* 1980;78:579–584.
Sood M, Booth I: Is prolonged rotavirus infection a common cause of protracted diarrhoea? *Arch Dis Child* 1999;80:309–310.

Eccessiva proliferazione batterica

Lichtman S: Bacterial overgrowth. In Walker WA, Goulet O, Kleinman RE, et al (editors): *Pediatric Gastrointestinal Disease,* 4th ed. Hamilton, Ontario, BC, Decker, 2004, pp 691–701.
Ruckebusch Y: Development of digestive motor patterns during perinatal life: Mechanism and significance. *J Pediatr Gastroenterol Nutr* 1986;5:523–536.

Sprue tropicale

Gray G: Tropical sprue: Chronic intestinal malabsorption in the tropics. In Blaser M, Smith P, Pavdin J, et al (editors): *Infections of the Gastrointestinal Tract.* New York, Raven Press, 1995, pp 333–341.

Malattie da immunodeficienza

Kotler DP, Francisco A, Clayton F, et al: Small intestinal injury and parasitic diseases in AIDS. *Ann Intern Med* 1990;113:444–449.
Weikel CS, Gaynes BN, Roche JK: Diarrheal disease in the immunocompromised host. In Guerrant R (editor): *Baillière's Clinical Tropical Medicine and Communicable Diseases,* vol 3. London, Baillière Tindall, 1988, p 401.
Winter H, Chang TI: Gastrointestinal and nutritional problems in children with immunodeficiency and AIDS. *Pediatr Clin North Am* 1996;43: 573–590.
Woroniecka M, Ballow M: Office evaluation of children with recurrent infection. *Pediatr Clin North Am* 2000;47:1211–1224.
Yolken RH, Hart W, Oung I, et al: Gastrointestinal dysfunction and disaccharide intolerance in children infected with human immunodeficiency virus. *J Pediatr* 1991;118:359–363.

Enteropatia autoimmune

Bousvaros A, Leichtner AM, Book L, et al: Treatment of pediatric autoimmune enteropathy with tacrolimus (FK506). *Gastroenterology* 1996;111: 237–243.
Russo PA, Brochu P, Seidman EG, Roy CC: Autoimmune enteropathy. *Pediatr Dev Pathol* 1999;2:65–71.

Malattia immunoproliferativa da intestino corto

Akbulut H, Soykan I, Yakaryilmaz F, et al: Five-year results of the treatment of 23 patients with immunoproliferative small intestinal disease: A Turkish experience. *Cancer* 1997;80:8–14.

Sindrome dell'intestino corto

Andorsky D, Lund D, Lillehei C, et al: Nutritional and other postoperative management of neonates with short bowel syndrome correlates with outcomes. *J Pediatr* 2001;139:27–31.
Bines J, Francis D, Hill D, et al: Reducing parenteral requirement in children with short bowel syndrome: Impact of an amino acid–based complete infant formula. *J Pediatr Gastroenterol Nutr* 1998;26:123–128.
Fishbein TM, Matsumoto CS: Intestinal replacement therapy: timing and indications for referral of patients to an intestinal rehabilitation and transplant program. *Gastroenterology* 2006;130:5147–5151.
Kauffman SS, Atkinson JB, Bianchi A, et al: Indications for pediatric intestinal transplantation: A position paper of the American Society of Transplantation. *Pediatr Transplant* 2001;5:80–87.
Kaufman SS, Loseke CA, Lupo JV, et al: Influence of bacterial overgrowth and intestinal inflammation on duration of parenteral nutrition in children with short bowel syndrome. *J Pediatr* 1997;131:356–361.
Kocoshis S: Evolving concepts and improving prospects for neonates with short bowel syndrome. *J Pediatr* 2001;139:5–7.
Sigalet DL: Short bowel syndrome in infants and children: An overview. *Semin Pediatr Surg* 2001;10:49–55.
Taylor SF, Sondheimer JM, Sokol RJ, et al: Noninfectious colitis associated with short gut syndrome in infants. *J Pediatr* 1991;119:24–28.
Vanderhoof JA, Young RJ, Thompson JS: New and emerging therapies for short bowel syndrome in children. *Paediatr Drugs* 2003;5:525–531.

Apparato digerente in condizioni di malnutrizione cronica

Durie PR, Forstner GG, Gaskin KJ, et al: Elevated serum immunoreactive pancreatic cationic trypsinogen in acute malnutrition: Evidence of pancreatic damage. *J Pediatr* 1985;106:233–238.
Romer H, Urbach R, Gomez MA, et al: Moderate and severe protein-energy malnutrition in childhood: Effects on jejunal mucosal morphology and disaccharidase activities. *J Pediatr Gastroenterol Nutr* 1983;2:459–464.

Carenze di disaccaridasi

Ament ME, Perera DR, Esther L: Sucrase-isomaltase deficiency: A frequently misdiagnosed disease. *J Pediatr* 1973;83:721–727.
Flatz G: The genetics of lactose digestion in humans. *Adv Hum Genet* 1987;16:1–77.
Heyman MB, Committee on Nutrition: Lactose intolerance in infants, children, and adolescents. *Pediatrics* 2006;118:1279–1286.
Newton T, Murphy MS, Booth IW: Glucose polymer as a cause of protracted diarrhea in infants with unsuspected congenital sucrase-isomaltase deficiency. *J Pediatr* 1996;128:753–756.
Ouwendijk J, Moolenaar CE, Peters WJ, et al: Congenital sucrase-isomaltase deficiency: Identification of a glutamine to proline substitution that leads to a transport block of sucrase-isomaltase in a pre-Golgi compartment. *J Clin Invest* 1996;97:633–641.

Treem WR: Congenital sucrase-isomaltase deficiency. *J Pediatr Gastroenterol Nutr* 1995;21:1–14.
Treem WR, McAdams L, Stanford L, et al: Sacrosidase therapy for congenital sucrase-isomaltase deficiency. *J Pediatr Gastroenterol Nutr* 1999;28:137–142.

Sindrome da ingestione di succhi

Hourihane JO, Rolles CJ: Morbidity from excessive intake of high energy fluids: The "squash drinking syndrome." *Arch Dis Child* 1995;72:141–143.

Malassorbimento di glucosio-galattosio

Evans L, Grasset E, Heyman M, et al: Congenital selective malabsorption of glucose and galactose. *J Pediatr Gastroenterol Nutr* 1985;4:878–886.
Fairclough PD, Clark ML, Dawson AM, et al: Absorption of glucose and maltose in congenital glucose-galactose malabsorption. *Pediatr Res* 1978;12:1112–1114.
Martin MG, Turk E, Lostao MP: Defects in Na^+/glucose cotransporter *(SGLT1)* trafficking and function cause glucose-galactose malabsorption. *Nat Genet* 1996;12:216–220.

Patologie epatiche e biliari

Argao EA, Heubi JE: Fat-soluble vitamin deficiency in infants and children. *Curr Opin Pediatr* 1993;5:562–566.
Hadorn B, Hess J, Troesch V, et al: Role of bile acids in the activation of trypsinogen by enterokinase: Disturbance of trypsinogen activation in patients with intrahepatic biliary atresia. *Gastroenterology* 1974;66:548–555.
Kooh SW, Jones G, Reilly BJ, et al: Pathogenesis of rickets in chronic hepatobiliary disease in children. *J Pediatr* 1979;94:870–874.

Malassorbimento primitivo degli acidi biliari

Heubi JE, Balistreri WF, Fondacaro JD, et al: Primary bile acid malabsorption: Defective in vitro ileal active bile acid transport. *Gastroenterology* 1982;83:804–811.
Oelkers P, Kirby LC, Heubi JE, et al: Primary bile acid malabsorption caused by mutations in the ileal sodium-dependent bile acid transporter gene *(SLC10A2)*. *J Clin Invest* 1997;99:1880–1887.

Abetalipoproteinemia, ipobetalipoproteinemia e malattia di Anderson

Levy E, Chouraqui JP, Ray CC: Steatorrhea and disorders of chylomicron synthesis and secretion. *Pediatr Clin North Am* 1988;35:53–67.
Narchi H, Amr SS, Mathew PM, El Jamil MR: Rickets as an unusual initial presentation of abetalipoproteinemia and hypobetalipoproteinemia. *J Pediatr Endocrinol Metab* 2001;14:329–333.
Rader DJ, Brewer B: Abetalipoproteinemia: New insights into lipoprotein assembly and vitamin E metabolism from a rare genetic disease. *JAMA* 1993;270:865–869.
Scott BB, Miller JP, Losowsky MS: Hypobetalipoproteinemia: A variant of the Bassen-Kornzweig syndrome. *Gut* 1979;20:163–168.

Malassorbimento della vitamina B_{12}

Hall CA: Congenital disorders of vitamin B12 transport and their contribution to concepts. *Gastroenterology* 1973;65:684–686.
Hitzig WH, Dohmann V, Pluss HJ, et al: Hereditary transcobalamin II deficiency: Clinical findings in a new family. *J Pediatr* 1974;85:622–628.
Imerslund O: Idiopathic chronic megaloblastic anaemia in children. *Acta Paediatr Suppl* 1960;49:1–115.
MacKenzie IL, Donaldson RM, Trier JS, et al: Ileal mucosa in familial selective vitamin B12 malabsorption. *N Engl J Med* 1972;286:1021–1025.

Malassorbimento dei folati

Malatack J, Moran M, Moughan B: Isolated congenital malabsorption of folic acid in a male infant: Insights into treatment and mechanism of defect. *Pediatrics* 1999;104:1133–1137.
Urbach J, Abrahamov A, Grossowicz N: Congenital isolated folic acid malabsorption. *Arch Dis Child* 1987;62:78–80.

Diarrea cloro-disperdente

Holmberg C, Perheentupa J, Launiala K, et al: Congenital chloride diarrhea. *Arch Dis Child* 1977;52:255–267.
Kere J, Lohi H, Höglund P: Genetic disorders of membrane transport III. Congenital chloride diarrhea. *Am J Physiol* 1999;276:G7–G13.

Diarrea congenita da sodio

Booth IW, Murer H, Strange G, et al: Defective jejunal brush border Na^+/H^+ exchange: A cause of congenital secretory diarrhea. *Lancet* 1985;1:1066–1069.
Holmberg C, Perheentupa J: Congenital Na^+ diarrhea: A new type of secretory diarrhea. *J Pediatr* 1985;106:56–61.

Ipokaliemia primitiva

Romero R, Meacham LR, Winn KT: Isolated magnesium malabsorption in a 10-year-old boy. *Am J Gastroenterol* 1996;91:611–613.
Stromme JH, Nesbakken R, Normann T, et al: Familial hypomagnesemia. *Acta Paediatr Scand* 1969;58:433–444.

Acrodermatite enteropatica

Bohane TD, Cutz E, Hamilton JR, et al: Acrodermatitis enteropathica, zinc and the Paneth cell. *Gastroenterology* 1977;73:587–592.
Moynahan EJ: Acrodermatitis enteropathica: A lethal inherited human zinc-deficiency disorder. *Lancet* 1974;2:399–400.

Sindrome di Menkes

Danks DM: Of mice and men, metals and mutations. *J Med Genet* 1986;23:99–106.
Jankov RP, Boerkoel CF, Hellman J, et al: Lethal neonatal Menkes' disease with severe vasculopathy and fractures. *Acta Paediatr* 1998;87:1297–1300.
Kodama H, Murata Y, Kobayashi M: Clinical manifestation and treatment of Menkes disease and its variants. *Pediatr Int* 1999;41:423–429.

Malassorbimento indotto da farmaci

Franklin JL, Rosenberg HH: Impaired folic acid absorption in inflammatory bowel disease: Effects of salicylazosulfapyridine (Azulfidine). *Gastroenterology* 1973;64:517–525.
Morijiri Y, Sato T: Factors causing rickets in institutionalised handicapped children on anticonvulsant therapy. *Arch Dis Child* 1981;56:446–449.
Rogers AL, Vloedman DA, Bloom EC, et al: Neomycin-induced steatorrhea. *JAMA* 1966;197:185–190.
Trier JS: Morphologic alterations induced by methotrexate in the mucosa of human proximal intestine: I. Serial observations by light microscopy. *Gastroenterology* 1962;42:295–305.

Capitolo 336 ■ Trapianto dell'intestino in età pediatrica Jorges Reyes

La pratica del trapianto intestinale è stata incentivata dall'introduzione del **tacrolimus** nel 1989, che ha portato a una sopravvivenza significativamente migliore sia del paziente sia dell'organo trapiantato nei casi di trapianto epatico in età pediatrica. Il successo di questo farmaco è dovuto non soltanto al controllo del rigetto, ma anche alla possibilità di sospendere la terapia immunosoppressiva a lungo termine riducendo quindi le infezioni e la tossicità da farmaci. L'evoluzione delle tecniche di **espianto multiorgano** ha reso possibile trapiantare l'intestino in associazione con altri organi intraddominali, in particolare il fegato. Il fatto che il fegato possa proteggere l'intestino da rigetto è stata suggerita da precedenti combinazioni di utilizzo contemporaneo di fegato e di altri organi, come il rene. Queste procedure si sono potute applicare a una popolazione molto varia di riceventi, il che ha permesso di eliminare quasi completamente il più complesso trapianto multiorgano, facilitando così l'assistenza perioperatoria. Uno sviluppo di fondamentale importanza è stato la dimostrazione dell'interazione (ospite vs. trapianto e trapianto vs. ospite) tra gli immunociti del ricevente e del donatore (permessa dall'allotrapianto) che, sotto la copertura dell'immunosoppressione, permette diversi gradi di accettazione dell'organo trapiantato e la riduzione al minimo della terapia farmacologica.

INDICAZIONI AL TRAPIANTO INTESTINALE

I successi del trapianto intestinale hanno fatto sì che si affermasse il concetto di **insufficienza intestinale**, per indicare i casi in cui i pazienti che hanno perduto la capacità di mantenere il supporto nutrizionale tramite l'intestino dipendono in permanenza dalla nutrizione parenterale completa (TPN, *Total Parenteral Nutrition*). La maggior parte di questi pazienti ha l'intestino corto a causa di un'alterazione funzionale dovuta a carenza congenita o a una patologia acquisita (vedi Capitolo 335.7), mentre in altri l'origine dell'insufficienza intestinale è l'alterazione funzionale della motilità o dell'assorbimento (Tab. 336-1). È raro che vengano sottoposti a trapianto intestinale i pazienti con neoplasie benigne, i quali possono essere sottoposti o meno a TPN. Tuttavia, a differenza di un'insufficienza a carico di altri tipi di organi, l'insufficienza intestinale è una sindrome di complicanze "satellitari" tra cui scarsità degli accessi venosi, infezioni potenzialmente fatali e colestasi epatica indotta dalla TPN. I pazienti che sviluppano queste complicanze presentano una mortalità nel primo anno del 70% circa e dovrebbero essere candidati al trapianto intestinale.

Scarsità degli accessi venosi. La somministrazione della TPN richiede l'inserimento di un catetere venoso centrale; i siti facilmente accessibili sono solo sei (le vene giugulari interne bilaterali, le succlavie e le iliache). La perdita di accessi venosi si verifica generalmente quando s'instaura una sepsi ricorrente da catetere; la perdita del 50% di questi siti mette a rischio il paziente, che non può essere trattato con TPN.

INFEZIONI POTENZIALMENTE FATALI. Anche se tali infezioni sono spesso correlate alla presenza di un catetere, dato che in questi casi l'intestino è corto, il problema può essere associato a una motilità anomala dell'intestino residuo (il che può provocare uno svuotamento sia ritardato sia troppo rapido) con vari gradi di eccessiva proliferazione batterica e possibile traslocazione batterica in seguito a perdita di funzionalità della barriera intestinale e/o perdita dell'immunità intestinale. Ciò può provocare epatopatia colestatica, insufficienza organica multisistemica e metastasi dei focolai infettivi nei polmoni, nei reni, nel fegato e nel cervello.

EPATOPATIE. Si sa che l'epatopatia colestatica indotta dalla TPN dipende dagli effetti tossici della TPN sugli epatociti. Gli effetti sul fegato includono la trasformazione dei grassi, steatoepatite e necrosi e poi colestasi. Lo sviluppo di ittero clinico (bilirubina totale >3 mg/dL) è un significativo fattore di rischio per un risultato insoddisfacente, poiché queste variazioni portano allo sviluppo di gastroenteropatia portale ipertensiva, ipersplenismo, coagulopatia ed emorragie incontrollabili.

INTERVENTO DI TRAPIANTO

SELEZIONE DEL DONATORE. I trapianti intestinali si ottengono di solito da donatori di cui è stata dichiarata la morte cerebrale, emodinamicamente stabili, ABO-identici, che non abbiano mostrato evidenze cliniche o di laboratorio suggestive di ischemia intraddominale. I criteri d'esclusione comprendono un'anamnesi di malignità, come pure evidenze d'infezione intraddominale, ma non le infezioni batteriche o virali sistemiche. La preparazione del donatore consiste semplicemente nella somministrazione di antibiotici sistemici ed enterici. La profilassi della malattia del trapianto contro l'ospite (GVHD, *Graft vs Host Disease*), che consiste nel pretrattamento del trapianto tramite irraggiamento o il ricorso ad anticorpi antilinfocitari monoclonali, è cambiata nel tempo e varia a seconda del centro che l'esegue.

TIPI DI TRAPIANTI INTESTINALI. Gli allotrapianti intestinali sono utilizzati sotto varie forme, come trapianto isolato dell'intestino tenue oppure come trapianto composito, comprendente anche il fegato, il duodeno, il pancreas e/o lo stomaco, laddove le combinazioni più comuni sono i trapianti di fegato e intestino e i trapianti multiviscerali. L'approvvigionamento di questi svariati tipi di trapianto si accentra soprattutto sul mantenimento dei vasi arteriosi delle arterie celiaca e /o mesenterica superiore, come pure sul mantenimento di un appropriato deflusso venoso che, nei trapianti compositi, dovrebbe comprendere la vena mesenterica superiore o le vene epatiche. Le varie eziologie che fanno precipitare l'insufficienza intestinale hanno stimolato lo sviluppo degli allotrapianti, dove gli organi interessati si possono rimuovere o lasciare in sede in base alle necessità cliniche del singolo paziente. I trapianti compositi di maggiore entità devono conservare le arterie celiache e mesenteriche superiori; tra questi si annoverano i trapianti multiviscerali, i trapianti fegato/intestino tenue e i trapianti multiviscerali modificati che non coinvolgono il fegato, ma l'intero apparato gastrointestinale, stomaco compreso. Nel trapianto intestinale isolato vengono conservate la vena e l'arteria mesenterica superiore; si possono mantenere anche i vasi afferenti del pancreas, qualora questo organo sia destinato a un altro ricevente. L'organo destinato a un determinato ricevente deve essere dissezionato *in situ* e rimosso dopo l'arresto cardiaco del donatore, sottoponendo gli organi a una procedura ECCS (*Emergency Core Cooling System*) tramite infusione di una soluzione conservante (Fig. 336-1).

INTERVENTI SUL RICEVENTE. Il trapianto intestinale è una sfida tecnica notevole, la cui entità tuttavia varia in base sia al grado di malattia del paziente (per es. se il bambino presenta epatopatia e ipertensione portale) sia all'anamnesi di interventi addominali precedenti. Un allotrapianto intestinale isolato implica l'esposizione del basso addome, dell'aorta infrarenale e della vena cava inferiore. Il posizionamento di trapianti vascolari delle arterie e delle vene iliache del donatore permette l'arterializzazione e il drenaggio venoso del trapianto intestinale. In pazienti che hanno conservato l'intestino e che subiscono un'enterectomia al momento del trapianto si può ricorrere all'utilizzo delle vene mesenteriche superiori native.

L'inserimento di un trapianto composito più grande (fegato più intestino o trapianti multiviscerali) richiede un'operazione di maggiori proporzioni, con una dissezione più estesa. In modo analogo, l'aorta infrarenale viene esposta, in vista del trapianto di

TABELLA 336-1. Cause dell'insufficienza intestinale che necessita di trapianto

INTESTINO CORTO	DISMOTILITÀ INTESTINALE	DISFUNZIONE ENTEROCITARIA	TUMORI
Enterocolite necrotizzante	Pseudo-ostruzione intestinale	Malattia da inclusione dei microvilli	Poliposi familiare
Gastroschisi	Aganglionosi intestinale (malattia di Hirschsprung)	Enteropatia a ciuffi (*tufting enteropathy*)	Pseudotumore infiammatorio
Volvolo		Enteropatia autoimmune	
Atresia intestinale			
Trauma			

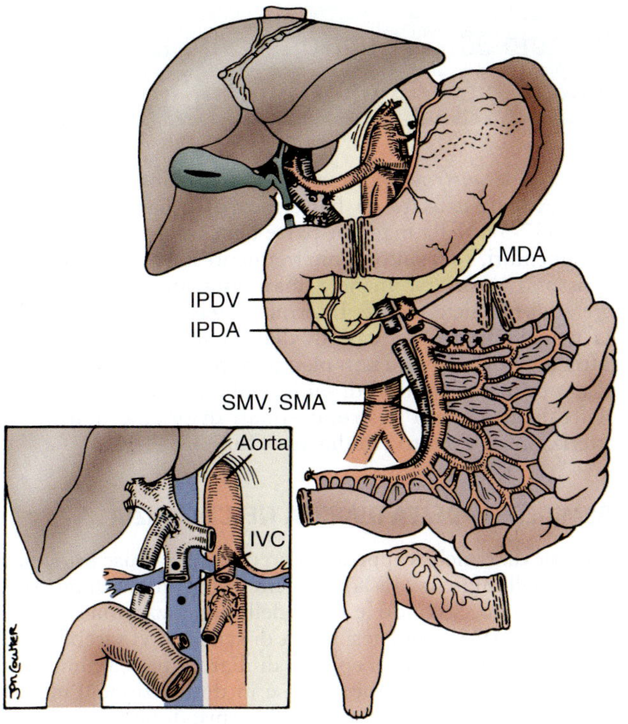

Figura 336-1. I vari organi addominali possono essere dissezionati *in situ*, in modo da fornire trapianti isolati o compositi adeguati ai bisogni dei singoli pazienti. È possibile separare l'intestino dal pancreas, preservando l'arteria (IPDA, *Inferior Pancreatico-Duodenal Artery*) e la vena (IPDV, *Inferior Pancreatico-Duodenal Vein*) pancreatico-duodenale inferiore. Il ricorso a trapianti vascolari dal donatore consente di collegarsi al peduncolo mesenterico superiore (SMA e SMV), all'aorta e alla vena cava inferiore (IVC) o alla vena porta (*riquadro più piccolo*). (Riprodotta per gentile concessione di Abu-Elmagd K, Fung J, Bueno J, et al: Logistics e technique for procurement of intestinal, pancreatic e hepatic transplants from the same donor. *Ann Surg* 2000;232:680-697.)

un dotto arterioso (aorta toracica del donatore), per l'arterializzazione del trapianto. Quando l'operazione implica la rimozione del fegato, il drenaggio venoso si ottiene attraverso il mantenimento delle vene epatiche, adattate in modo da creare un unico condotto per l'anastomosi del fegato allotrapiantato.

Si eseguono anastomosi intestinali all'intestino distale e prossimale nativo lasciando una stomia addominale dell'ileo allotrapiantato distale; quest'ultima in seguito sarà usata per i controlli post-trapianto di routine tramite endoscopia e biopsia, e infine richiusa 3-6 mesi dopo il trapianto (Fig. 336-2).

TRATTAMENTO POSTOPERATORIO

IMMUNOSOPPRESSIONE. L'immunosoppressione per il trapianto intestinale si è basata in passato sull'induzione con tacrolimus e corticosteroidi. Questa procedura richiedeva alti livelli di tacrolimus (nella gamma nefrotossica) e, nonostante all'inizio il tasso di successo fosse alto, in seguito si registravano percentuali di rigetto >80%, infezioni e tossicità tardiva da farmaci. Ciò comportava una graduale perdita dei pazienti e degli organi trapiantati nel giro di 10 anni. I protocolli successivi si sono basati sull'aggiunta di altri agenti, quali l'azatioprina, la ciclofosfamide, il micofenolato mofetil, la rapamicina, e sull'induzione con un antagonista anticorpale dell'interleuchina 2 (IL-2), portando a una minore incidenza della gravità del rigetto; tuttavia, la prerogativa di ridurre l'immunosoppressione più tardivamente non permetteva la stabilizzazione della sopravvivenza a lungo termine. L'introduzione del pretrattamento con anticorpi antilinfocitari e l'eliminazione della terapia con ormoni steroidei, nel ricevente, ha migliorato la sopravvivenza dei trapianti, con diminuzione significativa dell'incidenza dei rigetti e delle infezioni. Ciò ha permesso di ridurre il trattamento farmacologico immunosoppressivo nel giro di 3 mesi e ha portato a una diminuzione dei casi di tossicità da farmaci.

VALUTAZIONE DELL'ALLOTRAPIANTO. Non esistono strumenti di laboratorio semplici che consentano la valutazione dell'allotrapianto intestinale. In passato la regola aurea della diagnosi di rigetto di un allotrapianto intestinale era costituita da sorveglianza endoscopica seriale e biopsie attraverso l'ileostomia dell'allotrapianto. Segni e sintomi clinici di rigetto o infezione dell'allotrapianto possono sovrapporsi l'un l'altro, provocando una diarrea a rapida insorgenza o un ileo completo con sindromi di pesudo-ostruzione o emorragia gastrointestinale. Qualunque variazione dello status clinico dovrebbe richiedere un'accurata valutazione del rigetto tramite biopsie endoscopiche, come pure una valutazione delle infezioni opportunistiche, del malassorbimento e di altre infezioni enteriche.

La diagnosi di rigetto acuto si basa sul reperto della distruzione delle cellule epiteliali delle cripte a partire dall'apoptosi, in associazione con un infiltrato linfocitario misto. Questi risultati istologici possono essere o meno correlati a evidenze endoscopiche di una lesione, che può variare da un eritema diffuso e da friabilità fino alla formazione di ulcerazioni e, in caso di rigetto grave, esfoliazione della mucosa intestinale. Il rigetto cronico dell'allotrapianto si può diagnosticare soltanto attraverso una campionatura a pieno spessore dell'intestino che mostri la tipica vasculopatia, la quale può esitare in un'ischemia progressiva dell'allotrapianto.

RIGETTO. I tassi di rigetto di un allotrapianto intestinale sono significativamente più alti di quelli di un altro organo, pari a

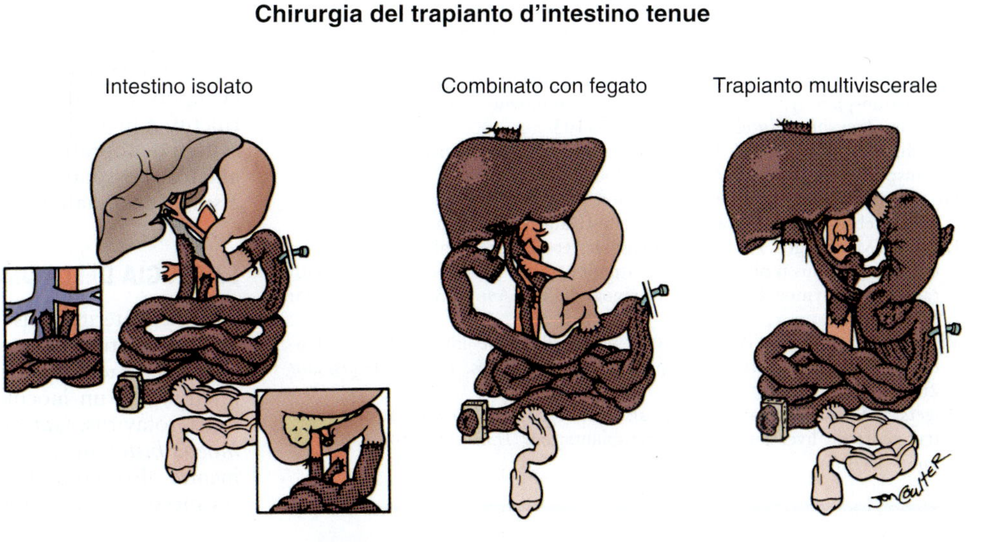

Figura 336-2. Le tre procedure fondamentali di trapianto intestinale (l'organo trapiantato è *ombreggiato*). Con il trapianto isolato di intestino, il deflusso venoso può portare alla vena porta (*figura principale*), alla vena cava inferiore (*riquadro più piccolo a sinistra*) o alla vena mesenterica superiore del ricevente (*riquadro più piccolo a destra*). Nel caso di trapianti compositi che includano il fegato, si ottiene l'arterializzazione a partire dall'aorta con un drenaggio venoso che vada dal fegato trapiantato alla vena cava inferiore del ricevente.

circa l'80-90%, e un rigetto grave che richieda il ricorso a preparati anticorpali antilinfocitari può arrivare al 30%. I regimi farmacologici tipici e il ricorso agli inibitori anticorpali dell'IL-2 hanno prodotto una significativa diminuzione dei tassi di rigetto; ciononostante, l'entità dell'immunosoppressione continua a essere incompatibile con il miglioramento della sopravvivenza a lungo termine sia del malato sia dell'organo trapiantato. Tassi di rigetto del 40% si possono raggiungere somministrando globulina antilinfocitaria. Questi protocolli inducono livelli variabili di "tolleranza" e quindi finiscono per ridurre al minimo l'immunosoppressione, diminuendo anche il rischio di tossicità da farmaci e infezioni.

INFEZIONI. Le infezioni più comuni in seguito a trapianto intestinale sono dovute alla necessità di utilizzare costantemente un catetere venoso fino a un anno dopo il trapianto. Le infezioni insorte come conseguenza di un trattamento farmacologico immunosoppressivo sono dovute al Cytomegalovirus (CMV) [22% d'incidenza], al virus di Epstein-Barr (EBV, *Epstein-Barr Virus*) [21% d'incidenza] e agli adenovirus, responsabili di enterite (40% d'incidenza). Un trattamento risolutivo di queste infezioni virali si raggiunge grazie all'identificazione precoce e alla terapia preventiva, sia nel CMV sia nell'EBV, prima che si sviluppi un'infezione grave e potenzialmente fatale. Questa procedura ha migliorato i tassi di guarigione da CMV, eliminando la mortalità nella popolazione pediatrica (vedi Capitoli 177, 251 e 252).

RISULTATI. Il trapianto intestinale è la cura standard per i bambini affetti da insufficienza intestinale e che soffrono delle complicanze della nutrizione parenterale totale. I dati dell'International Transplant Registry, e quelli dei singoli centri, hanno documentato miglioramenti graduali nella sopravvivenza a breve e a lungo termine relativamente ai trapianti effettuati dal 1990 al 2004. Negli Stati Uniti, Medicare riconosce il trapianto intestinale come terapia clinica standard. Attualmente i tassi di sopravvivenza dei trapianti intestinali sono pari al 97% e all'89% rispettivamente a 1 anno e a 3 anni. Si spera che, grazie alle strategie attualmente in uso, la sopravvivenza a lungo termine si stabilizzi, come sta avvenendo con i trapianti di altri organi.

Abu-Elmagd K, Fung J, Bueno J, et al: Logistics and technique for procurement of intestinal, pancreatic and hepatic grafts from the same donor. *Ann Surg* 2000;232:680–697.

Bond G, Reyes J, Mazariegos G, et al: The impact of positive T-cell lymphocytotoxic crossmatch on intestinal allograft rejection and survival. *Transplant Proc* 2000;32:1197–1198.

Fishbein TW, Matsumoto CS: Intestinal replacement therapy: timing and indications for referral of patients to an intestinal rehabilitation and transplant program. *Gastroenterology* 2006;130:S147–S151.

Grant D, Abu-Elmagd K, Reyes J, et al: 2003 report of the Intestine Transplant Registry: A new era has dawned. *Ann Surg* 2005;241:607–613.

Green M, Reyes J, Webber S, Rowe D: The role of antiviral and immunoglobulin therapy in the prevention of Epstein-Barr virus infection and post-transplant lymphoproliferative disease following solid organ transplantation. *Transplant Infect Dis* 2001;3:97–103.

Kauffman SS, Atkinson JB, Bianchi A, et al: Indications for pediatric intestinal transplantation. *Pediatr Transplant* 2001;5:80–87.

Organ Procurement and Transplantation Network data (liver, kidney, and lung) website: http://www.optn.org/latestData/rptData.asp.

Reyes J, Mazariegos GV, Abu-Elmagd K, et al: Intestinal transplantation under tacrolimus monotherapy after perioperative lymphoid depletion with rabbit anti-thymocyte globulin (thymoglobulin). *Am J Transplant* 2005;5:1430–1436.

Reyes J, Mazariegos GV, Bond GM, et al: Pediatric intestinal transplantation: Historical notes, principles and controversies. *Pediatr Transplant* 2002;6:193–207.

Rogers J, Bueno J, Shapiro R, et al: Results of simultaneous and sequential pediatric liver and kidney transplantation. *Transplantation* 2001;72:1666–1670.

Capitolo 337 ■ Gastroenterite acuta nei bambini

Zulfiqar Ahmed Bhutta

Con il termine *gastroenterite* ci si riferisce a infezioni del tratto gastrointestinale causate da batteri, virus e parassiti (Tabb. da 337-1 a 337-3). Nella maggior parte dei casi si tratta di tossinfezioni alimentari, i cui sintomi più frequenti sono diarrea e vomito, che possono associarsi anche a manifestazioni sistemiche come dolore addominale e febbre. Il termine "**gastroenterite**" raggruppa la maggior parte dei casi di diarrea infettiva. L'espressione **malattia diarroica** è usata con maggiore frequenza per indicare la diarrea infettiva in contesti di sanità pubblica, anche se sono noti diversi tipi di disturbi gastrointestinali di origine non infettiva caratterizzati da vomito e/o diarrea (Tab. 337-4).

EPIDEMIOLOGIA DELLA DIARREA NELL'INFANZIA

Le malattie diarroiche rappresentano una delle cause principali di morbilità nell'infanzia (18%), con circa 1,8 milioni di morti ogni anno nel mondo. Secondo le stime dell'Organizzazione Mondiale della Sanità (OMS), nei Paesi in via di sviluppo vi sarebbero ogni anno più di 700 milioni di episodi di diarrea nei bambini sotto i 5 anni di età. Mentre la mortalità è in diminuzione, l'incidenza complessiva resta invariata a circa 3,2 episodi per ogni bambino all'anno (Fig. 337-1). Negli Stati Uniti, ogni anno la gastroenterite determina circa 1,5 milioni di visite mediche, 200 000 ricoveri in ospedale e 300 decessi.

A livello mondiale, nel 1999 è stato stimato che nei bambini sotto i 5 anni di età le infezioni causate da *Shigella* determinino 600 000 decessi all'anno, o da un quarto a un terzo della mortalità da diarrea, sempre in questa fascia di età. I tassi di ospedalizzazione e di mortalità causati dall'infezione da *Shigella*, in particolare da *S. dysenteriae* di tipo 1, la forma più severa di shigellosi, sono in diminuzione; i dati più recenti indicano circa 160 000 decessi. Le infezioni da rotavirus (la forma virale più diffusa di gastroenterite nei bambini) è responsabile di almeno il 35% degli episodi di diarrea acquosa severa e potenzialmente fatale, con circa 500 000 decessi all'anno causati da infezioni da rotavirus in tutto il mondo.

La riduzione della mortalità dovuta a malattia diarroica, cui peraltro non corrisponde una diminuzione significativa dell'incidenza, è da imputarsi ai progressi compiuti nel trattamento della diarrea e nell'alimentazione dei lattanti e dei bambini. Tali interventi comprendono la reidratazione orale a domicilio e in ospedale e il miglioramento dell'approccio nutrizionale per il bambino che presenta diarrea.

La persistenza di elevati tassi di incidenza di diarrea tra i bambini piccoli, nonostante gli sforzi fatti per prevenirla, rappresenta un argomento di grande interesse. Esistono poche informazioni sugli effetti a lungo termine della malattia diarroica, in particolare sulla diarrea persistente o prolungata e sulla malnutrizione. Si tratta di una patologia che può avere conseguenze rilevanti sullo sviluppo psicomotorio e cognitivo dei bambini piccoli: episodi ripetuti e precoci di diarrea nell'infanzia nel periodo critico dello sviluppo, soprattutto se associati a malnutrizione, coinfezioni e anemia, possono avere effetti a lungo termine sull'accrescimento e sulla funzionalità fisica e cognitiva.

EZIOLOGIA DELLA DIARREA

La gastroenterite, causata da infezioni orofecali oppure da ingestione di alimenti o acqua contaminati, si associa a povertà, condizioni igieniche scadenti e bassi indici di sviluppo. Gli enteropatogeni infettivi con un inoculo ridotto (*Shigella*, *Escherichia coli*, norovirus, rotavirus, *Giardia lamblia*, *Cryptosporidium parvum*, *Entamoeba histolytica*) vengono trasmessi per contatto interpersonale, mentre altri, come l'agente causale del colera, sono solitamente trasmessi mediante alimenti o acqua contaminati (vedi Tabb. da

TABELLA 337-1. Tossinfezioni alimentari (batteriche)

CAUSA	PERIODO DI INCUBAZIONE	SEGNI E SINTOMI	DURATA DELLA MALATTIA	ALIMENTI ASSOCIATI	ESAMI DI LABORATORIO	TRATTAMENTO
Bacillus anthracis	Da 2 giorni a settimane	Nausea, vomito, malessere, diarrea ematica, dolore addominale acuto	Alcune settimane	Carne contaminata, cotta in modo insufficiente	Sangue	La penicillina è la prima scelta per l'antrace gastrointestinale acquisito in modo naturale. La ciprofloxacina è la seconda opzione
Bacillus cereus (enterotossina preformata)	1-6 ore	Rapido esordio di nausea severa e vomito, con o senza diarrea	24 ore	Riso o carne cotti o fritti, conservati in frigo in modo improprio	Di norma, diagnosi clinica. I laboratori clinici non identificano di routine questo microrganismo. Se indicato, inviare i campioni di feci e dei cibi a laboratori di riferimento per la coltura e l'identificazione della tossina	Terapia di supporto
Bacillus cereus (tossina diarroica)	10-16 ore	Crampi addominali, diarrea acquosa, nausea	24-48 ore	Carne, stufati, sugo di carne, crema alla vaniglia	Non necessari, perché la tossinfezione si autolimita (nell'epidemia, esame delle feci e dei cibi per la ricerca della tossina)	Terapia di supporto
Brucella abortus, B. melitensis e *B. suis*	7-21 giorni	Febbre, brividi, sudorazione, debolezza, cefalea, dolore muscolare e articolare, diarrea, feci ematiche, durante la fase acuta	Alcune settimane	Latte vaccino, formaggio di capra da latte non pastorizzato, carni contaminate	Emocoltura e sierologia positive	Fase acuta: rifampicina e doxiciclina ogni giorno per ≥6 settimane. Le infezioni complicate richiedono una terapia combinata con rifampicina, tetraciclina e aminoglicosidico
Campylobacter jejuni	2-5 giorni	Diarrea, crampi, febbre e vomito; la diarrea può essere sanguinolenta	2-10 giorni	Pollame crudo o poco cotto, latte non pastorizzato, acqua contaminata	Coprocoltura di routine; il *Campylobacter* per crescere richiede speciali terreni di coltura e un'incubazione a 42 °C	Terapia di supporto. Nei casi severi, gli antibiotici come l'eritromicina o i chinolonici possono essere indicati nelle fasi iniziali della malattia diarroica. La sindrome di Guillain-Barré può essere una sequela
Clostridium botulinum – bambini e adulti (tossina preformata)	12-72 ore	Vomito, diarrea, visione indistinta, diplopia, disfagia e debolezza muscolare progressiva	Variabile (da giorni a mesi). Possibili complicanze sono insufficienza respiratoria e decesso	Alimenti a basso contenuto acido inscatolati in casa, alimenti confezionati, pesce inscatolato in casa o fermentato, oli alle erbe, patate cotte in fogli di alluminio, crema di formaggio, aglio confezionato, cibi mantenuti a lungo al caldo (per es. nel forno)	Feci, siero e cibi possono essere esaminati per la ricerca della tossina. Le feci e gli alimenti possono inoltre essere sottoposti a coltura per la ricerca del microrganismo. Questi test possono essere eseguiti nei laboratori dei Dipartimenti di sanità e dei CDC	Terapia di supporto. L'antitossina botulinica è utile se somministrata precocemente nel corso della malattia. Contattare il Dipartimento di sanità pubblica degli Stati Uniti al numero (700) 488-7100, disponibile 24 ore su 24
Clostridium botulinum – lattanti	3-30 giorni	Nei lattanti sotto i 12 mesi, sonnolenza, debolezza, nutrizione ridotta, stipsi, ipotonia, scarso controllo della testa, riduzione dei riflessi di protezione delle via aeree e di suzione	Variabile	Miele, verdure e frutta in barattolo confezionate in casa, sciroppo di mais	Feci, siero e cibi possono essere esaminati per la ricerca della tossina. Le feci e gli alimenti possono inoltre essere sottoposte a coltura per la ricerca del microrganismo. Questi test possono essere eseguiti nei laboratori dei Dipartimenti di sanità e dei CDC	Terapia di supporto. Per ottenere negli Stati Uniti l'immunoglobulina contro il botulismo rivolgersi all'Infant Botulism Program, Health and Human Services , California (510-540-2646); tale tossina non è indicata per i lattanti
Clostridium perfringens tossina	8-16 ore	Diarrea acquosa, nausea, crampi addominali; la febbre è rara	24-48 ore	Carne, pollame, salse, alimenti essiccati o precotti, cibi trattati con tempi e/o temperature inadeguati	Le feci possono essere esaminate per la ricerca dell'enterotossina e la coprocoltura è utile per la ricerca del microrganismi. Poiché il *Clostridium perfringens* può essere trovato nelle feci, occorre effettuare colture quantitative	Terapia di supporto. Gli antibiotici non sono indicati
E. coli enteroemorragico (EHEC) incluso *E. coli* 0157:H7 e altre tossine *Shiga*-like prodotte da *E. coli* (STEC)	1-8 gg	Diarrea severa, spesso sanguinolenta, dolore addominale e vomito. Di solito febbricola o assenza di febbre. Più frequente nei bambini di età <4 anni	5-10 giorni	Manzo poco cotto (soprattutto hamburger), latte non pastorizzato e succhi di frutta, frutta e verdura cruda (per es. germogli), insaccati (raramente) e acqua contaminata	Coprocoltura; l'*E. coli* 0157:H7 richiede un terreno di coltura speciale per crescere. Se si sospetta questo batterio bisogna richiedere un esame specifico. Il test per la tossina *Shiga*-like può essere effettuato con il kit commerciale; i positivi devono essere inviati ai laboratori di sanità pubblica per la conferma e la sierotipizzazione	Terapia di supporto; attento monitoraggio della funzionalità renale, dell'emoglobina e delle piastrine. L'infezione da *E. coli* 0157:HT è associata anche alla sindrome emolitico-uremica (HUS), con complicanze a lungo termine. Gli studi indicano che l'uso degli antibiotici può promuovere la HUS
E. coli enterotossigeno (ETEC)	1-3 giorni	Diarrea acquosa, crampi addominali e talvolta vomito	Da 3 a >7 giorni	Acqua e alimenti contaminati con feci umane	Coprocoltura. L'ETEC necessita di speciali tecniche laboratoristiche per l'identificazione. Se si sospetta questo batterio, occorre richiedere test specifici	Terapia di supporto. Gli antibiotici di rado sono necessari, salvo che nei casi gravi. Tra quelli raccomandati, TMP-SMX e chinolonici
Listeria monocytogenes	9-48 ore per i sintomi gastrointestinali; 2-6 settimane per la malattia invasiva	Febbre, dolori muscolari, nausea o diarrea. In gravidanza si può avere una lieve sintomatologia simil-febbrile e l'infezione può portare a parto prematuro o a morte del neonato. Gli anziani e gli immunocompromessi possono presentare batteriemia o meningite	Variabile	Formaggi freschi morbidi, latte non adeguatamente pastorizzato, carne pronta, piatti di gastronomia, hot dog	Emocoltura e coltura del liquor. Considerare un tampone fecale, in casi asintomatici; di conseguenza, la coprocoltura non è utile. Gli anticorpi anti-listerolisina O possono essere utili per identificare retrospettivamente l'epidemia	Terapia di supporto e antibiotici; per la malattia invasiva sono indicati ampicillina, penicillina o TMP-SMX per via endovenosa
	Alla nascita e durante l'infanzia	I neonati infettati dalla madre sono a rischio per sepsi o meningite				

TABELLA 337-1. Tossinfezioni alimentari (batteriche) – *continua*

Salmonella spp.	1-3 giorni	Diarrea, febbre, dolore addominale, crampi, vomito. *S. typhi* e *paratyphi* sono gli agenti causali del tifo, malattia con esordio insidioso caratterizzato da febbre, cefalea, stipsi, malessere, brividi e mialgia; la diarrea non è frequente e il vomito di solito non è severo	4-7 giorni	Uova contaminate, pollame, latte non pastorizzato o succhi di frutta, formaggio, frutta e verdura cruda contaminate (germogli di erba medica, meloni). Le epidemie di *S. typhi* sono spesso legate a contaminazione fecale dell'acqua o dei cibi venduti per strada	Coprocoltura di routine	Terapia di sostegno. Tranne che nella *S. typhi* e *paratyphi*, gli antibiotici non sono utilizzati, a meno che non sia in atto una diffusione extraintestinale o non se ne presenti il rischio. Se indicato, valutare ampicillina, gentamicina, TMP-SMX o i chinoloni. Esiste un vaccino per *S. typhi*
Shigella spp.	24-48 ore	Crampi addominali, febbre e diarrea. Le feci possono contenere sangue e muco	4-7 giorni	Alimenti o acqua contaminati da materia fecale umana. Solitamente diffusione interpersonale, trasmissione orofecale. Cibi pronti manipolati da personale infetto, per es. verdura cruda, insalate, sandwich	Coprocoltura di routine	Terapia di sostegno. Se il microrganismo è suscettibile, è raccomandato TMP-SMX negli Stati Uniti. L'acido nalidico o altri chinoloni possono essere indicati se il microrganismo è resistente, soprattutto nei Paesi in via di sviluppo
Staphylococcus aureus (enterotossina preformata)	1-6 ore	Esordio improvviso di nausea severa e vomito. Crampi addominali. Possono essere presenti diarrea e febbre	24-48 ore	Carne non tenuta in frigo o mal conservata, patate e uova, insalate, dolci alla crema	Normalmente, diagnosi clinica. Feci, vomito e alimenti possono essere esaminati per la ricerca della tossina ed è indicata la coltura	Terapia di sostegno
Vibrio cholerae (tossina)	24-72 ore	Profusa diarrea acquosa e vomito che può condurre a disidratazione severa e morte nel giro di poche ore	3-7 giorni. Causa disidratazione che mette a rischio la vita	Acqua, pesce, molluschi contaminati, alimenti venduti per strada, per es. in America Latina o Asia	Coprocoltura; il *Vibrio cholerae* per crescere richiede terreni di coltura speciali. Se si sospetta questo batterio occorre richiedere il test specifico	Terapia di sostegno. Trattamento aggressivo con reidratazione orale o ev. Se il colera è confermato, si raccomandano tetraciclina o doxiciclina per gli adulti, TMP-SMX per i bambini (<8 anni)
Vibrio parahaemolyticus	2-48 ore	Diarrea acquosa, crampi addominali, nausea, vomito	2-5 giorni	Pesce e molluschi poco cotti o crudi	Coprocoltura; il *Vibrio parahaemoliticus* per crescere richiede terreni di coltura speciali. Se si sospetta questo batterio occorre richiedere il test specifico	Terapia di sostegno. Nei casi gravi sono raccomandati gli antibiotici: tetraciclina, doxiciclina, gentamicina e cefotaxima
Vibrio vulnificus	1-7 giorni	Vomito, diarrea, dolore addominale, batteriemia e infezioni delle ferite. Più frequente nei pazienti immunocompromessi o in quelli con epatopatia cronica (si presenta con lesioni cutanee bollose). In questi soggetti può essere fatale	2-8 giorni	Molluschi poco cotti o crudi, soprattutto ostriche, altri pesci contaminati e spesso ferite venute a contatto con acqua di mare	Coprocoltura, emocoltura e coltura delle ferite. Il *Vibrio vulnificus* per crescere necessita di terreni di coltura speciali. Se si sospetta questo batterio, occorre richiedere il test specifico	Terapia di sostegno e antibiotici; sono raccomandate tetraciclina, doxiciclina e ceftadizima
Yersinia enterocolitica e *Y. pseudotuberculosis*	24-48 ore	Sintomi simili a quelli dell'appendicite (diarrea e vomito, febbre e dolore addominale); colpisce essenzialmente i bambini più grandi e i giovani adulti. Può esserci rash scarlattiforme o eritema nodoso con *Y. pseudotuberculosis*	1-3 settimane; di solito si autolimita	Maiale poco cotto, latte non pastorizzato, tofu, acqua contaminata. L'infezione si verifica nei lattanti quando coloro che li accudiscono hanno manipolato le interiora di maiale	Coprocoltura, emocoltura e coltura del vomito. La *Yersinia* per crescere richiede terreni di coltura speciali. Se si sospetta questo batterio, occorre richiedere il test specifico. La sierologia è disponibile per la ricerca e in laboratori di riferimento	Terapia di sostegno. In caso di setticemia o malattia invasiva, terapia antibiotica con con gentamicina o cefotaxima (sono efficaci anche doxiciclina e ciprofloxacina)

CDC, Centers for Disease Control and Prevention; TMP-SMX, trimetoprim/sulfametoxazolo.
Da Department of Health and Human Services, Centers for Disease Control and Prevention: Diagnosis and management of foodbourne illnesses. *MMWR* 2004:53:7-9.

337-1 a 337-3). Negli Stati Uniti, i rotavirus e i norovirus (piccoli microrganismi rotondi come il virus Norwalk-like e i calicivirus) rappresentano i virus più comuni, seguiti dagli adenovirus enterici e dagli astrovirus (vedi Tab. 337-2). Negli Stati Uniti, le epidemie di diarrea da intossicazione alimentare in genere sono causate da *Salmonella* e *Campylobacter* spp., seguiti nell'ordine da *Shigella*, *Cryptosporidium*, *E. coli* 0157.H7, *Yersinia*, *Listeria*, *Vibrio* e *Cyclospora* spp., tutti agenti causali molto meno frequenti. Nei Paesi in via di sviluppo, i patogeni più frequentemente coinvolti nello sviluppo della diarrea sono *Salmonella*, *Shigella* e, soprattutto, diversi *E. coli* (vedi Tab. 337-1). Il *Clostridium difficile* (mediante la produzione di tossine) è responsabile di una forma associata a terapia antibiotica e a colite pseudomembranosa, sebbene nei bambini molti casi di diarrea associata ad antibioticoterapia non siano imputabili a questo microrganismo. Nell'adulto, la colite emorragica associata agli antibiotici non dovuta a *C. difficile* è imputabile a citotossine prodotte dalla *Klebsiella oxytoca*.

Nei Paesi industrializzati, gli episodi di diarrea infettiva possono svilupparsi in seguito a esposizione stagionale a microrganismi come i rotavirus o a esposizione a patogeni in condizioni di stretto contatto (per es. negli asili). Nelle aree in via di sviluppo, i bambini possono contrarre infezioni a opera di differenti tipi di batteri e parassiti, mentre sia i bambini dei Paesi in via di sviluppo sia i bambini dei Paesi sviluppati sono infettati da rotavirus e da altri virus enteropatogeni come *G. lamblia* e *C. parvum* tra il primo e il quinto anno di vita.

PATOGENESI DELLA DIARREA INFETTIVA

La patogenesi e la gravità della malattia batterica dipendono dai microrganismi responsabili (*Staphylococcus aureus*, *Bacillus cereus*): se hanno tossine preformate, se producono tossine o se si moltiplicano negli alimenti. Gli enteropatogeni possono scatenare una risposta di tipo tanto infiammatorio quanto non infiammatorio a livello della mucosa intestinale.

Gli enteropatogeni provocano una **diarrea non infiammatoria** mediante la produzione di **enterotossine** a opera di alcuni batteri, la distruzione dei villi enterocitari imputabile ad al-

TABELLA 337-2. Tossinfezioni alimentari (virali)

EZIOLOGIA	PERIODO DI INCUBAZIONE	SEGNI E SINTOMI	DURATA DELLA MALATTIA	ALIMENTI ASSOCIATI	ESAMI DI LABORATORIO	TRATTAMENTO
Epatite A	In media 28 giorni (15-50 giorni)	Diarrea, urine scure, ittero, sintomi simil-influenzali, per es. febbre, cefalea, nausea e dolore addominale	Variabile da 2 settimane a 3 mesi	Frutti di mare provenienti da acque contaminate, prodotti crudi, acqua da bere contaminata alla fonte, cibi non cotti e cotti che non sono stati riscaldati dopo contatto con personale infetto	Aumento ALT, bilirubina. Positività a IgM e anticorpi anti-epatite A	Terapia di supporto. Prevenzione con vaccinazione
Norovirus (e altri calicivirus)	12-48 ore	Nausea, vomito, crampi addominali, diarrea, febbre, mialgia, talora cefalea. La diarrea è più frequente negli adulti, mentre il vomito prevale tra i bambini. È possibile una secrezione asintomatica, prolungata	12-60 ore	Frutti di mare, cibi contaminati da materia fecale, cibi pronti toccati da personale infetto (insalate, sandwich, ghiaccio, biscotti, frutta)	RT-PCR e ME di routine su campione di feci fresche non conservate: diagnosi clinica, coltura batterica negativa. Le feci sono negative per leucociti	Terapia di supporto come reidratazione. Misure di igiene
Rotavirus	1-3 giorni	Vomito, diarrea acquosa, febbricola. Può esserci temporanea intolleranza al lattosio. Lattanti, bambini, anziani e soggetti immunocompromessi sono particolarmente vulnerabili	4-8 giorni	Cibi contaminati da materia fecale, cibi pronti toccati da personale infetto (insalate, frutta)	Identificazione del virus nelle feci mediante immunoassay	Terapia di supporto. La diarrea severa può rendere necessaria la reintegrazione di liquidi ed elettroliti
Altri agenti virali (astrovirus, adenovirus, parvovirus)	10-70 ore	Nausea, vomito, diarrea, malessere, dolore addominale, cefalea, febbre	2-9 giorni	Cibi contaminati da materia fecale, cibi pronti toccati da personale infetto. Alcuni frutti di mare	Identificazione del virus nel campione delle feci appena emesse. Il kit ELISA in commercio non è disponibile per adenovirus e astrovirus	Terapia di supporto; solitamente la tossinfezione è lieve, autolimitante. Misure di igiene

ALT, alanina aminotransferasi; ELISA (*Enzyme Linked Immunoserbent Assay*), saggio di immunoassorbimento enzimatico; ME, microscopia elettronica; IgM, immunoglobulina M; RT-PCR (*Reverse Transcriptase Polymerase Chain Reaction*), reazione a catena della polimerasi-transcriptasi inversa.
Da Department of Health and Human Services, Centers for Disease Control and Prevention: Diagnosis and management of foodbourne illnesses. *MMWR* 2004:53:9.

cuni virus, l'adesione da parte di parassiti, l'adesione e/o la traslocazione da parte di batteri. La **forma infiammatoria** è in genere dovuta a batteri che invadono direttamente l'intestino o producono citotossine con passaggio di liquidi, proteine e cellule (eritrociti, leucociti) nel lume intestinale. Alcuni enteropatogeni esplicano più di un meccanismo d'azione. Alcuni enterovirus, come i rotavirus, hanno come target l'estremità dei microvilli e possono entrare nell'enterocita mediante invasione diretta o mediante endocitosi calcio-dipendente; si viene così a determinare accorciamento dei villi e perdita della superficie di assorbimento legata all'appiattimento e alla distruzione dei microvilli (Fig. 337-2).

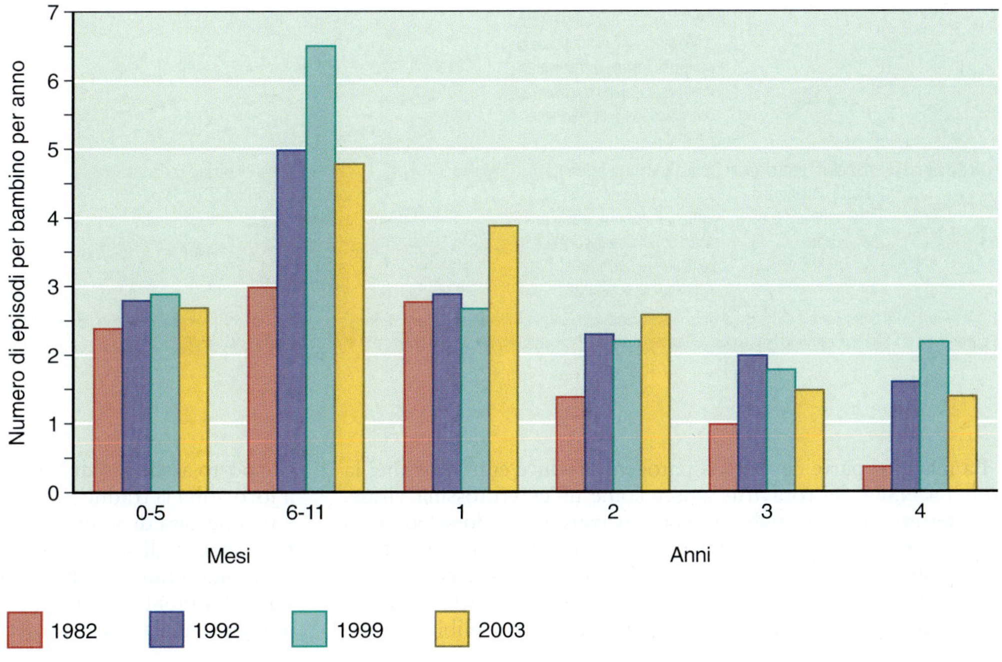

Figura 337-1. Andamento globale dell'incidenza della diarrea.

TABELLA 337-3. Tossinfezioni alimentari (parassiti)

EZIOLOGIA	PERIODO DI INCUBAZIONE	SEGNI E SINTOMI	DURATA DELLA MALATTIA	ALIMENTI ASSOCIATI	ESAMI DI LABORATORIO	TRATTAMENTO
Angiostrongylus cantonensis	Da 1 settimana a ≥1 mese	Cefalea severa, nausea, vomito, rigidità nucale, parestesia, iperestesia, convulsioni e altre anomalie neurologiche	Da diverse settimane a diversi mesi	Ospiti intermedi crudi o poco cotti (per es. lumache), ospite paratenico (trasporto) infetto (per es. granchi, gamberetti di acqua dolce), prodotti freschi contaminati con ospite intermedio o di trasporto	Esame del liquor per ipertensione e aumento delle proteine, dei leucociti e degli eosinofili; test sierologici che usano il metodo ELISA per la ricerca di anticorpi contro l'*Angiostrongylus cantonensis*	Terapia di supporto. Punture lombari ripetute e corticosteroidi per i pazienti più gravi
Cryptosporidium	2-10 giorni	Diarrea (solitamente acquosa), dolori gastrici crampiformi, disturbi gastrici, febbricola	Remissioni e ricadute per settimane/mesi	Cibi non cotti o contaminati dopo la cottura in seguito a manipolazione da soggetto infetto; acqua da bere	Esami specifici per l'esame delle feci per il *Cryptosporidium*. Può essere necessario esaminare l'acqua e gli alimenti	Terapia di supporto; la tossinfezione si autolimita. Se grave, considerare paromomicina per 7 giorni. Per i bambini di età compresa tra 1 e 11 anni, considerare nitazoxanide per 3 giorni
Cyclospora cayetanensis	1-14 giorni, solitamente almeno 1 settimana	Diarrea (solitamente acquosa), riduzione dell'appetito, calo ponderale notevole, dolori gastrici crampiformi, nausea, vomito, astenia	Remissioni e ricadute per settimane/mesi	Diversi tipi di prodotti freschi (bacche importate, lattuga)	Esami delle feci specifici per *Cyclospora*. Può essere necessario esaminare l'acqua e gli alimenti	TMP-SMX per 7 giorni
Entamoeba histolytica	Da 2 a 3 giorni a 1-4 settimane	Diarrea (spesso sanguinolenta), aumento della motilità intestinale, dolori addominali lievi	Può essere protratta (da diverse settimane e diversi mesi)	Cibi non cotti o contaminati dopo la cottura in seguito a manipolazione da soggetto infetto; acqua da bere	L'esame delle feci per la ricerca di cisti e parassiti necessita di almeno 3 campioni. Sierologia per l'infezione a lungo termine	Metronidazolo e agenti luminali (iodochinolo, paromomicina)
Giardia lamblia	1-2 settimane	Diarrea, crampi a livello gastrico, flatulenza, calo ponderale	Da giorni a settimane	Cibi non cotti o contaminati dopo la cottura in seguito a manipolazione da soggetto infetto; acqua da bere	L'esame delle feci per la ricerca di uova e parassiti necessita di almeno 3 campioni	Metronidazolo
Toxoplasma gondii	5-23 giorni	Generalmente asintomatico, il 20% può sviluppare linfoadenopatia cervicale e sintomatologia simil-influenzale. Nei soggetti immunocompromessi, spesso si hanno alterazioni a carico del sistema nervoso centrale (SNC), miocardite e polmonite	Alcuni mesi	Ingestione accidentale di sostanze contaminate (frutta e verdura presenti su suolo contaminato da feci di gatto), carne cruda o cotta parzialmente (soprattutto di maiale, agnello, cervo)	Isolamento del parassita dal sangue e altri liquidi corporei; osservazione del parassita mediante istologia o microscopia. Il rilevamento del microrganismo è raro; la sierologia può essere un'aggiunta utile (occorrono laboratori di riferimento). Le IgM persistono per 6-18 mesi, quindi non sono indicative di infezione recente. PCR dei liquidi corporei. Per l'infezione congenita: isolamento del *T. gondii* dalla placenta, cordone ombelicale o sangue del neonato. PCR dei leucociti, CSF o liquido amniotico o sierologia IgA e IgM eseguita da un laboratorio di riferimento	I soggetti asintomatici ma infetti non necessitano di alcun trattamento. Le donne gravide possono essere trattate con spiramicina o pirimetamina. In casi specifici, nei soggetti immunocompromessi può essere usata pirimetamina più sulfadiazina. Pirimetamina più sulfadiazina (con o senza corticosteroidi) per malattia oculare, quando indicato. Per combattere la soppressione del midollo osseo si usa acido folinico con pirimetamina più sulfadiazina
Toxoplasma gondii (infezione congenita)	Nei neonati, alla nascita	Il trattamento della madre può ridurre la gravità e/o l'incidenza dell'infezione congenita. La maggior parte dei neonati infetti ha pochi sintomi alla nascita. In seguito, generalmente sviluppano segni di toxoplasmosi congenita (ritardo mentale, gravi difetti visivi, paralisi cerebrale, convulsioni) se l'infezione non è trattata	Alcuni mesi	Trasmessa dalla madre (che contrae l'infezione in gravidanza) al bambino	Sierologia positiva o dimostrazione delle larve mediante biopsia muscolare. Aumento degli eosinofili	
Trichinella spiralis	1-2 giorni per i sintomi iniziali; altri iniziano 2-8 settimane dopo l'infezione	Forma acuta: nausea, diarrea, vomito, affaticamento, febbre, disturbi addominali seguiti da dolore muscolare, debolezza, complicanze cardiache e neurologiche occasionali	Alcuni mesi	Carne contaminata cruda o poco cotta, solitamente maiale o cacciagione (orso o cervo)		Terapia di supporto più mebendazolo o albendazolo

ELISA (*Enzyme Linked Immunoserbent Assay*), test di immunoassorbimento enzimatico; IgM, immunoglobulina M; PCR (*Polymerase Chain Reaction*), reazione a catena della polimerasi; TMP-SMX, trimetoprim/sulfametoxazolo.
Da Department of Health and Human Services, Centers for Disease Control and Prevention: Diagnosis and management of foodbourne illnesses. *MMWR* 2004:53:9-10.

La maggior parte dei batteri patogeni produce enterotossine; la proteina NSP4 dei rotavirus agisce come un'enterotossina virale. Le enterotossine batteriche possono attivare in modo selettivo, a livello degli enterociti, il segnale di transduzione intracellulare e anche influire sul riarrangiamento del citoscheletro, con conseguente alterazione del flusso di acqua ed elettroliti attraverso gli enterociti. L'*up-regulation* di questa via determina inibizione del trasporto associato di NaCl e incremento dell'efflusso di cloro, che a loro volta si traducono, in ultima istanza, in una secrezione netta e una perdita di acqua nel lume intestinale (Fig. 337-3). Il trasporto associato di sodio e glucosio e di sodio e aminoacidi è in gran parte inalterato. Anche la via dell'ossido nitrico può essere coinvolta dal momento che la produzione endogena di ossido nitrico è maggiore nella diarrea infettiva che in quella non infettiva.

TABELLA 337-4. Intossicazioni alimentari (non infettive)

EZIOLOGIA	PERIODO DI INCUBAZIONE	SEGNI E SINTOMI	DURATA DELLA MALATTIA	ALIMENTI ASSOCIATI	ESAMI DI LABORATORIO	TRATTAMENTO
Antimonio	Da 5 min a 8 ore, solitamente <1 ora	Vomito, sapore metallico	Di solito si autolimita	Contenitori metallici	Identificazione del metallo in bevande e alimenti	Terapia di supporto
Arsenico	Poche ore	Vomito, coliche, diarrea	Diversi giorni	Alimenti contaminati	Urine. Può causare eosinofilia	Lavanda gastrica, BAL (dimercaprolo)
Cadmio	Da 5 min a 8 ore, solitamente <1 ora	Nausea, vomito, mialgia, aumento della salivazione, epigastralgia	Di solito si autolimita	Frutti di mare, ostriche, vongole, aragoste, cereali, arachidi	Identificazione del metallo negli alimenti	Terapia di supporto
Avvelenamento da pesce (tossina ciguatera)	2-6 ore	Gastroenterologici: dolore addominale, nausea, vomito e diarrea Neurologici: parestesie, percezione alterata e opposta di caldo e freddo, dolore, debolezza Cardiovascolari: bradicardia, ipotensione, anomalie dell'onda T	Giorni, settimane, mesi	Diversi pesci di scoglio, cernia, snapper rossi (lutianidi), amberjack e barracuda (più frequenti)	Test radioimmunologico per la ricerca della tossina nel pesce o anamnesi dettagliata	Terapia di supporto, mannitolo ev. I bambini sono più vulnerabili
Rame	Da 5 min a 8 ore, solitamente <1 ora	Nausea, vomito, vomito blu o verde	Di solito si autolimita	Contenitori metallici	Identificazione del metallo in bevande e alimenti	Terapia di supporto
Mercurio	1 settimana o più	Riduzione della sensibilità, debolezza arti inferiori, paralisi spastica, alterazioni del visus, cecità, coma. Particolarmente vulnerabili la donna in gravidanza e il feto	Può essete protratta	Pesce esposto a mercurio organico, cereali trattati con fungicidi contenenti mercurio	Analisi sangue, capelli	Terapia di supporto
Tossine dei funghi, a breve durata d'azione (museinolo, muscarina, psilocibina, *Coprius artemetaris*, acido ibotenico)	<2 ore	Vomito, diarrea, confusione, disturbi del visus, salivazione, diaforesi, allucinazioni, reazione simil-disulfiram	Si autolimita	Funghi selvatici (la cottura può non distruggere le tossine)	Sindrome caratteristica e identificazione dei funghi o dimostrazione della tossina	Terapia di supporto
Tossine dei funghi, a lunga durata d'azione (amanitina)	4-8 ore per la diarrea; 24-48 ore per l'insufficienza epatica	Diarrea, crampi addominali, insufficienza epatica e renale	Spesso fatale	Funghi	Sindrome caratteristica e identificazione dei funghi e/o dimostrazione della tossina	Terapia di supporto, supporto respiratorio se a rischio di vita
Avvelenamento da nitriti	1-2 ore	Nausea, vomito, cianosi, cefalea, vertigini, perdita di forza, perdita di coscienza, sangue marrone cioccolato	Di solito si autolimita	Carni conservate, alcuni cibi contaminati, spinaci esposti a nitrificazione eccessiva	Analisi dei cibi e del sangue	Terapia di supporto, blu di metilene
Pesticidi (organofosforici o carbamati)	Pochi minuti o poche ore	Nausea, vomito, crampi addominali, diarrea, cefalea, irrequietezza, visione indistinta, contrazioni, convulsioni, salivazione e miosi	Di solito si autolimita	Alcuni cibi contaminati	Analisi cibi e sangue	Atropina; 2-PAM (pralidoxima) usata quando l'atropina non è in grado di controllare i sintomi ed è raramente necessaria nell'avvelenamento da carbammati
Pesce palla (tetrodotossina)	<20 min	Parestesie, vomito, diarrea, dolore addominale, paralisi ascendente, insufficienza respiratoria	Solitamente morte nel giro di 4-6 ore	Pesce palla	Riscontro della tetrodotossina nel pesce	Il paziente a rischio di morte può necessitare di supporto respiratorio
Scombroidi (istamina)	Da 1 min a 3 ore	Arrossamento, rash, sensazione di bruciore sulla cute, nel cavo orale e in gola, vertigini, orticaria, parestesie	3-6 ore	Pesce: tonno fresco e in scatola, marlin, maccarello, escolar e mahi mahi	Dimostrazione dell'istamina negli alimenti o diagnosi clinica	Terapia di supporto, antistaminici
Tossine dei molluschi (diarroica, neurotossica, amnesica)	Avvelenamento diarroico da molluschi: da 30 min a 2 ore Intossicazione neurotossica da molluschi: da pochi minuti a qualche ora Intossicazione amnesia da molluschi: 24-48 ore	Nausea, vomito, diarrea, dolore addominale, accompagnato da brividi, cefalea e febbre. Formicolio, insensibilità di labbra, lingua e gola, dolori muscolari, vertigini, percezione alterata e opposta di caldo e freddo, diarrea e vomito Vomito, diarrea, dolore addominale e alterazioni neurologiche come confusione, perdita della memoria, disorientamento, convulsioni, coma	Da ore a 2-3 giorni	Diversi frutti di mare, soprattutto cozze, ostriche, cappesante, e frutti di mare provenienti dalla costa della Florida e dal Golfo del Messico	Riscontro della tossina nei frutti di mare; cromatografia liquida ad alta pressione	Terapia di supporto, generalmente si autolimita. Gli anziani sono particolarmente sensibili a questo tipo di intossicazione
Tossine dei molluschi (intossicazione paralitica da molluschi)	Da 30 min a 3 ore	Diarrea, nausea, vomito, che conduce a parestesie di bocca e labbra, debolezza, disfasia, disfonia, paralisi respiratoria	Giorni	Cappesante, cozze, vongole, cockles ("cuori")	Riscontro della tossina negli alimenti e nell'acqua in cui era il pesce; cromatografia liquida ad alta pressione	Il paziente a rischio di morte può necessitare di supporto respiratorio
Floruro di sodio	Da pochi minuti a 2 ore	Sapore salato o simile a sapone, insensibilità della bocca, vomito, diarrea, pupille dilatate, spasmi, pallore, shock, collasso	Di solito si autolimita	Cibi disidratati (per es. latte in polvere, farina, lievito, preparato per dolci) contaminati con insetticidi e veleni per roditori contenenti fluoruro di sodio	Esame del vomito o lavanda gastrica. Analisi degli alimenti	Terapia di supporto
Tallio	Poche ore	Nausea, vomito, diarrea, parestesie dolorose, polineuropatia motoria, caduta dei capelli	Diversi giorni	Alimenti contaminati	Urine, capelli	Terapia di supporto
Stagno	Da 5 min a 8 ore, solitamente <1 ora	Nausea, vomito, diarrea	Di solito si autolimita	Contenitori metallici	Analisi degli alimenti	Terapia di supporto
Vomitotossina	Da pochi minuti a 3 ore	Nausea, cefalea, dolore addominale, vomito	Di solito si autolimita	Cereali come frumento, mais, orzo	Analisi degli alimenti	Terapia di supporto
Zinco	Poche ore	Crampi a livello gastrico, nausea, vomito, diarrea, mialgia	Di solito si autolimita	Contenitori metallici	Analisi degli alimenti sangue, feci, saliva, urine	Terapia di supporto

Da Department of Health and Human Services, Centers for Disease Control and Prevention: Diagnosis and management of foodbourne illnesses. *MMWR* 2004:53:11-12.

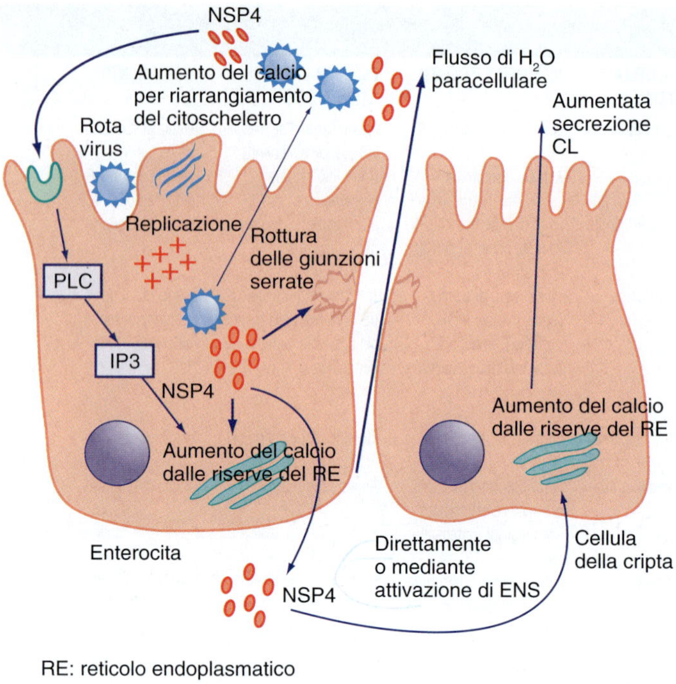

Figura 337-2. Patogenesi dell'infezione da rotavirus e diarrea. RE (*Endoplasmic Reticulum*), reticolo endoplasmatico. (Adattata da Ramig RF: Pathogenesis of intestinal and systemic rotavirus infection. *J Virol* 2004;78:10213-10220.)

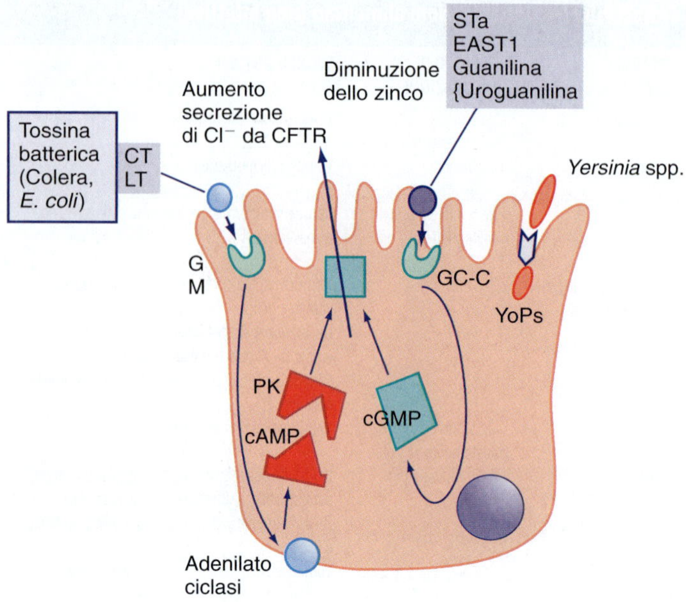

Figura 337-3. Meccanismo d'azione della tossina colerica. (Adattata da Thapar M, Sanderson IR: Diarrhoea in children: An interface between developing and developed countries. *Lancet* 2004;363:641-653; Montes M, DuPont HL: Enteritis, enterocolitis and infectious diarrhea syndromes. In Cohen J, Powderly WG, Opal SM, et al [ed]: *Infections Diseases*, 2nd ed. London, Mosby, 2004, pp 31-52.)

L'***E. coli*** **enterotossigeno** (**ETEC**, *EnteroToxigenic E. coli*) colonizza l'intestino tenue e aderisce ai suoi enterociti mediante le fimbrie (pili) di superficie, inducendo ipersecrezione di fluidi ed elettroliti attraverso una delle due tossine: l'enterotossina termolabile (LT) o quella termostabile. L'LT, simile dal punto di vista strutturale alla tossina del *Vibrio colera*, attiva l'adenilato ciclasi determinando un aumento di guanosin monofosfato ciclico (cGMP) intracellulare (vedi Fig. 337-3). Invece, le *Shigella* spp. danno luogo a gastroenterite attraverso l'invasione superficiale della mucosa del colon, attraverso le cellule M localizzate sulle placche del Peyer.

Successivamente alla fagocitosi si verifica una serie di eventi, tra cui l'apoptosi dei macrofagi, la moltiplicazione e diffusione dei batteri nelle cellule adiacenti, il rilascio dei mediatori della flogosi (interleuchina IL-1 e IL-8), la migrazione transepiteliale dei neutrofili nel lume del colon, la necrosi dei neutrofili e la degranulazione, un'ulteriore breccia nella barriera epiteliale e la distruzione della mucosa (Fig. 337-4).

FATTORI DI RISCHIO DELLA GASTROENTERITE

I principali fattori di rischio includono la contaminazione ambientale e una maggiore esposizione agli enteropatogeni. Altri fattori di rischio sono la giovane età, l'immunodeficienza, il morbillo, la malnutrizione e l'allattamento completamente o prevalentemente artificiale. La malnutrizione aumenta di diverse volte il rischio di diarrea e di mortalità associata. Il tasso di decessi da diarrea infettiva varia con la prevalenza dei deficit; è maggiore nell'Africa sub-sahariana, nell'Asia meridionale e nelle Ande, in America Latina. Il rischio è particolarmente elevato quando sussiste un deficit di micronutrienti; nei bambini con **carenza di vitamina A** il rischio di morire per diarrea, morbillo e malaria aumenta del 20-24%. Il rischio di mortalità per diarrea, polmonite e malaria aumenta del 13-21% in caso di **deficit di zinco**.

La maggior parte dei casi di diarrea si risolve in una settimana, ma una piccola percentuale persiste oltre le 2 settimane. Si definisce **diarrea persistente** un episodio di diarrea che insorge acutamente ma continua per più di 14 giorni. Queste forme includono dal 3 al 20% di tutti i casi di diarrea nei bambini al di sotto dei 5 anni di età e portano al 50% i casi di diarrea associata a decesso. Nei Paesi in via di sviluppo molti pazienti in età pediatrica (soprattutto lattanti e i bambini piccoli) vanno frequentemente incontro a episodi di diarrea acuta; nonostante siano pochi i casi che persistono per più di i 14 giorni, episodi frequenti di diarrea possono compromettere lo stato nutrizionale e predisporre allo sviluppo di diarrea persistente, malnutrizione calorico-proteico e infezioni secondarie.

MANIFESTAZIONI CLINICHE DELLA DIARREA

La maggior parte delle manifestazioni cliniche e delle sindromi cliniche diarroiche sono correlate a infezioni da patogeni e alla dose di inoculazione (vedi Tabb. da 337-1 a 337-3). Le altre manifestazioni dipendono dallo sviluppo di complicanze (come disidratazione e squilibrio elettrolitico) e dalla natura dell'agente infettivo (vedi Capitolo 55.1). Di solito l'ingestione di tossine preformate (come quelle dello *Staphylococcus aureus*) è associata a rapida insorgenza di nausea e vomito entro 6 ore, con possibile febbre, dolore addominale e diarrea entro 8-72 ore. Diarrea acquosa e dolori addominali dopo 8-16 ore di incubazione sono associate all'enterotossina prodotta da *Clostridium perfringens* e *Bacillus cereus*. Crampi addominali e diarrea acquosa dopo un periodo di incubazione di 16-48 ore possono essere dovuti a norovirus, diverse enterotossine batteriche, *Cryptosporidium* e *Cyclospora*. Diversi microrganismi, come *Salmonella*, *Shigella*, *Campylobacter jejuni*, *Yersinia enterocolitica*, *E. coli* enteroinvasiva e *Vibrio parahaemolyticus*, sono responsabili di una diarrea che può contenere sangue e leucociti fecali, associati a crampi addominali, tenesmo e febbre; queste caratteristiche sono indice di **dissenteria batterica** e febbre. Diarrea ematica e crampi addominali dopo 72-120 ore di incubazione sono indicativi di *Shigella* o produzione di tossina *Shiga-like* da parte di *E. coli* come *E. coli* 0157:H7. I microrganismi che determinano dissenteria o diarrea emorragica possono essere responsabili anche di diarrea acquosa isolata senza febbre o precedere una condizione più complessa che causa dissenteria.

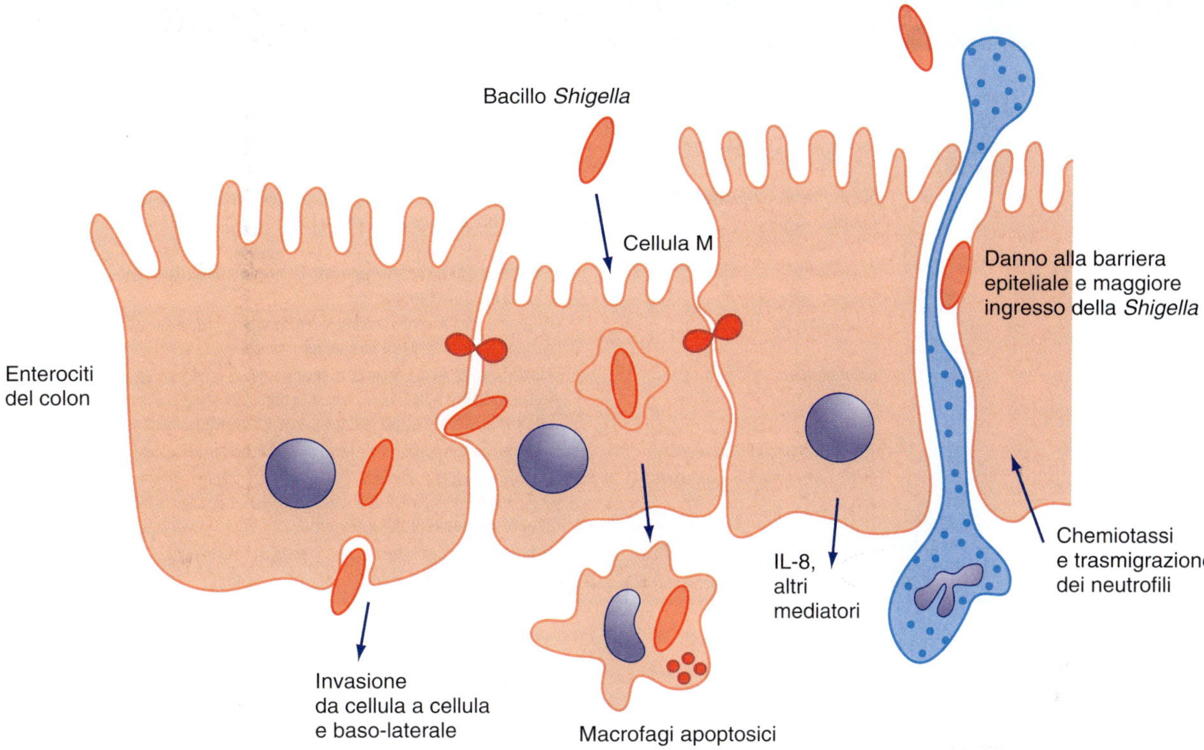

Figura 337-4. Patogenesi dell'infezione e diarrea da *Shigella*. (Adattata da Opal SM, Keusch GT: Host responses to infection. In Cohen J, Powderly WG, Opal SM, et al [ed]: *Infections Diseases*, 2nd ed. London, Mosby, 2004, pp 31-52.)

Sebbene nei bambini molti sintomi di gastroenterite acuta siano aspecifici, le caratteristiche cliniche possono essere d'aiuto per identificare la maggior parte dei tipi di diarrea, consentendo una tempestiva scelta della terapia antibiotica e dietetica specifica (vedi Tabb. da 337-1 a 337-3). C'è una sovrapposizione notevole nella sintomatologia. Se il valore predittivo positivo delle caratteristiche della diarrea è scarso, la predittività negativa dei microrganismi patogeni è molto migliore in assenza di segni di dissenteria. Quando possibile, se risulta facile e se le risorse lo consentono, l'eziologia deve essere verificata mediante le opportune indagini di laboratorio.

COMPLICANZE

La maggior parte delle complicanze associate alla gastroenterite è correlata al ritardo nella diagnosi e nella terapia. Se non vengono sottoposti a una reidratazione precoce e corretta, molti bambini con diarrea acuta sviluppano disidratazione con complicanze associate (vedi Capitoli 53, 54, 55 e 68), talvolta tali di mettere a rischio di vita i lattanti e i bambini piccoli. Una terapia non corretta può prolungare gli episodi di diarrea con conseguente malnutrizione e complicanze come infezioni secondarie e deficit di micronutrienti (ferro, zinco). Nei Paesi in via di sviluppo, una batteriemia associata è una complicanza riscontrata in bambini malnutriti con diarrea. Patogeni specifici sono associati a manifestazioni extraintestinali e complicanze; queste non sono patognomoniche di infezione né sono sempre in stretta associazione temporale con l'episodio diarroico (Tab. 337-5).

DIAGNOSI

La diagnosi di gastroenterite si basa sul riscontro clinico, su una tempestiva valutazione della sua severità e sulla conferma mediante indagini di laboratorio, se indicato.

VALUTAZIONE CLINICA DELLA DIARREA. Le manifestazioni più frequenti dell'infezione del tratto gastrointestinale nel bambino sono rappresentate da diarrea, crampi addominali e vomito. Le manifestazioni sistemiche sono varie e associate a diverse cause. La valutazione del bambino con diarrea acuta include:

- Valutazione del grado di disidratazione e acidosi, seguita da una rapida ristabilizzazione e rianimazione con liquidi per via orale o endovenosa, se necessario (Tabb. 337-6 e 337-7).
- Raccolta di un'anamnesi appropriata del contatto o dell'esposizione, comprendente informazioni sull'esposizione a contatti che hanno sintomi simili, l'ingestione di acqua o alimenti contaminati, frequenza di asili, viaggi recenti in aree dove la diarrea è endemica, uso di antibiotici.
- Determinazione dell'eziologia della diarrea dal punto di vista clinico per iniziare una pronta antibioticoterapia, se indicata. Nausea e vomito, pur essendo sintomi aspecifici, sono indicativi di infezione del tratto alto dell'intestino. La febbre, frequente nella diarrea infiammatoria, indica la presenza di un processo infiammatorio, ma si ha anche nella disidratazione o nelle coinfezioni (per es. infezione delle vie urinarie, otite media). Il dolore addominale severo e il tenesmo sono indicativi del coinvolgimento di colon e retto. Sintomi come nausea e vomito e assenza di febbre o febbricola con dolore periombelicale da lieve a moderato e diarrea acquosa sono indicativi di coinvolgimento del tenue e riducono la probabilità che sia presente un'infezione batterica grave.

L'approccio clinico alla diagnosi e alla gestione della diarrea nel bambino piccolo è una componente critica del programma di **gestione integrata delle malattie dell'infanzia** (IMCI, *Integrated Management of Childhood Illness*), che deve essere implementato nei Paesi in via di sviluppo con elevato tasso di decessi per diarrea (Fig. 337-5).

ESAME DELLE FECI. L'esame microscopico delle feci e la coprocoltura possono fornire importanti informazioni sull'eziologia della diarrea. Nel campione fecale si devono ricercare muco, sangue e leucociti. La presenza di leucociti nelle feci è indicativa di invasione batterica della mucosa del colon, sebbene alcuni pazienti con shigellosi abbiano pochi leucociti in una fase precoce dell'infezioni, come i pazienti infettati da tossina *Shiga-like* prodotta da *E. coli* ed *E. histolytica*. Nelle aree endemiche, l'esame microscopico delle feci deve includere la ricerca di parassiti, come *G. lamblia* ed *E. histolytica*.

La coprocoltura va effettuata nella fase iniziale della malattia, nei bambini con **diarrea ematica** in cui l'esame microscopico delle feci

TABELLA 337-5. Manifestazioni extraintestinali delle infezioni intestinali

MANIFESTAZIONI	PATOGENI ENTERICI ASSOCIATI	ESORDIO E PROGNOSI
Infezioni focali dovute a diffusione sistemica dei batteri patogeni, tra cui vulvovaginiti, infezioni del tratto urinario, endocardite, osteomieliti, meningiti, polmoniti, epatite, peritonite, corionamnionite, infezione dei tessuti molli e tromboflebite settica	Tutti i principali patogeni possono causare queste infezioni extraintestinali dirette, inclusi *Salmonella, Shigella, Yersinia, Campylobacter, Clostridium difficile*	Esordio solitamente durante l'infezione acuta, ma può presentarsi anche in seguito. La prognosi dipende dalla sede dell'infezione.
Artrite reattiva	*Shigella, Yersinia, Campylobacter, Cryptosporidium, Clostridium difficile*	Tipicamente esordisce 1-3 settimane dopo l'infezione. Le ricadute dopo l'infezione si hanno nel 15-50% delle persone, ma la maggior parte dei bambini guarisce entro 2-6 mesi dalla comparsa dei primi sintomi.
Sindrome di Guillain-Barré	*Campylobacter*	Solitamente si ha poche settimane dopo l'infezione originale. La prognosi è buona, nonostante il 15-20% possa avere sequele.
Glomerulonefrite	*Shigella, Campylobacter, Yersinia*	Può essere acuta, a esordio improvviso con un attacco infiammatorio acuto, oppure cronica, a inizio graduale. In molti casi il rene guarisce con il tempo.
Nefropatia da IgA	*Campylobacter*	Caratterizzata da episodi ricorrenti di ematuria, questa condizione deriva dalla deposizione di immunoglobuline A (IgA) nei glomeruli. La nefropatia ad IgA può progredire per anni senza sintomi notevoli. Gli uomini sono più predisposti a sviluppare questo disordine rispetto alle donne.
Eritema nodoso	*Yersinia, Campylobacter, Salmonella*	Sebbene doloroso, è solitamente benigno e più frequente nell'adolescenza. Si risolve in 4-6 settimane.
Sindrome uremico-emolitica	*Shigella dysenteriae* 1, *Escherichia coli* 0157:H7, altri	Esordio improvviso, insufficienza renale a breve termine. Nei casi gravi, l'insufficienza renale rende necessarie diverse sedute di dialisi per sostituire la funzionalità renale, ma la maggior parte dei bambini guarisce senza danni per la salute.
Anemia emolitica	*Campylobacter, Yersinia*	Complicanza relativamente rara che può avere un decorso cronico.

Da Department of Health and Human Services, Centers for Disease Control and Prevention: Managing acute gastroenteritis among children. *MMWR Recomm Rep* 2004; 53:1-33.

TABELLA 337-6. Sintomi associati alla disidratazione

SINTOMO	DISIDRATAZIONE MINIMA O ASSENTE (PERDITA <3% DEL PESO CORPOREO)	DISIDRATAZIONE DA LIEVE A MODERATA (PERDITA TRA IL 3 E IL 9% DEL PESO CORPOREO)	DISIDRATAZIONE SEVERA (PERDITA >9% DEL PESO CORPOREO)
Stato mentale	Buono; vigile	Normale, affaticato o irrequieto, irritabile	Apatia, letargia, incoscienza
Sete	Beve normalmente; può rifiutare i liquidi	Assetato; forte bisogno di bere	Beve poco oppure è incapace di bere
Frequenza cardiaca	Normale	Da normale ad aumentata	Tachicardia, con bradicardia nei casi più severi
Polso	Normale	Da normale a diminuito	Debole, esile o impalpabile
Respiro	Normale	Normale; veloce	Profondo
Occhi	Normali	Lievemente infossati	Profondamente infossati
Secrezione lacrimale	Presente	Ridotta	Assente
Labbra e lingua	Idratate (umide)	Secche	Inaridite
Pliche cutanee	Scomparsa istantanea	Scomparsa in <2 s	Scomparsa in >2 s
Tempo di riempimento capillare	Normale	Prolungato	Prolungato, minimo
Estremità	Calde	Fredde	Fredde, chiazzate, cianotiche
Volume urinario (diuresi)	Da normale a ridotto	Diminuito	Minimo

Fonte: Adattata da Duggan C, Santosham M, Glass RI: The management of acute diarrhea in children: Oral rehydration, maintenance, and nutritional therapy. *MMWR* 1992;41 (No.RR-16):1-20; and World Health Organization: The treatment of diarrhoea: a manual for physicians and other senior health workers. Geneva, Switzerland: World Health Organization, 1995. Available at http://www.who.int/child-adolescent-health/New_Publications/CHILD_HEALTH/WHO.CDR.95.3.htm.
Da Department of Health and Human Services, Centers for Disease Control and Prevention: Diagnosis and management of foodbourne illnesses. *MMWR* 2004:52;5.

TABELLA 337-7. Riepilogo del trattamento basato sul grado di disidratazione

GRADO DI DISIDRATAZIONE	TERAPIA REIDRATANTE	SOSTITUZIONE DELLE PERDITE	NUTRIZIONE
Disidratazione minima o assente	Non applicabile	<10 kg di peso corporeo: 60-120 mL di soluzione reidratante orale (ORS) per ogni scarica diarroica o episodio di vomito; >10 kg di peso corporeo: 120-240 mL ORS per ogni scarica diarroica o episodio di vomito	Continuare l'allattamento al seno o riprendere una dieta normale appropriata per l'età, compreso un intake calorico per il mantenimento*
Disidratazione da lieve a moderata	ORS, 50-100 mL/kg di peso corporeo per 3-4 ore	Uguale	Uguale
Disidratazione severa	Lattato di Ringer o soluzione fisiologica ev alla dose di 20 mL/kg finché non migliorano la perfusione e lo stato mentale; successivamente somministrare 100 mL/kg di peso corporeo di ORS in 4 ore o destrosio 5% ½ soluzione fisiologica ev a 2 volte i tassi di mantenimento dei fluidi	Uguale; se il paziente non riesce a bere, utilizzo del sondino nasogastrico o somministrazione destrosio 5% ¼ di soluzione salina con 20 mEq/L di cloruro di potassio endovena	Uguale

*Durante gli episodi diarroici acuti occorre evitare diete troppo severe. L'allattamento al seno deve essere continuato ad libitum anche durante la reidratazione acuta. I neonati troppo deboli per le poppate devono ricevere latte materno o in formula attraverso sondino nasogastrico. Le formule contenenti lattosio sono solitamente ben tollerate. Se compaiono segni sostanziali di malassorbimento di lattosio, si può ricorrere a formule prive di lattosio. Sono raccomandati: carboidrati complessi, frutta fresca, carne magra, yogurt e verdure. Le bevande gassate o i succhi di frutta in commercio con un'elevata concentrazione di zuccheri semplici devono essere evitate.

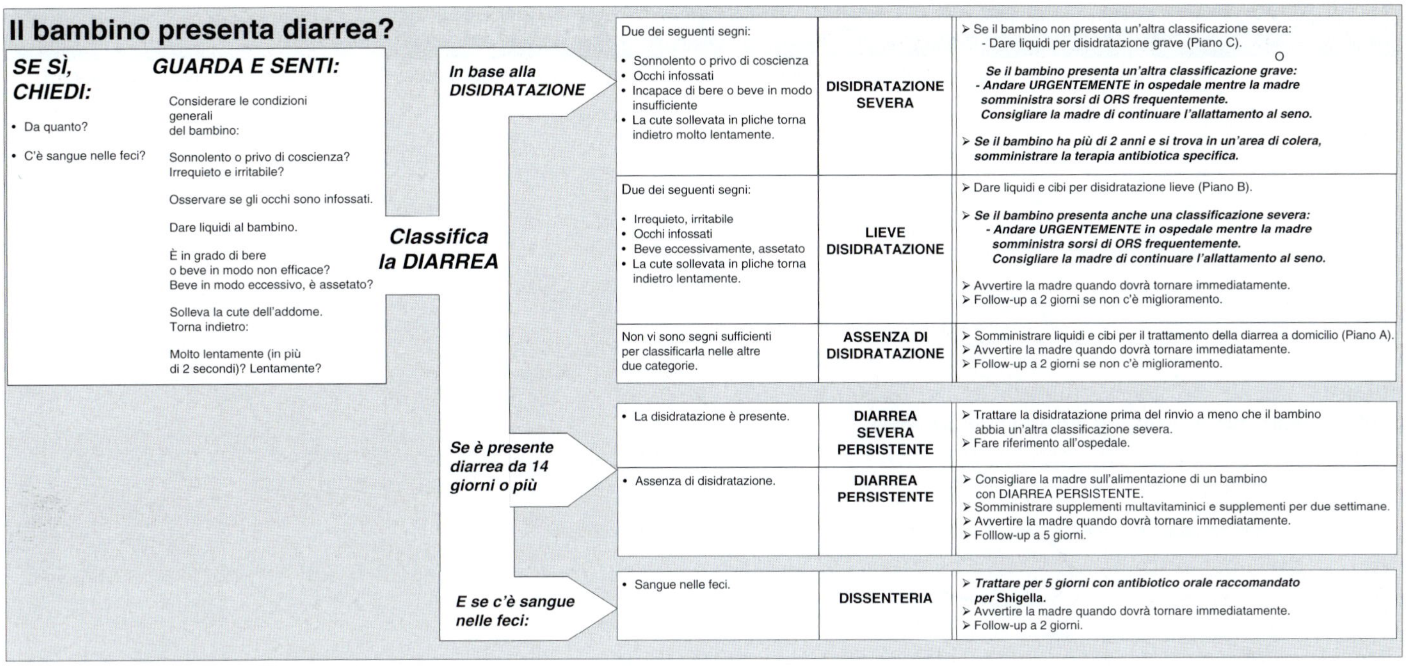

Figura 337-5. Approccio integrato al bambino malato (IMCI, *Integrated Management of Childhood Illness*) per il riconoscimento e la gestione della diarrea nei Paesi in via di sviluppo.

indica la presenza di **leucociti fecali**, se sono in atto **epidemie** con sospetto di **sindrome uremico-emolitica** (HUS, *Hemolytic-Uremic Syndrome*) e nei bambini **immunocompromessi** con diarrea. Il campione fecale deve essere posto rapidamente in coltura; se quest'ultima non è rapidamente disponibile, occorre trasportarlo in terreni di crescita specifici. Il risultato e la diagnosi di diarrea batterica possono essere migliorati in modo significativo usando tecniche di diagnostica molecolare come la reazione a catena della polimerasi (PCR, *Polymerase Chain Reaction*). Nella maggior parte dei bambini con diarrea acquosa non complicata e in precedenza sani, non occorrono indagini di laboratorio, se non per fini epidemiologici.

TRATTAMENTO

I principi generali su cui si basa la gestione della gastroenterite acuta nei bambini comprendono la reidratazione orale, la nutrizione enterale e la scelta della dieta, la supplementazione con zinco e terapie aggiuntive come quella con probiotici.

REIDRATAZIONE ORALE. I bambini, in particolare i lattanti, sono più sensibili alla disidratazione degli adulti per due motivi: a causa delle maggiori esigenze basali di liquidi ed elettroliti per chilogrammo di peso e anche poiché essi dipendono dagli altri per il soddisfacimento dei propri bisogni. Bisogna valutare rapidamente la **disidratazione** e correggerla entro 4-6 ore a seconda della sua gravità e del fabbisogno giornaliero stimato. Una minoranza di bambini, soprattutto quelli che presentano shock o che non tollerano liquidi per via orale, necessitano inizialmente di reidratazione endovenosa, anche se la via orale è quella preferita per reidratare e sostituire le perdite in atto (Tabb. 337-7 e 337-8). I rischi associati alla disidratazione severa che possono richiedere un intervento correttivo per via endovenosa includono: età <6 mesi, prematurità, malattie croniche, febbre >38 °C se il lattante ha meno di 3 mesi o >39 °C se ha tra 3 e 36 mesi, diarrea ematica, emesi persistente, urine concentrate, occhi infossati e depressione dello stato di coscienza. Sebbene, in linea generale, la soluzione reidratante orale dell'OMS (ORS, *Oral Rehydration Solution*) sia adeguata, la ridotta osmolarità delle soluzioni reidratanti orali può essere più efficace nel ridurre il volume delle feci. Tale soluzione reidratante (contenente 75 mEq di sodio e 75 mmol di glucosio per litro, con un'osmolarità totale di 245 mOsm/L), con il suo contenuto di sodio e glucosio minore rispetto a quelli dell'ORS standard, determina una ridotta produzione di feci, oltre a ridurre il vomito e il bisogno di liquidi per via endovenosa, senza aumentare sostanzialmente il rischio di iponatriemia.Ì

Le soluzioni reidratanti orali a base di cereali, utili nei bambini malnutriti, possono essere preparate a casa. I rimedi domestici, tra cui bevande con bicarbonato di sodio, succhi di frutta e tè, non sono adatti né per la reidratazione, né per la terapia di mantenimento, a causa dell'osmolalità elevata e della ridotta concentrazione di sodio. Nella Figura 337-5 e nella Tabella 337-7 sono illustrati un piano di valutazione clinica e la strategia di trattamento raccomandata per pazienti pediatrici con diarrea da moderata a severa. Nei lattanti e nei bambini piccoli la reidratazione orale, da effettuarsi lentamente, soprattutto in caso di emesi, può essere somministrata inizialmente mediante contagocce, cucchiaino da tè, siringa, a piccole quantità (5 mL alla volta); il suo volume va incrementato quando e se viene tollerata. La reintegrazione in caso di emesi o diarrea è presentata nella Tabella 337-7. La reidratazione orale può essere effettuata anche mediante sondino nasogastrico, se necessario; questa però non è la norma.

Le limitazioni alla terapia reidratante orale comprendono lo shock, l'invaginazione ileale, l'intolleranza ai carboidrati (rara), l'emesi severa e l'elevata produzione di feci (>10 mL/kg/24 ore).

NUTRIZIONE ENTERALE E SCELTA DELLA DIETA. Una nutrizione enterale protratta favorisce la guarigione dall'episodio diarroico; la norma è istituire, dopo la reidratazione, un'alimentazione adeguata per l'età. Sebbene l'orletto a spazzola della superficie intestinale e gli enzimi luminali possano presentare alterazioni nei bambini con diarrea prolungata, esistono prove che un soddisfacente assorbimento di carboidrati, proteine e grassi può aversi con diversi tipi di diete. Una volta portata a termine la reidratazione vanno reintrodotti i cibi, mentre la reidratazione orale può essere continuata per compensare le perdite legate all'emesi o alla diarrea e per il mantenimento. Il più presto possibile va ripreso l'allattamento al seno o quello con latte in formula non diluito. Sono tollerati alimenti contenenti carboidrati complessi (riso, frumento, pane e cereali), carne magra, yogurt, frutta e verdura. Cibi grassi o contenenti elevate percentuali di zucchero (succhi di frutta, bicarbonato di sodio) vanno invece evitati. La densità energetica delle diete utilizzate nella terapia della diarrea

TABELLA 337-8. Composizione delle soluzioni commerciali per la reidratazione orale (ORS) e bevande più usate

SOLUZIONE	CARBOIDRATI (G/L)	SODIO (MMOL/L)	POTASSIO (MMOL/L)	CLORO (MMOL/L)	BASE* (MMOL/L)	OSMOLARITÀ (MMOL/L)
ORS						
Organizzazione Mondiale della sanità (OMS) (2005)	13,5	75	20	65	10	245
OMS (2002)	13,5	75	20	65	30	245
OMS 1975)	20	90	20	80	30	311
European Society of Paediatric Gastroenterology, Hepatology and Nutrition	16	60	20	60	30	240
Enfalyte®[†]	30	50	25	45	34	200
Pedialyte®[§]	25	45	20	35	30	250
Rehydralyte[¶]	25	75	20	65	30	305
Ceralyte®[**]	40	50-90	20	NA[††]	30	220
BEVANDE DI USO COMUNE (NON ADATTE AL TRATTAMENTO DELLA DIARREA)						
Succo di mela[§§]	120	0,4	44	45	N/A	730
Coca-Cola® classica[¶¶]	112	1,6	N/A	N/A	13,4	650

*Bicarbonato normale o potenziato (per es. lattato, citrato o acetato).
[†]Mead-Johnson Laboratories, Princeton, New Jersey. Ulteriori informazioni sono disponibili sul sito: www.meadjohnson.com/products/cons-infant/enfalyte.html.
[§]Ross Laboratories (Abbott Laboratories), Columbus, Ohio. Data regarding Flavored and Freezer Pop Pedialyte are identical. Ulteriori informazioni sono disponibili sul sito www.pedialyte.com.
[¶]Ross Laboratories (Abbott Laboratories), Columbus, Ohio. Ulteriori informazioni sono disponibili sul sito: http://rpdcon40.ross.com/pn/PediatricProducts.NSF/web_Ross.com_XML_PediatricNutrition/96A5745B1183947385256A80007546E5?OpenDocument.
[**]Cera Products, L.L.C., Jessup, Maryland. Ulteriori informazioni sono disponibili sul sito: www.ceralyte.com/index.htm.
[††]Non applicabile.
[§§]Secondo i requisiti minimi previsti dall'U.S. Department of Agriculture.
[¶¶]Coca-Cola Corporation, Atlanta, Georgia. I dati non includono gli elettroliti che dovrebbero essere presenti nell'acqua locale utilizzata per imbottigliare. Base = fosfato.
Da Department of Health and Human Services, Centers for Disease Control and Prevention: Diagnosis and management of foodbourne illnesses. *MMWR* 2004;52:1-33.

deve essere di circa 1 kcal/g, per cercare di fornire un *intake* energetico minimo di 100 kcal/kg/die e un *intake* proteico di 2-3 g/kg/die. Nelle circostanze in cui risulta problematico raggiungere un introito adeguato di alimenti con una determinata densità energetica, può rivelarsi utile addizionare amilasi mediante tecniche di germinazione.

A parte piccoli sottogruppi che presentano intolleranza acuta al lattosio, la maggior parte dei bambini con diarrea è in grado di tollerare il latte e le diete contenenti lattosio. Non risulta quindi necessario eliminare il latte sostituendolo con formulazioni specifiche (e costose) prive di lattosio. Sebbene i bambini con diarrea persistente non siano intolleranti al lattosio, somministrare un carico di lattosio >5 g/kg/die può aumentare l'incidenza di diarrea e di insuccesso del trattamento. Strategie alternative per ridurre il carico di lattosio finché si alimenta il bambino malnutrito con diarrea prolungata includono aggiungere cereali nel latte o sostituire quest'ultimo con latticini fermentati come lo yogurt.

Raramente, quando l'intolleranza nutrizionale impedisce la somministrazione di formule di latte vaccino, può risultare necessario ricorrere a una dieta specifica priva di latte come diete a base di pollo tritato o frullato o formule elementari. Queste ultime, pur essendo talora efficaci, non sono facili da ottenere nei Paesi in via di sviluppo. Oltre a formule a base di riso e lenticchie, l'aggiunta di banane verdi o di pectina alla dieta si è dimostrata efficace nel trattamento della diarrea persistente. La Figura 337-6 illustra un algoritmo indicativo per il trattamento dei bambini che presentano diarrea prolungata nei Paesi in via di sviluppo.

SUPPLEMENTAZIONE DI ZINCO. Esistono importanti evidenze che la supplementazione a base di zinco nei bambini che presentano diarrea prolungata nei Paesi in via di sviluppo, riduca la durata e la gravità della diarrea ed è potenzialmente in grado di prevenire 300 000 decessi per questa causa. L'OMS e l'UNICEF raccomandano che tutti i bambini con diarrea acuta che vivono nelle aree a rischio ricevano zinco per via orale, in diverse forme, per 10-14 giorni durante e successivamente all'episodio diarroico (10 mg/die per lattanti di meno di 6 mesi di vita e 20 mg/die per quelli di età >6 mesi). Oltre a migliorare la diarrea, la somministrazione di zinco in contesti di comunità comporta un aumento dell'uso delle ORS e la riduzione dell'antibioticoterapia.

TERAPIE ALTERNATIVE. L'utilizzo di batteri non patogeni probiotici per prevenire e curare la diarrea si è rivelato positivo nei Paesi in via di sviluppo. Diversi sono i microrganismi (*Lactobacillus*, *Bifidobacterium*) che offrono garanzie di sicurezza; la terapia non è stata standardizzata e non è stato identificato il microrganismo piu efficace (e sicuro).

I **farmaci antispastici** (loperamide) sono controindicati nei pazienti pediatrici con dissenteria e probabilmente non c'è motivo di utilizzarli per il trattamento della diarrea acquosa acuta in bambini altrimenti sani. Allo stesso modo gli **antiemetici**, come le fenotiazine, hanno scarsa rilevanza a causa dei loro effetti collaterali potenzialmente gravi (sonnolenza, distonia, iperpiressia maligna). Tuttavia, tra questi, l'ondansetron è il farmaco che risulta più efficace e meno tossico. Qualora il vomito persistente ostacolasse la terapia reidratante orale, si può somministrare una compressa singola di ondansetron per via sublinguale (2 mg nei bambini di peso compreso tra 8 e 15 kg, 4 mg in quelli con peso ≥15-30 kg e 8 mg in quelli con peso >30 kg). La maggior parte dei bambini non necessita comunque di una terapia antiemetica specifica; di solito è sufficiente un'attenta terapia reidratante orale (vedi Capitolo 55.1).

Il **racecadotril**, un inibitore delle encefalinasi, si è dimostrato efficace per ridurre la produzione fecale nei pazienti con diarrea. Questo farmaco, non molto usato nei pazienti pediatrici, in genere non sembra necessario.

TERAPIA ANTIBIOTICA. In casi selezionati un terapia antibiotica tempestiva può ridurre la durata e la gravità della diarrea e prevenirne le complicanze (Tab. 337-9). Se è importante usare questi farmaci in casi specifici, occorre comunque ricordare che il loro uso esagerato e indiscriminato induce antibioticoresistenza. La **nitazoxanide**, farmaco antinfettivo, è risultato efficace nei confronti di diversi patogeni, tra cui *Cryptosporidium parvum*, *Giardia lamblia*, *Entamoeba histolytica*, *Blastocystis hominis*, *C. difficile* e rotavirus.

PREVENZIONE

In molti Paesi sviluppati la diarrea dovuta a patogeni come *Clostridum botulinum*, *E. coli* 0157:H7, *Salmonella*, *Shigella*, *V. cholerae*, *Cryptosporidium* e *Cyclospora* rappresenta una malattia

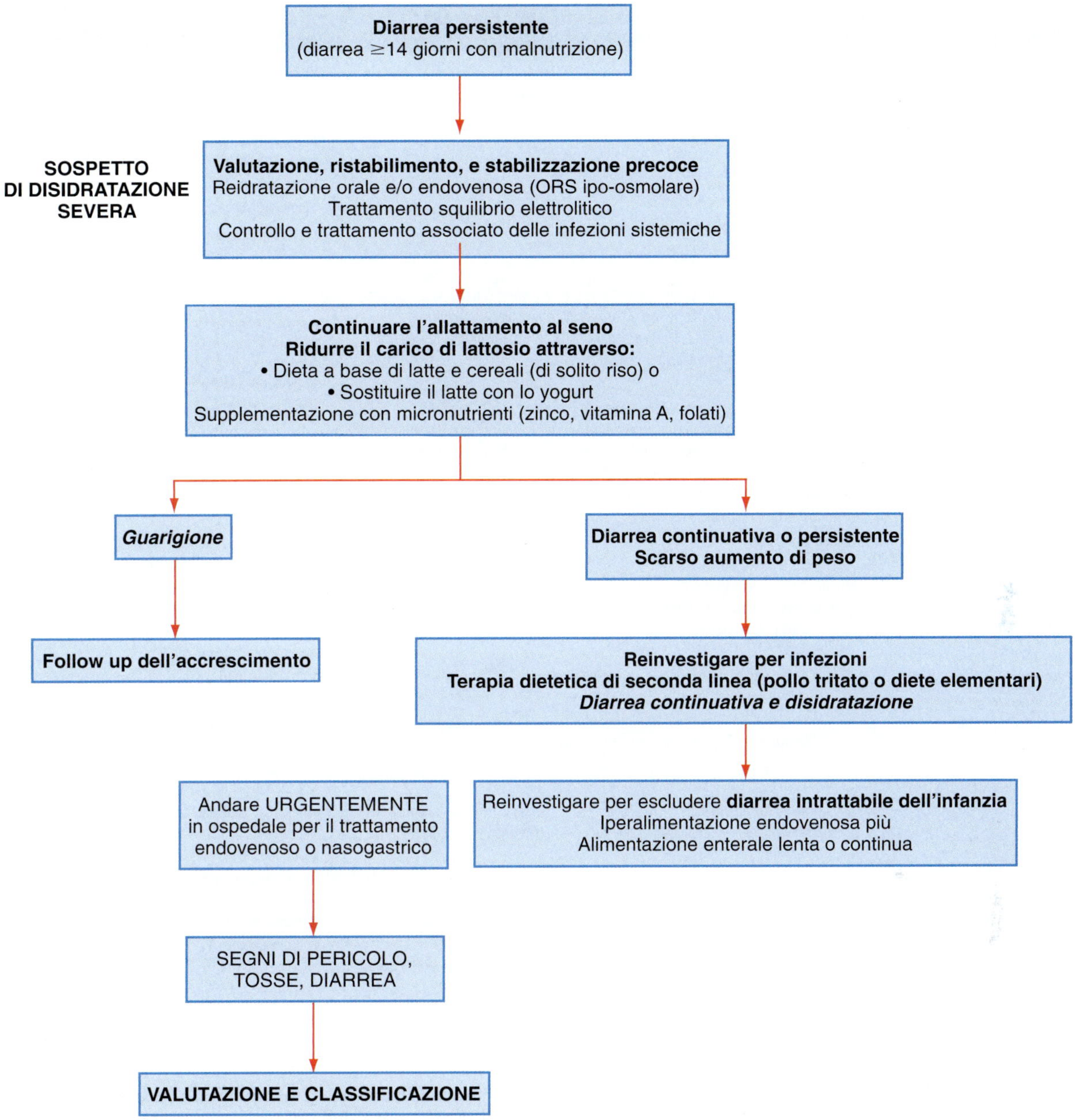

Figura 337-6. Diarrea persistente. NG, Sondino nasogastrico; ORS (*Oral Rehydration Solution*), soluzione reidratante orale.

notificabile e, di conseguenza, per prevenire le epidemie è importante identificare i contatti e risalire alla sorgente di infezione.

Molti Paesi in via di sviluppo si trovano a fronteggiare un numero enorme di casi di diarrea e ciò rende necessario un approccio più ampio alla prevenzione. Identificare strategie preventive è comunque importante sia per i Paesi sviluppati sia per quelli in via di sviluppo

PROMOZIONE DELL'ALLATTAMENTO ESCLUSIVO AL SENO. L'allattamento esclusivo al seno (senza somministrazione di altro liquido o alimento per i primi 6 mesi di vita) non è una pratica frequente. L'allattamento esclusivo protegge i lattanti dalla malattia diarroica non solo inducendo un'immunità passiva (vedi Capitoli 42 e 94), ma diminuendo l'introduzione di cibi e acqua potenzialmente contaminati. Il latte materno possiede tutti i nutrienti necessari nella prima infanzia; se si continua a somministrarlo anche durante l'episodio diarroico, riduce gli effetti collaterali sullo stato nutrizionale.

PERFEZIONAMENTO DELLE TECNICHE DI NUTRIZIONE COMPLEMENTARI. Esiste una forte associazione inversa tra alimentazione complementare appropriata e sicura e mortalità nei bambini di età compresa tra 6 e 11 mesi; la malnutrizione è un fattore di rischio indipendente per quanto riguarda la frequenza e la severità della malattia diarroica. I cibi complementari dovrebbero essere introdotti all'età di 6 mesi mentre l'allattamento al seno dovrebbe essere protratto fino a 1 anno (più a lungo nei Paesi in via di sviluppo). I cibi complementari nelle aree in via di sviluppo sono generalmente poveri dal punto di vista qualitativo e spesso molto contaminati, predisponendo così alla diarrea. Tale contaminazione potrebbe essere ridotta educando coloro che si prendono cura del bambino e migliorando la conservazione domestica dei cibi. L'integrazione con vitamina A riduce la mortalità infantile del 34%; un migliore status della vitamina A riduce la frequenza di diarrea severa.

VACCINAZIONE PER IL ROTAVIRUS. La maggior parte dei lattanti contrae, nei primi mesi di vita, una diarrea da rotavirus; una vaccinazione efficace contro questi ultimi ridurrebbe la mortalità per diarrea nei Paesi in via di sviluppo. Nel 1998 è stato messo in commercio negli Stati Uniti un vaccino tetravalente derivato da rotavirus Rhesus, poi ritirato perché aumentava il rischio di

TABELLA 337-9. Terapia antibiotica per la diarrea infettiva

MICRORGANISMO	FARMACO DI SCELTA	DOSE E DURATA DEL TRATTAMENTO
Shigella (dissenteria severa e dissenteria EIEC)	Ciprofloxacina, ampicillina, ceftriaxone o trimetoprim-sulfametoxazolo (TMP-SMX). La maggior parte delle specie è resistente a molti antibiotici.	Ceftriaxone ev, im 50-100 mg/kg/d qd, bid per 7 d Ciprofloxacina per os 20-30 mg/kg/d bid per 7-10 d 10 mg/kg/d di TMP e 50 mg/kg/d di SMX bid per 5 d Ampicillina per os, ev 50-100 mg/kg/d qid per 7 d
EPEC, ETEC, EIEC	TMP-SMX o ciprofloxacina	10 mg/kg/d di TMP e 50 mg/kg/d di SMX bid per 5 d Ciprofloxacina per os 20-30 mg/kg/d qid per 5-10 d
Salmonella	No antibiotici in caso di gastroenterite non complicata negli ospiti normali, causata da specie non tifoidi. **Trattamento** indicato nei lattanti di età <3 mesi e nei pazienti con neoplasie, malattia gastrointestinale cronica, colite severa, emoglobinopatie o infezioni da HIV e in altri soggetti non immunocompetenti. La maggior parte delle specie diventa resistente al trattamento antibiotico multiplo.	Vedi trattamento della *Shigella*
Aeromonas/Plesiomonas	TMP-SMX Ciprofloxacina	10 mg/kg/d di TMP e 50 mg/kg/d di SMX bid per 5 d Ciprofloxacina per os 20-30 mg/kg/d diviso bid per 7-10 d
Yersinia spp.	Gli antibiotici non sono solitamente necessari per la diarrea. La terapia con deferoxamina deve essere riservata a infezioni severe o batteriemia associate. Trattare la sepsi come per ospiti immunocompromessi, usando una terapia combinata con doxiciclina, aminoglicosidi. TMP-SMX o fluorochinoloni	
Campylobacter jejuni	Eritromicina o azitromicina	Eritromicina per os, 50 mg/kg/d diviso tid per 5 d Azitromicina per os, 5-10 mg/kg/d qid per 5 d
Clostridium difficile	Metronidazolo (prima scelta) Interrompere l'antibiotico iniziato Vancomicina (seconda scelta)	per os 30 mg/kg/d diviso tid per 5 d per os 40 mg/kg/d qid per 7 d
Entamoeba histolytica	Metronidazolo seguito da iodochinolo o paromomicina	per os 30-40 mg/kg/d tid per 7-10 d per os 30-40 mg/kg/d tid per 20 d per os 25-35 mg/kg/d tid per 7 d
Giardia lamblia	Furazolidone o metronidazolo o albendazolo o chinacrina	Furazolidone per os 25 mg/kg/d qid per 5-7 d Metronidazolo per os 30-40 mg/kg/d tid per 7 d Albendazolo per os 200 mg bid per 10 d
Cryptosporidium spp.	Il trattamento con nitazoxanide per os può non essere necessario negli ospiti normali. Negli immunocompromessi, immunoglobulina per os + trattare aggressivamente HIV ecc.	Bambini 1-3 anni: 100 mg bid per 3 d Bambini 4-11 anni: 200 mg bid Adulti: 500 mg bid
Isospora spp. *Cyclospora* spp. *Blastocystis hominis*	TMP-SMX TMP/SMX Metronidazolo o iodochinolo	per os 5 mg/kg/d e 25 mg/kg/d, rispettivamente, bid per 7-10 d per os 5 mg/kg/d e 25 mg/kg/d rispettivamente, bid per 7 d Metronidazolo per os 30-40 mg/kg/d tid per 7-10 d Iodochinolo per os 40 mg/kg/d tid per 20 d

bid, 2 volte al giorno; EIEC (*EnteroInvasive Escherichia coli*), *Escherichia coli* enteroinvasiva; EPEC (*EnteroPathogenic E. coli*), *E. coli* enteropatogeno; ETEC (*EnteroToxigenic E. coli*), *E. coli* enterotossigeno; im, intramuscolare; ev, endovena; per os, orale; d, giornaliero; qid, 4 volte al giorno SMX, sulfametoxazolo; tid, 3 volte al giorno; TMP, trimetoprim.

invaginazione intestinale. Più di recente sono stati approvati, sia per i Paesi sviluppati sia per quelli in via di sviluppo, vaccini in grado di ridurre significativamente il rischio di mortalità per diarrea (vedi Capitoli 170, 262).

Altri vaccini capaci di ridurre potenzialmente il carico di diarrea severa e mortalità nei bambini piccoli sono quelli contro la *Shigella* e l'ETEC.

MIGLIORAMENTO DELLE RISORSE IDRICHE E SANITARIE E PROMOZIONE DELL'IGIENE PERSONALE E DOMESTICA. La riduzione della prevalenza della diarrea, nei Paesi sviluppati, è per lo più attribuibile al miglioramento degli standard di igiene, miglioramento delle condizioni sanitarie ed erogazione dell'acqua. Inoltre l'abitudine di lavare le mani con sapone delicato, tra le mura domestiche, riduce l'incidenza di diarrea in tutti gli ambienti/condizioni. Le strategie messe in atto per promuovere un cambiamento comportamentale indicano che il lavaggio della mani e l'uso del sapone riducono il carico di diarrea nei Paesi in via di sviluppo.

MIGLIORAMENTO DELLA GESTIONE DEI CASI DI DIARREA. Il miglioramento della gestione della diarrea attraverso l'identificazione rapida e la terapia appropriata riduce significativamente la sua durata, il suo impatto sullo stato nutrizionale e il rischio di morte nell'infanzia. La migliore gestione della diarrea acuta è un fattore chiave per ridurre l'entità degli episodi di diarrea prolungata e persistente. Le linee guida dell'OMS/UNICEF, che raccomandano di usare ORS a bassa osmolalità e la supplementazione di zinco nel trattamento della diarrea, associate all'uso di antibiotici selezionati e appropriati, ha il potere di ridurre il numero di decessi per diarrea nella popolazione pediatrica.

337.1 • Diarrea del viaggiatore (vedi Capitolo 173) • Zulfiqar Ahmed Bhutta

La diarrea del viaggiatore è una complicanza che si presenta frequentemente in coloro che si recano nei Paesi in via di sviluppo ed è causata da diversi patogeni che possono variare in base alla stagione e alla regione visitata (Tab. 337-10). Questa patologia miete vittime soprattutto tra i viaggiatori provenienti da Paesi ad alto reddito, che durante l'estate visitano Paesi a clima più caldo, caratterizzati da un'elevata prevalenza di diarrea infettiva a livello locale. La diarrea del viaggiatore può manifestarsi con diarrea acquosa o dissenteria.

TRATTAMENTO. La diarrea del viaggiatore tende ad autolimitarsi ma richiede un'attenzione particolare per evitare il rischio di disidratazione. Per quanto riguarda i lattanti, è indicata la reidratazione (trattata nel Capitolo 337), seguita da una dieta standard. Gli adolescenti e gli adulti dovrebbero aumentare l'introito di liquidi ricchi di elettroliti. Non risultano essere efficaci le terapie a base di caolino-pectina, anticolinergici, *Lactobacillus*, salicilato

TABELLA 337-10. Distribuzione geografica dei più comuni microrganismi patogeni che causano diarrea del viaggiatore

	Asia	America Latina	Africa
BATTERICA			
E. coli enterotossigeno	6-37%	17-70%	8-42%
Altri *E. coli*	3-4%	7-22%	2-9%
Campylobacter jejuni	9-39%	1-5%	1-28%
Salmonella spp.	1-33%	1-16%	4-25%
Shigella spp.	0-17%	2-30%	0-9%
Plesiomonas shigelloides	3-13%	0-6%	3-5%
Aeromonas spp.	1-57%	1-5%	0-9%
VIRALE			
Rotavirus	1-8%	0-6%	0-36%
PARASSITARIA			
Entamoeba histolytica	5-11%	<1%	2-9%
Giardia lamblia	1-12%	1-2%	0-1%
Cryptosporidium spp.	1-5%	<1%	2%
Cyclospora cayetanensis	1-5%?	<1%?	<1%?
Nessun patogeno identificato	10-56%	24-62%	15-53%

Da Al-Abri SS, Beeching NJ, Nye FJ:Traveller's diarrhoea. *Lancet Infect Dis* 2005;5:349-360.

di bismuto. La loperamide, farmaco antispastico e antisecretivo, riduce la frequenza della diarrea nei bambini più grandi che presentano diarrea acquosa, ma va usato con molta cautela e non deve essere utilizzato in pazienti che presentano febbre o sepsi con dissenteria.

La terapia antibiotica con o senza loperamide riduce la frequenza di feci non formate. Una terapia breve (di durata <3 giorni) con fluorochinolonici, trimetoprim/sulfametoxazolo, azitromicina o rifaximina, è efficace; la scelta dell'antibiotico dipende dall'età del paziente, dal microrganismo potenziale e dai pattern di resistenza locale dell'organismo. Per aggiornamenti sui patogeni locali e i pattern resistenti, si rinvia al sito www.cdc.gov/travel.

PREVENZIONE. I viaggiatori dovrebbero bere bevande in bottiglia o in lattina e acqua bollita, evitando il consumo di ghiaccio e insalata, mentre per quanto riguarda la frutta è preferibile consumino solo quella che possono sbucciare da sé. Il cibo deve essere il più caldo possibile. Il pesce crudo o poco cotto rappresenta un rischio, come mangiare al ristorante o in una casa privata. Le piscine o altre strutture ricreative con giochi d'acqua possono essere contaminate.

Non è raccomandata di routine la chemioprofilassi per bambini o adulti altrimenti sani.

Al-Abri SS, Beeching NJ, Nye FJ: Traveller's diarrhoea. *Lancet Infect Dis* 2005;5:349–360.

American Medical Association, American Nurses Association–American Nurses Foundation, Centers for Disease Control and Prevention, et al: Diagnosis and management of foodborne illnesses: A primer for physicians and other health care professionals. *MMWR Recomm Rep* 2004;53:1–33.

Ashkenazi S: *Shigella* infections in children: New insights. *Semin Pediatr Infect Dis* 2004;15:246–252.

Bhatnagar S, Bahl R, Sharma PK, et al: Zinc with oral rehydration therapy reduces stool output and duration of diarrhea in hospitalized children: A randomized controlled study. *J Pediatr Gastroenterol Nutr* 2004;38:34–40.

Bhutta ZA, Ghishan F, Lindley K, et al: Persistent and chronic diarrhea and malabsorption: Working Group report of the Second World Congress of Pediatric Gastroenterology, Hepatology, and Nutrition. *J Pediatr Gastroenterol Nutr* 2004;39:S711–S716.

Bouckenooghe AR, Jiang ZD, de la Cabada FJ, et al: Enterotoxigenic *Escherichia coli* as cause of diarrhea among Mexican adults and US travelers in Mexico. *J Travel Med* 2002;9:137–140.

Caeiro JP, DuPont HL, Albrecht H, Ericsson CD: Oral rehydration therapy plus loperamide versus loperamide alone in the treatment of traveler's diarrhea. *Clin Infect Dis* 1999;28:1286–1289.

Cartwright RY: Food and waterborne infections associated with package holidays. *J Appl Microbiol* 2003;94:12S–24S.

Centers for Disease Control and Prevention: Ongoing multistate outbreak of *Escherichia coli* serotype 0157 : H7 infections associated with consumption of fresh spinach–United States, September 2006. *MMWR* 2006;55:1045–1046.

Centers for Disease Control and Prevention (CDC): Outbreak of cyclosporiasis associated with snow peas—Pennsylvania, 2004. *MMWR* 2004;53:876–878.

Centers for Disease Control and Prevention: Outbreaks of multidrug-resistant *Shigella sonnei* gastroenteritis associated with day care centers—Kansas, Kentucky, and Missouri, 2005. *MMWR* 2006;55:1068–1070.

Centers for Disease Control and Prevention: Preliminary food net data on the incidence of infection with pathogens transmitted commonly through food–10 states, United States, 2005. *MMWR* 2006;55:392–395.

Chouraqui JP, Van Egroo LD, Fichot MC: Acidified milk formula supplemented with *Bifidobacterium lactis*: Impact on infant diarrhea in residential care settings. *J Pediatr Gastroenterol Nutr* 2004;38:288–292.

De Bruyn G, Hahn S, Borwick A: Antibiotic treatment fot travellers' diarrhoea. *Cochrane Database Syst Rev* 2000;3:CD002242.

Denno DM, Stapp JR, Boster DR, et al: Etiology of diarrhea in pediatric outpatient settings. *Pediatr Infect Dis J* 2005;24:142–148.

Elliott EJ: Acute gastroenteritis in children. *BMJ* 2007;334:35–40.

Finley R, Reid-Smith R, Weese JS: Human health implications of Salmonella-contaminated natural pet treat and raw pet food. *CID* 2006;42:686–691.

Fonseca BK, Holdgate A, Craig JC: Enteral vs intravenous rehydration therapy for children with gastroenteritis. *Arch Pediatr Adolesc Med* 2004;158:483–490.

Freedman SB, Adler M, Seshadri R, Powell EC: Oral ondansetron for gastroenteritis in a pediatric emergency department. *N Engl J Med* 2006;354:1698–1705.

Fullerton KE, Ingram A, Jones TF, et al: Sporadic *Campylobacter* infection in infants: a population-based surveillance case-control study. *Pediatr Infect Dis J* 2007;26:19–24.

Guandalini S, Pensabene L, Zikri MA, et al: *Lactobacillus* GG administered in oral rehydration solution to children with acute diarrhoea: A multicenter European trial. *J Pediatr Gastroenterol Nutr* 2000;30:54–60.

Hahn S, Kim Y, Garner P: Reduced osmolarity oral rehydration solution for treating dehydration due to diarrhoea in children: Systematic review. *Br Med J* 2001;323:s81–s85.

Högenauer C, Langner C, Beubler E, et al: *Klebsiella oxytoca* as a causative organism of antibiotic-associated hemorrhagic colitis. *N Engl J Med* 2006;355:2418–2426.

Huang DB, Awasthi M, Le B, et al: The role of diet in the treatment of traveler's diarrhea: A pilot study. *Clin Infect Dis* 2004;39:468–771.

Jalava K, Hakkinen M, Valkonen M, et al: An outbreak of gastrointestinal illness and erythema nodosum from grated carrots contaminated with *Yersinia pseudotuberculosis*. *JID* 2006;194:1209–1216.

Jones TF, Angulo FJ: Eating in restaurants: a risk factor for foodbourne disease? *CID* 2006;43:1324–1328.

Kang G, Ramakrishna BS, Daniel J, et al: Epidemiological and laboratory investigations of outbreaks of diarrhoea in rural South India: Implications for control of disease. *Epidemiol Infect* 2001;127:107–112.

King CK, Glass R, Bresee JS, Duggan C; Centers for Disease Control and Prevention: Managing acute gastroenteritis among children: Oral rehydration, maintenance, and nutritional therapy. *MMWR Recomm Rep* 2003;52:1–16.

Kirkwood C: Viral gastroenteritis in Europe: A new norovirus variant? *Lancet* 2004;363:671–672.

Kosek M, Bern C, Guerrant RL: The global burden of diarrhoeal disease, as estimated from studies published between 1992 and 2000. *Bull World Health Organ* 2003;81:197–204.

Luby SP, Agboatwalla M, Painter J, et al: Effect of intensive handwashing promotion on childhood diarrhea in high-risk communities in Pakistan. *JAMA* 2004;291:2547–2554.

Maki DG: Don't eat the spinach—controlling foodborne infectious disease. *N Engl J Med* 2006;355:1952–1955.

Murata T, Katsushima N, Mizuta K, et al: Prolonged norovirus shedding in infants ≤6 months of age with gastroenteritis. *Pediatr Infect Dis J* 2007;26:46–49.

Musher DM, Musher BL: Contagious acute gastrointestinal infections. *N Engl J Med* 2004;351:2417–2427.

O'Ryan M, Diaz J, Mamani N, et al: Impact of rotavirus infections on outpatient clinic visits in Chile. *Pediatr Infect Dis J* 2007;26:41–45.

O'Ryan M, Prado V, Pickering L: A millennium update on pediatric diarrheal illness in the developing world. *Semin Pediatr Infect Dis* 2005;16:125–136.

Rossignol JF, Abu-Zakry M, Hussein A, Santoro MG: Effect of nitazoxanide for treatment of severe rotavirus diarrhoea: randomized double-blind placebo-controlled trial. *Lancet* 2006;368:124–129.

Shavit I, Brant R, Nijsen-Jordan C, et al: A novel imaging technique to measure capillary-refill time: improving diagnostic accuracy for dehydration in young children with gastroenteritis. *Pediatrics* 2006;118:2402–2408.

Spandorfer PR, Alessandrini EA, Joffe MD, et al: Oral versus intravenous rehydration of moderately dehydrated children: A randomized, controlled trial. *Pediatrics* 2005;115:295–301.

Stauffer WM, Konop RJ, Kamat D: Traveling with infants and young children. Part III: Traveler's diarrhea. *J Travel Med* 2002;9:141–150.

Swanson SJ, Snider C, Branden CR, et al: Multidrug-resistant *Salmonella enterica* serotype typhimurium associated with pet rodents. *N Engl J Med* 2007;356:21–28.

Taylor JA: Oral rehydration. *Arch Pediatr Adolesc Med* 2004;158:420–421.

Thapar M, Sanderson IR: Diarrhoea in children: An interface between developing and developed countries. *Lancet* 2004;363:641–653.

Thielman NM, Guerrant RL: Acute infectious diarrhea. *N Engl J Med* 2004; 350:38–47.

Turck D, Bernet JP, Marx J, et al: Incidence and risk factors of oral antibiotic-associated diarrhea in an outpatient pediatric population. *J Pediatr Gastroenterol Nutr* 2003;37:22–26.

Widdowson MA, Cramer EH, Hadley L, et al: Outbreaks of acute gastroenteritis on cruise ships and on land: Identification of a predominant circulating strain of norovirus—United States, 2002. *J Infect Dis* 2004;190:27–36.

337.2 • I PROBIOTICI NEI DISTURBI GASTROINTESTINALI • David Branski e Michael Wilschanski

I **probiotici** sono microrganismi vivi o componenti di cellule microbiche che esercitano effetti benefici sull'ospite. Essi sono principalmente bacilli produttori di acido lattico, in particolare *Lactobacilli* e *Bifidobacteria*, oltre al lievito *Saccharomyces boulardii.*

Un probiotico deve soddisfare i seguenti requisiti: essere di derivazione umana, non patogeno, sicuro; essere resistente all'acido gastrico, alla bile e alla digestione pancreatica; aderire e colonizzare gli enterociti. Inoltre, essi producono sostanze ad azione antimicrobica, esplicano un effetto di immunomodulazione e hanno la capacità di influenzare l'attività metabolica.

I **prebiotici**, atti a stimolare la proliferazione e lo sviluppo di microrganismi probiotici, includono sostanze come frutto-oligosaccaridi, galatto-oligosaccaridi, inulina, alimenti derivati da orzo germinato, psillio. I prebiotici devono passare indenni il tratto superiore dell'apparato digestivo ed essere un substrato per probiotici selettivi del colon.

Con il termine **simbiotici** si indica infine l'approccio combinato che utilizza prebiotici e probiotici per indurre effetti sinergici come la produzione nell'ospite di un habitat favorevole a livello intestinale.

MECCANISMI FISIOLOGICI

La risposta immune della mucosa ai commensali (flora batterica non patogena) è molto diversa rispetto a quella ai patogeni. Questa differenza si spiega per la produzione da parte dei patogeni di fattori virulenti, assenti nei commensali. Questa "tolleranza" immunologica verso i commensali permette loro di colonizzare il lume intestinale e di svilupparvisi. Inoltre, tra probiotici e sistema immunitario mucosale dell'ospite si stabilisce uno scambio di informazioni e segnali. Nell'epitelio intestinale i recettori *toll-like* (TLR, *Toll-Like Receptor*) e le isoforme NOD (*Nucleotide-binding Oligomerization Domain*) identificano i commensali come tali, impedendo così l'inizio della risposta immunitaria che altrimenti li eliminerebbe, avendoli riconosciuti come patogeni.

I probiotici esplicano un effetto benefico sull'ospite mediante un'azione di immunomodulazione a livello locale. Nell'intestino, essi competono con i patogeni per i nutrienti, producono batteriocine che fungono da antibiotici locali contro i patogeni e inducono la sintesi di peptici antimicrobici come la β-defensina 2 umana. Gli agenti probiotici riducono il fattore di virulenza dell'*E. coli* enteroaggregante mediante la *down-regulation* dell'espressione del regolatore della trascrizione aggR, in concomitanza con un'aumentata espressione dei batteri commensali.

Alcuni batteri probiotici producono acido lattico e acido acetico che possono inibire la crescita dei patogeni riducendo il pH intraluminale. Inoltre, i probiotici occupano i siti di legame della mucosa epiteliale, prevenendo l'adesione dei batteri patogeni alla mucosa. I probiotici inattivati o le sequenze ripetute di DNA isolate dai batteri probiotici possono modificare il recettore per la tossina.

Si è scoperto che il DNA ottenuto da un insieme di specie di probiotici attenua la colite in un modello animale, un effetto dipendente da TLR-9. Il DNA ottenuto da una combinazione di probiotici può inibire l'attivazione della trascrizione del fattore NF-πB (fattore nucleare πB) come la secrezione delle citochine proinfiammatorie nelle cellule epiteliali umane.

I probiotici possono migliorare l'integrità della funzione della barriera mucosa stimolando la produzione di mucina. Essi inibiscono l'aumentata permeabilità paracellulare indotta dai patogeni e hanno la proprietà di attenuare l'ipercontrattilità muscolare osservabile nella dismotilità intestinale postinfettiva.

Alcuni di essi riducono la sintesi di potenti citochine proinfiammatorie come il fattore di necrosi tumorale α (TNF-α, *Tumor Necrosis Factor α*), l'interferone ψ (IFN-ψ), l'interleuchina 12 (IL-12) e anche il fattore attivante le piastrine (PAF, *Platelet Activating Factor*), aumentando la produzione di citochine antinfiammatorie come IL-10. La maggiore produzione di IL-10 si accompagna a un aumento di fattore di crescita trasformante β (TGF-β, *Transforming Growth Factor β*) attraverso il legame di alcuni antigeni probiotici al TLR. I probiotici possono alterare l'equilibrio Th1/Th2 a favore di Th1, con conseguente *down-regulation* della risposta allergica mediata da Th2.

EFFETTI DEI PROBIOTICI IN ALCUNI DISTURBI

DIARREA INFETTIVA ACUTA. Alcune specie di probiotici possono contribuire alla gestione della diarrea acuta infettiva nei pazienti pediatrici sia dal punto di vista della profilassi sia per quanto riguarda l'aspetto terapeutico, riducendone incidenza e durata (vedi Capitolo 337). Nei bambini con gastroenterite da rotavirus trattati con i probiotici, non solo la diarrea è più breve e lieve, ma si osserva anche una maggiore produzione di immunoglobuline A (IgA). Questi batteri si sono rivelati benefici anche nella diarrea infettiva degli adulti.

DIARREA ASSOCIATA AGLI ANTIBIOTICI. La diarrea associata all'uso di antibiotici è un'evenienza frequente, manifestandosi in più di un terzo della popolazione ospedalizzata che riceve questi farmaci (vedi Capitoli 209 e 337). Essa può avere diversa gravità, presentandosi sotto forma di diarrea lieve, colite o enterocolite pseudomembranosa, che può essere ricorrente e fatale. La causa dell'enterocolite pseudomembranosa è multifattoriale (tossina prodotta dal *Clostridum difficile*, alterazione della flora intestinale da terapia antibiotica precedente e riduzione delle difese immunitarie dell'ospite). Dal momento che una delle ipotesi proposte per spiegare la diarrea associata all'uso degli antibiotici è l'alterazione della flora intestinale, gli agenti probiotici possono essere salutari; infatti, diversi agenti hanno dimostrato effetti di tipo preventivo. Il microrganismo più studiato a questo riguardo è il *Saccharomyces boulardii.*

ENTEROCOLITE NECROTIZZANTE NEONATALE. La flora batterica del colon dei neonati pretermine, soprattutto di quelli ricoverati nei reparti di terapia intensiva, è differente da quella dei neonati sani, nati a termine. *Bifidobacteria* spp., che si ritrovano generalmente nei neonati sani, a termine, allattati al seno, compaiono solo alcune settimane dopo la nascita. I neonati pretermine, che sono esposti tardivamente alla microflora materna, tendono a ricevere un ampio spettro di antibiotici e pasti sterili; di conseguenza il loro colon può ospitare microrganismi antibioticoresistenti potenzialmente dannosi. La somministrazione in via profilattica di probiotici per via orale a questa popolazione riduce l'incidenza e la severità dell'enterocolite necrotizzante neonatale (vedi Capitolo 102.2).

DEFICIT DI LATTASI. Il deficit di lattasi è un fenomeno frequente nei bambini con disturbi digestivi correlati al consumo di latte e derivati (vedi Capitolo 335.11). Questi disturbi comprendono flatulenza, diarrea e distensione addominale. I batteri probiotici sono in grado di digerire il lattosio che altrimenti resterebbe solo parzialmente digerito, alleviando di conseguenza i sintomi da deficit di lattasi nei soggetti suscettibili. Infatti, in questi pazienti lo yogurt (ma non il latte) contenente tali probiotici alleviava i sintomi, oltre a ridurre la concentrazione di idrogeno espirato.

SINDROME DELL'INTESTINO IRRITABILE. Questo disturbo digestivo di tipo funzionale comprende entità come la diarrea cronica aspecifica o "diarrea del bambino da 1 a 3 anni" e i dolori addominali ricorrenti che, in accordo con i criteri di Roma II, vanno sotto la definizione di *dolore addominale funzionale* (vedi Capitolo 339). Tale sindrome colpisce soprattutto i bambini di età >5 anni e gli adolescenti. Negli adulti che ne soffrono i batteri probiotici specifici migliorano i sintomi. Inoltre, il rapporto basale IL-10:IL-12, che è basso prima del trattamento con probiotici, si normalizza in seguito al loro utilizzo.

MALATTIA INFIAMMATORIA INTESTINALE. Si tratta di una patologia dall'eziologia complessa, a cui concorrono fattori sia ambientali sia genetici (vedi Capitolo 333) in grado di alterare la risposta immunitaria dell'ospite nei confronti della flora batterica. I roditori con disfunzioni a carico del sistema immunitario, che servono come modello di malattia infiammatoria intestinale, non sviluppano infiammazione quando tenuti in condizioni *germ-free*. Ciò implica che i batteri commensali dell'intestino esercitano un ruolo importante nello sviluppo di questa patologia. Le prove che testimoniano il ruolo importante svolto dalla flora luminale nella patogenesi della malattia infiammatoria intestinale hanno condotto a ipotizzare che la manipolazione della flora intestinale possa esercitare effetti benefici a livello terapeutico.

La somministrazione di probiotici a topi che presentano un deficit di IL-10 con infiammazione intestinale riduce i livelli di citochine proinfiammatorie TNF-α e IL-12 e attenua l'infiammazione intestinale. Nonostante i promettenti risultati ottenuti nel modello animale, l'efficacia dei probiotici nell'uomo non è chiara. L'unico disturbo associato a malattia infiammatoria intestinale in cui tali batteri si sono dimostrati efficaci è la pouchite. Una miscela probiotica con otto specie batteriche è efficace nel trattamento e nella prevenzione della pouchite che fa seguito alla creazione di una tasca ileoanale. Da studi in cui si somministrava una miscela probiotica a pazienti con colite ulcerosa non candidati al trattamento chirurgico è emersa un'induzione di remissione in più del 75% dei partecipanti. L'efficacia dei probiotici nella colite ulcerosa è comunque ancora oggetto di dibattito.

Sono stati condotti trial clinici nel morbo di Crohn, che hanno confrontato la mesalazina con i probiotici; questi ultimi si sono dimostrati in grado di ridurre la frequenza delle recidive. Il probiotico più utilizzato nei bambini è *Lactobacillus* GG (LGG), la cui aggiunta al prednisone ha ridotto l'attività della malattia in un piccolo studio condotto su bambini con morbo di Crohn. In uno studio più ampio, comunque, non si è emersa alcuna differenza nel tasso di remissione osservata al di sopra dei 2 anni.

MALATTIA CELIACA. La gliadina e le rispettive prolamine contengono le sequenze aminoacidiche "tossiche" responsabili dei sintomi dell'enteropatia glutine-sensibile in soggetti immunologicamente suscettibili (vedi Capitolo 335). Tali epitopi, inclusi i peptidi 33-mer corrispondenti al 57-89 della α-2 gliadina, sono molto resistenti alla digestione. *In vitro*, la prolina endopeptidasi dei batteri probiotici è in grado di digerire i peptidi 33-mer. Solo una miscela di varie specie di probiotici contiene l'intera gamma di peptidasi in grado di degradare le gliadine.

Una biotecnologia modificata di lievitazione del pane, che si avvale di lunghi tempi di fermentazione con bacilli probiotici selettivi e farine non tossiche aggiunte, riduce il grado di intolleranza al glutine nei celiaci. La prolil endopeptidasi batterica promuove la digestione delle proteine dei cereali, consentendo l'attacco agli epitopi dei linfociti T multipotenti, che possono quindi detossificare le sequenze "tossiche". Resta da stabilire a quale livello questo processo di digestione intraluminale detossifica i peptidi che altrimenti contribuirebbero agli effetti dannosi della gliadina sulla mucosa dell'intestino tenue prossimale.

IPERSENSIBILITÀ ALLE PROTEINE ALIMENTARI. La flora commensale stimola lo sviluppo del tessuto linfoide associato all'intestino ed è importante per lo sviluppo della tolleranza orale agli antigeni alimentari (vedi Capitoli 144 e 151). Si ipotizza che i microrganismi intestinali siano fondamentali nello sviluppo dei disturbi allergici in quanto creano uno squilibrio della risposta immune. La flora intestinale dei bambini atopici è molto diversa da quella dei controlli; per esempio, *Bifidobacteria* spp., che sono marker di uno sviluppo sano dei commensali, sono ridotti in tali soggetti ancor prima che sviluppino allergia. Alcuni batteri commensali stimolano i linfociti a produrre Th1, come IL-10, TGF-β e IFN-ψ. Sia *in vitro* sia nel modello animale i probiotici si sono dimostrati in grado di stimolare Th1 e la produzione di Th reg. Questo fenomeno è stato osservato in trial clinici condotti nei lattanti con eczema atopico e in quelli con ipersensibilità alle proteine del latte vaccino. LGG somministrato alle donne gravide con una forte storia di disturbi allergici riduce la frequenza di eczema atopico nei loro neonati, e questo risultato si mantiene per oltre 4 anni. I probiotici contrastano l'aumento di permeabilità intestinale e aumentano le risposte IgA-specifiche che sono generalmente deficitarie nei bambini con allergia alimentare.

HELICOBACTER PYLORI. Alcuni studi hanno evidenziato che i probiotici possono inibire o uccidere *Helicobacter pylori in vitro*. Un piccolo numero di studi clinici è stato condotto con risultati incoraggianti in adulti e bambini.

ALTRE CONDIZIONI. Il ruolo potenziale dei probiotici nella prevenzione e nel trattamento della stipsi, della diarrea del viaggiatore, della pancreatite acuta e dell'ipercolesterolemia deve essere oggetto di ulteriori ricerche e valutazioni.

APPROCCIO RAZIONALE ALL'USO DEI PROBIOTICI

Dopo aver dimostrato gli effetti benefici dei probiotici sull'ospite, ci si chiede se occorra raccomandarli come alimenti aggiuntivi o includerli nelle formule per neonati.

Per rispondere a questo interrogativo, bisogna per prima cosa considerare gli aspetti relativi alla sicurezza. Esistono studi che hanno documentato disturbi gastrointestinali come diarrea, flatulenza e cambiamenti dell'habitat intestinale con l'uso di probiotici. Ci sono inoltre rare descrizioni aneddotiche di batteriemie ed endocarditi nei bambini trattati con probiotici, soprattutto in quelli caratterizzati da uno stato di immunodeficienza o da alterazioni cardiache, e di fungemia, soprattutto negli adulti ricoverati nei reparti di terapia intensiva e trattati con *Saccharomyces cerevisia*. È importante sottolineare che le cellule epiteliali intestinali sotto stress metabolico percepiscono la stessa flora batterica commensale dell'ospite come agente offensivo, con conseguente aumento della sintesi di IL-8, riduzione della funzione di barriera degli enterociti e quindi aumento della traslocazione.

Un'altra importante considerazione è il potenziale trasferimento di fattori di virulenza e/o resistenza agli antibiotici dai microrganismi in materiale probiotico alla flora commensale dell'intestino. Questa eventualità deve essere tenuta presente, soprattutto se si considera di supplementare le formule per neonati con i probiotici. Quest'ultima supplementazione, infatti, può modulare la flora intestinale e contribuire alla prevenzione delle allergie. Due specie di *Lactobacilli*, tuttavia, causano un'elevata incidenza di mortalità nei topi neonati (ma non in quelli adulti) con atimia; se ne deduce che i probiotici potrebbero non essere sicuri nei neonati con immunodeficienza. Si raccomanda che le formule per neonati abitualmente commercializzate arricchite con probiotici siano usate solo in soggetti immunocompetenti di età >4-5 mesi.

Un altro potenziale effetto nocivo dei probiotici riguarda la carie dentale: alcuni *Lactobacilli* sono potenzialmente in grado di contribuirvi, presumibilmente a causa della loro proprietà di produrre acidi organici che decalcificano la matrice dentale.

È di estrema importanza definire in modo più preciso le specie più benefiche o la combinazione di specie probiotiche adatta per ciascun obiettivo. In una determinata situazione, un commensale può contribuire a un'immunomodulazione vantaggiosa, mentre in un'altra può non avere effetto o causare una stimolazione indiscriminata della risposta immune. Inoltre, una specie specifica può avere un effetto utile quando somministrata da sola ed essere inefficace quando inclusa in una miscela di probiotici.

Agostoni C, Axelsson I, Braegger C, et al: Probiotic bacteria in dietetic products for infants: A commentary by the ESPGHAN Committee on Nutrition. *J Pediatr Gastroenterol Nutr* 2004;38:365–374.

Bin-Nun A, Bromiker R, Wilschanski M, et al: Oral probiotics prevent necrotizing enterocolitis in very low birth weight neonates. *J Pediatr* 2005;147:192–196.

Di Marzio L, Russo FP, D'Alo S, et al: Apoptotic effects of selected strains of lactic acid bacteria on a human T leukemia cell line are associated with bacterial arginine deiminase and/or sphingomyelinase activities. *Nutr Cancer* 200;40:185–196.

Ezendam J, van Loveren H: Probiotics: Immunomodulation and evaluation of safety and efficacy. *Nutr Rev* 2006;64:1–14.

Gionchetti P, Rizzello F, Helwig U, et al: Prophylaxis of pouchitis onset with probiotic therapy: A double-blind, placebo-controlled trial. *Gastroenterology* 2003;124:1202–1209.

Kalliomaki M, Salminen S, Poussa T, et al: Probiotics and prevention of atopic disease: 4-year follow-up of a randomised placebo-controlled trial. *Lancet* 2003;361:1869–1871.

Rachmilewitz D, Karmeli F, Takabayashi K, et al: Immunostimulatory DNA ameliorates experimental and spontaneous murine colitis. *Gastroenterology* 2002;122:1428–1441.

Sazawal S, Hiremath G, Dhingra U, et al: Efficacy of probiotics in prevention of acute diarrhoea: A meta-analysis of masked, randomised, placebo-controlled trials. *Lancet Infect Dis* 2006;6:374–382.

Szajewska H, Setty M, Mrukowicz J, et al: Probiotics in gastrointestinal diseases in children: Hard and not-so-hard evidence of efficacy. *J Pediatr Gastroenterol Nutr* 2006;42:454–475.

Weizman Z, Asli G, Alsheikh A: Effect of a probiotic infant formula on infections in child care centers: Comparison of two probiotic agents. *Pediatrics* 2005;115:5–9.

Capitolo 338 ■ Diarrea cronica

Fayez K. Ghishan

(Vedi anche Capitoli 335 e 337.)

Nei Paesi in via di sviluppo la diarrea infantile è responsabile di 5 000 000 di decessi all'anno; negli Stati Uniti è causa del 10% di tutte le visite ambulatoriali e di 14 ricoveri ospedalieri all'anno ogni 1000 bambini di età <1 anno (vedi Capitolo 337).

DEFINIZIONE. La diarrea, definita come aumento del volume totale giornaliero di feci, è solitamente associata a un aumento del contenuto di acqua delle feci (vedi Capitoli 303 e 337). Per i lattanti e i bambini, è da considerarsi diarrea un volume fecale >10 g/kg/24 ore o più rispetto al limite dell'adulto di 200 g/24 ore. Quando la diarrea dura più di 2 settimane è definita cronica. La diarrea deriva da un'alterazione del meccanismo di trasporto intestinale di acqua ed elettroliti. La quantità di liquidi assorbita dal tratto gastrointestinale dei bambini è pari a circa 285 mL/kg/24 ore (liquidi introdotti più secrezioni intestinali) con un volume di feci di 5-10 g/kg/24 ore. I meccanismi efficienti responsabili di questa capacità di assorbimento sono dovuti alla funzione di diverse proteine di trasporto situate sull'orletto a spazzola delle cellule dell'intestino tenue e del colon. Il volume di feci del lattante e del bambino contengono circa 20-25 mEq di sodio, 50-70 mEq di potassio e 20-25 mEq di cloruro per litro. I normali meccanismi cellulari responsabili del trasporto dei nutrienti e degli elettroliti attraverso il tratto gastrointestinale sono illustrati nella Figura 338-1.

ANATOMIA FUNZIONALE DELLA MUCOSA INTESTINALE. Il villo, unità funzionale dell'intestino tenue, amplifica notevolmente la

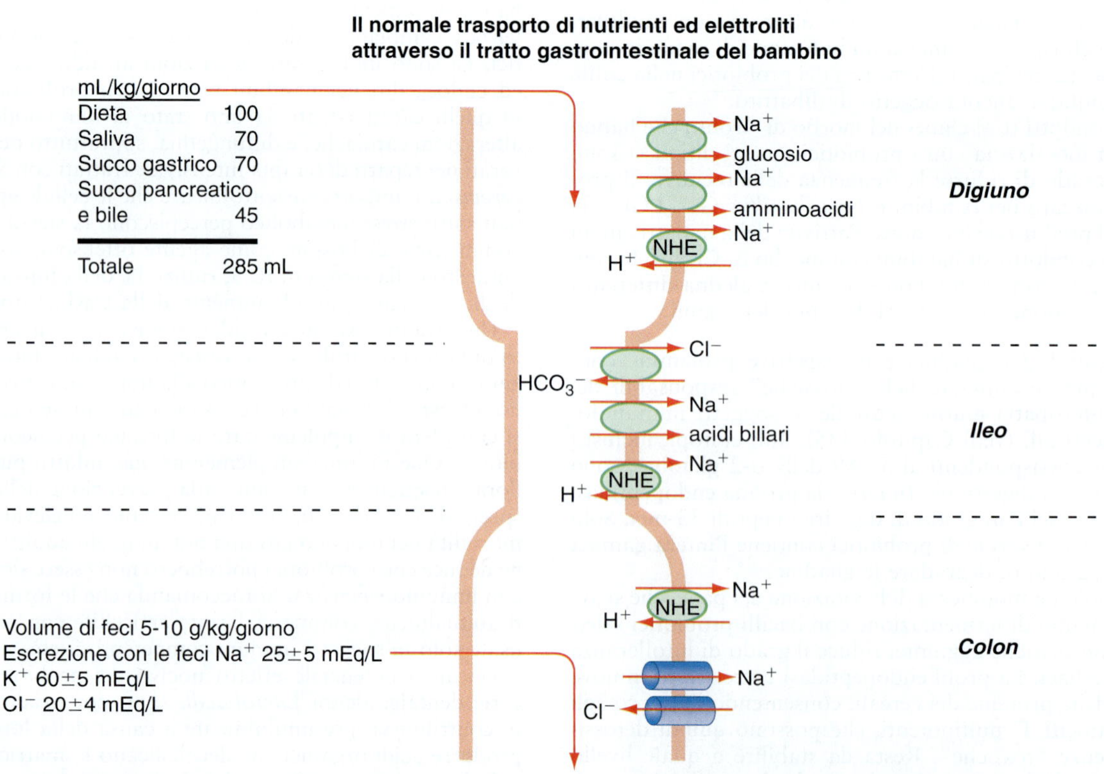

Figura 338-1. Il tratto gastrointestinale dei bambini assorbe 285 mL/kg/die di liquidi, introdotti con la dieta ed endogeni. La maggior parte dei nutrienti e dei liquidi viene assorbita mediante proteine di trasporto descritte qui in modo sintetico. NHE-2, NHE-3 e NHE-8 sono le isoforme 2, 3 e 8 degli scambiatori Na^+/H^+. Il colon assorbe soprattutto acqua ed elettroliti mediante la via elettricamente neutra del NaCl e il processo elettrogenico del Na^+.

superficie assorbente e digestiva della mucosa intestinale. La sua estremità è la sede delle cellule assorbenti altamente differenziate, mentre l'epitelio della cripta è formato da cellule secretorie indifferenziate. Le cellule epiteliali dell'estremità del villo vanno incontro a ricambio ogni 4-5 giorni a partire dalle cellule indifferenziate della cripta. Gli enzimi digestivi e le proteine di trasporto responsabili del passaggio degli elettroliti attraverso la mucosa intestinale sono localizzati sull'orletto a spazzola delle cellule dei villi. Gli epiteli del tratto gastrointestinale sono epiteli permeabili che regolano la quantità di liquidi presenti nel tenue. Le *tight junction* (giunzione serrata), strutture dinamiche situate tra le cellule epiteliali, sono responsabili del passaggio di acqua ed elettroliti. Il trasporto degli elettroliti attraverso l'epitelio intestinale avviene attraverso diversi meccanismi, tra cui quello della proteina di cotrasporto glucosio-sodio: quest'ultima necessita della presenza di un gradiente di sodio attraverso l'orletto a spazzola, che viene mantenuto attraverso la pompa adenosin trifosfato (ATPasi) del sodio e del potassio posta sulla membrana basolaterale degli enterociti. Il difetto di malassorbimento del glucosio-galattosio è dovuto a una mutazione *missense* del gene che codifica per la proteina di cotrasporto del sodio-glucosio (vedi Capitolo 335.11).

Un secondo meccanismo di trasporto degli elettroliti attraverso l'epitelio intestinale è la via elettricamente neutra accoppiata del sodio-cloro, basata su un doppio meccanismo di scambio sodio-idrogeno e cloro-bicarbonato. Tre scambiatori del sodio-idrogeno (NHE-2,-3 e -8) localizzati sulla membrana apicale sembrano coinvolti nel trasporto di sodio. Si ipotizza che alterazioni dei geni che codificano per gli scambiatori del sodio-idrogeno e del cloro-bicarbonato siano responsabili della diarrea congenita da sodio e da cloruro, rispettivamente. Il sodio è assorbito nel colon attraverso la via elettricamente neutra accoppiata del sodio-cloro e mediante un meccanismo elettrogenico regolato dell'aldosterone. Le secrezioni intestinali, prodotte principalmente dalle cellule della cripta, sono stimolate dall'aumento dei livelli intracellulari di adenosinmonofosfato ciclico (cAMP), guanosinmonofosfato ciclico (cGMP) e calcio. Questi mediatori inibiscono l'entrata neutra del sodio e del cloruro e permettono l'entrata del cloruro nelle cellule a livello della membrana basolaterale mediante la proteina di trasporto sodio-potassio-2 cloruro (NA^+-K^+-$2Cl^-$). Il cloro è successivamente secreto attraverso l'apertura dei canali del cloro (regolatore della conduttanza transmembrana della fibrosi cistica), situati sulla membrana apicale delle cellule della cripta. Il sodio e la conseguente secrezione di acqua provocano la diarrea secretoria. Il cotrasporto sodio-glucosio non è alterato dai mediatori intracellulari, e su questo principio si basa della terapia reidratante orale. La Figura 338-2 descrive un modello della secrezione intestinale indotta dall'enterotossina.

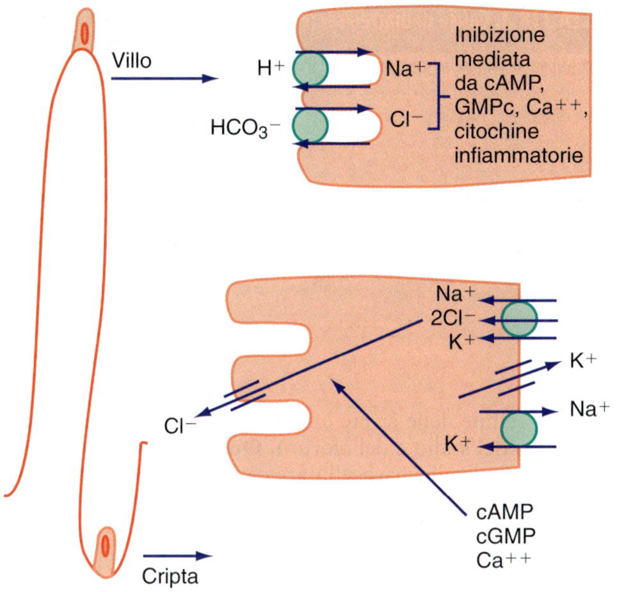

Figura 338-2. Modello di secrezione intestinale: le enterotossine aumentano i livelli dei mediatori intracellulari (cAMP, cGMP, Ca^{2+}) che determinano l'apertura dei canali del cloro delle cellule delle cripte e l'inibizione della via accoppiata neutra del NaCl delle cellule dei villi.

FISIOPATOLOGIA. I meccanismi fisiopatologici della diarrea includono diarrea osmotica, diarrea secretoria, alterazione delle proteine di trasporto della membrana apicale, riduzione della superficie anatomica, alterazione della motilità intestinale e inibizione del trasporto degli elettroliti attraverso mediatori della flogosi (vedi Tab. 303-4).

Diarrea osmotica. La diarrea osmotica è causata dalla presenza di soluti non assorbiti a livello del tratto gastrointestinale (Tab. 338-1). Un esempio classico è l'intolleranza al lattosio causata dal deficit dell'enzima lattasi per cui il lattosio, non assorbito nell'intestino tenue, raggiunge il colon intatto (vedi Capitolo 335.9); i batteri colici fermentano il lattosio non assorbito in acidi organici a catena corta, producendo un carico osmotico e accrescendo l'escrezione di acqua nel lume. Altri esempi sono l'ingestione di quantità eccessive di liquidi carbonati, che superano la capacità di trasporto soprattutto nei bambini molto piccoli, e l'introduzione di idrossido di magnesio e sorbitolo, che, non venendo assorbiti, determinano un carico osmotico. Il lattulosio, un disaccaride sintetico terapeutico, composto da galattosio e fruttosio, non viene digerito nell'intestino tenue e subisce un processo di fermentazione a opera dei batteri del colon con produzione di acidi grassi organici, determinando diarrea osmotica. Quest'ultima cessa con il digiuno, ha un pH basso ed è positiva alle sostanze riducenti. La somma del sodio e del potassio contenuti nelle feci, moltiplicata per due sarà inferiore all'osmolarità delle feci, reperto che indica la presenza di altre osmosi nelle feci. Le caratteristiche principali che differenziano la diarrea osmotica dalla diarrea secretoria sono illustrate nella Tabella 338-2.

Diarrea secretoria. Le cause principali di diarrea secretoria sono descritte nella Tabella 338-3. Tra i suoi meccanismi vi è l'attivazione dei mediatori intracellulari come cAMP, cGMP e il calcio intracellulare, che stimolano la secrezione attiva del cloruro da

TABELLA 338-1. Cause di diarrea osmotica

MALASSORBIMENTO DI NUTRIENTI SOLUBILI IN ACQUA
Malassorbimento glucosio-galattosio
Congenito
Acquisito
Deficit di disaccaridasi (lattasi e saccarasi-isomaltasi)
Congenito
Acquisito
ECCESSIVA INTRODUZIONE DI LIQUIDI CARBONATI
ECCESSIVA INTRODUZIONE DI SOLUTI NON ASSORBIBILI
Sorbitolo
Lattulosio
Idrossido di magnesio

TABELLA 338-2. Diagnosi differenziale tra diarrea osmotica e diarrea secretoria

	DIARREA OSMOTICA	DIARREA SECRETORIA
Volume delle feci	<200 mL/24 h	>200 mL/24 h
Risposta al digiuno	La diarrea termina	La diarrea continua
Na^+ fecale	<70 mEq/L	>70 mEq/L
Sostanze riducenti*	Positivo	Negativo
pH fecale	<5	>6

*Il saccarosio non è un agente riducente. Aggiungere 5 gocce di HCl 0,1 N al campione di feci prima di aggiungere l'agente riducente (compressa Clinitest®).

TABELLA 338-3. Cause di diarrea secretoria

ATTIVAZIONE DI ADENOSIN MONOFOSFATO CICLICO
Tossine batteriche: enterotossine del colera, *Escherichia coli* (termosensibile), *Shigella*, *Salmonella*, *Campylobacter jejuni*, *Pseudomonas aeruginosa*
Ormoni: peptici intestinali vasoattivi, gastrina, secretina
Surfattanti anionici: acidi biliari, acido ricinoleico
ATTIVAZIONE DEL GUANOSINMONOFOSFATO CICLICO
Tossine batteriche: enterotossina di *E. coli* (termostabile), tossina di *Yersinia enterocolitica*
CALCIO-DIPENDENTE
Tossine batteriche: enterotossina di *Clostridium difficile*
Neurotrasmettitori: acetilcolina, serotonina
Agenti paracrini: bradichinina

parte delle cellule delle cripte e inibiscono l'assorbimento accoppiato neutro del sodio e del cloruro. Questi mediatori alterano il flusso di ioni a livello paracellulare causando un danno tossinomediato a carico delle *tight junctions* (giunzioni serrate). Un esempio classico è la diarrea secretoria indotta dal colera e dalle enterotossine di *Escherichia coli* che si legano a specifici recettori di superficie degli enterociti (i monosialogangliosidi GM_1); un frammento della tossina entra nella cellula attivando l'adenilato ciclasi della membrana basolaterale, attraverso l'interazione con una proteina G stimolante; ne deriva un aumento del cAMP intracellulare. L'*E. coli* enterotossigeno causa diarrea secretoria mediante la produzione di una tossina termolabile (LT, *heat-Labile Toxin*) e una termostabile (ST, *heat-Stable Toxin*) nell'intestino tenue. La LT, la cui azione è simile a quella della tossina colerica, si lega allo stesso recettore di superficie GM_1. I pazienti più giovani sono particolarmente sensibili alla ST, dal momento che il numero di recettori per questa tossina sono maggiori nelle fasi precoci della vita che nell'adulto. Altre cause di diarrea secretoria includono i peptidi vasoattivi, che attivano i recettori accoppiati alla proteina G, determinando un aumento intracellulare dei mediatori che scatena una diarrea secretoria.

Quest'ultima è caratterizzata da elevato volume di feci, molto acquose, la cui analisi rivela un elevato contenuto di sodio e cloruro (>70 mEq/L). La diarrea secretoria persiste a digiuno.

Difetti di mutazione delle proteine di trasporto degli ioni. Difetti congeniti dello scambio sodio-idrogeno, cloruro-bicarbonato e delle proteine di trasporto sodio-acidi biliari si manifestano con una diarrea secretoria alla nascita. Alterazioni dello scambio cloruro-bicarbonato e delle proteine di trasporto sodio-acidi biliari sono causate da mutazione dei geni che codificano per le proteine di trasporto corrispettive. Il difetto dello scambio sodio-idrogeno si pensa sia dovuto all'alterazione della proteina di scambio apicale del sodio-idrogeno. I pazienti con questi deficit presentano diarrea secretoria e crescita stentata nel periodo neonatale. Il difetto dello scambio cloruro-bicarbonato, peraltro ben conosciuto, è più frequente rispetto di quello dello scambio di sodio-idrogeno e del trasportatore degli acidi biliari (vedi Capitolo 335.11). I pazienti con diarrea ricca di cloruro presentano alcalosi metabolica ipocloremica con basso livello sierico di cloruro, feci con elevato contenuto di cloruro associato ad assenza di cloruro nelle urine, livelli sierici di potassio bassi e di bicarbonato alti. Le madri possono presentare idramnios.

Riduzione della superficie anatomica. La sindrome dell'intestino corto è determinata da una resezione intestinale secondaria a indicazioni chirurgiche come enterocolite necrotizzante, volvolo o atresia intestinale (vedi Capitolo 335.7). La celiachia è caratterizzata dall'appiattimento della superficie mucosa dell'intestino prossimale, con spiccata diminuzione della funzionalità digestiva e di assorbimento dell'epitelio dei villi (vedi Capitolo 335.2). La diarrea è caratterizzata da perdita di liquidi, elettroliti, macronutrienti e micronutrienti.

Alterazioni della motilità intestinale. Le cause di un'alterata motilità intestinale includono malnutrizione, sclerodermia, sindromi intestinali pseudo-ostruttive e diabete mellito. La malnutrizione in genere determina ipomotilità, la quale predispone a un'eccessiva proliferazione batterica, che a sua volta conduce alla deconiugazione dei sali biliari, con conseguente aumento del mediatore intracellulare cAMP e diarrea secretoria.

EZIOLOGIA. Una classificazione semplice dell'eziologia della diarrea cronica è illustrata nella Tabella 338-4. A scatenare la diarrea sono principalmente fattori intraluminali e fattori mucosali. I primi sono coinvolti nel processo della digestione, mentre i secondi partecipano ai processi digestivi e al trasporto di nutrienti attraverso la mucosa. In molte situazioni, sia i fattori intraluminali sia quelli mucosali causano diarrea. I fattori intraluminali intervengono nelle alterazioni del pancreas, del fegato e dell'orletto a spazzola della membrana degli enterociti. In circa l'85% dei pazienti con **fibrosi cistica**, l'insufficienza pancreatica determina malassorbimento dei grassi e delle proteine. Una bassa statura, l'ipoplasia del pancreas esocrino, una normale concentrazione di cloruro nel sudore, neutropenia di vario grado e alterazioni scheletriche contraddistinguono la **sindrome di Shwachman** (vedi Capitolo 346). La **sindrome di Johannson-Blizzard** è caratterizzata da ano imperforato, agenesia della cartilagine nasale, alterazioni della peluria, ritardo mentale, sordità, ipotiroidismo e insufficienza pancreatica (vedi Capitolo 346). I deficit isolati degli enzimi pancreatici sono congeniti e determinano malassorbimento dei grassi o delle proteine, a seconda del tipo di deficit. Queste alterazioni comprendono i deficit congeniti di lipasi/colipasi e di tripsinogeno. I pazienti con **pancreatite cronica** possono presentare insufficienza pancreatica e diabete insulinodipendente. La **pancreatite familiare**, secondaria a mutazione del gene del tripsinogeno, può determinare pancreatite cronica o insufficienza pancreatica. La **sindrome di Pearson** è caratterizzata da anemia sideroblastica refrattaria con vacuolizzazione dei precursori del midollo osseo, insufficienza del pancreas esocrino, delezioni e duplicazioni del DNA mitocondriale. Alterazioni epatiche, come la colestasi, determinano una riduzione del pool di acidi biliari con malassorbimento dei grassi. La perdita di acidi biliari con malassorbimento di grassi può verificarsi in alcune patologie dell'ileo terminale, come il morbo di Crohn, o in seguito a resezione di questa parte dell'intestino. Il **malassorbimento primario**

TABELLA 338-4. Eziologia della diarrea cronica

FATTORI INTRALUMINALI	FATTORI MUCOSALI
PATOLOGIE PANCREATICHE	**ALTERAZIONE DELL'INTEGRITÀ DELLA MUCOSA**
Fibrosi cistica	Infezioni: batteriche, virali, fungine
Sindrome di Shwachman-Diamond	Infestazioni: parassiti
Sindrome di Johannson-Blizzard	Intolleranza alle proteine del latte vaccino e della soia
Deficit isolati di enzimi pancreatici	Malattia infiammatoria intestinale (colite ulcerosa, colite microscopica, morbo di Crohn)
Pancreatite cronica	
Sindrome di Pearson	**ALTERAZIONI DELLA FUNZIONE IMMUNITARIA**
PATOLOGIE DEGLI ACIDI BILIARI	Enteropatia autoimmune
Colestasi cronica	Gastroenteropatia eosinofila
Resezione dell'ileo terminale	AIDS
Eccessiva proliferazione batterica	Immunodeficienza combinata
Uso cronico di chelanti degli acidi biliari	Deficit di immunoglobuline A e G
Malassorbimento primario degli acidi biliari	**ALTERAZIONI FUNZIONALI**
PATOLOGIE INTESTINALI	Difetti di Cl^-/HCO_3, Na^+/H^+, acidi biliari, acrodermatite enteropatica, deficit selettivo di folati, abetaliproteinemia
Osmolarità intraluminale	
Malassorbimento dei carboidrati	**ALTERAZIONI DELLA FUNZIONE DIGESTIVA**
Deficit congeniti e acquisiti di saccarasi, lattasi	Deficit di enterochinasi
Deficit congeniti e acquisiti di monosaccaridasi	Deficit di glucoamilasi
Eccessiva assunzione di liquidi addizionali di anidride carbonica	**ALTERAZIONI DELL'AREA DI SUPERFICIE**
Eccessiva assunzione di sorbitolo, Mg $(OH)_2$, e lattulosio	Celiachia, sindrome postgastroenterica
	Malattia da inclusione nei microvilli
	Sindrome dell'intestino corto
	ALTERAZIONI DELLA FUNZIONE SECRETORIA
	Batteri produttori di enterotossine
	Tumori secernenti peptici vasoattivi
	ALTERAZIONI DELLE STRUTTURE ANATOMICHE
	Malattia di Hirschsprung
	Ostruzione parziale dell'intestino tenue
	Malrotazione

degli acidi biliari è un disturbo raro, dovuto alla mutazione del gene che codifica per la proteina di trasporto degli acidi biliari a livello dell'ileo. I pazienti presentano malassorbimento di grassi e diarrea. L'eccessiva proliferazione batterica a livello del tratto gastrointestinale determina deconiugazione e deidrossilazione dei sali biliari, responsabili della comparsa di diarrea. L'assunzione a lungo termine di chelanti degli acidi biliari, come la colestiramina, può portare a una diminuzione della quantità degli acidi biliari a causa della loro perdita continua con le feci. L'aumento dell'osmolarità intraluminale, dovuta al malassorbimento di carboidrati, determina diarrea osmotica. Il malassorbimento di carboidrati è dovuto a deficit di monosaccaridasi e disaccaridasi per cause congenite e acquisite. Un'assunzione eccessiva di liquidi carbonati, tale da superare la capacità di trasporto dell'intestino tenue dei bambini più piccoli, determina diarrea aspecifica. L'assunzione in eccesso di soluti poco assorbibili come sorbitolo, idrossido di magnesio e lattulosio scatena una diarrea osmotica.

I fattori mucosali responsabili di diarrea cronica possono essere secondari ad alterazioni dell'integrità secondarie a infezioni batteriche, virali, parassitarie. Le infestazioni da parassiti come *Giardia* o *Cryptosporidium* possono determinare diarrea cronica. Malattie infiammatorie intestinali come la rettocolite ulcerosa, il morbo di Crohn e le coliti microscopiche alterano l'integrità della mucosa, diminuendo dell'assorbimento di acqua ed elettroliti da parte del tratto gastrointestinale. L'intolleranza al latte vaccino e alle proteine della soia può presentarsi con diarrea secondaria ad atrofia parziale dei villi e alla colite allergica. Anche le alterazioni del sistema immunitario, come quelle dei pazienti con agammaglobulinemia, deficit isolato di immunoglobuline A (IgA) e immunodeficienza combinata, possono determinare diarrea. I pazienti con AIDS sono particolarmente suscettibili alle infezioni batteriche, virali e fungine. Anche l'**enteropatia autoimmune** e la **gastroenteropatia eosinofila** sono disturbi che si ritiene determinino alterazione immunitaria della mucosa intestinale, e che possono causare diarrea. Alterazioni a carico della funzione di trasporto della mucosa, come quelle delle malattie congenite che interessano lo scambio di sodio-idrogeno e cloruro-bicarbonato, il trasporto degli acidi biliari e del glucosio-galattosio, determinano diarrea che si manifesta precocemente nel periodo neonatale. Allo stesso modo, difetti dell'assorbimento dello zinco (come l'acrodermatite enteropatica) e del trasporto dei folati possono provocare diarrea.

L'abetalipoproteinemia è caratterizzata da malassorbimento di grassi, lesioni neurologiche e alterazioni oculari, come la retinite pigmentosa (vedi Capitolo 86.3). La diagnosi è confermata dal quadro ematologico di acantocitosi e dalla biopsia dell'intestino tenue, che evidenzia goccioline di lipidi a livello dell'apice degli enterociti. Alterazioni della funzione digestiva della mucosa comprendono deficit congeniti di enterochinasi, che incidono negativamente sull'attivazione del tripsinogeno a tripsina, con malassorbimento di proteine (vedi Capitolo 335.9). Il deficit di α-glucoamilasi, peraltro raro, determina una riduzione dell'idrolisi dei polimeri di glucosio.

Alterazioni della superficie mucosa sono presenti nella **celiachia**, nell'atrofia parziale dei villi secondaria alla sindrome da malassorbimento postgastroenteritica, nella sprue tropicale, nella malattia da inclusioni dei microvilli, nella malattia di Whipple e nella sindrome dell'intestino corto. Queste patologie sono caratterizzate da alterazioni dell'altezza e della struttura dei villi, tali da ridurre la capacità di assorbimento della superficie mucosa. La celiachia è secondaria a sensibilizzazione al glutine (vedi Capitolo 335.2). La sindrome postgastroenteritica è un disturbo nutrizionale che si verifica in seguito a un episodio prolungato di gastroenterite e ridotto introito energetico. La malattia da inclusioni dei microvilli si manifesta con diarrea, deficit di assorbimento e inclusioni all'interno dei microvilli, evidenti all'esame istologico (vedi Capitolo 335.3). La superficie mucosa è priva di orletto a spazzola o presenta microvilli appiattiti. La malattia di Whipple, che colpisce soprattutto gli adulti, è imputabile a un actinomicete, il *Tropheryma whippelii*, che provoca calo ponderale, diarrea e artropatie. La diagnosi si basa sulla biopsia dell'intestino tenue; i pazienti rispondono a somministrazione prolungata di trimetoprim/sulfametoxazolo. La sprue tropicale è più frequente tra i soggetti che vivono o tornano da Paesi in via di sviluppo (vedi Capitolo 335.4). I pazienti presentano diarrea e deficit nutrizionali, soprattutto di folati. Un'alterazione della struttura anatomica, come quella che si verifica nella malattia di Hirschsprung, nella malrotazione e nell'ostruzione parziale del tenue, può causare diarrea secondaria a eccessiva proliferazione batterica. Alterazioni della funzione secretoria della mucosa sono presenti in patologie batteriche producenti enterotossine e in tumori secernenti peptidi vasoattivi. La Tabella 338-5 riassume le cause più frequenti di diarrea cronica nelle diverse fasce di età.

VALUTAZIONE DEI PAZIENTI. La valutazione dei pazienti con diarrea cronica è presentata nella Tabella 338-6. Innanzitutto è importante stabilire se il paziente ha davvero diarrea, in quanto si ritiene erroneamente che i soggetti con encopresi presentino diarrea secondaria a perdita costante di feci. I primi passi della fase I sono rappresentati dall'anamnesi e dall'esame obiettivo, comprendente la valutazione dello stato nutrizionale. L'anamnesi clinica deve tener conto della quantità e del tipo di liquidi introdotti ogni giorno. Se l'anamnesi rivela l'assunzione di un volume di liquidi addizionati di anidride carbonica o di succhi di frutta >150 mL/kg/24 h, con parametri normali di crescita staturoponderale, si può considerare la diagnosi di **diarrea cronica aspecifica.** Una riduzione della quantità di liquidi a non più di 90 mL/kg/24 h dovrebbe determinare la scomparsa della diarrea. Se il paziente

TABELLA 338-5. Cause frequenti di diarrea cronica

PRIMA INFANZIA
Sindrome da malassorbimento post-gastroenteritica
Intolleranza al latte vaccino o alle proteine della soia
Deficit secondario di disaccaridasi
Fibrosi cistica
INFANZIA
Diarrea cronica aspecifica
Deficit secondario di disaccaridasi
Giardiasi
Sindrome da malassorbimento postgastroenteritica
Celiachia
Fibrosi cistica
ADOLESCENZA
Sindrome dell'intestino irritabile
Malattia infiammatoria intestinale
Giardiasi
Intolleranza al lattosio

TABELLA 338-6. Valutazione dei pazienti con diarrea cronica

FASE I
Anamnesi clinica inclusa la quantità specifica di liquidi assunta giornalmente
Esame obiettivo compresa la valutazione dello stato nutrizionale
Esame delle feci (pH, sostanze riducenti, striscio per la conta leucocitaria, grassi, uova e parassiti)
Coprocolture
Esame delle feci per la ricerca della tossina di *Clostridum difficile*
Esame ematochimici (conta leucocitaria con formula, velocità di eritrosedimentazione, elettroliti, azotemia, creatinina)
FASE II
Test del sudore
Determinazione dei grassi nelle feci delle 72 ore
Elettroliti e osmolarità delle feci
Ricerca di fenolftaleina, magnesio solfato e fosfati nelle feci
Breath test per H2
FASE III
Esami endoscopici
Biopsia del tenue
Sigmoidoscopia e colonscopia con biopsia
Esami con il bario
FASE IV
Studi ormonali per il peptide vasoattivo intestinale, gastrina, secretina, e acido 5-idrossindolacetico

sta assumendo una quantità eccessiva di nutrienti non assorbibili, come il sorbitolo, occorre modificare la sua dieta prima di effettuare ulteriori approfondimenti.

L'esame delle feci rappresenta un passo importante nella valutazione di un paziente con diarrea cronica. L'esame delle feci evacuate di recente, incluso il loro contenuto liquido, è utile ai fini diagnostici. Esistono diverse tecniche per la raccolta delle feci: per esempio, si può posizionare un contenitore per urine a livello anale o ricorrere a un pannolino monouso. Il campione deve essere conservato in frigorifero fino al momento in cui verrà esaminato. I campioni per la coprocoltura devono essere immediatamente trasportati al laboratorio di microbiologia per l'inoculazione nei terreni di coltura. L'esame macroscopico delle feci deve aiutare il medico a valutare se il paziente ha diarrea e se vi sono sangue o muco nelle feci, indici di una flogosi a livello del colon. Il colore delle feci è di scarsa utilità, a meno che non siano del colore del sangue. La ricerca del sangue occulto nelle feci è utile per stabilire se il paziente ha perdite ematiche microscopiche. Il malassorbimento dei carboidrati si evidenzia mediante l'analisi della componente liquida di un campione di feci fresche. Un pH <5 o una moderata quantità di sostanze riducenti indica la presenza di carboidrati riducenti (il saccarosio non è una sostanza riducente). Il campione fecale deve essere inviato in laboratorio per la determinazione degli elettroliti e dell'osmolarità, se si sospetta una diarrea secretoria (vedi Tab. 338-2).

L'esame microscopico delle feci è utile per evidenziare la presenza di globuli bianchi, indicativa di infiammazione del colon. Occorre inoltre procedere alla ricerca di uova e parassiti come *Giardia*, *Amoeba* o *Cryptosporidium*. La colorazione tricromica o quella acida rapida sono utili per l'identificazione di *Cryptosporidium*. Le feci devono essere esaminate per la ricerca dell'antigene di *Giardia*. La colorazione Sudan deve essere usata su un vetrino, con le feci soltanto o con l'aggiunta di acido acetico e calore, per evidenziare i trigliceridi e le goccioline di lipidi.

Se le indagini della fase I non hanno permesso di risalire alla causa, è indicato passare alla fase II, comprendente il test del sudore per la diagnosi di fibrosi cistica. Per determinare se il paziente ha malassorbimento dei grassi, se il test del sudore è negativo, occorre valutare i grassi nelle feci delle 72 ore. Si può inoltre esaminare il campione fecale alla ricerca di fenolftaleina, magnesio, solfato e fosfato, per valutare se la diarrea è secondaria all'uso di **lassativi** (diarrea fittizia). Il breath test all'idrogeno serve a determinare un malassorbimento specifico dei carboidrati. Un breath test all'idrogeno per il glucosio o il lattulosio è utile per la diagnosi di un'eccessiva proliferazione batterica.

Le indagini della fase III includono gli esami endoscopici dell'intestino tenue e le biopsie del colon. Gli esami con il bario, come il transito gastroesofageo e il clisma opaco, possono essere utilizzati per rivelare lesioni anatomiche del tratto gastrointestinale. Se nessuna di queste indagini ha permesso di arrivare alla diagnosi, le valutazioni della fase IV comprendono studi ormonali, neuro-ormonali e l'analisi dei neurotrasmettitori, come il peptide intestinale vasoattivo (VIP, *Vaso-active Intestinal Peptide*), la gastrina, la secretina e l'acido 5-idrossindolacetico.

TRATTAMENTO. La Figura 338-3 descrive l'approccio terapeutico generale per il trattamento della diarrea cronica. Il primo principio è garantire un adeguato apporto nutrizionale per permettere una crescita e uno sviluppo normali. È necessario valutare l'altezza, il peso e lo stato nutrizionale del paziente. Se i parametri nutrizionali (peso e altezza compresi) sono normali e l'esame delle feci non mostra la presenza di grassi, occorre considerare la

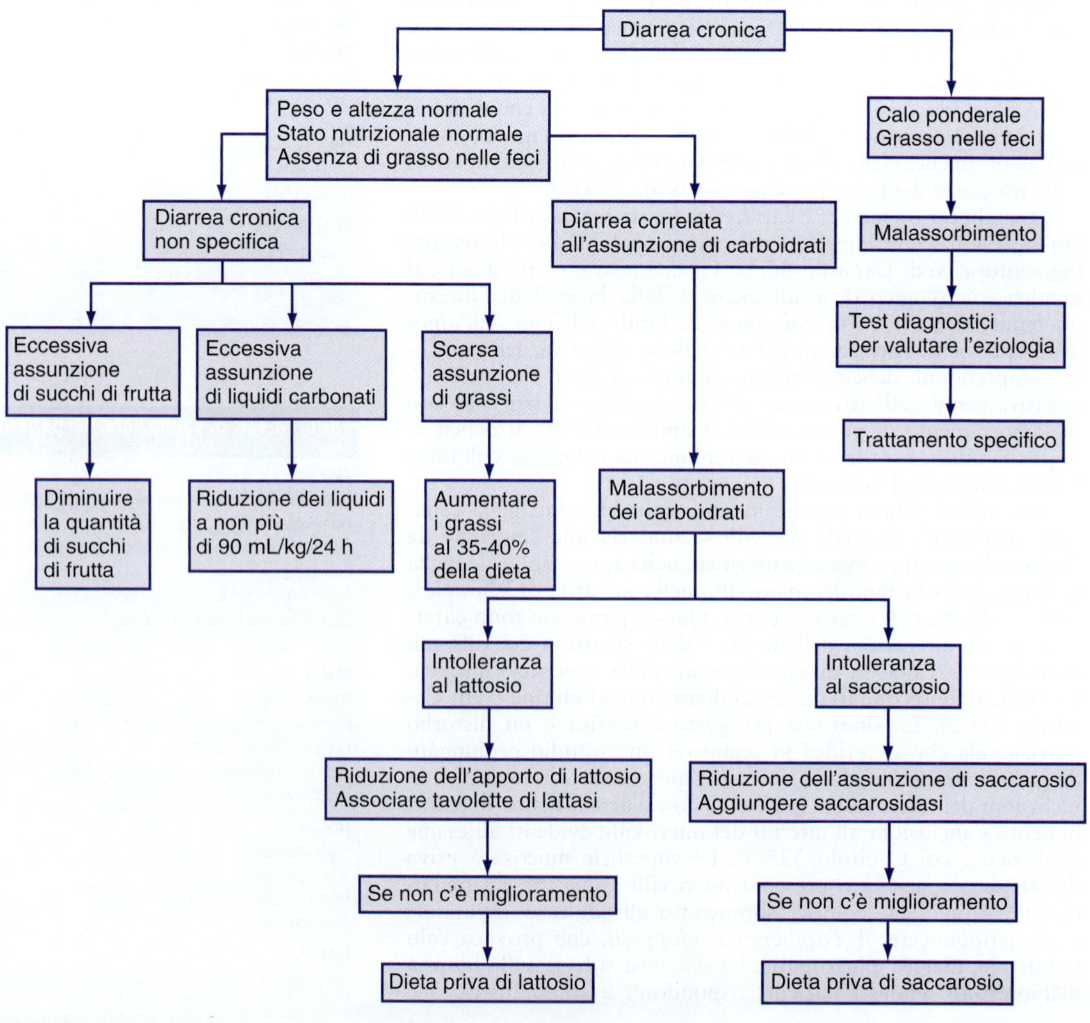

Figura 338-3. Approcci terapeutici generali per il trattamento della diarrea cronica.

possibilità di una diarrea cronica aspecifica. Nella patogenesi di questa condizione rientrano un'eccessiva introduzione di liquidi addizionati di anidride carbonica, malassorbimento di carboidrati non digeribili per consumo eccessivo di succhi di frutta e scarsa assunzione di grassi.

La **diarrea cronica aspecifica** di solito si presenta nei soggetti di 1-3 anni di età (toddler's diarrhea). La diarrea è spesso marrone e acquosa e talvolta contiene frammenti di cibo non digerito. Se l'introito di liquidi è >150 mL/kg/24 h, esso va ridotto in modo che non superi i 90 mL/kg/24 h. I genitori possono notare che il bambino è irritabile nei primi 2 giorni successivi alla riduzione dei liquidi; comunque, perseverando in questo approccio per diversi giorni si ottiene una riduzione del volume e della frequenza delle feci. Se dall'anamnesi alimentare emerge che il bambino assume una grande quantità di succhi di frutta, questi devono essere ridotti. Il sorbitolo, uno zucchero non assorbibile contenuto nei succhi di mela, pera e prugna, può causare diarrea nel bambino ai primi passi. Inoltre, i succhi di mela e pera hanno una quantità di fruttosio maggiore della concentrazione di glucosio, possibile causa della diarrea in questa fascia di età.

Anche la quantità di grassi introdotti con la dieta può avere un ruolo nella diarrea cronica. Se sono stati i genitori a limitare l'assunzione dei grassi da parte del bambino, l'assunzione di grassi deve essere aumentata al 40% delle calorie totali giornaliere.

Se la diarrea è secondaria a intolleranza ai carboidrati, occorre fare una prova, riducendo la quantità di lattosio o saccarosio per un certo periodo. La lattasi può essere utilizzata per facilitare la digestione del lattosio. Se la diarrea persiste, è indicato un periodo di prova con una dieta priva di lattosio o saccarosio. In alternativa, il breath test all'idrogeno può rivelare un'intolleranza al lattosio o al saccarosio. Il breath test al glucosio o lattulosio è utile per diagnosticare un'eccessiva proliferazione batterica.

Se il paziente presenta calo ponderale e l'esame delle feci dimostra la presenza di grassi, occorre prendere in esame la possibilità di diarrea cronica secondaria a sindrome da malassorbimento. La causa più frequente di diarrea cronica associata a malassorbimento è la sindrome da malassorbimento postgastroenteritica. Questi pazienti rispondono bene a preparati predigeriti. Qualora il paziente manifestasse intolleranza all'alimentazione orale con formule predigerite, andrebbe considerata l'ipotesi di somministrare mediante sondino naso-gastrico preparati elementari per 3-4 settimane.

Un paziente che si presenta all'attenzione del medico con il sospetto di un'eccessiva proliferazione batterica nell'intestino tenue deve essere valutato per una terapia chirurgica, medica e nutrizionale. Il trattamento chirurgico è indicato in caso di malrotazione o di ostruzione parziale del tenue. La terapia antibiotica solitamente si inizia con metronidazolo associato ad ampicillina o trimetoprim/sulfametoxazolo. La diarrea da *Giardia lamblia* può essere trattata con metronidazolo o nitazoxanide, quella da *Cryptosporidium parvum* con nitazoxanide.

Per i pazienti con diarrea secretoria, soprattutto durante il primo mese di vita, occorre valutare l'eventualità di un supporto nutrizionale perché la causa più probabile è un difetto congenito delle proteine di trasporto. Nei bambini più grandi con diarrea secretoria occorre innanzitutto individuarne la causa, su cui basarsi per formulare le ipotesi terapeutiche.

Acra S, Ghishan, FK: Electrolyte fluxes in the gut and oral rehydration solutions. *Pedriatr Clin North Am* 1996;43:433–449.

Bhutta ZA, Hendricks KM: Nutritional management of persistent diarrhea in childhood: A perspective from the developing world. *J Pediatr Gastroenterol Nutr* 1996;22:17–37.

Binder HJ: Causes of chronic diarrhea. *N Engl J Med* 2006;355:236–239.

Boissieu D, Chaussain M, Badoual J, et al: Small-bowel bacterial overgrowth in children with chronic diarrhea, abdominal pain, or both. *J Pediatr* 1996;128:203–207.

Castro-Rodriguez JA, Salazar-Lindo E, Leon-Barua R: Differentiation of osmotic and secretory diarrhea by stool carbohydrate and osmolar gap measurements. *Arch Dis Child* 1997;77:201–205.

Cutz E, Sherman PM, Davidson GP: Enteropathies associated with protracted diarrhea of infancy: Clinicopathological features, cellular and molecular mechanisms. *Pediatr Pathol Lab Med* 1997;17:335–368.

Dellert SF, Cohen MB: Diarrheal disease. *Pediatr Gasterol* 1994;23: 637–654.

Donowitz M, Kokke FT, Saidi R: Evaluation of patients with chronic diarrhea. *N Engl J Med* 1995;332:725–729.

Duggan C, Nurko S: Feeding the gut: The scientific basis for continued enteral nutrition during acute diarrhea. *J Pediatr* 1997;131:801–808.

Greene HL, Ghishan FK: Excessive fluid intake as a cause of chronic diarrhea in young children. *J Pediatr* 1983;102:836–840.

Kneepkens CM, Hoekstra JH: Chronic nonspecific diarrhea of childhood: Pathophysiology and management. *Pediatr Clin North Am* 1996;43: 375–390.

338.1 • Diarrea causata da tumori secernenti ormoni • Joel Shilyansky

Alcuni tumori che producono ormoni determinano un aumento marcato della secrezione intestinale, causando una grave diarrea acquosa (Tab. 338-7). La diarrea secretoria persiste anche quando si sospende l'assunzione di cibi. Questi tumori derivano da cellule del sistema APUD provenienti dalla cresta neurale (captazione e decarbossilazione dei precursori aminici) del sistema endocrino gastrenteropancreatico e delle sedi nervose surrenaliche ed extra-

TABELLA 338-7. Diarrea causata da tumori secernenti ormoni

NOME	SEDE	ORMONE	MANIFESTAZIONI	TERAPIA
Carcinoide	Cellule intestinali argentaffini	Serotonina	Diarrea, crampi addominali dolorosi, flushing, wheezing, danno delle valvole cardiache	Analoghi della somatostatina, resezione
	Appendice, ileo, colon, digiuno, retto Tratto bronchiale			
Gastrinoma	Pancreas	Gastrina	Ulcera peptica, diarrea	Farmaci anti-H_2, omeprazolo, resezione del tumore (gastrectomia)
Mastocitoma	Cute, intestino, fegato, milza	Istamina, VIP	Prurito, flushing, apnea, se VIP (+)-diarrea	Farmaci anti-H_1 e anti-H_2, cromolina, corticosteroidi, resezione se isolato
Carcinoma midollare	Tiroide	Calcitonina, VIP, prostaglandine	Diarrea acquosa	Tiroidectomia
Ganglioneuroma, ganglioneuroblastoma, neuroblastoma, feocromocitoma	Cellule cromaffini, soprattutto in sede addominale, extrasurrenale, surrene	Catecolamine, VIP	Ipertensione, tachicardia, sudorazione, diarrea acquosa†	Agente bloccante α-adrenergico per il controllo della PA, agente bloccante β-adrenergico per la tachicardia, resezione
Somatostatinoma	Pancreas	Somatostatina	Diarrea massiva	Resezione
VIPoma	Pancreas	VIP	Diarrea acquosa, acloridria, ipokaliemia	Analoghi della somatostatina, resezione

†*La diarrea è stata riscontrata solo in pazienti adulti con feocromocitoma.*

PA, pressione arteriosa; H_1, recettori per l'istamina di tipo 1; H_2, recettori per l'istamina di tipo 2; VIP (*Vaso-active Intestinal Polypeptide*), polipeptide intestinale vasoattivo.

surrenaliche. La diarrea, massiva, altera l'equilibrio dei liquidi e degli elettroliti, oltre a determinare calo ponderale. La diagnosi si basa sulla presenza di diarrea acquosa secretoria, manifestazioni di tipo extraintestinale, misurazioni dei livelli dell'ormone sospettato o dei suoi metabolici nel siero e nelle urine e diverse tecniche di imaging (TC, RM). La resezione del tumore, quando possibile, è il trattamento di scelta. La terapia farmacologica con antagonisti degli ormoni, come gli analoghi sintetici a lunga azione della somatostatina, può essere un palliativo (vedi Tab. 338-7). In un approccio terapeutico sperimentale è stata utilizzata somatostatina radiomarcata.

Dall'Igna P, Ferrari A, Luzzatto C, et al: Carcinoid tumor of the appendix in childhood: The experience of two Italian institutions. *J Pediatr Gastroenterol Nutr* 2005;40:216–219.

Doede T, Foss HD, Waldschmidt J: Carcinoid tumors of the appendix in children: Epidemiology, clinical aspects and procedure. *Eur J Pediatr Surg* 2000;10:372–377.

Oberg K: Chemotherapy and biotherapy in the treatment of neuroendocrine tumours. *Ann Oncol* 2001;12:S111–S114.

Soga J: Early-stage carcinoids of the gastrointestinal tract: An analysis of 1914 reported cases. *Cancer* 2005;103:1587–1595.

Capitolo 339 ■ Dolore addominale ricorrente dell'infanzia Robert Wyllie

Il dolore addominale cronico viene classificato in "organico" e "non organico", a seconda che sia individuata o meno una causa specifica. Il dolore non organico, o dolore addominale "funzionale", non ha una base strutturale, fisiologica o biochimica che lo giustifichi. Il dolore addominale ricorrente (RAP, *Recurrent Abdominal Pain*) nei bambini è definito come un episodio di dolore che ricorre almeno mensilmente per 3 mesi consecutivi ed è di tale gravità da interferire con le attività di routine/quotidiane. Il DAR colpisce circa il 15% dei ragazzi in età prescolare e scolare. Circa il 10% dei bambini in età scolare che ne soffre richiede una valutazione medica; la probabilità di ottenere l'attenzione del medico è proporzionale alla gravità e alla frequenza del dolore addominale e al suo impatto sulla frequenza scolastica.

I primi ricercatori avevano trovato una causa organica per il DAR nel 5-10% dei bambini. Grazie ai progressi compiuti nelle tecnologie mediche, tra cui l'endoscopia, il breath test all'idrogeno per il malassorbimento dei carboidrati e per la motilità intestinale e le indagini radiografiche, è diminuita la percentuale di dolore da causa inspiegata. Nella maggior parte degli adolescenti con DAR, le tecniche diagnostiche attualmente a disposizione non permettono di appurarne la causa; molti probabilmente andranno incontro a una diagnosi di sindrome dell'intestino irritabile.

Nei bambini con DAR, il dolore addominale è per lo più localizzato in sede periombelicale. Il dolore in sede epigastrica è spesso associato a sintomi come sazietà precoce, nausea, gonfiore o eruttazione e, in caso di valutazione negativa e di assente risposta alla terapia con antiacidi, viene considerato una manifestazione della *dispepsia non ulcerosa*. Il dolore al di sotto dell'ombelico è spesso accompagnato da crampi addominali, gonfiore, distensione e alterazione della motilità intestinale; questo complesso di sintomi è indicativo di sindrome dell'intestino irritabile (IBS, *Irritable Bowen Syndrome*) nella popolazione adulta. Una sintomatologia simile a quella dell'IBS è stata riscontrata nel 35% circa dei bambini con DAR. I criteri diagnostici Roma II per i sistemi tipo-IBS comprendono: dolore o fastidio per 12 settimane negli ultimi 12 mesi, più 3 dei seguenti criteri:

- **dolore addominale attenuato dalla defecazione**
- **esordio del dolore con cambiamento nella frequenza dell'evacuazione (>3 scariche/die o <3 scariche/settimana)**
- **esordio del dolore con cambiamento nella consistenza delle feci (granulose, liquide, dure), presenza di muco, gonfiore, anomalie della defecazione (difficoltosa, impellente, sensazione di evacuazione incompleta)**

La sintomatologia del tratto gastrointestinale è positivamente correlata sia ad ansia sia a depressione, in particolare nei bambini con sintomatologia tipo sindrome del colon irritabile. Il miglioramento della sintomatologia durante i weekend e le vacanze scolastiche suggerisce l'ipotesi di un dolore di tipo funzionale, ma l'assenza di tale modalità non permette di escludere questa diagnosi.

Gli studi sulle cause del DAR si sono focalizzati su alterazioni del sistema nervoso autonomo e della motilità intestinale. Le corna dorsali del midollo spinale regolano la conduzione degli impulsi dai recettori nocicettivi periferici al midollo spinale e al cervello, e l'esperienza del dolore è ulteriormente influenzata dai centri cognitivi ed emotivi. Il dolore periferico cronico può determinare un'aumentata attività neuronale dei centri superiori del sistema nervoso centrale, che a sua volta contribuisce a perpetuarlo. Lo stress psicosociale può influire sull'intensità e sulla qualità del dolore attraverso questi meccanismi. Gli studi manometrici e di svuotamento con radionuclidi indicano che l'alterazione della motilità, associata a una maggiore consapevolezza, può causare dolore addominale in alcuni bambini.

La risposta del piccolo paziente al dolore può essere influenzata dallo stress, dal tipo di personalità e dal rinforzo che i familiari forniscono alle sue turbe del comportamento. Una percentuale significativamente elevata di bambini con DAR ha parenti con disturbi da somatizzazione, alcolismo e comportamento antisociale. I genitori e i fratelli hanno maggiori probabilità di soffrire di dolore addominale, esaurimento nervoso ed emicrania. I bambini con dolore addominale funzionale hanno maggiore probabilità di sperimentare fattori stressanti. Abusi sessuali in età infantile possono essere associati con DAR. Questa evenienza deve essere sempre tenuta in considerazione, soprattutto nelle ragazze in cui i sintomi addominali iniziano in età prepubere o adolescenziale.

DIAGNOSI. Prima di effettuare una diagnosi di dolore funzionale occorre valutare un'ampia gamma di potenziali cause organiche di DAR (vedi Tab. 303-4). Tra le cause più frequenti vi sono la stipsi cronica, l'infezione parassitaria (*Giardia*), il reflusso gastroesofageo, la malattia infiammatoria intestinale e il deficit di lattasi. L'intolleranza al lattosio è così frequente che il suo riscontro può essere accidentale; i medici devono essere cauti nell'attribuire il dolore addominale cronico a questa condizione. Gli ossiuri sono raramente la causa di dolore addominale.

Il DAR esordisce caratteristicamente dopo i 6 anni di età, con dolore parossistico a livello della linea mediana per lo più periombelicale, ma anche localizzato in sede epigastrica o nell'area sovrapubica. Il dolore costringe il paziente a interrompere le sue attività consuete, ma di solito non c'è alcun rapporto con i pasti. I bambini con IBS lamentano tipicamente dolore addominale che si attenua con la defecazione. Essi possono presentare muco nelle feci e all'esordio del dolore feci più liquide o frequenti. Possono essere presenti gonfiore e sensazione di evacuazione incompleta.

I sintomi indicativi di un'eziologia organica comprendono età <6 anni, calo ponderale, sintomi di tipo articolare o anomalie della crescita. Il dolore organico è generalmente localizzato lontano dalla zona ombelicale e può svegliare il bambino dal sonno. Vomito, diarrea e sangue nelle feci sono suggestivi di una causa organica. I bambini con DAR hanno un esame obiettivo negativo, mentre quelli con eziologia organica hanno dolorabilità addominale, fissurazioni rettali o sangue occulto nelle feci. Occorre valutare le curve di accrescimento, se disponibili, dal momento che un rallentamento della crescita si accompagna spesso alle cause organiche di dolore addominale.

VALUTAZIONE. Le indagini di laboratorio, radiologiche o endoscopiche, da eseguire sui bambini con dolore addominale cronico devono essere individualizzate in base ai dati raccolti con un'anamnesi dettagliata e l'esame obiettivo. Gli esami di laboratorio possono non essere necessari se anamnesi ed esame obiettivo indicano chiaramente una diagnosi di dolore addominale funzionale. L'esame emocromocitometrico completo, la velocità di eritrosedimentazione, l'esame delle feci per la ricerca di parassiti (soprattutto *Giardia*) e l'analisi delle urine rappresentano test di screening ragionevoli. Se si sospetta una malattia infiammatoria intestinale, la velocità di eritrosedimentazione è spesso elevata. Il riscontro di una velocità di eritrosedimentazione anomala, o l'alterazione di altri reagenti della fase acuta, devono spingere il medico ad approfondire le indagini alla ricerca di un'eziologia organica del disagio. Quest'ultima è suggerita da livelli elevati di calprotectina nelle feci. Se indicata, un'ecografia addominale può fornire informazioni su reni, colecisti e pancreas; un dolore addominale più basso rappresenta un'indicazione all'ecografia pelvica. Radiografie seriate del tratto gastrointestinale alto sono indicate nel sospetto di un disturbo gastrico o dell'intestino tenue. L'infezione da *Helicobacter pylori* non sembra essere associata a DAR. Nei pazienti con sintomi indicativi di gastrite o ulcera, si può eseguire il test per *H. pylori* (sierico o fecale) per dimostrare l'infezione. Si consiglia l'esofagogastroduodenoscopia in presenza di sintomi indicativi di patologia persistente del tratto gastrointestinale superiore; in assenza di questo sospetto, tuttavia, tale indagine non è necessaria, in quanto è poco probabile che identifichi un'anomalia.

TRATTAMENTO. La famiglia e il bambino con DAR funzionale possono essere preoccupati dall'impossibilità di identificare una causa organica e non accettare una diagnosi di malattia non organica. Dopo un'anamnesi e un esame obiettivo accurati, l'aspetto più importante del trattamento è rassicurare sia il diretto interessato sia i suoi familiari; in particolare, occorre sottolineare che non ci sono evidenze di un disturbo grave sottostante. I bambini i cui genitori non accettano un causa psicologica dei sintomi probabilmente avranno un disagio somatico persistente e faranno molte assenze da scuola. Ai genitori occorre insegnare a non rafforzare i sintomi con conseguente vantaggio secondario. Inoltre se il bambino a causa del dolore ha fatto assenze da scuola o è stato distolto dalle attività consuete, è importante che tornino a condurre una vita normale. I farmaci sono generalmente inutili o al massimo possono esplicare un effetto placebo transitorio. I bloccanti degli acidi gastrici o i rilassanti della muscolatura intestinale (anticolinergici) possono essere usati empiricamente, ma sono spesso inutili in assenza di un'indicazione precisa. Nei bambini con dolore funzionale possono rivelarsi utili il biofeedback, l'immaginazione guidata e le tecniche di rilassamento.

Se si sospetta un'intolleranza alimentare, la diagnosi deve essere dimostrata con breath test all'idrogeno. La prescrizione di una dieta priva di lattosio determina risoluzione del dolore. I sintomi del reflusso gastroesofageo in genere si attenuano con l'uso di bloccanti degli acidi gastrici. Sintomi ricorrenti di solito rappresentano un'indicazione per eseguire test formali prima di istituire una terapia cronica. I bambini che presentano sintomi di intestino irritabile o feci liquide spesso beneficiano di un'integrazione a base di fibre. Gli anticolinergici o gli antidepressivi triciclici possono essere utili in alcuni pazienti. Gli adulti con IBS sono stati trattati con antagonisti dei recettori della 5-idrossitriptamina (se la predomina la diarrea) o agonisti (per la stipsi). Gli antagonisti dei recettori per $5HT_3$ (alosetrone), essendo associati alla colite ischemica, non sono raccomandati. Una stipsi cronica deve essere trattata con l'approccio standard (vedi Capitoli 22.4 e 329).

Il successo del trattamento dipende da uno stretto follow-up. I genitori devono adottare nuovi approcci ai sintomi del bambino, senza timore che il medico li stia abbandonando se sanno che è stato stabilito un follow-up telefonico o una visita ambulatoriale. Spesso è durante le visite di follow-up che il pediatra arriva a conoscere pienamente il bambino e i suoi sintomi. È possibile che un problema organico non sia evidente alla prima visita, ma che il complesso dei sintomi diventi più caratteristico con il tempo.

Questi approcci portano alla riduzione o all'eliminazione dei sintomi addominali. È probabile che i bambini con dolore addominale funzionale continuino a presentare disturbi funzionali da adulti, sebbene la natura di questi sintomi possa cambiare.

Ball TM, Shapiro DE, Monheim CJ, Weydert JA: A pilot study of the use of guided imagery for the treatment of recurrent abdominal pain in children. *Clin Pediatr (Phila)* 2003;42:527–532.

Ball TM, Weydert JA: Methodological challenges to treatment trials for recurrent abdominal pain in children. *Arch Pediatr Adolesc Med* 2003;157:1121–1127.

Biggs AM, Aziz Q, Tomenson B, Creed F: Effect of childhood adversity on health related quality of life in patients with upper abdominal or chest pain. *Gut* 2004;53:180–186.

Biggs AM, Aziz Q, Tomenson B, Creed F: Do childhood adversity and recent social stress predict health care use in patients presenting with upper abdominal or chest pain? *Psychosom Med* 2003;65:1020–1028.

Chang L, Ameen VZ, Dukes GE, et al: A dose-ranging, phase II study of the efficacy and safety of alosetron in men with diarrhea-predominant IBS. *Am J Gastroenterol* 2005;100:115–123.

Chitkara DK, Camilleri M, Zinsmeister AR, et al: Gastric sensory and motor dysfunction in adolescents with functional dyspepsia. *J Pediatr* 2005;146:500–505.

Crushell E, Rowland M, Doherty M, et al: Importance of parental conceptual model of illness in severe recurrent abdominal pain. *Pediatrics* 2003;112:1368–1372.

El-Matary W, Spray C, Sandhu B: Irritable bowel syndrome: The commonest cause of recurrent abdominal pain in children. *Eur J Pediatr* 2004;163:584–588.

Farthing MJG: Treatment of irritable bowel syndrome. *Br Med J* 2005;330: 429–430.

Faure C, Wieckowska A: Somatic referral of visceral sensations and rectal sensory threshold for pain in children with functional gastrointestinal disorders. *J Pediatr* 2007;150:66–71.

Ghandour RM, Overpeck MD, Huang ZJ, et al: Headache, stomachache, backache, and morning fatigue among adolescent girls in the United States: Associations with behavioral, sociodemographic, and environmental factors. *Arch Pediatr Adolesc Med* 2004;158:797–803.

Gremse DA, Greer AS, Vacik J, DiPalma JA: Abdominal pain associated with lactose ingestion in children with lactose intolerance. *Clin Pediatr (Phila)* 2003;42:341–345.

Haim A, Pillar G, Pecht A, et al: Sleep patterns in children and adolescents with functional recurrent abdominal pain: Objective versus subjective assessment. *Acta Paediatr* 2004;93:677–680.

Lindley KJ, Glaser D, Milla PJ: Consumerism in healthcare can be detrimental to child health: Lessons from children with functional abdominal pain. *Arch Dis Child* 2005;90:335–337.

Tibble JA, Sigthorsson G, Foster R, et al: Use of surrogate markers of inflammation and Rome criteria to distinguish organic from nonorganic intestinal disease. *Gastroenterology* 2002;123:450–460.

Walker LS, Lipani TA, Greene JW, et al: Recurrent abdominal pain: Symptom subtypes based on the Rome II Criteria for pediatric functional gastrointestinal disorders. *J Pediatr Gastroenterol Nutr* 2004;38:187–191.

Weydert JA, Ball TM, Davis MF: Systematic review of treatments for recurrent abdominal pain. *Pediatrics* 2003;111:e1–e11.

Capitolo 340 ■ Appendicite acuta

John J. Aiken e Keith T. Oldham

L'appendicite acuta, nonostante una riduzione dell'incidenza registratasi negli Stati Uniti nell'ultimo mezzo secolo, resta la condizione chirurgica acuta più frequente nei bambini e la maggiore causa di morbilità nell'infanzia. Attualmente più di 80 000 soggetti in età pediatrica ne sono colpiti ogni anno, a un tasso di 4/1000 bambini al di sotto dei 14 anni di età. Sebbene negli ultimi dieci anni vi sia stata una tendenza verso una durata minore del ricovero, l'appendicite è responsabile di più di 1 milione di giorni di ospedalizzazione all'anno. L'obiettivo principale è migliorare la diagnosi, per evitare le complicanze e la morbilità significativa associata alla perforazione. L'appendicite è più frequente nei bambini più grandi, con un picco di incidenza tra i 12 e i 18 anni; è rara nei bambini di età <5 anni (<5% dei casi) ed estremamente rara (<1% dei casi) in quelli di età <3 anni. Nel Regno Unito colpisce i maschi un po' più spesso delle femmine e la razza bianca più spesso di quella nera. In autunno e in primavera si registra un picco di incidenza stagionale. In alcuni casi può esserci una predisposizione familiare, soprattutto nei pazienti che sviluppano appendicite prima dei 6 anni. Malgrado i progressi compiuti nelle tecniche diagnostiche di immagine e i sistemi di valutazione/modelli di supporto decisionale computerizzati, una diagnosi accurata può essere difficoltosa e il tasso di perforazione riportato è >20%. Negli ultimi decenni la gestione dell'appendicite è cambiata notevolmente con l'uso degli antibiotici, il miglioramento delle tecniche d'immagine, il trattamento iniziale non chirurgico in casi selezionati, le procedure di drenaggio percutaneo mediante radiologia interventistica e laparoscopia. La mortalità è bassa, ma la morbilità resta elevata, soprattutto in caso di appendicite perforata, la cui incidenza è maggiore nei bambini appartenenti a minoranze etniche e con assicurazione sanitaria statale.

ANATOMIA PATOLOGICA

L'appendicite acuta è di solito una patologia a eziologia multipla, che culmina sempre nell'invasione batterica della parete dell'appendice. Il processo che porta all'appendicite acuta inizia con l'ostruzione del lume; materia fecale ispessita, iperplasia linfoide, corpi estranei ingeriti, parassiti e tumori sono tutti considerati fattori causali. L'ostruzione del lume appendicolare determina un aumento della pressione intraluminale a causa della proliferazione batterica e della continua secrezione di muco. L'aumento della pressione intraluminale, a sua volta, determina congestione venosa e linfatica ed edema, seguiti da insufficiente perfusione arteriosa, talora responsabile di ischemia della parete appendicolare, invasione batterica con infiltrato infiammatorio di tutti gli strati della parete dell'appendice e necrosi. Questa progressione è correlata, dal punto di vista clinico, con la progressione da appendicite semplice alla forma gangrenosa e, quindi, a perforazione dell'appendice. I follicoli linfoidi sottomucosi, che possono ostruire il lume appendicolare, sono numericamente scarsi alla nascita, sono in costante aumento durante l'infanzia, raggiungendo un picco nell'età adolescenziale, quando l'appendicite acuta è più frequente, e infine si riducono dopo i 30 anni. Sia i coproliti sia l'appendicite sono più frequenti nei Paesi industrializzati, dove la dieta abituale è a base di cibi raffinati e poveri di fibre, rispetto a quelli in via di sviluppo, dove l'alimentazione è ricca di fibre; non è stata definita una relazione causale tra carenza di fibre nelle dieta e appendicite. Poiché meno del 50% dei campioni provenienti da pazienti con appendicite acuta presenta ostruzione del lume all'esame istologico, sono stati ricercati altri fattori causali. Le infezioni intestinali probabilmente giocano un ruolo in molti casi, in associazione con ulcerazione della mucosa e invasione della parete dell'appendice da parte dei batteri. Sono stati chiamati in causa batteri come *Yersinia*, *Salmonella* e *Shigella* spp. e virus come quello della parotite epidemica, il Coxsackie B e l'adenovirus. Inoltre, sono stati dimostrati casi di appendicite da corpi estranei, in associazione a tumori carcinoidi dell'appendice o *Ascaris* o dopo traumi addominali chiusi. I bambini con fibrosi cistica hanno una maggiore incidenza di appendicite e la causa sembra essere l'alterazione della secrezione mucosa caratteristica della malattia. L'appendicite nei neonati è rara e giustifica la valutazione per un'eventuale fibrosi cistica e di malattia di Hirschsprung.

Uno degli obiettivi principali nella gestione dell'appendicite acuta è evitare la sepsi e le complicanze infettive di più frequente riscontro in associazione alla perforazione. È possibile prelevare i batteri dalla superficie mucosa dell'appendice prima che una perforazione microscopica o macroscopica e l'invasione batterica della vena mesenterica determinino una sepsi della vena porta (pileflebite) ed eventualmente un ascesso epatico. Una volta verificatasi la perforazione, la contaminazione microbica fecale può localizzarsi dall'omento alla fossa iliaca destra o allo scavo pelvico e alle anse ileali adiacenti, determinando un ascesso localizzato, una massa infiammatoria (flemmone) o ancora la contaminazione fecale; in alternativa, può diffondersi nella cavità peritoneale causando una peritonite diffusa. I bambini piccoli, che hanno un omento poco sviluppato, di solito non sono in grado di controllare l'infezione a livello locale. La perforazione o l'ascesso possono portare a formazione di una fistola in organi adiacenti, a una cellulite scrotale e a un ascesso attraverso un processo vaginale pervio (ernia inguinale indiretta congenita) o a occlusione dell'intestino tenue.

MANIFESTAZIONI CLINICHE

L'appendicite acuta può avere diverse "forme" prevedibili; i segni e i sintomi possono essere tipici o variabili in base al tempo di esordio, alla localizzazione dell'appendicite e alle differenziaioni individuali legate all'evoluzione della malattia. Pur essendo quella meglio descritta, la presentazione classica dell'appendicite si riscontra solo nella metà dei casi, mentre nella maggior parte si ha una presentazione "atipica". Nonostante i progressi della diagnostica per immagini, la diagnosi di appendicite acuta si basa essenzialmente su un'anamnesi completa e accurata del paziente e su un'attenta valutazione clinica. Una volta accertata la diagnosi, l'obiettivo primario consiste nel prestare attenzione all'evoluzione temporale della malattia in relazione ai segni e ai sintomi specifici.

L'appendicite acuta inizia tipicamente in forma insidiosa, con malessere generalizzato e anoressia. Il primo sintomo è il dolore addominale, che si manifesta a distanza di poche ore dall'esordio della malattia; inizialmente è vago, indistinto, non correlato all'attività o alla posizione, spesso colico e localizzato nell'area periombelicale, come esito dell'infiammazione viscerale di un appendice dilatata. La progressione della flogosi nelle successive 12-24 ore comporta il coinvolgimento della superficie parietale adiacente, suscitando dolore somatico localizzato in fossa iliaca destra. Il dolore, diventato fisso e più severo, viene esacerbato dai movimenti. Il bambino riferisce spesso un aumento del disagio durante il trasporto in ospedale, si muove con cautela e ha difficoltà a salire sul lettino dell'ambulatorio. Nausea e vomito si hanno in più della metà dei pazienti e quasi sempre fanno seguito di alcune ore all'esordio del dolore addominale. L'anoressia è il sintomo classico e più significativo dell'appendicite acuta, ma occasionalmente i pazienti possono anche non perdere l'appetito. Sono inoltre frequenti la diarrea e la sintomatologia a carico dell'apparato urinario, soprattutto in caso di appendice perforata, quando è probabile siano in atto un'infiammazione e un ascesso pelvico. La febbre è caratteristicamente bassa, in assenza di perforazione. La maggior parte dei pazienti presenta almeno una lieve tachicardia. La progressione temporale dei sintomi da un dolore lieve e impreciso, con malessere e anoressia, a dolore severo localizzato, accompagnato da febbre e vomito, avviene rapidamente, in 24-48 ore nella maggior parte dei casi. Se la diagnosi è ritardata oltre le 36-48 ore, il tasso di perforazione supera il 65%. Molti pazienti per un certo lasso di tempo dopo la perforazione sperimentano una riduzione del dolore addominale e della sintomatologia acuta, presumibilmente per effetto della minore pressione all'interno dell'appendice. Se l'omento o l'intestino adiacente è in grado di circoscrivere il processo infettivo, l'evoluzione della malattia è meno prevedibile ed è probabile un ritardo della presentazione. Se la perforazione causa peritonite diffusa, il bambino solitamente presenta dolore addominale diffuso progressivo e rapido sviluppo di segni di tossicità, evidenziata da segni di disidratazione e sepsi come: ipotensione, oliguria, acidosi e febbre elevata. A distanza di alcuni giorni dalla progressione dell'appendicite, i pazienti spesso sviluppano segni e sintomi che denotano l'insorgenza di un'occlusione intestinale. Se l'appendice è in sede retrocecale, si suppone che la patologia evolva più lentamente e i pazienti possono riferire di aver avuto 4-5 giorni di malattia prima della visita. Inoltre, il dolore sarà lateroposteriore e potrà ricordare i sintomi associati ad artrite settica dell'anca o ascesso dello psoas.

L'**esame obiettivo**, fondamentale per una diagnosi accurata dell'appendicite acuta, inizia con l'osservazione del comportamento del bambino e dell'aspetto dell'addome. I bambini con appendicite precoce appaiono lievemente sofferenti e si muovono in modo incerto, curvi in avanti, spesso con un'andatura leggermente zoppicante, generalmente a destra. Spesso rimangono supini, immobili, distesi sul lato destro, con le ginocchia flesse per rilassare la parete addominale, e quando gli si chiede di distendersi o alzarsi si muovono lentamente portandosi una mano al quadrante addominale inferiore destro come per proteggerlo. Inizialmente, nell'appendicite, l'addome è piatto; la distensione addominale segnala una fase della malattia più avanzata con perforazione o occlusione dell'intestino tenue. L'auscultazione, nella fase iniziale, può rivelare una peristalsi intestinale normale o aumentata, peristalsi che si riduce progredendo verso la perforazione. **Il segno isolato più affidabile nella diagnosi di appendicite acuta è la dolorabilità addominale localizzata.** Un uso cauto della morfina a scopo analgesico, usata negli Stati Uniti per alleviare il dolore addominale, non interferisce con l'accuratezza diagnostica e con la decisione di intervenire chirurgicamente, e il paziente dovrebbe ricevere misure adeguate per il controllo del dolore. Nel 1889, McBurney descrisse il classico punto di localizzazione dell'iperestesia nell'appendicite acuta, all'incontro tra il terzo laterale e il terzo medio di una linea che unisce la spina iliaca anteriore superiore destra e l'ombelico, ma l'iperestesia può anche essere localizzata in corrispondenza delle eventuali sedi anomale dell'appendice. Inoltre, l'iperestesia localizzata è un sintomo più tardivo e meno importante quando l'appendice è in posizione retrocecale. Accarezzare il braccio del bambino prima di iniziare l'esame obiettivo, rassicurandolo che la palpazione dell'addome sarà altrettanto delicata, può aiutare a creare un clima di fiducia e ad aumentare le possibilità di un esame affidabile e riproducibile. È meglio iniziare la palpazione dal quadrante addominale superiore sinistro, in modo da non causare dolore, e proseguire in senso antiorario verso il quadrante addominale superiore destro per poi terminare in quello inferiore destro. Questa manovra riduce l'ansia, permette un rilassamento della muscolatura addominale e aumenta la fiducia. L'esaminatore descrive alcuni "cerchi" sull'addome, aumentando via via la pressione. Un segno importante dell'appendicite acuta è la rigidità del muscolo retto sovrastante; questa può essere volontaria, per proteggere l'area dell'iperestesia dalla mano dell'esaminatore, oppure involontaria, imputabile alla peritonite che causa spasmo del muscolo sovrastante. I riscontri dell'esame obiettivo devono essere interpretati in base all'evoluzione temporale della malattia. L'iperestesia addominale può essere vaga o anche assente all'inizio, e spesso diffusa dopo la perforazione. La dolorabilità di rimbalzo e la dolorabilità di rimbalzo riferita (**segno di Rovsing**) sono aspetti importanti nell'appendicite acuta, anche se non sempre presenti. La dolorabilità di rimbalzo si manifesta quando il medico che sta effettuando la palpazione profonda dell'addome allontana all'improvviso la mano. Questa manovra, oltre a essere molto dolorosa per il bambino, ha una scarsa correlazione con la peritonite e quindi dovrebbe essere evitata. Una leggera percussione è il test migliore per indagare la presenza di irritazione peritoneale. L'esplorazione rettale è utile in casi specifici, per esempio quando la diagnosi è dubbia, quando si sospetta un'appendice pelvica o un ascesso o nelle adolescenti in cui si ipotizza una patologia ovarica. I segni dello psoas e dell'otturatore interno sono dolori da distensione passiva di questi muscoli. Il segno dello psoas, evocato dalla flessione attiva della coscia destra o dall'estensione passiva dell'articolazione dell'anca, è positivo in caso di appendice retrocecale. Il segno dell'otturatore, che consiste nella comparsa di dolore a livello dell'adduttore dopo rotazione interna della coscia flessa sull'addome, è caratteristicamente positivo in caso di appendice pelvica. L'esame obiettivo può rivelare una massa nel quadrante addominale inferiore destro, segno di flemmone infiammatorio intorno all'appendice o di ascesso localizzato.

INDAGINI DI LABORATORIO

Diversi esami di laboratorio sono stati utilizzati nella valutazione dei bambini con sospetto di appendicite. Ciascuno di essi, pur non essendo molto sensibile o specifico per l'appendicite, considerato singolarmente, può comunque aiutare il medico a decidere se eseguire a un'appendicectomia in urgenza, lasciar trascorrere un periodo di osservazione e di accertamenti oppure utilizzare altre tecniche diagnostiche d'immagine. I risultati devono essere interpretati prestando attenzione all'evoluzione temporale della malattia. Sono necessari un emocromo completo e un esame delle urine. La conta leucocitaria in un primo momento (<24 ore dall'inizio della malattia) può essere normale e tipicamente è appena elevata (11 000-16 000/mm^3) quando progredisce nelle prime 24-48 ore. Dal momento che una conta leucocitaria normale non allontana mai completamente il sospetto di appendicite, una conta <8000/mm^3 in un paziente con una storia di malattia che dura da più di 48 ore deve essere considerata come una preziosa opportunità di diagnosi alternativa. La conta leucocitaria può essere molto elevata (>20 000/mm^3) tanto nell'appendicite perforata quanto (seppur raramente) in quella non perforata; una conta leucocitaria molto elevata può sollevare il sospetto di una diagnosi alternativa. L'esame delle urine, che dimostra spesso pochi leucociti e poche emazie, a causa della prossimità dell'appendice infiammata all'uretere e alla vescica, non deve comunque rivelare la presenza di batteri. L'ematuria macroscopica non è frequente e suggerisce una patologia renale primitiva. Le urine sono spesso concentrate e contenenti corpi chetonici a causa della riduzione dell'introito alimentare e del vomito. Gli elettroliti e gli enzimi epatici di solito sono normali, a meno che un ritardo nella diagnosi non abbia condotto a grave disidratazione/o sepsi. L'amilasi e gli enzimi epatici servono soltanto a escludere la diagnosi alternativa di pancreatite e colecistite e non si ricercano se c'è un forte sospetto di appendicite. La proteina C reattiva aumenta in proporzione al grado di infiammazione dell'appendice, ma è aspecifica e non molto utilizzata. La proteina amiloide A sierica subisce un notevole aumento nei pazienti con appendicite acuta, con sensibilità e specificità rispettivamente dell'86 e dell'83%. Diversi studi hanno descritto sistemi di valutazione clinica e modelli decisionali computerizzati che incorporano elementi specifici dell'anamnesi, dell'esame obiettivo, e indagini di laboratorio mirate a migliorare l'accuratezza diagnostica dell'appendicite acuta. A tutt'oggi nessuno di essi ha comunque rivelato un'accuratezza superiore a quella del giudizio clinico.

INDAGINI RADIOLOGICHE.

Radiografia diretta. La radiografia addominale diretta, pur evidenziando alcuni segni caratteristici dell'appendicite acuta, tra cui l'ansa sentinella intestinale e l'ileo localizzato, la scoliosi da spasmo dello psoas, un livello idroaereo nel colon al di sopra della fossa iliaca destra (segno del cutoff) o coproliti (5-10% dei casi), è dotata di scarsa sensibilità per l'appendicite e non è solitamente indicata (Fig. 340-1). Essa è più utile nella valutazione dei casi complicati in cui si sospetta occlusione dell'intestino tenue o aria libera in cavità peritoneale.

Ecografia. L'ecografia, di uso frequente nella valutazione dell'appendicite acuta, ha dimostrato una sensibilità e una specificità >90% nei centri pediatrici specializzati in questa tecnica. La palpazione graduale dell'addome è utile per spostare il cieco e il colon ascendente e individuare l'appendice, che ha un aspetto caratteristico (Fig. 340-2). I criteri ecografici dell'appendicite comprendono spessore della parete ≥6 mm, distensione del lume, mancanza di comprimibilità, presenza di una massa complessa in fossa iliaca destra o presenza di coproliti. La localizzazione dell'appendice di solito coincide con la sede del dolore e dell'iperestesia. Segni ecografici indicativi di appendicite in fase avanzata comprendono asimmetria dello spessore della parete, presenza di ascesso, associazione di liquidi liberi a livello intraperitoneale, edema circostante e riduzione dell'iperestesia locale alla palpazione. Il limite maggiore dell'ecografia è l'incapacità di visualizzare l'appendice, cosa che accade in più del 20% dei casi. Per escludere ecograficamente l'appendicite occorre visualizzare un'appendice normale. Alcune condizioni, tra cui l'obesità, la distensione intestinale e il dolore, riducono la sensibilità e l'affidabilità dell'ecografia per l'appendicite. I vantaggi principali di

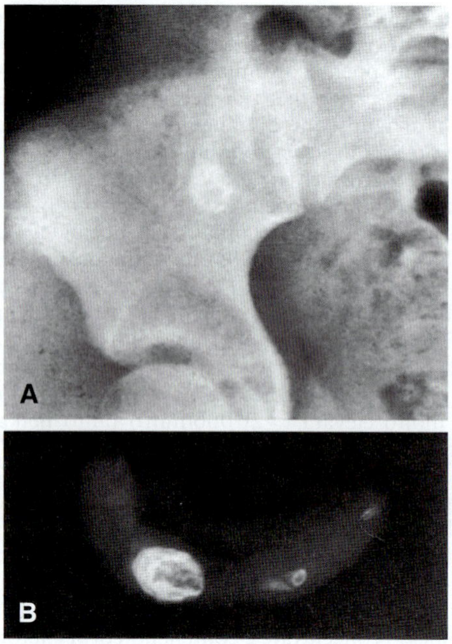

Figura 340-1. Appendicoliti calcificati osservati in una proiezione obliqua anteroposteriore del quadrante addominale inferiore destro e nell'appendice asportata di una bambina di 10 anni con appendicite acuta. (Da Kuhn JP, Slovis TL, Haller JO: *Caffrey's Pediatric Diagnostic Imaging*, vol 2, 10th ed. Philadelphia, Mosby, 2004, p 1682.)

questa metodica comprendono il basso costo e l'assenza di radiazioni ionizzanti. L'ecografia è inoltre particolarmente utile nelle adolescenti, per la sua capacità di valutare patologie dell'ovaio senza l'uso di radiazioni.

TC. Tra le tecniche per immagini, la TC rappresenta il *gold standard* per valutare i bambini con dolore addominale e sospetto di appendicite. Alcuni ne sostengono l'uso per valutare tutti i pazienti con sospetto di appendicite, al fine di facilitare il processo decisionale ed evitare il ricorso a un intervento chirurgico non necessario. Questa indagine può essere eseguita secondo diverse modalità: TC standard, con o senza mezzo di contrasto somministrato per os o endovena, la valutazione di addome e pelvi o della sola area pelvica, TC spirale dell'appendice e TC spirale dell'appendice con mezzo di contrasto rettale. Tutte queste tecniche hanno una sensibilità e una specificità >95% per l'appendicite acuta. I segni della TC indicativi di appendicite comprendono una parete appendicolare distesa e spessa, e flogosi del tessuto adiposo circostante, oppure un flemmone pericecale o un ascesso (Figg. 340-3 e 304-4). Gli appendicoliti si visualizzano meglio con la TC che con l'Rx diretta dell'addome. La TC è utile anche in caso di appendicite avanzata per identificare e guidare il drenaggio percutaneo della raccolta di liquidi e per individuare una massa infiammatoria, che può portare alla pianificazione di un primo trattamento non chirurgico. Gli svantaggi dell'uso di questa metodica comprendono i costi elevati, l'esposizione alle radiazioni, il possibile utilizzo di un mezzo di contrasto per via orale, endovenosa o rettale, e la possibilità che si renda necessaria la sedazione del paziente. Il mezzo di contrasto per via orale è particolarmente problematico se l'appendicite è stata confermata, a causa del rischio di aspirazione nella fase di induzione dell'anestesia. Poiché la presenza di grasso sottocutaneo è un elemento critico nella valutazione dell'appendicite mediante TC, quest'ultima è meno affidabile nei bambini magri con poca massa grassa; se ne deduce che il mezzo di contrasto somministrato per via rettale può aumentare l'accuratezza diagnostica in questo gruppo. Infine, la TC è utile per rivelare le cause di dolore addominale non legate ad appendicite.

RISONANZA MAGNETICA/SCINTIGRAFIA WBC. La risonanza magnetica (RM) ha dimostrato un'accuratezza diagnostica per l'appendicite almeno equivalente a quella della TC, senza esposizione alle radiazioni ionizzanti. L'utilizzo della RM nella valutazione dell'appendicite è limitato in quanto questa metodica, oltre a essere meno diffusa, comporta costi maggiori, richiede sedazione più frequentemente e non offre un accesso equivalente per drenare la raccolta di liquidi. La scintigrafia con i globuli bianchi (WBC, *White Blood Cell*) marcati, usata in alcuni centri per valutare i casi atipici di appendicite nei bambini, ha dimostrato un'elevata sensibilità (97%) e solo una modesta specificità (80%).

APPROCCIO DIAGNOSTICO

Soltanto nel 50-70% dei bambini la diagnosi di appendicite acuta viene effettuata durante la valutazione iniziale. In passato era invalsa la pratica di eseguire un intervento chirurgico precoce nei casi dubbi, poiché le complicanze e la morbilità aumentano in modo significativo con la perforazione dell'appendice. La negatività laparotomica del 10-20% era ritenuta accettabile per ridurre il tasso di perforazione. Di pari passo con il miglioramento delle tecniche diagnostiche d'immagine, si è prestata maggiore attenzione a migliorare l'accuratezza diagnostica e quindi a ridurre il tasso di perforazione e l'intervento chirurgico non necessario, quando l'appendice risulta normale. I dati di 36 centri pediatrici riportano un tasso negativo di appendicectomia del 3% soltanto. Alcuni medici non transigono sull'importanza di un'anamnesi accurata e dell'esame obiettivo e raramente fanno ricorso alle immagini diagnostiche. Nei casi dubbi, occorre mettere in atto un piano di "osservazione attiva". Molti clinici sostengono l'osservazione attiva con esami seriati, per un periodo di 12-24 ore nei casi dubbi, per migliorare l'accuratezza diagnostica solo mediante i criteri clinici, semplificando la decisione se procedere a un'appendicectomia o dimettere il paziente, e non riferiscono una correlazione tra la morbilità chirurgica e il momento dell'intervento. Questo approccio presenta un buon rapporto costo/beneficio e spesso evita le indagini radiologiche. Nei pazienti pediatrici, meno del 2% delle appendici andrà incontro a perforazione durante il periodo di osservazione. Altri clinici usano frequentemente le immagini radiologiche in aggiunta all'esame obiettivo e alcuni le raccomandano in **tutti** i casi atipici per ridurre la morbilità, oltre che per ottimizzare i piani di gestione e gli esiti clinici. I dati di 36 ospedali pediatrici riferiscono un tasso di appendicectomia negativa dell'1-2% grazie alla diagnostica d'immagine. È stato inoltre riportato che la probabilità di perforazione dell'appendice è influenzata da fattori socioeconomici come le possibilità di accesso ai servizi sanitari, il tipo di assicurazione e il modo in cui il paziente descrive i suoi sintomi.

Sembra probabile che, eseguendo indagini diagnostiche per immagini in tutti i pazienti con presentazioni dubbie e una malattia di breve durata (<24 ore), si assisterà a un aumento del tasso di falsi negativi. Le indagini strumentali forniscono il maggior beneficio e si rivelano particolarmente efficaci quando vengono usate selettivamente nei bambini in cui la diagnosi è dubbia, dopo un'anamnesi attenta e un esame obiettivo condotto da un medico esperto, e non troppo presto nell'ambito dell'evoluzione temporale della malattia. Un approccio ponderato nei casi dubbi consiste nell'utilizzare l'ecografia, se è disponibile e se il personale ospedaliero ha esperienza nell'uso degli ultrasuoni in caso di sospetta appendicite. Si preferisce invece la TC se l'ecografia non è disponibile o non ha chiarito i dubbi o come prima scelta nei pazienti obesi, in caso di probabile appendicite in fase avanzata o in caso di distensione gassosa dell'intestino. Questo approccio si è rivelato molto accurato ed economicamente vantaggioso.

DIAGNOSI DIFFERENZIALE

La diagnosi di appendicite acuta può trarre in inganno anche i clinici più esperti. La lista di patologie che possono mimare un'appendicite acuta è estesa e comprende anche condizioni frequenti

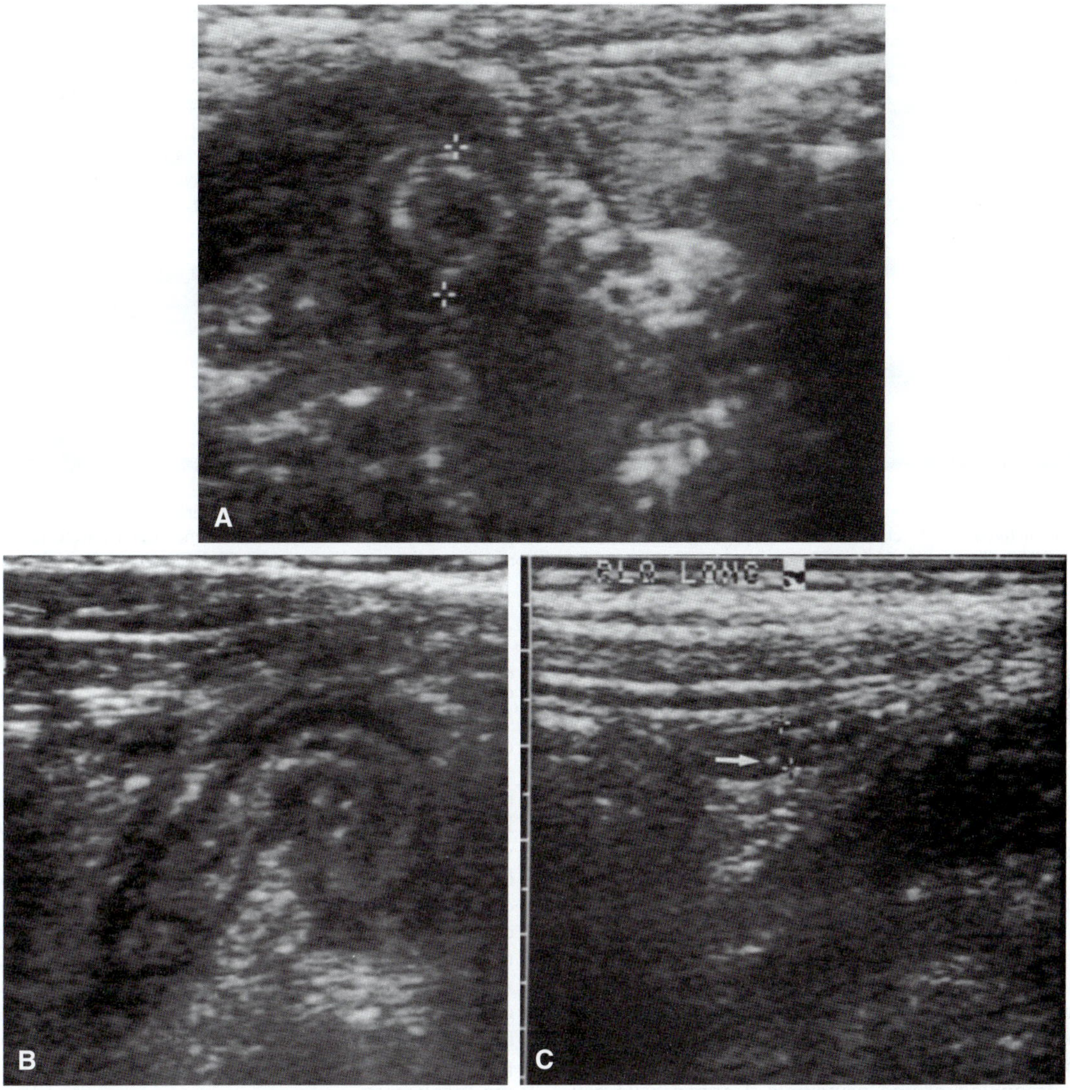

Figura 340-2. Valutazione ecografica di pazienti con appendicite. *A*, La scansione trasversale dell'appendice evidenzia il caratteritico segno "a bersaglio" o "a coccarda". In questo caso, la porzione interna è sonolucente, compatibile con la presenza di liquidi o pus. *B*, La scansione longitudinale, in un altro paziente, evidenzia l'alternanza di strati iper- e ipocecogeni; quello esterno, ipoecogeno, è suggestivo di liquido in sede periappendicolare. *C*, La scansione longitudinale ecografica della fossa iliaca destra mostra un'appendice dilatata, non comprimibile. L'eco luminoso all'interno dell'appendice rappresenta un appendicolita con ombra acustica (*freccia*). (Da Kuhn JP, Slovis TL, Haller JO: *Caffrey's Pediatric Diagnostic Imaging*, vol 2, 10th ed. Philadelphia, Mosby, 2004, p 1684.)

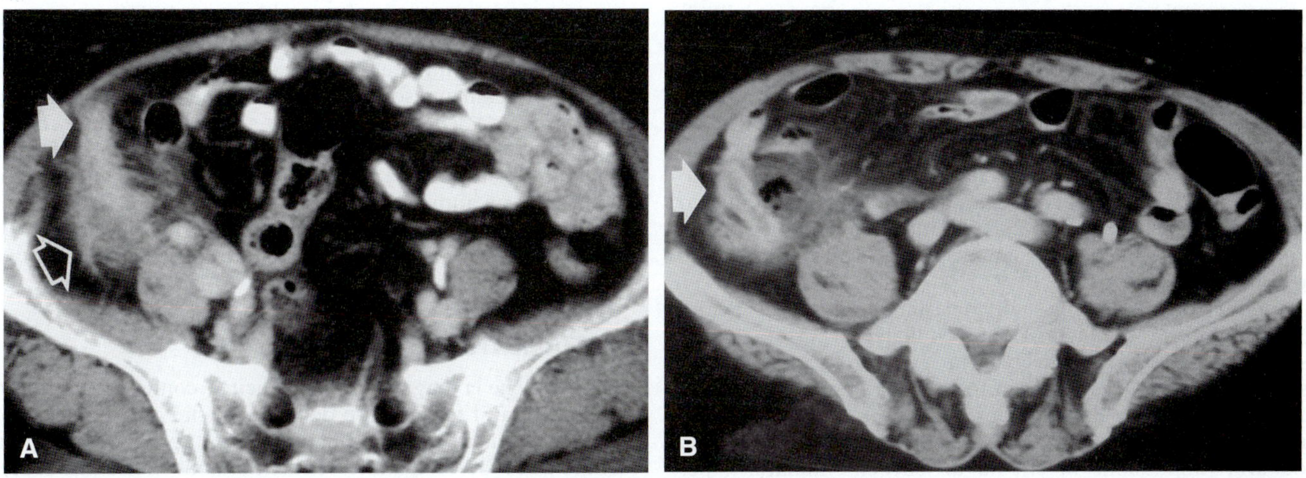

Figura 340-3. *A*, Flemmone (*freccia vuota*) intorno all'appendice dilatata (*freccia piena*), in un appendicite perforata. *B*, Presenza di aria extraluminale intorno alla parete ispessita dell'appendice (*freccia*), in un'appendicite perforata. (Da Yeung KW, Chang MS, Hsiao CP: Evaluation of perforated and nonperforated appendicitis with CT. *J Clin Imag* 2004;28:422-427.)

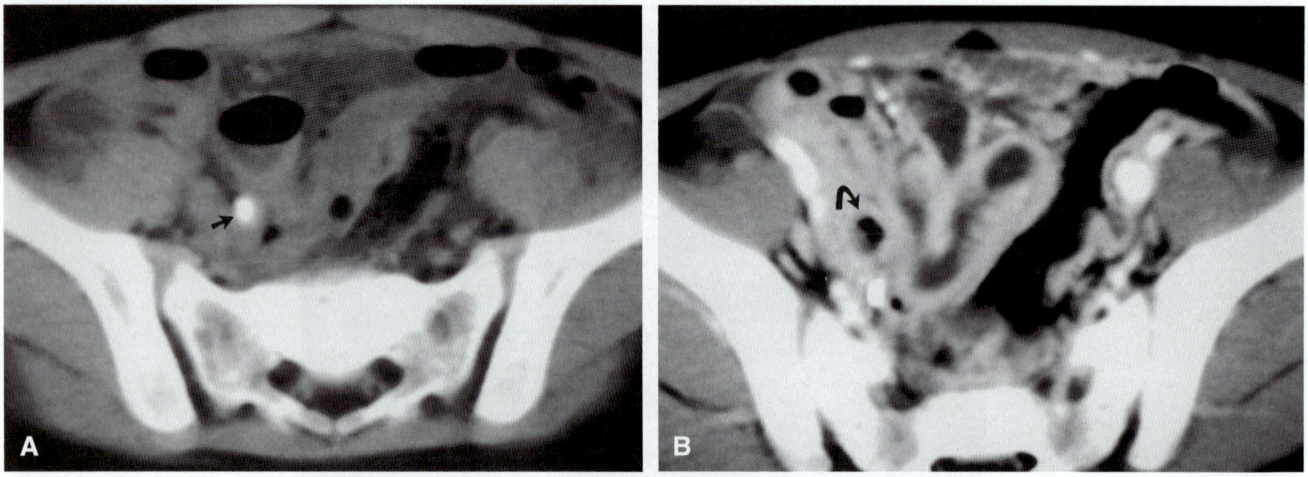

Figura 340-4. *A*, TC con pre-enhancement di contrasto che evidenzia un appendicolita (*freccia*), in un'appendicite perforata. *B*, TC con post-enhancement di contrasto (1 cm sotto il livello di A) che rivela una raccolta aerea intraluminale (freccia curva) associata a ispessimento della parete ileale, in un'appendicite perforata. (Da Yeung KW, Chang MS, Hsiao CP: Evaluation of perforated and nonperforated appendicitis with CT. *J Clin Imag* 2004;28:422-427.)

come: gastroenterite, adenite mesenterica, diverticolite di Meckel, malattia infiammatoria intestinale, polmonite, colecistite, pancreatite, infezioni delle vie urinarie, enteriti infettive e, nelle donne, torsione ovarica, gravidanza ectopica, rottura di cisti ovariche, malattia infiammatoria pelvica (ascesso salpingo-ovarico compreso). Anche i linfomi del tratto intestinale, i tumori dell'appendice (il carcinoide nei bambini) e i tumori ovarici possono mascherare un'appendicite acuta. I bambini di età <3 anni e le adolescenti sono a elevato rischio di ricevere una diagnosi non esatta. La cosa più importante è distinguere i pazienti con gastroenterite, la patologia più spesso responsabile di un errore diagnostico, da quelli con appendicite, a causa della morbilità significativa e dell'errore medico che caratterizza questa diagnosi differenziale. Il lasso di tempo che intercorre dall'inizio della malattia (ore, giorni, o settimane) alla sua presentazione è un aspetto critico dell'anamnesi. Il classico paziente con appendicite acuta descrive dolore addominale quale sintomo principale. L'appendicite acuta solitamente si manifesta in modo insidioso come malessere generalizzato o anoressia, ma vi è un esordio precoce del dolore addominale e la sintomatologia si acuisce tipicamente nelle prime 24-48 ore. Mentre la maggior parte dei pazienti presenta 1 o 2 episodi di vomito nelle prime 24-48 ore della malattia, più episodi non sono frequenti durante la fase precoce della patologia. Al contrario, quando la diagnosi è quella di gastroenterite, il dolore addominale può sembrare associato con episodi frequenti di diarrea e vomito, che rappresentano i principali sintomi di presentazione. Nei pazienti con esordio acuto (<72 ore dall'inizio della malattia), il vomito che precede il dolore, la diarrea e il vomito abbondanti, la febbre di grado elevato sono indicativi di gastroenterite. Inoltre, nei pazienti con appendicite, tipicamente la peristalsi è normale o diminuita, mentre la gastroenterite determina iperperistalsi intestinale. Nel caso tipico di un bambino con appendicite acuta che si presenta entro 48 ore dall'esordio della patologia, la conta leucocitaria può essere bassa, normale o elevata, ma raramente supera i 200 000 mm^3. La conta leucocitaria in questo range deve far propendere per diagnosi alternative e suggerire indagini ulteriori.

I bambini con un'anamnesi di malattia >3-4 giorni creano maggiori dubbi. Se la diagnosi è appendicite, la perforazione è probabile e la presentazione del paziente evidenzia segni e sintomi di ascesso/flemmone localizzato in fossa iliaca destra o peritonite diffusa. In questa fase della malattia, la conta leucocitaria deve essere elevata (>12 000) con spostamento a sinistra della formula leucocitaria (immissione in circolo di leucociti immaturi); per contro, una conta leucocitaria <7000 con linfocitosi dovrebbe essere chiaramente inusuale e più caratteristica della gastroenterite. Un emocromo normale associato a lesioni cutanee emorragiche, artrite e nefrite è indice di porpora di Schönlein-Henoch o sindrome emolitico-uremica. La torsione di un testicolo non disceso e l'epididimite, peraltro frequenti, devono essere individuate mediante esame obiettivo. Nella diverticolite di Meckel, una patologia poco frequente, la presentazione clinica ricorda molto l'appendicite e la diagnosi viene effettuata chirurgicamente. La peritonite primaria spontanea nelle ragazze in età prepubere viene spesso scambiata per appendicite. Occorre riconoscere che l'appendicite "non diagnosticata" è la causa più frequente di occlusione del tenue nei bambini che non hanno un'anamnesi di chirurgia addominale precedente. Ci si aspetta una presentazione atipica dell'appendicite in associazione con altre condizioni come la gravidanza, il morbo di Crohn, il trattamento con corticosteroidi o la terapia immunosoppressiva. L'appendicite in associazione con il morbo di Crohn spesso ha una presentazione protratta con modalità atipiche di dolore addominale, ricorrente ma localizzato.

La diagnosi di appendicite nelle adolescenti è particolarmente difficile e alcuni riportano un tasso negativo di appendicectomia del 30%. Le cisti ovariche sono spesso dolorose a causa della rottura, dell'aumento rapido di dimensioni o dell'emorragia. La rottura di un follicolo ovarico associata a ovulazione causa dolore lateralizzato a metà del ciclo (dolore basso addominale su un solo lato: *Mittelschmerz*), ma non c'è progressione della sintomatologia ed è assente una malattia sistemica. I tumori ovarici e la torsione possono mimare l'appendicite acuta, sebbene la torsione ovarica sia caratterizzata da esordio acuto di dolore severo associato a forte nausea e vomito, rispetto a quanto visto nelle fasi precoci dell'appendicite. Nella malattia infiammatoria pelvica, il dolore è tipicamente sovrapubico, bilaterale e di durata maggiore. Nelle donne si rende necessaria una diagnosi urgente in quanto l'appendicite perforata può predisporre la paziente a una futura gravidanza ectopica o a infertilità tubarica, nonostante i dati non dimostrino un aumento significativo dell'incidenza di infertilità in seguito a un'appendice perforata. Per queste ragioni, la maggior parte delle adolescenti deve essere sottoposta a ulteriori approfondimenti diagnostici (ecografia, TC o laparoscopia).

TRATTAMENTO

Una volta che la diagnosi di appendicite è confermata o fortemente sospettata, il trattamento dell'appendicite acuta consiste per lo più nell'appendicectomia. Gli antibiotici e i progressi compiuti nel campo della radiologia interventistica hanno consentito il drenaggio delle raccolte di liquidi e la gestione iniziale non operatoria come opzione alternativa nelle presentazioni tardive, in base sia alle condizioni generali del paziente sia allo stato dell'appendice.

La chirurgia d'urgenza è raramente indicata e la maggior parte dei pazienti necessita di mezzi di supporto preoperatori, onde garantire la sicurezza della procedura e il miglioramento degli esiti. Anche se l'approccio tradizionale consiste nel procedere all'intervento chirurgico non appena la diagnosi di appendicite è confermata, l'appendicectomia non dovrebbe essere effettuata di notte. Spesso patologie inattese (tumori dell'appendice, linfomi intestinali, anomalie congenite del rene, malattia infiammatoria intestinale complicata) possono essere scoperte al momento dell'operazione, rendendo quindi necessaria una consulenza intraoperatoria e una biopsia al criostato. Non esiste correlazione tra il momento in cui viene effettuato l'intervento chirurgico e il tasso di perforazione o la morbilità postoperatoria, se l'intervento viene effettuato entro 12-24 ore dalla diagnosi. Inoltre l'appendicectomia può essere un'operazione rischiosa, con possibili complicanze maggiori, tra cui danni all'intestino adiacente, ai vasi iliaci o all'uretere destro. L'operazione dovrebbe sempre avvenire entro 12-24 ore dalla diagnosi. I bambini con appendicite spesso presentano un certo grado di disidratazione e quindi necessitano di liquidi in fase preoperatoria per correggere l'ipovolemia e l'alterazione idroelettrolitica prima dell'anestesia. L'eventuale febbre dovrebbe essere trattata. Il trattamento del dolore viene effettuato anche prima della diagnosi definitiva; una volta che si è deciso di procedere all'intervento chirurgico, è opportuno richiedere una consulenza presso il servizio di controllo del dolore, se disponibile. Nella maggior parte dei casi, il trattamento preoperatorio può spesso essere condotto durante il periodo della valutazione diagnostica e può essere eseguita l'appendicectomia.

Nei pazienti in cui, al momento della diagnosi, si è individuata la presenza di un appendice perforata, l'intervento chirurgico è ancora meno urgente e una gestione corretta in fase preoperatoria ancora più importante. Quando la malattia raggiunge uno stadio avanzato, a causa di un ritardo nella diagnosi o nella presentazione, i pazienti possono manifestare alterazioni fisiologiche significative come disidratazione grave, ipotensione, acidosi e insufficienza renale. Questi pazienti necessitano di un periodo di stabilizzazione più lungo, con somministrazione di liquidi per compensare le perdite, antibiotici e talvolta ricovero in un reparto di terapia intensiva, prima di iniziare il trattamento definitivo. In base alle condizioni generali, ai risultati della TC e alla disponibilità di radiologi esperti, il piano di cura iniziale può prevedere il drenaggio della raccolta di liquidi mediante radiologia interventistica e la continuazione della somministrazione di liquidi. Un flemmone, in assenza di una raccolta liquida identificabile, può beneficiare di un iniziale trattamento non operatorio, con somministrazione di antibiotici. Il posizionamento di uno o più cateteri di drenaggio sotto guida ecografica o TC ha successo nell'80% dei pazienti. Nella maggior parte dei pazienti è ancora necessario ritardare l'appendicectomia (durante la stessa ospedalizzazione) o eseguire un'appendicectomia a distanza (4-6 settimane dopo la presentazione iniziale).

Se è presente peritonite diffusa, la maggior parte dei chirurghi procede tempestivamente all'intervento chirurgico, dopo un breve periodo di somministrazione di liquidi ev e di antibioticoterapia. Altri proseguono la gestione non operatoria affinché i pazienti vadano incontro a un miglioramento di parametri fisiologici come la stabilità emodinamica, il volume urinario, il controllo della temperatura e la riduzione della conta leucocitaria. Se il paziente presenta un miglioramento clinico con risoluzione della febbre, della sepsi e ripresa della funzionalità intestinale, si continua la terapia antibiotica per 2 settimane e si decide se effettuare l'appendicectomia a distanza nel giro di 6-8 settimane. Se il bambino non migliora in 24-72 ore occorre effettuare l'appendicectomia per controllare la sepsi. Si interviene chirurgicamente d'urgenza solo in circostanze occasionali, quando per ripristinare le condizioni fisiologiche si rende necessario un controllo urgente della sepsi peritoneale avanzata non ottenibile con il drenaggio dei fluidi o quando quest'ultimo non è disponibile.

ANTIBIOTICI. Gli antibiotici riducono l'incidenza di infezione postoperatoria della ferita e di ascesso intraperitoneale in un appendicite perforata, ma i risultati del loro impiego nell'appendicite semplice sono meno chiari. Il regime antibiotico deve essere diretto contro la flora batterica tipica rilevata a livello dell'appendice, compresi i microrganismi anaerobi (*Bacteroides*, *Clostridia* e *Peptostreptococcus* spp.) e i batteri aerobi Gram-negativi (*Escherichia coli*, *Pseudomonas aeruginosa*, *Enterobacter*, *Klebsiella* spp.). Poiché i microrganismi Gram-positivi sono di riscontro meno frequente nel colon, la necessità di una copertura antibiotica specifica (in primo luogo per gli enterococchi) è controversa. Diverse combinazioni hanno dimostrato efficacia equivalente in trial controllati, in termini di tasso di infezione della ferita, risoluzione della febbre, durata della degenza e incidenza delle complicanze. Per l'appendicite semplice non perforata, è sufficiente una dose di un unico antibiotico ad ampio spettro (cefoxitina) o di un farmaco equivalente in fase preoperatoria, sebbene molti chirurghi continuino la copertura per 24 ore. Nell'appendicite perforata o gangrenosa, la maggior parte dei chirurghi preferisce o la terapia tradizionale a tre antibiotici (ampicillina, gentamicina e clindamicina o metronidazolo) o una combinazione come ceftriaxone/metronidazolo o ticarcillina/acido clavulanico più gentamicina; la copertura antibiotica prosegue nella fase postoperatoria per 3-5 giorni. Poiché gli antibiotici per via orale hanno la stessa efficacia di quelli somministrati endovena, è possibile passare alla somministrazione per os non appena viene ripristinata la funzionalità intestinale.

APPENDICECTOMIA A DISTANZA. L'appendicite complicata da una massa infiammatoria o da un ascesso deve essere trattata senza appendicectomia immediata. Questa strategia si propone di evitare un elevato tasso di complicanze chirurgiche ed è spesso utile nei bambini in cui l'incidenza globale della perforazione è del 50% circa. Si discute sulla necessità di eseguire un'appendicectomia a distanza in questo gruppo di pazienti. Il rischio che si sviluppi un'appendicite ricorrente, se l'appendice non viene rimossa, è sconosciuto, ma gli studi pubblicati riportano percentuali tra il 10 e l'80%. La maggior parte dei casi di appendicite ricorrente si sviluppa entro 2 anni dall'inizio della malattia. Alcuni studiosi ritengono che l'appendicectomia a distanza non sia necessaria, considerato il basso rischio di appendicite ricorrente, mentre altri sono del parere che serva a prevenire l'appendicite ricorrente e a confermare la diagnosi iniziale, riportando un'incidenza di patologia inattesa nel 30% dei casi di appendicectomia a distanza. La maggior parte dei chirurghi pediatrici esegue questo intervento di routine dopo il trattamento non operatorio dell'appendicite perforata.

Tecnica chirurgica. L'appendicectomia si esegue solitamente attraverso l'incisione con sezione dei muscoli del quadrante addominale inferiore destro. L'intervento in laparoscopia è spesso usato dai chirurghi pediatrici sia per l'appendicite semplice sia per quella perforata. Gli studi che hanno posto a confronto l'approccio a cielo aperto con l'appendicectomia in laparoscopia hanno rilevato differenze per quanto riguarda sia i fattori di tipo amministrativo (costi, impiego delle risorse, durata della degenza) sia i parametri relativi agli esiti clinici (infezione della ferita, ascesso intra-addominale, necessità di un controllo analgesico, ritorno ad attività a tempo pieno), ma non sono riusciti a stabilire, sulla base di prove certe, quale approccio sia da preferire nei bambini. Nell'appendicite semplice, l'appendicectomia laparoscopica parrebbe connessa a un minor utilizzo di anestetico, a una ridotta morbilità della ferita e a un migliore risultato estetico, ma sembra comportare tempi e costi leggermente superiori in confronto alla procedura a cielo aperto. La durata dell'ospedalizzazione è simile. Il ruolo dell'intervento laparoscopico nell'appendicite perforata è meno chiaro. Non si dispone di dati convincenti per raccomandare un unico approccio per tutti i pazienti. La maggior parte dei chirurghi pediatrici li usa entrambi scegliendo l'uno o l'altro a seconda della situazione. L'approccio laparoscopico è più usato nei pazienti obesi, quando si sospettano diagnosi alternative, e nelle adolescenti, per valutare meglio patologie ovariche e la malattia infiammatoria pelvica, evitando le radiazioni ionizzanti legate alla TC. Da trial controllati randomizzati condotti sui bambini è emerso che l'iniezione di bupivacaina nella ferita riduce in modo significativo il dolore postoperatorio.

COMPLICANZE. Il **tasso di morbilità** per appendicite è molto variabile, oscillando dal 10 al 45%. Il principale fattore che incide sull'insorgenza di complicanze è la gravità dell'appendicite. Nell'appendicite acuta semplice, ci si attende un tasso globale di complicanze tra il 5-10%; in caso di appendicite gangrenosa o perforata, invece, il tasso sale al 15-30%. Le complicanze più frequenti sono l'infezione della ferita e gli ascessi intra-addominali, entrambi più frequenti dopo la perforazione. Il tasso di perforazione è >80% nei bambini al di sotto dei 5 anni di età. I pazienti con appendicite avanzata possono andare incontro a sepsi e insufficienza a carico di diversi organi, ma di solito rispondono rapidamente alla terapia antibiotica, alla somministrazione di liquidi e ad altre misure di sostegno. La **mortalità** dopo appendicite è rara (<0,3%) e riscontrabile soprattutto nei neonati e nei pazienti immunocompromessi. La perforazione e la formazione di un ascesso può portare a fistolizzazione negli organi adiacenti. Altre complicanze potenziali sono ileo postoperatorio, peritonite diffusa, pileflebite e occlusione adesiva dell'intestino tenue.

ASSISTENZA POSTOPERATORIA. In caso di appendicite semplice, la maggior parte dei chirurghi prosegue la terapia antibiotica per 24 ore; la dieta viene portata avanti. La maggior parte dei bambini viene dimessa nel giro di 24-48 ore. Nell'appendicite perforata, poiché è in atto un'infezione, la terapia antibiotica endovena prosegue per 3-5 giorni dopo l'intervento, seguita da un breve ciclo di antibiotici per via orale. Alcuni medici si avvalgono di criteri clinici e terminano l'antibioticoterapia quando il paziente resta senza febbre per 24 ore e presenta una conta leucocitaria normale. Gli antibiotici per via orale hanno la stessa efficacia di quelli somministrati per via endovenosa e i pazienti possono poi completare la terapia farmacologica a casa, non appena si verifica la ripresa della funzionalità intestinale e risultano soddisfatti gli altri criteri necessari alla dimissione.

Applegate, KE, Sivit CJ, Salvator AE, et al: Effect of cross-sectional imaging on negative appendectomy and perforation rates in children. *Radiology* 2001;220:103–107.

Benjamin IS, Patel AG: Managing acute appendicitis. *Br Med J* 2002; 325:505–506.

Brown CV, Abrishami M, Muller M, et al: Appendiceal abscess: Immediate operation or percutaneous drainage? *Am Surg* 2003;69:829–832.

Cappendijk VC, Hazebroek FWJ: The impact of diagnostic delay on the course of acute appendicitis. *Arch Dis Child* 2000;83:64–66.

Chong CF, Wang TL, Chen CC, et al: Preconsultation use of analgesics on adults presenting to the emergency department with acute appendicitis. *Emerg Med* 2004;21:41–43.

Garcia Pena BM, Taylor GA, Fishman SJ, Mandl KD: Costs and effectiveness of ultrasonography and limited computed tomography for diagnosing appendicitis in children. *Pediatrics* 2000;106:672–676.

Guillerman RP, Brody AS, Kraus SJ: Evidence-based guidelines for pediatric imaging: The example of the child with possible appendicitis. *Pediatr Ann* 2002;31:629–640.

Humes DJ, Simpson J: Acute appendicitis. *BMJ* 2006;333:530–534.

Kaiser S, Mesas-Burgos C, Soderman E, et al: Appendicitis in children–Impact of US and CT on the negative appendectomy rate. *Eur J Ped Surg* 2004; 14:260–264.

Kim MK, Strait RT, Sato TT, et al: A randomized clinical trial of analgesia in children with acute abdominal pain. *Acad Emerg Med* 2002;9:281–287.

Kokki H, Lintula H, Vanamo K, et al: Oxycodone vs placebo in children with undifferentiated abdominal pain. *Arch Pediatr Adolesc Med* 2005;159: 320–325.

Kosloske AM, Love CL, Rohrer JE, et al: The diagnosis of appendicitis in children: Outcomes of a strategy based on pediatric surgical evaluation. *Pediatrics* 2004;113:29–34.

Lee JH, Jeong YK, Hwang JC, et al: Graded compression sonography with adjuvant use of posterior manual compression technique in the sonographic diagnosis of acute appendicitis. *AJR Am J Roentgenol* 2002;178:863–868.

Lintula H, Kokki H, Vanamo K: Single-blind randomized clinical trial of laparoscopic versus open appendectomy in children. *Br J Surg* 2001;88: 510–514.

Lycopoulou L, Mamoulakis C, Hantzi E, et al: Serum amyloid A protein levels as a positive aid in the diagnosis of acute appendicitis in children. *Clin Chem Lab Med* 2005;43:49–53.

Martin AE, Vollman D, Adler B, et al: CT scans may not reduce the negative appendectomy rate in children. *J Pediatr Surg* 2004;39:886–890.

Mittal VK, Goliath J, Sabir M, et al: Advantages of focused helical computed tomographic scanning with rectal contrast only vs triple contrast in the diagnosis of clinically uncertain acute appendicitis. *Arch Surg* 2004;139: 495–500.

Morrow SE, Newman KD: Appendicitis. In Ashcraft KW, Holcomb, GW III, Murphy JP: *Pediatric Surgery,* 4th ed. Philadelphia, Elsevier Saunders, 2005, pp 577–585.

Nance ML, Adamson WT, Hedrick HL: Appendicitis in the very young child: A continuing diagnostic challenge. *Pediatr Emerg Care* 2000;16:160–162.

Newman K, Ponsky T, Little K, et al: Appendicitis 2000: Variability in practice, outcomes, and resource utilization at 30 pediatric hospitals. *J Pediatr Surg* 2003;38:372–379.

Ponsky TA, Huang ZJ, Kittle K, et al: Hospital and patient-level characteristics and the risk of appendiceal rupture and negative appendectomy in children. *JAMA* 2004;292:1977–1982.

Prommeger R, Obrist P, Ensinger C, et al: Retrospective evaluation of carcinoid tumors of the appendix in children. *World J Surg* 2002;26:1489–1492.

Sauerland S, Lefering R, Neugebauer EA: Laparoscopic versus open surgery for suspected appendicitis. *Cochrane Database Sys Rev* 2002:CD001546.

Smink DS, Finkelstein JA, Garcia Pena BM, et al: Diagnosis of acute appendicitis in children using a clinical practice guideline. *J Pediatr Surg* 2004;39:458–463.

Taylor, GA: Suspected appendicitis in children: In search of the single best diagnostic test. *Radiology* 2004;231:293–295.

Ziegler, MM: The diagnosis of appendicitis: An evolving paradigm. *Pediatrics* 2004;113:130–132.

Capitolo 341 ■ Patologie chirurgiche di ano, retto e colon

Michael D. Klein e Robert P. Thomas

341.1 • Malformazioni anorettali

Per comprendere lo spettro delle anomalie anorettali, è importante considerare l'importanza del complesso muscolare sfinterico, un insieme di fibre muscolari che circonda l'ano-retto (Fig. 341-1). Questo complesso è formato dall'insieme dei muscoli puborettale, elevatore dell'ano, sfintere esterno e interno e dalla parte superficiale dello sfintere esterno, che si incrociano a livello del retto. Le malformazioni anorettali, definite in base ai rapporti del retto con questo complesso, consistono in diversi gradi di stenosi fino all'atresia completa; l'incidenza è di 1/4000 nati. Le principali preoccupazioni a lungo termine riguardano il controllo dell'intestino e la funzionalità urinaria e sessuale.

EMBRIOLOGIA

La parte terminale dell'intestino (ano e retto) si forma precwocemente; corrisponde infatti a quella parte dell'intestino primitivo che si prolunga nella piega ventrale dell'estremità caudale del disco embrionario nella 2ª settimana di gestazione. Intorno al 13° giorno di gestazione si sviluppano il diverticolo ventrale, l'allantoide o vescica primitiva. L'unione dell'allantoide e della parte terminale dell'intestino determina la formazione della cloaca, in cui sboccano gli orifizi delle vie genitali, urinarie e intestinali. Essa è coperta dalla membrana della cloaca. Il setto urorettale scende a dividere questo canale comune formando pieghe laterali che crescono e si fondono a partire dalla metà della 7ª settimana. L'apertura della porzione posteriore della membrana (la membrana anale) si verifica durante l'8ª settimana. Le anomalie che si manifestano in qualunque fase di questo processo conducono allo spettro clinico delle alterazioni anogenitali.

L'**ano imperforato** comprende lesioni basse, in cui il retto è disceso attraverso il complesso sfinterico, e lesioni alte, in cui ciò non è avvenuto. La maggior parte dei pazienti con ano imperforato presenta una fistola. Esiste uno spettro di malformazioni, sia nei maschi sia nelle femmine (vedi Fig. 341-1). Nei maschi le lesioni basse si caratterizzano solitamente per la presenza di meconio in un punto qualunque del perineo lungo il rafe mediano (Fig. 341-2*A*). Anche le femmine con lesioni basse presentano uno spettro di anomalie, che vanno dall'ano leggermente anteriore sul corpo perineale a una fistola con la forchetta vaginale che si apre sulla mucosa dell'introitus distalmente all'imene (Fig. 341-3*A*). L'ano imperforato alto in un maschio non presenta né un'apertura cutanea apparente né una fistola, ma di solito si associa a una fistola nel tratto urinario, oppure a livello dell'uretra o della vescica (Fig. 341-2*B*). Sebbene nelle donne vi sia occasionalmente una fistola rettovaginale, le lesioni alte di solito sono alterazioni della cloaca in cui il retto, la vagina e l'uretra confluiscono in un canale comune, o canale della cloaca, di diversa lunghezza (Fig. 341-3*B*). I maschi con ano imperforato senza fistola sono soprattutto bambini con trisomia 21.

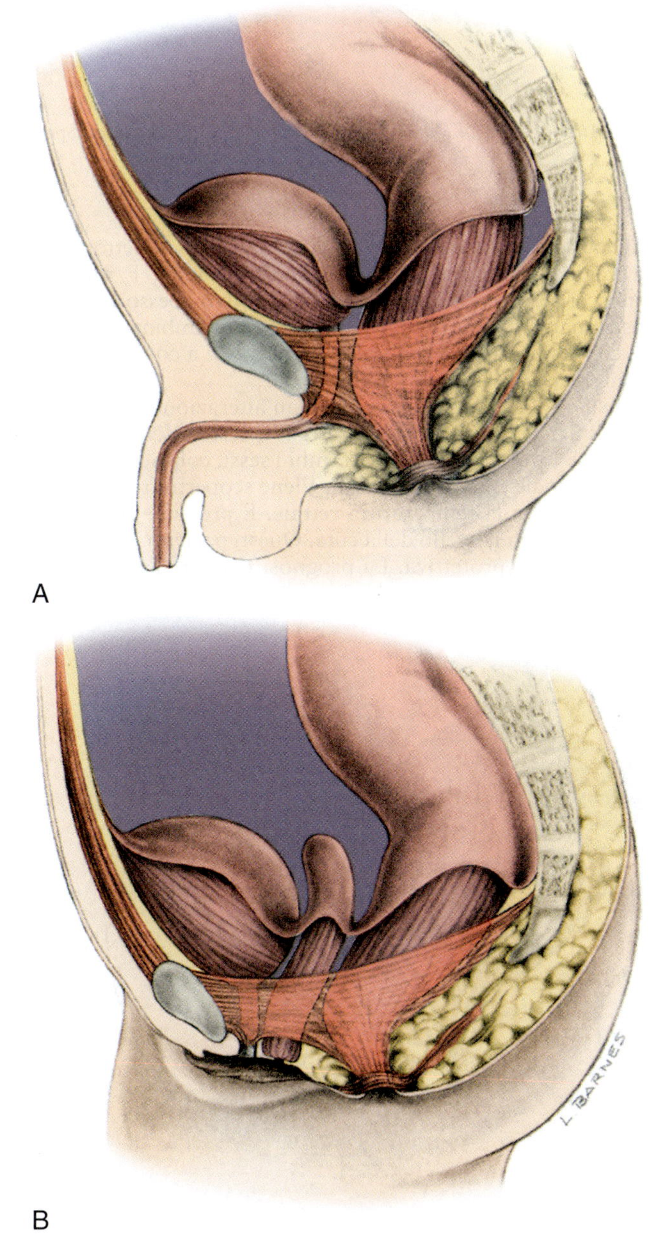

Figura 341-1. Anatomia anorettale normale in relazione alle strutture pelviche. *A*, Maschio. *B*, Femmina. (Da Peña A: *Atlas of Surgical Management of Anorectal Malformations*. Springer-Verlag, New York, 1989, p 3.)

ANOMALIE ASSOCIATE

Vi sono diverse anomalie associate alle malformazioni anorettali (Tab. 341-1); le più comuni sono a carico del rene e del tratto urinario, in associazione ad anomalie del sacro. Questo complesso è spesso indicato con il nome di **sindrome da regressione caudale**. I maschi con fistola rettovescicale e i pazienti con cloaca persistente hanno un rischio del 90% di avere alterazioni urologiche. Altre anomalie frequentemente associate sono quelle cardiache e l'atresia esofagea con o senza fistola tracheoesofagea, che possono raggrupparsi in diversi tipi di combinazioni. Quando combinate, esse si accompagnano spesso ad alterazioni dall'aspetto radiale dell'estremità superiore, nel qual caso vengono definite associazioni malformative VATERR (*Vertebral, Anal, Tracheal, Esophageal, Radial, Renal*, difetti vertebrali, anali, cardiaci, fistola tracheale, fistola esofagea, displasia radiale, difetti renali) o VACTERL (*Vertebral, Anal, Cardiac, Tracheal, Esophageal, Renal, Limb*, difetti vertebrali, anali, malformazione cardiaci, fistola tracheale, fistola esofagea, difetti renali, malformazione degli arti).

Esiste una buona correlazione tra il grado di sviluppo sacrale e la funzionalità renale. I pazienti con sacro assente di solito presentano incontinenza fecale e urinaria permanente. Le anomalie spinali e i diversi gradi di disrafismo sono spesso associati a questi difetti. Un tethered cord (midollo ancorato) si ha in circa il 25% dei pazienti con malformazioni anorettali. La diagnosi dei difetti spinali si può stabilire nei primi 3 mesi di vita mediante ecografia spinale; nei pazienti più grandi è necessaria la RM.

MANIFESTAZIONI E DIAGNOSI

LESIONI BASSE. La valutazione delle condizioni di un neonato include l'ispezione perineale. La mancanza dell'orifizio anale in posizione corretta rende necessarie ulteriori valutazioni. Le forme lievi di ano imperforato, solitamente definite stenosi o ano interiorizzato, consistono probabilmente in un ano imperforato con fistola perineale. La posizione normale dell'ano sul perineo è circa a metà (rapporto 0,5) tra il coccige e lo scroto o l'introitus vaginale. Sebbene i sintomi, in primo luogo la stipsi, siano attribuiti all'ano interiorizzato (rapporto <0,34 nelle femmine, <0,46 nei maschi), molti pazienti sono asintomatici.

Se non sono visibili l'ano o la fistola, ci può essere una lesione bassa o un "ano coperto". In questi casi si osservano glutei ben formati e spesso un rafe ispessito o "bucket handle" ("manico di secchio") (detto anche "black ribbon", nastro nero). Dopo 24 ore il rigonfiamento formato dal meconio appare blu o nero. In tal caso occorre effettuare una procedura perineale immediata, seguita da un programma di dilatazione.

Nel maschio, la fistola perineale (cutanea) può estendersi anteriormente lungo il rafe mediano attraverso lo scroto e anche nell'asta del pene. Si tratta di solito di un tragitto sottile, con un retto normale a pochi millimetri dalla cute. Anomalie extraintestinali si verificano in meno del 10% di questi pazienti.

Nelle femmine, una lesione bassa si apre nel vestibolo o nella forchetta (parte rivestita da epitelio mucoso sita all'esterno dell'imene, ma entro l'introitus). In questo caso il retto è disceso attraverso il complesso dello sfintere.

I bambini con lesioni basse possono essere trattati inizialmente con manipolazione e dilatazione perineale. Visualizzare le fistole basse è importante ai fini della valutazione e del trattamento in quanto permette di evitare il posizionamento del sondino nasogastrico nelle prime 24 ore, così da permettere all'addome e all'intestino di distendersi e da sospingere il meconio verso il retto distale.

LESIONI ALTE. In un bambino con ano imperforato alto il perineo appare distrofico. Si può verificare un passaggio di aria o meconio attraverso il pene (uretra) quando la fistola è alta, aprendosi nell'uretra bulbare o prostatica o anche nella vescica. Nella **fistola rettouretrale** (la più comune nei maschi) il meccanismo sfinterico è soddisfacente, il sacro può essere iposviluppato ed è presente

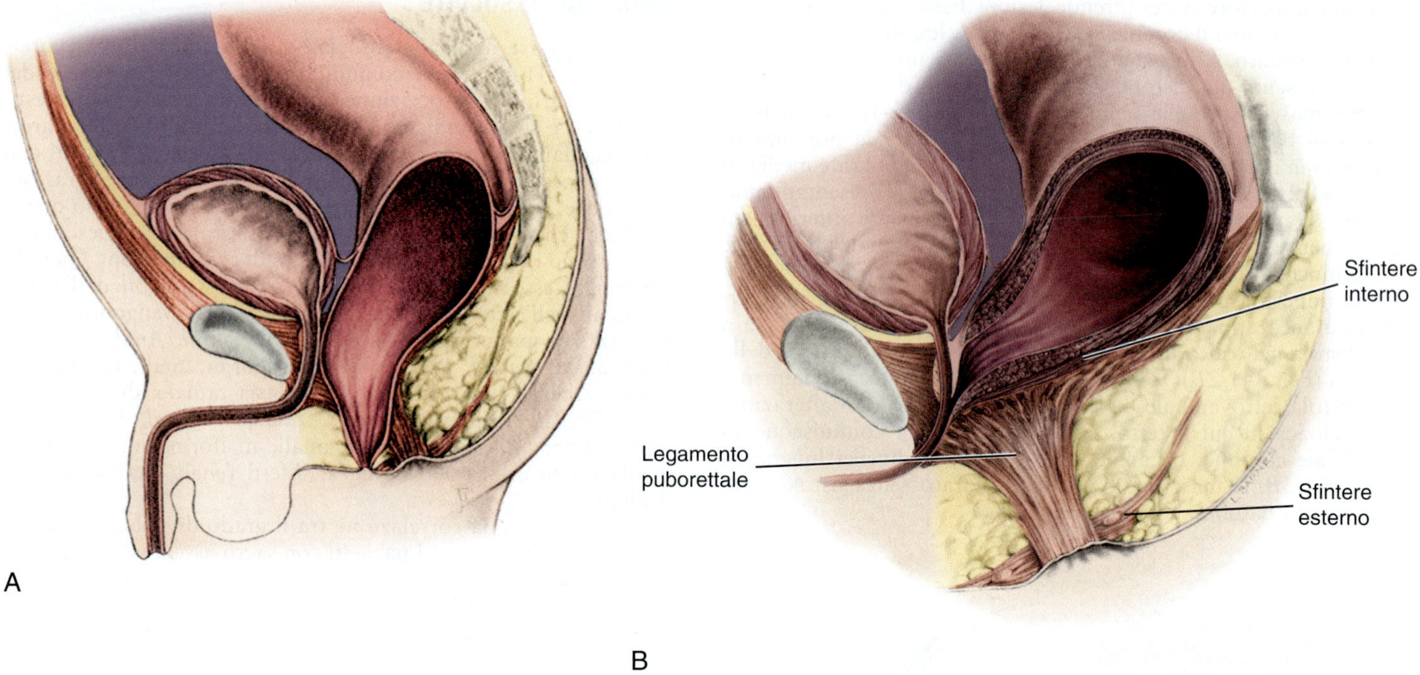

Figura 341-2. Ano imperforato nel maschio. *A*, Lesioni basse. *B*, Lesioni alte. (Da Peña A: *Atlas of Surgical Management of Anorectal Malformations*. Springer-Verlag, New York, 1989, pp 7, 26.)

una fossetta anale. Nella **fistola rettoprostatica** il sacro è poco sviluppato, lo scroto può essere bifido e la fossetta anale è vicino allo scroto. Nella **fistola rettovescicale** il meccanismo sfinterico è poco sviluppato, il sacro ipoplastico o assente. Nei bambini con trisomia 21 sono presenti tutte le caratteristiche di una lesione alta, ma non la fistola; il sacro e il meccanismo sfinterico sono solitamente ben sviluppati e la prognosi è buona.

Nelle bambine con ano imperforato alto vi può essere un'apparente fistola rettovaginale, mentre una fistola rettovaginale vera è rara. Nella maggior parte dei casi si tratta di fistole con il vestibolo, esterne all'orifizio dell'imene. Queste hanno una buona prognosi, con un sacro normale, una fossetta anale e una funzione sfinterica intatta.

Cloaca persistente. È una condizione in cui il retto, l'uretra e la vagina confluiscono in un canale comune. È importante riconoscerla, dato che l'intervento correttivo spesso richiederà l riposizionamento di uretra, vagina e retto. I bambini di entrambi i sessi con lesioni alte devono essere sottoposti a colostomia prima dell'intervento correttivo.

Atresia rettale. L'atresia rettale è un'alterazione rara, presente solo nell'1% delle anomalie anorettali. Questo difetto, che presenta le stesse caratteristiche in entrambi i sessi, colpisce pazienti con un canale anale e un ano normali. Viene scoperto frequentemente mentre si rileva la temperatura rettale. È presente un'ostruzione circa 2 cm sopra il livello della cute. Questi pazienti necessitano di una colostomia protettiva. La prognosi rispetto alla funzionalità

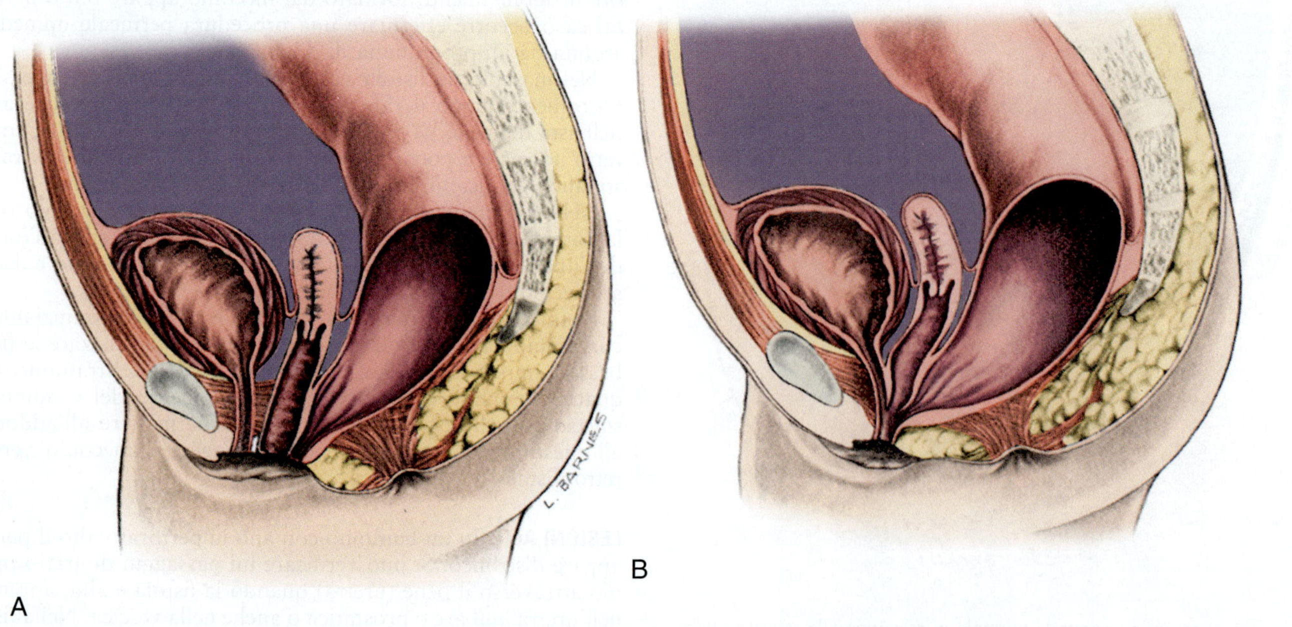

Figura 341-3. Ano imperforato nelle femmine. *A*, Fistola vestibolare. *B*, Cloaca. (Da Peña A: *Atlas of Surgical Management of Anorectal Malformations*. Springer-Verlag, New York, 1989, pp 50, 60.)

è eccellente, poiché il meccanismo sfinterico che risiede nel canale anale è normale (come pure la sensibilità).

APPROCCIO AL PAZIENTE

Nell'80-90% dei pazienti **maschi** una buona valutazione clinica e l'esame delle urine forniscono informazioni sufficienti per stabilire se sussiste la necessità di una colostomia. Se il bambino presenta una fistola perineale o rettourinaria, il meconio potrebbe non vedersi a livello del perineo o nelle urine prima che siano trascorse 16-24 ore dalla nascita. I muscoli sfinterici volontari circondano la parte più distale dell'intestino in presenza di fistole perineale e rettouretrale; la pressione intestinale intraluminale deve essere sufficientemente alta da superare il tono di questi muscoli prima che il meconio faccia la sua comparsa nelle urine o nel perineo. Poiché alla nascita l'intestino non è disteso, le valutazioni cliniche e radiologiche non sono affidabili durante le prime 16-24 ore di vita. Si pone un pezzo di garza attorno alla punta del pene, cercando di valutare se particelle di meconio siano filtrate attraverso di esso. La presenza di meconio nelle urine e il riscontro di glutei distrofici sono considerate indicazioni alla colostomia protettiva. Segni clinici indicativi di fistola perineale rappresentano un'indicazione per l'anoplastica senza colostomia protettiva. A volte nessuno dei segni clinici già descritti diventa evidente dopo 24 ore di osservazione; in tal caso è indicata la valutazione radiologica. Una radiografia laterale trasversale con il paziente in posizione prona, 16-24 ore dopo la nascita, è importante per determinare la posizione della tasca rettale; quando questa risulta separata dalla cute per più di 1 cm, il paziente necessita di una colostomia.

In più del 90% dei casi, per fare diagnosi nelle **femmine** occorre procedere all'ispezione perineale. Queste pazienti devono essere tenute sotto osservazione per le prime 16-24 ore di vita. La presenza di un unico orifizio perineale è significativo di cloaca, diagnosi avvalorata dal reperto di una massa pelvica palpabile (idrocolpo). La fistola vestibolare si diagnostica mediante attenta separazione delle labbra per esaminare il vestibolo. L'orifizio rettale è localizzato immediatamente dietro l'imene all'interno dei genitali femminili e nel vestibolo. La fistola perineale è facile da diagnosticare. L'orifizio rettale, localizzato tra i genitali femminili e il centro dello sfintere, è circondato dalla cute; l'espressione *ano anteriorizzato*, a volte usata per questo difetto, non è corretta, dato che sono orifizi di fistole anomale non circondate da un meccanismo sfinterico normale. Meno del 10% di queste pazienti non riesce ad evacuare il meconio attraverso i genitali o il perineo dopo 24 ore di osservazione; in tal caso può rendersi necessaria una radiografia laterale trasversale.

La valutazione consiste anche nell'identificare le anomalie associate (vedi Tab. 341-1). Un'ispezione attenta del perineo è importante per determinare la presenza o meno della fistola; se l'indagine dà esito positivo, la lesione è bassa. L'invertografia è poco utile, ma una radiografia diretta dell'intera zona sacrale, ali iliache comprese, è importante per identificare alterazioni del sacro e valutarne l'adeguatezza. Se vi sono anomalie o se il rapporto sacrale è <0,52 la prognosi, per quanto riguarda la continenza vera, non è buona; con un rapporto <0,3, non vi sono evidenze di un buon controllo intestinale. Occorre eseguire un'ecografia addominopelvica e una cistouretrografia minzionale (VCUG, *Voiding CystoUrethroGram*). È inoltre necessario posizionare il sondino nasogastrico per identificare un'atresia esofagea ed eseguire un'ecocardiografia. Nei bambini con lesioni alte, la VCUG spesso identifica la fistola rettourinaria. Nelle bambine con lesioni alte di frequente si rendono necessarie valutazioni più invasive, comprendenti la vaginografia e l'endoscopia, per una valutazione più dettagliata dell'alterazione della cloaca.

TABELLA 341-1. Malformazioni associate

GENITOURINARIE	**CARDIOVASCOLARI**
Reflusso vescicoureterale	Tetralogia di Fallot
Agenesia renale	Difetto del setto ventricolare
Displasia renale	Trasposizione dei grandi vasi
Duplicazione ureterale	Sindrome ipoplasica del cuore sinistro
Criptorchidismo	**GASTROINTESTINALI**
Ipospadia	Fistola tracheoesofagea
Utero bicorne	Atresia duodenale
Setto vaginale	Malrotazione
VERTEBRALI	Malattia di Hirshsprung
Disrafismo spinale	
Tethered cord (midollo ancorato)	
Masse presacrali	
Meningocele	
Lipoma	
Dermoide	
Teratoma	

CHIRURGIA CORRETTIVA

A volte, se la fistola perineale è aperta in una buona posizione, può essere trattata con la semplice dilatazione. Si comincia con dilatatori di Hegar di calibro 5 o 6; il bambino viene dimesso quando la madre può usare un dilatatore di calibro 8. Le dilatazioni vengono effettuate a casa due volte al giorno aumentando la dimensione di settimana in settimana fino ad arrivare al numero 14. A partire dall'anno di età le feci sono solitamente ben formate, pertanto non occorrono ulteriori dilatazioni. Raggiunta la dimensione di 14, l'esaminatore può inserire il dito mignolo. Se l'anello anale è morbido e duttile, è possibile eseguire la dilatazione con minore frequenza oppure addirittura sospenderla.

Talvolta non c'è una fistola visibile, ma è possibile assistere al riempimento del retto a opera del meconio che rigonfia il perineo; in caso contrario si sospetta un ano coperto. Se la radiografia diretta o l'ecografia del perineo confermano che il retto è a meno di 2 cm dalla cute, bisogna eseguire una procedura perineale minore per perforare la cute e quindi procedere con la dilatazione o effettuare un'anoplastica perineale semplice.

Quando l'orifizio della fistola è molto vicino all'introitus o allo scroto, è spesso indicato riposizionarlo chirurgicamente. Ciò richiede anche una dilatazione postoperatoria per prevenire la formazione di una strozzatura/restringimento. Questa procedura va eseguita sempre in un arco di tempo compreso tra il periodo neonatale e il compimento del primo anno di vita. È preferibile aspettare che siano trascorse diverse settimane dalla dilatazione e che il bambino sia più grande, perché in questi casi la dissezione dell'anoretto risulta più facile. L'approccio sagittale posteriore di Peña prevede un'incisione dapprima intorno alla fistola, poi sulla linea mediana della parete posteriore della nuova posizione. La dissezione si continua sulla linea mediana usando uno stimolatore muscolare per essere sicuri che su entrambi i lati vi sia muscolo a sufficienza. La fistola deve essere sezionata in senso cefalico per diversi centimetri, per permettere il posizionamento posteriore senza trazione. Se è necessario, si reseca una parte della fistola distale prima dell'anastomosi alla cute perineale.

I bambini con lesione alta vengono trattati con colostomia *double barrel*, con la quale si separa il passaggio delle feci dal tratto urinario. Questo approccio permette inoltre l'esecuzione di una colostografia ad alta pressione prima dell'intervento correttivo, per identificare la posizione precisa del retto distale e della fistola. L'intervento correttivo definitivo o anorettoplastica sagittale posteriore (PSARP, *Posterior Sagittal AnoRectoPlasty*) si esegue a circa 1 anno di età. Si effettua un'incisione sulla linea mediana, spesso selezionando il coccige e anche il sacro. Usando uno stimolatore nervoso e muscolare, il chirurgo si mantiene strettamente sulla linea mediana, separa il complesso dello sfintere e identifica il retto. Il retto è quindi aperto sulla linea mediana e la fistola viene individuata dal suo interno. Questo permette la divisione della fistola senza danneggiare le vie urinarie. Quindi si disseziona il retto prossimalmente finché non si ottiene una lunghezza sufficiente per suturarlo in posizione adeguata sul perineo. Infine si suturano muscoli del complesso sfinterico intorno (e soprattutto dietro) al retto.

Una procedura analoga può essere effettuata su femmine con anomalie alte, con alcune variazioni rispetto alla separazione della vagina e del retto dall'interno del canale anale. Quando il canale è più lungo di 3 cm, l'intervento è particolarmente difficile e la procedura risulta complessa.

Di solito si può chiudere la colostomia a distanza di 6 settimane o più dalla PSARP. Due settimane dopo qualsiasi procedura anale, un familiare deve eseguire la dilatazione due volte al giorno. Le dilatazioni frequenti, oltre a risultare meno dolorose, comportano un trauma minore a livello tissutale, minore infiammazione e una cicatrizzazione migliore.

PROGNOSI

I pazienti con lesioni basse è più probabile abbiano una continenza vera. Ciononostante, sono anche particolarmente predisposti alla stipsi, che porta a incontinenza massiva. È molto importante sottoporli tutti a uno stretto monitoraggio gestendo adeguatamente la stipsi e la dilatazione anale fino all'acquisizione del controllo sfinterico. Le Tabelle 341-2 e 341-3 mostrano gli esiti riguardo la continenza e la stipsi in relazione alle malformazioni osservate. I bambini con lesioni alte, specialmente i maschi con fistola uretrale rettoprostatica e le femmine con anomalie della cloaca, hanno scarse probabilità di essere continenti; ciononostante, possono raggiungere modalità di defecazione socialmente accettabili con un programma di gestione dell'intestino (senza colostomia), che spesso consiste in un clistere giornaliero per tenere il colon vuoto e il paziente pulito fino al clistere successivo. Se questo programma ha successo, l'esecuzione di una procedura che preveda un clistere per via anterograda (ACE, *Antegrade Continence Enema*, o procedura di Malone) può migliorare la qualità della vita del paziente. L'ACE consiste nell'utilizzare l'appendice per creare un canale non refluente tra la cute e il cieco, oppure nell'eseguire uno stoma nel quadrante addominale inferiore per accedere al cieco. Il paziente può quindi sedersi sulla toilette e praticarsi il clistere attraverso l'ACE, lavando così l'intero colon. La procedura anterograda garantisce un tasso di igiene personale/pulizia per 24 ore del 95%.

TABELLA 341-2. Esiti del trattamento chirurgico delle malformazioni anorettali: continenza totale*

BASSE	
Fistola perianale	100%
Atresia/stenosi rettale	88
Fistola vestibolare	55
ALTE	
Ano imperforato senza fistola	52
Fistola bulbouretrale	31
Cloaca con canale comune <3 cm	28
Fistola prostatica	20
Cloaca con canale comune >3 cm	17
Fistola al collo della vescica	0

*Motilità intestinale volontaria, assenza di *soiling* (imbrattamento).
Modificata da: Peña A, Hong A: Advances in the management of anorectal malformations. *Am J Surg* 2000;180:370-376.

TABELLA 341-3. Stipsi e tipi di malformazioni anogenitali*

Fistola vestibolare	61%
Fistola uretrale bulbare	59
Atresia/stenosi rettale	57
Ano imperforato senza fistola	55
Fistola perineale	50
Cloaca con canale comune >3 cm	48
Fistola prostatica	45
Cloaca con canale comune <3 cm	39
Fistola al collo della vescica	15

*Modificata da Peña A, Hong A: Advances in the management of anorectal malformations. *Am J Surg* 2000;180:370-376.

341.2 • RAGADI ANALI

La ragade anale è una lacerazione della giunzione mucocutanea dell'ano. Si tratta di una lesione acquisita a eziologia sconosciuta, probabilmente secondaria al passaggio violento di feci dure, osservata soprattutto nella più tenera infanzia, prima che il bambino abbia compiuto un anno. Le ragadi possono essere la conseguenza anziché la causa della stipsi.

MANIFESTAZIONI CLINICHE. È spesso presente una storia di stipsi. Il paziente può aver avuto una prima evacuazione dolorosa, con passaggio di feci dure e conseguente formazione di una ragade. Dopo questa esperienza, il bambino trattiene volontariamente le feci per non sentire dolore all'evacuazione, con il risultato di aggravare la stipsi e creare le condizioni per il transito di feci dure. Si possono osservare dolore alla defecazione e sangue rosso vivo sulla superficie delle feci. La diagnosi viene effettuata mediante l'ispezione dell'area anale: tenendo le anche del lattante in flessione estrema, si separano le natiche per espandere le pieghe della cute perineale; la ragade diventa così visibile come una piccola lacerazione. Talvolta, alla periferia della lacerazione, il paziente presenta una piccola appendice cutanea che rappresenta il tessuto granulomatoso epitelizzato causato dall'infiammazione cronica. All'esplorazione rettale è possibile apprezzare feci dure nell'ampolla e spasmo rettale.

TRATTAMENTO. I genitori devono conoscere l'origine della ragade e il circolo vizioso che porta alla stipsi. L'obiettivo è mantenere le feci fluide ed evitare una dilatazione eccessiva dell'ano. Il processo di guarigione può richiedere diversi giorni o anche settimane. Un singolo episodio di fecaloma è sufficiente a esacerbare il problema. È indicato l'uso di un emolliente delle feci: spetta ai genitori stabilire la dose in base alla risposta del paziente. Occorre trattare la causa primaria della stipsi, se identificata. Non esistono evidenze scientifiche a sostegno di altri tipi di trattamento, come la dilatazione dell'ano, la sfinterectomia anale "interna" o l'escissione della ragade.

Le ragadi anali croniche nei pazienti adulti, che sono state poste in associazione con la stipsi, un intervento chirurgico rettale effettuato in precedenza, il morbo di Crohn e la diarrea cronica, vanno trattate in fase iniziale con emollienti delle feci, come quelle dei bambini, aggiungendo l'utilizzo del semicupio. Il trinitrato di glicerina allo 0,2% per uso topico riduce lo spasmo anale e guarisce le ragadi. Anche gli anestetici locali come lidocaina al 10% o una pomata con prilocaina al 5% + lidocaina al 5% possono risultare efficaci. Nei pazienti che non rispondono a questi trattamenti si può iniettare localmente la tossina botulinica per tenere sotto controllo la contrazione associata dello sfintere.

341.3 • ASCESSI E FISTOLE PERIANALI

Gli ascessi e le fistole perianali possono osservarsi in due gruppi di pazienti pediatrici, con cause, patogenesi e trattamento diversi. Questi sono: 1) lattanti che non hanno condizioni predisponenti, e 2) bambini più grandi con fattori predisponenti. Questo disturbo è relativamente frequente nel primo gruppo, formato da bambini, solitamente maschi, di età <2 anni. Generalmente è una condizione benigna, autolimitantesi, che però può coinvolgere anche la cute circostante; l'ascesso è in comunicazione con una delle cripte della linea pettinata del canale anale. La cripta può rappresentare una fonte di contaminazione. L'ascesso drena attraverso un orifizio nell'area perianale, ma rimane una fistola che comunica tramite la cripta colpita con l'orifizio esterno perianale. La fistola diventa cronica, ma di solito scompare spontaneamente prima dei due anni di età. Essendo situata molto vicino al lume dell'ano, è una condizione benigna perché risparmia il meccanismo sfinterico.

I pazienti di età >2 anni con un ascesso perianale o perirettale presentano una condizione predisponente, come neutropenia indotta da farmaci o autoimmune, leucemia, AIDS, diabete mellito, morbo di Crohn, precedente chirurgia rettale (malattia di Hirschsprung, ano imperforato) o sequele da uso di farmaci immunoppressivi. La prognosi è strettamente correlata con quella della malattia predisponente. L'ascesso può essere profondo ed espandersi rapidamente dando luogo a gravi sintomi tossici, in particolare quando la malattia predisponente è associata a immunosoppressione o neutropenia. L'esame colturale del materiale che costituisce l'ascesso rivela una flora mista con aerobi (*Escherichia coli*, *Klebsiella pneumoniae*, *Staphylococcus aureus*) e anaerobi (*Bacteroides* spp., *Clostridium*, *Veillonella*). Dal 10 al 15% presenta una crescita pura di *E. coli*, *S. aureus* o *Bacteroides fragilis*. I pazienti neutropenici possono presentare anche una batteriemia associata in modo non costante all'ascesso.

MANIFESTAZIONI CLINICHE. I lattanti senza malattia predisponente hanno manifestazioni cliniche lievi, talvolta con febbricola, dolore rettale non molto accentuato e un'area di cellulite perianale. In seguito si forma una pustola e l'ascesso drena attraverso questo orifizio, fenomeno che allevia i sintomi. L'infiammazione scompare e la pustola guarisce. Una o diverse settimane più tardi, il drenaggio del pus si ripresenta e continua in modo intermittente e cronico. Questa condizione di solito guarisce spontaneamente prima dei 2 anni di età.

I bambini con malattie predisponenti hanno un decorso più grave, con o senza febbre a seconda del loro stato immnunologico. La cellulite può espandersi rapidamente con calore, eritema, indurimento, dolorabilità e fluttuazione della fossa ischiorettale. L'organismo può andare incontro a grave tossiemia e sviluppare setticemia. Talvolta i pazienti presentano i sintomi della malattia predisponente. La biopsia della parete ascessuale può evidenziare un granuloma, che rappresenta un segno del morbo di Crohn.

TRATTAMENTO. I lattanti senza malattia predisponente e con una condizione autolimitante in genere non necessitano di trattamento. È sufficiente una gestione di tipo conservativo (osservazione) poiché, nella maggior parte dei casi, la fistola scompare spontaneamente prima dei 2 anni di età. In questi casi, gli antibiotici non risultano utili. A volte, quando il disagio del paziente è notevole, è possibile drenare l'ascesso in anestesia locale. La valutazione mediante (retto-)sigmoidoscopia in anestesia permette di identificare la situazione anatomica e procedere all'incisione, al curretage e/o al drenaggio, se indicati. Un ascesso a livello del sopraelevatore può essere confermato dalla palpazione di una massa fluttuante sopra lo sfintere. Il semplice drenaggio può non essere efficace e danneggiare lo sfintere. Al suo posto si esegue quindi una sutura resistente, passata sopra la fistola, ripresa dall'ano e legata strettamente per separare a poco a poco lo sfintere.

Un altro approccio in caso di fistola cronica è la fistolectomia in anestesia generale. Dopo aver esposto mediante un divaricatore adatto il canale anale e la parte inferiore del retto, si passa una sonda per condotti lacrimali attraverso l'orifizio esterno della fistola, facendolo poi fuoriuscire attraverso una delle cripte. Il tessuto tra la fistola e il lume del canale anale viene separato mediante cauterizzazione. La ferita viene lasciata aperta perché possa guarire spontaneamente. Questo tipo di trattamento presenta in genere il 20% di probabilità di recidiva.

I bambini più grandi con condizioni predisponenti necessitano di un trattamento più aggressivo della fistola e della malattia sottostante. Occorre somministrare antibiotici il cui spettro d'azione comprenda la flora intestinale Gram-negativa, *S. aureus* e la flora anaerobica fecale. Sono obbligatori un'ampia escissione e il drenaggio in caso di sepsi e cellulite in espansione.

Nei pazienti più grandi le fistole sono solitamente associate a morbo di Crohn o a un'anamnesi di chirurgia per il trattamento della malattia di Hirschsprung. Queste fistole risultano difficili da trattare. La terapia è la stessa della malattia predisponente.

341.4 • EMORROIDI

Le emorroidi nei bambini sono generalmente benigne, anche se va sempre sospettata la presenza di ipertensione portale, condizione peraltro rara nei pazienti pediatrici. Le emorroidi si accompagnano a rettorragia, prurito e disagio. Se si esclude l'ipertensione portale, i bambini più grandi e gli adolescenti che lamentano un dolore acuto e lancinante in sede anale possono avere una trombosi di un'emorroide esterna preesistente. Questa va trattata con un'infiltrazione locale di bupivacaina 0,25%, con adrenalina 1:200 000, seguita da incisione della vena o del lembo di cute e dall'estrazione del coagulo. Dopo questa procedura, che dà un sollievo immediato, la recidiva è rara e non sono necessari follow-up. Ulteriori approcci alle emorroidi croniche refrattarie comprendono l'emorroidopessi con graffe, la coagulazione o l'escissione.

341.5 • PROLASSO RETTALE

Il prolasso rettale è la protrusione della mucosa rettale attraverso l'ano. Quando coinvolge tutte le tonache della parete rettale, evenienza peraltro inconsueta, prende il nome di **procidenza**. Nella maggior parte dei casi in cui si ha protrusione del tessuto rettale attraverso l'ano, si tratta di un prolasso e non di polipi, invaginazione o di altri tessuti.

Il prolasso, per lo più idiopatico, di solito esordisce tra 1 e 5 anni di età (media 3 anni): generalmente si manifesta quando il bambino inizia a stare in piedi e si risolve tra i 3 e i 5 anni di età, quando il sacro assume la struttura dell'adulto e il lume anale si orienta posteriormente. In questa fase dell'accrescimento l'intero peso dei visceri addominali non preme più sul retto come nelle fasi precoci dello sviluppo.

Altri fattori predisponenti comprendono parassitosi intestinali (soprattutto nelle aree endemiche), malnutrizione, diarrea, colite ulcerosa, sindrome di Ehlers-Danlos, meningocele (più spesso associato a procidenza a causa della mancanza del sostegno muscolare perineale), fibrosi cistica e stipsi cronica. I pazienti trattati chirurgicamente per l'ano imperforato possono presentare gradi diversi di prolasso rettomucosale, fenomeno particolarmente frequente in caso di scarso sviluppo sfinterico.

MANIFESTAZIONI CLINICHE. Il prolasso del retto si verifica solitamente durante la defecazione, soprattutto quando il bambino sta acquisendo il controllo sfinterico. In seguito si risolve spontaneamente o viene ridotto manualmente dal paziente stesso o dai genitori. Nei casi gravi, il retto prolassato è esteriorizzato cronicamente, diventando congesto ed edematoso, difficilmente riducibile. Il prolasso rettale di solito non è doloroso o si limita a dare un lieve fastidio. Se il retto si riduce dopo la defecazione, può subire traumi per sfregamento con la biancheria intima, con sanguinamento ed essudazione. Il retto esposto può ulcerarsi. La massa protrudente è di colore variabile dal rosso vivo al rosso scuro ed essere lungo anche 10-12 cm. Per la diagnosi differenziale con il polipo prolassato si rimanda al Capitolo 342.

TRATTAMENTO. La valutazione deve comprendere tutti i test necessari per escludere le condizioni predisponenti menzionate, in particolare la fibrosi cistica e le lesioni sacrali. Per agevolare la riduzione della protrusione si esercita una pressione con compresse tiepide. Un facile metodo di riduzione consiste nell'introdurre un dito, avvolto in un pezzo di carta igienica, nel lume della massa, spingerlo delicatamente nel retto del paziente e quindi ritirarlo immediatamente. La carta igienica aderisce alla mucosa, permettendo l'estrazione del dito; la carta, una volta ammorbidita, verrà eliminata.

Le misure generali devono includere un'accurata riduzione manuale del prolasso dopo la defecazione, i tentativi per evitare la pressione eccessiva durante l'evacuazione (con i piedi del paziente sollevati dal pavimento), l'uso di lassativi e di emollienti delle feci in caso di stipsi, il trattamento delle condizioni infiammatorie del retto e delle parassitosi intestinali, se presenti. Se tutti questi accorgimenti non hanno successo, è indicato il trattamento chirurgico. Nessuno degli interventi a disposizione del chirurgo è ritenuto ideale, dal momento che ognuno presenta rischi e svantaggi: di conseguenza, si raccomanda di tentare sempre il trattamento medico.

Il prolasso della mucosa rettale può essere trattato con la cauterizzazione lineare. In sala operatoria, si causa il prolasso esercitando una trazione sulla mucosa. Con una pistola di Bovie (elettrocauterio) si effettuano cauterizzazioni lineari quasi per tutto lo spessore della mucosa. Solitamente si eseguono 8 cauterizzazioni lineari all'esterno e 4 all'interno della mucosa. Il prolasso si può ripresentare nell'immediato periodo postperatorio, ma nelle settimane successive l'area cauterizzata si contrarrà, mantenendo la mucosa all'interno del canale anale.

341.6 • Seno pilonidale e ascesso pilonidale

Sono state formulate almeno tre ipotesi circa l'eziologia della malattia pilonidale. Una presuppone che il trauma da prolungata posizione seduta impatti i follicoli piliferi nel tessuto sottocutaneo, che quindi agiscono da focolai di infezione. Un'altra ipotesi parte dal presupposto che, in alcuni soggetti, si formino follicoli piliferi nel tessuto sottocutaneo, forse a causa di alterazioni embriologiche, e che nuovamente essi fungano da punti focali per l'infezione, soprattutto con la secrezione sebacea. Una terza ipotesi è che il movimento delle natiche interferisca con una piega interglutea particolarmente profonda, favorendo l'imprigionamento di batteri e peli sotto la cute. Questa teoria è nata dall'osservazione dell'apparente miglioramento, a breve e a lungo termine, ottenibile con l'intervento che chiude la lesione lungo la linea mediana, obliterando la fessura profonda presente alla nascita.

La malattia pilonidale di solito si presenta durante l'adolescenza o la prima età adulta con un accumulo di peli sulla parte mediale dell'area sacrale e coccigea, non correlato a malattia perineale. Oltre che sotto forma di un ascesso acuto con una tumefazione soffice, calda, eritematosa, fluttuante, può presentarsi come una o più aperture o tragitti che drenano piccole quantità di essudato sieroso, emorragico e/o purulento. Questa condizione non si risolve senza intervento chirurgico. L'ascesso acuto deve essere drenato e medicato lasciandolo aperto con opportuna anestesia. Gli antibiotici per os possono risultare utili; spetta ai familiari del paziente eliminare la medicazione, togliendone qualche centimetro ogni giorno. Una volta rimossa tutta la medicazione, l'area deve essere tenuta pulita mediante bagno o doccia. La ferita di solito guarisce completamente in 6 settimane. A guarigione avvenuta, occorre programmare l'escissione elettiva per evitare le recidive. Di solito, i pazienti che si presentano con aperture o tragitti possono essere trattati con un'unica escissione elettiva.

La maggior parte dei chirurghi, dopo aver valutato attentamente l'estensione di ogni tragitto, effettua un'escissione di tutta la cute e del tessuto sottocutaneo colpito fino alla fascia che ricopre il sacro e il coccige. Alcuni chiudono la sutura sulla linea mediana; altri la lasciano aperta e medicata per avere una guarigione per seconda intenzione, con formazione di tessuto di granulazione che va a colmare la ferita. Alcuni marsupializzano la ferita suturando i margini cutanei alla fascia esposta che ricopre sacro e coccige. Un successo maggiore sembra essere legato all'escissione e alla chiusura eseguite in modo che la linea di sutura non sia sulla linea mediana. Le recidive o i problemi di guarigione della ferita sono relativamente frequenti. Alcuni li hanno trattati con VAC (*Vacuum Assisted Closure*) con una medicazione di poliuretano, un sistema che applica una pressione negativa continua controllata attraverso una medicazione (spugna) porosa. La medicazione viene cambiata di solito ogni 3 giorni, operazione che può essere fatta a casa, con l'assistenza di un infermiere. I casi refrattari vengono trattati mediante un ampio lembo cutaneo a tutto spessore.

Nei bambini normali è relativamente frequente una fossetta semplice nella fessura mediana tra i glutei, a livello del coccige. Non c'è alcuna prova che questo piccolo seno pilonidale causi problemi al paziente. La degenerazione maligna della cisti del seno pilonidale è stata osservata solo in pazienti con infezioni e ascessi cronici. Un seno dermico aperto è una condizione benigna e solitamente asintomatica.

Ashcraft KW, Garred JL, Holder TM, et al: Rectal prolapse: 17 year experience with the posterior repair and suspension. *J Pediatr Surg* 1990;15:992–994.

Georgeson KE, Inge TH, Albanese CT: Laparoscopically assisted anorectal pull-through for high imperforate anus—A new technique. *J Pediatr Surg* 2000;35:927–930.

Levitt MA, Patel M, Rodriguez G, et al: The tethered spinal cord in patients with anorectal malformations. *J Pediatr Surg* 1997;32:462–468.

Levitt MA, Soffer SZ, Peña A: Continent appendicostomy in the bowel management of fecally incontinent children. *J Pediatr Surg* 1997;32:1630–1633.

Madoff RD, Fleshman JW: AGA technical review on the diagnosis and care of patients with anal fissure. *Gastroenterology* 2003;124:235–245.

Nelson RL: Treatment of anal fissure. *Br Med J* 2003;327:354–355.

Peña A: Anorrectal malformations. *Semin Pediatr Surg* 1995;4:35–47.

Peña A, Guardino K, Tovilla JM, et al: Bowel management for fecal incontinence in patients with anorectal malformations. *J Pediatr Surg* 1998; 33:133–137.

Peña A, Hong AR: Advances in the management of anorectal malformations. *Am J Surg* 2000;180:370–376.

Piazza DJ, Radhakrishnan J: Perianal abscess and fistula-in-ano in children. *Dis Colon Rectum* 1990;33:1014–1016.

Rakhimov S: Treatment of rectal prolapse in children. *Vestn Khir Im II Grek* 1989;142:72–74.

Rosen R, Buonomo C, Andrade R, Nurko S: Incidence of spinal cord lesions in patients with intractable constipation. *J Pediatr* 2004;145:409–411.

Sigalet DL, Laberge JM, Adolph VR, Guttman FM: The anterior sagittal approach for high imperforate anus: A simplification of the mollard approach. *J Pediatr Surg* 1996;31:625–629.

Smyth EF, Baker RP, Wilken BJ, et al: Stapled versus excision haemorrhoidectomy: Long-term follow up of a randomized controlled trial. *Lancet* 2003;361:1437–1438.

Sonmez K, Demirogullari B, Ekingen G, et al: Randomized, placebo-controlled treatment of anal fissures by lidocaine, EMLA and GTN in children. *J Pediatr Surg* 2002;37:1313–1316.

Torres R, Levitt MA, Tovilla JM, et al: Anorectal malformations and Down's syndrome. *J Pediatr Surg* 1998;33:194–197.

Tsakayannis DE, Shamberger RC: Association of imperforate anus with occult spinal dysraphism. *J Pediatr Surg* 1995;30:1010–1012.

Capitolo 342 ■ Tumori del tratto digerente

Joel Shilyansky

SINDROMI DELLA POLIPOSI FAMILIARE. Le sindromi familiari associate a polipi intestinali sono particolarmente importanti dal momento che aumentano il rischio di insorgenza del cancro (Tab. 342-1). I bambini devono essere seguiti in modo regolare e richiedono un piano di interventi appropriati pianificati con un certo anticipo. Inoltre, è necessario proporre test genetici per identificare i familiari a rischio.

SINDROMI DELLA POLIPOSI AMARTOMATOSA. I **polipi giovanili del colon**, noti anche come polipi infiammatori o da "ritenzione", sono i più comuni tumori intestinali dell'infanzia, presenti nell'1-3% dei soggetti di età <21 anni, ma poco frequenti al di sotto dei 15 anni. I polipi sono uniformemente distribuiti nel colon; anche se le forme solitarie sono frequenti, possono essere presenti anche due o più polipi. Tali lesioni sono per lo più eritematose, friabili, peduncolate e hanno dimensione compresa tra pochi millimetri e 3 centimetri. L'esame istologico evidenzia una proliferazione amartomatosa delle cellule ghiandolari mucose e degli elementi dello stroma, oltre a una marcata vascolarizzazione e infiltrazioni di linfociti, eosinofili, polimorfonucleati e plasma-

TABELLA 342-1. Caratteristiche generali delle sindromi neoplastiche ereditarie colorettali

SINDROME	QUADRO ISTOLOGICO DEL POLIPO	LOCALIZZAZIONE DEL POLIPO	ETÀ DI ESORDIO	RISCHIO DI NEOPLASIA DEL COLON	ALTERAZIONE GENETICA	MANIFESTAZIONI CLINICHE	LESIONI ASSOCIATE
Poliposi familiare adenomatosa	Adenoma	Colon	16 anni (8-34 anni)	100%	5q (gene *APC*)	Sanguinamento rettale, dolore addominale, occlusione intestinale	Desmoidi, CHRPE
Sindrome di Gardner	Adenoma	Intestino tenue e colon	16 anni (8-34 anni)	100%	5q (gene *APC*)	Sanguinamento rettale, dolore addominale, occlusione intestinale	Desmoidi, CHRPE
Sindrome di Peutz-Jeghers	Amartoma	Intestino tenue e colon	Prima decade di vita	Aumentato	19p (*STK11*)	Possibile sanguinamento rettale, dolore addominale, invaginazione	Pigmentazione melaninica orocutanea
Poliposi giovanile	Amartoma (raramente adenoma)	Intestino tenue e colon	Prima decade di vita	Circa 10-50%	*PTEN, SMAD4, BMPR1*	Possibile sanguinamento rettale, dolore addominale, invaginazione	Alterazioni congenite nel 20% delle forme non familiari
Tumore del colon ereditario non poliposico	Adenoma	Colon	40 anni (18-65 anni)	30%	Geni del mismatch repair*	Sanguinamento rettale, dolore addominale, occlusione intestinale	Altri tumori (per es. ovaio, uretere, pancreas, stomaco)

*Inclusi *hMSH2, hMSH3, hMSH6, hMLH1, hPMS1* e *hPMS2*.
CHRPE (*Congenital Hypertrophy of the Retinal Pigment Epithelium*), ipertrofia congenita dell'epitelio retinico pigmentato.
Da Goldman L, Ausiello D: *Cecil Textbook of Medicine*, 22nd ed. Philadelphia, WB Saunders, 2004, p 1213.

cellule. I polipi presentano formazioni ghiandolari cistiche mucose, ricoperte da uno strato epiteliale singolo e fragile. Il tipico polipo giovanile senza alterazioni adenomatose non ha potenziale di malignità. I polipi giovanili con variazioni adenomatose sono di raro riscontro.

Le **manifestazioni cliniche** comprendono un sanguinamento rettale rosso vivo e non doloroso durante o subito dopo l'evacuazione. L'emorragia massiva è rara; il sanguinamento spesso si arresta spontaneamente. Nel 30% dei bambini si riscontra anemia sideropenica, che però di rado costituisce il sintomo principale. I crampi e il dolore in regione addominale inferiore, peraltro non frequenti, sono associati a invaginazione. I polipi prolassati appaiono come masse rosso scuro, carnose, peduncolate, in contrasto con la mucosa rosa chiaro del prolasso rettale. Il prurito anale e la suppurazione della mucosa sono spesso associati al prolasso. Sono comuni l'infarcimento spontaneo del polipo e autoamputazione, mentre non sono frequenti la diarrea e l'occlusione. La **diagnosi differenziale** comprende le altre forme di poliposi intestinale, il diverticolo di Meckel, le ragadi anali, la malattia infiammatoria intestinale, la porpora di Schönlein-Henock e anomalie della coagulazione.

La **diagnosi** solitamente si effettua con la colonscopia. I polipi hanno l'aspetto di lesioni lisce e peduncolate. Nonostante il clisma opaco con contrasto gassoso possa dimostrarne la presenza, è ancora necessaria la colonscopia a fini terapeutici. Il **trattamento** include la rimozione del polipo durante la colonscopia con un'ansa per cauterizzazione o, raramente, la polipectomia transaddominale. Si dovrebbe sempre procedere al recupero dei polipi per la conferma istologica della diagnosi. Le recidive sono rare.

La **poliposi giovanile**, caratterizzata da polipi giovanili gastrointestinali multipli (>5), si manifesta in determinate famiglie come carattere dominante e può essere associata ad alterazioni congenite (il 20% dei nuovi casi è sporadico). In un sottogruppo di famiglie, mutazioni inattivanti del gene *MADH4* (*SMAD4*) e dei geni oncosoppressori per il recettore per la proteina morfogenetica dell'osso di tipo 1A (*BMPR1A, Bone Morphogenetic Protein Receptor 1A*) determinano un'interruzione del segnale intracellulare del fattore di crescita β trasformante (TGF-β). Questi polipi sono identici a quelli solitari; gli individui affetti hanno un rischio elevato di sviluppare una neoplasia gastrointestinale (10-50%). I bambini possono presentare sanguinamento non doloroso, invaginazione o, occasionalmente, arresto della crescita, malassorbimento, anemia, ipoalbuminemia e dolore addominale. Il rischio di neoplasia maligna è basso in soggetti senza storia familiare di cancro e con due polipi o meno, mentre è molto elevato negli individui con tre o più polipi. Di conseguenza, i pazienti con polipi giovanili multipli devono essere sottoposti a esofagogastroduodenoscopia, colonscopia e radiografia con mezzo di contrasto del tratto gastrointestinale alto, con controlli dell'intestino tenue ogni due anni. La frequenza dell'esame aumenta negli adulti. La capsula endoscopica è una modalità innovativa che potrà essere utilizzata in futuro per effettuare lo screening della poliposi giovanile.

La **sindrome di Cowden** e la **sindrome di Bannayan-Riley-Ruvalcaba** sono rare sindromi autosomiche dominanti associate con anomalie multiple, distinte, e amartomi a carico di cute (99% dei pazienti), mammella, tiroide, endometrio, cervello e tratto gastrointestinale (60% dei pazienti). Entrambe le patologie sono associate a mutazioni nel gene soppressore tumorale dell'omologo della proteina tirosina fosfatasi e della tensina PTEN (*Protein tyrosine phosphatase and TENsin homologue*). I soggetti interessati sono a rischio elevato di sviluppare una neoplasia della tiroide e della mammella, mentre il rischio di neoplasia gastrointestinale non è certo.

La **sindrome di Peutz-Jeghers** (**PJS**, *Peutz-Jeghers Syndrome*) è una sindrome ereditaria, autosomica dominante, rara, caratterizzata da pigmentazione della mucosa delle labbra e delle gengive, e da amatomi del tratto gastrointestinale. La sua incidenza è di 1/120 000. Lentiggini dai margini ben definiti, pigmentate in profondità, si osservano alla nascita o compaiono durante l'infanzia sulle labbra e sulla mucosa della cavità orale, oltre che intorno alla bocca (Fig. 342-1). Una lesione intestinale viene segnalata dal

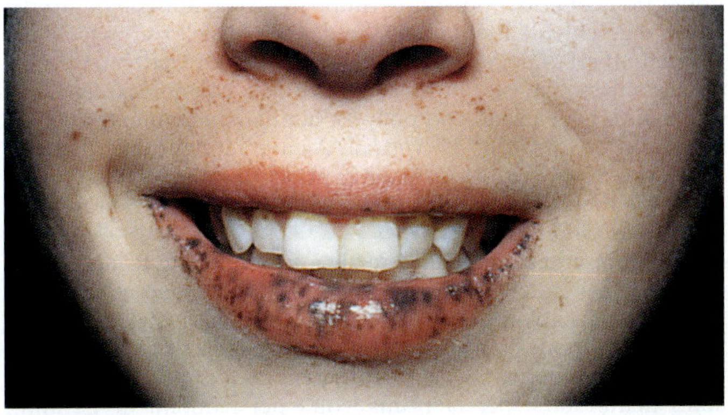

Figura 342-1. Sindrome di Peutz-Jeghers. Lesioni pigmentate. (Da Swartz MH: *Textbook of Physical Diagnosis: History and Examination*, 4th ed. Philadelphia, WB Saunders, 2002, p 295.)

sanguinamento o, più spesso, da crampi intestinali dolorosi associati a occlusione, a sua volta dovuta a invaginazioni ricorrenti.

I polipi della PJS sono amartomi benigni caratterizzati da un asse di tessuto stromale e da una muscolatura liscia "a fronda", rivestita da epitelio intestinale di aspetto normale. La lesione intestinale deve essere escissa se causa sintomi significativi e persistenti. Il coinvolgimento intestinale è solitamente troppo esteso perché si possano rimuovere tutti i polipi, sebbene tale intervento sia indicato in alcuni pazienti.

Gli studi familiari e la consulenza genetica possono rivelare parenti con manifestazioni parziali o complete della sindrome. Il 50% dei pazienti non ha familiari con questo disordine, a riprova del tasso elevato di nuove mutazioni. Nella patogenesi della sindrome sono coinvolte mutazioni inattivanti in un gene localizzato sul cromosoma 19p13.3, *LKB1* (*STK11*), che codifica per una serina/treonina chinasi. La PJS è la prima sindrome in grado di causare cancro identificata come risultato di mutazioni inattivanti la proteinchinasi. Il cancro colpisce fino al 50% dei pazienti con sindrome di Peutz-Jeghers, manifestandosi soprattutto negli adulti di mezza età. I tumori del colon-retto, della mammella e dell'apparato riproduttivo sono i più diffusi. Si raccomanda di cominciare a effettuare la mammografia, la visita ginecologica e la colonscopia nei pazienti alla fine della seconda decade di vita o all'inizio della terza.

POLIPOSI FAMILIARE ADENOMATOSA. Molte lesioni adenomatose del colon caratterizzano queste condizioni autosomiche dominanti preneoplastiche. Sono tutte causate da mutazioni della linea germinativa del gene della poliposi adenomatosa del colon (*APC*, *Adenomatous Polyposis Coli*), gene oncosoppressore localizzato sul cromosoma 5q21. Le mutazioni del gene *APC* determinano la presenza di proteine citoplasmatiche tronche, da cui dipende il legame e la regolazione della degradazione della catena β. L'accumulo intracellulare delle catene β svolge un ruolo importante nella proliferazione delle cellule epiteliali del colon e nella formazione dell'adenoma. L'incidenza della poliposi familiare adenomatosa è tra 1/5000 e 1/17 000 soggetti, con esordio in genere tradivo nella prima decade di vita o nell'adolescenza. **Per definizione**, sono presenti più di cinque polipi adenomatosi al momento della diagnosi. Solitamente più di 100 (spesso 1000) adenomi visibili sono presenti quando il paziente è nella seconda o terza decade di vita. L'ipertrofia congenita dell'epitelio retinico pigmentato è presente dalla nascita nella maggior parte dei pazienti. La variabilità delle caratteristiche cliniche, incluse quelle extracoliche, dipende dalla sede della mutazione del gene *APC*. Queste ultime sono responsabili anche della **sindrome di Gardner** (poliposi colorettale multipla, polipi periampollari, osteomi [mandibolari], lipomi, fibromi, cisti epidermoidi e tumori dermoidi) e di alcuni, ma non di tutti i casi di **sindrome di Turcot** (tumore primitivo dell'encefalo [medulloblastoma] e poliposi multipla colorettale). Le lesioni del tessuti molli (tumori dermoidi) e gli osteomi possono manifestarsi nell'infanzia, mentre i polipi intestinali possono non diventare evidenti fino all'adolescenza e alla prima età adulta. I polipi preneoplastici possono svilupparsi in qualunque punto del tratto digerente; le lesioni a livello del colon, dello stomaco e del duodeno (periampollari) sono quelle dominanti. Il rischio relativo di epatoblastoma, carcinoma della tiroide e colangiocarcinoma è aumentato nei pazienti con poliposi familiare adenomatosa (FAP, *Familial Adenomatous Polyposis*). Alcune famiglie che, pur non soddisfacendo i criteri per la FAP, presentano un'alta frequenza di polipi adenomatosi e di tumore del colon possono presentare mutazione del gene *APC*.

Nella **presentazione clinica** iniziale i polipi sono asintomatici; molti restano tali. Quando sono sintomatici, i polipi causano ematochezia, talvolta crampi o, raramente, diarrea. La presenza dei sintomi non è correlata con le alterazioni displasiche. Le neoplasie che derivano da polipi adenomatosi preesistenti possono manifestarsi per la prima volta nei bambini di 10 anni, sebbene queste lesioni di solito compaiano nei giovani adulti. La maggior parte dei soggetti affetti svilupperà il cancro a partire dai 40 anni.

La **diagnosi** deve essere sospettata in base all'anamnesi familiare e confermata mediante colonscopia. I polipi sono numerosi; la biopsia ne rivela la natura adenomatosa, in contrasto con il reperto infiammatorio e cistico dei polipi giovanili. Le mutazioni del gene *APC* si riscontrano nell'80-90% delle famiglie affette da poliposi familiare, diagnosi che in fase presintomatica necessita di esami associati a una consulenza genetica. Se si identifica una mutazione nel paziente indice, i familiari affetti possono essere differenziati dai non affetti mediante test genetici. Se il paziente indice appartiene al 10-20% dei soggetti affetti da questa malattia nei quali non si riesce a identificare la mutazione, i test genetici nei familiari possono essere utili per identificare nuove mutazioni nel gene *APC*. Poiché un risultato negativo può essere confondente, occorre cautela nell'effettuare la consulenza familiare. Un bambino con una diagnosi di FAP o con una storia familiare di FAP e test genetico positivo, deve essere seguito con una colonscopia ogni 6-12 mesi finché non si intraprende il trattamento chirurgico definitivo. Se il test genetico risulta negativo in un bambino proveniente da una famiglia in cui è stata identificata la mutazione, è probabile che tale bambino non soffra di FAP. Anche i pazienti con sindrome di Gardner devono essere sottoposti regolarmente a gastroduodenoscopia per l'asportazione dei polipi gastrici e duodenali. Le lesioni preneoplastiche dell'ampolla di Vater insorgono nell'età adulta e di solito vengono trattati con resezione locale, anche se può rendersi necessaria una pancreato-duodenectomia.

Il **trattamento** definitivo della FAP richiede la proctocolectomia profilattica per la prevenzione del tumore. Il ripristino della continuità intestinale tramite *pull-through* ileoanale dà risultati eccellenti. Nonostante si discuta su quale sia il momento più indicato per l'intervento chirurgico, il successo della ricostruzione ha permesso la resezione precoce allontanando il rischio della disseminazione neoplastica. I farmaci antinfiammatori non steroidei come il sulindac, e ancora più gli inibitori selettivi della ciclossigenasi 2 come il celecoxib, possono rallentare lo sviluppo del polipo; la loro efficacia nel prevenire la trasformazione neoplastica è sconosciuta e il loro uso è in fase di studio, specialmente alla luce della potenziale morbilità cardiaca.

CARCINOMA. Poiché i tumori epiteliali del tratto digerente sono rari nei bambini, è consigliabile un approccio diagnostico non aggressivo nei confronti di molti sintomi di tipo gastroenterico in questa fascia di età. Diverse sono le patologie dell'infanzia che predispongono allo sviluppo di un adenocarcinoma del tratto gastrointestinale all'inizio dell'età adulta, per esempio la poliposi adenomatosa familiare, il carcinoma del colon non poliposico ereditario (*Hereditary Non-Polyposis Colon Carcinoma*, HNPCC), la sindrome di Peutz-Jeghers, la poliposi giovanile, la colite ulcerosa, il morbo di Crohn, e disordini associati a rotture cromosomiche. La sede più frequente è il colon, ma sono riportate anche localizzazioni gastriche e duodenali. La diagnosi si basa sull'anamnesi familiare, sull'esame endoscopico e sul riscontro di sanguinamento gastrointestinale e occlusione. La sintomatologia è aspecifica: dolori addominali, massa in sede addominale, stipsi e, meno frequentemente, emorragia. I tumori sono relativamente indifferenziati e a elevata malignità. Il **trattamento** del carcinoma colorettale è essenzialmente chirurgico. La prognosi dipende dallo stadio del tumore. Il carcinoma del colon è raro nei bambini in assenza di fattori predisponenti noti. È importante disporre di un'anamnesi familiare e sottoporre a screening e consulenza genetica sia i pazienti con il cancro (casi indice) sia i suoi familiari per identificare i parenti a rischio. Le mutazioni del gene *PAC*, che conducono a FAP, e quelle dei geni implicati nella riparazione del *mismatch* DNA (*hMSH2*, *hMSH6*, *PMS1*, *PMS2* e *hMLH1*), che determinano HNPCC, sono frequentemente associate a carcinoma colorettale nei bambini e nei giovani adulti. La diagnosi di HNPCC deve essere sospettata in presenza di familiarità positiva per esordio precoce di carcinoma del colon e confermata mediante analisi genetiche. Sebbene gran parte dei pazienti con HNPCC non sviluppi cancro fino all'età adulta, gli adolescenti possono esserne colpiti. L'età per iniziare la sorveglianza endoscopica è controversa e deve essere scelta in modo individualizzato. Inoltre, è aumentato il rischio di carcinoma a carico di utero, ovaio, pancreas, vie biliari e stomaco. Quando si prende in esame l'eventualità di effettuare lo screening genetico, occorre considerare l'impatto etico, sociale e psicologico.

MALFORMAZIONI VASCOLARI (EMANGIOMI). Queste rare lesioni benigne possono causare emorragia massiva, anche fatale. La manifestazione clinica comune è un sanguinamento non doloroso che inizia durante l'infanzia. L'emorragia può essere subdola e cronica oppure improvvisa e massiva. Solitamente i pazienti non hanno altri sintomi intestinali, ma in caso di invaginazione possono essere presenti sintomi da occlusione. Circa il 50% dei pazienti presenta emangiomi cutanei o teleangiectasia e alcuni hanno un'anamnesi familiare per lesioni analoghe. Le malformazioni vascolari del tratto gastrointestinale possono essere associate a sindrome "blu rubber bleb nevus syndrome" o teleangiectasia emorragica ereditaria. Circa la metà di queste lesioni è a livello del colon, dove possono essere evidenziate con la colonscopia. Durante il periodo di sanguinamento l'arteriografia mesenterica selettiva può essere utile per la loro localizzazione. La chirurgia è il trattamento definitivo delle lesioni isolate.

LEIOMIOMA. Questo raro tumore benigno si presenta frequentemente a livello di stomaco, digiuno e ileo distale. Esso può rimanere asintomatico a lungo. I sintomi possono derivare da invaginazione, volvolo, necrosi centrale e occlusione. Può essere difficile differenziare un leiomioma da un leiomiosarcoma, un tumore maligno che si ha raramente nel tratto gastrointestinale nel bambino. I tumori originati dalla muscolatura liscia si hanno frequentemente nei bambini con AIDS o nei pazienti sottoposti a immunosoppressione dopo un trapianto.

LINFOMA. Il linfoma è il tumore maligno del tratto gastrointestinale più frequente nei bambini (vedi Capitolo 496). Circa il 30% dei pazienti pediatrici con linfoma non Hodgkin presenta un tumore addominale. I disordini che predispongono allo sviluppo del linfoma includono AIDS, atassia-teleangectasia, sindrome di Wiskott-Aldrich, agammaglobulinemia, sindrome da immunodeficienza combinata grave, trapianto di midollo osseo o di organi solidi e celiachia di vecchia data. Il linfoma può interessare lo stomaco, l'ileo distale, il cieco o l'appendice presentandosi con crampi addominali dolorosi, vomito, distensione addominale o massa addominale palpabile. La perforazione non è frequente. Occorre prendere in esame la diagnosi di linfoma intestinale in bambini di età <3 anni che presentano invaginazione acuta. Può essere difficile differenziare i sintomi del linfoma intestinale dal morbo di Crohn.

TUMORI CARCINOIDI. Questi tumori delle cellule enterocromaffini solitamente compaiono a livello dell'appendice, nei bambini, e presentano un basso grado di malignità. Il loro riscontro nell'appendice può essere accidentale, durante un'appendicectomia. La resezione completa con margini chirurgici definiti del tumore carcinoide dell'appendice di dimensioni <1 cm è solitamente curativa. I carcinoidi non situati nell'appendice (retto, stomaco, duodeno, ileo-digiuno e colon, in ordine di frequenza) di solito metastatizzano e le metastasi epatiche danno origine alla sindrome da carcinoide, causata dalla produzione di ormoni da parte del tumore. Questi ormoni sono responsabili di ipermotilità intestinale e diarrea, disturbi vasomotori (flushing), broncocostrizione (dispnea) e insufficienza cardiaca destra. Il più importante agente attivo è la serotonina. Elevati livelli urinari del metabolica della serotonina, l'acido 5-idrossi-indolacetico, sono solitamente diagnostici. Le neoplasie funzionali sono rare nei bambini. Il carcinoide può anche invadere il mesentere dell'intestino tenue, determinando fibrosi retroperitoneale e mesenterica. La resezione è l'indicazione terapeutica principale. La terapia con analoghi della somatostatina a lunga durata d'azione può essere un supporto palliativo.

IPERPLASIA NODULARE LINFOIDE. I follicoli linfoidi della lamina propria dell'intestino di norma si aggregano nella placche di Peyer, più numerose nell'ileo distale. I follicoli iperplasici appaiono come noduli sottomucosi alla radiografia con mezzo di contrasto e possono essere scambiati per anomalie. L'iperplasia nodulare linfoide colpisce il colon o l'intestino tenue. La forma diffusa a carico del tenue può manifestarsi in caso di deficit immunoglobulinico, con o senza infestazione da *Giardia lamblia*. I pazienti possono accusare sanguinamento rettale, diarrea e crampi addominali, ma i sintomi sono generalmente lievi. Nei neonati con ipersensibilità alle proteine alimentari, questa patologia può essere associata a enterocolite. L'iperplasia nodulare linfoide è stata riscontrata anche nella malattia infiammatoria intestinale e nella malattia di Castelman. La sua importanza risiede nella somiglianza delle sue manifestazioni con quelle di disordini più gravi. Essa solitamente si risolve spontaneamente e di rado richiede una terapia specifica. Per il sanguinamento massivo o il dolore addominale vengono utilizzati la ciproeptadina e il prednisone.

Amos CI, Keitheri-Cheteri MB, Sabripour M, et al: Genotype-phenotype correlations in Peutz-Jeghers syndrome. *J Med Genet* 2004;41:327–333.

Attard TM, Cuffari C, Tajouri T, et al: Multicenter experience with upper gastrointestinal polyps in pediatric patients with familial adenomatous polyposis. *Am J Gastroenterol* 2004;99:681–686.

Bisgaard ML, Ripa RS, Bulow S: Mutation analysis of the adenomatous polyposis coli (*APC*) gene in Danish patients with familial adenomatous polyposis (FAP). *Hum Mutat* 2004;23:522.

Bulow S, Bjork J, Christensen IJ, et al: Duodenal adenomatosis in familial adenomatous polyposis. *Gut* 2004;53:381–386.

Burt R, Neklason DW: Genetic testing for inherited colon cancer. *Gastroenterology* 2005;128:1696–1716.

Corredor J, Wambach J, Barnard J: Gastrointestinal polyps in children: Advances in molecular genetics, diagnosis, and management. *J Pediatr* 2001;138:621–628.

Durno CA, Aronson M, Bapat B, et al: Family history and molecular features of children, adolescents and young adults with colorectal carcinoma. *Gut* 2005;54:1146–1150.

Gupta SK, Fitzgerald JF, Croffie JM, et al: Experience with juvenile polyps in North American children: The need for pancolonoscopy. *Am J Gastroenterol* 2001;96:1695–1697.

Hampel H, Frankel WL, Martin E, et al: Screening for the Lynch syndrome (hereditary nonpolyposis colorectal cancer). *N Engl J Med* 2005; 352:1851–1860.

Howe JR, Sayed MG, Ahmed AF, et al: The prevalence of *MADH4* and *BMPR1A* mutations in juvenile polyposis and absence of *BMPR2*, *BMPR1B*, and *ACVR1* mutations. *J Med Genet* 2004;41:484–491.

Latchford AR, Phillips RK: Duodenal adenoma and cancer in FAP. *Gut* 2005;54:171.

Merg A, Howe JR; Genetic conditions associated with intestinal juvenile polyps. *Am J Med Genet C Semin Med Genet* 2004;129:44–55.

Molle ZL, Moallem H, Desai N, et al: Endoscopic features of smooth muscle tumors in children with AIDS. *Gastrointest Endosc* 2000;52:91–94.

Parc Y, Piquard A, Dozois RR, et al: Long-term outcome of familial adenomatous polyposis patients after restorative coloproctectomy. *Ann Surg* 2004;239:378–382.

Samowitz WS, Curtin K, Lin HH, et al: The colon cancer burden of genetically defined hereditary nonpolyposis colon cancer. *Gastroenterology* 2001;121:830–838.

Schreibman IR, Baker M, Amos C, McGarrity TJ: The hamartomatous polyposis syndromes: A clinical and molecular review. *Am J Gastroenterol* 2005;100:476–490.

Strate LL, Syngal S: Hereditary colorectal cancer syndromes. *Cancer Causes Control* 2005;16:201–213.

Tonelli F, Valanzano R, Monaci I, et al: Restorative proctocolectomy or rectum-preserving surgery in patients with familial adenomatous polyposis: Results of a prospective study. *World J Surg* 1997;21:653–658, discussion 659.

Vasen HFA: Clinical diagnosis and management of hereditary colorectal cancer syndromes. *J Clin Oncol* 2000;18:81–92.

Capitolo 343 ■ Ernie inguinali

John J. Aiken e Keith T. Oldham

Le ernie inguinali sono una delle patologie di più frequente riscontro nell'attività pediatrica. La frequenza di questa condizione, insieme con il potenziale rischio di danno ischemico a carico dell'intestino, del testicolo e dell'ovaio, rende molto importante, nell'ambito dell'attività quotidiana di pediatri e chirurghi pediatrici, la sua diagnosi e il piano di trattamento conseguente. Le ernie inguinali dei lattanti e dei bambini nella stragrande maggioranza dei casi sono ernie indirette congenite (99%), conseguenza di un processo vaginale che rimane pervio. Altri tipi di ernie inguinali sono quelle dirette o acquisite (0,5-1,5%) e le femorali (<0,5%). Circa la metà delle ernie inguinali si manifesta clinicamente nel corso del primo anno di vita, la maggior parte nei primi 6 mesi. I progressi compiuti nella terapia intensiva neonatale hanno aumentato la sopravvivenza dei prematuri con esposizione a fattori di rischio per lo sviluppo di ernia inguinale; questi neonati presentano un'incidenza di ernia inguinale del 30% circa. Inoltre, poiché il rischio di incarceramento e strangolamento dell'ernia è maggiore nel primo anno di vita (30-40%), sono necessari un'identificazione rapida e un intervento chirurgico correttivo per ridurre la morbilità e le complicanze.

EMBRIOLOGIA E PATOGENESI

Nella maggior parte dei casi le ernie inguinali di lattanti e bambini sono congenite e derivano da una pervietà persistente del dotto vaginale. La pertinente anatomia evolutiva delle ernie inguinali congenite indirette è correlata allo sviluppo delle gonadi e alla discesa del testicolo attraverso l'anello inguinale interno e, nelle fasi successive della gestazione, nello scroto. Le gonadi si formano nello stesso periodo dei reni, in conseguenza della migrazione delle cellule germinali primitive dal sacco vitellino alla cresta gonadica, e il loro sviluppo risulta completato nella 6ª settimana di gestazione. La differenziazione in testicoli o ovaie si verifica tra la 7ª e l'8ª settimana di gestazione sotto lo stimolo ormonale. I testicoli discendono dalla cresta urogenitale nel retroperitoneo, nell'area dell'anello inguinale interno, intorno alla 28ª settimana di gestazione. Il dotto vaginale è presente, nello sviluppo del feto, dalla 12ª settimana sotto forma di una protrusione diverticolare del peritoneo, che si estende attraverso l'anello inguinale interno e accompagna il testicolo nella sua uscita dall'addome e discesa nello scroto. Il gubernaculum testis si forma dal mesonefro, unito al polo inferiore del testicolo, guidando il testicolo nella discesa attraverso l'anello interno, il canale inguinale e nello scroto. Il testicolo attraversa il canale inguinale in pochi giorni, ma impiega 4 settimane per migrare dall'anello inguinale esterno allo scroto. Anche le ovaie scendono nella pelvi dalla piega genitale, ma non fuoriescono dalla cavità addominale. Nelle femmine, la parte superiore del gubernaculum si differenzia nel legamento ovarico, mentre la parte inferiore diventa legamento rotondo, che attraversa l'anello inguinale interno per raggiungere le grandi labbra. Il dotto vaginale si estende nelle grandi labbra attraverso il canale inguinale, noto come canale di Nuck.

L'influenza degli androgeni, la presenza di recettori sull'organo bersaglio, l'aumentata pressione intraddominale sono tutti fattori grazie ai quali si completa la discesa del testicolo attraverso il canale inguinale. I testicoli e le strutture spermatiche (vasi spermatici e deferenti), pur essendo localizzati nel retroperitoneo, sono colpiti dall'aumento della pressione intraddominale a causa del loro stretto rapporto con il dotto vaginale. Anche il nervo genitofemorale esercita un ruolo importante; innerva il muscolo cremastere che si sviluppa all'interno del gubernaculum e la divisione sperimentale, o la lesione di entrambi i nervi nel feto, ostacola la discesa dei testicoli. Le strutture funicolari del gubernaculum occasionalmente passano in sede ectopica (regionale perineale o femorale), determinando ectopia testicolare. Nelle ultime settimane di gestazione o subito dopo la nascita, le tonache del dotto vaginale si fondono chiudendo l'ingresso al canale inguinale in vicinanza dell'anello inguinale interno al testicolo. Anche il dotto vaginale si oblitera proprio al di sopra dei testicoli, con una parte del dotto vaginale che circonda il testicolo che diventa tonaca vaginale. Nelle femmine il dotto vaginale si oblitera precocemente, circa al 7° mese di gestazione. La mancata obliterazione del dotto vaginale permette la fuoriuscita di fluidi e visceri dalla cavità peritoneale ed è responsabile di gran parte delle anomalie inguinoscrotali dell'infanzia e dell'adolescenza (Fig. 343-1).

ANATOMIA PATOLOGICA

La pervietà del dotto vaginale dopo la nascita rappresenta un'ernia potenziale, ma non tutti coloro che la presentano sviluppano clinicamente un'ernia. Un'ernia inguinale insorge quando il contenuto intraddominale fuoriesce dalla cavità addominale entrando nella regione inguinale attraverso il dotto vaginale pervio. Dal punto di vista della loro posizione nel canale inguinale (laterale o inferiore ai vasi epigastrici), si tratta di ernie inguinali indirette, che però sono raramente associate a debolezza/lassità muscolare o difetti muscolari come avviene nell'adulto. In base all'estensione della pervietà della parte distale del dotto, l'ernia può essere confinata alla regione inguinale o scendere nello scroto. L'obliterazione incompleta del dotto predispone a un'ernia inguinale completa, caratterizzata da protrusione del contenuto addominale nel canale inguinale con possibile estensione nello scroto. L'obliterazione del dotto vaginale distalmente (intorno al testicolo) con pervietà prossimale determina la classica ernia inguinale indiretta con la protrusione nel canale inguinale.

L'**idrocele** si ha quando entrano solo i liquidi attraverso la pervietà del dotto vaginale e la tumefazione può essere presente solo a livello dello scroto (idrocele scrotale), solo lungo il funi-

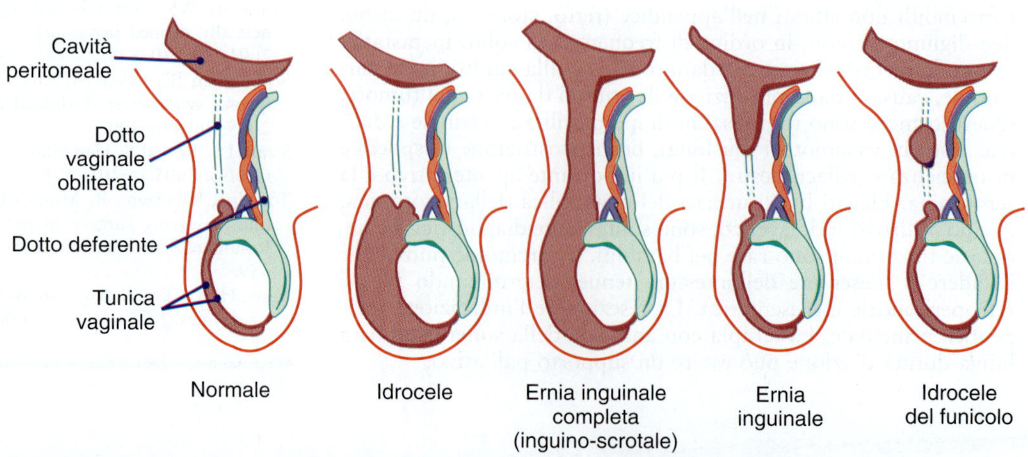

Figura 343-1. Ernie e idroceli. (Modificata da Scherer LR III, Grosfeld JL: Inguinal and umbilical anomalies. *Pediatr Clin North Am* 1993;40: 1121-1131.)

colo spermatico nella regione inguinale (idrocele del funicolo spermatico) o si estende dallo scroto attraverso il canale inguinale e anche nell'addome (idrocele addominoscrotale). Un idrocele si definisce *comunicante* se è di dimensioni variabili: spesso aumenta in seguito ad attività, mentre talvolta si riduce quando i fluidi defluiscono nella cavità peritoneale. Occasionalmente, l'idrocele nei bambini più grandi segue un trauma, un'infiammazione o tumori che colpiscono il testicolo. La mancata chiusura del dotto vaginale, di cui peraltro non sono note le cause, è più frequente in caso di testicolo non disceso e prematurità. Inoltre, la pervietà persistente del dotto vaginale è due volte più frequente a destra, presumibilmente in conseguenza della discesa tardiva del testicolo destro e dell'interferenza creata dallo sviluppo della vena cava inferiore e della vena iliaca esterna. I fattori di rischio identificati che contribuiscono allo sviluppo dell'ernia inguinale congenita, correlata alle condizioni che predispongono a insufficiente obliterazione del dotto vaginale, sono elencati nella Tabella 343.1. I pazienti con fibrosi cistica hanno un'incidenza di ernia inguinale pari a circa il 15%, che sembra correlata ad alterazioni nell'embriogenesi delle strutture del dotto di Wolff; tali alterazioni conducono ad assenza dei vasi deferenti nei maschi che presentano questa condizione. Si osserva inoltre un'aumentata incidenza di ernia inguinale in pazienti con sindrome della femminilizzazione testicolare e altre forme di ambiguità dei genitali. Il tasso di recidiva dopo intervento riparativo dell'ernia inguinale nei bambini con disordini del tessuto connettivo si avvicina al 50%. Avviene spesso che nei pazienti pediatrici la diagnosi di disordini del tessuto connettivo derivi dalle indagini compiute dopo lo sviluppo di un'ernia inguinale ricorrente.

INCIDENZA

L'incidenza dell'ernia inguinale indiretta nei neonati a termine è del 3,5-3%, mentre è assai più elevata nei pretermine e nei neonati di basso peso alla nascita (9-11%) e si avvicina al 30% nei soggetti di peso molto basso alla nascita (<1000 g) e nei pretermine (<28 settimane di gestazione). L'ernia inguinale è molto più frequente nei maschi che nelle femmine, con un rapporto di 6:1. Il 60% delle ernie inguinali interessa il lato destro, mentre nel 30% dei casi sono localizzate a sinistra e nel 10% sono bilaterali. L'incidenza di ernie bilaterali è più alta (pare intorno al 20-40%). La frequenza maggiore di ernie a destra è presumibilmente correlata alla discesa successiva del testicolo destro e all'interferenza esercitata sul processo di obliterazione del dotto vaginale dallo sviluppo della vena cava inferiore. Un'aumentata incidenza di ernia inguinale congenita è stata documentata nei gemelli e nei familiari di pazienti con ernia inguinale. Un'anamnesi familiare di ernia inguinale è emersa nell'11,5% dei pazienti.

TABELLA 343-1. Fattori che predispongono allo sviluppo di ernie

PREMATURITÀ
UROGENITALI
Criptorchidismo
Estrofia della vescica o della cloaca
Genitali ambigui
Ipospadia/Epispadia
AUMENTO DEL LIQUIDO INTRAPERITONEALE
Ascite
Shunt ventricoloperitoneale
Catetere per dialisi peritoneale
AUMENTO DELLA PRESSIONE INTRA-ADDOMINALE
Interventi riparativi di alterazioni della parete addominale
Ascite severa (chilosi)
Peritonite da meconio
MALATTIE RESPIRATORIE CRONICHE
Fibrosi cistica
DISORDINI DEL CONNETTIVO
Sindrome di Ehlers-Danlos
Sindrome di Hunter-Hurler
Sindrome di Marfan
Mucopolisaccaridosi

PRESENTAZIONE CLINICA

L'ernia inguinale si manifesta tipicamente come una tumefazione localizzata nella regione inguinale o che si estende attraverso la regione inguinale dentro lo scroto. Nel sesso femminile, si presenta tipicamente nella porzione superiore delle grandi labbra. La tumefazione o la massa è più visibile durante forti emozioni o di aumentata pressione intraddominale (pianto, sforzo, tosse). Essa si può presentare alla nascita oppure manifestarsi solo a distanza di settimane, mesi o persino anni. La tumefazione solitamente viene notata dai genitori oppure dal pediatra, durante la visita di routine. I genitori tipicamente riferiscono un'anamnesi di tumefazione a livello inguinale, labiale o scrotale che, pur riducendosi spontaneamente, a poco a poco si espande, si fa più persistente e diventa sempre più difficile da ridurre. I **segni patognomonici** di ernia inguinale all'esame obiettivo sono quelli di una massa liscia, fissa, che emerge attraverso l'anello inguinale esterno lateralmente al tubercolo pubico e si dilata quando la pressione intraddominale aumenta. Quando il bambino si rilassa l'ernia tipicamente va incontro a riduzione spontanea oppure può essere ridotta esercitando una lieve pressione, prima posteriormente, per liberarla dall'anello inguinale esterno, poi verso l'alto, in direzione della cavità peritoneale.

Le modalità utilizzate per dimostrare l'ernia mediante esame obiettivo dipendono dall'età del paziente. Se il bambino è tranquillo si può farlo sdraiare sul letto in posizione supina, con le gambe in estensione e le braccia sopra la testa, per mettere in tensione i muscoli addominali. Questa manovra di solito provoca il pianto, che a sua volta aumenta la pressione intraddominale determinando la fuoriuscita dell'ernia. Ai pazienti più grandi viene chiesto di eseguire la manovra del Valsalva gonfiando un pallone o tossendo. Il bambino più grande deve essere visitato in piedi e può essere utile procedere all'esame dopo svuotamento vescicale. Con l'aumento della pressione intraddominale, la massa che protrude risulta evidente all'esame della regione inguinale o può essere palpata dal dito dell'esaminatore che invagina lo scroto verso l'alto, palpando a livello dell'anello inguinale esterno. Nei neonati di sesso femminile, l'ovaio e le tube di Falloppio possono ritrovarsi nel sacco erniario, presentandosi come una massa fissa, distinta e non iperestesica a livello labiale. Un altro esame è quello del **"segno del guanto di seta"**, che descrive la sensazione data dagli strati del sacco erniario (processo vaginale) quando scorrono sulle strutture del fluido spermatico, con lo scorrimento del fluido spermatico sotto il dito indice a livello del tubercolo pubico. Se la massa è localizzata al di sotto del canale inguinale sulla parte mediale della coscia, bisogna sospettare un'ernia femorale. In assenza di tumefazione, riscontrare un aumento dello spessore delle strutture del canale inguinale può essere indicativo di ernia inguinale. Durante l'esame obiettivo è importante individuare la posizione dei testicoli, dal momento che i testicoli retrattili, frequenti nei lattanti e nei bambini piccoli, possono simulare l'ernia inguinale, con una tumefazione nella regione dell'anello inguinale esterno. Poiché nelle femmine il 20-25% delle ernie inguinali sono ernie da scivolamento (il contenuto del sacco erniario aderisce al sacco e quindi non è riducibile), è possibile palpare nel canale inguinale una tuba di Falloppio o un ovaio.

VALUTAZIONE DELLA TUMEFAZIONE ACUTA INGUINOSCROTALE

Talvolta può capitare che nel lattante compaia improvvisamente una massa a livello inguinoscrotale, associata a sensazione di disagio. La **diagnosi differenziale** comprende l'ernia inguinale incarcerata, l'idrocele acuto, la torsione di un testicolo non disceso, la linfoadenite inguinale suppurativa; le due forme che risulta più difficile distinguere l'una dall'altra sono l'ernia inguinale incarcerata e l'idrocele acuto. Il lattante o il bambino con ernia inguinale incarcerata con molta probabilità presenta in associazione segni di occlusione intestinale come dolore colico addominale, distensione addominale, vomito, mancata emissione delle feci, e può apparire sofferente. Il lattante con idrocele acuto può presentare disagio ma è consolabile e tollera l'alimentazione in assenza di segni e sintomi suggestivi di occlusione intestinale. Quando la diagnosi è di ernia inguinale incarcerata, la radiografia diretta evidenzia livelli idroaerei multipli. All'esame obiettivo del bambino con idrocele acuto, il medico riscontra una certa mobilità della massa. Inoltre, nell'area tra la massa sospettata di essere un idrocele e l'anello inguinale interno, le strutture funicolari possono sembrare solo lievemente ispessite. Nell'ernia incarcerata, si osservano mancanza di mobilità della massa inguinale e una tumefazione o massa marcata che si estende dalla massa scrotale attraverso l'area inguinale e verso l'alto, includendo l'anello inguinale interno. Un medico esperto può ricorrere alla tecnica di palpazione bimanuale per differenziare le anomalie inguinali. L'esaminatore palpa l'anello inguinale interno attraverso il retto, mentre con l'altra mano esercita una lieve pressione nella regione inguinale sopra l'anello inguinale interno. In caso di ernia inguinale indiretta, si può palpare un organo intraddominale che si estende attraverso l'anello inguinale. Un altro metodo è la **transilluminazione**, che però può essere fuorviante poiché lo spessore della parete intestinale del neonato talvolta è simile a quello dell'idrocele, nel qual caso l'indagine può dare esito positivo. Questo è anche il motivo per cui si scoraggia l'utilizzo dell'aspirazione per stabilire il contenuto di una massa a livello inguinale. L'**ecografia** può essere utile per distinguere tra ernia e idrocele. Una diagnosi rapida è importante per evitare le complicanze potenziali di un'ernia incarcerata, che si può sviluppare rapidamente. La laparoscopia diagnostica si è dimostrata uno strumento efficace e affidabile per quest'esigenza, ma richiede l'anestesia generale.

Un'adenopatia suppurativa che si manifesta nella regione inguinale può essere confusa con un'ernia inguinale incarcerata. L'esame obiettivo dell'area al limite con i linfonodi inguinali può rivelare una lesione superficiale infettata o ricoperta da una crosta. Inoltre, la tumefazione associata a linfoadenopatia inguinale è tipicamente situata più in basso e di lato rispetto alla massa dell'ernia inguinale e vi possono essere associati altri noduli nell'area. La torsione del testicolo non disceso può presentarsi coma una massa arrossata dolorosa a livello dell'inguine. L'assenza di gonadi nello scroto dallo stesso lato permette di confermare questa diagnosi.

ERNIA INCARCERATA. È un'ernia in cui non è possibile ridurre il contenuto del sacco erniario nella cavità addominale. Gli organi contenuti possono essere l'intestino tenue, l'appendice, l'omento, il colon o, seppure raramente, il diverticolo di Meckel. Nelle femmine, possono essere interessati l'ovaio, le tube di Falloppio o entrambi. Raramente nel lattante si può trovare l'utero. L'ernia si dice **incarcerata** se il suo passaggio attraverso il canale inguinale risulta fortemente costretto e quindi il contenuto erniato diviene ischemico o gangrenoso. Mentre gli adulti possono tollerare l'incarceramento per anni, la maggior parte delle ernie inguinali non riducibili nei bambini evolve rapidamente, se non trattata, verso lo strangolamento, con infarto potenziale del contenuto dell'ernia. Inizialmente, la pressione sui visceri erniati nel loro passaggio attraverso l'anello inguinale interno, il canale inguinale, e l'anello inguinale esterno conduce a un'alterazione della circolazione linfatica e venosa. Ne deriva una tumefazione dei visceri erniati che aumenta ulteriormente la compressione nel canale inguinale determinando occlusione totale della vascolarizzazione arteriosa dei visceri incarcerati. Si instaurano alterazioni ischemiche progressive con conseguente gangrena e/o perforazione dei visceri erniati. Anche il testicolo è a rischio di ischemia per la compressione delle strutture del funicolo spermatico da parte dell'ernia strangolata. Nelle femmine, l'erniazione dell'ovaio lo mette a rischio di strangolamento e torsione. L'incidenza di incarceramento di un'ernia inguinale va dal 12 al 17%. I due terzi delle ernie incarcerate si verificano nel primo anno di vita. Il rischio maggiore è durante la prima infanzia, con un'incidenza compresa tra il 25 e il 30% nei bambini al di sotto dei 6 mesi di vita. L'incidenza di incarceramento è lievemente inferiore nei prematuri, anche se la ragione non è chiara.

I sintomi dell'ernia incarcerata sono irritabilità, dolore inguinale e addominale, distensione addominale e vomito. Nella regione inguinale è presente una massa piuttosto tesa, non mobile, che può estendersi nello scroto o nelle grandi labbra. Tale massa, ben definita, può essere iperestesica e irriducibile. Con l'insorgenza delle alterazioni ischemiche, il dolore aumenta e il vomito diventa biliare o fecaloide. Si può riscontare sangue nelle feci. La massa è tipicamente iperestesica e spesso si osservano edema e arrossamento della cute che la riveste, con febbre e segni di occlusione intestinale. I testicoli possono essere o normali o tumefatti e duri sul lato affetto, a causa della congestione venosa imputabile alla massa erniata strangolata, che comprime le vene spermatiche e i vasi linfatici a livello dell'anello inguinale. La radiografia addominale evidenzia segni di occlusione intestinale parziale o completa; talvolta è possibile riscontrare aria nel segmento intestinale incarcerato del legamento inguinale o entro lo scroto.

GENITALI AMBIGUI. I lattanti con disturbi di intersessualità presentano con una certa frequenza l'ernia inguinale, spesso contenente una gonade, e necessitano di una particolare considerazione. Nelle femmine, in particolare se presentano masse inguinali bilaterali, va sospettata una **sindrome della femminilizzazione testicolare** poiché più del 50% dei pazienti che la presentano hanno un'ernia inguinale (vedi Capitolo 584). Viceversa, l'incidenza reale della femminilizzazione testicolare in tutte le neonate con ernia inguinale è di difficile determinazione (ma dovrebbe essere pari a circa l'1%). Nel fenotipo femminile, se si sospetta femminilizzazione testicolare in fase preoperatoria, il paziente deve essere sottoposto a screening per ricerca dei corpi di Barr nella mucosa orale e ad adeguata valutazione genetica prima dell'intervento di chirurgia riparativa dell'ernia. La diagnosi di femminilizzazione testicolare viene effettuata occasionalmente al momento dell'intervento, riscontrando una gonade anomala (il testicolo) all'interno del sacco erniario o l'assenza dell'utero all'ispezione rettale. Nella neonata normale, l'utero viene facilmente palpato all'ispezione rettale, come una struttura distinta sulla linea mediana, sotto la sinfisi pubica. La diagnosi preoperatoria di sindrome della femminilizzazione testicolare o altri disordini con intersessualità, come la disgenesia gonadica mista e lo pseudoermafroditismo, fa sì che sia effettuata una consulenza alla famiglia e la gonadectomia può essere realizzata al momento dell'intervento riparativo dell'ernia.

TRATTAMENTO

La presenza di un'ernia inguinale in età pediatrica è un'indicazione alla correzione chirurgica. Dal momento che essa non si risolve spontaneamente, un intervento precoce elimina il rischio di incarceramento e di complicanze potenziali, in particolar modo nei primi 6-12 mesi di vita. Il momento dell'intervento dipende da diversi fattori, tra cui l'età, le condizioni generali di salute e le comorbilità. Nei lattanti al di sotto dell'anno di età cui viene diagnosticata un'ernia inguinale, occorre procedere rapidamente all'intervento poiché ben il 70% delle ernie inguinali incarcerate che richiede l'intervento d'urgenza per la riduzione e la correzione si riscontra nel primo anno di vita. Inoltre, l'incidenza di atrofia testicolare dopo incarceramento nei lattanti al di sotto dei 3 mesi è del 30%. Nei bambini di età >1 anno il rischio di incarceramento è minore e la correzione può essere programmata con minore urgenza. Per le ernie riducibili, l'intervento deve essere programmato subito dopo la diagnosi. La correzione elettiva per ernia inguinale è eseguibile in modo sicuro a livello ambulatoriale, con guarigione totale nel giro di 48 ore. L'operazione deve essere eseguita in una struttura che permette il ricovero in unità ospedaliera, se necessario. Alcune condizioni obbligano a posticipare la chirurgia correttiva, come la forte prematurità, la polmonite intercorrente (specialmente da virus respiratorio sinciziale), altre infezioni o cardiopatie congenite. In caso di forte prematurità (1800-2000 g) la chirurgia correttiva va effettuata prima della dimissione dal reparto di terapia intensiva.

L'operazione è generalmente eseguita in anestesia generale, ma anche in anestesia spinale o caudale, se è preferibile evitare l'intubazione a causa di una pneumopatia cronica o una displasia broncopolmonare. La profilassi antibiotica non è utilizzata di routine, eccetto che per condizioni associate come le cardiopatie congenite o la presenza di shunt ventricoloperitoneale. I prematuri richiedono un'attenzione speciale, dal momento che sono a elevato rischio di apnea e bradicardia dopo l'anestesia generale (vedi Capitolo 76). I neonati al di sotto delle 44 settimane e quelli a termine al di sotto di 3 mesi di vita e con comorbilità vanno tenuti sotto osservazione durante la notte con monitor che rilevino l'apnea e i parametri cardiorespiratori.

Un'ernia incarcerata, irriducibile, senza segni di strangolamento, in un paziente clinicamente stabile deve inizialmente essere gestita in modo non chirurgico. Si può tentare una lieve compressione, ma la manovra va interrotta se il bambino piange o oppone resistenza. Prima di tentare la riduzione può essere utile utilizzare sedativi o analgesici, che riducono la pressione intraddominale e alleviano la pressione sul colletto del sacco erniario a livello dell'anello inguinale. L'assistenza è volta a evitare la depressione respiratoria, specialmente nel prematuro. Altre tecniche proposte per assistere la riduzione chirurgica di un'ernia inguinale incarcerata comprendono l'elevazione delle gambe e una breve applicazione della borsa del ghiaccio. Molti medici non adottano quest'ultima tecnica nei neonati per il rischio di ipotermia. La riduzione manuale inizia con una trazione dapprima in senso caudale e posteriormente, per liberare la massa dall'anello inguinale esterno, poi verso l'alto, per ridurre il contenuto nella cavità peritoneale. Se la riduzione ha avuto buon esito ma è stata difficoltosa, il paziente va tenuto sotto osservazione per assicurarsi che l'alimentazione sia tollerata e non vi sia il rischio che sia stato ridotto l'intestino necrotico. La chirurgia correttiva si esegue 24-48 ore dopo, quando c'è meno edema, maneggiare il sacco erniario è più facile e il rischio di complicanze è minore. Una presentazione frequente nelle femmine altrimenti asintomatiche è la presenza di un ovaio irriducibile nell'ernia inguinale. La massa inguinale è molle, non iperestesica a una manipolazione leggera, e non si riscontrano tumefazione o edema (il che significa che non vi sono segni evidenti di strangolamento). Questo rappresenta uno "scivolamento" dell'ernia con le tube di Falloppio e l'ovaio fusi alla parete posteromediale del sacco erniario. Accanirsi nel tentativo di ridurre l'ernia è ingiustificato e potenzialmente dannoso per tube e ovaio. Il rischio che l'incarceramento dell'ovaio in questa sede conduca allo strangolamento non è noto. La maggior parte dei chirurghi pediatrici raccomanda la chirurgia correttiva elettiva dell'ernia entro 48-72 ore. Per alcuni pazienti che presentano una storia prolungata di anamnesi di incarceramento, segni di irritazione peritoneale o occlusione dell'intestino tenue, bisogna ricorrere a chirurgia riduttiva e riparativa dell'ernia.

TRATTAMENTO OPERATORIO. Quando l'ernia non è riducibile o è incarcerata, è indicato un intervento chirurgico immediato per prevenire un danno ulteriore al contenuto del sacco erniario o ai testicoli. Se ci sono segni di occlusione intestinale o strangolamento, la gestione iniziale consiste nell'intubazione nasogastrica, nell'infusione di liquidi endovena e nella somministrazione di antibiotici a largo spettro. Una volta corretto lo squilibrio idroelettrolitico, se le condizioni del bambino sono soddisfacenti si inizia l'esplorazione. L'operazione si articola nelle seguenti fasi: riduzione del contenuto del sacco erniario, separazione di quest'ultimo dai vasi del funicolo spermatico e dal vaso deferente nel canale inguinale, legatura alta del sacco erniario all'anello inguinale interno. La resezione di strutture non vitali all'interno del sacco erniario o di un testicolo infartuato può essere indicata in base all'esperienza e al giudizio del chirurgo. È importante sottolineare che, sebbene il testicolo possa apparire ischemico, la maggior parte guarisce dopo la liberazione dall'incarceramento senza richiedere rimozione.

La chirurgia riparativa elettiva di un'ernia inguinale congenita indiretta è semplice e consiste nella legatura alta del sacco erniario (pervietà del dotto vaginale) a livello dell'anello inguinale interno, prevenendo la protrusione del contenuto addominale nel canale inguinale. Nel maschio è necessaria un'attenta separazione del sacco dalle strutture del funicolo spermatico, evitando di danneggiare queste strutture vitali. Nelle femmine la chirurgia riparativa è più semplice, poiché il sacco erniario e il legamento rotondo possono essere sottoposti a legatura senza rischiare di danneggiare l'ovaio e la sua vascolarizzazione, che generalmente resta all'interno dell'addome. La tuba di Falloppio viene visualizzata abitualmente per scoprire un'eventuale sindrome della femminilizzazione testicolare. Se la tuba e l'ovaio sono all'interno del sacco erniario e non risultano riducibili, solitamente si lega il sacco distalmente a queste strutture e si chiude l'anello inguinale interno dopo la riduzione del sacco e del suo contenuto nella cavità addominale.

ESPLORAZIONE INGUINALE CONTROLATERALE. Ancora si discute su quale sia il momento più adatto per procedere all'esplorazione della regione inguinale controlaterale. Nei lattanti e nei bambini con ernia inguinale indiretta unilaterale, effettuare un'esplorazione controlaterale serve a evitare lo sviluppo di un'ernia da quel lato in un momento successivo. L'incidenza di un processo vaginale persistentemente pervio controlateralmente è circa del 60% al secondo mese di vita e si riduce al 40% a 2 anni. Un processo pervio rappresenta solo un'ernia potenziale e molti fattori di rischio influenzano la probabilità che essa si sviluppi. L'esplorazione controlaterale comporta il vantaggio di evitare (1) la preoccupazione dei genitori e forse una seconda anestesia, (2) i costi di un altro intervento chirurgico, (3) il rischio di incarceramento controlaterale. Gli svantaggi comprendono (1) i danni potenziali delle strutture vascolari del funicolo spermatico e del testicolo, (2) una maggior durata dell'intervento chirurgico e (3) il fatto che, in molti neonati, è un intervento non necessario. I più importanti interrogativi suscitati da questo dibattito riguardano la frequenza di un'ernia controlaterale dopo la chirurgia correttiva da un lato e la relazione esistente tra questa, l'età, il sesso e il lato in cui l'ernia è clinicamente evidente. La maggior parte degli studi importanti finora compiuti ha riportato una possibilità di sviluppo dell'ernia controlaterale del 30-40% nei bambini al di sotto dei 2 anni di età: tali risultati hanno spinto la maggior parte dei chirurghi pediatrici a raccomandare che l'esplorazione controlaterale sia effettuata di routine in questa fascia di età. Nelle femmine, a causa della più elevata incidenza di ernia inguinale bilaterale e della mancanza di danno al funicolo spermatico e al testicolo, l'esplorazione controlaterale è stata raccomandata fino ai 5-6 anni. I lattanti e i bambini con fattori di rischio per lo sviluppo di ernia inguinale o con condizioni mediche che rendono rischiosa l'anestesia generale devono essere inizialmente gestiti con un'esplorazione controlaterale di routine. La laparoscopia permette una valutazione del lato controlaterale senza alcun rischio di danneggiare le strutture del funicolo spermatico o del testicolo. Questa procedura può essere eseguita attraverso un'incisione ombelicale o passando un laparoscopio obliquo a 30 o 70° attraverso il sacco erniario aperto subito prima della legatura del sacco erniario sul lato colpito. Se si dimostra una pervietà del lato controlaterale, il chirurgo procede alla chirurgia correttiva bilaterale dell'ernia; se il lato controlaterale viene obliterato in modo corretto, si evitano così l'esplorazione e le complicanze potenziali (Figg. 343-2 e 343-3).

ERNIA INGUINALE DIRETTA

Rare nei bambini, le ernie dirette appaiono come masse inguinali che si estendono verso i vasi femorali con gli sforzi, compresi quelli sportivi. L'eziologia risiede in un difetto o debolezza muscolare a livello del pavimento del canale inguinale, mediale ai vasi epigastrici. Le ernie inguinali dei bambini sono generalmente considerate acquisite. In un terzo dei casi il paziente ha un'anamnesi di intervento chirurgico per ernia sul lato dell'ernia diretta, suggerendo

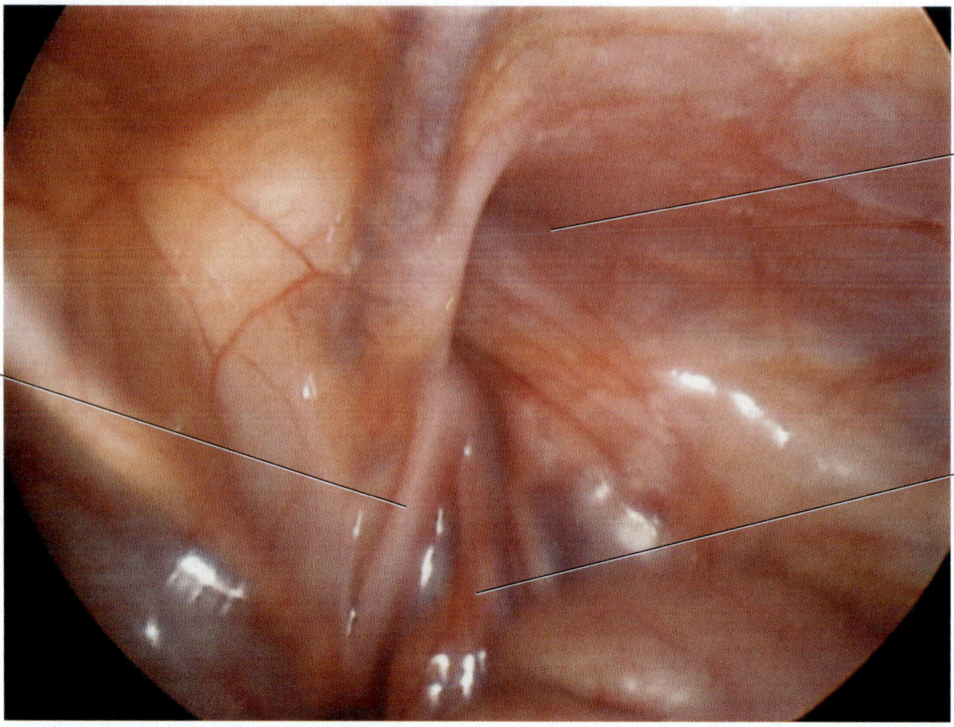

Figura 343-2. Immagine laparoscopica di pervietà del processo vaginale sul lato destro.

un possibile danno dei muscoli del pavimento del canale inguinale durante la precedente erniorrafia. Inoltre pazienti con **disordini del connettivo**, come quelli affetti da sindrome di Ehlers-Danlos, di Marfan, e con mucopolisaccaridosi, come la sindrome di Hunter-Hurler, hanno un rischio maggiore di sviluppare ernia inguinale diretta sia indipendentemente sia in seguito a chirurgia correttiva per ernia inguinale indiretta. La chirurgia correttiva dell'ernia inguinale diretta comporta il rafforzamento del pavimento del canale inguinale e ne sono state descritte diverse tecniche standard, simili a quelle riparative usate nell'adulto. La correzione può essere eseguita attraverso un'incisione singola e limitata; quindi la correzione laparoscopica non offre vantaggi significativi. La recidiva dopo la correzione, a differenza che nell'adulto, è molto rara. L'impianto prostetico per la correzione dell'ernia diretta o altri approcci, come la correzione preperitoneale, sono di raro impiego in età pediatrica. I bambini più grandi con ernia inguinale e connettivopatia possono rappresentare l'eccezione all'approccio laparoscopico e all'uso di materiale prostetico.

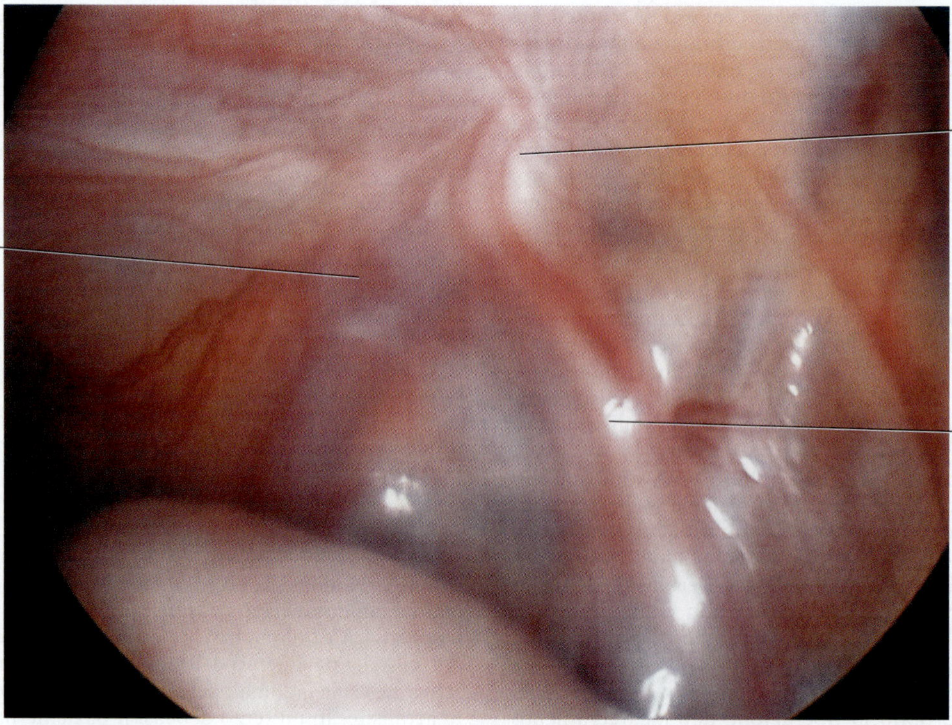

Figura 343-3. Immagine diagnostica laparoscopica di un processo vaginale obliterato sul lato sinistro.

ERNIA FEMORALE

Le ernia femorali sono rare nei bambini. Sono più frequenti nelle bambine che nei maschi, con un rapporto di 2:1. Esse rappresentano una protrusione attraverso il canale femorale. La tumefazione è situata sotto il legamento inguinale e si proietta tipicamente verso la parte mediale della coscia. Le ernie femorali, rispetto a quelle dirette, sfuggono più spesso all'osservazione durante l'esame obiettivo o al momento della chirurgia correttiva dell'ernia indiretta. La chirurgia riparativa dell'ernia femorale presuppone la chiusura delle alterazioni del canale femorale, generalmente suturando il ligamento inguinale a quello pettineo e alla fascia omonima.

COMPLICANZE

Le complicanze dopo chirurgia correttiva elettiva dell'ernia inguinale sono poco frequenti (1,5%) ma significativamente più alte in associazione con l'incarceramento (10%). Alcune sono dovute a fattori tecnici (recidive, criptorchidismo iatrogeno), mentre altre sono correlate al processo sottostante, come l'ischemia intestinale, l'infarto delle gonadi e l'atrofia testicolare, associati a ernia incarcerata. La maggior parte delle complicanze è correlata a episodi di incarceramento oppure insorge dopo chirurgia riduttiva o riparativa d'urgenza.

INFEZIONE DELLA FERITA. L'infezione della ferita si ha in meno dell'1% degli interventi correttivi per ernie inguinali nei lattanti e nei bambini, ma sale al 5-7% in associazione con l'incarceramento e la chirurgia d'urgenza. Il paziente sviluppa tipicamente febbre e irritabilità, 3-5 giorni dopo l'intervento. La ferita, che si presenta calda, eritematosa e fluttuante, va gestita con drenaggio, breve ciclo di antibiotici e medicazione giornaliera. I microrganismi più frequenti sono Gram-positivi (*Staphylococcus* e *Streptococcus* spp.) e occorre prestare attenzione alla copertura di *Staphylococcus aureus* meticillino-resistente; la ferita in genere guarisce in 1-2 settimane, con bassa morbilità e un buon risultato estetico.

ERNIA RECIDIVANTE. Il tasso di recidiva dell'ernia inguinale dopo chirurgia correttiva è generalmente dello 0,5-1% e del 2% nei prematuri. Il tasso di recidiva dopo intervento d'urgenza è significativamente maggiore, circa il 3-6%. L'incidenza reale di recidiva è sicuramente maggiore, considerando la difficoltà di effettuare un accurato follow-up a lungo termine. Nel gruppo di pazienti che sviluppa ernia inguinale recidivante, la recidiva è del 50% entro 1 anno dall'intervento iniziale e del 75% dopo 2 anni.

La recidiva di un'ernia indiretta è più probabilmente dovuta a problemi tecnici connessi alla procedura, come errori nell'identificazione del sacco, errori nel legame alto del sacco all'anello inguinale interno, o lacerazioni del sacco che lasciano una striscia di peritoneo lungo le strutture del funicolo. La recidiva di un'ernia diretta può derivare da una lesione del pavimento inguinale (fascia trasversale) durante l'intervento o errori nell'identificare l'ernia diretta durante la prima esplorazione. I pazienti con connettivopatie o condizioni che determinano aumento della pressione intraddominale (shunt ventricoloperitoneali, ascite, catetere peritoneale per dialisi) sono ad alto rischio di recidiva.

CRIPTORCHIDISMO IATROGENO. Il criptorchidismo iatrogeno indica un errato posizionamento del testicolo in seguito a intervento chirurgico correttivo per ernia inguinale. La complicanza è solitamente correlata all'interruzione del legame del testicolo o all'incapacità di riconoscere il testicolo non disceso durante l'intervento, con conseguente retrazione dello stesso nella regione dell'anello inguinale esterno. Al termine dell'intervento correttivo, il testicolo deve essere collocato in posizione intrascrotale dipendente. Se il testicolo non resta in questa posizione, occorre effettuata un'orchidopessi al momento della correzione dell'ernia.

INCARCERAMENTO. L'incarceramento di un'ernia inguinale può derivare da danni a intestino, tube di Falloppio e ovaio, o testicolo omolaterale. L'incidenza di incarceramento di un'ernia indiretta inguinale è dal 6 al 18%, e del 30% per i bambini di età >3 mesi. Il danno intestinale che necessita di resezione intestinale non è frequente, presentandosi nell'1-2% delle ernie incarcerate. In casi di incarceramento in cui l'ernia è ridotta in modo non chirurgico, la probabilità di danno intestinale è bassa, anche se questi pazienti devono essere tenuti sotto stretta osservazione per segni e sintomi persistenti di occlusione intestinale come febbre, vomito, distensione addominale o feci ematiche.

L'incidenza riportata di infarto testicolare e successiva atrofia con incarceramento va dal 4 al 12%, con un tasso più alto in caso di irriducibilità. Il danno testicolare può essere causato da compressione dei vasi gonadici da parte della massa erniata incarcerata o come risultato del danno insorto durante la chirurgia riparativa. I lattanti di pochi mesi sono a elevato rischio (l'infarto testicolare può colpire fino al 30% dei lattanti al di sotto dei 2-3 mesi di vita). Da questi problemi si deduce la necessità di una rapida riduzione dell'ernia incarcerata e una correzione precoce, non appena è nota la diagnosi, per evitare ripetuti episodi di incarceramento.

DANNO AI VASI DEFERENTI E INFERTILITÀ MASCHILE. Allo stesso modo dei vasi gonadici, quelli deferenti possono risultare danneggiati in conseguenza della compressione creata da un'ernia incarcerata o durante la chirurgia riparativa. Il danno è quasi sicuramente sottostimato poiché è improbabile riconoscerlo fino all'età adulta e anche in questo gruppo di pazienti si rende evidente solo se è bilaterale. Sebbene la vulnerabilità dei vasi deferenti sia stata documentata in molti studi, non esistono informazioni sull'incidenza attuale di questo problema. Una review ha riportato un'incidenza di danno dell'1,6% in base a segmenti di vasi deferenti dimostrati anatomopatologicamente nel sacco erniario; questo dato può essere esagerato, in quanto altri hanno dimostrato che piccole inclusioni ghiandolari trovate nel sacco erniario possono rappresentare resti del dotto di Müller, privi di rilevanza clinica. Non è nota la relazione tra fertilità maschile e un precedente intervento chirurgico riparativo sull'ernia inguinale. Sembra esserci un'associazione tra infertilità maschile con atrofia testicolare, e anomalie della conta degli spermatozoi e una precedente chirurgia riparativa dell'ernia. È stata riportata una relazione tra infertilità maschile e anticorpi autoagglutinanti spermatici e una precedente chirurgia riparativa dell'ernia. Si ipotizza, a livello eziologico, che il danno ai vasi deferenti durante l'intervento chirurgico correttivo dell'ernia possa determinare un'ostruzione dei vasi deferenti con diversione degli spermatozoi nei vasi linfatici testicolari e che questa breccia aperta nella barriera emato-testicolare produca uno stimolo antigenico determinando la formazione di anticorpi autoagglutinanti spermatici.

Gallagher TM: Regional anesthesia for surgical treatment of inguinal hernia in preterm babies. *Arch Dis Child* 1993;69:623–624.

Holcomb GW: Laparoscopic evaluation for a contralateral inguinal hernia or a nonpalpable testis. *Pediatr Ann* 1993;22:678–684.

Lobe TE, Schropp KP: Inguinal hernias in pediatrics: Initial experience with laparoscopic inguinal exploration of the asymptomatic contralateral side. *J Laparoendosc Surg* 1992;2:135–140.

Owings EF, Georgeson KE: A new technique for laparoscopic exploration to find contralateral patent processus vaginalis. *Surg Endosc* 2000; 14:114–116.

Rescorla FJ: Hernias and umbilicus. In Oldham KT, Colambani PM, Foglia RP, Skinner MA (editors): *Principles and Practice of Pediatric Surgery.* Philadelphia, Lippincott Williams and Wilkins, 2005, pp 1087–1101.

Rowe MI, Copelson LW, Clatworthy HW: The patent processus vaginalis and the inguinal hernia. *J Pediatr Surg* 1969;4:102–107.

Shier F, Montupet P, Esposito C: Laparoscopic inguinal herniorrhaphy in children: A three center experience with 933 repairs. *J Pediatr Surg* 2002;37:395–397.

Skandalakis JE, Gray SW: *Embryology for Surgeons: The Embryologic Basis for the Treatment of Congenital Anomalies,* 2nd ed. Baltimore, Williams and Wilkins, 1994, pp 184–241.

Stergman C, Sotelo-Avila C, Weber TR: The incidence of spermatic cord structures in inguinal hernia sacs from male children. *Am J Surg Pathol* 1999;23:883–885.

Tacket LD, Breuer CK, Luks FI, et al: Incidence of contralateral inguinal hernia: A prospective analysis. *J Pediatr Surg* 1999;34:684–687.

Weber TR, Tracy TF Jr, Keller MS: Groin hernias and hydroceles. In Ashcraft KW, Holcomb GW III, Murphy JP (editors): *Pediatric Surgery*, 4th ed. Philadelphia, WB Saunders, 2005, pp 697–705.

Wiener ES, Touloukian RJ, Rodgers BM, et al: Hernia survey of the Section on Surgery of the American Academy of Pediatrics. *J Pediatr Surg* 1996;31:1166–1169.

Sezione 5 — Pancreas esocrino — Steven L. Werlin

Capitolo 344 ■ Embriologia, anatomia e fisiologia

Il pancreas si sviluppa da un'invaginazione del duodeno primitivo, a partire dalla quinta settimana di gestazione. L'abbozzo dorsale, più grande, che dà origine alla coda, al corpo e a parte della testa del pancreas, si sviluppa direttamente dal duodeno. L'abbozzo ventrale, più piccolo, si sviluppa come una o due gemme dal fegato primitivo, per andare poi a formare la porzione principale della testa del pancreas. Intorno alla 17ª settimana di gestazione, i due abbozzi, dorsale e ventrale, si fondono, mentre si sviluppano le gemme e avviene la rotazione dell'intestino. Il dotto ventrale formerà la porzione prossimale del dotto pancreatico principale o di Wirsung, che si apre nella papilla di Vater. Il dotto dorsale formerà invece la porzione distale del dotto di Wirsung e il dotto accessorio di Santorini, che ha uno sbocco indipendente in circa il 15% della popolazione. Le possibili variazioni in questo processo di fusione possono causare anomalie di sviluppo del pancreas. L'agenesia pancreatica è stata associata alla delezione di una coppia di basi nel gene *ipf1* HOX, *PDX1*. Altri geni implicati nell'organogenesi pancreatica comprendono il gene *Sonic Hedgehog* e il gene del TGF 1β (*Transforming Growth Factor* 1β).

Il pancreas è situato trasversalmente nell'addome superiore a livello retroperitoneale, tra il duodeno e la milza. La testa, che appoggia sulla vena cava e sulla vena renale, è adiacente all'ansa a C del duodeno e circonda il dotto biliare comune distale. La coda del pancreas arriva, a sinistra, all'ilo splenico, passando superiormente al rene sinistro. Il piccolo omento separa la coda pancreatica dallo stomaco.

Intorno alla 13ª settimana di gestazione, possono già essere identificate le cellule esocrine ed endocrine. Gli acini primitivi, contenenti i granuli zimogeni immaturi, possono essere reperiti dalla 16ª settimana. I granuli zimogeni maturi, contenenti amilasi, tripsinogeno, chimotripsinogeno e lipasi, sono invece presenti dalla 20ª settimana. Le cellule centroacinari e duttali, responsabili della secrezione di acqua, elettroliti e bicarbonati, sono anch'esse presenti intorno alla 20ª settimana. La struttura finale tridimensionale del pancreas è costituita da una complessa serie di ramificazioni duttali, circondate da grappoli di cellule epiteliali. Le cellule che producono glucagone sono reperibili dall'8ª settimana, mentre le isole di Langerhans compaiono tra la 12ª e la 16ª settimana.

344.1 • Anomalie anatomiche

L'*agenesia pancreatica*, completa o parziale, è una condizione rara. L'agenesia completa è associata a un diabete neonatale grave e comporta generalmente la morte nei primi anni di vita. L'agenesia parziale o dorsale è spesso asintomatica, ma può associarsi a diabete, cardiopatie congenite, polisplenia e pancreatite ricorrente. L'agenesia pancreatica si associa inoltre a malassorbimento.

Il *pancreas anulare* può originare da un'incompleta rotazione dell'abbozzo sinistro (ventrale). I pazienti si presentano normalmente in età infantile con sintomi di ostruzione intestinale completa o parziale. Si trova spesso un'anamnesi di polidramnios materno. Alcuni bambini si presentano con vomito cronico, pancreatite o coliche biliari. Il trattamento di scelta è la duodenodigiunostomia. Non si pratica la divisione dell'anello pancreatico, poiché questo si accompagna spesso a un diaframma o a una stenosi del duodeno. Il pancreas anulare si può associare inoltre a sindrome di Down, atresia intestinale, ano imperforato, pancreatite e malrotazione.

In circa il 3% della popolazione sono presenti *residui pancreatici ectopici* a livello dello stomaco o dell'intestino tenue. Nella maggior parte dei casi (70%) sono localizzati nel tratto intestinale superiore; sono riconoscibili nelle radiografie con mezzo di contrasto baritato, per la tipica forma ombelicata, e presentano scarso significato clinico. Endoscopicamente appaiono come noduli giallastri irregolari, di 2-4 mm di diametro. Occasionalmente, un residuo pancreatico può essere il punto di inizio di un'intussuscezione, provocare emorragie o causare un'ostruzione intestinale.

Il *pancreas divisum*, presente nel 5-15% della popolazione, è la più frequente anomalia di sviluppo del pancreas. A causa della mancata fusione degli abbozzi pancreatici dorsali e ventrali, la coda, il corpo e parte della testa del pancreas sono drenati dal piccolo dotto accessorio di Santorini, invece che da quello principale di Wirsung. Questa anomalia può associarsi a pancreatite ricorrente quando è presente un'ostruzione del deflusso dal pancreas ventrale. In questi casi, il trattamento di scelta è l'inserzione endoscopica di uno stent endoprotesico. Se gli episodi cessano, è indicata la sfinterotomia chirurgica.

Le *cisti coledociche* sono dilatazioni del tratto biliare che causano generalmente sintomi collegati all'albero biliare, come ittero, dolore e febbre. Occasionalmente, tuttavia, si possono presentare con una pancreatite. La diagnosi è agevole con ecografia, TC o imaging del tratto biliare. Analogamente, il coledococele, una cisti coledocica intraduodenale, può esordire con una pancreatite. La diagnosi in questi casi può essere più difficile e necessita della colangiopancreatografia in risonanza magnetica (MRCP, *Magnetic Resonance ColangioPancreatography*) o della colangiopancreatografia retrograda endoscopica (ERCP, *Endoscopic Retrograde ColangioPancreatography*).

Esistono poi alcune condizioni rare, come la sindrome di Ivemark o la sindrome di Johanson-Blizzard, che comprendono, tra le loro caratteristiche, anche disgenesie o disfunzioni pancreatiche. In molte di queste sindromi, le anomalie pancreatiche si associano a disgenesia epatica o renale. L'assenza delle cellule delle isole pancreatiche, o l'agenesia pancreatica, comporta un diabete mellito permanente che insorge in epoca neonatale (vedi Capitolo 590).

Hill ID, Lebenthal E: Congenital abnormalities of the exocrine pancreas. In Go VLW, et al (editors): *The Exocrine Pancreas: Biology, Pathology, and Diseases*, 2nd ed. New York, Raven Press, 1993, pp 1029–1040.

Klein SD, Affronti JP: Pancreas divisum, an evidence-based review: Part I, pathophysiology. *Gastrointest Endosc* 2004;60:9–25.
Klein SD, Affronti JP: Pancreas divisum, an evidence-based review: Part II, patient selection and treatment. *Gastrointest Endosc* 2004;60:585–589.

344.2 • Fisiologia

L'unità funzionale del pancreas esocrino è l'acino; le cellule acinari sono disposte a semicerchio intorno al lume dei dotti che drenano gli acini, così che questi risultano contornati sia dalle cellule centroacinari che dalle cellule duttulari. Questa disposizione consente ai secreti delle diverse cellule di mescolarsi tra loro.

Le cellule acinari sintetizzano, accumulano e secernono più di 20 enzimi diversi, che si inglobano nei granuli zimogeni, alcuni di essi in forma inattiva. La concentrazione relativa dei vari enzimi nel succo pancreatico è influenzata, e forse anche controllata, dalla dieta, probabilmente per via della regolazione della sintesi di RNA messaggeri specifici. Una dieta ricca di lipidi aumenta la concentrazione di lipasi; una dieta a elevato contenuto proteico fa aumentare il contenuto di proteasi del succo pancreatico, mentre una dieta ricca di carboidrati porta a un aumento del contenuto di amilasi. Le amilasi scindono l'amido in maltosio, isomaltosio, maltotriosio e destrine. La tripsina e la chimotripsina, entrambe endopeptidasi, e la carbossipeptidasi, che è invece un'esopeptidasi, sono secrete dal pancreas sotto forma di proenzimi inattivi, rispettivamente tripsinogeno e chimotripsinogeno. Il tripsinogeno è attivato, nel lume intestinale, dall'enterochinasi, un enzima dell'orletto a spazzola. La tripsina può quindi attivare il tripsinogeno, il chimotripsinogeno e la procarbossipeptidasi nelle rispettive forme attive.

Le lipasi pancreatiche, per funzionare, necessitano della colipasi, un coenzima presente anch'esso nel succo pancreatico. Le lipasi liberano gli acidi grassi dalla posizione 1 e 3 dei trigliceridi, lasciando un monogliceride. Gli stimoli che sollecitano la secrezione esocrina possono essere sia di tipo ormonale sia nervoso. La fase cefalica è mediata dall'acetilcolina, mentre quella intestinale dalla colecistochinina (CCK). La CCK è secreta dalla mucosa duodenale per stimolazione degli aminoacidi e degli acidi grassi endoluminali. La regolazione a feedback della secrezione pancraetica è mediata dalle proteasi pancreatiche nel duodeno. La secrezione di CCK è inibita dalla digestione di un peptide rilasciante la CCK, sensibile alla tripsina, secreto nel lume dell'intestino tenue, oppure da un peptide rilasciato nel liquido pancreatico.

Le cellule centroacinari e duttali secernono acqua e bicarbonato. La secrezione di bicarbonato è sottoposta a un controllo a feedback, regolato dal pH duodenale intraluminale, ed è stimolata dalla secretina in associazione con la CCK. La secretina è prodotta da cellule presenti in grande quantità nel duodeno.

Sebbene il processo digestivo richieda una funzione pancreatica integra, occorre una considerevole riduzione della quota di funzione pancreatica perché si manifesti una maldigestione. La secrezione di lipasi e colipasi deve, per esempio, essere ridotta del 90-98% perché si verifichi una maldigestione dei lipidi.

Sebbene sia le amilasi sia le lipasi compaiano precocemente durante la gestazione, la secrezione di entrambi gli enzimi è scarsa in età neonatale e raggiunge i livelli adulti solo verso la fine del primo anno di vita. La digestione dell'amido, che si trova in diverse formule pediatriche, dipende in parte dai bassi livelli di amilasi salivari che raggiungono il duodeno. Questo può spiegare la diarrea che si osserva nei bambini nutriti con formulazioni ricche di polimeri glucidici o di amido. La secrezione neonatale di tripsinogeno e chimotripsinogeno è circa il 70% dei livelli osservati nel bambino di un anno. I bassi livelli di amilasi e lipasi nel lume duodenale in età neonatale possono essere parzialmente compensati dall'amilasi salivare e dalla lipasi linguale. Questo spiega anche la parziale intolleranza all'amido e ai grassi dei neonati prematuri.

Christian M, Edwards C, Weaver LT: Starch digestion in infancy. *J Pediatr Gastroenterol Nutr* 1999;29:116–124.
Werlin SL, Lee PC: Development of the exocrine pancreas. In Polin RA, Fox WW (editors): *Fetal and Neonatal Physiology,* 3rd ed. Philadelphia, WB Saunders, 2003, pp 1142–1151.

Capitolo 345 ■ Test di funzionalità pancreatica

La funzione pancreatica può essere misurata con metodiche dirette e indirette. Può essere effettuata una stimolazione diretta del pancreas con un pasto campione (di **Lundh**) o con olio di mais, latte in polvere scremato e destrosio, oppure con una combinazione di secretina e colecistochinina. Classicamente, si usa un sondino a tre vie per isolare le secrezioni pancreatiche nel duodeno. Sulle secrezione aspirate viene effettuata la misurazione della concentrazione di bicarbonati e dell'attività enzimatica (tripsina, chimotripsina, lipasi e amilasi). Il test diretto più utilizzato, attualmente, è la raccolta del succo pancreatico dopo stimolazione con secretina e colecistochinina, per via endoscopica.

La raccolta delle feci per 72 ore, per l'analisi quantitativa del contenuto di grassi, è il *gold standard* per la diagnosi di malassorbimento. La raccolta viene normalmente effettuata a casa, chiedendo ai genitori di registrare accuratamente la dieta del bambino, per poter calcolare l'importo lipidico. Si utilizza un contenitore di plastica prepesato, sigillabile, che i genitori devono tenere nel congelatore, sia per conservare il campione sia per evitare il cattivo odore. Ai bambini vengono fatti indossare pannolini usa e getta con il lato in plastica verso la cute, così da poter trasferire l'intero campione nel contenitore. L'assorbimento normale dei lipidi è >93% dell'introito. Inoltre, può essere misurata nelle feci l'attività degli enzimi pancreatici. L'esame qualitativo delle feci per la ricerca di globuli di grasso microscopici può dare risultati sia falsamente positivi sia falsamente negativi; il dosaggio dell'elastasi fecale, l'esame di screening standard per l'insufficienza pancreatica, ha invece una sensibilità e una specificità superiori al 90%. Si possono avere risultati falsamente alterati anche in molte enteropatie.

Gli elevati livelli sierici di tripsinogeno osservabili nei neonati con fibrosi cistica sono alla base dei nuovi test di screening che si sono resi recentemente disponibili. Con la progressione del danno pancreatico, i livelli sierici di tripsinogeno si riducono al di sotto dei valori normali.

La funzione pancreatica può anche essere misurata con vari test del respiro. Viene fatto ingerire un trigliceride marcato, normalmente la ^{14}C trioleina, che è digerito dalla lipasi pancreatica nel duodeno, liberando $^{14}CO_2$, rilevabile nell'aria espirata. A causa della radioattività e della lunga emivita del ^{14}C, questo test non è tuttavia adatto all'utilizzo in età pediatrica. La trioleina marcata con il ^{13}C, un isotopo stabile e non radioattivo, può essere usata con sicurezza nei bambini, ma questo test non ha ottenuto particolare riscontro a causa della poca sensibilità nel rilevare i casi di insufficienza pancreatica lieve, e perché per la rilevazione della $^{13}CO_2$ occorre uno spettrofotometro di massa, non sempre facilmente disponibile.

Beharry S, Ellis L, Corey M, et al: How useful is fecal pancreatic elastase 1 as a marker of exocrine pancreatic disease? *J Pediatr* 2002;141:84–90.
Del Rosario MA, Fitzgerald JF, Gupta SK, et al: Direct pancreatic measurement of pancreatic enzymes after stimulation with secretin versus secretin plus cholecystokinin. *J Pediatr Gastroenterol Nutr* 2000;31:28–32.

Capitolo 346 ■ Alterazioni del pancreas esocrino

ALTERAZIONI ASSOCIATE A INSUFFICIENZA PANCREATICA. A parte la fibrosi cistica, sono rare nell'infanzia le condizioni che causano insufficienza pancreatica. Queste comprendono la sindrome di Shwachman-Diamond, i deficit enzimatici isolati, il deficit di enterochinasi (vedi Capitolo 335), la pancreatite cronica e la malnutrizione proteico-calorica (vedi Capitolo 335).

Fibrosi cistica (vedi Capitolo 400). La fibrosi cistica è la più comune malattia genetica letale e la più frequente causa di malassorbimento nei bambini americani ed europei bianchi. Verso la fine del primo anno di vita, l'85-90% dei bambini affetti da fibrosi cistica ha sviluppato insufficienza pancreatica che, se non trattata, può portare a malnutrizione. Il trattamento di questa condizione, per contro, porta a un miglioramento dell'assorbimento e quindi della crescita e alla normalizzazione delle feci. Nei bambini con fibrosi cistica la funzione pancreatica può essere valutata con misurazioni seriali dell'elastasi fecale. Alcune mutazioni nel gene della fibrosi cistica sono state associate alla pancreatite cronica idiopatica.

Sindrome di Shwachman-Diamond (vedi Capitolo 130). La sindrome di Shwachman-Diamond è una sindrome autosomica recessiva (1/20 000 nati) che comporta insufficienza pancreatica, neutropenia (che può essere ciclica), difetti della chemiotassi neutrofila, disostosi metafisaria, mancato sviluppo e bassa statura. Alcuni pazienti affetti da sindrome di Shwachman-Diamond hanno anche un coinvolgimento epatico o renale, oppure presentano difficoltà di apprendimento. I pazienti si presentano generalmente nell'infanzia con problemi di crescita e feci untuose e maleodoranti, caratteristiche del malassorbimento. Questi bambini si differenziano facilmente da quelli con fibrosi cistica per i normali livelli di cloro nel sudore, per la mancanza del gene della fibrosi cistica, per le caratteristiche lesioni metafisarie e per la presenza di un pancreas grasso alla TC. Nonostante un'adeguata terapia sostitutiva pancreatica, spesso la crescita continua a essere scarsa. L'insufficienza pancreatica è spesso transitoria e la steatorrea può migliorare spontaneamente con l'età. Questi soggetti vanno frequentemente incontro a infezioni piogene ricorrenti (otiti medie, polmoniti, osteomieliti, dermatiti, sepsi) che rappresentano una frequente causa di morte. Nel 70% dei pazienti è presente trombocitopenia e nel 50% anemia. Può svilupparsi una *sindrome mielodisplasica* ed è stata osservata la trasformazione in *leucemia mieloide acuta* nel 33% e nel 24% dei pazienti, rispettivamente. Il gene della sindrome di Shwachman-Diamond si trova sul cromosoma 7. Dal punto di vista anatomopatologico, gli acini sono sostituiti da grasso, con scarsa fibrosi. Le isole e i dotti sono normali. Il pancreas grasso ha un caratteristico aspetto ipodenso alla TC e alla RM.

Sindrome di Pearson. Si tratta di una mutazione sporadica del DNA mitocondriale, che altera la fosforilazione ossidativa e che si manifesta nei bambini con grave anemia macrocitica e trombocitopenia di grado variabile. Nel midollo osseo si osservano vacuoli nei precursori delle cellule mieloidi ed eritroidi e sideroblasti ad anello. Oltre a svolgere un ruolo nella grave insufficienza midollare, l'insufficienza pancreatica contribuisce al ritardo di crescita. Esistono altre mutazioni del DNA mitocondriale che si associano a diabete mellito (sindrome di Kearns-Sayre, oftalmoplegia esterna cronica progressiva, diabete con sordità). Questo genere di mutazioni può essere sporadico o trasmesso per via materna a entrambi i sessi.

Deficit enzimatici isolati. Sono stati riportati in letteratura deficit isolati di tripsinogeno, enterochinasi, lipasi e colipasi. Sebbene l'enterochinasi sia un enzima dell'orletto a spazzola, un suo deficit causa insufficienza pancreatica per mancata attivazione delle proteasi pancreatiche. Il deficit di tripsinogeno o di enterochinasi si manifesta con mancato sviluppo, ipoproteinemia ed edema. Il deficit isolato di amilasi è tipicamente legato allo sviluppo e si risolve intorno ai 2-3 anni di età.

SINDROMI ASSOCIATE A INSUFFICIENZA PANCREATICA. L'agenesia pancreatica, la sindrome di Johanson-Blizzard (insufficienza pancreatica, sordità, basso peso alla nascita, microcefalia, difetti della linea mediana della cresta ectodermica, ritardo psicomotorio, ipotiroidismo, nanismo, assenza della dentatura permanente e aplasia delle ali nasali), l'ipoplasia pancreatica congenita e la rosolia congenita sono cause rare di insufficienza pancreatica. Alcuni bambini con paucità dei dotti biliari intraepatici, sia sindromici (Alagille) sia non, hanno un'insufficienza pancreatica associata all'epatopatia. L'insufficienza pancreatica è stata anche riportata nell'atresia e nella stenosi duodenale ed è stata anche osservata nei bambini con ipoglicemia iperinsulinemica familiare o non familiare (precedentemente chiamata nesidioblastosi), che richiedono una pancreatectomia del 95-100% per controllare l'ipoglicemia.

Boocock GR, Morrison JA, Popovic M, et al: Mutations in SBDS are associated with Shwachman-Diamond syndrome. *Nat Genet* 2003;33:97–101.
Toth T, Bokay J, Szonyi L: Detection of mtDNA deletion in Pearson syndrome by two independent PCR assays from Guthrie card. *Clin Genet* 1998;53:210–213.

Capitolo 347 ■ Trattamento dell'insufficienza pancreatica

Il trattamento dell'insufficienza pancreatica esocrina con enzimi sostitutivi per via orale corregge di solito la steatorrea, che però difficilmente si risolve completamente. Questo può essere dovuto alla variabilità dell'attività lipasica nelle diverse preparazioni commerciali, a dosaggio inadeguato, a orari di somministrazioni errati, a inattivazione della lipasi da parte del pH acido gastrico e al fatto che la chimotripsina nelle preparazioni enzimatiche digerisce e pertanto inattiva la lipasi. Nei supplementi enzimatici, la vera attività lipasica si è dimostrata anche il doppio del valore dichiarato. Le preparazioni più usate sono a base di pancrelipasi e sono tutte enterorivestite, perciò resistenti all'inattivazione da parte dell'acido gastrico. Le preparazioni enzimatiche generiche sono meno efficaci e dovrebbero essere evitate.

Il dosaggio degli enzimi sostitutivi, nei bambini, dipende dalla quantità di cibo assunto con la dieta ed è stabilito tramite tentativi e correzioni. Poiché questi prodotti contengono un eccesso di proteasi in rapporto alle lipasi, il dosaggio viene stimato in base al fabbisogno di lipasi di 500-1500 UI/kg/pasto. La dose adeguata è quella che viene seguita dalla normalizzazione del contenuto fecale di grassi, nonché della quantità, del colore e dell'odore delle feci. Gli enzimi sostitutivi dovrebbero essere somministrati all'inizio e durante il pasto; le tavolette devono essere masticate; la polvere e i granuli possono essere mescolati con un po' di cibo. Gli enzimi devono essere somministrati anche con gli snack. Un aumento del supplemento enzimatico oltre la dose raccomandata non solo non migliora l'assorbimento, ma può ritardare la crescita e causare colopatia fibrosante.

Se non viene ottenuto un adeguato assorbimento lipidico, la neutralizzazione dell'acido gastrico con un antagonista dei recettori H_2 o con un inibitore di pompa protonica riduce l'inattivazione degli enzimi da parte dell'acido gastrico e migliora l'apporto di lipasi all'intestino. L'involucro delle preparazioni enterorivestite protegge anch'esso la lipasi dall'inattivazione acida.

Gli effetti indesiderati della terapia enzimatica sostitutiva comprendono reazioni allergiche, aumento dei livelli di acido urico e nefrolitiasi. La colopatia fibrosante, che comporta fibrosi e stenosi del colon, insorge da 7 a 12 mesi dopo una terapia sostitutiva pancreatica a dosi elevate (da 6500 a 58 000 UI di lipasi/kg/pasto).

Baker SS, Borowitz D, Duffy D: Pancreatic enzyme therapy and clinical outcomes in cystic fibrosis. *J Pediatr* 2005;146:189–193.
Borowitz D, Baker RD, Stallings V: Census report in nutrition for pediatric patients with cystic fibrosis. *J Pediatr Gastroenterol Nutr* 2002;35:246–259.
Powell CJ: Colonic toxicity from pancreatins: A contemporary safety issue. *Lancet* 1999;353:911–915.

Capitolo 348 ■ Pancreatite

348.1 • PANCREATITE ACUTA

L'incidenza della pancreatite acuta, la patologia pancreatica più frequente in età infantile, è in aumento. Nei grandi centri pediatrici si osservano attualmente almeno 30-50 casi all'anno. Le eziologie più comuni sono i traumi addominali chiusi, le patologie multisistemiche, i calcoli biliari o la microlitiasi (*sludging*) e la tossicità da farmaci. L'acido valproico è la più comune causa di pancreatite da farmaci nei bambini. Altri casi compaiono in seguito a trapianto d'organo, infezioni o alterazioni metaboliche. Una minoranza di casi è idiopatica o dovuta ad altre cause (Tab. 348-1).

PATOGENESI. La teoria eziologica classica suggerisce che dopo un insulto iniziale, come la rottura o l'ostruzione duttale, le idrolasi lisosomiali si colocalizzino con i proenzimi pancreatici nella cellula acinare; si verifica allora una stasi pancreatica (concettualmente simile alla colestasi) con una sintesi continuativa di enzimi. Il tripsinogeno è attivato a tripsina, che attiva a sua volta gli altri proenzimi pancreatici, portando all'autodigestione della cellula, all'ulteriore attivazione enzimatica e al rilascio di proteasi attive. La lecitina è attivata dalla fosfolipasi A2 nel composto tossico lisolecitina; la profosfolipasi è instabile e può essere attivata da piccolissime quantità di tripsina. Un'altra teoria suggerisce che, dopo un insulto, il rilascio di citochine e la conseguente deplezione di antiossidanti causino la pancreatite e la progressiva attivazione dei proenzimi pancreatici.

Il pancreas sano è fisiologicamente dotato di diversi meccanismi di protezione: (1) le proteasi pancreatiche sono sintetizzate come proenzimi inattivi; (2) gli enzimi digestivi sono segregati nei granuli secretori a pH 6,2 con basse concentrazioni di calcio, con una minimizzazione dell'attività tripsinica; (3) la presenza di inibitori delle proteasi sia nel citoplasma sia nei granuli zimogeni; (4) la secrezione degli enzimi direttamente nel lume duttale. Da un punto di vista istopatologico, nelle fasi precoci compare edema interstiziale; successivamente, con la progressione dell'episodio pancreatitico, si possono sviluppare necrosi localizzata o confluente, distruzione dei vasi sanguigni con conseguente emorragia, e risposta infiammatoria peritoneale.

MANIFESTAZIONI CLINICHE. Il paziente con pancreatite acuta manifesta dolore addominale intenso, vomito persistente e febbre. Il dolore può essere localizzato a livello epigastrico oppure nei quadranti superiori, è fisso e porta spesso il bambino ad assumere una posizione antalgica con le cosce e le ginocchia flesse, seduto oppure coricato su un lato. Il bambino è molto sofferente, irritabile e presenta segni di patologia acuta. L'addome può essere disteso e dolente; talvolta può essere palpabile una massa. Il dolore aumenta di intensità in 24-48 ore, durante le quali il vomito può peggiorare e può essere necessaria l'ospedalizzazione, per correggere la disidratazione con terapia idroelettrolitica endovenosa. La prognosi per la risoluzione completa, nei casi acuti non complicati, è eccellente.

TABELLA 348-1. Eziologia della pancreatite acuta nei bambini

FARMACI E TOSSINE	**OSTRUTTIVE**
Sovradossaggio da paracetamolo	Patologia ampollare
Alcol	Ascaridiosi
5-aminosalicitato	Malformazioni del tratto biliare
L-asparaginasi	Cisti coledociche
Azatioprina	Coledococele
Cimetidina	Colelitiasi, microlitiasi e coledocolitiasi (calcoli o sabbia)
Corticosteroidi	Cisti da duplicazione
DDC	Complicazioni di colangiopancreatografia retrograda endoscopica
DDI	Pancreas divisum
Enalapril	Anomali duttali pancreatiche
Erithromicina	Postoperatorie
Estrogeni	Disfunzioni dello sfintere di Oddi
Furosemide	Tumori
Isoniazide	**PATOLOGIE SISTEMICHE**
6-Mercaptopurina	Deficit di α_1-antitripsina
Mesalamina	Trapianto di midollo osseo
Metildopa	Tumore cerebrale
Metronidazolo	Collagenopatie
Pentamidina	Morbo di Crohn
Sulfonamidi	Fibrosi cistica
Sulindac	Diabete mellito
Tetracicline	Traumi cranici
Tiazidici	Emocromatosi
Trimethoprim	Sindrome uremico-emolitica
Acido valproico	Iperlipidemia: tipo I, IV, V
Veleni (ragno, scorpione, lucertola eloderma)	Iperparatiroidismo/Ipercalcemia
Vincristina	Malattia di Kawasaki
PANCREATITE EREDITARIA	Malnutrizione
Gene del tripsinogeno cationico	Acidemia Organica
Gene della fibrosi cistica	Ulcera peptica
Gene *SPINK1*	Panarterite nodosa
INFETTIVE	Insufficienza renale
Ascaridiosi	Lupus eritematoso sistemico
Virus Coxsackie B	Trapianto: midollo osseo, cuore, fegato, rene, pancreas
Virus di Epstein-Barr	Vasculiti
Epatite A, B	**TRAUMATICHE**
Influenza A, B	Trauma chiuso
Leptospirosi	Ustioni
Malaria	Abuso infantile
Morbillo	Ipotermia
Parotite	Trauma chirurgico
Micoplasma	Ingessatura total body
Rosolia	
Rubeola	
Sindrome di Reye: varicella, influenza B	
Shock settico	

La **pancreatite acuta grave** è rara nei bambini. In questa temibile condizione, il quadro sintomatologico esordisce acutamente con nausea e vomito intensi e dolore addominale. Possono insorgere shock, iperpiressia, ittero, ipocalcemia e versamento pleurico. Può essere osservata una colorazione bluastra intorno all'ombelico (**segno di Cullen**) o a livello dei fianchi (**segno di Grey Turner**). Il pancreas va incontro a necrosi e può trasformarsi in una massa emorragico-infiammatoria. La mortalità, che si aggira intorno al 25%, è correlata alla risposta infiammatoria sistemica con conseguente disfunzione multiorgano (MOD, *Multiple Organ Disfunction*): shock, insufficienza renale, sindrome da distress respiratorio acuto, coagulazione intravascolare disseminata, emorragie digestive massive e infezioni endoaddominali o sistemiche. I fattori prognostici negativi sono rappresentati da un elevato punteggio APACHE II, alti livelli di proteina C reattiva (PCR), MOD persistente per più di 1 settimana, elevata percentuale di necrosi osservata alla TC e mancato *enhancement* del tessuto pancreatico alla TC (suggestivo di necrosi).

DIAGNOSI. La diagnosi di pancreatite acuta viene generalmente posta tramite la determinazione dei livelli di amilasi e lipasi nel siero. Le amilasi risultano tipicamente aumentate anche per 4 giorni. Tuttavia, molte altre condizioni possono causare iperamilasemia in assenza di pancreatite (Tab. 348-2). Un aumento dell'amilasi salivare, per esempio, può portare a un'errata diagnosi di pancreatite acuta in un bambino con dolore addominale, ma il laboratorio può differenziare gli isoenzimi dell'amilasi nelle frazioni salivare e pancreatica. Inizialmente, i livelli di amilasi misurati sono normali nel 10-15% dei pazienti. Le lipasi risultano più specifiche delle amilasi nella diagnosi di pancreatopatia infiammatoria acuta e dovrebbero sempre essere misurate qualora vi sia un sospetto di una pancreatite acuta, con amilasi normali. I livelli di lipasi aumentano in 4-8 ore, raggiungono il picco verso le 24-48 ore e restano elevate per 8-14 giorni più a lungo delle amilasi. Anch'esse, tuttavia, possono aumentare in corso di patologie extrapancreatiche.

Altre anomalie di laboratorio osservabili in corso di pancreatite acuta comprendono emoconcentrazione, coagulopatia, leucocitosi, iperglicemia, glicosuria, ipocalcemia, aumento della γ-glutamiltransferasi e iperbilirubinemia.

La radiografia del torace e dell'addome può mostrare reperti aspecifici. Alla radiografia del torace possono essere presenti atelectasia basale, infiltrati basali, elevazione dell'emidiaframma, versamento pleurico sinistro (o più raramente destro), versamento pericardico o edema polmonare. La radiografia del torace può dimostrare ansa sentinella, dilatazione del colon trasverso (segno "cutoff"), ileo, calcificazioni pancreatiche (nel caso di episodi ricorrenti), opacizzazione del margine dello psoas sinistro, pseudocisti, opacizzazione addominale diffusa per la presenza di ascite e bolle gassose extraluminali peripancreatiche.

L'ecografia e più specificamente la TC hanno un ruolo fondamentale nella diagnosi e nel follow-up dei bambini con pancreatite. I reperti possono comprendere allargamento del pancreas, pancreas ipoecogeno, sonolucente, edematoso, masse pancreatiche, raccolte e ascessi (Fig. 348-1); tuttavia, almeno il 20% dei bambini con pancreatite acuta presenta reperti di imaging normali nelle fasi iniziali. Negli adulti, i reperti TC sono alla base di un sistema prognostico universalmente accettato. La colangiopancreatografia retrograda endoscopica (*Endoscopic Retrograde Cholangiopancreatography*, ERCP) o più spesso la **colangiopancreatografia con risonanza magnetica** (MRCP, *Magnetic Resonance Cholangiopancreatography*) sono indagini essenziali nella pancreatite ricorrente, nel pancreas divisum, nella disfunzione dello sfintere di Oddi e nelle patologie associate a disturbi della colecisti. L'ecoendoscopia può anche svolgere un ruolo nella visualizzazione del sistema pancreatobiliare.

TABELLA 348-2. Diagnosi differenziale dell'iperamilasemia

PATOLOGIE PANCREATICHE
Pancreatite aucta o cronica
Complicazioni della pancreatite (pseudocisti, ascite, ascessi)
Pancreatite fittizia
PATOLOGIE DELLE GHIANDOLE SALIVARI
Parotite (parotite, *Staphylococcus aureus*, Cytomegalovirus, HIV, virus di Epstein-Barr)
Sialoadenite (calcolo, radiazioni)
Disturbi dell'alimentazioni (anoressia nervosa, bulimia)
PATOLOGIE INTRADDOMINALI
Patologie del tratto biliare (colelitasi)
Perforazione di ulcera peptica
Peritonite
Ostruzione intestinale
Appendicite
MALATTIE SISTEMICHE
Acidosi metabilica (diabete mellito, shock)
Insufficienza o trapianto renale
Ustioni
Gravidanza
Farmaci (morfina)
Traumi cranici
Bypass cardiopolmonare

TRATTAMENTO. Gli obiettivi della terapia medica sono il sollievo del dolore e il ripristino dell'omeostasi metabolica. Deve quindi essere fornita un'analgesia in dosi adeguate e deve essere compensato e mantenuto l'equilibrio idroelettrolitico. Il sondino nasogastrico può essere utile nei pazienti con vomito incoercibile, che devono essere mantenuti a digiugno. La somministrazione profilattica di antibiotici (imipenem/cilastatina) è controversa, ma è praticata comunque nei casi più gravi per prevenire l'infezione della necrosi pancreatica o per trattare un'infezione già in atto. La guarigione è generalmente completa nell'arco di 4-5 giorni. L'alimentazione può essere ripresa dopo la risoluzione del vomito, la riduzione dei livelli di amilasi e la risoluzione della sintomatologia.

Il trattamento della pancreatite acuta grave comprende antibiotici, inibitori dell'acidità gastrica e lavaggio peritoneale per ridurre il rischio di infezione secondaria. La terapia endoscopica può essere utile quando la pancreatite è causata da anomalie anatomiche, come stenosi o calcoli. L'alimentazione enterale è preferibile a quella parenterale; può essere praticata per via orale, tramite sondino nasogastrico o nasodigiunale (nei casi gravi o in quelli intolleranti alla nutrizione orale o nasogastrica) entro 2-3 giorni dall'esordio e ha dimostrato una riduzione della necessità di intervento, delle complicanze infettive e della durata dell'ospedalizzazione. In rari casi, la pancreatite acuta richiede il trattamento chirurgico, che può comprendere il drenaggio di materale necrotico o di ascessi.

PROGNOSI. I bambini con pancreatite acuta non complicata hanno un decorso favorevole e guariscono nell'arco di 4-5 giorni. Quando la pancreatite si associa a un trauma o a una patologia sistemica, la prognosi è tipicamente correlata alle condizioni mediche associate. È stato recentemente proposto un sistema prognostico pediatrico basato sulla valutazione di criteri clinici al momento del ricovero e dopo 48 ore, ma non è ancora stato validato da altri Autori.

DeBanto JR, Goday PS, Pedroso MRA, et al: Acute pancreatitis in children. *Am J Gastroenterol* 2002;97:1726–1731.

Johnson CD, Abu-Hilal M: Persistent organ failure during the first week as a marker of fatal outcome in acute pancreatitis. *Gut* 2004;53:1340–1344.

Lopez M: The changing incidence of acute pancreatitis in children: A single-institution perspective. *J Pediatr* 2002;140:622–624.

Makola D, Krenitsky J, Parrish C, et al: Efficacy of enteral nutrition for the treatment of pancreatitis using standard enteral formula. *Am J Gastroenterol* 2006;101:2347–2355.

Marik PE, Zaloga GP: Meta-analysis of parenteral nutrition versus enteral nutrition in patients with acute pancreatitis. *Br Med J* 2004;328:1407.

Mitchell RMS, Byrne MF, Baillie J: Pancreatitis. *Lancet* 2003;361:1447–1455.

Nathens AB, Curtis R, Beale RJ, et al: Management of the critically ill patient with severe acute pancreatitis. *Crit Care Med* 2004;32:2524–2536.

Swaroop VS, Chari ST, Clain JE: Severe acute pancreatitis. *JAMA* 2004;291:2865–2868.

Werlin SL, Kugathasan S, Frautschy B: Pancreatitis in children. *J Pediatr Gastroenterol Nutr* 2003;37:591–595.

348.2 • PANCREATITE CRONICA

La pancreatite cronica ricorrente nei bambini è frequentemente ereditaria o causata da anomalie del sistema duttale pancreatico o biliare. La pancreatite ereditaria (HP, *Hereditary Pancreatitis*) è generalmente trasmessa come tratto autosomico dominante a penetranza incompleta ed espressività variabile. I sintomi compaiono spesso nella primo decennio di vita, ma sono generalmente di lieve entità all'esordio. Sebbene gli attacchi si risolvano spontaneamente nell'arco di 4-7 giorni, gli episodi hanno la tendenza a diventare progressivamente più gravi. Clinicamente, la HP può essere diagnosticata per la presenza della patologia nel succedersi delle generazioni di una stessa famiglia. Una valuta-

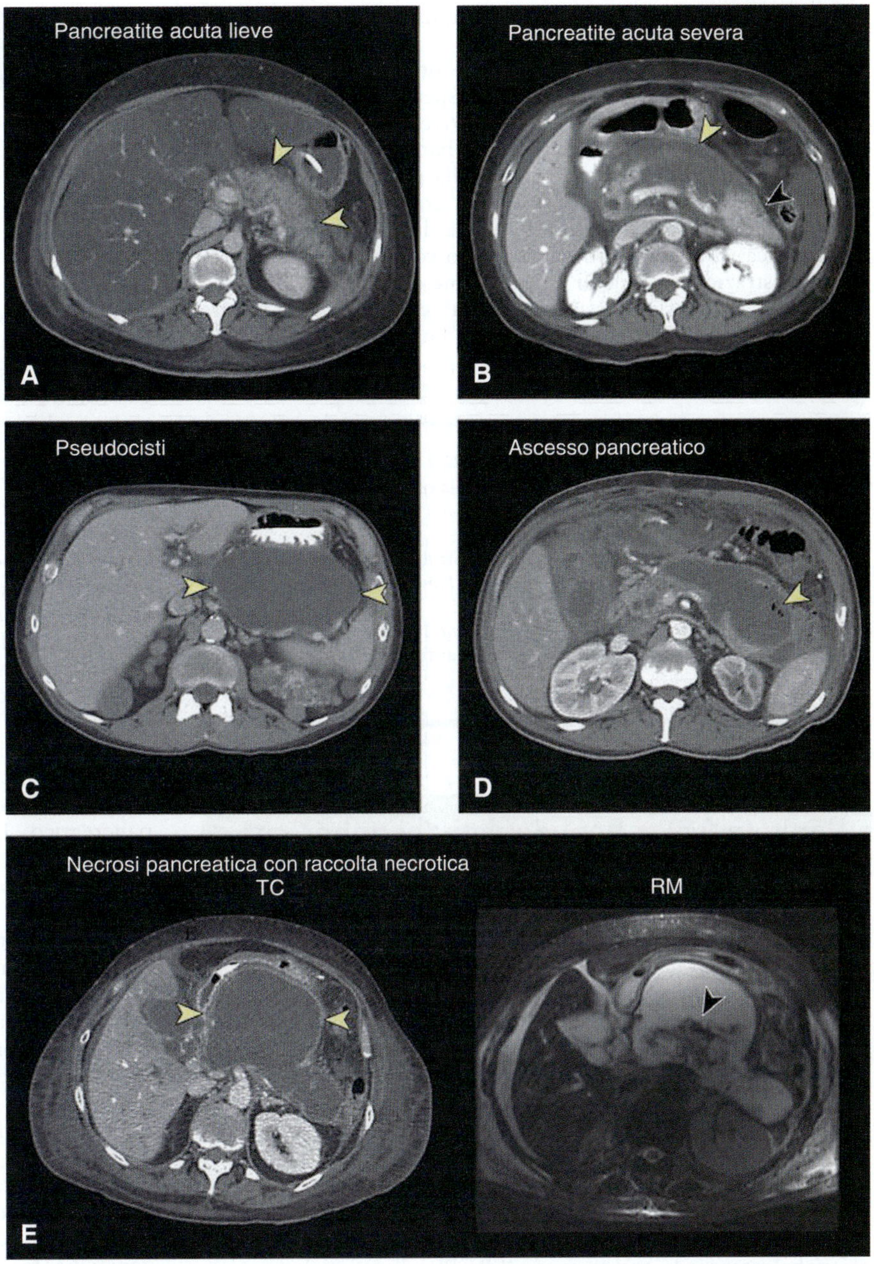

Figura 348-1. Aspetto in tomografia computerizzata (TC) e risonanza magnetica (RM) della pancreatite. Da *A* a *E (sinistra)*, immagini TC; *E (destra)*, RM. *A*. Pancreatite acuta lieve con normale *enhancement* del corpo del pancreas (*punte di freccia*) dopo somministrazione di contrasto endovena. *B*. Pancreatite acuta severa con necrosi pancreatica e aree pancreatiche che non prendono contrasto (*punte di freccia*) dopo somministrazione di mezzo di contrasto, rispetto alle zone normalmente perfuse (*punte di freccia nere*). *C*. Pseudocisti del pancreas (*punte di freccia*) a contenuto liquido, nella raccolta vicino al pancreas. *D*. Ascesso pancreatico con presenza di gas (*punta di freccia*) nella cavità. *E*. Necrosi pancreatica (raccolta necrotica) che appare in TC come una raccolta di liquido limpido (*punta di freccia gialla*). La stessa raccolta in RM appare formata da aree di detriti necritici (*punta di freccia nera*) non visibili in TC, una differenza che ha implicazioni prognostiche e terapeutiche. (Da Swaroop VS, Chari ST, Clain JE: Severe acute pancreatitis. *JAMA* 2004;291:2865–2868.)

zione durante il periodo asintomatico può non essere significativa fino allo sviluppo di calcificazioni, pseudocisti o insufficienza pancreatica esocrina ed endocrina. La pancreatite cronica è un fattore di rischio per l'insorgenza di un futuro carcinoma pancreatico. Il gene responsabile della HP è stato clonato e mappato a livello del gene del tripsinogeno cationico sul braccio lungo del cromosoma 7. Sono state descritte numerose mutazioni del gene HP associate a pancreatite ereditaria. Nei casi di pancreatite cronica non familiare, possono essere identificati altri alleli. Il tripsinogeno cationico che si autoattiva a tripsina ha un sito di clivaggio sensibile alla tripsina stessa. Nella HP, la perdita di questo sito di clivaggio nella proteina alterata permette l'attivazione incontrollata del tripsinogeno a tripsina, con conseguente autodigestione del pancreas. Sono state associate alla pancreatite cronica o ricorrente anche mutazioni in altri geni, tra cui l'eterozigosi per il gene della fibrosi cistica (*CFTR*), tipicamente nella regione promoter 5T, e nel gene *SPINK1* (inibitore della tripsina pancreatica). L'inibitore della tripsina agisce come meccanismo di difesa dall'autoattivazione incontrollata della tripsina. In caso di mutazioni del gene *SPINK1* questo meccanismo protettivo viene perso; questo gene potrebbe anche essere un gene modificante e non il fattore eziologico diretto. Le indicazioni al test genetico per le mutazioni del gene per il tripsinogeno cationico comprendono episodi ricorrenti di pancreatite acuta, pancreatite cronica, una storia familiare di pancreatite e una pancreatite inspiegata in un bambino.

Altre condizioni associate a pancreatite cronica ricorrente sono l'iperlipidemia (di tipo I, IV e V), l'iperparatiroidismo e l'ascaridiosi. In precedenza, molti casi di pancreatite ricorrente dell'infanzia erano considerati idiopatici; con la scoperta di almeno tre famiglie di geni associate a questa condizione, la situazione è cambiata. Le anomalie congenite del sistema duttale, come il pancreas divisum, sono probabilmente più frequenti di quanto si ritenesse un tempo.

È essenziale un'accurata valutazione diagnostica di tutti i bambini con più di un episodio di pancreatite. Devono essere determinati i livelli di lipidi, calcio e fosforo, le feci devono essere valutate per la ricerca di ascaridiosi e deve essere effettuato il test del sudore. Saranno effettuate radiografie addominali per la ricerca di calcificazioni pancreatiche, e successivamente un'ecografia o una TC per rilevare un'eventuale pseudocisti. Dovrà inoltre essere esclusa una litiasi dell'albero biliare. Dopo una consulenza genetica, potrà essere effettuata la genotipizzazione per i geni HP, *SPINK1* e *CFTR*.

La MRCP e la ERCP sono tecniche utilizzabili per definire l'anatomia della ghiandola e sono indispensabili se si pensa di ricorrere all'intervento chirurgico. Si dovrebbe effettuare uno di questi esami nella valutazione di tutti i bambini con pancreatite idiopatica, ricorrente o non tendente alla guarigione, poiché in questi casi la MRCP e la ERCP sono in grado di rilevare un difetto anatomico misconosciuto, passibile di terapia endoscopica o chirurgica. Il trattamento endoscopico comprende la sfinterotomia, l'estrazione di calcoli e l'inserzione di stent endoprotesici pancreatici o biliari. Questi trattamenti consentono di gestire per via non chirurgica condizioni che un tempo richiedevano invariabilmente l'intervento.

Kingsnorth A, O'Reilly D: Acute pancreatitis. *BMJ* 2006;332:1072–1076.

Stevens T, Conwell DL, Zuccaro G: Pathogenesis of chronic pancreatitis: An evidence-based review of past theories and recent developments. *Am J Gastroenterol* 2004;99:2256–2270.

Werlin SL, Taylor A: ERCP. In Howard ER, Stringer MD, Colombani PM (editors): *Surgery of the Liver, Bile Ducts and Pancreas in Children*, 2nd ed. London, STM Publishing, 2002, pp 509–520.

Whitcomb DC: Acute pancreatitis. *N Engl J Med* 2006;354:2142–2150.

Witt H, Becker M: Genetics of chronic pancreatitis. *J Pediatr Gastoenterol Nutr* 2002;34:125–136.

Capitolo 349 ■ Pseudocisti del pancreas

La formazione di una pseudocisti pancreatica è una sequela poco frequente della pancreatite acuta o cronica. Le pseudocisti sono raccolte delimitate da una parete fibrosa, nel piccolo omento. Possono aumentare di volume ed estendersi praticamente in ogni direzione, provocando quindi sintomi molto diversi (vedi Fig. 348-1).

Si deve sospettare la presenza di una pseudocisti pancreatica quando un episodio di pancreatite non si risolve o quando è seguito dalla formazione di una massa. Clinicamente, è caratterizzata da nausea, dolore e vomito. I segni più comuni sono una massa palpabile nel 50% dei pazienti e ittero nel 10%; altri reperti possono comprendere ascite e versamento pleurico, generalmente a sinistra.

Le indagini più utili sono l'ecografia, la TC, la colangiopancreatografia retrograda endoscopica (ERCP) e la colangiopancreatografia con risonanza magnetica (MRCP). L'ecografia è l'esame di prima scelta per la facile disponibilità e il basso costo. Studi ecografici sequenziali hanno dimostrato che le pseudocisti più piccole (<6 cm) si risolvono spontaneamente. È auspicabile che tutti i pazienti con pancreatite acuta siano sottoposti a ecografia 2-4 settimane dopo la risoluzione dell'episodio acuto, per escludere la formazione di un'eventuale pseudocisti.

Il drenaggio percutaneo o endoscopico della pseudocisti ha sostituito il drenaggio chirurgico a cielo aperto, salvo che per i casi complicati o ricorrenti. Mentre le pseudocisti devono essere lasciate maturare per 4-6 settimane prima di operare un drenaggio chirurgico, quello endoscopico o percutaneo può essere praticato più precocemente. Prima di un eventuale trattamento chirurgico, occorre sempre effettuare una MRCP o una ERCP, per permettere all'operatore di pianificare l'approccio e definire eventuali anomalie anatomiche.

Baillie J: Pancreatic pseudocysts (part 1). *Gastrointest Endosc* 2004;59:873–879.

Baillie J: Pancreatic pseudocysts (part 2). *Gastrointest Endosc* 2004; 60:105–113.

Capitolo 350 ■ Tumori pancreatici

NEOPLASIE. I tumori pancreatici possono essere di origine endocrina o non endocrina. I primi comprendono gli insulinomi e i gastrinomi. Questi, come altri tumori funzionanti, fanno parte della cosiddetta sindrome MEN-1 (*Multiple Endocrine Neoplasia type 1*, neoplasie endocrine multiple), a ereditarietà autosomica dominante. L'ipoglicemia associata a livelli relativamente elevati di insulina o la presenza di ulcere gastriche refrattarie (sindrome di Zollinger-Ellison) sono indici di un possibile tumore pancreatico (vedi Capitolo 342). La maggior parte dei gastrinomi è situata al di fuori del pancreas. Il trattamento di scelta è chirurgico. Se il tumore primitivo non può essere localizzato, o ha già metastatizzato, un trattamento radicale può non essere possibile; in questi casi è indicata una terapia con inibitori di pompa protonica per sopprimere la secrezione degli acidi gastrici.

La **sindrome diarrea acquosa-ipokaliemia-acidosi** è normalmente causata dalla secrezione di peptide intestinale vasoattivo (VIP, *Vasoactive Intestinal Peptide*) da parte di un tumore a cellule non-α (VIPoma) (vedi Tab. 342-2). I livelli di VIP nel siero risultano spesso, anche se non sempre, elevati. Il trattamento è la rimozione chirurgica del tumore. Se questo non è possibile, i sintomi possono essere controllati con octreotide acetato (somatostatina ciclica), un analogo sintetico della somatostatina. Sono stati inoltre descritti tumori pancreatici secernenti diversi altri ormoni, tra cui glucagone, somatostatina e polipeptide pancreatico. Il trattamento di scelta, ove possibile, è sempre chirurgico.

Il pancreatoblastoma, l'adenocarcinoma pancreatico, il cistoadenoma e il rabdomiosarcoma sono di rara osservazione. Il pancreatoblastoma, che è proprio dell'età infantile, è un tumore embrionale secernente α-fetoproteina, che può contenere elementi sia endocrini sia esocrini. Il comportamento clinico è maligno, ma non è ben caratterizzato, a causa della sua rarità. Nelle lesioni che non possono essere sottoposte a resezione primaria, deve essere presa in considerazione la chemioterapia prechirurgica. La resezione può essere curativa; seppur in mancanza di un'efficacia non ancora dimostrata, è stata utilizzata la chemioterapia adiuvante. Il carcinoma del pancreas esocrino è proprio dell'età adulta, rappresentando circa il 2% delle diagnosi e il 5% dei decessi per tumore, ma è molto raro nell'infanzia. Non è stata riconosciuta alcuna causa definita. Diverse sindromi genetiche, tra cui la pancreatite ereditaria e la MEN-1, causano un'aumentata incidenza di tumore del pancreas in età adulta. Il tumore di Frantz è un tumore cistico papillare che si osserva generalmente nelle ragazze e nelle giovani donne. I sintomi tipici di presentazione sono dolore addominale, masse o ittero. Il trattamento di scelta è l'asportazione chirurgica.

Gli insulinomi e l'ipoglicemia iperinsulinemica persistente dell'infanzia (nesidioblastosi) causano ipoglicemia sintomatica. Il trattamento di scelta è la pancreasectomia massiva totale o subtotale, in caso di fallimento del trattamento medico (vedi Capitolo 92). Questi bambini possono sviluppare in seguito insufficienza pancreatica e diabete, come complicanza iatrogena.

Le cisti del pancreas si sviluppano nella malattia di von Hippel-Lindau. I tumori papillari solidi e cistici imitano l'ontogenesi pancreatica. La loro storia naturale deve ancora essere definita; è stata riportata l'insorgenza di metastasi, ma la chemioterapia adiuvante, dopo l'asportazione chirurgica, non può ancora essere raccomandata. La diagnosi è suggerita dalle osservazioni alla TC. L'unica terapia dimostratasi efficace è quella chirurgica.

La prognosi per i tumori endocrini asportati completamente è buona, mentre è scadente per i carcinomi, anche se sottoposti a chirurgia radicale. I bambini che sopravvivono a una pancreasectomia parziale o totale possono avere una riserva pancreatica esocrina ed endocrina ridotta.

Shorter NA, Glick RD, Klimstra DS, et al: Malignant pancreatic tumors in childhood and adolescence: The Memorial Sloan-Kettering experience, 1967–present. *J Pediatr Surg* 2002;37:887–892.

Tomassetti P, Migliori M, Lalli S, et al: Epidemiology, clinical features and diagnosis of gastroenteropancreatic endocrine tumours. *Ann Oncol* 2001;12:S95–S99.

Sezione 6 — Fegato e vie biliari

Capitolo 351 ■ Morfogenesi del fegato e delle vie biliari

Michael D. Bates e William F. Balistreri

La morfogenesi del fegato e del vie biliari è un processo complesso; alterazioni di questo processo di sviluppo possono comportare conseguenze significative, tra cui disordini a impronta colestatica, come la sindrome di Alagille e la presentazione neonatale dell'atresia biliare. Durante il processo iniziale di gastrulazione dell'embrione, si formano i tre strati embrionali germinativi (endoderma, mesoderma, ectoderma). Il fegato e le vie biliari originano dalle cellule endodermiche dell'intestino anteriore ventrale; il loro sviluppo può essere diviso in tre fasi distinte (Fig. 351-1). Nella prima fase, con un meccanismo sconosciuto, l'endoderma dell'intestino anteriore ventrale acquisisce la *competenza* di ricevere i segnali provenienti dal mesoderma cardiaco. Tali segnali mesodermici, sotto forma di vari fattori di crescita fibroblastici (FGF, *Fibroblast Growth Factors*) e proteine morfogenetiche dell'osso (BMP, *Bone Morphogenetic Proteins*), portano alla *specializzazione* delle cellule che formeranno il fegato e all'attivazione di geni epatospecifici. Questa specializzazione si verifica, nei modelli animali, appena prima della gemmazione visibile del fegato. Nell'uomo, le cellule neospecializzate migrano quindi in direzione cranioventrale, verso il setto trasverso, intorno alla 4ª settimana di gestazione, per dare inizio alla *morfogenesi* epatica. La crescita e lo sviluppo del fegato in formazione richiedono l'interazione con le cellule endoteliali. Nei modelli animali sono state riconosciute proteine specifiche, essenziali per lo sviluppo epatico (Tab. 351-1).

Nel mesentere ventrale, la proliferazione delle cellule migrate forma il cordone epatico anastomotico, con la rete di epatociti primitivi, sinusoidi e mesenchima settale, strutturando così l'architettura fondamentale del lobulo epatico (Fig. 351-2). La porzione *craniale* solida del diverticolo epatico (*pars hepatis*) forma infine il parenchima epatico e i dotti biliari intraepatici; la porzione *caudale* (*pars cistica*) dà origine alla colecisti, al dotto cistico e al dotto biliare comune. I lobuli epatici sono identificabili, nell'uomo, a partire dalla 6ª settimana di gestazione. Le strutture canalicolari biliari, comprendenti i microvilli e i complessi giunzionali, sono aree specializzate della membrana epatocitaria che compaiono precocemente nel corso della gestazione; intorno alla 6ª-7ª settimana, sono già osservabili grossi canalicoli circondati da numerosi epatociti. I dotti biliari intraepatici derivano dalla ramificazione e dal rimodellamento del dotto epatico; la loro formazione è completa intorno al 3° mese. Il dotto cistico e la colecisti risultano completamente canalizzati verso la 7ª-8ª settimana (vedi Fig. 351-2C).

Nel sistema escretorio (biliare) epatico, i canalicoli biliari confluiscono nei duttuli biliari più piccoli, che a loro volta si uniscono a formare i dotti biliari interlobulari, che seguono le ramificazioni terminali della vena porta. A livello dell'ilo epatico, i dotti intraepatici lasciano i rami portali e si uniscono a formare il complesso delle vie biliari extraepatiche. I dotti dei lobi destro e sinistro confluiscono nel dotto epatico comune. Il dotto biliare comune, che deriva dalla fusione del dotto epatico comune e del dotto cistico, si estende lungo il margine destro del piccolo

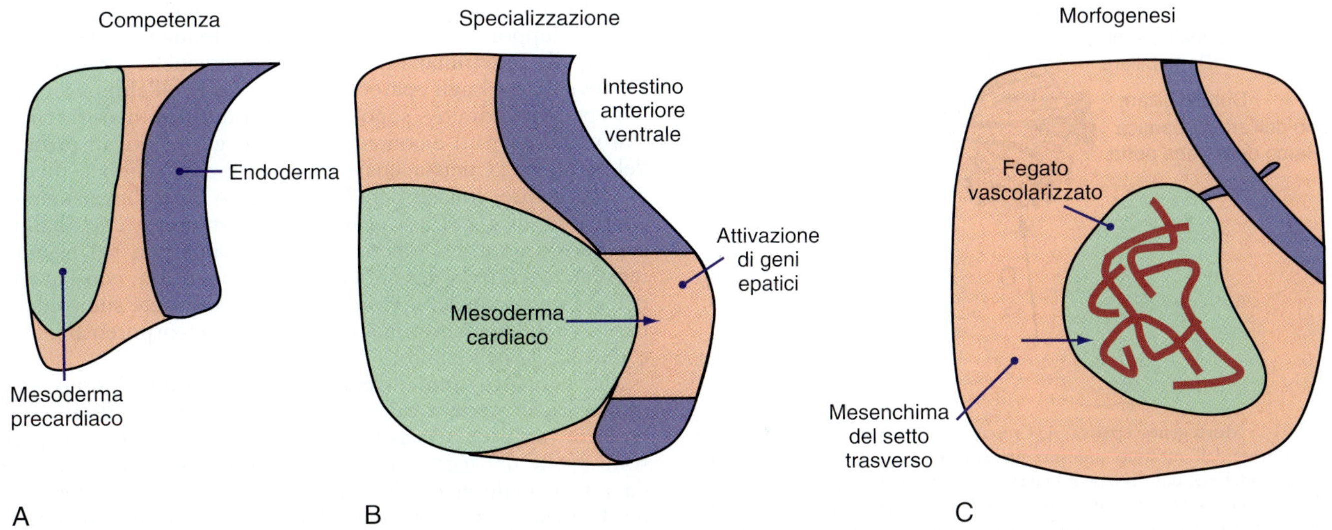

Figura 351-1. Processi coinvolti nello sviluppo epatico precoce. *A*, L'endoderma ventrale dell'intestino anteriore acquisisce la competenza a ricevere i segnali provenienti dal mesoderma cardiaco. *B*, Cellule specifiche dell'endoderma ventrale dell'intestino anteriore vanno incontro a specializzazione con l'attivazione di geni epatospecifici sotto l'influenza di segnali mesodermici. *C*, La morfogenesi epatica inizia quando le nuove cellule neospecializzate migrano nel setto trasverso sotto l'influenza di molecole di segnale e della matrice extracellulare, rilasciate dalle cellule mesenchimali del setto trasverso, e delle cellule endoteliali primitive. (Ristampata da Zaret KS: Liver specification and early morphogenesis. *Mech Dev* 92:83-88; © 2000, per gentile concessione di Elsevier Science.)

TABELLA 351-1. Proteine necessarie per un normale sviluppo epatico nei modelli animali

FATTORI DI CRESCITA E ALTRI LIGANDI
Proteine morfogenetiche dell'osso 2, 4, 7
Fattori di crescita fibroblastici 1, 2, 8
Fattori di crescita epatocitari
Jagged1
Famiglia Wnt
RECETTORI
Flk-1 (recettore del fattore di crescita dell'endotelio vascolare)
Met (recettore del fattore di crescita epatocitario)
Notch2 (recettore Jagged1)
PROTEINCHINASI
IκB chinasi γ (IKBKB; IKBKG o NEMO)
IκB chinasi β (IKBKB)
Proteinchinasi chinasi attivata da mitogeni 4
FATTORI DI TRASCRIZIONE
Foxa1 (fattore nucleare epatocitario-3α)
Foxa2 (fattore nucleare epatocitario-3β)
Foxf1
GATA-4
TCF2 (fattore nucleare epatocitario-1β)
Fattore nucleare epatocitario-4α
Fattore nucleare epatocitario-6
Hes1
Hex
Hlx
Jun/AP-1
Fattore di trascrizione di regolazione del metallo 1
NF-κB p65 subunità (RelA)
N-myc
Prox1
Proteina legante X-box 1

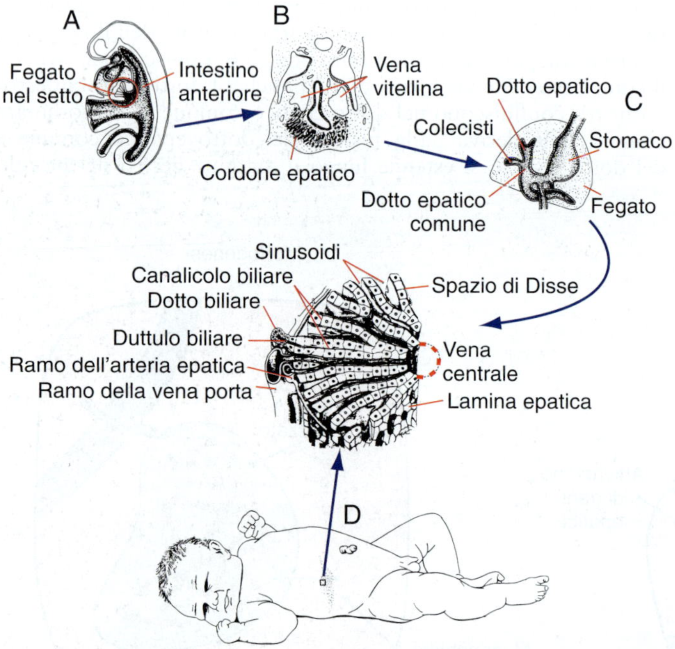

Figura 351-2. Morfogenesi epatica. *A*, Crescita ventrale del diverticolo epatico dall'endoderma dell'intestino anteriore nell'embrione di 3-5 settimane. *B*, Tra le due vene vitelline, dal diverticolo epatico che si sta sviluppando gemmano corde epiteliali (epatiche) che andranno a formare il parenchima epatico, intorno a cui si allinea l'endotelio dei capillari (sinusoidi) (embrione di 4 settimane). *C*, Emisezione di un embrione di 7,5 settimane che dimostra la canalizzazione del tratto biliare. *D*, Rappresentazione tridimensionale del lobulo epatico così come si presenta nel neonato. (Ristampata da Andres JM, Mathis RK, Walker WA: Liver disease in infants. Part I: Developmental hepatology and mechanisms of liver dysfunction. *J Pediatr* 1977;90:686-697.)

omento, terminando nel duodeno a livello della papilla intramurale di Vater. L'unione delle vie biliari con i dotti pancreatici forma l'ampolla di Vater, che, tramite lo sfintere di Oddi, regola il flusso di bile nell'intestino, impedisce il reflusso biliare nel dotto pancreatico e il reflusso di contenuto intestinale nei dotti.

Nel feto il flusso sanguigno epatico deriva dall'arteria epatica e dalle vena porta e ombelicale, che formano il seno portale. Il flusso venoso portale è diretto principalmente al lobo epatico destro, il flusso ombelicale soprattutto al sinistro. Il dotto venoso cortocircuita il sangue dalla vena porta e ombelicale verso la vena epatica, evitando così il sistema sinusoidale. Dopo la nascita, con l'inizio dell'alimentazione orale, il dotto venoso si oblitera. Poiché la saturazione di ossigeno, nel feto, è inferiore nel sangue portale rispetto a quello ombelicale, il lobo epatico destro riceve una minore ossigenazione e presenta una maggiore attività ematopoietica rispetto al sinistro. L'endotelio sinusoidale fetale è inoltre sede di grandi macrofagi che formeranno la rete di cellule di Kupffer (reticoloendoteliali).

Il trasporto e le attività metaboliche epatiche sono facilitate dalla struttura dei cordoni epatocitari, formati da file di epatociti, separate dai sinusoidi, che convergono verso rami tributari della vena epatica (vena centrale), situati al centro del lobulo (vedi Fig. 351-2*D*). Questa struttura determina il percorso e la direzione del flusso delle sostanze da e per il fegato. Oltre all'apporto arterioso della circolazione sistemica, il fegato riceve anche un apporto venoso dal tratto gastrointestinale, tramite il sistema portale. Il rilascio dei prodotti del sistema epatobiliare avviene per due vie diverse: attraverso la vena epatica nella circolazione sistemica, e attraverso il vie biliari di nuovo all'intestino. Le proteine plasmatiche e altri componenti del plasma sono secreti dal fegato. I nutrienti assorbiti ed entrati in circolo arrivano tramite la circolazione portale o l'arteria epatica e passano nella circolazione sistemica attraverso i sinusoidi e gli epatociti, a livello della vena centrale. I componenti della bile sono trasportati dai canalicoli biliari, tramite una serie di canali di diametro progressivamente maggiore, attraverso i duttuli biliari fino al dotto biliare comune.

La secrezione biliare si osserva a partire dalla 12ª settimana di gestazione. I componenti principali della bile variano a seconda dello stadio di sviluppo. In prossimità del parto, il contenuto di colesterolo e fosfolipidi è relativamente basso; la bassa concentrazione di acidi biliari, l'assenza di acidi di derivazione batterica (secondari) e la presenza di acidi biliari inusuali rispecchiano i bassi livelli di flusso biliare e l'immaturità della via sintetica degli acidi biliari.

Il fegato raggiunge le sue massime dimensioni relative verso la 9ª settimana, con il 10% circa del peso fetale. Nelle prime fasi dello sviluppo, quest'organo è una sede fondamentale di ematopoiesi; alla 7ª settimana le cellule ematopoietiche sono numericamente superiori agli epatociti funzionanti, nell'abbozzo epatico. Gli epatociti primitivi sono più piccoli di quelli maturi (circa 20 μm vs 30-35 μm) e contengono meno glicogeno. In prossimità del termine, la massa epatocitaria si espande fino a diventare predominante, con un parallelo aumento della dimensione e del contenuto di glicogeno cellulare. L'ematopoiesi è virtualmente assente durante il 2° mese di vita extrauterina, nel neonato a termine. Mentre la densità epatocitaria aumenta, con l'avanzare dell'età gestazionale, il volume relativo della rete sinusoidale diminuisce. Il fegato costituisce il 5% del peso corporeo alla nascita e solo il 2% nell'adulto.

Nel neonato sano, diversi processi metabolici sono ancora immaturi, in parte a causa del permanere di un'attività di tipo fetale in vari processi enzimatici. Nel feto molte funzioni epatiche sono svolte dal fegato materno, che fornisce i nutrienti e funge da via di smaltimento dei sottoprodotti metabolici e delle tossine. Il metabolismo del fegato fetale è volto principalmente alla produzione di proteine necessarie alla crescita. Prima del termine, le funzioni principali diventano la produzione e l'accumulo di nutrienti essenziali, l'escrezione di bile e la formazione di un processo di eliminazione. L'adattamento extrauterino richiede la sintesi di enzimi *ex novo*; la modulazione di tali processi dipende dall'apporto placentare di substrati e ormoni, dalla dieta e dagli stimoli ormonali nel periodo postnatale.

ULTRASTRUTTURA EPATICA

Gli epatociti presentano diverse caratteristiche ultrastrutturali che riflettono la loro funzione biologica (Fig. 351-3). Come le altre cellule epiteliali, essi sono polarizzati, ovvero la struttura e la funzione sono orientate in una data direzione. Una conseguenza di questo fenomeno è che le diverse zone della membrana plasmatica epatocitaria possiedono funzioni specializzate. A livello della superficie sinusoidale si verifica un trasporto bidirezionale, con l'entrata nell'epatocita dei substrati che raggiungono il fegato passando per il sistema portale, e l'uscita dei composti secreti a livello epatico. La membrana canalicolare degli epatociti adiacenti forma i canalicoli biliari, collegati tra loro tramite *tight junctions* (giunzioni serrate) in modo da impedire il reflusso nei sinusoidi dei composti secreti. All'interno degli epatociti, l'attività metabolica e sintetica è localizzata in diversi organuli subcellulari. L'ossidazione e il metabolismo di classi eterogenee di substrati, l'ossidazione degli acidi grassi, i processi chiave della gluconeogenesi e l'immagazzinamento e il rilascio di energia si svolgono nei numerosi mitocondri degli epatociti. Il reticolo endoplasmatico (RE), una rete continua formata da tubuli a superficie rugosa e liscia e da cisterne, è sede di vari processi, tra cui la sintesi di proteine e trigliceridi e il metabolismo dei farmaci. Alla bassa attività fetale degli enzimi del RE è dovuta l'insufficienza relativa del metabolismo degli xenobiotici (farmaci). L'apparato di Golgi svolge un'attività di ripiegamento delle proteine e forse anche di secrezione biliare. I perossisomi epatocitari, organuli citoplasmatici delimitati da una membrana singola, contengono enzimi quali ossidasi e catalasi, e partecipano al metabolismo di lipidi e acidi biliari. I lisosomi contengono numerose idrolasi, attive nella digestione intracellulare. Il citoscheletro epatocitario, composto di actina e altri filamenti, è distribuito in tutta la cellula ma si concentra soprattutto in prossimità della membrana plasmatica. I microfilamenti e i microtubuli entrano in gioco nell'endocitosi recettore-mediata, nella secrezione biliare e nel mantenimento dell'architettura e della motilità.

FUNZIONI METABOLICHE DEL FEGATO

METABOLISMO DEI CARBOIDRATI. Il fegato regola i livelli sierici di glucosio, immagazzinando i carboidrati in eccesso sotto forma di glicogeno, un polimero del glucosio che, nei periodi di digiuno, viene rapidamente idrolizzato a glucosio. Per mantenere adeguati livelli sierici di glucosio, gli epatociti producono glucosio libero grazie sia alla glicogenolisi, sia alla gluconeogenesi. Nei primi momenti dopo la nascita, il neonato dipende completamente dalla glicogenolisi epatica. L'attività gluconeogenetica è infatti presente a livelli molto bassi, nel fegato fetale, e aumenta rapidamente dopo la nascita. La sintesi di glicogeno, nel feto, inizia intorno alla 9ª settimana di gestazione, con un più rapido accumulo di depositi di glicogeno con l'approssimarsi del termine, quando il fegato contiene da due a tre volte la quantità di glicogeno del fegato adulto. La maggior parte del glicogeno accumulato è utilizzato nell'immediato periodo postnatale. L'accumulo riprende dalla 2ª settimana di vita extrauterina e i depositi raggiungono gli stessi livelli dell'adulto verso la 3ª settimana, nei neonati sani a termine. Le fluttuazioni dei livelli sierici di glucosio nei neonati pretermine sono in parte causate dal fatto che una regolazione efficiente della sintesi, dell'accumulo e della degradazione del glicogeno si sviluppa solo verso la fine di una gravidanza a termine. I carboidrati alimentari, come il galattosio, sono convertiti a glucosio, ma nei primi giorni di vita il neonato dipende sostanzialmente dalla gluconeogenesi, in particolare se i depositi di glicogeno sono limitati.

METABOLISMO PROTEICO. Durante la fase di rapida crescita fetale, rispetto al fegato maturo si osservano livelli più elevati di decarbossilasi specifiche, enzimi limitanti nei confronti della biosintesi di importanti poliamine. Durante lo sviluppo epatico, la velocità

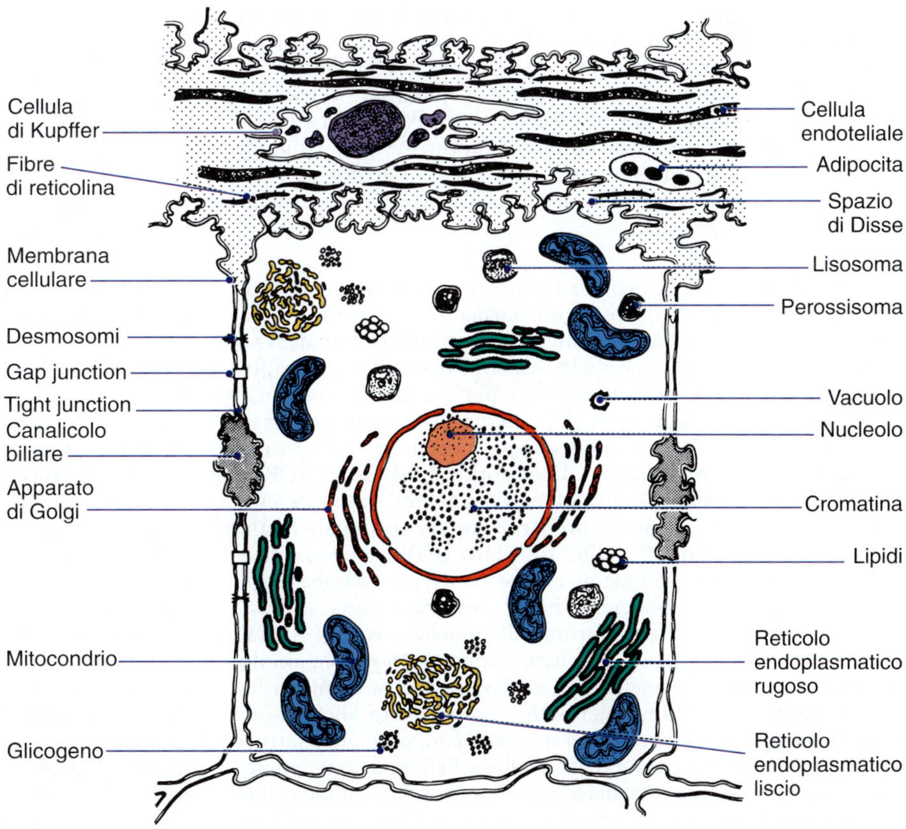

Figura 351-3. Veduta schematica dell'ultrastruttura e degli organuli epatocitari. (Ristampata da Sherlock S: Hepatic cell structure. In Sherlock S [editor]: *Diseases of the Liver and Biliary System*, 6th ed. Oxford, Blackwell Scientific, 1981, p 10; per gentile concessione di Blackwell Scientific.)

di sintesi dell'albumina e delle proteine secretorie è direttamente proporzionale alle variazioni quantitative del reticolo endoplasmatico. Nel feto umano la sintesi di albumina compare intorno alla 7ª-8ª settimana di gestazione e il suo aumento è inversamente proporzionale a quella di α-fetoproteina, che rappresenta la proteina fetale predominante. Intorno al 3°-4° mese di gestazione, il fegato fetale è in grado di produrre fibrinogeno, transferrina e lipoproteine a bassa densità. A partire da questo periodo, il plasma fetale contiene tutte le principali classi di proteine, a concentrazioni molto inferiori rispetto a quelle raggiunte con la maturità.

L'andamento *postnatale* della sintesi proteica varia a seconda del tipo di proteina. Le lipoproteine di tutte le classi aumentano bruscamente nella prima settimana dopo la nascita, fino a raggiungere livelli che poi rimarranno invariati fino alla pubertà. La concentrazione di albumina nel neonato è bassa (circa 2,5 g/dL), e raggiunge i livelli propri dell'adulto (circa 3,5 g/dL) dopo diversi mesi. I livelli di ceruloplasmina e di fattori del complemento aumentano lentamente, fino ai valori adulti, nel corso del primo anno. Al contrario, i livelli di transferrina alla nascita sono simili a quelli dell'età adulta, si riducono per 3-5 mesi e aumentano nuovamente fino a raggiungere la concentrazione finale. La scarsa attività di proteine specifiche si ripercuote sulla nutrizione del bambino; un'insufficiente attività della cistationina γ-liasi (cistationasi) compromette la via di trans-solforazione tramite la quale la metionina introdotta con gli alimenti viene convertita a cisteina; quest'ultima deve quindi essere fornita con la dieta. Analoghe necessità di supplementazione dietetica possono sussistere per altri aminoacidi contenenti zolfo, come la taurina.

METABOLISMO LIPIDICO. L'ossidazione degli acidi grassi fornisce la principale fonte di energia nei primi momenti di vita, insieme alla glicogenolisi e alla gluconeogenesi. I neonati sono relativamente intolleranti al digiuno prolungato, in parte a causa di una ridotta capacità di chetogenesi epatica. Nei primi giorni di vita si verifica una rapida maturazione della capacità epatica di ossidare gli acidi grassi. Nel neonato il latte rappresenta la principale fonte di calorie: questa dieta ricca di lipidi e povera di carboidrati necessita di un'attiva gluconeogenesi per mantenere adeguati livelli ematici di glucosio. In presenza di un apporto di glucosio limitato, la produzione di corpi chetonici a partire dagli acidi grassi endogeni può fornire l'energia per la gluconeogenesi epatica e un substrato alternativo per il metabolismo cerebrale. Quando i carboidrati sono in eccesso, il fegato produce trigliceridi. La concentrazione di lipidi e lipoproteine può risultare compromessa nel fegato immaturo o in corso di epatopatie, dal momento che i relativi processi metabolici avvengono prevalentemente a livello epatico.

BIOTRASFORMAZIONE. I neonati hanno una ridotta capacità di metabolizzare e detossificare alcuni farmaci, a causa di un insufficiente sviluppo della componente epatica microsomiale, che costituisce la sede delle specifiche reazioni di ossidazione, riduzione, idrolisi e coniugazione richieste per queste biotrasformazioni. I principali componenti del sistema delle monossigenasi, come il citocromo P450, la citocromo-*c* reduttasi e la forma ridotta del nicotinamide adenin dinucleotide difosfato (NADPH, *Nicotinamide-Adenine Dinucleotide Phosphate*) sono presenti a basse concentrazioni nelle preparazioni microsomiali fetali. Nei neonati a termine, l'uridina difosfato (UDP) glucoronosiltransferasi epatica e gli enzimi coinvolti nell'ossidazione degli idrocarburi aromatici policiclici hanno una bassissima attività. Sono riscontrabili differenze farmacodinamiche correlate all'età, che variano da un composto all'altro. L'emivita del paracetamolo nel neonato è simile a quella dell'adulto, mentre la teofillina ha un'emivita di circa 100 ore nel prematuro, rispetto alle 5-6 ore nell'adulto. Queste differenze nel metabolismo, così come fattori quali il legame alle proteine plasmatiche e l'eliminazione renale, determinano il dosaggio farmacologico appropriato, onde evitare fenomeni di tossicità. Esempi drammatici della suscettibilità dei neonati alla tossicità dei farmaci sono la risposta al cloramfenicolo (sindrome del bambino grigio) o all'alcol benzolico e ai suo prodotti metabolici, che comportano una coniugazione inefficiente del glucuronile e della glicina, rispettivamente. Le basse concentrazioni di antiossidanti (vitamina E, superossido dismutasi, glutatione perossidasi), nel fegato del feto e del neonato, comportano un'aumentata suscettibilità agli effetti nocivi dell'ossigeno e al danno ossidativo mediato dalla perossidazione lipidica.

Le reazioni di coniugazione, che convertono i farmaci o i metaboliti in forme idrosolubili, eliminabili con la bile, sono anch'esse catalizzate dagli enzimi microsomiali epatici. I neonati hanno una ridotta attività dell'UDP glucoroniltransferasi, che converte la bilirubina non coniugata nel coniugato glucuronico facilmente eliminabile e che costituisce l'enzima limitante nei confronti dell'escrezione di bilirubina. Dopo la nascita si assiste a un rapido sviluppo dell'attività della transferasi, indipendentemente dall'età gestazionale, fenomeno che suggerisce la predominanza di fattori correlati alla nascita, più che all'età gestazionale, nell'aumento postnatale dell'attività di tale enzima. L'attività dei microsomi può essere stimolata con la somministrazione di fenobarbital, rifampicina o altri induttori del citocromo P450. Al contrario, farmaci come la cimetidina possono inibire l'attività microsomiale del citocromo P450.

FUNZIONE ESCRETORIA EPATICA. La funzione escretoria epatica e la produzione di bile sono strettamente correlate all'escrezione e al ricircolo degli acidi biliari. Gli acidi biliari, il principale prodotto della degradazione del colesterolo, sono incorporati, con colesterolo e fosfolipidi, in micelle miste che fungono da veicolo per la solubilizzazione e l'assorbimento intestinale dei composti lipofilici, come i grassi alimentari e le vitamine liposolubili. La secrezione di acidi biliari è il principale determinante del flusso biliare, nell'animale maturo. Pertanto, la maturità dei processi metabolici relativi agli acidi biliari influenza la funzione escretoria epatica nel suo complesso, compresa l'escrezione biliare di composti endogeni ed esogeni.

Nell'uomo è a livello epatico che avviene la sintesi dei due acidi biliari primari, l'acido colico e l'acido chenodesossicolico. Questi ultimi, prima dell'escrezione, sono coniugati con glicina e taurina. In risposta al pasto, la contrazione della colecisti fa arrivare gli acidi biliari all'intestino per facilitare la digestione e l'assorbimento dei lipidi. Dopo aver mediato la digestione dei grassi, gli stessi acidi biliari sono riassorbiti nell'ileo terminale tramite processi di trasporto attivo specifico. Ritornano poi al fegato attraverso la circolazione portale, per essere captati dagli epatociti e nuovamente escreti nella bile. Nell'adulto, questa circolazione enteroepatica riguarda il 90-95% del pool di acidi biliari circolanti. Quelli che sfuggono al riassorbimento ileale raggiungono il colon, dove la flora batterica, tramite processi di deidrossilazione e deconiugazione, produce gli acidi biliari secondari, desossicolico e litocolico. Nell'adulto, la composizione della bile rispecchia l'escrezione non solo degli acidi biliari primari, ma anche di quelli secondari, riassorbiti nel tratto distale dell'intestino.

I neonati hanno un riassorbimento ileale di acidi grassi poco efficiente e una bassa velocità di eliminazione epatica dal sangue portale: di conseguenza, i soggetti sani presentano elevate concentrazioni di acidi biliari nel siero, spesso a livelli che sarebbero suggestivi di epatopatia in individui più grandi. Il pool di acidi biliari nel neonato è circa la metà di quello dell'adulto, e la concentrazione di acidi biliari nel lume dell'intestino prossimale è parimenti ridotta, a livelli spesso inferiori a quelli necessari per la formazione di micelle (2 mM); pertanto, l'assorbimento dei grassi alimentari e delle vitamine liposolubili è ridotto, sebbene non al punto da causare malassorbimento. Le fasi transitorie di "colestasi fisiologica" e di "steatorrea fisiologica" hanno un ruolo nella nutrizione dei neonati di basso peso, ma sono di minor importanza per i neonati sani a termine. Dopo il periodo neonatale, le alterazioni del metabolismo degli acidi grassi possono essere responsabili di diversi effetti sulla funzione epatobiliare e intestinale (Tab. 351-2).

TABELLA 351-2. Cause di alterato metabolismo degli acidi biliari e della circolazione enteroepatica

DEFICIT DELLA SINTESI E DEL TRASPORTO DEGLI ACIDI BILIARI
Errori congeniti della sintesi degli acidi biliari (deficit di reduttasi, deficit di isomerasi)
Colestasi intraepatica progressiva famigliare (PFIC, *Progressive Familial Intrahepatic Cholestasis*, 1, 2, 3)
Colestasi intraepatica (epatite neonatale)
Difetti acquisiti della sintesi degli acidi biliari secondari a danno epatico severo
ANOMALIE DEL TRASPORTO DEGLI ACIDI BILIARI ALL'INTESTINO
Malattia celiaca (contrazione lenta della colecisti)
Ostruzione extraepatica del dotto biliare (per es. atresia biliare, litiasi)
PERDITA DELLA CIRCOLAZIONE ENTEROEPATICA DEGLI ACIDI BILIARI
Fistola biliare esterna
Fibrosi cistica
Sindrome da contaminazione batterica dell'intestino tenue (con precipitazione degli acidi biliari, aumentato assorbimento digiunale e "corto circuito")
Intrappolamento degli acidi biliari nel lume intestinale indotto da farmaci (per es. colestiramina)
MALASSORBIMENTO DEGLI ACIDI BILIARI
Malassorbimento primario degli acidi biliari (assente o inefficace trasporto attivo ileale)
Malassorbimento secondario degli acidi biliari
Patologia o resezione dell'ileo
Fibrosi cistica
DEFICIT DELLA CAPTAZIONE O ALTERATO METABOLISMO INTRACELLULARE
Patologie parenchimali (epatite acuta, cirrosi)
Rigurgito cellulale
Shunt portosistemico
Colestasi

Bates MD, Balistreri WF: The gastrointestinal tract: Development of the human digestive system. In Fanaroff AA, Martin RJ (editors): *Neonatal-Perinatal Medicine: Diseases of the Fetus and Infant*, 7th ed. St. Louis, Mosby, 2002, pp 1255–1263.

Beath SV: Hepatic function and physiology in the newborn. *Semin Neonatol* 2003;8:337–346.

Costa RH, Kalinichencko VV, Holterman AL, Wang X: Transcription factors in liver development, differentiation, and regeneration. *Hepatology* 2003;38:1331–1347.

Desmet VJ: Congenital diseases of intrahepatic bile ducts: Variations on the theme "ductal plate malformation." *Hepatology* 1992;16:1069–1083.

Karpen SJ, Suchy FJ: Structural and functional development of the liver. In Suchy FJ, Sokol RJ, Balistreri WF (editors): *Liver Disease in Children*, 2nd ed. Philadelphia, Lippincott Williams and Wilkins, 2001, pp 3–21.

Lemaigre F, Zaret KS: Liver development update: New embryo models, cell lineage control, and morphogenesis. *Curr Opin Genet Dev* 2004;14:582–590.

Meier PJ, Stieger B: Molecular mechanisms of bile formation. *News Physiol Sci* 2000;15:89–93.

Rudolph AM: Hepatic and ductus venosus blood flows during fetal life. *Hepatology* 1983;3:254–258.

Shneider BL: Intestinal bile acid transport: Biology, physiology, and pathophysiology. *J Pediatr Gastroenterol Nutr* 2001;32:407–417.

Zaret KS: Regulatory phases of early liver development: Paradigms of organogenesis. *Nat Rev Genet* 2002;3:499–512.

Capitolo 352 ■ Manifestazioni delle epatopatie

Lynelle Boamah e William F. Balistreri

Le epatopatie spesso rappresentano un pericolo per la vita e un'insidia diagnostica. La presentazione clinica varia a seconda dell'eziologia e della gravità dell'insulto epatico. La conoscenza delle possibili manifestazioni, unitamente a un elevato indice di sospetto e all'impiego di capacità diagnostico-cliniche, sono il primo passo nell'identificazione di queste patologie in età pediatrica.

ANATOMIA PATOLOGICA

Le alterazioni della struttura e della funzione epatica possono essere acute o croniche, con diversi quadri di reazione epatica all'insulto cellulare. Il danno epatico può comportare l'infiltrazione da parte di cellule infiammatorie o la morte cellulare (necrosi), a sua volta seguita da processi riparativi con formazioni di cicatrici (fibrosi) e, potenzialmente, dalla formazione di noduli di rigenerazione. La cirrosi è il risultato finale di qualsiasi tipo di danno epatico progressivo.

L'insulto a carico dei singoli epatociti può essere dovuto a un'infezione virale, farmaci o tossine, ipossia, disordini immunologici o errori congeniti del metabolismo. Il processo evolutivo può portare alla riparazione, alla persistenza dell'insulto con alterazioni croniche, o, in rari casi, a un danno epatico massivo.

La **colestasi** è una risposta alternativa o concomitante al danno causato da ostruzione extraepatica o intraepatica al flusso biliare. Nel siero si accumulano sostanze normalmente escrete con la bile, come bilirubina coniugata, colesterolo, acidi biliari e oligoelementi. L'accumulo di pigmenti biliari, nel parenchima epatico, è visibile nei reperti bioptici. Nell'ostruzione extraepatica, il pigmento biliare può essere visibile nei dotti biliari intralobulari e in tutto il parenchima, sotto forma di laghi o infarti biliari. Nella colestasi intraepatica, un danno epatocitario o un'alterazione della fisiologia epatica comportano una riduzione della velocità di secrezione di soluti e acqua. Le cause più probabili sono alterazioni dell'attività di trasporto enzimatica o canalicolare, della permeabilità dell'apparato canalicolare biliare, degli organuli responsabili della secrezione biliare o dell'ultrastruttura del citoscheletro epatocitario. Il risultato finale può essere clinicamente indistinguibile dalla colestasi ostruttiva.

La **cirrosi**, definita istologicamente dalla presenza di bande di tessuto fibroso che collegano le aree portali e centrali formando noduli parenchimali, potenzialmente rappresenta lo stadio finale di qualunque epatopatia acuta o cronica. Può essere *postepatitica* (dopo un'epatite acuta o cronica) o *postnecrotica* (dopo un danno tossico), oppure derivare da un'ostruzione biliare cronica (*cirrosi biliare*). Se ne distinguono inoltre una forma macronodulare, con noduli di diverse dimensioni (fino a 5 cm) separati da larghi setti, o micronodulare, con noduli di dimensioni uniformi (<1 cm) separati da setti più fini; possono verificarsi anche forme miste. La progressiva cicatrizzazione caratteristica della cirrosi porta a un alterato flusso ematico, con conseguente aggravamento del danno funzionale epatocitario. Inoltre, l'aumentata resistenza al flusso ematico portale sfocia in un quadro di ipertensione portale.

I tumori primitivi del fegato sono trattati nel Capitolo 504. Quest'organo può essere coinvolto secondariamente in processi neoplastici (metastasi) o non neoplastici (malattie da accumulo, infiltrazione grassa), così come in numerose condizioni sistemiche e malattie infettive, oltre a essere interessato dalla congestione cronica passiva o dall'ipossia acuta, con danno epatocellulare.

MANIFESTAZIONI CLINICHE

EPATOMEGALIA. L'ingrandimento del fegato può essere causato da diversi meccanismi (Tab. 352-1). La stima delle dimensioni epatiche normali si basa su indici clinici correlati all'età, come il grado di estensione del margine epatico sotto il margine costale, l'ampiezza dell'ottusità alla percussione e la lunghezza dell'asse verticale del fegato, stimata mediante tecniche di imaging. Nei bambini, il bordo del fegato può essere palpato normalmente fino a 2 cm dal margine costale. Nel neonato, la sua estensione oltre i 3,5 cm al di sotto del margine costale, sulla linea emiclaverare mediana, è suggestiva di epatomegalia. L'ampiezza del fegato viene valutata tramite percussione, che permette di rilevare il margine superiore dell'ottusità, e mediante palpazione del margine inferiore, a livello della linea emiclaveare destra; questa stima può essere più affidabile della sola rilevazione dell'estensione del bordo epatico; tra le due misurazioni può esservi scarsa correlazione.

L'ampiezza del fegato aumenta linearmente con il peso corporeo e l'età in entrambi i sessi, andando da 4,5-5 cm a una

TABELLA 352-1. Cause di epatomegalia

AUMENTO DEL NUMERO O DELLE DIMENSIONI DELLE CELLULE EPATICHE INTRINSECHE

Accumulo

- Grasso: malnutrizione, obesità, malattie metaboliche del fegato (anomalie dell'ossidazione degli acidi grassi e malattie tipo sindrome di Reye), infusione di lipidi (nutrizione parenterale totale), fibrosi cistica, diabete mellito, farmaci, gravidanza
- Patologie da accumulo di lipidi specifici: malattie di Gaucher, Niemann-Pick, Wolman
- Glicogeno: glicogenosi (difetti enzimatici multipli); nutrizione parenterale totale; nati da madre diabetica; sindrome di Beckwith
- Altro: deficit di α_1-antitripsina, malattia di Wilson, ipervitaminosi A, emocromatosi neonatale

Infiammazione

- Aumento di volume degli epatociti (epatite)
  - Virale: acuta e cronica
  - Batterica: sepsi, ascessi, colangite
  - Tossica: farmaci
  - Autoimmune
- Aumento di volume delle cellule di Kupffer
  - Sarcoidosi
  - Lupus eritematoso sistemico
  - Sindrome da attivazione mastocitaria

INFILTRAZIONE CELLULARE

Tumori epatici primitivi

- Benigni
  - Epatocellulari
    - Iperplasia nodulare focale
    - Iperplasia nodulare rigenerativa
    - Adenoma epatocellulare
  - Mesodermici
    - Emangioendotelioma infantile
    - Amartoma mesenchimale
  - Masse cistiche
    - Cisti del coledoco
    - Cisti epatica
    - Ematoma
    - Cisti parassitaria
    - Ascesso piogenico o amebico
- Maligni
  - Epatocellulari
    - Epatoblastoma
    - Carcinoma epatocellulare
  - Mesodermici
    - Angiosarcoma
    - Sarcoma embrionario indifferenziato
  - Processi secondari o metastatici
    - Linfoma
    - Leucemia
    - Istiocitosi
    - Neuroblastoma
    - Tumore di Wilms

AUMENTO DI VOLUME DEL COMPARTO VASCOLARE

- Ostruzione intraepatica del deflusso venoso epatico
  - Malattia veno-occlusiva
  - Trombosi delle vene epatiche (sindrome di Budd-Chiari)
  - Stenosi delle vene epatiche
- Organi sovraepatici
  - Scompenso cardiaco congestizio
  - Malattie del pericardio
  - Tamponamento cardiaco
- Pericardite costrittiva
- Malattie ematologiche: anemia falciforme, talassemia

AUMENTO DI VOLUME DEL COMPARTO BILIARE

- Fibrosi epatica congenita
- Malattia di Caroli
- Ostruzione extraepatica

IDIOPATICA ("BENIGNA"?)

settimana di vita fino a 7-8 cm nei bambini e 6,0-6,5 cm nelle bambine di 12 anni. Il margine inferiore del lobo epatico destro si estende verso il basso (lobo di Riedel) ed è palpabile come una grande massa in alcuni individui normali. Talvolta nei pazienti con cirrosi è possibile palpare il lobo epatico sinistro, aumentato di volume, a livello epigastrico. Lo spostamento verso il basso del fegato, per la pressione esercitata dal diaframma (iperinflazione) o degli organi toracici, può creare un'erronea impressione di epatomegalia.

L'esame obiettivo del fegato deve valutare la consistenza, il contorno, la dolorabilità e la presenza di masse o soffi, oltre a comprendere una stima delle dimensioni della milza. È inoltre importante documentare la presenza di ascite o di altri segni di epatopatia cronica.

L'ecografia è utile per valutare dimensioni e consistenza del fegato e della colecisti. Nelle patologie metaboliche (glicogenosi) e nella steatosi epatica (obesità, malnutrizione, iperalimentazione, steroidi) si osserva iperecogenicità del parenchima epatico.

La lunghezza della colecisti varia di norma da 1,5-5,5 cm (in media 3,0) nei lattanti a 4-8 cm negli adolescenti; la larghezza va da 0,5 a 2,5 cm per tutte le età. Nei lattanti con sepsi si può osservare distensione della colecisti, che risulta invece assente nei soggetti con atresia biliare.

ITTERO. La colorazione giallastra delle sclera, della cute e delle mucose è un segno di iperbilirubinemia (vedi Capitolo 102.3). L'ittero clinicamente evidente, nei bambini e negli adulti, si verifica quando la concentrazione di bilirubina nel siero raggiunge valori di 2-3 mg/dL (85 μmol/L). L'ittero può essere il segno più precoce, e talvolta l'unico, di disfunzione epatica. Si deve sospettare un'epatopatia nel bambino che appare anche solo lievemente itterico, ma che presenta urine scure e feci chiare. In questi casi è indispensabile un'immediata valutazione diagnostica.

La misurazione della bilirubinemia totale consente di stimare la gravità dell'ittero. La bilirubina si trova nel plasma in quattro forme: forma non coniugata, strettamente legata all'albumina; forma libera o non legata (responsabile del kernittero, poiché può attraversare le membrane cellulari); forma coniugata (l'unica frazione che può essere presente nelle urine); frazione δ (bilirubina legata con legami covalenti all'albumina), che compare nel siero quando l'escrezione epatica della bilirubina coniugata è compromessa, in pazienti con patologie epatobiliari. Sebbene nell'uso comune le espressioni "bilirubina diretta e indiretta" e "bilirubina coniugata e non coniugata" si equivalgano, questo non è corretto dal punto di vista quantitativo, poiché la frazione diretta comprende sia la bilirubina coniugata sia la frazione δ. In presenza di colestasi di qualsiasi origine, spesso si osserva un aumento concomitante degli acidi biliari.

L'iter diagnostico della colestasi, in un lattante o in un bambino più grande, deve comprendere la determinazione dei livelli di bilirubina coniugata e non coniugata. Un'iperbilirubinemia prevalentemente non coniugata può essere indicativa di aumentata produzione, emolisi, ridotta eliminazione epatica o alterazioni del metabolismo della bilirubina (Tab. 352-2). L'aumento della bilirubina coniugata rispecchia invece una ridotta escrezione, a causa di un danno delle cellule parenchimali epatiche, o una patologia delle vie biliari, dovuta a ostruzione, sepsi, tossine, infiammazione, patologie genetiche o metaboliche (Tab. 352-3).

PRURITO. Un prurito intenso e generalizzato, spesso accompagnato da escoriazioni cutanee, può essere un sintomo di colestasi (aumento della bilirubina coniugata). Questo sintomo non è correlato con il grado di iperbilirubinemia; un paziente intensamente itterico può essere asintomatico. Sebbene i componenti della bile accumulati siano importanti, la patogenesi è verosimilmente multifattoriale, come dimostra la riduzione del prurito in risposta alla somministrazione di farmaci diversi, tra cui agenti sequestranti degli acidi biliari (colestiramina), coleretici (acido ursodesossicolico), antagonisti degli oppiacei, antistaminici e antibiotici. La diversione chirurgica della bile (diversione biliare esterna parziale) può dare sollievo al prurito refrattario alla terapia medica.

TABELLA 352-2. Diagnosi differenziale dell'iperbilirubinemia non coniugata

AUMENTATA PRODUZIONE DI BILIRUBINA NON CONIUGATA A PARTIRE DALL'EME
Emolisi (patologie ereditarie o acquisite)
Emolisi isoimmune (neonatale; reazione acuta o ritardata a trasfusioni; autoimmune)
Incompatibilità Rh
Incompatibilità ABO
Incompatibilità per altri gruppi sanguigni
Sferocitosi congenita
Ellissocitosi ereditaria
Picnocitosi infantile
Difetti enzimatici infantili
Emoglobinopatie
Anemia falciforme
Talassemia
Altre
Sepsi
Microangiopatie
Sindrome emolitico-uremica
Emangioma
Trauma meccanico (valvola cardiaca)
Eritropoiesi inefficace
Farmaci
Infezioni
Ematoma ritenuto
Policitemia
Diabete materno
Trasfusione fetale (ricevente)
Ritardata chiusura del cordone
RIDOTTO APPORTO DI BILIRUBINA NON CONIUGATA (NEL PLASMA) ALL'EPATOCITA
Scompenso cardiaco congestizio destro
Shunt portocavale
RIDOTTA CAPTAZIONE DELLA BILIRUBINA ATTRAVERSO LA MEMBRANA EPATOCITARIA
Deficit degli enzimi di trasporto (presunto)
Inibizione competitiva
Ittero da latte materno
Sindrome di Lucey-Driscoll
Inibizione da farmaci (mezzi di contrasto radiologici)
Altre
Ipotiroidismo
Ipossia
Acidosi
RIDOTTO ACCUMULO DI BILIRUBINA NON CONIUGATA NEL CITOPLASMA (RIDUZIONE DELLE PROTEINE Y E Z)
Inibizione competitiva
Febbre
RIDOTTA BIOTRASFORMAZIONE (CONIUGAZIONE)
Ittero neonatale (fisiologico)
Inibizione (farmaci)
Ereditaria (sindrome di Crigler-Najjar)
Tipo I (deficit enzimatico completo)
Tipo II (deficit parziale)
Morbo di Gilbert
Disfunzione epatocellulare
RICIRCOLO ENTEROEPATICO
Ittero da latte materno
Ostruzione intestinale
Atresia ileale
Morbo di Hirschsprung
Fibrosi cistica
Stenosi pilorica
Somministrazione di antibiotici

SPIDER NAEVI. Gli angiomi aracniformi (teleangectasie), caratterizzati da un'arteriola centrale pulsante da cui si irradiano venule filiformi, sono un segno caratteristico di epatopatia cronica; in genere più evidenti sul viso e sul torace, è probabile riflettano l'alterato metabolismo degli estrogeni conseguente alla disfunzione epatica.

ERITEMA PALMARE. Nei pazienti con epatopatia cronica si osserva anche un eritema maculare, più evidente sull'eminenza tenar e

TABELLA 352-3. Diagnosi differenziale della colestasi neonatale e infantile

INFETTIVA
Sepsi batterica generalizzata
Epatite virale
Epatite A, B, C (rara)
Cytomegalovirus
Virus della rosolia
Virus erpetici: HSV, HHV 6 e 7
Virus della varicella
Coxsackievirus
Echovirus
Reovirus di tipo 3
Parvovirus B19
HIV
Altre
Toxoplasmosi
Sifilide
Tuberculosi
Listeriosi
TOSSICA
Nutrizione parenterale
Sepsi (tratto urinario) con endotossinemia
Farmaci
METABOLICA
Alterazioni del metabolismo degli aminoacidi
Tirosinemia
Alterazioni del metabolismo lipidico
Malattia di Wolman
Malattia di Niemann-Pick (di tipo C)
Malattia di Gaucher
Alterazioni del metabolismo dei carboidrati
Galattosemia
Fruttosemia
Glicogenosi di tipo IV
Alterazioni della biosintesi degli acidi biliari
Altri difetti metabolici
Deficit di α_1-antitripsina
Fibrosi cistica
Ipopituitarismo idiopatico
Ipotiroidismo
Sindrome di Zellweger (cerebroepatorenale)
Emocromatosi neonatale
Cirrosi indiana infantile/sovraccarico infantile di rame
Alterazioni congenite della glicosilazione
Epatopatie mitocondriali
Deficit di citrina
GENETICA/ALTERAZIONI CROMOSOMICHE
Trisomia E
Sindrome di Down
SINDROMI COLESTATICHE INTRAEPATICHE
Epatite neonatale "idiopatica"
Sindrome di Alagille (displasia arterioepatica)
Colestasi intraepatica familiare progressiva
Colestasi intraepatica ricorrente benigna associata a linfedema (Aagenaes)
Fibrosi epatica congenita
Malattia di Caroli (dilatazione cistica dei dotti intraepatici)
Polimorfismo del gene per il recettore dell'endotossina CD14
PATOLOGIE EXTRAEPATICHE
Atresia biliare
Colangite sclerosante
Stenosi del dotto biliare
Anomalie della giunzione colodoco-dotto pancreatico
Perforazione spontanea del dotto biliare
Cisti del coledoco
Massa (neoplasia, calcolo)
Linfoistiocitosi emofagocitica
Tappi di bile/muco ("sabbia biliare")
ALTRO
Shock e ipoperfusione
Associata a enterite
Associata a ostruzione intestinale
Lupus eritematoso neonatale
Disordini mieloproliferativi (trisomia 21)

ipotenar e sulla punta delle dita. Può essere dovuto a vasodilatazione con aumentato flusso ematico.

XANTOMI. Il notevole aumento dei livelli sierici di colesterolo (>500 mg/dL) che accompagna la colestasi cronica può causare il deposito di lipidi nel derma e nel tessuto sottocutaneo. Possono svilupparsi noduli brunastri, in particolare sulla superficie estensoria delle estremità, mentre è raro che compaiano anche xantelasmi a livello palpebrale.

IPERTENSIONE PORTALE. La vena porta drena il sangue refluo dalla regione splancnica (la porzione addominale del tratto gastrointestinale, il pancreas e la milza) verso i sinusoidi epatici. Il normale gradiente pressorio, ovvero la differenza di pressione tra la vena porta e il sistema venoso sistemico (vene sovraepatiche o vena cava inferiore), è di 36 mmHg. L'ipertensione portale clinicamente significativa compare per gradienti >10 mmHg. L'ipertensione portale è la principale complicanza della cirrosi, direttamente responsabile di due delle sue conseguenze principali e potenzialmente letali: l'ascite e l'emorragia da varici esofagogastriche.

ASCITE. Lo sviluppo di ascite, in un bambino con epatopatia cronica, indica la presenza di due presupposti fondamentali: ipertensione portale e insufficienza epatica. L'ascite può associarsi anche a sindrome nefrosica o altre anomalie nefrologiche, malattie metaboliche (come la malattia dei lisosomi), cardiopatie congenite o acquisite e idrope fetale. I fattori che favoriscono l'accumulo endoaddominale di liquidi comprendono: ridotta pressione colloido-osmotica plasmatica, aumentata pressione idrostatica capillare, aumentata pressione colloido-osmotica nel liquido ascitico, ridotta pressione idrostatica dell'ascite. Si deve inoltre ricordare il ruolo svolto dalla ritenzione anomala renale di sodio (vedi Capitolo 367).

EMORRAGIA DA VARICI. Le varici esofagogastriche rappresentano i collaterali portosistemici più significativi dal punto di vista clinico, in quanto con la loro propensione alla rottura possono causare un'emorragia severa e potenzialmente letale. Tale emorragia è riconducibile a una pressione interna abnorme, in conseguenza della quale aumentano il diametro della varice e la tensione di parete. Quando la pressione supera la forza di parete del vaso, si verifica la rottura fisica della varice. Considerando l'elevato flusso ematico e l'alta pressione che caratterizzano il sistema dei collaterali portosistemici, unitamente alla mancanza di un meccanismo fisiologico di tamponamento dell'emorragia in questa sede, l'entità del sanguinamento da varici può essere impressionante.

ENCEFALOPATIA. L'encefalopatia epatica può coinvolgere qualsiasi funzione neurologica, essere eclatante oppure insorgere in maniera subdola con deterioramento delle prestazioni scolastiche, depressione o crisi emotive. La comparsa di encefalopatia epatica dipende dalla presenza di shunt portosistemici, da alterazioni della barriera ematoencefalica e da interazioni dei metaboliti tossici con il sistema nervoso centrale. Tra le cause ipotizzate, un'alterazione del metabolismo dell'ammonio, neurotossine che agiscono in sinergia o falsi neurotrasmettitori, con squilibri degli aminoacidi plasmatici.

ALTERAZIONI ENDOCRINE. Le alterazione endocrine associate a epatopatia sono più frequenti negli adulti che nei bambini, e riflettono anomalie delle funzioni epatiche relative alla sintesi, all'accumulo e al metabolismo, comprese quelle riguardanti il metabolismo epatico degli ormoni. Nel fegato hanno luogo la sintesi delle proteine plasmatiche che legano gli ormoni e la coniugazione degli ormoni steroidei che verranno escreti nell'urina: la perdita di tali funzioni può avere conseguenze clinicamente rilevanti. La causa di alcune alterazioni endocrine può inoltre essere ricercata nella malnutrizione o in deficit specifici.

DISFUNZIONE RENALE. Alcune malattie sistemiche e determinate tossine possono colpire contemporaneamente sia il fegato sia il rene; talora invece una malattia epatoparenchimale può portare a un'alterazione secondaria della funzione renale. Le patologie epatobiliari possono accompagnarsi ad alterazioni renali del metabolismo del sodio e dell'acqua, compromissione della capacità di concentrazione renale e squilibri del metabolismo del potassio. Lo sviluppo di ascite, nei pazienti con cirrosi, può essere correlato a un'inappropriata ritenzione di sodio da parte dei reni, con espansione del volume plasmatico, o a ritenzione di sodio mediata dalla riduzione del volume plasmatico effettivo. La **sindrome epatorenale** (HRS, *HepatoRenal Syndrome*) è definita come un'insufficienza renale funzionale, in pazienti con epatopatia terminale. La fisiopatologia di questa sindrome, non ancora completamente conosciuta, è caratterizzata da un'intensa vasocostrizione renale (mediata da meccanismi emodinamici, umorali o neurogeni) che si accompagna a vasodilatazione sistemica. La diagnosi è confermata dalla presenza di oliguria (<1 mL/kg/die), un quadro caratteristico di alterazione degli elettroliti urinari (sodio urinario <10 mEq/L, frazione di escrezione del sodio <1%, rapporto creatinina urinaria/plasmatica <10, sedimento urinario normale), dall'assenza di ipovolemia e dall'esclusione di altre patologie renali. Il miglior trattamento della sindrome epatorenale è il trapianto epatico precoce, che può consentire una completa ripresa della funzione renale.

COINVOLGIMENTO POLMONARE. La **sindrome epatopolmonare**, caratterizzata dalla tipica triade ipossiemia, dilatazione vascolare intrapolmonare ed epatopatia, comporta uno shunt di sangue intrapolmonare destro-sinistro, con conseguente desaturazione sistemica. Deve essere sospettata e ricercata nei bambini con epatopatia cronica, che si presentano con dispnea o intolleranza all'esercizio fisico, segni di cianosi all'esame obiettivo (in particolare labiale e digitale), ippocratismo digitale e ridotta saturazione dell'ossigeno (<96%), soprattutto in ortostatismo. Il trattamento di scelta è il trapianto epatico precoce, che porta generalmente alla risoluzione dei sintomi polmonari.

COLANGITE RICORRENTE. L'infezione ascendente delle vie biliari, un evento frequente nelle patologie colestatiche infantili, è per lo più causata da microrganismi intestinali Gram-negativi, come *Escherichia coli*, *Klebsiella*, *Pseudomonas* ed *Enterococcus*. Il trapianto epatico è il trattamento definitivo di scelta, nel bambino con epatopatia colestatica, in particolare nei casi resistenti alla terapia medica.

ALTRE MANIFESTAZIONI DI EPATOPATIA. I segni aspecifici di epatopatia acuta e cronica possono comprendere: anoressia, che spesso colpisce pazienti con epatite anitterica e con cirrosi associata a colestasi cronica; dolore o distensione addominale derivanti da ascite; peritonite batterica spontanea o visceromegalia; malnutrizione e alterazione della crescita; sanguinamenti, dovuti ad alterata sintesi dei fattori della coagulazione (ostruzione biliare con deficit di vitamina K o danno epatico massivo); ipertensione portale con ipersplenismo. In presenza di ipersplenismo, possono verificarsi una ridotta sintesi di specifici fattori della coagulazione, produzione di proteine qualitativamente alterate o riduzione del numero e della funzionalità piastrinica. Un alterato metabolismo dei farmaci può prolungare l'emivita biologica di farmaci di uso comune.

352.1 • VALUTAZIONE DEI PAZIENTI CON POSSIBILE DISFUNZIONE EPATICA

Una valutazione accurata di neonati, bambini o adolescenti con sospetta epatopatia deve comprendere un'anamnesi attenta e appropriata, un esame obiettivo accurato e una lucida interpretazione di segni e sintomi. In seguito, tale valutazione è supportata dalla scelta di test diagnostici, seguita dall'uso di tecniche di imaging adatte o dalla biopsia epatica. La maggior parte dei cosiddetti test di funzionalità epatica non misura specifiche funzioni epatiche: un aumento delle transaminasi rispecchia un danno epatocellulare, un aumento dei livelli di immunoglobuline indica una risposta immunologica a un insulto, mentre l'iperbilirubinemia può essere dovuta a una delle tante possibili alterazioni del metabolismo della bilirubina (vedi Tabb. 352-2 e 352-3). Ciascun esame biochimico considerato singolarmente è in grado di fornire informazioni limitate, che devono essere inserite nel contesto del quadro clinico globale. L'approccio più efficace deriva dalla conoscenza del razionale, delle implicazioni e delle limitazioni connesse a un gruppo selezionato di test, in grado di fornire risposte a quesiti specifici. I neonati con ittero colestatico devono essere valutati precocemente, per identificare quelli che necessitano di intervento chirurgico.

In un paziente con sospetta epatopatia, la valutazione diagnostica deve seguire il seguente iter logico: È presente una patologia epatica? Se sì, di che natura? Di quale gravità? È disponibile un trattamento specifico? Qual è la prognosi?

ESAMI DI LABORATORIO. Gli esami di laboratorio utilizzati nello screening e nella conferma di un sospetto di epatopatia comprendono: transaminasi, bilirubina (totale e frazionata), fosfatasi alcalina (ALP, *ALkaline Phosphatase*), determinazione del tempo di protrombina (PT, *Protrombine Time*) o dell'INR (*International Normalized Ratio*), e dei livelli di albumina. Questi esami sono complementari, forniscono una stima della funzione di sintesi ed escrezione epatica e possono dare indicazioni sulla natura del problema (infiammazione o colestasi).

Un danno epatocellulare acuto (patologia parenchimale), osservabile per esempio nell'epatite virale, nell'epatite da farmaci o da tossine, nello shock, nell'ipossiemia o nelle malattie metaboliche, è indicato da un marcato aumento delle transaminasi. La colestasi (patologia ostruttiva) comporta il passaggio nel siero di componenti della bile: i livelli sierici di bilirubina totale e coniugata, così come degli acidi biliari, risultano elevati. Anche aumenti dell'ALP, della 5′ nucleotidasi (5′NT) e della γ-glutamil transpeptidasi (GGT) sono indicatori sensibili di danno ostruttivo o infiammatorio del tratto biliare.

La gravità del danno epatico può essere desunta da segni clinici (presenza di encefalopatia, emorragia da varici, ittero ingravescente, apparente riduzione della massa epatica a causa di necrosi massiva o scompenso ascitico) oppure da alterazioni biochimiche (ipoglicemia, iperammoniemia, squilibri elettrolitici, iperbilirubinemia persistente, ipoalbuminemia severa o prolungamento del PT o dell'INR che non risponde alla somministrazione parenterale di vitamina K).

Il frazionamento del livello di bilirubinemia totale nelle forme coniugata e non coniugata permette di distinguere un aumento causato da emolisi da uno dovuto a danno epatico. L'aumento predominante della bilirubina coniugata è un indice relativamente sensibile di danno epatocellulare o di colestasi, mentre un aumento dei livelli di transaminasi è un indice ancora più sensibile di danno epatocellulare.

L'alanina aminotransferasi (ALT, o glutammato-piruvato transaminasi sierica) è epatospecifica, mentre l'aspartato aminotransferasi (AST, o transaminasi glutamico-ossalacetica sierica) può derivare anche da altri organi. Gli aumenti più spiccati di entrambi gli enzimi si verificano in corso di danno epatocellulare acuto; nell'epatite virale acuta, nel danno tossico, nell'ipossia o nell'ipoperfusione si osservano aumenti fino a mille volte i valori normali. Dopo un trauma addominale chiuso, un rialzo parallelo dei livelli di transaminasi può fornire un indice precoce di danno epatico. Un aumento o una riduzione differenziale dei livelli di AST e ALT può talora essere di utilità diagnostica. Nell'epatite acuta, il rialzo dell'ALT può essere più marcato di quello dell'AST, mentre nel danno epatico da alcol, nell'infezione fulminante da echovirus e in diverse malattie metaboliche si osserva un maggiore incremento dell'AST. Nell'epatopatia cronica e nell'ostruzione biliare intraepatica ed extraepatica, l'aumento di AST e ALT può essere meno marcato. La steatoepatite non alcolica e altre forme di steatosi non alcolica sono epatopatie croniche osservate nei bambini obesi, che presentano un aumento delle transaminasi. La caratteristica principale sono i reperti istologici simili a quelli del danno indotto da alcol, in assenza di potus.

La funzione di sintesi epatica è indicata dai livelli sierici di albumina e proteine, e dal PT o dall'INR. Può essere utile determinare la concentrazione sierica di proteine e la percentuale delle frazioni globuliniche. I pazienti con epatite autoimmune spesso hanno livelli elevati di gammaglobuline e titoli aumentati di anticorpi anti-muscolo liscio, antinucleo e anti-microsoma epatico e renale. In questi pazienti è inoltre possibile il riscontro di anticorpi antimitocondrio. Un aumento dei livelli di α-fetoproteina può suggerire un epatocarcinoma, un epatoblastoma o la tirosinemia ereditaria. L'ipoalbuminemia da ridotta sintesi rappresenta una possibile complicanza dell'insufficienza epatica grave e costituisce un fattore prognostico negativo. I pazienti con epatopatia severa o insufficienza epatica fulminante possono presentare deficit del fattore V e dei fattori della coagulazione vitamina K-dipendenti (I, VII, IX e X). Se il PT o l'INR sono prolungati per il malassorbimento intestinale di vitamina K (causato da colestasi) o per un ridotto introito di vitamina K con la dieta, la somministrazione parenterale della vitamina è in grado di correggere la coagulopatia e di normalizzare l'INR nell'arco di 12-24 ore. Una mancata risposta alla vitamina K suggerisce un danno epatico grave. La presenza di livelli persistentemente ridotti di fattore VII sono un indice prognostico negativo nell'insufficienza epatica fulminante.

Al momento di interpretare i risultati dei test biochimici relativi a struttura e funzione epatica occorre tenere conto delle variazioni correlate all'età. Il bambino con crescita normale ha livelli di ALP significativamente aumentati, a causa del passaggio nel siero dell'isoenzima osseo, fenomeno riscontrabile soprattutto negli adolescenti in rapida crescita. Pertanto, un aumento isolato dell'ALP non è di per sé indice di disfunzione epatica o biliare, in assenza di altre alterazioni biochimiche epatospecifiche. Gli altri enzimi, come la 5′NT e la GGT, aumentano in corso di colestasi e sono dunque indicatori più specifici di danno epatobiliare: la 5′NT, per esempio, non è presente nell'osso; l'attività enzimatica della GGT, maggiore nei primi mesi di vita, si riduce rapidamente con l'età. La concentrazione di colesterolo, che aumenta nel corso della vita, può essere molto elevata nei pazienti con colestasi intra- o extraepatica, o al contrario ridotta in corso di epatopatie acute severe come l'epatite.

L'interpretazione dell'ammoniemia deve sempre essere cauta, a causa della variabilità dei possibili fattori che la influenzano e della difficoltà intrinseca della misurazione di laboratorio.

BIOPSIA EPATICA. La biopsia epatica, combinata con i dati clinici, consente nella maggior parte dei casi di risalire alla causa di un'epatopatia. I campioni di tessuto epatico possono essere utilizzati per formulare una diagnosi istologica precisa nei pazienti con colestasi neonatale, epatite cronica attiva, malattie metaboliche, sospetta sindrome di Reye, colestasi intraepatica (paucità dei dotti biliari), fibrosi epatica congenita o ipertensione portale di origine ignota; per l'analisi enzimatica, nel sospetto di errori congeniti del metabolismo; per l'analisi di sostanze di accumulo, come ferro, rame o metaboliti specifici. La biopsia epatica può anche essere utile per monitorare la risposta alla terapia o per individuare eventuali complicanze, in corso di trattamento con agenti potenzialmente epatotossici come acido acetilsalicilico, antimicrobici (eritromicina, minociclina, chetoconazolo, isoniazide), antimetaboliti, antineoplastici o anticonvulsivanti.

Nei neonati e nei bambini, l'agobiopsia epatica è facilmente effettuabile per via percutanea. La quantità di tessuto che è possibile prelevare, anche nei neonati, è in genere sufficiente per l'interpretazione istologica e le analisi biochimiche, quando necessarie. La biopsia percutanea, procedura sicura anche nei soggetti di una settimana di vita, si effettua di norma in condizioni di anestesia locale con sedazione cosciente. Le controindicazioni comprendono un aumento del PT o dell'INR, trombocitopenia, sospetto di lesioni di natura vascolare, cistica o infettiva, lungo il tragitto dell'ago, e ascite tesa. Se non si riesce a correggere l'ipocoagulabilità o la trombocitopenia con la somministrazione di plasma fresco congelato o la trasfusione di piastrine, si possono tentare approcci alternativi a quello percutaneo. Si può prendere in considerazione l'approccio chirurgico laparotomico (a cuneo), eseguito da un chirurgo generale, o quello transgiugulare sotto guida fluoroscopica ed ecografica, affidato a un radiologo interventista pediatrico esperto, in una sala radiologica equipaggiata. Il rischio di complicanze quali emorragia, ematoma, formazione di fistole arterovenose, pneumotorace o peritonite biliare è scarso.

INDAGINI RADIOLOGICHE. Esistono numerose tecniche che possono aiutare a definire le dimensioni, la forma e l'architettura del fegato e l'anatomia delle vie biliari intraepatiche ed extraepatiche. Sebbene le tecniche di imaging non possano fornire una diagnosi istologica e biochimica ben precisa, possono tuttavia rispondere a quesiti specifici, per esempio se un'epatopatia sia causata da un accumulo di grasso o di glicogeno oppure da un tumore o una cisti. Queste indagini possono inoltre indirizzare verso ulteriori esami come la biopsia epatica e consentono di individuare rapidamente i pazienti con ostruzione biliare, che necessitano di un intervento. La scelta delle indagini radiologiche dovrebbe far parte di un approccio diagnostico studiato attentamente, onde evitare una ridondanza di informazioni desunte da tecniche d'indagine diverse.

La radiografia semplice può suggerire un'epatomegalia, ma un esame obiettivo attento può fornire una stima più affidabile delle dimensioni epatiche. Il fegato può apparire meno denso del normale nei pazienti con infiltrazione grassa e viceversa iperdenso in quelli con deposito di metalli pesanti come il ferro. Una massa nel fegato o nell'albero biliare può spostare un'ansa intestinale a contenuto aereo. Possono essere presenti calcificazioni a livello del fegato (parassitosi o neoplasie), del sistema vascolare (trombosi portale), della colecisti e dell'albero biliare (litiasi). È inoltre possibile osservare raccolte gassose nel fegato (ascessi), nel tratto biliare o nei vasi portali (enterocolite necrotizzante).

L'ecografia fornisce informazioni su dimensioni, composizione e flusso ematico del fegato. L'iperecogenicità è tipica dell'infiltrazione grassa; la tecnica consente inoltre di rilevare masse di diametro fino a 1-2 cm. L'ecografia ha sostituito la colangiografia nella diagnosi dei calcoli della colecisti e delle vie biliari. Persino nei neonati, questa indagine è in grado di valutare le dimensioni della colecisti, rilevare un'eventuale dilatazione delle vie biliari o individuare una cisti del coledoco. Nei lattanti con atresia biliare, i reperti ecografici possono comprendere una colecisti piccola o addirittura assente, mancata visualizzazione del dotto comune, presenza del segno del cordone triangolare, ovvero un'area di iperecogenicità di forma triangolare/tubulare alla biforcazione della vena porta, che rappresenta residui fibrosi dell'ilo epatico. Nei pazienti con ipertensione portale, l'eco-Doppler è in grado di verificare la pervietà della vena porta, dimostrare la presenza di collaterali, valutare le dimensioni della milza e l'entità dello scompenso ascitico. L'ecografia può rilevare un versamento ascitico anche di modesta entità. L'uso dell'eco-Doppler è inoltre utile nella valutazione della pervietà dei vasi, dopo il trapianto epatico.

La tomografia computerizzata (TC) fornisce informazioni simili a quelle ottenibili con l'ecografia, ma è meno indicata nei pazienti di età inferiore ai due anni, a causa delle piccole dimensioni delle strutture, della scarsità del contrasto fornito dal grasso endoaddominale e dalla necessità di una sedazione pesante, o addirittura dell'anestesia generale, per effettuare l'esame. La risonanza magnetica (RM) è una valida alternativa. La colangiorisonanza magnetica può essere utile nella diagnosi differenziale delle lesioni del tratto biliare. La TC e la RM si sono dimostrate più accurate dell'ecografia nella rilevazione di lesioni focali come tumori, cisti e ascessi. La TC con mezzo di contrasto può rilevare una massa neoplastica di densità molto simile a quella del parenchima normale. Nel sospetto di un tumore epatico, la TC è l'indagine migliore per definirne l'estensione anatomica, la natura solida o cistica e la vascolarizzazione. Può inoltre rivelare differenze minime nella densità del parenchima epatico, tenendo conto che il coefficiente medio di attenuazione del fegato è ridotto in caso di steatosi. Un aumento della densità può verificarsi per esempio in caso di accumulo diffuso di ferro o di glicogeno. Nella diagnosi differenziale della colestasi ostruttiva e non ostruttiva, la TC e la RM possono identificare con maggior precisione il livello dell'ostruzione, rispetto all'ecografia. Sia la TC sia l'ecografia trovano impiego per guidare la biopsia epatica percutanea, l'aspirazione di lesioni specifiche o la colangiografia.

La scintigrafia con radionuclide si basa sulla captazione selettiva di determinati radiofarmaci. Gli agenti più utilizzati sono: solfuri colloidali marcati con Tecnezio-99m (^{99m}Tc), che viene fagocitato dalle cellule di Kupffer; agenti a base di acido iminodiacetico marcato con ^{99m}Tc, che sono captati dagli epatociti ed escreti nella bile come la bilirubina; il Gallio-67, che si concentra nelle cellule infiammatorie e neoplastiche. La risoluzione anatomica ottenibile con la scintigrafia epatica è in genere inferiore a quella della TC, della RM e dell'ecografia.

La scintigrafia con colloidi marcati con ^{99m}Tc, in grado di rilevare lesioni focali (tumori, cisti e ascessi) di dimensioni >2-3 cm, può essere utile anche nella valutazione dei pazienti con probabile cirrosi e captazione epatica disomogenea e con spostamento della captazione di colloide dal fegato al midollo osseo.

I mezzi a base di acido iminodiacetico marcato con ^{99m}Tc possono aiutare a differenziare la colestasi intraepatica dall'ostruzione extraepatica, nei neonati. I risultati sono migliori se la scintigrafia è preceduta da un trattamento di 5-7 giorni con fenobarbital per stimolare il flusso biliare. Di norma l'isotopo è rilevabile nell'intestino a 1-2 ore di distanza dall'iniezione endovenosa. In presenza di ostruzione extraepatica, l'escrezione risulta ritardata e sono necessarie scintigrafie seriate fino a 24 ore dopo la somministrazione. Nelle fasi precoci dell'atresia biliare, la funzione epatocitaria è normalmente conservata; la captazione (clearance) avviene rapidamente, ma senza escrezione nell'intestino. Al contrario, la captazione è scarsa nelle epatopatie parenchimali, come l'epatite neonatale, mentre l'escrezione nella bile e nell'intestino alla fine avviene.

La colangiografia, ovvero la visualizzazione diretta del tratto biliare intraepatico ed extraepatico, previa iniezione di materiale radio-opaco, può rendersi necessaria in alcuni pazienti per valutare la causa, la localizzazione e l'estensione di un'ostruzione biliare. La colangiografia percutanea transepatica con ago sottile è la metodica di scelta nei lattanti e nei bambini piccoli. La probabilità di opacizzazione del tratto biliare è eccellente nei pazienti in cui la TC, la RM o l'ecografia ha dimostrato una dilatazione dei dotti biliari. La colangiografia percutanea transepatica è stata utilizzata per delineare il sistema duttale biliare.

Una metodica alternativa per lo studio dei dotti biliari nei bambini più grandi è la colangiografia retrograda endoscopica (ERCP, *Endoscopic Retrograde ColangioPancreatography*), che si esegue incannulando la papilla di Vater sotto controllo diretto endoscopico e iniettando il mezzo di contrasto nei dotti biliari e pancreatici, per definirne l'anatomia.

L'angiografia selettiva dell'arteria celiaca, mesenterica superiore o epatica può essere utile per visualizzare la circolazione epatica o portale. Si presta allo studio dei sistemi vascolari arterioso e venoso. L'angiografia, oltre a essere spesso richiesta per valutare la vascolarizzazione dei tumori prima dell'intervento chirurgico, si rivela utile nello studio dei pazienti con ipertensione portale nota o presunta. Permette di apprezzare la pervietà del sistema portale, l'estensione dei collaterali e il calibro dei vasi studiati per una procedura di shunt. La RM può fornire informazioni analoghe.

APPROCCIO DIAGNOSTICO AI BAMBINI CON ITTERO

La North American Society for Pediatric Gastroenterology, Hepatology and Nutrition ha pubblicato le linee guida per la valutazione dei neonati con ittero da 2 a 8 settimane di vita, utilizzate per differenziare l'ittero non colestatico da quello colestatico, che deriva in genere da disturbi più gravi. Un neonato di aspetto sano

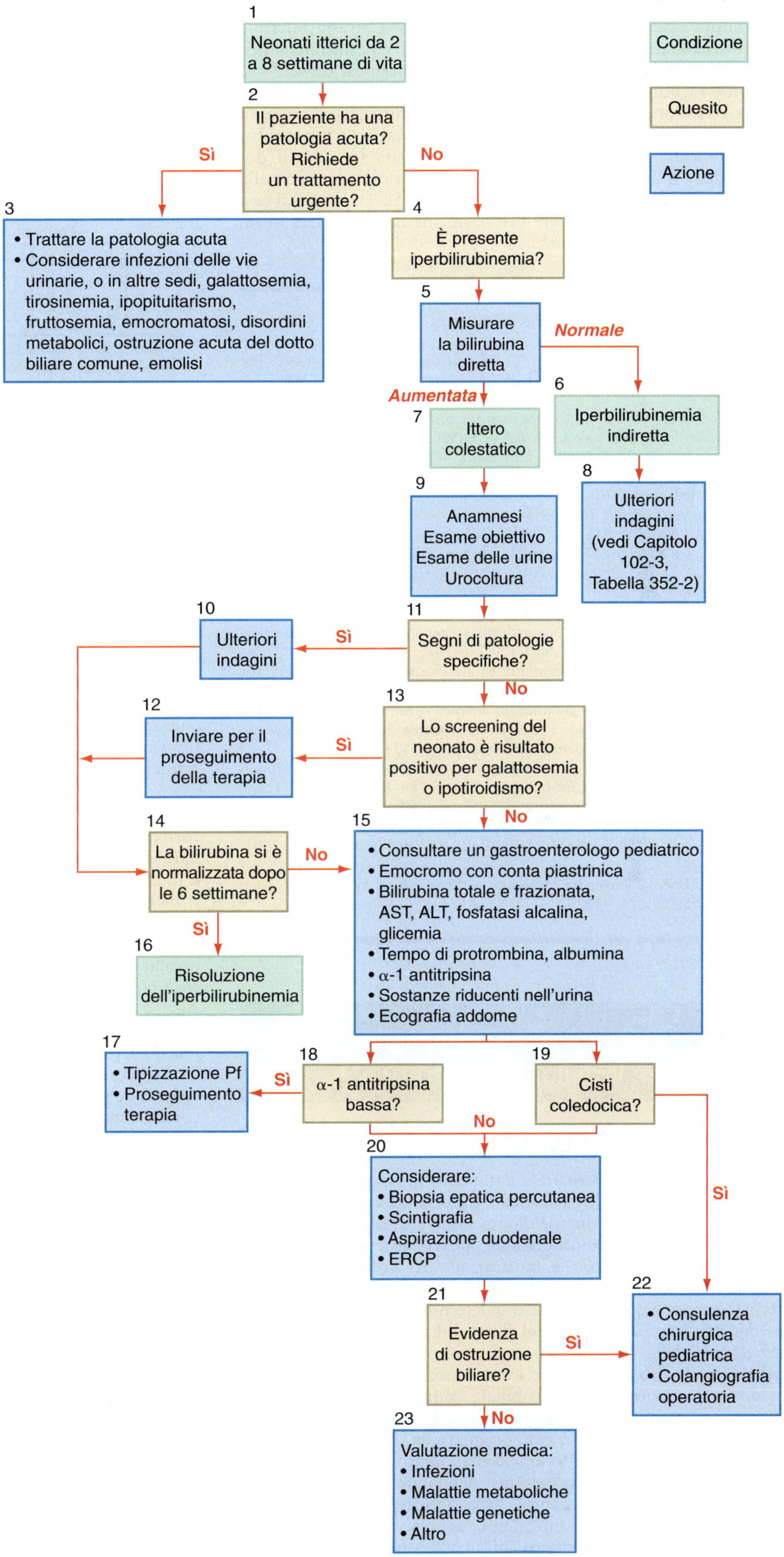

Figura 352-1. Linee guida per la pratica clinica in caso di colestasi. Algoritmo per pazienti da 2 a 8 settimane di vita. ALT, alanina aminotransferasi; AST, aspartato aminotransferasi; PT, tempo di protrombina (Moyer V, Freese DK, Whitington PF, et al; North American Society for Pediatric Gastroenterology, Hepatology and Nutrition: Guideline for the evaluation of cholestatic jaundice in infants: Recommendations of the North American Society for Pediatric Gastroenterology, Hepatology and Nutrition. *J Pediatr Gastroenterol Nutr* 2004;39:115-128.)

può talora essere affetto da ittero colestatico. L'atresia biliare e l'epatite neonatale sono le cause più comuni di colestasi nella prima infanzia. L'atresia biliare comporta una prognosi sfavorevole se non è identificata precocemente. I risultati migliori, in questa patologia, si ottengono con la ricostruzione chirurgica precoce (a 40-60 giorni di vita). L'anamnesi, l'esame obiettivo e il riscontro di iperbilirubinemia prevalentemente coniugata (tramite il dosaggio della bilirubina totale e diretta) sono il primo passo nella valutazione dell'ittero in età pediatrica (Fig. 352-1). In questi casi sarebbe opportuno richiedere precocemente la consulenza di un gastroenterologo pediatrico.

Balistreri WF: Pediatric hepatology. A half-century of progress. *Clin Liver Dis* 2000;4:191–210.

Balistreri WF: Bile acid therapy in pediatric hepatobiliary disease: The role of ursodeoxycholic acid. *J Pediatr Gastroenterol Nutr* 1997;24: 573–589.

Batres LA, Maller ES: Laboratory assessment of liver function and injury in children: In Suchy FS, Sokol RJ, Balistreri WF (editors): *Liver Disease in Children,* 2nd ed. Philadelphia, Lippincott, Williams and Wilkins, 2001, pp 155–170.

Bezerra JA, Balistreri WF: Cholestatic syndromes of infancy and childhood. *Semin Gastrointest Dis* 2001;12:54–65.

Feranchak AP, Ramirez RO, Sokol RJ: Medical and nutritional management of cholestasis: In Suchy FS, Sokol RJ, Balistreri WF (editors): *Liver Disease in Children,* 2nd ed. Philadelphia, Lippincott, Williams and Wilkins, 2001, pp 195–238.

Garcia-Tsao G: Current management of the complications of cirrhosis and portal hypertension: Variceal hemorrhage, ascites and spontaneous bacterial peritonitis. *Gastroenterology* 2001;120:726–748.

Moyer V, Freese DK, Whitington PF, et al; North American Society for Pediatric Gastroenterology, Hepatology and Nutrition: Guideline for the evaluation of cholestatic jaundice in infants: Recommendations of the North American Society for Pediatric Gastroenterology, Hepatology and Nutrition. *J Pediatr Gastroenterol Nutr* 2004;39:115–128.

Ryckman FC, Alonso MH: Causes and management of portal hypertension in the pediatric population. *Clin Liver Dis* 2001;5:789–818.

Ryckman FC, Alonso MH, Bucuvalas JC, Balistreri WF: Liver transplantation in children: In Suchy FS, Sokol RJ, Balistreri WF (editors): *Liver Disease in Children,* 2nd ed. Philadelphia, Lippincott, Williams and Wilkins, 2001, pp 949–974.

Trauner M, Meier PJ, Boyer JL: Molecular pathogenesis of cholestasis. *N Engl J Med* 1998;339:1217–1227.

Capitolo 353 ■ Colestasi Hassan H.A-Kader, William F. Balistreri

353.1 • Colestasi neonatale

Si definisce colestasi neonatale l'aumento protratto della bilirubinemia coniugata, oltre i primi 14 giorni di vita. L'ittero che compare dopo le 2 settimane di vita e non si risolve entro questo periodo, o addirittura progredisce, dovrebbe essere approfondito in primo luogo con la misurazione dei livelli di bilirubina coniugata. La colestasi, in un neonato, può presentare cause infettive, genetiche, metaboliche o indeterminate, che danno luogo a un'ostruzione *meccanica* del flusso biliare o a un'alterazione *funzionale* della funzione epatica escretoria e della secrezione biliare (vedi Tab. 352-3). Le lesioni meccaniche comprendono stenosi e ostruzione del dotto biliare comune; il prototipo delle alterazioni ostruttive è l'atresia biliare. Le anomalie funzionali della secrezione biliare possono originare da difetti congeniti, da danno epatocitario o da lesioni dell'apparato secretorio biliare. Le patologie che causano colestasi neonatale sono classificabili in extraepatiche e intraepatiche (Fig. 353-1). Le caratteristiche cliniche della colestasi sono simili, a prescindere dall'origine. Nei neonati affetti, la diagnosi di alcune affezioni come la galattosemia, la sepsi o l'ipotiroidismo è relativamente semplice. Nella maggior parte dei casi, tuttavia, individuare la causa della colestasi è più complesso; in particolare, la diagnosi differenziale tra l'atresia biliare, l'epatite idiopatica neonatale e la colestasi intraepatica può risultare molto difficile.

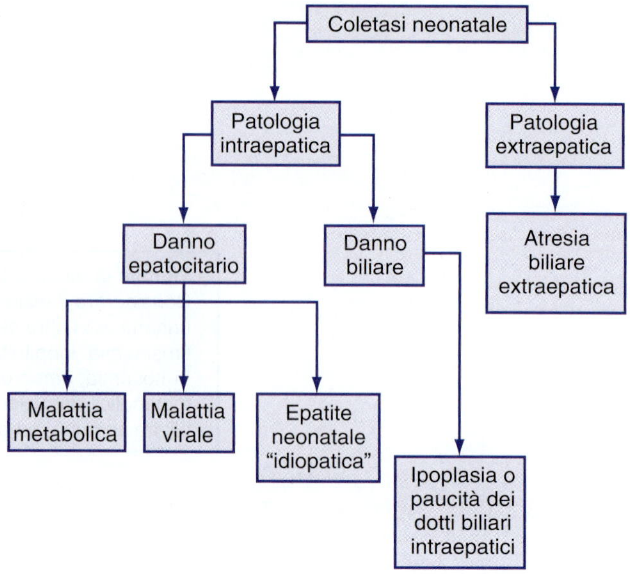

Figura 353-1. Colestasi neonatale. Approccio concettuale al gruppo di patologie che si presenta con colestasi nel neonato. Vi sono aree di sovrapposizione, ovvero pazienti con atresia biliare extraepatica possono avere un certo grado di danno intraepatico. I pazienti con epatite neonatale "idiopatica" potrebbero, in futuro, risultare portatori di un difetto metabolico primitivo o di una malattia virale.

MECCANISMI. Le patologie epatiche metaboliche, causate da errori congeniti del metabolismo o del trasporto degli acidi biliari, sono caratterizzate dall'accumulo di acidi biliari primitivi e dall'incapacità di produrre i normali acidi biliari coleretici e trofici. Le manifestazioni cliniche e istologiche sono aspecifiche e simili a quelle delle altre forme di danno epatobiliare neonatale. È inoltre possibile che in certe forme enigmatiche di danno epatico neonatale entrino in gioco meccanismi autoimmuni. Nel complesso, i meccanismi fisiopatologici non sono ancora ben conosciuti. Alcune manifestazioni istologiche di danno epatico neonatale non compaiono negli individui più grandi. La trasformazione gigantocellulare degli epatociti, per esempio, è un reperto comune nei lattanti con colestasi e può verificarsi in qualsiasi forma di danno epatico neonatale; tuttavia, è più frequente e severa nelle forme di colestasi intraepatica. Le manifestazioni cliniche e istopatologiche dell'epatite neonatale e dell'atresia biliare sono le più disparate; il processo di base è scatenato da un insulto non meglio precisato, che causa un'infiammazione degli epatociti o dei biliociti. Se la sede principale del danno è l'epitelio duttale, si sviluppa una colangite, che porta a sclerosi e restringimento progressivi delle vie biliari, fino alla completa obliterazione (atresia biliare). Un danno predominante a carico degli epatociti si manifesta invece con il quadro clinico e istologico dell'"epatite neonatale". Questo concetto non chiarisce il meccanismo preciso, ma offre una spiegazione per i casi, peraltro ben documentati, di evoluzione postnatale inaspettata di questi processi patologici; per esempio, un neonato con una diagnosi iniziale di epatite neonatale, con le vie biliari pervie alla colangiografia, può in seguito sviluppare un'atresia biliare.

Le anomalie funzionali della generazione del flusso biliare possono anch'esse svolgere un ruolo nella genesi della colestasi neonatale. Il flusso biliare dipende direttamente da un'efficiente escrezione epatica di acidi biliari.

Durante la fase di relativa inefficienza del trasporto epatocitario e del metabolismo degli acidi biliari, nei primi giorni di vita, insulti di entità anche lieve possono ridurre ulteriormente il flusso biliare, portando alla produzione di acidi biliari anomali, tossici. L'alterazione selettiva di una singola tappa, nella serie di eventi necessari per l'escrezione epatica, può provocare l'espressione manifesta di una sindrome colestatica. Nei bambini con colestasi intraepatica o con sindrome di Zellweger si possono trovare difetti specifici della sintesi degli acidi biliari. Le forme severe di colestasi familiare sono state associate all'emocromatosi neonatale e ad aberrazioni delle proteine contrattili che compongono il citoscheletro epatocitario. L'emocromatosi neonatale può insorgere anche come malattia gestazionale immunomediata, responsiva alle immunoglobuline somministrate alla madre per via endovenosa (IVIG, *IntraVenous ImmunoGlobulin*). La sepsi è una causa nota di colestasi, probabilmente mediata da un'endotossina prodotta dall'*Escherichia coli*.

VALUTAZIONE. La valutazione del neonato itterico deve seguire un percorso logico che tenga conto del rapporto costo-efficacia, con un processo a step successivi (Tab. 353-1). Sebbene nel neonato la colestasi possa essere la manifestazione iniziale di numerosi disturbi, la presentazione clinica è in genere molto simile e fornisce pochi indizi diagnostici. I bambini colpiti sono itterici, hanno urine scure, feci chiare o acoliche ed epatomegalia, a causa del ridotto flusso biliare causato da danno epatocitario o da ostruzione biliare. Una disfunzione della sintesi epatica può causare ipoprotrombinemia ed emorragie. La somministrazione di vitamina K dovrebbe essere il primo passo nella terapia dei bambini con colestasi, onde prevenire le emorragie.

Se l'iperbilirubinemia non coniugata può essere fisiologica, la colestasi (aumento della bilirubina coniugata di qualsiasi origine), nel neonato, è **sempre patologica** e impone una rapida diagnosi differenziale. Il primo passo è l'identificazione della colestasi. Successivamente occorre riconoscere eventuali cause di colestasi per cui esiste un trattamento specifico, al fine di prevenire la progressione del danno ed evitare le complicanze a lungo termine come la sepsi, le endocrinopatie (ipotiroidismo, panipopituitarismo), l'epatotossicità nutrizionale causata da malattie metaboliche specifiche (galattosemia) o altre malattie metaboliche (tirosinemia).

Il danno epatobiliare può rappresentare la manifestazione iniziale dell'omozigosi per il deficit di α_1-antitripsina o per la fibrosi cistica. La patologia epatica neonatale può associarsi anche alla sifilide congenita e a infezioni virali specifiche, in particolare da echovirus e herpesvirus, Cytomegalovirus compreso (CMV). I virus epatitici (A, B, C) sono cause rare di colestasi neonatale.

La tappa finale, e più critica, nella valutazione dei neonati con colestasi, è la differenziazione dell'atresia biliare extraepatica dall'epatite neonatale.

TABELLA 353-1. Significato degli esami specifici nella valutazione dei pazienti con sospetta colestasi neonatale

TEST	RAZIONALE
Bilirubina sierica frazionata	Documenta la presenza di colestasi
Valutazione del colore delle feci	Indice del flusso biliare nell'intestino
Misurazione degli acidi biliari nelle urine/nel siero	Conferma la colestasi; può indicare errori congeniti della biosintesi degli acidi biliari
Indici di sintesi epatica (albumina, coagulazione)	Indica la gravità della disfunzione epatica
Genotipo α_1-antitripsina	Suggerisce (o esclude) PiZZ
Tiroxina e TSH	Suggerisce (o esclude) un'endocrinopatia
Test del sudore/analisi delle mutazioni	Suggerisce (o esclude) la fibrosi cistica
Aminoacidi nelle urine/nel siero e sostanze riducenti	Suggerisce (o esclude) epatopatie metaboliche
Ecografia	Suggerisce (o esclude) cisti del coledoco; può visualizzare il segno della corda triangolare, suggerendo l'atresia biliare
Scintigrafia epatobiliare	Documenta la pervietà o l'ostruzione dei dotti biliari
Biopsia epatica	Differenzia l'atresia biliare dall'epatite neonatale; suggerisce diagnosi alternative

PiZZ, fenotipo inibitore delle proteasi ZZ; TSH, *Thyroid Stimulating Hormone*, ormone stimolante la tiroide.

COLESTASI INTRAEPATICA

EPATITE NEONATALE. L'espressione "epatite neonatale" implica la presenza di colestasi intraepatica (vedi Fig. 353-1), che a sua volta comprende diverse forme (Tabb. 353-2 e 353-3).

L'**epatite neonatale idiopatica**, che può insorgere in forma sia sporadica sia familiare, è una malattia a eziologia sconosciuta. I pazienti sono probabilmente affetti da una patologia metabolica o virale specifica, sebbene ancora non definita. I soggetti con deficit di α_1-antitripsina, che in passato erano inclusi in questa categoria, dopo la caratterizzazione del difetto metabolico specifico sono ora considerati (in modo più preciso) come un sottogruppo a sé stante.

Nel neonato l'epatite infettiva può essere causata da virus specifici dimostrabili, come herpes simplex, enterovirus, CMV o, raramente, virus dell'epatite B. Questi casi rappresentano una piccola percentuale delle sindromi epatitiche neonatali.

La **sindrome di Aagenaes** è una forma di colestasi intraepatica familiare idiopatica, associata a linfedema degli arti inferiori. La correlazione tra epatopatia e linfedema non è chiara, e può essere attribuibile a un ridotto flusso linfatico epatico o a ipoplasia linfatica epatica. I pazienti colpiti si presentano generalmente con colestasi episodica, associata ad aumento della transaminasi, della fosfatasi alcalina e degli acidi biliari. Nei periodi intercritici, i pazienti sono di norma asintomatici e gli indici biochimici tendono a migliorare. Il locus della sindrome di Aagenaes è stato mappato nell'intervallo 6.6cM, sul cromosoma 15q.

La **sindrome di Zellweger** (**cerebroepatorenale**) è una rara malattia genetica autosomica recessiva, caratterizzata da una degenerazione progressiva del fegato e dei reni (vedi Capitolo 86.2). L'incidenza è stimata di circa 1/10 000 nati; la malattia è in genere fatale entro 6-12 mesi. I neonati affetti presentano un'ipotonia severa generalizzata, una marcata compromissione delle funzioni neurologiche, con ritardo psicomotorio. Si osservano una forma anomala del capo e una facies particolare, epatomegalia, cisti renali corticali, calcificazioni puntiformi della rotula e del grande trocantere, anomalie oculari. Negli epatociti, all'osservazione ultrastrutturale, si nota l'assenza dei perossisomi.

TABELLA 353-2. Sottotipi di colestasi neonatale

A. Disturbi del trasporto e della secrezione di membrana
   1. Disturbi della secrezione canalicolare
      a. Trasporto degli acidi biliari – deficit della BSEP
         i. Persistente, progressiva (PFIC di tipo 2)
         ii. Ricorrente, benigna (BRIC di tipo 2)
      b. Trasporto dei fosfolipidi – deficit di MDR3 (PFIC di tipo 3)
      c. Trasporto di ioni – fibrosi cistica (CFTR)
   2. Disturbi complessi/multiorgano
      a. Deficit di FIC1
         i. Persistente, progressiva (PFIC di tipo 1, malattia di Byler)
         ii. Ricorrente, benigna (BRIC di tipo1)
      b. Colangite sclerosante neonatale (CLDN1)
      c. Artrogrifosi – insufficienza renale – sindrome colestatica (VPS33B)
B. Disturbi della biosintesi e coniugazione degli acidi biliari
   1. Deficit di 3-ossi-4-steroido 5β-riduttasi
   2. Deficit di 3β-idrossi-5-C27-steroido deidrogenasi/isomerasi
   3. Deficit di ossisterolo 7α-idrossilasi
   4. Deficit di BAAT (ipercolanemia familiare)
C. Disturbi dell'embriogenesi
   1. Sindrome di Alagille (difetto di Jagged1, paucità sindromica dei dotti biliari)
   2. Malformazione del piatto duttale (ARPKD, ADPLD, malattia di Caroli)
D. Non classificate ("epatite neonatale" idiopatica) – meccanismo sconosciuto

Nota: Il deficit di FIC1, il deficit di BSEP e alcuni disordini della biosintesi degli acidi biliari sono caratterizzati clinicamente da bassi livelli sierici di GGT, nonostante la presenza di colestasi. In tutti gli altri disturbi elencati, i livelli di GGT sono elevati.
ADPLD, *Autosomal Dominant Polycystic Liver Disease*, malattia del fegato policistico autosomica dominante (solo cisti epatiche); ARPKD, *Autosomal Recessive Polycystic Kidney Disease*, malattia del rene policistico autosomica recessiva (cisti epatiche e renali); BAAT, *Bile Acid Transporter*, trasportatore degli acidi biliari; BRIC, *Benign Recurrent Intrahepatic Cholestasis*, colestasi intraepatica ricorrente benigna; BSEP, *Bile Salt Export Pump*, pompa di secrezione degli acidi biliari; PFIC, *Progressive Familial Intrahepatic Cholestasis*, colestasi familiare intraepatica progressiva.
Da Balistreri WF, Bezerra JA, Jansen P, et al: Intrahepatic cholestasis: Summary of an American Association for the Study of Liver Diseases single-topic conference. *Hepatology* 2005;42:222-235.

TABELLA 353-3. Difetti molecolari che possono causare un danno epatico

GENE	PROTEINA	FUNZIONE, SUBSTRATO	DISTURBO
ATP8b1	FIC1	ATPasi di tipo P; traslocasi degli aminofosfolipidi che fa girare la fosfatidil serina e la fosfatidiletanolamina dal lato esterno a quello interno della membrana canalicolare	PFIC1 (malattia di Byler), BRIC1, GFC
ABCB11	BSEP	Proteina canalicolare con sito legante l'ATP (famiglia di proteine ABC); funziona come una pompa che trasporta gli acidi biliari attraverso il dominio canalicolare	PFIC 2, BRIC 2
ABCB4	MDR3	Proteina canalicolare con sito legante l'ATP (famiglia di proteine ABC); funziona da flippasi dei fosfolipidi del membrana canalicolare	PFIC3, ICP, colelitiasi
AKR1D1	5β-riduttasi	gene della 3-ossiΔ-4-steroide 5β-riduttasi; regola la sintesi degli acidi biliari	BAS: colestasi neonatale con epatite a cellule giganti
HSD3B7	C27-3β-HSD	Gene della3β-idrossi-5-C27-steroido ossido-riduttasi (C27-3β-HSD); regola la sintesi degli acidi biliari	BAS: colestasi intraepatica cronica
CYP7BI	CYP7BI	Ossisterolo 7α-idrossilasi; regola la via acidica della sintesi degli acidi biliari	BAS: colestasi neonatale con epatite a cellule giganti
JAG1	JAG1	Proteine transmembrana della superficie cellulare che interagiscono con i recettori Notch per regolare il destino delle cellule durante l'embriogenesi	Sindrome di Alagille
TJP2	Proteina delle *tight junctions*	Appartiene alla famiglia degli omologhi delle guanilato chinasi di membrana, coinvolti nell'organizzazione delle giunzioni intercellulari epiteliali ed endoteliali; regola la permeabilità paracellulare	FHC
BAAT	BAAT	Enzima che trasferisce la porzione di acidi biliari dal tioestere dell'acil coenzima A alla glicina oppure alla taurina	FHC
EPHX1	Epossido idrossilasi	L'epossido idrossilasi microsomiale regola l'attivazione e la detossificazione degli agenti chimici esogeni	FHC
ABCC2	MRP2	Proteina canalicolare con sito legante l'ATP (famiglia di proteine ABC); regola il trasporto canalicolare dei coniugati del GSH e l'arsenico	Sindrome di Dubin-Johnson
ATP7B	ATP7B	ATPasi di tipo P; funge da pompa di esportazione del rame	Malattia di Wilson
CLDN1	Claudina 1	Proteina delle *tight junctions*	NSC
CIRH1A	Cirina	Segnali cellulari?	NAICC
CFTR	CFTR	Canale del cloro con sito legante l'ATP (famiglia di proteine ABC); regola il trasporto di cloro	Fibrosi cistica
PKHD1	Fibrocistina	Proteina coinvolta nella funzione ciliare e nella tubulogenesi	ARPKD
PRKCSH	Epatocistina	Si assembla con la subunità II α delle glucosidasi nel reticolo endoplasmatico	ADPLD
VPS33B	Proteina vascolare sorting 33	Regola la fusione di proteine con la membrana cellulare	ARC

ADPLD, *Autosomal Dominant Polycystic Liver Disease*, malattia del fegato policistico autosomica dominante; ARC, *Arthrogryposis-Renal Dysfunction-Cholestasis Sindrome**, sindrome artrogrifosi, disfunzione renale, colestasi; ARPKD, *Autosomal Recessive Polycystic Kidney Disease*, malattia del rene policistico autosomica recessiva; BAAT, *Bile Acid Transporter*, trasportatore degli acidi biliari; BAS, *Bile Acid Synthetic Defect*, difetto di sintesi degli acidi biliari; BRIC, *Benign Recurrent Intrahepatic Cholestasis*, colestasi intraepatica ricorrente benigna; BSEP, *Bile Salt Export Pump*, pompa di esportazione degli acidi biliari; CFTF, *Cystic Fibrosis Transmembrane Conductance Regulator*, regolatore della conduttanza transmembrana della fibrosi cistica; FHC, *Familial HyperCholanemia*, ipercolanemia familiare; GFC, *Greenland Familial Cholestasis*, colestasi familiare della Groenlandia; GSH, *glutatione*; ICP, *Intrahepatic Cholestasis of Pregnancy*, colestasi intraepatica gravidica; NAICC, *North American Indian Childhood Cirrhosis*, cirrosi infantile degli Indiani del Nord America; NSC, *Neonatal Sclerosing Cholangitis*, colangite sclerosante neonatale con ictiosi, vacuoli dei leucociti e alopecia; PFIC, *Progressive Familial Intrahepatic Cholestasis*, colestasi intraepatica familiare progressiva*.

* bassi livelli di GGT (PFIC tipo 1 & 2, BRIC tipo 1 & 2, ARC).

Da Balistreri WF, Bezerra JA, Jansen P, et al: Intrahepatic cholestasis: Summary of an American Association for the Study of Liver Diseases single-topic conference. *Hepatology* 2005; 42:222-235.

L'**emocromatosi neonatale** (NISD, *Neonatal Iron Storage Disease*, malattia neonatale da accumulo di ferro) è una patologia rapidamente progressiva caratterizzata da accumulo di ferro nel fegato, nel cuore e nelle ghiandole endocrine, senza aumento dei suoi depositi nel sistema reticoloendoteliale. I pazienti sviluppano un'insufficienza multiorgano e hanno una sopravvivenza ridotta. Sono stati riportati casi familiari; la malattia può essere trasmessa per via autosomica recessiva o per via codominante. I dati di laboratorio comprendono ipoglicemia, iperbilirubinemia, ipoalbuminemia e grave ipoprotrombinemia. I livelli di transaminasi possono essere elevati nelle fasi iniziali e normalizzarsi con la progressione della malattia. La diagnosi è confermata dalla biopsia della mucosa orale o dalla RM, che evidenzia la siderosi extraepatica. La prognosi è scadente, anche se il trapianto epatico può essere curativo. Nonostante alcune segnalazioni iniziali incoraggianti, l'uso di una combinazione di antiossidanti e infusione di prostaglandine, associata alla terapia chelante, non ha dimostrato di aumentare uniformemente la sopravvivenza nei pazienti affetti da NISD.

In alcuni pazienti, la NISD può essere causata da un meccanismo alloimmune che si sviluppa in seguito alla sensibilizzazione materna, da parte di un primo feto, a un antigene fetale sconosciuto. Il trattamento della madre con 1 g/kg di IVIG alla settimana, a partire dalla 18ª settimana di gestazione, migliora l'esito di una successiva gravidanza.

DISTURBI DEL TRASPORTO, DELLA SECREZIONE, DELLA CONIUGAZIONE E DELLA BIOSINTESI DEGLI ACIDI BILIARI. La colestasi familiare progressiva di tipo 1 (PFIC1, *Progressive Familial Intrahepatic Cholestasis*) o malattia FIC1 (prima nota come **morbo di Byler**) è una forma severa di colestasi intraepatica. Questa malattia fu descritta per la prima volta nei bambini Amish di Jacob Baylor. I pazienti affetti presentavano steatorrea, prurito, rachitismo da deficit di vitamina D, sviluppavano progressivamente cirrosi epatica e avevano **bassi** livelli di γ-glutamiltranspeptidasi. La mancanza di paucità dei dotti biliari e le caratteristiche extraepatiche permettono di differenziare questo disturbo dalla sindrome di Alagille.

La **PFIC 1** (deficit di FIC1), mappata sul cromosoma 18q12, risulta da un deficit del gene F1C1 (ATP8B1; vedi Tab. 353-3). Il gene F1C1 è un'adenosina trifosfatasi (ATPasi) che funziona da flippasi di aminofosfolipidi, facilitando il trasferimento della fosfatidilserina e della fosfatidiletanolamina dallo strato esterno della membrana cellulare a quello interno. Il gene F1C1 può anche avere una funzione nell'assorbimento intestinale degli acidi biliari, come è suggerito dagli alti livelli di espressione nell'intestino. Il deficit di F1C1 può inoltre dare luogo a un'altra forma di colestasi intraepatica: la **colestasi intraepatica ricorrente benigna** (BRIC, *Benign Recurrent Intrahepatic Cholestasis*) **di tipo 1**. Questa patologia è caratterizzata da picchi ricorrenti di colestasi, ittero e prurito intenso, che durano da 2 settimane a 6 mesi, ma in rari casi possono protrarsi fino a 5 anni. La PFIC di tipo 1 può essere causata da mutazioni nonsense, frame-shift o da delezioni; le mutazioni missense o split portano invece alla BRIC di tipo 1. Tipicamente, i pazienti con BRIC di tipo 1 hanno normali livelli di colesterolo e di GGT. Sebbene sia considerato un disturbo benigno, alcuni casi possono sfociare in un danno epatico severo.

La **PFIC di tipo 2** (deficit di BSEP), che è stata mappata sul cromosoma 2q24, è simile alla PFIC 1, con la differenza che colpisce le famiglie non Amish (in particolare dell'Europa centro-orientale). È conseguenza di un difetto del trasportatore canalicolare ATP-dipendente BSEP (ABCB11). Il danno epatico progressivo risulta dall'accumulo di acidi biliari secondario alla compromessa secrezione canalicolare. Sono state descritte mutazioni del gene ABC11 anche in un altro disturbo, la BRIC di tipo 2, caratterizzata da episodi ricorrenti di colestasi associata a colelitiasi e diarrea acquosa.

Diversamente dalla PFIC 1 e 2, i pazienti con **PFIC di tipo 3** (MDR3) hanno livelli **elevati** di GGT. Questa malattia è causata da difetti della flippasi canalicolare dei fosfolipidi, MDR3 (ABCB4), che provoca un'alterazione della traslocazione della fosfatidilcolina attraverso la membrana canalicolare. Le madri eterozigoti per questo gene possono sviluppare una colestasi intraepatica durante la gravidanza.

L'**ipercolanemia familiare** (FHC, *Familial HyperCholanemia*) è caratterizzata da elevate concentrazioni di acidi biliari nel siero, prurito, mancato sviluppo e coagulopatia. La FHC è un tratto genetico complesso associato a una mutazione del coenzima A (CoA) degli acidi biliari, aminoacido N-aciltransferasi (codificata da BAAT), cos" come a mutazioni nella proteina 2 delle giunzioni serrate (codificata da TJP 2, altrimenti noto come ZO-2). Le mutazioni di BAAT, che è un enzima di coniugazione degli acidi biliari, ne azzerano l'attività enzimatica. I pazienti omozigoti per questa mutazione hanno nella bile solo acidi biliari non coniugati. Mutazioni concomitanti di BAAT e TJP 2 possono portare alla perdita del trasporto e del circolo degli acidi biliari. I pazienti con FHC rispondono in genere alla somministrazione di acido ursodesossicolico.

Si ritiene che un'*alterata biosintesi degli acidi biliari* possa essere un fattore in grado di scatenare o perpetuare i disturbi colestatici neonatali; l'ipotesi è che errori congeniti della biosintesi degli acidi biliari determinino l'assenza dei normali acidi biliari primari trofici o coleretici e l'accumulo di metaboliti (tossici) primitivi. Tali difetti congeniti possono essere causa di epatopatie acute e croniche; la diagnosi precoce permette di instaurare una terapia sostitutiva mirata degli acidi biliari mancanti, in grado di far regredire il danno epatico. Sono stati descritti numerosi difetti specifici, che sono elencati di seguito.

Il **deficit di Δ^4-3-ossisteroide-5β-riduttasi**, che rappresenta la quarta tappa nella via di degradazione del colesterolo ad acidi biliari primari, si manifesta con colestasi importante e insufficienza epatica, che si sviluppano rapidamente dopo la nascita, con coagulopatia e un danno epatico metabolico simile a quello della tirosinemia. L'istologia epatica è caratterizzata da disorganizzazione del lobulo, con cellule giganti, trasformazione pseudoacinare e stasi biliare canalicolare. La spettrometria di massa è necessaria per documentare l'aumentata escrezione urinaria degli acidi biliari e la predominanza degli acidi osso-idrossi e osso-deidrossi colenoici. Il trattamento con acido colico e ursodesossicolico si associa a normalizzazione degli indici biochimici, istologici e clinici.

Il **deficit di 3β-idrossi C_{27}-steroido deidrogenasi** (**3β-HSD**) isomerasi, la seconda tappa della biosintesi degli acidi biliari, causa una colestasi intraepatica familiare progressiva. I pazienti affetti hanno in genere ittero con aumento delle transaminasi, epatomegalia e **normali** livelli di GGT e di coliglicina sierica. L'aspetto istologico può variare da un'epatite a cellule giganti a un'epatite cronica. La diagnosi, suggerita dalla scoperta, mediante spettrometria di massa, di acidi biliari marcati con 24-C nelle urine, che mantiene la struttura 3β-idrossi-Δ^5, può essere confermata dalla determinazione dell'attività di 3β-HSD in colture di fibroblasti, usando il 7α-idrossi-Δ^5 colesterolo come substrato. La terapia con acidi biliari primari, somministrati per via orale per inibire l'attività della 7α-idrossilasi, limitare la produzione di acidi biliari 3β-idrossi-Δ^5 e favorire l'eliminazione epatica, si è dimostrata efficace nel far regredire il danno epatico.

ALTERAZIONI DELL'EMBRIOGENESI

La **sindrome di Alagille** (displasia arterioepatica) è la più frequente sindrome con paucità dei dotti biliari intraepatici. Prende il nome di "paucità dei dotti biliari" (spesso chiamata erroneamente atresia biliare) l'assenza o la netta riduzione del numero dei dotti biliari interlobulari nella triade portale, con rami portali e arteriola epatica di dimensioni normali. La biopsia effettuata in età precoce spesso mette in luce un processo infiammatorio a carico dei dotti biliari; dai campioni bioptici successivi emerge la risoluzione dell'infiammazione con una riduzione residua del numero e del diametro dei dotti biliari, analoga al quadro della sindrome da scomparsa dei dotti biliari (VBS, *Vanishing Bile duct Syndrome*), osservata in adulti affetti da patologie immunomediate. Valutazioni seriali dell'istologia epatica suggeriscono una distruzione progressiva dei dotti biliari. Le **manifestazioni cliniche** della sindrome di Alagille, che hanno diversi gradi di espressione e possono essere aspecifiche, comprendono una facies caratteristica (fronte ampia, occhi infossati e distanziati, naso lungo e diritto, ipoplasia mandibolare), cui possono associarsi anomalie oculari (embriotoxon posteriore), cardiovascolari (in genere stenosi periferica della polmonare, talora tetralogia di Fallot), difetti dell'arco vertebrale e mancata fusione dell'arco vertebrale anteriore (vertebre a farfalla), nefropatia tubulointerstiziale. Altre caratteristiche come il ritardo di crescita e il deficit della spermatogenesi possono rispecchiare carenze nutrizionali. La prognosi per la sopravvivenza a lungo termine è buona, ma i pazienti, se non trattati, sviluppano frequentemente prurito, xantomi, ipercolesterolemia severa e complicanze neurologiche da deficit di vitamina E. Sono state osservate mutazioni del gene umano Jagged1 (JAG1), che codifica per un ligando del recettore notch, associate alla sindrome di Alagille.

ATRESIA BILIARE

L'espressione "atresia biliare" è imprecisa, dal momento che l'anatomia dei dotti biliari alterati, nei pazienti affetti, presenta un'ampia variabilità. Una terminologia più appropriata dovrebbe riflettere la fisiopatologia, per esempio "colangiopatia obliterante progressiva". I pazienti possono presentare obliterazione dei dotti biliari segmentali distali con dotti extraepatici pervi fino all'ilo epatico. Si tratta di una lesione correggibile chirurgicamente, sebbene di raro riscontro. La forma più comune di atresia biliare, che si trova in circa l'85% dei casi, è l'obliterazione dell'intero albero biliare extraepatico a livello o al di là dell'ilo portale. In questa forma l'approccio chirurgico è più problematico. Nella maggior parte dei pazienti (85-90%) l'atresia biliare esordisce in epoca postnatale; l'esordio embrionale o fetale si presenta alla nascita ed è associato ad altre anomalie congenite, nell'ambito della polisplenia (atresia biliare e malformazioni spleniche [BASM, *Biliary Atresia Splenic Malformation*]) (Fig. 353-2) (vedi Capitolo 431.11).

INCIDENZA. L'atresia biliare è stata osservata in 1/10 000-15 000 nati vivi, l'epatite neonatale idiopatica in 1/5000-10 000. La paucità dei dotti biliari intraepatici è molto meno frequente, colpendo circa 1/50 000-75 000 nati vivi.

DISTINZIONE DELL'EPATITE NEONATALE DALL'ATRESIA BILIARE. Può essere difficile distinguere con chiarezza i neonati con atresia biliare, che necessitano di correzione chirurgica, da quelli con colestasi intraepatica (epatite neonatale) e dotti biliari pervi. Nessun esame o procedura, preso singolarmente, risulta pienamente soddisfacente; occorre quindi fare riferimento a schemi diagnostici che comprendano caratteristiche cliniche, anamnestiche, biochimiche e radiologiche.

L'epatite neonatale idiopatica ha un'incidenza familiare del 20% circa, mentre l'atresia biliare si ripresenta di rado nella stessa famiglia. Una minoranza di neonati, con esordio fetale di atresia biliare, ha un'aumentata incidenza di altre anomalie, come la sindrome polisplenica, con eterotassia addominale, malrotazione, levocardia e anomalie vascolari addominali. L'epatite neonatale sembra essere più frequente nei prematuri o nei nati piccoli per l'età gestazionale. La persistenza di feci acoliche suggerisce un'ostruzione biliare (atresia biliare), ma i pazienti con epatite neonatale severa possono presentare una compromissione severa, seppure transitoria, dell'escrezione biliare. La presenza di feci fortemente pigmentate e il riscontro di succo duodenale tinto di bile, all'intubazione duodenale, consentono di escludere l'atresia biliare. Nei pazienti con atresia biliare extraepatica il fegato può risultare di dimensioni o consistenza alterate, reperto che è invece meno frequente nell'epatite neonatale.

L'ecografia addominale è un'utile strumento diagnostico nella valutazione della colestasi neonatale, poiché identifica un'eventuale coledocolitiasi, perforazioni del dotto biliare o altre anomalie strutturali delle vie biliari, come una cisti coledocica. Nei pazienti con atresia biliare, l'ecografia può rilevare anomalie associate come polisplenia addominale e malformazioni vascolari. Nei pazienti con atresia biliare, la colecisti non è visualizzabile, o appare come una microcolecisti. I bambini con colestasi intra-

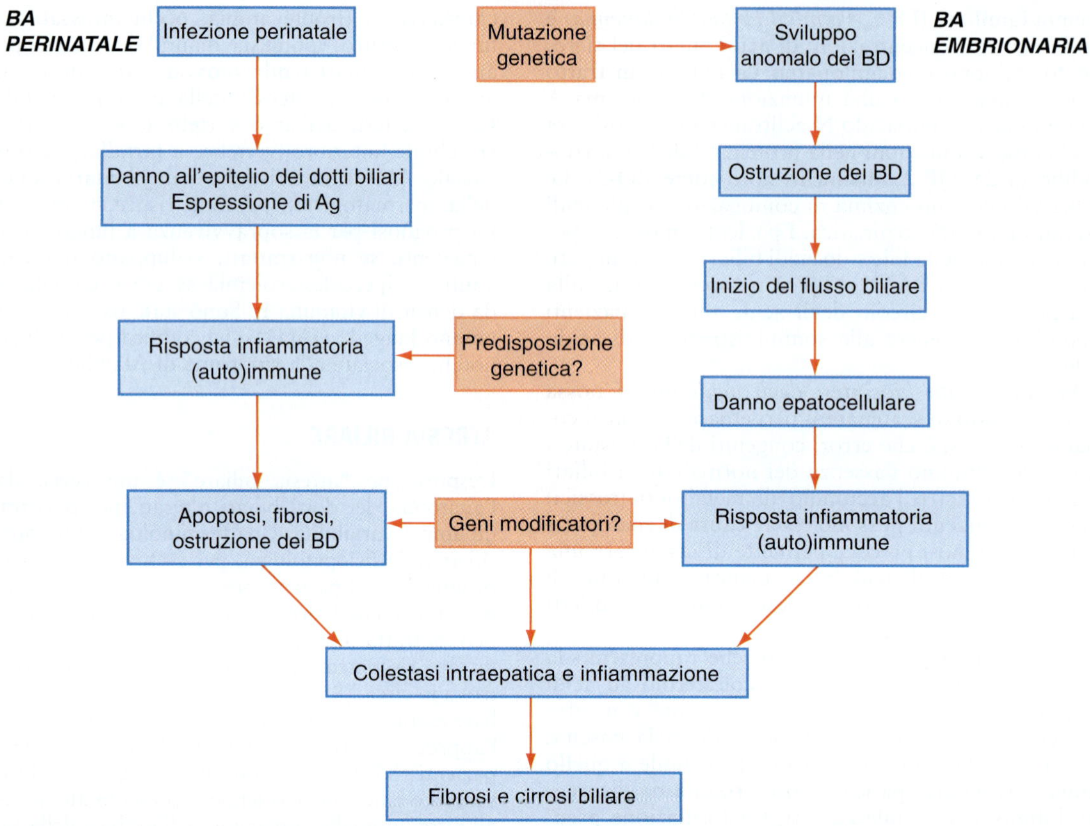

Figura 353-2. Algoritmo proposto per la patogenesi delle due forme di atresia biliare (BA, *Biliary Atresia*). La BA perinatale può insorgere quando un insulto perinatale, come un'infezione da virus colangiotropi, scatena un danno a carico dell'epitelio dei dotti biliari (BD, *Bile Duct*) con esposizione di autoantigeni di neoantigeni che elicitano la conseguente risposta immunitaria. L'infiammazione che ne risulta induce apoptosi e necrosi dell'epitelio dei BD extraepatici, che risulta in obliterazione fibrosa del lume e ostruzione del BD. I BD intraepatici possono diventare anch'essi bersaglio del persistente attacco (auto)immunitario TH1 e del danno colestatico, con conseguente fibrosi portale progressiva che culmina nella cirrosi biliare. La BA embrionale può essere il risultato di mutazioni di geni la cui funzione è controllare la normale formazione e differenziazione dei BD, che indurrebbero secondariamente una risposta infiammatoria/autoimmune nel dotto biliare comune e nel fegato, dopo l'inizio del flusso biliare verso la 11ª-13ª settimana di gestazione. Il danno secondario degli epatociti e dei BD intraepatici insorge o come risultato del danno colestatico o in quanto bersaglio della risposta (auto)immune che si sviluppa. Il risultato finale è la colestasi intraepatica e la fibrosi del tratto portale, che culminano nella cirrosi biliare. Altri fattori importanti possono essere la predisposizione genetica all'autoimmunità, geni modificatori che determinano l'estensione e il tipo di risposta cellulare e immunitaria, e lo sviluppo di fibrosi. (Da Mack CL, Sokol RJ: Unraveling the pathogenesis and etiology of biliary atresia. *Pediatr Res* 2005;57:87R-94R.)

epatica causata da epatite neonatale idiopatica, fibrosi cistica, o nutrizione parenterale totale, possono avere immagini ecografiche simili. Si può osservare il segno ecografico della corda triangolare, che rappresenta una massa fibrosa a forma di cono, situata cranialmente alla biforcazione della vena porta (Figg. 353-3 e 353-4). L'ecogenicità, che rappresenta un indice dei residui fibrosi all'ilo portale, osservati all'atto chirurgico nei pazienti con atresia biliare, può essere uno strumento diagnostico utile nella valutazione dei pazienti con colestasi neonatale.

La scintigrafia epatobiliare con derivati dell'acido iminodiacetico marcati con Tecnezio è utile per differenziare l'atresia biliare dalla colestasi non ostruttiva. Nei pazienti con atresia biliare la captazione epatica dell'agente è normale, mentre è assente l'escrezione intestinale. Sebbene la captazione possa risultare compromessa nei pazienti con epatite neonatale, l'escrezione intestinale alla fine avviene sempre. Una scintigrafia di follow-up dopo 24 ore è utile per determinare la pervietà delle vie biliari. È consigliabile somministrare fenobarbital (5 mg/kg/die) per 5 giorni, prima della scintigrafia, per aumentare l'escrezione biliare dell'isotopo. La scintigrafia epatobiliare è un esame sensibile per l'atresia biliare, ma manca di specificità e non è in grado di identificare altre anomalie strutturali delle vie biliari o del sistema vascolare. La mancanza di specificità e la necessità di aspettare 5 giorni rendono questa procedura poco pratica e di limitata utilità nella valutazione dei bambini con sospetta atresia biliare.

La biopsia epatica percutanea è la procedura più valida per la valutazione delle patologie epatobiliari neonatali, poiché fornisce le evidenze discriminanti più affidabili. L'atresia biliare è caratterizzata da proliferazione dei duttuli biliari, presenza di tappi biliari ed edema e fibrosi portali o perilobulari, con conservazione dell'architettura lobulare epatica fondamentale. Nell'epatite neonatale, si riscontra un danno epatocellulare severo e diffuso, con distorsione dell'architettura lobulare, spiccata infiltrazione di cellule infiammatorie e necrosi epatocellulare focale; i duttuli biliari, per contro, presentano scarse alterazioni. La trasformazione gigantocellulare, potendo essere caratteristica di entrambe le condizioni, è priva di specificità diagnostica.

Le altreazioni istologiche osservate nei pazienti con epatite neonatale idiopatica possono comparire anche in altre patologie, come il deficit di α_1-antitripsina, la galattosemia e varie forme di colestasi intraepatica. Sebbene la paucità dei duttuli biliari intraepatici sia rilevabile alla biopsia epatica già nelle prime settimane di vita, una biopsia più tardiva, in questi pazienti, può dimostrare un quadro più caratteristico.

TRATTAMENTO DEI PAZIENTI CON SOSPETTA ATRESIA BILIARE. Tutti i pazienti con sospetta atresia biliare andrebbero sottoposti a laparotomia esplorativa e colangiografia diretta per determinare la presenza e la sede dell'ostruzione. Nei pazienti con una lesione correggibile (che rappresentano la minoranza) sarebbe opportuno posizionare il drenaggio diretto. In mancanza di questo, un esame delle sezioni congelate ottenute dall'ilo epatico sezionato può identificare la presenza di epitelio biliare e determinare le dimensioni e la pervietà dei dotti biliari residui. In alcuni casi la

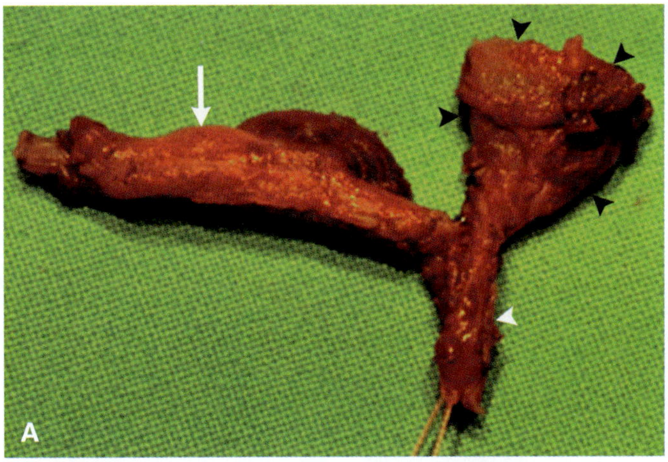

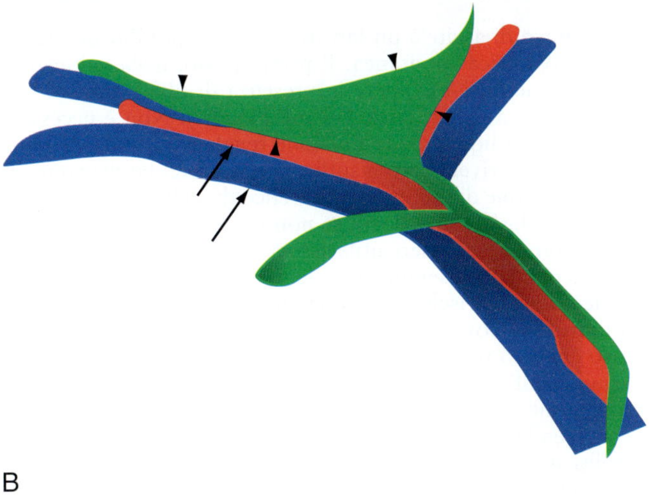

Figura 353-3. Reperti chirurgici nell'atresia biliare. *A*, Fotografia di un campione chirurgico di dotti biliari extraepatici ostruiti, che mostra il residuo duttale fibroso (punta di freccia nera) all'ilo portale, la colecisti atresica (freccia) e il dotto biliare comune fibroso (punta di freccia bianca). Il residuo duttale fibroso è una massa conica triangolare. *B*, Disegno schematico che rappresenta la relazione anatomica tra il residuo duttale fibroso e i vasi intorno all'ilo portale. Il residuo fibroso triangolare, conico (punte di freccia nere, zona verde) è posizionato anteriormente e appena superiormente alla vena porta (freccia lunga, zona blu) e all'arteria epatica (freccia corta, zona rossa). (Da Lee HJ, Lee SM, Park WH, Choi SO: Objective criteria of triangular cord sign in biliary atresia on US scans. *Radiology* 2003;229:395-400.)

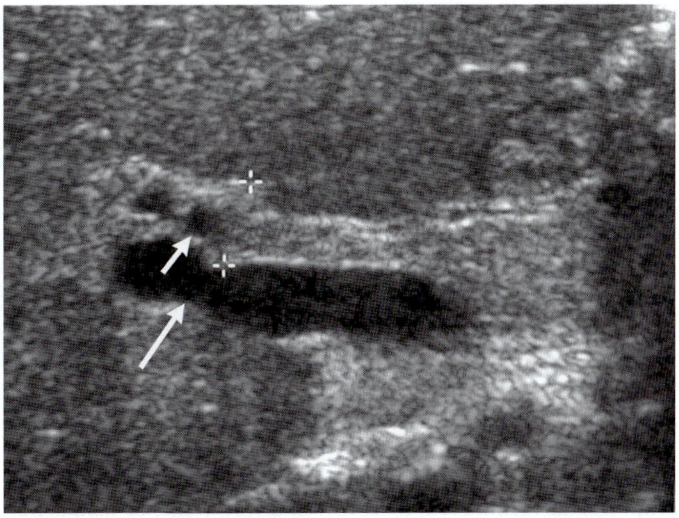

Figura 353-4. Rappresentazione del segno della corda triangolare (TC, *Triangular Cord*). La parete anteriore ecogena del ramo portale destro (EARPV, *Echogenic Anterior wall of the Right Portal Vein*) presentava uno spessore di 5,4 mm alla scansione ecografica longitudinale, in cui si osserva il segno TC (cursore) come un'area spessa, tubolare ed ecogena lungo il margine anteriore del ramo portale destro (freccia lunga). L'arteria epatica destra (freccia corta) si trova nella compagine dell'EARPV. (Da Lee HJ, Lee SM, Park WI I, Choi SO: Objective criteria of triangular cord sign in biliary atresia on US scans. *Radiology* 2003;229:395-400.)

colangiografia indica che l'albero biliare è pervio, ma di calibro ridotto, suggerendo che la colestasi non sia dovuta a obliterazione delle vie biliari, ma a paucità dei dotti biliari o a marcata riduzione del flusso in presenza di un danno intraepatico. In questi casi si dovrebbe evitare la transezione o un'ulteriore dissezione nell'ilo epatico.

Nei pazienti in cui non è reperibile alcuna lesione correggibile occorre procedere a un'**epatoportoenterostomia secondo Kasai.** Il razionale di questa operazione è che possano essere presenti piccoli residui dei dotti biliari, che rappresentano i canali residui, nella compagine del tessuto fibroso dell'ilo epatico; tali canali possono essere in diretta continuità con il sistema duttulare intraepatico. In tali casi, la transezione dell'ilo con anastomosi dell'intestino alla superficie prossimale della transezione può consentire il drenaggio biliare. Se il flusso non si ristabilisce rapidamente nel primo mese di vita, si instaura una progressiva obliterazione che esita in cirrosi epatica. Se si trovano canali microscopici pervi di diametro >150 µm, è probabile che nel postoperatorio si stabilisca il flusso biliare. Poiché la percentuale di successo nella ripresa del flusso biliare è molto maggiore (90%) quando l'intervento secondo Kasai viene effettuato prima dell'8ª settimana di vita, è di fondamentale importanza riconoscere e valutare precocemente i neonati con sospetta atresia biliare.

Alcuni soggetti con atresia biliare, anche del tipo "non correggibile", traggono un beneficio a lungo termine da interventi come la procedura di Kasai. Nella maggior parte dei casi persiste un certo grado di disfunzione epatica. Tali pazienti biliare hanno in genere un'infiammazione persistente delle vie biliari intraepatiche, che induce a pensare che l'atresia biliare rifletta un processo dinamico relativo all'intero sistema epatobiliare. Questa ipotesi potrebbe spiegare per quale motivo in fase terminale si sviluppino complicanze come l'ipertensione portale. I benefici a breve termine dell'epatoportoenterostomia sono una decompressione e un drenaggio sufficienti a posticipare l'insorgenza della cirrosi e a sostenere la crescita fino a quando possa essere effettuato con successo il trapianto epatico (vedi Capitolo 365).

TRATTAMENTO DELLA COLESTASI CRONICA

In tutte le forme di colestasi neonatale, che siano causate da epatite neonatale idiopatica, colestasi intraepatica o atresia biliare, i pazienti colpiti sono ad aumentato rischio di complicanze croniche. Queste ultime rispecchiano i diversi gradi di funzionalità epatica residua e sono correlate direttamente o indirettamente alla riduzione del flusso epatico. Tutte le sostanze normalmente escrete nella bile, come acidi biliari, bilirubina, colesterolo e oligoelementi, sono trattenute nel fegato, con conseguente accumulo nei tessuti e nel siero. Il ridotto afflusso di acidi biliari all'intestino tenue è causa di maldigestione e malassorbimento dei trigliceridi a catena lunga e delle vitamine liposolubili assunte con la dieta. La compromissione della funzione metabolica del fegato può incidere negativamente sull'equilibrio ormonale e sull'utilizzo dei nutrienti. Il danno epatico progressivo può esitare in cirrosi biliare, ipertensione portale e insufficienza epatica.

Il trattamento di questi pazienti è empirico e deve essere guidato da un attento monitoraggio (Tab. 353-4). Non si conosce una terapia efficace né per arrestare la progressione della colestasi, né per prevenire un ulteriore danno epatico e la cirrosi.

L'arresto della crescita è uno dei problemi più gravi, correlato in parte al malassorbimento e alla malnutrizione che derivano da una digestione e un assorbimento inefficaci dei grassi alimentari.

TABELLA 353-4. Trattamenti medici suggeriti per la colestasi persistente

DISTURBO CLINICO	TRATTAMENTO
Malnutrizione dovuta a malassorbimento dei trigliceridi a catena lunga provenienti dalla dieta	Sostituire con formule dietetiche o supplementi con trigliceridi a media catena
Malassorbimento di vitamine liposolubili	
Deficit di vitamina A (emeralopia, cute ispessita)	Terapia sostitutiva con 10 000-15 000 UI/die come Aquasol A (nome commerciale)
Deficit di vitamina E (degenerazione neuromuscolare)	Terapia sostitutiva con 50-400 UI/die come α-tocoferolo orale o TPGS
Deficit di vitamina D (osteopatia metabolica)	Terapia sostitutiva con 5000-8000 UI/die di vitamina D_2 o 3-5 μg/kg/die di 25-idrossicolecalciferolo
Deficit di vitamina K (ipoprotrombinemia)	Terapia sostitutiva con 2,5-5,0 mg a giorni alterni come derivato idrosolubile del menadione
Deficit di oligoelementi	Supplementi di calcio, fosfato, zinco
Deficit di vitamine idrosolubili	Supplementi con il doppio della dose massima raccomandata
Ritenzione di costituenti biliari come il colesterolo (xantomi)	Somministrare acidi biliari coleretici e acido ursodesossicolico, 15-20 mg/kg/die
Epatopatia progressiva; ipertensione portale (emorragia da varici, ascite, ipersplenismo)	Gestione delle complicanze (controllo dell'emorragia, restrizione salina; spironolattone)
Insufficienza epatica terminale	Trapianto epatico

TPGS, D-tocoferolo polietilen glicole 1000 succinato.

L'utilizzo di formule contenenti trigliceridi a catena media può migliorare il bilancio calorico.

In caso di colestasi cronica con sopravvivenza prolungata, i bambini affetti da malattie epatobiliari possono andare incontro a carenza di vitamine liposolubili (A, D, E, K). Il malassorbimento dei grassi e delle vitamine liposolubili può essere esacerbato dalla somministrazione di agenti sequestranti gli acidi biliari, come la colestiramina. Sono frequenti le osteopatie metaboliche.

La concentrazione sierica di vitamina A, che nei pazienti con colestasi cronica deve essere sottoposta a stretto controllo, può in genere essere mantenuta a livelli normali, con la supplementazione orale di esteri della vitamina A.

Nella colestasi cronica si può osservare una sindrome muscoloscheletrica degenerativa, causata dal malassorbimento e dal deficit di vitamina E; i bambini affetti presentano areflessia progressiva, atassia cerebellare, oftalmoplegia e ridotta sensibilità vibratoria. A livello del sistema nervoso centrale, dei nervi periferici e dei muscoli sono state riscontrate lesioni morfologiche specifiche, potenzialmente reversibili nei bambini più piccoli (di età <3-4 anni). I bambini colpiti hanno bassi livelli di vitamina E, aumentata emolisi da perossido di idrogeno e un basso rapporto tra concentrazione di vitamina E e lipidi totali (<0,6 mg/g per i soggetti di età inferiore a 12 anni e <0,8 mg/g per quelli più grandi). Il deficit di vitamina E può essere prevenuto con la somministrazione orale della vitamina stessa ad alte dosi (fino a 1000 UI/die); i pazienti che non riescono ad assorbirne una quantità adeguata possono richiedere la somministrazione di d-α-tocoferolo polietilenglicole 1000 succinato, per os. Occorre tenere sotto controllo i livelli sierici per monitorare l'efficacia della terapia.

Il prurito è una complicanza particolarmente problematica della colestasi cronica, spesso associata alla comparsa di xantomi. Entrambi sembrano correlati all'accumulo di colesterolo e acidi biliari nel siero e nei tessuti. L'eliminazione di questi composti è difficile in presenza di ostruzione dei dotti biliari, ma se persiste anche un minimo grado di pervietà dei dotti, la somministrazione di acido ursodesossicolico può aumentare il flusso biliare o interrompere la circolazione enteroepatica degli acidi biliari, riducendo gli xantomi e attenuando il prurito (vedi Tab. 353-4). La terapia con acido ursodesossicolico può inoltre ridurre i livelli di colesterolo. La dose iniziale consigliata è di 15 mg/kg/24 ore.

La biliostomia esterna parziale è un'opzione efficace in caso di prurito resistente alla terapia medica e consente un'evoluzione favorevole in un gruppo selezionato di pazienti con colestasi cronica che non hanno ancora sviluppato cirrosi epatica. La tecnica chirurgica consiste nella resezione di un segmento di intestino che verrà utilizzato come condotto per la bile. Un'estremità è anastomizzata alla colecisti, mentre l'altra viene abboccata alla cute, confezionando una stomia. Il risvolto negativo della procedura è la necessità di utilizzare un sacchetto da stomia per tutta la vita.

La fibrosi progressiva e la cirrosi conducono allo sviluppo di ipertensione portale, con conseguenti ascite ed emorragia da varici. Il riscontro di ascite è un fattore di rischio per l'insorgenza di peritonite batterica spontanea. Il primo passo, nella valutazione di questi pazienti, è escludere la presenza di PBS e ridurre l'apporto di sodio a 0,5 g (circa 1-2 mEq/kg/die). Non è necessaria la restrizione di liquidi se la funzione renale è normale. Qualora queste misure si rivelassero insufficienti, si potrebbe ricorrere alla somministrazione di diuretici. Il diuretico di scelta è lo spironolattone (3-5 mg/kg/die in 4 dosi); se non riesce a controllare l'ascite in monoterapia, può essere utile associare un altro diuretico come un tiazidico, o la furosemide. I pazienti con ascite ma senza edema periferico sono a rischio di riduzione del volume plasmatico e della diuresi, in corso di terapia con diuretici. L'ascite tesa altera il flusso ematico renale e l'emodinamica sistemica. La paracentesi, seguita dall'infusione endovena di albumina, può migliorare l'emodinamica, la perfusione renale e la sintomatologia. Il follow-up comprende il counseling dietologico e il monitoraggio degli elettroliti sierici e urinari (vedi Capitoli 361-364).

Nei pazienti con ipertensione portale sono frequenti l'emorragia da varici e lo sviluppo di ipersplenismo. È importante accertare sempre la causa del sanguinamento, poiché certi episodi di emorragia gastrointestinale, in soggetti con epatopatia cronica, possono essere dovuti a gastrite o a malattia ulcerosa. Dal momento che il trattamento di queste complicanze è diverso, è importante effettuare una diagnosi differenziale, mediante endoscopia, prima di iniziare la terapia (vedi Capitolo 364). Se il paziente ha subito una riduzione del volume plasmatico, si dovrebbe procedere a un'emotrasfusione, esercitando un attento controllo per evitare un'ipertrasfusione che potrebbe precipitare un ulteriore sanguinamento. L'utilizzo del tamponamento con palloncino non è consigliabile nei bambini, poiché può associarsi a complicanze significative. La scleroterapia o la legatura endoscopica delle varici sono misure palliative utili nell'emorragia da varici e possono rivelarsi addirittura superiori alle alternative chirurgiche.

Nei pazienti con epatopatia avanzata, il trapianto epatico ha una percentuale di successo >85% (vedi Capitolo 365). L'intervento, se tecnicamente fattibile, prolunga l'aspettativa di vita e corregge gli errori metabolici in patologie come il deficit di α_1-antitripsina, la tirosinemia e la malattia di Wilson. Il successo dipende dall'adeguatezza delle cure intraoperatorie, preoperatorie e postoperatorie, e da un uso attento della terapia immunosoppressiva. La scarsità di donatori di fegati di piccole dimensioni limita l'applicazione del trapianto epatico nei lattanti e nei bambini. L'utilizzo di trapianti di dimensioni ridotte e da donatore vivente aumenta la possibilità di trattare con successo i bambini più piccoli.

PROGNOSI

Nei pazienti con epatite neonatale idiopatica, la variabilità della prognosi rispecchia l'eterogeneità della malattia. Nei casi sporadici, il 60-70% dei pazienti guarisce senza evidenza di altreazioni epatiche strutturali o funzionali. Circa il 5-10% ha fibrosi o infiammazione persistenti, mentre una percentuale minore soffre di una patologia epatica più severa come la cirrosi. Nei lattanti il decesso avviene generalmente nel corso della malattia, a causa di emorragie o sepsi. Dei lattanti con epatite neonatale idiopatica familiare, il 20-30% guarisce, mentre il 10-15% sviluppa epatopatia cronica con cirrosi che può richiedere il trapianto epatico.

353.2 • Colestasi nei bambini più grandi

La maggior parte dei casi di colestasi che esordiscono dopo il periodo neonatale è causata da epatite virale o da farmaci epatotossici. Molte delle condizioni che causano colestasi neonatale possono portare a colestasi cronica anche nei pazienti più grandi. Gli adolescenti con iperbilirubinemia coniugata devono essere sottoposti a indagini per epatite acuta e cronica, deficit di α_1-antitripsina, malattia di Wilson, epatopatia associata a malattia infiammatoria cronica intestinale, epatite autoimmune e sindromi colestatiche intraepatiche. Altre possibili cause comprendono l'ostruzione causata da calcoli, tumori addominali, linfoadenomegalia o l'infiammazione epatica da ingestione di farmaci. Il trattamento della colestasi, nei bambini più grandi, è simile a quello proposto per la colestasi neonatale (vedi Tab. 353-4).

Aagenaes O: Hereditary recurrent cholestasis with lymphedema: Two new families. *Acta Pediatr Scand* 1974;63:465–471.

Alagille D, Estrada A, Hadchovel M, et al: Syndromic paucity of interlobular bile ducts (Alagille syndrome or arteriohepatic dysplasia): Review of 80 cases. *J Pediatr* 1987;110:195–200.

Balistreri WF, Bezerra JA, Jansen P, et al: Intrahepatic cholestasis: Summary of an American Association for the Study of Liver Diseases single-topic conference. *Hepatology* 2005;42:222–235.

Carlton VE, Harris BZ, Puffenberger EG, et al: Complex inheritance of familial hypercholanemia with associated mutations in TJP2 and BAAT. *Nat Genet* 2003;34:91–96.

Chardot C, Carton M, Spire-Bendelac N, et al: Is the Kasai operation still indicated in children older than 3 months diagnosed with biliary atresia? *J Pediatr* 2001;138:224–228.

Chardot C, Serinet MO: Prognosis of biliary atresia: What can be further improved. *J Pediatr* 2006;148:432–435.

Chen J, Raymond K: Nuclear receptors, bile-acid detoxification, and cholestasis. *Lancet* 2006;367:454–456.

Danks DM, Campbell PE, Smith AL, et al: Prognosis of babies with neonatal hepatitis. *Arch Dis Child* 1977;52:368–372.

Davenport M, De Ville de Goyet J, Stringer MD, et al: Seamless management of biliary atresia in England and Wales (1999–2002). *Lancet* 2004; 363:1354–1357.

Davenport M, Tizzard SA, Underhill J, et al: The biliary atresia splenic malformation syndrome: A 28-year single-center retrospective study. *J Pediatr* 2006;149:393–400.

Gissen P, Kelly D: New hope for treatment of neonatal haemochromatosis. *Lancet* 2004;364:1644–1645.

Hinds R, Davenport M, Mieli-Vergani G, et al: Antenatal presentation of the biliary atresia. *J Pediatr* 2004;144:43–46.

Jansen PLM, Muller M: The molecular genetics of familial intrahepatic cholestasis. *Gut* 2000;47:1–5.

Jansen PLM, Sturm E: Paediatric cholestasis: Is villin the villain? *Lancet* 2003;362:1090–1091.

Klomp LW, Vargas JC, van Mil SW, et al: Characterization of mutations in ATP8B1 associated with hereditary cholestasis. *Hepatology* 2004;40:27–38.

Lee HJ, Lee SM, Park WH, Choi SO: Objective criteria of triangular cord sign in biliary atresia on US scans. *Radiology* 2003;229:395–400.

Mack CL, Sokol RJ: Unraveling the pathogenesis and etiology of biliary atresia. *Pediatr Res* 2005;57:87R–94R.

Miga D, Sokol RJ, MacKenzie T, et al: Survival after first esophageal variceal hemorrhage in patients with biliary atresia. *J Pediatr* 2001;139:291–296.

Mowat AP, Psacharopoulos HT, Williams R: Extrahepatic biliary atresia versus neonatal hepatitis: Review of 137 prospectively investigated infants. *Arch Dis Child* 1976;51:763–770.

Nio M, Ohi R, Miyano T, et al: Five- and 10-year survival rates after surgery for biliary atresia: A report from the Japanese biliary atresia registry. *J Pediatr Surg* 2003;38:997–1000.

Oda T, Elkahloun AG, Pike BL, et al: Mutations in the human Jagged1 gene are responsible for Alagille syndrome. *Nat Genet* 1997;16:235–292.

Setchell KD, Schwarz M, O'Connell NC, et al: Identification of a new inborn error in bile acid synthesis: Mutation of the oxysterol 7alpha-hydroxylase gene causes severe neonatal liver disease. *J Clin Invest* 1998; 102:1690–1703.

Shih HH, Lin TM, Chuang JH, et al: Promotor polymorphism of the CD14 endotoxin receptor gene is associated with biliary atresia and idiopathic neonatal cholestasis. *Pediatrics* 2005;116:437–441.

Shneider BL, Brown MB, Haver B, et al: A multicenter study of the outcome of biliary atresia in the United States, 1997 to 2000. *J Pediatr* 2006;148: 467–474.

Sokol RJ, Heubi JE, Butler-Simon N, et al: Treatment of vitamin E deficiency during chronic childhood cholestasis with oral d-alpha-tocopheryl polyethylene glycol-1000 succinate. *Gastroenterology* 1987;93:975–985.

Stringer MD, Dhawan A, Davenport M, et al: Choledochal cysts: Lessons from a 20 year experience. *Arch Dis Child* 1995;73:528–531.

Utterson EC, Shepherd RW, Sokol RJ, et al: Biliary atresia: Clinical profiles, risk factors, and outcomes of 755 patients listed for liver transplantation. *J Pediatr* 2005;147:180–185.

van Mil SW, van der Woerd WL, van der Brugge G, et al: Benign recurrent intrahepatic cholestasis type 2 is caused by mutations in ABCB11. *Gastroenterology* 2004;127:379–384.

Whitington PF, Hibbard JU: High-dose immunoglobulin during pregnancy for recurrent neonatal haemochromatosis. *Lancet* 2004;364:1690–1698.

Yeh JN, Jeng YM, Chen HL, et al: Hepatic steatosis and neonatal intrahepatic choleostasis caused by citrin deficiency (NICCD) in Taiwanese infants. *J Pediatr* 2006;148:642–646.

Yoon PW, Bresee JS, Olney RS, et al: Epidemiology of biliary atresia: A population-based study. *Pediatrics* 1997;99:376–382.

Capitolo 354 ■ Malattie metaboliche del fegato

Rebecca G. Carey e William F. Balistreri

Dal momento che il fegato svolge un ruolo centrale nelle vie metaboliche di sintesi, degradazione e regolazione di carboidrati, proteine, lipidi, oligoelementi e vitamine, numerose anomalie metaboliche o difetti enzimatici specifici possono colpire quest'organo primitivamente o secondariamente (Tab. 354-1). Molte malattie metaboliche sono rilevabili con i nuovi programmi allargati di screening neonatale (vedi Capitolo 84). Può insorgere un'epatopatia quando l'assenza di un enzima provoca il blocco di una via metabolica, quando un substrato non metabolizzato si accumula a monte di un blocco, quando si sviluppa il deficit di una sostanza essenziale prodotta a valle di una reazione chimica alterata o quando si verifica la sintesi di metaboliti anomali. Lo spettro di alterazioni patologiche comprende: **danno epatocitario**, con conseguente alterazione delle altre funzioni metaboliche, che spesso esita in cirrosi, tumori epatici o entrambi; **accumulo** di lipidi, glicogeno o altri prodotti, che si manifesta con epatomegalia, spesso con complicanze specifiche a seconda del tipo di metabolismo alterato (ipoglicemia nella glicogenosi); assenza di alterazioni strutturali, nonostante la presenza di gravi **effetti metabolici**, come nei difetti del ciclo dell'urea. Le manifestazioni cliniche delle malattie metaboliche del fegato possono mimare infezioni, intossicazioni e malattie immunologiche ed ematologiche (Tab. 354-2). Si possono cercare indizi nell'anamnesi familiare o nell'osservazione della correlazione tra lo sviluppo dei sintomi e un cambiamento delle abitudini alimentari; per esempio, nei pazienti con intolleranza ereditaria al fruttosio, i sintomi si manifestano dopo l'ingestione di fruttosio. I dati clinici e di laboratorio spesso guidano la valutazione. La biopsia epatica consente uno studio morfologico e permette di effettuare test enzimatici, così come una valutazione quantitativa e qualitativa di vari altri costituenti. È inoltre disponibile la diagnosi genetica/molecolare. Tali studi richiedono la cooperazione di laboratori specializzati e una particolare attenzione nella raccolta e nell'utilizzo dei campioni.

TABELLA 354-1. Errori congeniti del metabolismo che colpiscono il fegato

DISTURBI DEL METABOLISMO DEI CARBOIDRATI
Disturbi del metabolismo del galattosio
Galattosemia
Disturbi del metabolismo del fruttosio
Intolleranza ereditaria al fruttosio (deficit di aldolasi)
Deficit di fruttosio-1,6 difosfatasi
Glicogenosi
Tipo I
Di von Gierke (Ia)
Tipo Ib
Tipo III (Cori/Forbes)
Tipo IV (Andersen)
Tipo VI (Hers)
Disturbi congeniti della glicosilazione (CGD, *Congenital Disorders of Glycosilation*)
DISTURBI DEL METABOLISMO DEGLI AMINOACIDI E DELLE PROTEINE
Disturbi del metabolismo della tirosina
Tirosinemia ereditaria (di tipo I)
Tirosinemia di tipo II
Difetti ereditari del ciclo enzimatico dell'urea
Deficit di CPS
Deficit di OTC (X-linked dominante)
Citrullinemia
Aciduria argininosuccinica
Argininemia
Deficit di N-AGS
DISTURBI DEL METABOLISMO LIPIDICO
Malattia di Wolman
Malattia da accumulo degli esteri colesterilici
Malattia di Gaucher
Malattia di Niemann-Pick di tipo C
DISTURBI DEL METABOLISMO DEGLI ACIDI BILIARI
Deficit di isomerasi
Deficit di riduttasi
Sindrome di Zellweger (cerebroepatorenale)
DISTURBI DEL METABOLISMO DEI METALLI
Malattia di Wilson
Sovraccarico epatico di rame
Cirrosi infantile indiana
Malattia da deposito neonatale di ferro (emocromatosi perinatale)
DISTURBI DEL METABOLISMO DELLA BILIRUBINA
Sindrome di Crigler-Najjar
Tipo I
Tipo II
Morbo di Gilbert
Sindrome di Dubin-Johnson
Sindrome di Rotor
ALTRE
Deficit di α_1-antitripsina
Fibrosi cistica
Protoporfiria eritropoietica
Deficit di citrina

CPS, *Citrin Carbamoyl Phosphate Synthetase*, citrina carbamolo fosfato sintetasi; N-AGS, N-acetiglutamato sintetasi; OTC, ornitina transcarbamoilasi.

TABELLA 354-2. Manifestazioni cliniche che suggeriscono la possibilità di una malattia metabolica

Vomito ricorrente, mancato accrescimento, bassa statura, caratteristiche dismorfiche, edema/anasarca
Ittero, epatomegalia (± splenomegalia), insufficienza epatica fulminante
Ipoglicemia, acidemia organica, acidosi lattica, iperammoniemia, sanguinamenti (coagulopatia)
Ritardo di sviluppo, ritardo psicomotorio, ipotonia, degenerazione neuromuscolare progressiva, convulsioni
Disfunzione o insufficienza cardiaca, odori strani, rachitismo, cataratta

354.1 • Difetti ereditari della coniugazione della bilirubina (iperbilirubinemia non coniugata familiare non emolitica)

La bilirubina è il metabolita finale dell'eme. Prima di essere escreta nella bile, viene glucuronata una prima volta dall'enzima bilirubina uridina difosfoglucuronato glucuronosiltransferasi (UDPGT), la cui attività risulta carente o alterata in tre malattie genetiche funzionalmente distinte (le sindromi di Crigler-Najjar di tipo I e II, e la sindrome di Gilbert), con conseguente iperbilirubinemia non coniugata congenita, non ostruttiva e non emolitica. L'UGT1A1 è l'isoforma primaria dell'enzima, necessaria per la glucuronazione della bilirubina, la cui assenza completa causa la sindrome di Crigler-Najjar (CN) di tipo I. La CN di tipo II è dovuta a una riduzione di attività dell'UGT1A1; la sindrome di Gilbert è causata da un polimorfismo della regione promoter della UGT1A1 che riduce anch'esso l'attività dell'enzima, ma solo del 30% circa. A differenza delle sindromi di Crigler-Najjar, la sindrome di Gilbert è benigna e non necessita di alcun trattamento; è la più frequente e si riscontra nel 5-10% della popolazione bianca.

SINDROME DI CRIGLER-NAJJAR DI TIPO 1 (DEFICIT DELLA GLUCURONIL TRANSFERASI). Questa forma, ereditata come tratto autosomico recessivo, è generalmente secondaria a mutazioni che causano un codone di stop prematuro o a mutazioni frameshift, che risultano nella soppressione dell'attività dell'UGT1A1. Ad oggi, sono state identificate più di 35 mutazioni. I genitori dei bambini colpiti hanno difetti parziali della coniugazione, come si può rilevare dai test enzimatici epatici o dalla misurazione della formazione del glucuronide; i loro livelli di bilirubina nel siero risultano normali.

Manifestazioni cliniche. I bambini omozigoti sviluppano nei primi tre giorni di vita una grave iperbilirubinemia non coniugata che, in assenza di trattamento, raggiunge livelli di 25-30 mg/dL nel corso del primo mese. Il kernittero, complicanza praticamente universale di questo disturbo, è osservabile normalmente già nel periodo neonatale precoce; alcuni bambini sottoposti a terapia sono sopravvissuti oltre l'età infantile senza sequele. La persistenza di livelli di bilirubina non coniugata >20 mg/dL oltre la prima settimana di vita, in assenza di emolisi, dovrebbe suggerire la presenza di questa sindrome.

Diagnosi. La diagnosi della sindrome di Crigler-Najjar di tipo I si basa sulla precocità dell'esordio e sugli elevati livelli di bilirubina, in assenza di emolisi. Nella bile, la concentrazione di bilirubina è <10 mg/dL, mentre le concentrazioni normali sono di 50-100 mg/dL; è inoltre assente la bilirubina glucuronide. La diagnosi definitiva è confermata dalla misurazione dell'attività della glucuronil transferasi epatica in un campione bioptico ottenuto da una biopsia a cielo coperto; la biopsia a cielo aperto va invece evitata in quanto l'anestesia chirurgica potrebbe precipitare il kernittero. È inoltre disponibile la diagnosi tramite analisi del DNA, talora preferibile. L'identificazione dello stato di eterozigosi nei genitori è altamente suggestivo per la diagnosi. La diagnosi differenziale dell'iperbilirubinemia non coniugata è trattata nel Capitolo 102.3.

Trattamento. La concentrazione sierica di bilirubina non coniugata deve essere mantenuta <20 mg/dL almeno per le prime 2-4 settimane di vita; nei neonati di basso peso, i livelli dovrebbero essere ancora più bassi. A tal scopo in genere si ricorre a ripetute trasfusioni di scambio e alla fototerapia. La terapia con fenobarbital deve essere presa in considerazione per determinare la responsività e per la diagnosi differenziale tra la forma di tipo I e quella di tipo II (vedi oltre). Anche se il rischio di kernittero persiste in età adulta, una volta passato il periodo neonatale, per provocare provocare un danno cerebrale sono necessari i livelli di bilirubinemia molto più elevati (in genere >35 mg/dL). Pertanto, la fototerapia è spesso continuata nei primi anni di vita. Nei bambini più grandicelli viene somministrata prevalentemente durante il sonno, per non interferire con le normali attività. Nonostante la somministrazione di intensità di luce crescenti, per periodi progressivamente più lunghi, la riduzione della bilirubina, in risposta alla fototerapia, diminuisce con l'età. La terapia adiuvante con agenti che legano i prodotti della fotobilirubina, come il calcio fosfato, la colestiramina o l'agar, può essere utile per interferire con la circolazione enteroepatica della bilirubina. Grazie a una terapia tempestiva in caso di infezioni intercorrenti, episodi febbrili e altre condizioni patologiche, è possibile prevenire lo sviluppo tardivo di kernittero, che può insorgere per livelli di bilirubina di 45-55 mg/dL. Tutti i pazienti con la CN di tipo I, giunti all'età giovane-adulta, hanno sviluppato kernittero, nonostante un trattamento continuo e vigoroso che ha mantenuto la normalità neurologica in età infantile. Il trapianto epatico ortotopico può risolvere la malattia e si è già dimostrato efficace in un piccolo numero di pazienti. In letteratura si trova menzione del trapianto di epatociti isolati eseguito su un paziente, il quale tuttavia ha dovuto in seguito essere sottoposto a trapianto epatico ortotopico. Altre possibilità terapeutiche comprendono la plasmaferesi e l'inibizione della produzione di bilirubina; quest'ultima opzione è possible grazie all'inibizione dell'eme ossigenasi, utilizzando una terapia con metalloporfirine. La terapia sostitutiva tramite enzimi corretti con tecniche di ingegneria genetica e la terapia genica epatodiretta sono opzioni terapeutiche ricche di potenzialità per il futuro, ma che finora sono state testate solo su modelli animali.

SINDROME DI CRIGLER-NAJJAR DI TIPO 2 (DEFICIT PARZIALE DI GLUCURONIL TRANSFERASI). Come la sindrome di Crigler-Najjar di tipo I, anche quella di tipo II è una malattia autosomica recessiva; è causata dall'omozigosi per una mutazione missense dell'UGT1A1 che comporta una ridotta (parziale) attività enzimatica. Ad oggi sono state identificate più di 18 mutazioni. La forma di tipo II si differenzia da quella di tipo I per il netto decremento della bilirubina sierica che si verifica in risposta al trattamento con fenobarbital, che dipende da un elemento inducibile di risposta al fenobarbital, sulla regione promoter dell'UGT1A1.

Manifestazioni cliniche. Quando il disturbo si presenta nel periodo neonatale, l'iperbilirubinemia compare in genere nei primi 3 giorni di vita; la concentrazione sierica di bilirubina può rientrare in un range compatibile con l'ittero fisiologico, oppure aumentare a livelli francamente patologici. Tale concentrazione rimane tipicamente elevata durante la terza settimana di vita, e oltre, mantenendosi in un range di 1,5-22 mg/dL; quando si assesta sui valori più bassi del range, può creare incertezza sulla presenza di iperbilirubinemia cronica. Lo sviluppo di kernittero è raro. Le feci sono di colore normale e i bambini non presentano segni clinici o sintomi di malattia. Sono assenti segni di emolisi.

Diagnosi. La concentrazione di bilirubina nella bile è quasi normale, nella sindromme di Crigler-Najjar di tipo II. I neonati e i bambini più piccoli affetti, che presentano ittero, rispondono prontamente a dosi di 5 mg/kg/die di fenobarbital, con una riduzione della bilirubina sierica pari a 2-3 mg/dL nell'arco di 7-10 giorni

Trattamento. Si può ottenere una riduzione a lungo termine della bilirubina sierica con la somministrazione continua di fenobarbital, alla dose di 5 mg/kg/die. È necessario soppesare benefici estetici e psicosociali rispetto ai rischi di una dose efficace del farmaco, poiché sussiste un basso rischio a lungo termine di kernittero anche in assenza di emolisi.

IPERBILIRUBINEMIA CONIUGATA EREDITARIA

L'iperbilirubinemia coniugata può essere causata di un numero ristretto di patologie rare, trasmesse per via autosomica recessiva e caratterizzate da ittero moderato. Il trasporto della bilirubina e degli altri anioni organici dal fegato alla bile risulta difettoso. L'iperbilirubinemia cronica, di lieve entità, viene in genere scoperta durante l'adolescenza o all'inizio dell'età adulta, ma può insorgere già nel secondo anno di vita. Gli esami di routine relativi alla funzionalità epatica risultano normali. L'ittero può essere esacerbato da infezioni, gravidanze, contraccettivi orali, consumo di alcol e interventi chirurgici. Non è presente in genere alcuna morbilità e l'aspettativa di vita è normale; tuttavia, questi disordini inizialmente possono porre seri problemi di diagnosi differenziale con patologie più gravi.

SINDROME DI DUBIN-JOHNSON. La sindrome di Dubin-Johnson, ereditata per via autosomica recessiva, è un difetto della secrezione epatocitaria della bilirubina glucuronide. Il difetto della funzione escretoria epatica riguarda non solo la bilirubina, ma anche numerosi anioni organici, normalmente escreti nella bile dalle cellule epatiche. Il difetto molecolare alla base della sindrome è l'assenza di funzione della proteina MRP2 (*Multiple Drug-Resistant Protein*, proteina della mutiresistenza farmacologica), un trasportatore canalicolare ATP (adenosin trifosfato)-dipendente. Sono state identificate circa 10 mutazioni diverse che possono colpire la localizzazione della MRP2, con conseguente aumento della degradazione, o alterarne l'attività di trasporto nella membrana canalicolare. L'escrezione e i livelli sierici di acidi biliari sono normali. Anche se l'escrezione urinaria di coproporfirina totale è quantitativamente normale, si registra un aumento della coproporfirina I, che può costituire fino all'80% del totale, con una concomitante riduzione dell'escrezione di coproporfirina III, che normalmente rappresenta più del 75% del totale. La colangiografia non permette di visualizzare le vie biliari e la radiografia della colecisti risulta anomala. Gli epatociti contengono un pigmento nerastro, simile a melanina.

SINDROME DI ROTOR. i pazienti affetti da questa sindrome presentano un ulteriore difetto, relativo alla captazione degli anioni organici. A differenza della sindrome di Dubin-Johnson, la coproporfirina urinaria totale è elevata, con un aumento relativo dell'isomero coproporfirina I. La colecisti è normale alla radiografia e gli epatociti non contengono pigmento. Sia nella sindrome di Dubin-Johnson sia in quella di Rotor l'escrezione di solfobromoftaleina risulta spesso alterata.

354.2 • MALATTIA DI WILSON

La malattia di Wilson (degenerazione epatolenticolare) è un disturbo autosomico recessivo caratterizzato da alterazioni degenerative dell'encefalo, da epatopatia e dall'anello corneale di Keyser-Fleischer. L'incidenza varia da 1/500 000 a 1/100 000 nascite. È una malattia progressiva e, se non trattata, fatale, per la quale è disponibile una terapia specifica ed efficace. La precoce ricerca della malattia di Wilson, nella valutazione di un paziente con qualsiasi forma di epatopatia, in particolare se di età >5 anni, non solo rende possibile iniziare precocemente la terapia specifica per questa patologia e il counseling genetico correlato, ma consente anche un trattamento appropriato di epatopatie diverse, una volta esclusa la tossicosi da rame.

PATOGENESI. Il gene anomalo della malattia di Wilson, localizzato sul braccio lungo del cromosoma 13 (13q14.3), codifica per un'ATPasi trasportatrice del rame, di tipo P (ATP7B). Questo enzima, espresso prevalentemente (ma non esclusivamente) negli epatociti, si ritiene svolga un ruolo critico nell'escrezione biliare del rame e nella sua incorporazione nella ceruloplasmina. L'assenza o il malfunzionamento dell'ATP7B comporta una riduzione dell'escrezione biliare di rame, con accumulo diffuso nel citoplasma degli epatociti. Quando le cellule epatiche sono saturate, il rame è redistribuito agli altri tessuti, tra cui il rene e il cervello, per i quali risulta particolarmente tossico, in quanto potente inibitore dei processi enzimatici. Il rame in forma ionica inibisce la piruvato ossidasi encefalica e l'ATPasi delle membrane, portando a una riduzione del contentuto tissutale di ATP-fosfocreatina e di potassio.

Dal momento che sono state identificate più di 250 mutazioni genetiche, la diagnosi tramite analisi delle mutazioni del DNA è un compito arduo, a meno che non si conosca la mutazione probanda. Nella maggior parte dei casi i pazienti sono eterozigoti composti. Le mutazioni che azzerano completamente la funzione genica si associano a un esordio precoce dei sintomi, già nel secondo o terzo anno di vita, quando la malattia di Wilson non viene generalmente considerata nella diagnosi differenziale delle epatopatie. Le mutazioni meno gravi possono associarsi a sintomi neurologici o a epatopatia tardivamente, fino a 70 anni di età. La clonazione del gene della malattia di Wilson renderà possibile una rilevazione presintomatica precisa della malattia, con inizio tempestivo della terapia, e, infine, di una terapia genica.

MANIFESTAZIONI CLINICHE. Le forme di epatopatia wilsoniana comprendono l'epatomegalia asintomatica (con o senza splenomegalia), l'epatite cronica o subacuta e l'insufficienza epatica fulminante. Lo spettro di manifestazioni cliniche della malattia di Wilson include la cirrosi criptogenetica, l'ipertensione portale, l'ascite, gli edemi, il sanguinamento da varici e altre conseguenze della disfunzione epatica (ritardo puberale, amenorrea, difetti della coagulazione).

La presentazione della malattia è variabile, con una tendenza a formare quadri familiari caratteristici. Più è giovane il paziente, più è probabile che la manifestazione predominante sia il coinvolgimento epatico. Il sesso femminile ha un rischio tre volte maggiore di presentare fin dall'esordio un'insufficienza epatica fulminante.

Dopo i 20 anni di età prevalgono i sintomi neurologici, che possono svilupparsi insidiosamente o improvvisamente, con tremore intenzionale, disartria, distonia, mancanza di coordinazione motoria, peggioramento del rendimento scolastico o cambiamenti comportamentali. L'anello di Keyser-Fleischer può essere assente nei pazienti più giovani con epatopatia, ma è sempre presente nei pazienti con sintomi neurologici. Le manifestazioni psichiatriche comprendono depressione, ansia o psicosi. Come presentazione iniziale si può riscontrare un'anemia emolitica Coombs-negativa, forse correlata al rilascio di grandi quantità di rame dagli epatociti danneggiati; questa forma di malattia di Wilson è generalmente fatale in assenza di trapianto. Durante gli episodi di emolisi, l'escrezione urinaria e i livelli sierici di rame (non legato alla ceruloplasmina) sono molto elevati. Possono essere presenti manifestazioni della sindrome di Fanconi a livello renale e di insufficienza renale progressiva, con alterazioni del trasporto tubulare di aminoacidi, glucosio e acido urico. Manifestazioni meno frequenti comprendono artrite, miocardiopatia ed endocrinopatie (ipoparatiroidismo).

ANATOMIA PATOLOGICA. Si possono osservare tutti i livelli di danno epatico, con steatosi, degenerazione balloniforme degli epatociti, granuli di glicogeno, minima infiammazione e ingrandimento delle cellule di Kupffer. Le lesioni possono essere indistinguibili da quelle dell'epatite autoimmune. Con la progressione del danno parenchimale si sviluppano fibrosi e, successivamente, cirrosi epatica. Le alterazioni ultrastrutturali a carico dei mitocondri comprendono aumentata densità della matrice, inclusioni di lipidi e materiale granulare, aumento dello spazio intracrestale con dilatazione dell'estremità delle creste. Il contenuto epatico di rame è aumentato.

DIAGNOSI. La malattia di Wilson dovrebbe essere considerata nei bambini e negli adolescenti con epatopatia acuta o cronica inspiegabile, sintomi neurologici inspiegabili, emolisi acuta, patologie psichiatriche, alterazioni comportamentali, sindrome di Fanconi o osteopatia di origine sconosciuta. Il sospetto clinico è confermato dallo studio degli indici del metabolismo rameico.

Il miglior test di screening è la misurazione dei livelli sierici di ceruloplasmina, che nella maggior parte dei pazienti con malattia di Wilson risultano ridotti. La mancata incorporazione del rame nella ceruloplasmina porta alla formazione di una proteina con emivita inferiore e, pertanto, con riduzione della concentrazione in circolo allo *steady state*. I livelli di ceruloplasmina devono essere interpretati con cautela, poiché possono aumentare in corso di infiammazione acuta e negli stati iperestrogenici come la gravidanza, la somministrazione di estrogeni esogeni o l'uso di contraccettivi orali. Il livello sierico di rame può essere elevato nelle fasi precoci della malattia; l'escrezione urinaria (normalmente <40 mcg/die) supera i 100 μg/die, spesso fino a raggiungere o addirittura superare i 1000 μg/die. Nei casi dubbi, la risposta dell'escrezione urinaria di rame alla terapia chelante può essere di aiuto diagnostico. Durante la raccolta delle 24 ore, si somministrano ai pazienti due dosi orali di D-penicillamina, di 500 mg, a distanza di 12 ore; i pazienti affetti hanno un'escrezione di 1200-2000 mg/die. Per individuare l'anello di Keyser-Fleischer, che peraltro può essere assente nei bambini più piccoli, l'oculista deve effettuare l'esame con lampada a fessura.

La biopsia epatica è utile per determinare l'estensione e la severità del danno epatico, oltre che per misurare il contenuto epatico di rame (normalmente <10 μg/g di peso secco). Nella malattia di Wilson, il contenuto epatico di rame supera i 250 μg/g di peso secco. Gli eterozigoti sani possono presentare livelli intermedi.

I familiari dei pazienti con malattia dimostrata devono essere sottoposti a screening per malattia di Wilson presintomatica. Lo screening deve comprendere la determinazione dei livelli sierici di ceruloplasmina e l'escrezione urinaria di rame. Se questi valori risultano anomali o dubbi, occorre effettuare una biopsia epatica per determinare la morfologia e il contenuto di rame del fegato. Lo screening genetico tramite analisi dei linkage o analisi diretta delle mutazioni del DNA è possibile, in particolare se la mutazione per il caso probando è conosciuta o se il paziente proviene da un'area geografica in cui è diffusa una mutazione speficica nota (per es., nell'Europa centrale e orientale la mutazione H1069Q è presente nel 50-80% dei pazienti).

TRATTAMENTO. Il principale obiettivo dovrebbe essere cercare di ridurre l'apporto di rame a meno di 1 mg/die. A tal scopo, occorre evitare cibi come fegato, molluschi, noci e cioccolato; se il contenuto di rame dell'acqua potabile è $>0,1$ mg/L, può essere necessaria la demineralizzazione. La somministrazione di agenti chelanti il rame, nei pazienti con malattia di Wilson, porta alla rapida escrezione dei depositi di rame in eccesso. La terapia chelante migliore consiste nella somministrazione orale di D-penicillamina (β,β-dimetilcisteina) alla dose di 1 g/die in due somministrazioni prima dei pasti, negli adulti, e di 20 mg/kg/die nei pazienti pediatrici. In risposta al farmaco, l'escrezione urinaria di rame aumenta nettamente e con la somministrazione a lungo termine i livelli di rame urinario possono arrivare a normalizzarsi, con un marcato miglioramento della funzione epatica e neurologica, e la scomparsa dell'anello di Keyser-Fleischer. Tuttavia, il 10-50% dei pazienti trattati inizialmente con penicillamina per i sintomi neurologici va incontro a un peggioramento. Gli effetti tossici della penicillamina, che compaiono nel 10-20% dei casi, consistono in reazioni di ipersensibilità (sindrome di Goodpasture, lupus eritematoso sistemico, polimiosite), interazione con il collagene e l'elastina, deficit di altri elementi come lo zinco, anemia aplastica e sindrome nefrosica. È necessario un supplemento di vitamina B_6, di cui la penicillamina è un antimetabolita. Nei pazienti intolleranti alla penicillamina, un'alternativa accettabile è rappresentata dalla trietilentetramina diidroclorito, alla dose di 0,5-2,0 g/die per gli adulti e di 20 mg/kg/die per i bambini. Un agente chelante alternativo è l'ammonio tetraidromolibdato, in corso di studio per i pazienti con patologia neurologica; i risultati iniziali suggeriscono che una percentuale significativamente inferiore di pazienti vada incontro a deterioramento neurologico con questo farmaco, in confronto alla penicillamina. La dose iniziale è di 120 mg/die (20 mg tra i pasti, due volte al giorno e 20 mg durante i pasti, due volte al giorno). Se il paziente mangia qualcosa durante la notte, deve assumere contemporaneamente altri 20 mg di farmaco. Gli effetti collaterali comprendono anemia, leucopenia, trombocitopenia e lieve aumento delle transaminasi. È stato anche utilizzato lo zinco come terapia adiuvante, di mantenimento o di prima scelta nei pazienti presintomatici, grazie alla sua capacità unica di alterare l'assorbimento gastrointestinale di rame. Lo zinco acetato viene somministrato sotto forma di elemento alla dose di 25-50 mg, tre volte al giorno, negli adulti e di 25 mg, tre volte al giorno, nei bambini di età superiore a 5 anni.

PROGNOSI. I pazienti con malattia di Wilson non trattati muoiono per le complicanze epatiche, neurologiche, renali o ematologiche. Quelli sottoposti a terapia precoce e continua con penicillamina hanno una prognosi variabile, che dipende dall'epoca di inizio e dalla risposta individuale alla terapia chelante. Il trapianto epatico dovrebbe essere preso in considerazione nei pazienti con epatopatia fulminante, cirrosi scompensata o degenerazione neurologica progressiva; quest'ultima indicazione, tuttavia, è controversa. Il trapianto epatico è curativo, con una sopravvivenza dell'85-90%. Nei fratelli asintomatici dei pazienti affetti, la somministrazione precoce della terapia chelante può prevenire l'espressione della patologia.

354.3 • Cirrosi indiana infantile

Il rame ha anche un ruolo in epatopatie diverse dalla malattia di Wilson, che colpiscono i bambini più piccoli, con altre anomalie genetiche, per la maggior parte sconosciute, che ne alterano il metabolismo. La cirrosi indiana infantile (ICC, *Indian Childhood Cirrhosis*), frequente nelle aree rurali dell'India, si presenta con ittero, prurito, letargia ed epatosplenomegalia. Istologicamente, è caratterizzata da necrosi epatocitaria, corpi di Mallory, fibrosi intralobulare e infiammazione. È presente un aumento del contenuto epatico di rame, in genere >700 μg/g di peso secco. L'ICC è stata correlata a un'eccessiva assunzione di rame con l'alimentazione, riconducibile in particolare agli utensili in questo materiale usati per la cottura e la somministrazione del latte ai bambini. Poiché le quantità ingerite da sole non bastano a spiegare un contenuto epatico di rame così elevato, si potrebbe ipotizzare una suscettibilità genetica alla tossicosi da rame. L'ICC, se non trattata, ha una mortalità del 45% entro 4 settimane. La somministrazione di penicillamina durante le fasi iniziali della malattia, a dosi simili a quelle previste per il trattamento della malattia di Wilson, riduce della metà la mortalità. Da quando è stata avviata una campagna volta a sensibilizzare le famiglie sull'associazione tra utensili in rame e ICC, l'incidenza di questa patologia si è ridotta. Sono state scoperte varianti della sindrome, che hanno preso il nome dalla popolazione in cui sono state descritte, come la cirrosi infantile del Tirolo, riportata anche in Medio Oriente, nell'Africa Occidentale e nell'America settentrionale e centrale.

354.4 • Malattia da deposito di ferro neonatale

La malattia da deposito di ferro neonatale (NISD, *Neonatal Iron Storage Disease*), nota anche con il nome di **emocromatosi neonatale**, è una rara forma di epatopatia fulminante che si manifesta nei primi giorni di vita. Sono presenti indici di danno intrauterino, come il fatto che i bambini colpiti siano spesso prematuri o presentino ritardo di crescita intrauterina. Numerosi neonati con NISD sono affetti anche da disgenesia renale. Clinicamente, la NISD è una malattia progressiva, rapidamente fatale, caratterizzata da epatomegalia, ipoglicemia, ipoprotrombinemia, ipoalbuminemia, iperferritinemia e iperbilirubinemia. La colagulopatia è refrattaria alla terapia con vitamina K. La diagnosi può essere confermata dalla documentazione di siderosi extraepatica (materiale bioptico delle ghiandole della mucosa orale sature di ferro) o dalla determinazione con RM dell'accumulo di ferro in organi come il pancreas.

La NISD ha un elevato tasso di ricorrenza in ambito familiare, con una probabilità dell'80% che i figli nati successivamente ne siano affetti. Potrebbe trattarsi di una malattia gestazionale alloimmune; si è ipotizzato che il bersaglio della risposta materna alloimmune sia un antigene epatico fetale. La ricorrenza della NISD potrebbe essere modificata dalla somministrazione di IVIG, una volta alla settimana, dalla 18ª settimana di gestazione fino al parto. La più ampia esperienza finora riguarda 18 donne, già madri di soggetti affetti da NISD, che hanno partorito 22 bambini (2 coppie di gemelli) dopo trattamento con IVIG. Tutti i bambini sono sopravvissuti con o senza terapia medica. La maggior parte di essi aveva un'evidenza biochimica di danno epatico con elevati livelli di α-fetoproteina e di ferritina. La biopsia epatica, eseguita su quattro pazienti, ha dimostrato la presenza di epatite severa con necrosi e depositi di ferro. Alcuni pazienti con NISD sono stati trattati con successo con agenti chelanti il ferro (deferoxamina) e una terapia antiossidante aggressiva. Questo approccio può essere efficace se iniziato molto precocemente. La possibilità di un trapianto epatico dovrebbe anche essere presa in esame precocemente.

354.5 • Altre malattie metaboliche del fegato

Deficit di α_1-antitripsina

Una piccola percentuale di individui omozigoti per il deficit del più importante inibitore sierico delle proteasi, l'α_1-antitripsina, manifesta colestasi neonatale o insorgenza più tardiva di cirrosi infantile. L'α_1-antitripsina, un inibitore delle proteasi sintetizzato dal fegato, protegge il tessuto alveolare polmonare dalla distruzione da parte dell'elastasi dei neutrofili (vedi Capitolo 389). È presente in più di 20 alleli codominanti, di cui solo alcuni associati a un inibitore delle proteasi difettoso. L'allele più comune del sistema inibitore delle proteasi (Pi) è M, e il genotipo normale è PiMM. L'allele Z predispone al deficit clinico; i pazienti con epatopatia hanno generalmente un genotipo PiZZ e presentano livelli di α_1-antitripsina <2 mg/mL (10-20% del normale). L'incidenza del genotipo PiZZ nella popolazione bianca è stimata intorno a 1/2000-4000. Anche gli eterozigoti composti PiZ-, PiSZ, PiZI sono stati associati a danno epatico, mentre il genotipo null non è associato a malattia epatica.

Il peptide di α_1-antitripsina neoformato, una volta entrato nel reticolo endoplasmatico, va incontro a modificazione enzimatica e a ripiegamento, prima del trasporto alla membrana plasmatica, dove verrà escreto sotto forma di glicoproteina di 55 kDa. Nei pazienti affetti con genotipo PiZZ, la velocità alla quale il peptide di α_1-antitripsina si ripiega è ridotta e questo ritardo permette la formazione di polimeri, che sono trattenuti nel reticolo endoplasmatico. Nelle biopsie epatiche dei pazienti, i peptidi di α_1-antitripsina polimerizzati possono essere osservati al microscopio elettronico e in immunoistochimica come glubuli PAS-positivi, diastasi-resistenti, principalmente negli epatociti periportali, ma anche nelle cellule di Kupffer e nelle cellule epiteliali biliari. Non è noto attraverso quale meccanismo i polimeri causino il danno epatico. Il quadro del danno epatico neonatale può essere molto variabile e la biopsia può rivelare necrosi epatocellulare, infiltrato di cellule infiammatorie, proliferazione dei dotti biliari, fibrosi periportale o cirrosi.

Nei pazienti affetti anche il decorso dell'epatopatia è molto variabile. Studi prospettici condotti in Svezia hanno dimostrato che solo 10% dei pazienti sviluppa un danno epatico clinicamente significativo entro la quarta decade di vita. Tratti genetici o fattori ambientali probabilmente influiscono sullo sviluppo della malattia negli individui con deficit di α_1-antitripsina. I neonati con epatopatia sono indistinguibili dagli altri con epatite neonatale "idiopatica", di cui costituiscono il 5-10% circa. L'ittero, presente nella prima settimana di vita in associazione con feci acoliche ed epatomegalia, si risolve normalmente in un lasso di tempo compreso tra il secondo e il quarto mese. Possono seguire risoluzione completa, epatopatia persistente o l'evoluzione in cirrosi. I bambini più grandi possono presentarsi con epatomegalia asintomatica o manifestazione di epatopatia cronica o cirrosi, con evidenza di ipertensione portale.

Il trapianto epatico può essere curativo.

Ala A, Walker AP, Ashkan K, et al: Wilson's disease. *Lancet* 2007;369: 397–408.

Bosma PJ: Inherited disorders of bilirubin metabolism. *J Hepatol* 2003; 38:107–117.

Bove KE, Daugherty CC, Tyson W, et al: Bile acid synthetic defects and liver disease. *Pediatr Dev Pathol* 2000;3:1–16.

Brewer GJ, Hedera P, Kluin KJ, et al: Treatment of Wilson disease with ammonium tetrathiomolybdate. *Arch Neurol* 2003;60:379–385.

Feranchak AP, Sokol RJ: Cholangiocyte biology and cystic fibrosis liver disease. *Semin Liver Dis* 2001;21:471–488.

Fox IJ, Chowdhury JR: Hepatocyte transplantation. *Am J Transplant* 2004;4:7–13.

Grabhorn E, Richter A, Burdelski M, et al: Neonatal hemochromatosis: Long-term experience with favorable outcome. *Pediatrics* 2006;118:2060–2065.
Grompe M: The pathophysiology and treatment of hereditary tyrosinemia type 1. *Semin Liver Dis* 2001;21:563–571.
Kadakol A, Ghosh SS, Sappal BS, et al: Genetic lesions of bilirubin uridine-diphosphoglucuronate glucuronosyltransferase (UGT1A1) causing Crigler-Najjar and Gilbert syndromes: Correlation of genotype to phenotype. *Hum Mutat* 2000;16:297–306.
Keitel V, Nies AT, Brom M, et al: A common Dubin-Johnson syndrome mutation impairs protein maturation and transport activity of MRP2 (ABCC2). *Am J Physiol Gastrointest Liver Physiol* 2003;284:G165–G174.
Kelley AL, Lunt PW, Rodrigues F, et al: Classification and genetic features of neonatal haemochromatosis: A study of 27 affected pedigrees and molecular analysis of genes implicated in iron metabolism. *J Med Genet* 2001;38:599–610.
Loudinos G, Gitlin JD: Wilson's disease. *Semin Liver Dis* 2000;20:353–364.
Mor-Cohen R, Zivelin A, Rosenberg N, et al: Identification and functional analysis of two novel mutations in the multidrug resistance protein 2 gene in Israeli patients with Dubin-Johnson syndrome. *J Biol Chem* 2001; 276:36923–36930.
Perlmutter DH: Alpha-1-antitrypsin deficiency: Diagnosis and treatment. *Clin Liver Dis* 2004;8:839–859.
Primhak RA, Tanner MS: Alpha-1 antitrypsin deficiency. *Arch Dis Child* 2001;85:2–5.
Schilsky ML: Wilson disease: New insights into pathogenesis, diagnosis, and future therapy. *Curr Gastroenterol Rep* 2005;7:26–31.
Taly AB, Meenakshi-Sundaram S, Sinha S, et al: Wilson disease. Description of 282 patients evaluated over 3 decades. *Medicine* 2007;82:112–121.
Tanner MS: Role of copper in Indian childhood cirrhosis. *Am J Clin Nutr* 1998;67:1074S–1081S.
Tao TY, Gitlin JD: Hepatic copper metabolism: Insights from genetic disease. *Hepatology* 2003;37:1241–1247.
Whitington PF, Malladi P: Neonatal hemochromatosis: Is it an alloimmune disease? *J Pediatr Gastroenterol Nutr* 2005;40:544–549.

Capitolo 355 ■ Epatite virale Nada Yazigi e William F. Balistreri

L'epatite virale è un problema di salute primario sia nei Paesi sviluppati sia in quelli in via di sviluppo. Può essere causata da almeno cinque dei virus patogeni epatotropi attualmente riconosciuti: i virus dell'epatite A, B, C, D ed E (Tab. 355-1). Molti altri virus possono causare epatite, in genere nell'ambito di un quadro patologico multisistemico; tra questi il virus dell'herpes simplex (HSV, *Herpes Simplex Virus*), il Cytomegalovirus (CMV), il virus di Epstein-Barr (EBV, *Epstein-Barr Virus*), il virus varicella-zoster, l'HIV, il virus della rosolia, gli adenovirus, gli enterovirus, il parvovirus B19 e gli arbovirus. Il virus dell'epatite G (HGV, *Hepatitis G Virus*) e il virus trasmissibile tramite trasfusione (TTV, *Transfusion Trasmissible Virus*) colpiscono spesso il fegato come coinfettanti, insieme ad altri virus epatotropi, e possono dare origine a viremia acuta o cronica, ma raramente sono in grado, da soli, di provocare un danno epatocellulare.

I virus epatotropi sono un gruppo eterogeneo di agenti infettivi che causano una patologia acuta e cronica simile. Nella maggior parte dei pazienti in età pediatrica, la fase acuta della malattia dà disturbi molto lievi oppure è asintomatica. La morbilità è correlata ai rari casi di **insufficienza epatica fulminante** che si instaura in pazienti suscettibili e alla condizione di malattia cronica, con le sue complicanze, che tre di questi virus (B, C, D) possono causare. L'epidemiologia di queste forme presentano un'estrema variabilità geografica e altrettanto variabile è il loro impatto clinico.

TABELLA 355-1. Caratteristiche dei virus epatotropi

	HAV	HBV	HCV	HDV	HEV	HGV*	TTV**
Virologia	**RNA**	**DNA**	**RNA**	**RNA**	**RNA**	**RNA**	**DNA**
Incubazione (gg)	15-19	60-180	14-160	21-42	21-63	?	?
Trasmissione							
Parenterale	Rara	Sì	Sì	Sì	No	Sì	Sì
Orofecale	Sì	No	No	No	Sì	Possibile	Possibile
Sessuale	No	Sì	Sì	Sì	No	Sì	Possibile
Perinatale	No	Sì	Rara	Sì	No	Sì	Sì
Infezione cronica	No	Sì	Sì	Sì	No	Sì	Sì
Malattia fulminante	Rara	Sì	Rara	Sì	Sì	No	No

HAV, *Hepatitis A Virus*, virus dell'epatite A; ?, sconosciuta.
*Anche detto GBV-C (causa raramente danno epatico, spesso coinfezione).
** *Transfusion Transmissible Virus*, virus trasmissibile con le trasfusioni (spesso coinfezione con altri virus epatitici, raramente causa epatopatia da solo).

CARATTERISTICHE COMUNI A TUTTE LE FORME DI EPATITE VIRALE

DIAGNOSI DIFFERENZIALE. Spesso il paziente giunge all'attenzione medica per l'ittero, che, nell'epatite, è dato da un'iperbilirubinemia mista o prevalentemente diretta (coniugata).

Nel **periodo neonatale**, le infezioni sono una causa comune di iperbilirubinemia diretta; la causa infettiva può essere un agente batterico (*Escherichia coli*, *Listeria*) o uno dei virus non epatotropi (HSV, enterovirus, CMV). Occorre sempre escludere cause metaboliche o anatomiche (tirosinemia, atresia biliare, cisti del coledoco) (vedi Capitolo 353.1).

Nell'**infanzia** devono essere escluse l'ostruzione extraepatica (calcoli, colangite sclerosante primitiva, patologia pancreatica), condizioni infiammatorie (epatite autoimmune, artrite reumatoide giovanile, malattia di Kawasaki, disregolazione immunitaria), patologie infiltrative (tumori maligni), tossine/farmaci, malattie metaboliche (malattia di Wilson, fibrosi cistica) e infezioni (EBV, varicella, malaria, leptospirosi, sifilide).

PATOGENESI. La risposta acuta del fegato ai virus epatotropi consiste sia nel danno citopatico diretto, sia in quello immunomediato. Tutto il fegato è coinvolto. La necrosi, quando presente, è generalmente più marcata nelle aree centrolobulari. L'infiltrato infiammatorio misto acuto predomina nelle aree portali, ma coinvolge anche i lobuli. L'architettura lobulare rimane intatta, sebbene la degenerazione balloniforme e la necrosi di singoli gruppi di cellule parenchimali siano frequenti. L'infiltrazione grassa è rara, salvo che nell'infezione da HCV. È comune la proliferazione dei dotti biliari, ma non il danno dei dotti stessi. Nei sinusoidi si osserva iperplasia diffusa delle cellule di Kupffer. I neonati spesso rispondono al danno epatico con la formazione di **cellule giganti**.

Nell'**epatite fulminante**, al quadro appena descritto si aggiunge il collasso del parenchima. Con la guarigione, il fegato ritorna alla normalità morfologica nell'arco di tre mesi dall'infezione acuta. Se si sviluppa un'epatite cronica, l'infiltrato infiammatorio si insedia nelle aree periportali, portando spesso alla progressiva cicatrizzazione; entrambi questi indici di epatite cronica sono tipici dell'infezione da HBV e da HCV.

PROFILI BIOCHIMICI COMUNI NELLA FASE DI INFEZIONE ACUTA. Il danno epatico acuto causato dai virus epatotropi si manifesta con tre principali profili degli esami biochimici di funzionalità epatica. Questi sono un'importante guida alla terapia di supporto e al monitoraggio della fase acuta dell'infezione, per tutti i virus.

1. **Come riflesso del danno citopatico agli epatociti, si verifica un aumento dei livelli sierici di alanino aminotransferasi (ALT, in passato chiamata transaminasi glutamico-ossalacetica sierica). L'entità dell'aumento enzimatico non correla con l'estensione della necrosi epatocellulare e ha scarso valore prognostico. Di solito si assiste a un lento miglioramento delle transaminasi, nel corso di diverse settimane, ma i livelli di AST/ALT si mantengono elevati più a lungo di quelli della bilirubina, che tende a normalizzarsi prima. Livelli di transaminasi che si riducono rapidamente possono essere predittivi di esito sfavorevole, in particolare se il fenomeno si verifica in concomitanza con un aumento dei livelli di bilirubina e del PT; questa combinazione indica generalmente lo sviluppo di un danno epatico massivo.**
2. **La colestasi, definita da elevati livelli sierici di bilirubina coniugata, è conseguenza di un anomalo flusso biliare a livello canalicolare e cellulare, causato dal danno epatocitario e dai**

mediatori dell'infiammazione. Si osserva un aumento della fosfatasi alcalina sierica (ALP, *ALkaline Phosphatase*), della 5′-nucleotidasi, della γ-glutamil transpeptidasi (GGT) e dell'urobilinogeno, che sono tutti marcatori di colestasi. Il miglioramento tende a seguire in parallelo la fase epatitica acuta. L'assenza di marcatori di colestasi non esclude la progressione alla cronicità nelle infezioni da HBV e da HCV.

3. Il più importante marcatore di danno epatico è l'alterazione della funzione di sintesi, il monitoraggio della quale dovrebbe quindi essere l'obiettivo principale del follow-up clinico per definire l'acuzie della malattia. Nella fase acuta, il grado di disfunzione della sintesi epatica fornisce indicazioni per il trattamento e aiuta a stabilire criteri di intervento. Una funzione sintetica anomala è un marcatore di insufficienza epatica e un indicazione al rapido invio a un centro trapianti. È necessaria una valutazione seriata, poiché la disfunzione epatica non ha una progressione lineare. Indici di alterata sintesi sono una sintesi proteica compromessa (prolungamento del tempo di protrombina, INR elevato, ridotti livelli sierici di albumina, ipoglicemia, acidosi lattica, iperammoniemia) o segni clinici come una ridotta eliminazione dei farmaci a metabolismo epatico, o un'alterazione del sensorio con aumento dei riflessi tendinei profondi (encefalopatia epatica; vedi Capitolo 361).

EPATITE A

Il virus dell'epatite A (HAV, *Hepatitis A Virus*) è quello a prevalenza più elevata, tra i cinque virus epatotropi, negli Stati Uniti e nel mondo. È inoltre responsabile della maggior parte delle epatiti acute e benigne; l'epatite fulminante, sebbene possibile, resta un evento raro e si verifica più spesso negli adulti che nei bambini.

EZIOLOGIA. L'HAV è un virus a RNA, membro della famiglia dei picornavirus. È stabile al calore e ha una gamma limitata di ospiti, ovvero l'uomo e gli altri primati.

EPIDEMIOLOGIA. L'infezione da HAV si verifica in tutto il mondo, ma ha una prevalenza maggiore nei Paesi in via di sviluppo. Negli Stati Uniti, il 30-40% della popolazione adulta ha un'evidenza di pregressa infezione da HAV. Si ritiene che l'epatite A sia responsabile del 50% circa di tutte le epatite virali acute, clinicamente evidenti, negli Stati Uniti. In conseguenza di un'aggressiva implementazione della campagna di vaccinazione infantile, la prevalenza dei casi sintomatici di HAV, negli Stati Uniti, si è significativamente ridotta. Tuttavia, picchi di incidenza nei centri di assistenza diurna (dove la diffusione da bambini piccoli infetti, non itterici, può avvenire facilmente), così come numerose epidemie causate da cibo e acqua contaminati, negli ultimi anni, hanno giustificato l'adozione di un programma di vaccinazione universale in diversi Stati.

L'HAV, altamente contagioso, si trasmette quasi sempre tramite contatto interpersonale, per via orofecale. La trasmissione parenterale è rara; non sono conosciute altre forme di trasmissione. L'infezione da HAV durante la gravidanza o al momento del parto non sembra provocare un aumento delle complicanze gestazionali, né una malattia clinica nel neonato. Negli Stati Uniti si osserva un aumentato rischio di infezione nei contatti con persone infette, negli asili, in ambito familiare. L'infezione è stata associata anche al contatto con cibo e acqua contaminati, dopo viaggi in aree endemiche. Si sono verificate epidemie da una fonte alimentare comune, in particolare molluschi, bacche surgelate e verdure crude contaminate; tuttavia, in circa la metà dei casi non è possibile identificarne l'origine. Il periodo medio di incubazione dell'HAV è di tre settimane. L'escrezione fecale del virus inizia tardivamente nel periodo di incubazione, raggiunge un picco poco prima dell'insorgenza dei sintomi e si risolve due settimane dopo l'esordio dell'ittero, nei pazienti più grandi. La durata dell'escrezione virale è più prolungata nei neonati. Il paziente è pertanto contagioso prima della comparsa dei sintomi clinici e resta tale finché non cessa il rilascio di virus.

MANIFESTAZIONI CLINICHE. L'HAV è responsabile solo di forme di epatite acuta. Spesso ha decorso anitterico, con sintomi clinici indistinguibili da quelli di altre forme di gastroenterite virale, in particolare nei bambini più piccoli. La patologia è sintomatica soprattutto nella tarda adolescenza o in età adulta, nei pazienti con disturbi epatici sottostanti e in quelli immunocompromessi. Si presenta caratteristicamente come una malattia febbrile acuta con insorgenza improvvisa di anoressia, nausea, malessere, vomito e ittero. La sua durata tipica è di 7-14 giorni (Fig. 355-1).

Durante l'infezione acuta da HAV possono essere coinvolti anche altri organi. Linfonodi regionali e milza possono aumentare di volume. Il midollo osseo può essere moderatamente ipoplastico e sono stati riportati casi di anemia aplastica. La mucosa dell'intestino tenue talvolta presenta cambiamenti della struttura villosa e possono svilupparsi ulcere del tratto digerente, in particolare nei casi fatali. Sono stati riportati casi di pancreatite acuta e di miocardite, per quanto rari, e possono svilupparsi nefrite, artrite, vasculite e crioglobulinemia a causa degli immunocomplessi circolanti.

DIAGNOSI. L'infezione acuta da HAV viene diagnosticata tramite la rilevazione degli anticorpi specifici, in particolare le immunoglobline (Ig) M anti-HAV, tramite *radioimmunoassay* o, raramente, mediante identificazione delle particelle virali nelle feci. È disponibile un test virale in PCR (*Polymerase Chain Reaction*, reazione a catena della polimerasi) a scopo di ricerca (Tab. 355-2). Gli anti-HAV sono rilevabili quando i sintomi sono clinicamente evidenti e restano positivi per 4-6 mesi dopo l'infezione acuta. A distanza di 8 settimane dell'esordio sintomatologico si trova normalmente un anticorpo neutralizzanne anti-HAV (IgG), che viene misurato insieme agli anti-HAV totali del siero e che conferisce protezione a lungo termine.

Il virus è escreto nelle feci da due settimane prima a una settimana dopo l'insorgenza della malattia. Altri reperti, come l'aumento di AST, ALT, bilirubina, 5′-nucleotidasi e GGT, sono pressoché universali e non sono di alcun aiuto nella diagnosi differenziale dell'epatite.

COMPLICANZE. Sebbene la maggior parte dei pazienti guarisca completamente, due sono le complicanze che possono insorgere:

1. L'insufficienza epatica acuta (ALF, *Acute Liver Failure*) da infezione HAV è rara ma possibile. I pazienti più a rischio sono gli adulti, ma anche gli individui immunocompromessi o con una sottostante epatopatia. L'entità della viremia HAV può essere correlata alla severità dell'epatite. Sebbene negli Stati Uniti l'epatite da HAV rappresenti meno dello 0,5% delle ALF in età pediatrica, è responsabile del 3% della mortalità nella popolazione adulta con ALF. Nelle aree endemiche, l'epatite da HAV costituisce fino al 40% di tutti i casi di ALF pediatrica.
2. L'epatite da HAV può evolvere in una sindrome colestatica prolungata ad andamento ondulante, nel corso di diversi mesi. Il prurito e il malassorbimento lipidico possono essere problematici e richiedono un supporto sintomatico con farmaci contro il prurito e vitamine liposolubili. Questa sidrome si verifica in assenza di disfunzione epatica e si risolve senza sequele.

TRATTAMENTO. Non esiste un trattamento specifico per l'epatite A. La terapia di supporto consiste nell'idratazione per via endo-

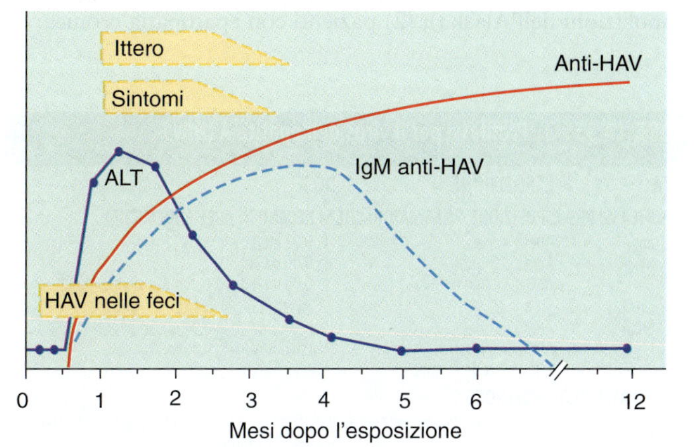

Figura 355-1. Andamento sierologico dell'epatite A acuta. ALT, alanino aminotransferasi; HAV, *Hepatitis A Virus*, virus dell'epatite A (Da Goldman L, Ausiello D: *Cecil Textbook of Medicine*, 22nd ed. Philadelphia, Saunders, 2004, p 913.)

TABELLA 355-2. Esami di laboratorio diagnostici: sierologia e PCR virali

	HAV	HBV	HCV	HDV	HEV
Acuta Infezione	Anti-HAV IgM (+) Blood PCR (+)*	Anti-HBc IgM (+) HBsAg (+) Anti-HBs HBV DNA (+) (PCR)	Anti-HCV (+) HCV RNA (+) (PCR)	Anti-HDV IgM (+) Blood PCR (+) (PCR) Anti-HBs (−)	Anti-HEV IgM (+) Blood PCR (+) HBsAg (+)
Infezione pregressa (guarita)	Anti-HAV IgG (+)	Anti-HBs (+) Anti-HBc IgG (+)	Anti-HCV (−) Blood PCR (−)	Anti-HDV IgG (+) Blood PCR (−)	Anti-HEV IgG (+) Blood PCR (−)
Infezione cronica	N/A	Anti-HBc IgG (+) HBsAg (+) Anti-HBs PCR (+) o (−)	Anti-HCV (+) Blood PCR (+)	Anti-HDV IgG (+) Blood PCR (−) HBsAg (+)	N/A
Risposta al vaccino	Anti-HAV IgG (+)	Anti-HBs (+) Anti-HBc (−)	N/A	N/A	N/A

*A scopo di ricerca.
HAV, *Hepatitis A Virus*, virus dell'epatite A; HBs, *Hepatitis B surface*, superficie del virus dell'epatite B HBsAg, *Hepatitis B surface Antigen*, antigene di superficie del virus dell'epatite B; Ig, immunoglobuline; PCR, *Polymerase Chain Reaction*, reazione a catena della polimerasi.

venosa, se necessario, e nella somministrazione di farmaci contro il prurito e di vitamine liposolubili, nella forma con colestasi prolungata. Il monitoraggio seriato per eventuali segni di insufficienza epatica acuta e il rapido invio a un centro trapianti possono salvare la vita ai pazienti nei casi a evoluzione più grave.

PREVENZIONE. I pazienti infettati dall'HAV sono contagiosi per 2 settimane prima e per circa 7 giorni dopo l'insorgenza dell'ittero; durante questo periodo non dovrebbero quindi frequentare scuole, asili o luoghi di lavoro. È necessaria un'attenta pulizia delle mani, in particolare dopo il cambio dei pannolini e prima di preparare o servire il cibo. In ambiente ospedaliero, le precauzioni standard e di contatto sono consigliate per una settimana dopo l'insorgenza dei sintomi.

Vaccini. La disponibilità di due vaccini per l'HAV inattivati, altamenti immunogeni e sicuri, ha avuto un impatto notevole sulla prevenzione dell'infezione. Tali vaccini, approvati entrambi per i bambini di età >1 anno, vengono somministrati per via intramuscolare in due dosi, a distanza di 6-12 mesi l'una dall'altra. Nei bambini, il tasso di sieroconversione supera il 90% dopo la dose iniziale e si avvicina al 100% dopo la seconda. Nei pazienti immunocompromessi, la risposta immunitaria può essere subottimale. Il vaccino per l'HAV può essere somministrato contemporaneamente ad altri vaccini, in sede separata. Per i soggetti di età >1 anno, il vaccino è preferibile alle immunoglobuline per la profilassi pre-esposizione (Tab. 355-3). Si riserva inoltre grande attenzione ad altri gruppi a rischio, tra cui: (1) bambini di età >1 anno che vivono in comunità chiuse, con tassi endemici o epidemie periodiche di infezione da HAV (per es. indiani d'America o popolazioni dell'Alaska); (2) pazienti con epatopatia cronica; (3) individui a rischio di esposizione occupazionale; (4) persone con disturbi della coagulazione o deficit immunitari. Negli Stati Uniti e in alcuni altri Paesi, la vaccinazione universale è consigliata per tutti i bambini di età >1 anno.

In caso di epidemie scolastiche si è fatto ricorso all'immunizzazione di massa dei bambini in età scolare. Il vaccino è efficace nell'arginare le epidemie di epatite A, anche quando viene somministrato dopo l'esposizione, grazie alla rapida sieroconversione e al lungo periodo di incubazione della malattia. Tuttavia, non si dispone ancora di dati sufficienti per consigliare il solo vaccino HAV per la profilassi postesposizione della malattia.

Immunoglobuline (Ig). Le indicazioni per la somministrazione intramuscolare di Ig comprendono la profilassi pre- e postesposizione (vedi Tab. 355-3). Le Ig endovena sono probabilmente efficaci contro l'infezione da HAV, ma la dose appropriata, l'efficacia e la durata della protezione non sono ancora state definite. Le Ig sono raccomandate per la profilassi pre-esposizione in tutti i viaggiatori ricettivi, che si recano in Paesi dove l'HAV è endemico. Per i bambini di età >2 anni, l'immunizzazione per l'HAV è preferibile se l'intervallo prima della partenza è >1 mese, dopo la prima dose. La profilassi postesposizione con Ig è indicata per: (1) familiari e partner sessuali dei casi di HAV; (2) neonati con madri infette; (3) personale di asili, così come impiegati, bambini e loro familiari; (4) epidemie in istituti o ospedali. L'utilizzo di Ig quando sono trascorse >2 settimane dall'esposizione non è indicato. Le Ig non sono consigliate di routine per l'esposizione sporadica in ambiente non familiare (per es. protezione del personale ospedaliero o dei bambini in età scolare).

TABELLA 355-3. Profilassi per il virus dell'epatite A (HAV)

ETÀ	ESPOSIZIONE	DOSE
PROFILASSI PRE-ESPOSIZIONE (VIAGGIATORI CHE SI RECANO IN AREE ENDEMICHE)		
<1 anno	Attesa <mesi	Ig 0,02 mL/kg
	Attesa 3-5 mesi	Ig 0,06 mL/kg
	Attesa a lungo termine	Ig 0,06 mL/kg alla partenza e ogni 5 mesi da allora in poi
≥1 anno	Attesa <3mesi	Vaccino HAV* o Ig 0,02 mL/kg
	Attesa 3-5 mesi	Vaccino HAV* o Ig 0,06 mL/kg
	Attesa a lungo termine	Vaccino HAV*
PROFILASSI POSTESPOSIZIONE		
	≤2 settimane dall'esposizione	Ig 0,02 mL/kg e vaccino HAV se >1 anno e probabile riesposizione futura
	>2 settimane dall'esposizione	Nessuna profilassi. Considerare il vaccino HAV se >1 anno e probabile riesposizione futura

*Due vaccini inattivati sono stati approvati in soggetti di età ≥1 anno.
Ig, immunoglobuline.

PROGNOSI. La prognosi è eccellente, priva di sequele a lungo termine. L'unica complicanza temibile è l'ALF. Tuttavia, l'infezione da HAV resta una causa importante di morbilità, e ha un elevato impatto socioeconomico durante le epidemie e nelle aree endemiche.

EPATITE B

EZIOLOGIA. Il virus dell'epatite B (HBV, *Hepatitis B Virus*) appartiene alla famiglia delle Hepadnaviridae, comprendente un gruppo di virus epatotropi a DNA. L'HBV ha un DNA circolare, parzialmente a doppia elica, composto da circa 3200 nucleotidi. Sono stati identificati quattro geni: S (superficie), C (core), X e P (polimero). La superficie del virus comprende particelle chiamate *antigeni di superficie dell'HBV* (HBsAg, *Hepatitis B surface Antigen*), caratterizzati da una particella sferica di 22 nm di diametro e una tubulare di lunghezza variabile, fino a 200 nm. La parte interna del virione contiene l'antigene core (interno) dell'epatite B (HBcAg), il nucleocapside che codifica per il DNA virale e un antigene non strutturale, detto antigene e dell'epatite B (HBe-

Ag), un antigene solubile non particolato, derivato dall'HBcAg tramite autoclivaggio proteolitico. L'HBeAg funge da marcatore di replicazione virale attiva e correla normalmente con i livelli di HBV DNA. La replicazione dell'HBV avviene principalmente nel fegato, ma anche nei linfociti, nella milza, nei reni e nel pancreas.

EPIDEMIOLOGIA. L'HBV è diffuso in tutto il mondo; circa 400 milioni di persone presentano un'infezione cronica. Le aree di maggior prevalenza sono l'Africa Subsahariana, la Cina, parte del Medio Oriente, il bacino amazzonico e le isole del Pacifico. Negli Stati Uniti, la popolazione eschimese, in Alaska, aveva il più alto tasso di prevalenza, prima dell'implementazione dei programmi di vaccinazione universale. Si stima che 1,25 milioni di persone, negli Stati Uniti, siano portatori cronici di HBV, con circa 300 000 nuovi casi di HBV ogni anno, con la maggior incidenza negli adulti tra i 20 e i 39 anni. Un portatore cronico su quattro sviluppa complicanze gravi nel corso della vita. Il numero di nuovi casi nei bambini, riportato ogni anno, è stimato piuttosto basso, ma è difficile da valutare, poiché molte infezioni nei bambini sono asintomatiche. Negli Stati Uniti, dal 1982, anno in cui fu introdotto il primo vaccino per l'HBV, l'incidenza globale di questa infezione si è ridotta di più della metà. Con l'implementazione di programmi di vaccinazione universale, sono stati fatti considerevoli passi avanti verso l'eliminazione dell'HBV nei bambini.

L'HBV è presente a concentrazioni elevate nel sangue, nel siero e negli essudati sierosi, a in concentrazioni più modeste nella saliva, nelle secrezioni vaginali e nello sperma; la modalità di trasmissione più efficiente è tramite contatto con il sangue o rapporti sessuali. I fattori di rischio per l'infezione da HBV, nei bambini e negli adolescenti, comprendono il contagio per via ematogena (iniezione di droga o trasfusioni, puntura con aghi o tatuaggi), contatto sessuale, ricovero in istituti e contatto intimo con portatori. Nel 40% circa dei casi non è identificabile alcun fattore di rischio. Non si ritiene che l'HBV si trasmetta per via indiretta, per esempio con la condivisione di giocattoli. Nei bambini, il fattore di rischio più importante per l'acquisizione dell'HBV resta l'esposizione perinatale a una madre HBsAg-positiva. Il rischio di trasmissione è maggiore se la madre è anche HHBeAg-positiva; in assenza di trattamento, fino al 90% dei figli può sviluppare infezione cronica; l'infezione intrauterina avviene nel 2,5% dei neonati. Nella maggior parte dei casi, i marcatori sierologici di infezione e antigenemia compaiono dal primo al terzo mese dopo la nascita, suggerendo che la trasmissione avvenga al momento del parto, tramite i virus contenuti nel liquido amniotico oppure nelle feci o nel sangue materno. L'immunoprofilassi di questi neonati è molto efficace per prevenire l'infezione, con un tasso di protezione >95%. Dei 22 000 neonati, nati ogni anno da madri HBsAg-positive negli Stati Uniti, più del 98% riceve un'immunoprofilassi e risulta pertanto protetto.

L'HBsAg è stato trovato in piccole quantità nel latte umano di madri infette. L'allattamento al seno di neonati non immunizzati, da parte di madri infette, non comporta tuttavia un rischio maggiore di epatite rispetto all'allattamento con formule artificiali.

Il rischio di sviluppare un'**infezione cronica da HBV**, definita dalla positività all'HBsAg per più di 6 mesi, è inversamente proporzionale all'età di acquisizione. Negli Stati Uniti, sebbene meno del 10% delle infezioni avvenga in età infantile, queste sono responsabili del 20-30% di tutti i casi cronici. Il rischio di infezione cronica è del 90% nei bambini di età inferiore a 1 anno; del 30% per quelli tra 1 e 5 anni e del 2% negli adulti. L'infezione cronica si associa allo sviluppo di epatopatia cronica e di epatocarcinoma. Il rischio di carcinoma è indipendente dalla presenza di cirrosi, e in passato era la causa di morte correlata a tumore a maggior prevalenza, nei giovani adulti, in Asia, dove l'HBV era endemico.

L'HBV ha otto genotipi (A-H). Il genotipo A è pandemico, il B e il C sono prevalenti in Asia, il D è presente nell'Europa meridionale, il genotipo E in Africa, quello F negli Stati Uniti, il G negli Stati Uniti e in Francia, l'H in America Centrale. Inoltre, alcune varianti genetiche hanno sviluppato resistenza nei confronti degli agenti antivirali. Dopo l'infezione, il periodo di incubazione dura da 45 a 160 giorni, con una media di 120.

PATOGENESI. La risposta acuta del fegato all'HBV è la stessa per tutti i virus epatotropi. La persistenza di alterazioni istologiche nei pazienti con epatite B indica l'insorgenza di un'epatopatia cronica. L'HBV, a differenza degli altri virus epatotropi, è principalmente un virus non citopatogeno, che causa un danno in prevalenza immunomediato. La severità del danno epatocitario riflette il grado della risposta immunitaria; pertanto, una risposta immunitaria completa è associata a una maggiore probabilità di eliminazione del virus e a un danno più severo a carico degli epatociti. Perché si instauri un'**epatite acuta** il primo passo è l'infezione degli epatociti da parte dell'HBV, che dà luogo all'espressione di antigeni virali sulla superficie cellulare. I più importanti potrebbero essere gli antigeni nucleocapsidici HBcAg e HBeAg, i quali, in combinazione con le proteine del complesso maggiore di istocompatibilità di classe I (MHC I, *Major Histocompatibility Complex* I), rendono la cellula un bersaglio di lisi per i linfociti T citotossici. Il meccanismo che conduce allo sviluppo di **epatite cronica** è meno conosciuto. Per consentire la persistente infezione degli epatociti, le proteine del core o le proteine MHC di classe I potrebbero non essere riconosciute, i linfociti T citotossici non attivati, o qualche altro meccanismo, ancora sconosciuto, potrebbe interferire con la distruzione degli epatociti. Questo fenomeno di **tolleranza** predomina nei casi di acquisizione perinatale, traducendosi in un'elevata incidenza dello stato di portatore cronico nei bambini con infiammazione epatica scarsa o assente. Sebbene sia raro che si sviluppi un'insufficienza epatica terminale, il rischio di carcinoma epatocellulare è molto elevato, in parte a causa dei cicli di replicazione virale incontrollata.

Inoltre, l'**ALF** è stata osservata nei neonati da madri portatrici croniche anti-HBe positive, o infettate con un ceppo di mutante precore. Questa evidenza conduce al postulato che l'esposizione in utero all'HBeAg dei figli di portatrici croniche induca tolleranza al virus in caso di esposizione postnatale. In assenza di questa tolleranza, il fegato è attaccato massivamente dai linfociti T e il paziente va incontro ad ALF.

Anche le **affezioni extraepatiche** che si possono associare all'infezione da HBV dipendono da meccanismi immunomediati. Possono essere presenti **immunocomplessi circolanti** in pazienti che sviluppano panarterite nodosa, glomerulonefrite membranosa o membranoproliferativa, polimialgia reumatica, vasculite leucocitoclastica e sindrome di Guillain-Barré.

MANIFESTAZIONI CLINICHE. Molti casi di infezione acuta da HBV, nei bambini, sono asintomatici, come si desume dall'elevata frequenza di positività dei marcatori sierici in persone senza un'anamnesi epatite acuta. Di norma, l'episodio sintomatico acuto è simile a quello delle infezioni da HAV o da HCV, ma può anche essere più grave e ha maggiore probabilità di causare un coinvolgimento cutaneo e articolare (Fig. 355-2). La prima evidenza biochimica di infezione da HBV è l'aumento dei livelli di ALT, che iniziano a salire poco prima della comparsa di letargia, anoressia e malessere, ovvero circa 6-7 settimane dopo l'esposizione. La malattia può essere preceduta, in alcuni bambini, da prodromi tipo malattia da siero, con artralgie o lesioni cutanee, tra cui orticaria, rash purpurici, maculari o maculopapulari. Può comparire acrodermatite papulare (sindrome di Gianotti-Crosti). Altre condizioni extraepatiche associate a infezione da HBV nei bambini comprendono panarterite, glomerulonefrite e anemia aplastica. L'ittero, che è presente nel 25% circa degli individui infetti, inizia a manifestarsi in genere 8 settimane circa dopo l'esposizione e dura per 4 settimane. Nel decorso abituale di HBV autorisolventesi, i sintomi persistono per 6-8 settimane. La percentuale di bambini con evidenza clinica di epatite è superiore per l'HBV che per l'HAV, e anche la frequenza di ALF è maggiore. La maggior parte dei pazienti guarisce, ma lo stato di "portatore cronico sano" complica fino al 10% dei casi acquisiti in età adulta. La frequenza di sviluppo di epatite cronica, che dipende in gran parte dalla modalità e dall'età

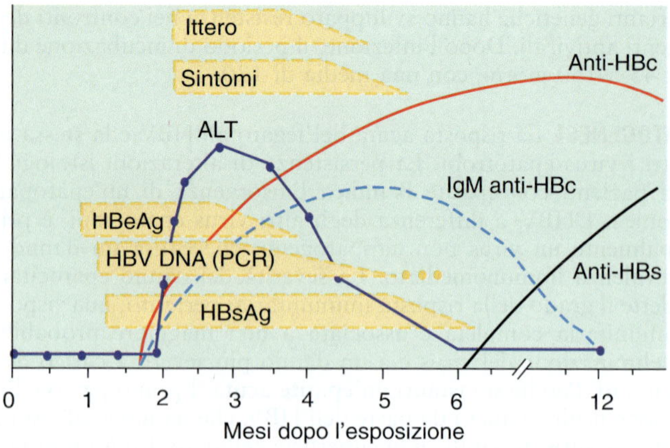

Figura 355-2. Andamento sierologico dell'epatite B acuta. HBc, *Hepatitis B core*, antigene core dell'epatite B; HBeAG, *Hepatitis B e Antigen*, antigene e dell'epatite B; HBs, *Hepatitis B surface*, superficie del virus dell'epatite B; HBsAg, *Hepatitis B surface Antigen*, antigene di superficie dell'epatite B; HBV, *Hepatitis B Virus*, virus dell'epatite B; PCR, *Polymerase Chain Reaction*, reazione a catena della polimerasi. (Da Goldman L, Ausiello D: *Cecil Textbook of Medicine*, 22nd ed. Philadelphia, Saunders, 2004, p 914.)

di acquisizione, raggiunge il 90% nei casi perinatali. L'infezione cronica può condurre a cirrosi ed epatocarcinoma.

All'esame obiettivo, l'infezione sintomatica comporta ittero cutaneo e mucoso. Il fegato risulta in genere ingrandito e dolente alla palpazione e alla percussione. Sono comuni splenomegalia e linfoadenomegalia. Occorre cercare attentamente segni clinici di alterazione del sensorio e di iperriflessività, poiché sono indici di encefalopatia e ALF (vedi Capitolo 361).

DIAGNOSI. Il profilo sierologico dell'infezione da HBV è più complesso di quello dell'HAV, ed è diverso a seconda che la malattia sia acuta oppure cronica (Fig. 355-3). Per la conferma della diagnosi di infezione acuta da HBV si utilizzano numerosi antigeni e anticorpi (vedi Tab. 355-2). Lo screening di routine per l'HBV comprende almeno tre marcatori sierologici (HBsAg, anti-HBc e anti-HBs). L'HBsAg, il primo marcatore sierologico di infezione a comparire, si può trovare in quasi tutti i soggetti affetti; il suo aumento è praticamente concomitante con l'esordio sintomatologico. Poiché i livelli di HBsAg crollano prima della scomparsa dei sintomi, gli anticorpi IgM diretti verso l'HBcAg (anti-HBc IgM) aiutano a identificare i casi di infezione acuta, in quanto aumentano precocemente dopo l'infezione e restano positivi per molti mesi, prima di essere sostituiti dagli antiHBc IgG, che persistono per anni. Gli anti-HBc sono il marcatore singolo più affidabile per la diagnosi di infezione acuta, poiché compaiono precocemente come l'HBsAg e continuano a persistere nelle fasi avanzate della malattia, quando l'HBsAg è già scomparso. Gli anti-HBs sono indicativi di guarigione sierologica e protezione. Nei pazienti immunizzati con il vaccino è presente solo l'HBsAg, mentre in quelli con infezione risolta si trovano sia gli anti-HBs sia gli anti-HBc. L'HBeAg, presente nell'infezione attiva acuta o nelle infezioni croniche, è un marcatore di infettività. Lo sviluppo di anti-HBe indica il miglioramento e rappresenta l'obiettivo della terapia nei pazienti con infezione cronica. L'HBV DNA può essere rilevato nel siero dei pazienti con infezione acuta e nei portatori cronici. Nei pazienti HBeAg-positivi si osservano elevati livelli di HBV DNA, che subiscono un brusco calo con lo sviluppo degli anti-HBe.

COMPLICANZE. L'**ALF**, con coagulopatia, encefalopatia ed edema cerebrale, si sviluppa più frequentemente con l'HBV che con gli altri virus epatotropi. Il rischio di sviluppare questa patologia risulta ulteriormente aumentato in caso di coinfezione o superinfezione con HDV. La mortalità da ALF supera il 30%. Il trapianto epatico è l'unico trattamento efficace; la terapia di supporto, volta a sostenere il paziente, e il precoce invio a un centro trapianti possono salvare la vita del bambino. L'infezione da HBV può condurre a **epatite cronica**, che a sua volta può portare a cirrosi, complicanze dell'insufficienza epatica terminale e **carcinoma epatocellulare** primitivo.

La **glomerulonefrite membranosa**, con deposito di complemento e HBeAg nei capillari glomerulari, è una complicanza rara dell'infezione da HBV.

TRATTAMENTO. Nessuna terapia medica finora disponibile ha un'efficacia garantita per la maggior parte dei pazienti con infezione da HBV. Il trattamento dell'infezione acuta è in gran parte di supporto. L'interferone α2b (IFN-α2b) e la lamivudina (analogo nucelosidico sintetico) sono le terapie attualmente approvate per il trattamento dell'epatite **cronica** B, negli adulti di età superiore ai 18 anni, con epatopatia compensata e replicazione HBV. L'IFN-α2b è stato utilizzato anche nei bambini, con tassi di eradicazione a lungo termine simili a quelle riportate negli adulti (25%). La terapia di combinazione con entrambi gli agenti, nei bambini, non sembra aumentare il tasso di risposta. Gli interferoni ricombinanti hanno effetti immunomodulatori e

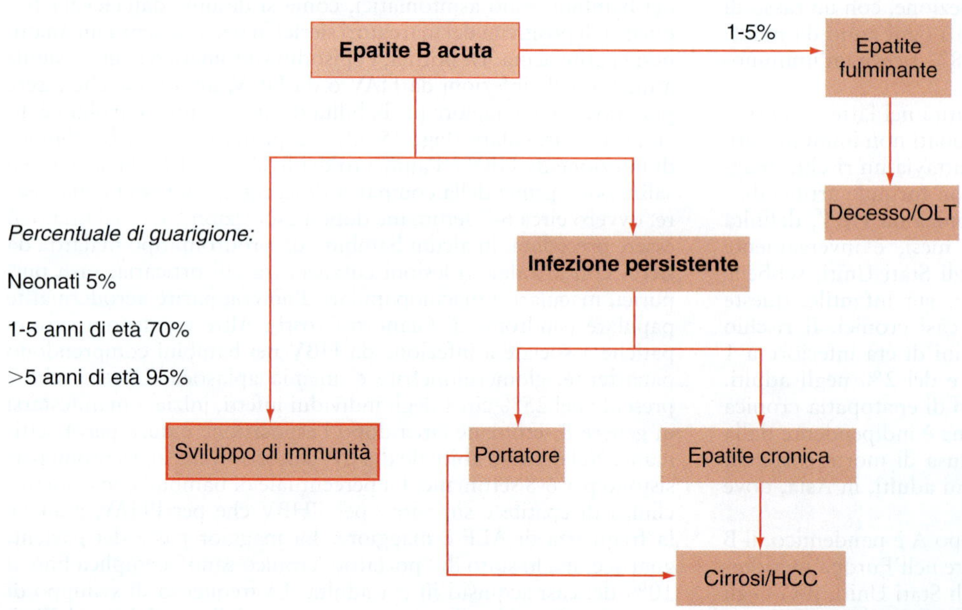

Figura 355-3. Storia naturale dell'infezione da virus dell'epatite B (HBV). HCC, *Hepato-Cellular Carcinoma*, epatocarcinoma; OLT, *Orthotopic Liver Transplant*, trapianto epatico ortotopico.

antivirali, mentre la lamivudina inibisce la trascrittasi inversa virale. I pazienti con maggior probabilità di rispondere hanno bassi titoli di HBV DNA circolante, sono HBeAg-positivi, presentano un'infiammazione epatica attiva (valori di ALT doppi rispetto al limite di normalità) e una patologia di recente acquisizione. Il peginterferone α2 e due nuovi analoghi nucleosidici (afefovir dipivoxil ed entecavir) sono stati approvati negli adulti, ma mancano dati sull'utilizzo in età pediatrica; sembrano avere una maggior efficacia e una ridotta percentuale di resistenze virali, rispetto all'IFN-α2b e alla lamivudina, nella popolazione adulta. Gli adulti portatori cronici, HBeAg-positivi, trattati con entecavir presentano un miglioramento più marcato rispetto a quello ottenibile con lamivudina. Nei bambini, il trattamento dell'infezione cronica da HBV dovrebbe essere individualizzato e condotto da un gastroenterologo pediatra, esperto in epatologia. L'obiettivo del trattamento è la cessazione della replicazione attiva, manifestata dalla sieroconversione HBeAg. La sieroconversione HBsAg avviene invece in una minoranza di casi.

PREVENZIONE. Il vaccino per l'epatite B e le IVIG sono disponibili per la prevenzione dell'infezione. Negli Stati Uniti esistono due vaccini ricombinanti, entrambi altamente immunogenici nei bambini. Il profilo di sicurezza del vaccino HBV è eccellente. Gli effetti collaterali più comuni comprendono dolore nella sede di iniezione (fino al 29% dei casi) e febbre (fino al 6% dei casi).

I soggetti esposti al virus in ambito familiare, per contatto sessuale o per condivisione di siringhe dovrebbero essere identificati e vaccinati, se ricettivi all'infezione da HBV. I pazienti dovrebbero essere informati sul rischio di trasmissione perinatale e tramite contatti intimi. L'HBV non si trasmette con l'allattamento, il bacio, gli abbracci, né con la condivisione di acqua o oggetti. Ai bambini con HBV non si dovrebbe impedire di frequentare la scuola, l'asilo o di giocare con i coetanei, a meno che non abbiano la tendenza a mordere. Un gruppo di supporto può aiutare i bambini a far fronte alla malattia. Tutti gli individui HBsAg-positivi devono essere segnalati al dipartimento di sanità locale o di stato, e viene posta diagnosi di cronicità se la positività persiste per più di 6 mesi.

Immunoglobuline per l'epatite B. Le IVIG sono indicate solo in circostanze specifiche di profilassi postesposizione e forniscono una protezione solo temporanea (3-6 mesi) (Tab. 355-4).

Vaccinazione universale. Nel 2005, il Comitato di Consulta sulle Pratiche di Immunizzazione del Centers for Disease Control and Prevention (CDC) ha rivisto i suoi consigli sulla vaccinazione per l'HBV. Queste raccomandazioni sono state incorporate nel programma vaccinale revisionato dell'American Academy of Pediatrics. Uno degli obiettivi principali è la **vaccinazione universale infantile**, a partire dalla nascita, per fornire una "rete di protezione" in grado di prevenire l'infezione perinatale, l'infezione in età infantile, facilitare l'implementazione di raccomandazioni per una vaccinazione universale e prevenire l'infezione negli adolescenti e negli adulti. L'obiettivo finale è l'eliminazione della trasmissione dell'HBV negli Stati Uniti, e l'integrazione della vaccinazione per l'HBV in un programma armonizzato di vaccinazioni infantili.

Sono stati approvati due vaccini a singolo antigene (Recombivax HB ed Engerix-B), per l'uso pediatrico, che sono le sole preparazioni approvate anche per i neonati di età inferiore ai 6 mesi. Tre vaccini di combinazione possono essere usati per le successive dosi di immunizzazione, che consentono l'integrazione del vaccino HBV nel regolare programma di vaccinazioni. La sieropositività, maggiore del 95% per tutti i vaccini, viene raggiunta dopo la seconda dose nella maggior parte dei pazienti. La terza dose serve come potenziamento e può avere l'effetto di prolungare l'immunità a lungo termine. Negli individui immunocompromessi e nei neonati di peso <2000 g si consiglia una quarta dose, oltre al controllo della sieroconversione. Nonostante il declino del titolo HBs nel tempo, la maggior parte degli individui vaccinati resta protetta dall'infezione HBV.

Le attuali raccomandazioni per la vaccinazione sono le seguenti (vedi Tab. 355-4):

1. Per tutti i neonati stabili dal punto di vista medico, di peso >2 kg alla nascita, e nati da madri HBsAg-negative, la prima dose di vaccino HBV deve essere somministrata prima della dimissione dall'ospedale; per la dose alla nascita si deve usare il vaccino antigenico a dose singola. Le dosi successive, per completare la serie, vengono somministrate dal primo al quarto mese, e dal sesto al diciottesimo mese di età. L'esame routinario postvaccinale dei neonati immunizzati nati da madri HBsAg negative, o con anti-HBs, non è raccomandato.
2. In rari casi (valutati singolarmente), la prima dose può essere posticipata (fino a 2 mesi) fino a dopo la dimissione dall'ospedale. Quando prende questa decisione, tuttavia, occorre registrare l'ordine medico di soprassedere alla dose vaccinale alla nascita, insieme a una copia del risultato originale del laboratorio che attesta che la madre è HBsAg-negativa.
3. I neonati pretermine di peso <2 kg alla nascita, con madri HBsAg-negative, devono ricevere la dose iniziale ritardata fino al primo mese di vita, o prima della dimissione ospedaliera.
4. Occorre migliorare la copertura vaccinale per i bambini e gli adolescenti non vaccinati in

TABELLA 355-4. Indicazioni e dosaggio del vaccino per l'epatite B e delle immunoglobuline per l'epatite B (HBIG)

	DOSE VACCINO		
	RECOMBIVAX HB® (μg)	ENGERIX-B® (μg)	PROGRAMMA
PROFILASSI UNIVERSALE			
Neonati da madri HBsAg-negative	5	10	Alla nascita, 1-2 e 6-18 mesi
Bambini e adolescenti (11-19 anni)	5	10	0, 1 e 6 mesi
PROFILASSI POSTESPOSIZIONE NEGLI INDIVIDUI RICETTIVI			
Contatto con fonte HBsAg-positiva			
Neonati da madri HBsAg (+)	5	10	Alla nascita* (+*HBIG*∫), 1 e 6 mesi
Contatto intimo o ematico identificabile			
0-19 anni di età	5	10	Esposizione (+*HBIG*∫), 1 e 6 mesi
>19 anni di età	10	20	Esposizione (+*HBIG*∫), 1 e 6 mesi
Familiare			
0-19 anni di età	5	10	Esposizione, 1 e 6 mesi
>19 anni di età	10	20	Esposizione, 1 e 6 mesi
Casuale	Nessuna	Nessuna	Nessuna
Immunocompromessi**	40	40	Esposizione (+*HBIG*∫), 1 e 6 mesi
Contatto con stato HBsAg ignoto			
Contatto intimo o ematico identificabile			
>19 anni di età	10	20	Esposizione, 1 e 6 mesi
Immunocompromessi**	40	40	Esposizione (+*HBIG*∫), 1 e 6 mesi

*Sia le HBIG, sia il vaccino devono essere somministrati entro 12 ore dalla nascita, ed entro 24 da un'esposizione identificabile. Le HBIG possono essere somministrate fino a 14 giorni dopo un'esposizione sessuale.

∫Dose HBIG: 0,5 μL per i neonati da madri HBsAg-positive, e 0,06 μL/kg per tutti gli altri casi, quando indicato.

**Nei pazienti immunocompromessi si deve controllare l'avvenuta sieroconversione 1-2 mesi dopo l'ultima dose di vaccino, e poi annualmente. Se il titolo anti-HBs è <10 mUI/mL si devono somministrare dosi di potenziamento. I pazienti non responsivi devono essere considerati ad alto rischio di acquisire l'HBV e informati sulle misure protettive adeguate.

HBs, *Hepatitis B surface*, superficie del virus dell'epatite B; HBsAg, *Hepatitis B surface antigen*, Antigene di superficie del virus dell'epatite B; HBV, *Hepatitis B Virus*, virus dell'epatite B.

precedenza. Per aumentare la copertura, molti stati hanno rischiesto l'immunizzazione per consentire l'accesso alle scuole medie inferiori.

5. Bisogna prevenire **la trasmissione perinatale** tramite il miglioramento dello screening materno e dell'immunoprofilassi dei neonati di madri HBsAg-positive. **I neonati da madri HBsAg-positive** dovrebbero ricevere il vaccino alla nascita, a 1-2 mesi, e al sesto mese di vita (vedi Tab. 355-4). La prima dose deve essere accompagnata dalla somministrazione di 0,5 mL di IGVI appena possibile subito dopo il parto (entro 12 ore), poiché la loro efficacia si riduce rapidamente con il passare del tempo, dopo la nascita. Il controllo postvaccinale per l'HBsAg e per l'anti-HBs deve essere effettuato verso i 9-18 mesi. Se il risultato è positivo per l'anti-HBs, il bambino è immune dal virus. Se è positivo solo per l'HBsAg, il genitore deve essere informato e il bambino valutato da un gastroenterologo pediatra. Se infine è negativo per entrambi, occorre somministrare un secondo ciclo completo di vaccino anti-HBV, seguito da un nuovo controllo per l'anti-HBs per valutare la necessità di ulteriori dosi. La somministrazione di quattro dosi di vaccino è possibile quando si usano vaccini di combinazione dopo la dose alla nascita; questo non aumenta la reattogenicità del vaccino.

Profilassi postesposizione. Le raccomandazioni per la profilassi postesposizione, per l'infezione da epatite B, dipendono dalle condizioni in cui questa è avvenuta (vedi Tab. 355-4). La vaccinazione non dovrebbe mai essere rimandata in mancanza di una documentazione scritta dell'anamnesi di immunizzazione dell'individuo esposto, che si dovrebbe comunque cercare di recuperare.

PROGNOSI. In generale, l'evoluzione dell'infezione acuta da HBV è favorevole, nonostante il rischio di ALF. Il rischio di sviluppare un'infezione cronica porta in primo piano il rischio di cirrosi epatica ed epatocarcinoma. La trasmissione perinatale che porta a cronicizzazione è responsabile dell'elevata incidenza di carcinoma epatocellulare nei giovani adulti, nelle aree endemiche. È importante ricordare che la vaccinazione è in grado di tenere sotto controllo l'infezione da HBV e le sue complicanze.

EPATITE C

EZIOLOGIA. Il virus dell'epatite C (HCV, *Hepatitis C Virus*) è la causa della maggior parte dei casi noti un tempo come "epatite trasfusionale non-A, non-B". Si tratta di un virus a RNA a singola elica, classificato in un genere separato all'interno della famiglia delle Flaviviridae, con una spiccata eterogenicità genetica. Ha sei genotipi principali e numerosi sottotipi e quasi-specie, che gli consentono di sfuggire alla sorveglianza immunitaria dell'ospite. La variazione genotipica può spiegare almeno in parte le differenze nel decorso clinico e nella risposta al trattamento. Il genotipo 1b è il più frequente negli Stati Uniti e il meno responsivo ai farmaci disponibili.

EPIDEMIOLOGIA. Negli Stati Uniti, l'infezione da HCV è la causa più comune di epatopatia cronica negli adulti, responsabile di 8000-10 000 decessi all'anno. Si ritiene che circa 4 milioni di persone negli Stati Uniti e 170 milioni nel mondo siano infetti da HCV. Circa l'85% degli adulti infetti sviluppa infezione cronica. Nei bambini, la sieroprevalenza dell'HCV è dello 0,2% in quelli di età inferiore a 11 anni, e dello 0,4% negli altri.

I fattori di rischio per la trasmissione dell'HCV, negli Stati Uniti, in passato comprendevano le trasfusioni di sangue come la più frequente via di infezione, ma, grazie alle attuali pratiche di screening, il rischio di trasmissione dell'HCV è ora dello 0,001% per unità trasfusa. L'uso di sostanze illecite per via endovenosa con esposizione al sangue o a prodotti ematici di individui infetti è responsabile di più della metà dei casi di infezione negli adulti, negli Stati Uniti. La trasmissione sessuale, in particolare attraverso partner sessuali multipli, è la seconda causa più frequente di infezione. Altri fattori di rischio comprendono la detenzione in carcere e l'occupazione professionale; circa il 10% delle nuove infezioni non ha una fonte di trasmissione identificabile. Nei bambini, la trasmissione perinatale è quella a maggior prevalenza (vedi Tab. 355-1). La trasmissione verticale si verifica nel 5% dei bambini nati da madri viremiche. La coinfezione con HIV e un'elevata viremia nella madre (HCV RNA-positiva) possono aumentare la probabilità di trasmissione portandola al 20%.

Il periodo di incubazione è di 7-9 settimane (range da 2 a 24 settimane).

PATOGENESI. Il quadro del danno epatico acuto è indistinguibile da quello di altri virus epatotropi. Nei casi cronici, si osservano aggregati o follicoli linfoidi nei tratti portali, sia isolati sia facenti parte di un infiltrato infiammatorio generalizzato. La steatosi è di frequente osservazione nei campioni bioptici. L'HCV sembra causare un danno principalmente tramite meccanismi citopatici, nonostante si possa verificare anche un danno immunomediato. La componente citopatica appare lieve, in quanto la malattia acuta è tipicamente la meno grave di tutte le infezioni da virus epatotropi.

MANIFESTAZIONI CLINICHE. L'infezione acuta da HCV tende a essere di lieve entità e a esordio insidioso (Fig. 355-4; vedi anche Tab. 355-1). L'insufficienza epatica acuta è rara. Tuttavia, l'HCV è il virus epatotropo che più spesso causa infezione cronica (Fig. 355-5). Degli adulti affetti, meno del 15% elimina il virus; gli altri sviluppano un'epatite cronica. Negli studi pediatrici, il 6-19% dei bambini ottiene l'eliminazione spontanea e persistente del virus durante un follow-up di 6 anni, a prescindere dalla modalità di acquisizione. L'epatite cronica C è clinicamente silente fino allo sviluppo di complicanze. I livelli sierici di transaminasi sono tipicamente fluttuanti e possono talora essere normali, ma l'infiammazione a livello istologico è sempre presente. La progressione della fibrosi epatica è lenta e avviene nel corso di diversi anni, a meno che non siano presenti fattori di comorbilità, in grado di accelerarne la progressione. Circa il 25% dei pazienti infetti sviluppa cirrosi epatica, insufficienza epatica e, occasionalmente, un epatocarcinoma primitivo (HCC, *HepatoCellular Carcinoma*), a 20-30 anni dall'infezione acuta. Sebbene la progressione avvenga raramente nell'arco dell'età pediatrica, sono stati riportati casi di cirrosi e di HCC da HCV, anche nell'infanzia. La morbidità a lungo termine costituisce il razionale per la diagnosi e il trattamento dei bambini con HCV.

L'infezione cronica da HCV, che si può associare a **vasculite dei piccoli vasi**, è una causa comune di crioglobulinemia mista essenziale. Altre manifestazioni extraepatiche, osservate soprattutto negli adulti, comprendono vasculite cutanea, neuropatia periferica, cerebrite, glomerulonefrite membranoproliferativa e sindrome nefrosica. Possono essere presenti anticorpi anti-muscolo liscio, antinucleo e bassi livelli di ormoni tiroidei.

DIAGNOSI. I test clinici disponibili per la rilevazione dell'infezione da HCV si basano sull'individuazione degli anticorpi diretti verso antigeni dell'HCV, oppure dell'RNA virale (vedi Tab. 355-2);

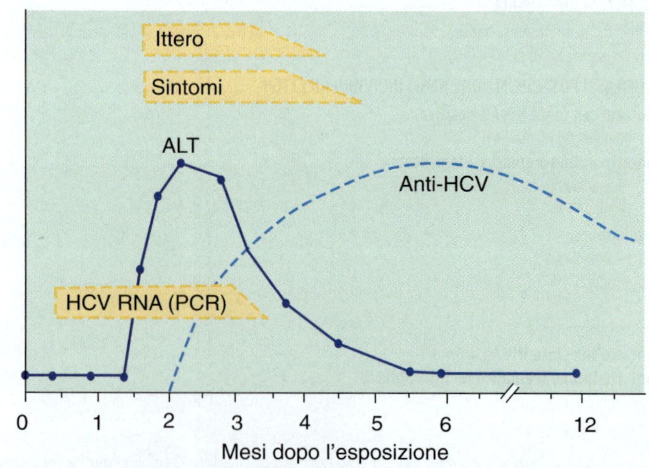

Figura 355-4. Andamento sierologico dell'epatite C acuta. HCV, *Hepatitis C Virus*, virus dell'epatite C; PCR, *Polymerase Chain Reaction*. (Da Goldman L, Ausiello D: *Cecil Textbook of Medicine*, 22nd ed. Philadelphia, Saunders, 2004, p 915.)

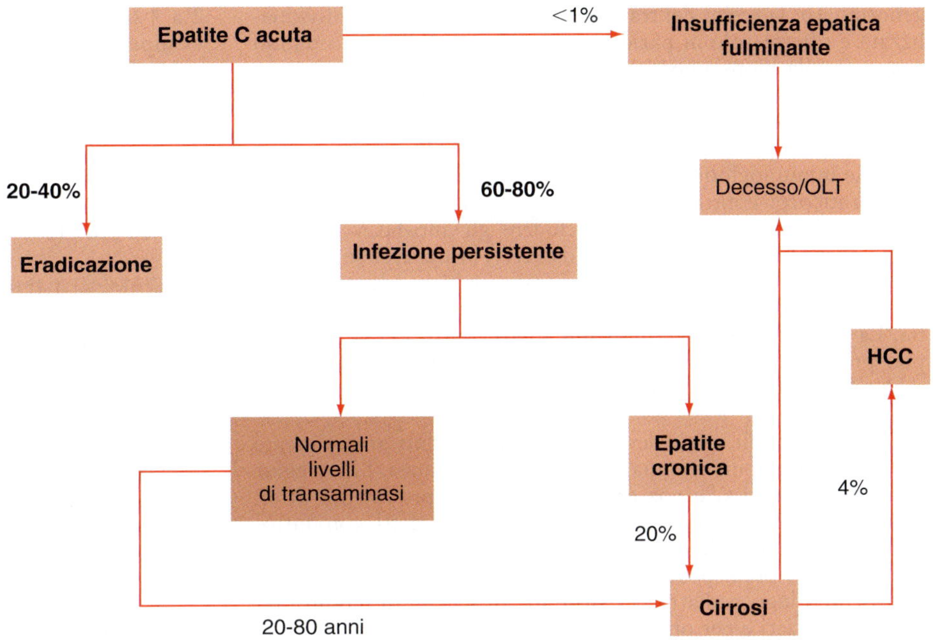

Figura 355-5. Storia naturale dell'infezione da virus dell'epatite C (HCV). HCC, *HepatoCellular Carcinoma*, epatocarcinoma; OLT, *Orthotopic Liver Transplant*, trapianto epatico ortotopico. (Da Hochman JA, Balistreri WF: Chronic viral hepatitis: Always be current! *Pediatr Rev* 2003;24:399-410.)

nessuno di essi permette di predire la gravità del danno epatico.

Il **test sierologico** di uso più comune è un test immunoenzimatico (EIA, *Enzyme ImmunoAssay*) per rilevare gli anti-HCV. Il valore predittivo di questo esame è più elevato nella popolazione a rischio, ma i falsi positivi possono arrivare al 50-60% nella popolazione a basso rischio. Possono anche verificarsi falsi negativi, poiché gli anticorpi restano negativi anche per 1-3 mesi, dopo l'esordio clinico della malattia. L'anti-HCV non è un anticorpo protettivo e non conferisce immunità; è presente contemporaneamente al virus.

Il **test virologico** più usato per l'HCV è un esame in PCR, che permette di individuare piccole quantità di **HCV RNA** nel siero e nei campioni tissutali, pochi giorni dopo l'infezione. Il test in PCR qualitativa, utile in particolare nei pazienti con infezione recente o perinatale, ipogammaglobulinemia o immunosoppressione, è molto sensibile. La PCR quantitativa aiuta a identificare i pazienti con maggiori probabilità di risposta alla terapia.

Lo **screening** per l'HCV dovrebbe includere tutti i pazienti con i seguenti fattori di rischio: anamnesi di consumo di sostanze stupefacenti per via endovenosa (anche solo una volta), terapia con fattori della coagulazione ricevuta prima del 1987 (quando furono introdotte procedure di inattivazione) o di derivati ematici prima del 1992, emodialisi, epatopatia idiopatica, e figli di donne infette da HCV (PCR qualitativa in età neonatale e dosaggio anti-HCV dopo i 12 mesi di età). Lo screening routinario di tutte le *gestanti* non è raccomandato.

Importante è anche la determinazione del **genotipo** dell'HCV, in particolare in previsione della terapia, in quanto la risposta agli attuali agenti terapeutici varia molto. Il genotipo 1 è più resistente, mentre i genotipi 2 e 3 rispondono meglio alla terapia (vedi oltre).

I livelli di transaminasi presentano tipiche fluttuazioni durante l'infezione da HCV e non correlano con il grado di fibrosi epatica.

La biopsia epatica è l'unico strumento di cui si dispone per valutare la presenza e l'estensione della fibrosi epatica, in assenza di segni conclamati di epatopatia. La biopsia è indicata solo prima dell'inizio del trattamento o per escludere altre cause di epatopatia.

COMPLICANZE. Il rischio di insufficienza epatica acuta da HCV è basso; in compenso, il rischio di **epatite cronica**, tra tutti i virus epatotropi, è il più elevato. Negli adulti, i fattori di rischio per la progressione verso la fibrosi epatica comprendono età avanzata, obesità, sesso maschile e consumo di quantità anche modiche di alcol (due bicchieri al giorno). Negli Stati Uniti, la progressione alla cirrosi o all'HCC rappresenta la causa principale di morbilità e l'indicazione più frequente per il trapianto epatico, negli adulti.

TRATTAMENTO. Negli adulti, la terapia più efficace è il peginterferone (una dose settimanale per via sottocutanea), combinato con la somministrazione quotidiana di ribavirina per via orale (combinazione che però non è attualmente approvata per i bambini). I pazienti con maggiori probabilità di risposta hanno un'epatite lieve, una minor durata di infezione e bassi livelli di viremia. I genotipi 2 e 3 sono i più sensibili al trattamento; i soggetti con genotipo 1, invece, rispondono meno. L'obiettivo del trattamento è ottenere una risposta virologica sostenuta (SVR, *Sustained Viral Response*), definita come l'assenza di viremia 6 mesi dopo la sospensione del trattamento; la SVR si associa al miglioramento istologico e alla riduzione del rischio di morbilità.

La storia naturale dell'infezione da HCV nei bambini è ancora da definire, ma i dati emergenti suggeriscono che i bambini abbiano una maggior probabilità di eliminazione spontanea del virus, così come un minor rischio di epatopatia avanzata o rapidamente progressiva. Queste caratteristiche giustificano l'attuale approccio di monitoraggio seriale, in attesa di nuove terapie più efficaci. Sono stati riportati rari casi di cirrosi, e perfino HCC, osservati nei bambini. La minor durata dell'infezione e la minor incidenza di comorbilità, rispetto agli adulti, sembrano implicare che i bambini siano i candidati migliori per il trattamento; a causa degli effetti collaterali delle terapie attualmente disponibili, tuttavia, gli Autori non raccomandano il trattamento al di fuori di studi clinici controllati.

Solo l'IFN-α2b e la ribavirina sono stati approvati dalla Food and Drug Administration (FDA) nei bambini di età superiore a 3 anni con epatite HCV. Studi condotti sull'IFN in monoterapia nei bambini hanno mostrato una SVR maggiore che negli adulti, con una miglior compliance e minori effetti collaterali. Da un singolo studio, che ha valutato la terapia di combinazione, è emersa una SVR del 49%. I fattori associati a una maggior probabilità di risposta sono l'età minore di 12 anni, i genotipi 2 e 3, e, nei pazienti con genotipo 1, una viremia <2 milioni di copie/mL. Gli effetti collaterali, che portano alla sospensione della terapia in un'elevata percentuale di pazienti, comprendono anemia, neutropenia e sintomi simil-influenzali.

Il trattamento dovrebbe essere preso in considerazione per tutti i bambini infetti con genotipo 2 e 3, che hanno maggiori probabilità di rispondere ai farmaci. Se il bambino ha un virus di genotipo 1b, la scelta del trattamento dovrebbe essere individualizzata e offerta solo ai pazienti con evidenza di fibrosi o danno avanzato alla biopsia epatica.

PREVENZIONE. Non sono disponibili vaccini per prevenire l'infezione da HCV. Le preparazioni di immunoglobuline non sono utili. Le immunoglobuline prodotte negli Stati Uniti non contengono anticorpi contro l'HCV, poiché il sangue e il plasma dei donatori sono selezionati per escludere gli anti-HCV positivi. Dopo aver identificato l'infezione da HCV, bisognerebbe controllare i pazienti annualmente con ecografia epatica e dosaggio dell'α-fetoproteina, per l'HCC, ed escludere segni clinici di epatopatia. La vaccinazione degli individui affetti contro l'HAV e l'HBV può prevenire la superinfezione con questi virus, che aumenterebbe il rischio di insufficienza epatica severa.

PROGNOSI. I titoli virali devono essere controllati annualmente per documentare un'eventuale remissione spontanea. La maggior parte dei pazienti sviluppa epatite cronica. La probabilità di un danno epatico progressivo è maggiore nei soggetti con fattori di comorbidità ulteriori, come consumo di alcol, variazioni genotipiche e predisposizione genetica. Si consiglia l'invio a un gastroenterologo pediatra per sfruttare gli schemi di monitoraggio più avanzati e per ottimizzare l'arruolamento in protocolli di trattamento, quando disponibili.

EPATITE D

EZIOLOGIA. Il virus dell'epatite D (HDV, *Hepatitis D Virus*), che con i suoi di 36 nm di diametro è il più piccolo virus animale conosciuto, viene considerato difettivo, non essendo in grado di provocare infezione in assenza di una concomitante infezione da HBV. È incapace di produrre le proprie proteine di superficie; il rivestimento esterno è composto dall'eccesso di HBsAg proveniente dall'HBV, mentre la sua porzione interna è costituita da un RNA circolare a singola elica, che esprime l'antigene HDV.

EPIDEMIOLOGIA. L'HDV non può provocare infezione in assenza dell'HBV, in qualità di adiuvante. L'HDV può infettare contemporaneamente alla prima infezione da HBV (**coinfezione**), oppure infettare una persona con una preesistente infezione da HBV (**superinfezione**). La trasmissione avviene in genere per contatti familiari o intimi in aree a elevata prevalenza, ovvero soprattutto nei Paesi in via di sviluppo (vedi Tab. 355-1). Nelle aree a bassa prevalenza, come gli Stati Uniti, è molto più comune la via parenterale. Negli Stati Uniti, l'infezione da HDV è poco frequente nei bambini, ma deve essere presa in considerazione nei casi di insufficienza epatica acuta. Il periodo di incubazione è di 2-8 settimane in caso di superinfezione, e simile a quello dell'HBV in caso di coinfezione.

PATOGENESI. L'istologia epatica, nell'epatite da HDV, non presenta caratteristiche peculiari, a parte il fatto che il danno è spesso di una certa gravità. Al contrario dell'HBV, l'HDV causa un danno diretto tramite meccanismi citopatici. Molti dei casi più severi di infezione HDV sembrano derivare dalla coinfezione con HBV e HDV.

MANIFESTAZIONI CLINICHE. I sintomi dell'epatite D sono simili a quelli dell'epatite da altri virus epatotropi, ma più severi. L'evoluzione dell'infezione da HDV dipende dal meccanismo dell'infezione. Nella coinfezione, l'epatite acuta, che è più severa di quella causata dal solo HBV, è comune, ma il rischio di cronicizzazione è basso. Nei casi di superinfezione, la malattia acuta è più rara e l'epatite cronica è frequente. Il rischio di ALF è maggiore nella superinfezione. L'epatite D dovrebbe essere esclusa in tutti i bambini con insufficienza epatica acuta.

DIAGNOSI. L'HDV non è stato isolato e non sono stati identificati antigeni circolanti. La diagnosi è effettuata tramite il riscontro degli anticorpi IgM verso l'HDV, che si sviluppano da 2 a 4 settimane dopo la coinfezione, e circa 10 settimane dopo la superinfezione.

Negli Stati Uniti il test per gli anticorpi anti-HDV è disponibile in commercio. I test in PCR per l'RNA virale è disponibile solo a scopo di ricerca (vedi Tab. 355-2).

COMPLICANZE. L'HDV deve essere escluso in tutti i casi di ALF. La coinfezione con questo virus può anche causare un danno cronico più grave.

TRATTAMENTO. Il trattamento si basa su misure di supporto, dopo l'identificazione dell'infezione. Attualmente non esiste un trattamento specifico contro l'HDV. La terapia si basa soprattutto sul controllo e sul trattamento dell'infezione da HBV, senza la quale l'HDV non può indurre epatite.

PREVENZIONE. Non esiste un vaccino per l'epatite D. Poiché la replicazione virale dell'HDV non è possibile in assenza di coinfezione con l'epatite B, l'immunizzazione verso l'HBV protegge anche dall'infezione da HDV. I vaccini per l'HBV e le IVIG sono utilizzati con le stesse indicazioni cliniche dell'epatite B.

EPATITE E

EZIOLOGIA. Il virus dell'epatite E (HEV, *Hepatitis E Virus*) non è stato isolato, ma clonato con tecniche molecolari. Questo virus a RNA ha una forma sferica, è privo di envelope ed è strutturalmente simile ai calicivirus.

EPIDEMIOLOGIA. L'epatite E è la forma epidemica di quella che un tempo era chiamata "epatite non-A, non-B". La trasmissione avviene per via orofecale (spesso la fonte è rappresentata da acque infette) e si associa al rilascio nelle feci di particelle di 27-34 nm di diametro (vedi Tab. 355-1). La prevalenza più alta di infezione da HEV è stata riportata nel subcontinente indiano, in Medio Oriente, nel Sudest Asiatico e in Messico, in particolare nelle aree con condizioni igieniche scadenti. Negli Stati Uniti, i soli casi riportati sono stati in persone che avevano fatto viaggi o erano emigrate da aree endemiche. Il periodo medio di incubazione è di circa 40 giorni (range 15-60 giorni).

PATOGENESI. L'HEV sembra agire come un virus citopatico. I reperti istologici sono simili a quelli degli altri virus epatitici.

MANIFESTAZIONI CLINICHE. La malattia clinica associata all'infezione da HEV è simile all'epatite da HAV, ma tende a essere più severa. Come nel caso dell'infezione da HAV, non cronicizza. Oltre a causare frequentemente un episodio di epatite più grave rispetto all'HAV, l'HEV tende a colpire pazienti di età superiore, con un picco tra i 15 e i 34 anni. L'HEV è un fattore patogeno importante nelle donne incinte, nelle quali può causare ALF con un'elevata mortalità.

COMPLICANZE. L'HEV si associa a un elevato rischio di morte nelle donne in gravidanza. Non sono state riconosciute altre complicanze associate a questo virus.

DIAGNOSI. La tecnologia del DNA ricombinante ha consentito lo sviluppo di anticorpi verso particelle dell'HEV e sono attualmente disponibili test IgG e IgM che permettono di distinguere l'infezione acuta da quella pregressa (vedi Tab. 355-2). Gli anticorpi IgM verso l'antigene virale si positivizza dopo la prima settimana di malattia. L'RNA virale può essere rilevato nelle feci e nel siero tramite PCR.

PREVENZIONE. Esiste un vaccino ricombinante contro l'epatite E, molto efficace negli adulti. Non esistono prove che le immunoglobuline siano utili per la prevenzione dell'infezione da HEV. Le immunoglobuline raccolte da pazienti in aree endemiche potrebbero dimostrarsi efficaci.

APPROCCIO ALL'EPATITE ACUTA E CRONICA

Sebbene siano in via di sviluppo nuove modalità di trattamento per l'epatite virale cronica, e i risultati delle terapia siano migliorati, per quanto riguarda la popolazione pediatrica il vero grande passo avanti è stato compiuto nell'ambito della prevenzione, grazie alla disponibilità di vaccini efficaci e sicuri per le infezione da HAV e da HBV. La messa a punto di strumenti diagnostici più sensibili e affidabili potrebbe portare al miglioramento delle terapie per i pazienti affetti. Il medico di base è in prima linea nella cura e nel controllo dei soggetti esposti a questi virus. Le strategie aggressive di immunizzazione perinatale, infantile e in età adolescenziale hanno già avuto un forte impatto nelle aree dove l'HAV e l'HBV sono endemici.

Uno dei principali contributi del pediatra di base consiste nell'identificazione del deterioramento del paziente con epatite acuta che sviluppa insufficienza epatica acuta (Fig. 355-6). Una volta diagnosticata un'ALF, il medico deve immediatamente inviare il paziente a un centro trapianti, iniziativa che può davvero salvare una vita.

Dopo aver identificato un'infezione cronica, invece, è d'obbligo uno stretto monitoraggio e l'invio a un gastroenterologo pediatra per arruolare il paziente negli studi di trattamento appropriati. Il trattamento dell'infezione da HBV e HCV nei bambini dovrebbe, se possibile, essere svolto all'interno di studi controllati, poiché le indicazioni, la scelta di quando iniziare, il regime e l'esito sono ancora da definire e non possono semplicemente essere estrapolati dai dati sulla popolazione adulta. Tutti i pazienti con epatite virale cronica devono evitare il più possibile ulteriori danni al fegato: è consigliabile il vaccino per l'HAV, l'astensione dal consumo di alcolici e una particolare attenzione nell'assunzione di nuovi farmaci, compresi quelli da banco e i preparati a base di erbe.

L'adozione internazionale e l'abitudine di viaggiare continuano a cambiare l'epidemiologia di questi virus. Negli Stati Uniti, l'epatite cronica da HBV e da HCV ha un'elevata prevalenza nei pazienti adottati di provenienza internazionale; è necessaria un'attenta vigilanza pe stabilire una diagnosi precoce e offrire un trattamento appropriato, oltre a misure profilattiche per limitare la diffusione del virus.

L'epatite cronica può essere una patologia colpevolizzante per i bambini e le loro famiglie. Il pediatra dovrebbe offrire, tramite un attivo coinvolgimento, un adeguato supporto ai pazienti e la necessaria educazione alle persone con cui vengono in contatto in ambito sociale. Dati scientifici e informazioni sui gruppi di supporto sono disponibili per le famiglie sul sito web dell'American Liver Foundation (www.liverfoundation-ne.org) e della North American Society for Pediatric Gastroenterology, Hepatology and Nutrition (www.naspghan.org), oltre che nei centri di gastroenterologia pediatrica americani.

Epatite A

Centers for Disease Control and Prevention (CDC): Multistate outbreak of hepatitis A among young adult concert attendees—United States, 2003. *MMWR Morb Mortal Wkly Rep* 2003;52:844–845.

Dagan R, Leventhal A, Anis E, et al: Incidence of hepatitis A in Israel following universal immunization of toddlers. *JAMA* 2005;294:202–210.

Nainan OV, Armstrong GL, Han XH, et al: Hepatitis A molecular epidemiology in the United States, 1996–1997: Sources of infection and implications of vaccination policy. *J Infect Dis* 2005;191:957–963.

Rein DB, Fiore AE, Bell BP: What's next for the hepatitis A vaccine? *Lancet* 2006;367:546–548.

Temte JL: Should all children be immunized against hepatitis A? *Br Med J* 2006;332:715–718.

Wheeler C, Vogt TM, Armstrong GL: An outbreak of hepatitis A associated with green onions. *N Engl J Med* 2005;353:890–897.

Epatite B

Aggarwal R, Ranjan P: Preventing and treating hepatitis B infection. *Br Med J* 2004;329:1080–1086.

Beeching NJ: Hepatitis B infections. *Br Med J* 2004;329:1059–1060.

Boxall EH, Sira J, Standish RA, et al: Natural history of hepatitis B in perinatally infected carriers. *Arch Dis Child Fetal Neonatal Ed* 2004;89:F456–F460.

Broderick A, Jonas MM: Management of hepatitis B in children. *Clin Liver Dis* 2004;8:387–401.

Centers for Disease Control and Prevention (CDC): Acute hepatitis B among children and adolescents, United States, 1990–2002. *MMWR Morb Mortal Wkly Rep* 2004;53:1015–1018.

Chang TT, Gish RG, de Man R, et al: A comparison of entecavir and lamivudine for HBeAg-positive chronic hepatitis B. *N Engl J Med* 2006;354:1001–1010.

D'Antiga L, Aw M, Mieli-Vergani G, et al: Combined lamuvidine/interferon alpha treatment in immunotolerant children perinatally infected with hepatitis B: A pilot study. *J Pediatr* 2006;148:228–233.

Ganem D, Prince AM: Hepatitis B virus infection—Natural history and clinical consequences. *N Engl J Med* 2004;350:1118–1129.

Hadziyannis SJ, Tassopoulos NC, Heathcoate EJ, et al: Long-term therapy with adefovir dipivoxil for HBeAg-negative chronic hepatitis B. *N Engl J Med* 2005;352:2673–2681.

Hadziyannis SJ, Tassopoulos NC, Heathcoate EJ, et al: Adefovir dipivoxil for the treatment of hepatitis B e antigen–negative chronic hepatitis B. *N Engl J Med* 2003;348:800–806.

Janssen HLA, van Zonneveld M, Senturk H, et al: Pegylated interferon alfa-2b alone or in combination with lamivudine for HBeAg-positive hepatitis B: A randomised trial. *Lancet* 2005;365:123–128.

Jonas MM, Kelley DA, Mizerski J, et al: Clinical trial of lamivudine in children with chronic hepatitis B. *N Engl J Med* 2002;346:1706–1713.

Kao JH, Chen DS: Hepatitis B vaccination: To boost or not to boost? *Lancet* 2005;366:1337–1338.

Kobak GE, MacKenzie T, Sokol RJ, et al: Interferon treatment for chronic hepatitis B: Enhanced response in children 5 years old or younger. *J Pediatr* 2004;145:340–345.

Lai CL, Ratziu V, Yuen MF, Poynard T: Viral hepatitis B. *Lancet* 2003; 362:2089–2094.

Lai CL, Shouval D, Lok AS, et al: Entecavir versus lamivudine for patients with HBeAg-negative chronic hepatitis B. *N Engl J Med* 2006;354:1011–1020.

Liaw YF, Sung JJY, Cheng Chow W, et al: Lamivudine for patients with chronic hepatitis B and advanced liver disease. *N Engl J Med* 2004;351:1521–1530.

Marcellin P, Chang TT, Gee Lim S, et al: Adefovir dipivoxil for the treatment of hepatitis B e antigen–positive chronic hepatitis B. *N Engl J Med* 2003;348:808–816.

The Medical Letter: Telbivudine *(Tyzeka)* for chronic hepatitis B. *Med Lett* 2007;49:11–12.

Poland GA, Jacobson RM: Clinical practice: Prevention of hepatitis B with the hepatitis B vaccine. *N Engl J Med* 2004;351:2832–2838.

Schildgen O, Sirma H, Funk A, et al: Variant of hepatitis B virus with primary resistance to adefovir. *N Engl J Med* 2006;354:1807–1812.

Yang HI, Lu SN, Liaw YF, et al: Hepatitis B e antigen and the risk of hepatocellular carcinoma. *N Engl J Med* 2002;347:168–174.

Epatite C

Bair RM, Baillargeon JG, Kelly PJ, et al: Prevalence and risk factors for hepatitis C virus infection among adolescents in detention. *Arch Pediatr Adolesc Med* 2005;159:1015–1018.

Cagle HH, Jacob J, Homan CE, et al: Results of a general hepatitis C lookback program for persons who received blood transfusions in a neonatal intensive care unit between January 1975 and July 1992. *Arch Pediatr Adolesc Med* 2007;161:125–130.

Carrat F, Bani-Sadr F, Pol S, et al: Pegylated interferon alfa-2b vs standard interferon alfa-2b, plus ribavirin, for chronic hepatitis C in HIV-infected patients. *JAMA* 2004;292:2839–2848.

Elisofon SA, Jonas MM: Hepatitis B and C in children: Current treatment and future strategies. *Clin Liver Dis* 2006;10:133–148.

Flamm SL: Chronic hepatitis C virus infection. *JAMA* 2003;289:2413–2417.

Fried MW, Shiffman ML, Reddy R, et al: Peginterferon alfa-2a plus ribavirin for chronic hepatitis C virus infection. *N Engl J Med* 2002;347:975–982.

Hoofnagle JH, Seeff LB: Peginterferon and ribavirin for chronic hepatitis C. *N Engl J Med* 2006;355:2444–2451.

Iorio R, Giannattasio A, Sepe A, et al: Chronic hepatitis C in childhood: An 18-year experience. *Clin Infect Dis* 2005;41:1431–1437.

Jara P, Resti M, Hierro L, et al: Chronic hepatitis C virus infection in childhood: Clinical patterns and evolution in 224 white children. *Clin Infect Dis* 2003;36:275–280.

Mast EE, Hwang LY, Seto DSY, et al: Risk factors for perinatal transmission of hepatitis C virus (HCV) and the natural history of HCV infection acquired in infancy. *J Infect Dis* 2005;192:1880–1889.

Patel K, Muir AJ, McHutchison JG: Diagnosis and treatment of chronic hepatitis C infection. *Br Med J* 2006;332:1013–1017.

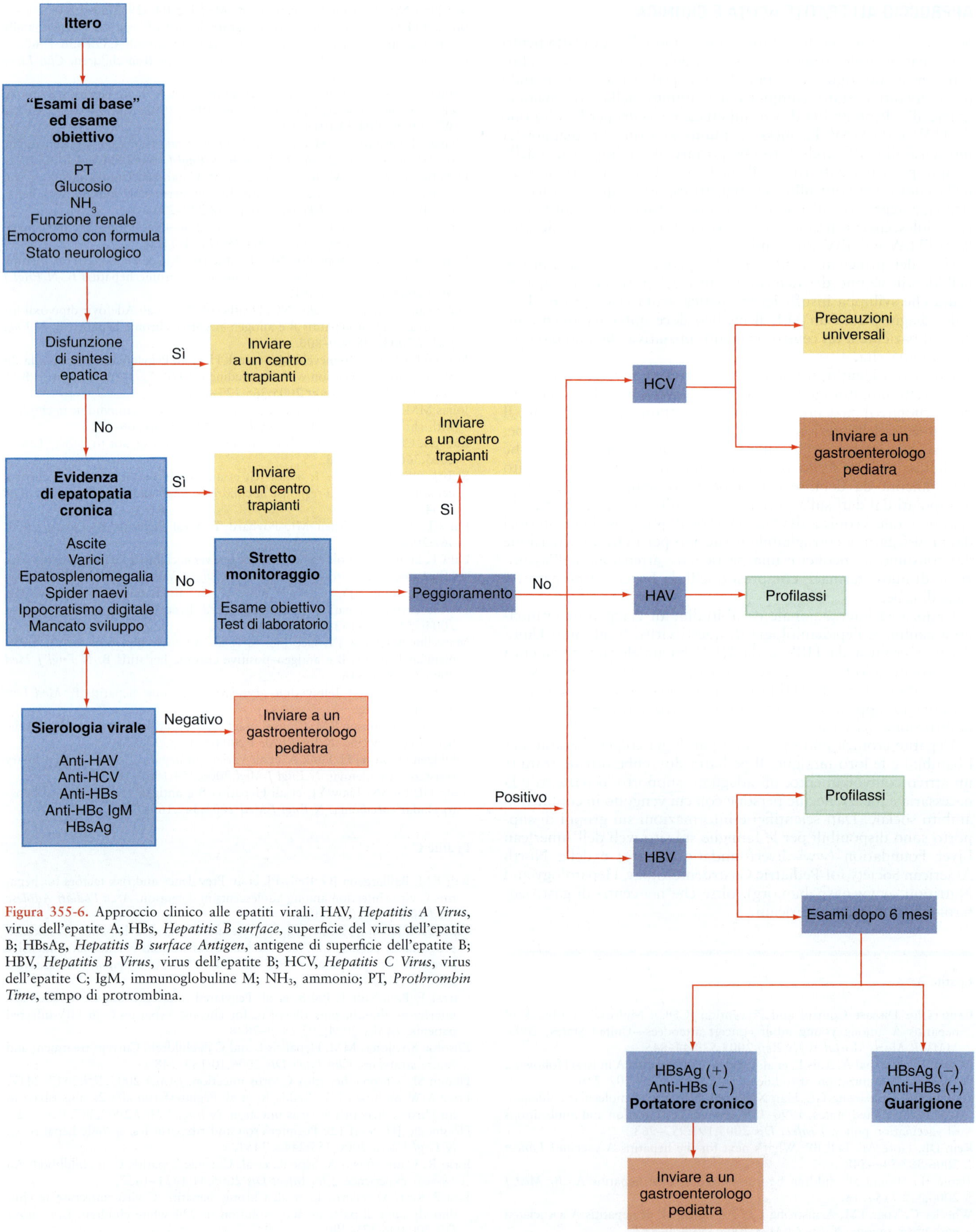

Figura 355-6. Approccio clinico alle epatiti virali. HAV, *Hepatitis A Virus*, virus dell'epatite A; HBs, *Hepatitis B surface*, superficie del virus dell'epatite B; HBsAg, *Hepatitis B surface Antigen*, antigene di superficie dell'epatite B; HBV, *Hepatitis B Virus*, virus dell'epatite B; HCV, *Hepatitis C Virus*, virus dell'epatite C; IgM, immunoglobuline M; NH_3, ammonio; PT, *Prothrombin Time*, tempo di protrombina.

Poynard T, Yuen MF, Ratziu V, Lai CL: Viral hepatitis C. *Lancet* 2003; 362:2095–2100.

Schiff ER: Prevention of mortality from hepatitis B and hepatitis C. *Lancet* 2006;368:896–897.

Vento S, Nobili V, Cainelli F: Clinical course of infection with hepatitis C. *Br Med J* 2006;332:374–375.

Wirth S, Pieper-Boustani H, Lang T, et al: Peginterferon alfa-2b plus ribavirin treatment in children and adolescents with chronic hepatitis C. *Hepatology* 2005;41:1013–1018.

Altri agenti virali

Chang MH, Hadzic D, Rouassant AH, et al: Asian Pan-Pacific Society for Pediatric Gastroenterology, Hepatology, and Nutrition: Acute and chronic hepatitis: Working Group report of the Second World Congress of Pediatric Gastroenterology, Hepatology, and Nutrition. *J Pediatr Gastroenterol Nutr* 2004;39:S584–S588.

Emerson SU, Purcell RH: Running like water—The omnipresence of hepatitis E. *N Engl J Med* 2004;351:2367–2368.

Kelly D, Skidmore S: Hepatitis C–Z: Recent advances. *Arch Dis Child* 2002;86:339–343.

Mehrishi JN, Bakács T: HIV and hepatitis G virus/GB virus C co-infection: Beneficial or not? *Lancet* 2005;5:464–466.

Shrestha MP, Scott RM, Joshi DM, et al: Safety and efficacy of a recombinant hepatitis 5 vaccine. *N Engl J Med* 2007;356:895–902.

Capitolo 356 ■ Ascesso epatico

Stavra A. Xanthakos e William F. Balistreri

Gli ascessi epatici piogeni sono rari nei bambini. Nei Paesi sviluppati, gli ascessi epatici compaiono prevalentemente in un contesto di immunosoppressione (40-60% dei casi); mentre nelle aree in via di sviluppo giocano un ruolo centrale la malnutrizione, la sepsi e le infezioni parassitarie. Gli ascessi epatici piogeni possono essere causati da: batteri che arrivano al fegato tramite la circolazione portale, nei casi di pileflebite, infezioni endoaddominali o ascessi secondari ad appendicite, a malattia infiammatoria intestinale, a sepsi generalizzata; colangite ascendente, associata a ostruzione delle vie biliari imputabile a calcoli o a colangite sclerosante, come complicanza di una procedura di Kasai o di una cisti coledocica; infezioni criptogenetiche delle vie biliari. In rari casi, un ascesso epatico può svilupparsi in seguito a una biopsia percutanea. Nei neonati può insorgere in seguito a sepsi, infezione o incannulamento della vena ombelicale. Negli adulti, il trapianto epatico si è dimostrato un importante fattori di rischio per l'ascesso epatico piogeno; non è noto se lo sia anche nei pazienti pediatrici.

Nei bambini, i patogeni più comuni sono *Staphylococcus aureus*, *Streptococcus* spp., *Escherichia coli*, *Salmonella* e organismi anaerobi; nei Paesi in via di sviluppo e nelle zone endemiche sono anche stati riportati casi di ascessi epatici associati a *Entamoeba histolytica* o *Toxocara canis*. Nei pazienti adulti, la *Klebsiella* spp., oltre a essersi rivelata una causa significativa di ascessi epatici piogeni, si associa a un aumentato rischio di endoftalmite settica metastatica, in particolare nei pazienti con diabete mellito. I microascessi sono spesso secondari a batteriemia, candidemia o malattia da graffio di gatto. Nella malattia da graffio di gatto e nelle patologie fungine, sono stati anche osservati granulomi infettivi epatici (e/o splenici) multipli.

I segni e i sintomi sono aspecifici e possono comprendere febbre, brividi, sudorazione notturna, malessere, astenia, nausea, dolore addominale con dolenzia del quadrante superiore destro e lieve epatomegalia; l'ittero è infrequente. La diagnosi, talvolta ardua, è spesso ritardata; nei bambini con fattori di rischio, pertanto, si rende necessario un elevato indice di sospetto. I livelli di transaminasi e di fosfatasi alcalina possono essere moderatamente elevati; la velocità di eritrosedimentazione risulta elevata e può essere presente leucocitosi; le emocolture possono anche risultare negative. La radiografia del torace può mostrare elevazione dell'emidiaframma destro con ridotta mobilità o versamento pleurico destro. L'ecografia o la TC in genere confermano la diagnosi (Figg. 356-1, 356-2 e 356-3). L'ascesso solitario del lobo epatico destro è più comune sia degli ascessi multipli, sia dell'ascesso solitario del lobo sinistro. Il **trattamento** richiede l'aspirazione percutanea ecoguidata o TC-guidata o, in alcuni casi, il drenaggio chirurgico a cielo aperto, in particolare in presenza di ascessi multipli o di grosse dimensioni. Sul liquido ascessuale occorre effettuare colture per aerobi e anaerobi. La terapia antibiotica deve essere inizialmente ad ampio spettro e in seguito ristretta sulla base dei risultati colturali sul liquido ascessuale. La terapia, somministrata per via endovenosa, va pro-

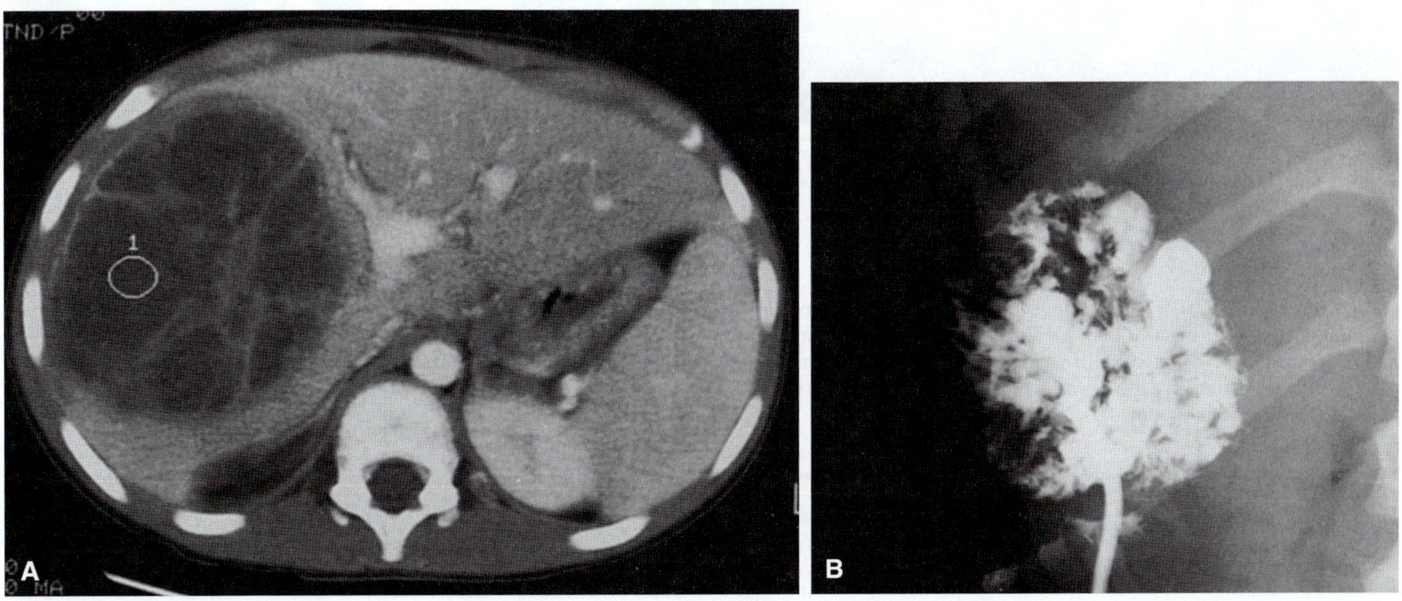

Figura 356-1. Ascesso epatico. *A*, TC con contrasto che mostra una massa settata, multiloculata, ipodensa, nel lobo epatico destro. Sono presenti non solo un'aumentata densità a livello dei setti, ma anche un edema appena visibile tra l'ascesso e il fegato normalmente contrastato. *B*, Iniezione di mezzo di contrasto previo drenaggio percutaneo di questo ascesso streptococcico, che dimostra la natura multiloculata della lesione e la sua parete dai margini irregolari. (Da Kuhn JP, Slovis TL, Haller JO: *Caffrey's Pediatric Diagnostic Imaging*, vol. 2, 10th ed. Philadelphia, Mosby, 2004, p 1470.)

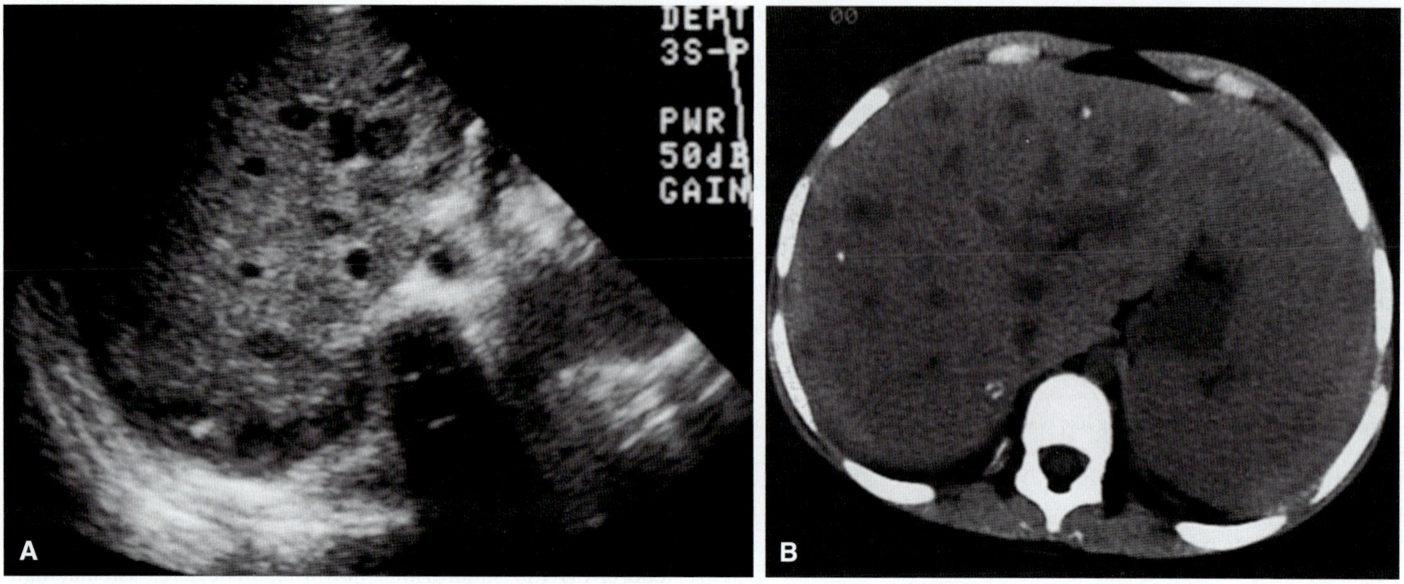

Figura 356-2. Candidosi epatica. Ecografia trasversa (*A*) e TC (*B*) dell'addome superiore, che dimostrano lesioni "a occhio di bue" a carico del lobo epatico destro, in un paziente immunocompromesso. Le calcificazioni osservabili con la TC sono probabilmente esiti di una pregressa infezione. La biopsia epatica ha dimostrato la candidosi. (Da Kuhn JP, Slovis TL, Haller JO: *Caffrey's Pediatric Diagnostic Imaging*, vol. 2, 10th ed. Philadelphia, Mosby, 2004, p 1472.)

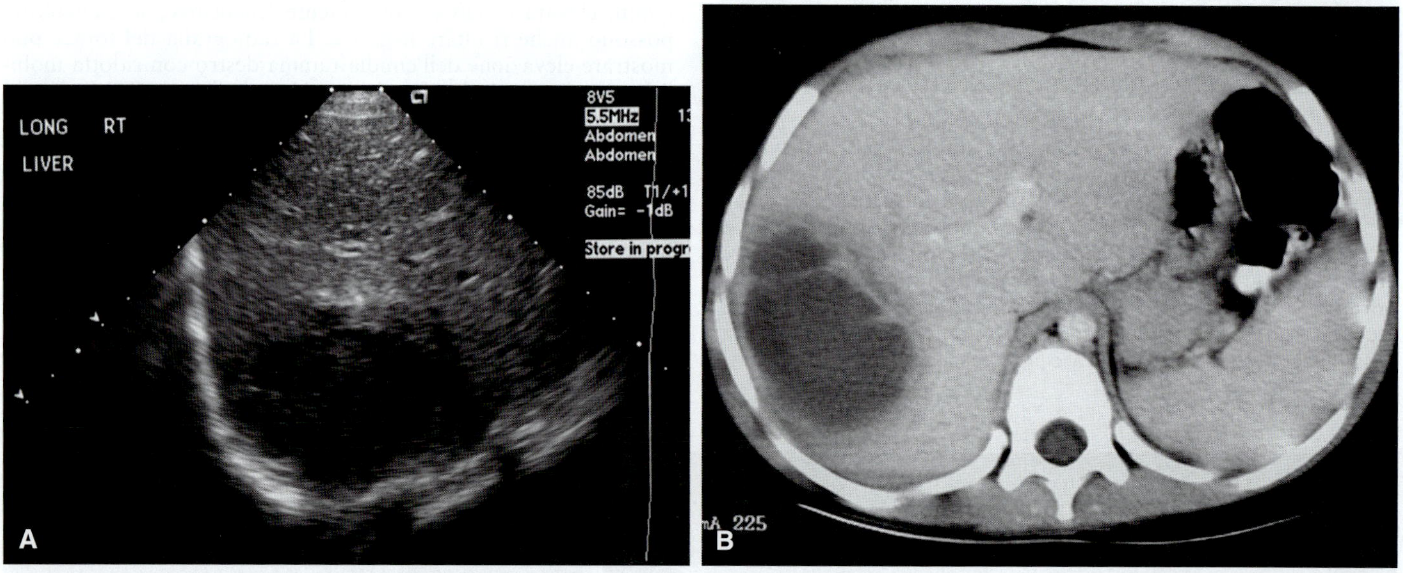

Figura 356-3. Ascesso amebico. *A*, Ecografia che dimostra una massa ipoecogena nel lobo epatico destro, contornata da un anello ancora più ipoecogeno. *B*, TC che rivela una massa ipodensa nel lobo epatico destro, con un alone accentuato. (Da Kuhn JP, Slovis TL, Haller JO: *Caffrey's Pediatric Diagnostic Imaging*, vol. 2, 10th ed. Philadelphia, Mosby, 2004, p 1473.)

lungata per almeno 4-8 settimane, sebbene non esistano evidenze sperimentali su cui basarsi per stabilire la durata del trattamento. La mortalità si è drasticamente ridotta negli ultimi trent'anni, grazie alla diagnosi precoce e alla tempestiva somministrazione di una terapia appropriata.

Fung CP, Change SC, Hu BS, et al: A global emerging disease of *Klebsiella pneumoniae* liver abscess: Is serotype K1 an important factor for complicated endopthalmitis? *Gut* 2002;50:420–424.

Kaplan GG, Gregson DB, Laupland KB: Population-based study of the epidemiology of and the risk factors for pyogenic liver abscess. *Clin Gastroenterol Hepatol* 2004;2:1032–1038.

Kumar A, Srinivasan S, Sharma AK: Pyogenic liver abscess in children—South Indian experiences. *J Pediatr Surg* 1998;33:417–421.

Margalit M, Elinav H, Ilan Y, et al: Liver abscess in inflammatory bowel disease: Report of two cases and review of the literature. *J Gastroenterol Hepatol* 2004;19:1338–1342.

Pereira FE, Musso C, Castelo JS: Pathology of pyogenic liver abscess in children. *Pediatr Dev Pathol* 1999;2:537–543.

Pineiro-Carrero VM, Andres JM: Morbidity and mortality in children with pyogenic liver abscess. *Am J Dis Child* 1989;143:1424–1427.

Capitolo 357 ■ Patologie epatiche associate a disturbi sistemici

Stavra A. Xanthakos e William F. Balistreri

Un'ampia varietà di malattie sistemiche può comportare coinvolgimento epatico, sia come risultato del processo patologico primitivo, sia come complicanza secondaria della patologia stessa o della terapia somministrata.

MALATTIE INFIAMMATORIE INTESTINALI (IBD, *INFLAMMATORY BOWEL DISEASE*). La colite ulcerosa e il morbo di Crohn (vedi Capitolo 333) si associano a patologie epatobiliari che comprendono processi autoimmuni e infiammatori correlati all'IBD (colangite sclerosante, epatite autoimmune), tossicità da farmaci (mercaptopurina, metotrexato, 6-tioguanina), malnutrizione e dismetabolismo (steatosi epatica, colelitiasi), traslocazione batterica e infezioni sistemiche (ascesso epatico, trombosi portale), ipercoagulabilità (infarto) e complicanze a lungo termine di queste epatopatie, come colangite ascendente, cirrosi, ipertensione portale e colangiocarcinoma.

La **colangite sclerosante** è una malattia epatobiliare piuttosto frequente, associata a IBD, che compare nel 2-8% dei pazienti adulti con colite ulcerosa e in una percentuale minore di pazienti con morbo di Crohn. Nei pazienti pediatrici con IBD, la diagnosi è posta tipicamente nella seconda decade di vita. La colangite sclerosante è caratterizzata da infiammazione e fibrosi progressive di segmenti di vie biliari intra- ed extraepatiche, che possono esitare nell'obliterazione duttale completa. È stata dimostrata una predisposizione genetica, associata a numerosi HLA (*Human Leukocyte Antigens*, alleli leucocitari umani). Molti pazienti sono asintomatici e inizialmente si giunge alla diagnosi grazie agli esami routinari di funzionalità epatica, da cui emergono elevati livelli di fosfatasi alcalina (ALP, *Alkaline Phosphatase*), 5'-nucleotidasi o γ-glutamiltranspeptidasi (GGT); possono inoltre essere presenti anticorpi antinucleo o anti-muscolo liscio. Dal 10 al 15% dei pazienti adulti si presenta con sintomi quali anoressia, calo ponderale, prurito, astenia, dolore al quadrante superiore destro e ittero; può insorgere anche una colangite acuta intermittente, accompagnata da febbre, ittero e dolore in ipocondrio destro. Con la progressione del danno, può svilupparsi ipertensione portale. Questi sintomi sono meno comuni nei bambini, in cui la malattia spesso viene scoperta per caso, grazie agli esami di screening della funzionalità epatica. Nei bambini accade occasionalmente che la colangite sclerosante costituisca la presentazione iniziale e che solo in seguito l'esame endoscopico permetta di diagnosticare un'IBD associata. La diagnosi definitiva di colangite sclerosante richiede la biopsia epatica, da cui emergono reperti tipici come fibrosi e infiammazione periduttali, colangite fibro-obliterante e fibrosi portale. La colangiografia può rivelare un aspetto irregolare o a grano di rosario dei dotti biliari intraepatici ed extraepatici.

Non esiste un trattamento medico definitivo per la colangite sclerosante; il trapianto epatico è l'unica opzione a lungo termine per la cirrosi avanzata, anche se nell'organo trapiantato può recidivare un danno autoimmune. La terapia a breve termine è volta a migliorare il drenaggio biliare e a rallentare il processo di obliterazione. L'acido ursodesossicolico, alla dose di 15 mg/kg/die, migliora il flusso biliare e i dati di laboratorio, ma non si è dimostrato in grado di incidere sull'evoluzione clinica. La vancomicina per via orale può migliorare i valori biochimici. Le stenosi biliari extraepatiche dominanti possono essere sottoposte a dilatazione per via endoscopica, con eventuale posizionalmento di uno stent. La terapia immunosoppressiva con corticosteroidi e/o azatioprina ha effetti positivi sul quadro biochimico, ma si è dimostrata deludente nel rallentare la progressione istologica a lungo termine. Occorre instaurare una terapia sintomatica in caso di prurito (rifampicina, acido ursodeossicolico, difenidramina), malnutrizione (supplementi enterali) e colangite ascendente (antibiotici), secondo le indicazioni. La colectomia totale non si è rivelata di alcun beneficio per prevenire o trattare le complicanze epatobiliari, nei pazienti con colite ulcerosa.

L'**epatite autoimmune** (AIH, *Autoimmune Hepatitis*) associata all'IBD può presentare molte analogie con la colangite sclerosante, tanto che si parla spesso di **sindrome da sovrapposizione** (*overlap syndrome*) o di colangite sclerosante autoimmune (ASC, *Autoimmune Sclerosing Cholangitis*). Questi pazienti presentano tipicamente ipergammaglobulinemia (marcato incremento dei livelli di immunoglobuline [Ig] G). In alcuni bambini dapprima viene diagnosticata un'AIH e solo in seguito si scopre una colangite sclerosante, mediante colangiografia; in altri casi l'AIH si presenta a distanza di anni dalla diagnosi di una colangite sclerosante associata a IBD. La biopsia epatica, nei pazienti con sindrome da sovrapposizione AIH/colangite sclerosante (ASC) presenta epatite dell'interfaccia (*Interface Hepatitis*), oltre al danno duttale associato alla colangite sclerosante. I farmaci immunosoppressori (corticosteroidi e/o azatioprina) sono il caposaldo della terapia dell'ASC; la risposta a lungo termine sembra tuttavia meno favorevole che nell'AIH. La sopravvivenza a lungo termine, nei bambini con ASC, appare simile a quella dei bambini con colangite sclerosante, con una sopravvivenza media (50%) globale, senza trapianto epatico, di 12,7 anni.

La steatosi epatica sembra avere una prevalenza maggiore nei pazienti adulti con IBD, variando dal 35 al 40%, in un'ampia serie studiata. I calcoli biliari sono più frequenti nei pazienti con morbo di Crohn (11%) che in quelli con colite ulcerosa (7,5%) e nei soggetti normali (5%). La reale prevalenza di queste malattie epatiche associate a IBD, nei pazienti pediatrici, è tuttavia sconosciuta.

SEPSI BATTERICA (VEDI CAPITOLI 109 E 176). La sepsi può mimare un danno epatico e dovrebbe sempre essere esclusa nei pazienti critici che sviluppano colestasi, in assenza di un marcato aumento delle transaminasi o dell'ALP, anche quando non sono presenti altri segni di infezione. I microrganismi isolati più di frequente in emocoltura sono batteri Gram-negativi, in particolare *Escherichia coli*, *Klebsiella pneumoniae* e *Pseudomonas aeruginosa*. È probabile che lipopolisaccaridi e altre endotossine batteriche interferiscano con la secrezione biliare, alterando direttamente la struttura o la funzione delle proteine di trasporto della membrana canalicolare biliare. La bilirubinemia è elevata, soprattutto la frazione coniugata. Non sempre le transaminasi e l'ALP risultano elevate. La biopsia epatica dimostra colestasi intraepatica con necrosi scarsa o assente. Sono frequenti l'iperplasia delle cellule di Kupffer e l'aumento delle cellule infiammatorie. Reperti simili possono comparire con l'urosepsi.

CARDIOPATIE. Talora un danno epatico può insorgere come complicanza di un grave scompenso cardiaco congestizio, acuto o cronico (vedi Capitolo 442), di una cardiopatia cianogena congenita (vedi Capitoli 429 e 430), e di uno shock ischemico acuto. In tutte queste condizioni, possono contribuire al danno epatico sia la congestione passiva, sia la ridotta gittata cardiaca. L'aumento della pressione venosa centrale, trasmessa alle vene epatiche, alle venule minori e infine agli epatociti circostanti, porta ad atrofia epatocellulare nella zona centrolobulare. A causa della gittata ridotta, inoltre, anche il flusso ematico nell'arteria epatica diminuisce, con conseguente ipossia centrolobulare. La necrosi epatica porta ad acidosi lattica, aumento dei livelli di transaminasi, colestasi, aumento del tempo di protrombina e, talora, ipoglicemia per la compromissione del metabolismo epatico. Possono insorgere ittero, epatomegalia dolente e, in alcuni casi, ascite e splenomegalia.

Dopo uno shock ipovolemico acuto le transaminasi possono subire un notevole aumento, ma in breve tempo ritornano ai valori normali con il miglioramento della perfusione e della funzione cardiaca. Nei neonati con sindrome del cuore sinistro ipoplasico e coartazione aortica può insorgere necrosi epatica o insufficienza epatica acuta. Anche l'elevata pressione venosa centrale dopo le procedure di Fontan può dar luogo a una disfunzione epatica, caratterizzata da un aumento del tempo di protrombina. In tutti i casi di epatopatia associata a malattia cardiaca, gli obiettivi della terapia sono il miglioramento della gittata cardiaca, la riduzione della pressione venosa sistemica e il controllo di eventuali altri segni di ipoperfusione, tramite uno stretto monitoraggio della funzione renale e dello stato mentale.

OBESITÀ. La steatosi epatica non alcolica (NAFLD, *NonAlcoholic Fatty Liver Disease*) rientra nell'ambito delle epatopatie strettamente associate all'obesità. Può presentarsi in varie forme, dalla sola steatosi epatica alla triade di infiltrazione grassa, infiammazione e fibrosi (NASH, *NonAlcoholic Steatohepatitis*, steatoepatite non alcolica), simile al danno da alcol, a fronte però di un'assunzione di etanolo minima o nulla. La NAFLD, un tempo considerata frequente soprattutto nei giovani adulti (in particolare di sesso femminile) con obesità centrale, insulinoresistenza e diabete di tipo II, oggi è di riscontro sempre più frequente anche nell'infanzia. La reale prevalenza nei bambini è ignota, poiché la diagnosi richiede la biopsia epatica. L'aumento dei livelli di transaminasi non è un marcatore sensibile né specifico di questa patologia; analogamente, non esistono indagini radiologiche che permettano di distinguerla dalla NASH. Globalmente, la prevalenza stimata negli adulti raggiunge il 15-20% per la NAFLD e il 2-4% per la NASH. I fattori di rischio, in coorti pediatriche, sono risultati l'obesità, il sesso maschile, l'etnia bianca o ispanica, l'ipertrigliceridemia e l'insulinoresistenza.

La steatosi epatica isolata talvolta è benigna, ma fino a un quarto degli individui con NASH può sviluppare fibrosi progressiva fino alla cirrosi epatica. Non si conosce la prognosi a lungo termine della NASH che si sviluppa in età infantile. Un calo ponderale graduale si rivela efficace per normalizzare i livelli di ALT e migliorare la NAFLD. Attualmente sono in corso studi relativi alla somministrazione nei bambini di vitamina E e metformina, che potrebbero rivelarsi utili per tenere sotto controllo le anomalie biochimiche; non è noto tuttavia se possano avere effetti positivi anche sull'istopatologia epatica. I tiazolidenedioni migliorano il quadro istologico negli adulti con NASH, ma non sono mai stati studiati nei bambini.

COLESTASI ASSOCIATA A NUTRIZIONE PARENTERALE TOTALE (NPT). La NPT può causare varie forme di danno epatico, tra cui steatosi, danno a carico della colecisti e dei dotti biliari, colelitiasi. Quest'ultima è la complicanza più severa, potendo portare a una progressiva fibrosi epatica, fino alla cirrosi, soprattutto nei neonati e nei bambini piccoli sottoposti a NPT per periodi prolungati. In quanto tale, costituisce il maggiore fattore limitante l'uso della NPT a lungo termine, tanto nei bambini quanto negli adulti. I fattori di rischio per la colestasi da NPT comprendono lunga durata della NPT, prematurità, basso peso alla nascita, sepsi, enterocolite necrotizzante e sindrome dell'intestino corto. La colestasi da NPT si sviluppa in quasi la metà dei neonati con peso <1000 g, nel 20% di quelli di peso compreso tra 1000 e 1500 g, e nel 5-10% di quelli tra 1500 e 2000 g.

La patogenesi della colestasi da NPT è multifattoriale. Diversi sono i fattori che possono contribuire al danno epatico, quali sepsi, eccessivo introito calorico, elevate quantità di proteine, grassi o carboidrati, tossicità da aminoacidi specifici, carenze di alcuni nutrienti, tossicità da oligoelementi come manganese, alluminio o rame. Il digiuno enterale prolungato altera l'integrità della mucosa e aumenta la traslocazione batterica, oltre a ridurre il rilascio di ormoni enterali, come la colecistochinina, che stimolano il flusso biliare. La sepsi, in particolare da batteri Gram-negativi, e l'endotossinemia associata possono aggravare il danno epatico.

I reperti istologici precoci comprendono steatosi macrovacuolare, colestasi canalicolare e infiammazione della triade portale, tutte alterazioni che possono regredire dopo la sospensione di una NPT a breve termine. La NPT di lunga durata è invece caratterizzata da proliferazione dei dotti biliari, fibrosi portale ed espansione della triade portale, danni che possono progredire fino alla cirrosi e all'insufficienza epatica terminale.

L'esordio clinico tipicamente consiste nell'insorgenza graduale di colestasi, dopo circa 2 settimane di NPT. Nei neonati di basso peso, la comparsa dell'ittero può sovrapporsi alla fase di iperbilirubinemia (non coniugata) fisiologica. La bilirubinemia frazionata andrebbe determinata in tutti i neonati itterici sottoposti a NPT per più di una settimana. In caso di durata maggiore, possono svilupparsi epatomegalia e splenomegalia e può aumentare la concentrazione di acidi biliari, mentre l'aumento delle transaminasi talvolta è un reperto tardivo. Un aumento dell'ALP può essere causato anche da rachitismo, una complicanza frequente della NPT nei neonati di basso peso alla nascita.

Oltre alla colestasi, le complicanze biliari della NPT (talvolta asintomatiche) comprendono colelitiasi e formazione di sabbia biliare, associata a un contenuto colecistico spesso e viscoso. La steatosi epatica o l'aumento delle transaminasi possono insorgere anche in assenza di colestasi, in particolare nei bambini più grandi; in questi casi di solito sono lievi e si risolvono con la sospensione della NPT. La bilirubinemia e i livelli di acidi biliari restano nella norma. Occorre prendere in esame anche altre cause di danno epatico, soprattutto se persistono segni di disfunzione epatica nonostante la sospensione della NPT e la ripresa dell'alimentazione enterale. Dal momento che i gruppi più a rischio, in cui la colestasi da NPT si sviluppa più facilmente, ricevono spesso derivati ematici o farmaci, occorre escludere anche malattie epatiche di origine virale o indotte da farmaci. Se i livelli di transaminasi o di ALP permangono elevati, può rendersi necessaria la biopsia epatica per una diagnosi accurata.

Il **trattamento** della colestasi associata a NPT si focalizza sulla prevenzione del danno epatico progressivo, tramite la limitazione della durata della NPT, ove possibile. Bisognerebbe iniziare l'alimentazione enterale non appena viene tollerata ed evitare il digiuno prolungato. Anche piccole quantità di nutrienti, somministrati tramite alimentazione orale intermittente o sondino nasogastrico continuo, possono sia stimolare il flusso biliare, la circolazione enteroepatica degli acidi biliari, la motilità intestinale, sia potenziare la funzione di barriera della mucosa intestinale, riducendo il rischio di traslocazione batterica. Migliorare le soluzioni somministrate nella NPT, adattandole alle necessità specifiche dei neonati, potrà prevenire le carenze ed evitare la tossicità. Al momento di valutare se proseguire o meno la NPT a tempo indefinito, bisognerebbe sempre considerare il rischio di danno epatico e si dovrebbe fare il possibile per portare avanti la nutrizione enterale, ove consentito dalla situazione. Il trattamento con acido ursodesossicolico può contribuire a ridurre l'ittero e l'epatosplenomegalia. Altre terapie, come l'impiego degli antibiotici per ridurre la crescita batterica endoluminale o la somministrazione orale di taurina o colecistochinina, restano opzioni sperimentali.

FIBROSI CISTICA (FC). La FC è causata da mutazioni nel gene CFTR (*Cystic Fibrosis Transmembrane Conductance Regulator*, regolatore di contuttanza transmembrana della fibrosi cistica), che alterano il trasporto del cloro attraverso la membrana apicale delle cellule epiteliali di numerosi organi (tra cui i colangiociti) (vedi Capitolo 400). La prevalenza di epatopatia in corso di FC è stimata del 37%, ma potrebbe essere in aumento, considerate le aumentate aspettative di vita di questi pazienti e le maggiori conoscenze di cui attualmente si dispone nel campo dell'epatopatia associata a FC.

Si ritiene che, nei pazienti con FC, il danno epatico sia in parte dovuto all'alterata funzione secretoria dell'epitelio biliare duttale; i dotti biliari contengono un materiale denso, granulare, eosinofilo, che porta alla cirrosi biliare focale. Si può verificare quindi una graduale progressione alla cirrosi multilobulare, con conseguenti ipertensione portale e insufficienza epatica. Il danno epatico tende a insorgere soprattutto nei pazienti con insufficienza pancreatica, ma le ragioni di questa associazione non sono ancora state chiarite. Il raggruppamento familiare dei casi suggerisce anche una predisposizione genetica; tuttavia, non sono state trovate associazioni specifiche genotipo-fenotipo, con determinate mutazioni CFTR. L'analisi mutazionale è oggi in grado di prevedere quali pazienti con FC svilupperanno un'epatopatia. I fattori di rischio clinici che possono associarsi a danno epatico comprendono età avanzata, insufficienza pancreatica, sesso maschile e, forse, un'anamnesi di ileo da meconio.

Il **trattamento** con acido ursodesossicolico (10-15 mg/kg/die) può essere utile per migliorare la funzione epatica, probabilmente per stimolazione del flusso biliare, ma sono necessari ulteriori studi per determinare se si tratta di un reale beneficio a lungo termine. Essendo difficile prevedere quali pazienti svilupperanno un'epatopatia, non è possibile praticare una terapia profilattica. La progressione del danno epatico è generalmente lenta; nei casi in cui evolve fino all'insufficienza epatica, il trapianto può rappresentare l'unica possibilità di sopravvivenza.

TRAPIANTO DI MIDOLLO OSSEO. Nei pazienti sottoposti a trapianto di cellule staminali emopoietiche (SCT, *Stem Cell Transplantation*) è di frequente riscontro un danno epatico, sia che le cellule trapiantate provengano dal midollo osseo, sia che provengano dal sangue periferico (vedi Capitoli 134-138). La patogenesi è variabile e comprende: infezioni (virali, batteriche o fungine); tossicità da farmaci, nutrizione parenterale, chemioterapia o radioterapia; malattia veno-occlusiva (VOD, *Veno-Occlusive Disease*); malattia da rigetto del trapianto verso l'ospite (GVHD, *Graft Versus Host Disease*); emosiderosi secondaria al sovraccarico di ferro, per le frequenti emotrasfusioni. La GVHD, la tossicità da farmaci e la sepsi sono le cause più frequenti di disfunzione epatica dopo trapianto allogenico di cellule staminali. La diagnosi è spesso ardua, per la compresenza di fattori di rischio multipli. Ai fini di un corretto iter diagnostico, occorre sempre considerare il decorso clinico, i sintomi e i segni, così come i risultati degli esami biochimici di funzionalità epatica e dei test virologici. Talvolta è necessario effettuare una biopsia epatica percutanea: l'esame istologico può mostrare un danno massivo dei dotti biliari nella GVHD, inclusioni virali nell'infezione da Cytomegalovirus o le caratteristiche lesioni endoteliali nella VOD. È importante diagnosticare accuratamente la causa, poiché il trattamento della GVHD è molto diverso da quello di altre patologie (in particolare, richiede che si instauri una terapia immunosoppressiva), e potrebbe peggiorare un'epatite su base infettiva.

La **GVHD epatica**, che può essere acuta o cronica, si associa spesso a GVHG in altri organi bersaglio, come la cute e l'intestino (vedi Capitolo 136). La GVHD epatica è causata da una reazione immunologica diretta contro l'epitelio dei dotti biliari, che porta a una colangite non suppurativa. Le caratteristiche istologiche comprendono perdita dei dotti biliari intralobulari, danno endoteliale delle venule epatiche e portali, necrosi epatocellulare.

L'esordio avviene tipicamente al momento dell'attecchimento del trapianto (14-21 giorni dopo l'SCT). Nella GVHD epatica acuta i livelli di transaminasi possono aumentare notevolmente, in assenza di iperbilirubinemia e di alterazione dei livelli di ALP e GGT, mimando un'epatite virale. La GVHD epatica acuta può insorgere precocemente (14-21 giorni) oppure tardivamente (più di 70 giorni) dopo un SCT allogenico. Nella malattia cronica, le transaminasi subiscono un rialzo più contenuto e sono più evidenti i segni di colestasi, con un netto aumento della bilirubina coniugata, della GGT e dell'ALP. Altri segni e sintomi comprendono dolorabilità epatica, urine scure, feci acoliche, prurito e anoressia.

La **VOD epatica** si sviluppa abitualmente nelle prime 3 settimane dopo un SCT. L'incidenza è minore del 10%, con una mortalità inferiore al 4%. I fattori di rischio comprendono traumi, coagulopatie, anemia falciforme, leucemia, policitemia vera, ascessi epatici, radioterapia e GVHD. La VOD è causata dall'obliterazione fibrosa delle venule epatiche terminali e delle piccole vene lobulari, con conseguente danno degli epatociti e dei sinusoidi circostanti. Non è associata alla formazione di trombi, diversamente dalla sindrome di Budd-Chiari, che comporta l'occlusione delle vene epatiche principali o della vena cava inferiore da parte di una rete, di una massa o di un trombo. La causa della VOD dopo trapianto di midollo osseo non è chiara; i fattori di rischio comprendono regimi di condizionamento a dosi elevate, radioterapia, leucemia, età avanzata ed epatopatia preesistente.

Il modo migliore per individuare le alterazioni patologiche nei pazienti con VOD è servirsi di colorazioni particolari (tricromica) che evidenziano le vene centrali. La lesione precoce è un restringimento concentrico del lume delle piccole vene centrali, causato da edema della zona subendoteliale. Nelle vene centrali è presente una banda di collagene continua, densa e ondulata, associata a necrosi emorragica centrolobulare. La lesione può essere focale. Nelle fasi successive di malattia, le venule epatiche possono risultare completamente obliterate.

I sintomi caratteristici comprendono ittero, epatomegalia dolente, rapido aumento ponderale e ascite. La VOD si risolve nella maggior parte dei pazienti, ma può anche esitare in insufficienza multiorgano, encefalopatia epatica e insufficienza epatica fulminante. Le forme meno gravi possono essere caratterizzate da ittero e ascite a lenta risoluzione; nei casi molto lievi, le alterazioni istologiche talvolta sono le uniche manifestazioni di malattia. La diagnosi si basa sull'esclusione di altre patologie, come la GVHD, la pericardite costrittiva e la sindrome di Budd-Chiari.

Non esiste una profilassi efficace, né una terapia specifica per la VOD. Sono attualmente in corso di studio agenti profilattici come l'eparina per via endovenosa, o a basso peso molecolare, la prostaglandina E_1 e l'acido ursodesossicolico. Quest'ultimo farmaco, somministrato per via orale, può ridurre l'incidenza di epatopatia severa nei pazienti sottoposti a SCT, ma non è chiaro se dia un beneficio diretto nella prevenzione della VOD. Il trattamento di supporto comprende il mantenimento dell'idratazione e della perfusione renale per via endovenosa. La VOD severa, nei pazienti adulti ad alto rischio, è stata trattata con difibrotide, un agente sperimentale con proprietà antitrombotiche e trombolitiche.

EMOGLOBINOPATIE. I pazienti con anemia falciforme (vedi Capitolo 462.1) o talassemia a cellule falciformi (Capitolo 462.1) possono soffrire di una disfunzione epatica causata da epatiti virali acute o croniche, emosiderosi derivante dalla frequente terapia trasfusionale, crisi epatiche correlate a grave colestasi intraepatica, sequestro o necrosi ischemica. Inoltre, è frequente la presenza di colelitiasi.

La **crisi falciforme epatica**, o "epatopatia falciforme", si verifica in circa il 10% dei pazienti con anemia falciforme. Si presenta con intenso dolore in ipocondrio destro, febbre, leucocitosi, dolorabilità al quadrante superiore destro dell'addome e ittero. I livelli di bilirubina possono essere molto elevati; l'ALP, per contro, può essere solo moderatamente aumentata. Dal momento che può essere difficile distinguere l'epatopatia dall'anemia falciforme dall'epatite virale o dalla colecistite/coledocolitiasi acuta, si devono sempre escludere queste condizioni. In genere la crisi falciforme epatica è autolimitante. La **colestasi intraepatica da anemia falciforme**, che si manifesta con epatomegalia, dolore addominale, iperbilirubinemia e coagulopatia, può progredire verso l'insufficienza epatica acuta; in tal caso, l'unica possibilità di sopravvivenza rimane il trapianto epatico, che peraltro comporta un rischio elevato di perdita dell'organo per le complicanze vascolari. Fortunatamente la colestasi intraepatica è un evento raro.

Talvolta i bambini con anemia falciforme presentano livelli di bilirubina >20 mg/dL, non accompagnati da dolore grave o da febbre. L'ematocrito e i reticolociti risultano normali e non è presente una crisi emolitica associata. Il decorso clinico, in questi casi, è benigno.

COLLAGENOPATIE. Le collagenopatie, nei bambini, si associano spesso ad anomalie degli enzimi epatici. Tali patologie comprendono il lupus eritematoso sistemico, l'artrite reumatoide e le collagenopatie miste. Sono stati riportati casi di arterite epatica, epatite reattiva aspecifica, epatite autoimmune, iperplasia nodulare rigenerativa, steatosi e infarto epatico. Occorre sempre escludere la tossicità da farmaci e l'epatite virale. In caso di anomalie biochimiche idiopatiche persistenti, per formulare una diagnosi specifica può rendersi necessaria la biopsia epatica.

Ahmad J, Slivka A: Hepatobiliary disease in inflammatory bowel disease. *Gastroenterol Clin North Am* 2002;31:329–345.

Bargiggia S, Maconit G, Elli M, et al: Sonographic prevalence of liver steatosis and biliary tract stones in patients with inflammatory bowel disease: Study of 511 subjects at a single center. *J Clin Gastroenterol* 2003;36:417–420.

Beale E, Nelson R, Bucciarelli R, et al: Intrahepatic cholestasis associated with parenteral nutrition in premature infants. *Pediatrics* 1979;64:342–347.

Buchanan GR, Glader BE: Benign course of extreme hyperbilirubinemia in sickle cell anemia: Analysis of six cases. *J Pediatr* 1977;91:21–24.

Chen CY, Tsao PN, Chen HL, et al: Ursodeoxycholic acid (UDCA) therapy in very-low-birth-weight infants with parenteral nutrition–associated cholestasis. *J Pediatr* 2004;145:317–321.

Colombo C, Battezzati PM, Podda M, et al: Ursodeoxycholic acid for liver disease associated with cystic fibrosis: A double-blind multicenter trial. The Italian Group for the Study of Ursodeoxycholic Acid in Cystic Fibrosis. *Hepatology* 1996;23:1484–1490.

Columbo C, Battezzati PM, Strazzabosco M, et al: Liver and biliary problems in cystic fibrosis. *Semin Liver Dis* 1998;18:227–235.

Debray D, Pariente D, Urvoas E, et al: Sclerosing cholangitis in children. *J Pediatr* 1994;124:49–56.

Feldstein AE, Perrault J, El-Youssif M, et al: Primary sclerosing cholangitis in children: A long-term follow-up study. *Hepatology* 2003;38:210–217.

Fujii N, Takenaka K, Shinagawa K et al: Hepatic graft-versus-host disease presenting as acute hepatitis after allogeneic peripheral blood stem cell transplantation. *Bone Marrow Transplant* 2001;27:1007–1010.

Giallourakis CC, Rosenberg P, Friedman LS: The liver in heart failure. *Clin Liver Dis* 2002;6:947–967.

Gregorio GV, Portmann B, Karani J, et al: Autoimmune hepatitis/sclerosing cholangitis overlap syndrome in childhood: A 16-year prospective study. *Hepatology* 2001;33:544–553.

Hong-Curtis J, Yeh MM, Jain D, et al: Rapid progression of autoimmune hepatitis in the background of primary sclerosing cholangitis. *J Clin Gastroenterol* 2004;38:906–909.

Kaufman SS: Prevention of parenteral nutrition-associated liver disease in children. *Pediatr Transplant* 2002;6:37–42.

Khurshid I, Anderson L, Downie GH, et al: Sickle cell disease, extreme hyperbilirubinemia, and pericardial tamponade: Case report and review of the literature. *Crit Care Med* 2002;30:2363–2367.

Kim BK, Chung KW, Sun HS: Liver disease during the first post-transplant year in bone marrow transplantation recipients: Retrospective study. *Bone Marrow Transplant* 2000;26:193–197.

Kwan V and George J: Liver disease due to parenteral and enteral nutrition. *Clin Liver Dis* 2004;8:893–913.

Lavine JE: Vitamin E treatment of nonalcoholic steatohepatitis in children: A pilot study. *J Pediatr* 2000;136:734–738.

Levine A, Maayan A, Shamir R, et al: Parenteral nutrition–associated cholestasis in preterm neonates: Evaluation of ursodeoxycholic acid treatment. *J Pediatr Endocrinol Metab* 1999;12:549–553.

Margalit M, Elinav H, Ilan Y, et al: Liver abscess in inflammatory bowel disease: Report of two cases and review of the literature. *J Gastroenterol Hepatol* 2004;19:1338–1342.

Matsumoto T, Kobayashi S, Shimizu H, et al: The liver in collagen diseases: Pathologic study of 160 cases with particular reference to hepatic arteritis, primary biliary cirrhosis, autoimmune hepatitis and nodular regenerative hyperplasia of the liver. *Liver* 2000;20:366–373.

Moseley RH: Sepsis and cholestasis. *Clin Liver Dis* 2004;8:83–94.

Narkewicz MR, Sondheimer HM, Ziegler JW, et al: Hepatic dysfunction following the Fontan procedure. *J Pediatr Gastroenterol Nutr* 2003;36: 352–357.

Ribaud P, Gluckman E: Hepatic veno-occlusive disease. *Pediatr Transplant* 1999;3:41–44.

Roberts EA: Nonalcoholic steatohepatitis in children. *Curr Gastroenterol Rep* 2003;5:253–259.

Ruutu T, Eriksson B, Juvonen E, et al: Ursodeoxycholic acid for the prevention of hepatic complications in allogeneic stem cell transplantation. *Blood* 2002;100:1977–1983.

Schubert TT: Hepatobiliary system in sickle cell disease. *Gastroenterology* 1986;90:2013–2021.

Schwimmer JB, Deutsch R, Kahen T, et al: Prevalence of fatty liver in children and adolescents. *Pediatrics* 2006;118:1388–1393.

Schwimmer JB, Deutsch R, Rauch JB, et al: Obesity, insulin resistance and other clinicopathological correlates of pediatric nonalcoholic fatty liver disease. *J Pediatr* 2003;143:500–505.

Strauss RS, Barlow SE, Dietz WH: Prevalence of abnormal serum aminotransferase values in overweight and obese adolescents. *J Pediatr* 2000;136: 727–733.

Wilschanski M, Rivlin J, Cohen S, et al: Clinical and genetic risk factors for cystic fibrosis–related liver disease. *Pediatrics* 1999;103:52–57.

Zakrzewski JL, Ballauff A, Wieland R: Differential diagnosis of cholestasis following allogeneic hematopoietic stem cell transplantation: The contribution of serum bile acid levels in relation to other liver tests. *Pediatr Hematol Oncol* 2004;21:697–705.

Capitolo 358 ■ Epatopatie mitocondriali

Rebecca G. Carey e William F. Balistreri

Gli epatociti sono ricchi di mitocondri, per la notevole quantità di energia richiesta dai processi metabolici, e risentono pertanto delle alterazioni della funzione mitocondriale. I difetti funzionali dei mitocondri possono portare a un'alterazione della fosforilazione ossidativa (OXPHOS, *OXidative PHOSphorylation*), a un aumento della produzione di specie reattive dell'ossigeno, a un'alterazione di altre vie metaboliche e a un'attivazione dei meccanismi di apoptosi. Le alterazioni mitocondriali possono essere suddivise in primitive, in cui il difetto mitocondriale è la prima causa del disturbo, e secondarie, in cui la funzione mitocondriale è alterata da un danno esogeno o da una mutazione in un gene non mitocondriale (vedi Capitolo 87.4). Le forme primitive possono essere causate da mutazioni sia del DNA mitocondriale (mtDNA), sia di geni nucleari che codificano per proteine o cofattori mitocondriali (Tab. 358-1). Le forme secondarie comprendono invece patologie a eziologia incerta, come la sindrome di Reye, malattie causate da tossine endogene o esogene, farmaci o metalli pesanti, e altre condizioni in cui un danno ossidativo a livello mitocondriale può concorrere alla patogenesi dell'insulto epatico.

EPIDEMIOLOGIA. Sono state identificate più di 200 mutazioni a carico del mtDNA o del DNA nucleare che codifica per proteine mitocondriali. La genetica dei mitocondri è unica, poiché questi organuli sono in grado di replicare, trascrivere e traslare autonomamente il proprio DNA. Il genoma mitocondriale codifica per due RNA ribosomiali, 22 RNA di trasferimento e 13 proteine del complesso I, III, IV e V della catena respiratoria. L'OXPHOS (il processo di produzione dell'adenosin trifosfato [ATP]) avviene nella catena respiratoria, localizzata nella membrana mitocondriale interna, e si articola in cinque complessi multienzimatici: il nicotinamide adenin dinucleotide ridotto (NADH) coenzima Q (CoQ) reduttasi (complesso I), la succinato-CoQ reduttasi

TABELLA 358-1. Epatopatie mitocondriali primitive

Difetti del trasporto di elettroni (catena respiratoria)
Insufficienza epatica neonatale: deficit del complesso I (NADH: ubiquinone ossidoreduttasi), deficit del complesso IV (citocromo-c ossidasi), deficit del complesso III (ubiquinolo: citocromo-c ossidoreduttasi), deficit di più di un complesso
Sindrome da deplezione del DNA mitocondriale (desossiguanosina chinasi)
Malattia di Alpers (deficit del complesso I, DNA polimerasi-γA)
Sindrome midollo-pancreas di Pearson (delezione di mtDNA)
Encefalomiopatia neurogastrointestinale mitocondriale (timidina fosforilasi, tRNA del triptofano)
Diarrea cronica (atrofia dei villi) con coinvolgimento epatico (deficit del complesso III)
Neuroepatopatia Navajo
Difetti della traslazione mitocondriale (fattore di allungamento G1)
Deficit della catena lunga dell'idrossiacil CoA deidrogenasi
Steatosi acuta gravidica
Difetti dell'ossidazione e del trasporto degli acidi grassi
Deficit di carnitina-palmitoil trasferasi I e II
Deficit di carnitina-acilcarnitina traslocasi
Deficit di enzimi del ciclo dell'urea
Deficit di flavoproteina trasportatore di elettroni (EFT, *Electron Transfer Flavoprotein*) e di EFT-deidrogenasi
Deficit di fosfoenolpiruvato carbossichinasi (PEPCK) (mitocondriale)
Iperglicemia non chetosica (deficit dell'enzima di clivaggio della glicina)

CoA, coenzima A; mtDNA, DNA mitocondriale; NADH, nicotinamide adenin dinucleotide.

(complesso II), la CoQ ridotto-citocromo c reduttasi (complesso III), la citocromo-c ossidasi (complesso IV) e l'ATP sintetasi (complesso V). I polipeptidi che formano questi complessi sono trascritti sia dal DNA mitocondriale, sia da quello nucleare; mutazioni in entrambi questi genomi possono comportare alterazioni dell'OXPHOS. L'espressione delle alterazioni mitocondriali è complessa e gli studi epidemiologici risentono delle difficoltà tecniche connesse alla raccolta e all'elaborazione dei campioni tissutali, necessarie per una diagnosi accurata, della variabilità della presentazione clinica e del fatto che la maggior parte dei disturbi presenta un'ereditarietà per via materna a penetranza variabile (vedi Capitolo 80). Inoltre, il mtDNA va incontro a mutazione 10 volte più spesso del DNA nucleare, a causa della mancanza di introni, di istoni protettivi e di un sistema di riparazione efficace all'interno dei mitocondri. La genetica mitocondriale presenta anche un effetto soglia, in quanto il tipo e la gravità della mutazione, necessari per l'espressione clinica, variano non solo da un individuo all'altro, ma anche da un apparato all'altro. Ciononostante, si è stimato che le malattie mitocondriali abbiano una prevalenza di 11,5 casi su 100 000 individui.

MANIFESTAZIONI CLINICHE. I difetti dell'OXPHOS possono colpire qualsiasi tessuto, seppure con un grado di severità variabile, in quanto i più vulnerabili sono gli organi a elevato metabolismo energetico. Si dovrebbe ipotizzare un'alterazione mitocondriale in un paziente di qualsiasi età, con coinvolgimento progressivo multisistemico che nessuna diagnosi specifica riesce a spiegare. I disturbi gastrointestinali comprendono vomito, diarrea, stipsi, mancato sviluppo e dolore addominale; alcune alterazioni mitocondriali hanno una presentazione gastrointestinale caratteristica. La sindrome midollo-pancreas di Pearson si presenta con anemia sideroblastica e insufficienza pancreatica esocrina, mentre l'encefalomiopatia neurogastrointestinale mitocondriale (MNGIE, *Mitochondrial NeuroGastroIntestinal Encephalomyopathy*) è caratterizzata da pseudo-ostruzione intestinale cronica e cachessia. Le manifestazioni epatiche vanno dalla colestasi cronica all'epatomegalia, alla steatosi, fino all'insufficienza epatica fulminante e al decesso.

EPATOPATIE MITOCONDRIALI PRIMITIVE

Una presentazione comune dei difetti della catena respiratoria è l'insufficienza epatica severa che si manifesta nei primi mesi di vita, caratterizzata da acidosi lattica, ittero, ipoglicemia, disfunzione renale e iperammoniemia. I sintomi sono aspecifici e comprendono letargia e vomito. La maggior parte dei pazienti presenta inoltre un coinvolgimento neurologico, che si manifesta con suzione debole, apnea ricorrente o epilessia mioclonica. La biopsia epatica mostra una steatosi prevalentemente microvescicolare, colestasi, proliferazione dei dotti biliari, deplezione delle riserve di glicogeno e sovraccarico di ferro. Con la terapia standard la prognosi è molto scadente, e la maggior parte dei pazienti muore nei primi mesi di vita per insufficienza epatica o infezioni. La **citocromo-*c* ossidasi** (complesso IV), un gene nucleare, è il gene più spesso colpito da deficit in questi neonati (vedi Tab. 358-1).

La **sindrome di Alpers** (sindrome di Alpers-Huttenlocher o poliodistrofia epatopatica di Alpers) si presenta anche in età neonatale con convulsioni, ipotonia, difficoltà ad alimentarsi e atassia. I pazienti sviluppano tipicamente epatomegalia e ittero e hanno una progressione verso l'insufficienza epatica più lenta rispetto a quelli con deficit della citocromo-*c* ossidasi. La malattia è trasmessa con modalità autosomica recessiva; in una famiglia con sindrome di Alpers sono state identificate mutazioni nella subunità catalitica del gene nucleare per la mtDNA polimerasi-γA.

SINDROME DA DEPLEZIONE DI DNA MITOCONDRIALE (MDS, *MITOCHONDRIAL DNA DEPLETION SINDROME*). La MDS, caratterizzata da una riduzione tessuto-specifica del numero di copie di mtDNA, si presenta con grande eterogeneità fenotipica e forme di malattia multisistemica oppure localizzata, che comprendono presentazioni miopatiche, epatocerebrali ed epatiche isolate. I neonati affetti dalla forma epatocerebrale si presentano con insufficienza epatica progressiva, anomalie neurologiche, ipoglicemia e acidosi lattica. Il decesso avviene di norma verso il primo anno di vita. È stata riportata la guarigione spontanea in un paziente con malattia esclusivamente epatica. L'ereditarietà è autosomica recessiva e in molti pazienti con MDS epatocerebrale sono state identificate mutazioni nel gene della **desossiguanosina chinasi** (**dGK**). Non è invece noto il difetto genetico specifico che dà luogo allla MDS epatica. La dGK è un gene nucleare il cui prodotto proteico fosforila la desossiguanosina a desossiguanosina monofosfato, confermando l'importanza dell'omeostasi del pool nucleotidico nella stabilità e nel mantenimento del mtDNA. Le biopsie epatiche dei pazienti con MDS mostrano steatosi microvescicolare, colestasi, necrosi citoplasmatica biliare focale, siderosi degli epatociti e delle cellule sinusoidali. Caratteristiche sono le alterazioni ultrastrutturali, tra cui trasformazione oncocitica dei mitocondri (che presentano creste sparse), matrice granulare e inclusioni dense o vescicolari. La **diagnosi** è confermata dalla dimostrazione di una basso rapporto tra mtDNA e DNA nucleare (<10%) nei tessuti colpiti e/o dall'analisi gentica. È importante sottolineare che la sequenza del genoma mitocondriale è normale.

NEUROEPATOPATIA NAVAJO (NNH, *NAVAJO NEUROHEPATOPATHY*). La NNH è una neuropatia sensitivo-motoria associata a epatopatia, trasmessa per via autosomica recessiva e riscontrata esclusivamente negli Indiani Navajo del Sudovest degli Stati Uniti. L'incidenza è di 1/1600 nati vivi. I criteri diagnostici sono stati definiti e comprendono: neuropatia sensitiva, neuropatia motoria, anestesia corneale, epatopatia, complicanze metaboliche o infettive (tra cui deficit di sviluppo, bassa statura, pubertà ritardata o infezioni sistemiche), evidenza di demielinizzazione del sistema nervoso centrale alle indagini radiologiche. La definizione di un caso richiede la positività di almeno quattro di questi criteri, oppure di tre in presenza di un fratello con diagnosi già accertata di NNH.

La NNH è stata divisa in tre varianti fenotipiche, in base all'età di presentazione e alle manifestazioni cliniche. Le diverse presentazioni sono state osservate anche all'interno della stessa famiglia. La **NNH classica** si presenta nell'infanzia con deterioramento neurologico grave e progressivo, le cui manifestazioni cliniche sono debolezza, ipotonia, perdita di sensibilità con associate mutilazioni delle estremità e ulcere corneali, crescita stentata. L'epatopatia, presente nella maggior parte dei pazienti, è secondaria e di gravità variabile, e può comportare aumento asintomatico degli enzimi epatici, episodi tipo sindrome di Reye, carcinoma epatocellulare, cirrosi. I livelli di γ-glutamil transpeptidasi (GGT) tendono a essere più elevati che nelle altre forme di NNH. La biopsia epatica può evidenziare infiammazione cronica dei tratti portali e cirrosi, mentre, rispetto alle altre forme di NNH, sono meno marcati la colestasi, la degenerazione balloniforme degli epatociti e la trasformazione gigantocellulare. La **NNH neonatale** si presenta in soggetti di 1-6 mesi di vita, con ittero e deficit di sviluppo, e progredisce fino all'insufficienza epatica e al decesso, verso i 2 anni di età. I pazienti hanno epatomegalia con un moderato aumento di AST, ALT e GGT. La biopsia epatica dimostra formazioni pseudoacinari, cellule giganti multinucleate, infiammazione portale e lobulare, colestasi canalicolare e steatosi microvescicolare. I sintomi neurologici progressivi non sono in genere evidenti alla presentazione, ma si sviluppano in seguito. La **NNH infantile** si presenta in soggetti di età compresa tra 1 e 5 anni, con l'insorgenza acuta di insufficienza epatica fulminante, che porta al decesso nell'arco di alcuni mesi. La maggior parte dei pazienti ha anche un'evidenza di neuropatia, al momento della presentazione. La biopsia epatica è simile a quella della NNH neonatale, tranne che per la possibile presenza di degenerazione balloniforme significativa, necrosi epatocitaria, proliferazione dei dotti biliari e cirrosi. La biopsia nervosa, in tutti i tipi, può rivelare una riduzione delle fibre nervose mieliniche di grande e piccolo calibro, oltre a degenerazione e rigenerazione delle fibre nervose non mieliniche. Non esiste un trattamento efficace per alcuna delle forme di NNH e i sintomi neurologici spesso impediscono di prendere in considerazione il trapianto epatico. Il difetto genetico alla base della malattia è sconosciuto, anche se sussiste il forte sospetto che l'origine vada ricercata a livello mitocondriale, a causa di alterazioni mitocondriali ultrastrutturali, degli elevati livelli di acido lattico sierico, dell'evidenza di deplezione mitocondriale e della ridotta attività di multipli enzimi della catena respiratoria.

EPATOPATIE MITOCONDRIALI SECONDARIE

Le epatopatie mitocondriali secondarie sono causate da metalli epatotossici, farmaci, tossine o metaboliti endogeni. In passato, la forma più frequente era la **sindrome di Reye**, la cui prevalenza registrò un picco negli anni '70, con una mortalità superiore al 40%. Anche se quest'ultima non è cambiata, la prevalenza si è ridotta da più di 500 casi nel 1980 a circa 35 casi/anno negli anni '90. In un individuo suscettibile geneticamente, è scatenata dall'interazione tra un'infezione virale (influenza, varicella) e l'uso di acido salicilico. Clinicamente, è preceduta da un'infezione virale che sembra in via di risoluzione, e dall'esordio acuto di vomito ed encefalopatia (Tab. 358-2). I sintomi neurologici possono rapidamente progredire fino alle convulsioni, al coma e alla morte. La disfunzione epatica è sempre presente quando compare il vomito, con coagulopatia ed elevati livelli di AST, ALT e ammoniaca. È importante notare che i pazienti restano anitterici e che i livelli di bilirubinemia sono normali. La biopsia epatica rivela steatosi microvescicolare, senza evidenza di infiammazione o necrosi epatica. Il decesso è in genere secondario all'ipertensione endocranica e alla conseguente erniazione. I pazienti che sopravvivono hanno una ripresa completa della funzione epatica, ma devono essere attentamente controllati per difetti dell'ossidazione e del trasporto degli acidi grassi (Tab. 358-3).

Le anomalie acquisite della funzione mitocondriale possono essere causate da numerosi farmaci e tossine, tra cui l'acido valproico, la cianide, l'amiodarone, il cloramfenicolo, il ferro, l'antimicina A, la tossina emetica del *Bacillus cereus* e gli analoghi nucleosidici. L'acido valproico è un acido grasso ramificato che può essere metabolizzato nella tossina mitocondriale acido 4-envalproico. I bambini con sottostanti difetti della catena respiratoria sembrano più sensibili agli effetti tossici di questo farmaco, che sembra inoltre poter precipitare l'insufficienza epatica nei pazienti con **sindrome di Alpers** e **deficit della citocromo-*c* ossidasi**. Gli analoghi nucleosidici inibiscono direttamente i complessi mitocondriali della catena respiratoria. La fialuridina, utilizzata nella terapia dell'epatite B, può causare un'acidosi lattica fatale con insufficienza epatica. Il meccanismo del danno mitocondriale comprende l'incorporazione diretta della fialuridina nel mtDNA, a sostituzione della timidina; questo fenomeno determina un'inibizione diretta della trascrizione del DNA, che a sua volta porta alla sindrome da deplezione acquisita del mtDNA. Gli inibitori della trascrittasi inversa zidovudina, didanosina, stavudina e zalcitabina, utilizzati nel trattamento dei pazienti con HIV, inibiscono la DNA polimerasi-γ dei mitocondri e possono bloccare l'allungamento del mtDNA, causando deplezione del mtDNA. Altre condizioni che possono portare a stress ossidativo mitocondriale comprendono la colestasi, la steatoepatite non alcolica, il deficit di α_1-antitripsina e la malattia di Wilson.

Nella maggior parte dei casi, non esiste una terapia efficace delle epatopatie mitocondriali; il danno neurologico spesso impedisce di procedere a un trapianto epatico ortotopico. Sono state proposte diverse associazioni farmacologiche, tra cui antiossidanti, vitamine, cofattori e accettori degli elettroni, tutti farmaci su cui tuttavia non è stato compiuto alcuno studio randomizzato controllato. Pertanto, le attuali strategie di trattamento sono solo di supporto.

TABELLA 358-2. Stadiazione clinica della sindrome di Reye

SINTOMI AL MOMENTO DEL RICOVERO	
I.	Paziente tranquillo, letargico, sonnolento, evidenza di disfunzione epatica agli esami di laboratorio
II.	Letargia profonda, confusione, delirio, combattività, iperventilazione, iperreflessia
III.	Ottundimento, coma lieve, con o senza convulsioni, rigidità decerebrata, reazione pupillare alla luce conservata
IV.	Convulsioni, coma più profondo, rigidità decerebrata, perdita dei riflessi oculocefalici, pupille fisse
V.	Coma, perdita dei riflessi tendinei profondi, arresto respiratorio, pupille fisse dilatate, flaccidità/posizione decerebrata (intermittente); elettroencefalogramma isoelettrico

TABELLA 358-3. Malattie che presentano un quadro clinico e anatomopatologico simile a quello della sindrome di Reye

Malattie metaboliche
- Aciduria organica
- Alterazioni della fosforilazione ossidativa
- Difetti del ciclo dell'urea (carbamol fosfato sintetasi, ornitina transcarbamilasi)
- Difetti del metabolismo ossidativo degli acidi grassi
- Deficit di Acyl-CoA deidrogenasi
- Deficit sistemico di carnitina
- Deficit di carnitina palmitoiltransferasi
- Deficit di 3-OH, 3-metilglutaril-CoA liasi
- Fruttosemia

Infezioni o intossicazioni del sistema nervoso centrale (meningiti), encefaliti, encefalopatia tossica

Shock emorragico con encefalopatia

Ingestione di farmaci o tossici (valproato, salicilato)

CoA, coenzima A.

Belay E, Bresee JS, Holman RC, et al: Reye's syndrome in the United States from 1981 through 1997. *N Engl J Med* 1999;340:1377–1382.

Bougneres PF, Rocchiccioli F, Koluraa S, et al: Medium-chain acyl-CoA dehydrogenase deficiency in two siblings with a Reye-like syndrome. *J Pediatr* 1985;106:918–921.

Casteels-Van Daele M, Van Geet C, Wounter C, et al: Reyes syndrome revisited: A descriptive term covering a group of heterogeneous disorders. *Eur J Pediatr* 2000;159:641–648.

Ducluzeau PH, Lachaux A, Bouvier R, et al: Progressive reversion of clinical and molecular phenotype in a child with liver mitochondrial DNA depletion. *J Hepatol* 2002:36:698–703.

Gillis LA, Sokol RJ: Gastrointestinal manifestations of mitochondrial disease. *Gastroenterol Clin North Am* 2003;32:789–817.

Holve S, Hu D, Shub M, et al: Liver disease in Navajo neuropathy. *J Pediatr* 1999;135:482–493.

Mancuso M, Filosto M, Tsujino S, et al: Muscle glycogenosis and mitochondrial hepatopathy in an infant with mutations in both the myophosphorylase and deoxyguanosine kinase genes. *Arch Neurol* 2003;60:1445–1447.

Rabinowitz SS, Gelfond D, Chen CK, et al: Hepatocerebral mitochondrial DNA depletion syndrome: Clinical and morphologic features of a nuclear gene mutation. *J Pediatr Gastroenterol Nutr* 2004;38:216–220.

Teitelbaum JE, Berde CB, Nurko C, et al: Diagnosis and management of MNGIE syndrome in children: Case report and review of the literature. *J Pediatr Gastroenterol Nutr* 2002;35:377–383.

Capitolo 359 ■ Epatiti croniche e autoimmuni Benjamin L. Shneider e Frederick J. Suchy

L'epatite autoimmune è un processo infiammatorio cronico a carico del fegato, che si manifesta con ipertransaminasemia, ipergammaglobulinemia e presenza di autoanticorpi sierici associati al fegato. I bersagli del processo infiammatorio possono essere sia gli epatociti, sia l'epitelio dei dotti biliari. La cronicità è determinata dalla durata dell'epatopatia (tipicamente superiore a 3-6 mesi), oppure dall'evidenza di danno epatico severo o di segni clinici di epatopatia cronica (ippocratismo digitale, teleangectasie aracniformi, epatosplenomegalia). La gravità è variabile: i bambini affetti possono avere solo un'evidenza biochimica di disfunzione epatica, oppure segni di danno epatico cronico o anche presentarsi già con insufficienza epatica.

Un'**epatite cronica** può anche essere causata da infezioni virali persistenti (vedi Capitolo 355), farmaci (vedi Capitolo 360), malattie metaboliche (vedi Capitolo 358) o fattori sconosciuti (Tab. 359-1). Circa il 15-20% dei casi è associato a infezione da epatite B; talvolta, una patologia particolarmente severa può essere causata dalla sovrainfezione da epatite D (un virus a RNA difettivo, che dipende dalla replicazione del virus dell'epatite B [HBV, *Hepatitis B Virus*]). Più del 90% delle infezioni da epatite B, acquisite nel primo anno di vita, vanno incontro a cronicizzazione, contro il 5-10% di quelle acquisite in età infantile più avanzata o adulta. L'epatite cronica si sviluppa in più del 50% delle infezioni acute da virus dell'epatite C. I pazienti che ricevono derivati ematici o che hanno subito trasfusioni massive corrono un rischio maggiore. I virus dell'epatite A ed E non causano epatite cronica. I **farmaci** usati comunemente nei bambini, che possono determinare un danno epatico cronico, comprendono isoniazide, metildopa, pemolina, nitrofurantoina, dantrolene, minociclina e sulfonamidi. Le **malattie metaboliche** che possono portare a epatite cronica sono, in particolare, il deficit di α_1-antitripsina, gli errori congeniti della biosintesi degli acidi biliari e la malattia di Wilson. La **steatoepatite**, in genere associata a obesità e insulinoresistenza, è un'altra frequente causa di epatite cronica; è relativamente benigna e risponde al calo ponderale e/o alla terapia con vitamina E. Negli adulti è stata descritta la progressione a cirrosi. Nella maggior parte dei casi, la causa dell'epatite cronica è sconosciuta; spesso un meccanismo autoimmune è suggerito dal riscontro di anticorpi antinucleo e anti-muscolo liscio e dal coinvolgimento multisistemico (artropatia, tiroidite, eruzioni cutanee, anemia emolitica Coombs-positiva).

I reperti istologici aiutano a caratterizzare le epatiti croniche. La suddivisione in forme persistenti e attive, sulla base delle caratteristiche istologiche, non è utile come si riteneva in passato. Il reperto di un'infiammazione contenuta entro la lamina limitante del tratto portale (epatite cronica persistente) e l'assenza di fibrosi/cirrosi suggeriscono un decorso più benigno. Il riscontro di attività istologica può essere predittivo di risposta alla terapia antivirale, se è presente un'infezione da virus B, ed è un criterio utilizzato nella diagnosi di epatite autoimmune. Le caratteristiche istologiche aiutano a identificare l'eziologia: nel deficit di α_1-antitripsina si osservano granuli caratteristici PAS-positivi, diastasi-resistenti, mentre l'accumulo di grasso neutro sia macrovescicolare, sia microvescicolare, all'interno degli epatociti, è una caratteristica della steatoepatite. Un danno a carico dei dotti biliari può far pensare a una colangiopatia autoimmune. L'analisi ultrastrutturale può suggerire tipi distinti di malattie da accumulo.

L'**epatite autoimmune** è una costellazione clinica che suggerisce un processo immunomediato; è responsiva alla terapia immunosoppressiva (Tab. 359-2). L'epatite autoimmune si riferisce tipicamente a un processo primitivo specifico degli epatociti, mentre la colangiopatia autoimmune e la colangite sclerosante sono caratterizzate da un danno prevalentemente a carico dei dotti biliari intra- ed extraepatici. Nei bambini è frequente la sovrapposizione di processi che coinvolgono sia il danno agli epatociti, sia quello diretto verso i dotti biliari. Un'epatite de novo è osservabile in una minoranza di pazienti sottoposti a trapianto epatico, la cui epatopatia di base non era di tipo autoimmune.

EZIOLOGIA. L'epatite autoimmune, la cui causa è sconosciuta, viene ritenuta il risultato di uno squilibrio tra l'attività dei linfociti CD4 e CD8; anche se è probabile che la predisposizione genetica giochi un ruolo importante nello sviluppo della malattia, l'evento scatenante potrebbe essere un'infezione virale o l'assunzione di farmaci tossici.

ANATOMIA PATOLOGICA. Le caratteristiche istologiche comuni dei casi non sottoposti a trattamento comprendono: (1) infiltrato infiammatorio, formato da linfociti e plamacellule che espandono le aree portali e spesso penetrano nel lobulo; (2) necrosi parcellare (*piecemeal necrosis*) degli epatociti moderata o severa, che si estende oltre la lamina limitante; (3) vari gradi di necrosi, fibrosi e zone di collasso parenchimale, che collegano triadi portali adiacenti, o una triade portale con la vena centrale (necrosi a ponte); (4) danno a carico dell'epitelio duttale di grado varia-

TABELLA 359-1. Malattie che causano epatite cronica

EPATITE VIRALI CRONICHE
Epatite B
Epatite C
Epatite D
EPATITI AUTOIMMUNI
Posività degli anticorpi antiactina
Positività degli anticorpi anti-microsoma epatico-renale (LKM)
Positività degli anticorpi anti-antigene solubile epatico
Altre (compresi anticorpi anti-lipoproteine epatospecifiche o asialoglicoproteina)
Sindrome da sovrapposizione con colangite sclerosante e autoanticorpi
Lupus eritematoso sistemico
Celiachia
EPATITI DA FARMACI
MALATTIE METABOLICHE ASSOCIATE A EPATOPATIA CRONICA
Malattia di Wilson
Deficit di α_1-antitripsina
Tirosinemia
Malattia di Niemann-Pick di tipo 2
Glicogenosi di tipo IV
Fibrosi cistica
Galattosemia
ANOMALIE DELLA BIOSINTESI DEGLI ACIDI BILIARI

TABELLA 359-2. Classificazione delle epatiti autoimmuni

VARIABILE	EPATITE AUTOIMMUNE DI TIPO 1	EPATITE AUTOIMMUNE DI TIPO 2
Autoanticorpi caratteristici	Anticorpi antinucleo* Anticorpi anti-muscolo liscio* Anticorpi antiactina† Anticorpi anti-antigene solubile epatico e anti-antigene epatopancreatico‡ Anticorpi atipici perinucleari anti-citoplasma dei neutrofili	Anticorpi anti-microsoma epatico-renale 1* Anticorpi anti-citoplasma epatico 1*
Distribuzione geografica	Ubiquitaria	Ubiquitaria; rara nel Nord America
Età di presentazione	Qualsiasi età	Prevalentemente infanzia e adolescenza
Sesso	Femminile nel 75% dei casi	Femminile nel 95% dei casi
Associazione con altre patologie autoimmuni	Comune	Comune§
Severità clinica	Ampia variabilità	Generalmente severa
Caratteristiche istopatologiche	Ampia variabilità	Generalmente severa alla presentazione
Fallimento terapeutico	Raro	Frequente
Recidiva dopo la sospensione dei farmaci	Variabile	Comune
Necessità di mantenimento a lungo termine	Variabile	Circa 100%

*Il metodo migliore per la rilevazione è l'immunofluorescenza.
†I test per questi autoanticorpi sono raramente disponibili nei laboratori.
‡Questi autoanticorpi sono rilevati tramite ELISA (*Enzyme-Linked Immunosorbent Assay*).
§La poliendocrinopatia-candidosi-distrofia ectodermica autoimmune si osserva solo nei pazienti con malattia di tipo 2.
Da Krawitt EL: Autoimmune hepatitis. *N Engl J Med* 2006;354:54-66.

bile. La distorsione dell'architettura epatica può essere marcata; al momento della diagnosi, nei bambini, può anche essersi già instaurata una cirrosi. Le caratteristiche istologiche, nei casi di insufficienza epatica acuta, sono talora mascherate dalla necrosi massiva.

MANIFESTAZIONI CLINICHE. Le caratteristiche e il decorso clinico dell'epatite autoimmune sono estremamante variabili. I segni e i sintomi al momento della presentazione comprendono un ampio spettro di manifestazioni, tra cui un considerevole numero di presentazioni asintomatiche e alcune a esordio acuto o addirittura fulminante. Nel 25-30% dei pazienti con epatite autoimmune, in particolare nei bambini, la malattia mima un'epatite virale acuta. Nella maggior parte dei casi l'esordio è insidioso. I pazienti possono essere asintomatici o accusare astenia, malessere, alterazioni comportamentali, anoressia e amenorrea, talora per molti mesi, prima che siano riconoscibili l'ittero o altri segni di epatopatia cronica. Le manifestazioni extraepatiche possono comprendere artriti, vasculiti, nefriti, tiroiditi, anemia emolitica Coombs-positiva e rash cutanei. In alcuni pazienti le manifestazioni cliniche iniziali rispecchiano la presenza di cirrosi epatica (ascite, sanguinamento da varici esofagee, encefalopatia epatica).

In genere è presente ittero da lieve a moderato, talora associato a teleangectasie aracniformi ed eritema palmare. Il fegato è spesso dolorabile e lievemente aumentato di volume, ma può anche non essere palpabile, nei pazienti con cirrosi. Nei casi più avanzati si possono riscontrare edemi periferici e ascite, come pure segni di coinvolgimento di altri sistemi e organi.

DATI DI LABORATORIO. I reperti sono correlati con la gravità della presentazione. In molti casi asintomatici le transaminasi sono a livelli compresi tra 100 e 300 UI/L, mentre nei pazienti giovani sintomatici si possono trovare livelli superiori a 1000 UI/L. La concentrazione di bilirubina (soprattutto la frazione diretta) è generalmente di 2-10 mg/dL. L'attività della fosfatasi alcalina (ALP, *ALkaline Phosphatase*) e della γ-glutamil transpeptidasi (GGT) è normale o appena aumentata, ma può andare incontro a maggiori alterazioni nella colangiopatia autoimmune. L'ipoalbuminemia è frequente. Il tempo di protrombina è aumentato, spesso in conseguenza del deficit di vitamina K, ma anche a causa dell'alterata funzione epatocellulare. Sono di frequente riscontro un'anemia normocromica, normocitica, leucopenia e trombocitopenia, che si aggravano con lo sviluppo di ipertensione portale e ipersplenismo.

La maggior parte dei pazienti presenta ipergammaglobulinemia. I livelli di immunoglobuline (Ig) G sono in genere >16 mg/L. Si riconoscono diversi sottogruppi di epatite autoimmune, in base a pattern caratteristici di **autoanticorpi** (vedi Tab. 359-2). Nel quadro più comune si ha la generazione di anticorpi non organo-specifici, come gli anticorpi antiactina (muscolo liscio), antinucleo e antimitocondrio. Circa il 50% di questi pazienti ha un'età compresa tra i 10 e i 20 anni. Elevati livelli di anticorpi anti-microsoma fegato-rene (LKM, *Liver-Kidney Microsome*) sono caratteristici di un'altra forma che colpisce normalmente i bambini da 2 a 14 anni di età. Un sottogruppo costituito prevalentemente da giovani donne può presentare autoanticorpi contro un antigene solubile epatico (SLA, *Soluble Liver Antigen*), ma non contro proteine nucleari o microsomiali. Gli anticorpi anticitoplasma dei neutrofili sono di più frequente riscontro nella colangiopatia autoimmune. Gli autoanticorpi sono rari nei bambini sani, pertanto anche titoli bassi, come di 1:40, devono essere considerati significativi. Fino al 20% dei pazienti con apparente epatite autoimmune può non avere autoanticorpi all'esordio. Gli anticorpi contro il citocromo P450, componente degli LKM, sono frequenti negli adulti con epatite cronica C, probabilmente a causa di omologie tra epitopi peptidici antigenici del virus dell'epatite C e del citocromo P450. Altri autoanticorpi meno comuni sono il fattore reumatoide, anticorpi anticellule parietali, anticorpi antitiroide. Può essere presente un'anemia emolitica Coombs-positiva.

DIAGNOSI. La diagnosi dell'epatite autoimmune è prevalentemente clinica e si basa su determinati criteri diagnostici; non esiste un test che possa porre diagnosi isolatamente. Negli adulti sono stati sviluppati criteri diagnostici basati su un punteggio, che, con alcune modifiche, sono stati utilizzati anche nei bambini. Le caratteristiche positive principali comprendono il sesso femminile, un aumento primitivo delle transaminasi e non dell'ALP, elevati livelli di gammaglobuline, presenza di autoanticorpi (più spesso antinucleo, anti-muscolo liscio o anti-LKM) e reperti istologici tipici (Fig. 359-1). Le caratteristiche negative principali consistono in assenza di marcatori virali (epatite B, C, D), assenza di pregressa tossicodipendenza o trasfusione di derivati ematici in anamnesi e consumo trascurabile di alcol.

È necessario escludere qualsiasi altra condizione che possa causare un'epatite cronica (vedi Tab. 359-1). La diagnosi differenziale comprende il deficit di α_1-antitripsina (vedi Capitolo 354) e la malattia di Wilson (vedi Capitolo 354.2). La prima patologia deve essere esclusa tramite la determinazione del fenotipo α_1-antitripsina, la seconda con la misurazione della ceruloplasminemia, dell'escrezione urinaria di rame nelle 24 ore e dei livelli epatici di rame. L'epatite cronica può anche complicare le malattie infiammatorie intestinali, ma la disfunzione epatica, in questi pazienti, è causata per lo più da una pericolangite o da una colangite sclerosante. La celiachia (vedi Capitolo 335.2) si associa a un'epatopatia simile all'epatite autoimmune, e dovrebbero essere effettuati i test sierologici appropriati, tra cui il test per la transglutaminasi tissutale. Si rende inoltre necessaria un'ecografia epatica per identificare eventuali cisti del coledoco o altre alterazioni strutturali delle vie biliari. La colangiorisonanza magnetica può essere molto utile per individuare una colangite sclerosante. La presenza di vene epatiche dilatate o obliterate all'ecografia suggerisce una possibile sindrome di Budd-Chiari.

TRATTAMENTO. Il prednisone, associato o meno ad azatioprina o 6-mercaptopurina, migliora le caratteristiche cliniche, biochimiche e istologiche nella maggior parte dei pazienti con epatite autoimmune, e prolunga la sopravvivenza nella maggior parte dei pazienti con malattia grave. Gli agenti coleretici come l'acido ursodesossicolico possono essere particolarmente utili nei soggetti con danno a impronta biliare.

Obiettivo del trattamento è arrestare o eliminare l'infiammazione epatica, riducendo al tempo stesso gli effetti collaterali. La somministrazione di prednisone, alla dose iniziale di 1-2 mg/kg/die, prosegue finché i valori di transaminasi non tornano a meno

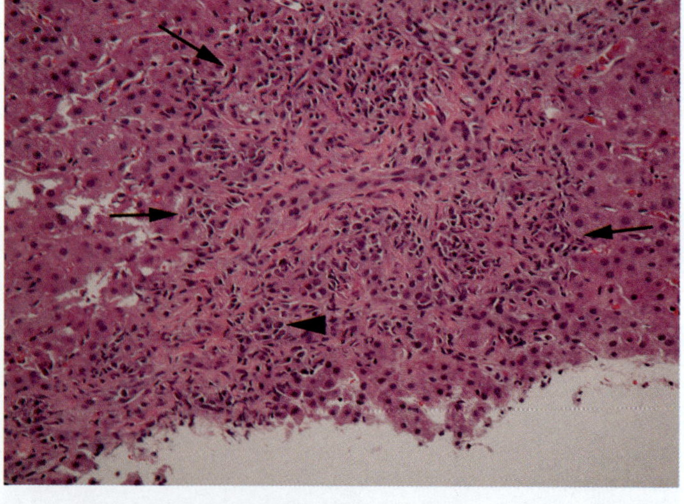

Figura 359-1. Epatite autoimmune. Biopsia epatica che mostra l'espansione fibrosa dei tratti portali con modesti infiltrati linfociti portali, ricchi di plasmacellule (punta di freccia). È presente un'estesa epatite dell'interfaccia (frecce). Ingrandimento originale 20×. (Per gentile concessione di Margret Magid, Mount Sinai School of Medicine.)

del doppio del limite superiore della norma. In seguito occorre ridurre la dose scalando di 5 mg per volta, nel corso 2-4 mesi, fino a raggiungere una dose di mantenimento di 0,1-0,3 mg/kg/die. Nei pazienti con scarsa risposta al prednisone, che accusano effetti collaterali severi o che non possono essere mantenuti in terapia con basse dosi di steroidi, si può aggiungere azatioprina (1,5-2-0 mg/kg/die, fino a 100 mg/die), con un monitoraggio frequente della funzione midollare. Il controllo dei metaboliti dell'azatioprina può essere utile per adattare la terapia al singolo paziente. La monoterapia con steroidi a giorni alterni deve essere utilizzata con cautela, sebbene associata all'azatioprina possa rivelarsi una strategia efficace per ridurre al minimo la tossicità da steroidi. Per i pazienti con presentazione lieve o asintomatica, alcuni Autori prediligono una dose iniziale di prednisone più bassa (10-20 mg) associata alla precoce somministrazione contemporanea di 6-mercaptopurina (1,0-1,5 mg/kg/die) o azatioprina (1,5-2,0 mg/kg/die). Alcuni studi aneddotici hanno dimostrato le potenzialità di ciclosporina, tacrolimus, micofenolato mofetile e sirolimus nel trattamento dei casi resistenti alla terapia convenzionale. La prescrizione di questi farmaci deve essere riservata a specialisti con notevole esperienza, a causa del basso rapporto tra dose terapeutica e dose tossica.

Il miglioramento istologico non necessita di una valutazione con biopsie seriate, sebbene la remissione biochimica non garantisca la risoluzione anche istologica. La biopsia epatica di follow-up è pertanto importante in quei pazienti in cui si ipotizza di sospendere la terapia steroidea. In caso di scomparsa dei sintomi e delle alterazioni biochimiche e risoluzione del processo necroinfiammatorio alla biopsia, è giustificato tentare una sospensione graduale del farmaco. La recidiva può richiedere il ripristino di una terapia immunosoppressiva ad alte dosi per controllare la malattia.

La terapia per l'epatite virale cronica differisce da quella per le patologie a eziologia autoimmune (vedi anche Capitolo 355). L'**epatite cronica B** è caratterizzata da livelli persistentemente elevati di HBV-DNA e dalla presenza dell'antigene di superficie dell'epatite B (HBsAg), con o senza antigene e dell'epatite B (HBeAg). Inoltre, si registra un costante aumento dei livelli di transaminasi, con evidenza istologica di un'epatite cronica. La terapia con interferone α (5-10 MU/m^2 di superficie corporea, sottocute, tre volte/settimana), per 4-6 mesi, induce la sieroconversione (ossia la conversione da HBeAg-positività ad antiHBe-positività) nel 25-40% dei bambini. Molto efficaci sono pure le preparazioni a base di interferone pegilato α2b, che prolungano l'emivita del farmaco, consentendo la somministrazione settimanale e il mantenimento di livelli ematici più costanti. Si ritiene che la sieroconversione si associ a una riduzione del rischio a lungo termine di sviluppare cirrosi epatica e/o carcinoma epatocellulare. Gli effetti collaterali dell'interferone α comprendono episodi simil-influenzali con coinvolgimento sistemico, alterazioni comportamentali e cognitive, sviluppo di autoanticorpi e aumentata suscettibilità alle infezioni batteriche. La lamivudina, un analogo nucleosidico orale che inibisce la DNA polimerasi, è meno tossica ed efficace nel rallentare la progressione della malattia, negli adulti.

L'**epatite cronica C** è caratterizzata dalla presenza di HCV-RNA nel sangue. Sono stati descritti anche nei bambini casi di progressione a insufficienza epatica terminale, e, pertanto, la presenza di transaminasi cronicamente elevate associate all'evidenza istologica di attività può rappresentare un'indicazione al trattamento. La terapia comprende la combinazione di interferone α (3 MU/m^2 di superficie corporea, sottocute, tre volte/settimana) e ribavirina (15 mg/kg divisi in due somministrazioni/die) per una durata di 6 mesi (genotipi 2 e 3) o 12 mesi (genotipo 1). L'eliminazione a lungo termine del virus è ottenuta nel 40-50% dei bambini trattati, con una risposta virologica sostenuta dell'80-90% nei soggetti con genotipo 2 e 3. L'utilizzo di interferone pegilato in età infantile è ancora in fase di studio.

PROGNOSI. Nell'epatite autoimmune, la risposta iniziale alla terapia è in genere rapida, con un tasso di remissione >75%. Le transaminasi e la bilirubina si riducono a livelli pressoché normali, spesso entro i primi 3 mesi. Se presenti, le alterazioni dei livelli di albumina e del tempo di protrombina rispondono in un periodo più lungo (3-9 mesi). Metà dei pazienti che rispondono ai criteri per la diminuzione e quindi la sospensione del trattamento (25-40% dei bambini) non necessita più di farmaci, mentre l'altra metà recidiva dopo un periodo variabile. Le recidive rispondono normalmente al ritrattamento. Molti bambini non raggiungono i criteri richiesti per un tentativo di interruzione della terapia immunosoppressiva e devono proseguire la terapia con la minima dose di prednisone in grado di ridurre l'attività biochimica della malattia. È necessario valutare continuamente il rapporto rischio-beneficio della terapia immunosoppressiva continuata e i rischi connessi alla progressione dell'epatite, facendo attenzione alle eventuali complicanze della terapia medica (mediante esame oculistico, misurazione della densità ossea, monitoraggio della pressione arteriosa). Eventuali riacutizzazioni intermittenti dell'epatite possono richiedere la ripetizione di cicli di terapia steroidea. Alcuni bambini hanno una forma di epatite relativamente steroidoresistente; in questi casi è necessaria una valutazione approfondita dell'eziologia del danno epatico, in particolare per escludere la presenza di una colangite sclerosante o della malattia di Wilson. La terapia corticosteroidea, nell'epatite autoimmune fulminante, può essere utile ma deve essere somministrata con cautela, per la vulnerabilità di questi pazienti alle infezioni sistemiche batteriche o fungine.

Il trapianto epatico ortotopico è stato praticato con successo nei pazienti con epatopatia terminale associata a epatite autoimmune (vedi Capitolo 365), sebbene la malattia possa recidivare. Le indicazioni all'intervento devono comprendere la presenza di scompenso epatico.

Alvarez F, Berg PA, Bianchi FB, et al: International Autoimmune Hepatitis Group Report: Review of criteria for diagnosis of autoimmune hepatitis. *J Hepatol* 1999;31:929–938.

Andries S, Casamayou L, Sempoux C, et al: Posttransplant immune hepatitis in pediatric liver transplant recipients: Incidence and maintenance therapy with azathioprine. *Transplantation* 2001;72:267–272.

Bahar R, Yanni G, Martin M, et al: Orthotopic liver transplantation for autoimmune hepatitis and cryptogenic cirrhosis in children. *Transplantation* 2001;72:829–833.

Carrat F, Bani-Sadr F, Pol S, et al: Pegylated interferon alfa-2b vs standard interferon alfa-2b, plus ribavirin, for chronic hepatitis C in HIV-infected patients. *JAMA* 2004;292:2839–2848.

Czaja AJ, Bianchi FB, Carpenter HA, et al: Treatment challenges and investigational opportunities in autoimmune hepatitis. *Hepatology* 2005;41:207–215.

Ebbeson RL, Schreiber RA: Diagnosing autoimmune hepatitis in children: Is the International Autoimmune Hepatitis Group Scoring System useful? *Clin Gastroenterol Hepatol* 2004;10:935–940.

Gregorio GV, Portmann B, Reid F, et al: Autoimmune sclerosing cholangitis overlap syndrome in childhood: A 16 year prospective study. *Hepatology* 2001;33:544–553.

Janssen HLA, van Zonneveld M, Senturk H, et al: Pegylated interferon alfa-2b alone or in combination with lamivudine for HBeAg-positive chronic hepatitis B: A randomised trial. *Lancet* 2005;365:123–128.

Krawitt EL: Autoimmune hepatitis. *N Engl J Med* 2006;354:54–66.

Oettinger R, Brunnberg A, Gerner P, et al: Clinical features and biochemical data of Caucasian children at diagnosis of autoimmune hepatitis. *J Autoimmun* 2005;24:79–84.

Rumbo C, Emerick KM, Emre S, et al: Azathioprine metabolite measurements in the treatment of autoimmune hepatitis in pediatric patients: A preliminary report. *J Pediatr Gastroenterol Nutr* 2002;35:391–398.

Sokal E, Conjeevaram H, Roberts E, et al: Interferon alfa therapy for chronic hepatitis B in children: A multinational randomized controlled trial. *Gastroenterology* 1998;114:988–995.

Squires RH: Autoimmune hepatitis in children. *Curr Gastroenterol Rep* 2004;6:225–230.

Wen L, Ma Y, Bogdanos DP, et al: Pediatric autoimmune liver diseases: The molecular basis of humoral and cellular immunity. *Curr Mol Med* 2001;3:379–389.

Capitolo 360 ■ Danno epatico da farmaci e tossine Frederick J. Suchy

Il fegato rappresenta la sede principale del metabolismo degli xenobiotici e pertanto è particolarmente suscettibile al danno strutturale e funzionale che deriva dall'ingestione, dalla somministrazione parenterale o dall'inalazione di agenti chimici, farmaci, derivati fitoterapici (cure fai-da-te), tossine ambientali. In tutti i bambini con disfunzione epatica si deve sempre prendere in esame la possibilità di un'esposizione a farmaci, tossine o sostanze d'abuso, a casa o sul posto di lavoro dei genitori. Lo spettro clinico della malattia può variare da anomalie biochimiche asintomatiche della funzione epatica all'insufficienza epatica fulminante. Il danno epatico può essere l'unica manifestazione clinica di una reazione avversa a un farmaco oppure associarsi a manifestazioni sistemiche di danno multiorgano.

Il metabolismo epatico dei farmaci e delle tossine è mediato da una sequenza di reazioni enzimatiche le quali, per la maggior parte, trasformano molecole lipofile, poco solubili, in composti meno tossici, idrosolubili, che possono essere facilmente escreti nelle urine o nella bile. Le dimensioni relative del fegato, il flusso ematico a livello epatico e l'entità del legame alle proteine sono tutti fattori che influiscono sul metabolismo degli xenobiotici. La fase 1 del processo prevede l'attivazione enzimatica del substrato in composti intermedi reattivi, contenenti un gruppo carbossilico, epossidico o idrossilico. Gli enzimi coinvolti in questo processo sono mono-ossigenasi a funzione mista, la citocromo-*c* riduttasi, varie idrolasi e il sistema del citocromo P450 (CYP). L'induzione aspecifica di queste vie enzimatiche, osservabile in corso di infezioni virali intercorrenti, durante un digiuno prolungato o con la somministrazione di alcune classi di farmaci come gli anticonvulsivanti, può alterare il metabolismo degli xenobiotici, aumentandone il potenziale epatotossico. Un singolo agente può essere metabolizzato da più di una reazione biochimica. I composti intermedi reattivi, potenzialmente tossici per le cellule, sono coniugati enzimaticamente, nelle reazioni di fase 2, con acido glucuronico, solfato, acetato, glicina o glutatione. Alcuni farmaci possono essere metabolizzati direttamente tramite queste reazioni di coniugazione, senza subire l'attivazione della fase 1. La fase 3 è l'escrezione attiva, energia-dipendente, dei metaboliti dei farmaci e dei loro coniugati, grazie a un sistema di trasportatori di membrana, come la proteina di resistenza multipla ai farmaci 1 (MDR-1, *Multiple Drug Resistant Protein*).

I percorsi di biotrasformazione sono espressi precocemente nel feto e nel neonato, ma molti enzimi della fase 1 e 2 sono immaturi, in particolare nel primo anno di vita. Il CYP3A4, il principale CYP epatico espresso in epoca postnatale, metabolizza più di 75 farmaci di uso comune, oltre a diversi inquinanti e agenti cancerogeni ambientali. L'attività del CYP3A4 epatico è scarsa nel feto, ma aumenta dopo la nascita, fino a raggiungere il 30% dei valori adulti nel primo mese, e il 50% dei valori adulti tra il 6° e il 12° mese. Il CYP3A4 può essere indotto da numerosi farmaci, tra cui fenitoina, fenobarbital e rifampicina. Un'aumentata produzione di metaboliti tossici può superare la capacità delle reazioni di fase 2. All'inverso, numerosi inibitori del CYP3A4, di diverse classi farmacologiche, come l'eritromicina e la cimetidina, possono portare ad accumuli tossici di substrati del CYP3A4. Per contro, il CYP2D6, pur essendo anch'esso regolato dallo sviluppo (raggiunge la maturazione verso i 10 anni di età), presenta un'attività che dipende più dai polimorfismi genetici che dalla sensibilità a sostanze inducenti o inibenti, poiché le sue oltre 70 varianti alleliche influenzano significativamente il metabolismo di molti farmaci. L'UDP-glucuronosiltransferasi 1A6, un enzima di glucuronazione di fase 2 che metabolizza il paracetamolo, è assente nel feto, è scarso nel neonato e raggiunge i livelli adulti solo verso i 10 anni di età. I meccanismi di captazione ed escrezione degli ioni organici possono anche essere ipoattivi, in epoca neonatale. All'alterato metabolismo dei farmaci, tramite le reazioni di fase 1 e 2, caratteristico dei primi mesi di vita, fa seguito un periodo di aumentato metabolismo di molti farmaci, nei bambini fino a 10 anni, rispetto agli adulti.

I polimorfismi genetici degli enzimi e dei trasportatori delle reazioni di fase 1, 2 e 3 possono associarsi anche ad alterato metabolismo degli xenobiotici, con aumento del rischio di epatotossicità. Alcuni casi di epatotossicità idiosincrasica possono insorgere in conseguenza di aberrazioni (polimorfismi) del metabolismo di fase 1, che causano prodotti intermedi a elevato potenziale epatotossico, in combinazione con un'inefficacia di sviluppo, acquisita o relativa delle reazioni di coniugazione di fase 2. I bambini possono essere più o meno suscettibili degli adulti alle reazioni epatotossiche; il danno epatico conseguente all'uso dell'anestetico alotano è raro nell'infanzia, così come la tossicità da paracetamolo è meno frequente che negli adolescenti, sebbene la maggior parte dei casi di epatotossicità fatale da acido valproico sia stata descritta proprio nei bambini. Una somministrazione eccessiva o prolungata di paracetamolo, combinata con una riduzione dell'apporto calorico o proteico, può tuttavia causare epatotossicità anche nei bambini. In questi casi, il metabolismo del farmaco può risultare alterato a causa della ridotta sintesi di metaboliti solfati o glucuronati e delle scarse riserve di glutatione. L'immaturità delle vie metaboliche epatiche può impedire la degradazione di un agente tossico; in altre circostanze, la stessa immaturità può limitare la formazione di metaboliti tossici.

L'epatotossicità chimica può essere (1) prevedibile o (2) idiosincrasica. L'epatotossicità prevedibile implica un'elevata incidenza di danno epatico negli individui esposti, con un meccanismo dose-dipendente. È comprensibile che solo pochi farmaci di uso clinico rientrino in questa categoria. Questi agenti, tra cui il tetracloruro di carbonio e il tricloroetilene, possono danneggiare l'epatocita direttamente, alterando i lipidi di membrana (perossidazione) o denaturando le proteine. Il danno indiretto può essere dovuto all'interferenza con vie metaboliche essenziali per l'integrità cellulare o alla distorsione di costituenti cellulari, tramite il legame covalente di metaboliti reattivi; ne sono responsabili, per esempio, il paracetamolo o antimetaboliti come il metotrexato e la 6-mercaptopurina.

L'epatotossicità idiosincrasica, rara e imprevedibile, è responsabile della maggior parte delle reazioni avverse. Il danno non è dose-dipendente e può verificarsi in qualsiasi momento durante l'esposizione alla sostanza. Le reazioni idiosincrasiche ai farmaci, in alcuni pazienti, possono riflettere aberrazioni delle vie metaboliche dei farmaci, talora legate a polimorfismi genetici, che portano alla produzione di intermedi tossici (l'isoniazide e il sodio valproato possono causare danno epatico con questo meccanismo). La durata dell'uso del farmaco, prima che si manifesti il danno epatico, è variabile (da alcune settimane a più di un anno) e la risposta alla riesposizione può essere ritardata.

Una reazione idiosincrasica può anche essere mediata da meccanismi immunologici, in conseguenza di una precedente sensibilizzazione (ipersensibilità); le manifestazioni extraepatiche di ipersensibilità possono comprendere febbre, rash cutanei, artralgia ed eosinofilia. La durata dell'esposizione prima della reazione è generalmente di 1-4 settimane, con una rapida recidiva del danno in caso di riesposizione. Gli studi indicano che gli ossidi arenici, prodotti dal metabolismo ossidativo (tramite il citocromo P450) degli anticonvulsivanti aromatici (fenitoina, fenobarbital, carbamazepina), possono scatenare la patogenesi di alcune reazioni da ipersensibilità. Gli ossidi arenici, formatisi *in vivo*, possono legarsi a macromolecole cellulari, perturbando la funzione cellulare e dando inizio al meccanismo immunologico del danno epatico.

L'attivazione delle cellule epatiche non parenchimali di Kupffer e l'infiltrato neutrofilo perpetuano il danno tossico indotto da molti farmaci, tramite il rilascio sia di specie reattive dell'ossigeno e dell'azoto, sia di citochine. Anche l'attivazione delle cellule stellate è potenzialmente in grado di portare alla fibrosi e alla cirrosi epatica.

TABELLA 360-1. Quadri diversi di danno epatico da farmaci

MALATTIA	FARMACO
Necrosi centrolobulare	Paracetamolo
	Alotano
Steatosi microvescicolare	Acido valproico
Epatite acuta	Isoniazide
	Sulfamidici
Ipersensibilità generalizzata	Fenitoina
Fibrosi	Metotrexato
Colestasi	Clorpromazina
Eritromicina	Estrogeni
Malattia veno-occlusiva	Radioterapia più busulfano
	Ciclofosfamide
Trombosi portale e delle vene epatiche	Estrogeni
	Androgeni
Sabbia biliare	Ceftriaxone
Adenoma epatico o epatocarcinoma	Contraccettivi orali
	Steroidi anabolizzanti

Lo spettro anatomopatologico del danno epatico indotto da xenobiotici è estremamente variabile, raramente specifico, e può mimare altre epatopatie (Tab. 360-1). Le epatotossine che causano un danno prevedibile, come il paracetamolo, provocano necrosi centrolobulare degli epatociti. La steatosi è una caratteristica importante della tossicità indotta da tetracicline (steatosi microvescicolare) ed etanolo (steatosi macrovescicolare). In caso di danno causato da eritromicina estolato e clorpromazina si può osservare un'epatite colestatica. La colestasi senza infiammazione può essere un effetto tossico degli estrogeni e degli steroidi anabolizzanti. L'utilizzo di contraccettivi orali e di androgeni è stato associato anche a tumori epatici benigni e maligni. Alcune reazioni idiosincrasiche ai farmaci possono provocare quadri di danno misto, con presenza sia di colestasi diffusa, sia di necrosi cellulare. Diversi agenti antineoplastici, così come alcuni rimedi erboristici, hanno causato una malattia veno-occlusiva epatica. Anche l'uso di metildopa e di nitrofurantoina è stato associato a epatite cronica. Alcuni preparati erboristici sono risultati associati a insufficienza epatica (Tab. 360-2).

Le **manifestazioni cliniche** possono essere lievi e aspecifiche, come febbre e malessere. Nei casi di ipersensibilità, la febbre, il rash cutaneo e le artralgie possono essere severi. Nei pazienti ospedalizzati per altre patologie talora risulta difficile distinguere i segni e sintomi della tossicità epatica imputabile ai farmaci da quelli della malattia di base. La diagnosi differenziale deve comprendere le epatiti virali acute e croniche, le patologie delle vie biliari, la setticemia, il danno epatico ischemico e ipossico, l'infiltrazione maligna e le malattie metaboliche epatiche ereditarie.

TABELLA 360-2. Integratori dietetici o erboristici potenzialmente epatotossici

Kava (*Kava kava, awa, kew*)
Chaparral (*Sarcobatus, Larrea tridentata*)
Ma Huang (*Ephedra*)
Foglie di *Synphitum* (*alcaloidi della pirrolizidina*)
Estratti di *Teucrium* (*Teucrium chamaedrys*)
Valeriana con scutellaria della Virginia
Funghi (*Amanita phalloides, Galerina*)
LipoKinetix (fenilpropanolamina, usinato di sodio, diiodontironina, yohimbina, caffeina)

Le **caratteristiche di laboratorio** del danno epatico da xenobiotici sono estremamente variabili. Il danno epatocitario può portare all'aumento delle transaminasi e della bilirubina, oltre che a un'alterata funzione, evidenziata dalla riduzione dei fattori della coagulazione e dell'albumina. In caso di insufficienza epatica o di inibizione selettiva del ciclo dell'urea (valproato di sodio), può insorgere iperammoniemia. Lo screening tossicologico dei campioni di sangue e di urine può essere d'aiuto per individuare un'esposizione a farmaci o tossine. La biopsia epatica percutanea talvolta si rende necessaria per distinguere il danno da farmaci da eventuali complicanze di una malattia sottostante, o da infezioni intercorrenti.

Un lieve aumento delle transaminasi (generalmente <2-3 volte i valori normali) può verificarsi durante la terapia con alcuni farmaci, in particolare gli anticonvulsivanti, in grado di indurre le vie microsomiali del metabolismo degli xenobiotici. La biopsia epatica rivela proliferazione del reticolo endoplasmatico liscio, in assenza di danno epatico significativo. Le anomalie degli esami epatici si risolvono spesso con la prosecuzione della terapia.

Il **trattamento** del danno epatico da farmaci o tossine è prevalentemente di supporto. Il contatto con l'agente responsabile dovrebbe essere evitato. I corticosteroidi possono avere un ruolo nelle malattie immunomediate. La terapia con N-acetilcisteina, stimolando la sintesi del glutatione, è efficace nella prevenzione dell'epatotossicità, se somministrata entro 16 ore da un'overdose acuta di paracetamolo, e sembra aumentare la sopravvivenza nei pazienti con danno epatico severo, anche a distanza di 36 ore dall'ingestione (vedi Capitolo 758). Il trapianto epatico può essere talora necessario, in caso di insufficienza epatica indotta da farmaci.

La prognosi dell'epatopatia da farmaci o tossine dipende dal tipo e dalla severità del danno. Le alterazioni sono in genere completamente reversibili con la sospensione del fattore epatotossico. La mortalità in caso di necrosi epatica submassiva con insufficienza epatica fulminante può, tuttavia, superare il 50%. Con l'uso continuativo di alcuni farmaci, come il metotrexato, gli effetti dell'epatotossicità possono progredire insidiosamente fino alla cirrosi epatica. Una terapia a lungo termine con androgeni può indurre lo sviluppo di neoplasie epatiche. La risomministrazione del farmaco sospettato di aver causato in precedenza danno epatico è raramente giustificata e può portare a necrosi epatica fatale.

Bessmertny O, Hatton RC, Gonzalez-Peralta RP: Antiepileptic hypersensitivity syndrome in children. *Ann Pharmacother* 2001;35:533–538.

Blake MJ, Castro L, Leeder JS, Kearns GL: Ontogeny of drug metabolizing enzymes in the neonate. *Semin Fetal Neonatal Med* 2005;10:123–138.

Clarkson A, Choonara I: Surveillance for fatal suspected adverse drug reactions in the UK. *Arch Dis Child* 2002;87:462–466.

Estes JD, Stolpman D, Olyaei A, et al: High prevalence of potentially hepatotoxic herbal supplement use in patients with fulminant hepatic failure. *Arch Surg* 2003;138:852–858.

Heubi JE, Barbacci MB, Zimmerman HJ: Therapeutic misadventures with acetaminophen: Hepatoxicity after multiple doses in children. *J Pediatr* 1998;132:22–27.

James LP, Wells E, Beard RH, Farrar HC: Predictors of outcome after acetaminophen poisoning in children and adolescents. *J Pediatr* 2002;140:522–526.

Kearns GL, Abdel-Rahman SM, Alander SW, et al: Developmental pharmacology—Drug disposition, action, and therapy in infants and children. *N Engl J Med* 2003;349:1157–1167.

Lee WM: Drug-induced hepatotoxicity. *N Engl J Med* 1995;333:1118–1127.

Leeder JS: Pharmacogenetics and pharmacogenomics. *Pediatr Clin North Am* 2001;48:765–781.

Navarro VJ, Senior JR: Drug-related hepatotoxicity. *N Engl J Med* 2006;354: 731–739.

Roberts EA: Drug-induced liver disease in children. In Suchy FJ, Sokol RJ, Balistreri WF (editors): *Liver Disease in Children,* 2nd ed. Philadelphia, Lippincott, William & Wilkins 2001, pp 463–492.

Russo MW, Galanko JA, Shrestha R, et al: Liver transplantation for acute liver failure from drug induced liver injury in the United States. *Liver Transpl* 2004;10:1018–1023.

Capitolo 361 ■ Insufficienza epatica fulminante Frederick J. Suchy

L'insufficienza epatica fulminante è una sindrome clinica che risulta dalla necrosi massiva o da un'alterazione funzionale severa degli epatociti. Le funzioni di sintesi, escrezione e detossificazione del fegato sono tutte gravemente compromesse. Negli adulti, l'encefalopatia epatica è considerata un criterio diagnostico essenziale. Questa rigida definizione può essere però problematica, poiché l'encefalopatia epatica precoce talvolta è difficile da rilevare nei neonati e nei bambini. La definizione attualmente in uso nei bambini comprende: (1) evidenza biochimica di danno epatico acuto (in genere di durata <8 settimane); (2) nessuna evidenza di epatopatia cronica; (3) coagulopatia su base epatica, caratterizzata da un tempo di protrombina (PT, *Prothrombin Time*) >15 s o un INR (*International Normalized Ratio*, Rapporto Internazionale Normalizzato) >1,5, non correggibile con la somministrazione di vitamina K, in presenza di encefalopatia epatica clinicamente evidente, o da un PT >20 s o un INR >2, indipendentemente dalla presenza di encefalopatia. L'insufficienza epatica, nel periodo perinatale, può associarsi a danno prenatale e persino a cirrosi. Gli esempi includono la malattia da accumulo di ferro neonatale (emocromatosi), la tirosinemia e alcuni casi di infezioni virali congenite. L'epatopatia può essere rilevata alla nascita o dopo vari giorni di salute apparente. Una malattia di Wilson fulminante può insorgere in bambini più grandi precedentemente asintomatici, ma per definizione affetti da un'epatopatia preesistente. Inoltre, in alcuni casi di insufficienza epatica, in particolare nelle forme idiopatiche, l'esordio di encefalopatia avviene tardivamente, da 8 a 28 settimane dopo l'insorgenza dell'ittero.

EZIOLOGIA. L'insufficienza epatica fulminante può insorgere come complicanza di un'epatite virale (A, B, D, E). Un rischio insolitamente elevato di insufficienza epatica fulminante si osserva nei giovani adulti con infezione combinata da HBV e virus dell'epatite D. La presenza di mutazioni nella regione precore e/o promoter dell'HBV-DNA è stata associata a epatite severa o fulminante. L'HBV è inoltre responsabile di alcuni casi di insufficienza epatica fulminante in cui, a fronte dell'assenza dei marcatori sierologici dell'infezione da HBV, si riscontra la presenza di HBV-DNA a livello epatico. È raro che i virus dell'epatite C ed E causino insufficienza epatica fulminante. I pazienti con epatite cronica C sono ad aumentato rischio in caso di sovrainfezioni da HAV. Le infezioni da virus di Epstein-Barr, herpes simplex, adenovirus, enterovirus, Cytomegalovirus, parvovirus B19 e varicella-zoster possono indurre un'epatite fulminante nei bambini. Un'altra causa può essere l'epatite autoimmune. Esiste infine una forma idiopatica, responsabile del 40-50% dei casi nei bambini. Tale patologia si verifica sporadicamente e, in genere, in assenza dei comuni fattori di rischio per l'epatite virale. L'eziologia, in questi casi, è probabilmente eterogenea, potendo comprendere virus varianti o non ancora identificati, oppure malattie metaboliche non diagnosticate.

Anche diversi farmaci e composti chimici epatotossici possono causare un'insufficienza epatica fulminante. Un danno epatico prevedibile si verifica per esposizione al tetracloruro di carbonio e al fungo *Amanita phalloides*, o per sovradosaggio di paracetamolo; quest'ultimo è una causa comune di insufficienza epatica nei bambini e negli adolescenti. Un danno idiosincrasico può far seguito all'utilizzo di farmaci come l'alotano o il valproato di sodio. L'ischemia e l'ipossia che risultano dall'occlusione vascolare epatica, dallo scompenso cardiaco congestizio, dalle cardiopatie congenite cianogene o dallo shock cardiocircolatorio possono provocare un'insufficienza epatica fulminante. Le malattie metaboliche associate a insufficienza epatica comprendono la malattia di Wilson, la steatosi acuta gravidica, la galattosemia, la tirosinemia ereditaria, l'intolleranza ereditaria al fruttosio, l'emocromatosi neonatale, i difetti della β-ossidazione degli acidi grassi e i deficit di traporto mitocondriale degli elettroni. Infine, un'altra causa di insufficienza epatica sono alcuni preparati erboristici (vedi Tab. 360-2).

ISTOLOGIA. La biopsia epatica rivela abitualmente necrosi massiva focale o confluente degli epatociti. La necrosi multilobulare o a ponte può associarsi a collasso della struttura di reticolina del fegato. I segni di rigenerazione epatocitaria possono essere scarsi o assenti. Con alcuni tipi di insulti si osserva un pattern di necrosi zonale (il danno centrolobulare è caratteristico della tossicità da paracetamolo o da shock circolatorio). Occasionalmente, il reperto istologico predominante è l'evidenza di disfunzione epatica severa, più che la necrosi cellulare (l'infiltrazione steatosica microvescicolare degli epatociti è tipica della sindrome di Reye, dei difetti della beta-ossidazione e della tossicità da tetracicline).

PATOGENESI. I meccanismi che portano all'insufficienza epatica fulminante sono poco conosciuti. Non è noto il motivo per cui solo l'1-2% dei pazienti con epatite virale va incontro a insufficienza epatica. La distruzione massiva degli epatociti può rappresentare sia un effetto citotossico diretto del virus, sia una risposta immunitaria agli antigeni virali. Da un terzo alla metà dei pazienti con insufficienza epatica da HBV si negativizza per l'antigene di superficie dell'epatite B sierico nell'arco di pochi giorni dalla presentazione e spesso non ha l'antigene HBV o l'HBV-DNA rilevabili nel siero. Questi reperti suggeriscono che una risposta iperimmune al virus possa sottostare allo sviluppo di necrosi epatica massiva. La formazione di metaboliti epatotossici, che legano covalentemente alcuni costituenti cellulari macromolecolari, è coinvolta nel danno epatico causato da farmaci come il paracetamolo e l'isoniazide; l'insufficienza epatica fulminante può far seguito alla deplezione di substrati intracellulari reponsabili della detossificazione, in particolare il glutatione. A prescindere dalla causa iniziale del danno epatico, alla patogenesi dell'insufficienza epatica possono contribuire diversi fattori, tra cui una ridotta rigenerazione epatocitaria, un'alterata perfusione parenchimale e una ridotta funzione epatica reticoloendoliale.

La patogenesi dell'encefalopatia può essere correlata all'aumento dei livelli di ammonio, di falsi neurotrasmettitori e di amine, all'aumentata attività del recettore dell'acido γ-aminobutirrico (GABA) o all'aumento dei livelli circolanti di composti endogeni simil-benzodiazepinici. La ridotta eliminazione epatica di questi substrati può provocare una grave disfunzione del sistema nervoso centrale.

MANIFESTAZIONI CLINICHE. L'insufficienza epatica fulminante può essere la presentazione iniziale di un'epatopatia o complicare una malattia epatica già nota. Un'anamnesi di ritardo di sviluppo e/o disfunzione neuromuscolare può indicare un sottostante difetto mitocondriale o della β-ossidazione. Di solito il bambino con insufficienza epatica fulminante in precedenza godeva di buona salute e spesso non presentava alcun fattore di rischio per epatopatia, come esposizione a farmaci o a emoderivati. Si osservano comunente ittero progressivo, fetor hepaticus, febbre, anoressia, vomito e dolore addominale. Una rapida riduzione delle dimensioni del fegato, in assenza di un miglioramento clinico, è un segno infausto. Possono svilupparsi diatesi emorragica e ascite. I pazienti devono essere strettamente monitorati per l'insorgenza di encefalopatia epatica, inizialmente caratterizzata da alterazioni minori della coscienza o della funzione motoria. Nei neonati l'irritabilità, difficoltà di alimentazione e un cambiamento del ritmo sonno-veglia possono essere gli unici reperti; nei bambini più grandi talvolta si evidenzia asterissi. I pazienti sono spesso sonnolenti, confusi o aggressivi al risveglio, e finiscono per reagire solo agli stimoli dolorosi, fino a progredire rapidamente verso stadi di coma più profondi, in cui compaiono solo i riflessi di estensione e postura decerebrata o decorticata. La frequenza respiratoria è in genere aumentata nelle fasi precoci, ma allo stadio IV del coma può insorgere insufficienza respiratoria (Tab. 361-1).

TABELLA 361-1. Stadi dell'encefalopatia epatica

	STADI			
	I	II	III	IV
Sintomi	Periodi di letargia, euforia; inversione del ritmo sonno-veglia; il paziente può essere vigile	Sonnolenza, comportamento inadeguato, agitazione, oscillazioni dell'umore, disorientamento	Stupor, ma risvegliabile, confusione, eloquio incorente	Coma IVa: reazione a stimoli dolorosi IVb: nessuna reazione
Segni	Difficoltà a disegnare figure, a effettuare operazioni mentali	Asterissi, fetor hepaticus, incontinenza	Asterissi, iperreflessia, riflessi in estensione, rigidità	Areflessia, non asterissi, flaccidità
Elettroencefalogramma	Normale	Rallentamento generalizzato, onde θ	Onde trifasiche marcatamente anormale	Rallentamento bilaterale marcatamente anomalo, onde δ, silenzio elettrocorticale

CARATTERISTICHE DI LABORATORIO. I livelli di bilirubina (diretta e indiretta) e delle transaminasi possono essere molto aumentati. I valori di transaminasi non si correlano con la severità del danno epatico e possono addirittura ridursi quando il paziente peggiora. La concentrazione di ammonio è in genere aumentata, ma l'insorgenza di coma epatico è possibile anche in pazienti con livelli di ammoniemia normali. Il PT, sempre allungato, spesso non migliora con la somministrazione parenterale di vitamina K. Può verificarsi ipoglicemia, in particolare nei neonati; possono inoltre svilupparsi ipokaliemia, iponatriemia, acidosi metabolica o alcalosi respiratoria.

TRATTAMENTO. Il trattamento dell'insufficienza epatica fulminante è di supporto. Non è nota alcuna terapia in grado di far regredire il danno epatico o promuovere la rigenerazione. Un neonato o un bambino più grande con insufficienza epatica acuta dovrebbero essere ricoverati in una struttura attrezzata per un eventuale trapianto epatico e ospitati in un reparto di terapia intensiva, sotto monitoraggio continuo delle funzioni vitali. Per evitare l'aspirazione, ridurre l'edema cerebrale da iperventilazione e facilitare la pulizia polmonare, può rendersi necessaria l'intubazione endotracheale. La ventilazione meccanica e la somministrazione di ossigeno sono spesso necessari nel coma avanzato. Nel paziente intubato è preferibile evitare la somministrazione di sedativi, se non strettamente necessari, poiché possono aggravare o precipitare l'encefalopatia. Occorre prendere in considerazione l'uso profilattico di antiacidi, H_2-antagonisti o entrambi, a causa dell'elevato rischio di sanguinamento gastrointestinale. L'ipovolemia deve essere prevenuta e trattata con caute infusioni di liquidi ed emoderivati. Una disfunzione renale può essere conseguenza di una disidratazione, di una necrosi tubulare acuta o di un'insufficienza renale funzionale (sindrome epatorenale). Occorre procedere alla somministrazione per via endovenosa di soluzioni glucosate ed elettrolitiche allo scopo di mantenere il flusso urinario, prevenire o correggere l'ipoglicemia e mantenere il potassio a concentrazioni normali. L'iponatriemia è comune, ma è in genere dovuta a diluizione, non a deplezione di sodio. Possono rendersi necessari supplementi parenterali di calcio, fosforo e magnesio. L'ipofosfatemia, che probabilmente indica la rigenerazione epatica, e la somministrazione precoce di fosforo si associano a una prognosi migliore, nell'insufficienza epatica acuta, mentre l'iperfosfatemia è un indice predittivo di mancata guarigione spontanea.

La coagulopatia deve essere trattata con la somministrazione parenterale di vitamina K; talvolta si richiede l'infusione di plasma fresco congelato e piastrine per far fronte a un sanguinamento clinicamente significativo; può anche insorgere coagulazione vascolare disseminata. La plasmaferesi consente una temporanea correzione della diatesi emorragica, senza comportare un sovraccarico di volume. Il fattore della coagulazione VIIa ricombinante, utilizzato per la correzione transitoria della coagulopatia refrattaria all'infusione di plasma fresco congelato, può facilitare l'esecuzione di procedure invasive, come il posizionamento di un accesso venoso centrale o il monitoraggio della pressione endocranica. L'emofiltrazione continua è utile per il trattamento del sovraccarico di liquidi e dell'insufficienza renale acuta.

È importante tenere i pazienti sotto stretto monitoraggio per rilevare eventuali infezioni, tra cui sepsi, polmonite e infezioni delle vie urinarie. Almeno il 50% dei pazienti contrae un'infezione grave. I patogeni più comuni sono i batteri Gram-positivi (*Staphylococcus aureus*, *S. epidermidis*), ma si osservano anche infezioni da Gram-negativi e miceti.

Le emorragie gastrointestinali, le infezioni, la stipsi, i sedativi, gli squilibri elettrolitici e l'ipovolemia devono essere prontamente individuati e corretti, in quanto possono precipitare l'encefalopatia. L'apporto proteico deve inizialmente essere limitato o abolito, a seconda del grado di encefalopatia. L'intestino deve essere ripulito con numerosi clisteri. Si deve somministrare lattulosio ogni 2-4 ore, per via orale o tramite sondino nasogastrico, in dosi sufficienti a causare diarrea (10-50 mL). In seguito, il dosaggio viene aggiustato in modo da ottenere numerose evacuazioni quotidiane di feci acide e non formate. Ogni 6 ore è inoltre possibile somministrare per via rettale sciroppo di lattulosio, diluito in 1-3 volumi di acqua. Il lattulosio, essendo un disaccaride non assorbibile, viene metabolizzato ad acidi organici dalla flora batterica del colon; probabilmente riduce i livelli di ammoniemia, diminuendo la produzione microbica di ammoniaca, che inoltre rimane intrappolata nel contenuto acido intestinale. La somministrazione per via orale o rettale di antibiotici non assorbibili, come la neomicina, può ridurre i batteri intestinali, responsabili della produzione di ammoniaca. Per diminuire l'ammoniemia, gli antibiotici orali sono probabilmente più efficaci del lattulosio. Il flumazenil, un antagonista delle benzodiazepine, può far regredire temporaneamente un'encefalopatia epatica in fase precoce. Una complicanza temibile dell'encefalopatia epatica è l'edema cerebrale, poco responsivo a misure come la somministrazione di corticosteroidi e diuretici osmotici. Il monitoraggio della pressione endocranica può essere utile per prevenire l'edema cerebrale grave, per mantenere la pressione di perfusione cerebrale e per stabilire l'indicazione a un eventuale trapianto epatico.

Studi controllati hanno dimostrato che i pazienti con insufficienza epatica fulminante, trattati con corticosteroidi, presentavano un esito peggiore. La terapia immunosoppressiva può essere utile nei casi di epatite autoimmune fulminante. Il farmaco antivirale picovir è la terapia di scelta per l'epatite enterovirale nel neonato.

Il supporto epatico temporaneo (il cosiddetto fegato artificiale) è tuttora in corso di valutazione, nei pazienti con insufficienza epatica, come una possibile fase di passaggio verso il trapianto epatico o la rigenerazione epatocitaria. I sistemi non biologici, costituiti essenzialmente da una forma di dialisi epatica con un dialisato contenente albumina, e le forme di supporto epatico biologico, che comprendono la perfusione del sangue del paziente attraverso una colonna contenente linee cellulari epatiche o epatociti porcini, migliorano le anomalie biochimiche sieriche e, in qualche caso, anche la funzione neurologica, ma non è stato dimostrato un aumento della sopravvivenza e solo pochi bambini, finora, hanno ricevuto questo trattamento.

Il trapianto epatico ortotopico (OLT, *Orthotopic Liver Transplantation*) può salvare la vita ai pazienti che si trovano in stadi avanzati di coma epatico. Gli allotrapianti di dimensioni ridotte e i trapianti da donatore vivente sono stati importanti passi avanti nel trattamento dei neonati con insufficienza epatica. Il trapianto ortotopico parziale ausiliario e il trapianto epatico eterotopico hanno avuto successo in un piccolo numero di bambini e, in alcuni casi, hanno consentito la rigenerazione del fegato nativo e la sospensione della terapia immunosoppressiva. L'OLT tuttavia non può essere effettuato nei pazienti con insufficienza epatica associata a disfunzione neuromuscolare secondaria a malattie mitocondriali, poiché è probabile che il deterioramento neuromuscolare progressivo continui anche dopo il trapianto.

PROGNOSI. Nonostante i bambini con insufficienza epatica possano avere un decorso talora migliore rispetto agli adulti, la mortalità complessiva, con la sola terapia di supporto, supera il 70%. La prognosi può variare moltissimo a seconda della causa dell'insufficienza epatica e dello stadio dell'encefalopatia. Con la terapia medica intensiva, la sopravvivenza è pari al 50-60% (anche se può arrivare fino al 90%) sia per l'insufficienza epatica da sovradosaggio di paracetamolo, sia per le infezioni fulminanti da HAV o HBV. Al contrario, la guarigione spontanea avviene solo nel 10-20% dei pazienti con insufficienza epatica acuta idiopatica o da esordio acuto di malattia di Wilson. Nei pazienti che raggiungono lo stadio IV del coma (vedi Tab. 361-1) la prognosi è gravissima. L'erniazione del tronco cerebrale è la causa di morte più comune. Le complicanze più frequenti, come la sepsi, l'emorragia severa o l'insufficienza renale, possono aumentare ulteriormente la mortalità. La prognosi è particolarmente grave nei pazienti con necrosi epatica e insufficienza multiorgano. I fattori associati a un'elevata mortalità sono risultati l'età <1 anno, l'encefalopatia di stadio IV e la necessità di dialisi prima del trapianto. La bilirubinemia e l'INR pretrapianto non sono predittivi della sopravvivenza post-trapianto. I bambini con insufficienza epatica acuta hanno maggiori probabilità di andare incontro a exitus in lista d'attesa, rispetto a quelli con altre diagnosi. Inoltre, data la gravità della patologia, la sopravvivenza a 6 mesi dal trapianto (pari al 75% circa) risulta significativamente inferiore a quella raggiunta nei bambini trapiantati per epatopatie croniche (attualmente >90%). I pazienti che sopravvivono a un'insufficienza epatica fulminante grazie alla sola terapia di supporto in genere non sviluppano cirrosi o epatopatia cronica. Nel 10% circa dei bambini con la forma idiopatica di insufficienza epatica fulminante, si instaura un'anemia aplastica spesso fatale.

Als-Nielsen B, Gluud LL, Gluud C: Non-absorbable disaccharides for hepatic encephalopathy: Systematic review of randomized trials. *Br Med J* 2004;328:1046–1050.

Baliga P, Alvarez S, Lindblad A, Zeng L: Posttransplant survival in pediatric fulminant hepatic failure: The SPLIT experience. *Liver Transpl* 2004;10:1364–1371.

Dhawan A, Cheeseman P, Mieli-Vergani G: Approaches to acute liver failure in children. *Pediatr Transplant* 2004;8:584–588.

Dubern B, Broue P, Dubuisson C, et al: Orthotopic liver transplantation for mitochondrial respiratory chain disorders: A study of 5 children. *Transplantation* 2001;71:633–637.

Emre S, Schwartz ME, Shneider B, et al: Living related liver transplantation for acute liver failure in children. *Liver Transpl Surg* 1999;5:161–165.

Gines P, Guevara M, Arroyo V, Rodes J: Hepatorenal syndrome. *Lancet* 2003;362:1819–1826.

Lee WM: Management of acute liver failure. *Semin Liver Dis* 1996;16: 369–378.

Shawcross D, Jalan R: Dispelling myths in the treatment of hepatic encephalopathy. *Lancet* 2005;265:431–433.

Shneider BL, Rinaldo P, Emre S, et al: Abnormal concentrations of esterified carnitine in bile: A feature of pediatric acute liver failure with poor prognosis. *Hepatology* 2005;41:717–721.

Singer AL, Olthoff KM, Kim H, et al: Role of plasmapheresis in the management of acute hepatic failure in children. *Ann Surg* 2001;234:418–424.

Squires RH, Shneider BL, Bucuvalus J, et al: Acute liver failure in children: The first 348 patients in the pediatric acute liver failure study group. *J Pediatr* 2006;148:652–658.

Teo EK, Ostapowicz G, Hussain M, et al: Hepatitis B infection in patients with acute liver failure in the United States. *Hepatology* 2001;33:972–976.

van de Kerkhove MP, Hoekstra R, Chamuleau RA, van Gulik TM: Clinical application of bioartificial liver support systems. *Ann Surg* 2004; 240:216–230.

Capitolo 362 ■ Patologia cistica delle vie biliari e del fegato Frederick J. Suchy

Le lesioni cistiche del fegato possono essere riconosciute precocemente durante la prima e la seconda infanzia. La fibrosi epatica può anche far parte di un difetto di sviluppo di base. La malattia cistica renale di solito è associata a quella epatica e spesso determina la presentazione clinica e la prognosi. Praticamente tutte le proteine codificate da geni mutati, nella malattia cistica combinata del fegato e del rene, sono almeno parzialmente localizzate nelle cilia primitive delle cellule tubulari renali e dei colangiociti.

CISTI DEL COLEDOCO. Sono dilatazioni congenite del dotto biliare comune, che causano una progressiva ostruzione biliare, fino alla cirrosi biliare. Le più comuni sono le cisti cilindriche e sferiche dei dotti extraepatici, ma si possono osservare anche dilatazioni segmentarie o diffuse. Una possibile variante è il diverticolo o la dilatazione della porzione intraduodenale del dotto comune (coledococele). La dilatazione cistica dei dotti biliari intraepatici può associarsi a una cisti del coledoco.

La patogenesi delle cisti del coledoco è ancora incerta. Alcuni studi hanno suggerito che la giunzione del dotto biliare comune e di quello pancreatico, prima della confluenza nello sfintere di Oddi, possa consentire il reflusso di enzimi pancreatici nel dotto biliare comune, causando infiammazione, debolezza localizzata e dilatazione del dotto. Si è inoltre ipotizzato che le cisti del coledoco rappresentino malformazioni del dotto comune o che possano svilupparsi nell'ambito dello spettro clinico di una malattia infettiva, comprendente l'epatite neonatale e l'atresia biliare. A sostegno di questa teoria, è stato identificato RNA di reovirus nel fegato e nei tessuti biliari di neonati con cisti del coledoco.

Circa il 75% dei casi compare in età infantile. Il bambino si presenta tipicamente con ittero colestatico; se l'ostruzione non si risolve, può insorgere rapidamente una grave disfunzione epatica con ascite e coagulopatia. Una massa addominale è raramente palpabile. La **classica triade** di dolore addominale, ittero e massa si osserva in meno del 33% dei bambini più grandi. Può talvolta essere presente il quadro tipico della colangite acuta (febbre, dolorabilità nei quadranti addominali superiori, ittero e leucocitosi). La diagnosi è effettuata tramite l'ecografia, che consente di identificare le cisti coledociche anche in epoca prenatale. La colangiorisonanza magnetica è utile per la valutazione preoperatoria dell'anatomia della cisti.

Il **trattamento di scelta** è l'escissione della cisti con il confezionamento di una coledocodigiunostomia su ansa a Y alla Roux. Il drenaggio semplice nell'intestino tenue è meno soddisfacente, per il rischio che si sviluppi un carcinoma nel tessuto cistico residuo. Il decorso postoperatorio può essere complicato da colangiti ricorrenti o stenosi dell'anastomosi.

DILATAZIONE CISTICA DEI DOTTI BILIARI INTRAEPATICI (MALATTIA DI CAROLI). Questa dilatazione sacculare congenita può presentarsi in diversi segmenti dei dotti biliari intraepatici; i dotti dilatati, delimitati da epitelio cuboide, sono in continuità con il sistema duttale principale, che è in genere normale. Caroli in realtà descrisse due varianti: la malattia di Caroli, caratterizzata da ectasie dei dotti biliari intraepatici, in assenza di altre anomalie, e la sindrome di Caroli, in cui la dilatazione duttale congenita si associa a un quadro di fibrosi epatica congenita e a lesioni renali tipiche della malattia policistica renale autosomica recessiva. La sindrome di Caroli è più comune, ma all'interno della stessa famiglia possono verificarsi entrambe le forme, trasmesse con modalità autosomica recessiva. Tavolta la malattia di Caroli si associa anche alle cisti del coledoco. Si osserva una spiccata predisposizione alla colangite ascendente e alla formazione di calcoli, all'interno dei dotti biliari anomali.

I pazienti affetti presentano generalmente i sintomi della colangite acuta, in età infantile o nella prima età adulta. Compaiono febbre, dolore addominale, ittero e prurito; è palpabile un fegato lievemente ingrandito e dolorabile. Durante gli episodi di infezioni acuta si osservano un aumento della fosfatasi alcalina (ALP, *ALkaline Phosphatase*), della bilirubinemia diretta e leucocitosi. Nei pazienti con sindrome di Caroli, le caratteristiche cliniche possono essere dovute a una combinazione di attacchi ricorrenti di colangite, che rispecchiano le anomalie dei dotti intraepatici, con il sanguinamento da ipertensione portale, conseguenza della fibrosi epatica. L'ecografia mostra dotti intraepatici dilatati, ma per la conferma diagnostica e la valutazione dell'estensione della malattia è necessaria la colangiografia, per via percutanea transepatica o endoscopica, oppure la colangiorisonanza magnetica.

La colangite e la sepsi richiedono l'appropriata antibioticoterapia. Può rendersi necessaria la rimozione chirurgica dei calcoli. L'epatectomia parziale può essere curativa nei casi di malattia confinata a un singolo lobo. Negli altri casi, la prognosi è riservata, per le difficoltà che il trattamento della colangite e della litiasi biliare comporta e per l'elevato rischio che si sviluppi un colangiocarcinoma. Il trapianto epatico può essere un'alternativa terapeutica.

FIBROSI EPATICA CONGENITA. Si tratta di una malattia autosomica recessiva caratterizzata istologicamente da una fibrosi diffusa periportale e perilobulare, in ampie bande che contengono strutture distorte simili a dotti biliari e che spesso comprimono o incorporano le vene centrali o sublobulari. Sono presenti isole irregolari di parenchima epatico contenenti epatociti di aspetto normale. La fibrosi epatica congenita può associarsi alla malattia di Caroli e alle cisti coledociche; circa il 75% dei pazienti presenta anche una nefropatia, in prevalenza la malattia policistica renale autosomica recessiva, raramente la nefronoftisi. La fibrosi epatica congenita rientra nel quadro della sindrome COACH (*Cerebellar vermis hypoplasia, Oligophrenia, congenital Ataxia, Coloboma, and Hepatic fibrosis*, ipoplasia del verme cerebellare, oligofrenia, atassia congenita, coloboma e fibrosi epatica), oltre a essere stata descritta in bambini con alterazioni congenite della glicosilazione, causate da mutazioni del gene per la fosfomannoso isomerasi (vedi Capitolo 87.6).

L'esordio clinico avviene generalmente in età infantile, con epatosplenomegalia o sanguinamento da ipertensione portale. Nei pazienti con associate anomalie dei dotti biliari può svilupparsi colangite.

La funzione epatocellulare è ben conservata. Le transaminasi e la bilirubina sono in genere normali; l'ALP può essere leggermente elevata. I livelli di albumina e il tempo di protrombina sono normali. Di norma la diagnosi richiede l'esecuzione della biopsia epatica.

Il **trattamento** di questa malattia deve focalizzarsi sul controllo del sanguinamento da varici esofagee. Gli episodi poco frequenti di sanguinamento lieve possono essere trattati con scleroterapia o legatura endoscopica delle varici. In caso di emorragia più severa, può essere necessaria un'anastomosi portocavale per ridurre l'ipertensione portale. La prognosi può essere molto migliorata da una procedura di shunt, ma in alcuni pazienti la sopravvivenza risulta limitata dall'insufficienza renale.

MALATTIA POLICISTICA AUTOSOMICA DOMINANTE DEL RENE (ADPKD, *AUTOSOMAL DOMINANT POLYCYSTIC KIDNEY DISEASE*) (VEDI CAPITOLO 521.3). L'ADPKD è una malattia ereditaria comune che colpisce 1/1000 nati vivi, caratterizzata dal progressivo sviluppo di cisti renali e da una costellazione di manifestazioni extrarenali. Nella sua espressione clinica si riscontra un grado elevato di variabilità intra- e interfamiliare.

L'ADPKD è causata da una mutazione nei geni *PKD1* o *PKD2*, responsabili rispettivamente dell'85-90% e del 10-15% dei casi. Le proteine da essi codificate, la policistina-1 e la policistina-2, sono espresse nelle cellule tubulari renali e nei colangiociti. La policisina-1 funge da meccanosensore nelle cilia, rilevando il movimento del liquido attraverso i tubuli e trasmettendo il segnale attraverso la policistina-2, che agisce come un canale del calcio.

L'ADPKD è stata associata a lesioni epatiche multiple, tra cui la malformazione della lamina duttale con elementi duttali comunicanti, cisti dilatate e apparentemente non comunicanti, microamartomi biliari (i cosiddetti complessi di von Meyenburg). È stata riportata anche una correlazione con la dilatazione segmentale dei dotti intraepatici (malattia di Caroli) e con la fibrosi epatica congenita. Circa il 50% dei pazienti con insufficienza renale ha cisti epatiche dimostrabili, che derivano dalle vie biliari, ma non sono in comunicazione con esse. Le cisti epatiche aumentano con l'età, ma sono estremamente rare prima dei 16 anni. La cistogenesi epatica sembra essere influenzata dagli estrogeni. Sebbene la frequenza delle cisti sia simile nei due sessi, lo sviluppo di cisti epatiche di grandi dimensioni è una complicanza più frequente nel sesso femminile. Le cisti epatiche sono spesso asintomatiche, ma possono causare dolore e, occasionalmente, complicarsi con emorragie, infezioni, ittero da compressione dei dotti biliari, ipertensione portale e sanguinamento da varici, oppure ostruzione al deflusso venoso epatico, da compressione meccanica delle vene epatiche, che causa epatomegalia dolente e ascite essudatizia. Può svilupparsi anche un colangiocarcinoma. Un sottogruppo selezionato di pazienti, con fegato policistico severo sintomatico e un'anatomia favorevole, può essere sottoposto con successo a resezione o a fenestrazione epatica.

Gli aneurismi arteriosi cerebrali associati possono dare origine a un'emorragia subaracnoidea.

MALATTIA POLICISTICA AUTOSOMICA DOMINANTE DEL FEGATO (ADPLD, *AUTOSOMAL DOMINANT POLYCYSTIC LIVER DISEASE*). L'ADPLD è un'entità clinicamente e geneticamente distinta, caratterizzata dallo sviluppo di cisti multiple, non associate a malattia cistica renale. Le cisti epatiche non sono in continuità con le vie biliari, pur originando da esse. Il sesso femminile è colpito con maggiore frequenza rispetto a quello maschile, e le cisti spesso aumentano di volume durante la gravidanza. Nei bambini le cisti sono di raro riscontro. Le complicanze sono correlate agli effetti locali di compressione, infezione, emorragia o rottura. I geni associati all'ADPLD sono *PRKCSH* e *SEC63*, che codificano rispettivamente per l'epatocistina e per Sec63. L'epatocistina, un substrato della proteinchinasi c adK-H che è stato localizzato nel reticolo endoplasmatico, contribuisce al corretto ripiegamento e alla maturazione delle glicoproteine. Il gene *SEC63* codifica per la proteina omonima, che è un componente del meccanismo di traslocazione delle proteine, nel reticolo endoplasmatico.

Per quanto si tratti di un'evenienza rara, nell'infanzia si può osservare lo sviluppo di una cisti solitaria, non parassitaria. Possono essere presenti dolore e distensione addominale e può essere palpabile una massa poco definita nel quadrante addominale superiore. Si consiglia di lasciare indisturbate queste lesioni benigne, a meno che non comprimano strutture adiacenti, o non siano sede di complicanze, come un'emorragia intracistica.

MALATTIA POLICISTICA AUTOSOMICA RECESSIVA DEL RENE (ARPKD, *AUTOSOMAL RECESSIVE POLYCYSTIC KIDNEY DISEASE*) (VEDI CAPITOLO 521.2). L'ARPKD si presenta prevalentemente in età infantile. L'aumento bilaterale delle dimensioni dei reni è causato da una dilatazione generalizzata dei tubuli collettori. La malattia si associa invariabilmente a fibrosi epatica congenita e a vari gradi di ectasia dei dotti biliari.

Il gene dell'ARPKD codifica una proteina chiamata fibrocistina o poliductina, che è stata localizzata sulle cilia del dominio apicale delle cellule collettrici renali e dei colangiociti. Il difetto primitivo, nella ARPKD, può essere una disfunzione ciliare correlata all'anomalia di questa proteina. Le cisti si sviluppano come espansioni ectasiche dei tubuli collettori e dei dotti biliari, che restano in continuità con le loro strutture di origine.

Di solito l'ARPKD insorge precocemente, spesso subito dopo la nascita, e in genere è più severa rispetto all'ADPKD. Questi pazienti, che possono morire nel periodo perinatale a causa dell'insufficienza renale o della disgenesia polmonare, di norma presentano reni molto ingranditi e non funzionanti. Si può instaurare insufficienza respiratoria dovuta alla compressione del torace da parte dei reni grossolanamente aumentati, alla ritenzione di liquidi o a un'ipoplasia polmonare concomitante. Le caratteristiche istologiche e cliniche tendono a ripresentarsi sempre uguali all'interno della stessa famiglia, sebbene sia stata osservata una certa variabilità per quanto riguarda gravità della malattia ed epoca di presentazione.

Il fegato presenta una fibrosi periportale di vario grado, iperplasia dei duttuli biliari e disgenesia biliare. L'epatopatia e le complicanze della fibrosi epatica tendono a essere clinicamente più significative nei soggetti con un grado di danno renale tale da consentire una più lunga sopravvivenza. Il problema clinico principale, nei pazienti più grandi con ARPKD e fibrosi epatica congenita, è l'ipertensione portale; sebbene il sanguinamento che ne consegue possa verificarsi già nel primo anno di vita, colpisce più spesso i bambini più grandi, con ematemesi o melena. È spesso presente epatomegalia compatta o di consistenza dura. Un altro reperto frequente è a splenomegalia, associata a ipersplenismo. A causa della dilatazione dei dotti biliari intraepatici, questi pazienti sono esposti a un rischio aumentato di colangite batterica. La malattia di Caroli o una dilatazione congenita, segmentaria o sacculare dei dotti biliari intraepatici possono coesistere con la fibrosi epatica congenita e l'ARPKD.

L'emorragia da varici esofagee può essere trattata inizialmente con scleroterapia o legatura endoscopica. Alcuni pazienti con funzione epatica ben conservata possono trarre beneficio da uno shunt portocavale selettivo. Il trattamento della sepsi biliare deve essere aggressivo. Le crisi ricorrenti di colangite batterica possono portare alla perdita progressiva della funzione epatica. È raro il coinvolgimento monolaterale, che può essere trattato con la resezione epatica. In caso di insufficienza epatica può rendersi necessario il trapianto.

Varie anomalie dei dotti biliari (dilatazioni irregolari, proliferazioni, cisti) e di fibrosi portale possono associarsi con la sindrome di Meckel, la trisomia 17 e 18, la sclerosi tuberosa e la distrofia toracica asfittica.

Cisti del coledoco

Miyano T, Yamataka A: Choledochal cysts. *Curr Opin Pediatr* 1997;9: 283–288.

Okada T, Sasaki F, Ueki S, et al: Postnatal management for prenatally diagnosed choledochal cysts. *J Pediatr Surg* 2004;39:1055–1058.

Stringer MD, Dhawan A, Davenport M, et al: Choledochal cysts: Lessons from a 20-year experience. *Arch Dis Child* 1995;73:528–531.

Malattia di Caroli

Asselah T, Ernst O, Sergent G, et al: Caroli's disease: A magnetic resonance cholangiopancreatography diagnosis. *Am J Gastroenterol* 1998;93: 109–110.

Desmet VJ: Ludwig symposium on biliary disorders—Part I. Pathogenesis of ductal plate abnormalities. *Mayo Clin Proc* 1998;73:80–89.

Keane F, Hadzic N, Wilkinson ML, et al: Neonatal presentation of Caroli's disease. *Arch Dis Child Fetal Neonatal Ed* 1997;77:F145–F146.

Fibrosi epatica congenita

Desmet VJ: What is congenital hepatic fibrosis? *Histopathology* 1992;20: 465–477.

Perisic VN: Long-term studies on congenital hepatic fibrosis in children. *Acta Paediatr* 1995;84:695–696.

Polycystic Diseases of the Liver and Kidney

Davila S, Furu L, Gharavi AG: Mutations in *SEC63* cause autosomal dominant polycystic liver disease. *Nat Genet* 2004;36:575–577.

Everson GT, Taylor MR: Management of polycystic liver disease. *Curr Gastroenterol Rep* 2005;7:19–25.

Guay-Woodford LM, Desmond RA: Autosomal recessive polycystic kidney disease: The clinical experience in North America. *Pediatrics* 2003;111:1072–1080.

Johnson CA, Gissen P, Sergi C: Molecular pathology and genetics of congenital hepatorenal fibrocystic syndromes. *J Med Genet* 2003;40:311–319.

Lina F, Satlinb LM: Polycystic kidney disease: The cilium as a common pathway in cystogenesis. *Curr Opin Pediatr* 2004;16:171–176.

Qian Q, Li A, King BF, et al: Clinical profile of autosomal dominant polycystic liver disease. *Hepatology* 2003;37:164–171.

Wilson PD: Polycystic kidney disease. *N Engl J Med* 2004;350:151–164

Capitolo 363 ■ Patologie della colecisti

Frederick J. Suchy

ANOMALIE. La colecisti è congenitamente assente nello 0,1% della popolazione. L'ipoplasia o l'assenza della colecisti si possono associare all'atresia dei dotti biliari extraepatici o alla fibrosi cistica. La duplicazione della colecisti è un'eventualità rara.

IDROPE ACUTA (TAB. 363-1). La distensione acuta, alitiasica, non infiammatoria della colecisti può verificarsi sia nei lattanti, sia nei bambini più grandi; è definita dall'assenza di calcoli, infezione batterica o anomalie congenite del sistema biliare. Questo disturbo può complicare infezioni di lunga durata, ma la causa spesso non viene individuata. L'idrope della colecisti può inoltre svilupparsi nei pazienti sottoposti a nutrizione parenterale a lungo termine, probabilmente in conseguenza di una stasi a livello della colecisti, nel periodo di digiuno enterale. L'idrope, che si distingue dalla colecistite alitasica per l'assenza di un processo infiammatorio significativo, ha una prognosi generalmente favorevole.

I pazienti affetti accusano dolore in ipocondrio destro e hanno generalmente una massa palpabile. Possono essere presenti febbre, vomito e ittero; è raro che si associ una malattia sistemica, come un'infezione streptococcica. L'ecografia mostra una colecisti molto distesa, priva di eco, senza dilatazione delle vie biliari. La terapia dell'idrope acuta è conservativa, con una particolare attenzione al trattamento di supporto e a quello delle malattie intercorrenti; la colecistectomia con drenaggio è raramente necessaria. La risoluzione spontanea, con il ripristino di una normale funzione della colecisti, di norma avviene nell'arco di alcune settimane. Nei casi in cui è necessaria una laparotomia, si osserva una colecisti edematosa, contenente bile bianca, gialla o verdastra. Occasionalmente, si osserva ostruzione del dotto cistico da parte di un'adenopatia mesenterica. Se la colecisti è gangrenosa, è necessaria la colecistectomia. L'esame istologico della colecisti asportata rivela edema con scarsa infiammazione. Le colture biliari risultano di norma sterili.

COLECISTITE E COLELITIASI. La colecistite acuta alitiasica, rara nei bambini, è in genere causata da processi infettivi. I patogeni più comuni comprendono gli streptococchi (gruppo A e B), i batteri Gram-negativi, in particolare *Salmonella* e *Leptospira interrogans*. Si possono osservare infestazioni parassitarie da ascaridi o da *Giardia lamblia*. La colecistite alitiasica può conseguire a un trauma addominale o a un'ustione, per quanto si tratti di un'evenienza rara, oppure associarsi a una vasculite sistemica come la panarterite nodosa.

Le caratteristiche cliniche comprendono dolore in sede epigastrica o in ipocondrio destro, vomito, febbre e ittero. Sono presenti difesa addominale e dolorabilità nel quadrante superiore

TABELLA 363-1. Condizioni che si associano a idrope della colecisti

Malattia di Kawasaki	Talassemia
Faringite streptococcica	Nutrizione parenterale totale
Infezione stafilococcica	Digiuno prolungato
Leptospirosi	Epatite virale
Ascaridiosi	Sepsi
Strongiloidiasi	Porpora di Schönlein-Henoch
Crisi di anemia falciforme	Adenite mesenterica
Febbre tifoidea	Enterocolite necrotizzante

destro. L'ecografia mostra una colecisti di dimensioni aumentate, con parete ispessita, senza calcoli. L'ALP e la bilirubina diretta sono aumentate; la leucocitosi è comune.

I pazienti guariscono normalmente con il trattamento dell'infezione sistemica e biliare. Dal momento che la colecisti può divenire gangrenosa, è necessario un monitoraggio ecografico quotidiano per controllarne la distensione e lo spessore di parete. La colecistectomia è indicata per coloro che non migliorano con il trattamento conservativo. Il drenaggio con colecistotomia è un approccio alternativo nei casi critici.

La colelitiasi è relativamente rara nei bambini che per il resto sono in buona salute, verificandosi più spesso in pazienti con diverse malattie predisponenti (Tab. 363-2). In età pediatrica, più del 70% dei calcoli colecistici è di tipo pigmentario, il 15-20% è di colesterolo, e i rimanenti sono misti, composti da colesterolo, matrice organica e bilirubinato di calcio. I calcoli pigmentari neri, formati prevalentemente da bilirubinato di calcio e matrice glicoproteica, sono una complicanza frequente delle anemie emolitiche croniche; quelli marroni si formano per lo più nei neonati, a causa di infezioni delle vie biliari. Il componente principale è la bilirubina non coniugata, prodotta dall'elevata attività beta-glucuronidasica della bile infetta. I calcoli di colesterolo possono essere composti da colesterolo puro, oppure contenere più del 50% di colesterolo, insieme a mucine della matrice glicoproteica e a bilirubinato di calcio. Nei bambini sono stati descritti anche calcoli di carbonato di calcio.

I pazienti con malattie emolitiche (tra cui anemia falciforme, talassemie, enzimopatie eritrocitarie) e quelli con malattia di Wilson hanno un rischio aumentato di colelitiasi da calcoli neri pigmentari. Nell'anemia falciforme i calcoli, che si possono sviluppare prima dei 4 anni di età, sono stati riportati nel 17-33% dei pazienti dai 2 ai 18 anni. La sindrome di Gilbert, causata da una variante genetica del promoter dell'uridina difosfato (UDP) glucuronosiltransferasi 1A1 (genotipi [TA]7/[TA]7 e [TA]7/[TA]8), consiste in una forma di iperbilirubinemia non coniugata cronica, che rappresenta un fattore di rischio per la formazione di calcoli pigmentari, in caso di anemia falciforme.

La cirrosi e la colestasi cronica aumentano il rischio di formazione di calcoli di pigmento. Anche i neonati prematuri malati possono sviluppare una colelitiasi; il trattamento, in questi casi, è spesso complicato da fattori come la resezione intestinale, l'enterocolite necrotizzante, la nutrizione parenterale totale prolungata, la colestasi, le trasfusioni frequenti e l'uso di diuretici. La colelitiasi nei neonati prematuri è spesso asintomatica e può risolversi spontaneamente. Nei neonati con ittero ostruttivo e infezione delle vie biliari intra- ed extraepatiche si trovano spesso calcoli di pigmento marroni, che in genere sono radiotrasparenti per via del basso contenuto di fosfato e carbonato di calcio, e di un maggior contenuto di colesterolo rispetto ai calcoli pigmentati neri. La discinesia biliare, un disturbo della contrattilità della colecisti, è una fattore anomalo che predispone alla formazione di calcoli alla fine dell'infanzia e in età adolescenziale.

La colelitiasi da colesterolo di interesse pediatrico colpisce soprattutto le adolescenti obese. I calcoli di colesterolo si osservano anche nei bambini con alterazioni della circolazione enteroepatica degli acidi biliari, compresi i pazienti con malattie ileali e malassorbimento degli acidi biliari, oltre a quelli con resezione ileale, morbo di Crohn ileale e fibrosi cistica. In questi casi possono formarsi anche calcoli di pigmento.

La formazione di calcoli di colesterolo sembra imputabile a un eccesso di colesterolo nella bile, in rapporto alla capacità legante delle micelle. La supersaturazione della bile con il colesterolo, che porta alla formazione di cristalli e di calcoli, può derivare da una riduzione del contenuto di acidi biliari, oppure da un aumento della concentrazione di colesterolo. Altri fattori scatenanti, che possono svolgere un ruolo nella formazione dei calcoli, sono la stasi biliare e la presenza nella bile di mucoproteine anomale o di pigmenti biliari anomali, che fungere da nuclei intorno a cui il colesterolo si cristallizza.

L'uso prolungato di ceftriaxone, una cefalosporina di terza generazione, è stato associato alla formazione di precipitati di sali di ceftriaxone di calcio (*pseudolitiasi biliare*) nella colecisti. In più del 40% dei bambini trattati con questo farmaco per almeno 10 giorni si possono rilevare sabbia biliare o colelitiasi. In rari casi il soggetto sviluppa ittero e dolore addominale; i precipitati si risolvono spontaneamente nel corso di diversi mesi dopo la sospensione del farmaco.

La colecistite acuta o cronica si associa spesso a colelitiasi. La forma acuta può essere precipitata dall'incuneamento di un calcolo nel dotto cistico. La proliferazione di batteri nel lume della colecisti ostruita può contribuire al processo e portare alla sepsi biliare. La colecistite cronica litiasica, più frequente, può svilupparsi insidiosamente o seguire una serie di attacchi di colecistite acuta. L'epitelio della colecisti diviene spesso ulcerato e cicatriziale.

La caratteristica clinica più importante della colelitiasi è il dolore addominale ricorrente, spesso di tipo colico, localizzato nel quadrante addominale superiore destro. I bambini più grandi possono presentare intolleranza ai cibi grassi. La colecistite acuta può essere la prima manifestazione, con febbre, dolore in ipocondrio destro, talora irradiato all'area sotto la scapola destra, e spesso una massa palpabile. L'ittero compare più frequentemente nei bambini che negli adulti. La radiografia diretta dell'addome può rivelare un calcolo radiopaco, mentre quelli radiotrasparenti (di colesterolo) non sono visibili. Pertanto la metodica di scelta, per la visualizzazione dei calcoli, è l'ecografia. La scintigrafia epatobiliare è un ausilio importante, in quanto l'impossibilità di visualizzare la colecisti è indice di colecistite.

La colecistectomia è curativa. La colecistectomia laparoscopia viene effettuata di routine nei lattanti e nei bambini con colelitiasi sintomatica. In età pediatrica i calcoli del dotto biliare comune sono rari, verificandosi nel 2-6% dei casi di colelitiasi, spesso in associazione con ittero ostruttivo e pancreatite. Durante l'intervento, occorre eseguire una colangiografia operatoria per rilevare la presenza di eventuali calcoli del dotto comune. La colangiografia retrograda endoscopica, con estrazione dei calcoli dal dotto comune, è un'opzione da considerare prima della colecistectomia laparoscopica, nei bambini più grandi e negli adolescenti.

I pazienti asintomatici con colelitiasi pongono problemi di trattamento maggiori. Dagli studi effettuati negli adulti è emerso che tra la formazione iniziale dei calcoli e lo sviluppo dei sintomi trascorre un intervallo superiore a un decennio. La risoluzione spontanea della colelitiasi è stata riportata sia nei lattanti, sia nei bambini più grandi. Se si decide di rimandare l'intervento chirurgico, occorre sempre informare i genitori sui segni e sintomi indicativi di colangite o di ostruzione del dotto biliare comune. Nei pazienti con emolisi cronica o malattia ileale, la colecistectomia può essere effettuata contestualmente ad altri interventi chirurgici. Dal momento che la chirurgia laparoscopia può essere intrapresa in tutta sicurezza anche nei bambini con anemia falciforme, la colecistecomia elettiva viene effettuata per lo più al momento della rilevazione dei calcoli, prima che si sviluppino sintomi o eventuali complicanze. Nei casi associati a epatopatia cronica, obesità grave o fibrosi cistica, il rischio chirurgico della colecistectomia, che può essere elevato, impone di valutare attentamente il rapporto rischio-beneficio connesso all'intervento.

TABELLA 363-2. Condizioni che si associano a colelitiasi
Malattie emolitiche croniche (anemia falciforme, sferocitosi)
Obesità
Resezione o patologia ileale
Fibrosi cistica
Epatopatia cronica
Morbo di Crohn
Nutrizione parenterale prolugata
Prematurità con decorso medico o chirurgico complicato
Digiuno prolungato o rapido calo ponderale
Trattamento dei tumori infantili
Chirurgia addominale
Gravidanza

Barton LL, Luisiri A, Dawson JE: Hydrops of the gallbladder in childhood infections. *Pediatr Infect Dis J* 1995;14:163–164.
Bor O, Dinleyici EC, Kebapci M, Aydogdu SD: Ceftriaxone-associated biliary sludge and pseudocholelithiasis during childhood: A prospective study. *Pediatr Int* 2004;46:322–324.
Chaar V, Keclard L, Diara JP, et al: Association of UGT1A1 polymorphism with prevalence and age at onset of cholelithiasis in sickle cell anemia. *Haematologica* 2005;90:188–199.
Lobe TE: Cholelithiasis and cholecystitis in children. *Semin Pediatr Surg* 2000;9:170–176.
Rescorla FJ: Cholelithiasis, cholecystitis, and common bile duct stones. *Curr Opin Pediatr* 1997;9:276–282.
Stringer MD, Taylor DR, Soloway RD: Gallstone composition: Are children different? *J Pediatr* 2003;142:435–440.
Suchy FJ: Anatomy, anomalies and pediatric disorders of the biliary tract. In Feldman M, Friedman LS, Sleisenger MH (editors): *Gastrointestinal and Liver Disorders,* 7th ed. Philadelphia, WB Saunders, 2002, pp 1019–1036.
Suell MN, Horton TM, Dishop MK, et al: Outcomes for children with gallbladder abnormalities and sickle cell disease. *J Pediatr* 2004;145:617–621.
Walker TM, Hambleton IR, Serjeant GR: Gallstones in sickle cell disease: Observations from the Jamaican Cohort study. *J Pediatr* 2000;136:80–85.

Capitolo 364 ■ Ipertensione portale e varici Frederick J. Suchy

L'ipertensione portale, definita come un aumento della pressione portale >10-12 mmHg, è la principale causa di morbilità e mortalità nei bambini con epatopatia. La pressione portale venosa normale è di circa 7 mmHg. Mentre le caratteristiche cliniche delle varie forme di ipertensione portale possono essere simili, le complicanze associate, il trattamento e la prognosi variano significativamente e dipendono dalla presenza o meno di insufficienza epatica.

EZIOLOGIA. L'ipertensione portale può dipendere da un'ostruzione del flusso ematico portale, in un punto qualsiasi lungo il tragitto del sistema venoso portale. Può svilupparsi in conseguenza di un'ostruzione pre-epatica, intraepatica o postepatica, comportando una serie di disturbi che sono indicati nella Tabella 364-1.

In età pediatrica una causa importante di ipertensione portale è l'ostruzione portale extraepatica, che può manifestarsi a qualsiasi livello della vena porta. L'infezione ombelicale (onfalite), con o senza una pregressa cateterizzazione della vena ombelicale, rappresenta una delle cause nei neonati. L'infezione può potenzialmente diffondersi dalla vena ombelicale al ramo portale sinistro e infine al tronco portale principale. Le infezioni endoaddominali, comprese l'appendicite acuta e la peritonite primitiva, possono essere un'altra causa nei bambini più grandi. La trombosi della vena porta è stata anche associata a condizioni di disidratazione neonatale e di infezione sistemica. Nei bambini più grandi, le malattie infiammatorie intestinali possono associarsi a uno stato di ipercoagulabilità che talvolta determina ostruzione portale. La trombosi portale, oltre a essere stata descritta in associazione con le infezioni delle vie biliari e la colangite sclerosante, può verificarsi anche in pazienti con stati di ipercoagulabilità, come il deficit di proteina C, proteina S o la mutazione del fattore V di Leyden. La vena porta può essere sostituita da residui fibrosi o contenenti trombi organizzati. Anomalie di sviluppo rare, che possono provocare ipertensione portale extraepatica, comprendono l'agenesia, l'atresia e la stenosi della vena porta; può inoltre verificarsi un'ostruzione da parte di una rete o di un diaframma. In almeno metà dei casi riportati, tuttavia, non si riconosce una causa definita.

Raramente, un'ipertensione presinusoidale può essere causata da un aumento del flusso portale risultante da una fistola artero-venosa congenita o acquisita.

TABELLA 364-1. Cause di ipertensione portale

IPERTENSIONE PORTALE EXTRAEPATICA
Agenesia, atresia, stenosi della vena porta
Trombosi o trasformazione cavernosa della vena porta
Trombosi della vena splenica
Aumento del flusso portale
Fistola arterovenosa
IPERTENSIONE PORTALE INTRAEPATICA
Malattia epatocellulare
Epatiti virali acute e croniche
Cirrosi
Fibrosi epatica congenita
Malattia di Wilson
Deficit di α_1-antitripsina
Glicogenosi di tipo IV
Epatotossicità
Metotrexato
Nutrizione parenterale
Patologie biliari
Atresia biliare extraepatica
Fibrosi cistica
Cisti del coledoco
Colangite sclerosante
Paucità dei dotti biliari intraepatici
Ipertensione portale idiopatica
Ostruzione postsinusoidale
Sindrome di Budd-Chiari
Malattia veno-occlusiva

Le cause intraepatiche di ipertensione portale sono numerose. L'ostruzione al flusso portale può svilupparsi sulla base di un processo presinusoidale, per esempio l'epatite acuta o cronica, la fibrosi epatica congenita e la schistosomiasi, ma anche l'infiltrazione portale da parte di cellule maligne o di granulomi può contribuire. È stata inoltre descritta una forma idiopatica, caratterizzata da splenomegalia, ipersplenismo e ipertensione portale, senza occlusione della vena porta o splenica e in assenza di una malattia epatica evidente. In alcuni pazienti è stata osservata una fibrosi portale non cirrotica.

La cirrosi è la causa principale di ipertensione portale, correlata all'ostruzione del flusso attraverso la vena porta. La cirrosi a sua volta può essere dovuta a varie cause, tra cui l'atresia biliare, l'epatite autoimmune, l'epatite virale cronica e le malattie epatiche metaboliche come il deficit di α_1-antitripsina, la malattia di Wilson, la glicogenosi di tipo IV, l'intolleranza al fruttosio ereditaria e la fibrosi cistica.

Nei bambini si osservano anche casi di ipertensione portale postsinusoidale. La sindrome di Budd-Chiari è caratterizzata da un'ostruzione delle vene epatiche, in qualsiasi punto tra le vene epatiche efferenti e la confluenza della vena cava inferiore nell'atrio destro. Sebbene nella maggior parte dei casi non si trovi una causa specifica, la trombosi può verificarsi nelle condizioni di ipercoagulabilità congenita o acquisita (per es. il deficit di antitrombina III, di proteina C o S, le mutazioni del fattore V di Leyden o della protrombina, l'emoglobinuria parossistica notturna, la gravidanza, l'assunzione di contraccettivi orali) e complicare il decorso di neoplasie epatiche primitive o secondarie, collagenopatie, infezioni e traumi. Altre cause di sindrome di Budd-Chiari comprendono la sindrome di Behçet, le malattie infiammatorie croniche intestinali, l'aspergillosi, la terapia con dacarbazina e le reti a livello della vena cava inferiore. La malattia veno-occlusiva, la causa più frequente di ostruzione delle vene epatiche nei bambini, comporta l'occlusione delle venule centro-lobulari o delle vene epatiche sublobulari e insorge in seguito alla radioterapia total body, con o senza chemioterapia, effettuata comunemente prima del trapianto di midollo osseo. Questa malattia è stata descritta anche in correlazione con l'ingestione di preparati erboristici contenenti alcaloidi della pirrolizidina, che talvolta entrano nella composizione di tisane medicinali.

FISIOPATOLOGIA. L'anomalia emodinamica primitiva, nell'ipertensione portale, consiste nell'aumento delle resistenze al flusso ematico portale. Questo accade sia che la resistenza al flusso portale abbia una causa intraepatica, come nel caso della cirrosi, sia che dipenda dall'ostruzione della vena porta. Lo shunt portosistemico dovrebbe decomprimere il sistema portale, riducendo significativamente la pressione portale. Nonostante lo sviluppo significativo di collaterali, che deviano il sangue portale nelle vene sistemiche, l'ipertensione portale è mantenuta da un aumento complessivo del flusso portale. Si sviluppa una condizione di circolazione iperdinamica, sostenuta da tachicardia, aumento della gittata cardiaca e riduzione delle resistenze vascolari sistemiche, spesso accompagnata da vasodilatazione splancnica. L'aumento del flusso portale si correla al contributo del flusso epatico e collaterale, mentre il flusso ematico portale reale che raggiunge il fegato è ridotto. È inoltre probabile che la disfunzione epatocellulare e gli shunt portosistemici portino alla degenerazione di vari fattori umorali che causano vasodilatazione e aumento del volume plasmatico.

Molte complicanze dell'ipertensione portale sono riconducibili allo sviluppo di un'importante circolazione collaterale. I vasi collaterali possono formarsi prevalentemente nelle zone in cui l'epitelio di assorbimento si unisce a quello stratificato, in particolare nell'esofago e nella regione anorettale. I collaterali sottomucosi superficiali, soprattutto quelli dell'esofago, dello stomaco e, in minor misura, quelli del duodeno, del colon o del retto, sono predisposti alla rottura e al sanguinamento, per effetto dell'aumentata pressione. Nell'ipertensione portale, anche la vascolarizzazione dello stomaco risulta anomala e dimostra comunicazioni arterovenose sottomucose prominenti tra la muscolaris mucosae e le vene e i capillari dilatati. La lesione risultante, un'ectasia vascolare nota come "gastropatia congestizia", contribuisce ad aumentare significativamente il rischio di sanguinamento gastrico.

MANIFESTAZIONI CLINICHE. Il sanguinamento da varici esofagee è la presentazione più frequente. Nei pazienti con una sottostante malattia epatica, all'esame obiettivo è possibile riscontrare ittero e altri segni di cirrosi, come eritema palmare e teleangectasie vascolari. Nei bambini cirrotici e, in misura minore, anche in quelli con ostruzione portale extraepatica isolata è frequente un ritardo della crescita. L'ascite può svilupparsi nei pazienti con ipertensione portale intraepatica e, transitoriamente, in quelli con ostruzione portale. A livello della regione periombelicale si rendono evidenti vasi cutanei collaterali dilatati, che convogliano il sangue dal sistema portale alla circolazione sistemica. In assenza di caratteristiche cliniche o biochimiche di epatopatia e in presenza di un fegato di dimensioni normali, la causa più probabile è l'ostruzione portale. In queste condizioni, non si può escludere completamente una cirrosi compensata. La colestasi con disfunzione epatica, caratterizzata da aumento della bilirubinemia e delle transaminasi, è una complicanza poco frequente dell'ostruzione portale, causata dalla compressione estrinseca sui dotti biliari da parte della trasformazione cavernosa della vena porta. Il reperto di un fegato aumentato di volume, di consistenza dura, con un'alterazione minima della funzionalità, suggerisce la possibilità di una fibrosi epatica congenita. L'emorragia, soprattutto nei bambini con ostruzione della vena porta, può essere precipitata da patologie febbrili intercorrenti minori. Il meccanismo spesso non è chiaro; l'uso di acido acetilsalicilico o di altri farmaci antinfiammatori non steroidei può contribuire a danneggiare l'integrità di una mucosa gastrica congesta, interferendo inoltre con la funzione piastrinica. Anche la tosse, nel corso di una malattia respiratoria, può aumentare la pressione endovariceale. Il sanguinamento può manifestarsi con ematemesi o melena. L'emorragia gastrointestinale può originare anche da una gastropatia congestizia o da varici gastriche, duodenali, peristomali o rettali. La splenomegalia, spesso associata a ipersplenismo, è la seconda complicanza dell'ostruzione portale in ordine di frequenza e può essere rilevata per prima nel corso di un esame obiettivo di routine. Poiché molti studi documentano che più della metà dei pazienti con ostruzione portale non va incontro a sanguinamento prima dei 6 anni di età, la diagnosi dovrebbe essere sospettata in un bambino senza epatopatia che ha avuto un decorso neonatale complicato e che ha sviluppato successivamente splenomegalia asintomatica.

I bambini con ipertensione portale, a prescindere dalla causa, possono avere crisi ricorrenti di emorragia imponente. Nei pazienti con ostruzione portale e funzione epatica normale, il sanguinamento tende a essere autolimitante, mentre in quelli con malattia intraepatica la coesistenza di una ridotta funzione sintetica epatica (coagulopatia) può rendere il sanguinamento difficile da controllare. Inoltre, l'emorragia da varici esofagee e la cirrosi possono avere effetti deleteri sul fegato, alterandone ulteriormente la funzione e talora precipitando l'ittero, l'ascite e l'encefalopatia.

Un'altra grave complicanza dell'ipertensione portale è la sindrome epatopolmonare, che si sviluppa in almeno il 10% dei pazienti con cirrosi. È definita come un difetto di ossigenazione arteriosa indotto da dilatazione microvascolare intrapolmonare, in conseguenza del rilascio nel circolo venoso di mediatori come l'ossido nitrico.

DIAGNOSI. Nei pazienti con malattia cronica stabilizzata o in quelli in cui si sospetta un'ostruzione portale, si dovrebbe effettuare un'ecografia accurata per dimostrare la pervietà della vena porta. Inoltre, l'eco-Doppler può indicare la direzione del flusso nel sistema portale. Il pattern del flusso correla con la gravità della cirrosi e dell'encefalopatia. L'inversione del flusso ematico portale (flusso epatofugo) è frequentemente associata a sanguinamento da varici. Anche l'ecografia è utile per rilevare la presenza di varici esofagee. Un'altra importante caratteristica dell'ostruzione portale extraepatica è la cosiddetta trasformazione cavernosa della vena porta, caratterizzata dallo sviluppo, nel sistema venoso paracoledocico ed epicoledocico, di un esteso complesso di piccoli vasi collaterali la cui funzione è di bypassare l'ostruzione. Altre tecniche di imaging possono concorrere a un'ulteriore definizione dell'anatomia portale, pur rendendosi necessarie in un minor numero di casi; la TC con contrasto e l'angiorisonanza magnetica forniscono informazioni simili a quelle dell'ecografia. L'arteriografia selettiva del tripode celiaco, dell'arteria mesenterica superiore e della vena splenica permette di definire la geografia vascolare extraepatica; questo non è richiesto per formulare la diagnosi, ma può essere utile al momento di pianificare la decompressione chirurgica dell'ipertensione portale.

In un paziente con ipossia (sindrome epatopolmonare), la dilatazione microvascolare intrapolmonare è dimostrabile con l'ecocardiografia con contrasto, che evidenzia il ritardo di comparsa nel cuore sinistro delle microbolle di soluzione fisiologica iniettata in una vena periferica.

L'endoscopia è il metodo più affidabile per rilevare le varici esofagee e identificare l'origine di un sanguinamento gastrointestinale. Sebbene l'emorragia da varici gastriche o esofagee sia la più comune nei bambini con ipertensione portale, fino a un terzo dei pazienti, in particolare quelli con cirrosi, può avere un sanguinamento da altre sedi, come una gastropatia congestizia ipertensiva o ulcere gastroduodenali. Esiste una forte correlazione tra le dimensioni delle varici valutate endoscopicamente e il rischio di emorragia. Le chiazze rossastre visibili sulla varice in endoscopia sono un importante fattore predittivo di emorragia imminente.

TRATTAMENTO. La terapia dell'ipertensione portale si articola nel trattamento di emergenza dell'emorragia potenzialmente letale e nel trattamento profilattico volto a prevenire un primo sanguinamento o una recidiva. È importante sottolineare che molti studi condotti in questo campo sono basati sull'esperienza con pazienti adulti.

Il trattamento dei pazienti con emorragia da varici si deve focalizzare sul ripristino del volume circolante, inizialmente tramite infusione di cristalloidi, poi mediante somministrazione di emazie concentrate. Può essere necessario correggere la coagulopatia con vitamina K oppure infusione di piastrine, plasma fresco congelato o entrambi. Occorre posizionare un sondino nasogastrico per documentare la presenza di sangue nella cavità gastrica e monitorare un'ulteriore emorragia in corso. Occorre somministrare per via endovenosa un bloccante del recettore H_2, come la ranitidina, per ridurre il rischio di sanguinamento da erosioni gastriche. Nella maggior parte dei pazienti, in particolare in quelli con ipertensione portale extraepatica e funzione di sintesi epatica normale, spesso accade che il sanguinamento si arresti spontaneamente. Occorre cautela nella somministrazione di liquidi dopo un'emorragia, onde evitare un aumento eccessivo della pressione venosa, che peggiorerebbe ulteriormente il sanguinamento.

Nei pazienti con emorragia persistente si può prendere in considerazione una terapia farmacologica volta a ridurre la pressione portale. La vasopressina (o uno dei suoi analoghi) è di uso comune; si pensa che agisca aumentando il tono vascolare splancnico, con il risultato di ridurre il flusso ematico portale. La vasopressina è somministrata dapprima in bolo, alla dose di 0,33 U/kg in 20 minuti, poi in infusione continua alla stessa dose su base oraria, oppure alla dose di 0,2 U/1,73 m^2/min. L'emivita del farmaco è di circa 30 minuti. Un limite al suo utilizzo è rappresentato dagli effetti collaterali di vasocostrizione, che può alterare la funzione cardiaca e la perfusione di cuore, intestino e reni, esacerbando, di conseguenza, la ritenzione di liquidi. La nitroglicerina, somministrata generalmente sotto forma di cerotto cutaneo, è stata utilizzata anche per ridurre la pressione portale e gli effetti indesiderati della vasopressina. L'octreotide, l'analogo della somatostatina, riduce il flusso splancnico con minori effetti collaterali e può essere somministrato in infusione endovenosa continua alla dose di 1,0-1,5 μg/kg/ora. Sebbene gli studi negli adulti siano promettenti, il suo uso e la sua efficacia in età pediatrica non sono ancora stati adeguatamente valutati.

Dopo un episodio di emorragia da varici non controllabile con la sola terapia medica, la sclerosi o la legatura endoscopica delle varici sono importanti opzioni terapeutiche. La sclerosi endoscopica consiste nell'iniezione di agenti sclerosanti o all'interno della varice o intorno a essa, fino all'arresto del sanguinamento. Sebbene l'emorragia acuta possa essere controllata nella maggior parte dei casi, sono in genere necessarie ulteriori sessioni di scleroterapia per ottenere un'obliterazione temporanea delle varici. Il trattamento può complicarsi con ulteriore sanguinamento, batteriemia, ulcerazione esofagea e formazione di stenosi. La maggior parte dei centri non effettua la scleroterapia delle varici a scopo profilattico, ma si serve di questa procedura per guadagnare tempo in attesa del trapianto epatico, o fino a quando non si sia sviluppato un circolo collaterale nell'ostruzione portale extraepatica. In studi condotti su pazienti adulti e pediatrici, la legatura elastica endoscopica delle varici si è dimostrata più efficace e associata a un minor numero di complicanze rispetto alla scleroterapia.

Nei pazienti che continuano a sanguinare nonostante il trattamento medico ed endoscopico, si può posizionare una sonda di Sengstaken-Blakemore, che arresta l'emorragia grazie alla compressione meccanica delle varici esofagee e gastriche. Talvolta questo è l'unico strumento in grado di controllare un'emorragia massiva, pur comportando un rischio significativo di complicanze e un elevato tasso di risanguinamento al momento della rimozione. In particolare sussiste un rischio elevato di aspirazione polmonare e la sonda non è tollerata nei bambini, in assenza di un'adeguata sedazione.

Sono state sviluppate varie procedure chirurgiche con lo scopo di deviare il flusso ematico portale e ridurre la pressione portale. Uno shunt portocavale devia quasi la totalità del flusso portale nella vena cava inferiore sottoepatica. Pur riducendo significativamente la pressione portale, quest'importante deviazione di sangue dal fegato può comportare un rischio significativo di encefalopatia epatica, nei pazienti con epatopatia parenchimale. Procedure di shunting più selettive, come lo shunt mesocavale o splenorenale distale, possono esercitare un'efficace decompressione del sistema portale, consentendo una maggior quantità di flusso al fegato. Le piccole dimensioni dei vasi rendono questi interventi tecnicamente ardui nei neonati e nei bambini più piccoli, con un rischio significativo di fallimento a causa di trombosi. La trombosi della vena porta viene trattata con lo shunt REX (bypass mesenterica-ramo portale sinistro), che ripristina il flusso portale fisiologico e l'apporto di fattori epatotropi.

Il trapianto epatico ortotopico rappresenta la terapia migliore dell'ipertensione portale da cause intraepatiche. Una pregressa procedura di shunt portosistemico non pregiudica la possibilità di un trapianto efficace, anche se rende l'intervento tecnicamente più difficile. Lo shunt portosistemico resta una valida alternativa nei bambini con ipertensione portale extraepatica, in particolare in quelli predisposti alle emorragie pericolose per la vita, non controllate efficacemente da altre misure, e che risiedono a una certa distanza da centri ospedalieri con un pronto soccorso. Lo shunt portosistemico intraepatico transgiugulare (TIPS, *Transjugular Intrahepatic Portosystemic Shunt*), eseguito da un radiologo, consiste nel posizionare uno stent tra la vena epatica destra e la vena porta destra o sinistra. Questa procedura, pur essendo talvolta utile per controllare l'ipertensione portale nei bambini, soprattutto in quelli che necessitano di un supporto in attesa del trapianto epatico, può aggravare l'encefalopatia epatica e la tendenza alla trombosi.

La terapia a lungo termine con β-bloccanti aspecifici, come il propranololo, è stata ampiamente utilizzata negli adulti con ipertensione portale. Questi farmaci agiscono verosimilmente tramite la riduzione della gittata cardiaca e della perfusione portale. I dati disponibili dimostrano che nei pazienti adulti i β-bloccanti riducono l'incidenza di emorragia da varici e migliorano la sopravvivenza a lungo termine. L'effetto terapeutico è ottenuto con una riduzione delle pulsazioni pari almeno al 25%. Tuttavia, al momento sono scarse le pubblicazioni relative all'uso di questi farmaci nei bambini.

PROGNOSI. L'ipertensione portale secondaria a malattie intraepatiche ha una prognosi severa, essendo in genere progressiva e spesso associata a deterioramento della funzione epatica. È imperativo adoperarsi sempre per instaurare un trattamento tempestivo del sanguinamento acuto e per prevenire le recidive emorragiche, con i metodi attualmente a disposizione. I pazienti con epatopatia progressiva e varici esofagee importanti necessitano, in ultima analisi, del trapianto epatico. Quest'ultimo, oltre a rappresentare l'unica terapia efficace della sindrome epatopolmonare, dovrebbe essere preso in considerazione anche in caso di ipertensione portale secondaria a ostruzione delle vene epatiche da malattia veno-occlusiva severa.

Nei pazienti con ostruzione portale, la frequenza e la gravità degli episodi di sanguinamento possono ridursi con l'età, in conseguenza dello sviluppo di un circolo collaterale. La maggior parte di essi può essere trattata conservativamente con scleroterapia o legatura endoscopiche, al bisogno. Alcuni tuttavia continuano a presentare anche in età adolescenziale emorragie significative, per le quali si rende infine necessario uno shunt portosistemico.

Botha JF, Campos, BD, Grant, WJ, et al: Portosystemic shunts in children: A 15-year experience. *J Am Coll Surg* 2004;199:179–185.

Gauthier-Villars M, Franchi S, Gauthier F, et al: Cholestasis in children with portal vein obstruction. *J Pediatr* 2005;146:568–573.

Gentil-Kocher S, Bernard O, Brunelle F, et al: Budd-Chiari syndrome in children: Report of 22 cases. *J Pediatr* 1988;113:30–38.

Heyman MB, LaBerge JM, Somberg KA, et al: Transjugular intrahepatic portosystemic shunts (TIPS) in children. *J Pediatr* 1997;131:914–919.

Hoeper MM, Krowka MJ, Strassburg CP: Portopulmonary hypertension and hepatopulmonary syndrome. *Lancet* 2004;363:1461–1468.

Lykavieris P, Gauthier F, Hadchouel P, et al: Risk of gastrointestinal bleeding during adolescence and early adulthood in children with portal vein obstruction. *J Pediatr* 2000;136:805–808.

Miga D, Sokol RJ, Mackenzie T, et al: Survival after first esophageal variceal hemorrhage in patients with biliary atresia. *J Pediatr* 2001;139: 291–296.
Narayanan Menon KV, Shah V, Kamath PS: The Budd-Chiari syndrome. *N Engl J Med* 2004;350:578–584.
Peter L, Dadhich SK, Yachha SK: Clinical and laboratory differentiation of cirrhosis and extrahepatic portal venous obstruction in children. *J Gastroenterol Hepatol* 2003;18:185–189.
Ryckman FC, Alonso MH: Causes and management of portal hypertension in the pediatric population. *Clin Liver Dis* 2001;5:789–818.
Sarin SK, Agarwal SR: Extrahepatic portal vein obstruction. *Semin Liver Dis* 2002;22:43–58.
Shashidhar H, Langhans N, Grand RJ: Propranolol in prevention of portal hypertensive hemorrhage in children: A pilot study. *J Pediatr Gastroenterol Nutr* 1999;29:12–17.

Capitolo 365 ■ Trapianto epatico

Melissa Hurwitz e Kenneth L. Cox

Il trapianto epatico è la terapia di scelta nei bambini con insufficienza epatica terminale, malattie metaboliche epatiche potenzialmente fatali, insufficienza epatica severa da farmaci (paracetamolo) o tossine (funghi) e tumori epatici localizzati. Con le attuali strategie di immunosoppressione e tecniche chirurgiche, i tassi di sopravvivenza a 1 anno e a 5 anni dal trapianto sono, per i bambini, dell'87% e del 77%, rispettivamente. Un terzo dei riceventi in età pediatrica ha meno di 1 anno di età al momento del trapianto e a 1 anno dall'intervento presenta una sopravvivenza significativamente inferiore (85%) rispetto ai bambini più grandi (90%). Negli Stati Uniti circa 500 bambini sono sottoposti ogni anno a trapianto epatico, di cui il 6% subisce un trapianto multiorgano, che comprende in genere il rene o l'intestino tenue (vedi Capitolo 336). L'indicazione più frequente al trapianto epatico è l'atresia biliare extraepatica, dopo il fallimento di una portoenterostomia (procedura di Kasai). Le malattie metaboliche e la necrosi epatica acuta occupano il secondo posto, in ordine di frequenza (Tab. 365-1). La decisione di effettuare un trapianto, nei pazienti con malattie metaboliche epatiche, si basa sulle seguenti valutazioni: la malattia è di origine epatica? È possibile trattarla con successo con la sola terapia medica? Sono presenti manifestazioni extraepatiche reversibili?

Il pronto invio a un centro trapianti è di fondamentale importanza per assicurare ai pazienti e alle loro famiglie una valutazione e un trattamento appropriati e tempestivi. Si valutano numerose caratteristiche mediche e psicologiche per determinare l'opportunità di procedere al trapianto, il trattamento ottimale e l'urgenza. L'età (<1 anno), il ritardo di crescita (definito come un peso o un'altezza inferiori al normale di 2 deviazioni standard), l'iperbilirubinemia, l'ipoalbuminemia e la coagulopatia, consistenti in un aumento dell'INR (*International Normalized Ratio*), si sono rivelati fattori predittivi di aumento della mortalità e morbilità da epatopatia, e rappresentano i criteri su cui ci si basa per determinare l'urgenza del trapianto. Altre variabili che indicano anch'esse la necessità del trapianto epatico sono l'ascite, l'encefalopatia, il sanguinamento da varici e l'insufficienza renale. Il pronto invio a un centro trapianti dei pazienti con insufficienza epatica fulminante è un fattore critico, poiché la maggior parte dei pazienti muore dopo poco tempo in assenza di trapianto. Il counseling familiare sulle particolari necessità dei bambini con malattia cronica migliora gli aspetti psicosociali. La valutazione precoce consente non solo di guadagnare tempo prezioso per la ricerca di un donatore, ma anche di informare adeguatamente le famiglie sul trapianto epatico. Il trattamento pretrapianto è fondamentale per il successo della procedura e per limitare la morbilità da epatopatia (vedi Capitoli 353, 361 e 364). Nei bambini con atresia biliare si dovrebbe effettuare una portoenterostomia, poiché questa procedura permette di rimandare il trapianto epatico e talvolta di farne a meno. Anche i lattanti con atresia biliare di età <3 mesi possono trarre beneficio da questa procedura.

Le aree di maggior importanza sono la nutrizione e l'immunizzazione. I pazienti con epatopatia hanno spesso malassorbimento e anoressia, che portano a un ritardo della crescita. Le formule contenenti trigliceridi a catena media sono utili, poiché non necessitano dei sali biliari per l'assorbimento. Il fabbisogno calorico può raggiungere le 150 kcal/kg/die. La nutrizione notturna con sondino nasogastrico e la nutrizione parenterale, soprattutto lipidica, possono rendersi necessarie a causa dell'anoressia e del malassorbimento.

Il deficit di vitamine liposolubili deve essere prevenuto con la somministrazione di supplementi vitaminici. Per ovviare alla carenza di vitamina E (atassia, neuropatia periferica, ritardo motorio grossolano) si ricorre alla somministrazione di preparazioni ben assorbite, idrosolubili, contenenti d-α-tocoferolo polietilenglicole succinato. L'osteopatia da deficit di vitamina D si previene con preparazioni orali di 25-idrossivitamina D_3. Carenze di vitamina A si manifestano precocemnte nella cornea e nella congiuntiva; si possono prevenire con preparati orali idrosolubili di vitamina A. Di frequente riscontro è la carenza di vitamina K, sotto forma di un aumento del tempo di protrombina che talvolta risponde alla supplementazione orale, ma spesso richiede la somministrazione parenterale di vitamina K. L'assorbimento delle vitamina e dei grassi può essere stimolato con acido ursodesossicolico, un acido biliare intraluminale ad azione coleretica (aumenta il flusso biliare all'intestino). Occorre monitorare i livelli sierici di vitamine E, D ed A, oltre al tempo di protrombina. La carenza di ferro, causata da perdite ematiche occulte, e quella di zinco possono verificarsi in associazione con diarrea cronica.

Si consiglia di immunizzare i pazienti per l'epatite A e B, per evitare la possibilità di un ulteriore danno epatico; i vaccini contenenti virus vivi (morbillo, rosolia, parotite, varicella) devono essere somministrati secondo il piano normale, poiché l'immunosoppressione post-trapianto potrebbe poi controindicarli.

Il trattamento medico deve anche essere volto anche al controllo del sanguinamento da varici, dell'ascite, dell'encefalopatia, della coagulopatia e della sepsi. In attesa del trapianto, la morbilità e la mortalità da insufficienza epatica possono essere ridotte con la diagnosi e il trattamento precoci di queste complicanze. Le probabilità che il trapianto abbia successo sono aumentate grazie al miglioramento delle tecniche di conservazione dell'organo (fino a 18 ore *ex vivo*, con <2% di non funzionamento primitivo), al perfezionamento delle tecniche chirurgiche, e ai progressi compiuti nel campo della terapia immunosoppressiva. La disponibilità di donatori per pazienti pediatrici è stata ampliata grazie

TABELLA 365-1. Indicazioni al trapianto epatico in età pediatrica

INDICAZIONI	PERCENTUALE DI TRAPIANTI (%)
Atresia biliare	39
Epatopatia metabolica	13
Deficit di α_1-antitripsina	5
Tirosinemia	1
Malattia di Wilson	1
Altre*	6
Necrosi epatica acuta	12
Ipoplasia biliare, sindrome di Alagille compresa	5
Epatopatia associata a TPN	5
Cirrosi idiopatica	4
Epatite autoimmune	3
Tumori, incluso l'epatoblastoma	3
Epatite neonatale	2
Fibrosi cistica	2
Colangite sclerosante primitiva	2
Fibrosi epatica congenita	1
Altre	9

*Inclusi i difetti del ciclo dell'urea.
I dati provengono dall'United Network for Organ Sharing Data Base per 8950 trapianti epatici pediatrici effettuati su bambini tra il 1° gennaio 1998 e il 31 ottobre 2004.

all'utilizzo di un lobo o di un segmento epatico da cadavere o da donatore vivente, e con l'uso di gruppi sanguigni ABO diversi. Anche la donazione da vivente del lobo epatico destro ha avuto successo con riceventi adolescenti e adulti. In genere, nei bambini più piccoli si collegano le vie biliari a un'ansa a Y alla Roux del digiuno e si effettuano anastomosi vascolari dirette. Occasionalmente si utilizzano trapianti di vene dal donatore, nei casi di trombosi portale pretrapianto.

La terapia standard per la prevenzione del rigetto prevede l'uso di steroidi con ciclosporina o tacrolimus. Rispetto alla ciclosporina, il tacrolimus è risultato associato a percentuali inferiori di rigetto acuto e cronico. La ciclosporina in formulazione idrosolubile microemulsionata è assorbita meglio della forma liposolubile, dipendente dagli acidi biliari, ed è paragonabile al tacrolimus nella prevenzione del rigetto. Gli effetti collaterali specifici comprendono irsutismo e iperplasia gengivale.

Le complicanze precoci nel periodo postoperatorio consistono in spostamento di liquidi, squilibri elettrolitici, disfunzione renale e ipertensione. L'insufficienza primitiva dell'organo trapiantato o le complicanze vascolari, come la trombosi dei vasi dell'organo, sono problemi drammatici che spesso conducono al decesso, se l'organo non viene sostituito al massimo entro 48 ore. Dopo questa fase precoce, i problemi più frequenti sono le infezioni e il rigetto d'organo. Le infezioni batteriche, compresa la colangite, sono le più comuni, seguite da quelle virali (Cytomegalovirus, adenovirus), fungine e, raramente, parassitarie (*Pneumocystis carinii*). La degenza media è di circa 2-3 settimane, ma può arrivare a diversi mesi. Possono insorgere complicanze tardive, come rigetto, disfunzione renale da ciclosporina o tacrolimus, malattia linfoproliferativa post-trapianto associata a virus di Epstein-Barr (EBV), che può evolvere in un linfoma. Il rigetto, nei bambini più grandi, è spesso legato a una ridotta compliance.

Quando il rigetto ha richiesto una terapia ad alte dosi con ciclosporina o tacrolimus, e/o l'uso continuativo di steroidi, l'azatioprina, il sirolimus, o il micofenolato mofetile possono controllare il fenomeno e consentire di ridurre le dosi dei farmaci più tossici. Sono stati usati anche anticorpi monoclonali murini anti-linfociti T (OKT3) per trattare i casi di rigetto grave e steroidoresistente. La timoglobulina, un preparato policlonale antilinfocitico meno tossico, trova impiego nel rigetto grave.

Le malattie linfoproliferative post-trapianto (PTLD, *Post-Transplant Lymphoproliferative Disease*) insorgono nel 4-11% dei bambini, sono associate a dosi elevate di terapia immunosoppressiva e a infezione da HBV, e hanno una mortalità complessiva del 10-20%. I gruppi EBV-naïve, più giovani di età, sono a rischio maggiore di sviluppare un'infezione primaria da EBV nel periodo post-trapianto. La morbilità e la mortalità da PTLD si sono ridotte grazie alla diagnosi precoce, consentita da un monitoraggio frequente della sierologia dell'EBV e dell'EBV-PCR, all'utilizzo del ganciclovir per via endovenosa nei periodo post-trapianto, nei pazienti ad alto rischio, e alla sospensione o riduzione dell'immunosoppressione non appena viene riscontrata l'infezione da EBV.

La pressione sanguigna e la clearance della creatinina devono essere sempre monitorate, poiché l'ipertensione arteriosa e l'insufficienza renale sono complicanze a lungo termine molto comuni, soprattutto nei bambini che ricevono ciclosporina o tacrolimus a dosi elevate.

La prognosi, per chi sopravvive alla fase precoce, è molto incoraggiante. La maggior parte dei bambini ha un miglioramento della crescita e dello sviluppo, mentre i segni della pregressa epatopatia cronica si risolvono progressivamente. I pazienti e le loro famiglie possono tornare a una vita normale. È sempre necessario uno stretto monitoraggio delle problematiche non solo mediche, ma anche psicosociali. Sebbene alcuni possano sviluppare tolleranza all'organo trapiantato e non necessitare di un'immunosoppressione a vita, la maggior parte va incontro a rigetto fino a 4 anni dopo la sospensione della terapia immunosoppressiva. I bambini vanno dunque sottoposti a immunosoppressione a tempo indefinito, in attesa di nuove metodologie in grado di identificare quelli che hanno sviluppato davvero tolleranza.

Bartosh, S, Thomas SE, Sutton MM, et al: Linear growth after pediatric liver transplantation. *J Pediatr* 1999;135:624–631.

Cacciarelli TV, Reyes J, Jaffe R, et al: Primary tacrolimus (FK506) therapy and the long-term risk of post-transplant lymphoproliferative disease in pediatric liver transplant recipients. *Pediatr Transplant* 2001;5:359–364.

Chardot C, Carton M, Spire-Bendelac N, et al: Is the Kasai operation still indicated in children older than 3 months diagnosed with biliary atresia? *J Pediatr* 2001;138:224–228.

Cherqui D, Soubrane O, Husson E, et al: Laparoscopic living donor hepatectomy for liver transplantation in children. *Lancet* 2002;359:392–396.

Cox K, Rodriguez-Baez N, Nasr A, et al: Mortality rate correlated with the number of pediatric liver transplants performed at a center. *Transplant Proc* 2001;33:1512–1513.

Hurwitz M, Desai DM, Cox KL, et al: Complete immunosuppressive drug withdrawal as a uniform approach to post-transplant lymphoproliferative disease in pediatric liver transplantation. *Pediatr Transplant* 2004;8:267–272.

McDiarmid SV: Liver transplantation: The pediatric challenge. *Clin Liver Dis* 2000;4:879–927.

Split Research Group: Studies of Pediatric Liver Transplantation (SPLIT): Year 2000 outcomes. *Transplantation* 2001;72:463–476.

United Network for Organ Sharing (UNOS) Scientific Registry data as of December 31, 2004. Available online at www.unos.org/data

Van Mourik IDM, Beath SV, Brook GA, et al: Long-term nutritional and neurodevelopmental outcomes of liver transplantation in infants aged less than 12 month. *J Pediatr Gastroenterol Nutr* 2000;30:269–275.

Wayman KI, Cox KL, Esquivel CO: Neurodevelopmental outcome of young children with extrahepatic biliary atresia 1 year after liver transplantation. *J Pediatr* 1997;131:894–898.

Sezione 7 — Peritoneo

Capitolo 366 ■ Malformazioni

Jeffrey S. Hyams

Le bande peritoneali congenite possono essere responsabili di occlusioni intestinali; durante lo sviluppo del peritoneo possono verificarsi anche molte altre anomalie, che tuttavia è raro risultino clinicamente significative. Raramente si sviluppano ernie intraddominali attraverso formazioni ad anello prodotte da bande peritoneali anomale. L'assenza o la duplicazione dell'omento è un'eventualità rara. Le cisti omentali, che si formano in canali linfatici ostruiti, all'interno dell'omento, possono essere congenite o post-traumatiche e sono in genere asintomatiche. Talvolta la compressione o la torsione dell'intestino tenue, per trazione da parte dell'omento, determinano dolore addominale o ostruzione parziale dell'intestino tenue.

Capitolo 367 ■ Ascite Jeffrey S. Hyams

L'ascite è un accumulo di liquido sieroso nella cavità peritoneale. Molte sono le cause possibili (Tab. 367-1); le più frequenti nei bambini sono le malattie epatiche, renali e cardiache.

La caratteristica tipica dell'ascite è la tensione addominale, che tuttavia può essere dovuta anche ad altre condizioni, come distensione gassosa, ritenzione fecale, masse tumorali, emorragia peritoneale, distensione estrema della vescica, gravidanza e obesità. Si può accumulare una notevole quantità di liquido prima che l'ascite si renda rilevabile tramite i cinque segni classici: fianchi prominenti, ottusità declive, ottusità mobile, onda liquida e segno della vibrazione (ridotta auscultazione delle vibrazioni a elevata frequenza nella parte centrale dell'addome, mentre si colpisce delicatamente il lato dell'addome, con il paziente appoggiato su mani e ginocchia). L'ascite tesa si può associare a ernia ombelicale. L'esame ecografico è in grado di rilevare anche un'ascite di piccola entità.

Il decorso, la prognosi e il trattamento dell'ascite variano a seconda della causa. I pazienti con ascite di qualsiasi origine presentano un rischio aumentato di sviluppare peritonite batterica spontanea.

TABELLA 367-1. Cause di ascite

EPATICHE	**GASTROINTESTINALI**
Cirrosi	Infarto intestinale
Fibrosi epatica congenita	Perforazione
Ostruzione della vena porta	**NEOPLASTICHE**
Insufficienza epatica fulminante	Linfomi
Sindrome di Budd-Chiari	Neuroblastoma
Malattia da accumulo lisosomiale	**GINECOLOGICHE**
RENALI	Tumori ovarici
Sindrome nefrosica	Torsione o rottura ovarica
Uropatia ostruttiva	**PANCREATICHE**
Perforazione delle vie urinarie	Pancreatite
Dialisi peritoneale	Rottura del dotto pancreatico
CARDIACHE	**MISTE**
Insufficienza cardiaca	Lupus eritematoso sistemico
Pericardite costrittiva	Shunt ventricoloperitoneale
Reti della vena cava inferiore	Ascite eosinofila
INFETTIVE	Ascite chilosa
Ascessi	Ipotiroidismo
Tubercolosi	
Chlamydia	
Schistosomiasi	

Sabri M, Saps M, Peters JM: Pathophysiology and management of pediatric ascites. *Curr Gastroenterol Rep* 2003;5:240–246.

367.1 • Ascite chilosa

L'ascite chilosa può risultare da un'anomalia, un danno o un'ostruzione della porzione addominale del dotto toracico. Sebbene sia rara, può insorgere a qualsiasi età. Le cause comprendono malformazioni congenite, bande peritoneali, linfangiomatosi generalizzata, processi infiammatori cronici dell'intestino, tumori, linfoadenomegalie, pregressa chirurgia addominale e traumi. Le anomalie congenite del sistema linfatico si possono associare alle sindromi di Turner, Nooan, dell'unghia gialla e di Klippel-Trenaunay-Weber.

Nei neonati, si nota una distensione addominale rapidamente progressiva, associata a scarso aumento ponderale e feci non formate. È frequente il riscontro di edemi periferici. L'ascite chilosa massiva può comportare edema scrotale, ernie inguinali e ombelicali, disfunzione respiratoria.

La diagnosi di ascite chilosa si basa sulla dimostrazione di liquido ascitico lattigginoso, ottenuto tramite paracentesi, dopo un pasto contenente lipidi. L'analisi del liquido rivela un abbondante contenuto proteico, trigliceridi elevati e linfocitosi. Se il paziente è a digiuno, il liquido può apparire sieroso. È frequente riscontrare ipoalbuminemia, ipogammaglobulinemia e linfopenia.

Il trattamento comprende la somministrazione di supplementi dietetici a elevato contenuto proteico e basso contenuto lipidico, con trigliceridi a catena media, che vengono assorbiti direttamente nella circolazione portale. Se lo stato nutritivo basato sull'alimentazione orale resta alterato può rendersi necessaria la nutrizione parenterale, che permette inoltre di ridurre il flusso linfatico facilitando così la guarigione del punto di dispersione della linfa. È stato utilizzato anche l'octreotide, un analogo della somatostatina. La paracentesi deve essere ripetuta solo quando la distensione addominale causa difficoltà respiratoria. La laparotomia può essere indicata per ricercare la sede della perdita, dopo il fallimento di un tentativo su base dietetica.

Aalami AO, Allen DB, Organ CH: Chylous ascites: A collective review. *Surgery* 2000;128:761–768.
Caty MG, Hilfiker ML, Azizkhan RG, et al: Successful treatment of congenital chylous ascites with somatostatin analogue. *Pediatr Surg Int* 1996;11:396–397.
Man DW, Spitz L: The management of chylous ascites in children. *J Pediatr Surg* 1985;20:72–75.

Capitolo 368 ■ Peritonite Elias S. Hyams e Jeffrey S. Hyams

L'infiammazione del peritoneo che delimita la cavità addominale può derivare da processi infettivi, autoimmuni, neoplastici o chimici. La peritonite infettiva può essere primitiva (spontanea) o secondaria. Nella forma primitiva, l'infezione origina all'esterno dell'addome e si dissemina attraverso la cavità peritoneale per via ematogena, linfatica o trasmurale; in quella secondaria si instaura nella cavità peritoneale a causa della rottura di un viscere endoaddominale o di un ascesso in un organo. La peritonite terziaria indica la malattia ricorrente diffusa o localizzata, che si associa a un esito meno favorevole rispetto a quella secondaria.

La peritonite del neonato può essere conseguenza di un'infezione transplacentare in utero, anche se più spesso è il risultato di un'infezione acquisita nel periodo perinatale. Può essere una manifestazione di setticemia, un'estensione diretta da un'infezione ombelicale, da una perforazione dell'intestino, da un'enterocolite necrotizzante o, raramente, la sequela di una perforzione dell'appendice o di un diverticolo di Meckel. La peritonite da meconio è descritta nei Capitoli 102.1 e 327.

Evans HL, Raymond DP, Pelletier SJ, et al: Tertiary peritonitis (recurrent diffuse or localized disease) is not an independent predictor of mortality in surgical patients with intra-abdominal infection. *Surg Infect* 2001;2: 255–263.

368.1 • Peritonite acuta primitiva

EZIOLOGIA ED EPIDEMIOLOGIA. Con l'espressione "peritonite primitiva" si intende un'infezione batterica della cavità peritoneale senza un focolaio di origine endoaddominale dimostrabile. La maggior parte dei casi si verifica in bambini con ascite da sindrome nefrosica o da cirrosi. L'infezione può risultare dalla traslocazione batterica dal lume intestinale o da una disfunzione immunitaria, mentre insorge di rado in bambini in buona salute. I patogeni responsabili identificati più spesso sono gli pneumococchi (i più frequenti), gli streptococchi di gruppo A, gli enterococchi, gli stafilococchi e gli enterobatteri Gram-negativi, in particolare l'*Escherichia coli* e la *Klebsiella pneumoniae*; sono invece di più raro riscontro il *Mycobacterium tuberculosis* e il *M. bovis*. I due sessi sono colpiti in egual misura; la maggior parte dei casi si verifica prima dei 6 anni di età.

MANIFESTAZIONI CLINICHE. L'esordio, che può essere insidioso o brusco, è caratterizzato da febbre, dolore addominale, vomito, diarrea e "aspetto tossico". È frequente l'ipotensione, accompagnata da tachicardia e respiro rapido e superficiale, a causa del dolore scatenato dal movimento dei muscoli respiratori. Alla palpazione addominale si possono riscontrare rigidità e dolorabilità di rimbalzo. I rumori peristaltici sono ridotti o assenti. Una precedente terapia steroidea può attenuare l'espressione clinica della peritonite, ritardando la diagnosi.

DIAGNOSI E TRATTAMENTO. La leucocitosi periferica, con una marcata predominanza di polimorfonucleati, è frequente, sebbene la conta leucocitaria possa essere influenzata da un ipersplenismo preesistente, nei pazienti con cirrosi. Nei soggetti con sindrome nefrosica e proteinuria la ridotta albuminemia si associa a un rischio più elevato di peritonite. La radiografia dell'addome rivela dilatazione dell'intestino tenue e del crasso, con aumento della distanza tra le anse, dovuto all'ispessimento della parete intestinale. Talora, nei pazienti senza un'anamnesi di cirrosi o sindrome nefrosica, può essere impossibile distinguere una peritonite primitiva da un'appendicite; pertanto, la diagnosi di peritonite primitiva viene posta tramite TC, laparoscopia o laparotomia. In un bambino con una malattia epatica o renale nota e ascite, la presenza di segni peritoneali dovrebbe indurre a eseguire una paracentesi diagnostica. Nei casi di infezione, il liquido ascitico presenta una conta leucocitaria $\geq$250 cellule/mm^3, con i polimorfonucleati che rappresentano $>$50%.

Altre caratteristiche del liquido ascitico suggestive di peritonite primitiva comprendono un pH $<$7,35, un gradiente del pH tra sangue arterioso e liquido ascitico $>$0,1 ed elevati livelli di lattato. La colorazione di Gram del liquido rivela tipicamente un'unica specie di batteri Gram-positivi o, meno frequentemente, Gram-negativi. La presenza di una flora batterica mista nel liquido ascitico o di aria libera alla radiografia dell'addome, nei bambini con sospetta peritonite primitiva, impone una laparotomia per localizzare un'eventuale perforazione come probabile origine dell'infezione. L'inoculazione del liquido ascitico, ottenuto con la paracentesi, direttamente nei flaconi da emocoltura aumenta la probabilità di positività delle colture. L'antibioticoterapia parenterale, con cefotaxima più un aminoglicoside, deve essere iniziata subito, con successive variazioni in base all'antibiogramma (usare la vancomicina per gli pneumococchi resistenti). La terapia dovrebbe durare almeno 10-14 giorni.

L'ascite neutrofilica, sterile alle colture, è una variante della peritonite primitiva che presenta una conta leucocitaria $>$500 cellule/mm^3, colture negative, assenza di focolai endoaddominali di infezione e assenza di pregresse terapie antibiotiche. Deve essere trattata come una normale peritonite primitiva.

Garcia-Tsao G: Spontaneous bacterial peritonitis: A historical perspective. *J Hepatology* 2004;41:522–527.

Hingorani SR, Weiss NS, Watkins SL: Predictors of peritonitis in children with nephrotic syndrome. *Pediatr Nephrol* 2002;17:678–682.

Runyon BA: Early events in spontaneous bacterial peritonitis. *Gut* 2004;53:782–784.

368.2 • PERITONITE ACUTA SECONDARIA

È causata dall'ingresso di batteri enterici nella cavità peritoneale, attraverso un'alterazione necrotica della parete intestinale o di altro viscere, imputabile a un'ostruzione, a un infarto o alla rottura di un ascesso di un viscere addominale. La causa più comune è la perforazione dell'appendice. Altre cause gastrointestinali comprendono ernie incarcerate, rottura di un diverticolo di Meckel, volvolo dell'intestino medio, intussuscezione, sindrome uremico-emolitica, ulcera peptica, malattie infiammatorie intestinali, colecistite necrotizzante, enterocolite necrotizzante, tiflite e perforazione traumatica. Nel periodo neonatale, la peritonite insorge generalmente come complicanza di un'enterocolite necrotizzante, ma si può associare anche a ileo da meconio o rottura spontanea (o indotta da indometacina) dello stomaco o dell'intestino. Nelle ragazze in età postpuberale, i batteri del tratto genitale (*Neisseria gonorrhoeae*, *Chlamydia trachomatis*) possono raggiungere la cavità peritoneale attraverso le tube di Falloppio, causando una peritonite secondaria. La presenza di corpi estranei, come un catetere ventricoloperitoneale o un catetere da dialisi peritoneale, può predisporre alla peritonite a opera di microrganismi cutanei, come *Staphylococcus epidermidis*, *S. aureus* e *Candida albicans*, che possono contaminare lo shunt. La peritonite secondaria si sviluppa in conseguenza sia dell'effetto tossico diretto dei batteri, sia del rilascio di mediatori infiammatori a livello sistemico, in risposta ai microrganismi e ai loro prodotti (LPS, endotossine). Lo sviluppo di sepsi dipende da vari fattori relativi all'ospite e al patogeno, così come dalla tempestività della terapia antibiotica e dell'intervento chirurgico.

MANIFESTAZIONI CLINICHE. Come nella peritonite primitiva, i sintomi caratteristici comprendono febbre ($\geq$39,5 °C), dolore addominale diffuso, nausea e vomito. I segni obiettivi di infiammazione peritoneale comprendono dolorabilità di rimbalzo, rigidità della parete addominale, limitazione dei movimenti (posizione supina, immobile) e rumori peristaltici ridotti o assenti a causa dell'ileo paralitico. La massiva essudazione di liquidi nella cavità peritoneale, insieme al rilascio sistemico di mediatori ad azione vasodilatatoria, può portare rapidamente allo sviluppo di shock. Sono comuni l'"aspetto tossico", l'irritabilità e l'irrequietezza. Si può sviluppare atelettasia basale, con effetto di shunt intrapolmonare e progressione alla sindrome da distress respiratorio acuto (ARDS, *Acute Respiratory Distress Syndrome*).

I dati di laboratorio mostrano una leucocitosi periferica $>$12 000 cellule/mm^3, con una netta predominanza dei polimorfonucleati. Le radiografie dirette dell'addome possono rivelare la presenza di aria libera nella cavità peritoneale, segni di ostruzione o di ileo, versamento peritoneale o offuscamento dell'ombra dello psoas.

TRATTAMENTO. Occorre instaurare immediatamente le misure di sostegno della volemia e della funzione cardiovascolare. È fondamentale stabilizzare il paziente prima dell'intervento chirurgico. L'antibioticoterapia deve coprire i patogeni prevalenti nella sede di origine presunta dell'infezione. Nei casi di perforazione del tratto intestinale inferiore, una combinazione di ampicillina, gentamicina e clindamicina può coprire adeguatamente le infezioni da *E. coli*, *Klebsiella*, *Bacteroides* spp. ed enterococchi. Un approccio alternativo può consistere nell'associazione di ticarcillina-acido clavulanico con un aminoglicoside. L'intervento chirurgico, per riparare un viscere perforato, deve essere effettuato solo con il paziente stabilizzato e dopo l'inizio della terapia antibiotica. Le colture intraoperatorie di liquido peritoneale potranno eventualmente indicare se occorra apportare modifiche alla terapia antibiotica. Il trattamento empirico nella peritonite correlata a catetere da dialisi peritoneale (DP) comprende cefazolina più ceftazidima, imipenem/cilastatina o vancomicina/ciprofloxacina. Di norma le infezioni più gravi da catetere per DP possono essere prevenute con una buona igiene del catetere stesso e la rapida rimozione o sostituzione, ai primi segni di infezione progressiva.

Anaya DA, Nathens AB: Risk factors for severe sepsis in secondary peritonitis. *Surg Infect (Larchmt)* 2003;4:355–362.
Goffin E, Herbiet L, Pouthier D, et al: Vancomycin and ciprofloxacin: Systemic antibiotic administration for peritoneal dialysis-associated peritonitis. *Perit Dial Int* 2004;24:433–439.
Leung CB, Szeto CC, Chow KM, et al: Cefazolin plus ceftazidime versus imipenem/cilastatin monotherapy for treatment of CAPD peritonitis—A randomized control trial. *Perit Dial Int* 2004;24:440–446.
Malangoni MA: Current concepts in peritonitis. *Curr Gastroenterol Rep* 2003;5:295–301.
Piraino B: New insights on preventing and managing peritonitis. *Pediatr Nephrol* 2004;19:125–127.

368.3 • Peritonite acuta secondaria localizzata (ascesso peritoneale)

EZIOLOGIA. Gli ascessi endoaddominali sono meno frequenti nei bambini e nei lattanti che negli adulti, ma possono svilupparsi sia negli organi viscerali endoaddominali (ascessi epatici, splenici, renali, pancreatici, tubo-ovarici), sia nello spazio interintestinale, sottodiaframmatico, sottoepatico, pelvico o retroperitoneale. Gli ascessi periappendicolari e pelvici originano per lo più da una perforazione dell'appendice. Nei bambini affetti da morbo di Crohn un'infiammazione transmurale, con la formazione di una fistola, può portare all'insorgenza di un ascesso.

MANIFESTAZIONI CLINICHE. Una febbre prolungata, con anoressia, vomito e stanchezza, suggerisce il possibile sviluppo di un ascesso endoaddominale. È presente leucocitosi periferica, con aumento della VES. Nei casi di ascesso appendicolare, si riscontrano una dolorabilità localizzata e una massa palpabile, nel quadrante addominale inferiore destro.

I segni che suggeriscono la presenza di un ascesso pelvico sono distensione addominale, tenesmo rettale, con o senza passaggio di feci mucose di piccole dimensioni, e irritabilità vescicale. L'esplorazione rettale può rivelare una massa dolente in posizione anteriore. Nei casi di ascesso sottodiaframmatico possono essere presenti raccolte di gas a livello subfrenico, atelettasia basale, elevazione di un emidiaframma e versamento pleurico. Un ascesso dello psoas si può sviluppare per estensione di un'infezione da un'appendice retrocecale, da un morbo di Crohn o da un ascesso perirenale o intrarenale. Mentre i reperti addominali possono essere minimi, la presentazione comprende spesso zoppia, dolore all'anca e febbre. Per la localizzazione degli ascessi addominali possono essere utili sia l'ecografia, sia la TC, sebbene quest'ultima abbia una maggior sensibilità e riesca a valutare anche lo spazio retroperitoneale.

TRATTAMENTO. È necessario drenare gli ascessi e instaurare un'appropriata terapia antibiotica. Il drenaggio può essere effettuato sotto controllo radiologico (ecoguidato o TC-guidato), lasciando in sede un catetere di drenaggio a permanenza. La copertura antibiotica, inizialmente ad ampio spettro, con ampicillina, gentamicina e clidamicina, in seguito va modificata in base ai risultati dell'antibiogramma. Il trattamento della rottura dell'appendice, complicata dalla formazione di un ascesso, può essere problematico, poiché la formazione di un flemmone intestinale rende la resezione chirurgica più difficile. Il trattamento abituale prevede una terapia antibiotica intensiva per 4-6 settimane, seguita da un'appendicectomia intervallare.

Brook I: Intra-abdominal, retroperitoneal, and visceral abscesses in children. *Eur J Pediatr Surg* 2004;14:265–273.
Wilson-Storey D, Scobie WG: Appendix masses—A 15-year review. *Pediatr Surg Int* 1989;4:168–170.

Capitolo 369 ■ Ernia epigastrica

John J. Aiken e Keith T. Oldham

Le ernie epigastriche sono ernie ventrali sulla linea mediana della parete addominale, tra il processo xifoideo e l'ombelico. Più spesso congenite che acquisite, derivano da difetti delle fibre decussanti della linea alba. Non se ne conosce la reale incidenza, in quanto sono per lo più di piccole dimensioni e asintomatiche, ma l'incidenza riportata in età infantile va da $<1\%$ al 5%. Le ernie epigastriche, singole o multiple, sono 2-3 volte più frequenti nei maschi che nelle femmine. Il difetto di parete contiene tipicamente solo grasso peritoneale, senza tratti di peritoneo o visceri addominali. Le ernie epigastriche (da incisione) possono insorgere anche nella sede di una pregressa incisione o associarsi al posizionamento di shunt ventricolo-peritoneali.

PRESENTAZIONE CLINICA. Le ernie epigastriche si presentano tipicamente nei bambini più piccoli come masse visibili o palpabili a livello della linea mediana, tra l'ombelico e il processo xifoideo, e sono notate dai genitori o dal medico di base. La massa è quasi sempre piccola (<1 cm) e asintomatica; è tipicamente sempre presente, ma diviene più evidente con il pianto o uno sforzo. Occasionalmente, la massa appare e scompare e il bambino riferisce dolore localizzato nella sede dell'ernia. L'esame obiettivo dimostra una massa dura, direttamente sulla linea mediana, in un punto qualunque tra il processo xifoideo e l'ombelico. Le ernie epigastriche contengono tipicamente solo tessuto grasso e non sono riducibili, a causa delle piccole dimensioni del difetto fasciale. È raro osservare un difetto fasciale in assenza di una massa palpabile. La massa può essere intermittente se il grasso si riduce con il rilassamento dei muscoli addominali. L'erniazione di tratti di intestino o di visceri addominali in un'ernia epigastrica è un evento assolutamente eccezionale. La massa può essere dolorabile alla palpazione, ma lo strangolamento del contenuto erniario è infrequente. Dal momento che l'esame obiettivo è quasi sempre diagnostico, non sono necessarie indagini radiologiche.

La storia naturale dell'ernia epigastrica prevede un graduale ingrandimento nel tempo, poiché sempre più grasso peritoneale viene estruso attraverso il difetto di parete, sotto sforzo o ogniqualvolta aumenti la pressione endoaddominale. Se non trattato, il difetto si può allargare consentendo l'erniazione di visceri addominali con il loro peritoneo.

Poiché le ernie epigastriche non si risolvono spontaneamente, l'intervento chirurgico è sempre raccomandato. La sede deve essere marcata attentamente nel preoperatorio, in quanto sia la massa, sia il difetto possono essere difficili da localizzare dopo l'induzione dell'anestesia. Si pratica un'incisione trasversa limitata sulla massa e si effettua una dissezione per delineare i margini del difetto fasciale. Se è presente del grasso erniato, lo si isola dal tessuto sottocutaneo affinché possa essere ridotto, legato o escisso. Il difetto viene chiuso con una sutura sottocuticolare riassorbibile. Le complicanze postoperatorie sono rare e il tasso di ricorrenza è basso.

Coats RD, Helikson MA, Burd RS: Presentation and management of epigastric hernias in children. *J Pediatr Surg* 2000;35:1754–1756.
Richards AT, Quinn TH, Fitzgibbons RJ Jr: Epigastric hernias. In Mulholland MW, Lillemoe KD, Doherty GM, et al (editors): *Greenfield's Surgery: Scientific Principles and Practice,* 4th ed. Philadelphia, Lippincott Williams and Wilkins, 2006, pp 1201–1202.
Skandalakis J, Gray SQW, Rickets R: The anterior abdominal wall. In Skandalakis JG (editor): *Embryology for Surgeons,* 2nd ed. Baltimore, Williams and Wilkins, 1994, pp 540–593.

369.1 • Ernie da incisione

La formazione di un'ernia nella sede di una pregressa laparotomia è un evento raro in età infantile. I fattori associati con un maggior rischio di ernia da incisione sono un'aumentata pressione endoaddominale, l'infezione della ferita e le incisioni della linea mediana. Le incisioni trasverse sono in genere preferite, per la maggior tenuta e il più elevato apporto di sangue, che riducono la probabilità di infezione e di ernie da incisione. Sebbene la maggior parte delle ernie di questo tipo necessiti della riparazione chirurgica, l'intervento dovrebbe essere rimandato fino a quando il bambino non sia nelle condizioni mediche ottimali. Alcune ernie incisionali possono risolversi, in particolare quelle che insorgono nei lattanti. Alcuni Autori raccomandano il bendaggio elastico per evitare l'aumento di dimensioni dell'ernia e favorire la guarigione spontanea. I neonati con difetti della parete addominale rappresentano il gruppo principale di bambini con ernie da incisione. Il trattamento iniziale deve essere conservativo; per la riparazione chirurgica occorrerà attendere che il paziente abbia raggiunto 1 anno di età. L'incarcerazione, peraltro molto rara, è un'indicazione all'intervento precoce.

Coats RD, Helikson MA, Burd RS: Presentation and management of epigastric hernias in children. *J Pediatr Surg* 2000;35:1754–1756.

Neblett KW, Holcomb TM: Umbilical and other abdominal wall hernias. In Ashcraft KW, Holder TM (editors): *Pediatric Surgery.* Philadelphia, WB Saunders, 1993, pp 557–561.

Parte XVIII ▪ Apparato respiratorio

Sezione 1 — Sviluppo e funzione

Capitolo 370 ▪ Fisiopatologia e regolazione della respirazione

Ashok P. Sarnaik e Sabrina M. Heidemann

I cambiamenti correlati all'età e allo sviluppo della fisiologia e dell'anatomia dei meccanismi di controllo del respiro, della dinamica delle vie aeree e delle caratteristiche del parenchima polmonare esercitano una profonda influenza sulle manifestazioni fisiopatologiche dei processi patologici. Le minori dimensioni delle vie aeree, la maggior compliance della parete toracica e uno stimolo ipossico ridotto rendono i lattanti più vulnerabili dei bambini più grandi, a parità di gravità della malattia. La principale funzione del sistema respiratorio è di fornire ossigeno in quantità sufficiente alla richiesta metabolica e di permettere l'eliminazione dell'anidride carbonica. In questo processo sono coinvolti svariati meccanismi, tra cui la ventilazione, la perfusione e la diffusione: un'anomalia in uno qualsiasi di essi può portare a insufficienza respiratoria. In un bambino per formulare la diagnosi di distress respiratorio ci si basa su segni come la cianosi, l'alitamento delle pinne nasali, il russamento, la tachipnea, i sibili, i rientramenti della parete toracica e lo stridore. Un'insufficienza respiratoria può essere presente anche in assenza di distress; un paziente con anomalie del sistema nervoso centrale (SNC) o malattie neuromuscolari può non essere in grado di compiere uno sforzo sufficiente da farlo apparire in condizioni di distress. Per contro, un bambino che appare in condizione di distress respiratorio può non avere una malattia respiratoria; per esempio, chi soffre di acidosi metabolica primitiva (chetoacidosi diabetica) o stati eccitatori del SNC (encefalite) può presentarsi con un distress respiratorio marcato, in assenza di patologie respiratorie.

370.1 • Volumi e capacità polmonari in condizioni normali e patologiche

Per tradizione i volumi polmonari si misurano con la spirometria (Fig. 370-1). Il **volume corrente** (V_T, *Tidal Volume*) rappresenta la quantità di aria che entra ed esce dai polmoni a ogni atto respiratorio. A riposo, è pari a circa 6-7 mL/kg di peso corporeo. La **capacità inspiratoria** (**IC**, *Inspiratory Capacity*) è la quantità di aria introdotta con un'inspirazione massima, dopo un'espirazione corrente. Il **volume di riserva espiratoria** (**ERV**, *Expiratory Reserve Volume*) è la quantità di aria espirata con il massimo sforzo espiratorio, dopo un'espirazione normale. Il volume di gas che resta nei polmoni dopo un'espirazione massima è il **volume residuo** (**RV**, *Residual Volume*). La **capacità vitale** (**VC**, *Vital Capacity*) viene definita come la quantità di aria che entra ed esce dai polmoni con la massima inspirazione ed espirazione. VC, IC ed ERV si riducono in corso di patologia polmonare, ma sono anche sforzo-dipendenti. La **capacità polmonare totale** (**TLC**, *Total Lung Capacity*) è il volume di gas che occupa i polmoni dopo una massima inspirazione.

La **capacità funzionale residua** (**FRC**, *Functional Residual Capacity*), ossia la quantità di aria che resta nei polmoni dopo un'espirazione corrente, ha importanti implicazioni fisiopatologiche. La composizione dell'aria alveolare varia durante le fasi inspiratorie ed espiratorie. Durante l'inspirazione, la **PO_2 alveolare** (P_AO_2) aumenta e la **PCO_2 alveolare** (P_ACO_2) si riduce, a mano a mano che nuova aria atmosferica entra nei polmoni. Durante l'espirazione, la P_AO_2 si riduce e la P_ACO_2 aumenta, mentre il sangue capillare polmonare continua a rimuovere ossigeno dagli alveoli, cedendo CO_2 (Fig. 370-2). La FRC agisce da tampone, riducendo al minimo le variazioni di P_AO_2 e P_ACO_2 durante l'inspirazione e l'espirazione. Essa rappresenta, per i capillari pomonari, l'ambiente disponibile per gli scambi gassosi in ogni fase respiratoria. Una sua riduzione è di frequente riscontro nelle malattie alveolari

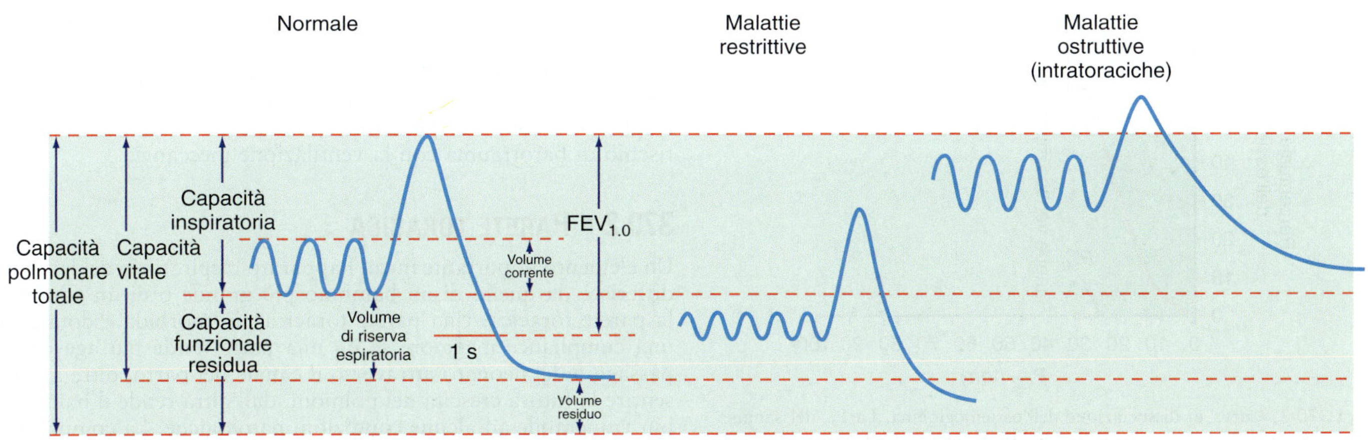

Figura 370-1. Spirometria che mostra i volumi e la capacità polmonari. La $FEV_{1.0}$ è il massimo volume espirato in un secondo, dopo un'inspirazione massima. Le malattie restrittive di solito si associano a riduzione dei volumi e delle capacità polmonari. L'ostruzione delle vie aeree intratoraciche si associa a intrappolamento di aria e a una capacità funzionale residua e un volume residuo abnormemente elevati. La $FEV_{1.0}$ e la capacità vitale sono ridotte sia nelle patologie restrittive sia in quelle ostruttive. Il rapporto tra $FEV_{1.0}$ e capacità vitale è normale nelle malattie restrittive, ma ridotto in quelle ostruttive. FEV (*Forced Expiratory Volume*), volume espiratorio forzato.

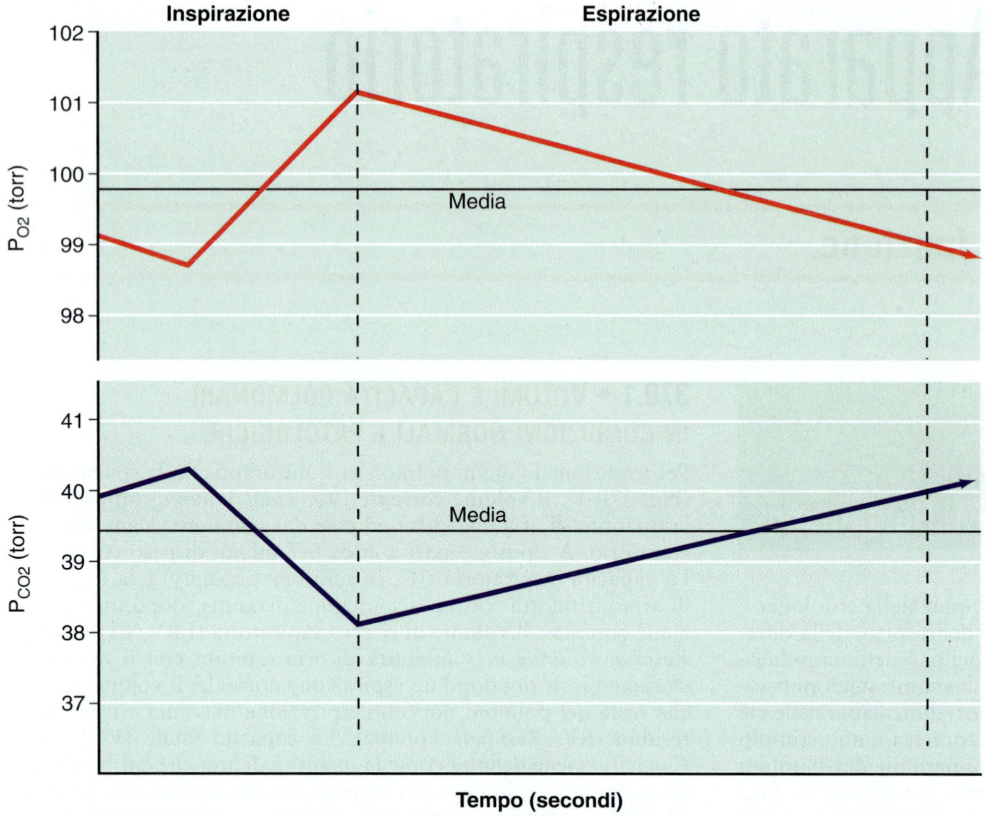

Figura 370-2. La PCO_2 alveolare aumenta e la PCO_2 diminuisce durante l'inspirazione, mentre nuova aria atmosferica entra nei polmoni. Durante l'espirazione, avvengono variazioni opposte, mentre il sangue capillare polmonare continua a rimuovere O_2 e ad apportare CO_2 all'alveolo, senza arricchimento atmosferico. Si noti che durante la fase precoce dell'inspirazione, la PO_2 alveolare continua a ridursi e la PCO_2 ad aumentare, a causa dell'inspirazione dello spazio morto che è occupato dall'aria precedentemente espirata. (Modificata da Comroe JH: *Physiology of Respiration*, 2nd ed. Chicago, Year Book Medical Publishers, 1974, p 12.)

interstiziali e nelle deformità toraciche. La principale conseguenza fisiopatologica della riduzione della FRC è l'**ipossiemia.** Una ridotta FRC, infatti, si traduce in un drastico declino della P_AO_2 durante l'espirazione, poiché è disponibile un volume limitato per gli scambi gassosi. La PO_2 del sangue capillare, pertanto, discende a livelli eccessivamente bassi durante l'espirazione, portando a una riduzione della **PO_2 arteriosa** (PaO_2). L'aumento della P_AO_2 (e quindi della PaO_2) durante l'inspirazione non riesce a compensare questa riduzione della PaO_2 durante l'espirazione. La ragione di ciò risiede nella particolare forma della curva di dissociazione dell'O_2-emoglobina, che è sigmoide (Fig. 370-3). Dal momento

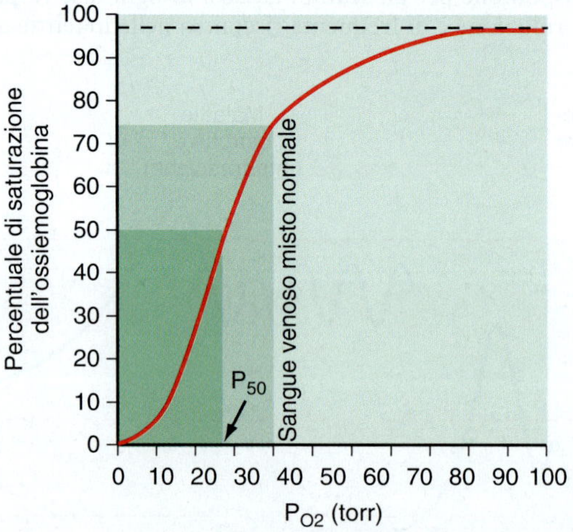

Figura 370-3. Curva di dissociazione dell'ossiemoglobina. La P_{50} del sangue adulto è di circa 72 torr. In condizioni basali, il sangue venoso misto ha una PO_2 di 40 torr e una saturazione di ossiemoglobina del 75%. Nel sangue arterioso, questi valori sono di 70 torr e 97,5%, rispettivamente. Si noti che vi è un ripido declino della saturazione dell'ossiemoglobina per PaO_2 <50 torr, mentre si ottiene un aumento relativamente basso della saturazione con PO_2 >70 torr.

che la maggior parte dell'ossigeno, nel sangue, è legata all'emoglobina, si fa la media della percentuale di **ossiemoglobina (SO_2)**, più che della PO_2. Mentre un aumento della PO_2 arteriosa non riesce ad aumentare la saturazione dell'ossiemoglobina oltre il 100%, avviene invece un drastica desaturazione dell'emoglobina per PO_2 inferiori a 50 torr; pertanto, la riduzione della SO_2 che si verifica durante l'espirazione, come risultato di una ridotta FRC, porta a una desaturazione complessiva con conseguente ipossiemia. Le conseguenze fisiopatologiche avverse di una ridotta FRC sono migliorabili con l'applicazione di una **pressione di fine espirazione positiva (PEEP,** *Positive End Expiratory Pressure*) e con l'aumento del tempo di inspirazione durante la ventilazione meccanica.

Il rapporto pressione-volume del polmone è fortemente influenzato dalla FRC (Fig. 370-4). La compliance polmonare si riduce per valori di FRC abnormemente bassi o elevati.

La FRC risulta eccessivamente elevata nell'ostruzione intratoracica delle vie aeree, che comporta un'espirazione incompleta, e abnormemente bassa nelle malattie alveolointerstiziali. In caso di FRC troppo elevate o troppo basse, la respirazione corrente richiede maggiori pressioni di inflazione rispetto a quelle richieste per una FRC normale: questo si traduce in un aumento del lavoro respiratorio con la respirazione spontanea, e in un aumento del rischio di barotrauma con la ventilazione meccanica.

370.2 • PARETE TORACICA

Un elemento importante in cui l'apparato respiratorio del lattante differisce da quello di un bambino più grande o di un adulto è la parete toracica. Una parete toracica più morbida e dotata di una compliance maggiore se da una parte rende più agevole il passaggio del neonato attraverso il canale del parto, oltre a consentire la futura crescita dei polmoni, dall'altra rende il bambino più vulnerabile ad alcune condizioni patologiche. La compliance della parete toracica è unr determinante maggiore della FRC. Dal momento che la parete toracica e i polmoni hanno forze elastiche che tendono in direzioni opposte, a riposo, la FRC è raggiunta nel punto in cui l'elasticità della gabbia toracica, diretta verso l'esterno, controbilancia esattamente quella dei polmoni, diretta

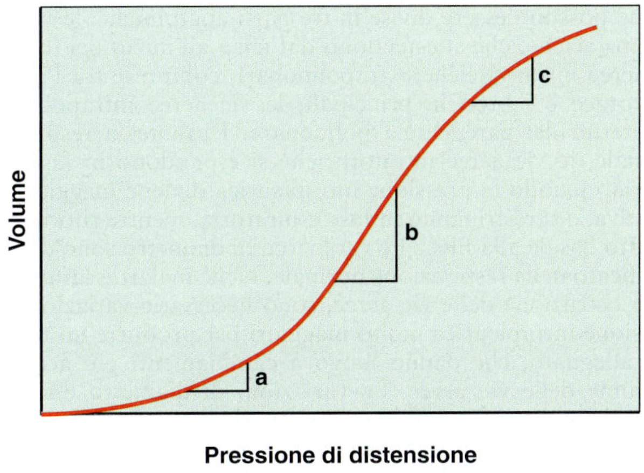

Figura 370-4. La compliance polmonare è influenzata significativamente dalla capacità funzionale residua (FRC). La stessa variazione di pressione si associa a una variazione inferiore del volume quando la FRC è troppo bassa (*a*) o troppo elevata (*c*), rispetto allo stato normale (*b*).

verso l'interno. Nei lattanti quest'equilibrio viene raggiunto a un volume polmonare inferiore che nei bambini più grandi, a causa dell'elevata compliance toracica (Fig. 370-5). Nel lattante non solo la FRC misurata è maggiore di quella attesa, poiché i muscoli respiratori mantengono la gabbia toracica in posizione leggermente inspiratoria in tutte le fasi, ma si verifica anche un intrappolamento d'aria durante l'espirazione nei bambini più piccoli.

L'elevata compliance toracica è uno svantaggio caratteristico dei bambini più piccoli, in diverse condizioni patologiche. Una riduzione del tono muscolare, come quella che si verifica durante il sonno REM (*Rapid Eye Movement*, movimento oculare rapido) o con la depressione del SNC, consente una maggior retrazione della gabbia toracica, a causa della minore resistenza alla forza elastica polmonare; in queste condizioni, la FRC si riduce. I muscoli respiratori dei lattanti non sono ancora allenati a sopportare un aumento del carico di lavoro e quindi si affaticano più facilmente, rispetto a quelli dei bambini più grandi, il che ne limita la capacità di mantenere un'adeguata ventilazione in caso di malattie polmonari. Nelle malattie con ridotta compliance polmonare (atelettasia, edema polmonare), un'eccessiva retrazione polmonare dà luogo a una maggiore retrazione della parete toracica cedevole, e a un'ulteriore perdita di FRC, rispetto ai bambini più grandi o agli adulti, che hanno una parete polmonare più rigida. L'aumento della pressione intratoracica negativa richiesto per superare la resistenza delle vie aeree, nelle pneumopatie ostruttive, provoca anche una più spiccata retrazione della parete toracica, con conseguente riduzione della FRC, nei bambini più piccoli. In questi casi, l'applicazione di una PEEP è utile per stabilizzare la parete toracica e ripristinare la FRC.

In alcune condizioni patologiche si possono riscontrare anomalie della parete toracica. L'instabilità della parete può essere conseguenza di un trauma (frattura costale, toracotomia) o di malattie neuromuscolari che indeboliscono i muscoli diaframmatici e intercostali. L'aumento della compliance della parete toracica rende questi lattanti più vulnerabili allo scompenso respiratorio quando devono affrontare queste patologie, rispetto ai bambini più grandi e agli adulti, la cui parete toracica è più rigida. I bambini con una parete toracica abnormemente rigida, priva di compliance (distrofia toracica asfissiante di Jeune [vedi Capitoli 416.3 e 698], acondroplasia [vedi Capitolo 416.4]) presentano una marcata riduzione dei volumi e delle capacità polmonari.

370.3 • Meccanica polmonare e lavoro respiratorio in condizioni normali e patologiche

Perché l'aria entri ed esca dai polmoni è necessario un adeguato gradiente pressorio tra gli alveoli e l'atmosfera, durante sia l'inspirazione, sia l'espirazione. Parte del gradiente pressorio è richiesta per superare l'elastanza polmonare e toracica; un'altra parte serve a superare la resistenza delle vie aeree. L'**elastanza**, ossia la proprietà di una sostanza di opporsi alla deformazione o allo stiramento, viene calcolata come variazione della pressione (ΔP) ÷ variazione di volume (ΔV). L'elasticità è la proprietà di una sostanza che le consente di ritornare al suo stato originario, quando non è più soggetto a una pressione. La **compliance** ($\Delta V \div \Delta P$) è l'inverso dell'elastanza. Nel contesto del parenchima polmonare, delle vie aeree e della parete toracica, la compliance indica la distensibilità. La **resistenza** viene definita come la quantità di pressione necessaria per generare un flusso di gas attraverso le vie aeree. In base alla *legge di Poiseuille*, la resistenza al flusso laminare si calcola come segue: $R = 8\, l\eta \div \Pi r^4$, in cui R indica la resistenza, l la lunghezza, η la viscosità e r il raggio. L'implicazione pratica del rapporto pressione-flusso è che la resistenza di una via aerea è inversamente proporzionale al suo raggio elevato alla quarta potenza. Ciò significa che se il lume è ridotto della metà, la resistenza aumenta di 16 volte. I neonati e i lattanti di pochi mesi, che hanno vie aeree più piccole, sono particolarmente inclini a un aumento marcato della resistenza delle vie aeree, a causa dell'infiammazione dei tessuti e delle secrezioni. In malattie che comportano un aumento della resistenza delle vie aeree, il flusso diviene spesso turbolento. La **turbolenza** dipende in gran parte dal *numero di Reynolds* (Re), un'entità priva di dimensioni, che si calcola nel modo seguente: $Re = 2rvd \div \eta$, in cui r è il raggio, v la velocità, d la densità e η la viscosità. La turbolenza, in un flusso gassoso, si verifica più facilmente quando Re supera 2000. La resistenza al flusso turbolento è strettamente correlata alla densità. Un gas a bassa densità, per esempio una miscela di elio e ossigeno, riduce la turbolenza nelle malattie respiratorie ostruttive come la laringotracheobronchite virale e l'asma. Poiché neonati e lattanti respirano prevalentemente con il naso, anche un grado minimo di ostruzione nasale risulta mal tollerato.

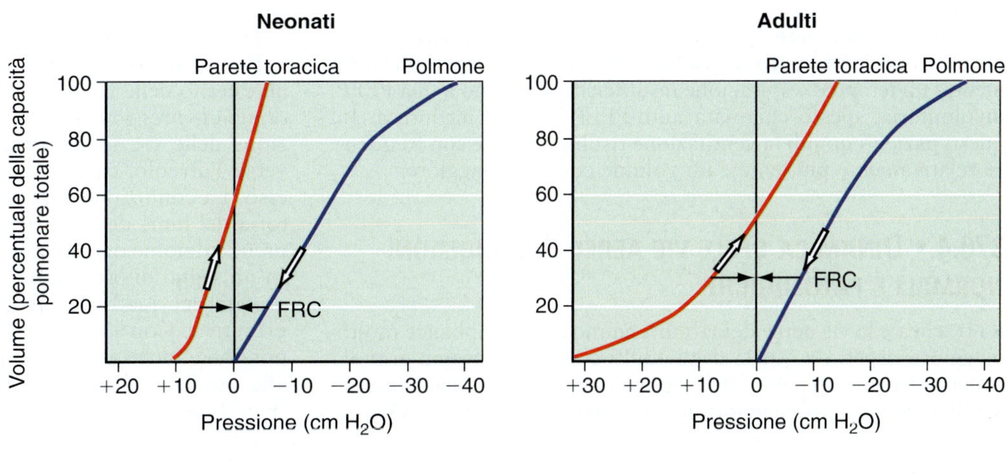

Figura 370-5. Rappresentazione schematica dell'interazione tra l'elasticità della parete toracica e quella del polmone nei neonati, rispetto agli adulti. La forza elastica di una parete toracica relativamente più compliante è controbilanciata dall'elasticità polmonare a un volume inferiore (FRC) nei neonati, rispetto agli adulti. FRC, capacità funzionale residua.

Il diaframma è il principale muscolo respiratorio. Quando è necessario incrementare il *lavoro respiratorio* (WOB, *Work of Breathing*), concorrono anche i muscoli intercostali e gli altri muscoli respiratori accessori. Il volume corrente e la frequenza respiratoria vengono corretti, in condizioni di salute come di malattia, per mantenere il volume minuto richiesto, con il minimo dispendio energetico. Il WOB totale (necessario per creare gradienti pressori che permettano il movimento dell'aria) si divide in due parti. La prima parte consiste nel superamento dell'elastanza del polmone e della parete toracica, e prende il nome di *lavoro elastico* (W_{elast}); la seconda è il superamento della resistenza delle vie aeree e dei tessuti, e viene chiamata *lavoro resistivo* (W_{resist}). Il W_{elast} è direttamente proporzionale al volume corrente, mentre il W_{resist} è determinato dalla frequenza del flusso aereo e quindi dalla frequenza respiratoria. Il WOB totale è ai livelli più bassi per frequenze di 35-40/min per i neonati, e di 14-16/min per i bambini più grandi e gli adulti. Un aumento sproporzionato del W_{elast} si verifica nelle malattie con ridotta compliance, mentre il W_{resist} risulta aumentato in presenza di ostruzione delle vie aeree. La respirazione è pertanto superficiale (basso V_T) e rapida nelle malattie con ridotta compliance, profonda e relativamente lenta (bassa frequenza respiratoria) nelle malattie con aumento della resistenza. Rispetto ai bambini più grandi, i neonati hanno un W_{elast} sproporzionatamente maggiore, poiché la pressione intrapleurica negativa, durante l'inspirazione, causa il collasso della parete toracica più retrattile (con maggiore compliance) ostacolando così l'ingresso dell'aria. I lattanti di pochi mesi di vita aumentano la frequenza respiratoria in caso di anomalia meccanica di qualunque origine. Altri esempi di svantaggio causato da una parete toracica con compliance eccessiva sono il lembo costale derivante da fratture costali, la toracotomia e la debolezza neuromuscolare. Uno degli effetti positivi della pressione positiva continua nelle vie aeree, in queste situazioni, è la stabilizzazione della parete toracica.

La *costante di tempo*, misurata in secondi, è il prodotto della compliance per la resistenza e rispecchia la quantità di tempo necessario per equilibrare la pressione delle vie aeree prossimali (e pertanto il volume) con la pressione alveolare. Occorrono 3 costanti di tempo per equilibrare il 95% della pressione e 5 costanti di tempo per il 99%. Poiché le vie aeree si espandono durante l'inspirazione e si contraggono durante l'espirazione, la costante di tempo espiratoria è maggiore di quella inspiratoria. Le malattie caratterizzate da ridotta compliance (polmonite, edema polmonare, atelettasia) si associano a una diminuzione della costante di tempo, e pertanto richiedono meno tempo per l'inflazione e la deflazione alveolari. Le malattie associate a un aumento della resistenza (asma, bronchiolite, sindrome da aspirazione), avendo una costante di tempo prolungata, richiedono un tempo maggiore per l'inflazione e la deflazione alveolare. Le alterazioni patologiche delle costanti di tempo hanno un significato pratico, in caso di ventilazione meccanica. I pazienti con costanti di tempo minori sono ventilati meglio con volumi correnti relativamente inferiori e frequenze più veloci, per ridurre al minimo i picchi di pressione di inflazione. Nei pazienti con incremento della resistenza delle vie aeree, una frequenza respiratoria rapida (e pertanto con un minor tempo) non consente di raggiungere una pressione sufficiente per equilibrare le vie aeree prossimali con gli alveoli. Un tempo di inspirazione inadeguato si traduce in volumi correnti inferiori, mentre un tempo di espirazione insufficiente dà luogo a una PEEP involontaria, spesso chiamata auto-PEEP o PEEP intrinseca. In questi pazienti quindi la ventilazione risulta migliore con frequenze relativamente più lente e un volume corrente maggiore.

370.4 • Dinamica delle vie aeree in condizioni normali e patologiche

La trachea e le vie aeree dei lattanti hanno una compliance molto maggiore rispetto a quella degli adulti e dei bambini più grandi, e pertanto le variazioni della pressione intrapleurica causano cambiamenti molto maggiori nel diametro delle vie aeree. Queste ultime possono essere divise in tre parti anatomiche: le vie aeree extratoraciche, che si estendono dal naso all'inizio del torace; le vie aeree intratoraciche-extrapolmonari, comprese tra l'ingresso del torace e i bronchi principali; le vie aeree intrapolmonari, all'interno del parenchima polmonare. Durante la respirazione normale, le vie aeree intratoraciche si espandono in fase inspiratoria, quando la pressione intrapleurica diviene maggiormente negativa, e si restringono in fase espiratoria, mentre ritornano allo stato basale alla FRC. Le variazioni di diametro sono di scarso significato nella respirazione normale. Nelle malattie caratterizzate da ostruzione delle vie aeree, sono necessarie variazioni della pressione intrapleurica molto maggiori per produrre un flusso di aria adeguato, che danno luogo a cambiamenti più accentuati del lume delle vie aeree. Le variazioni di diametro durante la respirazione sono accentuate nei neonati, che hanno vie aeree più morbide e con una compliance maggiore.

Nell'ostruzione delle vie aeree extratoraciche (atresia delle coane [vedi Capitolo 373], ascesso retrofaringeo, laringotracheobronchite [vedi Capitolo 382]), l'elevata pressione intrapleurica negativa durante l'inspirazione viene trasmessa alla sede dell'ostruzione, oltre la quale vi è una rapida dissipazione della pressione. Pertanto, le vie aeree extratoraciche che si trovano al di sotto della sede dell'ostruzione hanno una pressione negativa interna molto aumentata e vanno incontro a collasso, con conseguente peggioramento dell'ostruzione (Fig. 370-6*A*); ne derivano difficoltà dell'inspirazione, prolungamento dell'inspirazione e stridore inspiratorio. Inoltre, l'aumentata pressione intrapleurica negativa determina la retrazione della parete toracica. Durante l'espirazione, l'aumentata pressione intrapleurica positiva si trasmette nuovamente lungo le vie aeree fino alla sede dell'ostruzione, portando alla distensione delle vie aeree extratoraciche e al miglioramento dell'ostruzione (Fig. 370-6*B*).

L'aumento della pressione intrapleurica positiva fa sì che la parete toracica tenda a sporgere, causando la **classica respirazione paradossa,** in cui il torace si retrae durante l'inspirazione e sporge durante l'espirazione. Più il bambino è piccolo di età, più la parete toracica è cedevole, e più marcata è la respirazione paradossa, in caso di ostruzione delle vie aeree extratoraciche. Nei neonati e nei lattanti di pochi mesi può inoltre rendersi evidente un pattern respiratorio oscillante, poiché la parete toracica con un'elevata compliance viene risucchiata verso l'interno e l'addome si dilata durante l'inspirazione, mentre accade il contrario durante l'espirazione.

Nell'ostruzione delle vie aeree intratoraciche-extrapolmonari (anello vascolare [vedi Capitolo 383], tumori mediastinici) e delle vie aeree intrapolmonari (asma, bronchiolite), l'aumento della pressione negativa intrapleurica determina la distensione delle vie aeree intratoraciche durante l'inspirazione, attenuando così l'ostruzione (Fig. 370-7*A*).

Durante l'espirazione, l'aumentata pressione intratoracica positiva si trasmette alla sede dell'ostruzione, oltre la quale si dissipa rapidamente. Le vie aeree intratoraciche al di sopra della sede dell'ostruzione sono quindi soggette a una maggior pressione intrapleurica dall'esterno, che non può essere adeguatamente controbilanciata da una sufficiente pressione positiva dall'interno, risultando quindi nel collasso della via aerea al di sopra della sede dell'ostruzione (Fig. 370-7*B*).

Il punto in cui, durante l'espirazione, le pressioni all'interno e all'esterno delle vie aeree si equivalgono prende il nome di *punto di uguale pressione* (EPP, *Equal Pressure Point*). In caso di ostruzione delle vie aeree intratoraciche, l'EPP si sposta distalmente verso l'alveolo, causando il collasso delle vie aeree prossimali a esso. La condizione di marcata variazione inspiratoria ed espiratoria del lume delle vie aeree al di sopra dell'EPP, in un lattante, prende il nome di *trachea collassabile*. Il **collasso tracheale** è spesso un segno di ostruzione delle vie aeree, oltre a contribuire alla gravità del quadro clinico, ma raramente costituisce l'anomalia primitiva. Con l'ostruzione delle vie aeree intrapolmonari, una porzione anche maggiore di vie aeree intratoraciche va soggetta alle oscillazioni pressorie durante l'inspirazione e l'espirazione (Fig. 370-8).

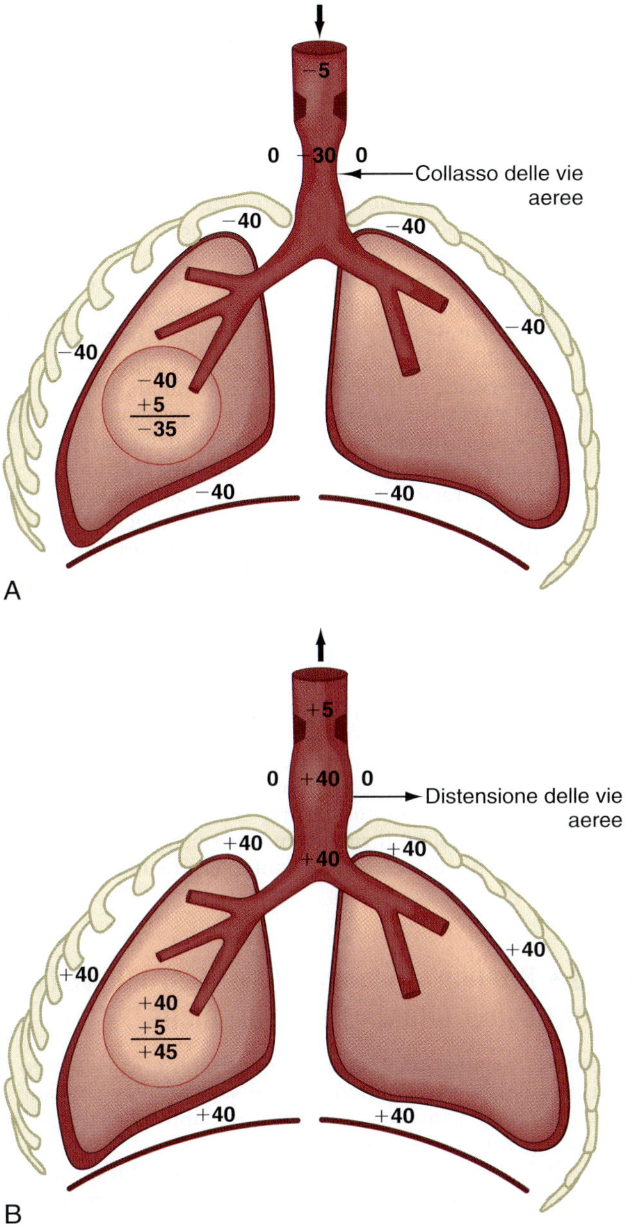

Figura 370-6. *A*, Nell'ostruzione delle vie aeree extratoraciche, l'aumentata pressione negativa durante l'inspirazione è trasmessa fino alla sede dell'ostruzione: si assiste quindi al collasso delle vie aeree extratoraciche al di sotto della sede dell'ostruzione e al conseguente peggioramento dell'ostruzione durante l'inspirazione. Si noti che la pressione è confrontata con la pressione atmosferica che è tradizionalmente rappresentata a 0 cm. La pressione delle vie aeree terminali è calcolata come (pressione intrapleurica + pressione di ritorno elastico polmonare). La pressione di ritorno elastico polmonare è arbitrariamente considerata di 5 cm per semplicità. *B*, Durante l'inspirazione, la pressione positiva al di sotto della sede dell'ostruzione porta alla distensione delle vie aeree extratoraciche e al miglioramento dei sintomi.

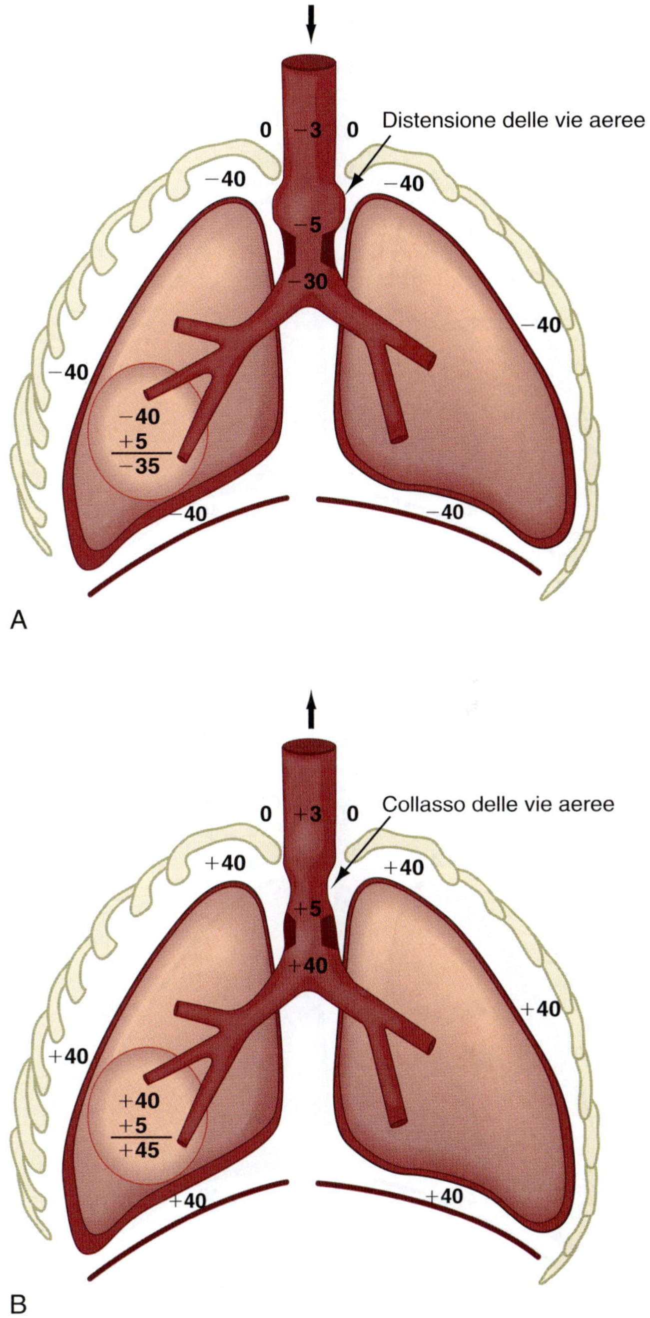

Figura 370-7. *A*, Nell'ostruzione delle vie aeree intratoraciche-extrapolmonari l'aumento della pressione negativa durante l'inspirazione è trasmessa fino alla sede dell'ostruzione; ne consegue una distensione delle vie aeree intratoraciche al di sopra della lesione poiché sono circondate da una pressione intrapleurica negativa anche maggiore. *B*, Durante l'espirazione, l'aumentata pressione positiva delle vie aeree si dissipa rapidamente al di sopra dell'ostruzione; si verifica così il collasso delle vie aeree intratoraciche al di sopra dell'ostruzione poiché sono sottoposte a una pressione intrapleurica positiva nettamente aumentata, che peggiora ulteriormente l'ostruzione durante l'espirazione.

Sia l'ostruzione delle vie aeree intratoraciche-extrapolmonari, sia quella delle vie aeree intrapolmonari si traducono in una difficoltà ingravescente durante l'espirazione, nel prolungamento dell'espirazione e in sibili espiratori. Qualsiasi ostruzione delle vie aeree all'interno del torace provoca sibili espiratori.

370.5 • Interpretazione dei segni clinici per la localizzazione della sede della patologia

La corretta interpretazione dei reperti clinici è il primo passo per la diagnosi delle malattie respiratorie. Una distress respiratorio può insorgere in assenza di malattie respiratorie, così come l'insufficienza respiratoria può sussistere in assenza di distress respiratorio significativo. Le malattie caratterizzate da eccitazione del SNC, come l'encefalite, e l'assunzione di sostanze neuroeccitatorie si associano a iperventilazione neurogena centrale. Analogamente, le patologie che provocano acidosi metabolica, come la chetoacidosi diabetica, il salicilismo e lo shock, causano iperventilazione come risposta compensatoria. Da un punto di vista clinico, i pazienti di entrambi i gruppi possono essere considerati affetti da distress respiratorio; essi si distinguono dai pazienti con

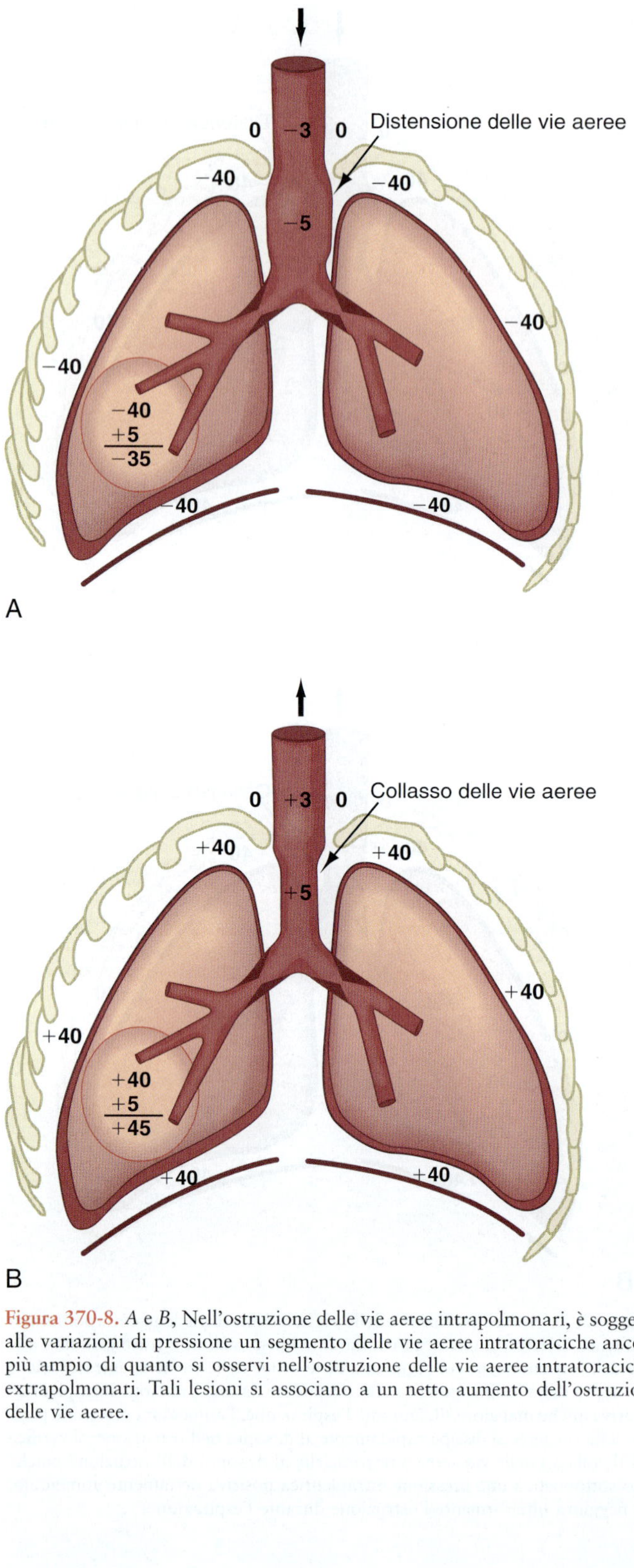

Figura 370-8. *A* e *B*, Nell'ostruzione delle vie aeree intrapolmonari, è soggetto alle variazioni di pressione un segmento delle vie aeree intratoraciche ancora più ampio di quanto si osservi nell'ostruzione delle vie aeree intratoraciche-extrapolmonari. Tali lesioni si associano a un netto aumento dell'ostruzione delle vie aeree.

malattia respiratoria dovuta all'aumento del volume corrente, oltre che della frequenza respiratoria. I loro valori all'emogasanalisi riflettono una $PaCO_2$ bassa e una PaO_2 normale. I pazienti con malattie neuromuscolari, come la sindrome di Guillain-Barré o la miastenia grave, e quelli con uno stimolo respiratorio anomalo possono andare incontro a insufficienza respiratoria severa, ma non sono in grado di sviluppare uno sforzo tale da apparire come distress respiratorio. In questi soggetti, gli atti respiratori sono inefficaci o possono anche apparire normali, in presenza di acidosi respiratoria e ipossiemia.

La frequenza e la profondità degli atti respiratori e la presenza di retrazioni, stridore, sibili e russamento sono segni importanti per la localizzazione della sede della patologia respiratoria (Tab. 370-1 e Fig. 370-9). Una respirazione rapida e superficiale (**tachipnea**) è caratteristica delle patologie parenchimali, in cui il lavoro respiratorio elastico aumenta in modo sproporzionato rispetto al lavoro respiratorio resistivo. I **rientramenti** della parete toracica, intercostali e soprasternali sono più eclatanti, con un'aumentata pressione intratoracica negativa, durante l'inspirazione, e si osservano nell'ostruzione delle vie aeree extratoraciche, così come nelle malattie con ridotta compliance. Lo **stridore** inspiratorio è una caratteristica dell'ostruzione delle vie aeree extratoraciche. I **sibili espiratori** sono tipici dell'ostruzione delle vie aeree intratoraciche, sia extrapolmonari, sia intrapolmonari. Il **russamento** è prodotto dall'espirazione contro una glottide parzialmente chiusa e rappresenta un tentativo di mantenere una pressione positiva nelle vie aeree durante l'espirazione per il maggior tempo possibile. Questo prolungamento della pressione positiva è di maggior beneficio nelle malattie alveolari che provocano una perdita diffusa della FRC, come l'edema polmonare, la malattia delle membrane ialine e la polmonite. Inoltre, nell'ostruzione delle piccole vie aeree (bronchiolite) il russamento permette di mantenere una pressione positiva più elevata durante l'espirazione, riducendo il collasso delle vie aeree.

370.6 • Rapporto ventilazione-perfusione (V/Q) in condizioni normali e patologiche

Durante la respirazione corrente, gli alveoli e le vie aeree nelle parti non declivi del polmone (i lobi superiori, in ortostatismo) sono sottoposti a una maggior pressione intrapleurica negativa, e restano pertanto più inflati, rispetto agli alveoli e alle vie aeree più declivi (i lobi inferiori, in ortostatismo). Questo avviene a causa della forza di gravità, che tende ad allontanare il polmone dalle regioni non declivi della pleura parietale. Gli alveoli non declivi hanno una minor compliance, essendo già più inflati. Durante un'inspirazione corrente, pertanto, la ventilazione avviene per lo più nelle regioni declivi del polmone, che si espandono più facilmente. Sebbene la perfusione sia persino maggiore nelle regioni declivi del polmoni, per la più elevata pressione idrostatica arteriosa polmonare, dovuta alla forza di gravità, nelle zone declivi il suo aumento è maggiore dell'aumento della ventilazione. Pertanto, il rapporto V/Q è a favore della ventilazione nelle

TABELLA 370-1. Interpretazione dei segni clinici delle patologie respiratorie

SEGNO	OSTRUZIONE DELLE VIE AEREE EXTRATORACICHE	OSTRUZIONE DELLE VIE AEREE INTRATORACICHE-EXTRAPOLMONARI	OSTRUZIONE DELLE VIE AEREE INTRAPOLMONARI	PATOLOGIA PARENCHIMALE
Tachipnea	+	+	++	++++
Retrazioni/rientramenti	++++	++	++	+++
Stridore	++++	++	–	–
Sibili	±	+++	++++	±
Russamento	±	±	++	++++

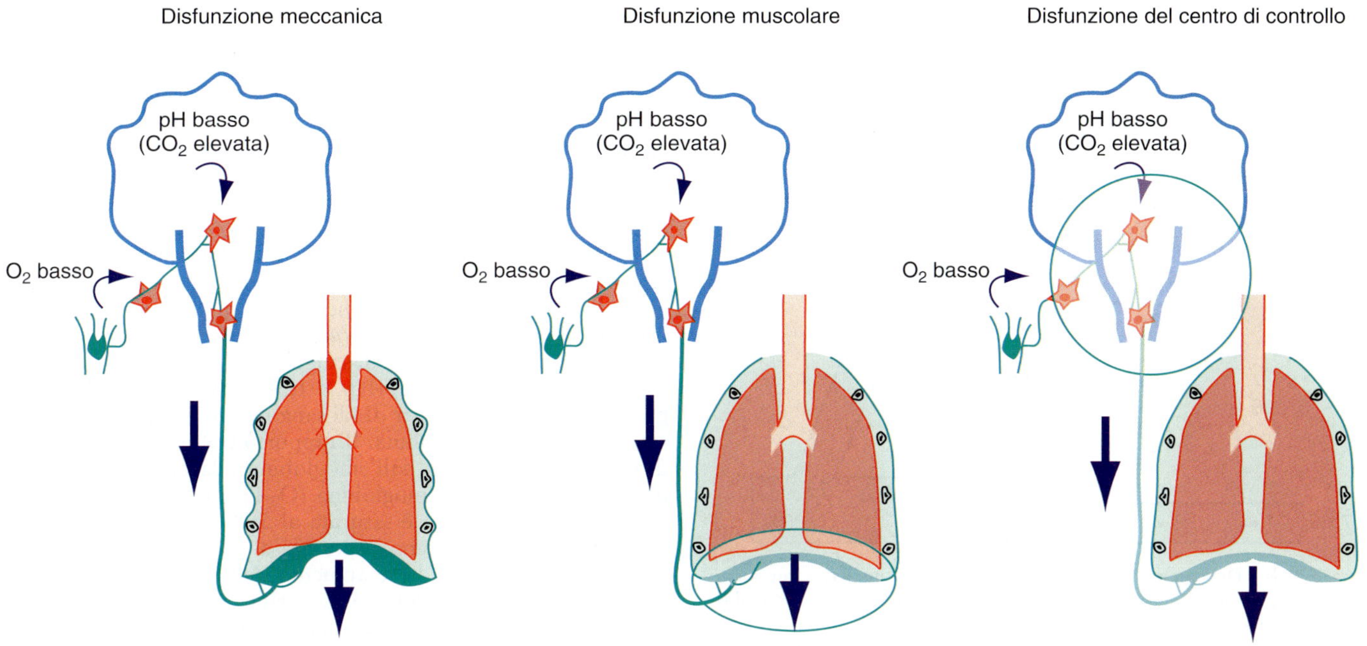

Figura 370-9. Profili di presentazione dell'insufficienza respiratoria in età infantile. Quando è presente una disfunzione meccanica (la circostanza di gran lunga più comune), l'ipossiemia arteriosa e l'ipercapnia (e pertanto il pH) vengono rilevate dai chemiocettori periferici (corpi carotidei) e centrali (midollo allungato) per poi essere integrate con le altre informazioni sensitive provenienti dai polmoni e dalla parete toracica; la successiva attivazione dei chemiocettori scatena un aumento degli impulsi nervosi ai muscoli respiratori (*frecce verticali*), che dà luogo ai segni clinici del distress respiratorio. Quando il problema risiede nei muscoli respiratori (o nella loro innervazione), avviene lo stesso aumento degli impulsi nervosi (*frecce*), ma i muscoli respiratori non riescono ad aumentare lo sforzo come richiesto; pertanto, i segni fisici di fatica sono più sfumati. Infine, quando il controllo della respirazione è esso stesso colpito da malattia, la risposta nervosa all'ipossiemia e all'ipercapnia è assente o attenuata e le anomalie dello scambio gassoso non sono accompagnate da distress respiratorio.

regioni non declivi, e a favore della perfusione in quelle declivi. Nelle zone declivi le vie aeree, essendo più strette, si chiudono prima durante l'espirazione. Il volume polmonare a cui le vie aeree declivi iniziano a chiudersi è chiamato *capacità di chiusura*. Nei bambini normali, *la FRC è maggiore della capacità di chiusura*. Durante la respirazione corrente, le vie aeree restano pervie sia nelle zone declivi del polmone, sia in quelle non declivi. Nei neonati, la capacità di chiusura è maggiore della FRC, dando luogo alla perfusione di alveoli scarsamente ventilati, durante la respirazione corrente; pertanto, i neonati normali hanno una PaO_2 inferiore rispetto ai bambini più grandi.

Diversi stati fisiopatologici incidono negativamente sul rapporto V/Q (Fig. 370-10). La cosiddetta **ventilazione dello spazio morto**, ossia il movimento dell'aria nelle zone scarsamente perfuse, si riscontra per esempio nella tromboembolia polmonare e nell'ipovolemia. La perfusione di alveoli poco ventilati, che si osserva nella polmonite, nell'asma e nella malattia delle membrane ialine, è chiamata shunt destro-sinistro intrapolmonare o commistione venosa. Nell'ostruzione delle vie aeree intrapolmonari, la capacità di chiusura è abnormemente aumentata e può superare la FRC. In queste condizioni, la perfusione di alveoli scarsamente ventilati, durante la respirazione corrente, si traduce nella commistione venosa.

370.7 • Scambi gassosi in condizioni normali e patologiche

La principale funzione del sistema respiratorio è di rimuovere l'anidride carbonica dai polmoni e aggiungere ossigeno al sangue venoso sistemico che vi affluisce. La composizione dell'aria inspirata, la ventilazione, la perfusione, la diffusione e il metabolismo tissutale hanno un influsso significativo sulla composizione dei gas nel sangue arterioso.

La pressione totale dell'atmosfera, a livello del mare, è di 760 torr. A mano a mano che l'altitudine aumenta, la pressione atmosferica diminuisce. La pressione atmosferica totale è uguale alla somma delle pressioni parziali esercitate da ognuno dei gas che la compongono. L'aria alveolare ha un'umidità del 100% e pertanto, per il calcolo dei gas alveolari, si suppone che il gas inspirato sia umidificato anch'esso al 100%. Alla temperatura di 37 °C e con un'umidità del 100%, il vapore acqueo esercita una pressione di 47 torr, a prescindere dall'altitudine. In un contesto naturale, l'atmosfera è formata per il 20,93% da ossigeno. La *pressione parziale d'ossigeno nell'aria inspirata* (PiO_2), a livello del mare, è pertanto (760 − 47) × 20,93% = 149 torr. Se si inspira ossigeno al 40% a livello del mare, la PiO_2 sarà: (760 − 47) × 40% = 285 torr. Ad altitudini maggiori, respirando concentrazioni diverse di ossigeno, la PiO_2 sarà inferiore rispetto al livello del mare, a seconda delle pressioni atmosferiche prevalenti. A Denver (altitudine di 1524 m e pressione barometrica di 632 torr), la PiO_2 in aria ambiente è (632 − 47) × 20,93% = 122 torr, e con ossigeno al 40% è (632 − 47) × 40% = 234 torr.

Il **volume minuto** è il prodotto del V_T e della frequenza respiratoria. Parte del V_T occupa le vie aeree di conduzione (spazio morto anatomico), che non contribuiscono allo scambio di gas negli alveoli. La **ventilazione alveolare** è il volume di aria atmosferica che entra negli alveoli ed è calcolata nel modo seguente: (V_T − spazio morto) × frequenza respiratoria. La ventilazione alveolare è inversamente proporzionale alla PCO_2 alveolare (P_ACO_2). Quando la ventilazione alveolare si riduce della metà, la P_ACO_2 raddoppia; all'inverso, se la ventilazione alveolare raddoppia, la P_ACO_2 diminuisce del 50%. La *PO_2 alveolare* (P_AO_2) è espressa dall'**equazione dell'aria alveolare** come segue: $P_AO_2 = PiO_2 - (P_A$-

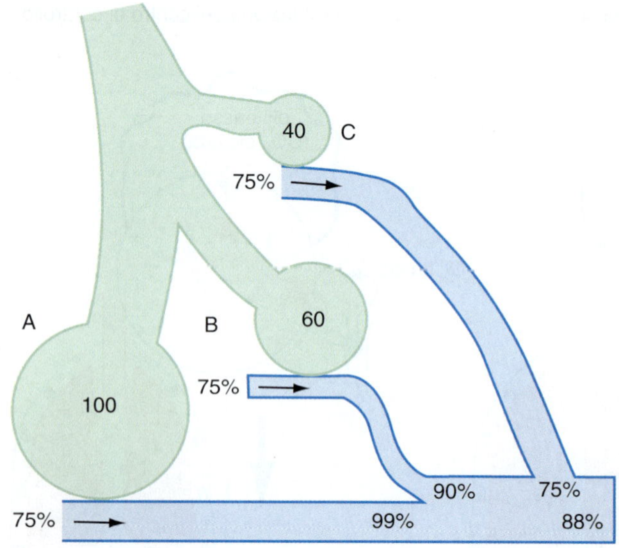

Figura 370-10. Diagramma che dimostra gli effetti di un basso rapporto ventilazione-perfusione sull'ossigenazione arteriosa nei polmoni. Sono illustrate tre unità alveolocapillari. L'unità A ha una ventilazione normale e una PO_2 alveolare di 100 mmHg (indicata dal numero a metà dello spazio). La saturazione arteriosa del sangue che circola attraverso quest'unità aumenta passando dal 75% (la saturazione del sangue venoso misto) al 99%. L'unità B ha un rapporto ventilazione-perfusione inferiore e una PO_2 inferiore, di 60 mmHg. Il sangue che circola attraverso quest'unità raggiunge una saturazione solo del 90%. Infine, l'unità C non è ventilata per nulla. La sua PO_2 alveolare è equivalente a quella del sangue venoso, che viaggia inalterato attraverso l'unità. La saturazione di ossigeno del sangue arterioso riflette i contributi bilanciati di queste tre unità. Partendo dal presupposto che ogni unità abbia lo stesso flusso sanguigno, il sangue arterioso avrebbe una saturazione solo dell'88%. Il mancato bilanciamento (*mismatch*) del rapporto ventilazione-perfusione è il meccanismo più comunemente responsabile di ipossiema arteriosa nelle patologie polmonari. La somministrazione di ossigeno aumenta la PO_2 arteriosa provocando un incremento della PO_2 alveolare nelle unità polmonari che, come la B, hanno un rapporto ventilazione-perfusione maggiore di zero.

$CO_2 \div R$), dove R è il quoziente respiratorio. A scopo pratico, la P_ACO_2 è sostituita dalla *PCO_2 arteriosa* ($PaCO_2$) e si assume che R sia 0,8. Secondo l'equazione dell'aria alveolare, per una data PiO_2, un aumento della $PaCO_2$ di 10 torr risulta in una diminuzione delle P_AO_2 di $10 \div 0,8$ o $10 \times 1,25$ o 12,5 torr. Pertanto si verificano variazioni proporzionalmente diverse della P_AO_2 di entità uguale a $1,25 \times$ la variazione della P_ACO_2 (o $PaCO_2$).

Una volta che la composizione dell'aria alveolare è stata determinata dalle condizioni dei gas inspirati e dai processi di ventilazione, lo scambio gassoso avviene tramite un processo di diffusione ed equilibrio tra gas alveolare e sangue polmonare capillare. La diffusione dipende dalla barriera alveolocapillare e dalla quantità di tempo disponibile per l'equilibrio. In condizioni normali, l'equilibrio del gas alveolare e del sangue capillare polmonare è completo sia per l'ossigeno sia per l'anidride carbonica. Nelle malattie in cui la barriera alveolocapillare è abnormemente aumentata (alveolopatie interstiziali) e/o quando il tempo disponibile per l'equilibrio è ridotto (aumento della velocità di flusso ematica), la diffusione risulta incompleta. Data la maggior solubilità nei mezzi liquidi, l'anidride carbonica è 20 volte più diffusibile dell'ossigeno. Pertanto, le malattie con difetti della diffusione sono caratterizzate da un marcato *gradiente alveoloarterioso di ossigeno* ($A - aO_2$) e da ipossiemia. I difetti della diffusione non danno luogo ad aumenti significativi della CO_2, a meno che non sussista una concomitante ipoventilazione.

Il sangue venoso che affluisce ai polmoni viene "arterializzato" dopo il completamento della diffusione. Al termine di questo processo di arterializzazione, il sangue venoso capillare dovrebbe avere la stessa PO_2 e PCO_2 degli alveoli. La composizione dei gas ematici arteriosi, tuttavia, differisce da quella degli alveoli, anche in condizioni normali, in quanto nel polmone normale si verifica ventilazione dello spazio morto, come pure commistione venosa. La ventilazione dello spazio morto fa sì che la $PaCO_2$ risulti maggiore della P_ACO_2, mentre la commistione venosa (o shunt destro-sinistro) dà luogo a una PaO_2 minore rispetto alla composizione del gas alveolare (vedi Fig. 370-10). La PaO_2 rispecchia la quantità di ossigeno dissolto nel sangue, che è una componente relativamente minore del contenuto totale di ossigeno del sangue. Per ogni 100 torr di PO_2, ci sono 0,3 mL di O_2 dissolti in 100 mL. Il contenuto totale di ossigeno del sangue è composto dall'ossigeno dissolto e da quello legato all'emoglobina. Ogni grammo di emoglobina trasporta 1,34 mL di O_2 con una saturazione di ossigeno del 100%; se ne deduce che 15 g di emoglobina trasportano 20,1 mL di ossigeno. Il *contenuto arterioso di ossigeno* (CaO_2), espresso come mL di O_2/dL di sangue, può essere calcolato con la formula: $(PaO_2 \times 0,003) + (Hb \times 1,34 \times SO_2)$, in cui Hb indica i grammi di emoglobina per dL di sangue, e SO_2 è la percentuale di saturazione dell'emoglobina. Il rapporto tra la PO_2 e la quantità di ossigeno trasportato dall'emoglobina è la base della curva di dissociazione dell'ossiemoglobina (O_2-Hb) (vedi Fig. 370-3). La PO_2 a cui l'emoglobina è saturata al 50% è chiamata P_{50}. A un pH normale, l'emoglobina è saturata al 94% a una PO_2 di 70, e si ottiene un ulteriore, lieve aumento della saturazione, per PO_2 più elevate. A valori di $PO_2 < 50$ si verifica un rapido declino della saturazione e, pertanto, del contenuto di ossigeno.

L'apporto di ossigeno ai tessuti è il prodotto del contenuto di ossigeno e della gittata cardiaca. Quando l'emoglobina è saturata quasi al 100%, il sangue contiene circa 20 mL di ossigeno per 100 mL, ovvero 2000 mL/L. In un adulto sano, la gittata cardiaca è di circa 5 L/min, l'apporto di ossigeno pari a circa 1000 mL/min e il consumo di ossigeno pari a 250 mL/min. Il sangue venoso misto che ritorna al cuore ha una PO_2 di 40 torr e una saturazione di ossigeno del 75%. Il contenuto di ossigeno nel sangue, la gittata cardiaca e il consumo di ossigeno sono elementi importanti, che influiscono sulla saturazione del sangue venoso misto. Per un contenuto ematico di ossigeno e un consumo di ossigeno fissi allo *steady state*, la saturazione del sangue venoso misto è un importante indicatore della gittata cardiaca. In questi casi, una riduzione della saturazione venosa mista indica una diminuzione della gittata cardiaca.

370.8 • Interpretazione dell'emogasanalisi

L'interpretazione dell'emogasanalisi è importante per localizzare la sede della lesione e stimarne la severità, in particolare quando viene integrata con le osservazioni cliniche (Tab. 370-2). Nell'ostruzione delle vie aeree al di sopra della carena (stenosi ipoglottica, anello vascolare), l'emogasanalisi riflette l'ipoventilazione alveolare complessiva. Questo si manifesta con un'elevata P_ACO_2 e una riduzione proporzionale della P_AO_2, come determinato dall'equazione dell'aria alveolare. Un aumento di 20 torr della P_ACO_2 provocherà una riduzione della P_AO_2 di $20 \times 1,25$ o 25 torr. In assenza di una malattia parenchimale significativa e di shunt intrapolmonare, queste lesioni rispondono molto bene alla somministrazione di ossigeno, che è in grado di risolvere l'ipossiemia. Questo tipo di emogasanalisi, che dimostra l'ipoventilazione alveolare e la risposta alla somministrazione di ossigeno, è osservabile nei pazienti con depressione del centro respiratorio e funzione neuromuscolare inefficace, che risultano in insufficienza respiratoria (vedi Fig. 370-9). È facile distinguere questi pazienti da quelli con ostruzione delle vie aeree, per lo scarso sforzo respiratorio che li caratterizza.

Nell'ostruzione delle vie aeree intrapolmonari (asma, bronchiolite), l'emogasanalisi riflette lo squilibrio ventilazione-perfusione e la commistione venosa. In queste malattie, l'ostruzione non è uniforme nell'ambito dei polmoni, ma dà luogo ad aree iperventilate e altre ipoventilate. Il sangue capillare polmonare proveniente dalle zone iperventilate ha una PO_2 più elevata e una PCO_2 più bassa, mentre quello che arriva dalle regioni ipoventilate ha una PO_2 più bassa e una PCO_2 più elevata. Un livello ematico di PCO_2 inferiore può compensare l'elevata PCO_2, poiché la curva di dissociazione

TABELLA 370-2. Interpretazione dell'emogasanalisi arteriosa (ABG, *Arterial Blood Gas*)

LESIONE	EFFETTO	ABG TIPICA
Ostruzione centrale (sopra la carena) o Depressione del centro del respiro o Funzione muscolare inefficace	Ipoventilazione alveolare uniforme	Aumento precoce della PCO_2 Riduzione proporzionale della PO_2 dipendente dall'equazione dell'aria alveolare Risposta alla somministrazione di ossigeno: eccellente
Ostruzione delle vie aeree intrapolmonari	Mismatch V/Q da commistione venosa	Lieve: ↓ PCO_2, ↓ PO_2 Moderata: PCO_2 "Normale", ↓↓ PO_2 Severa: ↑↑ PCO_2, ↓↓↓ PO_2 Risposta alla somministrazione di ossigeno: buona
Patologia alveolointerstiziale	Difetto di diffusione R ⟶L shunt	Riduzione precoce della PO_2 a seconda della gravità PCO_2 normale o bassa, ↑ PCO_2 se insorge fatica Risposta alla somministrazione di ossigeno: da modesta a scadente

V/Q, ventilazione-perfusione.

della carbossiemoglobina è relativamente lineare. Nelle patologie più lievi, le aree iperventilate predominano, configurando un quadro di ipocapnia. Una PaO_2 elevata nelle zone iperventilate non può compensare la riduzione della PaO_2 in quelle ipoventilate, a causa della forma della curva di dissociazione dell'ossiemoglobina, ma provoca commistione venosa, desaturazione arteriosa e riduzione della PaO_2 (vedi Fig. 370-10). A mano a mano che la gravità della patologia aumenta, sempre più aree sono soggette a ipoventilazione, fenomeno che determina la normalizzazione della $PaCO_2$ e un ulteriore declino della PaO_2. Una $PaCO_2$ normale o di poco aumentata, nell'asma, deve essere considerata con sospetto, in quanto potenziale indicatore di insufficienza respiratoria incombente. Nell'ostruzione severa delle vie aeree intrapolmonari predominano le zone ipoventilate, con conseguente ipercapnia, acidosi respiratoria e ipossiemia. Fino a che punto la somministrazione di ossigeno faccia aumentare la PaO_2 dipende dalla gravità della malattia e dal grado di commistione venosa.

Nelle malattie alveolari e interstiziali, l'emogasanalisi riflette sia lo shunt destro-sinistro intrapolmonare, sia l'alterata diffusione. L'ipossiema, caratteristica di queste condizioni, si verifica precocemente nel corso del processo patologico. La $PaCO_2$ può essere normale o ridotta. Un aumento della $PaCO_2$ si osserva solo tardivamente, quando la fatica e l'esaurimento muscolare conducono a ipoventilazione. Rispetto ad altre lesioni la risposta alla somministrazione di ossigeno è relativamente scadente, a causa dell'effetto shunt e delle alterazioni della diffusione.

La maggior parte dei quadri clinici si presenta con alterazioni miste. Un bambino con un anello vascolare può anche avere aree di atelettasia; l'emogasanalisi arteriosa mette in luce entrambi questi processi. L'emogasanalisi riflette la lesione predominante.

370.9 • Sistema vascolare del polmone in condizioni normali e patologiche

Durante lo sviluppo fetale intrauterino, la tonaca media delle arterie polmonari aumenta la sua componente muscolare nell'ultimo trimestre di gravidanza (vedi Capitolo 101.1). Fino al 90% del ritorno venoso sistemico è deviato dalla circolazione arteriosa polmonare attraverso il forame ovale e il dotto arterioso. Dopo la nascita, con la chiusura funzionale del forame ovale e del dotto arterioso e la dilatazione della circolazione arteriosa polmonare, con conseguente riduzione delle **resistenze vascolari polmonari** (PVR, *Pulmonary Vascular Resistance*), tutta la gittata del ventricolo destro passa attraverso il polmone. A 3 giorni dalla nascita le PVR sono pari a circa il 50% delle resistenze vascolari sistemiche. Nelle settimane successive, vi è un ulteriore declino delle PVR, e quindi della pressione arteriosa polmonare, con l'involuzione della muscolatura della tonaca media dell'arteria polmonare. Due-tre mesi dopo la nascita, le PVR e la pressione arteriosa polmonare sono circa il 15% dei valori sistemici, un rapporto che si mantiene inalterato durante l'infanzia e l'adolescenza. I vasi polmonari si costringono in risposta all'ipossiemia, all'acidosi e all'ipercapnia, mentre si dilatano con l'aumento della PO_2 alveolare e arteriosa, con l'alcalosi e l'ipocapnia. I lattanti di pochi mesi, che hanno arterie polmonari ancora relativamente muscolari, sono particolarmente suscettibili allo stimolo vasocostrittivo polmonare.

L'incapacità del sistema arterioso polmonare di dilatarsi dopo la nascita determina l'**ipertensione polmonare persistente del neonato** (**PPHN**, *Persistent Pulmonary Hypertension of the Newborn*; vedi Capitolo 101.8). Poiché le PVR si mantengono elevate, il sangue venoso sistemico, che ritorna al lato destro del cuore, continua a essere deviato, attraverso il forame ovale e il dotto arterioso, nella circolazione arteriosa sistemica: si instaura così un circolo vizioso di ipossiemia, acidosi e ulteriore vasocostrizione polmonare.

Le PVR relativamente elevate oppongono un eccessivo shunt sinistro-destro nei neonati a termine con difetti del setto ventricolare e dotto arterioso pervio (vedi Capitolo 426). Questi soggetti di solito non manifestano segni di insufficienza cardiaca fino a 2-3 mesi dopo la nascita, quando le PVR si sono sufficientemente ridotte. I neonati prematuri, con lesioni in grado di causare shunt sinistro-destro, possono sviluppare insufficienza cardiaca più precocemente, in quanto la muscolatura della tonaca media delle arterie è poco sviluppata e quindi le PVR sono inferiori. Lo shunt sinistro-destro persistente e a lungo termine comporta il rischio di evolvere in una malattia vascolare polmonare secondaria, caratterizzata dallo sviluppo postnatale di ipertrofia muscolare della tonaca media, seguito da proliferazione intimale e aumento delle PVR. Le alterazioni precoci dei vasi polmonari sono reversibili con la correzione del difetto cardiaco congenito responsabile dello shunt sinistro-destro. Le malattie polmonari vascolari avanzate sono caratterizzate invece da alterazioni irreversibili a carico dell'intima e della media. Quando le PVR aumentano fino a superare i livelli della circolazione sistemica, si verifica lo shunt destro-sinistro, caratterizzato da uno stato di cianosi (sindrome di Eisenmenger), che rende il difetto inoperabile, a meno che non si esegua contemporaneamente un trapianto polmonare (vedi Capitolo 433.2).

L'**ipertensione polmonare** può svilupparsi senza un'eziologia ben definita (ipertensione polmonare primitiva) o come conseguenza di una malattia sottostante (ipertensione polmonare secondaria) (vedi Capitolo 433). Gli effetti avversi dell'ipertensione polmonare sono correlati all'aumento del postcarico del ventricolo destro, alla riduzione della gittata cardiaca e all'insufficienza cardiaca, caratterizzata da aumentata pressione venosa sistemica, epatomegalia ed edema. Nelle situazioni acute, l'insufficienza ventricolare destra e la gittata cardiaca ridotta possono peggiorare il trasporto di ossigeno e l'ipossiemia. L'insufficienza ventricolare destra secondaria a patologie polmonari prende il nome di **cuore polmonare.** L'ipertensione polmonare secondaria è un evento comune nelle malattie polmonari ostruttive in stadio terminale, come la fibrosi cistica e la displasia broncopolmonare. Il coinvolgimento delle arterie polmonari è talvolta osservabile nelle collagenopatie vascolari come la sclerodermia (vedi Capitolo 159) e la dermatomiosite (vedi Capitolo 158). Anche l'ostruzione funzionale o strutturale delle vie aeree superiori può causare insufficienza ventricolare destra. Pure i bambini gravemente obesi vanno soggetti a ipoventilazione alveolare cronica e insufficienza ventricolare destra, che configurano la **sindrome di Pickwick**. Il trattamento della causa sottostante è obiettivo prioritario nei pazienti con ipertensione polmonare secondaria (vedi Capitolo 433).

370.10 • Risposta immunitaria del polmone all'insulto patologico

Sono molte le malattie, locali o sistemiche, potenzialmente in grado di indurre una risposta infiammatoria a livello polmonare. I fattori locali in grado di indurre una reazione infiammatoria a livello polmonare comprendono i processi infettivi, l'aspirazione, l'asfissia, la contusione polmonare e l'inalazione di sostanze chimiche irritanti; le malattie sistemiche comprendono la sepsi, lo shock, i traumi e il bypass cardiopolmonare. Questa risposta infiammatoria è mediata dal rilascio di citochine e altre sostanze. Nel polmone, i macrofagi alveolari sono i principali artefici della risposta citochinica, con la produzione del *fattore di necrosi tumorale* α (TNF-α, *Tumor Necrosis Factor* α) e *interleuchina 1*β (IL-1β). Queste citochine contribuiscono a innescare la cascata infiammatoria, che determina la produzione di altre citochine, prostaglandine, specie reattive dell'ossigeno e stimola la formazione di molecole di adesione cellulare che, a loro volta, portano alla migrazione dei leucociti nel tessuto polmonare. Le conseguenze fisiopatologiche della risposta infiammatoria consistono nel danneggiamento dell'endotelio capillare polmonare e delle cellule epiteliali alveolari. Un gran numero di citochine ed eicosanoidi provoca vasocostrizione polmonare, con conseguente ipertensione polmonare e aumento del postcarico ventricolare destro. Il danno dell'endotelio capillare risulta in un aumento della permeabilità con essudazione di liquido ricco di proteine nell'interstizio e negli alveoli polmonari. I detriti cellulari e la fibrina formano le caratteristiche membrane ialine eosinofile lungo le pareti dei dotti alveolari. Si verifica desquamazione degli pneumociti di tipo 1. L'edema interstiziale e alveolare comporta una ridotta FRC, un'alterata diffusione, lo shunt intrapolmonare destro-sinistro attraverso gli alveoli scarsamente ventilati e l'aumento del gradiente alveolo-arterioso di ossigeno (A-aO_2). Clinicamente, un gradiente A-aO_2 >200 è considerato *danno polmonare acuto*, mentre un gradiente >300 configura la **sindrome da distress respiratorio acuto (ARDS,** *Acute Respiratory Distress Syndrome*) [vedi Capitolo 69].

Il medico deve considerare i potenziali effetti avversi di determinati interventi terapeutici (somministrazione di ossigeno, intubazione endotracheale e ventilazione meccanica) come parte delle conseguenze fisiopatologiche dell'ARDS. Elevate concentrazioni di ossigeno nell'aria inspirata comportano il rischio di danno dei capillari e delle cellule epiteliali polmonari; non è stato stabilito il limite al di sotto del quale la concentrazione di ossigeno può essere ritenuta sicura. Oltre al potenziale sviluppo di polmonite nosocomiale, la ventilazione meccanica comporta il rischio di danno polmonare indotto da ventilazione a causa dello stress fisico subito dalle vie aeree terminali, dall'epitelio alveolare e dai capillari polmonari. Un volume corrente eccessivo, da solo, può causare un danno meccanico in grado di perpetuare la risposta infiammatoria. Se gli alveoli vanno incontro a una deflazione eccessiva durante l'espirazione, sono soggetti a un maggiore danno da stress da reclutamento e dereclutamento (*derecruitement*) alveolare. La strategia di ventilazione meccanica volta a minimizzare il danno indotto dal ventilatore, nell'ARDS, comprende il reclutamento alveolare e il mantenimento di una FRC adeguata, per tutto il ciclo respiratorio con una PEEP ottimale, e la ventilazione con volumi correnti relativamente bassi (6-8 mL/kg).

370.11 • Regolazione della respirazione

La principale funzione della respirazione è il mantenimento della normale omeostasi dei gas ematici e il soddisfacimento delle richieste metaboliche dell'organismo, con il minimo dispendio di energia. La frequenza respiratoria e il volume corrente sono regolati da una complessa interazione tra *controllori*, *sensori* ed *effettori*. Il centro di controllo della respirazione consiste in un gruppo di neuroni del SNC che, dopo aver ricevuto e integrato le informazioni afferenti dai sensori, invia impulsi motori agli effettori per iniziare e mantenere la respirazione. I sensori, costituiti da vari recettori localizzati in tutto il corpo, raccolgono le informazioni chimiche e fisiche, che poi inviano al centro di controllo per stimolarne o inibirne l'attività. Gli effettori sono i vari muscoli della respirazione che, sotto l'influenza del centro di controllo, permettono il flusso dell'aria dentro e fuori il polmone con un certo volume corrente e una certa frequenza. I meccanismi regolatori della respirazione vanno incontro a un processo di maturazione dal periodo neonatale alla prima infanzia. Gli **stati del sonno** esercitano potenzialmente una profonda influenza sul controllo della respirazione.

CENTRO DI CONTROLLO DEL RESPIRO. Il meccanismo di controllo della respirazione comprende due gruppi di neuroni funzionalmente e anatomicamente distinti, localizzati nel SNC: uno per il controllo volontario e uno per quello automatico. Queste aree, pur potendo funzionare indipendentemente, ma sono in grado anche di interagire tra loro.

Il **controllo volontario** della respirazione risiede nella corteccia cerebrale motoria e nelle strutture mesolimbiche. Il centro, dopo aver ricevuto dai neuroni sensitivi informazioni dolorifiche, tattili, termiche, olfattive, visive ed emozionali, invia impulsi direttamente ai muscoli respiratori attraverso i tratti corticobulbari e corticospinali. Il controllo volontario della respirazione è importante per proteggere dall'aspirazione e dall'inalazione di gas nocivi. Un certo livello di coscienza è necessario per esercitare un controllo volontario della respirazione. I pazienti con danni del SNC ed encefalopatie tossiche o metaboliche perdono il controllo volontario del respiro in grado variabile, a seconda dell'estensione della disfunzione del SNC.

Il **controllo automatico** della respirazione risiede nel tronco encefalico. Un gruppo di 150-200 neuroni, chiamato *complesso pre-Botzinger* (preBotC), localizzato nella regione midollare, è responsabile del mantenimento della ritmicità del respiro e può essere considerato il pacemaker dell'attività respiratoria automatica. I neuroni preBotC sono responsabili dei diversi pattern di respirazione, tra cui il gasping e il sospiro eupnoici, a seconda dell'impulso afferente. Questi neuroni hanno recettori specifici per i neurotrasmettitori, che possono stimolare, inibire o modificare la loro attività; tali recettori comprendono quelli per la sostanza P (neurochinina), l'acetilcolina (nicotinici), il glutamato e i recettori oppioidi μ. Diversi geni come gli Hox paralog e i geni Hox-regolanti kreisler/mafB e Krox20 regolano lo sviluppo embriogenico dei neuroni del tronco encefalico e le loro connessioni intrinseche. Un gruppo di neuroni localizzati nel ponte inferiore, denominato collettivamente *centro apneustico*, stimola il preBotC, dando luogo a prolungati gasp inspiratori (apneusi) interrotti da sforzi espiratori transitori. Un altro gruppo di neuroni nel ponte superiore, chiamato *centro pneumotassico*, è coinvolto nell'inibizione dell'attività del preBotC. I centri apneustico e pneumotassico permettono una regolazione più fine dell'attività respiratoria ritmica generata dai neuroni preBotC.

Le anomalie della respirazione sono comuni in corso di disfunzioni del SNC. Una depressione globale del SNC può manifestarsi con una respirazione lenta e superficiale, con conseguente ipoventilazione e acidosi respiratoria. Le patologie che colpiscono entrambi gli emisferi cerebrali e il diencefalo possono portare al **respiro di Cheyne-Stokes**, caratterizzato da periodi di apnea intervallati da iperventilazione. I danni della parte rostrale del tronco encefalico o del tegmento possono determinare iperventilazione centrale neurogena con alcalosi respiratoria. Le lesioni della parte intermedia e caudale del ponte possono risultare in un pattern di respirazione apneustica, caratterizzata da una pausa inspiratoria prolungata. Le lesioni midollari provocano un respiro atassico e irregolare, oppure apnea.

SENSORI. Diversi recettori, distribuiti in tutto il corpo, sono responsabili della captazione delle informazioni afferenti che modulano l'attività del centro di controllo del respiro. Tali terminazioni nervose, che rispondono a variazioni dell'ambiente circostante, sono chiamate *chemiocettori* o *meccanocettori* a seconda del tipo di stimolo a cui sono sensibili. I chemiocettori a loro volta si dividono in centrali e periferici, a seconda della loro localizzazione.

I **chemiocettori centrali**, così chiamati per la loro localizzazione all'interno del SNC, sono sensibili a variazioni della composizione chimica dei liquidi corporei con cui vengono in contatto. Distribuiti in una vasta area comprendente l'ipotalamo posteriore, il cervelletto, il locus coeruleus, il rafe e diversi nuclei all'interno del tronco encefalico, i chemiocettori centrali sono immersi nel liquido extracellulare encefalico e rispondono a variazioni della concentrazione di H^+. Un aumento della concentrazione di H^+ stimola la risposta ventilatoria del centro, mentre una riduzione la inibisce. Il liquido extracellulare encefalico, rappresentato dal liquido cefalorachidiano (CSF, *CerebroSpinal Fluid*), è separato dal sangue dalla barriera ematoencefalica, che è relativamente impermeabile agli ioni H^+ e HCO_3^-, ma relativamente permeabile alla CO_2. Un aumento della $PaCO_2$ si riflette rapidamente in un analogo aumento del CSF. La conseguente riduzione del pH del CSF, percepita dai chemiocettori centrali, si traduce nella stimolazione del centro di controllo e nell'aumento della ventilazione. Le variazioni della $PaCO_2$ comportano la stimolazione o l'inibizione della ventilazione tramite le variazioni del pH del CSF. Il pH del CSF in condizioni normali è circa 7,2. Rispetto al sangue, il CSF ha una capacità molto inferiore di tamponare la CO_2, a causa di una concentrazione di proteine molto minore. Di conseguenza, i cambiamenti di pH nel CSF sono più pronunciati rispetto a quelli nel sangue, a parità di variazione di $PaCO_2$. Con un aumento persistente della $PaCO_2$, il pH del CSF tende alla fine a normalizzarsi poiché il HCO_3^- si equilibra attraverso la barriera ematoencefalica. I pazienti con broncopneumopatia cronica ostruttiva hanno pertanto un pH relativamente normale nel CSF e non presentano la risposta ventilatoria che si osserva con un aumento acuto della $PaCO_2$.

L'ipossia può deprimere la funzione globale del SNC; ciononostante, diverse regioni encefaliche presentano una risposta eccitatoria all'ipossia, che contribuisce ad aumentare la ventilazione.

I **chemiocettori periferici** sono localizzati nei corpi carotidei, appena al di sopra della biforcazione delle arterie carotidi comuni, e nei corpi aortici, al di sopra e al di sotto dell'arco aortico; i corpi carotidei sono i più importanti nell'uomo. L'elemento più importante nel determinare l'attività dei corpi carotidei è la variazione di PaO_2. Sebbene i corpi carotidei abbiano un'attività metabolica relativamente elevata, ricevono un flusso molto alto in rapporto alle loro dimensioni, piuttosto piccole. Finché il flusso di sangue si mantiene normale, l'ossigeno disciolto riflesso dalla PaO_2 è sufficiente per il loro metabolismo. La stimolazione dei corpi carotidei, che determina un aumento della ventilazione, avviene quando l'apporto di ossigeno scende al sotto del loro fabbisogno metabolico. Questo si verifica in conseguenza di (1) una riduzione della PaO_2, (2) una riduzione del flusso di sangue (bassa gittata cardiaca) e (3) un alterato utilizzo dell'ossigeno (avvelenamento da cianuro). Nell'anemia, nell'avvelenamento da monossido di carbonio e nella metaemoglobinemia, i corpi carotidei non vengono stimolati finché PaO_2 e gittata cardiaca non sono compromesse. Il rapporto tra PaO_2 e stimolazione dei corpi carotidei è di tipo non lineare (Fig. 370-11).

I corpi carotidei sono attivati da livelli di PaO_2 <500 torr: a conferma di ciò, si assiste a una lieve ma chiara riduzione della ventilazione, negli individui normali che respirano ossigeno al 100%, quando la PaO_2 supera i 500 torr. Finché la PaO_2 non raggiunge i 100 torr si verifica un aumento relativamente lieve della ventilazione. Quando la PaO_2 è <100 torr, la stimolazione dei corpi carotidei aumenta significativamente. La frequenza di risposta dei recettori dei corpi carotidei è sufficientemente rapida da alterare la loro frequenza di scarica, durante il ciclo respiratorio, in conseguenza di piccole variazioni cicliche della PaO_2 durante l'inspirazione e l'espirazione. A livelli di PaO_2 <50 torr, la stimolazione dei corpi carotidei aumenta esponenzialmente. L'effetto più importante della stimolazione dei corpi carotidei è l'aumento della frequenza respiratoria e del volume corrente. Altri effetti comprendono vasocostrizione, bradicardia, ipertensione sistemica, rilascio di ormone antidiuretico e stimolazione della midollare e della corteccia surrenalica. L'effetto bradicardico della stimolazione dei corpi carotidei è mascherato dal riflesso polmonare, indotto dall'inflazione dei polmoni, che determina tachicardia. I pazienti in cui l'inflazione polmonare è impedita sono più a rischio di sviluppare bradicardia dopo stimolazione ipossica dei corpi carotidei. Esempi di questa situazione sono l'ipossia fetale, la depressione del SNC, il blocco neuromuscolare, le miopatie, le neuropatie e la ventilazione controllata. I chemiocettori periferici sono responsabili di quasi tutti gli aumenti della ventilazione che avvengono in risposta all'ipossiemia.

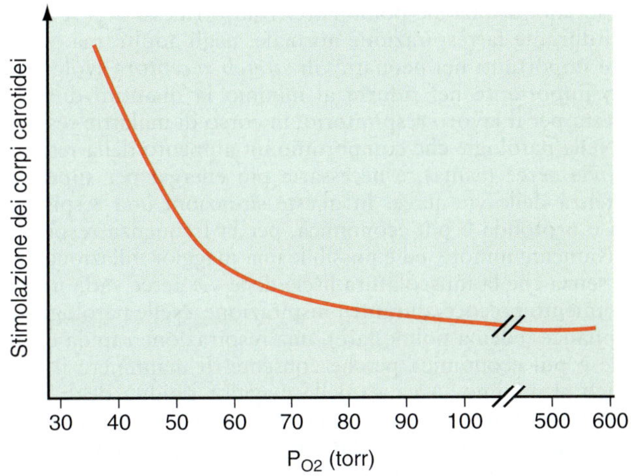

Figura 370-11. Una stimolazione significativa dei corpi carotidei si verifica per livelli di PaO_2 <100 torr. La sensazione soggettiva di dispnea non insorge, tuttavia, fino a quando la PaO_2 non è <50 torr, punto in cui la stimolazione dei corpi carotidei aumenta esponenzialmente.

Anche i chemiocettori periferici sono stimolati dall'aumento della $PaCO_2$; questa risposta richiede una variazione relativamente ampia della $PaCO_2$ e risulta in un aumento inferiore della ventilazione minuto, rispetto all'effetto della CO_2 sui chemiocettori centrali. I chemiocettori periferici, tuttavia, rispondono molto più rapidamente (nell'arco di un secondo), mentre quelli centrali possono impiegare alcuni minuti. Dunque i chemiocettori periferici sono importanti nell'aumento immediato della ventilazione, in risposta a un incremento imponente e improvviso della $PaCO_2$. Anche la riduzione del pH stimola i chemiocettori periferici; tale effetto si verifica a prescindere dall'origine respiratoria o metabolica dell'acidosi. La riduzione della PaO_2, l'aumento della $PaCO_2$ e la diminuzione del pH agiscono sinergicamente sui corpi carotidei. L'effetto combinato è maggiore della somma delle singole azioni.

Diversamente dai chemiocettori centrali, quelli periferici non vanno facilmente soggetti a depressione, per esempio per effetto dell'anestesia o degli oppiacei, e neppure si adattano a uno stimolo persistente come l'ipossia come fanno invece quelli centrali con l'ipercapnia. I chemiocettori centrali, nei pazienti ipossici, sono relativamente non responsivi alla CO_2 quando la respirazione è stimolata prevalentemente dagli effetti dell'ipossia sui chemiocettori periferici.

RECETTORI POLMONARI. Gli *stretch receptors* (recettori dello stiramento), localizzati nella muscolatura liscia delle vie aeree, sono stimolati dall'inflazione polmonare; l'impulso è condotto dal nervo vago. I principali effetti di questi recettori sono la riduzione della frequenza respiratoria (per inibizione dell'attività dei muscoli respiratori) e l'aumento del tempo di espirazione (cosiddetto riflesso di inflazione di Hering-Breuer). Il riflesso di deflazione di Hering-Breuer, invece, stimola l'attività dei muscoli inspiratori in risposta alla deflazione polmonare. Questi riflessi non sono operativi durante la respirazione normale, negli adulti, ma possono essere importanti nei neonati. Gli *stretch receptors* svolgono un ruolo importante nel ridurre al minimo la quantità di energia richiesta per il lavoro respiratorio, in corso di malattie respiratorie. Nelle patologie che comportano un aumento della resistenza delle vie aeree (asma), è necessaria più energia per superare la resistenza delle vie aeree. In queste situazioni una respirazione lenta e profonda è più economica, per la frequenza respiratoria relativamente minore, ed è possibile una maggior inflazione alveolare, senza che la muscolatura liscia delle vie aeree vada incontro a stiramento precoce, durante l'inspirazione. Nelle patologie della compliance (edema polmonare), una respirazione rapida e superficiale è più economica perché consente di mantenere il lavoro elastico al minimo. A causa della maggior rigidità degli alveoli, la pressione transpolmonare viene trasmessa ai muscoli lisci delle vie aeree più precocemente, durante l'inspirazione, stimolando gli *stretch receptors* e terminando l'inspirazione.

Gli *irritant receptors* (recettori dell'irritazione), presenti tra le cellule epiteliali della mucosa delle vie aeree, sono stimolati da particolati, gas nocivi e fumi chimici nell'aria inspirata, oltre che dall'aria fredda. Responsabile della conduzione dell'impulso è il nervo vago. La stimolazione di questi recettori dà luogo a broncocostrizione e iperpnea.

I *recettori J*, così denominati per la loro localizzazione "juxtacapillare", si trovano nelle pareti alveolari in prossimità dei capillari polmonari. La congestione dei capillari polmonari e l'edema interstiziale e della parete alveolare rappresentano lo stimolo per l'attivazione dei recettori J; quest'ultima dà luogo alla respirazione rapida e superficiale e alla dispnea osservabili nello scompenso cardiaco sinistro, nell'ARDS e nelle malattie interstiziali.

I *recettori muscolari* importanti per la regolazione della respirazione sono quelli del diaframma e dei muscoli intercostali. Lo stiramento dei muscoli percepito dal fuso muscolare permette di controllare la forza della contrazione. Un'eccessiva distorsione del diaframma e dei muscoli intercostali inibisce l'attività respiratoria quando è richiesta un'importante pressione intratoracica negativa per muovere l'aria, come nell'ostruzione delle vie aeree. Nei neonati e nei lattanti di pochi mesi la parete toracica è più flessibile e in quanto tale maggiormente soggetta alla distorsione; questi bambini possono rispondere all'ostruzione delle vie aeree superiori con la cessazione prematura dell'inspirazione e con l'apnea, invece che con il prolungamento dell'inspirazione richiesto per sospingere una sufficiente quantità di aria oltre l'ostruzione.

I *barocettori arteriosi* localizzati nell'arco aortico e nei seni carotidei possono influenzare la respirazione a seconda della pressione arteriosa. Una riduzione della pressione determina iperventilazione, mentre un aumento della pressione sanguigna causa ipoventilazione.

I *recettori termici e dolorifici* influenzano anch'essi la respirazione e hanno un ruolo particolarmente importante nei neonati e nei lattanti di pochi mesi. Uno stimolo doloroso induce il soggetto a trattenere il respiro, dopodiché subentra l'iperventilazione. L'aumento della temperatura cutanea causa iperventilazione, mentre l'ipotermia porta all'ipoventilazione. Nel contesto dello stimolo da freddo, l'area facciale è la più importante nel causare apnea.

EFFETTORI. Gli effettori della respirazione, di cui i più importanti sono il diaframma, i muscoli intercostali e quelli addominali, ricevono gli impulsi dal centro di controllo e provvedono alla ventilazione. In caso di necessità possono partecipare agli sforzi respiratori anche i muscoli accessori, come gli sternocleidomastoidei e i paraspinali. Gli effettori possono essere gravemente compromessi nella malnutrizione, nel danno spinale e nelle malattie neuromuscolari.

STATI DEL SONNO. La regolazione della respirazione è influenzata in modo considerevole dal sonno, che in generale riduce la chemiosensibilità centrale alla CO_2. La $PaCO_2$ è aumentata di pochi torr, rispetto a quella dello stato di veglia. Si distinguono due ampie categorie di stati del sonno: sonno *REM* (*Rapid Eye Movement*, movimento rapido degli occhi) e *non REM* (NREM) (vedi Capitolo 18). Il sonno NREM è caratterizzato da onde lente a elevato voltaggio all'elettroencefalogramma (EEG) e si associa ad attività mentale frammentaria. Non ha praticamente effetti sul tono muscolare e sui movimenti. Durante questa fase il cervello è relativamente inattivo mentre il corpo si muove. Il sonno REM è chiamato così per la presenza di momenti episodici di movimenti oculari rapidi; l'aspetto clinicamente più significativo è la marcata soppressione del tono muscolare posturale e la mancanza di movimenti spontanei. Durante questa fase a un cervello molto attivo fa riscontro un corpo "paralizzato". Responsabili della paralisi e dell'atonia caratteristiche, specifiche del sonno REM, sono gli assoni discendenti dalla regione del tegmento pontino. Il pattern predominante nei neonati prematuri è il sonno REM. Un neonato a termine ha il 50% di sonno REM. La maturazione del sonno avviene in gran parte nei primi sei mesi di vita. I bambini più grandi e gli adulti passano circa il 20% del sonno in stato REM. Le anomalie respiratorie correlate al sonno vengono osservate prevalentemente nella fase REM, durante la quale la depressione del tono muscolare ha due effetti principali. Innanzitutto, la parete toracica rilassata (e quindi dotata di maggiore compliance) si retrae verso l'interno in misura molto maggiore, durante l'inspirazione, rispetto a quanto farebbe una parete toracica con una compliance inferiore; questo fenomeno crea un impedimento al flusso aereo inspiratorio e porta a un pattern respiratorio paradosso (a onda), in cui l'addome e la parete toracica si muovono in modo asincrono. Il secondo effetto è il rilassamento dei muscoli genioglosso, palatino e di altri muscoli delle vie aeree superiori, con conseguente ostruzione delle vie aeree. Le anomalie respiratorie correlate al sonno REM sono di comune riscontro nei neonati prematuri e nei bambini in cui coesistono ostruzione anatomica delle vie aeree superiori, obesità e disfunzione neuromuscolare.

REGOLAZIONE DELLA RESPIRAZIONE IN SITUAZIONI PARTICOLARI.

Feto, neonato e lattante. Nei vari stadi dello sviluppo, la risposta alla stimolazione dei chemiocettori e dei meccanocettori e l'efficienza degli effettori sono marcatamente differenti. Al contrario degli adulti, che sviluppano una risposta immediata e sostenuta all'ipossiemia, caratterizzata da iperventilazione, il neonato presenta una risposta bifasica. Dopo un iniziale periodo di iperventilazione, piuttosto breve (1-2 minuti), se l'ipossiemia persiste, il neonato e il lattante sviluppano ipoventilazione e apnea. Questo spiega perché tali soggetti siano più inclini a sviluppare arresto respiratorio negli stati ipossici, rispetto ai bambini più grandi e agli adulti. Un'età gestazionale inferiore, nel neonato, si associa a una risposta apnoica all'ipossiemia più pronunciata e più precoce. L'attività respiratoria fetale, per esempio, è soppressa in situazioni di deprivazione di ossigeno. La maturazione dei chemocettori carotidei può spiegare le differenze nella risposta ipossica ai vari stadi di sviluppo. Anche la sensibilità dei sensori della CO_2 va incontro a maturazione. Rispetto agli adulti e ai bambini più grandi, i neonati e i lattanti hanno una ridotta responsività alla CO_2, misurata da un aumento della ventilazione alveolare minuto per un dato aumento di $PaCO_2$. La teofillina e la caffeina hanno dimostrato di aumentare la risposta ventilatoria dei chemiocettori centrali alla CO_2 e di diminuire il numero di periodi di apnea nei neonati prematuri.

I muscoli respiratori del neonato, non essendo allenati a sostenere pesanti carichi di lavoro, vanno più facilmente incontro a fatica rispetto a quelli dei bambini più grandi, e ciò limita significativamente la loro capacità di mantenere un'adeguata ventilazione nelle patologie polmonari. Inoltre, l'eccessiva retrazione verso l'interno della parete toracica, relativamente morbida nei lattanti, stimola gli *stretch receptors* dei muscoli intercostali, inviando impulsi inibitori al centro del respiro. I bambini molto piccoli sono quindi esposti a un rischio maggiore di sviluppare apnea, quando i muscoli respiratori sono soggetti a un elevato carico elastico, come nell'ostruzione delle vie aeree superiori.

Anche molti neurotrasmettitori coinvolti nella regolazione della respirazione vanno incontro a cambiamenti evolutivi e maturativi. I neuroni serotoninergici localizzati nei nuclei del rafe, dotati di proprietà chemiosensibili, rispondono alla riduzione del pH; negli animali, durante lo sviluppo, un loro aumento si associa a un aumento della chemiosensibilità. Sono state dimostrate autopticamente anomalie del nucleo arcuato (equivalente umano del rafe midollare del ratto e del gatto) nei bambini deceduti per sindrome da morte improvvisa del lattante (SIDS, *Sudden Infant Death Syndrome*; vedi Capitolo 372). Da studi di coorte compiuti su vittime della SIDS (giapponesi, afroamericani e bianchi) è emerso il coinvolgimento di un gene omozigote che codifica per l'allele lungo del promotore del trasportatore della serotonina. Le vittime della SIDS, rispetto ai controlli, hanno maggiori probabilità di esprimere l'allele lungo per il promotore del trasportatore della serotonina, e di non avere l'allele corto. Il ritardo di sviluppo dei neuroni serotoninergici o l'iperespressione dell'allele lungo del promotore del trasportatore della serotonina possono spiegare l'anomala risposta respiratoria a condizioni avverse, che sfocia nella SIDS. I chemiocettori centrali sono gravemente alterati anche nella sindrome da ipoventilazione centrale congenita.

Ipossia e ipercapnia croniche. Le malattie croniche alterano il meccanismo di controllo del respiro. Nei pazienti affetti da insufficienza respiratoria cronica con elevata $PaCO_2$, il pH del CSF si è normalizzato e i chemiocettori centrali sono divenuti non responsivi alla CO_2. Inoltre, il compenso renale determina ritenzione di bicarbonato con relativa normalizzazione del pH ematico. L'ipossiemia arteriosa rimane il principale stimolo alla ventilazione, che dipende prevalentemente dalla stimolazione dei chemiocettori periferici da parte della bassa PaO_2. La somministrazione di elevate concentrazioni di ossigeno, in questi pazienti, comporta il rischio di improvvisa eliminazione dello stimolo ipossico, con cessazione della respirazione ed esacerbazione dell'ipercapnia e della carbonarcosi, fino al coma. I pazienti con broncopneumopatia cronica ostruttiva e malattie neuromuscolari sono particolarmente suscettibili a questa complicanza. I bambini affetti da displasia broncopolmonare o distrofia muscolare che presentano elevate $PaCO_2$, con o senza ossigeno supplementare, possono sviluppare una grave ipoventilazione con acidosi respiratoria, quando la loro PaO_2 aumenta più dei loro valori basali, con la somministrazione di quantità maggiori di ossigeno.

I pazienti con ipossia cronica (per es. quelli che vivono ad altitudini elevate e quelli che soffrono di cardiopatie cianogene o pneumopatie interstiziali) hanno una funzione chemiorecettoriale attenuata e una scarsa risposta a un'ulteriore ipossiemia. Si tenga presente che i bambini con asma scarsamente controllato hanno anche una risposta ipossica attenuata; può quindi sembrare che abbiano una respirazione relativamente agevole, nonostante livelli di PaO_2 pericolosamente bassi. Chi si prende cura di questi bambini corre quindi il rischio di sottovalutare la gravità della malattia e questo atteggiamento può causare un ritardo nell'istituzione della terapia appropriata.

Abu-Shaweesh JM: Maturation of respiratory responses in the fetus and neonate. *Semin Neonatol* 2004;9:169–180.

Carskadon MA, Dement WC: Normal human sleep: An overview. In Kryger MH, Roth T, Dement WC (editors): *Principles and Practice of Sleep Medicine*. Philadelphia, W B Saunders, 2000, 3rd ed, pp 15–25.

Chokroverty S: Physiology of sleep. In Chokroverty S, Daroff RB (editors): *Sleep Disorders Medicine: Basic Science, Technical Considerations, and Clinical Aspects*. Boston, Butterworth-Heinemann, 2nd ed, 1999, pp 95–126.

Feldman JL, Mitchell GS, Nattie EE: Breathing: Rhythmicity, plasticity, chemosensitivity. *Annu Rev Neurosci* 2003;26:239–266.

Gozal D: New concepts in abnormalities of respiratory control in children. *Curr Opin Pediatr* 2004;19:305–308.

Polgar G, Weng T: The functional development of the respiratory system from the period of gestation to adulthood. *Am Rev Respir Dis* 1979;120:625–695.

Smith JC, Ellenberger HH, Ballanyi K, et al: Pre-Botzinger complex: A brain stem region that may generate respiratory rhythm in mammals. *Science* 1991;254:726–729.

West JB: *Respiratory Physiology: The Essentials*, 7th ed. Baltimore, Lippincott Williams and Wilkins, 2005.

Capitolo 371 ■ Approccio diagnostico alle patologie respiratorie

Gabriel G. Haddad e Thomas P. Green

La diagnosi appropriata, in un bambino che si presenta con segni e sintomi respiratori, dipende principalmente da un'anamnesi e da un esame obiettivo accurati. In alcuni pazienti sono necessari esami e tecniche diagnostiche complementari.

ANAMNESI

L'anamnesi deve includere domande sui sintomi respiratori (dispnea, tosse, dolore, sibili, russamento, apnea, cianosi), sulla cronicità, sul momento del giorno o della notte in cui si manifestano e sull'associazione con attività come lo sforzo fisico o l'assunzione di cibo. L'apparato respiratorio interagisce con molti altri apparati e le domande concernenti il sistema cardiovascolare, gastrointestinale, nervoso centrale, ematologico e immunitario possono essere rilevanti. Se il paziente va incontro a polmoniti ricorrenti, altrettanto importante potrebbe essere interrogarlo sul reflusso gastrointestinale o sullo stato immunitario. L'anamnesi familiare è essenziale e dovrebbe comprendere indagini sui fratelli e su altri parenti prossimi che presentino sintomi simili, o qualsiasi altra malattia cronica con una componente respiratoria.

ESAME OBIETTIVO

La disfunzione respiratoria di solito provoca alterazioni rilevabili nella modalità del respiro. I valori normali di frequenza respiratoria, presentati nella Tabella 66-3, dipendono da molti fattori, il più importante dei quali è l'età. Sono necessarie misurazioni ripetute della frequenza respiratoria, poiché questa, soprattutto nei bambini, è sensibile agli stimoli esogeni. La frequenza respiratoria durante il sonno è più riproducibile nei neonati, rispetto a quella ottenuta durante il pasto o l'attività. Questi valori variano da un individuo all'altro, ma sono in media di 40-50 atti/minuto nelle prime settimane e in genere $<$60 atti/minuto nei primi giorni di vita. Le anomalie del controllo del respiro nel bambino possono causare una respirazione lenta o periodica. Le anomalie meccaniche provocano alterazioni compensatorie volte in genere a mantenere o aumentare la ventilazione alveolare. Una riduzione della compliance polmonare richiede un aumento della forza muscolare e della frequenza respiratoria, che portano ad aumenti variabili dei rientramenti della parete toracica e dell'alitamento delle pinne nasali. Le escursioni respiratorie nei bambini con malattie respiratorie sono superficiali. Un grunting espiratorio è comune, poiché il soggetto cerca di aumentare la *capacità funzionale residua* (FRC, *Functional Residual Capacity*) chiudendo la glottide alla fine dell'espirazione.

I bambini con patologie ostruttive fanno respiri più lenti e profondi (vedi Capitolo 370). Quando l'ostruzione è **extratoracica** (dal naso a metà trachea), l'inspirazione è più prolungata dell'espirazione, e abitualmente si può udire uno stridore inspiratorio. Quando l'ostruzione è **intratoracica**, l'espirazione è più prolungata dell'inspirazione e il paziente deve spesso fare ricorso all'uso dei muscoli respiratori accessori.

La *percussione del polmone* ha un valore limitato nei lattanti di pochi mesi, poiché non riesce a discriminare tra i rumori che hanno origine da tessuti molto vicini l'uno all'altro. Negli adolescenti e negli adulti, la percussione in genere dà un suono ottuso nelle patologie polmonari restrittive e con versamento pleurico, nella polmonite e nell'atelettasia, e un suono timpanico nelle malattie ostruttive (asma, pneumotorace).

L'*auscultazione* conferma il prolungamento dell'inspirazione o dell'espirazione, e fornisce informazioni sulla simmetria e sulla qualità del movimento dell'aria. Inoltre, rileva spesso rumori anomali o patologici come **stridori** (un rumore monofonico prevalentemente inspiratorio), **crepitii** (suoni interrotti a elevata frequenza, udibili durante l'inspirazione e, più raramente, durante la fase precoce dell'espirazione, che denotano l'apertura di spazi aerei precedentemente chiusi), o **sibili** (suoni continui musicali, di solito causati dallo sviluppo di un flusso turbolento in vie aeree ristrette) (Tab. 371-1). L'**ippocratismo digitale** è un segno di ipossia cronica (Fig. 371-1), ma può essere dovuto anche a eziologie non polmonari (Tab. 371-2).

EMOGASANALISI

L'emogasanalisi arteriosa è probabilmente l'esame rapido più utile, da solo, per valutare la funzione polmonare. Questa indagine, pur non chiarendo la causa della condizione o la natura specifica del processo patologico, permette una valutazione complessiva dello stato funzionale del sistema respiratorio e fornisce indizi sulla patogenesi della malattia. Poiché il reperto di cianosi è influenzato dal colore della pelle, dalla perfusione e dalla concentrazione ematica di emoglobina, il riscontro clinico tramite ispezione è un segno poco affidabile di ipossiemia. L'ipertensione arteriosa, la tachicardia e la diaforesi sono segni tardivi e non esclusivi di ipoventilazione.

Per valutare in modo più corretto lo scambio gassoso nel sangue si esegue una misurazione diretta della PO_2, della PCO_2 e del pH arteriosi (vedi Capitoli 64, 101.4 e 370). Il campione di sangue dovrebbe essere raccolto in condizioni anaerobiche in una siringa eparinizzata, contenente solo la quantità di soluzione di eparina necessaria a spostare l'aria dalla siringa. Quest'ultima dovrebbe essere sigillata, posta nel ghiaccio e portata in laboratorio per l'analisi immediata. Sebbene queste misure siano insostituibili in molte condizioni, richiedono una puntura arteriosa e sono state in larga misura sostituite dal monitoraggio non invasivo.

Nell'interpretazione delle pressioni dei gas nel sangue, occorre considerare l'età e le condizioni cliniche del paziente. A eccezione dei neonati, valori di PO_2 arteriosa <85 mmHg in genere sono anomali per un bambino che respira in aria ambiente a livello del mare. Il calcolo del gradiente alveoloarterioso di ossigeno è utile nell'analisi dell'ossigenazione arteriosa, in particolare quando il paziente non sta respirando in aria ambiente, o in presenza di ipercapnia. Valori di PCO_2 arteriosa >45 mmHg indicano usualmente ipoventilazione o un grave squilibrio ventilazione-perfusione, a meno che non riflettano il compenso respiratorio di un'alcalosi metabolica (vedi Capitolo 52).

TABELLA 371-1. Nomenclatura dei suoni polmonari

	SUONI
DISCONTINUI	
Fini (elevata frequenza, bassa ampiezza, breve durata)	Crepitii fini
Grossolani (bassa frequenza, ampiezza elevata, lunga durata)	Crepitii grossolani
CONTINUI	
Elevata frequenza	Sibili
Bassa frequenza	Ronchi

Raccomandazioni dell'International Symposium on Lung Sounds, tenutosi a Tokyo nel 1985 per una nomenclatura unificata dei suoni polmonari. (Da Cugell DW: Lung sound nomenclature. *Am Rev Respir Dis* 1987;136:1016, per gentile concessione.)
Da Chernick V, Boat TF: *Kendig's Disorders of the Respiratory Tract in Children*, 6th ed. Philadelphia, WB Saunders, 1998, p 97.

TABELLA 371-2. Patologie non polmonari associate a ippocratismo digitale

CARDIACHE
Cardiopatie congenite cianogene
Endocardite batterica subacuta
Insufficienza cardiaca congestizia
EMATOLOGICHE
Talassemia
Metaemoglobinemia congenita (rara)
GASTROINTESTINALI
Morbo di Crohn
Colite ulcerosa
Dissenteria cronica, sprue
Poliposi del colon
Emorragia gastrointestinale severa
Linfoma dell'intestino tenue
Cirrosi epatica (compreso il deficit di α_1-antitripsina)
ALTRE
Deficit della tiroide (acropachia tiroidea)
Pielonefrite cronica (rara)
Tossiche (per es. arsenico, mercurio, berillio)
Granulomatosi linfomatoide
Morbo di Fabry
Morbo di Raynaud, sclerodermia
IPPOCRATISMO MONOLATERALE
Disordini vascolari (per es. aneurisma dell'arteria succlavia, fistola arterovenosa brachiale)
Sublussazione della spalla
Lesione del nervo mediano
Traumi locali

Da Chernick V, Boat TF: *Kendig's Disorders of the Respiratory Tract in Children*, 6th ed. Philadelphia, WB Saunders, 1998, p 102.

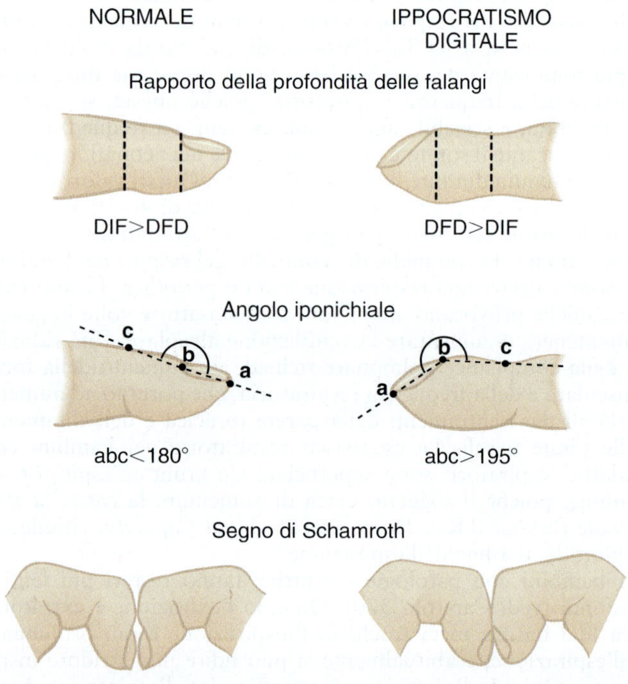

Figura 371-1. L'ippocratismo digitale può essere misurato in vari modi. Il rapporto tra il diametro falangeo distale (DPD, *Distal Phalangeal Diameter*) e il diametro interfalangeo (IPD, *InterPhalangeal Diameter*), o il rapporto di profondità delle falangi, è <1 nei soggetti normali, ma aumenta a >1 nell'ippocratismo digitale. Il rapporto DPD/IPD può essere misurato con i calibri o, più accuratamente, con calchi delle dita. L'angolo iponichiale può essere misurato dalle proiezioni laterali del contorno del dito su uno schermo ingrandente ed è di solito <180° nei soggetti normali, ma >195° nei pazienti con ippocratismo digitale. Per la valutazione clinica al letto del paziente, è utile il segno di Schamroth. La superficie dorsale delle falangi terminali di dita simili sono posizionate insieme. In caso di ippocratismo, la normale apertura o "finestra" a forma di rombo alla base del letto ungueale scompare, e si forma un angolo distale evidente tra i margini delle unghie. Nei soggetti normali, questo angolo è minimo o inesistente. (Da Chernick V, Boat TF: *Kendig's Disorders of the Respiratory Tract in Children*, 6th ed. Philadelphia, WB Saunders, 1998.)

TRANSILLUMINAZIONE DEL TORACE

Nei lattanti fino ai 6 mesi di età si può sovente diagnosticare uno pneumotorace tramite la transilluminazione della parete toracica, utilizzando una sonda luminosa a fibre ottiche. L'aria libera nello spazio pleurico spesso forma un alone insolitamente ampio di luce, nella cute che circonda la sonda. Il confronto con l'emitorace controlaterale è spesso molto utile nell'interpretazione dei risultati. Questo test non è affidabile nei pazienti più grandi o in quelli con enfisema sottocutaneo o atelettasia.

TECNICHE RADIOGRAFICHE

RADIOGRAFIA DEL TORACE. Quando possibile, si devono ottenere una proiezione anteroposteriore e una laterale (in ortostatismo e in massima inspirazione). Le lastre portatili, per quanto utili, possono fornire un'immagine alquanto distorta. Le lastre in espirazione possono essere mal interpretate, sebbene il confronto tra le immagini in espirazione e quelle in inspirazione possa essere utile nella valutazione di un bambino con sospetto corpo estraneo (un mancato svuotamento localizzato del polmone indica un'ostruzione bronchiale). Se si sospetta un versamento pleurico, sono indicate proiezioni in decubito. Le immagini ottenute in posizione supina sono difficili da interpretare se è presente un versamento nello spazio pleurico o una cavità.

RADIOGRAFIE DELLE VIE AEREE SUPERIORI. Una proiezione laterale del collo può fornire preziose informazioni sull'ostruzione delle vie aeree superiori e in particolare sulle condizioni degli spazi retrofaringeo, sovraglottico e sottoglottico (che devono essere visualizzati anche in proiezione anteroposteriore). Per un'interpretazione accurata è spesso essenziale conoscere la fase della respirazione durante la quale è stata ottenuta l'immagine. Le immagini ingrandite delle vie aeree sono spesso utili per delinea-re le vie aeree superiori. I pazienti con sospetta ostruzione non dovrebbero essere inviati senza sorveglianza medica in radiologia.

RADIOGRAFIA NASALE E DEI SENI PARANASALI. L'utilità dell'esame radiografico dei seni paranasali è incerta. Gli studi di imaging non sono necessari per confermare la diagnosi nei bambini di età <6 mesi. La TC è indicata nei casi in cui è richiesto un intervento chirurgico, in presenza di complicanze dovute a infezione dei seni, nei pazienti immuocompromessi e per le infezioni ricorrenti che non rispondono al trattamento medico.

TC E RM DEL TORACE. La TC delinea la struttura interna del torace con un dettaglio molto maggiore di quanto sia possibile con le radiografie semplici. I progressi tecnici hanno aumentato molto l'utilità di questa modalità diagnostica (spesso è possibile effettuare una ricostruzione tridimensionale) e hanno potenzialmente ridotto l'esposizione alle radiazioni. Le immagini TC sono di particolare importanza nella valutazione delle lesioni mediastiniche e pleuriche, delle lesioni parechimali solide o cistiche, dell'embolia polmonare e delle bronchiectasie. Durante la scansione si può iniettare del mezzo di contrasto per via endovenosa, per evidenziare le strutture vascolari, consentendo in tal modo di distinguere i vasi dagli altri tessuti molli in base alla loro densità. La RM può essere utile per le stesse entità patologiche della TC. La RM è una procedura eccellente per delineare l'anatomia ilare e vascolare associata ad anelli o a uno *sling* della polmonare.

FLUOROSCOPIA. La fluoroscopia è particolarmente utile per valutare lo stridore e i movimenti anomali del diaframma o del mediastino. Molte procedure, come l'agoaspirazione o la biopsia di una lesione periferica, vengono eseguite nel modo ottimale con l'ausilio della fluoroscopia, della TC o dell'ecografia. La videoregistrazione, che non aumenta l'esposizione alle radiazioni, può consentire uno studio dettagliato tramite la modalità di "riproduzione" durante una breve esposizione alla fluoroscopia.

STUDIO DEL TRANSITO ESOFAGEO CON BARIO. Questo studio, effettuato con fluoroscopia e immagini estemporanee, è indicato nella valutazione dei pazienti con polmonite ricorrente, tosse persistente da causa indeterminata, stridore o sibili persistenti. La tecnica può essere modificata utilizzando bario di diversa densità, da liquido a solido, per valutare la meccanica della deglutizione, la presenza di anelli vascolari e di fistole tracheoesofagee, specialmente quando si sospetta un'aspirazione. L'esofagogramma con contrasto è stato utilizzato nella valutazione dei neonati con sospetta atresia esofagea, ma questa procedura comporta un elevato rischio di aspirazione polmonare e di solito non è raccomandata. Gli esami di transito con bario sono utili nella valutazione del sospetto reflusso gastroesofageo, ma a causa dell'alta incidenza di reflusso asintomatico nei neonati, l'applicabilità dei risultati al problema clinico può essere complicata.

BRONCOGRAFIA. I dettagli dei bronchi più piccoli, difficilmente valutabili con la radiografia semplice e persino con la broncoscopia, possono essere delineati instillando il materiale di contrasto direttamente nelle vie aeree. Questa tecnica è stata utilizzata in passato per diagnosticare sospette bronchiectasie o anomalie delle vie aeree che possono richiedere un intervento chirurgico; la TC e la RM hanno ampiamente sostituito questa metodica di indagine, che richiede una sedazione e un'anestesia locale o generale.

ARTERIOGRAFIA POLMONARE E AORTOGRAFIA. L'arteriografia polmonare è stata utilizzata per consentire una valutazione dettagliata del sistema vascolare polmonare, oltre che per valutare il flusso ematico polmonare e diagnosticare le anomalie congenite come l'agenesia lobare, il polmone iperlucente monolaterale, gli anelli vascolari e le malformazioni arterovenose; talvolta è utile per valutare lesioni solide o cistiche. L'aortografia toracica visualizza l'arco aortico, i suoi vasi principali e la circolazione sistemica (bronchiale) polmonare. Serve inoltre per valutare gli anelli vascolari e il sospetto sequestro polmonare. Sebbene la maggior parte delle emottisi origini dalle arterie bronchiali, l'arteriografia bronchiale è raramente utile nella diagnosi o nel trattamento del sanguinamento intrapolmonare, nei bambini. L'ecocardiogradia real-time e con Doppler e la TC del torace con contrasto sono procedure non invasive che forniscono spesso informazioni simili e devono essere effettuate prima di ricorrere all'arteriografia.

SCINTIGRAFIA DEI POLMONI. La scintigrafia prevede l'iniezione endovenosa di materiale (come macroaggregati di albumina sierica umana marcata con ^{99m}Tc) che rimane intrappolato nel letto capillare polmonare. La distribuzione della radioattività, proporzionale al flusso di sangue nei capillari polmonari, è utile nella valutazione dell'embolia polmonare e dei difetti congeniti cardiovascolari e polmonari. Le variazioni acute nella distribuzione della perfusione polmonare possono riflettere alterazioni della ventilazione polmonare.

La distribuzione della ventilazione polmonare può anche essere determinata con una scansione, dopo che il paziente ha inalato un gas radioattivo come lo Xenon-133. Dopo l'iniezione endovenosa continua di Xenon-133 disciolto in soluzione salina, è possibile valutare sia la perfusione sia la ventilazione polmonari tramite la registrazione continua della velocità di comparsa e scomparsa dell'elemento radioattivo nel polmone. La comparsa dello xenon precocemente dopo l'iniezione è una misura della perfusione, mentre la velocità di eliminazione durante la respirazione è una misura della ventilazione, nella popolazione pediatrica. L'indicazione più importante a questo esame è la dimostrazione dei difetti di distribuzione delle arterie polmonari che si verificano in caso di malformazioni congenite o embolia polmonare. La **TC con ricostruzione spirale** con mezzo di contrasto è sempre più utilizzata per la valutazione della tromboembolia polmonare. Sono facilmente dimostrabili anche anomalie della ventilazione polmonare nell'enfisema lobare congenito, nella fibrosi cistica e nell'asma.

TEST DI FUNZIONALITÀ POLMONARE

Può essere difficile procedere alla misurazione della funzione polmonare nei lattanti e nei bambini più piccoli, che non sono in grado di cooperare. Sono stati fatti vari tentativi per ovviare a questa limitazione, creando test standard che non richiedono la partecipazione attiva del paziente. Tuttora i test di funzionalità respiratoria forniscono solo un'informazione parziale sui meccanismi delle patologie respiratorie, in età precoce.

Che si tratti di patologie restrittive o ostruttive, la maggior parte delle malattie respiratorie causa alterazioni del volume polmonare e delle sue suddivisioni (vedi Capitolo 370). Le malattie restrittive riducono tipicamente la **capacità polmonare totale** (TLC, *Total Lung Capacity*). La TLC include il volume residuo, che non è accessibile alla determinazione diretta e pertanto deve essere misurato indirettamente tramite metodiche di diluizione dei gas o, preferibilmente, con la **pletismografia.** Le malattie restrittive riducono anche la **capacità vitale** (VC, *Vital Capacity*). La VC può essere misurata con la **spirometria** (vedi Fig. 370-1) ed è usata comunemente al letto del paziente per valutare la progressione delle malattie neuromuscolari. Le malattie ostruttive provocano intrappolamento dell'aria e aumentano pertanto il volume residuo e la FRC, in particolare quando queste misurazioni sono considerate in relazione alla TLC.

Più di frequente per valutare l'ostruzione delle vie aeree si procede alla determinazione del flusso aereo nel corso di una manovra di espirazione forzata. Il **flusso di picco espiratorio** risulta ridotto nelle malattie ostruttive avanzate. L'ampia disponibilità di un semplice strumento che effettua questa misurazione al letto del paziente lo rende utile nella valutazione dei bambini con ostruzione delle vie aeree. La valutazione del flusso di picco richiede uno sforzo volontario, e questo valore può non risultare alterato quando l'ostruzione è da lieve a moderata. La misurazione del flusso di altri gas richiede che il bambino inali fino alla TLC e quindi espiri il più velocemente e il più a lungo possibile per alcuni secondi. Sono quindi necessarie cooperazione e una buona forza muscolare per rendere la misurazione riproducibile. Il **volume espiratorio forzato in 1 secondo** (FEV_1, *Forced Expiratory Volume in 1 second*) correla bene con la gravità delle malattie ostruttive. La **velocità massima di flusso espiratorio medio**, ovvero il flusso medio al 50% della capacità vitale forzata, è un indicatore più affidabile di ostruzione lieve delle vie aeree. La sua sensibilità alle variazioni del volume residuo e della capacità vitale, tuttavia, limitano ne limitano l'uso nei bambini con malattie più severe. La costruzione di una relazione flusso-volume durante le manovre di capacità vitale forzata supera alcune di queste limitazioni esprimendo il flusso espiratorio in funzione del volume polmonare (vedi Capitolo 370).

Per misurare la VC e le sue suddivisioni, oltre alle velocità di flusso espiratorio (o inspiratorio), si usa uno spirometro (vedi Fig. 370-1). Un semplice manometro può misurare la forza massimale inspiratoria ed espiratoria generata da un soggetto, normalmente di almeno 30 cm H_2O, che è utile per valutare la componente neuromuscolare della ventilazione. I valori normali attesi di VC, FRC, TLC e volume residuo sono ottenuti da equazioni di previsione basate sull'altezza.

Le velocità di flusso misurate dalla spirometria includono di solito la FEV_1 e la **velocità di flusso massima di flusso espiratorio medio.** Si può ottenere un numero ancora maggiore di informazioni dalla curva flusso-volume espiratoria massimale, in cui la velocità di flusso espiratorio è rapportata con il volume polmonare espirato (espresso in termini sia di VC sia di TLC). Le velocità di flusso per volumi inferiori al 75% della VC sono relativamente indipendenti dallo sforzo. Le velocità di flusso espiratorio per bassi volumi polmonari (<50% della VC) sono influenzate molto più dalle piccole vie aeree, rispetto alle velocità di flusso per volumi polmonari elevati (FEV_1). La velocità di flusso al 25% della VC (V_{25}) è un indice utile della funzione delle piccole vie aeree. Basse velocità di flusso a volumi elevati, associate a flusso normale a volumi bassi, suggeriscono un'ostruzione delle vie aeree superiori (vedi Capitolo 370).

La **resistenza delle vie aeree** (R_{AW}, *Airway Resistance*) è misurata da un pletismografo; in alternativa si può utilizzare il reciproco della R_{AW}, ovvero la **conduttanza delle vie aeree** (G_{AW}, *Airway Conductance*). Poiché la misurazione della resistenza delle vie aeree varia con il volume polmonare a cui viene effettuata, è più conveniente utilizzare la **resistenza specifica delle vie aeree,** SR_{AW} ($SR_{AW} = R_{AW}$/volume polmonare), che è quasi costante nei soggetti di età superiore ai 6 anni (normalmente <7 s/cm H_2O).

La **capacità di diffusione del monossido di carbonio** (DLCO, *Diffusing capacity of the Lung for Carbon Monoxide*) correla con la diffusione dell'ossigeno e si misura con la respirazione chiusa, in un contenitore con una concentrazione iniziale nota di monossido di carbonio, o utilizzando la tecnica del singolo respiro. Una riduzione della DLCO riflette una riduzione della superficie alveolocapillare effettiva, o una minore diffusibilità del gas attraverso la membrana alveolocapillare. Le anomalie primitive della diffusione sono rare in età pediatrica; pertanto, questo esame è utilizzato più di frequente nei bambini esposti a farmaci tossici per i polmoni (per es. i pazienti oncologici) o a radiazioni a livello della parete toracica. Lo scambio regionale del gas può essere adeguatamente valutato con la scintigrafia di ventilazione-perfusione allo xenon. Anche la determinazione dell'emogasanalisi arteriosa rivela l'efficacia dello scambio gassoso alveolare.

I test di funzionalità polmonare, sebbene portino raramente alla diagnosi, sono utili per definire il tipo di processo (ostruttivo o restrittivo) e il grado di compromissione funzionale, per seguire il decorso e il trattamento di una malattia e per stimare la prognosi. Sono inoltre preziosi per la valutazione preoperatoria e per confermare un'alterazione funzionale in pazienti con disturbi soggettivi ma esame obiettivo normale. Nella maggior parte dei pazienti con malattie ostruttive è necessario ripetere il test dopo la somministrazione di un broncodilatatore.

La maggior parte dei test richiede una certa cooperazione e la comprensione da parte del paziente; inoltre, l'interpretazione risulta molto facilitata se le condizioni del test e il comportamento del paziente durante l'esame sono noti. I lattanti e i bambini più piccoli che non sono in grado di cooperare con le procedure del test possono essere studiati con un numero limitato di modalità, che spesso richiedono la sedazione. Le velocità di flusso e le pressioni durante la respirazione corrente, con o senza interruzione transitoria del flusso, possono essere utili per valutare alcuni aspetti della resistenza o dell'ostruzione delle vie aeree, e per misurare la compliance dei polmoni e del torace. Le velocità di flusso espiratorio possono essere studiate nei lattanti sedati con la compressione passiva del torace e dell'addome con un giubbotto gonfiabile. I metodi di diluizione dei gas o la pletismografia possono anche essere utilizzati nei lattanti sedati, per misurare la FRC e la R_{AW}.

MICROBIOLOGIA: ESAME DELLE SECREZIONI POLMONARI

La diagnosi specifica delle infezioni del tratto respiratorio inferiore dipende dalla appropriata gestione di un campione adeguato ottenuto in un modo corretto. Le colture prelevate dal rinofaringe o dalla gola, pur essendo di frequente impiego, possono non correlare con le colture ottenute mediante tecniche più dirette dalle vie aeree inferiori. Sono preferibili i campioni di escreato, spesso ottenuti da pazienti che non espettorano tramite tampone profondo della gola immediatamente dopo la tosse, o tramite nebulizzazione di soluzione salina. I campioni possono anche essere ottenuti direttamente dall'albero tracheobronchiale mediante aspirazione nasotracheale (di solito fortemente contaminata), con aspirazione transtracheale attraverso la membrana cricotiroidea (utile negli adulti e negli adolescenti ma pericolosa in età pediatrica), e nei lattanti e nei bambini tramite o un catetere sterile inserito nella trachea durante la laringoscopia diretta, o un sondino endotracheale. Il campione si può prelevare anche in broncoscopia. L'unico modo per ottenere un campione assolutamente esente dalla flora batterica orale è un aspirato polmonare percutaneo o una biopsia a cielo aperto.

Un campione ottenuto con espettorazione diretta è considerato di origine tracheobronchiale, anche se spesso, specialmente nei bambini, non ha questa origine. La presenza di macrofagi alveolari (grandi cellule mononucleate) è indice di secrezioni di origine tracheobronchiale. Le secrezioni sia nasofaringee sia tracheobronchiali possono contenere cellule epiteliali ciliate, che sono di frequente riscontro nell'escreato. Le secrezioni rinofaringee e orali contengono spesso un gran numero di cellule epiteliali squamose. L'escreato può contenere cellule epiteliali sia ciliate sia squamose.

Durante il sonno, il trasporto mucociliare trasporta continuamente secrezioni tracheobronchiali alla faringe, dove sono inghiottite. Un aspirato gastrico eseguito al mattino, a digiuno, contiene spesso materiale del tratto tracheobronchiale adatto a colture per i bacilli acido-resistenti.

L'assenza di leucociti polimorfonucleati nello striscio di escreato o di liquido di **lavaggio broncoalveolare** (BAL, *BronchoAlveolar Lavage*) con colorazione di Wright, contenente un numero adeguato di macrofagi, rappresenta una prova significativa dell'assenza di un processo batterico infettivo nel tratto respiratorio inferiore, supponendo che il paziente abbia una funzione e una conta dei neutrofili normali. La presenza di eosinofili fa pensare a una malattia allergica. La colorazione per il ferro può rivelare granuli di emosiderina nei macrofagi, suggerendo un'emosiderosi polmonare. I campioni dovrebbero anche essere esaminati con colorazione di Gram. I batteri vicino o all'interno dei macrofagi e dei neutrofili possono essere significativi. La polmonite virale può essere accompagnata da corpi da inclusione intranucleari o citoplasmatici visibili agli strisci con colorazione di Wright, e le forme fungine possono essere identificate con la colorazione di Gram o argentica.

TEST DA SFORZO

Il test da sforzo (vedi Capitolo 423.5) è un approccio più diretto per rilevare un'alterazione della diffusione così come altre forme di malattie respiratorie. La misurazione della frequenza cardiaca e respiratoria, della ventilazione minuto, del consumo di ossigeno, della produzione di anidride carbonica e dell'emogasanalisi arteriosa durante carichi di esercizio aumentati progressivamente, fornisce spesso informazioni preziose sulla natura funzionale della malattia. Spesso una semplice valutazione della tolleranza allo sforzo del paziente, insieme ad altre forme più statiche di valutazione della funzione respiratoria, consente nei bambini la distinzione tra malattie respiratorie e non.

STUDIO DEL SONNO

Il sonno ha un'importante influenza sulla funzione respiratoria, in particolare nel neonato e nel lattante di pochi mesi (vedi Capitolo 18). Gli studi polisonnografici risultano spesso utili quando si sospettano anomalie del centro di controllo del respiro, disordini muscolari o complicanze respiratorie del **reflusso gastroesofageo**. La polisonnografia è attualmente considerata l'esame gold standard per l'apnea ostruttiva e l'ipoventilazione nel sonno. La pH-metria sonda è indicata, come esame complementare, nel sospetto di reflusso gastroesofageo. In questo esame si posiziona una sonda che valuta il pH nell'esofago e si effettua un monitoraggio prolungato (di solito della durata di diverse ore) (vedi Capitolo 320). Questi studi, che usualmente comprendono la contemporanea valutazione dello sforzo ventilatorio, del flusso di aria nelle vie aeree, dello scambio di gas e dello stato di sonno, sono utili anche nella diagnosi e nel trattamento dei disordini del centro di controllo del respiro e dell'ipossiemia e ipercapnia notturne, nei bambini con malattia respiratoria cronica (vedi Capitolo 370).

VISUALIZZAZIONE DEL POLMONE ED ESAME DIAGNOSTICO DI CAMPIONI

LARINGOSCOPIA. La valutazione dello stridore, dei problemi di vocalizzazione e di altre anomalie delle vie aeree superiori richiede in genere l'ispezione diretta. Sebbene la laringoscopia indiretta (con specchio) possa essere un approccio ragionevole nei bambini più grandi e negli adulti, raramente è effettuabile nei lattanti e nei bambini più piccoli. La laringoscopia diretta può essere effettuata con uno strumento sia rigido sia flessibile. Per un uso sicuro dello strumento rigido, durante l'esame delle vie aeree superiori, è necessaria l'anestesia locale associata alla sedazione o all'anestesia totale, mentre il modello flessibile può spesso essere utilizzato a livello ambulatoriale, con o senza sedazione. Altri vantaggi del laringoscopio flessibile comprendono la possibilità di valutare le vie aeree senza la distorsione che può essere introdotta dall'impiego di uno strumento rigido, e la possibilità di valutare più accuratamente la dinamica delle vie aeree. Data l'incidenza relativamente elevata di lesioni concomitanti nelle vie aeree superiori e inferiori, è spesso prudente esaminare le vie aeree sia sopra sia sotto la glottide, anche quando l'indicazione primaria riguarda le vie aeree superiori (stridore).

BRONCOSCOPIA E LAVAGGIO BRONCOALVEOLARE (BAL). La broncoscopia è l'ispezione delle vie aeree. Il BAL è una metodica utilizzata per ottenere un campione rappresentativo di liquidi e secrezioni dal tratto respiratorio inferiore, utile nella diagnosi microbiologica e citologica delle patologie polmonari, specialmente nei pazienti che non sono in grado di espettorare. Il BAL viene effettuato inserendo delicatamente la sonda in un bronco lobare, segmentario o subsegmentario e successivamente instillando e aspirando soluzione salina sterile non batteriostatica, in quantità sufficiente a far sì che una parte del liquido aspirato contenga materiale di origine alveolare. Nei pazienti intubati si può eseguire un BAL non broncoscopico (sebbene con minor accuratezza e, pertanto, con risultati meno affidabili), instillando e aspirando la soluzione salina attraverso un catetere inserito attraverso la via aerea artificiale senza controllo visivo nelle vie aeree distali. In entrambi i casi, la presenza di macrofagi alveolari testimonia l'ottenimento di un campione alveolare. Poiché i metodi utilizzati per il BAL comportano il passaggio degli strumenti attraverso le vie aeree superiori, sussiste il rischio di contaminazione del campione da parte delle secrezioni in esse presenti. Per la corretta interpretazione dei dati sono importanti un attento esame citologico e colture microbiologiche quantitative. Il BAL può spesso ovviare alla necessità di procedure più invasive, come la biopsia polmonare a cielo aperto, specialmente negli individui immunocompromessi.

Le indicazioni alla broncoscopia diagnostica e al BAL comprendono polmoniti o atelettasia ricorrenti o persistenti, sibili inspiegati o localizzati e persistenti, un sospetto corpo estraneo, emottisi, sospetto di anomalie congenite, masse, malattie interstiziali e polmoniti nel paziente immunocompromesso. Le indicazioni alla broncoscopia terapeutica e al BAL comprendono l'ostruzione bronchiale da parte di masse, corpi estranei o tappi mucosi, e la toeletta bronchiale generale e il lavaggio broncopolmonare. Gli individui sottoposti a broncoscopia ventilano intorno al broncoscopio flessibile, mentre se lo strumento utilizzato è rigido la ventilazione avviene attraverso la sonda. La broncoscopia rigida è indicata di preferenza per l'estrazione di corpi estranei, per la rimozione di masse di tessuto e nei pazienti con emottisi massiva. Negli altri casi, la sonda flessibile offre il vantaggio di poter essere inserita nei tubi endotracheali o da tracheostomia, di poter penetrare in bronchi che si diramano dalla via aerea ad angolo acuto e di poter essere utilizzata con sicurezza ed efficacia in anestesia locale con sedazione cosciente.

A prescindere dallo strumento prescelto, dalla procedura effettuata e dalla sue indicazioni, le complicanze più comuni sono correlate alla sedazione. Quelle più frequenti comprendono ipossiemia transitoria, laringospasmo, broncospasmo e aritmie cardiache. Le infezioni iatrogene, il sanguinamento, lo pneumotorace e lo pneumomediastino sono complicanze rare, ma riportate, della broncoscopia e del BAL. Nel contesto di un possibile ascesso polmonare, o di emottisi, la broncoscopia richiede una preparazione preliminare per il controllo definitivo delle vie aeree, ricordando la possibilità che del pus o del sangue possano inondare le vie aeree. L'edema sottoglottico è una complicanza più comune nella broncoscopia rigida che in quella flessibile, in cui si impiegano sonde più piccole, che hanno meno probabilità di danneggiare la mucosa. Il croup successivo a broncoscopia si tratta con ossigeno, nebulizzazione, aerosol di vasocostrittori e corticosteroidi, se necessario.

TORACOSCOPIA. La cavità pleurica può essere esaminata attraverso un toracoscopio, che è simile al broncoscopio rigido. Una volta inserito lo strumento attraverso uno spazio intercostale, il polmone viene parzialmente collassato, per dar modo all'operatore di vedere la superficie del polmone, la superficie pleurica del mediastino e del diaframma e la pleura parietale. È possibile inserire strumenti toracoscopici multipli, che permettono di effettuare biopsie pleuriche o polmonari, resezione di bolle, abrasioni parietali e legatura di anelli vascolari.

TORACENTESI. È possibile prelevare del liquido dallo spazio pleurico, a scopo diagnostico o terapeutico. Generalmente, bisognerebbe asportarne la maggior quantità possibile e si dovrebbe effettuare una radiografia del torace in ortostatismo, dopo la procedura. Le complicanze della manovra comprendono infezioni, pneumotorace e sanguinamento. La toracentesi del lato destro può essere complicata da rottura o lacerazione della capsula epatica, mentre quella sinistra dalla puntura o lacerazione della capsula splenica. I campioni ottenuti dovrebbero sempre essere sottoposti a coltura, esame microscopico per la ricerca di infezioni batteriche e valutazione delle proteine totali e dell'emocromo con formula. Può essere utile anche dosare la lattico deidrogenasi, il glucosio, il colesterolo, i trigliceridi (chilo) e le amilasi. Se si sospetta un tumore, è imperativo l'esame citologico.

Il trasudato, attribuibile a fattori meccanici che incidono sulla velocità di formazione o riassorbimento del liquido pleurico, generalmente non richiede ulteriori approfondimenti diagnostici. Gli essudati, dovuti a processi infiammatori o altre patologie della superficie pleurica e del polmone sottostante, richiedono invece una valutazione diagnostica più completa. In generale, i trasudati hanno valori di proteine totali <3g/dL, o un rapporto tra proteine pleuriche e plasmatiche $<0,5$, una conta leucocitaria totale inferiore a 2000/mm^3 con una predominanza di cellule mononucleate, e bassi livelli di lattico deidrogenasi. Gli essudati hanno elevati livelli di proteine e una predominanza di leucociti polimorfonucleati (sebbene gli essudati attribuibili a tumori o a tubercolosi possano avere una percentuale più alta di cellule mononucleate). Gli essudati complicati hanno un pH $<7,2$ e spesso necessitano di un tubo di drenaggio pleurico continuo. I versamenti tubercolari possono avere bassi livelli di glucosio e un contenuto di colesterolo elevato.

ASPIRATO POLMONARE. L'aspirato polmonare percutaneo, eseguito utilizzando una tecnica simile a quella della toracentesi, è il metodo più diretto per ottenere campioni batteriologici dal parenchima polmonare, oltre a essere l'unica tecnica (a parte la biopsia a cielo aperto) non associata a rischio anche basso di contaminazione da parte della flora orale. Dopo aver effettuato un'anestesia locale, si inserisce un ago unito a una siringa contenente soluzione salina sterile non batteriostatica, utilizzando tecniche asettiche, attraverso il lato inferiore di uno spazio intercostale, nella zona di interesse. L'ago è rapidamente spinto nel polmone; una volta iniettata e riaspirata la soluzione salina, si estrae l'ago. Queste procedure vanno effettuate il più velocemente possibile. Di solito la procedura appena descritta fornisce alcune gocce di liquido di origine polmonare, che devono essere sottoposte a coltura ed esame microscopico.

Le principali indicazioni all'aspirato polmonare sono gli infiltrati da causa indeterminata osservati radiograficamente, in particolare quelli non responsivi alla terapia, nei pazienti immuocompromessi, suscettibili a infezioni da microrganismi inusuali. Le complicanze sono le stesse della toracentesi, ma l'incidenza di pneumotorace è maggiore, e in qualche modo dipendente dalla natura della processo patologico sottostante. Nei pazienti con scarsa compliance polmonare, come i bambini con polmonite da *Pneumocystis*, la frequenza può arrivare al 30%, di cui il 5% necessita di drenaggio toracico. Il lavaggio broncopolmonare ha sostituito l'aspirato polmonare per la maggior parte delle indicazioni.

BIOPSIA POLMONARE. La biopsia polmonare può essere l'unico modo per stabilire una diagnosi, specialmente nelle malattie protratte, non infettive. Nei lattanti e nei bambini più piccoli, la toracoscopia e le biopsie chirurgiche a cielo aperto sono le procedure di scelta e, in mani esperte, hanno una bassa morbilità. La biopsia effettuata attraverso il broncoscopio pediatrico, del diametro di 3,5 mm, permette di prelevare solo un campione di piccole dimensioni, limitando le possibilità diagnostiche. Oltre ad assicurarsi di ottenere un campione adeguato, il chirurgo può ispezionare la superficie polmonare e scegliere la sede della biopsia. Nei bambini più grandi, si possono effettuare biopsie transbronchiali utilizzando una pinza flessibile inserita attraverso un broncoscopio, un tubo endotracheale, un broncoscopio rigido, in genere sotto guida fluoroscopica. Questa tecnica trova impiego in caso di patologie diffuse, come nella polmonite da *Pneumocystis*, o dopo rigetto di un polmone trapiantato. Le limitazioni diagnostiche correlate alle piccole dimensioni dei campioni bioptici possono essere compensate dalla possibilità di ottenere campioni multipli. Il rischio di pneumotorace correlato a broncoscopia aumenta quando la procedura comprende anche la biopsia transbronchiale; tuttavia, la possibilità di ottenere campioni bioptici in una procedura effettuata in anestesia locale e sedazione cosciente offre comunque dei vantaggi, in una popolazione selezionata, in cui questa procedura consente un ausilio diagnostico ragionevole.

TEST DEL SUDORE. Vedi Capitolo 400.

American Academy of Pediatrics, Subcommittee on Management of Sinusitis and Committee on Quality Improvement: Clinical practice guideline: Management of sinusitis. *Pediatrics* 2001;108:798–808.

Baughman RP (editor): *Bronchoalveolar Lavage*. St. Louis, Mosby–Year Book, 1992.

Goodman TR, McHugh K: The role of radiology in the evaluation of stridor. *Arch Dis Child* 1999;81:456–459.

Margolis P, Ferkol T, Marsocci S, et al: Accuracy of the clinical examination in detecting hypoxemia in infants with respiratory illness. *J Pediatr* 1994;124:552–560.

Saccomanno G: *Diagnostic Pulmonary Cytology*. Chicago, American Society of Clinical Pathologists Press, 1986.

Schechter MS: Snoring: Investigations guidelines. *Pediatr Pulmonol Suppl* 2004;26:172–174.

Schechter, MS; Section on Pediatric Pulmonology, Subcommittee on Obstructive Sleep Apnea Syndrome: Technical report: Diagnosis and management of childhood obstructive sleep apnea syndrome. *Pediatrics* 2002;109:e69.

Welsby PD, Earis JE: Some high pitched thoughts on chest examination. *Postgrad Med J* 2001;77:617–620.

Capitolo 372 ■ Sindrome della morte improvvisa del lattante

Carl E. Hunt e Fern R. Hauck

La sindrome della morte improvvisa del lattante (SIDS, *Sudden Infant Death Syndrome*) consiste nella morte improvvisa di un lattante, non prevedibile in base all'anamnesi e inspiegabile anche dopo accurato esame post mortem comprendente un'autopsia completa, l'analisi della scena del decesso e la revisione della storia clinica. L'autopsia, essenziale per identificare le cause naturali di morte improvvisa e inaspettata, come anomalie congenite o infezioni, e per diagnosticare l'abuso infantile traumatico (Tabb. 372-1, 372-2, 372-3), non permette invece di distinguere in modo affidabile la SIDS dal soffocamento intenzionale; tuttavia, la ricostruzione delle circostanze del decesso e la storia clinica spesso possono essere d'aiuto in caso di incongruenze palesi.

EPIDEMIOLOGIA. La SIDS è la terza causa principale di mortalità infantile negli Stati Uniti, responsabile dell'8% di tutti i decessi

TABELLA 372-1. Diagnosi differenziale dei decessi improvvisi e inaspettati nell'infanzia

CAUSA DI MORTE	CRITERI DIAGNOSTICI PRINCIPALI	FATTORI CONFONDENTI	FREQUENZA DI DISTRIBUZIONE
CHIARITA ALL'AUTOPSIA			
Naturale			18-20%*
Infezioni	Anamnesi, autopsia, coltura	Se reperti minimi: SIDS	35-46%†
Anomalie congenite	Anamnesi e autopsia	Se reperti minimi: SIDS o soffocamento intenzionale	14-24%†
Lesione non intenzionale	Anamnesi, analisi della scena, autopsia	Abuso traumatico infantile	15%*
Abuso traumatico infantile	Autopsia e analisi della scena	Lesione non intenzionale	13-24%*
Altre cause naturali	Anamnesi e autopsia	Se reperti minimi: SIDS o soffocamento intenzionale	12-17%*
NON CHIARITA ALL'AUTOPSIA			
Sindrome della morte improvvisa del lattante (SIDS)	Anamnesi, analisi della scena, assenza di cause spiegabili all'autopsia	Soffocamento intenzionale	80-82%
Soffocamento intenzionale (figlicidio)	Confessione del colpevole, assenza di cause spiegabili all'autopsia	SIDS	Sconosciuta

* Come percentuale di tutte le morti infantili inaspettate la cui causa è stata chiarita all'autopsia.
† Come percentuale di tutte le cause naturali di morte improvvisa inaspettata infantile la cui causa è stata chiarita all'autopsia.
Adattata da Hunt CE: Sudden infant death syndrome and other causes of infant mortality: Diagnosis, mechanisms and risk for recurrence in siblings. *Am J Respir Crit Care Med* 2001;164:346-357.

TABELLA 372-2. Condizioni che possono causare eventi apparentemente minacciosi per la vita o morte improvvisa

CAUSA	COMMENTO
SNC	Malformazioni arterovenose, convulsioni, ipoventilazione centrale congenita, disordini neuromuscolari (malattia di Werdnig-Hoffmann), crisi di Arnold-Chiari, sindrome di Leigh
Cardiache	Fibroelastosi subendocardica, stenosi aortica, anomalie delle arterie coronarie, miocarditi, miocardiopatia, aritmie (sindrome del QT lungo, sindrome di Wolff-Parkinson-White, blocco cardiaco congenito)
Polmonari	Ipertensione polmonare, paralisi delle corde vocali, aspirazione, malattia laringotracheale
Gastrointestinali	Pancreatite, diarrea e/o disidratazione, reflusso gastroesofageo, volvolo
Endocrino-metaboliche	Iperplasia surrenalica congenita, iperpiressia maligna, deficit di acil coenzima A a catena lunga o media, iperammoniemia (difetti enzimatici del ciclo dell'urea), glutaricaciduria, deficit di carnitina (sistemico o secondario), glicogenosi di tipo I, malattia delle urine a sciroppo d'acero, acidosi lattica congenita, deficit di biotinidasi
Infezioni	Sepsi, meningite, encefalite, ascesso encefalico, epatite, pielonefrite, bronchiolite (RSV), botulismo infantile, pertosse
Trauma	Abuso infantile, soffocamento, trauma fisico, sindrome di Munchausen per procura
Avvelenamento	Acido borico, monossido di carbonio, salicilati, barbiturici, ipecacuana, cocaina, insulina

SNC, sistema nervoso centrale; RSV, virus respiratorio sinciziale.
Da Kliegman RM, Greenbaum LA, Lye PS: *Practical Strategies in Pediatric Diagnosis and Therapy*, 2nd ed. Philadelphia, Elsevier Saunders, 2004, p 98.

TABELLA 372-3. Diagnosi differenziale della morte improvvisa del lattante ricorrente nei fratelli

Idiopatica	Vera sindrome da morte infantile improvvisa ricorrente
SNC	Ipoventilazione centrale congenita, disordini neuromuscolari, sindrome di Leigh
Cardiaca	Fibroelastosi endocardica, sindrome di Wolff-Parkinson-White, sindrome del Q-T lungo, blocco cardiaco congenito
Polmonare	Ipertensione polmonare
Endocrino-metabolica	Vedi Tabella 372-2
Infezioni	Disordini delle difese immunitarie dell'ospite
Abuso infantile	Figlicidio, infanticidio, sindrome di Munchausen per procura

SNC, sistema nervoso centrale
Da Kliegman RM, Greenbaum LA, Lye PS: *Practical Strategies in Pediatric Diagnosis and Therapy*, 2nd ed. Philadelphia, Elsevier Saunders, 2004, p 101.

in età infantile. È la causa più comune di mortalità infantile post-neonatale, responsabile del 40-50% di tutti i decessi dei lattanti di età compresa tra un mese e un anno. L'incidenza annuale di SIDS negli Stati Uniti era stabile a 1,3-1,4/1000 nati vivi (circa 7000 neonati/anno) prima del 1992, anno in cui l'American Academy of Pediatrics ha raccomandato che i neonati dormissero in posizione non prona per ridurre il rischio di SIDS. Da allora, in particolare dopo l'inizio della campagna "Back to Sleep" nel 1994, la frequenza della SIDS si è progressivamente ridotta per stabilizzarsi nel 2002 a 0,47/1000 nati vivi (2295 neonati). La diminuzione dei decessi da SIDS negli Stati Uniti e in altri Paesi del mondo è stato attribuito all'abitudine di distendere i lattanti in posizione supina durante il sonno. In molti Paesi la prevalenza del sonno in posizione prona è scesa a ≤2%, ma negli Stati Uniti nel 2004 il 13% dei bambini era ancora posto in posizione prona per dormire.

ANATOMIA PATOLOGICA. Non esistono reperti autoptici patognomonici di SIDS, né reperti richiesti per la diagnosi, sebbene ve ne siano alcuni comuni. Nel 68-95% dei casi si osservano emorragie petecchiali, più diffuse che nei casi di morte infantile da cause note. L'edema polmonare è spesso presente e può essere severo. La ragione di questi reperti è sconosciuta.

Le vittime della SIDS presentano varie alterazioni identificabili nei polmoni e negli altri organi, oltre che nella struttura e nella funzione del tronco encefalico. Quasi 2/3 delle vittime di questa sindrome ha evidenze strutturali di una preesistente asfissia cronica di basso grado, mentre altri studi hanno identificato marcatori biochimici di asfissia. Questi lattanti hanno inoltre un'elevata espressione nel liquido cefalorachidiano del fattore di crescita endoteliale vascolare (VEGF, *Vascular Endothelial Growth Factor*), che è stimolato dall'ipossia, reperto che fornisce una prova indipendente di eventi ipossici recenti singoli o multipli. I reperti a carico del tronco encefalico comprendono un aumento persistente delle spine dendritiche e un ritardo di maturazione delle sinapsi nei centri midollari di controllo del respiro, una ridotta immunoreattività della tirosina idrossilasi e una diminuzione dei neuroni catecolaminergici. L'immunoreattività dei recettori della 5-idrossitriptamina (5-HT) 1A e 2A appare ridotta nel nucleo dorsale del vago, nel nucleo solitario e nel midollo ventrolaterale, mentre è aumentata a livello della materia grigia periacqueduttale del mesencefalo. La diminuzione dell'immunoreattività recettoriale si accompagna a gliosi del tronco encefalico, e non è pertanto chiaro se sia secondaria all'ipossia o all'ischemia, oppure se rispecchi alterazioni primitive del metabolismo o del trasporto della 5-HT (vedi oltre la discussione sui polimorfismi della 5-HT).

In particolare, nelle vittime della SIDS il nucleo arcuato del midollo ventrale è stato oggetto di studi approfonditi. È una sede integrativa per le funzioni autonomiche, tra cui la respirazione e il risveglio, ed è integrato con altre regioni che regolano il risveglio e la funzione chemiosensoriale autonomica. Da studi anatomici quantitativi tridimensionali è emerso che alcune vittime della SIDS presentano un'ipoplasia del nucleo arcuato, e che fino al 60% di esse ha un'evidenza istopatologica di ipoplasia meno estesa, bilaterale o monolaterale. Considerando l'apparente sovrapposizione tra i meccanismi presunti della SIDS e della morte fetale tardiva inaspettata, è interessante che circa il 30% dei nati morti tardivi inaspettati e inspiegati abbia anche un'ipoplasia del nucleo arcuato.

Alcuni studi compiuti sui neurotrasmettitori del nucleo arcuato hanno identificato, in alcune vittime della SIDS, anomalie a carico di diversi tipi di recettori, importanti per il controllo autonomico stato-dipendente in generale e per la responsività ventilatoria e del risveglio in particolare. Questi deficit comprendono una significativa riduzione del legame ai recettori del kainato e ai recettori colinergici muscarinici e serotoninergici (5-HT). Questi lattanti, rispetto ai controlli, presentano livelli più elevati di interleuchina 1β (IL1-β) nei nuclei vagali dorsale e arcuato, fenomeno che forse contribuisce alle interazioni molecolari che influenzano le risposte cardiorespiratorie e di risveglio.

Dai dati post mortem qui riassunti non emerge alcun fattore di rischio genetico per la morte improvvisa inaspettata del lattante (SUDI, *Sudden Unexpected Death in Infants*), a esclusione dei fattori di rischio ambientali. Recenti studi genetici, tuttavia, hanno identificato diversi aspetti in cui i lattanti colpiti da SIDS differiscono geneticamente sia dai soggetti sani, sia da quelli che muoiono per altre cause (vedi il paragrafo "Fattori di rischio genetici" e la Tab. 372-4).

FATTORI DI RISCHIO AMBIENTALI. Nell'ultimo decennio si è registrata una diminuzione di oltre il 50% della frequenza di SIDS negli Stati Uniti e nel mondo, che può essere almeno in parte attribuita a una campagna di educazione nazionale volta a ridurre i fattori di rischio associati con questa sindrome. La riduzione del rischio sembra essere correlata principalmente alla diminuzione dell'abitudine di porre i lattanti in posizione prona per dormire e all'adozione della posizione supina. Anche vari altri fattori di rischio presentano associazioni significative con la SIDS (Tab. 372-5); nonostante molti non siano modificabili e la maggior parte di quelli modificabili non sia cambiata in modo apprezzabile, la prevalenza di fumo materno durante la gravidanza, autodichiarato, si è ridotta del 25% nell'ultimo decennio.

TABELLA 372-4. Geni identificati per i quali la distribuzione dei polimorfismi differisce nelle vittime di SIDS rispetto ai controlli

Geni per i canali ionici cardiaci del sodio e del potassio (*SCN5A*)
Regione promoter della proteina trasportatrice della serotonina (5-idrossitriptamina) (*5-HTT*)
Geni pertinenti allo sviluppo del sistema nervoso autonomo
Paired-like homeobox 2a (*PHOX2a*)
Fattore riarrangiato durante la transfezione (*RET*)
Enzima di conversione dell'endotelina-1 (*ECE1*)
Homeobox della leucemia T linfocitica (*TLX3*)
Engrailed-1 (*EN1*)
Gene *TSPYL*
Geni del complemento C4A e C4B
Polimorfismi del gene per l'interleuchina 10

Adattata da Hunt CE: Gene-environment interations: Implications for sudden unexpected deaths in infancy. *Arch Dis Child* 2005;90:48-53.

TABELLA 372-5. Fattori ambientali associati ad aumentato rischio di SIDS

FATTORI DI RISCHIO MATERNI E PRENATALI
Elevati livelli di α-fetoproteina nel secondo trimestre di gravidanza
Fumo
Consumo di alcol
Consumo di sostanze stupefacenti (cocaina, eroina)
Carenze nutrizionali
Cure prenatali inadeguate
Basso stato socioeconomico
Età molto giovane
Scarsa istruzione
Condizione di single
Breve intervallo intergestazionale
Ipossia intrauterina
Ridotta crescita fetale
FATTORI DI RISCHIO DEL LATTANTE
Età (picco a 2-4 mesi, ma talvolta anche prima)
Sesso maschile
Scarso accrescimento
Assenza del succhiotto
Prematurità
Posizioni prona e laterale nel sonno
Malattia febbrile recente
Esposizione al fumo (prenatale e postnatale)
Superficie di appoggio soffice, biancheria da letto morbida
Condivisione del letto con la mamma o entrambi i genitori
Stress termico, eccesso di riscaldamento
Stagione fredda, assenza di riscaldamento centrale

FATTORI DI RISCHIO NON MODIFICABILI. Sebbene la SIDS colpisca tutti gli strati sociali, un basso livello socioeconomico si associa a un rischio maggiore. Negli Stati Uniti, i neonati afroamericani, nativi Americani e nativi dell'Alaska hanno una probabilità da 2 a 3 volte maggiore dei neonati bianchi di morire di SIDS, mentre i neonati asiatici, delle Isole del Pacifico e ispanici hanno l'incidenza più bassa. Questa disparità può essere riconducibile almeno in parte all'elevata concentrazione di povertà e di altri fattori ambientali sfavorevoli osservata nelle comunità a maggior incidenza.

I soggetti più a rischio di andare incontro a SIDS sono quelli di circa 2-4 mesi, e la maggior parte dei decessi si è verificata entro i 6 mesi di vita. Questo dato caratteristico si è ulteriormente abbassato in alcuni Paesi, parallelamente al calo della SIDS, con decessi che si verificano più precocemente e un appiattimento del picco di incidenza. Analogamente, la predominanza stagionale invernale, di comune osservazione nella SIDS, si è ridotta o è scomparsa in alcuni Paesi, insieme alla riduzione della posizione prona, fenomeno che sembra avvalorare l'ipotesi di un'interazione tra la posizione del bambino nel sonno e fattori tipici dei mesi invernali (riscaldamento eccessivo, infezioni). I neonati maschi hanno il 30-50% di probabilità in più di essere colpiti, rispetto alle femmine.

FATTORI DI RISCHIO MODIFICABILI.

Fattori correlati alla gestazione. Numerosi fattori ostetrici si associano a un aumento del rischio di SIDS, suggerendo che l'ambiente intrauterino in questi casi sia subottimale. I lattanti colpiti da SIDS hanno spesso un ordine di nascita più alto, a prescindere dall'età materna, e sono nati da gestazioni dopo brevi periodi intergestazionali. Le madri di neonati colpiti da SIDS ricevono generalmente meno cure prenatali e in una fase più avanzata della gravidanza. Sono inoltre fattori di rischio il basso peso alla nascita, la nascita pretermine e una crescita intrauterina e postnatale più lenta.

Fumo di sigaretta. Esiste una forte associazione tra l'esposizione intrauterina al fumo di sigaretta e il rischio di SIDS. L'incidenza di SIDS risulta circa 3 volte maggiore nei figli delle fumatrici, negli studi condotti prima della campagna per la riduzione della SIDS negli Stati Uniti, e 5 volte maggiore in quelli successivi. Il rischio di morte aumenta progressivamente con l'aumento del consumo quotidiano di sigarette. Se invece a fumare sono il padre e altri membri della famiglia è più difficile interpretarne le conseguenze, a causa dell'elevata correlazione con il fumo materno. Sembra esservi un piccolo effetto indipendente del fumo paterno, ma i dati sui membri della famiglia finora non hanno portato a una conclusione univoca.

È molto difficile stabilire l'effetto indipendente dell'esposizione infantile al fumo passivo, poiché i comportamenti dei genitori relativi all'uso del tabacco durante e dopo la gravidanza sono strettamente correlati. Un aumento del rischio di SIDS si osserva anche nei lattanti la cui madre ha cominciato a fumare solo dopo il parto. Esiste una risposta dose-dipendente per il numero di familiari che fumano, per il numero di persone che fumano nella stessa stanza in cui si trova il lattante e per il numero di sigarette fumate. Il fumo materno è attualmente il più importante fattore di rischio per la SIDS.

Consumo di droga e alcol. Complessivamente, la maggior parte degli studi ha stabilito una correlazione tra l'abitudine della madre di consumare sostanze stupefacenti durante la gravidanza e un aumentato rischio di SIDS, mentre non ha trovato alcuna associazione tra il consumo materno di alcol (in epoca prenatale o postnatale) e la SIDS. In uno studio sugli Indiani delle Pianure del Nord, il consumo periconcezionale di alcol e il bere compulsivo nel primo trimestre si associavano a un aumento del rischio di SIDS rispettivamente di sei volte e di otto volte. I fratelli dei lattanti con la sindrome alcolica fetale hanno un rischio dieci volte maggiore di andare incontro a SIDS, rispetto ai controlli.

Ambiente del sonno del neonato. È stato dimostrato che il sonno in posizione prona aumenta il rischio di SIDS. Poiché la frequenza di questa posizione si è ridotta nella popolazione generale, sono aumentati gli odds ratio per i lattanti che dormono ancora proni. Il rischio di SIDS potrebbe essere più elevato nei neonati che abitualmente non dormono proni, ma che vengono messi in questa posizione nell'ultimo sonno ("proni non abituati") o che vengono trovati proni ("proni secondari"). La posizione dei "proni non abituati" si verifica con maggiore probabilità durante l'assistenza diurna o in altri contesti fuori casa; si sottolinea quindi la necessità di istruire tutti coloro che si prendono cura del lattante sulle posture appropriate durante il sonno.

Le raccomandazioni iniziali della campagna di riduzione del rischio di SIDS consideravano il sonno in posizione laterale quasi equivalente alla posizione supina, nel ridurre il rischio di SIDS. Studi successivi hanno indicato che, sebbene il decubito laterale sia più sicuro della posizione prona, i neonati che dormono distesi sul fianco hanno una probabilità doppia di morire di SIDS, rispetto a quelli che dormono supini. Questo aumento del rischio può essere correlato con la relativa instabilità della posizione, che porta alcuni neonati distesi su un fianco a rotolare in posizione prona. Le **raccomandazioni attuali** consigliano la **posizione supina** nel sonno per tutti i neonati, eccetto per quei pochi con problemi medici particolari, in cui può essere giustificato consigliare una postura diversa. All'inizio molti genitori manifestavano la preoccupazione che distendere il lattante in posizione supina comportasse conseguenze avverse, come disturbi del sonno, vomito o aspirazione; tuttavia, i dati suggeriscono che il rischio di rigurgito e di soffocamento sia maggiore per i lattanti che dormono in posizione prona. In alcuni casi il personale delle nursery neonatali continua ancora a privilegiare il decubito laterale, dando un esempio scorretto ai genitori. I neonati che dormono sul dorso non vanno incontro un maggior numero di episodi di cianosi o apnea; in Scandinavia i report di eventi apparentemente pericolosi per la vita si sono ridotti da quando si è diffusa l'abitudine di distendere i lattanti in posizione supina. Tra i neonati statunitensi che hanno mantenuto la stessa posizione durante il sonno a 1, 3 e 6 mesi di età, non sono più comuni sintomi clinici o richieste di visite domiciliari (dovute a febbre, tosse, sibili, disturbi della respirazione o del sonno, vomito, diarrea o malattie respiratorie) nei neonati che dormono supini o su un lato, rispetto a quelli che dormono proni. Tre sintomi sono in realtà meno comuni nei lattanti che dormono supini o su un lato: febbre al primo mese, rinite al sesto mese e disturbi del sonno al sesto mese. Le visite domiciliari per infezioni auricolari sono meno comuni al terzo e al sesto mese per i bambini che dormono supini, e ancor meno frequenti al terzo mese per quelli che dormono su un lato. Questi risultati dovrebbero rassicurare chi assiste il bambino e si spera porteranno alla generale accettazione della posizione supina come la più sicura e ottimale per il sonno, nei lattanti.

I materassi vecchi e troppo soffici, i cuscini imbottiti di fiocchi di polistirolo o la biancheria da letto più morbida si associano a un più alto rischio di SIDS, come pure le trapunte pesanti che possono finire per coprire la testa e il viso del lattante. Anche il surriscaldamento rappresenta un fattore di rischio, in base a indicatori come temperatura ambiente più alta, elevata temperatura corporea, sudorazione ed eccesso di vestiti o coperte. Da alcuni studi è emerso che l'eccessivo riscaldamento aumenta il rischio di SIDS solo quando i neonati dormono proni. Elevate temperature dell'ambiente esterno non si sono dimostrate associate a un'aumentata incidenza di SIDS negli Stati Uniti.

Diversi studi hanno indicato la condivisione del letto come un fattore di rischio per la SIDS, in particolare nei lattanti fino a 3 mesi di età, anche se la madre non è fumatrice. Questa abitudine è particolarmente rischiosa quando altri bambini dormono nello stesso letto, quando il genitore dorme con un neonato su un divano o su un'altra superficie di appoggio morbida o ristretta, e per i neonati di età inferiore a 4 mesi. Il rischio risulta aumentato anche in caso di condivisione del letto di durata prolungata, per tutta la notte; il ritorno del lattante nella sua culla non si associa ad aumento del rischio. Vi sono sempre più evidenze che la condivisione della stanza, ma non del letto, si associ a una minor frequenza di SIDS; sembra che per i lattanti il posto più sicuro in cui dormire sia il loro lettino, soprattutto se collocato nella stanza dei genitori.

Modalità di alimentazione dei lattanti. Numerosi studi hanno dimostrato un effetto protettivo dell'allattamento al seno che però non è presente dopo aggiustamento per fattori potenzialmente confondenti. Se ne deduce che l'allattamento al seno sta a segnalare uno stile di vita o uno stato socioeconomico, più che rappresentare un fattore indipendente. Sebbene i benefici di questa pratica siano molteplici, non si dispone di dati sufficienti per raccomandarla come strategia atta a ridurre il rischio di SIDS.

L'uso del succhiotto riduce il rischio di SIDS nella maggior parte degli studi, quando utilizzato per il sonno di riferimento o l'ultimo sonno. Secondo una metanalisi questo rischio ridotto corrisponde a un odds ratio corretto complessivo di 0,39 (intervallo di confidenza al 95% 0,31-0,50). Sebbene non sia noto se questo sia un effetto diretto del succhiotto stesso o di comportamenti associati del lattante o dei genitori, vi sono sempre più prove che l'uso e lo spostamento del succhiotto possa far sì che il lattante si risvegli più facilmente durante il sonno. La raccomandazione del succhiotto come mezzo per ridurre il rischio di SIDS ha suscitato perplessità e in particolare la preoccupazione che quest'abitudine possa comportare conseguenze negative sull'allattamento al seno. In alcuni studi ben costruiti, tuttavia, non sono state osservate associazioni tra l'uso del succhiotto e la durata dell'allattamento al seno. È stato riportato un modesto aumento dell'incidenza di otite media e di malattie respiratorie e gastrointestinali, negli utilizzatori di succhiotti, rispetto ai non utilizzatori. L'Olanda (per i bambini allattati artificialmente) e la Germania hanno consigliato l'uso del succhiotto come metodo potenzialmente utile per ridurre il rischio di SIDS. Le linee guida più recenti dell'American Academy of Pediatrics raccomandano l'uso del succhiotto dopo l'inizio dell'allattamento al seno.

Le infezioni delle vie respiratorie superiori non sono generalmente risultate un fattore di rischio indipendente per la SIDS, pur potendo concorrere, insieme ad altre infezioni minori, alla patogenesi della sindrome. Il rischio è risultato aumentato dopo una malattia, nei bambini che dormivano proni, in quelli avvolti in trapunte pesanti e in quelli che avevano avuto la testa coperta durante il sonno.

Non è emersa alcuna associazione tra le vaccinazioni e la SIDS. I neonati colpiti da SIDS hanno minori probabilità di essere stati vaccinati, rispetto ai controlli, e in quelli vaccinati, non è stata identificata alcuna correlazione temporale tra la somministrazione dei vaccini e la morte. Occorre quindi rassicurare i genitori che le vaccinazioni non comportano alcun rischio di SIDS.

La frequenza della SIDS resta elevata tra i Nativi Americani, i nativi dell'Alaska e gli Afroamericani. Questo può essere dovuto, almeno in parte, a differenze di gruppo nell'utilizzo della posizione supina nel sonno o in altri comportamenti di riduzione del rischio. Sono necessari ulteriori sforzi per affrontare questa persistente disparità e assicurare che la l'educazione alla riduzione del rischio di SIDS raggiunga tutti i genitori. Il messaggio deve arrivare a tutti coloro che si occupano del bambino, compresi i nonni, gli altri familiari e il personale degli asili.

FATTORI DI RISCHIO GENETICI. Gli studi di genetica hanno identificato molteplici aspetti per cui le vittime di SIDS differiscono dai neonati sani e da quelli che muoiono per altre cause (vedi Tab. 372-4): in particolare, difetti dei geni per i canali degli ioni sodio e potassio, del gene della proteina trasportatrice della serotonina (5-HTT), dei geni per lo sviluppo del sistema nervoso autonomo (SNA), del complemento C4 e dell'IL-10. La sindrome del QT lungo si associa a difetti del gene del canale del sodio (*SCN5A*). Pare che *SCN* sia il principale gene, codificante per un canale ionico, sospettato di avere una certa rilevanza nella SIDS: infatti, in uno studio su 93 casi di SIDS, il 2% dei bambini presentava un difetto distinto del canale *SCN5A*. Queste osservazioni suggeriscono che mutazioni nei canali ionici cardiaci costituiscano un substrato aritmogeno potenzialmente letale, in alcuni neonati a rischio di SIDS (Fig. 372-1).

I polimorfismi del gene *5-HTT* sono un esempio del modo in cui alterazioni a carico di singoli geni possono influire sul rischio di SIDS. La 5-HT è un neurotrasmettitore molto diffuso che influenza la respirazione, il controllo cardiovascolare, la temperatura e l'umore. Oltre a modulare l'attività dell'orologio circadiano, è il principale neurotrasmettitore del sonno non REM (*Rapid Eye Movement*, movimento rapido degli occhi). Molti sono i geni coinvolti nel controllo della sintesi, dell'accumulo, della captazione di membrana e del metabolismo della 5-HT. Sono stati identificati numerosi polimorfismi nella regione promoter del gene *5-HTT*, localizzato sul cromosoma 17. Le variazioni di tale regione promoter sembrano avere un ruolo nella captazione di membrana e nella regolazione della 5-HT. I lattanti bianchi, afroamericani e giapponesi colpiti da SIDS hanno maggiori probabilità, in confronto ai controlli, di avere l'allele lungo "L". È emersa anche un'associazione negativa tra SIDS e genotipo S/S. È stata inoltre osservata un'associazione tra la SIDS e un polimorfismo dell'introne 2 di *5-HTT*, che ne regola l'espressione differenziale. Questi polimorfismi del trasportatore porterebbero a ridotte concentrazioni di serotonina a livello delle terminazioni nervose con l'allele "L", rispetto all'allele "S". Il genotipo L/L si associa a un aumento dei trasportatori della serotonina negli studi di neuroimaging e negli studi di legame post mortem.

Gli studi di genetica molecolare hanno identificato mutazioni pertinenti allo sviluppo embriologico precoce del SNA nelle vittime della SIDS. I geni più importanti sono *MASH1* (*Mammalian Achaete-Scute Homolog*-1), la proteina morfogenica dell'osso-2 (BMP2, *Bone Morphogenic Protein*-2), *PHOX2a* (*paired-like homeobox* 2a), *PHOX2b*, il fattore riarrangiato durante la transfezione (RET), l'enzima di conversione dell'endotelina-1 (ECE1), l'endotelina-1 (EDN1), il gene homeobox della leucemia T linfocitica (TLX3) e il gene *engrailed*-1 (EN1).

Nei lattanti colpiti da SIDS, inoltre, sono state riportate alterazioni del gene della frazione C4 del complemento, in quanto quelli che prima della morte soffrivano di infezioni lievi delle vie respiratorie superiori avevano maggiori probabilità di presentare una delezione sia del gene C4A, sia del C4B, rispetto alle vittime della SIDS senza infezioni o rispetto ai controlli viventi. Questi dati suggeriscono che delezioni parziali del gene C4, se associate a un'infezione lieve delle vie respiratorie superiori, aumentino il rischio di SIDS.

Nelle vittime di SIDS è stato inoltre segnalato un polimorfismo nella regione promoter del gene dell'IL-10, una citochina antinfiammatoria. La morte improvvisa del lattante era fortemente associata al genotipo dell'IL-10, sia con l'aplotipo ATA, sia con la presenza degli alleli –592*A e –592*C. Questi polimorfismi dell'IL-10 si associano a ridotti livelli di IL-10 e possono quindi contribuire alla SIDS, ritardando l'inizio della produzione di anticorpi protettivi o per una ridotta capacità di inibire la produzione di citochine infiammatorie.

Una causa non comune di SIDS è legata a mutazioni del gene *TSPYL* (*Testis-Specific Y-Like*), che causano anche disgenesia testicolare.

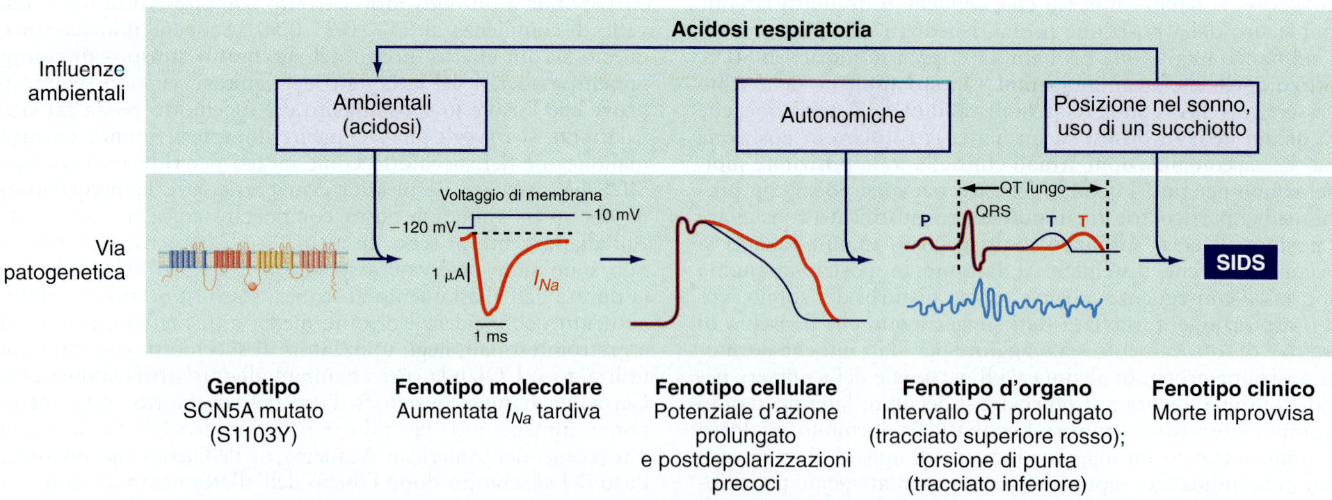

Figura 372-1. Via patogenetica aritmogena della sindrome della morte improvvisa del lattante (SIDS), dal genotipo del paziente al fenotipo clinico, con segnalazione delle influenze ambientali. L'anomalia genetica, in questo caso un polimorfismo del canale cardiaco del sodio SCN5A, causa un fenotipo molecolare di aumentata corrente tardiva del sodio (I_{Na}) per effetto di fattori ambientali come l'acidosi. Interagendo con altre correnti ioniche, che possono a loro volta essere alterate da fattori genetici e ambientali, la corrente tardiva del Na^+ causa un fenotipo cellulare con una prolungata durata del potenziale d'azione, e con postdepolarizzazioni precoci. Il prolungamento del potenziale d'azione, nelle cellule del miocardio ventricolare, e l'ulteriore interazione con fattori ambientali come l'innervazione autonomica che, a sua volta, può essere influenzata da fattori genetici, provocano un fenotipo, a livello del tessuto/organo, di prolungamento dell'intervallo QT all'elettrocardiogramma (ECG) e l'aritmia con torsione di punta in tutto il cuore. Se quest'ultima è prolungata o degenera in fibrillazione ventricolare, ne deriva il fenotipo clinico della SIDS. Molteplici fattori ambientali e genetici possono interagire a diversi livelli, determinando i fenotipi caratteristici a livello molecolare, cellulare, tissutale, dell'organo e clinico. (Da Makielski JC: SIDS: Genetic and environmental influences may cause arrhythmia in this silent killer. *J Clin Invest* 2006;116:297-299.)

INTERAZIONI TRA GENI E AMBIENTE. Il rischio reale di SIDS, nei singoli lattanti, è determinato da complesse interazioni tra fattori di rischio genetici e ambientali (vedi Fig. 372-1). Per esempio, sembra vi sia un'interazione tra il dormire in posizione prona e un'alterata responsività ventilatoria e di risveglio. Occasionalmente capita che i bambini abituati a giacere proni dormano a faccia in giù, circostanza che può dare luogo a episodi di ostruzione delle vie aeree e asfissia, in neonati sani a termine. I soggetti sani si svegliano prima che questi episodi divengano una minaccia per la vita, ma quelli con un'insufficiente risposta di risveglio all'asfissia possono essere a rischio di morte improvvisa. Potrebbe inoltre esservi un legame tra fattori di rischio modificabili, come l'uso di coperte soffici, la posizione prona nel sonno e lo stress termico, e un legame tra fattori di rischio genetici come le anomalie ventilatorie o del risveglio e i difetti di regolazione della temperatura o del metabolismo. I deficit del controllo cardiorespiratorio possono essere correlati, per esempio, ai polimorfismi di *5-HTT* o in geni pertinenti allo sviluppo del SNA. I lattanti affetti potrebbero essere ad aumentato rischio di ipossiemia correlata al sonno e, pertanto, più suscettibili agli effetti avversi associati a una posizione del sonno o all'uso di coperte poco sicure. I soggetti ad aumentato rischio di ipossiemia correlata al sonno potrebbero inoltre avere maggiori probabilità di sviluppare aritmie fatali, in presenza di polimorfismi del gene del canale ionico cardiaco del sodio o del potassio.

Una recente malattia febbrile, spesso correlata a infezioni delle vie respiratorie superiori (vedi Tab. 372-5), è stata osservata nel 50% o più delle vittime di SIDS. Sebbene in passato non siano state considerate di significato eziologico primario, queste infezioni, altrimenti benigne, possono aumentare il rischio di SIDS, interagendo con un'alterazione della risposta immunitaria geneticamente determinata dovuta, per esempio, a delezioni parziali del gene del complemento C4, a polimorfismi dell'interleuchina (vedi Tab. 372-4) o ad altri polimorfismi non ancora identificati. Anche l'interazione tra infezioni delle vie aeree superiori (o altre malattie minori) e altri fattori di rischio, come il sonno in posizione prona, può giocare un ruolo nella patogenesi della SIDS. Come meccanismo della SIDS è stata inoltre ipotizzata una scarsa risposta infiammatoria alle infezioni, e nelle vittime di questa sindrome è stata osservata la degranulazione dei mastociti, fenomeno che farebbe pensare a una reazione anafilattica a una tossina batterica; alcuni familiari dei lattanti colpiti da SIDS presentavano anch'essi un aumento del rilascio e della degranulazione dei mastociti, suggerendo che l'aumentata suscettibilità a una reazione anafilattica sia un altro fattore genetico in grado di predisporre i lattanti a un esito fatale in conseguenza di infezioni per altri versi di scarsa importanza.

Anche l'aumentato rischio di SIDS associato all'esposizione fetale e postnatale al fumo di sigaretta sembra dipendere, almeno in parte, da fattori genetici che influiscono sul controllo autonomico del tronco encefalico. Il fumo materno può accentuare l'iperplasia delle cellule neuroendocrine polmonari, e una disfunzione di queste cellule può contribuire alla fisiopatologia della SIDS. Sia gli studi clinici, sia quelli su animali indicano una ridotta responsività ventilatoria e di risveglio all'ipossia, dopo l'esposizione fetale, con un'alterata autorianimazione dopo l'apnea, in associazione all'esposizione postnatale alla nicotina. In ratti esposti in epoca prenatale al fumo di sigaretta è stata osservata una ridotta immunoreattività del tronco encefalico a isoforme selezionate della proteinchinasi C e all'ossido nitrico sintetasi neuronale, che potrebbe essere associata all'alterata risposta ventilatoria e di risveglio all'ipossia. Pertanto, l'attenuazione età-specifica delle difese ipossiche, dopo esposizione alla nicotina, sembra essere correlata, almeno in parte, a un alterato metabolismo delle catecolamine nel tronco encefalico, ma finora non sono stati identificati polimorfismi genetici che possano contribuire a queste alterazioni metaboliche correlate al fumo. Gli studi *in vitro* suggeriscono anche che il fumo aumenta il rischio di SIDS a causa di una maggior suscettibilità alle infezione virali e batteriche, e a un aumentato legame dei batteri dopo il rivestimento passivo delle superfici mucose con componenti del fumo: tutto questo induce a ipotizzare un'interazione tra il fumo, il controllo cardiorespiratorio e lo stato immunitario.

GRUPPI DI LATTANTI AD AUMENTATO RISCHIO DI SIDS

EVENTI INSPIEGATI APPARENTEMENTE PERICOLOSI PER LA VITA. I neonati con un evento inspiegato apparentemente minaccioso per la vita (ALTE, *Apparent Life-Threatening Event*) sono a rischio di SIDS. Un'anamnesi di ALTE inspiegato è stata riportata nel 5-9% delle vittime di SIDS, e il rischio sembra maggiore se gli eventi inspiegati sono due o più; tuttavia, non sono disponibili dati definitivi sull'incidenza. Rispetto ai soggetti sani di controllo, il rischio di SIDS può essere da 3 a 5 volte maggiore nei lattanti che hanno subito un ALTE. Sebbene nella maggior parte degli studi sugli ALTE non sia stata specificata l'età gestazionale, il 30% dei lattanti con ALTE nella Collaborative Home Infant Monitoring Evaluation era di ≤37 settimane alla nascita.

FRATELLI DI UNA VITTIMA DELLA SIDS, NATI SUCCESSIVAMENTE. I fratelli di un lattante deceduto per qualsiasi causa naturale non infettiva sono a rischio significativamente maggiore di morte neonatale dovuta alla stessa causa, compresa la SIDS. Il rischio relativo è di 9,1 per la recidiva di SIDS, rispetto all'1,6 per una causa di morte diversa. Il rischio relativo di ricorrenza della SIDS (range 5,4-5,8) è simile a quello riscontrato per cause di morte ricorrente diverse dalla SIDS (range 4,6-12,5). Il rischio di mortalità infantile ricorrente per la stessa causa del fratello indice, sembra quindi essere aumentato di un grado simile nei fratelli successivi, sia per le cause spiegate sia per la SIDS. L'aumentato rischio, nelle famiglie con casi di SIDS, è compatibile con l'interazione di fattori di rischio genetici e ambientali (vedi Tab. 372-2).

Ancora non è chiaro fino a che punto il rischio di SIDS possa essere maggiore nei fratelli nati successivamente, soprattutto perché in passato si è sottovalutato il ruolo dei fattori di rischio genetici, ma anche perché non si sa con quale frequenza il soffocamento intenzionale venga erroneamente classificato come SIDS. È difficile stabilire il ruolo del soffocamento intenzionale per la mancanza di criteri obiettivi da utilizzare nella diagnosi. Sebbene in passato alcuni operatori sanitari abbiano affermato che solo l'omicidio ricorre nelle famiglie e che tutti i casi successivi di morte infantile inaspettata devono essere indagati come possibili omicidi, esistono dati sostanziali a riprova che fattori genetici e ambientali concorrono ad aumentare il rischio di SIDS ricorrente in alcune famiglie. In Gran Bretagna, non solo le evidenze genetiche compatibili con un aumentato rischio di SIDS nei fratelli nati successivamente, ma anche i dati epidemiologici confermano che il decesso del secondo figlio, in determinati nuclei familiari, non è raro e che almeno l'80-90% dei casi è naturale. La percentuale dei casi di morte infantile ricorrente da SIDS, nei fratelli, era 5-9 volte maggiore rispetto alla percentuale dei probabili omicidi.

PREMATURITÀ. Molti studi hanno identificato una correlazione inversa tra il rischio di SIDS da una parte, e l'età gestazionale e il peso alla nascita dall'altra. I fattori di rischio ambientali, nei neonati pretermine, non sono sostanzialmente diversi da quelli osservati nei neonati a termine, comprese le posizioni prona e laterale nel sonno. L'età postnatale dei prematuri deceduti per SIDS è di 5-7 settimane maggiore rispetto a quella dei nati a termine, mentre l'età postconcezionale è di 4-6 settimane minore. Rispetto ai neonati con peso alla nascita >2500 g, i neonati con peso alla nascita di 1000-1499 g e 1500-2499 g hanno rispettivamente 4 e 3 volte più probabilità di morire per SIDS.

STUDI FISIOLOGICI. Studi fisiologici sono stati effettuati su soggetti sani nella prima infanzia, alcuni dei quali deceduti successivamente per SIDS. Analoghi studi sono stati condotti anche su gruppi di lattanti ad aumentato rischio per SIDS, in particolare soggetti che avevano subito un ALTE e fratelli di una vittima di SIDS. Nel complesso, questi studi sono indicativi di un'anomalia del tronco encefalico correlata alla neuroregolazione del controllo cardiorespiratorio e di altre funzioni autonomiche, e sono in accordo con i reperti autoptici, compresi gli studi genetici sulle vittime di SIDS (vedi i paragrafi "Anatomia patologica" e "Fattori di rischio genetici"). Le anomalie fisiologiche osservate riguardano i pattern respiratori, la sensibilità chemiorecettoriale, il controllo della frequenza e variabilità cardiaca e respiratoria, e la risposta di risveglio asfittica. Una scarsa risposta di risveglio può essere una condizione necessaria ma non sufficiente perché insorga la SIDS, in assenza di altri fattori di rischio genetici o ambientali. L'autorianimazione (*gasping*) è un componente critico della risposta di risveglio all'asfissia, e la sua mancanza, nelle vittime della SIDS, può essere il deficit fisiologico finale e più devastante. La maggior parte dei nati a termine di età <9 settimane reagisce a una lieve ipossia destandosi, mentre solo il 10-15% dei lattanti normali di età >9 settimane si sveglia. Da questi dati si deduce che a mano a mano che il lattante matura avvicinandosi al range di età a maggior rischio di SIDS, la sua capacità di svegliarsi a causa di stimoli ipossici lievi o moderati sembra ridursi.

La capacità di ridurre l'intervallo QT, aumentando la frequenza cardiaca, sembra essere alterata in alcune vittime della SIDS, suggerendo che questi lattanti possano essere predisposti ad aritmie ventricolari. Questo è in accordo con l'osservazione di polimorfismi nei geni dei canali ionici cardiaci, in altri soggetti deceduti per SIDS (vedi Tab. 372-4), ma non vi sono dati sull'intervallo QT ante mortem, nelle vittime della SIDS con dati genetici post mortem. I soggetti studiati dal punto di vista fisiologico, successivamente deceduti per SIDS, hanno una frequenza cardiaca maggiore in tutti gli stadi sonno-veglia, una ridotta variabilità della frequenza cardiaca durante lo stato di veglia e una variabilità significativamente inferiore della frequenza cardiaca con il ritmo respiratorio, in tutti i cicli sonno-veglia.

La ridotta variabilità e l'aumento della frequenza cardiaca, osservati nei lattanti in seguito deceduti per SIDS, possono essere correlati a una diminuzione del tono vagale, la quale sembra riconducibile, almeno in parte, a una neuropatia vagale o a una lesione del tronco encefalico, in aree responsabili del controllo cardiaco parasimpatico. Confrontando lo spettro di capacità di frequenza cardiaca prima e dopo le apnee ostruttive nei lattanti, si osserva che quelli destinati al decesso per SIDS non hanno la riduzione del rapporto tra capacità di bassa frequenza e di alta frequenza osservata nei soggetti di controllo. Alcune future vittime della SIDS hanno pertanto una diversa responsività autonomica all'apnea ostruttiva, che indica forse un alterato controllo del SNA, associato a una più elevata vulnerabilità a fattori di stress esterni o endogeni, e pertanto a una ridotta stabilità elettrica del cuore.

In alcuni lattanti con ALTE idiopatico, o vittime della SIDS, è stata osservata sudorazione durante il sonno, che potrebbe dipendere dal riscaldamento eccessivo, ma essere causata anche da ipoventilazione alveolare e asfissia secondaria, o da una disfunzione autonomica facente parte di un deficit più generalizzato della funzione del tronco encefalico.

Sebbene i sistemi di monitoraggio cardiorespiratorio domiciliari con capacità di memoria abbiano registrato gli eventi terminali in alcune vittime della SIDS, queste registrazioni non includevano la saturimetria e non consentivano di identificare gli atti respiratori con ostruzione, poiché si basavano sull'impedenza transtoracica per la rilevazione delle respirazioni. Nella maggior parte dei casi si è osservata l'improvvisa e rapida progressione di una severa bradicardia non associata ad apnea centrale, o verificatasi troppo precocemente per poter essere spiegata solo da questa. Queste osservazioni avvalorano l'ipotesi di un'anomalia del controllo autonomico della variabilità della frequenza cardiaca, o di un'ostruzione delle vie respiratorie associata a bradicardia o ipossiemia.

STRATEGIE CLINICHE

MONITORAGGIO. Allo stato attuale delle conoscenze non è possibile prevenire la SIDS nel singolo lattante, non essendo possibile identificarne prospetticamente le potenziali vittime; del resto, anche qualora ci fosse modo di individuare preventivamente i soggetti a rischio, finora non è emerso alcun intervento efficace da attuare. Gli studi sui pattern cardiorespiratori, o sulle altre anomalie autonomiche, non sono abbastanza sensibili e specifici da poter essere utili in ambito clinico come test di screening. La sorveglianza domiciliare con le apparecchiature elettroniche attualmente disponibili non si è dimostrata in grado di ridurre il rischio di SIDS. Sebbene il prolungamento dell'intervallo QT in un neonato possa essere trattato, quando diagnosticato, non sono stati determinati né il ruolo dell'elettrocardiogramma (ECG) eseguito di routine nello screening postnatale, né la sicurezza del trattamento (vedi Capitolo 435.5). È probabile che anche lo screening elettrocardiografico dei genitori sia inutile, poiché le mutazioni spontanee sono comuni.

RIDURRE IL RISCHIO DI SIDS. Le linee guida dell'American Academy of Pediatrics, per ridurre il rischio di SIDS nei neonati, sono appropriate per la maggior parte dei bambini, ma i medici e le altre figure sanitarie talvolta possono aver bisogno di adottare approcci alternativi. I punti principali sono elencati di seguito.

1. I neonati a termine e i prematuri devono essere posti a dormire in posizione supina, perché questa abitudine non ha effetti nocivi sulla salute. Non è invece consigliabile che i lattanti dormano in decubito laterale.
2. È consigliabile che il lattante dorma nella stessa stanza dei genitori, ma nel suo lettino o nella culla, vicino al letto della madre, per facilitare la cura e il contatto.
3. I neonati dovrebbero essere posti a dormire su un materasso rigido. Si raccomanda di non utilizzare letti ad acqua, divani, materassi morbidi o altre superfici soffici.
4. Bisognerebbe evitare di lasciare materiali soffici accanto al lattante addormentato. Questi comprendono cuscini, trapunte, coperte, pelli di pecora e pupazzi imbottiti. Dal momento che le coperte non tese possono essere pericolose, le lenzuola, se utilizzate, devono essere rimboccate sotto il materasso del lettino. Al posto delle lenzuola si possono utilizzare i sacchiletto.
5. Non infagottare il lattante, che dovrebbe indossare indumenti leggeri; si consiglia inoltre di regolare il termostato su una temperatura confortevole.
6. I lattanti dovrebbero essere lasciati un po' di tempo in posizione prona, da svegli e sotto osservazione. Cambiare la posizione della testa del bambino, così come il suo orientamento nel lettino, può inoltre minimizzare il rischio di appiattimento del cranio dovuto all'abitudine di dormire in posizione supina (plagiocefalia posizionale).
7. Gli strumenti pubblicizzati per mantenere la posizione del sonno, "proteggere" un bambino che condivide il letto con altri, o ridurre il rischio di rebreathing, non sono raccomandati.
8. Il monitoraggio domiciliare respiratorio, cardiaco e della saturazione di O_2 può essere utile in alcuni casi selezionati, con estrema instabilità, ma non vi sono evidenze che riduca l'incidenza di SIDS e non è pertanto raccomandato a questo scopo.
9. Porgere il succhiotto al lattante che sta per addormentarsi. Il succhiotto dovrebbe essere usato quando si adagia il bambino nella culla e non essere reinserito quando cade. Prima di introdurre questa abitudine attendere che l'allattamento al seno sia ben avviato.
10. Le madri non dovrebbero fumare durante la gravidanza e i lattanti non dovrebbero essere esposti al fumo passivo.
11. La campagna statunitense nazionale Back to Sleep dovrebbe continuare, essere ampliata per sottolineare quali caratteristiche deve avere un sano ambiente per dormire e concentrare l'attenzione sui gruppi che continuano ad avere un'elevata incidenza di SIDS. Le strategie educative dovrebbero essere individualizzate per raggiungere tutti i gruppi etnico-culturali. Questi messaggi non devono essere rivolti solo ai genitori, ma a tutti coloro che assistono il lattante, compresi il personale dei nidi, i nonni, i genitori adottivi e i babysitter. I professionisti sanitari, nelle terapie intensive e nelle normali nurseries neonatali, dovrebbero implementare queste raccomandazioni prima di una dimissione anticipata.

Ackerman MJ, Siu BL, Sturner WQ, et al: Postmortem molecular analysis of SCN5A defects in SIDS. *JAMA* 2001;286:2264–2269.

American Academy of Pediatrics Task Force on Infant Sleep Position and Sudden Infant Death Syndrome: The changing concept of sudden infant death syndrome: Diagnostic coding shifts, controversies regarding the sleeping environment, and new variables to consider in reducing risk. *Pediatrics* 2005;116:1245–1255.

Blair PS, Sidebotham P, Berry PJ, et al: Major epidemiological changes in sudden infant death syndrome: A 20-year population-based study in the UK. *Lancet* 2006;367:314–319.

Carpenter RG, Irgens LM, Blair PS, et al: Sudden unexplained infant death in 20 regions in Europe: Case control study. *Lancet* 2004;363:185–190.

Carpenter RG, Waite A, Coombs RC, et al: Repeat sudden unexpected and unexplained infant deaths: Natural or unnatural? *Lancet* 2005;365: 29–35.

Centers for Disease Control and Prevention: Release of sudden, unexplained infant death investigation reporting form. *MMWR* 2006;55:212–213.

Corwin MJ, Lesko SM, Heeren T, et al: Secular changes in sleep position during infancy: 1995–1998. *Pediatrics* 2003;111:52–60.

Gaultier C: Functional brain deficits in congenital central hypoventilation syndrome. *Pediatr Res* 2005;57:471–472.

Gordon AE, El Ahmer OR, Chan R, et al: Why is smoking a risk factor for sudden infant death syndrome? *Child Care Health Dev* 2002;28:23–25.

Hauck FR, Omojokun OO, Siadaty MS: Do pacifiers reduce the risk of sudden infant death syndrome? A meta-analysis. *Pediatrics* 2005;116: e716–e723.

Horn MH, Kinnamon DD, Ferraro N, Curley MAQ: Smaller mandibular size in infants with a history of an apparent life-threatening event. *J Pediatr* 2006;149:499–504.

Hunt CE: Gene-environment interactions: Implications for sudden unexpected deaths in infancy. *Arch Dis Child* 2005;90:48–53.

Hunt CE, Lesko SM, Vezina RM, et al: Infant sleep position and associated health outcomes. *Arch Pediatr Adolesc Med* 2003;157:469–474.

Immunization Safety Review Committee. Stratton K, Almario DA,Wizemann TM, McCormick MC (eds): Immunization safety review. Vaccinations and sudden unexpected death in infancy. Washington DC, National Academies Press, 2003. National Infant Sleep Position website (http://dc-cwww.bumc.bu.edu/ChimeNisp/Main_Nisp.asp), accessed April 8, 2005.

Iyasu S, Randall LL, Welty TK, et al: Risk factors for sudden infant death syndrome among northern plains Indians. *JAMA* 2002;288:2717–2723.

Jones KL, Krous HF, Nadeau J, et al: Vascular endothelial growth factor in the cerebrospinal fluid of infants who died of sudden infant death syndrome: Evidence for antecedent hypoxia. *Pediatrics* 2003;111:358–363.

Kadhim H, Kahn A, Sébire G: Distinct cytokine profile in SIDS brain: A common denominator in a multifactorial syndrome. *Neurology* 2003;61:1256–1259.

Kinney HC, Randall LL, Sleeper LA, et al: Serotonergic brainstem abnormalities in northern plains Indians with the sudden infant death syndrome. *J Neuropathol Exp Neurol* 2003;62:1178–1191.

Korachi M, Pravica V, Barson AJ, et al: Interleukin 10 genotype as a risk factor for sudden infant death syndrome: Determination of IL-10 genotype from wax-embedded postmortem samples. *FEMS Immunol Med Microbiol* 2004;42:125–129.

Li DK, Willinger M, Petitti DB, et al: Use of a dummy (pacifier) during sleep and risk of sudden infant death syndrome (SIDS): Population based case-control study. *Br Med J* 2006;332:18–21.

Makielski JC: SIDS: Genetic and environmental influences may cause arrhythmia in this silent killer. *J Clin Invest* 2006;116:297–299.

Matthews T: Sudden unexpected infant death: Infanticide or SIDS? *Lancet* 2005;365:3–4.

Matturri L, Biondo B, Suarez-Mier MP, et al: Brain stem lesions in the sudden infant death syndrome: Variability in the hypoplasia of the arcuate nucleus. *Acta Neuropathol (Berl)* 2002;104:12–20.

McGovern MC, Smith MBH: Causes of apparent life threatening events in infants: A systematic review. *Arch Dis Child* 2004;89:1043–1048.

Opdal SH, Rognum TO: New insight into sudden infant death syndrome. *Lancet* 2004;364:825–826.

Opdal SH, Rognum TO: The sudden infant death syndrome gene: Does it exist? *Pediatrics* 2004;114:e506–e512.

Ramanathan R, Corwin MJ, Hunt CE, et al: Collaborative Home Infant Monitoring Evaluation (CHIME) Study Group: Cardiorespiratory events recorded on home monitors: Comparison of healthy infants with those at increased risk for SIDS. *JAMA* 2001;285:2199–2207.

Skinner JR, Chung SK, Montgomery D, et al: Near-miss SIDS due to Brugada syndrome. *Arch Dis Child* 2005;90:528–529.

Smith GCS, Wood AM, Pell JP, et al: Second-trimester maternal serum levels of alpha-fetoprotein and the subsequent risk of sudden infant death syndrome. *N Engl J Med* 2004;351:978–986.

Van Wouwe J, HiraSing RA: Prevention of sudden unexpected infant death. *Lancet* 2006;367:277–278.

Weese-Mayer DE, Berry-Kravis EM, Zhou L, et al: Sudden infant death syndrome: Case-control frequency differences at genes pertinent to early autonomic nervous system embryologic development. *Pediatr Res* 2004;56:391–396.

Weese-Mayer DE, Zhou L, Berry-Kravis, et al: Association of the serotonin transporter gene with sudden infant death syndrome: A haplotype analysis. *Am J Med Genet A* 2003;122:238–245.

Willinger M, Ko C-W, Hoffman HJ, et al: Factors associated with caregivers' choice of infant sleep position, 1994–1998. The National Infant Sleep Position Study. *JAMA* 2000;283:2135–2142.

Sezione 2 — Malattie delle vie respiratorie

Capitolo 373 ■ Patologie congenite del naso Joseph Haddad Jr.

NASO NORMALE NEL NEONATO. Se bambini e adulti respirano di preferenza con il naso, in assenza di un'ostruzione, nella maggior parte dei neonati questa forma di respirazione è l'unica possibile; di conseguenza, un'ostruzione nasale severa che si presenti alla nascita, come l'atresia delle coane, può mettere in pericolo la vita del neonato, a meno che non si stabilisca una via alternativa. La congestione nasale con ostruzione è comune nel primo anno di vita e può incidere negativamente sulla qualità della respirazione durante il sonno; può associarsi a vie nasali strette, infezioni batteriche o virali, aumento di volume delle adenoidi o stimolazione estrogenica materna, responsabile di un quadro simile alla rinite gravidica. Le vie nasali raddoppiano di dimensioni nei primi sei mesi di vita, portando alla risoluzione dei sintomi nella maggior parte dei bambini. In questi casi è di beneficio una cura sintomatica con una siringa a bulbo e gocce di soluzione fisiologica per il naso, decongestionanti nasali topici e antibiotici, quando indicati.

FISIOLOGIA. Il naso, oltre a essere l'organo dell'olfatto, è responsabile del riscaldamento e dell'umidificazione dell'aria inspirata. Nella cavità nasale anteriore, il flusso aereo turbolento e i robusti peli favoriscono il deposito delle particelle solide più grandi; le restanti vie aeree nasali filtrano le particelle più piccole fino a un diametro di 6 µm. Nella zona dei turbinati, il flusso aereo diviene laminare e la via aerea si restringe dirigendosi superiormente; questo fa sì che il deposito delle particelle, il riscaldamento e l'umidificazione si intensifichino. Nella respirazione normale le vie aeree nasali contribuiscono alle resistenze totali per il 50%. L'alitamento delle pinne nasali, un segno di distress respiratorio, riduce le resistenze al flusso inspiratorio attraverso il naso e può migliorare la ventilazione.

Pur essendo più vascolarizzata rispetto alle vie aeree inferiori, specialmente nella zona dei turbinati, la mucosa nasale è simile all'epitelio di superficie delle vie aeree inferiori, con cellule ciliate, cellule caliciformi, ghiandole sottomucose e un rivestimento di muco. Le secrezioni nasali contengono lisozima, immunoglobuline A (IgA) secretorie (entrambi con attività antimicrobica), IgG, IgE, albumina, istamina, batteri, lattoferrina e detriti cellulari, oltre a glicoproteine mucose, dotate di proprietà viscoelastiche. Grazie alle cellule ciliate, il muco scorre verso il rinofaringe, dove le vie aeree si ampliano, l'epitelio diventa squamoso e le secrezioni vengono inghiottite. Lo strato di muco si ricostituisce ogni 10-20 minuti circa. La produzione giornaliera di muco, imputabile soprattutto alle ghiandole sottomucose, è stimata di 0,1-0,3 mg/kg/die.

ALTERAZIONI CONGENITE. Le *malformazioni nasali strutturali* congenite sono poco comuni rispetto alle anomalie acquisite. Se le ossa nasali sono congenitamente assenti, il ponte nasale non si sviluppa e si configura un quadro di *ipoplasia nasale*. L'assenza congenita del naso (*arinia*), la duplicazione completa o parziale, o una narice singola centrale, pur potendo verificarsi in forma isolata, in genere fanno parte di una sindrome malformativa. Raramente, nel naso si trovano *denti sovrannumerari* o sviluppatisi al suo interno dalla mascella.

Le ossa nasali possono essere talmente malformate da causare un grave restringimento delle vie nasali, spesso associato a un palato duro alto e stretto. I bambini con questi difetti possono presentare una significativa ostruzione al flusso aereo durante le infezioni delle vie aeree superiori e sono più suscettibili allo sviluppo di ipoventilazione cronica o ricorrente (vedi Capitolo 18). In rari casi le pinne nasali sono talmente sottili e prive di supporto da determinare un'ostruzione inspiratoria oppure può esservi un'ostruzione congenita del dotto nasolacrimale con estensione cistica nel rinofaringe, che causa distress respiratorio.

ATRESIA DELLE COANE. È la più comune anomalia congenita del naso e ha una frequenza di circa 1/7000 nati vivi. Consiste in un setto monolaterale o bilaterale osseo (90%) o membranoso (10%) tra il naso e la faringe; nella maggior parte dei casi si osserva una combinazione di atresia ossea e membranosa. Quasi il 50% dei pazienti affetti ha altre anomalie congenite, più frequenti nei casi bilaterali. La **sindrome CHARGE** (*Coloboma, Heart disease, Atresia choanae, Retarded growth and development or CNS anomalies or both, Genital anomalies or hypogonadism or both, and Ear anomalies or deafness or both*, coloboma, cardiopatia, atresia delle coane, ritardo della crescita e dello sviluppo e/o anomalie del SNC, anomalie genitali e/o ipogonadismo, anomalie dell'orecchio e/o sordità) è una delle anomalie più comuni associate ad atresia delle coane. La maggior parte dei pazienti con sindrome CHARGE presenta mutazioni nel gene CHD7, che è coinvolto nell'organizzazione della cromatina.

Manifestazioni cliniche. I neonati hanno una capacità variabile di respirare attraverso la bocca, pertanto l'ostruzione nasale non provoca gli stessi sintomi in tutti. Quando l'ostruzione è monolaterale, il neonato può essere asintomatico per un periodo prolungato, spesso fino alla prima infezione delle vie respiratorie, quando le secrezioni nasali monolaterali o l'ostruzione nasale persistente possono suggerire la diagnosi. I soggetti con atresia bilaterale delle coane che hanno difficoltà a respirare con la bocca faranno sforzi vigorosi nel tentativo di inspirare, spesso risucchiando le labbra e sviluppando cianosi. In seguito i bambini in queste condizioni di sofferenza piangono (il che diminuisce la cianosi) e si calmano, riprendendo un colorito cutaneo normale; non appena chiudono la bocca, però, il ciclo si ripete. I neonati in grado di respirare con la bocca da subito incontrano difficoltà quando succhiano e deglutiscono il latte, diventando cianotici nel tentativo di nutrirsi.

Diagnosi. È stabilita dall'impossibilità di far passare attraverso ogni narice, per 3-4 cm, un catetere rigido al fine di introdurlo nel rinofaringe. La lamina atresica può essere osservata direttamente in rinoscopia a fibre ottiche. La metodica migliore per valutare l'anatomia è la TC ad alta risoluzione (Fig. 373-1).

Trattamento. Il trattamento iniziale consiste nel rapido inserimento di una via aerea orale, nel mantenimento della bocca in posizione aperta o nell'intubazione. Si può utilizzare una via aerea orale standard (come quella impiegata in anestesia) oppure confezionare una tettarella per il latte dotata di grossi fori per rendere il passaggio dell'aria più agevole. Una volta stabilita una via aerea orale, è possibile alimentare il neonato con un sondino, finché non riesce a respirare e nutrirsi senza la via aerea assistita. Nei casi bilaterali, può essere indicata l'intubazione o, meno spesso, la tracheotomia. Se il neonato non ha altri problemi medici seri, si può procedere all'intervento chirurgico; il trattamento di scelta è la riparazione transnasale, previa introduzione di un piccolo endoscopio a ingrandimento e piccoli strumenti e trapani chirurgici. Di solito, dopo la riparazione, gli stent vengono lasciati in sede per alcune settimane onde evitare la richiusura o la stenosi. La tracheotomia dovrebbe essere presa in esame nei casi di atresia bilaterale in cui il bambino ha altri problemi potenzialmente pericolosi per la vita, e in cui una riparazione chirurgica precoce potrebbe non essere appropriata o fattibile. La correzione chirurgica dell'ostruzione monolaterale può essere rimandata di alcuni anni. Sia nei casi monolaterali, sia in quelli bilaterali, è comune una ristenosi, che può necessitare di dilatazione e/o di un reintervento. È stata utilizzata la mitomicina C per aiutare a prevenire lo sviluppo di tessuto di granulazione e di una nuova stenosi.

DIFETTI CONGENITI DEL SETTO NASALE. La **perforazione del setto** è per lo più acquisita dopo la nascita, in seguito a infezioni come la sifilide e la tubercolosi o a traumi; raramente è un difetto dello sviluppo. Le cannule per la pressione continua positiva delle vie aeree sono una causa di perforazione iatrogena. Il trauma da parto è la causa più comune di deviazione del setto osservata alla nascita che, se riconosciuta precocemente, può essere corretta con riallineamento immediato utilizzando sonde smusse, tamponi di cotone e anestesia locale. La correzione chirurgica, quando richiesta, è abitualmente rimandata per evitare di alterare lo sviluppo della parte centrale del viso.

Le **deviazioni lievi del setto** sono comuni e abitualmente asintomatiche; un'anomala formazione del setto è rara, a meno che non siano presenti altre malformazioni, come la labiopalatoschisi.

STENOSI DEL MEATO PIRIFORME. I neonati con quest'anomalia ossea del meato nasale anteriore si presentano con ostruzione nasale severa già alla nascita o poco dopo. La diagnosi è effettuata tramite TC del naso; può essere necessaria la riparazione chirurgica, tramite approccio anteriore sottolabiale, se il bambino non riesce a nutrirsi o a respirare normalmente.

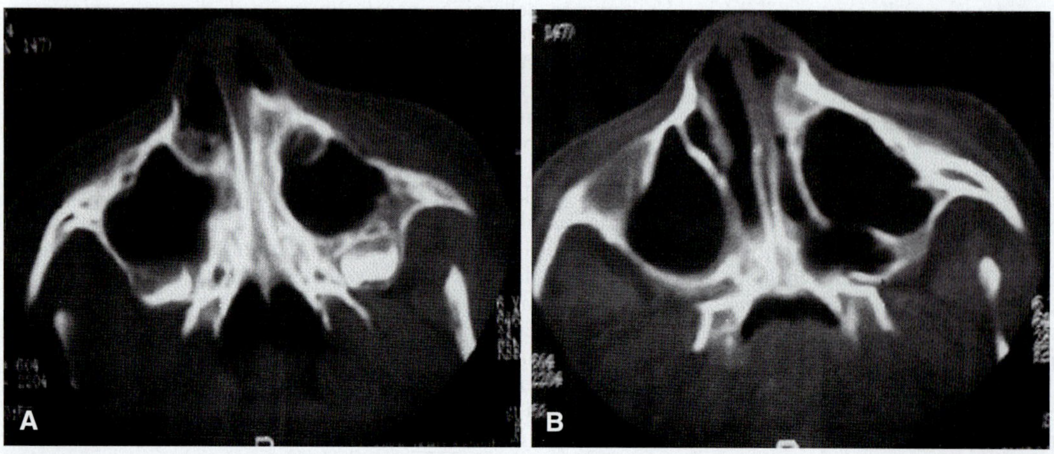

Figura 373-1. TC che mostra (a) cavità nasali ipoplasiche e (b) atresia delle coane ossea e mucosa. (Da Altuntas A, Yilmaz MD, Kahveci OK, et al: Coexistence of choanal atresia and Tessier's facial cleft number 2. *Int J Pediatr Otorhinolaryngol* 2004;68:1083.)

MASSE NASALI CONGENITE DELLA LINEA MEDIANA. I *dermoidi*, i *gliomi* e gli *encefaloceli* (in ordine di frequenza decrescente) possono essere intranasali o extranasali, e avere connessioni endocraniche. I dermoidi nasali sono spesso localizzati in una fossetta o una cavità sul dorso nasale, talvolta con presenza di peli, e possono predisporre a infezioni endocraniche, se sono presenti un seno o una fistola endocranica. Le infezioni ricorrenti delle cisti dermoidi sono comuni. I gliomi, o tessuti encefalici eterotopici, sono fissi, mentre l'encefalocele è morbido e aumenta di volume con il pianto o con la manovra di Valsalva. La diagnosi si basa sull'esame obiettivo e sui risultati delle indagini radiologiche. La TC fornisce il miglior dettaglio osseo, ma la RM consente vedute sagittali, che possono essere necessarie per definire ulteriormente l'estensione endocranica (Fig. 373-2). In genere è richiesta l'escissione chirurgica; il tipo e l'estensione dell'approccio chirurgico si basano sul tipo e sulle dimensioni della massa.

Altre masse nasali comprendono gli *emangiomi*, l'*ostruzione congenita del dotto nasolacrimale* (che può presentarsi come una massa nasale), i polipi nasali e i tumori come il rabdomiosarcoma (vedi Capitolo 500). I polipi nasali sono raramente presenti alla nascita, ma le altre masse si presentano spesso alla nascita o nella prima infanzia (vedi Capitolo 375).

Nella sindrome di Down, lo scarso sviluppo dei seni paranasali e le vie aeree nasali ristrette si associano a infezioni croniche o ricorrenti delle vie aeree superiori (vedi Capitolo 81).

DIAGNOSI E TRATTAMENTO. Nei bambini con alterazioni nasali congenite, si pratica una cura sintomatica delle vie aeree fino al momento della diagnosi; quest'ultima si effettua tramite endoscopia flessibile e studi radiologici, principalmente la TC. Nel caso di problemi congeniti correggibili chirurgicamente, come l'atresia delle coane, si procede all'intervento quando il bambino è giudicato sano ed esente da problemi pericolosi per la vita, come una cardiopatia congenita.

Aramaki M, Udaka T, Kosaki R, et al: Phenotypic spectrum of CHARGE syndrome with *CHD7* mutations. *J Pediatr* 2006;148:410–414.

Brown OE, Myer CM, Manning SC: Congenital nasal pyriform aperture stenosis. *Laryngoscope* 1989;99:86–91.

Giffon SD, Goncalves VM, Zanardi VA, gil-da-Silva Lopes VL: Cerebellar involvement in midline facial defects with ocular hypertelorism. *Cleft Palate Craniofac J* 2006;43:466–470.

Harley EH: Pediatric congenital nasal masses. *Ear Nose Throat J* 1991; 70:28–32.

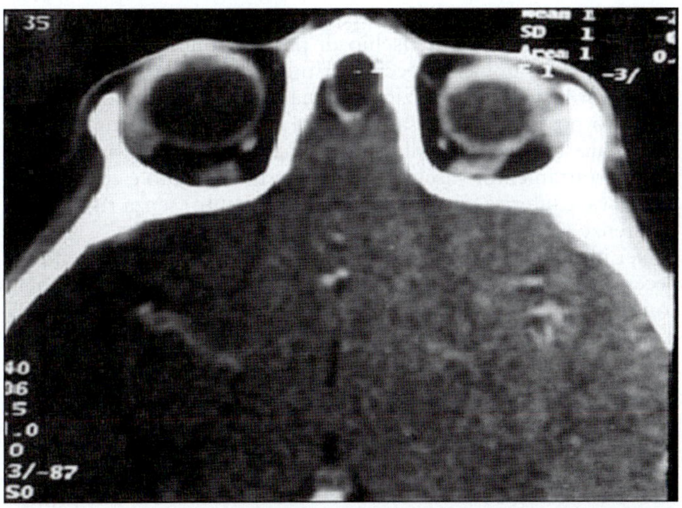

Figura 373-2. TC: proiezione assiale che mostra l'estensione di una cisti dermoide nasale nella fossa cranica anteriore attraverso un difetto della lamina cribriforme. (Da Meher R, Singh I, Aggarwal S: Nasal dermoid with intracranial extension. *J Postgrad Med* 2005;51:39.)

Jongmans MCJ, Admiraal RJ, vander Donk KP, et al: CHARGE syndrome: the phenotypic spectrum of mutations in the *CHD7* gene. *J Med Genet* 2006;43:306–314.

Khafagy YW: Endoscopic repair of bilateral congenital choanal atresia. *Laryngoscope* 2002;112:316–319.

Lusk RP, Lee PC: Magnetic resonance imaging of congenital midline nasal masses. *Otolaryngol Head Neck Surg* 1986;95:303–306.

Rahbar R, Jones DT, Nuss RC, et al: The role of mitomycin in the prevention and treatment of scar formation in the pediatric aerodigestive tract: Friend or foe? *Arch Otolaryngol Head Neck Surg* 2002;128:401–406.

Rohrich RJ, Lowe JB, Schwartz MR: The role of open rhinoplasty in the management of nasal dermoid cysts. *Plast Reconstr Surg* 1999;10:2163–2170.

Samadi DS, Shah UK, Handler SD, et al: Choanal atresia: A twenty-year review of medical comorbidities and surgical outcomes. *Laryngoscope* 2003;113:254–258.

Sanlaville D, Etehevers HC, Gonzales M, et al: Phenotypic spectrum of CHARGE syndrome in fetuses with *CHD7* truncating mutations correlates with expression during human development. *J Med Genet* 2006;43: 211–217.

Van Den Abbeele T, Triglia JM, Francois M, Narcy P: Congenital nasal pyriform aperture stenosis: Diagnosis and management of 20 cases. *Ann Otol Rhinol Laryngol* 2001;110:70–75.

Veruloed MPJ, Hoevenadrs-van den Boom MAA, Knoors H, et al: CHARGE syndrome: Relations between behavioral characteristics and medical conditions. *Am J Med Genet* 2006;140A:851–862.

Capitolo 374 ■ Patologie acquisite del naso

Joseph Haddad Jr.

GENERALI. Molte patologie acquisite del naso e dei seni paranasali, come i tumori e le perforazioni del setto, si presentano con epistassi. I traumi della parte centrale del volto o le fratture faciali possono essere accompagnati da epistassi. I traumi del naso possono causare un *ematoma settale* che, se il trattamento è ritardato, può portare a necrosi della cartilagine settale con conseguente *deformità del naso a sella*. Altre anomalie che possono incidere sulla forma del naso e delle ossa paranasali, con ostruzione e pochi altri sintomi, comprendono le *lesioni osteofibrose* (fibroma ossificante, displasia fibrosa, fibroma cementificante) e i *mucoceli dei seni paranasali*. Queste condizioni possono essere sospettate all'esame obiettivo e confermate dalla TC e dalla biopsia. Sebbene siano considerate lesioni benigne, possono tutte alterare in misura notevole l'anatomia delle strutture ossee circostanti e richiedono spesso l'intervento chirurgico.

374.1 • Corpi estranei

EZIOLOGIA. Spesso i bambini piccoli o con ritardo dello sviluppo introducono nel naso cibo, matite, piccoli giocattoli, gomme, palline di carta, perline, piselli, pietre, pezzi di spugna e altri corpi estranei. I sintomi iniziali comprendono ostruzione monolaterale, starnuti, fastidio relativamente modesto e, in rari casi, dolore. In uno studio retrospettivo, i sintomi clinici di presentazione comprendevano un'anamnesi di inserimento di corpi estranei (86%), secrezioni nasali mucopurulente (24%), secrezione nasale maleodorante (9%), epistassi (6%), ostruzione nasale (3%) e respirazione con la bocca (2%). L'irritazione determina edema della mucosa, poiché alcuni corpi estranei sono igroscopici e aumentano di volume assorbendo l'acqua; i segni di ostruzione locale e di fastidio possono aggravarsi nel tempo. Il paziente si può anche presentare con uno sgradevole odore corporeo (*bromidrosi*).

DIAGNOSI. L'ostruzione e la secrezione nasale monolaterale devono suggerire la presenza di un corpo estraneo, spesso visibile all'esame con uno speculo nasale o con un ampio otoscopio posizionato nel naso, previa rimozione delle secrezioni purulente; di frequente si rendono necessari una torcia frontale, l'aspirazione e decongestionanti topici. All'inizio di solito l'oggetto è situato anteriormente, ma a causa di tentativi inesperti di rimozione può essere spinto più in profondità all'interno del naso. Se presente da molto tempo, il corpo estraneo può essere avvolto da tessuto di granulazione o dalla mucosa e avere l'aspetto di una massa nasale. Una radiografia laterale del cranio aiuta nella diagnosi se si tratta di un oggetto metallico o radiopaco.

COMPLICANZE. Spesso insorgono infezioni che danno origine a secrezioni purulente, maleodoranti o ematiche. La lesione tissutale locale da corpo estraneo di lunga durata o il danno provocato dalle sostanze alcaline contenute nelle pile a disco possono portare a perdita di tessuto e distruzione della cartilagine. Possono quindi formarsi sinechie o bande cicatriziali, che causano ostruzione nasale. La perdita della mucosa e della cartilagine settali porterà alla perforazione del setto. Le pile a disco sono pericolose, quando inserite nel naso, in quanto rilasciano sostanze basiche che causano dolore e distruzione tissutale locale nell'arco di poche ore.

TRATTAMENTO. Si procede a un rapido esame del naso per determinare se è presente un corpo estraneo e se necessita di essere rimosso con urgenza. Si pianifica quindi l'estrazione del corpo estraneo, in sede ambulatoriale o in sala operatoria. La rimozione tempestiva, che minimizza il rischio di aspirazione e di necrosi tissutale locale, abitualmente può essere effettuata in anestesia locale, utilizzando una pinza a forcipe o l'aspirazione nasale. In presenza di edema importante, sanguinamento o crescita tissutale, può essere necessaria l'anestesia generale per rimuovere l'oggetto. Di solito l'infezione si risolve rapidamente dopo la rimozione dell'oggetto e non sono necessarie ulteriori terapie.

COMPLICANZE. Il tetano è una rara complicanza dei corpi estranei nasali di vecchia data, nei bambini non vaccinati. Altrettanto rara è la sindrome da shock tossico, che tuttavia, quando insorge in questo contesto, deriva per lo più dalle medicazioni nasali chirurgiche (vedi Capitolo 180.2).

PREVENZIONE. Si potrà consentire al bambino di maneggiare piccoli oggetti potenzialmente pericolosi, come perline, solo sotto la sorveglianza di un adulto. Le pile a disco vanno conservate fuori dalla portata dei bambini piccoli.

Figueiredo RR, Azevedo AA, Kos AO, Tomita S: Nasal foreign bodies: description of types and complications in 420 cases. *Rev Bras Otorrinolaringol* 2006;72:18–23.
Haddad J Jr: Foreign bodies of the ear, nose and pharynx. In Burg FD, Gershon A, Indelfinger JR, Polin RA (eds): *Current Pediatric Therapy,* 17th ed. Philadelphia, WB Saunders, 2002, p 23.
Lin VY, Daniel SJ, Papsin BC: Button batteries in the ear, nose and upper aerodigestive tract. *Int J Pediatr Otorhinolaryngol* 2004;68:473–479.
Ogunleye AO, Sogebi OA: Nasal foreign bodies in the African children. *Afr J Med Sci* 2004;33:225–228.

374.2 • Epistassi

La fuoriuscita di sangue dal naso è rara nei lattanti e comune nei bambini più grandi; la sua incidenza si riduce dopo la pubertà. La diagnosi e il trattamento dipendono dalla localizzazione e dalla causa del sanguinamento.

ANATOMIA. La più comune sede dell'epistassi è il plesso di Kiesselbach, un'area del setto anteriore in cui convergono i vasi dalla carotide interna (arterie etmoidali anteriori e posteriori) e dalla carotide esterna (rami sfenopalatini e terminali dell'arteria mascellare interna). Per la sua localizzazione anteriore questa zona, ricoperta da mucosa sottile, è particolarmente esposta all'aria secca e ai traumi.

EZIOLOGIA. Le cause più comuni di sanguinamento nasale dal setto anteriore comprendono il trauma digitale, i corpi estranei, l'aria secca e le infiammazioni, comprese le infezioni del tratto respiratorio superiore, le sinusiti e la rinite allergica. Anche l'uso cronico di spray nasali a base di steroidi, peraltro di comune impiego nei bambini, può associarsi a sanguinamento. I lattanti di pochi mesi con significativo reflusso gastroesofageo nel naso possono occasionalmente presentare epistassi, secondaria all'infiammazione della mucosa. È spesso presente un'anamnesi familiare di epistassi in età infantile. La suscettibilità aumenta durante le infezioni respiratorie e d'inverno, quando l'aria più secca irrita la mucosa nasale, provocando la comparsa di fissurazioni e croste. Un sanguinamento severo può essere osservato in presenza di anomalie vascolari congenite, come la *teleangectasia emorragica ereditaria* (vedi Capitolo 432.3), le varici, gli emangiomi e, nei bambini con trombocitopenia, deficit dei fattori della coagulazione, in particolare la malattia di von Willebrand, l'ipertensione, l'insufficienza renale o la congestione venosa. Anche i polipi e altre neoplasie nasali possono associarsi a epistassi. Un sanguinamento ricorrente e spesso severo può essere il sintomo di presentazione degli **angiofibromi nasali giovanili**, che insorgono negli adolescenti di sesso maschile. L'incidenza del sanguinamento dal plesso di Kiesselbach diminuisce nell'adolescenza.

MANIFESTAZIONI CLINICHE. Di solito l'epistassi insorge senza preavviso, con fuoriuscita lenta ma continua di sangue da una narice o, occasionalmente, da entrambe. Nei bambini con lesioni nasali, può manifestarsi in seguito a uno sforzo fisico. Quando si verifica di notte, il sangue può essere ingerito e rendersi evidente solo quando il bambino vomita o defeca. L'epistassi posteriore si manifesta con sanguinamento nasale anteriore; se però è copiosa, il paziente può vomitare sangue come sintomo iniziale.

TRATTAMENTO. Nella maggior parte dei casi l'epistassi si arresta spontaneamente dopo pochi minuti. Si raccomanda di comprimere le narici e di tenere il bambino il più tranquillo possibile, in posizione ortostatica, con la testa piegata in avanti per evitare che il sangue entri nella faringe. Può inoltre essere utile l'applicazione di impacchi freddi sul naso. Se queste misure non arrestano il sanguinamento, si consiglia l'applicazione locale di una soluzione di oximetazolina o di fenilefrina (0,25-1%). Se il sanguinamento persiste ancora, può essere necessario inserire un tampone nasale anteriore; se l'emorragia origina dalla cavità nasale posteriore, si rendono necessari il tamponamento anteriore e posteriore combinati. Una volta che l'emorragia è sotto controllo, dopo averne identificato la sede, si può procedere all'obliterazione tramite cauterizzazione con nitrato d'argento per prevenire ulteriori episodi. Poiché la cartilagine del setto viene nutrita dal mucopericondrio sovrastante, si raccomanda di cauterizzare solo un lato del setto alla volta, per ridurre il rischio di perforazione settale. Durante l'inverno, o in ambienti secchi, l'uso di un umidificatore ambientale, l'instillazione di soluzione salina e l'applicazione di vaselina nel setto possono aiutare a prevenire l'epistassi. Tre studi hanno esaminato diverse opzioni di trattamento (crema antisettica vs. nessun trattamento, vaselina vs. nessun trattamento e crema antisettica vs. cauterizzazione con nitrato d'argento) senza riscontrare differenze significative.

Nei pazienti con epistassi severa o ripetuta, possono rendersi necessarie trasfusioni di sangue. Per questi bambini, e per quelli con sanguinamento bilaterale o con emorragia che non origina dal plesso di Kiesselbach, è indicata la valutazione otorinolaringoiatrica. Nei casi di epistassi severa ricorrente, per giungere a una diagnosi definitiva si esegue una valutazione ematologica (per coagulopatia e anemia), oltre all'endoscopia nasale e a indagini di imaging. Talvolta occorre procedere alla sostituzione dei fattori della coagulazione deficitari nei pazienti con un problema ematologico sottostante (vedi Capitolo 476). Un'epistassi monolaterale profusa, associata a una massa nasale, in un soggetto di sesso maschile prossimo alla pubertà, può segnalare un **angiofibroma rinofaringeo giovanile.** Nonostante questo tumore piuttosto insolito sia stato riscontrato anche in bambini di 2 anni e in adulti di 30-40 anni, la sua incidenza raggiunge il picco nei maschi adolescenti e preadolescenti. Per la valutazione iniziale ci si avvale della TC con mezzo di contrasto e della RM; può essere necessario procedere all'arteriografia, all'embolizzazione o all'intervento chirurgico esteso.

L'intervento chirurgico può essere richiesto anche se l'emorragia origina dall'arteria mascellare interna o da altri vasi che causano l'ingresso del sangue nella cavità nasale posteriore.

PREVENZIONE. Per prevenire l'epistassi in molti casi è sufficiente scoraggiare l'abitudine di infilare le dita nel naso e umidificare adeguatamente la camera da letto, durante i mesi invernali più secchi. Prestare attenzione al minimo accenno di infezioni nasali e allergie è un'utile pratica di igiene nasale. Per prevenire ulteriori episodi di epistassi si consiglia di sospendere l'uso di spray nasali a base di steroidi.

Burton MJ, Doree CJ: Interventions for recurrent idiopathic epistaxis (nosebleeds) in children. *Cochrane Database Syst Rev* 2004;CD004461.

Makura ZG, Porter GC, McCormick MS: Paediatric epistaxis: Alder Hey experience. *J Laryngol Otol* 2002;116:903–906.

Wurman LH: Epistaxis. In Gates GA (ed): *Current Therapy in Otolaryngology–Head and Neck Surgery,* 5th ed. St Louis, Mosby, 1994, p 354.

Capitolo 375 ■ Polipi nasali

Joseph Haddad Jr.

EZIOLOGIA. I polipi nasali sono tumori peduncolati benigni formati da mucosa edematosa, in genere con infiammazione cronica. Si sviluppano comunemente dal seno etmoidale e si presentano nel meato medio; occasionalmente compaiono nell'antro mascellare e possono estendersi al rinofaringe (polipi antrocoanali) (Fig. 375-1). I polipi antrocoanali rappresentano solo il 4-6% di tutti i polipi nasali nella popolazione generale, ma circa il 33% nella popolazione pediatrica. I polipi di maggiori dimensioni o multipli possono ostruire completamente il passaggio nasale. Quelli che originano dal seno etmoidale tendono a essere piccoli e multipli, mentre quelli antrocoanali sono più grossi e in genere singoli.

La fibrosi cistica è la causa più comune di poliposi nasale in età pediatrica e dovrebbe essere sospettata in tutti i bambini di età inferiore a 12 anni con polipi nasali, anche in assenza dei sintomi respiratori e digestivi tipici; fino al 30% dei bambini con fibrosi cistica sviluppa polipi nasali. La poliposi nasale si associa anche alla sinusite cronica e alla rinite allergica. Nella rara triade di Samter, i polipi nasali si associano a sensibilità all'acido acetilsalicilico e asma.

MANIFESTAZIONI CLINICHE. La manifestazione clinica più importante è l'ostruzione delle vie aeree nasali, associata a timbro nasale e respirazione orale. Può inoltre essere presente una rinorrea profusa monolaterale, mucoide o mucopurulenta. L'esame delle vie nasali evidenzia masse di colore grigio lucente, disposte a grappolo, compresse tra i turbinati nasali e il setto.

DIAGNOSI E DIAGNOSI DIFFERENZIALE. Si effettua l'esame del naso esterno e la rinoscopia. I polipi etmoidali si distinguono facilmente dal tessuto ben vascolarizzato dei turbinati, che è di colore rosa o rosso; i polipi antrocoanali possono avere un aspetto più carnoso e prolassare nel rinofaringe; la rinofaringoscopia con strumento flessibile può aiutare a porre questa diagnosi. La presenza prolungata di polipi etmoidali, in un bambino, può comportare l'allargamento del ponte nasale e l'erosione delle strutture ossee adiacenti. I tumori del naso causano una distruzione locale e una distorsione dell'anatomia più severe. La TC del massiccio facciale è essenziale per la diagnosi e la pianificazione del trattamento chirurgico (Fig. 375-2).

TRATTAMENTO. I decongestionanti locali o sistemici di solito non riducono le dimensioni dei polipi, sebbene possano fornire un sollievo sintomatico all'edema della mucosa associato. Più efficaci in tal senso sono gli spray nasali a base di steroidi, e talvolta gli steroidi sistemici, che si sono dimostrati utili nei bambini con fibrosi cistica e negli adulti con polipi nasali. I polipi devono essere rimossi chirurgicamente se causano ostruzione completa, rinorrea incontrollata o deformità del naso. Se non è possibile eliminare il meccanismo patogenetico sottostante (fibrosi cistica), i polipi recidiveranno precocemente. La chirurgia endoscopica funzionale dei seni, oltre a permettere una rimozione più completa dei polipi, consente il trattamento di altre patologie nasali associate, in alcuni casi riducendo la necessità di interventi chirurgici frequenti. Gli spray nasali steroidei dovrebbero essere iniziati precocemente, dopo la guarigione postchirurgica.

I polipi antrocoanali non rispondono alle misure mediche e devono essere asportati chirurgicamente. Non associandosi in

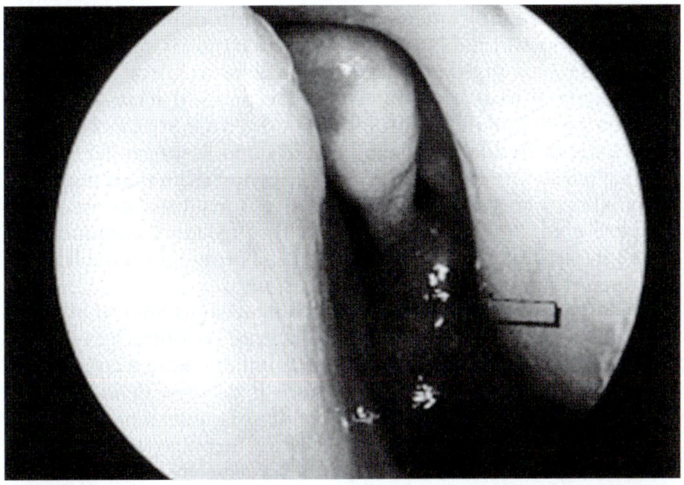

Figura 375-1. Visualizzazione endoscopica di un polipo antrocoanale (*freccia*). (Da Basak S, Karaman CZ, Akdilli A, Metin KK: Surgical approaches to antrochoanal polyps in children. *Int J Pediatr Otorhinolaryngol* 1998;46:197-205.)

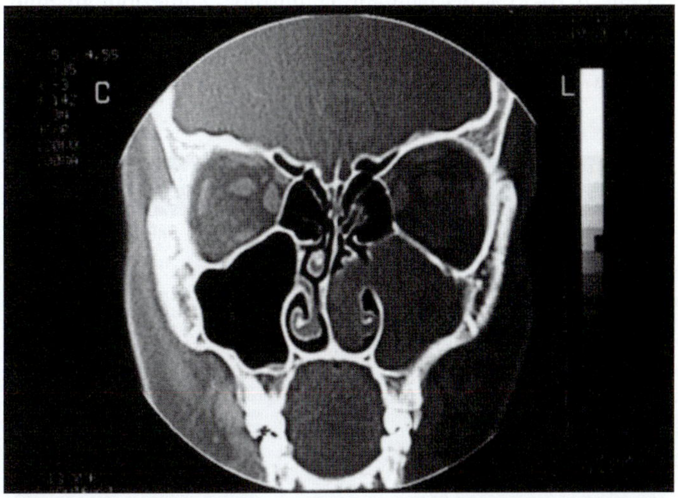

Figura 375-2. Tipica immagine TC di un polipo antrocoanale isolato, localizzato a sinistra. (Da Basak S, Karaman CZ, Akdilli A, Metin KK: Surgical approaches to antrochoanal polyps in children. *Int J Pediatr Otorhinolaryngol* 1998;46:197-205.)

genere ad altri processi patologici sottostanti, i polipi di questo tipo tendono a recidivare con minore frequenza.

Basik S, Karaman CZ, Akdilli A, Metin KK: Surgical approaches to antrochoanal polyps in children. *Int J Pediatr Otorhinolaryngol* 1998; 46:197–205.

Magit AE: Tumors of the nose, paranasal sinuses, and nasopharynx. In Bluestone CD, Stool SE, Kenna MA (eds): *Pediatric Otolaryngology,* 3rd ed. Philadelphia, WB Saunders, 1996, pp 893–904.

Orvidas LJ, Beatty CW, Weaver AL: Antrochoanal polyps in children. *Am J Rhinol* 2001;15:321–325.

Stjärne P, Mösges R, Jorissen M, et al: A randomized controlled trial of mometasonc furoate nasal spray for the treatment of nasal polyposis. *Arch Otolaryngol Head Neck Surg* 2006;132:179–185.

Capitolo 376 ■ Raffreddore comune

Ronald B. Turner e Gregory F. Hayden

Il raffreddore comune è una malattia virale, in cui predominano i sintomi di rinorrea e ostruzione nasale, mentre i sintomi e i segni sistemici come mialgie e febbre sono assenti o lievi. È spesso chiamato *rinite*, anche se sarebbe più corretto usare il termine *rinosinusite*, dal momento che comporta il coinvolgimento autolimitante della mucosa sinusale.

EZIOLOGIA. Anche se i patogeni più spesso associati al raffreddore comune sono i rinovirus (vedi Capitolo 260), la sindrome può essere causata da molti virus diversi (Tab. 376-1).

EPIDEMIOLOGIA. Il raffreddore può insorgere in qualsiasi momento dell'anno, ma la sua incidenza è maggiore dall'inizio dell'autunno fino a primavera inoltrata, riflettendo la prevalenza stagionale dei patogeni virali associati ai sintomi del raffreddore. L'incidenza più elevata delle infezioni da rinovirus si verifica all'inizio dell'autunno (da agosto a ottobre) e nella tarda primavera (aprile-maggio). L'incidenza stagionale dei virus parainfluenzali (vedi Capitolo 256) in genere raggiunge il picco alla fine dell'autunno, ed è maggiore tra dicembre e aprile per il virus respiratorio sinciziale (RSV, *Respiratory Syncytial Virus*; vedi Capitolo 257) e i virus influenzali (vedi Capitolo 255).

I bambini più piccoli hanno in media 6-8 raffreddori all'anno, ma il 10-15% dei bambini ha almeno 12 infezioni all'anno. L'incidenza delle malattie si riduce con l'età, arrivando a circa 2-3 episodi nell'adulto. I bambini che frequentano l'asilo nido durante il primo anno di vita hanno il 50% di raffreddori in più rispetto agli altri. La differenza di incidenza della malattia in questi gruppi di bambini si riduce via via che il tempo passato in ambito comunitario aumenta, sebbene l'incidenza di malattia rimanga maggiore nel gruppo che frequenta l'asilo per almeno i primi 3 anni di vita.

TABELLA 376-1. Patogeni associati al raffreddore comune

ASSOCIAZIONE	PATOGENO	FREQUENZA RELATIVA*
Agenti associati principalmente con il raffreddore	Rinovirus	Frequente
	Coronavirus	Occasionale
Agenti associati principalmente con altre sindromi cliniche	Virus respiratori sinciziali	Occasionale
	Metapneumovirus umani che causano anche i sintomi del raffreddore	Occasionale
	Virus influenzali	Non comune
	Virus parainfluenzali	Non comune
	Adenovirus	Non comune
	Enterovirus	Non comune
	Bocavirus	Non comune

*Frequenza relativa dei raffreddori causati dall'agente indicato.

PATOGENESI. I virus che causano il raffreddore comune si diffondono tramite nebulizzazione di microparticelle e macroparticelle o tramite contatto diretto. Sebbene sia probabile che i vari patogeni del raffreddore comune possano diffondersi attraverso uno qualsiasi di questi meccanismi, alcune vie di trasmissione sembrano essere più efficaci di altre per particolari virus. Gli studi compiuti sui rinovirus e sull'RSV suggeriscono che il contatto diretto sia un meccanismo di trasmissione efficiente per questi virus, sebbene possa anche aver luogo la trasmissione tramite aerosol di macroparticelle. Al contrario dei rinovirus e dell'RSV, i virus influenzali sembrano diffondersi più efficacemente tramite aerosol di microparticelle.

I virus respiratori hanno sviluppato diversi meccanismi per sfuggire alle difese dell'ospite. Le infezioni da rinovirus e adenovirus portano allo sviluppo di un'immunità protettiva sierotipo-specifica. Se si verificano infezioni ripetute da parte di questi patogeni è perché esistono numerosi sierotipi diversi per ogni virus. I virus influenzali hanno la capacità di mutare gli antigeni presentati sulla superficie virale e pertanto si comportano come se avessero sierotipi virali multipli. L'interazione tra i coronavirus (vedi Capitolo 261) e l'immunità dell'ospite non è stata ancora chiarita, ma sembra che ceppi multipli e distinti di coronavirus siano in grado di indurre almeno un'immunità protettiva a breve termine. I virus parainfluenzali e l'RSV hanno ciascuno un piccolo numero di sierotipi diversi. La reinfezione con questi virus è possibile, poiché dopo l'infezione l'organismo non sviluppa un'immunità protettiva a questi patogeni. Sebbene la reinfezione non possa essere prevenuta dalla risposta di adattamento dell'ospite a questi virus, la severità degli episodi di malattia successivi risulterà almeno limitata dall'immunità preesistente.

L'infezione virale dell'epitelio nasale può associarsi a distruzione del rivestimento epiteliale (virus influenzali e adenovirus) o non comportare alcun danno istologico evidente (rinovirus, RSV e coronavirus). A prescindere dal quadro istopatologico, l'infezione dell'epitelio nasale si associa a una risposta infiammatoria acuta, caratterizzata dal rilascio di una varietà di citochine infiammatorie e dall'infiltrazione della mucosa da parte di cellule infiammatorie. Questa risposta infiammatoria acuta sembra essere responsabile, almeno in parte, di molti dei sintomi associati al raffreddore comune. L'infiammazione può ostruire l'ostio sinusale o la tuba di Eustachio predisponendo alla sinusite batterica o all'otite media.

MANIFESTAZIONI CLINICHE. L'esordio dei sintomi del raffreddore comune avviene tipicamente da 1 a 3 giorni dopo l'infezione virale. Il primo sintomo è spesso rappresentano da fastidio o mal di gola, seguito rapidamente da ostruzione nasale e rinorrea. Il mal di gola si risolve in fretta e dal secondo al terzo giorno di malattia predominano i sintomi nasali. La tosse si associa a circa il 30% dei raffreddori e inizia di solito dopo l'esordio dei sintomi nasali. I virus influenzali, l'RSV e gli adenovirus hanno maggiore probabilità, rispetto ai rinovirus e ai coronavirus, di associarsi a febbre e ad altri sintomi sistemici. Il raffreddore comune dura circa una settimana, sebbene nel 10% si prolunghi, talvolta fino alle due settimane.

I reperti obiettivi del raffreddore comune sono limitati al tratto respiratorio superiore. Spesso l'esaminatore riscontra un evidente aumento delle secrezioni nasali. Variazioni di colore e consistenza delle secrezioni sono comuni durante il decorso della malattia e non sono indicativi di sinusite o di sovrainfezione batterica. L'esame delle cavità nasali può rivelare turbinati edematosi ed eritematosi, sebbene questo reperto sia aspecifico e di limitato valore diagnostico.

DIAGNOSI. Il compito più importante, per il medico che si occupa di un paziente con il raffreddore, è escludere altre condizioni che siano potenzialmente più gravi o trattabili. La diagnosi differenziale comprende malattie non infettive così come altre infezioni del tratto respiratorio superiore (Tab. 376-2).

LABORATORIO. Le indagini di laboratorio di routine non sono utili per la diagnosi e il trattamento del raffreddore comune. Lo striscio nasale per la ricerca degli eosinofili può essere d'aiuto nel sospetto di una rinite allergica (vedi Capitolo 142). La predominanza di leucociti polimorfonucleati nelle secrezioni nasali è caratteristica dei raffreddori non complicati e non indica una sovrainfezione batterica.

I patogeni virali associati al raffreddore comune sono rilevabili tramite coltura, ricerca degli antigeni, reazione a catena della polimerasi (PCR, *Polymerase Chain Reaction*) o metodiche sierologiche. Questi esami non sono generalmente indicati nei pazienti con il raffreddore, poiché una diagnosi eziologica specifica è utile solo quando si contempla un trattamento con un agente antivirale. Le colture batteriche o la ricerca degli antigeni sono utili solo nel sospetto di infezioni da streptococco di gruppo A (vedi Capitolo 182), da *Bordetella pertussis* (vedi Capitolo 194) o di difterite nasale. L'isolamento di altri patogeni batterici non è un'indicazione di infezione nasale batterica, né un fattore predittivo specifico dell'agente eziologico della sinusite.

TRATTAMENTO. Il trattamento del raffreddore comune consiste principalmente in misure sintomatiche.

Trattamento antivirale. Non è attualmente disponibile una terapia antivirale specifica per le infezioni da rinovirus. La ribavirina, che è stata approvata per le infezioni da RSV, non ha alcuna efficacia nel trattamento del raffreddore comune. Gli inibitori delle neuraminidasi oseltamivir e zanamivir hanno un effetto modesto sulla durata dei sintomi associati alle infezioni da virus influenzali nei bambini. L'oseltamivir riduce anche la frequenza di otite media associata a influenza. La difficoltà di distinguere i virus influenzali dagli altri patogeni del raffreddore comune e la necessità che la terapia sia iniziata precocemente nel corso della malattia (entro 48 ore dall'esordio dei sintomi) per essere efficace, sono limitazioni pratiche all'uso di questi agenti, nelle infezioni lievi del tratto respiratorio superiore. Altri agenti antivirali come il picovir per il trattamento delle infezioni da rinovirus sono in fase di sviluppo, sebbene il ruolo di questi agenti, se esiste, nel trattamento di routine del raffreddore comune sia ancora da determinare. La terapia antibatterica non è di alcun beneficio nel trattamento del raffreddore comune.

Trattamento sintomatico. L'uso di terapie sintomatiche nei pazienti pediatrici è controverso; sebbene alcuni di questi farmaci siano efficaci nell'adulto, mancano studi che dimostrino un effetto significativo nei bambini. Dal momento che i pazienti più piccoli non possono collaborare a queste valutazioni, in questi casi gli studi sul trattamento si sono generalmente basati sulle osservazioni dei genitori. L'uso di terapie sintomatiche in età pediatrica può basarsi solo sul presupposto che gli effetti di questi trattamenti siano simili negli adulti e nei bambini. La decisione di somministrare questi farmaci ai bambini deve essere valutata tenendo conto dei potenziali effetti avversi. I sintomi prevalenti o più fastidiosi del raffreddore variano nel corso della malattia e, pertanto, se si decide di instaurare un trattamento sintomatico, è ragionevole mirare ai sintomi che arrecano maggiore disturbo. Se si consiglia un trattamento sintomatico, ci si deve assicurare che chi si occupa del bambino capisca quale effetto si vuole ottenere e sia in grado di valutare il corretto dosaggio dei farmaci.

FEBBRE. La febbre si associa di rado al raffreddore comune non complicato e il trattamento antipiretico non è generalmente indicato.

OSTRUZIONE NASALE. Come decongestionanti nasali si possono somministrare agenti adrenergici topici o orali. Gli agenti adrenergici locali come la xilometazolina, l'oximetazolina o la fenilefrina sono in commercio sotto forma di gocce o spray nasali. Questi farmaci sono disponibili anche in formulazioni a basso dosaggio specifiche per l'uso pediatrico, sebbene non ne sia stato approvato l'utilizzo nei bambini di età inferiore a 2 anni. L'assorbimento sistemico delle imidazoline (oximetazolina e xilometazolina) è stato associato molto raramente a bradicardia, ipotensione e coma. L'uso prolungato di agenti adrenergici topici andrebbe evitato per prevenire lo sviluppo di una **rinite da farmaci**, un apparente effetto rebound che dà una sensazione di ostruzione nasale quando si sospende il farmaco. Gli agenti adrenergici orali sono meno efficaci delle preparazioni topiche e si associano occasionalmente a effetti sistemici con stimolazione del sistema nervoso centrale, ipertensione e palpitazioni.

RINORREA. Gli antistaminici di prima generazione riducono la rinorrea del 25-30%; tale prerogativa sembra essere correlata alle proprietà anticolinergiche, più che a quelle antistaminiche, di tali farmaci, e pertanto gli antistaminici di seconda generazione, meno sedativi, non hanno effetto sui sintomi del raffreddore comune. Il principale effetto indesiderato associato all'uso degli antistaminici è la sedazione, che tuttavia parrebbe meno fastidiosa nei bambini rispetto agli adulti. La rinorrea può essere trattata anche con ipratropio bromuro, un agente anticolinergico topico. I principali effetti indesiderati dell'ipratropio sono l'irritazione e il sanguinamento nasali.

MAL DI GOLA. Anche se il mal di gola tipico del raffreddore non è in genere intenso, il trattamento con analgesici blandi è occasionalmente indicato, in particolare se il paziente accusa anche mialgie e cefalea. L'uso di paracetamolo durante l'infezione da rinovirus è stato associato alla soppressione della riposta anticorpale neutralizzante, ma questa osservazione non sembra avere alcun significato clinico. L'acido acetilsalicilico non dovrebbe essere somministrato in caso di infezioni respiratorie, per il rischio che si sviluppi una sindrome di Reye nei bambini con influenza (vedi Capitolo 598).

TOSSE. La sedazione della tosse non è generalmente necessaria nei pazienti con raffreddore. In alcuni casi la tosse sembra dovuta all'irritazione del tratto respiratorio associata allo scolo postnasale ed è quindi più accentuata durante il periodo in cui predominano i sintomi nasali, durante il quale può essere utile somministrare antistaminici di prima generazione. Gocce o pasticche per la tosse contenenti zucchero possono dare un sollievo temporaneo. In altri pazienti, la tosse può essere il risultato di una **malattia reattiva delle vie aeree** indotta dal virus; se la tosse persiste per giorni o settimane, dopo la malattia acuta, l'inalazione di steroidi e broncodilatatori può essere benefica. La codeina e il destrometorfano idrobromuro non hanno effetto contro la tosse da raffreddore. Neppure gli agenti espettoranti come la guaifenesina sono efficaci.

Trattamenti inefficaci. La vitamina C, la guaifenesina e l'inalazione di aria calda e umida non si sono dimostrati più efficaci del placebo nel trattamento sintomatico del raffreddore.

Lo zinco, somministrato oralmente sotto forma di compresse, è stato valutato in diversi studi come trattamento sintomatico del raffreddore comune. Lo zinco inibisce la funzione della rinovirus proteasi 3C, un enzima essenziale per la replicazione dei rinovirus, ma non vi sono state evidenze di un suo effetto antivirale *in vivo*. Per quanto riguarda la sua efficacia contro i sintomi, i risultati ottenuti sono stati contraddittori: alcuni studi hanno riportato effetti eclatanti del trattamento (negli adulti) mentre

TABELLA 376-2. Condizioni che possono simulare il raffreddore comune

CONDIZIONE	CARATTERISTICHE DISTINTIVE
Rinite allergica	Prevalenza di prurito e starnuti
Corpo estraneo	Eosinofili nasali
	Secrezioni monolaterali maleodoranti
	Secrezioni nasali ematiche
Sinusite	Presenza di febbre, cefalea o algia faciale, o edema periorbitario o persistenza di rinorrea o tosse per più di 14 giorni
Infezione da streptococco	Secrezioni nasali che escoriano le narici
Pertosse	Esordio di tosse persistente o severa
Sifilide congenita	Rinorrea persistente che insorge nei primi 3 mesi di vita

altri che non hanno riscontrato alcun beneficio. È difficile trarre conclusioni da questi dati divergenti, ma sembra comunque poco probabile che lo zinco abbia un significativo impatto clinico sui sintomi del raffreddore comune nei bambini.

L'echinacea è un trattamento erboristico diffuso per il raffreddore comune. Sebbene gli estratti di echinacea abbiano dimostrato un effetto biologico, l'echinacea non è efficace come trattamento del raffreddore comune nei bambini. La mancanza di standardizzazione dei prodotti in commercio contenenti echinacea rappresenta anche un grosso ostacolo alla valutazione razionale o all'uso di questa terapia.

COMPLICANZE. La complicanza più comune è l'**otite media** (vedi Capitolo 639), che è stata riportata nel 5-30% dei bambini con raffreddore, con l'incidenza più elevata in quelli che frequentano l'asilo. Il trattamento sintomatico non ha alcun effetto sullo sviluppo dell'otite media, ma la terapia con oseltamivir può ridurre l'incidenza di questa complicanza, nei pazienti con influenza.

Un'altra complicanza è la **sinusite** (vedi Capitolo 377); un'infiammazione autolimitante dei seni fa parte della fisiopatologia del raffreddore comune, ma lo 0,5-2% delle infezioni virali delle vie aeree superiori negli adulti, e il 5-13% nei bambini, si complica con una sinusite batterica acuta. Distinguere i sintomi del raffreddore da quelli della sinusite può essere difficile. Si dovrebbe prendere in considerazione la diagnosi di sinusite batterica quando la rinorrea o la tosse diurna persistono senza miglioramenti per almeno 10-14 giorni, o si sviluppano segni di un coinvolgimento più severo dei seni, come febbre, algie faciali o edema faciale. Non vi sono evidenze che il trattamento sintomatico del raffreddore incida sulla frequenza di sviluppo della sinusite batterica.

L'esacerbazione dell'**asma** è una complicanza relativamente poco frequente, ma potenzialmente grave, del raffreddore. La maggior parte delle esacerbazioni asmatiche, nei bambini, si associa al raffreddore comune. Non vi sono evidenze che il trattamento sintomatico del raffreddore prevenga questa complicanza.

Sebbene non sia una complicanza, un'altra importante conseguenza del raffreddore comune è l'uso inappropriato degli antibiotici, che favorisce lo sviluppo di ceppi batterici resistenti. Negli Stati Uniti, si è stimato che vi furono 25 milioni di visite ambulatoriali dal medico di base per raffreddore comune, con il 30% di queste risultato in un'inappropriata prescrizione di antibiotici.

PREVENZIONE. Non sono generalmente disponibili una chemioprofilassi o un'immunoprofilassi per il raffreddore comune. La vaccinazione o la chemioprofilassi contro l'influenza possono essere utili per la prevenzione del raffreddore causato da questo patogeno, che però è responsabile solo di una piccola parte di tutti i casi di rinite comune. Vitamina C ed echinacea non hanno alcuna efficacia preventiva.

L'interruzione della catena di diffusione del virus tramite contatto diretto può prevenire il raffreddore. In ambiente ospedaliero, per impedire la trasmissione dei virus respiratori si è adottata la precauzione di far indossare al personale le mascherine protettive, che impediscono il contatto mano-occhi e mano-naso. Il sistema più semplice per prevenire la diffusione dei virus tramite contatto diretto è l'accurato lavaggio delle mani da parte dell'individuo affetto e/o delle persone con cui viene in contatto.

Arnold JC, Singh KK, Spector SA, Sawyer MA: Human bocavirus: prevalence and clinical spectrum at a children's hospital. *CID* 2006;43:283–288.

Butler CC, Kinnersley P, Hood K, et al: Clinical course of acute infection of the upper respiratory tract in children: Cohort study. *Br Med J* 2003; 327:1088–1089.

Eccles R: Efficacy and safety of over-the-counter analgesics in the treatment of common cold and flu. *J Clin Pharm Ther* 2006;31:309–319.

Gonzales R, Malone DC, Maselli JH, et al: Excessive antibiotic use for acute respiratory infections in the United States. *Clin Infect Dis* 2001;33:757–762.

Hampton T: New guidelines released for managing cough. *JAMA* 2006;295:746–747.

Hedrick JA, Barzilai A, Behre U, et al: Zanamivir for treatment of symptomatic influenza A and B infection in children five to twelve years of age: A randomized controlled trial. *Pediatr Infect Dis J* 2000;19:410–417.

Hrastinger A, Dietz B, Bauer R, et al: Is there clinical evidence supporting the use of botanical dietary supplements in children? *J Pediatr* 2005:146: 311–317.

Jackson JL, Peterson C, Lesho E: A meta-analysis of zinc salts lozenges and the common cold. *Arch Intern Med* 1997;157:2373–2376.

Kusel MMH, de Klerk NH, Holt PG, et al: Role of respiratory viruses in acute upper and lower respiratory tract illness in the first year of life. *Pediatr Infect Dis J* 2006;25:680–686.

Simon HK, Weinkle DA: Over-the-counter medications. Do parents give what they intend to give? *Arch Pediatr Adolesc Med* 1997;151:654–656.

Taylor JA, Weber W, Standish L, et al: Efficacy and safety of Echinacea in treating upper respiratory tract infections in children: A randomized controlled trial. *JAMA* 2003;290:2824–2830.

Turner RB: The treatment of rhinovirus infections: Progress and potential. *Antiviral Res* 2001;49:1–14.

Capitolo 377 ■ Sinusite

Diane E. Pappas e J. Owen Hendley

La sinusite è una malattia comune nell'infanzia e nell'adolescenza, caratterizzata da una significativa morbilità acuta e cronica, oltre che da complicanze potenzialmente gravi. Esistono due tipi di sinusite acuta: virale e batterica. Il raffreddore comune provoca una rinosinusite virale autolimitante (vedi Capitolo 376). Circa lo 0,5-2% delle infezioni virali delle vie aeree superiori, nei bambini e negli adolescenti, si complica con una sinusite acuta batterica. Alcuni bambini con condizioni predisponenti hanno una malattia cronica dei seni, che non sembra di origine infettiva. Le modalità per una diagnosi corretta e il trattamento ottimale della sinusite restano controverse.

Alla nascita sono presenti sia i seni **etmoidali**, sia i seni **mascellari**, ma solo i primi sono pneumatizzati (Fig. 377-1); i seni mascellari non sono pneumatizzati fino all'età di 4 anni. I seni **sfenoidali** sono presenti dall'età di 5 anni, mentre quelli **frontali** iniziano a svilupparsi all'età di 7-8 anni e non sono completi fino all'adolescenza. Gli osti che drenano i seni sono stretti (1-3 mm) e drenano nel complesso ostiomeatale, nel meato medio. Di norma i seni **paranasali** sono sterili, mantenuti tali dal sistema di clearance mucociliare.

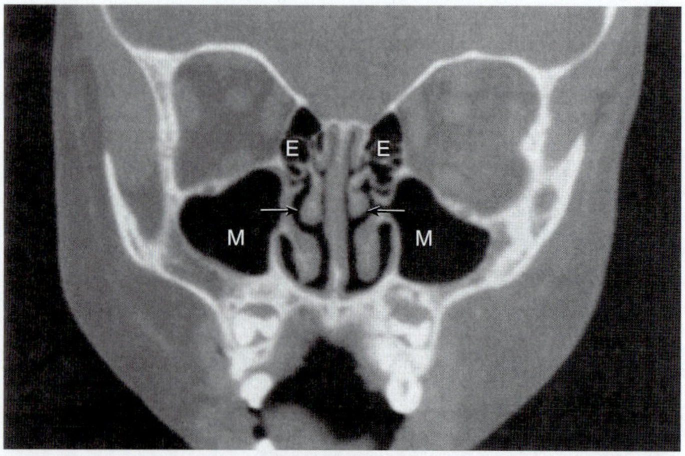

Figura 377-1. TC coronale normale di un bambino di 3 anni. Le *frecce* indicano il meato medio. E, seni etmoidali; M, seni mascellari. (Da Isaacson G: Sinusitis in childhood. *Pediatr Clin North Am* 1996;43:1297-1317.)

EZIOLOGIA. I batteri patogeni che causano sinusite acuta nei bambini e negli adolescenti comprendono *Streptococcus pneumoniae* (circa 30%), *Haemophilus influenzae* non tipizzabile (circa 20%) e *Moraxella catarrhalis* (circa 20%). Circa il 50% degli *H. influenzae* e il 100% delle *M. catarrhalis* sono β-lattamasi positivi. Circa il 25% degli *S. pneumoniae* può essere penicillino-resistente. *Staphylococcus aureus*, gli altri streptococchi e gli anaerobi sono cause non comuni di sinusite batterica acuta nei bambini. *H. influenzae*, gli streptococchi α- e β-emolitici, *M. catarrhalis*, *S. pneumoniae* e gli stafilococchi coagulasi-negativi sono di comune riscontro nei bambini con **sinusopatia cronica**.

EPIDEMIOLOGIA. La sinusite batterica acuta può insorgere a qualunque età. Le condizioni predisponenti comprendono le infezioni virali delle vie respiratorie superiori (associate con la frequentazione di asili o con la presenza di fratelli in età scolare), la rinite allergica e l'esposizione al fumo di sigaretta. I bambini con carenze del sistema immunitario, relative in particolare alla produzione di anticorpi (immunoglobuline G [IgG], sottoclassi di IgG e IgA) (vedi Capitolo 123), fibrosi cistica (vedi Capitolo 400), disfunzione ciliare (vedi Capitolo 401), anomalie della funzione fagocitica, reflusso gastroesofageo, difetti anatomici (palatoschisi), polipi nasali e corpi estranei nasali (compresi i sondini nasogastrici) possono sviluppare una malattia cronica dei seni. L'immunosoppressione per il trapianto di midollo osseo o un tumore con neutropenia e linfopenia accentuate predispongono a gravi sinusiti fungine (aspergilli, *Mucor*), spesso con estensione endocranica. I pazienti con intubazione nasotracheale o sondini nasogastrici possono andare incontro a ostruzione dell'ostio dei seni e sviluppare sinusiti dovute agli organismi multiresistenti dei reparti di terapia intensiva.

PATOGENESI. La sinusite batterica acuta tipicamente insorge in seguito a un'infezione virale delle vie respiratorie superiori, che inizialmente provoca una rinosinusite virale; la valutazione dei seni paranasali con RM rivela notevoli anomalie dei seni paranasali (ispessimento della mucosa, edema, infiammazione) nel 68% dei bambini sani, durante il normale decorso del raffreddore comune. È stato dimostrato che l'azione di soffiarsi il naso produce una forza sufficiente a spingere le secrezioni nasali nelle cavità sinusali. Di norma i batteri del rinofaringe che entrano nei seni vengono eliminati rapidamente, ma durante una rinosinusite virale, l'infiammazione e l'edema possono bloccare il drenaggio dei seni e alterare la clearance mucociliare dei batteri: si vengono così a creare condizioni favorevoli alla proliferazione batterica.

MANIFESTAZIONI CLINICHE. I bambini e gli adolescenti con sinusite possono presentare disturbi aspecifici, tra cui congestione nasale, secrezioni nasali purulente (mono- o bilaterali), febbre e tosse. Altri sintomi meno comuni comprendono alitosi, riduzione dell'olfatto ed edema periorbitario. È raro che i bambini lamentino cefalea o dolore faciale. Ulteriori sintomi comprendono fastidio ai denti dell'arcata mascellare, dolore o pressione che si esacerbano quando il soggetto si piega in avanti e iposmia. L'esame obiettivo può rivelare eritema ed edema della mucosa nasale, con secrezioni purulente. Negli adolescenti e negli adulti può essere rilevabile dolorabilità dei seni. La transilluminazione rivela un seno opaco che trasmette male la luce.

DIAGNOSI. La diagnosi clinica della sinusite batterica acuta si basa unicamente sull'anamnesi. Sintomi persistenti di infezione delle vie aeree superiori, tra cui la presenza di secrezioni nasali e tosse per più di 10-14 giorni senza miglioramento, o sintomi respiratori severi, tra cui una temperatura di almeno 39 °C e secrezioni nasali purulente per più di 3-4 giorni consecutivi, sono suggestivi di sinusite batterica acuta insorta come complicanza. Nel 70% dei bambini studiati, con questi sintomi severi o persistenti, si riscontrano batteri nell'aspirato del seno mascellare. I bambini con sinusite cronica hanno un'anamnesi di sintomi respiratori persistenti, tra cui tosse, secrezione o congestione nasale, che durano da più di 90 giorni.

La *coltura dell'aspirato sinusale* è l'unico metodo accurato per la diagnosi; non è di uso comune nei pazienti immunocompetenti, in quanto poco pratico, ma può rendersi necessario nei pazienti immunosoppressi con sospetta sinusite fungina. Negli adulti, l'*endoscopia nasale con strumento rigido* è una metodica meno invasiva che permette di prelevare dai seni materiale per l'esame colturale, ma che, rispetto all'aspirato, rileva un eccesso di colture positive. Con la *transilluminazione* delle cavità sinusali è possibile rilevare la presenza di liquido, ma non stabilire se sia di origine batterica o virale. Nei bambini, la transilluminazione è difficile da effettuare e inaffidabile. I reperti degli studi radiologici (radiografia semplice dei seni, TC), che comprendono l'opacizzazione, l'ispessimento della mucosa o la presenza di un livello idroaereo, non sono completamente diagnostici (Fig. 377-2); possono confermare la presenza di infiammazione sinusale, ma sono utili per stabilire se l'infiammazione è dovuta a cause virali, batteriche o allergiche.

A causa del quadro clinico aspecifico, la diagnosi differenziale comprende le infezioni delle vie aeree superiori, la rinite allergica, la rinite aspecifica e i corpi estranei nasali. Le infezioni virali delle vie aeree superiori sono caratterizzate da secrezioni chiare e in genere non purulente, tosse e febbre iniziale; di solito i sintomi non durano più di 10-14 giorni, sebbene alcuni bambini (10%) abbiano sintomi persistenti anche a distanza di 14 giorni. La rinite allergica può essere stagionale; la valutazione delle secrezioni nasali deve rivelare un'eosinofilia significativa.

TRATTAMENTO. Non è chiaro se il trattamento antimicrobico della sinusite batterica acuta, diagnosticata clinicamente, offra un beneficio effettivo. Da uno studio randomizzato, controllato con placebo, che ha posto a confronto amoxicillina e amoxicillina clavulanato, somministrati per 14 giorni a bambini con sinusite diagnosticata clinicamente, è emerso che la terapia antimicrobica non incideva sulla risoluzione dei sintomi, sulla durata o sul numero di giorni di assenza scolastica. Le linee guida dall'American Academy of Pediatrics raccomandano il trattamento antimicrobico, nella sinusite batterica acuta, per promuovere la risoluzione dei sintomi e prevenire le complicanze suppurative, sebbene il 50-60% dei bambini con sinusite batterica acuta guariscano senza terapia antimicrobica. La terapia iniziale con amoxicillina (45 mg/kg/die) è adeguata per la maggior parte dei bambini con sinusite batterica acuta non complicata. I trattamenti alternativi, per i pazienti allergici alle penicilline, comprendono il trimetoprim-sulfametoxazolo, la cefuroxima, la cefpodoxima, la claritromicina o l'azitromicina. Per i bambini a rischio di sviluppare specie batteriche resistenti (trattamento antibiotico nei precedenti 3 mesi, frequentazione di un asilo o età inferiore a 2 anni) e per quelli che non rispondono a una terapia iniziale con amoxicillina entro 72 ore,

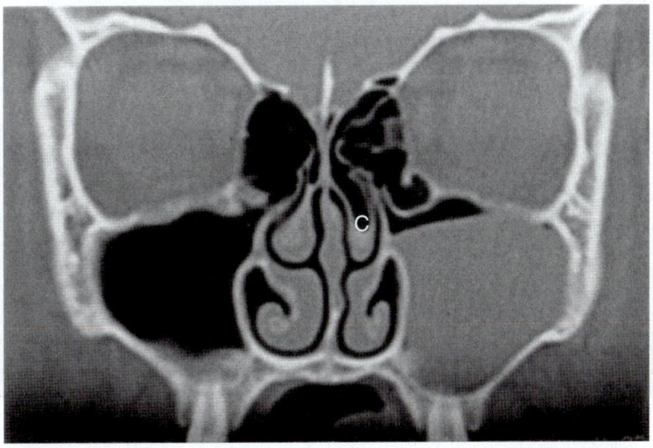

Figura 377-2. Sinusite mascellare acuta sinistra con un livello idroaereo. Si noti la conca bullosa (C). (Da Isaacson G: Sinusitis in childhood. *Pediatr Clin North Am* 1996;43:1297-1317.)

occorre iniziare un trattamento con amoxicillina clavulanato a dosi elevate (80-90 mg/kg/die di amoxicillina e 6-4 mg/kg/die di clavulanato). In alternativa, si può somministrare azitromicina (o, nei bambini più grandi, levofloxacina). Se il paziente non risponde a questo schema terapeutico si richiede la consulenza di un otorinolaringoiatra per un'ulteriore valutazione, poiché potrebbe essere necessaria l'aspirazione del seno mascellare per un esame colturale con antibiogramma. Ancora non è stata stabilita la giusta durata della terapia per la sinusite; si consiglia di individualizzare il trattamento e di interromperlo solo 7 giorni dopo la risoluzione dei sintomi.

La sinusite frontale, che può progredire rapidamente dando luogo a gravi complicanze endocraniche, richiede la tempestiva prescrizione di una terapia parenterale con ceftriaxone, da somministrare finché non si ottiene un miglioramento clinico sostanziale (Figg. 377-3 e 377-4). Il trattamento è quindi proseguito con un antibiotico per via orale.

L'applicazione intranasale di decongestionanti, antistaminici, mucolitici e corticosteroidi non è stata adeguatamente studiata nei bambini e non è raccomandata per il trattamento della sinusite batterica acuta non complicata. Analogamente, il lavaggio nasale con soluzione salina e gli spray nasali possono fluidificare le secrezioni e agiscono da blandi vasocostrittori, ma i loro effetti non sono stati valutati sistematicamente nei bambini.

COMPLICANZE. A causa della stretta prossimità dei seni paranasali con il cervello e gli occhi, da una sinusite acuta batterica possono svilupparsi e progredire rapidamente gravi complicanze a livello orbitario o endocranico. Le complicanze a carico dell'orbita, tra cui la *cellulite periorbitaria* e la *cellulite orbitaria* (vedi Capitolo 633), sono per lo più secondarie all'etmoidite batterica acuta. L'infezione può diffondersi direttamente attraverso la lamina papiracea, il sottile osso che forma la parete laterale del seno etmoidale. La cellulite periorbitaria provoca eritema ed edema dei tessuti circostanti il bulbo oculare, mentre la cellulite orbitaria coinvolge le struttura intraorbitarie provocando proptosi, chemosi, diminuzione dell'acuità visiva,

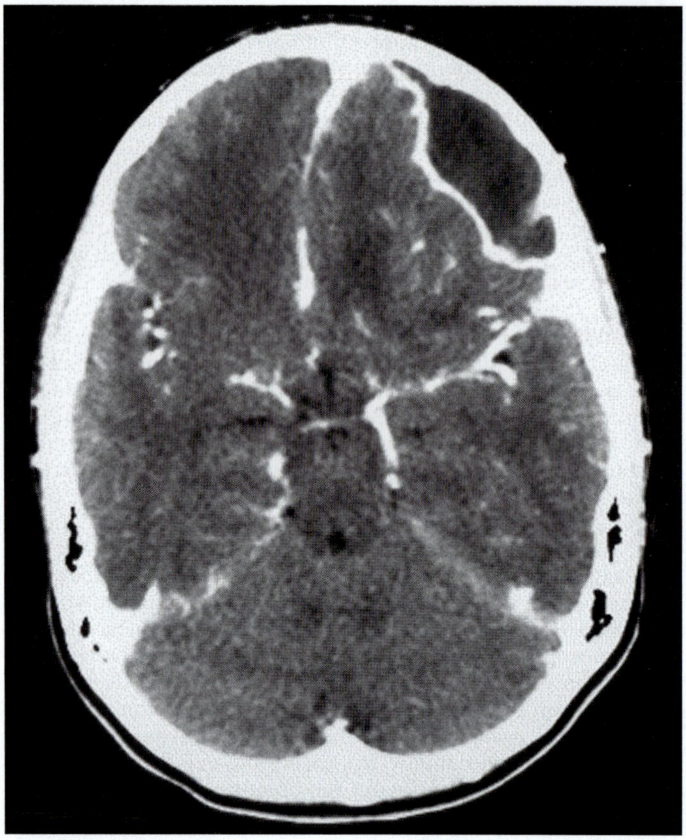

Figura 377-4. TC assiale con mezzo di contrasto eseguita, previa sedazione, in una bambina di 11 anni con ascesso del lobo sottofrontale secondario a una sinusite frontale. La TC rivela un cavità piena di liquido di forma ellittica, adiacente al lobo frontale, con uno spostamento in senso controlaterale della linea mediana. (Da Parikh SR, Brown SM: Image-guided frontal sinus surgery in children. *Operative Tech Otolaryngol Head Neck Surg* 2004;15:37-41.)

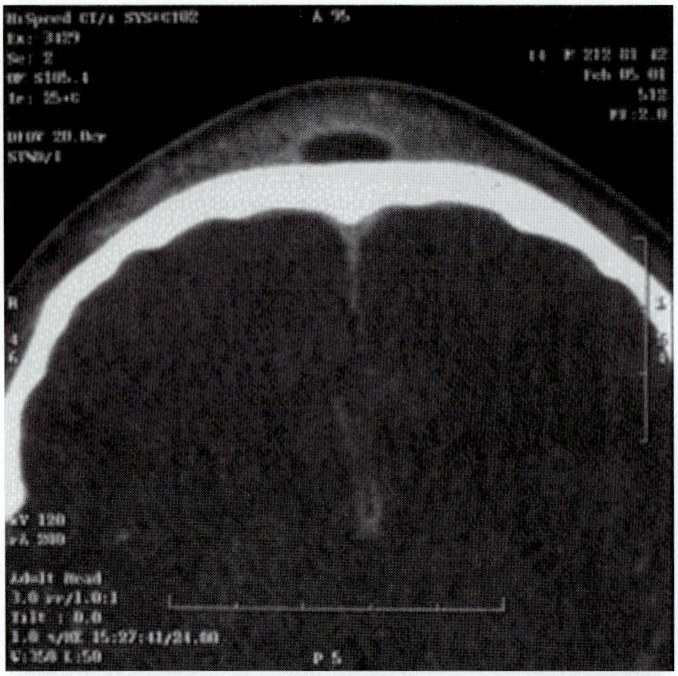

Figura 377-3. TC assiale con mezzo di contrasto di un bambino di 11 anni con un ascesso sottoperiostale frontale, secondario a una sinusite frontale acuta. La TC dimostra una zona ad anello a densità liquida sulla linea mediana, al di sopra dell'osso frontale. (Da Parikh SR, Brown SM: Image-guided frontal sinus surgery in children. *Operative Tech Otolaryngol Head Neck Surg* 2004;15:37-41.)

diplopia, alterazione dei movimenti extraoculari e dolore oculare. La valutazione deve comprendere la TC delle orbite e dei seni, con consulenza oculistica e otorinolaringoiatrica. Bisogna iniziare un trattamento con antibiotici per via endovenosa. La cellulite orbitaria può richiedere il drenaggio chirurgico dei seni etmoidali.

Le complicanze intracraniche possono comprendere ascessi epidurali, meningite, trombosi del seno cavernoso, empiema subdurale e ascesso cerebrale (vedi Capitolo 602). I bambini con alterazioni dello stato mentale, rigidità nucale o segni di ipertensione endocranica (cefalea, vomito) richiedono una TC immediata dell'encefalo, delle orbite e dei seni, per valutare la presenza di complicanze endocraniche di una sinusite batterica acuta. Il trattamento con antibiotici ad ampio spettro per via endovenosa (cefotaxima o ceftriaxone associati a vancomicina) deve essere iniziato immediatamente, in attesa dei risultati delle colture e dell'antibiogramma. Nel 50% degli ascessi è in atto un'infezione polimicrobica. Gli ascessi possono richiedere il drenaggio chirurgico. Altre complicanze comprendono l'osteomielite dell'osso frontale (**tumore di Pott**), caratterizzato da edema e gonfiore della fronte (vedi Fig. 377-3), e il **mucocele**, una lesione infiammatoria cronica comunemente localizzata nei seni frontali, che può espandersi causando lo spostamento dell'occhio con conseguente diplopia. È abitualmente richiesto il drenaggio chirurgico.

PREVENZIONE. Il metodo migliore per prevenire la sinusite consiste nel lavarsi spesso le mani e nell'evitare il contatto con persone raffreddate. Poiché la sinusite batterica acuta può complicare un'infezione influenzale, la profilassi dell'influenza tramite vaccinazione precoce può essere utile per prevenire alcuni casi di complicanze sinusitiche. L'immunizzazione o la chemioprofilassi contro l'influenza con oseltamivir o zanamivir può essere utile per prevenire i raffreddori causati da questi patogeni e le complicanze associate; bisogna tuttavia ricordare che l'influenza è responsabile solo di una piccola parte di tutti i raffreddori.

American Academy of Pediatrics, Subcommittee on Management of Sinusitis and Committee on Quality Improvement: Clinical practice guideline: Management of sinusitis. *Pediatrics* 2001;108:798–808.

Arroll B, Kenealy T: Are antibiotics effective for acute purulent rhinitis? Systematic review and meta-analysis of placebo controlled randomised trials. *BMJ* 2006;333:279–280.

Brook I, Gooch WM III, Jenkins SG, et al: Medical management of acute bacterial sinusitis: Recommendations of a clinical advisory committee on pediatric and adult sinusitis. *Ann Otol Rhinol Laryngol* 2000;109:1–20.

Butler C, Kinnersley P, Hood K, et al: Clinical course of acute infection of the upper respiratory tract in children: Cohort study. Br Med J 2003;327:1088–1089.

Chan KH, Abzug MJ, Coffinet L, et al: Chronic rhinosinusitis in young children differs from adults: A histopathology study. *J Pediatr* 2004;144:206–212.

Don DM, Yellon RF, Casselbrant ML, et al: Efficacy of a stepwise protocol that includes intravenous antibiotic therapy for the management of chronic sinusitis in children and adolescents. *Arch Otolaryngol Head Neck Surg* 2001;127:1093–1098.

Garbutt JM, Goldstein M, Gellman E, et al: A randomized, placebo-controlled trial of antimicrobial treatment for children with clinically diagnosed acute sinusitis. *Pediatrics* 2001;107:619–24.

Germiller JA, Monin DL, Sparano AM, et al: Intracranial complications of sinusitis in children and adolescents and their outcomes. *Arch Otolaryngol Head Neck Surg* 2006;132:969–976.

Goldsmith AJ, Rosenfeld RM: Treatment of pediatric sinusitis. *Pediatr Clin North Am* 2003;50:413–426.

Isaacson G: Sinusitis in childhood. *Pediatr Clin North Am* 1996;43:1297–1317.

Kristo A, Uhari M, Luotonen J, et al: Paranasal sinus findings in children during respiratory infection evaluated with magnetic resonance imaging. *Pediatrics* 2003;111:e586–e589.

[No authors listed]: Antimicrobial treatment guidelines for acute bacterial rhinosinusitis. Sinus and Allergy Health Partnership. *Otolaryngol Head Neck Surg* 2000;123:5–31.

Parikh SR, Brown SM: Image-guided frontal sinus surgery in children. *Operative Tech Otolaryngol Head Neck Surg* 2004;15:37–41.

Phipps CD, Wood WE, Gibson WS, et al: Gastroesophageal reflux contributing to chronic sinus disease in children: A prospective analysis. *Arch Otolaryngol Head Neck Surg* 2000;126:831–836.

Piccirillo JF: Acute bacterial sinusitis. *N Engl J Med* 2004;351:902–910.

Slavin RG, Spector RL, Bernstein IL: The diagnosis and management of sinusitis: A practice parameter update. *J Allergy Clin Immunol* 2005;116:S13–S47.

Steele RW: Rhinosinusitis in children. *Curr Allergy Asthma Rep* 2006;6:508–512.

Talbot G, Kennedy D, Scheld W, et al: Rigid nasal endoscopy versus sinus puncture and aspiration for microbiologic documentation of acute bacterial maxillary sinusitis. *Clin Infect Dis* 2001;33:1668–1675.

Capitolo 378 ■ Faringite acuta

Gregory F. Hayden e Ronald B. Turner

Le infezioni del tratto respiratorio superiore sono responsabili di un'elevata percentuale di visite pediatriche. Circa un terzo di queste patologie è caratterizzato dal mal di gola come sintomo principale.

EZIOLOGIA. Gli agenti più importanti che causano faringite sono i virus (adenovirus, coronavirus, enterovirus, rinovirus, virus respiratorio sinciziale [RSV, *Respiratory Syncytial Virus*], virus di Epstein-Barr [EBV, *Epstein-Barr Virus*], virus dell'herpes simplex [HSV, *Herpes Simplex Virus*], metapneumovirus) e gli streptococchi β-emolitici di gruppo A (SBEA). Altri microrganismi che possono talvolta associarsi alla faringite sono gli streptococchi di gruppo C, *Arcanobacterium haemolyticum*, *Francisella tularensis*, *Mycoplasma pneumoniae*, *Neisseria gonorrhoeae* e *Corynebacterium diphtheriae*.

Altri batteri, come *Haemophilus influenzae* e *Streptococcus pneumoniae*, possono essere isolati dai tamponi faringei di bambini con faringite, ma il loro ruolo come agenti causali non è stato definito.

EPIDEMIOLOGIA. Le infezioni virali delle vie aeree superiori si diffondono per contatto ravvicinato e si verificano più comunemente in autunno, inverno e primavera. La faringite streptococcica è rara prima dei 2-3 anni di età, ha un picco di incidenza nei primi anni di scuola e declina nella tarda adolescenza e in età adulta. La malattia insorge per lo più in inverno e in primavera, diffondendosi tra fratelli e compagni di scuola. La faringite da streptococco di gruppo C e da *A. haemolyticum* colpisce con maggiore frequenza adolescenti e adulti. L'infezione primitiva da HIV si manifesta anch'essa con una faringite e una sindrome simile alla mononucleosi.

PATOGENESI. La colonizzazione della faringe da parte degli SBEA può risultare sia nello stato di portatore cronico, sia nell'infezione acuta. La proteina M è il principale fattore di virulenza dello SBEA e facilita la resistenza alla fagocitosi da parte dei neutrofili polimorfonucleati. Durante l'infezione si sviluppa un'immunità tipo-specifica, che fornisce un'immunità protettiva verso successive infezioni con quel particolare sierotipo M.

La *scarlattina* è causata da SBEA che producono da una a tre esotossine eritrogeniche streptococciche (A, B e C) che possono indurre un fine rash papulare (vedi Capitolo 182). L'esotossina A sembra essere quella più strettamente associata alla scarlattina. L'esposizione a ogni esotossina conferisce immunità specifica solo verso quella tossina e, pertanto, uno stesso soggetto può ammalarsi di scarlattina fino a tre volte.

MANIFESTAZIONI CLINICHE. L'esordio della faringite streptococcica è spesso rapido, con importante mal di gola, assenza di tosse e febbre. La cefalea e i sintomi gastrointestinali (dolore addominale, vomito) sono frequenti. La faringe è arrossata, le tonsille aumentano di volume e classicamente si rivestono di un essudato giallo, tinto di sangue. Possono formarsi petecchie o lesioni "a ciambella" sul palato molle e sulla faringe posteriore, e l'uvula può essere rossa, puntinata ed edematosa. I linfonodi cervicali anteriori sono aumentati di volume e dolenti alla palpazione. Il periodo di incubazione è di 2-5 giorni. Alcuni pazienti presentano anche i segni della scarlattina: pallore periorale, lingua a fragola e un rash finemente papulare che alla palpazione ha una consistenza simile alla carta vetrata e nell'aspetto ricorda un'ustione solare associata a pelle d'oca (vedi Capitolo 182).

L'esordio della faringite virale può essere più graduale; i sintomi più frequenti comprendono rinorrea, tosse e diarrea. Un'eziologia virale è suggerita dalla presenza di congiuntivite, coriza, raucedine e tosse. La faringite da adenovirus può manifestarsi con congiuntivite e febbre (febbre faringocongiuntivale). La faringite da virus Coxackie può causare la comparsa di piccole (1-2 mm) vescicole grigiastre e ulcere nella faringe posteriore (herpangina), o noduletti (3-6 mm) bianco-giallastri nella faringe posteriore (faringite acuta linfonodulare). Nella faringite da EBV si può riscontrare un notevole aumento di volume delle tonsille con presenza di essudato, linfoadenite cervicale, epatosplenomegalia, rash e astenia generalizzata, che configurano una sindrome mononucleosica infettiva (vedi Capitolo 251). L'infezione primaria da HIV nei bambini più piccoli si presenta spesso con febbre elevata e gengivostomatite, ma può anche essere presente faringite (vedi Capitolo 249).

Le malattie attribuite allo streptococco di gruppo C e ad *A. hemoliticum* sono generalmente simili a quelle causate dagli SBEA. Le infezioni da *A. hemoliticum* sono talvolta accompagnate da un rash maculopapulare eritematoso desquamante. L'infezione faringea da gonococco è in genere asintomatica, ma può causare faringite acuta con febbre e linfoadenite cervicale.

DIAGNOSI. L'obiettivo di una diagnosi specifica è di identificare l'infezione da SBEA. Le presentazioni cliniche delle faringiti streptococciche e virali sono ampiamente sovrapponibili. I medici che si basano solo sul giudizio clinico spesso sopravvalutano la probabilità di un'eziologia streptococcica; pertanto, l'esame di laboratorio è utile per identificare i bambini che hanno maggiori probabilità di trarre beneficio da una terapia antibiotica. La coltura del tampone faringeo resta un gold standard imperfetto per la diagnosi di faringite streptococcica. Possono verificarsi colture falsamente positive, se altri microrganismi vengono erroneamente identificati come SBEA, e i bambini portatori dello streptococco possono anch'essi avere colture positive. I falsi negativi sono attribuibili a svariate cause, tra cui un tampone effettuato in modo non corretto e l'uso surrettizio di antibiotici da parte del paziente. La specificità dei test rapidi per rilevare l'antigene dello streptococco di gruppo A è elevata; pertanto, se un test rapido risulta positivo, il tampone faringeo è inutile e si consiglia di iniziare il trattamento appropriato, in particolare se vi è un elevato sospetto clinico di SBEA. Per rilevare *A. haemolyticum* sono necessari terreni di coltura speciali e un tempo di incubazione prolungato. Le colture virali spesso non sono disponibili e in genere sono troppo costose e lente per poter essere utili clinicamente. La reazione a catena della polimerasi (PCR, *Polymerase Chain Reaction*) virale è più rapida e può essere utile, pur non essendo sempre necessaria. Un emocromo con numerosi linfociti atipici e un test di agglutinazione su vetrino ("spot test") positivo possono aiutare a confermare la diagnosi clinica di mononucleosi infettiva da EBV.

TRATTAMENTO. La maggior parte degli episodi di faringite streptococcica si risolve senza sequele in pochi giorni, ma una terapia antibiotica precoce accelera la guarigione clinica di 12-24 ore. Il beneficio principale del trattamento è la prevenzione della febbre reumatica acuta, che è quasi sempre efficace se la terapia antibiotica è iniziata nei primi 9 giorni di malattia. La terapia antibiotica dovrebbe essere iniziata immediatamente, senza esami colturali, nei bambini con faringite sintomatica e un test rapido antigenico per lo streptococco positivo, diagnosi clinica di scarlattina, un familiare con faringite streptococcica documentata, anamnesi di pregressa febbre reumatica acuta o un familiare con un episodio recente di febbre reumatica acuta.

Diversi agenti antimicrobici possono essere efficaci. Gli SBEA restano universalmente sensibili alla penicillina, che ha uno spettro ridotto e pochi effetti collaterali. La penicillina V, poco costosa negli Stati Uniti, viene somministrata due o tre volte al dì per 10 giorni: 250 mg/dose nei bambini e 500 mg/dose negli adolescenti e negli adulti. Nei bambini è spesso preferibile somministrare l'amoxicillina per via orale, disponibile negli Stati Uniti in compresse masticabili dal sapore gradevole; 750 mg di amoxicillina orale somministrati una volta al dì per 10 giorni possono essere efficaci quanto 250 mg di penicillina due volte al dì per 10 giorni. Uno schema più breve (6 giorni) di amoxicillina per via orale (50 mg/kg/die divisi in due somministrazioni; dose per adulti 1 g due volte al dì) può avere la stessa efficacia di un trattamento di 10 giorni con penicillina V tre volte al dì. Se l'efficacia di questi schemi terapeutici sarà confermata, i vantaggi renderanno l'amoxicillina un'opzione efficace. Una singola dose intramuscolare di benzatinpenicillina (600 000 U per i bambini di peso <27 kg; 1,2 milioni di U per i bambini di peso superiore e per gli adulti) o una combinazione di benzatinprocaina e penicillina G è dolorosa, ma garantisce la compliance e adeguati livelli ematici per più di 10 giorni. Secondo alcuni studi un'elevata percentuale di pazienti trattati con penicillina per via orale o intramuscolare rimarrebbero positivi all'esame colturale dopo il trattamento, ma queste segnalazioni devono essere ulteriormente valutate. L'eritromicina (eritromicina etilsuccinato 40 mg/kg/die in due, tre o quattro somministrazioni, per via orale, per 10 giorni; o eritromicina estolato 20-40 mg/kg/die divisi in due, tre o quattro somministrazioni per 10 giorni; dose massima per entrambi i farmaci 1 g/die) è consigliata nei pazienti allergici agli antibiotici β-lattamici. L'azitromicina offre i vantaggi di una monosomministrazione giornaliera e di una minore durata della terapia, che possono aumentare la compliance, ma è più costosa; inoltre il sempre maggiore utilizzo di macrolidi si accompagna a un aumento della resistenza all'eritromicina negli streptococchi di gruppo A. In base alla percentuale di colture che permangono positive per lo SBEA dopo la terapia, le cefalosporine sembrano essere altrettanto efficaci della penicillina, se non di più, forse perché questi farmaci si rivelano più efficaci nell'eliminare lo stato di portatore streptococcico. Attualmente non si dispone di dati sufficienti per consigliare una terapia di routine con cefalosporine di durata inferiore.

Non sono necessarie colture di follow-up, a meno che non vi sia una recidiva dei sintomi. Alcuni pazienti trattati continuano a ospitare lo SBEA nella faringe e divengono portatori cronici. Lo stato di portatore comporta generalmente un basso rischio per il paziente e i suoi familiari, ma può confondere il risultato del test utilizzato per determinare l'eziologia di episodi successivi di mal di gola. Lo schema di trattamento più efficace per eradicare lo stato di portatore di streptococco è con clindamicina 2 mg/kg/die divisi in 3 dosi (dosaggio per gli adulti: 150-450 mg, due o tre volte al dì, dose massima giornaliera 1,8 g), per via orale, per 10 giorni.

Per la maggior parte delle faringiti virali non è disponibile una terapia specifica. In base ai dati sulla sensibilità *in vitro*, spesso si consiglia la somministrazione orale di penicillina nei pazienti in cui viene isolato uno streptococco di gruppo C e di eritromicina nei pazienti con *A. haemolyticum*, anche se il beneficio clinico di questo trattamento è incerto.

La terapia sintomatica, aspecifica, può essere una componente importante del piano complessivo di trattamento. Un agente antipiretico e analgesico per via orale (paracetamolo o ibuprofene) può ridurre la febbre e il mal di gola. Spesso i gargarismi con acqua tiepida e sale alleviano il fastidio, e gli spray e pastiglie anestetici (di solito a base di benzocaina, fenolo o mentolo) possono dare un beneficio locale.

FARINGITE RICORRENTE. La faringite streptococcica ricorrente può rappresentare una recidiva con un ceppo identico. In caso di scarsa compliance alla terapia antibiotica, si suggerisce la somministrazione intramuscolare di benzatin-penicillina. Si deve considerare la possibilità di una resistenza se era stato somministrato un trattamento non penicillinico, come l'eritromicina. Le recidive possono essere causate anche da ceppi diversi, in conseguenza di nuove esposizioni, o consistere in faringiti da altre cause, associate allo stato di portatore cronico dello streptococco. Quest'ultima possibilità è probabile se la malattia è lieve e atipica per una faringite streptococcica. Se si rileva uno SBEA in colture ripetute alcuni giorni dopo la fine del trattamento, si consiglia di effettuare la terapia per eradicare lo stato di portatore. Una faringite prolungata (>1-2 settimane) suggerisce un disturbo diverso, come la neutropenia o le sindromi febbrili ricorrenti.

La tonsillectomia riduce l'incidenza di faringite per 1-2 anni nei bambini con faringite ricorrente, positiva alla coltura per SBEA, severa e frequente (più di 7 episodi nell'anno precedente, o più di 5 in ciascuno dei 2 anni precedenti). Tuttavia, anche senza intervento chirurgico, la maggior parte dei pazienti ha sempre meno episodi con il passare del tempo; di conseguenza, occorre soppesare il beneficio clinico atteso tenendo conto dei rischi connessi all'anestesia e alla procedura stessa. Un'anamnesi non documentata di faringite ricorrente non è motivo sufficiente per consigliare la tonsillectomia.

Complicanze e prognosi. Le infezioni virali delle vie respiratorie possono predisporre alle infezioni batteriche dell'orecchio medio. Le complicanze della faringite streptococcica comprendono fenomeni suppurativi locali, come l'ascesso parafaringeo, e le malattie non suppurative tardive, come la febbre reumatica acuta (vedi Capitolo 182.1) e la glomerulonefrite acuta postinfettiva (vedi Capitolo 511.1).

Prevenzione. Sono in corso di sviluppo vaccini antistreptococcici polivalenti a base di peptidi della proteina M. La profilassi antimicrobica con somministrazione quotidiana di penicillina per via orale previene le infezioni ricorrenti da SBEA, ma è consigliabile solo per scongiurare le recidive della febbre reumatica acuta (vedi Capitolo 182.1).

Bisno AL: Are cephalosporins superior to penicillin for treatment of acute streptococcal pharyngitis? *Clin Infect Dis* 2004;38:1535–1537.
Bisno AL: Acute pharyngitis. *N Engl J Med* 2001;344:205–211.
Bisno AL, Gerber MA, Gwaltney JM Jr, et al: Practice guidelines for the diagnosis and management of group A streptococcal pharyngitis. *Clin Infect Dis* 2002;35:113–125.
Bisno AL, Robin FA, Cleary PP, Dale JB: Prospects for a group A streptococcal vaccine: rationale, feasibility, and obstacles—report of a NIAID workshop. *Clin Infect Dis* 2005;41:1150–1156.
Casey JR, Pichichero ME: Meta-analysis of cephalosporin versus penicillin treatment of group A streptococcal tonsillopharyngitis in children. *Pediatrics* 2004;113:866–882.
Clegg HW, Ryan AG, Dallas SD, et al: Treatment of streptococcal pharyngitis with once daily compared with twice daily amoxicillin: a mono-inferiority trial. *Pediatr Infect Dis J* 2006;25:761–767.
Gerber MA: Diagnosis and treatment of pharyngitis in children. *Pediatr Clin N Amer* 2005;52:729–747.
Gerber MA, Shulman ST: Rapid diagnosis of pharyngitis caused by group A streptococci. *Clin Microbiol Rev* 2004;17:571–580.
Jaggi P, Shulman ST: Group A streptococcal infections. *Pediatr Rev* 2006;27: 99–105.
Martin JM, Green M: Group A streptococcus. *Semin Pediatr Infect Dis* 2006;3:140–148.
McIsaac WJ, Kellner JD, Aufricht P, et al: Empirical validation of guidelines for the management of pharyngitis in children and adults. *JAMA* 2004;291:1587–1595.
Shulman ST, Gerber MA: So what's wrong with penicillin for strep throat? *Pediatrics* 2004;113:1816–1819.

Capitolo 379 ■ Ascesso retrofaringeo, ascesso faringeo laterale (parafaringeo) e ascesso/cellulite peritonsillare

Diane E. Pappas e J. Owen Hendley

Il collo contiene linfonodi localizzati in profondità, come quelli *retrofaringei* e *faringei laterali*, che drenano le superfici mucose delle vie aeree superiori e del tratto digerente. Questi linfonodi occupano lo *spazio retrofaringeo* (compreso tra la faringe e le vertebre cervicali ed esteso verso il basso fino al mediastino superiore) e lo *spazio faringeo laterale* (confinante con la faringe medialmente, la tunica carotidea posteriormente e i muscoli del processo stiloideo lateralmente), che sono interconnessi. I linfonodi situati in questi spazi profondi del collo comunicano tra loro, favorendo la diffusione di batteri provenienti da una cellulite o un ascesso linfonodale. Abitualmente l'interessamento linfonodale è conseguenza dell'estensione di un'infezione all'inizio localizzata nell'orofaringe. L'ascesso retrofaringeo può essere causato da un trauma penetrante dell'orofaringe, da infezioni dentarie e dall'osteomielite vertebrale. L'infezione linfonodale può attraversare tre stadi: *cellulite*, *flemmone* e *ascesso*: quella a carico degli spazi retrofaringeo e faringeo laterale richiede una diagnosi precoce, potendo compromettere la pervietà delle vie aeree o dar luogo a una mediastinite posteriore.

ASCESSO RETROFARINGEO E FARINGEO LATERALE. L'ascesso retrofaringeo è più comune nei bambini di età inferiore a 3-4 anni, soprattutto in quelli di sesso maschile. Fino al 67% dei pazienti ha un'anamnesi di infezione recente dell'orecchio, del naso o della gola. Dal momento che i linfonodi retrofaringei subiscono un'involuzione dopo i 5 anni di età, l'infezione nei bambini più grandi e negli adulti è meno comune.

Le *manifestazioni cliniche* dell'ascesso retrofaringeo sono aspecifiche e comprendono febbre, irritabilità, difficoltà dell'alimentazione e scialorrea. Possono inoltre essere presenti rigidità del collo, torcicollo e rifiuto di muovere il capo. Il bambino può lamentare mal di gola e dolore al collo. Altri segni possono comprendere afonia, stridore e distress respiratorio. L'esame obiettivo talvolta rivela una protrusione nella parete faringea posteriore, sebbene questa sia presente in meno del 50% dei bambini con ascesso retrofaringeo. È inoltre possibile riscontrare una linfadenopatia laterocervicale. L'ascesso faringeo laterale si presenta comunemente con febbre, disfagia e un'accentuata protrusione a livello della parete faringea posteriore, talora con dislocazione mediale della tonsilla.

La *diagnosi differenziale* comprende l'epiglottite acuta e l'aspirazione di un corpo estraneo. Nel bambino più piccolo con ridotta mobilità del collo bisogna considerare anche la meningite. Altre possibilità comprendono il linfoma, l'ematoma e l'osteomielite vertebrale.

L'incisione per il drenaggio e l'esame colturale di un linfonodo ascessualizzato fornisce la diagnosi definitiva, ma la TC può essere utile per identificare un ascesso retrofaringeo o laterofaringeo (Fig. 379-1). La TC permette di identificare e localizzare con precisione le infezioni profonde del collo, mentre l'identificazione degli ascessi è accurata solo nel 63% dei pazienti. Le radiografie dei tessuti molli del collo, effettuate in inspirazione con il collo in estensione, possono mostrare un aumento dell'ampiezza o un livello idroaereo nello spazio retrofaringeo. La TC con mezzo di contrasto può rivelare un'area centrale lucente, un'area di enhancement ad anello o la dentellatura delle pareti di un linfonodo. Si ritiene che la dentellatura della parete ascessuale sia un reperto tardivo e sia predittivo di formazione di un ascesso.

Le infezioni retrofaringee e laterofaringee sono per lo più polimicrobiche; i patogeni abituali comprendono lo streptococco di gruppo A (vedi Capitolo 182), i batteri orofaringei anaerobici (vedi Capitolo 210) e *Staphylococcus aureus* (vedi Capitolo 180.1). Alcuni studi hanno documentato un'aumentata incidenza di streptococchi di gruppo A reperiti in tali ascessi. Altri patogeni sono *Haemophilus influenzae*, *Klebsiella* e *Mycobacterium avium-intracellulare*.

Le *opzioni terapeutiche* comprendono l'uso di antibiotici per via endovenosa, con o senza drenaggio chirurgico. Le cefalosporine di terza generazione combinate con ampicillina-sulbactam o clindamicina, per fornire una copertura sugli anaerobi, sono efficaci. In base ad alcuni studi, più del 50% dei bambini con ascesso retrofaringeo o laterofaringeo identificati con la TC può essere trattato con successo senza drenaggio chirurgico; quest'ultimo tuttavia si rende necessario nei pazienti con distress respiratorio o che non hanno dato segno di miglioramento dopo un trattamento antibiotico endovena. La durata ottimale del trattamento non è nota; tipicamente si somministrano antibiotici per via endovenosa per diversi giorni, fino a quando il paziente non inizia a migliorare, dopodiché si prosegue con un ciclo di antibiotici per via orale.

Le *complicanze* dell'ascesso retrofaringeo e laterofaringeo comprendono un'ostruzione significativa delle vie aeree superiori, la rottura con conseguente polmonite da aspirazione e l'estensione al mediastino; possono verificarsi anche tromboflebite della vena giugulare interna ed erosione della tonaca carotidea.

Un'infezione non comune ma caratteristica dello spazio parafaringeo è la **malattia di Lemierre**, in cui un'infezione proveniente dall'orofaringe si estende fino a causare una tromboflebite settica della vena giugulare interna con ascessi polmonari metastatici (Fig. 379-2). Il patogeno responsabile è *Fusobacterium necrophorum*, un batterio anaerobo che fa parte della normale flora orofaringea. La presentazione tipica è quella di un adolescente o di un giovane adulto precedentemente sano, con un'anamnesi di malattia faringotonsillare recente, che sviluppa una malattia

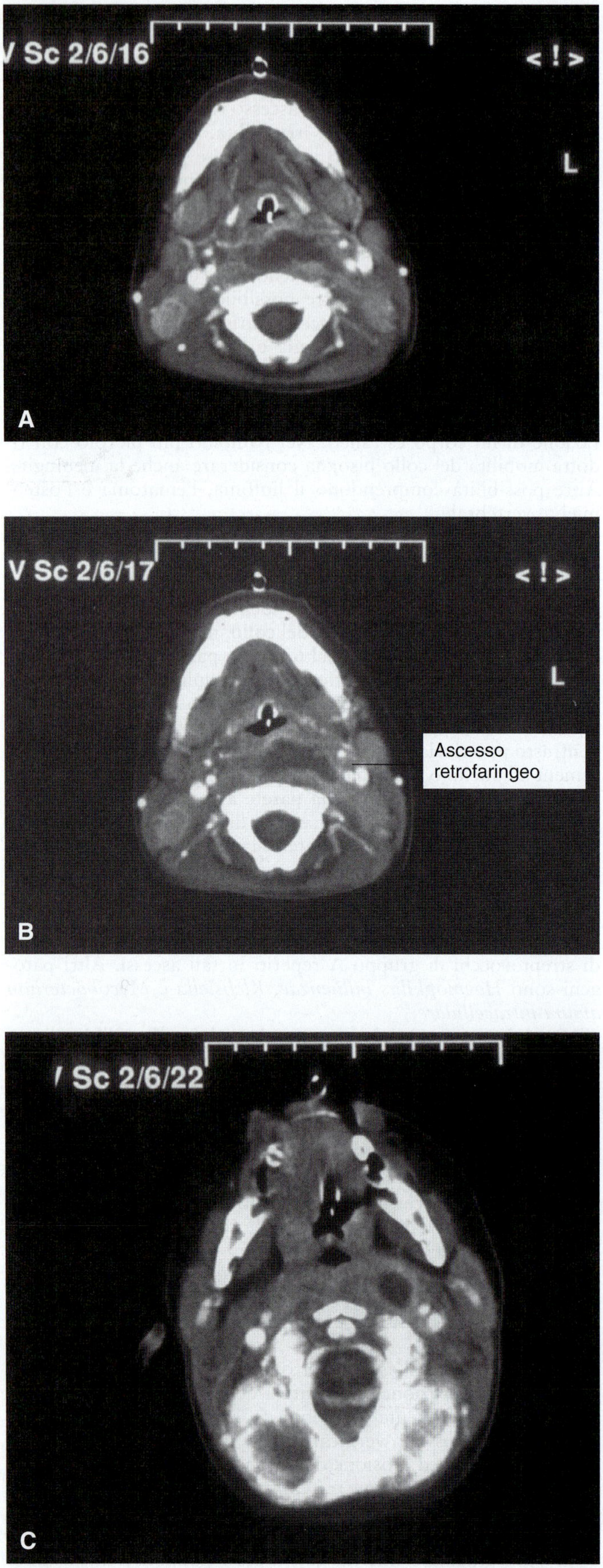

Figura 379-1. TC di un ascesso retrofaringeo. *A*, Immagine TC a livello dell'epiglottide. *B*, Sezione TC sequenziale che mostra una lesione con area di enhancement ad anello. *C*, Ulteriore sezione sequenziale che rivela l'estensione inferiore della lesione. (Da Philpott CM, Selvadurai D, Banerjee AR: Paediatric retropharyngeal abscess. *J Laryngol Otol* 2004;118:925.)

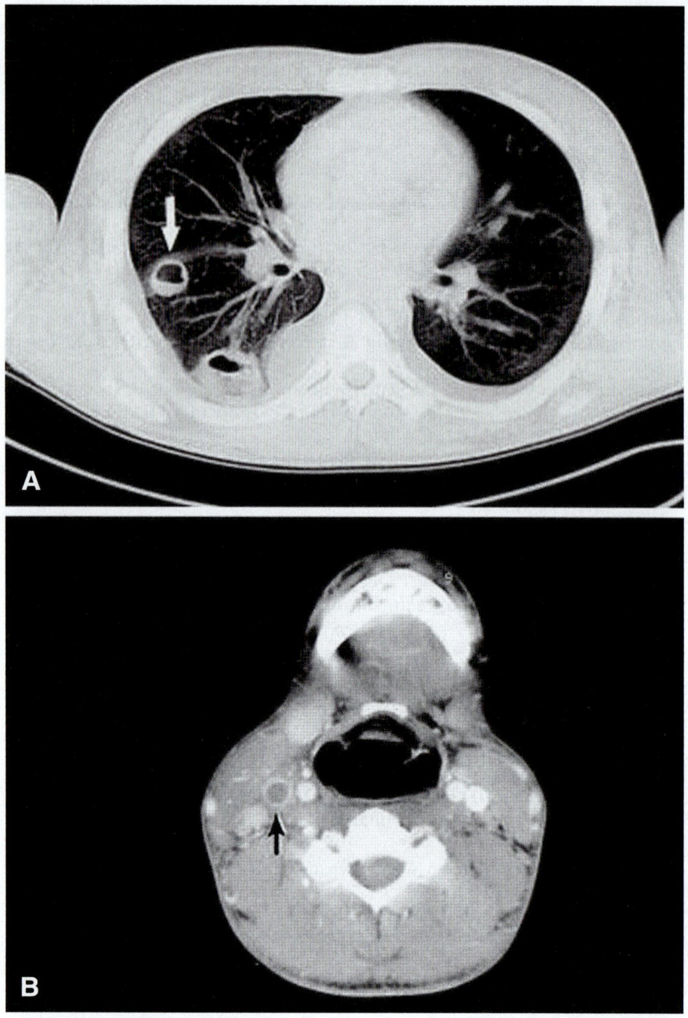

Figura 379-2. TC nella malattia di Lemierre. *A*, TC che evidenzia l'aspetto nodulare degli infiltrati polmonari (*frecce*). *B*, TC del collo che dimostra la trombosi della vena giugulare interna (*frecce*). (Da Plymyer MR, Zoccola DC, Tallarita G: An 18 year old man presenting with sepsis following a recent pharyngeal infection. *Arch Pathol Lab Med* 2004;128:813. Ristampata per gentile concessione da Archives of Pathology & Laboratory Medicine. Copyright 2004. College of American Pathologists.)

acuta caratterizzata da febbre e sintomi polmonari. La radiografia del torace dimostra noduli cavitari multipli, spesso bilaterali e accompagnati da versamento pleurico. L'emocoltura può essere positiva. Il trattamento consiste nella somministrazione endovenosa prolungata di penicillina o cefoxitina; può essere necessario il drenaggio chirurgico degli ascessi metastatici extrapolmonari.

ASCESSO/CELLULITE PERITONSILLARE. L'ascesso/cellulite peritonsillare, relativamente comune rispetto alle infezioni profonde del collo, è causato da un'invasione batterica attraverso la capsula tonsillare, che porta alla formazione di cellulite e/o di un ascesso nei tessuti circostanti. Il tipico paziente con ascesso peritonsillare è un adolescente con un'anamnesi recente di faringotonsillite acuta. Le *manifestazioni cliniche* comprendono mal di gola, febbre, trisma e disfagia. L'*esame obiettivo* rivela una massa tonsillare asimmetrica con dislocazione dell'uvula. Una massa tonsillare asimmetrica è diagnostica, ma la sua visibilità può essere compromessa dalla presenza del trisma. La TC è utile per identificare l'ascesso. I patogeni più comuni sono gli streptococchi di gruppo A e gli anaerobi orofaringei misti, con più di quattro isolati batterici per ascesso, recuperati caratteristicamente dall'agoaspirato.

Il *trattamento* comprende il drenaggio chirurgico e un'antibioticoterapia efficace contro gli streptococchi di gruppo A e gli anaerobi. Il drenaggio chirurgico può essere effettuato tramite agoaspirazione, incisione e drenaggio o tonsillectomia. Nel paziente non collaborante può essere necessaria l'anestesia generale. Circa il 95% degli ascessi peritonsillari si risolve dopo l'agospirazione (che solo in una piccola percentuale di pazienti deve essere ripetuta) e la terapia antibiotica. L'agoaspirazione può essere eseguita nelle porzioni superiori, intermedie e inferiori della tonsilla al fine di localizzare l'ascesso. Il 5% dei casi che non si risolve con l'aspirazione richiede l'incisione con drenaggio chirurgico. La tonsillectomia deve essere presa in considerazione se non si verifica un miglioramento 24 ore dopo l'inizio della terapia antibiotica e dell'aspirazione, se c'è un'anamnesi di tonsilliti ricorrenti o se sono presenti complicanze dell'ascesso peritonsillare. La complicanze più temuta, sebbene rara, è la rottura dell'ascesso con conseguente polmonite da aspirazione. L'ascesso peritonsillare ha un rischio di ricorrenza del 10%.

Azimi PH, Grossman M: Irritability and neck stiffness in a five-month-old infant. *Pediatr Infect Dis J* 2001;20:724, 728–729.
Blotter JW, Yin L, Glyn M, et al: Otolaryngology consultation for peritonsillar abscess in the pediatric population. *Laryngoscope* 2000;110:1698–1701.
Conway JH, Nyquist AC, Goldson E: Posterior mediastinal abscess caused by invasive group A Streptococcus infection. *Pediatr Infect Dis J* 1996;15:547–549.
Coticchia JM, Getnick GS, Yun RD, et al: Age-, site-, and time-specific differences in pediatric deep neck abscesses. *Arch Otolaryngol Head Neck Surg* 2004;130:201–207.
Friedman NR, Mitchell RB, Pereira KD, et al: Peritonsillar abscess in early childhood: Presentation and management. *Arch Otolaryngol Head Neck Surg* 1997;123:630–632.
Herzon FS: Peritonsillar abscess: Incidence, current management practices, and a proposal for treatment guidelines. *Laryngoscope* 1995;105:1–17.
Jousimies-Somer H, Savolainen S, Mäkitie A, et al: Bacteriologic findings in peritonsillar abscesses in young adults. *Clin Infect Dis* 1993;16:S292–S298.
Kirse DJ, Roberson DW: Surgical management of retropharyngeal space infections in children. *Laryngoscope* 2001;111:1413–1422.
Lee SS, Schwartz RH, Bahadori RS: Retropharyngeal abscess: Epiglottitis of the new millennium. *J Pediatr* 2001;138:435–437.
Moreno S, Garcia Altozano J, Pinilla JC, et al: Lemierre's disease: Postanginal bacteremia and pulmonary involvement caused by Fusobacterium necrophorum. *Rev Infect Dis* 1989;11:319–324.
Philpott CM, Selvadurai D, Banerjee AR: Paediatric retropharyngeal abscess. *J Laryngol Otol* 2004;118:919–926.
Plymyer MR, Zoccola DC, Tallarita G: An 18 year old man presenting with sepsis following a recent pharyngeal infection. *Arch Pathol Lab Med* 2004;128:813–814.
Vural C, Gungor A, Comerci S: Accuracy of computerized tomography in deep neck infections in the pediatric population. *Am J Otolaryngol* 2003;24:143–148.
Weinberg E, Brodsky L, Stanievich J, et al: Needle aspiration of peritonsillar abscess in children. *Arch Otolaryngol Head Neck Surg* 1993;119:169–172.

Capitolo 380 ■ Tonsille e adenoidi

Ralph Wetmore

ANATOMIA. L'*anello di Waldeyer* è formato da tessuto linfatico che circonda lo sbocco delle cavità orale e nasale nella faringe e comprende le tonsille palatine, la tonsilla faringea o adenoide, il tessuto linfatico che circonda l'orifizio della tromba di Eustachio nella parete laterale del rinofaringe, la tonsilla linguale alla base della lingua e tessuto linfatico sparso nelle altre parti di faringe, in particolare dietro i pilastri faringei posteriori e lungo la parete faringea posteriore. Il tessuto linfatico localizzato tra la piega palatoglossa (pilastro tonsillare anteriore) e la piega palatofaringea (pilastro tonsillare posteriore) forma la *tonsilla palatina*. Questo tessuto linfatico è separato dalla muscolatura faringea circostante da una spessa capsula fibrosa. Le *adenoidi* formano un unico aggregato di tessuto linfatico che occupa lo spazio tra il setto nasale e la parete faringea posteriore. Una sottile capsula fibrosa le separa dalle strutture sottostanti; le cripte delle adenoidi non sono molto meno complesse di quelle delle tonsille palatine. Il tessuto linfatico alla base della lingua forma la *tonsilla linguale* che contiene anch'essa cripte tonsillari semplici.

FUNZIONE NORMALE. Circa il 65% dei linfociti che formano il tessuto linfatico dell'anello di Waldeyer sono linfociti B, mentre il restante 35% è costituito da linfociti T e plasmacellule (vedi Capitolo 122). Il ruolo immunologico delle tonsille e delle adenoidi è di indurre l'immunità secretoria e regolare la produzione di immunoglobuline secretorie. Situate all'imboccatura della faringe, tonsille e adenoidi sono in posizione privilegiata per fornire una difesa primaria contro i fattori esterni. Nel tessuto tonsillare sono presenti profonde fessure che formano le cripte tonsillari, delimitate da epitelio squamoso ma dotate alla base di un'elevata concentrazione di linfociti. L'attività immunologica del tessuto linfatico dell'anello di Waldeyer è maggiore tra i 4 e i 10 anni di età, per poi subire una flessione dopo la pubertà. Non sono stati dimostrati deficit immunologici significativi dopo l'asportazione di entrambe le tonsille e delle adenoidi.

PATOLOGIA

INFEZIONE ACUTA. La maggior parte delle faringotonsilliti è causata da virus (vedi Capitolo 378). Gli streptococchi β-emolitici di gruppo A (SBEA) sono la causa più comune di infezione batterica della faringe (vedi Capitolo 182). Le infezioni batteriche possono inoltre essere dovute ad altre specie di streptococco β-emolitico (gruppo C), a *Staphylococcus aureus*, microrganismi Gram-negativi, *Mycoplasma pneumoniae* e, raramente, *Neisseria gonorrhoeae* e *Corynebacterium diphtheriae* (vedi Capitolo 186). Nei pazienti immunocompromessi o nei bambini trattati cronicamente con antibiotici o steroidi per via inalatoria, può insorgere candidosi orale.

INFEZIONE CRONICA. Le tonsille e le adenoidi possono essere infettate cronicamente da vari microrganismi, con un'elevata incidenza di batteri produttori di β-lattamasi. Prevalgono sia le specie aerobie, come gli streptococchi e *Haemophilus influenzae*, sia quelle anaerobie, come *Peptostreptococcus*, *Prevotella* e *Fusobacterium*. Nelle cripte tonsillari si possono accumulare cellule epiteliali desquamate, linfociti, batteri e altri detriti, responsabili della tonsillite criptica. Con il tempo, questi tappi criptici possono calcificare in concrezioni tonsillari, o tonsilloliti.

OSTRUZIONE DELLE VIE AEREE. Tanto le tonsille quanto le adenoidi sono una causa importante di ostruzione delle vie aeree, nel bambino. L'ostruzione delle vie aeree, in età pediatrica, si manifesta tipicamente con disturbi respiratori durante il sonno: apnea e ipopnea ostruttive e sindrome da resistenza delle vie aeree superiori (vedi Capitolo 18).

NEOPLASIE TONSILLARI. Nell'infanzia, un rapido aumento di volume di una sola tonsilla è altamente suggestivo di un tumore tonsillare, tipicamente un linfoma.

MANIFESTAZIONI CLINICHE

INFEZIONE ACUTA. I sintomi dell'infezione da SBEA comprendono odinofagia, secchezza della gola, malessere, febbre con brividi, disfagia, otalgia riferita, cefalea, algie muscolari e aumento di volume dei lifonodi cervicali. I segni comprendono lingua disidratata, tonsille eritematose e ingrandite, essudato tonsillare o faringeo, petecchie palatine e aumento e dolenzia dei linfonodi giugulogastrici (Fig. 380-1; vedi anche Capitoli 182 e 378).

INFEZIONE CRONICA. I bambini con tonsillite cronica o criptica spesso presentano alitosi, mal di gola cronico, sensazione di corpo estraneo o anamnesi di espulsione di frammenti di materiale

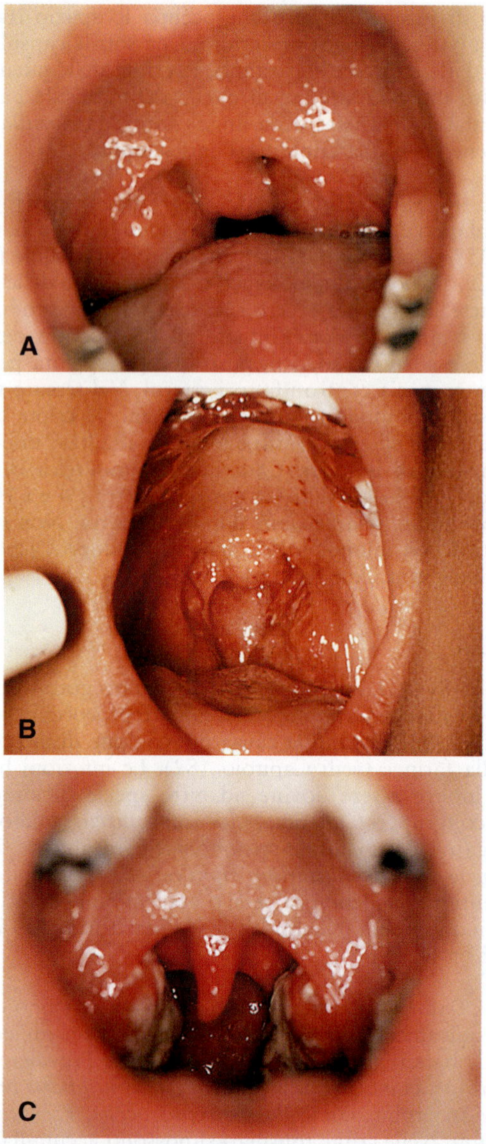

Figura 380-1. Faringotonsillite. Questa sindrome comune è causata da diversi agenti patogeni e presenta un ampio spettro di severità. *A*, Eritema tonsillare e faringeo diffuso, reperto aspecifico che può essere causato da diversi patogeni. *B*, Questo intenso eritema, osservato in associazione con aumento di volume acuto delle tonsille e petecchie del palato, è altamente suggestivo di infezione da β-streptococco di gruppo A, sebbene anche altri patogeni possano provocare un simile quadro. *C*, Tonsillite essudativa, osservata più comunemente in caso di infezione sia da β-streptococco di gruppo A, sia da virus di Epstein-Barr. (*B*, per gentile concessione di Michael Sherlock, Lutherville.) (Da Yellon RF, McBride TP, Davis HW: Otolaryngology. In Zitelli BJ, Davis HW [editors]: *Atlas of Pediatric Physical Diagnosis*, 4th ed. Philadelphia, Mosby, 2002, p 852.)

caseoso, maleodoranti e di sapore cattivo. L'esame può rivelare tonsille di qualunque dimensione, spesso contenenti copiosi detriti nelle cripte. Poiché in genere il patogeno responsabile non è lo SBEA, la coltura per lo streptococco è abitualmente negativa.

OSTRUZIONE DELLE VIE AEREE. In molti bambini, è possibile porre diagnosi di ostruzione delle vie aeree (vedi Capitoli 18 e 370) basandosi su anamnesi ed esame obiettivo. I sintomi diurni dell'ostruzione delle vie aeree, secondaria a ipertrofia adenotonsillare, comprendono respirazione orale cronica, ostruzione nasale, rinolalia, iposmia, diminuzione dell'appetito, rendimento scolastico scarso e, seppure raramente, sintomi di scompenso cardiaco destro. I sintomi notturni consistono in russamento sonoro, soffocamento, gasping, apnee franche, agitazione, posizioni anomale nel sonno, sonnambulismo, incubi, diaforesi, enuresi e tendenza a parlare nel sonno. Le radiografie laterali del collo o l'endoscopia con strumento flessibile permettono di valutare le dimensioni del tessuto adenoideo. Altri segni che possono contribuire all'ostruzione delle vie aeree comprendono la presenza di una sindrome craniofacciale o di ipotonia.

NEOPLASIA TONSILLARE. Il rapido aumento di volume monolaterale di una tonsilla, in particolare se si accompagna a segni sistemici come sudorazione notturna, febbre, calo ponderale e linfadenopatia, è altamente suggestivo di una neoplasia tonsillare. Inoltre, la diagnosi di neoplasia tonsillare deve essere presa in considerazione se la tonsilla appare grossolanamente anormale.

TRATTAMENTO

TERAPIA MEDICA. Il trattamento della faringotonsillite acuta è discusso nel Capitolo 378, mentre l'antibioticoterapia per lo SBEA è discussa nel Capitolo 182. Poiché i copatogeni come gli stafilococchi o gli anaerobi possono produrre β-lattamasi che inattivano la penicillina, l'uso di cefalosporine o di clindamicina può essere più efficace nel trattamento delle infezioni croniche della gola. Talvolta i bambini con tonsillite criptica sono in grado di espellere i tonsilloliti o i detriti manualmente, usando un applicatore con del cotone a un'estremità o un getto d'acqua. Le cripte tonsillari con infezione cronica possono essere cauterizzate utilizzando nitrato d'argento.

TONSILLECTOMIA. La tonsillectomia isolata viene effettuata abitualmente nella faringotonsillite ricorrente o cronica. Le indicazioni all'intervento restano incerte; vi sono ampie variazioni nella frequenza con cui si ricorre alla chirurgia nei diversi Paesi: 11/10 000 bambini in Olanda, 65/10 000 bambini in Gran Bretagna e 50/10 000 bambini negli Stati Uniti. Un criterio è rappresentato dalla ricorrenza di 7 o più episodi di infezione della gola trattati con antibiotici nell'anno precedente, 5 o più infezioni della gola trattate in ognuno dei due anni precedenti, o 3 o più infezioni della gola trattate con antibiotici in ognuno dei 3 anni precedenti. L'American Academy of Otolaryngology-Head and Neck Surgery ritiene che l'intervento chirurgico sia indicato nei pazienti con 3 o più infezioni delle tonsille e/o adenoidi all'anno, nonostante un'adeguata terapia medica, mentre lo Scottish Intercollegiate Tonsillectomy indica 5 o più episodi all'anno di tonsillite con sintomi altamente debilitanti, che durano per più di un anno. La tonsillectomia si è dimostrata efficace nel ridurre il numero di infezioni e i sintomi della tonsillite cronica, come l'alitosi, il mal di gola persistente o ricorrente e l'adenite cervicale ricorrente. Nei casi di tonsillite criptica resistente, la chirurgia può essere curativa. In età pediatrica è raro che la tonsillectomia possa essere indicata per la biopsia di una tonsilla aumentata di volume monolateralmente, al fine di escludere una neoplasia o di trattare un'emorragia ricorrente da vasi sanguigni tonsillari superficiali. Nei bambini con sintomi lievi l'intervento non sembra offrire un beneficio clinico maggiore rispetto al trattamento conservativo.

ADENOIDECTOMIA. L'adenoidectomia isolata può essere indicata per il trattamento delle infezioni nasali croniche (adenoidite cronica), delle infezioni sinusali croniche refrattarie alla terapia medica e degli episodi ricorrenti di otite media, compresi quelli nei bambini con tubi timpanostomici, che soffrono di otorrea ricorrente. Inoltre, l'adenoidectomia può essere utile nei bambini che soffrono di otite media con versamento cronico o ricorrente. La sola adenoidectomia può essere curativa nel trattamento dei pazienti con ostruzione nasale, respirazione orale cronica e russamento sonoro, suggestivo di un disturbo della respirazione nel sonno. Può inoltre essere indicata qualora si sospetti l'ostruzione delle vie aeree superiori a causa di anomalie di sviluppo craniofaciali o occlusive.

TONSILLECTOMIA E ADENOIDECTOMIA. I criteri per effettuare una tonsillectomia e un'adenoidectomia combinate in caso di infezioni ricorrenti sono gli stessi della tonsillectomia isolata. L'altra principale indicazione a effettuare le due procedure insieme è l'ostruzione delle vie aeree, secondaria a ipertrofia adenotonsillare che causa disturbi respiratori nel sonno, scarso accrescimento, anomalie di sviluppo craniofaciali o occlusive, alterazioni del linguaggio o, raramente, cuore polmonare.

COMPLICANZE

FARINGOTONSILLITE ACUTA. Le due principali complicanze dell'infezione da SBEA non trattata sono la glomerulonefrite post-streptococcica e la febbre reumatica acuta (vedi Capitoli 511 e 182).

INFEZIONE PERITONSILLARE. L'infezione peritonsillare può manifestarsi sotto forma di cellulite o di un vero e proprio ascesso nella regione superiore e laterale della capsula tonsillare (vedi Capitolo 379). Queste infezioni insorgono abitualmente nei bambini con un'anamnesi di infezioni tonsillari ricorrenti e sono polimicrobiche, comprendendo sia aerobi sia anaerobi. I sintomi di presentazione sono mal di gola monolaterale, otalgia riferita, scialorrea e trisma. La tonsilla colpita è spostata in basso e medialmente dall'edema del pilastro tonsillare anteriore e del palato. La diagnosi di ascesso può essere confermata con la TC o con l'agoaspirazione, il cui contenuto deve essere sottoposto a esame colturale. Per il trattamento, si rimanda al Capitolo 379.

INFEZIONE DELLO SPAZIO RETROFARINGEO. L'infezione dello spazio retrofaringeo si sviluppa nei linfonodi che drenano l'orofaringe, il naso e il rinofaringe. Vedi Capitolo 379.

INFEZIONE DELLO SPAZIO PARAFARINGEO. L'infezione tonsillare si può estendere allo spazio parafaringeo, causando sintomi come febbre, dolore e rigidità del collo, e segni come edema della parete faringea laterale e del collo, dal lato colpito. La diagnosi è confermata dalla TC con mezzo di contrasto, e il trattamento consiste nella somministrazione di antibiotici per via endovenosa e nell'incisione esterna con drenaggio, se la TC rivela la presenza di un ascesso (vedi Capitolo 379). La tromboflebite settica della vena giugulare, o **sindrome di Lemierre**, si presenta con febbre, stato tossico, dolore e rigidità cervicali, oltre a distress respiratorio dovuto ai numerosi emboli settici polmonari, ed è una complicanza delle infezioni dello spazio parafaringeo o delle infezioni odontogene da *Fusobacterium necrophorum*. Una concomitante mononucleosi da virus di Epstein-Barr può essere un evento predisponente prima dell'insorgenza acuta di febbre, brividi e distress respiratorio in un paziente adolescente. Il trattamento comprende la somministrazione endovenosa di antibiotici ad alto dosaggio (ampicillina-sulbactam, clindamicina, penicillina o ciprofloxacina) e l'eparinizzazione.

FARINGOTONSILLITE CRONICA O RICORRENTE. Vedi Capitolo 378.

OSTRUZIONE CRONICA DELLE VIE AEREE (VEDI ANCHE CAPITOLO 18). Sebbene raramente, i bambini con ostruzione cronica delle vie aeree da ipertrofia tonsillare possono presentare cuore polmonare.

Gli effetti dell'ostruzione cronica delle vie aeree e della respirazione con la bocca sullo sviluppo faciale restano oggetto di controversia. Gli studi sulla respirazione orale cronica, tanto nell'uomo quanto negli animali, hanno dimostrato alterazioni dello sviluppo faciale, tra cui l'aumento dell'altezza faciale anteriore totale e la tendenza alla retrognazia mandibolare (la cosiddetta "facies adeoidea"). L'adenotonsillectomia può risolvere alcune di queste anomalie. Altri studi hanno contestato questi risultati.

TONSILLECTOMIA E ADENOIDECTOMIA. Un'emorragia può insorgere nell'immediato periodo postoperatorio o manifestarsi più tardi, dopo la caduta dell'escara. L'edema della lingua e del palato molle possono portare a un'ostruzione acuta delle vie aeree nelle prime ore successive all'intervento. I bambini con una sottostante ipotonia o con anomalie craniofaciali presentano un rischio maggiore di andare incontro a questa complicanza. La disidratazione da odinofagia non è infrequente nella prima settimana postoperatoria. Le complicanze rare comprendono l'insufficienza velofaringea, la stenosi rinofaringea o orofaringea e problemi psicologici.

American Academy of Otolaryngology–Head and Neck Surgery. (2000.) Clinical indicators: Tonsillectomy, adenoidectomy, adenotonsillectomy. Available at www.entlink.net/practice/products/indicators/tonsillectomy.html.

Brook I, Shah K: Bacteriology of adenoids and tonsils in children with recurrent adenotonsillitis. *Ann Otol Rhinol Laryngol* 2001;110:844–848.

de Serres LM, Derkay C, Sie K, et al: Impact of adenotonsillectomy on quality of life in children with obstructive sleep disorders. *Arch Otolaryngol Head Neck Surg* 2002;128:489–496.

Ebert CS, Drake AF: The impact of sleep-disordered breathing on cognition and behavior in children: A review and meta-synthesis of the literature. *Otolaryngol Head Neck Surg* 2004;131:814–1826.

Gozal D: Sleep-disordered breathing and school performance in children. *Pediatrics* 1998;102:616–620.

Johnson RF, Stewart MG, Wright CC: An evidence-based review of the treatment of peritonsillar abscess. *Otolaryngol Head Neck Surg* 2003:128:332–343.

Paradise JL, Bluestone CD, Colborn DK, et al: Tonsillectomy and adenotonsillectomy for recurrent throat infection in moderately affected children. *Pediatrics* 2002;110:7–15.

Ramirez S, Hild TG, Rudolph CN, et al: Increased diagnosis of Lemierre syndrome and other *Fusobacterium necrophorum* infections at a children's hospital. *Pediatrics* 2003;112:e380–e385.

Scottish Intercollegiate Guidelines Network. (1999.) Management of sore throat and indications for tonsillectomy. Available at www.sign.ac.uk/guidelines.

van Staaij BK, van den Akker EH, Rovers MM, et al: Effectiveness of adenotonsillectomy in children with mild symptoms of throat infections or adenotonsillar hypertrophy: Open, randomised controlled trial. *Br Med J* 2004;329:651.

Capitolo 381 ■ Sintomi respiratori cronici o ricorrenti

Thomas F. Boat e Thomas P. Green

Sintomi respiratori, come la tosse, i sibili e lo stridore, si verificano frequentemente o per lunghi periodi in un numero considerevole di bambini; in altri si osservano invece infiltrati polmonari persistenti o ricorrenti, con o senza sintomi. Determinare la causa di questi reperti cronici è talvolta difficile, poiché i sintomi possono essere causati sia da una serie di infezioni acute del tratto respiratorio in rapida successione, non correlate tra loro, sia da un unico processo fisiopatologico; per molte condizioni respiratorie, acute e croniche, esistono pochi esami diagnostici specifici e di facile esecuzione. Gli sforzi diagnostici e terapeutici possono inoltre essere complicati dall'atteggiamento dei familiari del bambino che, preoccupati per i sintomi correlati alla respirazione, fanno pressione affinché il medico prescriva un rimedio rapido.

Un approccio sistematico alla diagnosi e al trattamento di questi pazienti si articola nei seguenti punti: valutare se i sintomi siano la manifestazione di un problema minore oppure di un processo potenzialmente fatale; determinare il meccanismo patogenetico sottostante più probabile; selezionare il trattamento più semplice ed efficace per la patologia sottostante, che spesso può essere solo sintomatico; valutare attentamente l'effetto della terapia. Se questo approccio non permette di identificare il processo patologico responsabile o di ottenere un miglioramento, si renderanno necessarie indagini diagnostiche più estese ed eventualmente invasive, compresa la broncoscopia.

GIUDICARE LA GRAVITÀ DEI SINTOMI RESPIRATORI CRONICI

Le manifestazioni cliniche indicative che una malattia del tratto respiratorio può essere potenzialmente fatale, o associata a disabilità cronica, sono elencate nella Tabella 381-1. Se non si rileva nessuno di questi reperti, l'affezione respiratoria cronica è probabilmente benigna. Quando un neonato attivo, in buono stato nutrizionale e con una crescita appropriata, presenta una respirazione rumorosa intermittente in assenza di altre anomalie fisiche o di laboratorio, è sufficiente prescrivere un trattamento sintomatico e rassicurare i genitori. Accade talvolta che sintomi in apparenza benigni, ma persistenti, siano precursori di un problema grave del tratto respiratorio inferiore; al contrario, alcuni bambini (quelli con asma correlato a infezioni) hanno episodi ricorrenti potenzialmente fatali, ma pochi o nessun sintomo negli intervalli. La ripetizione degli esami in un arco di tempo prolungato, sia quando il bambino appare in condizioni di benessere, sia quando è sintomatico, è spesso utile per determinare la gravità e la cronicità delle malattie polmonari.

TOSSE RICORRENTE O PERSISTENTE

La **tosse** è una risposta riflessa del tratto respiratorio inferiore alla stimolazione dei recettori dell'irritazione o della tosse, presenti nella mucosa delle vie aeree. Nei bambini la causa più comune del fenomeno è la reattività delle vie aeree (asma). Dal momento che i recettori dell'irritazione si trovano anche nella faringe, nei seni paranasali, nello stomaco e nel canale uditivo esterno, l'origine di una tosse persistente talvolta non deve essere ricercata solo nei polmoni. Gli stimoli specifici delle vie aeree inferiori comprendono l'eccesso di secrezioni, l'aspirazione di materiale estraneo, l'inalazione di particelle di polvere o di gas nocivi, e la risposta infiammatoria ad agenti infettivi o a processi allergici. Alcune delle condizioni responsabili di tosse cronica sono elencate nella Tabella 381-2.

Le caratteristiche della tosse che possono aiutare a distinguerne l'origine sono presentate nella Tabella 381-3. Altre informazioni utili comprendono un'anamnesi di atopia (asma, eczema, orticaria, rinite allergica), una variazione stagionale o ambientale nella frequenza e nell'intensità della tosse, e una forte familiarità per condizioni atopiche, che suggeriscono tutte una causa allergica; sintomi di malassorbimento, o un'anamnesi familiare indicativa di fibrosi cistica; sintomi correlati all'alimentazione, che suggeriscono l'aspirazione; un episodio di soffocamento, che fa pensare all'aspirazione di un corpo estraneo; cefalea o edema faciale associati a sinusite, e un'anamesi di fumo, nei bambini più grandi e negli adolescenti, o la presenza di un fumatore in casa (Tab. 381-4).

Durante l'esame obiettivo si possono ottenere informazioni importanti sulla causa della tosse cronica. Il drenaggio faringeo posteriore, associato a tosse notturna, suggerisce una malattia cronica delle vie aeree superiori, come una sinusite. L'iperinflazione del torace è indicativa di un'ostruzione cronica delle vie aeree, come nell'asma o nella fibrosi cistica. Un sibilo espiratorio, con o senza riduzione di intensità del murmure vescicolare, deve indurre a sospettare l'asma o la bronchite asmatica, ma può anche essere compatibile con una diagnosi di fibrosi cistica, anello vascolare, aspirazione di materiale estraneo o emosiderosi polmonare. Un'attenta auscultazione durante l'espirazione forzata può rivelare sibili espiratori, altrimenti non udibili, che talvolta rappresentano l'unico segno di una sottostante reattività delle vie aeree. I crepitii grossolani suggeriscono le bronchiectasie, inclusa la fibrosi cistica, ma possono anche insorgere con un'esacerbazione acuta o subacuta dell'asma. L'ippocratismo digitale è osservabile nella maggior parte dei pazienti con bronchiectasie, e solo in poche altre condizioni respiratorie con tosse cronica (vedi Fig. 371-1 e Tab. 371-2). La deviazione della trachea fa pensare all'aspirazione di un corpo estraneo o una massa mediastinica.

Durante l'esame, è essenziale avere a disposizione un tempo sufficiente per rilevare la tosse spontanea. Se non spontaneamente, la maggior parte dei bambini è in grado di tossire a richiesta, dall'età di 4-5 anni. Chiedendo al paziente di fare un'inspirazione massima e un'espirazione forzata ripetutamente, di solito si induce il riflesso della tosse. I bambini che tossiscono molto spesso, fino a diverse volte al minuto, con regolarità,

TABELLA 381-1. Indicatori di malattia cronica grave del tratto respiratorio inferiore nei bambini

Febbre persistente
Limitazione persistente dell'attività
Mancata crescita
Scarso aumento ponderale
Ippocratismo digitale
Tachipnea e ventilazione difficoltosa persistenti
Escreato purulento cronico
Ipossiemia importante e sostenuta
Infiltrati refrattari alla radiografia toracica
Anomalie persistenti della funzione polmonare
Anamnesi familiare di malattia polmonare ereditaria
Cianosi e ipercapnia

TABELLA 381-2. Diagnosi differenziale della tosse ricorrente e persistente nei bambini

TOSSE RICORRENTE
Reattività bronchiale, compreso l'asma allergico
Drenaggio dalle vie aeree superiori
Sindromi da aspirazione
Infezioni ricorrenti dell'apparato respiratorio in pazienti immunocompetenti o immunodeficienti
Emosiderosi polmonare idiopatica

TOSSE PERSISTENTE
Ipersensibilità dei recettori della tosse dopo un'infezione
Malattia da reattività della vie aeree (asma)
Sinusite cronica
Bronchite e tracheite causate da infezione cronica, fumo attivo o passivo
Bronchiectasie, comprese fibrosi cistica, discinesia ciliare primitiva, immunodeficienza
Aspirazione di corpo estraneo
Aspirazione ricorrente da incompetenza faringea, schisi tracheolaringoesofagea, fistola tracheoesofagea
Reflusso gastroesofageo, con o senza aspirazione
Sindrome da pertosse
Compressione estrinseca del tratto tracheobronchiale (anello vascolare, neoplasia, linfonodo, cisti polmonare)
Tracheomalacia, broncomalacia
Tumori endobronchiali o endotracheali
Tubercolosi endobronchiale
Tosse abituale
Polmonite da ipersensibilità
Infezioni fungine
Irritanti inalatori, compreso il fumo di tabacco
Irritazione del canale uditivo esterno

TABELLA 381-3. Caratteristiche della tosse cronica e loro significato eziologico

TIPO DI TOSSE	CONDIZIONE RESPONSABILE PIÙ PROBABILE
Grassa (discontinua), produttiva	Bronchite, bronchite asmatica, fibrosi cistica, bronchiectasie
Metallica	Tracheite, tosse abituale
Con stridore	Ostruzione laringea, pertosse
Parossistica (con o senza soffocamento)	Fibrosi cistica, sindrome da pertosse e corpo estraneo
Discontinua	Polmonite da *Chlamydia*
Notturna	Reazione allergica delle vie aeree superiori o inferiori, o entrambe, sinusite
Più severa al risveglio mattutino	Fibrosi cistica, bronchiectasie, bronchite cronica
Insorge con l'attività fisica intensa	Asma da sforzo, fibrosi cistica, bronchiectasie
Scompare nel sonno	Tosse abituale, stati ipersecretori lievi come nella fibrosi cistica e nell'asma
Chiusa (sibilante)	Reattività delle vie aeree

TABELLA 381-4. Indizi clinici sulla tosse

CARATTERISTICHE	PENSARE A
Discontinua, parossistica	Pertosse, fibrosi cistica, corpo estraneo, *Chlamydia* spp., *Mycoplasma* spp.
Seguita da un urlo	Pertosse
Tutto il giorno, mai di notte	Psicogena, abituale
Abbaiante, metallica	Croup, tosse psicogena, tracheomalacia, tracheite, epiglottite
Raucedine	Coinvolgimento laringeo (croup, interessamento del nervo laringeo ricorrente)
Esordio improvviso	Corpo estraneo, embolia polmonare
Segue l'attività fisica	Malattia da reattività delle vie aeree
Associata al mangiare e al bere	Aspirazione, reflusso gastroesofageo, fistola tracheoesofagea
Tendenza a schiarirsi la gola	Scolo postnasale
Produttiva (escreato)	Infezione
Tosse notturna	Sinusite, malattia reattiva delle vie aeree
Stagionale	Rinite allergica, malattia reattiva delle vie aeree
Paziente immunosoppresso	Polmonite batterica, *Pneumocystis carinii*, *Mycobacterium tuberculosis*, *Mycobacterium avium-intracellulare*, Cytomegalovirus
Dispnea	Ipossia, ipercapnia
Esposizione ad animali	*Chlamydia psittaci* (uccelli), *Yersinia pestis* (roditori), *Francisella tularensis* (conigli), febbre Q (pecore, bestiame), hantavirus (roditori), istoplasmosi (piccioni)
Geografica	Istoplasmosi (Mississippi, Missouri, River Valley in Ohio), coccidioidiomicosi (sud-est degli Stati Uniti), blastomicosi (nord e ovest degli Stati Uniti)
Nei giorni feriali e non in quelli festivi	Esposizione occupazionale

Da Kliegman RM, Greenbaum LA, Lyle PS: *Practical Strategies in Pediatric Diagnosis and Therapy*, 2nd ed. Philadelphia, Elsevier Saunders, 2004, p 19.

hanno probabilmente una tosse originata da abitudine (tic). Se la tosse è produttiva, si dovrebbe cercare in ogni modo possibile di ottenere un campione di escreato; molti bambini più grandicelli sono in grado di collaborare. È talvolta possibile prelevare piccoli campioni di escreato tramite un tampone faringeo inserito rapidamente nella faringe inferiore, mentre il paziente tossisce con la lingua che protrude. L'escreato mucoide chiaro è per lo più associato a reazioni allergiche o a bronchite asmatica. L'escreato torbido (purulento) suggerisce un'infezione del tratto respiratorio, ma può anche riflettere un'aumentata cellularità (eosinofilia) dovuta a un processo asmatico, mentre quello molto purulento è caratteristico delle bronchiectasie. L'espettorato maleodorante è indicativo di un'infezione polmonare da anaerobi. Nella fibrosi cistica l'escreato, anche quando è purulento, raramente ha un odore fetido.

Gli esami di laboratorio possono essere utili nella valutazione della tosse cronica. Solo i campioni di escreato contenenti macrofagi alveolari devono essere interpretati come un indice attendibile dei processi del tratto respiratorio inferiore. L'eosinofilia nell'escreato suggerisce l'asma, la bronchite asmatica o una reazione da ipersensibilità nel polmone, mentre una risposta cellulare polimorfonucleata fa pensare a un'infezione; se l'escreato non è disponibile, la presenza di eosinofilia nelle secrezioni nasali indica anch'essa una malattia su base atopica. Se la maggior parte delle cellule dell'escreato è costituita da macrofagi, si deve sospettare un'ipersensibilità postinfettiva dei recettori della tosse. I macrofagi contenuti nell'escreato possono essere sottoposti a colorazione per l'emosiderina, che è diagnostica di emosiderosi polmonare, o per i lipidi, che suggeriscono fortemente, sebbene non in modo specifico, un'aspirazione ripetuta. I bambini con tosse che persiste per più di 6 settimane devono essere valutati per la fibrosi cistica. La coltura dell'escreato è utile per la diagnosi della fibrosi cistica, ma meno per le altre condizioni, perché la flora del cavo orale può contaminare il campione.

Gli esami ematologici possono rivelare anemia, come risultato dell'emosiderosi, o un'eosinofilia che accompagna l'asma e le altre reazioni da ipersensibilità del polmone. La presenza di infiltrati alla radiografia polmonare suggerisce una fibrosi cistica, bronchiectasie, un corpo estraneo, una polmonite da ipersensibilità o la tubercolosi. Quando si sospetta una tosse da equivalente asmatico, un tentativo terapeutico con broncodilatatori può essere diagnostico. Se la tosse non risponde agli sforzi terapeutici iniziali, possono essere indicate procedure diagnostiche più specifiche, tra cui una valutazione immunologica o allergologica, immagini radiologiche del torace e dei seni paranasali, esofagogramma, esami per il reflusso gastroesofageo, studi microbiologici speciali tra cui test virologici rapidi, valutazione delle caratteristiche morfologiche delle ciglia, e la broncoscopia.

La **tosse da abitudine** ("tosse psicogena" o "tic della tosse") deve essere presa in considerazione in tutti i bambini con una tosse che perdura da settimane o mesi, refrattaria al trattamento, e che scompare nel sonno o quando il soggetto si distrae. Oltre a essere improvvisa e forte, ha una qualità aspra, gridata, "abbaiante". Ciò che colpisce è la tipica incongruenza tra l'intensità della tosse e l'atteggiamento del bambino. Questa tosse può essere assente quando il medico rivolge la sua attenzione a quel che avviene fuori dallo studio, ma quasi sicuramente comparirà non appena rivolgerà la sua attenzione al bambino e al sintomo. Il disturbo tipicamente compare in concomitanza con un'infezione delle vie aree superiori, ma poi si trascina. Il paziente perde molti giorni di scuola poiché la tosse interferisce con il normale svolgimento delle lezioni. Questo sintomo spinge a effettuare molte procedure mediche inutili e cicli di terapia non necessari. Il trattamento consiste nello spiegare che non è in atto alcun processo patologico a carico dei polmoni e che il bambino dovrebbe riprendere tutte le sue attività consuete, scuola compresa. Questa rassicurazione, insieme alle tecniche di logopedia, che allentano la tensione muscoloscheletrica a livello del collo e del torace, rendendo inoltre il bambino più cosciente della sensazione iniziale che scatena la tosse, ha avuto un grande successo. Tale approccio non si basa sull'inganno, a differenza di un'altra tecnica che consiste nell'avvolgere il torace di un bambino *molto suggestionabile* con una coperta per "rinforzare i muscoli indeboliti" finché la tosse non cessa. L'autoipnosi è un'altra valida terapia, spesso efficace con una sola seduta. L'espressione "tosse da abitudine" è preferibile a quella di "tosse psicogena" perché non presuppone un'accezione negativa e perché la maggior parte di questi bambini non ha in realtà problemi emotivi. Quando la tosse scompare, non riemerge sotto forma di un altro sintomo. Ciononostante, altri sintomi, come quella dell'intestino irritabile, possono essere presenti nel paziente o nei suoi familiari.

STRIDORE RICORRENTE O PERSISTENTE

Lo **stridore**, un suono inspiratorio aspro, di media frequenza, associato a ostruzione della zona laringea o della trachea extratoracica, si accompagna spesso a tosse da croup e a voce rauca. È di comune riscontro nei bambini con croup; anche i corpi estranei e i traumi possono causare uno stridore acuto. Un piccolo numero di bambini, tuttavia, acquisisce uno stridore ricorrente, o ha uno stridore persistente, dai primi giorni o settimane di vita (Tab. 381-5). Nella maggior parte delle anomalie congenite delle prime vie aeree che provocano stridore, i sintomi si manifestano subito dopo la nascita. L'aumento dello stridore in posizione supina suggerisce una laringomalacia o una tracheomalacia; la concomitante presenza di raucedine o afonia deve indurre a sospettare un coinvolgimento delle corde vocali.

L'esame obiettivo per lo stridore ricorrente o persistente di solito è poco significativo, sebbene debbano essere valutate le variazioni di gravità e di intensità correlate al cambio di posizione del corpo. Le radiografie anteroposteriori e laterali, l'esofagografia, la fluoroscopia, la TC e la RM sono tutti strumenti diagnostici che potrebbero rivelarsi utili. Nella maggior parte dei casi, è necessaria per la diagnosi l'osservazione diretta in laringoscopia. Con la laringoscopia a fibre ottiche si riescono a ottenere immagini non distorte della laringe.

TABELLA 381-5. Cause di stridore ricorrente o persistente nei bambini

RICORRENTE
Croup allergico (spastico)
Infezioni respiratorie in un bambino con restringimento, per altri aspetti asintomatico, delle vie aeree maggiori
Laringomalacia
PERSISTENTE
Ostruzione laringea
Laringomalacia
Papillomi, altri tumori
Cisti e laringoceli
Diaframmi laringei
Paralisi bilaterale degli abduttori delle corde vocali
Corpo estraneo
Malattia tracheobronchiale
Tracheomalacia
Diaframmi tracheali sottoglottici
Tumori endotracheali, endobronchiali
Stenosi tracheale sottoglottica
Congenita
Acquisita
Masse estrinseche
Masse mediastiniche
Anello vascolare
Enfisema lobare
Cisti broncogena
Aumento di volume della tiroide
Corpo estraneo esofageo
Fistola tracheoesofagea
ALTRO
Reflusso gastroesofageo
Macroglossia, sindrome di Pierre Robin
Sindrome del *cri-du-chat*
Stridore isterico
Ipocalcemia
Paralisi delle corde vocali
Crisi di Chiari

WHEEZING RICORRENTE O PERSISTENTE

I genitori si lamentano spesso che il loro bambino "fischia", intendendo riferirsi a suoni respiratori udibili senza fonendoscopio, che provocano una risonanza palpabile attraverso il torace e si verificano prevalentemente in inspirazione. Alcuni di questi soggetti hanno stridore, sebbene molti emettano suoni udibili quando la via aerea sovraepiglottica non è completamente libera da residui alimentari o secrezioni.

Per contro, il vero **wheezing** è una manifestazione relativamente frequente e particolarmente problematica di una malattia ostruttiva delle vie aeree inferiori nei bambini. La sede dell'ostruzione può essere in qualunque punto, dalla trachea intratoracica ai piccoli bronchi o ai bronchioli più grandi, ma il suono è prodotto dalla turbolenza nelle vie aeree più ampie che collassano con l'espirazione forzata. I bambini di età <2-3 anni sono particolarmente soggetti a sviluppare wheezing, poiché il broncospasmo, l'edema della mucosa e l'accumulo di secrezioni in eccesso hanno un effetto ostruttivo relativamente maggiore sulle loro vie aeree, di calibro minore. Inoltre, nei bambini più piccoli, la maggiore compliance fa sì che le vie aeree collassino più facilmente con l'espirazione attiva. Gli episodi isolati di insorgenza acuta di wheezing, riscontrabili nella bronchiolite, non sono infrequenti, ma il wheezing che si ripete o persiste per più di 4 settimane deve orientare verso altre diagnosi (vedi Tab. 388-2). La maggior parte dei casi di wheezing ricorrente o persistente, nei bambini, è conseguenza di una malattia da iperreattività delle vie aeree. Alcuni fattori ambientali aspecifici, come il fumo di sigaretta, possono contribuire in modo importante al fenomeno.

La presenza di wheezing che si ripete frequentemente, o persistente, iniziato poco dopo la nascita, suggerisce svariate diagnosi, tra cui anomalie strutturali congenite del tratto respiratorio inferiore o la tracheobroncomalacia. Il wheezing che accompagna la fibrosi cistica è più comune nel primo anno di vita. L'esordio improvviso di wheezing severo, in un bambino precedentemente sano, dovrebbe far sospettare l'aspirazione di un corpo estraneo.

Per verificare un'anamnesi di wheezing in un bambino con sintomi episodici, può essere necessaria l'osservazione ripetuta, volta a valutare il movimento dell'aria, l'adeguatezza della ventilazione e la presenza di segni di pneumopatie croniche, come un'iperinflazione fissa del torace, un ritardo della crescita e l'ippocratismo digitale: quest'ultimo suggerisce un'infezione polmonare cronica ed è raramente pronunciato nell'asma non complicato. Si dovrebbe cercare un'eventuale deviazione tracheale da aspirazione di un corpo estraneo. È essenziale escludere che il wheezing sia secondario a insufficienza cardiaca. Il riscontro di rinite allergica, orticaria, eczema o ittiosi volgare suggerisce una diagnosi di asma o bronchite asmatica. Si deve esaminare il naso per escludere la presenza di polipi, che possono accompagnare condizioni allergiche o la fibrosi cistica.

L'eosinofilia dell'escreato e livelli elevati di immunoglobuline E sieriche (IgE) sono indicativi di reazioni allergiche. Un FEV_1 (*Forced Expiratory Volume*, volume espiratorio forzato, in un secondo) che aumenta del 15% in risposta ai broncodilatatori conferma la diagnosi di reattività delle vie aeree. Se la risposta non è soddisfacente, occorre prendere in esame studi microbiologici appositi, speciali tecniche di imaging delle vie aeree e delle strutture cardiovascolari, indagini specifiche per la fibrosi cistica e la broncoscopia.

INFILTRATI POLMONARI RICORRENTI E PERSISTENTI

Infiltrati polmonari visibili alla radiografia del torace, causati da una polmonite acuta, si risolvono di solito in 1-3 settimane, anche se un certo numero di bambini, in particolare lattanti, non riesce a eliminarli completamente nel giro di 4 settimane. Questi pazienti possono essere febbrili o meno, e presentare un'ampia varietà di sintomi e segni respiratori. Gli infiltrati persistenti o ricorrenti rappresentano una sfida dal punto di vista diagnostico (Tab. 381-6).

I sintomi associati agli infiltrati polmonari cronici, nelle prime settimane di vita (ma non correlati alla sindrome da distress respiratorio neonatale), suggeriscono la presenza di infezioni acquisite in utero o durante il passaggio attraverso il canale del parto. La comparsa precoce di infiltrati cronici si può anche associare alla fibrosi cistica o ad anomalie congenite, che danno luogo ad aspirazione o ostruzione delle vie aeree. Un'anamnesi di infiltrati ricorrenti, sibili e tosse può riflettere una condizione di asma, anche nel primo anno di vita.

Una sindrome non comune ma caratteristica, che esordisce nel primo anno di vita con infiltrati polmonari ricorrenti, è l'emosiderosi polmonare correlata a ipersensibilità al latte vaccino, o da cause sconosciute. I bambini con un'anamnesi di displasia broncopolmonare hanno spesso episodi di distress respiratorio, accompagnati da sibili e nuovi infiltrati polmonari. Le polmoniti ricorrenti, in un bambino con frequenti otiti medie, rinofaringiti, adeniti o manifestazioni dermatologiche, suggeriscono una condizione di immunodeficienza, deficit del complemento o deficit della funzione fagocitaria (vedi Capitoli 123-126). Si deve prestare particolare attenzione alla possibilità che gli infiltrati rappresentino una polmonite interstiziale linfocitaria o un'infezione opportunistica associate a infezione da HIV (vedi Capitolo 273). Un'anamnesi positiva per tosse parossistica in un lattante è suggestiva di una sindrome da pertosse o fibrosi cistica. Gli infiltrati persistenti, specialmente se caratterizzati da perdita di volume, in un bambino ai primi passi, deve indurre a ipotizzare l'aspirazione di un corpo estraneo.

La presenza di iperinflazione e infiltrati suggerisce la fibrosi cistica o l'asma cronico. Un "torace silente" con infiltrati deve far sorgere il sospetto di proteinosi alveolare, infezione da *Pneumocystis carinii*, alterazioni genetiche della sintesi e della secrezione del surfattante che causano polmonite interstiziale, o tumori. Si deve valutare attentamente la crescita per determinare se l'affezione polmonare abbia ripercussioni a livello sistemico, indicando una marcata gravità e cronicità, come nella fibrosi cistica o nella

TABELLA 381-6. Malattie che si associano a infiltrati polmonari ricorrenti, persistenti o migranti, oltre il periodo neonatale

Asma
Aspirazione ripetuta
Polmonite da ipersensibilità
Emosiderosi polmonare
Corpo estraneo
Anemia falciforme
Fibrosi cistica
Infezione congenita
  Cytomegalovirus
  Rosolia
  Sifilide
Infezione acquisita
  Cytomegalovirus
  Tubercolosi
  HIV
  Altri virus
  Chlamydia
  Mycoplasma, Ureaplasma
  Pertosse
  Micosi
  Pneumocystis carinii
Infezione batterica trattata inadeguatamente
Anomalie congenite
  Cisti polmonari
  Sequestro polmonare
  Stenosi bronchiale
  Anello vascolare
  Cardiopatia congenita con shunt sinistro-destro
Aspirazione
  Incontinenza faringea (per es. palatoschisi)
  Laringotracheoesofagoschisi
  Fistola tracheoesofagea
  Reflusso gastroesofageo
  Corpo estraneo
  Aspirazione di lipidi
Immunodeficienza, deficit della funzione fagocitaria
  Stati di immunodeficienza umorale, cellulare o combinata
  Malattia granulomatosa cronica e difetti fagocitici correlati
  Deficit del complemento
Allergia-ipersensibilità
  Emosiderosi polmonare (correlata al latte vaccino, altre)
  Asma
  Polmonite da ipersensibilità (alveolite allergica)
Fibrosi cistica
Discinesia ciliare primitiva (sindrome di Kartagener)
Altre bronchiectasie
Sarcoidosi
Neoplasie (primitive, metastatiche)
Polmonite interstiziale e fibrosi
  Usuale
  Linfoide (AIDS)
  Alterazioni genetiche della sintesi e della secrezione del surfattante
  Desquamativa
  Acuta (di Hamman-Rich)
Proteinosi alveolare
Linfangectasia polmonare
Deficit di α1-antitripsina
Infiammazione e fibrosi indotte da farmaci o radiazioni
Collagenopatie vascolari
Polmonite eosinofila
Larva migrans viscerale
Istiocitosi
Leucemia

proteinosi alveolare. La presenza di cataratta, retinopatia o microcefalia suggerisce un'infezione intrauterina. La rinorrea cronica si può associare a malattie atopiche, intolleranza al latte vaccino, fibrosi cistica o sifilide congenita. L'assenza delle tonsille e dei linfonodi cervicali suggerisce una condizione di immunodeficienza.

Le indagini diagnostiche dovrebbero essere effettuate selettivamente, basandosi sulle informazioni ottenute dall'anamnesi e dall'esame obiettivo; loro presupposto fondamentale è una profonda conoscenza delle condizioni elencate nella Tabella 381-6. L'esame citologico dell'escreato, se disponibile, può essere utile. La TC del torace fornisce spesso dettagli anatomici più precisi sull'infiltrato. La broncoscopia è indicata per individuare i corpi estranei, le anomalie congenite o acquisite del tratto tracheobronchiale, e l'ostruzione da parte di masse endobronchiali o estrinseche. La broncoscopia permette il prelievo delle secrezioni, che possono così essere esaminate dal punto di vista citologico e microbiologico. Il liquido di lavaggio alveolare, oltre a essere diagnostico per la proteinosi alveolare e l'emosiderosi polmonare persistente, può suggerire sindromi da aspirazione. Se non si giunge a una diagnosi pur avendo effettuato tutte le indagini del caso, la biopsia polmonare può essere risolutiva.

Il trattamento medico e chirurgico ottimale degli infiltrati polmonari cronici dipende frequentemente da una diagnosi specifica, ma le condizioni croniche possono essere autolimitanti (infezioni virali severe e prolungate nei neonati); in questi casi, la terapia sintomatica può mantenere un'adeguata funzione polmonare in attesa che si verifichi un miglioramento spontaneo. Sono misure utili la terapia inalatoria e la fisioterapia per le secrezioni eccessive, gli antibiotici per le infezioni batteriche, la somministrazione di ossigeno nell'ipossiemia e il mantenimento di un'adeguata nutrizione. Poiché i polmoni di un bambino piccolo hanno un notevole potenziale di recupero, il trattamento finisce per ripristinare una funzione polmonare normale, nonostante la severità del danno polmonare che si verifica in età neonatale o nella prima infanzia.

Anbar RD, Hall HR: Childhood habit cough treated with self-hypnosis. *J Pediatr* 2004;144:213–217.

Blager F, Gay M, Wood R: Voice therapy techniques adapted to treatment of habit cough: A pilot study. *J Commun Disord* 1988;21:393–400.

Chang AB, Newman RG, Carlin JB, et al: Subjective scoring of cough in children: Parent-completed vs child-completed diary cards vs an objective method. *Eur Respir J* 1998;11:462–466.

De Jongste JC, Shields MD: Cough 2: Chronic cough in children. *Thorax* 2003;58:998–1003.

del Rosario JF, Orenstein SR: Evaluation and management of gastroesophageal reflux and pulmonary disease. *Curr Opin Pediatr* 1996;8:209–215.

Hay AD, Schroeder K, Fahey T: Acute cough in children. *Br Med J* 2004;328:1062–1063.

Irwin RS, Madison JM: The diagnosis and treatment of cough. *N Engl J Med* 2000;343:1715–1721.

Mamlock R: A cost-effective approach to the diagnosis and treatment of the wheezing infant. *Allergy Asthma Proc* 1997;18:149–152.

Mancuso RF: Stridor in neonates. *Pediatr Clin North Am* 1996;43:1339–1356.

Martinez FD, Wright AL, Taussig LM, et al: Asthma and wheezing in the first six years of life. *N Engl J Med* 1995;332:133–138.

Morgan WJ, Taussig LM: The child with persistent cough. *Pediatr Rev* 1987;8:249–253.

Nogee LM: Alterations of SP-B and SP-C expression in neonatal lung disease. *Ann Rev Physiol* 2004;66:601–623.

Capitolo 382 ■ Ostruzione acuta infiammatoria delle vie aeree superiori (croup, epiglottite, laringite e tracheite batterica)

Genie E. Roosevelt

CONSIDERAZIONI GENERALI. Poiché la resistenza delle vie aeree è inversamente proporzionale alla quarta potenza del raggio, piccole riduzioni dell'area di sezione, causate da edema della mucosa o da altri processi infiammatori, provocano un aumento esponenziale della resistenza delle vie aeree e un aumento significativo del lavoro respiratorio. La laringe si compone di quattro cartilagini maggiori (epiglottica, aritenoidea, tiroidea e cricoidea, dall'alto verso il basso) e dei tessuti molli che le circondano. La cartilagine cricoidea circonda la via aerea appena sotto le corde vocali e definisce la porzione più stretta delle vie aeree superiori, nei bambini di età <10 anni.

L'infiammazione che coinvolge le corde vocali e le strutture sottostanti è chiamata *laringite*, *laringotracheite* o *laringotracheobronchite*, mentre quella delle strutture soprastanti (ovvero, aritenoidi, pliche ariepiglottiche ["false corde"], epiglottide) prende il nome di *sovraglottite*. Con il termine **croup** si indica un gruppo eterogeneo di processi prevalentemente acuti e infettivi, caratterizzati da tosse abbaiante o metallica, che possono associarsi a raucedine, stridore inspiratorio e distress respiratorio. Lo **stridore** è un suono respiratorio aspro, acuto, udibile di solito durante l'inspirazione, ma che può essere bifasico, provocato da un flusso aereo turbolento; non è una diagnosi, ma un segno di ostruzione delle vie aeree superiori (vedi Capitolo 371). Il croup colpisce tipicamente la laringe, la trachea e i bronchi. Quando il coinvolgimento della laringe è sufficiente a provocare i sintomi, questi dominano il quadro clinico, sovrastando i segni tracheali e bronchiali. Tradizionalmente si usa fare una distinzione tra croup spastico, o ricorrente, e la laringotracheobronchite. Alcuni ritengono che il croup spastico possa avere una componente allergica e che migliori rapidamente senza trattamento, mentre la laringotracheobronchite è sempre associata a un'infezione virale del tratto respiratorio; secondo altri, invece, segni e sintomi sarebbero così simili da permettere di considerare queste due entità come facenti parte dello spettro di una singola malattia.

382.1 • Ostruzione delle vie aeree superiori di origine infettiva

EZIOLOGIA ED EPIDEMIOLOGIA. Gli agenti virali sono responsabili della maggior parte delle ostruzioni delle vie aeree superiori di origine infettiva; fanno eccezione la difterite, la tracheite batterica e l'epiglottite. I virus parainfluenzali (di tipo 1, 2 e 3; vedi Capitolo 256) sono responsabili del 75% circa dei casi; altri virus associati a questa patologia comprendono quelli dell'influenza A e B, l'adenovirus, il virus respiratorio sinciziale (RSV, *Respiratory Syncytial Virus*) e il morbillo. L'influenza di tipo A è stata associata a una laringotracheobronchite severa. *Mycoplasma pneumoniae*, raramente isolato da bambini con croup, può causare una malattia lieve (vedi Capitolo 220). La maggior parte dei pazienti con croup è di età compresa tra 3 mesi e 5 anni, con un picco nel secondo anno di vita. Le recidive sono frequenti dai 3 ai 6 anni di età e si riducono con la crescita delle vie aeree. Circa il 15% dei pazienti ha un'importante anamnesi familiare di croup.

In passato, l'*Haemophilus influenzae* di tipo b era l'agente eziologico isolato più comunemente nell'epiglottite acuta. Con la diffusione del vaccino HiB, la malattia invasiva causata da questo patogeno, nei pazienti pediatrici, si è ridotta dell'80-90% (vedi Capitolo 192). Pertanto, altri microrganismi, come *Streptococcus pyogenes*, *Streptococcus pneumoniae* e *Staphylococcus aureus*, sono attualmente responsabili di una percentuale maggiore di casi di epiglottite, nei bambini vaccinati. Prima dell'avvento del vaccino, il paziente tipico con epiglottite da *H. influenzae* di tipo b era un bambino di 2-4 anni di età, sebbene si osservassero casi nel primo anno di vita e in soggetti fino a 7 anni di età. Oggi il tipico paziente con epiglottite è un adulto con mal di gola, sebbene si verifichino ancora casi in bambini ipoimmunizzati; sono stati riportati casi di fallimento della vaccinazione.

MANIFESTAZIONI CLINICHE.

Croup (laringotracheobronchite). I virus sono la causa più comune di croup, la forma più frequente di ostruzione delle vie aeree superiori. Il termine *laringotracheobronchite* si riferisce a un'infezione virale della regione glottica e sottoglottica. Alcuni clinici usano il termine *laringotracheite* per indicare la forma più comune e più tipica di croup, mentre riservano il termine *laringotracheobronchite* alla forma più severa, considerata un'estensione della laringotracheite associata a sovrainfezione batterica, che si verifica dopo 5-7 giorni, nel decorso clinico.

La maggior parte dei pazienti ha un'infezione delle vie aeree superiori con una combinazione di rinorrea, faringite, tosse lieve e febbre non elevata per 1-3 giorni, prima che divengano evidenti i segni e i sintomi di ostruzione delle vie aeree superiori. Il bambino sviluppa quindi la caratteristica tosse "abbaiante", raucedine e stridore inspiratorio. Talvolta persiste una febbricola, sebbene la temperatura possa raggiungere anche i 39-40 °C e alcuni bambini siano apirettici. I sintomi peggiorano caratteristicamente di notte, spesso recidivano, diminuendo di intensità, per diversi giorni, e si risolvono completamente nell'arco di una settimana. L'agitazione e il pianto aggravano notevolmente segni e sintomi. Il bambino può preferire stare seduto nel letto o essere tenuto in posizione ortostatica. I bambini più grandi abitualmente non hanno una patologia severa. Altri membri della famiglia possono presentare una malattia respiratoria lieve con laringite. Nella maggior parte dei pazienti giovani con croup la malattia progredisce solo fino allo stridore e a una lieve dispnea, prima che inizi la guarigione.

L'esame obiettivo può rivelare raucedine, corizza, faringe normale o con infiammazione moderata, e una frequenza respiratoria lievemente aumentata. Il grado di distress respiratorio presenta variazioni sostanziali da un paziente all'altro. È raro che l'ostruzione delle vie aeree superiori progredisca accompagnandosi ad aumento della frequenza respiratoria, alitamento delle pinne nasali, retrazioni sovrasternali, sottosternali e intercostali, stridore continuo. Il croup è una malattia delle vie aeree superiori, in cui lo scambio gassoso a livello alveolare è in genere normale. Si osservano ipossia e riduzione della saturazione di ossigeno solo quando l'ostruzione completa delle vie aeree è imminente. Il bambino che si presenta ipossico, cianotico, pallido o letargico necessita di un immediato trattamento delle vie aeree. Talvolta può essere difficile distinguere il quadro della laringotracheobronchite severa da quello dell'epiglottite, nonostante l'esordio abitualmente più acuto e il decorso più rapido di quest'ultima.

Il croup è una diagnosi clinica e non richiede la radiografia del collo. Quest'ultima può mostrare il tipico restringimento sottoglottico o "segno della guglia" del croup, nella proiezione anteroposteriore (Fig. 382-1); tale segno, tuttavia, non solo può essere assente in pazienti con croup, ma può comparire in sog-

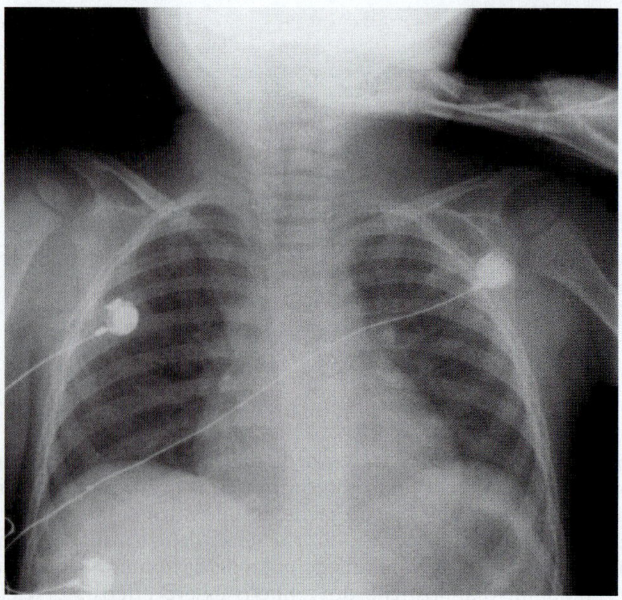

Figura 382-1. Radiografia delle vie aeree di un paziente con croup, che mostra il tipico restringimento sottoglottico ("segno della guglia").

contatto di età <12 mesi che non abbia ricevuto le vaccinazioni di base; o (3) qualsiasi bambino immunocompromesso appartenente al nucleo familiare.

L'**edema laringeo acuto su base allergica** risponde all'adrenalina (diluizione 1:1000 al dosaggio di 0,01 mL/kg fino a un massimo di 0,5 mL/dose) somministrata sottocute o all'adrenalina racemica (dose di 0,25-0,75 mL di adrenalina racemica al 2,25% in 3 mL di soluzione fisiologica) (vedi Capitolo 148). Spesso sono necessari i corticosteroidi (2-4 mg/kg/die di prednisone). Dopo la guarigione, il paziente e i parenti all'atto della dimissione dovrebbero essere muniti di una siringa precaricata di adrenalina, da usare in caso di emergenza. Nei bambini, l'edema reattivo della mucosa, lo stridore severo e il distress respiratorio non responsivo alla terapia inalatoria possono far seguito all'intubazione endotracheale per anestesia generale; in tal caso, l'adrenalina racemica e i corticosteroidi sono utili.

Tracheotomia e intubazione endotracheale. Con l'introduzione dell'intubazione nasotracheale di routine o, meno spesso, la tracheotomia per l'epiglottite, la mortalità per epiglottite si è quasi ridotta a zero. Entrambe le procedure dovrebbero essere sempre effettuate in sala operatoria o in un reparto di terapia intensiva, se il tempo a disposizione lo consente; l'intubazione e l'anestesia generale rendono più agevole la tracheotomia e riducono l'insorgenza di complicanze. Si raccomanda l'uso di un sondino nasotracheale di un calibro <0,5-1 mm rispetto a quello stimato per l'età, per facilitare l'intubazione e ridurre le sequele a lungo termine. La scelta fra tracheotomia e intubazione endotracheale andrà fatta in base all'esperienza e all'abilità del personale non solo in ciascuna delle due procedure, ma anche nelle cure postoperatorie che queste comportano.

L'intubazione endotracheale o la tracheotomia sono necessarie nella maggior parte dei pazienti con tracheite batterica e in tutti i pazienti in tenera età con epiglottite, mentre sono raramente richieste in caso di laringotracheobronchite, croup spastico o laringite. Durante alcune epidemie severe di morbillo e di virus dell'influenza A, sono state riportate forme severe di laringotracheobronchite con necessità di intubazione in un'elevata percentuale di pazienti. La decisione se eseguire o meno queste procedure richiede esperienza e capacità di giudizio, poiché per effettuare la scelta non bisogna attendere che compaiano cianosi e irrequietezza estrema (vedi Capitoli 64 e 69).

L'intubazione endotracheale o la tracheostomia devono restare in sede fino a quando l'edema e lo spasmo si sono risolti e il paziente è in grado di gestire le secrezioni in modo soddisfacente. Andrebbero rimosse il prima possibile, di solito nell'arco di alcuni giorni. Un'adeguata risoluzione dell'infiammazione epiglottica, confermata accuratamente dalla laringoscopia a fibre ottiche, che permette una più rapida estubazione, spesso avviene entro 24 ore. L'adrenalina racemica e il desametasone (0,5 mg/kg/dose ogni 6 ore, secondo necessità) possono essere utili nel trattamento del croup associato all'estubazione.

PROGNOSI. In generale, nei casi di ostruzione infettiva acuta delle vie aeree superiori, la durata dell'ospedalizzazione e la mortalità aumentano via via che l'infezione si estende, coinvolgendo porzioni sempre più ampie del tratto respiratorio; costituisce un'eccezione l'epiglottite, in cui anche un'infezione localizzata può di per sé essere fatale. La maggior parte dei decessi da croup è causata da ostruzione laringea o dalle complicanze della tracheotomia. Raramente, è stato riportato un arresto respiratorio fatale extraospedaliero da laringotracheobronchite virale, soprattutto nei lattanti e nei pazienti con un decorso complicato da tracheite batterica. L'epiglottite non trattata ha una mortalità del 6% in alcune casistiche, ma se si effettua la diagnosi e si instaura il trattamento appropriato prima che il paziente sia gravemente compromesso, la prognosi è eccellente. Eccellente è anche l'esito della laringotracheobronchite acuta, della laringite e del croup spastico. Complessivamente, coloro che richiedono il ricovero ospedaliero per croup presentano un certo aumento della reattività bronchiale, rispetto ai bambini normali, quando vengono esaminati dopo alcuni anni, ma la significatività di questo dato è incerta.

Laringotracheobronchite

Bjornson CL, Klassen TP, Williamson J, et al: A randomized trial of a single dose of oral dexamethasone for mild croup. *N Engl J Med* 2004;351:1306–1313.
Fogel JM, Berg IJ, Gerber MA, et al: Racemic epinephrine in the treatment of croup: Nebulization alone versus nebulization with intermittent positive pressure breathing. *J Pediatr* 1982;101:1028–1031.
Geelhoed GC, Turner J, MacDonald WB: Efficacy of a small single dose of oral dexamethasone for outpatient croup: A double blind placebo controlled trial. *Br Med J* 1996;313:140–142.
Kristjansson S, Berg-Kelly K, Winso E: Inhalation of racemic adrenaline in the treatment of mild and moderately severe croup: Clinical symptom score and oxygen saturation measurements for evaluation of treatment effects. *Acta Pediatr* 1994;83:1156–1160.
Ledwith CA, Shea LM, Mauro RD: Safety and efficacy of nebulized racemic epinephrine in conjunction with oral dexamethasone and mist in the outpatient treatment of croup. *Ann Emerg Med* 1995;25:331–337.
Luria JW, Gonzalez-del-Rey JA, DiBiulio GA, et al: Effectiveness of oral or nebulized dexamethasone for children with mild croup. *Pediatr Adolesc Med* 2001;155:1340–1345.
Rittichier KK, Ledwith CA: Outpatient treatment of moderate croup with dexamethasone: Intramuscular versus oral dosing. *Pediatrics* 2000;106:1344–1348.
Scolnik D, Coates AL, Stephens D, et al: Controlled delivery of high vs low humidity vs mist therapy for croup in emergency departments. *JAMA* 2006;295:1274–1280.
Waisman Y, Klein BL, Boenning DA, et al: Prospective randomized double-blind study comparing L-epinephrine and racemic epinephrine aerosols in the treatment of laryngotracheitis. *Pediatrics* 1992;89:302–306.
Walner DL, Ouanounou S, Donnelly LF, et al: Utility of radiographs in the evaluation of pediatric upper airway obstruction. *Ann Otol Rhinol Laryngol* 1999;108:378–383.
Weber JE, Chudnofsky CR, Younger JG, et al: A randomized comparison of helium-oxygen mixture (Heliox) and racemic epinephrine for the treatment of moderate to severe croup. *Pediatrics* 2001;107:E96.

Epiglottite

Adams WG, Deaver KA, Cochi SL, et al: Decline in childhood Haemophilus influenzae type b (HiB) in the HiB vaccine era. *JAMA* 1993; 269:221–226.
Frantz TD, Rasgon BM: Acute epiglottitis: Changing epidemiologic patterns. *Otolaryngol Head Neck Surg* 1993;109:457–460.
Gorelick MH, Baker MD: Epiglottitis in children, 1979 through 1992: Effects of *Haemophilus influenzae* type b immunization. *Arch Pediatr Adolesc Med* 1994;148:47–50.
Hickerson SL, Kirby RS, Wheeler JG, et al: Epiglottitis: A 9-year case review. *South Med J* 1996;89:487–490.
Kulick RM, Selbst SM, Baker MD, et al: Thermal epiglottitis after swallowing hot beverages. *Pediatrics* 1988;81:441–444.
Murrage KJ, Janzen VD, Ruby RR: Epiglottitis: Adult and pediatric comparisons. *J Otolaryngol* 1988;17:194–198.
Senior BA, Radkowski D, MacArthur C, et al: Changing patterns in pediatric epiglottis: A multi-institutional review, 1980 to 1992. *Laryngoscope* 1994;104:1314–1322.

382.2 • TRACHEITE BATTERICA

La tracheite batterica, un'infezione acuta delle vie aeree superiori, non coinvolge l'epiglottide ma, come l'epiglottite e il croup, è in grado di causare un'ostruzione delle vie aeree potenzialmente letale. Il patogeno isolato più comunemente è *Staphylococcus aureus*, ma sono stati implicati anche *Moraxella catarrhalis*, *H. influenzae* non tipizzabili e microrganismi anaerobi. In passato la maggior parte dei pazienti aveva meno di 3 anni di età, mentre nelle casistiche più recenti l'età media è risultata di 5-7 anni. L'incidenza e la severità non differiscono tra i due sessi. La tracheite batterica, dal momento che spesso si instaura in seguito a un'infezione virale delle vie respiratorie (specialmente una laringotracheite), può essere considerata una complicanza batterica di una malattia virale, più che una patologia batterica primitiva. Quest'entità nosologica potenzialmente fatale è più comune dell'epiglottite nella popolazione vaccinata.

MANIFESTAZIONI CLINICHE. Tipicamente, il bambino presenta una tosse metallica, che sembra rientrare nel quadro di una laringotracheobronchite virale. La febbre elevata e uno stato "tossico" con distress respiratorio possono insorgere immediatamente o dopo alcuni giorni di apparente miglioramento. Il paziente giace supino e non presenta né la scialorrea né la disfagia che si associano all'epiglottite. Il trattamento abituale del croup (adrenalina racemica) è inefficace. Possono essere necessarie l'intubazione o la tracheostomia, anche se, secondo le casistiche più recenti, solo il 50-60% dei pazienti ha richiesto l'intubazione nel corso del trattamento; i pazienti più giovani hanno maggiori probabilità di averne necessità.

La caratteristica patologica principale sembra essere l'edema della mucosa a livello della cartilagine cricodea, complicato da copiose secrezioni spesse, purulente, che talvolta portano alla formazione di pseudomembrane. L'aspirazione di queste secrezioni, sebbene occasionalmente possa fornire un sollievo temporaneo, non sostituisce la creazione di una via aerea artificiale, che è sempre necessaria.

DIAGNOSI. La diagnosi si basa sugli indizi di una malattia batterica delle vie aeree superiori, che comprendono febbre elevata, secrezioni purulente delle vie aeree e assenza dei reperti caratteristici dell'epiglottite. La radiografia, pur non essendo indispensabile, può mostrare reperti caratteristici (Fig. 382-3); durante l'intubazione endotracheale si nota materiale purulento al di sotto delle corde vocali (Fig. 382-4).

TRATTAMENTO. In qualsiasi paziente il cui decorso clinico suggerisca una tracheite batterica, occorre instaurare una terapia antimicrobica appropriata, che comprende abitualmente agenti antistafilococcici.

Quando la tracheite batterica viene diagnosticata tramite laringoscopia diretta o fortemente sospettata su base clinica, si deve prendere seriamente in considerazione il posizionamento di una via aerea artificiale. Può essere necessaria la somministrazione di ossigeno.

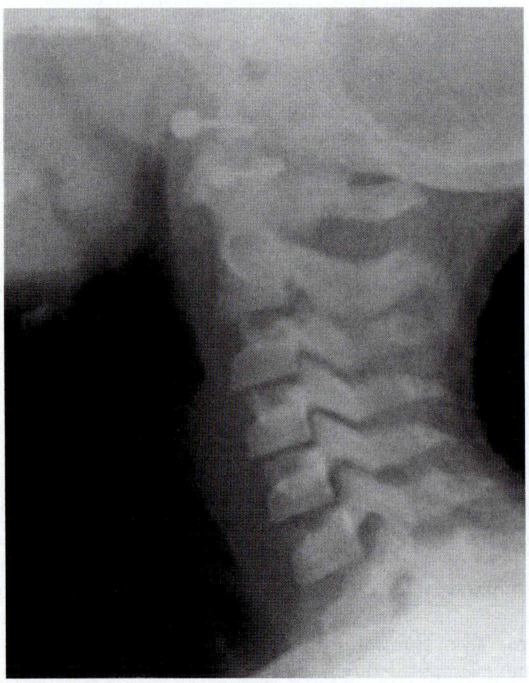

Figura 382-3. Radiografia laterale del collo di un paziente con tracheite batterica, che evidenzia il distacco di pseudomembrane nella trachea. (Da Stroud RH, Friedman NR: An update on inflammatory disorders of the pediatric airway: Epiglottitis, croup, and tracheitis. *Am J Otolaryngol* 2001;22:268-275. Per gentile concessione del Department of Radiology, University of Texas Medical Branch at Galveston.)

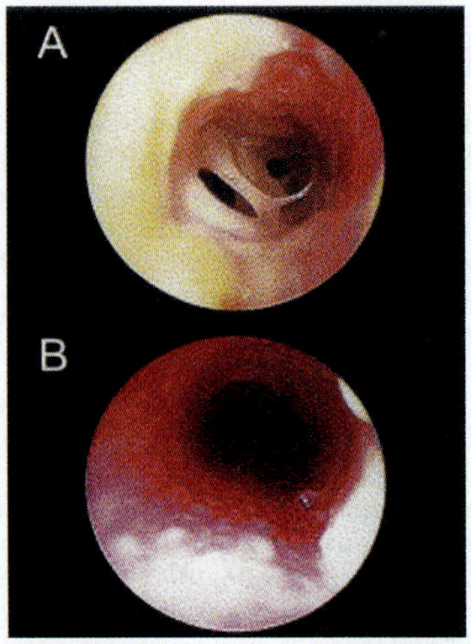

Figura 382-4. Alla broncoscopia con strumento rigido si osservano spesse membrane tracheali. La regione sovraglottica è normale. *A*, Secrezioni membranose spesse e adese. *B*, L'albero tracheobronchiale distale non presenta segni rilevanti. Contrariamente a quanto avviene nel croup, si osservano secrezioni tenaci in tutta la trachea, e, a differenza della bronchite, i bronchi non sono colpiti. (Da Salamone FN, Bobbitt DB, Myer CM, et al: Bacterial tracheitis reexamined: Is there a less severe manifestation? *Otolaryngol Head Neck Surg* 2004;131:871-876. © 2004 American Academy of Otolaryngology - Head and Neck Surgery Foundation, Inc.)

COMPLICANZE. Le radiografie del torace rivelano spesso infiltrati focali, e talvolta addensamenti localizzati. Di frequente è possibile dimostrare radiograficamente un restringimento sottoglottico e un'irregolarità della colonna aerea della trachea. Se la gestione delle vie aeree non è ottimale, può verificarsi un arresto cardiorespiratorio. La tracheite da stafilococco è stata associata alla sindrome da shock tossico (vedi Capitolo 180.2).

PROGNOSI. La prognosi è eccellente per la maggior parte dei pazienti, che abitualmente divengono apiretici entro 2-3 giorni dall'inizio della terapia antimicrobica appropriata, anche se può essere necessaria un'ospedalizzazione prolungata. Di recente sembra sia in atto una tendenza verso una minore morbilità di questa condizione. Con la riduzione dell'edema della mucosa e delle secrezioni purulente, il paziente può essere estubato senza correre rischi, ma deve rimanere sotto attenta osservazione, mentre si continua la terapia con antibiotici e ossigeno.

Berstein T, Brilli R, Jacobs B: Is bacterial tracheitis changing? A 14-month experience in a pediatric intensive care unit. *Clin Infect Dis* 1998;27:458–462.
Brook I: Aerobic and anerobic microbiology of bacterial tracheitis in children. *Pediatr Emerg Care* 1997;13:16–18.
Donnelly LF: *Diagnostic Imaging Pediatrics*. Salt Lake City, Amirys, 2005, p 17.
Eckel HE, Widemann B, Damm M, et al: Airway endoscopy in the diagnosis and treatment of bacterial tracheitis in children. *Int J Pediatr Otorhinolaryngol* 1993;27:147–157.
Faden H: The dramatic change in the epidemiology of pediatric epiglottitis. *Pediatr Emerg Care* 2006;22:443–444.
Salamone FN, Bobbitt DB, Myer CM, et al: Bacterial tracheitis reexamined: Is there a less severe manisfestation? *Otolaryngol Head Neck Surg* 2004;131:871–876.

Capitolo 383 ■ Anomalie congenite della laringe, della trachea e dei bronchi

Lauren D. Holinger

La laringe funge da passaggio per l'aria nella respirazione, da valvola di protezione dei polmoni e da organo principale per l'emissione dei suoni. Le anomalie laringee si manifestano con sintomi tipici, come ostruzione delle vie aeree, difficoltà di alimentazione e anomalie della fonazione. Nell'ostruzione delle vie aeree, la severità delle lesioni ostruenti rende necessarie procedure diagnostiche e interventi chirurgici. I sintomi ostruttivi variano da un lieve stridore a un'ostruzione severa con episodi di apnea, cianosi, retrazioni sovrasternali (*tirage* tracheale) e sottocostali, dispnea e tachipnea. L'ostruzione cronica può causare arresto della crescita.

Le anomalie congenite della trachea e dei bronchi possono creare gravi difficoltà respiratorie fin dai primi istanti di vita. Queste lesioni **intratoraciche**, che causano tipicamente sibili espiratori o stridore, sono spesso scambiate per manifestazioni dell'asma. I sibili espiratori contrastano con lo stridore inspiratorio causato dalle lesioni **extratoraciche** delle anomalie congenite laringee, in particolare la laringomalacia e la paralisi bilaterale delle corde vocali.

383.1 • Laringomalacia

MANIFESTAZIONI CLINICHE. Di tutte le anomalie laringee congenite riscontrate nei pazienti in età pediatrica che presentano stridore, il 60% è causato da laringomalacia, la più comune anomalia congenita laringea e la più frequente causa di stridore nei neonati e nei bambini. Tipicamente lo stridore, inspiratorio, di bassa frequenza, è esacerbato da qualsiasi attività (pianto, agitazione, alimentazione), dalla posizione supina e dalle infezioni virali delle vie aeree superiori. Esso risulta dal collasso delle strutture sovraglottiche verso l'interno, durante l'inspirazione. I sintomi di solito compaiono nelle prime 2 settimane di vita e aumentano di gravità anche fino ai 6 mesi, sebbene un graduale miglioramento possa iniziare in qualsiasi momento. La laringomalacia si associa comunemente a reflusso laringofaringeo.

DIAGNOSI. La diagnosi è confermata dalla laringoscopia con strumento flessibile, eseguita in ambulatorio. Quando il lavoro respiratorio è da moderato a severo, sono indicate le radiografie delle vie aeree e del torace. Se si associa disfagia, possono essere indicati uno studio della deglutizione con contrasto e l'esofagografia. Dal momento che il 15-60% dei neonati con laringomalacia presenta anomalie concomitanti delle vie aeree, nei pazienti con ostruzione moderata o severa si effettua la broncoscopia completa.

TRATTAMENTO. L'osservazione è indicata nella maggior parte dei neonati, poiché la maggior parte dei sintomi si risolve spontaneamente. Il reflusso laringofaringeo deve essere trattato aggressivamente. Per quei pochi pazienti che hanno un'ostruzione talmente severa da rendere inevitabile l'intervento chirurgico (pazienti con eventi potenzialmente fatali, cuore polmonare, cianosi, arresto della crescita), è possibile eseguire la sovraglottoplastica endoscopica, evitando così la tracheotomia.

383.2 • Stenosi sottoglottica congenita

La stenosi sottoglottica congenita è la seconda causa di stridore in ordine di frequenza. Lo stridore è bifasico o principalmente inspiratorio. Il croup ricorrente o persistente è tipico. I primi sintomi insorgono spesso in concomitanza con un'infezione delle vie respiratorie poiché l'edema e le secrezioni spesse del raffreddore comune riducono ulteriormente il calibro di una via area già compromessa (vedi Capitolo 385.1).

383.3 • Paralisi delle corde vocali

La paralisi delle corde vocali è la terza causa più comune di anomalie congenite laringee che causano stridore nei lattanti e nei bambini. Spesso si associano lesioni centrali congenite, come il mielomeningocele, la malformazione di Arnold-Chiari e l'idrocefalo. Essa può far seguito alla correzione chirurgica di anomalie cardiache congenite o di una fistola tracheoesofagea.

La paralisi bilaterale delle corde vocali provoca tipicamente un'ostruzione delle vie aeree che si manifesta con stridore inspiratorio a elevata frequenza: un suono fonatorio o un grido inspiratorio. La forma monolaterale causa aspirazione, tosse e soffocamento. Il pianto è debole e accompagnato da suoni respiratori, ma lo stridore e gli altri sintomi di ostruzione delle vie aeree sono meno comuni.

La diagnosi di paralisi delle corde vocali è effettuata tramite laringoscopia flessibile da svegli. È indicata un'accurata indagine delle cause sottostanti. A causa dell'associazione con altre lesioni congenite, la valutazione comprende la consulenza neurologica e cardiologica, così come l'endoscopia diagnostica della laringe, della trachea e dei bronchi.

La paralisi delle corde vocali nei neonati in genere si risolve spontaneamente nel giro di 6-12 mesi; se bilaterale, può richiedere la tracheotomia temporanea. Nei casi di paralisi monolaterale con aspirazione, la corda vocale paralizzata viene iniettata lateralmente, così che tocchi la corda sana medialmente, riducendo l'aspirazione e le relative complicanze.

383.4 • Atresia e diaframmi laringei congeniti

La maggior parte dei diaframmi laringei congeniti è glottica, con estensione sottoglottica e stenosi sottoglottica associata (Fig. 383-1). Il pianto può avere una tonalità elevata. L'ostruzione delle vie aeree, peraltro non sempre presente, può essere correlata alla stenosi sottoglottica. I diaframmi più spessi possono essere sospettati alla radiografia laterale delle vie aeree. La diagnosi è posta tramite laringoscopia diretta. Il trattamento può richiedere solo l'incisione o la dilatazione. I diaframmi con stenosi sotto-

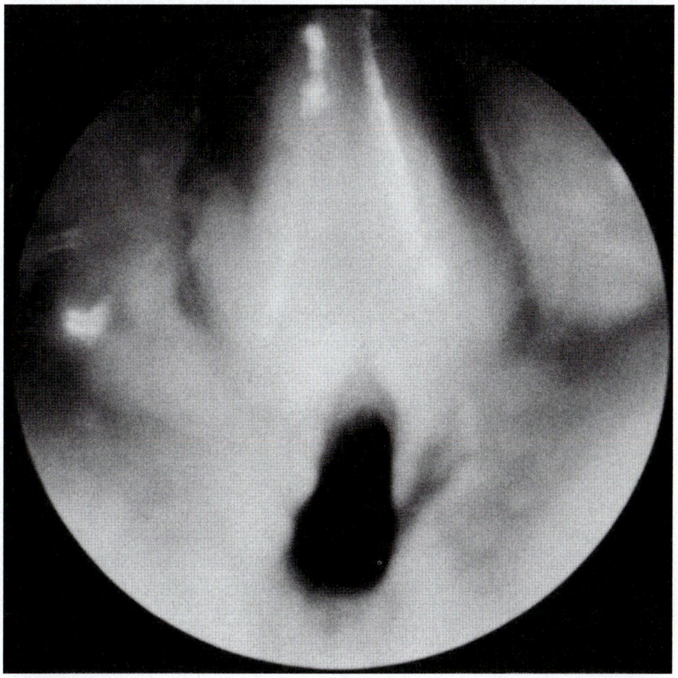

Figura 383-1. Diaframma glottico anteriore. Risulta coinvolta gran parte delle corde vocali vere membranose. (Da Milczuk HA, Smith JD, Everts EC: Congenital laryngeal webs: Surgical management and clinical embryology. *Int J Pediatr Otorhinolaryngol* 2000;52:4.)

glottica associata hanno più probabilità di richiedere l'intervento di aumento della cartilagine cricoidea (ricostruzione laringotracheale).

L'atresia laringea, che si sviluppa come un diaframma glottico completo, è comunemente associata ad agenesia della trachea e fistola tracheoesofagea; non è compatibile con la sopravvivenza a lungo termine.

383.5 • EMANGIOMA SOTTOGLOTTICO CONGENITO

I sintomi di ostruzione delle vie aeree insorgono tipicamente nei primi due mesi di vita. Lo stridore è bifasico, ma in genere più pronunciato durante l'inspirazione. Sono presenti tosse abbaiante, raucedine e sintomi di croup ricorrente o persistente. Le radiografie del collo e del torace possono mostrare il caratteristico restringimento asimmetrico della laringe sottoglottica. Il trattamento è discusso nel Capitolo 387.3.

383.6 • LARINGOCELE E CISTI SACCULARE

Il laringocele è una dilatazione anomala a contenuto aereo del sacculo laringeo. Comunica con il lume della laringe e quando si riempie in modo intermittente di aria causa raucedine e dispnea. La cisti sacculare (cisti congenita della laringe) si distingue dal laringocele in quanto ha il lume isolato dall'interno della laringe e contiene muco, anziché aria. La cisti sacculare può essere visibile radiograficamente, ma la diagnosi si effettua tramite laringoscopia. L'agoaspirato della cisti conferma la diagnosi, ma raramente è curativo. Può essere sufficiente l'escissione endoscopica con il laser a CO_2, anche se spesso si rende necessaria l'escissione esterna.

383.7 • LARINGOSCHISI POSTERIORE E LARINGOTRACHEOESOFAGOSCHISI

La rara laringoschisi posteriore (PLC, *Posterior Laryngeal Cleft*) è caratterizzata da un deficit della linea mediana nella laringe posteriore. Nei casi severi, la schisi si estende inferiormente al tratto cervicale o toracico della trachea, così che non vi è separazione tra la trachea e l'esofago, ovvero si configura una laringotracheoesofagoschisi (LTEC, *LaryngoTracheoEsophageal Cleft*). La schisi laringea può verificarsi con ricorrenza familiare ed essere associata ad agenesia della trachea, fistola tracheoesofagea e anomalie congenite multiple, come la sindrome G, la sindrome di Opiz-Frias e la sindrome di Pallister-Hall.

I sintomi iniziali sono aspirazione e difficoltà respiratoria. Il pianto può essere debole o assente. L'esecuzione dell'esofagogramma richiede estrema cautela. La conferma della diagnosi è ottenuta tramite laringoscopia diretta e broncoscopia. La stabilizzazione delle vie aeree rappresenta una priorità assoluta. Si deve controllare il reflusso gastroesofageo ed effettuare un'attenta valutazione per ricercare eventuali altre anomalie congenite.

383.8 • ANOMALIE VASCOLARI E CARDIACHE

L'arteria innominata aberrante è la causa più comune di tracheomalacia secondaria. Si verificano sibili espiratori e tosse e, raramente, apnea riflessa o "morte apparente". L'intervento chirurgico è raramente necessario. Nei neonati si segue una strategia di attesa, poiché il problema è autolimitante.

Con l'espressione *anello vascolare* si indicano le anomalie vascolari che risultano da un anomalo sviluppo del complesso dell'arco aortico (vedi Capitolo 432). L'anello vascolare completo più comune è il doppio arco aortico, che circonda sia la trachea sia l'esofago, comprimendo entrambi. Salvo rare eccezioni, questi pazienti divengono sintomatici verso il terzo mese di vita. I sintomi respiratori sono predominanti, ma può essere presente anche disfagia. La diagnosi è posta tramite esofagografia con bario, che mostra un'indentazione posteriore dell'esofago da parte dell'anello vascolare. La TC con mezzo di contrasto o la RM forniscono al chirurgo le informazioni di cui ha bisogno (vedi Capitolo 432).

Altre anomalie vascolari comprendono lo *sling* dell'arteria polmonare, che richiede anch'esso la correzione chirurgica. L'anello aperto (incompleto) più comune è l'arteria succlavia destra aberrante. Sebbene comune, è in genere asintomatico e riveste solo un interesse accademico.

I difetti cardiaci congeniti comprimono spesso il bronco principale sinistro o la parte inferiore sinistra della trachea. Qualsiasi condizione che provochi ipertensione polmonare significativa aumenta le dimensioni delle arterie polmonari che, a loro volta, causano compressione del bronco principale sinistro. La correzione della patologia di base, che ha lo scopo di migliorare l'ipertensione polmonare, risolve la compressione delle vie aeree.

383.9 • STENOSI, DIAFRAMMI A MEMBRANA E ATRESIA DELLA TRACHEA

Le stenosi congenite dei tessuti molli e i diaframmi a membrana sono rare. L'unico intervento richiesto può essere la dilatazione. Le stenosi tracheali congenite lunghe, con anelli tracheali completi, si presentano tipicamente nel primo anno di vita, di solito dopo una crisi precipitata da una malattia respiratoria acuta. La diagnosi può essere suggerita dalle radiografie semplici. La TC con contrasto delinea anomalie intratoraciche associate come uno *sling* dell'arteria polmonare, che è presente in un terzo dei pazienti; un quarto dei pazienti presenta anomalie cardiache associate. La broncoscopia è la metodica migliore per definire il grado e l'estensione della stenosi.

Se il diametro delle vie aeree è adeguato, l'intervento chirurgico non è necessario. Quando però la gravità dell'ostruzione impone l'intervento, la resezione del segmento ristretto e la rianastomosi sono sufficienti, nelle forme brevi. Per le forme lunghe di stenosi, con anelli tracheali completi, si effettua una tracheoplastica di scorrimento o un autotrapianto di tessuto tracheale libero, con bypass cardiopolmonare.

L'agenesia e l'atresia tracheali sono anomalie rare, incompatibili con la vita. Si associano spesso ad altre anomalie congenite, in particolare malformazioni laringee e fistola tracheoesofagea. La diagnosi può essere effettuata con la broncoscopia, in un neonato con distress respiratorio severo.

383.10 • CISTI DERIVANTI DALL'INTESTINO ANTERIORE

Le cisti broncogene, esofagee intramurali (duplicazione esofagea) ed enteriche possono tutte causare sintomi da ostruzione respiratoria e disfagia. La diagnosi può essere sospettata quando alla radiografia del torace o alla TC si identifica la massa e, nel caso delle cisti enteriche, le anomalie vertebrali associate. Il trattamento per tutte le forme di cisti derivate dall'intestino anteriore è l'escissione chirurgica.

383.11 • TRACHEOMALACIA E BRONCOMALACIA

Vedi Capitolo 386.

Backer CM, Mavroudis, C, Dunham ME, et al: Free tracheal autograft for long segment congenital tracheal stenosis. *J Pediatr Surg* 2000;35:813–819.

Civantos FJ, Holinger LD: Laryngoceles and saccular cysts in infants and children. *Arch Otolaryngol Head Neck Surg* 1992;118:296–300.

Holinger LD: Histopathology of congenital subglottic stenosis. *Ann Otol Rhinol Laryngol* 1999;108:101–111.

Hughes CA, Rezaee A, Ludemann JP, et al: Management of congenital subglottic hemangioma. *J Otolaryngol* 1999;28:223–228.
Mavroudis C, Backer CL: Vascular rings and pulmonary artery sling. In Mavroudis C, Backer CL (eds): *Pediatric Cardiac Surgery.* Chicago, Mosby, 1994, p 147.
Men S, Ikiz AO, Topcu I, et al: CT and virtual endoscopy findings in congenital laryngeal web. *Int J Pediatr Otorhinolaryngol* 2006;70(6): 1125–1127.
Milczuk HA, Smith JD, Everts EC: Congenital laryngeal webs: Surgical management and clinical embryology. *Int J Pediatr Otorhinolaryngol* 2000;52:1–9.
Moungthong G, Holinger LD: Laryngotracheoesophageal clefts. *Ann Otol Rhinol Laryngol* 1997;106:1002–1011.
Myer CM III, O'Connor DM, Cotton RT: Proposed grading system for subglottic stenosis based on endotracheal tube sizes. *Ann Otol Rhinol Laryngol* 1994;103:319–323.

Capitolo 384 ■ Corpi estranei delle vie aeree Lauren D. Holinger

EPIDEMIOLOGIA ED EZIOLOGIA

I lattanti e i bambini più piccoli usano la bocca per esplorare l'ambiente circostante. Sebbene vi sia stata una diminuzione nelle morti infantili da asfissia per ingestione di oggetti, l'incidenza dell'aspirazione di corpi estranei non è cambiata significativamente. Nella maggior parte dei casi le vittime di aspirazione di corpi estranei sono bambini più grandi o ai primi passi; quelli di età <3 anni rappresentano il 73% dei casi. I bambini non ancora in grado di camminare possono aspirare oggetti dati loro dai fratelli più grandi. Un terzo degli oggetti aspirati sono noccioline, in particolare arachidi; sono inoltre comuni i frammenti di carota cruda, di mela, fagioli secchi, popcorn e semi di girasole o di anguria, così come i piccoli giocattoli o parti di essi.

La complicanza più grave dell'aspirazione di corpi estranei è l'ostruzione completa delle vie aeree. Gli oggetti alimentari sferici o rotondi, come hotdog, acini d'uva, noccioline e caramelle, sono quelli più spesso responsabili. Gli hotdog si osservano raramente come corpo estraneo, poiché i bambini che si soffocano con gli hotdog muoiono di asfissia sul posto, se non si interviene immediatamente. L'ostruzione completa delle vie aeree si manifesta nel bambino cosciente come un improvviso distress respiratorio seguito da incapacità di parlare o tossire.

MANIFESTAZIONI CLINICHE

L'aspirazione di un oggetto nelle vie aeree può dare luogo a tra stadi sintomatologici:

1. **Evento iniziale:** violento parossismo di tosse, soffocamento, intasamento e possibile ostruzione delle vie aeree che si verificano immediatamente appena il corpo estraneo viene aspirato.
2. **Intervallo asintomatico:** il corpo estraneo si insedia, i riflessi si esauriscono e i sintomi irritativi iniziali scompaiono. Questo stadio è il più insidioso e può spiegare un'ampia percentuale di diagnosi ritardate e di sottostima di corpi estranei. È durante questo secondo stadio che il medico può trascurare la possibilità di un incidente da corpo estraneo, lasciandosi fuorviare dall'assenza di sintomi.
3. **Complicanze:** si sviluppano ostruzione, erosione o infezione che attirano nuovamente l'attenzione sulla possibilità di un corpo estraneo. In questo terzo stadio, le complicanze comprendono febbre, tosse, emottisi, polmonite e atelettasia.

Un'anamnesi positiva non deve mai essere ignorata; una negativa può essere fuorviante. Episodi di soffocamento o di tosse accompagnati da sibili sono altamente suggestivi di un corpo estraneo nelle vie aeree. Poiché i corpi estranei bronchiali più frequenti sono le noccioline, il medico interroga i genitori del bambino proprio a questo riguardo; se in famiglia c'è l'abitudine di consumare noccioline, si effettua rapidamente la broncoscopia.

La maggior parte dei corpi estranei si insedia in un bronco (quello destro nel 58% dei casi); la localizzazione laringea o tracheale si verificano nel 10% circa dei casi. Un corpo estraneo esofageo può comprimere la trachea ed essere scambiato per un corpo estraneo delle vie respiratorie. Il paziente è asintomatico e la radiografia normale nel 15-30% dei casi. I corpi estranei radiopachi rappresentano il 10-25% dei casi. La TC o la RM aiutano a definire i corpi estranei radiotrasparenti. Se vi è un elevato indice di sospetto, la broncoscopia deve essere effettuata nonostante la negatività delle indagini radiologiche.

TRATTAMENTO

Il trattamento di scelta per i corpi estranei delle vie aeree è la rapida rimozione endoscopica con strumento rigido. Prima di eseguire la broncoscopia si procede alle indagini preoperatorie e alla preparazione del paziente con un'adeguata idratazione e lo svuotamento dello stomaco. I corpi estranei delle vie aeree di solito vengono rimossi lo stesso giorno in cui si prende in considerazione la diagnosi per la prima volta.

384.1 • CORPI ESTRANEI NELLA LARINGE

L'ostruzione completa causa rapidamente asfissia, a meno che non sia risolta immediatamente con la manovra di Heimlich. Di

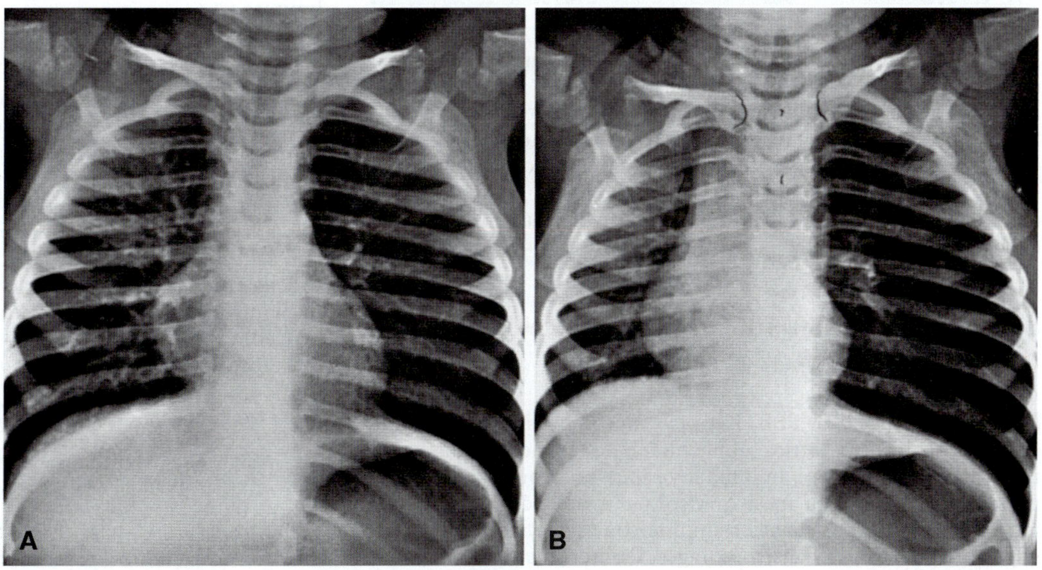

Figura 384-1. *A*, Radiografia normale del torace effettuata durante l'inspirazione in un bambino con un frammento di nocciolina nel bronco principale destro. *B*, Radiografia in espirazione dello stesso bambino che mostra il classico enfisema ostruttivo (intrappolamento d'aria) dal lato colpito (sinistro). L'aria esce dal lato normale, consentendo al polmone di svuotarsi. Il mediastino si sposta verso il lato non ostruito.

solito gli oggetti che provocano ostruzione parziale sono piatti e sottili; si incuneano tra le corde vocali sul piano sagittale, causando sintomi di croup, raucedine, tosse, stridore e dispnea.

384.2 • CORPI ESTRANEI NELLA TRACHEA

Il soffocamento e l'aspirazione si verificano nel 90% dei pazienti con corpi estranei tracheali, lo stridore nel 60% e i sibili nel 50%. Le radiografie anteroposteriori e laterali dei tessuti molli del collo (lastre delle vie aeree) sono anormali nel 92% dei bambini, mentre le radiografie del torace lo sono solo nel 58% dei casi.

384.3 • CORPI ESTRANEI NEI BRONCHI

La radiografia del torace in proiezione anteroposteriore e laterale rappresenta lo standard nella valutazione dei neonati e dei bambini con sospetta aspirazione di un corpo estraneo. L'addome è incluso. Una buona immagine anteroposteriore del torace in espirazione è la più utile. Durante l'espirazione, il corpo estraneo bronchiale ostacola la fuoriuscita dell'aria dal polmone ostruito, provocando un enfisema ostruttivo (intrappolamento d'aria) con inflazione persistente del polmone colpito e spostamento del mediastino verso il lato opposto (Fig. 384-1). L'intrappolamento d'aria è una complicanza immediata, a differenza dell'atelettasia che si sviluppa tardivamente. Le radiografie laterali declivi o la fluoroscopia possono fornire le stesse informazioni, ma non sono necessarie. Sono l'anamnesi e l'esame obiettivo, non le radiografie, a determinare l'indicazione alla broncoscopia, che è sia diagnostica sia terapeutica.

Babin E, Sigston E, Bigeon JY, et al: How we do it: Management of tracheobronchial foreign bodies in children. *Clin Otolaryngol Allied Sci* 2004;29:750–753.

Nova A, Muntz H, Clary R: Utility of conventional radiography in pediatric airway foreign bodies. *Ann Otol Rhinol Laryngol* 1998;107:834–838.

White DR, Zdanski CJ, Drake AF: Comparison of pediatric airway foreign bodies over fifty years. *South Med J* 2004;97:434–436.

Williams H: Inhaled foreign bodies. *Arch Dis Child Educ Pract Ed* 2005;90:ep31–ep33.

Capitolo 385 ■ Stenosi laringotracheale, stenosi sottoglottica Lauren D. Holinger

La stenosi laringotracheale è la causa più frequente di ostruzione delle vie aeree che richiede la tracheostomia nei lattanti. Anche la glottide (corde vocali) e la parte superiore della trachea sono compromesse nella maggior parte delle stenosi laringee, in particolare in quelle causate da intubazione endotracheale. La stenosi sottoglottica è considerata congenita quando non vi è altra causa apparente, come un'anamnesi di trauma laringeo o di intubazione.

385.1 • STENOSI SOTTOGLOTTICA CONGENITA (VEDI CAPITOLO 383.2)

MANIFESTAZIONI CLINICHE. Il tipico sintomo di presentazione della stenosi sottoglottica congenita è lo stridore, bifasico o inspiratorio. In questi bambini, si verifica un croup ricorrente o persistente all'età di 6 mesi o ancora più precocemente. L'edema di lieve entità, associato a un'infezione delle vie respiratorie superiori o a reflusso gastroesofageo, compromette le vie aeree già ristrette. La diagnosi è suggerita dalle radiografie delle vie aeree e confermata dalla laringoscopia diretta. Il trattamento dipende dalla gravità dell'ostruzione ed è lo stesso delle stenosi sottoglottiche acquisite. Poiché nella maggior parte dei casi la stenosi sottoglottica congenita è cartilaginea, la dilatazione o la chirurgia laser non sempre sono efficaci. La decompressione laringotracheale anteriore (**split cricoideo**) o la ricostruzione con trapianti di cartilagine abitualmente permettono di evitare la tracheostomia.

385.2 • STENOSI LARINGOTRACHEALE ACQUISITA

Il 90% delle stenosi acquisite è correlato all'intubazione endotracheale. Quando la pressione del tubo endotracheale contro la mucosa è maggiore della pressione capillare, si verifica ischemia, seguita da necrosi e ulcerazione. Con l'esposizione della cartilagine si sviluppa un'infezione secondaria con pericondrite. Intorno alle ulcerazioni si forma tessuto di granulazione. Queste alterazioni, insieme all'edema della laringe, si risolvono di solito spontaneamente dopo l'estubazione. Una piccola percentuale di casi sviluppa edema cronico e stenosi fibrosa.

I fattori che predispongono alla stenosi laringea comprendono: (1) reflusso laringofaringeo di acido e pepsina dallo stomaco, che esacerba il trauma provocato dal tubo endotracheale. Un ulteriore danno deriva dalle aree lasciate non protette, a causa della perdita di mucosa; (2) la stenosi sottoglottica congenita provoca un restringimento della laringe predisponendola ai traumi legati all'utilizzo di un tubo endotracheale di dimensioni appropriate per l'età; (3) altri fattori correlati al paziente comprendono sepsi e infezione, disidratazione, malnutrizione, disturbi infiammatori cronici e immunosoppressione; (4) la causa più comune di danno laringeo è l'utilizzo di un tubo di calibro eccessivo. Un tubo che consente un piccolo passaggio di aria alla fine del ciclo inspiratorio minimizza il potenziale trauma; (5) altri fattori estrinseci, come un'intubazione traumatica, reintubazioni multiple, uno spostamento del tubo endotracheale e la durata dell'intubazione, possono contribuire in grado variabile nei singoli pazienti.

Le manifestazioni cliniche delle stenosi acquisite e congenite (vedi Capitolo 383.2) sono simili. Il croup spastico, ossia l'esordio improvviso di croup severo nelle prime ore del mattino, in genere è dovuto a un episodio di reflusso laringofaringeo con laringospasmo transitorio e conseguente edema laringeo. Questi episodi, che spaventano molto, si risolvono rapidamente, spesso prima che i familiari e il bambino raggiungano il pronto soccorso.

DIAGNOSI. La diagnosi è confermata dalla laringoscopia diretta e dalla broncoscopia. La TC ad alta risoluzione ha un valore limitato.

TRATTAMENTO. Dipende dalla gravità, dalla localizzazione e dal tipo di stenosi (cartilaginea o dei tessuti molli). Nei casi lievi può non essere necessario un intervento operatorio poiché la via aerea tende a migliorare con la crescita del bambino. Le stenosi moderate dei tessuti molli si trattano in endoscopia usando dilatazioni delicate o il laser a CO_2. Le stenosi laringotracheali severe richiedono generalmente interventi chirurgici di espansione laringotracheale o la resezione della porzione stenosata della laringe o della trachea (resezione cricotracheale). Si cerca in ogni modo di evitare la tracheotomia, utilizzando tecniche endoscopiche o procedure chirurgiche a cielo aperto, come la decompressione laringotracheale anteriore (*split* o divisione cricoidea).

Benjamin B: Prolonged intubation injuries of the larynx: Endoscopic diagnosis, classification, and treatment. *Ann Otol Rhinol Laryngol Suppl* 1993;160:1–15.

Cotton RT, Gray SD, Miller RP, et al: Update of the Cincinnati experience in pediatric laryngotracheal reconstruction. *Laryngoscope* 1989;99:1111–1116.

Gerber M, Stern Y, Walner D, et al: Role of laryngoscopy, dual pH probe monitoring, and laryngeal mucosa biopsy in the diagnosis of pharyngoesophageal reflux. *Ann Otol Rhinol Laryngol* 2001;110:299–304.
Liu H, Chen J, Holinger L, et al: Histopathologic fundamentals of acquired laryngeal stenosis. *Pediatr Pathol Lab Med* 1995;15:655–677.

Capitolo 386 ■ Broncomalacia e tracheomalacia Jonathan D. Finder

La condromalacia della trachea o di un bronco principale è una causa comune di sibilo (*wheezing*) persistente nell'infanzia. In questi disturbi, non vi è una cartilagine sufficiente a mantenere la pervietà delle vie aeree durante il ciclo respiratorio. La tracheomalacia e la broncomalacia possono essere primitive o secondarie (Tab. 386-1). Sebbene le forme primitive siano di frequente riscontro nei neonati prematuri, la maggior parte dei pazienti affetti è nata a termine. La tracheomalacia e la broncomalacia vengono dette secondarie quando la via aerea centrale è compressa da strutture adiacenti (per es. un anello vascolare) o la mancanza di cartilagine è dovuta a una fistola tracheoesofagea. La laringomalacia può associarsi alla broncomalacia o alla tracheomalacia primitive (vedi anche Capitolo 383.1). È inoltre possibile osservare il coinvolgimento di tutte le vie aeree centrali (laringotracheobroncomalacia).

MANIFESTAZIONI CLINICHE. La tracheomalacia e la broncomalacia primitive sono principalmente disturbi dei lattanti, con un rapporto maschi:femmine di 2:1. Il reperto dominante, un sibilo monofonico a bassa frequenza, è più accentuato a livello delle vie aeree centrali. I genitori descrivono spesso una congestione respiratoria persistente anche in assenza di infezioni respiratorie virali. Quando la lesione coinvolge solo un bronco principale (per lo più il sinistro), il sibilo è più udibile da quel lato. In caso di tracheomalacia, il sibilo è più forte sulla trachea. Non si verificano iperinflazione e/o retrazioni sottocostali, a meno che il paziente non abbia anche l'asma o un'altra causa di ostruzione delle piccole vie aeree. In assenza di asma, i pazienti con tracheomalacia e broncomalacia non traggono beneficio dalla somministrazione di broncodilatatori. Le forme acquisite si osservano in associazione con anelli vascolari (nel qual caso possono persistere dopo la correzione chirurgica), fistole tracheoesofagee, cardiomegalia e dopo trapianto polmonare.

DIAGNOSI. La diagnosi definitiva di tracheomalacia e broncomalacia è stabilita tramite broncoscopia con strumento flessibile o rigido. La lesione è difficile da diagnosticare alla radiografia semplice, ma la fluoroscopia può dimostrare il collasso dinamico ed evitare l'utilizzo di tecniche diagnostiche invasive. I test di funzionalità polmonare possono mostrare un quadro di riduzione del picco di flusso espiratorio e l'appiattimento della curva flusso-volume. Altri strumenti diagnostici importanti comprendono la RM e la TC; la RM è particolarmente utile quando sussiste la possibilità di un anello vascolare, e dovrebbe essere effettuata qualora si osservasse un arco aortico destro alla radiografia semplice.

TABELLA 386-1. Classificazione della tracheomalacia

TRACHEOMALACIA PRIMITIVA
Assenza congenita delle cartilagini di supporto tracheali
TRACHEOMALACIA SECONDARIA
Atresia esofagea/fistola tracheoesofagea
Anelli vascolari (doppio arco aortico)
Compressione della trachea da parte di un'arteria innominata aberrante
Compressione della trachea da parte di masse mediastiniche
Cartilagini tracheali abnormemente morbide associate a malattie del connettivo
Ventilazione meccanica prolungata/pneumopatia cronica

DaMcNamara VM, Crabbe DC: Tracheomalacia. *Paediatr Respir Rev* 2004;5:147-154.

TRATTAMENTO. Il drenaggio posturale può aiutare a eliminare le secrezioni. Gli agenti β-adrenergici andrebbero evitati in assenza di asma. L'ipratropio bromuro nebulizzato può essere utile. Nei pazienti con forme severe sono stati utilizzati stent endobronchiali, che però presentano un'elevata incidenza di complicanze, dall'ostruzione delle vie aeree da parte di tessuto di granulazione all'erosione di strutture vascolari adiacenti. Nei casi più gravi può essere indicata la pressione positiva continua nelle vie aeree (CPAP, *Constant Positive Airway Pressure*), somministrata attraverso la tracheostomia. L'approccio chirurgico (artopessi e broncopessi) è raramente necessario e solo per i pazienti con apnea, cianosi e bradicardia (crisi cianotiche) da ostruzione delle vie aeree, potenzialmente fatali.

PROGNOSI. La broncomalacia e la tracheomalacia primitive hanno una prognosi eccellente, poiché il flusso aereo migliora con la crescita della via aerea. Il sibilo a riposo in genere si risolve entro i 3 anni di età. La prognosi delle forme secondarie e acquisite varia in base alla causa. I pazienti con asma associato necessitano di un importante trattamento di supporto.

Boogaard R, Huijsmans SH, Pijnenburg MW, et al: Tracheomalacia and bronchomalacia in children: incidence and patient characteristics. *Chest* 2005;128:3391–3397.
Carden KA, Boiselle PM, Waltz DA, et al: Tracheomalacia and tracheobronchomalacia in children and adults: An in-depth review. *Chest* 2005;127:984–1005.
Filler RM, Forte V, Chait P: Tracheobronchial stenting for the treatment of airway obstruction. *J Pediatr Surg* 1998;33:304–311.
Finder JD: Primary bronchomalacia in infants and children. *J Pediatr* 1997;130:59–66.
Masters IB, Chang AB, Patterson L, et al: Series of laryngomalacia, tracheomalacia, and bronchomalacia disorders and their associations with other conditions in children. *Pediatr Pulmonol* 2002;34:189–195.
McNamara VM, Crabbe DC: Tracheomalacia. *Paediatr Respir Rev* 2004;5:147–154.
Panitch HB, Keklikian EN, Motley RA, et al: Effect of altering smooth muscle tone on maximal expiratory flows in patients with tracheomalacia. *Pediatr Pulmonol* 1990;9:170–176.
Yalcin E, Dogru D, Ozcelik U, et al: Tracheomalacia and bronchomalacia in 34 children: clinical and radiologic profiles and associations with other diseases. *Clin Pediatr* 2005;44:777–781.

Capitolo 387 ■ Neoplasie della laringe, della trachea e dei bronchi Lauren D. Holinger

387.1 • Noduli delle corde vocali

Sebbene i noduli delle corde vocali non siano vere e proprie neoplasie, sono la causa più comune di raucedine cronica nei bambini. L'uso eccessivo o improprio delle corde vocali provoca la formazione di noduli, alla giunzione tra il terzo medio e anteriore del margine libero delle corde vocali. Queste tumefazioni simmetriche, bilaterali, interferiscono con la fonazione e causano ai bambini uno sforzo vocale. Tali noduli possono insorgere nei lattanti e sono esacerbati dal reflusso gastroesofageo.

La terapia vocale può essere efficace nei pazienti collaboranti, ma per la maggior parte di bambini ai primi passi e di quelli più grandi si rende necessaria la terapia comportamentale. I noduli di solito si risolvono nei primi anni dell'adolescenza, via via che il soggetto matura e impara a non abusare della voce. L'asportazione chirurgica è raramente indicata, ma può essere necessaria se il bambino non è in grado di comunicare adeguatamente, se si sviluppa afonia o se qualunque tentativo di esprimersi provoca tensione o sforzo.

Il reflusso laringofaringeo esacerba comunemente l'abuso vocale, peggiorando l'edema delle corde vocali. Quando il fattore principale è l'abuso vocale, la voce peggiora alla sera, mentre quando è il reflusso laringofaringeo, la raucedine è più accentuata al mattino. È indicata una terapia antireflusso (vedi Capitolo 320.1).

387.2 • Papillomatosi respiratoria ricorrente

EPIDEMIOLOGIA ED EZIOLOGIA. I papillomi sono le neoplasie più comuni delle vie respiratorie, nei bambini, con una frequenza di 4,3/100 000. Si tratta di semplici verruche, ossia tumori benigni, causate dal papillomavirus umano (HPV, *Human Papilloma Virus*) (vedi Capitolo 263); le stesse alterazioni anatomopatologiche si osservano nei condilomi acuminati (verruche vaginali). Gli HPV di tipo 6 e 11 si associano per lo più alla malattia laringea. Il 50% insorge nei bambini di età <5 anni, ma la diagnosi può essere fatta a qualsiasi età. Il 60% dei bambini con papillomatosi respiratoria ricorrente sono figli di madri con condilomi attivi. Sono stati riportati molti casi di PRR nei neonati, reperto che suggerisce la possibilità di una trasmissione intrauterina dell'HPV.

MANIFESTAZIONI CLINICHE. Queste lesioni squamose benigne possono provocare raucedine cronica nei lattanti. Per la maggior parte sono solitarie e insorgono nella laringe, in particolare sulle corde vocali, ma nel 31% dei casi colpiscono altre parti delle vie respiratorie: naso, faringe (specialmente l'uvula e il palato molle posteriore), trachea, bronchi e polmoni. Con la progressiva crescita sulle corde vocali, la raucedine peggiora e la comunicazione diviene difficoltosa. Può insorgere distress respiratorio. L'asportazione chirurgica è una scelta che ha effetti sulla qualità di vita, perché migliora la fonazione. L'intervento diviene una necessità medica quando l'ostruzione delle vie aeree progredisce. Spesso i sintomi insorgono per la prima volta nel sonno, con manifestazioni tipiche dell'apnea ostruttiva del sonno. Il distress respiratorio progressivo che si manifesta durante il sonno, l'esercizio, le attività quotidiane e, alla fine, anche a riposo, indica la necessità dell'intervento chirurgico.

TRATTAMENTO. Il trattamento della papillomatosi respiratoria ricorrente è la rimozione chirurgica endoscopica. La maggior parte dei chirurghi nel Nord America preferisce il *microdebrider*, mentre gli altri si avvalgono del laser a CO_2. La tracheostomia è raramente necessaria; la terapia medica, compresa l'iniezione di cidofovir, può essere di qualche beneficio nelle lesioni gravi e ricorrenti. Il reflusso laringofaringeo può richiedere il trattamento quando la laringite da reflusso è un fattore causale.

La vaccinazione per l'HPV può ridurre l'infezione materna e la sua trasmissione perinatale al neonato.

387.3 • Emangioma sottoglottico congenito

Gli emangiomi divengono sintomatici entro i primi 2 mesi di vita, e si presentano quasi sempre prima del sesto mese. Lo stridore è bifasico, ma abitualmente più pronunciato durante l'inspirazione. Il lattante può essere rauco, avere una tosse abbaiante e presentarsi con un croup. Il 50% di tutti gli emangiomi sottoglottici congeniti si associa a lesioni cutanee, spesso nella zona facciale mandibolare. Le radiografie delineano classicamente un restringimento sottoglottico asimmetrico. La diagnosi si effettua in laringoscopia diretta.

Il trattamento medico comprende l'uso di steroidi per via sistemica. Si somministra prednisone (2-4 mg/kg/die) per via orale, per 4-6 settimane, o anche meno se la lesione si stabilizza precocemente. Il dosaggio viene poi scalato. In assenza di risposta, si interrompe la terapia. È stato utilizzato anche l'interferone $\alpha 2a$ nel trattamento degli emangiomi pericolosi per la vita, corticoresistenti, che coinvolgono la via aerea e rischiano di compromettere massivamente le strutture vitali (vedi Capitolo 649).

Sebbene la tracheostomia stabilizzi una via aerea sicura, ci si dovrebbe sforzare in ogni modo di cercare un'alternativa. I corticosteroidi possono essere iniettati direttamente nella lesione. L'escissione endoscopica con il laser a CO_2 è efficace. La combinazione di diversi approcci aumenta la possibilità di evitare il ricorso alla tracheotomia. L'escissione chirurgica esterna è indicata per le lesioni rare.

387.4 • Anomalie vascolari

Le malformazioni vascolari non sono vere lesioni neoplastiche. Hanno una normale velocità di turnover e varie anomalie di canali. Sono classificate in base al tipo predominante (capillari, venose, arteriose, linfatiche o una combinazione di queste). Le malformazioni a flusso lento hanno componenti capillari, linfatiche o venose. In passato, furono chiamate erroneamente emangiomi capillari, igromi cistici o linfangiomi, ed emangiomi cavernosi, rispettivamente.

Le malformazioni linfatiche (igromi cistici) insorgono raramente nella laringe. Quando avviene, sono invariabilmente un'estensione di una malattia da un'altra sede, nella testa o nel collo. L'ostruzione aerea può richiedere la tracheostomia. La lesione può essere ridotta con il laser a CO_2.

387.5 • Altre neoplasie laringee

La *neurofibromatosi* (vedi Capitolo 596.1) coinvolge raramente la laringe. Quando a esserne colpito è un bambino, si effettua una resezione locale limitata per mantenere la pervietà della via aerea e ottimizzare la voce. L'eradicazione chirurgica completa è virtualmente impossibile senza una resezione disabilitante di strutture laringee vitali. La maggior parte dei chirurghi sceglie una chirurgia sintomatica meno aggressiva, a causa della natura infiltrante e scarsamente circoscritta di questi fibromi. Il *rabdomiosarcoma* (vedi Capitolo 500) e gli altri tumori maligni della laringe sono rari. I sintomi di raucedine e progressiva ostruzione respiratoria impongono una valutazione iniziale mediante laringoscopia ambulatoriale con strumento flessibile.

387.6 • Neoplasie tracheali

La maggior parte dei tumori tracheali è benigna; i due più comuni sono lo *pseudotumore infiammatorio* e l'*amartoma*. Lo pseudotumore infiammatorio è probabilmente una reazione a una precedente infezione tracheale o a un insulto traumatico. Il tumore è caratterizzato da crescita lenta e può avere un'invasività locale. Gli amartomi sono tumori di elementi tissutali primitivi, anormali per proporzione e struttura.

Le neoplasie tracheali, che si presentano con stridore, sibili, tosse o polmonite, è raro vengano diagnosticate prima che sia ostruito il 75% del lume. Poiché i loro sintomi mimano quelli dell'asma, avviene spesso che le neoplasie tracheali vengano scambiate per questa patologia. La radiografia del torace o della via aerea possono identificare l'ostruzione. Gli esami di funzionalità polmonare dimostrano una curva flusso-volume anomala. Una blanda risposta ai broncodilatatori può risultare fuorviante.

387.7 • Tumori bronchiali

I tumori bronchiali sono rari; due terzi di essi sono maligni. Gli "adenomi" sono i più comuni, rappresentando il 30% di tutti i tumori polmonari. Il carcinoma broncogeno è il secondo in ordine di frequenza, manifestandosi nel 20% circa dei casi. La diagnosi è confermata dalla broncoscopia e dalla biopsia; il trattamento dipende dall'istologia.

Derkay CS: Recurrent respiratory papillomatosis. *Laryngoscope* 2001;111: 57–67.

Desai DP, Maddalozzo J, Holinger LD: Granular cell tumor of the trachea. *Otolaryngol Head Neck Surg* 1999;120:595–598.

Desai DP, Mahoney EM, Miller RP, et al: Case report: Mucoepidermoid carcinoma of the trachea in a child. *Int J Pediatr Otorhinolaryngol* 1998;45:259–263.

Hughes CA, Rezaee A, Ludemann JP, et al: Management of congenital subglottic hemangioma. *J Otolaryngol* 1999;28:223–228.

Newhouse MT, Martin L, Kay JM, Miller JD: Laser resection of a pedunculated tracheal adenoma. *Chest* 2000;118:262–265.

Reeves WC, Ruparelia SS, Swanson KI, et al: National registry for juvenile-onset recurrent respiratory papillomatosis. *Arch Otolaryngol Head Neck Surg* 2003;129:976–982.

Ruparelia S, Unger ER, Nisenbaum R, et al: Predictors of remission in juvenile-onset recurrent respiratory papillomatosis. *Arch Otolaryngol Head Neck Surg* 2003;129:1275–1278.

Schraff S, Derkay CS, Burke B, Lawson L: American Society of Pediatric Otolaryngology members' experience with recurrent respiratory papillomatosis and the use of adjuvant therapy. *Arch Otolaryngol Head Neck Surg* 2004; 130:1039–1042.

Tasca RA, Clarke RW: Recurrent respiratory papillomatosis. *Arch Dis Child* 2006;91:689–691.

Vijavasekaram S, White DR, Hartley BB, et al: Open excision of subglottic hemangiomas to avoid tracheostomy. *Arch Otolaryngol Head Neck Surg* 2006;132:159–163.

Zacharisen MC, Conley SF: Recurrent respiratory papillomatosis in children: masquerader of common respiratory diseases. *Pediatrics* 2006;118: 1925–1931.

Capitolo 388 ■ Sibili, bronchiolite e bronchite

388.1 • Sibili nei lattanti: bronchiolite

Kimberly Danieli Watts e Denise M. Goodman

DEFINIZIONE E FISIOPATOLOGIA GENERALE

Un **sibilo** (*wheezing*) è un suono musicale e continuo che origina da oscillazioni in vie aeree ristrette. I sibili sono udibili prevalentemente in espirazione, per effetto di un'ostruzione critica delle vie aeree. Essi sono **polifonici** quando vi è un restringimento diffuso delle vie aeree (per es. nell'asma), che causa vari toni o livelli di ostruzione al flusso aereo. Vengono invece definiti **monofonici** quando hanno un solo tono e si producono nelle vie aeree di calibro maggiore durante l'espirazione, come nella tracheomalacia distale o nella broncomalacia. Quando l'ostruzione si verifica a livello delle vie aeree extratoraciche durante l'inspirazione, il suono è detto **stridore**.

I lattanti sono particolarmente inclini a sviluppare sibili a causa di meccanismi di tipo diverso, rispetto ai bambini più grandi e agli adulti. L'ostruzione al flusso è influenzata dal calibro delle vie aeree e dalla compliance del polmone. La resistenza al flusso aereo attraverso un tubo è inversamente proporzionale al raggio del tubo alla quarta potenza. Nei bambini di età <5 anni, il piccolo calibro delle vie aeree periferiche può contribuire fino al 50% della resistenza totale al flusso aereo. Un restringimento ulteriore, anche lieve, può limitare ancora di più il flusso, determinando l'insorgenza di sibili.

Quando la parete toracica ha un'elevata compliance, come avviene nei neonati, la pressione verso l'interno prodotta in espirazione porta la via aerea al collasso. Nei lattanti la limitazione al flusso è ulteriormente aggravata dalle differenze nella composizione della cartilagine tracheale e nel tono della muscolatura liscia, che determinano un ulteriore aumento della compliance delle vie aeree. La combinazione di tutti questi meccanismi rende il lattante più suscettibile al collasso delle vie aeree, all'aumento di resistenza e al conseguente sibilo. Molte di queste condizioni vengono superate con la crescita, già nel primo anno di vita.

Fattori immunologici e molecolari possono contribuire a influenzare la tendenza del lattante a sviluppare sibili. Rispetto ai bambini più grandi e agli adulti, i lattanti tendono ad avere livelli più elevati di linfociti e neutrofili, piuttosto che di mastociti ed eosinofili, nel liquido di broncolavaggio alveolare. Per spiegare i sibili in questi pazienti sono stati chiamati in causa anche svariati mediatori dell'infiammazione, come l'istamina, i leucotrieni e le interleuchine. Si può inoltre verificare una "programmazione" fetale e/o postnatale precoce, in cui la struttura e la funzione del polmone sono influenzate da fattori come la nutrizione fetale e l'esposizione fetale o neonatale al fumo materno.

EZIOLOGIA

Sebbene i sibili nei lattanti siano per lo più causati da un'infiammazione (generalmente bronchiolite), possono associarsi anche a molte altre entità (Tab. 388-1).

BRONCHIOLITE ACUTA E INFIAMMAZIONE DELLE VIE AEREE. Un'infezione può causare ostruzione al flusso per restringimento interno delle vie aeree.

La **bronchiolite acuta** è prevalentemente una malattia virale. Il virus respiratorio sinciziale (RSV) è responsabile di più del 50% dei casi (vedi Capitolo 257). Altri agenti comprendono i virus parainfluenzali (vedi Capitolo 256), gli adenovirus, il *Mycoplasma* e, occasionalmente, altri virus. Il metapneumovirus umano (vedi Capitolo 258) è un'importante causa primaria di infezione respiratoria virale, ma può anche dare luogo a una coinfezione insieme con l'RSV. Non vi sono evidenze di una causa batterica per la bronchiolite, sebbene la polmonite batterica sia talvolta confusa clinicamente con la bronchiolite e quest'ultima sia in casi rari seguita da una sovrainfezione batterica.

Circa 50 000-80 000 casi di ospedalizzazione all'anno, tra i bambini di età inferiore a un anno, sono attribuibili a infezione da RSV, con 200-500 decessi all'anno negli Stati Uniti. L'aumento del tasso di ospedalizzazione può riflettere una maggiore frequentazione di asili diurni da parte dei bambini, un cambiamento dei criteri di ricovero ospedaliero e/o un aumento della sopravvivenza dei neonati prematuri e di altri soggetti a rischio di malattia da RSV severa.

La bronchiolite è più comune nei maschi, nei bambini non allattati al seno e in quelli che vivono in condizioni di affollamento. I bambini più grandi e gli adulti della famiglia sono una comune fonte di infezione e possono accusare solo lievi sintomi respiratori. Le manifestazioni cliniche di malattia delle vie respiratorie inferiori (LRTI, *Lower Respiratory Tract Illness*) osservate nei lattanti possono essere minime nei pazienti più grandi, in cui l'edema bronchiolare è meglio tollerato.

Non tutti i lattanti colpiti dall'infezione sviluppano la LRTI. Sembra che fattori anatomici e immunologici legati all'ospite giochino un ruolo significativo, nella gravità della sindrome clinica. I lattanti che di base presentano vie aeree più piccole e una ridotta funzione polmonare hanno un decorso più severo. Inoltre, l'infezione da RSV stimola una risposta immunitaria complessa. Gli eosinofili degranulano e rilasciano la proteina cationica eosinofila, che svolge un'azione citotossica sull'epitelio delle vie aeree. Anche il rilascio di immunoglobuline E (IgE) può essere correlato all'insorgenza di sibili. Altri mediatori coinvolti nella patogenesi dell'infiammazione delle vie aeree comprendono chemiochine, come l'interleuchina 8 (IL-8), la proteina infiammatoria dei macrofagi (MIP, *Macrophage Inflammatory Protein*) 1α, e il RANTES (*Regulated on Activation, Normal T cell Expressed and Secreted*, regolato all'attivazione, espresso e secreto dai lin-

TABELLA 388-1. Diagnosi differenziale dei sibili nell'infanzia

INFEZIONI
- Virali
  - Virus respiratorio sinciziale
  - Metapneumovirus umano
  - Virus parainfluenzali
  - Adenovirus
  - Virus influenzali
  - Rinovirus
- Altre
  - *Chlamydia trachomatis*
  - Tubercolosi
  - Istoplasmosi
  - Papillomatosi

ASMA
- Sibili transitori
  - Il fattore di rischio iniziale è principalmente la ridotta dimensione del polmone
- Sibili persistenti
  - I fattori di rischio iniziali comprendono l'esposizione al fumo passivo, un'anamnesi di asma materno ed elevati livelli di immunoglobuline E (IgE) nel primo anno di vita
  - Ad aumentato rischio di sviluppare asma
- Sibili a esordio tardivo

ANOMALIE ANATOMICHE
- Anomalie delle vie aeree centrali
  - Laringo-, tracheo- e/o broncomalacia
  - Fistola tracheoesofagea (in particolare fistola a H)
  - Laringoschisi (con conseguente aspirazione)
- Anomalie estrinseche delle vie aeree che danno luogo a compressione del lume
  - Anello o sling vascolare
  - Linfadenopatia mediastinica da infezioni o tumori
  - Massa o tumore mediastinico
  - Corpo estraneo esofageo
- Anomalie intrinseche delle vie aeree
  - Emangioma o altro tumore delle vie aeree
  - Malformazione adenomatoide cistica
  - Cisti bronchiale o polmonare
  - Enfisema lobare congenito
  - Bronco tracheale aberrante
  - Sequestro
  - Cardiopatia congenita con shunt sinistro-destro (aumento dell'edema polmonare)
  - Corpo estraneo

STATI DI IMMUNODEFICIENZA
- Deficit di IgA
- Deficit dei linfociti B
- Discinesia ciliare primitiva
- AIDS
- Bronchiectasie

ALTERAZIONI DELLA CLEARANCE MUCOCILIARE
- Fibrosi cistica
- Discinesia ciliare primitiva
- Bronchiectasie

DISPLASIA BRONCOPOLMONARE

SINDROMI DA ASPIRAZIONE
- Reflusso gastroesofageo
- Disfunzione faringea e della deglutizione

PNEUMOPATIA INTERSTIZIALE, COMPRESA LA BRONCHIOLITE OBLITERANTE

INSUFFICIENZA CARDIACA

ANAFILASSI

DANNO DA INALAZIONE, USTIONI

fociti T normali). I neonati infettati da RSV che presentano sibili esprimono livelli più elevati di interferone-γ nelle vie aeree, così come di leucotrieni. La coinfezione da RSV e da metapneumovirus può essere più severa della monoinfezione.

La bronchiolite acuta è caratterizzata da ostruzione bronchiolare dovuta a edema, muco e detriti cellulari. Un ispessimento anche modesto della parete bronchiolare incide significativamente sul flusso aereo poiché la resistenza è inversamente proporzionale alla quarta potenza del raggio del passaggio bronchiolare. La resistenza nei piccoli passaggi aerei aumenta sia durante l'inspirazione sia durante l'espirazione, ma dal momento che il raggio delle vie aeree è minore durante l'espirazione, la risultante ostruzione respiratoria porta a intrappolamento d'aria e iperinflazione. Se l'ostruzione diviene completa, vi è riassorbimento dell'aria intrappolata distalmente, e il bambino sviluppa atelettasia.

L'ipossiemia è una conseguenza dell'alterazione del rapporto ventilazione-perfusione, che avviene precocemente nel decorso clinico. Con la malattia ostruttiva più grave e l'esaurimento dello sforzo respiratorio, si può sviluppare ipercapnia.

Le cause **infettive croniche** devono essere prese in considerazione per spiegare i sibili in quei neonati che non sembrano rientrare nel range di un decorso clinico normale. La fibrosi cistica è una di queste entità; il sospetto aumenta nei pazienti con sintomi respiratori persistenti, ippocratismo digitale, malassorbimento, arresto della crescita, anomalie elettrolitiche o resistenza al trattamento con broncodilatatori (vedi Capitolo 400).

L'**allergia** e l'**asma** sono importanti cause di sibili, quelle che probabilmente suscitano più interrogativi nei genitori. L'asma è caratterizzato da infiammazione delle vie aeree, iperreattività bronchiale e reversibilità dell'ostruzione (vedi Capitolo 143). I tre quadri identificati di sibili infantili sono: il sibilante precoce transitorio, che rappresenta il 19,9% della popolazione generale, ha avuto almeno un episodio di sibili con un'infezione delle vie respiratorie inferiori prima dell'età di 3 anni, ma in seguito non ha più presentato il disturbo; il sibilante persistente, corrispondente al 13,7% della popolazione generale, ha avuto episodi di sibili prima dell'età di 3 anni e ne presentava ancora all'età di 6 anni; il sibilante a esordio tardivo, ossia il 15% della popolazione generale, non ha avuto sibili prima dei 3 anni, ma li presentava all'età di 6 anni. L'altra metà dei bambini non ha mai avuto sibili all'età di 6 anni. Di tutti i lattanti che avevano sibili prima dei 3 anni di età, quasi il 60% non ha più sofferto del disturbo entro i 6 anni. I fattori di rischio per sibili persistenti comprendono l'asma materno, il fumo materno, la rinite persistente (a parte le infezioni acute delle vie respiratorie superiori) e l'eczema prima dell'età di un anno.

ALTRE CAUSE. Le **malformazioni congenite** delle vie respiratorie causano sibili nella prima infanzia. Questi reperti, che siano diffusi o focali, possono derivare da una compressione estrinseca o da un'anomalia intrinseca. La *compressione vascolare esterna* comprende gli anelli vascolari, in cui la trachea e l'esofago sono circondati da strutture vascolari, o lo *sling* (bretella) vascolare, in cui tale accerchiamento non è completo (vedi Capitolo 432). Le *cause cardiovascolari* dei sibili comprendono la dilatazione delle camere cardiache, inclusi la cardiomegalia massiva, l'ingrandimento atriale sinistro e la dilatazione delle arterie polmonari. Anche l'edema polmonare causato dall'insufficienza cardiaca può causare sibili per l'intasamento dei vasi linfatici e di quelli bronchiali, che porta a ostruzione ed edema dei bronchioli e al peggioramento dell'ostruzione (vedi Capitolo 442).

L'**aspirazione di un corpo estraneo** (vedi Capitolo 348) può causare sibili acuti o cronici. Si stima che il 78% di coloro che muoiono per aspirazione di un corpo estraneo sono di età compresa tra i 3 e i 4 anni. Anche i bambini in tenera età possono ingerire oggetti ricevuti da un'altra persona, per esempio da un fratello più grande. I lattanti con storie atipiche o reperti clinici o radiografici fuorvianti possono avere una diagnosi errata di asma o di altra patologia ostruttiva, poiché intorno al corpo estraneo si sviluppano infiammazione e granulazione. I corpi estranei esofagei possono comprimere la trachea membranosa, causando una compromissione del lume delle vie aeree.

Il **reflusso gastroesofageo** (vedi Capitolo 320.1) può causare sibili con o senza aspirazione diretta nell'albero tracheobronchiale. In assenza di aspirazione, si ritiene che il reflusso scateni un riflesso vagale o neurale, determinando un aumento della resistenza e della reattività delle vie aeree. Anche l'aspirazione da reflusso gastroesofageo o da aspirazione diretta di liquidi orali può dare luogo a sibili.

I **traumi e i tumori** sono cause molto più rare di sibili nei lattanti. Un trauma di qualsiasi tipo a carico dell'albero tracheobronchiale può causare ostruzione al flusso aereo. L'aspirazione, accidentale e non, le ustioni o le scottature dell'albero tracheobronchiale possono provocare infiammazione delle vie aeree e conseguenti sibili. Qualsiasi lesione occupante spazio, sia nel polmone stesso sia estrinseca al polmone, può determinare compressione tracheobronchiale e ostruzione al flusso aereo.

MANIFESTAZIONI CLINICHE

ANAMNESI ED ESAME OBIETTIVO. L'anamnesi iniziale di un lattante con sibili deve raccogliere informazioni sull'evento recente, come l'esordio, la durata e i fattori associati (Tab. 388-2). L'*anamnesi della nascita* comprende le settimane di gestazione, il ricovero nel reparto di terapia intensiva neonatale, un'anamnesi di intubazione o di necessità di ossigeno, le complicanze materne, tra cui infezioni, stato del virus dell'herpes simplex (HSV), stato HIV ed esposizione prenatale al fumo. L'anamnesi medica remota deve tenere conto di qualsiasi condizione di comorbilità, comprese le sindromi o la associazioni. Occorre raccogliere l'*anamnesi familiare* di fibrosi cistica, immunodeficienza, asma nei parenti di primo grado, o di qualsiasi altra affezione respiratoria ricorrente nei bambini. L'*anamnesi sociale* deve comprendere la storia ambientale, inclusi la presenza di fumatori in casa o fuori, la frequentazione di asili, il numero di fratelli, l'occupazione degli abitanti della casa, la presenza di animali domestici, l'esposizione alla tubercolosi e particolari riguardanti l'ambiente domestico (acari della polvere, polvere di costruzioni, tecniche di riscaldamento e condizionamento d'aria, muffe, scarafaggi).

Il primo passo dell'**esame obiettivo** consiste nella valutazione dei segni vitali del paziente, con una speciale attenzione alla frequenza respiratoria e al valore della saturazione di ossigeno determinato mediante pulsossimetria. Si raccomanda di procedere a un attento esame dello sviluppo del paziente, che deve essere paragonato con le curve di crescita, per individuare i segni di un arresto dell'accrescimento. I sibili provocano un suono espiratorio fischiante che può essere di natura polifonica o monofonica. Può essere presente un tempo di espirazione prolungato. In presenza di un'ampia e centrale ostruzione delle vie aeree, può insorgere un sibilo bifasico. La mancanza di sibili udibili non è rassicurante se il paziente mostra altri segni di distress respiratorio, poiché l'ostruzione completa al flusso aereo può eliminare la turbolenza, responsabile della risonanza del suono. Bisogna notare l'aerazione e tentare una terapia con broncodilatatori per valutare qualsiasi cambiamento nei sibili dopo il trattamento. L'auscultazione dei suoni respiratori sopra il collo può aiutare a distinguere i suoni provenienti dalle vie aeree superiori da quelli provenienti dalle vie aeree inferiori. L'assenza o la presenza di stridore deve essere notata e apprezzata in inspirazione. I segni di distress respiratorio comprendono la tachipnea, l'aumento dello sforzo respiratorio, l'alitamento delle pinne nasali, il tirage tracheale, le retrazioni sottocostali e intercostali, l'eccessivo utilizzo dei muscoli accessori. Nelle vie aeree superiori, i segni di atopia, tra cui turbinati purulenti e acciottolamento dell'orofaringe posteriore, sono valutabili nei bambini più grandi. È inoltre utile esaminare la cute del paziente alla ricerca di eczema e di emangiomi significativi; le lesioni della linea mediana possono essere associate a lesioni intratoraciche. Si raccomanda di prestare attenzione anche a un eventuale ippocratismo digitale (vedi Capitolo 371).

TABELLA 388-2. Anamnesi medica pertinente nei bambini con sibili

I sintomi sono esorditi alla nascita o successivamente?
Il bambino respira rumorosamente, e quando in particolare?
È presente una storia di tosse, oltre ai sibili?
Vi è stata una precedente infezione delle vie respiratorie inferiori?
Il bambino è mai stato portato al pronto soccorso oppure ricoverato in ospedale o in un reparto di terapia intensiva per distress respiratorio?
Ha mai sofferto di eczema?
Tossisce dopo il pianto oppure di notte?
Come sono la crescita e lo sviluppo del bambino?
È presente un associato deficit dell'accrescimento?
È presente un deficit dell'accrescimento senza difficoltà nella nutrizione?
Il bambino ha mai avuto squilibri elettrolitici?
Vi sono segni di malassorbimento intestinale, come evacuazioni frequenti di feci grasse o oleose?
La madre ha mai sofferto di infezione da virus dell'herpes simplex (HSV) genitale?
Qual era l'età gestazionale al momento del parto?
Il paziente è stato intubato appena nato?
Il bambino si alimenta al biberon nel letto o nella culla, specialmente in posizione appoggiata?
Sono presenti difficoltà della nutrizione, come soffocamento, ingozzamento, inarcamento o vomito?
Al paziente è stato somministrato qualche alimento nuovo?
Tra i familiari del paziente c'è un bambino ai primi passi, o può essersi verificata un'aspirazione di corpo estraneo sfuggita all'attenzione degli adulti?
C'è stato un cambiamento delle persone incaricate di seguire il bambino o sussiste la possibilità di un trauma non accidentale?

La **bronchiolite acuta** di solito è preceduta dall'esposizione a un contatto di età maggiore con una sindrome respiratoria di lieve entità, nella settimana precedente. Il lattante sviluppa dapprima un'infezione lieve delle vie respiratorie superiori, con starnuti e rinorrea limpida. Questi sintomi possono accompagnarsi a diminuzione dell'appetito e febbre di 38,5-39 °C, sebbene la temperatura possa essere da più bassa del normale a molto elevata. Gradualmente, si sviluppa distress respiratorio, con tosse sibilante parossistica, dispnea e irritabilità. Il paziente è spesso tachipnoico (il che può interferire con la nutrizione) e in genere non presenta altri sintomi sistemici, come diarrea o vomito. L'apnea può essere più pronunciata dei sibili, nella fase iniziale della malattia, in particolare nei bambini molto piccoli (meno di 2 mesi di vita) o nati prematuri.

Il reperto più evidente all'**esame obiettivo** è il sibilo. Il grado di tachipnea non correla sempre con il grado di ipossiemia o ipercapnia, pertanto è essenziale ricorrere alla pulsossimetria e alla determinazione non invasiva del biossido di carbonio. Lo sforzo respiratorio può essere molto aumentato, con alitamento delle pinne nasali e retrazioni. L'auscultazione può rivelare crepitii fini o sibili conclamati, con prolungamento della fase espiratoria. La presenza di suoni respiratori udibili a orecchio suggerisce una malattia con ostruzione bronchiolare quasi completa. L'iperinflazione polmonare può consentire la palpazione del fegato e della milza.

VALUTAZIONE DIAGNOSTICA. La valutazione diagnostica iniziale dipende dall'eziologia più probabile; una radiografia diretta del torace, in proiezione anteroposteriore e laterale, è necessaria in molti casi e indispensabile per qualsiasi bambino con distress respiratorio acuto. Gli infiltrati focali si osservano più spesso nei lattanti con sibili che hanno una saturazione di ossigeno <93%, grugniti, riduzione dei rumori respiratori, prolungamento del rapporto tra tempo di inspirazione e di espirazione, e crepitii. La radiografia del torace può anche essere utile nella valutazione dell'iperinflazione (comune nella bronchiolite e nella polmonite virale), dei segni di malattie croniche come le bronchiectasie o delle lesioni occupanti spazio che causano compressione delle vie aeree. Un tentativo con broncodilatatori può essere tanto diagnostico quanto terapeutico, poiché questi farmaci sono in grado di risolvere condizioni come la bronchiolite (occasionalmente) e l'asma, ma non influiranno su un'ostruzione fissa. Sussiste inoltre la possibilità che i broncodilatatori peggiorino un caso di sibili causati da tracheo- o broncomalacia. Il test del sudore per individuare la fibrosi cistica e la valutazione dello stato immunitario di base sono ragionevoli nei lattanti con sibili ricorrenti o decorsi complicati. Indagini più approfondite, come la radiografia con contrasto del tratto gastrointestinale (GI) superiore, la TC del torace, la broncoscopia, i test di funzione polmonare, i videostudi di deglutizione, e le sonde per il pH, possono essere considerate procedure diagnostiche di secondo o terzo livello, nei pazienti con complicanze.

Nella **bronchiolite acuta**, la radiografia del torace rivela i polmoni iperinflati con atelettasie focali. La conta leucocitaria e differenziale sono di solito normali. Gli esami virologici (in genere l'immunofluorescenza rapida, la reazione polimerasica a catena o le colture virali) sono utili se la diagnosi è incerta oppure a scopo epidemiologico. La diagnosi è clinica, in particolare nei lattanti precedentemente sani con un primo episodio di sibili durante un'epidemia nella comunità. Poiché un'infezione batterica concomitante (sepsi, polmonite, meningite) è altamente improbabile, la conferma della bronchiolite virale può ovviare alla necessità di una valutazione per la sepsi, in un lattante febbrile, e assistere con precauzioni respiratorie e isolamento, se il paziente richiede l'ospedalizzazione.

TRATTAMENTO

Il trattamento di un neonato con sibili dipende dall'eziologia sottostante. La risposta ai broncodilatatori è imprevedibile, a prescindere dalla causa, ma suggerisce una componente di iperreattività bronchiale. È appropriato somministrare un aerosol di albuterolo e osservare clinicamente la risposta. Per i bambini di età <3 anni, è accettabile continuare a somministrare farmaci per via inalatoria attraverso un MDI con maschera e spaziatore, se si dimostra un beneficio terapeutico. La terapia dovrebbe essere continuata in tutti i pazienti con esacerbazioni asmatiche causate da una malattia virale.

L'ipratropio bromuro, il cui uso in questa popolazione è controverso, sembra sia abbastanza efficace come terapia aggiuntiva, oltre a essere utile nei bambini con bronco- o tracheomalacia significative che possono essere peggiorate dai β-2 agonisti come l'albuterolo, per la conseguente riduzione del tono della muscolatura liscia.

Un tentativo con steroidi per via inalatoria può essere indispensabile in un paziente che ha risposto a multipli cicli di steroidi per via orale, ha sibili da moderati a severi, o un'anamnesi significativa di atopia, incluse allergie alimentari o eczemi. Gli steroidi inalatori sono appropriati nella terapia di mantenimento nei pazienti con reattività delle vie aeree nota, mentre sono controversi per le malattie acute o episodiche.

Gli steroidi orali sono generalmente riservati ai bambini atopici con sibili, che si ritiene abbiano un asma refrattario agli altri farmaci. Il loro utilizzo pediatrico in soggetti al primo episodio di sibili o in quelli che non necessitano di ospedalizzazione è controverso.

I lattanti affetti da **bronchiolite acuta** con distress respiratorio devono essere ricoverati; la terapia è principalmente di supporto. Se è ipossiemico, il bambino deve ricevere ossigeno fresco umidificato. I sedativi devono essere evitati poiché possono deprimere lo stimolo respiratorio. Talvolta il paziente sta meglio se viene fatto sedere con la testa e il torace sollevati di 30°, con il collo esteso. Il rischio di aspirazione di alimenti può essere elevato nei soggetti con bronchiolite, a causa della tachipnea e dell'aumentato lavoro respiratorio. La nutrizione può essere somministrata con sondino nasogastrico. Se sussiste anche il minimo rischio di scompenso respiratorio con potenziale necessità di intubazione tracheale, tuttavia, l'alimentazione orale va evitata, e il bambino deve ricevere liquidi per via parenterale. L'aspirazione frequente delle secrezioni orali e nasali spesso allevia la crisi respiratoria o la cianosi. L'ossigeno è indicato in tutti i bambini con ipossia.

Diverse sostanze sono state proposte come terapia di supporto per la bronchiolite. I broncodilatatori determinano un modesto miglioramento a breve termine delle caratteristiche cliniche, ma il miglioramento statistico nei sistemi di punteggio clinico non è sempre clinicamente significativo. Molti studi hanno incluso sia bambini con primo episodio di sibili sia quelli con sibili ricorrenti, rendendo più complessa l'interpretazione dei risultati. L'adrenalina nebulizzata può essere più efficace dei β-agonisti. Può essere ragionevole una dose trial di broncodilatatori inalatori, proseguendo o meno la terapia in base alla risposta del singolo paziente. I corticosteroidi, somministrati per via parenterale, orale o inalatoria, sono stati utilizzati nella bronchiolite nonostante i dati contrastanti e spesso negativi emersi dagli studi, la cui interpretazione peraltro è resa più complicata da differenze relative a criteri diagnostici, misurazioni dell'efficacia, tempi e modi di somministrazione e gravità della malattia. I corticosteroidi non sono raccomandati nei bambini precedentemente sani con infezione da RSV. La ribavirina, un agente antivirale somministrato per aerosol, è stato utilizzato nei lattanti con cardiopatie congenite o pneumopatie croniche. Non vi sono prove convincenti di un impatto positivo su esiti clinici importanti come la mortalità e la durata dell'ospedalizzazione. Gli antibiotici non hanno alcun ruolo, a meno non via sia una polmonite batterica secondaria. Analogamente, non vi sono dati a sostegno della somministrazione di immunoglobuline per l'RSV durante gli episodi di bronchiolite da questo virus.

PROGNOSI

I lattanti con **bronchiolite acuta** sono a maggior rischio di ulteriore compromissione respiratoria nelle prime 48-72 ore successive all'esordio della tosse e della dispnea; il bambino può apparire in condizioni di estrema sofferenza, con fame d'aria, apnea e acidosi respiratoria. Il tasso di mortalità è <1%, con decessi attribuibili ad apnea, acidosi respiratoria scompensata o disidratazione severa. I sintomi possono persistere anche oltre il periodo critico; la loro durata media nei pazienti ambulatoriali è di circa 12 giorni. I lattanti affetti da patologie come cardiopatie congenite, displasia broncopolmonare e immunodeficienze spesso hanno un decorso più grave, con mortalità e morbilità più elevate. Vi è una maggiore incidenza di sibili e asma nei bambini con un'anamnesi di bronchiolite inspiegabile alla luce della storia familiare o di altre sindromi atopiche. Non è chiaro se la bronchiolite susciti una risposta immunitaria che si manifesta successivamente sotto forma di asma, o se questi pazienti abbiano una predisposizione costituzionale all'asma che è solo svelata dall'episodio di infezione da RSV. In circa il 60% dei bambini con sibili, questi si risolvono.

PREVENZIONE

La riduzione della gravità e dell'incidenza di **bronchiolite acuta** da RSV può essere dovuta alla somministrazione di un pool di immunoglobuline iperimmuni contro l'RSV per via endovenosa (RSV-IVIG) e di palivizumab, un anticorpo monoclonale intramuscolare diretto contro la proteina F dell'RSV, prima e durante la stagione del RSV. Il palivizumab è consigliato nei bambini di età <2 anni con pneumopatie croniche (displasia broncopolmonare) o prematuri. Un lavaggio meticoloso delle mani è la miglior misura per prevenire la trasmissione nosocomiale.

388.2 • BRONCHITE • Denise M. Goodman

La bronchite è un'infiammazione bronchiale aspecifica che si associa a numerose patologie dell'infanzia. La *bronchite acuta* è una sindrome, in genere di origine virale, la cui caratteristica principale è la tosse.

Per indicare un coinvolgimento prevalente della trachea si usa l'espressione *tracheobronchite acuta*. Può anche essere presente una rinofaringite, imputabile a numerosi agenti virali e batterici, come quelli che causano influenza, pertosse e difterite. L'isolamento dall'escreato di batteri comuni, come lo pneumococco, lo *Staphylococcus aureus* e lo *Streptococcus pneumoniae*, può anche non implicare una causa batterica che renda necessaria l'antibioticoterapia.

BRONCHITE ACUTA

MANIFESTAZIONI CLINICHE. La bronchite acuta è spesso preceduta da un'infezione virale delle vie aeree superiori. È più comune in inverno, quando prevalgono le sindromi respiratorie virali. L'epitelio tracheobronchiale è invaso dall'agente infettivo, che porta all'attivazione delle cellule infiammatorie e al rilascio di citochine. Insorgono quindi i sintomi sistemici, come febbre e malessere. L'epitelio tracheobronchiale può essere significativamente danneggiato o ipersensibilizzato, portando a una tosse protratta che dura 1-3 settimane.

Il bambino si presenta la prima volta con sintomi aspecifici di infezione delle vie respiratorie superiori, come la rinite. Dopo 3 o

4 giorni, si sviluppa una tosse frequente, secca, stizzosa, che può essere o meno produttiva. Dopo qualche giorno l'escreato diviene purulento, reperto indicativo della migrazione dei leucociti ma non necessariamente di un'infezione batterica. Molti bambini lo ingoiano, e questo può provocare vomito. Il dolore toracico, che può rappresentare un sintomo importante nei bambini più grandi, è esacerbato dalla tosse. Il muco gradualmente si fa meno denso, in genere nel giro di 5-10 giorni, e la tosse a poco a poco si riduce. L'intero episodio dura complessivamente 2 settimane circa, e raramente supera le 3 settimane.

I reperti all'esame obiettivo variano in base all'età del paziente e allo stadio della malattia. I reperti precoci o sono assenti o consistono in febbricola e segni delle vie respiratorie superiori, come rinofaringite, congiuntivite e rinite. L'auscultazione del torace può non evidenziare nulla di significativo in questa fase iniziale. Con la progressione della sindrome e il peggioramento della tosse, i suoni polmonari divengono più aspri, con crepitii grossolani e fini e sibili sparsi ad alta frequenza. Le radiografie del torace sono normali o presentano un aumento della trama bronchiale.

L'obiettivo principale del clinico è escludere una polmonite, che richiederebbe una terapia antibiotica essendo imputabile per lo più a batteri. Questa patologia è poco probabile negli adulti che non presentano alterazioni dei segni vitali (tachicardia, tachipnea e febbre) e che risultano normali all'esame obiettivo del torace.

DIAGNOSI DIFFERENZIALE. La presenza di sintomi persistenti o ricorrenti dovrebbe far sospettare entità diverse dalla bronchite acuta. Molte sono le affezioni che si manifestano con la tosse come sintomo predominante (Tab. 388-3).

TRATTAMENTO. Non esiste una terapia specifica per la bronchite acuta. La malattia è autolimitante e gli antibiotici, sebbene siano prescritti frequentemente, non accelerano la guarigione. Cambiamenti frequenti della posizione possono facilitare il drenaggio polmonare, nei lattanti. L'umidità talvolta allevia i sintomi nei bambini più grandi, pur non accorciando il decorso della malattia. I sedativi della tosse possono dare un sollievo sintomatologico, ma anche aumentare il rischio di suppurazione e di ispessimento delle secrezioni e, pertanto, dovrebbero essere utilizzati con giudizio. Gli antistaminici asciugano le secrezioni e non sono utili; analogamente, gli espettoranti non sono indicati.

BRONCHITE CRONICA

La bronchite cronica, di facile riconoscimento negli adulti, viene definita come una tosse produttiva che duri più di 3 mesi all'anno, per almeno 2 anni. La malattia si può sviluppare insidiosamente, con episodi di ostruzione acuta alternati a periodi quiescenti. Numerosi fattori predisponenti possono portare alla progressione dell'ostruzione al flusso aereo o alla broncopneumopatia cronica ostruttiva (BPCO), primo tra tutti il fumo di sigaretta (fino all'80% dei pazienti ha un'anamnesi positiva a questo riguardo). Altre condizioni comprendono l'inquinamento atmosferico, l'esposizione in ambito lavorativo e le infezioni ripetute. Nei bambini bisogna escludere la fibrosi cistica, la displasia broncopolmonare e le bronchiectasie.

Non è chiaro fino a che punto questa definizione sia applicabile ai bambini. L'esistenza della bronchite cronica come entità distinta, nei pazienti pediatrici, è controversa. Come gli adulti, i bambini con malattie infiammatorie croniche o quelli con esposizione a sostanze tossiche possono sviluppare un danno all'epitelio polmonare. Pertanto, la tosse cronica o ricorrente deve spingere il pediatra a ricercare una sottostante malattia polmonare o sistemica (vedi Tab. 388-3).

TABELLA 388-3. Disturbi che si presentano con tosse come sintomo predominante

CATEGORIA	DIAGNOSI
Disturbi di origine infiammatoria	Asma
Malattie polmonari croniche	Displasia broncopolmonare, pneumopatia cronica
	Bronchiectasie postinfettive
	Fibrosi cistica
	Tracheo- o broncomalacia
	Anomalie ciliari
Altre malattie croniche o disturbi congeniti	Laringoschisi
	Disturbi della deglutizione
	Reflusso gastroesofageo
	Compressione delle vie aeree (come un anello vascolare o un emangioma)
	Cardiopatie congenite
Malattie infettive o alterazioni immunitarie	Immunodeficienze
	Tubercolosi
	Allergie
	Sinusite
	Tonsillite o adenoidite
	Chlamydia, *Ureaplasma* (neonati)
	Bordetella pertussis
	Mycoplasma pneumoniae
Problemi acquisiti	Aspirazione di un corpo estraneo (tracheale o esofageo)

FUMO DI SIGARETTA E INQUINAMENTO ATMOSFERICO

L'esposizione a irritanti ambientali, come il fumo di tabacco e l'inquinamento atmosferico, può stimolare o aggravare la tosse. Vi è un'associazione ben dimostrata tra l'esposizione al fumo di tabacco e le malattie polmonari, compresi la bronchite e i sibili. Questo può verificarsi anche con il fumo passivo. Il fumo di marijuana è un altro irritante che viene talora trascurato quando si raccoglie l'anamnesi. In base ad alcuni dati sembra che le donne possano sviluppare una particolare suscettibilità alle malattie polmonari a lungo termine per essere state esposte al fumo in età infantile.

Numerosi agenti inquinanti, tra cui sostanze particolate, ozono, vapori acidi e biossido di azoto, compromettono lo sviluppo dei polmoni e possono precipitare una malattia polmonare. Poiché tutte queste sostanze sono presenti nell'atmosfera, il contributo relativo di ognuna di esse allo sviluppo dei sintomi respiratori è difficile da determinare. I gas di scarico delle automobili sono un'importante fonte di questi inquinanti.

Sibili e bronchiolite

Bush A: Treatment options of asthma in infancy. *Pediatr Pulmonol Suppl* 2004;26:20–22.

Castro-Rodriguez JA, Rodrigo GJ: Beta agonists through metered-dose inhaler with valved holding chamber versus nebulizer for acute exacerbation of wheezing or asthma in children under five years of age: A systematic review with meta-analysis. *J Pediatr* 2004;172–177.

Covar RA, Spahn JD: Treating the wheezing infant. *Pediatr Clin North Am* 2003;50:631–654.

Frey U, Makkonen K, Wellman T, et al: Alterations in airway wall properties in infants with a history of wheezing disorders. *Am J Respir Crit Care Med* 2000;161:1825–1829.

Hartling L, Wiebe N, Russell K, et al: A meta-analysis of randomized controlled trials evaluating the efficacy of epinephrine for the treatment of acute viral bronchiolitis. *Arch Pediatr Adolesc Med* 2003;157:957–964.

Hofhuis W, van der Wiel EC, et al: Bronchodilation in infants with malacia or recurrent wheeze. *Arch Dis Child* 2003;88:246–249.

Joseph L, Goldberg S, Picard E: A randomized trial of home oxygen therapy from the emergency department for acute bronchiolitis. *Pediatrics* 2006; 118:1319–1320.

King VJ, Viswanathan M, Bordley WC, et al: Review: Commonly used pharmacological treatments for bronchiolitis in children do not seem to be effective. *Arch Pediatr Adolesc Med* 2004;158:127–137.

Klinnert MD, Liu AH, Pearson MR, et al: Short-term impact of a randomized multifaceted intervention for wheezing infants in low-income families. *Arch Pediatr Adolesc Med* 2005;159:75–82.

Klinnert MD, Price MR, Liu AH, Robinson JL: Morbidity patterns among low-income wheezing infants. *Pediatrics* 2003;112:49–57.

Kussman BD, Geva T, McGowan FX: Cardiovascular causes of airway compression. *Paediatr Anaesth* 2004;14:60–74.

Martinez FD, Wright AL, Taussig LM, et al: Asthma and wheezing in the first six years of life. *N Engl J Med* 1995;332:133–138.
Meates-Dennis M: Bronchiolitis. *Arch Dis Child* 2005;90:ep81–ep86.
Morton RL, Sheikh S, Corbett ML, Eid NS: Evaluation of the wheezy infant. *Ann Allergy Asthma Immunol* 2001;86:251–256.
Principi N, Esposito S: Emerging role of *Mycoplasma pneumoniae* and *Chlamydia pneumoniae* in paediatric respiratory tract infection. *Lancet* 2001;1:334–344.
Semple MG, Cowell A, Dove W, et al: Dual infection of infants by human metapneumovirus and human respiratory syncytial virus is strongly associated with severe bronchiolitis. *J Infect Dis* 2005;191:382–386.
Silvestri M, Sabatini F, Defilippi AC, Rossi GA: The wheezy infant—immunological and molecular considerations. *Paediatr Respir Rev* 2004;5:S–1–S87.
Smyth RL, Openshaw PJM: Bronchiolitis. *Lancet* 2006;368:312–322.
Subcommittee on Diagnosis and Management of Bronchitis: Diagnosis and management of bronchitis. *Pediatrics* 2006;118:1774–1793.
Tokar B, Ozkan R, Ilhan H: Tracheobronchial foreign bodies in children: Importance of accurate history and plain chest radiography in delayed presentation. *Clin Radiol* 2004;59:609–615.
Weinberger M: Corticosteroids for first-time young wheezers: Current status of the controversy. *J Pediatr* 2003;143:700–702.
Williams JV, Harris PA, Tollefson SJ, et al: Human metapneumovirus and lower respiratory tract disease in otherwise healthy infants and children. *N Engl J Med* 2004;350:443–450.

Bronchite

Arnold JC, Singh KK, Spector SA, et al: Human bocavirus: Prevalence and clinical spectrum at a children's hospital. *CID* 2006;43:283–288.
Arroll B, Kenealy T: Antibiotics for acute bronchitis. *Br Med J* 2001;322:939–940.
Gauderman WJ, Avol E, Gilliland F, et al: The effect of air pollution on lung development from 10 to 18 years of age. *N Engl J Med* 2004;351: 1057–1067.
Gergen PJ, Fowler JA, Maurer KR, et al: The burden of environmental tobacco smoke exposure on the respiratory health of children 2 months through 5 years of age in the United States: Third National Health and Nutrition Examination Survey, 1988 to 1994. *Pediatrics* 1998;101:e8.
Gonzales R, Sande MA: Uncomplicated acute bronchitis. *Ann Intern Med* 2000;133:981–991.
Irwin RS, Madison JM: The diagnosis and treatment of cough. *N Engl J Med* 2000;343:1715–1721.
Kim JJ, Smorodinsky S, Lipsett M, et al: Traffic-related air pollution near busy roads: The East Bay Children's Respiratory Health Study. *Am J Respir Crit Care Med* 2004;170:520–526.
Morice AH, et al: The diagnosis and management of chronic cough. *Eur Respir J* 2004;24:481–492.
Patel BD, Luben RN, Welch AA, et al: Childhood smoking is an independent risk factor for obstructive airways disease in women. *Thorax* 2004;59:682–686.
Peters JM, Avol E, Navidi W, et al: A study of twelve Southern California communities with differing levels and types of air pollution: I. Prevalence of respiratory morbidity. *Am J Respir Crit Care Med* 1999;159:760–767.
Peters JM, Avol E, Gauderman WJ, et al: A study of twelve Southern California communities with differing levels and types of air pollution: II. Effects on pulmonary function. *Am J Respir Crit Care Med* 1999;159:768–775.
Snow V, Mottur-Pilson C, Gonzales R, et al: Principles of appropriate antibiotic use for treatment of acute bronchitis in adults. *Ann Intern Med* 2001;134:518–520.

Capitolo 389 ■ Enfisema e iperinflazione

Steven R. Boas e Glenna B. Winnie

L'enfisema polmonare è una distensione degli spazi aerei, con distruzione irreversibile dei setti alveolari. Può essere generalizzato o localizzato, ovvero coinvolgere tutto il polmone o solo una parte. L'iperinflazione è una distensione con o senza rottura degli alveoli, spesso reversibile.

L'iperinflazione compensatoria, che può essere acuta o cronica, si verifica nel tessuto polmonare normalmente funzionante quando, per qualsiasi ragione, una porzione considerevole del polmone è rimossa o diviene parzialmente o completamente priva d'aria, come accade nella polmonite, nell'atelettasia, nell'empiema o nello pneumotorace.

L'iperinflazione ostruttiva è imputabile all'ostruzione parziale di un bronco o di un bronchiolo, in conseguenza della quale l'uscita di aria dagli alveoli diviene più difficile della sua entrata, e consiste in un graduale accumulo di aria distalmente all'ostruzione, la cosiddetta ostruzione tipo bypass, valvola globulare o valvola di non ritorno (vedi Capitolo 384).

IPERINFLAZIONE OSTRUTTIVA LOCALIZZATA

Quando un'ostruzione del tipo valvola globulare occlude un bronco principale, l'intero polmone va incontro a iperinflazione; quando l'ostruzione si verifica in un bronco lobare, a essere colpiti sono i singoli lobi. L'interessamento di segmenti o sottosegmenti è legato all'ostruzione dei loro bronchi individuali. Le ostruzioni localizzate responsabili di iperinflazione possono dipendere da corpi estranei e dalla reazione infiammatoria che la loro presenza scatena, da muco troppo denso (fibrosi cistica, vedi Capitolo 400), dalla tubercolosi endobronchiale o da un linfonodo tracheobronchiale (vedi Capitolo 212), oltre che da tumori endobronchiali o mediastinici. Quando è coinvolta la maggior parte di un lobo, alla percussione dell'area si apprezza un'eccessiva risonanza e il murmure vescicolare è di intensità ridotta. Il polmone iperdisteso può estendersi attraverso il mediastino fino all'emitorace opposto. All'esame fluoroscopico, durante l'espirazione l'area caratterizzata da iperinflazione non si riduce di dimensioni, e il cuore e il mediastino si spostano dal lato opposto poiché il polmone non ostruito si svuota normalmente.

Il **polmone iperlucente monolaterale** può associarsi a varie patologie infantili cardiache e polmonari, ma in alcuni pazienti insorge in assenza di una sottostante malattia attiva dimostrabile. Più della metà dei casi segue uno o più episodi di polmonite; in molti bambini è stato documentato un aumento del titolo anticorpale contro gli adenovirus (vedi Capitolo 259). Questa condizione, oltre a far seguito a una bronchiolite obliterante, può comprendere anche una vasculite obliterante: si spiega così la marcata riduzione della perfusione e della trama vascolare dal lato affetto.

I pazienti con polmone iperlucente monolaterale possono presentarsi con **caratteristiche cliniche** di polmonite, ma alcuni vengono individuati solo se sottoposti a radiografia del torace per un'altra ragione. Una piccola percentuale di pazienti ha emottisi. L'esame obiettivo può rilevare iperfonesi e un polmone piccolo, con spostamento del mediastino verso il polmone più anormale, condizione nota come **sindrome di Swyer-James** o **di Macleod**. Alcuni soggetti presentano uno spostamento del mediastino dal lato opposto alla lesione, durante l'espirazione. La TC o la broncoscopia possono dimostrare la presenza di bronchiectasie. In alcuni pazienti, le radiografie del torace effettuate in precedenza erano normali o rivelavano solo una polmonite acuta: tale osservazione fa pensare che il polmone iperlucente sia una lesione acquisita. Non esiste alcun trattamento specifico; la sintomatologia può ridursi con il passare del tempo.

L'**enfisema lobare congenito** (CLE, *Congenital Lobar Emphysema*) può dare luogo a distress respiratorio severo nella prima infanzia ed essere causato da un'ostruzione localizzata. È stata riportata una ricorrenza familiare, e nel 50% dei casi si può identificare una causa. Tra le possibili cause di ostruzione bronchiale e conseguente CLE sono stati indicati deficit congeniti della cartilagine bronchiale, compressione esterna da parte di vasi aberranti, stenosi bronchiale, ridondanza delle pliche mucose e angolatura del bronco causata da erniazione nel mediastino.

Le **manifestazioni cliniche** di solito si rendono evidenti nel periodo neonatale, ma nel 5% dei pazienti compaiono più tardi, quando il lattante ha raggiunto i 5-6 mesi di vita. Molte volte già l'ecografia prenatale permette di formulare la diagnosi, sebbene non sempre i casi diagnosticati in epoca prenatale siano sintomatici alla nascita. Alcuni pazienti restano non diagnosticati fino all'età scolare o anche oltre. I segni variano da una lieve tachipnea con sibili fino a dispnea severa e cianosi. Il CLE può colpire i lobi superiori e medi; la sede più comune è il lobo superiore sinistro. L'area affetta è essenzialmente non funzionante, a causa dell'iperinflazione che può portare ad atelettasia del polmone ipsilaterale normale. Con il progredire della distensione, il mediastino si sposta dal lato opposto, con possibile alterazione funzionale (Fig. 389-1). Spesso l'esame radiografico rivela il lobo radiolucente e lo spostamento del mediastino. La TC può dimostrare l'anatomia aberrante della lesione e la RM/ARM evidenzierà un'eventuale lesione vascolare che potrebbe causare compressione extraluminale. L'esame scintigrafico è utile per dimostrare difetti di perfusione nel lobo affetto. La Figura 389-2 illustra la valutazione di un bambino che si presenta con sospetto CLE. La diagnosi differenziale comprende la polmonite, con o senza versamento, e la malformazione adenomatoide cistica.

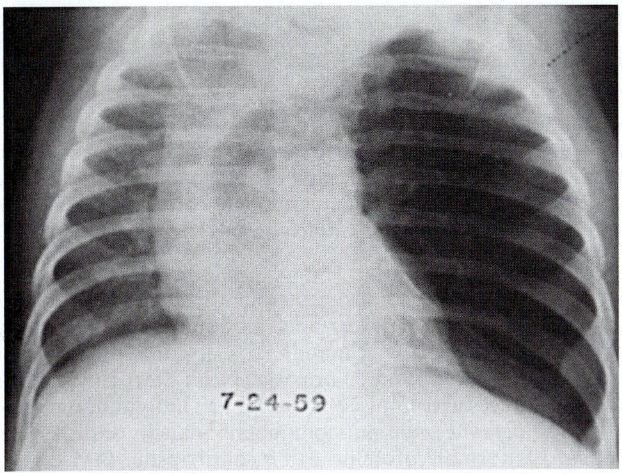

Figura 389-1. Enfisema congenito del lobo superiore sinistro. Si noti l'estensione del lobo enfisematoso nel lobo inferiore sinistro e lo spostamento del mediastino verso destra.

Il **trattamento** con intervento chirurgico immediato e asportazione del lobo può salvare la vita al paziente, quando sono presenti cianosi e distress respiratorio, ma alcuni rispondono al trattamento medico. L'intubazione selettiva del polmone sano può essere di beneficio. Alcuni bambini con apparente enfisema lobare congenito hanno un'iperinflazione reversibile, senza la classica rottura dei setti alveolari implicita nel termine *enfisema*. La broncoscopia può rivelare un'eventuale lesione endobronchiale.

L'iperinflazione di tutti e tre i lobi del polmone destro può essere causata da un'anomala localizzazione dell'arteria polmonare sinistra, che urta il bronco principale destro. L'iperinflazione si verifica anche nei pazienti affetti da tetralogia di Fallot, con assenza della valvola polmonare (vedi Capitolo 430.1) e dilatazione aneurismatica secondaria dell'arteria polmonare, che comprime parzialmente i bronchi principali. Alcuni neonati sviluppano iperinflazione lobare durante il trattamento della malattia delle membrane ialine con ventilazione assistita, fenomeno che suggerisce una causa acquisita. Il trattamento medico con l'intubazione selettiva del bronco non affetto, o con ventilazione ad alta frequenza, ha occasionalmente avuto successo, permettendo di evitare la lobectomia.

IPERINFLAZIONE OSTRUTTIVA GENERALIZZATA

L'iperinflazione ostruttiva generalizzata dei polmoni si instaura in seguito al coinvolgimento diffuso dei bronchioli ed è abitualmente reversibile. Più comune nei lattanti che nei bambini, può essere secondaria a numerose condizioni cliniche, tra cui asma, fibrosi cistica, bronchiolite acuta, polmonite interstiziale, forme atipiche di laringotracheobronchite, aspirazione di polvere di stearato di zinco, congestione passiva cronica secondaria a lesioni cardiache congenite, tubercolosi miliare.

ANATOMIA PATOLOGICA. Nell'iperinflazione cronica molti alveoli sono distrutti e comunicano tra loro, formando sacculi iperdistesi. L'aria può penetrare anche nel tessuto interstiziale (enfisema interstiziale), dando luogo a pneumomediastino e pneumotorace (vedi Capitoli 410 e 411).

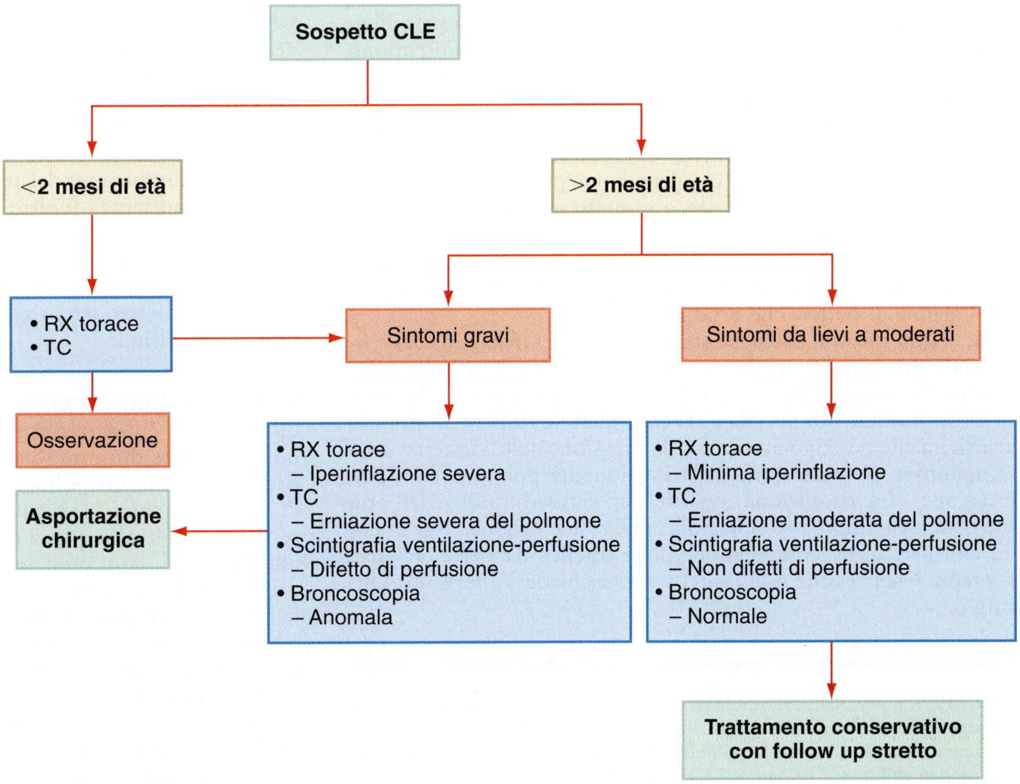

Figura 389-2. Algoritmo per la valutazione e il trattamento dell'enfisema lobare congenito. (Adattata da Senocak ME, Ciftci AO, et al: Congenital lobar emphysema: diagnostic and therapeutic considerations. *J Pediatr Surg* 1999;34:1347-1351. Citata in Chao MC, Karamzadeh AM, Ahuja G: Congenital lobar emphysema: An otolaryngologic perspective. *Int J Pediatr Otorhinolaryngol* 2005;69:553.)

MANIFESTAZIONI CLINICHE. L'iperinflazione ostruttiva generalizzata è caratterizzata da dispnea espiratoria. I polmoni vanno incontro a progressiva iperdistensione, e il torace resta espanso anche durante l'espirazione. Si riscontrano un aumento della frequenza e una riduzione dell'escursione respiratoria, derivanti dall'iperdistensione degli alveoli e dalla loro incapacità a svuotarsi normalmente attraverso i bronchioli ristretti. La fame d'aria è responsabile dei movimenti respiratori forzati. L'iperattività dei muscoli accessori della respirazione provoca retrazioni a livello del giugulo, degli spazi sovraclaveari, del margine inferiore del torace e degli spazi intercostali. A differenza del torace appiattito in inspirazione e in espirazione tipico dell'ostruzione laringea, durante l'espirazione il torace iperdisteso va incontro a riduzioni di dimensioni minime. Il suono alla percussione è iperfonetico. All'auscultazione la fase inspiratoria risulta di solito meno evidente di quella espiratoria, che è prolungata e aspra. Possono essere udibili crepitii medi o fini. La cianosi è più comune nei casi gravi.

DIAGNOSI. L'esame radiografico e fluoroscopico del torace aiuta a formulare la diagnosi. Entrambe le cupole diaframmatiche sono abbassate e appiattite, le costole sono più distanziate del normale e i campi polmonari meno densi. Il movimento del diaframma durante l'espirazione è ridotto e l'escursione del diaframma, basso e appiattito, è appena percettibile nei casi gravi. Il diametro anteroposteriore del torace è aumentato, e lo sterno può essere estroflesso.

Enfisema bolloso. Le bolle, o cisti, dell'enfisema bolloso (pneumatocele) sono conseguenza dell'iperdistensione e della rottura degli alveoli durante la nascita o poco dopo, ma possono anche essere sequele di polmoniti o di altre infezioni. Sono state osservate nelle lesioni tubercolotiche durante la terapia antibatterica specifica. Queste aree enfisematose presumibilmente derivano dalla rottura di alveoli distesi, che formano una cavità singola o multiloculata. La cisti può ingrandirsi e contenere del liquido; alla radiografia può essere dimostrabile un livello idroaereo. La cisti, che deve essere differenziata dagli ascessi polmonari, nella maggior parte dei casi scompare spontaneamente entro alcuni mesi, sebbene possa persistere anche per un anno o più. L'aspirazione o l'intervento non sono indicati, tranne che nei casi di grave compromissione cardiaca o respiratoria.

Enfisema sottocutaneo. L'enfisema sottocutaneo si instaura in seguito a qualsiasi processo che consenta l'entrata di aria libera nel tessuto sottocutaneo; le cause più comuni comprendono lo pneumomediastino e lo pneumotorace (vedi Capitolo 410 e 411). Inoltre, può rappresentare una complicanza delle fratture orbitarie, che permettono all'aria libera di fuoriuscire dai seni paranasali. Nel collo e nel torace, l'enfisema sottocutaneo può far seguito a una tracheotomia, un'ulcerazione profonda della regione faringea, una ferita esofagea o a qualsiasi lesione perforante della laringe o della trachea. Occasionalmente è una complicanza della toracentesi, dell'asma o degli interventi chirurgici addominali. Avviene di rado che l'aria si formi nei tessuti sottocutanei per l'azione di batteri che producono gas.

Le manifestazioni classiche sono dolorabilità nella sede dell'enfisema e una sensazione di "crepitio" alla palpazione della cute. L'enfisema sottocutaneo è un processo autolimitante che non richiede trattamento specifico. È consigliabile ridurre al minimo le attività che possono aumentare la pressione nelle vie aeree (tosse, manovre di valutazione della funzionalità polmonare ad alta pressione). La risoluzione avviene per riassorbimento dell'aria sottocutanea dopo l'eliminazione della sua origine. Raramente, una pericolosa compressione della trachea da parte dell'aria contenuta nei tessuti molli circostanti richiede l'intervento chirurgico.

Chao MC, Karamzadeh AM, Ahuja G: Congenital lobar emphysema: An otolaryngologic perspective. *Int J Pediatr Otorhinolaryngol* 2005;69:549–554.
Cumming GR, Macpherson RI, Chernick V: Unilateral hyperlucent lung syndrome in children. *J Pediatr* 1971;78:250–260.
Horak E, Bodner J, Gassner I, et al: Congenital cystic lung disease: Diagnostic and therapeutic considerations. *Clin Pediatr* 2003;42:251–261.
Karnak I, Senocak ME, Ciftci AO, et al: Congenital lobar emphysema: Diagnostic and therapeutic considerations. *J Pediatr Surg* 1999;34:1347–1351.
McKenzie SA, Allison DJ, Singh MP, et al: Unilateral hyperlucent lung: The case for investigation. *Thorax* 1980;35:745–750.
Mei-Zahar M, Konen O, Manson D, Langer JC: Is congenital lobar emphysema a surgical disease? *J Pediatr Surg* 2006;41:1058–1061.
Mura M, Zompatori M, Mussoni A, et al: Bullous emphysema versus diffuse emphysema: A functional and radiologic comparison. *Respir Med* 2005;99:171–178.

Capitolo 390 ■ Deficit di α_1-antitripsina ed enfisema

Glenna B. Winnie e Steven R. Boas

Il deficit omozigote di α_1-antitripsina (α-AT) è un'importante causa di sviluppo precoce di enfisema panacinare severo negli adulti, nella terza e quarta decade di vita, e un'importante causa di epatopatia nei bambini, ma raramente causa malattia polmonare in età pediatrica (vedi Capitolo 354.5).

PATOGENESI. Il tipo e la concentrazione dell'α_1-antitripsina sono ereditabili come una serie di alleli codominanti sul segmento cromosomico14q32.1. Si rimanda al Capitolo 354.5 per una trattazione su genotipi ed epatopatia. Negli Stati Uniti il deficit autosomico recessivo colpisce 1/1600-1800 individui, ovvero circa 100 000 persone, ed è più comune nei bianchi di discendenza europea. La normale proteina dell'α_1-antitripsina PiM è secreta in circolo dal fegato alla velocità di 34 mg/kg/die. La proteina mutante, che non è prodotta (*null*) o è arrangiata male (PiZ e altre), può polimerizzare nel reticolo endoplasmatico o essere degradata, con conseguenti bassi livelli sierici. L'enfisema dell'adulto a insorgenza precoce, associato al deficit di α_1-antitripsina, si manifesta per lo più con PiZZ (mutazione nel gene *SERPINA1*), sebbene siano stati associati a enfisema anche Pi (*null*) (*null*) e, in minor misura, altri mutanti di tipo Pi come SZ.

L'α_1-antitripsina e le altre antiproteasi sieriche sono importanti per l'inattivazione degli enzimi proteolitici, rilasciati nei polmoni da batteri morti o leucociti. Un deficit di queste antiproteasi porta ad accumulo degli enzimi proteolitici in quest'organo, che causa distruzione del tessuto polmonare e conseguente sviluppo di enfisema. Inoltre, le proteine mutanti polimerizzate nel polmone possono avere attività proinfiammatoria. Anche la concentrazione di proteasi (elastasi) nei leucociti del paziente può essere un importante fattore che contribuisce a determinare la severità clinica della malattia polmonare, per un dato livello di α_1-antitripsina.

MANIFESTAZIONI CLINICHE. La maggior parte dei pazienti con difetto PiZZ è caratterizzata da un danno polmonare minimo o non rilevabile durante l'infanzia. In alcuni si assiste all'esordio precoce di sintomi polmonari, tra cui dispnea, sibili e tosse, e l'enfisema panacinare è stato documentato alla biopsia polmonare; è probabile che questi reperti si verifichino secondariamente alle infezioni, causando infiammazione e conseguente malattia precoce. Il fumo aumenta molto il rischio di sviluppare enfisema nei mutanti di tipo Pi. Lo screening neonatale per identificare i bambini con fenotipo PiZZ, pur non inducendo i genitori a smettere di fumare, riduce la percentuale di tabagismo negli adolescenti affetti.

L'esame obiettivo nell'infanzia è in genere normale: avviene molto raramente che riveli ritardo dell'accrescimento, aumento del diametro anteroposteriore del torace con suono iperfonetico alla percussione, crepitii (se è presente un'infezione attiva) e ippocratismo digitale. Un enfisema severo può spostare in basso il diaframma, rendendo il fegato e la milza più facilmente palpabili.

ESAMI DI LABORATORIO. Dagli esami sierici di *immunoassay* emergono bassi livelli di α_1-antitripsina; i livelli sierici normali sono di 180-280 mg/dL. L'elettroforesi sierica rivela il fenotipo, mentre il genotipo è determinato tramite reazione polimerasica a catena. Nei rari pazienti che presentano malattia polmonare nell'adolescenza, la radiografia del torace mostra iperinflazione con depressione delle cupole diaframmatiche, e la TC del torace può rivelare una maggiore iperespansione delle regioni polmonari inferiori, con occasionali bronchiectasie.

TRATTAMENTO. La terapia per il deficit di α_1-antitripsina è la sostituzione con enzimi derivati da pool di plasma umano. Un livello di 80 mg/dL protegge dall'enfisema, e questo livello, obiettivo della terapia a scalare, corrisponde alla comparsa dell'antiproteasi trasfusa, nel liquido di lavaggio polmonare. Viene abitualmente ottenuto con dosi di 60 mg/kg ev alla settimana. La Food and Drug Administration ha approvato l'uso di enzima umano purificato derivato dal sangue, per i pazienti ZZ e *null-null*. Il beneficio di questa terapia non è stato ancora chiaramente dimostrato. La terapia sostitutiva sembra dare maggiori risultati nei pazienti con malattia polmonare ostruttiva moderata (volume espiratorio forzato in un secondo [FEV_1, *Forced Expiratory Volume in 1 s*] 30-65% dell'atteso) o in quelli con malattia polmonare lieve che vanno incontro a un rapido declino della funzione polmonare. Sono in corso di sviluppo forme ricombinanti di α_1-antitripsina che potrebbero essere utilizzate come terapia inalatoria, sebbene i prodotti attuali siano rapidamente rimossi dalla circolazione, quando somministrati per via endovenosa.

La terapia di supporto standard per la pneumopatia cronica comprende il trattamento aggressivo delle infezioni polmonari, l'uso routinario dei vaccini antipneumococcico e antinfluenzale, broncodilatatori, educazione sui gravi rischi del fumo. Questo trattamento è indicato anche per gli altri membri della famiglia in cui si riscontra un fenotipo PiZZ o *null-null*, anche se asintomatici. Le persone con fenotipo Pi MZ non hanno un rischio aumentato di sviluppare malattia polmonare. Il significato clinico del fenotipo Pi SZ è sconosciuto, ma un trattamento aspecifico è ragionevole. Tutti i soggetti con bassi livelli sierici di antiproteasi dovrebbero essere avvisati che l'eventuale sviluppo di enfisema è in parte correlato a fattori ambientali, tra cui l'esposizione a fumi industriali, le infezioni delle vie respiratorie e, soprattutto, il fumo di sigaretta. Sebbene l'identificazione degli individui affetti possa aiutare a prevenire lo sviluppo di malattia polmonare ostruttiva, i programmi di screening negli Stati Uniti sono attualmente sospesi, per la preoccupazione di possibili discriminazioni sul lavoro e da parte delle assicurazioni sanitarie.

Abboud RT, Ford GT, Chapman KR: Standards Committee of the Canadian Thoracic Society: Alpha1-antitrypsin deficiency: A position statement of the Canadian Thoracic Society. *Can Respir J* 2001;8:81–88.

Primhak RA, Tanner MS: Alpha 1-antitrypsin deficiency. *Arch Dis Child* 2001;85:2–5.

Sandhaus RA: Alpha1-antitrypsin deficiency: New and emerging treatments for alpha1-antitrypsin deficiency. *Thorax* 2004;59:904–909.

Stoller JK, Aboussouan LS: Alpha1-antitrypsin deficiency. *Lancet* 2005; 365:2225–2236.

Strange C, Moseley MA, Jones Y, et al: Genetic testing of minors for alpha 1-antitrypsin deficiency. *Arch Pediatr Adolesc Med* 2006;160:531–534.

von Ehrenstein OS, Maier EM, Weiland SK, et al: Alpha1 antitrypsin and the prevalence and severity of asthma. *Arch Dis Child* 2004;89:230–231.

Capitolo 391 ■ Altre malattie delle vie aeree distali Steven R. Boas

391.1 • Bronchiolite obliterante

EPIDEMIOLOGIA. La bronchiolite obliterante (BO) è una rara malattia cronica a carico dei bronchioli e delle piccole vie aeree. Nella popolazione pediatrica è più comune dopo infezioni respiratorie (adenovirus, *Mycoplasma*, morbillo, *Legionella*, influenza, pertosse), ma può essere causata anche da patologie infiammatorie (artrite reumatoide giovanile, lupus eritematoso sistemico, sclerodermia, sindrome di Stevens-Johnson), inalazione di fumi tossici (NO_2, NH_3), oltre a manifestarsi dopo trapianto osseo o polmonare. La BO colpisce tutti i gruppi di età, e la sua prevalenza in una serie autoptica pediatrica è risultata di 2/1000.

PATOGENESI. Dopo l'insulto iniziale, l'infiammazione che colpisce i bronchioli terminali, i bronchioli respiratori e i dotti alveolari può causare l'obliterazione del lume delle vie aeree. Il danno epiteliale, che risulta in riparazione anomala, è caratteristico della BO. L'ostruzione completa o parziale del lume può dare luogo a intrappolamento di aria o atelettasia. La polmonite organizzata da bronchiolite obliterante (BOOP, *Bronchiolitis Obliterans Organizing Pneumonia*) è una malattia polmonare fibrosante che comprende le caratteristiche istologiche della BO, con estensione del processo infiammatorio dai dotti alveolari distali agli alveoli, e proliferazione dei fibroblasti. La sindrome da bronchiolite obliterante (BOS, *Bronchiolitis Obliterans Syndrome*) è un'entità clinica che si correla a deterioramento dell'organo dopo trapianto polmonare, a causa di un danno progressivo delle vie aeree, che appare istologicamente simile alla BO. Di eziologia non chiara, potrebbe non essere correlata ai meccanismi responsabili della BO, nei pazienti non trapiantati.

MANIFESTAZIONI CLINICHE/DIAGNOSI. I primi segni di BO possono essere tosse, febbre, cianosi, dispnea, dolore toracico e distress respiratorio, seguiti da un miglioramento. In questa fase la BO è facilmente confusa con la polmonite, la bronchite o la bronchiolite. La malattia può quindi progredire, con dispnea ingravescente, tosse cronica, produzione di espettorato e sibili. I reperti dell'esame obiettivo, in genere aspecifici, comprendono sibili e crepitii. Le radiografie del torace possono essere relativamente normali, rispetto all'importanza dei segni obiettivi, ma dimostrare infiltrati radiolucenti e a chiazze. Occasionalmente si sviluppa una sindrome di Swyer-James (polmone iperlucente monolaterale; vedi Capitolo 389). Gli esami di funzionalità polmonare possono dare risultati variabili, ma tipicamente rivelano segni di ostruzione delle vie aeree. La scintigrafia ventilazione-perfusione mette in luce un tipico aspetto tarlato, con multipli difetti appaiati di ventilazione e perfusione. Alla TC del torace spesso si apprezzano aree focali iperlucenti e bronchiectasie. La biopsia polmonare a cielo aperto, oppure transbronchiale, resta la metodica migliore per formulare la diagnosi di BO o BOOP.

TRATTAMENTO. Non esiste una terapia definitiva per la BO. La somministrazione di corticosteroidi può essere efficace. Gli agenti immunomodulatori, come il sirolimus, il tacrolimus, la ciclosporina per aerosol e gli antibiotici macrolidi, sono stati utilizzati nei riceventi di trapianto polmonare con BO, con successo variabile. L'infliximab, un anticorpo monoclonale che si lega al fattore di necrosi tumorale-α (TNF-α, *Tumor Necrosis Factor alpha*), ha avuto successo in un paziente con BO dopo trapianto osseo. Per la BOOP, l'uso di corticosteroidi orali fino a un anno è stato considerato la terapia di prima scelta nei pazienti con malattia sintomatica e progressiva. Per i pazienti con BOOP asintomatica o non progressiva è possibile la semplice osservazione nell'arco del tempo.

PROGNOSI. Alcuni pazienti con BO vanno incontro a rapido deterioramento delle condizioni e muoiono entro alcune settimane dall'esordio dei sintomi; la maggior parte dei non trapiantati sopravvive con una disabilità cronica. A differenza di quanto avviene nella BO, il 60-80% dei soggetti con BOOP presenta una guarigione completa, sebbene quest'ultima dipenda dalla malattia sistemica di base. Possono verificarsi recidive, specialmente se il trattamento è di durata inferiore a un anno e comporta la somministrazione di cicli ripetuti di corticosteroidi orali. A differenza della più comune BOOP idiopatica, la BOOP progressiva, caratterizzata da sindrome da distress respiratorio acuto (ARDS, *Acute Respiratory Distress Syndrome*), è rara ma ha un decorso clinico aggressivo che porta alla morte.

Epler GR: Bronchiolitis obliterans organizing pneumonia. *Arch Intern Med* 2001;161;158–164.
Fullmer JJ, Fan LL, Dishop MK, et al: Successful treatment of bronchiolitis obliterans in a bone marrow transplant patient with tumor necrosis factor-a blockade. *Pediatrics* 2005;116:767–770.
Hardy KA, Schidlow DV, Zaeri N: Obliterative bronchiolitis in children. *Chest* 1988;93:460–466.
Kurland G, Michelson P: Bronchiolitis obliterans in children. *Pediatr Pulmonol* 2005;39:193–208.
Zhang L, Irion K, Kozakewich H, et al: Clinical course of postinfectious bronchiolitis obliterans. *Pediatr Pulmonol* 2000;29:341–350.

391.2 • Bronchite follicolare

La bronchite follicolare è una malattia polmonare linfoproliferativa, rara nei bambini, caratterizzata dalla presenza di follicoli linfoidi lungo le vie aeree (bronchi e bronchioli). Sebbene la causa sia sconosciuta, è stata proposta un'eziologia infettiva (virale). I sintomi si manifestano generalmente intorno alle 6 settimane di vita e raggiungono un picco tra i 6 e gli 8 mesi. I reperti clinici più comuni sono tosse, distress respiratorio moderato, febbre e crepitii fini; questi ultimi in genere persistono nel tempo, e la recidiva sintomatologica è comune. Le radiografie del torace all'inizio possono essere relativamente benigne (intrappolamento d'aria, ispessimento peribronchiale), ma evolvono nel tipico quadro interstiziale. La TC del torace può mostrare un pattern finemente reticolare. La diagnosi definitiva è effettuata tramite biopsia polmonare a cielo aperto. Alcuni individui con bronchite follicolare rispondono alla terapia con corticosteroidi. La prognosi è variabile: alcuni individui presentano una progressione significativa della patologia polmonare, mentre altri sviluppano solo una lieve malattia respiratoria ostruttiva. La diagnosi differenziale comprende le complicanze polmonari dell'infezione da HIV.

Bramson RT, Cleveland R, Blickman JG, et al: Radiographic assessment of follicular bronchitis in children. *AJR Am J Roentgenol* 1996;166:1447–1450.
Kinane BT, Mansell AL, Zwerdling RG, et al: Follicular bronchitis in the pediatric population. *Chest* 1993;104:1183–1186.
Yousem SA, Colby TV, Carrington CB: Follicular bronchitis/bronchiolitis. *Hum Pathol* 1985;16:700–706.

391.3 • Microlitiasi alveolare polmonare

Sono stati riportati circa 400 casi di questa rara malattia. La microlitiasi alveolare polmonare (PAM, *Pulmonary Alveolar Microlithiasis*), la cui causa è sconosciuta, consiste nella formazione di concrezioni lamellari di fosfato di calcio o "microliti" negli alveoli, che creano un pattern caratteristico apprezzabile alla radiografia (Fig. 391-1).

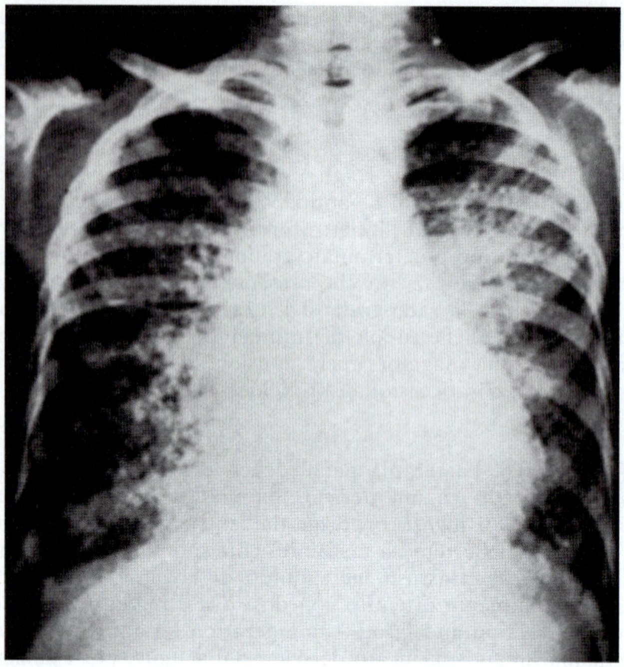

Figura 391-1. Radiografia del torace di un bambino di 7 anni con microlitiasi alveolare polmonare (Da Clark RB III, Johnson FC: Idiopathic pulmonary alveolar microlithiasis: A case report and brief review of the literature. *Pediatrics* 1961;28:650.)

EPIDEMIOLOGIA ED EZIOLOGIA. Sebbene l'età media al momento della diagnosi sia intorno alla metà della quarta decade, l'esordio della malattia può verificarsi in età infantile. In circa la metà dei casi riportati si osserva una forte associazione familiare, con un verosimile pattern di ereditarietà autosomico recessivo. In alcune famiglie si assiste a una rapida progressione della malattia. La frequenza è uguale nei due sessi. Una percentuale relativamente ampia di pazienti con PAM è di origine turca. La forma non familiare, o sporadica, sembra associata ad altre condizioni mediche, come la stenosi mitralica, la nefrolitiasi, la fibrosi polmonare, la sindrome latte-alcali, o fattori ambientali (sabbia).

MANIFESTAZIONI CLINICHE. Quando sintomatici, i pazienti con PAM lamentano dispnea da sforzo e tosse non produttiva. L'esame obiettivo dei polmoni può rivelare crepitii inspiratori fini e riduzione dei suoni respiratori. Può insorgere ippocratismo digitale, che tuttavia di solito rappresenta un segno più avanzato. È comune la discordanza tra le manifestazioni cliniche e radiologiche. I bambini sono spesso asintomatici alla presentazione iniziale. Sono state riportate complicanze come pneumotorace, aderenze e calcificazioni pleuriche, fibrosi pleurica, bolla apicale e sedi extrapolmonari di microlitiasi (reni, prostata, catena del simpatico e testicoli).

DIAGNOSI. La radiografia del torace rivela tipicamente infiltrati bilaterali con un aspetto finemente granulare o "a tempesta di sabbia" con una maggiore densità nei campi polmonari inferiori e medi (vedi Fig. 391-1). La TC del torace mostra diffuse densità calcificate micronodulari, con ispessimento dei microliti lungo i setti e intorno ai bronchioli distali, specialmente nelle regioni inferiori e posteriori. È stata riportata una diffusa captazione di ^{99m}Tc alla scintigrafia. La biopsia polmonare a cielo aperto, o transbronchiale, rivela concrezioni calcifiche laminari di 0,1-0,3 mm all'interno degli alveoli. Sebbene gli alveoli siano spesso normali nelle fasi iniziali, durante il decorso della malattia si ha progressione verso la fibrosi polmonare. L'espettorato può rivelare piccoli microliti, sebbene questo reperto non sia diagnostico di PAM e non si osservi tipicamente nei bambini. Gli esami di funzionalità polmonare rivelano una malattia restrittiva con alterazione della capacità di diffusione, con la progressione della malattia, mentre i test sotto sforzo dimostrano desaturazione arteriosa. La diagnosi differenziale comprende la sarcoidosi, la tubercolosi miliare, l'emosiderosi, l'istoplasmosi disseminata guarita, la calcinosi polmonare e le calcificazioni polmonari metastatiche.

TRATTAMENTO. Non esiste un trattamento specifico efficace, sebbene alcuni abbiano utilizzato i corticosteroidi, l'etidronato disodico e il lavaggio broncopolmonare con un successo limitato. Per questa condizione è stato effettuato il trapianto polmonare, sebbene non si sappia se la malattia recidivi dopo il trapianto.

PROGNOSI. Può esitare una malattia cardiopolmonare progressiva, che porta a cuore polmonare, sovrainfezioni e conseguente decesso nell'età adulta. A causa della natura famigliare di questa malattia, sono indicati il counseling e la radiografia del torace nei membri della famiglia.

Edelman, JD, Bavaria J, Kaiser LR, et al: Bilateral sequential lung transplantation for pulmonary alveolar microlithiasis. *Chest* 1997;112:1140–1144.
Erelel M, Kiyan E, Cuhadaroglu C, et al: Pulmonary alveolar lithiasis in two siblings. *Respiration* 2001;68:327–330.
Mariotta S, Ricci A, Papale M, et al: Pulmonary alveolar microlithiasis: report on 576 cases published in the literature. *Sarcoidosis Vase Diffuse Lung Dis* 2004;21(3):173–181.
Schmidt H, Lorcher U, Kitz R, et al: Pulmonary alveolar microlithiasis in children. *Pediatr Radiol* 1996;26:33–36.
Wallis C, Whitehead B, Malone M, et al: Pulmonary alveolar microlithiasis in childhood: Diagnosis by transbronchial biopsy. *Pediatr Pulmonol* 1996;21:62–64.

Capitolo 392 ■ Disordini congeniti del polmone Jonathan D. Finder e Peter H. Michelson

392.1 • Agenesia e aplasia polmonari

EZIOLOGIA E ANATOMIA PATOLOGICA. L'agenesia polmonare si differenzia dall'ipoplasia in quanto comporta l'assenza completa di un polmone, e dall'aplasia per l'assenza di un moncone bronchiale o della carena, con agenesia. La forma bilaterale, incompatibile con la vita, si presenta con grave distress e insufficienza respiratoria. Poiché sono stati riportati casi di pazienti con consanguineità dei genitori, si pensa che l'agenesia polmonare sia un tratto autosomico recessivo.

MANIFESTAZIONI CLINICHE E PROGNOSI. L'agenesia o l'ipoplasia unilaterali possono dare sintomi scarsi e aspecifici, tanto che solo un terzo dei pazienti viene diagnosticato nel corso della vita. I sintomi tendono a essere correlati a complicanze delle vie aeree centrali, come stenosi e/o tracheobroncomalacia. Se a essere assente è il polmone destro, l'aorta può comprimere la trachea e portare a sintomi di compressione delle vie aeree centrali; l'agenesia del polmone destro è contraddistinta da una mortalità e una morbilità più elevate rispetto a quella del polmone sinistro. L'agenesia polmonare si osserva spesso in associazione con altre anomalie congenite, come la sequenza VACTERL (*Vertebral anomalies, Anal atresia, Congenital heart disease, Tracheoesophageal fistola, Renal anomalies, and Limb anomalies*, anomalie vertebrali, atresia anale, cardiopatie congenite, fistola tracheoesofagea e anomalie degli arti), malformazioni facciali e scheletriche ipsilaterali, malformazioni cardiache e del sistema nervoso centrale. La crescita compensatoria del polmone superstite migliora lo scambio gassoso, ma lo spostamento del mediastino può portare a scoliosi e compressione delle vie aeree.

DIAGNOSI E TRATTAMENTO. Il riscontro alla radiografia del torace di un polmone solo, o di collasso lobare con spostamento delle strutture mediastiniche verso il lato colpito, può indurre all'invio dallo specialista per sospetta aspirazione di un corpo estraneo, occlusione da parte di tappi di muco o di altre masse bronchiali. La diagnosi richiede un elevato indice di sospetto per evitare gli inutili rischi di una broncoscopia, compresa la potenziale perforazione del bronco rudimentale. La TC del torace è diagnostica, sebbene la diagnosi possa essere suggerita da alterazioni croniche dell'aspetto della parete toracica e dell'espansione polmonare controlaterali, alla radiografia del torace. Generalmente si consiglia il trattamento conservativo, sebbene la chirurgia apporti benefici in casi selezionati.

392.2 • Ipoplasia polmonare

EZIOLOGIA E ANATOMIA PATOLOGICA. L'ipoplasia polmonare in genere è secondaria ad altre alterazioni intrauterine che influiscono sul normale sviluppo polmonare (vedi Capitolo 101). Condizioni come deformità della colonna dorsale e della cassa toracica (distrofia toracica), versamento pleurico con idrope fetale, malformazione adenomatoide cistica ed ernia diaframmatica congenita, comprimono il polmone nel corso dello sviluppo. Qualsiasi condizione che provochi oligoidramnios (insufficienza renale fetale o rottura prematura prolungata delle membrane) può inoltre portare a ridotta crescita polmonare. In queste situazioni, le vie aeree e le ramificazioni arteriose sono inibite, limitando così la capacità dell'area di scambio gassoso e capillare. Nell'ipoplasia polmonare sia gli alveoli sia le ramificazioni delle vie aeree risultano di numero ridotto. L'ipoplasia può essere bilaterale, per la presenza di una costrizione polmonare bilaterale, come quella riscontrabile nell'oligoidramnios o nella distrofia toracica. Grandi lesioni monolaterali, come un'ernia diaframmatica congenita e la malformazione adenomatoide cistica, possono spostare il mediastino e provocare così ipoplasia controlaterale, sebbene di solito non così severa come quella osservata ipsilateralmente.

MANIFESTAZIONI CLINICHE. L'ipoplasia polmonare è segnalata di solito nel periodo neonatale sia dall'insufficienza respiratoria sia dalla presentazione con ipertensione polmonare persistente. Nei lattanti con ipoplasia polmonare lieve è possibile osservare una presentazione tardiva (con tachipnea) in occasione di stress o di infezioni respiratorie virali.

TRATTAMENTO. La ventilazione meccanica e l'ossigeno possono essere necessari per sostenere lo scambio gassoso. Può essere utile una terapia specifica (per es. ossido nitrico inalatorio) per controllare l'ipertensione polmonare associata. Nei casi di ipoplasia severa, la limitata capacità di scambio gassoso del polmone può non essere sufficiente alla sopravvivenza. L'ossigenazione con membrana extracorporea consente lo scambio di gas durante il periodo critico permettendo talora la sopravvivenza. Sistemi di espansione costale possono migliorare la sopravvivenza dei pazienti con distrofia toracica (vedi Capitoli 678 e 692).

392.3 • Malformazione adenomatoide cistica

ANATOMIA PATOLOGICA. La malformazione adenomatoide cistica congenita (CCAM, *Congenital Cystic Adenomatoid Malformation*) è un'anomalia polmonare congenita comune (1-4/100 000 nati), consistente nella presenza di tessuto polmonare amartomatoso o displasico frammisto a tessuto polmonare più normale; è di solito limitata a un lobo. Sono stati descritti tre quadri istologici, sebbene la correlazione tra l'aspetto istologico e il decorso clinico sia controverso. Il **tipo 1** (50%) è macrocistico e consiste in una cisti singola o diverse cisti di grandi dimensioni (>2 cm di diametro), delimitate da epitelio ciliato pseudostratificato. La parete delle cisti contiene cellule muscolari lisce e tessuto elastico; un terzo dei casi ha cellule secernenti muco, mentre è raro che si osservi cartilagine. Questo tipo ha una buona prognosi per la sopravvivenza. Il **tipo 2** (40%) è microcistico e presenta piccole cisti multiple con istologia simile a quella delle lesioni del tipo 1. Si associa ad altre anomalie congenite e comporta una prognosi sfavorevole. Nel **tipo 3** (<10%) la lesione è solida, con strutture simil-bronchiolari, delimitate da epitelio cuboide ciliato e separate da aree di epitelio cuboide non ciliato. Questa lesione ha la prognosi peggiore e può essere fatale.

EZIOLOGIA. La lesione risulta probabilmente da un insulto embriologico, prima del 35° giorno di gestazione, con un alterato sviluppo delle strutture bronchiolari terminali. L'esame istologico rivela scarso tessuto polmonare normale e numerosi elementi ghiandolari. Le cisti sono molto comuni, mentre la cartilagine è rara; la sua presenza può indicare un insulto embriologico più tardivo, forse esteso alla 10ª-24ª settimana. Sebbene l'alterazione della morfogenesi della ramificazione polmonare sia stata attribuita a interazioni tra fattori di crescita e sistemi di segnalazione, il loro ruolo esatto nell'alterato sviluppo osservabile in questa patologia resta oscuro.

DIAGNOSI. La malformazione adenomatoide cistica può essere diagnosticata in utero tramite l'ecografia. In una casistica di 67 feti con diagnosi di anomalia polmonare cistica, di cui il 40% con malformazione adenomatoide cistica, il 14% con sequestro polmonare (vedi Capitolo 392.4) e il 26% con entrambe le alterazioni, l'età media alla diagnosi era di 21 settimane di gestazione. In questa casistica, il 7% aveva segni gravi di sofferenza fetale, tra cui idrope ($n = 4$), versamento pleurico ($n = 2$), polidramnios ($n = 1$), ascite ($n = 1$), ed edema facciale severo ($n = 1$); il 96% dei feti è nato vivo, ma due di essi sono morti nel periodo neonatale. Le caratteristiche ecografiche prenatali e l'aspetto macroscopico o istologico sono indicatori prognostici sfavorevoli. Le lesioni che causano idrope fetale hanno una prognosi infausta. Le lesioni più grandi, comprimendo il polmone adiacente, possono provocare ipoplasia polmonare dei lobi non affetti (vedi Capitolo 392.2). Anche le lesioni che sembrano più grandi nelle fasi precoci della gravidanza possono regredire considerevolmente o ridursi di dimensioni, e associarsi a una buona funzionalità polmonare nell'infanzia. La TC consente di determinare con precisione le dimensioni della lesione.

MANIFESTAZIONI CLINICHE. I pazienti che si presentano nel periodo neonatale o nella prima infanzia hanno distress respiratorio, infezioni respiratorie ricorrenti e pneumotorace. La lesione può essere confusa con un'ernia diaframmatica. I pazienti con lesioni più piccole sono asintomatici fino alla seconda infanzia, quando insorgono brevi episodi di infezione polmonare ricorrente o persistente, o dolore toracico relativamente acuto. I suoni respiratori possono essere ridotti; l'esame obiettivo evidenzia spostamento del mediastino dal lato opposto rispetto alla lesione. La radiografia del torace rivela una massa cistica, talvolta con spostamento mediastinico (Fig. 392-1). Occasionalmente, un livello idroaereo può suggerire un ascesso polmonare.

TRATTAMENTO. L'intervento prenatale nei pazienti affetti, seppure controverso, comprende l'asportazione del lobo affetto per le lesioni microcistiche, l'aspirazione delle lesioni macrocistiche e la chirurgia fetale a cielo aperto. Nel periodo postnatale, la chirurgia è indicata per tutti i pazienti sintomatici. Sebbene l'intervento possa essere rimandato nei lattanti asintomatici, poiché è stata riportata la risoluzione postnatale, una vera risoluzione sembra essere molto rara in caso di anomalie rilevabili alla TC o alla RM. È stata descritta una differenziazione (degenerazione) sarcomatosa o carcinomatosa nei pazienti con CCAM, pertanto si consiglia la resezione chirurgica entro il primo anno di vita, per limitarne il potenziale maligno. La mortalità è <10%.

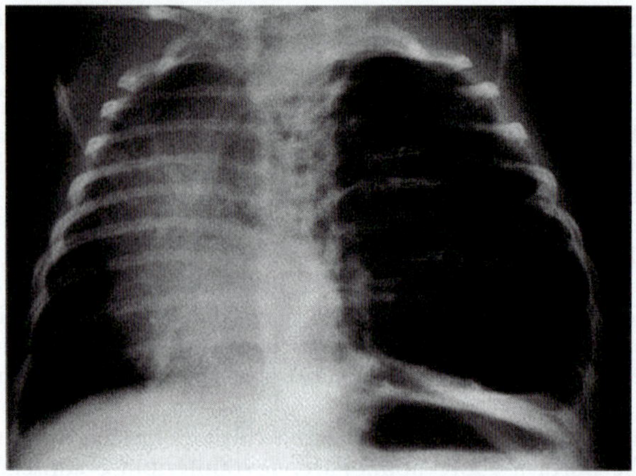

Figura 392-1. Radiografia toracica neonatale, che mostra una grande massa multicistica nell'emitorace sinistro, con spostamento del mediastino, da malformazione adenomatoide cistica congenita. (Da Williams HJ, Johnson KJ: Imaging of congenital cystic lung lesions. *Paediatr Resp Rev* 2002;3:120-127.)

392.4 • Sequestro polmonare

Il sequestro polmonare, un'anomalia congenita dello sviluppo polmonare, è classificabile come intrapolmonare o extrapolmonare, a seconda della sua localizzazione nell'ambito della pleura viscerale. La maggior parte dei casi è intrapolmonare.

FISIOPATOLOGIA. Il tessuto polmonare, in un sequestro, non è connesso a un bronco e riceve l'apporto arterioso dalle arterie sistemiche (comunemente dall'aorta), mentre il ritorno del sangue venoso al cuore destro avviene tramite la vena cava inferiore (se extralobare), o tramite le vene polmonari (se intralobare). Il sequestro si comporta come una lesione occupante spazio all'interno del torace; non ha una funzione di scambio gassoso e non contribuisce a uno shunt sinistro-destro, né allo spazio morto. Una comunicazione con le vie aeree può venire a formarsi in seguito all'ingresso di materiale infetto in una via aerea adiacente. Inoltre, può verificarsi ventilazione collaterale all'interno delle lesioni intrapolmonari, attraverso i pori di Kohn. Il sequestro polmonare può insorgere con lo stesso meccanismo patoembriologico come residuo di una crescita diverticolare dell'esofago. Secondo alcuni sarebbe una lesione acquisita, causata principalmente da infezioni e infiammazione, che porta ad alterazioni cistiche e all'ipertrofia di un'arteria sistemica che vascolarizza il sequestro. Tale ipotesi trova conferma nella rarità di questa lesione, nelle casistiche autoptiche di neonati. Nel sequestro si può rinvenire tessuto gastrico o pancreatico; possono anche essere presenti cisti. Non sono infrequenti altre anomalie, come la CCAM, l'ernia diaframmatica e le cisti esofagee. Alcuni, ritenendo che il sequestro intrapolmonare sia spesso la manifestazione di una malformazione adenomatoide cistica, hanno messo in dubbio l'esistenza del sequestro intrapolmonare come entità a sé stante.

MANIFESTAZIONI CLINICHE E DIAGNOSI. L'esame obiettivo, nei pazienti con sequestro, può rilevare un'area di ottusità alla percussione e di riduzione del murmure vescicolare in corrispondenza della lesione. In corso di infezione, si possono inoltre apprezzare crepitii. Può essere udibile un soffio continuo, o esclusivamente sistolico, sul dorso. Se l'aspetto della radiografia del torace di routine è compatibile con la diagnosi, si rendono necessari ulteriori approfondimenti prima dell'intervento chirurgico (Fig. 392-2). La TC con contrasto può dimostrare sia l'estensione della lesione, sia la sua vascolarizzazione. Anche l'angiorisonanza magnetica (ARM) può essere utile. L'ecografia aiuta a escludere un'ernia diaframmatica e a dimostrare le arterie sistemiche. È consigliata l'asportazione chirurgica. L'identificazione della vascolarizzazione prima dell'intervento scongiura il rischio che il chirurgo danneggi inavvertitamente le arterie sistemiche della lesione.

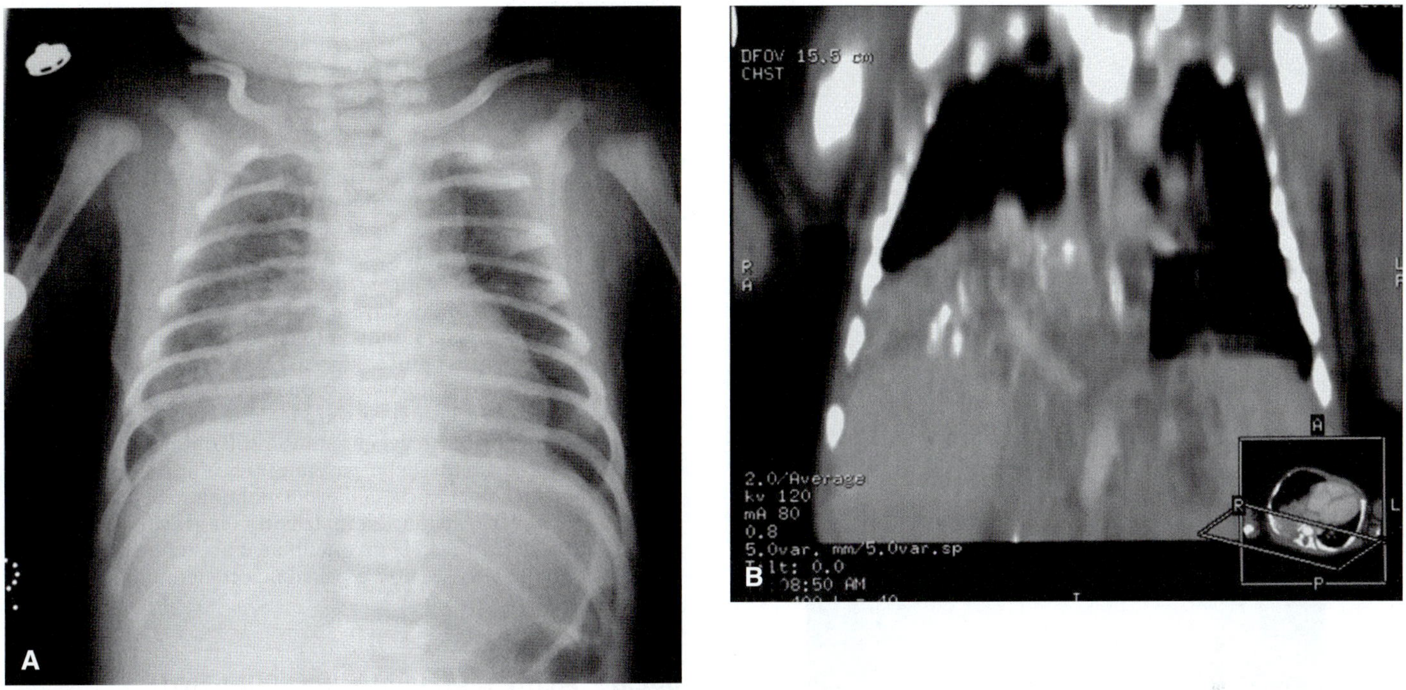

Figura 392-2. *A*, Radiografia toracica semplice, che mostra alterazioni della regione del lobo medio e inferiore destro del polmone. *B*, TC che rivela alterazioni del parenchima nel lobo inferiore destro del polmone, compatibili con un sequestro polmonare. (Da Corbett HJ, Humphrey GME: Pulmonary sequestration. *Paediatr Resp Rev* 2004;5:59-68.)

Il *sequestro intrapolmonare* è osservato generalmente in un lobo inferiore e non ha una pleura propria. I pazienti si presentano di solito con infezione. Nei bambini più grandi è comune l'emottisi. La radiografia del torace, effettuata in un periodo in cui non vi è infezione attiva, rivela una massa; può essere presente anche un livello idroaereo. Durante l'infezione, i margini della lesione possono essere sfumati. Non vi è differenza nell'incidenza della lesione nei due polmoni.

Il *sequestro extrapolmonare*, molto più comune nei maschi, colpisce quasi sempre il polmone sinistro. Questa lesione, circondata da un rivestimento pleurico, si associa a ernia diaframmatica e ad altre anomalie, come duplicazione del colon, anomalie vertebrali e ipoplasia polmonare. Molti di questi pazienti sono asintomatici, quando la massa è scoperta nel corso di una radiografia del torace di routine; altri presentano sintomi respiratori o insufficienza cardiaca. Il sequestro extrapolmonare sottodiaframmatico può manifestarsi come massa addominale all'ecografia prenatale. L'avvento dell'ecografia prenatale ha inoltre consentito di dimostrare che il sequestro polmonare fetale può regredire spontaneamente.

TRATTAMENTO. Il trattamento del sequestro intrapolmonare è la rimozione chirurgica della lesione, una procedura che richiede di solito l'asportazione di tutto il lobo coinvolto. Talvolta può essere sufficiente la resezione segmentaria. Se il sequestro è extrapolmonare si consiglia la resezione chirurgica dell'area coinvolta.

392.5 • Cisti broncogene

EZIOLOGIA E ANATOMIA PATOLOGICA. Le cisti broncogene derivano da gemme anomale del diverticolo tracheale dell'intestino primitivo, prima della 16ª settimana di gestazione, e in origine sono delimitate da epitelio ciliato. Si trovano più comunemente a destra e in vicinanza delle strutture della linea mediana (trachea, esofago, carena), anche se non sono infrequenti le cisti intrapolmonari periferiche del lobo inferiore e quelle peri-ilari. La diagnosi può essere accelerata da un aumento di dimensioni della cisti, che causa sintomi per compressione della via aerea adiacente. Quando la malattia viene individuata in ritardo, dopo l'insorgenza di un'infezione, l'epitelio ciliato può andare perduto e un'accurata diagnosi istopatologica diviene impossibile. È raro che le cisti siano dimostrabili alla nascita. In seguito, alcune possono divenire sintomatiche infettandosi o aumentando di volume, fino a compromettere la funzione delle vie aeree adiacenti.

MANIFESTAZIONI CLINICHE E TRATTAMENTO. I sintomi di presentazione più comuni sono febbre, dolore toracico e tosse produttiva. Può essere presente disfagia; alcune cisti broncogene sono asintomatiche. La radiografia del torace può rivelare la cisti, talvolta contenente un livello idroaereo (Fig. 392-3). Nella maggior parte dei casi si effettuano la TC o la RM per definire meglio l'anatomia e l'estensione della lesione, prima della resezione chirurgica. Il trattamento delle cisti sintomatiche è l'asportazione chirurgica dopo un trattamento antibiotico appropriato. In genere si asportano anche le cisti asintomatiche, che tendono a infettarsi con notevole frequenza.

392.6 • Linfangectasia polmonare congenita

EZIOLOGIA E ANATOMIA PATOLOGICA. Questa malattia, caratterizzata dalla presenza di dotti linfatici abnormemente dilatati in tutto il polmone, può insorgere in tre circostanze patologiche: (1) un'ostruzione venosa polmonare che produce un'elevata pressione transvascolare con ingorgo dei linfatici polmonari; (2) la linfangectasia generalizzata è una malattia sistemica di diversi organi e sistemi, compresi i polmoni e l'intestino, e si associa alla sindrome di Noonan; (3) la linfangectasia può essere limitata ai polmoni.

MANIFESTAZIONI CLINICHE E TRATTAMENTO. I bambini con ostruzione venosa polmonare o linfangectasia severa presentano dispnea e cianosi nel periodo neonatale. La radiografia del torace rivela addensamenti diffusi, radiopachi, reticolari, con strie B di Kerley. Se il coinvolgimento del polmone non è completo, le aree risparmiate appaiono iperlucenti. La respirazione è compromessa a causa dell'alterata diffusione e della ridotta compliance polmonare. La TC e il cateterismo cardiaco possono fornire indizi preziosi al medico, ma la diagnosi definitiva richiede la biopsia

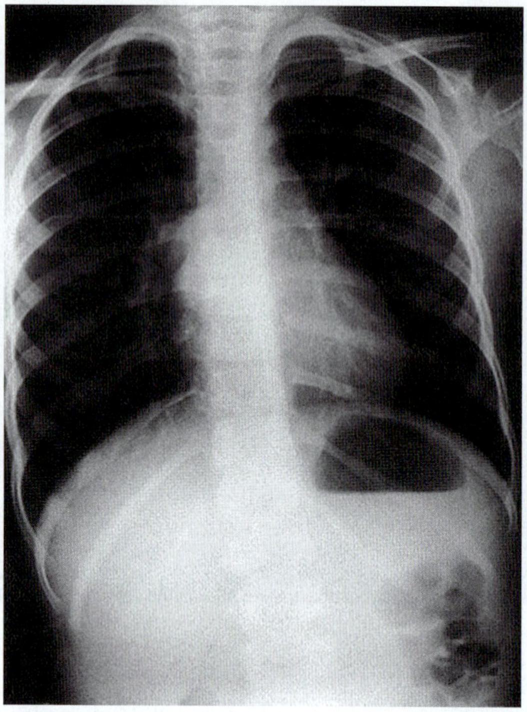

Figura 392-3. Radiografia del torace da cui emerge un addensamento ovoidale, ben definito, di tessuti molli, che causa l'allungamento della carena in conseguenza di una cisti broncogena. (Da Williams HJ, Johnson KJ: Imaging of congenital cystic lung lesions. *Paediatr Resp Rev* 2002;3:120-127.)

polmonare (sia toracoscopica sia a cielo aperto). Il trattamento è di supporto e comprende la somministrazione di ossigeno, la ventilazione meccanica, il supporto nutrizionale (compreso il posizionamento di una gastrostomia) e un accurato bilancio idrico, con somministrazione di diuretici. La linfangectasia polmonare primitiva può provocare una disfunzione polmonare così severa da richiedere la ventilazione meccanica a lungo termine; la sopravvivenza a lungo termine è possibile anche nei casi gravi. Talvolta l'ostruzione venosa polmonare è secondaria a lesioni cardiache sinistre, e la correzione di queste ultime si traduce in un miglioramento della disfunzione polmonare. La linfangectasia generalizzata provoca generalmente una disfunzione polmonare più lieve, e non è rara la sopravvivenza fino alla seconda infanzia e anche oltre.

392.7 • Ernia polmonare

EZIOLOGIA E ANATOMIA PATOLOGICA. Un'ernia polmonare è una protrusione del polmone oltre i suoi normali confini toracici. In circa il 20% dei pazienti è congenita; la maggior parte dei casi si manifesta dopo un trauma toracico o un intervento di chirurgia toracica, oppure in concomitanza con malattie polmonari come la fibrosi cistica o l'asma, che spesso causano tosse con aumento della pressione intratoracica. Una debolezza congenita delle membrane sovrapleuriche, o della muscolatura del collo, può giocare un ruolo nella sua comparsa. Più della metà delle ernie polmonari congenite e praticamente tutte quelle acquisite sono **cervicali**. Le ernie cervicali congenite di solito insorgono anteriormente, attraverso uno spazio tra i muscoli scaleno anteriore e sternocleidomastoideo, ma di norma il muscolo trapezio (posteriormente, a livello dell'ingresso del torace) e i tre muscoli scaleni (lateralmente) ne impediscono lo sviluppo.

MANIFESTAZIONI CLINICHE E TRATTAMENTO. Il segno di presentazione di un'ernia cervicale ("ernia di Sibson") è in genere una massa del collo, visibile quando il paziente fa uno sforzo o tossisce. Alcune lesioni sono asintomatiche e vengono rilevate solo al momento di effettuare una radiografia del torace per altre ragioni. I reperti all'esame obiettivo sono normali, tranne che durante la manovra di Valsalva, quando si può notare una tumefazione soffice nel collo. Anche se nella maggior parte dei casi non è necessario alcun trattamento, queste ernie possono causare problemi, durante i tentativi di posizionare un catetere venoso centrale nella vena giugulare o succlavia. Può verificarsi la risoluzione spontanea.

Le ernie paravertebrali o parasternali si associano di solito ad anomalie costali. Le ernie intercostali tendono a insorgere in posizione parasternale, dove è assente il muscolo intercostale esterno. Posteriormente, nonostante il muscolo intercostale interno sembri inadeguato, i muscoli paraspinali evitano normalmente l'erniazione. Gli sforzi, la tosse o suonare uno strumento musicale possono avere un ruolo nel causare le ernie intercostali, che tuttavia nella maggior parte dei casi sono probabilmente attribuibili a un difetto preesistente della parete toracica.

Il trattamento chirurgico dell'ernia polmonare è talvolta giustificato per motivi estetici. Nei pazienti con grave pneumopatia cronica e tosse cronica, e in quelli in cui è controindicata la soppressione della tosse, non è possibile ottenere una correzione permanente.

392.8 • Altre malformazioni congenite dei polmoni

ENFISEMA LOBARE CONGENITO E CISTI POLMONARI. Vedi Capitolo 389.

MALFORMAZIONE ARTEROVENOSA POLMONARE. Vedi Capitoli 432 e 444.

FISTOLA BRONCOBILIARE. Questa rara anomalia in genere comporta una serie di problemi che mettono a rischio la vita del paziente nella prima infanzia, anche se in alcuni casi la diagnosi è stata formulata con un certo ritardo, in età adulta. Il sesso femminile è il più colpito. La fistola broncobiliare consiste in un tragitto fistoloso tra il bronco lobare medio destro e il sistema duttale epatico sinistro. Tutti i pazienti hanno gravi infezioni broncopolmonari ricorrenti a partire dalla prima infanzia. La *diagnosi definitiva* richiede l'endoscopia e la broncografia, o l'intervento chirurgico esplorativo. Il *trattamento* comprende l'asportazione chirurgica di tutta la porzione intratoracica della fistola. Se la porzione epatica non comunica con il sistema biliare o con il duodeno, il segmento coinvolto può anche essere asportato. Una comunicazione broncobiliare può inoltre essere il risultato di lesioni acquisite, causate da malattie epatiche complicate da infezione.

Bentsianov BL, Goldstein NA, Giuste R, Har-El G: Unilateral pulmonary agenesis presenting as an airway lesion. *Arch Otolaryngol Head Neck Surg* 2000;126:1386–1389.

Calvert JK, Boyd PA, Chamberlain PC, et al: Outcome of antenatally suspected congenital cystic adenomatoid malformation of the lung: 10 years' experience 1991–2001. *Arch Dis Child* 2006;91:F26–F28.

Carpentieri DF, Guttenberg M, Quinn TM, Adzick NS: Subdiaphragmatic pulmonary sequestration: A case report with review of the literature. *J Perinatol* 2000;20:60–62.

Chung CJ, Fordham LA, Barker P, Cooper LL: Children with congenital pulmonary lymphangiectasia: After infancy. *AJR Am J Roentgenol* 1999;173:1583–1588.

Davenport M, Warne SA, Cacciaguerra S, et al: Current outcome of antenally diagnosed cystic lung disease. *J Pediatr Surg* 2004;39:549–556.

Garcia-Pena P, Lucaya J, Hendry GM, et al: Spontaneous involution of pulmonary sequestration in children: A report of two cases and review of the literature. *Pediatr Radiol* 1998;28:266–270.

Glenn C, Bonekat W, Cua A, et al: Lung hernia. *Am J Emerg Med* 1997;15:260–262.

Granata C, Gambini C, Balducci T, et al: Bronchioloalveolar carcinoma arising in congenital cystic adenomatoid malformation in a child: A case report

and review on malignancies originating in congenital cystic adenomatoid malformation. *Pediatr Pulmonol* 1998; 25:62–66.
Krivchenya DU, Dubrovin AG, Krivchenya TD, et al: Aplasia of the right lung in a 4-year-old child: Surgical stabilization of the mediastinum by diaphragm translocation leading to complete recovery from respiratory distress syndrome. *J Pediatr Surg* 2000;35:1499–1502.
Nicolette LA, Kosloske AM, Bartow SA, Murphy S: Intralobar pulmonary sequestration: A clinical and pathological spectrum. *J Pediatr Surg* 1993;28:802–805.
Riedlinger WF, Vargas SO, Jennings RW, et al: Bronchial atresia is common to extralobar sequestration, intralobar sequestration, congenital cystic adenomatoid malformation, and lobar emphysema. *Pediatr Dev Pathol* 2006;9:361–373.
Sauvat F, Michel JL, Benachi A, et al: Management of asymptomatic neonatal cystic adenomatoid malformations. *J Pediatr Surg* 2003; 38:548–552.
Schmittenbecher P: Congenital cystic adenomatoid malformation of the lung: Indications and timing of surgery. *J Pediatr Surg* 2005;40:891–892.
Schwartz D, Reyes-Mugica M, Keller M: Imaging of surgical diseases of the newborn chest. *Radiol Clin North Am* 1999;37:1067–1078.
Zach MS: Adult outcome of congenital lower respiratory tract malformations. *Thorax* 2001;56:65–72.

Capitolo 393 ■ Edema polmonare

Thomas Bahk, Robert Mazor e Thomas P. Green

L'edema polmonare consiste in un accumulo eccessivo di liquidi nell'interstizio e negli spazi aerei del polmone, che dà luogo a desaturazione di ossigeno e distress respiratorio. È un problema comune nel bambino con malattia acuta ed è una sequela di varie patologie.

FISIOPATOLOGIA. Sebbene l'edema polmonare sia tradizionalmente distinto in due categorie a seconda della causa (*cardiogeno* e *non cardiogeno*), il risultato finale di entrambi i processi è un accumulo netto di liquido negli spazi interstiziali e alveolari. L'edema polmonare non cardiogeno, nei suoi stadi più gravi, è anche noto come **sindrome da distress respiratorio acuto** (ARDS, *Acute Respiratory Distress Syndrome*) (vedi Capitolo 69).

La pressione e l'osmolarità sui due versanti di un capillare polmonare e la permeabilità capillare sono i fattori fisici che determinano il movimento dei liquidi attraverso la parete capillare. Le condizioni di base conducono a una filtrazione netta di liquido dallo spazio intravascolare verso l'interstizio. Questo liquido interstiziale in eccesso in condizioni normali viene riassorbito rapidamente dai linfatici polmonari. Le condizioni che portano a un'alterazione della permeabilità capillare, ad aumentata pressione capillare polmonare, o a una ridotta pressione oncotica intravascolare, aumentano il flusso netto di liquido che fuoriesce dai capillari (Tab. 393-1) e determinano quindi accumulo di acqua nei polmoni.

Per capire la concatenazione di eventi che porta all'accumulo di acqua nei polmoni, è utile considerare la sua distribuzione in quattro comparti distinti.

1. **Comparto vascolare:** questo comparto è formato da tutti i vasi sanguigni che partecipano allo scambio di liquidi nell'interstizio. Il comparto vascolare è separato dall'interstizio dalle cellule endoteliali capillari. Numerosi fattori infiammatori endogeni, così come tossine esogene, sono coinvolti nella patogenesi del danno endoteliale dei capillari polmonari, che porta allo "stravaso" osservato in numerosi processi sistemici.
2. **Comparto interstiziale:** questo spazio deriva la propria importanza dal fatto di essere interposto tra il comparto alveolare e quello vascolare. I liquidi che escono dal comparto vascolare si raccolgono nell'interstizio prima di diffondersi nello spazio aereo del comparto alveolare.
3. **Comparto alveolare:** questo comparto è delimitato da cellule epiteliali di tipo 1 e 2, che hanno un ruolo nel trasporto attivo del liquido dallo spazio alveolare.
4. **Comparto linfatico polmonare:** esiste un'estesa rete di linfatici polmonari. Il liquido in eccesso presente nei comparti alveolare e interstiziale è drenato dal sistema linfatico. I liquidi si accumulano quando il loro volume supera la capacità di drenaggio dei vasi linfatici.

TABELLA 393-1. Eziologia dell'edema polmonare

AUMENTO DELLA PRESSIONE CAPILLARE POLMONARE
Cardiogeno, come l'insufficienza ventricolare sinistra
Non cardiogeno, come la malattia veno-occlusiva polmonare, la fibrosi venosa polmonare, i tumori mediastinici
AUMENTO DELLA PERMEABILITÀ CAPILLARE
Polmoniti virali e batteriche
Sindrome da distress respiratorio acuto
Sostanze tossiche inalate
Tossine circolanti
Sostanze vasoattive come istamina, leucotrieni e trombossani
Sindrome da stravaso capillare diffuso, come nella sepsi
Reazioni immunologiche, come nelle reazioni trasfusionali
Inalazione di fumo
Polmonite da aspirazione
Annegamento o preannegamento
Polmonite da radiazioni
Uremia
INSUFFICIENZA LINFATICA
Congenita e acquisita
RIDOTTA PRESSIONE ONCOTICA
Ipoalbuminemia, come nelle malattie epatiche e renali, negli stati proteinodisperdenti e nella malnutrizione
AUMENTO DELLA PRESSIONE INTERSTIZIALE NEGATIVA
Lesioni ostruttive delle vie aeree superiori, come nel croup e nell'epiglottite
Edema polmonare da riespansione
CONDIZIONI VARIE O DA CAUSA SCONOSCIUTA
Edema polmonare neurogeno
Edema polmonare da altitudine elevata
Eclampsia
Pancreatite
Embolia polmonare
Edema da eroina (narcotici)

Modificata da Robin E, Carroll C, Zelis R: Pulmonary edema. *N Engl J Med* 1973;288:239, 292; Desphande J, Wetzel R, Rogers M: In Rogers M (ed): *Textbook of Pediatric Intensive Care*, 3rd ed. Baltimore, Williams & Wilkins, 1996, pp 432-442.

EZIOLOGIA. I reperti clinici specifici variano in base al meccanismo scatenante (vedi Tab. 393-1).

L'aumento della pressione vascolare polmonare (*pressione idrostatica capillare*) porta ad aumento del flusso di liquido proveniente dai vasi. I *processi cardiaci* che portano a insufficienza di pompa sinistra (miocardite) o ad aumento del reflusso sinistro (insufficienza mitralica) causano un aumento della pressione capillare polmonare. Inoltre, vi sono cause non cardiache, che comprendono anomalie delle vene polmonari che ostruiscono il drenaggio venoso, con conseguente *aumento della pressione capillare*.

L'aumento della permeabilità capillare è in genere secondario a un danno endoteliale; quest'ultimo può verificarsi secondariamente a danno diretto dell'epitelio alveolare o, indirettamente, tramite processi sistemici durante i quali vengono immessi in circolo mediatori infiammatori o tossine, che raggiungono i polmoni. A causa del consistente flusso ematico da cui sono interessati, i polmoni sono particolarmente esposti alle tossine circolanti. I mediatori dell'infiammazione (fattore di necrosi tumorale, leucotrieni, trombossani) e gli agenti vasoattivi (ossido nitrico, istamina), formati durante i processi polmonari e sistemici, giocano un ruolo nel danno endoteliale e nell'alterata permeabilità capillare che caratterizzano molti di questi processi patologici, di cui la sepsi è una causa comune.

L'omeostasi dei liquidi nei polmoni dipende in gran parte dal drenaggio attraverso i vasi linfatici. Sperimentalmente, l'edema polmonare si verifica per ostruzione del sistema linfatico. Negli stati edematosi cronici si riscontrano aumento del flusso linfatico e dilatazione dei vasi linfatici.

Riducendo le forze che promuovono il rientro dei liquidi nello spazio vascolare, la diminuzione della pressione oncotica intravascolare porta a edema polmonare; questo si verifica nei disordini da diluizione, come il sovraccarico di liquidi con soluzioni ipotoniche, e nelle malattie proteinodisperdenti, come la sindrome nefrosica e la malnutrizione.

L'aumento della pressione negativa interstiziale è considerato un fattore chiave nei disordini in cui è presente ostruzione delle vie aeree superiori, come il croup. Tuttavia, possono essere coinvolti anche altri meccanismi. Alcune teorie postulano una riduzione della pressione di CO_2, una riduzione della pressione di O_2 e un aumento estremo del postcarico cardiaco, che porta a insufficienza cardiaca transitoria.

Il meccanismo che causa l'edema polmonare neurogeno non è chiaro. Una scarica simpatica massiva, secondaria a un danno cerebrale, può provocare un aumento della vasocostrizione polmonare e sistemica, risultante in uno spostamento di sangue ai vasi polmonari, nell'aumento della pressione capillare e nella formazione di edema. Il meccanismo responsabile dell'edema polmonare da altitudine non è chiaro, ma può essere anch'esso correlato alla trasmissione simpatica, ad aumento della pressione vascolare polmonare e ad aumento della permeabilità capillare indotto dall'ipossia.

MANIFESTAZIONI CLINICHE. Le caratteristiche cliniche che ne derivano dipendono dal meccanismo della formazione dell'edema. In generale, l'edema interstiziale e alveolare impedisce l'espansione degli alveoli, portando ad atelettasia e a ridotta produzione di surfattante, che a loro volta si traducono in una diminuzione della compliance polmonare e del volume corrente. Per mantenere il volume corrente sono necessari un lavoro respiratorio più elevato e/o un aumento della frequenza respiratoria. I segni clinici più precoci comprendono un aumento dello sforzo respiratorio, sotto forma di tachipnea e dispnea. A causa dell'accumulo di liquidi nello spazio alveolare, l'ascultazione rivela crepitii fini e sibili, specialmente nelle regioni declivi del polmone. Nell'edema polmonare cardiogeno può essere presente un ritmo di galoppo, oltre a edemi periferici e distensione delle giugulari.

La radiografia del torace può fornire informazioni complementari utili, sebbene all'inizio possa essere normale. I segni radiologici precoci comprendono accentuazione del disegno peribronchiale e perivascolare, che indica l'accumulo dell'edema interstiziale. La presenza di striature diffuse riflette l'edema interlobulare e la distensione dei linfatici polmonari. Gli addensamenti diffusi, a chiazze, secondari al riempimento degli alveoli, sono un segno tardivo, compresa la classica descrizione dell'aspetto "a farfalla", che rappresenta infiltrati bilaterali interstiziali o alveolari. Nei casi attribuibili a una disfunzione ventricolare sinistra si osservano cardiomegalia e aumento del disegno vascolare. Le dimensioni del cuore sono di solito normali nell'edema polmonare non cardiogeno (Tab. 393-2). La TC del torace dimostra che l'edema si accumula nelle zone declivi del polmone. Pertanto, un cambiamento di posizione del paziente può incidere sulle differenze regionali della compliance e della ventilazione alveolare.

TABELLA 393-2. Caratteristiche radiografiche che possono essere utili per differenziare l'edema polmonare cardiogeno e non cardiogeno

CARATTERISTICHE RADIOGRAFICHE	EDEMA CARDIOGENO	EDEMA NON CARDIOGENO
Dimensioni del cuore	Normali o ingrandite	Di solito normali
Ampiezza del peduncolo vascolare*	Normale o superiore alla norma	Di solito normale o inferiore alla norma
Distribuzione vascolare	Equilibrata o invertita	Normale o equilibrata
Distribuzione dell'edema	Regolare o centrale	Irregolare o periferica
Versamento pleurico	Presente	Di solito non presente
Ispessimento peribronchiale	Presente	Di solito non presente
Linee settali	Presenti	Di solito non presenti
Broncogramma aereo	Di solito non presente	Di solito presente

* Per determinare l'ampiezza del peduncolo vascolare negli adulti si traccia una linea perpendicolare a partire dal punto in cui l'arteria succlavia sinistra si dirama dall'arco aortico, fino al punto in cui la vena cava superiore attraversa il bronco principale destro. Un'ampiezza del peduncolo vascolare >70 mm alla radiografia portatile anteroposteriore del torace, con paziente supino, è ottimale per differenziare un volume intravascolare elevato da uno normale o basso.

Da Ware LB, Matthay MA: Acute pulmonary edema. *N Engl J Med* 2005;353:2788-2796.

Il dosaggio del peptide natriuretico cerebrale (BNP, *Brain Natriuretic Peptide*), che è elevato in caso di cardiopatia, può aiutare a differenziare le cause cardiache di edema polmonare da quelle polmonari. Un livello di BPN >500 pg/mL suggerisce una patologia cardiaca, mentre uno <100 pg/mL è indicativo di una patologia polmonare.

TRATTAMENTO. Il trattamento di un paziente con edema polmonare non cardiogeno è in gran parte di supporto, con l'obiettivo principale di assicurare ventilazione e ossigenazione adeguate. La terapia aggiuntiva è rivolta alla causa sottostante. I pazienti dovrebbero ricevere un supplemento di ossigeno nel tentativo di aumentare la pressione alveolare di ossigeno e ridurre la vasocostrizione polmonare. I pazienti con cause cardiogene devono essere trattati con agenti inotropi e con vasodilatatori sistemici per ridurre il postcarico (vedi Capitolo 442). Un uso ragionevole dei diuretici è utile nel trattamento dell'edema polmonare associato a sovraccarico sistemico di liquidi corporei (sepsi, insufficienza renale). La morfina è spesso utile come vasodilatatore e blando sedativo.

La pressione positiva delle vie aeree aumenta efficacemente lo scambio gassoso nei pazienti con edema polmonare. La pressione positiva delle vie aeree può essere fornita come **pressione positiva di fine espirazione** (**PEEP**, *Positive End-Expiratory Pressure*) nei pazienti con intubazione tracheale, o nella forma non invasiva di pressione positiva continua delle vie aeree (CPAP, *Continuos Positive Airway Pressure*), con una maschera facciale o nasale. Il meccanismo attraverso il quale la pressione positiva nelle vie aeree migliora l'edema polmonare, pur non essendo del tutto chiaro, non sembra comunque avere alcun rapporto con la riduzione del liquido polmonare. La CPAP impedisce la chiusura degli alveoli e può riaprire le unità alveolari collassate. Questo fenomeno porta ad aumento della capacità funzionale residua (FRC, *Functional Residual Capacity*), miglioramento della compliance polmonare, miglioramento della funzione del surfattante e riduzione delle resistenze vascolari polmonari. L'effetto netto è la riduzione del lavoro respiratorio, l'aumento dell'ossigenazione e la diminuzione del postcarico cardiaco.

Quando si rende necessaria la ventilazione meccanica, specialmente nell'edema polmonare non cardiogeno, si deve porre attenzione a minimizzare il rischio di complicanze da barotrauma, tra cui lo pneumotorace, lo pneumomediastino e il danno alveolare primitivo (vedi Capitolo 70). Al fine di proteggere i polmoni si prevedono bassi volumi correnti, PEEP relativamente elevate e si consente un'ipercapnia permissiva.

L'edema polmonare da altitudine elevata (**HAPE**, *High Altitude Pulmonary Edema*) dovrebbe essere trattato con la discesa e la somministrazione di ossigeno. Una CPAP portatile o una camera iperbarica portatile possono essere utili. Anche la nifedipina (10 mg inizialmente, quindi 20-30 mg a lento rilascio ogni 12-24 ore) si rivela efficace negli adulti. Se vi è una storia di pregresso HAPE, la nifedipina e gli agonisti β-adrenergici (inalatori) possono prevenire le recidive.

Basnyat B, Murdoch DR: High-altitude illness. *Lancet* 2003;361:1967–1974.

Cotter G, Kaluski E, Moshkoviz Y, et al: Pulmonary edema: New insight on pathogenesis and treatment. *Curr Opin Cardiol* 2001;16:159–163.

Mahfood S, Hix WR, Aaron BL, et al: Reexpansion pulmonary edema. *Ann Thorac Surg* 1988;45:340–345.

Masip J, Roque M, Sanchez B, et al: Noninvasive ventilation in acute cardiogenic pulmonary edema. *JAMA* 2005;294:3124–3130.

Perina DG: Noncardiogenic pulmonary edema. *Emerg Med Clin North Am* 2003;21:385–393.

Peter JV, Moran JL, Phillips-Hughes J, et al: Effect of non-invasive positive pressure ventilation (NIPPV) on mortality in patients with acute cardiogenic pulmonary oedema: a meta-analysis. *Lancet* 2006;367:1155–1162.

Piantadosi C, Schwartz D: The acute respiratory distress syndrome. *Ann Intern Med* 2004;141:460–470.

Ware LB, Matthay MA: Acute pulmonary edema. *N Engl J Med* 2005;353:2788–2796.

Capitolo 394 ■ Sindromi da aspirazione

John L. Colombo

Lo gamma delle sindromi da aspirazione è vasta, andando da una condizione asintomatica a eventi acuti potenzialmente fatali, come nell'aspirazione massiva di contenuto gastrico o di idrocarburi. Altrove sono discusse l'ostruzione meccanica delle vie aeree di grande e di medio calibro (per es. imputabile a corpi estranei; vedi Capitolo 384) e le complicanze infettive dell'aspirazione e della microaspirazione ricorrente (vedi Capitolo 395), come quella che può verificarsi in caso di reflusso gastroesofageo (vedi Capitolo 320.1) o nella disfagia (vedi Capitolo 303). L'aspirazione occulta di secrezioni rinofaringee nel tratto respiratorio inferiore è un evento normale nelle persone sane, in genere privo di significato clinico.

CONTENUTO GASTRICO. L'aspirazione di grandi volumi di contenuto gastrico si verifica normalmente dopo il vomito; è una complicanza infrequente dell'anestesia generale, della gastroenterite e di un alterato livello di coscienza. Le conseguenze fisiopatologiche possono variare, principalmente a seconda del pH e del volume dell'aspirato, e della quantità di materiale particolato. Si nota un aumento della gravità clinica con aspirazione di volumi maggiori di circa 0,8 mL/kg e/o pH <2,5. Dopo un'aspirazione massiva insorgono rapidamente ipossiemia, polmonite emorragica, atelettasia, spostamento di liquidi intravascolari ed edema polmonare. Queste alterazioni insorgono più precocemente, sono più gravi e hanno durata maggiore con l'aspirazione acida. La maggior parte di esse compare da alcuni minuti a 1-2 ore dopo il momento dell'aspirazione. Nelle successive 24-48 ore si assiste a un marcato aumento degli infiltrati neutrofili parenchimali polmonari, distacco della mucosa e consolidamento alveolare, che spesso correlano con un aumento degli infiltrati alla radiografia del torace. Queste alterazioni tendono a verificarsi significativamente più tardi e sono più prolungate dopo aspirazione di materiale particolato. Di solito l'infezione non ha un ruolo nel danno polmonare iniziale, dopo aspirazione di contenuto gastrico; l'aspirazione può alterare le difese polmonari, predisponendo il paziente a polmonite batterica secondaria. In un paziente che va incontro a uno scadimento delle condizioni dopo un iniziale miglioramento clinico, specialmente se presenta febbre e leucocitosi, si deve sospettare una polmonite batterica secondaria.

Trattamento. Se un paziente che ha già una via aerea artificiale aspira una notevole quantità di materiale gastrico o una sostanza particolarmente tossica, è importante effettuare immediatamente l'aspirazione delle vie aeree. Qualora ciò non fosse possibile, l'aspirazione tardiva o la broncoscopia di solito hanno un valore terapeutico limitato. Fa eccezione il caso in cui si sospetti un'aspirazione significativa di materiale particolato. Non è consigliabile tentare di neutralizzare l'acido, poiché questo effetto viene svolto rapidamente dall'epitelio respiratorio. I pazienti con sospetta aspirazione di volumi elevati o di sostanze tossiche devono essere mantenuti in osservazione, con monitoraggio della saturazione di ossigeno tramite pulsossimetria o emogasanalisi, ed essere sottoposti a radiografia del torace anche se sono asintomatici. Se la radiografia del torace e la saturazione di ossigeno sono normali, e il soggetto rimane asintomatico, è sufficiente l'osservazione a domicilio, dopo un periodo di monitoraggio ospedaliero o ambulatoriale. Non è indicato alcun trattamento al momento, ma chi si occupa del paziente deve essere istruito a riportare il bambino dal medico se dovessero comparire sintomi respiratori o febbre. Ai pazienti che presentano o sviluppano alterazioni durante il periodo di osservazione si deve somministrare ossigeno per correggere l'ipossiemia. Nei casi più severi sono spesso necessari l'intubazione endotracheale e la ventilazione meccanica. Si può tentare con i broncodilatatori, che tuttavia in genere sono di beneficio limitato. Gli studi negli animali indicano che il trattamento con corticosteroidi non sembra apportare alcun beneficio, a meno che non sia somministrato quasi contemporaneamente all'evento di aspirazione; il loro utilizzo può aumentare il rischio di infezione secondaria. Gli antibiotici a scopo profilattico non sono indicati, sebbene nel paziente con riserva molto limitata possa essere indicata una copertura antibiotica precoce. Se si utilizzano, si devono scegliere farmaci che coprano anche i germi anaerobi. Se l'aspirazione avviene in un paziente ospedalizzato o con malattia cronica, si deve considerare anche la copertura contro lo *Pseudomonas* e i microrganismi enterici Gram-negativi. Se sono coinvolti 3 lobi, o meno, si osserva una mortalità ≤5%. A meno che non si sviluppino complicanze, come infezioni o barotraumi, la maggior parte dei pazienti guarisce in 2-3 settimane, sebbene possa persistere un danno polmonare prolungato, con cicatrizzazione e bronchiolite obliterante.

Prevenzione. La prevenzione dell'aspirazione dovrebbe sempre essere l'obiettivo primario ogniqualvolta si renda necessario predisporre le vie aeree per l'intubazione o altre procedure invasive. La nutrizione tramite sondini enterali introdotti attraverso il piloro e il sollevamento della testata del letto nei pazienti ventilati meccanicamente si sono dimostrati in grado di ridurre l'incidenza delle complicanze da aspirazione nei reparti di terapia intensiva.

ASPIRAZIONE DI IDROCARBURI. Le conseguenze più pericolose dell'ingestione di idrocarburi in genere sono l'aspirazione e la risultante polmonite (vedi Capitolo 58). Sebbene una polmonite significativa si verifichi in meno del 2% di tutte le ingestioni di idrocarburi, si stima che 20 decessi all'anno siano dovuti ad aspirazione di idrocarburi, tanto nei bambini quanto negli adulti. Alcuni di questi decessi sono in realtà suicidi. Gli idrocarburi con bassa tensione superficiale (benzina, trementina, naftalene) hanno un maggior potenziale di tossicità da aspirazione, rispetto agli oli minerali più pesanti o combustibili. L'ingestione di più di 30 mL (corrispondenti al volume di una deglutizione nell'adulto) di idrocarburi si associa a un aumentato rischio di polmonite severa. I reperti clinici di retrazione del torace, grunting, tosse e febbre possono insorgere precocemente, fino a 30 minuti dopo l'aspirazione, o presentarsi dopo diverse ore. Le alterazioni alla radiografia del torace compaiono usualmente entro 2-8 ore e raggiungono il picco circa 48-72 ore dopo. Possono insorgere pneumatocele e versamento pleurico. I pazienti che presentano tosse, dispnea o ipossiemia sono a rischio di polmonite. Possono essere presenti anomalie della funzionalità polmonare che persistono anche molti anni dopo l'aspirazione di idrocarburi. Altri apparati e organi, in particolare il fegato, il sistema nervoso centrale e il cuore, possono subire gravi danni. Possono insorgere aritmie cardiache, esacerbate dall'ipossia e dagli squilibri elettrolitici o dalle alterazioni dell'equilibrio acido-base.

Trattamento. Lo svuotamento gastrico è quasi sempre controindicato poiché il rischio di aspirazione è maggiore di qualsiasi tossicità sistemica. Il trattamento è generalmente di supporto, con ossigeno, liquidi e sostegno ventilatorio, se necessario. Il bambino asintomatico con una radiografia del torace normale deve essere tenuto sotto osservazione per 6-8 ore per garantirne una dimissione sicura. Alcuni idrocarburi hanno una maggiore tossicità sistemica intrinseca: particolarmente nocivi per i polmoni sono canfora, carburi idrogenati, idrocarburi aromatici e quelli associati a metalli e pesticidi (**CHAMP**, *Champhor, Halogenated carbons, Aromatic hydrocarbons, Metals and Pesticides*). I pazienti che ingeriscono questi composti in quantità superiore a 30 mL, come può avvenire con l'overdose intenzionale, possono trarre beneficio dallo svuotamento gastrico. Questa rimane una procedura ad alto rischio, che può comportare un'ulteriore aspirazione. Laddove sia possibile eseguire la procedura senza indurre il vomito, si dovrebbe prendere in esame l'eventualità di posizionare un tubo endotracheale cuffiato, specialmente in presenza di uno stato mentale alterato. Il trattamento dovrebbe comunque essere valutato caso per caso, con la guida di un centro antiveleni.

Altre sostanze che sono particolarmente tossiche e causano un danno polmonare significativo quando inalate o aspirate comprendono il borotalco, il cloro, la gommalacca, il berillio e i vapori di mercurio. L'esposizione ripetuta a basse concentrazioni di questi agenti può portare a una malattia polmonare cronica, come la polmonite interstiziale e la formazione di granulomi. I corticosteroidi possono aiutare a ridurre lo sviluppo di fibrosi e migliorare la funzione polmonare, sebbene vi siano evidenze limitate in tal senso.

Bynum L, Pierce A: Pulmonary aspiration of gastric contents. *Am Rev Respir Dis* 1976;114:1129–1136.

Colombo JL, Sammut PH: Aspiration syndromes: In Taussig LM, Landau LI (eds): *Pediatric Respiratory Medicine*. St. Louis, Mosby, 1999, pp 439–441.

DeLegge MH: Aspiration pneumonia: Incidence, mortality, and at-risk populations. *JPEN J Parenter Enteral Nutr* 2002;26:S19–S25.

Gleeson K, Eggli D, Maxwell S: Quantitative aspiration during sleep in normal subjects. *Chest* 1997;111:1266–1272.

Marik PE: Aspiration pneumonitis and aspiration pneumonia. *N Engl J Med* 2001;344:665–671.

Mickiewicz M, Gomez HF: Hydrocarbon toxicity: General review and management guidelines. *Air Med J* 2001;20:8–11.

Vale J, Kulig K: American Academy of Clinical Toxicology; European Association of Poisons Centres and Clinical Toxicologists: Position paper: Gastric lavage. *J Toxicol Clin Toxicol* 2004;42:933–943.

Warner MA, Warner ME, Warner DO, et al: Perioperative pulmonary aspiration in infants and children. *Anesthesiology* 1999;90:66–71.

Capitolo 395 ■ Aspirazione cronica ricorrente John L. Colombo

EZIOLOGIA. L'aspirazione ricorrente di piccole quantità di contenuto orale, gastrico o nasale può portare a diverse presentazioni cliniche, che comprendono bronchite o bronchiolite ricorrente, polmonite ricorrente, atelettasia, sibili, tosse, apnea e laringospasmo. Gli esiti istologici possono includere infiammazione granulomatosa, flogosi interstiziale, fibrosi, polmonite lipoidea e bronchiolite obliterante. La maggior parte dei casi, pur associandosi a una morbilità significativa, non giunge all'ispezione anatomopatologica, ma si manifesta clinicamente come infiammazione delle vie aeree. La Tabella 395-1 elenca i disturbi principali che si associano frequentemente ad aspirazione ricorrente. L'incoordinazione orofaringea è riportata come il problema di base più comune associato a polmonite ricorrente, nei bambini ospedalizzati. Secondo una casistica di bambini ospedalizzati con polmonite ricorrente, il 48% dei pazienti presentava disfagia come problema sottostante. La polmonite lipoidea può insorgere con l'uso di rimedi casalinghi o tradizionali, come la somministrazione orale o nasale di oli animali o vegetali per trattare varie malattie infantili. È infatti stata riportata come complicanza di queste pratiche in Medio Oriente, Asia, India, Brasile e Messico. La diagnosi può essere ritardata dalla malattia di base iniziale, da barriere linguistiche e dalla convinzione che tali rimedi non siano "medicine".

Tra le patologie di base che possono predisporre alla malattia da aspirazione ripetuta spesso figura anche il reflusso gastroesofageo (vedi Capitolo 320.1), che tuttavia è meno spesso associato a polmonite ricorrente. L'aspirazione è inoltre stata osservata nei lattanti con sintomi respiratori, senza altre anomalie apparenti. La microaspirazione ricorrente è stata riportata in neonati per altri aspetti apparentemente normali, soprattutto se prematuri. L'aspirazione rappresenta un rischio anche nei pazienti con malattie respiratorie acute dovute ad altre cause, specialmente nell'infezione da virus respiratorio sinciziale (vedi Capitolo 257). Questi pazienti, quando sottoposti allo studio della deglutizione con bario e videofluoroscopia, hanno dimostrato di avere

TABELLA 395-1. Condizioni che predispongono al danno polmonare da aspirazione nei bambini

ANATOMICHE E MECCANICHE
Fistola tracheoesofagea
Laringoschisi
Anello vascolare
Palatoschisi
Micrognazia
Macroglossia
Acalasia
Corpo estraneo esofageo
Tracheostomia
Tubo endotracheale
Sondino nasoenterico
Collagenopatie (sclerodermia, dermatomiosite)
Malattia da reflusso gastroesofageo
Obesità
NEUROMUSCOLARI
Alterazione dello stato di coscienza
Immaturità della deglutizione/prematurità
Disautonomia
Aumento della pressione endocranica
Idrocefalo
Paralisi delle corde vocali
Paralisi cerebrale
Distrofia muscolare
Miastenia grave
Sindrome di Guillain-Barré
Malattia di Werdnig-Hoffmann
Atassia-teleangectasia
Accidente cerebrovascolare
VARIE
Cattiva igiene orale
Gengivite
Ospedalizzazione prolungata
Ostruzione al deflusso gastrico o intestinale
Tecniche di alimentazione errate (biberon premuto contro la bocca, iperalimentazione, alimenti non appropriati per l'età)
Displasia broncopolmonare
Infezioni virali

un'aspirazione silente. Si sottolinea quindi la necessità di sospettare un'aspirazione ricorrente in ogni bambino con una malattia respiratoria acuta, alimentato per via enterale, che presenti un improvviso deterioramento.

DIAGNOSI. I fattori di base predisponenti (vedi Tab. 395-1) sono spesso evidenti da un punto di clinico, ma possono richiedere ulteriori valutazioni. Occorre chiedere alla persona che si occupa del bambino se quest'ultimo sputi spesso, vomiti, si inarchi o, nei bambini più grandi, se presenti un dolore epigastrico; è altrettanto importante stabilire il momento di insorgenza dei sintomi in rapporto ai pasti e alle variazioni posturali, e indagare sui sintomi notturni, come tosse o sibili. Si ricordi che la tosse o il gagging possono essere minimi o assenti in un bambino con una depressione del riflesso della tosse o del gagging. L'osservazione di un pasto è parte essenziale dell'esame, quando si prende in considerazione una diagnosi di aspirazione ricorrente. Si deve prestare particolare attenzione al reflusso nasofaringeo, alla difficoltà di suzione o di deglutizione, oltre che alla tosse e al soffocamento associati. Occorre ispezionare la cavità orale per escludere anomalie grossolane e stimolarla per valutare il riflesso faringeo. La scialorrea o l'accumulo eccessivo di secrezioni nella cavità orale suggerisce una disfagia. L'auscultazione polmonare può rivelare crepitii o sibili transitori dopo il pasto, in particolare nelle zone declivi del polmone.

La diagnosi di microaspirazione ricorrente è difficile, a causa della mancanza di esami con elevata sensibilità e specificità. La radiografia del torace semplice è la prima indagine abitualmente eseguita in un bambino con sospetta aspirazione ricorrente. Possono essere evidenti i reperti classici di infiltrati lobari o

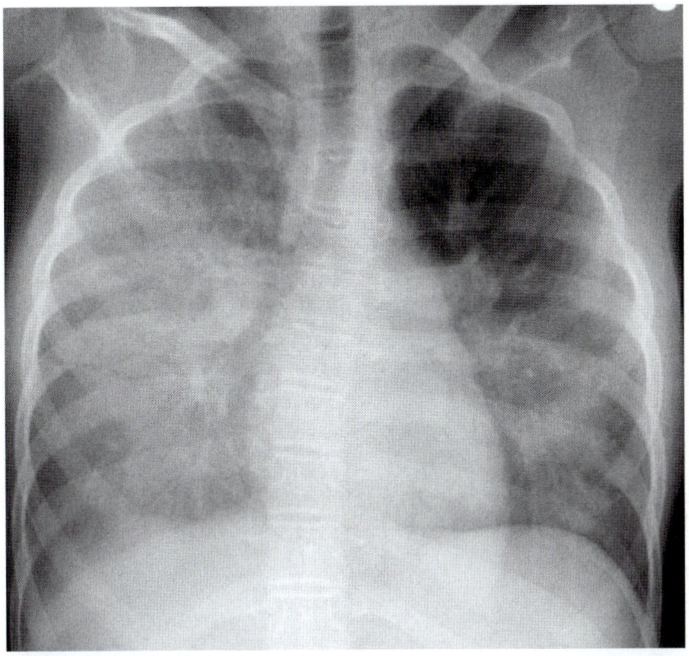

Figura 395-1. Radiografia del torace di un ragazzo di 15 anni con ritardo di sviluppo, con aspirazione cronica di formule orali. Si noti la distribuzione posteriore (aree declivi) con risparmio dei margini cardiaci.

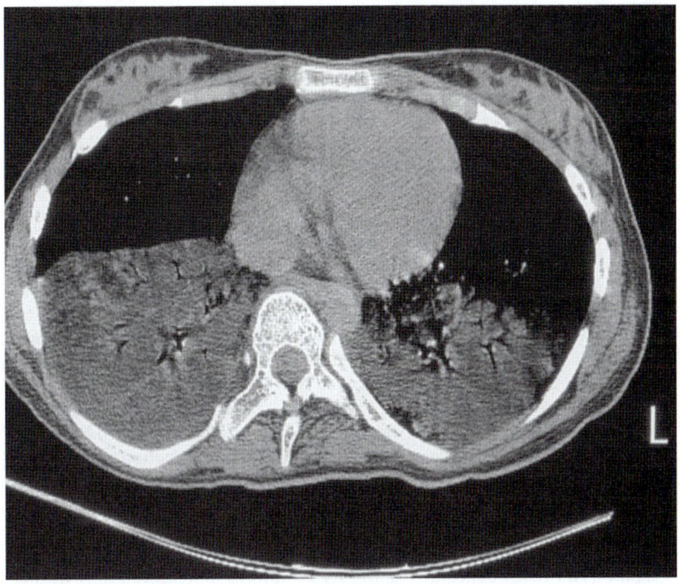

Figura 395-2. TC del torace dello stesso paziente della Figura 395-1. Si noti il consolidamento polmonare nella regione declive, della stessa densità del grasso sottocutaneo.

segmentari localizzati nelle zone declivi (Fig. 395-1), ma vi è un'ampia varietà di reperti radiografici, tra cui infiltrati diffusi, infiltrati lobari, ispessimento delle pareti bronchiali, iperinflazione e persino radiografie del torace di aspetto normale. Reperti radiologici compatibili con l'aspirazione possono essere scoperti accidentalmente, quando si esegue la radiografia per altre ragioni.

Un'esofagografia con bario, da effettuarsi con cautela, è utile per ricercare anomalie anatomiche, come anelli vascolari, stenosi, ernia iatale o fistola tracheoesofagea. Essa inoltre fornisce informazioni qualitative sulla motilità esofagea e, se estesa, sullo svuotamento gastrico. Questa indagine non è invece sensibile né specifica per l'aspirazione o il reflusso gastroesofageo.

Uno studio dinamico della deglutizione con bario, in videofluoroscopia, è considerato generalmente il gold standard per la valutazione del meccanismo di deglutizione. Lo studio è effettuato di preferenza con l'assistenza di un nutrizionista pediatra, e insieme alla persona che si occupa del bambino, per ricreare una situazione il più possibile simile a quella in cui il paziente abitualmente assume il cibo. Lo studio dinamico della deglutizione con bario rileva occasionalmente l'aspirazione in pazienti senza anomalie respiratorie evidenti.

La scintigrafia gastroesofagea con latte marcato offre vantaggi teorici rispetto allo studio della deglutizione con bario, essendo più fisiologica e fornendo una finestra di osservazione più prolungata, per rilevare l'aspirazione e il reflusso gastroesofageo. Questa procedura è un esame relativamente poco sensibile per rilevare l'aspirazione. Il "salivogramma", un altro studio scintigrafico, può essere utile per valutare l'aspirazione di contenuto esofageo, sebbene la sua sensibilità non sia stata ben studiata. È stato riportato che la valutazione della deglutizione tramite endoscopia a fibre ottiche, utilizzata con successo negli adulti, è utile anche nei pazienti pediatrici. Questa tecnica consente di osservare la deglutizione direttamente, senza esposizione a radiazioni. La reazione del bambino al posizionamento dell'endoscopio può incidere sulla valutazione della funzione, a seconda del grado di disagio o di collaborazione.

I reperti accidentali alla TC (generalmente non indicata per formulare la diagnosi di aspirazione) possono mostrare infiltrati con ridotta attenuazione, suggestivi di polmonite lipoidea (Fig. 395-2).

Per valutare l'aspirazione è possibile esaminare l'aspirato tracheobronchiale. Nei pazienti con una via aerea artificiale sono utili l'uso di un colorante orale e l'esame visivo delle secrezioni tracheali. Questo esame non dovrebbe essere effettuato ripetutamente, per la possibile tossicità del colorante. È importante utilizzare una quantità adeguata di colorante, ma anche così l'esame è relativamente poco sensibile, rispetto alla misurazione del lattosio o del glucosio nelle secrezioni respiratorie. La quantificazione dei macrofagi alveolari con infarcimento lipidico, nell'aspirato bronchiale, si è dimostrata un esame sensibile per l'aspirazione, nei bambini, sebbene gravato da falsi positivi, specialmente in caso di ostruzione endobronchiale, utilizzo di lipidi per via endovenosa, sepsi e sanguinamento polmonare. Anche il lavaggio bronchiale può essere esaminato alla ricerca di varie sostanze alimentari, tra cui lattosio, glucosio, fibre alimentari e antigeni del latte.

TRATTAMENTO. Se l'aspirazione cronica si associa a una condizione medica sottostante, il trattamento dovrebbe volto a eliminare il problema di base. Il livello di morbilità dato dai problemi respiratori dovrebbe incidere sull'entità dell'intervento. Spesso una disfagia lieve può essere trattata con il cambiamento della posizione durante il pasto, limitando la consistenza dei cibi a quella meglio tollerata all'esofagografia dinamica con bario (di solito i cibi più spessi) o somministrando quantità di cibo ridotte a ogni pasto. L'alimentazione con sondino nasogastrico può essere utilizzata temporaneamente durante i periodi di disfunzione transitoria delle corde vocali o di disfagia. Anche l'alimentazione post-pilorica può essere utile, specialmente se è presente reflusso gastroesofageo. Si possono prendere in esame varie procedure chirurgiche. La tracheostomia, sebbene talvolta predisponga all'aspirazione, nel complesso può garantire qualche beneficio, contribuendo a una migliore igiene bronchiale e offrendo la possibilità di aspirare. La fundoplicatio con sondino di nutrizione gastrostomico o digiunostomico riduce la probabilità di aspirazione delle vie aeree superiori. Il trattamento medico con anticolinergici, come il glicopirrolato, la scopolamina, o la tossina botulinica, possono ridurre significativamente la morbilità da aspirazione salivare, ma spesso presentano effetti collaterali. Nei casi più gravi e resistenti si può prendere in considerazione un intervento chirurgico aggressivo, con asportazione delle ghiandole salivari, legatura dei dotti, separazione laringotracheale o disconnessione esofagogastrica.

Celedon JC, Litonjua A, Ryan L, et al: Bottle feeding in the bed or crib before sleep time and wheezing in early childhood. *Pediatrics* 2002;110:e77.
Colombo JL, Hallberg TK: Pulmonary aspiration and lipid-laden macrophages: In search of gold (standards). *Pediatr Pulmonol* 1999;28:79–82.
Heuschkel RB, Fletcher K, Hill A, et al: Isolated neonatal swallowing dysfunction: A case series and review of the literature. *Dig Dis Sci* 2003; 48:30–35.
Hoffman LR, Yen EH, Kanne JP, et al: Lipoid pneumonia due to Mexican folk remedies. *Arch Pediatr Adolesc Med* 2005;159:1043–1048.
Khoshoo V, Ross G, Kelly B, et al: Benefits of thickened feeds in previously healthy infants with respiratory syncytial viral bronchiolitis. *Pediatr Pulmonol* 2001;31:301–302.
Link DT, Willging JP, Miller CK, et al: Pediatric laryngopharyngeal sensory testing during flexible endoscopic evaluation of swallowing: Feasible and correlative. *Ann Otol Rhinol Laryngol* 2000;109:899–905.
Mercado-Deane MG, Burton EM, Harlow SA, et al: Swallowing dysfunction in infants less than 1 year of age. *Pediatr Radiol* 2001;31:423–428.
Newman LA, Keckley C, Petersen MC, et al: Swallow function and medical diagnoses in infants suspected of dysphagia. *Pediatrics* 2001;108:E106.
Owayaed AF, Campbell DM, Wange GG: Underlying causes of recurrent pneumonia in children. *Arch Pediatr Adolesc Med* 2000;154:190–194.
Sheikh S, Allen E, Shell R, et al: Chronic aspiration without gastroesophageal reflux as a cause of chronic respiratory symptoms in neurologically normal infants. *Chest* 2001;120:1190–1195.
Takamizawa S, Tsugawa C, Nishijima E, et al: Laryngotracheal separation for intractable aspiration pneumonia in neurologically impaired children: Experience with 11 cases. *J Pediatr Surg* 2003;38:975–977.

Capitolo 396 ■ Malattie parenchimali con prevalente danno da ipersensibilità, infiltrazione eosinofila o mediato da tossine

Oren Lakser

396.1 • Ipersensibilità a materiali inalati

La polmonite da ipersensibilità (HP, *Hypersensitivity Pneumonitis*), o **alveolite allergica estrinseca**, è una malattia infiammatoria diffusa dell'interstizio polmonare, mediata da meccanismi immunologici, causata dall'inalazione di vari antigeni organici. Questi antigeni in genere sono di origine animale o vegetale e hanno tipicamente dimensioni di 1-5 μm, in virtù delle quali si depositano negli alveoli. Occasionalmente la HP può essere causata da antigeni reattivi, come alcuni farmaci o droghe.

EZIOLOGIA. Sebbene sia tipicamente una malattia degli adulti, la HP è stata riportata nei bambini e persino nei lattanti. Ne esistono diversi tipi, ciascuno correlato all'antigene causale. Le forme più comuni, negli Stati Uniti, comprendono il **polmone del contadino** (da fieno ammuffito; l'antigene è un actinomicete termofilo), il **polmone dell'allevatore di uccelli** (da feci o urine di un'ampia varietà di uccelli e altre specie animali), e la **HP da umidificatori** o condizionatori (da umidificatori o condizionatori contaminati, causata anch'essa da actinomiceti termofili). L'esposizione a piccioni (**malattia dell'allevatore di piccioni**) è la forma più comune in Turchia e in Messico. La maggior parte dei casi riportati nei bambini era imputabile ad antigeni inalati durante un'esposizione aviaria o a muffe. È stato riportato un caso di HP dopo esposizione ad antigene di pelo di gatto.

ANATOMIA PATOLOGICA E PATOGENESI. La HP si può presentare come malattia acuta, subacuta o cronica. Tale distinzione si basa sulle caratteristiche morfologiche del coinvolgimento polmonare. Nello stadio acuto, le pareti alveolari sono infiltrate da neutrofili, linfociti, plasmacellule e macrofagi (Fig. 396-1). Il lume alveolare

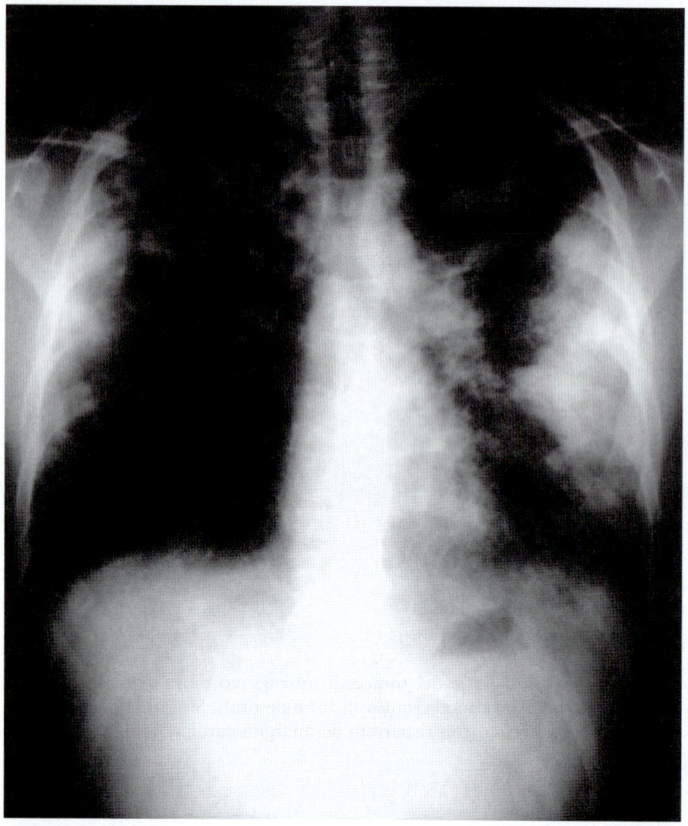

Figura 396-1. Radiografia del torace che mostra infiltrati irregolari bilaterali con consolidamento periferico. (Da Wubbel C, Fulmer D, Sherman J: Chronic eosinophilic pneumonia: A case report and national survey. *Chest* 2003;123:1763-1766.)

può contenere un essudato proteinaceo misto a cellule infiammatorie. L'esposizione ripetuta o continua può sfociare in una presentazione subacuta, caratterizzata dal classico granuloma non caseoso della HP. Spesso si associa una bronchiolite terminale e respiratoria; gli alveoli possono contenere macrofagi pallidi e schiumosi. La forma cronica dimostra un'ulteriore progressione dell'alveolite granulomatosa, che risulta in fibrosi interstiziale ed erosione, principalmente a carico dei lobi superiori.

Il meccanismo immunitario coinvolto nell'induzione di queste alterazioni morfologiche può comprendere ipersensibilità da immunocomplessi (di tipo III), soprattutto nella presentazione acuta, ipersensibilità cellulare ritardata (di tipo IV) e la via alternativa del complemento. Solo una piccola percentuale degli individui esposti va realmente incontro a sintomi clinici, suggerendo che a determinare la risposta dell'ospite sia un'interazione tra la natura dell'agente patogenetico, l'intensità e la durata dell'esposizione da una parte e fattori genetici dall'altra.

MANIFESTAZIONI CLINICHE. Gli attacchi acuti si verificano generalmente da 4 a 8 ore dopo l'esposizione. I sintomi tipici comprendono febbre, brividi, tosse, dispnea, mialgia e malessere, che possono persistere fino a 48 ore. L'esame obiettivo rivela di solito un bambino dispnoico, di aspetto sofferente, con crepitii bibasali o con un esame obiettivo polmonare nella norma. La radiografia del torace può essere normale oppure dimostrare un'opacità a vetro smerigliato bilaterale, che spesso risparmia gli apici e le basi polmonari, con fini nodularità. Questi pazienti, con un'esposizione continua o ricorrente, possono progredire verso la presentazione subacuta. La tosse peggiora, la dispnea si fa più pronunciata, e possono insorgere anoressia e calo ponderale. La radiografia del torace, in questo stadio, ha un aspetto maggiormente reticolonodulare. L'esposizione a lungo termine può portare alla presentazione cronica. La dispnea e la tosse sono severe, con calo ponderale, astenia e ipossiemia. Questi pazienti finiscono per sviluppare un'alveolite cronica con fibrosi, che può causare cuore polmonare. La radiografia del torace mostra infiltrati grossolani reticolonodulari e bronchiectasie, principalmente nelle zone superiori e intermedie del polmone. La TC ad alta risoluzione (HRCT, *High-Resolution Computed Tomography*) può essere più sensibile nella dimostrazione delle bronchiectasie.

DIAGNOSI. La diagnosi di HP si basa principalmente sulla presentazione clinica associata a un'esposizione sospetta. Poiché la presentazione clinica è aspecifica, è di importanza cruciale avere un alto indice di sospetto. I bambini con HP rientrano nella maggior parte dei criteri diagnostici proposti per gli adulti. I criteri maggiori comprendono sintomi compatibili con HP, evidenza di esposizione (studi anticorpali), radiografia o HRCT compatibili, linfocitosi nel liquido di broncolavaggio alveolare (BAL, *BronchoAlveolar Lavage*), alterazioni istologiche compatibili con HP e un test di provocazione antigenica positivo. I criteri minori comprendono crepitii bibasali, riduzione della capacità di diffusione e ipossiemia. La presenza di 4 criteri maggiori e di 2 minori è altamente suggestiva di HP, specialmente se sono state escluse altre malattie con presentazione simile. Numerosi esami di laboratorio possono rivelarsi utili per confermare un alto sospetto clinico. I pazienti con HP spesso presentano una modesta leucocitosi con neutrofilia e spostamento a sinistra della formula, e un moderato aumento della velocità di eritrosedimentazione. I livelli sierici di immunoglobuline (IgG, IgM e IgA) sono spesso elevati. I test cutanei per particolari antigeni mancano di sensibilità e specificità, così come le precipitine sieriche ad antigeni specifici. Entrambi questi test possono indicare l'esposizione, ma sono spesso positivi in individui senza malattia clinica. Negli adulti il liquido del BAL dimostra tipicamente una marcata linfocitosi (spesso più del 70%), in particolare dei linfociti T $CD8^+$ *suppressor*, sebbene nei bambini il rapporto CD4:CD8 non sia aumentato. Il liquido del BAL può inoltre contenere elevati livelli di immunoglobuline. I test di funzionalità polmonare dimostrano classicamente un **quadro restrittivo**, con alterazione dello scambio gassoso (capacità di diffusione). La presenza di alterazioni anche lievi di tipo ostruttivo, negli stadi acuti, è un indice prognostico negativo. Alcuni hanno proposto un test di provocazione inalatorio, da effettuarsi sia in laboratorio sia con la riesposizione ambientale. Tale test può essere pericoloso e pertanto deve essere effettuato solo in centri diagnostici appositamente attrezzati.

TRATTAMENTO. L'approccio terapeutico più efficace consiste nell'evitare l'antigene sospetto. Il prednisone (1-2 mg/kg/die) può essere utile, ma richiede trattamenti prolungati (fino a 6 mesi). In generale, la prognosi è piuttosto favorevole, ma se l'esposizione persiste, può insorgere fibrosi polmonare e il paziente può non recuperare la funzione polmonare di base.

Ceviz N, Kaynar H, Olgun H, et al: Pigeon breeder's lung in childhood: is family screening necessary? *Pediatr Pulmonol* 2006;41:279–282.

Fan LF: Hypersensitivity pneumonitis in children. *Curr Opin Pediatr* 2002;14:323–326.

Knutsen AP, Sotelo-Avila C, Albers GM: Hypersensitivity pneumonitis in children. *Pediatr Asthma Allergy Immunol* 2003;16:247–264.

Lacasse Y, Selman M, Costabel U, et al: Clinical diagnosis of hypersensitivity pneumonitis. *Am J Respir Crit Care Med* 2003;168:952–958.

Martinez-Cordero E, Aguilar Leon DE, Retana VN: IgM antiavian antibodies in sera from patients with pigeon breeder's disease. *J Clin Lab Anal* 2000;14:201–207.

Morell F, Roger A, Cruz MJ: Usefulness of specific skin tests in the diagnosis of hypersensitivity pneumonitis. *J Allergy Clin Immunol* 2002;110:939.

Nacar N, Kiper N, Yalcin E, et al: Hypersensitivity pneumonitis in children: Pigeon breeder's disease. *Ann Trop Paediatr* 2004;24:349–355.

Patel AM, Ryu JH, Reed CE: Hypersensitivity pneumonitis: Current concepts and future questions. *J Allergy Clin Immunol* 2001;108:661–670.

Ratjen F, Costabel U, Griese M, et al: Bronchoalveolar lavage fluid findings in children with hypersensitivity pneumonitis. *Eur Respir J* 2003;21:144–148.

Selman M: Hypersensitivity pneumonitis: A multifaceted deceiving disorder. *Clin Chest Med* 2004;25:531–547.

Stauffer Ettlin M, Pache JC, Renevey F, et al: Bird breeder's disease: A rare diagnosis in young children. *Eur J Pediatr* 2006;165:55–61. Epub 2005, Nov 4.

396.2 • Malattia dei riempitori di silos

La malattia dei riempitori di silos, conosciuta anche come **avvelenamento da gas dei silos** o **pneumoconiosi dei riempitori di silos**, è tipicamente causata dalla tossicità del biossido di azoto, che si produce nei silos (soprattutto in quelli di mais) già alcune ore dopo il riempimento e raggiunge una concentrazione massima nel giro di 2 giorni circa. In un silos chiuso, possono permanere concentrazioni pericolose di gas anche per due settimane. Chi entri in un silos senza adeguata protezione durante questo intervallo di tempo può sviluppare questa malattia in forma più o meno grave.

PATOGENESI. Il grado di danno polmonare dipende dalla durata dell'esposizione e dalla concentrazione di biossido di azoto. Poco dopo l'inalazione, il biossido di azoto è idrolizzato ad acido nitrico e nitroso, causando una polmonite chimica con edema polmonare, a carico prevalentemente degli pneumociti di tipo I e delle cellule ciliate che delimitano le vie aeree. I reperti bioptici o autoptici comprendono edema polmonare diffuso, iperplasia dell'epitelio delle vie aeree, allargamento dei setti intralobulari e bronchiolite obliterante. Se l'esposizione è stata di notevole entità, può insorgere metaemoglobinemia. Sono inoltre possibili alterazioni dell'attività macrofagica e della funzione immunitaria, che aumentano il rischio di infezioni.

MANIFESTAZIONI CLINICHE E DIAGNOSI. La maggior parte delle esposizioni determina sintomi lievi e autolimitanti. La tosse e la dispnea insorgono immediatamente all'entrata nel silos e si associano spesso a sibili, nausea, sensazione di soffocamento, irritazione oculare e stanchezza. In casi rari i sintomi si manifestano a distanza di giorni, o anche settimane, dall'esposizione. Le manifestazioni radiologiche comprendono edema polmonare nelle zone peri-ilari e alle basi. Alcuni pazienti guariscono e in tal caso l'edema polmonare scompare rapidamente. Spesso, tuttavia, questo stadio iniziale è seguito da un periodo di remissione di 2-3 settimane, destinato a lasciare il posto a una seconda fase di malattia, caratterizzata da febbre, dispnea progressiva, cianosi e tosse, associate a opacità miliari diffuse e sparse, che tendono a confluire acquistando un aspetto più irregolare e nodulare. Questi pazienti possono soffrire di metaemoglobinemia. Le complicanze comprendono l'infezione secondaria e la bronchiolite obliterante. La diagnosi richiede un'anamnesi medica e occupazionale accurata, poiché non è disponibile una conferma di laboratorio specifica per la malattia dei riempitori di silos.

TRATTAMENTO. È fondamentale prevenire la malattia dei riempitori di silos, evitando il più possibile l'esposizione nelle prime due settimane dopo il riempimento. Sebbene non sia stato condotto alcuno studio controllato, il prednisone ad alte dosi (fino a 30 mg/kg/die) è utile per ridurre la severità e la durata dei sintomi. Anche i broncodilatatori possono dare qualche beneficio, seppure limitato. La metaemoglobinemia, nei casi severi, è trattata con blu di metilene. Al contrario di ciò che si potrebbe supporre, è stato riportato che la terapia con ossido nitrico migliora l'ossigenazione in questi pazienti. La malattia dei riempitori di silos può essere fatale, andare incontro a una guarigione completa o provocare una pneumopatia cronica associata a fibrosi ed enfisema.

Dambro MR: Silo filler disease. In Griffith JA: *5 Minute Clinical Consult*. Philadelphia, Lippincott Williams and Wilkins, 2001.

Frampton MW, Boscia J, Roberts NJ Jr, et al: Nitrogen dioxide exposure: Effects on airway and blood cells. *Am J Physiol Lung Cell Mol Physiol* 2002;282:L155–L165.

Leavey JF, Dubin RL, Singh N, et al: Silo-filler's disease, the acute respiratory distress syndrome, and oxides of nitrogen. *Ann Intern Med* 2004; 141:410–411.

Rasmussen MD, Bascom R: Silo filler's disease. Available at emedicine website (www.emedicine.com).

396.3 • POLMONE DA PARAQUAT

Tra gli erbicidi dipiridilici, il paraquat è il più tossico. Le soluzioni concentrate (12-20%) tendono a essere più pericolose di quelle diluite. I suoi effetti tossici consistono nella produzione di superossidi e di altri radicali liberi altamente reattivi, che causano la perossidazione delle membrane cellulari e un danno mitocondriale selettivo, portando alla morte cellulare. Il paraquat si concentra selettivamente nei polmoni a causa di un processo di captazione delle amine che avviene nelle cellule epiteliali alveolari. Inoltre, il danno indotto da questa sostanza aumenta significativamente in presenza di concentrazioni di ossigeno elevate. Sebbene il suo impiego in alcuni Paesi sia proibito o soggetto a severe limitazioni, di questo diserbante si fa ancora ampio uso, soprattutto nei Paesi in via di sviluppo.

Dal punto di vista fisiopatologico, il paraquat provoca un danno diretto alla membrana alveolocapillare con perdita di surfattante, sindrome da distress respiratorio acuto, fibrosi progressiva intra-alveolare e insufficienza respiratoria.

MANIFESTAZIONI CLINICHE. Esistono tre gradi di intossicazione da paraquat, dose-correlati. I pazienti con avvelenamento lieve, dopo ingestione di meno di 20 mg di ione paraquat/kg di peso corporeo, sono di solito asintomatici, ma possono sviluppare anche vomito, diarrea e lieve alterazione dello scambio gassoso. Un avvelenamento da moderato a severo fa seguito all'ingestione di 20-40 mg/kg di ione paraquat; questi pazienti, che presentano tipicamente vomito, diarrea e lesioni da caustici alla mucosa orale o esofagea, possono sviluppare insufficienza renale, disfunzione epatica e fibrosi polmonare progressiva, fino all'insufficienza respiratoria e alla morte. L'ingestione di >40 mg/kg di ione paraquat provoca un avvelenamento acuto fulminante, con comparsa di gravi ulcere dell'orofaringe e dell'esofago e insufficienza multiorganica; la mortalità è del 100% entro alcune ore dall'ingestione. La misurazione della concentrazione plasmatica di paraquat può essere il miglior marcatore di esposizione e di severità (nomogrammi del paraquat), e per la previsione della prognosi.

TRATTAMENTO. Il trattamento è generalmente di supporto poiché non esiste un antidoto. La lavanda gastrica, il carbone attivo, l'emoperfusione e l'emodialisi sono di valore limitato nell'avvelenamento significativo. Vi sono state segnalazioni rare e isolate di successi ottenuti con terapia antiossidante, consistente nell'infusione di deferoxamina e acetilcisteina. Altri hanno riportato un certo successo con una terapia immunosoppressiva combinata a base di corticosteroidi endovena e ciclofosfamide, o cicli prolungati e ripetuti di corticoterapia. I risultati dopo trapianto polmonare sono scarsi, probabilmente in relazione all'accumulo a lungo termine del paraquat nei muscoli e al successivo riaccumulo nel polmone trapiantato. Un paziente è sopravvissuto grazie a un trapianto polmonare tardivo, eseguito più di 40 giorni dopo l'ingestione.

La prognosi complessiva è sfavorevole. I sopravvissuti soffrono generalmente di una malattia restrittiva, con alterazione della capacità di diffusione ai test di funzionalità polmonare.

Chen G, Lin J, Huang Y: Combined methylprednisolone and dexamethasone therapy for paraquat poisoning. *Crit Care Med* 2002;30:2584–2587.

Dalvie MA, White N, Raine R: Long-term respiratory health effects of the herbicide, paraquat, among workers in the Western Cape. *Occup Environ Med* 1999;56:391–396.

Eddleston M, Wilks MF, Buckley NA: Prospects for treatment of paraquat-induced lung fibrosis with immunosuppressive drugs and the need for better prediction of outcome: A systematic review. *Q J Med* 2003;96:809–824.

Ellenhorn MJ, Schonwald S, Ordog J, et al: Pesticides. In Ellenhorn MJ (ed): *Medical Toxicology: Diagnosis and Treatment of Human Poisoning,* 2nd ed. Baltimore, Williams and Wilkins, 1997.

Lo Sasso AA, Osterhoudt K, Meier FA, et al: A 16-year-old boy with rapidly progressing pulmonary fibrosis. *J Pediatr* 2002;140:270–275.

Schenker MB: Pulmonary function and exercise-associated changes with chronic low-level paraquat exposure. *Am J Respir Crit Care Med* 2004;170:773–779.

396.4 • PNEUMOPATIA EOSINOFILA (GIÀ SINDROME DI LÖFFLER)

Le pneumopatie eosinofile sono un gruppo eterogeneo di alterazioni, accomunate dal reperto di infiltrati polmonari ed eosinofilia circolante o tissutale. Molti Autori hanno adottato l'espressione **infiltrati polmonari con eosinofilia** (PIE, *Pulmonary Infiltrates with Eosinophilia*) come definizione più accurata per questi disordini. Esistono vari criteri di classificazione per questi tipi di pneumopatia. Le sindromi PIE possono essere distinte in eosinofilia polmonare semplice (sindrome di Löffler), eosinofilia polmonare protratta, eosinofilia polmonare tropicale, eosinofilia polmonare con asma, panarterite nodosa, polmonite eosinofila cronica e polmonite eosinofila acuta. Alcuni vi hanno incluso anche la **sindrome di Churg-Strauss**, l'**aspergillosi broncopolmonare allergica** (ABPA, *Allergic Bronchopulmonary Aspergillosis*) e la **sindrome da ipereosinofilia idiopatica.** Alcune pneumopatie, come la fibrosi polmonare idiopatica, il granuloma a cellule di Langerhans e altre forme interstiziali, pur potendo associarsi a eosinofilia, vengono classificate in altre categorie.

La **sindrome di Löffler**, la più comune sindrome PIE riportata nei bambini, è caratterizzata da infiltrati polmonari migranti accompagnati da eosinofilia periferica, con sintomi respiratori di minima entità. Questa dicitura è oggi poco utilizzata, ed è probabile che la maggior parte dei pazienti con questa diagnosi abbiano in realtà un'elmintiasi broncopolmonare allergica (parassitosi), reazioni a farmaci o un'ABPA.

EPIDEMIOLOGIA. Le sindromi PIE sembrano essere molto meno comuni nella popolazione pediatrica che in a quella adulta. In una casistica, solo il 6% dei pazienti era di età <20 anni. Sono stati riportati casi sporadici di polmonite eosinofila acuta e cronica nei bambini. I bambini precedentemente classificati come portatori di sindrome di Löffler rappresentano la maggioranza dei casi pediatrici. Dalla maggior parte dei *case report* pediatrici è emerso che la malattia colpisce in egual misura maschi e femmine; si possono tuttavia osservare differenze geografiche, poiché un gruppo ha riportato una preponderanza femminile nei bambini, come pure negli adulti con sindromi PIE. La presentazione avviene dalla prima infanzia all'adolescenza.

ANATOMIA PATOLOGICA E PATOGENESI. Nella popolazione pediatrica, l'eziologia più comune delle sindromi PIE comprende le infestazioni parassitarie e le reazioni ai farmaci. La prevalenza delle singole infestazioni parassitarie presenta differenze geografiche. Il parassita che causa più comunemente sindromi PIE negli Stati Uniti è l'*Ascaris lumbricoides*. Le larve nate dalle uova ingerite attraversano la parete intestinale e migrano nei polmoni, causando un'intensa reazione infiammatoria. Le cellule infiammatorie prevalenti sono i macrofagi alveolari, i linfociti, i neutrofili e gli eosinofili. Altri parassiti comuni comprendono *Strongyloides* spp., *Toxocara canis* (verme cilindrico del cane, larva migrans viscerale) e *Ancylostoma braziliense*. In Africa, in Sud America e nel Sudest Asiatico, i vermi filariformi *Wuche-*

reria bancrofti e *Brugia malayi* causano l'eosinofilia polmonare tropicale.

Anche molti farmaci possono essere responsabili di sindromi PIE: tra questi, la sulfasalazina, la penicillina, l'ampicillina, l'ibuprofene e il sodio cromoglicato, di uso comune nei pazienti pediatrici. Questi farmaci scatenano un'intensa reazione infiammatoria a livello polmonare, probabilmente a causa di meccanismi immunologici.

MANIFESTAZIONI CLINICHE. I pazienti con sindromi PIE causate da parassiti o da farmaci presentano malessere, tosse cronica, febbre intermittente, dispnea, sibili e, occasionalmente, dolore addominale, eruzioni cutanee, calo ponderale. La durata dei sintomi è variabile: nella polmonite eosinofila acuta di solito durano meno di un mese e tipicamente non recidivano una volta trattata, mentre nella polmonite eosinofila cronica sono presenti per più di 6 mesi e spesso si ripresentano nonostante un trattamento efficace. I reperti all'esame obiettivo variano, ma spesso mostrano tachipnea, crepitii e sibili.

DIAGNOSI. La diagnosi di sindrome PIE è formulata in base alle manifestazioni cliniche con eosinofilia periferica associata, e ai reperti della radiografia del torace. Radiologicamente, questi pazienti presentano infiltrati interstiziali, alveolari o misti aspecifici, che tendono a essere bilaterali e diffusi. Nei soggetti con polmonite eosinofila cronica si osservano infiltrati periferici con risparmio delle zone centrali ("negativo fotografico dell'edema polmonare"). Inoltre, le pneumopatie eosinofile possono essere diagnosticate in base alla presenza di infiltrati polmonari e di eosinofilia al broncolavaggio alveolare, o alla presenza di larve di parassiti nel lavaggio broncoscopico o gastrico. La biopsia polmonare può essere utile per formulare la diagnosi.

TRATTAMENTO. La terapia varia a seconda del tipo di sindrome PIE. Le forme indotte da parassiti o da farmaci hanno una buona prognosi e si risolvono spontaneamente con le cure di supporto e l'interruzione dell'esposizione. I farmaci per l'eradicazione dei parassiti sono indispensabili solo in rari casi. I pazienti con altre forme di pneumopatie eosinofile, tra cui la polmonite eosinofila acuta e cronica, possono richiedere un ciclo di terapia con corticosteroidi. Nella maggior parte delle forme di pneumopatia eosinofila la prognosi è buona. La polmonite eosinofila acuta, tuttavia, può essere potenzialmente fatale.

Allen JN, Magro CM, King MA: The eosinophilic pneumonias. *Semin Respir Crit Care Med* 2002;23:127–143.
O'Connor DL: Recognizing eosinophilic lung syndromes. *Resp Rev* 2001;6:6.
Oermann CM, Panesar KS, Langston C, et al: Pulmonary infiltrates with eosinophilia syndromes in children. *J Pediatr* 2000;136:351–358.
Savani DM, Sharma OP: Eosinophilic lung disease in the tropics. *Clin Chest Med* 2002;23:377–396.
Talmaciu I: Loffler syndrome. Available at emedicine website (www.emedicine.com).
Wubbel C, Fulmer D, Sherman J: Chronic eosinophilic pneumonia: A case report and national survey. *Chest* 2003;123:1763–1766.

Capitolo 397 ■ Polmonite

Theodore C. Sectish e Charles G. Prober

La polmonite è un'infiammazione del parenchima polmonare. Sebbene la maggior parte dei casi sia imputabile a microrganismi, le cause non infettive comprendono l'aspirazione di cibo o acido gastrico, di corpi estranei, idrocarburi e sostanze lipidiche, le reazioni da ipersensibilità, l'assunzione di determinati farmaci o l'esposizione alle radiazioni. L'infezione polmonare che colpisce neonati (vedi Capitolo 109) e pazienti immunocompromessi (vedi Capitolo 177) ha cause diverse rispetto a quella che si manifesta nei lattanti e nei bambini per altri aspetti sani.

EPIDEMIOLOGIA. La polmonite è una causa importante di morbilità e mortalità nei bambini (soprattutto in quelli di età <5 anni) in tutto il mondo, rivaleggiando con la diarrea come causa di morte nei Paesi in via di sviluppo. Con una stima di 146-159 milioni di nuovi episodi all'anno nei Paesi in via di sviluppo, si ritiene che la polmonite causi circa 4 milioni di decessi tra i bambini, in tutto il mondo. Attualmente, l'incidenza della polmonite acquisita in comunità, nei Paesi sviluppati, è stimata di 0,026 episodi per anno-bambino, rispetto a 0,280 episodi per anno-bambino nei Paesi in via di sviluppo.

Negli Stati Uniti, dal 1939 al 1996, la mortalità causata dalla polmonite nei bambini si è ridotta del 97%. Si ipotizza che questo declino sia attribuibile all'introduzione degli antibiotici, dei vaccini e all'estensione della copertura medico-assicurativa per i pazienti pediatrici. *Haemophilus influenzae* di tipo b (vedi Capitolo 192), che in passato era un'importante causa di polmonite batterica nei bambini piccoli, è diventato infrequente grazie all'uso routinario di vaccini orali. Negli Stati Uniti, l'introduzione del vaccino eptavalente coniugato antipneumococcico e il suo impatto sulla malattia da pneumococco (vedi Capitolo 181) hanno ridotto l'incidenza globale di polmonite nei lattanti e nei bambini del 30% circa nel primo anno di vita, del 20% circa nel secondo anno di vita e del 10% circa nei pazienti di età superiore a 2 anni.

EZIOLOGIA. La causa di polmonite nel singolo paziente è spesso difficile da determinare, poiché la coltura diretta di tessuto polmonare è una tecnica invasiva, praticata raramente. Le colture effettuate sull'escreato, ossia su campioni ottenuti dalle vie respiratorie superiori, generalmente non riflettono accuratamente la causa dell'infezione delle vie respiratorie inferiori. Utilizzando gli esami diagnostici attualmente disponibili, è possibile identificare una causa batterica o virale nel 40-80% dei bambini con polmonite acquisita in comunità. Il patogeno batterico più comune è *Streptococcus pneumoniae* (pneumococco), seguito da *Chlamydia pneumoniae* e *Mycoplasma pneumoniae*. Oltre allo pneumococco, altre cause batteriche di polmonite in bambini precedentemente sani, negli Stati Uniti, comprendono lo streptococco di gruppo A (*Streptococcus pyogenes*; vedi Capitolo 182) e *Staphylococcus aureus* (vedi Capitolo 180.1) (Tab. 397-1).

Nei Paesi in via di sviluppo *Streptococcus pneumoniae*, *Haemophilus influenzae* e *Staphylococcus aureus* sono le principali cause di ospedalizzazione e di morte da polmonite nei pazienti pediatrici, sebbene nei bambini con infezione da HIV debbano essere presi in considerazione anche *Mycobacterium tuberculosis* (vedi Capitolo 212), i micobatteri atipici, *Salmonella* (vedi Capitolo 195), *Escherichia coli* (vedi Capitolo 197) e *Pneumocistis jirovecii* (vedi Capitolo 241).

I patogeni virali sono una causa importante di infezioni delle vie respiratorie inferiori nei lattanti e nei bambini di età <5 anni. I virus sono responsabili del 45% degli episodi di polmonite identificati nei bambini ospedalizzati a Dallas. A differenza della bronchiolite, che ha un picco di incidenza nel primo anno di vita, la polmonite virale colpisce soprattutto tra i 2 e i 3 anni di età, dopodiché la sua frequenza si riduce lentamente. Tra i virus respiratori, il virus dell'influenza (vedi Capitolo 255) e il virus respiratorio sinciziale (RSV, *Respiratory Syncytial Virus*) (vedi Capitolo 257) sono i patogeni principali, specialmente nei bambini di età <3 anni. Altre cause comuni della polmonite sono i virus parainfluenzali, gli adenovirus, i rhinovirus e gli metapneumovirus. L'età del paziente aiuta a identificare i possibili patogeni (Tab. 397-2).

Negli Stati Uniti le affezioni delle vie respiratorie inferiori sono molto più comuni in autunno e in inverno, in relazione alle epidemie stagionali di infezioni respiratorie di origine virale, che avvengono ogni anno. Queste epidemie iniziano tipicamente

TABELLA 397-1. Cause di polmonite infettiva

Batteriche	
Comuni	
Streptococcus pneumoniae	
Streptococchi di gruppo B	Neonati
Streptococchi di gruppo A	
*Mycoplasma pneumoniae**	Adolescenti; epidemia in primavera-estate
*Chlamydia pneumoniae**	Adolescenti
Chlamydia trachomatis	Neonati
Anaerobi vari	Polmonite da aspirazione
Enterici Gram-negativi	Polmonite nosocomiale
Poco comuni	
Haemophilus influenzae di tipo B	Non vaccinati
Staphylococcus aureus	Pneumatoceli; neonati
Moraxella catarrhalis	
Neisseria meningitides	
Francisella tularensis	Animali, contatto con mosche o pulci
Nocardia spp.	Individui immunosoppressi
*Chlamydia psittaci**	Contatto con uccelli
Yersinia pestis	Peste
*Legionella spp.**	Esposizione ad acque contaminate; nosocomiale
Virali	
Comuni	
Virus respiratorio sinciziale	Bronchiolite
Virus parainfluenzali di tipo 1-3	Croup
Influenza A, B	Febbre alta, mesi invernali
Adenovirus	Può essere severa; spesso insorge tra gennaio e aprile
Metapneumovirus	Simile all'RSV
Poco comuni	
Rhinovirus	Rinorrea
Enterovirus	Neonati
Herpes simplex	Neonati
Cytomegalovirus	Lattanti, immunosoppressi
Morbillo	Rash, corizza, congiuntivite
Varicella	Adolescenti
Hantavirus	Stati Uniti sud-occidentali, roditori
Agente della SARS	Asia
Fungine	
Histoplasma capsulatum	Regioni geografiche; contatto con uccelli o pipistrelli
Cryptococcus neoformans	Contatto con uccelli
Aspergillus spp.	Immunosoppressi
Mucormicosi	Immunosoppressi
Coccidioides immitis	Regione geografica
Blastomyces dermatitides	Regione geografica
Da Rickettsie	
*Coxiella burnetii**	Febbre Q, esposizione ad animali (capra, pecora, besiame)
Rickettsia rickettsiae	Morso di zecca
Micobatteriche	
Mycobacterium tuberculosis	Paesi in via di sviluppo
Mycobacterium avium-intracellulare	Immunosoppressi
Parassiti	
Pneumocystis carinii	Immunosoppressi, steroidi
Eosinofilia	Parassiti vari (per es. *Ascaris Strongyloides* spp.)

*Sindrome da polmonite atipica; atipica in termini di manifestazioni extrapolmonari, febbre di basso grado, infiltrati irregolari diffusi, scarsa risposta alla terapia antibiotica con derivati penicillinici ed escreato negativo alla colorazione di Gram.
SARS (*Severe Acute Respiratory Syndrome*), sindrome respiratoria acuta severa.
Da Kliegman RM, Greenbaum LA, Lye PS: Practical *Strategies in Pediatric Diagnosis & Therapy*, 2nd ed, Philadelphia, Elsevier, 2004, p. 29.

in autunno con la comparsa delle infezioni parainfluenzali, che si manifestano per lo più con croup. Successivamente, durante l'inverno, l'RSV, gli metapneumovirus e i virus influenzali causano un'infezione diffusa, a carico delle vie aeree superiori, dei bronchioli e dei polmoni. L'RSV colpisce i lattanti e i bambini più piccoli, mentre il virus dell'influenza causa la malattia e un eccesso di ospedalizzazione da malattia respiratoria acuta in tutti i gruppi di età. Conoscere la prevalenza delle epidemie virali può aiutare a formulare una diagnosi iniziale di presunzione.

Lo stato vaccinale è importante, poiché i bambini completamente immunizzati contro *H. influenzae* di tipo b e *S. pneumoniae* hanno minori probabilità di essere infettati da questi patogeni. I bambini immunosoppressi o con una malattia sottostante possono essere a rischio di infezione da patogeni specifici (per es. *Pseudomonas* spp. nei pazienti con fibrosi cistica).

TABELLA 397-2. Agenti eziologici raggruppati in base all'età del paziente

GRUPPO DI ETÀ	PATOGENI COMUNI (IN ORDINE DI FREQUENZA)
Neonati (<1 mese)	Streptococco di gruppo B, *Escherichia coli*, altri bacilli Gram-negativi, *Streptococcus pneumoniae*, *Haemophilus influenzae* (di tipo b,* non tipizzabile)
1-3 mesi	
Polmonite febbrile	Virus respiratorio sinciziale, altri virus respiratori (parainfluenza, influenza, adenovirus), *S. pneumoniae*, *H. influenzae* (di tipo b,* non tipizzabile)
Polmonite afebbrile	*Chlamydia trachomatis*, *Mycoplasma hominis*, *Ureaplasma urealyticum*, Cytomegalovirus
3-12 mesi	Virus respiratorio sinciziale, altri virus respiratori (parainfluenza, influenza, adenovirus), *S. pneumoniae*, *H. influenzae* (di tipo b,* non tipizzabile), *C. trachomatis*, *Mycoplasma pneumoniae*, streptococco di gruppo A
2-5 anni	Virus respiratori (parainfluenza, influenza, adenovirus), *S. pneumoniae*, *H. influenzae* (di tipo b,* non tipizzabile), *M. pneumoniae*, *Chlamydophila pneumoniae*, *S. aureus*, streptococco di gruppo A
5-18 anni	*M. pneumoniae*, *S. pneumoniae*, *C. pneumoniae*, *H. influenzae* (di tipo b,* non tipizzabile), virus dell'influenza, adenovirus, altri virus respiratori
≥18 anni	*M. pneumoniae*, *S. pneumoniae*, *C. pneumoniae*, *H. influenzae* (di tipo b,* non tipizzabile), virus dell'influenza, adenovirus, Legionella pneumophila

**H. influenzae* di tipo b è poco comune con la vaccinazione universale contro *H. influenzae* di tipo b.
Da Kliegman RM, Marcdante KJ, Jenson HJ, Behrman RE: *Nelson Essentials of Pediatrics*, 5th ed Philadelphia, Elsevier, 2006, p. 504.

PATOGENESI. Di norma il tratto respiratorio inferiore è mantenuto sterile dai meccanismi di difesa fisiologici, che comprendono la clearance mucociliare, le proprietà delle secrezioni normali come le immunoglobuline A (IgA) secretorie e la pulizia delle vie aeree da parte della tosse. I meccanismi di difesa immunologica del polmone che limitano l'invasione da parte di organismi patogeni comprendono i macrofagi, presenti negli alveoli e nei bronchioli, le IgA secretorie e altre immunoglobuline.

La polmonite virale di solito fa seguito alla diffusione dell'infezione lungo le vie aeree, accompagnata dal danno diretto all'epitelio respiratorio, che porta all'ostruzione delle vie aeree da edema, secrezioni anomale e detriti cellulari. Il piccolo calibro delle vie aeree rende i bambini particolarmente suscettibili alle infezioni gravi nei primi mesi di vita. Spesso l'ostruzione delle vie aeree si associa ad atelettasia, edema interstiziale e alterazione del rapporto ventilazione-perfusione, con ipossiemia severa. L'infezione virale delle vie respiratorie può inoltre predisporre a un'infezione batterica secondaria, alterando i normali meccanismi di difesa dell'organismo, le secrezioni e la flora batterica.

Quando si instaura un'infezione batterica nel parenchima polmonare, il processo patologico varia in base al microrganismo responsabile. *M. pneumoniae* attacca l'epitelio respiratorio, inibendo l'azione ciliare e portando alla distruzione cellulare e a una risposta infiammatoria nella sottomucosa. Con la progressione dell'infezione, detriti cellulari prodotti dalla desquamazione, cellule infiammatorie e muco causano ostruzione delle vie aeree, con diffusione dell'infezione lungo l'albero bronchiale, come accade nella polmonite virale.

S. pneumoniae provoca un edema locale; quest'ultimo a sua volta favorisce la proliferazione di microrganismi e la loro diffusione nelle regioni adiacenti del polmone, che spesso danno luogo al caratteristico coinvolgimento lobare focale.

L'infezione delle vie respiratorie inferiori da streptococco di gruppo A risulta in un'infezione più diffusa, con polmonite interstiziale. Le alterazioni anatomiche comprendono necrosi della mucosa tracheobronchiale, formazione di grandi quantità di essudato, edema ed emorragia locale, con estensione nei setti interalveolari, coinvolgimento dei vasi linfatici e aumentata probabilità di coinvolgimento pleurico.

La polmonite da *S. aureus* si manifesta come broncopolmonite confluente, spesso monolaterale, caratterizzata dalla presenza di estese zone di necrosi emorragica e aree irregolari di cavitazione del parenchima polmonare, che provocano pneumatoceli, empiemi o, a volte, fistole broncopolmonari.

Si parla di **polmonite ricorrente** per indicare **due o più episodi** in un anno, o **tre o più** episodi in assoluto, con guarigione radiografica tra gli eventi. In un bambino che va soggetto a polmonite batterica ricorrente si deve ricercare una malattia di base sottostante (Tab. 397-3). Altri fattori che favoriscono l'infezione polmonare comprendono i traumi, l'anestesia e l'aspirazione.

Con l'espressione **polmonite a lenta risoluzione** si indica la persistenza dei sintomi o delle anomalie radiografiche oltre il decorso normalmente atteso. Il lasso di tempo varia a seconda del microrganismo coinvolto, dell'estensione della malattia e della presenza di complicanze associate.

MANIFESTAZIONI CLINICHE. Le polmoniti virali e batteriche sono spesso precedute da alcuni giorni di sintomi di infezione delle vie aeree superiori, tipicamente rinite e tosse. Nella polmonite virale è di solito presente febbre; la temperatura corporea in genere è più bassa che nella polmonite batterica. La tachipnea è la manifestazione clinica più importante della polmonite. È comune un aumento del lavoro respiratorio accompagnato da retrazioni intercostali, sottocostali e sovrasternali, alitamento delle pinne nasali e utilizzo dei muscoli accessori. L'infezione severa può essere accompagnata da cianosi e fatica respiratoria, specialmente nei lattanti. L'auscultazione del torace può rivelare crepitii e sibili, ma è spesso difficile localizzare l'origine di questi suoni patologici nei bambini molto piccoli con torace iperfonetico. Spesso non è possibile distinguere clinicamente una polmonite virale da una causata da *Mycoplasma* o da altri patogeni batterici.

L'esordio della polmonite batterica, negli adulti e nei bambini più grandi, è tipicamente improvviso, con brividi scuotenti seguiti da febbre elevata, tosse e dolore toracico. Nei bambini più grandi e negli adolescenti, un'affezione delle vie aeree superiori di breve durata è seguita dall'esordio improvviso di brividi scuotenti e febbre accompagnati da sonnolenza, con periodi intermittenti di irrequietezza, respiro rapido, tosse secca, stizzosa, non produttiva, ansia e, occasionalmente, delirio. Talvolta si osserva cianosi periorale. Molti bambini immobilizzano il lato affetto per ridurre al minimo il dolore pleuritico e migliorare la ventilazione; a tal fine, possono giacere su un lato con le ginocchia raccolte al torace.

I reperti dell'esame obiettivo dipendono dallo stadio della polmonite. Nelle fasi precoci della malattia, sono comunemente udibili sul campo polmonare affetto una riduzione del murmure vescicolare, crepitii sparsi e ronchi. Con il progressivo consolidamento o l'insorgenza di complicanze della polmonite, come versamenti, empiema o piopneumotorace, si percepisce ottusità alla percussione, e il murmure vescicolare può essere diminuito. Spesso dal lato affetto si verifica un ritardo dell'escursione respiratoria. La distensione addominale può essere notevole, a causa della dilatazione gastrica provocata dall'aria ingerita o da ileo. Il dolore addominale è comune nella polmonite lobare inferiore. Il fegato può sembrare aumentato di volume a causa dello spostamento verso il basso del diaframma, secondario all'iperinflazione dei polmoni, o dell'insufficienza cardiaca sovrapposta. Anche la rigidità nucale, in assenza di meningite, può essere pronunciata, specialmente con il coinvolgimento del lobo superiore destro.

I sintomi descritti negli adulti con polmonite pneumococcica possono presentarsi nei bambini più grandi, mentre sono di raro riscontro nei lattanti e nei bambini piccoli, in cui il quadro clinico ha una variabilità notevolmente maggiore. Nei lattanti, vi possono essere un'infezione prodromica delle vie aeree superiori e una riduzione dell'appetito, cui fa seguito la comparsa improvvisa di febbre, irrequietezza, ansia e distress respiratorio. In questi pazienti, dall'aspetto sofferente, il distress respiratorio si manifesta con grunting, alitamento delle pinne nasali, restrazioni delle zone sovraclaveari, intercostali e sottocostali, tachipnea, fame d'aria e spesso cianosi. I risultati dell'esame obiettivo possono essere fuorvianti, in particolare nei lattanti di pochi mesi, con reperti minimi rispetto al grado di tachipnea. Alcuni lattanti con polmonite batterica possono avere disturbi gastrointestinali associati (vomito, anoressia, diarrea e distensione addominale), secondari a ileo paralitico. La rapida progressione dei sintomi è caratteristica dei casi più severi di polmonite batterica.

TABELLA 397-3. Diagnosi differenziale della polmonite ricorrente

Malattie ereditarie
Fibrosi cistica
Anemia falciforme
Alterazioni immunitarie
AIDS
Agammaglobulinemia di Bruton
Deficit selettivo di sottoclassi di IgG
Sindrome da immunodeficienza comune variabile
Sindrome da immunodeficienza combinata severa
Alterazioni dei leucociti
Malattia granulomatosa cronica
Sindrome da iperimmunoglobulina E (sindrome di Job)
Difetti di adesione dei leucociti
Alterazioni ciliari
Sindrome delle ciglia immobili
Sindrome di Kartagener
Alterazioni anatomiche
Sequestro
Enfisema lobare
Reflusso esofageo
Corpo estraneo
Fistola tracheoesofagea (tipo a H)
Bronchiectasie
Aspirazione (incoordinazione orofaringea)

Da Kliegman RM, Marcdante KJ, Jenson HJ, Behrman RE: *Nelson Essentials of Pediatrics*, 5th ed, Philadelphia, Elsevier, 2006, p. 507.

DIAGNOSI. La radiografia del torace conferma la diagnosi di polmonite e può identificare una complicanza come un versamento pleurico o un empiema. La polmonite virale è in genere caratterizzata da iperinflazione con infiltrati interstiziali bilaterali e ispessimento peribronchiale (Fig. 397-1). Il consolidamento lobare confluente è tipico della polmonite pneumococcica (Fig. 397-2). L'aspetto radiografico da solo non è diagnostico e devono essere considerate altre caratteristiche cliniche. Non sono necessarie

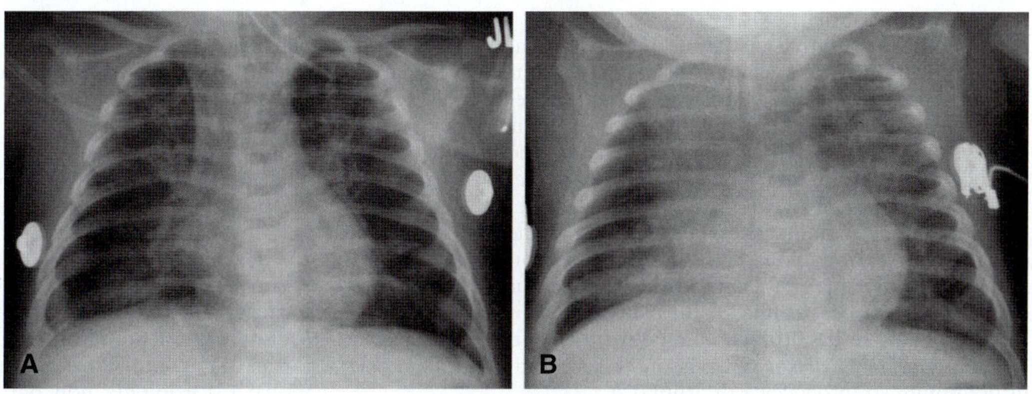

Figura 397-1. *A*, Aspetto radiologico caratteristico della polmonite da virus respiratorio sinciziale (RSV) in un neonato di 6 mesi con respiro rapido e febbre. La proiezione anteroposteriore del torace mostra iperespansione del polmone con malattia dei piccoli spazi aerei bilaterali e strie dense, che indicano la presenza sia di polmonite sia di atelettasia. È posizionato un tubo endotracheale. *B*, Il giorno successivo, la radiografia anteroposteriore del torace rivela una progressione della polmonite bilaterale.

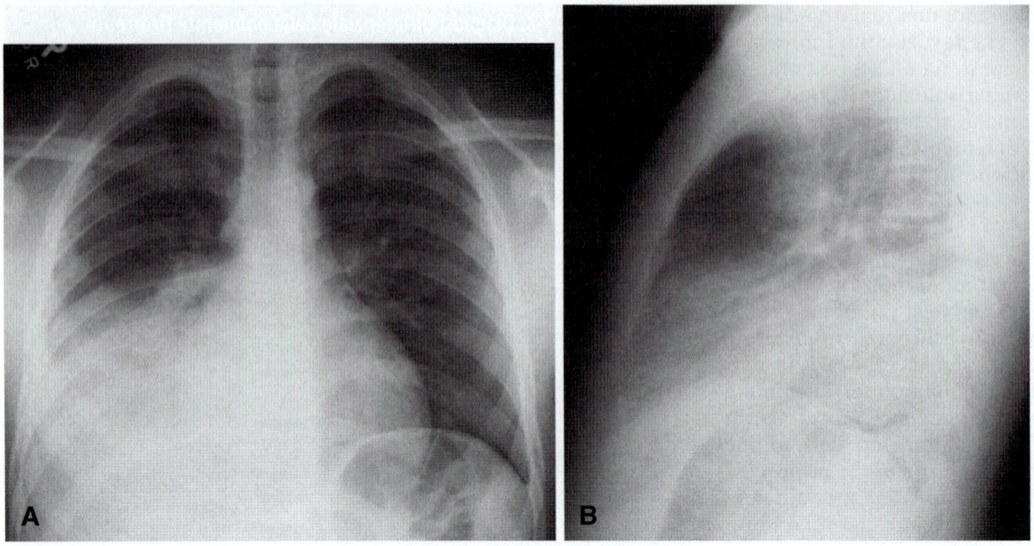

Figura 397-2. Aspetto radiografico caratteristico della polmonite da pneumococco in un ragazzo di 14 anni con tosse e febbre. Le radiografie anteroposteriori (*A*) e laterali (*B*) del torace rivelano il consolidamento del lobo superiore destro, fatto fortemente suggestivo di polmonite batterica.

radiografie seriate per confermare la guarigione nei pazienti con polmonite non complicata.

La conta leucocitaria periferica può essere utile per distinguere la polmonite batterica da quella virale. Nella forma virale, i leucociti possono essere normali o elevati (di solito non superiori a 20 000/mm^3), con una predominanza linfocitica. La forma batterica (occasionalmente la polmonite da adenovirus) si associa spesso a leucocitosi nel range di 15 000-40 000/mm^3 con predominanza di granulociti. Un versamento pleurico importante, il consolidamento lobare e la febbre elevata all'esordio della malattia sono altri reperti suggestivi di un'eziologia batterica. La **polmonite atipica** causata da *C. pneumoniae* o *M. pneumoniae* è difficile da distinguere dalla polmonite pneumococcica sulla base della radiografia e degli esami di laboratorio, e sebbene la polmonite pneumococcica si associ a livelli più elevati di leucocitosi, velocità di eritrosedimentazione (VES) e di proteina C reattiva (PCR), vi è una considerevole sovrapposizione.

La diagnosi definitiva di infezione virale si basa sull'isolamento di un virus o sul rilevamento del genoma o di un antigene virale nelle secrezioni respiratorie. La crescita di virus respiratori nelle colture tissutali di solito richiede 5-10 giorni. Sono disponibili test affidabili e precisi, al DNA o all'RNA, per l'identificazione rapida dell'RSV, dei virus influenzali, parainfluenzali e degli adenovirus. Gli esami sierologici, che possono essere anch'essi impiegati per diagnosticare un'infezione respiratoria virale recente, generalmente richiedono l'esame di campioni di siero durante la fase acuta e la convalescenza per rilevare un aumento del titolo anticorpale verso uno specifico agente virale. Queste tecniche sono laboriose, lente e nella maggior parte dei casi inutili dal punto di vista clinico poiché l'infezione di solito si risolve nell'arco di tempo necessario per ottenere la conferma sierologica. Gli esami sierologici possono tuttavia essere utili con strumento epidemiologico per definire l'incidenza e la prevalenza di vari patogeni respiratori virali.

La diagnosi definitiva di un'infezione batterica richiede l'isolamento di un microrganismo dal sangue, dal liquido pleurico o dal polmone. La coltura dell'escreato ha un valore limitato per la diagnosi di polmonite, nel bambino piccolo. Le emocolture sono positive solo nel 10% dei pazienti pediatrici con polmonite pneumococcica. In caso di infezione da *M. pneumoniae*, si trovano nel sangue agglutinine *a frigore* con titoli >1:64 nel 50% circa dei pazienti. Tali agglutinine tuttavia non sono specifiche, poiché anche altri patogeni, come i virus influenzali, possono causarne un aumento. L'infezione acuta causata da *M. pneumoniae* può essere diagnosticata in base a una PCR positiva o alla sieroconversione delle IgG. I dati sierologici, come il titolo antistreptolisinico (ASLO, *AntiStreptoLysin O*), possono essere utili nella diagnosi di polmonite streptococcica di gruppo A.

TRATTAMENTO. Il trattamento di una sospetta polmonite batterica dipende dalla causa presunta e dall'aspetto clinico del paziente (vedi Tabb. 397-1 e 397-2). Per i bambini con malattia lieve che non richiedono ospedalizzazione, si consiglia l'amoxicillina, che nelle comunità con percentuali elevate di pneumococchi penicillinoresistenti andrebbe prescritta ad alti dosaggi (80-90 mg/kg/die). Le alternative terapeutiche comprendono la cefuroxima axetil o l'amoxicillina/acido clavulanico. Nei bambini in età scolare e in quelli in cui si sospetta un'infezione da *M. pneumoniae* o da *C. pneumoniae* (polmoniti atipiche), un antibiotico macrolide, come l'azitromicina, è una scelta appropriata. Negli adolescenti con polmoniti atipiche, si può utilizzare un fluorochinolonico con attività sul sistema respiratorio (levofloxacina, gatifloxacina, moxifloxacina, gemifloxacina).

Il trattamento empirico della sospetta polmonite batterica, in un bambino ricoverato, richiede un approccio basato sulle manifestazioni cliniche al momento della presentazione. Il cardine della terapia è la somministrazione di cefuroxima (150 mg/kg/die), cefotaxima o ceftriaxone per via parenterale, quando si ipotizza un'eziologia batterica. Se le caratteristiche cliniche suggeriscono una polmonite stafilococcica (pneumatoceli, empiema), la terapia antimicrobica iniziale deve comprendere anche la vancomicina o la clindamicina.

Se si sospetta una polmonite virale, è ragionevole evitare la terapia antibiotica, specialmente nei pazienti affetti da malattia lieve, con evidenze cliniche che suggeriscono un'infezione virale e senza distress respiratorio. Fino al 30% dei pazienti con infezione virale nota può avere un patogeno batterico coesistente. Pertanto, se si prende la decisione di non effettuare una terapia antibiotica in base alla diagnosi presunta di infezione virale, bisogna prestare attenzione al deterioramento delle condizioni cliniche, che segnala la possibilità di un'infezione batterica sovrapposta e richiede quindi la somministrazione di antibiotici.

Le indicazioni al ricovero in ospedale sono elencate nella Tabella 397-4. Nei Paesi in via di sviluppo, lo zinco per via orale (20 mg/die) aiuta ad accelerare la guarigione in caso di polmonite severa.

RISPOSTA AL TRATTAMENTO. Tipicamente, i pazienti con polmonite batterica non complicata acquisita in comunità rispondono alla terapia con un miglioramento della sintomatologia clinica (febbre, tosse, tachipnea, dolore toracico) entro 48-96 ore dall'inizio degli antibiotici. L'evidenza radiografica del miglioramento si ottiene con notevole ritardo rispetto al dato clinico. Quando il paziente non risponde a una terapia antibiotica appropriata (**polmonite a lenta risoluzione**), occorre esaminare una serie di fattori: (1) complicanze, come un empiema; (2) resistenza batterica; (3) eziologia non batterica, come virus e aspirazione di

TABELLA 397-4. Fattori che suggeriscono la necessità dell'ospedalizzazione nei bambini con polmonite

Età <6 mesi
Anemia a cellule falciformi con sindrome toracica acuta
Coinvolgimento multilobare
Stato immnocompromesso
Aspetto tossico
Distress respiratorio severo
Necessità di somministrazione di ossigeno
Disidratazione
Vomito
Mancata risposta alla terapia antibiotica orale
Genitori con scarsa compliance

Adattata da Baltimore RS: Pneumonia. In Jenson HB, Baltimore RS (ed): *Pediatric Infectious Diseases: Principles and Practice*. Philadelphia, WB Saunders, 2002, p. 801.

corpi estranei o cibo; (4) ostruzione bronchiale da parte di lesioni endobronchiali, corpi estranei o tappi di muco; (5) malattie preesistenti, come immunodeficienza, discinesia ciliare, fibrosi cistica, sequestro polmonare o malformazione adenomatoide cistica; (6) altre cause non infettive (bronchiolite obliterante, polmonite da ipersensibilità, polmonite eosinofila, aspirazione e granulomatosi di Wegener). La ripetizione della radiografia del torace è il primo passo per determinare la ragione di un ritardo nella risposta al trattamento.

COMPLICANZE. Le complicanze della polmonite in genere sono la conseguenza della diffusione diretta dell'infezione batterica nella cavità toracica (versamento pleurico, empiema, pericardite) o di una batteriemia con diffusione ematogena (Fig. 397-3). La meningite, l'artrite suppurativa e l'osteomielite sono complicanze rare della diffusione ematogena dell'infezione da pneumococco o da *H. influenzae* di tipo b.

S. aureus, *S. pneumoniae* e *S. pyogenes* sono le cause più comuni di versamento parapneumonico e di empiema (Tab. 397-5). Il trattamento dell'empiema si basa sul suo stadio (essudativo, fibrinopurulento, organizzato): per determinarlo, si rivelano utili gli studi radiologici, tra cui l'ecografia e la TC. Il cardine del trattamento comprende la terapia antibiotica e il drenaggio con tubo di toracostomia. Ulteriori approcci comprendono l'uso di una terapia fibrinolitica (urochinasi, streptochinasi, alteplasi) e la toracoscopia selettiva videoassistita (VATS, *Video-Assisted Thoracoscopy*) per sbrigliare, lisare le aderenze e drenare le raccolte purulente saccate. La diagnosi e l'intervento precoci, in particolare con la VATS, possono ovviare alla necessità della toracotomia e dello sbrigliamento a cielo aperto.

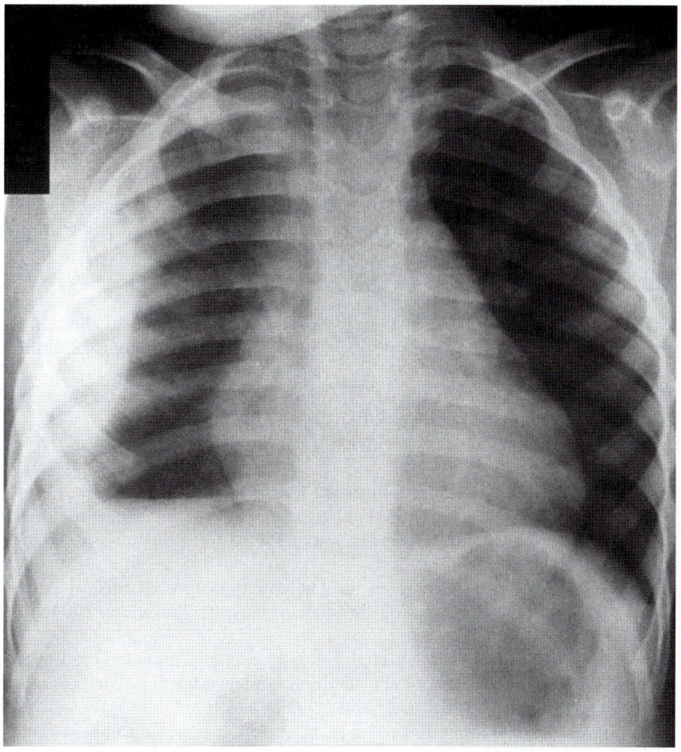

Figura 397-3. Empiema da pneumococco in un bambino di 3 anni con raffreddore e febbre per tre giorni. Si osserva una raccolta pleurica o extrapleurica dal lato destro. Il paziente, che aveva un tampone pleurico e un'emocoltura positivi per pneumococco, è guarito completamente in 3 settimane. (Da Kuhn JP, Slovis TL, Haller JO: *Caffrey's Pediatric Diagnostic Imaging*, vol 1, 10th ed. Philadelphia, Mosby/Elsevier, 2004, p 1002.)

Addo-Yoba E, Chisaka N, Hassan M, et al: Oral amoxicillin versus injectable penicillin for severe pneumonia in children aged 3 to 59 month: A randomized multicentre equivalency study. *Lancet* 2004;364:1141–1148.

Avansino JR, Goldman B, Sawin RS, Flum DR: Primary operative versus nonoperative therapy for pediatric empyema: A meta-analysis. *Pediatrics* 2005;115:1652–1659.

Baumer JH: Parapneumonic effusion and empyema. *Arch Dis Child* 2005;90:ep21–ep24.

Bhutta ZA: Childhood pneumonia in developing counries. *BMJ* 2006;333: 612–613.

Black SB, Shinefeld HR, Ling S, et al: Effectiveness of heptavalent pneumococcal conjugate vaccine in children younger than five years of age for prevention of pneumonia. *Pediatr Infect Dis J* 2002;21:810–815.

Bouros D, Antoniou KM, Light RW: Intrapleural streptokinase for pleural infection. *Br Med J* 2006;332:133–134.

Brooks WA, Yunus M, Santosham M, et al: Zinc for severe pneumonia in very young children: Double-blind placebo-controlled trial. *Lancet* 2004;363:1683–1688.

Duke T: Neonatal pneumonia in developing countries. *Arch Dis Child Fetal Neonatal Ed* 2005;90:F211–F219.

TABELLA 397-5. Diagnosi differenziale del liquido pleurico

	TRASUDATO	ESSUDATO	EMPIEMA COMPLICATO
Aspetto	Limpido	Torbido	Purulento
Leucociti	<1000	>1000	>5000
Tipo di cellule	Linfociti, monociti	PMN	PMN
LDH	<200 U/L	>200 U/L	>1000 U/L
Rapporto LDH siero/liquido pleurico	<0,6	>0,6	>0,6
Proteine >3 g	Inusuale	Comune	Comune
Rapporto proteine siero/liquido pleurico	<0,5	>0,5	>0,5
Glucosio*	Normale	Basso	Molto basso* (<40 mg/dL)
pH*	Normale (7,40-7,60)	7,20-7,40	<7,20, necessità di posizionamento di un drenaggio toracico
Colorazione di Gram	Negativa	Di solito positiva	>85% positiva, a meno che il paziente non abbia ricevuto una precedente terapia antibiotica

* Bassi livelli di glucosio o di pH possono essere osservati nei versamenti maligni, nella tubercolosi, nella rottura esofagea, nella pancreatite (amilasi pleurica positiva) e nelle malattie reumatologiche (per es. lupus eritematoso sistemico).
LDH, lattato deidrogenasi; PMN, polimorfonucleati neutrofili.
Da Kliegman RM, Greenbaum LA, Lye PS: *Practical Strategies in Pediatric Diagnosis & Therapy*, 2nd ed Philadelphia, Elsevier, 2004, p. 30.

Esposito S, Bosis S, Cavagna R, et al: Characteristics *of Streptococcus pneumoniae* and atypical bacterial infections in children 2–5 years of age with community-acquired pneumonia. *Clin Infect Dis* 2002;35:1345–1352.
File TM Jr: Community-acquired pneumonia. *Lancet* 2003;362:1991–2001.
Kusel MMH, de Klerk NH, Holt PG, et al: Role of respiratory viruses in acute upper and lower respiratory tract illness in the first year of life: a birth cohort study. *Pediatr Infect Dis J* 2006;25:680–686.
Lakhanpaul M, Atkinson M, Stephenson T: Community acquired pneumonia in children: A clinical update. *Arch Dis Child* 2004;89:ep29–ep34.
McCracken GH Jr: Diagnosis and management of pneumonia. *Pediatr Infect Dis J* 2000;19:924–928.
McIntosh K: Community-acquired pneumonia in children. *N Engl J Med* 2002;346:429–437.
Michelow IC, Olsen K, Lozana J, et al: Epidemiology and clinical characteristics of community-acquired pneumonia in hospitalized children. *Pediatrics* 2004;113:701–707.
Nelson JD: Community-acquired pneumonia in children: Guidelines for treatment. *Pediatr Infect Dis J* 2000;19:251–253.
Panitch HB: Evaluation of recurrent pneumonia. *Pediatr Infect Dis J* 2005;24:265–266.
Rudan I, Tomaskovic L, Boschi-Pinto C, Campbell H: WHO Child Health Epidemiology Reference Group: Global estimate of the incidence of clinical pneumonia among children under five years of age. *Bull World Health Organ* 2004;82:895–903.
Schultz KD, Fan LL, Oinsky J, et al: The changing face of pleural empyemas in children: Epidemiology and management. *Pediatrics* 2004;113: 1735–1740.
Tsolia MN, Psarras S, Bossios A, et al: Etiology of community-acquired pneumonia in hospitalized school-age children: Evidence for high prevalence of viral infections. *Clin Infect Dis* 2004;39:686–686.
Ulloa-Guiterrez R, Skippen P, Synnes A, et al: Life-threatening human metapneumovirus pneumonia requiring extracorporal membrane oxygenation in a preterm infant. *Pediatrics* 2004;114:e517–e519.
Wacogne I, Negrine RJS: Are follow up chest x ray examinations helpful in the management of children recovering from pneumonia? *Arch Dis Child* 2003;88:457–458.
Wardlaw T, Salama P, White Johansson E: Pneumonia: the leading killer of children. *Lancet* 2006;368:1048–1050.
Weinstein M, Restrepo R, Chait PG, et al: Effectiveness and safety of tissue plasminogen activator in the management of complicated parapneumonic effusions. *Pediatrics* 2004;113:e182–e185.
Zar HJ: Pneumonia in HIV-infected and HIV-uninfected children in developing countries: Epidemiology, clinical features, and management. *Curr Opin Pulm Med* 2004;10:176–182.

Capitolo 398 ■ Bronchiectasie

Oren Lakser

Le bronchiectasie, dilatazioni anomale e irreversibili dell'albero bronchiale, rappresentano probabilmente lo stadio finale comune di diversi eventi antecedenti, aspecifici e non correlati. La loro incidenza si è ridotta complessivamente nei Paesi industrializzati, ma continua a rappresentare un problema in quelli in via di sviluppo. In almeno una casistica di bambini con bronchiectasie (non dovute a fibrosi cistica) il rapporto maschi:femmine era di 2:1.

FISIOPATOLOGIA E PATOGENESI. Nel mondo industrializzato, la fibrosi cistica (vedi Capitolo 400) è la causa più comune di bronchiectasie significative; altre condizioni a esse associate comprendono la discinesia ciliare, le sindromi da immunodeficienza e le infezioni, in particolar modo la pertosse, il morbillo e la tubercolosi. Le bronchiectasie possono essere anche congenite, come nella *sindrome di Williams-Campbell*, in cui vi è assenza della cartilagine anulare bronchiale, e nella *sindrome di Marnier-Kuhn* (tracheobroncomalacia congenita), contraddistinta da un'alterazione del tessuto connettivo. Altre entità patologiche associate sono la *sindrome del lobo medio destro* (compressione estrinseca cronica del bronco lobare medio destro, da parte di linfonodi ilari) e la *sindrome dell'unghia gialla* (versamento pleurico, linfedema, colore anomalo delle unghie).

Nella patogenesi delle bronchiectasie entrano in gioco tre meccanismi di base. L'ostruzione può insorgere a causa di tumori, corpi estranei, muco impattato dovuto a una clearance mucociliare insufficiente, oppure a causa di compressione esterna, membrane bronchiali o atresia. Le infezioni provocate da *Bordetella pertussis*, virus del morbillo o della rosolia, togavirus, virus respiratorio sinciziale e *Mycobacterium tuberculosis* inducono un'infiammazione cronica, danno progressivo della parete bronchiale e dilatazione. L'infiammazione cronica contribuisce in modo analogo al meccanismo tramite il quale l'ostruzione conduce alle bronchiectasie. Tale meccanismo, nelle forme congenite, è probabilmente correlato a un'anomala formazione della cartilagine. La sequenza comune, nella patogenesi delle bronchiectasie, consiste nella difficoltà di eliminare le secrezioni che, sommata alle infezioni ricorrenti, produce un "circolo vizioso" di infezione e infiammazione, con conseguente danno alle vie aeree e rimodellamento.

Le bronchiectasie possono presentarsi in qualsiasi combinazione delle tre forme patologiche, che è possibile studiare grazie alla TC ad alta risoluzione (HRCT, *High Resolution Computer Tomography*). Nelle bronchiectasie cilindriche, il profilo bronchiale è regolare, ma si riscontra dilatazione diffusa dell'albero bronchiale. Il lume bronchiale termina bruscamente a causa dei tappi di muco. Nelle bronchiectasie varicose, il grado di dilatazione è maggiore e stenosi locali causano irregolarità del profilo, simili a vene varicose; possono essere presenti anche piccole sacculazioni. Nelle bronchiectasie sacculari (cistiche), la dilatazione bronchiale progredisce dando luogo a dilatazione a pallone dei bronchi, che terminano in cavità piene di liquido o muco. Tra tutte le forme di bronchiectasia, questa è la più grave. Le bronchiectasie fanno parte di un ampio spettro di malattie polmonari suppurative croniche dell'età pediatrica. Sono state proposte le seguenti definizioni: *prebronchiectasie* (infezioni endobronchiali croniche o ricorrenti con alterazioni aspecifiche alla HRCT), *bronchiectasie HRCT* (sintomi clinici con evidenza di dilatazione bronchiale alla HRCT; in tal caso la malattia può persistere, progredire oppure migliorare e risolversi), *bronchiectasie permanenti* (come la forma precedente, ma senza risoluzione entro 2 anni).

MANIFESTAZIONI CLINICHE. I sintomi più comuni lamentati dai pazienti con bronchiectasie sono la tosse e la produzione di un escreato abbondante e purulento. I bambini più piccoli possono ingoiare l'espettorato. Si osserva inoltre, con una certa frequenza, emottisi. Nel corso delle esacerbazioni infettive può insorgere febbre. Con il passare del tempo si verificano anoressia e scarso aumento ponderale. L'esame obiettivo rivela tipicamente crepitii localizzati nell'area colpita, sebbene possano essere presenti anche sibili, così come ippocratismo digitale. Nei casi severi insorgono ipossiema e dispnea. Gli studi di funzionalità polmonare dimostrano un quadro ostruttivo, restrittivo o misto. Tipicamente, l'alterazione della capacità di diffusione è un reperto tardivo.

DIAGNOSI. Nei pazienti con bronchiectasie, la radiografia del torace tende a essere aspecifica. I reperti tipici comprendono aumento di dimensione e perdita di definizione della trama broncovascolare, affastellamento bronchiale e perdita di volume polmonare. Nelle forme più severe si possono riscontrare aree cistiche, occasionalmente con livelli idroaerei e aspetto ad alveare. Talvolta è osservabile iperinflazione compensatoria del polmone controlaterale. La HRCT a sezione sottile rappresenta il *gold standard*, poiché ha un'ottima sensibilità e specificità. La TC fornisce ulteriori informazioni sulla localizzazione della malattia, sulla presenza di lesioni mediastiniche e sull'estensione del segmento coinvolto. L'aggiunta a questa indagine dell'inalazione di un aerosol radiomarcato può fornire ulteriori informazioni. I reperti TC, nei pazienti con bronchiectasie, comprendono tipicamente forme cilindriche ("a rotaie del tram", "aspetto ad anello con castone"), varicose (bronchi con "contorno a rosario"), cistiche (cisti "a catena e a grappolo") e forme miste (Fig. 398-1). Sono colpiti più comunemente i lobi inferiori.

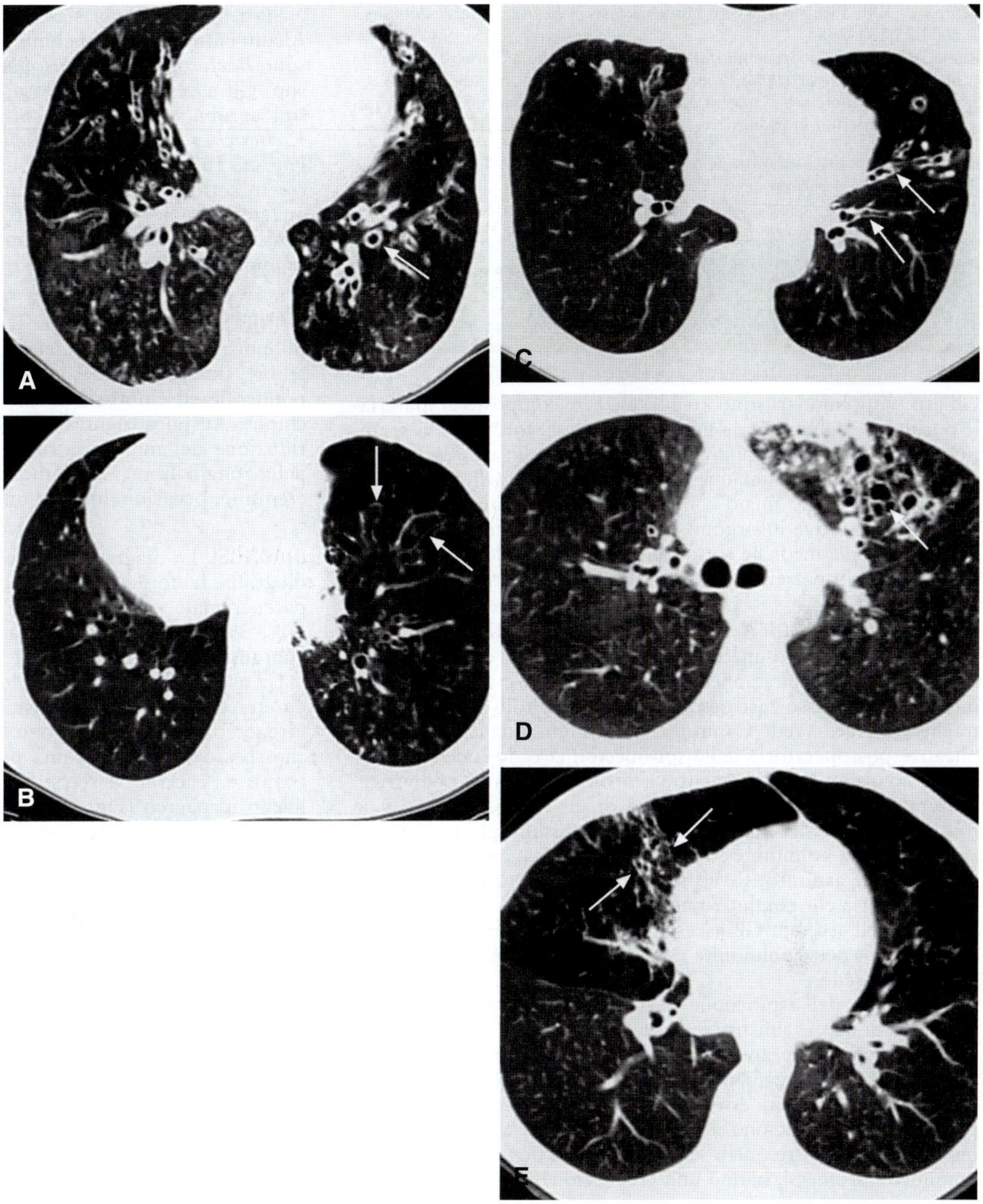

Figura 398-1. Immagini TC ad alta risoluzione di un polmone con bronchiectasie. Il riquadro *A* mostra le vie aeree dilatate e ispessite (*freccia*). Il riquadro *B* mostra le vie aeree che non si restringono verso la periferia (*frecce*), in un paziente con sindrome di Kartagener. Nel riquadro *C* sono evidenti le alterazioni varicose (vie aeree dilatate e a rosario [*frecce*]), mentre nel riquadro *D* si osservano cisti a grappolo o dilatazioni sacciformi (*frecce*), oltre a infiltrati periferici. Il riquadro *E* mostra bronchiectasie del lobo medio (*frecce*) in un paziente con infezione da *Mycobacterium avium*-complex. (Da Barker AF: Bronchiectasis. *N Engl J Med* 2002;346:1383.)

TRATTAMENTO. La terapia iniziale è medica, volta a ridurre l'ostruzione delle vie aeree e a controllare l'infezione. Sono essenziali la fisioterapia respiratoria (drenaggio posturale), gli antibiotici e i broncodilatatori. Spesso si rende necessario somministrare antibiotici parenterali per 2-4 settimane al fine di trattare adeguatamente le esacerbazioni acute. La scelta del farmaco dipende dall'identificazione e dalla sensibilità del microrganismo trovato all'esame colturale del tampone faringeo, dell'escreato (indotto o spontaneo) o del liquido di broncolavaggio alveolare. Possono essere utili antibiotici profilattici cronici per via orale (macrolidi) o nebulizzati. Quando le bronchiectasie localizzate divengono più severe o resistenti al trattamento medico, può essere necessaria la resezione segmentale o lobare. Nei pazienti con bronchiectasie una possibile opzione di trattamento è il trapianto polmonare.

PROGNOSI. Complessivamente, la prognosi per i pazienti con bronchiectasie è migliorata moltissimo negli ultimi decenni. Le possibili ragioni di questo successo sono il riconoscimento precoce o la prevenzione delle condizioni predisponenti, l'uso di antibiotici più potenti e a più ampio spettro e il miglioramento delle tecniche chirurgiche.

Barker AF: Bronchiectasis. *N Engl J Med* 2002;346:1383–1393.
Callahan CW, Redding GJ: Bronchiectasis in children: Orphan disease or persistent problem? *Pediatr Pulmonol* 2002;33:492–496.
Chang AB, Grimwood K, Mulholland EK, et al: Bronchiectasis in indigenous children in remote Australian communities. *Med J Aust* 2002;177:200–204.
Eastham KM, Fall AJ, Mitchell L, et al: The need to redefine non-cystic fibrosis bronchiectasis in childhood. *Thorax* 2004;59:324–327.
Evans DJ, Greenstone M: Long-term antibiotics in the management of non-CF bronchiectasis—do they improve outcome? *Respir Med* 2003;97:851–858.
Galvin JR, D'Alessandro MP: Electric diffuse lung: The diagnosis of diffuse lung disease, bronchiectasis. Available at University of Iowa Virtual Hospital website (www.vh.org).
Haciibrahimoglu G, Fazlioglu M, Olcmen A, et al: Surgical management of childhood bronchiectasis due to infectious disease. *J Thorac Cardiovasc Surg* 2004;127:1361–1365.
Karakoc GB, Yilmaz M, Altintas DU, et al: Bronchiectasis: Still a problem. *Pediatr Pulmonol* 2001;32:175–178.

Morrissey BM, Evans SJ: Severe bronchiectasis. *Clin Rev Allergy Immunol* 2003:25:233–248.
Rama M, Yousef E: Bronchiectasis and chronic asthma: How common in pediatrics? *Allergy Asthma Proc* 2006;27:354–358.
Santamaria F, Montella S, Camera L, et al: Lung structure abnormalities, but normal lung function in pediatric bronchiectasis. *Chest* 2006;130:480–486.

Capitolo 399 ■ Ascesso polmonare

Oren Lakser

Gli ascessi polmonari sono aree localizzate composte di materiale purulento, delimitate da una parete spessa, formatesi in seguito a un'infezione polmonare che ha portato alla distruzione del parenchima, con cavitazione e necrosi centrale. Gli ascessi polmonari sono molto meno comuni nei bambini che negli adulti. Le forme primitive insorgono in soggetti precedentemente sani, senza patologie mediche sottostanti, mentre quelle secondarie si manifestano in pazienti con condizioni di base predisponenti.

ANATOMIA PATOLOGICA E PATOGENESI. Numerose condizioni possono predisporre un bambino allo sviluppo di ascessi polmonari, tra cui aspirazione, polmonite, fibrosi cistica (vedi Capitolo 400), reflusso gastroesofageo (vedi Capitolo 320.1), fistola tracheoesofagea (vedi Capitolo 316), immunodeficienze, complicanze postoperatorie della tonsillectomia e dell'adenoidectomia, convulsioni e varie malattie neurologiche. In età pediatrica, l'aspirazione di materiale infetto o di un corpo estraneo è la fonte prevalente dei microrganismi che causano gli ascessi. Inizialmente, una polmonite compromette il drenaggio del liquido o del materiale aspirato; si verifica quindi un'ostruzione vascolare infiammatoria che conduce a necrosi tissutale, liquefazione e formazione dell'ascesso. Gli ascessi possono insorgere anche come conseguenza della polmonite e della disseminazione ematogena da un'altra sede.

Se l'evento dell'aspirazione si verifica in clinostatismo, i lobi superiori destro e sinistro e il segmento apicale del lobo inferiore destro sono le aree declivi più colpite. Se il bambino era in ortostatismo, i segmenti posteriori dei lobi superiori hanno maggiori probabilità di essere colpiti in quanto declivi. Gli ascessi polmonari primitivi sono di più frequente osservazione nel polmone destro, mentre quelli secondari, in particolare nei pazienti immuocompromessi, hanno una predilezione per il lato sinistro.

Sia i batteri aerobi sia gli anaerobi possono causare ascessi. Alcuni batteri anaerobi comuni che provocano ascessi polmonari sono *Bacteroides* spp., *Fusobacterium* spp. e *Peptostreptococcus* spp. Gli ascessi possono essere imputabili anche a microrganismi aerobi, come *Streptococcus* spp., *Staphylococcus aureus*, *Escherichia coli*, *Klebsiella pneumoniae* e *Pseudomonas aeruginosa*. Tutti i pazienti con un ascesso polmonare dovrebbero essere sottoposti a colture tanto per gli aerobi quanto per gli anaerobi, come parte del loro iter diagnostico. Anche i miceti possono causare ascessi polmonari, in particolare nei pazienti immunocompromessi.

MANIFESTAZIONI CLINICHE. I sintomi più comuni dell'ascesso polmonare, nella popolazione pediatrica, comprendono tosse, febbre, dolore toracico, vomito, produzione di espettorato, calo ponderale ed emottisi. L'esame obiettivo rivela tipicamente tachipnea, dispnea, rientramenti con utilizzo dei muscoli accessori, riduzione del murmure vescicolare e ottusità alla percussione nella zona colpita. All'esame dei polmoni possono essere udibili crepitii e, occasionalmente, un prolungamento dell'espirio.

DIAGNOSI. La diagnosi viene effettuata per lo più grazie alla radiografia del torace, che classicamente mostra un'infiammazione parenchimale con una cavità contenente un livello idroaereo (Fig. 399-1). La TC del torace offre una migliore definizione anatomica, che comprende la localizzazione e le dimensioni.

Un ascesso è in genere una lesione con una parete spessa e una parete centrale a bassa densità che progredisce verso un livello idroaereo. Gli ascessi devono essere distinti dagli pneumatoceli, che spesso complicano una polmonite batterica grave; caratterizzati da raccolte aeree sottili e a parete liscia, con o senza un livello idroaereo (Fig. 399-2), gli pneumatoceli spesso si risolvono spontaneamente con il trattamento della causa specifica della polmonite.

La determinazione dei batteri eziologici in un ascesso polmonare può essere molto utile per guidare la scelta dell'antibiotico. Sebbene la colorazione di Gram dell'escreato possa fornire un indizio precoce sulla classe di batteri coinvolta, le colture dell'escreato rivelano tipicamente una flora mista e pertanto non sempre sono attendibili. I tentativi di evitare la contaminazione da parte della flora orale comprendono la puntura diretta del polmone e l'aspirazione percutanea (TC guidata), broncoscopica e transtracheale. L'aspirazione broncoscopica deve essere effettuata con estrema cautela, in quanto può essere complicata da aspirazione intrabronchiale massiva. Per evitare procedure invasive in un ospite precedentemente sano, si può iniziare una terapia empirica, in assenza di materiale da sottoporre a coltura.

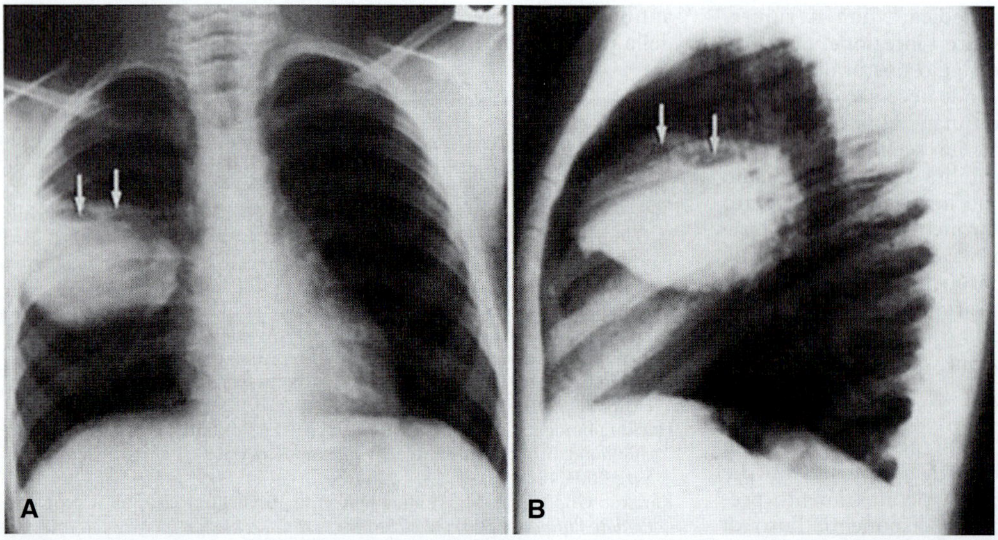

Figura 399-1. Ascesso polmonare multiloculato (*frecce*). (Da Brook I: Lung abscess and pulmonary infections due to anaerobic bacteria. In Chernick V, Boat TF, Wilmott RW, Bush A [ed]: *Kendig's Disorders of the Respiratory Tract in Children*, 7th ed. Philadelphia, Saunders, 2006, p 482.)

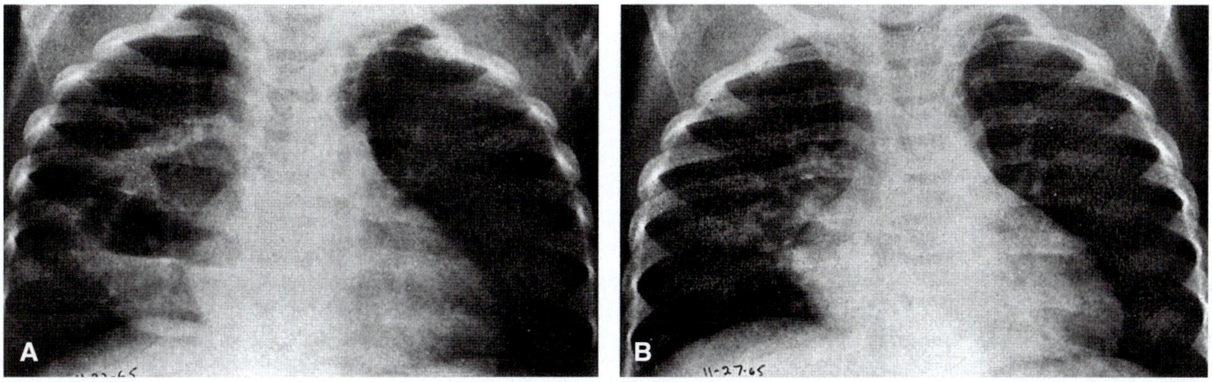

Figura 399-2. Aspetto, nell'arco di 5 giorni, di un grande pneumatocele multiloculato, in un segmento di consolidamento alveolare. *A*, È presente un'ampia cavità con due livelli idroaerei, in un segmento di polmonite alveolare, nel lobo superiore destro. *B*, Dopo 5 giorni la cavità e la maggior parte del consolidamento alveolare sono scomparsi. (Da Silverman FN, Kuhn JP: *Essentials of Caffrey's Pediatric X-Ray Diagnosis*. Chicago, Year Book Medical Publishers, 1990, p 303.)

TRATTAMENTO. Si consiglia un trattamento conservativo. La maggior parte degli esperti raccomanda un ciclo di terapia antibiotica parenterale per 2-3 settimane, nei casi non complicati, seguito da un ciclo di antibiotici per via orale, per un totale di 4-6 settimane. La scelta dell'antibiotico, pur essendo basata sulla colorazione di Gram e sull'esame colturale, inizialmente dovrebbe garantire una copertura sia sugli aerobi sia sugli anaerobi. Gli schemi di trattamento devono comprendere un agente penicillinasi-resistente attivo contro *S. aureus* e una copertura contro gli anaerobi, di solito con clindamicina o ticarcillina/acido clavulanico. Se si sospettano o si isolano batteri Gram-negativi, occorre aggiungere un aminoglicoside.

Nei pazienti con patologia grave o in quelli che non migliorano dopo 7-10 giorni di terapia antimicrobica appropriata, si deve considerare l'opzione chirurgica. L'intervento iniziale, spesso l'unico, viene praticato con tecniche percutanee minimamente invasive, spesso TC-guidate. Nei rari casi complicati può essere necessaria la toracotomia con lobectomia o decorticazione.

PROGNOSI. Complessivamente, la prognosi per i bambini con ascessi polmonari primitivi è eccellente. La presenza di organismi aerobi può essere un indice prognostico negativo, in particolare in quelli con ascessi polmonari secondari. La maggior parte dei pazienti pediatrici diviene asintomatica nell'arco di 7-10 giorni, sebbene la febbre possa persistere anche per 3 settimane. Le anomalie radiologiche di solito si risolvono in 1-3 mesi, ma possono anche persistere per anni.

Brook I: Anaerobic pulmonary infections in children. *Pediatr Emerg Care* 2004;20:636–640.
Chan PC, Huang LM, Wu PS, et al: Clinical management and outcome of childhood lung abscess: a 16-year experience. *J Microbiol Immunol Infect* 2005;38:183–188.
De A, Varaiya A, Mathur M: Anaerobes in pleuropulmonary infections. *Indian J Med Microbiol* 2002;20:150–152.
Mansharamani NG, Koziel H: Chronic lung sepsis: Lung abscess, bronchiectasis, and empyema. *Curr Opin Pulm Med* 2003;9:181–185.
Mueller PR, Berlin L: Complications of lung abscess aspiration and drainage. *AJR Am J Roentgenol* 2002;178:1083–1886.
Tseng YL, Wu MH, Lin MY, et al: Surgery for lung abscess in immunocompetent and immunocompromised children. *J Pediatr Surg* 2001;36:470–473.
Yen C, Tang R, Chen S, et al: Pediatric lung abscess: A retrospective review of 23 cases. *J Microbiol Immunol Infect* 2004;37:45–49.
Young CS: Cough, fever, a lung mass, and a complex history. *JAAPA* 2004;17:31–32, 37–39.

02/03/2017 corso Collevecchio Paolo!

Capitolo 400 ■ Fibrosi cistica

Thomas F. Boat e James D. Acton

La fibrosi cistica è una malattia ereditaria multisistemica del bambino e dell'adulto, caratterizzata principalmente da ostruzione e infezione delle vie aeree e da maldigestione, con le relative conseguenze. È il tratto genetico recessivo a prognosi sfavorevole più comune nei bianchi. La caratteristica patogenetica principale è una disfunzione delle superfici epitelizzate, che è responsabile di uno spettro ampio, variabile e spesso confondente di manifestazioni cliniche e complicanze.

La fibrosi cistica rappresenta la principale causa di pneumopatia cronica severa nei bambini ed è responsabile della maggior parte delle insufficienze pancreatiche esocrine nella prima fase della vita. È inoltre all'origine di molti casi di deplezione di sali, poliposi nasale, pansinusite, prolasso rettale, pancreatite, colelitiasi e iperglicemia insulinodipendente. Potendo presentarsi con mancato accrescimento e, occasionalmente, con cirrosi o un'altra forma di disfunzione epatica, questa malattia entra in diagnosi differenziale con molte condizioni pediatriche (Tab. 400-1).

GENETICA. La fibrosi cistica colpisce con maggiore frequenza la popolazione bianca del Nord Europa, del Nord America, dell'Australia e della Nuova Zelanda. La prevalenza varia da uno studio all'altro, ma in generale è di circa 1/3500 nati vivi. Sebbene sia meno frequente nelle popolazioni dell'Africa, del Medio Oriente e del Sud-Est Asiatico, con il miglioramento degli accertamenti, la prevalenza in questi gruppi è risultata notevolmente maggiore di quanto si stimasse in precedenza. A Toronto la prevalenza della fibrosi cistica nei bambini da 0 a 14 anni tra gli immigrati provenienti dell'Asia meridionale è solo di poco inferiore che nella popolazione generale (1/9200 vs 1/6600).

L'ereditarietà è autosomica recessiva. Il gene responsabile codifica per una proteina di 1480 aminoacidi, detta *regolatore transmembrana della fibrosi cistica* (CFTR, *Cystic Fibrosis Transmembrane Regulator*). Il CFTR è espresso abbondantemente nelle cellule epiteliali delle vie aeree, del tratto digerente (compresi il pancreas e il sistema biliare), nelle ghiandole sudoripare e nell'apparato genitourinario. Il canale ionico e le funzioni regolatorie di questo gene possono essere alterati in vario modo dalle diverse mutazioni. Sono stati associati alla sindrome della fibrosi cistica più di 1500 polimorfismi del CFTR. La delezione di un singolo residuo di fenilalanina a livello dell'aminoacido 508 (ΔF508), che rappresenta la mutazione a maggiore prevalenza, è responsabile

TABELLA 400-1. Complicanze della fibrosi cistica

RESPIRATORIE
Bronchiectasie, bronchite, bronchiolite, polmonite
Atelettasia
Emottisi
Pneumotorace
Polipi nasali
Sinusite
Reattività delle vie aeree
Cuore polmonare
Insufficienza respiratoria
Ostruzione dei bronchi da parte del muco
Aspergillosi broncopolmonare allergica
GASTROINTESTINALI
Ileo da meconio, tappi di meconio (neonati)
Peritonite da meconio (neonati)
Sindrome da ostruzione intestinale distale (ostruzione non neonatale)
Prolasso rettale
Intussuscezione
Volvolo
Colopatia fibrosante (stenosi)
Appendicite
Atresia intestinale
Pancreatite
Cirrosi biliare (ipertensione portale: varici esofagee, ipersplenismo)
Ittero ostruttivo neonatale
Steatosi epatica
Reflusso gastroesofageo
Colelitiasi
Ernia inguinale
Deficit di crescita (malassorbimento)
Deficit vitaminici (vitamine A, D, E, K)
Deficit di insulina, iperglicemia sintomatica, diabete
Tumori (rari)
ALTRE
Infertilità
Pubertà ritardata
Edema-ipoproteinemia
Osteoatropatia ipertrofica-artrite
Ippocratismo digitale
Diabete mellito

Silverman FN, Kuhn JP: *Essentials of Caffrey's Pediatric X-Ray Diagnosis*. Chicago, Year Book Medical Publishers, 1990, p 649.

dell'elevata incidenza della patologia nelle popolazioni del Nord Europa ed è molto meno frequente nelle altre popolazioni, per esempio in quelle dell'Europa meridionale e di Israele. Circa il 50% degli individui di origini nordeuropea con fibrosi cistica è omozigote per la ΔF508, e più del 70% è portatore di almeno un gene con questa mutazione. Gli altri pazienti hanno una vasta gamma di mutazioni, nessuna delle quali ha una prevalenza superiore a pochi punti percentuale, tranne che in popolazioni circoscritte; la mutazione W1282X è presente nel 60% degli Ebrei Ashkenazi con fibrosi cistica. La correlazione tra genotipo CFTR e fenotipo clinico, molto complessa, non è prevedibile nel singolo paziente. Le mutazioni etichettate come "gravi" (ΔF508) si associano quasi uniformemente a insufficienza pancreatica, ma solo in linea generale a una più rapida progressione della malattia polmonare. Sembra che polimorfismi di un gene modificatore siano responsabili di gran parte della variabilità della progressione della pneumopatia. L'associazione più stretta con forme di malattia più gravi è con una singola variazione nucleotidica nel gene del TGF-β1. Alleli varianti della lectina legante il mannosio, un fattore chiave dell'immunità innata sistemica, si associano a infezioni polmonari più gravi e a una sopravvivenza ridotta. Diverse mutazioni (3849 + 10 kb C > T) sono riscontrabili nei pazienti con normale secrezione di cloro nel sudore. Alcuni individui con polimorfismi di entrambi i geni CFTR hanno scarse manifestazioni della fibrosi cistica (o addirittura nessuna) fino all'adolescenza o all'età adulta, quando presentano pancreatite, sinusite, bronchiectasie diffuse o infertilità maschile. Mentre le mutazioni del CFTR sono una *conditio sine qua non* per la fibrosi cistica, due mutazioni del CFTR possono provocare disturbi che non rientrano nei criteri diagnostici di questa patologia e talvolta non causano neppure problemi clinici rilevabili.

L'insorgenza di epatopatia non può essere prevedibile in base al genotipo CFTR; questo suggerisce una componente ambientale maggiore (acquisita) prevalente nella disfunzione del sistema d'organo, e la presenza di altri geni in grado di modificare il fenotipo della fibrosi cistica.

Utilizzando sonde per le 30 mutazioni più frequenti è possibile accertare il genotipo dell'80-90% della popolazione americana, e aumentando il numero di sonde a 70 o più il riconoscimento delle mutazioni migliora solo di pochi punti percentuali. Alcuni laboratori hanno stabilito dei protocolli per uno screening completo di tutte le mutazioni conosciute del CFTR. In casi particolari, per determinare il genotipo è necessaria la sequenziazione del gene del CFTR.

Si è ipotizzato che l'elevata frequenza di mutazioni del CFTR sia ascrivibile alla resistenza alla morbilità e mortalità per colera, nei secoli passati. In coltura, le cellule epiteliali intestinali omozigoti per la mutazione ΔF508 non sono interessate dagli effetti secretori della tossina colerica.

PATOGENESI. Quattro osservazioni a lungo termine sono di fondamentale importanza dal punto di vista fisiopatologico: l'incapacità di eliminare le secrezioni mucose, uno scarso contenuto d'acqua nelle secrezioni mucose, un elevato contenuto di sali nel sudore e nelle altre secrezioni sierose e infezioni croniche limitate all'apparato respiratorio. Inoltre, vi è una maggior differenza di potenziale negativo attraverso l'epitelio respiratorio nei pazienti con fibrosi cistica, rispetto ai soggetti di controllo. In questi pazienti sono state dimostrate proprietà elettriche aberranti anche nell'epitelio duttale delle ghiandole sudoripare; le membrane delle cellule epiteliali non sono in grado di secernere ioni cloro in risposta a segnali mediati dall'adenosin monofosfato ciclico (cAMP, *cyclic Adenosine MonoPhosphate*) e, almeno nel tratto respiratorio, viene assorbita una quantità eccessiva di sodio attraverso queste membrane (Fig. 400-1). Tali difetti sono ascrivibili a una disfunzione del CFTR (Figg. 400-2 e 400-3).

La conduttanza per il cloro stimolata dall'AMP ciclico è una funzione del CFTR stesso, che risulta assente nelle cellule epiteliali con molte differenti mutazioni di tale gene. Le mutazioni del CFTR rientrano in 6 classi, sebbene con un certo grado di sovrapposizione (vedi Fig. 400-3). Gli individui con mutazioni delle classi I, II e III, in media, hanno una sopravvivenza ridotta rispetto a quelli con genotipi meno gravi (classi IV o V). L'importanza clinica di queste categorie funzionali è limitata, poiché non correlano uniformemente con caratteristiche cliniche specifiche o con la loro severità, quanto piuttosto con l'attività residua del CFTR. Gli individui con l'1% della normale attività del CFTR hanno malattia polmonare e insufficienza pancreatica; la funzione pancreatica è conservata con un'attività del 5%, mentre un'attività del 10% risulta in assenza congenita bilaterale isolata dei vasi deferenti o in pancreatite cronica idiopatica. Questi numeri dovrebbero essere considerati relativi, poiché è ancora in corso il dibattito su quale sia il livello assoluto di attività del CFTR necessario per preservare le funzioni dei vari organi.

La fisiopatologia che è stata postulata per l'epitelio delle vie aeree comprende l'incapacità di secernere sali e, secondariamente, acqua, in presenza di un eccessivo riassorbimento di entrambi. La conseguenza, secondo questa teoria, è che la quantità di acqua sulla superficie delle vie aeree risulta insufficiente a idratare le secrezioni; queste ultime divengono quindi più viscose ed elastiche (gommose) e sono più difficili da eliminare da parte del sistema mucociliare e degli altri meccanismi. L'alterata reologia del muco può essere aggravata da basse concentrazioni di HCO_3^- e da un pH più acido. Il ristagno di queste secrezioni causa ostruzione delle vie aeree a partire da quelle di calibro minore, i bronchioli. L'ostruzione al flusso a livello delle piccole vie aeree è l'anomalia fisiologica più precoce, osservabile nell'apparato respiratorio.

È plausibile che eventi fisiopatologici analoghi abbiano luogo nei dotti pancreatici e biliari (e nei vasi deferenti), con conseguen-

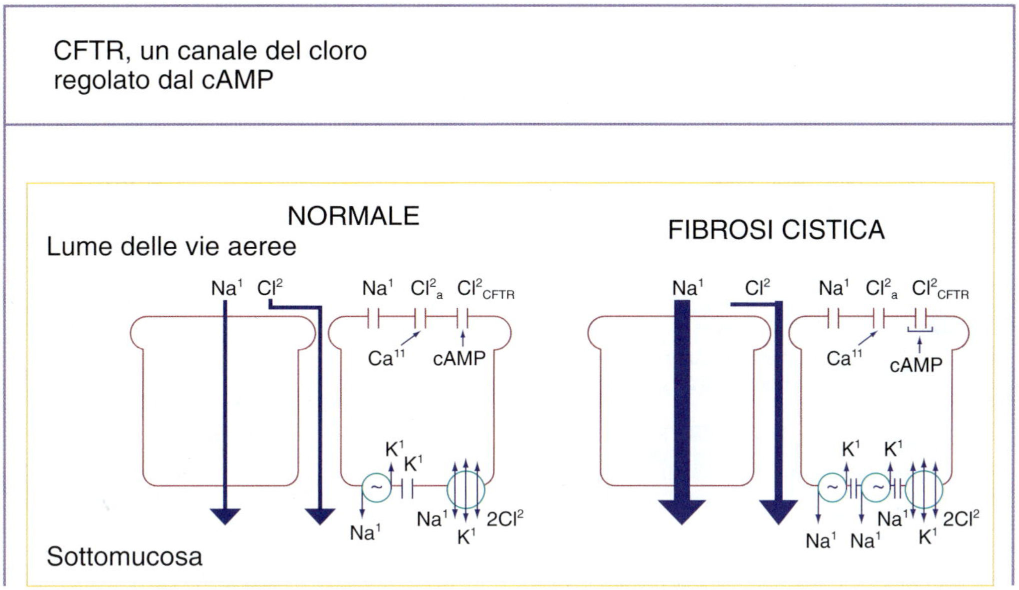

Figura 400-1. Flusso ionico netto attraverso l'epitelio respiratorio normale e quello affetto da fibrosi cistica, in condizioni basali (*frecce grandi*). Poiché l'acqua segue il movimento dei sali, il flusso netto di acqua previsto andrà dal lume delle vie aeree alla sottomucosa e sarà maggiore attraverso l'epitelio con fibrosi cistica. L'aumentato riassorbimento di Na^+ da parte delle cellule, nella fibrosi cistica, si associa a un aumento della conduttanza per il Na^+ sensibile all'amiloride attraverso la membrana apicale (luminale) e a un aumento dei siti Na^+, K^+-ATPasi sulla membrana basolaterale. La conduttanza del Cl^- cAMP-mediata della membrana apicale, associata al regolatore transmembrana della fibrosi cistica (CFTR, *Cystic Fibrosis Transmembrane Regulator*), non è funzionale nell'epitelio dei pazienti con fibrosi cistica; in compenso, è presente una conduttanza del Cl^- alternativa, attivata dal calcio, nelle cellule normali e in quelle con fibrosi cistica. Si postula che nella fibrosi cistica le cellule abbiano una capacità limitata di secernere il Cl^- e riassorbano il Na^+ in quantità eccessiva, limitando la disponibilità di acqua per idratare secrezioni che quindi possono essere eliminate dal lume delle vie aeree. ATP, adenosin trifosfato; cAMP, adenosin monofosfato ciclico. (Da Knowles MR: Contemporary perspectives on the pathogenesis of cystic fibrosis. *New Insights Cystic Fibrosis* 1993;1:1.)

te disidratazione delle secrezioni proteinacee e ostruzione. Poiché la funzione delle cellule duttali delle ghiandole sudoripare è di riassorbire, più che di secernere, il cloruro, i sali non vengono recuperati dal primitivo sudore isotonico, ma sono trasportati verso la superficie cutanea; questo fa sì che i livelli di cloruri e sodio siano elevati.

L'infezione cronica, nella fibrosi cistica, è limitata alle vie aeree. La spiegazione più verosimile di questo fenomeno è una sequenza di eventi che inizia con l'incapacità di eliminare rapidamente i batteri inalati per poi proseguire con la colonizzazione persistente e con una risposta infiammatoria nella parete delle vie aeree. Un'ipotesi alternativa è che il CFTR anomalo crei uno stato proinfiammatorio o amplifichi la risposta infiammatoria alle infezioni virali iniziali. L'evento infiammatorio colpisce per prime le vie aeree di piccolo calibro, forse perché in queste regioni la clearance delle secrezioni alterate e dei microrganismi è più difficile. Le prime manifestazioni polmonari sono la bronchiolite e la bronchite cronica, ma dopo mesi o anni le alterazioni strutturali della parete delle vie aeree provocano la formazione di bronchiolectasie e bronchiectasie.

Gli agenti responsabili del danno alle vie aeree comprendono i prodotti dei neutrofili, come radicali ossidativi e proteasi, e i prodotti delle reazioni immunitarie. Via via che la malattia polmonare progredisce, l'infezione può estendersi al parenchima polmonare peribronchiale. Numerosi prodotti dell'infiammazione, tra cui le proteasi, contribuiscono all'ipersecrezione di muco, caratteristica della malattia cronica delle vie aeree.

Un reperto non facilmente spiegabile è l'elevata prevalenza di colonizzazione delle vie aeree da parte di *Staphylococcus aureus* (vedi Capitolo 180.1), *Pseudomonas aeruginosa* (vedi Capitolo 202) e *Burkholderia cepacia* (vedi Capitolo 202), microrganismi che raramente infettano il polmone negli altri individui. Le cellule epiteliali o il liquido di superficie delle vie aeree, nella fibrosi cistica, possono creare un ambiente favorevole allo sviluppo di tali microrganismi. In questa patologia, l'epitelio respiratorio può subire una compromissione delle sue difese innate contro questi batteri, tramite alterazioni genetiche o acquisite. L'attività antimicrobica delle secrezioni risulta diminuita, verosimilmente in conseguenza dell'eccessiva acidità dei liquidi di superficie o di altri effetti sull'immunità innata. Un altro enigma è la propensione di *P. aeruginosa* ad andare incontro a trasformazione mucoide nelle vie aeree dei pazienti con fibrosi cistica. Il complesso polisaccaridico prodotto da questi microrganismi genera un biofilm che costituisce un ambiente ipossico e pertanto protegge *Pseudomonas* dagli antimicrobici.

Sebbene nell'infezione polmonare di grado avanzato possano verificarsi deficit dell'immunità cellulare, della funzione immune delle mucose e della via alternativa del complemento, nella fibrosi cistica il sistema immunitario sembra fondamentalmente integro. Tra i fattori che predispongono all'infezione delle vie respiratorie sono stati indicati deficit nutrizionali, tra cui la carenza di acidi grassi. Più specificamente, le concentrazioni di lipossine, molecole che sopprimono l'infiammazione neutrofila, appaiono ridotte nelle vie aeree dei pazienti con fibrosi cistica. Il 10-15% degli individui che conservano una funzione pancreatica esocrina sostanziale ha statisticamente valori inferiori di cloruro nel sudore, oltre a presentare una colonizzazione più tardiva da parte di *P. aeruginosa* e un deterioramento più lento della funzione polmonare. Sembra che i fattori nutrizionali siano solo in grado di contribuire, poiché il mantenimento della funzione pancreatica non impedisce lo sviluppo della malattia polmonare tipica.

ANATOMIA PATOLOGICA. Le ghiandole eccrine sudoripare e salivari, dotti compresi, non sono coinvolte dal punto di vista anatomopatologico, nonostante le anomalie del contenuto elettrolitico dei loro secreti.

La lesione anatomica più precoce, nel polmone, è la **bronchiolite** (tappi di muco e risposta infiammatoria nelle parete delle piccole vie aeree). Con il tempo, l'accumulo di muco e l'infiammazione si estendono alle vie aeree di calibro maggiore (**bronchite**). L'iperplasia delle cellule caliciformi e l'ipertrofia delle ghiandole sottomucose divengono l'espressione patologica principale di uno

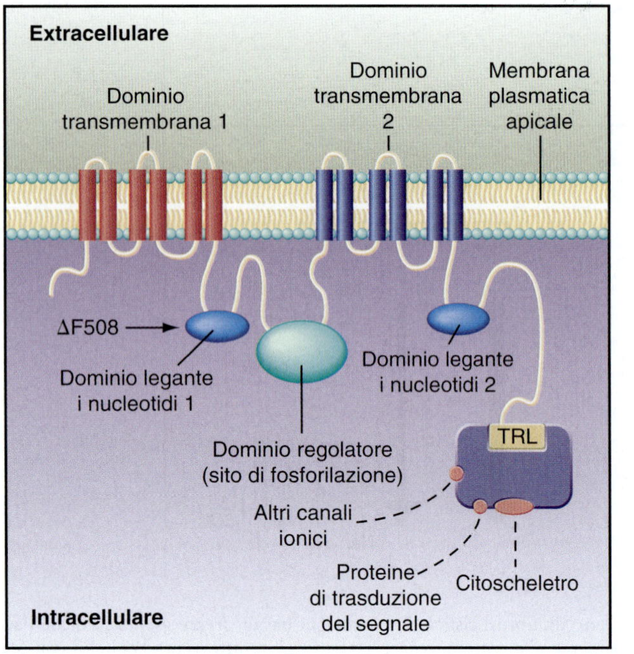

Figura 400-2. Struttura ipotizzata del regolatore transmembrana della fibrosi cistica (CFTR). La proteina contiene 1480 aminoacidi e numerosi domini globulari e transmembrana discreti. L'attivazione del CFTR si basa sulla fosforilazione, in particolare tramite la proteinchinasi A, ma probabilmente coinvolge anche altre chinasi. L'attività del canale è governata dai due domini leganti i nucleotidi, che regolano l'apertura del canale. Il terminale carbossilico (formato da treonina, arginina e leucina [TRL]) del CFTR è ancorato tramite un'interazione di legame tipo PDZ con il citoscheletro e mantenuto in stretta prossimità (*frecce spezzate*) con numerose proteine importanti. Queste proteine associate influiscono sulle funzioni del CFTR, tra cui la conduttanza, la regolazione degli altri canali, la trasduzione del segnale e la localizzazione sulla membrana plasmatica apicale. Ogni dominio che attraversa la membrana contiene 6 α-eliche che attraversano la membrana, alcune porzioni delle quali formano un poro di conduttanza per il cloro. Il dominio regolatore è un sito di fosforilazione della proteinchinasi A. La mutazione comune F508 interessa la superficie del dominio 1 legante i nucleotidi. (Da Rowe SM, Miller S, Sorscher EJ: Cystic fibrosis. *N Engl J Med* 2005;352:1992-2001.)

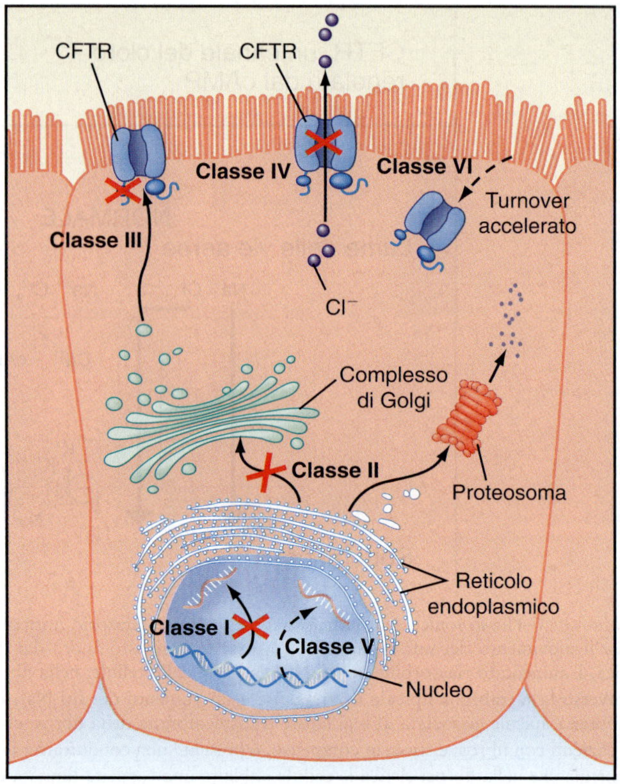

Figura 400-3. Categorie delle mutazioni del CFTR. I difetti del gene CFTR si classificano nel modo seguente: mancata sintesi (classe I); maturazione difettosa della proteina con degradazione prematura (classe II); alterata regolazione, per es. riduzione del legame con l'ATP e dell'idrolisi (classe III); difetto della conduttanza per il cloro o dell'apertura del canale (classe IV); riduzione del numero di trascritti del CFTR dovuta a un'anomalia del promoter o di splicing (classe V); e accelerato turnover dalla superficie cellulare (classe VI). CFTR (*Cystic Fibrosis Transmembrane Regulator*), regolatore transmembrana della fibrosi cistica; ATP, adenosin trifosfato. (Da Rowe SM, Miller S, Sorscher EJ: Cystic fibrosis. *N Engl J Med* 2005;352:1992-2001.)

stato ipersecretivo, che è probabilmente una risposta all'infezione cronica delle vie aeree. I microrganismi sembrano confinati nello spazio endobronchiale; l'infezione batterica invasiva non è caratteristica della fibrosi cistica. Se la malattia perdura a lungo, si accentuano i segni di distruzione delle vie aeree, come l'**obliterazione bronchiolare**, le **bronchioloectasie** e le **bronchiectasie**. Le indagini radiologiche dimostrano un aumento sia dello spessore della parete delle vie aeree, sia dell'area di sezione del lume, in una fase relativamente precoce della valutazione della malattia polmonare. Caratteristiche frequenti della patologia avanzata sono le cisti bronchiectasiche e le bolle enfisematose o subpleuriche, per lo più a carico dei lobi superiori. Questi spazi aerei di dimensioni aumentate possono rompersi e causare pneumotorace. La malattia interstiziale non è una caratteristica pronunciata, sebbene negli stadi avanzati possano comparire aree di fibrosi. L'enfisema vero può svilupparsi, ma non è un reperto patologico universale. Le arterie bronchiali sono dilatate e tortuose, contribuendo a predisporre all'**emottisi** le vie aeree bronchiectasiche. Le piccole arterie polmonari finiscono per presentare ipertrofia delle tonaca media, come ci si aspetterebbe nell'ipertensione polmonare secondaria.

I **seni paranasali** sono uniformemente ripieni di secrezioni contenenti prodotti infiammatori, e nell'epitelio di rivestimento si riscontrano elementi secretori iperplastici e ipertrofici. Sono state riportate lesioni polipoidi dei seni, mucopioceli ed erosioni ossee. La mucosa nasale può contenere cellule infiammatorie, essere edematosa e formare polipi di grandi dimensioni o multipli, di solito a partenza dall'ostio dei seni mascellari ed etmoidali.

Il **pancreas** è in genere piccolo, occasionalmente cistico, e spesso difficile da trovare all'esame postmortem. L'estensione del coinvolgimento alla nascita è variabile. Nei lattanti, gli acini e i dotti sono spesso distesi e ripieni di materiale eosinofilo. Nell'85-90% dei pazienti la lesione progredisce fino alla distruzione pressoché completa degli acini e alla loro sostituzione da parte di tessuto fibroadiposo. Non è frequente osservare focolai di calcificazione alla radiografia dell'addome. Le isole di Langerhans contengono cellule β di aspetto normale, sebbene a partire dalla seconda decade di vita possano presentare una distruzione dell'architettura da parte di tessuto fibroso.

Il **tratto digerente** mostra solo alterazioni minime. Le ghiandole esofagee e duodenali sono spesso distese con secrezioni mucose. Si possono formare concrezioni nel lume appendicolare o nel cieco. Le cripte dell'appendice o del retto possono essere dilatate e ripiene di secrezioni.

La **cirrosi biliare focale** secondaria al blocco dei dotti biliari intraepatici non è comune nei primi mesi di vita, sebbene sia responsabile di casi occasionali di ittero neonatale prolungato. Queste lesioni divengono più frequenti ed estese con l'età e si trovano nel 25% o più dei pazienti, all'esame autoptico. Raramente questo processo progredisce fino alla cirrosi biliare multilobulare sintomatica, il cui quadro distintivo è caratterizzato da grandi noduli parenchimali irregolari con bande interposte di tessuto fibroso. Circa il 30% dei pazienti presenta infiltrazione grassa del fegato, in alcuni casi nonostante una nutrizione in apparenza adeguata. All'autopsia è di frequente riscontro una congestione epatica, secondaria a cuore polmonare. La colecisti, che può essere ipoplasica e ripiena di materiale mucoide, spesso contiene calcoli. Il rivestimento epiteliale di frequente presenta un'estesa metaplasia mucosa. Sono state osservate atresia del dotto cistico e stenosi del dotto biliare comune.

Le ghiandole salivari secernenti muco sono abitualmente ingrandite, con ostruzione focale e dilatazione dei dotti.

Le ghiandole della **cervice uterina** sono distese da muco, che si raccoglie in grande quantità nel canale cervicale. L'endocervicite può essere comune nelle adolescenti e nelle donne giovani. In più del 95% dei maschi, il corpo e la coda dell'epididimo, i vasi deferenti e le vescicole seminali sono obliterati o atresici.

Raramente è stata riportata amiloidosi generalizzata (vedi Capitolo 163).

TABELLA 400-2. Caratteristiche di presentazione di più di 20 000 pazienti negli Stati Uniti

CARATTERISTICA	%
Sintomi respiratori acuti o persistenti	50,5
Scarso accrescimento, malnutrizione	42,9
Feci anomale	35,0
Ileo da meconio, ostruzione intestinale	18,8
Anamnesi familiare	16,8
Anomalie elettrolitiche e dell'equilibrio acido-base	5,4
Prolasso rettale	3,4
Polipi nasali, sinusopatia	2,0
Malattia epatobiliare	0,9
Altre*	1,0-2,0

*Comprendono azoospermia, rash simil-acrodermatite, stati di carenze vitaminiche, edema ipoproteinemico, ipoprotrombinemia con sanguinamento, sindrome da tappo da meconio.

Dati tratti dal Patient Registry, Cystic Fibrosis Foundation, Bethesda, MD.

MANIFESTAZIONI CLINICHE. L'eterogeneità delle mutazioni e dei fattori ambientali sembra responsabile dell'elevata variabilità del coinvolgimento dei polmoni, del pancreas e degli altri organi. L'elenco delle manifestazioni di esordio è lungo, sebbene le presentazioni polmonari e gastrointestinali siano quelle prevalenti (Tab. 400-2).

Apparato respiratorio. La tosse è il sintomo più costante del coinvolgimento polmonare: dapprima secca e stizzosa, può poi diventare grassa e produttiva. Nei bambini più grandi, la tosse peggiora al risveglio mattutino o dopo l'attività fisica. Il muco espettorato è di solito purulento. Alcuni pazienti restano asintomatici per lunghi periodi o sembrano avere infezioni respiratorie acute prolungate ma intermittenti; altri sviluppano una tosse cronica nella prima settimana di vita o sviluppano polmoniti ripetute. La bronchiolite diffusa è accompagnata da sibili, che sono un sintomo frequente durante il primo anno di vita. Con la lenta progressione della pneumopatia, si notano intolleranza allo sforzo, dispnea, deficit d'accrescimento staturoponderale. Le esacerbazioni dei sintomi polmonari, presumibilmente dovuti a infezioni più attive delle vie aeree, finiscono per richiedere ripetuti ricoveri ospedalieri per un trattamento efficace. Negli stadi avanzati subentrano cuore polmonare, insufficienza respiratoria e infine il decesso, a meno che non si effettui il trapianto polmonare. La colonizzazione da parte di *Burkholderia cepacia* e di altri microrganismi multiresistenti ai farmaci si può associare a un deterioramento polmonare particolarmente rapido e alla morte.

La velocità di progressione della malattia polmonare è il principale determinante della morbilità e della mortalità. Il decorso della pneumopatia, tuttavia, è in gran parte indipendente dal genotipo. Mutazioni severe tendono ad associarsi a una progressione più rapida. Alcune mutazioni (R117H) possono risparmiare sostanzialmente, o anche completamente, i polmoni. Anche il sesso maschile e la conservazione della funzione pancreatica esocrica si associano a un declino più lento della funzione polmonare. Gli insulti polmonari precoci (infezioni virali severe) giocano probabilmente un ruolo determinante nel decorso della malattia.

I **reperti obiettivi** precoci comprendono aumento del diametro anteroposteriore del torace, iperfonesi generalizzata, crepitii grossolani generalizzati o localizzati, ippocratismo digitale. Possono essere udibili sibili espiratori, in particolare nei bambini più piccoli. La cianosi è un segno tardivo. Le complicanze polmonari comuni, che di solito compaiono dopo la prima decade di vita, comprendono atelettasie, emottisi, pneumotorace e cuore polmonare.

Anche se virtualmente i seni paranasali appaiono sempre opacizzati alla radiografia, la sinusite acuta non è frequente. Comuni sono l'ostruzione nasale e la rinorrea, causate dalle membrane mucose infiammate ed edematose o, in alcuni casi, da poliposi nasale. I **polipi nasali** sono più problematici tra i 5 e i 20 anni di età.

Apparato digerente. Nel 15-20% dei neonati con fibrosi cistica l'ileo è completamente ostruito dal meconio (**ileo da meconio**). La frequenza è maggiore (circa 30%) tra i fratelli nati successivamente a un bambino con ileo da meconio, ed è particolarmente marcata nei gemelli monozigoti, riflettendo il contributo genetico di uno o più geni modificatori. Nelle prime 24-48 ore di vita si osservano distensione addominale, emesi e mancato transito del meconio (vedi Capitolo 102.1). Le radiografie addominali (Fig. 400-4) mostrano anse intestinali dilatate con livelli idroaerei e,

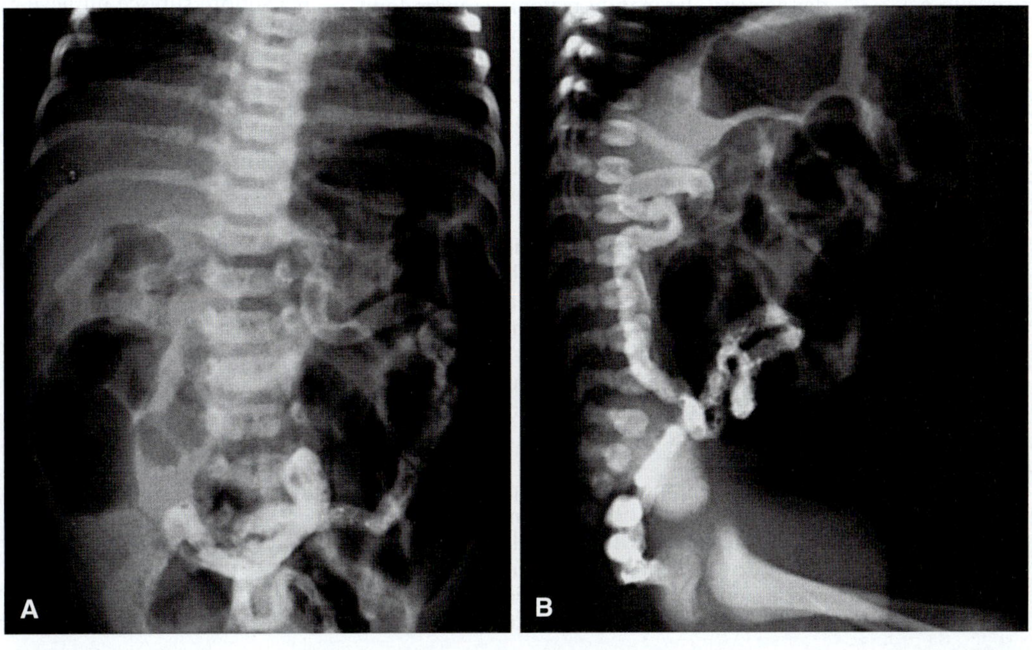

Figura 400-4. *A* e *B*, Clisma con contrasto in un neonato con distensione addominale e mancata evacuazione del meconio. Si notino il piccolo diametro del sigma e del colon ascendente e le anse dilatate e ripiene d'aria dell'intestino tenue. Nelle proiezioni laterali in ortostatismo si osservano numerosi livelli idroaerei nell'intestino tenue.

spesso, una raccolta di materiale granulare "a vetro smerigliato" nella parte centrale inferiore dell'addome. Per quanto si tratti di un'evenienza rara, la rottura intrauterina di una parete intestinale, riconoscibile radiograficamente dalla presenza di calcificazioni peritoneali o scrotali, può dare luogo a una **peritonite da meconio.** La **sindrome da tappo di meconio** si verifica con maggior frequenza nei lattanti affetti da fibrosi cistica, ma è meno specifica dell'ileo da meconio. L'ostruzione ileale da parte di materiale fecale (sindrome ostruttiva dell'intestino distale o equivalente dell'ileo da meconio) insorge nei bambini più grandi, causando dolore addominale crampiforme e distensione addominale.

Più dell'85% dei bambini affetti presenta disturbi digestivi riconducibili a insufficienza pancreatica esocrina. I sintomi comprendono evacuazioni frequenti di feci abbondanti e oleose, e mancato aumento ponderale, anche quando l'apporto di cibo sembra abbondante. Quasi il 40% dei pazienti presenta deficit nutrizionali, secondo il criterio di peso/altezza al di sotto del decimo percentile. Caratteristicamente, le feci contengono gocce lipidiche ben visibili. I segni fisici tipici sono addome globoso, riduzione della massa muscolare, crescita stentata e ritardo di maturazione. L'eccessiva flatulenza può rappresentare un problema. Numerose mutazioni si associano alla conservazione di un certo grado di funzione pancreatica esocrina, tra cui R117H e 3849 +10 kb C > T. Virtualmente, tutti gli individui omozigoti per ΔF508 soffrono di insufficienza pancreatica.

Le manifestazioni gastrointestinali meno comuni comprendono intussuscezione, ingombro fecale nel cieco con massa asintomatica nel quadrante inferiore destro e dolore epigastrico da infiammazione duodenale. Il reflusso acido o biliare con sintomi di esofagite è comune nei bambini più grandi e negli adulti. Sono stati descritti appendicite subacuta e ascesso periappendicolare. Il prolasso rettale, un evento abbastanza comune in passato, oggi si verifica molto meno frequentemente, in virtù della precocità della diagnosi e dell'inizio della terapia sostitutiva con enzimi pancreatici. Occasionalmente si assiste alla comparsa di ipoproteinemia con anasarca nei lattanti malnutriti, soprattutto se alimentati con preparati a base di soia. Possono insorgere disfunzioni neurologiche (demenza, neuropatia periferica) e anemia emolitica, dovute alla **carenza di vitamina E.** Talvolta si riscontrano sintomi da deficit delle altre vitamine liposolubili. L'**ipoprotrombinemia** da deficit di vitamina K può portare a diatesi emorragica. Sono state osservate manifestazioni cliniche di altre carenze di vitamine liposolubili, come una riduzione della densità ossea e cecità notturna. Il rachitismo è raro.

Vie biliari. I segni di disfunzione epatica, rilevati più frequentemente nei primi 15 anni di vita, possono manifestarsi anche nel 30% degli individui, sebbene la cirrosi biliare divenga sintomatica solo nel 2-3% dei pazienti. Le manifestazioni comprendono ittero, ascite, ematemesi da varici esofagee e segni di ipersplenismo. Sono stati riportati un quadro neonatale simil-epatitico e un'epatomegalia massiva da steatosi. Le coliche biliari da colelitiasi possono insorgere nella seconda decade di vita o successivamente. L'epatopatia è indipendente dal genotipo, ma si associa all'ileo da meconio e all'insufficienza pancreatica.

Pancreas. Oltre all'insufficienza pancreatica esocrina, possono comparire anche segni di iperglicemia e glicosuria, tra cui poliuria e calo ponderale, soprattutto nella seconda decade di vita. L'8% dei pazienti dagli 11 ai 17 anni e il 18% di quelli dai 18 ai 24 anni soffrono di diabete insulinodipendente. Di solito non si verifica chetoacidosi, ma sono state riportate complicanze oculari, renali e vascolari, nei pazienti che sopravvivono per più di 10 anni dopo aver sviluppato iperglicemia. La pancreatite acuta ricorrente si verifica occasionalmente negli individui con una funzione pancreatica residua, e può essere l'unica manifestazione di due mutazioni del CFTR.

Apparato genitourinario. Lo sviluppo sessuale è spesso ritardato, ma in media solo di 2 anni. Più del 95% dei maschi presenta azoospermia, a causa del mancato sviluppo delle strutture dei dotti di Wolff, ma la funzione sessuale è generalmente intatta. L'incidenza di ernia inguinale, idrocele e testicolo ritenuto è maggiore dell'atteso. Le adolescenti possono andare incontro ad amenorrea secondaria, specialmente con le esacerbazioni della malattia polmonare. Sono stati osservati cervicite e accumulo di muco tenace nel canale cervicale. La fertilità femminile è ridotta. La gravidanza, in genere ben tollerata dalle donne con una buona funzione polmonare, può accelerare la progressione della malattia polmonare in quelle con problemi respiratori moderati o severi.

Ghiandole sudoripare. L'eccessiva perdita di sali con il sudore predispone i bambini più piccoli alla deplezione salina, in particolare durante episodi di gastroenterite e nella stagione calda. Questi pazienti si presentano con **alcalosi ipocloremica.** Spesso i genitori notano piccole incrostazioni di sale sulla cute o avvertono un sapore salato quando baciano il bambino. Alcuni genotipi (3849 + 10 kb C > T) si associano a valori normali di cloruro nel sudore.

DIAGNOSI E VALUTAZIONE. La diagnosi della fibrosi cistica si basa sulla positività del test del sudore quantitativo ($Cl^- \geq 60$ mEq/L) insieme a uno o più dei seguenti criteri: malattia polmonare cronica ostruttiva tipica, insufficienza pancreatica cronica documentata o un'anamnesi familiare positiva. Sono stati consigliati criteri diagnostici che includano procedure di valutazione aggiuntive (Tab. 400-3).

Test del sudore. Il test del sudore, che utilizza la ionoforesi con pilocarpina per raccogliere il sudore e analizzarne chimicamente il contenuto, è l'approccio diagnostico standard. La procedura richiede attenzione e accuratezza. Si utilizza una corrente elettrica di 3 mA per veicolare la pilocarpina nella cute dell'avambraccio e stimolare localmente le ghiandole sudoripare. Dopo aver lavato il braccio con acqua distillata, si raccoglie il sudore su una carta da filtro o una garza (o con un tubo capillare) posizionati sulla cute stimolata e ricoperta, per evitare l'evaporazione. Dopo 30 minuti, la carta da filtro viene rimossa, pesata ed eluita in acqua distillata. Si consiglia l'uso di un clorurimetro per l'analisi del cloruro in questi campioni. La quantità di sudore raccolta dovrebbe essere misurata e annotata. Per risultati attendibili, sono necessari almeno 75 mg di sudore (la quantità ottimale sarebbe di 100 mg). L'esame può essere di difficile esecuzione nelle prime 2 settimane di vita a causa della scarsa traspirazione, ma è consigliato in qualsiasi momento dopo le prime 48 ore di vita. I risultati positivi devono ricevere conferma; in caso di risultato negativo, il test deve essere ripetuto se permane un sospetto diagnostico.

Valori di cloruro >60 mEq/L nel sudore sono diagnostici di fibrosi cistica quando sono presenti uno o più degli altri criteri. Sono stati suggeriti livelli soglia di 40 mEq/L nei lattanti. Valori compresi tra 40 e 60 mEq/L sono stati riportati a tutte le età, nei casi con coinvolgimento tipico. Negli adulti sani, il cloruro nel sudore subisce un lieve aumento, ma un valore di 60 mEq/L è ancora adeguato per differenziare la fibrosi cistica da altre patologie. La concentrazione di cloruro nel sudore è un po' più bassa nei pazienti che conservano la funzione pancreatica esocrina, ma rientrano comunque nel range diagnostico. Nei bambini con edema da ipoproteinemia si possono ottenere risultati falsi

TABELLA 400-3. Criteri diagnostici per la fibrosi cistica

Presenza delle caratteristiche cliniche tipiche (respiratorie, gastrointestinali o genitourinarie)
OPPURE
Anamnesi di fibrosi cistica in un fratello
OPPURE
Test di screening neonatale positivo
PIÙ
Evidenza di laboratorio di disfunzione del CFTR:
Due concentrazioni elevate di cloro nel sudore ottenute in due giorni separati
OPPURE
Identificazione di due mutazioni del CFTR
OPPURE
Una misurazione anomala della differenza di potenziale nasale

CFTR, *Cystic Fibrosis Transmembrane Regulator*, regolatore transmembrana della fibrosi cistica.

negativi; risultati falsi positivi possono invece verificarsi quando il test viene effettuato su cute affetta da eczema o contaminata con creme o lozioni.

Oltre alla fibrosi cistica, altre condizioni che si associano a elevate concentrazioni di elettroliti nel sudore sono l'insufficienza surrenalica non trattata, la displasia ectodermica, il diabete insipido nefrogenico ereditario, il deficit di glucosio-6-fosfatasi, l'ipotiroidismo, l'ipoparatiroidismo, la colestasi familiare, la pancreatite, le mucopolisaccaridosi, la fucosidosi e la malnutrizione. La maggior parte di esse può essere facilmente distinta dalla fibrosi cistica tramite criteri clinici.

Esame del DNA. Molti kit di laboratorio in commercio esaminano da 30 a 80 mutazioni del CFTR tra le più comuni. Questo test identifica più del 90% degli individui portatori di due mutazioni. Alcuni bambini con manifestazioni tipiche della fibrosi hanno una sola mutazione, o addirittura non presentano alcuna mutazione rilevabile con questa metodologia. Alcuni laboratori effettuano un'analisi genetica completa, facendo uno screening per tutte le oltre 1500 mutazioni identificate.

Altri test diagnostici. Il reperto di aumento della differenza di potenziale attraverso l'epitelio nasale, la perdita di questa differenza con l'applicazione di amiloride topica e l'assenza di una risposta di voltaggio ad agenti β-adrenergici sono stati utilizzati per confermare la diagnosi in pazienti con valori di cloro nel sudore equivoci o normali. Per caratterizzare varianti della fibrosi cistica è stata utilizzata anche la mancata emissione di sudore dopo l'iniezione nella cute di una combinazione di isoproterenolo e atropina.

Funzione pancreatica. La disfunzione pancreatica esocrina è clinicamente evidente in molti pazienti; è però consigliabile che sia documentata se sussistono dubbi sullo stato funzionale del pancreas. La stima del bilancio lipidico con la raccolta delle feci per 3 giorni, o con la documentazione diretta della secrezione enzimatica, dopo intubazione del duodeno e stimolazione con pancreozimina-secretina, fornisce una misura affidabile, ma questi metodi sono troppo complicati o invasivi per i bambini e quindi non vengono utilizzati di routine. La misurazione quantitativa dell'attività dell'elastasi-1 in un campione fresco di feci è un utile test di screening. Anche la misurazione del tripsinogeno immunoreattivo nel siero, in uso per lo screening neonatale, distingue accuratamente i pazienti affetti da fibrosi cistica, con e senza insufficienza pancreatica. Sono disponibili anche altre misurazioni indirette della secrezione enzimatica del pancreas, che tuttavia hanno un valore clinico limitato o non documentato. La disfunzione del pancreas endocrino potrebbe essere molto più diffusa di quanto si ritenesse in passato. Molti consigliano il monitoraggio annuale con un test di tolleranza al glucosio (OGTT, *Oral Glucose Tolerance Test*) a 2 ore modificato, dopo i 10 anni di età. Questo approccio è più sensibile della misurazione estemporanea dei livelli di glucosio nel sangue e nelle urine e dei livelli di emoglobina glicata.

Indagini radiologiche. I reperti radiologici polmonari suggeriscono la diagnosi senza tuttavia essere specifici. L'iperinflazione polmonare insorge precocemente e può essere sottostimata, in assenza di infiltrati o di strie di iperdensità. L'ispessimento e l'ostruzione bronchiale e le ombre ad anello, che suggeriscono le bronchiectasie, di solito compaiono dapprima nei lobi superiori; in seguito si assiste alla formazione di densità nodulari, atelettasie focali e infiltrati confluenti. I linfonodi ilari possono essere ingranditi. Nella malattia in stadio avanzato si osserva un'iperinflazione considerevole, con diaframma notevolmente appiattito, incurvamento anteriore dello sterno e assottigliamento dell'ombra cardiaca. Con la progressione della patologia spesso si evidenzia la formazione di cisti, bronchiectasie estese, dilatazione di segmenti dell'arteria polmonare e atelettasie lobari o segmentarie. La tipica progressione della malattia polmonare è presentata nella Figura 400-5. Nella maggior parte dei centri specializzati nella cura della fibrosi cistica si eseguono radiografie del torace (anteroposteriori [AP] e laterali) almeno una volta all'anno. È stato utilizzato un punteggio standardizzato delle alterazioni radiografiche per seguire nel tempo la progressione della malattia a livello polmonare. La TC del torace, che può individuare e localizzare l'ispessimento della parete bronchiale, i tappi di muco, l'iperinflazione focale e le bronchiectasie precoci (Fig. 400-6), in genere non viene usata per la valutazione di routine della pneumopatia. Molti bambini con funzione polmonare normale hanno bronchiectasie alla TC, a riprova che questa modalità di studio è sensibile alle alterazioni polmonari precoci.

Le radiografie dei seni paranasali rivelano una panopacizzazione e spesso il mancato sviluppo dei seni frontali. La TC visualizza le alterazioni sinusali con una miglior risoluzione, se questa informazione è richiesta dal punto di vista clinico. L'ecografia fetale può suggerire un'ostruzione ileale da meconio già nel secondo trimestre di gravidanza, ma questo reperto non è predittivo di ileo da meconio alla nascita.

Funzione polmonare. Gli studi standard di funzionalità polmonare non vengono effettuati prima dei 4-6 anni di età, quando molti pazienti presentano il tipico quadro di coinvolgimento polmonare ostruttivo (vedi Capitolo 381). La riduzione della velocità di flusso mesoespiratorio massimale è un'alterazione funzionale precoce, che rispecchia l'ostruzione delle piccole vie aeree. Questa lesione colpisce anche la distribuzione della ventilazione e aumenta il gradiente alveoloarterioso per l'ossigeno. I reperti di malattia ostruttiva delle vie aeree e di risposta modesta ai broncodilatatori sono compatibili con la diagnosi di fibrosi cistica a qualunque età. Il volume residuo e la capacità funzionale residua risultano aumentati già nei primi stadi della malattia polmonare. Le alterazioni restrittive, caratterizzate da diminuzione della capacità polmonare totale e della capacità vitale, correlano con un danno polmonare e una fibrosi estesa e sono un reperto tardivo. È consigliabile la valutazione a ogni visita clinica, per monitorare il decorso del coinvolgimento polmonare e intervenire precocemente non appena si rileva un deterioramento importante. Nonostante siano sempre di più i centri per la cura della fibrosi cistica attrezzati per misurare il quadro di funzionalità respiratoria nei neonati sedati, questa procedura è effettuata abitualmente nell'ambito di studi di ricerca. Alcuni pazienti raggiungono l'adolescenza o l'età adulta con una funzione polmonare normale e senza evidenza di iperinflazione.

Indagini microbiologiche. Il reperto di *S. aureus* o di *P. aeruginosa* nelle colture delle vie aeree inferiori (escreato) suggerisce fortemente una diagnosi di fibrosi cistica. Nei polmoni di pazienti con fibrosi cistica sono di riscontro particolarmente frequente le forme mucoidi di *P. aeruginosa*, come pure un'ampia varietà di altri microrganismi, soprattutto nella malattia polmonare avanzata, tra cui vari bacilli Gram-negativi, funghi e specie di micobatteri non tubercolari. La mancata risposta dei sintomi delle riacutizzazioni respiratorie ai soliti antibiotici induce a ricercare micoplasmi e virus. La broncoscopia a fibre ottiche è utilizzata per raccogliere secrezioni delle vie aeree inferiori nei lattanti e nei bambini piccoli che non sono in grado di espettorare.

Identificazione degli eterozigoti e diagnosi prenatale. L'analisi delle mutazioni dovrebbe essere completamente informativa quando esamina un portatore potenziale o un feto, perché le mutazioni all'interno della famiglia siano state precedentemente identificate. L'esame effettuato sul coniuge di un portatore, con una combinazione standard di sonde, ha una sensibilità di circa il 90%. Si sta rivalutando la raccomandazione, formulata da una Consensus Conference dei National Institutes of Health del 1977, di offrire l'indagine prenatale a tutte le coppie che desiderano avere un figlio, oltre agli individui con una storia familiare di fibrosi cistica. L'interruzione di gravidanza è un'opzione meno diffusa, poiché il decorso clinico non è prevedibile e l'aspettativa di vita attualmente si avvicina a una media di 40 anni.

Screening neonatale. La maggior parte dei neonati con fibrosi cistica è identificabile mediante la determinazione del tripsinogeno immunoreattivo e un test del DNA limitato su blood spot, unitamente all'analisi del sudore di conferma. Questo screening ha una sensibilità del 95% circa. Le diagnosi prenatali possono evitare i deficit nutrizionali precoci e migliorare la crescita a lungo termine, preservando la funzione cognitiva. La diagnosi precoce ha anche il vantaggio di consentire un counseling genetico alla

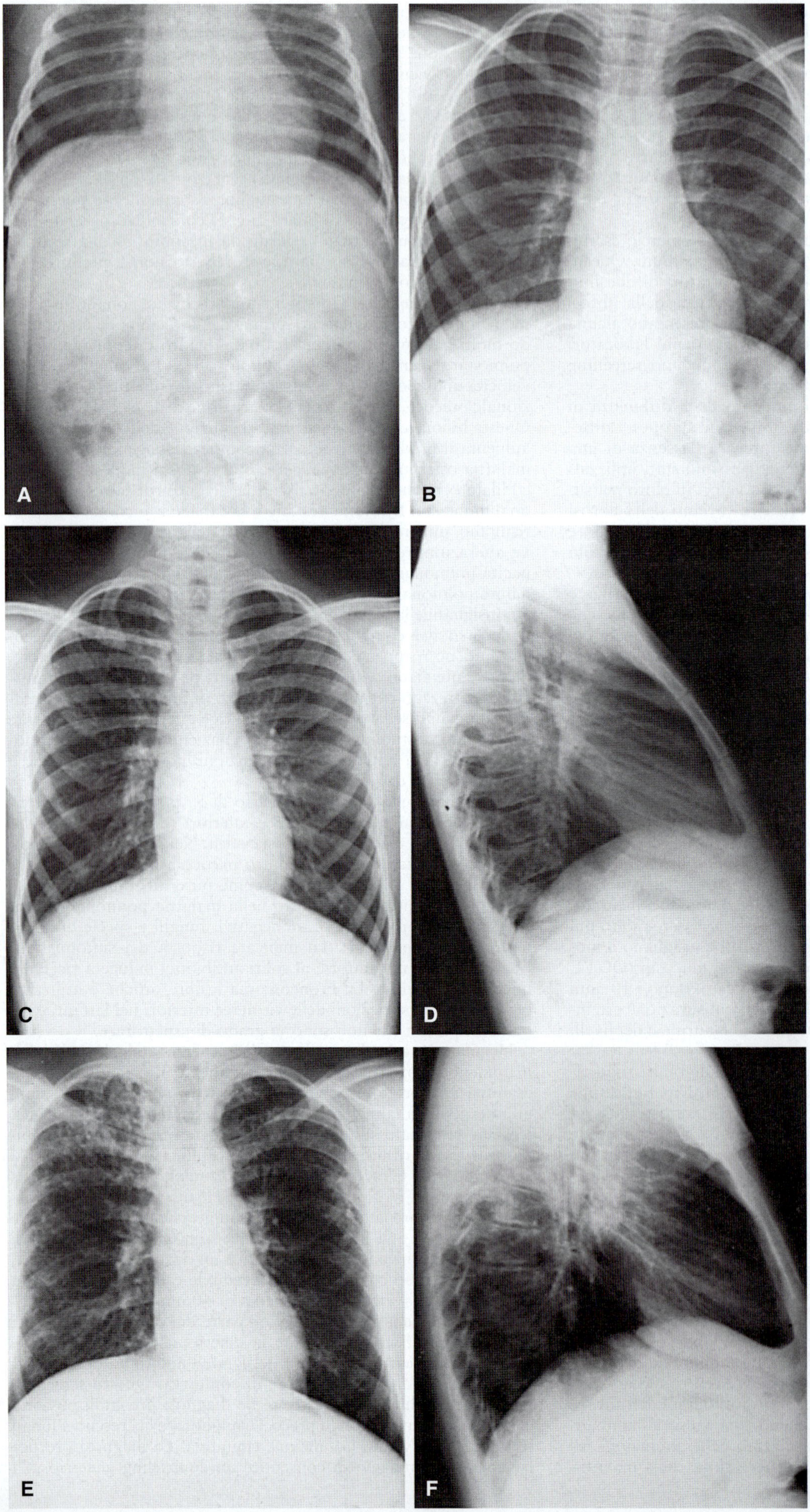

Figura 400-5. Progressione radiologica della malattia polmonare nella fibrosi cistica, dalla diagnosi in età infantile fino ai 18 anni di età. *A*, Il paziente all'età di 2 mesi presentava tosse e sibili, per i quali veniva ricoverato in ospedale. Si noti il lieve rinforzo della trama broncovascolare, soprattutto nei lobi superiori. *B*, All'età di 4 anni, la tosse era minima. La trama broncovascolare era lievemente aumentata e si osservava un certo miglioramento nei lobi superiori. I sibili non recidivarono mai. *C* e *D*, All'età di 13 anni, la tosse era minima, con produzione occasionale di escreato. La trama broncovascolare era ulteriormente aumentata, con alterazioni bronchiectasiche precoci nel lobo superiore destro. La proiezione laterale non è suggestiva di iperinflazione. *E* e *F*, Età: 18 anni. Durante l'adolescenza la tosse e la produzione di escreato aumentarono, nonostante l'intensificazione della terapia antibiotica ambulatoriale. Emottisi di scarsa entità, parossismi di tosse occasionali e calo ponderale, insieme ad aumento degli infiltrati nodulari (specialmente nel lobo superiore destro) e dell'iperinflazione (osservabile nella proiezione laterale) portarono al primo ricovero dopo l'infanzia. Il peso e l'altezza si mantennero nel 25°-50° percentile.

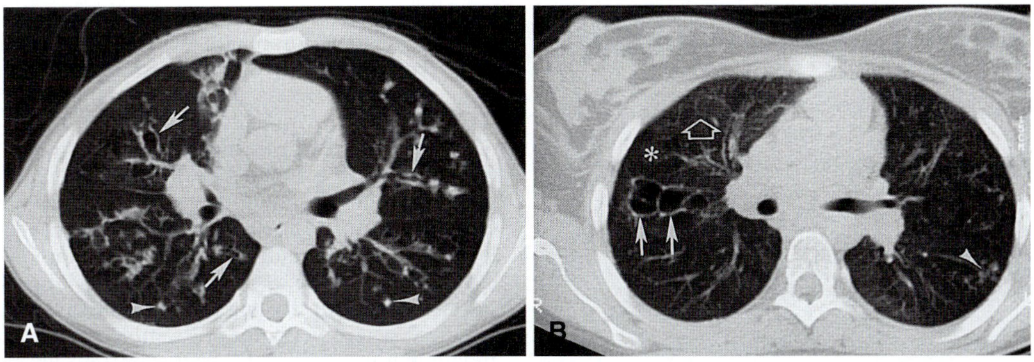

Figura 400-6. Immagini tomografiche del torace nella fibrosi cistica. *A*, Ragazzo di 12 anni con malattia polmonare moderata. Sono presenti alterazioni delle vie aeree e del parenchima in entrambi i polmoni. Si osservano aree multiple di bronchiectasia (*frecce*) con tappi di muco (*punte di freccia*). *B*, Una ragazza di 19 anni ha un polmone quasi normale con un'area di bronchiectasia sacculare nel lobo superiore destro (*frecce*) e un addensamento focale di muco nel lobo inferiore destro (*punta di freccia*). La densità polmonare è eterogenea, con aree di polmone normale (*freccia aperta*) e aree di bassa attenuazione indicative di intrappolamento d'aria segmentale e subsegmentale (*asterisco*).

famiglia e, in alcuni casi, evitare sforzi diagnostici protratti. *Non vi sono ancora prove definitive che la diagnosi precoce migliori la funzione polmonare e, pertanto, la sopravvivenza.* Lo screening neonatale può mettere i neonati con fibrosi cistica a maggior rischio di contrarre precocemente l'infezione da *P. aeruginosa* e altre affezioni respiratorie problematiche, se non viene praticato uno stretto controllo in tal senso. L'ansia dei genitori impone che sia effettuato rapidamente un test di conferma, in caso di positività del test di screening.

TRATTAMENTO. Il piano di trattamento dovrebbe essere globale, collegato a uno stretto monitoraggio e all'intervento precoce e aggressivo.

Approccio generale. Una volta formulata la diagnosi occorre adottare un approccio intensivo, comprendente una valutazione di base, l'inizio del trattamento, la determinazione del coinvolgimento polmonare e l'educazione del paziente e dei genitori. Le valutazioni successive sono previste ogni 2-3 mesi, poiché sono molti gli aspetti di questa patologia che richiedono un attento monitoraggio. A ogni visita occorre raccogliere l'anamnesi del periodo trascorso ed effettuare l'esame obiettivo. Si preleva un campione di escreato o, se questo non è disponibile, si esegue un tampone faringeo basso, durante o dopo una tosse forzata, per l'esame colturale e l'antibiogramma. Dal momento che la perdita irreversibile della funzionalità polmonare da infezioni di basso grado può insorgere gradualmente e in assenza di sintomi acuti, si sottolinea l'importanza di un'accurata anamnesi polmonare. La Tabella 400-4 elenca i sintomi e i segni che indicano la necessità di una terapia antibiotica e fisica più intensive. L'immunoprofilassi, in particolare contro la rosolia, la pertosse e l'influenza, è essenziale. In particolare si raccomanda la protezione verso *S. aureus* meticillino-resistente, *P. aeruginosa*, *B. cepacia* e altri Gram-negativi resistenti, senza trascurare le procedure di isolamento e un'accurata sterilizzazione dell'attrezzatura per la terapia inalatoria. Dovranno prendere parte al programma di cure un'infermiera, un fisioterapista respiratorio, un assistente sociale, un dietista e uno psicologo, a seconda dei bisogni del paziente. Dare indicazioni ai familiari del paziente e ai bambini più grandi, responsabilizzandoli e aiutandoli a prendere decisioni sulla propria salute, è molto importante perché in questo modo è possibile ottenere una miglior aderenza ai programmi di cure quotidiane. Migliori risultati a lungo termine sembrano ottenibili grazie alla standardizzazione della pratica dell'assistenza, da parte sia di chi fornisce le cure sia della famiglia, accompagnata da un attento monitoraggio e dall'intervento precoce in caso di sintomi nuovi o in peggioramento.

Poiché le secrezioni dei pazienti con FC non sono adeguatamente idratate, una particolare attenzione all'idratazione orale, nella prima infanzia, specialmente nella stagione calda o in caso di gastroenterite acuta, può ridurre al minimo le complicanze as-

TABELLA 400-4. Sintomi e segni associati a esacerbazioni dell'infezione polmonare nei pazienti con fibrosi cistica

SINTOMI
Aumento della frequenza e durata della tosse
Aumento della produzione di escreato
Cambiamento dell'aspetto del muco
Aumento della dispnea
Riduzione della tolleranza allo sforzo
Riduzione dell'appetito
Sensazione di congestione toracica aumentata
SEGNI
Aumento della frequenza respiratoria
Utilizzo dei muscoli accessori della respirazione
Retrazioni intercostali
Alterazioni all'auscultazione del torace
Declino degli esami di funzionalità polmonare compatibile con la presenza di malattia ostruttiva delle vie aeree
Febbre e leucocitosi
Calo ponderale
Nuovi infiltrati alla radiografia del torace

Da Ramsey B: Management of pulmonary disease in patients with cystic fibrosis. *N Engl J Med* 1996;335:179.

sociate con l'alterata clearance del muco. Per la stessa ragione, occorre iniziare quanto prima la terapia endovenosa reidratante.

L'obiettivo della terapia è il mantenimento di una condizione stabile per lunghi periodi. Nella maggior parte dei pazienti questo risultato viene raggiunto con valutazioni periodiche e aggiustamenti del programma di trattamento domiciliare. Alcuni bambini hanno infezioni polmonari acute episodiche oppure croniche di bassa entità che tendono a progredire; in tal caso sono indicati un ciclo di terapia inalatoria, fisioterapia respiratoria e antibiotici per via endovenosa, della durata di almeno 2 settimane. Nonostante il miglioramento sia più facile da ottenere in ambito ospedaliero, anche alcuni pazienti selezionati seguiti a domicilio hanno avuto un esito favorevole. La somministrazione di antibiotici per via endovenosa può essere necessaria a intervalli piuttosto distanziati oppure anche ogni 2-3 mesi. Obiettivo del trattamento è riportare i pazienti allo stato polmonare e funzionale precedente.

Il programma di cure quotidiane varia in base all'età del bambino, al grado di coinvolgimento dei polmoni e di altri organi o apparati e al tempo che si ha a disposizione per la terapia, anche se i suoi due capisaldi sono la terapia polmonare e nutrizionale. L'uso intensivo di farmaci spesso determina l'insorgenza di problemi iatrogeni, il cui monitoraggio fa parte integrante del trattamento (Tab. 400-5).

Terapia polmonare. Il suo scopo è l'eliminazione delle secrezioni dalle vie aeree e il controllo dell'infezione. L'efficacia dell'approccio nel suo complesso, comprendente la continuità delle cure,

TABELLA 400-5. Complicanze della terapia nella fibrosi cistica

COMPLICANZA	AGENTE
Emorragia gastrointestinale	Ibuprofene
Iperglicemia	Corticosteroidi (sistemici)
Ritardo della crescita	Corticosteroidi (sistemici, inalatori)
Disfunzione renale	
Tubulare	Aminoglicosidi
Nefrite interstiziale	Penicilline semisintetiche, FANS
Perdita dell'udito, disfunzione vestibolare	Aminoglicosidi
Neuropatia periferica o atrofia ottica	Cloramfenicolo (uso prolungato)
Ipomagnesiemia	Aminoglicosidi
Iperuricemia, stenosi colica	Estratti pancreatici (a dosi molto alte)
Gozzo	Espettoranti a base di iodio
Ginecomastia	Spironolattone
Ipoplasia o colorazione dello smalto	Tetracicline (nei primi 8 anni di vita)

Nota: le reazioni comuni da ipersensibilità ai farmaci non sono incluse.
FANS, farmaci antinfiammatori non steroidei.

valutazioni frequenti, interventi aggressivi e un atteggiamento ottimistico, è più importante delle variazioni nell'utilizzo delle misure individuali. Quando un bambino non sta bene, si deve considerare ogni aspetto della terapia potenzialmente utile.

Terapia inalatoria. La terapia con aerosol ha la funzione di veicolare i farmaci e idratare le vie aeree inferiori. Per somministrare agenti come i broncodilatatori e i corticosteroidi si impiegano erogatori spray predosati, muniti di un distanziatore per i bambini più piccoli. Il cardine della terapia è la somministrazione intermittente con un compressore collegato a un nebulizzatore manuale. La soluzione di base è la soluzione salina allo 0,9%. Nei pazienti con reattività delle vie aeree si aggiunge albuterolo o altri β-agonisti, anche se questi ultimi possono ridurre la Pa_{O_2} acutamente aumentando il mismatch ventilazione-perfusione, fenomeno che può destare preoccupazioni se la Pa_{O_2} è marginale.

In caso di patogeni delle vie aeree resistenti agli antibiotici orali, o quando l'infezione è difficile da controllare a domicilio, gli antibiotici per aerosol possono ridurre i sintomi, migliorare la funzionalità polmonare e ovviare alla necessità di ospedalizzazione (vedi il paragrafo "Terapia antibiotica per aerosol").

La DNasi umana ricombinante (2,5 mg), somministrata in dose singola quotidiana per aerosol, migliora la funzione polmonare, riduce il numero di esacerbazioni polmonari e promuove un senso di benessere nei pazienti con malattia moderata e secrezioni purulente. Un beneficio è stato documentato anche nei pazienti con valori normali di volume espiratorio forzato in un secondo (FEV_1, *Forced Expiratory Volume in 1 second*) e in quelli con malattia polmonare avanzata. Il miglioramento persiste per ≥12 mesi, con la terapia continuativa. Considerata la variabilità della risposta, occorre condurre un trial su base individuale per documentare il beneficio prima di intraprendere una terapia a lungo termine che comporta costi considerevoli. Un altro agente mucolitico, la *N*-acetilcisteina, è tossico per l'epitelio ciliato e la sua somministrazione ripetuta andrebbe quindi evitata.

È stato riportato che l'aerosol con soluzione salina ipertonica aumenta la clearance del muco e migliora la funzione polmonare. Il beneficio, quanto mai variabile, è comunque inferiore a quello ottenibile con la DNasi.

Terapia di clearance delle vie aeree. Questo trattamento, che consiste in genere nella percussione toracica associata al drenaggio posturale, si basa sul principio secondo cui se la tosse libera dal muco le vie aeree principali, sono necessarie vibrazioni per rimuovere le secrezioni dalle vie aeree di piccolo calibro, dove le velocità di flusso espiratorio sono inferiori. La **fisioterapia respiratoria** può essere particolarmente utile nei pazienti con fibrosi cistica, nelle cui vie aeree di piccolo calibro le secrezioni iniziano ad accumularsi ancor prima dell'esordio dei sintomi. Sebbene non sia generalmente dimostrabile un miglioramento immediato della funzione polmonare dopo questa terapia, la sua sospensione nei bambini con limitazione del flusso da lieve a moderata provoca un deterioramento della funzione polmonare nell'arco di 3 settimane e, per contro, la sua ripresa dà luogo a un rapido miglioramento. Essa è consigliata da 1 a 4 volte al giorno, a seconda della gravità della disfunzione polmonare. Dopo il "drenaggio" di ogni segmento polmonare si incoraggia il paziente a tossire, soffiare e compiere espirazioni forzate. Nei bambini più grandi possono essere utili percussori meccanici a giubbotto. Per eliminare il muco possono essere utili anche la tosse volontaria, le ripetute manovre di espirazione forzata con e senza pressione espiratoria positiva, il respiro programmato e l'uso di strumenti portatili per il *flutter* (pressione positiva espiratoria oscillante). Gli esercizi aerobici di routine sembrano rallentare il declino della funzione polmonare, ed è stato riportato un beneficio anche con l'allenamento con i pesi.

Terapia antibiotica. Gli antibiotici sono il cardine della terapia, in quanto non tengono sotto controllo l'infezione polmonare. L'obiettivo è attenuare l'infezione endobronchiale e rallentare la progressione del danno polmonare. I segni abituali delle infezioni respiratorie acute, come febbre, tachipnea o dolore toracico, sono spesso assenti; di conseguenza, per stabilire la frequenza e la durata della terapia occorre basarsi su tutti gli aspetti dell'anamnesi e dell'esame obiettivo del paziente, compresi l'anoressia, il calo ponderale e la riduzione delle attività. Lo schema del trattamento farmacologico varia da brevi cicli intermittenti con un solo antibiotico alla somministrazione quasi ininterrotta di uno o più antibiotici. Il dosaggio di alcuni di essi spesso risulta superiore di 2-3 volte alla dose raccomandata per le infezioni minori, poiché i pazienti con fibrosi cistica hanno in proporzione più massa magra e velocità di clearance più elevate per molti antibiotici, rispetto agli altri individui. Inoltre, per molti antimicrobici è difficile ottenere livelli farmacologici efficaci nelle secrezioni respiratorie.

TERAPIA ANTIBIOTICA ORALE. Le indicazioni comprendono la presenza di sintomi respiratori e l'identificazione di microrganismi patogeni nelle colture delle vie aeree. Quando possibile, la scelta dell'antibiotico dovrebbe essere guidata dall'esame della sensibilità in vitro. Si trovano con sempre maggior frequenza organismi comuni, come *S. aureus*, *Haemophilus influenzae* non tipizzabile e *P. aeruginosa*, *B. cepacia* e altri bacilli Gram-negativi. I primi due possono essere eradicati dalle vie respiratorie, nei pazienti con FC, ma *Pseudomonas* è più difficile da trattare. La durata abituale del trattamento è di due settimane, e sono consigliati dosaggi massimali. Gli antibiotici orali utili sono elencati nella Tabella 400-6. La tetraciclina deve essere evitata nei bambini di età inferiore a 9 anni. I chinoloni sono gli unici antibiotici ad ampio spettro efficaci nell'infezione da *Pseudomonas*, ma emerge rapidamente la resistenza. È stata documentata l'infezione da micoplasmi o da clamidie, che rappresenta il razionale per l'utilizzo dei macrolidi su base empirica per le riacutizzazioni sintomatologiche. I macrolidi possono ridurre le proprietà di virulenza di *P. aeruginosa* come la produzione di biofilm e contribuiscono all'effetto antifiammatorio. La terapia a lungo termine con azitromicina settimanalmente ha dimostrato di migliorare la funzione polmonare nei pazienti con infezione cronica da *P. aeruginosa*.

TERAPIA ANTIBIOTICA PER AEROSOL. *P. aeruginosa* e gli altri microrganismi Gram-negativi sono spesso resistenti agli antibiotici per via orale. Veicolando questi farmaci tramite aerosol si ha la possibilità di somministrare a domicilio agenti addizionali. La tobramicina inalatoria è stata la più studiata: grazie a questo farmaco, somministrato alla dose di 300 mg, due volte al giorno a mesi alterni, per 6 mesi, la densità di *Pseudomonas* nell'escreato si riduce, sono necessari meno ricoveri e la funzione polmonare può aumentare del 10% o più. La tossicità è trascurabile. Questa terapia può essere indicata per far fronte a un peggioramento dei sintomi o per migliorare la funzione a lungo termine nei pazienti con malattia da moderata a severa. Altri agenti antimicrobici come la colistina (75-100 mg) sono stati somministrati per aerosol 2-4 volte al giorno. L'uso di antibiotici inalatori può dar luogo a reazioni di sensibilizzazione o resistenza, che però sono sorprendentemente rare. Il broncospasmo può complicare la terapia

TABELLA 400-6. Antimicrobici per le infezioni polmonari, nella fibrosi cistica

VIA	MICRORGANISMI	FARMACI	DOSAGGIO (mg/kg/die)	DOSI/DIE
Orale	*Staphylococcus aureus*	Dicloxacillina	25-50	4
		Linezolide	20	2
		Cefalexina	50	4
		Clindamicina	25-40	3-4
		Amoxicillina/acido clavulanico	25-45	2-3
	Haemophilus influenzae	Amoxicillina	50-100	2-3
	Pseudomonas aeruginosa	Ciprofloxacina	15-30	2-3
	Burkholderia cepacia	Trimetoprim/sulfametoxazolo	20*	2-4
	Empirica	Azitromicina	10, giorno 1; 5, giorni 2-5	1
		Eritromicina	30-50	3-4
Endovenosa	*S. aureus*	Nafcillina	100-200	4-6
		Vancomicina	40	3-4
	P. aeruginosa	Tobramicina	8-20	1-3
		Amikacina	15-30	2-3
		Netilmicina	6-12	2-3
		Carbenicillina	400	4
		Ticarcillina	400	4
		Piperacillina	300-400	4
		Ticarcillina/acido clavulanico	400**	4
		Piperacillina/tazobactam	240-400***	3
		Meropenem	60-120	3
		Cefipime	150	3
		Imipenem/cilastatina	45-100	3-4
		Ceftazidima	150	3
		Aztreonam	150-200	4
	B. cepacia	Cloramfenicolo	50-100	4
Aerosol		Meropenem	60-120	3
		Tobramicina (inalatoria)	300⁺	2

*Quantità di trimetroprim.
**Quantità di ticarcillina.
***Quantità di piperacillina.
⁺ mg per dose.

con colistina. Un'altra indicazione alla terapia antibiotica tramite aerosol è l'emergenza di colonizzazione delle vie aeree da parte di *Pseudomonas*. L'infezione precoce può essere eliminata per mesi, o anche per diversi anni, con ciprofloxacina per via orale più colistina o tobramicina per aerosol, mentre l'infezione stabile è raramente eradicabile. Sempre più studiosi sono concordi nel ritenere che siano indicate la sorveglianza continua per *Pseudomonas* e una pronta terapia intensiva.

TERAPIA ANTIBIOTICA ENDOVENOSA. Nei pazienti con sintomi e segni progressivi o continui, nonostante misure domiciliari intensive, è indicata la terapia antibiotica endovenosa, la quale di solito viene iniziata in ospedale, ma può essere completata ambulatorialmente. Sebbene molti pazienti migliorino entro 7 giorni, in genere è consigliabile prolungare il periodo di trattamento per almeno 14 giorni. Può essere fornito un accesso venoso a lungo termine per i cicli di terapia prolungati o frequenti, in ospedale o a domicilio.

Da numerosi studi è emersa un'incidenza sorprendentemente elevata di trombofilia, sia genetica sia acquisita. Prima di utilizzare accessi endovenosi totalmente impiantabili, o in caso di problemi ricorrenti con i cateteri centrali, occorre procedere allo screening per la trombofilia.

Gli antibiotici comunemente utilizzati per via endovenosa sono elencati nella Tabella 400-6. In generale, il trattamento dell'infezione da *P. aeruginosa* richiede una terapia con due farmaci, anche se può essere necessario un terzo agente per una copertura ottimale contro *S. aureus* o altri microrganismi. La somministrazione simultanea di agenti antimicrobici per aerosol può aumentare le concentrazioni endobronchiali. Gli aminoglicosidi hanno un'emivita relativamente breve in molti pazienti con fibrosi cistica. La dose parenterale iniziale, indicata nella Tabella 400-6, viene somministrata generalmente ogni 8 ore. Dopo aver determinato i livelli ematici, occorre aggiustare la dose giornaliera totale. Sono auspicabili livelli di picco di 10-15 mg/L, mentre i livelli di mantenimento devono essere mantenuti <3 mg/L per ridurre al minimo il rischio di ototossicità e nefrotossicità. La somministrazione una o due volte al giorno può essere più vantaggiosa rispetto a quella ogni 8 ore. Qualunque variazione nella terapia andrà introdotta tenendo conto dei risultati dell'esame colturale o del mancato miglioramento. Se il paziente non migliora, si devono escludere complicanze come l'insufficienza cardiaca, la reattività delle vie aeree o l'infezione da virus, da *Aspergillus fumigatus* (vedi Capitolo 234), da micobatteri non tubercolari (vedi Capitolo 214) o da altri microrganismi inusuali. *B. cepacia* è il più frequente di una serie di bacilli Gram-negativi che possono essere particolarmente refrattari alla terapia antimicrobica.

Broncodilatatori. Molti bambini con fibrosi cistica sviluppano un'ostruzione reversibile delle vie aeree, talvolta associata ad asma franco o ad aspergillosi broncopolmonare acuta (vedi Capitolo 234). L'ostruzione reversibile è definita come un miglioramento ≥15% della velocità di flusso, dopo inalazione di un broncodilatatore. Anche se parecchi pazienti con fibrosi cistica possono migliorare solo del 5-10%, molti di essi riportano un beneficio soggettivo inalando agonisti β-adrenergici. Il sodio dicromoglicato e l'ipratropio cloridrato sono agenti alternativi, la cui efficacia tuttavia non è stata studiata sistematicamente.

Antinfiammatori. I corticosteroidi sono utili nel trattamento dell'aspergillosi broncopolmonare allergica e della malattia da iperreattività delle vie aeree severa, di riscontro occasionale nei bambini con fibrosi cistica. Il trattamento prolungato della malattia polmonare classica da fibrosi con uno schema a giorni alterni sembrò inizialmente migliorare la funzione polmonare e ridurre la frequenza di ospedalizzazione. Tuttavia, uno studio multicentrico in doppio cieco della durata di 4 anni, che ha testato questo schema nei pazienti con malattia da lieve a moderata, ha trovato solo un'efficacia modesta, a fronte di effetti collaterali proibitivi, tra cui ritardo della crescita, cataratta, alterata tolleranza al glucosio alla dose di 2 mg/kg e ritardo della crescita a 1 mg/kg. I corticosteroidi inalatori sembrano promettenti in linea teorica, ma vi sono pochi dati che ne documentino l'efficacia e la sicurezza. L'ibuprofene, somministrato cronicamente (dose aggiustata per raggiungere concentrazioni di picco sieriche di 50-100 mcg/mL) per 4 anni, si associa a un'impressionante rallentamento della progressione della malattia, in particolare nei pazienti più giovani con una forma lieve. Sono stati riscontrati gli effetti collaterali tipici dei farmaci antinfiammatori non steroidei (vedi Tab. 400-5) e questa terapia non ha ottenuto un'accettazione diffusa.

Endoscopia e lavaggio. Il trattamento delle vie aeree ostruite comprende talvolta l'aspirazione e il lavaggio tracheobronchiale, specialmente se sono presenti atelettasie o impattamento di muco. Il lavaggio broncopolmonare può essere effettuato con l'instillazione di soluzione salina o di un agente mucolitico tramite un broncoscopio a fibre ottiche. È inoltre possibile instillare antibiotici (in genere gentamicina o tobramicina) direttamente al momento del lavaggio, raggiungendo in via temporanea una concentrazione endobronchiale molto maggiore di quella ottenibile con la terapia endovenosa. Non vi sono prove che l'endoscopia o le procedure di lavaggio ripetute apportino un beneficio prolungato.

Altre terapie. Gli espettoranti come gli ioduri e la guaifenesina non sono di alcuna utilità per rimuovere le secrezioni dall'apparato respiratorio. L'allenamento dei muscoli inspiratori può potenziare il consumo massimo di ossigeno durante l'esercizio, così come la FEV_1.

TRATTAMENTO DELLE COMPLICANZE POLMONARI. Sono numerose le complicanze polmonari che richiedono un'attenzione particolare o misure speciali.

Atelettasia. L'atelettasia lobare, relativamente poco frequente, può essere asintomatica e venire notata solo in seguito all'esecuzione di una radiografia del torace di routine. La terapia endovenosa aggressiva con antibiotici e l'aumento della fisioterapia respiratoria diretta al lobo affetto possono essere efficaci. Se nel giro di 5-7 giorni non si riscontra alcun miglioramento, può essere indicato l'esame broncoscopico delle vie aeree. Se l'atelettasia non si risolve, è indicata la terapia domiciliare intensiva continuativa, poiché la guarigione può richiedere settimane o addirittura mesi. Un'atelettasia persistente può essere asintomatica. La lobectomia va presa in considerazione solo se non si ottiene l'espansione e il paziente peggiora a causa di febbre, anoressia e tosse incoercibile (vedi Capitolo 407).

Emottisi. Il sanguinamento endobronchiale in genere indica un'erosione della parete delle vie aeree, secondaria all'infezione. Con l'aumento del numero dei pazienti più grandi, l'emottisi è diventata una complicanza relativamente frequente. L'escreato screziato di sangue è particolarmente comune. Un'emottisi di scarsa entità (<20 mL) non dovrebbe scatenare il panico, ma di solito indica la necessità di intensificare la terapia antimicrobica e la fisioterapia respiratoria. Quando però persiste o si aggrava, è indicato il ricovero ospedaliero. L'**emottisi massiva**, corrispondente a una perdita totale di sangue ≥250 mL in un periodo di 24 ore, è rara nella prima decade di vita e insorge in <1% degli adolescenti, ma richiede uno stretto monitoraggio e la possibilità di reintegrare rapidamente le perdite di sangue. La fisioterapia respiratoria viene spesso sospesa per 12-24 ore dopo l'ultimo episodio di sanguinamento attivo, per poi essere reintrodotta gradualmente. Se il tempo di protrombina è alterato, i pazienti dovrebbero ricevere vitamina K. Durante le emottisi acute occorre rassicurare il bambino e i genitori che il sanguinamento si arresterà. La trasfusione di sangue non è indicata, a meno che non vi sia ipotensione o l'ematocrito non sia significativamente ridotto. La ticarcillina, i salicilati e i farmaci antinfiammatori non steroidei interferiscono con la funzione piastrinica e possono aggravare l'emottisi. È raro che la broncoscopia riveli la sede dell'emorragia. La lobectomia andrebbe evitata, se possibile, al fine di preservare la funzione polmonare. L'embolizzazione dell'arteria bronchiale può essere utile per controllare un'emottisi persistente e significativa.

Pneumotorace. Lo pneumotorace (vedi Capitolo 410) è riscontrato in <1% dei bambini e degli adolescenti con fibrosi cistica, ma è di più frequente riscontro nei pazienti più grandi e può essere pericoloso per la vita. L'episodio, pur potendo essere asintomatico, è spesso accompagnato da dolore al torace e alle spalle, dispnea o emottisi. Una piccola raccolta d'aria che non aumenta può essere tenuta sotto stretta osservazione. La terapia iniziale consiste spesso nel posizionamento di un tubo di drenaggio toracico, con o senza pleurodesi. Se la perdita di aria persiste occorre prendere in considerazione la toracotomia a cielo aperto o la toracoscopia videoassistita (VATS, *Video-Assisted Thoraco-Scopy*) con plicazione delle bolle, decorticazione pleurica apicale e abrasione pleurica basale. L'intervento chirurgico è di solito ben tollerato anche nei casi di malattia polmonare avanzata. La somministrazione di antibiotici per via endovenosa inizia al momento del ricovero. Il tubo di drenaggio toracotomico va rimosso appena possibile, di solito in seconda o terza giornata postoperatoria, dopodiché è possibile mobilizzare il paziente e instaurare di nuovo il drenaggio posturale completo. È raro che si osservi uno pneumotorace bilaterale simultaneo, nel qual caso bisogna ottenere immediatamente il controllo della perdita di aria, almeno da un lato. Il pregresso pneumotorace, con o senza pleurodesi, non è una controindicazione al successivo trapianto polmonare.

Aspergillosi allergica. Questa complicanza insorge nel 5-10% dei pazienti presentandosi con sibili, aumento della tosse, dispnea e marcata iperinflazione (vedi Capitoli 234 e 396). In alcuni casi la radiografia del torace rileva nuovi infiltrati focali. La presenza di escreato color ruggine, il riscontro dell'*Aspergillus* nell'escreato, la dimostrazione di immunoglobiline E (IgE) sieriche precipitanti e specifiche e di anticorpi IgG verso *A. fumigatus*, o la presenza di eosinofili in un campione di espettorato fresco, sono tutti elementi che supportano la diagnosi. I livelli sierici di IgE in genere sono elevati. Il trattamento mira al controllo della reazione infiammatoria con corticosteroidi orali e alla prevenzione delle bronchiectasie centrali. Nei casi refrattari può essere necessario l'itraconazolo per via orale.

Infezione da micobatteri non tubercolari (vedi Capitolo 214). Le vie aeree danneggiate e con ridotta clearance possono essere colonizzate da *Mycobacterium avium-complex*, ma anche da *M. abscessus* e *M. kansasii*. Distinguere la colonizzazione endobronchiale (frequente) da un'infezione invasiva (infrequente) è difficile. La febbre persistente e la presenza di nuovi infiltrati o di lesioni cistiche, insieme al riscontro di microrganismi acidoresistenti allo striscio dell'escreato, suggeriscono un'infezione. Il trattamento è prolungato e richiede agenti antimicrobici multipli. I sintomi possono migliorare, ma i micobatteri non tubercolari di solito non vengono eliminati dai polmoni.

Complicanze ossee e articolari. L'osteoartropatia ipertrofica causa un sollevamento del periostio a livello della porzione distale delle ossa lunghe, con dolore osseo, edema sovrastante e versamenti articolari. Il paracetamolo o l'ibuprofene possono dare qualche sollievo. Il controllo dell'infezione polmonare in genere riduce i sintomi. Occasionalmente può insorgere un'artropatia intermittente non correlata ad altri disturbi reumatologici, che non ha una patogenesi riconosciuta e risponde di solito agli antinfiammatori non steroidei. Il mal di schiena o le fratture costali da tosse vigorosa possono richiedere la terapia del dolore per consentire un'adeguata clearance delle vie aeree. Queste e altre fratture possono essere dovute a una riduzione della mineralizzazione ossea, a sua volta imputabile a ridotto assorbimento di vitamina D, terapia corticosteroidea, ridotta tolleranza agli esercizi con i pesi e, forse, altri fattori.

Alterata respirazione nel sonno. Gli individui affetti da fibrosi cistica, in particolare quelli con malattia polmonare avanzata e durante le esacerbazioni respiratorie, possono andare incontro a diversi risvegli notturni, accorciamento della fase REM (*Rapid Eye Movement*, movimento oculare rapido), ipossiemia notturna, ipercapnia e alterazioni neurocomportamentali associate. L'ipossiemia notturna può accelerare l'esordio dell'ipertensione polmonare e dello scompenso cardiaco sinistro. L'efficacia di interventi specifici non è stata valutata sistematicamente. Occorre considerare il rapido trattamento dei sintomi respiratori e, in casi selezionati, la somministrazione notturna di ossigeno o il supporto con pressione positiva a due livelli delle vie aeree (BiPAP, *Bilevel Positive Airway Pressure*).

Insufficienza respiratoria acuta. L'insufficienza respiratoria acuta (vedi Capitoli 69 e 370), peraltro rara nei pazienti con malattia polmonare da lieve a moderata, di solito è imputabile a un'infezione virale severa o a un'altra malattia infettiva. Poiché i pazienti con questa complicanza possono ritornare al loro stato precedente, è indicata una terapia aggressiva. Oltre all'aerosol, al drenaggio posturale e al trattamento antibiotico endovena, è necessario somministrare ossigeno per aumentare la Pa_{O_2}. Una P_{CO_2} in aumento può richiedere un'assistenza ventilatoria. L'aspirazione endotracheale o broncoscopica, talvolta necessaria per liberare le vie aeree dalle secrezioni ispessite, può essere ripetuta quotidianamente. Lo scompenso cardiaco destro deve essere trattato energicamente. La guarigione è spesso lenta. Una volta che il paziente è ritornato alle sue condizioni di base, occorre continuare la terapia antibiotica endovenosa intensiva e il drenaggio posturale per 1-2 settimane.

Insufficienza respiratoria cronica. I pazienti sviluppano insufficienza respiratoria cronica dopo un deterioramento prolungato della funzione polmonare. Sebbene questo fenomeno possa verificarsi a ogni età, è più frequente nei pazienti adulti. Poiché una Pa_{O_2} costantemente <50 mmHg predispone allo sviluppo di scompenso cardiaco destro, i pazienti di solito traggono beneficio dalla somministrazione di ossigeno a basso flusso finché la P_{O_2} arteriosa a non sale a ≥ 55 mmHg. L'aumento dell'ipercapnia può impedire l'utilizzo di una F_{IO_2} ottimale. La maggior parte dei pazienti va incontro a un certo miglioramento con una terapia antibiotica aggressiva e la fisioterapia respiratoria, e può quindi essere dimessa dall'ospedale. A domicilio, è necessaria la terapia con ossigeno a basso flusso, in particolare durante il sonno. Un supporto ventilatorio non invasivo, oltre a favorire lo scambio gassoso e a migliorare la qualità di vita, può essere particolarmente utile nei pazienti in attesa di trapianto polmonare. Questi soggetti, che presentano abitualmente cuore polmonare, dovrebbero seguire una dieta a ridotto apporto di sale e assumere diuretici. Si deve prestare attenzione a evitare l'alcalosi metabolica con soppressione della ventilazione, dovuta alla deplezione cloremica della fibrosi cistica e, in molti casi, alla ritenzione di bicarbonati indotta dai diuretici. Il dolore cronico (cefalea, dolore a carico del torace, dell'addome e degli arti) è frequente negli stadi terminali e risponde a un uso giudizioso degli analgesici, tra cui gli oppiacei. La dispnea migliora con il fentanil nebulizzato.

Il trapianto polmonare è una possibilità per i pazienti con malattia polmonare terminale (vedi Capitolo 443). I criteri per le indicazioni, tuttora oggetto di indagine, comprendono idealmente stime di longevità con e senza trapianto, basate sulla funzione polmonare e sui dati di tolleranza allo sforzo. L'infezione toracica da *B. cepacia* e l'artropatia sono indici prognostici negativi. La qualità della vita migliora generalmente nel postoperatorio. A causa della bronchiolite obliterante e di altre complicanze, i polmoni trapiantati non possono funzionare per tutta la vita del ricevente e sono sempre più frequenti i trapianti ripetuti. Poiché la domanda di donatori di polmone supera l'offerta, il numero dei candidati al trapianto e, di conseguenza, la durata dell'attesa sono in continuo aumento. Il protocollo con i criteri per l'assegnazione degli organi dei donatori ai riceventi è stato rivisto tenendo conto della gravità della malattia polmonare dei pazienti in lista d'attesa.

Scompenso cardiaco. Alcuni pazienti vanno incontro a scompenso cardiaco destro reversibile (vedi Capitoli 370 e 442) in conseguenza di un evento acuto come un'infezione virale o uno pneumotorace. Gli individui con malattia polmonare avanzata, di vecchia data, specialmente quelli con ipossiemia severa (Pa_{O_2} <50 mmHg) spesso sviluppano uno scompenso cardiaco destro cronico. I meccanismi patogenetici comprendono vasocostrizione arteriosa polmonare ipossica e perdita del letto polmonare vascolare. Le alterazioni della parete delle arterie polmonari contribuiscono all'aumento delle resistenze vascolari nel tempo. Spesso si riscontrano evidenze di una concomitante disfunzione ventricolare sinistra. Aiutano a confermare la diagnosi la presenza di cianosi, l'aggravamento della dispnea, l'ingrossamento del fegato con margine dolente, la presenza di edemi malleolari, di distensione delle vene giugulari, un aumento ponderale inusuale, l'aumento delle dimensioni cardiache alla radiografia del torace, o l'evidenza di ipertrofia del cuore destro all'elettrocardiogramma o all'ecocardiogramma. La diuresi indotta dalla furosemide (1 mg/kg endovena) conferma il sospetto di ritenzione idrica. Spesso sono richieste dosi ripetute a intervalli di 24-48 ore per ridurre l'accumulo di liquidi e i sintomi di accompagnamento. L'uso concomitante di spironolattone può proteggere dalla deplezione di potassio e promuovere la diuresi a lungo termine. L'alcalosi ipercloremica è una complicanza connessa all'uso cronico di diuretici dell'ansa. La digitale non è efficace nello scompenso cardiaco destro puro, ma può essere utile in caso di disfunzione sinistra associata. La P_{O_2} arteriosa deve essere mantenuta, se possibile, a livelli >50 mmHg. La terapia polmonare intensiva, comprendente la somministrazione di antibiotici per via endovenosa, rappresenta una priorità assoluta. Inizialmente l'apporto di sodio deve essere limitato. È necessario evitare il sovraccarico di volume, così come la somministrazione di antibiotici a elevato contenuto di sodio. Non è stato dimostrato un chiaro beneficio a lungo termine derivante dall'uso di vasodilatatori polmonari. La prognosi per lo scompenso cardiaco è scadente, ma un certo numero di pazienti sopravvive per ≥ 5 anni dopo la comparsa di scompenso cardiaco. Il trapianto polmonare o il trapianto cuore-polmone offrono le migliori possibilità di guarigione in caso di malattia polmonare avanzata (vedi Capitolo 443).

TERAPIA NUTRIZIONALE. Fino al 90% dei pazienti ha una perdita delle funzione pancreatica esocrina, oltre a una digestione e un assorbimento dei grassi e delle proteine inadeguati. Si rendono quindi necessari aggiustamenti dietetici, sostituzione di enzimi pancreatici e supplementi vitaminici. In generale, i bambini con fibrosi cistica richiedono un apporto calorico quotidiano maggiore del normale per crescere. L'obiettivo è stato fissato a 130 kcal/kg di peso corporeo. Occorre somministrare quotidianamente supplementi di vitamine liposolubili.

Dieta. Molti lattanti presentano carenze nutrizionali al momento della diagnosi. I neonati che si presentano con respiro sibilante e sono alimentati con formule a base di proteine della soia non utilizzano bene queste proteine e possono sviluppare ipoproteinemia con anasarca. I lattanti non necessitano routinariamente di formule contenenti proteine predigerite e trigliceridi a catena media. In passato, generalmente si consigliava una dieta a basso contenuto di lipidi e a elevato apporto calorico per i bambini più grandi. Alcuni pazienti, seguendo questa dieta, vanno però incontro a deficit di acidi grassi essenziali. Con l'avvento di prodotti migliori a base di enzimi pancreatici, sono di solito tollerati, e preferiti, quantitativi di lipidi normali o più elevati del normale. L'apporto di lipidi può essere ridotto se le feci contengono spesso grassi non digeriti. Non di rado l'interazione genitori-bambino al momento del pasto contribuisce a peggiorare il problema, e in tal caso un intervento comportamentale può migliorare l'introito calorico.

La maggior parte degli individui ha un fabbisogno calorico maggiore del normale a causa dell'aumentato lavoro respiratorio e forse anche dell'aumentata attività metabolica correlata al difetto di base. Quando sopravviene l'anoressia dell'infezione cronica, si verifica un calo ponderale. Incoraggiare il paziente a mangiare cibi molto calorici è importante, ma generalmente non basta per ottenere un aumento ponderale se l'infezione polmonare non è controllata. Via via che quest'ultima progredisce, la stabilizzazione o l'aumento del peso richiedono talvolta la nutrizione notturna con sondino nasogastrico, enterostomia percutanea o iperalimentazione endovenosa a breve termine. I benefici a lungo termine di questi interventi comprendono il miglioramento della qualità di vita e un maggiore benessere psicologico. Non è stato chiaramente documentato un miglioramento della funzione polmonare.

La terapia con ormone della crescita umano ricombinante, somministrato tre volte alla settimana, ha migliorato i parametri nutrizionali, sortendo anche un effetto positivo sul bilancio azotato e accelerando l'aumento di peso e altezza.

Sostituzione di enzimi pancreatici. Gli estratti di pancreas animale somministrati con il cibo riducono, ma non correggono completamente, le perdite fecali di grassi e azoto. Il dosaggio degli enzimi e il prodotto devono essere individualizzati per ogni paziente. Le microsfere enterorivestite contenenti enzimi, sensibili al pH, sono le più prescritte. Sono disponibili diversi dosaggi, fino a 20 000 UI di lipasi/capsula. Poiché la somministrazione di dosi troppo elevate è stata correlata a **stenosi coliche** tali da richiedere l'intervento chirurgico, la sostituzione enzimatica in genere non dovrebbe superare le 2500 unità di lipasi/kg/pasto. Nella maggior parte dei pazienti sono sufficienti da una a tre capsule a pasto; i lattanti necessitano di 2000-4000 unità di lipasi a pasto, che vengono somministrate più agevolmente se miscelate con polpa di mela; questa prescrizione vale anche gli spuntini. Le preparazioni a base di microsfere sono di solito sufficientemente efficaci da permettere una dieta libera, che dovrebbe comprendere latte omogeneizzato con vitamina D. Sebbene i bambini con fibrosi cistica presentino un malassorbimento dei sali biliari, le preparazioni enzimatiche contenenti sali biliari sono raramente necessarie. La dose degli enzimi richiesti di solito aumenta con l'età, ma alcuni adolescenti e giovani adulti in seguito possono avere una riduzione del loro fabbisogno.

Supplementi di vitamine e minerali. Dal momento che l'insufficienza pancreatica provoca malassorbimento delle vitamine liposolubili (A, D, E, K), si consiglia la supplementazione vitaminica. Per i pazienti con fibrosi cistica sono disponibili in commercio numerosi preparati contenenti tutte e quattro queste vitamine, che dovrebbero essere assunte quotidianamente. Possono essere necessarie dosi sostitutive quando si riscontrano bassi livelli sierici o quando il paziente è sintomatico. Sono stati riportati casi di lattanti con deficit di zinco e un rash simile all'acrodermatite enteropatica. Inoltre, si deve prestare attenzione allo stato marziale; in uno studio, almeno un terzo dei bambini con fibrosi cistica aveva basse concentrazioni di ferritina.

TRATTAMENTO DELLE COMPLICANZE INTESTINALI

Ileo da meconio. Nel sospetto di un ileo da meconio (vedi Capitolo 102.1), si posiziona un sondino nasogastrico per l'aspirazione e si idrata il neonato. In molti casi, un clisma contenente diatrizoato (Gastrografin®), con reflusso di mezzo di contrasto nell'ileo, non solo conferma la diagnosi, ma talvolta determina il transito di un tappo di meconio e la canalizzazione del tratto ostruito. L'utilizzo di questa soluzione ipertonica richiede un'attenta correzione delle perdite idriche a livello intestinale. I pazienti pediatrici in cui questa procedura fallisce richiedono l'intervento chirurgico. I bambini trattati con successo hanno generalmente un prognosi simile a quella dei pazienti più grandi con mutazioni severe della fibrosi cistica. I neonati con ileo da meconio devono essere trattati come se avessero la fibrosi cistica, in attesa che sia possibile effettuare un test diagnostico adeguato.

Sindrome da ostruzione intestinale distale (equivalente dell'ileo da meconio) e altre cause di sintomi addominali. Nonostante un'adeguata sostituzione di enzimi pancreatici, il 2-5% dei pazienti accumula materiale fecale nella porzione terminale dell'ileo e del cieco, potendo quindi sviluppare un'ostruzione parziale o completa. Per i sintomi intermittenti, occorre continuare la terapia con enzimi pancreatici sostitutivi o persino aumentarne il dosaggio, associandola alla somministrazione di emollienti fecali (polietilenglicole o docusato di sodio). Si consiglia inoltre un elevato introito di liquidi. La mancata risoluzione dei sintomi indica la necessità di un lavaggio intestinale con volumi elevati, con la somministrazione di una soluzione salina bilanciata contenente polietilenglicole, assunta per bocca o tramite sondino nasogastrico. Quando l'ostruzione è completa, può essere terapeutico un clisma di diatrizoato accompagnato da elevati volumi di liquidi endovena. Nella diagnosi differenziale devono essere presi in considerazione anche l'intussuscezione (vedi Capitolo 330.3) e il volvolo (vedi Capitolo 326.4). L'intussuscezione, di solito ileocolica, insorge a qualsiasi età, spesso dopo 1-2 giorni di stipsi; in molti casi può essere diagnosticata e ridotta con un clisma di diatrizoato. Se però l'intussuscezione non è riducibile o è presente un volvolo, si rende necessaria la laparotomia. Episodi ripetuti di intussuscezione possono rappresentare un'indicazione alla resezione cecale.

L'appendicite cronica, con o senza ascesso periappendicolare, può presentarsi con dolore addominale ricorrente o persistente, sollevando il dubbio sulla necessità di una laparotomia. La mancanza di tamponamento acido nel duodeno sembra predisporre alcuni bambini alla duodenite e alla formazione di ulcere. Il reflusso biliare viene osservato nei pazienti più grandi (vedi sezione seguente). Altre indicazioni all'intervento chirurgico sono il carcinoma del colon o delle vie biliari e la colopatia sclerosante.

Reflusso gastroesofageo (vedi Capitolo 320). Poiché diversi fattori possono aumentare la pressione endoaddominale, tra cui la tosse e l'ostruzione delle vie aeree, il reflusso gastroesofageo patologico non è raro e può esacerbare la malattia polmonare secondaria al broncospasmo riflesso e all'aspirazione ripetuta. Deve essere considerato il trattamento dietetico, posizionale e farmacologico. Gli agonisti colinergici sono controindicati poiché scatenano la secrezione di muco e una progressiva difficoltà respiratoria. La riduzione della secrezione acido-gastrica può essere d'aiuto, con l'uso di inibitori della pompa protonica che sono gli agenti più efficaci. La fundoplicatio è una procedura effettuata come extrema ratio.

Prolasso rettale (vedi Capitolo 341.5). Il prolasso, peraltro non comune, insorge più spesso nei lattanti e meno frequentemente nei bambini più grandi con fibrosi cistica. Di solito è correlato alla steatorrea, alla malnutrizione e alla tosse ripetuta. Il retto prolassato può essere ridotto manualmente esercitando una pressione delicata e continua, con il paziente in posizione fetale. Può essere utile la sedazione. Per prevenire la ricorrenza immediata, si può posizionare un cerotto per mantenere i glutei ravvicinati. Un miglioramento si ottiene grazie a un'adeguata terapia sostitutiva con enzimi pancreatici, alla riduzione dei lipidi e delle scorie nella dieta, all'uso di emollienti fecali e al controllo dell'infezione polmonare. Occasionalmente, un paziente può continuare ad avere prolasso rettale che richiede la scleroterapia o l'intervento chirurgico.

Malattia epatobiliare. Il trattamento con acido ursodesossicolico permette di ottenere un miglioramento in caso di anomalie della funzione epatica associate alla cirrosi biliare. Non è stato documentato chiaramente se gli acidi biliari siano in grado di prevenire la progressione della cirrosi. L'ipertensione portale con varici esofagee, ipersplenismo o ascite insorge in ≤2% dei bambini affetti da fibrosi cistica (vedi Capitolo 364). Il trattamento in acuto del sanguinamento da varici esofagee comprende l'aspirazione nasogastrica e il lavaggio con soluzione salina. La scleroterapia è raccomandata dopo un'emorragia iniziale. In passato, un sanguinamento significativo è stato trattato anche con successo con shunting portosistemico. L'anastomosi splenorenale è stata la procedura più efficace. Un ipersplenismo marcato può richiedere la splenectomia. La colelitiasi impone una consulenza chirurgica. Per il trattamento dell'ascite si rimanda al Capitolo 367.

L'ittero ostruttivo nei neonati con fibrosi cistica non richiede una terapia specifica. L'epatomegalia con steatosi impone una particolare attenzione alla nutrizione e può rispondere a supplementi di carnitina. Nonostante si tratti di un'evenienza rara, la cirrosi biliare può evolvere fino all'insufficienza epatocellulare, che dovrebbe essere trattata come nei pazienti più grandi con insufficienza epatica (vedi Capitoli 361 e 364). L'insufficienza epatica terminale è un'indicazione al trapianto epatico nei bambini con fibrosi cistica, soprattutto se la funzione polmonare è buona. Gli esiti sono stati incoraggianti.

Pancreatite. La pancreatite può essere precipitata da pasti grassi, ingestione di alcolici o terapia con tetracicline. I livelli di amilasi sieriche e di lipasi possono rimanere elevati per lunghi periodi. Il trattamento è discusso nel Capitolo 348.

Iperglicemia. L'esordio avviene per lo più nella prima decade di vita. Circa il 20% dei giovani adulti è trattato per l'iperglicemia, sebbene l'incidenza del diabete correlato alla fibrosi cistica possa essere elevata. La prevalenza è maggiore nelle femmine e negli omozigoti per la ΔF508. La chetoacidosi è di raro riscontrato. La patogenesi comprende sia un'alterata secrezione di insulina sia resistenza insulinica. Lo screening di routine consiste in un test di tolleranza al glucosio a 2 ore modificato, effettuato una volta all'anno, a partire dagli 8-10 anni di età. L'intolleranza al glucosio senza perdite urinarie di glucosio generalmente non viene trattata; i livelli di emoglobina glicata devono essere monitorati almeno una volta all'anno. Se la glicosuria è persistente e si manifestano sintomi, occorre instaurare la terapia insulinica. Gli ipoglicemizzanti orali, associati o meno a farmaci che riducano la resistenza all'insulina, possono essere efficaci. L'insufficienza pancreatica esocrina e il malassorbimento rendono difficile un controllo dietetico stretto dell'iperglicemia. La terapia steroidea deve essere evitata. Lo sviluppo di iperglicemia significativa favorisce l'acquisizione di *P. aeruginosa* e *B. cepacia* nelle vie aeree e può influire negativamente sulla funzione polmonare; pertanto, un attento controllo glicemico è un obiettivo fondamentale. Possono insorgere le complicanze vascolari a lungo termine del diabete, un motivo in più per tenere sotto controllo i livelli glicemici.

ALTRE TERAPIE

Polipi nasali. I polipi nasali (vedi Capitolo 375) insorgono nel 15-20% dei pazienti con fibrosi cistica e hanno una maggiore prevalenza nella seconda decade di vita. I corticosteroidi locali e i decongestionanti nasali talvolta forniscono qualche beneficio. In caso di completa ostruzione dei passaggi nasali, rinorrea costante o allargamento del ponte nasale, è indicata la rimozione chirurgica; i polipi, che possono recidivare rapidamente o dopo un intervallo di mesi o anni libero da sintomi, smettono inspiegabilmente di svilupparsi in molti adulti.

Rinosinusite. L'opacizzazione dei seni paranasali non è un'indicazione all'intervento. I sintomi acuti e cronici correlati ai seni paranasali sono trattati inizialmente con antimicrobici, con o senza aspirazione dei seni mascellari per l'esame colturale. La chirurgia endoscopica funzionale dei seni ha fornito qualche beneficio in casi aneddotici.

Deplezione di sali. Le perdite di sali con il sudore possono essere elevate, specialmente nei climi caldi e aridi. Occorre permettere ai bambini di consumare sale secondo le loro necessità e fare attenzione che i lattanti non indossino indumenti troppo pesanti. I supplementi di sali programmati non sono più prescritti, salvo che nei climi torridi. L'alcalosi ipocloremica deve essere sospettata in qualsiasi lattante con sintomi di gastroenterite e, al bisogno, occorre instaurare tempestivamente la terapia con liquidi ed elettroliti.

Crescita e maturazione. Il ritardo della crescita deve essere affrontato energicamente stimolando la nutrizione, trattando la malattia polmonare in modo più aggressivo, in casi selezionati, con una valutazione endocrinologica e talvolta con la somministrazione di ormone della crescita. Il rapporto rischio-beneficio degli steroidi anabolizzanti non depone a favore del loro utilizzo nei bambini affetti da fibrosi cistica con crescita stentata. È piuttosto frequente un ritardo della maturazione sessuale, spesso associato a bassa statura. Sebbene molti pazienti presentino infezioni polmonari severe o uno stato nutrizionale scadente, la pubertà ritardata colpisce anche quelli che per il resto hanno una malattia lieve, fenomeno che non è stato ancora completamente spiegato. Gli adolescenti con fibrosi cistica dovrebbero ricevere un counseling specifico negli anni dello sviluppo, in merito alla loro maturazione sessuale e al loro potenziale riproduttivo.

Chirurgia. Le procedure chirurgiche minori, comprese le cure dentarie, devono essere effettuate se possibile in anestesia locale. I pazienti con uno stato polmonare buono o eccellente possono tollerare l'anestesia generale senza misure polmonari intensive prima dell'intervento. Per quelli con infezione polmonare moderata o severa di solito si consiglia un ciclo di 1-2 settimane di terapia antibiotica intensiva e un aumento della terapia di clearance delle vie aeree, prima dell'intervento. Qualora questo non fosse possibile, è indicato iniziare la terapia antibiotica endovenosa non appena ci si rende conto della necessità di effettuare un intervento di chirurgia maggiore. La durata totale dell'anestesia dovrebbe essere la più breve possibile. Dopo l'induzione, è utile l'aspirazione tracheale, che andrebbe ripetuta almeno alla fine dell'intervento. I pazienti con malattia severa necessitano del monitoraggio dell'emogasanalisi e possono richiedere un'assistenza ventilatoria nell'immediato periodo postoperatorio.

Dopo un intervento chirurgico maggiore, bisogna incoraggiare la tosse e riprendere i trattamenti di clearance delle vie aeree il prima possibile, in genere nell'arco di 24 ore. Un'adeguata analgesia è importante se si deve instaurare rapidamente una terapia efficace. Per i pazienti con coinvolgimento polmonare significativo, gli antibiotici endovena vengono somministrati per 7-14 giorni dopo l'intervento. Dopo toracotomia a cielo aperto per il trattamento dello pneumotorace, o dopo lobectomia, il tubo di drenaggio toracico rappresenta il maggior ostacolo singolo a una terapia polmonare efficace e quindi dovrebbe essere rimosso il prima possibile per consentire la ripresa di una terapia di drenaggio posturale completa.

PROGNOSI. La fibrosi cistica resta tuttora una malattia con effetti negativi sulla durata della vita, sebbene negli ultimi 30-40 anni la sopravvivenza sia migliorata in misura notevole. Occasionalmente i lattanti con malattia polmonare severa soccombono, ma la maggior parte dei bambini sopravvive a questo periodo difficile e arriva all'adolescenza o all'età adulta in condizioni di salute relativamente buone. La lenta progressione della malattia, tuttavia, finisce sempre per avere esiti disabilitanti. I dati sulla durata di vita indicano attualmente una sopravvivenza cumulativa media che supera i 35 anni. La sopravvivenza maschile pare migliore di quella femminile, per ragioni che non sono facilmente comprensibili. I bambini di famiglie svantaggiate dal punto di vista socioeconomico hanno, in media, una prognosi peggiore.

I bambini con fibrosi cistica di solito hanno una buona frequenza scolastica e non dovrebbero essere limitati nelle loro attività. Un'elevata percentuale arriva a frequentare le scuole superiori e a diplomarsi; la maggior parte trova un impiego soddisfacente e un numero sempre maggiore si sposa. Il passaggio delle cure dai centri pediatrici agli ospedali per adulti, all'età di 21 anni, è un obiettivo importante e richiede un approccio attento e di sostegno, che oltre al pediatra coinvolga gli specialisti in medicina interna.

Con l'aumento dell'aspettativa di vita, sono emerse nuove considerazioni di ordine psicosociale, tra cui problemi riguardanti un senso di dipendenza-indipendenza, la cura di sé, i rapporti interpersonali, la sessualità, la riproduzione, l'abuso di sostanze, i progetti di vita, i costi delle cure mediche e altri oneri finanziari, oltre alle ansie relative alla prognosi della malattia. È preferibile affrontare molti di questi aspetti con un certo anticipo, prima ancora che si manifestino turbe psicologiche. Con un appropriato sostegno medico e psicologico, i bambini e gli adolescenti affetti da fibrosi cistica in genere riescono a convivere con la loro patologia. Il raggiungimento di una condizione di indipendenza e produttività nell'età adulta rappresenta un obiettivo realistico per molti pazienti.

Aaron SD, Vandemheen KL, Ferris W, et al: Combination antibiotic susceptibility testing to treat exacerbations of cystic fibrosis associated with multiresistant bacteria: A randomized, double-blind, controlled clinical trial. *Lancet* 2005;366:463–471.

Colombo C, Battezzati A: Growth failure in cystic fibrosis: A true need for anabolic agents? *J Pediatr* 2005;146:303–305.

Corey M, Edwards L, Levison H, et al: Longitudinal analysis of pulmonary function decline in patients with cystic fibrosis. *J Pediatr* 1997; 131:809–814.
Donaldson SH, Bennett WD, Zeman KL, et al: Mucus clearance and lung function in cystic fibrosis with hypertonic saline. *N Engl J Med* 2006;354: 241–250.
Drumm ML, Konstan MW, Schluchter MD, et al: Genetic modifiers of lung disease in cystic fibrosis. *N Engl J Med* 2005;353:1443–1453.
Elkins MR, Robinson M, Rose BR, et al: A controlled trial of long-term inhaled hypertonic saline on patients with cystic fibrosis. *N Engl J Med* 2006;354:229–240.
Emerson J, Rosenfeld M, McNamara S, et al: *Pseudomonas aeruginosa* and other predictors of mortality and morbidity in young children with cystic fibrosis. *Pediatr Pulmonol* 2002;34:91–100.
Eubanks V, Koppersmith N, Wooldridge N, et al: Effects of megestrol acetate on weight gain, body composition, and pulmonary function in patients with cystic fibrosis. *J Pediatr* 2002;140:439–444.
Ferkol T, Rosenfeld M, Milla CE: Cystic fibrosis pulmonary exacerbations. *J Pediatr* 2006;148:259–264.
FitzSimmons SC, Burkhart GA, Borowitz D, et al: High-dose pancreatic-enzyme supplements and fibrosing colonopathy in children with cystic fibrosis. *N Engl J Med* 1997;336:1283–1289.
Fuchs HJ, Borowitz DS, Christiansen DH, et al: Effect of aerosolized recombinant human DNase on exacerbations of respiratory symptoms and on pulmonary function in patients with cystic fibrosis. The Pulmozyme Study Group. *N Engl J Med* 1994;331:637–642.
Groman JD, Karczeki B, Sheridan M, et al: Phenotypic and genetic characterization of patients with features of nonclassic forms of cystic fibrosis. *J Pediatr* 2005;146:675–680.
Grosse SD, Rosenfeld M, Devine OJ, et al: Potential impact of newborn screening for cystic fibrosis on child survival: A systematic review and analysis. *J Pediatr* 2006;149:362–366.
Hardin DS, Rice J, Ahn C, et al: Growth hormone treatment enhances nutrition and growth in children with cystic fibrosis receiving enteral nutrition. *J Pediatr* 2005;146:324–328.
Kappler M, Griese M: Nutritional supplements in cystic fibrosis. *BMJ* 2006; 332:618–619.
Lenaerts C, Lapierre C, Patriqui H, et al: Surveillance for cystic fibrosis-associated hepatobiliary disease: Early ultrasound changes and predisposing factors. *J Pediatr* 2003;143:343–350.
Li Z, Kosorok MR, Farrell PM, et al: Longitudinal development of mucoid *Pseudomonas aeruginosa* infection and lung disease progression in children with cystic fibrosis. *JAMA* 2005;293:581–588.
Lion RG, Adler FR, Cahill BC, et al: Survival effect of lung transplantation among patients with cystic fibrosis. *JAMA* 2001;286:2683–2689.
McColley SA: Cystic fibrosis lung disease: When does it start, and how can it be prevented? J *Pediatr* 2004;145:6–7.
Moran A, Hardin D, Rodman D, et al: Diagnosis, screening and management of cystic fibrosis related diabetes mellitus: A consensus conference report. *Diabetes Res Clin Pract* 1999;45:61–73.
Poustie VJ, Russell JE, Watling, et al: Oral protein energy supplements for children with cystic fibrosis: CALICO multicentre randomized controlled trial. *BMJ* 2006;332:632–635.
Rajan S, Saiman L: Pulmonary infections in patients with cystic fibrosis. *Semin Respir Infect* 2002;17:47–56.
Rao S, Grigg J: New insights into pulmonary inflammation in cystic fibrosis. *Arch Dis Child* 2006;91:786–788.
Rowe SM, Miller S, Sorscher EJ: Cystic fibrosis. *N Engl J Med* 2005; 352:1992–2001.
Saiman L, Marshall BC, Mayer-Hamblett N, et al: Azithromycin in patients with cystic fibrosis chronically infected with *Pseudomonas aeruginosa:* A randomized controlled trial. *JAMA* 2003;290:1749–1756.
Sims EJ, McCormick J, Mehta G, Mehta A: Newborn screening for cystic fibrosis is associated with reduced treatment intensity. *J Pediatr* 2005; 147:306–311.
Smyth A, Tan KHV, Hyman-Taylor P, et al: Once versus three-times daily regimens of tobramycin treatment for pulmonary exacerbations of cystic fibrosis—the TOPIC study: A randomized controlled trial. *Lancet* 2005;365:573–578.
Smyth RL: Daily activity and disease status in cystic fibrosis: An important area for research. *J Pediatr* 2005;147:281–283.
Smyth RL: Diagnosis and management of cystic fibrosis. *Arch Dis Child* 2005;90:ep1–ep6.
Sun L, Jiang RZ, Steinbach S, et al: The emergence of a highly transmissible lineage of cbl+ *Pseudomonas (Burkholderia)* cepacia causing CF centre epidemics in North America and Britain. *Nat Med* 1995;1:661–666.
Texereau J, Marullo S, Hubert D, et al: Nitric oxide synthase 1 as a potential modifier gene of decline in lung function in patients with cystic fibrosis. *Thorax* 2004;59:156–158.
Vandenbussche HL, Klepser ME: Single daily tobramycin dosing in cystic fibrosis: Is it better for the patients or the bugs? *Lancet* 2005;365:547–548.
Wilschanski M, Yahav Y, Yaacov Y, et al: Gentamicin-induced correction of CFTR function in patients with cystic fibrosis and CFTR stop mutations. *N Engl J Med* 2003;349:1433–1441.
Zeitlin P: Can curcumin cure cystic fibrosis? *N Engl J Med* 2004;351:606–608.

Capitolo 401 ■ Discinesia ciliare primitiva (sindrome delle ciglia immobili)

Gabriel G. Haddad e Michael Kashgarian

La **discinesia ciliare primitiva** (**PCD**, *Primitive Ciliary Dyskinesia*) comprende quei disturbi respiratori che sono accomunati dal malfunzionamento delle ciglia delle vie aeree. Quest'anomalia dipende da vari difetti strutturali, primitivi ed ereditari, delle ciglia, che portano a infezioni ripetute e croniche dei polmoni e dei seni paranasali. Il malfunzionamento ciliare, nella PCD, non è conseguenza di ripetute infezioni polmonari acquisite, condizione in cui le anomalie ciliari, a differenza di quanto avviene nella PCD, sono reversibili. Circa il 50% dei pazienti con PCD ha la **sindrome di Kartagener**: situs viscerum inversus, sinusite e otite croniche e malattia respiratoria che conduce alla formazione di bronchiectasie. Circa il 25% dei pazienti con situs viscerum inversus ha anche PCD; il riscontro di situs inversus non è sufficiente per stabilire la presenza di PCD.

LOCALIZZAZIONE E STRUTTURA. Le ciglia sono strutture digitiformi che dalla superficie cellulare si proiettano verso il lume delle vie aeree. Esse misurano 0,25 micron di diametro e 306 micron di lunghezza. Ogni cellula ne presenta tipicamente circa 200 sulla sua superficie. Ogni ciglia è formata da un *tronco*, un *corpo basale*, punto di attacco delle ciglia alla cellula, e una *corona*, una struttura specializzata ritenuta importante per l'attacco al muco. Il tronco è costituito da una membrana cellulare esterna e da assonemi, o strutture proteiche del citoscheletro. Queste ultime formano una struttura circolare di 9 microtubuli in coppie, più due microtubuli singoli centrali (9 + 2 strutture). Ogni coppia periferica può attaccarsi all'altra tramite ponti o bracci di dineina. Anche i raggi sono proteine del citoscheletro, che collegano i microtubuli periferici a quelli centrali.

Le ciglia delle vie aeree sono localizzate sulle superfici epiteliali di naso, seni paranasali, orecchie e vie aeree. La loro densità è variabile: la maggior parte (50-80%) delle cellule delle vie aeree principali ne è dotata, mentre sono molto più scarse nelle vie aeree inferiori e non sono presenti negli alveoli e nei sacchi aerei. La frequenza del battito ciliare è di 1-20 Hz; i valori maggiori si riscontrano nelle vie aeree principali e correlano con la velocità del muco in diverse parti dell'albero tracheobronchiale.

Nell'uomo, vi sono almeno sei tipi di ciglia: *delle vie aeree*, *ventricolari*, *embrionali*, *olfattive*, *dei fotorecettori* e il *flagello spermatico*. Mentre le ciglia embrionali e quelle dei fotorecettori contengono 9 coppie di microtubuli e nessuna al centro (9 + 0 strutture), gli altri tipi di ciglia sono caratterizzati dalla stessa struttura periferica (9 coppie di microtubuli), ma hanno in più 2 microtubuli centrali singoli (9 + 2 strutture). Le ciglia delle vie aeree sospingono il muco nelle vie respiratorie; quelle ventricolari, localizzate sul rivestimento ependimale dei ventricoli cerebrali, sospingono invece il liquido cerebrospinale (LCS). In 4 fratelli maschi originari della Giordania è stata riportata un'associazione tra discinesia ciliare, idrocefalo e ritardo mentale, forse causata da una mutazione che colpisce la clearance polmonare, ostacolando il movimento del liquido nei polmoni e del LCS. Le ciglia embrionali, localizzate nel nodo embrionale, si suppone spingano morfogeni e stabiliscano, in questo stadio precoce, un gradiente morfogenico d'importanza cruciale per lo sviluppo della lateralità dell'embrione. Infatti, le anomalie delle ciglia nodali danno luogo a situs viscerum inversus.

FUNZIONE. Le ciglia vibrano e si muovono grazie allo scorrimento dei microtubuli. All'inizio del ciclo del battito, si piegano alla base e si spostano all'indietro, perpendicolarmente alla superficie, dopodiché si estendono ("scivolano") ruotando con un movimento in avanti. Questi movimenti di piegamento e di torsione (rotazioni tridimensionali in senso orario) sono resi possibili dall'idrolisi dell'adenosina trifosfato (ATP) e dai bracci di dineina, che sono ATPasi. La visualizzazione al microscopio rivela che le ciglia delle vie aeree coordinano la loro attività localmente, dando luogo a un *movimento a onda* (cui partecipano molte ciglia insieme).

La principale funzione delle ciglia delle vie aeree è di trasportare il muco verso la bocca, con i loro battiti. L'efficacia di questo meccanismo dipende dalla frequenza del battito, dalla composizione e dalla viscosità del liquido periciliare e dello strato di muco soprastante, oltre che dalla coordinazione dei movimenti ciliari. Numerosi sono i mediatori neurochimici che modulano il battito ciliare, aumentandone la frequenza, in particolare le sostanze β-adrenergiche, l'acetilcolina, le bradichinine e la serotonina. In alternativa, la riduzione dell'umidità delle vie aeree diminuisce significativamente la frequenza del battito ciliare, su cui influisce negativamente anche un aumento della carica batterica.

ANATOMIA PATOLOGICA. Si stima che la struttura ciliare contenga >250 polipeptidi, ed è probabile che la discinesia ciliare primitiva dipenda dall'assenza di una o più proteine del citoscheletro. A seconda del tipo di ciglia, si riscontra anche una certa variabilità delle proteine strutturali. Le anomalie strutturali sono osservabili mediante microscopia elettronica.

Le alterazioni ultrastrutturali delle ciglia, nella discinesia ciliare, comprendono la mancanza dei bracci di dineina, la trasposizione dei microtubuli, ciglia composte, orientamento casuale delle ciglia, anomalie della loro lunghezza, difetti dei legami di nexina e dei ponti radiali, assenza delle ciglia con metaplasia dell'orletto a spazzola. È importante distinguere le situazioni che causano difetti transitori, che riguardano soltanto un sottogruppo di ciglia (come l'infiammazione respiratoria acuta e cronica), dai difetti congeniti veri e propri. La PCD classica è caratterizzata dall'*assenza dei bracci di dineina sia interni sia esterni*, che si traduce in un deficit completo di tali bracci (Figg. 401-1 e 401-2). I *difetti parziali dei bracci di dineina* (in cui non sono visualizzabili i bracci interni, oppure quelli esterni) o i *difetti delle coppie centrali* non sono generalmente associati a situs inversus (vedi Capitolo 431.11) e sembrano insorgere come anomalie genetiche isolate. I *difetti dei ponti radiali*, peraltro molto più difficili da visualizzare, sono generalmente considerati un'entità autonoma, in questo spettro di anomalie ciliari. L'*aplasia ciliare* o *metaplasia dell'orletto a spazzola*, con assenza delle ciglia nell'epitelio, può in realtà essere il risultato di alterazioni infiammatorie croniche, in un individuo con anomalie ciliari preesistenti. L'*orientamento casuale delle ciglia* si verifica quando l'unico difetto ultrastrutturale presente è la coppia centrale orientata in modo casuale anziché in modo uniforme e parallelo.

Gli studi sulla motilità ciliare possono non correlare direttamente con i reperti ultrastrutturali. Le ciglia dei pazienti con la sindrome di Kartagener sono immobili. Al contrario, difetti di un singolo braccio possono presentare un movimento coordinato, sebbene la frequenza del battito ciliare sia più lenta del normale. L'orientamento casuale dell'asse delle ciglia dà luogo a un movimento scoordinato e disordinato. Tutti questi difetti strutturali sono responsabili di un malfunzionamento delle ciglia, consistente o in un battito anomalo, o nell'immobilità delle ciglia, che pertanto comportano un'alterata clearance mucociliare delle secrezioni respiratorie. La sequenza patogenetica più probabile è il ristagno di muco nelle vie aeree e l'incapacità di eliminare gli organismi patogeni, seguiti da infezioni croniche, o recidivanti con frequenza elevata, delle vie respiratorie e, infine, da danno alla parete delle vie aeree.

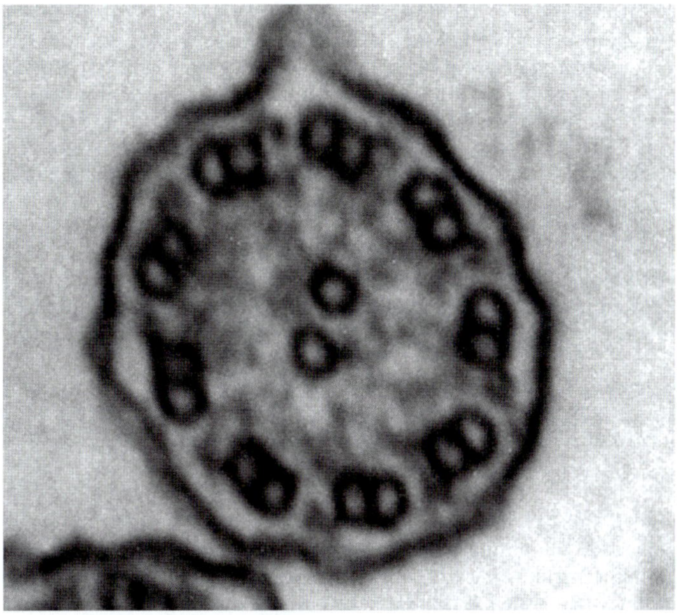

Figura 401-1. Ciglia normali alla microscopia elettronica, che rivela la normale configurazione 9 + 2 dell'assonema. Possono essere identificati sia i bracci interni sia quelli esterni della dineina, ma non sempre sulla stessa coppia di microtubuli. I bracci esterni in genere sono più facili da visualizzare e i raggi non sono chiaramente identificati.

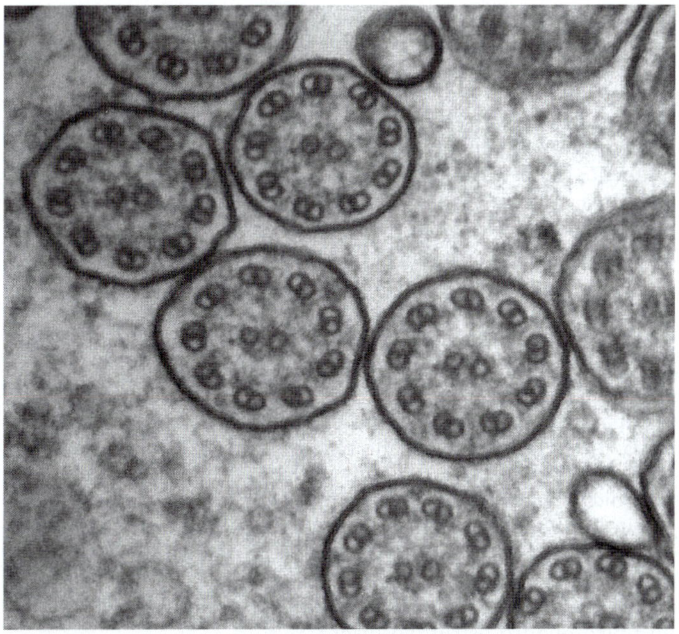

Figura 401-2. Ciglia di un paziente con sindrome di Kartagener. Sebbene l'assonema contenga le normali 9 + 2 coppie di microtubuli, sono assenti sia i bracci interni sia quelli esterni della dineina, in tutte le ciglia.

GENETICA. Le stime della prevalenza della PCD vanno da 1/15 000 a 1/60 000 nati vivi. È probabilmente la terza forma più comune di malattia cronica ereditaria delle vie respiratorie, nei bambini caucasici, dopo la fibrosi cistica (CF, *Cystic Fibrosis*) e gli stati di immunodeficienza. Sono stati riportati casi in diversi gruppi etnici e razziali, tra cui popolazioni del Giappone, della Cina e del Nord Africa. L'ereditarietà è per lo più autosomica recessiva, sebbene siano stati riportati casi di trasmissione autosomica dominante e persino X-linked.

Alla base della PCD sono stati ipotizzati vari geni. Il *DNAH5* è un gene della catena lunga della dineina assonemica, localizzato sul cromosoma 5p (5p14-5p15); molto lungo (79 esoni), codifica per una proteina di 4624 aminoacidi. È espresso nel polmone, nel rene e, in minor misura, nel cervello e nei testicoli. Nelle famiglie con PCD sono state riscontrate diverse mutazioni, omozigoti ed eterozigoti; un certo numero di individui presentava anche situs viscerum inversus.

Il *DNAI1*, un altro gene lungo sul cromosoma 9 (9p13-21), formato da 20 esoni, è altamente espresso nella trachea e nel testicolo. Codifica per una catena intermedia che si trova sui bracci esterni della dineina. Sono state trovate anche molte altre mutazioni, in altre famiglie con PCD, tra cui sostituzione di basi conservate e delezione di coppie di basi negli esoni. Alla PCD è stato associato infine un terzo gene (*DNAH11*), che codifica anche per una catena pesante di dineina nel braccio esterno, localizzato sul cromosoma 7 (7p21).

MANIFESTAZIONI CLINICHE. Il decorso è variabile. Gli individui con PCD possono avere distress respiratorio inspiegato durante il periodo neonatale, o sopravvivere fino all'età adulta senza una franca sinusite e senza sintomi respiratori. In uno studio sulla PCD, il 100% dei bambini aveva tosse produttiva, sinusite e otite. Molti si presentavano in età neonatale con congestione nasale, rinite e tosse. Una caratteristica che aiuta a differenziare la PCD dalla CF è la ricorrenza di episodi di otite media o otite cronica sierosa. I bambini diagnosticati dopo alcuni anni di vita sono spesso stati trattati con tubi timpanostomici; è comune una perdita di udito di tipo conduttivo. Spesso il posizionamento di un tubo timpanostomico è seguito da otorrea prolungata. Nel 20% circa dei pazienti, sono presenti ippocratismo digitale e polipi nasali. Molti bambini con PCD vanno incontro frequentemente a sibili e hanno una diagnosi iniziale di asma. Il sintomo caratteristico è la tosse cronica, spesso grassa o produttiva. Può insorgere polmonite, e la malattia delle vie aeree inferiori può progredire con calo ponderale, ridotta tolleranza all'esercizio e bronchiectasie. L'insufficienza respiratoria, nell'infanzia, è rara, così come le complicanze polmonari (per es. pneumotorace ed emottisi). È frequente l'atelettasia lobare. I maschi presentano spesso infertilità e una motilità assente o scarsa degli spermatozoi; le femmine sono ad aumentato rischio di gravidanza ectopica.

DIAGNOSI. La PCD deve essere sospettata in un bambino con sintomi cronici o ricorrenti delle vie respiratorie superiori e inferiori, specialmente in presenza di una malattia importante dell'orecchio medio. La presentazione avviene spesso in epoca neonatale. Le immagini radiografiche (o la TC) mostrano coinvolgimento dei seni paranasali. Le radiografie del torace possono rivelare iperinflazione, ispessimento della parete bronchiale e infiltrati peribronchiali. Sono spesso presenti atelettasia e consolidamento. La metodica migliore per individuare le **bronchiectasie** è la TC (vedi Capitolo 398). La localizzazione del cuore a destra, in un bambino con sintomi respiratori cronici, è virtualmente diagnostica, ma questa configurazione è presente solo nel 50% dei pazienti. I test di funzionalità polmonare, nei bambini più grandi, rivelano un tipico quadro ostruttivo (vedi Capitolo 371).

Nel bambino in grado di collaborare, è possibile valutare la clearance mucociliare misurando il tempo necessario per la percezione del sapore di una particella di saccarina, posta sul turbinato nasale inferiore (normalmente <30 min). Il raschiamento o il *brushing* (spazzolamento) della mucosa nasale possono essere esaminati direttamente alla luce, o meglio ancora al microscopio a contrasto di fase, per rilevare la motilità. Nella maggior parte dei campioni tissutali di PCD, si osserva una motilità ciliare scarsa o assente. Poiché è stata documentata una motilità importante nei campioni di numerosi individui con assenza dei bracci di dineina, l'esame del tessuto *in vivo*, al microscopio ottico, può essere utilizzato solo come strumento di screening. Il ***gold standard*** è la documentazione quantitativa di elementi strutturali anomali, come la mancanza dei bracci di dineina o l'orientamento casuale delle ciglia, nelle biopsie o nei campioni da raschiamento nasale o bronchiale, all'esame al microscopio elettronico. La concordanza delle anomalie ultrastrutturali nelle ciglia e negli spermatozoi non è completa. Per evitare le alterazioni ciliari acquisite, i campioni di mucosa non devono essere prelevati prima che siano trascorse 2 settimane da un'infezione acuta delle vie respiratorie. La valutazione ultrastrutturale deve essere riservata ai casi altamente sospetti. Alcune anomalie strutturali sono osservabili anche dopo che un'infezione virale o l'esposizione a biossido di zolfo (anidride solforosa) hanno danneggiato le cellule epiteliali ciliate. Per avere la prova definitiva che un'alterazione strutturale rappresenta una forma discreta di PCD occorre attendere l'identificazione delle mutazioni genetiche.

L'ossido nitrico (NO, *Nitric Oxyde*) espirato risulta nettamente diminuito nei pazienti con PCD, rispetto a quelli senza PCD, in particolare a quelli con fibrosi cistica, bronchiectasie idiopatiche, sinusite isolata e ai controlli normali. Un basso valore di NO può non essere diagnostico, ma un livello elevato suggerisce una patologia diversa dalla PCD.

TRATTAMENTO. La terapia è sintomatica. Si raccomanda di favorire la tosse. La fisioterapia respiratoria aiuta a eliminare il muco. Gli antibiotici devono essere prescritti in caso di evidenza di infezione dei seni o delle vie aeree inferiori. Se possibile, si raccomanda di scegliere il farmaco da utilizzare tenendo conto del microrganismo patogeno e della sua sensibilità: spesso si tratta di pneumococchi (vedi Capitolo 181) o *Haemophilus influenzae* non tipizzabili (vedi Capitolo 192). La somministrazione di antibiotici per via orale è abitualmente efficace. I broncodilatatori devono essere utilizzati nel broncospasmo sintomatico o se è stata documentata un'ostruzione reversibile delle vie aeree. I bambini vanno esaminati diverse volte all'anno e seguiti con radiografie periodiche del torace e con test di funzionalità polmonare seriati. I sintomi sinusali e dell'orecchio medio refrattari alla terapia medica devono essere sottoposti all'attenzione di un otorinolaringoiatra. L'intervento chirurgico può essere utile in casi selezionati. È altamente raccomandabile la prevenzione dell'infezione polmonare con i vaccini per morbillo, pertosse, influenza e, se possibile, pneumococco. Un'altra misura preventiva consiste nell'astensione del fumo di sigaretta e da altri irritanti delle vie aeree.

PROGNOSI. La progressione della malattia polmonare sembra molto più lenta nei pazienti con PCD, rispetto a quelli con CF. Con un adeguato trattamento, una malattia polmonare disabilitante può essere evitata per lunghi periodi. Una normale aspettativa di vita è possibile.

Afzelius BA: Cilia-related diseases. *J Pathol* 2004;204:470–477.

Al-Shroof M, Karnik AM, Karnik AA, et al: Ciliary dyskinesia associated with hydrocephalus and mental retardation in a Jordanian family. *Mayo Clin Proc* 2001;76:1219–1224.

Brueckner M: Cilia propel the embryo in the right direction. *Am J Med Genet* 2001;101:339–344.

Bush A, O'Callaghan C: Primary ciliary dyskinesia. *Arch Dis Child* 2002;87:363–365.

Bush A, Payne D, Pike S, et al: Mucus properties in children with primary ciliary dyskinesia: comparison with cystic fibrosis. *Chest* 2006;129(1): 118–123.

Chodhari R, Mitchison HM, Meeks M: Cilia, primary ciliary dyskinesia and molecular genetics. *Pediatr Respir Rev* 2004;5:69–76.

Noone PG, Leigh MW, Sannuti A, et al: Primary ciliary dyskinesia: Diagnostic and phenotypic features. *Am J Respir Crit Care Med* 2004;169:459–467.

Olbrich H, Haffner K, Kispert A, et al: Mutations in DNAH5 cause primary ciliary dyskinesia and randomization of left-right asymmetry. *Nat Genet* 2002;30:143–144.

Rutland J, de Iongh RU: Random ciliary orientation: A cause of respiratory tract disease. *N Engl J Med* 1990;323:1681–1684.

Wodehouse T, Kharitonov SA, Mackay IS, et al: Nasal nitric oxide measurements for the screening of primary ciliary dyskinesia. *Eur Respir J* 2003; 21:43–47.

Capitolo 402 ■ Pneumopatie interstiziali

Michelle S. Howenstine

L'espressione "pneumopatie interstiziali" (ILD, *Interstitial Lung Diseases*) nei lattanti e nei bambini indica un gruppo di malattie poco comuni, eterogenee, familiari o sporadiche, che causano alterazione dello scambio gassoso alveolare e sintomi di pneumopatia restrittiva. La conoscenza delle ILD in età pediatrica è limitata, a causa della loro rarità, della variabilità dello spettro patologico e della mancanza di studi clinici controllati che abbiano approfondito il processo patologico e le misure terapeutiche. La fisiopatologia è ritenuta più complessa di quella della malattia nell'adulto, poiché la lesione insorge durante il processo di crescita e differenziazione polmonare. Nelle ILD, l'insulto iniziale causa un danno all'epitelio alveolare e all'endotelio capillare. La riparazione anomala del tessuto danneggiato può essere più importante dell'infiammazione, nelle fasi iniziali dello sviluppo di ILD cronica. Alcuni casi familiari, ereditati come tratto autosomico dominante, possono essere dovuti a mutazioni dei geni delle proteine del surfattante, specificamente della proteina C del surfattante (SP-C, *Surfactant Protein*-C). Anche alcuni casi sporadici possono anche avere analoghe mutazioni genetiche della SP-C.

CLASSIFICAZIONE E ANATOMIA PATOLOGICA. Sebbene la classificazione delle ILD nei bambini non sia standardizzata, è comunque utile distinguere le patologie a eziologia nota da quelle a eziologia sconosciuta (Tab. 402-1). Le infezioni respiratorie causate da adenovirus (vedi Capitolo 259), virus influenzali (vedi Capitolo 255), *Chlamydia* (vedi Capitolo 222) e *Mycoplasma pneumoniae* (vedi Capitolo 220), pur essendo in genere malattie autolimitanti, sono state associate a danno polmonare prolungato e progressivo, spesso sotto forma di bronchiolite obliterante. L'**aspirazione** è una causa frequente di pneumopatia cronica, in età infantile. I bambini con ritardo di sviluppo o debolezza neuromuscolare sono ad aumentato rischio di aspirazione di cibo, saliva o corpi estranei, a causa di disfunzioni della deglutizione e/o di reflusso gastroesofageo. Anche una fistola tracheoesofagea non diagnosticata può dar luogo a complicanze polmonari, correlate all'aspirazione di contenuto gastrico e a polmonite interstiziale. I bambini che presentano un'esagerata risposta immunitaria alle polveri organiche, alle muffe o ad antigeni aviari possono contrarre una **polmonite da ipersensibilità**; quelli con tumori possono sviluppare una ILD correlata alla neoplasia di base, a infezioni opportunistiche o secondaria alla chemioterapia o alla radioterapia. Sono state descritte forme peculiari di ILD, in lattanti che presentano tachipnea cronica, retrazioni, crepitii e ipossiemia (Tab. 402-2). Alcuni difetti delle proteine del surfattante possono essere associati alle forme familiari o sporadiche di pneumopatia cronica. La prognosi di queste malattie è variabile.

La **polmonite interstiziale comune** è la forma più frequente di ILD negli adulti, mentre è rara nei bambini. La lesione polmonare è caratterizzata da una distribuzione mista di infiammazione persistente e fibrosi progressiva allo stadio terminale, irregolare ed eterogenea. Per la diagnosi ci si avvale della biopsia, in quanto non vi sono caratteristiche cliniche o radiologiche definitive. La diagnosi di *polmonite interstiziale desquamativa* (DIP, *Desquamative Interstitial Pneumonitis*) si basa sulla dimostrazione bioptica di un processo uniforme e omogeneo, caratterizzato da iperplasia delle cellule epiteliali alveolari con accumulo di grossi macrofagi negli spazi aerei. Di solito non si osserva fibrosi. In alcuni lattanti con istologia simile a quella della DIP è stata diagnosticata una carenza di surfattante B. È stata descritta una forma familiare nei bambini piccoli, insolitamente severa e spesso fatale.

La **polmonite interstiziale linfocitica** (LIP, *Lymphocytic Interstitial Pneumonitis*), la forma più comune di ILD in età pediatrica, è una forma di malattia linfoproliferativa polmonare. La LIP di solito si sviluppa in associazione a condizioni di alterata immunità, come una malattia autoimmune o un'immunodeficienza (infezione da HIV). L'interstizio polmonare è invaso da un infiltrato diffuso con linfociti maturi. La fibrosi è rara. L'infezione virale, come quella causata dal virus di Epstein-Barr (vedi Capitolo 251), spesso è un fattore che contribuisce allo sviluppo della LIP pediatrica.

TABELLA 402-1. Pneumopatie interstiziali in età pediatrica

PNEUMOPATIE INTERSTIZIALI A EZIOLOGIA NOTA
Sindromi da aspirazione
Infezioni croniche (virali, batteriche, fungine, parassitarie)
Ospite immunocompetente
Ospite immunocompromesso
Displasia broncopolmonare
Polmonite da ipersensibilità (da farmaci, ambientale o associata a esposizione occupazionale)*
Linfangioleiomiomatosi
Deficit di proteina B o C del surfattante
PNEUMOPATIE INTERSTIZIALI A EZIOLOGIA SCONOSCIUTA
Polmonite interstiziale comune
Polmonite desquamativa (DIP, *Desquamative Interstitial Pneumonitis*)
Polmonite interstiziale linfocitica (LIP, *Lymphocytic Interstitial Pneumonitis*) e disturbi correlati
Polmonite interstiziale aspecifica
Emosiderosi polmonare
Malattia di Goodpasture
Infiltrati polmonari con eosinofilia
Glicogenosi interstiziale polmonare
Iperplasia cellulare neuroendocrina dell'infanzia
Bronchiolite obliterante
Bronchiolite obliterante con polmonite organizzata
Proteinosi alveolare
Malattia vascolari polmonari (proliferative e congenite)
Malattie linfatiche polmonari
Microlitiasi polmonare
ALTRI DISTURBI CON COINVOLGIMENTO POLMONARE
Connettivopatie (artrite reumatoide, lupus eritematoso sistemico, dermatomiosite)
Tumori
Istiocitosi a cellule di Langerhans
Sindrome di Churg-Strauss
Sarcoidosi
Granulomatosi di Wegener
Sindromi neurocutanee (neurofibromatosi, sclerosi tuberosa)
Malattie da accumulo (morbo di Gaucher, morbo di Niemann-Pick)
Sindrome di Hermansky-Pudlak

*I farmaci comprendono antibiotici (penicillina, nitrofurantoina, cefalosporine, isoniazide, sulfamidici), terapia antineoplastica, sostanze stupefacenti, ossigeno, radiazioni e integratori dietetici. L'esposizione occupazionale o ambientale comprende polveri organiche e inorganiche, polmone del contadino, polmone dell'allevatore di uccelli, bagassosi, esalazioni (fumi, vapori), idrocarburi, resine e ossidi di azoto.

Modificata da Fan LL: Pediatric interstitial lung disease. In Schwartz MI, King TE (ed): *Interstitial Lung Disease*, 3rd ed. Toronto, BC Decker, 1998, p 103.

TABELLA 402-2. Forme di pneumopatia interstiziale peculiari dell'infanzia

Tachipnea persistente dell'infanzia
Bronchite/bronchiolite follicolare
Emosiderosi polmonare infantile
Polmonite cronica infantile
Malattie da deficit della proteina del surfattante
Polmonite interstiziale desquamativa familiare (DIP, *Desquamative Interstitial Pneumonitis*)
Fibrosi polmonare idiopatica dell'infanzia

Da Fan LL: Pediatric interstitial lung disease. In Schwarz MI, King TE (ed): *Interstitial Lung Disease*, 3rd ed. Toronto, BC Decker, 1998, p. 104.

La **polmonite interstiziale acuta**, anche nota come polmonite interstiziale rapidamente progressiva o sindrome di Hamman-Rich, è una forma distinta, rapidamente progressiva, di ILD. Il danno alveolare progredisce da un processo essudativo acuto a una fibrosi severa. Spesso non è identificabile un insulto antecedente; la fatalità è >50%.

MANIFESTAZIONI CLINICHE. È necessaria un'anamnesi dettagliata per valutare la gravità dei sintomi e la possibile presenza di una malattia sistemica sottostante. L'identificazione dei fattori precipitanti, come l'esposizione a muffe o a uccelli, o un'infezione severa delle vie aeree inferiori, è importante per stabilire la diagnosi e istituire misure di prevenzione. Un'anamnesi familiare positiva, specialmente in un lattante affetto, è suggestiva di una malattia genetica o familiare, come un deficit di proteina B o C del surfattante (vedi Capitoli 403 e 404). In più del 60% dei pazienti si riscontrano tachipnea, tosse, dispnea e intolleranza allo sforzo; la maggioranza ha una ridotta saturazione arteriosa di ossigeno. L'ipercapnia è una complicanza tardiva. I sintomi sono di solito insidiosi e insorgono con andamento continuo, non episodico. In più del 50% dei pazienti, sono presenti tachipnea e crepitii basali. Si osservano frequentemente retrazioni, mancato accrescimento, ippocratismo digitale e sibili. La presenza di cianosi e di un secondo tono cardiaco pronunciato sono indicativi di una malattia severa. L'anemia o l'emottisi suggeriscono una vasculopatia polmonare o l'emosiderosi polmonare. I rash o i disturbi articolari sono compatibili con una connettivopatia sottostante.

DIAGNOSI. Inizialmente si ricorre a esami non invasivi per valutare l'estensione e la gravità della malattia. Le anomalie riscontrabili alla radiografia del torace possono essere classificate in interstiziali, reticolari, nodulari, reticolonodulari o a nido d'ape. Il radiogramma del torace può anche essere normale, nonostante una compromissione clinica significativa, e avere una scarsa correlazione con l'estensione della malattia. La TC ad alta risoluzione (HRCT, *High Resolution Computed Tomography*) del torace definisce meglio l'estensione e la distribuzione della malattia e può fornire informazioni specifiche che aiutano il medico a scegliere una sede per la biopsia. Modalità più veloci, come la TC spirale, elicoidale o ultrarapida, possono offrire una risoluzione precisa dei quadri patologici nei lattanti tachipnoici. Può essere utile ottenere immagini HRCT in serie per monitorare la progressione e la gravità della malattia.

I test di funzionalità polmonare sono importanti per definire il grado di **pneumopatia restrittiva** e per seguire la risposta al trattamento. Nelle ILD, le anomalie della funzione polmonare denotano un deficit ventilatorio restrittivo con volumi polmonari ridotti. La capacità funzionale residua (FRC, *Functional Residual Capacity*) è diminuita, ma di solito in misura minore della capacità vitale (VC, *Vital Capacity*) e della capacità polmonare totale (TLC, *Total Lung Capacity*). Il volume residuo (RV, *Residual Volume*) è di solito conservato; pertanto i rapporti FRC:TLC e RV:TLC sono spesso aumentati. La capacità di diffusione del monossido di carbonio (DLCO, *Diffusion of Carbon Monoxide*) in genere risulta normale quando corretta per il ridotto volume alveolare. Un'alterazione della DLCO può suggerire una malattia vascolare. Il lavaggio broncoalveolare (BAL, *BronchoAlveolar Lavage*) può fornire informazioni utili su infezioni secondarie, sanguinamento o aspirazione, ma di solito non permette di determinare la diagnosi esatta. È tuttavia diagnostico per la **proteinosi polmonare alveolare**. La biopsia polmonare transtoracica, per l'esame istopatologico, di solito rappresenta l'ultimo passo necessario per una diagnosi conclusiva. Si utilizzano la toracotomia convenzionale o la toracoscopia videoassistita, per ottenere un campione di tessuto da un bambino con sospetta ILD. Può inoltre essere necessaria una valutazione per escludere eventuali malattie sistemiche.

TRATTAMENTO. Il trattamento di supporto è essenziale e comprende la somministrazione di ossigeno per l'ipossia e un'adeguata nutrizione per il deficit dell'accrescimento. Può essere necessario un trattamento antimicrobico per le infezioni intercorrenti. Alcuni pazienti sono responsivi ai broncodilatatori. Il trattamento antinfiammatorio con corticosteroidi rimane la terapia di scelta iniziale. Mancano studi controllati nei bambini, e la risposta clinica riportata negli studi sui casi singoli è variabile. La dose usuale di prednisone 1-2 mg/kg/die per 6-8 settimane, a scalare in base alla risposta clinica. Terapie alternative, sebbene non adeguatamente valutate, comprendono idrossiclorochina, azatioprina, ciclofosfamide, metotrexato, immunoglobuline endovena e boli di steroidi ad alte dosi. Il trattamento con idrossiclorochina ha avuto successo in alcuni bambini con ILD classica, in particolare in quelli con le alterazioni istopatologiche della DIP. Il trapianto polmonare per la ILD progressiva o terminale ha avuto successo in alcuni lattanti e bambini. È indicato il trattamento appropriato per le malattie sistemiche sottostanti. Le misure preventive consistono nell'evitare tutti gli irritanti inalatori, come il fumo di tabacco e, talvolta, le muffe e gli antigeni aviari. Possono essere utili programmi di riabilitazione polmonare supervisionati sotto controllo medico.

PROGNOSI. La mortalità complessiva da ILD dipende dalla diagnosi specifica e può raggiungere il 20% nei lattanti e nei bambini. La prognosi è variabile ed è infausta nei bambini con ipertensione polmonare, mancato accrescimento e fibrosi severa.

COUNSELING GENETICO. L'elevata incidenza di pneumopatie interstiziali in alcune famiglie induce a pensare che la predisposizione genetica giochi un ruolo tanto nell'insorgenza della malattia quanto nella sua gravità. Il counseling genetico può essere utile, se è presente un'anamnesi familiare di malattia.

Atival A, Godrey S, Maayan C, et al: Chloroquine treatment of interstitial lung disease in children. *Pediatr Pulmonol* 1994;18:356–360.

Cameron HS, Somaschini M, Carrera P, et al: A common mutation in the surfactant protein C gene associated with lung disease. *J Pediatr* 2005;146:370–375.

Clement A, ERS Task Force: Task force on chronic interstitial lung disease in immunocompetent children. *Eur Respir J* 2004;24:686–697.

Fan LL, Kozinetz CA, Wojtczak HA, et al: The diagnostic value of transbronchial, thoracoscopic and open lung biopsy in immunocompetent children with chronic interstitial lung disease. *J Pediatr* 1997;131:565–569.

Fan LL, Langston C: Chronic interstitial lung disease in children. *Pediatr Pulmonol* 1993;16:184–196.

Nogee LM: Genetics of pediatric interstitial lung disease. *Curr Opin Pediatr* 2006;18:287–292.

Shulenin S, Nogee LM, Annilo T, et at: ABCA3 gene mutations in newborns with fatal surfactant deficiency. *N Engl J Med* 2004;350:1296–1303.

Sondheimer HM, Lum Lung MC, Brugman SM, et al: Pulmonary vascular disorders masquerading as interstitial lung disease. *Pediatr Pulmonol* 1995;20:284–288.

Teirstein AS: The elusive goal of therapy for usual interstitial pneumonia. *N Engl J Med* 2004;350:181–183.

Capitolo 403 ■ Proteinosi alveolare polmonare

Aaron Hamvas, Lawrence M. Nogee, Stuart C. Sweet e F. Sessions Cole

La proteinosi alveolare polmonare (PAP) è una malattia caratterizzata dall'accumulo intra-alveolare di lipoproteine del surfattante polmonare. All'esame istopatologico, gli spazi aerei distali appaiono occupati da un materiale granulare, eosinofilo, positivo alla colorazione con l'acido periodico di Schiff e diastasi-resistente. Nei bambini, ne sono state descritte due forme, clinicamente distinte: una forma fulminante, spesso fatale, che si presenta poco dopo la nascita (**PAP congenita**), e un tipo gradualmente progressivo, che si presenta nei lattanti e nei bambini più grandi, simile alla PAP osservata negli adulti. La PAP negli individui più grandi è spesso classificata come primitiva, idiopatica (acquisita) o secondaria a numerose condizioni riconosciute (tumori, immunosoppressione, polveri inorganiche, fumi tossici, infezioni).

EZIOLOGIA E FISIOPATOLOGIA. Lo sviluppo precoce della forma neonatale di PAP, la sua incessante progressione fino al decesso e l'osservazione di casi familiari suggeriscono una base genetica. Alterazioni genetiche singole, che portano alla forma neonatale della PAP, comprendono mutazioni dei geni della proteina B del surfattante (SP-B), della proteina C del surfattante (SP-C), della catena β del recettore del fattore stimolante le colonie di granulociti e macrofagi (GM-CSF, *Granulocyte-Macrophage Colony-Stimulating Factor*), e dell'ABCA3 (*ATP-Binding Cassette Transporter*) (vedi Capitolo 404). Anche la proteinosi alveolare è stata riportata nei bambini, compresi quelli molto piccoli, come l'intolleranza alle proteine lisinurica (LPI, *Lysinuric Protein Intolerance*), una rara malattia autosomica recessiva causata da mutazioni nel trasportatore cationico degli aminoacidi SLC7A7. Questi pazienti presentano generalmente vomito, iperammoniemia e mancato sviluppo, sebbene la loro malattia polmonare possa rivelarsi fatale. La relazione tra il difetto di base e lo sviluppo di PAP non è chiara, sebbene un caso di recidiva della malattia dopo trapianto di polmone faccia pensare che la disfunzione dei macrofagi alveolari sia probabilmente importante nella patogenesi della PAP associata a LPI.

La **PAP primitiva (idiopatica)**, negli adulti, è una malattia autoimmune mediata da autoanticorpi diretti contro il GM-CSF. Il GM-CSF è essenziale nella regolazione della funzione macrofagica e della clearance del surfattante. Nel liquido di broncolavaggio alveolare (BAL, *BronchoAlveolar Lavage*) e nel siero di adulti con PAP primitiva si possono trovare elevati titoli di immunoglobuline (Ig) neutralizzanti IgG1 e autoanticorpi IgG2, diretti contro il GM-CSF. Questi autoanticorpi bloccano il legame del GM-CSF al suo recettore, inibendo così la funzione dei macrofagi alveolari e la clearance del surfattante. Essi sono stati trovati nei bambini più grandi con forme apparentemente primitive di PAP, ma non sono stati identificati nelle forme congenite di proteinosi alveolare.

La **proteinosi alveolare secondaria** può insorgere in associazione a infezioni, in particolare negli individui immunocompromessi. Anche l'esposizione ambientale a polveri, silice e agenti chimici è posta in relazione con lo sviluppo di proteinosi alveolare secondaria.

MANIFESTAZIONI CLINICHE. I lattanti con PAP congenita si presentano nell'immediato periodo postnatale e sviluppano rapidamente insufficienza respiratoria. Non si notano variazioni di frequenza nei due sessi. La PAP congenita è clinicamente e radiologicamente indistinguibile da disturbi più comuni del neonato che causano insufficienza respiratoria, come polmoniti, infezioni batteriche generalizzate, sindrome da distress respiratorio e ritorno venoso polmonare anomalo totale con ostruzione. La diagnosi differenziale comprende anche l'ipertensione polmonare primitiva del neonato, l'aspirazione di meconio e la displasia alveolocapillare, sebbene le caratteristiche radiologiche di queste malattie siano di solito differenti. L'incidenza della PAP congenita è sconosciuta; fu citata sul certificato di morte di 37 lattanti che morirono nel primo anno di vita, in una coorte di 1 052 554 nati in Missouri tra il 1979 e il 1992.

Altrettanto rara è la proteinosi alveolare idiopatica (acquisita) nei lattanti e nei bambini più grandi. I maschi sono colpiti tre volte più frequentemente delle femmine. Di solito è priva di un fattore eziologico identificabile (primitiva), ma può insorgere in associazione a tumori o infezioni, in particolare nel contesto di un'immunosoppressione sistemica o di un'immunodeficienza congenita, o dopo esposizione a diversi agenti, tra cui polvere o sostanze chimiche (secondaria). I lattanti più grandi e i bambini con PAP si presentano con dispnea, astenia, tosse, calo ponderale, dolore toracico o emottisi. Negli stadi avanzati, si possono osservare cianosi e ippocratismo digitale. Le alterazioni della funzione polmonare comprendono ridotta capacità di diffusione del monossido di carbonio (D_LCO), volumi polmonari con un quadro restrittivo ed emogasanalisi con marcata ipossiemia o acidosi respiratoria cronica.

DIAGNOSI. L'esame istopatologico dei campioni bioptici polmonari è il *gold standard* per la diagnosi, nei bambini. Nei pazienti con proteinosi alveolare causata da meccanismi diversi dal deficit di SP-B, la colorazione immunoistochimica rivela abbondanti quantità alveolari e intracellulari di proteine A e B del surfattante. I test di agglutinazione al lattice per la presenza degli anticorpi anti-GM-CSF nell'escreato o nel liquido del BAL, per le componenti del surfattante, sono stati usati a fini diagnostici nell'adulto, mentre non hanno ancora avuto convalida nei bambini. Nei protocolli di ricerca sono disponibili l'esame del sangue periferico e/o del midollo osseo per la stimolazione clonogena dei precursori dei monociti-macrofagi, per la ricerca del recettore del GM-CSF e dell'espressione del ligando e del legame del GM-CSF.

TRATTAMENTO. La proteinosi alveolare nei neonati, che dà luogo a un deficit di SP-B, è rapidamente fatale; a tutt'oggi non esiste alcuna terapia medica efficace. La storia naturale delle altre forme di PAP è significativamente più variabile, rendendo difficili le decisioni prognostiche e terapeutiche. Il lavaggio polmonare totale è stato associato a remissioni prolungate della PAP negli adulti, e rimane una possibilità terapeutica per i pazienti con forme a esordio tardivo. È invece inefficace nelle forme congenite della malattia, dovute a errori congeniti del metabolismo del surfattante. Il ruolo del BAL ripetuto, nel bambino, non è stato ben studiato; in alcune circostanze può aiutare a prendere tempo e dare beneficio nei pazienti con PAP autoimmune o secondaria. La somministrazione sottocutanea o per via inalatoria di GM-CSF ricombinante può migliorare la funzione polmonare in alcuni adulti con proteinosi alveolare idiopatica primitiva (autoimmune). I titoli di anticorpi anti-GM-CSF possono ridursi durante il trattamento con GM-CSF, suggerendo che questa terapia sia in grado di desensibilizzare il paziente. Questi interventi non hanno avuto successo nel trattamento a lungo termine dei neonati. Il trapianto di polmone è una possibilità terapeutica, il cui utilizzo è tuttavia limitato dai dubbi sulla recidiva di malattia in assenza di un meccanismo primitivo definito di danno polmonare.

Borsani G, Bassi MT, Sperandeo MP, et al: SLC7A7, encoding a putative permease-related protein, is mutated in patients with lysinuric protein intolerance. *Nat Genet* 1999;21:297–301.

de Blic J: Pulmonary alveolar proteinosis in children. *Paediatr Resp Rev* 2004;5:316–322.

Kitamura T, Uchida K, Tanaka N, et al: Serological diagnosis of idiopathic pulmonary alveolar proteinosis. *Am J Respir Crit Care Med* 2000; 162:658–662.

Mahut B, Delacourt C, Scheinmann P, et al: Pulmonary alveolar proteinosis: Experience with eight pediatric cases and a review. *Pediatrics* 1996; 97:117–122.

Seymour JF, Presneill JJ, Schoch OD, et al: Therapeutic efficacy of granulocyte-macrophage colony-stimulating factor in patients with idiopathic acquired alveolar proteinosis. *Am J Respir Crit Care Med* 2001; 163:524–531.

Trapnell BC, Whitsett JA, Nakata K: Pulmonary alveolar proteinosis. *N Engl J Med* 2003;329:2527–2539.

Uchida K, Nakata K, Trapnell BC, et al: High-affinity autoantibodies specifically eliminate granulocyte-macrophage colony-stimulating factor activity in the lungs of patients with idiopathic pulmonary alveolar proteinosis. *Blood* 2004;103:1089–1098.

Capitolo 404 ■ Disordini ereditari del metabolismo del surfattante

Aaron Hamvas, Lawrence M. Nogee e F. Sessions Cole

Il surfattante polmonare è una miscela di fosfolipidi e proteine sintetizzate, impacchettate e secrete dagli pneumociti di tipo II. Questa miscela forma un unico strato a livello dell'interfaccia aria-liquido, che abbassa la tensione di superficie al termine dell'espirazione, durante il ciclo respiratorio, impedendo così l'atelettasia e lo squilibrio del rapporto ventilazione-perfusione. Sono state descritte quattro proteine associate al surfattante: le proteine A e D (SP-A, SP-D) partecipano alla difesa dell'ospite nel polmone, mentre le B e C (SP-B, SP-C) contribuiscono all'attività di riduzione della tensione di superficie del surfattante polmonare. Due geni per la SP-A (*SFTPA1*, *SFTPA2*) e un gene per SP-D (*SFTPD*) sono localizzati sul cromosoma umano 10, mentre singoli geni localizzati sui cromosomi umani 2 e 8 codificano per SP-B (*SFTPB*) e SP-C (*SFTPC*), rispettivamente. Sebbene non siano stati identificati nell'uomo deficit ereditari di SP-A o SP-B, i topi geneticamente modificati, con deficit di queste proteine, vanno soggetti a infezioni virali e batteriche, e le linee con deficit di SP-D accumulano lipidi e macrofagi schiumosi nei polmoni, sviluppando enfisema con il passare del tempo. Nell'uomo sono state identificate alterazioni ereditarie di SP-B e SP-C. A3, il componente dell'ABCA3, è un trasportatore localizzato sulla membrana limitante dei corpi lamellari, gli organuli di accumulo del surfattante nelle cellule alveolari di tipo II. Mutazioni recessive nel gene ABCA3 (*ABCA3*), codificato sul cromosoma umano 16, sono state associate a un deficit letale del surfattante.

DEFICIT DI PROTEINA B DEL SURFATTANTE

GENETICA. Sono state identificate più di 30 mutazioni con perdita di funzione di *SFTPB*: la più comune è un'inserzione netta di 2 coppie di basi nel codone 121 (chiamata *121ins2*) che determina uno spostamento (*frameshift*), un trascritto SP-B instabile e la mancata produzione di proteina SP-B. L'inserzione dà luogo al polimorfismo di un frammento di restrizione (RFLP, *Restriction Fragment Polymophism*), utile per la diagnosi. Questa mutazione è responsabile del 60-70% degli alleli riscontrati finora, nei pazienti in cui è stato identificato un deficit di SP-B. La maggior parte delle altre mutazioni è famiglia-specifica.

ANATOMIA PATOLOGICA. Sebbene il deficit di SP-B sia stato il primo descritto in un paziente con esordio neonatale di proteinosi alveolare, questo quadro istologico non è né specifico per il deficit di SP-B, né universalmente presente nei polmoni dei bambini affetti. Numerosi pazienti con deficit di SP-B, omozigoti per la mutazione 121ins2, hanno caratteristiche istologiche più tipiche della **polmonite interstiziale desquamativa** (vedi Capitolo 402), con accumulo di macrofagi e scarsa proteinosi alveolare rilevabile al momento del trapianto polmonare. Altri reperti sono aspecifici e comprendono fibrosi interstiziale di grado variabile e iperplasia delle cellule alveolari. I reperti ultrastrutturali consistono in mancanza della mielina tubulare, disorganizzazione dei corpi lamellari e accumulo di corpi multivescicolari di aspetto anomalo, che suggeriscono un'alterazione della sintesi e della secrezione dei lipidi.

MANIFESTAZIONI CLINICHE. I lattanti con un deficit ereditario della SP-B si presentano nell'immediato periodo neonatale con insufficienza respiratoria. Questa malattia autosomica recessiva è simile, dal punto di vista clinico e radiologico, alla sindrome da distress respiratorio (RDS, *Respiratory Distress Syndrome*) dei nati prematuri (vedi Capitolo 101.4), ma colpisce tipicamente i nati a termine. Il grado iniziale di distress respiratorio è variabile, ma la malattia è progressiva, refrattaria alla ventilazione meccanica, alla terapia sostitutiva con surfattante, alla somministrazione di steroidi e all'ossigenazione a membrana extracorporea. Il deficit di SP-B è stato riconosciuto in diversi gruppi etnici e razziali. Quasi tutti i pazienti non sottoposti a trapianto polmonare sono deceduti; la sopravvivenza prolungata è possibile nei casi con deficit parziale di SP-B. Nell'uomo, gli eterozigoti per le mutazioni con perdita di funzione del gene SP-B sono clinicamente normali da adulti e hanno una funzione polmonare normale.

DIAGNOSI. È possibile formulare una diagnosi rapida e definitiva grazie all'analisi del DNA, per la ricerca delle mutazioni note di *SFTPB*, in particolare la mutazione 121ins2 (utilizzando l'analisi RFLP del DNA genomico amplificato tramite reazione a catena della polimerasi [PCR, *Polymerase Chain Reaction*]). La sensibilità della diagnosi genetica è limitata, poiché la malattia può risultare anche da mutazioni non ancora riconosciute. Nelle famiglie in cui è stata precedentemente identificata una mutazione, si può effettuare la diagnosi prenatale, con l'analisi molecolare del DNA da biopsia dei villi coriali o degli amniociti. Altri esami di laboratorio, ancora in fase sperimentale, comprendono l'analisi del fluido tracheale con test enzimatico ELISA (*Enzyme-Linked Immunosorbent Assay*) o *Western Blot* per la ricerca della proteina SP-B e di peptidi precursori proSP-B processati in modo aberrante, che sono stati trovati in lattanti e animali con deficit di SP-B. La diagnosi può essere supportata anche dalla colorazione immunoistochimica del tessuto proveniente da biopsia polmonare, per la ricerca delle proteine del surfattante, sebbene attualmente gli esami immunoistochimici per la SP-B e la SP-C siano disponibili solo in ambito di ricerca. In generale, la colorazione per la SP-B è assente, ma si osserva una spiccata colorazione extracellulare per la proSP-C dovuta a una processazione aberrante dei peptidi della proSP-C, diagnostica per il deficit di SP-B. Questi studi richiedono una biopsia polmonare in un bambino in condizioni critiche, ma possono essere effettuati anche sui campioni polmonari acquisiti al momento dell'autopsia, consentendo una diagnosi retrospettiva.

TRATTAMENTO. Virtualmente, tutti i pazienti con deficit di SP-B muoiono entro il primo anno di vita. Gli interventi convenzionali di terapia intensiva neonatale possono mantenere la funzione degli organi extrapolmonari per un tempo limitato (settimane o mesi). Il trattamento sostitutivo con i surfattanti disponibili in commercio è inefficace. Il trapianto polmonare è stato effettuato con successo, ma le cure mediche e chirurgiche necessarie prima, durante e dopo il trapianto sono altamente specialistiche e disponibili soltanto nei centri di trapianto polmonare pediatrico. Pertanto, è essenziale una diagnosi tempestiva se il paziente deve essere preso in considerazione per il trapianto polmonare. Il paziente più "anziano" vivente con deficit di SP-B, sopravvissuto grazie al trapianto polmonare, è nato nel 1994. La sopravvivenza a 5 anni dopo trapianto polmonare è del 50% circa, analoga quindi a quella per altre cause di trapianto polmonare infantile. Possono svilupparsi anticorpi anti SP-B, che però non hanno effetto sull'organo trapiantato. È importante il counseling genetico, per comunicare il rischio per gravidanze future e la disponibilità della diagnosi prenatale e delle opzioni terapeutiche. È utile anche una consulenza palliativistica.

ANOMALIE DELLA PROTEINA C DEL SURFATTANTE

La SP-C è una proteina a bassissimo peso molecolare, estremamente idrofobica, che, insieme alla SP-B, aumenta la prerogativa dei fosfolipidi del surfattante di ridurre la tensione di superficie. Deriva dal processamento proteolitico di una proteina precursore di dimensioni maggiori (proSP-C).

GENETICA. Sono state identificate più di 35 mutazioni a espressione dominante di *SFTPC*, in associazione a pneumopatie acute e croniche, in pazienti di età compresa tra il periodo neonatale e l'età adulta. Circa il 55% di queste mutazioni insorge spontaneamente, causando forme sporadiche di malattia; le rimanenti sono ereditarie. La sostituzione dell'isoleucina con la treonina, nel codone 73 (chiamata *I73T*), è responsabile del 25% dei casi identificati finora. Si ritiene che le mutazioni dell'*SFTPC* determinino la produzione di proSP-C con anomalie del ripiegamento, che si accumula negli pneumociti di tipo II causando danno cellulare. La frequenza delle mutazioni di *SFTPC* e della malattia che ne deriva è sconosciuta. Sono state identificate mutazioni in diversi gruppi etnici e razziali.

ANATOMIA PATOLOGICA. L'istopatologia del tessuto polmonare dei pazienti con mutazioni dell'*SFTPC* rientra nella categoria della **polmonite interstiziale**, con una varietà di diagnosi basate in gran parte sulla classificazione delle pneumopatie interstiziali negli adulti, comprendenti la polmonite interstiziale aspecifica, la polmonite interstiziale desquamativa, la fibrosi polmonare idiopatica, la proteinosi polmonare alveolare e la polmonite cronica dell'infanzia.

MANIFESTAZIONI CLINICHE. La presentazione clinica dei pazienti con mutazioni di *SFTPC* è alquanto variabile. Alcuni presentano alla nascita sintomi, segni e reperti radiologici tipici dell'RDS, mentre altri li sviluppano in seguito, dalla prima infanzia all'età adulta, con insorgenza graduale di insufficienza respiratoria, ipossiema, mancato sviluppo e pneumopatia interstiziale alla radiografia. L'età di esordio e la gravità della malattia variano anche all'interno delle famiglie con la stessa mutazione. Anche la storia naturale è piuttosto varabile: alcuni pazienti migliorano spontaneamente o con la terapia, alcuni sviluppano insufficienza respiratoria persistente e altri si aggravano al punto da richiedere il trapianto polmonare. Questa variabilità della gravità e del decorso della malattia, oltre a non sembrare correlata alla mutazione specifica, rende difficoltosa una valutazione accurata della prognosi.

DIAGNOSI. Al contrario del deficit di SP-B, non sono disponibili marcatori biochimici che consentano una diagnosi rapida. La sequenziazione del gene *SFTPC* è l'unico esame diagnostico definitivo, disponibile in alcuni laboratori clinici e di ricerca. Le dimensioni relativamente piccole del gene facilitano queste analisi, che sono abbastanza sensibili, ma poiché la maggior parte delle mutazioni *SFTPC* è di tipo *missense*, può essere difficile distinguere quelle responsabili della malattia dalle varianti benigne.

TRATTAMENTO. Non esiste un trattamento specifico per i pazienti con pneumopatia da mutazioni del gene SP-C. Gli approcci terapeutici utilizzati nelle pneumopatie interstiziali, come la somministrazione di chinolonici o corticosteroidi, sono stati utilizzati ma non valutati sistematicamente. Il trapianto polmonare è riservato ai pazienti con insufficienza respiratoria progressiva e refrattaria, che si qualificherebbero comunque per il trapianto polmonare, a prescindere dalla diagnosi. Il counseling genetico è importante al fine di definire il rischio per le gravidanze future.

MALATTIA CAUSATA DA MUTAZIONI DEL GENE ABCA3

GENETICA. Le mutazioni recessive di *ABCA3* sono state descritte per la prima volta in una serie di 20 lattanti con distress respiratorio letale. Vi è una considerevole eterogeneità allelica; sono state identificate più di 20 mutazioni sparse in tutto il gene, la maggior parte delle quali sono famiglia-specifiche. Finora non è stata individuata alcuna mutazione comune. La frequenza delle mutazioni e della malattia è sconosciuta, ma le mutazioni di *ABCA3*, identificate in diversi gruppi etnici e razziali, possono contribuire a una notevole percentuale di malattie polmonari fatali inspiegate, nei neonati a termine.

ANATOMIA PATOLOGICA. L'anatomia patologica polmonare dei neonati con mutazioni del gene *ABCA3*, peraltro simile a quella dei neonati con mutazioni *SFTPB*, comprende le alterazioni della polmonite interstiziale desquamativa e/o della proteinosi alveolare. All'esame ultrastrutturale, i corpi lamellari appaiono piccoli e contenenti inclusioni elettrondense posizionate eccentricamente, un reperto che può essere caratteristico delle mutazioni di *ABCA3* e che indica che la funzione di questo gene è necessaria per la biogenesi dei corpi lamellari.

MANIFESTAZIONI CLINICHE. I bambini con mutazioni di *ABCA3* hanno tipicamente presentato i primi sintomi nel periodo neonatale, con insufficienza respiratoria severa simile, sotto il profilo clinico e radiologico, a quella dei neonati con deficit di SP-B o dei prematuri con RDS, e refrattaria alle misure standard di terapia intensiva. Tuttavia, l'esperienza con questa malattia è limitata, e il primo gruppo di neonati sottoposti a studio era stato scelto deliberatamente per la gravità della natura della malattia polmonare. Il grado di variabilità fenotipica associato alle mutazioni di *ABCA3* è sconosciuto.

DIAGNOSI. Il sospetto clinico è cruciale per la diagnosi. Attualmente non esistono marcatori biochimici o istopatologici in grado di porre una diagnosi definitiva, sebbene la presenza delle inclusioni dense nei corpi lamellari, all'esame in microscopia elettronica del tessuto polmonare, sia in accordo con la diagnosi. Le dimensioni del gene *ABCA3* (80 kb con 30 esoni codificanti) e il grado di eterogeneità allelica limitano la diagnosi molecolare, che è attualmente disponibile solo a scopo di ricerca.

TRATTAMENTO. Non esiste un trattamento specifico per i pazienti con mutazioni del gene *ABCA3*. I lattanti con insufficienza respiratoria progressiva sono probabili candidati al trapianto polmonare. Il counseling genetico è importante per stabilire il rischio connesso alle gravidanze future.

Cameron HS, Somaschini M, Carrera P, et al: A common mutation in the surfactant protein C gene associated with lung disease. *J Pediatr* 2005;146:370–375.
Cole FS, Hamvas A, Nogee LM: Genetic disorders of neonatal respiratory function. *Pediatr Res* 2001;50:157–162.
Dunbar AE, Wert SE, Hamvas A, et al: Prolonged survival in hereditary surfactant protein B (SP-B) deficiency associated with a novel splicing mutation. *Pediatr Res* 2000;48:275–282.
Hamvas A: Surfactant protein B deficiency: Insights into inherited disorders of lung cell metabolism. *Curr Prob Pediatr* 1997;27:325–345.
Nogee LM, deMello DE, Dehner LP, et al: Pulmonary surfactant protein B deficiency in congenital pulmonary alveolar proteinosis. *N Engl J Med* 1993;328:406–410.
Nogee LM, Dunbar AE III, Wert SE, et al: A mutation in the surfactant protein C gene associated with familial interstitial lung disease. *N Engl J Med* 2001;344:573–579.
Nogee LM, Garnier G, Singer L, et al: A mutation in the surfactant protein B gene responsible for fatal neonatal respiratory disease in multiple kindreds. *J Clin Invest* 1994;93:1860–1863.
Nogee LM, Wert SE, Proffit SA, et al: Allelic heterogeneity in hereditary surfactant protein B (SP-B) deficiency. *Am J Respir Crit Care Med* 2000;161:973–981.
Palomar LM, Nogee LM, Sweet SC, et al: Long-term outcomes after infant lung transplantation for surfactant protein B deficiency related to other causes of respiratory failure. *J Pediatr* 2006;149:548–553.
Shulenin S, Nogee LM, Annilo T, et al: *ABCA3* gene mutations in newborns with fatal surfactant deficiency. *N Engl J Med* 2004;350:1296–1303.
Thomas AQ, Lane K, Phillips J, et al: Heterozygosity for a surfactant protein C gene mutation associated with usual interstitial pneumonitis and cellular nonspecific interstitial pneumonitis in one kindred. *Am J Respir Crit Care Med* 2002;165:1322–1328.

Capitolo 405 ■ Emosiderosi polmonare

Mary A. Nevin

L'emorragia polmonare è di raro riscontro nella popolazione pediatrica; quando presente, è spesso focale e di natura autolimitante. È raro che il sanguinamento rispecchi un'**emorragia alveolare diffusa** (**DAH**, *Diffuse Alveolar Hemorrage*); la diagnosi di emosiderosi polmonare si riferisce appunto a questo processo alveolare più cronico e diffuso. L'emosiderosi polmonare è classicamente caratterizzata dalla triade di anemia sideropenica, emottisi e infiltrati alveolari alla radiografia del torace. Può essere necessario un elevato livello di sospetto clinico, poiché tutte queste caratteristiche della malattia possono essere assenti in qualsiasi momento del decorso. L'emosiderosi polmonare può esistere in forma isolata, ma più comunemente insorge in associazione a una condizione sottostante. Non sempre si trova un'eziologia precisa per l'emorragia. Quando l'emorragia alveolare è isolata e una valutazione accurata per la ricerca di malattie di base risulta negativa, si dice che il paziente ha un'**emosiderosi polmonare idiopatica** (**IPH**, *Idiopathic Pulmonary Hemosiderosis*).

EZIOLOGIA. Alcune delle condizioni che possono associarsi a emorragie diffuse sono elencate nella Tabella 406-3. La maggior parte dei casi di DAH si associa a una malattia di base immunologica, reumatologica o vasculitica, ma possono essere presenti altre diagnosi, in caso di emorragia polmonare ricorrente o cronica.

L'emosiderosi polmonare può essere classificata come primitiva o secondaria. L'**emosiderosi polmonare primitiva** (**PPH**, *Primary Pulmonary Hemosiderosis*) è considerata comprensiva delle diagnosi di IPH, **sindrome di Goodpasture** (vedi Capitolo 517) e **sindrome di Heiner** (iperreattività al latte vaccino). Di queste eziologie, la sindrome di Goodpasture (o malattia degli anticorpi antimembrana basale) sembra essere la causa più comune di emorragia polmonare.

Con l'espressione **emosiderosi polmonare secondaria** si indica il rimanente gruppo di potenziali eziologie, piuttosto eterogeneo. Tra queste vi sono le cause cardiache di emosiderosi polmonare, come lo scompenso cardiaco congestizio, l'ipertensione polmonare e la stenosi mitralica. Le vasculiti e le collagenopatie come il lupus eritematoso sistemico (LES; vedi Capitolo 157), l'artrite reumatoide, la granulomatosi di Wegener (vedi Capitolo 166.4) e la porpora di Schönlein-Henoch (PSH; vedi Capitolo 166.1) sono un altro gruppo importante da considerare nella diagnosi differenziale. Si possono inoltre riscontrare coagulopatie, sia congenite sia acquisite. La prematurità è un altro fattore di rischio riconosciuto per l'emorragia. L'emosiderosi polmonare è stata ben descritta in associazione al morbo celiaco. Sono stati implicati anche processi postinfettivi, come la sindrome uremico-emolitica (vedi Capitolo 484.4) e le sindromi da immunodeficienza, compresa la malattia granulomatosa cronica (vedi Capitolo 129). Infine, sono stati riportati come potenziali eziologie numerosi farmaci, esposizioni ambientali, sostanze chimiche e allergeni alimentari.

EPIDEMIOLOGIA. La frequenza con cui la DAH si manifesta è difficile da quantificare; questo è dovuto in gran parte alla varietà di malattie che possono presentarsi con una componente di emorragia alveolare. Analogamente, la prevalenza della IPH è in gran parte sconosciuta. Di fatto, molti bambini e giovani adulti con una diagnosi di IPH effettuata in passato potrebbero avere oggi un'eziologia riconoscibile per le loro emorragie, se fossero studiati con metodi diagnostici nuovi e più avanzati. Le stime di prevalenza ottenute dalle analisi retrospettive svedesi e giapponesi vanno da 0,24 a 1,23 casi per milione. In generale, le manifestazioni di IPH si osservano prima dei 10 anni di età. Circa l'80% dei casi insorge in questo gruppo di età più precoce, mentre nel restante 20% dei pazienti adulti la diagnosi tipicamente viene effettuata prima dei 30 anni di età. Il rapporto tra maschi e femmine affetti è uguale nel gruppo con diagnosi in età pediatrica, mentre è leggermente superiore nei maschi del gruppo diagnosticato in età adulta.

ANATOMIA PATOLOGICA. In seguito a episodi ripetuti di emorragia polmonare, il tessuto polmonare acquisisce un colore brunastro, secondario alla presenza di **emosiderina**. Il reperto di sangue nelle vie aeree o negli alveoli è indicativo di un'emorragia recente. Nell'emorragia polmonare cronica o ricorrente, o nella fase di guarigione, si osservano macrofagi pieni di emosiderina. Devono passare 48-72 ore perché i macrofagi alveolari possano convertire il ferro degli eritrociti in emosiderina. I macrofagi pieni di emosiderina talvolta sono rilevabili per settimane, dopo un evento emorragico. Altre caratteristiche anatomopatologiche aspecifiche comprendono ispessimento dei setti alveolari e ipertrofia degli pneumociti di tipo II. Nella malattia cronica può essere osservata fibrosi (vedi anche Capitolo 413).

FISIOPATOLOGIA. Nella sindrome di Goodpasture, gli anticorpi antimembrana basale (ABMA, *Anti-Basement Membrane Antibody*) si legano alla membrana basale sia degli alveoli sia dei glomeruli. A livello alveolare, si verifica deposito di immunoglobuline (Ig) G, IgM e complemento nei setti alveolari. In microscopia elettronica, si osserva distruzione delle membrane basali e dell'integrità vascolare, che consente la fuoriuscita del sangue negli spazi alveolari.

L'emosiderosi associata all'**ipersensibilità al latte vaccino** fu riportata la prima volta da Heiner nel 1962. Questa condizione è caratterizzata da sintomi variabili di intolleranza al latte, i cui sintomi comprendono feci francamente ematiche o contenenti sangue occulto, vomito, mancato sviluppo, sintomi di reflusso gastroesofageo e/o congestione delle vie aeree superiori. I reperti patologici comprendono aumento delle IgE ed eosinofilia periferica, così come depositi alveolari di IgG, IgA e C3. Inoltre, nell'ipersensibilità al latte vaccino i titoli degli anticorpi contro le proteine del latte risultano elevati.

L'emorragia alveolare, osservata di rado in associazione al **LES**, è spesso severa e potenzialmente pericolosa per la vita. Possono essere assenti le caratteristiche anatomopatologiche della vasculite. Nonostante alcuni studi di immunofluorescenza abbiano rivelato depositi di IgG e C3 a livello dei setti alveolari, non è stato stabilito ancora un chiaro legame tra la formazione di immunocomplessi e l'emorragia alveolare.

Nella **PSH**, l'emorragia polmonare è una complicanza rara, ma riconosciuta. I reperti patologici comprendono infiltrazione neutrofila transmurale dei piccoli vasi, infiammazione dei setti alveolari ed emorragia intralveolare. Il meccanismo proposto per l'emorragia è un processo vasculitico.

La **granulomatosi di Wegener** è una causa di emorragia rara nei bambini. Si può apprezzare la formazione di granulomi polmonari (con o senza cavitazione) e la vasculite necrotizzante. Nei bambini, le presentazioni attribuibili alle vie aeree superiori, tra cui la stenosi subglottica, possono suggerire la diagnosi. La ricerca degli anticorpi anticitoplasma dei neutrofili (ANCA, *AntiNeutrophil Cytoplasmic Antibody*) è generalmente positiva.

Il decorso neonatale di un nato prematuro spesso è complicato da emorragia polmonare. Le reti alveolari e vascolari sono immature e particolarmente vulnerabili all'infiammazione e al danno da parte della ventilazione meccanica, dello stress ossidativo e delle infezioni. L'emorragia polmonare può non essere riconosciuta, se il sangue è in un volume insufficiente a raggiungere le vie aeree prossimali. I reperti dell'emorragia polmonare, alla radiografia del torace, possono essere apprezzati invece come un quadro progressivamente in peggioramento di sindrome da distress respiratorio, edema o infezione.

Esistono numerose altre patologie ed esposizioni associate, come accennato in precedenza. Queste si verificano di rado, nella popolazione pediatrica, e i meccanismi suggeriti per l'emorragia sono variabili. Si pone diagnosi di IPH quando vi è evidenza di un'emorragia diffusa cronica o ricorrente, e quando una valutazione esauriente per la ricerca di cause primitive o secondarie risulta negativa. Il campione bioptico non deve rivelare segni di malattie granulomatose, vasculiti, infezioni, infarto, deposito di immunocomplessi, tumori o di altre caratteristiche associate a condizioni primitive o secondarie.

MANIFESTAZIONI CLINICHE. La presentazione clinica dell'emosiderosi polmonare è quantomai variabile. I sintomi possono riflettere un processo patologico di base associato, anziché essere correlati specificamente all'emorragia polmonare. La presentazione può variare ampiamente, da una relativa assenza di sintomi allo shock e alla morte improvvisa. Un'emorragia significativa si può instaurare in assenza di sintomi importanti. Può non verificarsi emottisi. Occasionalmente il sanguinamento viene individuato dalla presenza di infiltrati alveolari, alla radiografia del torace. Si noti comunque che l'assenza di infiltrati non esclude che sia in atto un processo emorragico.

Poiché la presenza di sangue nei polmoni è una tipica fonte di irritazione e infiammazione significative, il paziente può presentarsi dopo un episodio di emorragia con sibili, tosse, dispnea e alterazioni dello scambio gassoso, che riflettono broncospasmo, edema, tappi di muco e infiammazione. All'esame obiettivo, il paziente può essere pallido con tachicardia e tachipnea. Durante un'esacerbazione acuta, i bambini sono spesso febbrili. L'esame del torace può rivelare retrazioni e ventilazione differenziale o ridotta, con crepitii o sibili. Il paziente può presentarsi in stato di shock, con insufficienza respiratoria da emottisi massiva. I bambini, in particolare, possono accusare sintomi di anemia cronica, come un deficit dell'accrescimento.

INDAGINI DI LABORATORIO E DIAGNOSI. L'emorragia polmonare si associa a una riduzione dell'emoglobina e dell'ematocrito. Il reperto classico è quello di un'anemia microcitica, ipocromica. La conta reticolocitaria è elevata. L'anemia della IPH può mimare un'anemia emolitica. L'assorbimento e la degradazione dell'emoglobina negli alveoli causano aumento della bilirubina plasmatica. La sideremia è ridotta. La capacità legante il ferro è generalmente elevata. Queste manifestazioni ematologiche possono essere del tutto o in parte assenti, in un quadro di emorragia recente.

Occorre valutare la conta e la formula leucocitaria per ricercare segni di infezione e l'eosinofilia. I campioni di feci possono essere positivi al sangue occulto, a causa del sangue ingerito. Devono essere controllate la funzione renale ed epatica. Si rende necessaria un'analisi delle urine per valutare eventuali segni di nefrite. Sono inoltre consigliati un profilo coagulativo, il dosaggio quantitativo delle immunoglobuline (comprese le IgE) e del complemento.

La ricerca degli ANCA, degli anticorpi antinucleo (ANA), anti-DNA a doppia elica, del fattore reumatoide, degli anticorpi antifosfolipidi e degli anticorpi antimembrana basale glomerulare (antiGBM, *Glomerular Basement Membrane*) valuta numerose condizioni primitive o secondarie che possono essere causa di DAH. L'aumento della velocità di eritrosedimentazione (VES) è un riscontro aspecifico.

Bisogna esaminare l'escreato, o le secrezioni polmonari, per la ricerca di sangue o di macrofagi pieni di emosiderina (HLM, *Hemosiderin-Laden Macrophages*). Anche le secrezioni gastriche possono rivelare la presenza di HLM. La broncoscopia flessibile fornisce una visualizzazione di qualsiasi area di sanguinamento attivo. Con il lavaggio broncoalveolare, le secrezioni polmonari possono essere inviate all'esame citologico e colturale. Le possibilità di effettuare una broncoscopia a fibre ottiche possono essere scarse, in presenza di grandi quantità di sangue o coaguli nelle vie aeree. Il modo più efficace per ventilare un paziente con insufficienza respiratoria può essere mediante broncoscopio rigido.

La biopsia polmonare è necessaria quando la DAH insorge senza un'eziologia riconoscibile, una malattia extrapolmonare o la presenza di ABMA circolanti. Il tessuto polmonare così ottenuto deve essere valutato per la ricerca di vasculiti, deposito di immunocomplessi e malattie granulomatose.

La radiografia del torace può rivelare segni di malattia acuta o cronica. È frequente riscontrare iperaerazione, soprattutto durante un'emorragia acuta. Gli infiltrati, tipicamente simmetrici, possono risparmiare gli apici polmonari. Talvolta è inoltre apprezzabile atelettasia. In caso di malattia cronica, si possono osservare linfoadenopatia e nodularità. I reperti alla TC possono rivelare un processo patologico subclinico che contribuisce al quadro clinico.

I test di funzionalità polmonare riveleranno probabilmente una malattia ostruttiva nel periodo acuto. Nella malattia cronica tendono a predominare la fibrosi e un quadro restrittivo. La saturazione di ossigeno può essere ridotta. I volumi polmonari possono rivelare intrappolamento d'aria acuto e riduzione cronica della capacità polmonare totale. La capacità di diffusione del monossido di carbonio (D_LCO) può essere bassa o normale nella fase cronica, ma è probabile risulti elevata nel contesto di un'emorragia acuta, in quanto il monossido di carbonio si lega all'emoglobina negli eritrociti stravasati.

TRATTAMENTO. La terapia di supporto comprende il ripristino del volume circolante, il supporto ventilatorio, la somministrazione di ossigeno e la trasfusione di derivati ematici al bisogno. Se esiste una condizione associata curabile, la terapia medica e chirurgica deve essere volta a trattare la patologia di base. Nella IPH, il trattamento precoce con corticosteroidi sistemici è la terapia di scelta. Generalmente si inizia con un dosaggio di 2-5 mg/kg/die, che viene ridotto a 1 mg/kg/die, a giorni alterni, dopo la risoluzione dei sintomi acuti. La somministrazione precoce di steroidi sembra ridurre gli episodi di emorragia; questa terapia può anche modulare l'afflusso dei neutrofili e l'infiammazione associati all'emorragia, riducendo così la progressione verso la fibrosi.

L'obiettivo di scalare in modo graduale gli steroidi sistemici può non essere tollerato. Inoltre, un sottogruppo di pazienti non risponde in modo ottimale agli steroidi da soli. In questi casi, sono stati utilizzati agenti immunosoppressori come la ciclofosfamide, l'azatioprina e la clorochina, di cui però rimangono poco chiare indicazioni ed efficacia a lungo termine. I numerosi effetti collaterali potenziali di una terapia a lungo termine con gli steroidi e gli altri farmaci immunosoppressori potrebbero costituire un ostacolo alla terapia.

Nella malattia cronica, è stata descritta la progressione verso una fibrosi polmonare debilitante. Nei pazienti con IPH refrattari alla terapia immunosoppressiva è stato effettuato il trapianto polmonare. In un caso riportato in letteratura, la IPH è recidivata dopo trapianto polmonare.

PROGNOSI. L'esito per i pazienti con DAH dipende in gran parte dal processo patologico sottostante. Alcune condizioni, come l'ipersensibilità al latte vaccino, rispondono bene all'eliminazione dell'agente causale, ma altre sindromi, soprattutto se sostenute da un meccanismo immunologico, tendono a comportare una prognosi più infausta. Nella IPH, la mortalità è spesso correlata alle emorragie massive o, in alternativa, alla fibrosi progressiva, all'insufficienza respiratoria e allo scompenso cardiaco destro.

La prognosi a lungo termine della IPH varia nei diversi studi. Le review delle casistiche iniziali hanno suggerito una sopravvivenza media dopo l'esordio dei sintomi di soli 2,5 anni. In queste revisioni iniziali, solo una minoranza di pazienti era trattata con steroidi. Una revisione più recente ha riportato una sopravvivenza a 5 anni dell'86%. Se questo miglioramento sia dovuto principalmente ai progressi complessivi delle cure o alla terapia immunosoppressiva a lungo termine non è stato ancora stabilito. Sono state documentate anche remissioni spontanee.

Boat TF: Pulmonary hemorrhage and hemoptysis. In Chernick V, Boat TF (editors): *Kendig's Disorders of the Respiratory Tract in Children.* Philadelphia, WB Saunders, 1998, pp 623–633.

Calabrese F, Giacometti C, Rea F, et al: Recurrence of idiopathic pulmonary hemosiderosis in a young adult patient after bilateral single-lung transplantation. *Transplantation* 2002;74:1643–1645.

Cohen S: Idiopathic pulmonary hemosiderosis. *Am J Med Sci* 1999; 317:67–74.

Dearborn DG: Pulmonary hemorrhage in infants and children. *Curr Opin Pediatr* 1997;9:219–224.

Godfrey S: Pulmonary hemorrhage/hemoptysis in children. *Pediatr Pulmonol* 2004;37:476–484.

Ioachimescu OC, Sieber S, Kotch A: Idiopathic pulmonary hemosiderosis revisited. *Eur Respir J* 2004;24:162–170.

Le Clainche L, Le Bourgeois M, Fauroux B, et al: Long-term outcome of idiopathic pulmonary hemosiderosis in children. *Medicine* 2000;79: 318–326.

McCoy KS: Hemosiderosis. In Taussig LM, Landau LI (eds): *Pediatric Respiratory Medicine.* St. Louis, Mosby, 1999, pp 835–841.

Moissidi SI, Chaidaroon D, Vichyanond P, Bahna SL: Milk-induced pulmonary disease in infants (Heiner Syndrome). *Pediatr Allergy Immunol* 2005;16(6):545–562.

Saeed MM, Woo MS, MacLaughlin EF, et al: Prognosis in pediatric idiopathic pulmonary hemosiderosis. *Chest* 1999;116:721–725.

Yao TC, Hung IJ, Jaing TH, et al: Pitfalls in the diagnosis of idiopathic pulmonary haemosiderosis. *Arch Dis Child* 2002;86:436–438.

Capitolo 406 ■ Embolia, infarto ed emorragia polmonare Mary A. Nevin

406.1 • Embolia e infarto polmonare

Sebbene i bambini siano considerati a minor rischio, rispetto agli adulti, per lo sviluppo di malattia tromboembolica venosa (VTE, *Venous Thromboembolic Disease*), quest'ultima si verifica ed è ben descritta in bambini e adolescenti, con o senza fattori di rischio (Tab. 406-1). La malattia embolica, nei pazienti pediatrici, può rappresentare una fonte significativa di morbilità e mortalità. Il miglioramento delle terapie per le malattie infantili e l'aumentata sopravvivenza con le patologie croniche possono aver contribuito all'aumento del numero di bambini che si presentano con eventi tromboembolici.

EZIOLOGIA. I fattori di rischio comunemente conosciuti per la malattia tromboembolica, negli adulti, comprendono l'immobilità, i tumori, la gravidanza, le infezioni e gli stati di ipercoagulabilità (vedi Tab. 406-1). Gli adulti possono anche avere una malattia tromboembolica in assenza di fattori di rischio identificabili. È stata descritta una malattia idiopatica anche nel 20% degli adulti con questa condizione. I bambini con trombosi venosa profonda (DVT, *Deep Venous Thrombosis*) ed embolia polmonare (PE, *Pulmonary Embolism*) hanno maggiori probabilità di avere una o più condizioni identificabili o circostanze che li rendono a rischio. In un'ampia casistica canadese, si è scoperto che il 96% dei pazienti pediatrici aveva un fattore di rischio e il 90% ne aveva due o più.

La malattia embolica ha varie eziologie, nei bambini. Oltre a un trombo, un embolo può contenere aria, liquido amniotico, materiale settico o tessuto neoplastico metastatico; tuttavia, i tromboemboli sono quelli di più frequente riscontro. Un fattore di rischio incontrato spesso per la DVT e la PE nella popolazione pediatrica è la presenza di un catetere venoso centrale. Il suo inserimento nel lume di un vaso e l'instillazione di farmaci attraverso di esso può infatti indurre un danno endoteliale favorendo la formazione di un trombo.

Anche i pazienti pediatrici con tumori maligni sono a rischio. Il rischio di PE è più significativo nei bambini con tumori solidi, rispetto a quelli con neoplasie ematologiche. La PE è stata descritta tanto nei bambini con tumore di Wilms, quanto in quelli con leucemia. Un paziente pediatrico con un tumore può avere numerosi fattori di rischio, correlati al processo patologico primitivo e agli interventi terapeutici. Le infezioni da immunosoppressione cronica possono interagire con l'ipercoagulabilità della neoplasia maligna e con gli effetti della chemioterapia sull'endotelio.

Nel periodo neonatale, la malattia tromboembolica e la PE sono spesso connesse all'inserimento di cateteri a permanenza, utilizzati per la nutrizione parenterale e la somministrazione dei farmaci. Gli emboli, in questo gruppo di età, possono riflettere occasionalmente fattori di rischio materni, come il diabete o la tossiemia gravidica. I soggetti con difetti congeniti omozigoti di antitrombina, proteina C e proteina S hanno anche elevate probabilità di manifestare alterazioni nel periodo neonatale.

Una malattia protrombotica può essere presente anche nei lattanti più grandi e nei bambini. La malattia può essere congenita o acquisita; la DVT/PE può essere la presentazione iniziale. La *mutazione del fattore V di Leiden* (vedi Capitolo 478), l'*iperomocisteinemia* (vedi Capitolo 85.3), la *mutazione 20210A della protrombina* (vedi Capitolo 478), gli *anticorpi anticardiolipina* ed elevati livelli di *lipoproteina A* sono tutti stati correlati alla malattia tromboembolica. I bambini con anemia a cellule falciformi sono anche ad aumentato rischio di embolia polmonare e infarto. Le malattie protrombotiche acquisite sono rappresentate dalla *sindrome nefrosica* (vedi Capitolo 527) e dalla *sindrome da anticorpi antifosfolipidi*. Dal 21 al 57% dei bambini con *lupus eritematoso sistemico* (vedi Capitolo 157) ha una malattia tromboembolica.

Altri fattori di rischio comprendono infezioni, cardiopatie, interventi chirurgici recenti e traumi. Il rischio chirurgico è ritenuto più significativo quando l'immobilità è una caratteristica importante della convalescenza. L'uso di contraccettivi orali apporta un rischio aggiuntivo, sebbene il livello di rischio nei pazienti che assumono questi farmaci sembri essere in riduzione, forse a causa del ridotto contenuto di estrogeni nelle attuali formulazioni.

Gli emboli settici, peraltro rari nei bambini, possono essere causati da osteomieliti, celluliti, infezioni delle vie urinarie, tromboflebite della vena giugulare o ombelicale, ed endocardite destra.

EPIDEMIOLOGIA. La giovane età sembra essere in una certa misura protettiva nei confronti della malattia tromboembolica. L'incidenza di DVT, in uno studio su bambini ospedalizzati, è stata di 5,3/10 000 ricoveri. In uno studio che ha analizzato i dati dal 1979 al 2001, vi sono stati 0,9 PE/100 000 bambini/anno, 4,2 DVT/100 000 bambini/anno e 4,9 VTE/100 000 bambini/anno (Tab. 406-2).

Le revisioni di autopsie pediatriche hanno stimato un'incidenza compresa tra l'1 e il 4%. Non tutti i reperti di embolia erano clinicamente significativi. La malattia tromboembolica polmonare spesso non viene riconosciuta e gli studi su viventi possono

TABELLA 406-1. Fattori di rischio per l'embolia polmonare

AMBIENTALI
Voli aerei di lunga durata
Obesità
Fumo di sigaretta
Ipertensione
Immobilità
SALUTE FEMMINILE
Contraccettivi orali, tra cui quelli con solo progesterone e la pillola di terza generazione
Gravidanza
Terapia ormonale sostitutiva
PATOLOGIE MEDICHE
Pregressa embolia polmonare o trombosi venosa profonda
Cancro
Scompenso cardiaco congestizio
Broncopneumopatia cronica ostruttiva
Diabete mellito
Malattia infiammatoria intestinale
Uso di farmaci antipsicotici
Catetere venoso centrale a permanenza
Pacemaker permanente
Defibrillatore intracardiaco
Ictus con paresi degli arti
Confinamento in una casa di cura protetta o ricoveri ospedalieri ripetuti
CHIRURGICHE
Traumi
Chirurgia ortopedica
Chirurgia generale
Neurochirurgia, specialmente craniotomia per tumori cerebrali
TROMBOFILICHE
Mutazione del fattore V di Leiden
Mutazione del gene della protrombina
Iperomocisteinemia (compresa la mutazione della metilene tetraidrofolato riduttasi)
Sindrome da anticorpi antifosfolipidi
Deficit di antitrombina III, di proteina C o di proteina S
Elevate concentrazioni di fattore VIII o XI
Aumento della lipoproteina a
NON TROMBOTICHE
Aria
Particelle estranee (per es. peli, talco, abuso di droghe per via endovenosa)
Liquido amniotico
Frammenti ossei o di midollo osseo
Grasso
Tumori (tumore di Wilms)

Modificata da Goldhaber SZ: Pulmonary embolism. *Lancet* 2004;363:1295-1305.

TABELLA 406-2. Malattia tromboembolica nei bambini: 1979-2001

		FREQUENZA DELLA DIAGNOSI/100 000 BAMBINI/ANNO		
	GRUPPO DI ETÀ	**Tutti**	**Maschi**	**Femmine**
PE	0-1	2,2*	—‡	—
	2-14	0,4	—	—
	15-17	2,0*	—	—
	Tutti	0,9	—	—
DVT	0-1	8,7†	9,3	8,0
	2-14	2,1	2,0	2,2
	15-17	9,9†	6,5	13,5
	Tutti	4,2	3,6	4,8
VTE	0-1	10,5†	11,3	9,7
	2-14	2,4	2,3	2,6
	15-17	11,4†	8,1	14,9
	Tutti	4,9	4,3	5,5

*$P < 0{,}05$ età 0-1 vs età 2-14, ed età 15-17 vs età 2-14.
†$P < 0{,}001$ età 0-1 vs età 2-14, ed età 15-17 vs età 2-14.
‡Dati insufficienti per l'interpretazione in base all'età e al sesso.
DVT (*Deep Venous Thrombosis*), trombosi venosa profonda; PE (*Pulmonary Embolism*), embolia polmonare; VTE, (*Venous Thromboembolic Disease*), malattia tromboembolica venosa.
Da Stein P, Kayali F, Olson R: Incidence of venous thromboembolism in infants and children: Data from the National Hospital Discharge Survey. *J Pediatr* 2004;145:564.

sottostimare la reale incidenza. I decessi pediatrici da emboli polmonari isolati sono rari. La maggior parte dei tromboemboli è correlata a cateteri venosi centrali. L'origine dell'embolo può essere a livello delle vene degli arti inferiori o superiori, così come della pelvi o del cuore destro. La sede più comune, per gli emboli non associati alla presenza di cateteri venosi a permanenza, è negli arti inferiori.

FISIOPATOLOGIA. Le condizioni che favoriscono la formazione di trombi comprendono il danno all'endotelio vascolare, l'emostasi e l'ipercoagulabilità. Una volta che l'embolo si è sviluppato e ha raggiunto il circolo polmonare, i sintomi di presentazione sono per lo più attribuibili a uno squilibrio del rapporto ventilazione/perfusione. L'occlusione del vaso coinvolto impedisce la perfusione delle unità alveolari distali, determinando così un aumento dello spazio morto e un'ipossia con elevato gradiente a-A O_2. La maggior parte dei pazienti ha un'ipocapnia secondaria all'iperventilazione, che spesso persiste anche dopo l'ottimizzazione dell'ossigenazione. Le anomalie dell'ossigenazione e della ventilazione sono probabilmente meno significative nella popolazione pediatrica, forse grazie alla minore incidenza di malattie cardiopolmonari di base e a una riserva maggiore. L'apporto vascolare al tessuto polmonare è abbondante e l'infarto polmonare da embolia polmonare è raro, anche se può derivare da un'occlusione arteriosa distale con emorragia alveolare. Nei rari casi di morte da embolia polmonare massiva, in genere sono presenti un marcato aumento delle resistenze vascolari polmonari e scompenso cardiaco. La maggior parte di questi esiti gravi è attesa nei pazienti con malattie cardiopolmonari preesistenti.

MANIFESTAZIONI CLINICHE. La presentazione è variabile e molti emboli polmonari sono silenti. È raro che la PE si presenti con insufficienza cardiopolmonare. I bambini è più probabile abbiano un processo patologico di base o fattori di rischio, ma possono comunque presentarsi asintomatici con gli emboli più piccoli. I sintomi e i segni comuni di PE comprendono ipossia (cianosi), tachipnea, dispnea, tosse, diaforesi e dolore toracico. Occasionalmente sono apprezzabili crepitii localizzati, all'esame obiettivo; si tratta di reperti aspecifici, in molti casi attribuibili a un processo patologico sottostante o una diagnosi non correlata o errata. È necessario un elevato livello di sospetto clinico, poiché è raro che nei pazienti pediatrici venga presa in considerazione la diagnosi di embolia polmonare. Molte altre diagnosi possono avere sintomi di presentazione simili; pertanto, una diagnosi clinica di PE deve essere seguita da esami di conferma.

INDAGINI DI LABORATORIO E DIAGNOSI. Le immagini radiografiche del torace sono spesso normali; tutte le anomalie osservabili alla radiografia del torace sono probabilmente aspecifiche. I pazienti con emboli settici possono avere aree multiple di nodularità e cavitazione, localizzate tipicamente alla periferia di entrambi i campi polmonari. Molti pazienti con PE presentano ipossiemia. La differenza tra la pressione alveolare e arteriosa di ossigeno, o gradiente a-A, è più sensibile nella rilevazione delle alterazioni dello scambio gassoso. Sono indispensabili l'esame emocromocitometrico completo, l'analisi delle urine e il profilo coagulativo. Le malattie protrombotiche devono essere fortemente sospettate sulla base dell'anamnesi patologica remota e familiare; pertanto, valutazioni di laboratorio ulteriori comprendono il dosaggio del fibrinogeno, della proteina C, della proteina S, dell'antitrombina III e l'analisi per la mutazione del fattore V di Leiden, oltre alla ricerca dell'anticoagulante lupico e degli anticorpi anticardiolipina.

L'elettrocardiogramma può rivelare alterazioni del tratto ST o segni di ipertensione polmonare con scompenso cardiaco destro (cuore polmonare). Queste alterazioni sono aspecifiche e non diagnostiche. L'ecocardiogramma può essere necessario per valutare la dimensione e la funzione ventricolare sinistra. L'ecocardiografia transtoracica va eseguita se si sospetta una trombosi intracardiaca o un'endocardite.

L'ecografia venosa non invasiva con Doppler può essere utile per confermare la presenza di DVT negli arti inferiori, ma talvolta non è in grado di rilevare i trombi nelle estremità superiori o nella pelvi. Nei pazienti con trombosi venosa significativa, il D-dimero di solito è elevato. Quando sussiste un elevato livello di sospetto clinico, occorre effettuare esami di conferma con la venografia. La DVT, ricorrente o multifocale che sia, può portare a episodi ripetuti di embolia polmonare.

Sebbene la scintigrafia di ventilazione-perfusione (V-Q) con radionuclide sia una metodica non invasiva e potenzialmente sensibile per l'identificazione dell'embolia polmonare, la sua interpretazione può essere problematica. La TC elicoidale o spirale con mezzo di contrasto endovenoso è molto utile e anzi costituisce l'esame diagnostico di scelta per rilevare una PE. La sua specificità supera il 90%. La sensibilità della TC può essere accettabile nell'identificazione degli emboli nei vasi lobari e segmentari, ma più scarsa nella valutazione dei basi polmonari subsegmentari. L'angiografia polmonare è il *gold standard* per la diagnosi di PE, ma con l'avvento dell'angioTC spirale multidetector non è più necessaria, salvo che in rari casi.

TRATTAMENTO. Il trattamento iniziale dovrebbe essere sempre diretto alla stabilizzazione del paziente. Un approccio attento alla ventilazione, alla somministrazione di liquidi e al supporto inotropo positivo è sempre indicato, poiché il miglioramento in un'area di scompenso può spesso esacerbare le patologie coesistenti.

Dopo aver stabilizzato il paziente con PE, il passo terapeutico successivo è la somministrazione di anticoagulanti. La valutazione per la ricerca di malattie protrombotiche deve precedere l'anticoagulazione. Generalmente si comincia con la somministrazione di eparina. La scoagulazione di solito si considera raggiunta quando il tempo di protrombina parziale attivata (*PTT, Partial Thromboplastine Time*) è 1,5-2 volte il controllo. La terapia a lungo termine con eparina deve essere evitata, ove possibile. Le complicanze di questo farmaco consistono in emorragie e nella trombocitopenia acquisita.

La terapia eparinica deve continuare per diversi giorni, prima dell'inizio del trattamento orale con warfarin. La terapia anticoagulante può essere necessaria per 3-6 mesi, in un quadro di malattia tromboembolica acuta. Nei pazienti con trombosi persistente sono richiesti trattamenti più prolungati. Occorre eseguire a intervalli regolari un profilo della coagulazione, che guidi la terapia con warfarin o eparina.

Negli adulti, l'eparina a basso peso molecolare (LMW, *Low Molecolar Weight*) è considerata equivalente alla terapia eparinica standard. L'emivita più lunga consente un dosaggio discontinuo e l'efficacia sembra analoga. È necessario un monitoraggio minimo, con la somministrazione del farmaco. Altri vantaggi possono comprendere il minor rischio sia di osteoporosi sia di trombocitopenia. Attualmente, l'eparina LMW è utilizzata anche in molti pazienti pediatrici.

La terapia trombolitica può essere combinata con gli anticoagulanti, nelle fasi iniziali del trattamento. I farmaci trombolitici comprendono l'urochinasi, la streptochinasi e l'attivatore tissutale del plasminogeno ricombinante. La terapia combinata può ridurre l'incidenza di tromboembolia progressiva, embolia polmonare e sindrome postflebitica. Sebbene la mortalità sembri invariata, con l'uso di ulteriori trattamenti il rischio aggiuntivo di emorragia limita l'utilizzo della terapia combinata in tutti i pazienti, salvo quelli più compromessi. L'uso di agenti trombolitici nei pazienti con emorragia attiva, accidenti cerebrovascolari recenti o traumi è controindicato.

L'embolectomia chirurgica, essendo invasiva e associata a una mortalità significativa, deve essere riservata ai pazienti con compromissione emodinamica persistente refrattaria alla terapia medica.

PROGNOSI. La mortalità nei pazienti pediatrici con PE è probabilmente attribuibile al processo patologico di base, più che all'embolia stessa. Le condizioni a prognosi peggiore comprendono i tumori, le infezioni e le cardiopatie. La mortalità da PE, nei bambini, è del 2,2%. La tromboembolia ricorrente può complicare la guarigione. Il medico deve condurre una valutazione completa per la ricerca di patologie di base, al fine di prevenire la progressione della malattia. La sindrome postflebitica è un'altra complicanza riconosciuta della malattia tromboembolica pediatrica. Il danno valvolare venoso, che può essere scatenato dalla presenza di DVT, talvolta porta a ipertensione venosa persistente con la deambulazione e a reflusso valvolare. I sintomi comprendono edema, dolore, iperpigmentazione e ulcere. I pazienti pediatrici affetti possono andare incontro a disabilità per tutta la vita.

Andrew M, David M, Adams M, et al: Venous thromboembolic complications (VTE) in children: First analysis of the Canadian registry of VTE. *Blood* 1994;83:1251–1257.

Bonduel M, Hepner M, Sciuccati G, et al: Prothrombotic abnormalities in children with venous thromboembolism. *J Pediatr Hematol Oncol* 2000;22:66–72.

Chan AK, Deveber G, Monagle P, et al: Venous thrombosis in children. *J Thromb Haemost* 2003;1:1443–1455.

Goldhaber SZ: Pulmonary embolism. *Lancet* 2004;363:1295–1305.

Holzer R, Peart I, Ciotti G, et al: Successful treatment with rTPA. *Pediatr Cardiol* 2002;23:548–552.

Hull RD: Diagnosing pulmonary embolism with improved certainty and simplicity. *JAMA* 2006;295:213–215.

Johnson AS, Bolte RG: Pulmonary embolism in the pediatric patient. *Pediatr Emerg Care* 2004;20:555–560.

Manco-Johnson MJ, Nuss R, Hays T, et al: Combined thrombolytic and anticoagulant therapy for venous thrombosis in children. *J Pediatr* 2000;136:446–453.

Perrier A, Roy PM, Sanchez O, et al: Multidetector-row computed tomography in suspected pulmonary embolism. *N Engl J Med* 2005;352:1760–1768.

Robinson GV: Pulmonary embolism in hospital practice. *Br Med J* 2006;332: 156–160.

Roy PM, Colombet I, Durieux P, et al: Systemic review and meta-analysis of strategies for the diagnosis of suspected pulmonary embolism. *Br Med J* 2005;331:259–263.

Stein PD, Fowler SE, Goodman LR: Multidetector computed tomography for acute pulmonary embolism. *N Engl J Med* 2006;354:2317–2326.

Stein P, Kayali F, Olson R: Incidence of venous thromboembolism in infants and children: Data from the National Hospital Discharge Survey. *J Pediatr* 2004;145:563–565.

van Belle A, Buller HR, Huisman MV, et al: Christopher Study Investigators: Effectiveness of managing suspected pulmonary embolism using an algorithm combining clinical probability, D-Dimer testing, and computed tomography. *JAMA* 2006;295:172–179.

Wells PS, Anderson DR, Rodger M, et al: Evaluation of d-dimer in the diagnosis of suspected deep-vein thrombosis. *N Engl J Med* 2003;349: 1227–1234.

Wong KS, Lin TY, Huang YC, et al: Clinical and radiographic spectrum of septic pulmonary embolism. *Arch Dis Child* 2002;87:312–315.

406.2 • Emorragia polmonare ed emottisi

L'emorragia polmonare è un'evenienza relativamente rara nella popolazione pediatrica, ma potenzialmente fatale. La sua incidenza può essere significativamente sottostimata, poiché molti bambini e giovani adulti ingoiano il muco invece di espettorarlo, abitudine che impedisce al medico di riconoscere l'emottisi, il sintomo di presentazione principale del disturbo. Inoltre, un sanguinamento lento e diffuso nelle vie aeree inferiori può diventare grave e presentarsi con anemia, astenia o compromissione respiratoria, senza che il paziente abbia mai avuto episodi di emottisi. Quest'ultima deve essere sempre distinta dagli episodi di ematemesi o epistassi, poiché tutti questi eventi possono avere manifestazioni simili nel paziente giovane.

EZIOLOGIA. Le condizioni che possono presentarsi con emorragia polmonare o emottisi, nei bambini, sono elencate nella Tabella 406-3. La presenza cronica (al contrario della presenza acuta) di un corpo estraneo può portare a infiammazione e/o infezione, inducendo così un'emorragia. Sebbene quest'ultima possa essere causata anche da infezioni acute come la bronchite o la broncopolmonite, è più comune che essa rispecchi un'infiammazione e un'infezione croniche, come si osserva nella fibrosi cistica con bronchiectasie o nella tubercolosi con cavitazione. Altre eziologie relativamente comuni comprendono le cardiopatie congenite e i traumi. L'irritazione o il danno traumatico delle vie aeree è spesso di natura accidentale. Il sanguinamento può anche essere correlato all'impiego di strumentazione per le vie aeree, come si osserva comunemente nei bambini con tracheostomia. È importante notare, tuttavia, che nei bambini che sono stati vittima di traumi non accidentali, o di soffocamento intenzionale, si rinviene del sangue anche nel cavo orale o nelle vie aeree. È meno frequente che le sindromi associate a disturbi vasculitici, autoimmuni e idiopatici si associno a emorragia alveolare diffusa (DAH, *Diffuse Alveolar Hemorrage*). I molteplici meccanismi della DHA sono discussi in maniera più approfondita nel Capitolo 405.

L'**emorragia polmonare acuta idiopatica** (AIPH, *Acute Idiopathic Pulmonary Hemorrage*) insorge nei lattanti di pochi mesi come entità a sé, ma occorre prendere in esame anche le malattie elencate nella Tabella 406-3.

EPIDEMIOLOGIA. La frequenza con cui l'emorragia polmonare si verifica nella popolazione pediatrica è difficile da stabilire. Questa difficoltà è dovuta in gran parte alla variabilità nella presentazione della malattia. Le bronchiectasie croniche, osservabili per esempio nella fibrosi cistica o nella discinesia ciliare, possono causare emottisi, ma di solito nei bambini di età >10 anni. L'AIPH è definita come un'evidenza di sangue nelle vie aeree, in un soggetto di età ≤1 anno, in assenza di condizioni mediche che predispongano all'emorragia polmonare, e in concomitanza con distress respiratorio severo che porta a insufficienza respiratoria. Questa entità può essere più comune di quanto si pensasse in passato. La maggior parte dei casi è idiopatica, ma talvolta è stata associata alla malattia di von Willebrand. Non sono emerse associazioni tra questa malattia e la contaminazione domestica da parte di muffe.

FISIOPATOLOGIA. L'emorragia polmonare può essere localizzata o diffusa. L'emorragia focale da una lesione bronchiale isolata è spesso secondaria a infezione o infiammazione cronica. L'erosione di una via aerea cronicamente infiammata, fino all'arteria bronchiale adiacente, è il meccanismo di una potenziale emorragia massiva. Il sanguinamento da queste lesioni è più probabilmente rosso vivo, profuso e secondario ad arterie bronchiali ingrandite e ad aumento della pressione arteriosa sistemica. La severità di

TABELLA 406-3. Eziologia dell'emorragia polmonare (emottisi)

EMORRAGIA FOCALE
- Bronchite e bronchiectasie (soprattutto se correlate a FC)
- Infezioni (acute o croniche)
- Tubercolosi
- Traumi
- Malformazione arterovenosa polmonare
- Corpo estraneo (cronico)
- Neoplasie, compreso l'emangioma
- Embolia polmonare con o senza infarto

EMORRAGIA DIFFUSA
- Idiopatica dell'infanzia
- Cardiopatie congenite (comprese l'ipertensione polmonare, la malattia veno-occlusiva e la CHF)
- Prematurità
- Iperreattività al latte vaccino (sindrome di Heiner)
- Sindrome di Goodpasture
- Collagenopatie vascolari (LES, artrite reumatoide)
- Porpora di Schönlein-Henoch e vasculiti
- Malattie granulomatose (Wegener)
- Celiachia
- Coagulopatia (congenita o acquisita)
- Tumori maligni
- Immunodeficienze
- Tossine esogene
- Emosiderosi polmonare idiopatica
- Sclerosi tuberosa
- Linfangiomiomatosi o linfangioleiomiomatosi
- Lesione o abuso fisici

CF (*Cistic Fibrosis*), fibrosi cistica; CHF (*Coronary Heart Failure*), scompenso cardiaco congestizio; LES, lupus eritematoso sistemico.

un'emorragia più diffusa può essere difficile da valutare. La perdita ematica può avvenire a un ritmo abbastanza lento, tale da non consentirle di raggiungere le vie aeree prossimali; di conseguenza, il paziente può non presentare emottisi. La diagnosi di emorragia polmonare è generalmente ottenuta grazie al riscontro di sangue o di emosiderina nel polmone. Entro 48-72 ore da un episodio di emorragia, i macrofagi alveolari convertono il ferro degli eritrociti in emosiderina. Perché questi macrofagi pieni di emosiderina vengano eliminati completamente dagli spazi alveolari possono essere necessarie settimane; questo fenomeno può consentire di differenziare le emorragie acute da quelle croniche. L'emorragia è spesso seguita dall'arrivo di neutrofili e altri mediatori dell'infiammazione. Se l'emorragia si ripete o diventa cronica, la fibrosi polmonare può diventare un reperto patologico predominante.

MANIFESTAZIONI CLINICHE. La gravità dei pazienti che si presentano con emottisi ed emorragia polmonare è quantomai variabile. I bambini più grandi e i giovani adulti con emorragia focale possono lamentare una sensazione di calore o di "bolle" nella parete toracica, elemento che in alcuni casi può aiutare il medico a localizzare l'area coinvolta. Una perdita rapida di grandi volumi ematici si presenta con sintomi di cianosi, distress respiratorio e shock. Una perdita cronica, subclinica, può presentarsi con anemia, astenia, dispnea o alterata tolleranza allo sforzo. Meno comunemente, i pazienti presentano infiltrati persistenti alla radiografia del torace o sintomi di malattia cronica come un ritardo di accrescimento staturale.

INDAGINI DI LABORATORIO E DIAGNOSI. Tutti i pazienti con sospetta emorragia devono essere sottoposti a esami di laboratorio con emocromo e profilo coagulativo. L'esame emocromocitometrico può dimostrare un'anemia microcitica ipocromica; altri reperti dipendono in gran parte dalla diagnosi di base. L'esame delle urine può rivelare segni di nefrite, nei pazienti con malattia polmonare e renale concomitanti. Il reperto classico, che definisce l'emorragia polmonare, è quello di macrofagi ripieni di emosiderina nelle secrezioni polmonari; questi ultimi possono essere ottenuti tramite analisi dell'espettorato con colorazione al blu di Prussia. La radiografia del torace può dimostrare densità bilaterali a batuffolo di cotone, come nell'AIPH della prima infanzia (Fig. 406-1). È inoltre possibile osservare infiltrati alveolari alla radiografia del torace, a riprova di un sanguinamento recente, per quanto la loro assenza non escluda la possibilità di un'emorragia. Gli infiltrati, quando presenti, sono spesso simmetrici e diffusi. La TC può essere indicata per valutare un processo patologico sottostante.

La broncoscopia con strumento flessibile e lavaggio broncoalveolare è spesso utilizzata per ottenere secrezioni polmonari, in un bambino o in un giovane adulto che non è in grado di espettorare. La biopsia polmonare è raramente necessaria, a meno che il sanguinamento non sia cronico o non si riconosca un'eziologia con le altre metodiche. I test di funzionalità polmonare, tra cui la determinazione dello scambio gassoso, sono importanti per valutare la gravità del difetto di ventilazione. Nei bambini più grandi, la spirometria può dimostrare segni prevalenti di malattia ostruttiva, nel periodo acuto. Le alterazioni restrittive, secondarie alla fibrosi, sono tipiche della malattia cronica.

TRATTAMENTO. In caso di perdita ematica massiva, si rende necessaria la rianimazione con somministrazione di liquidi e trasfusione di derivati ematici. Il mantenimento di un'adeguata funzione ventilatoria e circolatoria è essenziale. Si può ricorrere alla broncoscopia rigida per rimuovere i detriti o per applicare agenti vasocostrittori locali. Idealmente, il trattamento deve essere rivolto al processo patologico specifico responsabile dell'emorragia. Quando è presente una bronchiectasia nota ed è possibile localizzare l'arteria danneggiata, l'embolizzazione dell'arteria bronchiale è spesso la terapia di scelta. Se l'embolizzazione fallisce, può essere necessaria una lobectomia totale o parziale. In presenza di un'emorragia diffusa, i corticosteroidi e altri farmaci immunosoppressori hanno dimostrato un beneficio. La prognosi dipende in notevole misura dal processo patologico sottostante.

Brown CM, Redd SC, Damon SA: Centers for Disease Control and Prevention (CDC): Acute idiopathic pulmonary hemorrhage among infants: Recommendations from the Working Group for Investigation and Surveillance. *MMWR Recomm Rep* 2004;53:1–12.

Centers for Disease Control and Prevention (CDC): Investigation of acute idiopathic pulmonary hemorrhage among infants—Massachusetts, December 2002–June 2003. *MMWR Morb Mortal Wkly Rep* 2004;53:817–820.

Coss-Bu JA, Sachdeva RC, Bricker JT, et al: Hemoptysis: A 10-year retrospective study. *Pediatrics* 1997;100:E7.

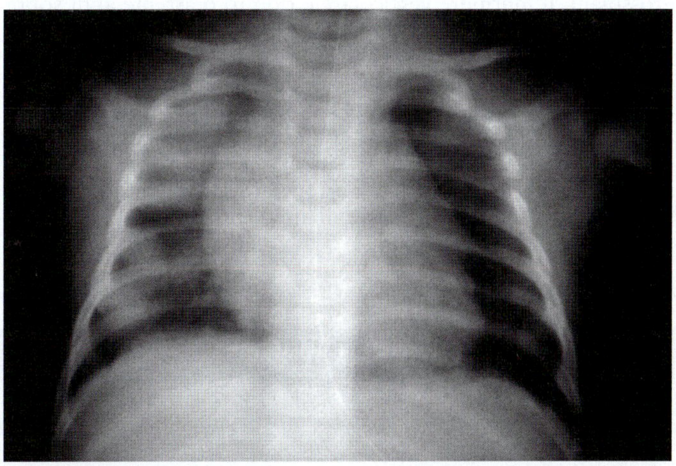

Figura 406-1. Aspetto radiografico di un'emorragia polmonare acuta idiopatica dell'infanzia. (Da Brown CM, Redd SC, Damon SA; Centers for Disease Control and Prevention (CDC): Acute idiopathic pulmonary hemorrhage among infants: Recommendations from the Working Group for Investigation and Surveillance. *MMWR Recomm Rep* 2004;53:1-12.)

Cottin V, Chinet T, Lavolé A, et al: Pulmonary arteriovenous malformations in hereditary hemorrhagic telagiectasia. A series of 126 patients. *Medicine* 2007;86:1–17.
Godfrey S: Pulmonary hemorrhage/hemoptysis in children. *Pediatr Pulmonol* 2004;37;476–484.

Capitolo 407 ■ Atelettasia

Ranna Rozenfeld

L'atelettasia, l'incompleta espansione o il collasso completo di tessuto contenente aria, è comune nei lattanti e nei bambini. Essa insorge quando l'ingresso di aria negli spazi alveolari risulta ostacolato. Il collasso segmentale, lobare o dell'intero polmone si associa all'assorbimento dell'aria contenuta negli alveoli, non più ventilati.

FISIOPATOLOGIA. Le sue cause possono essere divise in cinque gruppi (Tab. 407-1). Le infezioni virali nei bambini più piccoli, in particolare quella da virus respiratorio sinciziale (vedi Capitolo 257), possono causare aree multiple di atelettasia. I tappi di muco da qualsiasi causa sono un fattore predisponente comune. Il collasso massivo di uno o entrambi i polmoni spesso rappresenta una complicanza postoperatoria, ma occasionalmente è dovuto ad altre cause, come traumi, asma, polmonite, pneumotorace iperteso (vedi Capitolo 410), aspirazione di materiali estranei (vedi Capitoli 384 e 394), paralisi o estubazione. L'atelettasia massiva è provocata di solito da una combinazione di fattori, tra cui l'immobilizzazione o il ridotto uso del diaframma e dei muscoli respiratori, l'ostruzione dell'albero bronchiale e l'abolizione del riflesso della tosse.

MANIFESTAZIONI CLINICHE. I sintomi variano in base alla causa e all'estensione dell'atelettasia. Un'area piccola è in genere asintomatica. Quando invece è un'ampia zona di polmone precedentemente normale a diventare atelettasica, specialmente se all'improvviso, insorge dispnea accompagnata da atti respiratori rapidi e superficiali, tachicardia, tosse e spesso cianosi. Una volta rimossa l'ostruzione, i sintomi scompaiono rapidamente. In passato si riteneva che l'atelettasia da sola potesse causare febbre, ma alcuni studi hanno dimostrato che non vi è associazione tra i due fenomeni. I reperti obiettivi comprendono scarsa escursione toracica, riduzione di intensità del murmure vescicolare e crepitii grossolani. Il murmure vescicolare è ridotto o assente al di sopra delle zone atelettasiche estese.

L'atelettasia polmonare massiva si presenta di solito con dispnea, cianosi e tachicardia. Il bambino affetto è estremamente ansioso e, se abbastanza grande, lamenta dolore toracico. Il torace appare appiattito dal lato colpito, dove si notano riduzione dell'escursione respiratoria, ottusità alla percussione e rumori respiratori flebili o assenti. Nel postoperatorio, l'atelettasia si presenta in genere entro 24 ore dall'intervento, ma può insorgere anche dopo diversi giorni.

Il **collasso lobare acuto** è un'evenienza frequente nei pazienti sottoposti a cure intensive. Se non diagnosticato, può portare ad alterazioni dello scambio gassoso, infezione secondaria e conseguente fibrosi polmonare. Inizialmente, l'ipossiemia può derivare dall'alterazione del rapporto ventilazione-perfusione. Al contrario di quel che avviene nei pazienti adulti, in cui i lobi inferiori, e in particolare il sinistro, sono quelli più colpiti, il 90% dei casi nei bambini interessa i lobi superiori, e il 63% colpisce il lobo superiore destro. Anche nei reparti di terapia intensiva neonatale si osserva un'elevata incidenza di atelettasia dei lobi superiori, in particolare di collasso del lobo superiore destro, che può essere dovuto allo spostamento del tubo endotracheale nel bronco principale destro, con ostruzione o infiammazione del bronco fino al lobo superiore destro.

DIAGNOSI. In genere è possibile formulare la diagnosi di atelettasia sulla base della radiografia del torace. I reperti tipici comprendono perdita di volume e spostamento delle scissure. Le presentazioni atipiche comprendono un'atelettasia che si manifesta come un'opacità simile a una massa, o che presenta una localizzazione inusuale. L'atelettasia lobare può associarsi a pneumotorace.

Nei bambini asmatici alla radiografia del torace risulta una frequenza di anomalie del 44%, contro il 75% della TC ad alta risoluzione (HRCR, *High Resolution Computed Tomography*). I pazienti pediatrici con asma e atelettasie hanno un'aumentata incidenza di sindrome del lobo medio destro, esacerbazioni acute dell'asma, polmonite e infezioni delle vie aeree superiori.

Nell'aspirazione di corpi estranei, l'atelettasia è uno dei reperti radiografici più comuni. La sua sede in genere indica la localizzazione del corpo estraneo (vedi Capitolo 374.1). L'atelettasia è più comune quando la diagnosi viene formulata con più di 2 settimane di ritardo.

L'esame broncoscopico mostra un bronco principale collassato, quando l'ostruzione è a livello della giunzione tracheobronchiale, e può anche rivelare la natura dell'ostruzione.

L'atelettasia polmonare massiva è generalmente diagnosticabile con la radiografia del torace. I reperti tipici comprendono sollevamento del diaframma, restringimento degli spazi intercostali e spostamento delle strutture mediastiniche e del cuore verso il lato affetto (Fig. 407-1).

TRATTAMENTO. Il trattamento dipende dalla causa del collasso. Se a essere responsabile dell'atelettasia è un versamento o uno pneumotorace, innanzitutto occorre rimuovere la compressione esterna. Avviene spesso che i colpi di tosse vigorosi, la respirazione profonda e la percussione facilitino l'espansione. L'aspirazione con cateteri tracheali sterili può agevolare la rimozione dei tappi di muco. La pressione positiva continua delle vie aeree (CPAP, *Continuous Positive Airway Pressure*) può migliorare l'atelettasia.

L'esame broncoscopico è indicato nell'immediato, se l'atelettasia è conseguenza di un corpo estraneo o di qualsiasi altra ostruzione eliminabile. In caso di atelettasia bilaterale occorre effettuare immediatamente l'aspirazione broncoscopica, indicata anche quando un'area atelettasica isolata persiste per diverse settimane. Se non si trova una base anatomica, e non si ottiene materiale dall'aspirazione, l'introduzione di una piccola quantità di soluzione salina seguita da aspirazione consente il prelievo di secrezioni bronchiali per l'esame colturale ed eventualmente per quello citologico. Possono essere di beneficio cambi frequenti della

TABELLA 407-1. Cause anatomiche di atelettasia

CAUSE	ESEMPI CLINICI
Compressione esterna del parenchima polmonare	Versamento pleurico, pneumotorace, tumori intratoracici, ernia diaframmatica
Ostruzione endobronchiale che impedisce completamente l'ingresso di aria	Linfonodo ingrandito, tumore, cardiomegalia, corpo estraneo, tappi di muco, bronchiololitiasi
Ostruzione intraluminale di un bronco	Corpo estraneo, tessuto granulomatoso, tumori, secrezioni, tra cui tappi di muco, bronchiectasie, ascesso polmonare, asma, bronchite cronica, laringotracheobronchite acuta
Ostruzione intrabronchiale	Bronchiolite, polmonite interstiziale, asma
Compromissione o paralisi respiratoria	Anomalie neuromuscolari, deformità ossee, gessi o fasciature e strumentario chirurgico troppo compressivi, movimento deficitario del diaframma o restrizione dello sforzo respiratorio

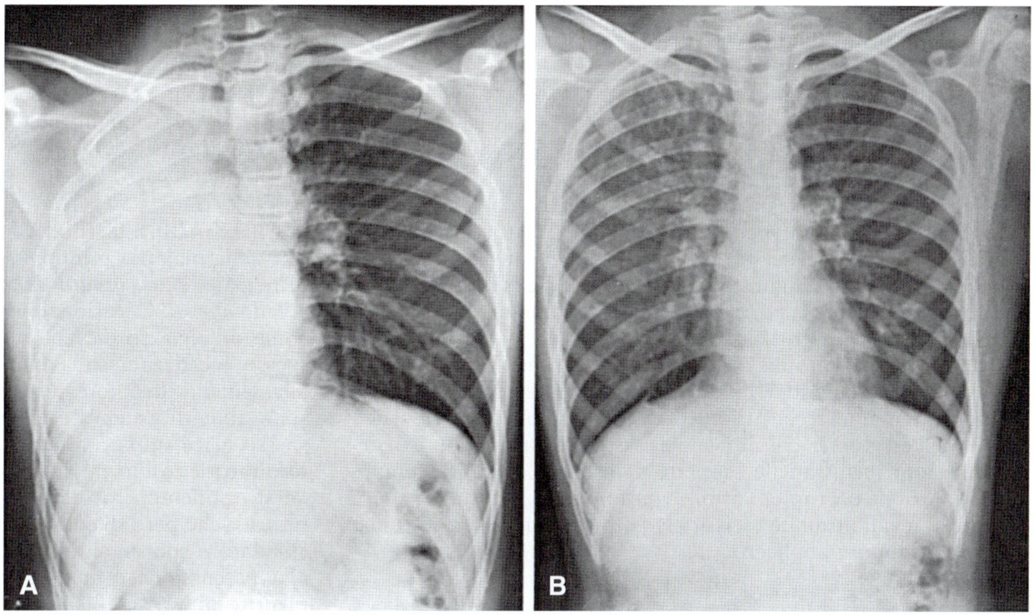

Figura 407-1. *A*, Atelettasia massiva del polmone destro, in un paziente asmatico. Il cuore e le altre strutture mediastiniche si spostano verso destra durante la fase atelettasica. *B*, Studio di confronto dopo la riespansione, successiva alla rimozione broncoscopica di un tappo di muco dal bronco principale destro.

posizione del bambino, respirazioni profonde e la fisioterapia respiratoria. La terapia con ossigeno è indicata in presenza di dispnea o desaturazione. La respirazione con pressione positiva intermittente e la spirometria incentiva sono consigliabili quando l'atelettasia non migliora dopo la fisioterapia respiratoria.

In alcune patologie, come l'asma, il trattamento con broncodilatatori e corticosteroidi può accelerare la risoluzione dell'atelettasia. La DNasi umana ricombinante (rhDNasi), che negli Stati Uniti è approvata solo per il trattamento della fibrosi cistica, è stata utilizzata *off label* per i pazienti senza fibrosi cistica, con atelettasie persistenti. Questo prodotto riduce la viscosità dei detriti bronchiali purulenti. Nei pazienti con asma severo, si verifica frequentemente ostruzione diffusa delle vie aeree da parte di secrezioni spesse e viscose, che dà luogo a un'atelettasia spesso refrattaria alla terapia convenzionale. La rhDNasi, utilizzata sia in forma nebulizzata nei pazienti non intubati sia in forma intratracheale negli asmatici intubati, ha determinato la risoluzione delle atelettasie non responsive alle terapie convenzionali per l'asma.

Per la discussione dell'atelettasia lobare nella fibrosi cistica si rimanda al Capitolo 400.

Anche gli individui affetti da malattie neuromuscolari possono sviluppare atelettasia. Questi pazienti tendono ad avere una tosse inefficace e difficoltà a espellere le secrezioni dalle vie respiratorie, che porta a polmonite e atelettasia. In tali casi sono disponibili diversi dispositivi di assistenza, tra cui la respirazione a pressione positiva intermittente, l'In-Exsufflator e la ventilazione non invasiva a pressione positiva bilivello con maschera nasale o facciale. I pazienti con malattie neuromuscolari che sono stati sottoposti a interventi chirurgici hanno un rischio importante di atelettasie postoperatorie e conseguente polmonite. L'**atelettasia migrante** del neonato è una presentazione rara e peculiare, che può essere secondaria a malattie neuromuscolari.

Vi è un'associazione tra lo sviluppo di collasso lobare e la necessità di ventilazione meccanica. Sebbene il collasso lobare sia raramente causa di morbilità a lungo termine, la sua insorgenza può richiedere il prolungamento della ventilazione meccanica o la reintubazione. Nei pazienti ventilati, in genere è indicata la pressione positiva di fine espirazione (PEEP, *Positive End Expiratory Pressure*) o la CPAP.

Ashizawa K, Hayashi K, Aso N, et al: Lobar atelectasis: Diagnostic pitfalls on chest radiography. *Br J Radiol* 2001;74:89–97.

Birnkrant DJ: The assessment and management of the respiratory complications of pediatric neuromuscular diseases. *Clin Pediatr* 2002;41:301–308.

Durward A, Forte V, Shemie SD: Resolution of mucus plugging and atelectasis after intratracheal rhDNase therapy in a mechanically ventilated child with refractory status asthmaticus. *Crit Care Med* 2000;28:560–562.

Engoren M: Lack of association between atelectasis and fever. *Chest* 1995;107:81–84.

Girardi G, Contador AM, Castro-Rodriguez JA: Two new radiological findings to improve the diagnosis of bronchial foreign-body aspiration in children. *Pediatr Pulmonol* 2004;38:261–264.

Miske LJ, Hickey EM, Kolb SM, et al: Use of the mechanical In-Exsufflator in pediatric patients with neuromuscular disease and impaired cough. *Chest* 2004;125:1406–1412.

Nuhoglu Y, Bahceciler N, Yuksel M, et al: Thorax high resolution computerized tomography findings in asthmatic children with unusual clinical manifestations. *Ann Allergy Asthma Immunol* 1999;82:311–314.

Scolieri P, Adappa ND, Coticchia JM: Value of rigid bronchoscopy in the management of critically ill children with acute lung collapse. *Pediatr Emerg Care* 2004;20:384–386.

Thomas K, Habibi P, Britto J, et al: Distribution and pathophysiology of acute lobar collapse in the pediatric intensive care unit. *Crit Care Med* 1999;27:1594–1597.

Tokar B, Ozkan R, Ilhan H: Tracheobronchial foreign bodies in children: Importance of accurate history and plain chest radiography in delayed presentation. *Clin Radiol* 2004;59:609–615.

Tsai SL, Crain EF, Silver EJ, et al: What can we learn from chest radiographs in hypoxemic asthmatics? *Pediatr Radiol* 2002;32:498–504.

Capitolo 408 ■ Tumori polmonari

Susanna A. McColley

EZIOLOGIA. I tumori primitivi del polmone sono rari nei bambini e negli adolescenti. Una stima accurata della loro frequenza è difficile, poiché la letteratura sull'argomento è limitata principalmente a case report e a casistiche. Inoltre, l'elevata incidenza di "pseudotumori infiammatori" confonde ulteriormente le statistiche. L'**adenoma bronchiale** e il **carcinoide** sono i tumori primitivi più comuni. Le lesioni metastatiche sono le forme più comuni di tumori polmonari nei bambini; i processi primitivi comprendono il tumore di Wilms, il sarcoma osteogenico e l'epatoblastoma (vedi Parte XXI). L'adenocarcinoma e l'istologia indifferenziata sono i reperti anatomopatologici più comuni nel tumore primitivo del polmone; il blastoma polmonare è più raro e spesso insorge nel quadro della pneumopatia cistica. Il coinvolgimento mediastinico da parte di un linfoma è più comune dei tumori polmonari maligni primitivi.

MANIFESTAZIONI CLINICHE E VALUTAZIONE. I tumori polmonari possono presentarsi con febbre, emottisi, sibili, tosse, versamento pleurico, dolore toracico, dispnea, oppure polmonite o atelettasia ricorrenti. Anche se la radiografia semplice del torace può far sorgere il sospetto, per una definizione anatomica precisa è necessaria una TC del torace. Occasionalmente le neoplasie bronchiali vengono diagnosticate nel corso di una broncoscopia a fibre ottiche, effettuata a causa di infiltrati polmonari persistenti o ricorrenti o di emottisi.

I pazienti con sintomi, o con una radiografia o altri reperti di laboratorio suggestivi di tumore polmonare, devono essere valutati attentamente per la ricerca di un tumore in altra sede, prima dell'escissione chirurgica. Sia le lesioni primitive isolate sia le lesioni metastatiche scoperte a distanza di molto tempo dalla rimozione del tumore primitivo, sono state asportate e sono trattate al meglio tramite escissione. La prognosi varia a seconda del tipo di tumore implicato.

Eggli KD, Newman B: Nodules, masses, and pseudomasses in the pediatric lung. *Radiol Clin North Am* 1993; 31:651–666.
Epstein DM, Aronchick JM: Lung cancer in childhood. *Med Pediatr Oncol* 1989;17:510–513.
Hancock BJ, Di Lorenzo M, Youssef S, et al: Childhood primary pulmonary neoplasms. *J Pediatr Surg* 1993;28:1133–1136.
Keita O, Lagrange JL, Michiels JF, et al: Primary bronchogenic squamous cell carcinoma in children: Report of a case and review of the literature. *Med Pediatr Oncol* 1995;24:50–52.
McCahon E: Lung tumours in children. *Pediatr Respir Rev* 2006;7(3): 191–196. E-pub 2006; Aug 4.
Roviaro Gc, Varoli F, Zannini P, et al: Lung cancer in the young. *Chest* 1985;87:456–459.
Tian DL, Liu HX, Zhang L, et al: Surgery for young patients with lung cancer. *Lung Cancer* 2003;42:215–220.

Capitolo 409 ■ Pleurite, versamento pleurico ed empiema pleurico

Glenna B. Winnie

La pleurite, o infiammazione della pleura, è spesso accompagnata da un versamento la cui causa più comune, nei bambini, è la polmonite batterica (vedi Capitolo 397), seguita dallo scompenso cardiaco (vedi Capitolo 442), dalle cause reumatologiche e dai tumori metastatici intratoracici maligni. A essere responsabili dei restanti casi sono molte altre malattie, tra cui la tubercolosi (vedi Capitolo 212), il lupus eritematoso (vedi Capitolo 157), la polmonite da aspirazione (vedi Capitolo 394), l'uremia, la pancreatite, l'ascesso sottodiaframmatico e l'artrite reumatoide. I maschi e le femmine sono affetti in egual misura.

I processi infiammatori della pleura possono essere di tre tipi: secchi o plastici, sierofibrinosi o sieroematici, e pleurite purulenta o empiema.

409.1 • Pleurite secca o plastica

EZIOLOGIA. La pleurite plastica può associarsi a infezioni polmonari batteriche o virali, oppure svilupparsi nel corso di una malattia delle vie respiratorie superiori. Questa patologia si associa inoltre alla tubercolosi e alle malattie del connettivo, come la febbre reumatica.

ANATOMIA PATOLOGICA E PATOGENESI. Il processo è di regola limitato alla pleura viscerale, con piccole quantità di liquido sieroso giallastro e aderenze tra le superfici pleuriche. Nella tubercolosi, le aderenze si sviluppano rapidamente e le pleure sono spesso ispessite. Occasionalmente, il deposito di fibrina e le aderenze sono di gravità tale da provocare un fibrotorace, che inibisce in misura significativa l'escursione polmonare.

MANIFESTAZIONI CLINICHE. I segni e i sintomi sono spesso eclissati dalla malattia primitiva. Il dolore, che costituisce il sintomo principale, è *accentuato dalla respirazione profonda, dalla tosse e dallo sforzo*. Occasionalmente, il dolore pleurico viene descritto come un'algia sorda, che non varia molto con la respirazione, spesso localizzata sulla parete toracica e riferita alla spalla o alla schiena. Il dolore suscitato dai movimenti del respiro è responsabile di grugniti e di difesa nella respirazione; il bambino spesso giace sul lato affetto nel tentativo di ridurre le escursioni respiratorie. All'inizio della malattia può essere udibile un rumore da sfregamento grossolano, simile a cuoio, inspiratorio ed espiratorio, che però di solito scompare rapidamente. Se lo strato di essudato è spesso, si apprezza talvolta un aumento dell'ottusità alla percussione e una riduzione del murmure vescicolare. La pleurite può essere asintomatica. La forma cronica è osservata occasionalmente in condizioni come atelettasie, ascessi polmonari, malattie del tessuto connettivo e tubercolosi.

INDAGINI DI LABORATORIO. La pleurite plastica si manifesta alle radiografie come un'opacità diffusa della superficie pleurica o come un'ombra densa, a margini netti; quest'ultimo reperto può essere indistinguibile da piccole quantità di essudato pleurico. La radiografia del torace può essere normale, ma l'ecografia o la TC saranno comunque positive.

DIAGNOSI DIFFERENZIALE. La pleurite plastica deve essere distinta da altre patologie, come la pleurodinia epidemica, i traumi della gabbia toracica (fratture costali), le lesioni dei gangli delle radici posteriori, i tumori della corda spinale, l'herpes zoster e la trichinosi. Anche se l'esame obiettivo o la radiografia non evidenziano segni di versamento pleurico, un tampone pleurico eco- o TC-guidato, nei casi sospetti, spesso permette di rilevare una piccola quantità di essudato che, quando sottoposto a coltura, può indicare la causa batterica sottostante, in pazienti con polmonite acuta. I pazienti con pleurite e polmonite devono sempre essere sottoposti a screening per la tubercolosi.

TRATTAMENTO. La terapia deve essere rivolta alla causa sottostante. Quando è presente una polmonite, non sono indicate né l'immobilizzazione del torace con gesso aderente, né la terapia con farmaci sedativi del riflesso della tosse. Se non è presente polmonite, o se è ben controllata, il bendaggio del torace per limitare l'espansione può alleviare il dolore. Può essere utile l'analgesia con farmaci antinfiammatori non steroidei.

409.2 • Pleurite sierofibrinosa o sieroematica

EZIOLOGIA. La pleurite sierofibrinosa è definita come un essudato fibrinoso sulla superficie pleurica e un versamento essudativo di liquido sieroso nello spazio pleurico. Si associa soprattutto a infezioni del polmone o a condizioni infiammatorie dell'addome o del mediastino, mentre è di riscontro meno frequente nelle malattie del tessuto connettivo, come il lupus eritematoso sistemico, la periarterite o l'artrite reumatoide. Occasionalmente, si osserva in caso di neoplasie primitive o metastatiche del polmone, della pleura o del mediastino; è comune l'associazione dei tumori con una pleurite emorragica.

PATOGENESI. Di norma, il liquido pleurico origina dai capillari della pleura parietale ed è assorbito dallo spazio pleurico, tramite gli stomi pleurici e i linfatici della pleura parietale. La velocità di formazione del liquido dipende dalla legge di Starling, secondo la quale il movimento di liquido è determinato dall'equilibrio tra la pressione idrostatica e oncotica nello spazio pleurico e nel letto capillare polmonare, e dalla permeabilità della membrana pleurica. Normalmente, sono presenti nello spazio pleurico solo 4-12 mL di liquido, ma se la formazione supera la clearance, si verifica un accumulo; vi può anche essere un'ostruzione dell'assorbimento linfatico.

MANIFESTAZIONI CLINICHE. Dal momento che la pleurite sierofibrinosa è spesso preceduta dalla forma plastica, i segni e i sintomi precoci possono essere quelli della pleurite plastica. Con l'accumulo del liquido, il dolore pleuritico talvolta scompare; il paziente può divenire asintomatico, se il versamento rimane di piccole dimensioni, oppure presentare solo segni e sintomi sfumati della malattia sottostante. Versamenti cospicui di liquido provocano tosse, dispnea, retrazioni, tachipnea, ortopnea e cianosi. L'esame obiettivo dipende in una certa misura dall'entità del versamento. Alla percussione si può apprezzare ottusità alle basi. Vi sono rumori respiratori ridotti o assenti, riduzione del fremito vocale tattile, spostamento del mediastino dal lato opposto a quello affetto e, occasionalmente, riempimento degli spazi intercostali. Se il liquido non è loculato, questi segni possono spostarsi quando il paziente cambia posizione. Nei lattanti, i segni obiettivi sono meno definiti; invece dei rumori respiratori ridotti o assenti, può essere udibile un soffio bronchiale. Se è presente una polmonite estesa, si possono apprezzare anche crepitii e ronchi. I rumori da sfregamento di solito sono rilevabili solo durante la fase iniziale o tardiva della pleurite plastica. Il processo è in genere monolaterale.

INDAGINI DI LABORATORIO. L'esame radiografico mostra una densità generalmente omogenea, che oblitera la normale trama del polmone sottostante. I versamenti di lieve entità possono causare obliterazione solo del seno costofrenico o cardiofrenico, o un ampiamento dei setti interlobari. L'esame va effettuato con il paziente sia supino sia in ortostatismo, per dimostrare lo spostamento del versamento con il cambio di posizione; la posizione in decubito può essere utile. L'esame ecografico è utile e può guidare la toracentesi, se il versamento è loculato. L'esame del liquido è essenziale per differenziare gli essudati dai trasudati e per determinare il tipo di essudato (vedi Capitolo 397). A seconda dello scenario clinico, il liquido pleurico viene sottoposto all'esame colturale per batteri, funghi e micobatteri, alla ricerca di antigeni, alla colorazione Gram o all'esame fisico-chimico, comprensivo di dosaggio di proteine, lattico deidrogenasi e glucosio, amilasi, peso specifico, conta cellulare totale e differenziale, esame citologico e pH. Di solito gli **essudati** hanno almeno una delle seguenti caratteristiche: livello di proteine >3,0 g/dL, con rapporto proteine del liquido pleurico/proteine sieriche >0,5, valori di lattico deidrogenasi >200 UI/L oppure rapporto tra lattico deidrogenasi del liquido pleurico e quella del siero >0,6. Un pH >7,2 fa pensare a un essudato. Il glucosio è usualmente <60 mg/dL nei tumori maligni, nella malattia reumatoide e nella tubercolosi; la presenza di molti piccoli linfociti e di un pH <7,2 suggerisce una tubercolosi. Il liquido della pleurite sierofibrinosa, limpido o appena torbido, contiene relativamente pochi leucociti e talvolta alcuni eritrociti. La colorazione di Gram può occasionalmente mostrare batteri; tuttavia, è raro che la colorazione acido-resistente riveli i bacilli tubercolari.

DIAGNOSI E DIAGNOSI DIFFERENZIALE. Quando è presente o si sospetta un versamento pleurico, occorre effettuare la toracentesi, a meno che il versamento non sia molto piccolo e il paziente non abbia la classica polmonite lobare pneumococcica. La toracentesi può permettere di differenziare la pleurite sierofibrinosa dall'empiema, dall'idrotorace, dall'emotorace e dal chilotorace. Gli essudati in genere sono associati a processi infiammatori. Nell'idrotorace, il liquido ha un peso specifico <1,015 e la valutazione rivela solo poche cellule mesoteliali, anziché leucociti. Il chilotorace e l'emotorace hanno in genere un liquido con un aspetto peculiare, ma distinguere una pleurite sierofibrinosa da una purulenta è praticamente impossibile, senza un esame microscopico del liquido. L'esame citologico può rivelare la presenza di cellule maligne. Il liquido sierofibrinoso può divenire rapidamente purulento.

COMPLICANZE. Se il liquido non diviene purulento, di solito scompare con relativa rapidità, in particolare grazie a un trattamento appropriato della polmonite batterica. Persiste un po' più a lungo nella tubercolosi e nelle malattie del tessuto connettivo e può recidivare o permanere per molto tempo in caso di neoplasie. Con l'assorbimento del liquido, spesso si sviluppano aderenze tra i due foglietti pleurici, che però in genere non compromettono il quadro clinico o lo influenzano solo lievemente. Può svilupparsi ispessimento pleurico, che talvolta viene scambiato per un versamento di lieve entità o per infiltrati polmonari persistenti. Pur potendo persistere per mesi, l'ispessimento pleurico di solito si risolve senza lasciare reliquati.

TRATTAMENTO. La terapia dovrebbe essere rivolta alla malattia sottostante, sebbene nei versamenti cospicui il drenaggio del liquido sia di beneficio per il paziente. Quando si effettua una toracentesi diagnostica, si dovrebbe raccogliere la maggior quantità possibile di liquido, a scopo terapeutico. La rapida rimozione di ≥1 L di liquido pleurico può associarsi allo sviluppo di edema polmonare da riespansione (vedi Capitolo 393). Se la malattia di base è trattata adeguatamente, di solito non è necessario un ulteriore drenaggio, ma se si riaccumula una quantità di liquido sufficiente a causare disordini della respirazione, si raccomanda di effettuarlo con un tubo toracico. Nei bambini più grandi, con sospetto versamento parapneumonico, si considera necessaria la toracostomia con tubo di drenaggio, se il pH del liquido pleurico è <7,2 o se il livello di glucosio nel liquido pleurico è <50 mg/dL. Se il liquido è francamente purulento, è indicato il tubo di drenaggio. L'acidosi sistemica fa sì che la misurazione del pH del liquido pleurico sia meno utile. I pazienti con versamento pleurico possono richiedere un'analgesia, in particolare dopo la toracentesi o l'inserimento di un tubo di drenaggio toracico. Quelli con polmonite acuta possono necessitare di ossigeno, oltre al trattamento antibiotico specifico.

409.3 • PLEURITE PURULENTA O EMPIEMA

EZIOLOGIA. L'empiema è un accumulo di pus nello spazio pleurico, per lo più associato alla polmonite da *Streptococcus pneumoniae*, sebbene lo *Staphylococcus aureus* sia più comune nei Paesi in via di sviluppo e nell'empiema post-traumatico (vedi Capitolo 397). L'incidenza relativa dell'empiema da *Haemophilus influenzae* si è ridotta dall'introduzione della vaccinazione Hib. Gli streptococchi di gruppo A, i microrganismi Gram-negativi, la tubercolosi, i funghi e i tumori sono cause meno comuni. La malattia può anche essere provocata dalla rottura di un ascesso polmonare nella cavità pleurica, dalla contaminazione introdotta da un trauma o da interventi di chirurgia toracica o, raramente, da una mediastinite o dall'estensione di un ascesso endoaddominale.

EPIDEMIOLOGIA. L'empiema è di frequente riscontro nei lattanti e nei bambini in età prescolare. Insorge nel 5-10% dei pazienti pediatrici con polmonite batterica.

ANATOMIA PATOLOGICA. L'empiema attraversa tre stadi: essudativo, fibrinopurulento e organizzativo. Durante lo *stadio essudativo*, si forma l'essudato fibrinoso sulle superfici pleuriche. Nello *stadio fibrinopurulento*, si formano setti fibrinosi, che causano la loculazione del liquido, con ispessimento della pleura parietale. Se il pus non viene drenato, può farsi strada, attraverso la pleura, nel parenchima polmonare, provocando fistole broncopleuriche e piopneumotorace, oppure nella cavità addominale. Raramente, il pus si fa strada attraverso la parete toracica (per es. empiema necessitatis). Durante lo *stadio organizzativo*, si verifica proliferazione dei fibroblasti e si possono sviluppare sacche di pus loculato nelle cavità ascessuali dalle pareti spesse; altrimenti, il polmone può collassare ed essere circondato da un involucro spesso e anelastico (corteccia).

MANIFESTAZIONI CLINICHE. I segni e i sintomi iniziali sono principalmente quelli della polmonite batterica. Nei bambini che non hanno ricevuto cure adeguate o hanno assunto antibiotici inappropriati può intercorrere un intervallo di alcuni giorni tra la fase della polmonite clinica e l'evidenza di empiema. La maggior parte dei pazienti è febbrile. Nei lattanti, vi può essere una moderata esacerbazione del distress respiratorio. Il bambino più grande appare in genere più prostrato e ha una maggiore difficoltà respiratoria. I segni obiettivi sono identici a quelli descritti per la pleurite sierofibrinosa, e le due condizioni sono differenziabili solo con la toracentesi, che dovrebbe essere sempre effettuata quando si sospetta un empiema.

INDAGINI DI LABORATORIO. Radiograficamente, tutti i versamenti pleurici sembrano simili, ma l'assenza di spostamento del liquido con il cambio di posizione indica un empiema loculato; la conferma della diagnosi può essere fornita dall'ecografia o dalla TC. Occorre asportare tramite toracentesi la massima quantità di liquido ottenibile, che va analizzato come descritto nel Capitolo 409.2. Il versamento è un empiema se risultano presenti batteri alla colorazione di Gram, se il pH è $<7{,}2$ e se vi sono $>100\,000$ neutrofili/μL. L'aspetto del pus prodotto dai diversi microrganismi non è distintivo; è sempre necessario effettuare le colture. Nell'empiema pneumococcico, la coltura è positiva nel 58% dei pazienti. Nei pazienti con coltura negativa per pneumococco, la PCR per lo pneumococco è più utile ai fini della diagnosi. Le emocolture hanno una resa elevata, talvolta persino superiore a quella del liquido pleurico. Si possono rilevare leucocitosi e aumento della velocità di eritrosedimentazione.

COMPLICANZE. Nelle infezioni da stafilococco si sviluppano comunemente fistole broncopleuriche e piopneumotorace. Altre complicanze locali comprendono pericardite purulenta, ascessi polmonari, peritonite secondaria a rottura attraverso il diaframma e osteomielite delle coste. Sono inoltre possibili complicanze settiche, come la meningite, l'artrite e l'osteomielite. La setticemia è di frequente riscontro nelle infezioni da *H. influenzae* e pneumococciche. Il versamento può organizzarsi in una spessa "corazza", che può limitare l'escursione polmonare e associarsi a febbre persistente.

TRATTAMENTO. Le opzioni di trattamento comprendono antibiotici, toracentesi, tubo di drenaggio toracico con o senza agenti fibrinolitici, chirurgia toracoscopica videoassistita (VATS, *Video-Assisted Thoracoscopic Surgery*) o decorticazione a cielo aperto (vedi Capitolo 397). Se l'empiema viene diagnosticato precocemente, con la toracentesi e il trattamento antibiotico si ottiene la guarigione completa. Al momento di prelevare del pus con la toracentesi, si deve posizionare immediatamente un tubo di drenaggio toracico chiuso, controllato da una valvola ad acqua o dall'aspirazione continua. Occorre inserire un catetere del massimo diametro interno possibile; talvolta sono necessari più tubi per drenare le aree loculate. Il drenaggio chiuso di solito rimane in sede per una settimana circa; i tubi che non drenano più devono essere rimossi. Non si devono tentare aspirazioni multiple della cavità pleurica invece del drenaggio chiuso continuo.

È inoltre necessaria una terapia antibiotica sistemica; la scelta del farmaco deve basarsi sullo studio di sensibilità *in vitro* del microrganismo responsabile. Si rimanda ai Capitoli 180, 181 e 192 per il trattamento delle infezioni rispettivamente da *Staphylococcus*, *Streptocccus pneumoniae* e *H. influenzae*. Nelle infezioni stafilococciche, che vanno incontro a una risoluzione molto lenta, è necessaria una terapia antibiotica sistemica per 3-4 settimane. Anche nell'empiema non stafilococcico la risposta clinica è lenta, nonostante un trattamento ottimale; il miglioramento può essere scarso anche per 2 settimane. L'instillazione di antibiotici nella cavità pleurica non solo non migliora i risultati ottenuti con la sola terapia antibiotica sistemica, ma si associa a reazioni locali.

L'instillazione di agenti fibrinolitici nella cavità pleurica può promuovere il drenaggio, ridurre la febbre, diminuire la necessità di interventi chirurgici e abbreviare l'ospedalizzazione; il farmaco e il dosaggio ottimali non sono stati determinati. La streptochinasi 15 000 U/kg in 50 mL di soluzione fisiologica, una volta al giorno per 3-5 giorni, e l'urochinasi 40 000 U in 40 mL di soluzione fisiologica, ogni 12 ore per 6 dosi, sono state studiate in studi randomizzati compiuti su pazienti pediatrici. La streptochinasi comporta il rischio di anafilassi ed entrambi i farmaci possono associarsi a emorragie e altre complicanze.

Anche se sulla superficie dei polmoni collassati possono essere presenti alterazioni fibrinose estese, le procedure di decorticazione chirurgica sono raramente indicate. Nel bambino che rimane febbrile e dispnoico per >72 ore dopo l'inizio della terapia con antibiotici endovena e con tubo di drenaggio toracico, la decorticazione chirurgica tramite **VATS** o, meno spesso, la toracotomia a cielo aperto possono accelerare la guarigione. Se si forma uno pneumatocele, non si deve fare alcun tentativo di trattarlo chirurgicamente o con aspirazione, a meno che non raggiunga una dimensione tale da causare difficoltà alla respirazione o infettarsi secondariamente. Di solito gli pneumatoceli si risolvono spontaneamente con il tempo. La prognosi clinica a lungo termine dell'empiema trattato adeguatamente è eccellente, e gli studi di follow-up della funzione polmonare suggeriscono che la malattia restrittiva residua sia poco comune, con o senza intervento chirurgico.

Jaffe A, Cohen G: Thoracic empyema: A role for primary video assisted thoracoscopic surgery? *Arch Dis Child* 2003;88:839–841.

Kohn GL, Walston C, Feldstein J, et al: Persistent abnormal lung function after childhood empyema. *Am J Respir Med* 2002;1:441–445.

Kurt BA, Winterhalter KM, Connors RH, et al: Therapy of parapneumonic effusions in children: video-assisted thoracoscopic surgery versus conventional thoracostomy drainage. *Pediatrics* 2006;118:e547–e553.

Le Monnier A, Carbonelle E, Zahar JR, et al: Microbiological diagnosis of empyma in children: comparative evaluations by culture, polymerase chain reaction, and pneumococcal antigen detection in pleural fluids. *CID* 2006;42:1135–1140.

Light RW: A new classification of parapneumonic effusions and empyema. *Chest* 1995;108:299–301.

Noppen M, DeWaele M, Li R, et al: Volume and cellular content of normal pleural fluid in humans examined by pleural lavage. *Am J Resp Crit Care Med* 2000;162:1023–1026.

Paganini H, Guinazu JR, Hernandez C, et al: Comparative analysis of outcome and clinical features in children with pleural empyema caused by penicillin-nonsusceptible and penicillin-susceptible Streptococcus pneumoniae. *Int J Infect Dis* 2001;5:86–88.

Redding GJ, Walund L, Walund D, et al: Lung function in children following empyema. *Am J Dis Child* 1990;144:1337–1342.

Singh M, Mathew JL, Chandra S, et al: Randomized controlled trial of intrapleural streptokinase in empyema thoracis in children. *Acta Paediatr* 2004;93:1443–1445.

Thompson AH, Hull J, Kumar MR, et al: Randomised trial of intrapleural urokinase in the treatment of childhood empyema. *Thorax* 2002; 57:343–347.

Yao CT, Wu JM, Liu CC, et al: Treatment of complicated parapneumonic pleural effusion with intrapleural streptokinase in children. *Chest* 2004;125:566–571.

Capitolo 410 ■ Pneumotorace

Glenna B. Winnie

Lo pneumotorace, poco comune nell'infanzia, consiste nell'accumulo di aria extrapolmonare nel torace. Più spesso, si forma in conseguenza della fuoriuscita di aria dal polmone, che a sua volta può essere primitiva o secondaria, spontanea, traumatica, iatrogena o catameniale (Tab. 410-1). Lo pneumotorace del periodo neonatale è discusso anche nel Capitolo 101.13.

TABELLA 410-1. Cause di pneumotorace nei bambini

SPONTANEO

Idiopatico primitivo, di solito risultante dalla rottura di bolle subpleuriche secondarie
Malattie polmonari congenite
Malformazione adenomatoide cistica congenita
Cisti broncogena
Ipoplasia polmonare
Condizioni associate ad aumento della pressione intratoracica
Asma
Bronchiolite
Sindrome da blocco dell'aria (*Air-block syndrome*) nei neonati
Fibrosi cistica
Corpo estraneo nelle vie aeree
Infezioni
Pneumatoceli
Ascessi polmonari
Fistola broncopleurica
Malattia polmonare diffusa
Istiocitosi a cellule di Langerhans
Sclerosi tuberosa
Sindrome di Marfan
Sindrome di Ehler-Danlos
Neoplasia metastatica, di solito osteosarcoma (raro)

TRAUMATICO

Non iatrogeno
Trauma penetrante
Trauma chiuso
Musica ad alto volume (pressione dell'aria)

Iatrogeno
Toracotomia
Toracoscopia, toracentesi
Tracheostomia
Puntura con tubo o con ago
Ventilazione meccanica

*Agenesia renale, ernia diaframmatica, perdita di liquido amniotico.
Da Kuhn JP, Slovis TL, Haller JO: *Caffey's Pediatric Diagnostic Imaging*, vol 1, 10th ed. Philadelphia, Mosby, 2004, p 885.

EZIOLOGIA ED EPIDEMIOLOGIA. Lo **pneumotorace spontaneo primitivo** insorge in individui senza traumi né malattie polmonari sottostanti. Lo pneumotorace spontaneo, con o senza sforzo (Valsalva), si manifesta occasionalmente negli adolescenti e nei giovani adulti, soprattutto nei maschi alti e magri che si ritiene abbiano bolle subpleuriche. Sono state descritte famiglie in cui molti membri hanno avuto pneumotoraci spontanei, con esordio in momenti diversi, dalla nascita all'età adulta. I pazienti con difetti della sintesi del collagene, come la malattia di Ehler-Danlos (vedi Capitolo 658) e la sindrome di Marfan (vedi Capitolo 700), sono raramente predisposti allo sviluppo pneumotorace.

Uno pneumotorace che insorge come complicanza di un disturbo polmonare sottostante, ma in assenza di traumi, è detto **pneumotorace spontaneo secondario**. Oltre a verificarsi in corso di polmonite, di solito con empiema, può anche essere secondario ad ascessi, gangrena o infarto polmonari, a rottura di una cisti o di una bolla enfisematosa (nell'asma), o a corpi estranei nel polmone. Nella polmonite stafilococcica del lattante, la sua incidenza è relativamente elevata. Si osserva nel 5% circa dei bambini asmatici ospedalizzati e si risolve abitualmente senza trattamento. Lo pneumotorace è una complicanza severa della fibrosi cistica (vedi Capitolo 400). Insorge anche nei pazienti con linfoma o altri tumori e nella malattia del trapianto verso l'ospite (GVHD, *Graft Versus Host Disease*) con bronchiolite obliterante.

I traumi toracici o addominali esterni, chiusi o penetranti, possono lacerare un bronco o un viscere addominale, con fuoriuscita di aria nello spazio pleurico. L'abuso di ecstasy (metilenediossimetamfetamina) è stato associato a pneumotorace.

Lo pneumotorace iatrogeno può complicare una tracheotomia, il posizionamento di una linea succlavia, una toracentesi, una biopsia transbronchiale o altre procedure diagnostico-terapeutiche. Può inoltre verificarsi dopo trattamento con agopuntura.

Lo **pneumotorace catameniale**, una rara condizione che è, per definizione, associata alle mestruazioni, è determinato dal passaggio di aria intraddominale attraverso difetti del diaframma.

Lo pneumotorace può associarsi a versamento sieroso (idropneumotorace) o purulento (piopneumotorace). La forma bilaterale è rara oltre il periodo neonatale, ma è stata riportata dopo trapianto polmonare, con l'infezione da *Mycoplasma pneumoniae* e con la tubercolosi.

FISIOPATOLOGIA. La tendenza del polmone a collassare (ritorno elastico) è controbilanciata, nel normale stato di riposo, dalla corrispondente tendenza della parete toracica a espandersi verso l'esterno; si crea così una pressione negativa nello spazio intrapleurico. Quando entra dell'aria nello spazio pleurico, il polmone collassa. Insorge ipossiemia, dovuta a ipoventilazione alveolare, alterazione del rapporto ventilazione-perfusione e shunt intrapolmonare. Nello pneumotorace semplice, la pressione intrapleurica è uguale a quella atmosferica e il polmone collassa fino al 30%; in quello complicato, o iperteso, la fuoriuscita continua produce un aumento della pressione nello spazio pleurico, con ulteriore compressione del polmone, spostamento delle strutture mediastiniche verso il lato opposto, ridotto ritorno venoso e riduzione della gittata cardiaca.

MANIFESTAZIONI CLINICHE. L'insorgenza è abitualmente improvvisa, e la severità dei sintomi dipende dall'estensione del collasso polmonare e dall'entità della malattia polmonare preesistente. Lo pneumotorace può causare dolore, dispnea e cianosi. Nei lattanti, i segni e i sintomi possono essere difficili da riconoscere. Uno pneumotorace moderato può causare un lieve spostamento degli organi intratoracici e sintomi scarsi o assenti. La gravità del dolore di solito non è direttamente proporzionale al grado di collasso.

Di solito si manifestano distress respiratorio, retrazioni e netta riduzione del murmure vescicolare sul polmone colpito. La percussione sull'area coinvolta produce un suono ipertimpanico. La laringe, la trachea e il cuore possono essere spostati verso il lato non colpito. Quando è presente anche versamento, di solito si apprezza un'area nettamente delimitata di timpania sopra un livello di ottusità alla percussione. La presenza di respirazione anforica o, quando è presente liquido nella cavità pleurica, di suoni gorgoglianti in sincrono con i movimenti del respiro suggerisce una fistola aperta in connessione con tessuti a contenuto aereo.

DIAGNOSI E DIAGNOSI DIFFERENZIALE. La diagnosi viene formulata abitualmente tramite l'esame radiografico (Figg. 410-1, 410-2, 410-3). La quantità di aria extrapolmonare varia nel tempo: una radiografia effettuata tempestivamente mostra un collasso polmonare minore di una ottenuta più tardi, se la perdita di aria continua. Le immagini in espirazione accentuano il contrasto tra la trama polmonare e la zona trasparente di pneumotorace (vedi Fig. 410-1). Quando si considera la possibilità di un'ernia diaframmatica, può essere necessaria una piccola quantità di bario per dimostrare che non si tratta di aria libera, ma di una porzione del tratto gastrointestinale erniata nella cavità toracica. Anche l'ecografia può essere utile a fini diagnostici.

Può essere difficile determinare se uno pneumotorace è sotto tensione. I **segni di tensione** comprendono lo spostamento delle strutture mediastiniche dal lato opposto a quello della perdita di aria. Tale spostamento può essere assente nelle situazioni in cui l'altro emitorace oppone resistenza, come nelle forme bilaterali. Quando entrambi i polmoni sono rigidi, come nella fibrosi cistica o nella sindrome da distress respiratorio, il polmone non colpito può non collassare facilmente e lo spostamento può non avvenire (vedi Fig. 410-3). Occasionalmente, la diagnosi di pneumotorace teso viene effettuata solo sulla base dei segni di compromissione del circolo, o sentendo il sibilo della rapida uscita dell'aria sotto pressione con l'inserzione del tubo toracostomico.

Lo pneumotorace deve essere differenziato dall'enfisema localizzato o generalizzato, dalle bolle enfisematose estese, dalle ampie cavità polmonari o dalla altre formazioni cistiche, dalle ernie

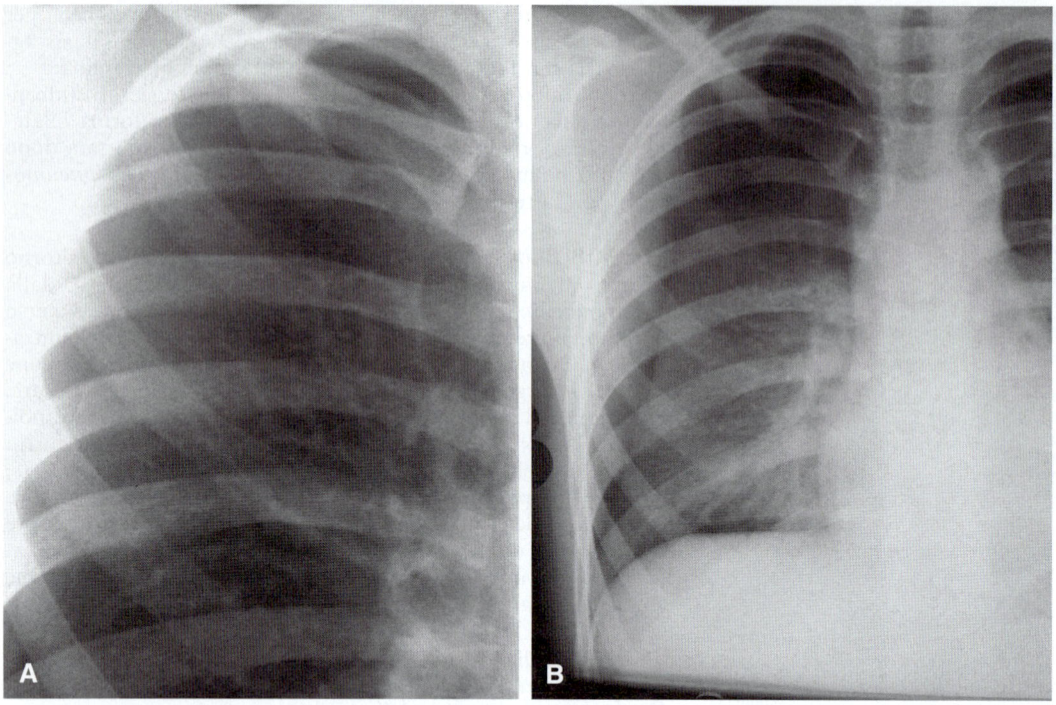

Figura 410-1. Utilità di un'immagine in espirazione ai fini di individuare lo pneumotorace. *A*, Adolescente con dolore toracico e lieve radiolucenza laterale nel lobo superiore destro. Il margine della pleura viscerale è appena visibile. *B*, Alla radiografia in espirazione, lo pneumotorace risulta evidente, poiché il polmone destro si è deflato ed è divenuto più opaco, fornendo un contrasto migliore con l'aria presente nello spazio pleurico. (Da Kuhn JP, Slovis TL, Haller JO: *Caffrey's Pediatric Diagnostic Imaging*, vol 1, 10th ed. Philadelphia, Mosby, 2004, p 885.)

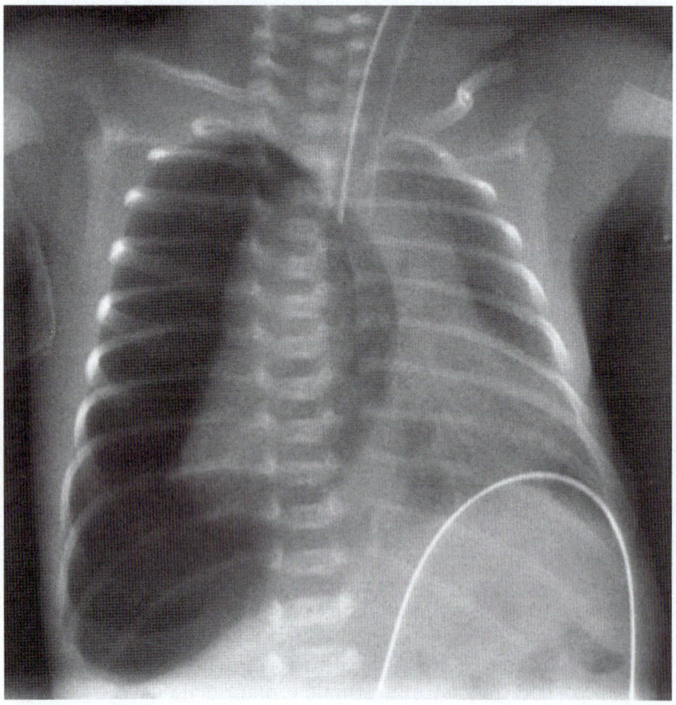

Figura 410-2. Pneumotorace destro, polmone collassato con compliance conservata. (Da Clark DA: *Atlas of Neonatology*, 7th ed. Philadelphia, WB Saunders, 2000, p 91.)

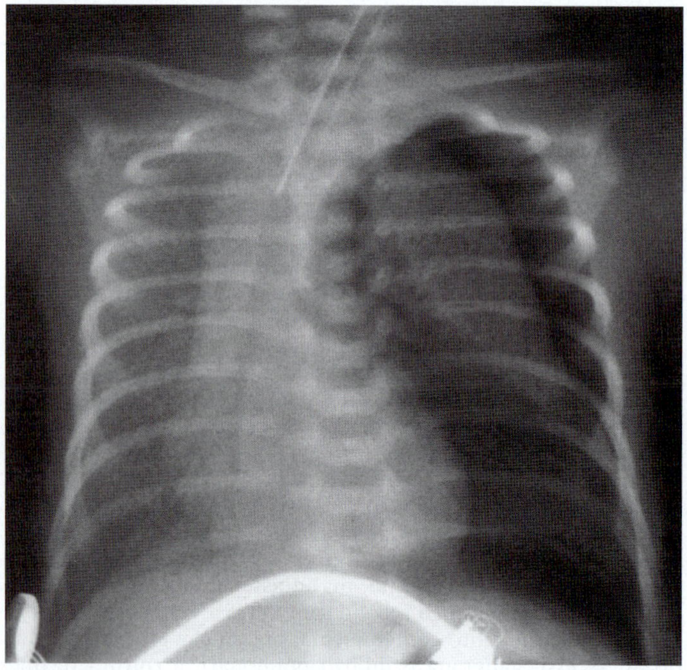

Figura 410-3. Pneumotorace sinistro, polmone con scarsa compliance. (Da Clark DA: *Atlas of Neonatology*, 7th ed. Philadelphia, WB Saunders, 2000, p 91.)

diaframmatiche, dall'iperespansione compensatoria dell'atelettasia controlaterale e dalla distensione gassosa dello stomaco. Nella maggior parte dei casi, si rivelano utili a tal fine la radiografia o la TC del torace.

TRATTAMENTO. Il trattamento varia in base all'entità del collasso e alla natura e severità della malattia di base. Uno pneumotorace sotto tensione può richiedere il drenaggio d'emergenza tramite toracostomia con ago; uno di piccole o medie dimensioni, in un bambino altrimenti normale, può risolversi senza un trattamento specifico, in genere nell'arco di una settimana. Anche un piccolo ($<5\%$) pneumotorace che complica l'asma può risolversi spontaneamente. La somministrazione di ossigeno al 100% può accelerare la guarigione. I pazienti con ipossiemia cronica devono essere sottoposti a uno stretto monitoraggio durante la somministrazione di ossigeno supplementare. Il dolore pleuritico richiede la terapia con analgesici. Se vi è un collasso $>5\%$ o se lo pneumotorace è ricorrente o sotto tensione, è necessario un tubo di drenaggio toracico. Poiché gli pneumotoraci che complicano la fibrosi cistica sono spesso ricorrenti, può essere giustificato un trattamento definitivo già dal primo episodio, anche con un collasso <5% (vedi Capitolo 400). Analogamente, se uno pneumotorace che complica un tumore, o il suo trattamento, non migliora rapidamente con l'osservazione, è spesso necessaria la pleurodesi chimica o la toracotomia aperta.

La toracotomia chiusa (semplice inserimento di un tubo toracico) e il drenaggio dell'aria intrappolata attraverso un catetere, la cui apertura esterna è mantenuta in posizione declive sott'acqua, è una misura adeguata per riespandere il polmone nella maggior parte dei pazienti; spesso si utilizzano cateteri *pigtail*. In caso di pneumotoraci pregressi, può essere indicato indurre la formazione di forti aderenze tra il polmone e la parete toracica tramite una procedura sclerosante, per prevenire le recidive. Questo risultato si può ottenere introducendo doxiciclina o talco nello spazio pleurico (**pleurodesi chimica**). Un altro trattamento efficace per lo pneumotorace ricorrente è la toracotomia aperta attraverso un'incisione limitata, con plicatura delle bolle, chiusura della fistola, decorticazione della pleura (usualmente nella parte apicale del polmone, dove il chirurgo ha una visione diretta) e abrasione della pleura basale. La decorticazione e l'abrasione della pleura lasciano superfici nude, infiammate, che guariscono con aderenze sigillanti. Il dolore postoperatorio è simile a quello della pleurodesi chimica, ma di solito il tubo toracico può essere rimosso in 24-48 ore, rispetto alle 72 ore minime richieste di regola per la toracotomia chiusa e la pleurodesi. La **chirurgia toracoscopica videoassistita** è la terapia preferita per la bullectomia, la decorticazione pleurica, lo spazzolamento pleurico e l'instillazione di agenti sclerosanti, con una morbilità in una certa misura inferiore rispetto alla toracotomia aperta tradizionale.

Le aderenze pleuriche estese aiutano a prevenire lo pneumotorace ricorrente, ma rendono più complicati gli interventi di chirurgia toracica. Nelle malattie in cui si prevede di poter considerare il trapianto polmonare tra le opzioni terapeutiche (per es. fibrosi cistica), è stato proposto un approccio di più fasi per il trattamento dello pneumotorace. Se il paziente sta bene e lo pneumotorace è piccolo, non è consigliato alcun intervento. Per le perdite più grandi o che non si risolvono, si può tentare la toracostomia semplice con tubo di drenaggio. Per le perdite che persistono, o si ripresentano, il passo successivo può essere la bullectomia toracoscopica senza abrasione pleurica. Solo se questi tentativi falliscono si dovrebbe ricorrere alla decorticazione e all'abrasione pleuriche complete più aggressive. A qualsiasi livello, durante questo approccio, si deve concedere al paziente e ai suoi familiari la possibilità di scegliere una procedura definitiva, purché capiscano che tale decisione può rendere il trapianto polmonare difficile o impossibile. Si deve anche ricordare che più a lungo un tubo di drenaggio resta in sede, maggiore sarà la possibilità di un deterioramento polmonare, in particolare in un paziente con fibrosi cistica, in cui sono importanti la tosse vigorosa, la respirazione profonda e il drenaggio posturale. Tutte queste manovre sono difficili da effettuare in presenza di un tubo toracico.

La terapia della malattia polmonare di base deve iniziare al momento del ricovero e proseguire per tutto il decorso del trattamento volto a risolvere la fuoriuscita di aria.

Liu CM, Hang LW, Chen WK, et al: Pigtail tube drainage in the treatment of spontaneous pneumothorax. *Am J Emerg Med* 2003;21:241–244.
Liu DM, Forkheim K, Rowan K, et al: Utilization of ultrasound for the detection of pneumothorax in the neonatal special-care nursery. *Pediatr Radiol* 2003;33:880–883.
Mathur NN, Kumar S, Bothra R, et al: Multi-lobulated cervical pneumatocoele communicating with pyopneumothorax and bronchopleural fistula. *Int J Pediatr Otorhinolaryngol* 2004;68:1525–1527.
Noppen M, Verbanck S, Harvey J, et al: Music: A new cause of primary spontaneous pneumothorax. *Thorax* 2004;59:722–724.
O'Connor AR, Morgan WE: Radiological review of pneumothorax. *Br Med J* 2005;330:1493–1497.
Ozcan C, McGahren ED, Rodgers BM: Thoracoscopic treatment of spontaneous pneumothorax in children. *J Pediatr Surg* 2003;38:1459–1464.
Ruddy RM: Trauma and the paediatric lung. *Paediatr Resp Rev* 2005;6:61–67.
Shaw KS, Prasil P, Nguyen LT, et al: Pediatric spontaneous pneumothorax. *Semin Pediatr Surg* 2003;12:55–61.
Wammanda RD, Ameh EA, Ali FU: Bilateral pneumothorax complicating miliary tuberculosis in children: Case report and review of the literature. *Ann Trop Paediatr* 2003;23:149–152.

Capitolo 411 ■ Pneumomediastino

Glenna B. Winnie

Lo pneumomediastino è la presenza di aria o gas nel mediastino.

EZIOLOGIA. In genere è causato dalla rottura alveolare nel corso di pneumopatie acute o croniche, ma può essere dovuto anche a un gruppo eterogeneo di entità nosologiche non respiratorie, e non sempre il polmone è la sede di origine dell'aria. Lo pneumomediastino è stato riportato dopo estrazioni dentarie, mestruazioni normali, parto ostetrico, diabete mellito con chetoacidosi, agopuntura e gastroenterite acuta, oltre a potere essere una conseguenza di perforazione esofagea, traumi toracici penetranti o inalazione di corpi estranei. Talvolta non si trova alcuna causa sottostante. L'asma acuto è la causa più comune di pneumomediastino nei bambini più grandi e negli adolescenti. In questi pazienti è raro uno pneumotorace simultaneo.

PATOGENESI. Dopo la rottura alveolare intrapolmonare, l'aria penetra tra i foglietti perivascolari e gli altri piani dei tessuti molli fino a raggiungere l'ilo e a penetrare nel mediastino.

MANIFESTAZIONI CLINICHE. La caratteristica principale dello pneumomediastino è un dolore toracico trafittivo, transitorio, che può irradiarsi al collo. Possono insorgere anche dolore addominale isolato o mal di gola. Il paziente può avere dispnea e tosse. Lo pneumomediastino è difficile da rilevare con il solo esame obiettivo. L'enfisema sottocutaneo, se presente, è diagnostico. L'ottusità cardiaca alla percussione può essere ridotta, ma molti di questi pazienti hanno un torace cronicamente iperinflato, ed è poco probabile che il clinico possa essere sicuro di queste osservazioni. Occasionalmente è udibile uno "scricchiolio" mediastinico (segno di Hamman), che però è facile confondere con un rumore da sfregamento.

INDAGINI DI LABORATORIO. La radiografia del torace rivela la presenza di aria nel mediastino, con un margine cardiaco più definito del normale (Figg. 411-1, 411-2, 411-3). Nelle proiezioni laterali, le strutture mediastiniche posteriori sono chiaramente definite, vi può essere un anello lucente intorno all'arteria polmonare destra e occasionalmente è osservabile aria retrosternale (vedi Fig. 411-2). Sono spesso visibili strie verticali nel mediastino e aria sottocutanea (vedi Fig. 411-1).

COMPLICANZE. È raro che lo pneumomediastino rappresenti un problema grave nei bambini più grandi, poiché è possibile depressurizzare il mediastino facendo fuoriuscire aria nel collo o nell'addome. Nel neonato, tuttavia, la velocità a cui l'aria può lasciare il mediastino non è elevata, e lo pneumomediastino può portare a una compromissione cardiovascolare o a uno pneumotorace pericolosi (vedi Capitoli 101.13 e 410).

TRATTAMENTO. È volto principalmente alla malattia polmonare ostruttiva di base o alle altre condizioni precipitanti. Talvolta si rendono necessari gli analgesici per il dolore toracico. Nonostante si tratti di un evenienza rara, l'enfisema sottocutaneo può causare una compressione tracheale tale da giustificare la trache-

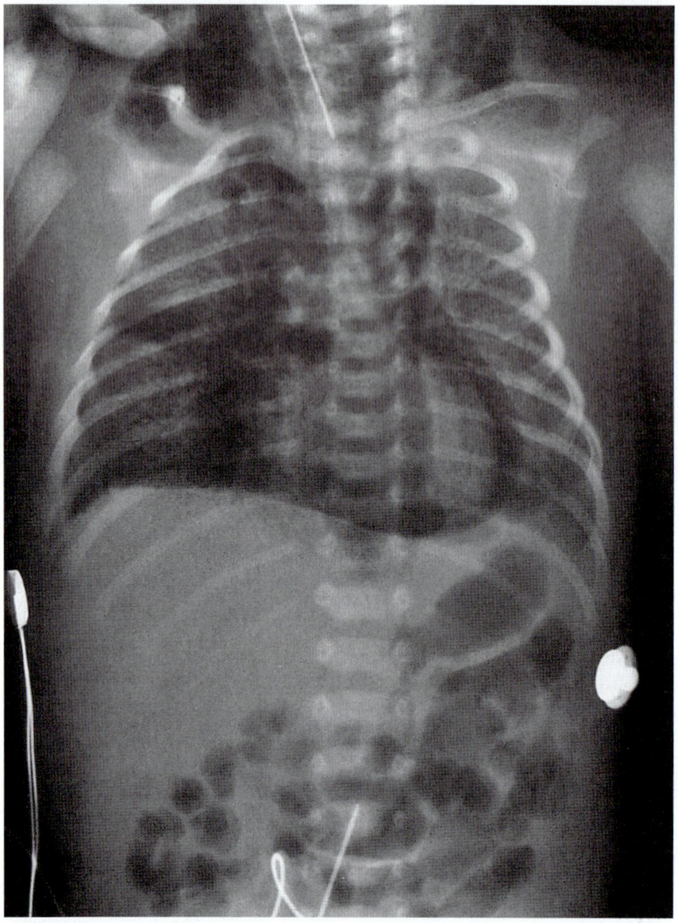

Figura 411-1. Importante pneumomediastino che circonda il cuore e penetra nel collo. (Da Clark DA: *Atlas of Neonatology*, 7th ed. Philadelphia, WB Saunders, 2000, p 94.)

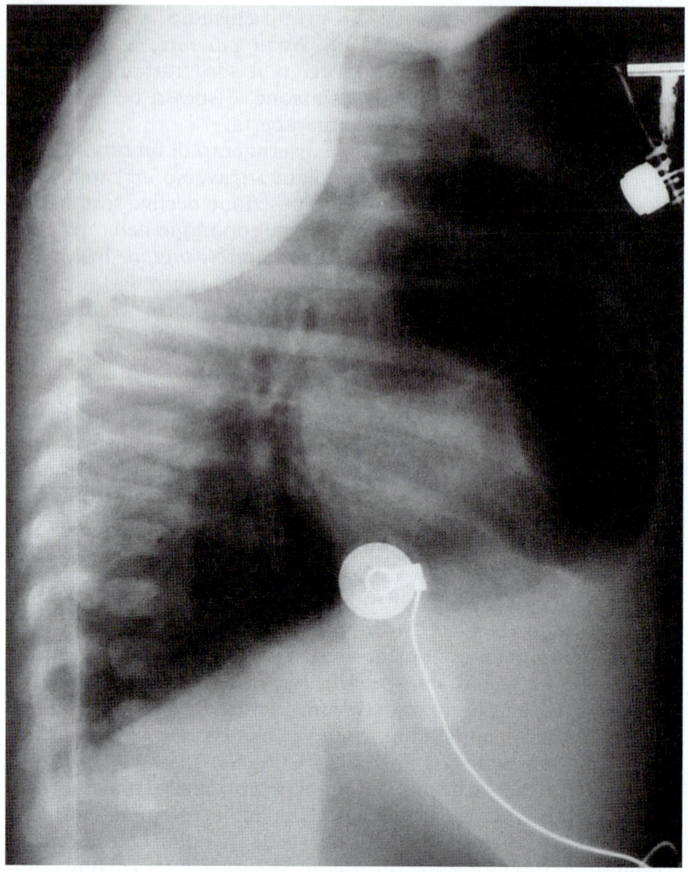

Figura 411-2. Radiografia laterale: aria nel mediastino superiore. (Da Clark DA: *Atlas of Neonatology*, 7th ed. Philadelphia, WB Saunders, 2000, p 94.)

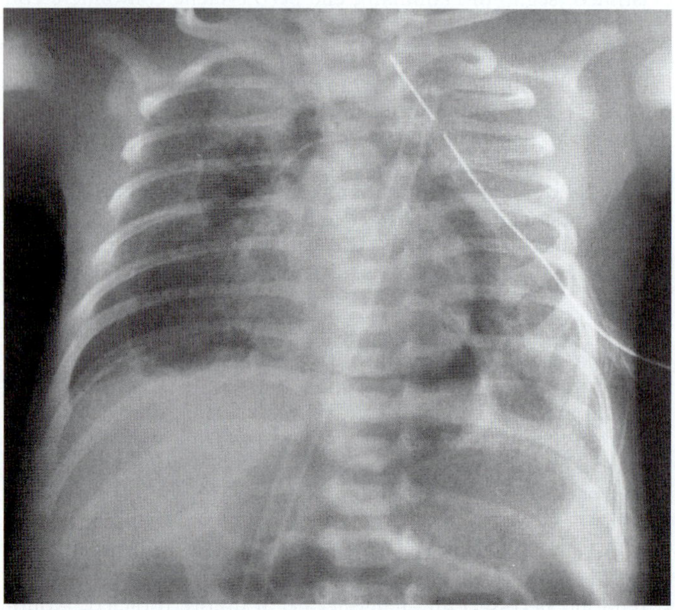

Figura 411-3. Segno della vela, sollevamento del timo. (Da Clark DA: *Atlas of Neonatology*, 7th ed. Philadelphia, WB Saunders, 2000, p 94.)

otomia; quest'ultima procedura decomprime anche il mediastino. La mediastinotomia a collare e il posizionamento di un catetere di drenaggio percutaneo sono altre modalità di trattamento.

Chalumeau M, Le Clainche L, Sayeg N, et al: Spontaneous pneumomediastinum in children. *Pediatr Pulmonol* 2001;31:67–75.

Chapdelaine J, Beaunoyer M, Daigneault P, et al: Spontaneous pneumomediastinum: Are we overinvestigating? *J Pediatr Surg* 2004;39:681–684.

Chau HH, Kwok PC, Lai AK, et al: Percutaneous relief of tension pneumomediastinum in a child. *Cardiovasc Intervent Radiol* 2003;26:561–563.

Damore DT, Dayan PS: Medical causes of pneumomediastinum in children. *Clin Pediatr* 2001;40:87–91.

Nounla J, Trobs R, Bennek J, et al: Idiopathic spontaneous pneumomediastinum: An uncommon emergency in children. *J Pediatr Surg* 2004; 39:E23–E24.

Capitolo 412 ■ Idrotorace

Glenna B. Winnie

L'idrotorace è un versamento pleurico trasudativo causato abitualmente da gradienti pressori anomali nel polmone.

EZIOLOGIA. L'idrotorace, associato per lo più a malattie cardiache, renali o epatiche, può anche essere la manifestazione di un edema nutrizionale severo, mentre è raro che dipenda da un'ostruzione venosa imputabile a neoplasie, aumento di volume dei linfonodi o aderenze. Inoltre, può insorgere nei portatori di shunt ventricoloperitoneale.

MANIFESTAZIONI CLINICHE. L'idrotorace è abitualmente bilaterale, ma nelle cardiopatie può essere anche limitato al lato destro, oppure essere maggiore dal lato destro rispetto al sinistro. I segni obiettivi sono gli stessi della pleurite sierofibrinosa (vedi Capitolo 409.2), ma nell'idrotorace vi uno spostamento più rapido del livello di ottusità con il cambio di posizione. Di solito si associa ad accumulo di liquidi anche in altre parti del corpo.

INDAGINI DI LABORATORIO. Il liquido non è infiammatorio, ha poche cellule e ha un peso specifico inferiore (<1,015) a quello dell'essudato sierofibrinoso. Il rapporto tra proteine del liquido pleurico e proteine sieriche totali è <0,5, quello tra lattico deidrogenasi del liquido pleurico e sierica è <0,6 e il livello di lattico deidrogenasi del liquido pleurico è meno di due terzi del livello normale di lattico deidrogenasi sierica.

TRATTAMENTO. La terapia è rivolta alla malattia di base; può essere necessaria l'aspirazione quando i sintomi dovuti alla pressione sono significativi.

Akyuz M, Ucar T, Goksu E: A thoracic complication of ventriculoperitoneal shunt: Symptomatic hydrothorax from intrathoracic migration of a ventriculoperitoneal shunt catheter. *Br J Neurosurg* 2004;18:171–173.
Cho HY, Lee BS, Kang CH, et al: Hydrothorax in a patient with Denys-Drash syndrome associated with a diaphragmatic defect. *Pediatr Nephrol* 2006; Aug 25 (e pub ahead of print).
Karakaya D, Baris S, Ustun E: Hydrothorax: A life threatening complication during thoracotomy. *Paediatr Anaesth* 2002;12:809–810.
Ortiz L, Hazley D, Seikaly MG: Thoracocentesis helps diagnose diaphragmatic defects in peritoneal dialysis patients. *Pediatr Nephrol* 2001;16:105–106.

Capitolo 413 ■ Emotorace
Glenna B. Winnie

L'emotorace, raro nei bambini, è un accumulo di sangue nella cavità pleurica.

EZIOLOGIA. Il sanguinamento nella cavità toracica insorge più comunemente dopo traumi toracici, sia chiusi sia penetranti. Può risultare da un trauma iatrogeno, tra cui le procedure chirurgiche e il posizionamento di una linea venosa centrale, oltre che dall'erosione di un vaso sanguigno associata a processi infiammatori come la tubercolosi e l'empiema. Può complicare varie anomalie congenite, tra cui il sequestro, la pervietà del dotto arterioso e la malformazione arterovenosa polmonare, ed è una manifestazione occasionale di neoplasie intratoraciche, discrasie ematiche, distesi emorragiche o terapia trombolitica. La rottura di un aneurisma è poco probabile in età pediatrica. L'emotorace può insorgere spontaneamente nei lattanti e nei bambini più grandi. Se associato a pneumotorace prende il nome di emopneumotorace.

MANIFESTAZIONI CLINICHE. Oltre ai sintomi e ai segni del versamento pleurico (vedi Capitolo 409.2), l'emotorace si associa a una compromissione emodinamica correlata all'entità e alla rapidità del sanguinamento.

DIAGNOSI. La diagnosi può essere fatta solo con la toracentesi. In ogni caso si deve cercare di determinare e trattare la causa.

TRATTAMENTO. Il trattamento iniziale è la toracostomia con tubo di drenaggio. Per controllare un sanguinamento attivo, può essere necessario l'intervento chirurgico ed essere indicata la trasfusione. Una rimozione inadeguata del sangue, nell'emotorace massivo, può portare a un'importante malattia restrittiva, secondaria all'organizzazione della fibrina, nel qual caso possono rendersi necessarie la terapia fibrinolitica o una procedura di decorticazione.

Ambrogi MC, Lucchi M, Dini P, et al: Videothoracoscopy for evaluation and treatment of hemothorax. *J Cardiovasc Surg* 2002;43:109–112.
Bagwell CE, Salzberg AM, Sonnino RE, et al: Potentially lethal complications of central venous catheter placement. *J Pediatr Surg* 2000;35:709–713.
Light RW, Broaddus VC: Pneumothorax, chylothorax, hemothorax and fibrothorax. In Murray RF, Nadel JA: *Textbook of Respiratory Medicine,* 3rd ed. Philadelphia, Elsevier Science, 2000, pp 2043–2055.
Shehata SM, Shabaan BS: Diaphragmatic injuries in children after blunt abdominal trauma. *J Pediatr Surg* 2006;41(10):1727–1731.

Capitolo 414 ■ Chilotorace
Glenna B. Winnie

Il chilotorace è una raccolta pleurica di liquido, dovuto alla fuoriuscita di chilo dal dotto toracico o dai linfatici, che si accumula nella cavità toracica.

EZIOLOGIA. Il chilotorace, nei bambini, insorge per lo più a causa di una lesione del dotto toracico, come complicanza di interventi cardiochirurgici. In altri casi si associa a lesioni del torace o a tumori intratoracici primitivi o metastatici, in particolare linfomi. Nei neonati, il rapido aumento della pressione venosa durante il parto può portare a rottura del dotto toracico. Cause meno comuni comprendono la linfangiomatosi, le pneumopatie restrittive, la trombosi del dotto, della vena cava superiore o della succlavia e le anomalie congenite del sistema linfatico. Il chilotorace può insorgere anche nei casi di abuso infantile (vedi Capitolo 36). Stabilirne l'eziologia è importante, poiché il trattamento varia in base alla causa. In alcuni pazienti non si identifica alcuna causa specifica.

MANIFESTAZIONI CLINICHE. I segni e i sintomi sono analoghi a quelli causati da un versamento pleurico della stessa entità. Dal momento che il chilo non è irritante, il dolore pleurico è poco comune. L'esordio è spesso graduale; tuttavia, dopo un trauma al dotto toracico, il chilo può accumularsi per giorni nel mediastino posteriore e quindi erompere nello spazio pleurico con insorgenza improvvisa di dispnea, ipotensione e ipossiemia. Circa il 50% dei neonati con chilotorace presenta distress respiratorio nel primo giorno di vita. Il chilotorace è raramente bilaterale e di solito insorge nel lato destro.

INDAGINI DI LABORATORIO. La toracentesi dimostra un versamento chiloso, ossia un liquido lattiginoso, giallo o ematico, contenente grassi, proteine, linfociti e altri costituenti del chilo. Nei neonati non ancora alimentati tale versamento può essere limpido. Nei versamenti sierosi cronici può essere presente un liquido lattiginoso pseudochiloso, in cui le sostanze grasse derivano dalle alterazioni degenerative del liquido stesso e non dalla linfa. Nel chilotorace, il livello di trigliceridi del liquido è >100 mg/dL, il rapporto tra trigliceridi del liquido pleurico e sierici è >1,0 e il rapporto tra colesterolo del liquido pleurico e sierico è <1,0; l'analisi delle lipoproteine rivela la presenza di chilomicroni. Le cellule sono principalmente linfociti T. Alle radiografie del torace si visualizza un versamento; la TC può mostrare un normale spessore pleurico e rivelare un linfoma come eziologia del chilotorace. Il linfangiogramma è in grado di localizzare la sede della perdita, nei casi refrattari in cui si contempla la possibilità della legatura chirurgica.

COMPLICANZE. Possono essere necessarie aspirazioni ripetute per migliorare i sintomi dovuti alla pressione. Il chilo si riaccumula in fretta e le toracentesi ripetute possono causare malnutrizione, con una perdita significativa di calorie, proteine ed elettroliti. Le toracentesi ripetute e croniche per il chilotorace sono state associate a immunodeficienze, incluse l'ipogammaglobulinemia e alterazioni della risposta immunitaria cellulomediata. La perdita di linfociti T si associa a un aumentato rischio di infezioni nei neonati; altrimenti, l'infezione non è comune, ma i pazienti non devono essere sottoposti a vaccinazione con virus vivi. La mancata risoluzione del chilotorace può portare a inanizione, infezioni e morte.

TRATTAMENTO. La guarigione spontanea avviene in più del 50% dei casi di chilotorace neonatale. La terapia iniziale comprende la nutrizione enterale con una dieta a basso contenuto di grassi (trigliceridi a catena media) e a elevato contenuto di proteine, oppure la nutrizione parenterale. In caso di necessità si effettuano toracentesi ripetute, per alleviare i sintomi da pressione; spesso si effettua una toracostomia con tubo di drenaggio. Se non vi è risoluzione in 1-2 settimane, si istituisce una nutrizione parenterale totale e, se quest'ultima misura fallisce, si prende in considerazione uno shunt pleuroperitoneale o la legatura del dotto toracico. La legatura viene effettuata tramite toracotomia a cielo aperto, oppure con chirurgia toracoscopica videoassistita. Nei casi di fallimento della chirurgia è stato utilizzato con successo l'octreotide parenterale. Altri approcci terapeutici comprendono la ventilazione a controllo pressorio, con pressione di fine espirazione positiva, la pleurodesi con talco e l'inalazione di ossido nitrico. Il trattamento è simile nel chilotorace traumatico. Nel chilotorace maligno si ricorre alla pleurodesi chimica o alla radioterapia.

Beghetti M, La Scala G, Belli D, et al: Etiology and management of pediatric chylothorax. *J Pediatr* 2000;136:653–658.
Cormack BE, Wilson NJ, Finucane K, et al: Use of Monogen for pediatric postoperative chylothorax. *Ann Thoracic Surg* 2004;77:301–305.
Coulter DM: Successful treatment with octreotide of spontaneous chylothorax in a premature infant. *J Perinatol* 2004;24:194–195.
Platis IE, Nwogu CE: Chylotherax. *Thorac Surg Clin* 2006;16(3):209–214.
Wasmuth-Pietzuch A, Hansmann M, Bartmann P, et al: Congenital chylothorax: Lymphopenia and high risk of neonatal infections. *Acta Paediatr* 2004;93:220–224.

Capitolo 415 ■ Displasia broncopolmonare Steven Lestrud

La displasia broncopolmonare (BPD, *BronchoPulmonary Dysplasia*), o pneumopatia cronica del periodo neonatale, è discussa in dettaglio nel Capitolo 101.4.

EPIDEMIOLOGIA. In passato la BPD si verificava caratteristicamente nei neonati prematuri con sindrome da distress respiratorio severa, trattati mediante ossigeno ad alte dosi e ventilazione meccanica prolungata, con elevate pressioni positive nelle vie aeree. Con l'aumentata sopravvivenza dei neonati con prematurità estrema (24-26 settimane di gestazione, peso alla nascita <1000 g), il gruppo a rischio è cambiato nonostante la disponibilità della terapia con surfattante; la percentuale di prematuri con BPD **severa** era del 9,7% nel 1994 e del 3,7% nel 2002. Le forme più lievi di BPD sono di riscontro frequente nei neonati con peso alla nascita molto basso, che non hanno sindrome da distress respiratorio iniziale o la presentano in forma lieve.

MANIFESTAZIONI CLINICHE. I reperti obiettivi variano in base alla gravità della malattia. La tachipnea è comune. L'esame del torace dimostra un aumento del diametro anteroposteriore che suggerisce intrappolamento d'aria. Sono frequentemente presenti retrazioni intercostali. Sebbene i suoni respiratori siano spesso normali in condizioni di benessere, e anomali solo durante le esacerbazioni acute, molti pazienti hanno sibili o crepitii grossolani di base. Nei soggetti con tendenza al sovraccarico idrico possono essere presenti crepitii fini.

I pazienti colpiti più gravemente necessitano di una ventilazione meccanica prolungata per ottenere uno scambio gassoso accettabile. I lattanti con pneumopatia significativa presenteranno un ritardo dell'accrescimento, dovuto al grande dispendio energetico richiesto per far fronte all'aumentata domanda metabolica. Molti hanno necessità basi di ossigeno inspiratorio, per mantenerne la saturazione oltre il 90%. L'insufficienza respiratoria cronica può essere evidente per l'aumento del bicarbonato o della CO_2 all'emogasanalisi.

Un'**esacerbazione polmonare** si manifesta tipicamente in corso di infezioni virali delle vie respiratorie superiori. Altri fattori scatenanti frequenti comprendono la sinusite, l'otite media, i cambiamenti meteorologici, l'esposizione al fumo di sigaretta e le esacerbazioni del reflusso gastroesofageo. Durante un'esarcerbazione, il lattante presenta un aumento del lavoro respiratorio, con peggioramento della tachipnea e delle retrazioni. La configurazione della parete toracica può cambiare, con aumento del diametro anteroposteriore. Anche se i sibili sono un reperto di base particolarmente accentuato, la scarsa entrata dell'aria durante un'esacerbazione può comportarne una riduzione.

I pazienti devono essere monitorati per lo sviluppo di cuore polmonare, specialmente se necessitano di ossigeno supplementare e hanno un'insufficienza respiratoria cronica. Altre condizioni che possono complicare il quadro sono la malattia da reflusso gastroesofageo (GERD, *Gastroesophageal Reflux Disease*) e l'aspirazione polmonare, in particolare durante un'esacerbazione, quando i lattanti sono per lo più tachipnoici e le meccaniche polmonari aumentano il rischio di GERD. Nei pazienti gravemente sofferenti e in quelli con una malattia non proporzionata rispetto al rischio di sviluppare una pneumopatia cronica, bisogna sospettare altre pneumopatie, come l'asma, la fibrosi cistica e la polmonite da aspirazione cronica. Gli episodi ricorrenti di distress respiratorio possono riflettere un'anomalia anatomica delle vie aeree come una stenosi sottoglottica e una malacia delle vie aeree.

TRATTAMENTO. Il trattamento è volto a ridurre il lavoro respiratorio e a normalizzare lo scambio gassoso, per permettere una crescita e uno sviluppo neurologico normali. I lattanti che necessitano di ossigeno supplementare oltre le 35 settimane di età postconcezionale hanno un'incidenza più elevata di ostruzione delle vie aeree inferiori e di responsività ai broncodilatatori e hanno maggiori probabilità di essere ospedalizzati durante i primi anni di vita. L'eziologia dei sibili, nella BPD, può essere un'infiammazione delle vie respiratorie inferiori, l'irritazione della muscolatura liscia bronchiale, l'ipertrofia della muscolatura liscia bronchiale e la malacia delle vie aeree. La somministrazione di broncodilatatori inalatori viene praticata frequentemente per valutare la risposta individuale. I β-agonisti per via inalatoria per lo più aumentano inizialmente il movimento d'aria e migliorano il comfort respiratorio. Nei pazienti che rispondono al trattamento, occorre proseguire la somministrazione del farmaco, soprattutto durante i periodi ad alto rischio, quando sono presenti fattori scatenanti, come infezioni delle vie aeree superiori, o nelle giornate calde e umide. I β-agonisti possono peggiorare lo scambio gassoso, in particolare nei neonati con BPD e concomitante malacia delle vie aeree. Le vie aeree, mantenute pervie dalla muscolatura liscia bronchiale in caso di malacia, vanno incontro a un collasso in seguito al rilasciamento della muscolatura liscia causato dalla somministrazione di β-agonisti. Questi pazienti possono trarre beneficio da broncodilatatori alternativi, come l'ipratropio per via inalatoria, o le metilxantine orali. Nei pazienti con frequenti esacerbazioni su base infiammatoria si può considerare la somministrazione di farmaci antinfiammatori in via preventiva, come i corticosteroidi inalatori e gli agenti modificanti i leucotrieni.

Un adeguato introito calorico può risultare difficile per svariati motivi, tra cui avversione al cibo, suzione e deglutizione incoordinate, GERD, aspirazione e aspirazione con GERD. Inoltre, la tachipnea, il distress respiratorio episodico, l'aumento del lavoro respiratorio e la necessità di ossigeno supplementare rendono il lattante al rischio di insufficiente accrescimento. Si rende necessario un elevato apporto calorico, con un fabbisogno medio di 120-160 kcal/kg/die, spesso associato a restrizione idrica. Per fornire un apporto calorico così elevato nel lattante compromesso, occorre considerare l'alimentazione supplementare tramite sondino nasogastrico o gastrostomia. È necessaria molta attenzione per mantenere il bilancio idrico.

Il reflusso gastroesofageo è comune e deve essere sospettato nei pazienti che non rispondono alla terapia e in quelli con esacerbazioni frequenti, specialmente in assenza di fattori scatenanti chiari. È necessaria una diagnosi definitiva poiché questi soggetti dovranno ricevere una terapia prolungata con procinetici e antiacidi (vedi Capitolo 320). Un'appropriata terapia antireflusso nei lattanti con GERD riduce le complicanze respiratorie. Il reflusso gastroesofageo con aspirazione polmonare o la sola aspirazione possono presentarsi con congestione toracica cronica, sibili ed episodiche crisi ipossiche. Nei pazienti non responsivi alla terapia si effettua la fundoplicatio con posizionamento di tubo gastrostomico. La valutazione e il trattamento da parte di un logopedista, di un pediatra pneumologo o di un otorinolaringoiatra possono ridurre il rischio che insorga una pneumopatia cronica associata ad aspirazione.

La prevenzione delle malattie respiratorie di origine virale è importante; è essenziale lavarsi spesso le mani, specialmente prima di toccare il neonato, ed evitare il contatto con bambini e adulti che presentino sintomi respiratori attivi. Si deve considerare l'immunoprofilassi per il virus respiratorio sinciziale in base alla gravità della pneumopatia, all'età gestazionale e all'età.

La prognosi per i lattanti con BPD è generalmente buona. In età scolare, la famiglia deve essere preparata a frequenti interazioni con il medico per episodi di distress respiratorio, spesso scatenati da semplici infezioni delle vie respiratorie superiori e cambiamenti del tempo. La funzione polmonare dei pazienti con malattia grave resterà ridotta, e potrà essere presente limitazione all'esercizio fisico a causa della dispnea. I pazienti colpiti in modo più grave trarranno beneficio dalle cure di un team multidisciplinare, composto da pediatri, pneumologi, logopedisti, nutrizionisti e specialisti dello sviluppo.

Ballard RA, Truog WE, Cnaan A, et al: Inhaled nitric oxide in preterm infants undergoing mechanical ventilation. *N Engl J Med* 2006;355:343–352.

Bott L, Béghin L, Devos P, et al: Nutritional status at 2 years in former infants with bronchopulmonary dysplasia influences nutrition and pulmonary outcomes during childhood. *Pediatr Res* 2006;60:340–344.

Clark RH, Gerstmann DR, Jobe AH, Moffitt ST: Lung injury in neonates: Causes, strategies for prevention, and long-term consequences. *J Pediatr* 2001;139:478–486.

Eber E, Zach MS: Long-term sequelae of bronchopulmonary dysplasia (chronic lung disease of infancy). *Thorax* 2001;56:317–323.

Halvorsen T, Skadberg BT, Eide GE, et al: Better care of immature infants; has it influenced long-term pulmonary outcome? *Acta Paediatr* 2006;95:547–554.

Kazzi SNJ, Quasney MW: Deletion allele of angiotensin-converting enzyme is associated with increased risk and severity of bronchopulmonary dysplasia. *J Pediatr* 2005;147:818–822.

Kinsella JP, Cutter GR, Walsh WF, et al: Early inhaled nitric oxide therapy in premature newborns with respiratory failure. *N Engl J Med* 2006;355:354–364.

Kinsella JP, Greenough A, Abman SH: Bronchopulmonary dysplasia. *Lancet* 2006;367:1421–1430.

Robin B, Kim YJ, Huth J, et al: Pulmonary function in bronchopulmonary dysplasia. *Pediatr Pulmonol* 2004;37:236–242.

Smith V, Zupancic J, McCormick M, et al: Trends in severe bronchopulmonary dysplasia rates between 1994 and 2002. *J Pediatr* 2005;146:469–473.

Capitolo 416 ■ Patologie scheletriche che influenzano la funzione polmonare

Steven R. Boas

Le anomalie della parete toracica possono portare a una malattia polmonare restrittiva o ostruttiva, ad alterazione della forza dei muscoli respiratori e a una ridotta funzione ventilatoria in risposta allo stress fisico. Le deformità congenite della parete toracica comprendono il pectus excavatum, il pectus carinatum, la sternoschisi, la sindrome di Poland e la displasia scheletrocartilaginea. Inoltre, le anomalie vertebrali come la cifoscoliosi possono alterare la funzione nei bambini e negli adolescenti.

416.1 • Pectus excavatum (petto a imbuto)

EPIDEMIOLOGIA. Il pectus excavatum è responsabile di oltre il 90% delle anomalie della parete toracica. L'incidenza è di circa 1/300 nati, con una preponderanza maschi:femmine di 9:1.

EZIOLOGIA. Il restringimento della cavità toracica a livello della linea mediana in genere è un'anomalia scheletrica isolata. La causa è sconosciuta. Il pectus excavatum può insorgere in forma isolata o in associazione con un'alterazione del tessuto connettivo (sindrome di Marfan [vedi Capitolo 700] o di Ehler-Danlos [vedi Capitolo 658]). Inoltre, può essere acquisita secondariamente a pneumopatie croniche, malattie neuromuscolari o traumi.

MANIFESTAZIONI CLINICHE. La deformità è presente alla nascita o poco dopo, ma abitualmente non si associa ad alcun sintomo in quel momento. Nel corso del tempo possono svilupparsi ridotta tolleranza allo sforzo, astenia, dolore toracico, palpitazioni, infezioni respiratorie ricorrenti, sibili, stridore e tosse. A causa delle conseguenze estetiche di questa deformità, i bambini possono andare incontro a uno stress psicologico significativo. L'esame obiettivo rivela depressione sternale, protrusione delle spalle, cifoscoliosi, movimento anomalo delle coste inferiori, rigidità della gabbia toracica, inclinazione in avanti della testa, scapole alate e perdita dei contorni delle vertebre (Fig. 416-1). I pazienti

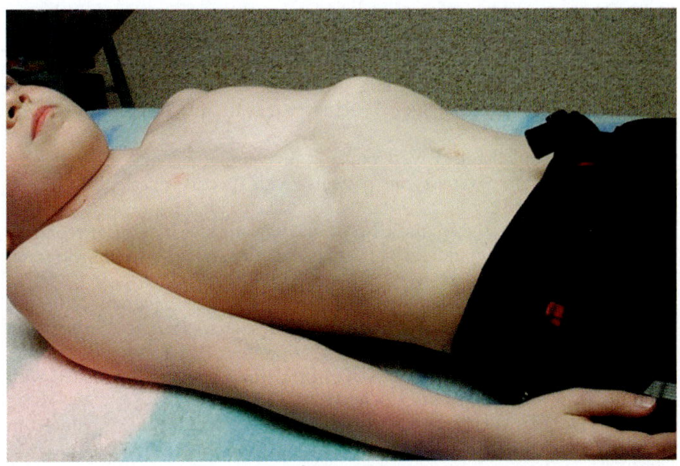

Figura 416-1. Pectus excavatum.

presentano movimento parossistico dello sterno e spostamento del punto di massimo impulso verso sinistra. Può essere udibile un soffio innocente.

INDAGINI DI LABORATORIO. Le radiografie laterali del torace mettono in luce la depressione sternale. L'uso dell'indice di Haller alla TC del torace (massimo diametro trasverso interno del torace diviso per il diametro anteroposteriore allo stesso livello), confrontato con i valori normativi appropriati in base all'età e al sesso, per valutare l'estensione della depressione, è diventato utile per determinare l'entità dell'anomalia anatomica. L'elettrocardiogramma può mostrare una deviazione a destra dell'asse o una sindrome di Wolff-Parkinson-White; l'ecocardiogramma può rivelare un prolasso della valvola mitrale e una compressione toracica. I risultati dei test di funzionalità polmonare statici talvolta sono normali, ma comunemente mostrano un difetto ostruttivo a livello delle vie aeree inferiori e, meno comunemente, un difetto restrittivo dovuto a una meccanica anomala della parete toracica. I test da sforzo possono essere indicativi di una tolleranza normale, o rivelare una limitazione dovuta a una disfunzione cardiopolmonare sottostante, che sembra associata alla severità del difetto. Le limitazioni della ventilazione sono di riscontro comune nei bambini piccoli e negli adolescenti, mentre le limitazioni cardiache secondarie ad alterazioni della gittata cardiaca sono di osservazione più comune nella tarda adolescenza e nella prima età adulta.

TRATTAMENTO. Il trattamento varia in base alla gravità della deformità e al grado di compromissione fisiologica. Le opzioni terapeutiche comprendono un'attenta osservazione, l'uso della fisioterapia per la compromissione muscoloscheletrica e la chirurgia correttiva. Nei pazienti con una compromissione fisiologica significativa, la correzione chirurgica può migliorare esteticamente la deformità e contribuire a minimizzare o anche a migliorare le alterazioni cardiopolmonari. I due principali interventi chirurgici consistono nelle procedure di Ravitch e di Nuss, sebbene la superiorità della prima non sia stata ancora dimostrata. Negli adolescenti con limitazioni all'esercizio fisico, la riparazione chirurgica può dar luogo a un miglioramento di questo parametro. Dopo l'intervento è stata inoltre osservata una normalizzazione della scintigrafia polmonare perfusionale e della ventilazione volontaria massima. Si esegue comunemente un trattamento continuo rivolto alle alterazioni muscoloscheletriche secondarie, sia nel preoperatorio sia nel postoperatorio.

Borowitz D, Cerny F, Zallen G, et al: Pulmonary function and exercise response in patients with pectus excavatum after Nuss repair. *J Pediatr Surg* 2003;38:544–547.

Daunt SW, Cohen JH, Miller SF: Age-related normal ranges for the Haller index in children. *Pediatr Radiol* 2004;34:326–330.

Haller JA Jr, Loughlin GM: Cardiorespiratory function is significantly improved following corrective surgery for severe pectus excavatum: Proposed treatment guidelines. *J Cardiovasc Surg* 2000; 41:125–130.

Koumbourlis AC, Stolar CJ: Lung growth and function in children and adolescents with idiopathic pectus excavatum. *Pediatr Pulmonol* 2004;38:339–343.

Malek MH, Fonkalsrud EW, Cooper CB: Ventilatory and cardiovascular responses to exercise in patients with pectus excavatum. *Chest* 2003;124:870–882.

Ohno K, Morotomi Y, Nakahira M, et al: Indications for surgical repair of funnel chest based on indices of chest wall deformity and psychologic state. *Surg Today* 2003;33:662–665.

Rowland T, Moriarty K, Banever G: Effect of pectus excavatum deformity on cardiorespiratory fitness in adolescent boys. *Arch Pediatr Adolesc Med* 2005;159:1069–1073.

Shamberger RC, Welch KJ, Sanders SP: Mitral valve prolapse associated with pectus excavatum. *J Pediatr* 1987;111:404–407.

Zhao L, Feinberg MS, Gaides M, et al: Why is exercise capacity reduced in subjects with pectus excavatum? *J Pediatr* 2000;136:163–167.

416.2 • Pectus carinatum e schisi sternale

PECTUS CARINATUM

EZIOLOGIA/EPIDEMIOLOGIA. Il pectus carinatum (petto di piccione) è una deformità sternale poco comune, responsabile del 5-15% delle anomalie congenite della parete toracica. La forma più comune consiste nello spostamento anteriore della parte media e inferiore dello sterno e delle cartilagini costali adiacenti, con protrusione della parte superiore dello sterno, mentre l'occasionale depressione della parte inferiore dello sterno si verifica solo nel 15% dei pazienti. È comune un'asimmetria dello sterno, con depressioni localizzate della parte inferiore anterolaterale del torace osservate di frequente. I maschi sono colpiti 4 volte più spesso delle femmine. Vi è un'ampia ricorrenza familiare e un'associazione comune con una scoliosi da media a moderata. Questa anomalia si può anche associare ad anomalie della valvola mitrale e dell'aorta.

MANIFESTAZIONI CLINICHE. Nella prima infanzia i sintomi sono di minima entità. Invece, i bambini in età scolare e gli adolescenti lamentano comunemente dispnea in seguito ad attività moderata, ridotta resistenza allo sforzo e wheezing indotti dall'esercizio fisico. L'incidenza di infezioni respiratorie e l'uso di farmaci per l'asma sono maggiori che nei pazienti non affetti. All'esame obiettivo, si nota un marcato aumento del diametro toracico anteroposteriore, con conseguente riduzione dell'escursione e dell'espansione toracica. L'aumento del volume residuo risulta in tachipnea e respirazione diaframmatica. Le radiografie del torace mostrano un aumento del diametro anteroposteriore del torace, polmoni di aspetto enfisematoso e un'ombra cardiaca stretta. Il *pectus severity score* (analogo all'indice di Haller) è ridotto.

TRATTAMENTO. Nei pazienti sintomatici, le nuove tecniche di correzione chirurgica non invasiva determinano un miglioramento dei sintomi clinici. L'intervento chirurgico è spesso effettuato per ragioni estetiche e psicologiche.

SCHISI STERNALE

Si tratta di rare malformazioni congenite che risultano nella mancata fusione dello sterno. Le schisi sternali parziali, più comuni, possono coinvolgere la parte superiore dello sterno in concomitanza con altre lesioni come displasie vascolari e rafe sovraombelicale, o le schisi sternali inferiori, che si associano spesso ad altri difetti della linea mediana (pentalogia di Cantrell). La schisi sternale completa con mancanza totale della fusione sternale è rara. Questi disordini possono insorgere anche in forma isolata. Il movimento paradosso degli organi toracici con il respiro può alterare la meccanica polmonare. È raro che si instaurino infezioni polmonari e anche una compromissione respiratoria significativa. È necessario procedere all'intervento in una fase precoce della vita, prima che si instaurino la fissazione e l'immobilità.

Fonkalsrud EW, Anselmo DM: Less extensive techniques for repair of pectus carinatum: The undertreated chest deformity. *J Am Coll Surg* 2004; 198:898–905.

Goretsky MJ, Kelly RE, Croitoru D, Nuss D: Chest wall anomalies: Pectus excavatum amd pectus carinatum. *Adolesc Med Clin* 2004;15:455–471.

Ohye RG, Rutherford JA, Bove EL: Congenital sternal clefts. *Pediatr Cardiol* 2002;23:472–473.

Waters P, Welch K, Micheli LJ, et al: Scoliosis in children with pectus excavatum and pectus carinatum. *J Pediatr Orthop* 1989;9:551–556.

Williams AM, Crabbe DC: Pectus deformities of the anterior chest wall. *Paediatr Resp Rev* 2003;4:237–242.

416.3 • Distrofia toracica asfissiante (distrofia toracico-pelvico-falangea)

PATOGENESI. Questa condizione, nota anche come sindrome di Jeune, è una malattia autosomica recessiva che risulta in una gabbia toracica ristretta e compressa, con condrodistrofia generalizzata. Possono essere coinvolti altri sistemi, incluse anomalie pelviche, falangee e neurologiche, insieme ad alterazioni epatiche e renali.

MANIFESTAZIONI CLINICHE. La maggior parte dei pazienti con questo disturbo muore poco dopo la nascita per insufficienza respiratoria, sebbene siano state riportate forme meno aggressive in bambini più grandi. Nei pazienti che sopravvivono al periodo neonatale, spesso esita un'insufficienza respiratoria progressiva, a causa dell'alterata crescita polmonare, di polmoniti ricorrenti e di atelettasie che originano dalla parete toracica rigida.

DIAGNOSI. L'esame obiettivo rivela un torace ristretto che, alla nascita, è molto più piccolo della circonferenza della testa. Le coste sono orizzontali e questi bambini hanno estremità più corte del normale. Le radiografie del torace dimostrano una gabbia toracica a forma di campana con coste corte, orizzontali e svasate, e clavicole alte.

TRATTAMENTO. Non esiste alcun trattamento, sebbene siano state tentate la toracoplastica per aumentare le dimensioni della parete toracica e la ventilazione meccanica. Le procedure di espansione delle coste hanno però comportato un prolungamento della sopravvivenza (vedi Capitoli 693-698).

PROGNOSI. In alcuni bambini, con il passare del tempo si assiste a un miglioramento delle anomalie ossee. Tuttavia i pazienti di età inferiore a un anno spesso vanno incontro a decesso a causa delle infezioni respiratorie e dell'insufficienza respiratoria. Spesso nei bambini più grandi insorgono malattie renali progressive. La vaccinazione contro i virus influenzali e altri patogeni respiratori è essenziale, così come l'uso aggressivo degli antibiotici per le infezioni respiratorie.

Davis JT, Long FR, Adler BH, et al: Lateral thoracic expansion for Jeune syndrome: Evidence of rib healing and new bone formation. *Ann Thorac Surg* 2004;77:445–448.

Kajantic E, Anderson S, Kaitila I: Familial asphyxiating thoracic dysplasia: Clinical variability and impact of improved neonatal intensive care. *J Pediatr* 2001;139:130–133.

Sharoni E, Erez E, Chorev G, et al: Chest reconstruction in asphyxiating thoracic dystrophy. *J Pediatr Surg* 1998;33:1578–1581.

Tahernia AC, Stamps P: "Jeune syndrome" (asphyxiating thoracic dystrophy): Report of a case, a review of the literature, and an editor's commentary. *Clin Pediatr* 1977;16:903–908.

Wiebicke W, Pasterkamp H: Long-term continuous positive pressure in a child with asphyxiating thoracic dystrophy. *Pediatr Pulmonol* 1988;4:54–58.

416.4 • Acondroplasia

Questa condizione, la cui patogenesi è sconosciuta, viene ereditata come tratto autosomico dominante che determina un'alterazione della crescita (vedi Capitolo 694).

MANIFESTAZIONI CLINICHE. L'acondroplasia si associa spesso a infezioni ricorrenti, cuore polmonare e dispnea. Vi un rischio aumentato di apnea ostruttiva notturna, sebbene la maggior parte dei pazienti non ne sia affetta. L'ipossiemia durante il sonno è una caratteristica comune. L'esordio della pneumopatia restrittiva può avvenire a un'età molto precoce. All'esame, il quadro respiratorio risulta rapido e superficiale, con respirazioni addominali associate. Il diametro anteroposteriore del torace è ridotto. Sono state messe a punto curve di crescita speciali per la circonferenza dei pazienti con acondroplasia, dalla nascita ai 7 anni di età. Esistono **tre fenotipi distinti**, di cui il gruppo 1 ha un'ipertrofia adenotonsillare relativa, il gruppo 2 ostruzione muscolare delle vie aeree superiori e idrocefalo, il gruppo 3 ostruzione delle vie aeree superiori senza idrocefalo. Durante l'infanzia si può sviluppare cifoscoliosi.

DIAGNOSI. I test di funzionalità polmonare rivelano una riduzione della capacità polmonare, più marcata nel maschio. I polmoni sono piccoli ma funzionalmente normali. Le radiografie del torace rivelano un ridotto diametro anteroposteriore insieme a un incurvamento delle coste. Il grado di coinvolgimento del forame magnum correla con il grado di disfunzione respiratoria.

TRATTAMENTO. Il trattamento dell'apnea ostruttiva, se presente, è di supporto (vedi Capitolo 18). La fisioterapia e l'uso di tutori possono ridurre al minimo le complicanze della cifosi e della lordosi severa. È indispensabile un trattamento aggressivo delle infezioni respiratorie e della scoliosi.

PROGNOSI. L'aspettativa di vita è normale per la maggior parte dei bambini con questa condizione, salvo il gruppo fenotipico con idrocefalo o con compressione spinale cervicale o lombare severa.

Hunter AG, Reid CS, Pauli RM, et al: Standard curves of chest circumference in achondroplasia and the relationship of chest circumference to respiratory problems. *Am J Med Genet* 1996;62:91–97.

Mogayzel PJ Jr, Carroll JL, Loughlin GM, et al: Sleep-disordered breathing in children with achondroplasia. *J Pediatr* 1998;132:667–671.

Stokes DC, Phillips JA, Leonard CO, et al: Respiratory complications of achondroplasia. *J Pediatr* 1983;102:534–541.

Stokes DC, Wohl ME, Wise RA, et al: The lungs and airways in achondroplasia: Do little people have little lungs? *Chest* 1990;98:145–152.

Tasker RC, Dundas I, Laverty A, et al: Distinct patterns of respiratory difficulty in young children with achondroplasia: A clinical, sleep, and lung function study. *Arch Dis Child* 1998;79:99–108.

416.5 • Cifoscoliosi: scoliosi idiopatica dell'adolescenza e scoliosi congenita

PATOGENESI. La scoliosi idiopatica dell'adolescenza (AIS, *Adolescent Idiopathic Scoliosis*), caratterizzata dall'incurvamento laterale della colonna vertebrale (vedi Capitolo 678), colpisce comunemente i soggetti in età pediatrica durante la pubertà e nei periodi di rapida crescita. La causa è sconosciuta. Rara è la scoliosi congenita, che colpisce le femmine più dei maschi e diviene evidente nel primo anno di vita.

MANIFESTAZIONI CLINICHE. Le manifestazioni polmonari della scoliosi possono comprendere restrizioni della parete toracica che portano a riduzione della capacità polmonare totale. L'angolo della deformità scoliotica è stato correlato al grado di compromissione polmonare solo nei pazienti con curve toraciche. La capacità vitale, il volume espiratorio forzato in un secondo (FEV_1, *Forced Expiratory Volume in 1 second*), la capacità di lavoro, la capacità di diffusione, la compliance della parete toracica e la Pa_{O_2} si riducono a mano a mano che aumenta la gravità delle curve toraciche. Queste alterazioni possono essere osservate anche nei casi da lievi a moderati di AIS (angolo di Cobb $<30°$), ma non insorgono nei casi con curve non toraciche. La riduzione della funzione dei muscoli periferici è stata associata all'AIS attraverso meccanismi intrinseci o di decondizionamento. Una compromissione severa, tale da portare a cuore polmonare o a insufficienza respiratoria, può insorgere prima dei 20 anni di età. I bambini con scoliosi severa, soprattutto i maschi, possono avere anomalie della respirazione durante il sonno, e i conseguenti periodi di ipossiemia possono contribuire allo sviluppo finale di ipertensione polmonare.

DIAGNOSI. L'esame obiettivo e la radiografia in ortostatismo in proiezione anteroposteriore con successiva misurazione dell'angolo di curvatura (tecnica di Cobb) restano il gold standard per la valutazione. Una curva >10° indica la presenza di scoliosi.

TRATTAMENTO. A seconda dell'estensione della curva e del grado di maturazione scheletrica, le opzioni di trattamento comprendono la rassicurazione, l'osservazione, l'uso di tutori e la chirurgia (fusione spinale). Si raccomanda di praticare la vaccinazione antinfluenzale, a causa del grado di compromissione respiratoria che può coesistere. Poiché la capacità vitale è un forte predittore per lo sviluppo di insufficienza respiratoria nell'AIS non trattata, gli obiettivi della chirurgia sono diminuire la curva scoliotica, mantenere la correzione e prevenire il deterioramento della funzione polmonare. Per stabilire quale sia il momento migliore per effettuare la correzione chirurgica si devono considerare le anomalie della capacità vitale, la capacità polmonare totale, l'intolleranza allo sforzo e la velocità con cui queste variabili cambiano nel tempo. La valutazione preoperatoria della funzione polmonare può aiutare a prevedere le difficoltà polmonari postchirurgiche. Molti pazienti sottoposti a correzione chirurgica possono essere trattati nel postoperatorio senza ventilazione meccanica. Anche i pazienti con scoliosi moderata possono presentare una compromissione polmonare immediatamente dopo la fusione spinale, secondaria al dolore e al un busto che limita i movimenti respiratori e interferisce con la tosse. Le procedure di espansione delle coste hanno avuto successo nei casi severi di scoliosi congenita (vedi Capitolo 416.5).

Chen S, Huang T, Lee Y, Hsu RW: Pulmonary function after thoracoplasty in adolescent idiopathic scoliosis. *Clin Orthop Related Res* 2002; 399:152–161.

Hedequist D, Emans J: Congenital scoliosis. *J Am Acad Orthop Surg* 2004;12:266–275.

Kearon C, Viviani GR, Killian KJ: Factors influencing work capacity in adolescent idiopathic thoracic scoliosis. *Am Rev Respir Dis* 1993;148:295–303.

Leech JA, Ernst P, Rogala EJ, et al: Cardiorespiratory status in relation to mild deformity in adolescent idiopathic scoliosis. *J Pediatr* 1985;106:143–149.

Mezon BL, West P, Israels J, et al: Sleep breathing abnormalities in kyphoscoliosis. *Am Rev Respir Dis* 1980;122:617–621.

416.6 • Anomalie costali congenite

MANIFESTAZIONI CLINICHE. I difetti isolati delle coste superiori e inferiori hanno conseguenze cliniche polmonari minime. La mancanza delle coste nella parte intermedia del torace si associa all'assenza dei muscoli pettorali, e la funzione polmonare può risultarne compromessa. Questo difetto può essere accompagnato da una cifoscoliosi e dalla presenza di emivertebre associate. Se il difetto costale è lieve, non si hanno conseguenze significative. Quando sono assenti anteriormente le coste dalla seconda alla quinta, si verificano un'ernia polmonare e un'anomalia respiratoria significativa. Il polmone è soffice e non dolente, e facilmente riducibile all'esame. Le possibili complicanze comprendono una restrizione polmonare severa (secondaria alla scoliosi), cuore polmonare e scompenso cardiaco congestizio. I sintomi, spesso minimi, possono comunque causare dispnea. Il distress respiratorio è raro nell'infanzia.

DIAGNOSI. La radiografia del torace dimostra l'assenza di coste o la loro deformità con scoliosi secondaria. La maggior parte delle anomalie costali è scoperta incidentalmente alle radiografie del torace.

TRATTAMENTO. Se i sintomi sono così severi da causare una compromissione clinica o un'ernia polmonare significativa, si può effettuare un trapianto costale omologo. Anche le procedure di espansione costale si rivelano preziose. Le adolescenti possono necessitare di un intervento di chirurgia estetica della mammella.

Bronsther B, Coryllos E, Epstein B, et al: Lung hernias in children. *J Pediatr Surg* 1968;3:544–550.

Mehta MH, Patel RV, Mehta LV, et al: Congenital absence of ribs. *Indian Pediatr* 1992;29:1149–1152.

Rickham PP: Lung hernia secondary to congenital absence of ribs. *Arch Dis Child* 1959;34:14–17.

Capitolo 417 ■ Malattie neuromuscolari con disfunzione respiratoria

David Gozal e Leila Kheirandish

La riduzione della forza e della resistenza muscolari dovuta ai disturbi neuromuscolari può colpire qualsiasi muscolo scheletrico, compresi quelli coinvolti nella funzione respiratoria. Sono di particolare interesse quei muscoli che mediano la pervietà delle vie aeree superiori, lo stimolo della tosse e l'inflazione polmonare. Un'insufficienza respiratoria acuta è spesso la presentazione clinica principale di diverse malattie neuromuscolari, come le lesioni alte del midollo spinale, la poliomielite, la sindrome di Guillain-Barré (vedi Capitolo 615) e il botulismo (vedi Capitolo 207). Lo sviluppo di disfunzione respiratoria, molto più insidiosa nel suo decorso, costituisce la causa principale di morbilità e mortalità nelle malattie neuromuscolari progressive (per es. distrofia muscolare di Duchenne [vedi Capitolo 608], atrofia muscolare spinale, distrofia miotonica congenita, miastenia grave [vedi Capitolo 611], malattia di Charcot-Marie-Tooth [vedi Capitolo 612]).

MANIFESTAZIONI CLINICHE. Il distress respiratorio acuto con dispnea, agitazione, diaforesi e cianosi è facilmente riconoscibile; questi segni impongono una valutazione e un trattamento immediati. La presenza di ipossiemia è documentata e monitorata con la pulsossimetria e la gravità dell'ipoventilazione alveolare può essere determinata con l'emogasanalisi su sangue arterioso o capillare. La valutazione radiografica può rivelare la presenza di atelettasia segmentale o lobare, talvolta difficile da distinguere da un infiltrato pneumonico, a cui spesso si associa. Nei bambini con malattie neuromuscolari progressive, la riduzione della capacità polmonare totale e della capacità vitale in genere sono strettamente correlate al grado di compromissione muscolare, e la malattia polmonare restrittiva è ulteriormente accentuata dalla comparsa e dalla progressione della cifoscoliosi. L'aumentato lavoro respiratorio è ulteriormente peggiorato dalla riduzione della parete toracica e della compliance polmonare imputabili alle alterazioni fibrose dei muscoli distrofici della parete toracica, all'accorciamento e all'irrigidimento dei tessuti non distensibili e ad alterazioni microatelettasiche diffuse. Nonostante la riduzione dei volumi polmonari, nei pazienti con malattie neuromuscolari si osserva di frequente un aumento del volume residuo, che riflette probabilmente un'eccessiva debolezza dei muscoli espiratori. Questa debolezza a carico soprattutto dei muscoli espiratori preclude, a sua volta, un'espirazione efficace a volumi polmonari al di sotto della capacità funzionale residua, con concomitante riduzione dell'efficienza della tosse e della clearance mucociliare. Poiché la debolezza muscolare riduce i flussi espiratori massimali, un'ostruzione vera al flusso aereo può essere mascherata durante le manovre spirometriche standard, e richiederà per la sua identificazione esami più sofisticati, come l'uso della tecnica di oscillazione forzata. La misurazione della forza dei muscoli respiratori è una componente importante della valutazione clinica dei pazienti neuromuscolari; risultano ridotte sia le pressioni massimali, sia inspiratorie sia espiratorie, sebbene in misura variabile. La principale implicazione di questa riduzione della forza respiratoria consiste nella mancata capacità di sviluppare una clearance efficiente delle secrezioni durante la tosse. In assenza di una clearance mucociliare competente, si formeranno tappi di muco con ulteriore compromissione della funzione polmonare, in particolare dopo lo sviluppo di un'infezione delle vie respiratorie superiori altrimenti benigna. Le infezioni ricorrenti o croniche e la fibrosi contribuiscono ad accelerare la perdita di parenchima polmonare funzionale, portando a ipossiemia, ipertensione polmonare e, infine, a cuore polmonare.

Durante il sonno (in particolare la fase REM [*Rapid Eye Movement*, movimento oculare rapido]) le normali riduzioni dello stimolo ventilatorio neurale centrale possono portare a un significativo aggravamento dell'ipoventilazione alveolare e dell'ipossiemia. Il ridotto tono motorio delle vie aeree superiori promuove ulteriormente lo sviluppo di ostruzione delle vie aeree superiori. I pazienti possono presentarsi con sonnolenza diurna, astenia, dispnea da sforzo, cefalea e ottundimento mattutino, vomito, difficoltà a tollerare la posizione supina e frequente necessità di cambiare posizione durante la notte. È necessario sviluppare una maggiore consapevolezza clinica dei disturbi correlati al sonno, o questi sintomi saranno erroneamente attribuiti alla malattia neuromuscolare.

TABELLA 417-1. Linee guida proposte per la valutazione iniziale e il follow-up dei pazienti con malattie neuromuscolari

VALUTAZIONE INIZIALE	INTERVENTO DI BASE/ALLENAMENTO
Anamnesi/esame obiettivo/antropometria	Consulenza e assistenza nutrizionale
Funzione polmonare e pressioni respiratorie massimali (PFT)	Fisioterapia toracica regolare
Emogasanalisi	Uso di strumenti per la percussione
Polisonnografia	Allenamento dei muscoli respiratori
Test sotto sforzo (in casi selezionati)	Vaccino antinfluenzale annuale
Se capacità vitale >60% dell'atteso o se pressioni respiratorie massimali >60 cmH_2O	Valutare PFT ogni 6 mesi CXR e polisonnografia annualmente
Se capacità vitale <60% dell'atteso o pressioni respiratorie massimali >60 cmH_2O	Valutare PFT ogni 3-4 mesi CXT, MIP/MEP ogni 6 mesi Polisonnografia a intervalli di 6 mesi o una volta all'anno

Si noti che se la polisonnografia non è facilmente disponibile, una registrazione multicanale che includa il flusso aereo oronasale, l'ossimetria notturna e i livelli di anidride carbonica di fine espirazione può rappresentare una valida alternativa.
CXR (*Chest X-Ray*), radiografia del torace; MEP (*Maximal Expiratory Pressure*), pressione espiratoria massima; MIP (*Maximal Inspiratory Pressure*), pressione inspiratoria massima.

TRATTAMENTO. Sebbene siano state sviluppate terapie genetiche per alcune malattie neuromuscolari, gli interventi terapeutici attualmente mirano soprattutto a fornire una terapia di supporto, più che a curare le anomalie sottostanti che portano a una data malattia neuromuscolare. È cruciale una stretta sorveglianza, tramite raccolta dell'anamnesi e dell'esame obiettivo, che permetteranno al medico di valutare la necessità di ulteriori esami di laboratorio. La comparsa di alterazioni della personalità, come irritabilità, difficoltà di concentrazione, astenia o sonnolenza, può indicare la presenza di anomalie dello scambio gassoso associate al sonno, e di frammentazione del sonno. Le alterazioni nelle caratteristiche della voce e del linguaggio, e l'uso delle pinne nasali e di altri muscoli respiratori accessori, durante la respirazione tranquilla a riposo, possono essere indicatori sensibili di disfunzione muscolare progressiva e di compromissione respiratoria. Sebbene la frequenza delle rivalutazioni periodiche vada stabilita caso per caso, di recente negli Stati Uniti sono state sviluppate alcune linee guida sperimentali per i pazienti con distrofia muscolare di Duchenne; un breve compendio di queste raccomandazioni, applicabili a tutti i bambini con malattie neuromuscolari, si trova nella Tabella 417-1.

L'esecuzione regolare della fisioterapia, del drenaggio posturale e di varie manovre per la tosse, manuali o assistite meccanicamente, si è dimostrata efficace sia per il trattamento delle esacerbazioni polmonari acute sia per la terapia a lungo termine di mantenimento. I genitori devono avere dimestichezza con questi interventi. Una clearance efficiente delle vie aeree nei pazienti con debolezza muscolare è fondamentale per prevenire le atelettasie e la polmonite. Una clearance inefficiente può accelerare lo sviluppo di insufficienza respiratoria e il decesso, mentre gli interventi precoci per migliorare la clearance possono evitare il ricovero in ospedale e ridurre l'incidenza di polmonite. Il ruolo di agenti mucolitici, come la *N*-acetilcisteina o la DNAsi inalatoria, resta poco chiaro. La terapia antibiotica orale o endovenosa deve essere istituita tempestivamente nel corso delle infezioni respiratorie, e i broncodilatatori per via inalatoria possono ulteriormente alleviare un broncospasmo sottostante. La somministrazione annuale del vaccino antinfluenzale è generalmente raccomandata e nei pazienti più giovani deve essere preso in seria considerazione il vaccino antipneumococcico. Il ruolo della teofillina, delle supplementazioni di creatina e della terapia con corticosteroidi resta sconosciuto.

Quando si sviluppa insufficienza respiratoria nel contesto di una malattia neuromuscolare, come evidenziato da pattern respiratori anomali durante il sonno o dall'insonnia, è necessario un supporto ventilatorio meccanico. La tracheotomia deve essere evitata il più a lungo possibile, poiché i dispositivi di ventilazione meccanica non invasiva con maschere nasali, orali o facciali hanno ormai dimostrato la loro superiorità rispetto a questo approccio ormai superato, e sono diventati il trattamento di prima linea nei quadri di insufficienza respiratoria acuta e cronica. Gli effetti benefici della ventilazione con maschera sui volumi polmonari, sull'architettura del sonno, sulla clearance mucociliare e sulla qualità globale della vita sono stati chiaramente dimostrati nei pazienti con malattie neuromuscolari. Possono rendersi necessarie dapprima la somministrazione di ossigeno per alleviare l'ipossiemia durante l'insufficienza respiratoria acuta o cronica, poi, in ultima istanza, la tracheotomia, se il paziente ha bisogno di aspirazioni frequenti delle secrezioni bronchiali o, più in particolare, se richiede più di 18 ore al giorno di supporto ventilatorio a lungo termine. Nonostante queste misure di supporto, la maggior parte delle malattie neuromuscolari croniche continua a seguire il suo decorso progressivo e irreversibile; per questo, nel trattamento multidisciplinare dei pazienti e delle loro famiglie occorre incorporare un'assistenza sociale e psicologica.

Bach JR, Ishikawa Y, Kim H: Prevention of pulmonary morbidity for patients with Duchenne muscular dystrophy. *Chest* 1997;112:1024–1028.

Finder JD, Birnkrant D, Carl J, et al: American Thoracic Society: Respiratory care of the patient with Duchenne muscular dystrophy: ATS consensus statement. *Am J Respir Crit Care Med* 2004;170:456–465.

Gozal D: Pulmonary manifestations of neuromuscular disease: Focus on Duchenne muscular dystrophy and spinal muscular atrophy. *Pediatr Pulmonol* 2000;29:141–150.

Hukins CA, Hillman DR: Daytime predictors of sleep hypoventilation in Duchenne muscular dystrophy. *Am J Respir Crit Care Med* 2000;161:166–170.

Simonds AK, Ward S, Heather S, et al: Outcome of paediatric domiciliary mask ventilation in neuromuscular and skeletal disease. *Eur Resp J* 2000;16:476–481.

Capitolo 418 ■ Malattie extrapolmonari con manifestazioni polmonari

Susanna A. McColley

Numerosi sono i sintomi respiratori che originano da processi patologici extrapolmonari. Il sistema respiratorio si adatta alla domanda metabolica ed è squisitamente responsivo allo stimolo corticale; pertanto, la **tachipnea** è comune in presenza di stress

TABELLA 418-1. Sintomi e segni respiratori che hanno origine fuori dell'apparato respiratorio

SEGNI/SINTOMI	CAUSE NON RESPIRATORIE	FISIOPATOLOGIA	INDIZI PER LA DIAGNOSI
Dolore toracico	Cardiopatie	Infiammazione (pericardite), ischemia	Dolore precordiale, sfregamenti all'auscultazione, dolore sotto sforzo
Dolore toracico	Malattia da reflusso gastroesofageo	Infiammazione esofagea e/o spasmo	Pirosi retrosternale, dolore addominale
Cianosi	Cardiopatie congenite	Shunt destro-sinistro	Esordio neonatale, mancata risposta all'ossigeno
Cianosi	Metaemoglobinemia	I livelli aumentati di metHb interferiscono con l'apporto di ossigeno ai tessuti	Esposizione a farmaci o tossine, mancata risposta all'ossigeno
Dispnea	Esposizione a tossine, effetti collaterali o sovradosaggio di farmaci	Variabile, ma spesso acidosi metabolica	Esposizione a farmaci o tossine confermata dall'anamnesi o dallo screnning tossicologico, Sp_{O_2} normale
Dispnea	Ansia, attacco di panico	Aumento dello stimolo ventilatorio e aumentata percezione degli sforzi respiratori	Insorge durante una situazione di stress, altri sintomi di ansia o depressione
Intolleranza allo sforzo	Anemia	Apporto di ossigeno ai tessuti inadeguato	Pallore, tachicardia, anamnesi di sanguinamento o di dieta inadeguata
Intolleranza allo sforzo	Mancanza di allenamento	Conseguenza diretta	Anamnesi di inattività, obesità
Emottisi	Fuoriuscita di sangue dal naso	Il flusso di sangue posteriore fa pensare erroneamente a un'origine polmonare	Anamnesi ed esame obiettivo suggestivi di origine nasale, esame polmonare e radiografia del torace normali
Sibili, tosse, dispnea	Cardiopatia congenita o acquisita	Iperafflusso polmonare, (ASD, VSP, PDA), disfunzione ventricolare sinistra	Murmure Refrettari ai broncodilatatori Alterazioni radiografiche (trama vascolare accentuata, edema polmonare)
Sibili, tosse	Malattia da reflusso gastroesofageo	Risposta laringea e bronchiale al contenuto gastrico Broncospasmo vagale (?)	Emesi, dolore, pirosi Refrattari ai broncodilatatori

ASD (*Atrial Septal Defect*), difetto settale atriale; PDA, pervietà del dotto arterioso; VSD (*Ventricular Septal Defect*), difetto del setto interventricolare.

TABELLA 418-2. Disordini con frequenti complicanze respiratorie

MALATTIA DI BASE	COMPLICANZE RESPIRATORIE	ESAMI DIAGNOSTICI
Malattie autoimmuni	Vasculopatie polmonari, pneumopatie restrittive, versamento pleurico (specialmente il lupus), malattia delle vie aeree superiori (granulomatosi di Wegener)	Spirometria, determinazione dei volumi polmonari, ossimetria, DL_{CO}, radiografia del torace, endoscopia delle vie aeree superiori e/o TC
Malattie del sistema nervoso centrale (stazionarie o progressive)	Aspirazione di contenuto orale o gastrico	Radiografia del torace, studio della deglutizione in videofluoroscopia, pHmetria esofagea
Immunodeficienze	Infezioni, bronchiectasie	Radiografia del torace, broncoscopia a fibre ottiche, TC del torace
Epatopatie	Versamento pleurico, sindrome epatopolmonare	Radiografia del torace, valutazione dell'ortodeossia
Tumori e terapie associate	Infiltrazione, metastasi, versamenti maligni o infettivi, infezioni parenchimali, malattia del trapianto contro l'ospite (GVHD, *Graft versus Host Disease*) (trapianto di midollo)	Radiografia del torace, TC del torace, broncoscopia a fibre ottiche, biopsia polmonare
Malattie neuromuscolari	Ipoventilazione, atelettasie, polmoniti	Spirometria, determinazione dei volumi polmonari, misurazione della forza polmonare
Obesità	Pneumopatia restrittiva, sindrome dell'apnea ostruttiva notturna	Spirometria, determinazione dei volumi polmonari, polisonnografia notturna

DL_{CO} (*Diffusing capacity of the Lung for Carbon monoxide*), capacità di diffusione polmonare per il monossido di carbonio.

metabolici come la febbre, mentre la dispnea può essere correlata all'ansia. La **tosse** è più comunemente imputabile a disturbi delle vie aeree superiori o inferiori, ma può anche avere origine dal sistema nervoso centrale (tosse psicogena o tic) e rappresentare un sintomo marcato in un bambino con malattia da reflusso gastroesofageo. Il **dolore toracico** non è comunemente dovuto a processi polmonari, in bambini per altri aspetti sani, ma ha per lo più un'eziologia neuromuscolare o infiammatoria. La **cianosi** può essere attribuita a malattie cardiache o ematologiche, mentre la **dispnea** e l'**intolleranza allo sforzo** possono avere numerose cause extrapolmonari. Tali disturbi possono essere sospettati in base all'anamnesi e all'esame obiettivo, o essere considerati nei bambini con reperti atipici agli esami diagnostici o una scarsa risposta alla terapia abituale. Le cause più comuni di questi sintomi sono elencate nella Tabella 418-1.

VALUTAZIONE. Nella valutazione di un bambino o di un adolescente con sintomi respiratori, è importante ottenere un'anamnesi medica remota dettagliata, l'anamnesi familiare e sottoporre a esame i vari apparati per valutare la possibilità di un'origine extrapolmonare. Anche un esame obiettivo esauriente è essenziale per raccogliere indizi che orientino verso malattie extrapolmonari.

Le patologie a carico di altri apparati e organi, così come molte malattie sistemiche, possono comportare un coinvolgimento respiratorio significativo. Sebbene sia più comune trovare queste complicanze in pazienti con diagnosi note, il disturbo respiratorio è talvolta l'unico sintomo o il sintomo più pronunciato al momento della presentazione. L'aspirazione acuta durante l'alimentazione può costituire la presentazione di una malattia neuromuscolare, in un lattante che inizialmente sembrava avere un tono muscolare e uno sviluppo normali. Le complicanze possono essere pericolose per la vita, in particolare nei pazienti immunocompromessi. L'esordio delle alterazioni respiratorie può essere insidioso: per esempio, nei pazienti con vasculite sistemica, il coinvolgimento dall'apparato vascolare polmonare può manifestarsi sotto forma di un'anomala capacità di diffusione polmonare del monossido di carbonio (DLCO, *Diffusion Lung capacity for Carbon monoxide*) prima dell'esordio sintomatologico. I disordini che comunemente causano complicanze respiratorie sono elencati nella Tabella 418-2.

Bowman CM: Hemoptysis. In Loughlin GM, Eigen H (editors): *Respiratory Disease in Children: Diagnosis and Management.* Baltimore, Williams and Wilkins, 1994, pp 201–205.

Loughlin GM: Chest pain. In Loughlin GM, Eigen H (editors): *Respiratory Disease in Children: Diagnosis and Management.* Baltimore, Williams and Wilkins, 1994, pp 207–214.

Methemoglobinemia. eMedicine Journal: Medicine, 2002.

Capitolo 419 ■ Insufficienza respiratoria cronica severa Zehava Noah e Cynthia Budek

I lattanti, i bambini e gli adolescenti con disturbi del controllo centrale della respirazione, malattie delle vie aeree, alterazioni polmonari residue dopo malattie respiratorie severe e disordini neuromuscolari possono sviluppare un'insufficienza respiratoria cronica ipercapnica e/o ipossiemica (vedi Capitolo 370). Sebbene sia generalmente possibile identificare la causa primitiva dell'insufficienza respiratoria, molti bambini hanno molteplici fattori causali. Meno dell'1% dei pazienti ricoverati nei reparti di terapia intensiva pediatrica necessita di assistenza ventilatoria invasiva o non invasiva a lungo termine.

EZIOLOGIE

Sindromi da apnea centrale e da ipoventilazione centrale. Le condizioni comuni comprendono le sindromi congenite da ipoventilazione centrale (CCHS, *Congenital Central Hypoventilation Syndrome*, maledizione di Ondina), una piccola percentuale di bambini con mielomeningocele, idrocefalo e malformazione di Arnold-Chiari, e coloro che sopravvivono a tumori del tronco encefalico. I bambini con questi disturbi non percepiscono l'ipercapnia e alcuni di essi non percepiscono l'ipossia. Sebbene alcuni possano essere gravemente bradipnoici o apnoici durante determinate fasi del sonno, il reperto classico nella CCHS è l'ipoventilazione in assenza di apnea o bradipnea (vedi Capitolo 370). La polisonnografia conferma la diagnosi documentando gli episodi di sforzo respiratorio scarso o assente e di flusso aereo scarso o assente durante il sonno.

Apnea ostruttiva notturna. Vedi Capitolo 18.

Malattie polmonari. Le patologie comuni includono la displasia broncopolmonare (BPD, *BronchoPulmonary Dysplasia*) e la sindrome da distress respiratorio acuto (ARDS, *Acute Repiratory Distress Syndrome*) in fase di remissione. I lattanti precedentemente prematuri e convalescenti dopo un'ARDS possono sviluppare una BPD (vedi Capitoli 101.4 e 415). Se estrema, la BPD può progredire fino all'insufficienza respiratoria.

Broncomalacia tracheale o bronchiale severa (malacia delle vie aeree). Le condizioni associate a malacia delle vie aeree comprendono le fistole tracheoesofagee, la compressione dell'arteria innominata e lo *sling* dell'arteria polmonare dopo riparazione chirurgica (vedi Capitolo 386).

Perdita di forza neuromuscolare. Gli stati patologici che determinano perdita di forza neuromuscolare comprendono l'atrofia muscolare spinale (vedi Capitolo 611.2), le malattie neurodegenerative, la miastenia grave, le lesioni del midollo spinale e le neuropatie postinfettive come la sindrome di Guillain-Barré (vedi Capitolo 615). I bambini che recuperano dopo una malattia grave nei reparti di terapia intensiva spesso hanno una perdita di forza neuromuscolare da nutrizione subottimale, che può essere devastante se associata all'effetto catabolico delle malattie severe e agli effetti residui di sedativi, analegesici e miorilassanti, in particolare se sono stati somministrati steroidi. I bambini con malattie neuromuscolari hanno una capacità limitata di aumentare la ventilazione, risultato che di solito ottengono aumentando la frequenza respiratoria. A causa della perdita di forza, le retrazioni possono non essere osservabili. Nelle malattie severe, alcuni di questi bambini rispondono all'aumentato carico respiratorio andando in apnea. Gli unici segni di insufficienza respiratoria possono essere un'espressione di panico, alterazioni dei segni vitali come una tachicardia o una bradicardia significative, e cianosi.

VALUTAZIONE. I bambini con insufficienza respiratoria cronica devono essere sottoposti a una valutazione accurata per determinare le caratteristiche e la severità della condizione e i suoi effetti sulle funzioni fisiche (vedi Capitolo 370). La valutazione deve includere un'anamnesi completa, l'esame obiettivo, gli esami radiologici, i test di funzionalità polmonare, una valutazione nutrizionale, dello sviluppo e l'analisi delle dinamiche familiari. La maggior parte dei bambini con insufficienza respiratoria cronica severa ha una combinazione di fattori che contribuiscono allo stato clinico complessivo.

VENTILAZIONE MECCANICA A LUNGO TERMINE

Alcuni bambini con insufficienza respiratoria cronica traggono beneficio da un supporto ventilatorio cronico, il cui obiettivo è mantenere una normale ossigenazione e ventilazione riducendo al minimo il lavoro respiratorio. La ventilazione a lungo termine a domicilio è una procedura complessa, costosa, impegnativa dal punto di vista tanto fisico quanto emotivo, che grava sia sulla famiglia sia sulla società. Oltre a incidere sullo stile di vita della famiglia, cambiando il sistema dei valori e delle priorità, può influire negativamente sulle relazioni intra- ed extrafamiliari.

La prognosi della malattia è un fattore di importanza fondamentale per decidere se sia opportuno iniziare la ventilazione a lungo termine. Il processo di dimissione con supporto ventilatorio deve iniziare appena il bambino è stabile dal punto di vista medico, con l'equipaggiamento che può essere utilizzato a domicilio. I bambini con malattie neuromuscolari degenerative, come l'atrofia muscolare spinale di tipo I (SMA, *Spinal Muscolar Atrophy*), vanno incontro a insufficienza respiratoria molto presto nel corso della vita, spesso in seguito a fattori scatenanti come una malattia delle vie aeree superiori. Alcuni genitori decidono di fornire solo un'assistenza palliativa terminale (vedi Capitolo 40) per i bambini con SMA, mentre altri scelgono il supporto a lungo termine, invasivo o non invasivo. I bambini più piccoli con pneumopatie croniche e malacia delle vie aeree hanno le potenzialità di migliorare la loro funzione polmonare e svezzarsi con successo dal supporto ventilatorio, se si predispongono un'adeguata ventilazione, una buona nutrizione e misure per promuovere il loro sviluppo e prevenire un ulteriore danno polmonare.

Il successo della dimissione a domicilio di un paziente sottoposto a ventilazione meccanica dipende dall'adeguatezza delle risorse destinate dalla comunità a sostegno della famiglia. Il programma in vigore in alcuni ospedali prevede che i bambini in fase di transizione con i ventilatori domiciliari usufruiscano dell'assistenza domiciliare con infermieri professionali ventiquattr'ore su ventiquattro. Questo dipende dalla disponibilità di fondi, oltre che di agenzie di infermieri nella comunità. Le caratteristiche dell'alloggio possono essere un ostacolo significativo alla dimissione, in quanto bisogna disporre di uno spazio adeguato per il bambino e gli assistenti, per l'equipaggiamento e le forniture; occorre inoltre garantire la sicurezza ambientale (in particolare che l'ambiente sia a norma per i codici elettrici e di costruzione) e introdurre modifiche dell'edificio per facilitare la mobilità, come rampe e ascensori.

Come reperire i fondi per finanziare l'assistenza domiciliare è spesso un problema di difficile soluzione, in questa popolazione di bambini. Anche se hanno un'assicurazione privata, la copertura per le cure domiciliari è spesso limitata. Negli Stati Uniti, nell'ambito di un programma di aiuti pubblici, la maggior parte degli stati ha stanziato fondi per venire incontro alle particolari esigenze dei bambini dipendenti dal ventilatore, sebbene l'estensione della copertura vari considerevolmente da una zona geografica all'altra.

STRUMENTAZIONE PER L'ASSISTENZA DOMICILIARE

Le modalità di supporto ventilatorio meccanico sono descritte nei Capitoli 70 e 70.1.

NON INVASIVO. L'ossigeno supplementare e la pressione positiva possono essere somministrati tramite cannula nasale. Questo sistema garantisce l'erogazione di gas riscaldati, ipersaturi, a flusso elevato. Sono disponibili numerose macchine per la somministrazione di una pressione positiva nelle vie aeree continua oppure bimodale. Queste apparecchiature sono connesse a maschere nasali o facciali totali oppure ad appoggio nasale, sono più adatte per il trattamento dell'apnea ostruttiva notturna. L'uso a lungo termine di questi strumenti, nei bambini piccoli, può dar luogo a displasia della parte centrale del volto. Occasionalmente possono venire impiegati per la somministrazione di pressione positiva tramite tracheostomia, nei lattanti con tracheobroncomalacia. Questo tipo di ventilazione è stato utilizzato anche nei pazienti meno gravi, con atelettasie ricorrenti, ipoventilazione notturna o entrambe.

LETTO OSCILLANTE. Un letto oscillante, al quale il bambino è assicurato mediante bretelle, oscilla con un movimento longitudinale a dente di sega a una velocità prestabilita. Il suo movimento promuove il movimento del diaframma. Il letto può essere un'opzione per i bambini con perdita di forza neuromuscolare lieve, per esempio quando sono in fase di recupero da una sindrome di Guillain-Barré. Questo strumento non dovrebbe essere introdotto in un'abitazione dove vivono bambini ai primi passi o poco più grandi, che rischierebbero di rimanere intrappolati nel suo meccanismo.

"CUIRASSE" (CORAZZA). È un apparecchio a pressione negativa simile a un guscio di tartaruga, progettato in modo da aderire a tenuta alla parte anteriore del torace. Attraverso un foro praticato in questa sorta di armatura si applica una pressione negativa ciclica al torace del bambino. Questi strumenti sono adatti solo per i lattanti e i bambini con perdita di forza neuromuscolare lieve. Sullo stesso principio si basa un dispositivo simile a una borsa di plastica che aderisce comodamente al torace.

POLMONE D'ACCIAIO. Il polmone d'acciaio è un'apparecchiatura ingombrante, che esercita una pressione negativa sul corpo del bambino. Il paziente è posto nel cilindro del polmone d'acciaio, in modo che solo la testa ne fuoriesca. Intorno al collo si posiziona una cuffiatura, per ridurre al minimo le perdite d'aria. La pressione negativa all'interno del polmone d'acciaio ha un andamento ciclico, facilitando il movimento della parete toracica. Quando si apre l'apparecchio per fornire le cure, la ventilazione si interrompe. Questo strumento è adatto ai bambini con perdita di forza neuromuscolare che necessitano di essere ventilati per una parte del giorno. Il suo principale vantaggio è che non richiede una tracheostomia; tuttavia, richiede un controllo costante in quanto sussiste sempre il rischio che si verifichi un'ostruzione delle vie aeree superiori. Di questo apparecchio esiste anche una versione più leggera, per gli spostamenti.

PACING (STIMOLATORE RITMICO) DIAFRAMMATICO. Il pacing diaframmatico può essere considerato nei bambini con ipoventilazione centrale e in quelli con lesioni alte del midollo spinale. Gli elettrodi vengono inseriti chirurgicamente sui nervi frenici, mentre il ricevitore è posizionato nel tessuto sottocutaneo. Il dispositivo esterno del pacing è piccolo e leggero, con antenne fissate esternamente sul ricevitore. Può essere necessaria una tracheostomia se non vi è coordinazione tra il ritmo di stimolazione e l'apertura della glottide. Qualsiasi problema nei cavi dell'elettrodo stimolatore o del ricevitore rende necessario un intervento chirurgico.

VENTILAZIONE A PRESSIONE POSITIVA. Idealmente, un ventilatore destinato all'utilizzo domiciliare dovrebbe essere leggero e di dimensioni contenute, essere in grado di usare l'aria della stanza, avere un flusso continuo e consentire un ampio range di regolazioni (pressione, volume, supporto di pressione e frequenza) che consentano la ventilazione dall'infanzia all'età adulta. Il supporto delle batterie per il ventilatore, sia interno sia esterno, deve essere sufficiente a consentire lo spostamento senza limiti sia tra le mura domestiche sia fuori. La strumentazione deve inoltre non risentire delle interferenze elettromagnetiche ed essere relativamente facile da gestire e da regolare. Sono disponibili svariati ventilatori, utilizzabili a domicilio, ed è necessaria una certa familiarità con questi apparecchi per scegliere l'opzione migliore per i bambini. Altri strumenti che possono essere utili nei pazienti con profonda debolezza sono quelli che favoriscono la mobilizzazione delle secrezioni, come il giubbotto a percussione, e gli apparecchi che facilitano la tosse del paziente.

PROCESSO DI DIMISSIONE

L'iter di dimissione di un bambino che dovrà usare un ventilatore a domicilio è complesso. È necessario un approccio multidisciplinare e coordinato, per sviluppare un piano complessivo che consideri i problemi medici, psicosociali, di sviluppo, di istruzione e di sicurezza. Il bambino ventilato deve presentare una certa stabilità medica per poter essere gestito in tutta sicurezza a domicilio; gli interventi per mantenere la stabilità devono essere minimi prima della dimissione. Il paziente deve attraversare una fase di transizione, con un ventilatore adatto all'uso domestico, che consenta lo spostamento e al tempo stesso una ventilazione adeguata. Il trattamento medico deve inoltre focalizzarsi sullo svezzamento dall'ossigeno e sulla regolazione di parametri ventilatori adeguati per l'assistenza domiciliare. A seconda del tipo di ventilazione impiegata, si può posizionare una tracheostomia per garantire una via aerea stabile e favorire il comfort, una volta deciso di ventilare cronicamente il paziente.

La nutrizione dovrebbe essere ottimizzata, per promuovere la crescita tenendo sotto controllo l'aumento ponderale e la produzione in eccesso di anidride carbonica. Le necessità nutrizionali di un bambino ventilato sono spesso ridotte a causa del supporto al lavoro respiratorio. Questo paziente non di rado ha problemi di deglutizione da incoordinazione e avversione orale secondaria all'intubazione. Bisognerebbe richiedere al più presto l'intervento del logopedista, per iniziare la terapia oromotoria e consentire la ripresa della deglutizione. In molti bambini occorre posizionare un tubo gastrostomico per sostituire l'apporto orale o integrarlo. Occorre inoltre procedere alla valutazione e alla gestione del reflusso e del rischio di aspirazione, che sono problemi comuni nei bambini ventilati. Dovrebbero far parte del progetto anche dispositivi di comunicazione, per migliorare la possibilità di parlare.

Nelle prime fasi della procedura di dimissione occorre istruire chi si prenderà cura del paziente; questo compito spetta a infermieri, personale addetto all'assistenza respiratoria, fisioterapisti, logopedisti e terapisti occupazionali. Tale formazione deve riguardare tutti gli aspetti della cura al bambino, comprese la gestione della tracheostomia e del ventilatore e la rianimazione cardiopolmonare. Occorre inoltre sottolineare la necessità che agiscano indipendentemente l'uno dall'altro sia quando prestano assistenza al letto sia durante il trasporto del bambino. In particolare bisogna concentrare l'attenzione sugli aspetti di sicurezza e di adeguata risposta in caso di emergenza. Si prepara una borsa di emergenza, contenente tutte le apparecchiature critiche, che dovrà accompagnare sempre il paziente. Gli assistenti devono dar prova della loro abilità prima della dimissione del bambino.

Bisogna inoltre identificare nel territorio le agenzie che forniscono servizi di supporto domiciliare, ivi compresa un'agenzia che fornisca assistenza privata. La cosa migliore sarebbe che gli infermieri destinati a prestare la loro opera a domicilio venissero istruiti sulla gestione del ventilatore e sulle cure da prestare al bambino prima della dimissione. È inoltre necessario scegliere un fornitore che fornisca l'equipaggiamento del ventilatore, la strumentazione e i servizi. Prima della dimissione si dovrebbe organizzare una riunione sull'assistenza cui partecipino il personale ospedaliero, le agenzie di finanziamento, le agenzie di fornitura dei servizi infermieristici, i fornitori di apparecchiature e i familiari. La riunione è importante per coordinare i dettagli dell'ultimo minuto e rendere così il ritorno a casa meno traumatico.

È molto importante fornire un continuo sostegno al bambino e alla famiglia dopo la dimissione. Il pediatra territoriale ha un ruolo centrale nel far sì che le cure siano coordinate, nell'assicurare una buona assistenza al bambino e nel far fronte ad altre necessità mediche, con la possibile eccezione della gestione del ventilatore. Altrettanto importante è stabilire linee di comunicazione con il centro medico e garantire ai familiari un immediato accesso a queste strutture per consigli e la risoluzione dei problemi durante gli intervalli tra le visite cliniche multidisciplinari.

Corrado A, Gorini M: Long-term negative pressure ventilation. *Respir Care Clin N Am* 2002;8:545–557.

Gilgoff RL, Gilgoff IS: Long-term follow-up of home mechanical ventilation in young children with spinal-cord injury and neuromuscular conditions. *J Pediatr* 2003;142:476–480.

Miske LJ, Hickey EM, Kolb SM, et al: Use of the mechanical in-exsufflator in pediatric patients with neuromuscular disease and impaired cough. *Chest* 2004;125:1406–1412.

Palfrey JS, Sofis LA, Davidson EJ, et al: The pediatric alliance for coordinated care: Evaluation of a medical home model. *Pediatrics* 2004;113:1507–1516.

Suchada S, Kun SS, Keens TG, et al: Initiation of home mechanical ventilation in children with neuromuscular diseases. *J Pediatr* 2003;142:481–485.

Talmaciu I: Pulmonary function in technology-dependent children two years and older with bronchopulmonary dysplasia. *Pediatr Pulmonol* 2002;33:181–188.

Trang H, Dehan M, Beaufils F, et al: French CCHS Working Group: The French Congenital Central Hypoventilation Syndrome Registry: General data, phenotype and genotype. *Chest* 2005;127:72–79.

Tzeng AC, Bach JR: Prevention of pulmonary morbidity for patients with neuromuscular disease. *Chest* 2000;118:1390–1396.

Waugh JB: An evaluation of two new devices for nasal high-flow gas therapy. *Respir Care* 2004;49:902–906.

Wright SE, VanDahm K: Long-term care of the tracheostomy patient. *Clin Chest Med* 2003;24:473–487.

Parte XIX ▪ Apparato cardiovascolare

Sezione 1 — Biologia dello sviluppo dell'apparato cardiovascolare — Daniel Bernstein

Capitolo 420 ▪ Sviluppo del cuore

È importante conoscere i meccanismi cellulari e molecolari dello sviluppo cardiaco per comprendere i difetti cardiaci congeniti e sviluppare strategie di prevenzione. I difetti cardiaci sono tradizionalmente raggruppati secondo caratteristiche morfologiche comuni: anomalie dei tratti di efflusso (lesioni conotroncali, come la tetralogia di Fallot e il tronco arterioso) e anomalie del setto atrioventricolare (difetto del setto atriale primum, difetto completo del canale atrioventricolare). Queste categorie morfologiche tuttavia non permettono di comprendere i meccanismi delle alterazioni genetiche sottese alle cardiopatie congenite.

420.1 • Morfogenesi cardiaca precoce

Nell'embrione presomitico allo stadio precoce, i primi precursori cardiaci identificabili sono ammassi di cellule angiogenetiche localizzati su entrambi i lati dell'asse centrale dell'embrione, che formano strutture tubulari cardiache appaiate a partire dal 18° giorno di gestazione. Le strutture tubulari appaiate si fondono sulla linea mediana sulla superficie ventrale dell'embrione, per formare il tubo cardiaco primitivo a partire dal 22° giorno. Le cellule premiocardiche, comprendenti le cellule epicardiche e quelle derivate dalla cresta neurale, continuano la loro migrazione nella regione del tubo cardiaco. La regolazione di questa fase precoce della morfogenesi cardiaca è controllata in parte dall'interazione di specifiche molecole di segnale o ligandi (di solito espressi da un tipo cellulare) con specifici recettori (di solito espressi da un altro tipo cellulare). L'informazione posizionale è inviata al mesoderma cardiaco in fase di sviluppo da fattori come i retinoidi (isoforme della vitamina A), che si legano a recettori nucleari specifici e regolano la trascrizione genetica. La migrazione delle cellule epiteliali nel tubo cardiaco in fase di sviluppo è diretta da proteine della matrice extracellulare (fibronectina) che interagiscono con recettori sulla superficie cellulare (integrine). L'importanza di questi ligandi è dimostrata dalla grande varietà di **effetti teratogeni** sul cuore causati dal farmaco simil-retinoide isotretinoina.

Attorno al 20°-22° giorno di gestazione, prima dello sviluppo della struttura ad anello del cuore, il cuore embrionale inizia a contrarsi e presenta fasi del ciclo cardiaco sorprendentemente simili a quelle del cuore maturo. Gli studiosi della morfologia cardiaca hanno identificato segmenti del tubo cardiaco che si riteneva corrispondessero a strutture del cuore maturo (Fig. 420-1): il seno venoso e l'atrio (atrio destro e sinistro), il ventricolo primitivo (ventricolo sinistro), il bulbo del cuore (ventricolo destro) e il tronco arterioso (aorta e arteria polmonare). Questo modello è eccessivamente semplificato. Solo le porzioni trabecolari (le più ricche dal punto di vista muscolare) del miocardio del ventricolo sinistro sono presenti nel tubo cardiaco primitivo; le cellule destinate a costituire la porzione di afflusso del ventricolo sinistro migrano nel tubo cardiaco in uno stadio successivo (dopo che è iniziata la formazione della struttura ad anello del cuore). In una fase ancora successiva compaiono le cellule primordiali che danno origine alle grandi arterie (tronco arterioso), comprese le cellule derivate dalla cresta neurale, che non sono presenti finché il processo di formazione della struttura ad anello del cuore non è completato. Alla differenziazione dei ventricoli destro e sinistro concorre la trascrizione di fattori specifici per le camere cardiache. Il fattore di trascrizione di base elica-loop-elica dHAND viene espresso nel ventricolo destro in fase di sviluppo; la soppressione di questo gene o di altri fattori trascrizionali come il fattore 2C enhancer dei miociti (MEF2C) nel topo porta all'ipoplasia del ventricolo destro. Il fattore di trascrizione eHAND, espresso dal ventricolo sinistro in fase di sviluppo e dal cono-tronco, è anch'esso fondamentale per il loro sviluppo.

420.2 • Ripiegamento ad anello delle strutture cardiache

Intorno alla 22ª-24ª giornata di gestazione il tubo cardiaco inizia a piegarsi ventralmente e verso destra (vedi Fig. 420-1) per effetto di forze biomeccaniche ancora sconosciute. Il ripiegamento ad anello porta il futuro ventricolo sinistro verso sinistra e in continuità con il seno venoso (futuri atrio sinistro e destro), mentre il futuro ventricolo destro viene portato verso destra e in continuità con il tronco arterioso (future aorta e arteria polmonare). Questo pattern di sviluppo spiega l'insorgenza relativamente comune di anomalie cardiache come un ventricolo destro con doppia via di efflusso o un ventricolo sinistro con doppia via di afflusso, come pure l'estrema rarità di un ventricolo sinistro con doppia via di efflusso e un ventricolo destro con doppia via di afflusso (vedi Capitolo 430.5). Il ripiegamento ad anello del cuore, una delle prime manifestazione dell'asimmetria destra-sinistra nell'embrione in fase di sviluppo, è critico per il corretto completamento della morfogenesi cardiaca. Quando questo processo presenta anomalie, l'incidenza di gravi malformazioni cardiache è elevata.

I meccanismi potenziali di ripiegamento ad anello del cuore comprendono diverse velocità di crescita dei miociti sulla superficie convessa rispetto a quella concava della curva, diversi tassi di morte cellulare programmata (apoptosi) e forze meccaniche generate nell'ambito delle cellule miocardiche dal loro citoscheletro di actina. Il segnale che ne indica la direzione può essere contenuto in un gradiente di concentrazione tra il lato destro e quello sinistro dell'embrione, per l'espressione di molecole di segnale critiche (famiglia TNF-β di fattori di crescita peptidici e peptidi dei fattori di crescita come *Sonic hedgehog*). In modelli murini di anomalo ripiegamento ad anello delle strutture cardiache, un difetto di questo tipo risiede nel gene della dineina.

420.3 • Formazione dei setti cardiaci

Quando il ripiegamento ad anello è completo, l'aspetto esterno del cuore è simile a quello del cuore maturo; internamente la struttura ricorda un tubo singolo, anche se presenta parecchi rigonfiamenti che portano alla formazione delle camere primitive. L'atrio comune (che comprende sia l'atrio destro sia quello sinistro) è connesso al ventricolo primitivo (il futuro ventricolo sinistro) tramite il canale atrioventricolare. Il ventricolo primitivo

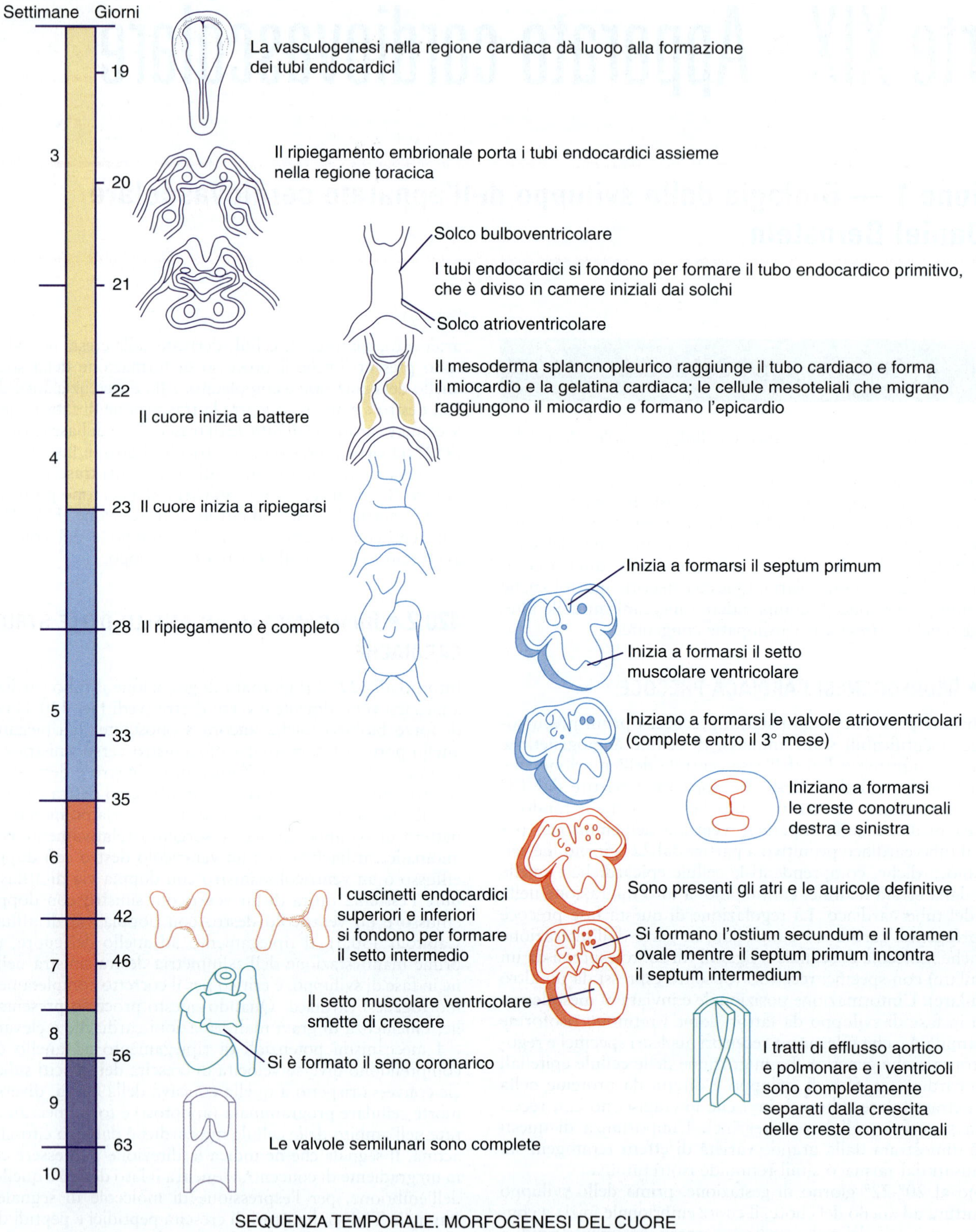

Figura 420-1. Sequenza temporale della morfogenesi cardiaca. (Da Larsen WJ: *Essentials of Human Embryology.* New York, Churchill Livingstone, 1998.)

è connesso al bulbo del cuore (futuro ventricolo sinistro) tramite il forame bulboventricolare. La porzione distale del bulbo è collegata al tronco arterioso tramite il segmento di efflusso (il cono).

Il tubo cardiaco ora è formato da parecchi strati di miocardio e da un unico strato di endocardio, separati da gelatina cardiaca, una matrice extracellulare acellulare secreta dal miocardio. La settazione del cuore inizia intorno alla 26ª giornata, con la crescita verso l'interno di grandi masse di tessuto, i cuscinetti endocardici, alle giunzioni atrioventricolari e conotroncali (vedi Fig. 420-1). Questi cuscinetti sono costituiti da protrusioni di gelatina cardiaca, le quali, oltre a svolgere un ruolo nello sviluppo, assolvono una funzione fisiologica di valvole cardiache primitive. Le cellule endocardiche si differenziano e migrano nella gelatina cardiaca nella regione dei cuscinetti endocardici, per poi trasformarsi in cellule mesenchimali destinate a formare parte delle valvole atrioventricolari.

La settazione completa del canale atrioventricolare avviene con la fusione dei cuscinetti endocardici. La maggior parte del tessuto delle valvole atrioventricolari deriva dal miocardio ventricolare, in un processo che comporta l'erosione delle pareti ventricolari. Poiché tale processo avviene in modo asimmetrico, l'anulus della valvola tricuspide risulta più vicino all'apice cardiaco rispetto all'anulus della valvola mitralica. La separazione fisica di queste due valvole produce il setto atrioventricolare, la cui assenza è il difetto primario comune in pazienti con **difetti del canale atrioventricolare** (vedi Capitolo 426.5). Se il processo di erosione è incompleto, una delle valvole atrioventricolari può non separarsi normalmente dal miocardio ventricolare, e questa è una possibile causa dell'**anomalia di Ebstein** (vedi Capitolo 430.7).

La settazione degli atri inizia verso il 30° giorno con la crescita del septum primum verso il basso, tra i cuscinetti endocardici (vedi Fig. 420-1). L'orifizio che rimane è l'ostium primum. In seguito i cuscinetti endocardici si fondono e, insieme al septum primum completo, dividono il canale atrioventricolare nei segmenti destro e sinistro. Nella porzione posteriore del septum primum compare una seconda apertura, l'ostium secundum, che permette a una parte del ritorno venoso fetale di passare dall'atrio destro al sinistro. Infine, il septum secundum cresce verso il basso, a destra del septum primum. Insieme a un lembo del septum primum, l'ostium secundum forma il forame ovale, attraverso cui il sangue fetale passa dalla vena cava inferiore all'atrio sinistro (vedi Capitolo 421).

La settazione dei ventricoli inizia verso il 25° giorno di vita embrionale, con protrusioni di endocardio in entrambi i segmenti cardiaci, quello di afflusso (ventricolo primitivo) e quello di efflusso (bulbo). Le protrusioni di afflusso si fondono nel setto bulboventricolare e si estendono posteriormente verso il cuscinetto endocardico inferiore, dove danno origine alle porzioni di afflusso e trabecolare del setto interventricolare. I difetti settali ventricolari possono verificarsi in qualsiasi punto del setto interventricolare in via di sviluppo (vedi Capitolo 426.6). Il setto di efflusso o conotruncale si sviluppa da creste di gelatina cardiaca, simili ai cuscinetti atrioventricolari, le quali si fondono a formare un setto spirale che porta la futura arteria polmonare in comunicazione con la parte anteriore e destra del ventricolo destro e la futura aorta in comunicazione con la parte posteriore e sinistra del ventricolo sinistro. Differenze della crescita cellulare del setto di efflusso portano a un allungamento del segmento del muscolo liscio al di sotto della valvola polmonare (cono), un processo che separa le valvole tricuspide e polmonare. Per contro, la scomparsa del segmento al di sotto della valvola aortica fa sì che si stabilisca la continuità fibrosa delle valvole mitralica e aortica. I difetti in questi processi sono responsabili dei **difetti conotruncali e dell'arco aortico** (tronco arterioso, tetralogia di Fallot, atresia polmonare, ventricolo destro a doppio efflusso, arco aortico interrotto), un gruppo di anomalie cardiache spesso associate a delezioni della regione critica DiGeorge del cromosoma 22q11 (vedi Capitoli 423 e 424). Si è ipotizzato che responsabile della sindrome di DiGeorge sia il fattore di trascrizione Tbx1.

420.4 • Sviluppo dell'arco aortico

L'arco aortico, i vasi di testa e collo, le arterie polmonari prossimali e il dotto arterioso si sviluppano dal sacco aortico, dagli archi arteriosi e dall'aorta dorsale. Quando si sviluppa il tubo cardiaco diritto, la porzione distale di efflusso si biforca nei primi archi aortici destri e sinistri, che collegano le aorte dorsali appaiate (Fig. 420-2). L'aorta dorsale si fonde formando l'aorta discendente. L'aorta prossimale dalla valvola aortica all'arteria carotide sinistra deriva dal sacco aortico. Il primo e il secondo arco in gran parte regrediscono entro il 22° giorno; il primo dà origine all'arteria mascellare, il secondo alle arterie stapedia e ioide. I terzi archi danno origine alle arterie anonima e succlavia destra, e il quarto arco di sinistra partecipa alla formazione del segmento dell'arco aortico tra l'arteria carotide interna sinistra e il dotto arterioso. Il quinto arco non è più presente come struttura principale nella circolazione matura. I sesti archi si connettono alle arterie polmonari più distalmente, con il sesto arco di destra che dà origine a una porzione dell'arteria polmonare destra prossimale, mentre il sesto arco di sinistra che dà origine al dotto arterioso. L'arco aortico tra il dotto arterioso e l'arteria succlavia sinistra si forma dall'aorta dorsale di sinistra, mentre l'arco aortico distalmente all'arteria succlavia sinistra deriva dalla fusione delle aorte dorsali destra e sinistra. Le anomalie di sviluppo degli archi aortici appaiati sono responsabili dell'**arco aortico destro**, del **doppio arco aortico** e degli **anelli vascolari** (vedi Capitolo 432.1).

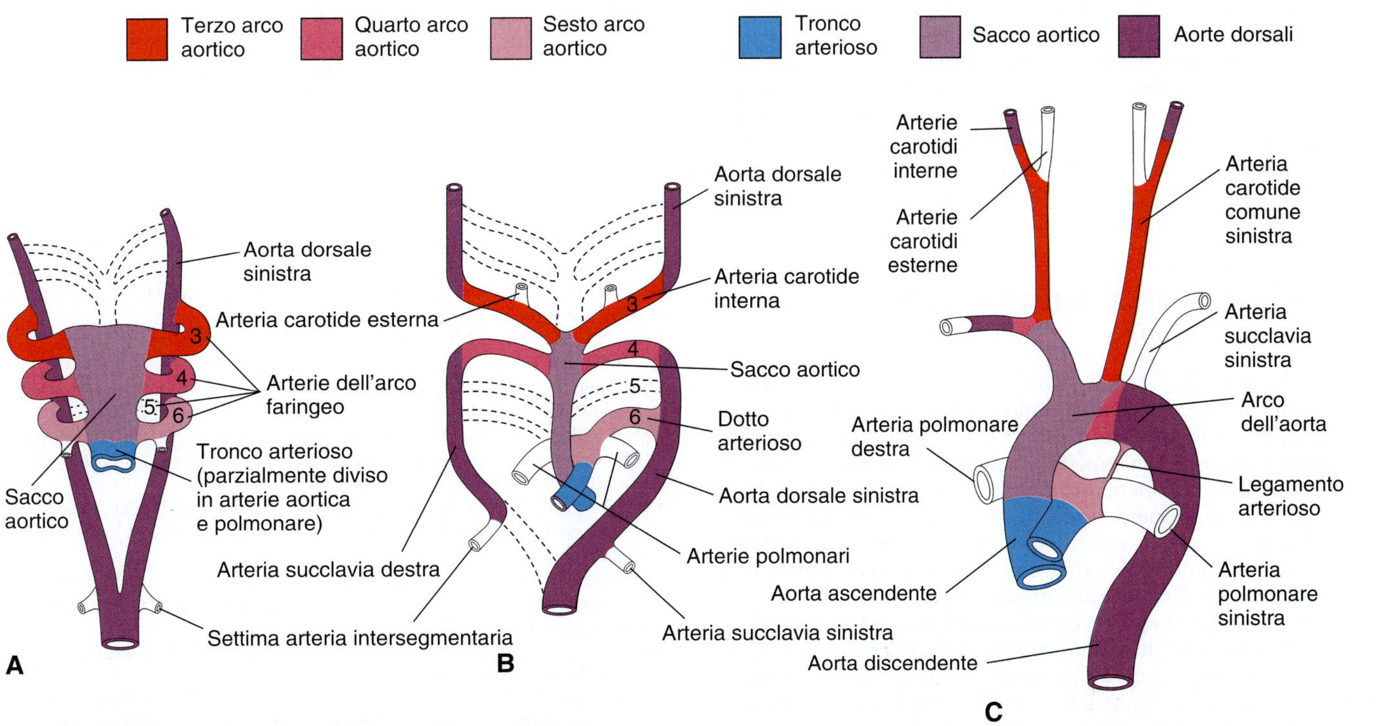

Figura 420-2. Schemi che illustrano i cambiamenti del pattern arterioso dell'adulto che si verificano durante la trasformazione del tronco arterioso, del sacco aortico e degli archi aortici. I vasi senza ombreggiature né colori non sono derivati da queste strutture. *A*, Arco aortico a 6 settimane; durante questo stadio le prime due paia di archi aortici sono in gran parte scomparse. *B*, Archi aortici a 7 settimane; le parti delle aorte dorsali e degli archi aortici che normalmente scompaiono sono indicate dalle linee tratteggiate. *C*, Vasi arteriosi in un neonato di 6 mesi. (Da Moore KL, Persaud TVN, Torchia M: *The Developing Human.* Philadelphia, Elsevier, 2007.)

420.5 • DIFFERENZIAZIONE CARDIACA

Il termine "differenziazione" indica il processo in virtù del quale le cellule totipotenti dell'embrione di fase precoce vengono indirizzate a formare specifiche linee cellulari. Le cellule precardiache mesodermiche si differenziano in cellule muscolari cardiache mature, dotate di un appropriato complemento di elementi contrattili cardiospecifici, proteine regolatorie, recettori e canali ionici. L'espressione della proteina contrattile miosina si verifica a uno stadio precoce dello sviluppo cardiaco, ancor prima della fusione dei primordi bilaterali del cuore. In queste cellule mesodermiche precoci la differenziazione è regolata da segnali dall'endoderma anteriore, attraverso un processo noto come induzione. Molte molecole di segnale precoce putative comprendono il fattore di crescita dei fibroblasti, l'attivina e l'insulina. Le molecole di segnale interagiscono con recettori sulla superficie cellulare; tali recettori attivano secondi messaggeri, i quali a loro volta attivano specifici fattori di trascrizione nucleare (GATA-4, MEF2, Nkx, bHLH e la famiglia dei recettori dell'acido retinoico) che inducono l'espressione di specifici prodotti genici per regolare la differenziazione cardiaca. Alcune delle principali patologie del muscolo cardiaco, le **cardiomiopatie**, possono essere in relazione con difetti di qualcuna di queste molecole di segnale (vedi Capitolo 439).

I processi di sviluppo sono camera-specifici. Nelle fasi precoci di sviluppo i miociti ventricolari esprimono isoforme sia ventricolari sia atriali di parecchie proteine, come il peptide natriuretico atriale (ANP, *Atrial Nutriuretic Peptide*) e la catena leggera della miosina (MLC, *Myosin Light Chain*). I miociti ventricolari maturi non esprimono ANP ed esprimono solo un'isoforma ventricolo-specifica della MLC (la 2v), mentre i miociti atriali esprimono ANP e un'isoforma di MLC atrio-specifica (la 2a). L'insufficienza cardiaca (vedi Capitolo 442), il sovraccarico di volume (vedi Capitoli 426 e 428) e l'ipertrofia da sovraccarico di pressione (vedi Capitolo 427) sono associati a una ripresa dei fenotipi delle cellule fetali, in cui i miociti maturi riesprimono le proteine fetali. Poiché le varie isoforme presentano comportamenti contrattili differenti (attivazione veloce/lenta, attività ATPasica elevata/bassa), l'espressione di isoforme diverse può avere importanti conseguenze funzionali.

Il quesito intorno al quale ruota la ricerca nel campo della cardiologia della rigenerazione è: fino a che punto le cellule staminali possano essere indotte a differenziarsi in cellule muscolari cardiache? Alcuni ricercatori ritengono che le cellule cardiache precursori note come miocardioblasti possano sostituire i miociti danneggiati e, se stimolate con gli opportuni fattori regolatori, possano essere indotte a rigenerare il muscolo cardiaco; altri ritengono che le cellule staminali circolanti o le cellule derivate dal midollo osseo contribuiscano alla rigenerazione cardiaca.

420.6 • CAMBIAMENTI DELLA FUNZIONE CARDIACA DURANTE LO SVILUPPO

Durante lo sviluppo, la composizione dei miocardio va incontro a profondi cambiamenti che portano a un aumento del numero e della dimensione dei miociti. Durante la vita prenatale, il processo comporta la divisione dei miociti (iperplasia), mentre dopo le prime settimane di vita post-natale la crescita cardiaca dipende dall'aumento della dimensione dei miociti (ipertrofia). Cambia anche la forma dei miociti, che da rotondi diventano cilindrici, e aumenta la proporzione di miofibrille (contenenti l'apparato contrattile), che diventano più regolari nel loro orientamento.

La membrana plasmatica (che nei miociti prende il nome di "sarcolemma") è la zona dove sono situati i canali ionici e i recettori transmembrana che regolano lo scambio di informazioni chimiche dalla superficie all'interno della cellula. I flussi ionici attraverso questi canali controllano i processi di depolarizzazione e ripolarizzazione. Cambiamenti durante lo sviluppo sono stati descritti per la pompa sodio-potassio, lo scambiatore sodio-idrogeno e i canali del calcio voltaggio-dipendenti. A mano a mano che il miocita matura, si sviluppano estensioni del sarcolemma verso l'interno della cellula (sistema dei tubuli T), che aumentano notevolmente la sua superficie e consentono l'attivazione rapida del miocita.

La regolazione dei recettori di membrana α e β-adrenergici con lo sviluppo aumenta la capacità del sistema nervoso simpatico di controllare la funzione cardiaca a mano a mano che il cuore matura.

Il reticolo sarcoplasmatico (SR, *Sarcoplasmic Reticulum*), un insieme di tubuli che circondano le miofibrille, controlla la concentrazione intracellulare di calcio. Una serie di pompe regola il rilascio del calcio alle miofibrille che dà inizio alla contrazione (canali del calcio rianodina-sensibili) e la captazione di calcio che dà inizio al rilassamento (pompa del calcio del SR ATP-dipendente). I cuori immaturi, in cui questo sistema di trasporto del cialcio nel SR non è altrettanto sviluppato, presentano una maggiore dipendenza dal trasporto di calcio dall'esterno della cellula per la contrazione. Nel cuore maturo, la maggior parte del calcio che serve ad attivare la contrazione deriva dal SR. Questo fenomeno che si verifica durante lo sviluppo può spiegare la sensibilità dei cuori dei bambini ai calcioantagonisti sarcolemmali, come il verapamil, che spesso determinano una marcata depressione della contrattilità e l'arresto cardiaco (vedi Capitolo 435).

Le principali proteine contrattili (miosina, actina, tropomiosina e troponina) sono organizzate nell'unità funzionale della contrazione cardiaca, il sarcomero. Ciascuna presenta diverse isoforme che sono espresse in maniera diversa a seconda della sede (atrio o ventricolo) e dello stadio di sviluppo (embrione, feto, neonato o adulto).

Le variazioni della struttura miocardica e la biochimica dei miociti portano a differenze facilmente quantificabili della funzione cardiaca con lo sviluppo. La funzione cardiaca fetale è scarsamente responsiva a cambiamenti sia del precarico (volume di riempimento) sia del postcarico (resistenze sistemiche). Nel feto l'aumento della frequenza cardiaca è il sistema più efficace per aumentare la funzione ventricolare. Dopo la nascita e con la successiva maturazione, il precarico e il postcarico giocano un ruolo sempre maggiore nella regolazione della funzione cardiaca. Anche la velocità di rilassamento cardiaco è regolata dallo sviluppo. La diminuita capacità della pompa del calcio nel SR immaturo di rimuovere il calcio dall'apparato contrattile si manifesta come una diminuita capacità del cuore fetale di aumentare il rilasciamento in risposta alla stimolazione simpatica. Questa incapacità del miocardio immaturo di utilizzare efficacemente il precarico può spiegare in parte la difficoltà che la maggior parte dei prematuri ha nel compensare lo shunt sinistro-destro attraverso un dotto arterioso pervio (vedi Capitoli 101.4 e 426.8).

Baldini A: DiGeorge syndrome: An update. *Curr Opin Cardiol* 2004;19:201–204.

Brand T: Heart development: Molecular insights into cardiac specification and early morphogenesis. *Dev Biol* 2003;258:1–19.

Chen JN, Fishman MC: Genetics of heart development. *Trends Genet* 2000;16:383–388.

Dimmeler S, Zeiher AM, Schneider MD: Unchain my heart: The scientific foundations of cardiac repair. *J Clin Invest* 2005;115:572–583.

Epstein JA, Buck CA: Transcriptional regulation of cardiac development: Implications for congenital heart disease and DiGeorge syndrome. *Pediatr Res* 2000;48:717–724.

Gittenberger-De Groot AC, Bartelings MM, Deruiter MC, et al: Basics of cardiac development for the understanding of congenital heart malformations. *Pediatr Res* 2005;57:169–176.

Kathiriya IS, Srivistava D: Left-right asymmetry and cardiac looping: Implications for cardiac development and congenital heart disease. *Am J Med Genet* 2000;97:271–279.

Person AD, Klewer SE, Runyan RB: Cell biology of cardiac cushion development. *Int Rev Cytol* 2005;243:287–335.

Srivastava D: HAND proteins: Molecular mediators of cardiac development and congenital heart disease. *Trends Cardiovasc Med* 1999;9:11–18.

Towbin JA, Belmont J: Molecular determinants of left and right outflow tract obstruction. *Am J Med Genet* 2000;97:297–303.

Capitolo 421 ■ Passaggio dalla circolazione fetale alla circolazione neonatale

421.1 • Circolazione fetale

La circolazione fetale e i suoi adattamenti dopo la nascita sono simili nell'uomo e negli altri grandi mammiferi, mentre la velocità di maturazione è diversa. Nella circolazione fetale i ventricoli destro e sinistro formano un circuito parallelo, anziché un circuito in serie come avviene nel neonato o nell'adulto (Fig. 421-1*A*). Nel feto lo scambio di gas e metaboliti avviene attraverso la placenta. Nei polmoni non avvengono gli scambi gassosi e i vasi nella circolazione polmonare sono costretti. Tre sono le strutture cardiovascolari presenti solo nel feto, importanti per il mantenimento di questa circolazione parallela: il dotto venoso, il forame ovale e il dotto arterioso.

Il sangue ossigenato di ritorno dalla placenta passa al feto attraverso la vena ombelicale, con una PO_2 di circa 30-35 mmHg. Circa il 50% del sangue venoso ombelicale entra nella circolazione epatica, mentre il resto aggira il fegato e raggiunge la vena cava inferiore attraverso il dotto venoso, dove si mescola parzialmente con il sangue povero di ossigeno della vena cava inferiore che proviene dalla parte inferiore del corpo fetale. Questo flusso ematico formato dalla combinazione di sangue dalla porzione corporea inferiore e di sangue venoso ombelicale (PO_2 di circa 26-28 mmHg) entra nell'atrio destro e si riversa preferenzialmente nell'atrio sinistro passando attraverso il forame ovale (vedi Fig. 421-1*B*); di qui passa nel ventricolo sinistro e viene spinto nell'aorta ascendente. Il sangue della vena cava superiore nel feto, che è assai più povero di ossigeno (PO_2 di 12-14 mmHg), entra nell'atrio destro, tende ad attraversare la valvola tricuspide anziché il forame ovale e affluisce principalmente al ventricolo destro, da cui viene sospinto nell'arteria polmonare. Poiché la circolazione arteriosa polmonare è vasocostretta, solo circa il 10% del sangue espulso dal ventricolo destro entra nei polmoni; la maggior parte di esso (caratterizzato da una PO_2 di circa 18-22 mmHg) bypassa i polmoni e scorre attraverso il dotto arterioso nell'aorta discendente per perfondere la parte inferiore del corpo del feto, dopodiché ritorna alla placenta tramite le due arterie ombelicali. Di conseguenza, la parte superiore del corpo fetale (comprese le arterie coronarie e cerebrali e quelle delle estremità superiori) è perfusa esclusivamente dal ventricolo sinistro con sangue la cui PO_2 è di poco più elevata di quella del sangue che perfonde la parte inferiore, il quale deriva principalmente dal ventricolo destro. Solo una piccola quantità di sangue dall'aorta ascendente (10% della gittata cardiaca fetale) passa all'aorta discendente attraverso l'istmo aortico.

La **gittata cardiaca fetale totale** (ossia la gittata combinata dei ventricoli sinistro e destro) è pari a circa 450 mL/kg/min. Circa il 65% del flusso ematico proveniente dall'aorta discendente ritorna alla placenta, mentre il restante 35% perfonde gli organi e i tessuti fetali. Nel feto di pecora, la gittata cardiaca destra è circa doppia rispetto a quella del ventricolo sinistro. Nel feto umano, in cui l'afflusso di sangue al cervello è di maggiore entità, la gittata cardiaca destra è probabilmente più vicina a 1,3 volte il flusso ventricolare sinistro. Perciò durante la vita fetale il ventricolo destro non solo pompa contro la pressione sanguigna sistemica, ma svolge anche un carico di lavoro maggiore rispetto al ventricolo sinistro.

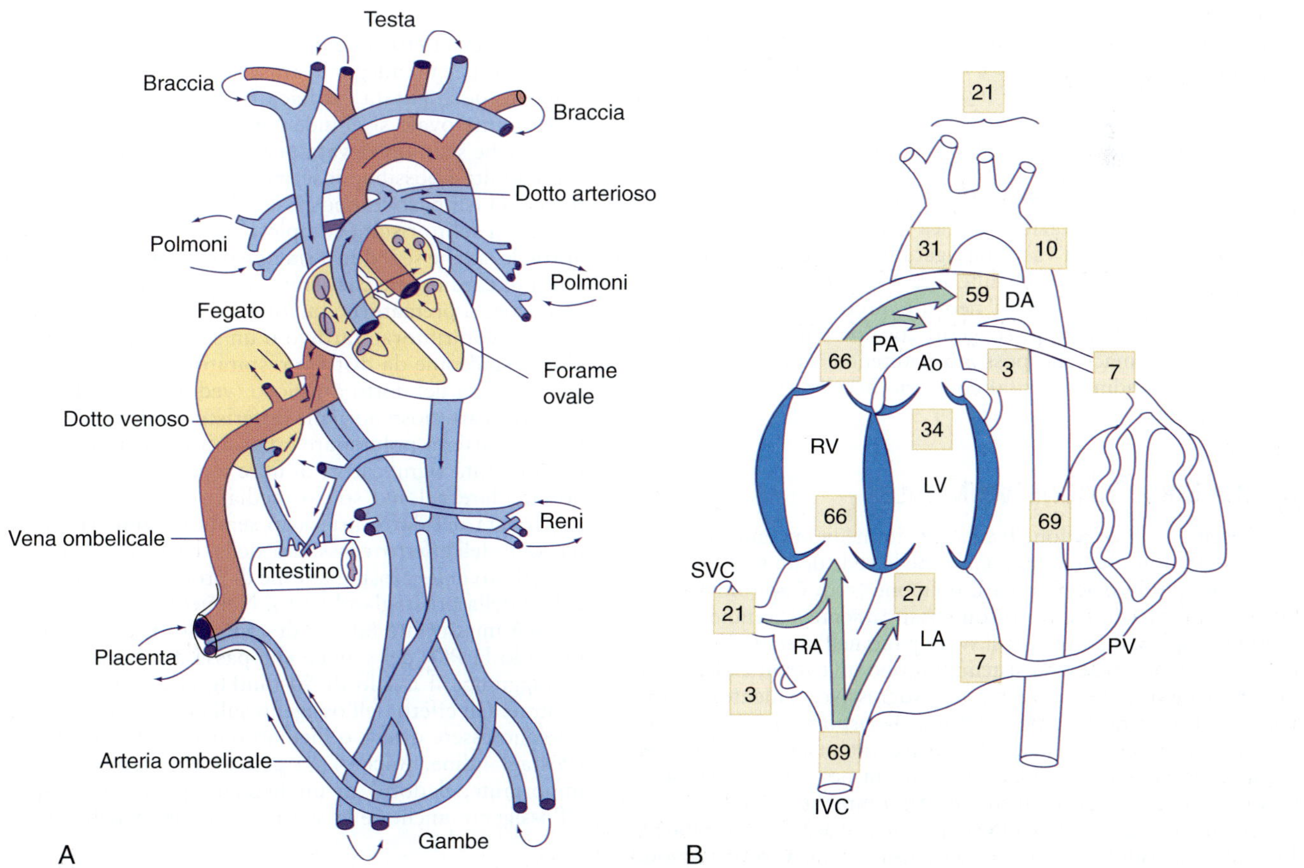

Figura 421-1. *A*, La circolazione umana prima della nascita (tratta in parte da Dawes). Il sangue ossigenato è rappresentato in *rosso*; le *frecce* indicano la direzione del flusso. Il sangue ricco di ossigeno proveniente dalla placenta fluisce dall'atrio destro all'atrio sinistro attraverso il forame ovale, bypassando così i polmoni. *B*, Percentuali della gittata ventricolare combinata che ritornano al cuore fetale, che vengono espulsi da ciascun ventricolo e che scorrono nei principali canali vascolari. Le figure sono state ricavate dallo studio di agnelli nella fase finale della gestazione. Ao, aorta; DA, dotto arterioso; IVC (*Inferior Vena Cava*), vena cava inferiore; LA (*Left Atrium*), atrio sinistro; LV (*Left Ventricle*), ventricolo sinistro; PA (*Pulmonary Artery*), arteria polmonare; PV (*Pulmonary Veins*), vene polmonari; RA (*Right Atrium*), atrio destro; RV (*Right Ventricle*), ventricolo destro; SVC (*Superior Vena Cava*), vena cava superiore. (Da Rudolph AM: *Congenital Diseases of the Heart.* Chicago, Year Book, 1974.)

421.2 • Circolazione di transizione

Alla nascita, l'espansione meccanica dei polmoni e un incremento della PO_2 arteriosa determinano una rapida diminuzione delle resistenze vascolari polmonari. La concomitante rimozione della circolazione placentare a bassa resistenza comporta un aumento delle resistenze vascolari sistemiche. Ora tutto il sangue espulso dal ventricolo destro entra nella circolazione polmonare e, poiché la resistenza vascolare polmonare è inferiore alla resistenza vascolare sistemica, lo shunt attraverso il dotto arterioso si inverte e diventa sinistro-destro. Nel corso di parecchi giorni, l'elevata PO_2 arteriosa funge da segnale per la costrizione del dotto arterioso che quindi si chiude, fino a trasformarsi nel legamento arterioso. Il maggior volume di sangue che fluisce attraverso i polmoni per poi ritornare all'atrio sinistro aumenta il volume e la pressione dell'atrio sinistro in modo tale da provocare la chiusura funzionale del forame ovale, anche se il forame può rimanere pervio al sondaggio.

La rimozione della placenta dalla circolazione ha inoltre come risultato la chiusura del dotto venoso. Il ventricolo sinistro ora è accoppiato alla circolazione sistemica a elevata resistenza, e spessore e massa della sua parete iniziano ad aumentare. Al contrario, il ventricolo destro è ora accoppiato alla circolazione polmonare a bassa resistenza e spessore e massa della sua parete diminuiscono leggermente. Il ventricolo sinistro, che nel feto pompava sangue solo alla parte superiore del corpo e al cervello, deve ora gestire l'intera gittata cardiaca sistemica (circa 350 mL/kg/min), con un aumento della gittata di quasi il 200%. Questo importante aumento del lavoro del ventricolo sinistro è determinato da una combinazione di segnali ormonali e metabolici, compreso un aumento delle catecolamine circolanti e dei recettori miocardici (β-adrenergici) attraverso cui le catecolamine espletano il loro effetto.

Quando a questi notevoli cambiamenti fisiologici si sovrappongono difetti cardiaci strutturali congeniti, spesso non può verificarsi una transizione graduale e il carico di lavoro del miocardio aumenta considerevolmente. Inoltre, a causa di un'incompleta chiusura alla nascita, il dotto arterioso e il forame ovale possono rimanere pervi in presenza di determinate lesioni cardiache congenite. La pervietà di queste vie fetali, che permettono al sangue di aggirare un difetto congenito (dotto arterioso pervio nell'atresia polmonare o nella coartazione aortica o forame ovale pervio nella trasposizione dei grossi vasi), può garantire la sopravvivenza del neonato o rappresentare un ulteriore stress per la circolazione (dotto arterioso pervio in un neonato prematuro, via per uno shunt destro-sinistro in un soggetto con ipertensione polmonare). Vi sono farmaci che possono mantenere aperte queste vie fetali (prostaglandina E_1) o al contrario accelerarne la chiusura (indometacina).

421.3 • Circolazione neonatale

Alla nascita, la circolazione fetale deve immediatamente adattarsi alla vita extrauterina dal momento che la sede dello scambio gassoso non è più la placenta ma il polmone (vedi Capitolo 101.1). Alcuni di questi cambiamenti sono praticamente istantanei, legati al primo respiro, mentre altri si sviluppano nell'arco di ore o giorni. La pressione sanguigna sistemica, dopo un calo iniziale, con il passare dei giorni va incontro a un progressivo aumento. La frequenza cardiaca rallenta per effetto della risposta dei barocettori a un aumento della resistenza vascolare sistemica, quando viene eliminata la circolazione placentare. In un neonato a termine la pressione centrale aortica media è 75/50 mmHg.

Con l'inizio della ventilazione la resistenza vascolare polmonare diminuisce sensibilmente in conseguenza di una vasodilatazione polmonare sia attiva (legata alla PO_2) sia passiva (legata a fattori meccanici). Nel neonato normale, la chiusura del dotto arterioso e la caduta della resistenza vascolare polmonare portano a una diminuzione della pressione arteriosa polmonare e ventricolare destra. Il principale calo della resistenza polmonare, che passa così dagli elevati livelli fetali ai bassi livelli propri dell'adulto, nel neonato a livello del mare si verifica entro i primi 2-3 giorni ma può prolungarsi per 7 giorni o più. Nelle prime settimane di vita, la resistenza vascolare polmonare diminuisce ulteriormente, in seguito al rimodellamento del sistema vascolare polmonare, che comprende l'assottigliamento del muscolo liscio vascolare e il reclutamento di nuovi vasi. Questa diminuzione della resistenza vascolare polmonare incide in modo significativo sul momento della manifestazione clinica di molte lesioni cardiache congenite che dipendono dalle resistenze vascolari relative sistemiche e polmonari. Lo shunt sinistro-destro attraverso un difetto settale ventricolare può essere minimo nella prima settimana dopo la nascita, quando la resistenza vascolare polmonare è ancora elevata. Nelle successive 1-2 settimane, durante le quali la resistenza polmonare diminuisce, il volume dello shunt sinistro-destro attraverso un difetto settale ventricolare che lascia liberamente passare il sangue aumenta e alla fine porta a sintomi di scompenso cardiaco.

Quelle elencate di seguito sono differenze significative tra la circolazione neonatale e quella dei bambini più grandi: (1) può persistere uno shunt destro-sinistro o sinistro-destro, attraverso il forame ovale; (2) in presenza di una patologia cardiopolmonare, la persistenza della pervietà del dotto arterioso può permettere uno shunt sinistro-destro, destro-sinistro o bidirezionale; (3) il sistema vascolare polmonare del neonato va incontro a una più spiccata costrizione in risposta all'ipossia, all'ipercapnia e all'acidosi; (4) lo spessore parietale e la massa muscolare dei ventricoli sinistro e destro nel neonato sono quasi uguali; (5) i neonati a riposo hanno un consumo di ossigeno relativamente elevato, associato a una gittata cardiaca anch'essa relativamente elevata. La gittata cardiaca del neonato (circa 350 mL/kg/min) diminuisce bruscamente nei primi 2 mesi di vita, fino a raggiungere i 150 mL/kg/min, poi più gradualmente fino a raggiungere la gittata cardiaca normale per l'adulto (circa 75 mL/mg/min). Dal momento che l'elevata percentuale di emoglobina fetale presente nel neonato può effettivamente interferire con il trasporto di ossigeno ai tessuti, per un adeguato trasporto di ossigeno è necessario un aumento della gittata cardiaca (vedi Capitolo 101.1).

Il forame ovale si chiude funzionalmente entro il 3° mese di vita, anche se in un'elevata percentuale di bambini e nel 15-20% degli adulti è possibile inserirvi una sonda facendola passare attraverso i lembi sovrapposti. La chiusura funzionale del dotto arterioso di solito risulta completa tra la 10ª-15ª ora in un neonato normale, anche se il dotto rimane pervio molto più a lungo in presenza di cardiopatie congenite, soprattutto se associate a cianosi. Nei neonati prematuri è talvolta percepibile un soffio sistolico in calando con rinforzo tardivo o un soffio continuo, e nel contesto di una sindrome da distress respiratorio bisognerebbe sospettare una pervietà del dotto arterioso (vedi Capitolo 101.4).

Il dotto arterioso normale differisce morfologicamente dall'aorta e dall'arteria polmonare adiacenti in quanto il dotto presenta una quantità significativa di fibre muscolari lisce disposte in modo circolare nel suo strato mediale. Nel corso della vita fetale, la pervietà del dotto arterioso sembra mantenersi per la combinazione dell'effetto rilassante della bassa tensione d'ossigeno e dell'effetto delle prostaglandine di produzione endogena, in particolare della prostaglandina E_2. Nel neonato a termine, l'ossigeno è il più importante fattore di controllo della chiusura del dotto. Quando la PO_2 del sangue che passa attraverso il dotto arterioso raggiunge il livello di 50 mmHg circa, la parete del dotto si contrae. Gli effetti dell'ossigeno sulla muscolatura liscia del dotto possono essere diretti o mediati dai suoi effetti sulla sintesi delle prostaglandine. Anche l'età gestazionale sembra avere un ruolo importante; il dotto di un neonato prematuro risponde meno all'ossigeno, anche se la sua muscolatura è sviluppata.

421.4 • Ipertensione polmonare persistente del neonato (persistenza delle vie della circolazione fetale)

Vedi Capitolo 101.8.

421.5 • Influenza dei fattori ambientali fetali sulle patologie cardiovascolari e metaboliche dell'adulto

L'ipotesi che la patologia dell'adulto abbia origine già nel feto suggerisce che fattori ambientali in utero, in particolare anomalie della nutrizione, possano "programmare" il soggetto a essere suscettibile, in età adulta, a patologie quali l'ipertensione e la sindrome metabolica (insulinoresistenza, diabete tipo 2, obesità). Questa ipotesi è supportata da studi tanto epidemiologici quanto sperimentali sull'animale, che esaminano gli adattamenti molecolari, metabolici ed endocrini legati alla deprivazione di nutrienti nel feto. I feti con basso peso alla nascita possono "programmare" il loro sviluppo cellulare per adattarsi a un ambiente nutrizionale uterino povero, divenendo "parsimoniosi". Dopo la nascita, la grande disponibilità di nutrienti può scatenare una sindrome metabolica, le cui complicanze si manifesteranno in età adulta. Ancora si discute sull'esatto contributo dei fattori fetali "epigenetici" rispetto ai fattori genetici tradizionali, e sulla loro relazione con l'ambiente postnatale.

Abman SH: Abnormal vasoreactivity in the pathophysiology of persistent pulmonary hypertension of the newborn. *Pediatr Rev* 1999;20:e103–e109.
Freed MD, Heymann MA, Lewis AB, et al: Prostaglandin E1 infants with ductus arteriosus-dependent congenital heart disease. *Circulation* 1981;64:899–905.
Gersony WM, Peckham GH, Ellison RC, et al: Effects of indomethacin in premature infants with patent ductus arteriosus: Results of a national collaborative study. *J Pediatr* 1983;102:895–906.
Konduri GG: New approaches for persistent pulmonary hypertension of newborn. *Clin Perinatol* 2004;31:591–611.
McMillen IC, Robinson JS: Developmental origins of the metabolic syndrome: Prediction, plasticity, and programming. *Physiol Rev* 2005;85:571–633.
Ozanne SE, Fernandez-Twinn D, Hales CN: Fetal growth and adult diseases. *Semin Perinatol* 2004;28:81–87.
Rudolph AM: *Congenital Diseases of the Heart: Clinical-Physiological Considerations,* 2nd ed. New York, Futura, 2001.
Trines J, Hornberger LK: Evolution of heart disease in utero. *Pediatr Cardiol* 2004;25:287–298.
Walsh MC, Stork EK: Persistent pulmonary hypertension of the newborn. Rational therapy based on pathophysiology. *Clin Perinatol* 2001;28:609–627.

Sezione 2 — Valutazione dell'apparato cardiovascolare — Daniel Bernstein

Capitolo 422 ■ Anamnesi ed esame obiettivo

Occorre sottolineare una volta di più l'importanza dell'anamnesi e dell'esame obiettivo nella valutazione dei lattanti e dei bambini in cui si sospetta una patologia cardiovascolare. Nel caso non si rendessero necessari un'ulteriore valutazione di laboratorio e un trattamento specifico, sarà possibile comunicare ai familiari che non sono emersi problemi significativi. Anche se la disponibilità dell'ecocardiografia può indurre il clinico a saltare queste fasi preliminari, è preferibile che un cardiologo esperto esegua una valutazione iniziale per varie ragioni: (1) l'esame obiettivo del cuore permette al cardiologo di guidare la valutazione ecocardiografica verso la conferma o l'esclusione di diagnosi specifiche, aumentandone così l'accuratezza; (2) poiché nella maggior parte dei casi i soffi cardiaci che si manifestano in età pediatrica sono innocenti, una valutazione da parte di un cardiologo pediatra può evitare esami di laboratorio non necessari e costosi; (3) la conoscenza e l'esperienza del cardiologo sono importanti per rassicurare i familiari del paziente e per evitare inutili restrizioni dell'attività fisica.

ANAMNESI. Un'anamnesi cardiologica esauriente consiste innanzitutto nel raccogliere informazioni sul periodo perinatale, con particolare riguardo alla presenza di cianosi, distress respiratorio o prematurità. Complicanze materne come il diabete gestazionale, l'assunzione di farmaci, il lupus eritematoso sistemico o l'abuso di sostanze possono essere associate a problemi cardiaci. Se i sintomi cardiaci compaiono nell'infanzia, occorre stabilire quando si sono verificati i primi sintomi perché questo dato fornisce importanti indizi sulle specifiche patologie cardiache.

Molti sintomi dell'**insufficienza cardiaca** in età pediatrica sono età-specifici. Nei lattanti, sono comuni le difficoltà di alimentazione. Bisognerebbe determinare la frequenza dell'allattamento e il volume di ciascuna poppata o il tempo di allattamento per ciascuna mammella. Un lattante con scompenso cardiaco spesso assume una minore quantità di latte per poppata e diviene dispnoico o diaforetico durante la suzione. Dopo essersi addormentato esausto, il bambino, inadeguatamente nutrito, si sveglia per la successiva poppata dopo breve tempo. Questo quadro, che si ripete nell'arco della giornata, deve essere accuratamente differenziato da malattie coliche o altre patologie legate all'allattamento. Ulteriori sintomi e segni sono quelli tipici del distress respiratorio: respirazione rapida, alitamento delle pinne nasali, cianosi e retrazione degli spazi intercostali al torace. Nei bambini più grandi lo scompenso cardiaco può manifestarsi come intolleranza all'esercizio fisico, difficoltà nel tenersi al passo con i compagni durante l'esercizio sportivo o bisogno di riposo al ritorno da scuola, e ritardo di crescita. Se emerge una storia di astenia in un bambino più grande è necessario porre domande riguardanti le attività specifiche per quell'età, compresi il salire le scale, il camminare, l'andare in bicicletta, le lezioni di educazione fisica e l'attività agonistica; è inoltre necessario indagare sull'eventuale comparsa di manifestazioni più gravi come l'ortopnea o la dispnea notturna.

La **cianosi** a riposo spesso viene sottovalutata dai genitori, che la scambiano per una normale variazione del colorito. Al contrario, se il fenomeno si verifica durante il pianto o l'attività fisica viene più spesso riconosciuto come anomalo. Molti lattanti e divezzi diventano "blu attorno alle labbra" quando piangono vigorosamente o quando trattengono a lungo il respiro; è necessario distinguere questa situazione dalle cardiopatie cianotiche facendo domande riguardo ai fattori scatenanti, alla lunghezza degli episodi e chiedendo se anche la lingua e le mucose apparivano cianotiche. I neonati presentano estremità cianotiche (acrocianosi) quando sono nudi ed esposti a basse temperature; questa risposta al freddo deve essere accuratamente differenziata dalla cianosi vera.

Il **dolore toracico** è una manifestazione non comune di patologia cardiaca nei pazienti pediatrici, anche se è una causa frequente di consulto cardiologico, specialmente negli adolescenti. Ciononostante, la raccolta di un'anamnesi accurata, l'esame obiettivo e, se indicati, esami di laboratorio o di imaging aiuteranno a identificarne la causa (Tab. 422-1).

La malattia cardiaca può essere una manifestazione di una sindrome malformativa congenita nota con reperti tipici all'esame obiettivo (Tab. 422-2) o di una patologia sistemica a carico del cuore e di altri organi e apparati (Tab. 422-3). Malformazioni extracardiache si riscontrano nel 20-45% dei bambini con

TABELLA 422-1. Diagnosi differenziale del dolore toracico nei pazienti pediatrici

MUSCOLOSCHELETRICO (COMUNE)
Traumi (accidentali, maltrattamenti)
Esercizio fisico, lesione da superlavoro (stiramenti, borsiti)
Costocondrite (sindrome di Tietze)
Herpes zoster (cutaneo)
Pleurodinia
Fibrosite
Slittamento costale
Crisi vaso-occlusive dell'anemia a cellule falciformi
Osteomielite (rara)
Tumori primari o metastatici (rari)
POLMONARE (COMUNE)
Polmonite
Pleurite
Asma
Tosse cronica
Pneumotorace
Infarto (anemia falciforme)
Corpi estranei
Embolia (rara)
Ipertensione polmonare (rara)
Tumori (rari)
Bronchiectasie
GASTROINTESTINALE (MENO COMUNE)
Esofagite (reflusso gastroesofageo, infettiva, da farmaci)
Corpo estraneo esofageo
Spasmo esofageo
Colecistite
Ascesso sottodiaframmatico
Periepatite (sindrome di Fitz-Hugh-Curtis)
Ulcera peptica
CARDIACO (MENO COMUNE)
Pericardite
Sindrome post-pericardiotomica
Endocardite
Miocardiopatia
Prolasso della valvola mitrale
Stenosi aortica o subaortica
Aritmie
Sindrome di Marfan (aneurisma aortico dissecante)
Malattia di Kawasaki
Consumo di cocaina o ingestione di sostanze simpaticomimetiche
Angina (ipercolesterolemia familiare, arteria coronaria anomala)
IDIOPATICO (COMUNE)
Ansia, iperventilazione
Attacchi di panico
ALTRE CAUSE (MENO COMUNI)
Compressione del midollo spinale o delle radici nervose
Patologie mammarie
Sindrome di Castleman (neoplasia nodosa linfatica)

cardiopatie congenite. Il 5-10% dei pazienti presenta anomalie cromosomiche; la genetica assumerà un'importanza sempre maggiore via via che aumenteranno le nostre conoscenze sui difetti genici specifici associati alle cardiopatie congenite. Un'accurata anamnesi familiare può inoltre rivelare storia di coronaropatia o ictus in giovane età (ipercolesterolemia familiare o trombofilia), malattie muscolari generalizzate (distrofia muscolare, dermatomiosite, miocardiopatia familiare o metabolica), o la presenza di parenti con cardiopatie congenite.

ESAME OBIETTIVO GENERALE. Dopo una valutazione generale del paziente, l'attenzione si concentra sulla presenza di cianosi, anomalie della crescita, segni di distress respiratorio. La valutazione di un soffio cardiaco va sempre effettuata tenendo conto degli altri reperti emersi dall'esame obiettivo. Spesso altri reperti associati, come la qualità del polso o la presenza di un itto ventricolare, forniscono indizi preziosi per la diagnosi di una patologia cardiaca specifica.

Si raccomanda un'accurata misurazione dell'altezza e del peso, che andranno poi riportati su una curva di crescita standard, in quanto sia l'insufficienza cardiaca sia la cianosi cronica determinano un **arresto della crescita**. Quest'ultimo di solito si manifesta con uno scarso aumento di peso; se finisce con l'avere ripercussioni anche sull'altezza o sulla circonferenza cranica, possono essere presenti ulteriori malformazioni congenite o malattie metaboliche.

Una cianosi lieve può essere difficile da evidenziare in fase precoce, e l'ippocratismo digitale alle mani e ai piedi di solito si manifesta tardivamente nel primo anno di vita, anche in presenza di grave desaturazione arteriosa di ossigeno. La **cianosi** è più evidente su letto ungueale, labbra, lingua e membrane mucose. Una cianosi differenziata, che si manifesta con estremità inferiori bluastre e arti superiori rosei (di solito il braccio destro) si osserva in caso di shunt destro-sinistro attraverso il dotto arterioso, in presenza di coartazione aortica o di arco aortico interrotto. Una cianosi periorale o un colorito bluastro della fronte possono dipendere da plessi venosi superficiali in queste aree, e non da una diminuita saturazione di ossigeno nel sangue arterioso. In età infantile spesso le estremità assumono un colorito cianotico quando il bambino è svestito ed esposto al freddo (acrocianosi) e questa condizione può essere distinta dalla cianosi centrale grazie all'esame della lingua e delle mucose.

Lo **scompenso cardiaco** nei lattanti e nei bambini comporta un certo grado di epatomegalia e talvolta di splenomegalia. Le aree di edema periferico sono età-dipendenti. Nei lattanti, l'edema di solito è visibile attorno agli occhi o sui fianchi, soprattutto al mattino, al risveglio. I bambini più grandi e gli adolescenti presentano edema sia periorbitale sia localizzato ai piedi; spesso questi pazienti si lamentano di non poter più indossare i propri vestiti.

Nei neonati la frequenza cardiaca è rapida e soggetta ad ampie fluttuazioni (Tab. 422-4). Tale valore, che in media oscilla dai 120 ai 140 battiti/min, può aumentare fino a 170 e più battiti/min durante il pianto e l'attività fisica, e scendere a 70-90 battiti/min durante il sonno. Con la crescita, la frequenza cardiaca media diminuisce e può abbassarsi fino a 40 battiti/min negli adolescenti che praticano sport. Una tachicardia persistente (>200 battiti/min nei neonati, 150 battiti/min nei lattanti o 120 battiti/min nei bambini più grandi), una bradicardia o un'irregolarità del battito cardiaco diversa dall'aritmia sinusale richiedono ulteriori accertamenti per escludere aritmie patologiche (vedi Capitolo 435).

Nell'ambito dell'esame obiettivo, un'attenta valutazione delle caratteristiche del **polso** è un elemento importante per la diagnosi di cardiopatia congenita. Un polso ampio con pulsazioni scoccanti può suggerire una lesione da fuoriuscita di sangue dall'aorta, come un dotto arterioso pervio, un'insufficienza aortica, una comunicazione arterovenosa o un aumento della gittata cardiaca secondario ad anemia, ansia o condizioni associate a ipersecrezione di catecolamine o ormoni tiroidei. La presenza di un polso piccolo a tutte le estremità è associata a tamponamento cardiaco, ostruzione all'efflusso ventricolare sinistro o miocardiopatia. Bisognerebbe sempre palpare i polsi radiali e femorali contemporaneamente. Di norma il polso femorale dovrebbe essere avvertito immediatamente prima del polso radiale. Nei bambini più grandi con coartazione dell'aorta, il flusso sanguigno diretto all'aorta discendente può essere deviato in vasi collaterali e questo fa sì che il polso femorale venga percepito in ritardo rispetto a quello radiale (**ritardo radiale-femorale**).

La **pressione sanguigna** dovrebbe essere misurata agli arti superiori e inferiori, e in questi ultimi almeno una volta per accertarsi che non vi sia una coartazione aortica. La palpazione del polso femorale o tibiale anteriore, o di entrambi, da sola, non consente di escludere completamente questa eventualità. Nei bambini più grandi, per misurare la pressione sanguigna si può utilizzare uno sfigmomanometro a mercurio con un bracciale che copra circa due terzi della parte superiore del braccio o della gamba. Un bracciale troppo piccolo porta a stime errate per eccesso, mentre un bracciale troppo grande registrerà valori leggermente ridotti. Gli ambulatori e le cliniche pediatriche dovrebbero essere dotati

TABELLA 422-2. Sindromi malformative congenite associate a cardiopatie congenite

SINDROME	CARATTERISTICHE
ANOMALIE CROMOSOMICHE	
Trisomia 21 (sindrome di Down)	Difetto dei cuscinetti endocardici, VSD, ASD
Trisomia 21p (sindrome dell'occhio di gatto)	Varie, ritorno venoso polmonare anomalo
Trisomia 18	VSD, ASD, PDA, coartazione aortica, aorta o polmonare bicuspide
Trisomia 13	VSD, ASD, PDA, coartazione aortica, aorta o polmonare bicuspide
Trisomia 9	Varie
XXXXY	PDA, ASD
Penta X	PDA, VSD
Triploidia	VSD, ASD, PDA
XO (sindrome di Turner)	Valvola aortica bicuspide, coartazione aortica
X Fragile	Prolasso mitralico, dilatazione dell'arco aortico
Duplicazione 3q2	Varie
Delezione 4p	VSD, PDA, stenosi aortica
Delezione 9p	Varie
Delezione 5p (sindrome del "cri du chat")	VSD, PDA, ASD
Delezione 10q	VSD, TOF, lesioni conotroncali*
Delezione 13q	VSD
Delezione 18q	VSD
SINDROMI COMPLESSE	
Associazione CHARGE (coloboma, cuore [*heart*], atresia delle coane, ritardo mentale, anomalie genitali e dell'orecchio [*ear*])	VSD, ASD, PDA, TOF, difetto dei cuscinetti endocardici
Sequenza di DiGeorge, CATCH 22 (difetti cardiaci, facies anomala, aplasia del timo, palatoschisi [*cleft palate*], e ipocalcemia [*hypocalcemia*])	Anomalie dell'arco aortico, anomalie conotroncali
Sindrome di Alagille (displasia arteriopatica)	Stenosi polmonare periferica
Associazione di VATER (anomalie vertebrali, anali, tracheali esofagee, radiali e renali)	VSD, TOF, ASD, PDA
FAVS (spettro facio-auricolo-vertebrale)	TOF, VSD
CHILD (*Congenital Hemidysplasia with Ichthyosiform erythroderma, Limb Defects* [emidisplasia congenita con eritrodermia ittiosiforme, difetti degli arti]	Varie
Nanismo Mulibrey (*muscle, liver, brain, eye* [muscolo, fegato, cervello, occhio])	Ispessimento pericardico, pericardite costrittiva
Sindrome da asplenia	Lesioni cardiache complesse con cianosi, riduzione del flusso polmonare, trasposizione delle grandi arterie, ritorno venoso polmonare anomalo, destrocardia, ventricolo unico, valvola atrioventricolare unica
Sindrome da polisplenia	Lesioni senza cianosi con aumento del flusso sanguigno polmonare, prosecuzione azygos della vena cava inferiore, parziale ritorno venoso polmonare anomalo, destrocardia, ventricolo unico, valvola atrioventricolare comune
Sindrome PHACE (*Posterior brain fossa anomalies, facial Hemangiomas, Arterial anomalies, Cardiac anomalies and aortic coarctation, Eye anomalies*) [anomalie della fossa cranica posteriore, emangiomi facciali, anomalie arteriose, anomalie cardiache e coartazione aortica, anomalie dell'occhio]	VSD, PDA, coartazione aortica, aneurismi arteriosi
AGENTI TERATOGENI	
Rosolia congenita	PDA, stenosi polmonare periferica
Sindrome fetale da idantoina	VSD, ASD, coartazione aortica, PDA
Sindrome fetoalcolica	ASD, VSD
Effetti sul feto del valproato	Coartazione aortica, ipoplasia delle camere cardiache di sinistra, stenosi aortica, atresia polmonare, VSD
Fenilchetonuria materna	VSD, ASD, PDA, coartazione aortica
Embriopatia da acido retinoico	Anomalie conotroncali
ALTRE	
Sindrome di Apert	VSD
Rene policistico autosomico dominante	Prolasso della valvola mitrale
Sindrome di Carpenter	PDA
Sindrome di Conradi	VSD, PDA
Malattia di Crouzon	PDA, coartazione aortica
Cutis laxa	Ipertensione polmonare, stenosi della polmonare
Sindrome di De Lange	VSD
Sindrome di Ellis-van Creveld	Atrio unico, VSD
Sindrome di Holt-Oram	ASD, VSD, blocco cardiaco di primo grado
Neonato di madre diabetica	Miocardiopatia ipertrofica, VSD, anomalie conotroncali
Sindrome di Kartagener	Destrocardia
Sindrome di Meckel-Gruber	ASD, VSD
Sindrome di Noonan	Stenosi polmonare, ASD, miocardiopatia
Sindrome di Pallister-Hall	Difetti dei cuscinetti endocardici
Sindrome di Rubinstein-Taybi	VSD
Sindrome della scimitarra	Ipoplasia del polmone destro, ritorno venoso polmonare anomalo alla vena cava inferiore
Sindrome di Smith-Lemli-Opitz	VSD, PDA
Sindrome TAR syndrome (trombocitopenia e assenza del radio)	ASD, TOF
Sindrome di Treacher Collins	VSD, ASD, PDA
Sindrome di Williams	Stenosi aortica sopravalvolare, stenosi polmonare periferica

*Conotroncali = TOF, atresia della polmonare, tronco arterioso, trasposizione delle grandi arterie.
ASD (*Atrial Septal Defect*), difetto settale atriale; PDA (*Patens Ductus Arteriosus*), dotto arterioso pervio; TOF (*Tetralogy Of Fallot*), tetralogia di Fallot; VSD (*Ventricular Septal Defect*), difetto settale ventricolare.

di bracciali da 3, 5, 7 e 12 cm per far fronte a tutte le esigenze dei pazienti pediatrici. Il primo tono di Korotkoff indica la pressione sistolica. A mano a mano che la pressione nel bracciale viene ridotta, i toni di solito si attenuano per poi scomparire. La pressione diastolica può essere registrata sia quando i toni si attenuano (di preferenza) sia quando scompaiono del tutto: nel primo caso il valore registrato è leggermente più elevato e nel secondo caso leggermente più basso della pressione diastolica effettiva. Per determinare la pressione sanguigna agli arti inferiori, si pone lo stetoscopio al di sopra dell'arteria poplitea. Di

TABELLA 422-3. Manifestazioni cardiache di patologie sistemiche

PATOLOGIA SISTEMICA	COMPLICANZE CARDIACHE
MALATTIE INFIAMMATORIE	
Sepsi	Ipotensione, disfunzione miocardica, versamento pericardico, ipertensione polmonare
Artrite reumatoide giovanile	Pericardite, raramente miocardite
Lupus eritematoso sistemico	Pericardite, endocardite di Libman-Sacks, arterite coronarica, aterosclerosi coronarica (con steroidi), blocco cardiaco congenito
Sclerodermia	Ipertensione polmonare, fibrosi miocardica, miocardiopatia
Dermatomiosite	Miocardiopatia, aritmie, blocco cardiaco
Malattia di Kawasaki	Aneurismi e trombosi delle arterie coronarie, infarto miocardico, miocardite, insufficienza valvolare
Sarcoidosi	Granuloma, fibrosi, amiloidosi, ipertrofia biventricolare, aritmie
Malattia di Lyme	Aritmie, miocardite
Sindrome ipereosinofila di Löffler	Endomiocardiopatia
ERRORI CONGENITI DEL METABOLISMO	
Malattia di Refsum	Aritmia, morte improvvisa
Sindrome Hunter-Hurler	Insufficienza valvolare, scompenso cardiaco, ipertensione
Malattia di Fabry	Insufficienza mitralica, coronaropatia con infarto miocardico
Malattia da accumulo di glicogeno IIa (malattia di Pompe)	Intervallo PR corto, cardiomegalia, scompenso cardiaco, aritmie
Deficit di carnitina	Scompenso cardiaco, miocardiopatia
Malattia di Gaucher	Pericardite
Omocistinuria	Trombosi coronarica
Alcaptonuria	Aterosclerosi, malattia valvolare
Sindrome di Morquio-Ullrich	Insufficienza aortica
Sindrome di Scheie	Insufficienza aortica
PATOLOGIE DEL TESSUTO CONNETTIVO	
Calcificazione arteriosa dell'infanzia	Calcinosi delle arterie coronarie e dell'aorta
Sindrome di Marfan	
Aracnodattilia contratturale congenita	Insufficienza o prolasso della mitrale
Sindrome di Ehlers-Danlos	Prolasso della valvola mitrale, dilatazione dell'arco aortico
Osteogenesi imperfetta	Insufficienza aortica
Pseudoxanthoma elasticum	Arteriopatia periferica
PATOLOGIE NEUROMUSCOLARI	
Atassia di Friedreich	Miocardiopatia
Distrofia di Duchenne	Miocardiopatia, scompenso cardiaco
Sclerosi tuberosa	Rabdomioma cardiaco
Sordità familiare	Talvolta aritmie, morte improvvisa
Neurofibromatosi	Stenosi della polmonare, feocromocitoma, coartazione aortica
Sindrome di Riley-Day	Ipertensione episodica, ipotensione posturale
Malattia di von Hippel-Lindau	Emangiomi, feocromocitoma
PATOLOGIE ENDOCRINOMETABOLICHE	
Morbo di Graves	Tachicardia, aritmie, scompenso cardiaco
Ipotiroidismo	Bradicardia, versamento pericardico, miocardiopatia, bassi voltaggi all'elettrocardiogramma
Feocromocitoma	Ipertensione, ischemia miocardica, fibrosi miocardica, miocardiopatia
Carcinoide	Fibrosi endocardica delle sezioni destre
Patologie ematologiche	
Anemia falciforme	Scompenso cardiaco ad alta gittata, miocardiopatia, ipertensione polmonare
Talassemia major	Scompenso cardiaco ad alta gittata, emocromatosi
Emocromatosi (I o II)	Miocardiopatia
ALTRE	
Inibitori dell'appetito (fenfluramina e dexfenfluramina)	Valvulopatia cardiaca, ipertensione polmonare
Sindrome di Cockayne	Aterosclerosi
Nanismo e nevi familiari	Miocardiopatia
Sindrome di Jervell e Lange-Nielsen	Intervallo QT prolungato, morte improvvisa
Sindrome di Kearns-Sayre	Blocco cardiaco
Sindrome LEOPARD (lentigginosi)	Stenosi polmonare, intervallo QT prolungato
Progerie	Aterosclerosi accelerata
Sindrome di Rendu-Osler-Weber	Fistole arterovenose (polmoni, fegato, membrane mucose)
Sindrome di Romano-Ward	Intervallo QI prolungato, morte improvvisa
Sindrome di Weill-Marchesani	Dotto arterioso pervio
Sindrome di Werner	Sclerosi vascolare, miocardiopatia

LEOPARD (*multiple lentigines, electrocardiographic conduction abnormalities, ocular hypertelorism, pulmonary stenosis, abnormal genitals, retardation of growth, sensorineural deafness*), lentiggini multiple, anomalie elettrocardiografiche di conduzione, ipertelorismo oculare, stenosi della polmonare, anomalie genitali, ritardo di crescita, sordità neurosensoriale).

norma, la pressione registrata agli arti inferiori con la tecnica del bracciale è di 10 mmHg più elevata rispetto a quella riscontrata agli arti superiori.

TABELLA 422-4. Frequenza cardiaca a riposo

ETÀ	LIMITI INFERIORI DELLA NORMA		MEDIA		LIMITI SUPERIORI DELLA NORMA	
Neonato	70/min		125/min		190/min	
1-11 mesi	80		120		160	
2 anni	80		110		130	
4 anni	80		100		120	
6 anni	75		100		115	
8 anni	70		90		110	
10 anni	70		90		110	
	FEMMINE	MASCHI	FEMMINE	MASCHI	FEMMINE	MASCHI
12 anni	70	65	90	85	110	105
14 anni	65	60	85	80	105	100
16 anni	60	55	80	75	100	95
18 anni	55	50	75	70	95	90

Nei lattanti, la pressione sanguigna può essere determinata per auscultazione, palpazione o con uno strumento oscillometrico che, se correttamente utilizzato, fornisce misurazioni precise tanto nei lattanti quanto nei bambini più grandi.

La pressione sanguigna, oltre a variare con l'età, è strettamente correlata all'altezza e al peso. Aumenti significativi si verificano durante l'adolescenza, e si registrano molte variazioni transitorie prima che siano raggiunti i livelli più stabili propri dell'adulto. L'esercizio fisico, l'eccitazione, la tosse, il pianto e gli sforzi possono aumentare la pressione sistolica di lattanti e bambini anche 40-50 mmHg al di sopra dei livelli abituali. Occorre aspettarsi una certa variabilità nella pressione sanguigna anche in bambini della stessa età e costituzione; inoltre, quando si valuta un paziente con ipertensione si consiglia di effettuare sempre più misurazioni in serie (Figg. 422-1 e 422-2).

L'ispezione delle **onde del polso venoso giugulare**, di scarsa utilità nei lattanti, si rivela invece preziosa nei bambini più grandi e collaboranti in quanto fornisce informazioni sulla pressione venosa centrale e sulla pressione nell'atrio destro. Le vene del collo dovrebbero essere ispezionate con il paziente seduto a 90°. La vena giugulare esterna non dovrebbe essere visibile al di sopra della clavicola, a meno che la pressione venosa centrale non sia elevata. Un'aumentata pressione venosa trasmessa alla vena giugulare interna può apparire come una pulsazione venosa apparentemente senza distensione; una simile pulsazione non è visibile nei bambini normali quando sono inclinati a un angolo di 45°. Poiché le grosse vene sono in comunicazione diretta con l'atrio destro, cambiamenti di pressione e di volume in questa camera si trasmettono anche alle vene; questo però non avviene nell'ostruzione della vena cava superiore, che comporta la perdita della pulsazione venosa.

ESAME OBIETTIVO DEL CUORE. Il cuore dovrebbe essere esaminato in modo sistematico, iniziando con l'ispezione e la palpazione. Una **bozza precordiale** a sinistra dello sterno con un'aumentata attività precordiale suggerisce un allargamento del cuore; tali bozze si possono meglio apprezzare quando il bambino è in posizione supina, con l'esaminatore ai suoi piedi. Un **impulso sottosternale** indica la presenza di ingrandimento ventricolare destro, mentre un itto apicale si registra in presenza di ipertrofia ventricolare sinistra. Un precordio iperdinamico suggerisce un sovraccarico di volume, come quello che si verifica in un ampio shunt sinistro-destro, anche se può essere normale in un paziente magro. Un precordio silente con un impulso apicale a malapena percepibile è indicativo di un versamento pericardico o una grave miocardiopatia, ma può essere normale in un paziente obeso.

Il rapporto tra l'**itto apicale** e la linea emiclaveare è altresì utile nella valutazione delle dimensioni del cuore: l'itto apicale si sposta lateralmente e verso il basso con l'ingrandimento del ventricolo sinistro. Itti della punta spostati verso destra indicano una destrocardia, uno pneumotorace iperteso o lesioni della parte sinistra del torace occupanti spazio (per es. ernia diaframmatica).

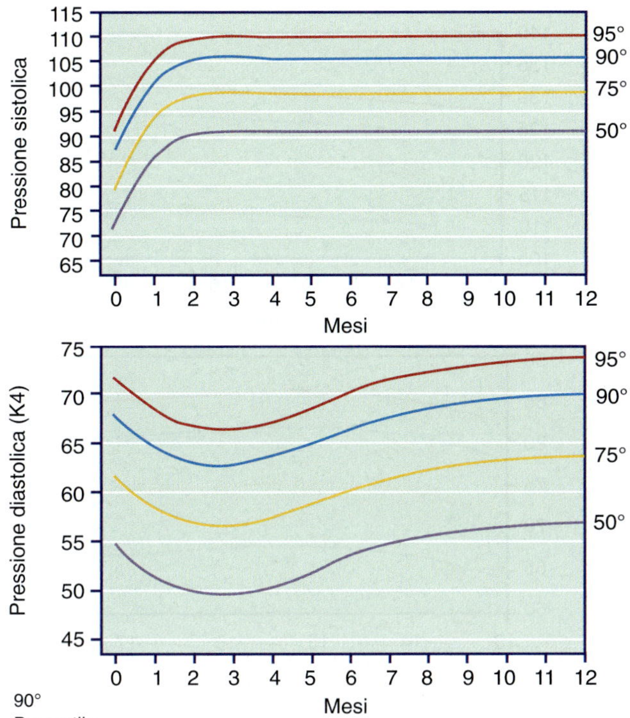

90° Percentile	0	1	2	3	4	5	6	7	8	9	10	11	12
Pr. sist.	87	101	106	106	106	105	105	105	105	105	105	105	105
Pr. diast.	68	65	63	63	63	65	66	67	68	68	69	69	69
Alt. cm	51	59	63	66	68	70	72	73	74	76	77	78	80
Peso kg	4	4	5	5	6	7	8	9	9	10	10	11	11

A

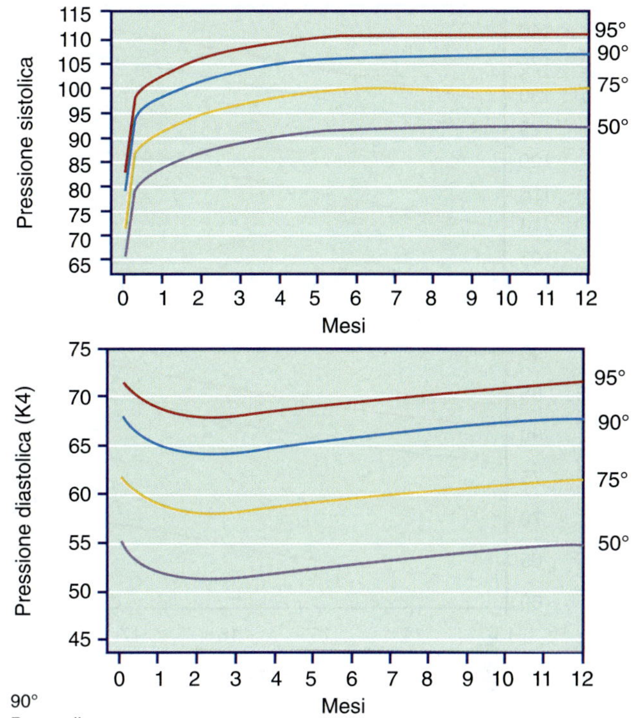

90° Percentile	0	1	2	3	4	5	6	7	8	9	10	11	12
Pr. sist.	76	98	101	104	105	106	106	106	106	106	106	105	105
Pr. diast.	68	65	64	64	65	65	66	66	66	67	67	67	67
Alt. cm	54	55	56	58	61	63	66	68	70	72	74	75	77
Peso kg	4	4	4	5	5	6	7	8	9	9	10	10	11

B

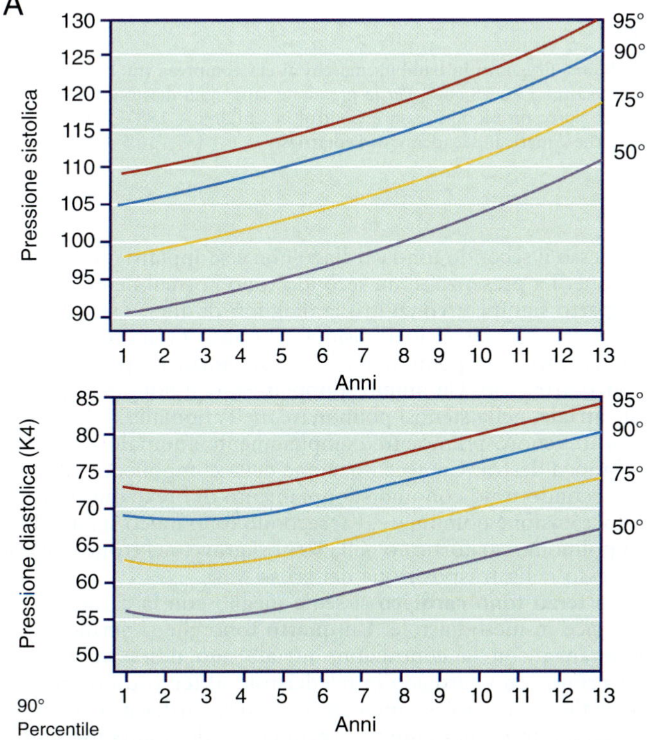

90° Percentile	1	2	3	4	5	6	7	8	9	10	11	12	13
Pr. sist.	105	106	107	108	109	111	112	114	115	117	119	121	124
Pr. diast.	69	68	68	69	69	70	71	73	74	75	76	77	79
Alt. cm	80	91	100	108	115	122	129	135	141	147	153	159	165
Peso kg	11	14	16	18	22	25	29	34	39	44	50	55	62

C

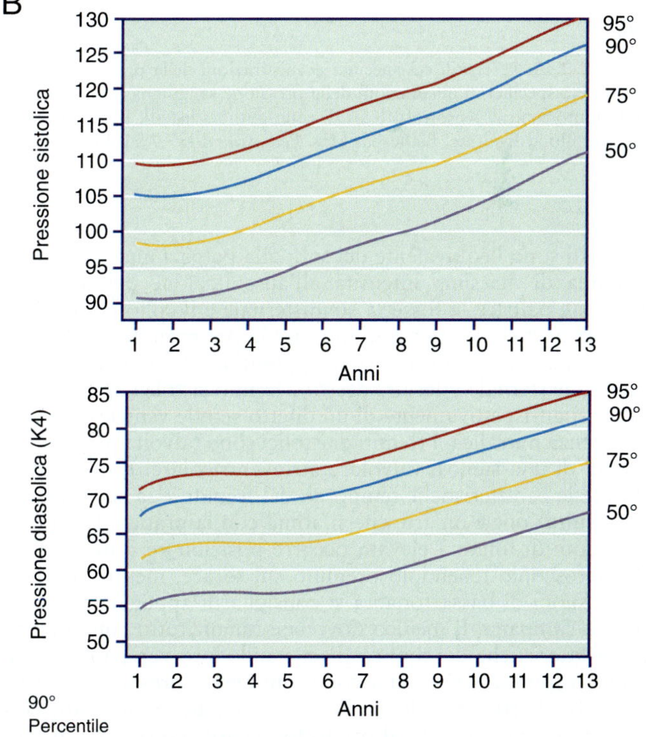

90° Percentile	1	2	3	4	5	6	7	8	9	10	11	12	13
Pr. sist.	105	105	106	107	109	111	112	114	115	117	119	122	124
Pr. diast.	67	69	69	69	69	70	71	72	74	75	77	78	80
Alt. cm	77	89	98	107	115	122	129	135	142	148	154	160	165
Peso kg	11	13	15	18	22	25	30	35	40	45	51	58	63

D

Figura 422-1. *A*, Percentili età-specifici di misurazioni della pressione sanguigna (BP, *Blood Pressure*) in bambini maschi dalla nascita al 12° mese di vita. *B*, Percentili età-specifici di misurazioni della pressione sanguigna in bambine dalla nascita al 12° mese di vita. *C*, Percentili età-specifici di misurazioni della pressione sanguigna in bambini maschi dalla nascita di età compresa da 1 e 13 anni. *D*, Percentili età-specifici di misurazioni della pressione sanguigna in bambine di età compresa tra 1 e 13 anni; per la pressione diastolica è stata utilizzata la fase IV di Korotkoff (K4). (Da [no authors listed]: Report of the Second Task Force on Blood Pressure Control in Children – 1987. National Heart, Lung, and Blood Institute, Bethesda, MD. *Pediatrics* 1987;79:1-25. Copyright 1987 by the American Academy of Pediatrics.)

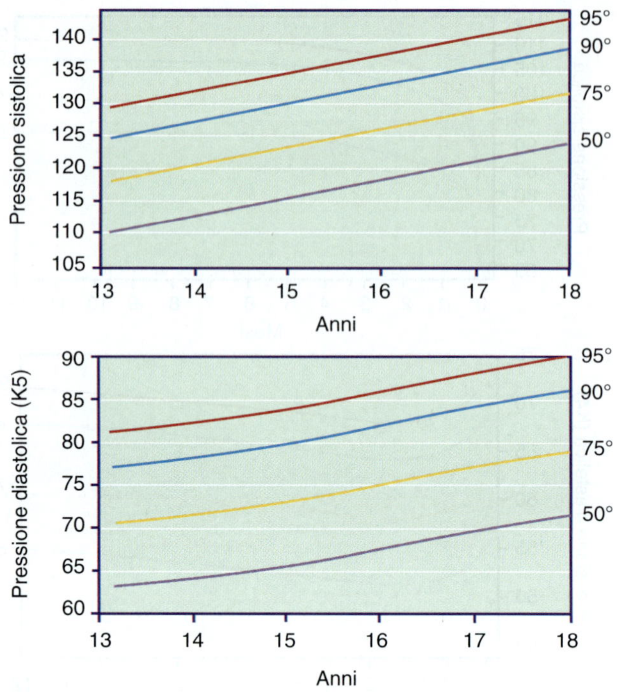

90° Percentile						
Pr. sist.	124	126	129	131	134	136
Pr. diast.	77	78	79	81	83	84
Altezza cm	165	172	178	182	184	184
Peso kg	62	68	74	80	84	86

A

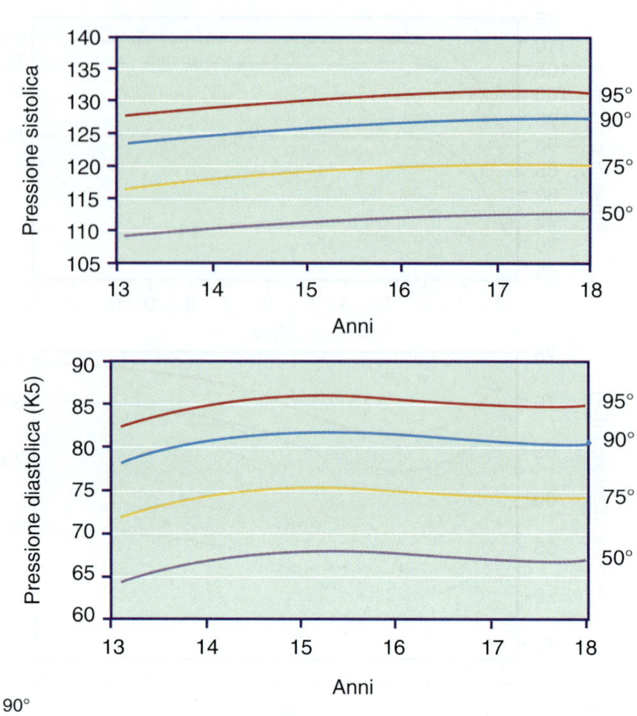

90° Percentile						
Pr. sist.	124	126	126	127	127	127
Pr. diast.	78	81	82	81	80	80
Altezza cm	165	168	169	170	170	170
Peso kg	63	67	70	72	73	74

B

Figura 422-2. *A*, Percentili età-specifici di misurazioni della pressione sanguigna (BP, *Blood Pressure*) in bambini maschi di età compresa tra 13 e 18 anni; *B*, Percentili età-specifici di misurazioni della pressione sanguigna in bambine di età compresa tra 13 e 18 anni. Per la pressione sanguigna diastolica è stato utilizzato il quinto tono di Koroftoff (K5). (Da [no authors listed]: Report of the Second Task Force on Blood Pressure Control in Children – 1987. National Heart, Lung, and Blood Institute, Bethesda, MD. *Pediatrics* 1987;79:1-25. Copyright 1987 by the American Academy of Pediatrics.)

I **fremiti** sono l'equivalente dei soffi alla palpazione e correlano con l'area di massima intensità all'auscultazione del soffio. È importante palpare la fossetta sovrasternale e il collo per evidenziare soffi aortici, che possono indicare la presenza di una stenosi aortica, o, se deboli, di una stenosi polmonare. Fremiti a livello del margine sternale inferiore destro e fremiti sistolici apicali sono caratteristici rispettivamente di un difetto settale ventricolare e di insufficienza mitralica. I fremiti diastolici sono talvolta palpabili in presenza di una stenosi valvolare atrioventricolare. È opportuno annotare le caratteristiche temporali del fremito e la sua sede.

L'**auscultazione** è un'arte che si affina con la pratica. Per ascoltare i suoni di tonalità elevata occorre posizionare il diaframma dello stetoscopio tenendolo premuto sul torace, mentre per percepire i suoni di bassa tonalità si consiglia di appoggiare leggermente la campana. Il medico dovrebbe innanzitutto concentrarsi sulle caratteristiche dei toni cardiaci e sulle loro variazioni legate agli atti respiratori, e in un secondo momento prestare attenzione ai soffi. Il paziente dovrebbe essere supino e rilassato, con una respirazione normale. Il **primo tono cardiaco** si sente meglio all'apice, mentre il secondo tono cardiaco dovrebbe essere valutato in corrispondenza dei margini sternali superiori sinistro e destro. Il primo tono cardiaco è causato dalla chiusura delle valvole atrioventricolari (mitrale e tricuspide); il **secondo tono** dipende invece dalla chiusura delle valvole semilunari (aortica e polmonare) (Fig. 422-3). Durante l'inspirazione, la diminuzione della pressione intratoracica provoca un maggiore riempimento della parte destra del cuore, che a sua volta aumenta il tempo di eiezione ventricolare destra determinando un ritardo di chiusura della valvola polmonare; di conseguenza, lo **sdoppiamento del secondo tono** cardiaco aumenta durante l'inspirazione e diminuisce durante l'espirazione.

Spesso il secondo tono cardiaco non è sdoppiato durante l'espirazione. La presenza di un secondo tono normalmente sdoppiato è reperto significativo contro la diagnosi di difetto settale atriale, di difetti associati a ipertensione arteriosa polmonare, di grave stenosi valvolare polmonare, di atresia aortica e polmonare e di tronco arterioso. Un ampio sdoppiamento si nota nel difetto settale atriale, nella stenosi polmonare, nell'anomalia di Ebstein, nel ritorno venoso polmonare completamente anomalo e nel blocco di branca destra. Un'accentuazione della componente polmonare del secondo tono con uno sdoppiamento di breve durata è segno di ipertensione polmonare. Un secondo tono unico si ha nell'atresia polmonare o aortica o nella stenosi grave, nel tronco arterioso e spesso nella trasposizione dei grossi vasi.

Un **terzo tono cardiaco** si sente meglio con la campana posta all'apice in mesodiastole. Un **quarto tono** che si verifica in concomitanza con la contrazione atriale può udirsi subito prima del primo tono cardiaco in telediastole. Il terzo tono può essere normale in un adolescente con frequenza cardiaca relativamente bassa, ma in un paziente con segni clinici di scompenso cardiaco e tachicardia può presentarsi come un ritmo di galoppo e fondersi con un quarto tono cardiaco, un reperto definito "galoppo di sommazione". Un ritmo di galoppo è attribuito alla scarsa compliance del ventricolo e l'accentuazione del terzo tono normale è associato al riempimento ventricolare.

I **click da eiezione**, udibili in protosistole, possono essere correlati a una dilatazione dell'aorta o dell'arteria polmonare, oppure a una valvola semilunare lievemente stenotica. Si percepiscono talmente a ridosso del primo tono cardiaco che possono essere scambiati per uno sdoppiamento del primo tono. I click da eiezione aortica, udibili soprattutto in corrispondenza del margine sternale superiore destro e di intensità costante, si verificano in

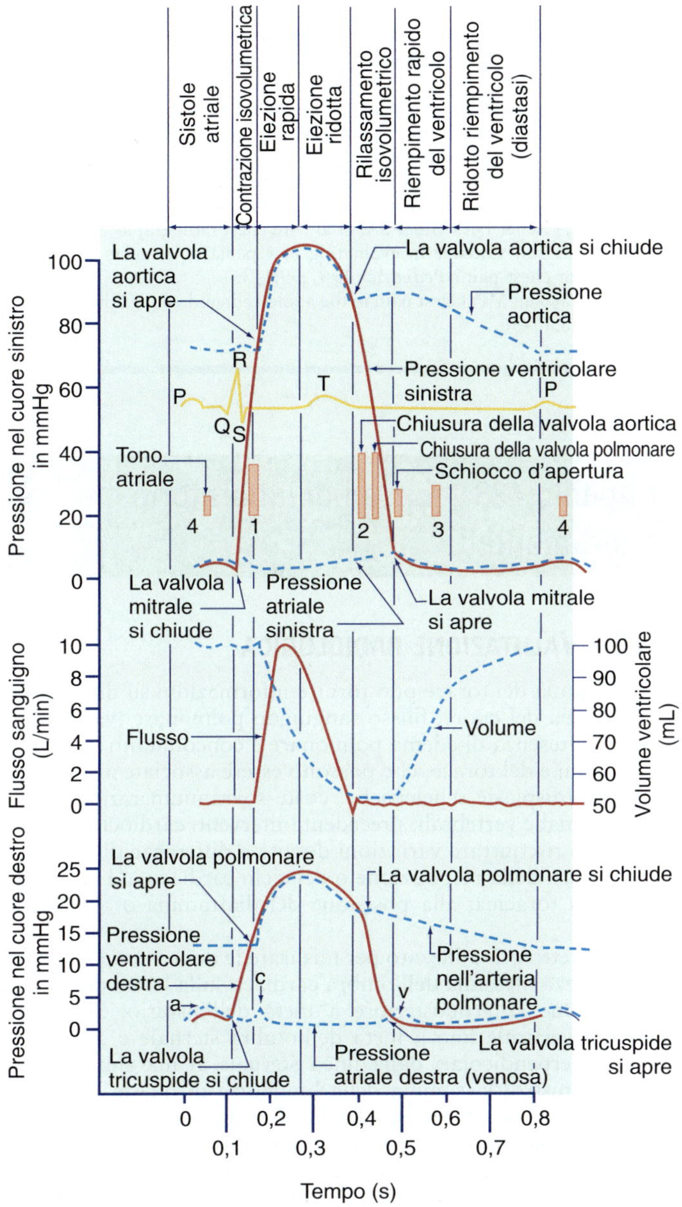

Figura 422-3. Diagramma ideale degli eventi temporali del ciclo cardiaco.

condizioni in cui la valvola aortica è stenotica o l'aorta è dilatata (tetralogia di Fallot, tronco arterioso). I click da eiezione polmonare, che sono associati a una stenosi polmonare lieve o moderata, si sentono meglio in corrispondenza del margine sternale superiore sinistro e variano con la respirazione, scomparendo spesso con l'inspirio. Uno sdoppiamento del primo tono cardiaco si avverte di solito in corrispondenza del margine sternale inferiore sinistro. Un click mesosistolico che si sente all'apice, e che spesso precede un soffio telesistolico, suggerisce un prolasso della valvola mitrale.

I **soffi** dovrebbero essere descritti in base alla loro intensità, alla loro tonalità, al momento in cui vengono percepiti (sistolici o diastolici), alla variazione di intensità, al tempo che impiegano a raggiungere la massima intensità, alla sede di massima intensità e alla loro irradiazione ad altre sedi. L'auscultazione dei soffi dovrebbe essere effettuata nel precordio superiore, lungo i margini sternali destro e sinistro, e fino all'apice cardiaco e all'ascella sinistra. L'auscultazione dovrebbe essere sempre effettuata in corrispondenza dell'ascella destra e a livello del dorso. I soffi sistolici possono essere da eiezione, olosistolici o telesistolici, a seconda di quando il soffio viene avvertito in rapporto al primo e al secondo tono cardiaco. L'intensità dei soffi sistolici viene così classificata: da 1/6 a 6/6: 1/6, appena udibile; 2/6, di media intensità; 3/6, forte ma senza fremito; 4/6, forte con fremito; 5/6, molto forte, ma per essere udito richiede che lo stetoscopio sia posizionato almeno parzialmente sul torace; 6/5, così forte da poter essere udito anche se lo stetoscopio non è a contatto con il torace.

I **soffi da eiezione sistolici** iniziano poco dopo un primo tono cardiaco ben udibile, aumentano di intensità e dopo aver raggiunto l'acme si attenuano; finiscono di solito prima del secondo tono. In pazienti con grave stenosi aortica o polmonare, tuttavia, il soffio può prolungarsi oltre la prima componente del secondo tono, coprendola. I **soffi pansistolici** od **olosistolici** iniziano quasi contemporaneamente al tono cardiaco e continuano per tutta la sistole, a volte divenendo via via decrescenti. È utile ricordare che dopo la chiusura delle valvole atrioventricolari (il primo tono cardiaco) vi è un breve lasso di tempo in cui la pressione ventricolare aumenta ma la valvola semilunare rimane chiusa (contrazione isovolumetrica; vedi Fig. 422-3). Perciò, i soffi olosistolici (che si sentono durante la contrazione isovolumetrica e la fase di eiezione della sistole) non possono essere causati dal flusso attraverso le valvole semilunari poiché queste ultime sono chiuse durante la contrazione isovolumetrica. Essi sono invece causati dal sangue che esce dal ventricolo in contrazione attraverso un'apertura anomala (un difetto settale ventricolare) o da un'insufficienza valvolare atrioventricolare (a carico della mitrale o della tricuspide). I soffi da eiezione sistolici di solito implicano un flusso più intenso o una stenosi in uno dei tratti di efflusso ventricolare (aortico o polmonare). Nei bambini con frequenza cardiaca elevata è spesso difficile distinguere i soffi da eiezione e quelli olosistolici. Se si apprezza un primo tono cardiaco chiaro e distinto, è più probabile che il soffio sia da eiezione.

Un **soffio continuo** è un soffio sistolico che perdura in diastole e indica un flusso continuo, come in presenza di un dotto arterioso pervio o di un'altra comunicazione aortopolmonare. Questo soffio dovrebbe essere distinto da un soffio "va-e-vieni", che indica che la componente sistolica del soffio finisce in corrispondenza o prima del secondo tono cardiaco e che il soffio diastolico inizia dopo la chiusura delle valvole semilunari (stenosi aortica o polmonare associata a insufficienza). Un soffio sistolico tardivo inizia ben oltre il primo tono cardiaco e continua fino alla fine della sistole. Tali soffi possono essere uditi dopo un click mesosistolico in pazienti con prolasso e insufficienza della valvola mitrale.

È possibile identificare diversi tipi di **soffi diastolici** (classificati da I a IV). Un soffio diastolico in decrescendo è un rumore soffiante lungo il margine sternale destro che inizia con S2 e diminuisce verso la mesodiastole. Se di tonalità elevata, è associato a insufficienza della valvola aortica o insufficienza polmonare correlata a ipertensione polmonare; se di tonalità bassa, è associato a insufficienza della valvola polmonare in assenza di ipertensione polmonare. Un soffio diastolico di bassa tonalità in decrescendo si nota tipicamente dopo riparazione chirurgica del tratto di efflusso polmonare in difetti come la tetralogia di Fallot o in pazienti con assenza delle valvole polmonari. Un soffio rullante mesodiastolico a livello del margine sternale medio e inferiore sinistro può essere dovuto a un aumento del flusso sanguigno attraverso la valvola tricuspide, come quello causato da un difetto settale atriale o, meno spesso, da un'effettiva stenosi di questa valvola. Il soffio, se percepito all'apice, è dovuto a un aumentato flusso attraverso la valvola mitrale, come avviene in ampi shunt sinistro-destro a livello dei ventricoli (difetti settali ventricolari) o dei grandi vasi (dotto arterioso pervio, shunt aorto-polmonari), oppure in concomitanza con un'insufficienza mitralica. Un soffio diastolico apicale rullante che, oltre a essere più lungo, si accentua alla fine della diastole (presistolico) di solito indica una stenosi anatomica della valvola mitrale.

In assenza di un soffio precordiale non si può comunque escludere una significativa cardiopatia congenita o acquisita. I difetti cardiaci congeniti, alcuni dei quali sono dotto-dipendenti, possono non essere caratterizzati da soffi se il dotto arterioso si chiude. Queste lesioni comprendono l'atresia della valvola polmonare o tricuspide e la trasposizione dei grandi vasi. I soffi possono sembrare insignificanti in pazienti con grave stenosi aortica, difetti settali atriali, ritorno venoso polmonare anomalo, difetti settali atrioventricolari, coartazione aortica o inserzione anomala di un'arteria coronaria. In questi casi, una scrupolosa attenzione ad altri aspetti dell'esame obiettivo (ritardo della crescita, cianosi, polsi periferici, itto precordiale, toni cardiaci) aumenta l'indice di sospetto di difetti cardiaci congeniti. Al contrario, forti soffi possono essere presenti in assenza di una cardiopatia strutturale, per esempio in pazienti con ampie malformazioni arterovenose non cardiache, con miocardite, con grave anemia o ipertensione.

Molti soffi, detti funzionali, normali, insignificanti o innocenti (quest'ultimo è il termine che si preferisce). non sono associati a significative anomalie emodinamiche. Più del 30% dei bambini può avere un soffio innocente una volta nella vita, riscontrato durante un'auscultazione di routine; questa percentuale aumenta quando l'auscultazione viene effettuata in circostanze non basali (elevata gittata cardiaca imputabile a febbre, infezioni, ansia). Il **soffio innocente più comune** è un soffio sistolico da eiezione di tonalità media, vibratorio o "musicale", relativamente breve, che si sente meglio lungo il margine sternale inferiore e medio sinistro, e non ha una significativa irradiazione all'apice, alla base o al dorso. È di più frequente riscontro in bambini di età compresa tra i 3 e i 7 anni. L'intensità del soffio spesso cambia con il respiro e con la posizione e può attenuarsi in posizione seduta o prona. I soffi innocenti polmonari, anch'essi comuni nei bambini e negli adolescenti, originano dalla normale turbolenza che si viene a creare nell'arteria polmonare durante l'eiezione. Sono di tonalità elevata, soffianti, brevi e presenti nella fase iniziale della sistole, di intensità 1-2/6 e meglio udibili in corrispondenza del secondo spazio parasternale con il paziente in posizione supina. Caratteristiche suggestive di cardiopatia comprendono soffi non olosistolici, di intensità 3/6 o superiore, aspri, localizzati in corrispondenza del margine sternale superiore sinistro e associati a un click proto- o mesosistolico o a un secondo tono anomalo.

Un **ronzio venoso** è un altro esempio di soffio innocente di comune riscontro durante l'infanzia. Tali ronzii, prodotti dalla turbolenza del sangue nel sistema venoso giugulare, non hanno significato patologico e sono percepibili a livello del collo o nella regione anterosuperiore del torace. Un ronzio venoso consiste in un lieve ronzio avvertibile sia in sistole sia in diastole; può essere accentuato o fatto scomparire cambiando posizione alla testa o può essere diminuito esercitando una lieve pressione sul sistema venoso giugulare a livello del collo. Queste semplici manovre sono sufficienti per differenziare un ronzio venoso dai soffi prodotti da patologie cardiovascolari organiche, in particolare un dotto arterioso pervio.

Bisognerebbe rassicurare i genitori del paziente, ribadendo che un soffio innocente è privo di significato clinico. È fondamentale fugare ogni loro timore poiché eventuali dubbi in proposito possono ripercuotersi sul modo in cui il bambino viene allevato, creando intorno a lui un'atmosfera iperprotettiva. Il medico dovrebbe spiegare che un soffio innocente è semplicemente un "rumore" e non presuppone la presenza di un difetto cardiaco significativo. Alla domanda "scomparirà?" la migliore risposta è affermare che questo non ha importanza, in quanto il soffio non ha alcun significato clinico. I genitori devono essere avvisati del fatto che l'intensità del soffio potrebbe aumentare durante una malattia febbrile (occasione in cui un altro medico visiterà il bambino). Con la crescita tuttavia i soffi cardiaci si attenuano e spesso scompaiono del tutto. Anche se talvolta possono essere indicati ulteriori esami per escludere un difetto cardiaco congenito, bisognerebbe evitare di sottoporre bambini sani con soffi innocenti a elettrocardiogrammi, radiografie del torace ed ecocardiogrammi "di routine".

Bhatikar SR, DeGroff C, Mahajan RL: A classifier based on the artificial neural network approach for cardiologic auscultation in pediatrics. *Artif Intell Med* 2005;33:251–260.

Biancaniello T: Innocent murmurs. *Circulation* 2005;111:e20–e22.

Hohn AR, Dwyer KM, Dwyer JH: Blood pressure in youth from four ethnic groups: The Pasadena Prevention Project. *J Pediatr* 1994;125:368–373.

Pelech AN: The physiology of cardiac auscultation. *Pediatr Clin North Am* 2004;51:1515–1535.

Pelech AN: The cardiac murmur. When to refer? *Pediatr Clin North Am* 1998;45:107–122.

Rosner B, Prineas RJ, Loggie MH, et al: Blood pressure nomograms for children and adolescents, by height, sex, and age, in the United States. *J Pediatr* 1993;123:871–886.

Steinberger J, Moller JH, Berry JM, et al: Echocardiographic diagnosis of heart disease in apparently healthy adolescents. *Pediatrics* 2000;105:815–818.

Swenson JM, Fischer DR, Miller SA, et al: Are chest radiographs and electrocardiograms still valuable in evaluating new pediatric patients with heart murmurs or chest pain? *Pediatrics* 1997;99:1–3.

Talner NS, Carboni MP: Chest pain in the adolescent and young adult. *Cardiol Rev* 2000;8:49–56.

Capitolo 423 ■ Esami di laboratorio e strumentali

423.1 • Valutazione radiologica

La radiografia del torace può fornire informazioni su dimensioni e morfologia del cuore, flusso sanguigno polmonare (vascolarizzazione), presenza di edema polmonare e concomitanti anomalie dei polmoni e del torace, che possono essere associate a sindromi congenite (displasie scheletriche, coste sovrannumerarie o mancanti, anomalie vertebrali, precedenti interventi cardiochirurgici). Si possono riscontrare variazioni dovute a differenze di corporatura, alle fasi della respirazione o del ciclo cardiaco, ad anomalie della cassa toracica, alla posizione del diaframma o a malattie polmonari.

Il parametro più utilizzato per misurare le dimensioni del cuore è la larghezza massima dell'ombra cardiaca sulla lastra del torace in proiezione anteroposteriore a metà dell'inspirio. Si traccia una linea verticale fino a metà dell'ombra sternale e si tracciano linee perpendicolari dalla linea sternale ai margini cardiaci destro e sinistro; la somma della lunghezza di queste linee è la larghezza cardiaca massima. La larghezza toracica massima si ottiene tracciando una linea orizzontale tra i margini interni destro e sinistro della cassa toracica a livello della parte più alta del diaframma destro. Quando la larghezza cardiaca massima è superiore alla metà della larghezza toracica massima (rapporto cardiotoracico >50%) il cuore è di solito dilatato. Le dimensioni del cuore andrebbero valutate solo quando la radiografia è stata effettuata in inspirio con il paziente in posizione eretta. Una diagnosi di "cardiomegalia" su radiogrammi effettuati in espirio o a paziente prono spesso porta a visite ed esami di laboratorio non necessari.

Il rapporto cardiotoracico è un indice di ingrandimento cardiaco meno utile nei bambini piccoli che in quelli più grandi, poiché la posizione orizzontale del cuore può aumentare il rapporto di più del 50% in assenza di un vero ingrandimento. Inoltre, il timo può sovrapporsi non solo alla base del cuore, ma anche all'intero mediastino, coprendo così la vera silhouette cardiaca.

Un radiogramma del torace in proiezione laterale può essere utile sia nei bambini piccoli sia in quelli più grandi con *pectus excavatum* o altre patologie che comportano una ridotta dimensione anteroposteriore del torace. In queste situazioni il cuore può apparire piccolo in proiezione laterale e suggerire che l'apparente ingrandimento nella proiezione posteroanteriore sia dovuto o all'immagine del timo (solo mediastino anteriore) o a un appiattimento delle camere cardiache, imputabile a un'anomalia strutturale del torace.

Nella proiezione posteroanteriore il margine sinistro dell'ombra cardiaca consiste in tre ombre convesse prodotte, dall'alto verso il basso, dall'arco aortico, da tronco polmonare e arteria polmonare sinistra e dal ventricolo sinistro (Fig. 423-1). In casi

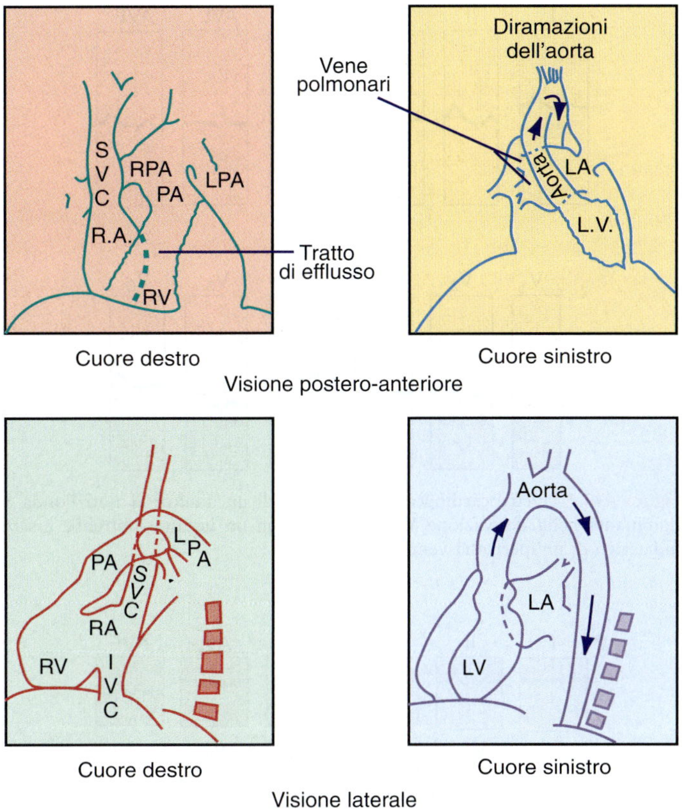

Figura 423-1. Diagrammi ideali che evidenziano la normale posizione delle camere cardiache e dei grandi vasi sanguigni. IVC (*Inferior Vena Cava*), vena cava inferiore; LA (*Left Atrium*), atrio sinistro; LPA (*Left Pulmonary Artery*), arteria polmonare sinistra; LV (*Left Ventricle*), ventricolo sinistro; PA (*Pulmonary Artery*), arteria polmonare; RA (*Right Atrium*), atrio destro; RPA (*Right Pulmonary Artery*), arteria polmonare destra; RV (*Right Ventricle*), ventricolo destro; SVC (*Superior Vena Cava*), vena cava superiore. (Adattata e ridisegnata da Dotter, Steinberg: *Radiology* 1949; 53:513.)

di ingrandimento atriale sinistro da moderato a marcato, l'atrio può proiettarsi tra l'arteria polmonare e il ventricolo sinistro. Il tratto di efflusso del ventricolo destro non contribuisce alle ombre formate dal margine sinistro del cuore. Visualizzare l'arco aortico nei lattanti e nei bambini non è facile come negli adulti. Spesso è possibile dedurre la posizione dell'arco aortico (a sinistra o a destra) considerando che, rispetto alla linea mediana, dovrebbe essere opposto al lato da cui si visualizza la trachea piena d'aria. Questa osservazione è importante poiché un arco aortico destro è spesso presente nelle cardiopatie congenite con cianosi, in particolare nella tetralogia di Fallot. Tre sono le strutture che contribuiscono al margine destro della silhouette cardiaca: dall'alto al basso, la vena cava superiore, l'aorta ascendente e l'atrio destro.

Un ingrandimento delle camere cardiache o delle arterie e vene principali porta alla sporgenza delle aree in cui queste strutture sono normalmente visualizzate sulla radiografia del torace. Al contrario, l'elettrocardiogramma (ECG) è un indice più sensibile e accurato per l'**ipertrofia ventricolare**.

Altrettanto importante è valutare il grado di vascolarizzazione polmonare. Studi angiocardiografici hanno dimostrato che le ombre ilari sono in prevalenza di origine vascolare. Un iperafflusso polmonare è di solito associato a lesioni con shunt sinistro-destro, mentre un ipoafflusso polmonare è associato a ostruzione del tratto di efflusso del ventricolo destro.

Poiché l'esofago è a stretto contatto con i grossi vasi, un'esofagografia con bario può aiutare a delineare queste strutture nella valutazione iniziale di sospetti anelli vascolari. L'esame ecocardiografico è quello più indicato per valutare le caratteristiche morfologiche delle camere cardiache, mentre la TC e la RMN definiscono meglio la morfologia vascolare extracardiaca.

423.2 • Elettrocardiogramma

CAMBIAMENTI LEGATI ALLO SVILUPPO

I notevoli cambiamenti che si verificano nella fisiologia cardiaca e nella dominanza delle camere cardiache durante il periodo di transizione perinatale (vedi Capitolo 421) si riflettono nell'evoluzione dell'ECG durante il periodo neonatale. Poiché nel feto a termine le resistenze vascolari nella circolazione polmonare e sistemica sono quasi uguali, il lavoro intrauterino del cuore porta i ventricoli destro e sinistro ad avere lo stesso volume. Dopo la nascita, la resistenza vascolare sistemica aumenta quando la circolazione placentare viene eliminata e la resistenza vascolare polmonare va incontro a una brusca diminuzione quando i polmoni si espandono. Questi cambiamenti trovano riscontro nell'ECG in quanto la parete del ventricolo destro inizia ad assottigliarsi.

L'ECG mette in luce queste caratteristiche anatomiche ed emodinamiche principalmente attraverso cambiamenti nelle caratteristiche morfologiche del QRS e dell'onda T. Nei pazienti pediatrici si raccomanda di eseguire un ECG a 13 derivazioni, comprendente anche le derivazioni V_3R o V_4R, che sono importanti per la valutazione di un'ipertrofia ventricolare destra. Talvolta la derivazione V_1 viene posizionata troppo a sinistra per poter riflettere accuratamente le forze ventricolari destre; questo problema si presenta in particolare nei prematuri, in cui il gel per gli elettrodi dell'elettrocardiografo può creare un contatto tra le derivazioni precordiali.

Durante il 1° giorno di vita, una deviazione assiale destra, ampie onde R e onde T positive sono la norma nelle derivazioni precordiali destre (V_3R o V_4R e V_1) (Fig. 423-2). Nei primi giorni dopo il parto, a mano a mano che la resistenza vascolare polmonare diminuisce, le onde T precordiali diventano negative; nella grande maggioranza dei casi questo fenomeno si verifica nelle prime 48 ore di vita. La persistenza di onde T positive nelle derivazioni V_3R, V_4R o V_1 oltre la prima settimana di vita è un reperto anomalo, che indica un'ipertrofia o un sovraccarico del ventricolo destro, anche in assenza di criteri di voltaggio del QRS. L'onda T in V_1 non dovrebbe mai essere positiva prima dei 6 anni di età e può restare negativa fino all'adolescenza. Questo reperto rappresenta una delle differenze più importanti, per quanto sottili, tra l'ECG pediatrico e quello dell'età adulta, e rappresenta una comune fonte di errore interpretativo.

In un neonato, l'**asse medio del QRS sul piano frontale** normalmente si mantiene tra 110 e 180°. Le derivazioni toraciche poste a destra rilevano un'onda positiva (R) maggiore di quella negativa (S) e possono restare tali per mesi o anni poiché il ventricolo destro rimane relativamente grande per tutta l'infanzia. Anche le derivazioni sinistre (V_5 e V_6) indicano una dominanza destra nel

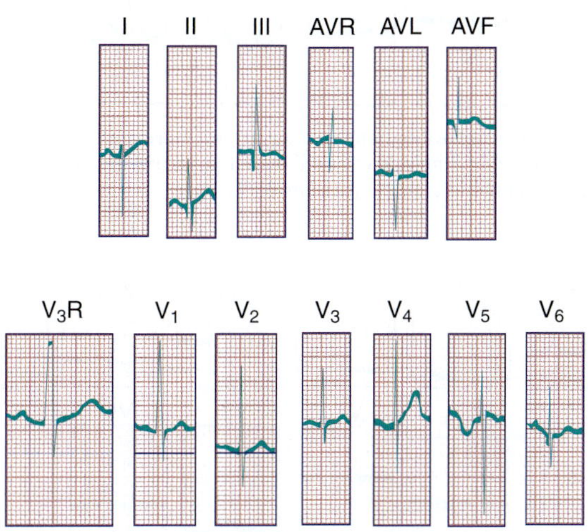

Figura 423-2. Elettrocardiogramma in un neonato normale con meno di 24 ore di vita. Si notino l'onda R dominante e le onde T positive nelle derivazioni V_3R e V_1 (velocità della carta in V_3R = 50 mm/s).

periodo neonatale, quando il rapporto R:S in queste derivazioni può essere <1. Nei primi giorni di vita si rende evidente un'onda R dominante che riflette le forze ventricolari sinistre (Fig. 423-3). Nel corso degli anni, l'asse QRS si sposta a sinistra e le forze ventricolari destre regrediscono lentamente. Le derivazioni V_1, V_3R e V_4R presentano un'onda R prominente fino al 6° mese-8° anno di età. La maggior parte dei bambini ha un rapporto R:S >1 nella derivazione V_4R fino ai 4 anni di età. Le onde T sono invertite nelle derivazioni V_4R, V_1, V_2 e V_3 durante l'infanzia e possono rimanere tali fino alla metà della seconda decade di vita e anche oltre. Il processo di assottigliamento del ventricolo destro e l'aumento del ventricolo sinistro si apprezzano in particolare sul pattern QRS-T, nelle derivazioni precordiali destre. Per formulare la diagnosi di ipertrofia ventricolare destra o sinistra in un paziente pediatrico è necessario conoscere la normale fisiologia dello sviluppo di queste camere dalla prima infanzia fino all'età adulta. Quando il ventricolo sinistro diventa dominante, l'ECG evolve fino a presentare le caratteristiche tipiche dei bambini più grandi (Fig. 423-4) e degli adulti (Fig. 423-5).

L'ipertrofia ventricolare può tradursi in un incremento di voltaggio delle onde R e S nelle derivazioni toraciche. L'altezza di queste deflessioni dipende da tre fattori: distanza dello specifico elettrodo dalla superficie del cuore, sequenza dell'attivazione elettrica attraverso i ventricoli (che può portare a gradi variabili di annullamento delle forze) e ipertrofia del miocardio. Poiché nei lattanti e nei bambini, come pure negli adolescenti, la parete toracica può essere relativamente sottile, la diagnosi di ipertrofia ventricolare destra non dovrebbe basarsi sui soli cambiamenti di voltaggio.

La diagnosi di ipertrofia ventricolare destra patologica è difficile nella prima settimana di vita, durante la quale un'ipertrofia ventricolare destra fisiologica è un reperto normale. Spesso si rendono necessari tracciati seriati per determinare se una marcata deviazione assiale destra e forze precordiali destre o onde T potenzialmente anomale persisteranno oltre il periodo neonatale (Fig. 423-6). Al contrario, il riscontro in un neonato di un pattern elettrocardiografico tipico dell'adulto (vedi Fig. 423-5) suggerisce un ingrandimento ventricolare sinistro. Il neonato prematuro costituisce un'eccezione, potendo presentare un ECG più "maturo" di quello di un nato a termine (Fig. 423-7) in conseguenza di una resistenza vascolare polmonare più bassa secondaria a iposviluppo dello strato muscolare mediale delle arteriole polmonari. Alcuni prematuri presentano un pattern di bassi voltaggi generalizzati su tutte le derivazioni precordiali.

L'ECG dovrebbe essere sempre valutato sistematicamente, per evitare il rischio di lasciarsi sfuggire un'anomalia minore ma importante. Un approccio corretto consiste nell'iniziare con la

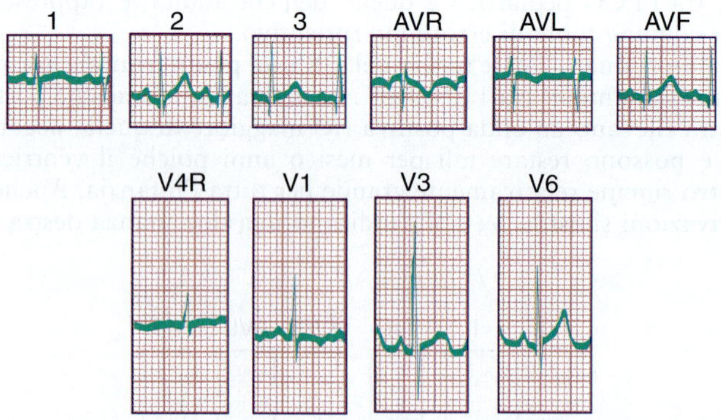

Figura 423-3. Elettrocardiogramma di un lattante normale. Si notino l'onda R alta, le piccole onde S in V_4R e V_1 e l'onda T invertita in queste derivazioni. Un'onda R dominante è altresì presente in V_6.

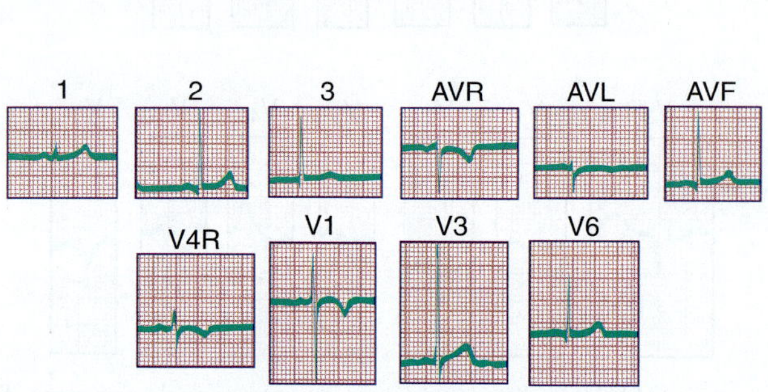

Figura 423-4. Elettrocardiogramma di un bambino normale. Si notino le onde R relativamente alte e l'inversione delle onde T in V_4R e V_1.

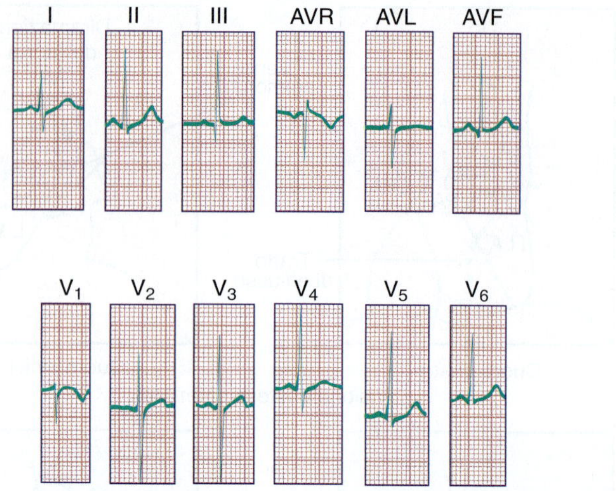

Figura 423-5. Elettrocardiogramma normale di un adulto. Si noti l'onda S dominante nella derivazione V_1, reperto che in un lattante potrebbe essere indicativo di un'ipertrofia ventricolare sinistra.

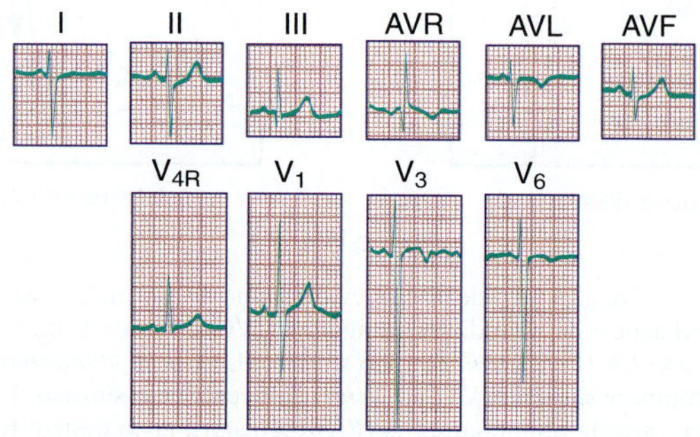

Figura 423-6. Elettrocardiogramma di un lattante con ipertrofia ventricolare destra (tetralogia di Fallot). Si notino le onde T alte nelle derivazioni precordiali destre e le profonde onde S in V_6. Anche le onde T positive in V_4R e V_1 sono caratteristiche dell'ipertrofia ventricolare destra.

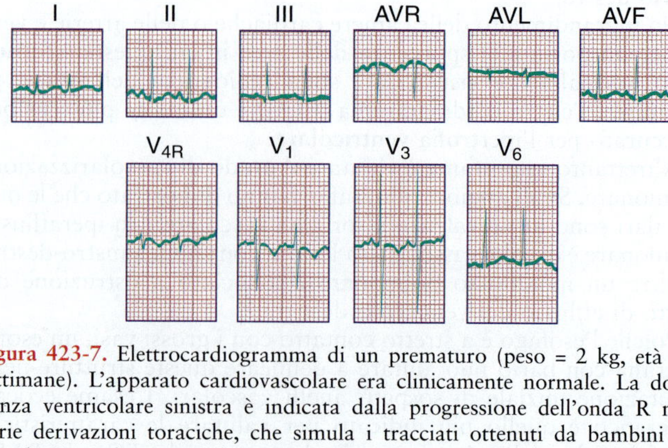

Figura 423-7. Elettrocardiogramma di un prematuro (peso = 2 kg, età = 5 settimane). L'apparato cardiovascolare era clinicamente normale. La dominanza ventricolare sinistra è indicata dalla progressione dell'onda R nelle varie derivazioni toraciche, che simula i tracciati ottenuti da bambini più grandi. Si confronti con il tracciato di un neonato normale, a termine (vedi Fig. 423-3).

valutazione della frequenza e del ritmo, per poi proseguire con il calcolo dell'asse medio del QRS sul piano frontale, la misurazione degli intervalli e dei voltaggi e infine la valutazione delle anomalie dell'ST e dell'onda T.

FREQUENZA E RITMO

Si consiglia di esaminare un breve tracciato per vedere se un'onda P precede sempre ogni complesso QRS. Si dovrebbe poi calcolare l'asse dell'onda P per appurare se il ritmo origina dal nodo del seno. Se gli atri sono situati normalmente nel torace, l'onda P dovrebbe essere positiva nelle derivazioni I e aVF, negativa nella derivazione aVR. Con l'inversione degli atri (*situs inversus*) l'onda P può essere negativa nella derivazione I. Onde P negative nelle derivazioni II e aVF si notano nei ritmi nodali o giunzionali indipendentemente dalla posizione degli atri. L'assenza di onde P indica che il ritmo ha un'origine più distale nel sistema di conduzione. In questo caso, le caratteristiche morfologiche dei complessi QRS sono importanti per distinguere un ritmo giunzionale (di solito con complesso QRS stretto) da un ritmo ventricolare (di solito con complesso QRS ampio).

ONDE P

Onde P alte (>2,5 mm), strette e appuntite, indicative di un **ingrandimento atriale destro**, si osservano nella stenosi polmonare congenita, nell'anomalia di Ebstein della valvola tricuspide, nell'atresia della tricuspide e talvolta nel cuore polmonare. Queste onde anomale sono più evidenti nelle derivazioni II, V_3R e V_1 (Fig. 423-8*A*). Onde simili si osservano a volte nella tireotossicosi. **Onde P ampie**, di solito **bifide** e a volte **bifasiche**, sono indicative di un ingrandimento atriale sinistro (Fig. 423-8*B*); si osservano in alcuni pazienti con ampio shunt sinistro-destro (difetto settale ventricolare, dotto arterioso pervio) e con grave stenosi o rigurgito mitralico. Onde P piatte possono riscontrarsi nell'iperkaliemia.

COMPLESSO QRS

Ipertrofia ventricolare destra. Per una valutazione quanto più accurata possibile dell'ipertrofia ventricolare, gli EGC pediatrici dovrebbero comprendere la derivazione precordiale destra V_3R o V_4R, o entrambe. La diagnosi di ipertrofia ventricolare destra si basa sulla presenza dei seguenti cambiamenti (vedi Fig. 423-6): (1) un aspetto qR nelle derivazioni di superficie del ventricolo destro; (2) un'onda T positiva nelle derivazioni V_3R-V_4R e V_1-V_3 in un arco di tempo che va dai 6 giorni di vita ai 6 anni di età; (3) un'onda R monofasica in V_3R, V_4R o V_1; (4) un aspetto rsR´ nelle derivazioni precordiali destre con la seconda onda R più alta della prima; (5) voltaggio aumentato, corretto per età, dell'onda R nelle derivazioni V_3R-V_4R o dell'onda S nelle derivazioni V_6-V_7, o in entrambe; (6) marcata deviazione assiale destra (>120° in pazienti oltre il periodo neonatale); (7) completa inversione del normale aspetto RS precordiale dell'adulto; (8) ingrandimento atriale destro. Dovrebbero essere presenti almeno due di questi cambiamenti per avvalorare la diagnosi di ipertrofia ventricolare destra.

Un sovraccarico ventricolare anomalo può essere sistolico (imputabile a un ostruzione del tratto di efflusso ventricolare destro come nella stenosi polmonare) o diastolico (attribuibile a un sovraccarico di volume, come nei difetti atriali settali). Questi due tipi di sovraccarico portano a diversi aspetti elettrocardiografici. Il **pattern da sovraccarico sistolico** è caratterizzato da onde R alte e pure nelle derivazioni precordiali destre. Nei bambini più grandi le onde T in queste derivazioni sono di solito positive e più tardi diventano negative. Nei lattanti e nei bambini di età inferiore a 6 anni, le onde T in V_3R-V_4R e V_1 sono anormalmente positive. Il **pattern da sovraccarico diastolico** (che si osserva tipicamente nei pazienti con difetto atriale settale) è caratterizzato da un aspetto rsR´ (Fig. 423-9) e da una durata del QRS lievemente aumentata (ritardo minore di conduzione ventricolare destra). I pazienti con stenosi polmonare da lieve a moderata possono inoltre presentare un aspetto rsR nelle derivazioni precordiali destre.

Ipertrofia ventricolare sinistra. Le seguenti caratteristiche indicano la presenza di ipertrofia ventricolare sinistra (Fig. 423-10): (1) depressione del tratto ST e inversione delle onde T nelle derivazioni precordiali sinistre (V_5, V6 e V_7), quadro noto come pattern da sovraccarico ventricolare sinistro (questi reperti suggeriscono la presenza di una lesione grave); (2) un'onda Q profonda nelle derivazioni precordiali sinistre; (3) un aumentato voltaggio dell'onda S in V_3R e V_1 o dell'onda R in V_6-V_7 o in entrambe queste derivazioni. È importante sottolineare che la valutazione di un'ipertrofia ventricolare sinistra non dovrebbe basarsi unicamente sui criteri di voltaggio. Anche i concetti di sovraccarico sistolico e diastolico, sebbene non sempre coerenti, sono utili per la valutazione di un ingrandimento ventricolare sinistro. Un grave sovraccarico sistolico del ventricolo sinistro è suggerito da uno stiramento dei tratti ST e da onde T invertite nelle derivazioni precordiali sinistre; un sovraccarico diastolico può manifestarsi con onde R alte, un'ampia onda Q e normali onde T nelle derivazioni precordiali sinistre. Infine, un lattante con un ECG che sarebbe considerato "normale" in un bambino più grande, potrebbe avere un'ipertrofia ventricolare sinistra.

Blocco di branca. Un blocco di branca destra completo può essere congenito o acquisito a seguito di un intervento chirurgico per una cardiopatia congenita, specialmente quando sia stata effettuata una ventricolotomia destra, come nella correzione della tetralogia di Fallot. Un blocco di branca sinistra congenito è raro; questo aspetto si osserva a volte nelle miocardiopatie. Un aspetto a blocco di branca può essere indicativo di un fascicolo di conduzione anomalo associato a una sindrome da pre-eccitazione (vedi Capitolo 435).

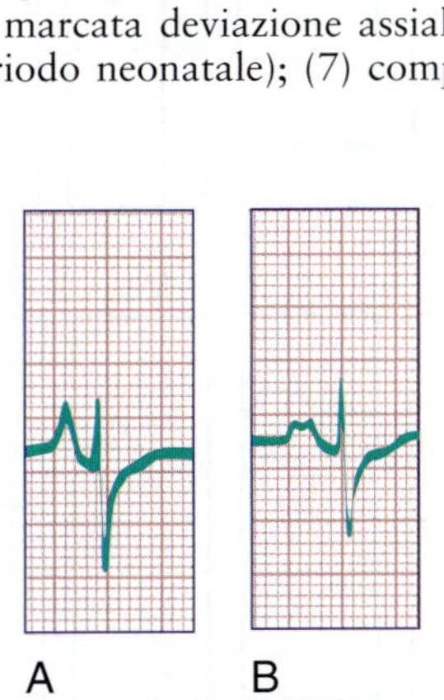

Figura 423-8. Ingrandimento atriale. *A*, Onde P strette e appuntite, caratteristiche dell'ingrandimento atriale destro. *B*, Onde P ampie, bifide e a forma di M, tipiche dell'ingrandimento atriale sinistro.

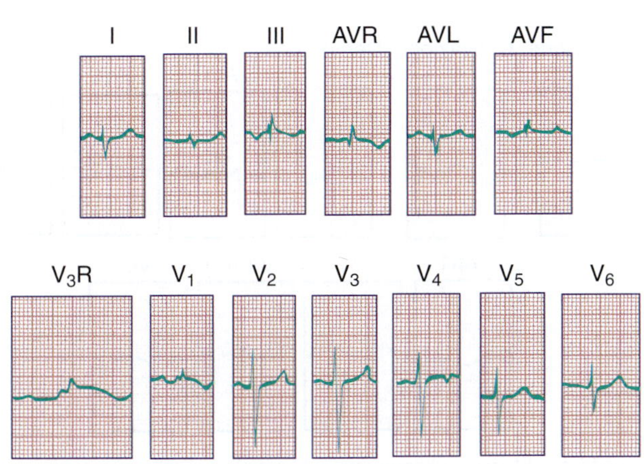

Figura 423-9. Elettrocardiogramma che evidenzia un ritardo di conduzione ventricolare destra caratterizzato da un aspetto rsR´ in V_1 e da un'onda S profonda in V_6 (velocità della carta in V_3R = 50 mm/s).

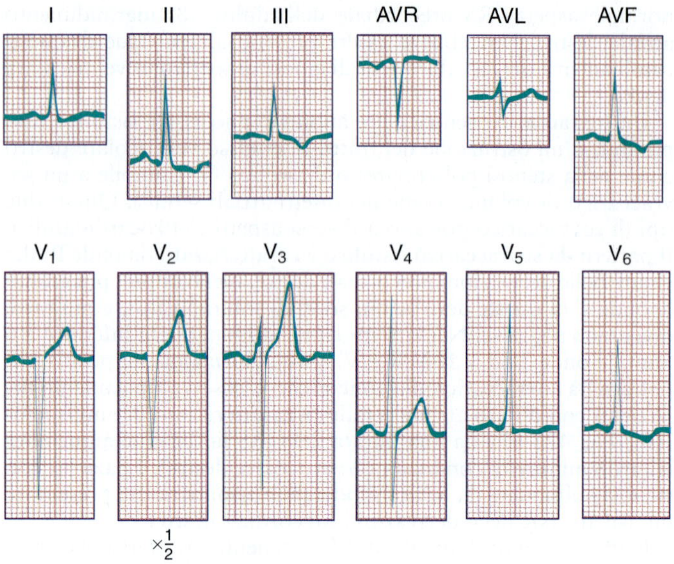

Figura 423-10. Elettrocardiogramma che evidenzia un'ipertrofia ventricolare sinistra in un bambino di 12 anni con stenosi aortica. Si notino la profonda onda S in V_1-V_3 e l'alta onda R in V_5. È inoltre presente un'inversione dell'onda T nelle derivazioni II, III, aVF e V_6.

INTERVALLI PR E QT

La durata dell'intervallo PR diminuisce via via che la frequenza cardiaca aumenta; perciò la sua valutazione dovrebbe basarsi su nomogrammi corretti per età e frequenza. Un intervallo PR lungo consente la diagnosi di **blocco atrioventricolare di primo grado**, che può essere congenito, postoperatorio, infiammatorio (miocardite, pericardite, febbre reumatica) o di origine farmacologica (digitale).

La durata dell'intervallo QT varia con la frequenza cardiaca; un intervallo QT corretto (QTc) può essere calcolato dividendo il valore misurato dell'intervallo QT per la radice quadrata dell'intervallo RR precedente. Il QTc, il cui valore normale dovrebbe essere $<0{,}45$, risulta spesso allungato in presenza di ipokaliemia e ipocalcemia; nel primo caso, può notarsi un'onda U alla fine dell'onda T (Fig. 423-11). Un intervallo QT prolungato congenito (Fig. 423-12) può osservarsi anche in bambini con una sindrome da QT lungo; questi pazienti presentano un elevato rischio di aritmie ventricolari, tra cui una forma di tachicardia nota come *torsades de pointes*, e di morte improvvisa (vedi Capitolo 435.5).

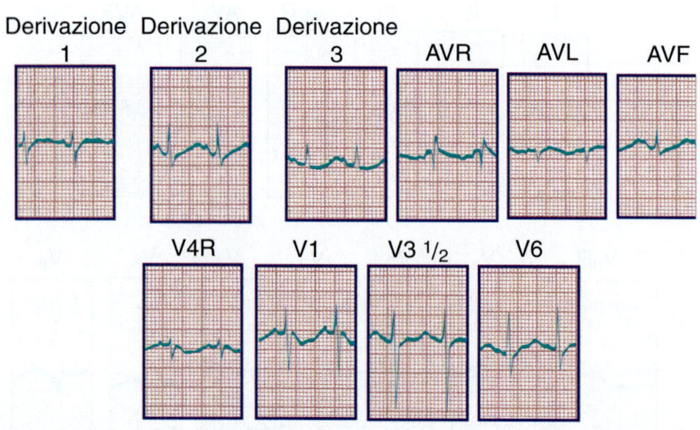

Figura 423-11. Elettrocardiogramma nell'ipokaliemia (potassio sierico = 2,7 mEq/L; calcio sierico = 4,8 mEq/L). Si noti il prolungamento della sistole elettrica, evidenziato tanto da onde TU allargate quanto da una depressione del tratto ST in V_4R, V_1 e V_6.

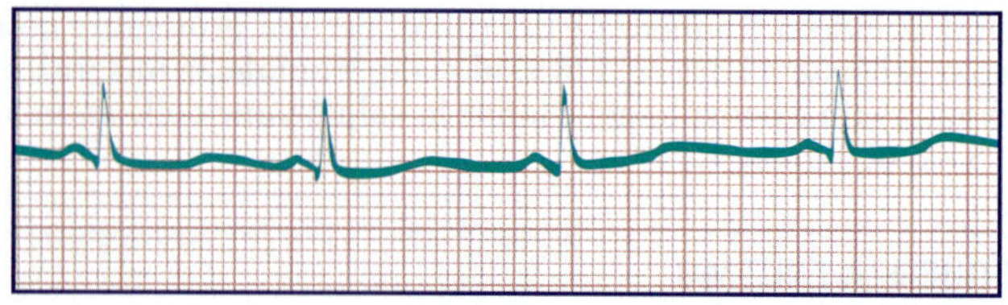

Figura 423-12. Intervallo QT prolungato in un paziente con sindrome del QT lungo.

ANOMALIE DEL TRATTO ST E DELL'ONDA T

In adolescenti normali può verificarsi un lieve sovraslivellamento del tratto ST, attribuibile a una ripolarizzazione precoce. Nella pericardite, l'irritazione dell'epicardio può causare un sovraslivellamento del tratto ST seguito da un'anomala inversione dell'onda T a mano a mano che il processo di guarigione progredisce. La somministrazione di digitale è a volte associata a un incurvamento del tratto ST verso il basso e a un'anomala inversione dell'onda T.

Un sottoslivellamento del tratto ST può anche verificarsi in qualsiasi condizione che provochi danno o ischemia miocardica, tra cui l'anemia grave, l'avvelenamento da monossido di carbonio, un'origine aberrante dell'arteria coronaria sinistra dall'arteria polmonare, malattie da accumulo di glicogeno che colpiscono il cuore, tumori miocardici e mucopolisaccaridosi. Un'origine aberrante dell'arteria coronaria sinistra dall'arteria polmonare può portare a quadri elettrocardiografici indistinguibili da quelli di un infarto miocardico acuto nell'adulto. Simili alterazioni possono verificarsi in pazienti con altre anomalie rare delle arterie coronarie, e in quelli con miocardiopatia, anche in presenza di arterie coronarie normali. Spesso questi pattern non vengono correttamente interpretati nella prima infanzia, in quanto i pediatri non hanno dimestichezza con questo quadro "da infarto", e perciò è necessario mantenere un elevato indice di sospetto di fronte a bambini con sintomi compatibili con ischemia coronarica.

L'inversione dell'onda T può avvenire nella miocardite e nella pericardite, oppure essere un segno di ipertrofia e sovraccarico destro o sinistro. L'ipotiroidismo può produrre onde T appiattite o invertite, in associazione con bassi voltaggi generalizzati. Nell'iperkaliemia, le onde T comunemente hanno un voltaggio elevato e una forma a tenda (Fig. 423-13).

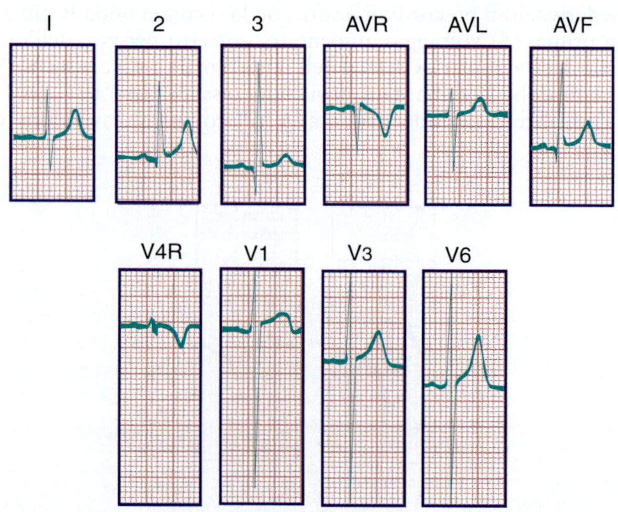

Fig. 423-13. Elettrocardiogramma nell'iperkaliemia (potassio sierico = 6,5 mEq/L; calcio sierico = 5,1 mEq/L). Si notino le onde T alte e a forma di tenda, specialmente nelle derivazioni I, II e V_6.

423.3 • Dati ematologici

In lattanti non cianotici con shunt sinistro-destro l'esordio dello scompenso cardiaco spesso coincide con il nadir della fisiologica anemia dell'infanzia. In questi pazienti, aumentare l'ematocrito a valori >40% può diminuire il volume dello shunt e portare a un miglioramento dei sintomi; questa forma di trattamento è riservata ai bambini che non sono per altri aspetti candidati alla chirurgia (neonati estremamente prematuri, o quelli con cardiopatie congenite estremamente complesse per i quali è possibile solo un intervento chirurgico palliativo). In questi soggetti selezionati, una regolare valutazione dell'ematocrito ed eventuali trasfusioni possono essere utili per migliorare la crescita. In alcuni pazienti, soprattutto se anemici ma emodinamicamente stabili, si può ricorrere all'eritropoietina per aumentare più gradualmente l'emoglobina e perciò la capacità di trasporto dell'ossigeno.

La **policitemia** è di frequente riscontro nei soggetti cianotici con shunt destro-sinistro. I pazienti con grave policitemia si trovano in equilibrio delicato tra il rischio di trombosi intravascolare e una diatesi emorragica. Le anomalie più frequenti comprendono fibrinolisi accelerata, trombocitopenia, anomala retrazione del coagulo, ipofibrinogenemia, tempo di protrombina prolungato e tempo di tromboplastina parziale prolungato. La preparazione di pazienti cianotici e policitemici per un intervento chirurgico elettivo, come un'estrazione dentaria, comprende la valutazione e il trattamento delle anomalie della coagulazione.

A causa dell'elevata viscosità del sangue tipica della policitemia (ematocrito >65%), i pazienti con cardiopatie congenite cianotiche sono a rischio di sviluppare trombosi vascolari, specialmente delle vene cerebrali. Poiché la disidratazione aumenta il rischio di trombosi, è necessario garantire un adeguato introito di fluidi in caso di temperature elevate o di concomitanti patologie gastrointestinali. I diuretici dovrebbero essere utilizzati con cautela in questi pazienti e potrebbe essere necessario ridurne la somministrazione qualora non fosse possibile garantire un adeguato introito di liquidi. I lattanti policitemici con concomitante **deficit di ferro** sono ancora più a rischio di incidenti cerebrovascolari, probabilmente a causa della minore deformabilità degli eritrociti microcitici. La terapia marziale produce un miglioramento, ma il trattamento chirurgico dell'anomalia cardiaca è la migliore terapia.

Pazienti con cianosi grave dovrebbero essere sottoposti a periodiche misurazioni dell'emoglobina e dell'ematocrito. Una policitemia ingravescente, spesso associata a cefalea, astenia, dispnea o a una combinazione di queste condizioni, è un'indicazione all'intervento chirurgico palliativo o correttivo. In caso di cianosi associata a patologie inoperabili può essere necessario ricorrere al salasso per trattare i pazienti il cui ematocrito abbia raggiunto livelli del 65-70%, di solito quando la policitemia è associata a sintomi come la cefalea. Questa proceduta non è esente da rischi, soprattutto in caso di estremo aumento della resistenza vascolare polmonare. Poiché questi pazienti non tollerano ampie fluttuazioni del volume ematico circolante, il sangue dovrebbe essere rimpiazzato con plasma fresco congelato o con albumina. È controverso se il salasso debba essere effettuato di routine nei policitemici asintomatici.

423.4 • Ecocardiografia

L'ecocardiografia riduce notevolmente la necessità di indagini invasive come il cateterismo cardiaco. L'esame ecocardiografico può essere utilizzato per valutare la struttura del cuore nelle cardiopatie congenite, per stimare le pressioni intracardiache e il gradiente attraverso valvole e vasi stenotici, per quantificare la funzione contrattile del cuore (sia sistolica sia diastolica), per determinare la direzione del flusso attraverso un difetto, per esaminare l'integrità delle arterie coronarie ed evidenziare la presenza di vegetazioni da endocardite, come anche la presenza di fluido pericardico, tumori cardiaci e trombi intracavitari. L'ecocardiografia può inoltre essere di ausilio nell'esecuzione di una pericardiocentesi, di una settostomia atriale con palloncino (vedi Capitolo 431.2), di una biopsia endocardica e nel posizionamento in arteria polmonare di cateteri di monitoraggio (Swan-Ganz) a flusso diretto. L'**ecocardiografia transesofagea** è utilizzata per monitorare la funzione ventricolare in pazienti nel corso di procedure chirurgiche complesse e non fornisce un'immediata valutazione del risultato della riparazione chirurgica delle lesioni cardiache congenite. L'**ecocardiografia fetale** può evidenziare la presenza di molte lesioni cardiache congenite, spesso fin dalla 17ª-19ª settimana di gestazione, ed è di grande valore nella valutazione delle aritmie cardiache fetali. Un esame ecocardiografico completo di solito si avvale della combinazione di imaging M-mode e bidimensionale, come anche di studi di flusso pulsato, continuo e color-Doppler. L'ecografia tridimensionale fornisce preziose informazioni aggiuntive sulla morfologia cardiaca.

ECOCARDIOGRAFIA M-MODE

L'ecocardiografia M-mode fornisce una visione unidimensionale, "a fetta", della struttura cardiaca e delle sue variazioni nel tempo (Fig. 423-14). Viene impiegata soprattutto per misurare

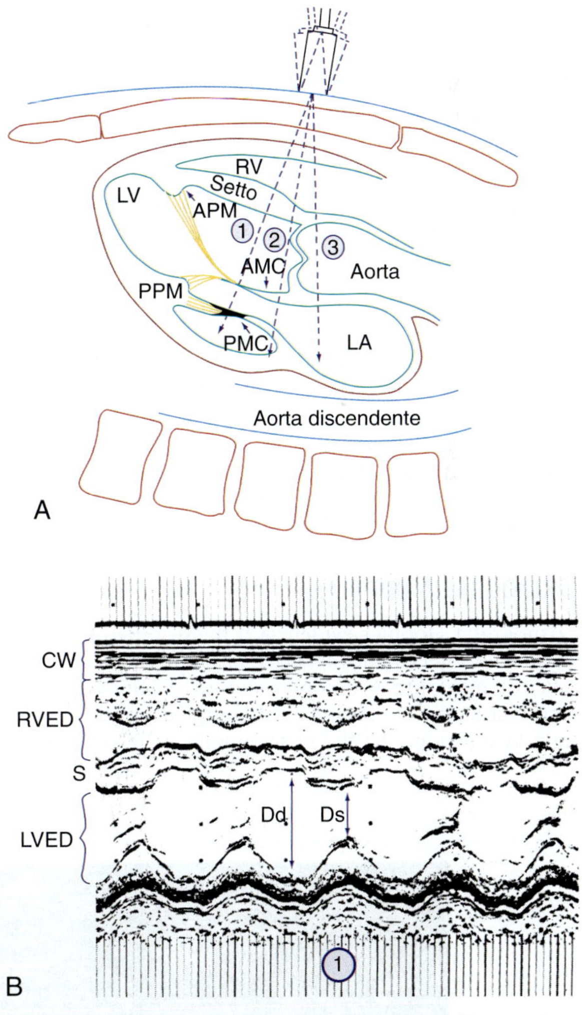

Fig. 423-14. Ecocardiogramma M-mode. *A*, Diagramma di una sezione sagittale del cuore, che evidenzia le strutture attraversate dal fascio di ultrasuoni mentre viene spostato superiormente nelle posizioni (1), (2) e (3). AMC (*Anterior Mitral Cusp*), cuspide anteriore della mitrale; APM (*Anterior Papillary Muscle*), muscolo papillare anteriore; LA (*Left Atrium*), atrio sinistro; LV (*Left Ventricle*), ventricolo sinistro; PMC (*Posterior Mitral Cusp*), cuspide posteriore della mitrale; PPM (*Posterior Papillary Muscle*), muscolo papillare posteriore; RV (*Right Ventricle*), ventricolo destro. *B*, Ecocardiogramma dalla posizione (1) del trasduttore; questa visione è la migliore per la misurazione delle dimensioni cardiache e dell'accorciamento frazionale. L'accorciamento frazionale è calcolato come (LVED – LVES)/LVED; CW (*Chest Wall*), parete toracica; Ds, dimensione del LV in sistole; LVED (*Left Ventricle End-Diastole*), dimensione del LV in telediastole (Dd); RVED (*Right Ventricle End-Diastole*), dimensione del RV in telediastole.

le dimensioni cardiache (spessore parietale e dimensioni delle camere) e la funzione cardiaca (accorciamento frazionale, ispessimento parietale), ma è utile anche per valutare il movimento delle strutture intracardiache (apertura e chiusura delle valvole, movimento delle pareti libere e dei setti) e l'anatomia delle valvole (Fig. 423-15). L'indice di funzione cardiaca più utilizzato nei bambini è l'accorciamento frazionale in percentuale (%), che è calcolato come (LVED – LVES)/LVED, dove LVED (*Left Ventricle at End-Diastole*) è la dimensione del ventricolo sinistro in telediastole e LVES (*Left Ventricle at End-Systole)* è la sua dimensione in telesistole. Il normale accorciamento frazionale è pari al 28-40%. Altri indici M-mode di funzione cardiaca comprendono la velocità media di accorciamento delle fibre (V_{CF} media), gli intervalli temporali sistolici (LVPEP [*Left Ventricle Pre-Ejection Period*] = periodo pre-eiettivo del ventricolo sinistro, LVET [*Left Ventricle Ejection Time*] = periodo di eiezione del ventricolo sinistro) e il tempo di contrazione isovolumetrico. Indici più sofisticati di funzione cardiaca possono essere determinati in modo non invasivo con l'assistenza dell'ecocardiografia (rapporto pressione-volume, rapporto stress-tensione parietale in telesistole); l'accuratezza è limitata a paragone con misurazioni analoghe effettuate nel laboratorio di emodinamica.

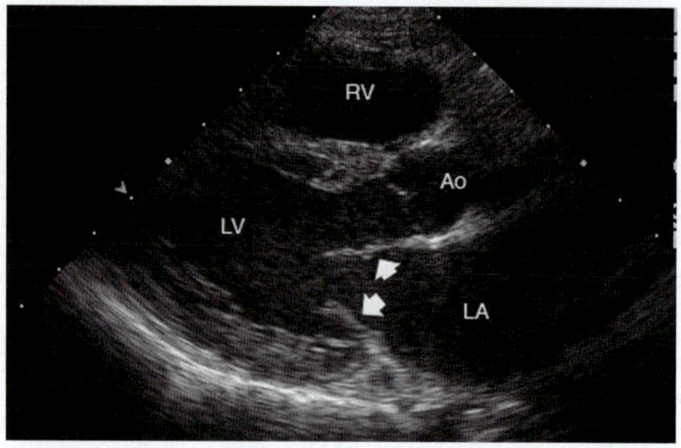

Figura 423-16. Normale finestra ecocardiografica parasternale asse lungo. Il trasduttore è angolato in direzione leggermente posteriore, in modo da visualizzare le strutture cardiache di sinistra. Se il trasduttore fosse angolato più anteriormente, verrebbero rappresentate le strutture del ventricolo destro. I lembi della valvola mitrale possono essere osservati in posizione parzialmente aperta in protodiastole (*punte di freccia*). I lembi valvolari aortici chiusi sono visibili appena al di sotto dell'abbreviazione Ao. Ao, aorta, LA, atrio sinistro; LV, ventricolo sinistro; RV, ventricolo destro.

ECOCARDIOGRAFIA BIDIMENSIONALE

L'ecocardiografia bidimensionale fornisce un'immagine in tempo reale delle strutture cardiache. La contrazione cardiaca è rappresentata in tempo reale utilizzando diverse proiezioni standard: finestra parasternale asse lungo (Fig. 423-16), la parasternale asse corto (Fig. 423-17), la quattro camere apicale (Fig. 423-18), la sottocostale (Fig. 423-19) e la sovrasternale (Fig. 423-20), ognuna delle quali evidenzia meglio strutture specifiche. L'ecocardiografia bidimensionale ha sostituito l'angiografia cardiaca per la diagnosi preoperatoria della maggior parte (ma non di tutte) le lesioni cardiache congenite; in particolare, si è dimostrata superiore nella rappresentazione delle valvole atrioventricolari e dell'impianto delle loro corde tendinee. Quando le informazioni ricavate dall'esame cardiaco non sono coerenti con quelle ottenute dall'ecocardiogramma, il cateterismo cardiaco è uno strumento importante per confermare la diagnosi anatomica e per valutare il grado di compromissione della fisiologia.

ECOCARDIOGRAFIA DOPPLER

L'ecocardiografia Doppler evidenzia il flusso sanguigno nelle camere cardiache e nei canali vascolari, basandosi sul cambiamento di frequenza impartita a un'onda sonora dal movimento degli eritrociti. Nel Doppler pulsato e nel Doppler a onda continua la velocità e la direzione del flusso sanguigno nella linea del fascio ultrasonoro cambiano la frequenza di riferimento del trasduttore. Questo cambiamento di frequenza può essere tradotto in dati di flusso volumetrico (L/min) per la stima del flusso ematico sistemico o polmonare e in dati di pressione (mmHg) per la stima di gradienti attraverso le valvole semilunari o atrioventricolari o attraverso difetti settali o comunicazioni vascolari come gli shunt. Il color-Doppler consente una valutazione molto accurata della presenza e della direzione degli shunt intracardiaci e permette l'identificazione di piccoli o multipli shunt sinistro-destro o destro-sinistro (Fig. 423-21). La gravità dell'insufficienza valvolare può essere valutata sia con il Doppler pulsato sia con il color-Doppler (Fig. 423-22).

Sofisticati metodi ecocardiografici M-mode, bidimensionali e Doppler per la valutazione della funzione sistolica e diastolica del ventricolo sinistro (per es. stress parietale telesistolico, ecostress con dobutamina, e imaging Doppler tissutale) si sono rivelati utili nella valutazione seriale di pazienti ad alto rischio di sviluppare una disfunzione ventricolare sia sistolica sia diastolica; in questa casistica rientrano i pazienti che assumono antracicline quale trattamento chemioterapico antineoplastico, quelli a rischio di sovraccarico marziale e quelli che vengono monitorati per un rigetto o una coronaropatia dopo trapianto cardiaco.

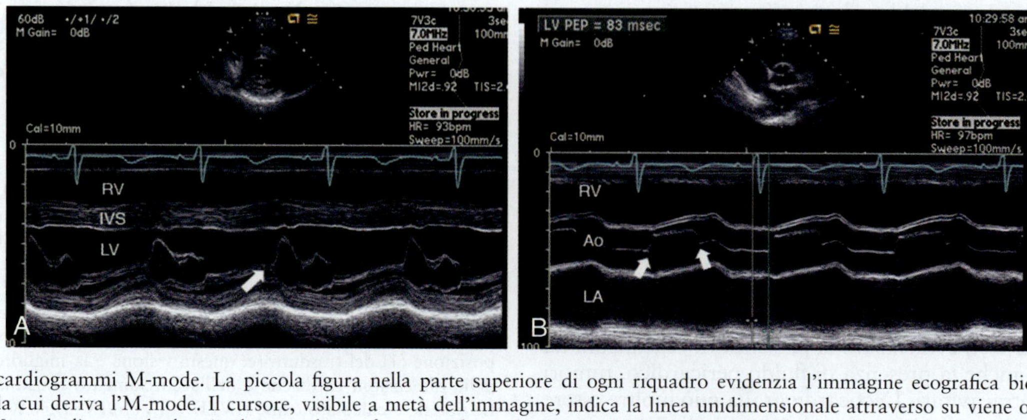

Figura 423-15. Ecocardiogrammi M-mode. La piccola figura nella parte superiore di ogni riquadro evidenzia l'immagine ecografica bidimensionale in parasternale asse corto da cui deriva l'M-mode. Il cursore, visibile a metà dell'immagine, indica la linea unidimensionale attraverso su viene ottenuto l'M-mode. *A*, Ecocardiogramma M-mode di una valvola mitrale normale. La *freccia* evidenzia l'apertura del lembo anteriore in protodiastole (vedi sopra il tracciato ECG come riferimento). *B*, Ecocardiogramma M-mode di una valvola aortica normale. L'apertura e la chiusura dei lembi aortici sono indicate dalle due *frecce*. Ao, aorta; IVS (*InterVentricular Septum*), setto interventricolare; LV, ventricolo sinistro; RV, ventricolo destro.

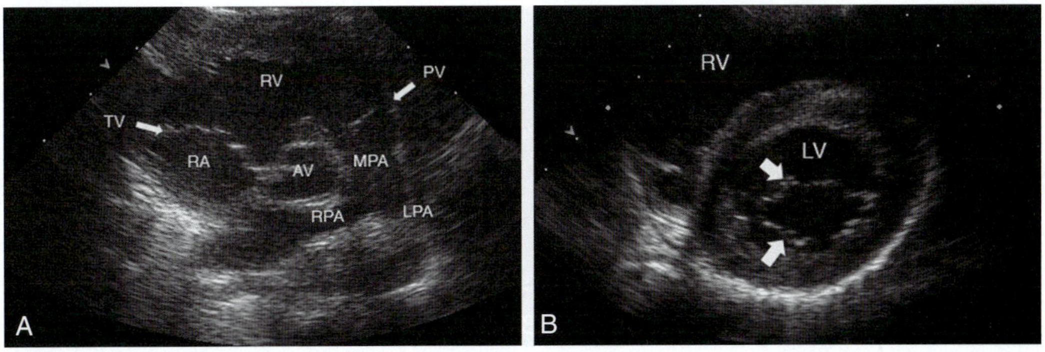

Figura 423-17. Normale finestra ecocardiografica parasternale asse corto. *A*, Con il trasduttore diretto verso l'alto a destra, viene visualizzata la valvola aortica (AV, *Aortic Valve*), circondata dai tratti di afflusso e di efflusso del ventricolo destro (RV). LPA (*Left Pulmonary Artery*), arteria polmonare sinistra; MPA (*Main Pulmonary Truncus*), tronco principale della polmonare; PV, valvola polmonare; RA, atrio destro; RPA, arteria polmonare destra; TV (*Tricuspid Valve*), valvola tricuspide. *B*, Con il trasduttore diretto verso il basso a sinistra, viene visualizzata la camera ventricolare sinistra con una sezione trasversale della valvola mitrale (*frecce*). LV, ventricolo sinistro; RV, ventricolo destro.

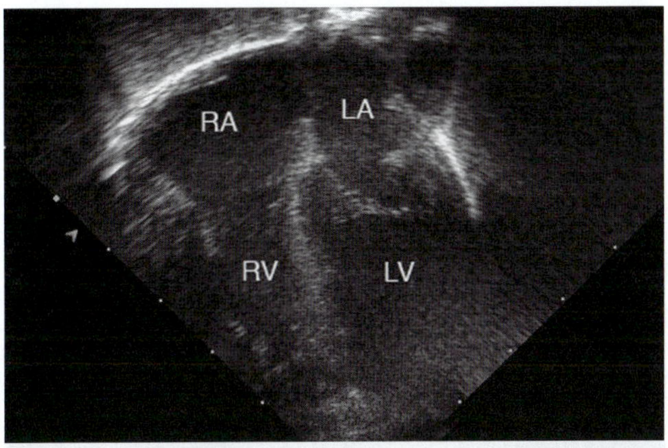

Figura 423-18. Normale finestra ecocardiografica a quattro camere che evidenzia tutte e quattro le camere cardiache ed entrambe le valvole atrioventricolari aperte in diastole. LA, atrio sinistro; LV, ventricolo sinistro; RA, atrio destro; RV, ventricolo destro.

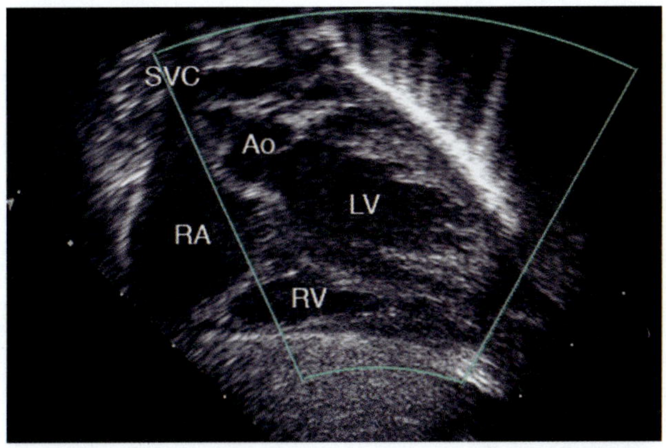

Figura 423-19. Normale finestra ecocardiografica sottocostale che evidenzia il tratto di efflusso ventricolare sinistro. Le strutture del cuore destro non sono rappresentate appieno in questa immagine. Ao, aorta ascendente; LV, ventricolo sinistro; RA, atrio destro; RV, ventricolo destro; SVC, vena cava superiore.

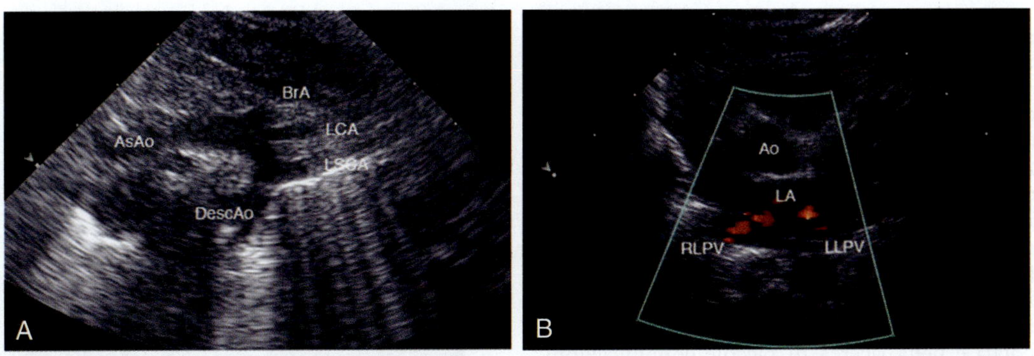

Figura 423-20. *A*, Normale finestra ecocardiografica sovrasternale che evidenzia l'arco aortico e le sue principali diramazioni. AsAo (*Ascending Aorta*), aorta ascendente; BrA, (*Brachiocefalic Artery*), arteria brachiocefalica; DescAo (*Descending Aorta*), aorta discendente; LCA (*Left Carotid Artery*), arteria carotide sinistra; LSCA (*Left SubClavian Artery*), arteria succlavia sinistra. *B*, Normale finestra parasternale alta che evidenzia l'immagine color-Doppler di un normale ritorno venoso polmonare all'atrio sinistro (LA) di entrambe le vene polmonari inferiori, destra (RLPV, *Right Lower Pulmonary Artery*) e sinistra (LLPV, *Left Lower Pulmonary Artery*).

ECOCARDIOGRAFIA TRIDIMENSIONALE

La ricostruzione ecocardiografica tridimensionale in tempo reale è utile per la valutazione della morfologia cardiaca (Fig. 423-23). L'eco 3-D consente di apprezzare i dettagli delle strutture valvolari e dei grandi vasi, le dimensioni e la sede di difetti settali, le anomalie del miocardio ventricolare, che potrebbero non essere altrettanto evidenti utilizzando l'imaging 2-D. La ricostruzione del quadro che il chirurgo si troverà ad affrontare in sala operatoria rende questa tecnica preziosa nell'imaging preoperatorio.

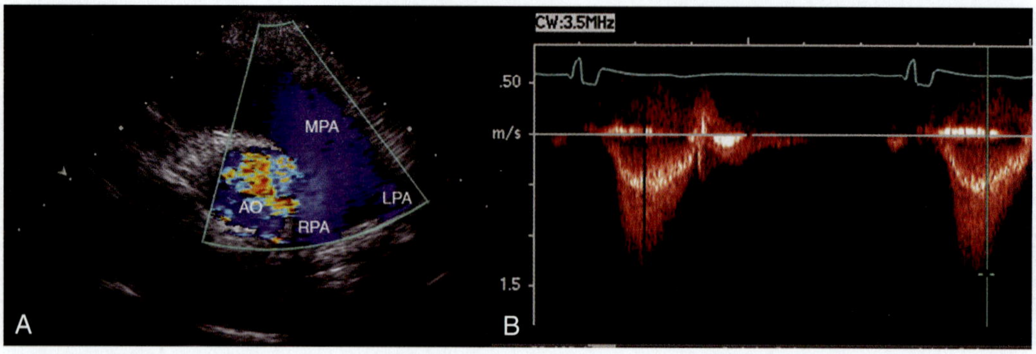

Figura 423-21. Valutazione con color-Doppler e Doppler pulsato del flusso in arteria polmonare. *A*, Valutazione color-Doppler di una proiezione parasternale asse corto che evidenzia un flusso normale attraverso la valvola polmonare fino all'arteria polmonare principale e alle sue diramazioni. Il flusso del color-Doppler è in blu, indicando che il flusso si allontana dal trasduttore (situato nella parte alta della figura, all'apice della finestra ecografica triangolare). Si tenga presente che il colore assegnato al segnale Doppler non indica la saturazione di ossigeno del sangue. Ao, aorta; LPA, arteria polmonare sinistra, MPA, tronco principale della polmonare; RPA, arteria polmonare destra. *B*, Pattern di flusso con Doppler a onda pulsata attraverso la valvola polmonare, che evidenzia una bassa velocità di flusso (<1,5 m/s), a indicare l'assenza di un gradiente di pressione attraverso la valvola. La rappresentazione grafica del segnale di flusso è al di sotto della linea, a indicare che il flusso si sta allontanando dal trasduttore.

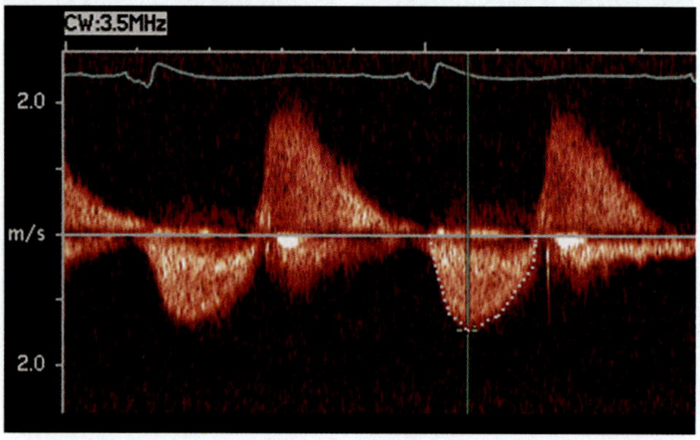

Figura 423-22. Valutazione Doppler di un paziente già sottoposto a correzione di una tetralogia di Fallot, che ha una lieve stenosi polmonare e un moderato rigurgito polmonare. Il tracciato evidenzia il flusso "va-e-vieni" attraverso la valvola polmonare con il segnale al di sotto della linea che rappresenta il flusso anterogrado in sistole (vedi il tracciato ECG come riferimento) e il segnale al di sopra della linea che rappresenta il rigurgito durante la diastole.

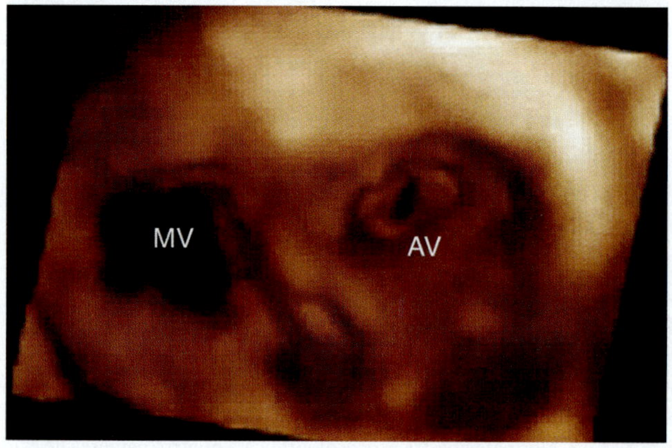

Figura 423-23. Ecocardiogramma 3-D che evidenzia una proiezione in asse corto del ventricolo sinistro. AV, valvola aortica; MV, valvola mitrale. (Per gentile concessione di Norman Silverman, Stanford University, Stanford, CA.)

ECOCARDIOGRAFIA TRANSESOFAGEA

L'ecocardiografia transesofagea è una tecnica di imaging estremamente sensibile che fornisce una visione più chiara di lesioni piccole come le vegetazioni dell'endocardite. È utile per visualizzare strutture a localizzazione posteriore, come gli atri, la radice aortica e le valvole atrioventricolari, oltre a rivelarsi preziosa come tecnica intraoperatoria per il monitoraggio della funzione cardiaca durante la chirurgia sia cardiaca sia non cardiaca e per lo screening di difetti cardiaci residui dopo bypass cardiopolmonare. Questa tecnica si è rivelata particolarmente utile nella valutazione del grado di rigurgito residuo dopo riparazione di difetti settali atrioventricolari e nella ricerca di piccole comunicazioni a livello della porzione muscolare che potrebbero essere sfuggite durante la chiusura di difetti più grandi.

ECOCARDIOGRAFIA FETALE

L'ecocardiografia fetale può essere utilizzata per valutare le strutture cardiache o le alterazioni del ritmo cardiaco (Fig. 423-24). I perinatologi spesso individuano anomalie macroscopiche nella struttura cardiaca all'ecografia ostetrica di routine o possono sottoporre all'esame il paziente a causa di un'idrope fetale non spiegata. Questa indagine è in grado di diagnosticare molte lesioni cardiache congenite fin dalla 17ª-19ª settimana di gestazione, per quanto la sua accuratezza in uno stadio così precoce sia ancora

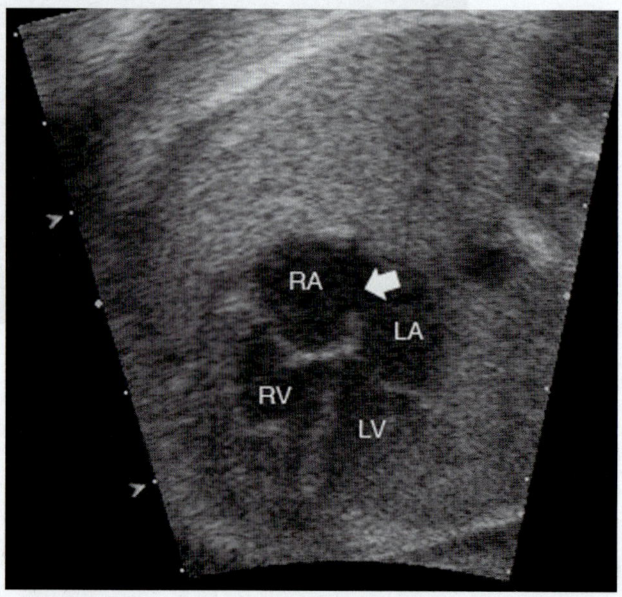

Figura 423-24. Normale visione ecocardiografica a quattro camere di un feto alla 20ª settimana di gestazione. Si può vedere il forame ovale (*freccia*) tra gli atri destro e sinistro. LA, atrio sinistro; LV, ventricolo sinistro; RA, atrio destro; RV, ventricolo destro.

limitata; i familiari dei pazienti dovrebbero quindi comprendere che questi studi non sono in grado di eliminare completamente la possibilità di presenza di una cardiopatia congenita; in compenso, possono evidenziare la progressione intrauterina di una lesione moderata (per es. stenosi aortica) in una più grave (per es. sindrome del cuore sinistro ipoplasico). L'ecocardiografia M-mode permette di diagnosticare disturbi del ritmo nel feto e di valutare l'efficacia di una terapia antiaritmica somministrata alla madre. Un ecocardiogramma fetale di screening è raccomandato per i pazienti con un precedente figlio o parente di primo grado affetto da cardiopatia congenita, per le donne che presentano un rischio aumentato di avere un figlio con una patologia cardiaca (diabetiche insulinodipendenti, gestanti che assumono farmaci teratogeni all'inizio della gravidanza) e per qualsiasi feto in cui si sospetti o sia confermata un'anomalia cromosomica.

423.5 • Test da sforzo

L'apparato cardiorespiratorio normale si adatta alle notevoli richieste legate all'attività fisica con un aumento considerevole del consumo di ossigeno e della gittata cardiaca. A causa dell'ampia capacità di riserva per lo sforzo, anomalie significative della prestazione cardiovascolare possono essere presenti in modo asintomatico a riposo o nel corso di attività comuni. Quando i pazienti vengono valutati a riposo, è possibile che non emergano significative anomalie nella funzione cardiaca o che comunque non ne vengano riconosciute le ripercussioni sulla qualità della vita. Spesso è sulla base di criteri puramente soggettivi che si permette ai bambini con patologia cardiovascolare di partecipare a vari tipi di attività fisica. Il test da sforzo gioca un ruolo importante nella valutazione dei sintomi e nella quantificazione della gravità delle anomalie cardiache, oltre a essere d'aiuto nella gestione clinica di questi pazienti, nella quale rientra anche la prescrizione di un programma razionale di attività fisica.

Nei bambini più grandi i test da sforzo vengono generalmente effettuati su un tapis-roulant graduato, con un aumento del livello di sforzo e della velocità a intervalli prestabiliti, mentre per i bambini piccoli ci si avvale di un cicloergometro. In molti laboratori è ora possibile misurare la gittata cardiaca e la funzione polmonare in modo non invasivo durante l'esercizio.

Con la crescita del bambino, la capacità di lavoro aumenta di pari passo con le dimensioni del corpo e della massa muscolare scheletrica. Non tutti gli indici di funzione cardiopolmonare aumentano in modo uniforme. Una risposta importante sotto sforzo è l'aumento della gittata cardiaca, che viene ottenuto principalmente attraverso un aumento della frequenza cardiaca, ma anche della gittata sistolica, del ritorno venoso sistemico e della pressione differenziale. La resistenza vascolare sistemica subisce una notevole diminuzione dal momento che i vasi sanguigni nei muscoli sotto sforzo si dilatano per far fronte alle maggiori richieste metaboliche. Via via che il bambino cresce in età e corporatura, la risposta della frequenza cardiaca all'esercizio rimane importante, ma la gittata cardiaca aumenta, perché aumentano la capacità volumetrica del cuore e, di conseguenza, la gittata sistolica. Le risposte allo sforzo dinamico non dipendono solo dall'età. Per ogni dato valore di superficie corporea, i maschi hanno una gittata sistolica maggiore delle femmine di pari dimensioni. Questo incremento è modificato anche dalla postura. L'aumento della gittata sistolica con lo sforzo dinamico in posizione eretta è facilitato dall'azione di pompa dei muscoli coinvolti, che vincono gli effetti statici della gravità e aumentano il ritorno venoso sistemico.

Il test da sforzo dinamico permette di valutare non solo la resistenza e la capacità d'esercizio, ma anche l'effetto di tale esercizio sul flusso sanguigno miocardico e sul ritmo cardiaco. Un significativo slivellamento del tratto ST rispecchia anomalie della perfusione miocardica, per esempio l'ischemia subendocardica che si verifica comunemente sotto sforzo in bambini con ventricolo sinistro ipertrofico. **L'ECG da sforzo** è considerato anormale se lo slivellamento del tratto ST è >2 mm e perdura per almeno 0,06 s dopo il punto J (inizio del segmento ST) in combinazione con un tratto ST orizzontale, ascendente o discendente. La provocazione dei disturbi del ritmo durante un test da sforzo è un importante metodo di valutazione di pazienti selezionati con patologie del ritmo note o sospette. In questo modo è possibile valutare anche gli effetti delle terapie farmacologiche.

423.6 • RM, MRA, TC e studi con radionuclidi

La **risonanza magnetica** (RM) e l'**angiografia con risonanza magnetica** (**MRA**, *Magnetic Resonance Angiography*) sono utilissime nella diagnosi e nella gestione dei pazienti con cardiopatie congenite. Queste tecniche producono immagini tomografiche del cuore in ogni proiezione (Fig. 423-25) con un'ottima risoluzione di contrasto di tessuto adiposo, miocardio e polmonare, oltre che del movimento del sangue rispetto alle pareti dei vasi sanguigni. La RM si è rivelata particolarmente utile nella valutazione di aree che vengono visualizzate in modo ottimale con l'ecocardiografia, come l'anatomia delle diramazioni distali dell'arteria polmonare e le anomalie del ritorno venoso sistemico e polmonare.

La MRA permette l'acquisizione di immagini in numerosi piani tomografici. In ogni piano, le immagini vengono ottenute durante le diverse fasi del ciclo cardiaco; perciò, quando vengono proiettate in formato "cinematografico" dinamico, è possibile evidenziare e analizzare alterazioni dello spessore parietale, del volume delle camere e della funzione valvolare. Possono essere calcolati la velocità e il volume del flusso sanguigno. La MRA è una tecnica eccellente per il follow-up dopo riparazione di cardiopatie congenite complesse, come la tetralogia di Fallot; in questi pazienti essa permette di valutare sia il volume e la massa del ventricolo destro, sia la quantità di rigurgito attraverso la valvola polmonare o tricuspide. La **spettroscopia RM** (**MRS**, *Magnetic Resonance Spectroscopy*), che allo stato attuale è principalmente uno stru-

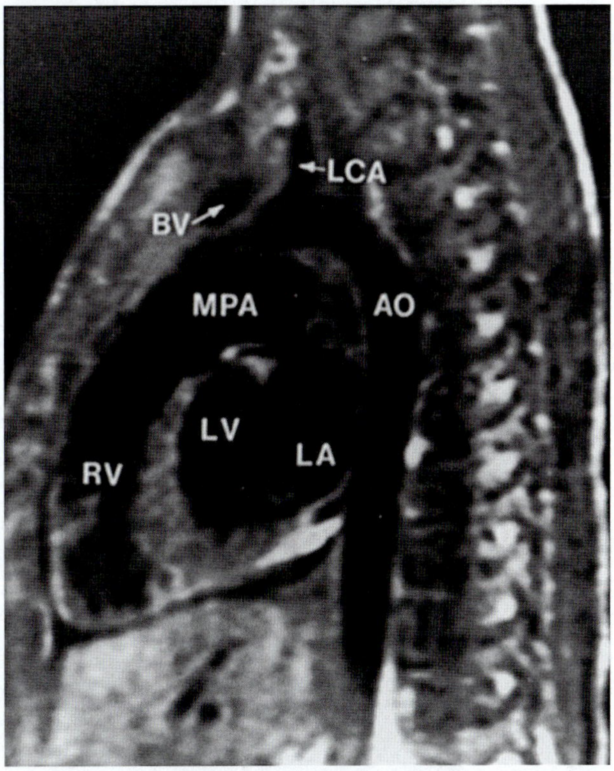

Figura 423-25. RMN normale in proiezione sagittale. Ao, aorta, BV (*Brachiocephalic Vein*), vena brachiocefalica; LA, atrio sinistro; LCA, arteria coronaria sinistra; MPA; tronco principale dell'arteria polmonare; RV, ventricolo destro. (Da Bisset GS III: Cardiac and great vessel anatomy. In El-Khoury GY, Bergman RA, Montgomery WJ [editors]: *Sectional Anatomy by MRI/CT*. New York, Churchill Livingstone, 1990.)

mento utilizzato nella ricerca, permette di dimostrare concentrazioni relative di metabolici ad alta energia (andenosin trifosfato, adenosin difosfato, fosfato inorganico e fosfocreatina) nelle varie regioni del miocardio.

L'**elaborazione computerizzata della MRA** consente una visualizzazione non invasiva dell'apparato cardiovascolare dall'interno del cuore o dei vasi, mediante la cosiddetta tecnica *fly-through*. Grazie a queste immagini il cardiologo può esplorare dall'interno varie strutture cardiovascolari (Fig. 423-26). Tale metodica si rivela particolarmente utile per la valutazione di complesse stenosi delle arterie periferiche, soprattutto dopo un tentativo di angioplastica a palloncino.

La **tomografia computerizzata a fascio di elettroni** (EBCT, *Electron Beam CT*) è utilizzata per ottenere immagini cardiache rapide e in sincrono con le fasi della respirazione in bambini con risoluzioni fino a 0,5 mm. La ricostruzione tridimensionale delle immagini EBCT (Fig. 423-27) è utile in particolar modo per valutare le ramificazioni delle arterie polmonari, le anomalie del ritorno venoso sistemico e polmonare, e le anomalie dei grossi vasi come la coartazione aortica.

L'**angiografia con radionuclidi** può essere utilizzata per evidenziare e quantificare gli shunt e per analizzare la distribuzione del flusso sanguigno a ogni polmone. Questa tecnica è particolarmente utile per quantificare la distribuzione del volume del flusso sanguino tra i due polmoni in pazienti con anomalie dell'albero vascolare polmonare o dopo un'operazione di shunt (Blalock-Taussig o Glenn), o per quantificare il successo di un'angioplastica con palloncino e di procedure di stenting intravascolare. L'angiografia all'equilibrio (*gated blood pool*) con radionuclidi può essere utilizzata per effettuare calcoli emodinamici, per quantificare il rigurgito valvolare e per evidenziare anomalie del movimento parietale regionale. Le immagini al tallio servono per valutare la perfusione del muscolo cardiaco. Questi metodi sono applicabili al letto di pazienti pediatrici gravemente malati e possono essere effettuati in serie, con minimo disagio e bassa esposizione alle radiazioni.

423.7 • Cateterismo cardiaco diagnostico e interventistico

Se l'ecocardiografia, la RMN e la TC sono ormai le tecniche standard per la diagnosi della maggior parte delle forme di cardiopatia congenita, il laboratorio di emodinamica è divenuto teatro di procedure interventistiche di alta tecnologia, che permettono una correzione minimamente invasiva o la palliazione di difetti cardiaci che un tempo richiedevano un intervento chirurgico a cuore aperto.

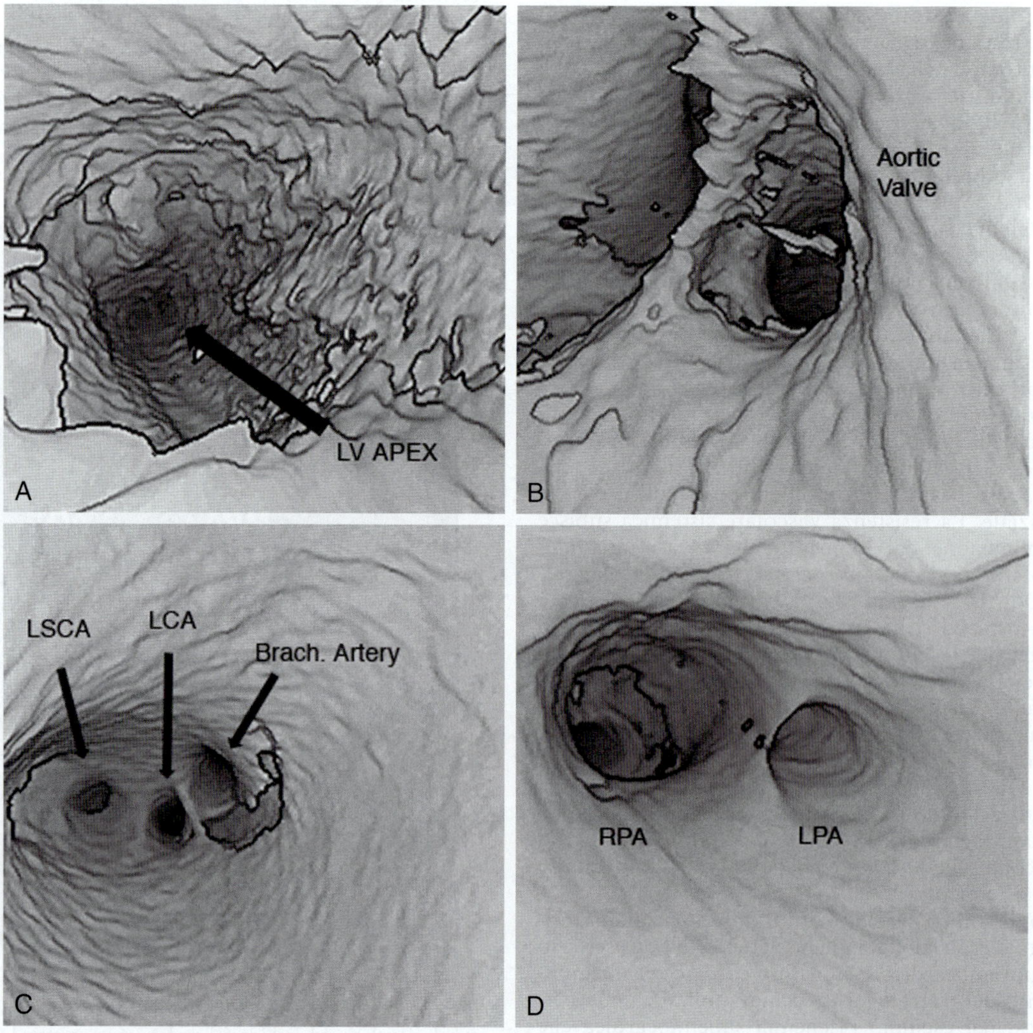

Figura 423-26. Immagine *fly-through* in un paziente con finestra aortopolmonare. Questa serie di immagini statiche evidenzia la progressione dalla camera del ventricolo sinistro (LV) (*A*), attraverso la valvola aortica (*B*) fino all'aorta ascendente (*C*), e poi attraverso il difetto fino alle diramazioni dell'arteria polmonare (*D*). Brach, arteria brachiocefalica; LCA, arteria carotide sinistra; LPA, arteria polmonare sinistra; LSCA, arteria succlavia sinistra; RPA, arteria polmonare destra; LV apex, apice del ventricolo sinistro; Aortic valve, valvola aortica.

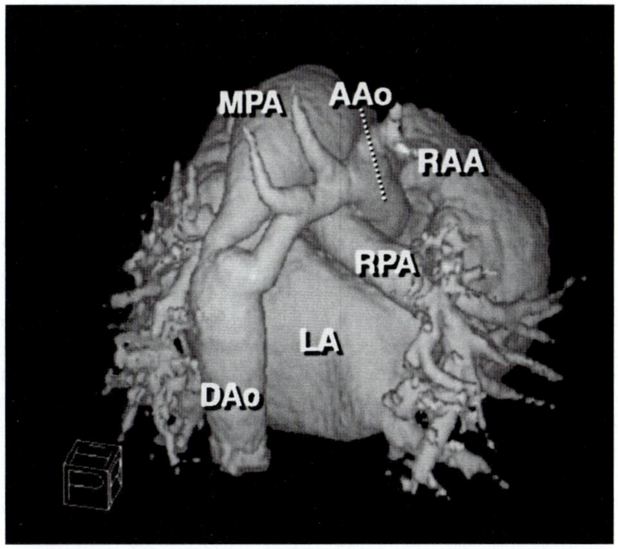

Figura 423-27. Ricostruzione tridimensionale di immagini TC con fascio di elettroni in un neonato con grave coartazione dell'aorta. Sulla sinistra è visibile il dotto arterioso pervio, che porta dal tronco principale dell'arteria polmonare all'aorta discendente. Il segmento coartato, tortuoso e ristretto, si trova immediatamente a destra rispetto al dotto. L'aorta traversa è anch'essa ipoplasica. AAo, aorta ascendente; LA, atrio sinistro; MPA, tronco principale dell'arteria polmonare; RAA (*Right Atrial Appendage*), appendice atriale destra; RPA, arteria polmonare destra. (Per gentile concessione di Paul Pitlick, Stanford University, Stanford, CA.)

CATETERISMO CARDIACO DIAGNOSTICO

Il cateterismo diagnostico viene ancora effettuato: (1) come ausilio nella diagnosi iniziale di alcune lesioni cardiache congenite complesse (tetralogia di Fallot con atresia della polmonare e importanti arterie collaterali aortopolmonari, atresia della polmonare con setto ventricolare intatto e sinusoidi coronarici); (2) in casi in cui altri studi di imaging non diano risultati chiari; (3) in pazienti per i quali la valutazione emodinamica è essenziale (per determinare le dimensioni di uno shunt sinistro-destro in casi borderline, o per determinare la presenza o l'assenza di una patologia vascolare polmonare in un paziente con shunt sinistro-destro); (4) tra gli stadi della riparazione di cardiopatie congenite complesse (sindrome del cuore sinistro ipoplasico); (5) per effettuare una biopsia miocardica nella diagnosi di miocardiopatia o nello screening del rigetto d'organo dopo trapianto cardiaco; (6) per studi elettrofisiologici nella valutazione delle aritmie cardiache (vedi Capitolo 435).

Il cateterismo cardiaco dovrebbe essere effettuato con il paziente quanto più possibile in condizione basale. La sedazione cosciente viene effettuata di routine; tuttavia, se si rende necessaria l'anestesia generale, occorre prestare attenzione nella scelta dell'agente anestetico per evitare di deprimere della funzione cardiovascolare e quindi alterare i parametri della gittata cardiaca, della resistenza vascolare polmonare e sistemica e dei rapporti di flusso negli shunt.

Il cateterismo cardiaco nei lattanti con cardiopatia congenita in condizioni critiche dovrebbe essere effettuato in un centro che disponga di un'équipe di chirurgia cardiovascolare pediatrica, nell'eventualità che si rendesse necessario un intervento chirurgico immediatamente dopo la procedura. Il tasso di complicanze del cateterismo cardiaco e dell'angiografia è molto elevato nei lattanti in condizioni critiche, che devono quindi essere studiati in un ambiente neutro dal punto di vista termico e trattati tempestivamente in caso di ipotermia, ipoglicemia, acidosi o emorragie massive.

Il cateterismo può essere limitato alle strutture del cuore destro o sinistro, oppure riguardare entrambi i lati del cuore. Il catetere viene introdotto nel cuore sotto guida fluoroscopica attraverso un punto d'ingresso percutaneo nella vena femorale o giugulare. Nei lattanti e in un certo numero di bambini più grandi, si può accedere al cuore sinistro inserendo il catetere attraverso un forame ovale pervio fino all'atrio sinistro e al ventricolo sinistro. Se il forame è chiuso, il cuore sinistro può essere raggiunto facendo passare il catetere per via retrograda attraverso un punto d'ingresso percutaneo in arteria femorale. Il catetere viene guidato attraverso i difetti intracardiaci (ASD, VSD). Si prelevano campioni di sangue per misurare la saturazione d'ossigeno e calcolare il volume degli shunt, si misurano le pressioni per calcolare i gradienti e le aree valvolari, e si inietta un mezzo di contrasto radio-opaco per delineare le struttura cardiache e vascolari. Ci si può avvalere di un catetere con sensore termico sulla punta per misurare la gittata cardiaca con il metodo della termodiluizione. Per misurare indici di funzione cardiaca più sofisticati possono essere indicati cateteri appositi: quelli con punte dotate di trasduttori di pressione servono per misurare la prima derivata della pressione ventricolare sinistra (dP/dt), mentre i cateteri di conduttanza sono utili per produrre loop pressione-volume, da cui si ricaveranno indici sia di contrattilità (elastanza telesistolica) sia di lusitropia (rilassamento). È possibile calcolare tutti i parametri emodinamici (Tab. 423-1), compresi la gittata cardiaca, gli

TABELLA 423-1. Valori normali e formule per la determinazione dei parametri emodinamici nel cateterismo cardiaco

1. Indice cardiaco: 3,0-5,0 L/min
2. Differenza arterovenosa d'ossigeno: 4,5 ± 0,7 mL/dL
3. Consumo d'ossigeno: 140-160 mL/m^2/min
4. Saturazione arteriosa d'ossigeno: 94-100%
5. Resistenza arteriolare polmonare: 50-150 dyn s cm^{-5} (1 U = 80 dyn)
6. Gittata cardiaca (Qs) mL/min = flusso sistemico =

$$\frac{\text{assunzione di } O_2 \text{ (mL/min)}}{\left\{\begin{array}{l}\text{contenuto in } O_2 \text{ del sangue arterioso (mL/dL)}\\ \text{meno contenuto in } O_2 \text{ del sangue venoso misto (mL/dL)}\end{array}\right.} \times 100$$

7. Indice cardiaco: gittata cardiaca (L/min)/m^2 di superficie corporea
8. Flusso in arteria polmonare (Qp) =

$$\frac{\text{assunzione di } O_2 \text{ (mL/min)}}{\left\{\begin{array}{l}\text{contenuto in } O_2 \text{ del sangue venoso polmonare (mL/dL)}\\ \text{meno contenuto in } O_2 \text{ del sangue arterioso polmonare (mL/dL)}\end{array}\right.} \times 100$$

Se non è disponibile un campione venoso polmonare, si presuppone che la saturazione sia al 95% della capacità

9. Flusso effettivo in arteria polmonare (Qep) =

$$\frac{\text{assunzione di } O_2 \text{ (mL/min)}}{\left\{\begin{array}{l}\text{contenuto in } O_2 \text{ del sangue venoso polmonare (100 mL/dL)}\\ \text{meno contenuto in } O_2 \text{ nel sangue venoso misto (100 mL/dL)}\end{array}\right.} \times 100$$

10. Shunt totale sinistro-destro: flusso in arteria polmonare meno flusso effettivo in arteria polmonare
11. Shunt totale destro-sinistro: flusso sistemico meno flusso effettivo in arteria polmonare
12. Resistenza arteriolare polmonare: $Rp = \frac{PA - PC}{Qp}$

dove R = resistenza arteriolare polmonare (unità di resistenza)
PA = pressione media in arteria polmonare in mmHg
PC = pressione media "capillare" polmonare in mmHg
Qp = flusso polmonare in L/min/m^2

shunt intracardiaci sinistro-destro e destro-sinistro e le resistenze vascolari sistemiche e polmonari. I normali parametri emodinamici sono illustrati nella Figura 423-28.

MISURAZIONE DELLA GITTATA CARDIACA CON IL METODO DELLA TERMODILUIZIONE

Il metodo della termodiluizione per la misurazione della gittata cardiaca prevede l'impiego di un catetere a flusso diretto, con una punta termosensibile, introdotto in arteria polmonare (catetere di Swan-Ganz). Viene provocata una nota modificazione della temperatura del sangue in un determinato punto del circolo (di solito nell'atrio destro o nella vena cava inferiore) e il risultante cambiamento di temperatura viene misurato in un punto a valle (di solito in arteria polmonare). La sostanza che viene iniettata è generalmente soluzione fisiologica a temperatura ambiente. Questo metodo viene utilizzato per misurare la gittata cardiaca nel laboratorio di emodinamica in pazienti senza shunt. Il monitoraggio della gittata cardiaca mediante termodiluizione può essere utile anche per la gestione di lattanti gravemente malati e di bambini ricoverati in terapia intensiva dopo intervento cardiochirurgico, o in presenza di shock. In questo caso, ci si avvale di un catetere a triplo lume per determinare la gittata cardiaca e misurare sia la pressione in arteria polmonare, sia la pressione di incuneamento capillare polmonare.

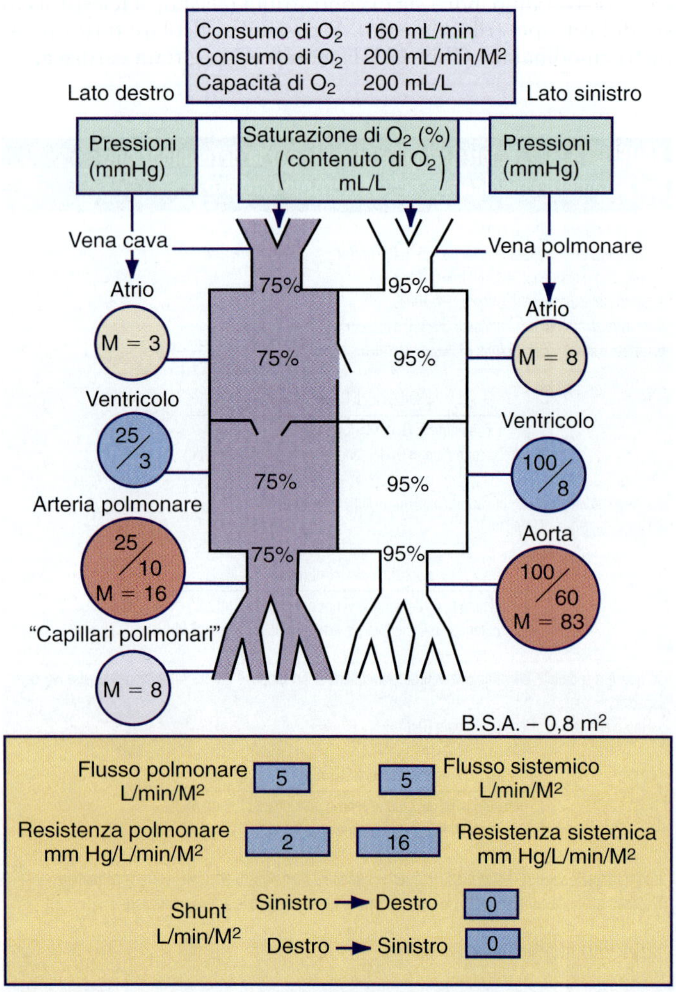

Figura 423-28. Diagramma dei normali parametri emodinamici con valori di pressione, contenuto in ossigeno e percentuali di saturazione. BSA (*Body Surface Area*), superficie corporea. (Modificata da Nadas AS, Fyler DC: *Pediatric Cardiology*, 3rd ed. Philadelphia, WB Saunders, 1972.)

ANGIOCARDIOGRAFIA

I principali vasi sanguigni e le singole camere cardiache possono essere visualizzati mediante angiocardiografia selettiva, o con l'iniezione di mezzo di contrasto nelle sedi specifiche. Questo metodo permette di identificare anomalie strutturali senza che le ombre sovrapposte di camere normali provochino interferenze. Per visualizzare il catetere mentre passa attraverso le varie camere cardiache ci si avvale della fluoroscopia. Una volta posizionato il catetere cardiaco nella camera da studiare, si inietta una piccola quantità di mezzo di contrasto con un iniettore a pressione e si acquisiscono cineangiogrammi con una frequenza che varia dalle 15 alle 60 immagini/s. La cineangiocardiografia biplanare permette la valutazione dettagliata di specifiche camere cardiache e dei vasi sanguigni in due piani simultaneamente previa iniezione di un unico bolo di mezzo di contrasto. Questa tecnica, che ormai è considerata lo standard nei laboratori di emodinamica cardiaca pediatrica, permette di ridurre al minimo il volume di mezzo di contrasto utilizzato e i relativi rischi. Ci si avvale di diversi angoli di visualizzazione (angolazione obliqua anteriore sinistra, craniale) per evidenziare nel modo migliore specifiche caratteristiche anatomiche delle singole lesioni. L'imaging digitale ha sostituito la radiografia standard per scopi sia diagnostici sia di archiviazione.

La rapida immissione in circolo di un mezzo di contrasto sotto pressione non è esente da rischi e ogni iniezione dovrebbe essere accuratamente programmata. Il mezzo di contrasto è costituito da soluzioni ipertoniche, alcune contenenti composti organici iodati che possono provocare complicanze come nausea, sensazione generalizzata di bruciore, sintomi a carico del sistema nervoso centrale, insufficienza renale e reazioni allergiche. In genere si evita l'iniezione intramiocardica, mediante il posizionamento accurato del catetere prima dell'iniezione. L'ipertonicità del mezzo di contrasto può provocare una transitoria depressione miocardica e un brusco calo della pressione sanguigna, presto seguiti da tachicardia, aumento della gittata cardiaca e richiamo di liquido interstiziale nella circolazione; quest'ultimo fenomeno può determinare un aggravamento transitorio dei sintomi di insufficienza cardiaca in pazienti critici.

CATETERISMO CARDIACO INTERVENTISTICO

Grazie alla miniaturizzazione dei sistemi di introduzione dei cateteri, molte di queste tecniche di cateterismo interventistico vengono oggi utilizzate senza rischi anche nel neonato e nel prematuro. Il trattamento mediante cateterismo è ormai la procedura standard per la maggior parte dei casi di stenosi isolate a carico delle valvole polmonari o aortiche (vedi Fig. 427-4) come anche per la recidiva di coartazione aortica. Uno speciale catetere con un palloncino a forma di salsiccia posizionato all'estremità distale viene fatto passare attraverso la valvola sede di ostruzione. Il rapido riempimento del palloncino con una miscela di mezzo di contrasto e soluzione fisiologica provoca la lacerazione del tessuto valvolare stenotico, di solito in corrispondenza del sito del rafe inappropriatamente fuso. La stenosi valvolare polmonare può essere trattata con successo mediante angioplastica a palloncino, la quale in molti pazienti viene utilizzata al posto della riparazione chirurgica come procedura di scelta iniziale. I risultati clinici di questa procedura sono simili a quelli ottenibili con la chirurgia a cuore aperto, ma senza la necessità di una sternotomia o di un'ospedalizzazione prolungata. La valvuloplastica a palloncino ha dato risultati eccellenti anche nella stenosi aortica; tuttavia quest'ultima spesso recidiva (come peraltro avviene con la chirurgia) quando il bambino cresce e perciò possono rendersi necessari vari interventi. Una complicanza sia della valvuloplastica sia dell'intervento chirurgico è la creazione di un'insufficienza valvolare. Questa complicanza presenta implicazioni più serie quando si verifica sul versante aortico della circolazione, anziché su quello polmonare, poiché il rigurgito è meno tollerato a livello delle pressioni arteriose sistemiche. L'angioplastica a palloncino è la procedura di scelta per pazienti con restenosi di coartazione aortica dopo un primo intervento chirurgico. È controverso se l'angioplastica sia la migliore procedura per la coartazione aortica nativa (non operata), poiché è stata riportata la successiva formazione di aneurismi. Altre applicazioni della tecnica comprendono il miglioramento della stenosi mitralica, la dilatazione dei condotti chirurgici (switch atriali di Mustard o Senning), la riduzione di restringimenti di diramazioni dell'arteria polmonare, la dilatazione di ostruzioni venose e la settostomia atriale a palloncino (procedura di Rashkind), da tempo utilizzata per la trasposizione delle grandi arterie (vedi Capitolo 431.2).

Le tecniche di cateterismo interventistico sono in via di adattamento in previsione di un loro utilizzo nel **feto** con lesioni come la stenosi aortica, nel tentativo di prevenirne la trasformazione in lesioni più complesse come la sindrome del cuore sinistro ipoplasico. In queste procedure, previa somministrazione di un'anestesia appropriata, viene introdotto un ago attraverso la parete addominale materna, la parete uterina e la parete toracica del feto, per raggiungere direttamente il ventricolo sinistro fetale (vedi Fig. 431-13). Viene fatto passare attraverso l'ago, e attraverso la valvola aortica stenotica, un catetere coronarico per angioplastica con palloncino, che viene poi dilatato. Una volta ristabilito un normale flusso sanguigno nel ventricolo sinistro, si spera che anche il normale potenziale di crescita del ventricolo sinistro venga ripristinato. I primi risultati ottenuti con questa tecnica in un numero limitato di pazienti sono incoraggianti.

In pazienti con stenosi di diramazioni dell'arteria polmonare, i precedenti risultati misti con l'angioplastica a palloncino sono stati migliorati grazie all'utilizzo di **stent intravascolari** (Fig. 423-29), introdotti su catetere a palloncino ed espansi all'interno del lume del vaso. Una volta posizionati, spesso possono dilatarsi fino a raggiungere dimensioni via via maggiori a mano a mano che il paziente cresce. Il posizionamento di stent in lattanti e bambini più grandi rimane problematico a causa della successiva crescita. Gli stent vengono utilizzati anche negli adolescenti e nei giovani adulti con coartazione aortica.

La chiusura di un dotto arterioso pervio di piccole dimensioni viene ora ottenuta di routine con spirali condotte in sede da un catetere (vedi Fig. 426-11), mentre un dotto arterioso più ampio può essere chiuso con una varietà di dispositivi "a sandwich". Le spirali consentono inoltre la chiusura di collegamenti vascolari anomali (fistole coronariche, collaterali veno-venosi in lesioni cardiache cianotiche). Il difetto atriale tipo "ostium secundum" (ASD) viene ora chiuso di routine con uno dei tanti dispositivi occlusivi a doppio disco attualmente disponibili (vedi Fig. 426-3); alcune versioni di questi dispositivi sono attualmente oggetto di trial clinici per la chiusura di VSD muscolari difficili da raggiungere chirurgicamente, oltre che per i più comuni VSD perimembranosi. I dispositivi collegati a catetere possono essere utilizzati anche in aggiunta a procedure di riparazione chirurgica complesse (dilatazione o stenting di diramazioni dell'arteria polmonare o stenosi delle vene polmonari o chiusura di un VSD muscolare in associazione a lesioni ostruttive del cuore sinistro). I pazienti ad alto rischio sottoposti a intervento di Fontan (vedi Capitolo 430.4) spesso presentano una piccola fenestrazione, creatasi tra la parte destra e quella sinistra della circolazione, che funge da "valvola di sfogo" per l'elevata pressione nella parte destra all'inizio dell'intervento chirurgico. I pazienti con queste "fenestrazioni di Fontan" sono i candidati ideali per la successiva chiusura con un dispositivo guidato da catetere.

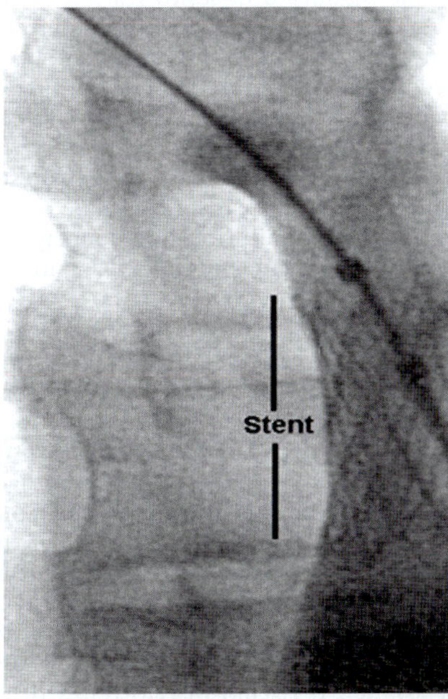

Figura 423-29. Stent intravascolare posizionato nell'aorta discendente per il trattamento di una coartazione aortica recidivante.

Elettrocardiogramma

Garson A: *The Electrocardiogram in Infants and Children: A Systematic Approach*. Philadelphia, Lea & Febiger, 1983.

Lipman BF, Massey EF: *Clinical Scalar Electrocardiography.* Chicago, Year Book, 1984.

Marriott H: *Rhythm Quizlets: Self Assessment.* Philadelphia, Lea & Febiger, 1987.

Schwartz PJ, Moss AJ, Vincent GM, et al: Diagnostic criteria for the long QT syndrome: An update. *Circulation* 1993;88:782–784.

Ecocardiografia

Alagarsamy S, Chhabra M, Gudavalli M, et al: Comparison of clinical criteria with echocardiographic findings in diagnosing PDA in preterm infants. *J Perinat Med* 2005;33:161–164.

Frommelt MA, Frommelt PC: Advances in echocardiographic diagnostic modalities for the pediatrician. *Pediatr Clin North Am* 1999;46:427–439.

Sahn DJ, Vick GW III: Review of new techniques in echocardiography and magnetic resonance imaging as applied to patients with congenital heart disease. *Heart* 2001;86(Suppl 2):II41–II53.

Stevenson JG: Role of intraoperative transesophageal echocardiography during repair of congenital cardiac defects. *Acta Paediatr Suppl* 1995;410:23–33.

Sullivan ID: Prenatal diagnosis of structural heart disease: Does it make a difference to survival? *Heart* 2002;87:405–406.

Todros T: Prenatal diagnosis and management of fetal cardiovascular malformations. *Curr Opin Obstet Gynecol* 2000;12:105–109.

Van Der Velde ME, Perry SB: Transesophageal echocardiography during interventional catheterization in congenital heart disease. *Echocardiography* 1997;14:513–528.

Test da sforzo

Braden DS, Strong WF: Cardiovascular responses to exercise in childhood. *Am J Dis Child* 1990;144:1255–1260.

James FW, Blomqvist CG, Freed MD, et al: Standards for exercise testing in the pediatric age group: American Heart Association Council on Cardiovascular Disease in the Young. Ad hoc committee on exercise testing. *Circulation* 1982;66:1377A–1397A.

Nixon PA, Joswiak ML, Fricker FJ: A six-minute walk test for assessing exercise tolerance in severely ill children. *J Pediatr* 1996;129:362–366.

Washington RL, van Gundy JC, Cohen C, et al: Normal aerobic and anaerobic exercise data for North American school-age children. J Pediatr 1988;112:223–233.

RM, MRA, TC e studi con radionuclidi

Nienaber CA, Rehders TC, Fratz S: Detection and assessment of congenital heart disease with magnetic resonance techniques. *J Cardiovasc Magn Reson* 1999;1:169–184.

Strife JL, Sze RW: Radiographic evaluation of the neonate with congenital heart disease. *Radiol Clin North Am* 1999;37:1093–1107.

Wolfson BJ: Radiologic interpretation of congenital heart disease. *Clin Perinatol* 2001;28:71–89.

Cateterismo cardiaco diagnostico e interventistico

Andrews RE, Tulloh RMR: Interventional cardiac catheterization in congenital heart disease. *Arch Dis Child* 2004;89:1168–1173.

Giardini A, Moore P, Brook M, et al: Effect of transcatheter atrial septal defect closure in children on left ventricular diastolic function. *Am J Cardiol* 2005;95:1255–1257.
Holzer R, Balzer D, Cao QL, et al: Device closure of muscular ventricular septal defects using the Amplatzer muscular ventricular septal defect occluder: Immediate and mid-term results of a U.S. registry. *J Am Coll Cardiol* 2004;43:1257–1263.
Knauth AL, Lock JE, Perry SB, et al: Transcatheter device closure of congenital and postoperative residual ventricular septal defects. *Circulation* 2004;110:501–507.
Kreutzer J: Transcatheter intervention in the neonate with congenital heart disease. *Clin Perinatol* 2001;28:137–157.
Masura J, Gavora P, Podnar T: Long-term outcome of transcatheter secundum-type atrial septal defect closure using Amplatzer septal occluders. *J Am Coll Cardiol* 2005;45:505–507.
Simpson JM, Moore P, Teitel DF: Cardiac catheterization of low birth weight infants. *Am J Cardiol* 2001;87:1372–1377.
Tworetzky W, Marshall AC: Fetal interventions for cardiac defects. *Pediatr Clin North Am* 2004;51:1503–1513.
Walsh KP: Interventional paediatric cardiology. *Br Med J* 2003;327:385–388.
Yew G, Wilson NJ: Transcatheter atrial septal defect closure with the Amplatzer septal occluder: Five-year follow-up. *Catheter Cardiovasc Interv* 2005;64:193–196.

Sezione 3 — Cardiopatie congenite — Daniel Bernstein

Capitolo 424 ■ Epidemiologia e basi genetiche delle cardiopatie congenite

PREVALENZA. Le cardiopatie congenite si osservano nello 0,5-0,8% dei nati vivi. L'incidenza è più elevata nei nati morti (3-4%), negli aborti spontanei (10-25%) e nei prematuri (circa il 2%, escludendo i pazienti con dotto arterioso pervio [PDA, *Patent Ductus Arteriosus*]). In questa incidenza globale non rientrano il prolasso della valvola mitrale, il PDA dei prematuri e la valvola aortica bicuspide (presente nell'1-2% degli adulti). I difetti cardiaci congeniti presentano un ampio spettro di gravità nei bambini: circa 2-3 lattanti su 1000 presenteranno sintomi di cardiopatia nel primo anno di vita. La diagnosi viene posta entro la prima settimana di vita nel 40-50% dei pazienti con cardiopatia congenita, ed entro il primo mese di vita nel 50-60%. Grazie ai progressi della chirurgia palliativa e correttiva, il numero di bambini con cardiopatia congenita che sopravvivono fino all'età adulta è aumentato in modo significativo; ciononostante, le cardiopatie congenite rimangono la causa principale di morte nei bambini con malformazioni congenite. La Tabella 424-1 riassume la frequenza relativa delle lesioni cardiache congenite più comuni.

La maggior parte dei difetti congeniti è ben tollerata nel feto a causa del funzionamento in parallelo della circolazione fetale. Anche i difetti cardiaci più gravi (sindrome del cuore sinistro ipoplasico) di solito sono ben compensati dalla circolazione fetale. In questo esempio, l'intera gittata cardiaca fetale verrebbe espulsa del ventricolo destro attraverso il dotto arterioso sia nell'aorta discendente sia in quella ascendente (quest'ultima con riempimento per via retrograda). Solo dopo la nascita, quando le vie fetali (dotto arterioso e forame ovale) si chiudono, si rende pienamente evidente l'impatto emodinamico dell'anomalia anatomica. Un'eccezione degna di nota è il caso delle gravi lesioni da rigurgito, per lo più a carico della valvola tricuspide. In queste lesioni (anomalia di Ebstein [vedi Capitolo 430.7]), la circolazione fetale in parallelo non è in grado di compensare il sovraccarico di volume imposto al cuore destro. Possono verificarsi uno scompenso cardiaco in utero, spesso con versamento pleurico e pericardico, e ascite generalizzata (idrope fetale non immune).

La circolazione, pur subendo i cambiamenti più significativi nell'immediato periodo prenatale, anche dopo la nascita continua ad andare incontro a modificazioni, che possono a loro volta avere un impatto emodinamico sulle lesioni cardiache e sulla loro incidenza apparente. Nelle prime settimane di vita, durante le quali la resistenza vascolare polmonare subisce un brusco calo, lo shunt sinistro-destro attraverso difetti intracardiaci aumenta e i sintomi diventano più evidenti. Perciò, in pazienti con difetto del setto interventricolare (VSD, *Ventricular Septal Defect*), lo scompenso cardiaco si rende manifesto di solito tra il 1° e il 3° mese di vita (vedi Capitolo 426.6). La gravità di vari difetti può anche cambiare drammaticamente con la crescita: alcuni VSD possono divenire più piccoli e addirittura chiudersi. In alternativa, la stenosi della valvola aortica o della valvola polmonare, che può essere lieve nel periodo neonatale, può peggiorare se la crescita dell'orifizio valvolare non va di pari passo con la crescita del paziente (vedi Capitolo 427-5). Il medico dovrebbe sempre prestare attenzione alla presenza di malformazioni congenite associate, che possono influire negativamente sulla prognosi del paziente (vedi Tab. 422-2).

TABELLA 424-1. Frequenza relativa delle principali cardiopatie congenite*

LESIONE	% DI TUTTE LE LESIONI
Difetto del setto interventricolare	35-30
Difetto del setto interatriale (tipo ostium secundum)	6-8
Dotto arterioso pervio	6-8
Coartazione aortica	5-7
Tetralogia di Fallot	5-7
Stenosi della valvola polmonare	5-7
Stenosi della valvola aortica	4-7
d-Trasposizione delle grandi arterie	3-5
Ventricolo sinistro ipoplasico	1-3
Ventricolo destro ipoplasico	1-3
Tronco arterioso	1-2
Ritorno venoso polmonare anomalo totale	1-2
Atresia della tricuspide	1-2
Ventricolo unico	1-2
Ventricolo destro a doppia uscita	1-2
Altre	5-10

*Esclusi il dotto arterioso pervio nei neonati pretermine, la valvola aortica bicuspide, la stenosi polmonare periferica e il prolasso della valvola mitrale.

EZIOLOGIA. La causa della maggior parte delle cardiopatie congenite è sconosciuta. In passato si riteneva che nella maggior parte dei casi le cardiopatie congenite fossero multifattoriali e risultassero dalla combinazione di una predisposizione genetica e di uno stimolo ambientale. Una piccola percentuale di lesioni cardiache congenite è correlata ad anomalie cromosomiche, in particolare trisomia 21, trisomia 13, trisomia 18 e sindrome di Turner; una cardiopatia si riscontra in più del 90% dei pazienti con trisomia 18, nel 50% dei pazienti con trisomia 21 e nel 40% di quelli con sindrome di Turner. Altri fattori genetici possono avere un ruolo nelle cardiopatie congenite; certi tipi di VSD (sopracristali) sono più comuni nei bambini asiatici. Il rischio di ricorrenza di una cardiopatia congenita aumenta se ne è affetto un parente di primo grado (genitore o fratello/sorella).

TABELLA 424-2. Genetica delle cardiopatie congenite

PATOLOGIA CARDIOVASCOLARE	LOCALIZZAZIONE CROMOSOMICA	GENE*
	Difetti cardiaci strutturali	
CATCH 22 (sindrome di DiGeorge, sindrome velocardiofaciale)	22q11.2	Tbx1
	11p13p14	Non noto
ASD familiare con blocco cardiaco	5q35	Nkx2.5
ASD familiare senza blocco cardiaco	8p22-23	GATA4
Sindrome di Alagille (ipoplasia dei dotti biliari, lesioni del cuore destro)	20p12	Jagged1
Sindrome di Holt-Oram (difetti degli arti, ASD)	12q2	TBX5
Trisomia 21 (difetto del setto AV)	21q22	Non noto
Difetto del setto AV isolato familiare (senza trisomia 21)	1p31-p21	Non noto
	3p25	CRELD1
TAPVR familiare	4p12-q12	Non noto
Sindrome di Noonan (stenosi polmonare, ASD, miocardiopatia ipertrofica)	12q24	PTPN11
Sindrome di Ellis-van Creveld (polidattilia, ASD)	4p16	EVC
Sindrome di Char (difetti craniofaciali e degli arti, PDA)	6p12-21.1	TFAP2B
Sindrome di Williams (stenosi aortica sopravalvolare, stenosi di una diramazione dell'arteria polmonare, ipercalcemia)	7q11	Elastina
Sindrome di Marfan (debolezza del tessuto connettivo, dilatazione della radice aortica)	15q21	Fibrillina
Anomalie di lato familiari (situs inversus, cardiopatie congenite complesse)	Xq24-2q7	ZIC3
	1q42	Non noto
	9p13-21	DNAI1
	Miocardiopatie	
Miocardiopatia ipertrofica	14q1	Catena pesante beta della miosina
	15q2	alfa-Tropomiosina
	1q31	Troponina T
	19p13.2-19q13.2	Troponina I
	11p13-q13	Proteina C legante la miosina
	12q23	Catena leggera regolatoria della miosina lenta cardiaca
	13p21	Catena leggera essenziale della miosina lenta ventricolare
	2q31	Titina
Miocardiopatia ipertrofica con sindrome di Wolf-Parkinson-White	7q3	Non noto
Miocardiopatia dilatativa	Xp21	Distrofina
Legata all'X	Xp28	G4.5
Autosomica recessiva	19p13.2-19q13.2	Troponina I
Autosomica dominante: sono stati identificati geni che codificano più proteine, comprese l'actina cardiaca, la desmina, il δ-sarcoglicano, la catena pesante della β-miosina, la troponina C e T cardiaca, l'α-tropomiosina, la titina, la metavinculina, la proteina C legante la miosina, la proteina muscolare LIM, l'α-actinina-2, il fosfolambano, il dominio 3 legante Cypher/Lim, la catena pesante dell'α-miosina, SUR2A (subunità regolatoria del canale K_{ATP}), e la lamina A/C.		
	Aritmie	
Blocco cardiaco completo	19q13	Non noto
Sindrome del QT lungo		
LQT1 (autosomica dominante)	11p15.5	KVLQT1 (canale del K^+)
LQT2 (autosomica dominante)	7q35	HERG (canale del K^+)
LQT3 (autosomica dominante)	3p21	SCN5A (canale del Na^+)
LQT4 (autosomica dominante)	4q25-27	Non noto
LQT5 (autosomica dominante)	21q22-q22	KCNE1 (canale del K^+)
LQT6	21q22.1	KCNE2 (canale del K^+)
Sindrome di Jervell e Lange-Nielsen (autosomica recessiva, sordità congenita)	11p15.5	KVLQT1 (canale del K^+)
Displasia aritmogena del ventricolo destro		
ARVD1	14q24.3	TGF-β3
ARVD2	1q42-q43	RyR2 (recettore della rianodina)
ARVD3	14q	Non noto
ARVD4	2q32.1-q32.3	Non noto
ARVD5	3p22-p25	SCN51 (canale del sodio)
ARVD8	6p24	Desmoplachina
Fibrillazione atriale familiare (autosomica dominante)	10q22-q24	Non noto
	11p15.5	KVLQT1 (canale del K^+)
	6q14-16	Non noto
Sindrome di Brugada (sindrome familiare delle morti notturne inspiegate)	3p21-p24	SCN5A

*In molti casi una mutazione di un singolo gene è stata strettamente correlata a una specifica patologia cardiovascolare, per esempio in seguito alla scoperta di un'elevata incidenza di mutazioni o delezioni di quel gene in un gruppo numeroso di pazienti. Questi reperti sono spesso confermati da studi nel topo, in cui la delezione o l'alterazione del gene induce un fenotipo cardiaco simile a quello riscontrato nella patologia dell'uomo. In altri casi, la mutazione di un gene può aumentare il rischio di una malattia cardiovascolare, ma con diminuita penetranza, suggerendo che possano essere coinvolti geni modificatori o fattori ambientali. Infine, in alcuni casi, le mutazioni genetiche sono state identificate solo in un piccolo numero di alberi genealogici e si attende la conferma dallo screening di un più grande numero di pazienti.

AS (*Aortic Stenosis*), stenosi aortica; ASD (*Atrial Septal Defect*), difetto del setto interatriale; AV, atrioventricolare; PDA (*Patent Ductus Arteriosus*), dotto arterioso pervio; PS (*Pulmonic Stenosis*), stenosi polmonare; RV (*Right Ventricle*), ventricolo destro; TAPVR (*Total Anomalous Pulmonary Venous Return*), ritorno venoso polmonare anomalo totale.

L'elenco delle lesioni cardiache congenite associate a specifiche anomalie cromosomiche continua ad allungarsi, e parecchie di esse sono state addirittura attribuite a difetti genici specifici. L'analisi con tecnica FISH (*Fluorescence In Situ Hybridization*) permette ai medici un rapido screening dei casi sospetti, una volta che sia stata identificata una specifica anomalia cromosomica.

Una causa genetica di cardiopatia congenita ben caratterizzata è la delezione di un'ampia regione (1,5-3 Mb) del cromosoma

22q11.2, nota come **regione critica di DiGeorge.** Almeno 30 geni sono stati mappati sulla regione deleta; Tbx1, un fattore di trascrizione coinvolto nelle prime fasi dello sviluppo del tratto di efflusso, è ritenuto la causa della sindrome di DiGeorge. La prevalenza stimata delle delezioni 22q11.2 è di 1 su 4000 nati vivi. Le lesioni cardiache associate alle delezioni 22q11.2 sono osservabili per lo più in concomitanza con la sindrome di DiGeorge o la **sindrome di Shprintzen (velocardiofaciale)**. L'acronimo *CATCH 22* riassume le principali componenti di queste sindromi (*Cardiac defect, Abnormal facies, Thymic aplasia, Cleft palate, Hypocalcemia*, difetti cardiaci, anomalie faciali, aplasia del timo, palatoschisi e ipocalcemia). Le specifiche anomalie cardiache sono difetti conotroncali (tetralogia di Fallot, tronco arterioso, ventricolo destro a doppia uscita, VSD sottoarterioso) e difetti degli archi branchiali (coartazione aortica, arco aortico interrotto, arco aortico destro). Talvolta sono presenti anomalie congenite delle vie aeree, come la tracheomalacia e la broncomalacia. Il rischio di ricorrenza, che è estremamente basso in assenza di delezione 22q11.2 nei genitori, risulta pari al 50% se uno dei genitori è portatore della delezione. Più del 90% dei pazienti con sindrome di DiGeorge ha una microdelezione a livello di 22q11.2. È stato identificato anche un secondo locus genetico sul braccio corto del cromosoma 10 (10p13p14), la cui delezione ha in comune alcune ma non tutte le caratteristiche fenotipiche della delezione 22q11.2; i pazienti con del(10p) presentano un'aumentata incidenza di ipoacusia neurosensoriale.

Altre lesioni cardiache strutturali che sono state associate a specifiche anomalie cromosomiche comprendono il **difetto del setto interatriale tipo ostium secundum familiare**, accompagnato da **blocco cardiaco** (fattore di trascrizione NKX2.5 sul cromosoma 5q35), il difetto del setto interatriale familiare senza blocco cardiaco (fattore di trascrizione GATA4), la sindrome di Alagille (Jagged1 sul cromosoma 20p12) e la sindrome di Williams (elastina sul cromosoma 7q11). È interessante notare che pazienti con VSD e difetti del setto atrioventricolare (AVSD, *AtrioVentricular Septal Defect*) hanno mutazioni NKX2.5 multiple in cellule isolate dai tessuti cardiaci malati, ma non in quelle provenienti dai tessuti cardiaci normali o dai linfociti circolanti, riscontro che induce a ipotizzare un coinvolgimento delle mutazioni somatiche che portano a un mosaicismo nella patogenesi dei difetti cardiaci congeniti. Le cause genetiche note di cardiopatia congenita sono elencate nella Tabella 424-2.

Sono stati compiuti grandi passi avanti nell'identificazione dell'origine genetica delle malattie cardiovascolari nella **miocardiopatia ipertrofica.** Sono state implicate mutazioni in 10 geni, che codificano tutte per componenti proteici del sarcomero cardiaco, componenti delle fibre spesse o sottili o subunità regolatorie associate. Le più comuni sono le mutazioni del gene della catena pesante della β-miosina cardiaca (cromosoma 14q1) e del gene della proteina C che lega la miosina (cromosoma 11q11) (vedi Tabb. 424-2 e 439-2), mentre meno comuni sono quelle a carico dei geni delle troponine cardiache T e I, dell'α-tropomiosina, delle catene leggere della miosina, regolatorie ed essenziali, e della catena pesante dell'α-miosina. Sono state identificate circa 200 mutazioni nei 10 geni più comuni, e alcuni pazienti possono essere portatori di mutazioni in più di un gene.

Notevoli progressi sono stati compiuti anche nell'identificazione delle basi genetiche della **miocardiopatia dilatativa**, che è familiare nel 20-50% dei casi. L'ereditarietà autosomica dominante è quella di riscontro di più comune, e finora sono stati identificati 16 geni (vedi Tab. 424-2). L'ereditarietà legata all'X rende conto del 5-10% dei casi di miocardiopatia dilatativa familiare. In questo gruppo le mutazioni più comuni sono quelle nel gene della distrofina (cromosoma Xp21). Mutazioni nel gene codificante TAZ (tafazzina) sono associate alla sindrome di Barth e ad alcuni casi di non compattazione isolata del ventricolo sinistro. L'ereditarietà autosomica recessiva è stata associata a una mutazione della troponina I cardiaca. Le miopatie mitocondriali possono essere dovute a mutazioni degli enzimi della catena di trasporto degli elettroni codificata dal DNA nucleare (che si trasmettono secondo gli schemi dell'ereditarietà mendeliana) o degli enzimi coinvolti nell'ossidazione degli acidi grassi codificati dal DNA mitocondriale (che vengono ereditate solo dalla madre).

Le basi genetiche delle **aritmie ereditarie**, in particolare delle **sindromi del QT lungo**, sono state associate a mutazioni di geni che codificano per subunità dei canali cardiaci del sodio e del potassio (vedi Tab. 424-2).

Dal 2 al 4% dei casi di cardiopatia congenita è associato a condizioni ambientali o materne avverse e influenze teratogene, tra cui diabete mellito, fenilchetonuria, lupus eritematoso sistemico, sindrome da rosolia congenita e assunzione di farmaci (litio, etanolo, warfarina, talidomide, antimetaboliti, derivati della vitamina A, anticonvulsivanti) (vedi Tab. 422-2). Malformazioni non cardiache associate, attribuibili a sindromi identificabili, si osservano in una percentuale di pazienti con cardiopatie congenite che può raggiungere il 25% (vedi Tab. 422-1).

Sono state identificate differenze di sesso nell'insorgenza di specifiche lesioni cardiache. La trasposizione delle grandi arterie e le lesioni ostruttive del cuore sinistro sono lievemente più comuni nei maschi (circa 65 %), mentre difetti del setto interatriale (ASD, *Atrial Septal Defect*), VSD, PDA e stenosi della polmonare sono più comuni nelle femmine. In generale, non sono emerse differenze di razza nell'incidenza delle lesioni cardiache congenite; per quanto riguarda lesioni specifiche, come la trasposizione delle grandi arterie, si è registrata un'incidenza maggiore nei bambini bianchi.

CONSULENZA GENETICA. Coloro che hanno un bambino affetto da cardiopatia congenita necessitano di una consulenza genetica volta a determinare la probabilità che una malformazione cardiaca si verifichi in un figlio successivo (vedi Capitolo 83). Con l'eccezione delle sindromi note dovute a mutazioni di un singolo gene, la maggior parte delle cardiopatie congenite è conseguenza di un quadro di ereditarietà multifattoriale, che dovrebbe comportare un basso rischio di ricorrenza. A mano a mano che si identificano nuove cause genetiche, tuttavia, è necessario aggiornare costantemente questi rischi. L'incidenza di una cardiopatia congenita nella popolazione è di circa l'0,8% ma sale al 2-6% in caso di una seconda gravidanza dopo la nascita di un bambino con cardiopatia congenita o se un genitore ne è affetto. Questo rischio di ricorrenza è strettamente dipendente dal tipo di lesione nel primo figlio. Quando due parenti di primo grado sono affetti da una cardiopatia congenita, il rischio per la prole successiva può raggiungere il 20-30%. Quando si riscontra una cardiopatia congenita in un secondo figlio, questa tenderà a essere simile alla lesione osservata nel parente di primo grado (lesioni conotroncali, lesioni ostruttive del cuore sinistro, difetti del setto atrioventricolare). Il grado di gravità può essere variabile, come anche la presenza di difetti associati. Un accurato screeening ecocardiografico dei parenti di primo grado spesso permette di scoprire forme lievi di cardiopatia congenita che erano clinicamente silenti. L'incidenza di una valvola aortica bicuspide è più che doppia (5% contro il 2% della popolazione generale) nei parenti di bambini con ostruzioni all'efflusso del ventricolo sinistro (stenosi aortica, coartazione aortica o sindrome del cuore sinistro ipoplasico). Un consulente genetico competente è la figura più indicata per fornire alla famiglia informazioni aggiornate riguardo al rischio di ricorrenza.

L'ecocardiografia fetale migliora la percentuale di identificazione di lesioni cardiache congenite in pazienti ad alto rischio (vedi Capitolo 96). La risoluzione e l'accuratezza di questa metodica sono eccellenti ma non perfette; le famiglie dovrebbero essere avvisate del fatto che un ecocardiogramma fetale normale non garantisce l'assenza di una cardiopatia congenita. È possibile che lesioni cardiache congenite si sviluppino nel corso della gravidanza e che una stenosi aortica moderata con un ventricolo sinistro di normali dimensioni alla 18ª settimana di gestazione evolva in atresia aortica con ventricolo sinistro ipoplasico entro la 34ª settimana, a causa della diminuzione del flusso attraverso atri, ventricoli e aorta nella seconda metà della gestazione. Questa progressione ha dato impulso a trial clinici di trattamento interventistico, come la valvuloplastica aortica con palloncino in epoca fetale, per la prevenzione della sindrome del cuore sinistro ipoplasico (vedi Capitolo 423.7).

Il principale fattore che determina se una **donna con cardiopatia congenita**, operata o meno, sarà in grado di portare a termine la gravidanza è il quadro cardiovascolare della madre. In presenza di un difetto cardiaco congenito lieve, o dopo riparazione a buon fine di una lesione più grave, è probabile una gestazione normale. In una donna con scarsa funzionalità cardiaca, tuttavia, l'aumentato carico emodinamico imposto dalla gravidanza può comportare un rischio significativamente aumentato sia per la gestante sia per il feto. L'incidenza di aborti spontanei in presenza di una grave cardiopatia congenita è elevata, specialmente quanto la madre è cianotica. Queste situazioni, che comportano un rischio elevato anche per la madre, dovrebbero essere gestite da un perinatologo esperto in collaborazione con un cardiologo che abbia dimestichezza con le cardiopatie congenite dell'adulto (vedi Capitolo 434.1). È importante discutere i vari metodi di controllo delle nascite con le giovani donne che sono state sottoposte a intervento correttivo o palliativo di lesioni cardiache congenite. Al momento del parto è inoltre indicata la profilassi antibiotica dell'endocardite.

Berend SA, Spikes AS, Kashork CD, et al: Dual-probe fluorescence in situ hybridization assay for detecting deletions associated with VCFS/DiGeorge syndrome I and DiGeorge syndrome II loci. *Am J Med Genet* 2000;91:313–317.
Boneva RS, Botto LD, Moore CA, et al: Mortality associated with congenital heart defects in the United States: Trends and racial disparities, 1979–1997. *Circulation* 2001;103:2376–2381.
Donnai D, Karmiloff-Smith A: Williams syndrome: From genotype through to the cognitive phenotype. *Am J Med Genet* 2000;97:164–171.
Epstein JA, Buck CA: Transcriptional regulation of cardiac development: Implications for congenital heart disease and DiGeorge syndrome. *Pediatr Res* 2000;48:717–724.
Ferencz C, Rubin JD, McCarter RJ, et al: Congenital heart disease: Prevalence at livebirth. The Baltimore-Washington Infant Study. *Am J Epidemiol* 1985;121:31–36.
Gill HK, Splitt M, Sharland G, et al: Patterns of recurrence of congenital heart disease: An analysis of 6,640 consecutive pregnancies evaluated by detailed fetal echocardiography. *J Am Coll Cardiol* 2003;42:923–929.
Goldmuntz E: The genetic contribution to congenital heart disease. *Pediatr Clin North Am* 2004;51:1721–1737.
Maslen CL: Molecular genetics of atrioventricular septal defects. *Curr Opin Cardiol* 2004;19:205–210.
Reamon-Buettner SM, Hecker H, Spanel-Borowski, et al. Novel NKX2-5 mutations in diseased heart tissues of patients with cardiac malformations. *Am J Pathol* 2004;164:2117–2125.
Schott JJ, Benson DW, Basson CT, et al: Congenital heart disease caused by mutations in the transcription factor NKX2-5. *Science* 1998;281:108–111.

Capitolo 425 ■ Valutazione del lattante o del bambino con cardiopatia congenita

La valutazione iniziale di una sospetta cardiopatia congenita consiste in un approccio sistematico a tre componenti principali. In primo luogo, i difetti cardiaci congeniti si dividono in due grandi gruppi a seconda della presenza o meno di cianosi, che può essere determinata dall'esame obiettivo con l'aiuto della pulsossimetria. Questi due gruppi possono essere ulteriormente suddivisi a seconda che dalla radiografia del torace emergano segni di una vascolarizzazione polmonare aumentata, normale o diminuita. Infine, l'elettrocardiogramma può tornare utile per determinare se vi sia un'ipertrofia ventricolare destra, sinistra o biventricolare. Il carattere dei toni cardiaci e la presenza e le caratteristiche di eventuali soffi restringe ulteriormente la diagnosi differenziale. La diagnosi finale riceve poi conferma dall'ecocardiografia, dalla TC o dalla RMN, oppure dal cateterismo cardiaco.

CARDIOPATIE CONGENITE NON CIANOGENE

Le lesioni cardiache congenite non cianogene sono classificabili in base al carico fisiologico predominante che impongono al cuore. Anche se molte cardiopatie congenite arrecano più di un disturbo fisiologico, è utile mettere a fuoco la primitiva anomalia di sovraccarico a fini classificatori. Le lesioni più comuni sono quelle che causano un sovraccarico di volume, in particolare quelle che comportano uno shunt sinistro-destro. Altre cause di sovraccarico di volume sono il rigurgito valvolare atrioventricolare (AV) e alcune miocardiopatie. La seconda classe principale di lesioni causa un sovraccarico di pressione, per lo più secondario a ostruzione all'efflusso ventricolare (stenosi valvolare aortica o polmonare) o a restringimento di uno dei grandi vasi (coartazione aortica). La radiografia del torace e l'elettrocardiogramma sono strumenti utili per differenziare queste classi principali di lesioni dal sovraccarico di volume o di pressione.

LESIONI CHE COMPORTANO UN SOVRACCARICO DI VOLUME. In questo gruppo le lesioni più comuni sono quelle che causano uno shunt sinistro-destro (vedi Capitolo 426): difetti del setto interatriale, difetti del setto interventricolare, difetti del setto atrioventricolare (canale AV) e dotto arterioso pervio. Il comune denominatore fisiopatologico è la comunicazione tra il versante sistemico e quello polmonare della circolazione, che porta allo shunt di sangue completamente ossigenato nei polmoni, quantificabile calcolando il rapporto tra il flusso sanguigno polmonare e quello sistemico, o Qp:Qs. Uno shunt 2:1 implica quindi un flusso sanguigno polmonare doppio rispetto al normale.

La direzione e l'entità dello shunt attraverso una simile comunicazione dipendono dalla grandezza del difetto e dalle pressioni, oltre che dalle resistenze vascolari relative, polmonari e sistemiche. Questi fattori sono dinamici e possono andare incontro a cambiamenti drammatici con l'età. Difetti intracardiaci possono diminuire di dimensioni con il tempo, e l'esposizione cronica della circolazione polmonare a una pressione elevata e a un elevato flusso sanguigno porta a un graduale aumento della resistenza vascolare polmonare (fenomeno di Eisenmenger, vedi Capitolo 433.2). Perciò, una lesione come un ampio VSD può essere associata a uno shunt piccolo e a scarsi sintomi durante le prime settimane di vita. Nelle settimane successive, quando la resistenza vascolare polmonare diminuisce, aumenta il volume dello shunt sinistro-destro e iniziano a comparire i sintomi.

L'aumento del volume di sangue nei polmoni riduce la compliance polmonare e incrementa il lavoro respiratorio. Il fluido si infiltra negli spazi interstiziali e negli alveoli causando edema polmonare. Il lattante manifesta i sintomi del cosiddetto **scompenso cardiaco**, come tachipnea, retrazione degli spazi intercostali del torace, alitamento delle pinne nasali e respiro affannoso. La dicitura *scompenso cardiaco*, tuttavia, non è del tutto corretta; la gittata totale del ventricolo sinistro è in realtà di molte volte superiore ai valori normali, pur rivelandosi in gran parte efficace poiché ritorna direttamente ai polmoni. Per sostenere questo elevato livello di gittata ventricolare sinistra, aumentano la frequenza cardiaca e la gittata sistolica, come pure l'attività del sistema nervoso simpatico. L'aumento delle catecolamine circolanti, in combinazione con un maggior lavoro respiratorio, porta a un innalzamento del consumo totale di ossigeno dell'organismo, spesso oltre la capacità di trasporto d'ossigeno della circolazione, che a sua volta si traduce in ulteriori sintomi: sudorazione, irritabilità e blocco della crescita. Si verifica un rimodellamento del cuore, con una maggior dilatazione e un minor grado di ipertrofia. Infine, se non trattata, la resistenza vascolare polmonare inizierà ad aumentare, e nell'arco di parecchi anni il volume dello shunt diminuirà e si invertirà, diventando destro-sinistro (fenomeno di Eisenmenger; vedi Capitolo 433.2).

Ulteriori lesioni che impongono un sopraccarico di volume al cuore comprendono le lesioni da rigurgito (vedi Capitolo 428) e le miocardiopatie (vedi Capitolo 439). Il rigurgito attraverso le valvole AV è di più frequente riscontro in pazienti con difetti AV parziali o completi (difetti atriosettali, canale AV). In queste lesioni, la combinazione di uno shunt sinistro-destro con un rigurgito valvolare AV aumenta il sovraccarico di volume per il cuore e porta a sintomi più gravi. Nell'anomalia di Ebstein si osserva un rigurgito isolato attraverso la valvola tricuspide (vedi Capitolo 430.7). Il rigurgito di una delle valvole semilunari è di solito associato a un certo grado di stenosi; tuttavia, un rigurgito aortico si può riscontrare in pazienti con un difetto del setto interventricolare (VSD, *Ventricular Septal Defect*) direttamente al di sotto della valvola aortica (VSD sovracristale) o con stenosi membranosa subaortica.

Al contrario di quanto avviene negli shunt sinistro-destri, in cui la funzione intrinseca del muscolo cardiaco è generalmente normale o aumentata, nelle miocardiopatie la funzione del muscolo cardiaco risulta diminuita. Le **cardiomiopatie** possono compromettere la contrattilità sistolica, il rilassamento diastolico, o entrambi. Una diminuita funzione cardiaca porta a un aumento delle pressioni di riempimento atriali e ventricolari, e l'edema polmonare si manifesta secondariamente all'aumento della pressione capillare. Le principali cause di miocardiopatia nei lattanti e nei bambini comprendono le miocarditi virali, le malattie metaboliche e i difetti genetici (vedi Capitolo 439).

LESIONI CHE COMPORTANO UN SOVRACCARICO DI PRESSIONE. Il comune denominatore fisiopatologico di queste lesioni è un'ostruzione al normale flusso sanguigno. Le più frequenti sono le ostruzioni all'efflusso ventricolare: stenosi valvolare polmonare, stenosi valvolare aortica e coartazione aortica (vedi Capitolo 427). Meno comuni sono le ostruzioni all'afflusso ventricolare: stenosi tricuspidalica o mitralica, e cor triatriatum. L'ostruzione all'efflusso ventricolare può essere localizzata a livello della valvola, al di sotto della valvola (ventricolo destro con doppia camera, membrana subaortica) o al di sopra di essa (stenosi di una diramazione dell'arteria polmonare o stenosi aortica sopravalvolare). A meno che l'ostruzione non sia grave, la gittata cardiaca sarà preservata e i sintomi clinici di scompenso cardiaco saranno sfumati o assenti. Il compenso consiste principalmente in un aumento dello spessore parietale del cuore (ipertrofia), ma in stadi più avanzati comprende anche la dilatazione.

Il quadro clinico è diverso quando l'ostruzione all'efflusso è grave, evenienza che si verifica nel primissimo periodo neonatale. Le condizioni del lattante possono diventare critiche già poche ore dopo la nascita. Una grave stenosi polmonare nel periodo neonatale (stenosi polmonare critica) dà luogo a segni di scompenso cardiaco destro (epatomegalia, edema periferico) come anche a cianosi per uno shunt destro-sinistro attraverso il forame ovale. Una grave stenosi aortica nel periodo neonatale (stenosi aortica critica) è caratterizzata da segni di scompenso cardiaco sinistro (edema polmonare, ipoperfusione) e destro (epatomegalia, edema periferico) e può progredire rapidamente fino al completo collasso circolatorio. Nei bambini più grandi, una grave stenosi polmonare determina sintomi di scompenso cardiaco destro ma non cianosi, a meno che non persista uno shunt destro-sinistro (per es. pervietà del forame ovale).

Nei bambini più grandi e negli adolescenti la coartazione aortica si manifesta di solito con ipertensione nel distretto superiore del corpo e iposfigmia dei polsi agli arti inferiori. Subito dopo la nascita, tuttavia, la diagnosi di coartazione aortica può essere ritardata dalla presenza di un dotto arterioso pervio. In questi pazienti l'estremità aortica del dotto può convogliare il flusso ematico, permettendogli di bypassare parzialmente l'ostruzione. Questi lattanti divengono quindi sintomatici, spesso in modo drammatico, quando il dotto alla fine si chiude.

CARDIOPATIE CONGENITE CIANOGENE

Questo gruppo di lesioni cardiache congenite può essere ulteriormente suddiviso in base alla fisiopatologia, a seconda che il flusso sanguigno polmonare sia diminuito (tetralogia di Fallot, atresia polmonare con un setto intatto, ritorno venoso polmonare anomalo totale con ostruzione) o aumentato (trasposizione dei grandi vasi, ventricolo unico, tronco arterioso, ritorno venoso polmonare anomalo totale senza ostruzione). La radiografia del torace è uno strumento prezioso per attribuire queste cardiopatie a una o all'altra categoria.

LESIONI CIANOGENE CON IPOAFLUSSO POLMONARE. Queste lesioni devono comprendere sia un'ostruzione al flusso sanguigno polmonare (a livello della valvola tricuspide, del ventricolo destro o della valvola polmonare), sia una via attraverso la quale il sangue venoso sistemico possa passare da destra a sinistra ed entrare nella circolazione sistemica (attraverso un forame ovale pervio, un difetto del setto interatriale o un VSD). All'interno di questo gruppo sono comuni l'atresia della tricuspide, la tetralogia di Fallot, e varie forme di ventricolo unico con stenosi polmonare (vedi Capitolo 430), lesioni in cui il grado di cianosi dipende dal grado di ostruzione al flusso sanguigno polmonare. Se l'ostruzione è lieve, la cianosi può essere assente a riposo. Questi pazienti possono avere crisi acute di cianosi se sottoposti a stress. Al contrario, se l'ostruzione è grave, il flusso sanguigno polmonare può essere dipendente dalla pervietà del dotto arterioso. Quando il dotto si chiude, nei primi giorni di vita, il neonato va incontro a grave ipossiemia e a shock.

LESIONI CIANOGENE CON IPERFLUSSO POLMONARE. Questo gruppo di lesioni non si associa a ostruzione al flusso sanguigno polmonare. La cianosi è causata o da connessioni anomale ventricolo-arteriose o da completo mescolamento di sangue venoso sistemico e sangue venoso polmonare nel cuore (vedi Capitolo 431). La trasposizione dei grandi vasi è la lesione più comune del primo gruppo. In questa condizione, l'aorta origina dal ventricolo destro e l'arteria polmonare dal ventricolo sinistro; il sangue venoso sistemico che ritorna all'atrio destro viene pompato direttamente nell'organismo, mentre il sangue ossigenato che ritorna dai polmoni all'atrio sinistro viene pompato di nuovo nei polmoni. Nel primissimo periodo neonatale la persistenza di vie fetali di circolo (forame ovale e dotto arterioso) fa sì che si verifichi un mescolamento di scarsa entità; quando il dotto inizia a chiudersi, questi lattanti sviluppano una cianosi accentuata.

Le lesioni con mescolamento totale comprendono difetti cardiaci con un atrio o un ventricolo comune, ritorno venoso polmonare anomalo totale e tronco arterioso (vedi Capitolo 431). In questo gruppo, il sangue venoso sistemico povero di ossigeno e il sangue venoso polmonare ossigenato si mescolano completamente nel cuore: ne consegue che la saturazione di ossigeno è uguale nell'arteria polmonare e nell'aorta. Se il flusso sanguigno polmonare non è ostruito, questi lattanti presentano un'associazione di cianosi e scompenso cardiaco. Se invece è presente una stenosi polmonare, hanno solo cianosi, simile a quella dei pazienti con tetralogia di Fallot.

Lister G, Moreau G, Moss M, et al: Effects of alterations of oxygen transport on the neonate. *Semin Perinatol* 1984;8:192–204.

Lister G, Pitt BR: Cardiopulmonary interactions in the infant with congenital heart disease. *Clin Chest Med* 1983;4:219–232.

Mair DD, Ritter DG: Factors influencing systemic oxygen saturation in complete transposition of the great arteries. *Am J Cardiol* 1973;31:742–748.

Weeks B, Friedman AH: Training pediatric residents to evaluate congenital heart disease in the current era. *Pediatr Clin North Am* 2004;51:1641–1651.

Capitolo 426 ■ Cardiopatie congenite non cianogene: lesioni con shunt sinistro-destro

426.1 • Difetto del setto interatriale

I difetti del setto interatriale (ASD, *Atrial Septal Defects*) possono presentarsi in qualsiasi punto del setto atriale (tipo ostium secundum, ostium primum o seno venoso), a seconda di quale struttura settale embrionale non si è sviluppata in modo normale (vedi Capitolo 420). Accade meno comunemente che il setto atriale sia quasi assente, con creazione di un atrio funzionalmente unico. Un difetto del setto interatriale tipo ostium secundum costituisce circa il 7% dei difetti cardiaci congeniti. La maggior parte dei casi di ASD è sporadica; l'ereditarietà autosomica dominante rientra nella sindrome di Holt-Oram (ipoplasia o assenza del radio, blocco cardiaco di pr grado, ASD), o in famiglie con ASD tipo ostium secundum e blocco cardiaco.

Un forame ovale pervio (PFO, *Patent Foramen Ovale*) isolato con incompetenza valvolare è un reperto ecocardiografico comune durante l'infanzia, di solito privo di significato emodinamico e non considerato un ASD, ma può giocare un ruolo importante se sono presenti altri difetti cardiaci strutturali. Se un'altra anomalia cardiaca (stenosi o atresia polmonare, anomalie della valvola tricuspide, disfunzione ventricolare destra) causa un aumento della pressione atriale destra, il sangue venoso può passare attraverso il PFO nell'atrio sinistro, con conseguente cianosi. Data la struttura anatomica del PFO, lo shunt sinistro-destro non è comune se non subito dopo la nascita. In presenza di un importante sovraccarico di volume o di un atrio sinistro ipertensivo (secondario a stenosi mitralica), il forame ovale può essere così dilatato da determinare uno shunt sinistro-destro significativo. Nel 15-30% degli adulti può essere presente un forame ovale con competenza valvolare ma pervio al sondaggio. Un PFO isolato non richiede trattamento chirurgico, pur potendo rappresentare un fattore di rischio per l'embolizzazione sistemica paradossa (da destra a sinistra). La chiusura di questi difetti viene presa in considerazione in adulti con anamnesi di ictus tromboembolico.

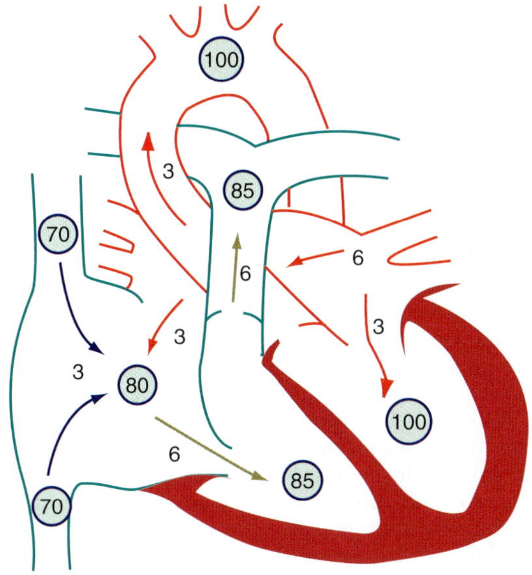

Figura 426-1. Fisiologia di un difetto del setto interatriale (ASD). I *numeri cerchiati* rappresentano i valori di saturazione di ossigeno. I *numeri accanto alle frecce* rappresentano i volumi del flusso ematico (in L/min/m^2). Questa illustrazione rappresenta un ipotetico paziente con un rapporto di flusso ematico polmonare/sistemico (Qp:Qs) pari a 2:1. Il sangue desaturato entra nell'atrio destro dalle vene cave a un volume di 3 L/min/m^2 e si mescola con altri 3 L di sangue completamente saturato che passa da sinistra a destra attraverso l'ASD; il risultato è un aumento della saturazione di ossigeno nell'atrio destro. Sei litri di sangue fluiscono attraverso la valvola tricuspide e causano un rullio mesodiastolico. La saturazione di ossigeno può essere leggermente più elevata nel ventricolo destro a causa di un mescolamento incompleto a livello atriale. Tutti i 6 L attraversano il tratto di efflusso del ventricolo destro provocando un soffio sistolico da eiezione. Sei litri ritornano all'atrio sinistro: 3 L vengono deviati da sinistra a destra attraverso il difetto e 3 L attraversano la valvola mitrale per poi essere eiettati dal ventricolo sinistro nell'aorta ascendente (gittata cardiaca normale).

426.2 • Difetto tipo ostium secundum

Un difetto tipo ostium secundum nella regione della fossa ovale è la forma più comune di ASD e si associa a valvole atrioventricolari strutturalmente normali. Il prolasso della valvola mitrale è stato descritto in associazione con questo difetto, ma è raro che abbia rilevanza clinica. ASD tipo ostium secundum possono essere singoli o multipli (setto atriale fenestrato) e aperture >2 cm di diametro sono comuni nei bambini più grandi sintomatici. Difetti ampi possono estendersi verso il basso (in direzione della vena cava inferiore e dell'ostio del seno coronario), verso l'alto (in direzione della vena cava superiore) o posteriormente. La popolazione femminile risulta più spesso colpita rispetto a quella maschile, con un rapporto di 3:1. Il ritorno venoso polmonare anomalo parziale, per lo più nella parte superiore destra della vena polmonare, può essere una lesione associata.

FISIOPATOLOGIA. Il grado di shunt sinistro-destro dipende dalle dimensioni del difetto, dalla compliance relativa dei ventricoli destro e sinistro e dalla resistenza vascolare relativa nelle circolazioni polmonare e sistemica. In difetti ampi si verifica un notevole shunt di sangue ossigenato che fluisce dall'atrio sinistro all'atrio destro (Fig. 426-1); questo sangue si aggiunge al normale ritorno venoso verso l'atrio destro ed è pompato dal ventricolo destro ai polmoni. In presenza di difetti ampi, il rapporto tra flusso ematico polmonare e sistemico (Qp:Qs) è di solito compreso tra 2:1 e 4:1. La scarsità di sintomi nei lattanti con ASD è correlata alla struttura del ventricolo destro nei primi giorni di vita, quando la parete muscolare è spessa e meno distensibile, condizione che limita lo shunt sinistro-destro. Quando il lattante cresce, e la resistenza vascolare polmonare cala, la parete ventricolare destra si assottiglia e lo shunt sinistro-destro attraverso l'ASD aumenta. L'importante flusso di sangue attraverso il lato destro del cuore comporta un ingrandimento dell'atrio destro e del ventricolo destro e una dilatazione dell'arteria polmonare. L'atrio sinistro può essere ingrandito, mentre il ventricolo sinistro e l'aorta sono di dimensioni normali. Nonostante l'abbondante flusso ematico polmonare, la pressione in arteria polmonare è di solito normale per la mancanza di comunicazione ad alta pressione tra le circolazioni polmonare e sistemica. La resistenza vascolare polmonare si mantiene bassa durante l'infanzia, anche se può iniziare a crescere in età adulta, fino a determinare un'inversione dello shunt e una cianosi clinicamente evidente.

MANIFESTAZIONI CLINICHE. Il bambino con ASD tipo ostium secundum è spesso asintomatico; può accadere che la lesione venga scoperta per caso durante una visita medica. Anche un ASD tipo ostium secundum estremamente ampio è raro che causi uno scompenso cardiaco clinicamente evidente nell'infanzia; nei lattanti può essere presente un lieve ritardo di crescita, mentre nei bambini più grandi possono notarsi vari gradi di intolleranza allo sforzo. Spesso tale limitazione può passare inosservata ai familiari fino alla correzione chirurgica, quando la crescita del bambino o il livello di attività aumentano in modo significativo.

I reperti obiettivi dell'ASD di solito sono caratteristici ma discretamente sfumati e richiedono un esame cardiaco scrupoloso, con particolare attenzione ai toni cardiaci. L'esame del torace può evidenziare una lieve bozza precordiale, a sinistra. Di solito è palpabile un sollevamento sistolico ventricolare destro a livello del margine sternale sinistro. Si possono udire un primo tono forte e, talvolta, un click di eiezione polmonare. Nella maggior parte dei pazienti il secondo tono cardiaco è caratteristicamente **ampiamente sdoppiato, con uno sdoppiamento fisso** in tutte le fasi del respiro. Di norma, la durata dell'eiezione dal ventricolo destro varia con il respiro: l'inspirio aumenta il volume ventricolare destro e ritarda la chiusura della valvola polmonare. Con un ASD, il volume ventricolare destro in diastole è costantemente aumentato e il tempo di eiezione è prolungato in tutte le fasi del respiro. Si riscontra un soffio sistolico da eiezione, di altezza media, senza caratteristiche di asprezza, raramente accompagnato da un fremito e meglio udibile a livello del margine sternale sinistro medio e superiore. Esso è prodotto non dal flusso a bassa pressione attraverso l'ASD, ma dall'aumento del flusso attraverso il tratto di uscita del ventricolo destro in arteria polmonare. A livello del margine sternale inferiore sinistro è spesso udibile un breve soffio rullante mesodiastolico, prodotto dal maggiore volume di sangue che attraversa la valvola tricuspide. Questo reperto, che può essere lieve e meglio apprezzabile con la campana dello stetoscopio, di solito indica un rapporto Qp:Qs di almeno 2:1.

DIAGNOSI. La radiografia del torace evidenzia vari gradi di ingrandimento del ventricolo e dell'atrio destro, a seconda delle dimensioni dello shunt. L'arteria polmonare è ampia e la vascolarizzazione polmonare appare aumentata. Questi segni variabili possono non essere importanti nei casi lievi. L'ingrandimento cardiaco spesso si apprezza meglio in proiezione laterale poiché il ventricolo destro protrude in avanti a mano a mano che il suo volume aumenta. L'elettrocardiogramma evidenzia un sovraccarico di volume del ventricolo destro; l'asse QRS può essere normale o presentare una deviazione assiale a destra, e può essere presente un lieve ritardo di conduzione ventricolare destra (aspetto rsR nelle derivazioni precordiali destre).

L'ecocardiogramma evidenzia reperti caratteristici di sovraccarico di volume del ventricolo destro, tra cui aumentate dimensioni del ventricolo destro in telediastole e un appiattimento e una motilità anomali del setto ventricolare (Fig. 426-2). Un setto normale si muove posteriormente durante la sistole e anteriormente durante la diastole. Con un sovraccarico ventricolare destro e una normale resistenza vascolare polmonare, il movimento del setto è invertito (impulso anteriore in sistole) o intermedio, cosicché il setto rimane diritto. Per apprezzare prontamente la sede e le dimensioni del difetto atriale si ricorre alla scansione bidimensionale, con una caratteristica iperecogenicità dell'immagine ecografia che si nota all'estremità del difetto (artefatto T). Lo shunt viene confermato con il Doppler pulsato e con il color-Doppler. I pazienti che presentano le classiche caratteristiche dell'ASD emodinamicamente significativo all'esame obiettivo e alla radiografia del torace, nei quali viene effettuata l'identificazione ecocardiografica di un ASD tipo ostium secundum isolato, non hanno bisogno di essere sottoposti a cateterismo cardiaco prima della chiusura chirurgica, a eccezione dei bambini più grandi, in cui vi può essere un problema di resistenza vascolare polmonare. Se sorge un sospetto in tal senso, il cateterismo cardiaco conferma la presenza del difetto e permette di misurare il rapporto dello shunt e della pressione polmonare.

All'atto del cateterismo il sangue proveniente dall'atrio destro avrà un contenuto di ossigeno molto più elevato rispetto a quello proveniente dalla vena cava superiore. Questa caratteristica non è diagnostica in modo specifico, poiché può verificarsi nel ritorno venoso polmonare anomalo parziale all'atrio destro, nel difetto del setto interventricolare (VSD, *Ventricular Septal Defect*) con insufficienza tricuspidale, nei difetti del setto atrioventricolare associati a shunt dal ventricolo sinistro all'atrio destro e nelle comunicazioni tra l'aorta e l'atrio destro (rottura di un aneurisma del seno di Valsalva). Le pressioni nella parte destra del cuore di solito sono normali, ma gradienti pressori da piccoli a moderati (<25 mmHg) possono essere misurati attraverso il tratto di efflusso ventricolare destro a causa di una stenosi funzionale correlata all'eccessivo flusso di sangue. Nei bambini e negli adolescenti la resistenza vascolare polmonare è quasi sempre normale. Lo shunt è variabile in base alla grandezza del difetto, ma può raggiungere un volume considerevole (fino a 20 L/min/m^2).

La cineangiografia, previo inserimento di un catetere nel difetto e nella vena polmonare superiore destra, evidenzia il difetto e la sede del drenaggio venoso polmonare superiore destro. In alternativa, l'angiografia polmonare dimostra il difetto nella fase sinistra (ritorno di contrasto sul lato sinistro del cuore dopo il passaggio attraverso i polmoni).

COMPLICANZE. Gli ASD tipo ostium secundum in genere sono isolati, anche se possono essere associati a ritorno venoso polmonare anomalo parziale, stenosi valvolare polmonare, VSD, stenosi di una diramazione dell'arteria polmonare e persistenza della vena cava superiore sinistra, oltre che a prolasso e insufficienza della valvola mitrale. Essi sono associati alla sindrome di Holt-Oram autosomica dominante, causata dal gene TBX5, appartenente alla famiglia trascrizionale T-box e situato nella regione 12q21-q22 del cromosoma 12. Una forma familiare di ASD tipo ostium secundum associata a ritardo di conduzione AV è stata collegata a mutazioni in un altro fattore di trascrizione, Nkx2.5. I pazienti con ASD familiare senza blocco cardiaco possono essere portatori di una mutazione nel fattore di trascrizione GATA4, situato sul cromosoma 8p22-23.

TRATTAMENTO. La tecnica di chiusura chirurgica o mediante cateterismo è consigliata per tutti i pazienti sintomatici e per i pazienti asintomatici con un rapporto Qp:Qs di almeno 2:1. Il momento opportuno per la chiusura in elezione è di solito dopo il primo anno e prima dell'inizio dell'età scolare. La chiusura effettuata mediante intervento chirurgico a cuore aperto è associata a un tasso di mortalità <1%. Si preferisce effettuare la riparazione

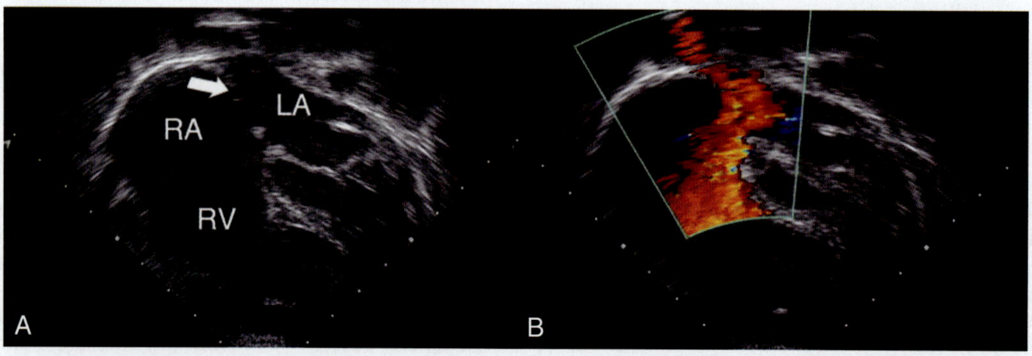

Figura 426-2. Reperti ecocardiografici in un difetto del setto interatriale (ASD) tipo ostium secundum. *A*, Ecocardiogramma bidimensionale (proiezione apicale a quattro camere) che evidenzia un ASD di dimensione moderata tipo ostium secundum (freccia). *B*, Flussimetria Doppler che rileva uno shunt sinistro-destro (il colore rosso rappresenta il sangue che si muove verso il trasduttore di ultrasuoni e non il livello di ossigenazione del sangue). LA (*Left Atrium*), atrio sinistro; RA (*Right Atrium*), atrio destro; RV (*Right Ventricle*), ventricolo destro.

nella prima infanzia, poiché mortalità chirurgica e morbilità sono significativamente maggiori nell'età adulta; il rischio a lungo termine di aritmie è anch'esso maggiore dopo la riparazione di un ASD negli adulti. I dispositivi per la chiusura dei difetti del setto interatriale vengono impiantati per via transvenosa nel laboratorio di emodinamica (Fig. 426-3). I risultati sono eccellenti e i pazienti vengono dimessi il giorno seguente. Grazie allo strumentario di ultima generazione, l'incidenza di complicanze gravi come l'erosione del dispositivo è dello 0,1% e può essere diminuita ulteriormente identificando i pazienti ad alto rischio (per es. quelli con un insufficiente bordo del setto attorno al dispositivo). In pazienti con un piccolo ASD tipo ostium secundum e minimo shunt sinistro-destro, vi è consenso generale sul fatto che la chiusura non è richiesta. Non è chiaro al momento attuale se la persistenza di un piccolo ASD in età adulta aumenti il rischio di ictus in modo tale da giustificare la chiusura profilattica di tutti questi difetti.

PROGNOSI. Gli ASD identificati nei bambini nati a termine possono chiudersi spontaneamente. Gli ASD tipo ostium secundum sono ben tollerati durante l'infanzia e i sintomi non compaiono di solito fino alla terza decade di vita o più tardi. Ipertensione polmonare, aritmie atriali, insufficienza tricuspidalica o mitralica e lo scompenso cardiaco sono manifestazioni tardive; questi sintomi possono inizialmente comparire durante un aumentato carico di volume dovuto a una gravidanza. L'endocardite infettiva è estremamente rara, e la profilassi antibiotica per un ASD tipo ostium secundum non è raccomandata.

I risultati dopo chiusura chirurgica o mediante dispositivo endovascolare in bambini con shunt da moderati ad ampi sono ottimi. I sintomi scompaiono rapidamente e la crescita viene spesso accelerata. La dimensione del cuore diminuisce fino alla normalità e l'elettrocardiogramma evidenzia una diminuzione delle forze ventricolari destre. Lo scompenso cardiaco destro tardivo e le aritmie sono meno frequenti nei pazienti sottoposti a riparazione chirurgica precoce, diventando più comuni in coloro che sono stati operati dopo i 20 anni di età. La chiusura con dispositivo intravascolare dà risultati a breve e a medio termine eccellenti, mentre i suoi effetti a lungo termine non sono ancora noti. Gli studi che riferiscono la scomparsa di attacchi di emicrania dopo chiusura con dispositivo intravascolare sono interessanti, in quanto inducono a ipotizzare una possibile eziologia tromboembolica; tuttavia, non mancano neppure casi paradossi di pazienti che hanno cominciato a soffrire di attacchi di emicrania dopo il posizionamento di uno di questi dispositivi.

426.3 • Difetto del setto interatriale tipo seno venoso

Un ASD tipo seno venoso è situato nella parte superiore del setto atriale, in stretta relazione con l'ingresso della vena cava superiore. Spesso una o più vene polmonari (di solito provenienti dal polmone destro) drenano il sangue in modo anomalo nella vena cava superiore. Quando quest'ultima è posta a cavallo del difetto, parte del sangue venoso sistemico entra nell'atrio sinistro, ma solo raramente causa una cianosi evidente. Il disturbo emodinamico, il quadro clinico, l'elettrocardiogramma e la radiografia del torace sono simili a quelli che si riscontrano nell'ASD tipo ostium secundum. Per la diagnosi ci si avvale dell'ecocardiografia bidimensionale. Se si procede al cateterismo cardiaco per definire meglio il drenaggio venoso, il catetere può entrare in una vena polmonare destra direttamente dalla vena cava superiore. La correzione anatomica richiede generalmente l'inserzione di un patch per chiudere il difetto, mentre si ricostruisce l'ingresso delle vene anomale nell'atrio sinistro. Se la vena anomala drena il sangue nella parte alta della vena cava superiore, è possibile lasciare la vena intatta e chiudere l'ASD incorporando l'imboccatura della cava nell'atrio sinistro. La vena cava superiore prossimamente all'entrata venosa viene staccata e anastomizzata direttamente all'atrio destro. I risultati chirurgici sono generalmente eccellenti. È raro che i difetti tipo seno venoso coinvolgano la vena cava inferiore.

426.4 • Ritorno venoso polmonare anomalo parziale

Una o più vene polmonari possono drenare il sangue in modo anomalo nella vena cava superiore o inferiore, nell'atrio destro o nel seno coronarico, producendo uno shunt sinistro-destro di sangue ossigenato. Il ritorno venoso polmonare anomalo parziale di solito coinvolge alcune o tutte le vene provenienti da un solo polmone, per lo più il destro. Quando vi si associa un ASD, quest'ultimo è in genere del tipo seno venoso (vedi Capitolo 426-3). Una volta rilevato un ASD tipo seno venoso con l'ecocardiogramma, si deve cercare la presenza di un ritorno venoso polmonare anomalo parziale a esso associato. L'anamnesi, i segni rilevabili all'esame obiettivo e i reperti elettrocardiografici e radiografici sono indistinguibili da quelli di un ASD isolato tipo ostium secundum. Talvolta alla radiografia del torace un drenaggio venoso anomalo nella vena cava inferiore assume l'aspetto di

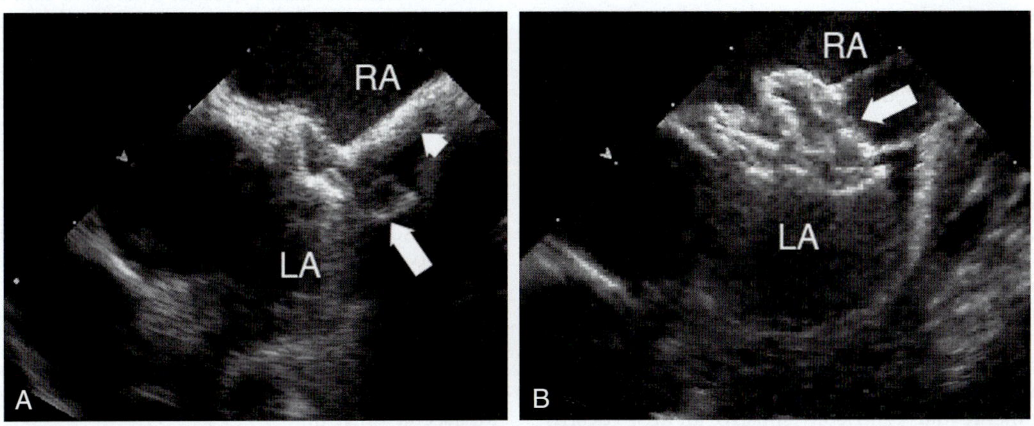

Figura 426-3. Immagine ecografica intravascolare di un'occlusione transcatetere di un difetto del setto interatriale. *A*, Un catetere (*freccia piccola*) è stato introdotto nel difetto atriale e il disco della parte sinistra del dispositivo (*freccia grande*) è stato fatto fuoriuscire dalla guaina nell'atrio sinistro (LA). *B*, Il disco atriale destro (*freccia*) è stato fatto uscire nell'atrio destro (RA). Le due metà del disco sono state unite e il catetere è stato distaccato dal dispositivo occludente e rimosso.

un'ombra di densità vascolare crescente lungo il margine destro dell'ombra cardiaca (**sindrome della scimitarra**); in questi casi di solito non è presente un ASD, mentre sono reperti comuni un **sequestro polmonare** e un apporto arterioso anomalo a quel lobo polmonare. Il ritorno venoso polmonare anomalo totale, una lesione associata a cianosi, è trattato nel Capitolo 431.7. L'ecocardiografia generalmente conferma la diagnosi. Anche RMN e TC sono utili per la definizione del drenaggio venoso polmonare. Se si procede al cateterismo cardiaco, la presenza di vene polmonari anomale è dimostrata dall'arteriografia polmonare selettiva.

La prognosi è eccellente, simile a quella degli ASD tipo ostium secundum. Quando è presente un ampio shunt sinistro-destro, si effettua la correzione chirurgica. L'ASD associato dovrebbe essere chiuso in modo tale che il ritorno venoso polmonare venga diretto all'atrio sinistro. Una singola vena polmonare anomala senza una comunicazione atriale può essere difficile da ricondurre all'atrio sinistro; se lo shunt è piccolo, si può evitare l'intervento chirurgico.

426.5 • DIFETTI DEL SETTO ATRIOVENTRICOLARE (OSTIUM PRIMUM E CANALE ATRIOVENTRICOLARE O DIFETTO DEI CUSCINETTI ENDOCARDICI)

Le anomalie che vanno sotto il nome di difetti del setto atrioventricolare (AV) sono considerate insieme poiché rappresentano uno spettro di anomalie accomunate dalla stessa base embriologica, un difetto del setto AV. Un difetto tipo **ostium primum** è situato nella porzione inferiore del setto atriale, al di sopra delle valvole mitrale e tricuspide. Nella maggior parte dei casi si nota anche una schisi del **lembo anteriore** della **valvola mitrale**. La valvola tricuspide è di solito funzionalmente normale, anche se in genere è presente qualche anomalia anatomica del lembo settale. Il setto interventricolare è intatto.

Un **difetto del setto AV**, altrimenti noto come **difetto tipo canale AV** o difetto dei cuscinetti endocardici, consiste in un difetto contiguo dei setti atriale e ventricolare; una valvola AV singola, comune a entrambi i ventricoli, è formata da due lembi, uno anteriore e l'altro posteriore, a ponte, collegati al setto ventricolare con un lembo laterale per ciascun ventricolo. La lesione, comune nei bambini con **sindrome di Down**, può talvolta verificarsi in associazione con la stenosi polmonare.

Sono inoltre possibili varianti transizionali di questi difetti, tra cui i difetti tipo ostium primum con schisi del lembo anteriore della mitrale e del lembo settale della valvola tricuspide, alterazioni minori del setto ventricolare e, meno frequentemente, difetti tipo ostium primum con valvole AV normali. In alcuni pazienti il setto atriale è intatto, ma l'ingresso del VSD simula quello riscontrabile nel difetto AV completo. Questi difetti sono inoltre comunemente associati a deformità delle valvole AV. Talvolta i difetti del setto AV sono associati a vari gradi di ipoplasia di uno dei ventricoli, condizione nota come difetti del setto AV a dominanza sinistra o destra. Se la camera ventricolare colpita è troppo piccola, l'intervento chirurgico palliativo, mirato a un'eventuale procedura di Fontan, è simile a quello per le sindromi del cuore sinistro o destro ipoplasico (vedi Capitoli 430.4 e 431.10).

FISIOPATOLOGIA. L'anomalia di base in pazienti con difetti tipo ostium primum è l'associazione tra shunt sinistro-destro attraverso il difetto atriale e insufficienza mitralica (o a volte tricuspidalica). Lo shunt è di solito moderato o ampio, il grado di insufficienza mitralica è generalmente lieve o moderato, e la pressione in arteria polmonare è tipicamente normale o solo leggermente aumentata. La fisiologia di questa lesione è perciò simile a quella di un ASD tipo ostium secundum.

Nel difetto del setto AV lo shunt sinistro-destro avviene a livello sia atriale sia ventricolare (Fig. 426-4). Un ulteriore shunt può svilupparsi direttamente dal ventricolo sinistro all'atrio destro a causa dell'assenza del setto AV. Sono comuni l'ipertensione polmonare e la tendenza precoce all'aumento della resistenza vascolare polmonare. L'insufficienza valvolare AV aumenta il carico di volume su uno o entrambi i ventricoli. Qualche shunt destro-sinistro si può inoltre verificare a livello sia atriale sia ventricolare, portando a una lieve ma significativa desaturazione arteriosa. Con il tempo, una vasculopatia polmonare progressiva aumenta lo shunt destro-sinistro cosicché si sviluppa una cianosi clinicamente evidente (fenomeno di Eisenmenger, vedi Capitolo 433.2).

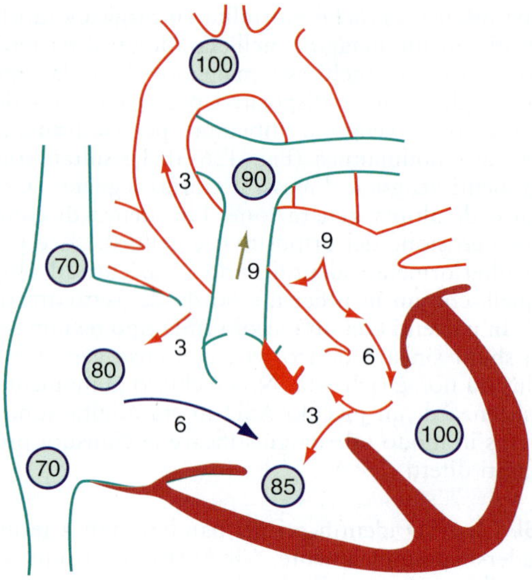

Figura 426-4. Fisiologia di un difetto del setto atrioventricolare (AVSD). I *numeri cerchiati* rappresentano i valori di saturazione d'ossigeno. I *numeri accanto alle frecce* rappresentano i volumi di flusso sanguigno (in L/min/m²). Questa illustrazione presenta il caso di un ipotetico paziente con un rapporto flusso sanguigno polmonare/sistemico (Qp:Qs) di 3:1. Il sangue desaturato entra nell'atrio destro dalle vene cave a un volume di 3 L/min/m² e si mescola con 3 L di sangue completamente saturo che viene deviato da sinistra a destra attraverso il difetto del setto interatriale; il risultato è un aumento della saturazione d'ossigeno nell'atrio destro. Sei litri di sangue fluiscono attraverso il lato destro della valvola AV comune, e a questi si aggiungono altri 3 L di sangue saturo che vengono deviati da sinistra a destra a livello ventricolare, aumentando ulteriormente la saturazione d'ossigeno nel ventricolo destro. Tutti i 9 L fluiscono attraverso il tratto di efflusso del ventricolo destro nei polmoni. Nove litri ritornano all'atrio sinistro: di questi, 3 L vengono deviati da sinistra a destra attraverso il difetto e 6 L attraversano il lato sinistro della valvola AV comune provocando un rullio mesodiastolico. Di questo volume, 3 L vengono deviati da sinistra a destra attraverso il VSD e altri 3 L vengono espulsi in aorta ascendente (normale gittata cardiaca).

MANIFESTAZIONI CLINICHE. Molti bambini con difetti tipo ostium primum sono asintomatici e l'anomalia viene scoperta durante una visita medica di routine. In pazienti con shunt moderato e lieve insufficienza mitralica i segni fisici sono simili a quelli dell'ASD tipo ostium secundum, ma con un ulteriore soffio apicale causato dall'insufficienza mitralica.

Può esservi un'anamnesi positiva per intolleranza allo sforzo, facile affaticabilità e polmoniti ricorrenti, soprattutto in lattanti con ampi shunt sinistro-destri e insufficienza mitralica grave. In questi pazienti l'ingrandimento cardiaco è moderato o marcato e il precordio iperdinamico. I segni ascultatori prodotti dallo shunt sinistro-destro comprendono un primo tono normale o rinforzato, uno sdoppiamento ampio e fisso del secondo tono, un soffio sistolico da eiezione polmonare talvolta preceduto da un click e un soffio di bassa tonalità, mesodiastolico, rullante, al margine sternale inferiore sinistro o all'apice, o in entrambe queste sedi, risultante dall'incremento del flusso che attraversa le valvole AV. L'insufficienza mitralica può manifestarsi come un soffio aspro (di solito di tonalità molto alta) olosistolico apicale che si irradia all'ascella sinistra.

Nel caso di difetti AV completi, lo scompenso cardiaco e le infezioni polmonari intercorrenti di solito si manifestano nell'infanzia. Durante questi episodi si può riscontrare una minima cianosi. Il fegato è ingrandito e il lattante presenta segni di ritardo di crescita. L'ingrandimento cardiaco è moderato o marcato, e spesso è palpabile un fremito a livello del margine sternale inferiore sinistro. Può essere anche presente una bozza e un sollevamento precordiale. Il primo tono è normale o rinforzato. Il secondo tono cardiaco è ampiamente sdoppiato se il flusso polmonare è massivo. È udibile un soffio di bassa tonalità, mesodiastolico, rullante, a livello del margine sternale inferiore sinistro, e un soffio sistolico da eiezione della polmonare viene prodotto dall'imponente flusso polmonare. Può essere presente anche l'aspro soffio olosistolico apicale tipico dell'insufficienza mitralica.

DIAGNOSI. Le radiografie del torace dei bambini con difetti AV completi spesso evidenziano un ingrandimento cardiaco da moderato a grave, causato dalla prominenza sia dei ventricoli sia degli atri. L'arteria polmonare è ingrandita, e si osserva un incremento della vascolarizzazione polmonare. Nei pazienti con difetto AV completo l'elettrocardiogramma è caratteristico. Le anomalie principali sono: (1) orientamento verso l'alto dell'asse medio del QRS sul piano frontale con deviazione assiale sinistra verso il quadrante superiore sinistro o superiore destro, (2) iscrizione antioraria del vettore QRS orientato verso l'alto, (3) segni di ipertrofia biventricolare o ventricolare destra isolata, (4) ritardo di conduzione ventricolare destra (aspetto RSR' nelle derivazioni V_3R e V_1), (5) onde P normali o alte e (6) talvolta prolungamento dell'intervallo PR (Fig. 426-5).

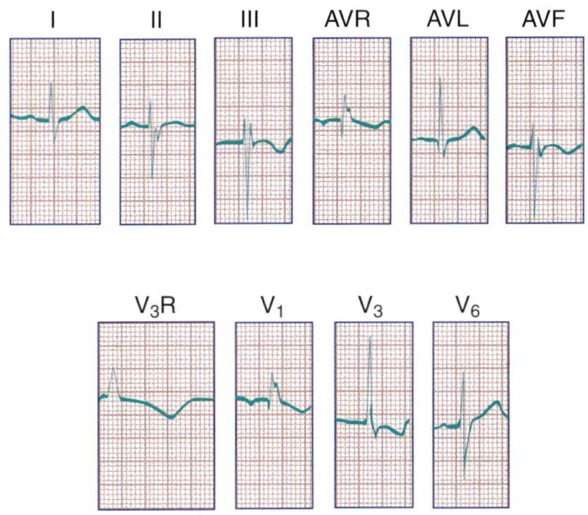

Figura 426-5. Elettrocardiogramma di un bambino con difetto del setto AV. Si notino l'asse del QRS a −60° e il ritardo di conduzione ventricolare destra con aspetto RSR' in V1 e V3R (velocità della carta in V3R = 50 mm/s).

L'ecocardiogramma (Fig. 426-6) è caratteristico ed evidenzia segni di ingrandimento ventricolare destro con invasione di echi della valvola mitrale sul tratto di efflusso ventricolare sinistro; la posizione abnormemente bassa delle valvole AV configura una deformità "a collo d'oca" del tratto di efflusso ventricolare sia all'ecocardiogramma sia all'angiografia. Nei cuori normali, la valvola tricuspide si inserisce un po' più verso l'apice rispetto alla valvola mitrale. Nel difetto del setto AV, entrambe le valvole si inseriscono allo stesso livello a causa dell'assenza del setto AV. Inoltre, nei difetti AV completi, l'eco del setto ventricolare è debole e si apprezza facilmente la valvola AV comune. L'ecocardiogramma con Doppler pulsato e color-Doppler evidenzierà uno shunt sinistro-destro a livello atriale, ventricolare o dal ventricolo all'atrio, e permetterà di calcolare in modo semiquantitativo il grado di insufficienza della valvola AV. L'ecocardiografia è utile per determinare i punti di inserzione delle corde della valvola AV comune e per valutare la presenza di lesioni associate, come il dotto arterioso pervio (PDA, *Patent Ductus Arteriosus*) o la coartazione aortica.

Ormai è raro che si rendano necessari il cateterismo cardiaco e l'angiocardiografia per la conferma della diagnosi, a meno che non sorga il sospetto di una patologia vascolare polmonare, per esempio in un paziente in cui la diagnosi è stata formulata dopo l'infanzia. Il cateterismo evidenzia l'ampiezza dello shunt sinistro-destro, il grado di aumento della resistenza vascolare polmonare e la gravità dell'insufficienza della valvola AV comune. Con l'ossimetria di solito è possibile dimostrare lo shunt sia a livello atriale sia a livello ventricolare. La saturazione arteriosa di ossigeno è normale o di poco ridotta, a meno che non sia presente una grave vasculopatia polmonare. I bambini con difetti tipo ostium primum generalmente hanno una pressione arteriosa polmonare normale o solo moderatamente elevata. D'altro canto, i difetti AV completi sono associati a ipertensione atriale destra e polmonare e, in pazienti più grandi, ad aumento delle resistenze vascolari polmonari (vedi Capitolo 433.2).

La ventricolografia sinistra selettiva evidenzierà la deformità della valvola mitrale o della valvola AV comune e la conseguente distorsione del tratto di efflusso ventricolare sinistro (deformità "a collo d'oca"). Il lembo anteriore della valvola mitrale, anomalo, è serrato, e si nota un'insufficienza mitralica, di solito con rigurgito di sangue negli atri sinistro e destro. Può essere dimostrato uno shunt diretto di sangue dal ventricolo sinistro all'atrio destro.

TRATTAMENTO. I difetti tipo ostium primum sono trattati chirurgicamente con un approccio che inizia con un incisione nell'atrio destro. La schisi a livello della valvola mitrale viene localizzata attraverso il difetto atriale e riparata mediante sutura diretta. Il difetto del setto atriale di solito viene chiuso mediante inserzione di un patch protesico. Il tasso di mortalità chirurgica per i difetti tipo ostium primum è molto basso. Più difficile è il trattamento chirurgico dei difetti AV completi, specialmente nei lattanti con scompenso cardiaco e ipertensione polmonare. A causa del rischio che si sviluppi una **patologia vascolare polmonare** dai 6-12

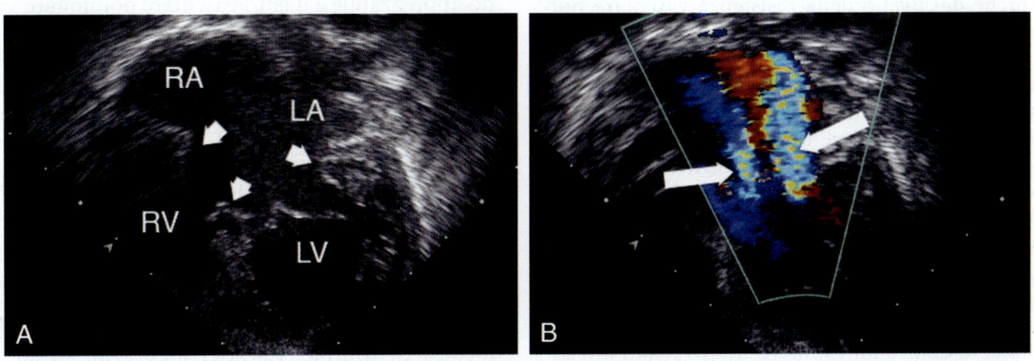

Figura 426-6. Ecocardiogramma di un difetto del setto atrioventricolare. *A*, Proiezione sottocostale a quattro camere da cui emerge che la valvola atrioventricolare comune (*frecce*) abbraccia i difetti del setto interatriale e interventricolare. *B*, Immagine Doppler che evidenzia due flussi di rigurgito attraverso il lato sinistro della valvola atrioventricolare comune (*frecce*). LA, atrio sinistro; LV, ventricolo sinistro; RA, atrio destro; RV, ventricolo destro.

mesi di età, l'intervento chirurgico deve essere effettuato nella prima infanzia. La correzione di questi difetti può essere ottenuta nell'infanzia e l'intervento palliativo mediante bendaggio dell'arteria polmonare è riservato a quel sottogruppo di pazienti che hanno altre lesioni associate, le quali renderebbero troppo rischiosa la correzione chirurgica precoce. I difetti atriali e ventricolari sono riparati mediante patch e le valvole AV vengono ricostruite. La complicanze comprendono il blocco cardiaco indotto chirurgicamente, che richiede il posizionamento di un pacemaker permanente, l'eccessivo restringimento del tratto di efflusso ventricolare sinistro, che impone la revisione chirurgica, e infine un peggioramento del rigurgito mitralico, che rende necessaria la sostituzione con protesi valvolare.

PROGNOSI. La prognosi per i difetti AV completi non sottoposti a correzione dipende dall'entità dello shunt sinistro-destro, dall'entità dell'aumento della resistenza vascolare polmonare e dalla gravità dell'insufficienza della valvola AV. La morte per insufficienza cardiaca durante l'infanzia era frequente prima dell'avvento della correzione chirurgica precoce. Nei pazienti non sottoposti a intervento chirurgico che sopravvivevano si sviluppava una patologia vascolare ostruttiva polmonare o, più raramente, una stenosi polmonare. La maggior parte dei pazienti con difetti tipo ostium primum e minimo coinvolgimento valvolare AV sono asintomatici o hanno solo sintomi minori e non progressivi fino al raggiungimento della 3ª-4ª decade di vita, presentando un decorso simile a quello dei pazienti con ASD tipo ostium secundum. Le complicanze postoperatorie tardive comprendono aritmie atriali e blocco cardiaco, progressivo restringimento del tratto di efflusso del ventricolo sinistro, che richiede la revisione chirurgica, e infine un peggioramento del rigurgito valvolare atrioventricolare (di solito dal lato sinistro), che impone la sostituzione con protesi valvolare.

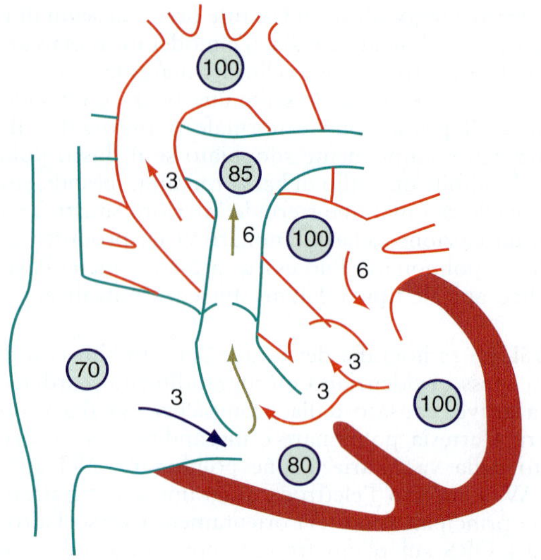

Figura 426-7. Fisiologia di un ampio VSD. I *numeri cerchiati* rappresentano i valori di saturazione d'ossigeno. I *numeri accanto alle frecce* rappresentano i volumi del flusso sanguigno (in L/min/m^2). Questa illustrazione rappresenta il caso di un ipotetico paziente con rapporto flusso sanguigno polmonare/sistemico (Qp:Qs) di 2:1. Il sangue desaturato entra nell'atrio destro dalla vena cava a un volume di 3 L/min/m^2 e attraversa la valvola tricuspide. Altri 3 L di sangue sono deviati da sinistra a destra attraverso il VSD, determinando un aumento della saturazione di ossigeno nel ventricolo destro. Sei litri di sangue vengono spinti nei polmoni. La saturazione arteriosa polmonare può essere ulteriormente aumentata a causa del mescolamento incompleto a livello del ventricolo destro. Sei litri ritornano all'atrio sinistro, attraversano la valvola mitrale e provocano un rullio mesodiastolico. Di questo volume, 3 L sono deviati da sinistra a destra attraverso il VSD e gli altri 3 L sono spinti nell'aorta ascendente (normale gittata cardiaca).

426.6 • DIFETTO DEL SETTO INTERVENTRICOLARE

Il VSD è la malformazione cardiaca più comune, che rende conto del 25% delle cardiopatie congenite. I difetti, per lo più di tipo membranoso, possono essere localizzati in qualsiasi porzione del setto ventricolare; si trovano in posizione posteroinferiore, anteriormente al lembo settale della valvola tricuspide. I VSD tra la cresta sopraventricolare e il muscolo papillare del cono possono essere associati a stenosi polmonare e ad altre manifestazioni della tetralogia di Fallot (vedi Capitolo 430.1). Meno comuni sono i VSD situati superiormente alla cresta sopraventricolare (sopracristali); localizzati appena al di sotto della valvola polmonare, possono estendersi al seno aortico e provocare un'insufficienza aortica. I VSD nella porzione intermedia o nella regione apicale del setto ventricolare sono di tipo muscolare e possono essere singoli o multipli (setto "a gruviera").

FISIOPATOLOGIA. La grandezza fisica del VSD è il determinante principale, ma non l'unico, dell'entità dello shunt sinistro-destro, la quale dipende anche dal livello della resistenza vascolare polmonare a confronto con la resistenza vascolare sistemica. Quando è presente una piccola comunicazione (di solito $<0,5$ cm^2), il VSD viene detto **restrittivo** e la pressione ventricolare destra è normale. La pressione più elevata del ventricolo sinistro determina uno shunt sinistro-destro; le dimensioni del difetto limitano l'ampiezza dello shunt. In ampi **VSD non restrittivi** (di solito $>1,0$ cm^2) le pressioni ventricolari destra e sinistra sono uguali; la direzione dello shunt e la sua ampiezza sono determinate dal rapporto tra resistenza vascolare polmonare e resistenza vascolare sistemica (Fig. 426-7).

Dopo la nascita, la presenza di un grande VSD può far sì che la resistenza vascolare polmonare si mantenga più elevata del normale e che l'ampiezza dello shunt sinistro-destro risulti inizialmente limitata. Nelle prime settimane dopo la nascita, a mano a mano che la resistenza vascolare polmonare continua a ridursi a causa della normale involuzione della tonaca media delle piccole arteriole polmonari, l'entità dello shunt sinistro-destro aumenta. Infine si sviluppa un ampio shunt sinistro-destro e i sintomi clinici divengono evidenti. Nella maggior parte dei casi durante la prima infanzia la resistenza vascolare polmonare è solo lievemente elevata e il principale contributo all'ipertensione polmonare è rappresentato da un flusso ematico polmonare molto abbondante. Tuttavia, in alcuni bambini con un VSD ampio lo spessore della tonaca media delle arteriole polmonari non diminuisce mai. La continua esposizione del letto vascolare polmonare a valori elevati di pressione sistolica e flusso comporta l'insorgenza di una vasculopatia polmonare ostruttiva. Quando il rapporto tra la resistenza polmonare e quella sistemica si avvicina a 1:1, lo shunt diviene bidirezionale, i segni di insufficienza cardiaca si attenuano e il paziente diventa cianotico (fenomeno di Eisenmenger, vedi Capitolo 433.2).

L'ampiezza degli shunt intracardiaci di solito è espressa dal rapporto Qp:Qs. Se lo shunt sinistro-destro è piccolo (Qp:Qs $<1,75:1$) le camere cardiache non risulteranno ingrandite in modo apprezzabile e il letto vascolare polmonare sarà probabilmente normale. Se lo shunt è ampio (Qp:Qs $>2:1$), si verificherà un sovraccarico di volume atriale e ventricolare sinistro, come anche un'ipertensione arteriosa polmonare e ventricolare destra. L'arteria polmonare principale, l'atrio sinistro e il ventricolo sinistro risultano ingranditi.

MANIFESTAZIONI CLINICHE. La presentazione clinica dei pazienti con VSD varia a seconda sia della grandezza del difetto, sia del flusso sanguigno e della pressione polmonare. Piccoli VSD con shunt sinistro-destro di poco conto e normali pressioni arteriose polmonari sono i più comuni. Questi pazienti sono asintomatici e di solito la lesione cardiaca viene scoperta durante una visita medica di routine. Caratteristico è un soffio olosistolico forte, aspro o soffiante, che si apprezza meglio a livello del margine sternale inferiore sinistro ed è frequentemente accompagnato da un fremito. In pochi casi il soffio si estingue prima del secondo tono, presumibilmente a causa della chiusura del difetto in telesistole. Un soffio sistolico breve, aspro, localizzato all'apice in un neonato è spesso un segno di un piccolo VSD muscolare. Subito dopo la nascita lo shunt sinistro-destro può essere minimo, a causa della pressione più elevata nelle sezioni destre, motivo per cui il soffio sistolico può non essere udibile durante i primi giorni di vita. Nei prematuri, il soffio può essere apprezzato precocemente poiché la resistenza vascolare polmonare diminuisce più rapidamente.

Nella prima infanzia, ampi VSD con flusso sanguigno eccessivo e ipertensione polmonare sono responsabili di dispnea, difficoltà di alimentazione, ritardo di crescita, sudorazione profusa, infezioni polmonari ricorrenti e scompenso cardiaco. La cianosi è di solito assente, ma talvolta si osserva un colorito cutaneo più scuro in corso di infezioni o durante il pianto. Sono comuni una prominenza del precordio di sinistra, un sollevamento parasternale palpabile, un itto apicale spostato lateralmente, un impulso apicale e un fremito sistolico. Il soffio olosistolico di un ampio VSD è generalmente meno aspro di quello di un VSD piccolo e di natura più soffiante per l'assenza di un significativo gradiente pressorio attraverso il difetto. Inoltre, è meno probabile apprezzarlo nel periodo neonatale. La componente polmonare del secondo tono cardiaco può essere aumentata come risultato di un'ipertensione polmonare. La presenza di un rullio mesodiastolico, a bassa tonalità all'apice, è riconducibile a un aumentato flusso sanguigno attraverso la valvola mitrale e indica un rapporto Qp:Qs ≥2:1. Il soffio si apprezza meglio con la campana dello stetoscopio.

DIAGNOSI. In pazienti con piccoli VSD, la radiografia del torace è di solito normale, anche se si può osservare una lievissima cardiomegalia e un incremento borderline della vascolarizzazione polmonare. L'elettrocardiogramma è generalmente normale, ma può suggerire un'ipertrofia ventricolare sinistra. La presenza di un'ipertrofia ventricolare destra sta a indicare che il difetto non è piccolo e che il paziente ha un'ipertensione polmonare o una lesione associata come una stenosi polmonare. In VSD ampi, la radiografia del torace evidenzia una macroscopica cardiomegalia con prominenza di entrambi i ventricoli, dell'atrio sinistro e dell'arteria polmonare (Fig. 426-8). I segni di vascolarizzazione polmonare sono aumentati e può essere presente un franco edema polmonare, con versamento pleurico. L'elettrocardiogramma evidenzia un'ipertrofia biventricolare e le onde P possono essere indentate o appuntite.

L'ecocardiogramma bidimensionale (Fig. 426-9) evidenzia la posizione e la dimensione del VSD. I difetti piccoli, specialmente quelli del setto muscolare, possono essere difficili da visualizzare e vengono evidenziati solo dal color-Doppler. Nei difetti del **setto membranoso**, una sottile membrana (detta **aneurisma del setto interventricolare**, anche se è formata da tessuto della valvola tricuspide) può coprire parzialmente il difetto e limitare il volume dello shunt sinistro-destro. L'ecocardiografia, inoltre, è utile per la stima dell'entità dello shunt, rilevando il grado di sovraccarico di volume dell'atrio e del ventricolo sinistri; in assenza di lesioni associate, l'entità del loro aumento di dimensioni riflette

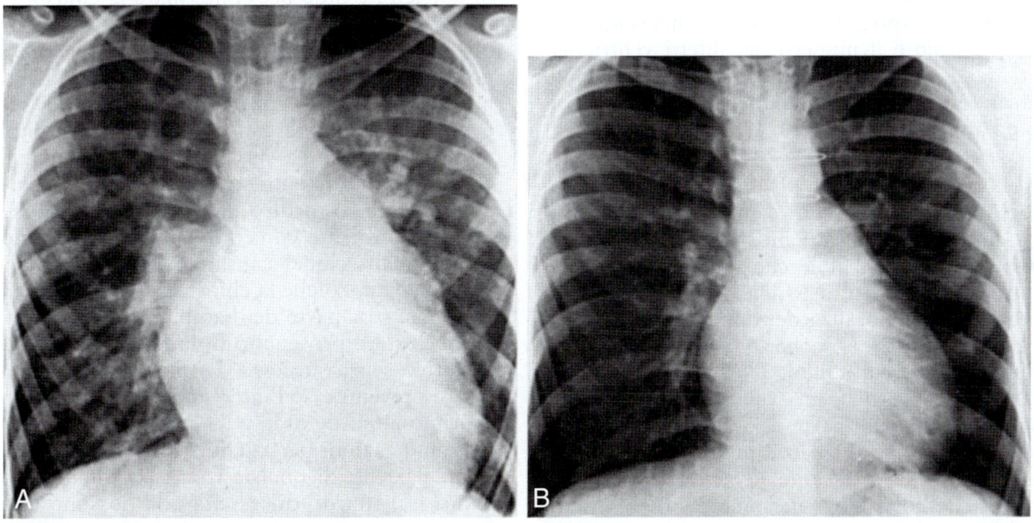

Figura 426-8. *A*, Radiogramma preoperatorio di un paziente che presenta un VSD con ampio shunt sinistro-destro e ipertensione polmonare. Sono evidenti una significativa cardiomegalia, una prominenza del tronco dell'arteria polmonare e un iperafflusso polmonare. *B*, Tre anni dopo la chiusura chirurgica del difetto, le dimensioni del cuore risultano marcatamente diminuite e la vascolarizzazione polmonare è normale.

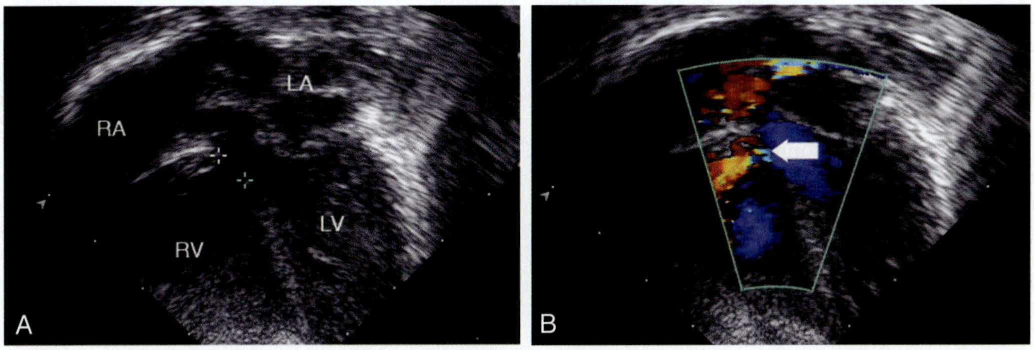

Figura 426-9. Ecocardiogramma in un paziente con un VSD perimembranoso. *A*, Proiezione apicale a quattro camere che mostra la sede del difetto (evidenziato tra i due *marcatori*) al di sotto della valvola aortica. *B*, L'immagine color-Doppler mostra lo shunt sinistro-destro (*freccia*) attraverso il difetto (il colore rosso indica il sangue che si muove verso il trasduttore di ultrasuoni e non il livello di ossigenazione del sangue). LA (*Left Atrium*), atrio sinistro; LV (*Left Ventricle*), ventricolo sinistro; RA (*Right Atrium*), atrio destro; RV (*Right Ventricle*), ventricolo destro.

la grandezza dello shunt sinistro-destro. L'esame con il Doppler pulsato mostra se il VSD è restrittivo per quanto concerne la pressione, calcolando il gradiente pressorio attraverso il difetto. Tale calcolo permette di stimare la pressione ventricolare destra e aiuta a stabilire se il paziente è a rischio di sviluppare una precoce patologia vascolare polmonare. L'ecocardiogramma può essere utile anche per determinare la presenza di un'insufficienza valvolare aortica o di un prolasso dei lembi valvolari in caso di VSD sovracristali.

Le caratteristiche emodinamiche di un VSD possono essere dimostrate mediante cateterismo cardiaco, che tuttavia oggi viene eseguito solo quando l'entità dello shunt non è chiara dopo una valutazione clinica completa, quando i dati di laboratorio non coincidono con i reperti clinici o quando si sospetta una patologia vascolare polmonare. L'ossimetria evidenzia un aumento del contenuto di ossigeno nel ventricolo destro; poiché alcuni difetti spingono il sangue quasi direttamente nell'arteria polmonare (a getto), questo aumento talvolta appare evidente solo quando si procede a un campionamento di sangue arterioso polmonare. Piccoli VSD restrittivi sono associati a normali pressioni nelle sezioni destre e normale resistenza vascolare polmonare. Ampi VSD non restrittivi sono associati a pressioni polmonari e sistemiche uguali o quasi uguali. Il flusso sanguigno polmonare può essere da due a quattro volte più elevato di quello sistemico. In pazienti con una tale "**ipertensione polmonare iperdinamica**" la resistenza vascolare polmonare sarà solo minimamente elevata, poiché la resistenza è uguale alla pressione diviso il flusso. Se è presente il fenomeno di Eisenmenger, le pressioni sistolica e diastolica in arteria polmonare sono elevate, il grado di shunt sinistro-destro è minimo e si verifica una desaturazione del sangue nel ventricolo sinistro. L'ampiezza, la sede e il numero dei difetti ventricolari sono evidenziati dalla ventricolografia sinistra. Il mezzo di contrasto passa attraverso il difetto (o i difetti) opacizzando il ventricolo sinistro e l'arteria polmonare.

TRATTAMENTO. Il decorso naturale del VSD dipende in gran parte dalle dimensioni del difetto. Un numero significativo (30-50%) di piccoli difetti si chiude spontaneamente, per lo più durante i primi 2 anni di vita. È più probabile che si chiudano piccoli VSD muscolari (fino all'80%) piuttosto che VSD membranosi (fino al 35%). La grande maggioranza dei difetti che si chiudono avviene prima dei 4 anni di età, anche se sono stati riportati casi di chiusura spontanea in età adulta. I VSD che si chiudono spesso hanno un aneurisma del setto ventricolare che limita l'ampiezza dello shunt. La maggior parte dei bambini con piccoli difetti rimane asintomatica, senza evidenza né di ingrandimento cardiaco, né di aumento della pressione in arteria polmonare o delle resistenze. Un rischio a lungo termine è rappresentato dall'endocardite infettiva. Alcuni studi a lungo termine su adulti con piccoli VSD non operati evidenziano una maggiore incidenza di aritmie, stenosi subaortica e intolleranza allo sforzo. Secondo il Council on Cardiovascular Disease in the Young dell'American Heart Association, un VSD isolato, piccolo ed emodinamicamente non significativo non è un'indicazione all'intervento chirurgico. Il rischio sempre minore correlato alla chirurgia cardiaca ha condotto altri a suggerire la chiusura di tutti i VSD in elezione a partire dalla media infanzia.

È meno comune che VSD di dimensioni moderate o grandi si chiudano spontaneamente, anche se difetti abbastanza ampi da determinare scompenso cardiaco possono ridursi fino al punto di chiudersi (evenienza che si verifica nell'8% dei casi). È più comune che bambini con ampi difetti abbiano ripetuti episodi di infezioni respiratorie e scompenso cardiaco, nonostante una gestione medica ottimale. Lo scompenso cardiaco può manifestarsi in molti di questi soggetti come un ritardo di crescita. L'ipertensione polmonare insorge come risultato di un elevato flusso sanguigno polmonare. Questi pazienti sono a rischio di sviluppare con il tempo una patologia vascolare polmonare se il difetto non viene riparato.

I pazienti con VSD sono anche a rischio di un rigurgito valvolare aortico, soprattutto se hanno un VSD sopracristale (vedi Capitolo 426.7). Un piccolo numero di pazienti con VSD presenta una **stenosi infundibolare polmonare acquisita**, che protegge la circolazione polmonare dagli effetti a breve termine della sovracircolazione e dagli effetti a lungo termine della patologia vascolare polmonare. In questi pazienti il quadro clinico passa da un VSD con ampio shunt sinistro-destro a un VSD con stenosi polmonare. Lo shunt può ridursi di dimensioni, diventare bilanciato o trasformarsi in un netto shunt destro-sinistro. Questi pazienti devono essere distinti da quelli che sviluppano il fenomeno di Eisenmenger (vedi Capitolo 433.2).

Se il paziente ha un VSD piccolo, occorre rassicurare i genitori sulla relativa benignità della lesione e incoraggiare il bambino a condurre una vita normale, senza restrizioni dell'attività fisica. La correzione chirurgica non è al momento raccomandata. Come protezione contro l'endocardite infettiva, è importante salvaguardare l'integrità della dentatura decidua e permanente; andrebbe effettuata la profilassi antibiotica per le visite odontoiatriche (comprese le sedute di igiene dentale), gli interventi di tonsillectomia e adenoidectomia e altre procedure chirurgiche orofaringee, come anche per manovre strumentali del tratto genitourinario e del tratto terminale dell'intestino (vedi Capitolo 437). Questi pazienti possono essere monitorati con esami clinici e test di laboratorio non invasivi finché il VSD non si chiude spontaneamente. L'elettrocardiogramma può essere utilizzato per lo screening di una possibile ipertensione polmonare o stenosi polmonare, segnalata da un'ipertrofia ventricolare destra. L'ecocardiografia, oltre a permettere lo screening dello sviluppo di una patologia del tratto di efflusso del ventricolo sinistro (membrana subaortica o rigurgito aortico), è utile per confermare la chiusura spontanea.

Nei bambini con un VSD ampio la gestione medica mira a due obiettivi: controllare lo scompenso cardiaco e prevenire lo sviluppo di una patologia vascolare polmonare. Le misure terapeutiche hanno lo scopo di controllare i sintomi di scompenso cardiaco e assicurare una crescita normale (vedi Capitolo 442). Se il trattamento precoce ha successo, lo shunt può ridursi di grandezza con un miglioramento spontaneo, specialmente durante il primo anno di vita. Il medico deve porre attenzione a non confondere un miglioramento clinico dovuto a una riduzione del difetto con cambiamenti clinici causati dallo sviluppo di un fenomeno di Eisenmenger. Poiché la chiusura chirurgica comporta scarsi rischi nella maggior parte dei bambini, il trattamento medico non dovrebbe essere proseguito in lattanti sintomatici dopo un iniziale tentativo senza successo. La patologia vascolare polmonare può essere prevenuta se l'intervento chirurgico viene effettuato entro il primo anno di vita.

Le indicazioni per la chiusura chirurgica di un VSD comprendono pazienti di qualsiasi età con difetti ampi in cui i sintomi clinici e il ritardo di crescita non possono essere controllati con la terapia medica; i lattanti di 6-12 mesi di vita con ampi difetti associati a ipertensione polmonare, anche se i sintomi sono controllati dalla terapia medica; i pazienti di età superiore a 24 mesi con un rapporto Qp:Qs superiore a 2:1. I pazienti con VSD sopracristali di qualsiasi dimensione di solito sono candidati all'intervento chirurgico a causa dell'elevato rischio di rigurgito valvolare aortico (vedi Capitolo 426.7). Una grave vasculopatia polmonare è una controindicazione alla chiusura di un VSD.

PROGNOSI. I risultati della riparazione chirurgica primaria sono eccellenti e le complicanze che portano a problemi a lungo termine (shunt ventricolari residui che richiedono un reintervento o un blocco cardiaco che richiede l'impianto di pacemaker) sono rare. Il bendaggio palliativo dell'arteria polmonare con riparazione nella tarda infanzia è riservato a casi complicati o a neonati molto prematuri. I rischi chirurgici sono più elevati per difetti del setto muscolare, in particolare difetti apicali e VSD multipli (tipo "gruviera"). Questi pazienti, se sintomatici, possono necessitare di un bendaggio dell'arteria polmonare, con riparazione dei VSD multipli in età più avanzata. I **cateteri di occlusione** sono attualmente sottoposti a valutazione come metodi di chiusura di VSD apicali muscolari, mentre altri dispositivi vengono testati per la chiusura di difetti perimembranosi più comuni. Dopo la chiusura chirurgica dello shunt sinistro-destro, il cuore iperdinamico si acquieta, le dimensioni cardiache diminuiscono fino a tornare alla normalità (vedi Fig. 426-8), fremiti e soffi scompaiono e l'ipertensione arteriosa polmonare regredisce. La condizione clinica del paziente migliora notevolmente. La maggior parte dei bambini inizia a crescere e la farmacoterapia non è più necessaria. Nel giro dei successivi 1-2 anni la maggior parte dei pazienti raggiunge peso e altezza normali. In alcuni casi dopo un intervento chirurgico condotto con successo, i soffi sistolici da eiezione di basse intensità persistono per mesi. La prognosi a lungo termine dopo l'intervento chirurgico è eccellente. I pazienti con un piccolo VSD e quelli sottoposti a chiusura chirurgica completa sono considerati a rischio standard per quanto riguarda l'aspettativa di vita e l'assicurazione vita.

426.7 • Difetto del setto interventricolare sopracristale con insufficienza aortica

Il VSD sopracristale è complicato da prolasso della valvola aortica nel difetto e insufficienza aortica, che possono manifestarsi nel 50-90% dei pazienti. Pur colpendo il 5% circa di tutti i pazienti, ha un'incidenza più elevata nei bambini asiatici. Il VSD, che può essere piccolo o medio, è situato anteriormente e direttamente al di sotto della valvolare polmonare nel setto di efflusso, al di sopra della cresta sopraventricolare. L'insufficienza aortica è talvolta associata a VSD situati nel setto membranoso. La cuspide aortica destra o, meno spesso, quella non coronarica prolassa nel difetto fino a occluderlo, parzialmente o completamente. Tale occlusione può limitare l'entità dello shunt sinistro-destro e dare la falsa impressione che il difetto non sia ampio. Nella maggior parte dei casi l'insufficienza aortica non viene riconosciuta finché il bambino non ha compiuto i 10 anni o anche oltre.

È raro che si verifichi uno scompenso cardiaco precoce, secondario a un ampio shunt sinistro-destro, ma se non si interviene chirurgicamente possono far seguito una grave insufficienza aortica e uno scompenso ventricolare sinistro. Il soffio di un VSD sopracristale, che di solito si ode in corrispondenza del margine sternale medio-superiore, anziché in corrispondenza del margine sternale inferiore sinistro, viene spesso confuso con quello della stenosi polmonare. I segni fisici di insufficienza aortica (soffio diastolico ed elevata pressione differenziale), quando presenti, si aggiungono a quelli del VSD. Questi reperti clinici devono essere distinti dal PDA o da altri difetti associati a insufficienza aortica.

Le manifestazioni cliniche variano ampiamente, da un banale rigurgito aortico con piccoli shunt sinistro-destri in bambini asintomatici a un'insufficienza aortica florida e a una spiccata cardiomegalia in adolescenti sintomatici. La chiusura di tutti i VSD ventricolari sopracristali al momento della diagnosi è comunemente raccomandata per prevenire lo sviluppo di un rigurgito aortico, anche in un bambino asintomatico. I pazienti che hanno già una significativa insufficienza aortica necessitano di intervento chirurgico volto a prevenire una disfunzione ventricolare sinistra irreversibile. Le opzioni chirurgiche, scelte in base all'entità del danno riportato dalla valvola, comprendono la valvuloplatica per un coinvolgimento lieve e la sostituzione con una protesi o un omograft oppure la traslocazione aortopolmonare (vedi Capitolo 427.5) per i quadri più gravi.

426.8 • Dotto arterioso pervio

Durante la vita fetale la maggior parte del sangue arterioso polmonare viene deviato nell'aorta attraverso il dotto arterioso (vedi Capitolo 421). Normalmente tale dotto va incontro a chiusura funzionale poco dopo la nascita, ma se questo non avviene quando la resistenza vascolare polmonare si riduce, il sangue aortico viene deviato in arteria polmonare. L'estremità aortica del dotto è appena distale all'origine dell'arteria succlavia sinistra, e il dotto entra nell'arteria polmonare alla sua biforcazione. Il PDA, più frequente nelle femminile che nei maschi (rapporto pari a 2:1), è inoltre associato all'infezione materna da rosolia durante i primi mesi di gestazione. È un problema comune nei prematuri, in cui può causare squilibri emodinamici di notevole entità e gravi sequele (vedi Capitolo 101.4).

Nel neonato a termine con PDA la parete del dotto è priva sia dello strato endoteliale mucoide sia della tonaca media muscolare, mentre nel prematuro il PDA di solito ha una struttura normale; la pervietà è il risultato di ipossia e immaturità. Perciò, è raro che un PDA che persiste oltre le prime settimane di vita in un neonato a termine si chiuda spontaneamente o in seguito a un trattamento farmacologico; nel prematuro invece, se non è richiesto un precoce intervento farmacologico o chirurgico, nella maggior parte dei casi si verifica la chiusura spontanea. Il PDA si osserva nel 10% dei pazienti con altre cardiopatie congenite e spesso gioca un ruolo critico nel provvedere al flusso sanguigno polmonare quando il tratto di efflusso del ventricolo destro è stenotico o atresico (vedi Capitolo 427.6) o al flusso sanguigno sistemico in presenza di una coartazione o di un'interruzione aortica (vedi Capitolo 427.8).

FISIOPATOLOGIA. In conseguenza della più elevata pressione aortica, il sangue viene deviato da sinistra a destra attraverso il dotto, dall'aorta all'arteria polmonare. L'entità dello shunt dipende dalla grandezza del dotto e dal rapporto tra la resistenza vascolare polmonare e quella sistemica. In casi estremi, il 70% della gittata ventricolare può essere deviato attraverso il dotto nella circolazione polmonare. Se il PDA è piccolo, la pressione in arteria polmonare, nel ventricolo destro e nell'atrio destro è normale; se invece è grande, la pressione in arteria polmonare può essere così elevata da uguagliare quella sistemica, sia durante la sistole sia durante la diastole. I pazienti con un ampio PDA sono a rischio elevatissimo di sviluppare una patologia vascolare polmonare se non operati. La pressione differenziale è ampia, a causa dell'ingresso del sangue in arteria polmonare durante la diastole.

MANIFESTAZIONI CLINICHE. Un dotto pervio di scarsa entità di solito è asintomatico. Un ampio PDA porterà a uno scompenso cardiaco analogo a quello riscontrabile nei bambini con un ampio VSD. Il ritardo di crescita può essere una delle manifestazioni principali nei bambini con shunt ampi.

Un ampio PDA porterà a evidenti segni fisici attribuibili all'ampia pressione differenziale, e in particolare a polsi arteriosi periferici scoccanti. Il cuore è di dimensioni normali quando il dotto è piccolo, ma presenta un ingrandimento moderato o importante in casi di ampia comunicazione. L'itto apicale è prominente e, quando si instaura una dilatazione cardiaca, è palpabile un suo innalzamento. È spesso presente un fremito, che è massimo nel secondo spazio intercostale, e che può irradiarsi verso la clavicola sinistra, in basso, lungo il margine sternale inferiore sinistro o verso l'apice. È di solito sistolico, ma può essere palpato anche durante tutto il ciclo cardiaco. Il classico soffio continuo è descritto come "a locomotiva" o rombante. Si manifesta subito dopo l'inizio del primo tono, raggiunge la massima intensità alla fine della sistole e svanisce in telediastole. Può essere localizzato a livello del secondo spazio intercostale sinistro o irradiarsi verso il basso, lungo il margine sternale sinistro, o verso la clavicola sinistra. Quando si verifica un aumento della resistenza vascolare polmonare, la componente diastolica del soffio può essere meno marcata o assente. In pazienti con ampio shunt sinistro-destro può essere apprezzabile un soffio di bassa tonalità mitralico mesodiastolico all'apice, per effetto del maggior volume di sangue che attraversa la valvola mitrale.

DIAGNOSI. Se lo shunt sinistro-destro è piccolo, l'elettrocardiogramma è normale; se il dotto è ampio, è presente ipertrofia ventricolare sinistra o biventricolare. La diagnosi di PDA isolato e non complicato è insostenibile quando si nota un'ipertrofia ventricolare destra.

Studi radiografici nei paziente con PDA ampi evidenziano un'arteria polmonare prominente con aumentati segni di iperafflusso polmonare. Il cuore può avere dimensioni normali oppure essere moderatamente o marcatamente ingrandito, a seconda del grado di shunt sinistro-destro. Le camere coinvolte sono l'atrio sinistro e il ventricolo sinistro. L'arco aortico è normale o sporgente.

L'aspetto ecocardiografico delle camere cardiache è normale se il dotto arterioso è piccolo. Con shunt ampi le dimensioni dell'atrio sinistro e del ventricolo sinistro risultano aumentate. Per calcolare le dimensioni dell'atrio sinistro di solito si fa riferimento alla grandezza della radice aortica (rapporto LA:Ao [atrio sinistro: radice aortica]). La proiezione radiografica dall'incisura sovrasternale permette la visualizzazione diretta del dotto. Il color-Doppler e il Doppler pulsato evidenziano un flusso turbolento sistolico o diastolico (o entrambi) retrogrado in arteria polmonare e un flusso aortico retrogrado in diastole (Fig. 426-10).

Il quadro clinico è sufficientemente caratteristico da permettere una diagnosi accurata mediante metodi non invasivi nella maggior parte dei pazienti. In presenza di reperti atipici o quando si sospettano lesioni cardiache associate può essere indicato il cateterismo cardiaco, che evidenzia una pressione in ventricolo destro e in arteria polmonare normale o elevata, a seconda delle dimensioni del dotto. La presenza di sangue ossigenato nell'arteria polmonare conferma uno shunt sinistro-destro. Attraverso il dotto, il catetere può passare dall'arteria polmonare all'aorta discendente. L'iniezione di mezzo di contrasto nell'aorta ascendente evidenzia un'opacizzazione dell'arteria polmonare dall'aorta e identifica il dotto.

Nella diagnosi differenziale, bisogna ricordare che anche altre condizioni possono dare origine a soffi sistolici e diastolici nell'area della polmonare in assenza di cianosi. Le caratteristiche di un soffio venoso sono descritte nel Capitolo 422. È raro che una **finestra aortopolmonare** risulti clinicamente indistinguibile da un dotto pervio, anche se nella maggior parte dei casi il soffio è solo sistolico e si ode meglio in corrispondenza del margine sternale destro piuttosto che sinistro. Un aneurisma del seno di Valsalva che si sia rotto nelle sezioni destre del cuore o in arteria polmonare, fistole arterovenose coronariche e un'arteria coronaria sinistra aberrante con grandi collaterali dalla coronaria destra presentano dinamiche simili a quelle di un PDA con un soffio continuo e un'ampia pressione differenziale. Anche un tronco arterioso con un flusso polmonare torrenziale presenta un "rigurgito aortico" fisiologico. La stenosi di una diramazione della polmonare può associarsi a soffi sistolici e diastolici, ma la pressione differenziale è normale. Anche una fistola arterovenosa periferica determina un'ampia pressione differenziale, ma il soffio caratteristico di un PDA non è presente. Un VSD con insufficienza aortica e un'insufficienza reumatica combinata aortica e mitralica possono essere confusi con il PDA, ma i soffi dovrebbero essere differenziati per la loro caratteristica di "va e vieni" piuttosto che continua. La combinazione di un ampio VSD e di un PDA dà luogo a reperti più simili a quelli di un VSD isolato. L'ecocardiografia dovrebbe mettere in condizione di escludere queste alternative diagnostiche. Se vi è il sospetto clinico di un PDA, ma questo non viene visualizzato all'ecocardiografia, di solito è indicato il cateterismo cardiaco.

PROGNOSI E COMPLICANZE. I pazienti con un PDA piccolo possono avere una normale aspettativa di vita con sintomi cardiaci scarsi o assenti, anche se sussiste sempre la possibilità che si verifichino manifestazioni tardive. La chiusura spontanea del dotto è estremamente rara dopo l'infanzia. Lo scompenso cardiaco in età pediatrica si manifesta per lo più in presenza di un dotto ampio, ma può presentarsi a un'età più avanzata, anche con una comunicazione di dimensioni moderate. Con gli anni il sovraccarico cronico di volume del ventricolo sinistro è sempre meno tollerato.

L'endoarterite infettiva può insorgere a qualsiasi età. Possono verificarsi embolizzazioni polmonari o sistemiche. Complicanze rare comprendono dilatazioni aneurismatiche dell'arteria polmonare o del dotto, calcificazioni del dotto, trombosi non infettive del dotto con embolizzazione ed embolie paradosse. L'ipertensione polmonare (fenomeno di Eisenmenger) di solito si sviluppa in pazienti con un ampio PDA che non vengono sottoposti a intervento chirurgico (vedi Capitolo 433.2).

TRATTAMENTO. A prescindere dalla loro età, i pazienti con PDA necessitano della chiusura del difetto per via chirurgica o tramite catetere. Se il PDA è piccolo, il razionale per la chiusura consiste nella prevenzione dell'endocardite batterica o di altre complicanze tardive. Nel caso di PDA moderati o ampi, la chiusura viene effettuata per trattare lo scompenso cardiaco o prevenire lo sviluppo di una vasculopatia polmonare, o per entrambi questi motivi. Laddove sia fatta diagnosi di PDA moderato o ampio, il trattamento non dovrebbe essere ritardato eccessivamente, una volta che sia stata istituita un'adeguata terapia medica per lo scompenso cardiaco.

La chiusura di un PDA transcatetere viene effettuata di routine nel laboratorio di emodinamica (Fig. 426-11). I PDA piccoli vengono generalmente chiusi mediante spirali intravascolari, mentre per quelli moderati o ampi si utilizzano un sacchetto, introdotto mediante catetere in cui vengono rilasciate più spirali, o un dispositivo a ombrello. La chiusura chirurgica di un PDA può essere effettuata in toracotomia sinistra tradizionale o con tecniche di toracoscopia. Poiché il tasso di mortalità con il trattamento interventistico o chirurgico è di molto inferiore all'1% e il rischio in assenza di intervento è maggiore, la chiusura del dotto è indicata nei pazienti asintomatici, preferibilmente prima del primo anno di vita. L'ipertensione polmonare non è una controindicazione alla chirurgia a qualsiasi età, se è possibile dimostrare mediante cateterismo cardiaco che il flusso dello shunt è ancora prevalentemente sinistro-destro e che non è presente una vasculopatia polmonare grave. Dopo la chiusura, i sintomi di scompenso cardiaco franco o incipiente scompaiono rapidamente. Bambini con ritardo di crescita di solito presentano un immediato miglioramento dello sviluppo fisico. La frequenza cardiaca e la pressione sanguigna ritornano normali, e il soffio "a locomotiva" scompare. Talvolta persiste un soffio sistolico funzionale sul focolaio della polmonare, che può rappresentare

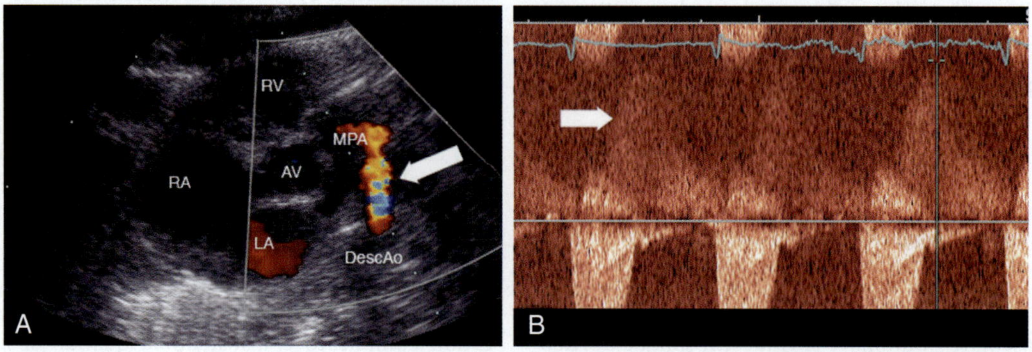

Figura 426-10. Ecocardiogramma in un neonato con PDA di dimensioni medio-piccole. *A*, Color-Doppler effettuato in proiezione parasternale asse corto, che evidenzia il flusso (*freccia*) dall'aorta nel tronco principale dell'arteria polmonare. *B*, La valutazione Doppler evidenzia un flusso diastolico retrogrado in arteria polmonare. AV, valvola aortica; DescAo, aorta discendente; LA, atrio sinistro; MPA (*Main Pulmonary Artery*), tronco principale dell'arteria polmonare; RA (*Right Atrium*), atrio destro; RV (*Right Ventricle*), ventricolo destro.

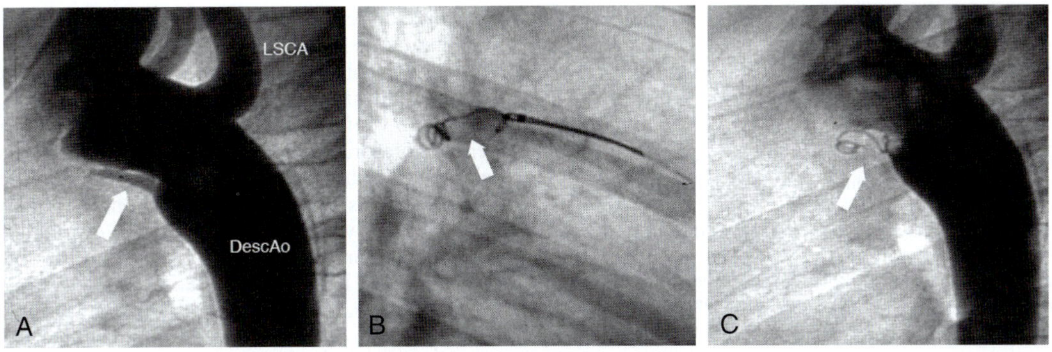

Figura 426-11. Chiusura transcatetere di un piccolo dotto arterioso pervio, effettuata utilizzando una spirale. *A*, Angiogramma dell'aorta traversa e discendente, che evidenzia un piccolo PDA (*freccia*). *B*, La spirale (*freccia*) è stata espulsa dalla guaina e posizionata nel lume del dotto. *C*, Angiogramma che mostra la totale occlusione del PDA da parte della spirale (*freccia*). DescAo, aorta discendente; LSCA (*Left SubClavian Artery*), arteria succlavia sinistra.

la turbolenza in un'arteria polmonare persistentemente dilatata. I segni radiografici di ingrandimento cardiaco e di iperafflusso polmonare scompaiono nell'arco di parecchi mesi e l'elettrocardiogramma diventa normale.

Dotto arterioso pervio in neonati con basso peso: vedi Capitolo 101.4.

426.9 • Finestra aortopolmonare

La finestra aortopolmonare è un difetto consistente in una comunicazione tra l'aorta ascendente e il tronco principale dell'arteria polmonare. La presenza delle valvole polmonare e aortica e di un setto ventricolare intatto distingue questa anomalia dal tronco arterioso (vedi Capitolo 431.8). I sintomi di scompenso cardiaco compaiono nella prima infanzia; a volte è presente una cianosi di minima entità. Il difetto è di solito ampio e il soffio cardiaco è sistolico con un rullio mesodiastolico per effetto di aumento del flusso ematico attraverso la valvola mitrale. Nella rara eventualità in cui la comunicazione sia più piccola e l'ipertensione polmonare assente, i reperti all'esame obiettivo possono simulare quelli del PDA (ampia pressione differenziale e un soffio continuo in corrispondenza dei margini sternali superiori). L'elettrocardiogramma evidenzia un'ipertrofia ventricolare sinistra o biventricolare. Gli studi radiografici mostrano un ingrandimento cardiaco, una prominenza dell'arteria polmonare e un'accentuazione della vascolarizzazione intrapolmonare. L'ecocardiogramma evidenzia un ingrandimento delle camere cardiache di sinistra; l'indagine che permette di visualizzare il difetto a finestra in modo ottimale è la flussimetria color-Doppler. Anche l'angioRM (MRA, *Magnetic Resonance Angiography*) può essere utilizzata per visualizzare il difetto (vedi Fig. 423-20).

Il cateterismo cardiaco evidenzia uno shunt sinistro-destro a livello dell'arteria polmonare, come pure un'ipertensione polmonare ipercinetica poiché il difetto è quasi sempre ampio. L'angiografia selettiva con iniezione di mezzo di contrasto nell'aorta ascendente evidenzia la lesione; anche la manipolazione del catetere dal tronco principale della polmonare direttamente in aorta ascendente è diagnostica.

La finestra aortopolmonare viene corretta chirurgicamente in età pediatrica con un bypass cardiopolmonare. Se non viene effettuato l'intervento chirurgico nell'infanzia, i pazienti che sopravvivono sono a rischio di una patologia vascolare polmonare ostruttiva progressiva, simile a quella dei pazienti che presentano ampie comunicazioni intracardiache o tra i grandi vasi.

426.10 • Fistola arterovenosa coronarica (fistola coronarocamerale)

Può esservi una fistola congenita tra un'arteria coronaria e un atrio, un ventricolo (specialmente il destro) o l'arteria polmonare. Talvolta vi sono fistole multiple. Indipendentemente della camera coinvolta, i segni clinici sono simili a quelli del PDA, anche se il soffio "a locomotiva" può essere più frequente. Se il flusso è di una certa entità, l'arteria coronaria coinvolta può essere dilatata o aneurismatica. L'anomalia anatomica è di solito dimostrabile con la flussimetria color-Doppler e, in corso di cateterismo, con l'iniezione di mezzo di contrasto nell'aorta ascendente. Piccole fistole possono essere emodinamicamente insignificanti, e addirittura chiudersi spontaneamente. Se lo shunt è ampio, il trattamento consiste nell'embolizzazione transcatetere con spirali o, in caso di lesioni non raggiungibili dal catetere, nella chiusura chirurgica della fistola.

426.11 • Rottura di aneurisma del seno di Valsalva

Quando uno dei seni di Valsalva dell'aorta è indebolito da una patologia congenita o acquisita, può formarsi un aneurisma soggetto a rottura, di solito nell'atrio destro o nel ventricolo. Questa condizione è estremamente rara nell'infanzia. L'esordio è di solito improvviso. La diagnosi dovrebbe essere sospettata nei pazienti che sviluppano sintomi di scompenso cardiaco acuto in associazione all'insorgenza di un nuovo soffio "va e vieni" ad alta tonalità. L'ecocardiografia color-Doppler e il cateterismo cardiaco evidenziano lo shunt sinistro-destro a livello atriale o ventricolare. È generalmente richiesta la riparazione chirurgica d'urgenza. Questa condizione è spesso associata a un'endocardite infettiva della valvola aortica.

Difetto del setto interatriale

Amin Z, Hijazi ZM, Bass JL, et al: Erosion of Amplatzer septal occluder device after closure of secundum atrial septal defects: Review of registry of complications and recommendations to minimize future risk. *Catheter Cardiovasc Interv* 2004;63:496–502.

Beda RD, Gill EA Jr: Patent foramen ovale: Does it play a role in the pathophysiology of migraine headache? *Cardiol Clin* 2005;23:91–96.

Benson DW, Silberbach GM, Kavanaugh-McHugh A, et al: Mutations in the cardiac transcription factor NKX2.5 affect diverse cardiac developmental pathways. *J Clin Invest* 1999;104:1567–1573.

Masura J, Gavora P, Podnar T: Long-term outcome of transcatheter secundum-type atrial septal defect closure using Amplatzer septal occluders. *J Am Coll Cardiol* 2005;45:505–507.

Radzik D, Davignon A, van Doesburg N, et al: Predictive factors for spontaneous closure of atrial septal defects diagnosed in the first 3 months of life. *J Am Coll Cardiol* 1993;22:851–853.

Riggs T, Sharp SE, Batton D, et al: Spontaneous closure of atrial septal defects in premature vs full term neonates. *Pediatr Cardiol* 2000;21:129–134.

Swartz EN: Is transcatheter device occlusion as good as open heart surgery for closure of atrial septal defects? *Arch Dis Child* 2004;89:687–688.

Yew G, Wilson NJ: Transcatheter atrial septal defect closure with the Amplatzer septal occluder: Five-year follow-up. *Catheter Cardiovasc Interv* 2005;64:193–196.

Difetti del setto atrioventricolare

Clapp SK, Perry BL, Farooki ZQ, et al: Surgical and medical results of complete atrioventricular canal: A ten-year review. *Am J Cardiol* 1987;59:454–458.
Drinkwater DC Jr, Laks H: Unbalanced atrioventricular septal defects. *Semin Thorac Cardiovasc Surg* 1997;9:21–25.
Marino B, Vairo U, Corno A, et al: Atrioventricular canal in Down syndrome. *Am J Dis Child* 1990;144:1120.
Murphy DJ Jr: Atrioventricular canal defects. *Curr Treat Options Cardiovasc Med* 1999;1:323–334.
Sigfusson G, Ettedgui JA, Silverman NH, et al: Is a cleft in the anterior leaflet of an otherwise normal mitral valve an atrioventricular canal malformation? *J Am Coll Cardiol* 1995;26:508–515.

Difetto del setto interventricolare

Glen S, Burns J, Bloomfield P: Prevalence and development of additional cardiac abnormalities in 1448 patients with congenital ventricular septal defects. *Heart* 2004;90:1321–1325.
Holzer R, Balzer D, Cao QL, et al: Device closure of muscular ventricular septal defects using the Amplatzer muscular ventricular septal defect occluder: Immediate and mid-term results of a U.S. registry. *J Am Coll Cardiol* 2004;43:1257–1263.
Hornberger LK, Sahn DJ, Krabill KA, et al: Elucidation of the natural history of ventricular septal defects by serial Doppler color flow mapping studies. *J Am Coll Cardiol* 1989;13:1111–1118.
Knauth AL, Lock JE, Perry SB, et al: Transcatheter device closure of congenital and postoperative residual ventricular septal defects. *Circulation* 2004;110:501–507.
Ramaciotti C, Keren A, Silverman NH: Importance of pseudoaneurysms of the ventricular septum in the natural history of isolated perimembranous ventricular septal defects. *Am J Cardiol* 1986;57:268–272.
Roos-Hesselink JW, Meijboom FJ, Spitaels SE, et al. Outcome of patients after surgical closure of ventricular septal defect at young age: Longitudinal follow-up of 22–34 years. *Eur Heart J* 2004;25:1057–1062.

Dotto arterioso pervio

Alagarsamy S, Chhabra M, Gudavalli M, et al: Comparison of clinical criteria with echocardiographic findings in diagnosing PDA in preterm infants. *J Perinat Med* 2005;33:161–164.
Bergwerff M, DeRuiter MC, Gittenberger-de Groot AC: Comparative anatomy and ontogeny of the ductus arteriosus, a vascular outsider. *Anat Embryol (Berl)* 1999;200:559–571.
Gittenberger-de Groot AC, Van Ertbruggen I, Moulaert A, et al: The ductus arteriosus in the preterm infant: Histologic and clinical observations. *J Pediatr* 1980;96:88–93.
Rothman A, Lucas VW, Sklansky MS, et al: Percutaneous coil occlusion of patent ductus arteriosus. *J Pediatr* 1997;130:447–454.

Fistola arterovenosa coronarica

Velvis H, Schmidt KG, Silverman NH, et al: Diagnosis of coronary artery fistula by two-dimensional echocardiography, pulsed Doppler ultrasound, and color flow imaging. *J Am Coll Cardiol* 1989;14:968–976.

Capitolo 427 ■ Cardiopatie congenite non cianogene: lesioni ostruttive

427.1 • Stenosi della valvola polmonare con setto interventricolare integro

Delle varie forme di ostruzione all'efflusso ventricolare destro con setto interventricolare integro, la più comune è la stenosi isolata della valvola polmonare, che rappresenta il 7-10% di tutte le cardiopatie congenite. Le cuspidi valvolari sono deformate in misura variabile e di conseguenza la valvola si apre in modo incompleto durante la sistole. La valvola può essere bicuspide o tricuspide e i lembi possono essere parzialmente fusi tra loro con un orifizio eccentrico. La fusione può essere così grave da lasciare sono un piccolo foro centrale. Se la valvola non è gravemente ispessita, durante la sistole si produce un'ostruzione a cupola all'efflusso ventricolare destro. La stenosi infundibolare isolata, la stenosi polmonare sopravalvolare e la stenosi di una diramazione dell'arteria polmonare sono di riscontro meno comune. Nei casi in cui la stenosi della valvola polmonare è associata a un difetto del setto interventricolare (VSD, *Ventricular Septal Defect*) ma senza deviazione anteriore del setto infundibolare, è più corretto classificare la condizione come stenosi polmonare con VSD che come tetralogia di Fallot (vedi Capitolo 430.1). Talvolta si riscontrano difetti associati come la stenosi polmonare e un difetto del setto interatriale (ASD, *Atrial Septal Defect*). I reperti clinici e laboratoristici rispecchiano la lesione dominante, ma è importante escludere la diagnosi di queste anomalie associate. La stenosi polmonare dovuta a displasia della valvola è l'anomalia cardiaca più comune nella **sindrome di Noonan** (vedi Capitolo 81) ed è associata in circa il 50% dei casi a una mutazione nel gene *PTPN11*, che codifica la proteina tirosin fosfatasi SHP-2 sul cromosoma 12. Il meccanismo che porta all'insorgenza della stenosi polmonare non è noto, anche se sono stati suggeriti un difetto di sviluppo della porzione distale del *bulbus cordis* e le sequele di un'endocardite fetale. La stenosi polmonare, che sia a carico della valvola o di una diramazione dell'arteria polmonare, è un reperto comune in pazienti con displasia arteriopatica, altrimenti nota come **sindrome di Alagille**. In questa sindrome e in alcuni pazienti con stenosi polmonare isolata, è presente una mutazione nel gene *Jagged1*.

FISIOPATOLOGIA. L'ostruzione all'efflusso dal ventricolo destro all'arteria polmonare comporta un aumento della pressione sistolica e dello stress parietale, che finisce per determinare un'ipertrofia ventricolare destra (Fig. 427-1). La gravità di queste anomalie dipende dalle dimensioni dell'apertura della valvola stenotica.

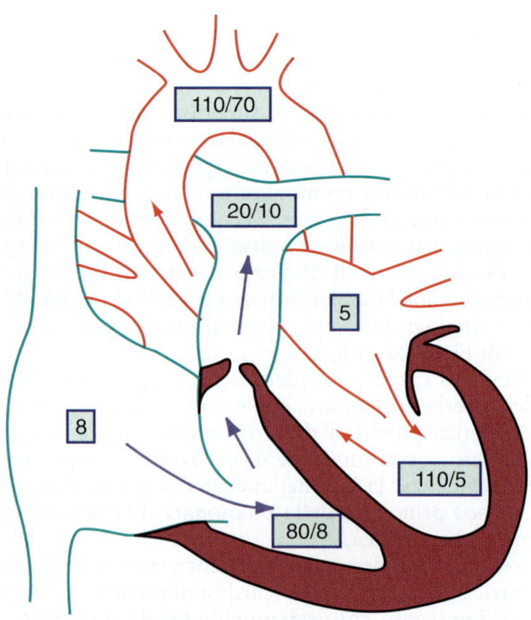

Figura 427-1. Fisiologia della stenosi della valvola polmonare. I numeri nelle caselle rappresentano la pressione espressa in mmHg. A causa dell'assenza di uno shunt destro-sinistro o sinistro-destro, il flusso ematico attraverso tutte le camere cardiache è normale (3 L/min/m^2). Il rapporto tra flusso sanguigno polmonare e sistemico (Qp:Qs) è 1:1. La pressione atriale destra è lievemente aumentata per la diminuita compliance del ventricolo destro. Il ventricolo destro è ipertrofico, le pressioni sistolica e diastolica sono aumentate. Il gradiente pressorio attraverso la valvola polmonare ispessita è di 60 mmHg. La pressione nel tronco principale dell'arteria polmonare è leggermente bassa, ed è presente una dilatazione post-stenotica. La pressione nel cuore sinistro è normale. A meno che non si sviluppi uno shunt destro-sinistro attraverso un forame ovale pervio, la saturazione d'ossigeno del paziente sarà normale.

In casi gravi, la pressione ventricolare destra può essere più elevata della pressione arteriosa sistemica, mentre in presenza di ostruzioni più lievi, la pressione ventricolare destra subisce solo un aumento lieve o moderato. La pressione in arteria polmonare è diminuita. La saturazione arteriosa d'ossigeno sarà normale anche in casi di stenosi grave, a meno che una comunicazione intracardiaca come un VSD o un ASD non permetta al sangue di passare dalle sezioni destre a quelle sinistre. Quando una grave stenosi polmonare si verifica in un neonato, la marcata diminuzione della compliance del ventricolo destro può portare a cianosi a causa di uno shunt destro-sinistro attraverso un forame ovale pervio, una condizione definita "stenosi polmonare critica".

MANIFESTAZIONI CLINICHE E INDAGINI DI LABORATORIO. I pazienti con stenosi lieve o moderata di solito non hanno sintomi. La crescita e lo sviluppo sono nella maggior parte dei casi normali; i lattanti e i bambini sembrano ben sviluppati e sani. Se la stenosi è grave, possono manifestarsi segni di scompenso ventricolare destro come epatomegalia, edema periferico e intolleranza allo sforzo. Nel neonato o lattante con stenosi polmonare critica possono essere più evidenti i segni di scompenso ventricolare destro, e la cianosi è spesso presente a causa dello shunt a livello del forame ovale.

Nella **stenosi polmonare lieve**, la pressione venosa e la frequenza cardiaca sono normali. Il cuore non è ingrandito, l'itto apicale è normale e l'impulso ventricolare destro non è palpabile. Durante l'espirazione si ode chiaramente un click da eiezione polmonare subito dopo il primo tono cardiaco, a livello del margine sternale superiore sinistro. Il secondo tono cardiaco è sdoppiato, con una componente polmonare di intensità normale che può essere lievemente ritardata. Un soffio da eiezione sistolica relativamente breve, di tonalità bassa o media, viene meglio percepito in corrispondenza del focolaio polmonare e si irradia bilateralmente ai campi polmonari in misura ridotta. L'elettrocardiogramma è normale o presenta le caratteristiche di una lieve ipertrofia ventricolare destra; si può assistere a un'inversione delle onde T nelle derivazioni precordiali destre (si ricordi che l'onda T nella derivazione V_1 dovrebbe essere invertita almeno fino ai 6-8 anni di età, motivo per cui un'onda T positiva in un bambino piccolo è segno di ipertrofia ventricolare destra). L'unica anomalia dimostrabile radiograficamente è di solito una dilatazione post-stenotica dell'arteria polmonare. L'ecocardiografia bidimensionale evidenzia un'ipertrofia ventricolare destra e una valvola polmonare lievemente ispessita, che si incurva in sistole; gli studi Doppler evidenziano un gradiente ≤ 30 mmHg tra ventricolo destro e arteria polmonare.

Nella **stenosi polmonare moderata**, la pressione venosa può subire un lieve aumento; nei bambini più grandi, si può notare un'onda *a* prominente al polso giugulare. Può essere palpabile un sollevamento del ventricolo destro a livello del margine sternale inferiore sinistro. Il secondo tono cardiaco è sdoppiato, con una componente polmonare ritardata e ridotta. A mano a mano che la motilità della valvola diminuisce per effetto di gradi più severi di stenosi, possono non udirsi più il click da eiezione polmonare e il secondo tono polmonare. Con l'aumento della gravità della stenosi, il picco del soffio sistolico da eiezione si prolunga nella sistole, oltre a farsi più forte e aspro (frequenza maggiore). Il soffio si irradia più facilmente a entrambi i campi polmonari.

L'elettrocardiogramma evidenzia ipertrofia ventricolare destra, talvolta con onde P prominenti e appuntite. Radiograficamente il cuore può presentare dimensioni normali o essere lievemente ingrandito, con uno spostamento verso l'alto dell'apice a causa della prominenza del ventricolo destro; la vascolarizzazione intrapolmonare può essere normale o di poco ridotta. L'ecocardiogramma rivela una valvola polmonare ispessita con un diminuito movimento sistolico. L'esame Doppler mostra un gradiente pressorio tra ventricolo destro e arteria polmonare tra 30 e 60 mmHg. L'eventuale presenza di un lieve rigurgito mitralico costituisce la conferma al Doppler della pressione sistolica ventricolare destra.

Nella **stenosi grave**, si può notare una cianosi da lieve a moderata in pazienti con comunicazione interatriale (difetto del setto interatriale o forame ovale pervio). La presenza di epatomegalia ed edema periferico è indice di scompenso ventricolare destro. È comune l'aumento della pressione venosa, causato da un'ampia onda *a* giugulare presistolica. Il cuore è moderatamente o marcatamente ingrandito, ed è presente un notevole sollevamento ventricolare destro parasternale, che spesso si estende fino alla linea emiclaveare. La componente polmonare del secondo tono di solito non è udibile. Un soffio sistolico da eiezione ad alta tonalità, prolungato e aspro, di solito accompagnato da un fremito, è udibile soprattutto sul focolaio polmonare e può irradiarsi all'intero precordio, a entrambi i campi polmonari, al collo e al dorso. Il picco del soffio si verifica nella parte finale della sistole, quando l'apertura valvolare si riduce. Il soffio frequentemente si sovrappone alla componente aortica del secondo tono, ma non è preceduto da un click da eiezione.

L'elettrocardiogramma evidenzia una macroscopica ipertrofia ventricolare destra, spesso accompagnata da un'onda P alta e appuntita. Gli studi radiografici confermano l'ingrandimento cardiaco con prominenza del ventricolo e dell'atrio destri. La prominenza del segmento del tronco principale dell'arteria polmonare è apprezzabile a causa della dilatazione post-stenotica (Fig. 427-2). La vascolarizzazione intrapolmonare è diminuita (Fig. 427-3). Negli stadi tardivi della malattia, si può notare una disfunzione sistolica del ventricolo destro, nel qual caso il ventricolo può dilatarsi, con marcato rigurgito tricuspidalico. Gli studi Doppler evidenziano un elevato gradiente (>60 mmHg) attraverso la valvola polmonare. Fortunatamente, grazie alla loro correzione precoce, i reperti classici della stenosi polmonare grave nei bambini grandi sono di raro riscontro. Segni di stenosi polmonare critica, con tutte le caratteristiche della stenosi polmonare grave con cianosi associata, si osservano di solito nel periodo neonatale.

Il cateterismo cardiaco di solito non è richiesto per scopi diagnostici, ma viene effettuato nel contesto di una procedura di **valvuloplastica con catetere a palloncino**. Il cateterismo evidenzia un brusco gradiente pressorio attraverso la valvola polmonare. La pressione in arteria polmonare è normale o bassa. Per valutare la gravità della stenosi ci si basa sul rapporto tra la pressione sistolica ventricolare destra e la pressione sistolica sistemica o sul gradiente pressorio tra ventricolo destro e arteria polmonare: il gradiente è di 10-30 mmHg nei casi lievi, 30-60 mmHg nelle forme moderate e >60 mmHg o con pressione ventricolare destra superiore alla pressione sistemica nei casi gravi. Se la gittata cardiaca è bassa o esiste un significativo shunt destro-sinistro attraverso il setto atriale, il gradiente pressorio può sottostimare

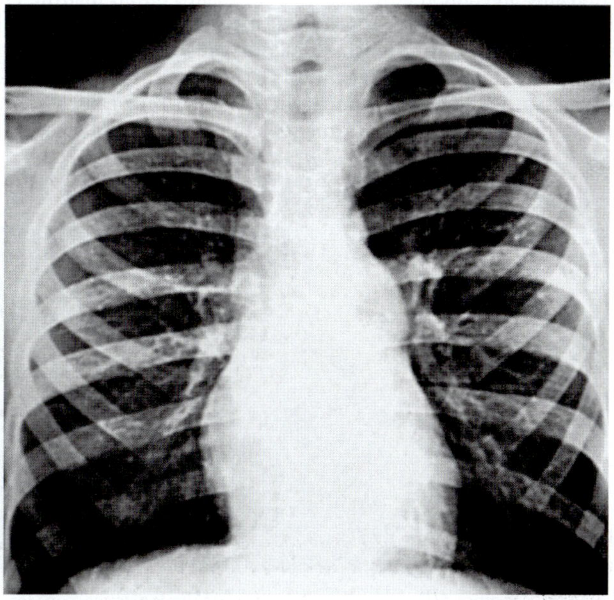

Figura 427-2. Radiografia del torace in un paziente con stenosi valvolare polmonare e radice aortica normale. Il cuore ha dimensioni nei limiti della norma, ma è presente una dilatazione post-stenotica dell'arteria polmonare.

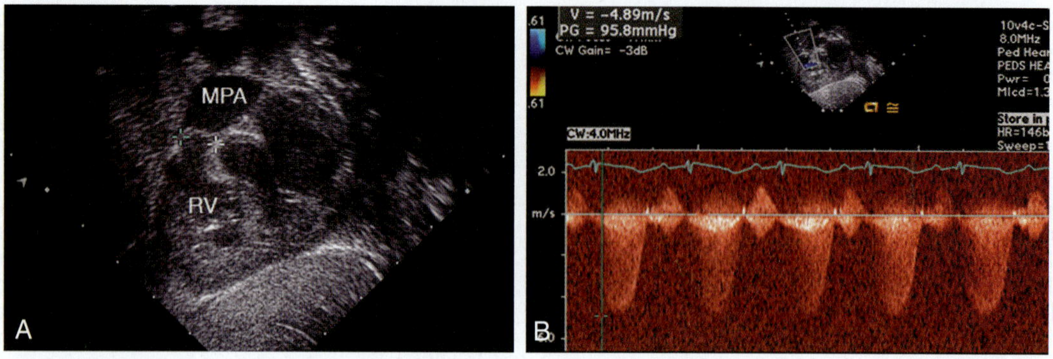

Figura 427-3. Ecocardiogramma che evidenzia una stenosi valvolare polmonare. *A*, Proiezione sottocostale da cui emergono ispessimenti dei lembi valvolari polmonari (tra gli indicatori). *B*, Esame Doppler che indica un gradiente pressorio di 95 mmHg al picco attraverso la valvola stenotica. MPA (*Main Pulmonary Artery*), tronco principale dell'arteria polmonare; RV (*Right Ventricle*), ventricolo destro.

il grado di stenosi valvolare. La ventricolografia destra selettiva evidenzia una valvola ispessita e poco mobile. Nella stenosi da lieve a moderata, l'incurvamento della valvola in sistole è facilmente visibile. Il mezzo di contrasto, passando attraverso la valvola stenotica nella sistole ventricolare, produce uno stretto getto che riempie l'arteria polmonare dilatata. Talvolta può essere presente un'ipertrofia sottovalvolare che contribuisce ad aggravare l'ostruzione. L'angiografia indica anche se il setto interventricolare è intatto.

TRATTAMENTO. I pazienti con stenosi polmonare isolata di grado moderato o severo richiedono una correzione dell'ostruzione. Nella maggior parte dei casi il trattamento di scelta iniziale è la valvuloplastica con catetere a palloncino (Fig. 427-4). I pazienti con valvole polmonari gravemente ispessite, fenomeno comune soprattutto in caso di sindrome di Noonan, possono necessitare di un intervento chirurgico. In un neonato con stenosi polmonare critica è imperativo il trattamento urgente, che consiste nella valvuloplastica con catetere a palloncino o nella valvulotomia chirurgica.

Nella maggior parte dei casi si ottengono risultati eccellenti. Il gradiente attraverso la valvola polmonare si riduce notevolmente o scompare. Nel periodo immediatamente successivo alla valvuloplastica con catetere a palloncino può permanere un gradiente residuo da lieve a moderato (dovuto a un restringimento muscolare infundibolare), che però quasi sempre si risolve con il tempo. Può essere udibile un soffio diastolico breve, in decrescendo, a livello del margine sternale medio-superiore, causato da un'insufficienza della valvola polmonare. Il grado di insufficienza non è di solito significativo dal punto di vista clinico. Non sono emerse differenze nel follow-up a lungo termine tra i pazienti sottoposti a valvuloplastica o a intervento chirurgico; la ricorrenza della stenosi non è comune dopo un trattamento condotto con successo.

PROGNOSI E COMPLICANZE. Lo scompenso cardiaco si verifica solo nei casi gravi, per lo più durante il primo mese di vita. Lo sviluppo di cianosi, a causa di uno shunt destro-sinistro attraverso un forame ovale pervio, si osserva esclusivamente nel periodo neonatale, quando la stenosi è grave. Sussiste inoltre il rischio di un'endocardite infettiva, che tuttavia non è comune nell'infanzia.

I bambini con stenosi lieve possono condurre una vita normale, ma devono essere sottoposti a controlli a intervalli regolari. I pazienti con un gradiente piccolo raramente vanno incontro a una progressione della stenosi e non necessitano dell'intervento, ma è più probabile che il gradiente aumenti nei pazienti pediatrici con stenosi moderata per effetto della crescita. Il peggioramento dell'ostruzione può essere dovuto anche allo sviluppo di un'ipertrofia sottovalvolare secondaria, costituita di tessuto muscolare e fibroso. Nella stenosi grave e non trattata, il decorso può peggiorare bruscamente con lo sviluppo di una disfunzione ventricolare destra e di scompenso cardiaco. I lattanti con stenosi polmonare critica devono essere sottoposti d'urgenza a valvuloplastica con catetere a palloncino o a valvulotomia chirurgica. L'insorgenza di uno scompenso ventricolare destro molti anni dopo una valvuloplastica polmonare con catetere a palloncino non è comune. Tuttavia, si consiglia di seguire i pazienti periodicamente per essere pronti a individuare un eventuale peggioramento dell'insufficienza della valvola polmonare e della dilatazione del ventricolo destro.

427.2 • Stenosi polmonare infundibolare e ventricolo destro a doppia camera

La stenosi polmonare infundibolare è causata da un'ostruzione muscolare o fibrosa al tratto di efflusso del ventricolo destro. La sede dell'ostruzione può essere vicina alla valvola polmonare o

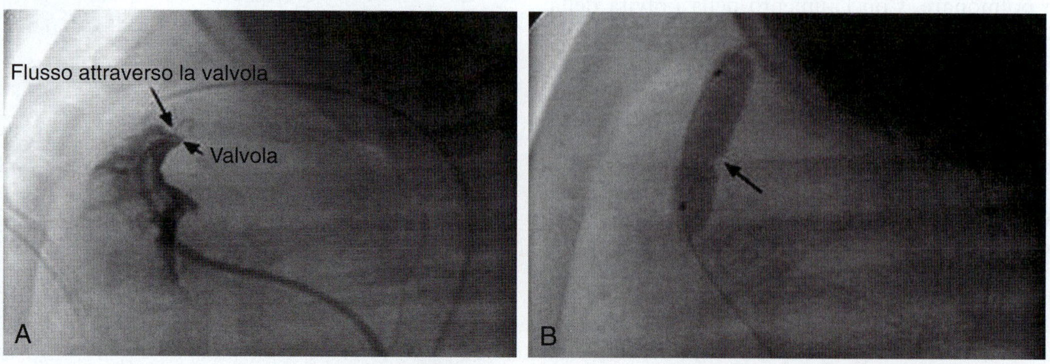

Figura 427-4 Stenosi della valvola polmonare e valvuloplastica con catetere a palloncino. *A*, Angiogramma del ventricolo destro che evidenzia una valvola polmonare gravemente stenotica con un sottile getto di sangue che fluisce attraverso di essa. *B*, Insufflazione del palloncino guidato dal catetere, che permette di osservare l'indentazione (*freccia*) prodotta dal palloncino a partire dalla valvola stenotica. (Per gentile concessione di Jeffrey Feinstein, Stanford University, Stanford, CA.)

ben al di sotto di essa; può essere presente una camera infundibolare tra la cavità del ventricolo destro e la valvola polmonare. In molti casi, può essere stato presente inizialmente un VSD che poi si è chiuso spontaneamente. Quando anche la valvola polmonare è stenotica, il difetto combinato viene classificato come stenosi valvolare con secondaria ipertrofia infundibolare. Le caratteristiche emodinamiche e le manifestazioni cliniche dei pazienti con stenosi infundibolare polmonare isolata sono in gran parte simili a quelle già descritte in relazione alla stenosi valvolare polmonare isolata (vedi Capitolo 427.1).

Una variante comune dell'ostruzione all'efflusso ventricolare destro al di sotto della valvolare polmonare è rappresentata dal ventricolo destro a doppia camera. Questa condizione è caratterizzata dalla presenza, nella regione medioventricolare, di una banderella muscolare, che divide la camera in due parti e crea un'ostruzione tra le porzioni di afflusso e di efflusso. Spesso si nota un VSD associato, che può chiudersi spontaneamente. L'ostruzione di solito passa inosservata nei primi mesi di vita, ma può progredire rapidamente, in modo simile all'ostruzione infundibolare progressiva che si osserva nella tetralogia di Fallot (vedi Capitolo 430.1).

Per formulare la diagnosi di stenosi infundibolare ventricolare destra isolata o di ventricolo destro a doppia camera ci si avvale dell'ecocardiogramma, del cateterismo cardiaco con angiografia, o di entrambi questi metodi. Occorre valutare accuratamente il setto interventricolare per determinare se sia presente un VSD associato. Per i casi non trattati di grave ostruzione all'efflusso del ventricolo destro la prognosi è simile a quella della stenosi valvolare polmonare. Se l'ostruzione è moderata o grave, è indicato l'intervento chirurgico, che porta alla scomparsa del gradiente pressorio o a una sua marcata riduzione, con prognosi a lungo termine eccellente.

427.3 • Stenosi polmonare associata a shunt intracardiaco

Le stenosi polmonari valvolare o infundibolare, o entrambe, possono essere associate ad ASD o a VSD. In questi pazienti le caratteristiche cliniche dipendono dal grado della stenosi polmonare, che determina la direzione dello shunt, se sinistro-destro o destro-sinistro.

La presenza di un ampio shunt sinistro-destro a livello atriale o ventricolare è segno che la stenosi polmonare è lieve. Questi soggetti presentano sintomi simili a quelli dei pazienti con ASD o VSD isolato. Con la crescita, il peggioramento dell'ostruzione può limitare lo shunt e portare a un graduale miglioramento dei sintomi. Un ulteriore aggravamento dell'ostruzione può infine portare allo shunt destro-sinistro e alla cianosi, soprattutto in pazienti con stenosi polmonare e VSD. Dinanzi a un elettrocardiogramma che mostra segni di miglioramento dell'insufficienza cardiaca e di un aumento della forza del ventricolo destro, in un paziente con un VSD, bisogna distinguere tra sviluppo di una stenosi polmonare e insorgenza di una patologia vascolare polmonare (sindrome di Eisenmenger, vedi Capitolo 433.2).

Queste anomalie vengono facilmente corrette con l'intervento chirurgico, consistente nella chiusura dei difetti del setto atriale o ventricolare e nella correzione della stenosi polmonare con resezione del muscolo infundibolare e/o valvulotomia polmonare, a seconda dell'indicazione. I pazienti con uno shunt destro-sinistro predominante hanno sintomi simili a quelli tipici della **tetralogia di Fallot** (vedi Capitolo 430.1).

427.4 • Stenosi periferica dell'arteria polmonare

Stenosi singole o multiple possono verificarsi in qualsiasi punto lungo le principali diramazioni delle arterie polmonari. Che siano lievi o gravi, localizzate o estese, sono spesso associate ad altri tipi di cardiopatie congenite, come la stenosi della valvola polmonare, la tetralogia di Fallot, il dotto arterioso pervio (PDA, *Patent Ductus Arteriosus*), il VSD, l'ASD e la stenosi aortica sopravalvolare. È stata riconosciuta una familiarità in alcuni pazienti con stenosi polmonare periferica. Un'elevata incidenza si riscontra in bambini con sindrome da rosolia congenita. Un quadro di stenosi aortica sopravalvolare con stenosi di una diramazione dell'arteria polmonare, ipercalcemia idiopatica dell'infanzia, facies a elfo e ritardo mentale è noto come **sindrome di Williams**, condizione associata a delezione del gene dell'elastina nella regione 7q11.23 sul cromosoma 7. La stenosi polmonare periferica è riscontrabile anche nella **sindrome di Alagille**, che può essere associata a una mutazione nel gene *Jagged1*.

Una stenosi lieve ha pochi effetti sulla circolazione polmonare. In presenza di stenosi multiple, invece, aumenta la pressione nel ventricolo destro e nell'arteria polmonare, prossimamente alla sede dell'ostruzione. Quando l'anomalia è isolata, la diagnosi viene sospettata dalla presenza di soffi diffusi al torace, anteriormente o posteriormente. Questi soffi sono di solito sistolici ed eiettivi come qualità, ma possono essere continui. Nella maggior parte dei casi i segni fisici sono dominati dall'anomalia associata, per esempio la tetralogia di Fallot (vedi Capitolo 430.1).

Subito dopo la nascita può essere presente una forma lieve e transitoria di stenosi polmonare periferica. In genere l'unico reperto fisico è un lieve soffio sistolico da eiezione, apprezzabile su uno o entrambi i campi polmonari. Depone a sostegno di questa diagnosi l'assenza di altri reperti obiettivi di stenosi della valvola polmonare (sollevamento ventricolare destro, secondo tono polmonare ridotto, click da eiezione, soffio più forte a livello del margine sternale superiore sinistro). Il soffio di solito scompare entro il 1°-2° mese di vita.

Se la stenosi è grave, l'elettrocardiogramma evidenzia un'ipertrofia ventricolare e atriale destra, mentre la radiografia del torace mostra cardiomegalia e prominenza del tronco principale dell'arteria polmonare. La vascolarizzazione polmonare è di solito normale; in alcuni casi, tuttavia, si riscontrano piccole ombre vascolari intrapolmonari, che rappresentano aree di dilatazione post-stenotica. L'ecocardiografia ha una capacità limitata di visualizzare le diramazioni distali dell'arteria polmonare. L'esame Doppler evidenzia l'accelerazione del flusso sanguigno attraverso le stenosi e, in presenza di un rigurgito tricuspidalico, permette una stima della pressione sistolica ventricolare destra. La RMN e la TC sono estremamente utili per delineare le ostruzioni distali; se si sospetta una patologia da moderata a grave, la diagnosi è di solito confermata dal cateterismo cardiaco.

Una grave ostruzione del tronco principale dell'arteria polmonare e delle sue principali diramazioni può essere risolta durante un intervento chirurgico volto a correggere lesioni associate come la tetralogia di Fallot o una stenosi della valvola polmonare. La stenosi polmonare periferica, se isolata, può essere trattata mediante dilatazione con catetere a palloncino. Quando però l'ostruzione periferica colpisce i vasi intrapolmonari distali, di solito non è affrontabile chirurgicamente. Queste ostruzioni, spesso multiple, vengono trattate nel modo migliore con ripetute angioplastiche con catetere a palloncino, anche se il tasso di recidiva è alto. Gli stent intravascolari espandibili, introdotti tramite catetere nei rami distali dell'arteria polmonare e poi dilatati con palloncino fino a raggiungere la dimensione voluta, possono prevenire la recidiva della stenosi (vedi Fig. 423-29).

427.5 • Stenosi aortica

FISIOPATOLOGIA. La stenosi aortica congenita rappresenta circa il 5% delle malformazioni cardiache riconosciute nell'infanzia; una valvola aortica bicuspide, una delle lesioni cardiache congenite più frequenti, viene identificata fino nel 2% degli adulti ed è di solito asintomatica nell'infanzia. La stenosi aortica è più frequente nei maschi (3:1). Nella sua forma più comune, la stenosi aortica valvolare, i lembi sono ispessiti e le commissure sono fuse in misura variabile. La pressione sistolica ventricolare sinistra è aumentata in conseguenza dell'ostruzione all'efflusso. La parete ventricolare sinistra va incontro a ipertrofia compensatoria; a mano a mano che la sua compliance diminuisce, anche la pressione telediastolica aumenta.

La **stenosi sottovalvolare** (**subaortica**), con un discreto "scalino" fibromuscolare al di sotto della valvola aortica, è anch'essa un'importante forma di ostruzione del tratto di efflusso del ventricolo sinistro. Questa lesione, spesso associata ad altre forme di cardiopatia congenita, può andare incontro a un rapido aggravamento. Viene diagnosticata meno comunemente durante la prima infanzia, e può svilupparsi anche se in precedenza non è stato documentato alcun segno di ostruzione del tratto di efflusso del ventricolo sinistro. La stenosi aortica sottovalvolare può rendersi evidente dopo un intervento chirurgico riuscito per altri difetti cardiaci congeniti (coartazione aortica, PDA, VSD), svilupparsi in associazione con lievi lesioni che non sono state corrette chirurgicamente o manifestarsi come anomalia isolata. Può inoltre essere anche dovuta a marcata ipertrofia del setto interventricolare, associata a miocardiopatia ipertrofica (vedi Capitolo 439.2).

La **stenosi aortica sopravalvolare**, il tipo meno comune, può essere sporadica, familiare o associata alla **sindrome di Williams**, che comprende ritardo mentale, facies da elfo (viso pieno, fronte ampia, sella nasale appiattita, labbro superiore sporgente, guance rotonde) e ipercalcemia idiopatica dell'infanzia (vedi Capitolo 81). Nei pazienti con questo difetto può svilupparsi un restringimento degli osti delle arterie coronarie ed essere presente una stenosi di altre arterie, in particolare di diramazioni dell'arteria polmonare. È stato dimostrato che la sindrome di Williams è dovuta a una delezione che coinvolge il gene dell'elastina sul cromosoma 7q11.23.

MANIFESTAZIONI CLINICHE. Nei pazienti con stenosi aortica i sintomi dipendono dalla gravità dell'ostruzione. Una forma grave nella prima infanzia è definita **stenosi aortica critica** ed è associata a scompenso ventricolare sinistro e segni di bassa gittata cardiaca. Lo scompenso cardiaco, la cardiomegalia e l'edema polmonare sono gravi, i polsi sono deboli a tutti gli arti e la cute può essere pallida o grigiastra. Il flusso urinario può essere ridotto. Se la gittata cardiaca è significativamente diminuita, l'intensità del soffio a livello del margine sternale superiore destro può essere minima. Il soffio viene di solito scoperto durante una visita medica di routine. In un bambino più grande con ostruzione all'efflusso ventricolare sinistro non diagnosticata in precedenza possono svilupparsi astenia, angina, capogiri o episodi sincopali, per quanto si tratti di un'evenienza rara. Nonostante ne siano stati riportati casi associati a stenosi aortica, la morte improvvisa di solito avviene in pazienti con grave ostruzione all'efflusso ventricolare sinistro in cui la correzione chirurgica è stata ritardata.

I reperti all'esame obiettivo dipendono dal grado di ostruzione all'efflusso ventricolare sinistro. Nella stenosi lieve, i polsi, le dimensioni del cuore e l'impulso apicale sono normali. Via via che la gravità aumenta, i polsi diminuiscono d'intensità e il cuore può essere ingrandito, con un impulso ventricolare sinistro. Una stenosi aortica valvolare da lieve a moderata è di solito associata a un click sistolico da eiezione precoce, che si percepisce meglio all'apice e a livello del margine sternale sinistro. A differenza del click che si riscontra nella stenosi polmonare, la sua intensità non varia nelle varie fasi del ciclo respiratorio. I click sono infrequenti nella stenosi aortica più grave o nella stenosi subaortica discreta. Se alla stenosi è grave, il primo tono cardiaco può essere ridotto a causa della minore compliance del ventricolo sinistro ispessito. Un normale sdoppiamento del secondo tono cardiaco è presente nell'ostruzione da lieve a moderata. In pazienti con ostruzione grave, l'intensità della chiusura della valvola aortica è ridotta e (reperto raro nei bambini) vi può essere uno sdoppiamento paradosso del secondo tono (che diventa più ampio in espirazione). In caso di ostruzione grave può essere udibile un quarto tono cardiaco.

L'intensità, il tono e la durata del soffio sistolico da eiezione sono altre indicazioni di gravità. Più il soffio è forte, aspro (di tonalità più alta) e prolungato, maggiore è il grado di ostruzione. Il soffio tipico è udibile soprattutto a livello del margine sternale superiore destro e si irradia al collo, fino al margine mediosternale sinistro; di solito è accompagnato da un fremito a livello dell'incisura soprasternale. Nei pazienti con stenosi aortica sottovalvolare, può essere più accentuato lungo il margine sternale sinistro o anche all'apice. Un soffio diastolico lieve, in decrescendo, indicativo di insufficienza aortica, è spesso presente in caso di ostruzione sottovalvolare o in pazienti con valvola aortica bicuspide. Talvolta è udibile un breve rullio apicale mesodiastolico, anche in presenza di una valvola mitralica normale; questo soffio dovrebbe sempre far insorgere il sospetto di una stenosi mitralica associata.

INDAGINI DI LABORATORIO E DIAGNOSI. Di solito è possibile formulare la diagnosi basandosi sull'esame obiettivo; la gravità dell'ostruzione può poi ricevere conferma dai test di laboratorio. Se il gradiente pressorio attraverso la valvola è piccolo, è probabile che l'elettrocardiogramma sia normale. Anche se quest'ultimo può risultare normale anche in caso di ostruzione più grave, in genere mostra segni di ipertrofia e sovraccarico ventricolare sinistro (onde T invertite nelle derivazioni precordiali sinistre) se la stenosi grave è presente da molto tempo. La radiografia del torace spesso evidenzia un'aorta ascendente prominente, ma un cappuccio aortico normale. Tipicamente il cuore ha dimensioni normali. Calcificazioni valvolari sono state riscontrate solo nei bambini più grandi o negli adulti. L'ecocardiografia fornisce informazioni sia sulla sede sia sulla gravità dell'ostruzione. Le immagini bidimensionali evidenziano un'ipertrofia ventricolare sinistra e una valvola aortica ispessita e a cupola (Fig. 427-5). Questa indagine permette inoltre di valutare il numero di lembi valvolari e la loro morfologia, ma anche di visualizzare una membrana subartica o una stenosi sopravalvolare, se presenti. L'incidenza di anomalie associate della valvola mitrale o dell'arco aortico oppure di VSD o PDA può raggiungere il 20% dei casi. In assenza di scompenso ventricolare sinistro, la frazione di accorciamento del ventricolo

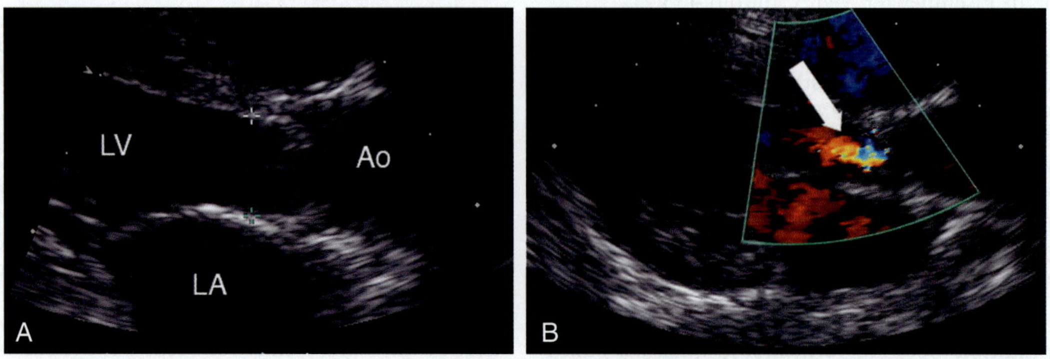

Figura 427-5. Ecocardiogramma che evidenzia una stenosi valvolare aortica con rigurgito. *A*, In questa proiezione parasternale asse lungo, è visibile la valvola aortica stenotica che si incurva a cupola in sistole. Gli indicatori racchiudono l'anulus aortico. *B*, Esame Doppler che mostra la presenza di rigurgito aortico (*freccia*). Ao, aorta; LA (*Left Atrium*), atrio sinistro; LV (*Left Ventricle*), ventricolo sinistro.

sinistro può risultare aumentata perché il ventricolo è ipercontrattile. Nel lattante con stenosi aortica critica, la frazione di accorciamento del ventricolo sinistro di solito risulta diminuita e l'endocardio può essere brillante, a testimoniare lo sviluppo di una cicatrizzazione fibrosa endocardica detta **fibroelastosi endocardica**. L'esame Doppler indica la sede specifica dell'ostruzione, oltre a determinare il picco e i gradienti mediosistolici del tratto di efflusso del ventricolo sinistro. Quando un'ostruzione aortica grave si associa a disfunzione ventricolare sinistra, il gradiente valvolare calcolato con metodo Doppler può sottostimare gravemente la gravità dell'ostruzione a causa della bassa gittata cardiaca.

La prova da sforzo graduata è utile per valutare la gravità dell'ostruzione del tratto di efflusso del ventricolo sinistro nei bambini più grandi. Via via che la gravità dei gradienti aumenta, la capacità di lavoro diminuisce, la pressione sistolica non aumenta adeguatamente, la pressione sanguigna diastolica può aumentare e può verificarsi un sottoslivellamento del tratto ST. Poiché il pazienti con stenosi aortica grave talvolta non riferiscono sintomi e presentare elettrocardiogrammi e radiografie del torace normali, ecocardiogrammi seriati e test da sforzo graduati possono essere preziosi per determinare il momento in cui effettuare il cateterismo cardiaco e la valvuloplastica chirurgica o con catetere a palloncino.

Il cateterismo cardiaco sinistro permette di valutare l'entità del gradiente pressorio dal ventricolo sinistro all'aorta. La curva di pressione aortica è anomala se l'ostruzione è grave. In pazienti con ostruzione grave e diminuita compliance ventricolare sinistra, la pressione in atrio sinistro è aumentata e può essere presente un'ipertensione polmonare. La metodica migliore per identificare la sede dell'ostruzione è la ventricolografia sinistra selettiva. La maggior parte dei lattanti con stenosi aortica critica non necessita di cateterismo cardiaco per la diagnosi, ma di solito viene sottoposta a tale procedura in corso di valvuloplastica con catetere a palloncino. Quando un lattante in condizioni critiche, con ostruzione del tratto di efflusso del ventricolo sinistro, viene sottoposto a cateterismo cardiaco, la funzione ventricolare sinistra è spesso marcatamente depressa. Come avviene con l'ecocardiogramma, il gradiente misurato attraverso la valvola stenotica può sottostimare il grado dell'ostruzione a causa della bassa gittata cardiaca; per questo possono essere utili la misurazione dell'effettiva gittata cardiaca con il metodo della termodiluizione e il calcolo dell'area valvolare aortica.

TRATTAMENTO. La valvuloplastica con catetere a palloncino è indicata per il bambini con stenosi valvolare aortica moderata o grave, per prevenire una progressiva disfunzione ventricolare sinistra e il rischio di sincope e morte improvvisa. Tutti concordano sul fatto che la valvuloplastica debba essere consigliata quando il gradiente picco-picco sistolico tra il ventricolo sinistro e l'aorta è >60-70 mmHg a riposo, supponendo che la gittata cardiaca sia normale, o per gradienti inferiori quando sono presenti sintomi o alterazioni elettrocardiografiche. Per lesioni ostruttive subaortiche più rapidamente progressive, un gradiente di 40-50 mmHg o la presenza di insufficienza aortica sono considerati indicazioni all'intervento chirurgico. Grazie allo sviluppo di palloncini e cateteri più piccoli che provocano meno danni alle arterie periferiche, questa metodica è divenuta la procedura di scelta anche nel periodo neonatale. Il trattamento chirurgico è di solito riservato alle valvole aortiche stenotiche che non sono adatte alla terapia con catetere a palloncino, in genere perché estremamente ispessite, ai pazienti che hanno anche una stenosi sopravalvolare o sottovalvolare.

Le stenosi subaortiche discrete possono essere sottoposte a resezione senza alcun danno per la valvola aortica, il lembo anteriore della valvola mitrale o il sistema di conduzione. Questo tipo di ostruzione di solito non si presta al trattamento con catetere. La correzione di una stenosi sopravalvolare, che di solito è chirurgica, dà risultati eccellenti se l'area dell'ostruzione è isolata e non associata a un'aorta ipoplasica. In associazione con una stenosi aortica sopravalvolare, una o più coronarie possono essere stenotiche all'origine, a causa di una spessa cresta fibrosa sovra-aortica. Per i pazienti con stenosi aortica associata a una grave ostruzione subaortica "a tunnel", il tratto di efflusso del ventricolo sinistro può essere allargato "prendendo in prestito" un po' di spazio anteriormente dal tratto di efflusso del ventricolo destro (procedura di Konno).

Che il trattamento sia chirurgico o consista nella valvuloplastica con catetere, è probabile si verifichi un'insufficienza aortica o una calcificazione con recidiva della stenosi a distanza di anni o persino decenni dall'intervento, e che possano rendersi necessari un reintervento e, spesso, la sostituzione della valvola aortica. Quando si sviluppa una recidiva, questa può non essere associata a sintomi precoci. Segni di stenosi ricorrente comprendono reperti elettrocardiografici di ipertrofia ventricolare sinistra, un aumento del gradiente all'ecocardiogramma Doppler, un deterioramento degli indici ecocardiografici di funzione ventricolare sinistra e il ripresentarsi di segni e sintomi durante il test da sforzo graduato su tapis roulant. Il rigurgito aortico è segnalato da sintomi di scompenso cardiaco, ingrandimento cardiaco alla radiografia del torace e dilatazione ventricolare sinistra all'ecocardiogramma. La scelta della procedura di riparazione dipende dal grado relativo di stenosi e rigurgito.

Quando è necessaria la **sostituzione della valvola aortica**, la scelta della procedura spesso dipende dall'età del paziente. Le valvole homograft tendono a calcificare più rapidamente nei bambini piccoli, ma non richiedono una terapia anticoagulante cronica, al contrario delle protesi valvolari meccaniche che, pur essendo più durevoli, sono di difficile gestione nei lattanti. Nelle adolescenti prossime all'età fertile, gli effetti teratogeni del warfarin possono giustificare l'utilizzo di una valvola omograft. Nessuna di queste opzioni è perfetta per un bambinho piccolo che deve essere sottoposto a sostituzione valvolare, poiché né le valvole homograft né quelle meccaniche crescono con il paziente. Un'operazione alternativa è la **traslocazione aortopolmonare (procedura di Ross)**, che consiste nella rimozione della valvola polmonare del paziente e nel suo utilizzo al posto della valvola aortica anomala; un homograft viene poi posizionato a livello polmonare. I vantaggi di questa procedura sono la possibilità di crescita della valvola "neoaortica" traslocata e la maggiore longevità della valvola homograft quando viene posizionata nel circolo polmonare a bassa pressione. Il successo a lungo termine di questo intervento, specialmente nei bambini piccoli, è ancora in corso di valutazione. Le valvole stent, che sono valvole tissutali cucite all'interno di uno stent di metallo espandibile, sono al momento oggetto di studi clinici. Esse possono venire impiantate nel laboratorio di emodinamica mediante approccio percutaneo. Le valvole di tessuto ingegnerizzato utilizzate per la sostituzione, fatte crescere in laboratorio a partire dalle stesse cellule endoteliali del paziente, rappresentano la migliore speranza per la palliazione a lungo termine e sono al momento in fase di sviluppo su modelli animali.

PROGNOSI. I neonati con stenosi aortica critica possono andare incontro a grave scompenso cardiaco e deterioramento rapido, che li porta a sviluppare uno shock a bassa portata. L'intervento chirurgico di emergenza o la valvuloplastica con catetere a palloncino sono salvavita, ma il rischio connesso alla mortalità non va sottovalutato. I neonati che muoiono di stenosi aortica critica spesso hanno una significativa fibroelastosi ventricolare sinistra. Quelli che sopravvivono possono sviluppare segni di disfunzione muscolare diastolica del ventricolo sinistro (miocardiopatia restrittiva) negli anni successivi (vedi Capitolo 439.3).

Nei lattanti dopo i primi mesi e nei bambini più grandi con stenosi aortica lieve o moderata, la prognosi è ragionevolmente buona, anche se è comune la progressione della malattia nell'arco di 5-10 anni. I pazienti con gradienti valvolari aortici <40-50 mmHg sono considerati affetti da malattia lieve; quelli con gradienti di 40-70 mmHg (che corrispondono a una malattia moderata) di solito rispondono bene al trattamento (chirurgico o di valvuloplastica), anche se spesso si rendono necessari reinterventi sulla valvola aortica nell'infanzia o in età adulta e molti finiscono per richiedere una sostituzione valvolare. Nei pazienti non operati con ostruzione grave, la morte improvvisa costituisce un rischio significativo e spesso avviene durante o subito dopo uno sforzo. La stenosi aortica è una delle cause di morte cardiaca improvvisa nel gruppo in età pediatrica.

I pazienti con stenosi aortica di grado moderato o grave non dovrebbero prendere parte attiva a sport agonistici. In quelli con malattia più lieve, le limitazioni relative all'attività sportiva sono meno rigide; tuttavia, i pazienti dovrebbero essere incoraggiati a partecipare ad attività fisiche poco impegnative. Bisognerebbe sottoporre a valutazione la forma fisica di ciascun paziente almeno su base annuale e consigliare l'intervento se si riscontrano segni o sintomi di progressione. È necessaria la profilassi contro l'endocardite infettiva per tutta la vita.

427.6 • Coartazione aortica

Stenosi dell'aorta di grado variabile possono essere presenti a qualsiasi livello, dall'arco trasversale alla biforcazione iliaca, ma il 98% è situato al di sotto dell'origine dell'arteria succlavia sinistra, all'origine del dotto arterioso (coartazione iuxtaduttale). L'anomalia è due volte più frequente nei maschi che nelle femmine. La coartazione aortica può essere una caratteristica della **sindrome di Turner** (vedi Capitoli 81 e 587.1) ed è associata a una valvola aortica bicuspide in più del 70% dei pazienti. Potenziali lesioni associate sono anomalie della valvola mitrale (un anello mitralico sopravalvolare o una valvola mitrale a paracadute) e la stenosi. Quando tutte queste lesioni ostruttive del cuore sinistro si verificano insieme, configurano il cosiddetto **complesso di Shone.**

FISIOPATOLOGIA. La coartazione aortica può presentarsi come un'ostruzione iuxtaduttale ben delimitata o come ipoplasia tubulare dell'aorta trasversale che inizia a livello di uno dei vasi della testa o del collo e si estende all'area duttale (in passato chiamata coartazione preduttale o di tipo infantile; Fig. 427-6). Spesso sono presenti entrambe le componenti. Si ipotizza che la coartazione possa iniziare a svilupparsi durante la vita fetale in presenza di un'anomalia cardiaca che comporti una riduzione del flusso ematico anterogrado attraverso la valvola aortica (per es., valvola aortica bicuspide, VSD). In alternativa, la coartazione può essere dovuta a un'estensione anomala del tessuto duttale contrattile nella parete aortica.

In pazienti con coartazione iuxtaduttale semplice, il sangue in aorta ascendente fluisce attraverso il segmento stenotico per poi raggiungere l'aorta discendente, pur dando luogo a ipertrofia e ipertensione ventricolare sinistra. Nei primi giorni di vita, il PDA può servire ad ampliare l'area iuxtaduttale dell'aorta e ad alleviare l'ostruzione, almeno in via temporanea. In questi bambini non cianotici si sviluppa uno shunt duttale netto sinistro-destro. Con una coartazione iuxtaduttale più grave, o in presenza di un'ipoplasia dell'arco trasversale, il sangue dal ventricolo destro viene spinto attraverso il dotto per rifornire l'aorta discendente. La perfusione della parte inferiore del corpo dipende quindi dalla gittata ventricolare destra (vedi Fig. 427-6). In questa situazione, i polsi femorali sono palpabili e la pressione sanguigna differenziale può non essere utile ai fini della diagnosi. Lo shunt duttale destro-sinistro si manifesta con cianosi differenziale, con le estremità superiori rosee e quelle inferiori blu.

Questi lattanti possono avere una grave ipertensione polmonare e un'elevata resistenza vascolare polmonare. I segni di scompenso cardiaco sono evidenti. A volte, i segmenti gravemente ipoplasici dell'istmo aortico diventano completamente atresici portando a interruzione dell'arco aortico, con l'arteria succlavia sinistra che origina prossimamente o distalmente rispetto all'ostruzione. La coartazione associata a ipoplasia dell'arco in passato veniva definita di tipo infantile, poiché la sua gravità di solito faceva sì che la patologia venisse scoperta nella prima infanzia. Il tipo adulto indicava la coartazione iuxtaduttale isolata, che se lieve di solito veniva diagnosticata solo nella tarda infanzia. Queste definizioni

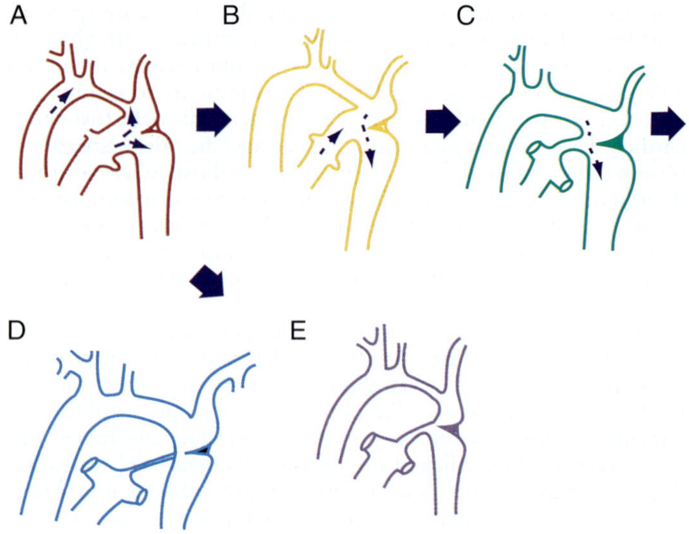

Figura 427-6. Evoluzione della coartazione. *A*, Prototipo fetale senza ostruzione al flusso. *B*, Gravidanza avanzata. Il ventricolo aortico aumenta la sua gittata e dilata il segmento ipoplasico. Il flusso aortico anterogrado scavalca il restringimento attraverso l'orifizio duttale. *C*, Neonato. Il restringimento del dotto dà inizio all'ostruzione rimuovendo il bypass e aumentando il flusso anterogrado nell'arco aortico. *D*, Stenosi iuxtaduttale matura. Il bypass è completamente chiuso e l'ipoplasia intimale alla sommità dell'ostruzione aggrava la stenosi. Si sviluppa un circolo collaterale. *E*, Persistenza del prototipo fetale nel tipo infantile. Un'ostruzione intracardiaca del cuore sinistro impedisce un incremento del flusso aortico anterogrado prima o dopo la nascita. Sono presenti sia ipoplasia dell'istmo sia un'ostruzione controduttale. Il flusso ematico agli arti inferiori spesso dipende dalla pervietà del dotto. (Da Gersony WM: Coarctation of the aorta. In Adams FH, Emmanouilides GC, Riemenshneider T [editors]: *Moss Heart Disease in Infants, Children, and Adolescents*, 4th ed. Baltimore, Williams & Wilkins, 1989.)

sono state sostituite da una terminologia anatomica più corretta, che descrive la sede e la gravità del difetto.

La pressione sanguigna è elevata nei vasi che originano prossimamente alla coartazione; a valle della stenosi, invece, sono più basse sia la pressione sanguigna sia quella differenziale. L'ipertensione non è dovuta soltanto all'ostruzione meccanica, ma coinvolge anche meccanismi neuroumorali. Se non operata nell'infanzia, la coartazione aortica di solito porta allo sviluppo di un'estesa circolazione collaterale, prevalentemente dai rami della succlavia, dalle arterie intercostali superiori e mammarie interne, che permette al sangue arterioso di aggirare l'area della coartazione. I vasi che contribuiscono al circolo collaterale possono andare incontro a marcata dilatazione e divenire tortuosi all'inizio dell'età adulta.

MANIFESTAZIONI CLINICHE. La coartazione aortica riconosciuta dopo l'infanzia non è di solito associata a sintomi significativi. Alcuni bambini o adolescenti lamentano di debolezza e/o dolore agli arti inferiori dopo uno sforzo fisico, ma in molti casi anche pazienti con coartazione grave sono asintomatici. È frequente che bambini più grandi giungano all'attenzione del cardiologo perché risultati ipertesi a una visita medica di routine.

Il segno classico della coartazione aortica è la disparità di polso e pressione sanguigna tra arti superiori e inferiori. I polsi femorali, poplitei, tibiali posteriori e pedidi sono deboli (o assenti in una percentuale di pazienti che può raggiungere il 40%), in contrasto con i polsi scoccanti delle braccia e dei vasi carotidei. I polsi radiali e femorali dovrebbero essere sempre palpati simultaneamente alla ricerca di un ritardo radiale-femorale. Normalmente, il polso femorale si palpa un po' prima del polso radiale. Un ritardo radiale-femorale si verifica quando il flusso sanguigno all'aorta discendente dipende dalle collaterali, nel qual caso il polso femorale si apprezza dopo il polso radiale. Nelle persone normali (a eccezione dei neonati) la pressione sanguigna sistolica misurata agli arti inferiori con il bracciale è di 10-20 mmHg più elevata di quella degli arti superiori. Nella coartazione aortica, la pressione sanguigna nelle gambe è più bassa che nelle braccia e spesso difficile da misurare. Questa differenza di pressione sanguigna è comune in pazienti con coartazione di età superiore a 1 anno; di questi, il 90% circa ha un'ipertensione sistolica a un arto superiore maggiore del 95° percentile per l'età. È importante misurare la pressione sanguigna in entrambi gli arti superiori; una pressione più alta nel destro rispetto al sinistro suggerisce un coinvolgimento dell'arteria succlavia sinistra nell'area della coartazione. A volte, l'arteria succlavia destra può originare in modo anomalo al di sotto dell'area della coartazione, portando a una pressione più elevata nel braccio sinistro che nel destro. Con l'esercizio fisico, si verifica un aumento più evidente della pressione sanguigna sistemica, e il gradiente pressorio tra gli arti superiori e quelli inferiori aumenterà.

L'itto precordiale e i toni cardiaci sono di solito normali; la presenza di un click sistolico da eiezione o di un fremito in corrispondenza dell'incisura sovrasternale suggerisce una valvola aortica bicuspide (presente nel 70% dei casi). Spesso è udibile un breve soffio sistolico lungo il margine sternale sinistro, a livello del terzo e del quarto spazio intercostale. Tale soffio è ben irradiato all'area sottoscapolare sinistra e talvolta al collo. Di frequente si avverte il tipico soffio da stenosi aortica lieve a livello del terzo spazio intercostale. Occasionalmente si riscontrano gradi più significativi di ostruzione attraverso la valvola aortica. La presenza di un soffio a bassa tonalità mesodiastolico all'apice suggerisce una stenosi della valvola mitrale. In pazienti più grandi con un flusso sanguigno collaterale ben sviluppato si possono percepire soffi sistolici o continui ai lati sinistro e destro del torace, lateralmente e posteriormente. In questi pazienti può talvolta apprezzarsi un fremito palpabile negli spazi intercostali sul dorso.

I neonati o i lattanti con una coartazione più grave, che di solito comporta una certa ipoplasia dell'arco aortico trasversale, inizialmente hanno segni di ipoperfusione nella parte inferiore del corpo, acidosi e grave scompenso cardiaco. Questi segni possono manifestarsi giorni o settimane dopo la chiusura del dotto arterioso. Se individuati prima della chiusura del dotto, i pazienti possono presentare una cianosi differenziale, che è possibile rilevare grazie soprattutto all'ossimetria simultanea degli arti superiori e inferiori. All'esame obiettivo, si riscontra ingrandimento cardiaco e si percepisce un soffio sistolico lungo il margine sternale sinistro, con un secondo tono elevato.

DIAGNOSI. I reperti che emergono dall'esame radiografico dipendono dall'età del paziente e dagli effetti dell'ipertensione e del circolo collaterale. L'ingradimento cardiaco e la congestione polmonare si apprezzano in lattanti con coartazione grave. Durante l'infanzia i reperti non sono particolarmente evidenti fino alla prima decade di vita, quando il cuore tende a essere lievemente o moderatamente ingrandito a causa della prominenza del ventricolo sinistro. L'arteria succlavia sinistra allargata produce un'ombra evidente nel mediastino superiore sinistro. La presenza di **incisure nel margine inferiore delle coste**, dovute all'erosione da pressione da parte dei vasi collaterali ingranditi, è comune fino alla fine dell'infanzia. Nella maggior parte dei casi l'aorta discendente presenta un'area di dilatazione post-stenotica.

L'elettrocardiogramma è di solito normale nei bambini piccoli, ma presenta segni di ipertrofia ventricolare sinistra nei pazienti più grandi. I neonati e i lattanti presentano ipertrofia ventricolare destra o biventricolare. In genere è possibile visualizzare il segmento coartato mediante ecocardiografia bidimensionale (Fig. 427-7); possono inoltre venire alla luce anomalie associate delle valvole mitrale e aortica. L'aorta discendente è ipopulsante. L'esame color-Doppler è utile per identificare la sede precisa dell'ostruzione. Studi con Doppler pulsato e ad onda continua determinano il gradiente pressorio proprio in corrispondenza dell'area di coartazione; in presenza di un PDA, tuttavia, la gravità della stenosi può essere sottovalutata. La TC e la RMN sono strumenti non invasivi, utili per la valutazione della coartazione quando l'ecocardiogramma non è chiaro. Il cateterismo cardiaco con ventricolografia sinistra selettiva e aortografia è utile in alcuni pazienti con altre anomalie e come metodo di visualizzazione del flusso sanguigno collaterale. In casi ben definiti mediante l'ecocardiografia, la TC o la RMN, il cateterismo cardiaco non è di solito necessario prima dell'intervento chirurgico.

TRATTAMENTO. In neonati con grave coartazione aortica, la chiusura del dotto spesso determina ipoperfusione, acidosi e rapido deterioramento delle condizioni cliniche. Questi pazienti dovrebbero essere sottoposti a infusione di **prostaglandina E_1** per riaprire il dotto e ripristinare un adeguato flusso sanguigno agli arti inferiori. Una volta confermata la diagnosi e stabilizzato il paziente, occorre procedere alla riparazione chirurgica. I bambini più grandi con scompenso cardiaco ma buona perfusione dovrebbero essere trattati con misure anticongestive per migliorarne le condizioni cliniche prima dell'intervento chirurgico. Di solito non vi è ragione di rimandare l'intervento chirurgico aspettando che il paziente sia cresciuto, dal momento che sono state effettuate con successo correzioni anche in piccoli prematuri.

Bambini più grandi con coartazione aortica significativa dovrebbero essere trattati relativamente presto dopo la diagnosi. Non è giustificato attendere, soprattutto perché a partire dalla seconda decade di vita l'operazione potrebbe avere esiti meno favorevoli a causa di una diminuita funzione ventricolare sinistra e di alterazioni degenerative in atto nella parete aortica. Ciononostante, se la riserva cardiaca è sufficiente, una correzione soddisfacente è possibile fino alla mezza età.

La procedura di scelta per la coartazione aortica iuxtaduttale isolata è oggetto di controversie. Nella maggior parte dei centri l'intervento chirurgico resta il trattamento di elezione, per il quale vengono utilizzate svariate tecniche chirurgiche. Si può

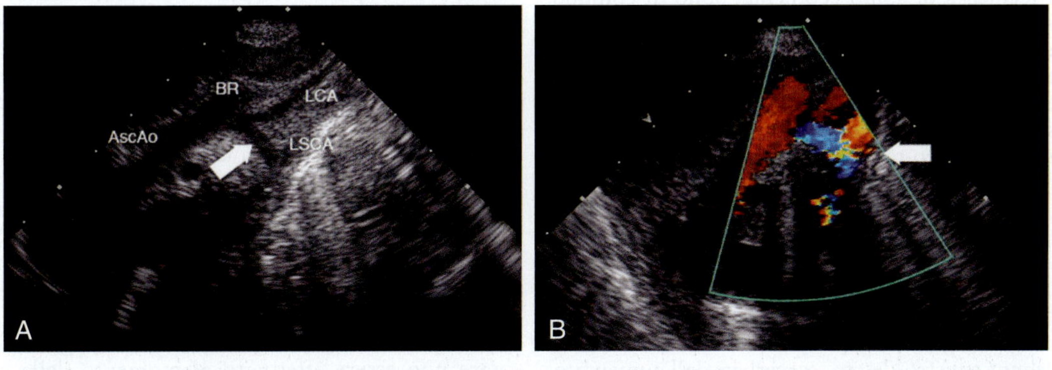

Figura 427-7. Ecocardiogramma che evidenzia una coartazione aortica con arco trasversale ipoplasico. *A*, Ecocardiogramma bidimensionale dall'incisura sovrasternale, da cui si evince un marcato restringimento che inizia subito distalmente rispetto all'arteria brachiocefalica. *B*, Il color-Doppler evidenzia un flusso turbolento nell'area iuxtaduttale (*freccia*). AscAo, aorta ascendente; BR, arteria brachiocefalica, LCA (*Left Carotid Artery*), arteria carotide sinistra; LSCA (*Left SubClavian Artery*), arteria succlavia sinistra.

procedere all'escissione dell'area della coartazione per poi effettuare una re-anastomosi primaria. Spesso l'aorta trasversale viene aperta e si effettua un'anastomosi "estesa termino-terminale" per aumentare la superficie trasversale effettiva della riparazione. Alcuni si avvalgono della procedura con lembo di succlavia, che consiste nella divisione dell'arteria succlavia sinistra e nella sua incorporazione nella parete della coartazione riparata, anche se questa metodica ha perso consensi a causa di un più elevato grado di stenosi residue. Altri preferiscono un'aortoplastica con patch, in cui l'area della coartazione viene allargata con un tetto di materiale protesico. L'utilizzo dell'angioplastica primaria per le coartazioni native rimane oggetto di discussione, anche se è utile quando l'intervento chirurgico può essere associato a un rischio aumentato, in pazienti con grave disfunzione ventricolare sinistra.

Dopo l'intervento chirurgico, si assiste a un impressionante aumento dell'ampiezza dei polsi agli arti inferiori. Nell'immediato periodo postoperatorio, un'**ipertensione rebound** è comune e richiede terapia medica. Quest'ipertensione acuta esagerata regredisce gradualmente e nella maggior parte dei pazienti è possibile sospendere la somministrazione dei farmaci antipertensivi. Sono comuni soffi residui, che possono essere dovuti ad anomalie cardiache associate, a turbe del flusso sanguigno residuo attraverso l'area sottoposta a correzione, o al flusso sanguigno collaterale. Rari problemi operatori comprendono danni al midollo spinale imputabili al clampaggio dell'aorta se le collaterali sono poco sviluppate, sviluppo di un chilotorace, danni al diaframma e lesione del nervo laringeo. Se si utilizza un lembo di succlavia sinistra, il polso radiale e la pressione sanguigna nell'arto superiore sinistro sono diminuiti o assenti.

SINDROME POST-COARTECTOMIA. Un'**arterite mesenterica** postoperatoria può essere associata a ipertensione acuta e dolore addominale nell'immediato periodo postoperatorio. Il dolore può avere diversa intensità e manifestarsi in associazione ad anoressia, nausea, vomito, leucocitosi, emorragia intestinale, necrosi intestinale e ostruzione dell'intestino tenue. Si ottiene un beneficio con farmaci antipertensivi (nitroprussiato, esmololo, captopril) e decompressione intestinale; l'esplorazione chirurgica è raramente necessaria per l'ostruzione o l'infarto intestinale.

PROGNOSI. Anche se una recidiva della stenosi nei bambini più grandi dopo un intervento di coartectomia è rara, un numero significativo di lattanti operati entro il primo anno di vita deve essere sottoposto a una revisione successivamente, durante l'infanzia. Tutti i pazienti dovrebbero essere monitorati attentamente per individuare lo sviluppo di una nuova coartazione e di un aneurisma aortico. Nel caso si verificasse una coartazione, l'angioplastica con catetere a palloncino è la procedura di scelta. In questi pazienti, il tessuto cicatriziale risultante dal precedente intervento chirurgico rende il reintervento più difficile, ma rende sicura l'**angioplastica con catetere a palloncino**, per la più bassa incidenza di formazione di aneurismi. La risoluzione dell'ostruzione con questa tecnica è di solito eccellente. Sono di comune utilizzo gli **stent intravascolari**, soprattutto negli adolescenti e nei giovani adulti, generalmente con risultati eccellenti.

La riparazione della coartazione nella seconda decade di vita od oltre può essere associata a una più elevata incidenza di patologie cardiovascolari premature, anche in assenza di anomalie cardiache residue. Nell'adulto può verificarsi un esordio precoce di un'ipertensione cronica, anche in pazienti con coartazione adeguatamente resecata.

Anomalie della valvola aortica sono presenti nella maggior parte dei pazienti. La valvole aortiche bicuspidi sono comuni, ma non causano generalmente segni clinici a meno che la stenosi non sia significativa. L'associazione di PDA e coartazione aortica è altresì comune. Può sorgere il sospetto di VSD e ASD in presenza di segni di shunt sinistro-destro, esacerbati dall'aumentata resistenza al flusso attraverso la parte sinistra del cuore. Talvolta si riscontrano anomalie della valvola mitrale, come pure stenosi aortiche sottovalvolari.

Per quanto si tratti di un'evenienza rara, possono verificarsi un grave danno neurologico o persino la morte a causa di un'associata patologia cerebrovascolare. Un'emorragia subaracnoidea o intracerebrale può derivare dalla rottura di aneurismi congeniti del circolo di Willis, dalla rottura di altri vasi con difetti del tessuto elastico e della tonaca media, o dalla rottura di vasi normali; questi incidenti sono secondari all'ipertensione. Bambini con la **sindrome PHACE** (*Posterior brain fossa anomalies, facial Hemangiomas, Arterial anomalies, Cardiac anomalies and aortic coarctation, Eye anomalies*, anomalie della fossa cranica posteriore, emangiomi faciali, anomalie arteriose, anomalie cardiache e coartazione aortica, anomalie oculari) possono andare incontro a ictus (vedi Tab. 422-2). Anomalie delle arterie succlavie possono comprendere il coinvolgimento dell'arteria succlavia sinistra nell'area della coartazione, la stenosi dell'orifizio dell'arteria succlavia sinistra e l'origine anomala dell'arteria succlavia destra.

In assenza di trattamento, la grande maggioranza dei pazienti adulti con coartazione aortica muore in età compresa tra i 20 e i 40 anni, mentre alcuni sopravvivono fino alla mezz'età senza gravi disabilità. Le complicanze gravi, peraltro comuni, sono correlate all'ipertensione sistemica, che può portare a una coronaropatia prematura, allo scompenso cardiaco, all'encefalopatia ipertensiva o all'emorragia intracranica. Lo scompenso cardiaco può essere peggiorato da anomalie associate. L'endocardite o l'endoarterite infettiva sono complicanze significative nell'adulto. Possono inoltre svilupparsi aneurismi dell'aorta discendente o dei vasi collaterali ingrossati.

427.7 • COARTAZIONE CON DIFETTO DEL SETTO INTERVENTRICOLARE

La coartazione in presenza di un VSD causa a un aumento sia del precarico sia del postcarico sul ventricolo sinistro; i pazienti con questa combinazione di difetti saranno identificati alla nascita o nel primo mese di vita e spesso avranno uno scompenso cardiaco intrattabile. L'entità dello shunt sinistro-destro attraverso un VSD dipende dal rapporto tra la resistenza vascolare polmonare e quella sistemica. In presenza di una coartazione, la resistenza all'efflusso nella circolazione sistemica è aumentata dall'ostruzione, e il volume dello shunt va incontro a marcato aumento. Il quadro clinico è quello di un bambino molto malato, con tachipnea, ritardo di crescita e i tipici reperti dello scompenso cardiaco. Spesso la differenza di pressione sanguigna tra arti superiori e inferiori non è molto marcata poiché la gittata cardiaca può essere bassa. Il trattamento medico dovrebbe servire a stabilizzare il paziente, almeno inizialmente, mentre non dovrebbe essere utilizzato per ritardare di molto l'intervento correttivo.

Nella maggior parte dei casi la coartazione è l'anomalia principale responsabile di gravi sintomi e la resezione del segmento coartato comporta un notevole miglioramento. In molti centri si riparano di routine sia il VSD sia la coartazione nel corso dello stesso intervento, mediante una sternotomia mediana, utilizzando un bypass cardiopolmonare. Alcuni riparano la coartazione attraverso una toracotomia laterale sinistra e nello stesso tempo posizionano un bendaggio dell'arteria polmonare per diminuire lo shunt a livello ventricolare. Altri non effettuano il bendaggio dell'arteria polmonare inizialmente, poiché un certo numero di pazienti migliora al punto da rendere inutile un successivo intervento chirurgico durante la prima infanzia. Se lo scompenso cardiaco rende difficile la gestione di questi bambini dopo l'intervento chirurgico, spesso poco dopo si procede alla riparazione del VSD. Una volta accertata la presenza di un VSD complicato (multiplo, muscolare apicale), il bendaggio dell'arteria polmonare può essere effettuato al momento della riparazione della coartazione onde evitare un intervento chirurgico a cuore aperto durante la prima infanzia per queste anomalie complesse del setto interventricolare.

427.8 • Coartazione associata ad altre anomalie cardiache e a interruzione dell'arco aortico

Spesso la coartazione si presenta nell'infanzia in associazione con altre importanti anomalie cardiache, tra cui un cuore sinistro ipoplasico, una grave patologia valvolare mitralica o aortica, la trasposizione delle grandi arterie e varianti del doppio efflusso o del ventricolo unico. Una grave coartazione può essere associata anche a fibroelastosi endocardica. Le manifestazioni cliniche dipendono dagli effetti delle malformazioni associate, oltre che dalla coartazione stessa.

La coartazione aortica con grave valvulopatia mitralica e aortica può necessitare di trattamento nel contesto della sindrome del cuore sinistro ipoplasico (vedi Capitolo 431.10), anche se la camera ventricolare sinistra non è gravemente ipoplasica. Tali pazienti di solito hanno un lungo segmento di arco aortico trasversale ristretto, con o senza coartazione isolata a livello del dotto arterioso. La coartazione dell'aorta con trasposizione delle grandi arterie o il ventricolo singolo possono essere riparati da soli o in combinazione con altre misure palliative.

L'interruzione completa dell'arco aortico è la forma di coartazione più grave, di solito associata a un'altra patologia intracardiaca. L'interruzione può interessare qualsiasi livello, anche è di più comune riscontro tra l'arteria succlavia sinistra e l'inserzione del dotto arterioso (tipo A), seguita come frequenza dalle interruzioni tra l'arteria succlavia sinistra e l'arteria carotide sinistra (tipo B). Nei neonati con arco aortico interrotto, il dotto arterioso è l'unico responsabile dell'apporto ematico all'aorta discendente, e si può osservare una disparità di saturazione di ossigeno tra il braccio destro (saturazione normale) e gli arti inferiori (diminuita). Quando il dotto inizia a chiudersi, in questi bambini possono svilupparsi un grave scompenso cardiaco congestizio, un'ipoperfusione delle estremità inferiori, anuria e uno stato di shock. I pazienti con interruzione dell'arco aortico possono essere sottoposti a terapia di supporto con prostaglandine per mantenere pervio il dotto in attesa della correzione chirurgica. In quanto malformazione conotroncale, l'interruzione dell'arco aortico può essere associata allo spettro di lesioni noto come **CATCH22** (*Cardiac defect, Abnormal facies, Thymic hypoplasia, Cleft palate, Hypocalcemia*, difetti cardiaci, facies anomala, aplasia del timo, palatoschisi, ipocalcemia). La CATCH22 comprende pazienti con caratteristiche cliniche della sindrome di DiGeorge (ipocalcemia, ipoplasia timica, lievi anomalie facciali) e della sindrome di Shprintzen velocardiofacciale (anomalie faciali, palatoschisi). L'analisi citogenetica mediante tecnica FISH (*Fluorescence In Situ Hybridization*) evidenzia la delezione di un segmento del cromosoma 22q11 noto come regione critica di DiGeorge, contenente il gene Tbx1, un fattore di trascrizione, che è stato chiamato in causa nella sindrome.

427.9 • Stenosi mitralica congenita

La stenosi mitralica congenita è un'anomalia rara che può essere isolata o associata ad altri difetti, i più comuni dei quali sono la stenosi aortica e la coartazione aortica (**complesso di Shone**). La valvola mitrale può avere una forma a imbuto, con lembi ispessiti e corde tendinee accorciate e deformate. Altre anomalie della valvola mitrale associate a stenosi comprendono la valvola mitrale a paracadute, causata dalla presenza di un unico muscolo papillare, e la valvola mitrale con doppio orifizio.

I sintomi compaiono di solito entro i primi 2 anni di vita. Questi bambini sono sottosviluppati e generalmente presentano una spiccata dispnea, secondaria a scompenso cardiaco; sono comuni la cianosi e il pallore. In alcuni pazienti, in cui il sintomo predominante è il respiro affannoso, è possibile sia stata posta diagnosi di patologia reattiva delle vie aeree. È comune l'ingrandimento cardiaco, imputabile a dilatazione e ipertrofia del ventricolo destro e dell'atrio sinistro. La maggior parte dei pazienti ha un rullio apicale diastolico seguito da un primo tono forte, ma i reperti auscultatori possono essere relativamente poco chiari. Il secondo tono è forte e sdoppiato. Può essere presente uno schiocco d'apertura della valvola mitrale. L'elettrocardiogramma evidenzia un'ipertrofia ventricolare destra con onde P normali, bifide o appuntite, indicative di ingrandimento atriale sinistro. Le radiografie del torace di solito rivelano un ingrandimento atriale sinistro e ventricolare destro e congestione polmonare. L'ecocardiogramma presenta reperti caratteristici: lembi della valvola mitrale ispessiti, una diminuita pendenza EF all'ecocardiogramma mitralico M-mode e un atrio sinistro ingrandito con un ventricolo sinistro normale o piccolo. L'esame ecocardiografico bidimensionale evidenzia una significativa riduzione dell'orifizio della valvola mitrale in diastole. Gli studi Doppler mostrano un gradiente pressorio medio attraverso l'orifizio mitralico. Al cateterismo cardiaco si osserva un aumento delle pressioni nel ventricolo destro e in arteria polmonare e un aumento della pressione di incuneamento capillare polmonare. Emerge inoltre la presenza di anomalie associate, come la stenosi aortica e la coartazione. L'angiocardiografia evidenzia un ritardato svuotamento dell'atrio sinistro e l'orifizio mitralico di piccole dimensioni.

In assenza di trattamento, la prognosi è infausta. Molteplici sono stati i risultati dell'intervento chirurgico; di solito è richiesto il posizionamento di una protesi valvolare mitralica, la quale però va sostituita a mano a mano che il bambino cresce. Dal momento che questi pazienti devono assumere warfarin, un farmaco anticoagulante, le complicanze connesse a un sovra- o sottodosaggio sono abbastanza comuni nell'infanzia. La valvuloplastica con catetere a palloncino è stata utilizzata da numerosi centri come procedura palliativa con risultati variabili, a seconda dell'anatomia della valvola e dei muscoli papillari.

427.10 • Ipertensione venosa polmonare

Molte sono le lesioni che possono dare origine a un'ipertensione venosa polmonare cronica, la quale a sua volta, se estrema, porta a ipertensione arteriosa polmonare e scompenso cardiaco destro. Queste lesioni comprendono la stenosi mitralica congenita, l'insufficienza mitralica, il ritorno venoso polmonare anomalo totale con ostruzione, i mixomi dell'atrio sinistro, il *cor triatriatum* (stenosi di un vena polmonare comune), la stenosi di una singola vena polmonare e la presenza di anelli o membrane mitraliche sopravalvolari. I sintomi precoci possono essere confusi con quelli di una patologia polmonare cronica come l'asma, per la mancanza di reperti specifici all'esame obiettivo. Possono essere presenti segni sfumati di ipertensione polmonare. L'elettrocardiogramma evidenzia un'ipertrofia ventricolare destra con onde P appuntite, mentre le radiografie del torace mostrano un ingrandimento cardiaco e la prominenza delle vene polmonari nella regione ilare, del ventricolo e dell'atrio destri, e del tronco principale dell'arteria polmonare; l'atrio sinistro è di dimensioni normali o solo lievemente ingrandito.

L'ecocardiogramma può evidenziare un mixoma atriale sinistro, un *cor triatriatum*, la stenosi di una o più vene polmonari, o un'anomalia della valvola mitrale. Il cateterismo cardiaco esclude la presenza di uno shunt e rivela ipertensione polmonare con un'elevata pressione arteriosa polmonare di incuneamento. La pressione atriale sinistra è normale se la lesione è a livello delle vene polmonari, mentre risulta elevata se la lesione si trova a livello della valvola mitrale. L'arteriografia polmonare selettiva caratterizza la lesione dal punto di vista anatomico. Il *cor triatriatum*, il mixoma atriale sinistro e le reti mitraliche sopravalvolari sono condizioni che possono essere tutte trattate con successo per via chirurgica.

La **diagnosi differenziale** comprende la patologia veno-occlusiva polmonare, un processo idiopatico di eziologia incerta che causa lesioni ostruttive a carico delle vene polmonari, in bambini e giovani adulti. Sebbene si riscontri di solito dopo riparazione di un ritorno venoso polmonare anomalo totale con ostruzione (vedi Capitolo 431.7), può insorgere anche in assenza di una cardiopatia congenita. Il paziente inizialmente presenta uno scompenso cardiaco sinistro sulla base di una congestione polmonare con un apparente edema polmonare. Sono comuni la dispnea, l'astenia e i versamenti pleurici; altri reperti talvolta presenti sono la cianosi, l'ippocratismo digitale e l'emottisi. La pressione atriale sinistra è normale, ma la pressione di incuneamento arteriosa polmonare di solito risulta elevata. Una pressione di incuneamento normale può essere attribuita alla formazione di collaterali o alla valutazione di un segmento non coinvolto. Dal punto di vista angiografico, le vene polmonari ritornano normalmente all'atrio sinistro, ma alcune di esse sono ristrette, a livello locale o diffusamente.

La biopsia polmonare evidenzia un coinvolgimento polmonare venoso e a volte arterioso. Le vene e le venule polmonari presentano un restringimento fibroso o un'occlusione, e nell'arteria polmonare possono essere presenti trombi. La terapia è deludente e la sopravvivenza variabile: non supera alcune settimane o mesi nel lattante, mentre può prolungarsi di qualche anno nell'adulto. Tentativi di riparazione chirurgica, di dilatazione con catetere a palloncino e di stenting mediante catetere non hanno migliorato significativamente la prognosi di questi pazienti. Sono attualmente in corso trial clinici riguardanti la somministrazione della chemioterapia antiproliferativa. Il trapianto combinato cuore-polmoni (vedi Capitolo 443.2) rimane l'unica opzione terapeutica con qualche probabilità di successo.

Stenosi polmonare

Crosnier C, Lykavieris P, Meunier-Rotival M, et al: Alagille syndrome. The widening spectrum of arteriohepatic dysplasia. *Clin Liver Dis* 2000; 4:765–778.

Krantz ID, Smith R, Colliton RP, et al: Jagged 1 mutations in patients ascertained with isolated congenital heart defects. *Am J Med Genet* 1999; 84:56–60.

Moller JH: Exercise responses in pulmonary stenosis. *Prog Pediatr Cardiol* 1993;2:8–13.

Phoon CK: Estimation of pressure gradients by auscultation: An innovative and accurate physical examination technique. *Am Heart J* 2001;141: 500–506.

Rosales AM, Lock JE, Perry SB, et al: Interventional catheterization management of perioperative peripheral pulmonary stenosis: Balloon angioplasty or endovascular stenting. *Catheter Cardiovasc Interv* 2002;56:272–277.

Yoshida R, Hasegawa T, Hasegawa Y, et al: Protein-tyrosine phosphatase, nonreceptor type 11 mutation analysis and clinical assessment in 45 patients with Noonan syndrome. *J Clin Endocrinol Metab* 2004;89:3359–3364.

Stenosi aortica

Doyle EF, Arumugham P, Lara E, et al: Sudden death in young patients with congenital aortic stenosis. *Pediatrics* 1974;53:481–489.

Freed MD: Recreational and sports recommendations for the child with heart disease. *Pediatr Clin North Am* 1984;31:1307–1320.

Jahangiri M, Nicholson IA, del Nido PJ, et al: Surgical management of complex and tunnel-like subaortic stenosis. *Eur J Cardiothorac Surg* 2000;17: 637–642.

Laudito A, Brook MM, Suleman S, et al: The Ross procedure in children and young adults: A word of caution. *J Thorac Cardiovasc Surg* 2001;122: 147–153.

Leichter DA, Sullivan I, Gersony WM: "Acquired" discrete subvalvular aortic stenosis: Natural history and hemodynamics. *J Am Coll Cardiol* 1989;14: 1539–1544.

Marino BS, Bridges ND, Paridon SM: Aortic insufficiency: Indications for surgery in children. *Semin Thorac Cardiovasc Surg Pediatr Card Surg Annu* 1998;1:147–156.

Ohye RG, Gomez CA, Ohye BJ, et al: The Ross/Konno procedure in neonates and infants: Intermediate-term survival and autograft function. *Ann Thorac Surg* 2001;72:823–830.

Pessotto R, Wells WJ, Baker CJ, et al: Midterm results of the Ross procedure. *Ann Thorac Surg* 2001;71(5 Suppl):S336–S339.

Rocchini A, Beekman RH, Ben Shachar G, et al: Balloon aortic valvuloplasty: Results of the valvuloplasty and angioplasty of congenital anomalies registry. *Am J Cardiol* 1990;65:784–789.

Tweddell JS, Pelech AN, Frommelt PC, et al: Complex aortic valve repair as a durable and effective alternative to valve replacement in children with aortic valve disease. *J Thorac Cardiovasc Surg* 2005;129:551–558.

Coartazione aortica

Daniels SR: Repair of coarctation of the aorta and hypertension: Does age matter? *Lancet* 2001;358:89.

Hamdan MA, Maheshwari S, Fahey JT: Endovascular stents for coarctation of the aorta: Initial results and intermediate-term follow-up. *J Am Coll Cardiol* 2001;38:1518–1523.

Ing FF, Starc TJ, Griffiths SP, et al: Early diagnosis of coarctation of the aorta in children: A continuing dilemma. *Pediatrics* 1996;98:378–382.

Markham LW, Knecht SK, Daniels SR, et al: Development of exercise-induced arm-leg blood pressure gradient and abnormal arterial compliance in patients with repaired coarctation of the aorta. *Am J Cardiol* 2004;94:1200–1202.

Metry DW, Dowd CF, Barkovich J, et al: The many faces of PHACE syndrome. *J Pediatr* 2001;139:117–123.

O'Sullivan JJ, Derrick G, Darnell R: Prevalence of hypertension in children after early repair of coarctation of the aorta: A cohort study using casual and 24 hour blood pressure measurement. *Heart* 2002;88:163–166.

Shone JD, Sellers RD, Anderson RC, et al: The developmental complex of "parachute mitral valve," supravalvar ring of left atrium, subaortic stenosis, and coarctation of the aorta. *Am J Cardiol* 1963;11:714–725.

Stenosi mitralica

Moore P, Adatia I, Spevak PJ, et al: Severe congenital mitral stenosis in infants. *Circulation* 1994;89:2099–2106.

Capitolo 428 ■ Cardiopatie congenite non cianogene: lesioni con rigurgito

428.1 • Insufficienza valvolare polmonare e assenza congenita della valvola polmonare

L'insufficienza valvolare polmonare nella maggior parte dei casi si associa ad altre patologie cardiovascolari o può essere secondaria a una grave ipertensione polmonare. L'incompetenza della valvola è un risultato atteso dopo intervento chirurgico per un'ostruzione del tratto di efflusso del ventricolo destro, per esempio una valvulotomia polmonare in pazienti con stenosi valvolare polmonare o una valvulotomia con resezione infundibolare in pazienti con tetralogia di Fallot. Un'insufficienza congenita isolata della valvola polmonare è rara e generalmente lieve, tanto che questi pazienti sono per lo più asintomatici.

Il segno obiettivo più evidente è un soffio diastolico in decrescendo a livello del margine sternale medio e superiore di sinistra, che ha una tonalità più bassa del soffio da insufficienza aortica a causa di una pressione inferiore. Dalle radiografie del torace emergono la prominenza del tronco principale dell'arteria polmonare e, se l'insufficienza è grave, una dilatazione del ventricolo destro. L'elettrocardiogramma è normale o evidenzia una minima ipertrofia del ventricolo destro. Il Doppler pulsato e il color-Doppler evidenziano un flusso retrogrado dall'arteria polmonare al ventricolo destro durante la diastole. La diagnosi può essere posta all'atto del cateterismo cardiaco, se necessario. La pressione arteriosa diastolica polmonare è bassa. L'arteriografia polmonare selettiva mostra l'incompetenza valvolare, ma è difficile da valutare in casi lievi in quanto il catetere che attraversa la valvola di solito determina un'insufficienza iatrogena durante l'iniezione. L'angiografia con risonanza magnetica o angioRM (MRA, *Magnetic Resonance Angiography*) è utile per quantificare sia il volume del ventricolo destro sia la frazione rigurgitante. L'insufficienza valvolare polmonare isolata in genere è ben tollerata e non richiede un trattamento chirurgico; nei casi gravi, specialmente se si associa una significativa insufficienza tricuspidalica, può rendersi necessaria la sostituzione con una valvola homograft per preservare la funzione ventricolare destra.

L'assenza congenita della valvola polmonare è di solito associata a un difetto del setto interventricolare, spesso nel contesto della tetralogia di Fallot (vedi Capitolo 430.1). In molti di questi neonati, le arterie polmonari vanno incontro a notevole dilatazione finendo per comprimere i bronchi, con conseguenti episodi di dispnea, collasso polmonare e polmoniti. La presenza e il grado della cianosi sono variabili. L'incompetenza florida della valvola polmonare può non essere ben tollerata al punto che può subentrare la morte a causa di una combinazione di compressione bronchiale, ipossiemia e scompenso cardiaco. La correzione comprende la plicatura delle arterie polmonari massivamente dilatate, la chiusura del difetto del setto interventricolare e il posizionamento di un homograft attraverso il tratto di efflusso del ventricolo destro.

428.2 • Insufficienza mitralica congenita

L'insufficienza mitralica congenita può essere isolata, ma più spesso è associata ad altre anomalie, tra cui dotto arterioso pervio, coartazione aortica, difetto del setto interventricolare, trasposizione corretta dei grossi vasi, origine anomala dell'arteria coronaria sinistra dall'arteria polmonare o sindrome di Marfan. L'insufficienza mitralica, comune in associazione con difetti del setto atrioventricolare (vedi Capitolo 426.5), può riscontrarsi anche in pazienti con miocardiopatia dilatativa (vedi Capitolo 439.1) secondariamente a dilatazione dell'anello valvolare.

Nell'insufficienza mitralica isolata, l'anello valvolare mitralico è di solito dilatato, le corde tendinee sono corte e possono avere un'inserzione anomala e i lembi valvolari sono deformati. Quando l'insufficienza mitralica è abbastanza grave da causare sintomi clinici, l'atrio sinistro si dilata in conseguenza del flusso da rigurgito, e il ventricolo sinistro diventa ipertrofico e dilatato. La pressione venosa polmonare aumenta fino a causare ipertensione polmonare e pertrofia del ventricolo destro con dilatazione. Le lesioni lievi rimangono asintomatiche; l'unico segno anomalo è il soffio olosistolico dell'incompetenza mitralica. Un rigurgito grave provoca sintomi che possono comparire a qualsiasi età, quali scarso sviluppo fisico, frequenti infezioni respiratorie, scarsa tolleranza allo sforzo ed episodi di edema polmonare o scompenso cardiaco congestizio. In molti casi sarà stata posta una diagnosi di patologia reattiva delle vie aeree a causa della somiglianza dei sintomi polmonari.

Tipico dell'insufficienza mitralica è un soffio a tonalità elevata, apicale e olosistolico. Se l'insufficienza è moderata o grave, è di solito caratterizzata da un rullio a bassa tonalità, apicale e mediodiastolico, indicativo di un aumento del flusso diastolico attraverso la valvola mitrale. La componente polmonare del secondo tono sarà accentuata in presenza di ipertensione polmonare. L'elettrocardiogramma evidenzia onde P bifide, segni di ipertrofia ventricolare sinistra e a volte segni di ipertrofia ventricolare destra. Le radiografie del torace mostrano ingrandimento dell'atrio sinistro, talvolta massivo. Il ventricolo sinistro è prominente e la vascolarizzazione polmonare è normale o accentuata. L'ecocardiogramma evidenzia un ingrandimento dell'atrio e del ventricolo sinistri. Il color-Doppler permette di valutare l'entità dell'insufficienza e il Doppler pulsato delle vene polmonari evidenzia il flusso retrogrado quando l'insufficienza mitralica è grave. Il cateterismo cardiaco rileva un'elevata pressione in atrio sinistro. Può essere presente un'ipertensione polmonare di gravità variabile. La ventricolografia sinistra selettiva permette di determinare la gravità del rigurgito mitralico.

La **valvuloplastica mitralica** può portare a un notevole miglioramento dei sintomi e delle dimensioni cardiache, ma in alcuni pazienti talvolta è necessario posizionare una protesi mitralica meccanica. Prima dell'intervento chirurgico, occorre identificare eventuali anomalie associate. Nei bambini di età superiore ai 3-4 anni può essere difficile escludere la febbre reumatica come causa di insufficienza mitralica.

428.3 • Prolasso della valvola mitrale

Il prolasso della valvola mitrale deriva da un anomalo meccanismo della valvola mitrale che porta alla protrusione di uno o entrambi i lembi mitralici, specialmente della cuspide posteriore, nell'atrio sinistro verso la fine della sistole. L'anomalia è per lo più congenita, ma può passare inosservata fino all'adolescenza o all'età adulta. Il prolasso della valvola mitrale, di solito sporadico, è più comune nelle ragazze e può essere ereditato come tratto autosomico dominante con espressività variabile. È di frequente riscontro in pazienti con sindrome di Marfan, sindrome della schiena diritta, *pectus excavatum*, scoliosi, sindrome di Ehler Danlos, osteogenesi imperfetta e *pseudoxanthoma elasticum*. Il soffio apicale è telesistolico e può essere preceduto da un click, ma questi segni variano nello stesso paziente e quindi talvolta è udibile solo il click. In posizione eretta o seduta, il click può verificarsi più precocemente durante la sistole e il soffio essere più marcato in telesistole. Eventuali aritmie consistono prevalentemente in contrazioni ventricolari premature unifocali o multifocali.

L'elettrocardiogramma è di solito normale ma può anche evidenziare onde T bifasiche, soprattutto nelle derivazioni II, III, aVF e V_6; le anomalie dell'onda T possono variare nel tempo nello stesso paziente. Le radiografie del torace sono normali. L'ecocardiogramma evidenzia un caratteristico movimento posteriore del lembo posteriore della mitrale durante la meso- o la telesistole, oppure un prolasso olosistolico di entrambi i lembi mitralici, anteriore e posteriore, si tratta di reperti che all'ecocardiogramma M-mode vanno interpretati con cautela, poiché la presenza di un minimo prolasso mitralico può rappresentare una variante normale. Un'interpretazione più precisa si avrà in presenza di un prolasso di uno o due lembi di >2 mm oltre il piano anulare in asse lungo, con o senza ispessimento dei lembi. Il prolasso con ispessimento valvolare >5 mm è "classico", mentre quello di grado inferiore non lo è. L'ecocardiografia bidimensionale in tempo reale evidenzia che sia l'estremità libera sia il corpo dei lembi valvolari si muovono posteriormente in sistole verso l'atrio. Il Doppler può valutare la presenza e la gravità del rigurgito mitralico.

Non è indicata alcuna terapia specifica per questa lesione, che non è progressiva nell'infanzia. Il paziente può essere a rischio di sviluppare un'endocardite infettiva. La profilassi antibiotica è raccomandata durante gli interventi chirurgici e le procedure dentarie (vedi Capitolo 437).

Gli adulti (soprattutto maschi) con prolasso della valvola mitrale sono a rischio di complicanze cardiovascolari (morte improvvisa, aritmie, incidenti cerebrovascolari, progressiva dilatazione valvolare, scompenso cardiaco ed endocardite) in presenza di lembi valvolari **ispessiti** (>5 mm) e **ridondanti.** Fattori di rischio per la morbilità comprendono anche una scarsa funzione ventricolare, un rigurgito mitralico da moderato a grave e un ingrandimento dell'atrio sinistro.

Spesso vi è confusione riguardo alla diagnosi di prolasso della valvola mitralico. L'elevata frequenza di un lieve prolasso all'ecocardiogramma in assenza di reperti clinici suggerisce che in questi casi non sia presente una vera sindrome da prolasso della valvola mitrale. Su questo punto andrebbero rassicurati pazienti e genitori; si consiglia inoltre di non raccomandare né trattamenti speciali, né indagini di laboratorio troppo frequenti. La profilassi per l'endocardite è indicata solo in casi ben documentati, ossia quelli con insufficienza mitralica.

428.4 • Rigurgito tricuspidale

Il rigurgito tricuspidale isolato è generalmente associato all'**anomalia di Ebstein** della valvola tricuspide. Tale anomalia può essere acianotica o dar luogo a cianosi di grado variabile, a seconda della gravità del rigurgito tricuspidale e della presenza di una comunicazione a livello atriale (forame ovale pervio o difetto del setto interatriale). I bambini più grandi tendono ad avere la forma acianotica, mentre se scoperta nel periodo neonatale, l'anomalia di Ebstein è di solito associata a cianosi grave (vedi Capitolo 430.7).

Il rigurgito tricuspidale è spesso associato a una **disfunzione ventricolare destra**. Quando il ventricolo destro si dilata a causa del sovraccarico di volume e/o di una miocardiopatia intrinseca, anche l'anulus tricuspidale si allarga, dando luogo a insufficienza valvolare. Questa forma di rigurgito può migliorare se la causa della dilatazione ventricolare destra viene corretta, oppure richiedere la plicatura chirurgica dell'anulus valvolare. Il rigurgito tricuspidale viene diagnosticato anche nei neonati con **asfissia perinatale**; questa causa può essere correlata a una maggiore suscettibilità del muscolo papillare al danno ischemico, sua volta responsabile di disfunzione transitoria del muscolo papillare.

Assenza della valvola polmonare

McDonnell BE, Raff GW, Gaynor JW, et al: Outcome after repair of tetralogy of Fallot with absent pulmonary valve. *Ann Thorac Surg* 1999;67:1391–1395.

Pinsky WW: Absent pulmonary valve syndrome. In Garson A, Bricker JT, Fisher DJ, Neish SR (editors): *The Science and Practice of Pediatric Cardiology.* Baltimore, Williams & Wilkins, 1998, pp 1413–1419.

Anomalie delle valvola mitrale

American Academy of Pediatrics Committee on Sports Medicine and Fitness: Mitral valve prolapse and athletic participation in children and adolescents. *Pediatrics* 1995;95:789–790.

Bouknight DP, O'Rourke RA: Current management of mitral valve prolapse. *Am Fam Physician* 2000;61:3343–3350, 3353–3354.

Hayek E, Gring CN, Griffin BP: Mitral valve prolapse. *Lancet* 2005;365:507–518.

Jacobs W, Chamoun A, Stouffer GA: Mitral valve prolapse: A review of the literature. *Am J Med Sci* 2001;321:401–410.

Maron BJ, Ackerman MJ, Nishimura RA, et al: Task Force 4: HCM and other cardiomyopathies, mitral valve prolapse, myocarditis, and Marfan syndrome. *J Am Coll Cardiol* 2005;45:1340–1345.

Capitolo 429 ■ Cardiopatie congenite cianogene: valutazione del neonato in condizioni critiche con cianosi e distress respiratorio

Vedi anche Capitolo 101.

Un neonato gravemente malato con distress cardiorespiratorio e cianosi rappresenta una sfida diagnostica. Il medico deve effettuare una rapida valutazione per determinare se la causa sottostante è una cardiopatia congenita, in modo da poter poi mettere in atto misure salvavita. La diagnosi differenziale della cianosi neonatale è presentata nella Tabella 101.1.

PATOLOGIE CARDIACHE. Una cardiopatia congenita causa cianosi quando l'ostruzione all'efflusso ventricolare destro provoca uno shunt intracardiaco destro-sinistro o quando difetti anatomici complessi, non associati a stenosi polmonare, provocano un mescolamento del ritorno venoso polmonare e sistemico nel cuore. Una cianosi da edema polmonare, per quanto in genere di minore entità, si può inoltre sviluppare in pazienti con scompenso cardiaco causato da shunt sinistro-destro. La cianosi può essere causata anche dalla persistenza di vie fetali, per esempio uno shunt destro-sinistro attraverso il forame ovale e il dotto arterioso in presenza di ostruzione del tratto di efflusso polmonare o di ipertensione polmonare persistente del neonato (vedi Capitolo 101.8).

DIAGNOSI DIFFERENZIALE. La valutazione iniziale di un bambino cianotico inizia con l'osservazione del pattern respiratorio. Un respiro debole o irregolare è spesso associato a un riflesso di suzione debole e a problemi riguardanti il sistema nervoso centrale (SNC). Convulsioni e uno stato di depressione generale sono reperti significativi che inducono a sospettare un'eziologia a carico del SNC. Per contro, il lattante con patologia primitiva cardiaca o polmonare presenta atti respiratori vigorosi o affaticati con tachipnea.

Il **test dell'iperossia** è una delle metodiche impiegate per distinguere una cardiopatia congenita cianogena da una patologia polmonare. I neonati con cardiopatie congenite cianogene di solito non presentano un significativo aumento della Pa_{O_2} arteriosa durante somministrazione di ossigeno al 100%; se quindi in queste condizioni la Pa_{O_2} aumenta fino a superare i 150 mmHg, si può escludere uno shunt intracardiaco, anche se in alcuni pazienti con cardiopatie cianogene questo valore può subire un rialzo transitorio oltre i 150 mmHg a causa di particolari potenziali di flusso intracardiaci. Invece, nei pazienti con patologia polmonare la Pa_{O_2} di solito aumenta significativamente a mano a mano che gli squilibri di ventilazione-perfusione vengono superati grazie alla somministrazione di ossigeno. In bambini con problemi del SNC, la Pa_{O_2} si normalizza completamente durante la ventilazione artificiale. L'ipossia è profonda e costante in molte lesioni cardiache, mentre nelle patologie respiratorie e nell'ipertensione polmonare persistente del neonato la pressione parziale di ossigeno arteriosa non è altrettanto bassa e spesso varia con il tempo o con i cambiamenti nella gestione della ventilazione. L'iperventilazione migliora l'ipossia nei neonati con ipertensione polmonare persistente, mentre è più raro che questo avvenga nei neonati con cardiopatie cianotizzanti.

Anche se un significativo soffio cardiaco di solito suggerisce una causa cardiaca della cianosi, molte tra le più gravi cardiopatie congenite (trasposizione dei grossi vasi) possono non essere inizialmente associate a un soffio. La radiografia del torace può essere utile per distinguere una patologia polmonare da una cardiopatia; in quest'ultimo caso, indica se il flusso sanguigno polmonare è aumentato, normale o diminuito.

L'ecocardiografia bidimensionale è il test non invasivo che permette di determinare in via definitiva la presenza di una cardiopatia congenita. Per esaminare strutture che non sono facilmente visibili con questa metodica di solito si fa ricorso al cateterismo cardiaco, che permette di valutare: le diramazioni distali dell'arteria polmonare o le arterie collaterali aortopolmonari in pazienti con tetralogia di Fallot con atresia della polmonare (vedi Capitolo 430.2); le arterie coronarie e i sinusoidi del ventricolo destro in pazienti con atresia della polmonare e setto interventricolare intatto (vedi Capitolo 430.3). Se l'ecocardiografia non è immediatamente disponibile, il medico che ha in carico un neonato con sospetta cardiopatia cianogena non dovrebbe esitare a somministrare prostaglandine in infusione (per la possibilità di una lesione dotto-dipendente). Dal momento che l'infusione di prostaglandine comporta un rischio di ipoventilazione, si rende necessaria la presenza di un medico esperto nell'intubazione endotracheale neonatale.

Capitolo 430 ■ Cardiopatie congenite cianogene: lesioni associate a ipoafflusso polmonare

430.1 • Tetralogia di Fallot

La tetralogia di Fallot è una lesione cardiaca conotroncale, in cui il difetto primario è una deviazione anteriore del setto infundibolare (il setto muscolare che separa l'efflusso aortico da quello polmonare). Le conseguenze di questa deviazione sono: (1) ostruzione all'efflusso ventricolare destro (stenosi polmonare), (2) difetto del setto interventricolare (VSD, *Ventricular Septal*

Defect), (3) destroposizione dell'aorta a cavallo del setto interventricolare e (4) ipertrofia ventricolare destra (Fig. 430-1). L'ostruzione al flusso dell'arteria polmonare si verifica a livello tanto dell'infundibolo ventricolare destro (area sottopolmonare) quanto della valvola polmonare. L'arteria polmonare principale è spesso più piccola della norma e può essere presente una stenosi di grado variabile a carico dei rami dell'arteria polmonare. L'ostruzione completa dell'efflusso ventricolare destro (atresia polmonare con VSD) è classificata come una forma estrema di tetralogia di Fallot (vedi Capitolo 430.2). Il grado di ostruzione dell'efflusso polmonare è variabile, e dalla sua severità dipende l'entità della cianosi.

FISIOPATOLOGIA. L'anulus della valvola polmonare può avere dimensioni quasi normali o piuttosto ridotte. La valvola stessa è spesso bicuspide e a volte costituisce l'unica sede della stenosi. Più comunemente, l'ipertrofia del muscolo sottopolmonare o infundibolare (cresta sopraventricolare) contribuisce alla stenosi sottovalvolare e porta a una camera infundibolare di dimensioni e contorno variabili. Quando il tratto di efflusso ventricolare destro è completamente ostruito (**atresia polmonare**), l'anatomia dei rami dell'arteria polmonare è estremamente variabile; un segmento del tronco principale dell'arteria polmonare può essere assente. Talvolta i rami dell'arteria polmonare possono essere discontinui. In questi casi più gravi, il flusso ematico ai polmoni può essere fornito da un dotto arterioso pervio (PDA, *Patent Ductus Arteriosus*) e da più **arterie aortopolmonari collaterali principali** (MAPCA, *Major AortoPulmonary Collateral Arteries*) che originano dall'aorta ascendente e discendente.

Il VSD, di solito non restrittivo e ampio, è situato subito al di sotto della valvola aortica ed è in relazione con le cuspidi aortiche posteriore e destra. È raro che si trovi nella porzione di afflusso del setto interventricolare (difetto del setto atrioventricolare). Di solito è mantenuta la normale continuità fibrosa delle valvole aortica e mitrale. L'arco aortico è situato a destra nel 20% dei casi e la radice aortica in genere è ampia e posta a cavallo del VSD in misura variabile. Quando l'aorta è a cavallo del VSD per più del 50% e vi è una porzione muscolare che separa la valvola aortica dall'anulus mitralico (cono subaortico), questo difetto è di solito classificato come una forma di ventricolo destro a doppia uscita; tuttavia la fisiopatologia è la stessa che caratterizza la tetralogia di Fallot.

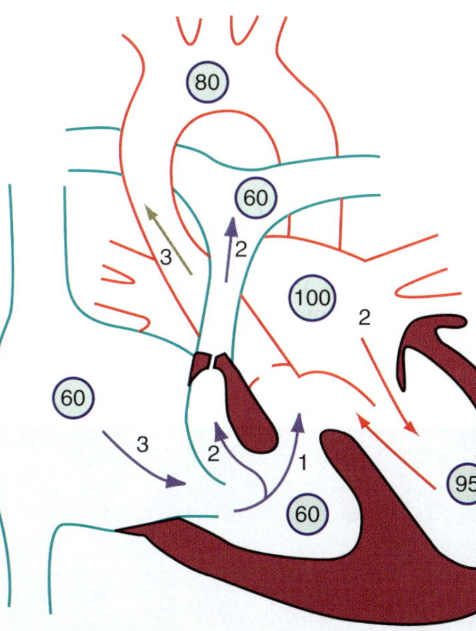

Figura 430-1. Fisiologia della tetralogia di Fallot. I numeri cerchiati rappresentano i valori di saturazione di ossigeno. I numeri accanto alle frecce rappresentano i volumi di flusso sanguigno (in L/min/m^2). La saturazione di ossigeno atriale (sangue venoso misto) è bassa a causa dell'ipossiemia sistemica. Un volume di sangue desaturato pari a 3 L/min/m^2 entra nell'atrio destro e attraversa la valvola tricuspide. Due litri attraversano il tratto di efflusso del ventricolo destro e raggiungono i polmoni, mentre 1 L viene deviato da destra a sinistra attraverso il difetto del setto interventricolare (VSD, *Ventricular Septal Defect*) nell'aorta ascendente. Il flusso sanguigno polmonare è quindi per 2/3 normale (Qp:Qs [rapporto tra il flusso sanguigno polmonare e sistemico] = 7:1). Il sangue che ritorna all'atrio sinistro è pienamente saturato. Solo 2 L di sangue attraversano la valvola mitrale. La saturazione di ossigeno nel ventricolo sinistro può risultare lievemente diminuita a causa dello shunt destro-sinistro attraverso il VSD. Due litri di sangue ventricolare sinistro saturo misti a 1 L di sangue ventricolare destro desaturato vengono sospinti in aorta ascendente. La saturazione aortica è ridotta e la gittata cardiaca è normale.

Il ritorno venoso sistemico all'atrio destro e al ventricolo destro è normale. Quando il ventricolo destro si contrae in presenza di una stenosi polmonare marcata, il sangue viene deviato attraverso il VSD in aorta, dando luogo a desaturazione arteriosa persistente e cianosi. Il flusso sanguigno polmonare, se gravemente ostacolato dall'ostruzione all'efflusso ventricolare destro, può essere supplementato dalla circolazione collaterale bronchiale (MAPCA) e, nel neonato, da un PDA. I picchi pressori sistolici e diastolici sono simili in ciascun ventricolo e a livello sistemico. Si verifica un ampio gradiente pressorio attraverso il tratto di efflusso ventricolare destro ostruito e la pressione arteriosa polmonare è normale o più bassa. Il grado di ostruzione all'efflusso ventricolare destro determina il momento dell'insorgenza dei sintomi, la gravità della cianosi e la gravità dell'ipertrofia ventricolare destra. Se l'ostruzione all'efflusso ventricolare destro è lieve o moderata, ed è presente uno shunt bilanciato attraverso il VSD, il paziente può non essere visibilmente cianotico (**tetralogia di Fallot acianotica o "rosa"**). In caso di ostruzione grave, la cianosi, già presente alla nascita, peggiorerà quando il dotto inizierà a chiudersi.

MANIFESTAZIONI CLINICHE. Bambini con ostruzione all'efflusso ventricolare destro di grado lieve possono presentare inizialmente uno scompenso cardiaco causato da uno shunt sinistro-destro a livello ventricolare. La cianosi spesso non è presente alla nascita, ma si instaura più tardi, nel primo anno di vita, con l'aumento dell'ipertrofia dell'infundibolo ventricolare destro e la crescita del paziente. È più evidente a livello delle membrane mucose delle labbra e della bocca e delle unghie di mani e piedi. In soggetti con grave ostruzione all'efflusso ventricolare destro la cianosi si nota immediatamente, già nel periodo neonatale. In questi casi, il flusso sanguigno polmonare può essere dipendente dal flusso attraverso il dotto arterioso. Quando il dotto inizia a chiudersi, nelle prime ore o nei primi giorni di vita, possono verificarsi grave cianosi e collasso circolatorio. I bambini più grandi con cianosi da lungo tempo che non sono stati sottoposti a intervento chirurgico possono presentare cute bluastra e scura, sclere grigie con vasi sanguigni congesti e marcato ippocratismo digitale a mani e piedi. Le manifestazioni extracardiache di una cardiopatia congenita con cianosi di vecchia data sono descritte nel Capitolo 434.

La dispnea si verifica in occasione di uno sforzo fisico. Lattanti e bambini piccoli giocano attivamente per poco tempo e poi si siedono o si distendono. Bambini più grandi possono essere in grado di camminare per un isolato circa prima di doversi fermare per riposare. Caratteristicamente i bambini assumono una posizione di *squatting* (accucciata) per trovare sollievo dalla dispnea causata dallo sforzo fisico; il bambino è di solito in grado di riprendere l'attività fisica nel giro di pochi minuti. Questi reperti si trovano più spesso in pazienti con significativa cianosi a riposo.

Gli **attacchi parossistici di ipercianosi** (**attacchi ipossici "blu"** transitori) sono un problema particolare durante i primi 2 anni di vita. Il lattante diventa iperpnoico e irrequieto, la cianosi aumenta, la respirazione diviene ansimante e può seguire una sincope. Questi accessi si verificano con maggiore frequenza al mattino, al risveglio, o dopo episodi di pianto vigoroso. La scomparsa temporanea o la diminuzione d'intensità del soffio sistolico è comune quando il flusso attraverso il ventricolo destro diminuisce. Le crisi, che possono durare da pochi minuti a qualche ora, raramente sono fatali. A episodi di breve durata fanno seguito debolezza generalizzata e sonno; gli episodi gravi possono progredire fino allo stato di incoscienza e talvolta alle convulsioni e all'emiparesi.

Gli attacchi, dall'esordio in genere spontaneo e imprevedibile, sono associati all'ulteriore riduzione di un flusso sanguigno polmonare già compromesso, che, se prolungata, provoca grave ipossia sistemica e acidosi metabolica. I bambini che presentano solo una lieve cianosi a riposo sono più inclini a sviluppare crisi ipossiche perché non hanno acquisito i meccanismi omeostatici necessari per tollerare un rapido calo della saturazione arteriosa d'ossigeno (per es. una policitemia).

A seconda della frequenza e della gravità degli attacchi di ipercianosi, occorrerà mettere in atto una o più delle seguenti procedure, nell'ordine indicato: (1) distendere il bambino sull'addome, in posizione ginocchia-torace, accertandosi che non indossi abiti costrittivi; (2) somministrare ossigeno (anche se una maggiore ispirazione di ossigeno non farà scomparire la cianosi causata dallo shunt intracardiaco); (3) iniettare morfina per via sottocutanea in dose non superiore a 0,2 mg/kg. Calmare il bambino tenendolo in posizione ginocchia-torace può essere sufficiente per arrestare la progressione di una crisi in fase iniziale. Tentativi prematuri di prelevare campioni di sangue possono aggravare l'agitazione del lattante e quindi essere controproducenti.

Poiché l'acidosi metabolica si sviluppa quando la PO_2 è <40 mmHg, è necessaria una rapida correzione (entro qualche minuto) con somministrazione endovenosa di bicarbonato di sodio se la crisi è insolitamente grave e il bambino non sembra rispondere ad altri trattamenti. La ripresa dopo la crisi è di solito rapida, una volta che il pH si è normalizzato. Talvolta si rendono necessarie ripetute misurazioni del pH sanguigno, poiché può verificarsi una rapida recidiva dell'acidosi. Per le crisi refrattarie a questa terapia, i farmaci che aumentano la resistenza vascolare sistemica, come la fenilefrina per via endovenosa, possono migliorare l'efflusso ventricolare destro, diminuire lo shunt destro-sinistro e attenuare i sintomi. Altrettanto utile è il blocco β-adrenergico, mediante somministrazione endovenosa di propranololo (0,1 mg/kg somministrato lentamente fino a un massimo di 0,2 mg/kg).

La crescita e lo sviluppo possono essere rallentati in caso di grave tetralogia di Fallot non trattata, in particolare quando la saturazione di ossigeno è cronicamente <70%. Anche la pubertà può essere ritardata nei pazienti che non vengono sottoposti a intervento chirurgico.

La frequenza cardiaca è di solito normale, come pure la pressione venosa e quella arteriosa. L'emitorace anteriore sinistro può protrudere anteriormente a causa dell'ipertrofia del ventricolo destro. Il cuore è generalmente di dimensioni normali e si percepisce un impulso ventricolare destro sottosternale. In circa la metà dei casi si apprezza un fremito sistolico lungo il margine sternale sinistro a livello del terzo e quarto spazio parasternale. Il soffio sistolico è di solito forte e aspro; può essere ampiamente irradiato, specialmente ai polmonari, ma è più intenso in corrispondenza del margine sternale. Il soffio è generalmente di tipo eiettivo a livello del margine sternale superiore, ma può essere più olosistolico verso il margine sternale inferiore. Talvolta preceduto da un click, è causato dalla turbolenza attraverso il tratto di efflusso ventricolare. Tende a divenire più forte, più prolungato e più aspro a mano a mano che aumenta la gravità della stenosi polmonare, da lieve a moderata; tuttavia può diventare meno evidente in caso di ostruzione grave, soprattutto durante una crisi di ipercianosi. Il secondo tono è singolo o la componente polmonare è dolce. Per quanto si tratti di un'evenienza poco frequente, può accadere che si percepisca un soffio continuo, specialmente se sono presenti collaterali importanti.

DIAGNOSI. Dal punto di vista radiografico, la configurazione tipica nella proiezione anteroposteriore consiste in una base stretta, in una concavità del margine sinistro del cuore nell'area di solito occupata dall'arteria polmonare e in dimensioni cardiache normali. In conseguenza dell'ipertrofia del ventricolo destro l'ombra dell'apice è arrotondata e spostata verso l'alto, addirittura al di sopra del diaframma. La silhouette cardiaca è stata paragonata a quella di una scarpa o zoccolo di legno (*coeur en sabot*) (Fig. 430-2). Le aree ilari e i campi polmonari sono relativamente chiari, a causa del diminuito flusso polmonare e/o delle piccole dimensioni delle arterie polmonari. L'aorta è di solito ampia, e in circa il 20% dei pazienti l'arco aortico curva a destra, fenomeno che determina un'incisura dell'ombra tracheobronchiale piena d'aria, posta a sinistra in visione anteroposteriore.

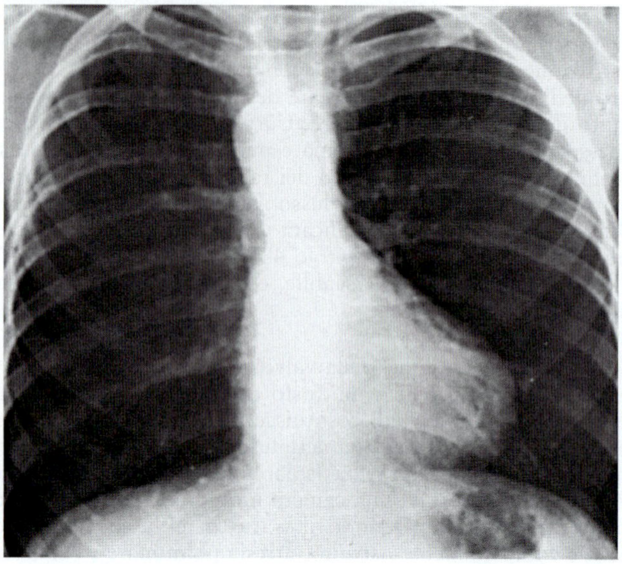

Figura 430-2. Radiografia del torace di un bambino di 8 anni con tetralogia di Fallot. Si notino le dimensioni normali del cuore, una certa elevazione dell'apice cardiaco, la concavità in corrispondenza del tronco principale dell'arteria polmonare, l'arco aortico a destra e la ridotta vascolarizzazione polmonare.

All'elettrocardiogramma si apprezzano la deviazione a destra dell'asse e segni di ipertrofia del ventricolo destro. Compare un'onda R dominante nelle derivazioni toraciche precordiali destre (Rs, R, qR, qRs) o un quadro RSR'. In alcuni casi, inizialmente l'unico segno di ipertrofia ventricolare destra è un'onda T positiva nelle derivazioni V_3R e V_1. L'onda P è alta, appuntita o talvolta bifida (vedi Fig. 423-8).

L'ecocardiografia bidimensionale permette di stabilire la diagnosi (Fig. 430-3) e fornisce informazioni sull'estensione della posizione dell'aorta a cavallo del setto, sulla sede e sul grado di ostruzione del tratto di efflusso del ventricolo destro, sulla dimensione delle diramazioni principali dell'arteria polmonare e sulla sede (destra o sinistra) dell'arco aortico. Questa indagine è utile anche per determinare se un PDA contribuisce in parte al flusso sanguigno polmonare. Nei pazienti senza atresia polmonare,

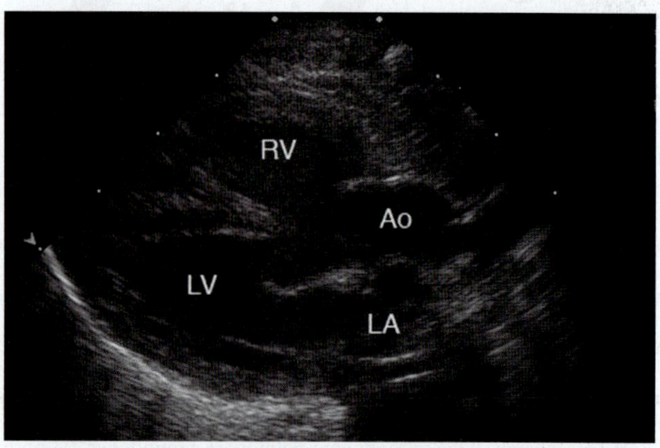

Figura 430-3. Ecocardiogramma in un paziente con tetralogia di Fallot. Questa proiezione parasternale asse lungo bidimensionale evidenzia uno spostamento anteriore del setto interventricolare di efflusso che ha portato a una stenosi del tratto subpolmonare di efflusso del ventricolo destro, a un'aorta a cavaliere e a un associato difetto del setto interventricolare. Ao, aorta a cavaliere; LA (*Left Atrium*), atrio sinistro; LV (*Left Ventricle*), ventricolo sinistro; RV (*Right Ventricle*), ventricolo destro.

l'ecocardiografia di solito rende inutile procedere al cateterismo cardiaco prima della riparazione chirurgica.

Il cateterismo cardiaco evidenzia una pressione sistolica in ventricolo destro uguale alla pressione sistemica. Se si entra in arteria polmonare, si assiste a una marcata riduzione della pressione, anche se oltrepassare il tratto di efflusso del ventricolo destro, specialmente nei casi gravi, può precipitare una crisi ipossica. Di solito la pressione arteriosa polmonare è inferiore alla norma, compresa tra 5 e 10 mmHg. Il livello di saturazione arteriosa di ossigeno dipende dalla grandezza dello shunt destro-sinistro; nelle "crisi rosa" la saturazione sistemica può essere normale, mentre in un paziente moderatamente cianotico a riposo di solito è del 75-85%.

La ventricolografia destra è la metodica che meglio evidenzia l'anatomia della tetralogia di Fallot. Il mezzo di contrasto delinea il ventricolo destro con una trabecolatura notevolmente sviluppata. La stenosi infundibolare varia per lunghezza, larghezza, contorno e dilatabilità (Fig. 430-4). La valvola polmonare è di solito ispessita e l'anulus può essere piccolo. In pazienti con atresia polmonare e VSD, l'anatomia dei vasi polmonari può essere estremamente complessa, per esempio è possibile riscontrare una discontinuità tra le arterie polmonari destra e sinistra. È importante ottenere informazioni complete e accurate riguardo all'anatomia delle arterie polmonari e dei vasi collaterali (MAPCA) quando si valutano questi pazienti come candidati all'intervento chirurgico.

La ventricolografia sinistra permette di valutare le dimensioni del ventricolo sinistro, la posizione del VSD e l'aorta a cavaliere; conferma inoltre la continuità mitroaortica, escludendo perciò la diagnosi di ventricolo destro a doppia uscita. L'aortografia o l'arteriografia coronarica delineano il decorso delle arterie coronarie. Nel 5-10% dei pazienti con tetralogia di Fallot, una coronaria principale aberrante attraversa il tratto di efflusso del ventricolo destro; questa arteria non deve essere sezionata durante la riparazione chirurgica. È importante verificare la presenza di arterie coronarie normali quando si valuta se sottoporre a intervento chirurgico bambini piccoli che possono necessitare di un patch attraverso l'anulus della valvola polmonare. Di solito l'ecocardiografia è in grado di delineare l'anatomia delle arterie coronarie; l'angiografia va riservata ai casi dubbi.

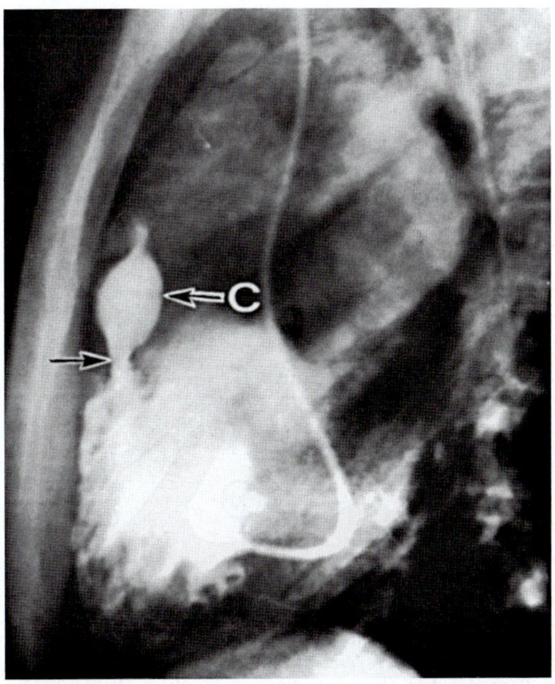

Figura 430-4. Proiezione laterale di un ventricologramma destro selettivo in un paziente con tetralogia di Fallot. La *freccia* indica una stenosi infundibolare al di sotto della camera infundibolare (C). Si noti il ristretto orifizio della valvola polmonare, all'estremità distale della camera infundibolare.

COMPLICANZE. Prima della correzione, i pazienti con tetralogia di Fallot sono suscettibili a molte complicanze gravi. Fortunatamente si tratta di complicanze rare, in quanto molti bambini vengono sottoposti a intervento palliativo o (più spesso) a riparazione completa in tenera età. Le **trombosi cerebrali**, che colpiscono le vene cerebrali o i seni durali e talvolta le arterie cerebrali, sono comuni in presenza di un'estrema policitemia e disidratazione. Esse si verificano con maggior frequenza nei pazienti di età inferiore ai 2 anni, talvolta affetti da anemia sideropenica, frequentemente con livelli di emoglobina ed ematocrito nei limiti della norma (ma troppo bassi per una cardiopatia cianogena). La terapia consiste in un'adeguata idratazione e in misure di supporto. Il salasso e la ricostituzione del volume plasmatico con albumina o soluzione fisiologica sono indicati in pazienti sintomatici con **policitemia** estrema.

Gli **ascessi cerebrali**, di per sé meno comuni degli eventi cerebrovascolari, sono estremamente rari quando la maggior parte dei pazienti è sottoposta a correzione in età precoce. I pazienti con ascesso cerebrale in genere sono di età superiore ai 2 anni. L'esordio della malattia è spesso insidioso e consiste in una febbricola e/o in un cambiamento comportamentale graduale. Alcuni pazienti presentano un esordio acuto dei sintomi che possono svilupparsi dopo una recente storia di cefalea, nausea e vomito. Possono insorgere convulsioni; i segni neurologici localizzati dipendono dalla sede e dalle dimensioni dell'ascesso, oltre che dall'aumento della pressione intracranica. La TC o la RMN confermano la diagnosi. Anche se la terapia antibiotica può aiutare a mantenere localizzata l'infezione, di solito è necessario il drenaggio chirurgico dell'ascesso (vedi Capitolo 603).

Un'**endocardite batterica** può verificarsi a livello dell'infundibolo ventricolare destro oppure delle valvole polmonare, aortica o (raramente) tricuspide. L'endocardite può complicare shunt palliativi o, in pazienti sottoposti a chirurgia correttiva, una stenosi polmonare residua o un VSD. La profilassi antibiotica è essenziale prima e dopo le estrazioni dentali e alcune procedure chirurgiche associate a elevata incidenza di batteriemia (vedi Capitolo 437).

Lo scompenso cardiaco non è una caratteristica comune nei pazienti con tetralogia di Fallot. Ciononostante, può verificarsi nei lattanti con tetralogia di Fallot "rosa" o acianotica. A mano a mano che il grado di ostruzione polmonare peggiora con l'età, i sintomi di scompenso cardiaco si risolvono e insorge la cianosi, spesso entro il 6°-12° mese di vita; questi pazienti sono ad alto rischio di sviluppare attacchi di ipercianosi.

ANOMALIE ASSOCIATE. Può essere presente un PDA associato e i difetti del setto interatriale sono di occasionale riscontro. Un arco aortico destro è presente in circa il 20% dei pazienti con tetralogia di Fallot, e possono osservarsi altre anomalie delle arterie polmonari e dell'arco aortico. Si può notare la persistenza di una vena cava superiore sinistra che drena nel seno coronario. Talvolta sono presenti VSD multipli, che devono essere diagnosticati prima dell'intervento chirurgico correttivo. È infine possibile la compresenza di tetralogia di Fallot e un difetto del setto atrioventricolare, spesso associato a sindrome di Down.

L'**assenza congenita della valvola polmonare** causa una sindrome distinta, di solito caratterizzata da segni di ostruzione delle vie aeree superiori (vedi Capitolo 428.1). La cianosi può essere assente, lieve o moderata; il cuore è dilatato e iperdinamico; è presente un forte soffio di tipo "va e vieni". Una marcata dilatazione aneurismatica del tronco principale della polmonare e delle sue diramazioni porta a compressione dei bronchi e produce un respiro stridulo o ansimante e polmoniti ricorrenti. Se l'ostruzione delle vie aeree è grave, può essere necessaria la ricostruzione della trachea al momento dell'intervento cardiochirurgico correttivo per alleviare i sintomi.

L'**assenza di una diramazione dell'arteria polmonare**, per lo più la sinistra, dovrebbe essere sospettata se l'immagine della vascolarizzazione polmonare alla radiografia del torace è diversa nei due lati. È importante riconoscere l'assenza di un'arteria polmonare, spesso associata a ipoplasia del polmone affetto, poiché l'occlusione dell'arteria polmonare rimanente, durante l'intervento chirurgico, compromette seriamente il già ridotto flusso polmonare.

In quanto malformazione conotroncale, la tetralogia di Fallot può essere associata allo spettro di lesioni note come **CATCH22** (*Cardiac defect, Abnormal facies, Thymic hypoplasia, Cleft palate, Hypocalcemia*, difetti cardiaci, anomalie faciali, ipoplasia timica, palatoschisi, ipocalcemia). In questa categoria rientrano pazienti con le caratteristiche cliniche della sindrome di DiGeorge (ipocalcemia, ipoplasia timica, lievi anomalie faciali) e della **sindrome di Shprintzen velocardiofacciale** (anomalie faciali, palatoschisi). L'analisi genetica con tecnica FISH (*Fluorescence In Situ Hybridization*) evidenzia la delezione di un ampio segmento del cromosoma 22q11, denominato "regione critica di DiGeorge". La delezione o la mutazione del gene che codifica per il fattore di trascrizione *Tbx1* sono state implicate come una possibile causa della sindrome di DiGeorge.

TRATTAMENTO. Il trattamento delle tetralogia di Fallot dipende dalla gravità dell'ostruzione all'efflusso nel ventricolo destro. I lattanti con una tetralogia grave richiedono un trattamento medico e chirurgico nel periodo neonatale. La terapia mira a determinare un immediato incremento del flusso sanguigno polmonare per prevenire le sequele di una grave ipossia. I pazienti dovrebbero essere trasportati in un centro medico adeguatamente equipaggiato per la valutazione e il trattamento di neonati con cardiopatie congenite. Durante il trasferimento è essenziale assicurare l'ossigenazione e mantenere la temperatura corporea entro valori normali. Un'ipossia prolungata e grave, oltre a determinare shock, insufficienza respiratoria e acidosi intrattabile, ridurrà significativamente le probabilità di sopravvivenza anche in presenza di lesioni trattabili chirurgicamente. Il freddo aumenta il consumo di ossigeno, che provoca un ulteriore stress nel bambino cianotico, il cui trasporto di ossigeno è già limitato. Si raccomanda di monitorare i livelli glicemici, poiché l'ipoglicemia ha maggiore probabilità di svilupparsi nei bambini con cardiopatie cianogene.

I neonati con marcata ostruzione all'efflusso ventricolare destro possono andare incontro a un rapido peggioramento poiché quando il dotto inizia a chiudersi il flusso sanguigno polmonare viene ulteriormente compromesso. La somministrazione endovenosa di prostaglandina E_1 (0,01-0,20 μg/kg/min), un potente e specifico rilassante della muscolatura liscia del dotto, provoca la dilatazione del dotto arterioso e di solito assicura un flusso sanguigno polmonare adeguato in attesa che sia possibile effettuare l'intervento chirurgico. Questa sostanza dovrebbe essere somministrata per via endovenosa non appena sorge il sospetto clinico di una cardiopatia congenita cianogena, e continuata sia per tutto il periodo preoperatorio, sia durante il cateterismo cardiaco.

I bambini con ostruzioni del tratto di efflusso del ventricolo destro meno gravi, che sono stabili e in attesa dell'intervento chirurgico, richiedono un'attenta osservazione. È importante prevenire la disidratazione, o trattarla tempestivamente, per evitare l'emoconcentrazione e possibili episodi trombotici. Attacchi parossistici di dispnea nel lattante o nel bambino piccolo possono essere precipitati da una relativa carenza di ferro; la terapia marziale può diminuirne la frequenza, migliorando anche la tolleranza allo sforzo e il benessere generale. Il numero di globuli rossi deve rimanere nel range normale. In passato, per ridurre la frequenza e la gravità delle crisi ipercianotiche, si faceva ricorso più spesso al propranololo per via orale (0,5-1 mg/kg ogni 6 ore), ma oggi, con la possibilità di un efficace intervento chirurgico, viene posta indicazione alla chirurgia non appena iniziano le crisi.

I bambini sintomatici che presentano cianosi grave nel 1° mese di vita hanno una marcata ostruzione del tratto di efflusso del ventricolo destro o un'atresia polmonare. In questi casi sono disponibili due opzioni. La prima, praticata soprattutto in passato, consiste nella creazione di uno shunt arterioso palliativo sistemico-polmonare al fine di aumentare il flusso sanguigno in arteria polmonare. Il razionale di questo intervento chirurgico, che in precedenza era l'unica opzione per questi pazienti, è diminuire l'ipossia e aumentare non solo la crescita lineare, ma anche lo sviluppo delle diramazioni dell'arteria polmonare. La seconda opzione è l'intervento chirurgico correttivo a cuore aperto, effettuato nella prima infanzia e anche nel periodo neonatale quando il paziente è in condizioni critiche. Questo approccio, che gode di ampio consenso, offre eccellenti risultati sia a breve sia a lungo termine e comporta un ulteriore vantaggio, almeno in linea teorica: una precoce correzione fisiologica dovrebbe infatti favorire la crescita delle diramazioni dell'arteria polmonare. Nei lattanti con cianosi meno grave, che presentano un buon accrescimento e non vanno soggetti ad attacchi di ipercianosi, la riparazione primaria viene effettuata in elezione tra il 4° e il 6° mese di vita.

Lo shunt modificato di Blalock-Taussig è attualmente la procedura di shunt aortopolmonare più comune e consiste in un condotto di Gore-Tex anastomizzato latero-lateralmente dall'arteria succlavia alla branca omolaterale dell'arteria polmonare (Fig. 430-5). A volte lo shunt viene effettuato direttamente dall'aorta ascendente al tronco principale dell'arteria polmonare, e in tal caso prende il nome di "shunt centrale". L'intervento di Blalock-Taussig non solo può essere effettuato con successo nel periodo neonatale, con shunt di 3-4 mm di diametro, ma è stato eseguito con successo anche nei prematuri.

La complicanze postoperatorie dopo shunt di Blalock-Taussig comprendono il chilotorace, la paralisi diaframmatica e la sindrome di Horner. Il chilotorace può richiedere toracentesi ripetute e talvolta un reintervento per legare il dotto toracico. La paralisi diaframmatica da lesione del nervo frenico comporta un decorso postoperatorio più difficile; possono essere necessari un prolungato supporto ventilatorio e una vigorosa terapia fisica, ma di solito nell'arco di 1-2 mesi si assiste al recupero della funzione del diaframma, a meno che il nervo non sia stato completamente sezionato. Può essere indicata la plicatura chirurgica del diaframma. In genere la sindrome di Horner è temporanea e non richiede trattamento. Lo scompenso cardiaco postoperatorio può essere causato da un ampio shunt; il suo trattamento è descritto nel Capitolo 442. A parte una diminuzione del polsi radiali e una disparità a lungo termine tra arti inferiori e superiori, altri problemi vascolari si osservano raramente negli arti superiori riforniti dall'arteria succlavia utilizzata per l'anastomosi.

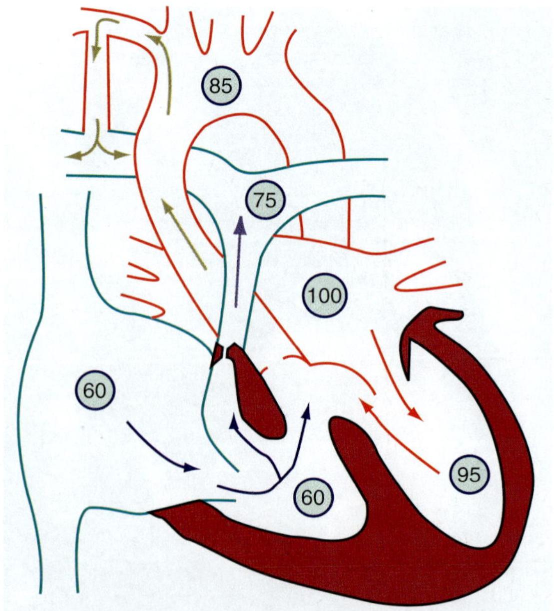

Figura 430-5. Fisiologia di uno shunt di Blalock-Taussig in un paziente con tetralogia di Fallot. I *numeri cerchiati* rappresentano i valori di saturazione di ossigeno. Il quadro degli shunt intracardiaci è come quello descritto nella Figura 430-1. Il sangue passa da sinistra a destra attraverso lo shunt dall'arteria succlavia destra all'arteria polmonare destra, aumentando il flusso polmonare totale e determinando una saturazione di ossigeno più elevata di quella che vi sarebbe senza lo shunt (vedi Fig. 430-1).

Dopo una procedura di shunt ben riuscita, la cianosi diminuisce. Lo sviluppo di un soffio continuo a livello dei campi polmonari dopo l'operazione indica un'anastomosi funzionante. Fino a parecchi giorni dopo l'intervento chirurgico potrebbe non udirsi un bel soffio continuo da shunt. La durata del sollievo sintomatico è variabile. A mano a mano che il bambino cresce, si rende necessario un flusso polmonare sempre maggiore, cosicché lo shunt finisce per diventare inadeguato. Quando si sviluppa una cianosi ingravescente, si raccomanda di effettuare un intervento correttivo se l'anatomia lo permette. Se ciò non è possibile (a causa di diramazioni dell'arteria polmonare ipoplasiche) o se il primo shunt è durato solo per un breve periodo nel lattante, potrebbe essere richiesta una seconda anastomosi aortopolmonare dall'altro lato.

La **terapia chirurgica correttiva** consiste nella correzione dell'ostruzione del tratto di efflusso del ventricolo destro rimuovendo i fasci muscolari che ne sono responsabili e mediante chiusura del VSD con patch. Se la valvola polmonare è stenotica, si procede a una valvulotomia. Se l'anulus della valvola polmonare è piccolo o la valvola è estremamente ispessita, si può effettuare una valvulectomia: una volta aperto l'anello della valvola polmonare, si posiziona un patch transanulare attraverso l'anello stesso. Un eventuale shunt sistemico-polmonare confezionato in precedenza deve essere legato e diviso prima della riparazione completa. Il rischio chirurgico della correzione totale nei centri più importanti è <5%. In passato l'approccio standard era la ventricolotomia destra; tuttavia, per ridurre i rischi a lungo termine di questa procedura, si adotta di routine un approccio **transatriale-transpolmonare**. Un intenso sanguinamento nell'immediato periodo postoperatorio può contribuire a complicare il quadro in pazienti estremamente policitemici.

PROGNOSI. Dopo una correzione completa effettuata con successo, i pazienti sono generalmente asintomatici e sono in grado di condurre una vita normale, senza troppe limitazioni. Nell'immediato postoperatorio, alcuni problemi (peraltro non comuni) sono lo scompenso ventricolare destro, il blocco cardiaco transitorio, un VSD residuo con shunt sinistro-destro e l'infarto del miocardio dovuto a interruzione di un'arteria coronaria aberrante. Uno scompenso cardiaco postoperatorio (in particolare in pazienti con patch nel tratto di efflusso transanulare) può richiedere la terapia con diuretici e agenti inotropi positivi come la digossina. Gli effetti a lungo termine di un'insufficienza valvolare polmonare isolata e chirurgicamente indotta non sono noti, ma l'insufficienza generalmente è ben tollerata. La maggior parte dei pazienti sottoposti a correzione della tetralogia e di quelli sottoposti a riparazione con patch transanulare presentano un soffio di tipo "va e vieni" a livello del margine sternale sinistro, di solito indicativo di una lieve ostruzione dell'efflusso e di un'insufficienza polmonare lieve-moderata. I pazienti con insufficienza valvolare polmonare più marcata presentano anche un ingrandimento cardiaco moderato o marcato. I pazienti con un notevole gradiente residuo a livello dell'efflusso del ventricolo destro possono necessitare di un reintervento, ma un'ostruzione lieve e moderata è quasi sempre presente e non richiede altri interventi.

Dal follow-up dei pazienti 5-20 anni dopo l'intervento emerge che il marcato miglioramento della sintomatologia viene generalmente mantenuto. Ciononostante, i pazienti asintomatici hanno una capacità di eseguire esercizi fisici, una frequenza cardiaca massimale e una gittata cardiaca inferiori alla norma. Questi reperti anomali sono più comuni in coloro che sono stati sottoposti a posizionamento di un patch transanulare nel tratto di efflusso, e possono essere meno frequenti quando l'intervento chirurgico è stato effettuato precocemente. Una volta entrati nell'adolescenza e nell'età adulta, alcuni di questi pazienti (più comunemente quelli con patch transanulari) svilupperanno una dilatazione ventricolare destra a causa di un grave rigurgito polmonare. È importante un attento follow-up per tutta la vita da parte di uno specialista in cardiopatie congenite dell'adulto. Ecocardiogramma e angiografia con risonanza magnetica (MRA) seriati sono strumenti utili per valutare il grado di dilatazione del ventricolo destro, la presenza di un disfunzione ventricolare destra e la frazione di rigurgito. La sostituzione valvolare è indicata per i pazienti con una patologia ingravescente a carico del ventricolo destro.

Dopo l'intervento chirurgico possono verificarsi disturbi della conduzione. Il nodo atrioventricolare e il fascio di His e le sue diramazioni, che sono in stretta vicinanza al VSD, possono essere lesi durante l'intervento chirurgico. Un blocco cardiaco permanente dopo intervento chirurgico è raro; quando si verifica, dovrebbe essere trattato con l'impianto di un pacemaker permanente. Altrettanto raro nell'immediato periodo postoperatorio è un blocco cardiaco completo transitorio, che può essere associato a una maggiore incidenza di blocco cardiaco completo a insorgenza tardiva e a morte improvvisa. Un blocco di branca destra completo dopo ventriculotomia destra è piuttosto comune all'elettrocardiogramma postoperatorio. La durata dell'intervallo QRS si è dimostrato un fattore di cui tenere conto per predire sia la presenza di residue alterazioni emodinamiche sia il rischio a lungo termine di morte improvvisa. Sono in corso ricerche per determinare l'efficacia del pacing biventricolare (in cui viene utilizzato un pacemaker per risincronizzare l'attivazione dei ventricoli destro e sinistro) nel migliorare le condizioni emodinamiche dei pazienti con lunghi ritardi di conduzione ventricolare.

Un certo numero di bambini presenta battiti ventricolari prematuri dopo la riparazione della tetralogia di Fallot. Questi battiti suscitano preoccupazione in pazienti con anomalie emodinamiche residue; si raccomanda di effettuare un monitoraggio elettrocardiografico nelle 24 ore (Holter) per accertarsi che non si verifichino brevi episodi occulti di tachicardia ventricolare. Il test da sforzo può essere utile per provocare aritmie cardiache che non sono evidenti a riposo. In presenza di aritmie ventricolari complesse o di gravi anomalie emodinamiche residue, si impone una terapia antiaritmica profilattica. Un secondo intervento correttivo è indicato se è presente una residua, significativa ostruzione all'efflusso ventricolare destro o una grave insufficienza polmonare.

430.2 • TETRALOGIA DI FALLOT CON ATRESIA DELLA POLMONARE

FISIOPATOLOGIA. Una forma estrema di tetralogia di Fallot è quella che si accompagna ad atresia della polmonare. La valvola polmonare è atresica, rudimentale o assente e il tronco polmonare è atresico o ipoplasico. L'intera gittata del ventricolo destro viene espulsa nell'aorta. Il flusso sanguigno polmonare è quindi dipendente dal un PDA o da vasi collaterali (MAPCA). La prognosi globale dipende dal grado di sviluppo delle diramazioni dell'arteria polmonare, che deve essere valutato con cateterismo cardiaco. Se le arterie polmonari sono gravemente ipoplasiche e non sono in grado di crescere dopo procedure palliative di shunt, il trapianto cuore-polmoni può essere l'unica terapia (vedi Capitolo 433.2). L'atresia della polmonare con VSD è inoltre associata alla delezione CATCH22 e alla sindrome di DiGeorge. L'associazione di una grave **tracheomalacia** o **broncomalacia** con queste gravi forme di tetralogia/atresia della polmonare può complicare il recupero postoperatorio.

MANIFESTAZIONI CLINICHE. I pazienti con atresia della polmonare e VSD presentano reperti simili a quelli della tetralogia di Fallot grave. La cianosi di solito appare poche ore dopo la nascita; il forte soffio sistolico associato alla tetralogia è di solito assente; il primo tono cardiaco è frequentemente seguito da un click da eiezione causato dalla radice aortica ingrandita; il secondo tono è moderatamente forte e non sdoppiato e si possono udire soffi continui derivanti dal flusso in un PDA o in collaterali bronchiali sull'intero precordio, sia anteriormente sia posteriormente. La maggior parte dei pazienti presenta cianosi moderata e viene inizialmente stabilizzata tramite infusione di prostaglandina E_1 in attesa del cateterismo cardiaco. Nel caso dei pazienti con MAPCA numerose e ampie, che possono essere meno cianotici, è possibile sospendere il trattamento con prostaglandine in attesa dell'intervento chirurgico palliativo, una volta che la diagnosi è stata confermata. Alcuni pazienti presentano addirittura uno scompenso cardiaco causato da un aumento del flusso ematico polmonare attraverso questi vasi collaterali.

DIAGNOSI. La radiografia del torace evidenzia un cuore di dimensioni inferiori o superiori alla norma (a seconda del grado del flusso sanguigno polmonare), una concavità a livello del segmento arterioso polmonare e spesso il pattern reticolare del flusso collaterale bronchiale. L'elettrocardiogramma rivela un'ipertrofia ventricolare destra, oltre a identificare l'aorta posta a cavaliere, un ispessimento della parete ventricolare destra e l'atresia della valvola polmonare. Le indagini ecocardiografiche con Doppler pulsato e color-Doppler evidenziano l'assenza di un flusso anterogrado attraverso la valvola polmonare, con un flusso polmonare derivante dal dotto arterioso o dalle MAPCA. All'atto del cateterismo cardiaco, la ventricolografia destra evidenzia un'aorta ampia, che si opacizza immediatamente al passaggio del mezzo di contrasto attraverso il VSD, ma senza ingresso di contrasto nei polmoni attraverso il tratto di efflusso ventricolare destro. È possibile seguire il percorso del flusso sanguigno polmonare dall'aorta ai polmoni (attraverso il dotto o i vasi collaterali). Per programmare l'intervento chirurgico è necessario valutare accuratamente entrambe le arterie polmonari native, per stabilire se sono continue o discontinue, e visualizzare dell'arborizzazione di tutte le MAPCA, previa iniezione selettiva di mezzo di contrasto.

TRATTAMENTO. Al momento di scegliere della procedura chirurgica occorre valutare se il tronco principale dell'arteria polmonare è o meno adeguato e considerare le dimensioni delle diramazioni dell'arteria polmonare. Se queste arterie sono ben sviluppate, si può procedere alla riparazione chirurgica a uno stadio con un condotto homograft tra il ventricolo destro e le arterie polmonari e alla chiusura del VSD. Se le arterie polmonari sono ipoplasiche, la prognosi è più cauta e può essere necessaria una ricostruzione estesa, che comporta numerosi atti chirurgici in sequenza, a partire dalla prima infanzia, con i quali si stabilisce una connessione tra l'aorta e le arterie polmonari principali ipolasiche (utilizzando o una finestra aortopolmonare o uno shunt centrale tipo Blalolck-Taussig) per indurne la crescita. Le numerose MAPCA vengono riunite (procedura di unifocalizzazione) e infine incorporate nella riparazione finale insieme alle arterie polmonari native.

Per essere candidate alla riparazione completa, le arterie polmonari devono avere dimensioni tali da accettare l'intero volume ematico della gittata ventricolare destra. La riparazione completa consiste nella chiusura del VSD e nel posizionamento di un condotto homograft tra il ventricolo destro e l'arteria polmonare. Al momento dell'intervento chirurgico correttivo, vengono rimossi i precedenti shunt. Poiché il paziente cresce e il calibro dell'homograft si restringe per la proliferazione di tessuto intimale e le calcificazioni, con il tempo di solito si rende necessaria la sostituzione del condotto homograft; talvolta anzi sono richieste molte sostituzioni. I pazienti spesso presentano malformazioni delle ramificazioni distali delle arterie polmonari. Questi vasi, la cui ricostruzione chirurgica è spesso difficoltosa, vengono trattati con un approccio transcatetere con dilatazione con palloncino ed eventuale stenting di stenosi multiple dell'arteria polmonare.

L'atresia totale acquisita del tratto di efflusso del ventricolo destro può verificarsi dopo un'anastomosi con shunt aortopolmonare per tetralogia di Fallot. Il soffio sistolico che deriva dalla stenosi polmonare si attenua per poi scomparire. L'ostruzione completa può essere confermata dall'ecocardiografia o dalla ventricolografia destra. L'intervento chirurgico correttivo del tratto di efflusso del ventricolo destro può essere effettuato con una procedura non dissimile da quella utilizzata per l'atresia congenita della polmonare.

430.3 • Atresia della polmonare con setto interventricolare intatto

FISIOPATOLOGIA. Nell'atresia della polmonare con setto interventricolare intatto, i lembi della valvola polmonare sono completamente fusi a formare una membrana e il tratto di efflusso del ventricolo destro è atresico. Poiché non è presente un VSD, non vi è fuoriuscita di sangue dal ventricolo destro. La pressione nell'atrio destro aumenta e il sangue viene deviato attraverso il forame ovale nell'atrio sinistro, dove si mescola con il ritorno venoso polmonare prima di entrare nel ventricolo sinistro (Fig. 430-6). La gittata ventricolare combinata, sinistra e destra, viene pompata unicamente dal ventricolo sinistro in aorta. Nel neonato con atresia della polmonare, l'unica fonte del flusso ematico polmonare è il **PDA**. Il ventricolo destro è di solito ipoplasico, anche se il grado di ipoplasia varia notevolmente. I pazienti con una cavità ventricolare destra di piccole dimensioni hanno anche un piccolo anulus tricuspidale, che limita l'afflusso al ventricolo destro; inoltre possono presentare, nell'ambito della parete ventricolare destra, **sinusoidi coronarici** in comunicazione diretta con il circolo arterioso coronarico. L'elevata pressione ventricolare destra fa sì che il sangue desaturato fluisca in senso retrogrado attraverso i collaterali nelle arterie coronarie e nell'aorta. Nei pazienti con questi sinusoidi la prognosi è cauta, soprattutto se a essi si associa una stenosi prossimale delle arterie coronarie. Pazienti con cavità ventricolare di dimensione media o grande possono avere un'insufficienza tricuspidale che serve a decomprimere il ventricolo destro.

MANIFESTAZIONI CLINICHE. Quando il dotto arterioso si chiude, nelle prime ore o primi giorni di vita, i neonati con atresia della polmonare e setto interventricolare integro sviluppano una cianosi marcata. In assenza di trattamento, la maggior parte dei

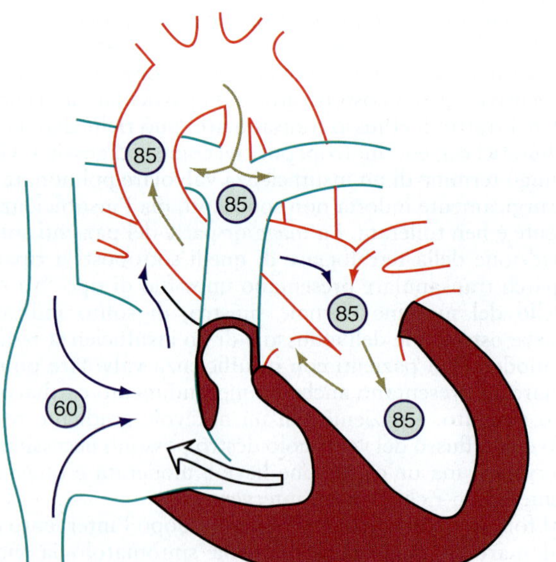

Figura 430-6. Fisiologia di un'atresia polmonare con setto interventricolare intatto. I *numeri cerchiati* rappresentano i valori di saturazione di ossigeno. La saturazione di ossigeno nell'atrio destro (sangue venoso misto) è ridotta a causa di un'ipossia sistemica. Una piccola quantità del sangue che entra nell'atrio destro può attraversare la valvola tricuspide, che spesso è anch'essa stenotica. La cavità ventricolare destra è ipertrofica e può essere ipoplastica. Non c'è fuoriuscita dal ventricolo destro a causa dell'atresia della valvola polmonare; perciò, il sangue che entra nel ventricolo destro ritorna all'atrio destro attraverso il rigurgito tricuspidale. La maggior parte del sangue desaturato viene deviato da destra a sinistra attraverso il forame ovale nell'atrio sinistro, dove si mescola con il sangue completamente saturo che ritorna dai polmoni. Il dotto arterioso pervio è l'unica fonte del flusso ematico polmonare. Le saturazioni arteriose di ossigeno aortica e polmonare saranno identiche (definizione di una lesione con mescolamento totale).

pazienti muore entro la prima settimana di vita. L'esame obiettivo evidenzia grave cianosi e distress respiratorio. Il secondo tono cardiaco è singolo e alto. Spesso non si percepiscono soffi, ma a volte è possibile auscultare un soffio sistolico o continuo, secondario al flusso di sangue nel dotto.

DIAGNOSI. L'elettrocardiogramma evidenzia un asse QRS sul piano frontale tra 0 e 90°, che risulta tanto più deviato a sinistra quanto maggiore è il grado di ipoplasia del ventricolo destro. Onde P alte e appuntite indicano un ingrandimento dell'atrio destro. I voltaggi del QRS sono coerenti con una dominanza o un'ipertrofia del ventricolo sinistro; la diminuzione delle forze ventricolari destre è proporzionale alla riduzione delle dimensioni della cavità ventricolare destra. La maggior parte dei pazienti con ventricolo destro piccolo presenta forze ventricolari destre diminuite; talvolta pazienti con cavità ventricolari destre grandi e ispessite possono presentare segni di ipertrofia del ventricolo destro. La radiografia del torace evidenzia una diminuzione della vascolarizzazione polmonare, di grado variabile a seconda delle dimensioni delle ramificazioni del tronco della polmonare, dalla pervietà del dotto o delle dimensioni dei collaterali bronchiali (peraltro molto meno comuni che nell'atresia della polmonare con VSD). Il cuore può essere di dimensioni variabili. L'ecocardiogramma bidimensionale è utile per valutare le dimensioni del ventricolo destro e dell'anulus tricuspide, parametri che si sono dimostrati di valore prognostico. L'ecocardiografia può spesso suggerire la presenza di sinusoidi, se sono ampi. Il cateterismo cardiaco, indispensabile per una valutazione completa, rileva ipertensione a livello dell'atrio e del ventricolo di destra. La ventricolografia indica la grandezza della cavità ventricolare destra, il tratto di efflusso ventricolare destro atresico, il grado del rigurgito tricuspidale e la presenza o assenza di sinusoidi intramiocardici che riempiono i vasi coronarici. L'aortografia dimostra il riempimento delle arterie polmonari attraverso il PDA ed è utile per determinare le dimensioni e il pattern di ramificazione del letto arterioso polmonare. L'aortogramma serve a valutare la presenza di stenosi prossimale delle arterie coronarie (dipendente dalla circolazione coronaria ventricolare destra); la presenza di queste lesioni influenza negativamente la prognosi.

TRATTAMENTO. L'infusione di prostaglandina E_1 (0,01-0,20 μg/kg/min) è di solito efficace per mantenere aperto il dotto arterioso prima dell'intervento, riducendo così l'ipossiemia e l'acidosi. Quando possibile, si procede a una valvulotomia polmonare chirurgica per alleviare l'ostruzione all'efflusso. Per garantire un adeguato flusso ematico polmonare, si effettua uno shunt aortopolmonare durante la medesima procedura. Spesso il tratto di efflusso ventricolare destro viene allargato con un patch. Un approccio alternativo è rappresentato dal cateterismo interventistico, che consiste nel pungere la valvola polmonare non perforata con un filo o un catetere per ablazione mediante radiofrequenze, per poi effettuare una valvuloplastica con palloncino. Se si opta per questa procedura, possono passare giorni o addirittura settimane prima che il muscolo ventricolare destro regredisca abbastanza perché il paziente possa essere svezzato dalla prostaglandina, e in alcuni casi si renderà necessario intervenire chirurgicamente. Lo scopo dell'intervento chirurgico o del cateterismo interventistico è promuovere la crescita della camera ventricolare destra permettendo un certo flusso anterogrado attraverso la valvola polmonare mentre si utilizza lo shunt per assicurare un adeguato flusso sanguigno polmonare. In seguito, se l'anulus della valvola tricuspide e la camera ventricolare destra raggiungono dimensioni adeguate, lo shunt viene rimosso e qualsiasi shunt a livello atriale viene chiuso. Se la camera ventricolare destra rimane ipoplasica, una **procedura di Fontan** modificata (vedi Capitolo 430.4) permetterà al sangue di aggirare il ventricolo destro ipoplasico affluendo alle arterie polmonari direttamente dalle vene cave. Quando sono presenti stenosi delle arterie coronarie e si verifica una perfusione coronarica dal ventricolo destro attraverso i sinusoidi miocardici, la prognosi può essere grave poiché sono comuni aritmie, ischemia coronarica e morte improvvisa. Alcuni di questi bambini traggono beneficio dal trapianto cardiaco.

430.4 • Atresia della tricuspide

FISIOPATOLOGIA. Nell'atresia della tricuspide non si verifica un efflusso dall'atrio destro al ventricolo destro; l'intero ritorno venoso sistemico entra nel cuore sinistro attraverso il forame ovale o un difetto del setto interatriale associato (Fig. 430-7). Il sangue ventricolare sinistro di solito fluisce nel ventricolo destro attraverso un VSD. Il flusso polmonare (oltre al grado di cianosi) dipende dalla grandezza del VSD, dalle presenza di stenosi polmonare e dalla sua gravità. Il flusso polmonare può essere reso maggiore, o totalmente dipendente, dal PDA. La porzione di afflusso del ventricolo destro è sempre assente in questi pazienti, mentre la porzione di efflusso ha dimensioni variabili. Se il setto interventricolare è intatto, il ventricolo destro è completamente ipoplasico ed è presente un'atresia della polmonare (vedi Capitolo 430.3). Nella maggior parte dei pazienti l'atresia della tricuspide viene riconosciuta nei primi mesi di vita, segnalata da una diminuzione del flusso ematico polmonare e dalla cianosi. In alternativa, un ampio VSD in assenza di ostruzione all'efflusso ventricolare destro può portare a un flusso polmonare elevato; questi pazienti hanno una lieve cianosi, segni di aumentata circolazione polmonare e scompenso cardiaco. Una variante dell'atresia della tricuspide è associata alla **trasposizione delle grandi arterie**. In questo caso, il sangue ventricolare sinistro fluisce direttamente in arteria polmonare, mentre il sangue sistemico deve attraversare il VSD e il ventricolo destro per raggiungere l'aorta. In questi pazienti il flusso ematico polmonare di solito subisce un notevole aumento e lo scompenso cardiaco si sviluppa precocemente. Se il VSD è restrittivo, il flusso aortico può essere compromesso.

MANIFESTAZIONI CLINICHE. La cianosi è di solito evidente alla nascita e la sua gravità dipende dall'entità dell'impedimento al flusso ematico polmonare. Si può notare un impulso ventricolare

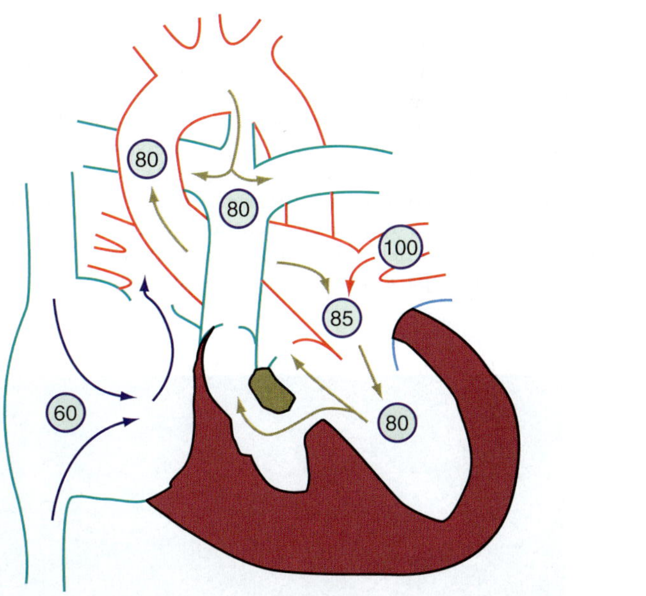

Figura 430-7. Fisiologia di un'atresia della tricuspide con grandi vasi normalmente posizionati. I numeri cerchiati rappresentano i valori di saturazione di ossigeno. La saturazione di ossigeno nell'atrio destro (sangue venoso misto) è ridotta in conseguenza dell'ipossia sistemica. La valvola tricuspide non è pervia e il ventricolo destro presenta gradi variabili di ipoplasia. L'unica uscita dall'atrio destro consiste nel passaggio da destra a sinistra attraverso un difetto del setto interatriale o un forame ovale pervio fino all'atrio sinistro. Qui, il sangue desaturato si mescola con il ritorno venoso polmonare, che invece è saturato. Il sangue entra nel ventricolo sinistro e viene spinto nel ventricolo destro attraverso l'aorta o un difetto del setto interventricolare (VSD). In questo esempio, parte del flusso sanguigno polmonare deriva dal ventricolo destro, il resto da un dotto arterioso pervio (PDA, *Patent Ductus Arteriosus*). Nei pazienti con atresia della tricuspide è possibile che il PDA si chiuda o che il VSD diventi più piccolo, comportando un notevole calo della saturazione di ossigeno sistemica.

sinistro aumentato, a differenza di quanto si verifica nella maggior parte delle altre cause di cardiopatia con cianosi, in cui in genere ad aumentare è impulso ventricolare destro. La maggior parte dei pazienti presenta soffi olosistolici udibili lungo il margine sternale sinistro; il secondo tono cardiaco è di solito singolo. La diagnosi viene sospettata nell'85% dei pazienti prima del secondo mese di vita. Nei bambini più grandi si verificano cianosi, policitemia, facile affaticabilità, dispnea da sforzo e a volte episodi ipossici dovuti alla compromissione del flusso sanguigno polmonare. I pazienti con atresia della tricuspide sono a rischio di chiusura spontanea del VSD, che può verificarsi rapidamente e portare a un marcato aumento della cianosi.

DIAGNOSI. Le radiografie del torace evidenziano o una diminuzione della circolazione polmonare (di solito in pazienti con grossi vasi normalmente posizionati) o un suo aumento (di solito in pazienti con trasposizione dei grossi vasi). Generalmente all'elettrocardiogramma si riscontrano una deviazione dell'asse verso sinistra e un'ipertrofia ventricolare sinistra (tranne che nei casi con trasposizione delle grandi arterie), caratteristiche che permettono di distinguere l'atresia della tricuspide dalla maggior parte delle altre lesioni cardiache con cianosi. La combinazione di cianosi e deviazione dell'asse a sinistra è altamente suggestiva di atresia della tricuspide. Nelle derivazioni precordiali destre l'onda R normalmente prominente è sostituita da un complesso rS. Le derivazioni precordiali sinistre presentano un complesso qR, seguito da un'onda T normale, piatta, bifasica o invertita. La R in V_6 è normale o alta, e la S in V_1 è generalmente profonda. Le onde P sono di solito bifasiche, con la componente iniziale alta e appuntita in D_2. L'ecocardiografia bidimensionale rivela la presenza di una membrana fibromuscolare al posto della valvola tricuspide, un ventricolo destro di dimensioni più o meno ridotte, un VSD e il ventricolo sinistro e l'aorta ingranditi (Fig. 430-8). Il grado di ostruzione a livello del VSD o del tratto di efflusso del ventricolo destro può essere determinato mediante misurazione diretta e con l'esame Doppler. È possibile determinare il rapporto tra i grossi vasi (normali o trasposti). Per valutare il flusso sanguigno attraverso un dotto pervio si ricorre al color-Doppler e al Doppler pulsato.

Il cateterismo cardiaco, indicato se rimangono dei dubbi dopo l'ecocardiogramma, evidenzia una pressione in atrio destro normale o lievemente elevata, con un'onda *a* pronunciata. Se si entra nel ventricolo destro attraverso il VSD, la pressione può essere inferiore a quella del ventricolo sinistro a causa della natura restrittiva del VSD. L'angiografia atriale destra evidenzia un'immediata opacizzazione dell'atrio sinistro attraverso l'atrio destro, seguita dal riempimento del ventricolo sinistro e dalla visualizzazione dell'aorta. L'assenza di un flusso diretto al ventricolo destro si traduce in un difetto di riempimento angiografico tra l'atrio destro e il ventricolo sinistro.

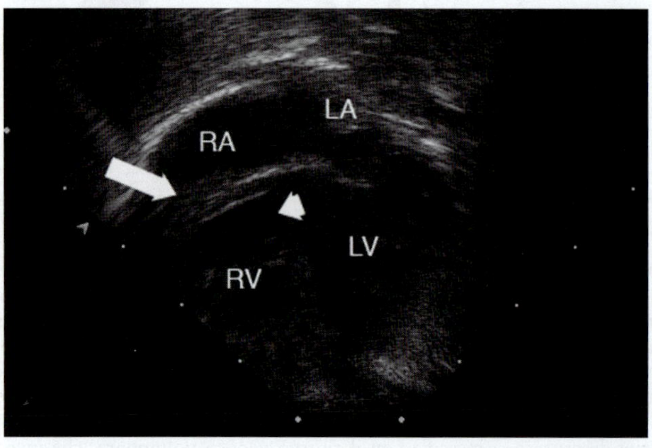

Figura 430-8. Ecocardiogramma che evidenzia un'atresia della tricuspide. Il pavimento dell'atrio destro è formato da una membrana fibromuscolare (*freccia grande*) al posto del normale apparato valvolare tricuspidale. Si noti l'ampio difetto del setto interatriale tipo ostium secundum tra gli atri destro e sinistro. Le punte di freccia indicano il difetto del setto interventricolare. LA (*Left Atrium*), atrio sinistro; LV (*Left Ventricle*), ventricolo sinistro; RA (*Right Atrium*), atrio destro; RV (*Right Ventricle*), ventricolo destro.

TRATTAMENTO. La gestione dei paziente con atresia della tricuspide dipende dall'adeguatezza del flusso sanguigno polmonare. I neonati gravemente cianotici dovrebbero essere tenuti sotto infusione endovenosa di prostaglandina E_1 (0,01-0,20 μg/kg/min) finché non sia possibile effettuare una procedura di shunt aortopolmonare per aumentare il flusso sanguigno polmonare. L'anastomosi preferita è la procedura di Blalock-Taussig (vedi Capitolo 430.1) o una sua variante. Alcuni pazienti con comunicazioni restrittive a livello atriale beneficiano anche di una settostomia atriale con catetere a palloncino secondo Rashkind (vedi Capitolo 431.2) o di una settostomia chirurgica.

I lattanti con aumentato flusso sanguigno polmonare dovuto a un tratto di efflusso polmonare non ostruito (nella maggior parte dei casi pazienti con trasposizione aortopolmonare) vanno sottoposti a un bendaggio dell'arteria polmonare, utile per diminuire i sintomi dello scompenso cardiaco e proteggere il letto polmonare dall'insorgenza di una vasculopatia polmonare. I bambini con un flusso sanguigno polmonare adeguato e un buon bilancio tra cianosi e sovracircolazione polmonare possono essere tenuti sotto stretta osservazione per lo sviluppo di una cianosi progressiva; quest'ultima può verificarsi quando il VSD inizia a ridursi e costituisce un'indicazione all'intervento chirurgico.

Lo stadio successivo di procedure palliative per pazienti con atresia della tricuspide comprende la creazione di un'anastomosi tra la vena cava superiore e le arterie polmonari (**shunt bidirezionale di Glenn**; Fig. 430-9*A*). Prima di questo intervento il paziente deve aver presentato segni suggestivi del fatto che un precedente shunt aortopolmonare sta diventando troppo piccolo, di solito tra i 4 e gli 8 mesi di vita. Lo shunt di Glenn, oltre a essere connesso a una minore probabilità che si sviluppi in futuro una disfunzione ventricolare sinistra, ha il vantaggio di ridurre il sovraccarico di volume sul ventricolo sinistro. Secondo alcuni Autori sarebbe opportuno effettuare l'anastomosi di Glenn in età ancora più precoce (2-4 mesi) per ridurre il carico di volume sul ventricolo sinistro; tuttavia, il beneficio a lungo termine di questo approccio non è stato ancora confermato.

L'**intervento di Fontan modificato** è la tecnica preferita per il trattamento chirurgico tardivo. Viene effettuato tra i 18 mesi e i 3 anni di vita, di solito quando il paziente è in grado di camminare. Inizialmente questa procedura veniva effettuata anastomizzando l'atrio destro o l'appendice atriale direttamente all'arteria polmonare. Una modifica, nota come "procedura di isolamento della cavità polmonare", comporta l'anastomosi della vena cava inferiore alle arterie polmonari attraverso un diaframma lungo la parete laterale dell'atrio destro (Fig. 430-9*B*) o attraverso un condotto homograft o di Gore-Tex che decorre al di fuori del cuore. Il vantaggio di questo approccio è che il sangue fluisce per una via più diretta nelle arterie polmonari, rendendo meno probabile una dilatazione atriale destra e diminuendo sensibilmente l'incidenza di versamenti pleurici postoperatori, che erano comuni con il metodo precedente. In questa complessa riparazione, il sangue desaturato fluisce da entrambe le vene cave direttamente nelle arterie polmonari. Il sangue ossigenato ritorna all'atrio sinistro, entra nel ventricolo sinistro e da qui viene sospinto nella circolazione sistemica. Il ventricolo sinistro non è più soggetto al sovraccarico di volume e lo shunt destro-sinistro viene abolito. Essendo basata sul riempimento passivo della circolazione polmonare, la procedura di Fontan è controindicata in caso di elevata resistenza vascolare polmonare, ipoplasia dell'arteria polmonare e disfunzione ventricolare sinistra. Il paziente deve essere in ritmo sinusale e non presentare un'insufficienza mitralica significativa.

I problemi postoperatori connessi alla procedura di Fontan comprendono un marcato aumento della pressione venosa sistemica, ritenzione idrica e versamenti pleurici o pericardici. In passato, i versamenti pleurici costituivano un problema nel 30-40% dei pazienti sottoposti alla procedura standard di Fontan, ma

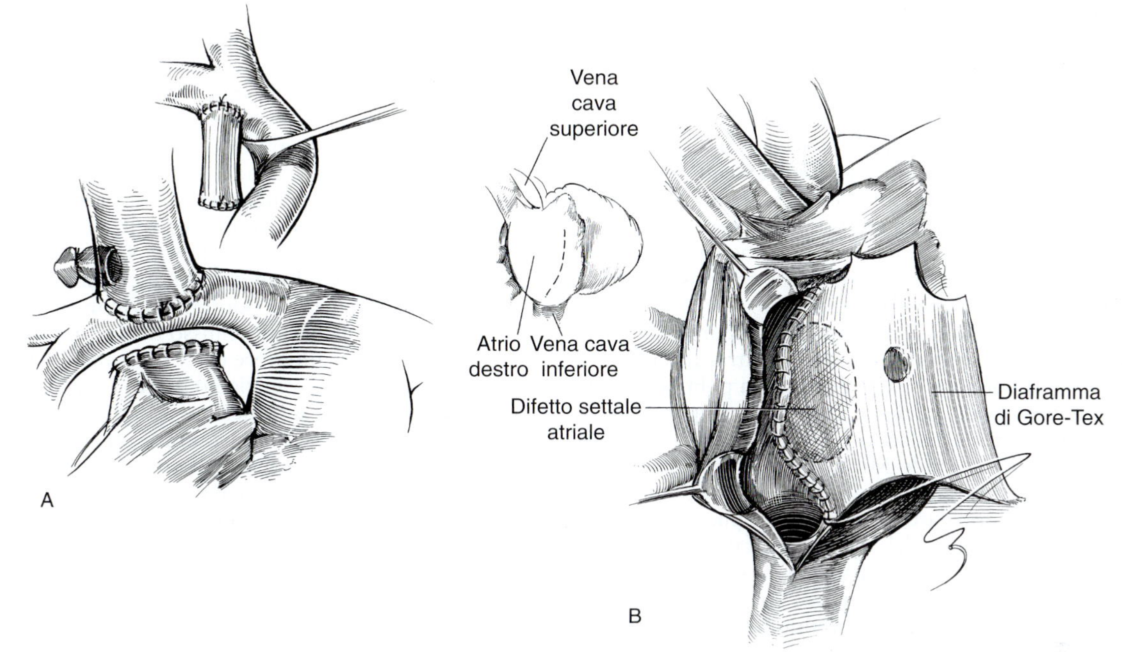

Figura 430-9. *A*, Shunt bidirezionale di Glenn che evidenzia l'anastomosi tra vena cava superiore e polmonare destra. *B*, Una procedura di Fontan modificata (isolamento della cavità polmonare) viene completata con il posizionamento di un diaframma per convogliare il sangue dalla vena cava inferiore lungo la parete laterale dell'atrio destro verso l'orifizio della vena cava superiore. Talvolta si effettua una fenestrazione di 4 mm sulla parte mediale del diaframma di politetrafluoroetilene. (Da Castañeda AR, Jonas RA, Mayer JE Jr, Hanley FL: Single-ventricle tricuspid atresia. In *Cardiac Surgery of the Neonate and Infant*. Philadelphia, WB Saunders, 1994.)

la procedura di isolamento della cavità polmonare ora in uso riduce questo rischio al 5% circa. Complicanze tardive sono l'ostruzione del diaframma, che causa una sindrome della vena cava superiore o inferiore, la tromboembolia della vena cava o dell'arteria polmonare, l'enteropatia protidodisperdente e le aritmie sopraventricolari (flutter atriale, tachicardia parossistica atriale), talvolta associate a morte improvvisa. La disfunzione ventricolare sinistra può verificarsi tardivamente, spesso in adolescenti o giovani adulti. Il trapianto cardiaco è un'opzione di trattamento che ha successo nei pazienti pediatrici con circuiti di Fontan "falliti".

430.5 • Ventricolo destro a doppia uscita con stenosi della polmonare

Un'aorta e un'arteria polmonare che originano entrambe dal ventricolo destro caratterizzano il ventricolo destro a doppia uscita con stenosi della polmonare; l'efflusso dal ventricolo sinistro è un VSD nel ventricolo destro. Le valvole aortica e mitralica sono separate di un cono muscolare liscio simile a quello visibile sotto la valvola polmonare normale. L'aorta può essere a cavaliere del VSD in misura variabile, ma occupa il ventricolo destro per almeno il 50%. Questo difetto può essere considerato complementare rispetto alla tetralogia di Fallot, a seconda del grado di sovrapposizione aortica. Fisiologia, anamnesi, esame obiettivo, elettrocardiogramma e radiografie del torace sono simili a quelli della tetralogia di Fallot (vedi Capitolo 430.1). L'ecocardiogramma bidimensionale rivela che entrambi i grandi vasi originano dal ventricolo destro e mette in luce una discontinuità della valvola mitrale-ortica. Durante il cateterismo cardiaco, l'angiografia dimostra che le valvole aortica e polmonare giacciono sul medesimo piano orizzontale e che l'aorta, spostata anteriormente, origina prevalentemente o esclusivamente dal ventricolo destro. La correzione chirurgica consiste nella creazione di un tunnel intraventricolare affinché il ventricolo sinistro possa sospingere il sangue attraverso il VSD, attraverso il tunnel, e in aorta. Per ovviare all'ostruzione polmonare si ricorre a un patch all'efflusso o a un condotto omograft dal ventricolo destro all'arteria polmonare (**operazione di Rastelli**). Nei bambini piccoli, la palliazione con uno shunt aortopolmonare assicura un miglioramento sintomatologico e permette un'adeguata crescita prima che venga effettuato l'intervento correttivo.

430.6 • Trasposizione delle grandi arterie con difetto del setto interventricolare e stenosi della polmonare

Questa combinazione di anomalie può simulare la tetralogia di Fallot per quando riguarda le caratteristiche cliniche (vedi Capitolo 430.1). A causa della trasposizione dei grandi vasi, il sito dell'ostruzione è nel ventricolo sinistro anziché nel destro. L'ostruzione può essere valvolare o sopravalvolare, e quest'ultima a sua volta può essere dinamica, correlata al setto interventricolare o al tessuto valvolare atrioventricolare, oppure acquisita, come nei pazienti con trasposizione e VSD dopo bendaggio dell'arteria polmonare.

Le manifestazioni cliniche possono cominciare a comparire poco dopo la nascita o comunque nella prima infanzia, a seconda del grado di stenosi polmonare. I reperti clinici comprendono cianosi, diminuita tolleranza allo sforzo e scarso sviluppo fisico, simile a quello descritto per la tetralogia di Fallot, sebbene il cuore possa presentare una dilatazione maggiore. La vascolarizzazione polmonare vista alla radiografia del torace dipende dal grado di ostruzione polmonare, ma spesso è normale. L'elettrocardiogramma evidenzia di solito una deviazione dell'asse a destra, un'ipertrofia dei ventricoli destro e sinistro e talvolta onde P alte e appuntite. L'ecocardiografia conferma la diagnosi ed è utile per la valutazione sequenziale del grado e della progressione dell'ostruzione del tratto di efflusso ventricolare. Il cateterismo cardiaco, se necessario, evidenzia che la pressione arteriosa polmonare è bassa e che la saturazione di ossigeno in arteria polmonare è più elevata che in aorta. La ventricolografia selettiva destra e sinistra mostra l'origine dell'aorta dal ventricolo destro, l'origine dell'arteria polmonare dal ventricolo sinistro, il VSD e la sede e la gravità della stenosi polmonare.

Nei neonati con cianosi occorre iniziare un'infusione di prostaglandina E_1 (0,01-0,20 μg/kg/min). Il trattamento chirurgico preferito in soggetti ipossici è uno shunt aortopolmonare (vedi Capitolo 430.1). Se necessario, viene effettuata una settostomia atriale con palloncino per migliorare il mescolamento a livello atriale e decomprimere l'atrio sinistro (vedi Capitolo 431.2). Il paziente può poi essere monitorato clinicamente finché non avrà raggiunto un'età maggiore, quando sarà preferibile eseguire l'intervento di Rastelli. La procedura di Rastelli permette di ottenere la correzione fisiologica e anatomica (1) mediante chiusura con patch del VSD, con un flusso ventricolare sinistro diretto in aorta; (2) con connessione del ventricolo destro all'arteria polmonare mediante legatura dell'arteria polmonare prossimale e posizionamento di un condotto homograft extracardiaco tra il ventricolo destro e la porzione distale dell'arteria polmonare (Fig. 430-10). Con la crescita del paziente tale condotto può divenire stenotico o funzionalmente ristretto e richiedere una revisione. La correzione chirurgica secondo Mustard (vedi Capitolo 431.2), che comporta la chiusura simultanea del VSD e la correzione dell'ostruzione all'efflusso ventricolare sinistro, può essere un'alternativa quando la posizione del VSD non è favorevole per un intervento di Rastelli. I pazienti con una stenosi polmonare più lieve, trattabile con valvulotomia semplice, possono essere sottoposti alla correzione completa con procedura di switch arterioso (vedi Capitolo 431.2).

430.7 • Anomalia di Ebstein della valvola tricuspide

FISIOPATOLOGIA. L'anomalia di Ebstein consiste nello spostamento verso il basso di una valvola tricuspide anomala all'interno del ventricolo destro. Il difetto può dipendere da un errore nel normale processo che porta la valvola tricuspide a separarsi dal miocardio del ventricolo destro (vedi Capitolo 420). La cuspide anteriore della valvola mantiene alcuni punti di attacco all'anello valvolare, ma gli altri lembi sono aderenti alla parete del ventricolo destro. Il ventricolo destro è così diviso in due parti dalla valvola tricuspide anomala: la prima, una porzione "atrializzata" dalla parete sottile, è in continuità con la cavità dell'atrio destro; la seconda, spesso più piccola, è costituita da normale miocardio ventricolare. L'atrio destro è enorme, e la valvola tricuspide è di solito rigurgitante, anche se il grado di rigurgito è estremamente variabile. La gittata effettiva del lato destro del cuore risulta diminuita a causa del ventricolo sinistro piccolo e dalla funzione ridotta, del rigurgito della valvola tricuspide e dell'ostruzione all'efflusso del ventricolo destro, prodotta dall'ampio lembo anteriore della tricuspide, a forma di vela. Talvolta la funzione del ventricolo destro è così compromessa che la forza prodotta non è sufficiente ad aprire la valvola polmonare in sistole: si viene così a instaurare un'atresia polmonare "funzionale". Alcuni lattanti hanno una vera atresia anatomica della polmonare. L'aumentato volume di sangue atriale destro viene deviato attraverso il forame ovale all'atrio sinistro, causando cianosi (Fig. 430-11).

MANIFESTAZIONI CLINICHE. La gravità dei sintomi e della cianosi sono altamente variabili e dipendono dal grado di spostamento della valvola tricuspide e dalla gravità dell'ostruzione all'efflusso ventricolare destro. In molti pazienti, i sintomi sono lievi e non sono evidenti fino alla pubertà o all'inizio dell'età adulta; all'inizio il paziente può presentare astenia o palpitazioni, riconducibili alle aritmie cardiache. Uno shunt destro-sinistro attraverso il forame ovale è responsabile di cianosi e policitemia. La pressione venosa centrale può essere normale o aumentata in caso di insufficienza della tricuspide. Alla palpazione, il precordio è in quiete. È udibile un soffio olosistolico sulla maggior parte del lato anteriore sinistro del torace, causato dal rigurgito della tricuspide. È

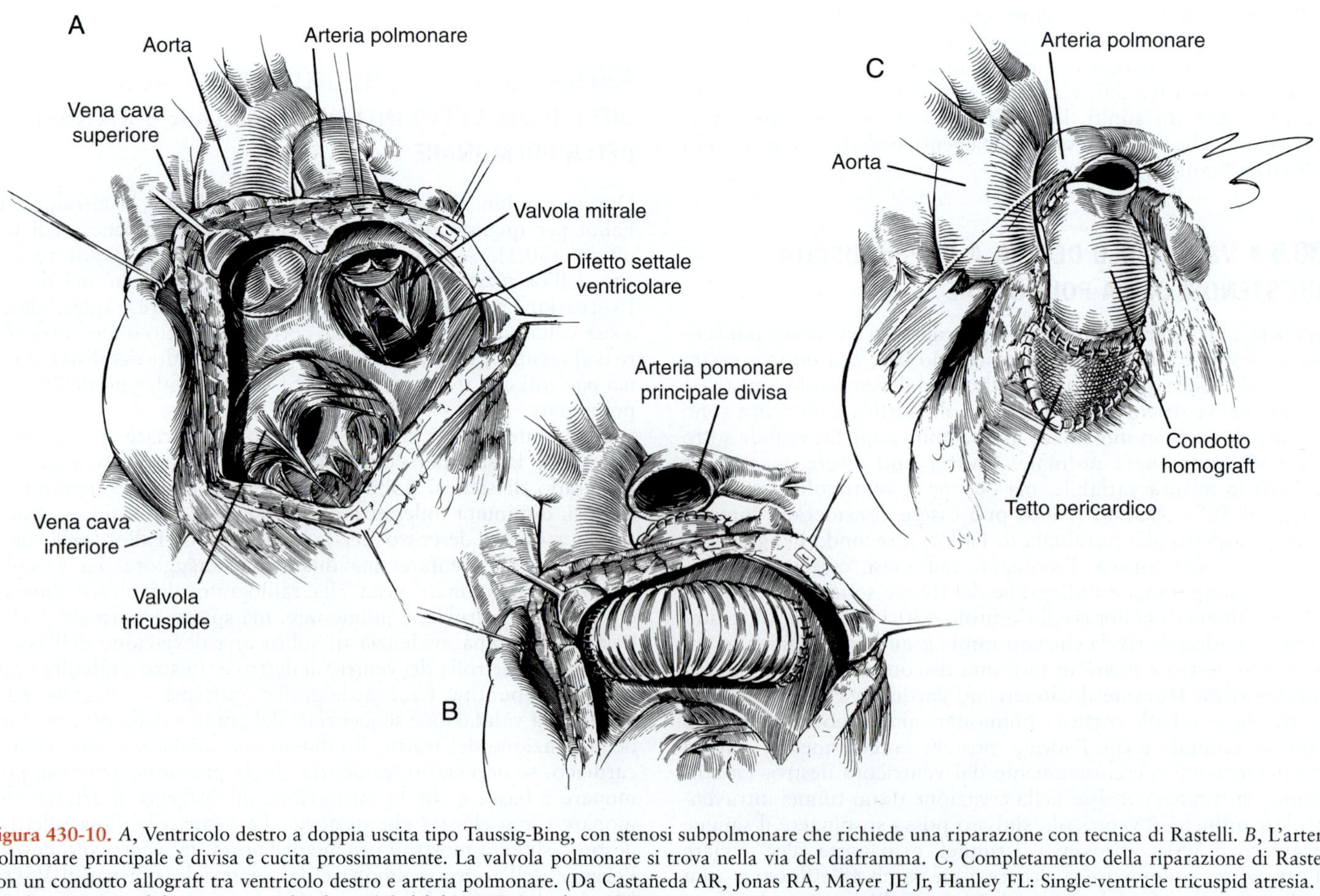

Figura 430-10. *A*, Ventricolo destro a doppia uscita tipo Taussig-Bing, con stenosi subpolmonare che richiede una riparazione con tecnica di Rastelli. *B*, L'arteria polmonare principale è divisa e cucita prossimamente. La valvola polmonare si trova nella via del diaframma. *C*, Completamento della riparazione di Rastelli con un condotto allograft tra ventricolo destro e arteria polmonare. (Da Castañeda AR, Jonas RA, Mayer JE Jr, Hanley FL: Single-ventricle tricuspid atresia. In *Cardiac Surgery of the Neonate and Infant*. Philadelphia, WB Saunders, 1994.)

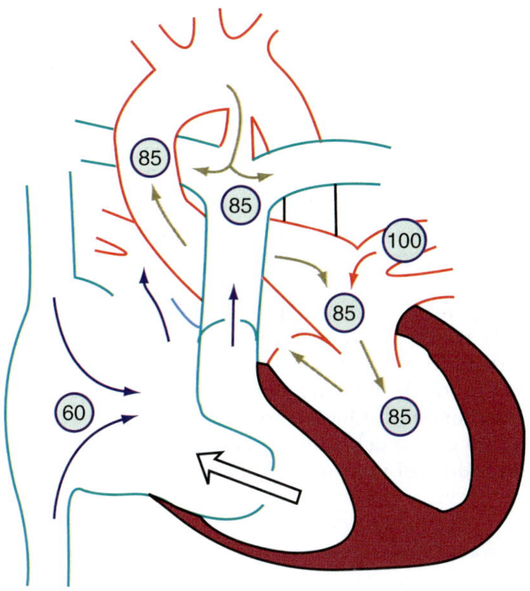

Figura 430-11. Fisiologia di un'anomalia di Ebstein della valvola tricuspide. I *numeri cerchiati* rappresentano i valori di saturazione di ossigeno. In seguito allo spostamento verso il basso dei lembi tricuspidali nel ventricolo destro si è formato un segmento di ventricolo destro dalla parete sottile, a bassa pressione e "atrializzato". La valvola tricuspide è grossolanamente insufficiente (*freccia chiara*). Il flusso sanguigno atriale destro viene deviato verso sinistra attraverso un difetto del setto interatriale o un forame ovale pervio nell'atrio sinistro. Una piccola quantità di sangue può attraversare il tratto di efflusso del ventricolo destro ed entrare in arteria polmonare; tuttavia, nei casi gravi, il ventricolo destro è incapace di produrre una forza sufficiente a provocare l'apertura della valvola polmonare: ne risulta un'"atresia polmonare funzionale". Nell'atrio sinistro, il sangue desaturato si mescola con il ritorno venoso polmonare saturo. Il sangue entra nel ventricolo sinistro ed è sospinto in aorta. In questo esempio, parte del flusso sanguigno polmonare deriva dal ventricolo destro, il resto da un dotto arterioso pervio (PDA). I neonati con una grave anomalia di Ebstein svilupperanno una marcata cianosi quando il PDA si chiuderà.

comune un ritmo di galoppo, spesso associato con click multipli a livello del margine sternale inferiore sinistro. Un soffio diastolico aspro può inoltre apprezzarsi a livello del margine sternale sinistro; si tratta di un soffio superficiale che può simulare uno sfregamento pericardico.

I neonati con forme gravi di anomalia di Ebstein hanno una cianosi marcata, una cardiomegalia massiva e soffi sistolici prolungati; la morte può avvenire per scompenso cardiaco e ipossiemia. Un miglioramento spontaneo può verificarsi in alcuni neonati quando la resistenza vascolare polmonare diminuisce fino a raggiungere livelli normali e migliora la capacità del ventricolo destro di provvedere al flusso sanguigno polmonare. La maggior parte dei pazienti è dipendente dalla presenza di un PDA perché sia presente un flusso sanguigno polmonare, e quindi è dipendente dall'infusione di prostaglandina.

DIAGNOSI. L'elettrocardiogramma di solito evidenzia un blocco di branca destro senza aumento del voltaggio nelle derivazioni precordiali, onde P normali o alte e ampie, e un intervallo PR normale o prolungato. Può essere presente la **sindrome di Wolff-Parkinson-White** (vedi Capitolo 435); i pazienti possono presentare episodi di tachicardia sopraventricolare. All'esame radiografico, le dimensioni del cuore variano dalla normalità a una cardiomegalia massiva, "a forma di scatola", causata dall'ingrandimento dell'atrio e del ventricolo destri. La vascolarizzazione polmonare può essere normale o ridotta. L'ecocardiografia evidenzia il grado di spostamento dei lembi valvolari tricuspidalici, un atrio destro dilatato e l'eventuale presenza di un'ostruzione del tratto di efflusso del ventricolo destro (Fig. 430-12). Il Doppler pulsato e il color-Doppler permettono di valutare il grado di rigurgito tricuspidale. Nei casi gravi, la valvola polmonare appare immobile e il flusso sanguigno polmonare proviene unicamente dal dotto arterioso. Può essere difficile distinguere un'atresia polmonare vera da una forma funzionale. Il cateterismo cardiaco, peraltro non sempre necessario, conferma la presenza di un atrio sinistro grande, di una valvola tricuspide anomala e di un eventuale shunt destro-sinistro a livello atriale. Il rischio di aritmia è significativo durante il cateterismo e gli studi angiografici.

PROGNOSI E COMPLICANZE. La prognosi dell'anomalia di Ebstein è estremamente variabile e dipende dallo spetto di gravità che si osserva. La prognosi è di solito infausta per neonati o lattanti con sintomi intrattabili e cianosi. I pazienti con una patologia più lieve di solito sopravvivono bene fino all'età adulta. Nel 18% dei pazienti l'anomalia di Ebstein è associata alla cardiomiopatia ventricolare sinistra (non compattazione isolata).

TRATTAMENTO. I neonati con grave ipossia e prostaglandina-dipendenti sono stati trattati con lo shunt aortopolmonare da solo,

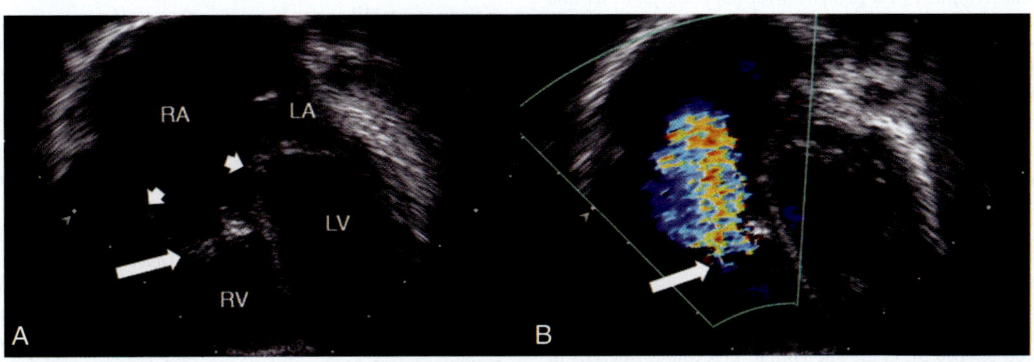

Figura 430-12. Dimostrazione ecocardiografica dell'anomalia di Ebstein della valvola tricuspide. *A*, Proiezione sottopostale quattro-camere bidimensionale che evidenzia un grave spostamento dei lembi della valvola tricuspide (*freccia grande*) verso il basso, all'interno del ventricolo destro. La sede dell'anulus tricuspidale è evidenziata dalle due punte di freccia. La porzione del ventricolo destro tra l'anulus valvolare e i lembi valvolari è la componente "atrializzata". *B*, L'esame color-Doppler evidenzia un grave rigurgito della valvola tricuspide displastica. Si noti che il flusso turbolento rigurgitante (*freccia*) inizia a metà strada nella camera ventricolare destra, a livello dei lembi valvolari spostati. LA (*Left Atrium*), atrio sinistro; LV (*Left Ventricle*), ventricolo sinistro; RA (*Right Atrium*), atrio destro; RV (*Right Ventricle*), ventricolo destro.

mediante riparazione della valvola tricuspide o sua chiusura chirurgica con patch, con settostomia atriale e con posizionamento di uno shunt aortopolmonare (**procedura di Starnes**). Molti lattanti con anomalia di Ebstein che sono stati sottoposti a riparazione valvolare avranno ancora un rigurgito tale da richiedere in seguito uno shunt di Glenn, eseguito per ridurre il carico di volume sul ventricolo destro (vedi Capitolo 430.4). Nei bambini più grandi con malattia lieve o moderata, è di primaria importanza tenere sotto controllo le alterazioni del ritmo sopraventricolari; il trattamento chirurgico può non essere necessario fino all'adolescenza o all'inizio età adulta. Nei pazienti con grave rigurgito tricuspidale, in seguito si procede alla riparazione o alla sostituzione della valvola tricuspide anomala insieme alla chiusura del difetto settale atriale. In alcuni pazienti più grandi si effettua anche uno shunt bidirezionale di Glenn, con l'anastomosi della vena casa alle arterie polmonari. Questa procedura riduce il volume di sangue che il lato destro del cuore (la cui funzione è alterata) deve pompare, creando così una riparazione ventricolare "uno-e-mezzo".

Tetralogia di Fallot

Boudjemline Y, Fermont L, Le Bidois J, et al: Prevalence of 22q11 deletion in fetuses with conotruncal cardiac defects: A 6-year prospective study. *J Pediatr* 2001;138:520–524.

Dubin AM, Feinstein JA, Reddy VM, et al: Electrical resynchronization: A novel therapy for the failing right ventricle. *Circulation* 2003;107:2287–2289.

Hanley FL: Management of the congenitally abnormal right ventricular outflow tract—what is the right approach? *J Thorac Cardiovasc Surg* 2000;119:1–3.

McCaughan BC, Danielson GK, Driscoll DJ, et al: Tetralogy of Fallot with absent pulmonary valve: Early and late results of surgical treatment. *J Thorac Cardiovasc Surg* 1985;89:280–287.

Pacifico AO, Saro ME, Bargeron LM Jr, et al: Transatrial-transpulmonary repair of tetralogy of Fallot. *J Thorac Cardiovasc Surg* 1987;74:382–395.

Parry AJ, McElhinney DB, Kung GC, et al: Elective primary repair of acyanotic tetralogy of Fallot in early infancy: Overall outcome and impact on the pulmonary valve. *J Am Coll Cardiol* 2000;36:2279–2283.

Reddy VM, McElhinney DB, Amin Z, et al: Early and intermediate outcomes after repair of pulmonary atresia with ventricular septal defect and major aortopulmonary collateral arteries: Experience with 85 patients. *Circulation* 2000;101:1826–1832.

Schultz AH, Wernovsky G: Late outcomes in patients with surgically treated congenital heart disease. *Semin Thorac Cardiovasc Surg Pediatr Card Surg Annu* 2005;8:145–156.

Atresia della polmonare con setto interventricolare intatto

Hanley FL, Sade RM, Blackstone EH, et al: Outcomes in neonatal pulmonary atresia with intact ventricular septum. A multiinstitutional study. *J Thorac Cardiovasc Surg* 1993;105:406–423.

Latson LA: Nonsurgical treatment of a neonate with pulmonary atresia and intact ventricular septum by transcatheter puncture and balloon dilatation of the atretic valve membrane. *Am J Cardiol* 1991;68:277–279.

L'Ecuyer TJ, Poulik JM, Vincent JA: Myocardial infarction due to coronary abnormalities in pulmonary atresia with intact ventricular septum. *Pediatr Cardiol* 2001;22:68–70.

Atresia della tricuspide

Anderson RH, Cook AC: Morphology of the functionally univentricular heart. *Cardiol Young* 2004;14(Suppl 1):3–12.

Donnelly JP, Rosenthal A, Castle VP, et al: Reversal of protein-losing enteropathy with heparin therapy in three patients with univentricular hearts and Fontan palliation. *J Pediatr* 1997;130:474–478.

Freedom RM, Hamilton R, Yoo SJ, et al: The Fontan procedure: Analysis of cohorts and late complications. *Cardiol Young* 2000;10:307–331.

Gelatt M, Hamilton R, McCrindle W, et al: Risk factors for atrial tachyarrhythmias after the Fontan operation. *J Am Coll Cardiol* 1994;24:1735–1741.

Hess J: Long-term problems after cavopulmonary anastomosis: Diagnosis and management. *Thorac Cardiovasc Surg* 2001;49:98–100.

Mair DD, Puga FJ, Danielson GK: The Fontan procedure for tricuspid atresia: Early and late results of a 25-year experience with 216 patients. *J Am Coll Cardiol* 2001;37:933–939.

Petrossian E, Reddy VM, McElhinney DB, et al: Early results of the extracardiac conduit Fontan operation. *J Thorac Cardiovasc Surg* 1999;117:688–696.

Shirai LK, Rosenthal DN, Reitz BA, et al: Arrhythmias and thromboembolic complications after the extracardiac Fontan operation. *J Thorac Cardiovasc Surg* 1998;115:499–505.

van den Bosch AE, Roos-Hesselink JW, Van Domburg R, et al: Long-term outcome and quality of life in adult patients after the Fontan operation. *Am J Cardiol* 2004;93:1141–1145.

Anomalia di Ebstein della valvola tricuspide

Kiziltan HT, Theodoro DA, Warnes CA, et al: Late results of bioprosthetic tricuspid valve replacement in Ebstein's anomaly. *Ann Thorac Surg* 1998;66:1539–1545.

Marianeschi SM, McElhinney DB, Reddy VM, et al: Alternative approach to the repair of Ebstein's malformation: Intracardiac repair with ventricular unloading. *Ann Thorac Surg* 1998;66:1546–1550.

Schreiber C, Cook A, Ho SY, et al: Morphologic spectrum of Ebstein's malformation: Revisitation relative to surgical repair. *J Thorac Cardiovasc Surg* 1999;117:148–155.

Starnes VA, Pitlick PT, Bernstein D, et al: Ebstein's anomaly appearing in the neonate. *J Thorac Cardiovasc Surg* 1991;101:1082–1087.

Capitolo 431 ■ Cardiopatie congenite cianogene: lesioni associate ad aumentato flusso sanguigno polmonare

431.1 • D-TRASPOSIZIONE DELLE GRANDI ARTERIE

La trasposizione dei grandi vasi, un'anomalia congenita associata a cianosi, costituisce circa il 5% di tutte le cardiopatie congenite. In questa anomalia, le vene sistemiche sboccano nell'atrio destro e le vene polmonari nell'atrio sinistro, come avviene di norma. Le connessioni tra gli atri e i ventricoli sono anch'esse normali (concordanza atrioventricolare). L'aorta origina dal ventricolo destro e l'arteria polmonare dal ventricolo sinistro (Fig. 431-1). Quando i grandi vasi sono normalmente in relazione l'uno con l'altro, l'aorta è posteriore e sita alla destra dell'arteria polmonare, mentre nella d-trasposizione delle grandi arterie (d-TGA, *d-Transposition of the Great Arteries*) essa è sita anteriormente e a destra dell'arteria polmonare (la *d* indica la destroposizione dell'aorta). Il sangue desaturato che dal corpo ritorna al cuore destro fuoriesce di nuovo in modo errato dall'aorta e viene pompato nell'organismo mentre il sangue venoso polmonare ossigenato che ritorna al cuore sinistro viene sospinto nuovamente ai polmoni. Le circolazioni sistemica e polmonare consistono di due circuiti paralleli. A consentire la sopravvivenza di questi neonati sono il forame ovale e il dotto arterioso, che rendono possibile un certo mescolamento di sangue ossigenato e deossigenato. Circa il 50% dei pazienti con TGA ha anche un difetto del setto interventricolare (VSD, *Ventricular Septal Defect*), che permette un miglior mescolamento. I reperti clinici ed emodinamici variano in relazione alla presenza o all'assenza di difetti associati. La TGA è più comune in bambini di madri diabetiche e nei maschi (3:1). Specialmente quando accompagnata da altri difetti cardiaci come la stenosi polmonare o l'arco aortico destro, può essere associata a delezione del cromosoma 22q11 (**CATCH22** [*Cardiac defects, Abnormal facies, Thymic aplasia, Cleft palate, Hypoplasia*, difetti cardiaci, anomalie facciali, aplasia del timo, palatoschisi, ipoplasia], sindrome di DiGeorge). Prima dell'era moderna della chirurgia correttiva o palliativa, la mortalità era >90% nel primo anno di vita.

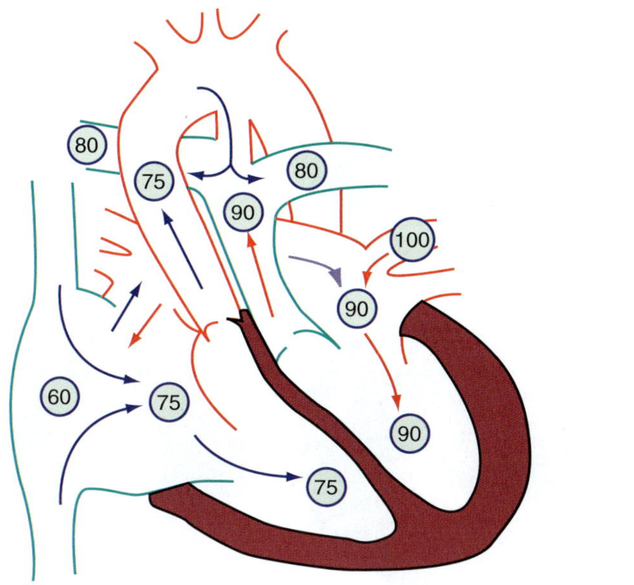

Figura 431-1. Fisiologia della d-trasposizione delle grandi arterie (d-TGA, *d-Transposition of the Great Arteries*). I *numeri cerchiati* rappresentano i valori di saturazione dell'ossigeno. La saturazione di ossigeno atriale destra (sangue venoso misto) è diminuita in conseguenza dell'ipossia sistemica. Il sangue desaturato entra nell'atrio destro, fluisce attraverso la valvola tricuspide nel ventricolo destro e viene sospinto nell'aorta trasposta, con una conseguente grave desaturazione in aorta. Il sangue venoso polmonare completamente saturo fluisce nell'atrio sinistro, giunge nel ventricolo sinistro attraverso la valvola mitrale e nei polmoni attraverso l'arteria polmonare trasposta. Ne deriva un aumento della saturazione di ossigeno polmonare. Questa lesione non sarebbe compatibile con la vita se il sangue non potesse essere deviato attraverso due vie fetali: il forame ovale pervio (PFO, *Patent Foramen Ovale*) e il dotto arterioso pervio (PDA, *Patent Ductus Arteriosus*). Il sangue può essere deviato da sinistra a destra o bidirezionalmente a livello del PFO. Poiché la resistenza vascolare sistemica tende a essere più elevata della resistenza vascolare polmonare, il sangue viene deviato attraverso il PDA principalmente dall'aorta all'arteria polmonare. Se la resistenza polmonare diminuisce nelle prime settimane di vita, il flusso sanguigno polmonare aumenterà gradualmente in pazienti con d-TGA.

431.2 • d-Trasposizione delle grandi arterie con setto interventricolare intatto

La d-TGA con setto ventricolare intatto è detta anche TGA semplice o isolata. Prima della nascita, l'ossigenazione del feto è quasi normale, ma una volta che il dotto inizia a chiudersi, il minimo mescolamento di sangue sistemico e polmonare attraverso il forame ovale pervio è di solito insufficiente e si instaura una grave ipossiemia, generalmente entro i primi giorni di vita.

MANIFESTAZIONI CLINICHE. La cianosi e la tachipnea vengono riconosciute per lo più nelle prime ore di vita. In assenza di trattamento, la vasta maggioranza di questi bambini non sopravvivrebbe oltre il periodo neonatale. L'ipossiemia è di solito grave, ma lo scompenso cardiaco è meno comune. Questa condizione è un'emergenza medica; solo una diagnosi precoce e un intervento mirato evitano lo sviluppo di un'ipossiemia grave e prolungata e di un'acidosi, che possono portare alla morte. I reperti fisici associati a cianosi possono essere aspecifici. L'impulso precordiale può essere normale, oppure può essere presente un sollevamento parasternale. Il secondo tono cardiaco di solito è singolo e forte, anche se a volte può essere sdoppiato. Talvolta sono assenti soffi, mentre in altri casi può notarsi un soffio sistolico da eiezione a livello del margine sternale medio sinistro.

DIAGNOSI. L'elettrocardiogramma mostra il normale pattern neonatale di dominanza destra. Le radiografie del torace possono evidenziare una lieve cardiomegalia, un mediastino stretto (e perciò un cuore a forma di uovo) e un flusso sanguigno polmonare normale o aumentato. Nel primissimo periodo postnatale la radiografia del torace è generalmente normale. Quando la resistenza vascolare polmonare cala durante la 1ª-2ª settimana di vita, diventa evidente l'aumento del flusso sanguigno polmonare. La PO_2 arteriosa è bassa e non aumenta in modo apprezzabile quando si somministra ossigeno al 100% (test dell'iperossigenazione), anche se questo test può non essere del tutto affidabile. L'ecocardiografia conferma le connessioni ventricoloarteriose della trasposizione (Fig. 431-2). È inoltre possibile visualizzare la dimensione della comunicazione interatriale e il dotto arterioso; il grado di mescolamento viene valutato mediante esame Doppler pulsato e color-Doppler. Può essere altresì valutata la presenza di qualsiasi lesione associata, come un'ostruzione del tratto di efflusso ventricolare sinistro o un VSD. Di solito è possibile visualizzare le origini delle arterie coronarie, anche se l'ecocardiografia non è accurata quanto il cateterismo per questo scopo. Il cateterismo cardiaco viene talora effettuato in pazienti per cui l'imaging non invasivo è inconcludente dal punto di vista diagnostico o in quelli che necessitano di una settostomia atriale con palloncino in emergenza (vedi oltre). Tale indagine dimostrerà che la pressione ventricolare destra è sistemica poiché questo ventricolo supporta la circolazione sistemica. Il sangue nel ventricolo sinistro e nell'arteria polmonare ha una saturazione di ossigeno più elevata che nell'aorta. A seconda dall'età del paziente al momento del cateterismo, le pressioni nel ventricolo sinistro e in arteria polmonare possono andare da livelli sistemici a valori <50% della pressione a livello sistemico. La ventricolografia destra evidenzia l'aorta posizionata anteriormente e a destra, che origina dal ventricolo destro, oltre al setto ventricolare intatto. Nel 10-15% dei pazienti si riscontrano **arterie coronarie anomale**. Alla ventricolografia sinistra risulta che l'arteria polmonare origina esclusivamente dal ventricolo sinistro.

TRATTAMENTO. Quando si sospetta una trasposizione, si dovrebbe iniziare immediatamente un'infusione di prostaglandina E_1 per mantenere la pervietà del dotto arterioso e migliorare l'ossigenazione (dosaggio: 0,01-0,20 mcg/kg/min). Dal momento che sussiste il rischio di apnea associata all'infusione di prostaglandina, dovrebbe essere disponibile un medico esperto in intubazione endotracheale neonatale. L'ipotermia intensifica l'acidosi metabolica che deriva dall'ipossiemia; pertanto, il paziente dovrebbe essere tenuto al caldo. Una tempestiva correzione dell'acidosi e dell'ipoglicemia è essenziale.

I bambini che rimangono gravemente ipossici o acidotici nonostante l'infusione di prostaglandina dovrebbero essere sottoposti

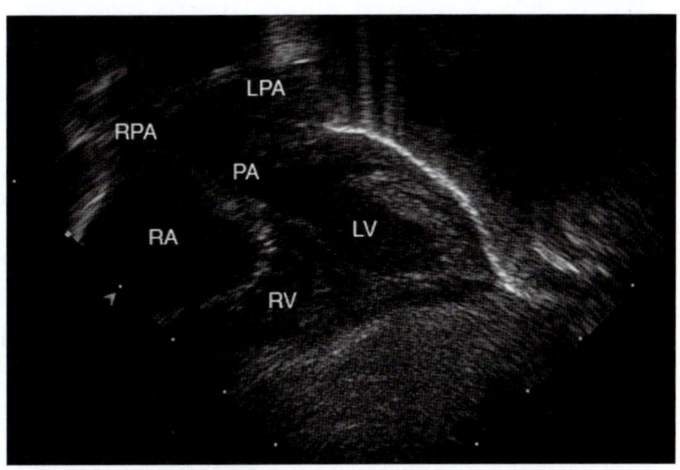

Figura 431-2. Dimostrazione di una d-trasposizione delle grandi arterie in una proiezione ecocardiografia bidimensionale sottocostale a quattro camere. È visibile l'arteria polmonare (PA, *Pulmonary Artery*), che origina direttamente dal ventricolo sinistro (LV, *Left Ventricle*). L'immediata biforcazione di questo grande vaso nelle diramazioni delle arterie polmonari la differenzia dall'aorta, che si ramifica più distalmente dal cuore. LPA (*Left Pulmonary Artery*), arteria polmonare sinistra; RA (*Right Atrium*), atrio destro; RPA (*Right Pulmonary Artery*), arteria polmonare destra; RV (*Right Ventricle*), ventricolo destro.

a **settostomia atriale con palloncino sec. Rashkind** (Fig. 431-3). Una settostomia atriale sec. Rashkind viene di solito effettuata in tutti i pazienti in cui è necessario posticipare significativamente l'intervento chirurgico. Nella maggior parte dei centri, l'intervento di switch arterioso (**procedura di Jantene**) viene effettuato nelle prime 2 settimane di vita: in questo modo è spesso possibile evitare il cateterismo e la settostomia atriale.

Una settostomia atriale sec. Rashkind condotta con successo dovrebbe portare a un aumento della Pa_{O_2} fino a 35-50 mmHg e all'eliminazione di qualsiasi gradiente pressorio attraverso il setto atriale. Alcuni pazienti con TGA e VSD possono richiedere una settostomia atriale con palloncino a causa di uno scarso mescolamento di sangue, anche se il VSD è ampio. Altri possono trarre beneficio da una decompressione dell'atrio sinistro che allevi i sintomi di un aumentato flusso sanguigno polmonare e di uno scompenso cardiaco sinistro.

La **procedura di switch arterioso (Jantene)**, che rappresenta il **trattamento chirurgico di scelta** per i neonati con d-TGA e un setto ventricolare intatto, di solito viene effettuata nelle prime 2 settimane di vita. Il motivo di quest'urgenza è che quando la resistenza vascolare polmonare diminuisce dopo la nascita, la pressione nel ventricolo sinistro (connesso al letto vascolare polmonare) diminuisce di pari passo. Questo calo pressorio porta a una diminuzione della massa ventricolare sinistra nelle prime settimane di vita. Se l'intervento di switch arterioso viene tentato dopo che la pressione ventricolare sinistra ha subito un'eccessiva diminuzione, il ventricolo sinistro sarà incapace di produrre una pressione adeguata per pompare il sangue nella circolazione sistemica. L'intervento consiste nel dividere l'aorta e l'arteria polmonare subito al di sopra dei seni e nell'eseguire la loro rianastomosi nella corretta posizione anatomica. Le arterie coronarie vengono poi rimosse dalla vecchia radice aortica insieme a un bottone di parete aortica e reimpiantate sulla vecchia radice polmonare ("neoaorta"). Utilizzando un bottone di tessuto dei grandi vasi, il chirurgo evita di effettuare una sutura direttamente sull'arteria coronaria (Fig. 431-4). Raramente viene utilizzata una procedura di switch arterioso a due stadi, con il posizionamento iniziale di una banderella di arteria polmonare, in pazienti con più di 3-4 settimane di vita, che hanno già una riduzione della massa muscolare e della pressione ventricolare sinistra.

La procedura di switch arterioso ha un tasso di sopravvivenza del 90-95% per la d-TGA non complicata. Essa ripristina i normali rapporti fisiologici del flusso sanguigno sistemico e polmonare, senza le complicanze a lungo termine della procedura di switch atriale.

Approcci ormai superati alla d-TGA consistono nelle **procedure di switch atriale** (interventi di **Mustard** o di **Senning**). In bambini più grandi, queste procedure comportavano un'eccellente sopravvivenza nell'immediato (circa 85-90%), ma una significativa morbilità a lungo termine. Le procedure di switch atriale invertono i pattern di flusso sanguigno a livello atriale mediante

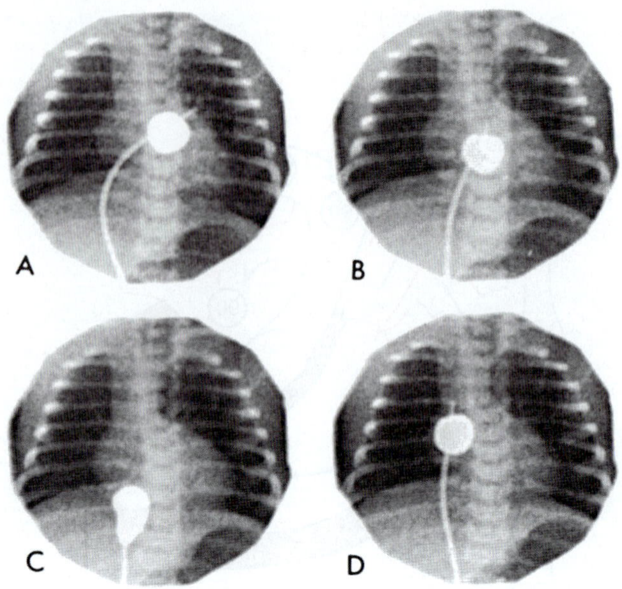

Figura 431-3. Settostomia atriale con palloncino sec. Rashkind. Quattro immagini tratte da un cineangiogramma continuo documentano la creazione di un difetto settale atriale in un neonato ipossiemico, con trasposizione delle grandi arterie e setto ventricolare intatto. *A*, Palloncino gonfiato nell'atrio sinistro. *B*, Il catetere viene ritirato improvvisamente, cosicché il palloncino rompe di forame ovale. *C*, Palloncino nella vena cava inferiore. *D*, Catetere fatto avanzare nell'atrio destro per sgonfiare il palloncino. Il tempo intercorso tra *A* e *C* è <1 s.

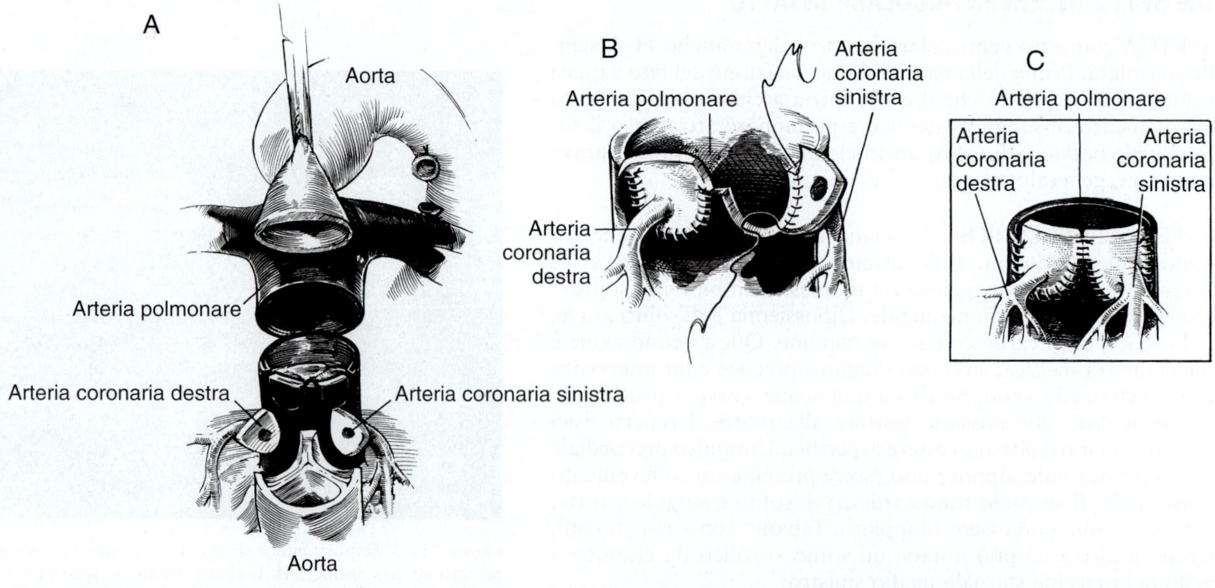

Figura 431-4. Metodo per traslocare le arterie coronarie nella procedura di switch arterioso (Jantene). *A*, L'aorta (anteriore) e l'arteria polmonare (posteriore) sono state sezionate per permettere la visualizzazione delle arterie coronarie sinistra e destra. Le coronarie sono state escisse dai loro rispettivi seni, compreso un ampio lembo (bottone) di parete arteriosa. Segmenti equivalenti della parete dell'arteria polmonare (che diverrà la neoaorta) sono stati altresì rimossi. *B*, I bottoni aortocoronarici vengono suturati nella porzione prossimale della neoaorta. Con questa tecnica tutte le suture sono posizionate nel bottone della parete aortica anziché direttamente sulle arterie coronarie. *C*, Anastomosi completata delle arterie coronarie sinistra e destra alla neoaorta. (Adattata da Castañeda AR, Jonas RA, Mayer JE Jr, Hanley FL: *Cardiac Surgery of the Neonate and Infant*. Philadelphia, WB Saunders, 1994.)

la creazione chirurgica di un diaframma intra-atriale che permette al sangue venoso sistemico di affluire all'atrio sinistro e al ventricolo sinistro per poi passare, attraverso l'arteria polmonare, nei polmoni. Il medesimo diaframma permette anche al sangue venoso polmonare ossigenato di giungere all'atrio destro, al ventricolo destro e all'aorta. La procedure di switch atriale consistono in un significativo intervento chirurgico atriale e possono portare allo sviluppo tardivo di disturbi della conduzione atriale, alla sindrome del seno malato con bradiaritmie e tachiaritmie, al flutter atriale, alla morte improvvisa, alla sindrome della vena cava superiore o inferiore, a edema, ascite e aenteropatia protidodisperdente. La procedura di switch atriale lascia il ventricolo destro come camera di pompaggio sistemica e spesso questi ventricoli destri sistemici iniziano a scompensarsi nella prima età adulta. Gli interventi di switch atriale sono riservati ai pazienti che per motivi anatomici non sono candidati alla procedura di switch arterioso (TGA e grave stenosi polmonare).

431.3 • Trasposizione delle grandi arterie con difetto del setto interventricolare

Se il VSD associato alla TGA è piccolo, le manifestazioni cliniche, i reperti di laboratori e il trattamento sono simili a quelli già descritti per la trasposizione con setto interventricolare intatto. Un soffio sistolico aspro, udibile a livello del margine sternale inferiore sinistro, deriva dal flusso di sangue che attraversa il difetto. Molti di questi piccoli difetti finiscono per chiudersi spontaneamente e spesso non vengono toccati al momento dell'intervento chirurgico.

Quando il VSD è ampio e non restrittivo per quanto attiene all'eiezione ventricolare, si verifica di solito un mescolamento significativo di sangue ossigenato e deossigenato e si osservano le manifestazioni cliniche dello scompenso cardiaco. L'insorgenza della cianosi può essere insidiosa e frequentemente ritardata, e la sua intensità è variabile. La cianosi generalmente viene riconosciuta nel primo mese di vita, ma in alcuni bambini può restare non diagnosticata per parecchi mesi. Il soffio è olosistolico e indistinguibile da quello prodotto da un ampio VSD in pazienti con grandi arterie normalmente posizionate. Il cuore di solito è significativamente ingrandito.

La cardiomegalia, un mediastino stretto e un aumento della vascolarizzazione polmonare vengono evidenziati alla radiografia del torace. L'elettrocardiogramma rileva onde P prominenti e un'ipertrofia ventricolare destra isolata o un'ipertrofia biventricolare. Talvolta è presente una dominanza del ventricolo sinistro. Anche se di solito l'asse del QRS è verso destra, talora può anche essere normale o deviato a sinistra. La diagnosi viene confermata con l'ecocardiografia; è inoltre possibile valutare l'entità del flusso sanguigno polmonare dal grado di ingrandimento dell'atrio sinistro e del ventricolo sinistro. Nei casi dubbi, la diagnosi viene confermata dal cateterismo cardiaco. La ventricolografia destra e sinistra, oltre a indicare la presenza di una trasposizione arteriosa, evidenzia la sede e le dimensioni del VSD. La pressione di picco sistolico è uguale nei due ventricoli, in aorta e nell'arteria polmonare. La pressione atriale sinistra può essere molto più elevata della pressione atriale, un reperto indicativo di una comunicazione restrittiva a livello atriale. All'atto del cateterismo cardiaco si può procedere a una settostomia atriale con palloncino sec. Rashkind per decomprimere l'atrio sinistro, anche quando vi è un adeguato mescolamento a livello ventricolare.

Si raccomanda di effettuare il trattamento chirurgico subito dopo la diagnosi, di solito entro il primo mese di vita, poiché lo scompenso cardiaco e il ritardo di crescita sono difficili da gestire e la vasculopatia polmonare potrebbe svilupparsi con insolita rapidità. Il trattamento comprende la somministrazione di diuretici e, se possibile, digitale per alleviare i sintomi dello scompenso cardiaco in attesa della correzione chirurgica.

I pazienti con TGA e VSD senza stenosi polmonare possono essere trattati con una procedura di switch arterioso combinata con la chiusura del VSD. In questi bambini l'intervento di switch arterioso può essere effettuata in sicurezza dopo le prime 2 settimane di vita poiché il VSD porta a un'uguale pressione in entrambi i ventricoli e previene la regressione della massa muscolare del ventricolo sinistro. Nei centri più importanti, tuttavia, non vi è motivo di ritardare la riparazione, da momento che i risultati sono comunque eccellenti, che l'intervento sia effettuato nel periodo neonatale o più tardi.

In assenza di trattamento, la prognosi è infausta: la maggior parte dei pazienti muore nel primo anno di vita per lo scompenso cardiaco, l'ipossiemia e l'ipertensione polmonare. In passato, alcuni sopravvivevano oltre l'infanzia con la sola terapia medica, ma spesso si sviluppava una patologia vascolare polmonare. Il quadro clinico e il trattamento di questi pazienti sono simili a quelli descritti per la sindrome di Eisenmenger secondaria a un ampio VSD isolato (vedi Capitolo 433.2).

431.4 • L-Trasposizione delle grandi arterie (trasposizione corretta)

Nella l-trasposizione, i rapporti atrioventricolari sono discordanti, con l'atrio destro connesso al ventricolo sinistro e l'atrio sinistro al ventricolo destro (inversione ventricolare). Le grandi arterie sono anch'esse trasposte, con l'aorta che origina dal ventricolo destro e l'arteria polmonare dal ventricolo sinistro. L'aorta origina alla sinistra dell'arteria polmonare (la *l* sta appunto a indicare la levotrasposizione). L'aorta può essere situata anteriormente all'arteria polmonare; di solito sono quasi l'una accanto all'altra. Il sangue venoso sistemico desaturato ritorna a un atrio destro normalmente posizionato, per poi passare, attraverso una valvola atrioventricolare bicuspide (mitrale), in un ventricolo situato a destra che ha architettura e caratteristiche morfologiche tipiche della parete liscia del normale ventricolo

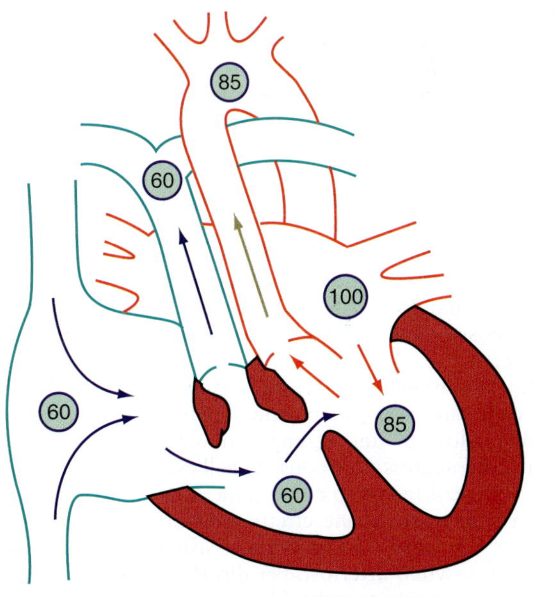

Figura 431-5. Fisiologia di una l-trasposizione, o trasposizione corretta delle grandi arterie (l-TGA) con un difetto del setto interventricolare e stenosi polmonare (VSD + PS). I *numeri cerchiati* rappresentano i valori di saturazione dell'ossigeno. La saturazione di ossigeno atriale destra (sangue venoso misto) è diminuita secondariamente all'ipossia sistemica. Il sangue dall'atrio destro fluisce attraverso la valvola mitrale nel ventricolo sinistro "invertito". Il ventricolo sinistro è, tuttavia, attaccato all'arteria polmonare trasposta. Perciò, nonostante le anomalie, il sangue desaturato viene sospinto nella circolazione polmonare. Il sangue saturo ritorna all'atrio sinistro, attraversa la valvola tricuspide fino a giungere nel ventricolo destro "invertito" e viene pompato nell'aorta trasposta. Questa circolazione sarebbe totalmente "corretta" se non fosse per la frequente associazione di altre anomalie congenite, in questo caso VSD + PS. A causa della valvola polmonare stenotica, parte del flusso sanguigno ventricolare sinistro attraversa il VSD e passa nel ventricolo destro e in aorta ascendente, con conseguente desaturazione sistemica.

sinistro (Fig. 431-5). Poiché è presente anche la trasposizione, il sangue desaturato espulso da questo ventricolo sinistro entra nell'arteria polmonare trasposta e fluisce nei polmoni. Il sangue venoso polmonare ossigenato ritorna da un atrio sinistro normalmente posizionato, passa attraverso una valvola atrioventricolare tricuspide in un ventricolo situato a sinistra che ha le caratteristiche morfologiche trabecolate di un ventricolo destro normale, e viene poi sospinto nell'aorta trasposta. La doppia inversione dei rapporti atrioventricolari e ventricoloarteriosi porta il sangue desaturato dell'atrio destro ai polmoni, mentre il sangue venoso ossigenato polmonare fluisce in modo corretto in aorta. La circolazione è fisiologicamente **"corretta"**. In assenza di altri difetti, le caratteristiche emodinamiche sarebbero quasi normali. Nella maggior parte dei pazienti, tuttavia, coesistono anomalie associate: VSD, anomalie tipo Ebstein della valvola atrioventricolare (tricuspide) situata a sinistra, stenosi polmonare valvolare o sottovalvolare (o entrambe) e disturbi della conduzione atrioventricolare (blocco cardiaco completo, vie di conduzione accessorie come la sindrome di Wolff-Parkinson-White).

MANIFESTAZIONI CLINICHE. I sintomi e i segni sono ampiamente variabili in quanto dipendono dalle lesioni associate. Se il flusso polmonare non è ostruito, i segni clinici sono simili a quelli di un VSD isolato; se invece la TGA è associata a stenosi polmonare e VSD, sono analoghi a quelli della tetralogia di Fallot.

DIAGNOSI. La radiografia del torace può indicare la posizione anomala delle grandi arterie; l'aorta ascendente occupa il margine sinistro della silhouette cardiaca e ha un profilo diritto. Oltre ai disturbi della conduzione atrioventricolare, l'elettrocardiogramma può evidenziare onde P anomale, onde Q assenti in V_6, onde Q presenti in modo anomalo nelle derivazioni III, aVR, aVF e V_1, onde T positive nelle derivazioni precordiali. L'ecocardiogramma è diagnostico. Le caratteristiche del ventricolo destro (banda moderatrice, trabecolatura più grossolana, valvola tricuspide situata più in basso rispetto alla valvola mitrale bicuspide, e un cono muscolare liscio o un infundibolo che separa la valvola atrioventricolare dalla valvola semilunare) permettono all'ecocardiografista di determinare la presenza della discordanza atrioventricolare (atrio destro connesso al ventricolo sinistro, atrio sinistro al ventricolo destro).

Il trattamento chirurgico delle anomalie associate (per lo più il VSD) è complicato dalla posizione del fascio di His, che può essere lesionato al momento dell'intervento e portare al blocco cardiaco. L'identificazione del decorso tipico del fascio nella trasposizione corretta (decorre superiormente al difetto) è stata ottenuta mappando il sistema di conduzione in modo tale che il chirurgo possa evitare il fascio di His durante la riparazione a cuore aperto.

Poiché la semplice correzione chirurgica lascia il ventricolo destro come camera di pompaggio sistemica e perciò soggetto allo sviluppo tardivo di uno scompenso ventricolare, l'approccio è diventato più aggressivo e consiste nell'eseguire interventi che lascino il ventricolo sinistro come camera di pompaggio sistemica. Questo risultato si ottiene effettuando un'operazione di switch atriale per dirottare i ritorni venosi sistemico e polmonare, seguita da uno switch arterioso per dirottare l'efflusso ventricolare (**procedura di doppio switch**). I benefici a lungo termine di questo approccio, volto a preservare la funzione ventricolare sistemica, non sono ancora noti.

431.5 • VENTRICOLO DESTRO A DOPPIA USCITA SENZA STENOSI DELLA POLMONARE

Nel ventricolo destro a doppia uscita senza stenosi della polmonare, tanto l'aorta quanto l'arteria polmonare originano dal ventricolo destro. L'unica uscita dal ventricolo sinistro è attraverso un VSD. Le manifestazioni cliniche simulano quelle di un VSD non complicato con un ampio shunt sinistro-destro, anche se può essere presente una lieve desaturazione sistemica a causa del mescolamento del sangue ossigenato e deossigenato nel ventricolo destro. L'elettrocardiogramma di solito evidenzia un'ipertrofia biventricolare. L'ecocardiografia è diagnostica ed evidenzia l'origine ventricolare destra di entrambi i grandi vasi e il loro rapporto anteroposteriore, come pure la posizione del VSD. Il cateterismo cardiaco rivela la prossimità del VSD all'aorta, che porta la maggior parte del sangue ventricolare sinistro a essere sospinto direttamente nella circolazione sistemica. L'angiogramma, oltre a confermare la mancanza di una continuità fibrosa mitroaortica, evidenzia come la valvola aortica sia spostata verso l'alto, venendosi a trovare allo stesso livello della valvola polmonare. È importante differenziare questa condizione da un VSD semplice.

La correzione chirurgica consiste nella creazione di un tunnel intracardiaco. Il sangue viene quindi pompato dal ventricolo sinistro in aorta attraverso il VSD. Nella prima infanzia può essere necessario il bendaggio dell'arteria polmonare, seguito dalla correzione chirurgica, da eseguirsi quando il bambino è più grande. Quando è presente una stenosi della polmonare, la cianosi è più marcata e il flusso sanguigno polmonare è diminuito (vedi Capitolo 430).

431.6 • VENTRICOLO DESTRO A DOPPIA USCITA CON TRASPOSIZIONE DELLE GRANDI ARTERIE (ANOMALIA DI TAUSSIG-BING)

Nel ventricolo destro a doppia uscita con TGA, il VSD è situato al di sopra della cresta sopraventricolare (VSD subarterioso) ed è sottopolmonare o in rapporto sia con la valvola polmonare sia con la valvola aortica (VSD con doppia relazione). I pazienti, che vanno incontro a scompenso cardiaco nella prima infanzia, sono a rischio di sviluppo di vasculopatia polmonare e cianosi. La cardiomegalia è comune, ed è udibile un soffio sistolico eiettivo parasternale, talvolta preceduto da un click da eiezione e da una chiusura rumorosa della valvola polmonare. Sono frequenti le lesioni ostruttive del cuore sinistro, compresi la coartazione aortica, l'interruzione dell'arco aortico e un VSD restrittivo, che ostacola l'eiezione ventricolare sinistra. L'elettrocardiogramma evidenzia una deviazione assiale destra e un'ipertrofia ventricolare destra, sinistra o biventricolare. La radiografia del torace mostra una cardiomegalia, un atrio sinistro grande e la sporgenza dell'arteria polmonare con aumento della vascolarizzazione polmonare. Il modo migliore per apprezzare le caratteristiche anatomiche dell'anomalia e le anomalie associate è una combinazione di ecocardiografia e ventricolografia selettiva destra e sinistra. La palliazione può essere ottenuta con il bendaggio dell'arteria polmonare nell'infanzia e con la correzione chirurgica a un'età maggiore, mediante procedura di Rastelli (vedi Capitolo 430) o switch arterioso (vedi Capitolo 431.2).

431.7 • RITORNO VENOSO POLMONARE ANOMALO TOTALE

FISIOPATOLOGIA. L'anomalo sviluppo delle vene polmonari può portare a un drenaggio anomalo, parziale o completo, nella circolazione venosa sistemica. Il ritorno venoso polmonare anomalo parziale di solito non è associato a cianosi (vedi Capitolo 426.4), al contrario del ritorno venoso polmonare anomalo totale (TAPVR, *Total Anomalous Pulmonary Venous Return*), che permette il mescolamento completo del flusso sanguigno sistemico e polmonare nel cuore.

Nel TAPVR, il cuore non ha una connessione venosa polmonare diretta con l'atrio sinistro. Le vene polmonari possono drenare il sangue al di sopra del diaframma direttamente nell'atrio destro, nel seno coronario o nella vena cava superiore attraverso una "vena verticale" o possono drenarlo al di sotto del diaframma e unirsi a una "vena discendente" che entra nella vena cava inferiore o in una delle sue maggiori tributarie, spesso attraverso il dotto venoso. Quest'ultima forma di drenaggio venoso anomalo è più comunemente associata a ostruzione, di solito quando il dotto venoso si chiude poco dopo la nascita, anche se le vene sopracardiache anomale possono andare incontro anche a ostruzione. Talvolta il drenaggio è misto, con alcune vene che drenano al di sopra e altre al di sotto del diaframma.

Tutte le forme di TAPVR consistono in un mescolamento di sangue ossigenato e deossigenato prima dell'atrio destro o a questo livello (lesioni con mescolamento totale). Il sangue dall'atrio destro passa nel ventricolo destro e in arteria polmonare, oppure fa ingresso nell'atrio sinistro attraverso un difetto settale atriale (ASD) o un forame ovale pervio. L'atrio destro, il ventricolo destro e l'arteria polmonare sono generalmente ingranditi, mentre l'atrio e il ventricolo di sinistra possono essere normali o di piccole dimensioni. Le manifestazioni del TAPVR dipendono dalla presenza o dall'assenza di ostruzione dei canali venosi (Tab. 431-1). Se il ritorno venoso polmonare è ostruito, si sviluppano una grave congestione polmonare e un'ipertensione polmonare; in assenza di intervento chirurgico si assiste a un rapido deterioramento del quadro. Il TAPVR rappresenta un'emergenza cardiochirurgica pediatrica poiché la terapia con prostaglandina di solito non è efficace.

MANIFESTAZIONI CLINICHE. Si osservano tre principali pattern clinici di TAVPR. Alcuni si manifestano nel periodo neonatale come grave ostruzione al ritorno venoso polmonare, con una particolare prevalenza nel gruppo infracardiaco (vedi Tab. 431-1). Si riscontrano cianosi e un'importante tachicardia, ma possono non essere presenti soffi. I bambini sono gravemente sofferenti e non rispondono alla ventilazione meccanica. Una diagnosi e una correzione chirurgica rapide sono necessarie per la sopravvivenza. Un altro gruppo è caratterizzato da scompenso cardiaco nelle prime fasi di vita, con ostruzione solo lieve o moderata al ritorno venoso polmonare e un ampio shunt sinistro-destro. Poiché è presente un'ipertensione arteriosa polmonare, questi bambini sono gravemente sofferenti. Sono udibili soffi sistolici lungo il margine sternale sinistro e può essere presente un ritmo di galoppo. Talvolta si apprezza un soffio continuo lungo il margine sternale superiore sinistro sul focolaio della polmonare. La cianosi è lieve. Il terzo gruppo è formato dai bambini con TAVPR, in cui si osserva un mescolamento totale di sangue venoso sistemico e venoso polmonare e un ampio shunt sinistro-destro, in assenza di un'ostruzione venosa polmonare. L'ipertensione polmonare è assente e questi pazienti sono meno inclini a sviluppare sintomi durante l'infanzia. La cianosi clinicamente evidente è di solito lieve.

TABELLA 431-1. Ritorno venoso polmonare anomalo

% E SEDE DELLA CONNESSIONE	% CON OSTRUZIONE GRAVE
Sopracardiaca (50)	
Vena cava superiore sinistra (40)	40
Vena casa superiore destra (10)	75
Cardiaca (25)	
Seno coronario (20)	10
Atrio destro (5)	5
Infracardiaca (20)	95-100
Mista (5)	

DIAGNOSI. L'elettrocardiogramma evidenzia un'ipertrofia ventricolare destra (di solito un pattern qR in V_3R e V_1; le onde P sono spesso alte e appuntite). I radiogrammi del torace sono patognomonici nei bambini più grandi se le vene polmonari anomale entrano nella vena anonima e nella vena cava superiore sinistra persistente (Fig. 431-6). Può notarsi un'ampia ombra sovracardiaca, che insieme alla normale ombra cardiaca forma un aspetto a "**pupazzo di neve**". Questo reperto non è utile per la diagnosi nella prima infanzia a causa del timo. Nella maggior parte dei casi senza ostruzione, il cuore è ingrandito, l'arteria polmonare e il ventricolo destro sono sporgenti e la vascolarizzazione polmonare è aumentata. In neonati con marcata ostruzione venosa polmonare, la radiografia del torace evidenzia un pattern peri-ilare di edema polmonare e un cuore piccolo, aspetto che può essere confuso con una patologia polmonare primitiva. La diagnosi differenziale comprende l'ipertensione polmonare persistente del neonato, la sindrome da distress respiratorio, la polmonite batterica, l'inalazione di meconio, la linfangectasia polmonare e altri difetti cardiaci (sindrome del cuore sinistro ipoplasico).

L'ecocardiogramma evidenzia un ventricolo destro grande e di solito identifica il pattern delle connessioni venose polmonari anomale (Fig. 431-7). La dimostrazione in addome di un vaso con il flusso venoso, evidenziato con metodica Doppler, che si allontana dal cuore è patognomonico di TAVPR al di sotto del diaframma. Lo shunt si verifica quasi esclusivamente da destra a sinistra a livello atriale.

Il cateterismo cardiaco evidenzia che la saturazione di ossigeno in entrambi gli atri, in entrambi i ventricoli e in aorta è più o meno simile, indicativa di una lesione con mescolamento totale. Un aumento nella saturazione venosa sistemica si verifica nel punto di entrata dei canali venosi polmonari anomali. Nei pazienti più

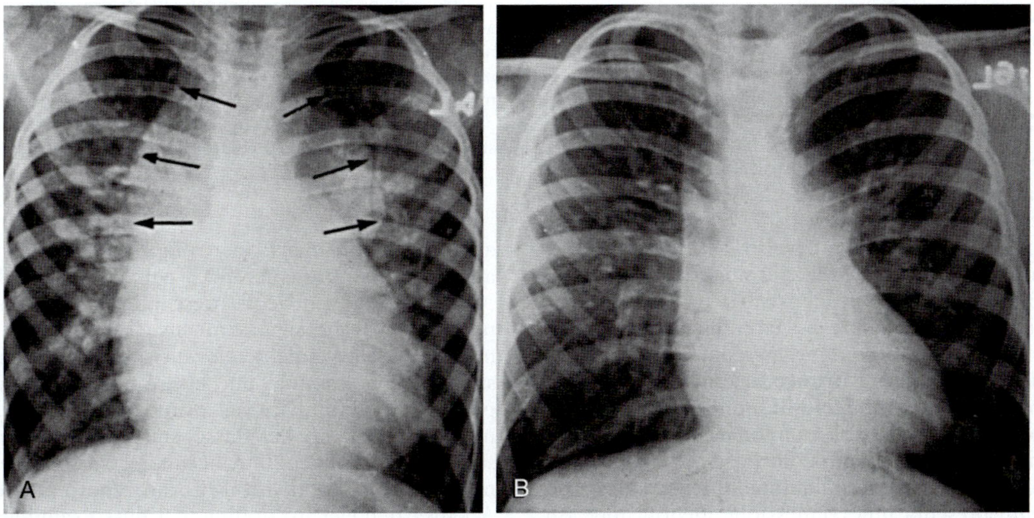

Figura 431-6. Radiografia del torace di un ritorno venoso polmonare anomalo totale alla vena cava superiore. *A*, Immagine preoperatoria. Le frecce indicano l'ombra sopracardiaca, che produce la figura a pupazzo di neve o la configurazione a 8. Sono evidenti la cardiomegalia e l'aumentata vascolarizzazione polmonare. *B*, Immagine postoperatoria che evidenzia la diminuzione di dimensione del cuore e dell'ombra sopracardiaca.

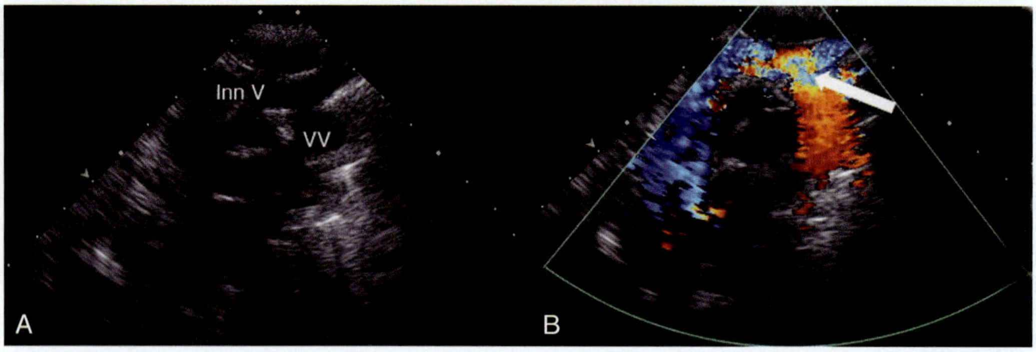

Figura 431-7. Proiezioni ecocardiografiche bidimensionali soprasternali che evidenziano un ritorno venoso polmonare anomalo totale sopracardiaco (tipo I). *A*, Si può notare l'ampia vena ascendente verticale che entra nella vena anonima. Vi è un moderato restringimento nel punto in cui la vena anonima entra nel sistema venoso della parte superiore del corpo. *B*, L'esame color-Doppler evidenzia un segnale di flusso venoso (*colore rosso*) indicando che il sangue si sta allontanando dal trasduttore e quindi dal cuore (tutto il flusso venoso dovrebbe normalmente tornare verso il cuore), aspetto diagnostico di un ritorno venoso polmonare anomalo. Si noti l'accelerazione turbolenta di flusso nel punto in cui la vena verticale entra nella vena anonima (*freccia*). Inn V, vena anonima; VV, vena verticale.

grandi, la pressione arteriosa polmonare e la pressione in ventricolo destro possono essere solo moderatamente elevate, ma nei bambini con ostruzione venosa polmonare di solito vi è ipertensione polmonare. L'arteriografia polmonare selettiva evidenzia l'anatomia delle vene polmonari e il loro punto di ingresso nella circolazione venosa sistemica. La RM e la TC possono essere metodi alternativi per confermare la diagnosi.

TRATTAMENTO. La correzione chirurgica di un TAPVR è indicata durante l'infanzia. Prima dell'intervento chirurgico si può stabilizzare il bambino con prostaglandina E_1 per dilatare il dotto venoso e il dotto arterioso, anche se in presenza di un'ostruzione significativa questa terapia non è di solito efficace. Se non è possibile effettuare l'intervento chirurgico in urgenza, può essere richiesta un'ossigenazione con membrana extracorporea (ECMO, *ExtraCorporeal Membrane Oxygenation*) per mantenere l'ossigenazione. Dal punto di vista chirurgico, si anastomizza il tronco venoso polmonare comune direttamente all'atrio sinistro, si chiude l'ASD e si interrompe la connessione al circuito venoso sistemico. I risultati a breve termine sono generalmente buoni, anche nei neonati critici. Il periodo postoperatorio può essere complicato da crisi ipertensive vascolari polmonari. In alcuni pazienti, specialmente in quelli in cui la diagnosi è stata ritardata o l'ostruzione era grave, può verificarsi una stenosi recidivante o una malattia veno-occlusiva polmonare. Sono stati effettuati tentativi di trattare le stenosi ricorrenti con la chirurgica, l'angioplastica con palloncino, stent e chemioterapia antiproliferativa. Al momento, la prognosi a lungo termine in questi pazienti è infausta, e il **trapianto cuore-polmone** rappresenta l'unica opzione (vedi Capitolo 443.2).

431.8 • Tronco arterioso comune

FISIOPATOLOGIA. Nel tronco arterioso comune, un singolo tronco arterioso (il "truncus") che origina dal cuore rifornisce le circolazioni sistemica, polmonare e coronarica. È sempre presente un VSD, con il truncus che è posto a cavallo del difetto e riceve sangue sia dal ventricolo destro sia da quello sinistro (Fig. 431-8). Il numero di cuspidi valvolari del truncus varia da due a sei. Le arterie polmonari possono originare assieme dal lato posteriore sinistro del tronco arterioso comune, per poi dividersi nelle arterie polmonari sinistra e destra (**tronco arterioso tipo I**). Nel tronco arterioso persistente **tipo II** e **tipo III**, non è presente un'arteria polmonare principale, e le arterie polmonari destra e sinistra originano da orifizi separati nelle porzioni posteriore (**tipo II**) o laterale (**tipo III**) del tronco arterioso comune. Il tronco arterioso comune **tipo IV** non presenta una connessione identificabile tra il cuore e le arterie polmonari, e il flusso sanguigno polmonare deriva dalle principali arterie collaterali aortopolmonari che originano dall'aorta traversa o discendente; questa forma, chiamata

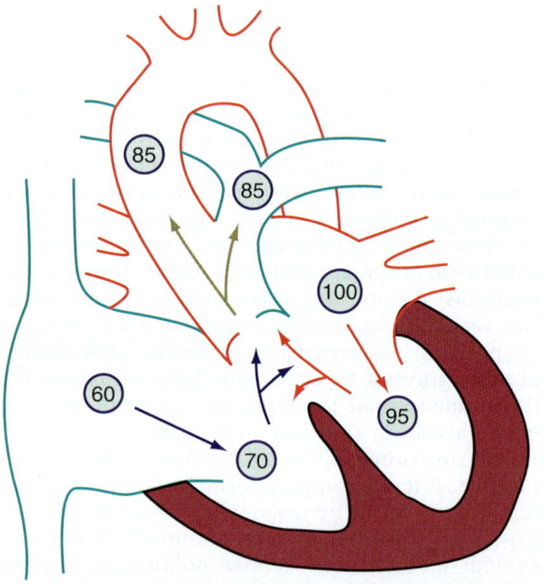

Figura 431-8. Fisiologia di un tronco arterioso comune. I *numeri cerchiati* rappresentano i valori di saturazione dell'ossigeno. La saturazione dell'ossigeno in atrio destro (sangue venoso misto) diminuisce secondariamente all'ipossia sistemica. Il sangue desaturato entra nell'atrio destro, fluisce attraverso la valvola tricuspide nel ventricolo destro e viene sospinto nel tronco arterioso comune. Il sangue saturo che ritorna dall'atrio sinistro entra nel ventricolo sinistro e viene anch'esso pompato nel tronco arterioso comune. Il tronco aortopolmonare comune dà origine all'aorta ascendente e all'arteria polmonare principale o alle sue diramazioni. La saturazione di ossigeno è di solito uguale nell'aorta e nelle arterie polmonari (definizione di una lesione con mescolamento totale). Se la resistenza vascolare polmonare diminuisce nelle prime settimane di vita, anche il flusso sanguigno polmonare diminuisce drasticamente, dando luogo a cianosi lieve e scompenso cardiaco.

anche pseudotruncus, in realtà è essenzialmente una forma di atresia polmonare con VSD (vedi Capitolo 430.2).

Entrambi i ventricoli presentano una pressione sistemica e pompano il sangue nel truncus. Se la resistenza vascolare polmonare è relativamente elevata subito dopo la nascita, il flusso sanguigno polmonare può essere normale; se però la resistenza polmonare diminuisce nel primo mese di vita, ne consegue un notevole aumento del flusso ematico ai polmoni e subentra lo scompenso cardiaco. Il tronco arterioso comune è una lesione con mescolamento totale tra il ritorno venoso polmonare e sistemico. A causa dell'elevato volume del flusso sanguigno polmonare, la cianosi clinica è di solito minima. Se la lesione non viene trattata, la resistenza polmonare alla fine aumenta, il flusso sanguigno polmonare diminuisce e la cianosi diventa più evidente (fenomeno di Eisenmenger, vedi Capitolo 433.2). La valvola del truncus è talvolta incompetente, il che complica significativamente la gestione medica e chirurgica.

MANIFESTAZIONI CLINICHE. I segni clinici del tronco arterioso comune variano con l'età e dipendono dal livello della resistenza vascolare polmonare. Nel primissimo periodo dopo la nascita i segni di scompenso cardiaco sono di solito assenti; un soffio e una cianosi minima rappresentano i segni iniziali. Nei bambini più grandi, il flusso sanguigno polmonare è torrenziale e il quadro clinico è dominato dallo scompenso cardiaco. La cianosi è minima. Il flusso di sangue che esce dal truncus per entrare nella circolazione polmonare può portare a un'ampia pressione differenziale e a polsi scoccanti. Questi reperti possono essere ulteriormente accentuati da un'insufficienza valvolare truncale. Il cuore è di solito ingrandito, e il precordio è iperdinamico. Il secondo tono cardiaco è forte e unico. È generalmente udibile un soffio sistolico da eiezione, talora accompagnato da un fremito, lungo il margine sternale sinistro. Il soffio è frequentemente preceduto da un precoce click da eiezione sistolica. In presenza di un'insufficienza valvolare truncale, si ode un soffio a elevata tonalità, protodiastolico in decrescendo, a livello del margine mediosternale sinistro. Un soffio rullante apicale mediodiastolico, causato da un aumentato flusso attraverso la valvola mitrale, è apprezzabile con la campana dello stetoscopio. Nei bambini più grandi con restrizione al flusso sanguigno polmonare secondaria a una patologia vascolare polmonare ostruttiva, si sviluppano cianosi progressiva, policitemia e ippocratismo digitale. Il tronco arterioso comune, una malformazione conotruncale, può essere associato alla **sindrome di DiGeorge**, che è stata correlata a una delezione del cromosoma 22q11.

DIAGNOSI. L'elettrocardiogramma evidenzia un'ipertrofia ventricolare destra, sinistra o combinata. La radiografia del torace presenta anch'essa considerevoli variazioni. L'ingrandimento cardiaco è dovuto a prominenza di entrambi i ventricoli. Il tronco comune può produrre un'ombra sporgente che segue il normale decorso dell'aorta ascendente e il bottone aortico; l'arco aortico è a destra nel 50% dei pazienti. Talvolta una notevole sporgenza a sinistra del bottone aortico è prodotta dall'arteria polmonare principale o dall'arteria polmonare sinistra. La vascolarizzazione polmonare è aumentata dopo le prime settimane di vita. L'ecocardiografia evidenzia l'ampia arteria del truncus posta a cavallo del VSD e il pattern di origine delle diramazioni delle arterie polmonari (Fig. 431-9). Si possono notare anomalie associate come un arco aortico interrotto. Si ricorre a studi con il Doppler pulsato e il colorDoppler per valutare il rigurgito valvolare truncale. Se richiesto, il cateterismo cardiaco rivela uno shunt sinistro-destro a livello ventricolare, con uno shunt destro-sinistro nel truncus. La pressione sistolica in entrambi i ventricoli e nel truncus è simile. L'angiografia evidenzia l'ampio tronco arterioso comune e definisce con maggior precisione l'origine delle arterie polmonari.

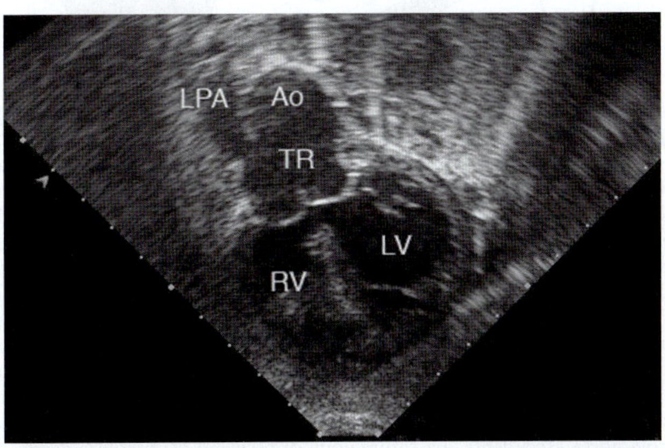

Figura 431-9. Dimostrazione mediante ecocardiogramma bidimensionale sottocostale di un tronco arterioso comune. L'ampia valvola truncale si può notare a cavallo del difetto settale ventricolare. In questo caso, solo l'arteria polmonare sinistra (LPA, *Left Pulmonary Artery*) origina dal tronco comune (TR). Le arterie polmonari sono discontinue e l'arteria polmonare destra origina dall'aorta discendente attraverso il dotto arterioso (non mostrato). Ao, Aorta; LV (*Left Ventricle*), ventricolo sinistro; RV (*Right Ventricle*), ventricolo destro.

PROGNOSI E COMPLICANZE. Se non sottoposti a intervento chirurgico, molti di questi pazienti muoiono durante l'infanzia o entro il primo o il secondo anno di vita. Se il flusso sanguigno polmonare è limitato dall'insorgenza di una malattia vascolare polmonare, il paziente può sopravvivere fino all'inizio dell'età adulta. I risultati della chirurgia sono stati molto buoni, e molti sono i pazienti sottoposti a riparazione del tronco arterioso comune che stanno raggiungendo l'età adulta. Quando il tronco arterioso comune è associato alla sindrome di DiGeorge, le conseguenti anomalie endocrinologiche, immunologiche, facciali e polmonari possono complicare il recupero.

TRATTAMENTO. Nelle prime settimane di vita, molti di questi bambini possono essere trattati con diuretici; quando la resistenza vascolare polmonare diminuisce, i sintomi di scompenso cardiaco peggiorano ed è indicato l'intervento chirurgico, di solito nelle settimane seguenti. Ritardarlo oltre le 4-8 settimane aumenta la probabilità che si instauri una malattia vascolare polmonare; in alcuni centri si raccomanda di eseguire la riparazione nel periodo neonatale, al momento della diagnosi. All'atto dell'intervento chirurgico, viene chiuso il VSD, le arterie polmonari sono separate dal tronco arterioso comune e viene stabilita una continuità tra il ventricolo destro e le arterie polmonari con un condotto omograft (**riparazione di Rastelli**). I risultati nell'immediato sono eccellenti, ma dopo la riparazione il condotto deve essere sostituito, spesso più volte, a mano a mano che il bambino cresce. Nei pazienti più grandi che hanno già un'ostruzione vascolare polmonare, il trattamento chirurgico di routine è controindicato e il **trapianto cuore-polmone** è l'unica opzione.

431.9 • VENTRICOLO UNICO (VENTRICOLO A DOPPIA ENTRATA, CUORE MONOVENTRICOLARE)

FISIOPATOLOGIA. In presenza di un ventricolo unico, entrambi gli atri si svuotano attraverso una valvola atrioventricolare comune o attraverso due valvole separate in un'unica camera ventricolare, con un mescolamento totale del ritorno venoso sistemico e polmonare. Questa camera può avere caratteristiche anatomiche di un ventricolo sinistro, destro o indeterminate. L'aorta e l'arteria polmonare originano entrambe da quest'unica camera, anche se uno dei grandi vasi può originare da una camera di efflusso rudimentale. L'aorta può essere posteriore, anteriore (malposizione) o affiancata all'arteria polmonare, a destra o a sinistra. La stenosi o l'atresia della polmonare sono comuni.

MANIFESTAZIONI CLINICHE. Il quadro clinico è variabile e dipende dalle anomalie intracardiache associate. Se l'efflusso polmonare è ostruito, i reperti possono essere simili a quelli della tetralogia di Fallot: cianosi marcata senza scompenso cardiaco. Se l'efflusso polmonare non è ostruito, i reperti sono gli stessi della trasposizione con VSD: minima cianosi con marcato scompenso cardiaco.

In pazienti con stenosi della polmonare, la cianosi è presente nei primi anni di vita e aumenta d'intensità durante l'infanzia, quando compaiono ippocratismo digitale e policitemia. La dispnea e l'astenia sono frequenti, la cardiomegalia è lieve o moderata, è palpabile un sollevamento parasternale sinistro ed è comune un fremito sistolico. Il soffio sistolico da eiezione è di solito forte; può essere udibile un click da eiezione, e il secondo tono cardiaco è unico e forte.

I pazienti con efflusso polmonare non ostruito hanno un flusso sanguigno polmonare torrenziale e si presentano all'attenzione del medico nella prima infanzia con tachipnea, dispnea, ritardo di crescita e infezioni polmonari ricorrenti. La cianosi è solito lieve o moderata. La cardiomegalia è generalmente marcata ed è palpabile un sollevamento parasternale sinistro. Il soffio sistolico da eiezione di solito non è intenso; il secondo tono cardiaco è forte e strettamente sdoppiato. È comune un terzo tono cardiaco, che può essere seguito da un breve soffio rullante mesodiastolico, causato da un aumento del flusso attraverso le valvole atrioventricolari. Alla fine lo sviluppo di una patologia vascolare polmonare riduce il flusso sanguigno polmonare cosicché la cianosi aumenta e i segni di scompenso cardiaco sembrano migliorare (fenomeno di Eisenmenger; vedi Capitolo 433.2).

DIAGNOSI. I reperti all'elettrocardiogramma sono aspecifici. Le onde P sono normali, appuntite o bifide. Il pattern delle derivazioni precordiali suggerisce un'ipertrofia ventricolare destra, un'ipertrofia ventricolare combinata o a volte una dominanza ventricolare sinistra. Le forze iniziali del QRS sono di solito dirette a sinistra e anteriormente. L'esame radiografico conferma il grado di cardiomegalia. Se presente, una rudimentale camera di efflusso può produrre una bozza sul margine superiore sinistro della silhouette cardiaca in proiezione posteroanteriore. In assenza di stenosi della polmonare, la vascolarizzazione polmonare è aumentata, mentre in presenza di stenosi della polmonare, la vascolarizzazione polmonare è diminuita. L'assenza o la quasi assenza di un setto ventricolare è il principale segno ecocardiografico. L'ecocardiogramma può di solito determinare se il ventricolo unico ha caratteristiche di ventricolo destro, sinistro o miste. Può essere identificata la presenza di un rudimentale camera di efflusso al di sotto di uno dei grandi vasi e il Doppler pulsati può essere utilizzato per determinare se il flusso attraverso questa comunicazione (forame bulboventricolare) è ostruito.

Se viene effettuato un cateterismo cardiaco, si vede come la saturazione di ossigeno sia diminuita in presenza di grave stenosi della polmonare o di un'ipertensione polmonare ostruttiva, ma può essere quasi normale quando il flusso sanguigno polmonare non è ostacolato. La pressione nella camera ventricolare è a livelli sistemici; può essere dimostrato un gradiente attraverso l'entrata della rudimentale camera di efflusso. Le misure della pressione e l'angiografia dimostrano se sia presente o meno una stenosi della polmonare. Una grave ipertensione polmonare può essere dimostrata in pazienti più grandi in assenza di stenosi della polmonare.

PROGNOSI E COMPLICANZE. In assenza di intervento chirurgico, alcuni pazienti muoiono durante l'infanzia per scompenso cardiaco; altri sopravvivono fino all'adolescenza e all'inizio dell'età adulta, ma infine muoiono per gli effetti dell'ipossiemia cronica o, in assenza di stenosi della polmonare, per gli effetti della malattia vascolare polmonare. I pazienti con stenosi polmonare moderata hanno la prognosi migliore poiché il flusso sanguigno polmonare, sebbene ostacolato, è ancora adeguato.

TRATTAMENTO. Se la stenosi della polmonare è grave, è indicato uno **shunt aortopolmonare di Blalock-Taussig** (vedi Capitolo 430.1). Se il flusso sanguigno polmonare non è ostruito, si ricorre al bendaggio dell'arteria polmonare per controllare lo scompenso cardiaco e prevenire una vasculopatia polmonare progressiva. Lo **shunt bidirezionale di Glenn**, seguito da **intervento di Fontan modificato** (procedura di isolamento cavopolmonare, vedi Capitolo 430.4), è l'ultimo trattamento di scelta. In presenza di una stenosi subaortica causata da una connessione restrittiva con una camera di efflusso rudimentale, può essere fornito sollievo chirurgicamente effettuando un'anastomosi dell'arteria polmonare prossimale con un lato dell'aorta ascendente (**operazione di Damus-Stansyl Kaye**).

431.10 • Sindrome del cuore sinistro ipoplasico

FISIOPATOLOGIA. Con l'espressione "cuore sinistro ipoplasico" si indica un gruppo di anomalie correlate consistenti nell'iposviluppo della parte sinistra del cuore (atresia dell'orifizio aortico o mitralico) e nell'ipoplasia dell'aorta ascendente. Il ventricolo sinistro può essere piccolo e non funzionale o totalmente atresico; quello destro mantiene sia la circolazione polmonare sia quella sistemica (Fig. 431-10). Il sangue venoso polmonare passa attraverso un difetto atriale o un forame ovale dilatato dalla parte sinistra del cuore a quella destra, dove si mescola con il sangue venoso sistemico (**lesione con mescolamento totale**). Quando il setto ventricolare è intatto, cosa che si verifica di solito, tutto il sangue ventricolare destro viene spinto nel tronco comune dell'arteria polmonare, mentre l'aorta discendente è rifornita attraverso il dotto arterioso, e il flusso di sangue dal dotto riempie anche l'aorta ascendente e le arterie coronarie in modo retrogrado. In presenza di un VSD e di un orifizio aortico pervio ma piccolo il sangue ventricolare destro viene spinto nel ventricolo sinistro piccolo e in aorta ascendente, oltre che in arteria polmonare. Le principali anomalie emodinamiche sono un inadeguato mantenimento della circolazione sistemica e, a seconda dell'entità della comunicazione a livello atriale, un'ipertensione venosa polmonare (forame ovale restrittivo) o un'ipercircolazione polmonare (ASD moderato o grande).

MANIFESTAZIONI CLINICHE. Anche se la cianosi può non essere sempre palese nelle prime 48 ore di vita, è precocemente evidente un colorito cutaneo blu-cinereo che denota un misto di cianosi e scarsa perfusione. Nella maggior parte dei bambini la condizione

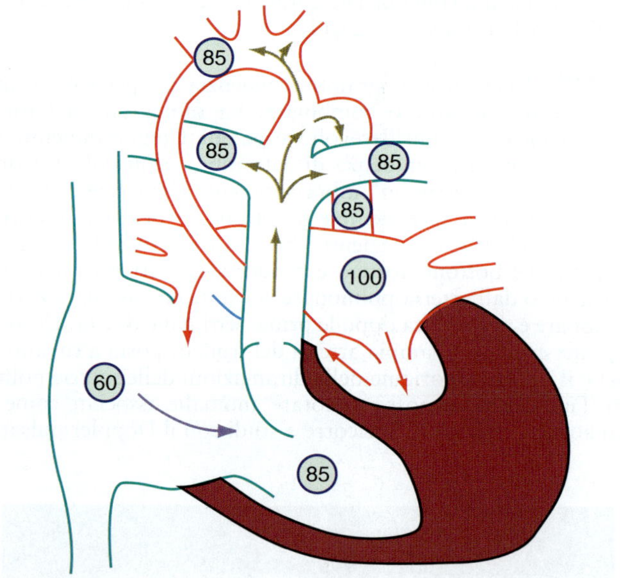

Figura 431-10. Fisiologia della sindrome del cuore sinistro ipoplasico (HLHS, *Hypoplastic Left Heart Syndrome*). I *numeri cerchiati* rappresentano i valori di saturazione dell'ossigeno. L'HLHS non è una lesione singola, ma una costellazione di diversi gradi di ipoplasia delle strutture del cuore sinistro. Questo disegno evidenzia una valvola mitrale pervia, una cavità ventricolare sinistra piccola e un'aorta ascendente di dimensioni inferiori alla norma. La saturazione di ossigeno in atrio destro (sangue venoso misto) è diminuita a causa dell'ipossia sistemica. Il sangue desaturato entra nell'atrio destro, fluisce attraverso la valvola tricuspide nel ventricolo destro e viene sospinto in arteria polmonare. A causa della compliance marcatamente ridotta del ventricolo sinistro, la maggior parte del sangue venoso polmonare che ritorna all'atrio sinistro viene deviato da sinistra a destra a livello atriale. Una piccola quantità di sangue atriale sinistro attraverserà la valvola mitrale e sarà pompato nella piccola aorta ascendente. La saturazione di ossigeno ventricolare destra rappresenta un mescolamento di sangue venoso sistemico desaturato e di sangue venoso polmonare saturo. Il sangue arterioso polmonare fluisce nelle arterie polmonari, come anche da destra a sinistra, attraverso il dotto arterioso pervio (PDA, *Patent Ductus Arteriosus*) in aorta. Il sangue duttale fluisce in modo anterogrado all'aorta discendente come anche in modo retrogrado all'aorta ascendente, dove rifornisce i vasi di testa e collo oltre alle arterie coronarie (che originano dalla piccola aorta ascendente). La chiusura del PDA porta a una grave ipossia e al collasso circolatorio.

viene diagnosticata nelle prime ore o nei primi giorni di vita. Se il dotto arterioso si chiude parzialmente, predominano i segni di ipoperfusione sistemica e shock. I segni di scompenso cardiaco, che di solito compaiono nei primi giorni o settimane di vita, comprendono dispnea, epatomegalia e bassa gittata cardiaca. Tutti i polsi periferici possono essere deboli o assenti. L'ingrandimento cardiaco è comune, con un sollevamento parasternale ventricolare destro palpabile. È generalmente udibile un soffio sistolico non caratteristico. Possono essere presenti anomalie extracardiache, in particolare a carico dei reni e del sistema nervoso centrale.

DIAGNOSI. Alla radiografia del torace, il cuore è di dimensione variabile nei primi giorni di vita, ma si sviluppa rapidamente una cardiomegalia associata a un'aumentata vascolarizzazione polmonare. L'elettrocardiogramma inizialmente può evidenziare solo la normale dominanza destra con bassi voltaggi ventricolari, ma in seguito le onde P diventano prominenti ed è comune l'ipertrofia ventricolare destra. L'ecocardiogramma, che è diagnostico, evidenzia l'assenza o l'ipoplasia della valvola mitrale e della radice aortica, un atrio e ventricolo sinistro piccoli in misura variabile e un atrio destro e un ventricolo destro di grandi dimensioni (Fig. 431-11). L'entità della comunicazione atriale, attraverso cui il sangue venoso polmonare lascia l'atrio sinistro, può essere valutata direttamente e mediante il Doppler pulsato e il color flow. La proiezione soprasternale identifica la piccola aorta ascendente e il piccolo arco aortico traverso, oltre a poter evidenziare una discreta coartazione dell'aorta nell'area iuxtaduttale. L'ecocardiografia Doppler evidenzia l'assenza di flusso anterogrado nell'aorta ascendente, che è rifornita dal flusso retrogrado attraverso il dotto arterioso. La diagnosi di sindrome del cuore sinistro ipoplasico può essere formulata di solito senza il cateterismo cardiaco. Qualora però quest'ultimo si rendesse necessario, l'aorta ascendente ipoplasica può essere evidenziata con l'angiografia.

PROGNOSI E COMPLICANZE. I pazienti non trattati nella maggior parte dei casi muoiono durante i primi mesi di vita, di solito già nella 1ª-2ª settimana. I pazienti non operati sopravvivono talvolta per mesi o, raramente, per anni. Un terzo dei bambini con sindrome del cuore sinistro ipoplasico presenta segni di un'anomalia maggiore o minore del sistema nervoso centrale. Altre caratteristiche dismorfiche si riscontrano in una percentuale di pazienti che può raggiungere il 40%. Perciò, si dovrebbe effettuare un'attenta valutazione preoperatoria (genetica, neurologica e oculistica) nei candidati alla terapia chirurgica standard o al trapianto cardiaco.

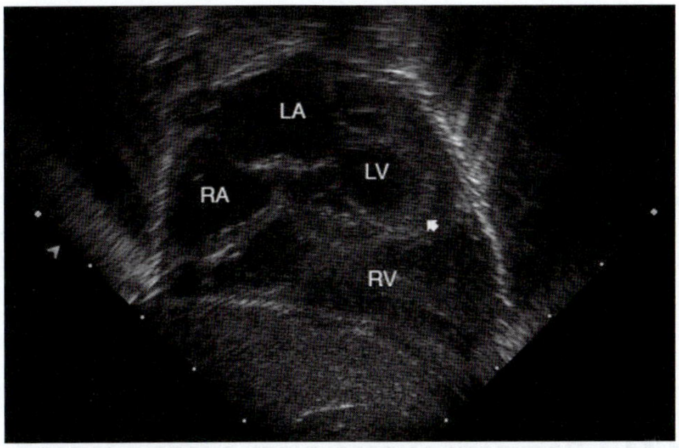

Figura 431-11. Diagnosi mediante ecocardiogramma bidimensionale sottocostale della sindrome del cuore sinistro ipoplasico. Si può vedere la piccola camera ventricolare sinistra, il cui apice (*punta di freccia*) non forma l'apice del cuore. Si noti che il setto atriale si piega da sinistra a destra, indicando che la comunicazione tra i due atri è restrittiva quanto a pressione. LA (*Left Atrium*), atrio sinistro; LV (*Left Ventricle*), ventricolo sinistro; RA (*Right Atrium*), atrio destro; RV (*Right Ventricle*), ventricolo destro.

TRATTAMENTO. La terapia chirurgica per la sindrome del cuore sinistro ipoplasico è stata associata a tassi di sopravvivenza che raggiungono il 95% per la palliazione di primo livello in molti centri. Le opzioni di trattamento comprendono la **procedura di Norwood** (Fig. 431-12) o la **procedura di Sano**, che è simile alla prima, con la differenza che, invece di utilizzare uno shunt di Blalock-Taussig per fornire un flusso sanguigno polmonare, il chirurgo inserisce un omograft che collega il ventricolo destro all'arteria polmonare, essenzialmente creando un ventricolo destro a doppia uscita. Il trapianto cardiaco primario, in precedenza sostenuto da numerosi centri, è ora meno comune, dal momento che le percentuali di sopravvivenza dopo chirurgia tradizionale sono sostanzialmente migliorate.

Se occorre effettuare una procedura di Norwood o di Sano, il trattamento medico preoperatorio comprende la correzione dell'acidosi e dell'ipoglicemia, il mantenimento della pervietà del dotto con prostaglandina E_1 (0,01-0,20 μg/kg/min) per supportare il flusso sanguigno sistemico, e la prevenzione dell'ipotermia. Il trattamento preoperatorio dovrebbe evitare un eccessivo flusso sanguigno polmonare, e spesso i pazienti sono trattati in aria ambiente con una FIO_2 del 18% con azoto gassoso miscelato nella sorgente di ossigeno. La dilatazione con palloncino del setto atriale può essere indicata se l'intervento chirurgico viene rimandato.

La procedura di Norwood si articola di solito in tre stadi. Lo **stadio I** (vedi Fig. 431-12) consiste in una settostomia atriale con transezione e legatura della porzione distale del tronco principale dell'arteria polmonare; in seguito, la porzione prossimale dell'arteria polmonare viene connessa all'arco aortico ipoplasico, aperta trasversalmente a formare una neoaorta, e il segmento coartato dell'aorta viene riparato. Uno shunt aortopolmonare sintetico connette l'aorta all'arteria polmonare principale per fornire un flusso sanguigno polmonare controllato. Nella modifica di Sano, si utilizza un omograft tra il ventricolo destro e l'arteria polmonare per assicurare il flusso sanguigno polmonare, creando temporaneamente un ventricolo destro a doppia uscita. Il rischio operatorio per queste procedure di stadio I si è notevolmente ridotto nei due decenni passati, e i migliori risultati evidenziano una percentuale di sopravvivenza del 90-95%.

Lo **stadio II** consiste in un'anastomosi di Glenn, eseguita per connettere la vena cava inferiore alle arterie polmonari attraverso un diaframma intra-atriale o esterno. Dopo lo **stadio III**, tutto il ritorno venoso sistemico entra direttamente nella circolazione polmonare. Il flusso venoso polmonare, una volta entrato nell'atrio sinistro, viene diretto attraverso il setto atriale alla valvola tricuspide e successivamente al ventricolo destro (ora sistemico). Il sangue lascia il ventricolo destro attraverso la neoaorta, che alimenta la circolazione sistemica. La vecchia radice aortica ora attaccata alla neoaorta fornisce il flusso sanguigno coronarico. Il rischio associato agli stadi II e III è addirittura inferiore a quello dello stadio I; i risultati a lungo termine delle procedure di Norwood e di Sano restano da dimostrare.

Una terapia alternativa è il **trapianto cardiaco**, eseguito nell'immediato periodo dopo la nascita, evitando pertanto lo stadio I della procedura di Norwood, o dopo uno stadio I della procedura di Norwood condotto a termine con successo come ponte verso il trapianto. Dopo il trapianto, i pazienti di solito presentano una funzione cardiaca normale, senza sintomi di scompenso cardiaco, ma in compenso hanno un rischio cronico di rigetto d'organo e di una terapia immunosoppressiva per tutta la vita (vedi Capitolo 443.1). La carenza di donatori e i risultati sempre migliori ottenibili con le procedure chirurgiche standard hanno fatto sì che molti centri non raccomandino più il trapianto, se non nei casi in cui le lesioni associate rendano la procedura di Norwood una procedura a rischio eccezionalmente elevato.

PREVENZIONE. Studi ecocardiografici fetali seriati evidenziano come in alcuni feti la sindrome del cuore sinistro ipoplasico possa essere una lesione progressiva, che inizia con una semplice stenosi valvolare aortica nella parte intermedia della gestazione. Il diminuito flusso attraverso la valvola aortica stenotica ridu-

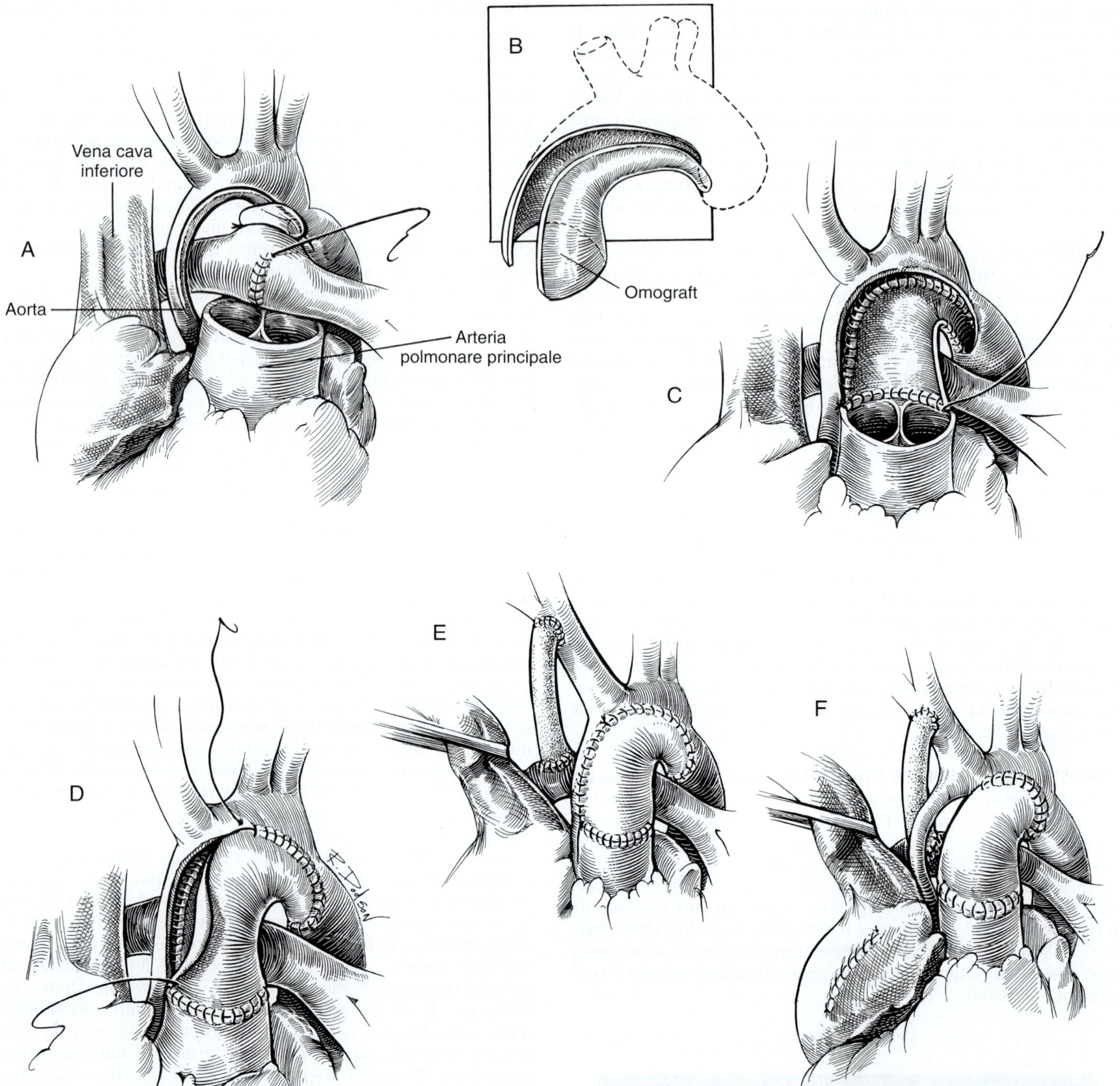

Figura 431-12. La procedura di Norwood, una delle due tecniche correntemente in uso per la palliazione di stadio I della sindrome del cuore sinistro ipoplasico. *A*, Le incisioni utilizzate per la proceduta incorporano un risvolto di parete arteriosa allograft. La parte distale dell'arteria polmonare divisa può essere chiusa per sutura diretta o con patch. *B*, Dimensioni del risvolto della parete arteriosa allograft. *C*, La parete arteriosa allograft viene utilizzata per integrare l'anastomosi tra la parte prossimale divisa dell'arteria polmonare principale e l'aorta ascendente, l'arco aortico e l'aorta prossimale discendente. *D* e *E*, Completamento della procedura con una settostomia atriale e uno shunt modificato di Blalock di 35 mm. *F*, Quando l'aorta ascendente è particolarmente piccola, un'alternativa consiste nel posizionamento di un tubo completo di allograft arterioso. La piccola aorta ascendente può essere lasciata *in situ*, come indicato, o impiantata in un lato della neoaorta. (Da Castañeda AR, Jonas RA, Mayer JE Jr, Hanley FL: Single-ventricle tricuspid atresia. In *Cardiac Surgery of the Neonate and Infant*. Philadelphia, WB Saunders, 1994.)

ce il flusso attraverso il ventricolo sinistro durante lo sviluppo, risultando in una graduale ipoplasia della camera ventricolare. È stata dimostrata la possibilità di prevenire questa ipoplasia effettuando una valvuloplastica aortica con palloncino in utero, nei feti nella parte intermedia della gestazione (Fig. 431-13). I primi risultati sono incoraggianti, anche se questa procedura è considerata sperimentale.

431.11 • Posizioni anomale del cuore e sindromi eterotassiche (asplenia, polisplenia)

La classificazione e la diagnosi della posizione anomala del cuore sono meglio effettuate con approccio segmentale, identificando prima la posizione dei visceri e degli atri, poi dei ventricoli e infine dei grandi vasi. La determinazione del **situs visceroatriale**

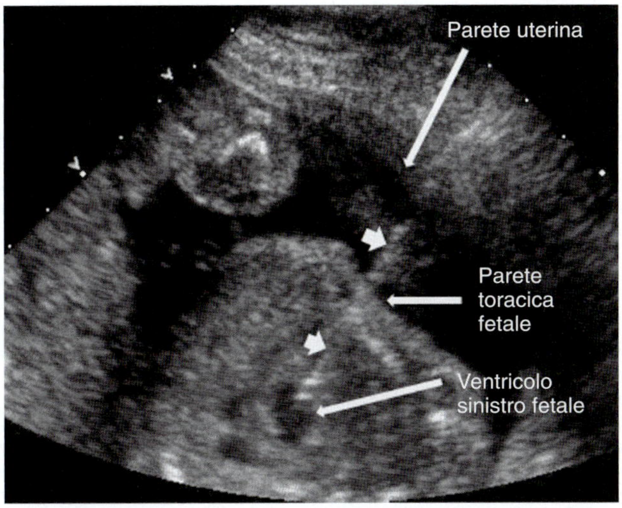

Figura 431-13. Trattamento fetale della stenosi aortica critica per prevenire lo sviluppo di una sindrome del cuore sinistro ipoplasico. L'ecografia fetale evidenzia l'inserimento di un ago (*punte di freccia*) attraverso la parete addominale materna, attraverso l'utero e la parete toracica del feto, nel ventricolo sinistro fetale. Un palloncino guidato da catetere viene poi inserito attraverso l'ago nella camera ventricolare sinistra e nella valvola aortica stenotica. Una volta gonfiato il palloncino per dilatare la valvola, si rimuovono il catetere e l'ago. (Figura per gentile concessione di Stanton Peny, Stanford University, Stanford, CA).

può essere effettuata con la dimostrazione radiografica della posizione degli organi addominali e della biforcazione tracheale per il riconoscimento dei bronchi destro e sinistro e con l'ecocardiografia. Il situs atriale è correlato al situs dei visceri e dei polmoni. Nel situs solitus, i visceri sono in posizione normale (stomaco e milza a sinistra, fegato a destra), il polmone destro trilobato è a destra e il polmone sinistro bilobato a sinistra; l'atrio destro è a destra e l'atrio sinistro a sinistra. Quando gli organi addominali e la locazione dei polmoni sono invertiti, si ha una condizione chiamata situs inversus, in cui l'atrio sinistro è a destra e l'atrio destro a sinistra. Se il situs visceroatriale non è immediatamente determinabile, si è in presenza di una condizione nota come situs indeterminato o eterotassia. Le due varianti principali sono (1) **sindrome da asplenia** (isomerismo destro), associata a un fegato situato centralmente, assenza di milza e due polmoni morfologicamente destri; (2) **sindrome da polisplenia** (isomerismo sinistro), associata a piccole milze multiple, assenza della porzione intraepatica della vena cava inferiore e morfologia polmonare sinistra bilateralmente (in entrambi i polmoni). Le sindromi da eterotassia sono di solito associate a gravi cardiopatie congenite: ASD, VSD, difetto settale atrioventricolare, stenosi o atresia della polmonare e ritorno venoso sistemico o polmonare anomali (Tab. 431-2).

Il passo successivo è la localizzazione dei ventricoli, che dipende dalla direzione in cui la struttura ad anello embrionale si è sviluppata. La protrusione iniziale dell'anello verso destra (*d-loop*) porta il futuro ventricolo destro a destra, mentre il ventricolo sinistro rimane a sinistra. Nel situs solitus, questa organizzazione porta a normali connessioni atrioventricolari (atrio destro che si connette al ventricolo destro, atrio sinistro al ventricolo sinistro). La protrusione dell'anello verso sinistra (*l-loop*) sposta il futuro ventricolo destro a sinistra e il ventricolo sinistro a destra. In questo caso, in presenza di un situs solitus, l'atrio destro si connette al ventricolo sinistro e l'atrio sinistro al ventricolo destro (inversione ventricolare).

La tappa finale è quella dei grandi vasi. Con ogni tipo di anello cardiaco, le relazioni ventricoloarteriose possono essere considerate normali (ventricolo destro connesso all'arteria polmonare, ventricolo sinistro all'aorta) o trasposte (ventricolo destro connesso all'aorta, ventricolo sinistro all'arteria polmonare). Un'ulteriore classificazione può basarsi sulla posizione dell'aorta (di norma a destra e posteriormente) in relazione all'arteria polmonare. Nella trasposizione, l'aorta è di solito posta anteriormente e a destra dell'arteria polmonare (d-trasposizione) o a sinistra (l-trasposizione). Queste relazioni segmentarie sono determinabili tramite studi ecocardiografici e angiografici che dimostrano le relazioni sia atrioventricolari sia ventricoloarteriose. Le manifestazioni cliniche di queste sindromi da anomala posizione cardiaca sono determinate primariamente dalle loro anomalie cardiovascolari associate.

La **destrocardia** si verifica quando il cuore è nella parte destra del torace, mentre si parla di levocardia (situazione normale) quando il cuore è nella parte sinistra del torace. La destrocardia senza un situs inversus associato e la levocardia in presenza di un situs inversus sono per lo più complicate da gravi malformazioni, consistenti in varie combinazioni di ventricolo unico, trasposizione arteriosa, stenosi della polmonare, ASD e VSD, difetti del setto atrioventricolare, ritorno venoso polmonare anomalo, atresia della tricuspide e ipoplasia o atresia dell'arteria polmonare. Studi

TABELLA 431-2. Confronto tra le sindromi cardiospleniche eterotassiche

CARATTERISTICA	ASPLENIA (ISOMERISMO DESTRO)	POLISPLENIA (ISOMERISMO SINISTRO)
Milza	Assente	Multiple
Sede (isomerismo)	Bilaterale destra	Bilaterale sinistra
Polmoni	Bilaterale trilobare con bronchi epiarteriosi	Bilaterali bilobare con bronchi ipoarteriosi
Sesso	Maschile (65%)	Femminile ≥ maschile
Stomaco a destra	Sì	Meno comune
Fegato simmetrico	Sì	Sì
Rotazione intestinale parziale	Sì	Sì
Destrocardia (%)	30-40	30-40
Flusso sanguigno polmonare	Diminuito (di solito)	Aumentato (di solito)
Grave cianosi	Sì	No
Trasposizione delle grandi arterie (%)	60-75	15
Ritorno venoso polmonare anomalo totale (%)	70-80	Raro
Valvola atrioventricolare comune (%)	80-90	20-40
Ventricolo unico (%)	40-50	10-15
Assenza della vena cava inferiore con continuazione azygos	No	Caratteristica
Vena cava superiore bilaterale	Sì	Sì
Altri difetti comuni	Atresia polmonare, stenosi polmonare	Ritorno venoso polmonare anomalo parziale, difetto settale ventricolare, ventricolo destro a doppia uscita
Rischio di sepsi	Sì	No
Corpi di Howell-Jolly e di Heins, eritrociti "pitted"; assenza della colecisti; atresia biliare	No	Sì

PA (*Pulmonary Atresia*), arteria polmonare; PS (*Pulmonary Stenosis*), stenosi polmonare.

su bambini più grandi e adulti indicano che la destrocardia con situs inversus e grandi arterie con rapporti normali (destrocardia "a specchio") è spesso associata a un cuore funzionalmente normale, anche se è comune una cardiopatia congenita di natura meno grave.

Le anomalie anatomiche o funzionali dei polmoni, del diaframma e della cassa toracica possono portare allo spostamento del cuore verso destra (destroposizione). In tal caso, tuttavia, l'apice cardiaco è diretto normalmente a sinistra. Questa posizione anatomica è meno spesso associata con cardiopatie congenite, anche se l'ipoplasia di un polmone può essere accompagnata da un ritorno venoso polmonare anomalo da quel polmone (**sindrome della scimitarra**).

L'elettrocardiogramma è di difficile interpretazione in presenza di lesioni con discordanze anatomiche atriali, ventricolari e dei grandi vasi. La diagnosi di solito richiede indagini dettagliate, effettuate mediante ecocardiografia e cateterismo cardiaco. La prognosi e il trattamento dei pazienti con una delle anomalie cardiache di posizione dipendono dai difetti sottostanti. L'asplenia aumenta il rischio di infezioni gravi come le sepsi batteriche e perciò richiede una profilassi antibiotica giornaliera.

Trasposizione delle grandi arterie

Bellinger DC, Wypij D, duDuplessis AJ, et al: Neurodevelopmental status at eight years in children with dextro-transposition of the great arteries: The Boston Circulatory Arrest Trial. *J Thorac Cardiovasc Surg* 2003;126:1385–1396.
Blume ED, Wernovsky G: Long-term results of arterial switch repair of transposition of the great vessels. *Semin Thorac Cardiovasc Surg Pediatr Card Surg Annu* 1998;1:129–138.
Dearani JA, Danielson GK, Puga FJ, et al: Late results of the Rastelli operation for transposition of the great arteries. *Semin Thorac Cardiovasc Surg Pediatr Card Surg Annu* 2001;4:3–15.
Dunbar-Masterson C, Wypij D, Bellinger DC, et al: General health status of children with D-transposition of the great arteries after the arterial switch operation. *Circulation* 2001;104(Suppl 1):I138–I142.
Hayes CJ, Gersony WM: Arrhythmias after the Mustard operation for transposition of the great arteries: A long-term study. *J Am Coll Cardiol* 1986;7:133–137.
Hovels-Gurich HH, Konrad K, Wiesner M, et al: Long term behavioural outcome after neonatal arterial switch operation for transposition of the great arteries. *Arch Dis Child* 2002;87:506–510.
Losay J, Touchot A, Serraf A, et al: Late outcome after arterial switch operation for transposition of the great arteries. *Circulation* 2001;104(Suppl 1):I121–I126.

Ritorno venoso polmonare anomalo totale

Choe YH, Lee HJ, Kim HS, et al: MRI of total anomalous pulmonary venous connections. *J Comput Assist Tomogr* 1994;18:243–249.
Duff DG, Nihill MR, McNamara DG: Infradiaphragmatic total anomalous pulmonary venous return. Review of clinical and pathological findings and results of operation in 28 cases. *Br Heart J* 1977;39:619–626.
Huhta J, Gutgesell HP, Nihill MR: Cross sectional echocardiographic diagnosis of total anomalous pulmonary venous connection. *Br Heart J* 1985;53:525–534.
Kirshbom PM, Flynn TB, Clancy RR, et al: Late neurodevelopmental outcome after repair of total anomalous pulmonary venous connection. *J Thorac Cardiovasc Surg* 2005;129:1091–1097.

Tronco arterioso comune

Reddy VM, Hanley F: Late results of repair of truncus arteriosus. *Semin Thorac Cardiovasc Surg Pediatr Card Surg Annu* 1998;1:139–146.
Reddy VM, McElhinney DB, Sagrado T, et al: Results of 102 cases of complete repair of congenital heart defects in patients weighing 700 to 2500 grams. *J Thorac Cardiovasc Surg* 1999;117:324–331.
Thompson LD, McElhinney DB, Reddy M, et al: Neonatal repair of truncus arteriosus: Continuing improvement in outcomes. *Ann Thorac Surg* 2001;72:391–395.
Wilson DI, Burn J, Scambler P, et al: DiGeorge syndrome: Part of CATCH 22. *J Med Genet* 1993;30:852–856.

Sindrome del cuore sinistro ipoplasico

Chiavarelli M, Gundry SR, Razzouk AJ, et al: Cardiac transplantation for infants with hypoplastic left heart syndrome. *JAMA* 1993;270:2944–2947.
Connor JA, Arons RR, Figueroa M, et al: Clinical outcomes and secondary diagnoses for infants born with hypoplastic left heart syndrome. *Pediatrics* 2004;114:e160–e165.
Daebritz SH, Nollert GD, Zurakowski D, et al: Results of Norwood stage I operation: Comparison of hypoplastic left heart syndrome with other malformations. *J Thorac Cardiovasc Surg* 2000;119:358–367.
Forbess JM, Visconti KJ, Bellinger DC, et al: Neurodevelopmental outcomes in children after the Fontan operation. *Circulation* 2001;104(Suppl 1):I127–I132.
Sano S, Ishino K, Kado H, et al: Outcome of right ventricle-to-pulmonary artery shunt in first-stage palliation of hypoplastic left heart syndrome: A multi-institutional study. *Ann Thorac Surg* 2004;78:1951–1958.
Theilen U, Shekerdemian L: The intensive care of infants with hypoplastic left heart syndrome. *Arch Dis Fetal Neonatal Ed* 2005;90:F97–F102.
Tworetzky W, Wilkins-Haug L, Jennings RW, et al: Balloon dilation of severe aortic stenosis in the fetus: Potential for prevention of hypoplastic left heart syndrome: Candidate selection, technique, and results of successful intervention. *Circulation* 2004;110:2125–2131.

Destrocardia e levocardia

Britz-Cunningham SH, Shah MM, Zuppan CW, et al: Mutation of the connexin 43 gap-junction gene in patients with heart malformations and defects of laterality. *N Engl J Med* 1995;332:1323–1329.
Rose V, Izukawa T, Moes CAF: Syndromes of asplenia and polysplenia: A review of cardiac and non-cardiac malformations in 60 cases with special reference to diagnosis and prognosis. *Br Heart J* 1975;37:840–852.
Wa MH, Wang JK, Lue HC: Sudden death in patients with right isomerism (asplenism) after palliation. *J Pediatr* 2002;140:93–96.

Capitolo 432 ■ Altre cardiopatie congenite e malformazioni vascolari

432.1 • Anomalie dell'arco aortico

ARCO AORTICO DESTRO

In quest'anomalia, l'aorta curva a destra e se scende alla destra della colonna vertebrale è di solito associata ad altre malformazioni cardiache. Oltre a trovarsi nel 20% dei casi di tetralogia di Fallot, è frequente nel tronco arterioso comune. Un arco aortico destro senza altre anomalie cardiache non è associato a sintomi. Spesso è visualizzabile alla radiografia del torace. La trachea è deviata a sinistra della linea mediana anziché a destra, come in presenza di un normale arco aortico a sinistra. All'esofagogramma con bario, l'esofago è indentato nel margine destro, a livello dell'arco aortico.

ANELLI VASCOLARI

La anomalie congenite dell'arco aortico e delle sue principali diramazioni portano alla formazione di anelli vascolari attorno alla trachea e all'esofago, con gradi variabili di compressione (Tab. 432-1). Per apprezzare meglio l'origine di queste lesioni occorre riconsiderare l'embriologia dell'arco aortico (vedi Fig. 420-2). Le anomalie più comuni comprendono: (1) un arco aortico doppio (Fig. 432-1*A*), (2) un arco aortico destro con legamento arterioso sinistro, (3) un'arteria anonima anomala che origina più a sinistra del normale, sull'arco, (4) un'arteria carotide sinistra anomala che origina più a destra del solito e passa anteriormente alla trachea e (5) un'arteria polmonare sinistra anomala (banderella vascolare). In quest'ultima anomalia il vaso anomalo, che origina da un'arteria polmonare principale allungata o dall'arteria polmonare destra, decorre tra la trachea e l'esofago comprimen-

TABELLA 432-1. Anelli vascolari

LESIONE	SINTOMI	RADIOGRAFIA STANDARD	ESOFAGO BARITATO	BRONCOSCOPIA	RM/ECOCARDIOGRAFIA	TRATTAMENTO
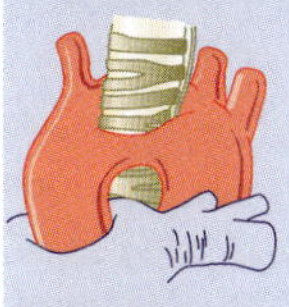 Arco aortico doppio	Stridore Distress respiratorio Disfunzione della deglutizione Apnea riflessa	AP – base cardiaca più ampia Lat. – trachea stenotica, spostata in avanti a livello di C_3-C_4	Indentazione bilaterale dell'esofago	Compressione tracheale bilaterale – pulsatile da entrambi i lati	Diagnostiche	Legatura e divisione dell'arco più piccolo (di solito il sinistro)
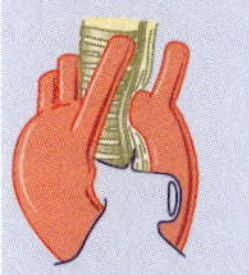 Arco aortico destro e legamento/dotto arterioso	Distress respiratorio Disfunzione della deglutizione	AP – deviazione tracheale a sinistra (arco aortico destro)	Indentazione bilaterale dell'esofago (dx > sx)	Compressione tracheale bilaterale – pulsatile a destra	Diagnostiche	Legatura del legamento o del dotto
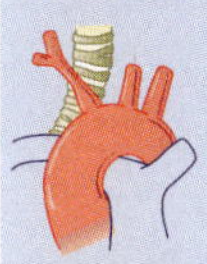 Arteria anonima anomala	Tosse Stridore Apnea riflessa	AP – normale Lat. – compressione tracheale anteriore	Normale	Compressione tracheale anteriore pulsatile	Non necessarie	Conservativo. Se apnea, allora sospensione
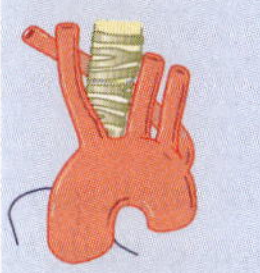 Arteria succlavia destra aberrante	Occasionale disfunzione della deglutizione	Normale	AP – difetto obliquo in alto a destra Lat. – piccolo difetto sulla parete posteriore destra	Di solito normale	Diagnostiche	Legatura dell'arteria
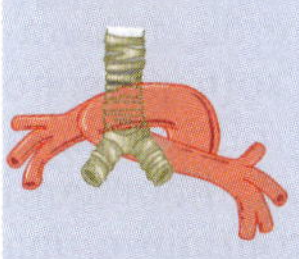 Banderella polmonare	Stridore espiratorio Distress respiratorio	AP – ilo basso, enfisema/atelettasia Lat. – bronco anteriore e trachea piegati in avanti	± indentazione anteriore al di sopra della carina tra l'esofago e la trachea	Deviazione della trachea verso sinistra Compressione del bronco principale destro	Diagnostiche	Distacco e reanastomosi all'arteria polmonare principale al davanti della trachea

AP, anteroposteriore; sx, sinistra; L e l, laterale; RM, risonanza magnetica; dx, destra.
Da Kliegman RM, Greenbaum LA, Lye PS: *Practical Strategies in Pediatric Diagnosis and Therapy*, 2nd ed. Elsevier, Philadelphia, 2004, p 88.

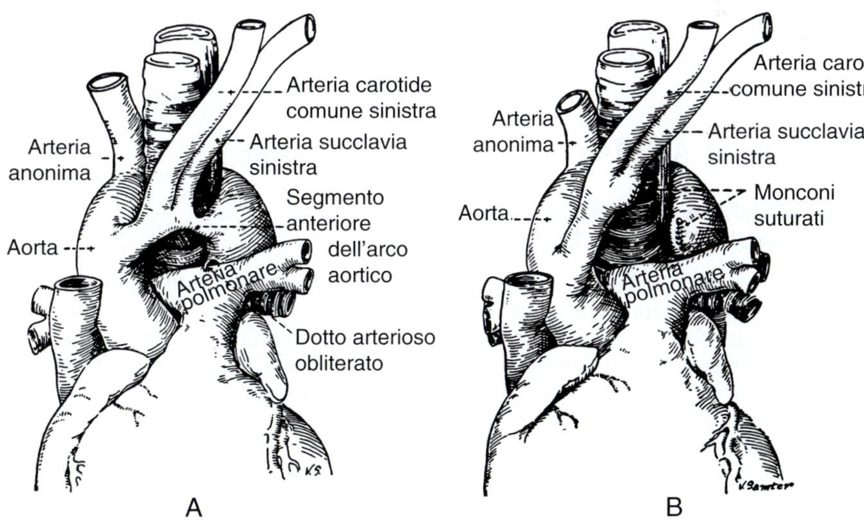

Figura 432-1. Arco aortico doppio. *A*, Piccolo segmento anteriore dell'arco aortico doppio (il tipo più comune). *B*, Procedura operatoria per il rilascio dell'anello vascolare.

doli. Può essere presente una cardiopatia congenita associata nel 5-50% dei pazienti, a seconda dell'anomalia vascolare.

MANIFESTAZIONI CLINICHE. Se l'anello vascolare produce una compressione della trachea e dell'esofago, spesso i sintomi sono presenti durante l'infanzia. Un affaticamento respiratorio cronico è esacerbato dal pianto, dalla suzione e dalla flessione del collo. L'estensione del collo tende a migliorare la respirazione rumorosa. Può essere presente anche vomito. I bambini colpiti possono avere una tosse secca, polmoniti o morte improvvisa da aspirazione.

DIAGNOSI. La radiografia dell'esofago riempito dal mezzo di contrasto (Fig. 432-2) e l'aortografia identificano l'anomalia. Un'arteria succlavia destra aberrante è di comune riscontro, ma non causa compressione della trachea. La diagnosi è confermata dall'ecocardiografia bidimensionale, dalla RM o dalla TC. Il cateterismo cardiaco è riservato ai pazienti con anomalie associate o

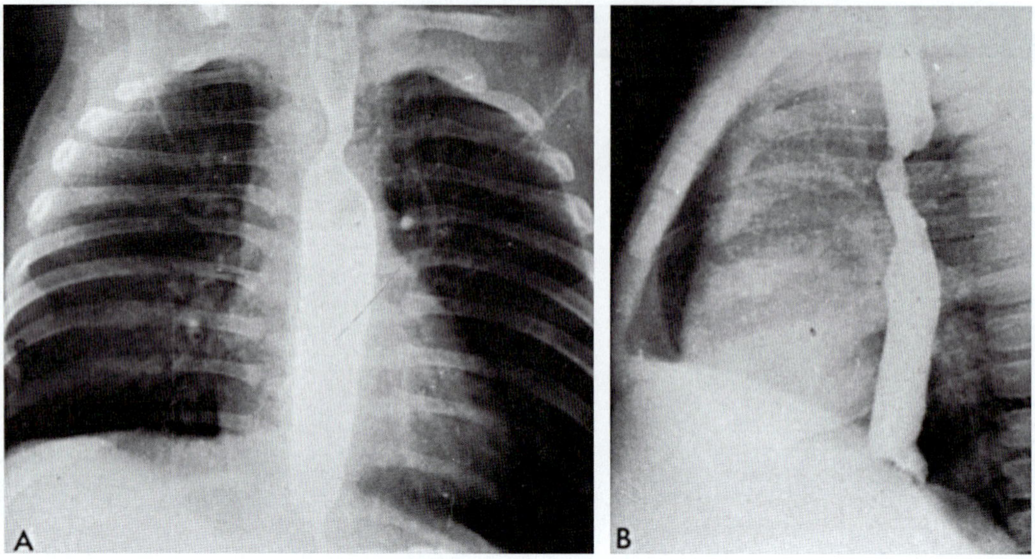

Figura 432-2. Arco aortico doppio in un lattante di 5 mesi. *A*, Proiezione anteroposteriore. L'esofago riempito di bario è stenotico su entrambi i lati. *B*, Proiezione laterale. L'esofago è spostato in avanti. L'arco aortico anteriore era il più piccolo ed è stato diviso all'atto dell'intervento chirurgico.

ai rari casi in cui queste altre modalità d'esame non sono diagnostiche. La broncoscopia è utile nei casi più gravi per determinare l'entità della stenosi delle vie aeree.

TRATTAMENTO. È consigliato l'intervento chirurgico per i pazienti sintomatici che hanno evidenza radiologica di compressione tracheale. Il vaso anteriore è di solito diviso nei soggetti con doppio arco aortico (vedi Fig. 432-1*B*). La compressione prodotta da un arco aortico destro e da un legamento arterioso sinistro viene risolta con la divisione di quest'ultimo. Arterie anonime o carotidi anomale non possono essere divise; l'attacco dell'avventizia di questi vasi allo sterno di solito risolve la compressione tracheale. Per correggere un'arteria polmonare sinistra anomala la si divide all'origine e si effettua la re-anastomosi dell'arteria polmonare principale dopo averla portata davanti alla trachea. Una grave tracheomalacia, se presente, può richiedere anche la ricostruzione della trachea.

432.2 • ORIGINE ANOMALA DELLE ARTERIE CORONARIE

ORIGINE ANOMALA DELL'ARTERIA CORONARIA SINISTRA DALL'ARTERIA POLMONARE (ALCAPA)

Nell'origine anomala dell'arteria coronaria sinistra dall'arteria polmonare il flusso ematico che rifornisce il miocardio ventricolare sinistro è gravemente compromesso. Poco dopo la nascita, quando la pressione arteriosa polmonare cala, la pressione di perfusione in arteria coronaria sinistra diventa inadeguata; ne risultano ischemia miocardica, infarto e fibrosi. In alcuni casi si sviluppano anastomosi collaterali interatriali tra le arterie coronarie destra e sinistra. Il flusso sanguigno nell'arteria coronaria sinistra è quindi invertito e si riversa nell'arteria polmonare, una condizione nota come **"sindrome da furto miocardico"**. Il ventricolo sinistro si dilata, e la sua funzione risulta diminuita. L'insufficienza mitralica è una complicanza frequente, secondaria a un anello valvolare dilatato o all'infarto di un muscolo papillare. Possono inoltre svilupparsi aneurismi localizzati nella parete ventricolare sinistra libera. A volte alcuni pazienti hanno un adeguato flusso sanguigno miocardico durante l'infanzia e, successivamente, un soffio continuo e un piccolo shunt sinistro-destro attraverso il sistema coronario dilatato (aorta → coronaria destra → coronaria sinistra → arteria polmonare).

MANIFESTAZIONI CLINICHE. I segni di scompenso cardiaco diventano evidenti nei primi mesi di vita, spesso precipitati da un'infezione respiratoria. Si verificano attacchi ricorrenti di malessere generale, agitazione, irritabilità, sudorazione, dispnea e pallore con o senza lieve cianosi, che probabilmente rappresentano segni di angina pectoris. L'ingrandimento cardiaco è da moderato a notevole. È comune un ritmo di galoppo. I soffi possono essere di tipo aspecifico ed eiettivo, oppure olosistolici a causa dell'insufficienza mitralica. I pazienti più grandi con abbondanti anastomosi intercoronariche possono avere soffi continui e una minima disfunzione ventricolare sinistra. Durante l'adolescenza, possono andare incontro a episodi di angina da sforzo. È raro che pazienti con un'arteria coronaria destra anomala presentino reperti clinici analoghi.

DIAGNOSI. L'esame radiografico conferma la cardiomegalia. L'elettrocardiogramma produce un pattern simile a quello descritto per l'infarto miocardico della parete laterale negli adulti. nelle derivazioni I e aVL si nota un pattern QR seguito da onde T invertite. Le derivazioni di superficie del ventricolo sinistro (V_5 e V_6) possono altresì evidenziare profonde onde Q e presentare un sopraslivellamento del tratto ST e onde T invertite (Fig. 432-3). Nei bambini più grandi, un test da sforzo può essere utile quando si verificano cambiamenti del tratto ST o dell'onda T o il paziente è sintomatico. Anche se l'ecocardiografia bidimensionale di solito può suggerire la diagnosi, l'ecocardiografia non sempre è affidabile nella diagnosi di questa condizione. Con il solo imaging bidimensionale, può sembrare che l'arteria coronaria sinistra origini dall'aorta. L'esame eco-color-Doppler, che ha migliorato l'accuratezza della diagnosi di questa lesioni, può evidenziare un flusso retrogrado nell'arteria coronaria sinistra. La TC o la RM possono essere utili per confermare l'origine delle arterie coronarie. Il cateterismo cardiaco è diagnostico; l'aortografia evidenzia l'immediata opacizzazione della sola arteria coronaria destra, un vaso ampio e tortuoso. Dopo il riempimento delle anastomosi intercoronariche, si opacizza l'arteria coronaria sinistra, e si può vedere l'ingresso del contrasto in arteria polmonare. L'arteriografia polmonare può anche opacizzare l'origine dell'arteria coronaria sinistra anomala. La ventricolografia selettiva sinistra di solito evidenzia un ventricolo sinistro dilatato che si svuota poco.

TRATTAMENTO E PROGNOSI. In assenza di trattamento, la morte avviene per scompenso cardiaco entro i primi 6 mesi di vita. I pazienti che sopravvivono generalmente hanno abbondanti anastomosi collaterali intercoronariche. Il trattamento medico comprende la terapia standard per lo scompenso cardiaco (diure-

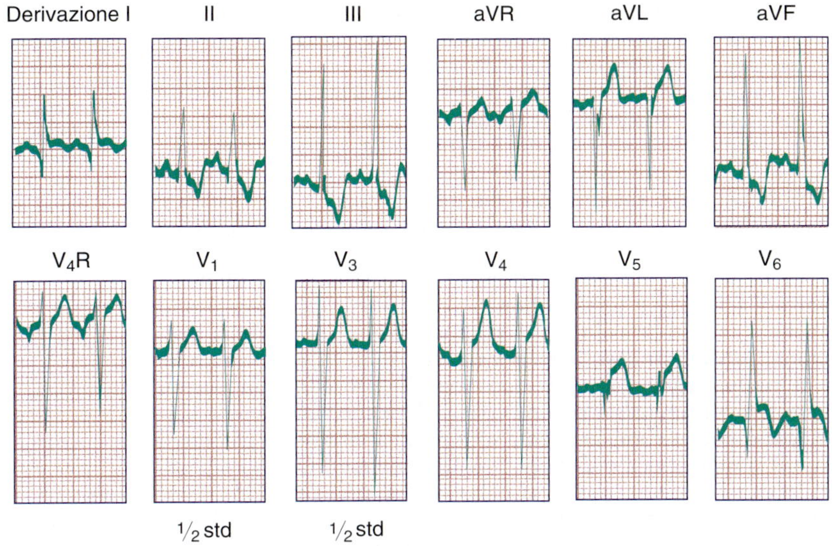

Figura 432-3. Elettrocardiogramma di un lattante di 3 mesi con origine anomala dell'arteria coronaria sinistra dall'arteria polmonare. È presente un infarto miocardio laterale, come evidenziato da onde Q abnormemente ampie e profonde nelle derivazioni I, V_5 e V_6, da un segmento ST sopraslivellato in V_5 e V_6 e dall'inversione dell'onda T in V_6.

tici, digossina, captopril) e per il controllo dell'ischemia (nitrati, β-bloccanti).

Il trattamento chirurgico consiste nel distacco dell'arteria coronaria anomala dall'arteria polmonare e nella sua anastomosi all'aorta per ristabilire una normale perfusione miocardica. Un bambino gravemente malato con un'arteria coronaria sinistra sottile può presentare un problema di difficoltà tecnica. La legatura dell'arteria coronaria anomala sinistra all'origine in passato veniva effettuata per impedire la fuoriuscita di sangue dal circuito coronarico e per aumentare, se possibile, la perfusione del miocardio da parte del circolo collaterale. Via via che l'esperienza chirurgica è aumentata nello switch di arterie coronarie nei neonati, questa opzione è in gran parte stata abbandonata. In pazienti che sono già andati incontro a un significativo infarto miocardio, il trapianto cardiaco può essere l'opzione migliore.

ORIGINE ANOMALA DELL'ARTERIA CORONARIA DESTRA DALL'ARTERIA POLMONARE

L'origine anomala dell'arteria coronaria destra dall'arteria polmonare si manifesta raramente nella prima infanzia. L'arteria coronaria sinistra è dilatata, mentre quella destra presenta una parete sottile e solo lievemente dilatata. Nella prima infanzia la perfusione dell'arteria coronaria destra avviene dall'arteria polmonare, mentre in seguito si verifica dalle collaterali dei vasi della coronaria sinistra. Possono insorgere episodi anginosi o morte improvvisa nell'adolescenza o nell'età adulta. Quest'anomalia, una volta riconosciuta, dovrebbe essere corretta mediante reanastomosi dell'arteria coronaria destra all'aorta.

ORIGINE ECTOPICA DELL'ARTERIA CORONARIA DALL'AORTA CON DECORSO PROSSIMALE ABERRANTE

Nell'origine ectopica dell'arteria coronaria dall'aorta con decorso prossimale aberrante, l'arteria aberrante può essere un'arteria coronaria sinistra, destra o una diramazione principale di un'arteria coronaria. La sede d'origine può essere un seno di Valsalva scorretto o un'arteria coronaria prossimale. L'ostio può essere ipoplasico, a fessura o di calibro normale. Il vaso aberrante può passare anteriormente, posteriormente o tra l'aorta e il tratto di efflusso ventricolare destro; può inoltre passare a tunnel nel tessuto settale conale o interventricolare. L'ostruzione che deriva dall'ipoplasia degli osti, il passaggio a tunnel tra l'aorta e il tratto di efflusso ventricolare destro o il setto interventricolare e l'angolo acuto che forma producono una fibrosi miocardica focale o un infarto miocardico. I vasi non ostruiti non danno luogo a sintomi. I pazienti con quest'anomalia estremamente rara giungono all'osservazione inizialmente con un grave infarto miocardico, aritmie ventricolari, angina pectoris o sincope; può insorgere la morte improvvisa, soprattutto nei giovani atleti.

La diagnosi dovrebbe comprendere un elettrocardiogramma, un test da sforzo, un'ecocardiografia bidimensionale, una TC o RM e un cateterismo cardiaco con angiografia coronaria selettiva.

Il trattamento è indicato per i vasi ostruiti e consiste in un'aortoplastica con reanastomosi del vaso aberrante, o talvolta nel bypass coronarico. Il trattamento dei bambini asintomatici con queste forme di origine ectopica delle coronarie rimane controverso.

432.3 • FISTOLA ARTEROVENOSA POLMONARE

Le comunicazioni vascolari fistolose nei polmoni possono essere ampie e localizzate o multiple, sparse e piccole. La forma più frequente di questa condizione peraltro non comune è la **sindrome di Osler-Weber-Rendu** (teleangectasia ereditaria emorragica tipo I), associata ad angiomi delle membrane mucose di naso e bocca, del tratto gastrointestinale o del fegato. Sono causa di questa sindrome mutazioni del gene dell'endoglina, una componente di superficie del complesso recettoriale del fattore di crescita trasformante β. La comunicazione che si instaura di solito è tra l'arteria polmonare e una vena polmonare; una comunicazione diretta tra l'arteria polmonare e l'atrio sinistro è estremamente rara. Il sangue desaturato in arteria polmonare viene deviato attraverso la fistola in una vena polmonare, aggirando così i polmoni, per poi entrare nel cuore sinistro; questa direzione di flusso aberrante porta a una desaturazione arteriosa sistemica e talora alla cianosi clinica. Lo shunt attraverso la fistola è a bassa pressione e resistenza, cosicché la pressione arteriosa è normale; la cardiomegalia e lo scompenso cardiaco non sono presenti.

Le manifestazioni cliniche dipendono dalla grandezza dello shunt. Ampie fistole sono associate a dispnea, cianosi, ippocratismo digitale, a un soffio continuo e a policitemia. L'emottisi è rara, ma quando si verifica può essere massiva. Le caratteristiche della sindrome di Osler-Weber-Rendu, riscontrabili in circa il 50% dei pazienti (o di altri membri della famiglia), comprendono epistassi ricorrenti e sanguinamenti dal tratto gastrointestinale. Transitori capogiri, diplopia, afasia, debolezza motoria o convulsioni possono derivare da una trombosi cerebrale, da un ascesso o da un'embolia paradossa. Soffi sistolici dolci o continui possono essere udibili sulla sede della fistola. L'elettrocardiogramma è normale. L'esame radiografico del torace può evidenziare opacità prodotte da ampie fistole; piccole fistole multiple possono essere visualizzate mediante fluoroscopia (come pulsazioni anomale), TC o RM. L'arteriografia polmonare selettiva evidenzia la sede, l'estensione e la distribuzione delle fistole.

Il **trattamento**, consistente nell'escissione delle lesioni solitarie o localizzate, mediante lobectomia o resezione a cuneo, porta alla completa scomparsa dei sintomi. Nella maggior parte dei casi le fistole sono così estese da rendere impossibile l'intervento chirurgico. La comunicazione diretta tra l'arteria polmonare e l'atrio sinistro, se presente, può essere chiusa mediante divisione e sutura.

I pazienti che sono stati sottoposti ad anastomosi **cavopolmonare di Glenn** per una cardiopatia congenita con cianosi sono anche a rischio di sviluppo di malformazioni arterovenose polmonari. In questi casi, le malformazioni sono di solito multiple e il rischio aumenta nel tempo dopo la procedura di Glenn. Queste malformazioni raramente si sviluppano dopo che la cardiopatia è stata completamente sottoposta a intervento palliativo con il completamento dell'operazione di Fontan. Questo reperto induce a ipotizzare che la circolazione polmonare richieda un fattore epatico ancora indeterminato per sopprimere lo sviluppo di malformazioni arterovenose. Il segno distintivo dello sviluppo di queste malformazioni è una diminuzione della saturazione di ossigeno del paziente. La diagnosi spesso può essere fatta con ecocardiografia con contrasto, e il cateterismo cardiaco è l'esame definitivo. Il completamento del circuito di Fontan, cosicché il flusso sanguigno della vena cava inferiore (contenente il drenaggio venoso epatico) venga dirottato attraverso i polmonari, di solito comporta un miglioramento o la risoluzione delle malformazioni.

432.4 • Ectopia cordis

Nella forma toracica più comune di ectopia cordis, lo sterno è diviso e il cuore protrude al di fuori del torace. In altre forme, il cuore penetra attraverso il diaframma nella cavità addominale o può essere situato nel collo. Sono comuni anomalie intracardiache associate. La morte subentra nei primi giorni di vita, di solito a causa di infezioni, scompenso cardiaco o ipossiemia. La terapia chirurgica per i neonati che non hanno gravi e irreparabili anomalie cardiache consiste nel coprire il cuore di cute senza compromettere il ritorno venoso o l'eiezione ventricolare. È inoltre necessaria la palliazione dei difetti associati. Alcuni pazienti con il tipo addominale di ectopia cordis sono sopravvissuti fino all'età adulta.

432.5 • Diverticolo del ventricolo sinistro

In questa rara anomalia, un diverticolo del ventricolo sinistro protrude in epigastrio. La lesione può essere isolata o associata a complesse anomalie cardiovascolari. Una massa pulsante è visibile e palpabile in epigastrio. Soffi sistolici o sistodiastolici prodotti dal flusso di sangue in entrata e in uscita dal diverticolo possono udirsi sulla parte inferiore dello sterno e in corrispondenza della massa. L'elettrocardiogramma evidenzia un pattern di blocco di branca sinistra, completo o incompleto. Le radiografie del torace possono evidenziare o meno la massa. Anomalie associate comprendono difetti dello sterno, della parete addominale, del diaframma e del pericardio. Il trattamento chirurgico del diverticolo e dei difetti cardiaci associati è possibile in casi selezionati. Occasionalmente capita che un diverticolo sia piccolo e non associato a segni o sintomi clinici. Questi piccoli diverticoli vengono diagnosticati al momento di un esame ecocardiografico effettuato per altri motivi.

Anelli vascolari

Azarow KS, Pearl RH, Hoffman MA, et al: Vascular ring: Does magnetic resonance imaging replace angiography? *Ann Thorac Surg* 1992;53:882–885.

Bertrand J-M, Chartrand C, Lamarre A, et al: Vascular ring: Clinical and physiological assessment of pulmonary function following surgical correction. *Pediatr Pulmonol* 1986;2:378–383.

Kussman BD, Geva T, McGowan FX: Cardiovascular causes of airway compression. *Paediatr Anaesth* 2004;14:60–74.

Murdison KA, Andrews BA, Chin AJ: Ultrasonographic display of complex vascular rings. *J Am Coll Cardiol* 1990;15:1645–1653.

van Son JA, Julsrud PR, Hagler DJ, et al: Imaging strategies for vascular rings. *Ann Thorac Surg* 1994;57:604–610.

Arteria coronaria anomala

Chang RR, Allada V: Electrocardiographic and echocardiographic features that distinguish anomalous origin of the left coronary artery from pulmonary artery from idiopathic dilated cardiomyopathy. *Pediatr Cardiol* 2001;22:3–10.

Frommelt PC, Berger S, Pelech AN, et al: Prospective identification of anomalous origin of left coronary artery from the right sinus of Valsalva using transthoracic echocardiography: Importance of color Doppler flow mapping. *Pediatr Cardiol* 2001;22:327–332.

Johnsrude CL, Perry JC, Cecchin F, et al: Differentiating anomalous left main coronary artery originating from the pulmonary artery in infants from myocarditis and dilated cardiomyopathy by electrocardiogram. *Am J Cardiol* 1995;75:71–74.

Schmidt KG, Cooper MJ, Silverman NH, et al: Pulmonary artery origin of the left coronary artery: Diagnosis by two-dimensional echocardiography, pulsed Doppler ultrasound and color flow mapping. *J Am Coll Cardiol* 1988;11:396–402.

Fistola arterovenosa polmonare

Feinstein JA, Moore P, Rosenthal DN, et al: Comparison of contrast echocardiography versus cardiac catheterization for detection of pulmonary arteriovenous malformations. *Am J Cardiol* 2002;89:281–285.

Freedom RM, Yoo SJ, Perrin D: The biological "scrabble" of pulmonary arteriovenous malformations: Considerations in the setting of cavopulmonary surgery. *Cardiol Young* 2004;14:417–437.

Marchuk DA: Genetic abnormalities in hereditary hemorrhagic telangiectasia. *Curr Opin Hematol* 1998;5:332–338.

Paterson A: Imaging evaluation of congenital lung abnormalities in infants and children. *Radiol Clin North Am* 2005;43:303–323.

Srivastava D, Preminger T, Lock JE, et al: Hepatic venous blood and the development of pulmonary arteriovenous malformations in congenital heart disease. *Circulation* 1995;92:1217–1222.

Capitolo 433 ■ Ipertensione polmonare

433.1 • Ipertensione polmonare primitiva

FISIOPATOLOGIA. L'ipertensione polmonare primitiva è caratterizzata da una malattia vascolare polmonare ostruttiva e da uno scompenso cardiaco destro. Si verifica a ogni età, anche se nei pazienti pediatrici la diagnosi viene posta nell'adolescenza. In età adulta, le femmine sono più colpite rispetto ai maschi, con un rapporto di 1.7:1; nei pazienti più giovani, entrambi i sessi sono colpiti in ugual misura. Alcuni pazienti hanno segni di una patologia immunologica o di uno stato di ipercoagulabilità. Sono state identificate mutazioni nel gene per il recettore 2 per la proteina morfogenetica dell'osso (BMPR-2, appartenente della famiglia del recettore per il fattore di crescita trasformante β) sul cromosoma 2q33, in pazienti con ipertensione polmonare primitiva familiare autosomica dominante (nota come PPH1). Questa variante genetica presenta una preponderanza nel sesso femminile e si ritrova fin nel 25% dei pazienti con la malattia sporadica. Sono stati identificati altri geni che potrebbero essere coinvolti nella malattia, compresi i cromosomi 2q31 (PPH2) e 12q13 (ALK1). Si è ipotizzato che le infezioni virali, in particolare quella dovuta all'herpesvirus umano vasculotropico 8 (HHV8), possano agire da fattore scatenante in molti pazienti. Sono stati inoltre implicati i farmaci dimagranti, in particolare la fenfluramina. L'ipertensione polmonare è associata a ostruzione precapillare del letto vascolare polmonare, in conseguenza dell'iperplasia dei tessuti muscolare ed elastico e di un ispessimento dell'intima delle piccole arterie e arteriole polmonari. Alterazioni aterosclerotiche possono ritrovarsi nelle arterie polmonari più grandi. Nei bambini, la patologia veno-occlusiva può rendere conto di alcuni casi di ipertensione polmonare primitiva. È necessario escludere altre cause di elevata pressione polmonare (patologia parenchimale polmonare cronica, ostruzione persistente delle vie aeree superiori, malformazioni cardiache congenite, embolie polmonari ricorrenti, displasia capillare alveolare, epatopatia, malattia autoimmune e malattia Moyamoya). Nella Tabella 433-1 è riportato un sistema di classificazione. L'ipertensione polmonare impone sul ventricolo destro un precarico aumentato, che porta all'ipertrofia ventricolare destra. È presente dilatazione dell'arteria polmonare e può verificarsi un'insufficienza valvolare polmonare. Negli stadi più avanzati della malattia, il ventricolo destro si dilata, si sviluppa un'insufficienza tricuspidalica e la gittata cardiaca diminuisce. Sono comuni aritmie, sincopi e morte improvvisa.

MANIFESTAZIONI CLINICHE. I sintomi predominanti comprendono l'intolleranza allo sforzo fisico e l'affaticabilità; talvolta il paziente accusa un dolore toracico precordiale, capogiri, sincope o cefalea. Può essere presente una cianosi periferica, specialmente in caso di forame ovale pervio attraverso cui il sangue può essere deviato da destra a sinistra; negli stadi più avanzati di malattia, i pazienti possono avere estremità fredde e un colorito cinereo, associato alla bassa gittata cardiaca. La saturazione arteriosa di ossigeno è di solito normale, a meno che non vi sia uno shunt intracardiaco associato. Se è sopravvenuto uno scompenso cardiaco destro, la pressione venosa giugulare è elevata, e si manifestano epatomegalia ed edemi. Sono presenti onde venose giugulari *a*, e nei soggetti con insufficienza tricuspidale funzionale sono evidenti una marcata onda giugulare *cv* e pulsazioni epatiche sistoliche. Il cuore è moderatamente ingrandito e può notarsi un sollevamento del ventricolo destro. Il primo tono cardiaco è spesso seguito da un click da eiezione proveniente dall'arteria polmonare dilatata. Il secondo tono cardiaco, strettamente sdoppiato, forte, talvolta di qualità esplosiva, è spesso palpabile a livello del margine sternale superiore sinistro. Può essere udibile un ritmo di galoppo presistolico a livello del margine sternale inferiore sinistro. Il soffio sistolico, dolce e breve, talvolta è seguito da un soffio diastolico soffiante in decrescendo causato da un'insufficienza polmonare. Negli stadi più avanzati, si apprezza un soffio olosistolico da insufficienza tricuspidale a livello del margine sternale inferiore sinistro.

TABELLA 433-1. Classificazione riveduta dell'ipertensione polmonare secondo l'Organizzazione Mondiale della Sanità (OMS)

- Gruppo I. Ipertensione arteriosa polmonare
  - Idiopatica (primitiva)
  - Familiare
    - Condizioni correlate: collagenopatie, shunt sistemico-polmonari congeniti, ipertensione portale, infezione da HIV, farmaci e sostanze tossiche (per es. anoressizzanti, olio di colza, L-triptofano, metanfetamina e cocaina); altre patologie: tireopatie, malattie da accumulo di glicogeno, malattia di Gaucher, teleangectasia emorragica ereditaria, emoglobinopatie, patologie mieloproliferative, splenectomia
  - Associata a un significativo coinvolgimento venoso o capillare
    - Malattia veno-occlusiva polmonare
    - Emangiomatosi polmonare-capillare
  - Ipertensione polmonare persistente del neonato
- Gruppo II. Ipertensione venosa polmonare
  - Cardiopatia atriale o ventricolare sinistra
  - Valvulopatia del cuore sinistro
- Gruppo III. Ipertensione polmonare associata a ipossiemia
  - Broncopneumopatia cronica ostruttiva
  - Patologia polmonare interstiziale
  - Malattia delle apnee notturne
  - Patologia da ipoventilazione alveolare
  - Esposizione cronica ad altitudini elevate
  - Anomalie dello sviluppo
- Gruppo IV. Ipertensione polmonare dovuta a patologia trombotica cronica, patologia embolia o entrambe
  - Ostruzione tromboembolica delle arterie polmonari prossimali
  - Ostruzione tromboembolica delle arterie polmonari distali
  - Embolia polmonare neoplastica, da parassiti, da materiale estraneo
- Gruppo V. Varie
  - Sarcoidosi, istiocitosi polmonare a cellule di Langerhans, linfangiomatosi, compressione dei vasi polmonari (adenopatie, tumori, mediastinite fibrosante)

Da Farber HW, Loscalzo J: Pulmonary arterial hypertension. *N Engl J Med* 2004;351:1655-1666.

DIAGNOSI. Le radiografie del torace evidenziano un'arteria polmonare e un ventricolo destro sporgenti (Fig. 433-1). La vascolarizzazione polmonare nelle aree ilari può essere accentuata, in contrasto con quella dei campi polmonari periferici in cui i segni polmonari sono diminuiti. L'elettrocardiogramma evidenzia un'ipertrofia ventricolare destra, spesso con onde P appuntite.

Al cateterismo cardiaco questa condizione deve essere distinta dalla sindrome di Eisenmenger (vedi Capitolo 433.2), che è associata a una comunicazione tra le sezioni sinistra e destra del cuore o delle grandi arterie, come pure a lesioni ostruttive del cuore sinistro (stenosi venosa polmonare, stenosi mitralico) responsabili di ipertensione venosa polmonare (vedi Capitolo 427). La presenza di un'ipertensione arteriosa polmonare con una normale pressione di incuneamento capillare è diagnostica di ipertensione polmonare primitiva. Se la pressione di incuneamento è elevata e la pressione telediastolica ventricolare sinistra è normale, si deve sospettare un'ostruzione a livello delle vene polmonari, dell'atrio sinistro o della valvola mitrale. I rischi associati al cateterismo cardiaco sono aumentati in pazienti in condizioni critiche con ipertensione polmonare primitiva.

PROGNOSI E TRATTAMENTO. L'ipertensione polmonare primitiva è progressiva, e non è attualmente disponibile alcuna cura. Sono stati riportati successi con una terapia a base di calcioantagonisti per via orale come la nifedipina, in bambini che presentano una vasoreattività polmonare quando questi farmaci vengono somministrati durante il cateterismo. L'infusione endovenosa continua di prostaciclina (prostaglandina I_2) allevia i sintomi fintanto che viene continuata. Pur essendosi dimostrata efficace per ridurre i sintomi e migliorare la qualità di vita, la prostaciclina rallenta, ma non arresta, la progressione della malattia. La somministrazione continua di ossido nitrico per cannula nasale, quella di prostaciclina in forma nebulizzata e di vasodilatatori per os (bosentan, un antagonista dei recettori dell'endotelina, o sildenafil, un inibitore

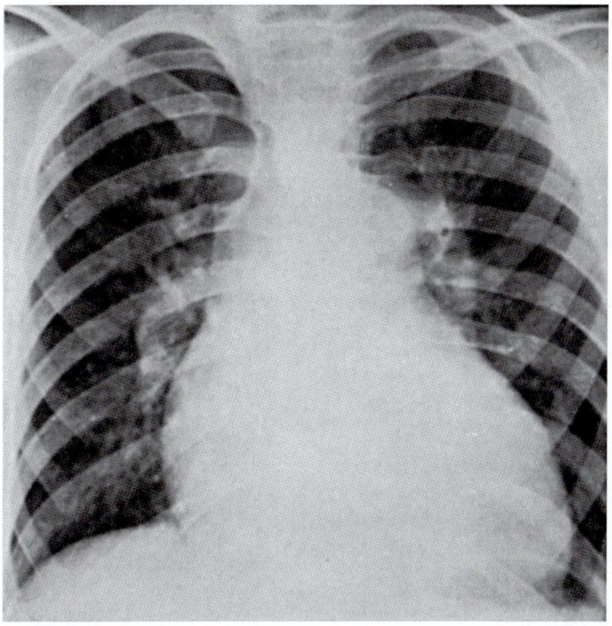

Figura 433-1. Radiografia di un'ipertensione polmonare primitiva. Si notino il moderato ingrossamento cardiaco, la dilatazione dell'arteria polmonare e relativa limitata vascolarizzazione nei due terzi esterni dei campi polmonari.

della fosfodiesterasi tipo 5) sono tutte oggetto di studio (Tab. 433-2). L'anticoagulazione può essere utile in pazienti con pregressa tromboembolia polmonare, alcuni dei quali risponderanno positivamente all'angioplastica con palloncino di segmenti di arteria polmonare stenotici. Nonostante i notevoli progressi compiuti, la terapia definitiva è ancora rappresentata dal trapianto (cuore-polmone o polmone) (vedi Capitolo 443.2). In pazienti con grave ipertensione polmonare e bassa gittata cardiaca, l'exitus è spesso improvviso e correlato a un'aritmia letale. Quelli con ipertensione polmonare primitiva diagnosticata nell'infanzia spesso hanno una progressione rapida di malattia e una mortalità elevata.

433.2 • Vasculopatia polmonare (sindrome di Eisenmenger)

FISIOPATOLOGIA. Si considerano affetti da **sindrome di Eisenmenger** i pazienti con un difetto del setto interventricolare in cui il sangue viene deviato parzialmente o totalmente da destra a sinistra in conseguenza dello sviluppo di una malattia vascolare polmonare. Quest'anomalia fisiologica può verificarsi anche con un difetto del setto interatriale, un difetto del setto atrioventricolare, un dotto arterioso pervio o qualsiasi altra comunicazione tra l'aorta e l'arteria polmonare. La malattia vascolare polmonare associata a un difetto del setto interatriale isolato, oltre a essere meno comune, non si verifica prima dell'età adulta.

Nella sindrome di Eisenmenger, la resistenza vascolare polmonare dopo la nascita rimane elevata o, dopo essere diminuita durante la prima infanzia, aumenta a causa di uno stress provocato dall'aumento del flusso nelle arteriole polmonari. I fattori che accelerano lo sviluppo della malattia vascolare polmonare comprendono una pressione arteriosa polmonare elevata, un aumentato flusso sanguigno polmonare e la presenza di ipossia o ipercapnia. Allo stadio iniziale della malattia, l'ipertensione polmonare (pressione elevata nelle arterie polmonari) è il risultato di un flusso sanguigno polmonare marcatamente aumentato (ipertensione polmonare ipercinetica). Questa forma di ipertensione polmonare diminuisce con la somministrazione di vasodilatatori polmonari, di ossigeno o di entrambi. Con lo sviluppo della sindrome di Eisenmenger, l'ipertensione polmonare è il risultato di una malattia vascolare polmonare (eventi patologici ostruttivi nei vasi polmonari). Questa forma di ipertensione polmonare di solito è minimamente responsiva ai vasodilatatori polmonari o all'ossigeno, o non lo è affatto.

ANATOMIA PATOLOGICA E FISIOPATOLOGIA. I cambiamenti patologici della sindrome di Eisenmenger si verificano nelle piccole arteriole polmonari e nelle arterie muscolari (<300 mm) e sono classificati in base alle loro caratteristiche istologiche (classificazione di Heath-Edwards): il **grado I** consiste nella sola ipertrofia della media, il **grado II** nell'ipertrofia della media e nell'iperplasia dell'intima, il **grado III** nell'obliterazione del lume vascolare, il **grado IV** nella dilatazione arteriosa, i **gradi V e VI** in lesioni plessiformi, formazioni angiomatoidi e necrosi fibrinoide. I gradi IV-VI corrispondono a una vasculopatia polmonare irreversibile. Si definisce fenomeno di Eisenmenger un aumento assoluto della resistenza arteriosa polmonare >12 unità Wood (unità di resistenza corrette per la superficie corporea) o un rapporto tra resistenza polmonare e sistemica ≥1,0.

La vasculopatia polmonare si sviluppa più rapidamente in pazienti con trisomia 21 che hanno uno shunt sinistro-destro, oltre a complicare la storia naturale di pazienti con pressione venosa polmonare elevata secondaria a stenosi mitralica o disfunzione ventricolare sinistra, soprattutto se associata a miocardiopatia restrittiva (vedi Capitolo 439.3). La vasculopatia polmonare può verificarsi anche in qualsiasi paziente con trasmissione della pressione sistemica alla circolazione polmonare attraverso uno shunt a livello interventricolare o dei grandi vasi, e in soggetti cronicamente esposti a bassa PO_2 (a causa dell'altitudine elevata). A rischio particolarmente elevato sono coloro che soffrono di cardiopatie congenite con cianosi associate a un flusso sanguigno polmonare non sottoposto a limitazioni.

MANIFESTAZIONI CLINICHE. I sintomi non si sviluppano di solito fino alla seconda o terza decade di vita, anche se può verificarsi un decorso più fulminante. Molti pazienti sopravvivono per decenni con sintomi minimi. Comunicazioni intracardiache o extracardiache che normalmente porterebbero il sangue a deviare da sinistra a destra sono convertite in shunt da destra a sinistra quando la resistenza vascolare polmonare diventa più elevata della resistenza vascolare sistemica. Insorge la cianosi e iniziano a manifestarsi dispnea, astenia e tendenza alle aritmie. Negli stadi avanzati della malattia, possono osservarsi scompenso cardiaco, dolore toracico, cefalea, sincope ed emottisi. L'esame obiettivo evidenzia un sollevamento del ventricolo destro e un secondo tono strettamente sdoppiato con una forte componente polmonare. Può essere presente una pulsazione palpabile dell'arteria polmonare a livello del margine sternale superiore sinistro. Talvolta è udibile un soffio olosistolico da rigurgito tricuspidalico lungo il margine sternale sinistro. Si può inoltre auscultare un precoce soffio diastolico in decrescendo da insufficienza polmonare lungo il margine sternale sinistro. Il grado di cianosi dipende dallo stadio della malattia.

DIAGNOSI. I pazienti cianotici hanno vari gradi di policitemia che dipendono dalla gravità e dalla durata dell'ipossia. Dal punto di

TABELLA 433-2. Quadro riassuntivo dei farmaci utilizzati per il trattamento dell'ipertensione polmonare

FARMACO E MECCANISMO D'AZIONE	DOSAGGI UTILIZZATI NEGLI STUDI IN PEDIATRIA	EFFETTI COLLATERALI COMUNI
Epoprostenolo ([prostaciclina PGI_2], un potente vasodilatatore, che inoltre inibisce l'aggregazione piastrinica)	1 nanogrammo/kg/min inizialmente, da aumentare tenendo conto del decorso clinico e della tolleranza, fino a 20-50 nanogrammi/kg/min. Alcuni pazienti possono richiedere anche dosi più elevate. Va somministrato per infusione continua senza interruzioni	Flushing, cefalea, nausea, diarrea, ipotensione, dolore toracico, dolore alla mandibola
Iloprost (analogo sintetico della prostaciclina PGI_2)	2,5-5,0 μg 6-9 volte al giorno (non più frequentemente di ogni 2 ore) per inalazione	Flushing, cefalea, diarrea, ipotensione, dolore alla mandibola, esacerbazione di sintomi polmonari (tosse, dispnea)
Treprostinil (analogo sintetico della prostaciclina)	Dosi simili a quelle dell'epoprostenolo anche se i pazienti possono richiedere dosi massime più elevate del 25% circa. Somministrato ev o sc o per infusione continua. Emivita più lunga rispetto all'epoprostenolo	Flushing, cefalea, diarrea, ipotensione, dolore alla mandibola. Dolore nei sito di infusione quando somministrato sc
Bosentan (antagonista dei recettori ETA e ETB dell'endotelina)	10-20 kg: 31,25 mg al giorno per 4 settimane, poi aumento a 32,5 mg due volte al giorno. 20-40 kg: 31,25 mg due volte al giorno per 4 settimane, poi aumento a 62,5 mg due volte al giorno. >40 kg: 625 mg due volte al giorno per 4 settimane, poi aumento a 125 mg due volte al giorno. Altri antagonisti selettivi dell'endotelina sono al momento oggetto di trial clinici	Flushing, cefalea, diarrea, ipotensione, ritenzione idrica, esacerbazione dello scompenso cardiaco, anemia, incremento degli indici di funzionalità epatica, palpitazioni
Sildenafil (inibitore della fosfodiesterasi PDE_5 cGMP-specifica)	Dose di 0,5-1,0 mg/kg somministrata 3-4 volte al giorno. Dose per l'adulto 20 mg 3 volte al giorno. Inibitori della PDE_5 a più lunga durata d'azione sono al momento oggetto di trial clinici	Flushing, cefalea, diarrea, mialgie, ipotensione, priapismo, disturbi visivi (visione blu)
Calcioantagonisti (per es. diltiazem, nifedipina)	Ampiamente utilizzati in passato. Ora indicati solo per i pazienti che presentano una risposta al farmaco durante il cateterismo cardiaco (diminuzione della pressione sistolica in arteria polmonare <40 mmHg). La dose dipende dal principio attivo utilizzato	Flushing, cefalea, edema, aritmie, cefalea, ipotensione, rash, nausea, stipsi, incremento degli indici di funzionalità epatica

sc, sottocute. Nota: questi farmaci dovrebbero essere somministrati solo su indicazione di uno specialista in ipertensione polmonare.

vista radiografico, il cuore può risultare da normale a notevolmente ingrandito; quest'ultima situazione di solito si verifica tardivamente nel decorso della malattia. L'arteria polmonare principale è di solito sporgente, analogamente a quanto si verifica nell'ipertensione polmonare primitiva (vedi Fig. 433-1). I vasi polmonari, dilatati nelle zone ilari, diventano affusolati rapidamente nelle ramificazioni periferiche. Il ventricolo destro e l'atrio destro sono sporgenti. L'elettrocardiogramma evidenzia una marcata ipertrofia ventricolare destra. L'onda P può essere alta e appuntita.

L'ecocardiogramma evidenzia un ventricolo destro dalle pareti ispessite e la lesione cardiaca congenita sottostante. L'ecocardiografia bidimensionale aiuta a escludere lesioni come un'ostruzione delle vene polmonari, una membrana sovramitralica e una stenosi mitralica. L'ecocardiogramma della valvola polmonare evidenzia una caratteristica chiusura mesosistolica, il "segno della W". Il Doppler mostra la direzione dello shunt e la presenza di una tipica forma d'onda nell'arteria polmonare principale; in questa indagine il rigurgito tricuspidale e polmonare può servire per stimare la pressione arteriosa polmonare.

Il cateterismo cardiaco di solito evidenzia uno shunt bidirezionale nella sede del difetto. La pressione sistolica è generalmente uguale nelle circolazioni sistemica e polmonare. La pressione di incuneamento capillare è normale, a meno che l'ipertensione arteriosa polmonare non sia causata da una lesione ostruttiva del cuore sinistro o uno scompenso ventricolare sinistro. La saturazione arteriosa di ossigeno è diminuita, a causa della grandezza dello shunt destro-sinistro. La risposta al trattamento vasodilatatore (ossigeno, calcioantagonisti, prostaciclina, ossido nitrico) permette di identificare i pazienti con ipertensione polmonare iperdinamica. Anche se l'angiocardiografia selettiva è in grado di localizzare la sede dello shunt, di solito viene evitata in questi pazienti a causa dell'aumentato rischio connesso alla proceduta e dell'accuratezza dell'ecocardiografia. Possono essere necessarie iniezioni selettive in arteria polmonare se si sospetta un'ostruzione venosa polmonare a causa di un'elevata pressione di incuneamento e di una bassa pressione telediastolica ventricolare sinistra.

TRATTAMENTO. Per i pazienti a rischio di sviluppare una vasculopatia polmonare tardiva l'approccio migliore è la prevenzione, consistente nell'eliminazione chirurgica, durante l'infanzia, di ampie comunicazioni intracardiache o tra i grandi vasi. Alcuni pazienti possono sfuggire all'attenzione del medico non avendo presentato manifestazioni cliniche precoci. La resistenza vascolare polmonare non diminuisce mai sostanzialmente alla nascita in alcuni di questi bambini, che perciò non acquisiscono mai uno shunt sinistro-destro tale da rendersi evidente clinicamente. Un tale riconoscimento tardivo è un rischio in particolare nei soggetti con cardiopatie congenite che vivono ad altitudini elevate e nei bambini con trisomia 21, che hanno una predisposizione a uno sviluppo più precoce della vasculopatia polmonare. A causa dell'elevata incidenza di cardiopatie congenite associate alla trisomia 21, molti medici raccomandano un ecocardiogramma di routine al momento della diagnosi iniziale, anche in assenza di altri reperti clinici.

Il trattamento medico della sindrome di Eisenmenger è principalmente sintomatico (Tab. 433-3). I bambini più grandi e gli adolescenti con policitemia sintomatica possono trarre giovamento da salassi accorti e ripetuti, con rimpiazzo di volume. Trial clinici hanno descritto i benefici derivanti dall'utilizzo cronico di calcioantagonisti o dalla terapia endovenosa con prostaciclina. Il trapianto combinato cuore-polmone o di polmone bilaterale è l'unica opzione chirurgica per molti di questi pazienti (vedi Capitolo 443.2).

Barst RJ: Medical therapy of pulmonary hypertension. An overview of treatment and goals. *Clin Chest Med* 2001;22:509–515.

Cool CD, Rai PR, Yeager ME, et al: Expression of human herpesvirus 8 in primary pulmonary hypertension. *N Engl J Med* 2003;349:1113–1122.

Farber HW, Loscalzo J: Pulmonary arterial hypertension. *N Eng J Med* 2004;351:1655–1666.

Feinstein JA, Goldhaber SZ, Lock JE, et al: Balloon pulmonary angioplasty for treatment of chronic thromboembolic pulmonary hypertension. *Circulation* 2001;103:10–13.

Ford K: Pulmonary artery hypertension: New drug treatment in children. *Arch Dis Child* 2005;90:ep15–ep20.

Galié N, Ghofrani HA, Torbicki A, et al: Sildenafil citrate therapy for pulmonary arteral hypertension. *N Engl J Med* 2005;353:2148–2157.

Gammie JS, Keenan RJ, Pham SM, et al: Single- versus double-lung transplantation for pulmonary hypertension. *J Thorac Cardiovasc Surg* 1998;115:397–402.

Ghofrani HA, Wiedemann R, Rose F, et al: Sildenafil for a treatment of lung fibrosis and pulmonary hypertension: A randomized controlled trial. *Lancet* 2002;360:895–900.

Mandegar M, Thistlethwaite PA, Yuan JX: Molecular biology of primary pulmonary hypertension. *Cardiol Clin* 2004;22:417–429.

McCann UD, Seiden LS, Rubin LJ, et al: Brain serotonin neurotoxicity and primary pulmonary hypertension from fenfluramine and dexfenfluramine. A systemic review of the evidence. *JAMA* 1997;278:666–672.

McLaughlin VV, Shillington A, Rich S: Survival in primary pulmonary hypertension. The impact of epoprostenol therapy. *Circulation* 2002;106:1477–1482.

McLaughlin VV, Sitbon O, Badesch DB, et al: Survival with first-line bosentan in patients with primary pulmonary hypertension. *Eur Respir J* 2005;25:244–249.

Mikhail G, Gibbs J, Richardson M, et al: An evaluation of nebulized prostacyclin in patients with primary and secondary pulmonary hypertension. *Eur Heart J* 1997;18:1499–1504.

Newman JH, Wheeler L, Lane KB, et al: Mutation in the gene for bone morphogenetic protein receptor II as a cause of primary pulmonary hypertension in a large kindred. *N Engl J Med* 2001;345:319–324.

Widlitz A, Barst RJ: Pulmonary arterial hypertension in children. *Eur Respir J* 2003;21:155–176.

TABELLA 433-3. Complicanze extracardiache delle cardiopatie congenite cianogene e del fenomeno di Eisenmenger

PROBLEMA	EZIOLOGIA	TERAPIA
Policitemia	Ipossia persistente	Salasso
Anemia relativa	Deficit nutrizionali	Supplementazione di ferro
Ascesso del SNC	Shunt destro-sinistro	Antibiotici, drenaggio
Ictus tromboembolico del SNC	Shunt destro-sinistro o policitemia	Salasso
CID subacuta, trombocitopenia	Policitemia	Nessuna per la CID, a meno che non vi sia sanguinamento, poi salasso
Emottisi	Infarto polmonare, trombosi o rottura di una lesione plessiforme di un'arteria polmonare	Embolizzazione
Patologia gengivale	Policitemia, gengivite, sanguinamento	Igiene dentale
Gotta	Policitemia, uso di diuretici	Allopurinolo
Artrite, ippocratismo digitale	Artropatia ipossica	Nessuna
Complicanze della gravidanza: aborti, ritardo di crescita fetale, aumento della prematurità, malattie materne	Scarsa perfusione placentare, scarsa capacità di aumentare la gittata cardiaca	Riposo a letto, counseling per la prevenzione della gravidanza
Infezioni	Asplenia associata, sindrome di DiGeorge, endocardite	Antibiotici
	Polmonite fatale da RSV con ipertensione polmonare	Ribavirina; immunoglobuline anti-RSV (prevenzione)
Ritardo di crescita	Aumentato consumo di ossigeno, diminuito apporto di nutrienti	Trattamento dello scompenso cardiaco; precoce correzione del difetto; aumentato apporto calorico
Difficoltà di adattamento psicosociale	Attività limitata, aspetto cianotico, malattia cronica, numerosi ricoveri ospedalieri	Counseling

SNC: sistema nervoso centrale; CID, coagulazione intravascolare disseminata; RSV (*Respiratory Syncytial Virus*), virus respiratorio sinciziale.

Capitolo 434 ■ Principi generali di trattamento delle cardiopatie congenite

La maggior parte dei pazienti che hanno una cardiopatia congenita lieve non richiede trattamento. Il diretto interessato e i suoi genitori devono essere informati che è prevista una vita normale e che non è necessaria alcuna limitazione delle attività. Genitori iperprotettivi possono prendere a pretesto una lieve cardiopatia congenita o anche un soffio cardiaco funzionale per esercitare un eccessivo controllo sulle attività del figlio. Anche se talvolta i timori non vengono espressi apertamente, il bambino può sviluppare ansia, temendo una morte precoce o un deterioramento precoce delle capacità fisiche, specialmente quando un membro adulto della famiglia viene colpito da una cardiopatia sintomatica. Poiché i familiari possono essere tormentati dal timore inespresso di una morte precoce, occorre sottolineare la rarità di questa manifestazione in discussioni volte ad aumentare la comprensione della cardiopatia congenita del bambino. Bisogna insistere sulla differenza che intercorre tra una cardiopatia congenita e una patologia coronarica degenerativa negli adulti. Si dovrebbero incoraggiare uno stile di vita sano, comprendente una dieta ben bilanciata e "benefica per il cuore", l'esercizio fisico aerobico e l'astensione dal fumo.

Neppure i pazienti con malattia moderata o grave hanno necessità di una marcata restrizione dell'attività fisica. L'**educazione fisica** dovrebbe essere opportunamente modificata per adattarsi alle possibilità del bambino. In genere, il modo migliore per stabilire l'entità di tali modifiche è l'esecuzione del test da sforzo. Si dovrebbe sconsigliare a questi soggetti di praticare sport competitivi. Del resto, i pazienti con cardiopatia grave e scarsa tolleranza allo sforzo fisico di solito tendono ad autolimitare la propria attività. Dispnea, cefalea e affaticabilità in pazienti cianotici possono essere un segno di un aumento dell'ipossiemia e richiedere una qualche limitazione dell'attività nei casi in cui non fosse disponibile uno specifico trattamento medico o chirurgico. Si raccomanda di effettuare le **vaccinazioni di routine**, compreso il vaccino antinfluenzale; i probabili candidati al trapianto di cuore o cuore-polmone non dovrebbero ricevere vaccini vivi nel periodo immediatamente precedente il trapianto.

Anche se le infezioni batteriche andrebbero trattate aggressivamente, la presenza di una cardiopatia congenita non è un buon motivo per l'utilizzo indiscriminato di antibiotici. Si dovrebbe effettuare la profilassi contro l'endocardite batterica durante procedure odontoiatriche, durante manovre strumentali del tratto urinario e prima di procedure a carico del tratto gastrointestinale inferiore (vedi Tab. 437-2).

I pazienti cianotici devono essere monitorati per evidenziare l'eventuale presenza di manifestazioni non cardiache di mancanza di ossigeno (Tab. 434-1). Il trattamento dell'anemia ferropriva è importante in soggetti con cianosi che presentano un miglioramento della tolleranza all'esercizio fisico e del benessere generale grazie a livelli di emoglobina adeguati. Questi pazienti devono inoltre essere controllati attentamente alla ricerca di una policitemia eccessiva. Essi dovrebbero evitare situazioni in cui si possa verificare una disidratazione, che porterebbe a una maggiore viscosità e aumenterebbe il rischio di ictus. I diuretici possono essere diminuiti secondo necessità o temporaneamente sospesi durante episodi di gastroenterite acuta. Si dovrebbero evitare altitudini elevate e cambiamenti improvvisi della temperatura ambientale. Il salasso con rimpiazzo di volume andrebbe effettuato in pazienti sintomatici con grave **policitemia** (ematocrito >65%), in quanto il suo utilizzo di routine in assenza di sintomi è controverso. Pazienti con una grave cardiopatia congenita o storia di disturbi del ritmo cardiaco dovrebbero essere attentamente monitorati durante l'anestesia anche per procedure chirurgiche di routine. Le donne con gravi cardiopatie congenite non sottoposte a correzione andrebbero informate sui rischi associati a una gravidanza, sull'uso di contraccettivi o sulla legatura delle tube. Una gravidanza può essere pericolosa in presenza di cianosi cronica o ipertensione arteriosa polmonare. Donne con cardiopatie da lievi a moderate e molte pazienti che sono state sottoposte a intervento chirurgico correttivo possono avere gravidanze normali, anche se quelle con alterazioni emodinamiche residue o con ventricolo destro sistemico sarebbe auspicabile fossero seguite da un perinatologo specializzato in gravidanze ad alto rischio e da un cardiologo esperto in cardiopatie congenite dell'adulto.

GESTIONE POSTOPERATORIA. Dopo un intervento chirurgico a cuore aperto condotto con successo, influenzano il decorso del paziente la gravità della cardiopatia congenita, l'età e le condizioni (status nutrizionale) del soggetto prima dell'intervento, gli eventi in sala operatoria e la qualità del trattamento postoperatorio. I fattori intraoperatori che influiscono sulla sopravvivenza e che dovrebbero essere annotati quando il paziente torna dalla sala operatoria comprendono la durata del bypass cardiopolmonare, la durata del clampaggio aortico (il tempo in cui il cuore non è perfuso) e la durata dell'ipotermia profonda (generalmente utilizzata nei bambini: il periodo in cui l'intero corpo non è perfuso).

Le cure immediatamente successive all'intervento dovrebbero essere prestate in un reparto di terapia intensiva e affidate a un team di medici, infermieri e tecnici esperti dei problemi peculiari che si incontrano dopo un intervento chirurgico a cuore aperto. Nella maggior parte dei grandi centri, questo avviene in un reparto di terapia intensiva specializzata in cardiochirurgia pediatrica. La preparazione per il monitoraggio postoperatorio inizia in sala operatoria, dove l'anestesista o il chirurgo posiziona un catetere arterioso al fine di effettuare misure dirette della pressione arteriosa e procedere alla raccolta di campioni di sangue arterioso per l'emogasanalisi. Viene posizionato anche un catetere venoso centrale per la misurazione della pressione venosa centrale e per l'infusione di farmaci cardioattivi. Nei casi più complessi, si possono inserire cateteri direttamente in atrio sinistro o in arteria polmonare, per effettuare il monitoraggio delle pressioni. Talvolta si utilizzano cateteri flusso-diretti (di Swan-Ganz) per il monitoraggio con il metodo della termodiluizione, per controllare la pressione di incuneamento capillare e l'indice cardiaco. Cateteri per il pacing temporaneo vengono posizionati nell'atrio, nel ventricolo o in entrambi, nel caso si verificasse un blocco cardiaco temporaneo. L'ossimetria transcutanea consente il monitoraggio continuo della saturazione arteriosa di ossigeno.

Gravi alterazioni della funzionalità di un organo o apparato possono causare profondi cambiamenti fisiologici e biochimici in altri organi o apparati (vedi Tab. 434-1). L'insufficienza respiratoria, per esempio, porta all'ipossia, all'acidosi e all'ipercapnia, che a loro volta compromettono la funzione cardiaca, vascolare e renale. Questi ultimi problemi non possono essere trattati con successo fino a che non viene ristabilita un'adeguata ventilazione. Perciò è necessario che venga identificata la causa prima di ogni problema postoperatorio.

L'**insufficienza respiratoria** è una grave complicanza postoperatoria che si incontra dopo chirurgia a cuore aperto. Un bypass cardiopolmonare effettuato in presenza di congestione polmonare porta a una diminuita compliance polmonare, a copiose secrezioni tracheali e bronchiali, ad atelettasia e a un aumentato sforzo respiratorio. Data la possibilità che possano seguire rapidamente fatica respiratoria e, di conseguenza, ipoventilazione e condizione di acidosi, si può proseguire la ventilazione endotracheale meccanica a pressione positiva dopo chirurgia a cuore aperto per un minimo di qualche ora in pazienti relativamente stabili e fino a 2-3 giorni o più in pazienti critici, specialmente nei bambini piccoli. I pazienti con determinate cardiopatie congenite, in particolare quelli con sindrome di Di George, possono anche avere anomalie delle vie aeree (tracheomalacia, broncomalacia) tali da rendere l'estubazione più difficile.

Il monitoraggio elettrocardiografico dovrebbe essere continuo durante il periodo postoperatorio. Una variazione della frequenza cardiaca può essere la prima indicazione di una grave com-

TABELLA 434-1. Approccio per sistemi alle cure postoperatorie dopo un intervento chirurgico per cardiopatia congenita

SISTEMA E PROBLEMA	EZIOLOGIA	TRATTAMENTO O PREVENZIONE
SISTEMA NERVOSO CENTRALE		
Coma	Ischemia globale	Monitoraggio e trattamento dell'aumentata pressione intracranica
	Effetto anestetico prolungato	Reversione dell'anestesia
	Ipoglicemia	Glucosio
Lesioni focali	Embolia (aria, trombi)	
Convulsioni	Alterazioni metaboliche (iponatriemia, ipoglicemia), ischemiche, emboliche	Fenitoina, correzione delle alterazioni metaboliche
Paralisi del diaframma	Lesione a carico del nervo frenico	Cure respiratorie
Paralisi delle corde vocali	Trazione sul nervo laringeo ricorrente	Cure respiratorie
Sindrome di Horner	Dissezione dell'arteria succlavia con danno alla catena del simpatico	Nessuno
Paraplegia	Riparazione post-coartazione con ischemia dell'arteria spinale	Evitare l'ischemia
Dolore	Trauma chirurgico	Fentanil, morfina
Ansia	Stress	Midazolam, diazepam
APPARATO RESPIRATORIO		
Sindrome ARDS dopo circolazione extracorporea	Non nota; possibile rilascio di sostanze vasoattive da bypass cardiopolmonare	PEEP, ventilazione meccanica, ossigeno
Edema polmonare	Scompenso cardiaco, ostruzioni del cuore sinistro, sovraccarico di fluidi	Diuretici, PEEP, ventilazione meccanica, agenti inotropi
Versamenti pleurici	Emotorace	Toracentesi
	Versamento sieroso precoce	Toracentesi
	Sindrome post-pericardiotomica ritardata	Farmaci antinfiammatori
Chilotorace	Lesione a carico del dotto toracico	Digiuno o dieta con trigliceridi a catena media
		Raramente, legatura chirurgica del dotto toracico
Atelettasia	Ipoventilazione, ridotta capacità di tossire	Fisioterapia toracica, PEEP
Polmonite	Aspirazione, nosocomiale, batteriemia	Identificare la causa batterica o virale (virus respiratorio sinciziale); terapia antimicrobica specifica
Ipertensione polmonare	Riparazione di TAVPR, primo stadio di Norwood, trisomia 21; ipertensione polmonare preesistente all'intervento chirurgico	Iperventilazione, iperossigenazione, ossido nitrico, ECMO
Stridore respiratorio	Edema delle corde vocali, paralisi delle corde vocali	Steroidi, raramente tracheotomia
APPARATO CARDIOVASCOLARE		
Bradicardia, sindrome del seno malato, blocco atrioventricolare	Danno al sistema di conduzione interatriale o interventricolare	Atropina, isoproterenolo, pacemaker
Blocco di branca destra	Ventricolotomia destra	Approccio atriale per la riparazione di un difetto del setto interventricolare o della tetralogia di Fallot
Tachiaritmie	Tachicardia sopraventricolare, giunzionale	Farmaci antiaritmici
	Tachicardia ventricolare	Defibrillazione, farmaci antiaritmici
Bassa gittata cardiaca	Cardiogena – ventricolotomia destra o "stordimento" cardiaco (prolungata circolazione extracorporea o lungo tempo di clampaggio) o infarto	Agenti inotropi, supporto al precarico, riduzione del postcarico, dispositivi di assistenza al ventricolo sinistro, ECMO
Tamponamento cardiaco	Versamento pericardico, emorragia acuta	Pericardiocentesi
	Sindrome sierosa post-pericardiotomica	Farmaci antinfiammatori
Ipertensione	Stress o dolore	Analgesia
	Sindrome post-coartectomia	Nitroprussiato
Arterite mesenterica	Sindrome post-coartectomia	Digiuno, nitroprussiato
SISTEMA RENALE-METABOLICO		
Oliguria prerenale	Ipovolemia	Somministrazione di fluidi
	Bassa gittata cardiaca	Agenti inotropi
Insufficienza renale	Ipotensione, circolazione extracorporea prolungata – tempo di clampaggio prolungato, necrosi tubulare acuta	Miglioramento della pressione sanguigna, diuretici, dialisi
Edema	Somministrazione di elevate quantità di fluidi, perdite dai capillari, bassa gittata cardiaca, pressione venosa sistemica elevata	Diuretici, agenti inotropi
Iponatriemia	Sindrome da diluizione per inappropriata secrezione di AHD	Restrizione di fluidi
	Diuretici	Restrizione di fluidi
Iperglicemia	Ipotermia, inibizione dell'insulina	Nessuna terapia necessaria (di solito), insulina
Ipoglicemia	Rebound dopo iperglicemia, insufficienza epatica	Infusione di glucosio
SISTEMA EMATOLOGICO		
Emorragia	Valori anomali di PT e PTT, trombocitopenia	Correzione della coagulopatia
	Perdita chirurgica	Reintervento, sutura
Trombosi dello shunt	Bassa gittata cardiaca, ipovolemia	Fluidi, eparina, reintervento
Anemia (che di solito rispecchia un ridotto volume di sangue)	Emorragia, emolisi	Trasfusione di emazie concentrate
Reazione del trapianto verso l'ospite (graft versus host disease)	Infusione di leucociti vivi in pazienti con sindrome di Di George	Emoderivati irradiati
MALATTIE INFETTIVE		
Infezione delle ferita (cutanea, costocondrale, sternotomia, mediastinite, accessi vascolari, drenaggi toracici)	Contaminazione in sala operatoria	Antibiotici
Endocardite	*Staphylococcus epidermidis*, *Corynebacterium*, contaminazione in sala operatoria	Antibiotici
Cistite, pielonefrite	Contaminazione di catetere urinario a dimora	Antibiotici, rimozione del catetere
Epatite	Da contatto con sangue infetto: Cytomegalovirus, virus di Epstein-Barr, virus dell'epatite B e C	Controllo degli emoderivati
Sindrome postperfusionale (febbre, epatosplenomegalia, linfociti atipici, linfoadenopatia, rash transitorio)	Cytomegalovirus, virus di Epstein-Barr	Controllo degli emoderivati
PROBLEMI PSICOSOCIALI		
Ansia, separazione	Legate all'età, paura ecc.	Prontezza nel seguire il paziente (videocassette, teatrino); visite da parte dei genitori, sedazione

ARDS (*Acute Respiratory Distress Syndrome*), sindrome da distress respiratorio acuto; ECMO (*ExtraCorporeal Membrane Oxygenation*), ossigenazione mediante membrana extracorporea; PEEP (*Positive End-Expiratory Pressure*), pressione positiva di fine espirazione; PT (*Prothrombin Time*), tempo di protrombina; PTT (*Partial Thromboplastin Time*), tempo di tromboplastina parziale; TAPVR (*Total Anomalous Pulmonary Venous Return*), ritorno venoso polmonare anomalo totale.

plicanza, come un'emorragia, l'ipotermia, un'ipoventilazione o uno scompenso cardiaco. I **disturbi del ritmo cardiaco** devono essere diagnosticati rapidamente, poiché un'aritmia prolungata non trattata può imporre al cuore un carico gravoso dal punto di vista emodinamico nel primo periodo postoperatorio, che rappresenta un momento critico (vedi Capitolo 435). Un danno al sistema di conduzione del cuore durante l'intervento chirurgico può portare a un blocco cardiaco completo nel postoperatorio. Questa complicanza, di solito temporanea, viene trattata con cateteri per pacing posizionati chirurgicamente, che in seguito possono essere rimossi. Talvolta il blocco cardiaco completo è permanente. Se il blocco cardiaco persiste per più di 10-14 giorni dopo l'intervento, è richiesto il posizionamento di un pacemaker definitivo. Le tachiaritmie sono un problema più comune nei pazienti appena operati. La tachicardia ectopica giunzionale può essere un disturbo del ritmo particolarmente difficile da trattare (vedi Capitolo 435), anche se di solito risponde alla somministrazione endovenosa di amiodarone.

Lo **scompenso cardiaco** con bassa gittata cardiaca (vedi Tab. 434-1) dopo chirurgia cardiaca può essere secondario a insufficienza respiratoria, gravi aritmie, danno miocardico, perdite ematiche, ipo- o ipervolemia, oppure ancora a una significativa anomalia emodinamica residua. Dovrebbe essere istituito un trattamento specifico a seconda della causa. Catecolamine, inibitori della fosfodiesterasi, nitroprussiato e altri agenti che riducono il postcarico e diuretici sono i farmaci cardioattivi più utilizzati in pazienti con disfunzione miocardica nel primo periodo postoperatorio (vedi Capitolo 442). L'ipertensione polmonare postoperatoria può essere trattata con l'iperventilazione e l'inalazione di ossido nitrico. Per coloro che non rispondono al trattamento farmacologico standard sono disponibili vari dispositivi di assistenza ventricolare, a seconda della corporatura del paziente. Se la funzione polmonare è adeguata, si può utilizzare un dispositivo di sostegno alla funzione ventricolare sinistra; in caso contrario, si può ricorrere all'ossigenazione mediante membrana extracorporea (ECMO, *ExtraCorporeal Membrane Oxygenation*). Queste misure straordinarie sono utili per mantenere la circolazione fino al miglioramento della funzione cardiaca, che si verifica di solito nel giro di 2-3 giorni. Inoltre, sono state utilizzate con un certo successo come "ponte" verso il trapianto in pazienti con scompenso cardiaco intrattabile postoperatorio.

L'acidosi secondaria a bassa gittata cardiaca, l'insufficienza renale o l'ipovolemia devono essere prevenute o prontamente corrette. Viene effettuato un monitoraggio seriato dell'emogasanalisi e delle concentrazioni di lattato. Un pH $<7,3$ può portare alla diminuzione della gittata cardiaca con un aumento della produzione di acido lattico e preludere a una serie di aritmie o ad arresto cardiaco.

Una **funzione renale** già ridotta a causa di uno scompenso cardiaco congestizio può essere ulteriormente compromessa da un bypass cardiopolmonare (vedi Tab. 434-1). Il rimpiazzo di sangue e di fluidi, gli agenti cardiaci inotropi e, talvolta, vasodilatatori di solito ristabiliscono il normale flusso urinario in pazienti con ipovolemia o scompenso cardiaco. La dopamina è un agente inotropo utile, perché aumenta direttamente anche il flusso sanguigno renale. Un'insufficienza renale secondaria a danno tubulare può richiedere una dialisi peritoneale o un'emofiltrazione temporanea.

Anomalie neurologiche possono svilupparsi dopo un bypass cardiopolmonare, specialmente nel periodo neonatale. Quando il paziente si sveglia dalla sedazione possono insorgere convulsioni, di solito controllabili con la somministrazione di fenitoina o fenobarbital. In assenza di altri segni neurologici, convulsioni isolate nell'immediato periodo postoperatorio di solito sono associate a una buona prognosi. Eventi tromboembolici e ictus sono rare ma gravi complicanze di interventi chirurgici a cuore aperto. A lungo termine, possono svilupparsi disturbi dell'apprendimento sia lievi sia più sostanziali. I bambini che sono stati sottoposti a una procedura chirurgica comprendente l'esecuzione di un bypass cardiopolmonare, specialmente nel periodo neonatale, dovrebbero essere seguiti con attenzione nei primi anni di scuola per evidenziare eventuali disturbi dell'apprendimento, che sono spesso correggibili con un intervento precoce. Il rischio è maggiore in pazienti che sono stati sottoposti a riparazione con arresto circolatorio totale in ipotermia.

La **sindrome postpericardiotomica** può verificarsi verso la fine della prima settimana postoperatoria o manifestarsi a distanza di settimane o mesi dall'intervento chirurgico. Questa malattia febbrile è caratterizzata da febbre, calo dell'appetito, torpore, nausea e vomito. Poiché il dolore toracico non sempre è presente, occorre mantenere un elevato indice di sospetto in qualsiasi paziente operato di recente. L'ecocardiografia è diagnostica. Nella maggior parte dei casi, la sindrome post-pericardiotomica si autolimita; tuttavia, quando il fluido pericardico si accumula rapidamente, bisogna tener conto del potenziale pericolo rappresentato da un tamponamento cardiaco (vedi Capitolo 440). Seppure raramente, possono verificarsi aritmie. I pazienti sintomatici di solito rispondono ai salicilati o all'indometacina e al riposo a letto. Talvolta si rendono necessarie una terapia steroidea o la pericardiocentesi. Possono verificarsi delle recidive tardive, che però sono meno frequenti.

Dopo la riparazione di alcuni difetti cardiaci, per esempio a carico del setto atrioventricolare, o dopo l'inserimento di una protesi valvolare meccanica, è raro osservare un'emolisi di origine meccanica, dovuta a un'insolita turbolenza di sangue ad alta pressione. Un reintervento può essere necessario nei rari casi di pazienti con grave e progressiva emolisi che richiedono frequenti trasfusioni di sangue, ma il più delle volte il problema regredisce lentamente.

Le infezioni sono un altro grave problema postoperatorio. Di solito si somministra un antibiotico ad ampio spetto nel primo periodo postoperatorio. Siti potenziali di infezione sono i polmoni (generalmente in relazione a un'atelettasia postoperatoria), i tessuti sottocutanei nel sito di incisione, lo sterno e il tratto urinario (specialmente dopo posizionamento di un catetere a dimora). La sepsi con endocardite infettiva è una complicanza non frequente, ma che può essere difficile da trattare (vedi Capitolo 437).

Booth KL, Roth SJ, Thiagarajan RR, et al: Extracorporeal membrane oxygenation support of the Fontan and bidirectional Glenn circulations. *Ann Thorac Surg* 2004;77:1341–1348.

Dunbar-Masterson C, Wypij D, Bellinger DC, et al: General health status of children with D-transposition of the great arteries after the arterial switch operation. *Circulation* 2001;104(Suppl 1):I138–I142.

Hoffman TM, Bush DM, Wernovsky G, et al: Postoperative junctional ectopic tachycardia in children: Incidence, risk factors, and treatment. *Ann Thorac Surg* 2002;74:1607–1611.

Hoffman TM, Wernovsky G, Atz AM, et al: Efficacy and safety of milrinone in preventing low cardiac output syndrome in infants and children after corrective surgery for congenital heart disease. *Circulation* 2003; 107:996–1002.

Limperopoulos C, Majnemer A, Shevell MI, et al: Predictors of developmental disabilities after open heart surgery in young children with congenital heart defects. *J Pediatr* 2002;141:51–58.

Limperopoulos C, Majnemer A, Shevell MI, et al: Functional limitations in young children with congenital heart defects after cardiac surgery. *Pediatrics* 2001;108:1325–1331.

Mou SS, Giroir BP, Molitor-Kirsch EA, et al: Fresh whole blood versus reconstituted blood for pump priming in heart surgery in infants. *N Engl J Med* 2004;351:1635–1644.

Nieminen H, Sairanen H, Tikanoja T, et al: Long-term results of pediatric cardiac surgery in Finland: Education, employment, marital status, and parenthood. *Pediatrics* 2003;112:1345–1350.

Ravishankar C, Tabbutt S, Wernovsky G: Critical care in cardiovascular medicine. *Curr Opin Pediatr* 2003;15:443–453.

Todd JL, Todd NW: Conotruncal cardiac anomalies and otitis media. *J Pediatr* 1997;131:215–219.

Visconti KJ, Bichell DP, Jonas RA, et al: Developmental outcome after surgical versus interventional closure of secundum atrial septal defect in children. *Circulation* 1999;100(Suppl):II145–II150.

Wernovsky G, Stiles KM, Gauvreau K, et al: Cognitive development after the Fontan operation. *Circulation* 2000;102:883–889.

434.1 • Il paziente adulto con cardiopatia congenita • Daniel Murphy

Lo straordinario successo della riparazione chirurgica dei difetti cardiaci congeniti ha migliorato notevolmente la prognosi dei bambini con una cardiopatia congenita. Prima dell'avvento della riparazione chirurgica, più del 50% di essi moriva prima di raggiungere l'età adulta. Ora possono esservi più adulti che bambini viventi con cardiopatia congenita negli Stati Uniti, e il loro numero è destinato ad aumentare, grazie al miglioramento dei risultati della chirurgia. Via via che è aumentato il numero delle persone adulte affette da cardiopatia congenita, è sorta una nuova sottospecialità a cui afferiscono la cardiologia pediatrica, la medicina interna a indirizzo cardiologico e le discipline chirurgiche cardiovascolari. Gli esperti cardiovascolari nazionali e internazionali, riconoscendo le esigenze peculiari di questa popolazione di pazienti, hanno pubblicato una serie di raccomandazioni riguardanti la formazione dei medici, la regionalizzazione delle cure, il follow-up e altri argomenti pertinenti.

Tutti i pazienti nati con difetti cardiaci congeniti richiedono sia cure mediche di base sia un follow-up cardiaco di routine. La coordinazione delle cure tra chi assicura quelle di primo livello e chi fornisce quelle specialistiche è particolarmente importante durante l'adolescenza, a causa dell'insorgenza di nuovi problemi medici e sociali che influiscono sulle cure mediche.

RUOLO DEL PEDIATRA

Alla pari dei soggetti con patologie croniche che necessitano di cure mediche per tutta la vita, gli adolescenti con cardiopatia congenita dovrebbero avere accesso a una "Medical Home", come definita dalla "Medical Home Policy Statement" dell'AAP. Alcuni aspetti della Medical Home sono importanti per la popolazione di adolescenti con cardiopatia congenita, soprattutto per coloro che soffrono di problemi medici multipli. Nella Tabella 434.2 sono elencati alcuni esempi di problemi che possono insorgere nei pazienti con cardiopatia congenita, richiedendo un coordinamento delle cure.

Una buona forma fisica e l'attività fisica sono in genere raccomandati per tutti i pazienti. Tuttavia, alcuni pazienti devono sottostare ad alcune limitazioni, relative a sport competitivi e ad attività aerobiche molto intense. Esistono documenti pubblicati che riassumono il consenso dell'opinione medica riguardo alla partecipazioni ad attività atletiche competitive (vedi Capitolo 685). Queste raccomandazioni fungono da punto di partenza per un dialogo tra chi fornisce le cure mediche di base, lo specialista cardiologo e il paziente. La partecipazione ad attività atletiche competitive non dovrebbe essere approvata senza una preventiva raccomandazione in tal senso da parte del cardiologo.

Come sempre dovrebbe avvenire quando il paziente è un adolescente, le questioni della contraccezione e della gravidanza vanno affrontate all'età appropriata e nel contesto più adatto. Per alcuni pazienti con cardiopatia congenita, determinati metodi contraccettivi potrebbero essere preferibili ad altri, come l'evitare l'utilizzo di dispositivi intrauterini a causa del rischio aumentato di endocardite infettiva. Anche se per la maggior parte delle giovani donne con cardiopatia congenita è possibile portare a termine con successo una gravidanza, vi sono patologie, come le cardiopatie congenite con cianosi persistente o l'ipertensione polmonare, in cui i rischi associati alla gestazione risultano significativamente aumentati (Tab. 434-3). Oltre alla lesione cardiaca originaria e alla storia chirurgica, eventi cardiaci precedenti, una bassa classe funzionale o una disfunzione ventricolare possono essere tutti criteri utili per prevedere la prognosi materna e neonatale. Per molte donne con cardiopatia congenita una gravidanza è possibile, ma comporta maggiori rischi e richiede una programmazione preconcezionale e/o una valutazione e una sorveglianza molto accurate durante la gestazione. La consulenza anticipata e l'educazione delle pazienti sono aspetti chiave da tenere presenti quando si consigliano le adolescenti in merito alla contraccezione e alla gravidanza.

Il medico di base dovrebbe tenere un archivio centrale facilmente accessibile ed esauriente, che contenga tutte le informazioni pertinenti riguardo al bambino, salvaguardandone la privacy. In preparazione alla transizione dell'adolescenza all'età adulta, l'archivio medico deve accompagnare il paziente nel trasferimento al nuovo luogo dove questi riceverà le cure mediche. Il medico coordinatore dovrebbe inoltre trasmettere i report del medico di base e dei sottospecialisti ad altri sanitari, al paziente e alla sua famiglia. Il processo di condivisione delle informazioni mediche è essenziale per evitare che più specialisti lavorino in modo indipendente, senza essere a conoscenza dell'attività l'uno dell'altro. Il coinvolgimento del paziente e della sua famiglia e la loro educazione sono una garanzia contro il frazionamento delle cure mediche.

PASSAGGIO DALL'ADOLESCENZA ALL'ETÀ ADULTA

Oltre a una coerente gestione medica di base, la Medical Home policy raccomanda che "le transizioni, compresa quella verso l'età adulta, siano programmate e organizzate con il bambino e la famiglia". La realizzazione di questo aspetto della Medical Home richiede una programmazione della transizione verso la gestione medica per adulti e l'identificazione dei professionisti che si occuperanno dell'assistenza sia di base sia cardiologica. Il processo dovrebbe essere intrapreso dal pediatra in collaborazione con il cardiologo pediatrico che ha in carico il caso. Ormai è generalmente riconosciuto che, nel contesto dell'acquisizione dell'indipendenza, adolescenti e giovani adulti debbano imparare ad affrontare i propri problemi medici con lungimiranza e autonomia di giudizio. Per i cardiopatici in età pediatrica, il processo di transizione deve iniziare nella prima adolescenza e dovrebbe essere incoraggiato sia dal medico di base sia dal cardiologo pediatrico, ai quali spetta individuare un appropriato programma

TABELLA 434-2. Aspetti che richiedono una coordinazione delle cure tra il cardiologo e il medico di base

Profilassi antibiotica per l'endocardite
Farmaci e interazioni farmacologiche
Anticoagulazione in presenza di protesi valvolari
Esercizio fisico e partecipazione all'attività sportiva
Programmazione dell'istruzione e della formazione professionale
Contraccezione e gravidanza
Uso di droghe, consumo di alcol e tabacco
Programmazione di interventi chirurgici non cardiaci
Problemi riguardanti l'anestesia
Nuovi sintomi o malattie acute
Problemi medici coesistenti
Viaggi

TABELLA 434-3. Rischi connessi a specifiche lesioni che la madre o il feto sviluppino complicanze in gravidanza

Nessun rischio aggiunto	Piccoli difetti settali
	ASD, VSD e PDA chiusi chirurgicamente
	Rigurgito aortico da lieve a moderato
	Stenosi polmonare da lieve a moderata
Rischio lievemente aumentato	Dopo riparazione chirurgica della tetralogia di Fallot
	Trasposizione delle grandi arterie, dopo procedura di switch arterioso
Rischio moderato	Trasposizione delle grandi arterie, dopo procedura di switch atriale
	Trasposizione congenitamente corretta delle grandi arterie
	Ventricolo unico, dopo procedura di Fontan
Rischio elevato	Cardiopatie congenite con cianosi non operate o sottoposte a palliazione
	Sindrome di Marfan
	Protesi valvolari
	Lesioni ostruttive, compresa la coartazione
Gravidanza controindicata	Grave ipertensione polmonare
	Gravi lesioni ostruttive
	Sindrome di Marfan, radice aortica >40 mm

ASD (*Atrial Septal Defect*), difetto del setto interatriale; PDA (*Patent Ductus Arteriosus*), dotto arterioso pervio; VSD (*Ventricular Septal Defect*), difetto del setto interventricolare.

per adulti con cardiopatie congenite verso cui possa essere effettuata la transizione nel momento opportuno.

Un processo di transizione condotto con successo comprende i seguenti elementi.

- **Sviluppo di un programma di transizione scritto, che dovrebbe iniziare entro e non oltre i 14 anni di età.**
- **Poiché gli adolescenti e i giovani adulti sono spesso all'oscuro dei dettagli della propria diagnosi e anamnesi cardiaca, un record medico completo, conciso e portatile, che contenga tutti gli aspetti pertinenti delle cure cardiache, dovrebbe essere messo a disposizione degli adolescenti e delle loro famiglie, e pronto per essere trasmesso alla destinazione finale dove il paziente diventato adulto riceverà le cure mediche.**
- **Il medico di base e il cardiologo devono tenere presenti i problemi medici peculiari dell'adolescenza nel momento in cui hanno ripercussioni sull'apparato cardiovascolare. Oltre ai problemi medici, andrebbero discussi con gli adolescenti e le loro famiglie l'istruzione, la programmazione della formazione professionale, argomenti di interesse psicosociale e problemi riguardanti l'accesso alle cure mediche.**

Anche se la maggior parte degli adolescenti e dei giovani adulti nati con difetti cardiaci congeniti completi viene sottoposta a "riparazione" chirurgica durante l'infanzia, è raro che tali individui "guariscano" dall'anomalia cardiaca sottostante. In realtà questa popolazione di pazienti deve affrontare un gran numero di residui e sequele che causano svariati problemi medici durante la vita adulta (Tab. 434-4). È perciò indispensabile riconoscere la necessità di portare avanti cure mediche di base con costanza e un follow-up cardiaco durante tutta l'adolescenza e fino alla prima età adulta. I giovani adulti hanno la tendenza a sottrarsi alle cure mediche a causa di una mancanza di educazione, di una reazione psicologica di negazione della propria malattia o di difficoltà di accesso al sistema sanitario. Perciò un obiettivo critico del processo di transizione consiste nell'identificare la sede appropriata dove il paziente possa proseguire le cure mediche e nell'assicurare la redazione dei record medici e la continuità delle cure per il giovane adulto. I giovani adulti affetti da cardiopatia congenita possono essere curati nell'ambito di un programma o una struttura medica pediatrica, oppure in un centro specializzato per adulti con cardiopatie congenite. I problemi critici sono la continuità delle cure, la preparazione del paziente e il suo coinvolgimento in questo iter.

TABELLA 434-4. Rischi per individui adulti con cardiopatia congenita

DISTURBI DEL RITMO
Tachicardia sopraventricolare
Blocco di branca destra
Blocco cardiaco
Tachicardia ventricolare
Morte improvvisa
COARTAZIONE AORTICA
Ipertensione essenziale
Recidiva della coartazione
Formazione di aneurisma
LESIONI RESIDUE (SHUNT)
VSD
ASD
PDA
LESIONI ACQUISITE
Endocardite batterica subacuta
Stenosi sottovalvolare
Stenosi sopravalvolare
Insufficienza valvolare
Restenosi valvolare
COMPLESSO DI EISENMENGER
RISCHIO LEGATO ALLA GRAVIDANZA
Vedi Tabella 434-3

ASD (*Atrial Septal Defect*), difetto del setto interatriale; PDA (*Patent Ductus Arteriosus*), dotto arterioso pervio; VSD (*Ventricular Septal Defect*), difetto del setto interventricolare.

American Academy of Pediatrics: Medical Home Initiatives for Children with Special Needs Project Advisory Committee. Policy statement: The Medical Home. *Pediatrics* 2004;113:1545–1547.

American Academy of Pediatrics: A consensus statement of health care transitions for young adults with special health care needs. *Pediatrics* 2002;110:1304–1306.

Deanfield J, Thaulow E, Warnes C, et al: Management of grown up congenital heart disease. *Eur Heart J* 2003;24:1035–1084.

Maron BJ, Zipes DP: 36th Bethesda Conference: Eligibility recommendations for competitive athletes with cardiovascular abnormalities. *J Am Coll Cardiol* 2005;45:1313–1375.

Perloff JK, Warnes CA: Challenges posed by adults with repaired congenital heart disease. *Circulation* 2001;103:2637–2643.

Siu SC, Sermer M, Colman JM, et al: Prospective multicenter study of pregnancy outcomes in women with heart disease. *Circulation* 2001;104:515–521.

Therrien J, Webb G: Clinical update on adults with congenital heart disease. *Lancet* 2003;362:1305–1313.

Tong EM, Kools S: Health care transitions for adolescents with congenital heart disease: Patient and family perspectives. *Nurs Clin North Am* 2004;39:727–740.

Webb GD, Williams RG: 32nd Bethesda Conference: Care of the adult with congenital heart disease. *J Am Coll Cardiol* 2001;37:1161–1198.

Sezione 4 — Aritmie cardiache — Anne Dubin

Capitolo 435 ■ Disturbi della frequenza e del ritmo cardiaco

Le aritmie pediatriche possono essere transitorie o permanenti, congenite (in un cuore strutturalmente normale o anomalo) o acquisite (febbre reumatica, miocardite), causate da una tossina (difterica) o da farmaci proaritmici o antiaritmici. Possono essere sequele di una correzione chirurgica di una cardiopatia congenita, il risultato di malattie metaboliche congenite dei mitocondri o causate da un'infiammazione fetale come nel lupus eritematoso sistemico materno (LES). Il principale rischio di qualsiasi aritmia è che insorga una grave forma di tachicardia o bradicardia, con conseguente diminuzione della gittata cardiaca o degenerazione in un'aritmia più pericolosa come la fibrillazione ventricolare. Queste complicanze possono portare a sincopi, già di per sé potenzialmente pericolose in determinate circostante (nuotando, guidando), o alla morte improvvisa. Quando un paziente ha un'aritmia, è di vitale importanza stabilire se questo particolare ritmo sarà incline a degenerare in una tachiaritmia o una bradiaritmia tali da mettere a repentaglio la vita del paziente. Alcune anomalie del ritmo, come battiti prematuri atriali e ventricolari isolati, sono comuni in bambini non affetti da alcuna patologia cardiaca e nella vasta maggioranza dei casi non rappresentano alcun rischio per il paziente.

Per il trattamento delle aritmie negli adulti si hanno a disposizione numerosi e potenti agenti farmacologici, molti dei quali non sono stati studiati in modo approfondito nei bambini. Rimangono interrogativi in merito alla frequenza di somministrazione, alla compliance, agli effetti collaterali, alle interazioni farmacologiche e alla variabilità della risposta, e la scelta di un farmaco appropriato è in parte empirica. Fortunatamente, la maggior parte dei disturbi del ritmo nei bambini può essere controllata in modo affidabile con un singolo farmaco (Tab. 435-1). L'ablazione transcatetere con radiofrequenze è utilizzata non solo per le tachiaritmie resistenti ma anche per il trattamento elettivo definitivo delle aritmie. In presenza di bradiaritmia, i pacemaker impiantabili sono abbastanza piccoli da essere utilizzabili anche nei prematuri. I defibrillatori-cardioversori impiantabili (ICD, *Implantable Cardioverter-Defibrillators*) sono disponibili per l'utilizzo in pazienti con aritmie ventricolari maligne e alto rischio di morte improvvisa.

435.1 • Principi di terapia antiaritmica

Quando si prende in considerazione una terapia farmacologica nella popolazione pediatrica, è importante tenere presente che vi sono notevoli differenze nella farmacocinetica nei bambini rispetto alla popolazione adulta. I bambini hanno un sistema di assorbimento immaturo, un lento svuotamento gastrico e dimensioni diverse dei compartimenti tissutali in relazione ai farmaci, il che influisce sul volume di distribuzione. Il metabolismo epatico e l'escrezione renale possono essere molto diversi nelle varie popolazioni pediatriche (neonati prematuri e a termine, lattanti, bambini, adolescenti), come anche rispetto agli adulti. Nel considerare una terapia antiaritmica in particolare, è importante rendersi conto che il substrato alla base dell'aritmia è estremamente diverso nei pazienti pediatrici e nella popolazione adulta, e che sono implicati meccanismi differenti.

Sono numerosi i farmaci antiaritmici disponibili per il controllo del ritmo, ma la maggior parte di essi non è stata approvata dalla Food and Drug Administration statunitense (FDA) per l'uso pediatrico. I cardiologi pediatrici hanno testato questi farmaci, tuttavia, e vi sono delle linee guida relativamente ben riconosciute riguardanti dosaggio, sicurezza ed efficacia.

Da quando si sono rese disponibili procedure di ablazione potenzialmente curative, la terapia medica è divenuta più complicata: i medici sono meno disposti a tollerare gli effetti collaterali e si aspettano una più elevata efficacia dei farmaci. Effetti collaterali inaccettabili, oltre al potenziale proaritmico, possono rappresentare gravi limiti alla terapia medica e porteranno il medico e la famiglia verso una procedura di ablazione potenzialmente curativa.

Gli antiaritmici vengono comunemente classificati secondo il sistema di Vaughan Williams, comprendente quattro classi: la classe I è costituita da farmaci che bloccano i canali del sodio, la classe II dai β-bloccanti, la classe III da agenti che bloccano la ripolarizzazione e la classe IV da farmaci calcioantagonisti. La classe I è suddivisa in sottoclassi in base alla dipendenza dall'uso e ai cambiamenti nell'elettrocardiogramma (ECG) (vedi Tab. 435-1).

435.2 • Aritmie sinusali ed extrasistoli

L'**aritmia sinusale** rappresenta una normale variazione fisiologica nella scarica di impulsi dal nodo del seno in relazione al ciclo respiratorio. La frequenza cardiaca diminuisce durante l'espirazione e accelera durante l'inspirazione. A volte, se la frequenza sinusale diventa abbastanza lenta, insorge un battito di scappamento dalla regione della giunzione atrioventricolare (AV) (Fig. 435-1). Irregolarità nel ritmo cardiaco, e in particolare una bradicardia associata ad apnea periodica, sono di comune riscontro nei prematuri. L'aritmia sinusale è accentuata durante le malattie febbrili e aggravata da farmaci che aumentano il tono vagale; di solito scompare durante l'attività fisica.

La **bradicardia sinusale** è dovuta a una lenta scarica di impulsi dal nodo del seno. Rientra in questa definizione una frequenza sinusale <90 battiti/min nei neonati e <60 battiti/min nelle età successive. È un reperto comune negli atleti ben allenati; negli individui sani è priva di significato. Una bradicardia sinusale può insorgere in corso di malattie sistemiche, per esempio nel mixedema, e si risolve quando la malattia è sotto controllo. È importante distinguerla dal blocco senoatriale o AV. I bambini con bradicardia sinusale sono in grado di aumentare la loro frequenza cardiaca con l'esercizio fino a valori molto elevati, pari a 100 battiti/min, mentre i pazienti con blocco AV di solito non hanno questa capacità. I bambini con basso peso alla nascita presentano ampie variazioni nella frequenza sinusale. La bradicardia sinusale è comune in questi soggetti, in associazione ad apnea, e può essere associata a battiti di scappamento giunzionali. Sono frequenti anche contrazioni atriali premature. Queste variazioni del ritmo cardiaco, soprattutto la bradicardia, compaiono più comunemente durante il sonno e non sono associate a sintomi. Di solito non è necessaria alcuna terapia.

La **sindrome da pacemaker atriale migrante** (Fig. 435-2) è definita come uno spostamento intermittente del segnapassi cardiaco dal nodo senoatriale a un'altra parte dell'atrio. Non è infrequente nell'infanzia e di solito rappresenta una variante normale, ma si può osservare anche in pazienti con disturbi del sistema nervoso centrale, per esempio un'emorragia subaracnoidea.

Le **extrasistoli** sono prodotte da una scarica proveniente da un focus ectopico, che può essere situato in qualsiasi sede a livello del tessuto atriale, giunzionale o ventricolare. Di solito extrasistoli isolate non hanno alcun significato clinico o prognostico. In determinate circostanze, tuttavia, battiti prematuri possono essere dovuti a una patologia cardiaca organica (infiammazione, ischemia o fibrosi) o a tossicità da farmaci, specialmente da digitale.

I **complessi atriali prematuri** sono comuni nell'infanzia, anche in assenza di una patologia cardiaca. A seconda del grado di prematurità del battito (intervallo di accoppiamento) e dell'intervallo R-R precedente (lunghezza del ciclo), i complessi atriali prematuri possono portare a complessi QRS normali, prolungati (aberranza) o assenti (complesso atriale prematuro bloccato). Quest'ultimo caso si verifica quando l'impulso prematuro è condotto al ventricolo mentre il sistema specializzato di conduzione ventricolare è parzialmente refrattario (Fig. 435-3). Le extrasistoli atriali devono essere distinte dai complessi ventricolari prematuri (PVC, *Premature Ventricular Complexes*). Per la diagnosi è essenziale un'accurata ricerca nell'elettrocardiogramma di un'onda P prematura che precede il QRS, la quale ha un aspetto diverso da quello di altre onde P sinusali. I complessi atriali prematuri spesso resettano il segnapassi del nodo del seno (mancanza di una pausa compensatoria), ma questa caratteristica non è considerata un metodo affidabile per differenziare i complessi prematuri atriali da quelli ventricolari.

I **PVC**, che possono insorgere in qualsiasi zona dei ventricoli, consistono in complessi QRS prematuri, allargati, bizzarri, che non sono preceduti da un'onda P (Fig. 435-4). Quando tutti i battiti prematuri hanno una forma identica, sono classificati come di origine unifocale. Quando le PVC variano di forma, sono definite multifocali. Le extrasistoli ventricolari sono spesso (ma non sempre) seguite da una pausa compensatoria. La presenza di battiti di fusione, ossia complessi con caratteristiche morfologiche intermedie tra quelle dei normali battiti sinusali e quelle dei PVC, è un indizio dell'origine ventricolare dell'extrasistole. Le extrasistoli producono una gittata sistolica e un polso inferiori al normale e, se abbastanza premature, possono non essere udibili con uno stetoscopio o palpabili al polso radiale. Se frequenti, le extrasistoli possono assumere un ritmo definito, per esempio in alternanza a battiti normali (**bigeminismo**) o un'extrasistole dopo due battiti normali (**trigeminismo**). La maggior parte dei pazienti non percepisce contrazioni ventricolari premature isolate, anche se alcuni possono avvertire la "mancanza di un battito" in regione precordiale. Questa sensazione è dovuta all'aumentata gittata sistolica del battito normale dopo una pausa compensatoria. L'ansia, una malattia febbrile o l'ingestione di vari farmaci o stimolanti possono causare battiti ventricolari prematuri.

È importante distinguere i PVC benigni da quelli che hanno una probabilità di degenerare in aritmie più gravi. I primi di solito

TABELLA 435-1. Farmaci antiaritmici comunemente utilizzati nei pazienti pediatrici, divisi per classe di appartenenza

FARMACO	INDICAZIONI	POSOLOGIA	EFFETTI COLLATERALI	INTERAZIONI FARMACOLOGICHE	RANGE TERAPEUTICO
CLASSE IA: INIBITORI DEI CANALI RAPIDI DEL NA$^+$, CHE PROLUNGANO LA RIPOLARIZZAZIONE					
Chinidina	SVT, fibrillazione atriale, flutter atriale, VT, blocco nodale AV (digossina, verapamil, propranololo); deve essere somministrata per prima onde prevenire una conduzione 1:1 nel flutter atriale	Orale: 20-60 mg/kg/24 h, divisi ogni 6 ore (solfato) o ogni 8 h (gluconato) Dose max: 2,4 g/24 h	Nausea, vomito, diarrea, febbre, cinconismo, prolungamento del QRS e del QT, blocco nodale AV, sincope con asistolia, trombocitopenia, anemia emolitica, LES, disturbi della visione, convulsioni, reazioni allergiche, esacerbazione di paralisi periodica	Aumenta i livelli plasmatici della digossina; può aumentare il PTT quando somministrata con il warfarin	2-7 μg/mL
Procainamide	SVT, fibrillazione atriale, flutter atriale, VT	Orale: 15-50 mg/kg/24 h, divisi ogni 4 ore Dose max: 4 g/24 h ev: 3-6 mg/kg in 5 min, ripetibili fino a 15 mg/kg, carico seguito da 20-80 μg/kg/min	Prolungamento degli intervalli PR, QRS e QT, anoressia, nausea, vomito, rash, febbre, agranulocitosi, trombocitopenia, anemia emolitica Coombs-positiva, LES, ipotensione, esacerbazione di paralisi periodica, effetti proaritmici	Tossicità aumentata da amiodarone e cimetidina	4-10 μg/mL
Disopiramide	SVT, fibrillazione atriale, flutter atriale	Orale: <2 anni: 20-30 mg/kg/24 h, divisi ogni 6 h o ogni 12 h (forma a lunga durata d'azione); 2-10 anni: 9-24 mg/kg/24 h, divisi ogni 6 h o 12 h (forma a lunga durata d'azione); 11 anni: 5-13 mg/kg/24 h, divisi ogni 6 h o ogni 12 h (forma a lunga durata d'azione) Dose max: 1,2 g/24 h	Effetti anticolinergici, ritenzione urinaria, disturbi della visione, secchezza delle fauci, prolungamento del QT e del QRS, tossicità epatica, effetti isotropi negativi, agranulocitosi, psicosi, ipoglicemia, effetto proaritmico		2-5 μg/mL
CLASSE IB: INIBITORI DEI CANALI RAPIDI DEL NA$^+$, CHE ACCORCIANO LA RIPOLARIZZAZIONE					
Lidocaina	PVC, VT, VF	ev: 1 mg/kg, ripetibile ogni 5 min per 2 volte, seguito da 20-50 μg/kg/min (dose max: 3 mg/kg)	Effetti sul SNC, confusione, convulsioni, blocco AV di grado elevato, asistolia, coma, parestesie, insufficienza respiratoria	Propranolo La cimetidina ne aumenta la tossicità	1-5 μg/mL
Mexiletina	VT, PVC	Orale: 6-15 mg/kg/24 h, divisi ogni 8 h	Disturbi gastrointestinali, rash cutaneo, disturbi neurologici	Cimetidina	
Fenitoina	Intossicazione digitalica	Orale: 3-6 mg/kg/24 h, divisi ogni 8 h Dose max: 600 mg ev: 10-15 mg/kg in un'ora (carico)	Rash, iperplasia gengivale, atassia, letargia, vertigini, tremore, anemia macrocitica, bradicardia quando iniettata in bolo rapido	Amiodarone, anticoagulanti orali, cimetidina, nifedipina, disopiramide ne aumentano la tossicità	10-20 μg/mL
CLASSE IC: INIBITORI DEL CANALE DEL NA$^+$					
Flecainide	SVT, tachicardia atriale, VT	Orale: 3-10 mg/kg/24 h, divisi ogni 8 h	Visione offuscata, nausea, diminuzione della contrattilità, effetto proaritmico	L'amiodarone ne aumenta la tossicità	0,2-1 μg/mL
Propafenone	SVT, tachicardia atriale, fibrillazione atriale, VT	Orale: 150-300 mg/m^2/24 h, divisi ogni 8 h	Ipotensione, diminuzione della contrattilità, tossicità epatica, parestesie, cefalea, effetto proaritmico	Aumenta i livelli di digossina	0,2-1 μg/mL
CLASSE II: β-BLOCCANTI					
Propranololo	SVT, PVC, QT lungo	Orale: 1-4 mg/kg/24 h, divisi ogni 6 h Dose max: 60 mg/24 h ev: 0,1-0,5 mg/kg in 5 min Dose max: 10 mg	Bradicardia, perdita della capacità di concentrazione, broncospasmo, ipoglicemia, ipotensione, blocco cardiaco, scompenso cardiaco	L'utilizzo in associazione alla disopiramide esacerba o precipita lo scompenso cardiaco	
CLASSE III: PROLUNGANO LA RIPOLARIZZAZIONE					
Amiodarone	SVT, tachicardia giunzionale ectopica, VT	Orale: 10 mg/kg/24 h in 1-2 dosi per 4-14; ridurre a 5 mg/kg/24 h per parecchie settimane; in assenza di recidive, ridurre a 2,5 mg/kg/24 h, che possono essere somministrati 5 giorni su 7	Ipotiroidismo o ipertiroidismo, aumento dei trigliceridi, tossicità epatica, fibrosi polmonare	Digossina (aumenta i livelli), flecainide, procainamide, chinidina, warfarin, fenitoina	0,5-2,5 mg/l
CLASSE IV: VARIE					
Digossina	SVT (non nella sindrome di WPW), flutter atriale, fibrillazione atriale	Orale: Carico: Prematuri: 20 μg/kg Neonati: 30 μg/kg 6 mesi: 40 μg/kg Dare ½ dose seguita da ¼ ogni 8-12 ore per due volte Mantenimento: 10 μg/kg/24 h, divisi ogni 12 h Dose max: 0,5 mg ev: ¾ della dose orale Dose max: 0,5 mg	PAC, PVC, bradicardia, blocco AV, nausea, vomito, anoressia, prolungamento dell'intervallo PR	Chinidina Amiodarone e verapamil ne aumentano i livelli	1-2 mg/mL
Verapamil	SVT (non nella sindrome di WPW)	Orale: 2-7 mg/kg/24 h, divisi ogni 8 h Dose max: 480 mg ev: 0,1-0,2 mg/kg ogni 20 min per 2 volte Dose max: 5-10 mg	Bradicardia, asistolia, blocco AV di grado elevato, prolungamento dell'intervallo PR, ipotensione, scompenso cardiaco	L'utilizzo in associazione con un β-bloccante o la disopiramide esacerba lo scompenso cardiaco; aumenta i livelli e la tossicità della digossina	
Adenosina	SVT	ev: 50-300 μg/kg, iniziando con 50 μg/kg e aumentando di 50-100 μg/kg/dose; se non si ottiene alcun effetto, è necessario un bolo rapido ev Dose max: 12 mg	Dolore toracico, flushing, dispnea, broncospasmo, bradicardia, asistolia		

AV, atrioventricolare; SNC, sistema nervoso centrale; ev, endovena; PAC (*Premature Atrial Contractions*), contrazione atriale prematura; PTT (*Partial Thromboplastin Time*), tempo di tromboplastina parziale; PVC (*Premature Ventricular Contractions*), contrazioni premature ventricolari; LES, patologia simile lupus eritematoso sistemico, con positività degli anticorpi anti-nucleo; SVT (*SupraVentricular Tachycardia*), tachicardia sopraventricolare; VT (*Ventricular Tachycardia*), tachicardia ventricolare; WPW, Wolff-Parkinson-White.

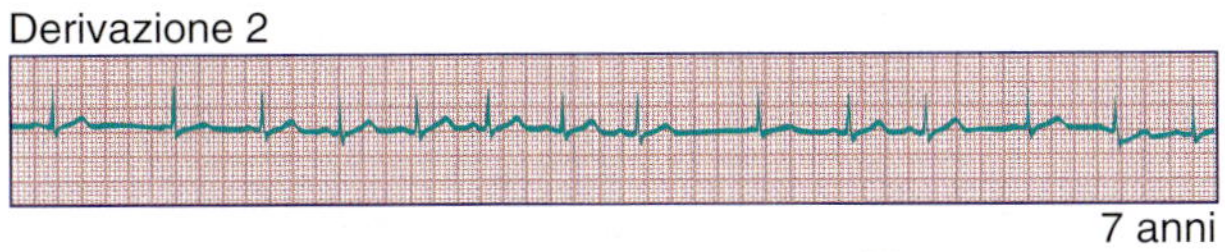

Figura 435-1. Aritmia sinusale con battito di scappamento giunzionale. Si noti la variazione dell'intervallo P-P con pochi cambiamenti nella morfologia dell'onda P o dell'intervallo P-R. Quando la frequenza sinusale è abbastanza bassa, la giunzione atrioventricolare subentra producendo battiti di scappamento. Questo ritmo è normale.

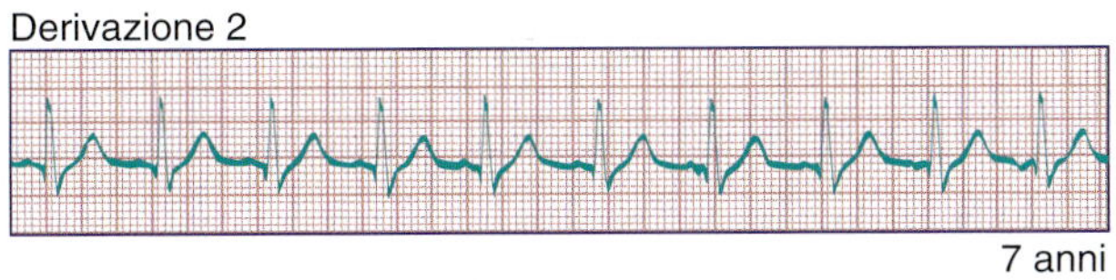

Figura 435-2. Pacemaker atriale migrante. Si noti il cambiamento della configurazione dell'onda P nel settimo, nono e decimo battito. La settima onda P può rappresentare una fusione tra l'onda P sinusale e il segnapassi atriale ectopico che si osserva nel decimo battito.

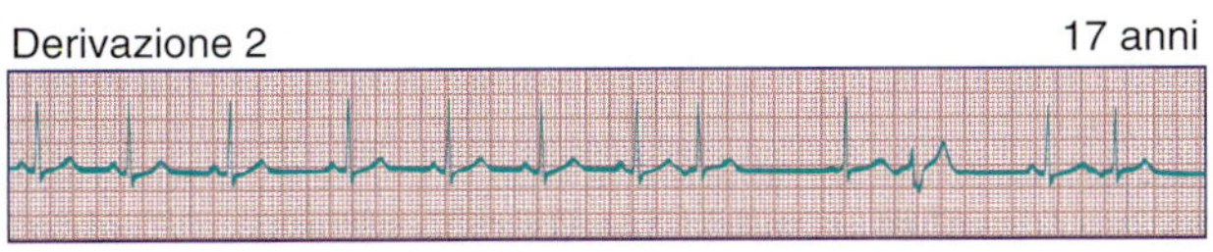

Figura 435-3. Contrazione atriale prematura (PAC, *Premature Atrial Contraction*). I complessi QRS (l'ottavo, il decimo e l'ultimo) in questo tracciato sono preceduti da un'onda P invertita, indicativa di un'origine ectopica della depolarizzazione atriale. Si noti che l'ottavo e l'ultimo complesso QRS assomigliano a quelli di origine sinusale, mentre il decimo è condotto con aberranza. Questo spostamento dell'origine dei complessi è in funzione della lunghezza del ciclo precedente, che influenza il periodo refrattario delle branche. Il fatto che la pausa dopo la PAC sia più lunga di quella tra due intervalli P-P implica che la depolarizzazione atriale prematura ha invaso e scaricato il nodo del seno per poi resettarlo in modo che scarichi in modo ritardato.

scompaiono durante la tachicardia indotta dall'esercizio fisico. Se persistono o divengono più frequenti durante l'esercizio fisico, l'aritmia può avere un significato più importante. I seguenti criteri sono indicazioni per approfondire gli accertamenti nel sospetto di PVC che potrebbero richiedere una **terapia soppressiva:** (1) due o più battiti ventricolari prematuri in sequenza, (2) origine multifocale, (3) aumentata attività ectopica ventricolare con l'esercizio fisico, (4) aspetto R su T (la depolarizzazione ventricolare prematura avviene sull'onda T del battito precedente), (5) presenza di una cardiopatia sottostante. Il cardine della terapia per i PVC benigni è la rassicurazione del paziente, al quale occorre spiegare che l'aritmia non rappresenta una minaccia per la vita. I PVC maligni sono di solito secondari a un altro problema medico (squilibrio elettrolitico, ipossia, tossicità da farmaci, danno cardiaco o presenza di un catetere intraventricolare). Un trattamento efficace consiste nella correzione dell'anomalia sottostante. Un bolo endovenoso di lidocaina seguito da infusione è la terapia di prima linea, mentre farmaci più potenti come l'amiodarone sono riservati ai casi refrattari o a pazienti con compromissione emodinamica.

435.3 • TACHICARDIA SOPRAVENTRICOLARE

La tachicardia sopraventricolare (SVT, *SupraVentricular Tachycardia*) coinvolge componenti del sistema di conduzione nel fascio di His o al di sopra di esso e può essere divisa in tre principali categorie: tachicardie da rientro che utilizzano una via accessoria, tachicardie da rientro senza una via accessoria e tachicardie ectopiche o con automatismo. Il rientro che utilizza una via accessoria

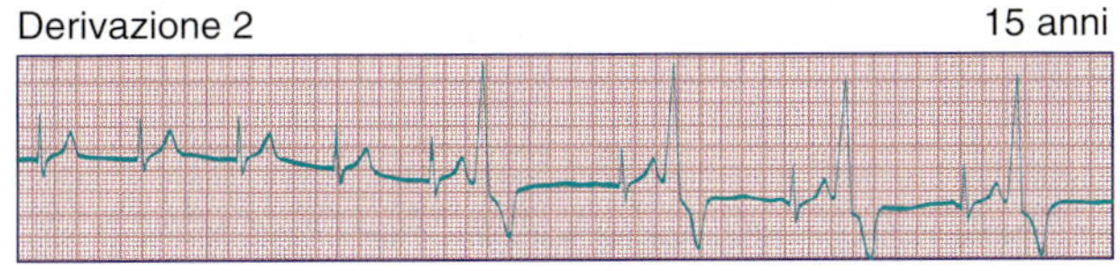

Figura 435-4. Contrazioni ventricolari premature (PVC, *Premature Ventricular Contractions*) indotte dall'iperventilazione. Si noti che il battito prematuro è ampio e ha una morfologia completamente diversa da quella di un battito sinusale. Il fatto che il battito prematuro non sia preceduto da un'onda P e che la pausa seguente sia completamente compensatoria (ossia, l'intervallo P-P che contiene la PVC è uguale a due cicli sinusali) indica che il meccanismo sinusale non è stato disturbato dai battiti prematuri.

è il meccanismo più comune di SVT nei bambini, con un'aumentata incidenza di rientro nodale AV nell'infanzia. La tachicardia viene iniziata da un battito atriale prematuro che è nella maggior parte dei casi condotto al ventricolo attraverso la normale via nodale AV (**conduzione ortodromica**). La risposta ventricolare trova la via nodale AV refrattaria, ma il tratto bypass, prontamente in grado di condurre l'impulso in via retrograda, ritorna all'atrio come battito eco, che a sua volta si trasmette di nuovo al ventricolo, e così via (Fig. 435-5). Le tachicardie ectopiche atriali e giunzionali sono per lo più associate ad anomalie cardiache (miocardiopatie) o al periodo postoperatorio nelle cardiopatie congenite.

MANIFESTAZIONI CLINICHE. La SVT da rientro è caratterizzata da un esordio brusco e da un'altrettanto brusca cessazione; può essere scatenata da un'infezione acuta e di solito di verifica quando il paziente è a riposo. L'attacco può durare solo pochi secondi o persistere per ore. La frequenza cardiaca di solito è >180 battiti/min e talvolta può arrivare fino a 300 battiti /min (Fig. 435-6). L'unico disturbo può essere rappresentato dalla percezione consapevole dell'elevata frequenza cardiaca. Molti bambini tollerano benissimo questi episodi, ed è improbabile che brevi parossismi rappresentino un rischio per la vita. Se la frequenza cardiaca è eccezionalmente rapida o l'attacco è prolungato, possono sopravvenire un fastidio precordiale o uno scompenso cardiaco. Una SVT può verificarsi in presenza di una cardiopatia congenita non operata (anomalia di Ebstein). Nei bambini, può essere precipitata dall'esposizione ad amine simpaticomimetiche contenute in farmaci decongestionanti da banco.

Nei bambini piccoli, la diagnosi può essere più difficoltosa a causa dell'incapacità dei pazienti di comunicare i loro sintomi. La frequenza cardiaca a quest'età di norma è elevata, e anche in assenza di una tachiaritmia aumenta in modo importante con il pianto. I lattanti con SVT giungono di solito all'osservazione con

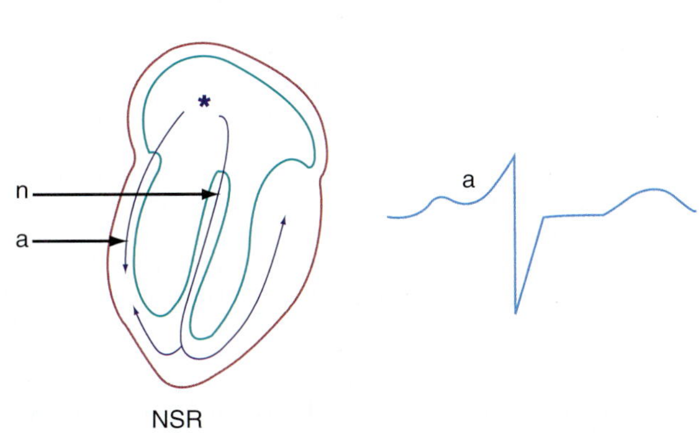

Figura 435-5. Rappresentazione schematica del cuore con una via anomala a destra. L'*asterisco* indica l'iniziazione del battito sinusale. Le *frecce* indicano la direzione e la diffusione dell'eccitazione. Il complesso elettrocardiografico riportato rappresenta un battito di fusione che combina l'attivazione delle vie normale (*n*) e accessoria (*a*). Quest'ultima iscrive l'onda delta. NSR (*Normal Sinus Rhythm*), ritmo sinusale normale.

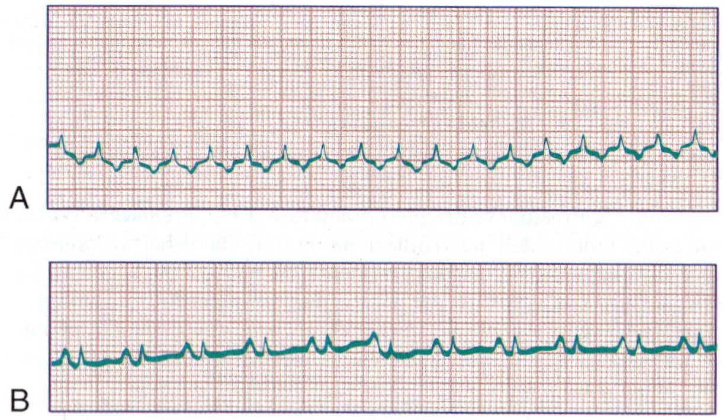

Figura 435-6. *A*, Tachicardia parossistica sopraventricolare o atriale con frequenza ventricolare di 230 battiti/min. *B*, Ritmo sinusale dopo cardioversione elettrica. Si noti che durante la tachicardia l'onda T è deformata da un'onda P invertita, presumibilmente retrograda. La morfologia del QRS rimane invariata durante la tachicardia. Il basso voltaggio è dovuto a edema periferico in un neonato di 1 giorno che aveva una tachicardia intrauterina e idrope fetale.

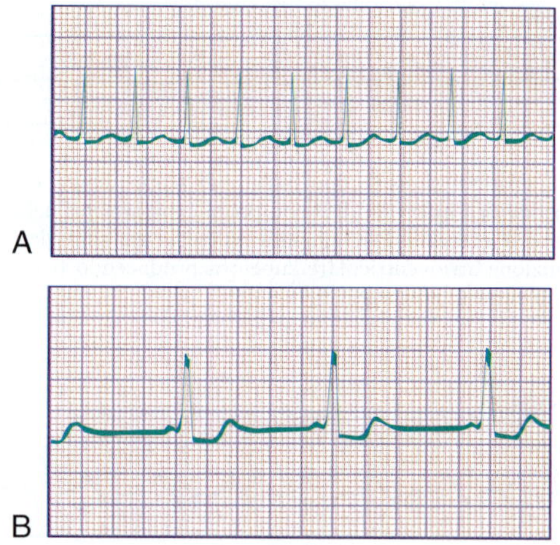

Figura 435-7. *A*, Tachicardia sopraventricolare in un bambino con sindrome di Wolff-Parkinson-White (WPW). Si notino i normali complessi QRS durante la tachicardia. *B*, In seguito, sono evidenti le caratteristiche tipiche della sindrome di WPW (intervallo P-R corto, onda delta, QRS ampio).

scompenso cardiaco, poiché la tachicardia non viene riconosciuta per lungo tempo. La frequenza cardiaca durante i parossismi è spesso compresa tra 200 e 300 battiti/min. Se l'attacco dura da 6 a 24 ore o più con una frequenza cardiaca estremamente elevata, il bambino può presentare i segni di una patologia acuta, avere colorito cinereo, essere irrequieto e irritabile. Tachipnea ed epatomegalia sono segni evidenti di scompenso cardiaco, e possono essere presenti febbre e leucocitosi. Quando la tachicardia si verifica nel feto, può causare un grave scompenso cardiaco e idrope fetale.

Nei neonati, la SVT si manifesta di solito con un complesso QRS stretto (<0,08 s). L'onda P è visibile all'elettrocardiogramma standard solo nel 50-60% dei neonati con SVT, ma è riconoscibile con una derivazione transesofagea nella maggior parte dei pazienti. **Può essere difficile differenziarla da una tachicardia sinusale**; se la frequenza è >230 battiti/min con un asse dell'onda P anomalo (un'onda P normale è positiva nelle derivazioni I e aVF), è più probabile che si tratti di una SVT. La frequenza cardiaca in una SVT, inoltre, tende a rimanere stabile, mentre nella tachicardia sinusale varia con i cambiamenti del tono vagale e simpatico. La distinzione tra una SVT e una tachicardia ventricolare è fondamentale, poiché la digossina può precipitare la fibrillazione ventricolare in pazienti con tachicardia ventricolare. L'assenza di conduzione ventricolare-atriale (e perciò onde P solo intermittenti), la presenza di battiti di fusione e complessi QRS ampi, diversi dal complesso QRS presente durante il ritmo sinusale, permettono di formulare la diagnosi di tachicardia ventricolare.

La tachicardia da rientro AV utilizza un tratto bypass che può essere in grado di condurre per via anterograda (**sindrome di Wolff-Parkinson-White [WPW]**) o che rimane nascosto. I pazienti con sindrome di WPW hanno un rischio basso ma concreto di morte improvvisa. Se la via accessoria conduce rapidamente in modo anterogrado il paziente è a rischio di fibrillazione atriale che ingenera una fibrillazione ventricolare. La stratificazione del rischio, comprendente un monitoraggio Holter nelle ventiquattr'ore e un test da sforzo, può aiutare a differenziare i pazienti a rischio più elevato di morte improvvisa da WPW. Allo stesso tempo, qualsiasi paziente con sincope e sindrome di WPW dovrebbe essere sottoposto a studio elettrofisiologico.

Le caratteristiche elettrocardiografiche tipiche della sindrome di WPW si osservano di solito quando il paziente non presenta la tachicardia. Esse comprendono un intervallo P-R corto e un lento innalzamento del QRS (onda delta) (Fig. 435-7). Anche se presente nella maggior parte dei casi in pazienti con cuore normale, questa sindrome può anche essere associata ad anomalia di Ebstein e ad altre lesioni cardiache congenite. I substrati anatomici compresi nel circuito di rientro sono il nodo AV e una via accessoria di pre-eccitazione, consistente in un ponte muscolare che connette l'atrio al ventricolo, a destra o a sinistra dell'anello AV (vedi Fig. 435-5). Durante il ritmo sinusale, l'impulso viene condotto attraverso sia il nodo AV sia la via accessoria, producendo un certo grado di fusione dei due fronti di depolarizzazione, che porta a un QRS anomalo. Durante la tachicardia, un impulso è condotto di solito in modo anterogrado attraverso il nodo AV (**conduzione ortodromica**), il che porta a un normale complesso QRS, e in modo retrogrado attraverso la via accessoria all'atrio, con il risultato di perpetuare la tachicardia. In questi casi, è solo dopo la cessazione della tachicardia che si riconoscono le caratteristiche tipiche della sindrome di WPW (vedi Fig. 435-7). Quando si verifica una rapida conduzione anterograda attraverso la via di pre-eccitazione durante la tachicardia e la via di rientro retrograda all'atrio è attraverso il nodo AV (**conduzione antidromica**), i complessi della tachicardia sono ampi ed è più elevata la possibilità che si verifichino aritmie più gravi (fibrillazione ventricolare), specialmente se insorge una fibrillazione atriale.

La **tachicardia nodale AV da rientro**, osservabile più comunemente nell'adolescenza, comporta l'utilizzo di due vie nel nodo AV. È una delle poche SVT a essere frequentemente associata a sincope. Questa aritmia è di solito sensibile alla terapia antiaritmica, per esempio con digossina o propranololo, o all'ablazione mediante radiofrequenze.

TRATTAMENTO. La stimolazione vagale ottenuta immergendo il volto in soluzione fisiologica ghiacciata (nei bambini più grandi) o posizionando una borsa del ghiaccio sul volto (nei bambini più piccoli) può stroncare l'attacco. Per abolire il parossismo, ai bambini più grandi possono essere insegnate manovre vagotoniche come la manovra di Valsalva, la manovra di forzatura, il trattenere il respiro, il bere acqua ghiacciata o l'adottare una particolare postura. Se queste misure falliscono, sono disponibili numerose alternative farmacologiche (vedi Tab. 435-1). Nei pazienti stabili, l'adenosina per bolo endovenoso rapido è il **trattamento di scelta** per la sua rapida azione e per i minimi effetti sulla contrattilità cardiaca. Può essere necessario ripetere la dose. Altri farmaci che sono stati utilizzati per il trattamento della SVT comprendono infusioni di fenilefrina o di edrofonio, con un aumento del tono vagale tramite il riflesso mediato dai barocettori, oltre che di agenti antiaritmici come la chinidina, la procainamide e il propranololo. Anche i calcioantagonisti come il verapamil sono stati utilizzati nel trattamento iniziale della SVT nei bambini più grandi. Il verapamil, potendo ridurre la gittata cardiaca e produrre ipotensione e arresto cardiaco nei pazienti di età <1 anno, è controindicato in questo gruppo di età. In situazioni urgenti, quando si sono già sviluppati i sintomi di grave scompenso cardiaco, è raccomandata come trattamento iniziale (vedi Capitolo 66) la cardioversione elettrica sincronizzata (0,5-2 W-s/kg).

Una volta effettuata la cardioversione a ritmo sinusale, si sceglie un farmaco a maggiore durata d'azione per la terapia di mantenimento. In pazienti senza una via accessoria anterograda, il cardine della terapia è rappresentato dalla digossina o dal propranololo. In bambini con evidenza di pre-eccitazione (sindrome di WPW), la digossina o i calcioantagonisti possono aumentare il grado di conduzione anterograda degli impulsi attraverso il tratto bypass e andrebbero quindi evitati. Questi pazienti sono di solito trattati a lungo termine con propranololo. In caso di tachicardia resistente, sono stati usati procainamide, chinidina, flecainide, propafenone, sotalolo e amiodarone. Occorre ricordare che la maggior parte dei farmaci antiaritmici potrebbe avere effetti proaritmici e inotropi negativi; la flecainide, in particolare, dovrebbe essere utilizzata solamente in pazienti con cuori per altri aspetti sani.

Se si sviluppa uno scompenso cardiaco a causa di una tachicardia prolungata in un bambino con un cuore normale, la funzione cardiaca di solito ritorna alla normalità una volta ripristinato il ritmo sinusale, anche se possono essere necessari giorni o settimane. I lattanti con SVT diagnosticata nei primi 3-4 mesi di vita hanno una più bassa incidenza di recidive di quelli in cui la prima diagnosi viene formulata a un'età maggiore. Questi pazienti hanno una probabilità di risoluzione del 40%; se è necessaria una terapia medica, questa può essere diminuita progressivamente fino alla sospensione nel giro di un anno, dopodiché il paziente può essere tenuto sotto osservazione per un'eventuale recidiva dell'aritmia.

Le **registrazioni elettrocardiografiche per ventiquattr'ore (Holter)** sono utili per il monitoraggio del decorso della terapia e per rilevare brevi run di tachicardia in assenza di sintomi. È possibile effettuare una breve valutazione del controllo dell'aritmia al letto del paziente con il **pacing transesofageo**. In pazienti con SVT refrattarie sono spesso indicati **studi elettrofisiologici** più dettagliati, eseguiti nel laboratorio di emodinamica. Durante queste indagini, numerosi elettrodi con catetere, posizionati in diverse sedi del cuore, possono aiutare a evidenziare un focus ectopico o un tratto bypass. Il pacing può indurre l'aritmia, e si può testare la capacità di diversi agenti farmacologici di inibirla. Questi studi sono prerequisiti necessari all'ablazione con radiofrequenze.

L'**ablazione con radiofrequenze** di una via accessoria è un'altra opzione di trattamento di comune impiego nei pazienti con ritmi da rientro. Spesso viene utilizzata selettivamente in bambini e adolescenti, come pure in pazienti che necessitano di più farmaci o trovano intollerabili i loro effetti collaterali, o nei quali il controllo dell'aritmia è scarso. Il tasso di successo complessivo iniziale va dall'80 al 95%, a seconda della sede del tratto o dei tratti bypass. Anche l'ablazione chirurgica dei tratti bypass può essere efficace in pazienti selezionati.

La **tachicardia atriale ectopica**, non comune nell'infanzia, è caratterizzata da una frequenza cardiaca variabile (raramente >200 battiti/min), da onde P identificabili con un asse anomalo e dalla cronicità, sia nella forma sostenuta sia in quella intermittente. Questa tachicardia atriale ha un singolo focus di automatismo anziché il più tipico meccanismo di rientro. Nell'identificazione di questo meccanismo risulta di aiuto il monitoraggio dell'elettrocardiogramma mentre si inizia una manovra vagale o una terapia farmacologica. Le tachicardie da rientro cessano improvvisamente, mentre quelle da automatismo dapprima rallentano, poi aumentano gradualmente la loro frequenza. Le tachicardie atriali ectopiche sono di solito più difficili da controllare farmacologicamente rispetto alle più comuni tachicardie da rientro. Se la terapia farmacologica con un unico principio attivo non ha successo, si suggerisce l'ablazione mediante catetere, che ha una tasso di successo >90%.

Le **tachicardie atriali caotiche o multifocali** sono caratterizzate da tre o più onde P ectopiche con tre o più cicli ectopici diversi P-P, da frequenti onde P bloccate e da intervalli R-R variabili di battiti condotti. Questa aritmia si verifica più spesso nei bambini di età <1 anno, di solito in assenza di una patologia cardiaca, anche se vi sono dati che suggeriscono un'associazione con la miocardite virale. Il trattamento farmacologico può non essere efficace, e sono spesso necessari più farmaci. Fortunatamente, quando questa aritmia si verifica nell'infanzia, di solito si risolve spontaneamente entro il terzo anno di età.

La **tachicardia giunzionale ectopica accelerata** è un'aritmia da automatismo (non da rientro) in cui la frequenza giunzionale è superiore a quella del nodo del seno, cosicché ne risulta una dissociazione AV. Principalmente riconosciuta nel primo periodo postoperatorio dopo chirurgia cardiaca, può essere difficilissima da controllare. La riduzione della velocità di infusione delle catecolamine e il controllo dell'iperpiressia sono fattori aggiuntivi importanti da gestire. La tachicardia giunzionale ectopica accelerata in assenza di un precedente intervento chirurgico è associata a una prognosi più cauta. Una tachicardia giunzionale può anche essere un segno di intossicazione da digitale; in tal caso, il farmaco va sospeso. L'amiodarone per via endovenosa è efficace nel trattamento della tachicardia giunzionale ectopica nel periodo postoperatorio. I pazienti che necessitano di una terapia cronica possono rispondere all'amiodarone o al sotalolo.

Il **flutter atriale**, detto anche tachicardia intra-atriale rientrante, è una tachicardia regolare o regolarmente irregolare caratterizzata da un'attività atriale di frequenza pari a 250-400 battiti/min. Si ritiene che queste contrazioni siano dovute a un ritmo rientrante o circolare: quest'ultimo origina negli atri coinvolgendo un microcircuito di rientro nell'ambito del tessuto atriale e alcune forme di ostacolo anatomico, che creano una discontinuità nella conduzione (fibrosi, sito di sutura chirurgica, anulus valvolare). Poiché il nodo AV non è in grado in trasmettere impulsi tanto rapidi, è virtualmente sempre presente un qualche grado di **blocco AV**, e i ventricoli rispondono ogni 2°-4° battito atriale. A volte la risposta è variabile e il ritmo appare irregolare.

Nei bambini più grandi, il flutter atriale si verifica nel contesto di una cardiopatia congenita; i neonati spesso hanno cuori normali. Il flutter atriale, pur potendo verificarsi durante malattie febbrili acute, si osserva per lo più in pazienti con atri grandi e distesi, come quelli associati a insufficienza mitralica o tricuspidalica di lunga data, atresia della tricuspide, anomalia di Ebstein o stenosi mitralica reumatica. Può inoltre manifestarsi dopo chirurgia palliativa o correttiva intra-atriale. Un flutter atriale incontrollato è in grado di far precipitare uno scompenso cardiaco. Le manovre vagali (come la pressione sul seno carotideo o l'immersione del volto in soluzione salina) o l'adenosina generalmente producono un temporaneo rallentamento della frequenza cardiaca. La **diagnosi** è confermata dall'elettrocardiografia, che evidenzia le onde di flutter, rapide e regolari, a dente di sega. Il flutter atriale di solito si converte immediatamente in ritmo sinusale con la **cardioversione elettrica sincronizzata**, che è nella maggior parte dei casi il **trattamento di scelta**. I pazienti con flutter atriale cronico nel contesto di una cardiopatia congenita possono essere ad aumentato rischio di **tromboembolismo** e ictus e dovrebbero essere sottoposti ad anticoagulazione prima della cardioversione in elezione. La digitale rallenta la risposta ventricolare nel flutter atriale, prolungando il tempo di conduzione attraverso il nodo AV. Dopo la digitalizzazione, è di solito necessario un farmaco di classe I come la chinidina o la procainamide per mantenere un adeguato controllo. I farmaci di classe III come l'amiodarone e il sotalolo si sono dimostrati promettenti e possono essere utili in pazienti refrattari ai farmaci di classe I. Altre modalità di trattamento, comprese l'ablazione a radiofrequenze e l'ablazione chirurgica, sono state utilizzate in pazienti più grandi con cardiopatie congenite, con moderato successo. I neonati con cuori normali che rispondono alla digossina vengono trattati per 6-12 mesi, dopodiché è spesso possibile sospendere il farmaco.

La **fibrillazione atriale** è molto meno comune nei bambini e rara nei lattanti. L'eccitazione atriale, caotica e più rapida (300-700 battiti/min), produce una risposta ventricolare e un polso irregolarmente irregolari (Fig. 435-8). Questo disturbo del ritmo è nella maggior parte dei casi dovuto a un miocardio atriale cronicamente disteso. La fibrillazione atriale si verifica principalmente nei bambini più grandi con valvulopatia mitralica reumatica. Per quanto raramente, si osserva anche come complicanza della chirurgia intra-atriale, in pazienti con ingrandimento

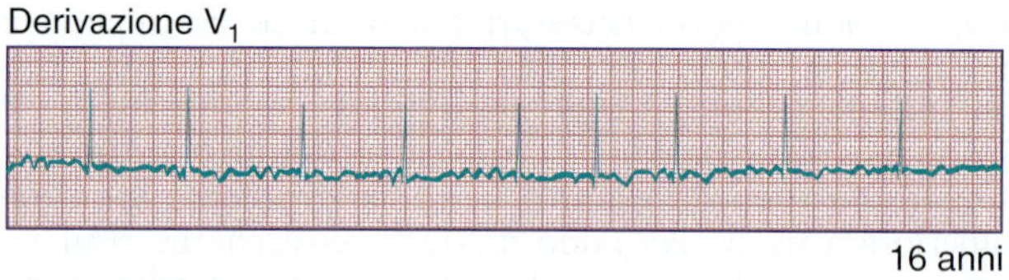

Figura 435-8. Fibrillazione atriale, caratterizzata dall'assenza di onde P; presenza di onde da fibrillazione, che sono rapide ondulazioni grossolanamente irregolari; risposta ventricolare irregolare. Le onde da fibrillazione possono non essere visibili in tutte le derivazioni e dovrebbero essere accuratamente ricercate in ogni tracciato con intervalli R-R irregolari (la coesistenza di qR in V_1 è diagnostica di ipertrofia ventricolare destra in questo paziente con sindrome di Eisenmenger).

atriale sinistro secondario a insufficienza valvolare AV del cuore sinistro, in condizioni che causano flutter atriale, e in pazienti con sindrome di WPW. La fibrillazione atriale può essere familiare. Il miglior trattamento iniziale è la **digitalizzazione**, che ripristina la frequenza ventricolare a valori normali, anche se la fibrillazione atriale di solito persiste. La digossina non viene somministrata se è presente una sindrome di WPW. Il normale ritmo sinusale può essere poi ripristinato con un farmaco di classe I (chinidina o procainamide), con l'amiodarone o con la cardioversione elettrica. I pazienti con fibrillazione atriale cronica, essendo a rischio di sviluppare tromboembolismo e ictus, dovrebbero essere sottoposti a trattamento anticoagulante con warfarin. Gli anticoagulanti andrebbero somministrati anche ai pazienti che vengono trattati con cardioversione elettrica in elezione.

435.4 • Tachiaritmie ventricolari

La **tachicardia ventricolare** (VT, *Ventricular Tachycardia*), meno comune della SVT nei pazienti pediatrici, per definizione consiste in almeno tre PVC a una frequenza >120 battiti/min. Che sia parossistica o sostenuta, può essere associata a miocardite, origine anomala di un'arteria coronaria, displasia aritmogena del ventricolo destro, prolasso della valvola mitrale, tumori cardiaci primitivi o miocardiopatia. È stata osservata in presenza di un intervallo Q-T prolungato da cause congenite o acquisite (farmaci proaritmici), nella sindrome di WPW e nell'uso di droghe (cocaina, anfetamine). Può svilupparsi anni dopo un intervento chirurgico intraventricolare (tetralogia di Fallot, difetto settale ventricolare) o verificarsi in assenza di un'evidente patologia cardiaca organica. La VT deve essere distinta dalla SVT condotta con aberranza o con conduzione rapida lungo una via accessoria (Tab. 435-2). La presenza di battiti di cattura e di fusione aiuta a confermare la diagnosi. Anche se alcuni bambini tollerano frequenze ventricolari elevate per molte ore, questa aritmia dovrebbe essere trattata rapidamente poiché può dar luogo a ipotensione e a una degenerazione in fibrillazione ventricolare. Nei pazienti emodinamicamente stabili, i farmaci di scelta iniziali sono l'amiodarone per via endovenosa, la lidocaina o la procainamide. Se il trattamento ha successo, è indispensabile ricercare e correggere qualsiasi anomalia sottostante come squilibri elettrolitici, ipossia o tossicità da farmaci. L'amiodarone è il **trattamento di scelta** durante l'arresto cardiaco (vedi Capitolo 66.1). Anche il pacing ventricolare overdrive può essere efficace, sebbene talvolta possa far sì che l'aritmia degeneri in fibrillazione ventricolare. Nel periodo neonatale, la VT può essere associata a un'arteria coronaria sinistra anomala (vedi Capitolo 433.2) o a un tumore miocardico.

A meno che non venga identificata una causa chiaramente reversibile, è indicato uno studio elettrofisiologico per i pazienti in cui si è sviluppata una VT.

La **fibrillazione ventricolare** è un'aritmia caotica che porta alla morte se non viene rapidamente ristabilito un efficace battito ventricolare. Un pugno precordiale può talvolta ripristinare il ritmo sinusale. Di solito è necessario il massaggio cardiaco esterno con ventilazione artificiale e defibrillazione. Se la defibrillazione è inefficace o vi è una recidiva di fibrillazione, è possibile somministrare amiodarone o lidocaina per via endovenosa, e ripetere la defibrillazione (vedi Capitolo 66). Una volta che la fibrillazione ventricolare si è risolta, si dovrebbe avviare una ricerca della causa sottostante. Di solito uno **studio elettrofisiologico** è indicato per i pazienti in cui si è sviluppata una fibrillazione ventricolare, a meno che non venga identificata una causa chiaramente reversibile. Se si riscontra una sindrome di WPW, occorre procedere a un'ablazione. Per i pazienti in cui non si individua alcuna anomalia correggibile, si dovrebbe considerare seriamente l'impianto di un ICD, a causa dell'alto rischio di morte improvvisa.

435.5 • Sindromi da Q-T lungo

Le sindromi da Q-T lungo (LQTS, *Long Q_T Syndromes*) sono anomalie genetiche della ripolarizzazione ventricolare, che presentano un intervallo Q-T lungo all'ECG di superficie e sono associate ad aritmie ventricolari maligne (*torsade de pointes*). Sono una causa di sincope e morte improvvisa e possono essere associate alla sindrome della morte infantile improvvisa o all'annegamento. Circa il 50% dei casi è familiare: la sindrome di Romano-Ward è una forma comune di LQTS che presenta una trasmissione autosomica dominante con bassa penetranza. Una forma non comune di LQTS è la sindrome di Jervell e Lange-Nielsen, che ha una trasmissione autosomica recessiva ed è associata a sordità congenita. I rimanenti casi sono sporadici. Non tutti i pazienti asintomatici (presintomatici) portatori della mutazione genetica hanno un intervallo Q-T prolungato. Questo può divenire evidente con l'esercizio fisico o durante infusione di catecolamine.

Gli studi genetici hanno identificato mutazioni nei canali cardiaci del sodio e del potassio. Nella LQT1 il gene è sul cromosoma 11p5.5 e codifica per un canale del potassio (KVLQT1). Il gene LQT2 è sul cromosoma 7q35-36, che codifica per HERG (*Human-Ether-a-go-go-Related Gene*), un canale del potassio. LQT3 è un difetto sul cromosoma 3p21-24 e codifica per un canale del sodio (SCN5A). La causa di LQT4 è sconosciuta. LQT5 è una mutazione sul cromosoma 21q22.1 e codifica per un regolatore (minK) dei canali del potassio. LQT6 è sul cromosoma 21q22 ed è un peptide correlato a minK. La sindrome di Jervell e Lange-Nielsen è stata osservata in pazienti che hanno mutazioni in omozigosi di KVLQT1 e minK, mentre lo stato di eterozigosi si

TABELLA 435-2. Diagnosi delle tachiaritmie

REPERTI ELETTROCARDIOGRAFICI

	FREQUENZA CARDIACA (BATTITI/MIN)	ONDA P	DURATA DEL QRS	REGOLARITÀ
Tachicardia sinusale	<225	Asse normale sempre presente	Normale	La frequenza varia con il respiro
Tachicardia atriale	180-320	Presente – 50% Asse superiore comune	Normale o prolungato (aspetto a RBBB)	Regolare
Fibrillazione atriale	120-180	Onde da fibrillazione	Normale o prolungato (aspetto a RBBB)	Irregolarmente irregolare
Flutter atriale	Atriale: 250-400 Risposta ventricolare variabile: 100-320	Onde di flutter a dente di sega	Normale o prolungato (aspetto a RBBB)	Risposta ventricolare regolare (per es. 2:1, 3:1, 3:2 e così via)
Tachicardia ventricolare	120-240	Assente, o dissociazione atrioventricolare	Di solito prolungato	Lievemente irregolare

RBBB (*Right Bundle Branch Block*), blocco di branca destra.

manifesta come sindrome di Romano-Ward. Il genotipo consente di predire le manifestazioni cliniche; per esempio, **gli eventi nella LQT1 sono indotti dallo stress**, mentre gli eventi nella LQT3 **avvengono durante il sonno** e quelli nella LQT2 hanno un pattern intermedio. La LQT3 comporta la più elevata probabilità di morte improvvisa, seguita dalla LQT2 e poi dalla LQT1. I farmaci possono prolungare l'intervallo Q-T direttamente (terfenadina, astemizolo, cisapride, droperidolo) ma più spesso questo effetto si verifica quando il loro metabolismo viene inibito da principi attivi come l'eritromicina o il ketoconazolo.

La **manifestazione clinica** delle LQTS nei bambini è nella maggior parte dei casi un episodio sincopale scatenato dall'esercizio fisico, da uno spavento o da una sorpresa improvvisa; alcuni eventi avvengono durante il sonno (LQT3). I pazienti possono giungere all'osservazione del medico con convulsioni, presincope o palpitazioni; circa il 10% è inizialmente in arresto cardiaco. La diagnosi si basa su criteri elettrocardiografici e clinici. Non tutti i pazienti con intervalli Q-T prolungati hanno una LQTS; d'altra parte, pazienti con intervalli Q-T normali all'elettrocardiogramma a riposo possono avere una LQTS. Un intervallo Q-T corretto per la frequenza cardiaca >0,47 s è altamente indicativo, mentre un intervallo Q-T >0,44 s è suggestivo. Altre caratteristiche comprendono onde T indentate, alternanza dell'onda T, una bassa frequenza cardiaca per l'età, un'anamnesi di sincopi (specialmente da stress) e una storia familiare di LQTS o di morte improvvisa inspiegata. Il monitoraggio Holter delle ventiquattr'ore e il test da sforzo aiutano nella diagnosi.

Il **trattamento** delle LQTS comprende l'utilizzo di **β bloccanti** a dosi che rallentano la frequenza cardiaca in risposta all'esercizio fisico. Alcuni pazienti necessitano di un **pacemaker** a causa dell'estrema bradicardia indotta dai farmaci. Se gli episodi sincopali continuano a ripresentarsi nonostante la terapia, è indicato il posizionamento di un defibrillatore impiantabile per quei pazienti che non rispondono alla terapia β-bloccante e per quelli che sono andati incontro ad arresto cardiaco.

435.6 • Disfunzione del nodo del seno

Un **arresto sinusale** e un **blocco senoatriale** possono provocare un'improvvisa interruzione del battito cardiaco. Il primo fenomeno è presumibilmente causato dalla mancata formazione dell'impulso a livello del nodo del seno, e il secondo da un blocco tra l'impulso sinusale e l'atrio circostante. Queste aritmie sono rare nell'infanzia, tranne quando sono manifestazioni di intossicazione digitalica o si presentano dopo un esteso intervento chirurgico a carico degli atri.

La **sindrome del seno malato** dipende da anomalie nel nodo del seno o nelle vie di conduzione atriali, o in entrambi. Si può manifestare in assenza di una cardiopatia congenita e sono stati riportati casi in fratelli, ma si osserva più comunemente dopo correzione chirurgica di difetti cardiaci congeniti, in particolare dopo intervento di switch atriale (Mustard e Senning) per trasposizione delle grandi arterie. Le manifestazioni cliniche dipendono dalla frequenza cardiaca. La maggior parte dei pazienti rimane asintomatica in assenza di terapia, ma possono manifestarsi capogiri e sincope durante periodi di marcato rallentamento sinusale senza che vi sia un ritmo di scappamento giunzionale (Fig. 435-9). L'impianto di un pacemaker è indicato in pazienti sintomatici.

I pazienti con disfunzione del nodo del seno possono anche avere episodi di SVT (**sindrome bradicardia-tachicardia**) ed essere sintomatici per palpitazioni, intolleranza allo sforzo, capogiri. Il trattamento deve essere individualizzato. La terapia farmacologica per controllare le tachiaritmie (propranololo, chinidina, procainamide) può sopprimere la funzione del nodo del seno e del nodo AV al punto da determinare una bradicardia sintomatica; perciò, è di solito necessario l'impianto di un pacemaker in combinazione con una terapia farmacologica per i pazienti sintomatici.

435.7 • Blocco AV

Il blocco AV si può manifestare in tre forme. Nel **blocco di primo grado**, l'intervallo P-R è prolungato ma tutti gli impulsi atriali sono condotti al ventricolo. Nel **blocco di secondo grado** alcuni impulsi non sono condotti al ventricolo. In una variante del blocco di secondo grado, nota come **tipo Wenckebach** (o **tipo Mobitz I**), l'intervallo P-P rimane costante e l'intervallo P-R aumenta progressivamente finché un'onda P non è condotta; nel ciclo successivo al battito mancante, l'intervallo P-R è di nuovo più breve (Fig. 435-10). Nel **tipo Mobitz II**, l'intervallo P-R non cambia, ma a volte un battito atriale non conduce al ventricolo. Questo difetto di conduzione non è comune ma ha una maggiore probabilità di causare sincope e può essere progressivo. Nel **blocco di terzo grado** (**blocco cardiaco completo**) nessun impulso dagli atri raggiunge i ventricoli.

Il **blocco AV completo congenito** in età pediatrica è causato nella maggior parte dei casi da un danno autoimmune al sistema di conduzione fetale, imputabile ad anticorpi IgG derivati dalla madre (anti-SSA-Ro, anti-SSb-La), quando la madre è affetta da LES conclamato o (più spesso) asintomatico, oppure da sindrome di Sjögren. Le patologie autoimmuni costituiscono il 60-70% di tutti i casi di blocco cardiaco completo congenito e circa l'80% dei casi in cui il cuore è strutturalmente normale. Il blocco cardiaco completo si osserva anche in pazienti con cardiopatia congenita complessa e anomalo sviluppo embrionale del sistema di conduzione. È stato associato a tumori miocardici e miocardite. Oltre a essere stato osservato nelle anomalie genetiche, comprese le LQTS e la sindrome di Kearn-Sayre, rappresenta una complicanza dell'ascesso miocardico secondario a endocardite e delle correzioni di cardiopatie congenite.

L'incidenza del blocco cardiaco completo congenito è di 1/20 000-25 000 nati vivi; un'elevata perdita fetale può tuttavia indurre a sottostimare la sua reale incidenza. In alcuni bambini nati da madri affette da LES, il blocco cardiaco completo non è presente alla nascita, ma si sviluppa nei primi 3-6 mesi di vita. L'aritmia, spesso diagnosticata nel feto (secondariamente alla dissociazione tra le contrazioni atriali e ventricolari osservate all'ecocardiografia fetale), può causare idrope fetale. I bambini

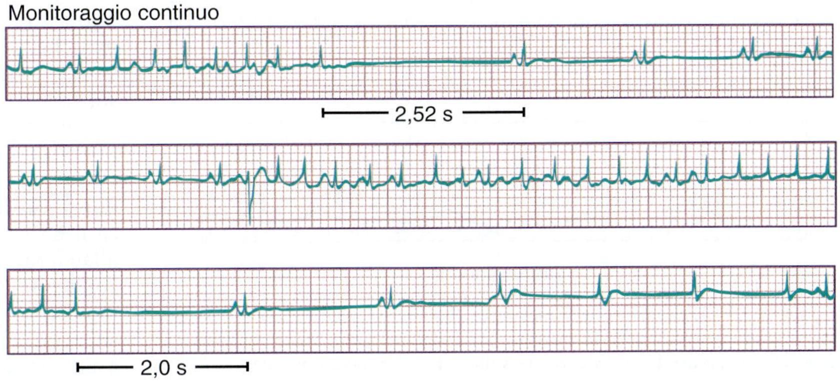

Figura 435-9. Blocco atrioventricolare (AV) completo. La frequenza ventricolare è regolare, 53 battiti/min. La frequenza atriale andava da 65 a 95 battiti/min. La morfologia del QRS è normale, come avviene di solito nel blocco AV congenito.

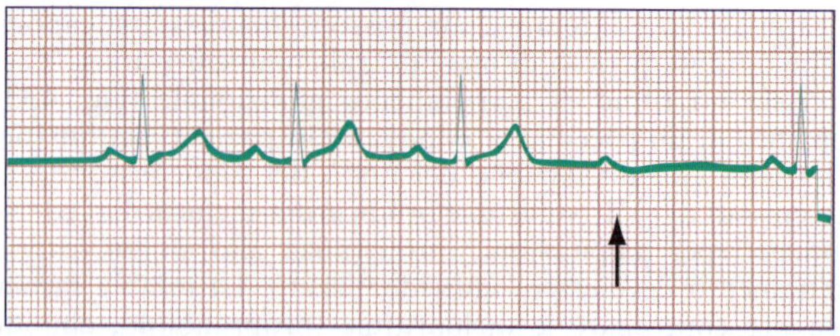

Figura 435-10. Sindrome del seno malato con bradi-tachicardia. Si notino i parossismi di tachicardia sopraventricolare, probabilmente di origine multifocale, seguiti da lunghi periodi di arresto sinusale e di bradicardia sinusale.

con cardiopatia congenita e scompenso cardiaco associati hanno un elevato tasso di mortalità.

Nei bambini più grandi con un cuore per altri aspetti normale, la condizione è comunemente asintomatica, anche se si possono verificare sincope e morte improvvisa. I lattanti e i bambini piccoli possono avere paure notturne, stanchezza con frequenti assopimenti e irritabilità. Il polso periferico è scoccante in conseguenza dell'ampia gittata sistolica ventricolare compensatoria e della vasodilatazione periferica; la pressione venosa sistolica è elevata. Le pulsazioni venose giugulari si verificano irregolarmente e possono essere evidenti quando l'atrio si contrae mentre la valvola tricuspide è chiusa (onda cannone). L'esercizio fisico e l'atropina possono produrre un'accelerazione della frequenza cardiaca ≥10-20 battiti/min. Sono spesso udibili soffi sistolici lungo il margine sternale sinistro e non sono infrequenti soffi apicali mesodiastolici. Il blocco cardiaco porta a un ingrandimento cardiaco sulla base di un maggiore riempimento diastolico ventricolare.

La **diagnosi** è confermata dall'elettrocardiogramma; le onde P e i complessi QRS non hanno un rapporto costante tra loro (Fig. 435-11). La durata del QRS può essere prolungata o anche normale, se il battito prende inizio nella zona alta del nodo AV o del fascio di His.

La **prognosi** per il blocco cardiaco completo congenito è di solito favorevole; i pazienti che sono giunti all'osservazione all'età di 30-40 anni hanno condotto una vita normale e attiva. Alcuni hanno episodi di intolleranza allo sforzo, capogiri e sincopi (attacchi di Stokes-Adams), sintomo che richiede l'impianto di un pacemaker cardiaco definitivo. L'impianto di pacemaker dovrebbe essere preso in considerazione quando si sviluppano sintomi quali un ingrandimento cardiaco progressivo, pause prolungate o frequenza cardiaca durante la veglia ≤40 battiti/min.

Il **pacing cardiaco** è raccomandato in neonati con basse frequenze ventricolari (≤50 battiti/min), segni di scompenso cardiaco, ritmi a complessi larghi o cardiopatie congenite. L'isoproterenolo, l'atropina o l'adrenalina possono essere utilizzati per cercare di aumentare temporaneamente la frequenza cardiaca in attesa che possa essere predisposto l'impianto di un pacemaker. Nei lattanti sono stati tradizionalmente utilizzati impianti di pacemaker epicardici transtoracici; il posizionamento transvenoso di pacemaker è disponibile per bambini piccoli.

Un blocco AV completo postoperatorio può verificarsi a seguito di qualsiasi procedura che richieda una sutura in vicinanza delle valvole AV o della cresta del setto ventricolare. Esso viene inizialmente trattato con elettrodi per pacing temporaneo. La probabilità di ripristino del ritmo sinusale dopo 10-14 giorni è bassa, e una volta trascorso questo lasso di tempo è raccomandato un pacemaker definitivo.

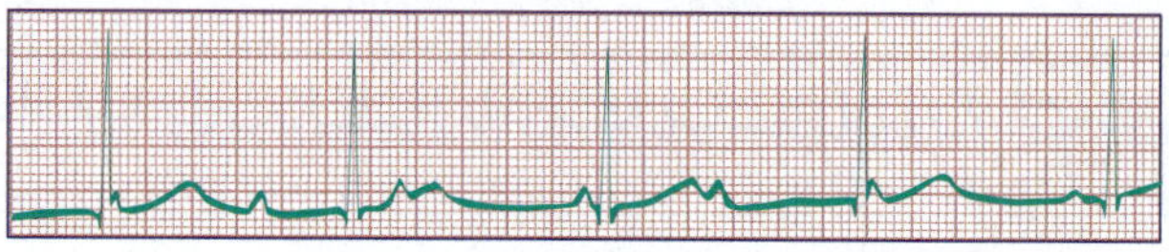

Figura 435-11. Fenomeno di Wenckebach (Mobitz I). L'intervallo P-R si allunga gradualmente finché la quarta onda P del ciclo non viene condotta al ventricolo (*freccia*). Il successivo intervallo P-R è di nuovo normale.

Ackerman MJ: Molecular basis of congenital and acquired long QT syndromes. *J Electrocardiol* 2004;37(Suppl):1–6.

Bar-Cohen Y, Walsh EP, Love BA, Cecchin F: First appropriate use of automated external difibrillator in an infant. *Resuscitation* 2005;67:135–137.

Benson DW Jr, Smith WM, Dunnigan A, et al: Mechanisms of regular, wide QRS tachycardia in infants and children. *Am J Cardiol* 1982;49:1778–1788.

Buyon JP, Friedman DM: Autobody associated congenital heart block: The clinical perspective. *Curr Rheumatol Rep* 2003;5:374–378.

Chun TU, Van Hare GF: Advances in the approach to treatment of supraventricular tachycardia in the pediatric population. *Curr Cardiol Rev* 2004;6:322–326.

Delacrètaz E: Superventricular tachycardia. *N Engl J Med* 2006;354:1039–1050.

Dunnigan A, Benson DW Jr, Banditt DG: Atrial flutter in infancy: Diagnosis, clinical features, and treatment. *Pediatrics* 1985;75:725–729.

Eronen M, Siren MK, Ekblad H, et al: Short- and long-term outcome of children with congenital complete heart block diagnosed in utero as a newborn. *Pediatrics* 2000;106:86–91.

Esberger D, Jones S, Morris F, et al: Junctional tachycardias. *Br Med J* 2002;324:662–665.

Goldberger Z, Lampert R: Implantable cardioverter-defibrillators. *JAMA* 2006;295:809–818.

Goodacre S, McLeod K: Paediatric electrocardiography. *Br Med J* 2002;324:1382–1385.

Kaultman H, Shah M: Evaluation of the child with an arrhythmia. *Pediatr Clin North Am* 2004;51:1537–1551.

Kirk CR, Gibbs JL, Thomas R: Cardiovascular collapse after verapamil in supraventricular tachycardia. *Arch Dis Child* 1987;62:1265–1266.

Miller MD, Porter CJ, Ackerman MJ: Diagnostic accuracy of screening electrocardiograms in long QT syndrome I. *Pediatrics* 2001;108:8–12.

Perry JC, Garson A Jr: Supraventricular tachycardia due to Wolff-Parkinson-White syndrome in children: Early disappearance and late recurrence. *J Am Coll Cardiol* 1990;16:1215–1220.

Roden DM: Drug-induced prolongation of the QT interval. *N Engl J Med* 2004;350:1013–1022.

Trohman RG, Kim MH, Pinski SL: Cardiac pacing: The state of the art. *Lancet* 2004;364:1701–1718.

Van Hare GF, Dubin AM, Collins KK: Invasive electrophysiology in children: State of the art. *J Electrocardiol* 2002;35(Suppl):165–174.

Walsh EP, Cecchin F: Recent advances in pacemaker and implantable defibrillator therapy for young patients. *Curr Opin Cardiol* 2004;19:91–96.

Wellens HJJ: Catheter ablation for cardiac arrhythmias. *N Engl J Med* 2004;351:1172–1174.

Capitolo 436 ■ Morte improvvisa

La morte improvvisa, eccettuata la sindrome della morte improvvisa del lattante (SIDS, *Sudden Infant Death Syndrome*; vedi Capitolo 372), è rara nei bambini di età <18 anni. Essa può avere origine traumatica o non traumatica. Le cause traumatiche, le più comuni nei bambini, comprendono incidenti stradali, morti violente, decessi durante un'attività sportiva o sul lavoro. Le morti improvvise non traumatiche sono spesso dovute a specifiche cause cardiache. L'incidenza di morte improvvisa va dallo 0,8 al 6,2 per 100 000 all'anno nei bambini e negli adolescenti, in contrasto con la più elevata incidenza di morte cardiaca improvvisa negli adulti, che è di 1 su 1000. Circa il 65% delle morti improvvise è dovuto a problemi correlati alla sfera cardiaca in pazienti con cuori normali o con anomalie congenite (corrette, sottoposte a palliazione o non trattate con intervento chirurgico). Gli sport competitivi praticati nelle scuole superiori (pallacanestro, calcio) sono fattori ambientali associati a un rischio elevato. La causa più comune di morte negli atleti che praticano sport competitivi è la miocardiopatia ipertrofica. Altre cause potenziali sono elencate nella Tabella 436-1; queste possono essere classificate come anomalie strutturali (stenosi aortica e anomalie delle arterie coronarie comprese), patologie miocardiche come le miocarditi, patologie del sistema di conduzione, come la sindrome del QT lungo (LQTS), e cause varie, tra le quali l'ipertensione polmonare e la commotio cordis. I sintomi possono essere assenti prima dell'evento; in caso contrario, comprendono sincope, dolore toracico, dispnea e palpitazioni. I pazienti possono avere un'anamnesi familiare positiva per cardiopatia (miocardiopatia dilatativa o ipertrofica, intervallo Q-T lungo, displasia del ventricolo destro, prolasso della valvola mitrale, sindrome di Marfan) o per morte improvvisa. Il decesso fa spesso seguito a un esercizio o uno sforzo fisico.

MECCANISMI ALLA BASE DELLA MORTE IMPROVVISA

Tre sono i meccanismi responsabili della morte improvvisa: aritmico, cardiaco non aritmico (cause circolatorie e vascolari) e non cardiaco. La fibrillazione ventricolare (VF, *Ventricular Fibrillation*), che è una delle più comuni cause finali di morte improvvisa negli adulti, rappresenta la causa finale solo nel 10-20% dei bambini con morte improvvisa di origine cardiaca. Più comunemente, una bradicardia porta alla VF o all'asistolia (vedi Capitolo 435).

TABELLA 436-1. Potenziali cause di morte improvvisa in lattanti, bambini e adolescenti

SIDS E PATOLOGIE CHE "MIMANO" LA SIDS
SIDS
Sindromi da Q-T lungo*
Errori congeniti del metabolismo
Abuso su minori
Miocarditi
Cardiopatie congenite dotto-dipendenti
CARDIOPATIE CONGENITE CORRETTE O NON OPERATE
Stenosi aortica
Tetralogia di Fallot
Trasposizione dei grandi vasi (dopo operazione di switch atriale)
Prolasso della valvola mitrale
Sindrome del cuore sinistro ipoplasico
Sindrome di Eisenmenger
PATOLOGIE A CARICO DELLE ARTERIE CORONARIE
Origine anomala*
Tratto anomalo (a tunnel)
Malattia di Kawasaki
Periarterite
Dissezione arteriosa
Sindrome di Marfan (rottura dell'aorta)
Infarto miocardico
MIOCARDIOPATIE
Miocarditi
Miocardiopatia ipertrofica*
Miocardiopatia dilatativa
Displasia aritmogena del ventricolo destro
ANOMALIE DEL SISTEMA DI CONDUZIONE/ARITMIE
Sindromi del Q-T lungo
Sindrome di Brugada
Farmaci proaritmici
Sindromi da pre-eccitazione
Blocco cardiaco
Commotio cordis
Fibrillazione ventricolare idiopatica
Displasia aritmogena del ventricolo destro
Tumore cardiaco
VARIE
Ipertensione polmonare
Embolia polmonare
Colpo di calore
Cocaina
Anoressia nervosa
Alterazioni elettrolitiche

*Comune.
SIDS (*Sudden Infant Death Syndrome*), sindrome della morte improvvisa del lattante.

CARDIOPATIE CONGENITE

La **stenosi valvolare aortica** è il difetto congenito più spesso associato a morte improvvisa in età pediatrica. Circa il 5% di bambini con questa patologia muore. Una storia di sincopi, dolore toracico e segni di grave ostruzione e ipertrofia ventricolare sinistra rappresentano fattori di rischio (vedi Capitolo 427.5).

Anche le **anomalie delle arterie coronarie** sono comunemente associate a morte improvvisa in bambini e adolescenti. Di queste, la più comune è l'origine della coronaria principale sinistra dal seno destro di Valsalva. L'arteria coronaria perciò decorre tra l'aorta e l'arteria polmonare. L'esercizio fisico porta a un aumento della pressione in arteria polmonare e in aorta, che comprimono la coronaria principale sinistra e causano ischemia.

MIOCARDIOPATIE

Tutti e tre i principali tipi di miocardiopatia (ipertrofica, dilatativa e restrittiva) sono associati a morte improvvisa nella popolazione pediatrica; anzi, la morte improvvisa può essere proprio la manifestazione iniziale della miocardiopatia (vedi Capitolo 439).

La **miocardiopatia ipertrofica** è la causa più comune di morte improvvisa negli adolescenti sportivi. Il rischio di morte improvvisa nei giovani affetti da questa patologia è del 2% all'anno. Fattori di rischio comprendono un'anamnesi familiare di morte improvvisa, la presenza di sintomi, aritmie ventricolari e una presentazione precoce. Molti pazienti con miocardiopatia ipertrofica presentano un'ostruzione del tratto di efflusso del ventricolo sinistro. Il meccanismo della morte improvvisa può essere secondario allo sviluppo di un'ostruzione dinamica con l'esercizio fisico e al brusco calo della gittata cardiaca che ne consegue, oppure essere correlato a un'ischemia cardiaca.

Le **miocardiopatie dilatative** sono anch'esse associate a morte cardiaca improvvisa. La displasia aritmogena del ventricolo destro è una forma specifica di miocardiopatia dilatativa associata ad aritmie ventricolari indotte dall'esercizio fisico e a morte improvvisa. La diagnosi può essere difficile; si utilizzano la RM o la biopsia endomiocardica, che però hanno un'affidabilità limitata. I cambiamenti patologici comprendono la sostituzione dei miociti del ventricolo destro con tessuto adiposo, con aree circoscritte di fibrosi.

Una **miocardite** è stata riscontrata all'esame istologico fin nel 42% dei pazienti deceduti improvvisamente. I sintomi, molto variabili, possono comprendere uno scompenso cardiaco franco oppure essere insidiosi, come un'elevata frequenza cardiaca. I pazienti pediatrici possono avere un blocco cardiaco completo o aritmie ventricolari nel corso di questa patologia.

ARITMIE CARDIACHE

Una patologia primitiva del sistema di conduzione può portare alla morte improvvisa. Le cause comprendono la sindrome di Wolff-Parkinson-White (WPW) e la sindrome del QT lungo. Oltre a causare tachicardia sopraventricolare (SVT, *SupraVentricular Tachycardia*), la sindrome di WPW può determinare una fibrillazione atriale a rapida conduzione attraverso la via accessoria, che porta alla fibrillazione ventricolare e alla morte improvvisa (Fig. 436-1) (vedi Capitolo 435). Questa evenienza, tuttavia, è estremamente rara nei pazienti pediatrici, con un'incidenza di morte improvvisa in pazienti asintomatici di 1 su 1000 pazienti all'anno. Dal momento che la digossina e il verapamil possono aumentare la conduzione attraverso le vie accessorie, questi farmaci sono controindicati nella sindrome di WPW.

La sindrome del Q-T lungo (vedi Capitolo 435), un gruppo di patologie dei canali che influiscono sulla ripolarizzazione ventri-

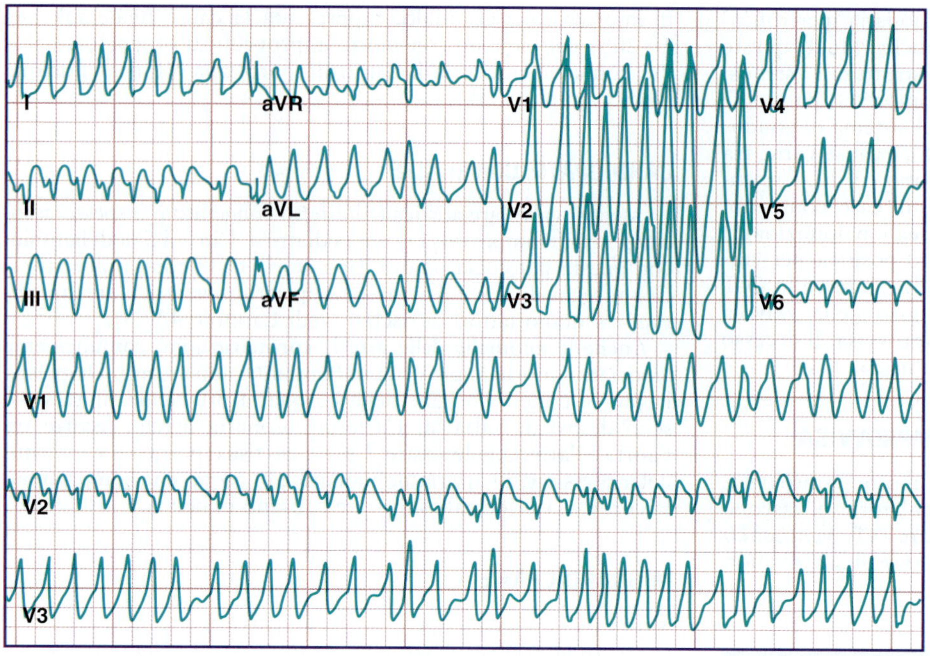

Figura 436-1. Fibrillazione atriale in un paziente con sindrome di Wolff-Parkinson-White (WPW) e conduzione rapida al ventricolo. Si noti il ritmo irregolarmente irregolare.

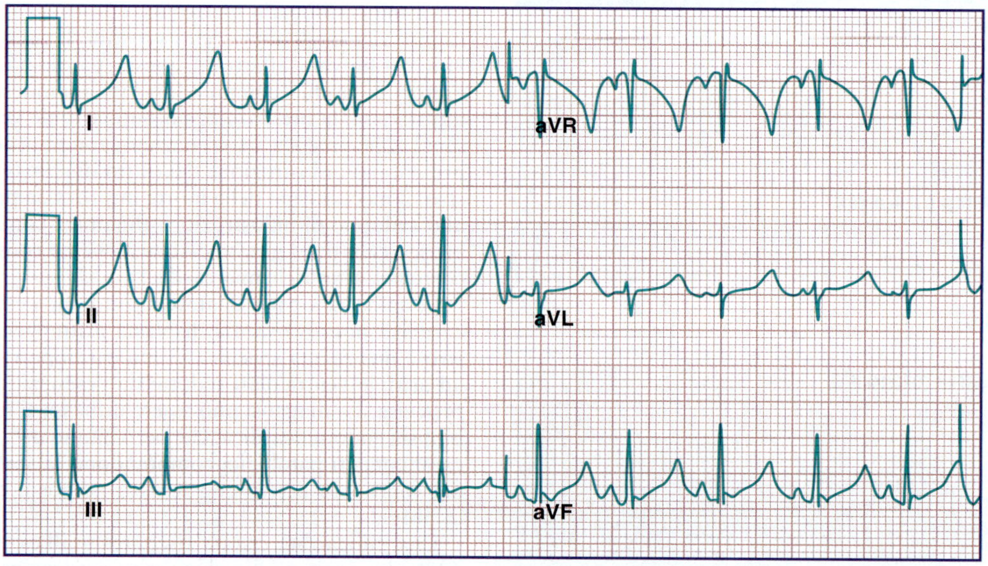

Figura 436-2. Sindrome del Q-T lungo in un neonato. Il QTc è marcatamente prolungato. Le onde T, inoltre, sono appuntite.

colare, è anch'essa associata a morte improvvisa (Fig. 436-2). Il meccanismo che conduce al decesso è una VT polimorfa (*torsade de pointes*) (Fig. 436-3). La morte cardiaca improvvisa costituisce la presentazione iniziale della patologia nel 9% dei pazienti; si raccomanda perciò il trattamento dei pazienti asintomatici con intervallo Q-T lungo all'elettrocardiogramma (ECG) e storia familiare positiva.

Intervalli Q-T lunghi acquisiti si possono osservare in pazienti con notevoli anomalie elettrolitiche, danni al SNC o *starvation* (termine inglese più ampio del nostro "digiuno": indica uno stato dovuto non solo alla mancata introduzione di alimenti, ma anche a tutte quelle condizioni che provocano riduzione dell'apporto, come la ridotta assimilazione e l'aumento delle perdite, *N.d.C.*) (comprese la bulimia e l'anoressia). Anche alcuni farmaci possono portare a un prolungamento dell'intervallo Q-T. Questi pazienti vanno inoltre soggetti ad aritmie ventricolari maligne, e la correzione del problema sottostante può essere necessaria per ridurre il rischio di morte improvvisa.

CAUSE VARIE

La **commotio cordis** è una condizione quasi sempre fatale che fa seguito a un trauma toracico chiuso (per es. colpo inferto con una mazza da baseball o da hockey). A volte traumi toracici apparentemente banali occorsi nell'ambiente domestico o su un campo da gioco possono essere fatali. I pazienti presentano immediatamente una fibrillazione ventricolare in assenza di un trauma cardiaco identificabile (contusione, ematoma, lacerazione di un'arteria coronaria). Nell'85-90% dei bambini la causa di morte è una fibrillazione ventricolare che non risponde ai tentativi di rianimazione.

VALUTAZIONE E TERAPIA PER I PAZIENTI IN RIANIMAZIONE

È importante intraprendere trattamenti mirati alle potenziali cause reversibili di morte improvvisa. Questi comprendono la

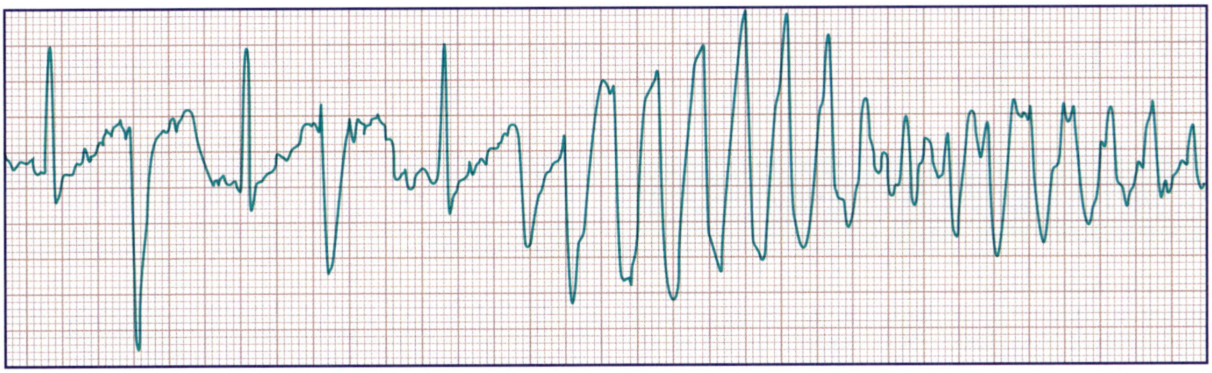

Figura 436-3. Episodi di *torsades de pointes* in un paziente con sindrome del Q-T lungo.

correzione dei principali difetti emodinamici, il pacing per i pazienti con bradicardia o la terapia di supporto per le miocarditi. Purtroppo è raro riscontrare cause reversibili nei giovani pazienti sopravvissuti a un arresto cardiaco. A questo dilemma si aggiunga la limitata capacità di prevedere la risposta ai farmaci antiaritmici o il rischio di recidiva. Perciò, il posizionamento di un defibrillatore impiantabile è divenuto il **trattamento di scelta** per i sopravvissuti a una morte improvvisa di natura aritmica.

PREVENZIONE DELLA MORTE IMPROVVISA

Per un paziente giovane che è andato incontro ad arresto cardiaco in ambiente extraospedaliero, la probabilità di sopravvivere e essere dimesso dall'ospedale è <20%. La presenza di defibrillatori esterni immediatamente trasportabili sul luogo, in combinazione con la rianimazione cardiopolmonare standard sul campo (palestra, campo di atletica, stadio di pallacanestro o di calcio), può migliorare sostanzialmente la sopravvivenza. Perciò, l'identificazione dei pazienti a rischio è di estrema importanza.

Molte delle più comuni cause di morte improvvisa nei bambini e negli adolescenti possono essere identificate dall'anamnesi del paziente (sintomi prodromici), dall'anamnesi familiare e dall'esame obiettivo.

È fondamentale che il paziente eviti i fattori ad alto rischio (uso di cocaina, anoressia nervosa) e acquisisca conoscenze riguardo agli effetti collaterali dei farmaci (antidepressivi triciclici) o delle interazioni farmacologiche (terfenadina ed eritromicina). I dispositivi di protezione del torace non sempre prevengono la commotio cordis. Una pronta rianimazione cardiopolmonare e una rapida defibrillazione con un defibrillatore automatico esterno o da parte di un'équipe medica d'emergenza migliorano la sopravvivenza. I familiari di pazienti sopravvissuti a morte improvvisa dovrebbero essere sottoposti a valutazione per la ricerca di cause genetiche come una LQTS e la miocardiopatia ipertrofica.

Atkins DL, Kenney MA: Automated external defibrillators: Safety and efficacy in children and adolescents. *Pediatr Clin North Am* 2004;51:1443–1462.
Bar-Cohen Y, Walsh EP, Love BA, Cecchin F: First appropriate use of automated external defibrillator in an infant. *Resuscitation* 2005;67:135–137.
Behr E, Wood DA, Wright M, et al: Cardiological assessment of first-degree relatives in sudden arrhythmic death syndrome. *Lancet* 2003;362:1457–1459.
Chun TU, Collins KK, Dubin AM: Implantable cardioverter defibrillators in children. *Expert Rev Cardiovasc Ther* 2004;2:561–571.
Doolan A, Langlois N, Semsarian C: Causes of sudden cardiac death in young Australians. *Med J Aust* 2004;180:110–112.
Geddes LA, Roeder RA: Evolution of our knowledge of sudden death due to commotio cordis. *Am J Emerg Med* 2005;23:67–75.
Gemayel C, Pelliccia A, Thompson PD: Arrhythmogenic right ventricular cardiomyopathy. *J Am Coll Cardiol* 2001;38:1773–1781.
Kumpf M, Sieverding L, Gass M, et al: Anomalous origin of left coronary artery in young athletes with syncope. *BMJ* 2006;332:1139–1141.
Kusumoto FM, Goldschlager N: Device therapy for cardiac arrhythmias. *JAMA* 2002;287:1848–1852.
Lee A, Ackerman MJ: Sudden unexplained death: Evaluation of those left behind. *Lancet* 2003;362:1429–1430.
Maron BJ: Sudden death in young athletes. *New Eng J Med* 2003;349:404–10.
Maron BJ, Gohman TE, Kyle SB, et al: Clinical profile and spectrum of commotio cordis. *JAMA* 2002;287:1142–1146.
Plunkett A, Hulse JA, Gill MJ: Variable presentation of Brugada syndrome: Lesions from three generations with syncope. *Br Med J* 2003;326:1078–1079.
Shaddy RA: Cardiomyopathies in adolescents: Dilated, hypertrophic and restrictive. *Adolesc Med* 2001;12:35–45.
Thompson PD, Levine BD: Protecting athletes from sudden cardiac death. *JAMA* 2006;296:1648–1650.
Towbin JA: Molecular genetic basis of sudden cardiac death. *Pediatr Clin North Am* 2004;51:1229–1255.
Weinstock J, Maron BJ, Song C, et al: Failure of commercially available chest wall protectors to prevent sudden cardiac death induced by chest wall blows in an experimental model of commotio cordis. *Pediatrics* 2006;117:e656–e662.
Williams RG, Chen AY: Identifying athletes at risk for sudden death. *J Am Coll Cardiol* 2003;42:1964–66.
Wren C: Sudden death in children and adolescents. *Heart* 2002;88:426–431.

Sezione 5 — Cardiopatie acquisite — Daniel Bernstein

Capitolo 437 ■ Endocardite infettiva

L'endocardite infettiva comprende sia l'endocardite batterica, acuta e subacuta, sia quella non batterica, causata da virus, funghi e altri agenti microbiologici. È una significativa causa di morbilità e mortalità nei bambini e negli adolescenti, nonostante i progressi compiuti nella gestione e nella profilassi della malattia mediante gli agenti antimicrobici. L'incapacità di eradicarla con la prevenzione o il trattamento precoce deriva da diversi fattori. La natura del microrganismo infettante può cambiare; medici, dentisti e persone comuni non sono abbastanza consapevoli del rischio di endocardite infettiva e delle misure preventive disponibili; la diagnosi può essere difficile quando ritardata; inoltre, sono emersi gruppi particolarmente a rischio, come gli utilizzatori di droghe per via endovenosa, i sopravvissuti a interventi cardiochirurgici, i pazienti che assumono farmaci immunosoppressori e quelli che necessitano di cateteri intravascolari per lungo tempo. Molti pazienti sviluppano un'endocardite su quella che era ritenuta una valvola nativa in precedenza sana. Inoltre, una forma sostenuta da batteri presenti nella flora orale può svilupparsi in assenza di una precedente procedura odontoiatrica.

EZIOLOGIA. Gli streptococchi viridanti (streptococchi α-emolitici) e lo *Staphylococcus aureus* sono i principali agenti causali di endocardite nei pazienti pediatrici. Altri microrganismi sono coinvolti meno frequentemente, e nel 6% circa dei casi le emocolture sono negative per qualsiasi tipo di microrganismo (Tab. 437-1). Molti pazienti affetti da endocardite con emocolture negative hanno la febbre Q (*Coxiella burnetii*) o un'infezione da varie specie di *Bartonella*. Non esiste alcuna relazione tra il microrganismo infettante e il tipo di difetto congenito, la durata della malattia o l'età del bambino. L'endocardite stafilococcica è più comune in soggetti senza una cardiopatia sottostante; l'infezione da streptococchi viridanti è più comune dopo procedure odontoiatriche; gli enterococchi di gruppo D si osservano per lo più dopo procedure invasive sul tratto terminale dell'intestino o dell'apparato genitourinario; *Pseudomonas aeruginosa* o *Serratia marcescens* si osservano più frequentemente nei soggetti che fanno uso di droghe per via endovenosa; inoltre, i miceti si riscontrano dopo la chirurgia a cuore aperto. Gli stafilococchi coagulasi-negativi sono comuni in presenza di un catetere venoso centrale a dimora.

TABELLA 437-1. Agenti batterici responsabili delle endocarditi infettive in età pediatrica

COMUNI: VALVOLE NATIVE O ALTRE LESIONI CARDIACHE
Streptococchi viridanti (*S. mutans*, *S. sanguis*, *S. mitis*)
Staphylococcus aureus
Streptococco di gruppo D (enterococco) (*S. bovis*, *S. faecalis*)
NON COMUNI: VALVOLE NATIVE O ALTRE LESIONI CARDIACHE
Streptococcus pneumoniae
Haemophilus influenzae
Stafilococchi coagulasi-negativi
Coxiella burnetii (febbre Q)*
Neisseria gonorrhoeae
*Brucella**
*Chlamydia psittaci**
*Chlamydia trachomatis**
*Chlamydia pneumoniae**
*Legionella**
*Bartonella**
Gruppo HACEK†
*Streptobacillus moniliformis**
*Pasteurella multocida**
Campylobacter fetus
Coltura negativa (6% dei casi)
VALVOLE PROTESICHE
Staphylococcus epidermidis
Staphylococcus aureus
Streptococchi viridanti
Pseudomonas aeruginosa
Serratia marcescens
Batteri difteroidi
Legionella spp.*
Gruppo HACEK†
Funghi‡

*Questi batteri esigenti, insieme ad alcuni funghi, possono causare endocardite con coltura negativa. Il loro isolamento richiede un terreno di coltura speciale, un'incubazione di durata superiore ai 7 giorni o test sierologici.

†Il gruppo HACEK comprende *Haemophilus* spp. (*H. paraphrophilus*, *H. parainfluenzae*, *H. aphrophilus*), *Actinobacillus actinomycetemcomitans*, *Cardiobacterium hominis*, *Eikenella corrodens* e *Kingella* spp.

‡*Candida* spp., *Aspergillus* spp., *Pseudoallescheria boydii*, *Histoplasma capsulatum*.

EPIDEMIOLOGIA. L'endocardite infettiva, pur essendo spesso una complicanza di una cardiopatia congenita o reumatica, può colpire anche bambini che non presentano anomalie valvolari né malformazioni cardiache. Nei Paesi sviluppati, le cardiopatie congenite sono i fattori predisponenti di gran lunga prevalenti. L'endocardite è rara nei lattanti, gruppo d'età nel quale fa di solito seguito a un intervento chirurgico a cuore aperto o è associata alla presenza di un accesso venoso centrale.

I pazienti con cardiopatie congenite in cui il sangue viene sospinto ad alta velocità attraverso un foro o un orifizio stenotico sono i più suscettibili a sviluppare un'endocardite. Le vegetazioni di solito si formano nella sede dell'erosione endocardica o intimale che risulta dal flusso turbolento. I bambini con difetti del setto interventricolare (VSD, *Ventricular Septal Defects*), valvulopatie del cuore sinistro come la stenosi aortica, la tetralogia di Fallot e comunicazioni arteriose sistemico-polmonari (dotto arterioso pervio o shunt di Blalock-Taussig) presentano il rischio più elevato. Nei pazienti di età maggiore, le valvole aortiche congenitamente bicuspidi e il prolasso della valvola mitrale con rigurgito rappresentano un rischio aggiuntivo. La correzione chirurgica di una cardiopatia congenita può ridurre ma non elimina il rischio di endocardite, con l'eccezione della riparazione di un difetto del setto interatriale semplice o di un dotto arterioso pervio. I bambini che sono stati sottoposti a sostituzione valvolare o a riparazione di condotto provvisto di valvola sono anch'essi a rischio elevato.

In circa il 30% dei pazienti con endocardite infettiva si riconosce un fattore predisponente. Una procedura chirurgica o odontoiatrica può essere implicata in circa il 65% dei casi in cui viene identificata una potenziale sorgente di batteriemia. Una scarsa igiene dentale in bambini con cardiopatia cianogena comporta un aumento del rischio. Un altro fattore (rischio del 10%) è costituito da una batteriemia primitiva da *Staphylococcus aureus*. È relativamente raro che un'endocardite si verifichi subito dopo un intervento cardiochirurgico, mentre spesso è un evento antecedente.

MANIFESTAZIONI CLINICHE (TAB. 437-2). Le manifestazioni iniziali sono di solito lievi, specialmente quando gli organismi infettanti sono streptococchi viridanti. Una febbre prolungata senza altre manifestazioni (tranne, talvolta, calo ponderale), persistente anche per parecchi mesi, può essere l'unico sintomo. In alternativa, l'esordio può essere acuto e grave, con febbre elevata, intermittente e prostrazione. Di solito l'esordio e di decorso variano tra questi due estremi. I sintomi, spesso aspecifici, consistono in febbricola con puntate pomeridiane, astenia, mialgie, artralgie, cefalea e a volte brividi, nausea e vomito. Sono comuni **soffi cardiaci nuovi**

TABELLA 437-2. Manifestazioni di endocardite infettiva

ANAMNESI	
Storia di cardiopatia congenita o reumatica	
Pregressa procedura odontoiatrica, sul tratto urinario o intestinale	
Utilizzo di droghe per via endovenosa	
Catetere venoso centrale	
Protesi valvolare cardiaca	
SINTOMI	
Febbre	
Brividi	
Dolore toracico e addominale	
Artralgie, mialgie	
Dispnea	
Malessere generale	
Sudorazione notturna	
Calo ponderale	
Manifestazioni a carico del SNC (ictus, convulsioni, cefalea)	
SEGNI	
Temperatura elevata	
Tachicardia	
Fenomeni embolici (macchie di Roth, petecchie, emorragie ungueali a scheggia, noduli di Osler, lesioni a carico del SNC o oculari)	
Lesioni di Janeway	
Soffio cardiaco di nuovo riscontro o modificato rispetto al passato	
Splenomegalia	
Artrite	
Scompenso cardiaco	
Aritmie	
Infezione metastatica (artrite, meningite, aneurisma arterioso micotico, ascessi, embolie polmonari settiche)	
Ippocratismo digitale	
LABORATORIO	
Emocolture positive	
Velocità di eritrosedimentazione elevata (può tuttavia essere bassa in presenza di insufficienza cardiaca o renale)	
Proteina C reattiva elevata	
Anemia	
Leucocitosi	
Immunocomplessi	
Ipergammaglobulinemia	
Ipocomplementemia	
Crioglobulinemia	
Fattore reumatoide	
Ematuria	
Insufficienza renale, elevata creatinina (glomerulonefrite)	
Radiografia del torace: infiltrati bilaterali, noduli, versamenti pleurici	
Evidenza ecocardiografia di vegetazioni valvolari, di disfunzione o insufficienza della protesi valvolare, di ascessi miocardici o di insufficienza valvolare di nuovo riscontro	

SNC, sistema nervoso centrale.

o modificati, in particolare con un associato scompenso cardiaco. La splenomegalia e le petecchie sono relativamente comuni. Gravi complicanze neurologiche come ictus embolici, ascessi cerebrali, aneurismi micotici ed emorragie sono per lo più associati a malattia streptococcica e possono costituire manifestazioni tardive. Meningismo, aumento della pressione intracranica, alterazione del sensorio e segni neurologici focali sono manifestazioni di queste complicanze. In corso di malattia stafilococcica talvolta si sviluppano ascessi miocardici, che possono danneggiare il sistema di conduzione del cuore, causando blocco cardiaco, o rompersi nel pericardio, provocando una pericardite purulenta. Embolie polmonari o altre embolie sistemiche sono infrequenti, tranne che in caso di malattia micotica. Tali manifestazioni comprendono i **noduli di Osler** (noduli intradermici dolenti, della grandezza di un pisello, sui polpastrelli delle dita delle mani e dei piedi), le **lesioni di Janeway** (piccole lesioni indolenti, eritematose o emorragiche, sul palmo delle mani e sulla pianta dei piedi) e **lesioni a scheggia** (lesioni lineari sotto le unghie). Questi fenomeni possono essere indicativi di una vasculite, prodotta da complessi antigene-anticorpo circolanti.

L'identificazione di un'endocardite infettiva è nella maggior parte dei casi basata su un elevato indice di sospetto durante la valutazione di un'infezione in bambini con un sottostante fattore contribuente.

DIAGNOSI. L'informazione fondamentale per il corretto trattamento di un'endocardite infettiva si ottiene dalle emocolture; tutti gli altri dati di laboratorio sono di importanza secondaria (vedi Tab. 437-2). I campioni di sangue da inviare per le colture andrebbero prelevati al più presto, anche se il bambino si sente bene e non presenta altri reperti all'esame obiettivo. Si dovrebbero ottenere da tre a cinque campioni di sangue separati, dopo accurata preparazione del sito di prelievo. La contaminazione rappresenta un problema particolare, in quanto i batteri che si trovano sulla cute possono essi stessi essere causa di endocardite infettiva. Il momento in cui viene effettuato il prelievo non è importante, poiché si suppone che la batteriemia sia relativamente costante. Nel 90% dei casi di endocardite, l'agente causale si scopre dalle prime due emocolture. Il laboratorio dovrebbe essere avvertito del sospetto di endocardite, in modo che, se necessario, sia possibile porre il sangue in coltura su terreni arricchiti per un periodo di tempo più lungo del normale (>7 giorni) per evidenziare la presenza di batteri e funghi nutrizionalmente carenti ed esigenti. Un pretrattamento antimicrobico del paziente riduce i risultati delle colture al 50-60%. Se il paziente ha assunto antibiotici il laboratorio di microbiologia dovrebbe esserne avvertito, cosicché vengano impiegati metodi più sofisticati per identificare l'agente responsabile. Altri campioni che possono essere posti in coltura comprendono materiale ottenuto per raschiamento da lesioni cutanee, urina, fluido sinoviale, ascessi e, in presenza di manifestazioni di meningite, liquido cerebrospinale. La diagnosi sierologica è necessaria in pazienti con infezione da microrganismi insoliti o esigenti (Tab. 437-3).

L'indice di sospetto dovrebbe essere elevato quando si valuta un'infezione in un bambino con un fattore predisponente sottostante. La combinazione di ecocardiogramma transtoracico e trasesofageo aumenta la capacità di diagnosticare un'endocardite. L'ecocardiografia bidimensionale è in grado di identificare la dimensione, la forma, la sede e la mobilità della lesione; in combinazione con studi Doppler, rende possibile determinare la presenza di una disfunzione valvolare (rigurgito, ostruzione) e quantificarne gli effetti sulla funzione ventricolare sinistra. L'ecocardiografia può essere utile anche per predire complicanze emboliche, dato che lesioni >1 cm e masse vegetanti comportano il rischio più elevato di embolizzazione. Le vegetazioni, la cui assenza peraltro non esclude l'endocardite, spesso non sono visualizzate nelle fasi precoci della malattia o in pazienti con cardiopatie congenite complesse.

I **criteri di Duke** aiutano nella diagnosi di endocardite. I **criteri maggiori** comprendono (1) emocolture positive (due colture separate per patogeni comuni, due o più per patogeni meno tipici) e (2) evidenza di endocardite all'ecocardiografia (massa intracardiaca su una valvola o in altra sede, flusso rigurgitante vicino a una protesi, ascesso, deiscenza parziale di valvole protesiche o nuovo flusso da rigurgito valvolare). I **criteri minori** consistono in condizioni predisponenti, febbre, segni di embolie vascolari, fenomeni da immunocomplessi (glomerulonefrite,

TABELLA 437-3. Approccio diagnostico a patogeni non comuni come causa di endocardite

PATOGENO	PROCEDURA DIAGNOSTICA
Brucella spp.	Emocolture; sierologia; coltura, immunoistologia e PCR sul materiale chirurgico
C. burnetii	Sierologia (IgG fase I >1 su 800); coltura tissutale, immunoistologia e PCR sul materiale chirurgico
Bartonella spp.	Emocolture; sierologia; coltura, immunoistologia e PCR sul materiale chirurgico
Chlamydia spp.	Sierologia; coltura, immunoistologia e PCR sul materiale chirurgico
Mycoplasma spp.	Sierologia; coltura, immunoistologia e PCR sul materiale chirurgico
Legionella spp.	Emocolture; sierologia; coltura, immunoistologia e PCR sul materiale chirurgico
T. whipplei	Istologia e PCR sul materiale chirurgico

PCR (*Polymerase Chain Reaction*), reazione a catena della polimerasi.
Da Moreillon P, Que YA; Infective endocarditis. *Lancet* 2004;363:139-148.

artrite, fattore reumatoide, noduli di Osler, macchie di Roth), un'unica emocoltura positiva o evidenza sierologica di infezione e segni ecocardiografici che non rientrano nei criteri maggiori. Due criteri maggiori, un criterio maggiore e tre minori o cinque criteri minori suggeriscono una precisa diagnosi di endocardite. Una modifica ai criteri di Duke può aumentare la sensibilità senza perdere la specificità. I seguenti criteri minori vanno aggiunti a quelli già elencati: la presenza di un ippocratismo digitale di nuova diagnosi, splenomegalia, emorragie a scheggia e petecchie; una velocità di eritrosedimentazione elevata; valori elevati di proteina C reattiva; presenza di accessi vascolari centrali chiusi, accessi vascolari periferici ed ematuria microscopica.

PROGNOSI E COMPLICANZE. Nell'era preantibiotica, l'endocardite infettiva era una malattia mortale. Nonostante l'uso degli antibiotici, la mortalità si aggira tuttora intorno al 20-25%. Una grave morbilità si verifica nel 50-60% dei bambini con endocardite infettiva documentata; la complicanza più comune è lo scompenso cardiaco, causato da vegetazioni che coinvolgono la valvola aortica o mitrale. Ascessi miocardici e miocarditi tossiche possono altresì portare allo scompenso cardiaco senza i caratteristici cambiamenti nei reperti auscultatori e, talvolta, ad aritmie minacciose per la vita. Le embolie sistemiche, spesso con manifestazioni a carico del sistema nervoso centrale, rappresentano una grave minaccia. Un'embolia polmonare può verificarsi in bambini con VSD e tetralogia di Fallot, anche se è rara un'embolizzazione polmonare massiva minacciosa per la vita. Altre complicanze comprendono aneurismi micotici, rottura di un seno di Valsalva, ostruzione di una valvola secondariamente alla presenza di ampie vegetazioni, VSD acquisiti e blocco cardiaco dovuto a un coinvolgimento (ascesso) del sistema di conduzione. Ulteriori complicanze comprendono meningite, osteomielite, artrite, ascessi renali e glomerulonefrite mediata da immunocomplessi.

TRATTAMENTO. Una volta fatta diagnosi definitiva, bisognerebbe intraprendere la terapia antibiotica immediatamente. Se l'endocardite è causata da microrganismi virulenti, anche un piccolo ritardo può portare a un progressivo danno endocardico e le probabilità di gravi complicanze sono più elevate. La scelta degli antibiotici, il metodo di somministrazione e la durata del trattamento sono delineati nelle Tabelle da 437-3 a 437-13. Elevati livelli sierici battericidi devono essere mantenuti abbastanza a lungo da eradicare microrganismi che stanno proliferando in vegetazioni avascolari relativamente inaccessibili. Per distruggere i batteri che stanno crescendo al centro di queste lesioni occorre raggiungere, nel sito dell'infezione, una concentrazione 5-20 volte maggiore rispetto alla concentrazione minima inibente *in vitro*. Devono trascorrere parecchie settimane prima che una vegetazione si organizzi completamente; il trattamento va continuato per tutto questo periodo, al fine di evitare una recrudescenza della malattia. Si raccomandano 4-6 settimane di terapia, con livelli sierici microbicidi per diluizione in provetta di almeno 1:8 dopo una dose di antibiotico. A seconda delle risposte cliniche e di laboratorio, la terapia antibiotica può richiedere alcune modifiche e in alcuni casi è necessario un trattamento più prolungato. Nel caso di infezioni da streptococchi viridanti altamente sensibili, sono stati raccomandati regimi abbreviati che comprendono penicillina per via orale per parte del trattamento. Nella malattia non sostenuta da stafilococchi, la batteriemia di solito si risolve in 24-48 ore, mentre la febbre scompare in 5-6 giorni con un'appropriata terapia antibiotica. In caso di malattia stafilococcica la guarigione richiede più tempo.

Per il trattamento dello scompenso cardiaco sono stati utilizzati la digitale, la restrizione salina e i diuretici. L'intervento chirurgico per l'endocardite infettiva è indicato in caso di grave coinvolgimento della valvola aortica o mitralica, con scompenso cardiaco intrattabile. È raro che un aneurisma micotico, la rottura di un seno aortico o la deiscenza di un patch intracardiaco richiedano

TABELLA 437-4. Terapia dell'endocardite su valvola nativa causata da streptococchi viridanti e *Streptococcus bovis* altamente sensibili alla penicillina

REGIME	DOSAGGIO* E VIA DI SOMMINISTRAZIONE	DURATA, IN SETTIMANE	COMMENTI
Penicillina G sodica acquosa cristallina	12-18 milioni di U/24 h ev in infusione continua o in 4-6 dosi ugualmente suddivise	4	Preferita in pazienti con compromissione della funzione dell'VIII nervo cranico o della funzione renale
o			
Ceftriaxone sodico	2 g/24h ev/im in 1 dose ***Dose pediatrica:***† penicillina 200 000 U/kg per 24 h ev in 4-6 dosi ugualmente suddivise; ceftriaxone 100 mg/kg per 24 h ev/im in 1 dose	4	
Penicillina G sodica acquosa cristallina	12-18 milioni U/24 h ev in infusione continua o in 6 dosi a intervalli regolari	2	Regime di 2 settimane non rivolto a pazienti con noti ascessi cardiaci o extracardiaci, o per quelli con clearance della creatinina <20 mL/min, compromissione della funzione dell'VIII nervo cranico o infezione da *Abiotrophia*, *Granulicatella* o *Gemella* spp.; il dosaggio di gentamicina dovrebbe essere adeguato per ottenere una concentrazione di picco sierica di 3-4 μg/mL e concentrazioni a valle <1 μg/mL quando vengono somministrate 3 dosi divise; viene utilizzato un nomogramma per un unico dosaggio giornaliero
o			
Ceftriaxone sodico	2 g/24h ev/im in 1 dose	2	
più			
Gentamicina solfato‡	3 mg/kg per 24 h ev/im in 1 dose, o in 3 dosi ugualmente suddivise ***Dose pediatrica:*** penicillina 200 000 U/kg per 24 h ev in 4-6 dosi ugualmente suddivise; ceftriaxone 100 mg/kg per 24 h ev/im in 1 dose; gentamicina 3 mg/kg per 24 h ev/im in 1 dose o in 3 dosi ugualmente suddivise‖	2	
Vancomicina idrocloruro¶	30 mg/kg per 24 h ev in 2 dosi ugualmente divise, senza superare i 2 g/24 h, a meno che le concentrazioni sieriche non siano inappropriatamente basse ***Dose pediatrica:*** 40 mg/kg per 24 h ev in 2-3 dosi ugualmente suddivise	4	Terapia con vancomicina raccomandata solo per pazienti che non tollerano la penicillina o il ceftriaxone; il dosaggio della vancomicina dovrebbe essere aggiustato per ottenere una concentrazione sierica di picco (1 h dopo il completamento dell'infusione) di 30-45 μg/mL e una concentrazione a valle di 10-15 μg/mL

Concentrazione minima inibitori ≤0,12 μg/mL.
*I dosaggi raccomandati sono per pazienti con normale funzione renale.
†La dose pediatrica non dovrebbe essere superiore a quella per un adulto normale.
‡Altri farmaci potenzialmente nefrotossici (per es. farmaci antinfiammatori non steroidei) dovrebbero essere utilizzati con cautela in pazienti che ricevono terapia con gentamicina.
‖Vi sono dati sul dosaggio in monosomministrazione giornaliera di aminoglicosidi nei bambini, ma non riguardano il trattamento dell'endocardite infettiva.
¶Le dosi di vancomicina dovrebbero esser infuse in almeno un'ora per ridurre il rischio della sindrome da "uomo rosso", dovuta al rilascio di istamina.

Da Baddour LM, Wilson WR, Bayer AS, et al: Infective endocarditis: Diagnosis, antimicrobial therapy, and management of complications. *Circulation* 2005;111:e394-e433 and correction *Circulation* 2005;112:2373.

TABELLA 437-5. Terapia dell'endocardite su valvola nativa causata da ceppi di streptococchi viridanti e *Streptococcus bovis* relativamente resistenti alla penicillina

REGIME	DOSAGGIO* E VIA DI SOMMINISTRAZIONE	DURATA, IN SETTIMANE	COMMENTI
Penicillina G sodica acquosa cristallina	24 milioni U/24 h ev in infusione continua o in 4-6 dosi ugualmente suddivise	4	Pazienti con endocardite causata da ceppi penicillino-resistenti (MIC >0,5 μg/mL) dovrebbero essere trattati con il regime raccomandato per l'endocardite enterococcica (vedi Tab. 437-9)
o			
Ceftriaxone sodico	2 g/24h ev/im in 1 dose	4	
più			
Gentamicina solfato†	3 mg/kg per 24 h ev/im in 1 dose o in 3 dosi ugualmente suddivise ***Dose pediatrica:***‡ penicillina 300 000 U/24 h ev in 4-6 dosi ugualmente suddivise; ceftriaxone 100 mg /kg per 24 h ev/ im in 1 dose; gentamicina 3 mg/kg per 24 h ev/im in 1 dose o in 3 dosi ugualmente suddivise	2	
Vancomicina idrocloruro‡	30 mg/kg per 24 h ev in 2 dosi ugualmente suddivise, senza superare i 2 g/24 h a meno che le concentrazioni sieriche non siano inappropriatamente basse ***Dose pediatrica:*** 40 mg/kg 24 h in 2 o 3 dosi ugualmente suddivise	4	Terapia con vancomicina§ raccomandata solo per i pazienti che non tollerano la terapia con penicillina o ceftriaxone

Concentrazione minima inibitoria (*MIC, Minimum Inibitory Concentration*) >0,12 μg/mL — ≤0,5 μg/mL.
*I dosaggi raccomandati si riferiscono a pazienti con normale funzione renale.
†Vedi Tabella 437-4 per il dosaggio appropriato della gentamicina.
‡La dose pediatrica non dovrebbe eccedere quella per un adulto normale.
§Vedi Tabella 437-4 per il dosaggio appropriato della vancomicina.
Da Baddour LM, Wilson WR, Bayer AS et al: Infective endocarditis: Diagnosis, antimicrobial therapy, and management of complications. *Circulation* 2005;111:e394-e433 and correction *Circulation* 2005;112:2373.

un intervento d'emergenza. Altre indicazioni chirurgiche comprendono l'incapacità di sterilizzare il sangue nonostante adeguati livelli di antibiotico, ascessi miocardici, embolie ricorrenti, blocco cardiaco di nuova insorgenza e un aumento delle dimensioni delle vegetazioni durante la somministrazione della terapia. Anche se la terapia antibiotica dovrebbe essere somministrata il più a lungo possibile prima dell'intervento chirurgico, l'infezione attiva non rappresenta una controindicazione se il paziente è in condizioni critiche come conseguenza di un grave deterioramento emodinamico derivante dall'endocardite infettiva. La rimozione delle vegetazioni e in alcuni casi la sostituzione valvolare possono essere salvavita, e una prolungata somministrazione di antibiotici

TABELLA 437-6. Terapia per endocardite su valvola protesica o altro materiale protesico, causata da streptococchi viridanti e *Streptococcus bovis*

REGIME	DOSAGGIO* E VIA DI SOMMINISTRAZIONE	DURATA, IN SETTIMANE	COMMENTI
CEPPI SENSIBILI ALLA PENICILLINA (CONCENTRAZIONE MINIMA INIBITORIA ≤ 0,12 μG/ML)			
Penicillina G sodica acquosa cristallina	24 milioni U/24 h in infusione continua o in 4-6 dosi ugualmente suddivise	6	Penicillina o ceftriaxone in associazione a gentamicina non hanno dimostrato percentuali di guarigione superiori in confronto alla monoterapia con penicillina o ceftriaxone per i pazienti con infezione da ceppi altamente sensibili; la terapia con gentamicina non dovrebbe essere somministrata in pazienti con clearance della creatinina <30 mL/min
o			
Ceftriaxone	2 g/24h ev/im in 1 dose	6	
con o senza			
Gentamicina solfato†	3 mg/kg in 24 h ev/im in 1 dose o in 3 dosi ugualmente suddivise ***Dose pediatrica:***‡ penicillina 300 000 U/kg per 24 h ev in 4-6 dosi ugualmente suddivise; ceftriaxone 100 mg/kg ev/im una volta al giorno; gentamicina 3 mg/kg per 24 h ev/im in 1 dose o in 3 dosi ugualmente suddivise	2	
Vancomicina idrocloruro§	30 mg/kg per 24 h ev in 2 dosi ugualmente suddivise ***Dose pediatrica:*** 40 mg/kg per 24 h ev o in 2 o 3 dosi ugualmente suddivise	6	Terapia con vancomicina raccomandata solo per pazienti che non tollerano la penicillina o il ceftriaxone
CEPPI RELATIVAMENTE O DEL TUTTO RESISTENTI ALLA PENICILLINA (CONCENTRAZIONE MINIMA INIBITORIA >0,12 μG/ML)			
Penicillina sodica acquosa cristallina	24 milione U/24 h ev in infusione continua o in 4-6 dosi ugualmente suddivise	6	
o			
Ceftriaxone	2 g/24 h ev/im in 1 dose	6	
più			
Gentamicina solfato	3 mg/kg per 24 h ev/im in 1 dose ***Dose pediatrica:*** penicillina 300 000 U/kg per 24 h ev in 4-6 dosi ugualmente suddivise	6	
Vancomicina idrocloruro	30 mg/kg per 24 h ev in 2 dosi ugualmente suddivise ***Dose pediatrica:*** 40 mg/kg per 24 h ev in 2 o 3 dosi ugualmente suddivise	6	Terapia con vancomicina raccomandata solo per pazienti che non tollerano la penicillina o il ceftriaxone

*I dosaggi raccomandati si riferiscono a pazienti con normale funzione renale.
†Vedi Tabella 437-4 per il dosaggio appropriato della gentamicina.
‡La dose pediatrica non dovrebbe superare quella per un adulto normale.
§Vedi testo e Tabella 437-4 per il dosaggio appropriato della vancomicina.
Da Baddour LM, Wilson WR, Bayer AS, et al: Infective endocarditis: Diagnosis, antimicrobial therapy, and management of complications. *Circulation* 2005;111:e394-e433 and corrections *Circulation* 2005;112:2373.

TABELLA 437-7. Terapia per l'endocardite infettiva causata da stafilococchi in assenza di materiale protesico

REGIME	DOSAGGIO* E VIA DI SOMMINISTRAZIONE	DURATA	COMMENTI
CEPPI OXACILLINA-SENSIBILI			
Nafcillina o oxacillina[†]	12 g/24h ev in 4-6 dosi ugualmente suddivise	6 settimane	Per endocardite infettiva complicata del cuore destro e per endocardite infettiva del cuore sinistro; per endocardite infettiva non complicata del cuore destro, 2 settimane
con			
Aggiunta opzionale di gentamicina solfato[‡]	3 mg/kg per 24 h ev/im in 2 o 3 dosi ugualmente suddivise ***Dose pediatrica:***[§] nafcillina o oxacillina 200 mg/kg per 24 h ev in 4-6 dosi ugualmente suddivise; gentamicina 3 mg/kg per 24 h ev/im in 3 dosi ugualmente suddivise	3-5 giorni	Il beneficio clinico degli aminoglicosidi non è stato stabilito
Per pazienti allergici alla penicillina (reazioni di tipo non anafilattoide):			Considerare test cutanei per stafilococchi sensibili alla penicillina e un'anamnesi discutibile di ipersensibilità di tipo immediato alla penicillina
Cefazolina	6 g/24 h ev in 3 dosi ugualmente suddivise	6 settimane	Le cefalosporine dovrebbero essere evitate in pazienti con ipersensibilità di tipo anafilattoide ai β-lattamici; in questi casi si dovrebbe utilizzare la vancomicina
con			
Aggiunta opzionale di gentamicina solfato	3 mg/kg per 24 h ev/im in 2 o 3 dosi ugualmente suddivise ***Dose pediatrica:*** nafcillina o oxacillina 200 mg/kg per 24 h ev in 4-6 dosi ugualmente suddivise; gentamicina 3 mg/kg per 24 h ev/im in 3 dosi ugualmente suddivise	3-5 giorni	Il beneficio clinico degli aminoglicosidi non è stato stabilito
CEPPI OXACILLINA-RESISTENTI			
Vancomicina[‖]	30 mg/kg per 24 h ev in 2 dosi ugualmente suddivise ***Dose pediatrica:*** 40 mg/kg per 24 h ev in 2 o 3 dosi ugualmente suddivise	6 settimane	Aggiustare i dosaggi di vancomicina per ottenere una concentrazione sierica a 1 ora di 30-45 μg/mL e una concentrazione a valle di 10-15 μg/mL

*I dosaggi raccomandati si riferiscono a pazienti con normale funzione renale.
[†]La penicillina G 24 milioni U/24 h ev in 4-6 dosi ugualmente suddivise può essere utilizzata al posto della nafcillina o dell'oxacillina se il ceppo è sensibile alla penicillina (concentrazione minima inibitoria ≤0,1 μg/mL) e non produce β-lattamasi.
[‡]La gentamicina dovrebbe essere somministrata a poca distanza dalla vancomicina, dalla nafcillina o dall'oxacillina.
[§]La dose pediatrica non dovrebbe essere superiore a quella per un adulto normale.
[‖]Per specifici aggiustamenti di dose e questioni riguardanti la vancomicina, vedi note alla Tabella 437-4.
Da Baddour LM, Wilson WR, Bayer AS, et al: Infective endocarditis: Diagnosis, antimicrobial therapy, and management of complications. *Circulation* 2005;111:e394-433 and corrections *Circulation* 2005;112:2373.

TABELLA 437-8. Terapia per endocardite su valvola protesica causata da stafilococchi

REGIME	DOSAGGIO* E VIA DI SOMMINISTRAZIONE	DURATA, IN SETTIMANE	COMMENTI
Ceppi oxacillina-sensibili	12 g/24 h in 6 dosi ugualmente suddivise	≤6	La penicillina G 24 milioni U/24 h ev in 4-6 dosi ugualmente suddivise può essere utilizzata al posto della nafcillina o dell'oxacillina se il ceppo è penicillino-sensibile (concentrazione minima inibitoria ≤0,1 μg/mL) e non produce β-lattamasi; la vancomicina dovrebbe essere utilizzata in pazienti con reazioni da ipersensibilità immediata agli antibiotici β-lattamici (vedi Tab. 437-4)
più			
Rifampicina	900 mg per 24 h ev/per os in 3 dosi ugualmente suddivise	≥6	
più			
Gentamicina[†]	3 mg/kg per 24 h ev/im in 2 o 3 dosi ugualmente suddivise ***Dose pediatrica:***[‡] nafcillina o oxacillina 200 mg/kg per 24 h ev in 4-6 dosi ugualmente suddivise; rifampicina 20 mg/kg per 24 h ev/per os in 3 dosi ugualmente suddivise; gentamicina 3 mg/kg per 24 h ev/im in 3 dosi ugualmente suddivise	2	
CEPPI OXACILLINA-RESISTENTI			
Vancomicina	30 mg/kg 24 h in 2 dosi ugualmente suddivise	≥6	Aggiustare la vancomicina per ottenere una concentrazione sierica a 1 h di 30-45 μg/mL e una concentrazione a valle di 10-15 μg/mL (vedi testo per alternative alla gentamicina)
più			
Rifampicina	900 mg/24 h ev/per os in 3 dosi ugualmente suddivise	≥6	
più			
Gentamicina	3 mg/kg per 24 h ev/im in 2 o 3 dosi ugualmente suddivise ***Dose pediatrica:*** vancomicina 40 mg/kg per 24 h ev in 2 o 3 dosi ugualmente suddivise; rifampicina 20 mg/kg per 24 h ev per os in 3 dosi ugualmente suddivise (fino alla dose prevista per l'adulto); gentamicina 3 mg/kg per 24 h ev o im in 3 dosi ugualmente suddivise	2	

*I dosaggi raccomandati si riferiscono a pazienti con normale funzione renale.
[†]La gentamicina dovrebbe essere somministrata a poca distanza dalla vancomicina, dalla nafcillina o dall'oxacillina (vedi Tab. 437-4).
[‡]La dose pediatrica non dovrebbe superare quella per un adulto normale.
Da Baddour LM, Wilson WR, Bayer AS, et al: Infective endocarditis: Diagnosis, antimicrobial therapy, and management of complications. *Circulation* 2005;111:e394-e433 and corrections *Circulation* 2005;112:2373.

TABELLA 437-9. Terapia per l'endocardite enterococcica su valvola nativa o protesica causata da ceppi sensibili a penicillina, gentamicina e vancomicina

REGIME	DOSAGGIO* E VIA SOMMINISTRAZIONE	DURATA, IN SETTIMANE	COMMENTI
Ampicillina sodica	12 g/24 h ev in 6 dosi ugualmente suddivise	4-6	Valvola nativa: raccomandate 4 settimane per pazienti con sintomi di malattia da 3 mesi o meno; terapia di 6 settimane raccomandata per pazienti con sintomi da più di 3 mesi
o			
Penicillina G acquosa cristallina	18-30 milioni U /24 h in infusione continua o in 6 dosi ugualmente suddivise	4-6	Valvola protesica o altro materiale protesico cardiaco: raccomandate minimo 6 settimane di terapia
più			
Gentamicina solfato[†]	3 mg/kg per 24 h ev/im in 3 dosi ugualmente suddivise ***Dose pediatrica:***[‡] ampicillina 300 mg/kg per 24 h ev in 4-6 dosi ugualmente suddivise; penicillina 300 000 U/kg per 24 h ev in 4-6 dosi ugualmente suddivise; gentamicina 3 mg/kg per 24 h ev/im in 3 dosi ugualmente suddivise		
Vancomicina idrocloruro[§]	30 mg/kg 24 h in 2 dosi ugualmente suddivise	6	Terapia con vancomicina raccomandata solo per pazienti che non tollerano la penicillina o l'ampicillina
più			
Gentamicina solfato	3 mg per 24 h ev/im in 3 dosi ugualmente suddivise ***Dose pediatrica:*** vancomicina 40 mg/kg per 24 h ev in 2 o 3 dosi ugualmente suddivise; gentamicina 3 mg/kg per 24 h ev/im in 3 dosi ugualmente suddivise	6	Raccomandate 6 settimane di terapia con vancomicina a causa della diminuita attività contro gli enterococchi

*I dosaggi raccomandati si riferiscono a pazienti con normale funzione renale.
[†]I dosaggi di gentamicina dovrebbero essere aggiustati per ottenere una concentrazione di picco sierica di 3-4 μg/mL e una concentrazione a valle <1 μg/mL (vedi Tab. 437-4 per il dosaggio della gentamicina).
[‡]La dose pediatrica non dovrebbe superare quella per un adulto normale.
[§]Vedi Tabella 437-4 per il dosaggio appropriato della vancomicina.
Da Baddour LM, Wilson WR, Bayer AS, et al: Infective endocarditis: Diagnosis, antimicrobial therapy, and management of complications. *Circulation* 2005;111:e394- e433 and corrections *Circulation* 2005;112:2373.

TABELLA 437-10. Terapia per l'endocardite enterococcica su valvola nativa o protesica causata da ceppi sensibili a penicillina, streptomicina e vancomicina, e resistenti a gentamicina

REGIME	DOSAGGIO* E VIA DI SOMMINISTRAZIONE	DURATA, IN SETTIMANE	COMMENTI
Ampicillina sodica	12 g/24 h in 6 dosi ugualmente suddivise	4-6	Valvola nativa: raccomandate 4 settimane di terapia nei pazienti con sintomi di malattia da meno di 3 mesi; raccomandate 6 settimane di terapia nei pazienti con sintomi da più di 3 mesi
o			
Penicillina G sodica acquosa cristallina	24 milioni U/24 h ev in infusione continua o in 6 dosi ugualmente suddivise	4-6	
più			
Streptomicina solfato	15 mg/kg per 24 h ev/im in 2 dosi ugualmente suddivise ***Dose pediatrica:***[‡] ampicillina 300 mg/kg per 24 h ev in 4-6 dosi ugualmente suddivise; penicillina 300 000 U/kg per 24 h ev in 4-6 dosi ugualmente suddivise; streptomicina 20-30 mg/kg per 24 h ev/im in 2 dosi ugualmente suddivise	4-6	Valvola protesica o altro materiale cardiaco protesico: raccomandate minimo 6 settimane di terapia
Vancomicina idrocloruro[‡]	30 mg/kg per 24 h in 2 dosi ugualmente suddivise	6	Terapia con vancomicina raccomandata solo per pazienti che non tollerano la penicillina o l'ampicillina
più			
Streptomicina solfato	15 mg/kg per 24 h ev/im in 2 dosi ugualmente suddivise ***Dose pediatrica:*** vancomicina 40 mg/kg per 24 h ev in 2 o 3 dosi ugualmente suddivise; streptomicina 20-30 mg/kg per 24 h ev/im in 2 dosi ugualmente suddivise	6	

*I dosaggi raccomandati si riferiscono a pazienti con normale funzione renale.
[†]Vedi Tabella 437-4 per il dosaggio appropriato della vancomicina.

Da Baddour LM, Wilson WR, Bayer AS et al: Infective endocarditis: Diagnosis, antimicrobial therapy, and management of complications. *Circulation* 2005;111:e394-e433 and corrections *Circulation* 2005;112:2373.

nella maggior parte dei casi preverrà la reinfezione. La sostituzione di protesi valvolari infette è associata a un rischio maggiore.

L'endocardite fungina, oltre a essere difficile da gestire, ha una prognosi peggiore. Si riscontra dopo interventi cardiochirurgici, in pazienti gravemente debilitati o immunosoppressi e in quelli in terapia antibiotica da molto tempo. I farmaci di scelta sono l'amfotericina B (preparazione liposomiale o standard) e la 5-fluorocitosina. Talvolta si tenta un intervento chirurgico di l'escissione del tessuto infetto, anche se spesso con limitato successo. L'attivatore tissutale del plasminogeno ricombinante può aiutare a lisare le vegetazioni intracardiache e a evitare l'intervento chirurgico in alcuni pazienti ad alto rischio.

PREVENZIONE. La profilassi antimicrobica prima di varie procedure e interventi odontoiatrici può ridurre l'incidenza di endocardite infettiva in pazienti suscettibili (Tabb. 437-14 e 437-15). È importante un'educazione continua riguardo alla profilassi, specialmente negli adolescenti e nei giovani adulti, che spesso hanno una scarsa conoscenza della propria cardiopatia congenita. Un'adeguata cura dei denti e una corretta igiene orale sono della massima importanza per diminuire il rischio di endocardite infettiva negli individui suscettibili. Anche un trattamento aggressivo di sepsi e infezioni localizzate e un'accurata asepsi durante interventi cardiochirurgici e cateterismo ne riducono l'incidenza.

TABELLA 437-11. Terapia per l'endocardite su valvola nativa o protesica causata da ceppi resistenti alla penicillina e sensibili agli aminoglicosidi ed alla vancomicina

REGIME	DOSAGGIO* E VIA DI SOMMINISTRAZIONE	DURATA, IN SETTIMANE	COMMENTI
CEPPI PRODUTTORI DI β-LATTAMASI			
Ampicillina/sulbactam	12 g/24 h ev in 4 dosi ugualmente suddivise	6	Improbabile che il ceppo sia sensibile alla gentamicina; se il ceppo è gentamicina-resistente, saranno necessarie più di 6 settimane di terapia con ampicillina/sulbactam
più			
Gentamicina solfato[†]	3 mg/kg per 24 h ev/im in 3 dosi ugualmente suddivise ***Dose pediatrica:***[‡] ampicillina/sulbactam 300 mg/kg per 24 h ev in 4 dosi ugualmente suddivise; gentamicina 3 mg/kg per 24 h ev/im in 3 dosi ugualmente suddivise	6	
Vancomicina idrocloruro[§]	30 mg/kg per 24 h ev in 2 dosi ugualmente suddivise	6	Terapia con vancomicina raccomandata solo per pazienti che non tollerano l'ampicillina/sulbactam
più			
Gentamicina solfato[†]	3 mg/kg per 24 ev/im in 3 dosi ugualmente suddivise ***Dose pediatrica:*** vancomicina 40 mg/kg per 24 h in 2 o 3 dosi ugualmente suddivise; gentamicina 3 mg/kg per 24 h ev/im in 3 dosi ugualmente suddivise	6	
RESISTENZA INTRINSECA ALLA PENICILLINA			
Vancomicina idrocloruro[‡]	30 mg/kg ev in 2 dosi ugualmente suddivise	6	Raccomandata consulenza di uno specialista in malattie infettive
più			
Gentamicina solfato[†]	3 mg/kg per 24 h ev/im in 3 dosi ugualmente suddivise ***Dose pediatrica:*** vancomicina 40 mg/kg per 24 h ev in 2 o 3 dosi ugualmente suddivise; gentamicina 3 mg/kg per 24 h ev/im in 3 dosi ugualmente suddivise	6	

*I dosaggi raccomandati si riferiscono a pazienti con funzione renale normale.
[†]Vedi Tabella 437-4 per il dosaggio appropriato della gentamicina.
[‡]La dose pediatrica non dovrebbe superare quella per un adulto normale.
[§]Vedi Tabella 437-4 per il dosaggio appropriato della vancomicina.
Da Baddour LM, Wilson WR, Bayer AS et al: Infective endocarditis: Diagnosis, antimicrobial therapy, and management of complications. *Circulation* 2005;111:e394-e433 and corrections *Circulation* 2005;112:2373.

TABELLA 437-12. Terapia per endocardite su valvola nativa o protesica causata da ceppi resistenti a penicillina, aminoglicosidi e vancomicina

REGIME	DOSAGGIO* E VIA DI SOMMINISTRAZIONE	DURATA, IN SETTIMANE	COMMENTI
E. faecium			
Linezolid	1200 mg/24 h ev/per os in 2 dosi ugualmente suddivise	≥8	I pazienti con endocardite causata da questi ceppi dovrebbero essere trattati dopo consulenza con uno specialista in malattie infettive; può essere necessaria per la cura batteriologica la sostituzione della valvola cardiaca; la percentuale di guarigione con la sola terapia antimicrobica può essere <50%; può verificarsi una grave trombocitopenia, di solito reversibile, con l'utilizzo di linezolid, specialmente dopo 2 settimane di terapia; quinopristina-dafopristina sono efficaci solo contro *E. faecium* e possono provocare gravi mialgie, richiedono la sospensione del trattamento; è riportato solo un piccolo numero di pazienti trattati con imipenem/cilastatina-ampicillina o ceftriaxone + ampicillina
o			
Quinopristina/dalfopristina	22,5 mg/kg per 24 h ev in 3 dosi ugualmente suddivise	≥8	
E. faecium			
Imipenem/cilastatina	2 g/24 h ev in 4 dosi ugualmente suddivise	≥8	
più			
Ampicillina sodica	12 g/24 h ev in 6 dosi ugualmente suddivise	≥8	
o			
Ceftriaxone sodico	4 g/24 h ev/im in 2 dosi suddivise	≥8	
più			
Ampicillina sodica	12 g /24 h ev in 6 dosi ugualmente suddivise ***Dose pediatrica:***[†] linezolid 30 mg/kg per 24 h ev/per os in 3 dosi ugualmente suddivise; quinopristina/dalfopristina 22,5 mg/kg per 24 h ev in 3 dosi ugualmente suddivise; imipenem/cilastatina 60-100 mg/kg per 24 h ev in 4 dosi ugualmente suddivise; ampicillina 300 mg/kg per 24 h ev in 4-6 dosi ugualmente suddivise; ceftriaxone 100 mg/kg per 24 h ev/im in 2 dosi ugualmente suddivise	≥8	

Ordine di preferenza decrescente, basato sui dati pubblicati.
*I dosaggi raccomandati si riferiscono a pazienti con normale funzionalità renale.
[†]La dose pediatrica non dovrebbe superare quella per un adulto normale.
Da Baddour LM, Wilson WR, Bayer AS et al: Infective endocarditis: Diagnosis, antimicrobial therapy, and management of complications. *Circulation* 2005;111:e394-e433 and correction *Circulation* 2005;112:2373.

TABELLA 437-13. Terapia per endocardite su valvola nativa e prostatica causata da microrganismi HACEK

REGIME	DOSAGGIO E VIA DI SOMMINISTRAZIONE	DURATA, IN SETTIMANE	COMMENTI
Ceftriaxone[†] sodico	2 g/24 h ev/im in 1 dose	4	Può essere sostituito da cefotaxime o da un'altra cefalosporina di terza o quarta generazione
o			
Ampicillina/sulbactam[‡]	12 g/24 h ev in 4 dosi ugualmente suddivise	4	
o			
Ciprofloxacina[§]	1000 mg/24 h per os o 800 mg/24 h ev in 2 dosi ugualmente suddivise ***Dose pediatrica:***[‖] ceftriaxone 100 mg/kg per 24 h ev/im una volta al giorno; ampicillina-sulbactam 300 mg/kg per 24 h suddivisi in 4-6 dosi uguali; ciprofloxacina 20-30 mg/kg per 24 h ev/per os in 2 dosi ugualmente suddivise	4	La terapia con fluorochinolonici è raccomandata solo per pazienti che non tollerano la terapia con cefalosporine e ampicillina; può essere sostituito da levofloxacina, gatifloxacina o moxifloxacina; i fluorochinolonici non sono in genere raccomandati per i pazienti di età <18 anni Valvola protesica: i pazienti con endocardite che coinvolge una valvola cardiaca protesica o altro materiale cardiaco protesico dovrebbero essere trattati per 6 settimane

**Haemophilus parainfluenzae, H. aphrophilus, Actinobacillus actinomuycetemcomitans, Cardiobacterium hominis, Eikenella corrodens* e *Kingella kingae*.
[†]I pazienti dovrebbero essere informati del fatto che l'iniezione im di ceftriaxone è dolorosa.
[‡]Dosaggio raccomandato per pazienti con normale funzionalità renale.
[§]I fluorochinoloni sono altamente attivi in vitro contro i microrganismi HACEK. I dati pubblicati sull'uso dei fluorochinolonici per la terapia dell'endocardite causata dai batteri del gruppo HACEK sono pochissimi.
[‖]La dose pediatrica non dovrebbe essere superiore a quella per un adulto normale.
Da Baddour LM, Wilson WR, Bayer AS et al: Infective endocarditis: Diagnosis, antimicrobial therapy, and management of complications. *Circulation* 2005;111:e394-e433 and correction *Circulation* 2005;112:2373.

TABELLA 437-14. Raccomandazioni per la profilassi contro l'endocardite batterica

PROCEDURE ODONTOIATRICHE E SUL CAVO ORALE O CHIRURGIA DEL TRATTO RESPIRATORIO SUPERIORE O DELL'ESOFAGO		PROCEDURE CHIRURGICHE E STRUMENTARI SUL TRATTO GASTROINTESTINALE E GENITOURINARIO	
Per la maggior parte dei pazienti	Amoxicillina per os Adulti 2,0 g, bambini 50 mg/kg 1 ora prima della procedura	Pazienti ad alto rischio	Ampicillina im o ev Adulti 2,0 g, bambini 50 mg/kg *più* Gentamicina im o ev 1,5 mg/kg (dose massima 120 mg) somministrati almeno 30 minuti prima della procedura *e 6 ore dopo* Ampicillina im o ev o amoxicillina per os Adulti 1 g, bambini 25 mg/kg
Per i pazienti non in grado di assumere farmaci per os	Ampicillina im o ev Adulti 2,0 g, bambini 50 mg/kg somministrati almeno 30 minuti prima dell'inizio della procedura	Pazienti ad alto rischio allergici all'ampicillina e all'amoxicillina	Vancomicina ev Adulti 1,0 g, bambini 20 mg/kg somministrati in 1-2 h *più* Gentamicina im o ev 1,5 mg/kg (dose massima 120 mg); completare l'iniezione/infusione almeno 30 minuti prima dell'inizio della procedura
Pazienti allergici all'ampicillina e all'amoxicillina	Clindamicina per os Adulti 600 mg, bambini 20 mg/kg 1 ora prima della procedura *o* Cefalexina* o cefadroxil* per os Adulti 2,0 g, bambini 50 mg/kg 1 ora prima della procedura *o* Azitromicina o claritromicina per os Adulti 500 mg, bambini 15 mg/kg 1 ora prima della procedura		
Pazienti allergici all'ampicillina e all'amoxicillina, non in grado di assumere farmaci per via orale	Clindamicina ev Adulti 600 mg, bambini 20 mg/kg somministrati almeno 30 minuti prima della procedura *o* Cefazolina ev Adulti 1,0 g, bambini 25 mg/kg somministrati almeno 30 minuti prima della procedura		

*Le cefalosporine non dovrebbero essere utilizzate in pazienti con reazione da ipersensibilità di tipo immediato alle penicilline.
Pazienti ad alto rischio: protesi valvolari cardiache (compresi gli homograft), precedente endocardite, cardiopatia congenita complessa con cianosi non sottoposta a correzione (per es. trasposizione dei grandi vasi, tetralogia di Fallot, ventricolo unico), shunt o condotti arteriosi sistemico-polmonari. Difetti cardiaci congeniti sottoposti a riparazione con materiale protesico (chirurgia o posizionamento di catetere) 6 mesi dopo la procedura. Cardiopatie congenite sottoposte a correzione con difetti residui. Trapianto cardiaco, se si sviluppa una valvulopatia.
Pazienti a rischio trascurabile (profilassi non raccomandata): ASD isolato tipo ostium secundum; correzione chirurgica di ASD, VSD o PDA (senza difetti residui e oltre 6 mesi dalla correzione); pregresso bypass arterioso coronarico; soffi cardiaci funzionali; pregressa malattia di Kawasaki o febbre reumatica senza disfunzione valvolare; pacemaker cardiaci; defibrillatori impiantabili.
Il rischio associato a prolasso mitralico è oggetto di controversie. Il prolasso mitralico con rigurgito o lembi valvolari ispessiti, o entrambe queste caratteristiche, è considerato a rischio moderato; il prolasso valvolare mitralico senza rigurgito è considerato a rischio trascurabile.
ASD (*Atrial Septal Defect*), difetto del setto interatriale; im, intramuscolo; ev, endovena; PDA (*Patent Ductus Arteriosus*), dotto arterioso pervio; VSD (*Ventricular Septal Defect*), difetto del setto interventricolare.
Adattata da Dajani AS, Taubert KA, Wilson W et al: Prevention of bacterial endocarditis. Recommendations by the American Heart Association. *JAMA* 1997; 277:1794-1801 e Wilson W, Taubert KA, Gewitz M et al: Prevention of infective endocarditis. Guidelines from the American Heart Association. *Circulation* 2007;DOI:10.1161/circulationaha.106.183095.

TABELLA 437-15. Procedure e profilassi contro l'endocardite

PROFILASSI CONTRO L'ENDOCARDITE RACCOMANDATA*

Procedure odontoiatriche

Estrazioni dentarie
Procedure peridontali, inclusa la chirurgia, il livellamento e la limatura delle radici, il sondaggio e le cure di mantenimento
Procedure di impianto dentario e reimpianto di avulsioni dentarie
Procedure strumentali o chirurgiche di endodonzia (cure canalari) solo oltre l'apice
Posizionamento sottogengivale di fibre o banderelle antibiotiche
Posizionamento iniziale di elastici ortodontici, ma non di apparecchi
Iniezioni anestetiche locali intraligamentarie
Pulizia profilattica di denti o impianti quando ci si aspetta un sanguinamento

Tratto respiratorio

Tonsillectomia o adenoidectomia, o entrambi
Operazioni chirurgiche che coinvolgono la mucosa respiratoria
Broncoscopia con broncoscopio rigido o biopsia

Tratto gastrointestinale†

Scleroterapia per varici esofagee
Dilatazione di stenosi esofagee
Colangiografia retrograda endoscopica in presenza di ostruzione biliare
Chirurgia sul tratto biliare
Operazioni chirurgiche che coinvolgono la mucosa intestinale

PROFILASSI CONTRO L'ENDOCARDITE NON RACCOMANDATA

Procedure odontoiatriche

Interventi dentistici di ricostruzione‡ (operatori e prostodontici), con o senza corda di retrazione§
Iniezioni per anestesia locale (non intraligamentaria)
Trattamento endodontico endocanalare, dopo posizionamento e costruzione
Posizionamento di chiusure gengivali
Rimozione postoperatoria di suture
Posizionamento di dispositivi prostodontici o ortodontici rimovibili
Calchi dentari
Trattamenti con fluoro
Radiografie dentarie
Sistemazione di apparecchi ortodontici
Caduta dei denti decidui

Tratto respiratorio

Intubazione endotracheale
Broncoscopia con broncoscopio flessibile senza biopsia§
Inserzione di tubo per timpanostomia

Tratto gastrointestinale

Ecocardiografia transesofagea§
Endoscopia con o senza biopsia gastrointestinale§

Tratto genitourinario

Cistoscopia
Parto vaginale§
Taglio cesareo
In tessuti non infetti:
- Cateterismo uretrale
- Dilatazione uterina e curettage
- Aborto terapeutico
- Procedure di sterilizzazione
- Inserzione o rimozione di dispositivi intrauterini

Altre procedure

Cateterismo cardiaco, compresa angioplastica con palloncino
Impianto di pacemaker cardiaci, di defibrillatori impiantabili e posizionamento di stent coronarici
Incisione o biopsia di cute detersa per intervento chirurgico
Circoncisione

*La profilassi è raccomandata per pazienti con patologie cardiache a rischio elevato o moderato.
†La profilassi è raccomandata per i pazienti ad alto rischio; è opzionale per i pazienti a medio rischio.
‡Comprende la ricostruzione di denti cariati (otturazioni) e la sostituzione di denti mancanti.
§La profilassi è opzionale per i pazienti ad alto rischio.

Ashrafian H, Bogle RG: Antimicrobial prophylaxis for endocarditis: emotion or science? *Heart* 2007;93:5–6.

Ayres NA, Miller-Hance W, Fyfe DA, et al: Indications and guidelines for performance of transesophageal echocardiography in the patient with pediatric acquired or congenital heart disease: Report from the task force of the Pediatric Council of the American Society of Echocardiography. *J Am Soc Echocardiogr* 2005;18:91–98.

Baddour LM, Wilson WR, Bayer AS, et al: Infective endocarditis: Diagnosis, antimicrobial therapy, and management of complications. *Circulation* 2005;111:e394–e433.

Bouza E, Menasalvas A, Munoz P, et al: Infective endocarditis—a prospective study at the end of the twentieth century. *Medicine (Baltimore)* 2001;80:298–307.

Dajani AS, Taubert KA, Wilson W, et al: Prevention of bacterial endocarditis. Recommendations by the American Heart Association. *JAMA* 1997;277:1794–1801.

Ellis ME, Al-Abdely H, Sandridge A, et al: Fungal endocarditis: Evidence in the world literature, 1965–1995. *Clin Infect Dis* 2001;32:50–62.

Ferrieri P, Gewitz MH, Berger M, et al: Unique features of infective endocarditis in childhood. *Pediatrics* 2002;109:931–943.

Hartzell JD, Torres D, Kim P, et al: Incidence of bacteremia after routine tooth brushing. *Am J Med Sci* 2005;329:178–180.

Hoen B, Alla F, Selton-Suty C, et al: Changing profile of infective endocarditis. Results of a 1-year survey in France. *JAMA* 2002;288:75–80.

Houpikian P, Raoult D: Blood culture-negative endocarditis in a reference center: Etiologic diagnosis of 348 cases. *Medicine (Baltimore)* 2005;84:162–173.

Lamas CC, Eykyn SJ: Blood culture negative endocarditis: Analysis of 63 cases presenting over 25 years. *Heart* 2003;89:258–262.

Levitas A, Zucker N, Zalzstein E, et al: Successful treatment of infective endocarditis with recombinant tissue plasminogen activator. *J Pediatr* 2003;143:649–652.

Martin JM, Neches WH, Wald ER: Infective endocarditis: 35 years of experience at a children's hospital. *Infect Dis* 1997;24:669–675.

Milazzo AS Jr, Li JS: Bacterial endocarditis in infants and children. *Pediatr Infect Dis J* 2001;20:799–801.

Moreillon P, Que YA: Infective endocarditis. *Lancet* 2004;363:139–148.

Morris CD, Reller MD, Menashe VD: Thirty-year incidence of infective endocarditis after surgery for congenital heart disease. *JAMA* 1998;279:599–603.

Tissieres P, Gervaix A, Beghetti M, et al: Value and limitations of the von Reyn, Duke, and modified Duke criteria for the diagnosis of infective endocarditis in children. *Pediatrics* 2003;112:e467.

Valente AM, Jain R, Scheurer M, et al: Frequency of infective endocarditis among infants and children with *Staphylococcus aureus* bacteremia. *Pediatrics* 2005;115:e15–e19.

Wilson W, Taubert KA, Gewitz M, et al: Prevention of infective endocarditis. Guidelines from the American Heart Association. *Circulation* 2007;DOI: 10.1161/circulationaha.106.183095.

Capitolo 438 ■ Cardiopatia reumatica

Il coinvolgimento reumatico delle valvole e dell'endocardio è la manifestazione più importante della febbre reumatica (vedi Capitoli 156 e 182.1). Le lesioni valvolari si presentano inizialmente come piccole verruche, composte da fibrina e cellule ematiche, lungo i bordi di una o più valvole cardiache. La valvola mitrale è quella più spesso colpita, seguita dalla valvola aortica; manifestazioni a carico del cuore destro sono rare. Quando l'infiammazione recede, le verruche tendono a scomparire lasciando un tessuto cicatriziale. Ripetuti attacchi di febbre reumatica portano alla formazione di nuove verruche accanto alle precedenti, con coinvolgimento dell'endocardio murale e delle corde tendinee.

PATTERN DI MALATTIA VALVOLARE

INSUFFICIENZA MITRALICA

Fisiopatologia. L'insufficienza mitralica è il risultato di alterazioni strutturali che di solito comprendono una certa perdita di sostanza valvolare e l'accorciamento e l'ispessimento delle corde tendinee. Durante la febbre reumatica acuta con un grave coinvolgimento cardiaco lo scompenso cardiaco è causato dall'insufficienza mitralica unita a una patologia infiammatoria del pericardio, del miocardio, dell'endocardio e dell'epicardio. A causa dell'elevato carico di volume e del processo infiammatorio, il ventricolo sinistro si dilata. Anche l'atrio sinistro va incontro a dilatazione quando il sangue rigurgita in questa camera. L'aumentata pressione atriale sinistra porta a congestione polmonare e sintomi di scompenso cardiaco sinistro. Con il tempo si assiste a un miglioramento spontaneo, anche in pazienti in cui l'insufficienza mitralica è grave fin dall'esordio. La lesione cronica che ne risulta è nella maggior parte dei casi di entità lieve o moderata, e il paziente è asintomatico. Più della metà dei pazienti con insufficienza mitralica acuta non ha più il soffio mitralico a distanza di un anno. In pazienti con grave insufficienza mitralica cronica, la pressione arteriosa polmonare subisce un notevole aumento, il ventricolo destro e l'atrio destro si dilatano e di conseguenza si sviluppa un'insufficienza del cuore destro.

Manifestazioni cliniche. I reperti obiettivi di insufficienza mitralica dipendono dalla sua gravità. Con una malattia lieve, non sono presenti segni di scompenso cardiaco, il precordio è in quiete e l'auscultazione rivela un soffio olosistolico di tonalità elevata all'apice, che si irradia all'ascella. Se invece l'insufficienza mitralica è grave, possono notarsi segni di scompenso cardiaco cronico. Il cuore è dilatato, con un sollevamento palpabile dell'apice ventricolare sinistro e spesso un fremito sistolico apicale. Si ode un soffio olosistolico all'apice, irradiato all'ascella. Un breve soffio rullante mesodiastolico è causato da un aumento del flusso attraverso la valvola mitrale, come risultato dell'insufficienza. L'auscultazione di un soffio diastolico non implica necessariamente che sia presente una stenosi mitralica. Quest'ultima lesione impiega molti anni a svilupparsi ed è caratterizzata da un soffio diastolico di lunghezza maggiore con rinforzo presistolico.

L'elettrocardiogramma e la radiografia del torace sono normali se la lesione è lieve. In un'insufficienza più grave, l'elettrocardiogramma evidenzia onde P prominenti e bifide, segni di ipertrofia ventricolare sinistra e un'associata ipertrofia ventricolare destra se è presente ipertensione polmonare. Dal punto di vista radiografico, si può osservare la sporgenza dell'atrio sinistro e del ventricolo sinistro. Inoltre, può essere evidente una congestione dei vasi peri-ilari, un segno di ipertensione venosa polmonare. Una calcificazione della valvola mitrale è rara nei bambini. L'ecocardiografia evidenzia ingrandimento dell'atrio sinistro e del ventricolo sinistro, mentre le indagini Doppler permettono di stimare la gravità del rigurgito mitralico. Il cateterismo cardiaco e la ventricolografia sinistra vengono presi in considerazione solo se le procedure non invasive non sono sufficienti a chiarire i quesiti diagnostici. Il grado di opacizzazione dell'atrio sinistro durante la ventricolografia sinistra permette la valutazione qualitativa della gravità dell'insufficienza mitralica.

Complicanze. Talvolta una grave insufficienza mitralica porta a uno scompenso cardiaco che può essere precipitato dalla progressione del processo reumatico, dall'esordio di una fibrillazione atriale o da un'endocardite infettiva. Gli effetti di un'insufficienza mitralica cronica, che possono rendersi evidenti dopo molti anni, comprendono uno scompenso ventricolare destro e aritmie atriali e ventricolari.

Trattamento. In pazienti con lieve insufficienza mitralica, è sufficiente la profilassi contro le recidive di febbre reumatica. Il trattamento di uno scompenso cardiaco che insorge come complicanza (vedi Capitolo 442) di aritmie (vedi Capitolo 435) e di un'endocardite infettiva (vedi Capitolo 437) è descritto altrove. I farmaci che diminuire il post-carico (ACE-inibitori) possono ridurre il volume di sangue rigurgitante e preservare la funzione ventricolare sinistra. Il trattamento chirurgico è indicato per pazienti che, nonostante un'adeguata terapia medica, hanno ricorrenti episodi di scompenso cardiaco, dispnea in occasione di sforzi moderati e progressiva cardiomegalia, spesso con ipertensione polmonare. Anche se l'anuloplastica dà buoni risultati in alcuni bambini e adolescenti, può essere richiesta la sostituzione valvolare. La profilassi contro l'endocardite batterica è d'obbligo in questi pazienti, in occasione di procedure odontoiatriche o chirurgiche di altro tipo. I normali antibiotici assunti da questi soggetti per la profilassi della febbre reumatica non sono sufficienti a prevenire l'endocardite.

STENOSI MITRALICA

Fisiopatologia. La stenosi mitralica di origine reumatica deriva dalla fibrosi dell'anello mitralico, dall'adesione delle commessure valvolari e dalla contrazione, nel tempo, dei lembi valvolari, delle corde tendinee e dei muscoli papillari. Sono necessari 10 anni o più perché la lesioni si instauri completamente, anche se il processo talvolta può essere accelerato. La stenosi mitralica reumatica si riscontra raramente prima dell'adolescenza e di solito non viene riconosciuta prima dell'età adulta. Una significativa stenosi mitralica comporta un'aumentata pressione con ingrandimento e ipertrofia dell'atrio sinistro, un'ipertensione venosa polmonare, un'aumentata resistenza vascolare polmonare e un'ipertensione polmonare. Ne derivano una dilatazione e un'ipertrofia ventricolare destra e atriale destra, a loro volta seguite da uno scompenso cardiaco destro.

Manifestazioni cliniche. Generalmente, sussiste una certa correlazione tra sintomi e gravità dell'ostruzione. I pazienti con lesioni lievi sono asintomatici. Gradi maggiori di ostruzione sono associati a intolleranza allo sforzo e dispnea. Lesioni critiche possono causare ortopnea, dispnea parossistica notturna ed edema polmonare franco, oltre ad aritmie atriali. Una volta che si sia sviluppata un'ipertensione polmonare, una dilatazione ventricolare destra può portare a insufficienza tricuspidalica funzionale, epatomegalia, ascite ed edema. Può verificarsi emottisi, causata da rottura di vene bronchiali o pleuroilari e talvolta da un infarto polmonare.

La pressione venosa giugulare è aumentata in parecchie patologie con scompenso cardiaco, patologia valvolare tricuspidalica o grave ipertensione polmonare. Nelle patologie di grado lieve il cuore ha dimensioni normali, mentre in caso di stenosi mitralica grave di solito si osserva una moderata cardiomegalia. L'ingrandimento cardiaco può essere massivo quando sopravvengono una fibrillazione atriale e uno scompenso cardiaco. Un sollevamento ventricolare destro parasternale risulta palpabile quando la pressione polmonare è elevata. I principali reperti auscultatori sono un primo tono cardiaco forte, uno schiocco d'apertura della valvola mitrale e un soffio diastolico mitralico lungo, a bassa tonalità, rullante, con rinforzo presistolico all'apice. Il soffio diastolico mitralico può essere virtualmente assente in pazienti che hanno uno scompenso cardiaco. È talvolta udibile un soffio olosistolico secondario a insufficienza tricuspidalica. In presenza di ipertensione polmonare, la componente polmonare del secondo tono cardiaco è accentuata. Un soffio diastolico precoce può essere causato da un'associata insufficienza aortica o da un'insufficienza valvolare polmonare secondaria.

Gli elettrocardiogrammi e le radiografie del torace sono normali se la lesione è lieve; con l'aumentare della gravità, divengono evidenti sia onde P prominenti e indentate, sia gradi variabili di ipertrofia ventricolare destra. La fibrillazione atriale è una manifestazione tardiva comune. Lesioni moderate o gravi sono associate a segni radiografici di ingrandimento dell'atrio sinistro e prominenza dell'arteria polmonare e delle camere del cuore destro; possono notarsi calcificazioni nella regione della valvola mitrale. Un'ostruzione grave è associata a redistribuzione del flusso sanguigno polmonare cosicché gli apici del cuore hanno una maggiore perfusione (contrariamente al normale). L'ecocardiografia evidenzia un evidente restringimento dell'orifizio mitralico durante la diastole e un ingrandimento atriale sinistro; il Doppler può stimare il gradiente pressorio transimitralico. Il cateterismo cardiaco quantifica il gradiente diastolico attraverso la valvola mitrale, permette il calcolo dell'area valvolare e valuta il grado di aumento della pressione arteriosa polmonare.

Trattamento. Un intervento è indicato in pazienti con segni clinici ed evidenza emodinamica di ostruzione severa, ma prima che insorgano le gravi manifestazioni sopraelencate. La valvulotomia chirurgica o la valvuloplastica mitralica con catetere e palloncino generalmente danno buoni risultati; si tende invece a evitare la sostituzione valvolare, a meno che non sia assolutamente necessaria. La valvuloplastica con palloncino è indicata in presenza di sintomi e di valvole stenotiche, flessibili e non calcifiche, in pazienti senza aritmie atriali né trombi atriali.

INSUFFICIENZA AORTICA. Nell'insufficienza aortica cronica di origine reumatica, la sclerosi della valvola aortica porta alla distorsione e alla retrazione delle cuspidi. Il rigurgito di sangue determina sovraccarico di volume e ipertrofia del ventricolo sinistro. Un'insufficienza combinata, mitralica e aortica, è più comune del coinvolgimento della sola valvola aortica.

Manifestazioni cliniche. Di solito non vi sono sintomi, tranne che nell'insufficienza aortica grave. L'elevato volume sistolico e le potenti contrazioni ventricolari sinistre possono causare palpitazioni. Un'eccessiva sudorazione e l'intolleranza al caldo sono correlate alla vasodilatazione. Una dispnea da sforzo può progredire fino all'ortopnea e all'edema polmonare; un'angina può essere precipitata dall'esercizio fisico intenso. Possono inoltre verificarsi attacchi notturni di sudorazione, tachicardia, dolore toracico e ipertensione.

La pressione differenziale è ampia con polsi periferici scoccanti. La pressione sanguigna sistolica è elevata, mentre quella diastolica è più bassa del normale. Nell'insufficienza aortica grave il cuore è ingrandito, con un sollevamento apicale ventricolare sinistro. Può essere presente un fremito diastolico. Il soffio tipico inizia immediatamente con il secondo tono cardiaco e continua fino alla parte finale della diastole. Il soffio si ode a livello del margine sternale superiore e medio di sinistra, con irradiazione all'apice e al focolaio aortico. Caratteristicamente di tipo soffiante e di tonalità elevata, è facilmente udibile al termine dell'espirio forzato, con il diaframma dello stetoscopio posto saldamente sul torace e il paziente piegato in avanti. Un soffio sistolico da eiezione è frequente a causa della gittata sistolica aumentata. Talvolta si ode un soffio apicale presistolico (**soffio di Austin Flint**) simile a quello da stenosi mitralica, conseguenza dell'ampio flusso aortico rigurgitante in diastole, che impedisce alla valvola mitrale di aprirsi completamente.

Le radiografie del torace evidenziano un ingrandimento del ventricolo sinistro e dell'aorta. L'elettrocardiogramma può essere normale, ma nei casi avanzati rivela segni di ipertrofica ventricolare sinistra e di sovraccarico con onde P prominenti. L'elettrocardiogramma evidenzia un ventricolo sinistro grande e una vibrazione o oscillazione della valvola mitrale causata dal flusso di rigurgito che colpisce i lembi valvolari. Le indagini Doppler rivelano il grado di reflusso aortico nel ventricolo sinistro. L'angiorisonanza magnetica può essere utile per quantificare il volume rigurgitante. Il cateterismo cardiaco è necessario solo quando i dati ecocardiografici sono equivoci.

Prognosi e trattamento. Le lesioni lievi e moderate sono ben tollerate. Molti adolescenti con grave rigurgito sono asintomatici e tollerano lesioni avanzate fino alla terza-quarta decade di vita. A differenza dell'insufficienza mitralica, quella aortica non regredisce. I pazienti con lesioni combinate durante l'episodio di febbre reumatica acuta possono avere, 1-2 anni più tardi, solo un coinvolgimento aortico. Il trattamento consiste nell'utilizzo di farmaci che riducono il postcarico (ACE-inibitori) e nella profilassi contro le recidive di febbre reumatica acuta e lo sviluppo di un'endocardite infettiva. L'intervento chirurgico (sostituzione valvolare) dovrebbe essere effettuato ben prima dell'insorgenza di scompenso cardiaco, edema polmonare o angina, o quando divengono evidenti segni di diminuzione della funzione miocardica, manifestandosi con un aumento delle dimensioni del ventricolo sinistro all'ecocardiogramma. L'intervento chirurgico viene preso in considerazione quando sono presenti sintomi precoci, quando si notano cambiamenti del tratto S-T e dell'onda T all'elettrocardiogramma, o si manifestano segni di diminuzione della frazione di eiezione del ventricolo sinistro.

VALVULOPATIA TRICUSPIDALICA. Il coinvolgimento primitivo della valvola tricuspide è raro dopo febbre reumatica. L'insufficienza tricuspidale è più comune quando secondaria a dilatazione ventricolare destra risultante da lesioni del cuore sinistro non sottoposte a riparazione. I segni prodotti da un'insufficienza tricuspidalica comprendono pulsazioni ampie delle vene giugulari, pulsazioni sistoliche del fegato e un soffio olosistolico soffiante a livello del margine sternale inferiore sinistro, che aumenta d'intensità durante l'inspirio. Sono frequenti segni concomitanti di valvulopatia mitralica o aortica, con o senza fibrillazione atriale. I segni di insufficienza tricuspidalica diminuiscono o scompaiono quando lo scompenso cardiaco causato da lesioni del cuore sinistro viene trattato con successo. In rari casi può essere necessaria una valvuloplastica della tricuspide.

VALVULOPATIA POLMONARE. L'insufficienza polmonare di solito è su base funzionale, secondaria a ipertensione polmonare, e costituisce un reperto tardivo in casi di stenosi mitralica grave. Il soffio (soffio di Graham Steel) è simile a quello dell'insufficienza aortica, ma i segni arteriosi periferici (polsi scoccanti) sono assenti. Per avere conferma che la diagnosi è corretta si ricorre all'ecocardiografia bidimensionale e al Doppler.

Camara EJ, Neubauer C, Camara GF, et al: Mechanisms of mitral valvar insufficiency in children and adolescents with severe rheumatic heart disease: An echocardiographic study with clinical and epidemiological correlations. *Cardiol Young* 2004;14:527–532.

Cilliers A: Treating acute rheumatic fever. *Br Med J* 2003;327:631–632.

Fesslova V, Bardare M: Rheumatic fever in the 21st century. *Cardiol Young* 2004;14:465; author reply 465–466.

Figueroa FE, Fernandez MS, Valdes P, et al: Prospective comparison of clinical and echocardiographic diagnosis of rheumatic carditis: Long term follow up of patients with subclinical disease. *Heart* 2001;85:407–410.

Griffiths SP, Gersony WM: Acute rheumatic fever in New York City (1969 to 1988): A comparative study of two decades. *J Pediatr* 1990;116:882–887.

Holmes DR, Nishimura RA, Reeder GS: Aortic and mitral balloon valvuloplasty: Emergence of a new percutaneous technique. *Int J Cardiol* 1987;16:227–233.

Narula J, Chandrasekhar Y, Rahimtoola S: Diagnosis of active rheumatic carditis. *Circulation* 1999;100:1576–1581.

Stollerman GH: Rheumatic fever in the 21st century. *Clin Infect Dis* 2001;33:806–814.

Sezione 6 — Patologie del miocardio e del pericardio — Daniel Bernstein

Capitolo 439 ■ Patologie del miocardio

Nella maggior parte dei bambini con cardiopatia congenita, la funzione miocardica è relativamente non compromessa nei primi tempi di vita. In alcune lesioni congenite, come nello shunt sinistro-destro, il miocardio può anche funzionare a un livello superiore al normale (**stato iperdinamico**). I bambini con cardiopatie congenite non operate, tuttavia, e quelli con una precedente correzione chirurgica o palliazione e residue anomalie emodinamiche, possono andare incontro a un sovraccarico di volume o di pressione o a ipossia cronica per lungo tempo. Tali residui possono alla fine portare allo sviluppo di disfunzione miocardica; questo è vero soprattutto per i pazienti con ventricolo destro sistemico, in particolare quando raggiungono l'adolescenza e la prima età adulta. Perciò la preservazione della funzione miocardica è uno degli obiettivi chiave della gestione medica e chirurgica delle cardiopatie congenite.

Vi sono altri bambini con patologie primitive del miocardio, note con il nome generale di miocardiopatie. Le **miocardiopatie** si suddividono, in base all'eziologia (Tab. 439-1), in **primitive** (che derivano da anomalie genetiche del muscolo cardiaco) e **secondarie** (dovute a infezioni, endocrinopatie, patologie metaboliche e nutrizionali, patologie neuromuscolari, patologie del sangue e tumori). Altre miocardiopatie sono classificate come **idiopatiche**; i progressi compiuti nel campo della diagnostica molecolare hanno permesso ai cardiologi di identificare cause specifiche in molti pazienti che erano stati precedentemente classificati come "idiopatici". In alcuni pazienti, gli studi di genetica hanno identificato

TABELLA 439-1. Eziologia delle patologie miocardiche

FAMILIARI-EREDITARIE
- Miocardiopatia dilatativa familiare
- Miocardiopatia ipertrofica familiare
- Miocardiopatia restrittiva familiare
- Non compattamento isolato del ventricolo sinistro
- Distrofie muscolari
  - Distrofia muscolare di Duchenne
  - Altre distrofie muscolari (Becker, distrofia dei cingoli)
- Distrofia miotonica
- Sindrome di Kearns-Sayre (oftalmoplegia esterna progressiva)
- Atassia di Friedreich
- Emocromatosi
- Malattia di Fabry
- Fibroelastosi endocardica primitiva
- Displasia aritmogena del ventricolo destro (familiare e non familiare)
- Sindrome di Noonan
- Sindrome di Barth

INFETTIVE
- Miocarditi virali: adenovirus, Coxsackievirus A e B, HIV, echovirus, rosolia, varicella, influenza, parotite, virus di Epstein-Barr, morbillo, poliomielite, vaccino per la varicella
- Rickettsie: psittacosi, Coxiella, febbre maculosa delle Montagne Rocciose, tifo
- Batteri: difterite, micoplasmi, meningococco, leptospirosi, malattia di Lyme, febbre tifoide, tubercolosi, streptococco, listeriosi
- Parassiti: malattia di Chagas, toxoplasmosi, *Loa loa*, *Toxocara canis*, schistosomiasi, cisticercosi, echinococco, trichinosi
- Funghi: istoplasmosi, coccidioidomicosi, actinomicosi

PATOLOGIE METABOLICHE, NUTRIZIONALI, ENDOCRINE
- Patologie dell'ossidazione degli acidi grassi a livello mitocondriale
  - Trasportatore della carnitina (OCTN2), carnitin-palmitil-transferasi (CPT-I), carnitin-traslocasi (CACT), carnitin-palmitoil-tranferasi-II (CPT-II), deidrogenasi degli acil-CoA a catena corta (SCAD), deidrogenasi degli acil-CoA a catena molto lunga (VLCAD), ETF deidrogenasi (ETF-DH), flavoproteina-α e β di trasporto degli elettroni (α e β-ETF), deidrogenasi degli L-3 idrossiacil CoA a catena corta (SCHAD), proteina trifunzionale mitocondriale (MTP, *Mitochondrial Trifunctional Protein*), tiolasi dei 3-chetoacil-CoA a catena lunga (LKAT, *Long-Chain 3-ketoacyl-CoA Thiolase*)
  - Malattia di Pompe (malattia da accumulo di glicogeno)
- Mucopolisaccaridosi
- Beriberi (deficit di tiamina)
- Malattia di Kashan (deficit di selenio)
- Kwashiorkor
- Ipertiroidismo
- Carcinoide
- Feocromocitoma
- Ipercolesterolemia
- Figlio di madre diabetica
- Sindrome di Beckwith-Wiedemann
- Sfingolipidosi
- Acidosi propionica
- Aciduria 3-metilglutaconica tipo II

PATOLOGIE DEL TESSUTO CONNETTIVO – GRANULOMATOSE – INFILTRATIVE
- Lupus eritematoso sistemico (LES)
- Figli di madre affetta da LES
- Sclerodermia
- Vasculite di Churg-Strauss
- Artrite reumatoide
- Febbre reumatica
- Sarcoidosi
- Amiloidosi
- Dermatomiosite
- Periarterite nodosa
- Leucemia

FARMACI – TOSSICI
- Doxorubicina (adriamicina)
- Ciclofosfamide
- Clorochina
- Ipecacuana (emetico)
- Sulfamidici
- Mesalazina
- Cloramfenicolo
- Reazione di ipersensibilità
- Alcol
- Avvelenamenti
- Irradiazione
- Rimedi erboristici (erba perenne)

CORONAROPATIE
- Malattia di Kawasaki
- Necrosi della media
- Coronaria sinistra anomala con origine dall'arteria polmonare
- Altre anomalie coronarie congenite (coronaria destra anomala, stenosi coronaria ostiale)

ALTRE PATOLOGIE
- Anemia
- Anemia a cellule falciformi
- Sindrome ipereosinofilica (sindrome di Löffler)
- Fibrosi endomiocardica
- Ischemia-ipossia
- Miocardiopatia peripartum
- Anomalia ventricolare destra di Uhl
- Miocardiopatia istocistoide (oncocitica, lipidotica)
- Miocardite acuta necrotizzante eosinofila
- Miocardiopatia restrittiva
- Tachiaritmie croniche

*Elenco delle patologie degli acidi grassi adattato da Shekhawat PS, Matern D, Strauss AW: Fetal fatty acid oxidation disorders, their effect on maternal health and neonatal outcome: Impact of expanded newborn screening on their diagnosis and management. *Pediatr Res* 2005;57:78R-86R.

difetti genetici ben precisi; in altri, è stata utilizzata la reazione a catena della polimerasi (PCR, *Polymerase Chain Reaction*) per evidenziare la presenza di genoma virale, suggerendo una pregressa miocardite virale. Un secondo schema utile per la classificazione delle miocardiopatia è basato sulle anomalie strutturali e funzionali predominanti (Tab. 439-2): **miocardiopatia dilatativa** (disfunzione primariamente sistolica), **miocardiopatia ipertrofica** (disfunzione primariamente diastolica) e **miocardiopatia restrittiva** (disfunzione primariamente diastolica, spesso combinata a disfunzione sistolica). L'incidenza annua è di poco più di 1 su 100 000 bambini, più elevata nei maschi che nelle femmine e nei bambini di età <1 anno. La prevalenza di una miocardiopatia nel periodo neonatale è di 10/100 000 nati vivi, mentre in tutti i bambini la prevalenza è di 36/100 000 per la miocardiopatia dilatativa e di 2/100 000 per la miocardiopatia ipertrofica e quella restrittiva.

439.1 • Miocardiopatia dilatativa

FISIOPATOLOGIA. La miocardiopatia dilatativa è caratterizzata da gradi variabili di dilatazione dei ventricoli, in particolare il sinistro. Può essere presente anche una componente di ipertrofia ventricolare compensatoria, che si ritiene dovuta a fattori di crescita indotti nei miociti dall'aumentato stress parietale. Nella maggior parte dei casi pediatrici la causa è sconosciuta (miocardiopatia dilatativa idiopatica), ma una percentuale (in aumento) è su base genetica o rappresenta le sequele di una miocardite virale.

Nel 20-50% dei casi la patologia è riconosciuta come **familiare**. L'ereditarietà autosomica dominante è quella che si riscontra più frequentemente e sono state identificate mutazioni in numerosi geni cardiaci strutturali o metabolici (vedi Tab. 439-2) In pazienti con miocardiopatia dilatativa associata a **difetti di conduzione**, sono state implicate mutazioni nel gene della lamina A/C. L'ereditarietà X-linked rende conto del 5-10% dei casi di miocardiopatia dilatativa familiare. Mutazioni nel gene della distrofina, che causano le distrofie muscolari, sono le più comuni in questo gruppo. Mutazioni nel gene che codifica per *tafazzin* sono associate alla **sindrome di Barth**, come anche a casi di non compattamento isolato del ventricolo sinistro, una forma di miocardiopatia dilatativa. L'ereditarietà autosomica recessiva è stata associata a una mutazione della troponina I cardiaca.

Le **miopatie mitocondriali** possono essere dovute a mutazioni degli enzimi della catena di trasporto degli elettroni o di quelli dell'ossidazione degli acidi grassi, che seguono un pattern di ereditarietà recessivo. Alcune patologie dell'ossidazione degli acidi grassi si presentano con alterazioni del metabolismo (ipoglicemia ipochetosica, acidosi, disfunzione epatica), altre con miopatia periferica e neuropatia, e altre ancora con morte improvvisa, attribuita erroneamente alla sindrome della morte improvvisa del lattante (SIDS, *Sudden Infants Death Syndrome*). Se la madre è eterozigote per il difetto enzimatico, possono insorgere complicanze durante la gravidanza, tra le quali una scarsa crescita fetale in utero e preeclampsia, steatoepatite acuta della gravidanza o la combinazione di emolisi, enzimi epatici elevati e piastrinopenia (sindrome HELLP [*Hemolysis, Elevated Liver enzyme, and Low Platelets*]) nella madre (vedi Capitolo 86).

Una **pregressa miocardite virale** è una delle cause principali di miocardiopatia dilatativa. Poiché i titoli virali sono di solito non diagnostici, nella maggior parte dei casi (spesso classificati in precedenza come idiopatici) il genoma virale viene evidenziato in un campione ottenuto mediante biopsia endomiocardica utilizzando la PCR. Dall'anamnesi può emergere una remota patologia virale. Una miocardite attiva viene identificata soltanto in una minoranza (2-15%) dei pazienti.

I pazienti con miocardiopatia dilatativa possono avere cause infettive di natura diversa da quella virale, patologie endocrine

TABELLA 439-2. Miocardiopatie

	DILATATIVA	IPERTROFICA	DISPLASIA ARITMOGENA DEL VENTRICOLO DESTRO	RESTRITTIVA
Prevalenza	50/100 000	1/500	Non nota	Non nota
Familiarità	25-50%, AD, AR, X-L, Mt	50% AD	30% AD, raramente AR (malattia di Naxos)	Non nota
Geni	AD: astina cardiaca, desmina, δ-sarcoglicano, catena pesante della β-miosina, troponina cardiaca C e T, α-tropomiosina, titina, metavinculina, proteina C legante la miosina, proteina muscolare LIM, α-actinina-2, fosfolambano, dominio3 legante cypher/LIM, catena pesante dell'α-miosina, SUR2A (subunità regolatoria del canale KATP), lamina A/C X linked: distrofina, tafazzina AR: troponina I	Catena pesante della β-miosina, troponina T o I, α-tropomiosina, proteina C che lega la miosina, catene leggere 1 o 2 della miosina, titina, PRKAG2, 2 α-galattosidasi	Placoglobina, desmoplachina, recettore della rianodina	Troponina I cardiaca Desminopatie (α-B-cristallina)
Morte improvvisa	Sì	Dipende dal gene. 0,7-11%/anno, associata all'esercizio fisico	Sì	1,5%/anno
Aritmie	Atriali, ventricolari, e disturbi di conduzione	Atriali e ventricolari	Ventricolari e disturbi di conduzione	Fibrillazione atriale
Funzione sistolica	Disfunzione sistolica e diastolica	Disfunzione diastolica Ostruzione dinamica all'efflusso sistolico	Funzione sistolica da normale a ridotta Funzione diastolica ridotta	Funzione diastolica gravemente ridotta Funzione sistolica da normale a ridotta
Diagnosi	Cavità ventricolare sinistra dilatata con spessore valvolare normale o assottigliato	Ipertrofia ventricolare sinistra asimmetrica, concentrica o apicale	Sostituzione fibrolipidica del ventricolo destro alla RM o alla biopsia, dilatazione ventricolare destra	Cavità ventricolare di dimensione normale o ridotta, marcato ingrandimento biatriale
Trattamento medico	ACE inibitori Diuretici (furosemide, spironolattone) Digitale β_2-bloccanti	Propranololo Pacemaker	β_2-bloccanti Antiaritmici di classe III	Accorto utilizzo di diuretici, milrinone
Trattamento chirurgico e interventistico	ICD, resincronizzazione, pacing biventricolare	ICD Miomectomia settale, ablazione mediante alcolizzazione (negli adulti)	Ablazione con catetere ICD	ICD
	Trapianto	Trapianto	Trapianto	Trapianto

ACE (*Angiotensin-Converting Enzyme*), enzima di conversione dell'angiotensina. AD, ereditarietà autosomica dominante; AR, ereditarietà autosomica recessiva; ICD (*Implantable Cardioverter-Defibrillator*), defibrillatore-cardioversore impiantabile; Mt, ereditarietà mitocondriale; X-L, ereditarietà X-linked.

come l'ipotiroidismo, patologie metaboliche come patologie da accumulo, deficit nutrizionali, esposizione ad agenti cardiotossici come la doxorubicina e patologie sistemiche come quelle a carico del tessuto connettivo. Cause prettamente cardiache di miocardiopatia dilatativa comprendono anomalie congenite e acquisite (malattia di Kawasaki) delle arterie coronarie, tachiaritmie e ipercolesterolemia familiare.

MANIFESTAZIONI CLINICHE. Possono essere colpiti pazienti di tutti i gruppi di età. Di solito l'esordio è insidioso, ma a volte i sintomi di scompenso cardiaco si manifestano improvvisamente. Sono comuni irritabilità, anoressia, dolore addominale, tosse dovuta alla congestione polmonare e dispnea da sforzo. Lattanti e bambini piccoli tendono ad avere sintomi respiratori e ritardo di crescita, mentre quelli più grandi e gli adolescenti spesso lamentano inizialmente disturbi addominali come nausea e anoressia. Anche se il tipico segno di edema polmonare è la presenza di rantoli, i bambini più piccoli possono presentare un respiro sibilante. Quando la malattia è conclamata, la cute è fredda e pallida, il polso arterioso diminuito, la pressione differenziale bassa ed è presente tachicardia. La pressione venosa giugulare è aumentata, e sono comuni epatomegalia ed edema. Il cuore è ingrandito; possono inoltre essere presenti soffi olosistolici da insufficienza mitralica e tricuspidalica. È di solito udibile un ritmo di galoppo di sommazione.

Nel periodo neonatale, un coinvolgimento sistemico (ipoglicemia, acidosi, insufficienza epatica) suggerisce la presenza di un errore congenito del metabolismo. Nei pazienti più grandi, un coinvolgimento muscolare periferico fa pensare o una distrofia muscolare o a una patologia mitocondriale. Un'anamnesi familiare di insufficienza cardiaca inspiegata, morte improvvisa o SIDS suggerisce una patologia genetica/metabolica.

DIAGNOSI. L'elettrocardiogramma evidenzia una combinazione di ingrandimento atriale, gradi variabili di ipertrofia ventricolare sinistra o destra e anomalie aspecifiche dell'onda T. La radiografia del torace, oltre a confermare la presenza di cardiomegalia, permette di valutare il grado di congestione polmonare e la presenza di versamenti pleurici. Spesso la diagnosi iniziale di miocardiopatia dilatativa viene sospettata quando si sottopone a radiografia del torace un bambino con distress respiratorio per valutare una sospetta polmonite. L'ecocardiogramma, che è diagnostico, evidenzia una dilatazione dell'atrio sinistro e del ventricolo sinistro e una scarsa contrattilità (Fig. 439-1). Anche il ventricolo destro può essere colpito. Le indagini Doppler evidenziano una diminuita velocità di flusso attraverso la valvola aortica e un rigurgito mitralico. Nei casi di vecchia data, può esservi evidenza di ipertensione polmonare.

Una **biopsia miocardica** nelle prime fasi della malattia può essere utile; è raro trovare una causa specifica quando si prelevano campioni bioptici dopo malattia di lunga durata, nel qual caso i reperti istologici consistono principalmente in aree di fibrosi e di ipertrofia compensatoria. L'origine virale di molti di questi casi "idiopatici" può essere evidenziata con la PCR. Un'anamnesi familiare completa è importante e, a meno che non venga confermata una diagnosi virale, i familiari di primo grado devono essere sottoposti a screening mediante ecocardiogramma per la presenza di una miocardiopatia subclinica. I fratelli/sorelle con ecocardiogramma normale dovrebbero essere sottoposti a esami ripetuti a intervalli regolari, dal momento che la presentazione della disfunzione ventricolare può variare considerevolmente nel tempo anche all'interno della stessa famiglia. Gli studi sul DNA dei membri affetti e non affetti della famiglia può aiutare a determinare lo specifico difetto genetico. Lo screening neonatale, eseguito mediante spettrometria di massa in tandem, è disponibile per evidenziare patologie mitocondriali dell'ossidazione degli acidi grassi.

PROGNOSI E TRATTAMENTO. Il decorso della malattia è di solito progressivamente ingravescente, anche se alcuni pazienti possono rimanere stabili per anni. Un trattamento aggressivo dello scompenso cardiaco (vedi Capitolo 442) può portare a una remissione temporanea, ma le recidive sono comuni e con il tempo i pazienti tendono a sviluppare resistenza alla terapia. A questo punto, la prognosi per la sopravvivenza a più di un anno è infausta. Complicanze gravi comprendono aritmie ventricolari che portano a sincope e morte improvvisa, embolie polmonari o sistemiche a partire da trombi intracardiaci e lo sviluppo di una patologia vascolare polmonare, imputabile alla pressione atriale sinistra cronicamente elevata. I pazienti con funzione miocardica gravemente depressa dovrebbero essere sottoposti a stretto monitoraggio per la comparsa di aritmie e, se queste sono presenti, trattati aggressivamente con agenti antiaritmici o sottoposti a impianto di defibrillatore-cardioversore (ICD, *Implantable Cardioverter-Defibrillator*). Dovrebbero anche essere sottoposti a terapia anticoagulante sistemica, preferibilmente con warfarin. L'utilizzo di β-bloccanti adrenergici come il metoprololo e il carvedilolo negli adulti con miocardiopatia ha portato a un miglioramento della resistenza allo sforzo e alla riduzione dell'ospedalizzazione e della mortalità. L'esperienza iniziale con questi farmaci nei bambini è incoraggiante. Può valer la pena di effettuare un tentativo con carnitina per via orale (100-200 mg/kg/die) in attesa dei risultati dei test definitivi di screening metabolico. Quando la terapia medica fallisce, il trapianto di cuore è molto efficace nei lattanti e nei bambini con miocardiopatia dilatativa (vedi Capitolo 443.1). A causa della scarsità di donatori di organi in età pediatrica, i pazienti con miocardiopatia dovrebbero essere indirizzati a un centro di trapianto cardiaco pediatrico per una valutazione iniziale nelle prime fasi della malattia.

MALATTIE NEUROMUSCOLARI. Nei pazienti con atassia di Friedreich (vedi Capitolo 597.1) è comune una cardiopatia, che colpisce prevalentemente il ventricolo sinistro portando a una miocardiopatia dilatativa o restrittiva. In alcuni pazienti i sintomi iniziali sono

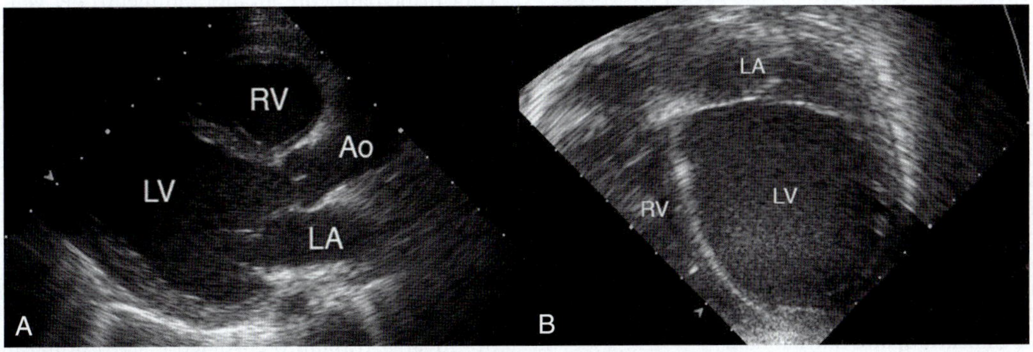

Figura 439-1. Ecocardiogramma di una paziente con miocardiopatia dilatativa. *A*, Proiezione parasternale asse lungo, che evidenzia il ventricolo sinistro dilatato. *B*, Proiezione apicale quattro camere, nella quale si osserva il grande ventricolo sinistro che comprime il ventricolo destro. Ao, aorta ascendente. LA (*Left Atrium*), atrio sinistro; LV (*Left Ventricle*); ventricolo sinistro; RV (*Right Ventricle*), ventricolo destro.

stati intolleranza allo sforzo, dolore toracico e scompenso cardiaco. Possono inoltre verificarsi aritmie, consistenti in tachicardia atriale, fibrillazione atriale o extrasistoli. Nella distrofia muscolare di Duchenne (vedi Capitolo 608.1) almeno il 50% dei bambini ha un'evidenza autoptica di un coinvolgimento miocardico simile a quello che si riscontra nel muscolo striato. I sintomi cardiaci erano in precedenza posti in ombra dai problemi muscolari e polmonari; grazie ai recenti miglioramenti nel supporto polmonare, si identifica un numero maggiore di pazienti con scompenso cardiaco. Stabilire una distinzione tra disabilità causata da uno scompenso cardiaco e quella dovuta a complicanze muscolari periferiche o polmonari può essere difficile. L'elettrocardiogramma può evidenziare una tachicardia, anomalie delle onde P, un intervallo P-R corto, onde Q e T anomale. Possono anche notarsi minimi segni di ipertrofia ventricolare destra o sinistra. Nelle forme meno gravi di distrofia muscolare (distrofia di Becker) il coinvolgimento cardiaco può essere più evidente, e costituire la causa principale di intolleranza allo sforzo e dei sintomi respiratori. Sono state descritte altre miocardiopatie dilatative legate all'X, cui non era associato un coinvolgimento del muscolo scheletrico. L'esperienza nel campo del trapianto di cuore, in pazienti con distrofia di Becker più lieve, è piuttosto limitata.

MALATTIA DI KAWASAKI (VEDI CAPITOLO 165). L'arterite associata alla malattia di Kawasaki all'inizio coinvolge le piccole arteriole, ma nella seconda e terza settimana di malattia si infiammano le arterie di medio calibro e può verificarsi una dilatazione aneurismatica delle arterie coronarie. Durante la fase di guarigione, possono residuare aree di dilatazione e stenosi coronarica, responsabili di un successivo infarto miocardico e morte. La miocardite è una sequela meno comune della malattia di Kawasaki, ma quando presente si manifesta con scompenso cardiaco nelle prime fasi della malattia.

MALATTIE AUTOIMMUNI. La cardite reumatica è descritta nei Capitoli 156 e 438. Le manifestazioni cardiovascolari di artrite reumatoide giovanile, lupus eritematoso sistemico, periarterite nodosa, dermatomiosite e sclerodermia sono descritte nei Capitoli 157-159. Lattanti nati da madri affette da malattie autoimmuni come il lupus eritematoso sistemico possono sviluppare una miocardiopatia, di solito associata a persistenza di anticorpi anti-Ro e anti-La.

ENDOCRINOPATIE. L'**ipertiroidismo** (vedi Capitolo 569) causa tachicardia, vasodilatazione, ampia pressione differenziale, ingrandimento cardiaco e talvolta fibrillazione atriale. L'**ipotiroidismo** può causare una disfunzione cardiaca negli adulti, mentre è raro che determini un macroscopico coinvolgimento cardiaco nei bambini. L'elettrocardiogramma è caratterizzato da bradicardia, bassi voltaggi di tutti i complessi (specialmente delle onde P e T), deviazione assiale sinistra e sistole elettrica prolungata. Questi segni di solito scompaiono nel giro di un mese dopo l'inizio di un'adeguata terapia ormonale. La miocardiopatia diabetica è rara nei bambini; tuttavia, lattanti nati da madri diabetiche possono andare incontro a ipertrofia e dilatazione cardiaca. La miocardiopatia può essere causata dall'esposizione cronica a elevati livelli di catecolamine in pazienti con feocromocitoma.

PATOLOGIE METABOLICHE E NUTRIZIONALI. Tra le malattie da carenza vitaminica, il **beri-beri** (vedi Capitolo 46) porta ai danni cardiaci più gravi. In pazienti con manultrizione come il **kwashiorkor**, i deficit sono spesso multipli e può essere difficile separare la lesione cardiaca di una malattia nutrizionale da quella di un'altra (vedi Capitolo 43). Altre cause nutrizionali e metaboliche di disfunzione cardiaca comprendono i deficit di **selenio** (vedi Capitolo 51), taurina e carnitina (vedi Capitolo 86.1). Anche in bambini che soffrono di malassorbimento, a causa della loro patologia primitiva, possono svilupparsi miocardiopatie nutrizionali.

PATOLOGIE EMATOLOGICHE. In lattanti e bambini, una grave anemia può essere associata a un coinvolgimento cardiaco. Anche se la gittata cardiaca aumenta quando il contenuto di emoglobina è <7 g/dL circa, si verifica un significativo ingrandimento cardiaco con un'estrema riduzione dell'emoglobina (≤3-4 g/L). La frequenza cardiaca è elevata, la pressione differenziale ampia e la pressione venosa aumentata. È usuale un soffio sistolico all'apice o lungo il margine sternale sinistro; soffi diastolici possono riscontrarsi nella stessa sede, ed è comune anche un ritmo di galoppo. Le anomalie elettrocardiografiche consistono in sottoslivellamenti del tratto S-T e onde T piatte. In pazienti con lesioni cardiache congenite, l'anemia può imporre un ulteriore stress sulla capacità del cuore di mantenere un adeguato apporto di ossigeno, portando a un considerevole peggioramento dei sintomi di insufficienza cardiaca. Il trattamento è diretto alla causa dell'anemia. Se sono indicate trasfusioni di sangue in presenza di cardiomegalia o scompenso cardiaco, si dovrebbero somministrare solo piccoli volumi (5 mL/kg) di eritrociti concentrati alla volta, seguiti da una dose di diuretico (vedi Capitolo 470). Talvolta può essere prudente ricorrere a un'exsanguinotrasfusione per evitare un aumento improvviso del volume ematico.

PATOLOGIE DELLE ARTERIE CORONARIE. L'origine anomala dell'arteria coronaria sinistra dall'arteria polmonare è una delle cause principali di ischemia miocardica nei lattanti (vedi Capitolo 432.2). L'origine anomala di una delle coronarie dall'aorta può portare a un suo decorso tra l'aorta e l'arteria polmonare ("coronaria suicida") e causare ischemia e infarto miocardico con l'esercizio fisico. La calcinosi coronarica è una rara patologia dei lattanti e dei bambini in cui le arterie coronarie sono tortuose e calcifiche. Altri vasi sanguigni possono presentare un coinvolgimento analogo. L'esordio dello scompenso cardiaco è improvviso; la morte di solito avviene nell'infanzia. Rare malformazioni delle arterie coronarie comprendono stenosi ostiali delle coronarie e una stenosi arteriosa coronarica nel contesto di una stenosi aortica sopravalvolare (vedi Capitolo 427.5). I pazienti con ipercolesterolemia familiare omozigote possono presentare una predisposizione all'aterosclerosi coronarica in età precoce. I pazienti che sono stati sottoposti a trapianto cardiaco sono a rischio di sviluppo di una coronaropatia a carico dell'organo trapiantato (vedi Capitolo 443.1).

CARDIOTOSSICITÀ DA DOXORUBICINA (ADRIAMICINA). Questo farmaco chemioterapico causa occasionalmente una miocardite acuta e più spesso una miocardiopatia dilatativa cronica. La manifestazione più comune è una miocardiopatia grave, cronica, dose-dipendente, che colpisce circa il 30% dei pazienti quando la dose totale cumulativa è >550 mg/m^2, ma si può talvolta osservare in pazienti dopo dosi più basse, fino a 200 mg/m^2. Uno studio ha evidenziato anomalie negli indici ecocardiografici di funzione ventricolare sinistra (stress parietale) fin nel 65% dei bambini che ricevono dosi >220 mg/m^2. Quando la terapia radiante è abbinata alla doxorubicina, il rischio di danno cardiaco è ancora maggiore.

La miocardiopatia può divenire manifesta mesi o anche anni dopo il trattamento con doxorubicina. La cardiomegalia è dovuta principalmente all'ingrandimento del ventricolo e dell'atrio sinistri. L'appiattimento o l'inversione dell'onda T sono un segno aspecifico di coinvolgimento cardiaco. Cambiamenti elettrocardiografici acuti, compreso un intervallo Q-T lungo, possono essere presenti nel 40% dei pazienti subito dopo un'unica dose. Alterazioni precoci della funzione cardiaca, anche in assenza di sintomi, possono essere evidenziati mediante ecocardiogramma seriati o indagini con radionuclidi (MUGA, *MUlti-Gate Acquisition*), ma nessun metodo è in grado di predire con sicurezza quali pazienti siano a rischio. La condizione del bambino può rimanere clinicamente stabile per molti anni, anche con un diminuito accorciamento frazionale. Una volta che si sviluppano i sintomi di insufficienza cardiaca, la percentuale di fatalità è elevata, fino al 30-50%. Il trapianto cardiaco è stato utilizzato con successo in questi pazienti (vedi Capitolo 443.1).

La miocardite acuta da doxorubicina, meno comune, tipicamente si presenta durante la somministrazione del farmaco. È spesso reversibile, e la prognosi a lungo termine può essere in un certo senso migliore. Il trattamento di supporto consiste nella somministrazione di antiedemigeni come la digossina, i diuretici e i farmaci che riducono il postcarico.

TOSSICITÀ CARDIACA DA IPECACUANA. Si può avere cardiotossicità da abuso cronico intenzionale di ipecacuana, secondario ad anoressia o bulimia nervose. Le sue manifestazioni comprendono dolore toracico, tachicardia, dispnea, ipotensione, aritmie, appiattimento e inversione delle onde T, anomalie del tratto ST, prolungamento degli intervalli Q-T e P-R, scompenso cardiaco e, potenzialmente, morte. Può essere difficile differenziare le anomalie cardiaca causate dall'ipecacuana da quelle del digiuno, di diete sbilanciate e di anomalie elettrolitiche.

439.2 • MIOCARDIOPATIA IPERTROFICA

FISIOPATOLOGIA. Le miocardiopatie ipertrofiche nei bambini possono essere primitive, dovute a una mutazione in uno dei numerosi geni che codificano per componenti proteiche del sarcomero, o secondarie, dovute alle sequele di cardiopatie congenite ostruttive (stenosi aortica critica, coartazione aortica), o a un errore congenito del metabolismo (malattia da accumulo di glicogeno o mucopolisaccaridosi). La miocardiopatia ipertrofica familiare o primitiva è la più comune patologia cardiovascolare genetica, che colpisce circa 1 individuo su 500.

La miocardiopatia ipertrofica primitiva è caratterizzata da un'ipertrofia ventricolare anomala di grado variabile, che si può incontrare in numerose varianti anatomiche. Il caso più comune comporta un coinvolgimento sproporzionato del setto ventricolare rispetto alla parete libera ventricolare, condizione definita anche miocardiopatia ipertrofica ostruttiva, stenosi subartica ipertrofica idiopatica o ipertrofia settale asimmetrica. Molti pazienti hanno un'ipertrofia ventricolare sinistra concentrica, una variante meno comune che colpisce in prevalenza l'apice ventricolare. Alcuni bambini, in particolare lattanti, possono avere un coinvolgimento sia del ventricolo sinistro sia di quello destro. La valvola mitrale è spostata anteriormente dall'ipertrofia dei muscoli papillari e la cavità ventricolare sinistra è distorta dalla massiva ipertrofia generalizzata. Possono essere presenti gradi variabili di fibrosi miocardica. Dal punto di vista microscopico, aree "a zolle" di fibre muscolari abnormemente spesse e corte sono disposte in modo circolare e sparse tra fibre muscolari normali e ipertrofiche. La microscopia elettronica evidenzia un disarrangiamento di miofibrille e miofilamenti.

Poiché il muscolo ipertrofico e fibrotico ha una **minore distensibilità (compliance)**, si verifica una resistenza al riempimento ventricolare sinistro; la funzione sistolica di pompa rimane intatta (o può essere addirittura iperdinamica) fino agli stadi avanzati della malattia. Nel 25% dei pazienti si sviluppa un'ostruzione all'efflusso ventricolare sinistro. Sono comuni anche gradi variabili di insufficienza della valvola mitrale.

EPIDEMIOLOGIA E GENETICA. La miocardiopatia ipertrofica viene nella maggior parte dei casi ereditata con pattern autosomico dominante, con ampia variabilità quanto a penetranza; molti casi rappresentano mutazioni *de novo*. Le manifestazioni si possono avere a qualsiasi età. I fratelli/sorelle del probando possono non essere colpiti da bambini, ma presentare segni della malattia quando raggiungono l'adolescenza e l'età adulta. Finora sono state implicate mutazioni in 10 geni, che codificano tutti per proteine del sarcomero cardiaco, essendo o componenti delle fibre spesse o sottili oppure subunità regolatorie associate. Le più comuni sono le mutazioni dei geni che codificano per la catena pesante della β-miosina e della proteina C che lega la miosina (vedi Tab. 439-2). Altre mutazioni note dei geni sarcomerici comprendono i geni che codificano per le troponine cardiache T e I, per l'α-tropomiosina, per le catene leggere regolatoria ed essenziale della miosina, per la titina e per la catena pesante dell'α-miosina. Le mutazioni nelle proteine non sarcomeriche comprendono la subunità regolatoria γ-2 della proteinchinasi attivata dall'AMP (PRKAG) e della proteina di membrana galattosidasi 2α associata ai lisosomi, che è responsabile della malattia di Danon, dovuta ad accumulo di glicogeno. Sono state identificate più di 200 mutazioni nei 10 geni più comuni e alcuni pazienti sono portatori di mutazioni in più di un gene. I test genetici sono disponibili e, in associazione all'anamnesi familiare, possono aiutare a predire quali pazienti hanno maggiore probabilità di avere aritmie e andare incontro a morte improvvisa.

Quando diagnosticata nella prima infanzia (malattia a esordio precoce), la miocardiopatia ipertrofica è associata a scompenso cardiaco più grave e aumentata mortalità. Al contrario, molti pazienti con comprovate mutazioni genetiche avranno ecocardiogrammi normali nell'infanzia, per manifestare i primi segni di ipertrofia solo nella media-tarda adolescenza. Alcuni pazienti, infine, non presenteranno segni di ipertrofia fino alla mezza età (malattia a esordio tardivo).

MANIFESTAZIONI CLINICHE. Molti bambini sono asintomatici e circa il 50% dei casi giunge alla valutazione iniziale a causa della presenza di un soffio cardiaco o poiché un altro membro della famiglia si è rivolto al medico. Nei bambini sintomatici, il quadro clinico è dominato da debolezza, astenia, dispnea da sforzo, palpitazioni, angina pectoris, capogiri e sincopi. Anche i bambini asintomatici sono a rischio di morte improvvisa. Il polso può essere forte a causa della precoce eiezione sistolica di sangue dal ventricolo. Possono riscontrarsi un evidente sollevamento ventricolare sinistro e un doppio impulso apicale. Il primo e il secondo tono cardiaco sono di solito normali. La rarità dei click da eiezione sistolica aiuta a differenziare la miocardiopatia ipertrofica dalla stenosi valvolare aortica. Il soffio sistolico, di tipo elettivo e di media intensità, si ode soprattutto al margine sternale sinistro e all'apice. Il soffio può aumentare brevemente dopo che l'esercizio fisico è stato interrotto, durante la **manovra di Valsalva** o all'assunzione della posizione eretta.

DIAGNOSI. L'elettrocardiogramma (ECG) evidenzia un'ipertrofia ventricolare sinistra con gradi variabili di sottoslivellamento del tratto S-T e inversione dell'onda T. Le anomalie elettrocardiografiche possono precedere i reperti ecocardiografici. Possono essere presenti segni della **sindrome di Wolff-Parkinson-White** e altri difetti di conduzione intraventricolare. Le radiografie evidenziano una lieve cardiomegalia, con sporgenza del ventricolo sinistro. L'ecocardiogramma rileva un'ipertrofia ventricolare sinistra che è asimmetrica, concentrica o apicale (Fig. 439-2). Vi è di solito un movimento sistolico anteriore del lembo anteriore della valvola mitrale. Le indagini Doppler dimostrano la presenza di un gradiente a livello del tratto di efflusso del ventricolo sinistro, che di solito è presente in meso-telesistole, quando l'ostruzione muscolare all'efflusso è massimale. Gli studi di flusso mediante Doppler possono evidenziare una disfunzione diastolica prima dello sviluppo dell'ipertrofia.

L'ecocardiografia ha sostituito il cateterismo cardiaco per la diagnosi iniziale, anche se il cateterismo può essere utile per stabilire se un paziente è un probabile candidato all'intervento chirurgico. Molti pazienti che non hanno un gradiente a livello del tratto di efflusso del ventricolo sinistro a riposo possono acquisirne uno significativo dopo somministrazione di isoproterenolo, nitrito di amile o nitroglicerina. La ventricolografia sinistra evidenzia un'invasione nella cavità ventricolare sinistra da parte del muscolo ipertrofico, specialmente da parte del setto interventricolare. L'obliterazione mesosistolica della cavità si verifica nei casi più gravi. È comune un'insufficienza mitralica. Occorre escludere la presenza di una discreta ostruzione subaortica con ipertrofia muscolare secondaria, poiché il trattamento chirurgico della stenosi subartica discreta è molto più efficace (vedi Capitolo 427.5).

La prognosi della miocardiopatia ipertrofica nel singolo paziente è imprevedibile. I pazienti asintomatici possono restare stabili per anni. Alcuni progrediscono verso lo scompenso cardiaco cronico, mentre altri sono a rischio di morte improvvisa da

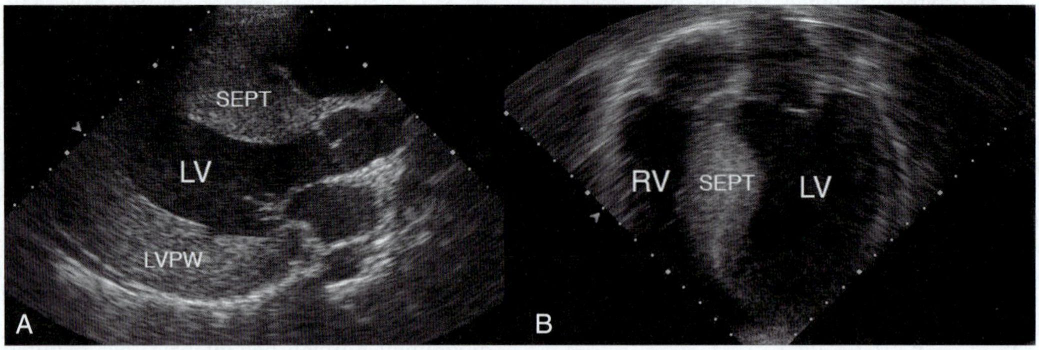

Figura 439-2. Ecocardiogrammi che evidenziano una miocardiopatia ipertrofica. *A*, Proiezione parasternale asse lungo di un paziente con grave ipertrofia ventricolare sinistra concentrica. *B*, Proiezione quattro camere di una paziente con ipertrofia settale asimmetrica. LV (*Left Ventricle*), ventricolo sinistro; LVPW (*Left Ventricular Posterior Wall*), parete posteriore del ventricolo sinistro; RV (*Right Ventricle*), ventricolo destro; SEPT, setto.

aritmie. Il decorso clinico degli altri membri della famiglia affetti dalla malattia e i risultati dei test genetici possono avere una certa utilità nella stratificazione del rischio per un bambino affetto.

TRATTAMENTO. Non è stato stabilito alcun trattamento standardizzato che senza dubbio protegga i pazienti dal rischio di morte improvvisa. Gli sport competitivi e l'attività fisica intensa dovrebbero essere proibiti, poiché la maggior parte delle morti improvvise si verifica durante o immediatamente dopo uno sforzo intenso, soprattutto negli adolescenti o nei giovani adulti. La digitale o una terapia diuretica aggressiva sono **controindicate** nella maggior parte dei pazienti a causa della loro potenziale capacità di aumentare l'ostruzione all'efflusso dal ventricolo sinistro. Andrebbe inoltre evitata l'infusione di isoproterenolo o di altri agenti isotropi, tranne che per scopi diagnostici, nell'ambiente controllato del laboratorio di emodinamica. I β-bloccanti adrenergici (propranololo) e i calcioantagonisti (verapamil, nifedipina) vengono utilizzati con un certo successo per diminuire il grado di ostruzione all'efflusso e possono rallentare lo sviluppo dell'ipertrofia ventricolare; questi farmaci non influiscono necessariamente sulla prognosi a lungo termine e non si sono rivelati in grado di ridurre l'incidenza di morte improvvisa. I calcioantagonisti non dovrebbero essere utilizzati durante l'infanzia, a causa dell'aumentato rischio di collasso cardiovascolare. I pazienti con aritmie documentate o storia di sincopi inspiegate vanno trattati in modo aggressivo, di solito con un **defibrillatore-cardioversore impiantabile** (**ICD**, *Implantable Cardioverter-Defibrillator*). In alcuni pazienti sono stati utilizzati pacemaker per alterare la depolarizzazione settale, anche se questa modalità è meno efficace nel ridurre i gradienti di efflusso ed è generalmente riservata agli adulti di età maggiore che sono a elevato rischio chirurgico. Il **trattamento chirurgico**, effettuando una **miotomia settale** ventricolare, è stato utilizzato in un sottogruppo di pazienti con angina invalidante o sincopi associate a ostruzione del tratto di efflusso del ventricolo sinistro (gradiente a riposo o provocato ≥50 mmHg). La riduzione chirurgica del gradiente a livello del tratto di efflusso, pur potendo migliorare i sintomi, non si è dimostrata in grado di ridurre il rischio di morte improvvisa. Se non è possibile alleviare l'ostruzione, in rari casi può rendersi necessaria la sostituzione della valvola mitrale. Negli adulti, alcuni centri effettuano procedure di ablazione ventricolare settale, in cui la branca dell'arteria coronaria che rifornisce il setto viene alcolizzata. Questa metodica non è stata utilizzata nei bambini.

Quando si ottiene un'anamnesi familiare positiva, lo screening consiste in un ECG e un ecocardiogramma, da ripetere a distanza di qualche anno nei bambini di età <12 anni, poi annualmente nei pazienti di età compresa tra 12 e 18-21 anni, che è il periodo in cui il rischio di malattia è massimo. In seguito lo screening può essere effettuato ogni 5 anni o a intervalli più frequenti se l'anamnesi familiare suggerisce un fenotipo particolarmente maligno. I test genetici, disponibili in qualche laboratorio, saranno un'utile aggiunta a questi studi clinici; tuttavia, fino al 20% dei casi di miocardiopatia ipertrofica non presenterà mutazioni nel pannello di geni comunemente testato.

MIOCARDIOPATIA IPERTROFICA IN LATTANTI FIGLI DI MADRE DIABETICA. Nei lattanti figli di madre diabetica si può riscontrare una forma transitoria di miocardiopatia ipertrofica, con o senza ostruzione del tratto di efflusso del ventricolo sinistro. L'aumentata massa ventricolare sinistra di solito regredisce nel giro di parecchi mesi (vedi Capitolo 107.1).

CORTICOSTEROIDI NEI PREMATURI. I neonati prematuri che ricevono corticosteroidi per una patologia polmonare cronica possono anch'essi andare incontro a una miocardiopatia ipertrofica transitoria, che di solito si risolve rapidamente con l'interruzione della terapia steroidea, anche se può recidivare se la terapia con steroidi viene ripresa.

MALATTIE DA ACCUMULO DI GLICOGENO. Sia il muscolo cardiaco sia la muscolatura scheletrica sono colpiti nella forma generalizzata di malattia da accumulo di glicogeno nota come tipo II o malattia di Pompe (vedi Capitolo 87.1). La cardiomegalia è massiva, ma i soffi sono insignificanti. È comune un'atelettasia polmonare con infezione secondaria, dovuta alla compressione esercitata dal cuore ingrandito. L'elettrocardiogramma è caratteristico ed evidenzia onde P prominenti, un intervallo P-R corto, voltaggi del QRS notevolmente aumentati, segni di ipertrofia sinistra isolata o di ipertrofia biventricolare, ritardi di conduzione intraventricolare. Le radiografie del torace confermano l'impressionante cardiomegalia con prominenza del ventricolo sinistro. L'ecocardiogramma evidenzia una grave ipertrofia ventricolare. La prognosi è infausta. La terapia sostitutiva con enzima ricombinante sembra promettente nel miglioramento della prognosi.

439.3 • Miocardiopatia restrittiva

Nella miocardiopatia restrittiva, oltre a una scarsa compliance ventricolare, che rappresenta la principale anomalia, si osserva un inadeguato riempimento delle cavità ventricolari durante la diastole, responsabile di manifestazioni cliniche che simulano da vicino quelle della pericardite costrittiva (vedi Capitolo 440). La funzione sistolica può essere preservata fino agli stadi avanzati della malattia. La miocardiopatia restrittiva determina dispnea, edema, ascite, epatomegalia, aumento della pressione venosa e congestione polmonare. A causa delle elevate pressioni di riempimento atriale sinistro, questi pazienti sono a rischio di sviluppare una patologia vascolare polmonare, spesso abbastanza rapidamente dopo la diagnosi. Il cuore è lievemente o moderatamente ingrandito e i soffi sono aspecifici. Se vi è ipertensione polmonare, la componente polmonare del secondo tono cardiaco è forte. L'elettrocardiogramma evidenzia onde P marcatamente prominenti, un voltaggio del QRS spesso normale, un sottoslivellamento del tratto S-T e un'inversione dell'onda T. Le radiografie del torace evidenziano una cardiomegalia da lieve a moderata. All'ecocardiogramma gli atri risultano marcatamente ingranditi (da due a tre volte può grandi dei ventricoli) mentre i ventricoli sono piccoli o di dimensioni normali, con una funzione sistolica spesso conservata ma caratteristiche di riempimento nettamente anomale all'ecocardiografia Doppler (Fig. 439-3). È essenziale, sebbene difficile, una diagnosi differenziale con la pericardite costrittiva, poiché quest'ultima si presta al trattamento chirurgico. La RM può essere utile per diagnosticare un pericardio ispessito in quest'ultima condizione. La miocardiopatia restrittiva può essere **idiopatica** oppure associata a una **patologia sistemica** come la sclerodermia, l'amiloidosi o la sarcoidosi, un errore congenito del metabolismo (**mucopolisaccaridosi**), la sindrome ipereosinofila, neoplasie maligne o radioterapia. Può anche derivare da un'anomalia congenita, come il **non compattamento isolato del miocardio ventricolare sinistro**. La prognosi per la miocardiopatia restrittiva è infausta e il peggioramento clinico può essere rapido. Il **trattamento** mira alla risoluzione dello scompenso cardiaco, anche se questi pazienti possono presentare una scarsa risposta al trattamento standard dello scompenso cardiaco (vedi Capitolo 442). I diuretici, utilizzati con giudizio, possono migliorare la ritenzione di liquidi nelle fasi precoci della malattia. I farmaci antiaritmici sono utilizzati in base alla necessità, e l'anticoagulazione con warfarin o l'antiaggregazione con acido acetilsalicilico sono indicate per lesioni come il non compattamento con un aumentato rischio di trombosi murale e ictus. Il trapianto cardiaco è stato utilizzato con successo in pazienti con miocardiopatia restrittiva, sempre che non sia presente un coinvolgimento multiorgano dovuto a una patologia sistemica. Una volta posta la diagnosi di miocardiopatia restrittiva, si dovrebbe provvedere immediatamente al trasferimento in un centro trapianti, dal momento che questi pazienti possono sviluppare rapidamente una patologia vascolare polmonare progressiva o un peggioramento clinico.

SINDROME IPEREOSINOFILICA DI LÖFFLER. Questa patologia causa una grave disfunzione multisistemica (a carico di cute, polmoni, sistema nervoso, fegato); la principale causa di morte è la miocardiopatia restrittiva con fibrosi endocardica delle valvole mitrale e tricuspide e dei ventricoli destro e sinistro. La successiva formazione di trombi endocardici porta all'embolizzazione. La sindrome di Löffler dovrebbe essere distinta dalla miocardite acuta eosinofilica necrotizzante non restrittiva e non fibrotica, una patologia acuta rapidamente fatale, e dalla **miocardite da ipersensibilità** (caratterizzata da febbre, rash, tachicardia, eosinofilia, allergia a farmaci e aritmie). Farmaci steroidei e citotossici possono portare a un beneficio nelle sindromi ipereosinofile. La terapia anticoagulante può ridurre l'incidenza di tromboembolismo.

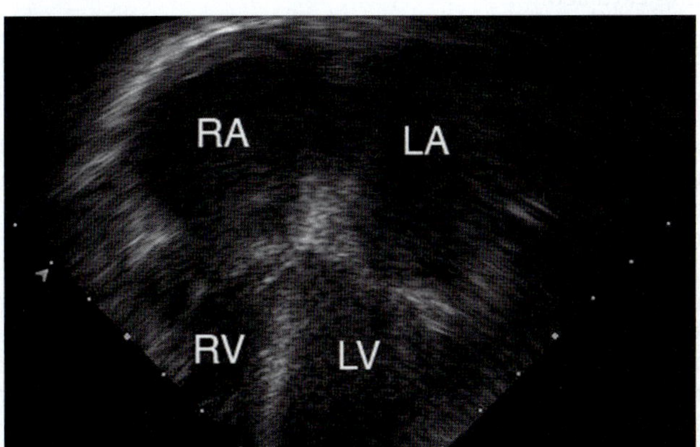

Figura 439-3. Ecocardiogramma di un paziente con miocardiopatia restrittiva. La proiezione apicale quattro camere evidenzia gli atri destro e sinistro marcatamente dilatati, in confronto alle camere ventricolari sinistra e destra di dimensioni normali. LA (*Left Atrium*), atrio sinistro; LV (*Left Ventricle*), ventricolo sinistro; RA (*Right Atrium*), atrio destro; RV (*Right Ventricle*), ventricolo destro.

MUCOPOLISACCARIDOSI. In queste patologie, la più comune delle quali è la sindrome di Hurler, i mucopolisaccaridi si accumulano in molti organi, compresi il cuore e i grossi vasi (vedi Capitolo 88). Le lesioni più gravi si trovano a carico delle valvole e delle arterie coronarie, ma non sono rare le anomalie del pericardio e dell'aorta. Il cuore può essere moderatamente ingrandito, con segni elettrocardiografici di ipertrofia ventricolare sinistra. I soffi cardiaci possono derivare da insufficienza e stenosi delle valvole mitralica e aortica. Talvolta sono interessate anche le valvole polmonare e tricuspide. La patologia a carico delle arterie coronarie può portare ad angina, che spesso spiega il frequente verificarsi di morte improvvisa. La prognosi è infausta.

NON COMPATTAMENTO ISOLATO DEL VENTRICOLO SINISTRO. Questa miocardiopatia da causa ignota presenta elementi sia di dilatazione sia di restrizione ventricolare sinistra. La condizione può essere diagnosticata a qualsiasi età, dall'infanzia alla prima età adulta, e la gravità dello scompenso cardiaco varia. L'ecocardiogramma è diagnostico ed evidenzia uno specifico pattern di ipertrofia ventricolare destra con profonde cripte muscolari. I pazienti possono essere a rischio di aritmie ventricolari e morte improvvisa, come pure di trombosi murali e ictus. Anche se alcuni pazienti possono rimanere stabili per anni, altri peggiorano rapidamente. Il trapianto cardiaco è stato utilizzato con successo in questo gruppo di pazienti.

439.4 • Miocarditi

Il termine "miocardite" si riferisce a infiammazione, necrosi o miocitolisi, causate da numerosi processi infettivi, connettivopatie, patologie granulomatose, cause tossiche o idiopatiche che colpiscono il miocardio con o senza manifestazioni sistemiche associate del processo patologico o coinvolgimento dell'endocardio o del pericardio (vedi Tab. 439-1). Una patologia coronarica è uniformemente assente. La manifestazione più comune è lo scompenso cardiaco, anche se le aritmie e la morte improvvisa possono essere i primi segni riscontrabili. Le infezioni virali sono la causa più comune.

EZIOLOGIA ED EPIDEMIOLOGIA. La reale incidenza della miocardite virale nei bambini è sconosciuta, poiché i casi lievi non vengono riconosciuti. La miocardite virale è tipicamente una patologia sporadica, ma talvolta assume proporzioni epidemiche. Le sue manifestazioni sono fino a un certo grado età-dipendenti: nella prima infanzia spesso si manifesta come una malattia acuta e fulminante; nei lattanti e nei bambini piccoli assume la forma di una miopericardite acuta ma meno fulminante, mentre nei bambini più grandi e negli adolescenti è spesso asintomatica e giunge all'attenzione clinica principalmente come precursore di una miocardiopatia dilatativa idiopatica. Gli agenti causali più comuni nei bambini sono gli adenovirus, i Coxackievirus B e altri enterovirus, anche se sono stati implicati quasi tutti gli agenti virali noti.

FISIOPATOLOGIA. La miocardite virale acuta può causare un processo infiammatorio fulminante caratterizzato da infiltrati cellulari, degenerazione e necrosi cellulare e successiva fibrosi. La miocardite virale può anche diventare un processo cronico, con persistenza dell'RNA o del DNA virale (ma non delle particelle virali infettive) nel miocardio. L'infiammazione cronica poi si perpetua per azione della risposta immune dell'ospite, che comprende linfociti T attivati diretti contro le alterazioni antigeniche virus-ospite. Tali linfociti citotossici e cellule natural killer, in associazione con la replicazione virale persistente e talvolta difettiva, può compromettere la funzione dei miociti senza un'evidente citolisi. In alternativa, un'infezione virale persistente può alterare l'espressione degli antigeni del complesso maggiore di istocompatibilità, con una conseguente esposizione di neoantigeni al sistema immunitario. Inoltre, alcune proteine virali possono avere in comune con le cellule dell'ospite epitopi antigenici, il che porta a un danno autoimmune a carico del miocita correlato all'antigene. Possono essere rilasciate citochine, come il fattore di necrosi tumorale α e l'interleuchina 1, le quali contribuiscono a dare inizio alla risposta immune alterata. Il risultato finale netto di un'infiammazione cronica associata a virus è spesso una **miocardiopatia dilatativa**.

MANIFESTAZIONI CLINICHE. I segni e i sintomi dipendono dall'età del paziente e dalla natura acuta o cronica dell'infezione. Un neonato può inizialmente avere febbre, grave scompenso cardiaco, distress respiratorio, cianosi, toni cardiaci parafonici, polso debole, tachicardia sproporzionata all'entità della febbre, insufficienza mitralica causata dalla dilatazione dell'anulus valvolare, ritmo di galoppo, acidosi e shock. Possono essere presenti segni di epatite virale, meningite asettica e un rash associato. Nella forma più fulminante, la morte si verifica 1-7 giorni dopo l'esordio dei sintomi. La radiografia del torace evidenzia un cuore enormemente ingrandito ed edema polmonare; l'elettrocardiogramma rileva tachicardia sinusale, ridotto voltaggio del complesso QRS, anomalie del tratto S-T e dell'onda T. Le aritmie, che possono essere la prima manifestazione clinica, in presenza di febbre e di un cuore ingrandito sono altamente suggestive di miocardite acuta.

Un paziente più grande con miocardite acuta può anche giungere all'osservazione con scompenso cardiaco acuto; tuttavia è più comune che i pazienti presentino un esordio graduale di scompenso cardiaco o un esordio improvviso di aritmie ventricolari. In questi pazienti, la fase infettiva acuta è di solito passata ed è presente una miocardiopatia dilatativa idiopatica (vedi Capitolo 439.1).

DIAGNOSI. La velocità di eritrosedimentazione, gli enzimi cardiaci (creatin fosfochinasi, lattico deidrogenasi) e il peptide natriuretico tipo B (BNP, *Brain Natriuretic Peptide*) possono essere elevati nella miocardite acuta o cronica. Se positivi, i titoli virali nel siero sono utili; una sierologia negativa non esclude la diagnosi. Studi appaiati che comprendono la PCR da biopsia ventricolare e campioni di siero hanno evidenziato che il genoma virale è presente di routine dei campioni cardiaci, ma assente nel sangue periferico. L'ecocardiografia rileva una scarsa funzione ventricolare sinistra e spesso un versamento pericardico, un rigurgito valvolare mitralico e l'assenza di lesioni arteriose coronariche o di altre cardiopatie congenite. La miocardite può essere confermata dalla biopsia endomiocardica. La biopsia, che viene effettuata durante una cateterismo cardiaco, è utilizzabile anche per individuare altre cause di miocardiopatia (malattie da accumulo, difetti mitocondriali). La PCR può identificare specifici RNA o DNA virali.

DIAGNOSI DIFFERENZIALE. Le principali patologie che mimano una miocardite acuta comprendono il deficit di carnitina, i difetti mitocondriali ereditari, la miocardiopatia dilatativa idiopatica, la pericardite, la fibroelastosi dell'endocardio e l'origine anomala dell'arteria coronaria sinistra (vedi Tab. 439-1).

TRATTAMENTO. L'approccio al trattamento della miocardite acuta comprende misure di supporto per lo scompenso cardiaco grave o per lo shock cardiogeno (vedi Capitolo 442). La dopamina, l'adrenalina e il milrinone possono essere utili nei pazienti con bassa gittata cardiaca e ipoperfusione sistemica. Tutti gli agenti inotropi, compresa la digossina, dovrebbero essere utilizzati con cautela, poiché i pazienti con miocardite sono sensibili agli effetti proaritmici di questi farmaci. Quando utilizzata, la digossina viene iniziata a un dosaggio che è la metà del normale. La pericardiocentesi andrebbe effettuata in pazienti con evidenza di tamponamento cardiaco, e la coltura del fluido pericardico può evidenziare l'agente virale responsabile. Le aritmie vanno trattate aggressivamente e possono richiedere l'utilizzo di amiodarone per via endovenosa per ottenere un adeguato controllo. In lattanti e i bambini con shock cardiogeno, si può procedere all'ossigenazione mediante membrana extracorporea (ECMO, *ExtraCorporeal Membrane Oxygenation*). Si può effetuare l'impianto di un dispositivo di assistenza ventricolare sinistra, che funge da ponte verso il trapianto di cuore, il **trattamento di scelta** nei pazienti con scompenso cardiaco refrattario (vedi Capitolo 443.1). Il ruolo di trattamenti specifici per la miocardite virale è controverso. Sono state utilizzate immunoglobuline per via endovenosa a un dosaggio di 2 g/kg. Si è inoltre fatto ricorso ai corticosteroidi e, in piccoli gruppi di pazienti pediatrici, un trattamento con prednisone (2 mg/kg al giorno, scalato fino a 0,3 mg/kg al giorno nell'arco di 3 mesi) è stato efficace nel ridurre l'infiammazione miocardica e nel migliorare la funzione cardiaca. Sono state osservate recidive quando l'immunosoppressione è stata sospesa in alcuni pazienti. Tuttavia, trial clinici in pazienti adulti hanno dato risultati variabili. È in fase di valutazione una terapia antivirale specifica per le infezione da enterovirus (picovir) o da virus di Epstein-Barr (aciclovir).

PROGNOSI. La prognosi per i neonati sintomatici con miocardite virale acuta è finora infausta. I pazienti con sintomi meno gravi hanno una prognosi migliore, ed è stata descritta una risoluzione completa. La prognosi per i bambini più grandi con progressione verso una miocardiopatia dilatativa cronica è altresì infausta in assenza di terapia. Questi pazienti continuano ad avere dilatazione, fibrosi e una funzione cardiaca in peggioramento. In vari studi condotti su adulti la risoluzione spontanea si è verificata nel 10-15% dei casi. Fino al 50% dei pazienti più anziani non trattati muore entro 2 anni dalla diagnosi, e l'80% entro 8 anni, a meno che non vengano sottoposti a trapianto cardiaco.

439.5 • Cause non virali di miocardite

INFEZIONI BATTERICHE. Nella difterite (vedi Capitolo 186) la tossina del bacillo può produrre uno scompenso circolatorio periferico o una miocardite tossica entro le prime 2 settimane di malattia. In aggiunta alla terapia per la difterite, è essenziale il trattamento dello shock cardiogeno. La miocardite causata dalla tossina difterica è caratterizzata dallo sviluppo di blocco atrioventricolare, blocco di branca o extrasistoli. Lo scompenso cardiaco, che avviene in un secondo momento, è caratterizzato da ingrandimento cardiaco e ritmo di galoppo. Oltre all'aritmia, l'elettrocardiogramma evidenzia un sottoslivellamento del tratto ST e un'inversione dell'onda T nella maggior parte delle derivazioni. La prognosi a brevissimo termine è infausta (mortalità del 50%). Il trattamento comprende un rigoroso riposo a letto fino alla scomparsa di tutti i segni di miocardite, come anche il trattamento della ritenzione di fluidi e delle aritmie, compreso il pacing cardiaco.

In molte infezioni batteriche sistemiche, il miglioramento circolatorio si manifesta come un collasso circolatorio periferico o una miocardite tossica. Una miocardite tossica, segnalata da tachicardia, ritmo di galoppo e ingrandimento cardiaco, può complicare una polmonite, un'endocardite infettiva e una setticemia. Un fattore con azione depressiva sul miocardio può produrre una miocardiopatia tossica acuta. La prognosi dipende alla capacità di controllare l'infezione primitiva.

MALATTIA DA RICKETTSIE. La febbre maculosa delle Montagne Rocciose (vedi Capitolo 225.1) può essere complicata da ipotensione e collasso vascolare periferico. Questa complicanza è stata attribuita alla vasculite generale caratteristica della malattia, ma una miocardite acuta può essere un fattore contribuente.

INFEZIONI PARASSITARIE E FUNGINE. Sono state descritte lesioni nel miocardio in associazione a istoplasmosi, coccidioidomicosi, toxoplasmosi e trichinosi. In queste patologie, la lesione cardiaca raramente produce segni clinici di miocardite. L'actinomicosi può coinvolgere il pericardio e il miocardio per stretta contiguità con un ascesso polmonare. Si possono riscontrare a una radiografia del torace di routine cisti idatidee del pericardio, che di solito causano sintomi solo in caso di rottura. La schistosomiasi può portare a ipertensione polmonare e cor polmonare. La tripanosomiasi di Cruz (malattia di Chagas) può provocare una miocardite acuta o subacuta ed è una causa importante di miocardiopatia dilatativa cronica nell'America centrale e meridionale.

439.6 • FIBROELASTOSI ENDOCARDICA

La fibroelastosi endocardica (EFE, *Endocardial FibroElastosis*) è stata chiamata endocardite fetale, fibrosi endocardica, fibroelastosi prenatale, iperplasia del tessuto elastico e sclerosi endocardica. Nell'EFE primitiva non si riscontrano evidenti lesioni valvolari predisponenti né altre anomalie cardiache congenite. In quella secondaria è presente una grave cardiopatia congenita del cuore sinistro di tipo ostruttivo (stenosi o atresia aortica, forme della sindrome del cuore sinistro ipoplasico o grave coartazione aortica). Nella forma secondaria la cavità ventricolare è spesso contratta, mentre nella malattia primitiva si osserva una cavità ventricolare sinistra dilatata, di solito durante l'infanzia; nei giovani adulti, tuttavia, è stata osservata una forma contratta di EFE primitiva. Non è stata stabilita alcuna causa di EFE primitiva, anche se è stata implicata un'associazione con l'infezione da virus della parotite attraverso l'analisi mediante PCR di campioni di miocardio affetto.

Dal punto di vista patologico, è presente un ispessimento opaco fibroelastico dell'endocardio (di solito nel ventricolo sinistro), che frequentemente copre la trabecolatura delle superfici interne delle camere cardiache. La lesione, che può diffondersi fino a coinvolgere le valvole, da punto di vista microscopico consiste in un ispessimento fibroelastico dell'endocardio e può portare a una degenerazione subendocardica o a necrosi muscolare con vacuolizzazione delle fibre muscolari. I lembi valvolari coinvolti sono caratterizzati da una proliferazione mixomatosa con un aumento degli elementi collagene.

Le manifestazioni cliniche sono variabili. I lattanti, di solito quelli di età >6 mesi fino a quel momento apparentemente stati in buona salute, vanno incontro a scompenso cardiaco congestizio, spesso precipitato da un'infezione respiratoria. I bambini colpiti possono manifestare dispnea, tosse, anoressia, splenomegalia, edemi, ritardo della crescita e infezioni polmonari ricorrenti. Lo scompenso cardiaco cronico può essere controllato per qualche tempo dalla digitale e dai diuretici; tuttavia la maggior parte dei pazienti finisce per andare incontro a morte. I lattanti nei quali sono predominanti lesioni valvolari o difetti cardiovascolari congeniti associati, di solito muoiono nel primo mese di vita. Le radiografie del torace confermano un significativo ingrandimento cardiaco (Fig. 439-4). L'elettrocardiogramma è anormale, con cambiamenti indicativi di ipertrofia dell'atrio e del ventricolo sinistri con sovraccarico. L'ecocardiogramma evidenzia una superficie endocardica dall'aspetto brillante e un ventricolo sinistro dilatato, con funzione depressa. La RM può anche delineare la superficie endomiocardica fibrotica.

Il trattamento mira ad alleviare lo scompenso cardiaco congestizio e a prevenire le infezioni intercorrenti. L'EFE allo stadio terminale, con segni di scompenso cardiaco nonostante un trattamento medico massimale, è un indicazione al trapianto di cuore (vedi Capitolo 443.1).

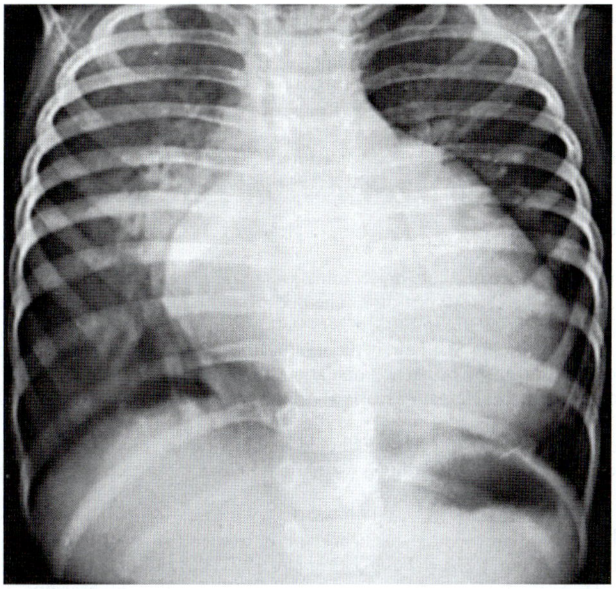

Figura 439-4. Radiografia del torace di una bambina di 7 anni con fibroelastosi endocardica. Si notino l'ingrandimento cardiaco, senza un contorno distinto, e i campi polmonari chiari.

Miocardiopatie (generale)

Lipshultz SE, Sleeper LA, Towbin JA, et al: The incidence of pediatric cardiomyopathy in two regions of the United States. *N Engl J Med* 2003;348:1647–1655.

Maron BJ, Chaitman BR, Ackerman MJ, et al: Recommendations for physical activity and recreational sports participation for young patients with genetic cardiovascular diseases. *Circulation* 2004;109:2807–2816.

Nugent AW, Daubeney PEF, Chondros P, et al: The epidemiology of childhood cardiomyopathy in Australia. *N Engl J Med* 2003;348:1639–1646.

Miocardiopatia dilatativa

Barbaro G, Lipshultz SE: Pathogenesis of HIV-associated cardiomyopathy. *Ann N Y Acad Sci* 2001;946:57–81.

Brown CA, O'Connell JB: Myocarditis and idiopathic dilated cardiomyopathy. *Am J Med* 1995;99:309–314.

Burkett EL, Hershberger RE: Clinical and genetic issues in familial dilated cardiomyopathy. *J Am Coll Cardiol* 2005;45:969–981.

Forleo C, Resta N, Sorrentino S, et al: Association of β-adrenergic receptor polymorphisms and progression to heart failure in patients with idiopathic dilated cardiomyopathy. *Am J Med* 2004;117:451–458.

Lipshultz SE, Colan SD, Gelber RD, et al: Late cardiac effects of doxorubicin therapy for acute lymphoblastic leukemia in childhood. *N Engl J Med* 1991;324:808–815.

Schonberger J, Seidman CE: Many roads lead to a broken heart: The genetics of dilated cardiomyopathy. *Am J Hum Genet* 2001;69:249–260.

Shaw T, Elliott P, McKenna WJ: Dilated cardiomyopathy: A genetically heterogeneous disease. *Lancet* 2002;360:654–655.

Shekhawat PS, Matern D, Strauss AW: Fetal fatty acid oxidation disorders, their effect on maternal health and neonatal outcome: Impact of expanded newborn screening on their diagnosis and management. *Pediatr Res* 2005;57:78R–86R.

Towbin JA, Solaro RJ: Genetics of dilated cardiomyopathy: More genes that kill. *J Am Coll Cardiol* 2004;44:2041–2043.

Weiford BC, Subbarao VD, Mulhern KM: Noncompaction of the ventricular myocardium. *Circulation* 2004;109:2965–2971.

Miocardiopatia ipertrofica

Elliott P, McKenna WJ: Hypertrophic cardiomyopathy. *Lancet* 2004;363:1881–1891.

MacRae CA, Ellinor PT: Genetic screening and risk assessment in hypertrophic cardiomyopathy. *J Am Coll Cardiol* 2004;44:2326–2328.

Maron BJ: Hypertrophic cardiomyopathy. *JAMA* 2002;287:1308–1320.

Maron BJ, Seidman JG, Seidman CE: Proposal for contemporary screening strategies in families with hypertrophic cardiomyopathy. *J Am Coll Cardiol* 2004;44:2125–2132.

Roberts R, Sigwart U: New concepts in hypertrophic cardiomyopathies, part II. *Circulation* 2001;104:2249–2252.

Watkins H, McKenna WJ, Thierfelder L, et al: Mutations in the genes for cardiac troponin T and alpha-tropomyosin in hypertrophic cardiomyopathy. *N Engl J Med* 1995;332:1058–1064.

Miocardiopatia restrittiva

Cetta F, O'Leary PW, Seward JB, et al: Idiopathic restrictive cardiomyopathy in childhood: Diagnostic features and clinical course. *Mayo Clin Proc* 1995;70:634–640.

Chen SC, Balfour IC, Jureidini S: Clinical spectrum of restrictive cardiomyopathy in children. *J Heart Lung Transplant* 2001;20:90–92.
Denfield SW, Rosenthal G, Gajarski RJ, et al: Restrictive cardiomyopathies in childhood. *Tex Heart J* 1997;24:38–44.
Kushwaha SS, Fallon JT, Fuster V: Restrictive cardiomyopathy. *N Engl J Med* 1997;336:267.
Taur Y, Frishman WH: The cardiac ryanodine receptor (RyR2) and its role in heart disease. *Cardiol Rev* 2005;13:142–146.

Miocarditi

Batra AS, Lewis AB: Acute myocarditis. *Curr Opin Pediatr* 2001;13:234–239.
Chen RT, Lane JM: Myocarditis: The unexpected return of smallpox vaccine adverse events. *Lancet* 2003;362:1345–1346.
Drucker NA, Colan SD, Lewis AB, et al: Gamma-globulin treatment of acute myocarditis in the pediatric population. *Circulation* 1994;89:252–257.
Feldman AM, McNamara D: Myocarditis. *N Engl J Med* 2000;343:1388–1398.
Hrobon P, Kuntz KM, Hare JM: Should endomyocardial biopsy be performed for detection of myocarditis? A decision analytic approach. *J Heart Lung Transplant* 1998;17:479–486.
Kleinert S, Weintraub RG, Wilkinson JL, et al: Myocarditis in children with dilated cardiomyopathy: Incidence and outcome after dual therapy immunosuppression. *J Heart Lung Transplant* 1997;16:1248–1254.
Levi D, Alejos J: Diagnosis and treatment of pediatric viral myocarditis. *Curr Opin Cardiol* 2001;16:77–83.
Liu PP, Mason JW: Advances in the understanding of myocarditis. *Circulation* 2001;104:1076–1082.

Capitolo 440 ■ Malattie del pericardio

Le principali patologie che coinvolgono il pericardio sono elencate nella Tabella 440-1. In alcuni casi il coinvolgimento pericardico rappresenta una manifestazione di una malattia generalizzata, la cui l'entità varia a seconda della patologia sottostante.

TABELLA 440-1. Eziologia delle patologie del pericardio

ANOMALIE CONGENITE
Assenza (parziale, completa)
Cisti
Nanismo Mulibrey (muscolo, fegato, cervello, occhio) con ispessimento pericardico congenito e costrizione
INFETTIVE
Virali (Coxsackievirus B, virus di Epstein-Barr, influenza, adenovirus)
Batteriche (streptococco, pneumococco, stafilococco, meningococco, micoplasma, tularemia, listeriosi, leptospirosi)
Da immunocomplessi (meningococco, *Haemophilus influenzae*)
Tubercolosi
Fungine (istoplasmosi, actinomicosi)
Parassitarie (toxoplasmosi, echinococcosi)
MALATTIE DEL TESSUTO CONNETTIVO
Artrite reumatoide
Febbre reumatica
Lupus eritematoso sistemico
Sclerosi sistemica
Sarcoidosi
Granulomatosi di Wegener
PATOLOGIE METABOLICHE ED ENDOCRINE
Uremia
Ipotiroidismo
Chilopericardio
PATOLOGIE EMATOLOGICHE-ONCOLOGICHE
Diatesi emorragica
Neoplasie maligne (primitive, metastatiche)
Post-radioterapia
ALTRE
Traumi (penetranti o chiusi)
Cause iatrogene (correlate a presenza di cateteri)
Postpericardiectomia (cardiochirurgia)
Dissezione aortica
Cause idiopatiche
Febbre mediterranea familiare
Vaccinazione contro la varicella
Pancreatine
Sindrome di Löffler

440.1 • PERICARDITE ACUTA

FISIOPATOLOGIA. L'infiammazione pericardica porta a un accumulo nello spazio pericardico di un liquido che, a seconda della causa della pericardite, può essere sieroso, fibrinoso, purulento o emorragico. Il **tamponamento cardiaco** si verifica quando la quantità di fluido pericardico raggiunge un livello tale da compromettere la funzione cardiaca. In un bambino sano 10-15 mL di liquido nello spazio pericardico sono un reperto normale, mentre in un adolescente con pericardite se ne possono accumulare fino a 1000 mL o più. A ogni piccolo aumento di fluido anche la pressione pericardica aumenta, seppure lentamente; una volta raggiunto un livello critico, la pressione cresce rapidamente culminando in una grave compressione cardiaca. Possono esservi inibizione del riempimento ventricolare durante la diastole, elevate pressioni venose sistemiche e polmonari e allo stadio terminale, in assenza di trattamento, compromissione della gittata cardiaca e shock.

MANIFESTAZIONI CLINICHE. Il primo sintomo di una patologia del pericardio è spesso un dolore precordiale. Il disturbo di cui il paziente si lamenta in particolare è un dolore acuto, trafittivo, in corrispondenza del precordio e spesso della spalla sinistra e del dorso; il dolore può essere esacerbato dalla posizione supina e alleviato da quella seduta, specialmente con il busto in avanti. A causa dell'assenza di un'innervazione sensitiva del pericardio, il dolore è probabilmente di tipo riferito, da irritazione diaframmatica e pleurica. Possono anche esservi tosse, dispnea, dolore addominale, vomito e febbre. Nei bambini più piccoli questi sintomi atipici possono essere predominanti. La presenza di sintomi o segni associati a coinvolgimento di altri organi dipende dalla causa della pericardite.

Molti dei reperti riscontrati all'esame obiettivo sono correlati alla quantità di liquido accumulato nel sacco pericardico. La presenza di **sfregamenti** è un segno utile ma variabile nella pericardite acuta; di solito diventa evidente quando il versamento è piccolo. Quando il versamento è più abbondante, gli unici reperti auscultatori sono i toni cardiaci parafonici. Un polso piccolo, tachicardia, distensione delle vene del collo e un aumento del polso paradosso suggeriscono un significativo accumulo di liquido.

Il **polso paradosso** è causato dal lieve decremento della pressione arteriosa sistolica che si verifica normalmente durante l'inspirio. In caso di tamponamento cardiaco, questo fenomeno normale è esagerato, probabilmente a causa del diminuito riempimento del cuore sinistro durante la fase inspiratoria del ciclo respiratorio. Per determinare il grado del polso paradosso di utilizza un manometro a mercurio. Al paziente viene chiesto di respirare normalmente, senza esagerare. Sgonfiando lentamente il manometro, il primo tono di Korotkoff si udirà inizialmente in modo intermittente (variando con gli atti del respiro). Dopo aver preso nota del primo punto, si sgonfia il manometro finché non si percepisce il primo tono di Korotkoff in modo continuo. La differenza tra queste due pressioni sistoliche è il polso paradosso. Un polso paradosso >20 mmHg in un bambino con pericardite è indicativo della presenza di tamponamento cardiaco; un cambiamento di 10-20 mmHg non è dirimente. Un aumento del polso paradosso si può osservare anche in pazienti con grave dispnea da qualsiasi causa, in quelli con patologia polmonare (enfisema o asma), in soggetti obesi o in pazienti ventilati con respiratore a pressione positiva. In tutti questi soggetti il polso paradosso è dovuto a un marcato aumento della pressione intratoracica. La causa di un polso paradosso in un bambino ventilato artificialmente dopo intervento cardiochirurgico può perciò essere difficile da valutare.

DIAGNOSI. I reperti specifici dipendono dalla patologia sottostante. La pericardite ha più di un effetto sull'elettrocardiogramma. Un basso voltaggio del QRS deriva da un effetto di attenuazione da parte del liquido pericardico. La pressione esercitata sul miocardio dal liquido o dall'essudato produce una corrente di lesione che porta a un lieve sopraslivellamento dei tratti ST. Un'inversione generalizzata delle onde T si verifica come conseguenza di un'associata infiammazione miocardica. Le alterazioni del tratto ST e dell'onda T in caso di pericardite sono più generalizzate di quelle che si osservano in caso di infarto miocardico e i sopraslivellamenti del tratto ST tendono a precedere i cambiamenti dell'onda T. Può essere presente un'**alternanza elettrica**, dimostrata da una variabile ampiezza del complesso QRS. Durante la fase acuta della malattia, prima della diagnosi, può verificarsi un intervallo in cui l'elettrocardigramma è in fase transizionale e sembra normale. In alcuni casi non vengono mai identificate chiare e nette anomalie elettrocardiografiche.

Deve essere presente un versamento pericardico relativamente importante perché si produca un ingrandimento dell'ombra cardiaca con la tipica configurazione "a fiasco" alla radiografia del torace (Fig. 440-1). Nella maggior parte dei casi, i campi polmonari sono chiari. In caso di patologia pericardica costrittiva, il cuore è relativamente piccolo e possono essere presenti calcificazioni pericardiche.

L'ecocardiogramma è la tecnica più sensibile per la valutazione della dimensione e della progressione dei versamenti pericardici (Fig. 440-2). Di norma il pericardio è strettamente aderente all'epicardio e i due strati possono essere separati solo di poco dal fascio di ultrasuoni. In pazienti con versamento pericardico si registra uno spazio vuoto, ecoprivo, tra epicardio e pericardio. Un versamento posteriore si registra posteriormente rispetto all'epicardio ventricolare sinistro e finisce alla giunzione tra ventricolo sinistro e atrio sinistro; quello anteriore si registrerà invece tra la parete toracica e la parete ventricolare anteriore destra. La presenza di un versamento sia anteriore sia posteriore generalmente indica un'ampia raccolta di fluido. L'appiattimento del movimento del setto e il collasso dell'efflusso ventricolare destro durante la diastole sono segni di tamponamento cardiaco.

DIAGNOSI DIFFERENZIALE.

Pericardite virale e pericardite acuta benigna. Queste entità sono considerate sinonimi poiché la maggior parte delle pericarditi acute benigne fa seguito a patologie virali o si manifesta in concomitanza con esse. I virus riconosciuti come causa di pericardite comprendono i Coxsackievirus B, i virus influenzali, gli echovirus e gli adenovirus. La patogenesi non è chiara, ma può essere correlata a una reazione di ipersensibilità alla malattia virale. L'infiammazione pericardica non è necessariamente il precursore di un processo infiammatorio generalizzato. La maggior parte dei casi è lieve e la guarigione avviene nel giro di qualche settimana. È indicato solo il trattamento sintomatico, di solito con farmaci antinfiammatori non steroidei (FANS) come l'indometacina. In rari casi, le condizioni cliniche del paziente sono gravi e può instaurarsi un tamponamento cardiaco. Inoltre, in alcuni pazienti può verificarsi una malattia cronica recidivante. La diagnosi differenziale tra questi pazienti e quelli affetti da collagenovasculopatie può essere difficile. Questi ultimi pazienti presentano una notevole risposta ai corticosteroidi o ai FANS; le forme più lievi possono essere controllate con l'acido acetilsalicilico. Il decorso clinico può durare da qualche mese a 1-2 anni, periodo di tempo durante il quale i pazienti sono dipendenti dalla terapia farmacologica per la soppressione della pericardite. Alla fine si assiste a un miglioramento e la prognosi è buona.

La diagnosi differenziale clinica tra pericardite acuta e miocardite può essere difficile; di solito, ciascuna delle due patologie comprende una componente dell'altra. Il trattamento di queste condizioni è abbastanza differente: nella prima sono appropriati un trattamento antinfiammatorio e una risposta urgente al tamponamento cardiaco, mentre nella seconda è richiesta una terapia per lo scompenso cardiaco. L'ecocardiogramma, oltre a indicare le dimensioni del versamento pericardico, può mettere in luce la presenza di disfunzione miocardica.

Pericardite purulenta. Questa condizione è nella maggior parte dei casi associata a infezioni batteriche come polmonite, epiglottite, meningite o osteomielite. Generalmente sono presenti i segni e i sintomi dell'infezione primaria. Una volta instauratosi un processo purulento, in assenza di trattamento il decorso è fulminante ed esita in tamponamento cardiaco acuto e morte. È richiesto un drenaggio pericardico aperto in associazione con appropriati antibiotici per via endovenosa. Anche se una pericardiocentesi fornisce un campione di essudato per scopi diagnostici e può essere salvavita di fronte a una grave compressione cardiaca, senza un drenaggio aperto e la rimozione delle aderenze il tamponamento recidiva quasi invariabilmente. Il drenaggio pericardico aperto ha significativamente aumentato la sopravvivenza. In rari casi, nelle infezioni identificate in modo estremamente precoce e in presenza di un liquido pericardico con caratteristiche più di trasudato che di essudato, ha avuto successo la creazione di più aperture nel pericardio con il posizionamento di un drenaggio, associato a terapia antibiotica. I microrganismi più comuni responsabili di pericardite purulenta sono lo *Staphylococcus aureus*, l'*Haemophilus influenzae* tipo b e la *Neisseria meningitidis* (per il trattamento antimicrobico, vedi Capitoli 180, 192 e 190, rispettivamente). La pericardite tubercolare si verifica raramente nei bambini. Si deve trattare con chemioterapia antitubercolare per diversi mesi (vedi Capitolo 212). Una pericardite mediata da immunocomplessi (sterile)

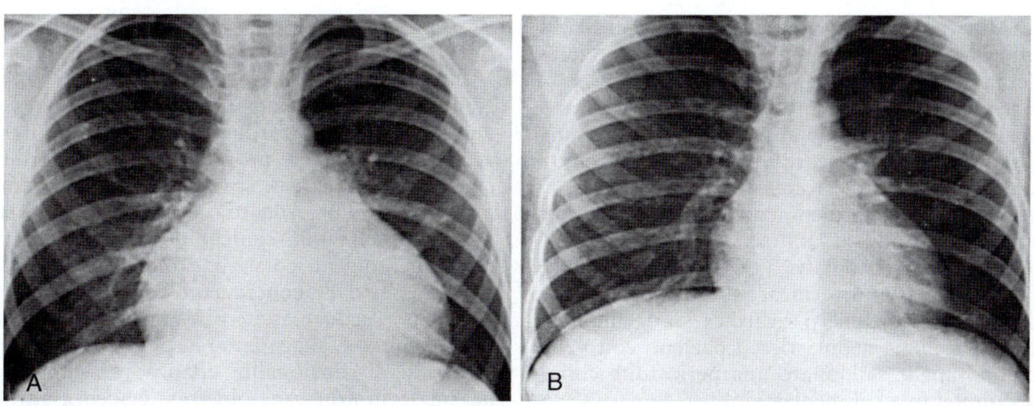

Figura 440-1. Radiografie del torace in un caso di pericardite acuta aspecifica. *A*, Ingrandimento dell'ombra cardiopericardica causata da versamento pericardico. *B*, Un mese dopo completa guarigione.

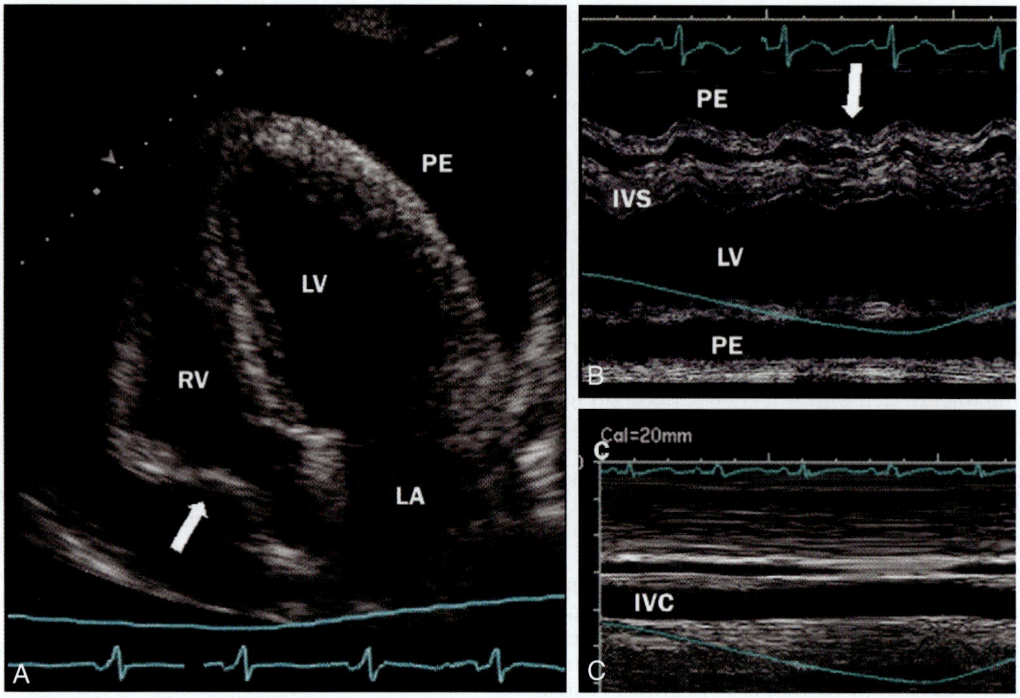

Figura 440-2. Immagini ecocardiografiche di un abbondante versamento pericardico con caratteristiche di tamponamento. *A*, Proiezione apicale quattro camere di ventricolo sinistro, atrio sinistro e ventricolo destro, che evidenzia un abbondante versamento pericardico con collasso diastolico dell'atrio destro (*freccia*). *B*, Immagine M-mode con cursore posizionato attraverso il ventricolo destro, il setto interventricolare e il ventricolo sinistro in parasternale asse lungo. La proiezione evidenzia un versamento pericardico circonferenziale con collasso diastolico della parete libera del ventricolo destro (*freccia*) in espirio. *C*, Immagine M-mode da finestra sottocostale nello stesso paziente, che evidenzia dilatazione della vena cava inferiore senza collasso in inspirio. IVC (*Inferior Vena Cava*), vena cava inferiore; IVS (*InterVentricular Septum*), setto interventricolare; LA (*Left Atrium*), atrio sinistro; LV (*Left Ventricle*), ventricolo sinistro; PE (*Pericardial Effusion*), versamento pericardico; RV (*Right Ventricle*), ventricolo destro. (Da Troughton RW, Asher CR, Klein AL: Pericarditis. *Lancet* 2004;363:717-727.)

può verificarsi 5-7 giorni dopo l'inizio del trattamento per una grave infezione sistemica o meningea da meningococco o *H. influenzae* tipo b. La terapia comprende farmaci antinfiammatori e pericardiocentesi se si sviluppa un tamponamento.

Febbre reumatica acuta. La pericardite si verifica nella febbre reumatica acuta come una componente della pancardite (vedi Capitoli 156, 182.1 e 430) ed è associata a una valvulite acuta. La pericardite e altre manifestazioni di pancardite reumatica acuta rispondono alla terapia con steroidi. Il tamponamento cardiaco è estremamente raro.

Artrite reumatoide giovanile. La pericardite è una manifestazione comune dell'artrite reumatoide giovanile (vedi Capitolo 154). Raramente può essere l'unica manifestazione e precedere l'esordio dell'artrite di mesi o anche di anni. Distinguere una pericardite reumatoide da quella che si osserva in altre collagenovasculopatie, in particolare nel lupus eritematoso sistemico, può essere difficile. Il trattamento consiste nell'utilizzo di steroidi e salicilati, che possono essere necessari per una terapia a lungo termine.

Uremia. La pericardite uremica, che si verifica solo in presenza di una grave insufficienza renale prolungata, deriva da un'irritazione chimica del pericardio secondaria ad anomalie metaboliche. Può culminare in un tamponamento cardiaco o provocare un'ipotensione ricorrente durante emodialisi. Se non si ottiene un ragionevole miglioramento della pericardite uremica con l'emodialisi, è raccomandata la pericardiectomia.

Neoplasie. Un versamento pericardico neoplastico, osservabile in pazienti con morbo di Hodgkin, linfosarcoma e leucemia, deriva da una diretta invasione neoplastica del pericardio. Nelle fasi avanzate della malattia si può verificare un tamponamento cardiaco. È raro che un'infiltrazione pericardica sia la manifestazione iniziale della patologia neoplastica. I pazienti con neoplasie maligne possono anche sviluppare una pericardite come conseguenza della radioterapia sul mediastino.

Sindrome post-pericardiotomica (vedi Capitolo 434). Si possono osservare versamenti pericardici per 1-2 settimane o più dopo intervento cardiochirurgico a cuore aperto e in alcune casistiche ecocardiografiche vengono diagnosticati nel 15-23% dei pazienti nel postoperatorio. La sindrome è una reazione da ipersensibilità aspecifica al trauma sul pericardio e sulla superficie epicardica del cuore. Sono stati riportati titoli elevati di anticorpi anti-cuore in relazione ai segni clinici della sindrome. I pazienti possono inizialmente presentare febbricola, letargia, perdita dell'appetito o dolore addominale. Può essere presente o meno un dolore toracico precordiale o pleurico. Occorre associare un elevato indice di sospetto a ogni malattia acuta che insorga in un bambino nelle prime 4-6 settimane dopo intervento cardiochirurgico. Nella maggior parte dei casi pediatrici, la sindrome risponde bene al trattamento con acido acetilsalicilico o altri FANS. Talvolta nei casi più gravi si rendono necessari i corticosteroidi e in assenza di trattamento si può assistere a una progressione verso il tamponamento cardiaco. La terapia viene continuata per 1-3 mesi, ma possono osservarsi recidive fino a un anno dopo l'intervento chirurgico, che richiedono la ripresa del trattamento.

440.2 • Pericardite costrittiva

Nella maggior parte dei casi, la costrizione si verifica mesi o anni dopo l'iniziale pericardite, ma a volte può essere un processo acuto e rapidamente progressivo. La pericardite costrittiva nella maggior parte dei casi si verifica in assenza di una patologia immediatamente precedente o di una malattia sistemica.

Le manifestazioni cliniche derivano dalla compromissione del riempimento ventricolare diastolico e della contrattilità miocardica, oltre che dalla conseguente depressione della funzione cardiaca. Epatomegalia e ascite possono essere sproporzionate agli altri segni e sintomi, suggerendo la presenza di un'epatopatia cronica. Gli studi di funzionalità epatica presentano solo lievi anomalie; un accurato esame obiettivo evidenza altri sfumati reperti di costrizione, compresi la distensione delle vene del collo, polso piccolo, precordio in quiete, toni cardiaci parafonici, un debole sfregamento pericardico e un aumento del polso paradosso. I reperti tipici diventano evidenti gradualmente e all'inizio possono passare inosservati. Le manifestazioni più evidenti sono la presenza all'auscultazione di un precoce knock pericardico e il reperto alle radiografie del torace di calcificazioni a carico del pericardio. Si può osservare un'enteropatia protidodisperdente con ipopoproteinemia e linfopenia in associazione a una grave costrizione.

La pericardite costrittiva può essere difficile da distinguere da una miocardiopatia restrittiva (vedi Capitolo 439.3). In entrambe le condizioni si ha una compromissione della funzione miocardica. La patologia miocardica della pericardite costrittiva è di solito reversibile con la pericardiectomia. Talvolta è possibile porre una diagnosi definitiva solo mediante toracotomia esplorativa ed esame diretto del pericardio.

La pericardiectomia radicale con decorticazione del pericardio comprendente un'ampia superficie cardiaca, comprese le vene sistemiche e polmonari, è l'unico trattamento efficace per la pericardite costrittiva. Nella maggior parte dei pazienti l'intervento chirurgico porta a una rapida risposta, caratterizzata da un aumento della gittata cardiaca e da pronta diuresi. La prognosi a lungo termine è di solito eccellente.

Demmler GJ: Infectious pericarditis in children. *Pediatr Infect Dis J* 2006;25: 165–166.

Goldstein JA: Cardiac tamponade, constrictive pericarditis, and restrictive cardiomyopathy. *Curr Probl Cardiol* 2004;29:503–567.

Lange RA, Hillis LD: Clinical practice. Acute pericarditis. *N Engl J Med* 2004;351:2195–2202.

Levy PY, Corey R, Berger P, et al: Etiologic diagnosis of 204 pericardial effusions. *Medicine* 2003;82:385–391.

Rienmuller R, Groll R, Lipton MJ: CT and MR imaging of pericardial disease. *Radiol Clin North Am* 2004;42:587–601.

Sinzobahamvya N, Ikeogu MO: Purulent pericarditis. *Arch Dis Child* 1987;62:696–699.

Troughton RW, Asher CR, Klein AL: Pericarditis. *Lancet* 2004;363:717–727.

Capitolo 441 ■ Tumori del cuore

I tumori primitivi del cuore sono rari nell'infanzia e nella maggior parte dei casi benigni. Le manifestazioni cliniche dipendono principalmente dalla sede del tumore, e in misura minore dal tipo istologico.

I tumori cardiaci benigni più comuni nei bambini sono i **rabdomiomi**, i fibromi e i mixomi. I rabdomiomi sono noduli singoli o, di solito, multipli, situati all'interno delle pareti delle camere cardiache. Spesso non acquisiscono mai un'importanza clinica e regrediscono con l'età, ma possono causare ostruzione meccanica, scompenso cardiaco o aritmie. Possono essere familiari e spesso si trovano in associazione con la sindrome di Gorlin o la sclerosi tuberosa. La maggior parte dei rabdiomiomi si osserva in bambini di età <1 anno. Una tachicardia ventricolare incessante in un bambino di età <2 anni dovrebbe far insorgere il sospetto di un piccolo rabdiomioma endocardico o epicardico o di un tumore a cellule di Purkinje. I fibromi, di solito noduli solitari e non capsulati, sono situati nei ventricoli; possono essere di notevoli dimensioni. Il trattamento dei rabdiomiomi e dei fibromi dipende dalla loro sede e dimensione. Piccoli tumori asintomatici localizzati nella parete miocardica o nel setto ventricolare possono essere tenuti sotto osservazione, per tenere sotto controllo una loro eventuale crescita o regressione. I rabdomiomi associati a **sclerosi tuberosa** spesso si risolvono con la crescita del bambino. Tumori più grandi che danno segno di ostruzione al flusso sanguigno e quelli che causano aritmie ventricolari andrebbero asportati. Tumori voluminosi e diffusi possono interferire con la funzione cardiaca, ma la loro rimozione spesso difficile poiché può rimanere un'insufficiente quantità di miocardio normale. Il trapianto cardiaco talvolta rappresenta l'unica soluzione per pazienti con tumori estesi.

I **mixomi**, che si sviluppano in sede intracavitaria, per lo più nell'atrio sinistro (75%), sono più frequenti nel sesso femminile (75%). Si tratta di masse solide, lisce, peduncolate (1-8 cm), che si attaccano al setto interatriale, protrudono nella camera atriale e, per la loro posizione rispetto alla valvola mitrale o tricuspide, causano un'ostruzione intermittente e un quadro clinico compatibile con stenosi (sincope, scompenso cardiaco, fibrillazione atriale). Bisognerebbe prendere in considerazione la presenza di un mixoma in pazienti con sincopi ricorrenti, un soffio di tipo posizionale (in posizione supina più che eretta), oppure segni di embolizzazione sistemica o polmonare. I mixomi atriali possono anche causare febbre, malessere generale, artralgie ed embolie sistemiche che mimano un'**endocardite**, una febbre reumatica o il lupus eritematoso sistemico. I reperti laboratoristici comprendono un'elevata velocità di eritrosedimentazione, ematuria ed evidenza del tumore all'ecocardiogramma. I mixomi atriali possono essere associati a multiple lesioni cutanee pigmentate (lentigginosi), fibroadenomi mixoidi della mammella, mixomi cutanei, noduli surrenalici pigmentati. Alcuni sono associati a varie lesioni cutanee e del tessuto connettivo, oltre che a tumori testicolari o adenomi ipofisari (sindrome di Carney). Il trattamento consiste nell'escissione chirurgica, che deve comprendere l'intera base del tumore per prevenire una recidiva.

Altri tumori benigni sono i papillomi, attaccati ai lembi valvolari, che possono verificarsi nei neonati, i lipomi, situati nelle pareti ventricolari, e i mesoteliomi, che possono coinvolgere il nodo atrioventricolare e causare anomalie della conduzione elettrica, compreso il blocco cardiaco completo.

I tumori cardiaci maligni primitivi nei bambini sono quasi esclusivamente sarcomi. Questi tumori sono di solito situati nel cuore destro, nel setto atriale, nella parete atriale destra o nella radice dell'arteria polmonare. Possono estendersi nella camera adiacente e causare ostruzione al flusso sanguigno, oppure nella cavità pericardica e produrre un versamento o un tamponamento cardiaco. Il cuore può essere anche coinvolto dalla disseminazione metastatica di una neoplasia non cardiaca, come un leucemia o un linfoma, oppure, nel caso del tumore di Wilms, dall'estensione diretta del tumore nell'atrio destro attraverso la vena cava inferiore. L'esame obiettivo può dare indicazioni sulla sede e sulla dimensione del tumore se questo interferisce con il flusso sanguigno. Il coinvolgimento del sistema di conduzione è valutabile con l'elettrocardiogramma. L'ecocardiogramma bidimensionale è diagnostico, e permette un'eccellente visualizzazione della sede e dell'estensione del tumore. Le indagini Doppler valutano l'entità dell'ostruzione al flusso sanguigno causata dal tumore. Il cateterismo cardiaco può fornire ulteriori informazioni sull'anatomia del tumore e sui suoi effetti emodinamici. Quando indicato, l'intervento chirurgico si prefigge come obiettivi la completa asportazione del tumore, alla rimozione dell'ostruzione e al controllo di qualsiasi aritmia. La prognosi a lungo termine dipende dal tipo di tumore, dalla radicalità dell'intervento chirurgico e dall'integrità postchirurgica delle strutture del cuore normale e del miocardio. Per i tumori che non sono resecabili a causa dell'impossibilità di separarli dal tessuto cardiaco normale, il trapianto di cuore è un trattamento efficace.

Butany J, Nair V, Naseemuddin A, et al: Cardiac tumours: Diagnosis and management. *Lancet* 2005;6:219–228.

Isaacs H Jr: Fetal and neonatal cardiac tumors. *Pediatr Cardiol* 2004;25: 252–273.

Shapiro LM: Cardiac tumours: Diagnosis and management. *Heart* 2001;85: 218–222.

Stratakis CA, Kirschner LS, Carney JA: Clinical and molecular features of the Carney complex: Diagnostic criteria and recommendations for patient evaluation. *J Clin Endocrinol Metab* 2001;86:4041–4046.

Sezione 7 — Terapia cardiaca — Daniel Bernstein

Capitolo 442 ■ Scompenso cardiaco

Lo scompenso cardiaco si manifesta quando il cuore non riesce a fornire un'adeguata gittata cardiaca per far fronte alle necessità metaboliche dell'organismo. Nei primi stadi dello scompenso cardiaco, subentrano vari meccanismi compensatori per mantenere una normale funzione metabolica. Quando però questi meccanismi divengono inefficaci, ne risultano manifestazioni cliniche progressivamente ingravescenti (vedi Capitolo 68).

FISIOPATOLOGIA. Il cuore può essere considerato una sorta di pompa, con una gittata proporzionale al suo volume di riempimento e inversamente proporzionale alla resistenza contro cui pompa. Quando il volume ventricolare telediastolico aumenta, un cuore sano incrementa la gittata cardiaca fino a raggiungere un massimo che non può essere superato (principio di Frank-Starling; Fig. 442-1). L'aumento della gittata sistolica che si ottiene in questo modo è dovuta all'allungamento delle fibre miocardiche, ma anche alla maggiore tensione di parete, che fa aumentare il consumo miocardico di ossigeno. Cuori che lavorano sotto vari tipi di stress funzionano lungo differenti curve di Frank-Starling. Un muscolo cardiaco con una contrattilità intrinseca compromessa richiede un più elevato grado di dilatazione per produrre un aumento della gittata sistolica e non raggiunge la stessa gittata cardiaca massimale di un miocardio normale. Se una camera cardiaca è già dilatata a causa di una lesione che determina un incremento del precarico (per es. uno shunt sinistro-destro o un'insufficienza valvolare), vi è poco spazio per un'ulteriore dilatazione e per l'aumento della gittata cardiaca. La presenza di lesioni che portano a un aumentato postcarico per il ventricolo (stenosi aortica o polmonare, coartazione aortica) diminuisce la performance cardiaca, comportando di conseguenza un depresso rapporto di Frank-Starling. La capacità di un cuore immaturo di

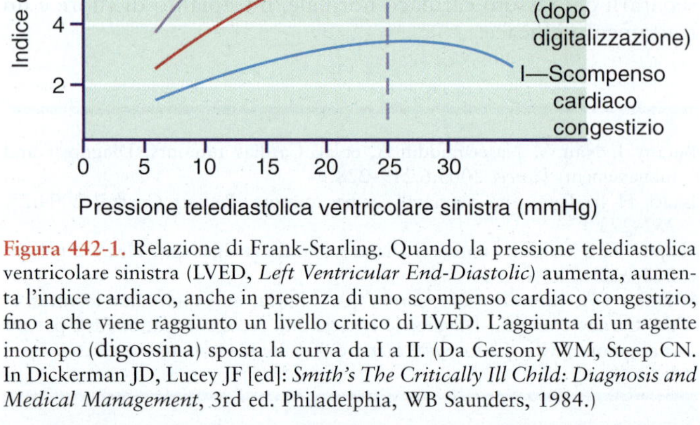

Figura 442-1. Relazione di Frank-Starling. Quando la pressione telediastolica ventricolare sinistra (LVED, *Left Ventricular End-Diastolic*) aumenta, aumenta l'indice cardiaco, anche in presenza di uno scompenso cardiaco congestizio, fino a che viene raggiunto un livello critico di LVED. L'aggiunta di un agente inotropo (digossina) sposta la curva da I a II. (Da Gersony WM, Steep CN. In Dickerman JD, Lucey JF [ed]: *Smith's The Critically Ill Child: Diagnosis and Medical Management*, 3rd ed. Philadelphia, WB Saunders, 1984.)

aumentare la gittata cardiaca in risposta a un maggiore precarico è inferiore a quella di un cuore maturo. I prematuri sono più compromessi da una shunt sinistro-destro rispetto ai neonati a termine.

Il **trasporto sistemico di ossigeno** è il prodotto della gittata cardiaca e del contenuto sistemico di ossigeno, mentre la **gittata cardiaca** è il prodotto della frequenza cardiaca e della gittata sistolica. I principali determinanti della gittata sistolica sono il postcarico (lavoro di pressione), il precarico (lavoro di volume) e la contrattilità (funzione miocardica intrinseca). Anomalie della frequenza cardiaca possono altresì compromettere la gittata cardiaca e causare tanto bradiaritmie quanto tachiaritmie; queste ultime accorciano l'intervallo di tempo diastolico disponibile per il riempimento ventricolare. Condizioni che alterano la capacità di trasporto di ossigeno del sangue (per es. anemia o ipossiemia) portano anch'esse a una diminuzione del trasporto di ossigeno sistemico e, se i meccanismi compensatori sono inadeguati, possono essere responsabili di un minor apporto di substrati ai tessuti.

Anche se in alcuni casi di scompenso cardiaco la gittata cardiaca è normale o aumentata, a causa di un diminuito contenuto di ossigeno sistemico (secondario ad anemia) o di maggiori richieste di ossigeno (secondarie a iperventilazione, ipertiroidismo o ipermetabolismo), la quantità di ossigeno fornita risulta insufficiente a far fronte alle richieste dell'organismo. Questa condizione, scompenso cardiaco ad alta portata, porta allo sviluppo di segni e sintomi di scompenso cardiaco quando non vi è alcuna anomalia di base nella funzione miocardica e la gittata cardiaca è più elevata del normale. Si osserva anche in presenza di ampie fistole arterovenose sistemiche. Queste condizioni riducono la resistenza vascolare periferica e il postcarico cardiaco, oltre ad aumentare la contrattilità miocardica. Lo "scompenso" cardiaco si instaura quando la richiesta di gittata cardiaca è superiore alla capacità del cuore di farvi fronte. Un grave scompenso cardiaco cronico a elevata gittata può infine condurre a una diminuzione della performance miocardica quando le richieste metaboliche del miocardio non sono soddisfatte.

Vari sono i meccanismi compensatori che l'organismo mette in atto per adattarsi allo scompenso cardiaco cronico. Alcuni sono mediati a livello molecolare/cellulare, come l'up- o la downregulation di vari componenti di vie metaboliche che portano a cambiamenti nell'efficienza di utilizzo dell'ossigeno e di altri substrati; altri sono mediati da neuro-ormoni come il sistema renina-angiotensina e l'asse simpatico-adrenergico. Uno dei principali meccanismi per aumentare la gittata cardiaca è un aumento del tono simpatico secondario alla secrezione surrenalica di adrenalina circolante e all'aumentato rilascio nervoso di noradrenalina. Gli iniziali effetti benefici della stimolazione simpatica comprendono un aumento della frequenza cardiaca e della contrattilità miocardica, mediato dall'azione di questi ormoni sui recettori β-adrenergici cardiaci; entrambi questi fattori servono ad aumentare la gittata cardiaca. A causa della vasocostrizione localizzata, mediata dall'azione di questi ormoni sui recettori arteriosi α-adrenergici periferici, il flusso sanguigno può essere ridistribuito al cuore e al cervello dai letti vascolari cutaneo, viscerale e renale. Se in parte questi effetti in acuto sono benefici, una stimolazione simpatica cronicamente elevata può avere conseguenze deleterie: ipermetabolismo, aumento del postcarico, effetti proaritmogeni e un aumento delle richieste di ossigeno da parte del miocardio. La vasocostrizione periferica può portare a una diminuzione della funzionalità renale, epatica e gastrointestinale. L'esposizione cronica alle catecolamine circolanti, oltre a causare una diminuzione del numero di recettori cardiaci β-adrenergici (downregulation o tachifilassi), danneggia direttamente le cellule miocardiche. Perciò gli agenti terapeutici per lo scompenso cardiaco mirano al ripristino dell'equilibrio di questi sistemi neuroendocrini. Singole differenze nucleotidiche (note come polimorfismi) nei geni che codificano per proteine coinvolte nella trasmissione del segnale simpatico possono alterare la risposta dei pazienti alla terapia medica e predire il rischio di progressione dello scompenso cardiaco, ospedalizzazione o morte. Questi studi farmacologici potranno presto permetterci di scegliere terapie individualizzate per ogni paziente, basandosi sulle caratteristiche genetiche individuali.

MANIFESTAZIONI CLINICHE. Le manifestazioni cliniche di scompenso cardiaco dipendono dal grado della riserva cardiaca del paziente in età pediatrica. Un bambino in condizioni critiche o che ha esaurito i meccanismi compensatori, giungendo al punto in cui la gittata cardiaca non è più sufficiente a far fronte alle necessità metaboliche basali dell'organismo, sarà sintomatico a riposo. Altri pazienti possono essere asintomatici a riposo ma incapaci di aumentare la gittata cardiaca in risposta a un'attività anche lieve senza lamentare sintomi significativi. D'altro canto, può essere necessario un esercizio fisico anche intenso per compromettere la funzione cardiaca in bambini che hanno una cardiopatia meno grave. La raccolta di un'anamnesi accurata è estremamente importante per fare diagnosi di scompenso cardiaco e per valutarne le possibili cause. I genitori che osservano il bambino tutti i giorni possono non riconoscere quei cambiamenti appena percettibili che si verificano nel giro di giorni o settimane. Un graduale peggioramento della perfusione o una cianosi ingravescente potrebbero non venire riconosciuti come reperti anomali. L'edema può essere scambiato per un normale aumento di peso e l'intolleranza all'esercizio fisico per mancanza di interesse verso una determinata attività. L'anamnesi di un bambino piccolo dovrebbe riguardare anche l'alimentazione (vedi Capitolo 422). Un bambino con scompenso cardiaco spesso assume un volume minore di latte a ogni poppata, diviene dispnoico durante la suzione e può sudare profusamente. Ricavare un'anamnesi di astemia in un bambino più grande richiede domande dettagliate sul grado di attività e sul suo decorso nell'arco di parecchi mesi.

Nei pazienti pediatrici i segni e i sintomi di scompenso cardiaco, consistenti in astenia, intolleranza allo sforzo fisico, anoressia, dolore addominale, dispnea e tosse, possono essere simili a quelli degli adulti. Molti bambini, tuttavia, specialmente gli adolescenti, possono lamentare principalmente sintomi addominali a fronte di una sorprendente mancanza di sintomi respiratori. Un problema al sistema cardiovascolare può giungere all'attenzione del medico solo dopo che una radiografia dell'addome ha inaspettatamente evidenziato un ingrandimento della porzione inferiore del cuore. Ortopnea e rantoli alle basi sono incostantemente presenti; l'edema è di solito evidenziabile nelle zone declivi del corpo, o può essere presente anasarca. Si riscontra invariabilmente una cardiomegalia. Un ritmo di galoppo è comune; quando la dilatazione ventricolare è avanzata, può udirsi il soffio olosistolico da rigurgito valvolare mitralico o tricuspidalico.

Nei lattanti lo scompenso cardiaco può essere difficile da identificare. Le manifestazioni evidenti comprendono tachipnea, difficoltà nell'allattamento, scarso aumento di peso, eccessiva sudorazione, irritabilità, pianto flebile e respirazione rumorosa e affaticata, con retrazione degli spazi intercostali e sottocostali, oltre ad alitamento delle pinne nasali. I segni di congestione polmonare indotta da un problema cardiaco possono essere indistinguibili da quelli di una bronchiolite; il respiro sibilante è ben udibile. È comune una polmonite con o senza atelettasia, specialmente nei lobi medio e inferiore di destra, dovuta alla compressione dei bronchi da parte del cuore ingrandito. Di solito si riscontra epatomegalia ed è invariabilmente presente una cardiomegalia. Nonostante una notevole tachicardia, spesso è apprezzabile un ritmo di galoppo. Gli altri segni auscultatori sono quelli prodotti dalla lesione cardiaca sottostante. La valutazione clinica della pressione venosa giugulare nei lattanti può essere difficile a causa del collo corto e della difficoltà di osservarli in uno stato di completa rilassamento. L'edema può essere generalizzato; coinvolge di solito le palpebre come anche il sacro, meno spesso le gambe e i piedi. La diagnosi differenziale è età-dipendente (Tab. 442-1).

DIAGNOSI. Le radiografie del torace evidenziano un ingrandimento cardiaco. La vascolarizzazione polmonare è variabile a seconda della causa dello scompenso cardiaco. I lattanti e i bambini con ampi shunt sinistro-destro presentano un'accentuazione del disegno dei vasi arteriosi polmonari alla periferia dei campi polmonari, mentre i pazienti con miocardiopatia possono avere un letto vascolare polmonare relativamente normale nelle prime fasi della malattia. Una disegno vascolare sfumato peri-ilare suggestivo di congestione venosa ed edema polmonare acuto si osserva solo nei casi più gravi di scompenso cardiaco. L'ingrandimento cardiaco si nota spesso come reperto inaspettato a una radiografia del torace effettuata per valutare una possibile infezione polmonare, una bronchiolite o un'asma.

Un'ipertrofia cardiaca evidenziata dall'elettrocardiogramma può essere utile per determinare la causa di scompenso cardiaco, ma non permette di formulare la diagnosi. Nelle miocardiopatie, cambiamenti ischemici ventricolari sinistri o destri possono correlare bene con parametri clinici e non invasivi di funzione ventricolare. Caratteristiche morfologiche di un QRS di voltaggio ridotto con anomalie del tratto ST e dell'onda T possono altresì suggerire una patologia infiammatoria del miocardio, nonostante siano talora riscontrabili anche in caso di pericardite. L'elettrocardiogramma è lo strumento migliore per la valutazione dei disordini del ritmo come potenziali cause di scompenso cardiaco.

TABELLA 442-1. Eziologia dello scompenso cardiaco
NEL FETO
Grave anemia (emolisi, trasfusione materno-fetale, anemia indotta da parvovirus B19, anemia ipoplasica)
Tachicardia sopraventricolare
Blocco cardiaco completo
Grave anomalia di Ebstein o altre gravi lesioni del cuore destro
Miocardite
NEL PREMATURO
Sovraccarico di liquidi
Dotto arterioso pervio
Difetto settale ventricolare
Cor polmonare (displasia broncopolmonare)
Ipertensione
Miocardite
Miocardiopatia su base genetica
NEL NEONATO A TERMINE
Miocardiopatia asfittica
Malformazione arterovenosa (vena di Galeno, epatica)
Lesioni ostruttive del cuore sinistro (coartazione aortica, sindrome del cuore sinistro ipoplasico)
Ampi difetti cardiaci con mescolamento (ventricolo unico, tronco arterioso comune)
Miocardite
Miocardiopatia su base genetica
NEL LATTANTE
Shunt cardiaco sinistro-destro (difetto settale ventricolare)
Emangioma (malformazione arterovenosa)
Arteria coronaria sinistra anomala
Miocardiopatia su base genetica o metabolica
Ipertensione acuta (sindrome emolitico-uremica)
Tachicardia sopraventricolare
Malattia di Kawasaki
Miocardite
NEL BAMBINO-ADOLESCENTE
Febbre reumatica
Ipertensione acuta (glomerulonefrite)
Miocardite
Tireotossicosi
Emocromatosi-emosiderosi
Terapia antineoplastica (radiazioni, doxorubicina)
Anemia a cellule falciformi
Endocardite
Cor polmonare (fibrosi cistica)
Miocardiopatia genetica o metabolica (ipertrofica, dilatativa)

Le tecniche **ecocardiografiche** sono di particolare utilità nella valutazione della funzione ventricolare. Il parametro più comunemente usato nei bambini è la frazione di accorciamento (un'unica dimensione variabile), determinato come la differenza tra i diametri telesistolico e telediastolico divisa per il diametro telediastolico. Una frazione di accorciamento normale è compresa tra il 28 e il 40%. Negli adulti, il parametro più comunemente utilizzato è la frazione di eiezione (che calcola un volume tridimensionale a partire da dati bidimensionali), di norma compresa tra il 55 e il 65%. Nei bambini con ingrandimento ventricolare destro o altre patologie cardiache che portano all'appiattimento del setto interventricolare, ci si avvale della frazione di eiezione, dal momento che la frazione di accorciamento non è accurata. Le indagini Doppler sono in grado di stimare la gittata cardiaca. L'angiorisonanza magnetica (MRA, *Magnetic Resonance Angiography*) può essere utile per quantificare sia la massa sia la funzione ventricolare sinistra e destra. Se è presente un rigurgito valvolare, la MRA può quantificare la frazione rigurgitante.

I livelli arteriosi di ossigeno talvolta vanno incontro a diminuzione quando si verificano discrepanze ventiloperfusorie secondarie a edema polmonare. Se lo scompenso cardiaco è grave, possono essere presenti un'acidosi respiratoria o metabolica, o entrambe. I lattanti con scompenso cardiaco spesso presentano iponatremia come conseguenza della ritenzione renale di sodio. Un trattamento cronico con diuretici può diminuire ulteriormente i livelli sierici di sodio. I livelli sierici di **peptide natriuretico tipo B** (**BNP**, *B Natriuretic Peptide*), un neurormone cardiaco rilasciato in risposta all'aumentata tensione parietale ventricolare, sono elevati nei pazienti adulti con scompenso cardiaco congestizio. In età pediatrica, il BNP può essere elevato in pazienti con scompenso cardiaco dovuto a disfunzione sistolica (miocardiopatia) oltre che in quelli con sovraccarico di volume (shunt sinistro-destro come un difetto del setto interventricolare).

TRATTAMENTO. La condizione che sta alla base dello scompenso cardiaco va eliminata o alleviata, se possibile. Se la causa è un'anomalia cardiaca congenita aggredibile chirurgicamente, il trattamento medico è indicato in preparazione all'intervento chirurgico e nel primo periodo postoperatorio, mentre il cuore si sta riprendendo dagli effetti del bypass cardiopolmonare. Grazie agli eccellenti risultati ottenuti con la riparazione chirurgica primaria dei difetti cardiaci congeniti, anche nel periodo neonatale, pochi bambini richiedono un trattamento aggressivo dello scompenso cardiaco per raggiungere un'età più opportuna per l'intervento chirurgico. D'altro canto, se la causa dello scompenso cardiaco è una miocardiopatia, il trattamento medico fornisce un sollievo temporaneo dai sintomi e può favorire la guarigione se l'insulto è reversibile (miocardite). Se invece la lesione non è reversibile, il trattamento dello scompenso cardiaco di solito permette al bambino di tornare alle normali attività per un certo periodo e al medico di posticipare, a volte di anni, la valutazione per un eventuale trapianto di cuore.

Misure generali. Anche se un tassativo riposo a letto si rende necessario solo in rari casi, è comunque importante che il bambino si riposi durante il giorno ogniqualvolta ne avverta la necessità e dorma adeguatamente di notte. Alcuni pazienti più grandi dormono meglio in posizione semiseduta, utilizzando più cuscini (ortopnea). Per i lattanti con scompenso cardiaco, può essere consigliabile un seggiolone. Una volta che i pazienti hanno iniziato a rispondere al trattamento, la restrizione alle attività fisiche spesso può essere modificata nel contesto della diagnosi specifica e della capacità del paziente. Gli sport agonistici e intensi sono di solito controindicati. Un test da sforzo cardiopolmonare formale può essere utilizzato per valutare la capacità del paziente di sostenere sforzi in un ambiente controllato ed è utile per prescrivere una limitazione dell'esercizio fisico su basi razionali. In presenza di edema polmonare, può essere necessaria una ventilazione a pressione positiva, in associazione con la terapia farmacologica. Nei pazienti con scompenso cardiaco a bassa gittata, la ventilazione a pressione positiva può ridurre significativamente il consumo totale di ossigeno dell'organismo, eliminando il lavoro respiratorio, e aiutare a risolvere un'acidosi metabolica. Gli agonisti β-adrenergici come la dopamina, l'adrenalina e la dobutamina, di solito vengono utilizzati in combinazione con inibitori della fosfodiesterasi come il milrinone. Se la pressione sanguigna lo permette, i farmaci che riducono il postcarico (nitroprussiato, inibitori dell'enzima di conversione dell'angiotensina [ACE, *Angiotensin-Converting Enzyme*]) possono apportare un beneficio. La somministrazione di questi farmaci inizia di solito in terapia intensiva, con un appropriato monitoraggio invasivo della pressione venosa centrale e della pressione arteriosa.

Dieta. I lattanti con scompenso cardiaco possono presentare una crescita stentata a causa delle maggiori richieste metaboliche e del minor apporto calorico. Aumentare le calorie giornaliere è un aspetto importante del trattamento. Aumentare il numero di calorie per 30 grammi di latte in polvere (o utilizzare supplementi al latte materno) può apportare beneficio. Molti lattanti non tollerano un aumento superiore a 24 calorie/30 grammi a causa della diarrea, o poiché queste formule forniscono un carico di soluti eccessivo per reni già compromessi.

Lattanti in gravi condizioni possono non avere la forza di effettuare una suzione efficace a causa di estrema astenia, tachipnea e debolezza generalizzata. In queste circostanze, può essere utile l'alimentazione tramite sondino nasogastrico. In molti bambini con ingrandimento cardiaco il reflusso gastroesofageo è un problema importante. L'utilizzo di una nutrizione continua mediante sondino nasogastrico durante la notte, somministrata in pompa, può migliorare l'apporto calorico e nel contempo diminuire i problemi associati al reflusso. A volte, soprattutto nei bambini con scompenso cardiaco dovuto a una cardiopatia congenita complessa, è necessario un intervento medico o chirurgico per correggere il reflusso (fundoplicatio di Nissen). Una malnutrizione prolungata può essere un fattore importante che influisce nella decisione di anticipare l'intervento chirurgico in pazienti con cardiopatie congenite operabili o di mettere in lista per il trapianto i pazienti con miocardiopatia.

L'utilizzo di formule iposodiche nel trattamento di routine di bambini con scompenso cardiaco non è raccomandato, poiché queste preparazioni sono spesso scarsamente tollerate e possono peggiorare un'iponatriemia indotta da diuretici. Il latte materno è la sorgente nutritiva iposodica ideale. L'utilizzo di diuretici più potenti permette di utilizzare formule nutrizionali più appetibili controllando nel contempo il bilancio di sodio e di acqua con la somministrazione cronica di questi farmaci. Nella maggior parte dei casi è possibile trattare i bambini più grandi con diete "prive di sodio" e con l'astinenza da cibi che ne contengano grandi quantità. È raro che si renda necessaria una dieta severamente iposodica.

Digitale. La digossina, che una volta rappresentava il cardine della terapia dello scompenso cardiaco sia nei bambini sia negli adulti, è attualmente meno utilizzata, come conseguenza dell'introduzione di terapie più nuove e della scoperta della sua potenziale tossicità. Molti cardiologi somministrano la digitale in aggiunta agli ACE-inibitori e ai diuretici in pazienti con scompenso cardiaco sintomatico, mentre altri non la usano più. Nonostante numerosi studi clinici, condotti prevalentemente sugli adulti, l'utilità della digitale rimane un argomento controverso.

La digossina è il glicoside digitalico di più comune impiego nei pazienti pediatrici. La sua emivita è di 36 ore, abbastanza lunga da permetterne la somministrazione una o due volte al giorno, e abbastanza corta da contenere gli effetti tossici da sovradosaggio. È ben assorbita dal tratto gastrointestinale (60-85%) anche nei lattanti. L'assorbimento è maggiore con lo sciroppo che con le compresse. Un primo effetto si può osservare già a distanza di 30 minuti dalla somministrazione, e il picco si ottiene circa 2-6 ore dopo la sua assunzione per os. Quando invece il farmaco viene somministrato per via endovenosa, un primo effetto si osserva dopo 15-30 minuti, e il picco a 1-4 ore. Il farmaco attraversa la placenta ed è quindi possibile trattare un feto con scompenso cardiaco (secondario ad aritmia) mediante somministrazione di digossina alla madre. Poiché viene eliminata dai reni, il dosaggio deve essere aggiustato a seconda della funzionalità renale del paziente. Il tasso di escrezione è proporzionale alla velocità di filtrazione glomerulare. Dopo somministrazione endovenosa, il 50-70% viene escreto nelle urine senza subire modifiche. L'emivita della digossina può durare fino a 6 giorni nei pazienti anurici, nei quali vengono utilizzate vie di escrezione epatica più lente.

La digitalizzazione rapida nei lattanti e nei bambini con scompenso cardiaco può essere effettuata per via endovenosa. La dose dipende dall'età del paziente (Tab. 442-2). Lo schema di digitalizzazione raccomandato consiste nel somministrare metà della dose totale immediatamente, seguita da due dosi da un quarto a intervalli di 12 ore. Occorre monitorare strettamente l'elettrocardiogramma e ottenere tracciati elettrocardiografici prima di ciascuna delle tre dosi di digitale. Si raccomanda di sospendere la digossina se si nota l'insorgenza di un nuovo disturbo del ritmo. Un prolungamento dell'intervallo P-R non è necessariamente un'indicazione alla sospensione della digitale, ma bisognerebbe prendere in considerazione la possibilità di ritardare la somministrazione della dose seguente o di ridurre il dosaggio, a seconda delle condizioni cliniche del paziente. La determinazione dei livelli sierici di digossina è utile quando si sospetta una tossicità da digitale, anche se può essere meno attendibile nei lattanti. Con la somministrazione di digitale si riscontrano comunemente cambiamenti del tratto ST o dell'onda T, che non dovrebbero quindi influire sul regime di digitalizzazione. Si raccomanda di misurare i livelli di base degli elettroliti sierici prima e dopo la digitalizzazione. Un'ipokaliemia e un'ipercalcemia esacerbano la tossicità da digitale. Poiché l'ipokaliemia è relativamente comune in concomitanza con un trattamento diuretico, i livelli di potassio dovrebbero essere strettamente monitorati nei pazienti che assumono diuretici potassio-disperdenti (per es. furosemide) insieme con la digitale. Nei pazienti con miocardite attiva, alcuni cardiologi raccomandano di evitare del tutto la digitalizzazione e di iniziare la digitale di mantenimento a metà del dosaggio normale, a causa dell'aumentato rischio di aritmie.

TABELLA 442-2. Dosaggio dei farmaci comunemente utilizzati per il trattamento dello scompenso cardiaco congestizio

FARMACO	DOSAGGIO
	DIGOSSINA
Digitalizzazione (1/2 inizialmente, seguita da 1/4 ogni 12 h per 2 volte)	Prematuro: 20 μg/kg Neonato a termine (fino a 1 mese): 20-30 μg/kg Lattante o bambino: 25-40 μg/kg Adolescente o adulto: 0,5-1 mg in dosi suddivise N.B.: queste dosi sono per os; la dose ev è il 75% della dose per os
Digossina – mantenimento	5-10 μg/kg/die, suddivisi ogni 12 ore Livelli sierici terapeutici: 1-5-3,0 ng/mL se età <6 mesi; 1-2 ng/mL se età >6 mesi N.B.: queste dosi sono per os; la dose ev è il 75% della dose per os
	DIURETICI
Furosemide	ev: 1-2 mg/dose quando necessario per os: 1,4 mg/kg/giorno, divisi ogni giorno 3 volte al giorno
Bumetanide	ev: 0,01-0,1 mg/kg/dose per os: 0,005-0,1 mg/kg/die suddivisi ogni 6-8 h
Clorotiazide	per os: 20-40 mg/kg/die suddivisi in 2 o 3 somministrazioni al giorno
Spironolattone	per os: 20-40 mg/kg/die suddivisi di 2 o 3 somministrazioni al giorno
Nesiritide (peptide netriuretico tipo B)	ev: 0,001-0,03 μg/kg/min
	AGONISTI ADRENERGICI (TUTTI EV)
Dobutamina	2-20 μg/kg/min
Dopamina	2-30 μg/kg/min
Isoproterenolo	0,01-0,5 μg/kg/min
Adrenalina	0,1-1,0 μg/kg/min
Noradrenalina	0,1-2,0 μg/kg/min
	INIBITORI DELLA FOSFODIESTERASI (TUTTI EV)
Amrinone	3-10 μg/kg/min
Milrinone	0,25-1,0 μg/kg/min
	AGENTI CHE RIDUCONO IL POSTCARICO
Captopril, solo per os	Prematuri: iniziare a 0,01 mg/kg/dose Lattanti: 0,1-0,5 mg/kg/dose ogni 8-12 h (massimo 4 mg/kg/die) Bambini: 0,1-2 mg/kg/die ogni 8-12 ore (dose nell'adulto: 6-25-25 mg/dose)
Enalapril, solo per os	0,08-0,5 mg/kg/dose ogni 12-24 h (massimo 0,5/mg/kg/die)
Idralazina	ev: 0,1-0,5 mg/kg/dose (massimo 20 mg) per os: 0,25-1,0 mg/kg/dose ogni 6-8 ore (massimo 200 mg/die)
Nitroglicerina	ev: 0,25-5 μg/kg/min
Nitroprussiato	ev: 0,5-8 μg/kg/min
Prazosin	per os: 0,005-0,025 mg/kg/die ogni 6-8 h (massimo 0,1 mg/kg/dose)
	BLOCCANTI β-ADRENERGICI
Carvedilolo	per os: dose iniziale 0,1 mg/kg/die (massimo 6,5 mg) divisi in 2 volte al giorno; aumentare gradualmente (di solito a intervalli di 2 settimane) fino a un massimo di 0,5-1 mg/kg/die nel giro di 8-12 settimane, in base alla tolleranza del paziente; dose massima nell'adulto 50-100 mg/die
Metoprololo	per os, forma a rilascio non prolungato: 0,2 mg/kg/die divisa in 2 volte al giorno; aumentare gradualmente (di solito a intervalli di 2 settimane) fino alla dose massima di 1-2 mg/kg/die per os, forma a rilascio prolungato, viene somministrata una volta al giorno; dose iniziale nell'adulto 25 mg/die, dose massima 200 mg/die

N.B.: le dosi pediatriche basate sul peso corporeo non dovrebbero essere superiori a quelle nell'adulto. Poiché le indicazioni possono cambiare, queste dosi dovrebbero essere sempre ricontrollate. Possono inoltre rendersi necessari aggiustamenti in pazienti con disfunzione renale o epatica.

La terapia digitalica di mantenimento inizia circa 12 ore dopo una digitalizzazione piena. Il dosaggio quotidiano viene diviso in due e somministrato a intervalli di 12 ore per ottenere livelli nel sangue più costanti e maggiore flessibilità in caso di tossicità. Il dosaggio ammonta a un quarto della dose totale utilizzata per la digitalizzazione. I pazienti a cui la viene inizialmente somministrata per via endovenosa possono assumere la digossina di mantenimento per via orale non appena sono in grado di tollerare l'alimentazione per os. Poiché l'assorbimento attraverso il tratto gastrointestinale è meno sicuro, la dose di mantenimento per via orale è di solito del 20-25% più elevata rispetto a quella consigliata per la somministrazione parenterale (vedi Tab. 442-2). La dose quotidiana normale di digossina per i bambini più grandi (età >5 anni), calcolata per peso corporeo, non dovrebbe superare gli 0,2-0,5 mg/24 h, ossia la normale dose per adulti.

Ai pazienti non critici è possibile somministrare la digitale per via orale fin dall'inizio; nella maggior parte dei casi la digitalizzazione viene completata nel giro 24 ore. Quando è preferibile una digitalizzazione lenta, per esempio nell'immediato periodo postoperatorio, iniziare uno schema di mantenimento senza effettuare un precedente carico fa sì che si ottenga una completa digitalizzazione in 7-10 giorni. Spesso lo schema può essere completato in sede ambulatoriale.

Misurare i **livelli sierici di digossina** è utile in varie circostanze: (1) quando ne è stata somministrata o ingerita accidentalmente una quantità non nota; (2) se la funzionalità renale è compromessa o se sono possibili interazioni farmacologiche; (3) quando sorgono dubbi sulla compliance; (4) quando si sospetta una reazione da tossicità. Il prelievo di sangue viene effettuato immediatamente prima di una dose, ma a un minimo di 4 ore di distanza dall'ultima dose, per essere sicuri che si sia già instaurato un equilibrio tessuti-plasma. Un appropriato livello ematico è di circa 2-4 ng/mL nei lattanti e 1-2 ng/mL nei bambini più grandi. Livelli più elevati non sono generalmente più utili nel trattamento dello scompenso cardiaco, ma aumentano solo il rischio di tossicità. In caso di sospetto, elevati livelli sierici di digossina non sono di per sé diagnostici di tossicità ma devono essere interpretati insieme con altri reperti clinici ed elettrocardiografici (disturbi del ritmo e della conduzione). Nausea e vomito sono meno frequenti nei pazienti pediatrici. Ipokaliemia, ipomagnesiemia, ipercalcemia, un'infiammazione cardiaca secondaria a miocardite e la prematurità possono potenziare la tossicità da digitale. Un'aritmia cardiaca che si sviluppa in un bambino che in terapia digitalica può essere correlata alla patologia cardiaca di base più che al farmaco. Qualsiasi tipo di aritmia che si verifichi dopo l'istituzione della terapia digitalica deve essere imputata al farmaco fino a prova contraria. È necessario sospendere le dosi successive fino alla risoluzione del problema.

Diuretici. Questi farmaci interferiscono con il riassorbimento di acqua e sodio da parte dei reni, il che porta a una riduzione del volume di sangue circolante e perciò riduce il sovraccarico di fluidi nei polmoni e la pressione di riempimento ventricolare. I diuretici sono nella maggior parte dei casi utilizzati in associazione con la terapia digitalica in pazienti con grave scompenso cardiaco congestizio.

La **furosemide**, il diuretico più utilizzato in pazienti con scompenso cardiaco, inibisce il riassorbimento di sodio e cloro nei tubuli distali e nell'ansa di Henle. Ai pazienti che necessitano di una diuresi immediata andrebbe somministrata per via endovenosa o intramuscolare al dosaggio iniziale di 1-2 mg/kg, che di solito porta a una rapida diuresi e a un rapido miglioramento della condizione clinica, in particolare se sono presenti sintomi di congestione polmonare. Viene poi prescritta una terapia cronica a base di furosemide al dosaggio di 1-4 mg/kg/24 h, somministrati da 1 a 4 volte al giorno. In caso di trattamento a lungo termine con questo farmaco, bisogna effettuare un accurato monitoraggio degli elettroliti, perché sussiste la possibilità di una significativa perdita di potassio. È di solito necessaria una supplementazione di cloruro di potassio, a meno che non venga somministrato contemporaneamente spironolattone, un diuretico risparmiatore di potassio. Quando la furosemide viene somministrata a giorni alterni, la supplementazione dietetica di potassio può essere adeguata per mantenere nella norma i livelli sierici di potassio. La somministrazione cronica di furosemide può causare contrazione del compartimento dei fluidi extracellulari e portare a un'"alcalosi da contrazione" (vedi Capitolo 52.7). Un'iponatremia indotta da diuretici può diventare difficile da gestire in pazienti con grave scompenso cardiaco.

Lo **spironolattone** è un inibitore dell'aldosterone e aumenta la ritenzione di potassio, spesso eliminando la necessità di una supplementazione di potassio per via orale, che a volte è poco tollerata. Questo farmaco viene di solito somministrato per via orale in due o tre dosi suddivise di 2-3 mg/kg/24 h. Per praticità, si utilizzano comunemente combinazioni di spironolattone e clorotiazide. Negli adulti con scompenso cardiaco si osserva un miglioramento della sopravvivenza quando il regime terapeutico comprende un inibitore dell'aldosterone.

Talvolta nei bambini con scompenso cardiaco cronico meno grave si utilizza come diuretico la **clorotiazide**. Dotata di un'azione meno immediata e meno potente della furosemide, agisce sul riassorbimento degli elettroliti solo nei tubuli renali. La dose standard è 20-40 mg/kg/24 h suddivisa in due dosi. È spesso richiesta una supplementazione di potassio se questo farmaco viene utilizzato da solo.

Farmaci che riducono il postcarico e ACE-inibitori. I farmaci appartenenti a questo gruppo riducono il postcarico ventricolare diminuendo la resistenza vascolare periferica e perciò migliorando la performance miocardica. Alcuni di essi diminuiscono anche il tono venoso sistemico, con il risultato di ridurre significativamente il precarico. I farmaci che riducono il postcarico sono utili soprattutto nei bambini con scompenso cardiaco secondario a miocardiopatia e nei pazienti con insufficienza mitralica o aortica gravi, ma possono rivelarsi efficaci anche in pazienti con scompenso cardiaco causato da shunt sinistro-destro. Non sono in genere utilizzati in presenza di lesioni stenotiche del tratto di efflusso ventricolare sinistro. Gli ACE-inibitori possono avere altri effetti benefici sul rimodellamento cardiaco, che sono indipendenti dalla loro azione sul postcarico. Negli adulti con miocardiopatia dilatativa, l'aggiunta di un ACE-inibitore al trattamento medico standard riduce sia la morbilità sia la mortalità. I farmaci che riducono il postcarico e gli ACE-inibitori nella maggior parte dei casi vengono impiegati in associazione con altri farmaci per lo scompenso come la digossina e i diuretici.

I farmaci somministrati per via endovenosa, come il nitroprussiato, dovrebbero essere utilizzati solo in unità di terapia intensiva e per il minor tempo possibile. La breve emivita del nitroprussiato ev lo rende ideale per gli aggiustamenti della dose in pazienti critici. Gli effetti principali sono la vasodilatazione arteriosa periferica e la riduzione del postcarico, ma può essere utile anche la venodilatazione che provoca una diminuzione del ritorno venoso al cuore. La pressione sanguigna deve essere costantemente monitorata poiché può verificarsi un'improvvisa ipotensione. Il nitroprussiato è controindicato in pazienti con ipotensione preesistente. Durante il metabolismo del farmaco si producono piccole quantità di cianato circolante, poi detossificato nel fegato a tiocianato, il quale viene escreto con l'urina. Quando vengono somministrate dosi elevate di nitroprussiato per parecchi giorni, possono insorgere sintomi correlati a un avvelenamento da tiocianato (astenia, nausea, disorientamento, acidosi e spasmi muscolari). In caso di uso prolungato del nitroprussiato, si dovrebbero monitorare i livelli di tiocianato; valori >10 g/dL sono coerenti con la presenza di sintomi da tossicità. Anche gli inibitori della fosfodiesterasi (vedi oltre) sono eccellenti per la riduzione del postcarico.

Il captopril, un ACE-inibitore attivo per via orale, determina una dilatazione arteriosa bloccando la produzione di angiotensina II, portando così a una significativa riduzione del postcarico. Sono stati riportati anche una venodilatazione e una conseguente riduzione del precarico. Inoltre, questo farmaco interferisce con la produzione di aldosterone aiutando a controllare la ritenzione di sale e di acqua. Gli ACE-inibitori hanno ulteriori effetti benefici sulla struttura e sulla funzione cardiaca che possono essere indipendenti dal loro effetto sul postcarico. La dose orale è 0,3-6 mg/kg/24 h, suddivisa in due o tre dosi. Reazioni avverse al captopril consistono nell'ipotensione e nelle sue sequele (sincopi, debolezza, capogiri, iperkaliemia). Anche se nel 5-8% dei pazienti si manifesta un rash maculopapuloso, quest'ultimo scompare spontaneamente con il tempo ed è quindi possibile proseguire l'assunzione del farmaco. Possono verificarsi anche neutropenia, tossicità renale e tosse cronica. L'enalapril è un ACE-inibitore ad azione più prolungata, che viene assunto una o due volte al giorno. Di recente sono stati introdotti nei protocolli di trattamento per adulti con scompenso cardiaco farmaci che bloccano il recettore per l'angiotensina II; tuttavia i dati riguardanti il loro utilizzo nei bambini con scompenso cardiaco sono limitati.

Agonisti α e β-adrenergici. Questi farmaci di solito vengono somministrati nei reparti di terapia intensiva, dove la dose può essere accuratamente aggiustata in base alla risposta emodinamica. Si tengono sotto monitoraggio continuo la pressione arteriosa e la frequenza cardiaca; la misurazione della gittata cardiaca al letto del paziente con il metodo della termodiluizione polmonare con catetere (Swan-Ganz) può anch'essa essere utile per valutare l'efficacia del farmaco. Sebbene gli agonisti adrenergici siano estremamente efficaci nei reparti di terapia intensiva, vi sono prove che la loro somministrazione a lungo termine possa in certi casi aumentare la mordilità e la mortalità in pazienti con scompenso cardiaco.

La **dopamina** è prevalentemente un agonista dei recettori β-adrenergici, ma ha effetti α-adrenergici a dosi elevate. Oltre ad avere meno effetti cronotropi e proaritmogeni dell'isoproterenolo, un agonista puro β-adregenergico, porta a una vasodilatazione renale selettiva a causa della sua interazione con i recettori dopaminergici renali, il che è particolarmente utile in pazienti con compromissione della funzione renale, peraltro spesso associata a bassa gittata cardiaca. A una dose di 2-10 μg/kg/min, la dopamina aumenta la contrattilità con pochi effetti di vasocostrizione periferica. Se la dose viene aumentata oltre i 15 μg/kg/min, i suoi effetti α-adrenergici possono indurre vasocostrizione. Il fenoldopam, un agonista recettoriale dopaminergico DA1, è utilizzato a un basso dosaggio (0,03 μg/kg/min) per aumentare il flusso sanguigno renale e il flusso urinario. Dal momento che può causare ipotensione, si raccomanda di monitorare accuratamente la pressione arteriosa.

La **dobutamina**, un derivato della dopamina, è utile nel trattamento della bassa gittata cardiaca. Causa effetti isotropi diretti con una moderata riduzione della resistenza vascolare periferica. Può essere utilizzata in associazione alla terapia con dopamina per evitare gli effetti vasocostrittori che quest'ultimo farmaco ha a dosaggio elevato. Rispetto all'isoproterenolo, la dobutamina ha minori probabilità di causare disturbi del ritmo. La dose standard è 2-20 μg/kg/min.

L'**isoproterenolo** è un agonista β-adrenergico puro, dal marcato effetto cronotropo; efficace soprattutto in pazienti con basse frequenze cardiache, dovrebbe essere utilizzato con cautela in presenza di una significativa tachicardia. I bambini sottoposti a terapia con questo farmaco dovrebbero essere accuratamente monitorati per la possibile insorgenza di aritmie.

L'**adrenalina** è un agonista recettoriale misto α- e β-adrenergico, di solito riservato a pazienti con shock cardiogeno e bassa pressione arteriosa. Anche se può aumentare significativamente la pressione sanguigna, aumenta anche la resistenza vascolare sistemica e, di conseguenza, il post-carico contro cui il cuore deve lavorare.

Inibitori della fosfodiesterasi. Il **milrinone** è utile nel trattamento di pazienti con bassa gittata cardiaca che sono refrattari alla terapia standard e si è dimostrato altamente efficace nel trattamento degli stati di bassa gittata nei bambini sottoposti a intervento cardiochirurgico a cuore aperto. Agisce inibendo la fosfodiesterasi, che impedisce la degradazione del cAMP intracellulare. Il milrinone ha sia effetti inotropi positivi sul cuore sia significativi effetti vasodilatatori periferici, ed è stato in genere utilizzato in associazione a dopamina o dobutamina nei reparti di terapia intensiva. Viene somministrato per infusione endovenosa continua a 0,25-1 μg/kg/min, a volte con una dose da carico iniziale di 50 μg/kg. Un importante effetto collaterale è l'ipotensione secondaria a vasodilatazione periferica, specialmente quando viene somministrata una dose da carico. L'ipotensione può generalmente essere trattata con la somministrazione di fluidi per via endovenosa al fine di ripristinare un adeguato volume intravascolare. L'amrinone, un altro inibitore della fosfodiesterasi, può causare trombocitopenia, la cui gravità sembra essere correlata sia alla velocità di infusione sia alla durata della terapia. Tale effetto è reversibile alla sospensione del farmaco.

Trattamento cronico con β-bloccanti. Studi su adulti con miocardiopatia dilatativa evidenziano come i farmaci β-bloccanti, introdotti gradualmente nell'ambito di un trattamento globale per lo scompenso cardiaco, migliorino la tolleranza allo sforzo, diminuiscano i ricoveri ospedalieri e riducano la mortalità globale. I farmaci più utilizzati sono il metoprololo, un antagonista recettoriale selettivo β_1-adrenergico, e il carvedilolo, dotato di proprietà sia α- sia β-bloccanti, che funge inoltre da "scavenger"nei confronti dei radicali liberi. I β-bloccanti sono utilizzati per il trattamento cronico dei pazienti con scompenso cardiaco e non dovrebbero essere somministrati quando i pazienti si trovano ancora nella fase acuta (per es. in corso di infusione endovenosa di agonisti adrenergici). Studi preliminari non controllati compiuti sui bambini evidenziano come i β-bloccanti siano ben tollerati e sembrino efficaci; è da poco giunto al termine un trial multicentrico controllato sul carvedilolo in pazienti pediatrici.

APPROCCI ELETTROFISIOLOGICI AL TRATTAMENTO DELLO SCOMPENSO CARDIACO. In pazienti adulti con miocardiopatia si sono ottenuti significativi miglioramenti nella sintomatologia e nella capacità funzionale utilizzando il pacing con risincronizzazione biventricolare (BiVP, *BiVentricular resynchronization Pacing*). Questa tecnica migliora la gittata cardiaca ripristinando una normale sincronia tra la contrazione ventricolare destra e quella sinistra, che spesso va perduta in pazienti con miocardiopatia dilatativa (i quali di solito presentano un blocco di branca sinistro all'elettrocardiogramma). L'esperienza con la BiVP nei bambini è limitata; tuttavia, piccoli campioni hanno riportato un precoce successo in pazienti con scompenso ventricolare sinistro (nel contesto di una miocardiopatia), scompenso ventricolare destro (nel contesto di una tetralogia di Fallot in precedenza sottoposta a correzione) e scompenso di ventricolo singolo (nel contesto di una cardiopatia congenita complessa).

Una delle cause principali di morte improvvisa in pazienti con grave miocardiopatia (sia dilatativa sia ipertrofica) è un'aritmia. Anche se i farmaci antiaritmici possono talvolta ridurre questo rischio, per i pazienti a rischio particolarmente elevato (quelli che sono già sopravvissuti a un episodio di "morte improvvisa"), l'utilizzo di un cardioversore-defibrillatore impiantabile (ICD, *Implantable Cardioverter-Defibrillator*) può essere salvavita (vedi Capitolo 435).

442.1 • SHOCK CARDIOGENO

Lo shock cardiogeno (vedi Capitolo 68) può verificarsi come complicanza di (1) una grave disfunzione cardiaca prima o dopo intervento cardiochirurgico, (2) una setticemia, (3) gravi ustioni, (4) anafilassi, (5) una miocardiopatia, (6) una miocardite, (7) un infarto o "stordimento" miocardico e (8) patologie acute del sistema nervoso centrale. Caratterizzato da una bassa gittata cardiaca e da ipotensione, comporta un'inadeguata perfusione tissutale.

Scopi del trattamento sono il ripristino di una gittata cardiaca e una perfusione periferica adeguate, per prevenire gli effetti indesiderati sugli organi vitali di un'ischemia prolungata, e l'eliminazione della causa sottostante. In condizioni fisiologiche, la gittata cardiaca aumenta in conseguenza di una scarica simpatica, che incrementa la frequenza cardiaca. In presenza di uno shock cardiogeno con marcata tachicardia, tuttavia, la frequenza cardiaca non aumenterà ulteriormente, e la gittata cardiaca può essere ridotta a causa di un diminuito tempo di riempimento diastolico. La gittata cardiaca deve essere aumentata aumentando la gittata sistolica. Se la somministrazione di fluidi avviene a un ritmo più rapido, la pressione venosa centrale e la pressione di riempimento ventricolare (precarico) aumentano, e il meccanismo di Frank-Starling determina un incremento della gittata sistolica. La pressione di riempimento ottimale è variabile e dipende da un certo numero di fattori extracardiaci, tra cui il supporto ventilatorio con pressione positiva tele-espiratoria, pressione di picco inspiratorio e pressione intraddominale elevate. Si dovrebbe tenere presente l'aumentata pressione necessaria a riempire un ventricolo relativamente non compliante, in particolare dopo intervento chirurgico a cuore aperto. Se un'oculata somministrazione di fluidi in quantità incrementali non porta a un miglioramento della gittata cardiaca, un'anomala contrattilità miocardica o un postcardico anormalmente elevato o entrambi questi fattori devono essere implicati come causa della bassa gittata cardiaca.

La contrattilità miocardica migliora non appena si inizia a trattare la causa di base dello shock, si elimina l'ipossia e si corregge l'acidosi. La dopamina, l'adrenalina e la dobutamina migliorano la contrattilità cardiaca, aumentano la frequenza cardiaca e, da ultimo, aumentano la gittata cardiaca.

L'utilizzo di glicosidi cardiaci per trattare stati acuti di bassa gittata cardiaca andrebbe evitato. La digossina ha un effetto più lento rispetto alle catecolamine, anche con la somministrazione endovenosa. Inoltre, possono insorgere effetti avversi, secondari a dosi più elevate; la tossicità è meno prevedibile in quanto dipende dai livelli miocardici e sierici di potassio e calcio. Nei pazienti in shock cardiovascolare la funzionalità renale è spesso compromessa, perciò la somministrazione di digossina può portare a livelli ematici persistentemente elevati poiché sono i reni che provvedono all'escrezione del farmaco. Quando è necessario somministrare il farmaco a questi pazienti, si dovrebbe utilizzare un dosaggio più basso e una frequenza di somministrazione inferiore; inoltre, si raccomanda di monitorarne frequentemente i livelli sierici.

I pazienti in shock cardiogeno possono avere un marcato incremento della resistenza vascolare sistemica, che porta a un elevato postcardico e a una scarsa perfusione periferica. Se la resistenza vascolare sistemica si mantiene elevata e la somministrazione di agenti inotropi positivi da sola non migliora la perfusione tissutale, l'utilizzo di un catetere per termodiluizione polmonare, al fine di misurare l'indice cardiaco e calcolare la resistenza vascolare sistemica, può essere indispensabile per guidare le decisioni terapeutiche.

La valutazione sequenziale e il trattamento dello shock cardiogeno sono essenziali (vedi Capitolo 68). La Tabella 442-3 elenca i principi di trattamento generali validi nella maggior parte dei casi di scompenso cardiocircolatorio acuto. Il trattamento di lattanti e bambini con bassa gittata cardiaca dopo intervento cardiochirurgico dipende dal tipo di procedura operatoria e dalle condizioni del paziente dopo l'intervento (vedi Capitolo 434).

I pazienti con shock cardiogeno ingravescente possono trarre beneficio da un dispositivo di assistenza ventricolare sinistra

TABELLA 442-3. Trattamento dello shock cardiogeno*

	DETERMINANTI DELLA GITTATA SISTOLICA		
	Precarico	**Contrattilità**	**Postcarico**
Parametri misurati	PVC, pressione di incuneamento capillare polmonare, pressione in atrio sinistro, dimensione delle camere cardiache all'ecocardiogramma	Gittata cardiaca, pressione sanguigna, frazione di accorciamento all'elettrocardiogramma, saturazione di O_2 nel sangue venoso misto	Pressione sanguigna, perfusione periferica, resistenza vascolare sistemica
Anomale manifestazioni fisiologiche	Basse PVC, pressione di incuneamento capillare polmonare, pressione in atrio sinistro Diminuita gittata cardiaca Diminuita pressione sanguigna	Elevate PVC, pressione di incuneamento capillare polmonare o pressione in atrio sinistro; bassa saturazione di O_2 nel sangue venoso misto Diminuita gittata cardiaca Diminuita pressione sanguigna	Elevate PVC, pressione di incuneamento capillare polmonare, pressione in atrio sinistro o resistenza vascolare periferica Diminuita gittata cardiaca Pressione sanguigna normale o elevata
Trattamento per migliorare la gittata cardiaca	Espansione di volume (cristalloidi, colloidi)	Agonisti β-adrenergici, inibitori della fosfodiesterasi	Farmaci che riducono il post-carico; nitroprussiato, ACE-inibitori

*L'obiettivo è di migliorare la perfusione periferica aumentando la gittata cardiaca: gittata cardiaca = frequenza cardiaca × gittata sistolica.

PVC, pressione venosa centrale. Gittata cardiaca misurata con catetere per termodilatazione. Pressione atriale sinistra misurata con catetere in atrio sinistro. Saturazione di O_2 nel sangue venoso misto misurata mediante catetere venoso centrale. Resistenza vascolare sistemica calcolata a partire dalla gittata cardiaca e dalla pressione sanguigna media.

(LVAD, *Left Ventricular Assist Device*). Gli LVAD sono stati utilizzati con successo nei bambini e negli adolescenti come ponte verso il trapianto di cuore. Alcuni di essi sono di dimensioni così ridotte da essere in grado di supportare bambini piccoli. In alcuni casi, è necessario un dispositivo ventricolare sia destro sia sinistro (BiVAD). Una volta impiantati, i dispositivi di assistenza permettono ai pazienti di riprendersi al punto da poter essere estubati, incominciare a camminare e spesso lasciare il reparto di terapia intensiva in attesa del trapianto. Pazienti con insufficienza ventricolare reversibile, per esempio quelli nell'immediato stato postoperatorio o quelli con miocardite acuta, possono trarre beneficio anche dall'ossigenazione tramite membrana extracorporea (ECMO, *ExtraCorporeal Membrane Oxygenation*). Se non si prevede che la funzione ventricolare migliori, si dovrebbe prendere in esame il trapianto di cuore (vedi Capitolo 443.1).

Aurigemma GP, Gaasch WH: Diastolic heart failure. *N Engl J Med* 2004;351:1097–1105.
Bristow M: Antiadrenergic therapy of chronic heart failure: Surprises and new opportunities. *Circulation* 2003;107:1100–1102.
Bristow MR, Saxon LA, Boehmer J, et al: Cardiac-resynchronization therapy with or without an implantable defibrillator in advanced chronic heart failure. *N Engl J Med* 2004;350:2140–2150.
Bruns LA, Chrisant MK, Lamour JM, et al: Carvedilol as therapy in pediatric heart failure: An initial multicenter experience. *J Pediatr* 2001;138:505–511.
Clark BJ III: Treatment of heart failure in infants and children. *Heart Dis* 2000;2:354–361.
Dubin AM, Berul CI, Bevilacqua LM, et al: The use of implantable cardioverter-defibrillators in pediatric patients awaiting heart transplantation. *J Card Fail* 2003;9:375–379.
Hoffman TM, Wernovsky G, Atz AM, et al: Efficacy and safety of milrinone in preventing low cardiac output syndrome in infants and children after corrective surgery for congenital heart disease. *Circulation* 2003;107:996–1002.
Jessup M, Brozena S: Heart failure. *N Engl J Med* 2003;348:2007–2018.
Kay JD, Colan SD, Graham TP Jr: Congestive heart failure in pediatric patients. *Am Heart J* 2001;142:923–928.
Liggett SB: Polymorphisms of beta-adrenergic receptors in heart failure. *Am J Med* 2004;117:525–527.
Maisel AS, Krishnaswamy P, Nowak RM, et al: Rapid measurement of B-type natriuretic peptide in the emergency diagnosis of heart failure. *N Engl J Med* 2002;347:161–166.
McMurphy JJV: Heart failure. *Lancet* 2005;365:1877–1889.
Murphy MB, Murray C, Shorten GD: Fenoldopam—a selective peripheral dopamine-receptor agonist for the treatment of severe hypertension. *N Engl J Med* 2001;345:1548–1557.
Neubauer S: The failing heart: an engine out of fuel. *N Engl J Med* 2007; 356:1140–1150.
Port JD, Bristow MR: Altered beta-adrenergic receptor gene regulation and signaling in chronic heart failure. *J Mol Cell Cardiol* 2001;33:887–905.
Rosenthal D, Chrisant MR, Edens E, et al: International Society for Heart and Lung Transplantation: Practice guidelines for management of heart failure in children. *J Heart Lung Transplant* 2004;23:1313–1333.
Shaddy RE: Optimizing treatment for chronic congestive heart failure in children. *Crit Care Med* 2001;29(Suppl):237–240.
Westerlind A, Wahlander H, Lindstedt G, et al: Clinical signs of heart failure are associated with increased levels of natriuretic peptide types B and A in children with congenital heart defects or cardiomyopathy. *Acta Paediatr* 2004;93:340–345.

Capitolo 443 ■ Trapianto di cuore e di cuore-polmone in età pediatrica

443.1 • TRAPIANTO DI CUORE IN ETÀ PEDIATRICA

Il trapianto di cuore è la terapia standard per i bambini con miocardiopatia in stadio terminale e altre lesioni non suscettibili di correzione chirurgica. Nel 2004, più di 5300 trapianti di cuore sono stati effettuati su bambini negli Stati Uniti, con circa 325 trapianti all'anno. I tassi di sopravvivenza in età pediatrica sono paragonabili a quelli tra gli adulti (78% a 1 anno e 68% a 5 anni). La sopravvivenza a 1 anno è del 75% nei bambini sottoposti a trapianto tra il 1982 e il 1988, del 90% in quelli operati dopo il 1999; durante gli stessi periodi, la sopravvivenza al 50% (il tempo in cui il 50% dei pazienti è ancora in vita) è migliorata, passando da 8,3 anni a 11,0 anni (Fig. 443-1). Un crescente numero di pazienti pediatrici raggiunge il 15°, 20° e 25° anno dopo il trapianto.

INDICAZIONI. Il trapianto di cuore viene effettuato in lattanti e bambini con miocardiopatia allo stadio terminale che sono divenuti refrattari alla terapia medica, in pazienti con cardiopatie congenite precedentemente sottoposte a riparazione o palliazione che hanno sviluppato una disfunzione ventricolare o altre complicanze tardive non operabili, e (meno frequentemente) in pazienti con cardiopatie congenite complesse (atresia della polmonare con setto intatto e stenosi delle arterie coronarie, alcune forme di sindrome del cuore sinistro ipoplasico), per cui le procedure chirurgiche standard comporterebbero un rischio estremamente elevato. Le miocardiopatie rendono conto di più del 50% dei trapianti di cuore in pazienti pediatrici di età <1 anno, anche se la percentuale di pazienti con lesioni congenite complesse precedentemente sottoposte a riparazione (30% circa) sta a poco a poco aumentando. In lattanti di età <1 anno, le cardiopatie congenite rappresentavano in passato più dell'80% dei trapianti, ma questo dato è sceso al 65% quando i risultati della chirurgica per le cardiopatie congenite complesse (sindrome del cuore sinistro ipoplasico) sono migliorati.

SELEZIONE DEL RICEVENTE E DEL DONATORE. I potenziali riceventi di trapianto di cuore devono essere esenti da gravi problemi medici non cardiaci come malattie neurologiche, infezioni si-

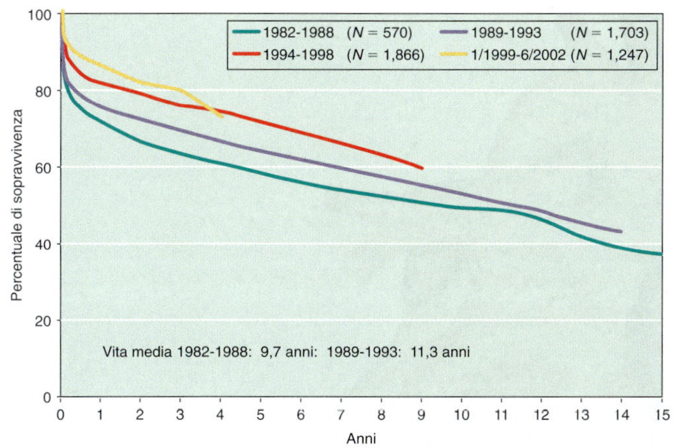

Figura 443-1. Sopravvivenza dopo trapianto di cuore in età pediatrica, confrontando l'epoca attuale con quelle passate, basata su più di 5300 pazienti che sono stati operati dal 1982 al 2002, come riportato nella lista del Registry of the International Society for Heart and Lung Transplantation. La sopravvivenza era significativamente migliorata con il passare del tempo: negli anni 1999-2002 rispetto a tutti gli altri periodi (p <0,0001); negli anni 1982-1988 vs 1994-1998 (p <0,0001); negli 1989-1993 vs 1994-1998 (p <0,0001). (Adattata da Boucek et al: Registry for the International Society for Heart and Lung Transplantation: Seventh official pediatric report 2004. *J Heart Lung Transplant* 2004;23:933-947. © 2004 International Society for Heart and Lung Transplantation.)

stemiche, gravi patologie epatiche o renali, malnutrizione grave. Molti bambini con disfunzione ventricolare possono avere un'ipertensione polmonare o anche una vasculopatia polmonare che precluderebbe il trapianto di cuore; la resistenza vascolare polmonare deve essere misurata all'atto del cateterismo cardiaco, sia a riposo sia in risposta a vasodilatatori. I pazienti con resistenza vascolare polmonare elevata e fissa (>6-8 unità Wood) sono a rischio più elevato per trapianto cardiaco e possono essere considerati candidati per trapianto cardiaco eterotopico (vedi oltre) o trapianto cuore-polmone (vedi Capitolo 443.2). Una consulenza globale da parte dei servizi sociali è una componente importante della valutazione del ricevente. A causa del complesso regime medico dopo il trapianto, la famiglia deve avere una storia di buona aderenza alla terapia. È necessario far firmare il modulo del consenso informato.

La carenza di donatori è un problema serio sia per gli adulti sia per i bambini. Nel registro nazione dei riceventi di trapianto negli Stati Uniti (United Network for Organ Sharing [UNOS]), gli allograft sono abbinati secondo il gruppo sanguigno ABO e il peso corporeo. L'abbinamento HLA non viene attualmente utilizzato e non è facilmente realizzabile per il trapianto di cuore; con l'immunosoppressione disponibile al giorno d'oggi, può offrire solo un vantaggio minimo. L'abbinamento ABO non è richiesto per i lattanti; non è stata ancora determinata l'età esatta in cui si sviluppa la tolleranza ABO. **Controindicazioni** alla donazione d'organi comprendono un arresto cardiaco prolungato con una grave disfunzione cardiaca in corso, patologie o infezioni sistemiche in corso, grave patologia cardiaca preesistente. I medici che hanno in carico un potenziale donatore dovrebbero sempre contattare il coordinatore per la donazione d'organi presso la propria sede, il quale, oltre a essere più di ogni altro grado di giudicare se la donazione d'organi sia possibile, ha esperienza nell'interazione con le famiglie dei donatori. Una storia di rianimazione isolata o di cardiopatia congenita riparabile non implica l'esclusione automatica dalla donazione.

La decisione riguardante il momento in cui inserire un paziente in lista d'attesa per trapianto si basa su molti fattori, compresa una funzione ventricolare estremamente scarsa (frazione d'accorciamento del ventricolo sinistro <10%; normale da 28 a 40%), scarsa tolleranza allo sforzo, determinata mediante test da sforzo cardiopolmonare (vedi Capitolo 423.5), scarsa risposta alla terapia per lo scompenso, numerosi ricoveri ospedalieri per scompenso cardiaco, aritmie, progressivo deterioramento della funzione renale o epatica, stadi iniziali di malattia vascolare polmonare e status nutrizionale scadente. Tra i pazienti che attendono il trapianto, quelli con scarsa funzione ventricolare sinistra (frazione di accorciamento <15%) di solito iniziano il trattamento anticoagulante, preferibilmente con warfarin, per ridurre il rischio di trombosi murale e tromboembolismo. I pazienti con shock cardiogeno non responsivo alla terapia farmacologica standard possono essere candidati al posizionamento di dispositivi di assistenza ventricolare sinistra (LVAD, *Left Ventricular Assist Device*) o biventricolare (BiVAD), o al supporto mediante ossigenazione con membrana extracorporea (ECMO, *ExtraCorporeal Membrane Oxygenation*), che può stabilizzare i parametri emodinamici e fungere da ponte verso il trapianto (vedi Capitolo 442).

TRATTAMENTO PERIOPERATORIO. Nell'intervento classico, sia il cuore del donatore sia quello del ricevente vengono escissi in modo che le porzioni posteriori degli atri contenenti le vene cave e le vene polmonari di sinistra rimangano intatte. L'aorta e l'arteria polmonare sono divise sopra il livello delle valvole semilunari. La porzione anteriore degli atri del donatore viene poi connessa alla rimanente porzione posteriore degli atri del ricevente, evitando così la necessità di una delicata sutura delle vene cave o delle vene polmonari. I grandi vasi del donatore e del ricevente vengono connessi con anastomosi termino-terminali. Di solito si utilizza un'anastomosi bicavale, che lascia intatto l'atrio destro del donatore; la connessione atriale sinistra viene ancora effettuata come nella procedura classica. Il **trapianto cardiaco eterotopico** è stato utilizzato per pazienti con miocardiopatia ventricolare sinistra ed elevata resistenza vascolare polmonare. In questo intervento i cuori del donatore e del ricevente vengono connessi in parallelo, cosicché il ventricolo destro del ricevente (che con il tempo è diventato ipertrofico a causa delle elevate pressioni polmonari) pompa principalmente ai polmoni, mentre il ventricolo sinistro del donatore pompa principalmente all'organismo (Fig. 443-2). Questo intervento è preferibile al trapianto cuore-polmone in candidati appropriati (pazienti con ipertensione polmonare ma senza patologie polmonari parenchimali, senza evidenza di insufficienza ventricolare destra e senza gravi cardiopatie congenite), dal momento che è associato a una più elevata sopravvivenza a tutti i controlli seriati eseguiti nel tempo, dopo il trapianto,

Nell'immediato periodo postoperatorio, l'**immunosoppressione** viene ottenuta comunemente con un regime a base di tre farmaci, anche se alcuni centri utilizzano schemi che non comprendono gli steroidi. Le combinazioni più comuni sono un inibitore della calcineurina (ciclosporina o tacrolimus), un inibitore enzimatico dei leucociti (mofetil micofenolato o azatioprina) e prednisone. Alcuni centri al posto del micofenolato utilizzano un inibitore del ciclo cellulare che agisce sulla proteina mTOR (bersaglio della rapamicina), per il suo potenziale effetto benefico sulla riduzione della coronaropatia nell'organo trapiantato. In molti centri nella prima settimana viene aggiunto un preparato antilinfocitario, una globulina anti-timociti, un anticorpo monoclinale murina anti-linfociti T umani (OKT3) o uno degli anticorpi umanizzati anti-recettore per l'interleuchina 2 (declizumab, basiliximab). Nei bambini che non vanno incontro a un significativo rigetto d'organo, gli steroidi possono essere gradualmente eliminati dopo i primi 6-12 mesi. In centri che non utilizzano steroidi di routine, questi vengono somministrati come trattamento in bolo per episodi acuti di rigetto.

La maggior parte dei riceventi di trapianto di cuore può essere estubata entro le prime 48 ore dopo il trapianto e scende dal letto entro 3-4 giorni. Questi pazienti vengono spesso dimessi nelle prime 2 settimane dopo il trapianto. Se però sussistono fattori di rischio preesistenti, il recupero postoperatorio può essere notevolmente prolungato. Per i pazienti con ipertensione polmonare preoperatoria, l'utilizzo di ossido nitrico (NO) nel periodo postoperatorio può far guadagnare tempo per permettere al ventricolo destro del donatore di ipertrofizzarsi in risposta alle elevate pressioni arteriose polmonari. Talvolta questi pazienti richiederanno un supporto con dispositivi di assistenza ventricolare destra (RVAD, *Right Ventricular assist Device*).

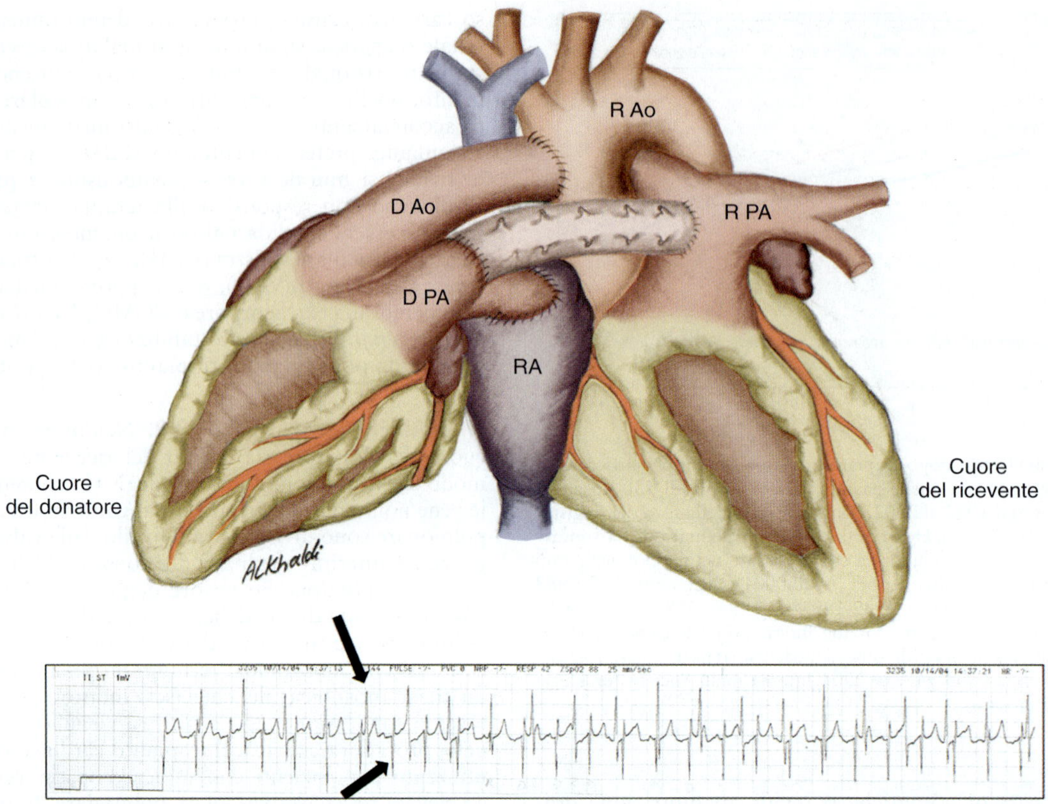

Figura 443-2. Trapianto cardiaco eterotopico. Il cuore del donatore e quello del ricevente sono connessi in parallelo: i due atri vengono attaccati; l'arteria polmonare del donatore viene anastomizzata all'arteria polmonare del ricevente; i due atri sinistri vengono attaccati; l'aorta del donatore viene anastomizzata all'aorta del ricevente. RA (*Right Atrium*), atrio destro; D PA (*Donor Pulmonary Artery*), arteria polmonare del donatore; R PA (*Recipient Pulmonary Artery*), arteria polmonare del ricevente; R Ao (*Recipient Aorta*), aorta del ricevente. Nella parte bassa della figura vi è l'elettrocardiogramma di un lattante di 22 mesi dopo trapianto cardiaco eterotopico. Si possono vedere i complessi QRS separati del donatore e del ricevente (*frecce*). (Illustrazione per gentile concessione di Aziz Alkhaldi, Stanford University, Stanford, CA.)

DIAGNOSI E TRATTAMENTO DEL RIGETTO ACUTO DELL'ORGANO TRAPIANTATO. Il trattamento successivo al trapianto consiste nell'aggiustare la terapia per controbilanciare il rischio di rigetto e gli effetti collaterali di un'eccessiva immunosoppressione. Con le infezioni, il rigetto acuto d'organo è una delle cause principali di morte nei riceventi di età adulta e pediatrica. La sua incidenza è massima nei primi 3 mesi dopo il trapianto e diminuisce significativamente nel periodo successivo. Molti pazienti pediatrici vanno incontro ad almeno un episodio di rigetto acuto nei primi 2 anni dopo il trapianto, anche se i moderni schemi di immunosoppressione hanno diminuito la frequenza di episodi di rigetto gravi. Poiché i sintomi di rigetto possono mimare molte patologie pediatriche comuni (polmonite, gastroenterite), è assolutamente necessario che il centro trapianti sia avvertito tutte le volte che un paziente trapiantato viene visitato dal pediatra o al pronto soccorso per qualsiasi patologia acuta.

Le manifestazioni cliniche del **rigetto acuto** possono comprendere astenia, ritenzione di liquidi, febbre, diaforesi, sintomi addominali e ritmo di galoppo. L'elettrocardiogramma talvolta rileva voltaggi ridotti, aritmie atriali o ventricolari, blocco cardiaco, ma di solito non è diagnostico. L'esame radiografico può evidenziare un ingrandimento cardiaco, versamenti o edema polmonare, ma di solito solo negli stadi più avanzati di rigetto. La maggior parte degli episodi di rigetto si verifica in assenza di sintomi clinici obiettivi. All'ecocardiografia, gli indici di funzione sistolica ventricolare sinistra possono essere ridotti; tuttavia, questi non si deteriorano finché il rigetto non è da moderato a grave. Le tecniche volte alla valutazione dell'ispessimento parietale e della funzione diastolico-ventricolare sinistra, che sembravano promettenti, non si sono dimostrate in grado di predire un rigetto precoce. La maggior parte dei centri trapianti non si affida alla sola ecocardiografia per la sorveglianza del rigetto.

La **biopsia miocardica** è il metodo più attendibile per il monitoraggio del rigetto nei trapiantati. I campioni bioptici vengono ottenuti dal lato ventricolare destro del setto interventricolare e possono essere prelevati in modo relativamente sicuro, anche nei bambini piccoli. Nei bambini più grandi le biopsie miocardiche possono essere effettuate in modo ravvicinato anche ogni 1-4 settimane nei primi 3-6 mesi dopo il trapianto; la frequenza viene poi ridotta a 2-4 biopsie all'anno, a meno che il paziente non abbia un episodio di rigetto. Nei lattanti le biopsie di controllo di solito sono effettuate con frequenza inferiore (talvolta solo una o due all'anno). I bambini possono avere episodi insospettati di rigetto anche 5-10 anni dopo il trapianto; la maggior parte dei centri trapianto continuano a effettuare di routine biopsie di controllo, anche se a intervalli meno frequenti (ogni 6-12 mesi).

I criteri per il **grading del rigetto cardiaco** si basano su un sistema sviluppato dalla International Society for Heart and Lung Transplantation (ISHLT); questi criteri prendono in considerazione il grado di infiltrato cellulare e l'eventuale presenza di necrosi dei miociti. I gradi di rigetto 1A, 1B e 2 ISHLT sono abbastanza lievi da non richiedere un trattamento immediato, e più del 50% di questi episodi si può risolvere spontaneamente. Di solito dopo qualche settimana la biopsia viene ripetuta. Nei pazienti con rigetto di grado 3A ISHLT viene istituita una terapia con metilprednisolone per via endovenosa o prednisone per via orale, partendo da una dose elevata per poi diminuire. I pazienti che 3 mesi dopo il trapianto sono asintomatici e hanno un ecocardiogramma normale sono spesso trattati ambulatorialmente. I pazienti con gradi 3B o 4, o qualsiasi paziente con instabilità emodinamica, vengono ricoverati per la somministrazione endovenosa di steroidi e una terapia antirigetto potenzialmente più aggressiva. Per gli episodi di rigetto resistenti alla trattamento steroideo, regimi terapeutici aggiuntivi comprendono cicli ripetuti di preparazione antilinfocitaria (daclizumab, OKT3, globulina anti-timociti), metotrexato o irradiazione linfatica totale. I pazienti con ripetuti episodi di rigetto possono inoltre trarre beneficio dal passaggio dalla ciclosporina al tacrolimus (o viceversa). Rari pazienti con rigetto refrattario possono richiedere un ritrapianto.

Alcuni episodi di rigetto non sono associati a un infiltrato cellulare alla biopsia. Questi casi di rigetto acellulare o umorale sono presumibilmente mediati da anticorpi circolanti e possono essere evidenziati dall'immunocolorazione del campione bioptico per la componente C4d del complemento o per altri marker immunitari. Il rigetto umorale, meno responsivo all'immunosoppressione standard (steroidi in bolo), è stato trattato con plasmaferesi, fotoferesi, immunoglobuline per via endovenosa, metotrexato e l'anticorpo monoclinale anti-CD20 rituximab.

COMPLICANZE DELL'IMMUNOSOPPRESSIONE.

Infezione. Le infezioni sono una delle due principali cause di morte nei pazienti pediatrici trapiantati (Fig. 443-3). La loro incidenza è massima nei primi 3 mesi dopo il trapianto, quando le dosi degli immunosoppressori sono più elevate. Le più comuni sono le infezioni virali, specialmente da Cytomegalovirus, responsabile di una percentuale di episodi infettivi che può raggiungere il 25%. L'infezione da Cytomegalovirus può verificarsi come infezione primitiva in pazienti senza precedente esposizione al virus, o sotto forma di riattivazione. Se grave, può essere disseminata o associata a polmonite, e provocare un episodio di rigetto acuto o una malattia coronarica nell'organo trapiantato. Molti centri utilizzano il ganciclovir per via endovenosa o le immunoglobuline anti-Cytomegalovirus o entrambi, come profilassi in qualsiasi paziente che riceva un cuore da un donatore positivo al Cytomegalovirus o in chiunque abbia un'evidenza sierologica di una precedente patologia da Cytomegalovirus. La reazione a catena della polimerasi (PCR, *Polymerase Chain Reaction*) aumenta la capacità di diagnosticare l'infezione da questo virus e di monitorare serialmente l'efficacia del trattamento. Sono disponibili preparazioni orali di ganciclovir con profili di assorbimento migliorati per la terapia in cronico.

Nella maggior parte dei casi le normali patologie virali dell'infanzia sono ben tollerate e di solito non richiedono un trattamento specifico. L'otite media e le comuni infezioni del tratto respiratorio superiore possono essere trattate ambulatorialmente, anche se una febbre o sintomi che durino più a lungo del normale decorso della malattia richiedono ulteriori accertamenti. Una gastroenterite, specialmente con vomito, può portare a una marcata riduzione dell'assorbimento dei farmaci immunosoppressori e provocare un episodio di rigetto. In questo contesto, si raccomanda di monitorare strettamente i livelli farmacologici e di prendere in esame la somministrazione per via endovenosa. L'esposizione al virus della varicella viene trattata con immunoglobuline antivaricella; se invece il paziente acquisisce un'infezione clinica, un trattamento con aciclovir per via endovenosa attenua la malattia.

Le infezioni batteriche sono le seconde in ordine di frequenza; il polmone è il sito più comunemente interessato (35%), seguito dal sangue, dal tratto urinario e, meno spesso, dal sito di sternotomia. Altre sorgenti di infezione post-trapianto sono miceti (14%) e protozoi (6%). Molti centri utilizzano la nistatina in collutorio per diminuire la colonizzazione fungina e una profilassi con trimetoprim/sulfametoxazolo per prevenire l'infezione da *Pneumocystis carinii*. L'incidenza di infezioni gravi è più bassa in bambini che possono essere trattati senza steroidi.

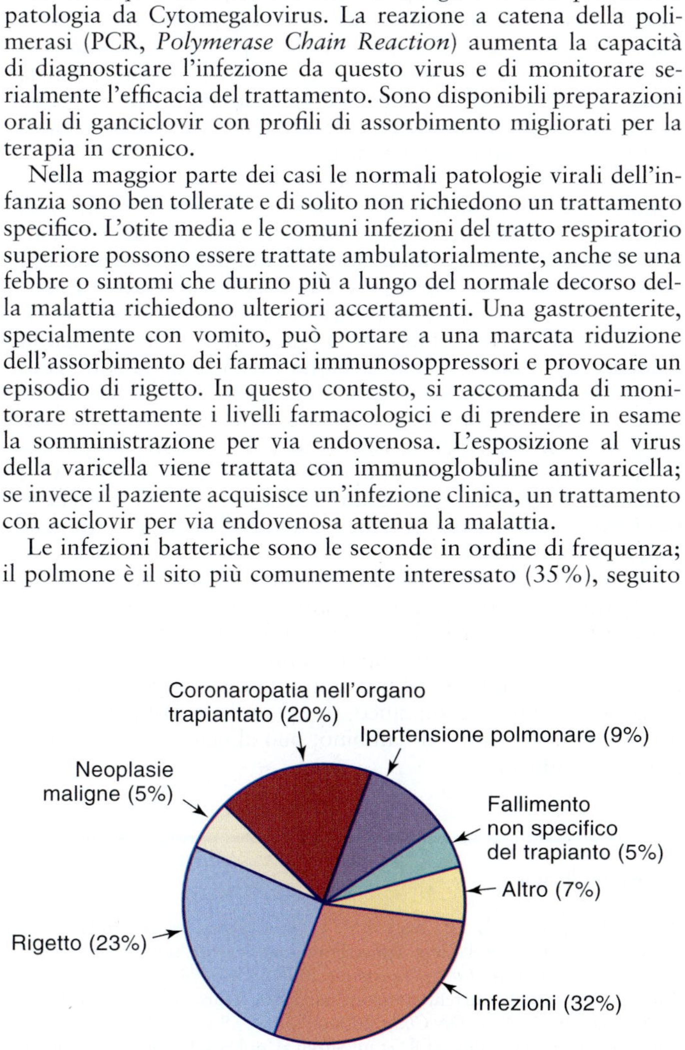

Figura 443-3. Principali cause di morte dopo trapianto di cuore in età pediatrica (Dati da Stanford University, Stanford, CA.)

Ritardo di crescita. I pazienti che necessitano della somministrazione cronica di steroidi di solito presentano una diminuita crescita lineare; per questo, la maggior parte dei programmi di trapianto pediatrici mira a un'immunosoppressione che non preveda l'utilizzo di questi agenti nei primi 1-2 anni successivi al trapianto. In quei pazienti che vanno incontro a rigetto quando gli steroidi vengono sospesi, un regime di steroidi a giorni alterni porta a un miglioramento della crescita lineare. L'irradiazione linfatica totale sembra promettente come protocollo che non prevede steroidi. I pazienti che sopravvivono a lungo termine dopo aver subito il trapianto di cuore in età pediatrica hanno una crescita normale nel 75% dei casi.

Ipertensione. L'ipertensione, comune nei pazienti trattati con ciclosporina, è dovuta a una combinazione di espansione del volume plasmatico e deficit di escrezione renale di sodio. I corticosteroidi di solito potenziano l'ipertensione indotta dalla ciclosporina. I pazienti vengono tipicamente trattati con un diuretico e un vasodilatatore in associazione. I farmaci che agiscono tramite il blocco dei canali del calcio (calcioantagonisti) potrebbero avere l'ulteriore vantaggio di attenuare lo sviluppo di coronaropatia nell'organo trapiantato. L'incidenza dell'ipertensione può essere leggermente più bassa in pazienti trattati con tacrolimus.

Funzionalità renale. La somministrazione cronica di ciclosporina o tacrolimus può causare una nefropatia tubulointerstiziale negli adulti, ma una grave disfunzione renale è rara nei bambini. La maggior parte dei pazienti pediatrici presenta un graduale aumento della creatinina sierina nel primo anno dopo il trapianto; se insorge una disfunzione renale, questa di solito risponde a una diminuzione del dosaggio di ciclosporina. I pazienti nel lungo termine raramente necessitano di trapianto renale.

Complicanze neurologiche. Gli effetti collaterali neurologici della ciclosporina e del tacrolimus comprendono tremore, mialgie, parestesie e raramente convulsioni. Queste complicanze possono essere trattate con una riduzione del dosaggio dei farmaci e a volte con supplementi orali di magnesio. Le infezioni intracraniche rappresentano un rischio significativo, specialmente perché alcuni dei segni più frequenti (rigidità nucale) possono essere assenti in pazienti immunosoppressi. Microrganismi potenzialmente responsabili comprendono *Aspergillus*, *Cryptococcus neoformans* e *Listeria monocytogenes*. alcuni giorni o settimane dopo somministrazione di OKT3 si può osservare una meningite asettica, che di solito si autolimita.

Tumori. Una delle complicanze gravi che influiscono negativamente sulla sopravvivenza a lungo termine dei pazienti pediatrici sottoposti a trapianto di cuore è il rischio di patologia neoplastica. La più comune è la malattia linfoproliferativa post-trapianto (PTLD, *Post-Tranplant Lymphoproliferative Disease*), una condizione associata a infezione da virus di Epstein-Barr. La PTLD di solito risponde a una riduzione dell'immunosoppressione e a un trattamento antivirale con aciclovir; solo in alcuni casi richiede la chemioterapia. Un anticorpo monoclonale diretto contro l'antigene CD20 sui linfociti attivati (rituximab) sembra promettente contro alcune forme di PTLD. Un aumentato rischio di cancro della pelle impone di adottare le opportune precauzioni prima di esporre i bambini alla luce del sole.

Rigetto cronico. La **coronaropatia nell'organo trapiantato** (CAD, *Coronary Artery Disease*) è una manifestazione di rigetto cronico del trapianto che si verifica nel 20% dei bambini. La causa è ancora poco chiara, anche se si ritiene che sia una forma di danno vascolare immunomediato. L'ipercolesterolemia e l'iperglicemia aumentano il rischio di questa patologia. A differenza dell'aterosclerosi su coronarie native, la CAD nel cuore trapiantato è un processo diffuso, con un grado elevato di coinvolgimento di vasi distali. Poiché il cuore trapiantato è stato denervato, i pazienti non hanno sintomi come l'angina pectoris durante gli episodi ischemici, e la manifestazione iniziale può essere un collasso cardiovascolare o la morte improvvisa. La maggior parte dei centri effettua su base annuale un'angiografia coronarica come screening per evidenziare anomalie coronariche; in alcuni centri si esegue invece un'ecografia coronarica intravascolare (IVUS, *IntraVascular UltraSound*). Le procedure standard di bypass coronarico non sono di solito utili a causa della natura diffusa del processo, anche se lo stenting transcatetere talvolta è efficace per lesioni isolate. Per i casi gravi, un nuovo trapianto di cuore si è dimostrato l'unico trattamento efficace. Perciò la maggior parte della ricerca attuale si concentra sulla prevenzione. Si è visto che gli inibitori del ciclo cellulare sirolimus ed everolimus diminuiscono l'ispessimento arterioso intimale coronarico 2 anni dopo il trapianto, in pazienti adulti. Altri farmaci con i quali è stata osservata una riduzione del rischio di coronaropatia nel cuore trapiantato comprendono i calcioantagonisti (come il diltiazem) e gli ipocolesterolemizzanti inibitori dell'HMG-CoA (3-idrossi 3-metil-coenzima A) reduttasi (pravastatina o l'atorvastatina).

Altre complicanze. I corticosteroidi di solito causano facies cushingoide, acne da steroidi e strie. La ciclosporina può causare lievi alterazioni delle caratteristiche del volto, come ipertricosi e iperplasia gengivale. Queste caratteristiche estetiche possono essere particolarmente spiacevoli per le adolescenti e rappresentare un motivo di mancata compliance alla terapia. Molte di queste complicanze sono dose-correlate e migliorano quando vengono gradualmente sospesi i farmaci immunosoppressori. L'osteoporosi e la necrosi ossea asettica sono ulteriori ragioni per ridurre il dosaggio degli steroidi il prima possibile. Il diabete e la pancreatite sono complicanze rare ma gravi.

Riabilitazione. Nonostante i potenziali rischi dell'immunosoppressione, le prospettive di riabilitazione dei pazienti pediatrici sottoposti a trapianto di cuore è eccellente. Più del 95% dei pazienti pediatrici sottoposti a trapianto cardiaco non ha limitazioni funzionali nella vita quotidiana. La maggior parte di essi non richiede ulteriori ricoveri ospedalieri per problemi correlati al trapianto.

I bambini sottoposti a trapianto cardiaco possono frequentare l'asilo o la scuola e partecipare a sport competitivi che non prevedano contatto fisico e ad altre attività appropriate per l'età. Le misure standardizzate della funzione ventricolare sono vicine alla normalità. Poiché il cuore trapiantato è denervato, l'aumento della frequenza cardiaca e della gittata cardiaca durante l'esercizio fisico è più lento, e le risposte della frequenza cardiaca massimale e della gittata cardiaca sono lievemente attenuate: sottili anomalie che di cui raramente il paziente si accorge.

La crescita del cuore trapiantato è eccellente, anche se è comune un'ipertrofia ventricolare e settale di rado lieve, anche a distanza di anni dal trapianto. Le sedi delle anastomosi degli atri e dei grandi vasi crescono senza sviluppare ostruzioni. Nei neonati sottoposti a trapianto per sindrome del cuore sinistro ipoplasico, tuttavia, può esservi una recidiva di coartazione aortica iuxtaduttale.

L'adattamento psicologico al trapianto cardiaco, valutato mediante test psicologici standardizzati, è di solito buono nei bambini. Tuttavia, in età adolescenziale possono insorgere gravi problemi di non compliance da cui può derivare un rigetto che mette in pericolo la vita del paziente. Un precoce intervento da parte di assistenti sociali, consulenti e psicologi permette di ridurre questo rischio.

443.2 • TRAPIANTO DI CUORE-POLMONE E DI POLMONE

Negli Stati Uniti sono stati effettuati più di 700 trapianti di cuore-polmone e di polmone (singolo o doppio) su bambini, con circa 60 procedure effettuate all'anno. Le indicazioni primarie per il trapianto di cuore-polmone sono la fibrosi cistica, l'ipertensione polmonare primitiva, le cardiopatie congenite complesse con ipoplasia polmonare o sindrome di Eisenmenger, le anomalie polmonari congenite e le patologie polmonari parenchimali allo stadio terminale (displasia broncopolmonare, pneumopatie croniche e fibrosi interstiziale). Molti di questi pazienti con cuori normali possono anche essere candidati al trapianto di polmone singolo o doppio se la funzione ventricolare destra è preservata. In alcuni soggetti con sindrome di Eisenmenger, il doppio trapianto di polmone può essere effettuato in combinazione con la riparazione di difetti intracardiaci. Chi è affetto da fibrosi cistica non è candidato al trapianto di polmone singolo, a causa del rischio di infezione dal polmone malato controlaterale. Molti dei criteri previsti per la selezione dei pazienti sono gli stessi che vengono applicati ai riceventi di trapianto di cuore (vedi Capitolo 443.1).

L'immunosoppressione post-trapianto si ottiene di solito con uno schema a tre farmaci, simile a quello utilizzato per il trapianto di cuore. A differenza di quanto avviene nel trapianto cardiaco isolato, pochi pazienti con trapianto di polmone possono essere completamente svezzati dalla terapia steroidea. La profilassi contro l'infezione da *Pneumocystis carinii* consiste nella somministrazione di trimetoprim-sulfametoxazolo o pentamidina in aerosol. Il ganciclovir e la profilassi con immunoglobuline anti-Cytomegalovirus vengono utilizzati come nei pazienti sottoposti a trapianto cardiaco (vedi Capitolo 443.1).

Il rigetto di polmone è comune nei pazienti sottoposti a trapianto di cuore-polmone, mentre il rigetto di cuore si riscontra meno spesso che nei pazienti sottoposti al solo trapianto di cuore. I sintomi di un rigetto di polmone possono comprendere febbre e astenia, anche se molti episodi sono minimamente sintomatici. La sorveglianza per un eventuale rigetto viene effettuata monitorando la funzione polmonare (capacità vitale forzata, volume espiratorio forzato in 1 s [FEV_1, *Forced Expiratory Volume in 1 s*], flusso espiratorio forzato, fase medioespiratoria [FEF, *Forced Expiratory Fase*, 25-75%]), la pressione parziale arteriosa sistemica di ossigeno, la radiografia del torace, e mediante biopsie transbronchiali seriate. A causa di limitazioni tecniche, le biopsie non vengono di solito effettuate nei lattanti, che vengono monitorati in base ai soli criteri clinici.

I tassi di sopravvivenza dopo trapianto di cuore-polmone o di polmone nei bambini sono al momento del 75% a 1 anno e del 50% a 5 anni; i progressi compiuti nella selezione dei pazienti e nella gestione postoperatoria stanno continuamente migliorando queste statistiche di sopravvivenza. Il fallimento del trapianto e le infezioni sono le cause principali di morte precoce, mentre una forma di rigetto cronico nota come **bronchiolite obliterante** rende conto di quasi il 50% della mortalità tardiva. Altre cause di morbilità e mortalità precoce comprendono complicanze tracheali, ostruzione venosa polmonare, disfunzione del polmone del donatore, emorragie e rigetto acuto. Ulteriori complicanze tardive consistono nello sviluppo di stenosi delle vie aeree, CAD accelerata dell'organo trapiantato (anche se meno comune che nel trapianto di cuore isolato) e altri effetti collaterali dell'immunosoppressione cronica.

Nel postoperatorio gli indici di funzione cardiopolmonare e la capacità di esercizio fisico vanno incontro a un significativo miglioramento. Più del 95% dei pazienti non presenta limitazioni dell'attività fisica al follow-up a 2 anni. La disponibilità di donatori è ancora minore nel trapianto di polmone. Il trapianto da donatore vivente consanguineo, in cui un lobo polmonare viene donato da un genitore al bambino, può almeno in parte ovviare a questo problema.

Trapianto di cuore

Boucek MM, Edwards LB, Keck BM, et al: Registry for the International Society for Heart and Lung Transplantation: Seventh official pediatric report—2004. *J Heart Lung Transplant* 2004;23:933–947.

Burch M, Aurora P: Current status of paediatric heart, lung, and heart-lung transplantation. *Arch Dis Child* 2004;89:386–389.

Canter C, Naftel D, Caldwell R, et al: Survival and risk factors for death after cardiac transplantation in infants. A multi-institutional study. The Pediatric Heart Transplant Study. *Circulation* 1997;96:227–231.

Chin C, Gamberg P, Miller J, et al: Efficacy and safety of atorvastatin after pediatric heart transplantation. *J Heart Lung Transplant* 2002; 21:1213–1217.
Fan X, Ang A, Pollock-Barziv SM, et al: Donor-specific B-cell tolerance after ABO-incompatible infant heart transplantation. *Nat Med* 2004; 10:1227–1233.
Hornung TS, de Goede C, O'Brien C, et al: Renal function after pediatric cardiac transplantation: The effect of early cyclosporine dosage. *Pediatrics* 2001;107:1346–1350.
Hotson JR, Enzmann DR: Neurologic complications of cardiac transplantation. *Neurol Clin* 1988;6:349–365.
Mazariegos GV, Reyes J, Webber SA, et al: Cytokine gene polymorphisms in children successfully withdrawn from immunosuppression after liver transplantation. *Transplantation* 2002;73:1342–1345.
Pahl E, Zales VR, Fricker FJ, et al: Posttransplant coronary artery disease in children. A multicenter national survey. *Circulation* 1994;90:II56–II60.
Pollock-BarZiv SM, Anthony SJ, et al: Quality of life and function following cardiac transplantation in adolescents. *Transplant Proc* 2003;35: 2468–2470.
Ringewald JM, Gidding SS, Crawford SE, et al: Nonadherence is associated with late rejection in pediatric heart transplant recipients. *J Pediatr* 2001;139:75–78.
Rosenthal DN, Chin C, Nishimura K, et al: Identifying cardiac transplant rejection in children: Diagnostic utility of echocardiography, right heart catheterization and endomyocardial biopsy data. *J Heart Lung Transplant* 2004;23:323–329.
Russo LM, Webber SA: Pediatric heart transplantation: Immunosuppression and its complications. *Curr Opin Cardiol* 2004;19:104–109.
Schowengerdt KO, Naftel DC, Seib PM, et al: Infection after pediatric heart transplantation: Results of a multi-institutional study. The Pediatric Heart Transplant Study Group. *J Heart Lung Transplant* 1997;16:1207–1216.
Shirali GS, Ni J, Chinnock RE, et al: Association of viral genome with graft loss in children after cardiac transplantation. *N Engl J Med* 2001;344:1498–1503.
Sigfusson G, Fricker FJ, Bernstein D, et al: Long term survivors of pediatric heart transplantation: A multicenter report of 68 children who have survived greater than five years. *J Pediatr* 1997;130:862–871.
Webber SA: Immunology of pediatric heart transplantation: A clinical update. *Semin Thorac Cardiovasc Surg Pediatr Card Surg Annu* 2001;4:158–184.
Webber SA, Naftel DC, Fricker FJ, et al: Lymphoproliferative disorders after pediatric heart transplantation: a multi-institutional study. *Lancet* 2006;367:233–239.
West LJ, Pollock-Barziv SM, Dipchand AI, et al: ABO-incompatible heart transplantation in infants. *N Engl J Med* 2001;344:793–800.

Trapianto di polmone

Conte JV, Robbins RC, Reichenspurner H, et al: Pediatric heart-lung transplantation: Intermediate-term results. *J Heart Lung Transplant* 1996;15:692–699.
Mendeloff EN, Huddleston CB, Mallory GB, et al: Pediatric and adult lung transplantation for cystic fibrosis. *J Thorac Cardiovasc Surg* 1998;115:404–413.
Moffatt SD, Demers P, Robbins RC, et al: Lung transplantation: A decade of experience. *J Heart Lung Transplant* 2005;24:145–151.
Sritippayawan S, Keens TG, Horn MV, et al: What are the best pulmonary function test parameters for early detection of post-lung transplant bronchiolitis obliterans syndrome in children? *Pediatr Transplant* 2003;7:200–203.
Starnes VA, Bowdish ME, Woo MS, et al: A decade of living lobar lung transplantation: Recipient outcomes. *J Thorac Cardiovasc Surg* 2004;127: 114–122.
Sweet SC, Spray TL, Huddleston CB, et al: Pediatric lung transplantation at St. Louis Children's Hospital, 1990–1995. *Am J Respir Crit Care Med* 1997;155:1027–1035.
Webber SA, McCurry K, Zeevi A: Heart and lung transplantation in children. *Lancet* 2006;368:53–68.

Sezione 8 — Malattie del sistema vascolare periferico — Daniel Bernstein

Capitolo 444 ■ Malattie dei vasi sanguigni (aneurismi e fistole)

444.1 • Malattia di Kawasaki (vedi anche il Capitolo 165)

Aneurismi delle arterie coronarie o delle arterie sistemiche possono complicare la malattia di Kawasaki e sono le principali cause di morbilità in questa patologia (Figg. 444-1 e 444-2). Tranne che nella malattia di Kawasaki, gli aneurismi non sono comuni nei bambini e colpiscono con maggior frequenza l'aorta, in associazione alla coartazione dell'aorta, al dotto arterioso pervio e alla sindrome di Marfan, e i vasi intracranici (vedi Capitolo 601). Possono anche essere secondari a un embolo infetto, a un'infezione contigua a un vaso sanguigno, a un trauma, ad anomalie congenite delle strutture vascolari, specialmente della tonaca media, e ad arterite, per esempio la poliartrite nodosa e l'arterite di Takayasu (vedi Capitolo 166.2).

444.2 • Fistole arterovenose

Le fistole arterovenose possono consistere in piccoli emangiomi cavernosi o essere estese (vedi Capitoli 505 e 649). Le sedi più comuni nei lattanti e nei bambini sono cranio, fegato, polmone, arti e vasi nel contesto o in prossimità della parete toracica. Queste fistole, sebbene di solito siano congenite, possono derivare da un trauma o essere la manifestazione di una teleangectasia ereditaria emorragica (malattia di Olser-Weber-Rendu). Le fistole arterovenose femorali sono una rara complicanza del cateterismo femorale percutaneo.

MANIFESTAZIONI CLINICHE. I sintomi clinici si verificano solo in associazione ad ampie comunicazioni arterovenose quando il sangue arterioso fluisce in un sistema venoso a bassa pressione; la pressione venosa locale è aumentata, mentre il flusso arterioso distale alla fistola è diminuito. La resistenza arteriosa sistemica cala, a causa della fuoriuscita di sangue attraverso la fistola. Meccanismi compensatori comprendono tachicardia e aumento della gittata sistolica, cosicché la gittata cardiaca aumenta. Il volume di sangue totale è altresì aumentato. Nelle fistole ampie si verificano una dilatazione ventricolare sinistra, una più ampia pressione differenziale e scompenso cardiaco. L'iniezione di mezzo di contrasto in un'arteria prossimale rispetto alla fistola conferma la diagnosi.

Nei neonati molto spesso si osservano ampie fistole arterovenose intracraniche in associazione a una **malformazione di una vena di Galeno**. L'ampio shunt intracranico sinistro-destro porta a uno scompenso cardiaco secondario alla richiesta di un'elevata gittata cardiaca. Pazienti con comunicazioni più piccole possono non avere manifestazioni cardiovascolari, essere predisposti a sviluppare in seguito un idrocefalo (vedi Capitolo 592.11) o convulsioni. I neonati con un'ampia fistola arterovenosa intracranica sintomatica hanno una prognosi infausta; alcuni sopravvivono con la terapia medica, ma sono soggetti a complicanze tardive

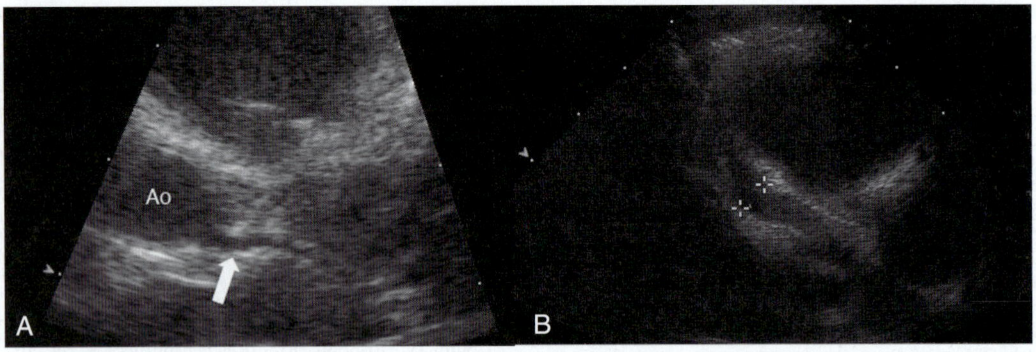

Figura 444-1. Ecocardiogramma bidimensionale che confronta un'arteria coronaria sinistra normale (*freccia* nella figura a sinistra) con un aneurisma gigante di un'arteria coronaria (evidenziato dalle *crocette* nella figura a destra) in un paziente con malattia di Kawasaki. Ao, aorta.

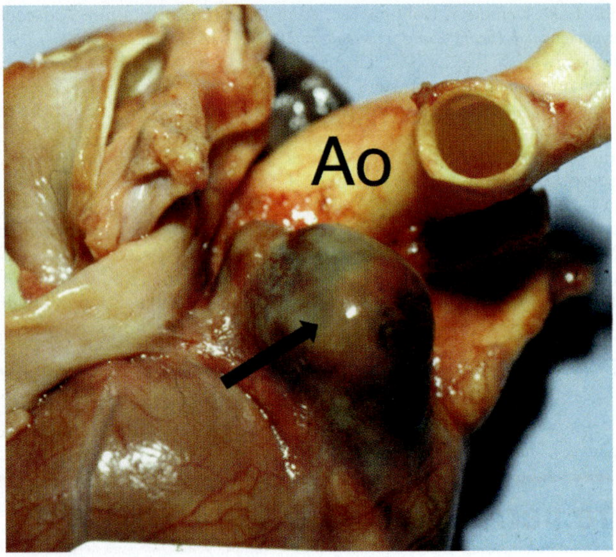

Figura 444-2. Campione patologico in cui è visibile un aneurisma gigante dell'arteria coronaria sinistra principale (*freccia*). Ao, aorta ascendente.

causate dalla massa intracranica. Per la diagnosi spesso ci si avvale dell'auscultazione di un soffio continuo al livello del cranio. I bambini più grandi con malformazioni arterovenose intracraniche più diffuse sono riconoscibili sulla base di calcificazioni intracraniche ed elevata gittata cardiaca senza scompenso cardiaco.

Fistole arterovenose epatiche, generalizzate o localizzate, possono essere emangioendoteliomi o emangiomi cavernosi. La fistola può essere situata tra l'arteria epatica e il dotto venoso o la vena porta. Può inoltre essere presente una teleangectasia congenita emorragica. Ampie fistole arterovenose sono associate a un aumento della gittata cardiaca e a scompenso cardiaco. Di solito è presente un'epatomegalia e possono essere udibili a livello del fegato soffi sistolici o continui.

Fistole arterovenose periferiche, generalmente a carico delle estremità, sono associate ad alterazioni dell'aspetto, gonfiore delle estremità ed emangiomi visibili. Alcune sono situate in aree che portano a un'ostruzione delle vie aeree superiori. Poiché solo un piccola minoranza determina un'abbondante fuoriuscita di sangue arterioso, lo scompenso cardiaco non è comune.

TRATTAMENTO. Il trattamento medico dello scompenso cardiaco può essere utile all'inizio, nei neonati con queste patologie; con il tempo, le dimensioni dello shunt talvolta diminuiscono e i sintomi possono regredire spontaneamente. Gli emangiomi epatici spesso finiscono per scomparire completamente. Ampi emangiomi epatici sono stati trattati con steroidi, acido ε-aminocaproico, interferone, compressione locale, embolizzazione o irradiazione locale; gli effetti benefici di queste opzioni di trattamento non sono chiari, poiché i singoli pazienti presentano notevoli variazioni nel decorso clinico in assenza di trattamento. L'embolizzazione tramite catetere sta diventando il trattamento di scelta per molti pazienti con fistole arterovenose sintomatiche. Sono stati utilizzati agenti embolizzanti, come palloncini staccabili, spirali di acciaio (Gianturco) e adesivi tissutali liquidi (cianoacrilati). Spesso sono necessarie più procedure prima che il flusso subisca una riduzione significativa. Nei pazienti con grave scompenso cardiaco che non migliorano con il trattamento medico si può tentare la rimozione chirurgica di un'ampia fistola. Il trattamento chirurgico può essere controindicato o non avere successo quando la lesione è estesa, diffusa oppure situata in una posizione in cui il tessuto circostante può essere leso durante l'intervento chirurgico o le procedure correlate.

Abernethy LJ: Classification and imaging of vascular malformations in children. *Eur Radiol* 2003;13:2483–2497.

Faughnan ME, Thabet A, Mei-Zahav M, et al: Pulmonary arteriovenous malformations in children: Outcomes of transcatheter embolotherapy. *J Pediatr* 2004;145:826–831.

Fong LV, Lee SH, Salmon AP: Diagnosis of cerebral arteriovenous malformations by colour Doppler examination. *Eur Heart J* 1992;13:415–417.

Ford EG, Stanley P, Tolo V, et al: Peripheral congenital arteriovenous fistulae: Observe, operate, or obturate? *J Pediatr Surg* 1992;27:714–719.

Friedman DM, Verma R, Madrid M, et al: Recent improvement in outcome using transcatheter embolization techniques for neonatal aneurysmal malformations of the vein of Galen. *Pediatrics* 1993;91:583–586.

Capitolo 445 ■ Ipertensione sistemica

L'ipertensione sistemica colpisce comunemente gli adulti, e in assenza di trattamento è uno dei principali fattori di rischio per infarto miocardico, ictus e insufficienza renale. In un'analisi raggruppata di diversi studi sull'ipertensione nell'adulto, un aumento di 5 mmHg della pressione sanguigna diastolica incrementa il rischio di coronaropatia del 20% e di ictus del 35%. L'ipertensione è implicata nell'eziologia di circa il 50% dei casi nefropatia allo stadio terminale nell'adulto. La prevalenza di ipertensione aumenta con l'età, andando dal 15% nei giovani adulti al 60% nei soggetti di età >65 anni.

Nei lattanti e nei bambini piccoli, l'ipertensione sistemica non è comune, con una prevalenza <1%, ma quando presente è di solito indicativa di un processo patologico sottostante (ipertensione secondaria). D'altro canto, gli adolescenti possono sviluppare un'ipertensione primitiva o essenziale (senza una causa sottostante). Un'ipertensione essenziale nell'infanzia può trascinarsi fino all'età adulta, come dimostrato da numerosi studi clinici su vasta scala. Bambini con pressione sanguigna >90° percentile hanno un rischio 2-4 volte maggiore di soffrire di ipertensione da adulti. Analogamente, circa la metà degli adulti ipertesi ha una pressione sanguigna >90° percentile in età pediatrica. Vi è anche una correlazione tra una precoce ipertensione nell'infanzia e una precoce aterosclerosi.

Accurate misurazioni della pressione sanguigna dovrebbero far parte dell'annuale visita medica di routine di tutti i bambini di età >3 anni. Occorre raccogliere un'anamnesi familiare completa per quanto riguarda l'ipertensione. Un'adeguata misurazione della pressione sanguigna richiede molta attenzione al comfort del paziente e dipende moltissimo dall'adeguato utilizzo dell'apparecchiatura, sia essa un semplice sfigmomanometro o un dispositivo automatico all'avanguardia. Effettuare una misurazione accurata della pressione sanguigna nei lattanti è spesso la parte più difficile dell'esame obiettivo, quella che richiede più tempo. Pazienti di qualsiasi età possono sviluppare ansia al momento di sottoporsi alla misurazione della pressione sanguigna, il che può portare a una falsa diagnosi di ipertensione. La pressione sanguigna può essere misurata a paziente seduto o supino: i lattanti devono essere tenuti in grembo da un genitore. Misure successive effettuate per confronto dovrebbero essere ottenute con il paziente nella medesima posizione. È necessaria una particolare attenzione alla dimensione del bracciale, per evitare una sovrastima. Dovrebbe essere disponibile un'ampia varietà di bracciali in qualsiasi ambulatorio medico dove vengono visitati di routine pazienti in età pediatrica. Il bracciale dovrebbe circondare completamente la parte superiore del braccio, per assicurare una compressione uniforme; la camera gonfiabile dove coprire almeno 2/3 della lunghezza della parte superiore del braccio e l'80-100% della sua circonferenza. Un bracciale troppo corto o troppo stretto aumenta artificialmente i valori pressori riscontrati. Si raccomanda di misurare la pressione sanguigna a tutte e quattro le estremità per evidenziare un'eventuale coartazione dell'aorta (vedi Capitolo 427.6).

La pressione sistolica è indicata dalla comparsa del primo tono di Korotkoff; quella diastolica è stata unanimemente definita come il quinto (e non il quarto) tono di Korotkoff. La palpazione è utile per una valutazione rapida della pressione sistolica sanguigna, anche se la pressione palpatoria in genere è di 10 mmHg inferiore a quella ottenuta per via auscultatoria. Il Doppler è un metodo estremamente accurato per la misurazione della pressione sanguigna sistolica; lo è meno per la pressione diastolica. Le tecniche oscillometriche sono usate frequentemente nei lattanti e nei bambini piccoli, ma non sono esenti da artefatti e risultano più attendibili per la misurazione della pressione media.

La pressione sanguigna aumenta gradualmente con l'età; i primi nomogrammi legati all'età sono stati sviluppati dai National Heart Lung and Blood Institutes nel 1977 e poi sottoposti a revisione (l'ultima volta nel 1996) per tenere conto delle differenze dovute a sesso ed età. Perciò sono necessari nomogrammi standard per l'interpretazione dei valori della pressione sanguigna (vedi Figg. 422-1 e 422-2). Se si riscontra un'ipertensione lieve, è imperativo che la misurazione venga ripetuta altre due volte in un periodo di 6 settimane. L'ansia di solito diminuisce quando il paziente prende confidenza con la procedura; perciò sono necessarie misurazioni ripetute per evitare di classificare un paziente come iperteso quando in realtà non lo è affatto. Una pressione sanguigna costantemente al di sopra del 95° percentile per l'età richiede ulteriori valutazioni. Un monitoraggio pressorio nelle ventiquattr'ore può essere particolarmente utile negli adolescenti che hanno un'ipertensione borderline, quando visitati in ambulatorio.

EZIOLOGIA E FISIOPATOLOGIA. La pressione sanguigna è il prodotto della gittata cardiaca e della resistenza vascolare periferica. Un aumento della gittata cardiaca o della resistenza periferica porta a un rialzo della pressione sanguigna; se uno di questi fattori aumenta mentre l'altro diminuisce, la pressione sanguigna può non aumentare. Quando l'ipertensione è la conseguenza di un altro processo patologico, è definita **ipertensione secondaria**, mentre in mancanza di una causa identificabile prende il nome di **ipertensione primitiva** o **essenziale**. Molti fattori, tra cui l'ereditarietà, la dieta, lo stress e l'obesità, possono giocare un ruolo nello sviluppo dell'ipertensione essenziale.

L'ipertensione secondaria è la più comune nei lattanti e nei bambini piccoli. Molte patologie dell'infanzia possono essere responsabili di un aumento acuto e cronico della pressione sanguigna (Tabb. 445-1 e 445-2). Le cause più probabili variano con l'età. L'ipertensione nel **neonato** è nella maggior parte dei casi associata a cateterismo dell'arteria ombelicale e trombosi dell'arteria renale, mentre nella **prima infanzia** può essere dovuta a una patologia renale, a una coartazione aortica, a endocrinopatie o a farmaci. Negli **adolescenti**, l'ipertensione essenziale è sempre più comune. La gravità dell'ipertensione è inoltre utile per distinguere l'ipertensione secondaria dal quella primitiva; bambini e adolescenti con ipertensione essenziale di solito hanno valori pressori solo pari o di poco superiori al 95° percentile per l'età.

L'**ipertensione renale** e **nefrovascolare** rende conto della maggior parte dei casi pediatrici di ipertensione secondaria. Un'anamnesi positiva per infezioni del tratto urinario è presente nel 25-50% di questi pazienti ed è spesso collegata a una lesione ostruttiva nel tratto urinario. Un'ipertensione nefrovascolare può essere associata a ritenzione di sodio e aumentata secrezione di renina. Altre lesioni renali parenchimali associate a ipertensione sono elencate nelle Tabelle 445-1 e 445-2. La ridotta velocità di filtrazione

TABELLA 445-1. Condizioni associate a ipertensione transitoria o intermittente nei bambini

RENALI
Glomerulonefrite acuta postinfettica
Porpora anafilattoide (Schönlein-Henoch) con nefrite
Sindrome emolitico-uremica
Necrosi tubulare acuta
Dopo trapianto di rene (immediatamente e durante gli episodi di rigetto)
Dopo trasfusione di sangue in pazienti con azotemia elevata
Ipervolemia
Dopo procedure chirurgiche sul tratto genitourinario
Pielonefrite
Traumi renali
Infiltrazione leucemica del rene
Uropatia ostruttiva associata a morbo di Crohn
FARMACI E SOSTANZE TOSSICHE
Cocaina
Contraccettivi orali
Agenti simpaticomimetici
Anfetamine
Fenciclidina
Corticosteroidi e ormone adrenocorticotropo
Trattamento con ciclosporina o sirolimus dopo trapianto
Liquirizia (acido glicirrizico)
Piombo, mercurio, cadmio, tallio
Sospensione di farmaci antipertensivi (clonidina, metildopa, propranololo)
Intossicazione da vitamina D
SISTEMA NERVOSO CENTRALE E AUTONOMO
Aumentata pressione endocranica
Sindrome di Guillain-Barré
Ustioni
Disautonomia familiare
Sindrome di Stevens-Johnson
Lesioni della fossa cranica posteriore
Porfiria
Poliomielite
Encefalite
VARIE
Preeclampsia
Fratture delle ossa lunghe
Ipercalcemia
Dopo riparazione di coartazione
Trasfusione di leucociti
Ossigenazione mediante membrana extracorporea
Ostruzione cronica delle vie aeree superiori

TABELLA 445-2. Condizioni associate a ipertensione cronica nei bambini

RENALI
Pielonefrite cronica
Glomerulonefrite cronica
Idronefrosi
Displasia renale congenita
Rene multicistico
Cisti renale solitaria
Nefropatia da reflusso vescica-ureterale
Ipoplasia segmentale (rene Ask-Upmark)
Ostruzione ureterale
Tumori renali
Traumi renali
Danno da rigetto a seguito di trapianto
Danno conseguente a radioterapia
Lupus eritematoso sistemico (altre malattie del tessuto connettivo)
VASCOLARI
Coartazione dell'aorta toracica o addominale
Lesioni dell'arteria renale (stenosi, displasia fibromuscolare, trombosi, aneurismi)
Cateterismo dell'arteria ombelicale con formazione di un trombo
Neurofibromatosi (intrinseca o estrinseca, che determina stenosi del lume vascolare)
Trombosi della vena renale
Vasculiti
Shunt arterovenoso
Sindrome di Williams-Beuren
Malattia Moyamoya
Arterite di Takayasu
ENDOCRINE
Ipertiroidismo
Iperparatiroidismo
Iperplasia surrenalica congenita (deficit di 11-β-idrossilasi e di 17-idrossilasi)
Sindrome di Cushing
Iperaldosteronismo primitivo
Iperaldosteronismo sopprimibile dal desametasone
Feocromocitoma
Altri tumori della cresta neurale (neuroblastoma, ganglioneuroblastoma, ganglioneuroma)
Nefropatia diabetica
Sindrome di Lille
SISTEMA NERVOSO CENTRALE
Massa intracranica
Emorragia
Sequele di danno cerebrale
Tetraplegia
IPERTENSIONE ESSENZIALE
A bassa renina
A renina normale
A elevata renina

glomerulare nei pazienti con nefrite porta a ritenzione di sali e acqua, mentre lesioni formanti massa (cisti, tumori solidi, ematomi) possono compromettere la perfusione renale e stimolare la produzione di renina da parte dell'apparato iuxtaglomerulare. Sia il tumore di Wilms sia il tumore a cellule iuxtaglomerulari (emangiopericitoma) possono secernere renina o altre sostanze che inducono ipertensione senza controllo a feedback.

Lesioni come una stenosi dell'arteria renale possono causare un'ipertensione attraverso la stimolazione del sistema renina-angiotensina-aldosterone. La renina è un enzima proteolitico secreto dalle cellule iuxtaglomerulari che converte l'angiotensinogeno in angiotensina I. La sua secrezione dipende dalla pressione di perfusione dell'arteriola afferente nel rene, dalla concentrazione di sodio nel plasma e nell'urina nei tubuli, dall'attivazione del sistema nervoso simpatico e da altri fattori come le prostaglandine, l'introito di potassio e i peptidi natriuretici. L'angiotensina I possiede scarsa attività fisiologica e viene rapidamente convertita in angiotensina II dall'enzima convertente l'angiotensina (ACE, *Angiotensin-Converting Enzyme*), il quale è responsabile anche della degradazione metabolica delle chinine vasodilatatrici. L'angiotensina II, oltre a essere un potente vasocostrittore, stimola la secrezione di aldosterone, che porta alla ritenzione di sodio e acqua.

Numerose **endocrinopatie** sono associate a ipertensione, di solito quelle che coinvolgono la tiroide, le paratiroidi e le ghiandole surrenaliche. Ipertensione sistolica e tachicardia sono comuni nell'ipertiroidismo; la pressione diastolica di solito non è elevata. L'ipercalcemia, secondaria a iperparatiroidismo o ad altre cause, spesso porta a un lieve aumento della pressione sanguigna, dovuto a un aumento del tono vascolare. Le malattie della corticale del surrene (tumori secernenti aldosterone, iperplasia surrenalica congenita, sindrome di Cushing) possono causare ipertensione in pazienti con aumentata secrezione di mineralcorticoidi. I feocromocitomi sono tumori secernenti catecolamine che danno luogo a ipertensione a causa degli effetti cardiaci e vascolari periferici dell'adrenalina e della noradrenalina. I bambini con feocromocitoma di solito hanno un'ipertensione sostenuta anziché intermittente o indotta dall'esercizio fisico (vedi Capitolo 581). Il feocromocitoma si sviluppa in circa il 5% dei pazienti con neurofibromatosi. Un alterato tono simpatico può essere responsabile di un aumento acuto o intermittente della pressione sanguigna nei bambini con sindrome di Guillain-Barré, poliomielite, ustioni e sindrome di Stevens-Johnson. Il rilascio simpatico dal sistema nervoso centrale è influenzato anche da lesioni intracraniche.

Negli adolescenti un certo numero di **sostanze stupefacenti**, farmaci e tossine può causare ipertensione. La cocaina può provocare un rapido aumento della pressione sanguigna provocando convulsioni o emorragia intracranica. La fenciclidina causa un'ipertensione transitoria che può divenire persistente in chi ne abusa cronicamente. Anche il consumo di tabacco può aumentare la pressione sanguigna. I simpaticomimetici utilizzati come decongestionanti nasali, anoressizzanti e stimolanti per pazienti affetti da sindrome da deficit d'attenzione producono vasocostrizione e stimolazione cardiaca di grado variabile. Ciascun individuo presenta una suscettibilità individuale a questi effetti. I contraccettivi orali dovrebbero essere sospettati quale causa di ipertensione nelle adolescenti, anche se l'incidenza è bassa con l'utilizzo di preparazioni a basso contenuto di estrogeni. Farmaci immunosoppressori come la ciclosporina e il tacrolimus causano ipertensione nei pazienti sottoposti a trapianto d'organo, e i loro effetti sono esacerbati dalla contemporanea somministrazione di steroidi. La pressione sanguigna può essere elevata in pazienti con avvelenamento da metalli pesanti.

L'ipertensione essenziale, la forma più comune negli adulti, viene riconosciuta più spesso negli adolescenti che nei bambini piccoli. È spesso accompagnata da una forte storia familiare. La sua causa è probabilmente multifattoriale: sono stati chiamati in causa l'obesità, alterazioni genetiche del trasporto di calcio e sodio, un'iperreattività della muscolatura liscia vascolare, il sistema renina-angiotensina e la resistenza all'insulina. Bambini normotesi figli di genitori ipertesi possono presentare anomale risposte fisiologiche, simili a quelle dei loro genitori. Quando sottoposti a stress o a incarichi competitivi, i figli di adulti ipertesi, come gruppo, reagiscono con un aumento della frequenza cardiaca e della pressione sanguigna maggiore rispetto ai bambini di genitori normotesi. Analogamente, alcuni bambini figli di genitori ipertesi possono presentare un'escrezione urinaria di metaboliti delle catecolamine più elevata del normale oppure rispondere al carico di sodio con maggiori aumenti di peso e della pressione sanguigna rispetto a quelli senza storia familiare di ipertensione. La risposta anomala in bambini con genitori affetti da ipertensione tende a essere maggiore tra i neri rispetto ai bianchi. Il trasporto eritrocitario di sodio, la concentrazione di calcio libero nelle piastrine e nei leucociti, l'escrezione urinaria di callicreina e i recettori simpatici del sistema nervoso centrale sono stati studiati come altri possibili marker di un successivo sviluppo di ipertensione.

La classificazione dell'ipertensione essenziale in base ai livelli di attività della renina plasmatica (elevata, normale, bassa) si è rivelata utile per la comprensione della fisiopatologia e per lo sviluppo di schemi terapeutici per pazienti adulti; studi analoghi su ampia scala non sono stati invece condotti su adolescenti con ipertensione primitiva. Moltissimi pazienti adulti con ipertensione essenziale sembrano essere particolarmente sensibili all'assunzione di sodio. Il meccanismo della sodio-sensibilità non è chiaro e potrebbe riguardare lo ione cloro anziché il sodio. Un sottogruppo di soggetti sodio-sensibili sembra avere una compromissione della capacità di escrezione urinaria di un carico di sodio. I peptici natriuretici atriali stimolano l'escrezione di sodio da parte dei reni; è oggetto di studio il loro ruolo nel mantenimento di una normale pressione sanguigna e nello sviluppo di ipertensione.

Il tracking della pressione sanguigna è il processo mediante il quale i soggetti mantengono il loro livello di pressione sanguigna nel tempo rispetto a individui di pari età. Bambini e adolescenti con pressione sanguigna >90° percentile per l'età hanno una probabilità quasi tre volte maggiore di divenire adulti ipertesi rispetto ai bambini con pressione sanguigna al 50° percentile. Gli adolescenti con ipertensione essenziale possono progredire da un'elevata gittata cardiaca e normale resistenza vascolare sistemica al pattern adulto di normale gittata cardiaca con elevata resistenza vascolare sistemica. Sono emerse differenze razziali: adulti di razza nera affetti da ipertensione hanno un maggiore aumento della resistenza periferica, mentre adulti ipertesi di razza bianca prevalentemente presentano un aumento della gittata cardiaca.

MANIFESTAZIONI CLINICHE. I bambini e gli adolescenti con ipertensione essenziale di solito sono asintomatici; l'aumento della pressione sanguigna in genere è lieve e viene riscontrato durante una visita medica di routine o durante una valutazione per la partecipazione ad attività sportive. Questi soggetti possono presentare un'obesità lieve o moderata.

I bambini con ipertensione secondaria possono andare incontro ad aumenti della pressione sanguigna da lievi a gravi. A meno che la pressione non sia costantemente elevata o aumenti rapidamente, l'ipertensione di solito rimane asintomatica. Perciò le manifestazioni cliniche della malattia sottostante, come un ritardo di crescita in bambini con nefropatia cronica, sono i motivi più frequenti per i quali viene riscontrata l'ipertensione. Le caratteristiche utili a fini diagnostici, riscontrabili all'esame obiettivo, sono elencate nella Tabella 445-3. Con un'ipertensione sostanziale possono verificarsi cefalea, capogiri, epistassi, anoressia, disturbi del visus e convulsioni. Vomito, temperatura elevata, atassia, stupor e convulsioni sono indicativi di un'**encefalopatia ipertensiva**. Indipendentemente dalla sua causa, una marcata ipertensione dà luogo a una disfunzione degli organi bersaglio (cuore e rene).

Bambini piccoli e lattanti con scompenso cardiaco inspiegato o convulsioni dovrebbero essere sottoposti a misurazione della pressione arteriosa. Tali pazienti non sono in grado di riferire i propri sintomi, per esempio la cefalea, e il loro comportamento può non essere considerato anomalo finché non si manifestano le complicanze dell'ipertensione. Dopo che la pressione sanguigna è stata abbassata, i genitori di lattanti affetti da ipertensione spesso riferiscono retrospettivamente che il bambino ha sviluppato una crescente irritabilità prima che l'ipertensione venisse alla luce.

TABELLA 445-3. Reperti da ricercare all'esame obiettivo

REPERTI OBIETTIVI	POTENZIALE RILEVANZA
GENERALI	
Pallore delle mucose, edema, ritardo di crescita	Nefropatia cronica
Facies a elfo, scarsa crescita, ritardo mentale	Sindrome di Williams
Pliche del collo, impianto basso dell'attaccatura dei capelli, capezzoli molto distanziati, gomito valgo	Sindrome di Turner
Facies a luna piena, gibbo di bufalo, irsutismo, obesità truncale, strie	Sindrome di Cushing
HABITUS	
Magrezza	Feocromocitoma, nefropatia, ipertiroidismo
Virilizzazione	Iperplasia surrenalica congenita
Rachitismo	Nefropatia cronica
CUTE	
Macchie caffelatte, neurofibromi	Neurofibromatosi, feocromocitoma
Tuberosità, macchie "a foglia di frassino"	Sclerosi tuberosa
Rash	LES, vasculiti (porpora di Schönlein-Henoch), impetigine con nefrite acuta
Pallore, flushing evanescente, sudorazione	Feocromocitoma
Segni di puntura	Abuso di droghe
Ecchimosi, strie	Sindrome di Cushing
OCCHI	
Paralisi dei muscoli extraoculari	Aspecifica, cronica, grave
Cambiamenti del fundus	Aspecifici, cronici, gravi
Proptosi	Ipertiroidismo
TESTA E COLLO	
Gozzo	Patologia tiroidea
SEGNI CARDIOVASCOLARI	
Assenza o diminuzione dei polsi femorali, pressione più bassa negli arti inferiori che in quelli superiori	Coartazione aortica
Dimensione del cuore, frequenza, ritmo; soffi; difficoltà respiratoria, epatomegalia	Coartazione aortica, scompenso cardiaco congestizio
Soffio a livello dei grandi vasi	Arterite o arteriopatia
Sfregamenti	Versamento pericardico secondario a nefropatia cronica
SEGNI POLMONARI	
Edema polmonare	Scompenso cardiaco congestizio, nefrite acuta
Quadro di displasia broncopolmonare	Ipertensione associata a displasia broncopolmonare
ADDOME	
Soffio epigastrico	Patologia nefrovascolare primitiva, o in associazione a sindrome di Williams, neurofibromatosi, displasia fibromuscolare o arterite
Masse addominali	Tumore, di Wilms, neuroblastoma, feocromocitoma, reni policistici, idronefrosi
SEGNI NEUROLOGICI	
Deficit neurologici	Ipertensione cronica o acuta grave con ictus
GENITALI	
Ambigui, virilizzazione	Iperplasia surrenalica congenita

LES, lupus eritematoso sistemico. Da Kliegman RM, Greenbaum LA, Lye PS: *Practical Strategies in Pediatric Diagnosis and Therapy*, 2nd ed, Philadelphia, Elsevier, 2004, p 200.

DIAGNOSI. La diagnosi di ipertensione essenziale è suggerita dall'età del paziente (di solito adolescente), dall'entità dell'aumento della pressione sanguigna (di solito lieve), dal peso corporeo (obesità da lieve a moderata) e dalla scarsità di segni e sintomi di una patologia sottostante. Non è comune fare diagnosi in bambini di età <10 anni. L'obesità è associata all'ipertensione essenziale, ma è raro che i pazienti con ipertensione secondaria siano obesi, a meno che non abbiano patologie della corticale del surrene. Anche l'ereditarietà è un importante fattore che influisce sulla pressione sanguigna; perciò è poco probabile che un adolescente con lieve aumento della pressione e forte storia familiare di ipertensione essenziale abbia una patologia sottostante. Se la pressione sanguigna continua ad aumentare nel giro di settimane o mesi dall'osservazione, sono indicate ulteriori procedure diagnostiche per escludere la possibilità di una causa di ipertensione secondaria.

La diagnosi di ipertensione secondaria è suggerita anche dall'età del paziente (giovane), dall'entità dell'aumento pressorio (da lieve a estremo) e dalla presenza di sintomi. L'anamnesi talvolta comprende malattie febbrili intermittenti, che possono suggerire un'intercorrente infezione del tratto urinario (nefropatia da reflusso). Occorre raccogliere un'anamnesi familiare mirata a patologie renali o patologie cardiovascolari in età prematura. È importante procedere ad accurate misurazioni di altezza e peso, parametri che sono spesso inferiori alla norma nei bambini con malattie croniche. L'esame obiettivo dovrebbe determinare la presenza di masse al fianco o di soffi addominali. L'esame obiettivo dovrebbe sempre comprendere la palpazione dei polsi a tutte le estremità e la misurazione della pressione sanguigna in entrambe le braccia e a una gamba, per valutare la possibile presenza di una coartazione aortica. Nei bambini la pressione sistolica agli arti inferiori dovrebbe essere di 10-20 mmHg superiore a quella riscontrata negli arti superiori. I **test di screening** dovrebbero comprendere un emocromo completo, l'esame delle urine, il dosaggio degli elettroliti sierici, l'azotemia, la creatininemia, il calcio e i livelli di acido urico. Si consiglia di eseguire l'urinocoltura anche se l'esame del sedimento urinario non presenta alterazioni. Un profilo lipidico è indicato se l'anamnesi familiare è suggestiva o si sospetta un'ipertensione primitiva. L'ecocardiogramma è utile nella valutazione della cronicità dell'ipertensione, che, se di vecchia data, dovrebbe portare a un'ipertrofia ventricolare.

L'ecografia renale permette di confrontare le dimensioni dei due reni e visualizzare l'anatomia del sistema di escrezione. Una scintigrafia è utile per rilevare variazioni nella perfusione o la presenza di eventuali cicatrici nei due reni. L'eco-Doppler renale e l'angiografia renale possono evidenziare lesioni a carico delle arterie principali o delle branche segmentarie; se si effettua un'angiografia, si dovrebbero prelevare campioni di sangue venoso da entrambe le vene renali e dalla vena cava inferiore per il dosaggio dell'attività reninica plasmatica. L'eco-Doppler può evidenziare un anomalo flusso sanguigno arterioso e venoso.

La determinazione dell'attività della renina plasmatica su sangue periferico è un utile test di screening per le patologie nefrovascolari e per quelle del parenchima renale. I valori normali diminuiscono gradualmente con l'età e variano da un laboratorio all'altro. Un valore basso suggerisce un effetto mineralcorticoide eccessivo, mentre uno elevato è associato a un coinvolgimento renale o nefrovascolare. Si raccomanda inoltre di dosare le catecolamine urinarie, come pure gli steroidi plasmatici e urinari. Un approccio all'adolescente con ipertensione è riassunto nella Figura 445-1. Un test di gravidanza può essere utile in una giovane donna sessualmente attiva in cui viene riscontrata un'ipertensione (preeclampsia). Nella Figura 445-2 viene presentato un approccio diagnostico iniziale all'ipertensione.

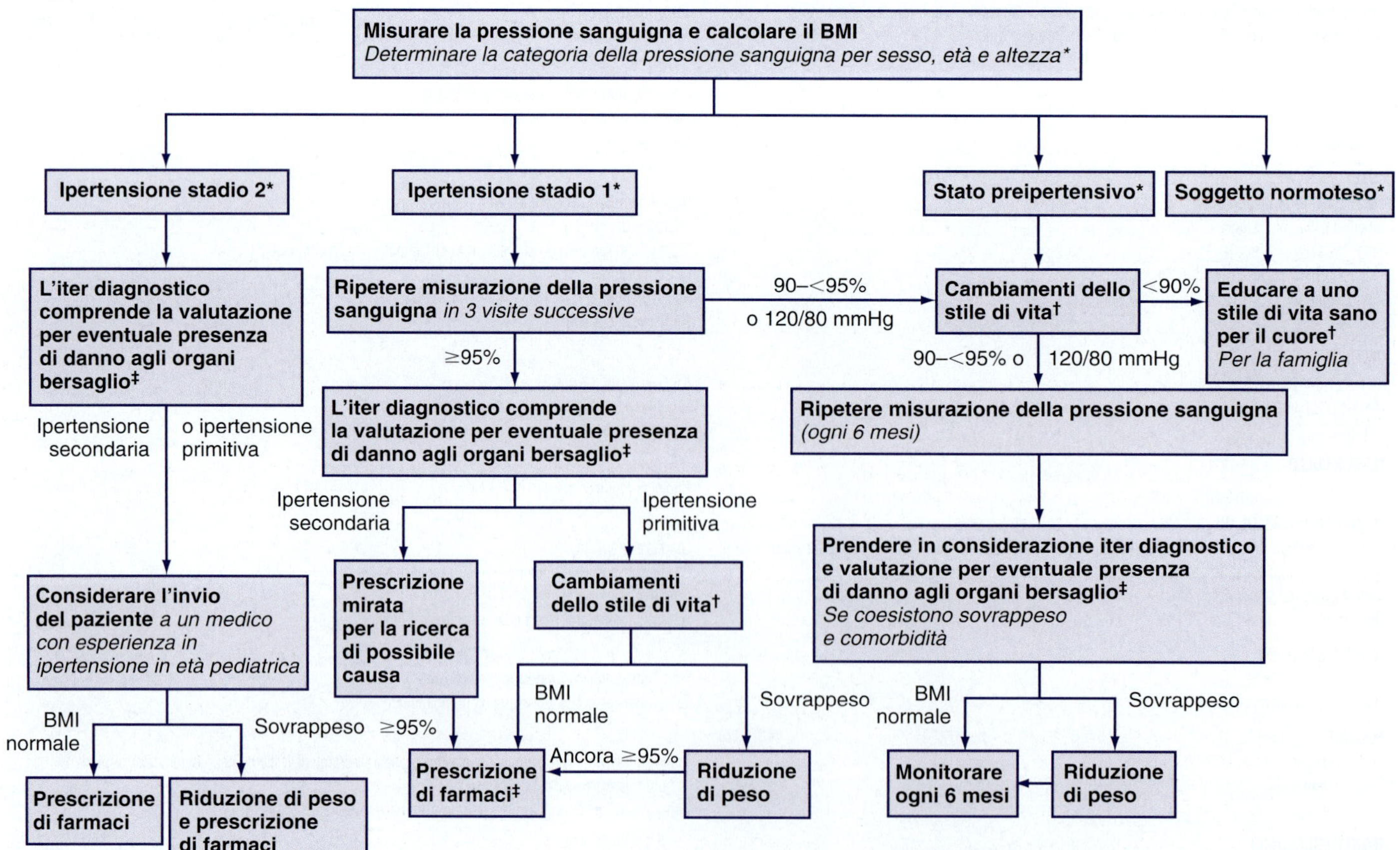

Figura 445-1. Algoritmi gestionali. BMI (*Body Mass Index*), indice di massa corporea; †modificazione della dieta e attività fisica; ‡specialmente nei bambini più piccoli, se la pressione sanguigna è molto elevata, se vi è una storia familiare scarsa o nulla, nei diabetici o in presenza di altri fattori di rischio. (Da National High Blood Pressure Education Program Working Group on High Blood Pressure in Children and Adolescents: The fourth report on the diagnosis, evaluation, and treatment of high blood pressure in children and adolescents. *Pediatrics* 2004;114:555-576.)

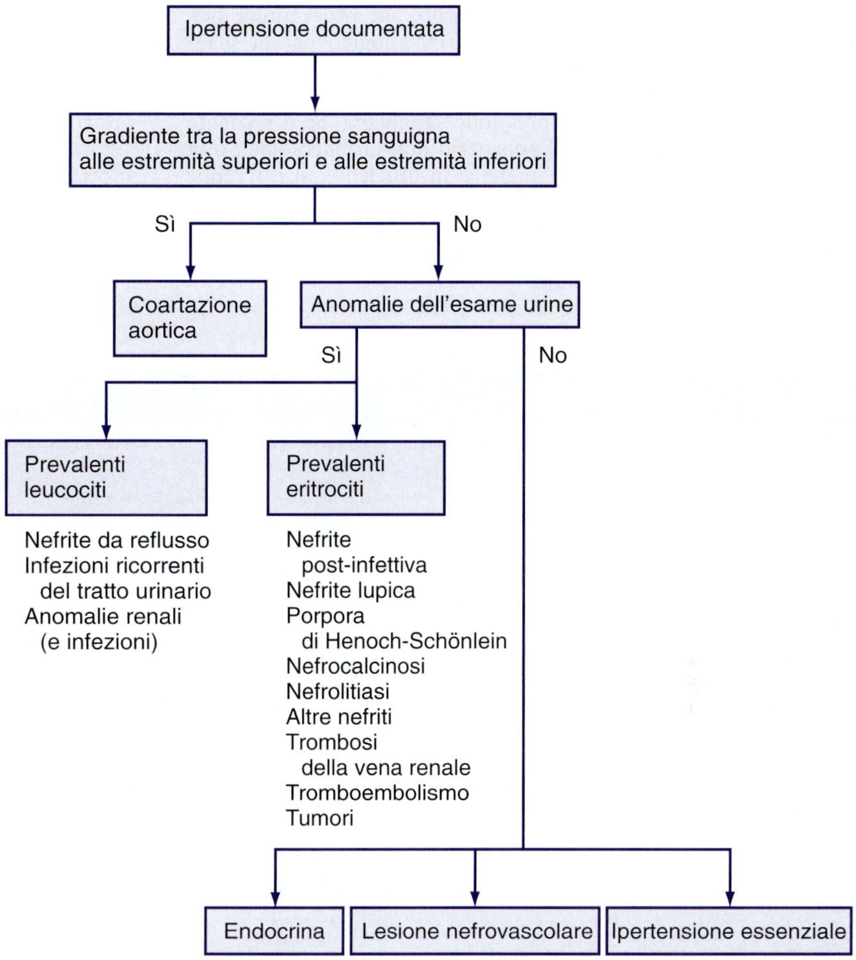

Figura 445-2. Algoritmo diagnostico iniziale nella valutazione dell'ipertensione. Da Kliegman RM, Greenbaum LA, Lye PS: *Practical Strategies in Pediatric Diagnosis and Therapy*, 2nd ed., Philadelphia, Elsevier, 2004, p. 222

DECORSO E PROGNOSI. La storia naturale dell'ipertensione essenziale che viene inizialmente riscontrata nell'infanzia o nell'adolescenza è oggetto di studio in studi di popolazione su vasta scala e a lungo termine. Molti di questi bambini continuano ad avere un'ipertensione essenziale da adulti, anche se la correlazione non è perfetta. Negli adulti con ipertensione essenziale, la terapia farmacologia si è rivelata efficace nel ridurre l'incidenza di scompenso cardiaco congestizio, insufficienza renale e ictus.

La prognosi per un bambini con ipertensione secondaria è determinata principalmente dalla natura della malattia sottostante e dalla risposta di questa alla terapia specifica. La sopravvivenza in un paziente con nefropatia sottostante dipende dalla risposta alla dialisi e dal successo del trapianto renale. In presenza di una patologia nefrovascolare, il grado di incremento dell'attività reninica nella vena renale può aiutare a predire la risposta alla terapia. Una discrepanza nella secrezione di renina tra i due reni >1,5:1 significa che il rene che produce il livello più alto è il principale responsabile dell'ipertensione. In questo caso, la correzione chirurgica ha elevate probabilità di ottenere un notevole miglioramento o una risoluzione dell'ipertensione. La prognosi dopo riparazione chirurgica della coartazione aortica è variabile e parzialmente dipendente dall'età a cui viene effettuata la correzione. La maggior parte dei pazienti operati durante la prima infanzia presenta valori pressori sistemici stabilmente normali dopo l'intervento chirurgico, a meno che non vi sia una recidiva della coartazione; i pazienti in cui viene fatta la diagnosi durante l'adolescenza, tuttavia, sono a rischio di persistenza di valori pressori elevati. La prognosi a lungo termine è favorevole per i neonati che sviluppano ipertensione come complicanza di un cateterismo dell'arteria ombelicale. Pochi tra questi bambini richiedono una terapia oltre i 12 mesi di vita e la maggior parte di essi presenta un notevole miglioramento della perfusione renale.

PREVENZIONE. La prevenzione dell'ipertensione può essere considerata parte integrante della prevenzione delle patologie cardiovascolari e dell'ictus, le principali cause di morte negli Stati Uniti. Altri fattori di rischio per patologie cardiovascolari comprendono obesità, elevati livelli di colesterolo sierico, elevato apporto dietetico di sodio, uno stile di vita sedentario e il consumo di alcol e tabacco. A partire dall'infanzia e per tutta l'adolescenza è particolarmente importante scoraggiare il fumo di sigaretta, a causa delle conseguenze polmonari e cardiovascolari. L'aumento della rigidità della parete arteriosa e della viscosità ematica che è associato a esposizione a componenti del tabacco può causare o peggiorare l'ipertensione. Approcci per la prevenzione dell'ipertensione essenziale comprendono una riduzione dell'apporto di sodio e un aumento dell'attività fisica tramite programmi scolastici.

TRATTAMENTO. Lo scopo della terapia antipertensiva dovrebbe essere la riduzione della pressione sanguigna al di sotto del 95° percentile per l'età. Per il trattamento di bambini con pressione sanguigna elevata sono utili sia gli approcci non farmacologici sia quelli farmacologici. Negli adolescenti con ipertensione essenziale la scelta migliore consiste nell'iniziare con una terapia non farmacologica. L'intervento dovrebbe essere focalizzato sui fattori di rischio più importanti citati nel paragrafo "Prevenzione". Poiché molti pazienti con lieve aumento della pressione sono obesi, una riduzione di peso può portare a una diminuzione della pressione sistolica di 5-10 mmHg. Una riduzione dell'introito di sodio spesso ottiene un effetto analogo, anche se è meno efficace nei bambini che negli adulti. Un programma coerente di esercizi aerobici riduce la pressione sanguigna nei pazienti con ipertensione essenziale lieve. Tale programma deve essere continuato per essere efficace a lungo termine. In considerazione di questi benefici e degli effetti indesiderati di molti farmaci antipertensivi, dovrebbe essere preferibilmente prescritto un programma ben supervisionato di trattamento non farmacologico per la maggior parte dei giovani pazienti con ipertensione essenziale. Gli adolescenti dovrebbero essere avvertiti circa gli effetti negativi del tabacco e dell'alcol sulla pressione sanguigna. Se il paziente non è in grado di attenersi all'approccio non farmacologico o la riduzione della pressione sanguigna è insufficiente, si dovrebbe prendere in esame un trattamento farmacologico antipertensivo. Gli adolescenti che non riescono a cambiare il proprio stile di vita è molto probabile che saranno poco inclini a seguire un regime farmacologico a lungo termine.

Per molti bambini con ipertensione secondaria e per pazienti selezionati con ipertensione essenziale, si rende necessaria una terapia farmacologica. Vi è un consenso generale sulla necessità di trattare i pazienti pediatrici con ipertensione essenziale in cui i valori della pressione sanguigna si mantengono persistentemente >99° percentile. Minore è invece l'accordo sull'approccio da adottare nel caso di bambini con ipertensione essenziale i cui valori di pressione sanguigna siano compresi tra il 95° e il 99° percentile. Sono disponibili numerosi farmaci antipertensivi sia per le emergenze ipertensive sia per la terapia in cronico (Tab. 445-4). È difficile determinare l'efficacia a lungo termine della

TABELLA 445-4. Farmaci antipertensivi

FARMACO	MECCANISMO D'AZIONE	RANGE DI DOSAGGIO	VIA DI SOMMINISTRAZIONE	DURATA D'AZIONE	EFFETTI COLLATERALI
VASODILATATORI ARTERIOSI	Rilassano il muscolo liscio delle arteriole	0,1-0,4 mg/kg/dose	ev	4-6 h	Tachicardia, nausea
		0,25-1 mg/kg/dose e aumentare fino a un massimo di 200 mg/24 h	per os	6-12 h	Lupus indotto da farmaci
		0,25-1 mg/kg/dose e aumentare fino a un massimo di 200 mg/24 h			
Nitroprussiato di sodio	Dilatazione di arteriole e venule	0,3-8,0 μg/kg/min	ev	Finché dura l'infusione	Produzione di tiocianati, raramente ipotiroidismo
Minoxidil	Dilatazione arteriolare	Dose iniziale 0,1-0,2 mg/kg/2 h, max 5 mg. Aumentare gradualmente a 0,25-1,0 mg/kg/24 h fino a un massimo di 50 mg	per os	12-24 h	Ipertricosi, ritenzione idrica
BLOCCANTI ADRENERGICI					
Esmololo	Bloccante β-adrenergico	50-300 μg/kg/min	ev	Finché dura l'infusione	Ipotensione, broncospasmo
Fentolamina	Bloccante i recettori α	0,05-0,1 mg/kg/dose fino a un massimo di 20 mg	ev	1-2 h	Tachicardia, Capogiri, congestione nasale, dolore toracico
Fenossibenzamina	Bloccante i recettori α	0,2-2,0 mg/kg/24 h, singola dose max 40 mg	per os	8-12 h	Congestione nasale, capogiri, tachicardia, aritmie
Prazosin	Bloccante i recettori α	0,005-0,1 mg/kg/dose	per os	6-12 h	Ipotensione ortostatica da prima dose
Propranololo	Bloccante i recettori β Riduce il rilascio di renina	0,01-0,1 mg/kg/dose 0,5-8,0 mg/kg/24 h	ev in bolo lento per os	6-8 h	Broncospasmo, bradicardia, sogni vividi
Atenololo	β-bloccante	1-2 mg/kg/24 h	per os	24 h	Broncospasmo, tachicardia
Labetalolo	α- e β-bloccante	0,2-1,0 mg/kg/dose (dose max 20 mg) 0,25-2,0 mg/kg/h 1-3 mg/kg/24 h	ev in bolo ev in infusione continua per os	Per tutta la durata dell'infusione 6-12 h	Ipotensione ortostatica, capogiri, broncospasmo
Clonidina	Agonista α-2 a livello del SNC	0,005-0,025 mg/kg/24 h inizialmente Max 0,9 mg/24 h	per os	6-12 h	Sedazione, stipsi, rebound da sospensione, ipertensione
INIBITORI DEL SISTEMA RENINA-ANGIOTENSINA					
Captopril	Inibizione dell'enzima di conversione dell'angiotensina (ACE)	Neonati <2 mesi: 0,05-0,1 mg/kg/dose fino a 0,5 mg/kg/dose	per os	8-24 h	Proteinuria, neutropenia, rash, disgeusia, tosse cronica
		Lattanti e bambini: 0,15-0,5 mg/kg/dose fino a 6 mg/kg/24 h	per os	8-12 h	
		Bambini più grandi e adolescenti: 6,25-25 mg/dose fino a 450 mg/24 h	per os	8-12 h	
Enalaprilat	ACE-inibitore	0,005-0,010 mg/kg/dose; adulti 0,625-1,25 mg/dose	ev in 5 minuti	8-24 h	Ipotensione transitoria
Enalapril	ACE-inibitore	Bambini: 0,1-0,5 mg/kg/24 h Adolescenti: 2,5-5 mg/24 h fino a 40 mg/24 h	per os	12-24 h	Ipotensione
CALCIOANTAGONISTI					
Nifedipina	Calcioantagonista	Bambini: 0,25-0,5 mg/kg/dose, max 5 mg/dose, max 1-2 mg/kg/24 h	per os, sl	Ripetere ogni 4-6 h	Flushing al viso, tachicardica
Nicardipina	Calcioantagonista	1-3 μg/kg/min	ev	Per tutta la durata dell'infusione	Tachicardia, ipotensione, cefalea
Amlodipina	Calcioantagonista	0,1-0,6 mg/kg/24 h, max 5 mg/24 h	per os	24 h	Edema , capogiri, flushing, palpitaszioni
DIURETICI					
Idroclorotiazide	Diuretico	1-2 mg/kg/24 h, max 200 mg/24 h	per os	12-24 h	Ipokaliemia iperuricemia, ipercalcemia
Furosemide	Diuretico	1 mg/kg/dose 1-2 mg/kg/dose fino a 6 mg/kg/24 h	ev per os	4-6 h 6-12 h	Ipokaliemia, alcalosi
Bumetanide	Diuretico	0,015-0,1 mg/kg/dose, max 10 mg/24 h	per os	6-24 h	Ipokaliemia, iperglicemia, iperuricemia

Nota: le dosi pediatriche basate sul peso corporeo non dovrebbero essere superiori alle dosi previste per l'adulto. Dal momento che le indicazioni possono cambiare, questi dosaggi dovrebbero essere sempre ricontrollati. Inoltre è necessario modificarli in pazienti con disfunzione renale o epatica.
ev, via endovenosa; sl, sublinguale.

terapia antipertensiva negli adolescenti, dato il follow-up di decenni richiesto per esaminare gli effetti sulle patologie cardiovascolari. Possono dimostrarsi utili numerosi end-point surrogati, come l'ipertrofia ventricolare sinistra, la disfunzione endoteliale, lo spessore mediointimale dell'arteria carotide, la presenza di calcificazioni delle arterie coronarie (alla TC) e il reperto di microalbuminuria. Al momento di decidere se iniziare o meno una terapia farmacologica, si dovrebbe ricordare che non è noto se instaurare tale trattamento nei primi anni di vita anziché nell'età adulta riduca il rischio di successive patologie cardiovascolari. La maggior parte dei farmaci antipertensivi non è stata testata sui bambini in maniera approfondita, mentre è proprio in questo gruppo di età che il rischio connesso all'utilizzo di tali farmaci può essere più elevato, data la più lunga durata di somministrazione e l'esposizione del paziente ai farmaci proprio durante la crescita e lo sviluppo.

In risposta a una **crisi ipertensiva**, è importante scegliere un farmaco con un inizio d'azione rapido e prevedibile, e monitorare attentamente la pressione sanguigna mentre è in corso la sua riduzione. Poiché l'encefalopatia ipertensiva è una possibile complicanza di emergenze ipertensive, si dovrebbe optare per agenti antipertensivi con minimi effetti collaterali a carico del sistema nervoso centrale, per evitare che si crei confusione tra i sintomi della malattia e gli effetti collaterali del farmaco stesso. Spesso si preferisce la somministrazione endovenosa cosicché il calo della pressione sanguigna possa essere accuratamente modulato. Poiché una riduzione troppo rapida della pressione sanguigna può interferire con la perfusione dei vari organi, si dovrebbe programmare una riduzione graduale della pressione. In generale, la pressione andrebbe ridotta per un terzo nelle prime 6 ore e dei restanti due terzi nelle successive 48-72 ore.

Nella maggior parte delle emergenze ipertensive, i **farmaci di scelta** sono il **labetalolo**, il **nitroprussiato di sodio** o la **nifedipina** sublinguale. Il labetalolo blocca i recettori α e β-adrenergici; con una singola dose seguita dall'infusione continua si può ottenere una riduzione controllata della pressione sanguigna. Un simile controllo è possibile con un'infusione di nitroprussiato. La nifedipina ha un inizio d'azione rapido, ma si deve prevedere una breve durata d'azione. Poiché tale farmaco è disponibile solo in forma liquida all'interno di una capsula, la somministrazione ai bambini più piccoli ha presentato qualche difficoltà. Anche se spesso è stata somministrata per via sublinguale al fine di ottenere un rapido assorbimento, anche l'assorbimento gastrointestinale è abbastanza rapido da rendere la nifedipina efficace in caso di crisi ipertensiva. Altri farmaci utili per le emergenze ipertensive comprendono l'esmololo e la nicardipina. La maggior parte dei bambini con crisi ipertensive ha una nefropatia acuta o cronica; in questi pazienti la gestione della pressione sanguigna richiede anche una particolare attenzione al bilancio di fluidi e alla diuresi. La furosemide per via endovenosa è di solito efficace, anche se può essere compromessa la filtrazione glomerulare.

Per poter scegliere il regime farmacologico in vista di un utilizzo a lungo termine, è utile comprendere il meccanismo fisiopatologico sottostante. Dal momento che sono disponibili farmaci con differenti siti e meccanismi d'azione, il trattamento può essere mirato alla condizione patologica specifica. Per esempio, un'eccessiva attività del sistema renina-angiotensina-aldosterone può essere trattata efficacemente con un farmaco β-bloccante (propranololo) per la soppressione della secrezione di renina, con un ACE-inibitore (captopril o enalapril) o, raramente, con un antagonista dell'aldosterone (per es. spironolattone). Gli ACE-inibitori sono utili non solo nei pazienti con ipertensione associata a elevata renina, secondaria a una patologia nefrovascolare o parenchimale renale, ma anche in quelli con ipertensione essenziale a elevata renina. Un'eccessiva produzione di angiotensina è la causa probabile della maggior parte dei casi di ipertensione nei neonati dopo l'occlusione parziale di un vaso renale da parte di un trombo. Il captopril o l'enalapril sono agenti efficaci nella maggior parte di questi pazienti, ma devono essere utilizzati con particolare attenzione alla funzionalità renale. Gli α-bloccanti adrenergici (fentolamina, fenoxibenzamina) apportano beneficio ai pazienti con tumori della cresta neurale che hanno elevati livelli circolanti di catecolamine. In tali pazienti sono necessari anche farmaci β-bloccanti per controllare la frequenza cardiaca, o è possibile utilizzare un farmaco con duplice azione bloccante (labetalolo). Il blocco simpatico con labetalolo è ugualmente efficace in pazienti che presentano una marcata stimolazione del sistema cardiovascolare da overdose di cocaina.

I pazienti giovani con ipertensione essenziale che richiedono una terapia farmacologica possono inizialmente essere trattati con un diuretico o un β-bloccante. Quelli con ipertensione volume-dipendente di solito presentano un'adeguata risposta ai diuretici, mentre quelli con elevata renina ed elevata gittata cardiaca rispondono meglio ai β-bloccanti. L'utilizzo cronico di diuretici può portare a un aumento dei lipidi sierici, che a sua volta aumenta il rischio di cardiopatia ischemica in adulti affetti da ipertensione. Non sono disponibili studi a lungo termine di questo effetto collaterale su pazienti pediatrici. I farmaci β-bloccanti sono stati associati anche a cambiamenti nei lipidi sierici, e alcuni studi suggeriscono una lieve riduzione della tolleranza allo sforzo in pazienti trattati con propranololo. Gli individui affetti da una patologia reattiva delle vie aeree spesso non sono in grado di tollerare un β-bloccante.

A causa di questi effetti collaterali, per la terapia iniziale di un adolescente con significativa ipertensione possono essere presi in considerazione gli ACE-inibitori o i calcioantagonisti. Anche se il captopril è stato utilizzato più spesso nei pazienti giovani, l'enalapril ha una più lunga durata d'azione e perciò richiede una somministrazione meno frequente.

In soggetti con ipertensione di vecchia data o poco controllata, il meccanismo fisiopatologico sottostante è spesso complesso. In tali pazienti a volte è necessario fare più di un tentativo con varie combinazioni di farmaci antipertensivi per controllare una pressione notevolmente elevata o in labile controllo. Il principio di base è la somministrazione combinata di farmaci con diverse sedi o meccanismi d'azione. Poiché la compliance può diventare un problema, il regime farmacologico dovrebbe essere il più semplice possibile e sfruttare i farmaci a maggiore durata d'azione che possano essere somministrati una o due volte al giorno, quando disponibili. Un calendario farmacologico, la supervisione dei genitori e una buona comunicazione medico-paziente, inoltre, aiutano ad assicurare una buona compliance.

L'angioplastica percutanea mediante palloncino può curare fino al 50% dei pazienti con stenosi dell'arteria renale secondaria a displasia fibromuscolare, mentre non ha successo per la stenosi dell'arteria renale dovuta a placche aterosclerotiche Se l'angioplastica fallisce, può essere indicato il posizionamento di uno stent intravascolare o un intervento chirurgico.

Bartosh SM, Aronson AJ: Childhood hypertension. An update on etiology, diagnosis, and treatment. *Pediatr Clin North Am* 1999;46:235–252.

Blaszak RT, Savage JA, Ellis EN: The use of short-acting nifedipine in pediatric patients with hypertension. *J Pediatr* 2001;139:34–37.

Chesney RW, Jones DP: Is there a role for β-adrenergic blockers in treating hypertension in children? *J Pediatr* 2007;150:121–122.

Choi Y, Kang BC, Kim KJ, et al: Renovascular hypertension in children with moyamoya disease. *J Pediatr* 1997;131:258–263.

Egger DW, Deming DD, Hamada N, et al: Evaluation of the safety of short-acting nifedipine in children with hypertension. *Pediatr Nephrol* 2002;17:35–40.

Flynn JT: What's new in pediatric hypertension? *Curr Hypertens Rep* 2001;3:503–510.

Flynn JT, Pasko DA: Calcium channel blockers: Pharmacology and place in therapy of pediatric hypertension. *Pediatr Nephrol* 2000;15:302–316.

Kay JD, Sinaiko AR, Daniels SR: Pediatric hypertension. *Am Heart J* 2001;142:422–432.

Lurbe E, Sorof JM, Daniels SR: Clinical and research aspects of ambulatory blood pressure monitoring in children. *J Pediatr* 2004;144:7–16.

[no authors listed]: Athletic participation by children and adolescents who have systemic hypertension. American Academy of Pediatrics Committee on Sports Medicine and Fitness. *Pediatrics* 1997;99:637–638.

[no authors listed]: Initial therapy of hypertension. *Med Lett Drugs Ther* 2004;46:53–55.

[no authors listed]: Update on the 1987 Task Force Report on High Blood Pressure in Children and Adolescents: A working group report from the National High Blood Pressure Education Program. National High Blood Pressure Education Program Working Group on Hypertension Control in Children and Adolescents. *Pediatrics* 1996;98:649–658.

Sinaiko AR: Hypertension in children. *N Engl J Med* 1996;335:1968–1973.

Tyagi S, Kaul UA, Satsangi DK, et al: Percutaneous transluminal angioplasty for renovascular hypertension in children: Initial and long-term results. *Pediatrics* 1997;99:44–49.

Wolfish NM, Delbrouck NF, Shanon A, et al: Prevalence of hypertension in children with primary vesicoureteral reflux. *J Pediatr* 1993;123:559–563.

Parte XX ■ Malattie del sangue

Sezione 1 — Il sistema emopoietico

Capitolo 446 ■ Sviluppo del sistema emopoietico Robin K. Ohls e Robert D. Christensen

La regolazione del sistema emopoietico nel feto umano è diversa da quella nell'adulto. Nell'adulto, l'omeostasi è una funzione primaria della regolazione emopoietica; nell'embrione e nel feto, invece, tutte le fasi dell'emopoiesi sono caratterizzate da una crescita costante e marcata. Durante l'eritropoiesi fetale, la costante crescita del feto e il conseguente bisogno di aumentare la massa di globuli rossi richiedono uno straordinario sforzo eritropoietico. Inoltre, le concentrazioni di ossigeno relativamente basse, rispetto agli elevati tassi metabolici dei tessuti fetali, impongono la necessità di un sistema di distribuzione dell'ossigeno molto diverso da quello operante negli adulti. Durante la granulopoiesi fetale, l'ambiente intra-amniotico, in quanto sterile, è caratterizzato da una scarsa richiesta di neutrofili, dei quali non è dunque necessaria un'ampia riserva.

L'emopoiesi fetale si suddivide in tre fasi, distinte secondo le sedi anatomiche di produzione: fase mesoblastica, fase epatica e fase mieloide. L'**emopoiesi mesoblastica**, che avviene nelle strutture extraembrioniali (principalmente nel sacco vitellino), ha inizio tra il 10° e il 14° giorno di gestazione. Alla 6ª-8ª settimana di gestazione il fegato sostituisce il sacco vitellino come principale sede di produzione dei globuli rossi, così che tra la 10ª e la 12ª settimana l'emopoiesi extraembrionale è sostanzialmente terminata. L'**emopoiesi epatica** avviene nel fegato durante tutto il resto della gestazione, benché incominci a diminuire durante il secondo trimestre, a mano a mano che aumenta l'**emopoiesi nel midollo osseo** (**emopoiesi mieloide**). Il fegato rimane l'organo emopoietico predominante fino alla 20ª-24ª settimana di gestazione.

Ciascun organo emopoietico ospita distinte popolazioni di cellule emopoietiche. Alla 18ª-20ª settimana di gestazione, l'85% delle cellule emopoietiche del fegato fetale appartiene alla serie eritroide, senza che siano, in pratica, presenti neutrofili. Viceversa, allo stesso tempo, <40% delle cellule all'interno del midollo osseo è costituito da cellule della serie eritroide e ≤15% da neutrofili. Anche la sottopopolazione di leucociti presente nel fegato e nel midollo osseo subisce dei mutamenti nel corso della gestazione. I macrofagi precedono i granulociti sia nel fegato, sia nel midollo e il rapporto tra macrofagi e granulociti diminuisce con il procedere della gestazione. Indipendentemente dall'età gestazionale o dalla sede anatomica, la produzione di tessuti emopoietici ha inizio con **cellule staminali pluripotenti**, in grado sia di riprodursi, sia di maturare e formare cloni relativi a tutte le linee cellulari del sangue. Le **cellule progenitrici** si differenziano in base all'influenza dei fattori di crescita emopoietica (Tab. 446-1) prodotti dal feto (Fig. 446-1). La produzione del fattore di crescita emopoietica del feto è indipendente dalla produzione del fattore di crescita materno.

Gli indici relativi alle cellule ematiche eritroidi e granulocitiche cambiano durante la gestazione e continuano a cambiare durante il primo anno di vita. Le concentrazioni di eritrociti e di

TABELLA 446-1. Caratteristiche dei fattori di crescita emopoietici

FATTORI DI CRESCITA	MASSA MOLECOLARE (KD)	POSIZIONE NEI CROMOSOMI	PRINCIPALE CELLULA BERSAGLIO
ERITROPOIETINA	30-39	7q11-12	CFU-E, BFU-E fetale
FATTORI STIMOLANTI LE COLONIE			
G-CSF	18-22	17q11,2-21	CFU-G, CFU-MIX, neutrofilo maturo
GM-CSF	18-30	5q23-31	CFU-MIX, CFU-GM, BFU-E, monocito, neutrofilo maturo
M-CSF	45-70 dimero di 2 subunità	5q33.1	CFU-M, macrofago
SCF	36	12	CFU-MIX, BFU-E, CFU-GM, mastocita
INTERLEUCHINE			
IL-1	17	Alfa 2q13 Beta 2q13-21	Epatocita, macrofago, linfocita
IL-2	15-20	4q26-27	Cellula T, linfocita citotossico
IL-3	14-30	5q23-31	CFU-MIX, CFU-Meg, CFU-GM, BFU-E, Macrofago
IL-4	16-20	5q23-31	Linfocita T, linfocita B
IL-5	46 (dimero di 2 subunità)	5q23-31	CFU-Eo, linfocita B
IL-6	19-26	7p21-24	CFU-MIX, CFU-GM, BFU-E, monocito, linfocita B, linfocita T, linfocita citotossico
IL-7	35	8q12-13	Cellula B
IL-8	8-10	4	Neutrofilo, cellula endoteliale, linfocita T
IL-9	16	5q31-32	BFU-E, CFU-MIX
IL-10	18.7	1	Macrofago, linfocita
IL-11	23	19q13	CFU-Meg, cellula B, cheratinocito
IL-12	70-75 dimero di subunità	p35/p40	Cellule T 3 (p35) e 11 (p40), cellule NK, macrofagi
IL-13	9	5q23-31	Linfocita pre-B, macrofago
IL-14	53	5q31	Linfocita B
IL-15	14-15	4q25-35	Linfocita B, Linfocita T
IL-16	12-14		Linfocita T
IL-17	20-30	2q31	Cellule stromali del midollo
IL-18	24	9p13	Linfocita T CD4+, cellule NK
IL-21			Linfocita T
IL-23	Dimero di subunità	19/IL-12p40	Linfocita T CD4+
TROMBOPOIETINA	35-38	3q27-28	Cellule progenitrici dei megacariociti, megacariociti

BFU-E (*Burst-forming units-erythroid*, precursori eritroidi formanti colonia a esplosione); CFU-E (*Colony-forming units-erythroid*, unità formanti colonie eritroidi); CFU-Eo (*Colony-forming units-eosinophil*, unità formanti colonie eosinofile); CFU-G (*Colony-forming units-granulocyte*, unità formanti colonie granulocitiche); CFU-GM (*Colony-forming units-granulocyte macrophage*, unità formanti colonie di granulociti-macrofagi); CFU-M (*Colony-forming units-macrophage*, unità formanti colonie di macrofagi); CFU-Meg (*Colony-forming units-megakaryocyte*, unità formanti colonie megacariocitiche); CFU-MIX (*Colony-forming units-mixed*, unità formanti colonie miste); G-CSF (*Granulocyte colony-stimulating factor*, fattore stimolante le colonie di granulociti); GM-CSF (*Granulocyte-macrophage colony-stimulating factor*, fattore stimolante le colonie di granulociti-macrofagi); IL (interleuchina); M-CSF (*Macrophage colony-stimulating factor*, fattore stimolante le colonie di macrofagi); NK (*natural killer*); SCF (*Stem cell factor*, Fattore delle cellule staminali).

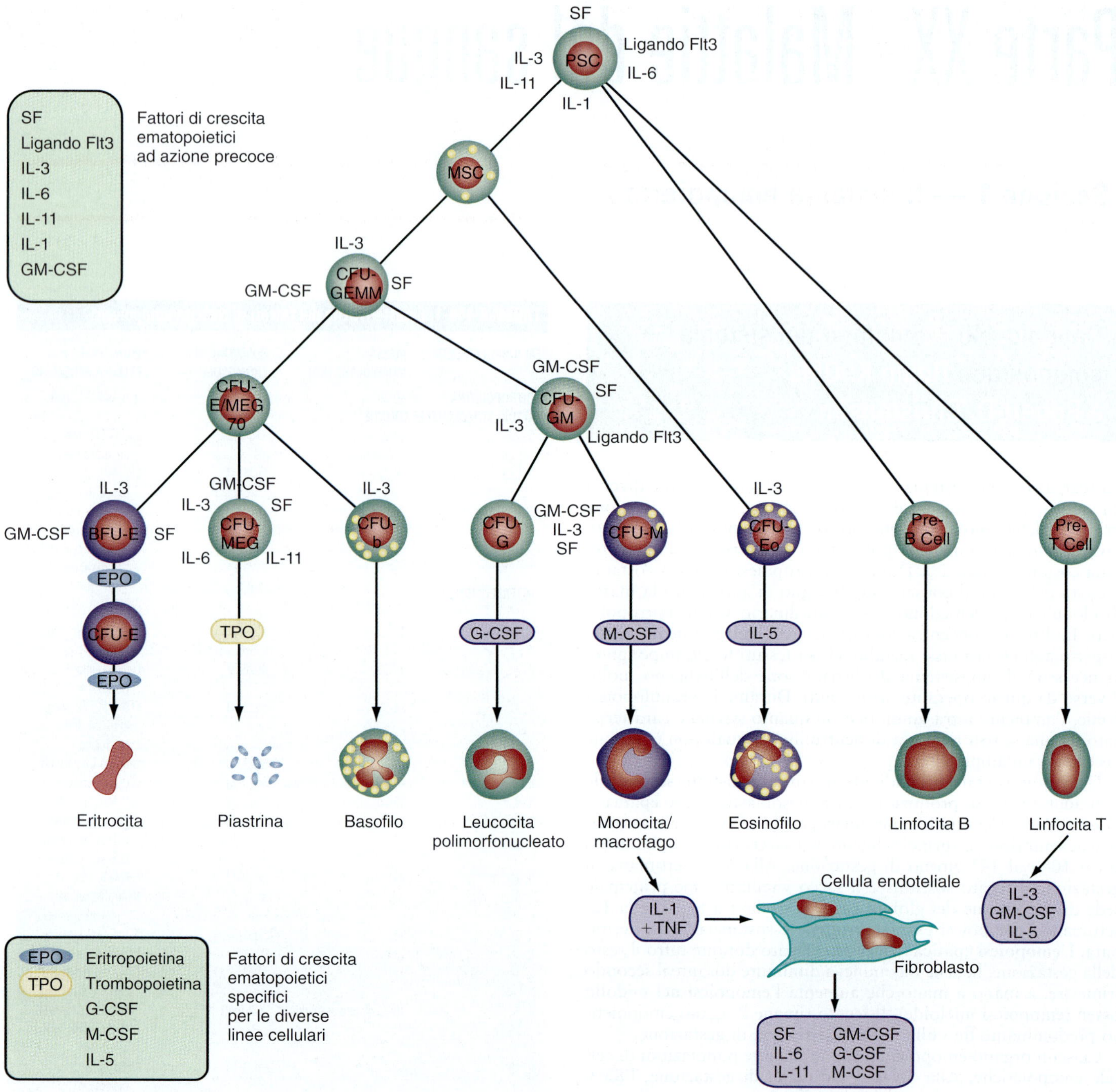

Figura 446-1. Principali fonti di citochine e attività di promozione dell'emopoiesi. Le cellule del microambiente del midollo osseo, come i macrofagi, le cellule endoteliali e i fibroblasti reticolari, producono, dopo la stimolazione, il fattore M-CSF (*Macrophage Colony-Stimulating Factor*, fattore stimolante le colonie di macrofagi), il fattore GM-CSF (*Granulocyte-Macrophage Colony-Stimulating Factor*, fattore stimolante le colonie di granulociti-macrofagi) e il fattore G-CSF (*Granulocyte Colony-Stimulating Factor*, fattore stimolante le colonie di granulociti). Durante la differenziazione emopoietica, fra queste citochine (accanto ad altre elencate nel testo) si attuano interazioni sovrapposte, come indicato. Per lo sviluppo ottimale di tutte le linee cellulari, è necessaria una combinazione di fattori con azione precoce e tardiva. BFU (*Burst Forming Unit*), cellula formante colonie a esplosione; CFU (*Colony Forming Unit*), cellula formante colonie; EPO (*Erythropoietin*), eritropoietina; MSC (*Myeloid Stem Cells*), cellule staminali mieloidi; PSC (*Pluripotent Stem Cell*), cellula staminale pluripotente. (Da Sieff CA, Nathan DG, Clark SC: The anatomy and physiology of hematopoiesis. In Orkin SH, Nathan DG [curatori]: *Hematology of Infancy and Childhood*, 5th ed. Philadelphia, WB Saunders, 1998, p 168.)

granulociti aumentano gradualmente durante il secondo e il terzo trimestre di gravidanza (Tab. 446-2). Parallelamente all'aumento della concentrazione di eritrociti, si verifica anche un aumento del valore ematocrito dal 30-40% durante il secondo trimestre, con progressivo aumento fino al termine della gravidanza, nel corso dell'ultima parte del terzo trimestre. A termine, il valore ematocrito è compreso tra il 50% e il 63%, con una variabilità dipendente dal momento del clampaggio del cordone ombelicale e dalla sede di prelievo. A differenza delle concentrazioni ematiche di eritrociti e di neutrofili, le concentrazioni di piastrine rimangono costanti a partire dalla 18ª settimana di gestazione fino al termine, con un intervallo compreso tra 150 000 e 450 000 per μL.

I volumi cellulari medi sono, in genere, inversamente proporzionali alla durata della gestazione e al ciclo di vita della cellula. Il *volume cellulare medio* (*Mean Cell Volume*, MCV) degli

TABELLA 446-2. Indici relativi agli elementi figurati del sangue durante la gestazione e alla nascita

SETTIMANE DI GESTAZIONE	CONTA LEUCOCITI TOTALE * ($\times 10^9$/L)	CONTA LEUCOCITI CORRETTA ($\times 10^9$/L)	PIASTRINE ($\times 10^9$/L)	RBC ($\times 10^{12}$/L)	HB (g/dL)	(%) HCT	(fL) MCV
18-21	4,68 ± 2,96	2,57 ± 0,42	234 ± 57	2,85 ± 0.36	11,69 ± 1.27	37,3 ± 4.3	131,1 ± 11,0
22-25	4,72 ± 2,84	3,73 ± 2,17	247 ± 59	3,09 ± 0.34	12,2 ± 1.6	38,6 ± 3.9	125,1 ± 7,8
26-29	5,16 ± 2,53	4,08 ± 0,84	242 ± 69	3,46 ± 0.41	12,91 ± 1.38	40,9 ± 4.4	118,5 ± 8,0
>30	7,71 ± 4,99	6,40 ± 2,99	232 ± 87	3,82 ± 0,64	13,64 ± 2,21	43,6 ± 7,2	114,4 ± 9,3
Termine		18,1 (9,0-30,0)	290 ± 100	4,70 ± 0,40	16,5 ± 1,5	51,0 ± 4,5	108,0 ± 5,0

*compresi i normoblasti.
Hb, emoglobina; Hct, ematocrito; MCV (*Mean Cell Volume*), volume cellulare medio; RBC (*Red Blood Cell*), globuli rossi.
Adattata da Forestier F, Daffors F, Catherine N, et al: Developmental hematopoiesis in normal human fetal blood. Blood 1991; 77:2361.

eritrociti, che nell'embrione è >180 fL, scende a circa 130 fL a metà gestazione, poi diminuisce a 110 fL alla 40ª settimana di gestazione (vedi Tab. 446-2). Il *volume piastrinico medio* (*Mean Platelet Volume*, MPV) varia da 8 a 10 fL alla nascita; questo valore può talora essere utile per stabilire se la piastrinopenia è principalmente causata dalla ridotta produzione (MPV normale) o dall'aumentata distruzione (MPV elevato).

GRANULOCITOPOIESI. Nel feto umano, la comparsa di neutrofili si può rilevare a distanza di circa 5 settimane dal concepimento. I neutrofili si presentano come piccoli grappoli cellulari, disposti attorno all'aorta. Queste cellule contengono mieloperossidasi e maturano formando cellule con nuclei segmentati, ma non sono state evidenziate altre similitudini tra esse e i neutrofili degli adulti. Il midollo osseo fetale incomincia a svilupparsi attorno all'8ª settimana dopo il concepimento. Tra l'8ª e la 10ª settimana lo spazio occupato dal midollo osseo aumenta, ma, in questa sede, non si riscontra la presenza di neutrofili fino a 10 settimane e mezzo di gestazione. Questi primi neutrofili del midollo hanno nuclei rotondi, contengono mieloperossidasi e presentano le caratteristiche di membrana dei **mieloblasti** e dei **promielociti.** Dalla 14ª settimana al termine, il tipo di granulocito maggiormente rappresentato nel midollo osseo fetale è il neutrofilo.

Nei bambini e negli adulti, i neutrofili e i macrofagi hanno origine da una cellula progenitrice comune. Non è chiaro se tale origine sia la stessa anche nel feto, poiché i neutrofili e i macrofagi compaiono in momenti diversi e in diverse sedi anatomiche. I macrofagi compaiono nel sacco vitellino, nel fegato, nei polmoni e nel cervello, prima che si formino le cavità del midollo osseo.

È probabile che siano coinvolti il **fattore stimolante le colonie di granulociti** (*Granulocyte Colony-Stimulating Factor*, G-CSF) e il **fattore stimolante le colonie di macrofagi** (*Macrophage Colony-Stimulating Factor*, M-CSF), come negli adulti, poiché entrambi i fattori sono espressi, nel corso dello sviluppo del midollo osseo, già dalla 6ª settimana dopo il concepimento e nel fegato fetale già dall'8ª settimana (vedi Fig. 446-1). Anche il **fattore stimolante le colonie di granulociti-macrofagi** (*Granulocyte-Macrophage Colony-Stimulating Factor*, GM-CSF) e il **fattore di crescita delle cellule staminali** (*Stem Cell Factor*, SCF) sono diffusamente distribuiti nei tessuti del feto umano. Tuttavia, nessun cambiamento nell'espressione dell'mRNA di nessuno di questi fattori, né dei relativi recettori specifici o nelle concentrazioni di proteine (secondo quanto risulta dalle colorazioni immunoistochimiche) sembra essere il segnale per la produzione fetale di neutrofili o di macrofagi. I segnali precisi non sono ancora stati identificati.

Prima del terzo trimestre si riscontra la presenza di pochi neutrofili nella circolazione sanguigna. Il numero dei neutrofili in circolo è, in media, pari a 190/mm^3 (con una variabilità compresa fra 0 e 490/mm^3 e con valore di moda di concentrazioni uguale a zero) nei feti alla 20ª settimana di gestazione. Nel sangue del feto, benché i neutrofili maturi siano scarsi, le cellule progenitrici dotate della capacità di generare cloni di neutrofili sono relativamente abbondanti. Quando queste cellule progenitrici fetali sono coltivate in vitro in presenza di G-CSF ricombinante, maturano in grandi colonie di neutrofili. Si ritiene che il ruolo fisiologico del G-CSF, comprendente la stimolazione della produzione dei neutrofili, non vari nel feto, nel neonato e nell'adulto. Di conseguenza, le scarse quantità di neutrofili circolanti e di riserva nel feto umano a metà della gestazione, possono dipendere, in parte, da una scarsa produzione del G-CSF. Quando sono stimolati da una varietà di mediatori infiammatori quali il **lipopolisaccaride batterico** (*Bacterial Lipopolysaccharide*, LPS) o l'**interleuchina-1** (*Interleukin-1*, IL-1), i monociti isolati dal sangue degli adulti producono il G-CSF. Viceversa, i monociti isolati dal sangue del cordone ombelicale dei neonati pretermine, come pure dal fegato e dal midollo osseo di aborti fino alla 24ª settimana di gestazione, producono solo piccole quantità (10-100× in meno per cellula) di proteina G-CSF e di mRNA a essa corrispondente, dopo stimolazione con LPS o IL-1. Nonostante tale ridotta capacità di produrre G-CSF, i recettori G-CSF presenti sulla superficie dei neutrofili dei neonati sono uguali (per numero e per affinità) a quelli presenti sui neutrofili degli adulti.

Nel feto, le azioni dei fattori G-CSF, M-CSF, GM-CSF e SCF non sono limitate all'emopoiesi. I recettori per ciascuno di questi fattori si trovano in aree diverse del sistema nervoso centrale e del tubo digerente del feto, dove si esprimono con modalità variabili in base alla fase dello sviluppo fetale. Questi fattori svolgono importanti ruoli nello sviluppo, oltre a quelli noti riguardo all'emopoiesi.

TROMBOPOIESI. Il compartimento del midollo pertinente ai megacariociti si può considerare costituito da due gruppi di cellule: i progenitori dei megacariociti e i megacariociti. I **megacariociti** sono identificati dalle proprie caratteristiche morfologiche, poiché subiscono l'**endoriduplicazione,** che genera grandi cellule con nuclei poliploidi.

I progenitori dei megacariociti possono essere suddivisi in due popolazioni: le cellule BFU-MK (*Burst-Forming Unit-Megakaryocytes,* precursori megacariocitici formanti colonie a esplosione), che sono i progenitori dei megacariociti primitivi, e le CFU-MK (*Colony-Forming Unit-Megakaryocytes,* precursori megacariocitici formanti colonie), che sono cellule più differenziate. Le cellule BFU-MK producono grandi colonie multifocali contenenti almeno 50 megacariociti, mentre le CFU-MK generano colonie monofocali più piccole (3-50 cellule/colonia). Le BFU-MK esprimono CD34, ma non HLA-DR, mentre le CFU-MK esprimono sia CD34 sia HLA-DR. Le colonie generate dalle BFU-MK di origine fetale contengono una quantità significativamente superiore di megacariociti rispetto alle colonie di origine adulta; su questa base, si ritiene che rappresentino cellule un po' più primitive.

I megacariociti, a differenza delle cellule loro progenitrici, non hanno la capacità di generare cloni. Essi subiscono, invece, una maturazione, trasformandosi da piccole cellule mononucleate in grandi cellule poliploidi. La ploidia modale dei megacariociti nel midollo di un adulto normale è 16N, mentre nel feto e nel neonato è minore, così com'è inferiore la dimensione dei megacariociti. Il sangue del cordone ombelicale presenta, tuttavia, una maggiore concentrazione di megacariociti rispetto al sangue dell'adulto. I megacariociti più grandi generano più piastrine rispetto a quelli più piccoli; di conseguenza, si suppone che i megacariociti dei neonati producano meno piastrine rispetto alle cellule corrispondenti dell'adulto.

I processi concernenti la produzione e il rilascio di piastrine dai megacariociti non sono ben noti. Un'ipotesi prevede che i megacariociti del midollo formino piccole estroflessioni della membrana (*buds*) e che queste siano liberate dal midollo come piastrine. Un'altra possibilità è che le piastrine siano liberate principalmente dai megacariociti presenti nei polmoni, come conseguenza dell'azione di forze di trazione. Questa teoria è corroborata dal riscontro di un gran numero di megacariociti nei polmoni.

La **trombopoietina** (*Thrombopoietin*, TPO), che è il regolatore fisiologico della produzione di piastrine, agisce come potente stimolatore di tutte le fasi di crescita e di sviluppo dei megacariociti. Il gene che codifica la TPO si trova nel braccio lungo del cromosoma 3 umano. Il TPO-mRNA è espresso principalmente nel fegato e nel rene e, in minor misura, nello stroma del midollo osseo. La TPO svolge una funzione regolatrice preminente, ma non esclusiva, in rapporto alla produzione di piastrine. La TPO stimola la proliferazione e la sopravvivenza non solo dei progenitori dei megacariociti, ma anche dei progenitori eritroidi, mieloidi e pluripotenti. Gli esperimenti sull'uomo (fasi I e II) hanno dimostrato che la rTPO stimola la produzione di piastrine, sia negli adulti non trombocitopenici, sia nei pazienti con trombocitopenia indotta dalla chemioterapia. La TPO ricombinante supporta la crescita delle colonie di megacariociti nei neonati e nei bambini. Nei neonati pretermine, le cellule progenitrici sono più sensibili alla rTPO rispetto a quanto avviene nei neonati a termine.

Non si sa nulla su eventuali vantaggi e rischi della somministrazione della rTPO nei neonati e nei bambini. Recenti studi clinici hanno dimostrato la produzione di anticorpi anti-TPO nei pazienti sottoposti a terapia con rTPO; ulteriori studi sono in corso a tale proposito.

ERITROPOIESI. L'eritropoiesi, nel corso della vita intrauterina, è controllata solo dai fattori di crescita eritroidi prodotti dal feto. Poiché l'eritropoietina (EPO) non oltrepassa la barriera placentare nell'uomo, la stimolazione della produzione di EPO nella madre non favorisce la produzione di globuli rossi fetali. Inoltre, la soppressione dell'eritropoiesi materna tramite l'ipertrasfusione non riduce l'eritropoiesi fetale.

Non è chiaro se nel feto o nel neonato prematuro sussista lo stesso meccanismo di regolazione eritropoietica tipico dell'eritropoiesi adulta. La produzione di globuli rossi è governata da una varietà di fattori di crescita prodotti da diverse altre cellule (macrofagi, linfociti e cellule stromali). Queste cellule, insieme ai fattori di crescita, costituiscono il microambiente eritropoietico e stimolano la maturazione, la crescita e la differenziazione di cellule eritrocitiche, nei loro vari stadi. Nessuno dei fattori che stimolano l'eritropoiesi svolge un ruolo regolatorio più importante dell'EPO. L'**EPO** è una glicoproteina del peso di 30-39 kd che si lega a specifici recettori sulla superficie dei precursori eritroidi e stimola la loro differenziazione e la loro maturazione clonale in eritrociti maturi. Nella regolazione dell'espressione del gene EPO è coinvolto un meccanismo di rilevamento della concentrazione dell'ossigeno, così che l'eritropoiesi è stimolata sia dall'ipossia, sia dall'anemia, che favoriscono trascrizione di mRNA e la produzione di EPO. La produzione di EPO-mRNA è regolata da *cis-acting elements* nel promotore e da regioni 3′ *enhancer*, sensibili all'ipossia. Due fattori, il fattore nucleare epatico 4 (HNF-4) e il fattore inducibile dall'ipossia 1 (*Hypoxic Inducible Factor*, HIF-1), mostrano di attivare la trascrizione del gene EPO e di altri geni inducibili dall'ipossia. È stato dimostrato che l'HNF-4 si lega in modo specifico alle regioni *promoter* ed *enhancer* del gene EPO ed è espresso nel rene, nel fegato e nelle cellule Hep3B. HIF-1 è un fattore di trascrizione *helix-loop-helix* basico, composto dalle subunità HIF-1α e HIF-1β che si legano ai *cis-acting elements* di risposta all'ipossia e inducono la trascrizione del gene EPO. HIF-1, espresso in molte cellule, è coinvolto nell'*upregulation* di varie proteine regolate dall'ipossia, incluso il VEG-F. Sembra che sia espresso costituzionalmente e vada incontro a una rapida degradazione in condizioni normossiche. La regolazione della proteina eterodimerica HIF-1 avviene attraverso il legame del DNA e la stabilizzazione della proteina. La stabilità dell'RNA dipende dal sistema di degradazione proteasomale mediato dall'ubiquitina; l'inibizione di questo sistema porta all'aumento di HIF-1 e di EPO, anche in condizioni normossiche. Nei modelli sperimentali di topi esposti all'ipossia, le concentrazioni di HIF-1α mRNA non presentano cambiamenti significativi. Sembra che l'HIF-1α operi in modo simile nel feto.

Il fegato del feto produce l'EPO durante il primo e il secondo trimestre di gestazione, principalmente a opera di cellule originate da monociti/macrofagi. La produzione di globuli rossi raggiunge il minimo dopo la nascita, sia nei bambini a termine, sia in quelli pretermine. In seguito, la sede anatomica della produzione di EPO sembra spostarsi dal fegato al rene. Lo stimolo specifico per tale cambiamento è sconosciuto, ma potrebbero essere in causa i mutamenti significativi della concentrazione arteriosa di ossigeno, che si verificano alla nascita. Nei modelli animali, la sensibilità del meccanismo di rilevamento epatico dell'ipossia appare inferiore alla sensibilità renale. Sembra, inoltre, che il fegato richieda un'ipossia più prolungata perché si attivi una risposta EPO. L'EPO-mRNA e la corrispondente proteina si possono trovare nel rene fetale umano, ma non si sa se tale produzione sia biologicamente rilevante. Tuttavia, sembra che la produzione renale di EPO non sia essenziale per l'eritropoiesi fetale normale, come dimostrato dal fatto che, nei feti con agenesia renale, i valori di concentrazione di EPO nel siero e l'ematocrito sono normali.

Quando le cellule del midollo osseo vengono poste in mezzi di coltura semisolidi per 5-7 giorni, i precursori sensibili all'EPO, denominati **unità eritroidi formanti colonie** (*Colony-Forming Units-Erythroid*, CFU-E), vanno incontro a maturazione clonale formando aggregati contenenti 30-100 normoblasti (Fig. 446-1). Le cellule progenitrici specifiche della serie eritroide, che sono meno ben differenziate delle CFU-E e sono, di conseguenza, cellule più primitive, sono denominate **precursori eritroidi formanti colonie a esplosione** (*Burst-Forming Units-Erythroid*, BFU-E). Dopo 12-14 giorni dall'inizio della coltura, le cellule BFU-E danno luogo a grandi aggregati di normoblasti, ciascuno contenente 200-10 000 cellule. Le cellule BFU-E dei feti umani rispondono in modo leggermente diverso, rispetto alle cellule BFU-E isolate degli adulti. In particolare, le cellule BFU-E di origine fetale si sviluppano in cloni eritroidi in modo generalmente più rapido e, di solito, danno luogo a un numero maggiore di normoblasti rispetto alle cellule BFU-E di origine adulta. Perché avvenga la maturazione clonale, le cellule BFU-E del midollo osseo adulto richiedono l'associazione di EPO e di altri fattori di crescita, quali l'IL-3 o il GM-CSF; per molte cellule BFU-E fetali, invece, è sufficiente la sola presenza dell'EPO.

EMOGLOBINA. Nel corso dell'evoluzione, la formazione di proteine in grado di legare l'ossigeno, le **emoglobine**, ha accresciuto la capacità del sangue di trasportare l'ossigeno. Il legame tra l'ossigeno e l'emoglobina, così come la sua dissociazione, non necessita di energia metabolica.

L'emoglobina è una proteina complessa, costituita da gruppi eme contenenti ferro e da una proteina, la globina. Un'interazione dinamica tra l'eme e la globina fornisce all'emoglobina le sue proprietà peculiari concernenti il trasporto reversibile di ossigeno. La molecola dell'emoglobina è un tetramero costituito da due coppie di catene polipeptidiche, a ognuna delle quali è legato un gruppo eme. Le catene polipeptidiche di varie emoglobine si presentano chimicamente eterogenee. L'emoglobina principale di un adulto normale (Hb A) è costituita da una coppia di catene polipeptidiche alfa (α) e da una coppia beta (β), rappresentate come $\alpha_2\beta_2$. La principale emoglobina presente nel feto (Hb F), costituita da due catene di globina α e due γ, è rappresentata come $\alpha_2\gamma_2$.

La sintesi delle varie catene di globina, distinte per numero e per sequenza di aminoacidi, è regolata da geni separati (Fig. 446-2). Due gruppi di geni relativi alle catene α sono posizionati nel cromosoma umano 16. Due coppie di alleli forniscono le informazioni genetiche per la struttura della catena α. I geni β, γ, δ sul cromosoma 11 sono strettamente collegati.

All'interno della componente eritrocitaria (*Red Blood Cells*, RBC) di un embrione, di un feto, di un bambino o di un adulto

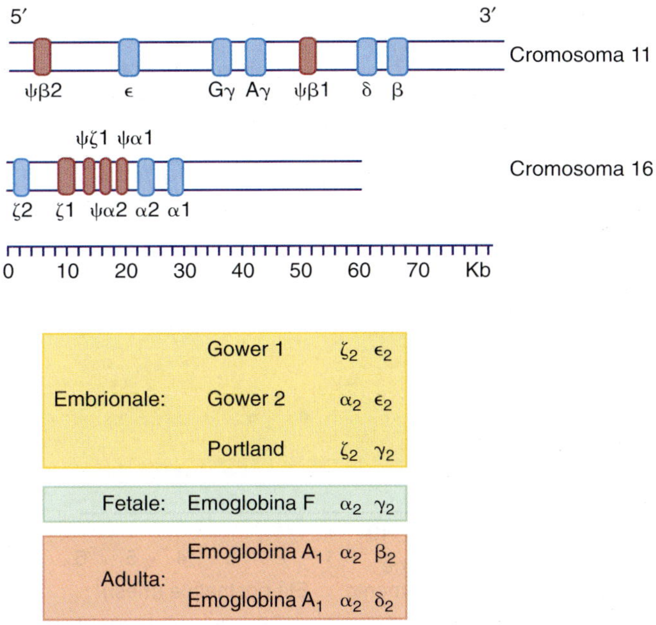

Figura 446-2. Organizzazione dei geni della globina. La linea in basso rispecchia la scala in chilobasi. Il segmento superiore rappresenta i geni beta della globina sul cromosoma 11, mentre il segmento inferiore mostra i geni alfa sul cromosoma 16. Le regioni geniche che codificano per le più importanti globine sono indicate come segmenti *blu* e le regioni che indicano gli pseudogeni ("ψ", residui non espressi) sono indicate come segmenti *rosa*. È elencata la composizione delle emoglobine embrionali, fetali e adulte. α, alfa; β, beta; γ, gamma; δ, delta; ϵ, epsilon; ζ, zeta.

è possibile rilevare, normalmente, sei emoglobine differenti: le **emoglobine embrionali,** Gower-1, Gower-2 e Portland; l'**emoglobina fetale,** Hb F; e le **emoglobine adulte,** Hb A e Hb A_2. La mobilità elettroforetica delle emoglobine varia col variare della loro struttura chimica. I momenti della comparsa delle diverse emoglobine e i loro rapporti quantitativi sono determinati da processi complessi inerenti allo sviluppo (Fig. 446-3).

Emoglobine embrionali. Il sangue degli embrioni umani nel primo periodo di gestazione contiene due emoglobine a migrazione lenta, *Gower-1* e *Gower-2*, e l'emoglobina *Portland*, che ha una mobilità simile all'Hb F. Le catene theta (θ) delle Hb Portland e Gower-1 sono strutturalmente alquanto simili alle catene α. Entrambe le emoglobine Gower contengono un unico tipo di catena polipeptidica, la catena epsilon (ε). L'Hb Gower-1 ha la struttura $\theta_2\varepsilon_2$ mentre la Gower-2 ha la struttura $\alpha_2\varepsilon_2$. L'Hb Portland ha struttura $\theta_2\gamma_2$. Negli embrioni di 4-8 settimane di gestazione, predominano le emoglobine Gower, le quali, tuttavia, incominciano a scomparire dal 3° mese.

Emoglobina fetale. L'Hb F contiene catene di polipeptidi gamma al posto delle catene β dell'Hb A. La sua resistenza alla denaturazione da parte di basi forti permette di determinare la presenza di emazie fetali nella circolazione materna (**test Kleihauer-Betke**). Dopo l'8ª settimana di gestazione, l'Hb F è l'emoglobina predominante; alla 24ª settimana di gestazione questa costituisce il 90% dell'emoglobina totale, che, durante il 3° trimestre, diminuisce gradualmente, così che alla nascita l'Hb F costituisce, in media, solo il 70% del totale. Poiché la sintesi dell'Hb F diminuisce rapidamente dopo la nascita, tra i 6 e i 12 mesi di età questa emoglobina è presente solo in tracce. Nei bambini più grandi e negli adulti, mediante denaturazione alcalina, può essere rilevata una percentuale inferiore al 2,0%. L'Hb F è eterogenea a causa

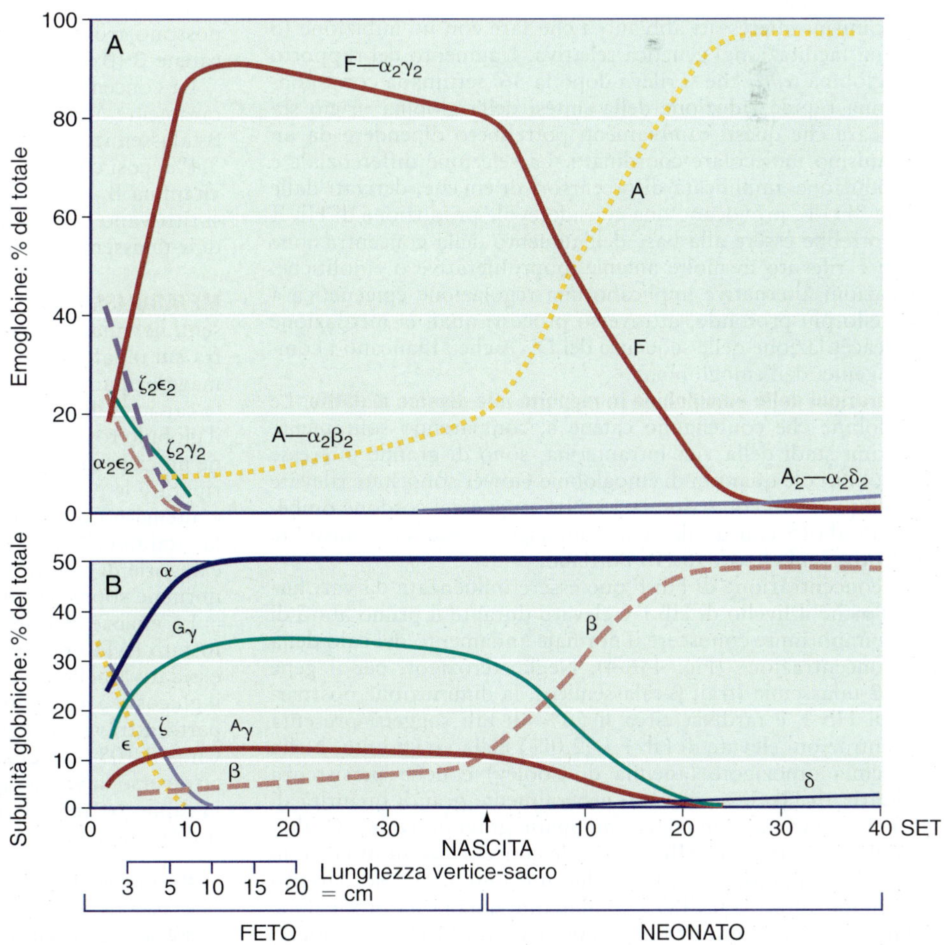

Figura 446-3. Cambiamenti nei tetrameri dell'emoglobina *(A)* e nelle subunità di globina *(B)* durante lo sviluppo umano dall'embrione alla prima infanzia. (Da Polin RA, Fox WW: *Fetal and Neonatal Physiology,* 2nd ed. Philadelphia, WB Saunders, 1998, p 1769.)

di due tipi di catene γ, la cui sintesi è regolata da due gruppi di geni. Le catene differiscono nella posizione 136 per la presenza di un residuo di glicina (catena Gγ) o di alanina (catena Aγ). Nei neonati, il rapporto fra Gγ e Aγ è pari a 3:1.

Emoglobine adulte. Tracce di Hb A ($\alpha_2\beta_2$) possono essere rilevate persino negli embrioni più piccoli. Di conseguenza, già tra la 16ª e la 20ª settimana di gestazione, è possibile formulare una diagnosi prenatale delle emoglobinopatie che vedono coinvolta la catena β principale, come la talassemia maior (vedi Capitolo 462.9). La diagnosi prenatale è basata su tecniche che permettono di valutare la sintesi delle catene β o la struttura delle catene β neoprodotte. Se la causa delle emoglobinopatie consiste in difetti strutturali del DNA, è possibile la diagnosi precoce mediante tecniche di biologia molecolare, applicate a campioni istologici di villi coriali o al liquido amniotico. Le alterazioni geniche da delezione, come la talassemia α, possono essere rilevate utilizzando lo stesso metodo.

Alla 24ª settimana di gestazione, la percentuale di Hb A è compresa fra il 5% e il 10%. Segue un aumento costante, cosicché, a termine, l'Hb A raggiunge in media il 30%. Tra il 6° e il 12° mese di età, compare il normale profilo di Hb A. L'Hb A meno rappresentata, vale a dire l'Hb A_2, contiene catene delta (δ) e ha la struttura $\alpha_2\delta_2$. Essa è rilevabile solo quando sono presenti quantità significative di Hb A. Alla nascita, l'Hb A_2 è inferiore all'1,0% ma a 12 mesi di età si rileva la normale quota del 2,0-3,4%. Nel corso della vita, il rapporto normale tra Hb A e Hb A_2 è di circa 30:1.

Rapporti normali tra le emoglobine. Durante la vita fetale e la prima infanzia, i tassi di sintesi delle catene γ e β e le quantità di Hb A e Hb F si trovano in un rapporto di proporzionalità inversa. Tale rapporto è stato attribuito a un "meccanismo di sostituzione" (switch) simile al meccanismo di regolazione genetica presente nei batteri. Non sono chiari, tuttavia, i processi genetici, biologici e di sviluppo che regolano il passaggio dalla predominanza della sintesi della catena γ *in utero* alla predominanza della sintesi della catena β dopo la nascita. Non è sicuro se i meccanismi interessati abbiano a che fare con un'inibizione (o con una facilitazione) genetica selettiva. L'aumento del rapporto della globina α_1/α_2 che si rileva dopo la 36ª settimana corrisponde a una rapida riduzione della sintesi della globina γ: ciò sta a indicare che questi cambiamenti potrebbero dipendere da un meccanismo molecolare coordinato. La selezione differenziale e la produzione amplificata di precursori di emazie, derivati dalle cellule BFU-E, provocano una considerevole produzione di Hb F. Ciò potrebbe essere alla base dell'aumento della concentrazione di Hb F rilevato in molte anemie ipoproliferative o emolitiche. Spiegazioni alternative implicano una regolazione epigenetica a un livello più profondo, attraverso processi quali la metilazione e la deacetilazione delle sequenze del DNA che affiancano i complessi genici dell'emoglobina.

Alterazioni delle emoglobine in rapporto alle diverse malattie. Le emoglobine che contengono catene ε, comparendo solitamente nei primi stadi della vita intrauterina, sono di grande interesse teorico. Piccole quantità di emoglobine Gower sono state rilevate in alcuni neonati con trisomia 13. Nel sangue del cordone ombelicale di aborti con α-talassemia omozigote sono state misurate concentrazioni elevate di Hb Portland.

La concentrazione di Hb F può essere influenzata da vari fattori. Poiché il livello di Hb F è elevato durante il primo anno di vita, è importante conoscere il normale andamento del calo della sua concentrazione (Fig. 446-4). Negli eterozigoti per il gene della β-talassemia (trait β-talassemico), la diminuzione postpartum di Hb F è tardiva; circa il 50% di tali soggetti presenta concentrazioni elevate di Hb F (>2,0%) nella vita adulta. Nella talassemia omozigote (anemia di Cooley) e nella persistenza ereditaria di Hb F, si rilevano generalmente grandi quantità di Hb F. Nei pazienti con emoglobinopatie gravi derivanti da alterazioni della catena β (Hb SS, SC), le concentrazioni di Hb F in genere aumentano, soprattutto durante l'infanzia. Nei lattanti pretermine curati con EPO ricombinante umana, la produzione di Hb F aumenta durante l'eritropoiesi attiva. Moderati aumenti

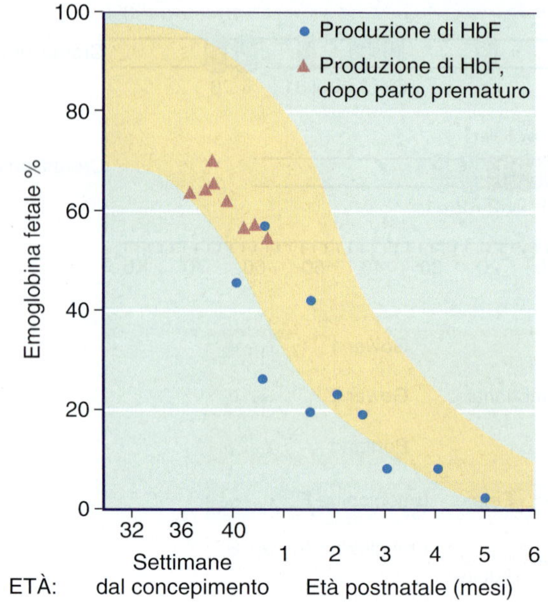

Figura 446-4. Cambiamenti prenatali e postnatali nella percentuale di emoglobina totale rappresentata dall'emoglobina fetale (Hb F) (in *giallo*). I *triangoli* rappresentano la produzione postnatale a partire dai reticolociti nei bambini prematuri e i *cerchi* rappresentano i reticolociti del sangue del cordone ombelicale e postnatali nei neonati a termine. (Da Brown MS: Fetal and neonatal erythropoiesis. In Stockman JA, Pochedly C [curatori]: *Developmental and Neonatal Hematology*. New York, Raven Press, 1988.)

di Hb F possono verificarsi in molte malattie accompagnate da stress ematologico, come le anemie emolitiche, la leucemia e l'anemia aplastica, a causa di una minore popolazione di emazie contenenti maggiori quantità di Hb F. Nei casi di α-talassemia possono trovarsi tetrameri delle catene γ (γ_4 o Hb di Bart) o catene β (β_4, Hb H) .

La concentrazione di Hb A_2 (2,0-3,4%) nell'adulto normale è raramente alterata. Nella maggior parte delle persone con trait β-talassemico si trovano concentrazioni di Hb A_2 superiori al 3,4%, così come nei casi di anemia megaloblastica da carenza di vitamina B_{12} e di acido folico. Concentrazioni inferiori di Hb A_2 si ritrovano nei casi di anemia da carenza ferro (Capitolo 455) e di α-talassemia (Capitolo 462).

METABOLISMO DEL GLOBULO ROSSO. Gli eritroblasti nucleati presenti nel midollo osseo partecipano a varie funzioni metaboliche, fra cui un'attiva sintesi proteica. Dopo l'estrusione del nucleo, la maggior parte di queste attività metaboliche va perduta, inclusa la capacità di sintetizzare le proteine. La perdita del nucleo rende il globulo rosso un miglior trasportatore di ossigeno, ma gli impone un ciclo di vita limitato, poiché la cellula non può sostituire o riparare le proprie proteine enzimatiche vitali. Le emazie mature contengono oltre 40 enzimi, molti dei quali sono essenziali per la vitalità cellulare; eventuali deficit genetici che interessino altre categorie di enzimi (per es. la catalasi) non interferiscono con la normale sopravvivenza.

Le emazie mature sono prive di mitocondri; l'adenosina trifosfato (ATP) non può, così, essere generata dalla fosforilazione ossidativa nelle reazioni del ciclo di Krebs, in assenza del quale il glucosio è assorbito e l'acido lattico è prodotto, per la maggior parte, attraverso la glicolisi anaerobia (*via di Embden-Meyerhof*). Circa il 10% del glucosio va incontro a fosforilazione ossidativa attraverso la via dei pentoso fosfati. Per la normale vita cellulare, in rapporto all'ATP generato dal metabolismo del glucosio, sono necessarie almeno 5 funzioni:

- **Mantenimento dei gradienti elettrolitici. Il principale catione intracellulare presente nelle emazie è il potassio, mentre il principale catione presente nel plasma è il sodio. L'inversione della tendenza costante del sodio a penetrare nei globuli rossi e del potassio a fuoriuscirne,** con conservazione dei gradienti ionici normali, è ottenuta per opera di un meccanismo di membrana, la pompa cationica, dipendente dall'energia fornita dall'ATP. Quando la pompa cationica non funziona correttamente, sodio e acqua penetrano nei globuli rossi, causandone la dilatazione e, infine, la lisi. Inoltre, è necessaria una certa quantità di energia per mantenere bassi i livelli intracellulari dello ione calcio.

- Inizio della produzione di energia. Per la reazione iniziale della glicolisi, che implica la fosforilazione del glucosio a formare glucosio-6-fosfato, è necessaria la presenza di ATP.
- Mantenimento della struttura della membrana e della forma delle emazie. Per mantenere la complessa struttura fosfolipidica della membrana dei globuli rossi, è necessaria energia. Probabilmente, anche il mantenimento della tipica forma biconcava richiede energia.
- Mantenimento del ferro dell'eme nella forma ridotta (ferrosa). I potenziali ossidativi all'interno dell'emazia possono causare l'ossidazione del ferro dell'emoglobina. L'emoglobina contenente ferro ferrico (metemoglobina) non è in grado di trasportare ossigeno. Se i perossidi e altri ossidanti non fossero inattivati, l'emoglobina potrebbe denaturarsi e precipitare. Le cellule contenenti tale emoglobina denaturata (corpi di Heinz) vengono rapidamente rimosse dalla circolazione. La protezione dei globuli rossi dagli effetti dell'ossidazione dipende, infine, dal NADPH e dal NADH. Questi composti sono continuamente rigenerati dalle attività della via glicolitica e dal ciclo dei pentosi. In molti deficit enzimatici, su base genetica, della via glicolitica e di quella dei pentosi, si manifesta emolisi a causa dell'impossibilità di generare l'energia per svolgere queste funzioni vitali.
- Mantenimento all'interno delle emazie delle normali concentrazioni di fosfati organici, come il 2,3-difosfoglicerato e l'ATP. Questi composti interagiscono con l'emoglobina e hanno effetti importanti sull'affinità dell'ossigeno.

CICLO DI VITA DEL GLOBULO ROSSO. Le differenze delle proprietà fisiche delle emazie, rilevate nei neonati pretermine e in quelli a termine, possono spiegare, in parte, la diminuzione della sopravvivenza delle emazie neonatali nella circolazione. La vita media di un globulo rosso neonatale è di 60-90 giorni, ovvero 1/2-1/3 circa la durata della vita di un globulo rosso nell'adulto. Le emazie neonatali, a causa di peculiarità intrinseche, presentano sopravvivenza più breve quando vengono trasfuse negli adulti. Si ritiene che, al contrario, le cellule trasfuse da donatori adulti sopravvivano normalmente nei neonati. Quanto maggiore è la prematurità, tanto più breve è la durata di vita del globulo rosso (fino a 35-50 giorni). La minor durata di vita delle emazie dei neonati pretermine e di quelli a termine può essere spiegata da alcune caratteristiche specifiche di tali cellule: un rapido declino dell'attività enzimatica intracellulare e della disponibilità di ATP, la riduzione della superficie della membrana a causa dell'internalizzazione dei lipidi di membrana, la diminuzione delle concentrazioni intracellulari di carnitina, la maggiore suscettibilità dei lipidi e delle proteine della membrana alla perossidazione e, infine, la maggiore fragilità meccanica causata dall'aumentata deformabilità della membrana.

Bain BJ: Diagnosis from the blood smear. *N Engl J Med* 2005;353:498–507.
Calhoun DA, Christensen RD: Human developmental biology of granulocyte colony-stimulating factor. *Clin Perinatol* 2000;27:559–576.
Dame C, Juul S: The switch from fetal to adult erythropoiesis. *Clin Perinatol* 2000;27:507–526.
Deutsch VR, Toner A: Megakaryocyte development and platelet production. *Br J Haematol* 2006;134:453–466.
Kaushansky K: Lineage-specific hematopoietic growth factors. *N Engl J Med* 2006;354:2034–2045.
Kaushansky K: Thrombopoietin and hematopoietic stem cell development. *Ann NY Acad Sci* 1999;30:314–341.
Ohls RK, Li Y, Abdel-Mageed A, et al: Neutrophil pool sizes and granulocyte colony-stimulating factor production in human mid-trimester fetuses. *Pediatr Res* 1995;37:806–811.
Slayton WB: Development of the immune system in the human fetus. In Christensen RD (editor): *Hematologic Problems of the Neonate.* Philadelphia, WB Saunders, 2000, pp 21–42.
Sola MC, Dame C, Christensen RD: Toward a rational use of recombinant thrombopoietin in the neonatal intensive care unit. *J Pediatr Hematol Oncol* 2001;23:179–184.
Szilvassy SJ: Haematopoietic stem and progenitor cell-targeted therapies for thrombocytopenia. *Expert Opin Bio Ther* 2006;6:983–992.
Vats A, Bielby RC, Tolley NS, et al: Stem cells. *Lancet* 2005; 366:592–602.

Capitolo 447 ■ Anemie

Bertil Glader

L'anemia è definita come una riduzione del volume dei globuli rossi o della concentrazione di emoglobina al di sotto dei livelli di riferimento riscontrati in persone sane. La Tabella 447-1 elenca i valori medi e il livello di riferimento dell'emoglobina e dell'ematocrito, suddivisi in base all'età di bambini sani. Su questo punto sembrano esserci differenze razziali nei livelli di emoglobina. I bambini neri hanno livelli circa 0,5 g/dL più bassi rispetto ai bambini bianchi e orientali della stessa età e stato socioeconomico, forse, in parte, come risultato dell'elevata incidenza di α-talassemia nella razza nera.

Benché una riduzione della quantità di emoglobina circolante diminuisca la capacità del sangue di trasportare ossigeno, si verificano pochi disturbi clinici finché il livello emoglobina non scende sotto 7-8 g/dL. Al di sotto di questo livello compare il pallore a carico delle mucose. Gli adattamenti fisiologici dell'anemia includono aumento della gittata cardiaca, aumento dell'estrazione di ossigeno (aumento della differenza arterovenosa di ossigeno) e una deviazione del flusso sanguigno verso gli organi e i tessuti vitali. Inoltre, la concentrazione di 2,3-difosfoglicerato (2,3-DPG) aumenta all'interno dei globuli rossi. Il risultante "spostamento a destra" della curva di dissociazione dell'ossigeno, riducendo l'affinità dell'emoglobina per l'ossigeno, causa un trasferimento più completo di ossigeno ai tessuti. Lo stesso spostamento nella curva di dissociazione dell'ossigeno può comparire anche ad altitudini elevate. Quando un'anemia abbastanza severa si sviluppa lentamente possono manifestarsi, sorprendentemente, pochi sintomi o reperti obiettivi. Astenia, tachipnea, dispnea da sforzo,

TABELLA 447-1. Valori ematologici durante le età pediatriche

	EMOGLOBINA (g/dL)		EMATOCRITO (%)		RETICOLOCITI (%)	MCV (fL)	LEUCOCITI (numero/mm³)		NEUTROFILI (%)		LINFOCITI (%)	EOSINOFILI (%)	MONOCITI (%)
ETÀ	Media	Range	Media	Range	Media	Limite inferiore	Media	Range	Media	Range	Media*	Media	Media
Sangue del cordone	16,8	13,7-20,1	55	45-65	5,0	110	18 000	(9000-30 000)	61	(40-80)	31	2	6
2 settimane	16,5	13,0-20,0	50	42-66	1,0		12 000	(5000-21 000)	40		63	3	9
3 mesi	12,0	9,5-14,5	36	31-41	1,0		12 000	(6000-18 000)	30		48	2	5
6 mesi-6 anni	12,0	10,5-14,0	37	33-42	1,0	70-74	10 000	(6000-15 000)	45		48	2	5
7-12 anni	13,0	11,0-16,0	38	34-40	1,0	76-80	8000	(4500-13 500)	55		38	2	5
Adulti													
Femmine	14	12,0-16,0	42	37-47	1,6	80	7500	(5000-10 000)	55	(35-70)	35	3	7
Maschi	16	14,0-18,0	47	42-52		80							

*Intervallo relativamente ampio.
fL, femtolitri; MCV, volume corpuscolare medio.

tachicardia, dilatazione cardiaca e infine insufficienza cardiaca congestizia sono causati da un'anemia ingravescente, indipendentemente dalla sua causa.

Quando si riduce il rilascio di ossigeno dagli eritrociti ai tessuti, diversi meccanismi, comprendenti un aumento della gittata cardiaca, un aumento di produzione di 2,3-DPG da parte dei globuli rossi, aumentati livelli di eritropoietina (EPO), aiutano il corpo a compensare la carenza. La produzione di globuli rossi da parte del midollo osseo in risposta all'EPO può aumentare numerose volte, compensando quindi riduzioni da medie a moderate della emivita dei globuli rossi. In alcune forme di anemia, il midollo osseo perde la sua usuale capacità di produzione prolungata ed espansione della massa di eritrociti; e, in questi casi, diminuisce il numero assoluto di reticolociti nel sangue periferico. La percentuale normale di reticolociti rispetto al totale di eritrociti, durante la maggior parte dell'infanzia, è circa 1%, con un numero assoluto di reticolociti pari a 25 000-75 000/mm^3. In presenza di anemia, la produzione di EPO e il numero assoluto di reticolociti dovrebbero aumentare. Un basso numero assoluto o percentuale di reticolociti in risposta all'anemia indica un'insufficienza relativa midollare oppure un'eritropoiesi inefficace (per esempio anemia megaloblastica, talassemia). La misura nel siero del livello del recettore transferrinico (TfR) o l'esame del midollo osseo permette di distinguere tra queste possibilità, poiché il TfR è elevato nei casi di eritropoiesi inefficace (o di carenza di ferro) e diminuisce nei casi di ipoproduzione dei globuli rossi nel midollo.

L'anemia non rappresenta un'entità specifica ma, piuttosto, il risultato di diversi processi patologici sottostanti. Le dimensioni dei globuli rossi cambiano con l'età; prima che un'anemia possa essere caratterizzata in maniera specifica secondo il volume degli

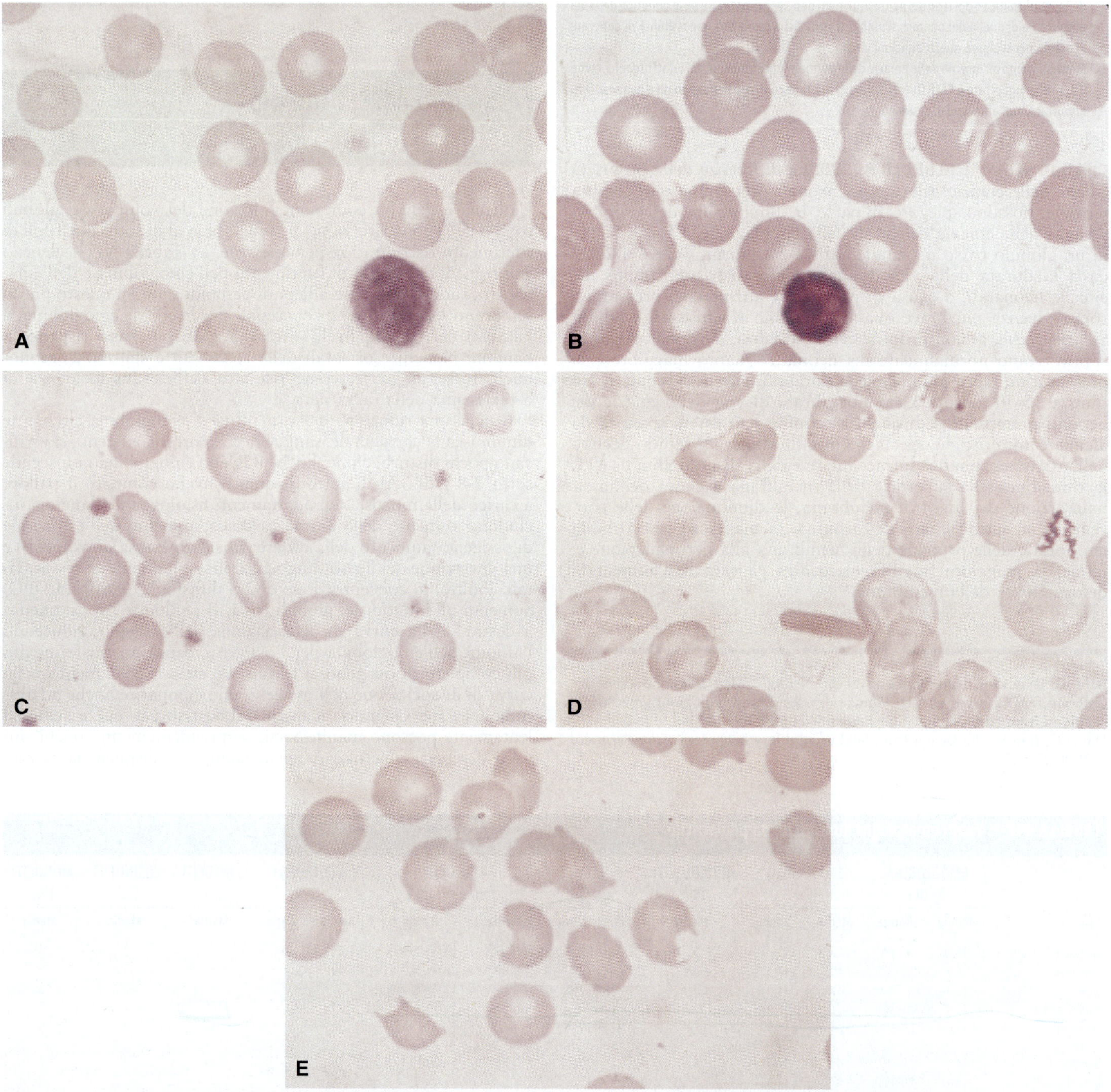

Figura 447-1. Anomalie morfologiche del globulo rosso. *A*, Normale. *B*, Macrociti (carenza di acido folico o vitamina B_{12}). *C*, Microciti ipocromici (carenza di ferro). *D*, Cellule bersaglio (malattia Hb CC). *E*, Schistociti (sindrome uremico-emolitica). (Per gentile concessione del Dr. E. Schwartz.)

eritrociti, devono essere compresi i normali cambiamenti evolutivi del volume corpuscolare medio (MCV) (vedi Tab. 447-1). È importante per i pediatri saper riconoscere le variazioni del valore di MCV nell'infanzia, poiché molti laboratori utilizzano solo i valori di riferimento per l'adulto, che differiscono in maniera considerevole da quelli del bambino. Per ogni bambino con anemia significativa è altrettanto essenziale esaminare l'aspetto dei globuli rossi dallo striscio del sangue periferico (Fig. 447-1). Caratteristiche morfologiche specifiche possono indicare la diagnosi sottostante. Inoltre, la presenza di policromatofilia, che generalmente correla con il grado di reticolocitosi, indica che il midollo osseo è in grado di rispondere alla perdita o distruzione di eritrociti.

CAUSE COMUNI DI ANEMIA. La Figura 447-2 presenta un utile approccio per stabilire le comuni cause di anemia nei bambini.

ASSOCIAZIONE DELL'ANEMIA AD ALTRI DISORDINI EMATOLOGICI. Trombocitopenia, anomalie nel numero dei globuli bianchi o la presenza di leucociti anomali spesso indicano un'insufficienza del midollo osseo causata da anemia aplastica, leucemia o altre patologie maligne a carico del midollo. Tutti questi disordini possono essere differenziati sulla base di un'attenta valutazione degli screening ematologici e di una particolare attenzione alla storia clinica e all'esame obiettivo del bambino.

ASSOCIAZIONE DI ANEMIA E RETICOLOCITOSI. Nei bambini anemici con un'appropriata risposta reticolocitaria, l'anemia generalmente è conseguente a un sanguinamento o un'emolisi in corso. L'aspetto più caratteristico di un'emolisi è la reticolocitosi con iperbilirubinemia indiretta e, spesso, aumentati livelli sierici di lattico deidrogenasi come indicatori di un'accelerata distruzione

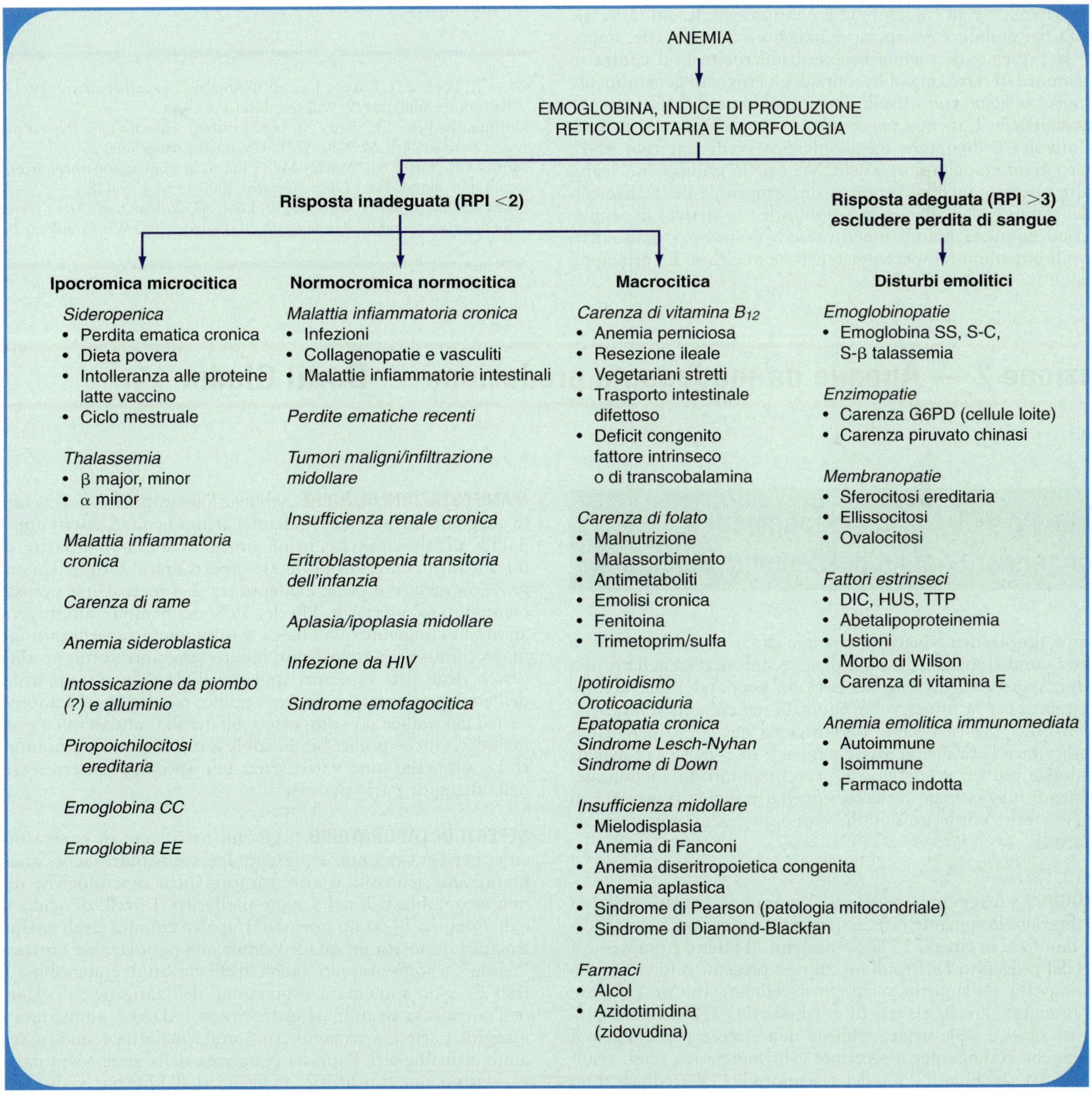

Figura 447-2. Utilizzo della conta cellulare completa, conta reticolocitaria e dello striscio periferico per la diagnosi di anemia. DIC (*Disseminated Intravascular Coagulation*), coagulazione intravascolare disseminata; G6PD (*Glucose-6-Phosphate Dehydrogenase*), glucosio-6-fosfato deidrogenasi; HUS (*Hemolytic Uremic Syndrome*), sindrome uremico-emolitica; RPI (*Reticulocyte Production Index*), indice di produzione reticolocitaria; TTP (*Thrombotic Thrombocytopenic Purpura*), porpora trombotica trombocitopenica. (Da Kliegman RM, Marcdante KJ, Jenson HJ, et al: *Nelson Essentials of Pediatrics,* 5th ed. Philadelphia, Elsevier/Saunders, 2006, p 694.

dei globuli rossi. La valutazione dello striscio di sangue periferico per identificare eritrociti morfologicamente anomali (per es. sferociti, aspetto falciforme, microangiopatie) è spesso utile per accertare le cause dell'emolisi.

ASSOCIAZIONE DI ANEMIA E RETICOLOCITOPENIA. L'anemia nei bambini con una risposta reticolocitaria inadeguata riflette un difetto nel normale processo di eritropoiesi; in questo caso risulta particolarmente utile l'analisi delle dimensioni dei globuli rossi (volume corpuscolare medio [MCV]).

Presenza di microcitemia. Quasi tutti i bambini con anemia e reticolocitopenia hanno difetti di sintesi emoglobinica legati a *carenza di ferro* (vedi Capitolo 455), *trait talassemico*, *malattie dell'emoglobina E o C* (vedi Capitolo 462). Il trait talassemico e altre emoglobinopatie sono prese in considerazione nei pazienti provenienti dal Mediterraneo, dal Medio Oriente, dall'Africa o dall'Asia. Una caratteristica distintiva delle patologie legate al trait talassemico e all'emoglobina E è rappresentato dal fatto che la conta dei globuli rossi spesso è maggiore del normale, nonostante la presenza di anemia lieve e di microcitosi, al contrario della carenza di ferro, in cui la conta degli eritrociti generalmente diminuisce insieme con i livelli di emoglobina e di MCV.

Macrocitemia. L'anemia nei bambini con globuli rossi macrocitici talvolta è di natura megaloblastica (vedi Capitolo 454), risultato di difetti nella sintesi del DNA e nello sviluppo nucleare, e risulta alterato anche il processo di formazione delle altre cellule del sangue. Nell'anemia megaloblastica lo striscio di sangue periferico contiene grandi macrovalociti e spesso i granulociti neutrofili mostrano un'ipersegmentazione nucleare. Le principali cause di anemia megaloblastica comprendono carenza di folati e di vitamina B_{12} oltre a rari disturbi congeniti del metabolismo. Tuttavia, non tutte le anemie macrocitiche sono anche megaloblastiche; una di queste nel bambino è rappresentata dalla malattia di Diamond-Blackfan.

Normocitemia. Un'anemia normocitica, una conta reticolocitaria bassa e livelli normali di bilirubinemia caratterizzano una grande varietà di anemie. L'*anemia delle malattie croniche* (vedi Capitolo 451) è generalmente normocitica. Solo occasionalmente può essere lievemente microcitica e, in questi casi, c'è di solito un'evidenza clinica di malattie croniche o infiammatorie associate. L'anemia nell'insufficienza renale è normocitica ed è causata da una ridotta produzione di eritropoietina. Immancabilmente è anche evidente, da un punto di vista clinico e di laboratorio, un'importante nefropatia. La causa più comune di aplasia pura eritrocitaria acquisita nei pazienti pediatrici è rappresentata dall'eritroblastopenia transitoria dell'infanzia, un tipo di anemia normocitica.

Greer JP, Foerster J, Lukens J, et al: *Wintrobe's Clinical Hematology,* 11th ed. Baltimore, Williams & Wilkins, 2004.

Hoffman R, Benz EJ, Shattil SJ, et al (editors): *Hematology: Basic Principles and Practice,* 4th ed. New York, Churchill Livingstone, 2005.

Morris CR, Singer ST, Walters MC: Clinical hemoglobinopathies: iron, lungs and new blood. *Curr Opin Hematol* 2006;13(6):407–418.

Nathan DG, Orkin SH, Ginsburg O, Look AT: *Nathan and Oski's Hematology of Infancy and Childhood,* 6th ed. Philadelphia, WB Saunders, 2003.

Sezione 2 — Anemie da inadeguata produzione — Bertil Glader

Capitolo 448 ■ Anemia ipoplastica congenita (anemia di Diamond-Blackfan)

L'anemia ipoplastica congenita (anemia di Diamond-Blackfan) è una rara condizione che di solito diviene sintomatica nella prima infanzia, spesso con pallore nel periodo neonatale, ma talvolta viene notata per la prima volta più tardi nel corso dell'infanzia. Oltre il 90% dei casi viene riconosciuto nel corso del primo anno di vita e l'età media alla diagnosi è di 3 mesi. Gli aspetti ematologici più caratteristici sono rappresentati da anemia, generalmente macrocitica, reticolocitopenia e deficit o assenza di precursori eritroidi in un midollo osseo altrimenti con normale cellularità.

EZIOLOGIA. La maggior parte dei casi è sporadica, benché modalità di ereditarietà dominante o recessiva siano suggeriti da una ricorrenza familiare in circa il 15% dei pazienti. Il difetto primitivo è a carico dei progenitori eritroidi, in cui ne è presente uno intrinseco che comporta un'aumentata apoptosi cellulare (morte cellulare programmata). Livelli elevati di eritropoietina (EPO) sono presenti nel siero e nelle urine, sebbene una ricerca per mutazioni nel gene che codifica per il recettore eritropoietinico siano risultate negative. In circa il 25% dei casi sporadici ed ereditari sono state riscontrate mutazioni in un gene (DBA1), codificante per la proteina ribosomiale S19, mappato sul cromosoma 19q13. Un secondo gene per l'*anemia di Diamond-Blackfan* è stato collegato al cromosoma 8p e probabilmente molte altre anomalie genetiche saranno identificate in futuro.

MANIFESTAZIONI CLINICHE. Sebbene l'ematopoiesi sia generalmente adeguata durante la vita fetale, alcuni neonati affetti appaiono pallidi alla nascita o nei primi giorni di vita dopo il parto; si manifesta raramente idrope fetale (vedi Capitolo 103). Un'anemia grave in genere diviene evidente tra 2-6 mesi d'età, occasionalmente un po' più tardi. Più del 50% dei bambini affetti presenta anomalie congenite quali bassa statura, dimorfismi cranio-facciali (naso camuso, ipertelorismo, labbro superiore sottile) o difetti a carico degli arti superiori (polso radiale debole, appiattimento dell'eminenza tenar), compreso pollice trifalangeo. Le anomalie a carico del pollice possono essere bilaterali o unilaterali e possono includere anche pollici bifidi, sublussati, assenti o soprannumerari. Le anomalie sono varie, senza uno specifico pattern d'esordio nella maggior parte dei casi.

REPERTI DI LABORATORIO. I globuli rossi sono in genere macrocitici per l'età ma non è presente ipersegmentazione a carico dei granulociti neutrofili o altre caratteristiche morfologiche di anemia megaloblastica nel sangue periferico. I livelli di acido folico e di vitamina B_{12} sono normali. L'analisi chimica degli enzimi eritrocitari dimostra un quadro simile alla popolazione eritrocitaria "fetale", e sono presenti anche livelli elevati di emoglobina fetale (Hb F) e un'aumentata espressione dell'antigene "i". L'attività dell'adenosina deaminasi eritrocitaria (ADA) è aumentata nella maggior parte dei pazienti con questa malattia e questo reperto aiuta a distinguere l'aplasia congenita della serie rossa dalla *eritroblastopenia transitoria acquisita dell'infanzia* (vedi Capitolo 450). Poiché livelli elevati di attività dell'ADA non rappresentano una peculiarità dei globuli rossi fetali, il dosaggio di questo enzima può aiutare nella diagnosi di anemia di Diamond-Blackfan nei lattanti molto piccoli. Inizialmente possono anche essere presenti trombocitosi o, di rado, trombocitopenia e talvolta neutropenia. Nonostante la severa anemia i reticolociti raramente sono tipicamente molto bassi. I precursori eritroidi nel midollo sono marcatamente ridotti nella maggior parte dei pazienti, mentre gli altri elementi cellulari midollari sono normali e i livelli di ferro sierico elevati. Gli studi sui cromosomi del midollo osseo sono normali e, al contrario dell'anemia di Fanconi, non c'è un aumentata rottura cromosomica quando i linfociti vengono sottoposti a stress con agenti alchilanti.

DIAGNOSI DIFFERENZIALE. L'anemia ipoplastica congenita deve essere differenziata dalle altre forme di anemia con bassa conta reticolocitaria. L'anemia della malattie emolitica del neonato può avere un decorso protratto e, occasionalmente, può associarsi a una marcata riduzione nell'eritropoiesi. Questa di solito termina spontaneamente a 5-8 settimane di vita. Crisi di anemia aplastica, caratterizzate da reticolocitopenia e diminuito numero dei precursori eritroidi, causate frequentemente da infezioni da parvovirus B19, possono complicare diversi tipi di malattie emolitiche croniche, ma generalmente dopo i primi mesi di vita (vedi Capitolo 450). Infezioni da parvovirus B19 (vedi Capitolo 248) in utero possono causare aplasia pura della serie rossa durante l'infanzia, anche con idrope fetale alla nascita. L'assenza del parvovirus B19 documentata mediante PCR (*Polymerase Chain Reaction*) è una caratteristica fondamentale per stabilire la diagnosi di anemia di Diamond-Blackfan nel piccolo lattante. La sindrome dell'eritroblastopenia transitoria dell'infanzia può essere differenziata dalla sindrome di Diamond-Blackfan per il suo esordio relativamente tardivo, anche se può svilupparsi talora in bambini più piccoli di 6 mesi (vedi Capitolo 450). Nei lattanti molto piccoli in cui i globuli rossi presentano caratteristiche "fetali", la determinazione degli elevati livelli eritrocitari di attività dell'ADA è particolarmente utile, perché l'aumentata attività di questo enzima non è una caratteristica degli eritrociti fetali.

TRATTAMENTO. La terapia con corticosteroidi è efficace in 3/4 dei pazienti che inizialmente risponde. Il meccanismo del suo effetto è sconosciuto. Inizialmente viene utilizzato il prednisone in tre dosi divise, per un totale di 2 mg/kg/24 ore. Dopo 1-3 settimane dall'inizio della terapia si può vedere un aumento dei precursori eritroidi nel midollo osseo a cui fa seguito una reticolocitosi periferica. L'emoglobina può raggiungere livelli normali in 4-6 settimane, anche se il grado di risposta è alquanto variabile. Una volta che si è stabilito che la concentrazione di emoglobina sta salendo, la dose di corticosteroidi dovrebbe essere ridotta gradualmente, riducendo a poco a poco le singole dosi e poi eliminandole tutte tranne una singola dose minima efficace giornaliera. Questa dose dovrebbe poi essere raddoppiata, somministrata a giorni alterni e ridotta ulteriormente in seguito, mantenendo la concentrazione di emoglobina a 9 g/dL o sopra. In alcuni pazienti possono essere sufficienti quantità molto piccole di prednisone, anche solo 2,5 mg due volte alla settimana, per mantenere un'eritropoiesi adeguata. Tuttavia, il 60% dei bambini con anemia di Diamond-Blackfan inizialmente trattati con corticosteroidi, smette di assumere il farmaco generalmente per effetti collaterali inaccettabili dei corticosteroidi o per sviluppo di refrattarietà a dosi accettabili di corticosteroidi. Talvolta si verifica remissione spontanea dell'anemia.

Per i pazienti che non rispondono alla terapia corticosteroidea sono necessarie trasfusioni a intervalli di 4-8 settimane per sostenere le normali attività e lo sviluppo del bambino. La terapia chelante per il sovraccarico di ferro con deferoxamina, somministrata per via sottocutanea tramite pompa portabile, viene iniziata quando l'eccesso di ferro accumulato è riflesso dai livelli di ferritina >1500 mg/dL. Il deferasirox ha completato i clinical trial ed è stato approvato dalla FDA come chelante del ferro da usare negli stati di sovraccarico di ferro. Questo agente si può sciogliere in acqua o succo di frutta e assunto come una bibita. Alcuni Autori hanno anticipato che l'uso del deferasirox per via orale sostituirà nel tempo l'utilizzo della deferoxamina per via parenterale. Altre terapie, compresi androgeni, ciclosporina, ciclofosfamide, la globulina antitimocita (ATG), immunoglobuline ad alte dosi per via endovenosa, metilprednisolone ad alte dosi, EPO e l'interleuchina 3 (IL-3) non hanno dimostrato benefici significativi e possono presentare un'elevata incidenza di effetti collaterali. La splenectomia può raramente risultare necessaria per diminuire il fabbisogno trasfusionale, se si sviluppa un ipersplenismo o un'isoimmunizzazione. Il **trapianto di cellule staminali** da un donatore familiare istocompatibile ha un ruolo nei bambini che non rispondono al trattamento corticosteroideo e che hanno necessitato per molti anni di trasfusioni di emazie. I risultati di sopravvivenza ottenuti con donatori familiari compatibili appaiono incoraggianti, ma le risposte sono state considerevolmente meno soddisfacenti utilizzando fratelli solo parzialmente compatibili o donatori compatibili non familiari.

PROGNOSI. La sopravvivenza media probabilmente supera i 40 anni, anche se mancano dati conclusivi a riguardo. Il Diamond-Blackfan Anemia Registry (DBAR) sta raccogliendo dati per verificare la risposta alla terapia e la sopravvivenza (http://www.dbar.org/). L'esito è migliore in quei pazienti che rispondono alla terapia corticosteroidea. Circa la metà dei pazienti risponde a lungo termine. Per gli altri la sopravvivenza dipende dalle trasfusioni. Alcuni bambini in ciascuno dei due gruppi talvolta possono andare incontro a una remissione spontanea (circa il 20%), e la maggior parte di queste remissioni si verifica nella prima decade di vita. Nei bambini che ricevono trasfusioni regolarmente i livelli di ferro totale aumentano e può verificarsi emosiderosi. Le complicanze delle trasfusioni croniche nell'anemia di Diamond-Blackfan sono simili a quelle della β-talassemia major, perciò la prevenzione e il trattamento del sovraccarico di ferro dovrebbe essere ugualmente aggressiva in entrambi i gruppi di pazienti trasfusi. L'anemia di Diamond-Blackfan può essere una sindrome premaligna, con la comparsa di leucemia acuta (generalmente di tipo mieloide) e mielodisplasia in una piccola proporzione di pazienti (<5%). Alcuni Autori riportano anche tumori maligni solidi, soprattutto l'osteosarcoma. Altre cause importanti di morte includono le complicanze associate al trapianto di cellule staminali, alla terapia corticosteroidea (infezioni opportunistiche) e sovraccarico di ferro.

Costa LD, Willig TN, Fixler J, et al: Diamond-Blackfan anemia. *Curr Opin Pediatr* 2001;13:10.

Freedman MH: Diamond-Blackfan anemia. *Baillieres Clin Haematol* 2000;13:391.

Gazda HT, Sieff CA: Recent insights into the pathogenesis of Diamond-Blackfan anaemia. *Br J Haematol* 2006 Oct;135:149–157. Epub 2006 Aug 31.

Gustavsson P, Willig TN, van Haeringen A, et al: Diamond-Blackfan anaemia: Genetic homogeneity for a gene on chromosome 19q13 restricted to 1.8 Mb. *Nat Genet* 1997;16:368.

Lipton JM: Diamond blackfan anemia: New paradigms for a "not so pure" inherited red cell aplasia. *Semin Hematol* 2006;43:167–177.

Vlachos A, Klein GW, Lipton JM: The Diamond Blackfan anemia registry: Tool for investigating the epidemiology and biology of Diamond-Blackfan anemia. *J Pediatr Hematol Oncol* 2001;23:377–382.

Willig TN, Niemeyer CM, Leblanc T, et al: Identification of new prognosis factors from the clinical and epidemiologic analysis of a registry of 229 Diamond-Blackfan anemia patients. *Pediatr Res* 1999;46:553.

Capitolo 449 ■ Sindrome midollare-pancreatica di Pearson

La sindrome midollare-pancreatica di Pearson è una forma di anemia ipoplastica che inizialmente può essere confusa con la sindrome di Diamond-Blackfan o con l'eritrobalstopenia transitoria dell'infanzia. L'insufficienza midollare generalmente compare nel periodo neonatale e si caratterizza per anemia macrocitica e, talvolta, neutropenia e trombocitopenia. I livelli di emoglobina F sono elevati. Nel midollo sono presenti eritroblasti e mieloblasti vacuolati. Questa rara malattia è considerata una variante particolare dell'anemia sideroblastica congenita poiché il midollo contiene anche sideroblasti ad anello. Altre caratteristiche cliniche sono rappresentate da: scarsa crescita, fibrosi pancreatica con diabete insulino dipendente e insufficienza pancreatica esocrina, compromissione muscolare e neurologica e, frequentemente, morte precoce. Questa patologia multiorgano è causata da delezioni nel DNA mitocondriale, con eterogeneità nei diversi tessuti e tra i diversi pazienti. Questa eterogeneità è responsabile delle diverse presentazioni cliniche e un cambiamento nelle proporzioni dei tipi di DNA mitocondriale (mtDNA) nei tessuti può portare, nel tempo, a un miglioramento spontaneo della ipoproduzione di globuli rossi (vedi Capitoli 80 e 346). La terapia comprende trasfusioni di emazie al bisogno. Il filgrastim (G-CSF, *Granulocyte Colony-Stimulating Factor*, fattore stimolante le colonie di granulociti) può far superare gli episodi di grave neutropenia.

Fleming MD: The genetics of inherited sideroblastic anemias. *Semin Hematol* 2002;39:270–281.

Knerr I, Metzler M, Niemeyer CM, et al: Hematologic features and clinical course of an infant with Pearson syndrome caused by a novel deletion of mitochondrial DNA. *J Pediatr Hematol Oncol* 2003;25:948–951.

Rotig A, Bourgeron T, Chretien D, et al: Spectrum of mitochondrial DNA rearrangements in the Pearson marrow-pancreas syndrome. *Hum Mol Genet* 1995;4:1327–1330.

Capitolo 450 ■ Anemie acquisite isolate della serie rossa

ERITROBLASTOPENIA TRANSITORIA DELL'INFANZIA. L'eritroblastopenia transitoria dell'infanzia (TEC, *Transient Erythrobalstopenia of Childhood*), la forma più comune di aplasia acquisita della serie rossa che si manifesta nel bambino, è più comune dell'anemia congenita ipoplastica. Questa sindrome di grave anemia ipoplastica transitoria si verifica soprattutto in bambini sani di età compresa tra 6 mesi e 3 anni e la maggior parte di loro ha più di 12 mesi di vita all'esordio. Solo il 10% ha più di 3 anni. La causa di questa diminuita produzione di eritrociti risiede in una soppressione immunologia transitoria dell'eritropoiesi. Questo spesso consegue a una malattia virale, anche se nessun virus specifico è ancora stato individuato. Le infezioni da parvovirus B19 (vedi Capitolo 248), che possono causare l'ipoplasia nei bambini con anemie emolitiche croniche (vedi Capitolo 469), non sono responsabili della TEC. I reticolociti e i precursori midollari eritroidi sono marcatamente diminuiti, anche se l'esame del midollo osseo è raramente necessario per la diagnosi. Diversi livelli di neutropenia possono manifestarsi nel 20% dei casi mentre il numero delle piastrine è normale o elevato. Come si è osservato nell'anemia da carenza di ferro e in altre ipoplasie della serie rossa, la trombocitosi è presumibilmente causata da aumentati livelli di eritropoietina, che si è visto avere una certa omologia con la trombopoietina. Il volume corpuscolare medio (MCV) è tipicamente normale per l'età e i livelli di emoglobina F (Hb F) sono normali prima della fase di guarigione. I livelli di adenosina deaminasi (ADA) eritrocitaria sono normali in questa patologia, mentre sono elevati nella maggior parte dei bambini con anemia ipoplastica congenita (Tab. 450-1). La diagnosi differenziale con questa ultima patologia può risultare difficile, ma possono risultare utili le differenze di età di esordio, i valori di MCV correlati all'età, i livelli di Hb F e ADA. Il picco di incidenza della TEC coincide con quello dell'anemia ferropriva nei lattanti che ricevono il latte come fonte calorica principale; le differenze nei valori di MCV distinguono chiaramente queste due patologie.

TABELLA 450-1. Confronto tra l'anemia di Diamond-Blackfan e l'eritrobalstopenia transitoria dell'infanzia

	DBA	TEC
N. di pazienti riportati	>700	>500
Maschi/femmine	1,1	1,3
Età alla diagnosi, maschi (mesi)		
Media	10	26
Mediana	2	23
Range	0-408	1-120
Età alla diagnosi, femmine (mesi)		
Media	14	26
Mediana	3	23
Range	0-768	1-192
Maschi >1 anno	9%	82%
Femmine >1 anno	12%	80%
Eziologia	Congenita	Acquisita
Storia precedente	Nessuna	Malattia virale
Esame obiettivo anormale	25%	0%
Laboratorio		
Emoglobina (g/dL)	1,2-14,8	2,2-12,5
GB < 5000/μL	15%	20%
Piastrine > 400 000/μL	20%	45%
Adenosina deaminasi	Aumentata	Normale
MCV aumentato alla diagnosi	80%	5%
Durante guarigione	100%	90%
In remissione	100%	0%
Hb F aumentata alla diagnosi	100%	20%
Durante guarigione	100%	100%
In remissione	85%	0%
Antigene "i" aumentato	100%	20%
Durante guarigione	100%	60%
In remissione	90%	0%

DBA, *Diamond-Blackfan Anemia*; Hb F, emoglobina fetale; MCV, volume corpuscolare medio; TEC, eritroblastopenia transitoria dell'infanzia; GB, globuli bianchi.

Da Nathan DG, Orkin SH, Ginsburg D, et al (editors): *Nathan and Oski's Hematology of Infancy and Childhood*, 6th ed., Vol. 1. Philadelphia, WB Saunders, 2003, p 329. Adattata da Alter BP: The bone marrow failure syndromes. In Nathan DG, Oski FA (editors): *Hematology of Infancy and Childhood*, 3rd ed. Philadelphia, WB Saunders, 1987, p 159; and Link MP, Alter BP: Fetal erythropoiesis during recovery from transient erythroblastopenia of childhood (TEC). *Pediatr Res* 1981; 15:1036.

Virtualmente tutti i bambini guariscono entro 1 e 2 mesi. Trasfusioni di emazie possono rendersi necessarie in caso di anemia severa senza segni di miglioramento precoce. L'anemia si sviluppa lentamente e sintomi marcati si sviluppano solo in caso di anemia severa. In questa malattia la terapia con corticosteroidi non è di alcun valore. Ogni bambino con presunta TEC che richieda più di una trasfusione dovrebbe essere rivalutato per altre possibili diagnosi. In rare situazioni, un caso prolungato di TEC può essere causato da un'aplasia eritrocitaria parvovirus indotta e compare in bambini con immunodeficienze congenite o acquisite.

APLASIA DELLA SERIE ROSSA ASSOCIATA A EMOLISI CRONICA. Il parvovirus B19 è la causa virale più documentata di aplasia della serie rossa nel feto, nei pazienti immunocompromessi o in quelli con emolisi cronica; esso è la causa della quinta malattia o eritema infettivo (vedi Capitolo 248). Il virus è particolarmente infettivo e citotossico nei progenitori eritrocitari intramidollari e interagisce, nello specifico, con l'antigene P eritrocitario come recettore. Con la microscopia a luce trasmessa è possibile vedere, nel midollo osseo, caratteristiche inclusioni nucleari negli eritrobalsti e nei promonoblasti giganti. Dal momento che l'infezione di questo virus è transitoria, con una guarigione in meno di 2 settimane, l'anemia non si presenta o non viene riconosciuta in quei bambini normali in cui la vita media dei globuli rossi è di 100-120 giorni. Tuttavia, nei pazienti con emolisi, causata da sferocitosi congenita o anemia falciforme, nei quali la vita media degli RBC è molto più breve, un momentaneo blocco delle eritropoiesi causata dal parvovirus può provocare un'anemia severa, le cosiddette **crisi aplastiche** che si verificano in queste patologie. La guarigione da forme di anemia da moderata a severa generalmente è spontanea, preannunciata da un aumento di emazie nucleate e successivamente reticolociti nel sangue periferico. Talvolta è necessaria una trasfusione di globuli rossi in caso di sintomi marcati provocati dall'anemia. Nei bambini con emolisi cronica, le crisi aplastiche indotte dal parvovirus generalmente compaiono una sola volta. Nelle famiglie con più di un bambino affetto da una malattia emolitica, i genitori dovrebbero essere avvertiti che un episodio di aplasia eritrocitaria simile può verificarsi negli altri bambini se questi non sono mai stati esposti prima al parvovirus.

APLASIA DELLA SERIE ROSSA ASSOCIATA A IMMUNODEFICIENZA. La persistenza di un'infezione da parvovirus raramente può verificarsi nei pazienti che non sono in grado di montare un'adeguata risposta anticorpale al virus, come i bambini con immunodeficienze congenite, quelli trattati con farmaci immunosoppressori e quelli con AIDS. La conseguente aplasia della serie rossa può essere severa e spesso si ritiene che i bambini affetti abbiano una TEC. Questo tipo di aplasia dei globuli rossi differisce dalla TEC in cui non c'è guarigione spontanea e si rende necessaria più di una trasfusione. La diagnosi di infezione da parvovirus viene effettuata mediante l'identificazione delle particelle virali (attraverso la *Polymerase Chain Reaction*, PCR, reazione a catena della polimerasi) dal momento che le abituali risposte sierologiche sono difettose in questi bambini immunodeficienti. L'infezione virale nei pazienti cronicamente affetti può essere trattata con alte dosi di immunoglobuline per via endovenosa (IVIG, *Intravenous Immunoglobulin*), che contengono anticorpi in grado di neutralizzare il virus.

APLASIA DELLA SERIE ROSSA CON ABORTO E IDROPE FETALE. Diverse manifestazioni cliniche di infezione da parvovirus e distruzione dei precursori eritroidi si hanno con le infezioni in utero, in cui si verifica un aumento della perdita fetale nel primo e secondo trimestre e i neonati possono nascere con idrope fetale (vedi Capitolo 103) e viremia. La presenza di infezione da parvovirus congenita persistente è dimostrata mediante PCR del DNA estratto dal sangue periferico e/o dal midollo osseo, perché la tolleranza immunologica al virus può ostacolare l'abituale sviluppo di anticorpi specifici.

ALTRE FORME DI APLASIA DELLA SERIE ROSSA NEI BAMBINI. Le forme di aplasia della serie rossa dell'adulto sono generalmente forme croniche mediate da anticorpi e spesso sono associate a patologie come la leucemia linfatica cronica, il timoma, il linfoma, i disturbi linfoproliferativi e il lupus eritematoso sistemico. Questa forma cronica di aplasia della serie rossa mediata da anticorpi è estremamente rara nell'infanzia. L'alemtuzumab (anticorpo umanizzato anti CD52) è stato utilizzato per trattare l'aplasia pura della serie rossa a esordio in età adulta quando il trattamento con corticosteroidi e altri agenti immunosoppressori si era rivelato inutile. Alcuni farmaci, come il cloramfenicolo, possono inibire l'eritropoiesi in maniera dose dipendente. Reticolocitopenia, ipoplasia eritroide e pronormoblasti vacuolati nel midollo sono effetti reversibili di questo farmaco e questi effetti sono distinti dal raro sviluppo di natura idiosincrasica di anemia aplastica in chi ha ricevuto il cloramfenicolo.

L'aplasia pura acquisita della serie rossa anticorpo mediata è una rara complicanza che si è vista in pazienti cronicamente trattati con eritropoietina ricombinante umana soprattutto per insufficienza renale cronica. Il trattamento comprende immunosoppressione e trapianto di rene così come sospensione dell'EPO.

ANEMIE DISERITROPOIETICHE CONGENITE. (VEDI CAPITOLO 452).

Au WY, Lam CCK, Chim CS, et al: Alemtuzumab induced complete remission of therapy-resistant pure red cell aplasia. *Leukemia Res* 2005;29: 1213–1215.

Bennett CL, Luminari S, Nissenson AR, et al: Pure red-cell aplasia and epoetin therapy. *N Engl J Med* 2004;351:1403–1408.

Cherrick I, Karayalcin G, Lanzkowsky P: Transient erythroblastopenia of childhood. *Am J Pediatr Hematol Oncol* 1994;16:320.

Heimpel H: Congenital dyserythropoietic anemias: Epidemiology, clinical significance, and progress in understanding their pathogenesis. *Ann Hematol* 2004; 83:613–621.

Intalapaporn P, Poovorawan Y, Suankratay C: Immune reconstitution syndrome associated with parvovirus B19-induced pure red cell apalasia during highly active antiretroviral therapy. *J Infect* 2006;53:e79–e82.

Verhelst D, Rossert J, Casadevall N, et al: Treatment of erythropoietin-induced pure red cell aplasia: A retrospective study. *Lancet* 2004;363:1768–1771.

Wickramasinghe SN, Wood WG: Advances in the understanding of the congenital dyserythropoietic anemias. *Brit J Haematol* 2005;131:431–446.

Capitolo 451 ■ Anemia delle malattie croniche e delle patologie renali

451.1 • Anemia da malattie croniche

L'anemia delle malattie croniche (ACD, *Anemia of Chronic Disease*) complica un numero di patologie croniche sistemiche associate a infezione, infiammazione, danno tissutale, come le infezioni piogeniche croniche (per es. bronchiectasie, osteomielite) e processi infiammatori cronici (per es. artrite reumatoide, lupus eritematoso sistemico, colite ulcerosa). Nonostante le diverse cause sottostanti, le anomalie eritrocitarie sono simili, anche se non completamente comprese. L'emivita dei globuli rossi è lievemente diminuita, ma questa aumentata emolisi non rappresenta il problema principale. È più importante l'insufficienza relativa del midollo osseo a rispondere adeguatamente all'anemia. Questa difettosa risposta eritropoietica è associata a una ridotta risposta all'eritropoietina (EPO), nonostante il fatto che i livelli di EPO siano modestamente aumentati. Una caratteristica importante dell'ACD è la diminuita disponibilità di ferro. Il ferro sierico è basso nonostante i macrofagi tissutali abbiano abbondante ferro e si ritenga che queste anomalie siano dovute non solo al sequestro del ferro nei macrofagi, ma anche a un diminuito assorbimento intestinale di esso. Un'ipotesi è stata che la condizione medica sottostante causi il rilascio di citochine infiammatorie, interleuchina 1 (IL-1), fattore di necrosi tumorale (TNF) e interleuchina 6 (IL-6), che inducono la produzione di interferone β (IFN-β) e γ (IFN-γ). Quest'ipotesi è sostenuta dall'osservazione che IFN-β e IFN-γ, quando somministrati ad animali da esperimento, causano un'alterazione simile all'anemia delle malattie croniche. Alcuni studi hanno trovato che IL-6 induce la produzione dell'epcidina, una proteina regolatrice del ferro che sembra essere responsabile di molte delle maggiori caratteristiche di questa patologia. L'epcidina, che viene prodotta nel fegato, diminuisce l'assorbimento intestinale del ferro e blocca anche il rilascio del ferro da parte dei macrofagi.

MANIFESTAZIONI CLINICHE. Anche se i sintomi e segni importanti sono relativi alla malattia sottostante, l'anemia da lieve a moderata che la accompagna può compromettere la qualità di vita del paziente.

REPERTI DI LABORATORIO. La concentrazione di emoglobina è generalmente pari a 6-9 g/dL. L'anemia è in genere normocromica e normocitica, anche se alcuni pazienti possono presentare modesta ipocromia e microcitosi. La conta assoluta dei reticolociti è normale o bassa e la leucocitosi è comune. La sideremia è ridotta, senza incremento della capacità totale di legare il ferro (transferrina sierica) come si osserva nella carenza di ferro. Questa riduzione della sideremia e capacità totale legante il ferro (transferrina sierica) ridotta o normale sono una caratteristica costante, utile per la diagnosi. La ferritinemia può essere elevata. Il midollo osseo ha una cellularità normale; i precursori eritroidi sono da ridotti ad adeguati, l'emosiderina midollare può essere aumentata e può essere presente iperplasia granulocitaria. Una difficoltà clinica comune è quella di identificare una concomitante carenza di ferro in pazienti con una patologia infiammatoria. Il dosaggio del rapporto TfR/ferritina può essere utile, poiché esso è elevato nei pazienti con deficit di ferro (vedi Capitoli 447 e 455). Anche un tentativo terapeutico a base di ferro può aiutare a risolvere questo problema, sebbene possa non esserci risposta qualora persista l'infiammazione causata dalla malattia di base.

TRATTAMENTO E PROGNOSI. Poiché queste forme di anemia sono secondarie ad altri processi patologici, esse non rispondono a una terapia con ferro o derivati a meno che non ci sia una carenza concomitante. Le trasfusioni aumentano la concentrazione di emoglobina temporaneamente, ma sono raramente indicate. Se la malattia sottostante può essere controllata, l'anemia si risolve. L'EPO ricombinante umana può aumentare i livelli di emoglobina e migliorare l'attività e il senso di benessere nei pazienti con neoplasie e in quelli con l'anemia della flogosi cronica. Il trattamento con ferro è di solito necessario per un effetto ottimale dell'EPO.

451.2 • Anemia da nefropatia

Sebbene l'anemia che si vede nelle nefropatie croniche mostri alcune caratteristiche comuni alle anemie delle malattie croniche, come un grado lieve di emolisi, la componente maggiore di questa anemia è la diminuita produzione di EPO a causa di un danno alle cellule renali che producono questo ormone. La concentrazione di emoglobina è variabile (6-10 g/dL), a seconda del grado di uremia. L'anemia è in genere normocitica, e la conta reticolocitaria assoluta è normale o bassa. Il bilancio marziale è normale. È presente un'evidenza di laboratorio di insufficienza renale. L'EPO ricombinante umana è utile somministrata insieme al ferro.

Andrews NC: Anemia of inflammation: The cytokine-hepcidin link. *J Clin Invest* 2004;113:1251–1253.

Cazzola M, Ponchio L, de Benedetti F, et al: Defective iron supply for erythropoiesis and adequate endogenous erythropoietin production in the anemia associated with systemic-onset juvenile chronic arthritis. *Blood* 1996;87:4824–4830.

Means RT: Hepcidin and anaemia. *Blood Reviews* 2004;18:219–225.

Weiss G, Goodnough LT: Anemia of chronic disease. *N Engl J Med* 2005; 352:1011–1023.

Capitolo 452 ■ Anemie diseritropoietiche congenite

Le anemie diseritropoietiche congenite (CDA, *Congenital Dyserythropoietic Anemias*) sono una classe di disordini emolitici caratterizzati da anomalie morfologiche uniche negli eritroblasti midollari: nucleo multiplo, frammenti nucleari anomali e ponti intracromatinici tra le cellule. La glicosilazione delle proteine di membrana è difettosa e i pazienti presentano un accumulo dei glicolipidi eritrocitari. La causa di entrambe queste anomalie si ritiene essere una carenza di N-acetil-glucosaminiltransferasi II, un enzima eritrocitario responsabile della glicosilazione delle proteine di membrana. Clinicamente, queste patologie si caratterizzano per gradi diversi di anemia, nonostante il fatto che ci sia un aumento dell'attività eritroide midollare (eritropoiesi inefficace). La CDA è stata riportata in neonati con idrope fetale. Sono stati definiti tre tipi di CDA (tipo I, II e III) (Tab. 452-1).

La **CDA di tipo I** è una rara patologia autosomica recessiva, in cui l'esordio dell'anemia macrocitica e/o l'ittero possono essere notati a qualsiasi età, sebbene la maggior parte dei casi venga riconosciuta per la prima volta nel periodo neonatale. Alcuni pazienti presentano anomalie ossee, soprattutto la sindattilia. La conta reticolocitaria è meno di quanto ci si può aspettare per il grado di anemia. I globuli bianchi e la piastrine sono normali. I livelli di bilirubina indiretta sono lievemente aumentati, i livelli di aptoglobina sono ridotti e la transferrina è satura di ferro (i livelli di ferro sierico sono prossimi alla capacità totale legante il ferro). Il midollo mostra iperplasia eritroide, dimostrata da eritroblasti megaloblastici in assenza di deficit di vitamina B_{12} o folati. Un piccolo numero di eritroblasti manifesta caratteristiche diseritropoietiche con ponti intercromatinici tra le cellule. Il **trattamento** di questa patologia è stato privo di successo con i normali stimolanti la eritropoiesi (vitamine e corticosteroidi), ma alcuni miglioramenti sono stati ottenuti con l'interferone-α. Anche se la splenomegalia è comune, la splenectomia non è d'aiuto. La più importante complicanza a lungo termine è l'emosiderosi causata dall'aumentato assorbimento intestinale di ferro e l'eritropoiesi inefficace. Il gene per la CDA di tipo I è stato mappato nel cromosoma 15q15.1; il gene *CDAN1* è stato clonato e numerose diverse mutazioni sono state identificate. Il ruolo cellulare della codanina-1, codificata dal gene *CDAN1*, è invece sconosciuto.

La **CDA di tipo II**, una patologia autosomica recessiva, è la variante di CDA più comune. Il gene per la CDA di tipo II è stato mappato sul cromosoma 20q11.2. Le caratteristiche cliniche e di laboratorio sono simili a quelle del tipo I, ma l'anemia è in genere più severa. Molti più eritroblasti midollari maturi (fino al 50%) possono essere anormali, come dimostrato dalla binuclearità, multinuclearità e lobulazioni anomale. Il reperto patognomonico nella CDA di tipo II è il fatto che i globuli rossi del paziente vengono lisati dall'acidificazione del siero. La CDA di tipo II è conosciuta con l'acronimo **HEMPAS** (*Hereditary Erythroblastic Multinuclearity with a Positive Acidified Serum test*) poiché essa è caratterizzata sia da eritrobalsti multinucleati sia da globuli rossi sensibili alla lisi da siero normale acidificato. I pazienti con anemia grave richiedono trasfusioni di sangue. Il sovraccarico di ferro consegue sia alle trasfusioni sia all'aumentato assorbimento intestinale (anche nei pazienti non trasfusi) e la terapia chelante del ferro dovrebbe essere considerata clinicamente indicata. Al contrario della CDA di tipo I, la splenectomia è utile nei pazienti con CDA di tipo II, e, come nella sferocitosi ereditaria, la sopravvivenza dei globuli rossi è normale dopo la splenectomia nonostante gli eritrociti anormali continuino a circolare. La sple-

TABELLA 452-1. Tipo di anemie diseritropoietiche congenite

ASPETTO	TIPO I	TIPO II	TIPO III
Pazienti riferiti	130	200	60
Rapporto maschi:femmine	1:1	0:9	0:8
Anemia	Lieve-moderata	Moderata	Lieve-moderata
Dimensioni dei GR	Macrocitici	Normo-macrocitici	Macrocitici
Eritroblasti Midollari	Megaloblasti, binucleati (2-5%), ponti cromatina	Bi e multinucleati (10-40%), carioressi	Gigantoblasti (10-40%)
Ereditarietà	Recessiva	Recessiva	Dominante
Emolisi siero acido	Negativa	Positiva	Negativa
Reazione			
Anti-i	Debole	Forte	Debole
Anti-I	Debole	Forte	Debole
Effetto della splenectomia	50%	96%	100%
Locus gene*	15q15.1-15.3	20q11.2	15q21-25
Nomenclatura gene	*CDAI*	*CDAII*	*CDAIII*

* Locus genetico per alcuni ma non tutti i pazienti in ogni categoria.

Da Nathan DG, Orkin SH, Ginsburg D, et al: *Nathan and Oski's Hematology of Infancy and Childhood*, 6th ed., Vol. 1. Philadelphia, WB Saunders, 2003, p 332.

nectomia non previene un ulteriore sovraccarico di ferro, anche in quei pazienti in cui l'emoglobina si normalizza; si ritiene che tutto questo rifletta la perdurante eritropoiesi inefficace nel midollo osseo. La maggior parte dei pazienti può condurre una vita normale e ha una normale aspettativa di vita se le complicanze e le loro conseguenze vengono trattate in modo appropriato.

La **CDA di tipo III**, il tipo meno comune, è un'anemia macrocitica da lieve a moderata. Le trasfusioni non sono in genere richieste. In contrasto con altri tipi di CDA, il sovraccarico di ferro non è un problema clinicamente importante; questa malattia è ereditata come difetto autosomico dominante. Un aspetto caratteristico del midollo osseo è l'iperplasia eritroide, con molti eritroblasti multinucleati contenenti fino a 12 nuclei. Il gene per la CDA di tipo III è stato mappato sul cromosoma15q21 vicino al gene CDAN1.

Chrobak L: Successful treatment of iron overload with phlebotomies in two siblings with congenital dyserythropoietic anemias-type II (CDA II). *Acta Medica (Hradee Krabue)* 2006;49:193–195.

Heimpel H, Wilts H, Hirschmann WD, et al: Aplastic crisis as a complication of Congenital Dyserythropoietic Anemia Type II. *Acta Haematol* 2006;117:115–118.

Wickramasinghe SN, Wood WB: Advances in the understanding of the congenital dyserythropoietic anaemias. *Br J Haematol* 2005;131:431–446.

Capitolo 453 ■ Anemia fisiologica del lattante

DESCRIZIONE ED EZIOLOGIA. Sebbene i neonati sani a termine abbiano alti livelli di emoglobina ed ematocrito con globuli rossi di dimensioni maggiori rispetto ai bambini più grandi e agli adulti, durante la prima settimana di vita inizia un progressivo calo nei livelli di emoglobina, che persiste per 6-8 settimane. Il risultato di tale declino è in genere conosciuto come **anemia fisiologica del lattante**. Sono coinvolti moltissimi fattori. Alla nascita, con l'inizio della respirazione, è disponibile molto più ossigeno per legare l'emoglobina, la saturazione aumenta dal 50 al 95% o anche oltre. Il normale cambiamento di sintesi dell'emoglobina da fetale ad adulta sostituisce in modo attivo l'emoglobina fetale, a elevata affinità per l'ossigeno, con quella adulta, a minore affinità per l'ossigeno, la quale è in grado di distribuire ai tessuti una percentuale maggiore dell'ossigeno che le è legato. Immediatamente dopo la nascita, l'aumento del contenuto dell'ossigeno nel sangue e del rilascio di esso ai tessuti abbassano la produzione di eritropoietina (EPO) e, di conseguenza, viene soppressa l'eritropoiesi. In assenza di quest'ultima, i livelli di emoglobina si riducono, dal momento che i globuli rossi più vecchi non vengono sostituiti come avviene di norma quando essi vengono rimossi dalla circolazione. Il ferro proveniente dai globuli rossi degradati viene depositato per la futura sintesi emoglobinica. La concentrazione di emoglobina continua a diminuire finché il fabbisogno di ossigeno dei tessuti non supera l'ossigeno a essi fornito. Di solito, questo punto viene raggiunto tra le 8-12 settimane di vita, quando la concentrazione emoglobinica è pari a 9-11 g/dL. Una volta che l'ipossia viene riconosciuta dai sensori renali o epatici, aumenta la produzione di EPO e ricomincia l'eritropoiesi. Il ferro dapprima depositato nel reticoloendotelio può essere in seguito utilizzato. Il ferro immagazzinato è sufficiente per la sintesi di emoglobina anche in assenza di assunzione di ferro con la dieta, fino a circa 20 settimane di vita. Questa "anemia" può essere vista come un adattamento fisiologico alla vita extrauterina, e riflette l'eccessiva capacità di rilascio di ossigeno rispetto alle richieste dei tessuti. Non vi è nessun problema ematologico e non è necessaria alcuna terapia.

Anche i *neonati prematuri* sviluppano un'anemia fisiologica, ma l'abbassamento dei livelli di emoglobina è più importante e più rapido. Livelli minimi di emoglobina di 7-9 g/dL sono comunemente raggiunti attorno alle 3-6 settimane di vita e possono essere anche più bassi nei prematuri estremamente piccoli (vedi Capitoli 97 e 103.1). L'eziologia di quest'anemia dipende da molti fattori. Sono coinvolti, ma in modo molto più importante, gli stessi fattori presenti nel neonato a termine. Una componente rilevante da considerare nelle primissime settimane di vita è la perdita di sangue in seguito a prelievo per i principali test di laboratorio, esami che sono necessari a stabilizzare la condizione clinica, in particolare dei neonati con problemi cardiorespiratori. La risposta eritropoietica all'anemia è inoltre subottimale e questo è un problema serio, poiché la richiesta di eritropoiesi è incrementata dalla ridotta sopravvivenza degli eritrociti del neonato prematuro (40-60 giorni al contrario dei 120 giorni dell'adulto) e dal rapido aumento della massa eritrocitaria che accompagna la crescita. La base di questa eritropoiesi subottimale nel prematuro sembra essere l'insufficiente produzione di EPO in risposta all'ipossia. Poiché è il fegato la sorgente principale di EPO durante la vita fetale, alcuni Autori hanno proposto che l'insensibilità relativa dei sensori epatici per l'ossigeno all'ipossia possa spiegare la ridotta risposta eritropoietinica che si riscontra nel neonato prematuro. La risoluzione spontanea dell'anemia che si verifica a circa 40 settimane gestazionali è dovuta al passaggio, legato alla crescita, dai recettori epatici all'ossigeno relativamente insensibili ai sensori renali, i quali sono estremamente sensibili all'ipossia, dal momento che a quest'età la sede principale per la sintesi dell'EPO è spostata ai reni.

L'entità dell'anemia fisiologica dell'infanzia può essere modificata da altri processi intercorrenti. Un'anemia iporigenerativa tardiva, con assenza di reticolociti, può verificarsi in bambini con una forma lieve di anemia emolitica del neonato, che richiede solo la fototerapia per ridurre in maniera efficace la concentrazione di bilirubina. La persistenza di anticorpi materni antieritrociti nel circolo del neonato può portare a un'anemia emolitica di basso grado per molte settimane e questo può aggravare l'anemia fisiologica del lattante. Inoltre può anche riflettere una difettosa risposta eritropoietinica. Un'altra osservazione riguarda l'emoglobina più bassa dell'atteso al nadir "fisiologico" che si vede nei neonati dopo trasfusioni intrauterine o neonatali di globuli rossi. Quando i prematuri vengono trasfusi con sangue dell'adulto contenente Hb A, lo spostamento della curva di dissociazione dell'ossigeno, come risultato della presenza dell'Hb A, facilita il rilascio di ossigeno ai tessuti. Pertanto, la definizione di anemia e la necessità di trasfondere i neonati prematuri devono essere basate non solo sui livelli di emoglobina, ma anche sulle richieste di ossigeno e sulla capacità dell'emoglobina neonatale circolante di rilasciarlo.

Anche fattori dietetici possono aggravare l'anemia fisiologica. La carenza di acido folico in aggiunta al processo fisiologico può portare a un'anemia molto più severa. La carenza di vitamina E e la conseguente terapia non sembrano avere un ruolo nell'anemia del prematuro, nonostante in passato si pensasse il contrario. Uno studio in cieco controllato sulla somministrazione orale di vitamina E (25 UI/dL di α-tocoferolo, soluzione colloidale acquosa) a neonati di peso inferiore a 1500 g non mostrò differenze nei livelli di emoglobina, reticolociti, morfologia delle emazie o conta piastrinica. L'allattamento al seno e le attuali formule per neonati sembrano fornire adeguate dosi di vitamina E (vedi Capitolo 49). La supplementazione orale di vitamina C (50 mg/24 ore) non causa emolisi nei neonati prematuri, mentre quella di ferro iniziando dalla dose di 4 mg/kg/24 h dalle 4-8 settimane di vita per neonati pretermine e dal 4° mese nei neonati a termine non causa una significativa emolisi legata all'ossidazione.

A meno che non ci sia stata un'importante perdita perinatale di sangue, la carenza di ferro non dovrebbe essere considerata una causa di anemia nei neonati a termine nei primi 4 mesi di vita. Assumendo che un bambino sia nato con adeguate riserve di ferro, la carenza dietetica non può essere causa di anemia finché tali riserve non vengono esaurite. In assenza di perdite di sangue, ciò non si può verificare finché il peso della nascita non si sia all'incirca raddoppiato.

TRATTAMENTO. L'anemia fisiologica non richiede alcun trattamento se non l'assicurarsi che la dieta del neonato contenga nutrienti essenziali per la normale eritropoiesi, soprattutto acido folico e ferro. Non sono stati stabiliti livelli ottimali di ematocrito per i prematuri (vedi Capitolo 470). I neonati prematuri che si stanno alimentando bene e che stanno crescendo normalmente di rado richiedono trasfusioni, a meno che non si siano verificate significative perdite di sangue iatrogene. Nei prematuri sani, livelli di emoglobina bassi fino a 6,5 g/dL sono di solito ben tollerati. La valutazione delle condizioni cliniche generali, inclusa la crescita, e il monitoraggio dell'ematocrito sono i migliori indicatori per capire quando è necessaria una trasfusione di emazie, la quale non sembra influenzare il corso delle crisi di apnea e bradicardia. Quando sono necessarie le trasfusioni, è consigliato un volume di emazie di 10-15 mL/kg. Il numero di donatori per un neonato dovrebbe essere minimo. Nei prematuri di peso inferiore a 1250 g, l'emivita dei globuli rossi trasfusi è di circa 30 giorni.

L'anemia nei prematuri molto piccoli per età gestazionale può essere correlata alla relativa carenza di EPO e trial clinici indicano che i prematuri senza gravi patologie, trattati con EPO ricombinante umana (rHuEPO) e ferro nelle prime 6 settimane di vita, richiedono meno trasfusioni. I tempi migliori di inizio trattamento con la rHuEPO e il dosaggio ottimale non sono ancora stati stabiliti. Per ottenere i risultati migliori devono essere somministrate dosi orali di ferro di almeno 4-6 mg/kg/die. I costi del trattamento con rHuEPO al momento attuale sono maggiori rispetto a quelli delle trasfusioni di emazie; comunque il trattamento con l'EPO svolge un ruolo importante nella presa in cura del neonato i cui genitori rifiutano le trasfusioni di sangue per motivi religiosi.

Bednarek FJ, Weisberger S, Richardson DK, et al: Variations in blood transfusions among newborn intensive care units. *J Pediatr* 1998;133:601–607.

Fain J, Hilsenrath P, Widness JA, et al: A cost analysis comparing erythropoietin and red cell transfusions in the treatment of anemia of prematurity. *Transfusion* 1995;35:936–943.

Meyer MP, Haworth C, Meyer JH: A comparison of oral and intravenous iron supplementation in preterm infants receiving recombinant erythropoietin. *J Pediatr* 1996;129:258–263.

Ohls RK: The use of erythropoietin in neonates. *Clin Perinatol* 2000;27: 681–696.

Capitolo 454 ■ Anemie megaloblastiche

Le anemie megaloblastiche hanno in comune alcune anomalie nella morfologia e della maturazione dei globuli rossi. A ogni stadio di sviluppo i globuli rossi sono più grandi del normale, hanno la cromatina nucleare aperta, finemente dispersa, e un'asincronia tra la maturazione del nucleo e quella del citoplasma, con un ritardo nella progressione nucleare che diventa molto più evidente nelle divisioni cellulari successive. Nel midollo sono anche presenti metamielociti giganti e con nucleo a banderella. Tutte le anemie megaloblastiche sono caratterizzate da eritropoiesi inefficace, un termine cinetico che descrive un'eritropoiesi attiva con morte prematura delle cellule, diminuita fuoriuscita dei globuli rossi dal midollo e, di conseguenza, anemia. Nel sangue periferico, i globuli rossi sono grossi (aumento del volume corpuscolare medio [MCV]) e spesso ovaliformi. Anche i neutrofili ipersegmentati sono caratteristici, molti con >5 lobi. Quasi tutti i casi di anemia megaloblastica dell'infanzia si sviluppano in seguito a una carenza di acido folico o vitamina B_{12}, ma raramente questi possono essere causati da errori congeniti del metabolismo. Sia la vitamina B_{12} sia i folati sono richiesti per la sintesi delle nucloproteine, la loro carenza causa un deficit di sintesi del DNA e, in misura minore, dell'RNA e delle proteine. Le anemie megaloblastiche conseguenti a malnutrizione sono relativamente poco comuni negli Stati Uniti ma sono importanti in tutto il mondo (vedi Capitoli 1 e 43).

454.1 • Carenze di acido folico

I folati sono abbondanti in molti cibi, inclusi gli ortaggi verdi, la frutta e gli organi animali (per es. il fegato, il rene). I folati sono labili al calore e solubili in acqua e, di conseguenza, riscaldare o bollire una sorgente di folati porta a diminuirne la quantità di vitamine. I folati che si possono trovare in natura sono in forma di poliglutammati e vengono assorbiti meno efficacemente di quelli monoglutammati (per es. l'acido folico). L'attività della folato coniugasi, nell'orletto a spazzola intestinale, induce la conversione dei poliglutammati in monoglutammati e pertanto aumenta l'assorbimento. L'acido folico è assorbito lungo tutto il piccolo intestino ed è presente un'attiva circolazione entero-epatica. La maggior parte del folato nel plasma è debolmente legato all'albumina. L'acido folico non è biologicamente attivo. Esso viene ridotto dalla diidrofolato reduttasi in tetraidrofolato, il quale viene poi trasportato all'interno delle cellule dei tessuti e poliglutammato. Le riserve dell'organismo di folato sono limitate e l'anemia megaloblastica si verifica dopo 2-3 mesi di dieta priva di folati.

MANIFESTAZIONI CLINICHE. L'anemia megaloblastica lieve è stata riscontrata in lattanti di peso molto piccolo alla nascita ed è consigliata la supplementazione con acido folico. Sebbene attualmente rara, l'anemia megaloblastica legata a carenza di folati presenta un picco di incidenza a 4-7 mesi di vita, un po' prima rispetto alla anemia sideropenica, anche se entrambe le condizioni possono essere presenti contemporaneamente nei neonati malnutriti. Nonostante mostrino i soliti tratti dell'anemia, i neonati affetti da carenza di folati sono irritabili, hanno una curva di crescita inadeguata e diarrea cronica. Emorragie da trombocitopenia si manifestano nei casi più avanzati. Nei bambini più grandi con carenza di folati, i segni e sintomi sono correlati all'anemia e a qualsiasi sottostante processo patologico responsabile della carenza vitaminica. La carenza di acido folico può accompagnare il kwashiorkor, il marasma o la sprue.

EZIOLOGIA. La carenza di acido folico può verificarsi come conseguenza di un inadeguato apporto di folati, diminuito assorbimento di folati oppure di disordini acquisiti o congeniti del metabolismo.

Apporto inadeguato di folati. L'anemia dovuta a diminuito apporto di folati si rende di solito evidente in presenza di condizioni cliniche che presentino richieste aumentate di vitamina (per es. la gravidanza, la crescita nell'infanzia, l'emolisi cronica). Il fabbisogno giornaliero normale per un lattante è di 25-30 μg/die. Il fabbisogno basato sul peso è maggiore nei bambini rispetto agli adulti perché nei bambini è più elevato il bisogno legato alla crescita. Il latte materno, il latte vaccino pastorizzato e le formule per neonati forniscono quantità adeguate di acido folico. Il latte di capra è carente, pertanto integrazioni di acido folico devono essere forniti quando questo costituisce l'alimento principale del bambino. Senza la supplementazione, anche il latte in polvere può essere una sorgente povera di acido folico.

Il fabbisogno di folati aumenta notevolmente durante la gravidanza, in parte per andare incontro alle necessità fetali. Diminuzioni dei livelli di folato nel siero e nei globuli rossi si verificano in circa il 25% delle donne a termine gravidanza e può essere aggravato da infezioni. Supplementazioni di folati di almeno 400 μg/die sono raccomandate sin dall'inizio della gravidanza per prevenire i difetti del tubo neurale e per andare incontro ai bisogni della crescita del feto. Madri con carenza di folati possono generare bambini con riserve normali di folati, a seguito del trasferimento selettivo dei folati al feto attraverso i relativi recettori placentari.

Diminuito assorbimento di folati. Lo scarso assorbimento dovuto a stati di diarrea cronica o malattie infiammatorie sistemiche può portare a carenza dei folati. L'anemia megaloblastica per carenza di acido folico può verificarsi in presenza di morbo celiaco o enteriti infettive croniche e in associazione a fistole enteroenteriche. Sia in corso di malattie infiammatorie intestinali sia in corso di diarrea, parte del diminuito assorbimento del folato può dipendere da un difetto di attività della folato coniugasi. La diarrea cronica interferisce anche con la circolazione enteroepatica del folato, incrementando così la perdita di esso a causa di un rapido transito intestinale. Inoltre, precedenti interventi chirurgici intestinali sono un'altra potenziale causa di diminuito assorbimento del folato.

Alcuni farmaci anticonvulsivanti (per es. fenitoina, primidone, fenobarbital) possono interferire con l'assorbimento dell' acido folico e molti pazienti trattati con questi farmaci hanno bassi livelli sierici di acido folico. Tuttavia un'anemia megaloblastica franca è rara e risponde alla terapia con acido folico anche se la somministrazione dei farmaci responsabili viene continuata.

Disordini congeniti nel metabolismo dei folati. L'anemia megaloblastica dovuta a carenza congenita di diidrofolato reduttasi è una patologia molto rara che è dovuta all'incapacità di produrre tetraidrofolato biologicamente attivo. I soggetti affetti hanno sviluppato un'anemia megalobalastica severa fin dalla prima infanzia. Questi pazienti sono stati trattati con successo con grandi dosi di acido folico o folinico. La carenza di metilene tetraidrofolato reduttasi è stata descritta in alcuni pazienti con omocistinuria senza anomalie ematologiche.

Disordini nel metabolismo dei folati indotti da farmaci. Un certo numero di farmaci presenta un'attività anti-acido folico come primo effetto farmacologico e regolarmente provoca anemia megaloblastica. Il methotrexate si lega alla diidrofolato reduttasi e impedisce la formazione di tetraidrofolato, la forma attiva. La pirimetamina, utilizzata nella terapia della toxoplasmosi, e il trimethoprim, impiegato nel trattamento di diverse infezioni, possono indurre carenza di acido folico e, talvolta, anemia megaloblastica. La terapia con acido folinico (5-formiltetraidrofolato) apporta, di solito, beneficio.

REPERTI DI LABORATORIO. L'anemia è macrocitica (volume corpuscolare medio >100 fL) e variazioni nella dimensione e nella forma dei globuli rossi sono comuni (vedi Fig. 447-1B). La conta dei reticolociti è bassa ed eritroblasti con morfologia megaloblastica sono spesso presenti nel sangue. Raramente può essere presente neutropenia e trombocitopenia, in particolare in pazienti con gravi carenze e di lunga durata. I neutrofili sono di grandi dimensioni, alcuni con nucleo ipersegmentato. I livelli normali di acido folico nel siero sono 5-20 ng/mL; in presenza di una carenza i livelli sono <3 ng/mL. I livelli del folato eritrocitario sono un indicatore migliore di una deficienza cronica. I normali livelli eritrocitari di folato sono pari a 150-160 ng/mL di globuli rossi concentrati. I livelli di ferro e vitamina B_{12} nel siero sono in genere normali o aumentati. L'attività sierica della lattico deidrogenasi (LDH), marker di eritropoiesi inefficace, è notevolmente aumentata. Il midollo osseo è ipercellulare a causa dell'iperplasia eritroide, e i cambiamenti megaloblastici sono molto evidenti. Si notano anche neutrofili di grandi dimensioni con anomali morfologiche (metamielociti giganti) con vacuoli citoplasmatici.

TRATTAMENTO. Quando viene accertata la diagnosi di carenza di folato, l'acido folico dovrebbe essere somministrato per via orale o parenterale alla dose di 0,5-1 mg/die. Se la diagnosi specifica è incerta, dosi minori di folato (0,1 mg/die) dovrebbero essere utilizzate per una settimana come test diagnostico, poiché ci si può aspettare una risposta ematologica entro 72 ore. Dosi di folato >0,1 mg/die possono correggere l'anemia da carenza di vitamina B_{12} ma possono aggravare qualsiasi anomalia neurologica associata. Nella maggior parte degli ambienti medici nei Paesi sviluppati, questa prova terapeutica per distinguere le diverse cause di anemia megaloblastica è raramente necessaria perché i livelli plasmatici di vitamina B_{12} e acido folico sono in genere velocemente disponibili. Le trasfusioni sono indicate solo quando l'anemia è severa o il bambino è gravemente malato. La terapia con acido folico (0,5-1 mg/die) dovrebbe essere continuata per 3-4 settimane finché non compare una definitiva risposta ematologica. La terapia di mantenimento con un multivitaminico (contenente 0,2 mg di folato) è adeguata.

454.2 • CARENZE DI VITAMINA B_{12} (COBALAMINA)

La vitamina B_{12} deriva dalla cobalamina degli alimenti (prevalentemente di origine animale), a seguito della produzione da parte dei microrganismi, poiché gli esseri umani non sono in grado di sintetizzarla. Le cobalamine vengono rilasciate nell'ambiente acido gastrico e si combinano con le proteine R e il fattore intrinseco (*Intrinsic Factor*, IF), attraversano il duodeno, dove le proteasi pancreatiche digeriscono le proteine R, e vengono assorbite nell'ileo distale attraverso recettori specifici per il complesso IF-cobalamina. Inoltre, una parte di vitamina B_{12} somministrata in grandi dosi può diffondere attraverso la mucosa dell'intestino e della bocca. Nel plasma, la cobalamina si lega a una proteina di trasporto, il transcobalamina II (TC-II), che trasporta la vitamina B_{12} al fegato, al midollo osseo e ad altri siti di deposito tissutale. Il TC-II entra nelle cellule attraverso un processo di endocitosi mediata da recettore e la cobalamina viene convertita in forme attive (metilcobalamina e adenosilcobalamina) importanti per il trasferimento di gruppi metile e per la sintesi del DNA. Il plasma contiene anche altre due proteine leganti la vitamina B_{12}, la transcobalamina I e la III (TC-I e TC-III). Queste ultime due forme non hanno alcuno specifico ruolo di trasporto, ma si sa che riflettono i depositi tissutali di vitamina B_{12}. Quasi tutta la vitamina B_{12} nel plasma, infatti, è legata alla TC-I e alla TC-III e perciò la concentrazione sierica di B12 riflette i suoi depositi. Al contrario dei depositi di folato, i bambini più grandi e gli adulti hanno depositi di vitamina B_{12} sufficienti per 3-5 anni. Tuttavia, nei piccoli lattanti nati da mamme con bassi depositi di vitamina B_{12}, i segni clinici della carenza di cobalamina possono divenire evidenti nei primi 6-18 mesi di vita.

EZIOLOGIA. La carenza di vitamina B_{12} può derivare da un inadeguato apporto di vitamina con la dieta, da mancata produzione di IF nello stomaco, da un difettoso assorbimento intestinale del complesso IF-cobalamina o da assenza delle proteina di trasporto della vitamina B_{12}.

Inadeguato apporto di vitamina B_{12}. Poiché la vitamina B_{12} è presente in molti cibi, la carenza alimentare è rara. Può verificarsi nei casi di restrizioni dietetiche estreme (per es. vegetariani stretti o vegani) in cui non viene consumato alcun prodotto di origine animale. La carenza di vitamina B_{12} non è comune nel kwashiorkor o nel marasma infantile. Nei bambini, l'anemia megaloblastica da inadeguato apporto di vitamina B_{12} si verifica nei neonati allattati al seno le cui madri sono vegane o presentano anemia perniciosa loro stesse. L'anemia perniciosa materna si può manifestare con ridotta vitamina B_{12} sierica con o senza anemia macrocitica materna. Questa causa di anemia megaloblastica può comparire nel corso del primo anno di vita.

Mancanza di fattore intrinseco. L'anemia perniciosa congenita è un raro disturbo autosomico recessivo dovuto all'incapacità di produrre l'IF gastrico o dovuto alla produzione di un IF funzionalmente anomalo. È differente dalla malattia tipica dell'adulto in cui lo stomaco produce una normale acidità ed è istologicamente normale. Non sono presenti anticorpi contro le cellule parietali e disturbi endocrini associati. I sintomi dell'anemia perniciosa giovanile diventano importanti attorno a 1 anno di vita. Questo intervallo corrisponde all'esaurimento delle scorte di vitamina B_{12} acquisite in utero. Quando l'anemia diventa severa si manifestano debolezza, irritabilità, anoressia e svogliatezza. La lingua è liscia, rossa e dolente. Le manifestazioni neurologiche comprendono atassia, parestesie, iporeflessia, riflesso di Babinski e clonie. L'anemia perniciosa giovanile è un'altra rara patologia che si presenta nei bambini più grandi. È un disturbo immunologico simile al tipo di anemia perniciosa dell'adulto, che si può manifestare con atrofia della mucosa gastrica, acloridria e presenza di anticorpi nel siero contro l'IF e le cellule parietali. Questi bambini possono presentare anomalie immunologiche associate, candidiasi cutanea, ipoparatiroidismo e altri difetti endocrini. Un risultato anomalo del test di Schilling è corretto da supplementazione di IF esogeno. A questi pazienti dovrebbe essere somministrata regolarmente vitamina B_{12} per via parenterale. La chirurgia gastrica può portare a carenza di fattore intrinseco e gli individui suscettibili necessitano di supplementazioni parenterali di vitamina B_{12} per tutta la vita.

Difettoso assorbimento di vitamina B_{12}. Pazienti con malattie infiammatorie come enteriti regionali o enterocolite necrotizzante neonatale possono presentare un assorbimento difettoso della vitamina B_{12}. Quando l'ileo terminale è stato rimosso chirurgicamente e c'è l'evidenza che la vitamina B_{12} non venga assorbita, questa dev'essere somministrata per tutta la vita per via parenterale. Una crescita eccessiva di batteri intestinali nei diverticoli o duplicazioni del piccolo intestino possono causare carenza di vitamina B_{12} per consumo della (o competizione con la) vitamina o anche per scissione del suo complesso con l'IF. In questi casi, la risposta ematologica può far seguito a un'appropriata terapia antibiotica. Meccanismi analoghi possono verificarsi quando il *Diphyllobothrium latum* infesta la prima parte del piccolo intestino. Quando si verifica in queste situazioni l'anemia megaloblastica, i livelli di vitamina B_{12} sierica sono bassi, il succo gastrico contiene il fattore intrinseco e il risultato anormale del test di Schilling non è corretto dall'aggiunta di IF esogeno.

Rari casi di anemia megaloblastica dovuti a carenza di vitamina B_{12} sono stati riportati come risultato di difetti del recettore per il complesso IF-B_{12} nell'ileo terminale, in alcuni casi associato a proteinuria (sindrome di Imerslund-Grasbeck). Questa patologia autosomica recessiva è dovuta a difetti nel gene CUBN nel cromosoma 10p12.1, che comporta una diminuita espressione del recettore per il complesso IF-B_{12}, detto cubilina. Il trattamento parenterale con vitamina B_{12} mensile corregge la carenza.

Assenza della proteina di trasporto per la vitamina B_{12}. La carenza della transcobalamina II (TC-II) è una rara causa di anemia megaloblastica dovuta a un diminuito utilizzo della cobalamina. La TC-II è il principale veicolo di trasporto fisiologico della vitamina B_{12} e il suo ruolo nel trasporto è simile a quello della transferrina (Tf) per il ferro; recettori specifici per la TC-II e la Tf esistono nelle cellule che necessitano di vitamina B_{12} o di ferro. Una carenza congenita è ereditata come una condizione autosomica recessiva, con insufficienza di assorbimento e trasporto della vitamina B_{12}. La maggior parte dei pazienti non possiede la TC-II, ma alcuni ne presentano forme funzionalmente difettose: sono normali i livelli di vitamina B_{12} sierica perché le forme di deposito della cobalamina, TC-I e TC-III non sono colpite. Questa malattia in genere si presenta durante le prime settimane di vita. Tipicamente, si manifestano scarsa crescita, diarrea, vomito, glossite, anomalie neurologiche e anemia megaloblastica. La diagnosi di questo disturbo è suggerita dalla presenza di una grave anemia megaloblastica con normali livelli sierici di vitamina B_{12} e di folato senza evidenza di alcun altro errore congenito del metabolismo. La diagnosi è effettuata con test specifici per la TC-II. I livelli di vitamina B_{12} sierici devono essere mantenuti elevati per utilizzare la cobalamina; pertanto, la terapia per questa patologia è rappresentata da alte dosi parenterali di vitamina B_{12} somministrate due volte la settimana per tutta la vita. Tali alte e frequenti dosi di cobalamina sembrano superare il difetto nel trasporto. La maggior parte dei bambini con questo disturbo muore se il trattamento non viene iniziato durante l'infanzia.

MANIFESTAZIONI CLINICHE. I bambini con carenza di cobalamina spesso presentano manifestazioni non specifiche come debolezza, affaticabilità, scarsa crescita o irritabilità. Altri reperti comuni includono pallore, glossite, vomito, diarrea e ittero. Si possono manifestare anche sintomi neurologici che possono includere parestesie, deficit sensitivi, ipotonia, crisi, difetti di sviluppo, regressioni comportamentali e cambiamenti neuropsichiatrici. I problemi neurologici legati alla carenza di vitamina B_{12} possono manifestarsi in assenza di qualsiasi anomalia ematologica.

REPERTI DI LABORATORIO. Le manifestazioni ematologiche della carenza di folato e di cobalamina sono identiche. L'anemia conseguente alla carenza di cobalamina è macrocitica, con importante macro-ovalocitosi dei globuli rossi (vedi Fig. 447-1B). I neutrofili possono essere grandi e ipersegmentati. Nei casi avanzati, si può verificare neutropenia e trombocitopenia, simulando un'anemia aplastica o una leucemia. I livelli sierici di vitamina B_{12} sono ridotti mentre le concentrazioni sieriche dell'acido metilmalonico e dell'omocisteina sono di solito elevate, come sono normali o elevate le concentrazioni sieriche di ferro e di acido folico. L'attività dell'LDH sierica è marcatamente aumentata, riflesso di un'eritropoiesi inefficace. Si possono trovare anche aumenti moderati (2-3 mg/dL) dei livelli di bilirubina sierica. Un'escrezione eccessiva di acido metilmalonico nelle urine (quantità normale, 0-3,5 mg/24 ore) è un sensibile e affidabile indice della carenza di vitamina B_{12}.

DIAGNOSI. La causa specifica della carenza di vitamina B_{12} è spesso evidente dalla storia clinica. Nei casi in cui ci sia una spiegazione ragionevole per un ridotto assorbimento della vitamina B_{12} (precedente alla chirurgia gastrica o ileale) può essere opportuno dare inizio a un'appropriata terapia senza ulteriori valutazioni. Nei bambini molto piccoli in cui l'insufficienza alimentare si può considerare una causa, la valutazione della madre per anemia e vitamina B_{12} sierica spesso è di aiuto. Se non c'è alcuna causa ovvia per una diminuzione della vitamina B_{12} sierica, l'assorbimento della vitamina B_{12} può essere valutato mediante il test di Schilling. Quando una persona normale ingerisce una piccola quantità di vitamina B_{12} in cui sia stato incorporato del cobalto 57 (Co^{57}), la vitamina radioattiva si combina con l'IF nelle secrezioni gastriche e passa nell'ileo terminale, dove si verifica l'assorbimento. Poiché la vitamina assorbita è legata alla TC-II e incorporata nei tessuti, solo una piccola quantità o niente viene eliminata con le urine. Se una dose alta (1 mg) di vitamina B_{12} non radioattiva viene iniettata per via parenterale dopo 2 ore (o "bolo rapido"), il 10-30% della precedente vitamina radioattiva assorbita compare nelle urine entro 24 ore. I bambini con anemia perniciosa di solito eliminano $\leq 2\%$ in queste condizioni. Per confermare che l'assenza dell'IF costituisce la base del malassorbimento della vitamina B_{12}, l'IF viene somministrato in associazione a una seconda dose di vitamina B_{12} radioattiva. Una quota normale di vitamina dovrebbe quindi essere assorbita ed eliminata con le urine. Tuttavia, quando lo scarso assorbimento della vitamina B_{12} consegue all'assenza dei siti recettoriali ileali o ad altre cause intestinali, non si verificano miglioramenti nell'assorbimento con l'IF. Il risultato del test di Schilling rimane anormale nei pazienti con anemia perniciosa, anche quando la terapia ha completamente normalizzato le manifestazioni ematologiche e neurologiche della malattia.

TRATTAMENTO. Una pronta risposta ematologica segue la somministrazione parenterale di vitamina B_{12} (1 mg), generalmente con una reticolocitosi in 2-4 giorni, senza che ci siano malattie infiammatorie concomitanti. Il fabbisogno fisiologico di vitamina B_{12} è di 1-5 µg/die, e sono state osservate risposte ematologiche con queste piccole dosi, che indicano che la somministrazione di una minidose può essere usata come prova terapeutica quando la diagnosi di carenza di vitamina B_{12} è incerta. Se c'è evidenza di un coinvolgimento neurologico, 1 mg dovrebbe essere somministrato per via intramuscolare quotidianamente per almeno 2 settimane. È necessaria una terapia di mantenimento durante tutta la durata di vita del paziente ed è sufficiente la somministrazione intramuscolo mensile di 1 mg di vitamina B_{12}. La terapia orale è in grado di avere successo per la diffusione mucosale a dosi elevate, ma non è generalmente consigliabile, a causa dell'assorbimento incerto.

454.3 • ALTRE ANEMIE MAGALOBLASTICHE RARE

L'**oroticoaciduria** è una rara patologia autosomica recessiva che di solito compare durante i primi anni di vita ed è caratterizzata da scarsa crescita, ritardo di sviluppo, anemia megaloblastica e aumento dell'escrezione urinaria di acido orotico (vedi Capitolo 89). Questo difetto, il più comune errore metabolico nella sintesi de novo delle pirimidine, colpisce quindi la sintesi degli acidi nucleici. La forma usuale dell'aciduria orotica ereditaria è dovuta a una carenza (in tutti i tessuti del corpo) sia dell'oro-tico-fosforibosil-transferasi (OPT), sia dell'orotidina-5-fosfato decarbossilasi (ODC), due tappe enzimatiche sequenziali nella sintesi del nucleotide pirimidina. La diagnosi di questa malattia è suggerita dalla presenza di una severa anemia megaloblastica con livelli normali di vitamina B_{12} e folati, senza evidenza di una carenza di TC-II. Una diagnosi ipotetica viene fatta dal riscontro di aumentati livelli urinari di acido orotico. La conferma della diagnosi, comunque, richiede il dosaggio enzimatico della transferasi e della decarbossilasi negli eritrociti del paziente. Un ritardo fisico e mentale spesso accompagna questa condizione. L'anemia è refrattaria alla vitamina B_{12} o all'acido folico ma risponde prontamente alla somministrazione di uridina (100-150 μg/kg/24 ore). L'anemia megaloblastica può anche presentarsi nella sindrome di Lesch-Nyhan, in cui la rigenerazione dei nucleotidi purine è bloccata (vedi Capitolo 89).

L'**anemia megaloblastica tiamino-responsiva** (TRMA) è caratterizzata da anemia megaloblastica, sordità neurosensoriale, diabete mellito e, talvolta, miocardiopatia e atrofia del nervo ottico. È stato precedentemente osservato che l'anemia megaloblastica in alcuni pazienti risponde a dosi elevate di tiamina, è oggi noto che il difetto in questa patologia è legato a un'anomalia nel gene per il trasporto della tiamina localizzato sul cromosoma 1. La TRMA è una patologia autosomica recessiva che si presenta nell'infanzia e si verifica in popolazioni etnicamente distinte.

La carenza di adenosilcobalamina e di metilcobalamina insieme ad anemia megaloblastica è stata riscontrata in pochi bambini con incapacità di convertire la cobalamina ai suoi metabolici attivi biologicamente. Queste patologie sono caratterizzate da anomalie neurologiche e metilmalonicoaciduria, omocisteinuria o entrambe. Le anomalie vengono di solito notate nelle prime settimane di vita e includono scarsa crescita, letargia, ipotonia, macrocitosi con alterazioni megaloblastiche nel midollo osseo, anemia o pancitopenia e disfunzione epatica. Le alterazioni megaloblastiche possono scomparire e altri sintomi possono migliorare con un trattamento a base di idrossicobalamina, inizialmente alla dose di 1 mg/24 ore intramuscolo e gradualmente modificata da una dose due o tre volte alla settimana e quindi a una volta al mese.

Carmel R, Green R, Rosenblatt DS, et al: Update on cobalamin, folate and homocysteine. *Hematology Am Soc Hematol Educ Program* 2003;62–81.
Grasbeck R: Imerslund-Grasbeck syndrome (selective vitamin B12 malabsorption with proteinuria). *Orphanet J Rare Dis* 2006 19;1:17.
Monagle PT, Tauro GP: Infantile megaloblastosis secondary to maternal vitamin B_{12} deficiency. *Clin Lab Haematol* 1997;19:23–25.
Rasmussen SA, Fernhoff PM, Scanlon KS: Vitamin B_{12} deficiency in children and adolescents. *J Pediatr* 2001;138:10–17.
Rosenblatt DS, Whitehead VM: Cobalamin and folate deficiency: Acquired and hereditary disorders in children. *Semin Hematol* 1999;36:19–34.
Xu D, Kozyraki R, Newman TC, et al: Genetic evidence of an accessory activity required specifically for cubilin brush-border expression and intrinsic factor–cobalamin absorption. *Blood* 1999;94:3604–3606.

Capitolo 455 ■ Anemia sideropenica

L'anemia che risulta da una mancanza di ferro sufficiente alla sintesi emoglobinica è la più comune patologia ematologica dell'infanzia e dell'età pediatrica. Si stima che il 30% della popolazione mondiale soffra di anemia sideropenica e che la maggior parte di questi soggetti affetti viva nei Paesi in via di sviluppo. L'anemia sideropenica è associata a numerose condizioni dannose per la salute (Tab. 455-1) (vedi Capitolo 51).

TABELLA 455-1. Giudizio collettivo sulla forza dell'evidenza causale che rapporta la sideropenia o l'anemia alle condizioni finali di salute e di sviluppo

Una significativa evidenza causale esiste per:*
1. Anemia sideropenica e produttività lavorativa
2. Anemia grave e mortalità infantile
3. Anemia grave e mortalità materna
4. Anemia sideropenica e sviluppo del bambino
Manca un'evidenza causale o è contradditoria per:
Anemia sideropenica e basso peso alla nascita, inclusi i prematuri
Anemia sideropenica e malattie infettive, per effetto sia protettivo sia avverso
Anemia lieve-moderata e mortalità materna
Anemia lieve-moderata e mortalità infantile

*I numeri riflettono la forza relativa di evidenza, non la grandezza potenziale dell'effetto del ferro in termini di salute pubblica.

Da Stoltzfus RJ: Iron-deficiency anemia: Reexamining the nature and magnitude of the public health problem: Summary. Implications for research and programs. *J Nutr* 2001; 131(2 Suppl 2): 698S.

La frequenza di anemia sideropenica è legata ad alcuni aspetti basilari del metabolismo del ferro e alla nutrizione; per mantenere un bilancio di ferro positivo nell'età pediatrica, dovrebbe essere assorbito quotidianamente circa 1 mg di ferro. Il corpo di un neonato contiene circa 0,5 g di ferro, mentre si ritiene che il contenuto di un adulto sia 5 g. Per andare da un livello all'altro una media di 0,8 mg di ferro dovrebbe essere assorbita ogni giorno durante i primi 15 anni di vita. Oltre a questo fabbisogno per la crescita, ne è necessaria una piccola quantità per bilanciare le normali perdite di ferro dalle cellule.

L'assorbimento del ferro alimentare si assume essere circa il 10%; una dieta contenente 8-10 mg di ferro al giorno è indispensabile per una nutrizione ottimale. Il ferro viene assorbito nel piccolo intestino prossimale, in parte mediato da una varietà di proteine duodenali. Il ferro viene assorbito da 2 a 3 volte più efficacemente dal latte umano rispetto al latte vaccino. I lattanti allattati al seno possono avere bisogno, quindi, di meno ferro proveniente dagli altri alimenti. Durante il primo anno di vita, poiché sono assunte relativamente poche quantità di cibi ricchi di ferro, è spesso difficile raggiungere adeguati apporti di ferro. Per questo motivo, la dieta dovrebbe includere cibi come i cereali o formule che siano stati supplementate con ferro, poiché entrambi sono molto efficaci nel prevenirne la carenza. Le formule con 7-12 mg Fe/L per neonati a termine e prematuri, e quelle con 15 mg/L per neonati di peso inferiore a 1800 g alla nascita sono efficaci. I lattanti esclusivamente allattati al seno dovrebbero ricevere supplementi di ferro a partire dal 4° mese di vita. Un lattante è in una situazione precaria per quanto riguarda il ferro. Qualora la dieta dovesse diventare inadeguata o si verificassero perdite di sangue, l'anemia insorgerebbe rapidamente.

Anche gli adolescenti sono suscettibili alle carenze di ferro a causa delle elevate richieste dovute alla crescita, alle carenze dietetiche e alle perdite di sangue legate ai cicli mestruali. Negli Stati Uniti circa il 9% dei bambini tra 1-2 anni di età presenta carenza di ferro; il 3% ha anemia. Delle adolescenti femmine, il 9% presenta carenza di ferro, mentre il 2% anemia.

EZIOLOGIA. Un basso peso alla nascita e un'emorragia perinatale superiore alla norma sono associate a diminuzioni nella massa emoglobinica neonatale e nelle riserve di ferro. Siccome l'alta concentrazione di emoglobina del neonato diminuisce durante i primi 2-3 mesi di vita, una notevole quantità di ferro è recuperata e immagazzinata. Queste scorte richieste sono generalmente sufficienti per la produzione di sangue nei primi 6-9 mesi di vita nei neonati a termine. Nei neonati di basso peso alla nascita o in quelli con perdita di sangue perinatale, il ferro immagazzinato può essere rimosso prima e le risorse alimentari diventano di notevole importanza. Una ritardata legatura del cordone ombelicale (circa 2 min) nei Paesi in via di sviluppo può ridurre l'incidenza della carenza di ferro. Nei neonati a termine, l'anemia causata unicamente da un'inadeguata quantità di ferro alimentare è insolita prima dei 6 mesi e di solito si verifica tra i 9-24 mesi di età. Dopo questo periodo, ciò è relativamente poco comune. Le tipiche abitudini dietetiche osservate nei lattanti con anemia sideropenica sono il consumo prolungato di grandi quantità di latte vaccino (>700 mL/die) e di alimenti non supplementati con ferro.

La perdita di sangue deve essere considerata come una possibile causa in tutti i casi di anemia sideropenica, soprattutto nei bambini più grandi. L'anemia sideropenica cronica da sanguinamento occulto può essere causata da lesioni del tratto gastrointestinale, come le coliti infiammatorie indotte dalle proteine del latte vaccino, l'ulcera peptica, il diverticolo di Meckel, i polipi, gli emangiomi o le malattie intestinali infiammatorie. In alcune aree geografiche, l'infestazione da vermi uncinati rappresenta un'importante causa di carenza di ferro; in altre, essa è associata a infezione da *Helicobacter pylori*. L'emosiderosi polmonare può essere correlata a sanguinamenti non riconosciuti del polmone e a ricorrente sideropenia dopo trattamento con ferro. La diarrea cronica nella prima infanzia può essere legata a importanti perdite non riconosciute di sangue. Negli Stati Uniti, alcuni bambini con anemia sideropenica severa hanno perdite di sangue intestinale croniche indotte dall'esposizione a una proteina labile al calore contenuta nel latte vaccino. La perdita di sangue nelle feci ogni giorno può essere prevenuta sia riducendo la quantità di latte vaccino intero a <500 mL/24 ore, utilizzando latte riscaldato o evaporato, sia utilizzando un sostituto del latte. Questa reazione gastrointestinale non è correlata ad anomalie enzimatiche nella mucosa, come la carenza di lattasi o la tipica allergia al latte. Talvolta, la colite indotta dal latte vaccino si presenta con edema e anemia; l'edema è dovuto a **enteropatia proteino-disperdente**. I neonati interessati sviluppano caratteristicamente l'anemia che è più severa e si verifica più precocemente di quanto ci si aspetti semplicemente da un inadeguato apporto di ferro.

Le anomalie istologiche della mucosa del tratto gastrointestinale, come l'appiattimento dei villi, sono presenti nell'anemia sideropenica avanzata e possono provocare perdita di sangue e diminuzione dell'assorbimento di ferro, ampliando ancora di più il problema.

La pratica di esercizi fisici intensi, come si verifica negli atleti agonisti nelle scuole superiori, può portare a una carenza di ferro nelle ragazze, ma ciò si verifica meno comunemente nei ragazzi.

MANIFESTAZIONI CLINICHE. Il più importante segno della carenza di ferro è il pallore; l'Organizzazione Mondiale della Sanità raccomanda, infatti, l'utilizzo del pallore palmare come metodo di screening per l'anemia. Tuttavia c'è alta incidenza di risultati falsi positivi e falsi negativi per il pallore palmare, del letto ungueale, congiuntivale, che variano in rapporto ai livelli di anemia. Nelle carenze di ferro lievi e moderate (per es. livelli di emoglobina 6-10 g/dL), meccanismi di compenso, inclusi gli aumentati livelli di 2,3-difosfoglicerato (2,3-DPG) e lo spostamento della curva di dissociazione dell'emoglobina, possono essere così efficaci che sono evidenti pochi sintomi di anemia, anche se i bambini affetti possono essere irritabili. Può essere presente la **pagofagia**, cioè il desiderio di ingerire sostanze insolite come il ghiaccio o la sporcizia. In alcuni bambini l'ingestione di sostanze contenenti il piombo può portare a concomitante **intossicazione da piombo** (vedi Capitolo 709). Quando i livelli di emoglobina scendono <5 g/dL, irritabilità e anoressia si fanno evidenti. Si verificano tachicardia e dilatazione cardiaca e sono spesso presenti soffi sistolici.

I bambini con anemia sideropenica possono essere obesi o sottopeso, con altri segni di malnutrizione. L'irritabilità e l'anoressia, tipiche dei casi avanzati, possono riflettere carenze di ferro tissutale, poiché la terapia con ferro spesso produce significativi miglioramenti nel comportamento prima che siano notati importanti miglioramenti ematologici.

La carenza di ferro può avere effetti sulle funzioni neurologiche e intellettuali. L'anemia sideropenica, come anche la carenza di ferro senza importante anemia, colpisce la durata dell'attenzione, la prontezza e l'apprendimento sia nel bambino sia nell'adolescente. Le ragazze adolescenti con livelli di ferritina ≤12 ng/L ma senza anemia hanno mostrato migliore apprendimento verbale e capacità mnemoniche dopo aver assunto ferro per 8 settimane.

REPERTI DI LABORATORIO. Nella sideropenia progressiva, di verifica una sequenza di eventi ematologici e biochimici. Per prima cosa, le riserve di ferro tissutale, rappresentate dall'emosiderina nel midollo osseo, scompaiono. I livelli di **ferritina sierici**, la proteina di deposito del ferro, forniscono una stima relativamente accurata delle riserve di ferro in assenza di patologie infiammatorie. I normali range sono età-dipendenti e livelli diminuiti accompagnano la carenza di ferro. In seguito, il livello di ferro sierico diminuisce (in modo età-dipendente), aumenta la capacità legante il ferro sierica (transferrina sierica) e la percentuale di saturazione (saturazione della transferrina) scende sotto i valori normali. Quando la disponibilità del ferro diviene limitante per la sintesi emoglobinica, si accumula la protoporfirina eritrocitaria libera (*Free Erythrocyte Protoporphyrins*, FEP). A mano a mano che la carenza progredisce, gli eritrociti diventano più piccoli del normale e il loro contenuto in emoglobina diminuisce. Le caratteristiche morfologiche dei globuli rossi sono meglio quantificate dalla determinazione dell'emoglobina corpuscolare media (*Mean Corpuscolar Hemoglobin*, MCH) e del volume corpuscolare medio (*Mean Corpuscolar Volume*, MCV). I cambiamenti dell'MCV con lo sviluppo richiedono l'uso di standard correlati all'età per la diagnosi di microcitosi (vedi Tab. 447-1). Con carenze importanti, i globuli rossi diventano deformati e presentano caratteristiche di microcitosi, ipocromia, poichilocitosi e aumento dell'ampiezza di distribuzione (*Red Cells Distribution Width*, RDW) (vedi Fig. 447-1C). La percentuale di reticolociti può essere normale o moderatamente elevata, ma la conta assoluta reticolocitaria indica una risposta insufficiente all'anemia. Gli eritroblasti sono talora visti nel sangue periferico se l'anemia è severa. La conta dei globuli bianchi è normale. Talvolta si evidenzia un'importante trombocitosi (600 000-1 milione/mm^3), la quale si ritiene sia dovuta ad aumentati livelli di eritropoietina ed è noto presenti alcune omologie strutturali con la trombopoietina. L'anemia sideropenica severa può occasionalmente essere associata alla trombocitopenia e ciò può portare a confondere la diagnosi con le patologie da insufficienza midollare. Il midollo osseo è ipercellulare con l'iperplasia eritroide. I normoblasti possono avere citoplasma scarso e frammentato con scarsa emoglobinizzazione. I leucociti e i megacariociti sono normali. Non è presente ferro colorabile nelle cellule del reticoloendotelio. In circa un terzo dei casi, può essere riscontrato nelle feci sangue occulto.

DIAGNOSI DIFFERENZIALE. La carenza di ferro deve essere differenziata dalle altre anemie microcitiche ipocromiche. Lo scenario più comune è la necessità di distinguere la sideropenia dal tratto α- e β-talassemico e dalle altre emoglobinopatie, in particolare l'emoglobina E (vedi Capitolo 462). Una semplice caratteristica distintiva di queste ultime condizioni è il fatto che la conta eritrocitaria è spesso superiore al normale, nonostante la presenza di una lieve anemia e microcitosi: questo dato è in netto contrasto con la carenza di ferro, in cui la conta dei globuli rossi è in genere diminuita insieme alla riduzione dell'emoglobina e del MCV. Un'altra differenza tra il trait α- e β-talassemico e la sideropenia è il fatto che il **RDW è elevato nella carenza di ferro**.

Il trait β-talassemico si presenta in persone provenienti dall'area del Mediterraneo, dell'Africa e dell'Asia. È una lieve anemia microcitica caratterizzata da elevati livelli di emoglobina A_2 e/o aumento della concentrazione di emoglobina fetale; il ferro sierico, la capacità totale legante il ferro (transferrina) e la ferritina sono normali; e all'elettroforesi non è visibile emoglobina anomala. La β-talassemia omozigote (o talassemia major), con la sua pronunciata eritroblastosi e grave componente emolitica, non rappresenta un problema diagnostico.

Il trait α-talassemico si presenta in persone di provenienza africana, cinese e del Sud-est asiatico. Questa lieve patologia microcitica è dovuta alla delezione di 2 dei 4 geni che regolano la produzione α-globulinica. Nelle presentazioni cliniche abituali, la diagnosi del tratto α-talassemico può essere fatta quando un paziente con familiarità per anemia microcitica ipocromica ha risultati normali negli studi sul ferro (inclusa la ferritina), livelli normali di Hb A_2 e Hb F e una normale elettroforesi emoglobinica. Nelle abituali presentazioni cliniche, il tratto α-talassemico rappresenta una diagnosi di esclusione tranne nel periodo perinatale, in cui i neonati con tratto α-talassemico presentano il 3-10% di emoglobina di Bart (γ_4) [vedi Capitolo 462]. Una diagnosi specifica per le patologie α-talassemiche è possibile se si utilizzano tecniche di diagnostica molecolare, ma questi studi in genere vengono effettuati solo quando tale informazione è necessaria per il counseling genetico e per la diagnosi prenatale.

La malattia da Hb H, un'altra forma di α-talassemia, consegue alla delezione di 3 dei 4 geni α-globinici. È anche caratterizzata da ipocromia e microcitosi, ma presenta inoltre una lieve componente emolitica dovuta all'instabilità dei tetrametri delle catene β (Hb H) dovuta alla carenza di catene α. Oltre l'infanzia, l'Hb H è rapidamente identificata attraverso l'elettroforesi emoglobinica. Nel periodo neonatale, la carenza di α-globinica moderatamente grave permette l'accumulo di più catene γ e la concentrazione dell'emoglobina di Bart è >20%. In molti Paesi, lo screening neonatale per le Hbpatie identifica i bambini con la malattia da Hb H e questa informazione viene trasmessa al medico del paziente.

L'anemia delle malattie croniche (ACD) e delle infezioni è in genere normocitica, anche se talvolta può essere lievemente microcitica (vedi Capitolo 451). Al contrario dell'anemia sideropenica, in queste condizioni infiammatorie, sia il livello di ferro sierico sia la capacità legante il ferro (transferrina) sono ridotte e il livello di ferritina sierico è normale o elevato (la ferritina è una proteina di fase acuta). Il livello del recettore sierico della transferrina (TfR) è utile per distinguere tra anemia sideropenica e anemia delle malattie croniche, poiché non è influenzato dall'infiammazione. La concentrazione del TfR è elevata nella carenza di ferro e rientra nel range normale nell'anemia delle patologie croniche.

L'intossicazione da piombo (vedi Capitolo 709) e l'anemia sideropenica sono entrambe associate con gli aumenti della protoporfirina eritrocitaria (FEP). Nei casi di avvelenamento da piombo associati a carenza di ferro, i globuli rossi non sono morfologicamente simili, ma sono spesso evidenti grossolane granulazioni basofile negli eritrociti. Sono presenti elevati livelli di piombo nel sangue, FEP e livelli di coproporfirina urinaria.

TRATTAMENTO. La normale risposta dell'anemia sideropenica ad adeguate quantità di ferro è un importante caratteristica diagnostica e terapeutica. La somministrazione orale di semplici sali ferrosi (per es. solfato, gluconato, fumarato) offre una terapia non costosa ed efficace. Non ci sono evidenze che l'aggiunta di qualsiasi oligoelemento, vitamina o altra sostanza ematinica aumenti significativamente la risposta ai semplici sali ferrosi. Un problema incontrato nella somministrazione di ferro orale ai bambini piccoli è il fatto che il $FeSO_4$ ha un gusto sgradevole, ma talvolta esso può essere camuffato dall'aggiunta di sciroppo aromatizzato. Sono disponibili altri preparati da banco con un gusto migliore, che però sono molto più costosi del semplice $FeSO_4$ liquido. A parte il gusto sgradevole, l'intolleranza al ferro orale è poco comune nel bambino piccolo, sebbene i bambini più grandi e gli adolescenti alcune volte presentino disturbi gastrointestinali. I problemi legati alla stipsi possono essere ridotti aumentando il consumo di acqua e fibre. Per alcuni bambini, il dolore addominale può essere abbassato dalla somministrazione del ferro con i cibi, pur riconoscendo che questo può per certi versi diminuire l'assorbimento del ferro. La dose terapeutica dovrebbe essere calcolata in termini di ferro elementare; il ferro solfato rappresenta il 20% del ferro semplice rispetto al peso. Una dose totale giornaliera di 4-6 mg/kg di ferro elementare in 3 dosi suddivise produce una quantità ottimale di ferro da usare per il midollo osseo stimolato. Una preparazione parenterale di ferro (ferro destano) è una forma efficace di ferro quando viene dato in dosi adeguatamente calcolate, ma la risposta al ferro parenterale non è più veloce o più completa rispetto a quella ottenuta con una giusta somministrazione orale di ferro, a meno che non ci sia una condizione di malassorbimento. Una complicanza occasionale del ferro è stata l'anafilassi. Il rischio di anafilassi è molto minore con il ferro gluconato per via ev, la forma parenterale di scelta.

Mentre viene somministrata un'adeguata terapia a base di ferro, la famiglia deve essere istruita sulla dieta del paziente e il consumo di latte dovrebbe essere limitato a una quantità ragionevole, preferibilmente 500 mL/24 ore o meno. Questa riduzione ha un duplice effetto: la quantità di cibi ricchi di ferro è aumentata e si riduce la perdita di sangue da intolleranza alle proteine del latte vaccino. Quando la rieducazione del bambino e dei genitori non ha successo, la terapia parenterale con il ferro può raramente essere indicata. La carenza di ferro può essere prevenuta nella popolazione ad alto rischio dalla somministrazione di formule o di cereali fortificati in ferro durante l'infanzia. La sideropenia nelle adolescenti secondaria a perdite di sangue con il flusso mestruale viene trattata con ferro o terapia ormonale (vedi Capitolo 115).

Entro 72-96 ore dopo la somministrazione di ferro nel bambino anemico, si nota una reticolocitosi periferica (Tab. 455-2). La misura di questa risposta è inversamente proporzionale alla severità dell'anemia. La reticolocitosi è seguita da un aumento dei livelli di emoglobina che può aumentare di 0,5 g/dL/24 ore. La terapia con ferro dovrebbe essere proseguita per 8 settimane dopo che i valori ematici sono tornati alla norma. I fallimenti della terapia con ferro si verificano quando un bambino non riceve la terapia prescritta, quando il ferro viene somministrato in forma poco assorbibile o quando vi sia una persistente perdita di sangue non riconosciuta, come nel caso della perdita intestinale o polmonare oppure nella perdita legata ai cicli mestruali. Il fallimento terapeutico della terapia con ferro può indicare che la diagnosi originale di carenza di ferro non era corretta.

Poiché una rapida risposta ematologica può essere strettamente prevista nelle sideropenie tipiche, la trasfusione di sangue è indicata solo quando l'anemia è molto severa o se un'infezione sovrapposta può interferire con la risposta. In genere non è necessaria la correzione rapida di un'anemia grave mediante trasfusioni; la procedura può essere pericolosa vista l'elevata associazione di insufficienza cardiaca. Globuli rossi centrifugati o concentrati dovrebbero essere somministrati lentamente in quantità sufficiente a portare l'emoglobina a valori di sicurezza in cui ci si possa aspettare una risposta al trattamento con ferro. In generale, a bambini gravemente anemici con valori di emoglobina <4 g/dL dovrebbero essere somministrati solo 2-3 mL/kg emazie concentrate in un'unica volta (dovrebbe anche essere somministrata furosemide come diuretico). Se c'è evidenza di insufficienza cardiaca franca, dovrebbe essere considerata un'exsanguino-trasfusione con emazie fresche concentrate, sebbene diuretici seguiti da una lenta infusione di globuli rossi concentrati possano risultare sufficienti.

Baggett HC, Parkinson AJ, Muth PT, et al: Endemic iron deficiency associated with *Helicobacter pylori* infection among school-aged children in Alaska. *Pediatrics* 2006;117:e396–404.

Brotanek JM, Halterman JS, Auinger P, et al: Iron deficiency, prolonged bottle-feeding and racial/ethnic disparities in young children. *Arch Pediatr Adolesc* 2005;159:1038–1042.

Chaparro CM, Neufeld LM, Alvarez GT, et al: Effect of timing of umbilical cord clamping on iron status in Mexican infants: a randomized controlled trial. *Lancet* 2006;367:1997–2004.

Galloway MJ, Smellie WS: Investigating iron status in microcytic anaemia. *BMJ* 2006;333:791–793.

TABELLA 455-2. Risposte alla terapia con ferro nell'anemia sideropenica

PERIODO SUCCESSIVO ALLA SOMMINISTRAZIONE DI FERRO	RISPOSTA
12-24 ore	Sostituzione degli enzimi ferrosi intracellulari; miglioramento soggettivo; diminuita irritabilità; aumento dell'appetito
36-48 ore	Risposta iniziale del midollo osseo; iperplasia eritroide
48-72 ore	Reticolocitosi, picco in 5-7 giorni
4-30 giorni	Aumento dei livelli di emoglobina
1-3 mesi	Ripristino delle riserve

Lozoff B, Jimenez E, Smith JB: Double burden of iron deficiency in infancy and low socioeconomic status. *Arch Pediatr Adoless Med* 2006;160:1108–1112.

Mercer J, Erickson-Owens D: Delayed cord clamping increases infants' iron stores. *Lancet* 2006;367:1956–1957.

Moy RJ: Prevalence, consequences and prevention of childhood nutritional iron deficiency: a child public health perspective. *Clin Lab Haematol* 2006;28:291–298.

Panagiotou JP, Douros K: Clinicolaboratory findings and treatment of iron-deficiency anemia in childhood. *Pediatr Hematol Oncol* 2004;21:521–534. Review.

Sutcliffe TL, Khambalia A, Westergard S, et al: Iron depletion is associated with daytime bottle-feeding in the second and third years of life. *Arch Pediatr Adolesc Med* 2006;160:1114–1120.

Capitolo 456 ■ Altre anemie microcitiche

ANEMIE SIDEROBLASTICHE. Le anemie sideroblastiche risultano da patologie acquisite o ereditarie della sintesi dell'eme. Le anemie sono caratterizzate da eritrociti microcitici ipocromici mescolati a globuli rossi normali: ciò produce un'immagine di insieme di una popolazione eritrocitaria dimorfica e la conta completa delle cellule ematiche indica un'ampiezza di distribuzione dei globuli rossi estremamente elevata (*Red Cells Distribution Width*, RDW). La concentrazione di ferro sierico è generalmente elevata e la saturazione della transferrina con il ferro è aumentata. In tutti i casi di anemia sideroblastica, a prescindere dalla causa specifica, la sintesi difettosa dell'eme conduce alla ritenzione del ferro all'interno dei mitocondri. Da un punto di vista morfologico, questo è visibile nei globuli rossi nucleati midollari con granuli di ferro (aggregati di ferro nei mitocondri) che presentano una distribuzione perinucleare. Queste cellule inusuali, note come sideroblasti ad anello (Fig. 456-1), si ritrovano solo negli stati patologici e si distinguono dai sideroblasti (precursori eritrocitari che contengono diffusi granuli citoplasmatici di ferritina) nel midollo di soggetti normali. Le anemie sideroblastiche più comunemente si presentano nell'età adulta e queste patologie acquisite possono essere idiopatiche o secondarie a farmaci, ad alcol oppure a patologie mielodisplastiche. Poche sono le anemie sideroblastiche visibili nel bambino.

Anemie sideroblastiche congenite. L'anemia sideroblastica congenita è rara e presenta un'ereditarietà legata al cromosoma X.

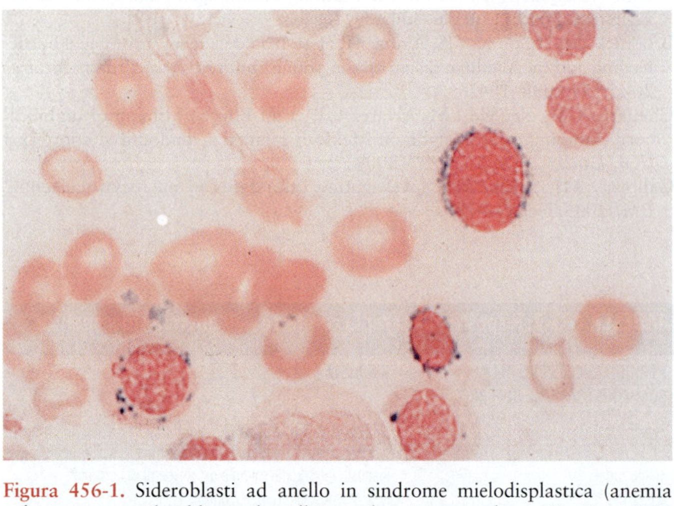

Figura 456-1. Sideroblasti ad anello in sindrome mielodisplastica (anemia refrattaria con sideroblasti ad anello) – colorazione per ferro. (Da Ryan DH, Cohen HJ: Bone marrow examination. In Hoffman R, Benz EJ Jr, Shattil SJ, et al [editors]: *Hematology*, 4th ed. Philadelphia, Churchill Livingstone, 2005.)

Si presenta generalmente nei maschi, sebbene una lionizzazione sbilanciata si sia verificata in femmine affette. Si verificano anche casi autosomici dominanti e sporadici. Le anemie sideroblastiche ereditarie conseguono ad anomalie dell'isozima eritrocitario per la 5-acido aminolevulinico sintetasi (ALAS), enzima che limita la velocità di reazione nella sintesi dell'eme. Un importante cofattore dell'ALAS è il piridossal-fosfato. Il gene per l'ALAS eritrocitario specifico (*ALAS2*) è localizzato sul cromosoma X e sono state identificate >25 mutazioni missense differenti. Si verificano centinaia di queste mutazioni vicino il sito di legame per il piridossal-fosfato.

Le anemie gravi sono state riconosciute nell'infanzia e nel bambino piccolo, mentre casi più blandi non diventano evidenti fino alla prima età adulta o più tardi. I **reperti clinici** includono pallore, ittero e modesta splenomegalia e/o epatomegalia. La gravità dell'anemia è così variabile che alcuni pazienti non necessitano di terapia mentre altri richiedono regolari trasfusioni di emazie. Un sottogruppo di pazienti con anemia sideroblastica ereditaria manifesta una risposta ematologica a dosi terapeutiche di piridossina. Il sovraccarico di ferro manifestato dall'elevata ferritina sierica, dall'elevata sideremia e dall'aumentata saturazione della transferrina è una complicanza maggiore di questa patologia. Segni clinici del sovraccarico di ferro (per es. diabete mellito, disfunzione epatica) possono ritrovarsi in alcuni pazienti che non hanno o hanno una modesta anemia. Il trapianto di cellule staminali è stato impiegato per trattare bambini affetti che erano dipendenti dalle trasfusioni di emazie.

Una variante unica di anemia sideroblastica congenita è la **sindrome di Pearson**, caratterizzata da un esordio precoce di anemia trasfusione-dipendente, neutropenia e trombocitopenia. Oltre alle frequenti anomalie midollari dell'anemia sideroblastica, i bambini con questa sindrome presentano anche una vacuolizzazione dei precursori eritroidi e mieloidi. A differenza delle altre anemie sideroblastiche, che sono microcitiche, questa è una anemia macrocitica e, di conseguenza, è talvolta confusa con l'anemia di Diamond-Blackfan (vedi Capitoli 489 e 506).

AVVELENAMENTO DA PIOMBO. Vedi Capitolo 709.

RARE FORME DI ANEMIA MICROCITICA IPOCROMICA. Sono conosciuti casi isolati di anemia ipocromica microcitica con altre anomalie del metabolismo del ferro; alcuni pazienti hanno presentato difetti di mobilizzazione o riutilizzazione del ferro. L'assenza congenita della proteina legante il ferro (atransferrinemia) è una patologia molto rara con anemia ipocromica grave, nonostante il sovraccarico di ferro, e richiede infusioni di apo-tranferrina e terapia chelante il ferro, anche se questa ultima può essere evitata se le infusioni di transferrina vengono iniziate precocemente. Il ferro viene assorbito normalmente e in seguito depositato negli organi interni piuttosto che nel midollo osseo.

Molti individui hanno mostrato un'anemia ipocromica refrattaria associata a tumori linfatici o iperplasia linfoide: in questi pazienti, la correzione dell'anemia seguiva la rimozione del tessuto linfatico anomalo (vedi Capitoli 489 e 506).

Alcindor T, Bridges KR: Sideroblastic anaemias. *Br J Haematol* 2002;116: 733–743.

Ayas M, Al-Jefri A, Mustafa MM, et al: Congenital sideroblastic anaemia successfully treated using allogeneic stem cell transplantation. *Br J Haematol* 2001;113:938.

Chalco JP, Huicho L, Alamo C, et al: Accuracy of clinical pallor in the diagnosis of anemia in children: A meta-analysis. *BMC Pediatrics* 2005;5: 46.

Fleming MD: The genetics of inherited sideroblastic anemias. *Semin Hematol* 2002;39:270–281.

Moy RJ: Prevalence, consequences and prevention of childhood nutritional iron deficiency: a child public health perspective. *Clin Lab Haematol* 2006;28:291–298.

Panagiotou JP, Douros K: Clinicolaboratory findings and treatment of iron-deficiency anemia in childhood. *Pediatr Hematol Oncol* 2004;21:521–534, Review.
Sandoval C, Jayabose S, Eden AN: Trends in diagnosis and management of iron deficiency during infancy and early childhood. *Hematol Oncol Clin North Am* 2004;18:1423–1438, x.
Walter T: Effect of iron-deficiency anemia on cognitive skills and neuromaturation in infancy and childhood. *Food Nutr Bull* 2003;24(4 Suppl): S104–S110.

Sezione 3 — Anemie emolitiche

Capitolo 457 ■ Definizione e classificazione delle anemie emolitiche

George B. Segel

L'**emolisi** è definita come la distruzione precoce degli eritrociti. L'anemia si verifica quando il grado di distruzione supera la capacità del midollo di produrre globuli rossi. La normale sopravvivenza dei globuli rossi è 110-120 giorni (vita media, 55-60 giorni) e circa lo 0,85% della maggior parte dei globuli rossi senescenti è rimosso e sostituito ogni giorno. Durante l'emolisi, la sopravvivenza degli eritrociti è ridotta, la conta eritrocitaria diminuisce, l'eritropoietina è aumentata e la stimolazione dell'attività midollare porta a un'aumentata produzione dei globuli rossi e ciò si riflette in un'elevata percentuale di reticolociti nel sangue. Pertanto, l'emolisi dovrebbe essere sospettata come causa di anemia se è presente una conta reticolocitaria elevata. La conta reticolocitaria può anche essere elevata come risposta a una perdita acuta di sangue o per un breve periodo dopo terapia di ripristino per la carenza di ferro, di vitamina B_{12} o di folato. Il midollo può aumentare la sua produzione di 2-3 volte in acuto, con un massimo di 6-8 volte se l'emolisi è duratura. La percentuale dei reticolociti può essere corretta per misurare l'entità della produzione midollare in risposta all'emolisi, come segue:

$$\text{Indice reticolocitario} = \text{reticolociti \%} \times \frac{\text{ematocrito osservato}}{\text{ematocrito normale}} \times \frac{1}{\mu}$$

dove μ è un fattore di maturazione da 1 a 3 correlato alla gravità dell'anemia (Fig. 457-1). L'indice reticolocitario normale è 1,0; quindi l'indice misura l'aumento in fold nell'eritropoiesi (per es. 2-fold, 3-fold).

Non appena l'anemia diventa meno severa, aumenta la concentrazione dell'eritropoietina e precocemente vengono rilasciati i reticolociti dal midollo; essi sono identificabili come reticolociti nel sangue per >1 giorno. Poiché l'indice reticolocitario è essenzialmente una misura della produzione giornaliera dei globuli rossi, il fattore di maturazione μ permette questa correzione (vedi Fig. 457-1). L'abituale risposta midollare nell'anemia emolitica acuta è evidenziata da un indice reticolocitario di 2-3, mentre nelle emolisi croniche di lunga durata, l'aumento nell'eritropoiesi è pari a circa 6 volte.

L'iperplasia eritroide risultante dall'anemia emolitica cronica nei bambini, soprattutto nella talassemia, può essere così estesa che gli spazi midollari possono espandersi a spese dell'osso corticale. Questi cambiamenti possono essere evidenti all'esame fisico o alle radiografie del cranio e delle ossa lunghe (Fig. 462-7). Può anche verificarsi una propensione alla frattura delle ossa lunghe.

Una valutazione diretta della gravità dell'emolisi richiede la misura del tempo di sopravvivenza eritrocitario utilizzando globuli rossi marcati con il radioisotopo $Na_2{}^{51}CrO_4$. La normale emivita del cromo 51 è pari a 25-35 giorni. Questo valore è inferiore a quello atteso di 50-60 giorni a causa della diluizione del cromo 51 da parte dei globuli rossi marcati al tasso di circa 1% al giorno. Le tecniche per valutare la sopravvivenza degli eritrociti utilizzando la biotina eritrocitaria marcata è stata testata negli animali e non richiede l'uso di isotopi.

Diverse altre alterazioni plasmatiche, urinarie e fecali evidenziano la presenza di un'emolisi. L'aumento del catabolismo dell'emoglobina conduce a un'aumentata escrezione biliare dei derivati del pigmento biliare e a un aumento dell'urobilinogeno urinario e fecale (vedi Fig. 457-2). Calcoli costituiti da bilirubi-

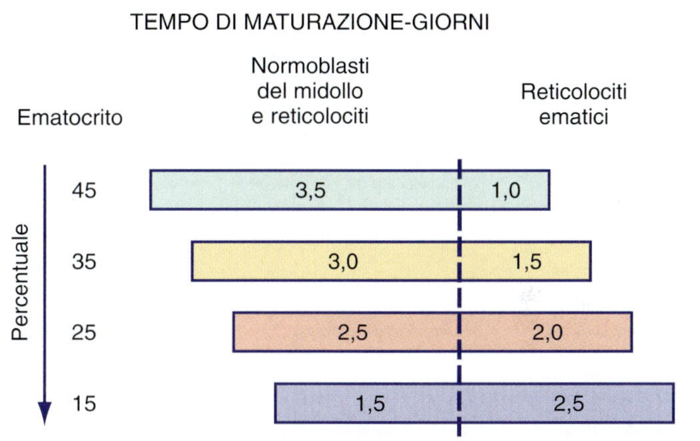

Figura 457-1. Numero di giorni necessari per la maturazione dei reticolociti nel midollo e nel sangue. La durata della maturazione in reticolociti ematici è espressa come μ, che è usato nella correzione dell'equazione in questo capitolo. (Modificata da: Hilman RS, Finch Ca: Red Cell Manual. *Philadelphia*, FA Davis, 1983).

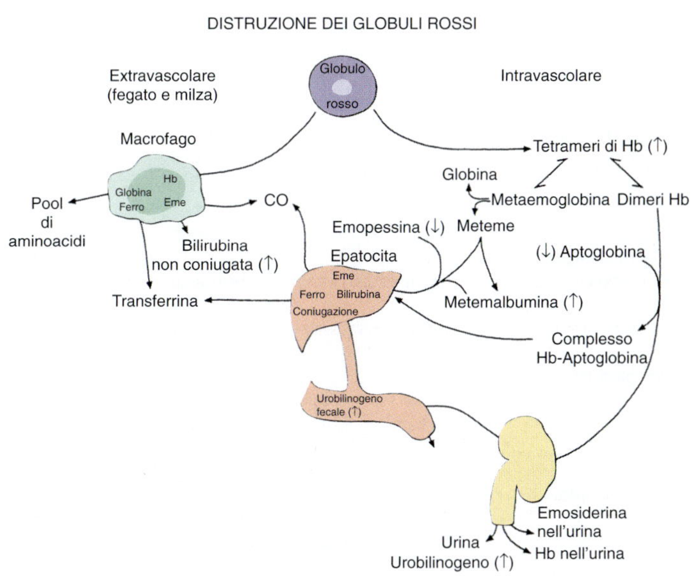

Figura 457-2. Distruzione dei globuli rossi e catabolismo dell'emoglobina (Hb) basata sulla descrizione fornita da Hillmane Finch. Fe, ferro. (Da Hillman RS, Finch CA: *Red Cell Manual*. Philadelphia, FA Davis, 1983.)

TABELLA 457-1. Anemie emolitiche e loro trattamento

DIAGNOSI	DIFETTO	TEST DI LABORATORIO	TRATTAMENTO
DIFETTI CELLULARI			
Difetti di membrana			
Sferocitosi ereditaria	Difetti della proteina del citoscheletro, frequentemente coinvolge interazioni verticali spettrina-anchirina, proteina 3	Sferociti nello striscio ematico I test di Coombs negativi eliminano l'emolisi immune, fragilità osmotica aumentata, analisi della proteina citoscheletrica aumentata.	Se Hb >10 g/dL e la conta reticolocitaria <10% – nessuno Se anemia severa, scarsa crescita, crisi aplastiche, ed età <2 anni – trasfusioni, acido folico 1 mg qd
Ellissocitosi ereditaria	Difetti della proteina citoscheletrica Frequentemente coinvolge le interazioni orizzontali della spectrina proteina 4.1, e glicoforina C	Ellissocitosi nello striscio ematico Lieve sensibilità al calore dei globuli rossi Analisi della proteina citoscheletrica anomala	Nella tipologia lieve – nessun trattamento Emolisi cronica – splenectomia e trasfusioni come raccomandato per sferocitosi (vedi sopra) Acido folico, 1 mg qd
Piropoichilocitosi ereditaria	Difetti della proteina citoscheletrica Anomala omozigosi o doppia eterozigoti in interazioni orizzontali dell'α spectrina	Variazione estrema nella dimensione e forma del globulo rosso Sensibilità termica – frammentazione a 45 °C per 15 min	Trasfusione e splenectomia come raccomandato per la sferocitosi (vedi sopra) Acido folico, 1 mg qd
Stomatocitosi ereditaria	Difetti della proteina citoscheletrica Proteina 7.2b diminuita (1 sottoserie) Anomalo contenuto in acqua e cationi dei globuli rossi	Stomatociti allo striscio di sangue	La splenectomia dovrebbe essere evitata (vedi testo) Acido folico, 1 mg qd
Emoglobinuria parossistica notturna	Disordine midollare primario acquisito Globuli rossi insolitamente sensibili alla lisi mediata dal complemento	Diminuzione dei GB CD55 e CD59 o dei globuli rossi CD59 con la citometria di flusso Test di Ham, test di lisi al sucrosio Aspirato midollare e biopsia per stabilire la cellularità Decadimento diminuito del fattore di accelerazione – per carenza di ferro secondaria	Acido folico, 1 mg qd Citopenia lieve – nessun trattamento Emolisi cronica e alter citopenie-prednisone, inizialmente 60 mg qd poi scalare se possibile; terapia di mantenimento 15-40 mg qd Androgeni – fluoximesterone Antocoagulanti Trapianto di midollo per pancitopenia
Deficit enzimatico			
Deficit piruvato chinasi	Enzima diminuito o anomalo	Saggio per piruvato chinasi – diminuita V_{max} o raramente variante elevata con km	Se anemia grave con sintomi, scarsa crescita ed età <2 anni – trasfusioni Splenectomia >6 anni di età, ma prima se necessario Acido folico, 1 mg qd
Carenza di G6PD	Tipo A$^-$: enzima labile con l'età Tipo Mediterraneo: no attività enzimatica nei globuli rossi circolanti	G6PD	Evitare lo stress ossidativi ai globuli rossi Trasfusioni se l'anemia acuta è sintomatica
Anomalie dell'emoglobina (*Per la discussione delle emoglobinopatie, vedi la sessione a riguardo*)			
DIFETTI EXTRACELLULARI			
Autoimmuni			
Anemia emolitica autoimmune	Alterazione nell'antigene di superficie di memebrana (Rh) o anomala risposta dei linfociti B, che causa produzione di autoanticorpi	Sferociti allo striscio ematico Test di Coombs diretto positivo per anticorpi IgG "caldi" di un autoanticorpo diretto contro i globuli rossi	Se Hb <10 g/dL e la conta reticolocitaria >10% – nessuno Anemia severa può richiedere trasfusione
Autoanticorpi "caldi"		Test di Coombs indiretto positivo e anticorpo riscontrabile nel plasma Ampiezza termica 35-40 °C Qualche frammento del complemento (C3b) nei globuli rossi Esami per una sottostante malattia	Prednisone, 2 mg/kg/24 h IVIG Danazolo Splenectomia Immunosoppressori Acido folico, 1 mg/24 h se cronica
Autoanticorpi "freddi"	Autoanticorpo "freddo" o IgM diretto contro l' antigene I/i	Agglutinazione o *rouleaux* allo striscio di sangue Positività del test di Coomb diretto, per il complemento (C3b) Test per la patologia sottostante Sierologia per mononucleosi infettiva; anti-I presente Sierologia per *Mycoplasma pneumoniae*; anti-I presente	Se Hb >10 g/dL e conta reticolocitaria <10% – nessuno L'anemia severa può richiedere trasfuzioni Evitare l'esposizione al freddo Se severa – immunosoppressori e plasmaferesi Prednisone è meno efficace La splenectomia non è utile Acido folico, 1 mg/24 h se cronica
Emolisi da frammentazione			
DIC, TTP, HUS	Danno diretto alla membrane dei globuli rossi	Frammenti sullo striscio di sangue	Trattare la patologia sottostante Trasfusione, ma le cellule trasfuse avranno comunque una durata di vita abbreviata
Ossigenazione extracorporea tramite membrana	Danno diretto alla membrane del globulo rosso	Frammenti sullo striscio di sangue	Di sostegno Trasfusione finché ECMO è interrotto
Protesi valvolare cardiaca	Danno diretto alla membrane del globulo rosso	Frammenti sullo striscio di sangue	Acido folico, 1 mg/24 h Ferro per la carenza di ferro secondaria
Ustioni-danno termico	Danno diretto alla membrane del globulo rosso	Sferociti sullo striscio di sangue	Di supporto Trasfusione
Ipersplenismo			
	Effetti del sequestro, ↓ pH, lipasi e altri enzimi, e macrofagi e dei globuli rossi	Trombocitopenia e neutropenia	Trattare la patologia sottostante-citopenie di solito lievi Splenectomia se complica altre condizioni anemiche (per es. talassemia major) Acido folico, 1 mg/24 h
Fattori plasmatici			
Epatopatia	Alterazione del colesterolo e fosfolipidi nel plasma Test di funzionalità epatica alterati	Cellule bersaglio o picnociti sullo striscio di sangue Trasfusione, ma le cellule transfuse avranno comunque durata di vita ridotta	Trattare la patologia sottostante Acido folico, 1 mg/24 h

TABELLA 457-1. Anemie emolitiche e loro trattamento – *continua*

DIAGNOSI	DIFETTO	TEST DI LABORATORIO	TRATTAMENTO
Abetalipoproteinemia	Assenza dell'apolipoproteina β Carenza di vitamina E e aumentata sensibilità a danno ossidativo	Acantociti allo striscio ematico Assenti chilomicroni, VLDL, e LDL	Vitamina E (A, K, e D) Acido folico, 1 mg/24 h Restrizione dietetica di trigliceridi
Infezioni	Effetto tossico sui globuli rossi	Sintomi e segni associati Colture	Antibiotici Di supporto
Malattia di Wilson	Effetto del rame sulla membrane del globulo rosso, in genere autolimitantesi	Sferociti allo striscio ematico Rame, ceruloplasmina Test di eliminazione con penicillamina ed escrezione urinaria di rame	Penicillamina Di supporto Trasfusione se l'anemia acuta è sintomatica

DIC, *Disseminated Intravascular Coagulation* (coaugulazione intravascolare disseminata); ECMO, *Extracorporeal Membrane Oxygenation* (ossigenazione extracorporea attraverso membrana); G6PD, glucosio-6-fosfato deidrogenasi; Hb, emoglobina; HUS, *Hemolytic Uremic Syndrome* (sindrome uremico emolitica); IVIG, immunoglobuline G endovenose; LDL, *Low Density Lipoprotein* (lipoproteina a bassa densità); TTP, *Thrombotic Thrombocytopenic Purpura* (porpora trombotica trombocitopenica); VLDL, *Very Low Density Lipoprotein* (lipoproteina a densità molto bassa); GB, globuli bianchi.
Modificata da Asselin BL, Segel GB: In Rakel R (ed): *Conn's Current Therapy*. Philadelphia, WB Saunders, 1994, pp 338-339.

nato di calcio possono formarsi in bambini di 4 anni con emolisi cronica. Anche aumenti della bilirubina non coniugata sierica e della lattico deidrogenasi possono accompagnare l'emolisi.

Tre proteine leganti l'eme nel plasma sono alterate nell'emolisi (vedi Fig. 457-2). L'emoglobina si lega all'aptoglobina e all'emopessina: entrambe vengono eliminate più rapidamente come coniugate e la loro concentrazione plasmatica è diminuita. L'eme ossidato si lega all'albumina per formare metemalbumina, che è aumentata nel plasma. Quando la capacità legante di queste molecole viene superata, l'emoglobina libera compare nel plasma e si può vedere un colore rosa se il plasma è separato dopo centrifugazione in un tubo capillare da ematocrito. Se presente l'emoglobina libera nel plasma rappresenta una prima evidenza di emolisi intravascolare. L'emoglobina libera si dissocia in dimeri e viene filtrata dai reni. Quando la capacità di riassorbimento tubulare dei reni per l'emoglobina viene superata, l'emoglobina libera compare nelle urine. Anche in assenza di emoglobinuria, la perdita di ferro può essere evidenziata dall'emoglobina riassorbita e dalla perdita delle cellule dell'epitelio renale in cui il ferro dell'emoglobina è immagazzinato come emosiderina. Ciò può condurre alla carenza di ferro durante l'emolisi cronica intravascolare. Quando l'emoglobina viene degradata si spezza un ponte α-metene nell'anello tetrapirrolico dell'eme, con il rilascio di monossido di carbonio (CO) (vedi Fig. 457-2). La quantità di CO nel sangue o nell'aria espirata produce una misura dinamica del grado di emolisi; il CO di fine espirazione (*end-tidal*) non è disponibile nella maggior parte dei laboratori clinici per misurare l'emolisi.

Il livello dell'ematocrito dipende dalla severità dell'emolisi e dalla risposta eritropoietica. La durata ridotta della vita dei globuli rossi assieme all'aumentata produzione eritrocitaria porta a una notevole suscettibilità alle crisi aplastiche o ipoplastiche, caratterizzate da insufficienza eritroide midollare e reticolocitopenia, che si accompagnano a una rapida caduta dell'emoglobina e dell'ematocrito a livelli molto bassi. La più comune causa di crisi aplastica è il parvovirus B19, che è eritrocitotropico (vedi Capitoli 248, 450, 458 e 462.1). Una crisi aplastica può produrre un precipitoso declino dell'ematocrito, pericoloso per la vita e che generalmente si protrae per 10-14 giorni. Tale insufficienza della eritropoiesi midollare transitoria ha un lieve effetto su chi presenta una normale durata di vita dei globuli rossi, ma ha un effetto proporzionalmente maggiore se la durata di vita dei globuli rossi viene ridotta dall'emolisi. Una seconda infezione da parvovirus è poco comune, ma altre infezioni possono compromettere la eritropoiesi midollare, producendo differenti gradi di crisi ipoplastiche o di ipoplasia.

Le anemie emolitiche possono essere classificate sia come (1) cellulari, causate da anomalie intrinseche delle membrane, degli enzimi o dell'emoglobina, sia come (2) extracellulari, causate da anticorpi, da fattori meccanici o da fattori plasmatici. La maggior parte dei difetti cellulari è ereditaria (l'emoglobinuria parossistica notturna è acquisita), mentre la maggior parte dei difetti extracellulari è acquisita (abetalipoproteinemia con acantocitosi è ereditaria). La Tabella 457-1 mostra le forme più comuni di anemie emolitiche, i loro difetti sottostanti, gli esami di laboratorio e le attuali raccomandazioni per il trattamento.

Capitolo 458 ■ Sferocitosi ereditaria

George B. Segel

La sferocitosi ereditaria è una causa comune di emolisi e anemia emolitica, con un ampio spettro di gravità e con una prevalenza di circa 1:5000 in persone di provenienza nordeuropea ed è la forma più comune di anomalia ereditaria della membrana dei globuli rossi. Gli individui affetti possono essere asintomatici, senza anemia o con una minima emolisi oppure possono presentare una grave anemia emolitica. La sferocitosi ereditaria è stata descritta nella maggior parte dei gruppi etnici, ma è più comune tra le persone di origine nordeuropea.

EZIOLOGIA. La sferocitosi ereditaria è generalmente trasmessa con carattere autosomico dominante e meno frequentemente come una patologia recessiva. Circa il 25% dei pazienti non ha un'anamnesi familiare precedente. Di questi, la maggior parte possiede nuove mutazioni e solo pochi casi conseguono a un'ereditarietà recessiva o rappresentano una non paternità. Il difetto molecolare più comune è costituito da anomalie a carico della spectrina o dell'ankirina, che sono le principali componenti del citoscheletro responsabili del mantenimento della forma del globulo rosso. Un difetto recessivo è stato descritto nell'α-spectrina; difetti dominanti nella β-spectrina e nella proteina 3 e difetti dominanti e recessivi nell'ankirina (Tab. 458-1). Un deficit di spectrina, proteina 3 o ankirina produce un accoppiamento difettoso nelle interazioni "verticali" del doppio strato lipidico di membrana e una perdita di microvescicole di membrana (Fig. 458-1). La perdita di un'area di superficie di membrana senza una perdita proporzionale di volume cellulare causa la sfericità del globulo rosso a un associato aumento di permeabilità ai cationi,

TABELLA 458-1. Mutazioni genetiche comuni nella sferocitosi ereditaria (SE)

PROTEINA	BANDA NEL GEL	GENE	PROPORZIONE DI PAZIENTI CON SE	EREDITARIETÀ
Ankirina	2,1	*ANK1*	50-67%	Dom e Rec
Banda 3	3	*AE1 (SLC4A1)*	15-20%	Per lo più Dom
β-spectrina	2	*SPTB*	15-20%	Dom
α-spectrina	1	*SPTA1*	<5%	Rec
Proteina 4,2	4,2	*EPB42*	<5%	Rec

Dom, dominante; Rec, recessiva.

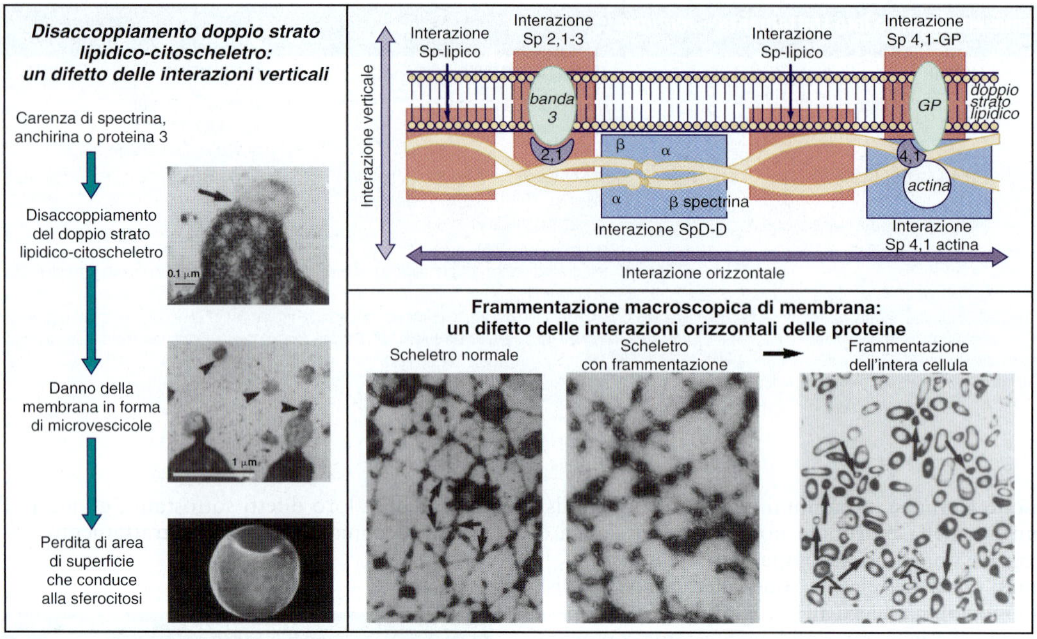

Figura 458-1. Interazioni verticali e orizzontali delle proteine di membrana e patobiologia delle lesioni dei globuli rossi nella sferocitosi ereditaria (SE) e nella ellissocitosi ereditaria/piropoichilocitosi ereditaria (EE/PE). A sinistra: un difetto delle interazioni verticali o trasversali come esemplificato dalla lesione della membrana dei globuli rossi nella SE. Carenze parziali della spectrina, ankirina (banda 2.1) o banda 3 portano a disaccoppiamento del doppio strato lipidico di membrana dal sottostante citoscheletro (*freccia*) seguito dalla formazione di microvescicole libere da spectrina che hanno un diametro di 0,2-0,5 μm (*punta della freccia*). Queste vescicole possono essere visualizzate tramite microscopia elettronica, ma non vengono riscontrate all'esame dello striscio di sangue. La perdita successiva della superficie cellulare e una riduzione del rapporto superficie/volume porta alla sferocitosi. A destra: un difetto delle interazioni orizzontali o parallele delle proteine del citoscheletro, come esemplificato dalla lesione della membrana nelle forme emolitiche della EE collegata a un difetto dell'autoassociazione spectrina-eterodimero. La lesione molecolare, che coinvolge una debole autoassociazione dell'eterodimero di spectrina in tetrameri, rappresenta un difetto orizzontale delle interazioni della proteina contro lo stress. Essa dà luogo a una distruzione del reticolo dello strato intermedio della membrana e di conseguenza della destabilizzazione dell'intera cellula, seguita dalla frammentazione del globulo rosso e della poichilocitosi. Tali frammenti sono immediatamente osservabili allo striscio ematico. Sp, spectrina; Sp-D, dimero di spectrina; GP, glicoforina. (Modificata da Palek J, Jarolim P: Clinical expression and laboratory detection of red blood cell membrane protein mutations. *Semin Hematol* 1993;30:249.)

di trasporto di cationi, di utilizzo dell'adenosina trifosfato e della glicolisi. La ridotta deformabilità dei globuli rossi influenza il loro passaggio dai cordoni ai sinusoidi splenici e gli eritrociti sferici vengono prematuramente distrutti nella milza. La splenectomia aumenta notevolmente la durata di vita dei globuli rossi e cura l'anemia.

MANIFESTAZIONI CLINICHE. La sferocitosi ereditaria può essere una causa di malattia emolitica nel neonato e si può presentare con un'anemia e un'iperbilirubinemia sufficientemente severe da richiedere la fototerapia o l'exsanguinotrasfusione. L'emolisi può essere predominante nel neonato perché l'emoglobina F lega in modo debole il 2,3-difosfoglicerato e gli aumentati livelli di 2,3-difosfoglicerato libero destabilizzano le interazioni tra spectrina-actina-proteina 4.1 nella membrana del globulo rosso (vedi Fig. 458-1). La gravità dei sintomi nei lattanti e nei bambini è variabile. Alcuni bambini rimangono asintomatici fino all'età adulta, ma altri possono manifestare un'anemia grave, con pallore, ittero, affaticabilità e intolleranza all'esercizio fisico. Casi gravi possono essere individuati attraverso l'aumento dello spessore della diploe cranica e della regione midollare di altre ossa, ma in misura minore che nella talassemia major. Dopo l'infanzia, la milza in genere aumenta il suo volume e calcoli biliari pigmentati (bilirubina) possono formarsi già a 4-5 anni. Almeno il 50% dei pazienti non splenectomizzati forma calcoli, anche se alle volte asintomatici. A causa dell'elevato ricambio dei globuli rossi e dell'aumentata attività eritroide midollare, i bambini con sferocitosi ereditaria sono suscettibili alle crisi aplastiche, prima di tutto come risultato dell'infezione da parvovirus e delle crisi ipoplastiche in associazione a varie altre infezioni (Fig. 458-2). L'insufficienza eritroide midollare può portare rapidamente a una grave anemia (ematocrito <10%), insufficienza cardiaca ad alta gittata, ipossia, collasso cardiovascolare e morte. Anche la conta dei globuli bianchi e delle piastrine può essere diminuita (vedi Fig. 458-2).

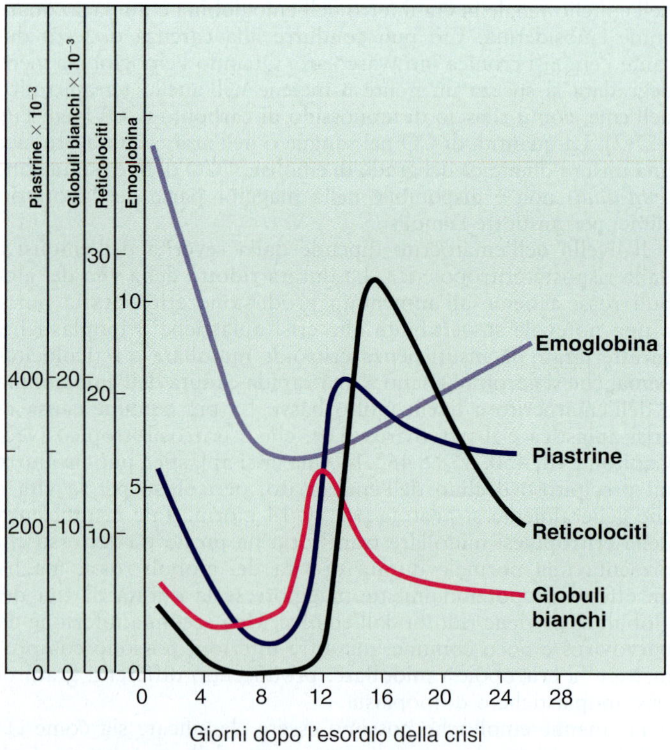

Figura 458-2. Crisi aplastica indotta da parvovirus. Viene mostrata la progressione dei cambiamenti nella conta dei globuli rossi per un paziente con sferocitosi ereditaria e infezione da parvovirus. Va notato che la caduta della reticolocitosi è associata a un rapido calo dei livelli di emoglobina. Anche i globuli bianchi e le piastrine sono affetti. (Modificata da Nathan DG, Orkin SH, Ginsburg D, et al [edit]: *Hematology of Infancy and Childhood*, 6th ed. Philadelphia, WB Saunders, 2003).

REPERTI DI LABORATORIO. Segni di emolisi evidente comprendono la reticolocitosi e l'iperbilirubinemia indiretta. Il livello di emoglobina in genere è pari a 6-10 g/dL, ma può rientrare anche nel range di norma. La percentuale dei reticolociti spesso è aumentata al 6-20% con un valore medio di circa 10%. Il volume corpuscolare medio è normale, mentre la concentrazione media di emoglobina corpuscolare è spesso aumentata (36-38 g/dL di globuli rossi). I globuli rossi allo striscio di sangue variano per dimensioni e presentano reticolociti policromatofili e sferociti (Fig. 458-3*A*). Gli sferociti sono più piccoli per diametro e appaiono ipercromici allo striscio di sangue come risultato dell'elevata concentrazione di emoglobina. Il pallore centrale è meno cospicuo che nelle cellule normali. Gli sferociti possono essere le cellule predominanti o possono essere relativamente rari a seconda della gravità della malattia, ma in genere, quando è presente un'anemia emolitica, rappresentano oltre il 15-20% delle cellule. L'iperplasia eritroide è evidente all'aspirato o alla biopsia midollare. L'espansione midollare può essere evidente all'esame radiografico di routine. Altre evidenze di emolisi possono includere la diminuzione dell'aptoglobina e la presenza di calcoli all'ecografia.

La diagnosi di sferocitosi ereditaria è in genere stabilita clinicamente attraverso lo striscio di sangue, che mostra molti sferociti e reticolociti, l'anamnesi familiare e la splenomegalia. La presenza degli sferociti nel sangue periferico può essere confermata con il test della fragilità osmotica (Fig. 458-4). I globuli rossi vengono incubati in diluizioni progressive di una soluzione fisiologica tamponata isosmotica. L'esposizione a soluzioni saline ipotoniche causa il rigonfiamento dei globuli rossi e gli sferociti vanno incontro a lisi più rapidamente rispetto alle cellule biconcave in soluzioni ipotoniche. Questa caratteristica è accentuata deprivando le cellule di glucosio durante la notte a 37 °C, un test noto come *test di fragilità osmotica dopo incubazione*. Purtroppo questo test non è specifico per la sferocitosi ereditaria e può risultare anormale anche nelle forme autoimmuni o in altre tipologie di anemia. Un test normale può inoltre essere ritrovato in circa il 10-20% dei pazienti. Altri test, come il test di crioemolisi, l'ectacitometria a gradiente osmotico, il test alla eocina-5-maleimide, possono essere più sensibili ma non sono ancora disponibili. La scoperta di una popolazione di globuli rossi iperdensi utilizzando uno strumento a laser o un contatore Coulter può essere una prova diagnostica più idonea.

La specifica proteina anomala può essere identificata nell'80% di questi pazienti attraverso l'analisi delle proteine di membrana dei globuli rossi utilizzando l'elettroforesi a gel e la quantizzazione densitometrica. Le anomalie proteiche sono più evidenti in pazienti che sono stati sottoposti a splenectomia. Studi per definire i sottostanti difetti nel citoscheletro possono richiedere la valutazione della sintesi proteica, della stabilità, dell'assemblaggio e del legame alle altre proteine di membrana. Anche la diagnosi molecolare è possibile. La maggior parte dei pazienti presenta mutazioni private familiari specifiche che possono essere identificate grazie all'analisi del DNA. Mutazioni *ex novo* nel

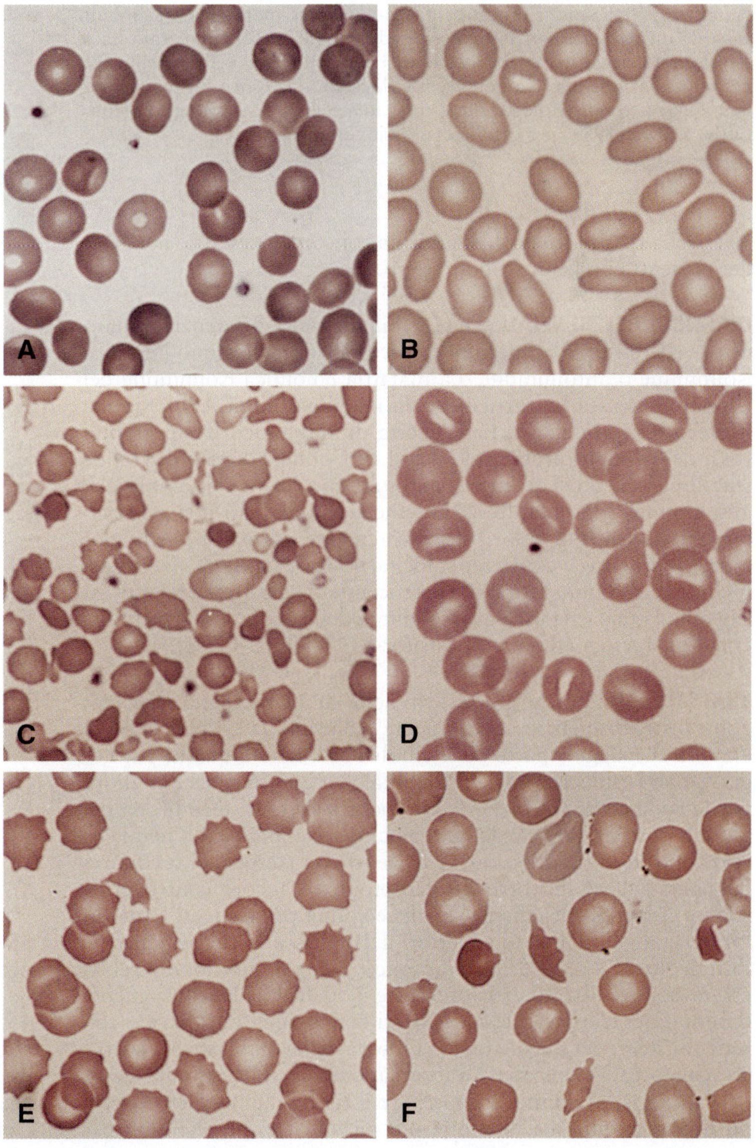

Figura 458-3. Morfologia dei globuli rossi anomali. *A*, Sferocitosi ereditaria; *B*, ellissocitosi ereditaria; *C*, piropoichilocitosi ereditaria; *D*, stomatocitosi ereditaria; *E*, acantocitosi; *F*, emolisi da frammentazione.

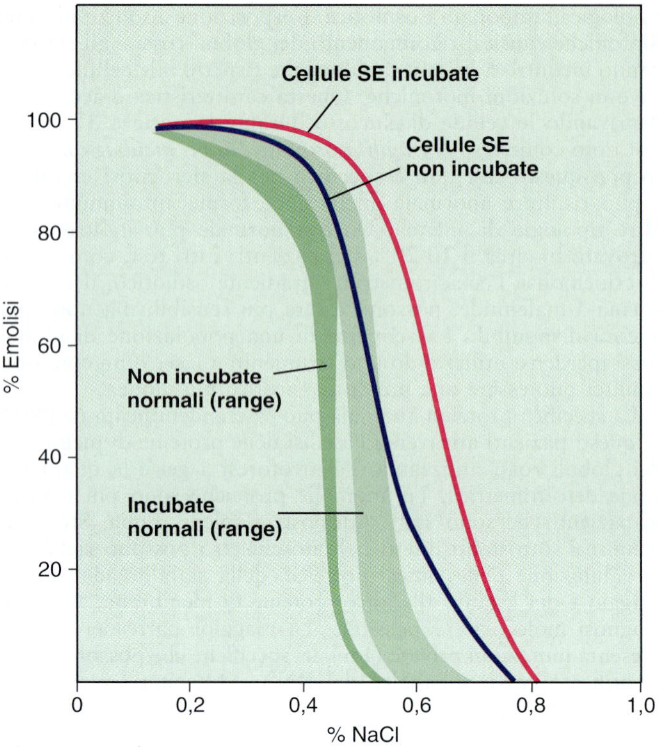

Figura 458-4. Fragilità osmotica dei globuli rossi normali e di globuli rossi da un paziente con sferocitosi ereditaria (SE). Viene mostrata l'accentuazione della sensibilità osmotica, in particolare delle cellule SE, dopo incubazione per una notte senza glucosio. (Da Reich PR [edit]: Hematology: *Pathophysiologic Basis for Clinical Practice*, 2nd ed. Boston, Little, Brown, 1984, per gentile concessione.)

gene della β-spectrina e dell'ankirina sono state descritte nel 50% dei pazienti con genitori non affetti.

DIAGNOSI DIFFERENZIALE. Le possibili diagnosi differenziali quando si vede un gran numero di sferociti allo striscio sono l'emolisi isoimmune o autoimmune. La malattia emolitica isoimmune del neonato, causata in particolare da incompatibilità ABO, simula la sferocitosi ereditaria. La scoperta di autoanticorpi sui globuli rossi del neonato utilizzando il test di Coombs diretto dovrebbe stabilire la diagnosi di emolisi autoimmune. Le anemie emolitiche autoimmuni sono caratterizzate anche da sferociti e si possono trovare evidenze di valori precedentemente normali per emoglobina, ematocrito e conta reticolocitaria. Rare cause di sferocitosi includono il danno termico, la setticemia da clostridi con esotossinemia, la malattia di Wilson, ognuna delle quali può presentarsi come un'anemia emolitica transitoria (vedi Tab. 457-1).

TRATTAMENTO. Poiché gli sferociti nella sferocitosi ereditaria vengono distrutti quasi esclusivamente nella milza, la splenectomia elimina la maggior parte delle emolisi associate a questa patologia. Dopo la splenectomia, la fragilità osmotica in genere migliora per le condizioni spleniche e la minore perdita di membrana dei globuli rossi; l'anemia, la reticolocitosi e l'iperbilirubinemia si risolvono in seguito. Se tutti i pazienti con sferocitosi ereditaria debbano andare incontro a splenectomia è ancora controverso. Alcuni Autori sconsigliano la splenectomia per pazienti i cui valori di emoglobina sono superiori a 10 g/dL e la cui percentuale di reticolociti è <10%. L'acido folico, 1 mg al giorno, dovrebbe essere somministrato per prevenire il deficit e la conseguente diminuita eritropoiesi. Per i pazienti con anemia più grave e con reticolocitosi, per quelli con crisi ipoplastiche o aplastiche, scarsa crescita o cardiomegalia è raccomandata la splenectomia dopo l'età di 5-6 anni, in modo da evitare il rischio aumentato di sepsi post-splenectomia nei bambini più piccoli. La splenectomia per via laparoscopica riduce i tempi di ospedalizzazione e ha sostituito la splenectomia a cielo aperto per molti pazienti. Vaccini (coniugati e/o capsulati) per gli organismi capsulati, come il pneumococco, il meningococco e l'*Haemophilus influenzae* di tipo b, dovrebbero essere somministrati prima della splenectomia, come anche la penicillina V orale in via profilattica (età <5 anni, 125 mg due volte al giorno; età 5 anni fino all'età adulta, 250 mg due volte al giorno) somministrata in seguito. Una trombocitosi post-splenectomia è comunemente osservata, ma non necessita di un trattamento, e di solito si risolve spontaneamente. Anche una splenectomia parziale può essere utile nei bambini più piccoli di 5 anni e può produrre alcuni aumenti nell'emoglobina nonché riduzione della conta reticolocitaria, con un potenziale mantenimento della funzione fagocitica e immune splenica.

Bader-Meunier B, Gauthier F, Archambaud F, et al: Long-term evaluation of the beneficial effect of subtotal splenectomy for management of hereditary spherocytosis. *Blood* 2001;97:399–403.

Bolton-Maggs PBH, Stevens RF, Dodd NJ, et al: Guidelines for the diagnosis and management of hereditary spherocytosis. *Br J Haematol* 2004;126: 455–474.

Delhommeau F, Cynober T, Schischmanoff PO, et al: Natural history of hereditary spherocytosis during the first year of life. *Blood* 2000;95:393–397.

Eber S, Lux SE: Hereditary spherocytosis: Defects in proteins that connect the membrane skeleton to the lipid bilayer. *Semin Hematol* 2004;41:118–141.

Iolascon A, Perrotta S, Stewart GW: Red cell membrane defects. *Rev Clin Exp Hematol* 2003;7:22–56.

Minkes RK, Lagzdins M, Langer JC, et al: Laparoscopic versus open splenectomy in children. *J Pediatr Surg* 2000;35:699–700.

Capitolo 459 ■ Ellissocitosi ereditaria

George B. Segel

L'ellissocitosi ereditaria è una patologia meno comune della sferocitosi che anche varia notevolmente in termini di gravità. L'ellissocitosi ereditaria lieve non produce sintomi; le forme più severe possono condurre a poichilocitosi neonatale (variazioni di forma) e a emolisi, anemia emolitica cronica o sporadica, oppure piropoichilocitosi ereditaria (*Hereditary PyroPoikilocitosis*, HPP), che è una patologia grave con microsferocitosi e poichilocitosi. L'ellissocitosi ereditaria è rara nelle popolazioni occidentali, mentre è più comune nell'Africa occidentale.

EZIOLOGIA. L'ellissocitosi ereditaria è ereditata come una patologia dominante. Nei rari esempi in cui vengono ereditati due alleli anormali (HPP), il paziente evidenzia un'anemia particolarmente grave. Diversi difetti molecolari sono stati descritti nell'ellissocitosi ereditaria, che producono anomalie di α e di β-spectrina e difetti dell'autoassociazione degli eterodimeri difettivi di spectrina (vedi Fig. 458-1). Le anomalie (mutazioni nella spectrina) possono produrre resistenza all'infezione malarica. Questi difetti nelle interazioni orizzontali delle proteine producono frammentazione grossolana della membrana, in particolare nell'HPP omozigote. Meno comunemente, le mutazioni nella proteina 4.1 e nella glicoforina C possono dare luogo a ellissocitosi.

MANIFESTAZIONI CLINICHE. L'ellissocitosi può essere un reperto occasionale all'esame dello striscio di sangue e può non venire associata a un'emolisi clinicamente significativa (vedi Fig. 458-3*B*). La diagnosi di ellissocitosi ereditaria viene stabilita dai riscontri sullo striscio di sangue periferico, dal pattern di ereditarietà autosomica dominante e dall'assenza di altre cause di ellissocitosi, come il deficit di ferro, di acido folico o di vitamina B_{12}. L'ellissocitosi emolitica può produrre ittero neonatale, anche se la caratteristica ellissocitosi può non essere evidente a quell'età. Il sangue del neonato affetto può mostrare poichilocitosi e picnocitosi. Un aumento transitorio della frammentazione e l'emolisi nel neonato possono risultare dalla presenza di emoglobina F, che lega debolmente all'intermedio glicolitico 2,3-difosfoglicerato. L'aumentato 2,3-difosfoglicerato tende a destabilizzare il complesso spectrina-actina-proteina 4.1, portando a instabilità di membrana (vedi Fig. 458-1). Le caratteristiche usuali del processo emolitico cronico con ellissocitosi si manifestano più tardi come anemia, ittero, splenomegalia e alterazioni ossee. La colelitiasi può verificarsi nell'infanzia; sono state riportate crisi aplastiche. La forma più severa è HPP, che è caratterizzata da un'estrema microcitosi (volume corpuscolare medio, 50-60 fL/cellula), un'importante variazione di dimensione e di forma cellulare e da cellule all'inizio microsferocitiche e in seguito ellittiche (vedi Fig. 458-3*C*). Questi pazienti in genere ereditano una spectrina mutata da un genitore, che non presenta un'ellissocitosi, o l'ha in forma lieve, e una parziale carenza di spectrina da parte dell'altro genitore, che è ematologicamente normale.

Gli **ovalociti**, al contrario degli ellissociti, sono meno allungati e possono riflettere una malattia nota come *ovalocitosi del Sud-est asiatico* (OSA). L'OSA viene associata a una proteina 3 anomala, che funziona come uno scambiatore di anioni. Questa patologia può causare iperbilirubinemia neonatale, ma causa in seguito una modesta emolisi. Essa offre protezione nei confronti di della malaria da *Plasmodium falciparum* poiché la proteina 3 è uno dei recettori per la malaria. La proteina 3 è un trasportatore di anioni espresso anche nelle cellule del tubulo renale e può causare un'acidosi tubulare renale distale se associata a OSA.

REPERTI DI LABORATORIO. Lo striscio di sangue periferico è il test più importante per diagnosticare l'ellissocitosi ereditaria (vedi Fig. 458-3*B*). I globuli rossi mostrano diversi livelli di allungamento e possono presentare una forma a bastoncello. Nell'ellissocitosi ereditaria, possono essere presenti altre anomalie della forma dei globuli rossi, a seconda della gravità dell'emolisi. Queste includono microciti, sferociti e altri poichilociti. La percentuale di reticolociti riflette la gravità dell'emolisi; un'iperplasia eritroide e un'iperbilirubinemia indiretta possono essere presenti. L'instabilità termica aumentata è caratteristica della HPP; da qui il suo nome. La spectrina anomala si denatura e le cellule vanno incontro a lisi a 45-46 °C invece degli abituali 49-50 °C. L'anomalia della proteina specifica può essere stabilita mediante la separazione proteica e le tecniche di analisi. I difetti molecolari sono definiti solo in laboratori di ricerca.

TRATTAMENTO. Se l'ellissocitosi ereditaria rappresenta un'anomalia morfologica nello striscio di sangue senza evidenti segni di emolisi, non è necessario alcun trattamento. I pazienti con emolisi cronica dovrebbero ricevere acido folico, 1 mg al giorno, per prevenire una carenza di acido folico secondaria. La splenectomia riduce l'emolisi e dovrebbe essere presa in considerazione se l'emoglobina è <10 g/dL e la conta reticolocitaria è >10%. I globuli rossi allo striscio di sangue periferico possono essere anormali dopo la splenectomia, sebbene aumenti l'emoglobina e diminuiscano i reticolociti. Le caratteristiche ematologiche dell'OSA non richiedono un trattamento dopo il periodo neonatale.

Benet A, Khong TY, Uru A, et al: Placental malaria in women with southeast Asian ovalocytosis. *Am J Trop Med Hyg* 2006;75:597–604.
Gallagher PG: Hereditary elliptocytosis: Spectrin and protein 4.1R. *Semin Hematol* 2004;41:142–164.
Vasuvattakul S, Yenchitsomanus PT, Vachuanichsanong P, et al: Autosomal recessive distal renal tubular acidosis associated with Southeast Asian ovalocytosis. *Kidney Int* 1999;56:1674–1682.

Capitolo 460 ■ Stomatocitosi ereditaria

George B. Segel

La stomatocitosi ereditaria è una condizione rara in cui i globuli rossi sono a forma di tazza. All'esame dello striscio di sangue periferico si presentano con una fessura a forma di bocca al posto della consueta area centrale circolare di pallore (vedi Fig. 458-3*D*). La stomatocitosi acquisita può essere vista in numerose condizioni, soprattutto nelle epatopatie. La stomatocitosi acquisita è associata con un'aumentata permeabilità della membrana degli eritrociti al Na^+ e al K^+ e ad alterazioni nello stato di idratazione del globulo rosso. La varietà **idrocitica** o **sovraidratata** è si solito la più grave. Essa è associata a una diminuzione della proteina 7.2, o "stomatica"; il gene è posto sul cromosoma 9. Un'alterazione della trascrizione del promotore produce una riduzione della stomatina, che può rendere difettoso il trasporto dei cationi. La stomatocitosi ereditaria **deidratata** è il tipo più comune; è eterogenea per severità e può essere associata alla sindrome dell'**edema perinatale** e con **ascite**. La sindrome dell'edema perinatale è transitoria e rimane non spiegata. Il difetto nella stomatina può anche essere presente in casi più gravi in pazienti con il tipo deidratato. Una terza tipologia, *crioidrocitosi*, è la forma più lieve di stomatocitosi. I globuli rossi in questa condizione vanno incontro a lisi durante raffreddamento *in vitro* e si può associare a "pseudoiperkaliemia" qualora venga misurato il potassio sierico. Un'anemia emolitica severa può accompagnarsi alla stomatocitosi ereditaria, ma la splenectomia non è raccomandata perché è inefficace; mentre una trombocitosi persistente sintomatica può seguire la splenectomia quando l'emolisi non è diminuita. Alcuni pazienti hanno una tendenza, con conseguenze negative per la vita, a una trombosi *in situ* dopo la splenectomia, a causa dell'anomala adesione dei globuli rossi stomatocitici all'endotelio vascolare associata alla trombocitosi post-splenectomia.

Delaunay J: The hereditary stomatocytoses: Genetic disorders of the red cell membrane permeability to monovalent cations. *Semin Hematol* 2004;41:165–172.
Delaunay J, Stewart G, Iolascon A: Hereditary dehydrated and overhydrated stomatocytosis: Recent advances. *Curr Opin Hematol* 1999;6:110–114.
Stewart GW, Amess JA, Eber SW, et al: Thrombo-embolic disease after splenectomy for hereditary stomatocytosis. *Br J Haematol* 1997;93:301–310.

Capitolo 461 ■ Altri difetti di membrana

George B. Segel

EMOGLOBINURIA PAROSSISTICA NOTTURNA

EZIOLOGIA. L'emoglobinuria parossistica notturna (*Paroxysmal Nocturnal Hemoglobinuria*, PNH) riflette un'anomalia della cellula staminale midollare che colpisce ogni linea cellulare del sangue. La malattia non è ereditaria, ma è una patologia acquisita dell'ematopoiesi caratterizzata da un difetto nelle proteine della membrana cellulare, che rende i globuli rossi e altre cellule suscettibili al danno provocato da normali proteine del complemento del plasma. Le proteine di membrana che vengono a mancare o sono deficitarie sono il fattore pro-invecchiamento, la proteina legante il CD8 e altre proteine che normalmente impediscono la lisi mediata dal complemento a diversi livelli. Il difetto sottostante coinvolge il glicolipide di ancoraggio che mantiene queste proteine protettive sulla superficie cellulare. Nei pazienti con

PNH sono state identificate diverse mutazioni nel gene *PIGA*, che è coinvolto nella biosintesi del glicosilfosfatidilinositolo. In un singolo paziente si verifica spesso più di una mutazione nel gene *PIGA*, suggerendo una mutliclonalità. Inoltre le cellule con carenza di glicosilfosfatidilinositolo si trovano con bassa frequenza in persone normali. Questo indica che il danno alle cellule staminali midollari produce un vantaggio selettivo per i cloni PNH nella genesi di questa patologia.

MANIFESTAZIONI CLINICHE. Soprattutto nei bambini, la PNH è una patologia rara, ma 26 pazienti di età media pari a 13 anni (range, 0,8-21,4 anni) sono stati diagnosticati presso il Duke University Medical Centre tra il 1966 e il 1991. Circa il 60% di questi pazienti presentava insufficienza midollare e i rimanenti presentavano anemia intermittente o cronica, spesso con una notevole emolisi intravascolare. Emoglobinuria notturna e diurna è un reperto classico negli adulti se l'emolisi è peggiore durante il sonno. Tuttavia, l'emolisi cronica è più comune nella PNH, a dispetto del nome. Oltre all'emolisi cronica, sono spesso caratteristiche una trombocitopenia e una leucopenia. La **trombosi** e i fenomeni **tromboembolici** rappresentano gravi complicanze, che sembrano essere collegate a glicoproteine alterate sulla superficie delle piastrine e che ne producono attivazione. Un dolore addominale, alle spalle e alla testa può essere il sintomo predominante. Una **pancitopenia** aplastica o ipoplastica può precedere o seguire l'esordio della PNH; la PNH raramente progredisce in leucemia acuta mielogena. Di 220 pazienti di tutte le età identificate in centri medici francesi dal 1950 al 1995 al momento della presentazione il 93% mostrava alcune anomalie a livello ematico (inclusi 33% con sola anemia, 17% con anemia e trombocitopenia, 7% con anemia e neutropenia e 32% con pancitopenia), il 13% dolore addominale e il 6% trombosi. La mortalità della PNH è legata principalmente allo sviluppo di anemia aplastica o complicanze trombotiche. Il tasso di sopravvivenza predetto per i bambini è dell'80% a 5 anni, 60% a 10 anni e 28% a 20 anni.

REPERTI DI LABORATORIO. La diagnosi di PHN è stabilita tipicamente con una risposta positiva sia al test del siero acidificato (Ham) sia al test di lisi al saccarosio. Questi test attivano, rispettivamente, la via alternativa e la via classica di lisi del complemento. L'emosiderinuria è comune e riflette l'emolisi cronica intravascolare. Inoltre si riscontrano livelli marcatamente ridotti di attività dell'acetilcolinesterasi eritrocitaria e del fattore di pro-invecchiamento. La **citometria di flusso** rappresenta il test diagnostico di scelta per la PNH. Utilizzando l'anti-CD59 per gli eritrociti e gli anti-CD55 e anti-CD59 per i granulociti, la citometria a flusso è più sensibile dei classici test di lisi dei globuli rossi nell'evidenziare il ridotto legame glicolipidico alle proteine della membrana cellulare. Il test della proteina aerolisina fluoresceinata può aumentare la sensibilità diagnostica poiché si lega selettivamente al sito di ancoraggio glicosilfosfatidilinositolo.

TRATTAMENTO. La splenectomia non è indicata. I glucocorticoidi, come il prednisone (2 mg/kg/24 h), sono stati usati per trattare gli episodi emolitici; il loro dosaggio dovrebbe essere ridotto non appena sia cessata l'emolisi. Una terapia anticoaugulante prolungata può essere di beneficio quando si verificano le trombosi; l'eparina e l'eparina a basso peso molecolare possono inibire l'emolisi mediata dal complemento. A causa della perdita urinaria cronica di ferro sottoforma di emosiderina, una terapia a base di ferro può essere necessaria. Gli androgeni, come il fluoximesterone, la globulina antitimocita, la ciclosporina, e i fattori di crescita, come l'eritropoietina e il fattore promuovente le colonie granulocitarie, sono stati usati per trattare l'insufficienza midollare. Il trapianto di midollo osseo ha successo nel trattamento di alcuni casi; il trapianto non mieloablativo può ridurre la mortalità e la morbilità trapianto-relata. L'eculizumab, un anticorpo monoclonale umanizzato diretto contro la proteina C5 del complemento, stabilizza i livelli di emoglobina, riduce il numero di trasfusioni e diminuisce il grado di emolisi negli adulti con PHN trattati. Il trasferimento retrovirale del gene *PIGA* ripristina il glicolipide di ancoraggio nelle cellule coltivate e può rappresentare la base per una futura terapia genetica.

ACANTOCITOSI

L'acantocitosi è caratterizzata da globuli rossi con proiezioni irregolari circonferenziali allungate (vedi Fig. 458-3*E*). Questo reperto morfologico è riscontrato assieme ad alterazioni del rapporto colesterolo/fosfolipidi in alcuni pazienti con epatopatie e nella abetalipoproteinemia congenita legata a malassorbimento, anomalie neuromuscolari e retinite pigmentosa (vedi Capitoli 86.3 e 629). È anche associata con la rara sindrome di McLeod, correlata al cromosoma X, che comprende l'assenza dell'antigene Kx (Kell), miopatie di tarda comparsa, anomalie neurologiche come corea, splenomegalia ed emolisi con acantocitosi.

Brodsky RA: New insights into paroxysmal nocturnal hemoglobinuria. *Hematology Am Soc Hematol Educ Program* 2006;24–28.

Gold MM, Shifteh K, Bello JA, et al: Chorea–acanthocytosis: A mimicker of Huntington disease. Case report and review of the literature. *Neurologist* 2006;12:327–329.

Hillmen P, Young NS, Shubert J, et al: The complement inhibitor eculizumab in paroxysmal nocturnal hemoglobinuria. *N Engl J Med* 2006;355: 1233–1243.

Rosse WF, Nishimura J: Clinical manifestations of paroxysmal nocturnal hemoglobinuria: Present state and future problems. *Int J Hematol* 2003;77:113–120.

Smith LJ: Paroxysmal nocturnal hemoglobinuria. [Review.] *Clin Lab Sci* 2004;17:172–177.

Socie G, Mary JY, de Gramont A, et al: Paroxysmal nocturnal haemoglobinuria: Long-term follow-up and prognostic factors. *Lancet* 1996;348: 573–577.

Suenaga K, Kanda Y, Niiya H, et al: Successful application of nonmyeloablative transplantation for paroxysmal nocturnal hemoglobinuria. *Exp Hematol* 2001;29:639–642.

Van den Heuvel-Eibrink MM, Bredius RG, te Winkel ML, et al: Childhood paroxysmal nocturnal hemoglobinuria (PHH): A report of 11 cases in the Netherlands. *Br J Haematol* 2005;128:571–577.

Capitolo 462 ■ Emoglobinopatie

Michael R. DeBaun e Elliott Vichinsky

L'emoglobina è un tetramero costituito da due paia di catene globiniche. Le anomalie in queste proteine sono note come **emoglobinopatie**. Esistono circa 800 varianti emoglobiniche. La classificazione più comune e clinicamente più utile delle emoglobinopatie è basata su una nomenclatura associata all'alterazione a carico della catena globinica coinvolta. Due gruppi di geni emoglobinici sono coinvolti nella produzione dell'emoglobina e sono localizzati rispettivamente all'estremità del braccio corto del cromosoma 16 e del cromosoma 11. Il loro controllo è complesso e comprende a monte un locus della regione di controllo in ciascun cromosoma così come un sito di controllo sul cromosoma X. Sul cromosoma 16 ci sono 3 geni all'interno del cluster del gene alfa (α): zeta (ζ) e 2 geni alfa (α_1, α_2). Sul cromosoma 11 ci sono 5 geni all'interno del cluster beta (β): epsilon (ε), delta (δ) e due geni gamma (γ). L'ordine dell'espressione genica dentro ogni cluster segue rigidamente l'ordine di espressione durante il periodo embrionale, il periodo fetale ed eventualmente l'infanzia. Dopo 8 settimane di vita gestazionale, le emoglobine embrionali sono formate: Gower-1 ($\zeta_2\varepsilon_2$), Gower-2 ($\alpha_2\varepsilon_2$) e Portland ($\zeta_2\gamma_2$). A 9 settimane di vita gestazionale l'emoglobina (Hb) maggiore è Hb F ($\alpha_2\gamma_2$). A circa un mese di vita fetale compare l'Hb A ($\alpha_2\beta_2$), ma l'Hb A non diviene predominante fino a dopo la nascita, quando i livelli di Hb F iniziano a diminuire. Un'emoglobina minore, Hb A_2 ($\alpha_2\delta_2$), compare poco prima della nascita e rimane a bassi livelli subito dopo. La distribuzione finale del pattern emoglobinico che si presenta nell'età pediatrica non viene raggiunta fino all'età di 6 mesi, ma qualche volta anche più tardi. Il pattern emoglobinico normale è $\geq$95% Hb A, $\leq$3,5% Hb A_2, <2,5% Hb F.

462.1 • Emoglobinopatia a cellule falciformi

L'emoglobina S (Hb S) è il risultato del cambiamento di un singolo paio di basi, timina per adenina, al sesto codone del gene β-globinico. Questo cambiamento codifica una valina anziché una glutammina alla posizione 6 nella molecola β-globinica. L'**anemia a cellule falciformi**, l'omozigosi Hb S, si verifica quando entrambi i geni β-globinici presentano la mutazione delle cellule falciformi. L'**emoglobinopatia a cellule falciformi** si riferisce non solo agli individui con anemia a cellule falciformi, ma anche ai casi eterozigoti in cui una mutazione del gene β-globinico comprende la mutazione delle cellule falciformi e la seconda β-globina include una mutazione nel gene della β-globina diversa da quella della drepanocitosi, come una mutazione associata a Hb C, Hb β-talassemia, Hb D e Hb O Arab. Nell'anemia falcifome, l'Hb S è in genere pari al 90% dell'emoglobina totale, mentre nell'emoglobinopatia a cellule falciformi, l'Hb S costituisce oltre il 50%.

Negli Stati Uniti l'emoglobinopatia a cellule falciformi è la patologia genetica più comune identificata attraverso il programma di screening neonatale voluto dallo Stato, che si verifica in 1/2647 nati, che supera l'incidenza dell'ipotiroidismo primario congenito (1/3000), della fibrosi cistica (1/3900) e dell'iperfenilalaninemia clinicamente significativa (1/14 000). L'emoglobinopatia a cellule falciformi negli Stati Uniti si verifica tra gli afroamericani con un tasso di 1/396 nati; tra gli ispanici a un tasso di 1/36 000 nati; tra i discendenti dei mediorientali non sono stati identificati casi tra i 22 000 sottoposti a screening tra gli indiani asiatici a un tasso di 1/16 000 dei sottoposti a screening.

I bambini con l'emoglobinopatia a cellule falciformi dovrebbero essere seguiti da esperti nel trattamento di questa malattia, che sono molto spesso gli ematologi pediatrici. Terapie mediche complete, con strategie basate sull'evidenza fornite da esperti in emolobinopatie a cellule falciformi, assieme a una corretta informazione ai genitori sulle più comuni complicanze, hanno notevolmente diminuito la mortalità e la morbilità correlate all'emoglobinopatia a cellule falciformi nel corso degli ultimi 20 anni. Le terapie mediche prescritte da ematologi pediatri si associano a una diminuzione delle visite presso i reparti di emergenza e a una minore durata del ricovero in ospedale, se comparate con pazienti che non sono stati visti da un ematologo pediatra nell'ultimo anno. Quando possibile, i bambini con emoglobinopatia a cellule falciformi dovrebbero essere seguiti da esperti di malattie a cellule falciformi o da medici di famiglia che si occupano della terapia medica della malattia in cogestione con un ematologo pediatra.

Anemia falciforme (omozigosi dell'emoglobina S) o S β-talassemia

MANIFESTAZIONI CLINICHE E TRATTAMENTO. I lattanti affetti da anemia falciforme hanno una funzione immune anormale. Precocemente, al sesto mese di età, alcuni bambini presentano un'asplenia funzionale, mentre la maggior parte lo diviene entro i 5 anni. La sepsi batterica è una delle cause più importanti di morbilità e di mortalità in questa popolazione. Bambini con anemia falciforme mostrano anche bassi livelli di opsonine sieriche della via alternativa del complemento contro i pneumococchi. Indipendentemente dall'età, tutti i pazienti con anemia falciforme sono a rischio maggiore per infezioni e morte come conseguenza di infezioni batteriche, in particolare con organismi capsulati, come lo *Streptococcus pneumoniae* (vedi Capitolo 181) e l'*Haemophilus influenzae* di tipo B (vedi Capitolo 192). I bambini con anemia falciforme dovrebbero ricevere penicillina VK orale in profilassi almeno fino a 5 anni di età (125 mg due volte al giorno fino all'età di 3 anni, poi 250 mg due volte al giorno). Non esistono linee guida stabilite per la profilassi penicillinica sotto i 5 anni di età. Alcuni medici la prolungano, altri raccomandano di interromperla. La continuazione della profilassi con penicillina dovrebbe essere presa in considerazione per bambini sotto i 5 anni di età, qualora vi sia una precedente diagnosi di infezione pneumococcica tenendo condo del rischio aumentato di infezioni ricorrenti. Un'alternativa per bambini che sono allergici alla penicillina è l'eritromicina-etilsuccinato 10 mg/kg due volte al giorno. Oltre alla profilassi con penicillina, sono molto raccomandate le vaccinazioni di routine dell'infanzia e la somministrazione annuale del vaccino antinfluenzale.

Il **parvovirus umano** B19 (vedi Capitolo 248) espone a un rischio particolare i bambini con anemia falciforme perché questo tipo di infezione limita la produzione di reticolociti. Ogni bambino con reticolocitopenia dovrebbe essere considerato come se avesse il parvovirus B19, finché non è provato il contrario. L'infezione acuta con il parvovirus B19 si accompagna di solito all'aplasia della serie rossa (**episodio aplastico**), febbre e dolore, oltre al sequestro splenico, alla sindrome toracica acuta (*Acute Chest Syndrome*, ACS), alla glomerulonefrite e all'infarto. Il **trattamento** richiede per l'instabilità emodinamica la trasfusione di emazie concentrate.

La **gestione della febbre** in un bambino con anemia falciforme rappresenta un'emergenza medica che richiede un'immediata valutazione e la somministrazione di antibiotici, a causa dell'elevato rischio di infezione batterica e il concomitante elevato tasso di mortalità nel caso di infezione. Sono state sviluppate numerose strategie cliniche di gestione: esse vanno dal far entrare in terapia antimicrobica ev tutti i pazienti con un episodio febbrile alla somministrazione di cefalosporine di 3ª generazione a lunga durata per via parenterale in ambiente esterno a pazienti febbrili ma clinicamente in buone condizioni, che non abbiano alcuno dei precedenti fattori di rischio stabiliti per batteriemia (Tab. 462-1). Considerando che è stato osservato che il tempo necessario per un'emocoltura patogeneticamente positiva è <20 ore in bambini con anemia falciforme, il ricovero per 24 ore è probabilmente la strategia più prudente per i bambini provenienti da famiglie con un'anamnesi di scarsa compliance o privi di telefono o di mezzi di trasporto. Per pazienti con emocoltura positiva, si deve iniziare la terapia mirata (dapprima empirica, poi basata sulla sensibilità). Se si verifica batteriemia da *Salmonella* e da *Staphylococcus*, bisogna prestare una grande attenzione alla ricerca dell'osteomielite con una scintigrafia ossea o una risonanza magnetica (RM), a causa del rischio elevato di osteomielite in bambini con anemia falciforme rispetto alla popolazione generale.

TABELLA 462-1. Fattori clinici associati a un rischio aumentato di batteriemia che richiede il ricovero dei bambini febbrili con anemia falciforme

Aspetto seriamente malato
Ipotensione (pressione sistolica <70 mmHg a 1 anno di età o <70 mmHg + 2 × età in anni per i bambini più grandi)
Scarsa perfusione (tempo di refill capillare >4 secondi)
Temperatura >40 °C
Conta leucocitaria corretta >30 000mm³ o <500 mm³
Conta piastrinica <100 000 mm³
Anamnesi di sepsi pneumococcica
Dolore severo
Disidratazione (scarso turgore cutaneo, mucose asciutte, anamnesi di scarsa assunzione di liquidi o diminuita escrezione di urine)
Infiltrato di un segmento o di una porzione più grande del polmone
Livelli di emoglobina <5 g/dL

Adattata da Wilimas JA, Flynn PM, Harris S, et al: A randomized study of outpatient treatment with ceftriaxone for selected febrile children with sickle cell disease. *N Engl J Med* 1993;329:472-476.

La **dattilite**, spesso riferita alla *sindrome mano-piede*, è frequentemente la prima manifestazione di dolore nei bambini con anemia falciforme, e si verifica nel 50% dei bambini dai 2 anni di età e spesso si presenta con gonfiore simmetrico delle mani e/o dei piedi (Fig. 462-1). Una dattilite unilaterale può essere confusa con l'osteomielite e richiede un'attenta considerazione con valutazioni nel tempo, poiché il trattamento della prima richiede un trattamento sintomatico con farmaci per il dolore, spesso paracetamolo con codeina, mentre l'osteomielite necessita di un ciclo di almeno 4-6 settimane di antibiotici endovena (vedi Capitolo 683).

Il **sequestro splenico** acuto è una complicanza che mette in pericolo la vita, che si verifica soprattutto nei lattanti e che può presentarsi precocemente già a 5 settimane di vita. Circa il 30% dei bambini con anemia falciforme ha importanti episodi di sequestro splenico; nonostante la presentazione possa essere variabile, una significativa percentuale di casi può essere mortale. L'eziologia degli episodi di sequestro splenico è ignota. Clinicamente, essi sono associati alla congestione splenica, con conseguente aumento di dimensioni della milza, evidenza di ipovolemia, e una diminuzione nell'emoglobina di almeno 2 g/dL dai valori di base. Possono essere presenti reticolocitosi e diminuzione della conta piastrinica. Questi eventi possono essere accompagnati da infezioni delle alte vie respiratorie, batteriemia o infezione virale. Il **trattamento** prevede un intervento precoce e il mantenimento della stabilità emodinamica, che può richiedere l'infusione sia di liquidi isotonici sia di sangue. Episodi ripetuti di sequestro splenico sono comuni e si verificano in circa il 50% dei pazienti. La maggior parte delle ricorrenze si verifica entro 6 mesi dall'evento precedente. La splenectomia profilattica praticata dopo che si è risolto l'episodio acuto è l'unica strategia efficace per prevenire episodi futuri che possono mettere a rischio la vita. È possibile insegnare ai genitori a palpare la milza quando il bambino sembra malato e a ricorrere alle cure mediche se essa è ingrossata. La terapia trasfusionale è stata utilizzata per prevenire episodi successivi, ma l'evidenza indica che questa strategia non riduce il rischio degli episodi di sequestro splenico ricorrente rispetto all'assenza di trattamento.

La principale caratteristica clinica dell'anemia falciforme è il dolore per **episodi vaso-occlusivi.** Non ci sono definizioni scritte che possano descrivere l'aspetto di un bambino affetto da anemia falciforme e che presenta dolore. Il dolore è caratterizzato da un malessere persistente che può coinvolgere ogni parte del corpo, ma più spesso si verifica al torace, all'addome o agli arti. Questi episodi dolorosi sono spesso improvvisi e possono compromettere le attività della vita quotidiana e causare angoscia nel paziente e nei familiari. L'unica misura dell'intensità del dolore è il paziente. Anche se le scale del dolore si sono rivelate utili per alcuni bambini, altri richiedono criteri prestabiliti che determinino quando la terapia con oppioidi dovrebbe essere iniziata, ridotta o interrotta. Il fatto di dormire durante la notte può rappresentare un'indicazione per diminuire il trattamento del dolore del 20% il mattino dopo. La maggior parte degli episodi dolorosi nei pazienti con anemia falciforme è trattata a casa con misure di comfort (coperta riscaldata, tecniche di rilassamento, massaggio) e terapia per il dolore. Un paziente con anemia falciforme in genere ha circa un episodio all'anno che richiede interventi medici.

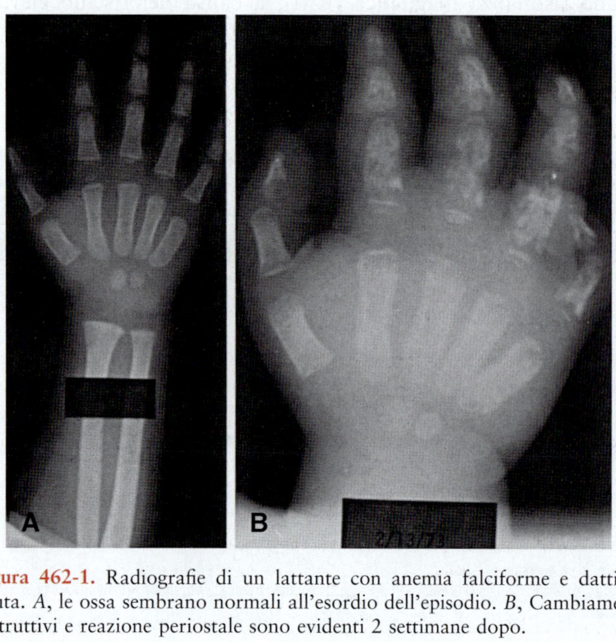

Figura 462-1. Radiografie di un lattante con anemia falciforme e dattilite acuta. *A*, le ossa sembrano normali all'esordio dell'episodio. *B*, Cambiamenti distruttivi e reazione periostale sono evidenti 2 settimane dopo.

La patogenesi del dolore è la compromissione del flusso ematico a livello della microcircolazione da parte delle cellule falciformi, che comporta un'ischemia tissutale. Le cause precipitanti degli episodi dolorosi possono includere stress fisico, infezioni, disidratazione, ipossia, acidosi locale o sistemica, esposizione al freddo e il nuoto in acqua non riscaldata per periodi prolungati. Un trattamento efficace degli episodi dolorosi richiede l'istruzione di entrambi, genitori e paziente, circa i sintomi e la strategia di gestione. Vista l'assenza di alcun reale parametro oggettivo di laboratorio oppure clinico associato al dolore, la fiducia tra paziente e medico che lo tratta è fondamentale per una strategia di gestione clinica efficace. Le terapie specifiche per il dolore variano, ma in genere, negli Stati Uniti, includono l'uso di paracetamolo o di un agente non steroideo precocemente durante il dolore, seguiti da paracetamolo con codeina e oppioidi per via orale a breve e lunga durata di azione o dal ricovero in ospedale con somministrazione di morfina o suoi derivati (vedi Capitolo 77). Il progressivo aumento o diminuzione nell'uso di farmaci per alleviare il dolore va posto grossomodo in parallelo con le 8 fasi associate a una cronologia di dolore e comfort (Tab. 462-2). In fase 1 (di base) il paziente è libero da dolore. La fase 2 non comprende il dolore, ma il bambino può mostrare segni e sintomi prodromici agli episodi dolorosi, come ittero sclerale o affaticamento. Durante questa fase, possono essere adottate misure di comfort. Le fasi 3-7 includono aumenti e poi diminuzioni dei livelli di dolore, compreso il punto di inizio del dolore, fase 3, quando possono essere utilizzati il paracetamolo con codeina o agenti antinfiammatori non steroidei. Un aggravamento del dolore, fase 4, è spesso trattato con la somministrazione di derivati della morfina a breve e lunga durata di azione. L'esperienza del picco di dolore, fase 5, è il momento in cui può essere iniziata la morfina endovena e il paziente viene spesso ricoverato in ospedale. La durata dell'ospedalizzazione per bambini ricoverati per dolore è di 3-5 giorni. Il dolore inizia a diminuire durante le fasi 6 e 7 e anche il trattamento del dolore viene ridotto lentamente. In generale, la riduzione degli oppioidi del 20% rispetto alla dose iniziale dovrebbe essere attuata nelle prime ore del mattino, quando il *caregiver*, il medico o lo staff del reparto sono in grado di determinare gli effetti del cambiamento della dose. La diminuzione della somministrazione di oppioidi nel pomeriggio o a tarda notte non è consigliabile, perché il dolore notturno è spesso maggiore e il responsabile principale delle cure di solito non è disponibile per determinare l'effetto nel cambiamento della dose da somministrare. Nella fase 8, la risoluzione del dolore, il dolore diminuisce a un livello gestibile così che il bambino può essere dimesso dall'ospedale. Le raccomandazioni dell'American Pain Society sono complete e rappresentano un punto di inizio per il trattamento del dolore (www.ampainsoc.org/pub/sc.htm).

Esistono molti miti sul trattamento del dolore nell'anemia falciforme. Il concetto che gli episodi dolorosi nei bambini debbano essere gestiti senza il ricorso a oppioidi è senza fondamento, anzi provoca un'inutile sofferenza al paziente. Non c'è evidenza che la terapia con trasfusioni di sangue durante un episodio doloroso in atto diminuisca la sua intensità o durata. Le trasfusioni di sangue dovrebbero essere riservate a pazienti con un calo dell'emoglobina, che causa una compromissione emodinamica, e ai pazienti con distress respiratorio o con una caduta della concentrazione di emoglobina senza aspettare che si raggiunga il livello minimo di sicurezza. L'idratazione non risolve e non previene il dolore ed è

TABELLA 462-2. Riassunto della cronologia del dolore nei bambini con emoglobinopatia a cellule falciformi

FASE	CARATTERISTICHE DEL DOLORE	MISURE DI COMFORT SUGGERITE UTILIZZATE
1(Di base)	Non dolore vaso-occlusivo. Dolore o complicanze possono essere presenti, come quelle collegate alla necrosi avascolare dell'anca.	Non sono usate misure di comfort.
2 (Pre-dolore)	Non dolore vaso-occlusivo. Dolore o complicanze possono essere presenti, possono comparire segni prodromici di un episodio vaso-occlusivo incombente, esempio, "occhi gialli" e/o affaticamento.	Sono usate misure di comfort. I caregiver possono incoraggiare il bambino ad aumentare i fluidi.
3 (Dolore all'esordio)	Compare il primo segno di dolore vaso-occlusivo, in genere in forma lieve.	Viene spesso somministrato un analgesico orale lieve e vengono aumentati i fluidi. Il bambino in genere mantiene le normali attività.
4 (Accentuazione del dolore)	L'intensità del dolore aumenta da lieve a moderata. Alcuni bambini possono saltare questo livello o passare rapidamente dalla fase 3 alla fase 5.	Vengono somministrati analgesici orali forti. Massaggi, calore o altre attività vengono spesso usate. Il bambino in genere sta a scuola finché il dolore non si fa più severo, poi sta a casa e limita le attività. Il bambino è in genere a letto.
5 (Esperienza di picco doloroso)	Il dolore perviene a un livello alto moderato o severo e raggiunge un plateau. Il dolore può rimanere elevato per un periodo lungo. L'aspetto del bambino, il comportamento, e l'umore sono significativamente alterati.	A casa sono somministrati analgesici orali. Viene usato un insieme di misure di comfort. La famiglia può rifiutare di andare all'ospedale. Se il dolore è molto intenso per il bambino, il genitore può portarlo in ospedale. Dopo che il bambino viene ricoverato, le famiglie spesso lasciano le attività di comfort ai caregiver e aspettano di vedere se gli analgesici funzionano. I familiari sono spesso stanchi, a causa della fatica di curare il bambino per molti giorni senza o con poco riposo.
6 (Punto d'inizio della diminuzione del dolore)	Il dolore finalmente inizia a diminuire di intensità dal picco doloroso.	I familiari diventano di nuovo attivi nel confortare il bambino, ma non così intensamente come in fase 4 e 5.
7 (Declino costante del dolore)	Il dolore diminuisce più rapidamente e diventa più tollerabile per il bambino. Il bambino e la famiglia sono più rilassati	I medici curanti iniziano a svezzare il bambino dagli analgescici endovena. Vengono dati oppioidi orali, e viene iniziato un programma di dimissione. I bambini possono essere dimessi prima di essere liberi dal dolore
8 (Risoluzione del dolore)	L'intensità del dolore è a un livello tollerabile e il cambiamento è imminente. Il bambino appare e si comporta come "il suo solito". L'umore migliora.	Il bambino può ricevere analgesici orali.

Adattata da Beyer JE, Simmons LE, Woods GM, et al: A Chronology of pain and comfort in children with sickle cell disease. *Arch Pediatr Adolesc Med* 1999;153:913-920.

appropriata quando il paziente è disidratato o non riesce a bere in conseguenza a un grave dolore. La dipendenza da oppioidi nei bambini con anemia falciforme non deve mai essere usata come motivo per non trattare il bambino per il dolore. I pazienti con episodi dolorosi multipli che richiedono il ricovero in ospedale nell'arco di un anno o quelli i cui episodi dolorosi richiedono un'ospedalizzazione più lunga di 7 giorni dovrebbero essere valutati per comorbilità e per fattori di stress psicosociale che possono contribuire alla frequenza e alla durata del dolore.

L'idrossiurea, un agente mielosoppressore, è l'unico farmaco di provata efficacia per ridurre la frequenza degli episodi dolorosi. L'idrossiurea innalza i livelli di Hb F e i livelli di emoglobina. L'idrossiurea in genere abbassa la frequenza di episodi dolorosi del 50%; essa inoltre diminuisce la frequenza di episodi di ACS e le trasfusioni di sangue di circa il 50% negli adulti. Nei bambini con anemia falciforme è stato condotto soltanto un trial di sicurezza e praticabilità sull'idrossiurea. Questo studio ha dimostrato che l'idrossiurea era sicura e ben tollerata in bambini con più di 5 anni. Non sono stati identificati eventi clinici avversi. La principale tossicità di laboratorio era limitata alla mielosoppressione, che si risolveva alla sospensione del farmaco. Considerato il profilo di sicurezza a breve termine dell'idrossiurea nel bambino e la sua dimostrata efficacia nell'adulto, essa è comunemente utilizzata in bambini con episodi multipli di dolore. Il trattamento con idrossiurea iniziato durante l'infanzia può preservare la funzione splenica, migliorare la crescita e ridurre l'incidenza di ACS. La tossicità a lungo termine associata all'idrossiurea nei bambini non è stata stabilita e ci sono problemi teorici sul potenziale rischio di leucemia e di complicanze sconosciute. La dose tipica di inizio dell'idrossiurea è 15-20 mg/kg/die, con un aumento di dose ogni 8 settimane di 2,5-5 mg/kg, se non si verifica tossicità, fino a una dose massima di 35 mg/kg. L'effetto terapeutico dell'idrossiurea può richiedere numerosi mesi di trattamento. Il monitoraggio dei bambini che stanno ricevendo idrossiurea è molto impegnativo, con visite inizialmente ogni due settimane e poi mensilmente, dopo che la dose terapeutica è stata identificata. Un monitoraggio stretto del paziente richiede un impegno da parte dei genitori e del paziente così come attenzione da parte del medico nel monitorare la tossicità.

Il **priapismo**, un problema comune nell'anemia falciforme, consiste in un'erezione involontaria del pene che dura più di 30 minuti. La persistenza di un'erezione dolorosa dopo diverse ore è suggestiva per la diagnosi di priapismo. Sebbene tipicamente la porzione ventrale del pene e del glande non siano coinvolte, qualora lo siano si dovrebbe ricorrere alla consulenza urologica basata sulla prognosi sfavorevole per una risoluzione spontanea. Il priapismo si realizza in due modi, **intermittente** e **refrattario**, ed entrambi si presentano nei pazienti dalla prima infanzia fino all'età adulta. Non sono state stabilite definizioni formali per questi temini, ma in genere il *priapismo intermittente* è definito come attacchi autolimitantisi intermittenti di priapismo con numerosi episodi in un periodo limitato. Il *priapismo refrattario* è definito come un priapismo prolungato che dura per molte ore. Circa il 20% dei pazienti tra 5-20 anni riportano di aver avuto almeno un episodio di priapismo della durata pari almeno a 30 minuti. La maggior parte degli episodi si verifica tra le 3.00 di notte e le 9.00 di mattina. L'età media al primo episodio è 12 anni, il numero medio di episodi per paziente è circa 16 e la durata media di un episodio è circa 2 ore. La probabilità reale per un paziente di incorrere nel priapismo è di circa il 90% a partire dai 20 anni di età. Non si sa quale sia il **trattamento** migliore, ma le strategie terapeutiche possono essere suddivise in trattamenti acuti e di prevenzione. Per il trattamento acuto del priapismo, è comunemente usata la terapia di supporto, come un semicupio o farmaci per il dolore. Se il priapismo dura più di 4 ore, allora l'aspirazione di sangue dai corpi cavernosi, seguita da irrigazione con adrenalina diluita, è efficace per produrre un'immediata e stabile detumescenza. Per iniziare questa procedura è necessaria una consulenza urologica con un appropriato consulto ematologico. Sebbene la terapia trasfusionale con sangue (sia semplice sia exanguino) sia stata citata per il trattamento acuto del priapismo, solo limitati dati ematologici supportano questo approccio e alcune evidenze mostrano che l'exsanguinotrasfusione non è efficace per ottenere la detumescenza. Per la prevenzione del priapismo ricorrente, l'**idrossiurea** sembra promettente; tuttavia non esistono trial che dimostrino i benefici dell'idrossiurea rispetto al non praticare alcun trattamento. L'effetto a lungo termine degli episodi di priapismo ricorrente o prolungato nei bambini prepubere non è conosciuto, ma nei pazienti più vecchi può produrre disfunzioni sessuali.

Le **complicanze neurologiche** associate all'anemia falciforme sono varie e complesse. Tra i bambini con anemia falciforme, circa l'11% e il 20% possono avere, rispettivamente, eventi ischemici sia **silenti** sia **evidenti**, prima del 18° compleanno. Un'*ischemia* *evidente* è definita come un deficit focale neurologico che dura >24 ore; questa definizione è sorpassata perché molti individui con anemia falciforme vengono trattati con terapia trasfusionale che può accelerare il ritorno alle condizioni basali. Una definizione più funzionale è la presenza di un deficit neurologico focale che dura >24 ore e/o lesioni cerebrali a livello T_2 pesate in RM indicative di un infarto cerebrale e corrispondenti al deficit neurologico focale (Fig. 462-2). Un'*ischemia silente* è l'assenza di deficit neurologici focali che durino >24 ore in presenza di lesioni in T_2 pesate in una RM indicativa di infarto cerebrale. La presentazione dell'ischemia può verificarsi già all'età di un anno. Le ischemie possono presentarsi in famiglie particolari. Altre complicanze neurologiche includono la cefalea, che può essere o non essere legata all'anemia falciforme, convulsioni, trombosi venosa cerebrale e la sindrome leucoencefalopatica posteriore reversibile (SRPL).

Per pazienti che si presentano con un deficit neurologico focale è raccomandata l'immediata valutazione neurologica. Il **trattamento** delle ischemie include la somministrazione di ossigeno per mantenere la saturazione di ossigeno >96% e trasfusioni semplici di sangue il più velocemente e in sicurezza possibile con un *optimum* trasfusionale entro un'ora dalla presentazione e con un *optimum* di aumento dell'emoglobina a massimo 11 g/dL. Superare questo valore di emoglobina può infatti limitare il rilascio di ossigeno al cervello, perché l'iperviscosità del sangue è in grado di ridurre la cessione di ossigeno. Successivamente, deve essere fortemente considerata la exsanguinotrasfusione, sia manualmente sia con l'eritrocitoferesi, che riduca l'Hb S almeno <50%, se non 30%. La TC per escludere un'emorragia cerebrale dovrebbe essere effettuata il prima possibile; se disponibile la RM cerebrale con immagini pesate diffuse dovrebbe essere eseguita per distinguere tra un infarto ischemico e la SRPL (Fig. 462-3). La flebografia RM è altrettanto utile per la possibilità di trombosi venose cerebrali. La presentazione clinica della SRPL o della trombosi venosa cerebrale può simulare quella dell'ischemia. Le diagnosi di SRPL e di trombosi venosa cerebrale richiedono diversi tipi di trattamento rispetto all'ischemia. Sia per la SRPL sia per la trombosi venosa cerebrale, non è stato stabilito quale sia il migliore trattamento nei pazienti con anemia falciforme; gli interventi necessitano di una consulenza con un neurologo pediatra e con un ematologo per la gestione del caso.

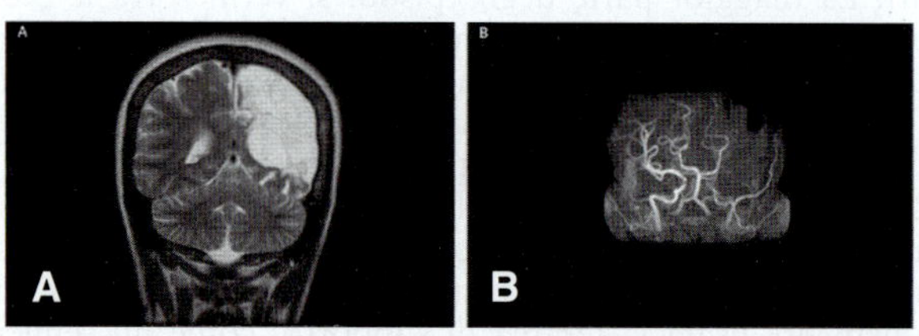

Figura 462-2. RM pesate in T_2 e angiografia RM del cervello. *A*, RM pesata in T_2 mostra pregresso infarto del territorio dell'arteria cerebrale anteriore sinistra e arteria cerebrale media. *B*, Angiografia RM che mostra occlusione del sifone distale dell'arteria carotide interna sinistra fino all'origine dell'arteria oftalmica.

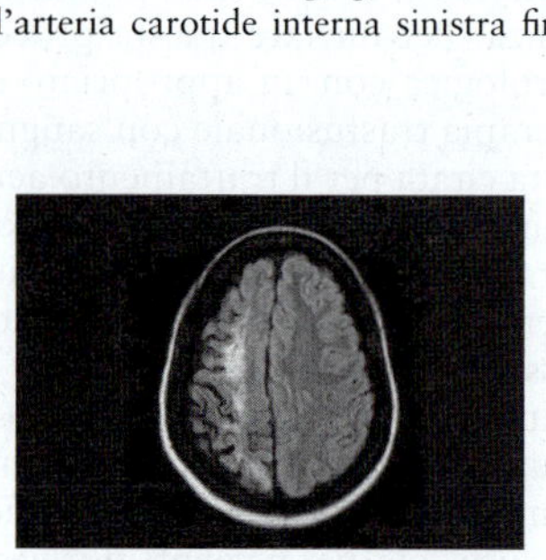

Figura 462-3. Sequenza RM veloce di inversione-recupero attenuata dal liquido (FLAIR) del cervello che mostra infarto nella zona di confine dell'emisfero destro in un bambino con anemia falciforme. (Da Switzer JA, Hess DC, Nichols F, et al: Pathophysiology and treatment of stoke in sickle-cell disease: Present and future. *Lancet Neurol* 2006;5:501-512.)

La **prevenzione primaria dell'ischemia** può essere attuata dalla determinazione mediante Doppler transcranico (*TransCranial Doppler*, TCD) della velocità del flusso sanguigno nella porzione terminale della carotide interna e nella porzione prossimale dell'arteria cerebrale media. Nei pazienti con velocità massima di flusso ematico medio ≥200 cm/s, valore soglia per la trasfusione, una terapia trasfusionale di sangue a scopo di profilassi viene istituita per mantenere i livelli di Hb S <30%. Questa strategia porta a ridurre la frequenza di ischemie evidenti dell'85%. Una volta iniziata, i pazienti possono ricevere questa terapia per un periodo indefinito. L'età migliore per iniziare e concludere la misurazione TCD nei bambini con anemia falciforme non è stata stabilita; molti ematologi iniziano lo screening con TCD intorno ai 2-3 anni, età in cui la maggior parte dei bambini non necessita di sedazione. Se la misura media massima calcolata nel tempo è <200 cm/s, ma ≥180 cm/s, valore di soglia condizionale, si consiglia una misura ripetuta dopo molti mesi a causa dell'elevata frequenza di conversione a una velocità di flusso ematico >200 cm/s.

Una **prevenzione secondaria dell'ischemia** si attua con una terapia trasfusionale di sangue che mantenga la concentrazione massima di Hb S a <30% nei primi 2 anni dopo l'ischemia e <50% in seguito. Nonostante una regolare terapia trasfusionale di sangue, circa il 20% dei pazienti avrà un secondo stroke e il 30% un terzo stroke. Il più importante effetto collaterale della trasfusione è l'accumulo di Fe, che può portare a danni d'organo irreversibili e a morte prematura. Un'unità di sangue contiene circa 200 mg di ferro. Negli Stati Uniti il più comune agente chelante del ferro utilizzato è stata la deferoxamina. La dose ottimale è 40 mg/kg sottocute per 5-7 notti per 10 ore. Un agente chelante orale (deferasirox) è stato approvato dalla FDA per pazienti >2 anni di età con emosiderosi trasfusionale. La dose iniziale di 20 mg/kg/die è modificata dopo 3-6 mesi di terapia, basandosi sui livelli di ferritina (se ferritina <500, il farmaco può essere temporaneamente sospeso). Sono disponibili 3 metodi per la terapia trasfusionale con sangue: eritrocitoferesi, exanguinotrasfusione normale (salasso di una quantità stabilita di sangue seguita da rapida infusione di sangue) e la semplice trasfusione. Di tutti questi metodi l'**eritrocitoferesi** è quello preferito, seguito dall'exsanguinotrasfusione manuale. La semplice terapia trasfusionale è la meno preferibile perché la strategia porta al più alto bilancio positivo di ferro a seguito della procedura. Nonostante sia il metodo preferito, l'eritrocitoferesi è praticata meno frequentemente a causa della necessità di esperienza nella tecnica, di accessi venosi di grandi dimensioni e dell'accesso a una macchina per l'aferesi. La terapia con idrossiurea può rappresentare un'alternativa valida per i pazienti che non vogliono o non possono continuare le trasfusioni per prevenire strokes successivi. Prima che la terapia trasfusionale ematica venga sostituita con l'idrossiurea nei bambini con strokes, la tossicità e l'efficacia dell'idrossiurea come possibilità di prevenzione secondaria degli strokes devono essere stabilite in un nuovo trial clinico. Il trapianto di midollo osseo da un fratello HLA compatibile come donatore è un approccio razionale per i pazienti con strokes, sebbene pochi bambini abbiano donatori compatibili.

La **malattia polmonare** nei bambini con anemia falciforme è il secondo motivo di ricovero in ospedale e una frequente causa di morte. La **sindrome toracica acuta** (*Acute Chest Syndrome*, **ACS**) consiste in un insieme di reperti che includono una nuova radiopacità alla radiografia del torace, febbre, distress respiratorio e dolore che spesso si presentano al torace, ma possono riguardare solo la schiena e/o l'addome. Anche quando non sono presenti sintomi respiratori, tutti i pazienti con febbre dovrebbero eseguire una radiografia toracica per identificare l'ACS perché l'esame clinico da solo non è sufficiente a identificare pazienti con nuove radiopacità alla radiografia del torace; inoltre, la scoperta precoce dell'ACS potrebbe modificare la gestione clinica. I reperti radiografici nell'ACS sono variabili e possono progredire abbastanza rapidamente. Le radiografie possono mostrare un coinvolgimento di un solo lobo polmonare, più spesso il lobo inferiore sinistro, e quando sono coinvolti più lobi, di solito entrambi i lobi inferiori

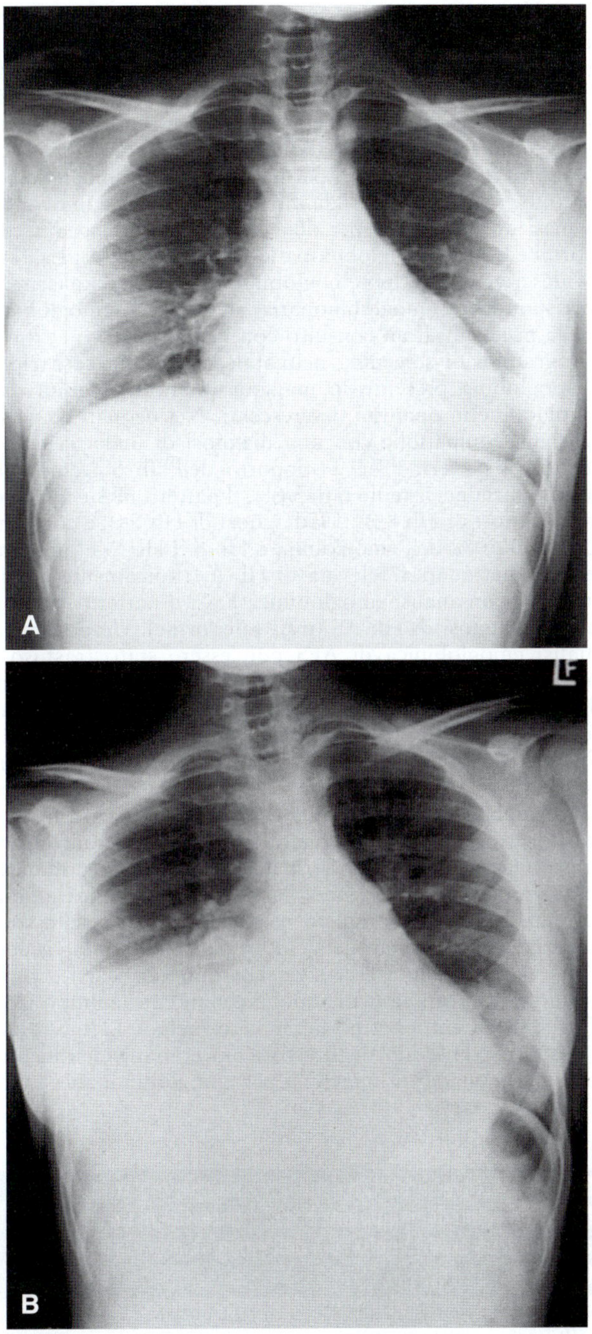

Figura 462-4. Probabile infarto polmonare in un quindicenne con anemia falciforme. *A*, Radiografia antero-posteriore mostra consolidamento e piccolo versamento pleurico posteriormente nel lobo inferiore destro. *B*, Radiografia ottenuta <24 ore dopo mostra un consolidamento massivo del lobo medio destro e inferiore con versamento. Non si è potuto coltivare alcun organismo. La diagnosi di un probabile infarto polmonare è stata stabilita clinicamente. (Per gentile concessione del Dr. Thomas L. Slovis, Children's Hospital of Michigan, Detroit, MI. Da Kuhn JP, Slovis TL, Haller JO: *Caffey's Pediatric Diagnostic Imaging*, Vol. 1, 10th ed. Philadelphia, Mosby, 2004, p 1087.)

sono interessati. Versamenti pleurici, sia unilaterali sia bilaterali, possono non essere presenti inizialmente (o possono essere di piccole dimensioni), ma possono progredire rapidamente fino a un completo sfocamento (Fig. 462-4).

Considerata la sovrapposizione clinica tra l'ACS e le comuni complicanze polmonari, come la bronchiolite, l'asma (che è anche comune nei bambini con anemia falciforme) e la polmonite, è stato utilizzato un ampio range di strategie terapeutiche. Il **trattamento** dell'ACS include la somministrazione di ossigeno e la semplice exsanguinotrasfusione (manuale o automatizzata). L'ossigeno dovrebbe essere somministrato quando la saturazione di ossigeno è <90%. La decisione su quando debba essere usato il sangue e quando invece l'exsanguinotrasfusione o la trasfusione semplice è poco definita. La trasfusione di sangue viene praticata quando si verifica almeno una delle seguenti condizioni cliniche: diminuzione della saturazione di ossigeno; aumento del lavoro respiratorio; rapido cambiamento dello sforzo respiratorio, con o senza peggioramento della radiografia del torace; oppure un'anamnesi di grave ACS che richieda il ricovero in unità di terapia intensiva.

La maggior parte dei pazienti con ACS non presenta una causa identificabile, anche se si pensa che l'infezione sia la causa più comunemente individuabile. La patologia più comune che precede l'ACS è un episodio doloroso che richiede gli oppioidi. Il tipo di oppioidi (la morfina presenta un rischio maggiore rispetto alla nalbufina idrocloride) e la frequenza di somministrazione dell'oppioide (orale a richio maggiore che per via endovenosa) sono direttamente associati a un aumento del rischio di ACS. La somministrazione di oppioidi non deve essere limitata in qualunque circostanza allo scopo di prevenire l'ACS; deve piuttosto essere posta attenzione per prevenire il verificarsi dell'ACS. Nei pazienti con dolore toracico, l'uso regolare dello **spirometro con incentivazione** può ridurre significativamente la frequenza dei nuovi episodi di dolore toracico acuto; l'uso di 10-12 respiri ogni 2 ore è un metodo efficace per prevenire l'ACS. Emboli grassosi sono anche stati implicati come causa di ACS. Gli emboli di grasso si ritiene derivino dal midollo osseo infartuato e possono essere pericolosi per la vita se una grande quantità di grasso viene rilasciata dal polmone.

Come risultato della sovrapposizione clinica tra la polmonite e l'ACS, tutti gli episodi dovrebbero essere trattati prontamente con una terapia antimicrobica che includa almeno un macrolide e una cefalosporina di 3ª generazione per trattare i patogeni più comuni associati all'ACS (*S. pneumoniae*, *Mycoplasma pneumoniae*, *Chlamydia pneumoniae*). Una precedente diagnosi di asma dovrebbe indurre a un trattamento con steroidi e broncodilatatori, anche se il paziente non presenta sibili o fischi (Tab. 462-3).

L'**ipertensione polmonare** è un fattore di rischio maggiore di morte in adulti con anemia falciforme. Circa il 60% degli adulti con anemia falciforme può presentare una malattia vascolare obliterante polmonare clinicamente insospettata. L'ipertensione polmonare è stata anche riportata in altre forme di anemia emolitica cronica (talassemia, sferocitosi ereditaria, emoglobinuria parossistica notturna), suggerendo che l'emolisi da sola contribuisca ai cambiamenti vascolari polmonari, forse mediante la ridotta disponibilità di ossido nitrico, indipendentemente dagli episodi vaso-occlusivi

TABELLA 462-3. Strategie di insieme per la gestione della sindrome toracica acuta

PREVENZIONE
Spirometria incentivata e deambulazione periodica in pazienti ricoverati per crisi vaso-occlusive, chirurgia o episodi febbrili
Attesa vigile in ciascun bambino ricoverato in ospedale o adulto ospedalizzato con malattia a cellule falciformi (monitoraggio della pulsossimetria e frequenti valutazioni respiratorie)
Evitare l'iperidratazione
Educazione intensa e cure ottimali per i pazienti con anemia falciforme e asma
TEST DIAGNOSTICI E MONITORAGGIO DI LABORATORIO
Emocolture
Campioni nasofaringei per colture virali (virus respiratorio sinciziale, influenza)
Esami ematologici quotidiani e biochimici secondo necessità
Pulsossimetria continua
Radiografie del torace
TRATTAMENTO
Trasfusioni di sangue (semplici o exsanguino)
Supplemento di O_2 e caduta della pulsossimetria del 4% dei valori di base, o per valori <90%
Antibiotici empirici (cefalosporine e macrolidi)
Terapia respiratoria continua (spirometria incentivata e fisioterapia respiratoria, se necessario)
Broncodilatatori e steroidi per i pazienti con asma
Controllo ottimale del dolore e gestione dei fluidi

polmonari. La storia naturale dell'ipertensione polmonare in bambini con anemia falciforme è sconosciuta; pertanto la migliore strategia terapeutica e diagnostica per l'ipertensione polmonare non è ancora stata identificata. Livelli elevati di N-terminale del peptide natriuretico procerebrale sono associati a ipertensione polmonare emolisi-relata in adulti con anemia falciforme. Il trattamento con ossido nitrico inalato delle crisi vaso-occlusive può avere un ruolo nella gestione dell'ipertensione polmonare.

La **malattia renale** in pazienti con anemia falciforme è una condizione di comorbilità maggiore che può condurre a morte prematura. Sono state identificate sette nefropatie correlate ad anemia falciforme: (1) ematuria grossolana, (2) necrosi papillare, (3) sindrome nefrosica, (4) infarto renale, (5) ipostenuria, (6) pielonefrite e (7) carcinoma midollare renale. La presentazione di tali patologie può includere ematuria, proteinuria, insufficienza renale, difetti di concentrazione o ipertensione. Gli ACE-inibitori (enzima di conversione dell'angiotensina) sono utili nella gestione dei pazienti con proteinuria. Il sospetto di carcinoma midollare renale, una neoplasia epiteliale maligna aggressiva, è importante perché la maggior parte dei pazienti si presenta con malattia disseminata allo stadio terminale, poco responsiva alla chemioterapia e alla terapia radiante.

Come per tutti i bambini con malattie croniche, il mantenimento di un buono stato di salute deve includere una valutazione psicologica e sociale. Una valutazione costante della famiglia e delle risorse disponibili per far fronte a una patologia cronica è critica per una gestione ottimale. Bambini con anemia falciforme sono a forte rischio di insuccesso accademico e presentano una percentuale di laureati molto bassa (circa 20%); circa un terzo dei bambini con anemia falciforme ha avuto infarti cerebrali, sia silenti sia evidenti. I bambini con infarti cerebrali richiedono costanti valutazioni cognitive e della performance scolastica, cosicché le risorse educazionali possano essere dirette a ottimizzare il rendimento educativo. L'importanza di gruppi di supporto e la frequenza ad attività di gruppo, come i campi-scuola per bambini con anemia falciforme, possono avere un beneficio diretto nel migliorare l'autostima e nello stabilire relazioni con i coetanei.

Oltre a tutte le disfunzioni d'organo precedentemente citate, i pazienti con anemia falciforme possono presentare altre complicanze importanti. Queste complicanze includono la retinopatia dell'anemia falciforme, ritardo puberale, necrosi avascolare della testa del femore e dell'omero e ulcere alle gambe. Il trattamento migliore per ciascuna di queste entità non è stato stabilito e la gestione individuale richiede la consulenza con lo specialista specifico per la patologia, un ematologo e il medico di famiglia.

La **preparazione chirurgica** per i bambini con anemia falciforme richiede lo sforzo coordinato di un ematologo, del chirurgo e di chi provvede alle cure primarie. Le complicanze postoperatorie più comuni sono il dolore e l'ACS, e questo ultimo è un fattore di rischio importante per morte postoperatoria. La trasfusione di sangue prima della chirurgia in bambini con anemia falciforme è prevista per raggiungere un livello di emoglobina preoperatorio desiderabile di 10 g/dL; tuttavia ottenere un livello almeno pari a 10 g/dL non è necessario per un bambino che trae beneficio da una semplice trasfusione. Quando un bambino è stato preparato alla chirurgia con una trasfusione di sangue semplice, deve essere prestata attenzione per evitare innalzamenti dell'emoglobina sopra 10,5 g/dL per il rischio di sindrome da iperviscosità. L'exsanguinotrasfusione prima della chirurgia non ha un grande beneficio rispetto alla trasfusione di sangue semplice e comporta un rischio significativamente aumentato di alloimmunizzazione verso globuli rossi.

DIAGNOSI DI EMOGLOBINOPATIA A CELLULE FALCIFORMI. Virtualmente tutti gli Stati americani hanno creato programmi di screening neonatale per l'emoglobinopatia a cellule falciformi. Questi programmi identificano i neonati malati, permettono una pronta diagnosi e linee guida anticipatorie per i genitori e rendono possibile l'inizio del trattamento con penicillina prima del 4° mese di vita.

Le procedure di diagnosi neonatali più comunemente utilizzate includono la cromatografia liquida ad alta risoluzione e la focalizzazione isolettrica su strato sottile. È raccomandato un sistema a due livelli in cui tutti i reperti inizialmente anormali vengono ritestati durante la prima visita clinica e di nuovo dopo il 6° mese di età per determinare il fenotipo emoglobinico finale. Un esame emocromocitometrico completo così come l'analisi dell'emoglobina è raccomandata per entrambi i genitori in modo da confermare la diagnosi e permettere un possibile *counseling* genetico. Nei pazienti affetti, la morfologia dei globuli rossi dopo i 3-6 mesi di vita è utile per diagnosticare la malattia a cellule falciformi e le altre emoglobinopatie (vedi Fig. 462-3). La Tabella 462-4 descrive il fenotipo emoglobinico iniziale alla nascita, con la corrispondente emoglobinopatia, il range di emoglobina di base e la necessità di un consulto con l'ematologo.

I programmi di screening neonatale per prima cosa riportano l'emoglobina presente in maggior quantità, seguita da altre emoglobine in quantità descrescenti. Nei neonati con analisi emoglobina compatibile con una diagnosi di malattia a cellule falciformi, il pattern FS è a supporto dell'Hb SS, emoglobina fetale ereditaria persistente (Hb S/β^0). Il pattern FSA è a supporto di una diagnosi di Hb S/β^+. La diagnosi di Hb S/β^+ è confermata se almeno il 50% dell'emoglobina è Hb S, l'Hb A è presente ed è presente una quantità elevata di Hb A_2 (tipicamente >3,5%). Nei neonati con analisi emoglobinica FSC, il pattern è a supporto di una diagnosi di Hb AS (**trait falciforme**). Un neonato con un'analisi emoglobinica di AFS può essere stato trasfuso con globuli rossi prima degli esami di laboratorio perché la quantità di Hb A è maggiore della quantità di Hb F oppure può essere stato fatto un errore. Il paziente può presentare sia la malattia a cellule falciforme (Hb SS o Hb S/β^+) sia il trait falciforme e dovrebbe ricevere una profilassi con penicillina fino a che non venga formulata la diagnosi finale. Date le implicazioni di una diagnosi sia di malattia a cellule falciformi sia di trait falcemico in un neonato, l'importanza di ripetere l'analisi emoglobinica nel paziente, come anche l'ottenere l'analisi emoglobinica e l'esame emocromocitometrico completo per la valutazione dello striscio e dei parametri eritrocitari nei genitori per il *counseling* genetico, non può essere ritenuta eccessiva. Possono verificarsi errori nei programmi di screening neonatale. Neonati con fenotipo iniziale di Hb FS, ma il cui fenotipo finale vero include l'Hb S/β^+, sono stati descritti come uno degli errori più comuni identificati nei programmi neonatali di screening per emoglobinopatie.

TABELLA 462-4. Diversi risultati degli screening per malattia a cellule falciformi con valori di emoglobina basali e necessità di un ematologo pediatrico o di un esperto nella cura dell'emoglobinopatia a cellule falciformi

RISULTATI DEGLI SCREENING NEONATALI: EMOGLOBINOPATIA A CELLULE FALCIFORMI	POSSIBILE FENOTIPO* DELL'EMOGLOBINA	EMOGLOBINA LIVELLI DI BASE: RANGE	NECESSITÀ DI ESPERIENZA IN TERAPIA EMATOLOGICA
FS	SCD-S	6-11 g/dL	Sì
	SCD-S/β^0 tal	6-10 g/dL	Sì
	SCD-S/β^+ tal	9-12 g/dL	Sì
	SCD-S/$\delta\beta^+$ tal	10-12 g/dL	Sì
	S HPFH	12-14 g/dL	Sì
FSC	SCD-SC	10-15 g/dL	Sì
FSA	SCD-S/β^0 tal	6-10 g/dL	Sì
FS altre	SCD-SD, SO^{Arab}, SC^{Harlem}, S Lepare	6-10 g/dL, 6-9 g/dL, 7-13 g/dL	Sì
AFS	SCD-SS, SCD-S/β^+ tal, SCD-S/β^0tal (impossibile determinare la diagnosi perché il neonato riceve una trasfusione di sangue prima del test)	Variabile	Sì

*Richiede un'analisi emoglobinica di conferma dopo almeno 6 mesi di età e, se possible, l'analisi emoglobinica di entrambi i genitori per una diagnosi accurate del fenotipo emoglobinico.

ALTRE SINDROMI A CELLULE FALCIFORMI. Le sindromi a cellule falciformi che si verificano più comunemente accanto all'Hb SS sono l'Hb SC, l'Hb S/β^0-talassemia e l'Hb S/β^+-talassemia. Le altre sindromi, SD, SO, Arab, persistenza ereditaria dell'emoglobina fetale (*Hereditary Persistence of Fetal Hemoglobin*, HPFH) e altre varianti sono molto meno comuni. Individui con Hb S/β^0-talassemia pres+entano un corso clinico simile a quello dell'Hb SS. I globuli rossi con Hb SC non polimerizzano come l'Hb SS, ma i cristalli di Hb C interagiscono con il trasporto di ioni di membrana, disidratando la cellula e inducendo la falcizzazione. Bambini che hanno la malattia a Hb SC possono presentare gli stessi sintomi e complicanze di quelli con malattia Hb SS severa, ma la frequenza è minore. I bambini con l'Hb SC presentano anche un'incidenza aumentata di retinopatia, ipersplenismo cronico, sequestro splenico e carcinoma midollare renale. La storia naturale di ognuna di queste sindromi a cellule falciformi è variabile e difficile da prevedere a causa della mancanza di valutazioni sistematiche. Attualmente, non c'è un modello valido che possa fare prevedere il corso clinico di un individuo con malattia a cellule falciformi. La gestione di una disfunzione terminale d'organo nei bambini con sindromi a cellule falciformi richiede gli stessi principi generali come la gestione dei pazienti con anemia falciforme; ogni situazione dovrebbe essere gestita caso per caso e richiede il consulto con un ematologo pediatra.

462.2 • Trait falciforme (Hb AS)

La prevalenza del **trait falciforme** varia in tutto il mondo; negli Stati Uniti l'incidenza è del 7-10% degli afroamericani. La quantità di Hb S in soggetti con il trait falcemico è <50%. La durata di vita delle persone con tratto falcemico è normale e le complicanze gravi sono rare. L'esame emocromocitometrico è all'interno dei range normali. L'analisi emoglobinica è diagnostica, rivelando una predominanza di Hb A, tipicamente >50%. Le complicanze del trait falcemico includono la morte improvvisa durante un esercizio intenso, l'infarto splenico a elevate altitudini, ematuria, ipostenuria e batteriuria, suscettibilità di danno oculare con la formazione di un ifema e il carcinoma midollare renale. Il carcinoma midollare renale associato al tratto falciforme si verifica soprattutto in giovani adulti e in bambini. I bambini con trait falcemico non dovrebbero avere alcuna restrizione nelle attività.

462.3 • Altre emoglobinopatie

EMOGLOBINA C. La mutazione per l'Hb C è nello stesso sito dell'Hb S, con una lisina invece di una valina sostituita per la glutammina. Negli Stati Uniti, l'Hb AC si presenta in 1/50 e l'Hb CC in 1/5000 afroamericani. L'Hb AC è asintomatica. L'Hb CC può causare un'anemia lieve, splenomegalia e colelitiasi; sono stati riportati raramente casi di rottura splenica spontanea. Non si verifica falcizzazione. Questa condizione è in genere diagnosticata attraverso i programmi di screening neonatale. L'Hb C cristallizza, distruggendo la membrana dei globuli rossi.

EMOGLOBINA E. L'emoglobina E/β è la seconda causa più comune di mutazione globinica nel mondo. In California, l'Hb E/β talassemia si ritrova quasi esclusivamente nei soggetti del Sud-est asiatico, con una prevalenza di 1/2600 nascite.

EMOGLOBINA D. Esistono almeno 16 varianti di Hb D; solo 1, D Punjab (Los Angeles), insieme con l'Hb S, produce i sintomi della malattia falciforme. Questa emoglobina rara è vista nell'1-3% degli indiani occidentali e in alcuni europei con un legame all'India. L'eterozigote D è clinicamente silente. L'omozigosi D produce un'anemia lieve-moderata con splenomegalia.

462.4 • Anomalie da emoglobine instabili

Sono state identificate almeno 200 rare emoglobine instabili; la più comune è l'Hb Köln. La maggior parte dei soggetti sembra presentare mutazioni *de novo* piuttosto che patologie ereditarie dell'emoglobina. Le più studiate sono quelle le cui mutazioni causano legame instabile all'eme che eventualmente conduce alla denaturazione della molecola emoglobinica. L'emoglobina denaturata può essere scoperta durante un'emolisi grave o dopo la splenectomia come corpi di Heinz. A differenza dei corpi di Heinz che sono visibili dopo l'esposizione ai tossici, nelle emoglobine instabili, i corpi di Heinz sono presenti nei reticolociti e negli eritrociti più vecchi (vedi Fig. 462-5*D*). Gli eterozigoti sono asintomatici.

I bambini con mutazioni geniche omozigoti possono presentarsi nella prima infanzia con anemia e splenomegalia o con un'anemia emolitica inspiegabile. L'emolisi è aumentata dalle patologie febbrili e con alcune emoglobine instabili e l'ingestione di farmaci ossidanti (simili alla glucosio-6-fosfato deidrogenasi). Se la milza è funzionale, lo striscio di sangue può sembrare quasi del tutto normale o può presentare solo un'ipocromasia e una punteggiatura basofila. Una diagnosi può essere fatta attraverso la dimostrazione dei corpi di Heinz, dell'instabilità emoglobinica, o di analisi anormali (sebbene alcune emoglobine instabili presentino una motilità normale).

Il **trattamento** è di supporto. Possono rendersi necessarie trasfusioni durante gli episodi emolitici nei casi gravi. Farmaci ossidanti dovrebbero essere evitati e dovrebbe essere garantito un supplemento di folati. È stata praticata la splenectomia, ma le complicanze della splenectomia, inclusa la sepsi e la possibile ipertensione polmonare, andrebbero considerate prima che tale terapia venga somministrata.

462.5 • Emoglobine anomale con aumentata affinità per l'ossigeno causanti poliglobulia

Sono state caratterizzate più di 110 emoglobine ad alta affinità. Queste mutazioni colpiscono lo stato di configurazione dell'emoglobina durante la fase di ossigenazione e deossigenazione. L'emoglobina cambia la struttura quando è in stato ossigenato rispetto a quando è in stato deossigenato. Lo stato deossigenato è definito lo stato T (tensione) ed è stabilizzato dal 2,3-difosfoglicerato. Quando completamente ossigenata, l'emoglobina assume lo stato R (rilassato). Le esatte interazioni molecolari tra questi due stati non sono conosciute. Le emoglobine ad alta affinità contengono mutazioni che contemporaneamente stabilizzano la forma R e destabilizzano la forma T. Le interazioni tra queste due forme sono complesse e i meccanismi di mutazione sono sconosciuti. Nella maggior parte dei casi, le emoglobine possono essere identificate dall'analisi emoglobinica; circa il 20% deve essere caratterizzato dalla misura della P_{50}, che sarà inferiore rispetto al normale (normale, 23-29 mmHg). A causa della diminuzione della P_{50}, la maggior parte di queste emoglobine causa una poliglobulia di 17-20 g/dL di emoglobina. La P_{50} è la tensione di ossigeno che si ha a metà saturazione del sangue con ossigeno. Minore è la P_{50}, maggiore è l'affinità per l'ossigeno. I livelli di eritropoietina e 2,3-difosfoglicerato sono normali. I pazienti sono di solito asintomatici e non necessitano di salassi. Se viene praticato il salasso, il rilascio di ossigeno può essere problematico a causa della diminuzione dell'emoglobina.

462.6 • Emoglobine anomale causanti cianosi

Queste varianti emoglobiniche sono rare. Il gruppo maggiore è quello delle emoglobine M: ne esistono 7. Le varianti di emoglobina M presentano mutazioni sia nella catena α sia nella β, tutte nel complesso dell'eme della molecola emoglobinica. Delle 7 varianti, 6 hanno un residuo di tiroxina che si lega covalentemente con il ferro dell'eme, stabilizzandolo nella forma ossidata. Queste emoglobine instabili conducono ad anemia emolitica che si presenta più pronunciata nella forma β. Questi bambini sono cianotici dalla nascita senza altri segni o sintomi di malattia se la tiroxina è nella catena α (Hb M Boston, Milwaukee). Le emoglobine anomale sono autosomiche dominanti e vengono diagnosticate attraverso l'analisi emoglobinica utilizzando tecniche speciali e la cromatografia liquida a elevata prestazione. Non c'è un trattamento; i bambini con la forma β dovrebbero evitare i farmaci ossidanti.

Le emoglobine a bassa affinità sono associate a un minor grado di cianosi rispetto alle emoglobine M. La sostituzione aminoacidica destabilizza l'ossiemoglobina e porta alla diminuzione della saturazione di ossigeno. Le forme meglio caratterizzate sono l'Hb Kansas e l'Hb Beth Israel.

462.7 • METEMOGLOBINEMIA EREDITARIA

Il ferro contenuto nell'emoglobina è normalmente allo stato ferroso (Fe^{2+}), che è essenziale per la sua funzione di trasporto dell'ossigeno. In condizioni fisiologiche, c'è una lenta, costante perdita di elettroni all'ossigeno rilasciato e la forma ferrica (Fe^{3+}) si combina con l'acqua, producendo la metemoglobina (MHg). Il meccanismo intracellulare predominante per la riduzione della MHg è la citocromo 5b. Questo meccanismo è >100 volte più efficiente della produzione di MHg e solo l'1% dell'emoglobina si trova normalmente allo stato ferrico.

Un aumento della MHg nei globuli rossi può realizzarsi come risultato dell'esposizione a sostanze tossiche (Tab. 462-5) o dell'assenza di vie riduttive (deficit di nicotinammide-adenina dinucleotide [NADH] citocromo b5 reduttasi). La metemoglobinemia tossica è molto più comune della forma ereditaria. I lattanti sono particolarmente vulnerabili all'ossidazione emoglobinica, perché essi possiedono il 50% in meno della citocromo b5 reduttasi rispetto agli adulti, l'emoglobina fetale è più suscettibile all'ossidazione dell'Hb A, e il tratto gastrointestinale del lattante molto più alcalino può promuovere la crescita di batteri Gram-negativi producenti nitriti. La metemoglobinemia è stata descritta in lattanti che hanno ingerito cibi e acqua molto ricchi in nitrati, in quelli che sono stati esposti a dentifrici con anilina o altri prodotti chimici e in alcuni lattanti con gastroenterite grave e acidosi. Un livello di MHg del 15% è associato a cianosi visibile; un livello del 70% di MHg è letale. Il livello è in genere riportato come la percentuale di emoglobina normale e il livello tossico è minore a livello di emoglobina più basso. MHg può colorare il sangue di marrone (Fig. 462.5). La saturazione di ossigeno sarà bassa, ma il sangue arterioso presenterà una Pao_2 normale o elevata (se riceve un trattamento con ossigeno) alla emogasanalisi.

TABELLA 462-5. Eziologie note di metemoglobinemia acquisita

FARMACI
Benzocaina
Clorochina
Dapsone
EMLA® (*Eutectic Mixture of Local Anesthetics*, insieme eutettico di anestetici locali) anestetici topici (lidocaina 2,5% e prilocaina 2,5%)
Flutamide
Lidocaina
Metoclopramide
Nitrati
Ossido nitrico
Nitroglicerina
Nitroprussiato
Ossido nitroso
Fenazopiridina
Prilocaina
Primachina
Riluzole
Nitrato di argento
Nitrato di sodio
Sulfonamidi
CONDIZIONI MEDICHE
Gastroenteriti infettive pediatriche, sepsi
Sovradosaggio con farmaci contenenti nitrato di amile ("automatici")
Malattia falciforme-episodi dolorosi correlati
MISCELLANEA
Coloranti all'anilina
Inalazione di fumi (scarico delle automobili, legno e plastica bruciati)
Erbicidi
Prodotti chimici industriali: nitrobenzene, nitroetano (che si trova nello smalto per unghie, resine, adesivi in gomma)
Pesticidi
Benzina arricchita in ottani

Da Ash-Bernal R, Wise R, Wright SM: Acquired methemoglobinemia. *Medicine* 2004; 83: 265-273.

METEMOGLOBINEMIA EREDITARIA CON CARENZA DI NADH CITOCROMO B5 REDUTTASI. La metemoglobina ereditaria con carenza di NADH citocromo b5 reduttasi è una patologia rara che è classificata in 4 tipi. Nel **tipo I** (il più comune), l'NADH citocromo b5 reduttasi è carente solo nei globuli rossi. Nel **tipo II** la carenza enzimatica è presente in tutti i tessuti ed è caratterizzata nell'età del lattante da encefalopatia, ritardo mentale, spasticità, microcefalia e ritardo di crescita. Nel **tipo III**, la carenza si verifica in leucociti, piastrine e globuli rossi e nel **tipo IV** c'è un deficit solo a carico del citocromo b5 eritrocitario.

La cianosi può variare in intensità con le stagioni e la dieta. Il sangue appare marrone. Varia anche il tempo di esordio della cianosi; in alcuni pazienti compare alla nascita, mentre in altri compare nella tarda adolescenza. Sebbene il 50% circa dell'emoglobina totale circolante possa essere in forma di MHg non funzionale, questi pazienti presentano poco o nessun distress cardiorespiratorio, se non durante l'esercizio.

Un trattamento orale quotidiano con acido ascorbico (200-250 mg al giorno in dosi suddivise) riduce gradualmente la MHg di circa il 10% dell'Hb totale e allevia la cianosi finché si continua la terapia. Dosi elevate croniche di acido ascorbico sono state associate all'iperossaluria e alla formazione di calcoli renali. L'acido ascorbico non dovrebbe essere usato per il trattamento della metemoglobinemia tossica. Il **blu di metilene** somministrato per via endovenosa (1-2 mg/kg all'inizio) è usato per trattare la metemoglobinemia tossica. Una dose orale può essere assunta (3-5 mg/kg/die) come terapia di mantenimento. Il blu di metilene non dovrebbe essere usato in pazienti con deficit di glucosio-6-deidrogenasi. Questo trattamento è inefficace e può causare una grave emolisi da ossidanti.

462.8 • SINDROME DA PERSISTENZA EREDITARIA DELL'EMOGLOBINA FETALE

Le sindromi da persistenza ereditaria dell'emoglobina fetale (*Hereditary Persistence of Fetal Hemoglobin*, HPFH) sono una forma di talassemia; una mutazione è associata a una diminuzione nella produzione sia di β sia di α globina. È presente uno squilibrio nel rapporto α/non-α (vedi Capitolo 462.9) tipico della talassemia. Sono state descritte oltre 20 varianti dell'HPFH, tra cui delezionali, $\delta\beta^0$, (neri, ghaniani, italiani), non delezionali (tunisini, giapponesi, australiani), legata al cluster dei geni della β-globina (britannici, italocinesi, neri) oppure non legate al cluster dei geni della β-globina (Atlanta, Repubblica Ceca, Seattle). Le forme $\delta\beta^0$ presentano delezioni dell'intera sequenza genica della δ- e della β-globina, con il tipo più comune negli Stati Uniti costituito dalla variante nera (HPFH-1). Come risultato delle delezioni del gene δ e β, è presente la produzione solo della γ-globina e la formazione di Hb F. Nella forma omozigote, non ci sono manifestazioni di talassemia, ma c'è solo l'Hb F, con un'anemia molto lieve e una leggera microcitosi. Quando ereditata con altre varianti emoglobiniche, l'Hb F è elevata fino a un range di 20-30%; quando ereditata con l'Hb S, è presente un miglioramento dell'emoglobinopatia falcemica con molte meno complicanze.

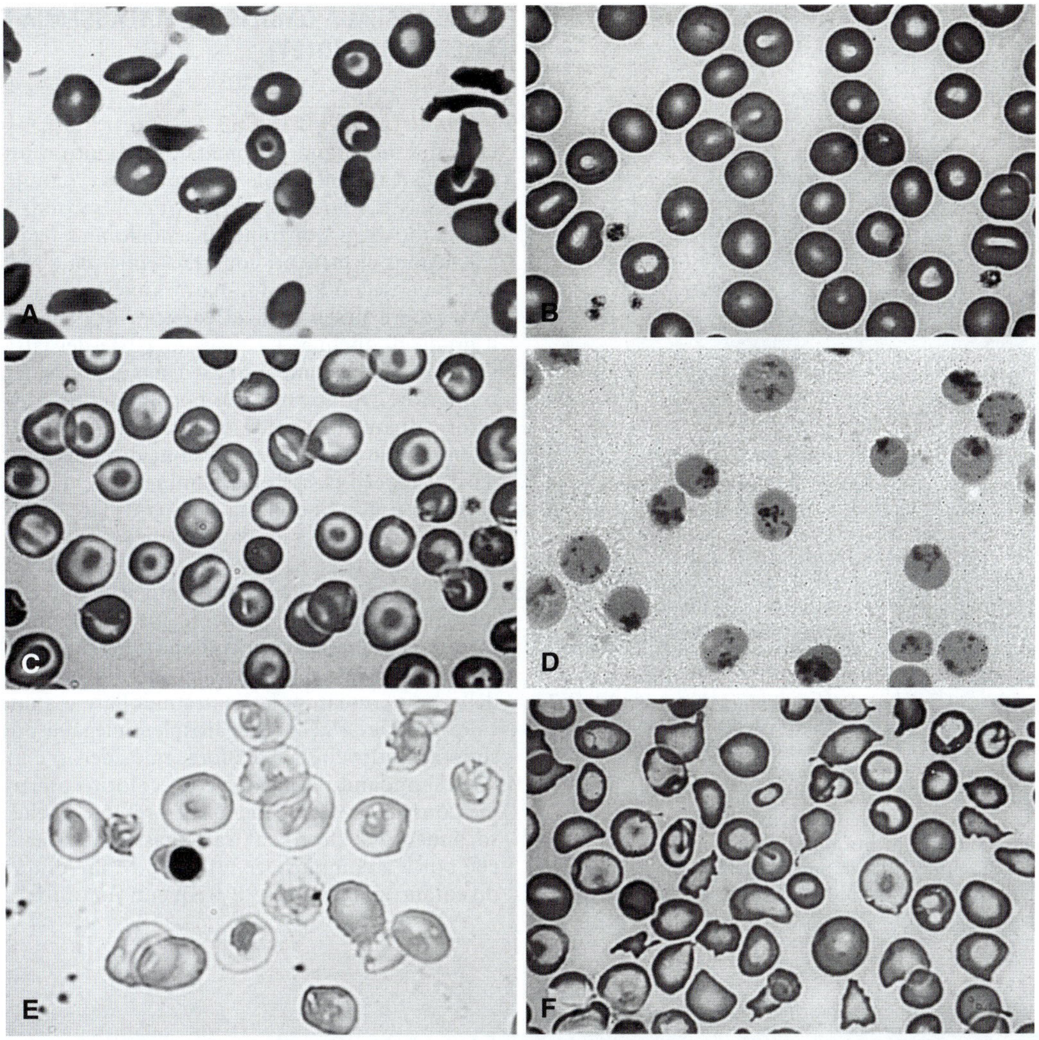

Figura 462-5. Morfologia dei globuli rossi associata alle emoglobinopatie. *A*, Anemia falciforme (Hb SS): cellule bersaglio e cellule fisse (irreversibilmente a falce). *B*, Tratto falcemico (Hb AS): morfologia dei globuli rossi normale. *C*, Emoglobina CC: cellule a bersaglio e occasionali sferociti. *D*, Anemia congenita a corpi di Heinz (emoglobina instabile): eritrociti colorati con colorazioni sopravitali (blu brillante di cresile) mostrano inclusioni intracellulari. *E*, Omozigosi β^0-talassemia: ipocromia severa con eritrociti deformati e normoblasti. *F*, Malattia dell'emoglobina F (α-talassemia): anisopoichilocitosi con cellule bersaglio. (Per gentile concessione del Dr. John Bolles, The ASH Collection, University of Washington, Seattle.)

462.9 • SINDROMI TALASSEMICHE

Le **talassemie** sono patologie genetiche della produzione delle catene globiniche. Negli individui con **β-talassemia** è presente o una completa assenza di produzione del gene della β-globina (β^0-talassemia) oppure una parziale riduzione (β^+-talassemia). Nell'**α-talassemia**, la produzione del gene dell'α globina è o assente o parzialmente ridotto. Il danno primario nelle talassemie è causato dalla quantità di produzione del gene globinico, mentre nell'emoglobinopatia a cellule falciformi, il danno primitivo risiede nella qualità della produzione globinica.

EPIDEMIOLOGIA. Sebbene la β-talassemia presenti >200 mutazioni, la maggior parte di queste è rara. Circa 20 alleli comuni costituiscono l'80% delle talassemie note al mondo; il 3% della popolazione mondiale porta il gene per la β-talassemia, e nel Sud-est asiatico, il 5-10% della popolazione porta il gene per l'α-talassemia. In un'area particolare esistono pochissimi alleli comuni. Negli Stati Uniti si stima che 2000 individui siano affetti da β-talassemia.

FISIOPATOLOGIA. Due caratteristiche maggiori contribuiscono alla patogenesi delle sequele della β-talassemia: inadeguata produzione del gene β-globinico, che conduce a diminuiti livelli di emoglobina normale (Hb A), e uno squilibrio nella produzione delle catene α- e β-globiniche. Caratteristiche selezionate delle talassemie sono illustrate nella Tabella 462-6. Nel midollo osseo, le mutazioni talassemiche compromettono la maturazione dei globuli rossi, causando un'eritropoiesi inefficace; il midollo è iperattivo, ma il paziente possiede relativamente pochi reticolociti e un'anemia grave. Nelle β-talassemie è presente un eccesso di catene α-globiniche in confronto alle γ- e alle β-; si formano tetrameri di α-globina (α_4), e queste inclusioni interagiscono con la membrana del globulo rosso e riducono la sopravvivenza eritrocitaria, portando all'anemia e a un'aumentata eritropoiesi. Le catene γ-globiniche sono prodotte in quantità crescenti, portando a un aumento dell'Hb F ($\alpha_2\gamma_2$). Le catene δ-globiniche sono anche prodotte in quantità aumentate, portando a un aumento dell'Hb A2 ($\alpha_2\delta_2$) nella β-talassemia.

Nell'α-talassemia ci sono relativamente poche catene α-globiniche e un eccesso di catene β- e γ-globiniche. Questo eccesso di catene produce l'**emoglobina di Bart** (γ_4) nella vita fetale e l'Hb H (β_4) dopo la nascita. Questi tetrameri anormali non sono egualmente tossici ma conducono a un'emolisi extravascolare. Prima della nascita un feto con α-talassemia può diventare sintomatico perché l'Hb F richiede una sufficiente produzione di catene α, mentre dopo la nascita, lattanti con β-talassemia diventano sintomatici perché l'Hb A richiede un'adeguata produzione di catene β.

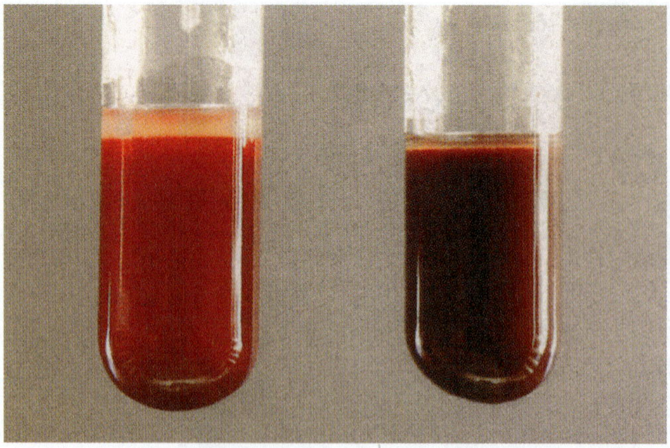

Figura 462-6. Sangue arterioso normale vs metemoglobinemia. Il sangue intero arterioso con l'1% di metemoglobina (*sinistra*) con sangue intero arterioso con il 72% di metemoglobina (*destra*) (metodi descritti in seguito). Da notare il caratteristico colore marrone cioccolato del preparato con un elevato livello di metemoglobina. Entrambi i preparati sono stati brevemente esposti al 100% di ossigeno e agitati. Questa veloce analisi è un buon test di base per la metemoglobinemia. Il preparato a *sinistra* cambia in rosso brillante, mentre il preparato a *destra* rimane di colore marrone cioccolato. Metodi: Tutti i campioni ematici sono stati preparati nello stesso momento dalla stessa persona. La concentrazione misurata dell'emoglobina era 11,7 g/dL. La concentrazione calcolata di metemoglobina: 11,7 g/dL × 0,01 = 0,117 g/dL (*sinistra*) e 11,7 g/dL × 0,72 = 8,42 g/dL (*destra*). Un elevato livello di metemoglobina è stato creato in vitro aggiungendo 0,1 mL di una soluzione 0,144 molare di sodio nitrato (*destra*), e 0,1 mL di una soluzione fisiologica aggiunti per controllo (*sinistra*). Misurazioni di co-ossimetria sono state ottenute in entrambi i campioni poco dopo che il sangue era stato preparato e 20 minuti dopo l'aggiunta della soluzione di sodio nitrato. Entrambi i campioni di sangue erano stati esposti al 100% di ossigeno prima della seconda misura. (Protocollo basato sulla comunicazione personale con il Dr. Ali Mansouri, Dicembre 2002.)

β-TALASSEMIA OMOZIGOTE (TALASSEMIA MAJOR, ANEMIA DI COOLEY)

MANIFESTAZIONI CLINICHE. Se non trattati, i bambini con β-talassemia diventano sintomatici in seguito a un'anemia emolitica progressiva, con debolezza profonda e scompenso cardiaco durante il secondo semestre di vita. A seconda della mutazione e del grado di produzione di emoglobina fetale, sono necessarie trasfusioni in pazienti con talassemia major nel secondo mese di vita o nel secondo anno, ma raramente più tardi. La decisione di trasfondere dipende dalla capacità del bambino di compensare il grado di anemia. La maggior parte dei lattanti e dei bambini manifesta uno scompenso cardiaco quando l'emoglobina è 4 g/dL o inferiore. Affaticamento, poco appetito e letargia sono reperti tardivi di anemia severa in un lattante o in un bambino ed erano comuni prima che le trasfusioni diventassero una terapia standard. I reperti classici nei bambini con talassemia severa, inclusi la facies tipica (iperplasia del mascellare, naso appiattito, bozze frontali), fratture ossee patologiche, epatosplenomegalia marcata, cachessia, si riscontrano soprattutto nei Paesi in via di sviluppo. La milza può diventare così grande che può causare un ingombro meccanico e secondariamente ipersplenismo. Caratteristiche di eritropoiesi inefficace includono aumento degli spazi midollari (con massiccia espansione del midollo nelle ossa della faccia e del cranio), ematopoiesi extramidollare e aumentato fabbisogno calorico (Fig. 462-7). L'epatosplenomegalia può interferire con il supporto nutrizionale. Pallore, emosiderosi e ittero possono combinarsi andando a produrre un colorito marrone-verdastro. Come conseguenza dell'anemia, è presente anche un aumentato assorbimento del ferro dal tratto gastrointestinale, con una tossicità che porta a complicanze ulteriori. Molte di queste caratteristiche diventano meno severe e frequenti con la terapia trasfusionale,

TABELLA 462-6. Le talassemie

TALASSEMIA	GENOTIPO GLOBINICO	CARATTERISTICHE	ESPRESSIONE	ELETTROFORESI EMOGLOBINICA
α-TALASSEMIA				
Delezione di 1 gene	-,α/α, α	Normale	Normale	Neonati: Bart 1-2%
Delezione di 2 geni trait	-,α/-,α-,-/α, α	Microcitosi, ipocromia lieve	Normale, lieve anemia	Neonato: Bart 5-10%
Delezione di 3 geni emoglobina H	-,-/-,α	Microcitosi, ipocromia	Anemia lieve, trasfusioni non richieste	Neonato: Bart 20-30%
Delezione di 2 geni + Constant Spring	-,-/α, $\alpha^{Constant\ Spring}$	Microcitosi, ipocromia	Anemia moderata-grave, trasfusioni, splenectomia	2-3% Constant Spring, 10-15% emoglobina H
Delezione di 4 geni	-,-/-,-	Anisocitosi, poichilocitosi	Idrope fetale	Neonato: 89-90% Bart con Gower 1 e 2 e Portland
Non delezioni	α,α /α,$\alpha^{variante}$	Microcitosi, lieve anemia	Normale	1-2% emoglobina variante
β-TALASSEMIA				
Eterozigote β^0 o β^+: trait	β^0/A, β^+/A	Microcitosi variabile	Normale	Elevata A_2, aumento variabile della F
β^0-Talassemia	β^0/β^0, β^+/β^0, E/β^0	Microcitosi, eritroblasti	Trasfusione-dipendente	F 98%, A_2 2% E 30-40%
β^+-Talassemia grave	β^+/β^+	Microcitosi, eritroblasti	Trasfusione-dipendente/talassemia intermedia	F 70-95%, A_2 2%, tracce A
Silente	β^+/A	Microcitosi	Normale con sola microcitosi	A_2 3,3-3,5%
	β^+/β^+	Ipocromia, microcitosi	Anemia lieve-moderata	A_2 2-5%, F 10-30%
Dominante (rara)	β^0/A	Microcitosi, globuli rossi anormali	Anemia moderatamente severa, splenomegalia	Aumentata F e A_2
δ-Talassemia	A/A	Normale	Normale	A_2 assente
$(\delta\beta)^0$-Talassemia	$(\delta\beta)^0$/A	Ipocromia	Anemia lieve	F 5-20%
$(\delta\beta)^+$-Talassemia Lepore	β^{Lepore}/A	Microcitosi	Anemia lieve	Lepore 8-20%
Lepore	$\beta^{Lepore}/\beta^{Lepore}$	Microcitica, ipocromica	Talassemia intermedia	F 80%, Lepore 20%
γδβ-Talassemia	$(\gamma^A\delta\beta)^0$/A	Microcitosi, microcitica, ipocromica	Anemia moderata, splenomegalia, omozigote: talassemia intermedia	Diminuita F e A_2 rispetto a δβ-talassemia
γ-Talassemia	$(\gamma^A\gamma^G)^0$/A	Microcitosi	Insignificante se non omozigote	Diminuita F
PERSISTENZA EREDITARIA DELL'EMOGLOBINA FETALE				
Delezionale	A/A	Microcitica	Lieve anemia	F 100% omozigote
Non delezionale	A/A	Normale	Normale	F 20-40%

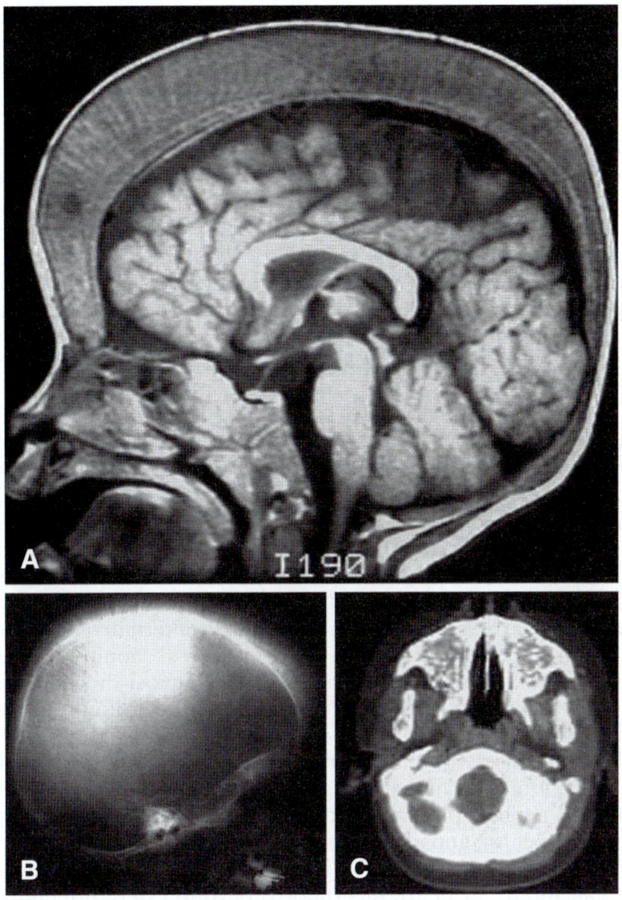

Figura 462-7. Eritropoiesi inefficace in un paziente di 3 anni non trasfuso con talassemia major. *A*, Allargamento massivo dello spazio diploico del cranio come visto alla RM. *B*, Aspetto radiografico delle trabecole come visto sulle radiografie standard. *C*, Obliterazione dei seni mascellari con tessuto ematopoietico come visto alla TC.

ma la presenza di eccessivi depositi di ferro associati a emosiderosi è uno dei maggiori problemi nei soggetti con β-talassemia. Molte delle complicanze della talassemia presenti nei Paesi in via di sviluppo oggi sono il risultato dell'aumentato deposito di ferro a causa delle continue trasfusioni di sangue. Le complicanze possono essere evitate attraverso il regolare utilizzo di un chelante del ferro. Comunque la terapia chelante ha anche complicanze associate. Patologie endocrine e cardiache sono spesso associate a eccessivi depositi di ferro in pazienti con talassemia major che sono stati cronicamente trasfusi. Le disfunzioni endocrine possono includere ipotiroidismo, insufficienza gonadica, ipoparatiroidismo e diabete mellito. L'insufficienza cardiaca congestizia e le aritmie cardiache sono complicanze potenzialmente letali delle emosiderosi in individui con β-talassemia.

REPERTI DI LABORATORIO. Il neonato nasce solo con l'Hb F o, in alcuni casi, Hb F e Hb E (eterozigosi per β^0-talassemia). Alla fine, i pazienti con β-talassemia presentano anemia grave, pochi reticolociti, numerosi globuli rossi nucleati, microcitosi, con quasi tutte i globuli rossi di apparenza anomala allo striscio (vedi Fig. 462-5*E*). Il livello di emoglobina scende progressivamente a livelli <5 g/dL senza che siano fatte trasfusioni. La conta reticolocitaria è comunemente <8% ed è inappropriatamente bassa se comparata al grado di anemia a causa della eritropoiesi inefficace. Il livello della bilirubina non coniugata sierica è in genere elevato, ma altri valori possono essere normali in uno stadio precoce. Anche se il paziente non è trasfuso, c'è alla fine un accumulo di ferro, con un elevato livello di ferritina sierica e di transferrina satura. L'iperplasia del midollo osseo può essere vista alle radiografie (vedi Fig. 462-7).

TRATTAMENTO. Prima che sia iniziata una terapia trasfusionale cronica, la diagnosi di β^0-talassemia dovrebbe essere confermata e i genitori informati sulla terapia a vita. L'inizio delle trasfusioni e della terapia chelante può essere difficile per i genitori da affrontare precocemente nella vita del bambino. Prima che inizi la terapia trasfusionale si deve ottenere il fenotipo dei globuli rossi; prodotti del sangue leucodepleti, tipizzati e compatibili con gli antigeni Rh e di Kell sono necessari per la trasfusione. Se c'è la possibilità di un trapianto di midollo osseo, il sangue dovrebbe essere negativo per il Cytomegalovirus e irradiato. La terapia trasfusionale migliora la salute generale e lo stato di benessere ed evita conseguenze della eritropoiesi inefficace. Un programma trasfusionale in genere richiede trasfusioni mensili, con il livello di emoglobina pretrasfusione >9,5 e <10,5 g/dL. In pazienti con cardiopatia, livelli elevati di emoglobina pretrasfusionali possono essere di beneficio. Alcune banche del sangue hanno programmi per i donatori che accoppiano donatori e riceventi, diminuendo l'esposizione ad antigeni eritrocitari multipli.

L'**emosiderosi trasfusionale** causa molte delle complicanze della talassemia major. Una valutazione accurata degli eccessivi depositi di ferro è essenziale per una terapia ottimale. Il livello di ferritina sierica è utile nella determinazione del bilancio del ferro ma non valuta accuratamente le quantità di ferro di riserva. Un sottotrattamento o un sovratrattamento di depositi presunti eccessivi di ferro si può verificare quando un paziente è gestito solo sulla base del livello di ferritina sierica. La misura del livello di ferro attraverso la biopsia epatica è il metodo standard per la determinazione accurata dei depositi di ferro. Un ferritometro e un software specifico per RM costituiscono alternative emergenti alla biopsia epatica. Anche se la misura quantitativa del ferro epatico guida in maniera accurata l'uso dei chelanti del ferro, essa non riflette l'accumulo di ferro cardiaco. I pazienti possono avere un sovraccarico di ferro cardiaco contemporaneamente a un livello sicuro di ferro epatico. Molti centri per le talassemie monitorano il ferro cardiaco con RM pesate in T_2, ma l'applicazione di routine di questa tecnologia non è stata implementata in tutti i centri.

L'emosiderosi trasfusionale può essere prevenuta attraverso l'uso della deferoxamina. La deferoxamina chela il ferro e alcuni altri cationi divalenti, permettendo la loro escrezione nelle urine e nelle feci. La deferoxamina viene somministrata per via sottocutanea per 10-12 ore, 5-6 giorni alla settimana. Effetti collaterali includono l'ototossicità con elevata frequenza di perdita di udito, cambiamenti retinici e displasia ossea con accorciamento del tronco. Il numero di ore in cui la deferoxamina viene impiegata ha più importanza della dose giornaliera. Le infusioni a dose elevata e in tempi brevi aumentano la tossicità, perdendo di efficacia. Il ferro plasmatico non legato alla transferrina (*Non Transferrin Bound Iron*, NTBI) è più il probabile responsabile del danno serio legato al ferro. Quando la deferoxamina viene somministrata, lega il NTBI. Quando invece viene sospesa, ci sono aumenti di rimbalzo dei livelli di NTBI, con rischio di danno. L'infusione di deferoxamina nelle 24 ore si è dimostrata in grado di recuperare la cardiomiopatia nei pazienti con eccessivi depositi di ferro nel cuore che comportano un'insufficienza cardiaca congestizia sintomatica.

Il deferiprone è un nuovo chelante del ferro approvato dalla U.S. Food and Drug Administration per bambini di età >2 anni (vedi Capitolo 462.1). Il deferiprone non può essere così efficace come la deferoxamina nella chelazione del ferro in tutto il corpo, ma risulta maggiormente efficace nel rimuovere il ferro cardiaco. Effetti collaterali includono la neutropenia, e sono necessari esami emocromocitometrici settimanali. Altri chelanti del ferro sono stati studiati per l'utilizzo orale e sottocutaneo. L'ICL670 è un chelante orale che sembra efficace nei trial di fase III e potrà essere approvato per l'uso negli Stati Uniti nel prossimo futuro.

Il trapianto di midollo osseo ha guarito >1000 pazienti che hanno la talassemia major. La maggior parte dei successi si è avuta nei soggetti con meno di 15 anni senza eccessivi depositi di ferro ed epatomegalia che hanno fratelli HLA-compatibili. A tutti i bambini che hanno un fratello HLA-compatibile dovrebbe essere offerta l'opzione del trapianto di midollo osseo.

ALTRE SINDROMI β-TALASSEMICHE

Le sindromi β-talassemiche sono suddivisibili in 6 gruppi: β-talassemia, δβ-talassemia, γ-talassemia, δ-talassemia, εγδβ-talassemie, e la sindrome HPFH. La maggior parte di queste talassemie è relativamente rara e alcune si ritrovano solo in gruppi familiari. Le β-talassemie possono anche essere clinicamente classificate come trait talassemico e come talassemia minima, minor, intermedia e major a seconda del grado di anemia. La classificazione genetica non definisce necessariamente il fenotipo e il livello di anemia non sempre predice la classificazione genetica.

La **talassemia intermedia** può essere dovuta a una qualunque combinazione delle mutazioni della β-talassemia ($\beta^0/\beta^+, \beta^0/\beta^{variante}$, E/β^0), che produrranno a un fenotipo di anemia microcitica con un livello di emoglobina di circa 7 g/dL. C'è controversia sul fatto di trasfondere o meno questi bambini. Essi potrebbero avere un certo grado di iperplasia midollare, emosiderosi nutrizionale che può richiedere la terapia chelante, splenomegalia, e altre complicanze della talassemia associate a eccessivi depositi di ferro. L'ematopoiesi extramidollare può verificarsi nel canale vertebrale, comprimendo il midollo spinale e causando sintomi neurologici; questi ultimi rappresentano un'emergenza medica che richiede l'immediata terapia radiante locale per bloccare l'eritropoiesi. Anche se le trasfusioni potrebbero alleviare le manifestazioni talassemiche, la decisione di trasfondere deve essere valutata contro il futuro bisogno di terapia chelante.

La splenectomia può essere indicata per i pazienti con talassemia intermedia che hanno un livello di emoglobina basale che scende e per i pazienti trasfusi con un fabbisogno trasfusionale aumentato. La splenectomia può avere serie complicanze infettive. Tutti i pazienti dovrebbero essere immunizzati efficacemente contro i batteri capsulati prima della splenectomia, e successivamente dovrebbero ricevere una profilassi a lungo termine con penicillina con appropriate istruzioni per la gestione della febbre.

Le **talassemie** classificate come **minima** e **minor** sono in genere eterozigoti (β^0/β, β^+/β^+) con un fenotipo più severo rispetto al trait talassemico, ma non così severo come la talassemia intermedia. Il genotipo dovrebbe essere determinato e questi bambini dovrebbero essere monitorati per l'accumulo di ferro. Le β-talassemie sono influenzate dalla presenza dell'α-talassemia, con un trait α-talassemico che porta a un anemia meno severa. I geni α duplicati (ααα/α α) comportano una talassemia più grave. Frequentemente questi individui richiedono trasfusioni nell'adolescenza e nell'età adulta; alcuni possono essere candidati per la chemioterapia, per esempio con idrossiurea.

Il **trait talassemico** viene spesso confuso con la sideropenia nei bambini perché i due sono ematologicamente simili e la sideropenia è decisamente più comune. Un piccolo ciclo di ferro e una rivalutazione è quanto è richiesto per identificare i bambini che necessiteranno di una successiva valutazione. I bambini che presentano il tratto β-talassemico hanno una distribuzione di globuli rossi persistentemente larga, e all'analisi dell'emoglobina presentano elevata Hb F e Hb A_2 elevata in maniera diagnostica. Esistono forme "silenti" di trait talassemico e, se l'anamnesi familiare è suggestiva, possono essere indicate indagini ulteriori.

α-TALASSEMIA

I neonati sono identificati nel periodo neonatale per l'aumentata produzione dell'**emoglobina di Bart** (γ_4) durante la vita fetale e per la sua presenza alla nascita. Queste talassemie si verificano più frequentemente nel Sud-est asiatico. Le mutazioni da delezione sono comuni nell'α-talassemia. Oltre a queste delezioni, ci sono mutazioni non delezionali del gene α-globinico, la più comune è rappresentata dalla Constant Spring ($\alpha^{CS}\alpha$). Ci sono quattro geni α-globinici e quattro fenotipi delezionali di α-talassemia.

La delezione di un gene α-globinico (trait silente) non è ematologicamente identificabile. Non si notano alterazioni nel volume corpuscolare medio e nell'emoglobina corpuscolare media. Gli individui con questa delezione sono in genere diagnosticati dopo la nascita di un bambino con la delezione di due geni o Hb H (β_4). Durante il periodo neonatale, tipicamente si osserva <3% di emoglobina di Bart. La delezione di un gene α è comune negli afroamericani.

La delezione di due geni α-globinici comporta il trait α-talassemico. I geni globinici possono essere persi in *trans*, come -α/-α, o in *cis*, come $\alpha,\alpha/^{-SEA}$. Le mutazioni in *cis* o in *trans*, insieme con altre mutazioni, possono portare all'HB H, o α-talassemia major. In soggetti provenienti dall'Africa o di discendenza africana, la delezione genetica dell'α-globina più comune è in *trans*, mentre negli individui dall'Asia o dell'area mediterranea la delezione in *cis* è più comune. Il trait α-talassemico si presenta come un'anemia microcitica che può essere scambiata per anemia sideropenica (vedi Fig. 462-5*F*). L'analisi emoglobinica è normale, tranne durante il periodo neonatale, quando l'emoglobina di Bart è comunemente <8% ma >3%. Bambini con delezione di due geni α-globinici sono comunemente considerati come se avessero una carenza di ferro, vista la presenza sia di un basso volume corpuscolare medio sia di una bassa emoglobina corpuscolare media. La via più semplice per distinguere tra la carenza di ferro e il tratto α-talassemico è con una buona anamnesi alimentare. I bambini con un'anemia sideropenica spesso presentano una dieta che è a basso contenuto di ferro. In alternativa, un breve ciclo di supplementazione con ferro insieme al monitoraggio dei parametri eritrocitari può permettere la diagnosi di sideropenia oppure può essere necessaria l'analisi della delezione del gene α-globinico.

La delezione di tre geni α porta alla diagnosi di malattia dell'Hb H. In California, che ha una grande popolazione asiatica, circa 1/15 000 neonati presenta la malattia dell'Hb H. Il metodo più semplice per diagnosticare la malattia dell'Hb H è durante il periodo neonatale, quando il livello di Hb Bart è comunemente >25%. Inoltre evidenze di supporto devono essere ottenute dai genitori (almeno un genitore deve avere il trait α-talassemico). Più tardi nel corso dell'infanzia si manifesta un eccesso di tetrameri di catene β-globinici che comporta l'Hb H. La diagnosi definitiva della malattia Hb H richiede l'analisi del DNA con prova a supporto. Il blu brillante di cresile può individuare l'Hb H, ma è raramente utilizzato per la diagnosi. Individui con malattia Hb H presentano una marcata microcitosi, anemia, splenomegalia lieve e, talvolta, ittero sclerale e colelitiasi. La trasfusione non è comunemente usata per la terapia perché il range di emoglobina è 7-11 g/dL, con un volume corpuscolare medio di 51-73 fL.

La delezione di tutti e 4 i geni α-globinici causa una severa anemia durante la vita fetale, comportando idrope fetale; il gene ζ-globinico deve essere presente per la sopravvivenza fetale. Non ci sono emoglobine normali presenti alla nascita (per prima cosa emoglobina di Bart, con Gower-1, Gower-2 e Portland). Se il feto sopravvive, un'exsanguinotrasfusione immediata è indicata. Questi neonati con α-talassemia major sono trasfusione-dipendenti e l'unica terpia è il trapianto di midollo osseo.

La presenza di una mutazione α-globinica non delezionale con delezione di 2 geni comporta un'anemia più grave rispetto all'α-talassemia tipo delezione globinica, maggiore epatosplenomegalia, ittero più intenso e un decorso molto più severo clinicamente rispetto alla malattia Hb H. La Constant Spring è la forma più comune ($\alpha^{CS}\alpha$).

Il **trattamento** delle sindromi da delezione α-talassemiche comprende supplementazione di folati, una possibile splenectomia (con i rischi connessi), trasfusioni occasionali durante anemia grave per la malattia Hb H non deletiva, e trasfusioni croniche o trapianto di midollo osseo per i sopravvissuti a idrope fetale. Questi bambini non dovrebbero essere esposti ai farmaci ossidanti.

Anemia falciforme

Alonso MH: Gallbladder abnormalities in children with sickle cell disease: Management with laparoscopic cholecystectomy. *J Pediatr* 2004;145:580–581.

Beyer JE, Simmons LE, Woods GM, et al: A chronology of pain and comfort in children with sickle cell disease. *Arch Pediatr Adolesc Med* 1999; 153:913–920.

Boyd JH, Strunk RC, Morgan WJ: The outcomes of sickle cell disease in adulthood are clear, but the origins and progression of sickle cell anemia-induced problems in the heart and lung in childhood are not. *J Pediatr* 2006;149:3–4.

Buchanan ID, Woodward M, Reed GW: Opioid selection during sickle cell pain crisis and its impact on the development of acute chest syndrome. *Pediatr Blood Cancer* 2005;45:716–724.

Claster S, Vichinsky EP: Managing sickle cell disease. *BMJ* 2003;327: 1151–1155.

De Montalembert M, Maunoury C, Acar P, et al: Myocardial ischaemia in children with sickle cell disease. *Arch Dis Child* 2004;89:359–362.

Dhar M, Bellevue R, Carmel R: Pernicious anemia with neuropsychiatric dysfunction in a patient with sickle cell anemia treated with folate supplementation. *N Engl J Med* 2003;348:2204–2207.

Driscoll MC, Hurlet A, Styles L, et al: Stroke risk in siblings with sickle cell anemia. *Blood* 2003;101:2401–2404.

Geva A, Clark JJ, Zhang Y, et al: Hemoglobin Jamaica plain: A sickling hemoglobin with reduced oxygen affinity. *N Engl J Med* 2004;351:1532–1538.

Gladwin MT, Sachdev V, Jison ML, et al: Pulmonary hypertension as a risk factor for death in patients with sickle cell disease. *N Engl J Med* 2004; 350:886–895.

Hankins JS, Ware RE, Rogers ZR, et al: Long-term hydroxyurea therapy for infants with sickle cell anemia: The HUSOFT extension study. *Blood* 2005;106:2269–2275.

Henderson JN, Noetzel MJ, McKinstry RC, et al: Reversible posterior leukoencephalopathy syndrome and silent cerebral infarcts are associated with severe acute chest syndrome in children with sickle cell disease. *Blood* 2003;101:415–419.

Kizito ME, Mworozi E, Ndugwa C, Serjeant GR: Bacteraemia in homozygous sickle cell disease in Africa: Is pneumococcal prophylaxis justified? *Arch Dis Child* 2007;92:21–23.

Kopecky EA, Jacobson S, Joshi P, et al: Systemic exposure to morphine and the risk of acute chest syndrome in sickle cell disease. *Clin Pharmacol Ther* 2004;75:140–146.

Machado RF, Anthi A, Steinberg MH, et al: N-terminal pro-brain natriuretic peptide levels and risk of death in sickle cell disease. *JAMA* 2006;296:310–318.

Makis AC, Hatzimichael EC, Stebbing J: The genomics of new drugs in sickle cell disease. *Pharmacogenomics* 2006;7:909–917.

McCarthy LJ, Vattuone J, Weidner J, et al: Do automated red cell exchanges relieve priapism in patients with sickle cell anemia? *Ther Apher* 2000;4:256–258.

Morris CR, Kato GJ, Poljakovic M, et al: Dysregulated arginine metabolism hemolysis-associated pulmonary hypertension, and mortality in sickle cell disease. *JAMA* 2005;294:81–90.

Neumayr L, Lennette E, Kelly D, et al: *Mycoplasma* disease and acute chest syndrome in sickle cell disease. *Pediatrics* 2003;112:87–95.

Norris CF, Smith-Whitley K, McGowan KL: Positive blood cultures in sickle cell disease: Time to positivity and clinical outcome. *J Pediatr Hematol Oncol* 2003;25:390–395.

Optimizing Primary Strike Prevention in Sickle Cell Anemia (STOP2) Investigators: Discontinuing prophylactic transfusions used to prevent stroke in sickle cell disease. *N Engl J Med* 2005;353:2769–2778.

Panepinto JA, Brousseau DC, Hillery CA, et al: Variation in hospitalization and hospital length of stay in children with vaso-occlusive crises in sickle cell disease. *Pediatr Blood Cancer* 2005;44:182–186.

Pirich LM, Chou P, Walterhouse DO: Prolonged survival of a patient with sickle cell trait and metastatic renal medullary carcinoma. *J Pediatr Hematol/Oncol* 1999;21:67–69.

Powars DR, Chan LS, Hiti A, et al: Outcome of sickle cell anemia: A 4-decade observational study of 1056 patients. *Medicine* 2005;84:363–376.

Quinn CT, Rogers ZR, Buchanan GR: Survival of children with sickle-cell disease. *Blood* 2004;103:4023–4027.

Qureshi N, Lubin B, Walter MC: The prevention and management of stroke in sickle cell anemia. *Expert Opin Biol Ther* 2006;6:1087–1098.

Saad ST, Lajolo C, Gilli S, et al: Follow-up of sickle cell disease patients with priapism treated by hydroxyurea. *Am J Hematol* 2004;77:45–49.

Scothorn DJ, Price C, Schwartz D, et al: Risk of recurrent stroke in children with sickle cell disease receiving blood transfusion therapy for at least five years after initial stroke. *J Pediatr* 2002;140:348–354.

Sebire G, Tabarki B, Saunders DE, et al: Cerebral venous sinus thrombosis in children: Risk factors, presentation, diagnosis and outcome. *Brain* 2005; 128:477–489; Epub 2005 Feb 7.

Smith LA, Oyeku SO, Homer C, Zuckerman B: Sickle cell disease: a question of equity and quality. *Pediatrics* 2006;117:1763–1770.

Smith-Whitley K, Zhao H, Hodinka RL, et al: Epidemiology of human parvovirus B19 in children with sickle cell disease. *Blood* 2004;103:422–427.

Strouse JJ, Hulbert ML, DeBaun MR, et al: Primary hemorrhagic stroke in children with sickle cell disease is associated with recent transfusion and use of corticosteroids. *Pediatrics* 2006;118:1916–1924.

Stuart MJ, Nagel RL: Sickle cell disease. *Lancet* 2004;364:1343–1360.

Switzer JA, Hess DC, Nichols FT, et al: Pathophysiology and treatment of stroke in sickle-cell disease: Present and future. *Lancet Neurol* 2006;5:501–512.

Sylvester KP, Patey RA, Milligan P, et al: Impact of acute chest syndrome on lung function of children with sickle cell disease. *J Pediatr* 2006;149:17–22.

Talano JAM, Hillery CA, Gottschall JL, et al: Delayed hemolytic transfusion reaction/hyperhemolysis syndrome in children with sickle cell disease. *Pediatrics* 2003;111:e661–e665.

Uong EC, Henderson Boyd J, DeBaun MR: Daytime pulse oximeter measurements do not predict incidence of pain and acute chest syndrome episodes in sickle cell anemia. *J Pediatr* 2006;149:707–709.

Vargas-Gonzalez R, Sotelo-Avila C, Coria AS: Case report: Renal medullary carcinoma in a six-year-old boy with sickle cell trait. *Pathol Oncol Res* 2003;9:193–195.

Vichinsky EP, Neumayr LD, Earles AN, et al: Causes and outcomes of the acute chest syndrome in sickle cell disease. *N Engl J Med* 2000;342:1855–1865.

Ware RE, Zimmerman SA, Sylvestre PB, et al: Prevention of secondary stroke and resolution of transfusional iron overload in children with sickle cell anemia using hydroxyurea and phlebotomy. *J Pediatr* 2004;145:346–352.

Weiner DL, Hibberd PL, Betit P, et al: Preliminary assessment of inhaled nitric oxide for acute vaso-occlusive crisis in pediatric patients with sickle cell disease. *JAMA* 2003;289:1136–1142.

Zarrouk V, Habibi A, Zahar JR, et al: Bloodstream infection in adults with sickle cell disease. *Medicine* 2006;85:43–48.

Metemoglobinemia

Ash-Bernal R, Wise R, Wright SM: Acquired methemoglobinemia: A retrospective series of 138 cases at 2 teaching hospitals. *Medicine* 2004;83: 265–273.

Moore TJ, Walsh CS, Cohen MR: Reported adverse event cases of methemoglobinemia associated with benzocaine products. *Arch Intern Med* 2004;164:1192–1196.

Rehman HU: Methemoglobinemia. *West J Med* 2001;175:193–196.

Sanchez-Echaniz J, Benito-Fernandez J, Mintegui-Raso S: Methemoglobinemia and consumption of vegetables in infants. *Pediatrics* 2001;107:1024–1028.

Talassemia

Aessopos A, Tsironi M, Vassiliadis I, et al: Exercise-induced myocardial perfusion abnormalities in sickle beta-thalassemia: Tc-99m tetrofosmin gated SPECT imaging study. *Am J Med* 2001;111:355–360.

Berkovitch M, Bistritzer T, Milone SD, et al: Iron deposition in the anterior pituitary in homozygous beta-thalassemia: MRI evaluation and correlation with gonadal function. *J Pediatr Endocrinol Metab* 2000;13:179–184.

Chen FE, Ooi C, Ha SY, et al: Genetic and clinical features of hemoglobin H disease in Chinese patients. *N Engl J Med* 2000;343:544–550.

Chern JP, Lin KH, Lu MY, et al: Abnormal glucose tolerance in transfusion-dependent beta-thalassemic patients. *Diabetes Care* 2001;24:850–854.

Chui DHK, Fuchareon S, Chan V: Hemoglobin H disease: Not necessarily a benign disorder. *Blood* 2003;101:791–800.

Eldor A, Rachmilewitz EA: The hypercoagulable state in thalassemia. *Blood* 2002;99:36–43.

Gallanello R, Piga A, Forri GL, et al: Phase II clinical evaluation of defarasirov, a once-daily oral chelating agent in pediatric patients with beta-thalassemia major. *Hematologica* 2006;91:1343–1351.

Gulati R, Bhatia V, Agarwal SS: Early onset of endocrine abnormalities in beta-thalassemia major in a developing country. *J Pediatr Endocrinol Metab* 2000;13:651–656.

Hahalis G, Manolis AS, Gerasimidou I, et al: Right ventricular diastolic function in beta-thalassemia major: Echocardiographic and clinical correlates. *Am Heart J* 2001;141:428–434.

Kattamis AC, Antoniadis M, Manoli I, et al: Endocrine problems in ex-thalassemic patients. *Transfus Sci* 2000;23:251–252.

Lorey F, Cunningham G, Vichinsky EP, et al: Universal newborn screening for Hb H disease in California. *Genet Test* 2001;5:93–100.

Rund D, Rachmilewitz E: β-Thalassemia. *N Engl J Med* 2005;353:1135–1146.

Telfer PT, Prestcott E, Holden S, et al: Hepatic iron concentration combined with long-term monitoring of serum ferritin to predict complications of iron overload in thalassaemia major. *Br J Haematol* 2000;110:971–977.

Weatherall DJ: Introduction to the problem of hemoglobin E–beta thalassemia. *J Pediatr Hematol Oncol* 2000;22:551.

Winichagoon P, Fucharoen S, Chen P, et al: Genetic factors affecting clinical severity in beta-thalassemia syndromes. *J Pediatr Hematol Oncol* 2000;22:573–580.

Wonke B: Clinical management of beta-thalassemia major. *Semin Hematol* 2001;38:350–359.

Disturbi da sovraccarico di ferro

Andrews NC: Inherited iron overload disorders. *Curr Opin Pediatr* 2000; 12:596–602.
Deferasirox (Exjade): A new iron chelator. *Med Lett Drugs Ther* 2006;48:35–36.
McCullen MA, Crawford DH, Hickman PE: Screening for hemochromatosis. *Clin Chim Acta* 2002;315:169–186.
Murray KF, Kowdley KV: Neonatal hemochromatosis. *Pediatrics* 2001;108: 960–964.
Roy CN, Andrews NC: Recent advances in disorders of iron metabolism: Mutations, mechanisms and modifiers. *Hum Mol Genet* 2001;10: 2181–2186.
Sanchez AM, Schreiber GB, Bethel J, et al: Prevalence, donation practices, and risk assessment of blood donors with hemochromatosis. *JAMA* 2001; 286:1475–1481.
Vohra P, Haller C, Emre S, et al: Neonatal hemochromatosis: The importance of early recognition of liver failure. *J Pediatr* 2000;136:537–541.

Capitolo 463 ■ Difetti enzimatici

George B. Segel

DEFICIT DI ENZIMI DELLA VIA GLICOLITICA

Una varietà di difetti enzimatici dei globuli rossi produce anemie emolitiche, le quali, in genere, non presentano alterazioni morfologiche importanti. Sono stati descritti deficit ereditari della maggior parte degli enzimi sia nella via anaerobica di Embden-Meyerhof sia nello shunt ossidativo degli esoso monofosfati (pentosi) (Fig. 463-1). Il più comune difetto enzimatico glicolitico come causa di anemia emolitica è la rara condizione di deficit di piruvato chinasi (*Pyruvate Kinasi*, PK).

463.1 • Deficit di piruvato chinasi

L'anemia emolitica congenita si verifica in soggetti omozigoti per un gene autosomico recessivo che causa o una riduzione marcata della PK o la produzione di un enzima anomalo con diminuita attività. La produzione di adenosina trifosfato (ATP) all'interno dei globuli rossi è alterata e si notano diminuiti livelli di ATP, di piruvato e della forma ossidata del nicotinamide adenindinucleotide (NAD^+) (vedi Fig. 463-1). La concentrazione di 2,3-difosfoglicerato è aumentata; il 2,3-difosfoglicerato è di aiuto, perché facilita il rilascio dell'ossigeno dall'emoglobina, ma riduce le capacità inibitorie dell'esochinasi e degli enzimi dello shunt degli esoso monofosfati. Inoltre, si verifica un'inspiegata diminuzione nella somma dell'adenina (ATP, adenosina di fosfato e adenosina monofosfato) e della piridina (NAD^+ e la forma ridotta del NAD); questo compromette ulteriormente la glicolisi. Come conseguenza della diminuzione dell'ATP, i globuli rossi non possono mantenere il contenuto di potassio e di acqua; le cellule diventano rigide e la loro durata di vita è considerevolmente ridotta.

EZIOLOGIA. Ci sono due geni per la PK nei mammiferi, ma solo il gene *PKLR* è espresso nei globuli rossi. Il gene umano *PKLR* è localizzato sul cromosoma 1q21; sono riportate 133 mutazioni in questo gene strutturale, che codifica per una proteina costituita da 574-amminoacidi che produce un tetramero funzionale. La maggior parte dei pazienti affetti è eterozigote composto per difetti di 2 differenti geni della PK. Le molte combinazioni possibili spiegano probabilmente la variabilità della gravità clinica. Le mutazioni 1456 C-T e 1529 G-A sono le più comuni mutazioni della popolazione bianca.

MANIFESTAZIONI CLINICHE E REPERTI DI LABORATORIO. Le manifestazioni cliniche variano da un'anemia emolitica neonatale grave a una lieve, un'emolisi ben compensata notata per la prima volta nell'età adulta. Ittero severo e anemia possono verificarsi nel periodo neonatale; è stato riportato kernittero. L'emolisi nei bambini più grandi e negli adulti varia in gravità, con valori di emoglobina compresi tra 8 e 12 g/dL associati a modesto pallore, ittero e splenomegalia. Questi pazienti in genere non richiedono trasfusioni. Una forma grave di malattia presenta un'incidenza relativamente alta tra gli Amish degli Stati Uniti medioccidentali.

La policromatofilia e la macrocitosi lieve riflettono l'elevata conta reticolocitaria. Gli sferociti sono poco comuni, ma si ritrovano pochi **picnociti** spiculati. La fragilità osmotica senza incubazione è normale. La diagnosi si basa sulla dimostrazione di una marcata riduzione dell'attività della PK eritrocitaria o sull'aumento della costante di dissociazione di Michaeli-Menten (K_m) per il suo substrato, il fosfoenolpiruvato. Altre attività enzimatiche eritrocitarie sono normali o aumentate, riflettendo la reticolocitosi. Non si notano alterazioni dell'emoglobina. I globuli bianchi presentano un'attività normale della PK e devono essere rigorosamente esclusi dagli emolisati usati per misurare l'attività della PK. I portatori eterozigoti in genere hanno livelli moderatamente ridotti dell'attività della PK.

TRATTAMENTO. Le exsanguinotrasfusioni possono essere indicate per l'iperbilirubinemia nei neonati. Le trasfusioni di emazie concentrate sono necessarie per l'anemia grave o per le crisi aplastiche. Se l'anemia è costantemente severa o se sono richieste frequenti trasfusioni, la splenectomia dovrebbe essere eseguita dopo i 5-6 anni di età. Anche se non curativa, la splenectomia può essere seguita da livelli più elevati di emoglobina e da reticolocitosi sorprendentemente alte (30-60%). La morte conseguente a una fulminante sepsi pneumococcica può conseguire alla splenectomia; quindi, l'immunizzazione con vaccini per germi incapsulati dovrebbe essere eseguita prima della splenectomia, mentre dopo la splenectomia dovrebbe essere somministrata la profilassi penicillinica.

463.2 • Altri deficit di enzimi della via glicolitica

Anemie emolitiche croniche non sferocitiche di diversa gravità sono state associate a deficit di altri enzimi della via glicolitica, inclusa l'esochinasi, la glucosio fosfato isomerasi e l'aldolasi che sono ereditate come patologie autosomiche recessive. Il **deficit di fosfofruttochinasi** si verifica soprattutto negli ebrei ashkenaziti degli Stati Uniti e comporta l'emolisi associata a una miopatia classificata come glicogenosi di tipo VII (vedi Capitolo 87.1). Clinicamente l'anemia emolitica è complicata da debolezza muscolare, intolleranza all'esercizio, crampi e possibile mioglobinuria. I saggi enzimatici per la fosfofruttochinasi sono bassi nei globuli rossi e nel muscolo.

Il **deficit della trioso fosfato isomerasi** (*Triose Phosphate Isomerase*, **TPI**) è una patologia autosomica recessiva che colpisce molti sistemi. I pazienti affetti presentano anemia emolitica, anomalie cardiache e danni al motoneurone inferiore e al tratto piramidale, con o senza evidenza di ritardo mentale. Essi di solito muoiono nella prima infanzia. Il gene per la TPI è stato clonato e sequenziato e si trova nel cromosoma 12.

La **fosfoglicerato chinasi** (*PhosphoGlycerate Kinase*, **PGK**) è il primo step ATP-generatore della glicolisi. Sono state descritte almeno 23 famiglie con deficit di PGK. La PGK è l'unico enzima glicolitico ereditato con il cromosoma X. I maschi affetti presentano una malattia extrapiramidale progressiva, miopatia, crisi e ritardo mentale grave assieme all'anemia emolitica. Nove pazienti giapponesi avevano sintomi neurologici, miopatici con emolisi: 6 avevano emolisi isolata, 7 avevano sintomi neurologici o miopatici isolati e uno non presentava sintomi. Il gene per la PGK è particolarmente grande, costituito da 23 kb, e diverse anomalie genetiche, incluse

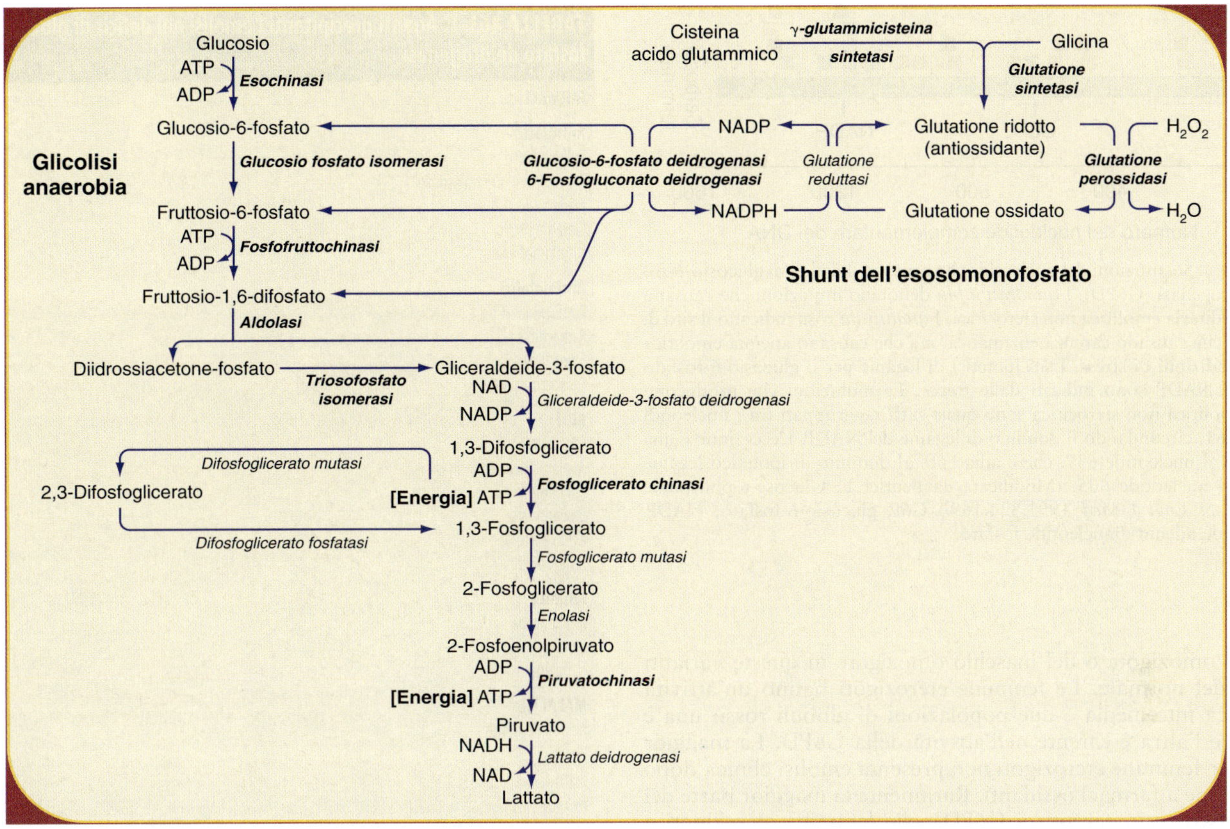

Figura 463-1. Metabolismo del globulo rosso. Glicolisi e via dell'esosomonofosfato. Le carenze enzimatiche associate chiaramente all'emolisi sono mostrate in grassetto. ATP, adenosina trifosfato; ADP, adenosina difosfato; NADP, nicotinamide adenin dinucleotide fosfato; forma ridotta del NADP.

le sostituzioni nucleotidiche, le delezioni geniche, i missense, le mutazioni dello *splicing*, comportano il deficit di PGK.

DEFICIT DEGLI ENZIMI DELLA VIA DEGLI ESOSO MONOFOSFATI

La più importante funzione della via degli esoso monofosfati è di mantenere il glutatione in stato ridotto (GSH) come protezione contro l'ossidazione dei globuli rossi (vedi Fig. 463-1). Circa il 10% del glucosio assorbito dai globuli rossi passa attraverso questa via per fornire la forma ridotta del nicotinamide adenin dinucleotide fosfato (NADPH) necessaria per la conversione del glutatione ossidato a GSH. Il mantenimento del GSH è essenziale per l'inattivazione fisiologica dei composti ossidanti, come il perossido di idrogeno, che si generano all'interno dei globuli rossi. Se il glutatione, o un qualunque composto o enzima necessario per mantenerlo allo stato ridotto, è diminuito, i gruppi SH della membrana del globulo rosso sono ossidati e l'emoglobina si denatura precipitando in **inclusioni eritrocitarie chiamate corpi di Heinz**. Una volta che i corpi di Heinz si sono formati, dal danno della membrana eritrocitaria causata dall'emoglobina precipitata, dall'agente ossidante e dall'azione della milza può derivare un'emolisi acuta. I globuli rossi danneggiati sono rapidamente rimossi dal circolo.

463.3 • DEFICIT DI GLUCOSIO-6-FOSFATO DEIDROGENASI E CORRELATI

Il deficit di glucosio-6-fosfato deidrogenasi (G6PD) è la più importante malattia della via degli esoso monofosfati ed è responsabile di due sindromi cliniche, un'anemia emolitica episodica indotta dalle infezioni, da taluni farmaci o più raramente dalle fave, e un'anemia emolitica spontanea cronica non sferocitica. Questa carenza enzimatica correlata all'X colpisce più di 200 milioni di persone nel mondo; rappresenta un esempio di "polimorfismo bilanciato" in cui è presente un vantaggio evolutivo di resistenza alla malaria da falciparum nelle femmine eterozigoti che bilanciano il piccolo effetto negativo dei maschi affetti emizigoti.

La carenza è causata dall'eredità di uno qualsiasi di un ampio numero di alleli anormali del gene responsabile della sintesi della proteina G6PD. Il gene della G6PD è stato clonato e sequenziato. Un database accessibile nel web cataloga le mutazioni della G6PD (www.bioinf.org.uk/g6pd) Alcune di queste mutazioni che causano emolisi episodica vs cronica sono mostrate nella Figura 463-2. Una malattia più lieve è associata con le mutazioni vicino all'estremità amino-terminale della molecola della G6PD e l'anemia emolitica cronica non sferocitica è associata a mutazioni localizzate vicino l'estremità carbossi-terminale. L'enzima normale che si trova nella maggior parte della popolazione è designato come G6PD B$^+$. Una variante normale, chiamata G6PD A$^+$, è comune nella popolazione afroamericana. Più di 100 distinte varianti enzimatiche della G6PD sono associate a un ampio spettro di malattia emolitica.

ANEMIE EMOLITICHE EPISODICHE O INDOTTE

EZIOLOGIA. La G6PD, un enzima centrale nello shunt degli esoso monofosfati del metabolismo glucidico, catalizza la conversione del glucosio-6-fosfato in acido 6-fosfogluconico per produrre NADPH e mantenere il glutatione in stato ridotto (vedi Fig. 463-1).

La sintesi del G6PD eritrocitario è determinata da un gene sul cromosoma X. Le malattie coinvolgenti questo enzima si verificano, perciò, più frequentemente nei maschi rispetto alle femmine. Circa il 13% dei maschi afroamericani ha un enzima mutante (**G6PD A$^-$**) che comporta una deficit dell'attività della G6PD eritrocitario (≤5-15% del normale). Italiani, greci e altri gruppi etnici mediterranei, mediorientali, africani e asiatici hanno un'elevata incidenza che va dal 5 al 40% di una variante designata **G6PD B$^-$ (G6PD mediterranea)**. L'attività G6PD della

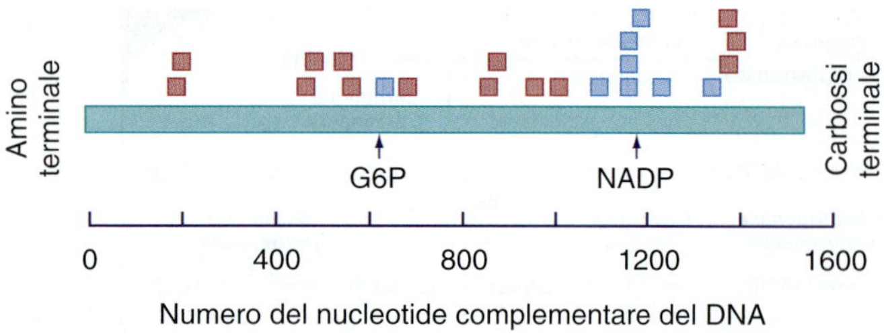

Figura 463-2. Sostituzioni del nucleotide che causano il deficit di glucosio-6-fosfato deidrogenasi (G6PD). I *quadratini blu* denotano mutazioni che causano anemia ereditaria emolitica non sferocitica. I *quadratini rosa* indicano il sito di mutazioni che causano carenza enzimatica, ma che causano anemia emolitica solo in condizioni di stress. I siti ipotetici di legame per il glucosio-6-fosfato (G6P) e il NADP sono indicati dalle *frecce*. Le mutazioni che producono anemia emolitica non sferocitica sono quasi tutti raggruppati tra i nucleotidi 1089 e 1361, circondando il dominio di legame del NADP. L'eccezione è una mutazione al nucleotide 637, che è adiacente al dominio di ipotetico legame del G6P al nucleotide 605. (Modificata da Beutler E: Glucose-6-phosphate deficiency. *N Engl J Med* 1991;324:169.) G6P, glucosio-6-fosfato; NADP, nicotinamide adenin dinucleotide fosfato.

femmina omozigote o del maschio omozigote in queste varianti è <5% del normale. Le femmine eterozigoti hanno un'attività enzimatica intermedia e due popolazioni di globuli rossi: una è normale e l'altra è carente nell'attività della G6PD. La maggior parte delle femmine eterozigoti non presenta emolisi clinica dopo l'esposizione a farmaci ossidanti. Raramente la maggior parte dei globuli rossi sono carenti di G6PD nelle femmine eterozigoti a causa dell'inattivazione casuale (ipotesi di Lyon) del cromosoma X normale.

Variazioni considerevoli nel difetto sono notate in diversi gruppi razziali. Il difetto negli americani di discendenza africana è meno grave che nei discendenti di americani ed europei malati. Negli afroamericani la variante enzimatica, elettroforeticamente distinta, è instabile in vivo e la sua attività è diminuita soprattutto nei globuli rossi circolanti più vecchi. L'attività enzimatica dei globuli rossi contenenti la variante enzimatica (G6PD B$^-$) negli americani di discendenza europea è molto bassa, spesso <1% del normale. Un terzo tipo comune di enzima mutante, con attività marcatamente ridotta (**G6PD Canton**) si verifica in circa il 5% della popolazione cinese. Un gran numero di altre rare varianti enzimatiche è stata associato all'emolisi indotta dai farmaci.

MANIFESTAZIONI CLINICHE. Nelle forme comuni di deficit di G6PD, i sintomi si sviluppano 24-48 ore dopo che un paziente ha ingerito sostanze con proprietà ossidanti. I farmaci che possiedono queste proprietà includono l'acido acetilsalicilico e gli antimalarici, come la primachina (Tab. 463-1). In alcuni pazienti, l'ingestione di fave, un ingrediente di base della dieta mediterranea, può anche produrre una sindrome emolitica acuta grave chiamata *favismo*. Questo deriva dai prodotti ossidativi derivati da due composti glicosidici, vicina e convicina, che sono idrolizzati in divicina e isouramile, che infine producono perossido di idrogeno e altri prodotti reattivi dell'ossigeno.

Il grado di emolisi varia con l'agente, la quantità ingerita e la gravità della carenza enzimatica. Nei casi gravi si verifica ittero ed emoglobinuria e la concentrazione emoglobinica può cadere precipitosamente, mettendo così a rischio la vita. Nella **varietà A$^-$** (afroamericani), la stabilità del dimero proteico è difettosa, e questo difetto è accentuato mano a mano che i globuli rossi invecchiano. Quindi, si possono osservare remissioni spontanee dell'emolisi sebbene la somministrazione del farmaco sia continuata. Questa remissione è il risultato della labilità età-dipendente dell'enzima, che è abbondante e più stabile negli eritrociti più giovani. La reticolocitosi associata compensa il processo emolitico. L'infezione può essere la causa più comune di emolisi e un'emolisi importante ma insidiosa può verificarsi in pazienti

TABELLA 463-1. Agenti precipitanti l'emolisi nel deficit di glucosio-6-fosfato deidrogenasi

FARMACI

Antibiotici
Sulfonamidici
Trimetoprim-sulfametoxazolo
Acido nalidixico
Cloramfenicolo
Nitrofurantoina

Antimalarici
Primachina
Pamachina
Clorochina
Quinacrina

Altri
Fenacetina
Analoghi della vitamina K
Blu di metilene
Probenecid
Acido acetilsalicilico
Fenazopiridina

CHIMICI
Fenilidrazina
Benzene
Naftalene

MALATTIE
Acidosi diabetica
Epatiti
Sepsi

Da Asselin BL, Segel GB. In Rakel R (editor): *Conn's Current Therapy*. Philadelphia, WB Saunders, 1994, p 341.

ricoverati in ospedale per altre patologie, anche quando non può essere documentata esposizione ai farmaci. Nel deficit di G6PD A$^-$, emolisi spontanee si possono verificare nei neonati prematuri, ma non in quelli a termine. Nei neonati greci e cinesi con **varietà G6PD B$^-$ e Canton** il deficit della G6PD è una causa importante di iperbilirubinuria e potenziale kernittero. In un gruppo di neonati femmine eterozigoti di ebrei sefarditi, è presente un'aumentata iperbilirubinemia, in particolare se è presente la variante del promotore (*UGT1A1*) dell'uridin-5-difosfato-glucuronil transferasi presente nella sindrome di Gilbert. Quando una donna incinta ingerisce farmaci ossidanti, essi possono essere trasmessi al feto G6PD carente e ittero e anemia emolitica possono essere presenti alla nascita.

REPERTI DI LABORATORIO. L'esordio dell'emolisi acuta produce una caduta precipitosa dell'emoglobina e dell'ematocrito. Se l'episodio è grave, le proteine leganti l'emoglobina, come l'aptoglobina, sono saturate e può comparire emoglobina libera nel plasma e in seguito nelle urine (vedi Fig. 457-2). Globuli rossi non colorati o dopo colorazione sopravitale rivelano i **corpi di Heinz** (emoglobina precipitata), che non sono visibili negli strisci di sangue con colorazione di Wright. Poiché le cellule contenenti queste inclusioni sono rapidamente rimosse dalla circolazione, esse non si vedono dopo i primi 3-4 giorni di malattia. Lo striscio di sangue rivela poche cellule frammentate e policromatofile (globuli rossi grandi e brunastri) che rappresentano i reticolociti, che possono essere significativamente aumentati (5-15%).

DIAGNOSI. La diagnosi dipende dalla dimostrazione diretta o indiretta della ridotta attività della G6PD nei globuli rossi. Attraverso misure dirette l'attività enzimatica nelle persone affette è ≤10% del normale e la riduzione dell'attività enzimatica è più importante negli americani di discendenza europea e negli asiatici rispetto agli afroamericani. Test di screening soddisfacenti sono basati su riduzione del blu di metilene, sulla riduzione della metemoglobina o sulla fluorescenza del NADPH. Immediatamente dopo un episodio emolitico, predominano i reticolociti e gli eritrociti giovani. Queste cellule giovani hanno un'attività enzimatica significativamente più elevata rispetto alle cellule più vecchie nella varietà A^-. I test devono essere perciò differiti di alcune settimane prima che si possa dimostrare un basso livello diagnostico di enzima. La diagnosi può essere sospettata quando l'attività della G6PD rientra nel range normale-basso in presenza di una conta reticolocitaria normale. Le varianti G6PD possono essere anche scoperte attraverso l'analisi elettroforetica.

PREVENZIONE E TRATTAMENTO. La prevenzione dell'emolisi costituisce la misura terapeutica più importante. Quando possibile i maschi appartenenti a gruppi etnici con incidenza importante di deficit di G6PD (per es. greci, italiani del sud, ebrei sefarditi, filippini, cinesi del Sud, afroamericani e thailandesi) dovrebbero essere indagati per il difetto prima che vengano somministrati i farmaci ossidanti noti. Le dosi abituali di acido acetilsalicilico e trimetoprim-sulfametoxazolo non causano un'emolisi clinicamente rilevante nella varietà A^-. Tuttavia, l'acido acetilsalicilico somministrato nelle dosi usate per la febbre reumatica (60-100 mg/kg/24 h) può produrre un'emolisi grave. Quando si sia verificata l'emolisi, la terapia di supporto può richiedere trasfusioni di sangue, anche se la guarigione è la regola quando l'agente ossidante viene sospeso.

ANEMIE EMOLITICHE CRONICHE ASSOCIATE A DIFETTO DI G6PD O A FATTORI CORRELATI

L'anemia emolitica cronica non sferocitica è stata associata a grave deficit di G6PD causata da varianti enzimatiche, in particolare quelle carenti in quantità, attività o stabilità. I difetti genici che portano all'emolisi cronica sono posti in primo luogo nella regione del sito di legame del NADP vicino all'estremità carbossi terminale della proteina (vedi Fig. 463-2). Queste includono le varianti Loma Linda, Tomah, Iowa, Beverly Hills, Nashville, Riverside, Santiago de Cuba e Andalus. Persone con deficit dell'enzima G6PD B^- (Mediterranea) occasionalmente presentano emolisi croniche e il processo emolitico può peggiorare dopo l'ingestione di farmaci ossidanti. La splenectomia è di scarsa utilità in questo tipo di emolisi cronica.

Altri difetti enzimatici possono compromettere la rigenerazione del GSH come una sostanza ossidante (vedi Fig. 463-1). Un'anemia cronica lieve non sferocitica è stata riportata in associazione a diminuzione del GSH eritrocitario, a causa dei deficit di γ-glutamilcisteina o di glutatione sintetasi. Il deficit di 6-fosfogluconato deidrogenasi (6PDG) è stato associato in primo luogo all'emolisi indotta dai farmaci, ed emolisi con iperbilirubinemia è stata correlata al deficit di glutatione perossidasi in neonati.

Beutler E: Glucose-6-phosphate dehydrogenase deficiency. *N Engl J Med* 1994;331:169–173.

Fujii H, Miwa S: Other erythrocyte enzyme deficiencies associated with non-haematological symptoms: Phosphoglycerate kinase and phosphofructokinase deficiency. *Baillieres Best Pract Res Clin Haematol* 2000;13:141–148.

Kaplan M, Beutler E, Vreman HJ, et al: Neonatal hyperbilirubinemia in glucose-6-phosphate dehydrogenase-deficient heterozygotes. *Pediatrics* 1999;104:68–74.

Kaplan M, Muraca M, Hammerman C, et al: Bilirubin conjugation, reflected by conjugated bilirubin fractions, in glucose-6-phosphate dehydrogenase-deficient neonates: A determining factor in the pathogenesis of hyperbilirubinemia. *Pediatrics* 1998;102:E37.

Martinov MV, Plotnikov AG, Vitvitsky VM, et al: Deficiencies of glycolytic enzymes as a possible cause of hemolytic anemia. *Biochim Biophys Acta* 2000;1474:75–87.

McMullin MF: The molecular basis of disorders of red cell enzymes. *J Clin Pathol* 1999;52:241–244.

Min-Oo G, Gros P: Erythrocyte variants and the nature of their malaria protective effect. *Cell Microbiol* 2005;7:753–763.

Valentin C, Pissard S, Martin J, et al: Triose phosphate isomerase deficiency in 3 French families: Two novel null alleles, a frameshift mutation (TPI Alfortville) and an alteration in the initiation codon (TPI Paris). *Blood* 2000;96:1130–1135.

Zanella A, Bianchi P: Red cell pyruvate kinase deficiency: From genetics. *Baillieres Best Pract Res Clin Haematol* 2000;13:57–81.

Zanella A, Fermo E, Bianchi P, Valentini G: Red cell pyruvate kinase deficiency: Molecular and clinical aspects. *Br J Haematol* 2005;130:11–25.

Capitolo 464 ■ Anemie emolitiche conseguenti a fattori extracellulari

George B. Segel

ANEMIE EMOLITICHE AUTOIMMUNI

Un certo numero di agenti esterni e di patologie può condurre a distruzione prematura dei globuli rossi (vedi Tab. 457-1). Tra quelli meglio definiti ci sono gli anticorpi associati ad anemie emolitiche immuni. Il segno distintivo di questo gruppo di patologie è la positività del test di Coombs, che evidenzia la presenza di immunoglobuline o fattori del complemento sulla superficie dei globuli rossi. La patologia emolitica immune più importante nella pratica pediatrica è la malattia emolitica del neonato (eritroblastosi fetale), causata dal trasferimento transplacentare di anticorpi materni diretti contro i globuli rossi del feto, cioè l'anemia emolitica isoimmune (vedi Capitolo 103.2). Diverse altre anemie emolitiche immuni sono autoimmuni (Tab. 464-1) e possono essere idiopatiche o correlate a diverse infezioni (virus di Epstein Barr, raramente HIV, Citomegalovirus e micoplasma), malattie immunomediate (lupus eritematoso sistemico [LES], artrite reumatoide), immunodeficienze (agammaglobulinemia, patologie linfoproliferative autoimmuni, disgammaglobulinemia), neoplasie (linfoma, leucemia, malattia di Hodgkin) o farmaci (metildopa, L-dopa). Altri farmaci (penicilline, cefalosporine) causano emolisi immune che non è "autoimmune". Gli anticorpi sono "farmaco-dipendenti" e in genere (anche se non sempre) non hanno "specificità" per gli antigeni di membrana del globulo rosso.

ANEMIE EMOLITICHE AUTOIMMUNI ASSOCIATE AD AUTOANTICORPI "CALDI"

EZIOLOGIA. Nelle anemie emolitiche autoimmuni anticorpi anomali sono diretti contro i globuli rossi, ma i meccanismi patogenetici sono incerti. L'autoanticorpo può essere prodotto come risposta immune inappropriata a un antigene eritrocitario o a un altro epitopo antigenico simile a un antigene eritrocitario, noto come *mimetismo molecolare*. In alternativa un agente infettivo può alterare la membrana eritrocitaria così che diventa "estranea" o antigenica per l'ospite. Gli anticorpi di solito reagiscono a epitopi (antigeni) che sono "pubblici" o comuni a tutti i globuli rossi umani, come le proteine Rh.

In molti casi di emolisi da anticorpi caldi, non può essere trovata alcuna causa sottostante; questo è il tipo primario o idiopatico (vedi Tab. 464-1). Se l'emolisi autoimmune è associata a una patologia sottostante, come una patologia linfoproliferativa, il LES o l'immunodeficienza, essa è secondaria. In circa il 20% dei casi di emolisi immune, i farmaci possono essere implicati (Tab. 464-2).

I farmaci (penicillina o talvolta cafalosporine) che causano emolisi tramite il meccanismo degli "apteni" (immune ma non autoimmune) si legano strettamente alla membrana eritrocitaria (vedi Tab. 464-1). Anticorpi contro il farmaco, neoformati o preesistenti, si legano alle molecole del farmaco sui globuli rossi mediando la loro distruzione nella milza. In altri casi alcuni farmaci, come il chinino e la chinidina, non si legano sui globuli

TABELLA 464-1. Malattie caratterizzate da distruzione immunomediata del globulo rosso

ANEMIA EMOLITICA AUTOIMMUNE DOVUTA AD ANTICORPI CALDI
Primaria (idiopatica)
Secondaria
 Patologie linfoproliferative
 Malattie del tessuto connettivo (soprattutto il lupus eritematoso sistemico)
 Neoplasie non linfoidi (per es. tumori ovarici)
 Malattie infiammatorie croniche (per es. colite ulcerosa)

ANEMIA EMOLITICA AUTOIMMUNE DOVUTA AD AUTOANTICORPI FREDDI (SINDROMI EMOLITICHE CRIOPATICHE)
Malattia da agglutinine fredde primaria (idiopatica)
Malattia da agglutinine fredde secondaria
 Patologie linfoproliferative
 Infezioni (*Mycoplasma pneumoniae*, virus di Epstein-Barr)
Emoglobinuria parossistica a frigore
 Primaria (idiopatica)
 Sindromi virali (più comuni)
 Sifilide congenita o terziaria

ANEMIA EMOLITICA IMMUNE FARMACO-INDOTTA (VEDI TAB. 464-2)
Aptene/Adsorbimento di farmaci (per es. penicillina)
Complesso ternario (immune) (per es. chinina o chinidina)
Induzione autoanticorpi vera (per es. metildopa)

Modificata da Packman CH: Autoimmune hemolytic anemias. In Rakel R (editor): *Conn's Current Therapy*. Philadelphia, WB Saunders, 1995, p 305.

TABELLA 464-2. Farmaci selezionati che causano emolisi immuno-mediata

MECCANISMO	ASSORBIMENTO DEL FARMACO (APTENE)	COMPLESSO IMMUNE	AUTOANTICORPO
Test dell'antiglobulina diretto	Positività anti-IgG	Positività anti-C3	Positività anti-IgG
Sito di emolisi	Extravascolare	Intravascolare	Extravascolare
Farmaci	Penicillina	Chinidina	α-Metildopa
	Ampicillina	Fenacetina	Acido mefenamico (Ponstel)
	Meticillina	Idroclorotiazide	L-dopa
	Carbenicillina	Rifamcina (Rifadin)	Procainamide
	Cefalotina*	Sulfonamidi	Ibuprofene
	Cefaloridina*	Isoniazide	Diclofenac
		Chinina	Interferone α
		Insulina	Melfalan
		Tetracicline	
		Paracetamolo	
		Idralazina	
		Probenecid	
		Clorpromazina	
		Streptomicina	
		Fluorouracile	
		Sulindac	

* Non disponibile negli Stati Uniti.
Adattata per gentile concessione dell'American Family Physician (vedi sotto) da Schwartz RS, Berkman EM, Silberstein LE: Autoimmune hemolytic anemias. In Hoffman R, Benz EJ Jr, Schattil SJ, et al (editors): *Hematology: Basic Principles and Practice*, 3rd ed. Philadelphia, Churchill Livingstone, 2000, p 624. Riprodotta per gentile concessione di Dhaliwal G, Cornett PA, Tierney LM: Hemolytic anemia. *Am Family Physician* 2004; 69:2603.

rossi ma piuttosto formano parte di un "complesso ternario", formato dal farmaco, un antigene di membrana eritrocitario e un autoanticorpo che riconosce entrambi (vedi Tab. 464-1). La metildopa e qualche volta le cefalosporine possono, attraverso meccanismi sconosciuti, stimolare autoanticorpi veri contro antigeni di membrana dei globuli rossi, così che la presenza del farmaco non è richiesta per causare l'emolisi.

MANIFESTAZIONI CLINICHE. Anemie emolitiche autoimmuni possono presentarsi secondo due quadri clinici generali. Il primo, un tipo acuto transitorio che dura 3-6 mesi e si verifica soprattutto in bambini di età tra i 2 e i 12 anni, riguarda il 70-80% dei pazienti. È frequentemente preceduto da un'infezione, in genere respiratoria. L'esordio può essere acuto, con prostrazione, pallore, ittero, febbre ed emoglobinuria, o più graduale soprattutto con affaticamento e pallore. La milza è in genere aumentata ed è il sito primitivo di distruzione dei globuli rossi rivestiti dalle immunoglobuline G (IgG). Patologie sistemiche sottostanti sono poco comuni. Un'ottima risposta alla terapia corticosteroidea, un basso tasso di mortalità e la piena guarigione sono tipiche della forma acuta.

L'altro quadro clinico presenta un decorso prolungato e cronico, che è più frequente nei lattanti e nei bambini più grandi di 12 anni. L'emolisi può continuare per molti mesi o anni. Le anomalie che coinvolgono altri elementi del sangue sono comuni, e la risposta ai glucocorticoidi è variabile e non prevedibile. Il tasso di mortalità è di circa il 10% e la morte è spesso da attribuire a una malattia sistemica sottostante.

REPERTI DI LABORATORIO. In molti casi l'anemia è grave con livelli di emoglobina <6 g/dL. Sono presenti un'importante sferocitosi e policromasia. Più del 50% dei globuli rossi circolanti può essere costituita da reticolociti, e di solito sono presenti eritroblasti. In alcuni casi, può esserci una bassa conta reticolocitaria, soprattutto all'esordio dell'episodio. La leucocitosi è comune. La conta piastrinica è di solito normale, ma talvolta compare una porpora trombocitopenica immune concomitante (**sindrome di Evans**). La prognosi per i pazienti con la sindrome di Evans è infausta, perché molti hanno malattie croniche, inclusi LES o patologie linfoproliferative autoimmuni.

Il test di Coombs diretto è fortemente positivo, e anticorpi liberi possono talvolta essere dimostrati nel siero (test di Coombs indiretto). Questi anticorpi sono attivi a 35-40 °C (anticorpi "caldi") e molto spesso appartengono alla classe IgG. Essi non richiedono il complemento per l'attività e in genere non producono l'agglutinazione *in vitro*; questa ultima caratteristica viene indicata come anticorpi *incompleti*. Anticorpi sierici e quelli eluiti dai globuli rossi reagiscono con i globuli rossi di molte persone, oltre che dei pazienti. Essi spesso sono stati definiti come panagglutinine aspecifiche, ma attenti studi hanno rivelato la specificità per gli antigeni eritrocitari del sistema Rh nel 70% dei pazienti (circa il 50% degli adulti). Il complemento, in particolare il C3b, può essere riscontrato sui globuli rossi insieme con le IgG. Il risultato del test di Coombs è occasionalmente negativo a causa della limitata sensibilità della reazione di Coombs. Un minimo di 260-500 molecole di IgG per cellula sulla membrana eritrocitaria è necessario per produrre una reazione positiva. Test speciali sono richiesti per scoprire l'anticorpo nei casi di anemia emolitica autoimmune "Coombs negativa". L'emolisi da anticorpi caldi può essere IgG-positiva, positiva sia per IgG sia per complemento (C3b), o solo complemento-positiva se le IgG sono inferiori al limite soglia per il reattivo di Coombs anti-IgG.

TRATTAMENTO. Le trasfusioni in genere producono un miglioramento solo transitorio, ma possono essere richieste inizialmente a causa della severità dell'anemia finché compaiono gli effetti degli altri trattamenti. Può essere molto difficile trovare sangue compatibile; dovrebbe essere scelto il sangue in cui i globuli rossi danno *in vitro* una reazione minore positiva al test di Coombs. È necessario qualche volta infondere sangue che è "incompatibile" come valutato con le reazioni crociate. La mancata trasfusione a un lattante o a un bambino profondamente anemico può portare a una grave morbilità e anche alla morte.

I pazienti con malattia lieve ed emolisi compensata possono non richiedere alcun trattamento. Se l'emolisi è grave e comporta un'anemia importante o sintomi, viene iniziato un trattamento con glucocorticoidi. I glucocorticoidi diminuiscono la velocità di emolisi bloccando la funzione dei macrofagi attraverso un meccanismo di *downregulation* dell'espressione del recettore Fcγ, diminuendo la produzione anticorpale e forse migliorando la eluizione degli anticorpi dai globuli rossi. Il prednisone o il suo equivalente è somministrato alla dose di 2 mg/kg/24 h. In alcuni pazienti con emolisi severa possono essere richieste dosi di prednisone fino a 6 mg/kg/24 h per ridurre il grado di emolisi. Il trattamento dovrebbe essere continuato finché l'emolisi non diminuisca e in seguito la dose viene gradualmente ridotta. Se si verifica una ricaduta, può essere necessario il ripristino del dosaggio pieno. La malattia tende a remissione spontanea entro poche settimane o mesi. Il risultato del test di Coombs può rimanere positivo anche dopo che l'emolisi ha subito una forte diminuzione. Quando l'anemia emolitica rimane grave nonostante la terapia glucocorticoidea, o se alte dosi sono necessarie per mantenere un accettabile valore di emoglobina, si può provare con immunoglobuline endovena. Il rituximab, un anticorpo monoclonale che ha per bersaglio i linfociti B, i produttori di anticorpi, si è rivelato utile in casi cronici refrattari alla terapia convenzionale. È stata usata la plasmaferesi nei casi refrattari, ma in genere non è utile. La splenectomia può essere di beneficio, ma è complicata da un elevato rischio di infezione da organismi capsulati, in particolare in pazienti di età inferiore ai 2 anni. È indicata la profilassi con vaccini appropriati (pneumoccoccico, meningococcico e *Haemophilus influenzae* tipo b) prima della splenectomia e con penicillina per via orale dopo la splenectomia.

DECORSO E PROGNOSI. La malattia emolitica idiopatica acuta autoimmune nell'infanzia varia in gravità, ma è autolimitantesi; la mortalità per anemia intrattabile è rara. Circa il 30% dei pazienti presenta emolisi cronica spesso associata a una patologia sottostante, come LES, linfoma o leucemia. Negli adulti, la presenza di anticorpi antifosfolipidi in pazienti con emolisi immune predispone alla trombosi. La mortalità nei casi cronici dipende dalla patologia primitiva.

ANEMIE EMOLITICHE AUTOIMMUNI ASSOCIATE AD ANTICORPI "FREDDI"

Gli anticorpi "freddi" sono anticorpi eritrocitari che sono più attivi alle basse temperature e agglutinano i globuli rossi a temperature <37 °C. Essi sono soprattutto di classe IgM e richiedono il complemento per essere attivi. Il range di temperatura associato all'agglutinazione dei globuli rossi è detto *ampiezza termica*. Un'ampiezza termica più elevata causa emolisi con esposizioni meno severe al freddo. Elevati titoli anticorpali sono associati a un'elevata ampiezza termica.

MALATTIA DELLE AGGLUTININE FREDDE. Gli anticorpi freddi in genere hanno specificità per gli antigeni oligosaccaridici del sistema I/i. Essi possono presentarsi nella malattia delle agglutinine fredde primaria o idiopatica, secondaria a infezioni come quelle da *Mycoplasma pneumoniae* e virus di Epstein Barr, o secondaria a patologie linfoproliferative. Dopo infezione da *M. pneumoniae* i livelli di anti-I possono aumentare molto, e talvolta possono verificarsi grandi aumenti fino a titoli ≥1:30 000. L'anticorpo ha specificità per l'antigene I e quindi reagisce poco con i globuli rossi del cordone ombelicale umano che esprimono l'antigene i e bassi livelli di antigene I. Pazienti con mononucleosi infettiva in alcune occasioni presentano agglutinine a freddo e gli anticorpi in questi pazienti hanno spesso una specificità anti-i. Questo anticorpo causa meno emolisi negli adulti rispetto ai bambini perché gli adulti presentano meno molecole i sui loro globuli rossi. Un'agglutinazione eritrocitaria spontanea viene osservata con il freddo e gli aggregati eritrocitari sono presenti allo striscio di sangue. Il volume corpuscolare medio può essere falsamente aumentato a causa dell'agglutinazione cellulare. La gravità dell'emolisi è associata all'ampiezza termica dell'anticorpo, esso stesso parzialmente dipendente dal titolo anticorpale IgM.

Quando sono presenti elevati titoli di anticorpi freddi e attivi a temperature simili a quella corporea, può verificarsi un'emolisi grave intravascolare con emoglobinemia ed emoglobinuria e aumentare con l'esposizione del paziente al freddo (temperatura esterna o alimenti ingeriti). Ogni molecola IgM ha il potenziale di attivare una molecola C1 così che una grande quantità di complemento si trova sui globuli rossi nella malattia delle agglutinine fredde. Questi eritrociti sensibilizzati possono andare incontro a lisi intravascolare mediata dal complemento o a distruzione nella milza e nel fegato.

La malattia da agglutinine fredde è meno comune nei bambini rispetto agli adulti e più frequentemente comporta un episodio acuto autolimitantesi di emolisi. I glucocorticoidi sono molto meno efficaci nella malattia da agglutinine fredde rispetto alla malattia con anticorpi caldi. I pazienti dovrebbero evitare l'esposizione al freddo e dovrebbero essere trattati per la patologia sottostante. Nei pochi pazienti con malattia emolitica grave il trattamento include l'immunosoppressione e la plasmaferesi. Il trattamento di successo della malattia da agglutinine fredde è stato riportato con l'anticorpo monoclonale rituximab, che riduce significativamente i linfociti B. La splenectomia non è utile nella malattia da agglutinine fredde.

EMOGLOBINURIA PAROSSISTICA A FRIGORE. Questa forma di anemia emolitica è mediata dall'emolisina di Donath-Landsteiner, che è un autoanticorpo IgG reattivo al freddo con specificità anti-P. Questo anticorpo fissa una grande quantità di complemento con il freddo e i globuli rossi lisano a mano a mano che la temperatura aumenta. La maggior parte dei casi riportati è autolimitante e in genere associata a infezioni virali non specifiche. Essi sono attualmente ritrovati raramente in associazione alla sifilide congenita o acquisita. Questa patologia può rendere conto del 30% degli episodi immuni emolitici tra i bambini. Il trattamento include la trasfusione per l'anemia grave e l'evitare ambienti freddi.

Flores G, Cunningham-Rundles C, Newland AC, et al: Efficacy of intravenous immunoglobulin in the treatment of autoimmune hemolytic anemia: Results in 73 patients. *Am J Hematol* 1993;44:237–242.

Gehrs BC, Friedberg RC: Autoimmune hemolytic anemia. *Am J Hematol* 2002;69:258–271.

King KE, Ness PM: Treatment of hemolytic anemia. *Semin Hematol* 2005;42:131–136.

Packman CH: Acquired hemolytic anemia due to warm-reacting autoantibodies. In Beutler E, Lichtman MA, Coller BS, et al (editors): *Williams Manual of Hematology*, 6th ed. New York, McGraw-Hill, 2001, pp 639–648.

Petz L: Treatment of autoimmune hemolytic anemias. *Curr Opin Hematol* 2001;8:411–416.

Ramanathan S, Koutts J, Hertzberg MS: Two cases of refractory warm autoimmune hemolytic anemia treated with rituximab. *Am J Hematol* 2005;78:123–126.

Sparling TG, Andricevic M, Wass H: Remission of cold hemagglutinin disease induced by rituximab therapy. *CMAJ* 2001;164:1405.

Capitolo 465 ■ Anemie emolitiche secondarie ad altri fattori extracellulari

George B. Segel

EMOLISI DA FRAMMENTAZIONE. Vedi Tabella 457-1. La distruzione del globulo rosso può verificarsi nelle anemie emolitiche a causa del danno meccanico nel momento in cui le cellule attraversano un letto vascolare danneggiato. Il danno può essere microvascolare, quando i globuli rossi sono danneggiati dalla fibrina nei capillari durante la coagulazione intravascolare o quando una malattia renovascolare accompagna la sindrome uremico-emolitica (vedi Capitolo 518) o la porpora trombotica trombocitopenica. Possono essere coinvolti i grandi vasi nella sindrome di Kasabach-Merritt (emangioma gigante e trombocitopenia; vedi Capitolo 505) o quando una sostituzione di una valvola cardiaca è male epitelizzata. Lo striscio di sangue mostra molti "schistociti", o cellule frammentate, così come la policromatofilia, che riflette la reticolocitosi (vedi Fig. 458-3*F*). Una sideropenia secondaria può complicare l'emolisi intravascolare a causa della perdita di ferro con l'emoglobina urinaria e l'emosiderina (vedi Fig. 457-2). Il trattamento dovrebbe essere diretto alla condizione sottostante e la prognosi dipende dalla sua efficacia. Il beneficio della trasfusione è transitorio perché le cellule trasfuse sono distrutte tanto velocemente quanto quelle prodotte dal paziente.

DANNO TERMICO. Ustioni estese possono direttamente danneggiare i globuli rossi e causare l'emolisi che comporta la formazione di sferociti. La perdita di sangue e la soppressione midollare possono contribuire all'anemia e richiedere trasfusioni di sangue. L'eritropoietina (EPO) è stata usata come trattamento per la diminuita produzione di globuli rossi.

PATOLOGIA RENALE. L'anemia dell'uremia ha un'origine multifattoriale. La produzione di EPO può essere diminuita e il midollo soppresso dai metabolici tossici. Inoltre, la vita dei globuli rossi è spesso accorciata a causa della ritenzione di metabolici e dell'acidemia organica. L'uso dell'EPO nella patologia renale cronica ha marcatamente diminuito il bisogno di trasfusioni di sangue.

PATOLOGIA EPATICA. Un cambiamento nel rapporto colesterolo/fosfolipidi nel plasma può portare cambiamenti nella composizione della membrana del globulo rosso e riduce la durata di vita dei globuli rossi. Alcuni pazienti affetti da epatopatia hanno molti eritrociti a bersaglio allo striscio periferico, mentre altri mostrano una preponderanza di acantociti.

TOSSINE E VELENI. La sepsi batterica dovuta all'*Haemophilus influenzae*, agli stafiloccocchi e agli streptococchi può essere complicata da un'emolisi di accompagnamento. Un'anemia emolitica particolarmente grave è stata osservata nelle infezioni da Clostridi e consegue a una tossina emolitica del Clostridium. Un grande numero di sferociti può essere identificato sullo striscio di sangue. L'emolisi sferocitica può anche essere notata dopo il morso di diversi serpenti, inclusi il cobra, le vipere e il serpente a sonagli, il cui veleno contiene fosfolipasi. Anche molti morsi di insetti, come le api, le vespe e i calabroni, possono causare un'emolisi sferocitica con un meccanismo simile (vedi Capitolo 714).

MALATTIA DI WILSON. Vedi Capitolo 354.2. Un episodio acuto e autolimitantesi di anemia emolitica può precedere di anni l'esordio dei sintomi epatici e neurologici della malattia di Wilson. Questo si verifica come risultato dell'effetto tossico del rame libero sulla membrana eritrocitaria. Lo striscio di sangue spesso (ma non sempre) mostra un gran numero di sferociti e il risultato del test di Coombs è negativo. Poiché la diagnosi precoce della malattia di Wilson permette un trattamento profilattico con la penicillamina e la prevenzione di patologie epatica e neurologica, è importante una valutazione corretta di questo raro tipo di emolisi.

Grudeva-Popova JG, Spasova MI, Chepileva KG, Zaprianov ZH: Acute hemolytic anemia as an initial clinical manifestation of Wilson's disease. *Folia Med (Plovdiv)* 2000;42:42–46.
Sakuri J, Nagahama M, Oda M: Clostridium perfringens alpha-toxin: Characterization and mode of action. *J Biochem (Tokyo)* 2004;136:569–574.

Sezione 4 — Policitemia (eritrocitosi) — Karen Burns e Bruce M. Camitta

Capitolo 466 ■ Policitemia primaria (policitemia rubra vera)

La policitemia si verifica quando la conta eritrocitaria, il livello emoglobinico e il volume totale eritrocitario eccedono i limiti superiori alla norma. Nei soggetti post-pubere una massa eritrocitaria di oltre il 25% del valore medio normale (basato sulla superficie corporea) o un ematocrito >60 (nei maschi) o >56 (nelle femmine) indica un'eritrocitosi assoluta. Una diminuzione del valore plasmatico, come si verifica nella disidratazione acuta e nelle ustioni, può comportare valori elevati di emoglobina. Queste situazioni sono meglio designate come *emoconcentrazione*, perché la massa eritrocitaria non è aumentata e la normalizzazione del volume plasmatico riportano l'emoglobina a livelli normali.

PATOGENESI. La policitemia primaria vera o primaria, un disordine panmieloproliferativo, è stata riportata solo in pochi bambini. È stata dimostrata una mutazione che causa un difetto di funzione di *JAK2* nel 75% dei pazienti affetti. Il recettore per l'eritropoietina è normale e le colture *in vitro* dei precursori eritroidi delle persone affette non richiedono eritropoietina aggiunta per stimolare la crescita. I livelli di eritropoietina sierica appaiono normali o bassi. I criteri diagnostici sono elencati nella Tabella 466-1.

MANIFESTAZIONI CLINICHE. I pazienti con policitemia vera in genere presentano epatosplenomegalia. L'eritrocitosi può causare ipertensione, cefalea, respiro corto o sintomi neurologici. La granulocitosi può causare diarrea o prurito per il rilascio di istamina. La trombocitosi (con o senza disfunzione piastrinica) può causare trombosi o emorragia.

TABELLA 466-1. Diagnosi di policitemia vera

CRITERI MAGGIORI
1. Aumento della massa eritrocitaria (vedi testo)
2. Saturazione arteriosa di O_2 ≥92%*
3. Splenomegalia palpabile
CRITERI MINORI
1. Conta piastrinica >400 × 10^9/L
2. Leucocitosi >12 × 10^9/L
3. Aumento della fosfatasi alcalina leucocitaria
4. Aumento della vitamina B_{12} (>900 pg/mL) o della capacità di legame della B_{12} libera (>2200 pg/mL)
DIAGNOSI
Tutti e 3 i criteri maggiori
1, 2 e 2 criteri minori

*Assenza di cause di policitemia secondaria.

TRATTAMENTO. Il salasso è il trattamento di scelta iniziale. Integrazioni di ferro dovrebbero essere somministrate per prevenire i problemi di viscosità derivanti dalla microcitosi. Gli agenti antipiastrinici (acido acetilsalicilico) possono ridurre il rischio di trombosi e di sanguinamento grave in pazienti con trombocitosi marcata. Se questo non ha successo, i trattamenti antiproliferativi (idrossiurea, anagrelide, interferone-α) possono essere di aiuto. Il rischio di trasformazione della malattia in mielofibrosi o in leucemia acuta è diminuito dopo la sospensione dell'utilizzo degli agenti alchilanti e del fosforo radioattivo. Una sopravvivenza prolungata non è inusuale.

Cario H: Childhood polycythemias/erythrocytoses: Classification, diagnosis, clinical presentation, and treatment. *Ann Hematol* 2005;84:137–145. Epub 2004 Dec 15.

Gregg XT, Prchal JT: Recent advances in the molecular biology of congenital polycythemias and polycythemia vera. *Current Hematol Rep* 2005;4: 238–242.

Klippel S, Strunck E, Temprinac S, et al: Quantification of PRV-1 mRNA distinguishes polycythemia vera from secondary erythrocytosis. *Blood* 2003;102:3569–3574.

Kralovics R, Passamonti F, Buser AS, et al: A gain of function mutation of *JAK2* in myeloproliferative disorders. *N Engl J Med* 2005;352:1779–1790.

Kwaan HC, Wang I: Hyperviscosity in polycythemia vera and other red cell abnormalities. *Semin Thromb Hemostasis* 2003;29:451–458.

Schaefer AI: Molecular basis of the diagnosis and treatment of polycythemia vera and essential thrombocythemia. *Blood* 2006;107:4214–4222.

Spivak JL: Polycythemia vera: Myths, mechanisms, and management. *Blood* 2002;100:4272–4290.

Capitolo 467 ■ Policitemia secondaria

PATOGENESI. La policitemia secondaria è diagnosticata quando la policitemia vera è causata da altri processi fisiologici (Tab. 467-1). La policitemia può essere presente in ogni situazione clinica associata a desaturazione arteriosa cronica di ossigeno. I difetti cardiovascolari con shunt destro-sinistri e patologie polmonari che interferiscono con la corretta ossigenazione sono le cause più comuni di policitemia ipossica. I reperti clinici in genere includono la cianosi, l'iperemia delle sclere e delle membrane mucose e le dita ippocratiche. Quando l'ematocrito raggiunge valori >65% le manifestazioni cliniche di iperviscosità, come la cefalea e l'ipertensione, possono richiedere il salasso (vedi Capitolo 103.3). Il fatto di vivere a elevate altitudini può

TABELLA 467-1. Diagnosi differenziale di policitemia

POLICITEMIA VERA
SECONDARIA
Familiare
Emoglobinopatie
Varianti di elevate affinità per l'ossigeno
Deficit di metemoglobina reduttasi
Esposizione cronica al monossido di carbonio
Ormonale
Patologia surrenale
Iperplasia virilizzante, sindrome di Cushing
Terapia steroidea anabolizzante
Tumori maligni
Renali, cerebellari, epatici, altro
Patologia renale
Cisti, idronefrosi
Ipossia
Altitudine
Cardiopatia
Malattia polmonare
Ipoventilazione centrale
Metabolica
Carenza di 2,3-difosfoglicerato
Neonatale
Ambiente intrauterino normale
Emorragia gemello-gemello o materno-fetale
Neonati di madri diabetiche
Ritardo di crescita intrauterina
Trisomia 13, 18 o 21
Iperplasia surrenalica
Tireotossicosi
SPURIA (riduzione del volume plasmatico)

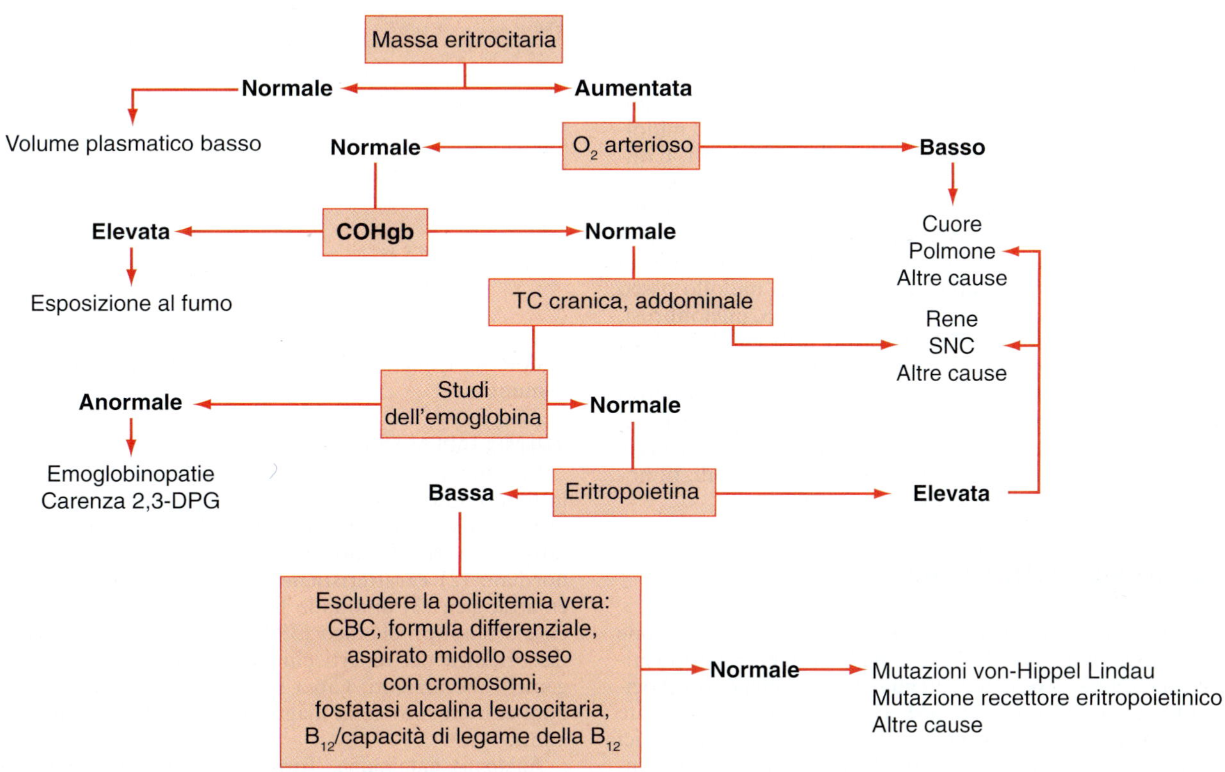

Figura 467-1. Studi sequenziali per valutare la policitemia. COHgb, carbossiemoglobina; SNC, sistema nervoso centrale; 2,3-DPG, 2,3-difosfoglicerato; CBC, conta ematica completa.

anche causare una policitemia ipossica; il livello di emoglobina aumenta di circa il 4% per ogni 1000 m di altitudine. Una parziale stenosi dell'arteria renale raramente comporta una policitemia.

Forme più insidiose di ipossia possono anche causare policitemia. La metemoglobinemia congenita causata dalla carenza della citocromo b5 reduttasi può portare a cianosi e policitemia (vedi Capitolo 462.7). Questa condizione è trasmessa come un trait autosomico recessivo. La maggior parte degli individui affetti è asintomatica. Anomalie neurologiche possono essere presenti in pazienti in cui il deficit enzimatico non è limitato alle cellule ematopoietiche. La policitemia trasmessa come carattere dominante è causata dalle emoglobine che hanno un'alterata affinità per l'ossigeno. La cianosi può verificarsi in presenza di metemoglobina in piccola quantità pari a 1,5 g/dL, ma è poco comune nelle altre varianti emoglobiniche a meno che l'iperviscosità non comporti un'ipossiemia localizzata (vedi Capitolo 103.3).

La policitemia è stata associata anche a tumori benigni e maligni che producono eritropoietina. Un eccesso di steroidi anabolizzanti esogeni o endogeni può causare anche la policitemia. Le policitemie sono state trasmesse come condizioni dominanti o recessive. In alcune famiglie, c'è un'anomalia del recettore dell'eritropoietina o del gene di von Hippel Lindau.

DIAGNOSI. Indagini sequenziali per valutare la policitemia sono elencati nella Figura 467-1.

TRATTAMENTO. Per la forma lieve, l'osservazione è sufficiente. Quando l'ematocrito è >65-70% (emoglobina >23 g/dL), la viscosità del sangue aumenta marcatamente. Un salasso periodico può prevenire o diminuire i sintomi. Il sangue rimosso dovrebbe essere reintegrato con plasma o soluzione salina, in modo da prevenire l'ipovolemia in pazienti abituati a volumi totali di sangue cronicamente elevati. Un'aumentata richiesta di produzione eritrocitaria può causare un deficit di ferro. I globuli rossi microcitici ferro-carenti sono più rigidi, aumentando poi il rischio di trombosi intracraniche e altre in pazienti con policitemia. Dovrebbero essere realizzate determinazioni periodiche dello stato del ferro, con trattamento della sideropenia.

Cario H: Childhood polycythemias/erythrocytoses: Classification, diagnosis, clinical presentation, and treatment. *Ann Hematol* 2005;84:137–145.

Pappas A, Delaney-Black V: Differential diagnosis and management of polycythemia. *Pediatr Clin North Am* 2004;51:1063–1086.

Percy MJ, McMullin MF, Jowit TT, et al: Chuvash-type congenital polycythemia in 4 families of Asian and Western European ancestry. *Blood* 2003;102:1097–1099.

Prchal JT: Pathogenetic mechanisms of polycythemia vera and congenital polycythemia disorders. *Semin Hematol* 2001;38(Suppl 2):10–20.

Van Maerken T, Hunnick K, Callewaert L, et al: Familial and congenital polycythemias: A diagnostic approach. *J Pediatr Hematol Oncol* 2004;26: 407–416.

Sezione 5 — Pancitopenie

Capitolo 468 ■ Pancitopenie costituzionali Melvin H. Freedman

La **pancitopenia** si riferisce a una riduzione dei valori delle tre linee cellulari del sangue periferico al di sotto dei valori normali: leucociti, piastrine ed eritrociti. La pancitopenia richiede esami microscopici della biopsia del midollo osseo e dell'aspirato midollare per determinare la cellularità completa e la morfologia. Il **midollo ipocellulare** alle biopsie è visibile nelle sindromi da insufficienza midollare costituzionale (ereditarie), nell'anemia aplastica acquisita di diversa eziologia (vedi Capitolo 469) e nella variante ipoplastica della sindrome mielodisplasica (MDS; vedi Capitolo 134). Il **midollo cellulare** è visibile in malattie del midollo osseo primitive: leucemia acuta (vedi Capitolo 495), MDS, mielofibrosi, osteopetrosi (vedi Capitolo 697) e linfoistiocitosi emofagocitica (vedi Capitolo 507). Il midollo cellulare è presente anche secondariamente a malattie sistemiche: autoimmuni (lupus eritematoso sistemico; vedi Capitolo 157), deficit di vitamina B_{12} o di folati (vedi Capitolo 46), malattie da accumulo (malattie di Gaucher e Neimann-Pick; vedi Capitolo 86), infezioni incontrollabili, tumori solidi metastatici, sarcoidosi e ipersplenismo.

LE PANCITOPENIE COSTITUZIONALI

La *pancitopenia costituzionale* è definita come una diminuzione della produzione midollare delle tre principali linee ematopoietiche su base ereditaria, che causa anemia, neutropenia e trombocitopenia. Queste condizioni (Tab. 468-1) possono essere ereditate in modalità mendeliana da geni mutati con schemi autosomici dominanti, autosomici recessivi o legati al cromosoma X. Anche fattori acquisiti possono essere implicati. Le pancitopenie costituzionali riguardano circa un terzo dei casi di insufficienza midollare. L'anemia di Fanconi è la patologia costituzionale più comune.

TABELLA 468-1. Sindromi pancitopeniche costituzionali (ereditarie)

Anemia di Fanconi
Sindrome di Shwachman-Diamond
Discheratosi congenita
Trombocitopenia amegacariocitica
Altre sindromi genetiche
Sindrome di Down
Sindrome di Dubowitz
Sindrome di Seckel
Disgenesia reticolare
Displasia immuno-ossea di Schimke
Anemia aplastica familiare (non-Fanconi)
Sindrome di Pearson
Disgenesia reticolare
Sindrome di Noonan

ANEMIA (APLASTICA) DI FANCONI

Eziologia ed epidemiologia. La sindrome di Fanconi è ereditata in modo autosomico recessivo in quasi tutti i casi; si verifica in ogni gruppo razziale ed etnico. Alla presentazione, i pazienti possono avere: (1) anomalie fisiche tipiche ma reperti ematologici normali; (2) caratteristiche fisiche normali ma anomali reperti ematologici; (3) anomalie fisiche e anomali reperti ematologici, cioè il fenotipo classico (39% dei casi). Ci può essere una lieve discordanza nei reperti clinici ed ematologici, anche in caso di gemelli monozigoti. Circa il 75% dei pazienti ha tra i 3 e i 14 anni al momento della diagnosi (età media, 8-9 anni; range, 0-48 anni).

Anatomia patologica. Tutti i pazienti presentano un'anormale fragilità cromosomica vista nelle preparazioni in metafase dei linfociti del sangue periferico coltivate con fitoemagglutinina e accentuate con l'aggiunta di un agente clastogenico come il **diepossibutano** (DEB). La fusione cellulare delle cellule di Fanconi con quelle normali oppure con le cellule provenienti da soggetti non correlati che hanno l'anemia di Fanconi produce un effetto correttivo sulla fragilità cromosomica, processo chiamato *complementazione*. Questo permette di suddividere i pazienti in gruppi di complementazione distinti. Sono stati identificati dodici gruppi di complementazione, che portano alla clonazione di 11 geni mutanti di Fanconi (*FANC*). I prodotti proteici dei geni *FANC* del ceppo selvaggio sono coinvolti nella via di riparazione biochimica del danno del DNA. Le proteine del gene mutato portano all'instabilità genomica, alla fragilità cromosomica e all'anemia di Fanconi. L'incapacità della cellula di Fanconi di rimuovere i radicali liberi dell'ossigeno, che comporta un danno ossidativo, è un fattore contribuente nella patogenesi. Fattori addizionali sono pure implicati. La lunghezza del telomero leucocitario è significativamente ridotta, ma l'attività della telomerasi è aumentata, suggerendo un tasso di proliferazione dei progenitori midollari elevato che porta alla fine al loro prematuro invecchiamento. Si verifica un aumento dell'apoptosi cellulare midollare mediata da Fas, un recettore glicoproteico di membrana contenente un dominio integrale di morte programmata. Un reperto costante è la diminuzione della produzione dell'interleuchina 6 e un aumento di produzione del TNF α.

Manifestazioni cliniche. L'anomalia più comune è l'iperpigmentazione del tronco, del collo e dell'area intertriginosa, così come macchie color caffellatte e vitiligine, isolate o insieme (Figura 468-1 e Tab. 468-2). La maggior parte dei pazienti presenta una statura bassa. La scarsa crescita può essere associata a un'anomala secrezione dell'ormone della crescita o all'ipotiroidismo. Sono comuni l'assenza del radio e pollici ipoplastici, in sovrannumero, bifidi o assenti. Sono visibili anomalie dei piedi, lussazione congenita

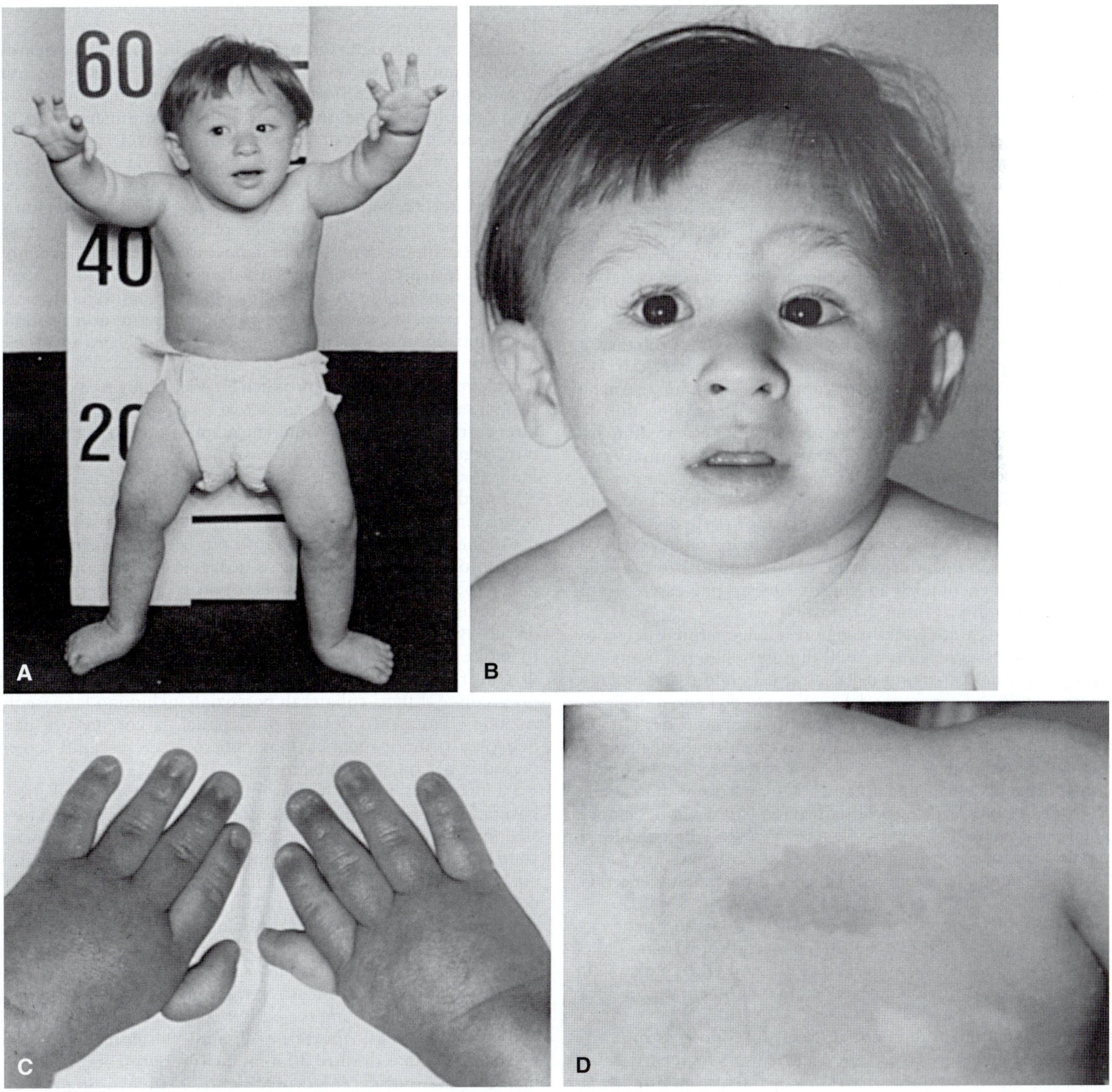

Figura 468-1. Un maschio di 3 anni con anemia di Fanconi che mostra molte caratteristiche fenotipiche classiche. *A*, Vista di fronte. *B*, Faccia. *C*, Mani. *D*, Spalla destra. Le caratteristiche da rilevare includono la statura piccola, lussazione delle anche, microcefalia, base del naso allargata, epicanto, micrognazia, pollici attaccati da un'appendice e macchie caffellatte con al di sotto aree ipopigmentate. (Da Nathan DC, Orkin SH, Ginsburg D, et al [editors]: *Nathan and Oski's Hematology of Infancy and Childhood*, 6th ed., Vol. I. Philadelphia, WB Saunders, 2003, p 285.)

TABELLA 468-2. Anomalie fisiche caratteristiche nell'anemia di Fanconi

ANOMALIA	FREQUENZA APPROSSIMATA (% DEI PAZIENTI)
Discromie cutanee	65
Bassa statura	60
Anomalie dell'arto superiore (pollici, mani, radio, ulna)	50
Alterazioni ipogonadiche e genitali (soprattutto maschi)	40
Altri reperti scheletrici (testa/faccia, collo, colonna vertebrale)	30
Occhio/palpebra/anomalie della piega epicantale	25
Malformazione renale	25
Anomalie delle orecchie (esterne e interne), sordità	10
Anomalie dell'anca, gamba, piede, dito del piede	10
Malformazioni gastrointestinali/cardiopolmonari	10

dell'anca e anomalie degli arti inferiori. I maschi possono avere un pene iposviluppato; testicoli ritenuti, atrofici o assenti; ipospadia o fimosi; le femmine, invece, malformazioni della vagina, dell'utero e dell'ovaio. Molti pazienti presentano la facies da Fanconi, inclusa la microcefalia, gli occhi piccoli, epicanto e anomalie di aspetto, dimensione o posizione delle orecchie (vedi Fig. 468-1). Circa il 10% dei pazienti è mentalmente ritardato. Reni ectopici, pelvici o a ferro di cavallo sono scoperti con le tecniche di imaging, così come organi duplicati, ipolastici, displastici oppure assenti.

Reperti di laboratorio. L'insufficienza midollare in genere esordisce alla prima decade di vita. Inizialmente di solito compare la trombocitopenia, con successivo sviluppo della granulocitopenia e poi dell'**anemia microcitica**. Una grave aplasia si sviluppa nella maggior parte dei casi, ma la sua piena espressione è variabile e insorge dopo un periodo che va da mesi ad anni. Il midollo diventa progressivamente ipocellulare e steatosico, come nelle anemie aplastiche acquisite. La fragilità cromosomica è indicata dal verificarsi spontaneamente di rotture cromatiniche, riarrangiamenti, gap, endoduplicazioni e scambio di cromatina. Anche i fibroblasti cutanei in coltura lo dimostrano, sottolineando la natura costituzionale della patologia. La fragilità è marcatamente più alta nei pazienti rispetto ai controlli se alle colture viene aggiunto il DEB. Rotture cromosomiche anomale possono essere ricreate sulle cellule del liquido amniotico o sulla biopsia dei villi coriali per una diagnosi prenatale. La maggior parte dei pazienti presenta livelli stabili elevati nel siero di α-fetoproteina espressi costitutivamente, indipendentemente dalle complicanze epatiche e da alcune terapie, come gli androgeni. Questo può essere usato come test rapido di screening diagnostico.

Complicanze. La caratteristica maggiore a lungo termine del fenotipo è la predisposizione al tumore. Il tumore solido più frequente è rappresentato dai carcinomi della testa, del collo e dell'esofago superiore, seguiti dai carcinomi della vulva e/o dell'ano o dell'esofago inferiore. Alcuni pazienti presentano neoplasie orali dopo trapianto di midollo osseo. Si verificano neoplasie epatiche maligne e benigne (epatomi, adenomi) e sono in genere associate alla terapia con androgeni dell'anemia aplastica. Gli androgeni sono anche coinvolti nell'eziologia della **peliosis hepatis** (spazi vuoti riempiti di sangue nel fegato). La peliosis hepatis è reversibile quando la terapia androgenica è sospesa e i tumori possono regredire. Circa il 15% dei pazienti con anemia di Fanconi presenta una leucemia acuta o MDS.

Diagnosi. Reperti ematologici anormali e anomalie fisiche caratteristiche suggeriscono la diagnosi, che viene confermata dallo studio della fragilità cromosomica che utilizza il DEB. Nessun'altra pancitopenia costituzionale è associata ad aumentata fragilità cromosomica.

Trattamento. Un ematologo che utilizza un approccio multidisciplinare dovrebbe supervisionare il paziente. Se i reperti ematologici sono stabili e non c'è necessità di trasfusioni è indicata l'osservazione. Consulenze specifiche possono essere programmate in questo intervallo. Se la velocità di crescita è al di sotto delle aspettative, è opportuna una valutazione endocrinologica per identificare un deficit di ormone della crescita o l'ipotiroidismo. L'intolleranza glucosidica e l'iperinsulinemia dovrebbe essere controllata annualmente oppure ogni due anni, a seconda del grado di iperglicemia individuato negli esami iniziali. I pazienti dovrebbero essere esaminati per tumore almeno una volta all'anno.

Il trapianto di cellule staminali ematopoietiche (*Hematopoietic Stem Cell Transplantation*, HSCT; vedi Capitolo 134) è l'unica terapia curativa per le anomalie ematologiche. Un paziente con anemia di Fanconi che viene sottoposto al trapianto con un fratello donatore HLA-identico ha una probabilità di sopravvivenza libera da malattia a 5 anni, che corrisponde a circa il 75%. Per i pazienti che non possiedono un fratello donatore compatibile, dovrebbe essere iniziata una ricerca per un donatore non parente compatibile (inclusa la ricerca nella banca del sangue del cordone ombelicale). A causa della più grave reazione del trapianto contro l'ospite nei pazienti con l'anemia di Fanconi, la percentuale di sopravvivenza e di guarigione non è stata così buona come nell'HSCT con i donatori fratelli compatibili (circa il 30% di sopravvivenza). La tecnologia molecolare ha portato a una diagnosi genetica di preimpianto sui blastomeri di derivazione genitoriale, per trovare fratelli donatori HLA compatibili senza anemia di Fanconi.

La potenzialità della terapia con il fattore (citochina) di crescita ricombinante non è stato definito. Il fattore stimolante colonie granulocitarie (G-CSF) può in genere indurre un aumento nella conta assoluta dei neutrofili e talvolta può aumentare la conta piastrinica e i livelli di emoglobina. Tuttavia, può esserci un rischio aumentato di espansione clonale della cellula midollare con monosomia del cromosoma 7. La terapia combinata con il G-CSF quotidianamente oppure ogni due giorni per via sottocutanea con l'eritropoietina per via sottocutanea o endovenosa tre volte la settimana comporta un aumento della conta dei neutrofili in quasi tutti i pazienti, una crescita sostanziale della conta piastrinica e un miglioramento dei livelli di emoglobina in circa un terzo dei pazienti, che però per la maggior parte non rispondono più dopo un anno, a causa della progressione dell'insufficienza del midollo osseo.

Il ricorso ad androgeni produce un effetto positivo nel 50% dei casi, si manifesta nella reticolocitosi e nell'aumento dell'emoglobina entro 1-2 mesi. La conta leucocitaria può in seguito aumentare, seguita da quella piastrinica, ma possono essere necessari molti mesi per ottenere la risposta massima.

Quando la risposta raggiunge il plateau, gli androgeni possono essere lentamente ridotti ma non completamente sospesi. L'ossimetolone per via orale è utilizzato più frequentemente una volta al giorno. Il prednisone a basso dosaggio per via orale ogni due giorni può essere aggiunto per opporsi all'accelerazione della crescita indotta dagli androgeni e per prevenire il sanguinamento dovuto alla trombocitopenia favorendo la stabilità vascolare. In molti pazienti che stanno assumendo androgeni, la malattia diventa refrattaria a mano a mano che l'insufficienza midollare progredisce. Effetti collaterali potenziali includono la mascolinizzazione e l'aumento degli enzimi epatici, la colestasi, la peliosis hepatis e i tumori epatici. Dovrebbero essere eseguiti screening periodici per questi cambiamenti.

La premessa per la terapia genica nell'anemia di Fanconi è basata sul presupposto che le cellule ematopoietiche corrette possiedono un vantaggio di crescita. I tentativi di terapia genetica sono stati deludenti, possibilmente a causa del tipo di vettore, ma anche a causa della fragilità e della difettosa capacità proliferativa dei progenitori ematopoietici. Dati preclinici incoraggianti che si basano su vettori lentovirali danno la speranza che la terapia genica si rivelerà un trattamento sicuro ed efficace per l'anemia di Fanconi. I trasposoni sono vettori non virali impiegati con successo per il trasferimento genico nei modelli murini e può rappresentare una promessa per gli esseri umani.

Prognosi. Dai casi riportati negli anni '90, la media di sopravvivenza stimata è di oltre 30 anni e ciò rappresenta un miglioramento rispetto al decennio precedente. I successi ottenuti grazie all'HSCT hanno molto migliorato l'aspettativa di vita. Anche un controllo attento per individuare le complicanze conosciute, in particolare i tumori, e l'intervento tempestivo hanno contribuito ad aumentare il tasso di sopravvivenza.

SINDROME DI SHWACHMAN-DIAMOND.

Eziologia ed epidemiologia. La sindrome di Shwachman-Diamond (*Shwachman-Diamond Syndrome*, SDS) è ereditata in maniera autosomica recessiva; si verifica in tutti i gruppi etnici e razziali. I criteri diagnostici essenziali sono rappresentati dall'insufficienza pancreatica esocrina e da citopenie ematologiche variabili causate dall'insufficienza midollare (vedi Capitolo 346). I cromosomi sono normali e non è presente un aumento delle rotture in seguito allo stress test clastogenico al DEB.

Patologia. Il gene mutato *SBDS* mappa sul cromosoma 7q11 ed è responsabile del fenotipo multisistemico pleiotropico nel 90% dei casi. Il prodotto della proteina del gene del ceppo selvaggio è coinvolto nel metabolismo del RNA e/o nella biogenesi dei ribosomi. L'insufficienza pancreatica è dovuta all'insufficiente sviluppo degli acini pancreatici. La sostituzione grassa del tessuto pancreatico è notevole. L'insufficienza midollare è caratterizzata da una disfunzione generalizzata della cellula midollare e del microambiente che non supporta e mantiene la normale ematopoiesi.

Manifestazioni cliniche. Anche se la maggior parte dei pazienti mostra sintomi di malassorbimento dei grassi fin dalla nascita a causa dell'insufficienza pancreatica, l'assenza della steatorrea non esclude una diagnosi di SDS. Circa il 50% dei pazienti sembra mostrare un modesto miglioramento nella secrezione degli enzimi pancreatici con l'aumentare dell'età. La bassa statura è una caratteristica importante della sindrome; la maggior parte dei pazienti mostra una velocità di crescita normale, ma che rimane notevolmente inferiore al 3° percentile per altezza e peso. L'adulto occasionalmente raggiunge il 25° percentile di altezza. L'aspetto clinico può essere dominato dalle complicanze della citopenia ematologica. La pancitopenia è diagnosticata all'età media di 7 anni e mezzo (range, 0-35 anni). Possono verificarsi infezioni batteriche e fungine secondarie a neutropenia e disfunzione neutrofila e immunodeficienza. Anche se le anomalie scheletriche sono variabili, reperti classici sono un ritardo di maturazione ossea, displasia delle metafisi ossee, coste piccole o brillanti, distrofia toracica e pollice bifido. La maggior parte dei pazienti presenta anomalie dentali e scarsa salute orale e molti hanno problemi neurocognitivi nonché scarse capacità sociali.

Reperti di laboratorio. La neutropenia è presente in tutti i pazienti virtualmente in almeno un'occasione. Essa può essere cronica, ciclica o intermittente. È stata identificata in alcuni neonati durante un episodio di sepsi. L'anemia, la trombocitopenia e la pancitopenia sono viste nel 66, 60 e 40% dei casi, rispettivamente. La pancitopenia può essere grave, come risultato dell'anemia aplastica completamente espressa. I campioni di biopsia del midollo osseo e gli aspirati in genere mostrano vari livelli di ipoplasia midollare e steatosi. La steatosi pancreatica può essere visualizzata alla TC o all'ecografia. Il malassorbimento dei grassi è confermato dal bilancio dei grassi fecali per 72 ore. Gli studi di funzionalità pancreatica mostrano una marcata compromissione della secrezioine enzimatica, ma la pervietà duttale è conservata. I livelli sierici di tripsinogeno e di isoamilasi sono ridotti. I neutrofili possono mostrare un marcato difetto nella mobilità, migrazione, e chemiotassi a causa di alterazioni nel citoscheletro del neutrofilo o della funzione microtubulare. I pazienti possono anche presentare uno o più dei seguenti difetti delle cellule B: basse immunoglobuline G o sottoclassi di immunoglobuline G, bassa percentuale di linfociti B circolanti, diminuzione della proliferazione *in vitro* delle cellule B e mancanza di produzione di anticorpi specifici. Si può anche registrare una bassa percentuale di cellule T circolanti, sottopopolazioni, o cellule natural killer, e diminuzione della proliferazione *in vitro* delle cellule T.

Diagnosi. L'analisi delle mutazioni dell'*SBDS* è definitiva nel 90% dei casi. La **sindrome di Pearson** (anemia sideroblastica refrattaria, vacuolizzazione citoplasmatica dei precursori midollari, acidosi metabolica, mutazioni del DNA mitocondriale e insufficienza pancreatica esocrina) è simile alla SDS, ma il decorso clinico e le caratteristiche morfologiche del midollo osseo sono differenti. L'anemia grave che richiede trasfusioni, diversamente dalla neutropenia, è presente dalla nascita fino al 1° anno di età. I pazienti con sindrome di Pearson mostrano anomalie del DNA mitocondriale (mtDNA). La SDS condivide alcune manifestazioni dell'anemia di Fanconi, come una disfunzione midollare e scarsa crescita, ma i pazienti con SDS sono facilmente distinguibili per: insufficienza pancreatica con malassorbimento dei grassi; steatosi del corpo pancreatico, che può essere visualizzata attraverso le tecniche di imaging; anomalie caratteristiche scheletriche non presenti nell'anemia di Fanconi; risultati normali al test di stress clastogenico al DEB.

Complicanze. I pazienti con SDS sono predisposti alle MDS e alla trasformazione leucemica. L'incidenza di MDS o di leucemia acuta nei pazienti con SDS è dell'8-33%. Il cambiamento clonale è spesso accompagnato all'isocromosoma 7 [i(7q)] nelle cellule midollari. Questo è particolarmente comune e suggerisce che ci sia un chiaro e specifico marker clonale della SDS probabilmente collegato alla presenza del gene mutato per la SDS sul cromosoma 7q11. Altre anomalie cromosomiche clonali includono la monosomia del 7, la i(7q) unita alla monosomia del 7, delezioni o traslocazioni che coinvolgono parte del 7q e le delezioni del 20q (20q).

Trattamento. Il malassorbimento dei grassi risponde alla somministrazione di enzimi pancreatici e ai supplementi di vitamine liposolubili, secondo linee guida simili a quelle della fibrosi cistica (vedi Capitolo 400). Un programma a lungo termine dovrebbe essere iniziato per monitorare i cambiamenti dell'esame emocromocitometrico che richiede un'azione correttiva e per individuare precocemente una trasformazione maligna mieloide. Quest'ultima richiede aspirati del midollo osseo seriati per la morfologia e le analisi citogenetica, oltre alla biopsia midollare. È raccomandata l'esecuzione dei test midollari ogni anno.

Il G-CSF giornaliero sottocutaneo per la grave neutropenia è efficace nell'indurre un sostanziale aumento dei neutrofili. Alcuni pazienti richiedono un supporto trasfusionale per gestire l'anemia grave o la trombocitopenia. L'esperienza con l'eritropoietina è limitata. Un piccolo numero di pazienti è stato trattato con i corticosteroidi, con un miglioramento sul piano ematologico in circa il 50% dei casi. Alcuni pazienti che hanno ricevuto androgeni e steroidi hanno migliorato l'emocromocitometrico. L'unica possibilità di trattamento per l'insufficienza midollare severa nella SDS è l'HSCT allogenico, sebbene l'esperienza sia limitata. Circa il 50% dei pazienti con SDS trapiantati è morto per le complicanze collegate al condizionamento per HSCT. È stato riportato un rischio di cardiotossicità.

Prognosi. Circa il 50% dei pazienti corregge spontaneamente l'insufficienza pancreatica in un livello di funzione sufficiente grazie al miglioramento della secrezione enzimatica pancreatica. La terapia sostitutiva enzimatica non è più necessaria. Sebbene tutti i pazienti evidenzino un qualche grado di citopenia periferica, questa nella maggior parte dei soggetti è lieve-moderata e non richiede interventi terapeutici. Una neutropenia grave risponde bene al G-CSF, ma esiste il problema che la predisposizione alle MDS e alle leucemie acute può essere aumentata da uno stimolo di crescita potente alle cellule midollari. L'HSCT per l'insufficienza midollare grave ottiene un tasso di sopravvivenza del 50%. La trasformazione midollare maligna è infausta.

DISCHERATOSI CONGENITA

Eziologia ed epidemiologia. La discheratosi congenita (DC) è una patologia ereditaria del sistema mucocutaneo ed ematopoietico associata ad anomalie somatiche. La triade ectodermica diagnostica è rappresentata dalla pigmentazione reticolare della parte superiore del corpo, dalla leucoplachia mucosa e dalla distrofia ungueale (vedi Fig. 468-2). I reperti cutanei e ungueali in genere diventano evidenti nei primi 10 anni di vita, mentre la leucoplachia orale si verifica più tardi. Queste manifestazioni tendono a progredire mano a mano che il paziente cresce. La DC è una pancitopenia costituzionale; l'anemia aplastica si verifica in circa il 50% dei casi, in genere nella seconda decade di vita. I pazienti presentano anche una predisposizione ai tumori e alle MDS. Circa l'85% dei pazienti è di sesso maschile, compatibile con l'ereditarietà recessiva legata all'X. Circa il 15% dei pazienti sembra possedere la modalità di ereditarietà autosomica dominante o recessiva.

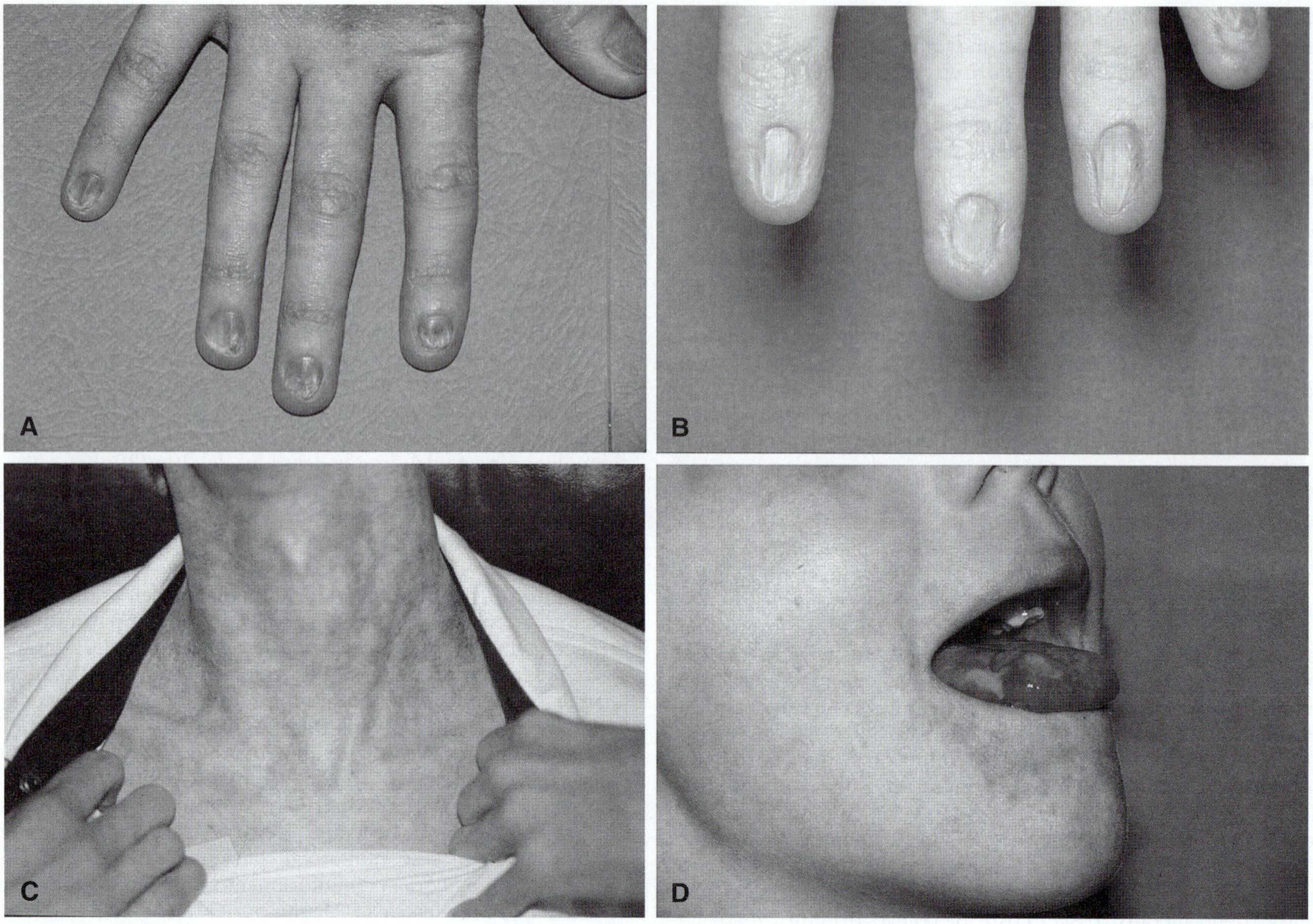

Figura 468-2. Reperti fisici in pazienti con discheratosi congenita. *A* e *B*, Unghie distrofiche in due diversi pazienti. *C*, Pigmentazione reticolare merlettata. *D*, Leucoplachia sulla lingua. (Da Nathan DG, Orkin SH, Ginsburg D, et al [editors]: *Nathan and Oski's Hematology of Infancy and Childhood*, 6th ed., Vol. I. Philadelphia, WB Saunders, 2003, p 300.)

Patologia. La forma di DC X-recessiva è mappata sul cromosoma Xq28, e sono state identificate molte mutazioni nel gene *DKC1*, che codifica per la proteina nucleare discherina, la quale può essere coinvolta nell'assemblaggio ribosomiale e nella produzione dell'RNA. La forma autosomica dominante è dovuta a mutazioni del gene *TERC* che codifica per componenti della RNA telomerasi che sono responsabili del mantenimento del telomero. Sono stati dimostrati telomeri corti nel sangue periferico dei pazienti con forme autosomiche dominanti e recessive legate all'X che rappresentano indicatori di insufficienza midollare. Il gene mutato autosomico recessivo non è stato identificato. L'insufficienza midollare può essere legata a progressiva usura e deplezione di cellule staminali, che si manifesta come pancitopenia. In alternativa, la disfunzione midollare può rappresentare un'insufficiente replicazione e/o maturazione delle cellule staminali.

Manifestazioni cliniche. Pigmentazioni cutanee e alterazioni ungueali compaiono caratteristicamente per prime, leucoplachia mucosa ed eccessiva lacrimazione oculare fanno la comparsa in seguito, e nella prima adolescenza insorgono insufficienza midollare e neoplasie maligne. Molte femmine mostrano le stesse caratteristiche dei maschi, ma nei maschi i reperti cutanei rappresentano la caratteristica più importante. Una pigmentazione cutanea merlettata reticolata a carico del volto, del collo, del torace e delle braccia è un reperto comune (89%). Il grado di pigmentazione aumenta con l'età e può coinvolgere l'intera superficie cutanea. Ci può anche essere una componente eritemato-teleangectasica. La distrofia ungueale delle mani e dei piedi è il reperto più comune (88%). In genere inizia con solcature longitudinali, fessurazione, formazione di uno pterigium e può progredire fino alla completa perdita ungueale. La leucoplachia in genere coinvolge la mucosa orale (78%), soprattutto la lingua, ma anche la congiuntiva e la mucosa anale, uretrale o genitale. L'iperidrosi del palmo della mano e della pianta dei piedi è comune e talvolta è presente la caduta dei capelli. Anomalie oculari sono osservate in circa il 50% dei casi. Una lacrimazione eccessiva (epifora) secondaria a ostruzione del dotto nasolacrimale è comune. Altre manifestazioni oftalmologiche includono congiuntiviti, blefariti, perdita delle ciglia, strabismo, cataratte e atrofia ottica. Un aumento della frequenza di caduta precoce dei denti e carie dentali sono comuni. Anomalie scheletriche, come osteoporosi, necrosi avascolare, anomalie della trabecolazione ossea, scoliosi, ipoplasia mandibolare sono presenti in circa il 20% dei casi. Le anomalie genitourinarie includono testicoli ipoplastici, ipospadia, fimosi, stenosi uretrali e rene a ferro di cavallo. I reperti gastrointestinali, come stenosi esofagee, epatomegalia o cirrosi, sono presenti nel 10% dei casi. Un piccolo gruppo di pazienti presenta complicanze polmonari, con una ridotta capacità di diffusione dell'ossigeno e/o difetti restrittivi. Nei casi mortali, il tessuto polmonare mostra fibrosi polmonare e anomalie della vascolarizzazione polmonare.

Reperti di laboratorio. L'alterazione ematologica inziale è in genere la trombocitopenia, l'anemia o entrambe, seguite da una completa pancitopenia causata dall'anemia aplastica. I globuli rossi sono spesso macrocitici e l'emoglobina fetale può essere inizialmente elevata. Le biopsie del midollo osseo possono essere ipercellulari, ma con il tempo compare una diminuzione simmetrica di tutte le linee ematopoietiche.

Alcuni pazienti presentano anomalie immunologiche, inclusi livelli ridotti o elevati delle immunoglobuline, ridotta conta dei linfociti B e/o T, e assente risposta proliferativi alle fitoemagglutinine. Non c'è differenza significativa nelle rotture cromosomiche nei linfociti stimolati con mitogeni con o senza esposizione al

DEB o alla mitomicina C tra pazienti e controlli. Comunque i fibroblasti cutanei in coltura presentano caratteristiche morfologiche anomale e frequenza di duplicazioni e mostrano numerosi riarrangiamenti cromosomici sbilanciati, come cromosomi dicentrici, tricentrici e traslocazioni in assenza di un agente clastogenico. Questi reperti producono evidenza di un difetto che predispone le cellule del paziente ai riarrangiamenti e al possibile danno al DNA.

Diagnosi. Le seguenti anomalie sono presenti nei pazienti con la DC ma non in quelli con l'anemia di Fanconi: distrofia ungueale, leucoplachia, anomalie dentali, iperidrosi del palmo delle mani o della pianta dei piedi e perdita dei capelli. Ci sono sindromi da sovrapposizione che condividono alcune delle caratteristiche della DC. La **sindrome di Hoyerall-Hreidarsson** è una patologia multisistemica che colpisce i ragazzi con anemia aplastica, immunodeficienza, microcefalia, ritardo della crescita, e ipoplasia cerebellare. La sindrome è causata dalla mutazione del gene DKC1 e quindi è una variante della DC. La **sindrome di Revesz** consiste di unghie distrofiche, leucoplachia, anemia aplastica, ipoplasia cerebellare, ritardo di crescita, microcefalia e retinopatia essudativa bilaterale. La mutazione non è stata identificata.

Complicanze. Il cancro si sviluppa in circa il 10-15% dei pazienti, in genere nella 3ª e 4ª decade di vita. I pazienti con DC sono predisposti alle MDS così come ai tumori solidi. La maggior parte dei tumori è costituita da carcinomi a cellule squamose o da adenocarcinomi, e l'orofaringe e il tratto gastrointestinale sono coinvolti più frequentemente.

Trattamento. Gli androgeni, di solito combinati con il prednisone in basse dosi, possono indurre un miglioramento della funzione midollare in circa il 50% dei pazienti. Quando la risposta è massima, la dose degli androgeni può essere lentamente ridotta, ma non sospesa. I pazienti possono diventare refrattari agli androgeni a mano a mano che l'anemia aplastica progredisce. Non esistono informazioni in letteratura sull'utilizzo della terapia immunosoppressiva in questa patologia. Anche se i casi riportati sono scarsi, la terapia citochinica con il fattore stimolante le colonie granulocito-macrofagiche o con il G-CSF da solo o con l'eritropoietina sembra offrire potenziali benefici, almeno a breve termine, soprattutto aumentando il numero dei neutrofili.

L'HSCT allogenico è stato utilizzato per correggere l'insufficienza midollare, con un tasso di sopravvivenza del 50%. Le lesioni vascolari e le fibrosi che coinvolgono diversi organi si verificano sia nel periodo precoce sia in quello tardivo dopo il trapianto e comportano un elevato tasso di mortalità. I pazienti con DC possono essere più suscettibili al danno endoteliale che si verifica dopo HSCT, come risultato di diversi fattori, inclusi il regime di condizionamento, le patologie infettive e la reazione del trapianto contro l'ospite. Fino al 40% dei pazienti con DC va incontro a complicanze polmonari precoci e tardive mortali dopo il trapianto. Fattori addizionali con effetti negativi dopo HSCT sono il lieve grado di instabilità cromosomica nella DC con una predisposizione al riarrangiamento cromosomico e il peculiare accorciamento dei telomeri che caratterizza la DC, insieme con l'accorciamento accelerato dei telomeri che si verifica dopo HSCT.

Sebbene i geni mutati per le forme recessive legate all'X e per le autosomiche dominanti siano noti, i presupposti per una terapia genica non sono ancora vicini.

Prognosi. I pazienti con malattia autosomica dominante presentano manifestazioni più lievi; quelli con malattia autosomica recessiva sembrano avere più anomalie fisiche e un'incidenza più elevata di anemia aplastica e tumore. L'età media di morte per i pazienti con la DC è di circa 30 anni e le principali cause sono l'insufficienza midollare, le complicanze dell'HSCT, il tumore e i problemi polmonari fatali.

TROMBOCITOPENIA AMEGACARIOCITICA

Eziologia ed epidemiologia. La trombocitopenia amegacariocitica congenita (*Congenital Amegakaryocytic Thrombocytopenia*, CAT o CAMT) è la più rara delle quattro maggiori pancitopenie costituzionali. È ereditata in maniera autosomica recessiva. La CAT si presenta nell'infanzia con una trombocitopenia isolata dovuta a magacariociti midollari ridotti o assenti, con conservazione iniziale delle linee granulocitopoietiche ed eritroidi. La pancitopenia dovuta all'**anemia aplastica** si completa successivamente in circa il 45% dei pazienti; l'età media all'esordio è 3-5 anni (range, 0,4-12,5 anni). Il difetto nella CAT è direttamente correlato alle mutazioni nel gene per il recettore trombopoietinico *c-mpl*, che mappa sul cromosoma 1p35. I portatori del difetto genetico hanno caratteristiche ematologiche normali; gli individui affetti presentano mutazioni in entrambi gli alleli. Senza la funzione del recettore che si vede nelle mutazioni del *c-mpl* frameshift o nonsense, l'effetto promuovente la crescita della trombopoietina è abolito e cessano così la crescita e lo sviluppo dei megacariociti. Poiché la trombopoietina ha anche un effetto antiapoptotico sulle cellule staminali, la compromissione della sopravvivenza della cellula staminale rende ragione dell'evoluzione della CAT nell'anemia aplastica. Le mutazioni missense del *c-mpl* sono associate a un decorso più lieve. I livelli di trombopoietina plasmatici nei pazienti con la CAT sono costantemente elevati e il materiale immunoreattivo ritrovato mantiene la piena attività biologica.

Manifestazioni cliniche. I pazienti presentano rash petecchiali, lividi e sanguinamento alla nascita o nel corso del primo anno di vita. Circa il 50% dei pazienti presentano **anomalie fisiche** caratteristiche; gli altri hanno un aspetto fisico e di imaging normale. Alcuni familiari presentano reperti fisici sia normali sia anormali nella stessa famiglia. Le anomalie più comuni sono quelle neurologiche e cardiache. I reperti correlati all'atrofia cerebellare e cerebrale sono frequenti, e il ritardo dello sviluppo è una caratteristica importante. I pazienti possono anche presentare microcefalia e facies anomala. Si verificano cardiopatie congenite, inclusi i difetti settali atriali, i difetti settali ventricolari, pervietà del dotto arterioso, tetralogia di Fallot e coartazione dell'aorta, alcune di queste in combinazione. Altre anomalie includono anomalie di anche o piedi, malformazioni renali, anomalie oculari e un palato con schisi o ogivale.

Reperti di laboratorio. La trombocitopenia è il maggiore reperto di laboratorio, inizialmente con livelli di emoglobina e conta dei globuli bianchi normali. Le piastrine del sangue periferico sono ridotte o completamente assenti. Come in altre sindromi ereditarie di insufficienza midollare, i globuli rossi possono essere macrocitici. L'emoglobina F può essere elevata e può esserci un'aumentata espressione dell'antigene i. Gli aspirati midollari e i preparati bioptici mostrano una cellularità normale, con megacariociti marcatamente ridotti o assenti. Nei pazienti che hanno un'anemia aplastica, la cellularità midollare è ridotta con steatosi; le linee eritroidi e granulocitarie sono anche simmetricamente ridotte.

Diagnosi. Se la CAT insorge dopo il periodo neonatale, sono la biopsia e l'aspirato midollare a portare alla diagnosi, che può essere confermata dall'analisi mutazionale. Se la CAT si presenta alla nascita o poco dopo, deve essere distinta dalle altre cause di trombocitopenia neonatale acquisite o ereditarie (vedi Capitolo 484). Un'aumentata distruzione delle piastrine si verifica anche nei neonati con emangiomi giganti benigni della cute, del fegato o della milza-sindrome di Kasabach-Merritt (vedi Capitolo 505).

Complicanze. In alcuni pazienti, la CAT evolve in leucemia. Il rischio di incidenza della trasformazione maligna è difficile da stabilire per la rarità della patologia e la scarsità dei dati pubblicati.

Terapia e prognosi. La mortalità nei pazienti con mutazioni del *c-mpl* frameshift o nonsense per sanguinamento trombocitopenico, per le complicanze dell'anemia aplastica o per la trasformazione mieloide maligna è stata molto vicina al 100%. L'HSCT è l'unica opzione di trattamento. La maggior parte dei pazienti con la CAT che riceve l'HSCT guarisce. La trasfusione piastrinica pretrapianto dovrebbe essere utilizzata con discrezione. La conta piastrinica non dovrebbe essere la sola indicazione; il sanguinamento clinico è un motivo più appropriato. Si preferiscono le piastrine filtrate da un unico donatore per ridurre la sensibilizzazione e, se l'HSCT è una possibilità, tutti i prodotti trasfusionali dovrebbero essere privi di

Cytomegalovirus. I corticosteroidi non sembrano efficaci per il trattamento della trombocitopenia. Per l'anemia aplastica, gli androgeni insieme con i corticosteroidi possono indurre una risposta temporanea parziale, ma l'effetto è di breve durata e non previene la mortalità. Dati sperimentali suggeriscono che l'interleuchina 3 possa essere un'importante aggiunta alla gestione medica della CAT. La trombopoietina non è stata testata nel trattamento della CAT e potrebbe fallire, perché i livelli endogeni di trombopoietina sono marcatamente aumentati e la forma di CAT autosomica recessiva presenta il recettore *c-mpl* mutato.

ALTRE SINDROMI GENETICHE

L'insufficienza del midollo osseo si verifica in moltissime sindromi non ematologiche, come anche in ambiti familiari che non corrispondono esattamente alle entità finora descritte.

SINDROME DI DOWN. La sindrome di Down (vedi Capitolo 81), o trisomia 21, presenta una tipica associazione con reperti ematologici anormali. Oltre alla predisposizione per le leucemie acute linfoblastiche e mieloblastiche, sono stati riportati pochi casi di pazienti con la pancitopenia causata dall'anemia aplastica.

SINDROME DI DUBOWITZ. La sindrome di Dubowitz è una patologia autosomica recessiva caratterizzata da una facies peculiare, eczema infantile, piccola statura e lieve microcefalia. Il viso è piccolo, con una bassa cresta sovraorbitaria, naso schiacciato allo stesso livello della fronte, rime piccole palpebrali, ptosi variabile e micrognazia. Predisposizione al tumore e alla disfunzione del midollo osseo si evidenzia in questi pazienti. Circa il 10% presenta patologie ematopoietiche, incluse anemia ipoplastica, moderata pancitopenia e anemia aplastica completa.

SINDROME DI SECKEL. La sindrome di Seckel, qualche volta chiamata "nanismo con testa di uccello", è una patologia autosomica recessiva dello sviluppo caratterizzata da un'importante deficit di crescita e ritardo mentale, microcefalia, faccia ipoplasica con naso prominente e orecchie malformate e/o con attaccatura bassa. Circa il 25% dei pazienti presenta anemia aplastica o tumori maligni. Un locus per la sindrome è mappato sul 3q22.1-q24. Un secondo locus mappa sul 18p11.31-q11.2, fatto che dimostra un'eterogeneità genetica.

DISGENESIA RETICOLARE. La disgenesia reticolare (vedi Capitolo 125) è una sindrome da immunodeficienza correlata ad agranulocitosi congenita. La modalità di ereditarietà è probabilmente autosomica recessiva, ma in alcuni casi è possibile anche una modalità legata all'X. La patologia è una variante dell'immunodeficienza combinata in cui l'immunità cellulo-mediata e umorale è assente e i pazienti mostrano inoltre una severa linfopenia e neutropenia, e possono anche essere presenti l'anemia e la trombocitopenia. I preparati del midollo osseo sono ipocellulari, con elementi linfoidi e mieloidi marcatamente ridotti. L'unica terapia curativa è l'HSCT.

DISPLASIA IMMUNO-OSSEA DI SCHIMKE. La displasia immuno-ossea di Schimke è una patologia autosomica recessiva causata da mutazioni nel rimodellamento cromatinico della proteina SMARCAL1. I pazienti hanno una displasia spondiloepifiseale con una lordosi lombare esagerata e un addome prominente. Ci sono alterazioni pigmentarie della cute e denti anomali per colore e posizione. La disfunzione renale può essere problematica, con proteinuria e sindrome nefrosica. Circa il 50% dei pazienti presenta ipotiroidismo, il 50% ischemia cerebrale e il 10% presenta insufficienza del midollo osseo con neutropenia, trombocitopenia e anemia. La linfopenia e l'alterata immunità cellulare sono presenti in quasi tutti i pazienti. In un caso pubblicato, un paziente è stato sottoposto a un trapianto di midollo osseo con successo.

ANEMIA APLASTICA FAMILIARE. L'insufficienza del midollo osseo può raggrupparsi nelle famiglie, ma molti di questi casi non possono essere rapidamente classificati in entità diagnostiche distinte, come l'anemia di Fanconi. Il fenotipo di queste condizioni può essere complesso, con diverse combinazioni di anormalità ematologiche, immunodeficienza, malformazioni fisiche e predisposizione alla leucemia. Sono state osservate entrambe le ereditarietà autosomiche dominanti e autosomiche recessive; entrambi i pattern si verificano con o senza anomalie fisiche associate. Un tipo X-dipendente è descritto con anomalie fisiche; inoltre, la sindrome linfoproliferativa legata all'X, virus di Epstein Barr correlato, si associa alla pancitopenia.

Alter BP: Inherited bone marrow failure syndromes. In Nathan DG, Orkin SH, Ginsburg D, et al (editors): *Hematology of Infancy and Childhood*, 6th ed. Philadelphia, WB Saunders, 2003, pp 280–365.

Dokal I: Dyskeratosis congenita in all its forms. *Br J Haematol* 2000;110: 768–779.

Dror Y, Freedman, MH: Shwachman-Diamond syndrome. *Br J Haematol* 2002;118:701–713.

Freedman MH: Inherited forms of bone marrow failure. In Hoffman R, Benz EJ, Shattil SJ, et al (editors): *Hematology: Basic Principles and Practice*, 5th ed. Philadelphia, Elsevier Churchill Livingstone, 2007, in press.

Kuijpers TW, Nannenberg E, Alders M, et al: Congenital aplastic anemia caused by mutations in the SBDS gene: A rare presentation of Shwachman-Diamond syndrome. *Pediatrics* 2004;114:e387–e391.

Landmann E, Bluetters-Sawatzki R, Schindler D, et al: Fanconi anemia in a neonate with pancytopenia. *J Pediatr* 2004;145:125–127.

Levitus M, Joenje H, de Winter JP: The Fanconi anemia pathway of genomic maintenance. *Cell Oncol* 2006;28:3–29.

Lieberman L, Dror Y: Advances in understanding the genetic basis for bone-marrow failure. *Curr Opin Pediatr* 2006;18:15–21.

Mathew CG: Fanconi anaemia genes and susceptibility to cancer. *Oncogene* 2006;25:5875–5884.

Tischkowitz M, Dokal I: Fanconi anaemia and leukaemia: Clinical and molecular aspects. *Br J Haematol* 2004;126:176–191.

Vulliamy T, Dokal I: Dyskeratosis congenita. *Semin Hematol* 2006;43: 157–166.

Xia B, Dorsman JC, Ameziane N, et al: Fanconi anemia is associated with a defect in the BRCA2 partner PALB2. *Nat Genet* 2007;39:159–161.

Capitolo 469 ■ Pancitopenie acquisite

Jeffrey D. Hord

EZIOLOGIA ED EPIDEMIOLOGIA. Farmaci, prodotti chimici, tossine, agenti infettivi possono portare a una pancitopenia, attraverso la distruzione diretta dei progenitori ematopoietici e del microambiente del midollo o la soppressione immunomediata degli elementi midollari (Tab. 469-1). Dovrebbe essere ottenuta da ciascun bambino che si presenta con pancitopenia un'attenta anamnesi dell'esposizione ai fattori di rischio conosciuti. Anche in assenza dei classici reperti fisici associati, la possibilità di una predisposizione genetica all'insufficienza del midollo osseo dovrebbe essere sempre considerata (vedi Capitolo 468). La maggior parte dei casi di insufficienza midollare acquisita nell'infanzia è "idiopatica" e non ne è identificato alcun agente causale. C'è probabilmente una distruzione dei progenitori midollari immunomediata attraverso i linfociti T attivati e le citochine. L'incidenza totale dell'anemia aplastica acquisita è relativamente bassa, con un'incidenza approssimativa sia nei bambini sia negli adulti, negli Stati Uniti e in Europa, di 2-6 casi/milione/anno. L'incidenza è più alta in Asia, con 14 casi/milione/anno in Giappone.

Una severa soppressione del midollo osseo può svilupparsi dopo l'esposizione a molti farmaci differenti e prodotti chimici, inclusi alcuni agenti chemioterapici, insetticidi, antibiotici, anticonvulsivanti e agenti antinfiammatori non steroidei. Alcuni

TABELLA 469-1. Eziologia dell'anemia aplastica acquisita

FARMACI RADIANTI E PRODOTTI CHIMICI
Prevedibile: chemioterapia, benzene
Idiosincrasica: cloramfenicolo, antiepilettici, oro
VIRUS
Cytomegalovirus
Epstein-Barr
Epatite B
Epatite C
Epatite non-A, non-B, non-C (epatiti sieronegative)
Immunodeficienza umana (HIV)
MALATTIE IMMUNITARIE
Fascite eosinofila
Ipoimmunoglobulinemia
Timoma
GRAVIDANZA
EMOGLOBINURIA PAROSSISTICA NOTTURNA
SOSTITUZIONE MIDOLLARE
Leucemia
Mielodisplasia
Mielofibrosi
PATOLOGIE AUTOIMMUNI
ALTRE
Discheratosi congenita criptica (non stigmate fisiche)
Aploinsufficienza della trascrittasi inversa telomerasica

degli agenti più noti sono il benzene, il cloramfenicolo e l'oro. La severità e la durata della pancitopenia dipende dall'entità dell'esposizione a tali agenti. Una predisposizione genetica può esistere e può aumentare la probabilità della pancitopenia dopo esposizione.

Un certo numero di virus può direttamente o indirettamente comportare un'insufficienza del midollo osseo. Il parvovirus B19 è tipicamente associato all'aplasia isolata della serie rossa, ma in pazienti con emoglobinopatia a cellule falciformi o con immunodeficienza può portare a una pancitopenia transitoria (vedi Capitoli 248 e 462). Una pancitopenia prolungata può verificarsi dopo l'infezione con molti dei virus delle epatiti, gli herpes virus, il virus di Epstein Barr (vedi Capitolo 251), il Cytomegalovirus (vedi Capitolo 252) e l'HIV (vedi Capitolo 273).

I pazienti con segni di insufficienza del midollo osseo dovrebbero essere valutati anche per l'emoglobinuria parossistica notturna (*Paroxysmal Nocturnal Hemoglobinuria*, PNH; vedi Capitolo 461) e le connettiviti associate a vasculiti, sebbene queste siano cause poco comuni di pancitopenia nell'infanzia. La pancitopenia senza blasti periferici può essere causata dalla sostituzione del midollo osseo con blasti leucemici o cellule del neuroblastoma.

ANATOMIA PATOLOGICA E PATOGENESI. Il carattere distintivo dell'anemia aplastica è la pancitopenia periferica, associata a midollo osseo ipoplastico o aplastico. La gravità del decorso clinico è legata al livello di mielosoppressione. L'**anemia aplastica grave** è definita come una condizione in cui due o più componenti cellulari sono seriamente compromesse (conta assoluta dei neutrofili [*Absolute Neutrophil Count*, ANC] $<500/mm^3$, conta piastrinica $<20\,000/mm^3$, conta reticolocitaria $<1\%$ dopo la correzione per l'ematocrito) in un paziente il cui materiale bioptico midollare è moderatamente o gravemente ipocellulare. Circa due terzi dei pazienti che si presentano inizialmente con una **forma più moderata di anemia aplastica** (ANC 500-1500/mm^3, conta piastrinica 20 000-100 000/mm^3, conta reticolocitaria $<1\%$) e che vengono osservati progrediranno probabilmente fino a soddisfare i criteri per la forma grave. L'insufficienza del midollo osseo può essere una conseguenza di un effetto diretto citotossico sulle cellule staminali ematopoietiche, dovuto a un farmaco o un prodotto chimico o può conseguire dalla citotossicità cellulo-mediata o anticorpo dipendente. C'è una forte evidenza che molti casi di anemia aplastica idiopatica siano causati da un processo immuno-mediato, con un aumento dei linfociti T attivati circolanti producenti citochine (interferone-α) che sopprimono l'ematopoiesi. Una ridotta lunghezza dei telomeri nei precursori granulocitici e un'aumentata espressione sulla superficie cellulare del ligando Flt3 (un membro della classe III recettoriale della famiglia delle tirosinchinasi) nei linfociti dei pazienti con anemia aplastica suggeriscono che l'apoptosi precoce dei progenitori ematopoietici possa giocare un ruolo nella patogenesi della malattia.

MANIFESTAZIONI CLINICHE, REPERTI DI LABORATORIO E DIAGNOSI DIFFERENZIALE. La pancitopenia comporta un aumentato rischio di insufficienza cardiaca, infezioni, sanguinamento e affaticamento. La pancitopenia acquisita è tipicamente caratterizzata da anemia, leucopenia e trombocitopenia in un contesto di livelli elevati di citochine sieriche. Altre patologie trattabili, come le neoplasie, le patologie vascolari del collagene, la PNH o le infezioni che possono rispondere a terapie specifiche (immunoglobuline per via endovenosa per il parvovirus), dovrebbero essere considerate nella diagnosi differenziale. Un esame attento dello striscio di sangue periferico per la morfologia di globuli rossi, leucociti e piastrine è importante. Dovrebbe essere effettuata una conta reticolocitaria per determinare l'attività eritropoietica midollare. Nei bambini, la possibilità di una pancitopenia congenita deve sempre essere considerata, come anche si dovrebbe eseguire l'analisi per la fragilità cromosomica per valutare l'anemia di Fanconi (vedi Capitolo 468). La presenza di emoglobina fetale potrebbe suggerire una pancitopenia congenita, ma non è diagnostica. Per determinare la possibilità della PNH, l'analisi citometrica a flusso degli eritrociti per il CD48 e il CD59 è il test più sensibile. L'esame del midollo osseo dovrebbe includere sia l'aspirato sia la biopsia e il midollo dovrebbe essere attentamente valutato per le caratteristiche morfologiche, la cellularità e i reperti citogenetici.

TRATTAMENTO. Il trattamento dei bambini con pancitopenia acquisita richiede terapie integrate di supporto insieme con un tentativo terapeutico per l'insufficienza midollare sottostante. Per pazienti con un fratello donatore di midollo HLA-compatibile, il trapianto di midollo allogenico (*Bone Marrow Transplantation*, BMT) offre il 90% di probabilità di sopravvivenza a lungo termine. I rischi associati a questo approccio includono le complicanze immediate del trapianto, il rigetto e la malattia del trapianto contro l'ospite. Effetti avversi tardivi associati con il trapianto possono includere tumori secondari, cataratta, bassa statura, ipotiroidismo e disfunzione gonadica (vedi Capitoli 136 e 138). Il problema del rigetto del trapianto con conseguenze negative per la vita è diminuito con l'incorporazione della globulina anti-timocita (ATG) e della ciclofosfamide nel regime di condizionamento del trapianto. Solo un paziente su cinque ha un fratello donatore HLA-compatibile, quindi il BMT allogenico non è un'alternativa possibile per la maggior parte dei soggetti.

Per i pazienti senza un fratello donatore, la migliore forma di terapia è l'immunosoppressione con ATG insieme con la ciclosporina, con un tasso di risposta del 60-80%. Circa il 25-30% di coloro che rispondono ha una ricaduta dopo la sospensione della terapia immunosoppressiva e alcuni pazienti devono continuare la ciclosporina per molti anni per preservare la risposta ematologica. C'è un rischio aumentato di malattia clonale del midollo osseo, come la leucemia, la mielodisplasia (MDS) o la PNH, dopo l'immunosoppressione. Il rischio esatto di malattia clonale dopo l'immunosoppressione è probabilmente $<10\%$, e i cariotipi anormali coinvolgono più frequentemente i cromosomi 6, 7 e 8. Per accelerare il recupero dei neutrofili, un fattore stimolante le colonie ematopoietiche (per es. il fattore stimolante colonie granulocitarie, il fattore stimolante colonie granulocito-macrofagiche) è talvolta aggiunto all'ATG e alla ciclosporina nel trattamento dei pazienti con neutropenia severa ($<200/mm^3$). Per quelli che non rispondono all'immunosoppressione o che hanno una ricaduta dopo l'immunosoppressione, donatori non familiari compatibili per il BMT e alte dosi di ciclofosfamide rimangono l'opzione principale. Altre terapie che sono state usate in passato con risultati scarsi includono gli androgeni, i corticosteroidi e la plasmaferesi. Continuano a essere studiate alternative al trapianto di midollo come gli interventi correttivi dell'anemia aplastica refrattaria.

COMPLICANZE. Le complicanze principali di una pancitopenia grave sono collegate soprattutto al rischio di sanguinamento, che mette a repentaglio la vita, a causa di una prolungata trombocitopenia o di infezioni secondarie alla neutropenia protratta. I pazienti con neutropenia prolungata dovuta a insufficienza del midollo osseo sono a rischio non solo di infezioni batteriche gravi, ma anche di micosi invasive. I principi generali della terapia di supporto, sviluppati per la mielosoppressione chemioterapia-collegata per il trattamento dei soggetti con tumori maligni, dovrebbero essere estesi del tutto alla cura dei pazienti con pancitopenia acquisita (vedi Capitolo 177).

PROGNOSI. Una guarigione spontanea si verifica raramente. Una pancitopenia grave, lasciata senza trattamento, presenta una mortalità complessiva di circa il 50% a 6 mesi dalla diagnosi e di >75% complessivamente, con infezioni ed emorragie come cause principali morbilità e mortalità. La maggior parte dei bambini con anemia aplastica acquisita severa risponde al trapianto di midollo osseo allogenico o all'immunosoppressione e alle citochine, lasciandoli con esami emocromocitometrici normali o vicini al normale. Per quelli che non rispondono alla terapia di prima linea la prognosi resta sfavorevole.

PANCITOPENIA CAUSATA DA SOSTITUZIONE MIDOLLARE

I processi che infiltrano o sostituiscono il midollo osseo possono presentarsi con pancitopenia acquisita. Questo può verificarsi prima o durante le neoplasie maligne (tipicamente il neuroblastoma o la leucemia) o come conseguenza di mielofibrosi, MDS o osteoporosi. Anche se poco comuni, i segni dell'anemia aplastica possono precedere, generalmente di pochi mesi, l'esordio della leucemia acuta. Questo è importante per riconoscere il valore della valutazione e del monitoraggio dei bambini che si presentano con quella che sembra essere un'anemia aplastica acquisita. L'esame morfologico del sangue periferico e del midollo osseo, così come gli studi citogenetici midollari, sono criticamente importante nel valutare la diagnosi di leucemia, mielofibrosi e MDS.

Anche se molto rara nei bambini, quando si verifica la MDS presenta un decorso clinico più aggressivo rispetto alla stessa categoria di MDS negli adulti. Circa la metà dei bambini dei casi pubblicati di MDS ha presentato anomalie clonali coinvolgenti il cromosoma 7 (in genere monosomia del 7). Il tempo di transizione dalla MDS pediatrica alla leucemia acuta è relativamente breve, 14-26 mesi, pertanto un trattamento aggressivo come il BMT deve essere considerato immediatamente dopo la diagnosi. Con la chemioterapia convenzionale con ATG, c'è un 20-25% di sopravvivenza a lungo termine, ma con il BMT allogenico, il tasso di sopravvivenza aumenta fino a circa il 50%. Un'eccezione può essere rappresentata dalla MDS e dalla leucemia acuta mieloide nei bambini con sindrome di Down, perché tale patologia in questa specifica popolazione è molto responsiva alla chemioterapia convenzionale, con una sopravvivenza a lungo termine superiore all'80%. Trial clinici attualmente in uso stanno studiando moltissime nuove terapie per le MDS, inclusi inibitori dell'angiogenesi, molecole che colpiscono l'apoptosi, agenti ipometilanti e inibitori della farnesil-transferasi.

Ades L, Mary JY, Robin M, et al: Long-term outcome after bone marrow transplantation for severe aplastic anemia. *Blood* 2004;103:2490–2497.

Bacigalupo A, Bruno B, Saracco P, et al: Antilymphocyte globulin, cyclosporine, prednisolone, and granulocyte colony-stimulating factor for severe aplastic anemia: An update of the GITMO/EBMT on 100 patients. *Blood* 2000;95:1931–1934.

Brodsky RA, Chen AR, Brodsky I, et al: High-dose cyclophosphamide as salvage therapy for severe aplastic anemia. *Exp Hematol* 2004;32:435–440.

Brodsky RA, Jones RJ: Aplastic anaemia. *Lancet* 2005;365:1647–1656.

Howard SC, Naidu PE, Hu XJ, et al: Natural history of moderate aplastic anemia in children. *Pediatr Blood Cancer* 2004;43:545–551.

Maciejewski JP, Selleri C: Evolution of clonal cytogenetic abnormalities in aplastic anemia. *Leuk Lymphoma* 2004;45:433–440.

Marsh JCW, Gordon-Smith EC: Insights into the autoimmune nature of aplastic anaemia. *Lancet* 2004;364:308–309.

Risitano AM, Maciejewski JP, Green S, et al: In-vivo dominant immune responses in aplastic anaemia: Molecular tracking of putatively pathogenetic T-cell clones by TCR beta-CDR3 sequencing. *Lancet* 2004;364:355–364.

Rosenfeld R, Follman D, Nunez O, et al: Antithymocyte globulin and cyclosporine for severe aplastic anemia. *JAMA* 2003;289:1130–1135.

Torres HA, Bodey GP, Rolston KVI, et al: Infections in patients with aplastic anemia. *Cancer* 2003;98:86–93.

Yamaguchi H, Calado RT, Ly H, et al; Mutations in *TERT*, the gene for telomerase reverse transcriptase, in aplastic anemia. *N Engl J Med* 2005;352: 1413–1424.

Young NS: *Bone Marrow Failure Syndromes*. Philadelphia, WB Saunders, 2000.

Sezione 6 — Trasfusioni di componenti ematiche — Ronald G. Strass

Capitolo 470 ■ Trasfusioni di globuli rossi e terapia eritropoietinica

I globuli rossi (GR) sono trasfusi per aumentare la capacità di trasporto dell'ossigeno nel sangue e per mantenere un'ossigenazione tissutale soddisfacente. Le linee guida per la trasfusione di GR nei bambini e negli adolescenti sono simili a quelle per gli adulti (Tab. 470-1). Tuttavia, le trasfusioni possono essere eseguite seguendo criteri più restrittivi nei bambini, perché i livelli normali di emoglobina sono più bassi nei bambini sani che negli adulti e, tranne in determinate circostanze, i bambini non presentano le sottostanti malattie cardiorespiratorie e vascolari che si sviluppano con l'età negli adulti. Pertanto, i bambini dovrebbero essere maggiormente in grado di compensare una perdita di GR. Nel periodo perioperatorio, per esempio, per la maggior parte dei bambini non è necessario mantenere i livelli di emoglobina di 80 g/dL o più alti, un livello che invece di solito è desiderabile per gli adulti. È opportuno che ci sia una valida ragione per ciascuna trasfusione di emazie postoperatoria, perché molti bambini (senza sanguinamento continuato) sono in grado, nel tempo, di rigenerare la massa eritrocitaria con la terapia a base di ferro. La più importante misura nel trattamento dell'emorragia acuta è il controllo dell'emorragia e il ripristino del volume di sangue circolante, la perfusione tissutale con soluzioni cristalloidi e/o colloidi. Se la perdita di sangue stimata è >25% del volume circo-

TABELLA 470-1. Linee guida per le trasfusioni di globuli rossi*

BAMBINI E ADOLESCENTI	
Perdita acuta di >25% del volume di sangue circolante	
Emoglobina <8 g/dL† nel periodo preoperatorio	
Emoglobina <13 g/dL e malattia cardiopolmonare *severa*	
Emoglobina <8 g/dL e anemia cronica *sintomatica*	
Emoglobina <8 g/dL e *insufficienza midollare*	
NEONATI ENTRO IL 4° MESE DI VITA	
Emoglobina <13 g/dL e malattia polmonare *severa*	
Emoglobina <10 g/dL e malattia polmonare *moderata*	
Emoglobina <13 g/dL e cardiopatia *severa*	
Emoglobina <10 g/dL e chirurgia *maggiore*	
Emoglobina <8 g/dL e anemia *sintomatica*	

* Le parole in *corsivo* devono essere definite in linee guida locali per la trasfusione.
† Ematocrito stimato attraverso Hb g/dL ×3.

lante (>17 mL/kg) e la condizione del paziente rimane instabile, le trasfusioni di GR possono essere indicate. Nei bambini gravemente malati, con una malattia polmonare severa che richiede un'assistenza ventilatoria, è comune la pratica di mantenere il livello di emoglobina vicino ai range normali, sebbene l'efficacia di tale tecnica non sia stata documentata da studi scientifici controllati. In realtà, alcuni medici negli ambienti di terapia intensiva preferiscono trasfondere GR in modo abbastanza conservativo e permettere una modesta anemia, perché i pazienti con livelli molto vicini al range normale hanno un'evoluzione meno favorevole. Gli studi condotti in adulti criticamente ammalati hanno dimostrato migliori risultati quando il target emoglobinico era 7-9 g/dL rispetto a 10-12 g/dL. Tuttavia, gli adulti anemici con insufficienza cardiaca congestizia cronica hanno migliori risultati con emoglobina di 13 g/dL contro i 10 g/dL.

Nel caso di anemia cronica, la decisione di trasfondere i GR non dovrebbe essere basata solo sui livelli ematici di emoglobina, perché i bambini compensano bene e possono risultare asintomatici nonostante i livelli bassi di emoglobina. I pazienti con anemia sideropenica sono spesso trattati con successo con ferro per via orale da solo, anche con livelli emoglobinici <5 g/dL. Altri fattori, oltre alla concentrazione emoglobinica, che devono essere considerati nella decisione di trasfondere i GR includono: (1) i sintomi, i segni e le capacità funzionali del paziente; (2) la presenza di patologie cardiorespiratorie, vascolari e del sistema nervoso centrale; (3) la causa e il decorso previsto dell'anemia; (4) terapie alternative, come la terapia con eritropoietina (EPO) ricombinante umana, che è nota per ridurre la necessità di trasfusioni ematiche e per migliorare la condizione complessiva dei bambini con insufficienza renale cronica (vedi Capitolo 535.2). Nelle anemie che probabilmente saranno permanenti, è importante anche bilanciare l'effetto dannoso dell'anemia sulla crescita e sullo sviluppo rispetto alla potenziale tossicità associata alle trasfusioni ripetute. Le trasfusioni di GR per patologie come l'anemia falciforme e la talassemia sono discusse nei Capitoli 462.1 e 462.9.

Per i neonati, non esistono indicazioni chiaramente stabilite e accettate per le trasfusioni dei GR, che si basano sui risultati degli studi scientifici controllati. In genere, i GR vengono somministrati per mantenere il valore emoglobinico che si ritiene più desiderabile per lo stato clinico di ciascun neonato (vedi Tab. 470-1). Questo approccio clinico è impreciso, ma più indicazioni fisiologiche, come la misura della massa eritrocitaria, calcoli disponibili del rilascio di ossigeno e di estrazione tissutale, e imaging della perfusione tissutale sono troppo complicati per la pratica clinica. Poiché i dati disponibili sono limitati, è importante che i pediatri valutino in modo critico la necessità di trasfusioni neonatali di GR alla luce dell'esigenza fisiopatologica.

Durante le prime settimane di vita, tutti i neonati sperimentano un calo della massa eritrocitaria circolante causata sia da fattori fisiologici sia, nei neonati malati prematuri, dalla perdita di sangue con i prelievi. Nei neonati sani a termine, il valore del nadir emoglobinico raramente scende <11 g/dL all'età di 10-12 settimane. Questa caduta "fisiologica" dei GR non richiede trasfusioni. Al contrario, il declino compare prima ed è più pronunciato nei neonati prematuri, anche in quelli senza complicanze patologiche, in cui la concentrazione media emoglobinica scende a circa 8 g/dL nei neonati di 1-1,5 kg di peso alla nascita, mentre a 7 g/dL in quelli che pesano meno di 1 kg. La maggior parte dei neonati con peso alla nascita inferiore a 1 kg necessita di trasfusioni di emazie. Una valida ragione che spiega perché i valori emoglobinici di nadir siano minori in quei neonati a termine in questo ultimo gruppo sono i livelli di EPO plasmatici in risposta all'anemia relativamente ridotti (vedi Capitoli 103.1 e 446). I meccanismi responsabili per i bassi livelli dell'EPO nel plasma sono solo parzialmente definiti. Un fattore è costituito dal fatto che il fegato dei neonati pretermine è il sito primario di produzione dell'EPO durante le prime settimane di vita. Il fegato è meno responsivo dei reni all'anemia e all'ipossia. I neonati pretermine mostrano una risposta lenta dell'EPO al calo dei valori di ematocrito. I bassi livelli plasmatici dell'EPO offrono un razionale per l'uso dell'EPO ricombinante nel trattamento dell'anemia del prematuro. Dosi appropriate di EPO e ferro stimolano efficacemente l'eritropoiesi neonatale. Tuttavia, l'efficacia della terapia con EPO per ridurre significativamente il bisogno di trasfusioni di emazie non è stata dimostrata con certezza, in particolare nei neonati malati molto prematuri, e l'EPO ricombinante non è stata uniformemente accettata come trattamento per l'anemia del prematuro (vedi Capitolo 103.1). In casi rari, alcune preparazioni di EPO si sono associate allo sviluppo di anticorpi anti-EPO che hanno comportato un'anemia severa.

A causa delle controversie sulla terapia con EPO ricombinante, molti neonati pretermine di basso peso alla nascita necessitano di trasfusioni di GR (vedi Tab. 470-1). Nei pazienti neonati con una patologia respiratoria grave, definiti come quelli che richiedono quantità relativamente grandi di ossigeno e un supporto ventilatorio, è consuetudine mantenere l'emoglobina ematica >13 g/dL (ematocrito >40%). Alcuni studiosi ritengono che i GR trasfusi che contengono emoglobina adulta, la quale ha una maggiore interazione con il 2,3-difosfoglicerato e un migliore rilascio di ossigeno rispetto all'emoglobina fetale, garantiscono una disponibilità probabilmente ottimale di ossigeno durante il periodo in cui la funzione polmonare è ridotta. Anche se questa pratica è uniformemente raccomandata, c'è una scarsa evidenza disponibile per stabilire fermamente la sua efficacia o il suo utilizzo migliore (il livello di emoglobina migliore per ogni grado di disfunzione polmonare). I lattanti con una malattia cardiopolmonare meno grave possono richiedere un supporto meno vigoroso; quindi, un livello di emoglobina più basso è indicato per coloro che hanno solo una forma moderata. Coerentemente con il razionale per il rilascio di ossigeno nei neonati con malattia respiratoria grave, sembra appropriato mantenere il valore dell'emoglobina >13 g/dL (ematocrito >40%) nei neonati con una grave cardiopatia che può portare a cianosi o a insufficienza cardiaca congestizia.

Il livello di emoglobina ottimale per i neonati che necessitano di interventi chirurgici maggiori non è stato stabilito con studi definitivi. Tuttavia, sembra ragionevole mantenere il livello di emoglobina >10 g/dL (ematocrito >30%) a causa della limitata capacità del cuore, dei polmoni e del sistema vascolare del neonato di compensare l'anemia; il minore rilascio di ossigeno per le diminuite interazioni tra l'emoglobina fetale e il 2,3-difosfoglicerato; e l'incompleto sviluppo della funzione renale, epatica e neurologica neonatale. Questa linea guida per la trasfusione deve essere applicata con flessibilità ai singoli neonati che vanno incontro a diversi tipi di chirurgia.

I neonati stabili non richiedono trasfusioni di GR, indifferentemente dal loro livello di emoglobina ematico, a meno che non mostrino problemi clinici attribuibili all'anemia. Coloro che propongono le trasfusioni di emazie per l'anemia sintomatica ritengono che la ridotta massa eritrocitaria contribuisca alla tachipnea, alla dispnea, alla tachicardia, all'apnea e alla bradicardia, alle difficoltà di alimentazione e alla letargia, le quali possono essere alleviate dalla trasfusione di GR. Tuttavia l'anemia è solo una delle moltissime cause possibili di questi problemi e le trasfusioni dei globuli rossi dovrebbero essere effettuate solo quando i problemi clinici sono attribuibili esclusivamente all'anemia.

Il prodotto eritrocitario di scelta per bambini e adolescenti è costituito dalla sospensione standard di GR separati dal sangue intero mediante centrifugazione e risospesi, in una soluzione di stoccaggio anticoaugulante/conservativa a un livello di ematocrito del 60%. La dose abituale è 10-15 mL/kg, ma i volumi da trasfondere variano molto, a seconda delle circostanze cliniche (sanguinamento continuato vs arrestato, emolisi). Ai neonati, molti centri trasfondono lo stesso prodotto eritrocitario come indicato per bambini più grandi, mentre altri preferiscono globuli rossi concentrati (ematocrito di 70-90%). Entrambi vengono trasfusi lentamente (oltre le 2-4 ore) alla dose di circa 15 mL/kg. Grazie alla minore quantità di fluido extracellulare somministrata con questi valori relativamente alti di ematocrito e alla ridotta velocità di trasfusione, il tipo di soluzione anticoaugulante/conservativa usata non pone a rischio di neonati prematuri. Il confezionamento dei globuli rossi attraverso la centrifugazione nel momento in cui la sacca è distribuita per la trasfusione assicura che una dose adeguata di globuli rossi venga infusa con ciascuna trasfusione, ma non è indispensabile ed è impraticabile per alcune banche del sangue.

L'impiego tradizionale di globuli rossi relativamente freschi (<7 giorni di deposito) è stato sospeso in molti centri per facilitare l'esposizione a un numero minore di donatori, utilizzando una singola unità di globuli rossi da cui ricavare le aliquote da trasportare a ogni neonato per la durata di stoccaggio permessa per la stessa unità di sangue (42 giorni attualmente). I neonatologi che insistono nel trasfondere solo GR freschi in genere temono l'aumento del livello di potassio (K^+) nel plasma che si verifica nelle unità di eritrociti conservate per lungo tempo. Dopo 42 giorni di deposito, i livelli di K^+ plasmatici sono circa 50 mEq/L (0,05 mEq/mL), un valore che, a prima vista, sembra alto a livelli allarmanti. Tuttavia, la dose attuale di K^+ trasfuso nel fluido extracellulare è molto ridotta. Un neonato che pesa 1 kg, a cui viene effettuata una trasfusione di 15 mL/kg di globuli rossi concentrati (ematocrito 80%), riceverà 3 mL di fluidi extracellulare che contengono solo 0,15 mEq di K^+ e saranno trasfusi lentamente. Tuttavia, la sicurezza dei GR conservati non si può applicare ai grandi volumi (>25 mL/kg) trasfusionali infusi rapidamente, in cui dosi maggiori di K^+ possono essere nocive.

Per i bambini che pesano >30-40 kg che devono essere sottoposti a interventi chirurgici, le trasfusioni di GR autologhi possono costituire un'altra alternativa ai GR allogenici dei donatori. Le raccolte di sangue **autologo predepositate** dal paziente vengono effettuate poche settimane prima della chirurgia. **L'emodiluizione acuta normovolemica** viene praticata nel periodo preoperatorio, in cui il sangue viene prelevato dal paziente e sostituito con soluzione salina. **Sangue autologo di recupero** è ottenuto dalle perdite di sangue durante interventi chirurgici, ma è meno preferibile a causa delle complicanze.

Bratton SL, Annich GM: Packed red blood cell transfusions for critically ill pediatric patients: When and for what conditions? *J Pediatr* 2003;142: 95–97.

Desmet L, Lacroix J: Transfusion in pediatrics. *Crit Care Clin* 2004;20: 299–311.

Guay J, de Moerloose P, Lasne D: Minimizing perioperative blood loss and transfusions in children. *Can J Anaesth* 2006;53:559–567.

Hebert PC, McDonald BJ, Tinmouth A: Clinical consequences of anemia and red cell transfusion in the critically ill. *Crit Care Clin* 2004;20:225–235.

Hume HA, Limoges P: Perioperative blood transfusion therapy in pediatric patients. *Am J Ther* 2002;9:396–405.

Ross SD, Allen IE, Henry DH, et al: Clinical benefits and risks associated with epoetin and darbepoetin in patients with chemotherapy-induced anemia: A systematic review of the literature. *Clin Ther* 2006;28:801–831.

Savakis EC, Strauss RG: Meta-analysis of controlled clinical trials studying the efficacy of recombinant human erythropoietin in reducing blood transfusions in the anemia of prematurity. *Transfusion* 2001;41:406.

Strauss RG: Controversies in the management of the anemia of prematurity using single-donor red blood cell transfusion and/or recombinant human erythropoietin. *Transfus Med Rev* 2006;20:34–44.

Capitolo 471 ■ Trasfusioni di piastrine

Le linee guida per le trasfusioni piastriniche (*Platelet*, PLT) nei bambini e negli adolescenti con patologie piastriniche quantitative e qualitative sono simili a quelle per gli adulti (Tab. 471-1), nei quali il pericolo di sanguinamento che metta a rischio la vita a seguito di una ferita o che si verifichi spontaneamente può essere proporzionale alla gravità della trombocitopenia. Le trasfusioni piastriniche dovrebbero essere eseguite nei pazienti con conte piastriniche $<50 \times 10^9$/L quando stanno sanguinando o sono in lista per una procedura invasiva. Gli studi di pazienti con trombocitopenia che conseguono a un'insufficienza del midollo osseo indicano che un sanguinamento spontaneo aumenta marcatamente quando i livelli piastrinici scendono $<20 \times 10^9$/L, se complicanze serie (infezioni, insufficienza d'organo, anomalie della coagulazione o anemia) sono presenti. In queste circostanze, le trasfusioni piastriniche di profilassi sono effettuate per mantenere la conta piastrinica $>20 \times 10^9$/L. Questo è stato messo in discussione da studi sui pazienti adulti; una soglia trasfusionale bassa di 5-10 $\times 10^9$/L è raccomandata nei pazienti stabili. Tuttavia, nella pratica, una grave trombocitopenia si verifica comunemente in associazione alle complicanze della febbre, della terapia antibiotica e del sanguinamento in atto, nonché alla necessità di una procedura invasiva, alla coagulazione intravascolare disseminata e ad altre gravi anomalie della coagulazione; casi in cui vengono effettuate le trasfusioni piastriniche per mantenere conte piastriniche relativamente alte. Nonostante il desiderio di alcuni medici, che sono spesso quelli che preparano il paziente per una procedura invasiva, di portare la conta piastrinica a un livello $\geq 70 \times 10^9$/L, non ci sono dati definitivi per giustificare un reale beneficio da una conta piastrinica $>50 \times 10^9$/L.

I disordini piastrinici qualitativi possono essere ereditari o acquisiti (nell'insufficienza epatica o renale avanzata o dopo bypass cardiopolmonare). In questi pazienti, le trasfusioni piastriniche sono giustificate solo se si verifica un significativo sanguinamento. Poiché la disfunzione piastrinica ereditaria può essere presente a lungo e le trasfusioni ripetute possono portare all'alloimmunizzazione e alla refrattarietà, le trasfusioni piastriniche di profilassi sono raramente giustificate, a meno che non sia in programma una procedura invasiva. In questi casi, un tempo di sanguinamento di oltre il doppio rispetto al limite normale di laboratorio o un risultato anormale con l'utilizzo di un sistema di funzione piastrinica più moderno può essere assunto come evidenza diagnostica di disfunzione piastrinica, ma il tempo di sanguinamento o qualsiasi altro risultato dei test di laboratorio è poco predittivo del rischio emorragico o del bisogno di trasfusioni piastriniche. Terapie alternative, in particolare la desmopressina acetato, dovrebbero essere considerate per evitare le trasfusioni di piastrine, mentre farmaci antipiastrine (farmaci antinfiammatori non steroidei) dovrebbero essere evitati in questi pazienti.

Nei neonati, l'emostasi è quantitativamente e qualitativamente differente da quella dei bambini più grandi, ed esiste un potenziale di rischio per emorragie o trombosi gravi. Circa il 25% dei neonati trattati nelle unità di terapia intensiva mostrano una conta piastrinica $<150 \times 10^9$/L in qualche occasione durante il ricovero. Meccanismi patogenetici multipli sono coinvolti in questi neonati malati, prevalentemente accelerata distruzione piastrinica associata a diminuita produzione piastrinica, come evidenziato dai ridotti numeri di progenitori megacariocitari e livelli di trombopoietina relativamente bassi nei neonati trombocitopenici, rispetto ai bambini e agli adulti trombocitopenici.

Le conte piastriniche nel sangue di $<100 \times 10^9$/L comportano rischi clinici significativi per i neonati prematuri. Il tempo di sanguinamento può essere prolungato a conte piastriniche $<100 \times 10^9$/L in neonati con peso alla nascita <1,5 kg, mentre la disfunzione piastrinica è suggerita dai tempi di sanguinamento, che sono sproporzionatamente lunghi per il grado di trombocitopenia, inoltre il rischio di emorragia può essere maggiore nei neonati trombocitopenici. L'incidenza di emorragia intracranica nei neonati trombocitopenici con peso alla nascita <1,5 kg è del 78% rispetto al 48% dei neonati non trombocitopenici di peso simile. Inoltre, l'entità dell'emorragia e della morbilità neurologica è maggiore nel gruppo trombocitopenico. Tuttavia, in un trial randomizzato, trasfondere le piastrine per via profilattica quando la conta piastrinica scende $<150 \times 10^9$/L per mantenere quella media $>200 \times 10^9$/L, rispetto al trasfondere le piastrine solo quando la conta piastrinica scende $<50 \times 10^9$/L per mantenere la conta piastrinica media a circa 100×10^9/L, non diminuisce l'incidenza dell'emorragia intracranica (28% rispetto a 26%). Quindi, non è stato dimostrato un beneficio nel trasfondere le piastrine in caso di trombocitopenia lieve (conta piastrinica <150 ma $>100 \times 10^9$/L) al fine di sostenere la conta piastrinica di sangue nel range normale. Anche se le questioni basilari circa i rischi relativi dei diversi livelli di trombocitopenia in diverse situazioni cliniche presentano solo risposte scarse, ci sono linee guida accettabili per molti neonatologi, elencate nella Tabella 471-1.

L'obiettivo della maggior parte delle trasfusioni piastriniche è di raggiungere una conta piastrinica $>50 \times 10^9$/L e di aumentarla nei neonati a valori $>100 \times 10^9$/L. Ciò può essere raggiunto in modo consistente in bambini che pesano fino a 30 kg attraverso l'infusione di 10 mL/kg di concentrati piastrinici standard (non modificati), ottenuti dalla processazione delle unità di sangue intero oppure attraverso la piastrinoferesi. Per i bambini con peso superiore, la dose appropriata è 3-6 unità riunite da più donatori di piastrine derivate da sangue intero oppure un'unità di aferesi. I concentrati piastrinici dovrebbero essere trasfusi il più rapidamente possibile compatibilmente con le condizioni generali del paziente, sicuramente entro 2 ore. I pazienti che richiedono trasfusioni di piastrine ripetute dovrebbero ricevere prodotti di sangue privati di leucociti, inclusi i concentrati piastrinici, per diminuire l'alloimmunizzazione e la refrattarietà piastrinica nonché ridurre il rischio di infezioni da Cytomegalovirus trasmesse con le trasfusioni.

La riduzione del volume dei concentrati piastrinici per i neonati e i bambini piccoli attraverso la centrifugazione addizionale è necessaria e prudente. La trasfusione di 10 mL/kg di un concentrato piastrinico immodificato è adeguato perché aggiunge 10×10^9 piastrine a 70 mL di sangue (il volume di sangue di un neonato di 1 kg), un numero calcolato (tenendo in considerazione l'ematocrito usuale e i valori di incremento delle piastrine post-trasfusione) per aumentare la conta piastrinica a 100×10^9/L. L'incremento calcolato è compatibile con quello attuale. Inoltre, 10 mL/kg non costituiscono un volume trasfusionale eccessivo, posto che l'assunzione di altri fluidi endovena, farmaci e nutrienti venga monitorato e regolato. È importante ridurre le trasfusioni ripetute di piastrine di gruppo 0 a riceventi di gruppo A o B perché gli anti-A o gli anti-B passivi nel plasma di gruppo 0 possono portare all'emolisi. Anche se esistono metodi testati per ridurre il volume dei concentrati piastrinici quando ciò sia veramente necessario (per es. quando sono previste molte trasfusioni, in cui la quantità di anti-A o anti-B passivi può condurre all'emolisi o all'inefficacia di 10 mL/kg di concentrati piastrinici non modificati nell'aumentare la conta piastrinica), trattamenti addizionali dovrebbero essere praticate con moltissima attenzione per la probabile perdita di piastrine, dall'agglutinazione, e le disfunzioni provocate dall'eccessivo trattamento: ciascuno di questi fattori infatti può diminuire l'efficacia e aumentare la tossicità delle trasfusioni piastriniche.

TABELLA 471-1. Linee guida per le trasfusioni pediatriche di piastrine*

BAMBINI E ADOLESCENTI
PLT $<50 \times 10^9$/L e sanguinamento
PLT $<50 \times 10^9$/L e una procedura *invasiva*
PLT $<20 \times 10^9$/L e *insufficienza midollare* con fattori di rischio emorragico
PLT $<10 \times 10^9$/L e *insufficienza midollare* senza fattori di rischio emorragici
PLT a qualsiasi conta, ma con disfunzione piastrinica con sanguinamento o una procedura invasiva
LATTANTI ENTRO IL 4° MESE DI VITA
PLT $<100 \times 10^9$/L e sanguinamento
PLT $<50 \times 10^9$/L e una procedura invasiva
PLT $<20 \times 10^9$/L e *clinicamente stabile*
PLT $<100 \times 10^9$/L e *clinicamente instabile*
PLT a qualsiasi conta, ma con disfunzione piastrinica più sanguinamento o una procedura invasiva

* Le parole in *corsivo* devono essere definite nelle linee guida per le trasfusioni locali.
PLT, piastrine.

Chakravorty S, Murray N, Roberts I: Neonatal thrombocytopenia. *Early Hum Dev* 2005;81:35–41.

Murray NA: Evaluation and treatment of thrombocytopenia in the neonatal intensive care unit. *Acta Paediatr Suppl* 2002;91:74–81.

Strauss RG: Low-dose prophylactic platelet transfusions: Time for further study, but too early for routine clinical practice. *Transfusion* 2004;44: 1680–1682.

Capitolo 472 ■ Trasfusioni di neutrofili (granulociti)

Le linee guida per le trasfusioni di granulociti (*Granulocyte Transfusion*, GTX) sono elencate nella Tabella 472-1. Anche se le GTX è stata moderatamente impiegata in passato, la capacità di raccogliere numeri notevolmente elevati di neutrofili da donatori stimolati con il fattore ricombinante stimolante le colonie granulocitarie (G-CSF) ha portato a rinnovato interesse, in particolare nei riceventi di un trapianto di progenitori ematopoietici. Le GTX dovrebbe essere riconsiderata dalle istituzioni in cui i pazienti neutropenici continuano a morire per infezioni progressive batteriche e fungine nonostante l'uso ottimale di agenti antibiotici e fattori ricombinanti di crescita mieloide.

Il ruolo delle GTX associate agli antibiotici per pazienti con neutropenia grave ($<0,5 \times 10^9$/L) dovuta a insufficienza del midollo osseo è simile per adulti e bambini. I pazienti neutropenici infetti in genere rispondono agli antibiotici da soli, producendo una ripresa della funzione del midollo osseo precocemente durante l'infezione. Poiché i bambini con una leucemia diagnosticata di recente rispondono rapidamente alla chemioterapia di induzione, essi sono di rado candidati per le GTX. Al contrario, i bambini con infezioni con insufficienza grave del midollo osseo (neoplasie maligne resistenti al trattamento, anemia aplastica e i riceventi un trapianto di progenitori ematopoietici) possono trarre beneficio quando le GTX vengono aggiunte agli antibiotici. L'utilizzo delle GTX per la sepsi batterica non rispondente agli antibiotici nei pazienti con neutropenia grave ($<0,5 \times 10^9$/L) è supportata da molti studi controllati (vedi Capitolo 177).

I bambini con difetti qualitativi dei neutrofili (disfunzione dei neutrofili) in genere presentano numeri adeguati di neutrofili ematici ma sono suscettibili a infezioni gravi, perché le loro cellule uccidono i microrganismi patogenetici inefficacemente. Le sindromi da disfunzione dei neutrofili sono rare e non ci sono studi definitivi che abbiano stabilito l'efficacia delle GTX. Tuttavia, molti pazienti con infezioni progressive con rischio per la vita

TABELLA 472-1. Linee guida per le trasfusioni pediatriche di granulociti*

BAMBINI E ADOLESCENTI
Neutrofili $<0,5 \times 10^9$/L e infezione batterica non risponsiva alla terapia antibiotica appropriata
Difetto qualitativo dei neutrofili e infezioni (batteriche o fungine) *non risponsiva* all'appropriata terapia antibiotica
LATTANTI NEI PRIMI 4 MESI DI VITA
Neutrofili $<3,0 \times 10^9$/L (prima settimana di vita) o $<1 \times 10^9$/L (in seguito) e infezione batterica *fulminante*

* Le parole in *corsivo* devono essere definite in linee guida locali per la trasfusione.

hanno migliorato in modo sorprendente con l'associazione delle GTX alla terapia antibiotica. Queste patologie sono croniche e a causa del rischio di indurre l'alloimmunizzazione, le GTX sono raccomandate solo quando le infezioni sono chiaramente poco rispondenti ai farmaci antibiotici.

I neonati sono in genere suscettibili alle infezioni batteriche severe, e un numero di difetti delle difese organiche neonatali possono essere fattori promuoventi (vedi Capitolo 109). Queste anomalie sono accentuate nei neonati malati prematuri, ed è logico considerare le GTX. I neonati che mostrano una sepsi fulminante, una neutropenia relativa ($<3 \times 10^9$/L durante la prima settimana di vita e $<1 \times 10^9$/L in seguito) e una severa diminuzione della riserva midollare di neutrofili (con <10% di neutrofili postmitotici fra gli elementi nucleati midollari) sono a rischio particolarmente elevato di morte se trattati solo con antibiotici. Anche se alcuni studi hanno mostrato un significativo beneficio dalle GTX, esse vengono raramente utilizzate. Al contrario, alcuni neonatologi considerano terapie alternative, incluse le immunoglobuline endovena e i fattori di crescita mieloidi ricombinanti (G-CSF o fattore stimolante colonie granulocito-macrofagiche). I risultati degli studi che valutano le immunoglobuline endovena sono contrastanti, ma la metanalisi ha trovato un beneficio significativo per i neonati con sepsi dimostrata. I dati disponibili sono insufficienti a determinare se i fattori di crescita ricombinanti mieloidi abbiano un ruolo nel trattamento di questi neonati, anche se è stato dimostrato che sia il G-CSF sia il fattore stimolante colonie granulocito-macrofagiche aumentano la mielopoiesi e incrementano la conta dei neutrofili nei neonati. È importante ricordare che il G-CSF è efficace per il trattamento di molti tipi di neutropenia congenita grave.

Una volta che la decisione di effettuare una GTX è stata presa, un'adeguata dose di cellule fresche da leucoferesi deve essere trasfusa. I neonati e i bambini di peso <10 kg dovrebbero ricevere 1-2 $\times 10^9$/kg di neutrofili per GTX. Bambini e neonati più grossi dovrebbero ricevere una dose totale di almeno 1×10^{10} neutrofili per GTX; la dose preferibile per gli adolescenti è 5-8 $\times 10^{10}$ per ogni GTX, una dose che richiede donatori stimolati con G-CSF, le GTX dovrebbero essere effettuate quotidianamente finché l'infezione non si risolve o la conta dei neutrofili non superi il valore di 1×10^9/L per pochi giorni.

Dale DC, Liles WC: Return of granulocyte transfusions. *Curr Opin Pediatr* 2000;12:18–22.

Stravss RG: Rebirth of granulocyte transfusions: Should it involve pediatric oncology and transplant patients? *J Pediatr Hematol Oncol* 1999;21: 475–478.

Capitolo 473 ■ Trasfusioni di plasma fresco congelato

Le linee guida per la trasfusione di plasma fresco congelato (PFC) nei bambini (Tab. 473-1) sono simili a quelle degli adulti. Il PFC è trasfuso per sostituire deficit clinicamente significativi delle proteine plasmatiche, per le quali non sono disponibili concentrati maggiormente purificati. Le quantità richieste di PFC variano a seconda dello specifico fattore che deve essere sostituito, ma una dose iniziale di 15 mL/kg è in genere soddisfacente. La trasfusione di PFC è efficace nel trattamento dei deficit dei fattori della coagulazione II, V, X e XI. I deficit del fattore XIII e del fibrinogeno sono trattati con il crioprecipitato. La trasfusione di PFC non è raccomandata per il trattamento dei pazienti con emofilia grave A o B o per il deficit del fattore VII, dal momento che sono disponibili concentrati più sicuri di fattore VII, VIII e IX. Inoltre, l'emofilia A lieve-moderata e alcuni tipi di malattia di von Willebrand possono essere trattati con la desmopressina (vedi Capitolo 477). Un'indicazione importante di PFC è per ottenere la rapida correzione degli effetti del warfarin in pazienti che presentano un sanguinamento attivo o che richiedono una chirurgia di emergenza (in cui i deficit funzionali dei fattori II, VII, IX e X non possono essere rapidamente corretti dalla vitamina K). I risultati di test di screening della coagulazione (protrombina, tromboplastina parziale attivata e tempo di trombina) non dovrebbero essere considerati da soli per riflettere l'integrità del sistema della coagulazione. Per giustificare la trasfusione di PFC, i risultati del test della coagulazione devono essere ricondotti alla condizione clinica del paziente. La trasfusione di PFC in pazienti con epatopatia cronica e tempo di coagulazione prolungato non è raccomandata, a meno che non sia presente sanguinamento o sia in programma una procedura invasiva, perché la correzione del deficit dei fattori della coagulazione è di breve durata.

TABELLA 473-1. Linee guida per le trasfusioni pediatriche di plasma fresco congelato*

NEONATI, BAMBINI E ADOLESCENTI
Grave deficit dei fattori della coagulazione e sanguinamento
Grave deficit dei fattori della coagulazione e una procedura invasiva
Correzione di emergenza degli effetti del warfarin
Coagulopatia da diluizione e sanguinamento
Sostituzione della proteina anticoaugulante (antitrombina III, proteine C e S)
Sostituzione dei fluidi per plasmaferesi per la porpora trombotica trombocitopenica

* Le parole in *corsivo* devono essere definite da linee guida locali per la trasfusione.

Il PFC contiene anche molte proteine anticoaugulanti (antitrombina III, proteina C e proteina S) le cui carenze sono associate a trombosi. In situazioni particolari, il PFC può essere appropriato come terapia sostitutiva, insieme con un trattamento anticoagulante, in pazienti con queste patologie. Tuttavia, quando disponibili, i concentrati purificati sono da preferire. Altre indicazioni per il PFC includono il ripristino di fluidi durante la plasmaferesi in pazienti con porpora trombotica trombocitopenica o altre patologie in cui il PFC è probabilmente efficace (plasma-exchange in un paziente con sanguinamento e coagulopatia grave). PFC non è indicato per la correzione dell'ipovolemia o come terapia sostitutiva immunoglobulinica, perché esistono alternative più sicure (albumina o soluzioni saline e immunoglobuline endovena, rispettivamente).

Nei neonati, la trasfusione di PFC merita considerazioni speciali. I tempi di coagulazione sono "fisiologicamente" prolungati, a causa del deficit di sviluppo delle proteine della coagulazione, pertanto il PFC dovrebbe essere trasfuso solo dopo riferimento ai normali valori attesi in base al peso neonatale e all'età del neonato. Le indicazioni per il PFC nei neonati includono: (1) ricostituzione dei concentrati di globuli rossi (GR) per simulare il sangue intero per l'utilizzo in trasfusioni massive (per es. exsanguinotrasfusioni o chirurgia cardiovascolare); (2) emorragia secondaria alla carenza di vitamina K; (3) coagulazione disseminata intravascolare con sanguinamento; (4) sanguinamento nella carenza congenita dei fattori coagulativi quando un trattamento più specifico è non disponibile oppure è inappropriato. L'uso delle trasfusioni di PFC a scopo di profilassi per prevenire l'emorragia intraventricolare nei neonati prematuri non è raccomandato. Il PFC non dovrebbe essere usato come agente di sospensione per normalizzare i valori di ematocrito dei concentrati di GR prima di trasfusioni di GR di piccolo volume nei neonati, perché non offre alcun beneficio medico dimostrabile rispetto all'utilizzo di soluzioni sterili. Allo stesso modo, l'uso di PFC nell'exsanguinotrasfusioni parziali per il trattamento della sindrome da iperviscosità neonatale non è necessaria, perché cristalloidi o soluzioni colloidi più sicure sono disponibili.

Nel trattamento dei neonati con sanguinamento, il crioprecipitato è spesso considerato per il suo piccolo volume di infusione. Tuttavia, il crioprecipitato contiene solo fibrinogeno e fattori VIII e XIII. Pertanto, esso non è efficace nel trattamento della condizione clinica abituale nei neonati con sanguinamento con deficit di fattori multipli della coagulazione, nonostante l'interesse e la convenienza dell'infusione di volumi ridotti. In studi preliminari, le infusioni di volumi veramente piccoli di fattore VII ricombinante attivato si è rivelato salvavita in pazienti con emorragia dovuta a diversi meccanismi. Poiché l'efficacia e la tossicità del fattore VIIa non è stata completamente definita in questi impieghi non registrati (non approvati dalla Food and Drug Administration), deve essere considerata una terapia sperimentale in questo momento.

Felderhoff-Mueser U, Buhrer C: Clinical measures to preserve cerebral integrity in preterm infants. *Early Hum Dev* 2005;81:237–244.

Goldenberg NA, Manco-Johnson MJ: Pediatric hemostasis and use of plasma components. *Best Pract Res Clin Haematol* 2006;19:143–155.

O'Shaughnessy DF, Atterbury C, Bolton Maggs P, et al: Guidelines for the use of fresh-frozen plasma, cryoprecipitate and cryosupernatant. *Br J Haematol* 2004;126:11–28.

Stanworth SJ, Brunskill SJ, Hyde CJ, et al: Is fresh frozen plasma clinically effective? A systematic review of randomized controlled trials. *Br J Haematol* 2004;126:139–152.

Capitolo 474 ■ Rischi nelle trasfusioni di sangue

Anche se i rischi delle trasfusioni di sangue allogenico sono bassi, le trasfusioni devono essere praticate con giudizio. Prendendo in considerazione il test di amplificazione degli acidi nucleici (*Nucleic acid Amplification Test*, NAT) e tutte le altre attività di screening nel donatore (screening anticorpale ed epidemiologico), una stima attuale del rischio dell'HIV associato alla trasfusione è circa 1/2 000 000 esposizione a donatori, con stime che variano da 1/800 000 a 1/4 000 000 esposizione a donatori. Allo stesso modo, mediante il NAT, il rischio di epatite virale C è 1/1 600 000 donatori esposti. Il NAT identifica i geni virali circolanti nel periodo finestra prima che si sviluppino gli anticorpi ed è disponibile per l'HIV, l'epatite C e il virus West Nile. Il Cytomegalovirus associato alle trasfusioni può essere eliminato precocemente attraverso la trasfusione di prodotti ematici deleucocitati o attraverso una selezione del sangue dai donatori che sono negativi per gli anticorpi anti-Cytomegalovirus. Entrambi i metodi presentano effetti compatibili e non c'è un vantaggio documentato nel praticarli entrambi (usando sangue deleucocitato prelevato da donatori sieronegativi). Rischi infettivi aggiuntivi includono altri tipi di epatite (B, E) e retrovirus (virus linfotropico T umano di tipo I e II e l'HIV-2), la sifilide, il parvovirus B19, il virus di Epstein Barr, l'herpesvirus umano 8, il virus West Nile, la malaria, la babesiosi e la malattia di Chagas. Una variante della malattia di Creutzfeldt-Jacob è anche stata trasmessa attraverso le trasfusioni di sangue tra esseri umani.

I rischi associati alle trasfusioni di natura non infettiva che possono verificarsi includono le reazioni trasfusionali emolitiche e non emolitiche, il sovraccarico di fluidi, la reazione del trapianto contro l'ospite, gli squilibri elettrolitici e acido-base, il sovraccarico di ferro se sono necessarie trasfusioni croniche ripetute, l'aumentata suscettibilità al danno ossidativo, l'esposizione ai plastici, l'emolisi da attivazione delle cellule T contro l'antigene eritrocitario, la porpora post-trasfusione, il danno polmonare acuto, l'immunosoppressione e l'alloimmunizzazione. L'immunomodulazione può essere dimunita con la riduzione del numero di leucociti. Le reazioni trasfusionali e l'alloimmunizzazione agli antigeni eritrocitari e leucocitari sembrano essere poco comuni nei lattanti. Effetti avversi si registrano solo con trasfusioni massive, come l'exsanguinotrasfusione, il trauma o la chirurgia, quando quantità di sangue relativamente grandi sono necessarie, mentre sono rare quando vengono praticate trasfusioni di piccolo volume. Inoltre, errori medici, come il trasfondere sangue di gruppo sbagliato, si verificano in circa 1/25 000 unità.

I neonati prematuri sono noti per presentare una disfunzione immunitaria, ma il loro rischio relativo di reazione del trapianto contro l'ospite post-trasfusionale è controverso. L'età postnatale del neonato, il numero di linfociti immunocompetenti nel prodotto trasfusionale, il grado di compatibilità dell'antigene leucocitario umano tra donatore e ricevente, e altri fenomeni poco descritti determinano quali neonati sono veramente a rischio. Le trasfusioni in utero presentano un elevato rischio di reazione del trapianto contro l'ospite. D'altra parte, molti centri che si prendono cura dei neonati prematuri trasfondono solamente prodotti cellulari γ-irradiati. Donazioni dirette di sangue prelevato da consanguinei devono sempre essere irradiate per il rischio di attecchimento con i leucociti aploidentici HLA-omozigoti trasfusi. I prodotti cellulari ematici somministrati in utero e le exsanguinotrasfusioni dovrebbero essere γ-irradiati, come lo sono le trasfusioni per pazienti con immunodeficienze congenite gravi (sindrome di DiGeorge che richiede la cardiochirurgia) e per i riceventi i trapianti di progenitori ematopoietici. Altri gruppi che sono potenzialmente a rischio, ma per i quali non sono disponibili dati conclusivi, sono i pazienti che ricevono una terapia con anticorpi anticellule T (globulina anti-timocita o OKT3), quelli con allotrapianti di organo, quelli che ricevono regimi farmacologici immunosoppressori e i pazienti infetti con HIV.

La pratica clinica attuale utilizza la γ-irradiazione da cesio, cobalto o sorgenti lineari di accelerazione a dosi variabili da 2500 a 5000 cGy; è necessaria una dose minima di 2500 cGy. Tutte le componenti cellulari ematiche dovrebbero essere irradiate, ma i prodotti "acellulari" congelati, come il plasma e il crioprecipitato, non lo richiedono. La filtrazione per rimuovere i leucociti non può essere sostituita con la γ-irradiazione per prevenire la risposta del trapianto contro l'ospite.

Arendt A, Carmean J, Koch E, et al: Fatal bacterial infections associated with platelet transfusions–United States, 2004. *MMWR* 2005;57:168.

Blajchman MA, Vamvakas EC: The continuing risk of transfusion-transmitted infections. *N Engl J Med* 2006;355:1303–1305.

Bolton-Maggs PHB, Murphy MF: Blood transfusions. *Arch Dis Child* 2004; 89:4–7.

Busch MP, Kleinman SH, Nemo GJ: Current and emerging infectious risks of blood transfusions. *JAMA* 2003;289:959–962.

Chakravorty S, Murray N, Roberts I: Neonatal thrombocytopenia. *Early Hum Dev* 2005;81:35–41.

College of American Pathologists Task Force: Practice parameter for the use of fresh-frozen plasma, cryoprecipitate, and platelets. *JAMA* 1994;271: 777.

Goodnough LT, Shander A, Brecher ME: Transfusion medicine: Looking to the future. *Lancet* 2003;361:161–169.

Hladik W, Dollard SC, Mermin J, et al: Transmission of human herpes virus 8 by blood transfusion. *N Engl J Med* 2006;355:1331–1338.

Mohan P, Brocklehurst P: Granulocyte transfusions for neonates with confirmed or suspected sepsis and neutropenia. *Cochrane Database Syst Rev* 2003;4:CD003956.

Murray NA: Evaluation and treatment of thrombocytopenia in the neonatal intensive care unit. *Acta Paediatr Suppl* 2002;91:74–81.

Savakis EC, Strauss RG: Meta-analysis of controlled clinical trials studying the efficacy of recombinant human erythropoietin in reducing blood transfusions in the anemia of prematurity. *Transfusion* 2001;41:406.

Stramer SL, Glynn SA, Kleinman SH, et al: Detection of HIV-1 and HCV infections among antibody-negative blood donors by nucleic acid amplification testing. *N Engl J Med* 2004;351:760–768.

Strauss RG: Low-dose prophylactic platelet transfusions: Time for further study, but too early for routine clinical practice. *Transfusion* 2004;44: 1680–1682.

Strauss RG: Data-driven blood banking practices for neonatal RBC transfusions. *Transfusion* 2000;40:1528–1540.

Wilson K, Ricketts MN: A third episode of transfusion-derived VCJD. *Lancet* 2006;368:2037–2038.

Sezione 7 — Patologie emorragiche e trombotiche — J. Paul Scott e Robert R. Montgomery

Capitolo 475 ■ Emostasi

L'emostasi è il processo attivo che coagula il sangue in aree di danno vascolare e che contemporaneamente limita l'entità del coagulo solo alle aree di lesione. Nel tempo, il coagulo viene lisato dal sistema fibrinolitico e si ripristina il normale flusso ematico. Se la coagulazione è difettosa si verificano le emorragie, se invece la coagulazione è eccessiva si presentano complicanze trombotiche. La risposta di emostasi deve essere rapida e regolata, in modo che il trauma non scateni una reazione sistemica, ma dia inizio a una risposta immediata e localizzata. La chiave della velocità e della coordinazione della risposta risiede nel fatto che, quando una piastrina aderisce a un sito di danno vascolare, la superficie piastrinica favorisce una superficie reattiva alla quale si legano i fattori della coagulazione. L'enzima attivo viene portato a contatto con il substrato, accelerando la velocità di reazione e fornendo i prodotti attivati per la reazione con i fattori della coagulazione a valle nella cascata coagulativa. La coagulazione attiva è controllata mediante feedback negativi che inibiscono il processo coagulativo quando il processo procoagulante viene a contatto con l'endotelio intatto. Le maggiori componenti del processo di emostasi sono la **parete vasale**, le **piastrine**, le **proteine coagulative**, le **proteine anticoagulanti** e il **sistema fibrinolitico**. Le maggiori componenti dell'emostasi sono multifunzionali; il fibrinogeno funziona come ligando tra le piastrine durante l'aggregazione piastrinica e serve anche come substrato per la trombina che forma il coagulo di fibrina. Le piastrine permettono la superficie reattiva su cui si realizza la reazione coagulativa, formano il coagulo sul sito di danno vascolare e si contraggono per costringere e limitare la dimensione del coagulo.

IL PROCESSO. L'endotelio vascolare intatto è la prima barriera contro l'emorragia. Le cellule endoteliali che rivestono la parete vascolare normalmente inibiscono la coagulazione, e formano una superficie liscia che permette un flusso ematico rapido.

Dopo un danno vascolare, si verifica una vasocostrizione e il flusso di sangue entra in contatto con la matrice sottoendoteliale (Fig. 475-1). Nel flusso di sangue, quando esposto alle proteine della matrice sottoendoteliale, il fattore di von Willebrand (*von Willebrand Factor*, VWF) cambia conformazione e produce una specie di colla con cui lega il recettore piastrinico per il VWF. Dopo l'aderenza, le piastrine si attivano e rilasciano i granuli di deposito che contengono l'adenosina di fosfato (ADP), il trombossano A_2 e altre proteine immagazzinate, che scatenano l'aggregazione e il reclutamento di altre piastrine per formare il tappo piastrinico. L'aggregazione coinvolge l'interazione di recettori specifici sulla superficie piastrinica con proteine dell'emostasi plasmatica, soprattutto il fibrinogeno. Una delle proteine della matrice subendoteliale che è esposta dopo il danno vascolare è il fattore tissutale. Non appena le proteine esposte della matrice subendoteliale legano il VWF, il fattore tissutale è pure esposto, lega il fattore VII e attiva la cascata coagulativa come mostrato nella Figura 475-2. Nella cascata, si attivano i fattori della coagulazione inattivi, evidenziati con la numerazione romana. Il fattore della coagulazione attivato in seguito inizia l'attivazione del fattore della coagulazione successivo in modo sistematico. Le

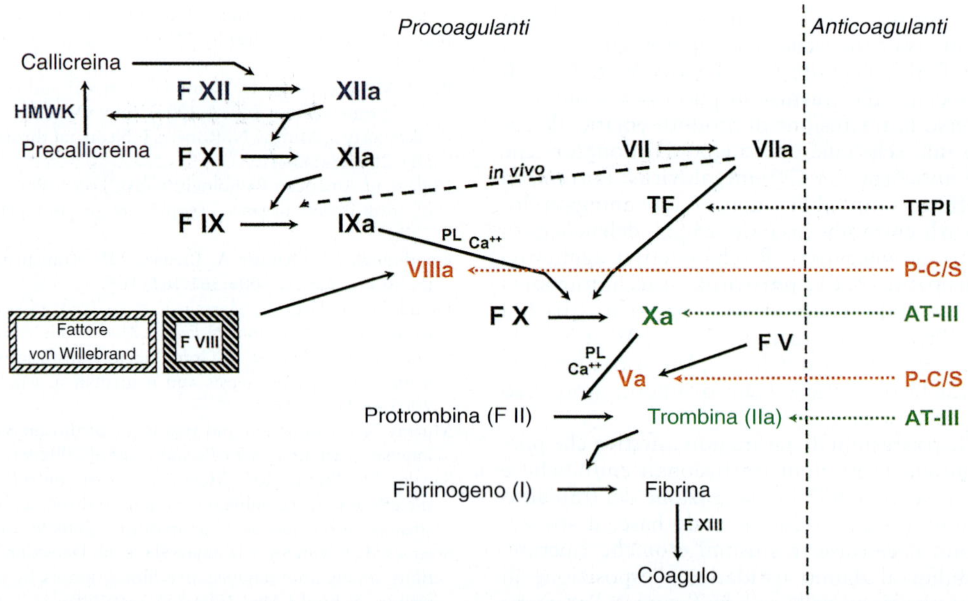

Figura 475-1. La cascata coagulativa, con attivazione sequenziale e amplificazione della formazione del coagulo. Molti dei fattori sono attivati dal fattore che li precede nella cascata. I fattori attivati (F) sono indicati mediante l'aggiunta di una *a*. Sul *lato destro*, sono mostrati i principali anticoagulanti e i siti da essi regolati (l'inibitore della via del fattore tissutale [TFPI] regola il fattore tissutale [TF] e il fattore VIIa; la proteina C e la proteina S [P-C/S] regolano i fattori VIII e V; e l'antitrombina III (AT-III) regola il fattore Xa e la trombina [factor IIa]). La *linea tratteggiata* mostra che, in vivo, il TF e il fattore VIIa attivano entrambi i fattori IX e X, ma in vitro, viene misurata solo l'attivazione del fattore X. Il fattore inattivato VIII, quando legato alla sua proteina di trasporto, il fattore di von Willebrand, è protetto dall'inattivazione mediata dalla proteina C. Quando la trombina, o fattore Xa, attiva il fattore VIII, si stacca dal fattore di von Willebrand e può partecipare con il fattore IXa all'attivazione del fattore X in presenza di fosfolipidi (PL) e calcio (Ca^{2+}). Il fattore XIIIa forma legami crociati con il coagulo di fibrina e lo rende quindi più stabile. La precallicreina, il chininogeno ad alto peso molecolare (HMWK) e il fattore XII sono mostrati in *blu* perché, anche se contribuiscono al tempo di coagulazione nel tempo di tromboplastina parziale (PTT), non hanno un ruolo fisiologico nella coagulazione.

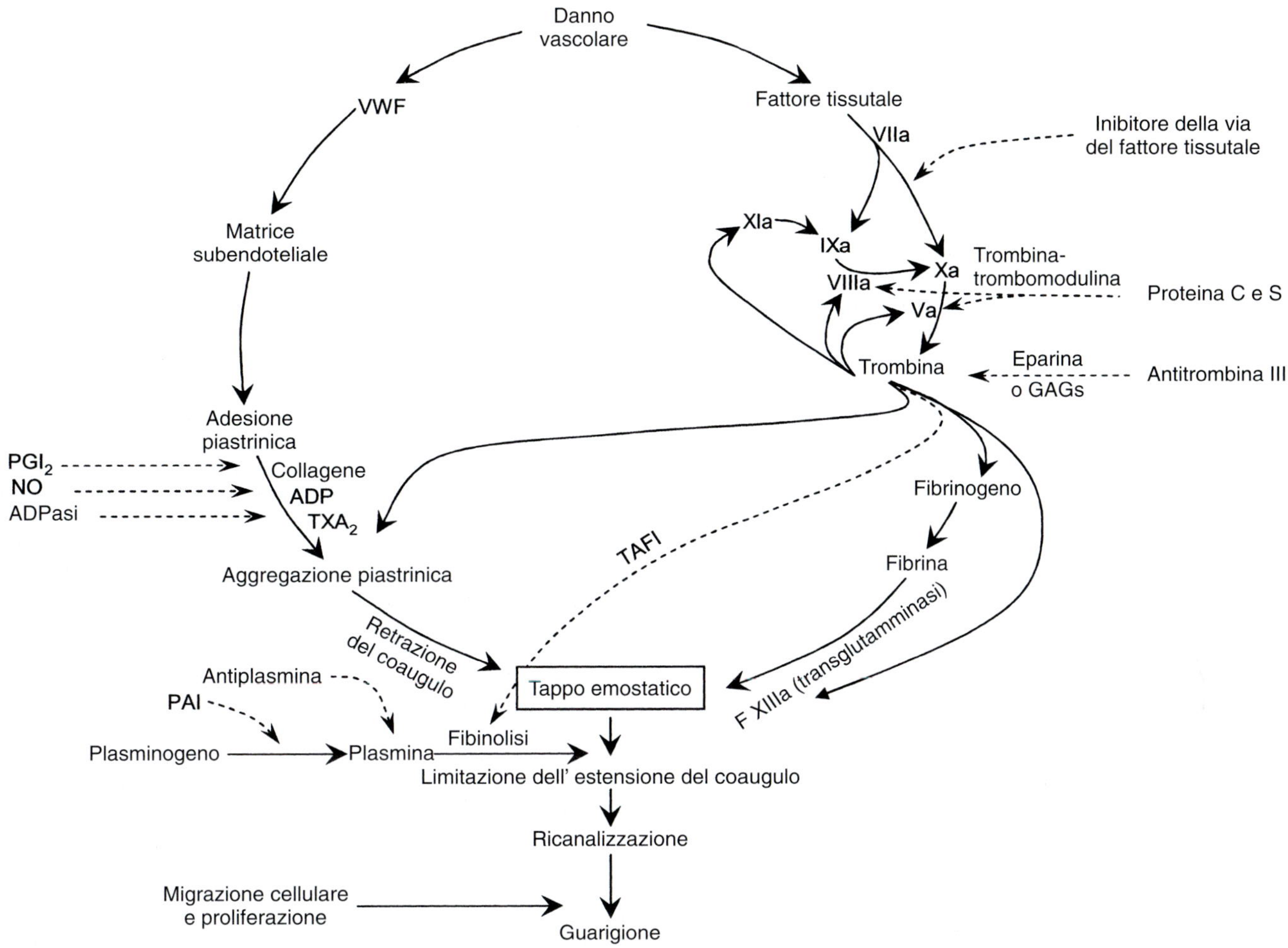

Figura 475-2. Il meccanismo emostatico. ADP, *Adenosine DiPhosphate* (adenosina difosfato); GAG, glicosaminoglicani; NO, ossido nitrico; PGI_2, prostaciclina; PAI, *Plasminogen Activator Inhibitor* (inibitore dell'attivatore del plasminogeno); TAFI, *Thrombin-Activated Fibrinolytic Inibitor* (inibitore della fibrinolisi attivata dalla trombina); TXA_2, trombossani A_2; VWF, *von Willebrand Factor* (fattore di von Willebrand).

proteine nella cascata sono divise in due gruppi: serin-proteasi zimogene che vengono attivate in enzimi funzionali e cofattori che aiutano a catalizzare le reazioni della coagulazione. Durante il processo di attivazione piastrinica, i fosfolipidi piastrinici presenti all'interno (soprattutto fosfatidilserina) vengono secreti e interagiscono a due livelli specifici che limitano la velocità nel processo coagulativo, coinvolgenti i cofattori del fattore VIII (il complesso X-asi) e il fattore V (complesso protrombinasi). Entrambe queste reazioni sono localizzate sulla superficie piastrinica e portano insieme l'enzima attivato, un cofattore attivato e lo zimogeno, che formeranno l'enzima successivo attivo della cascata. Ciò comporta un'amplificazione del processo, che fornisce un impulso coagulativo quando sia fisiologicamente necessario. *In vivo*, l'autocatalisi del fattore VII genera piccole quantità di fattore VIIa continuamente, così il sistema è sempre pronto ad agire. Vicino alla fine della cascata, si forma l'enzima multipotente trombina. La trombina trasforma il fibrinogeno in fibrina, attiva il fattore V, VIII e XI e fa aggregare le piastrine. La trombina attiva anche il fattore XIII. Il tappo stabile di fibrina e piastrine è infine formato attraverso la retrazione del coagulo e il legame crociato del coagulo di fibrina al fattore XIIIa.

Virtualmente tutte le proteine procoaugulanti sono equilibrate da proteine anticoagulanti che regolano o inibiscono le funzioni procoagulanti. Sono quattro gli anticoagulanti clinicamente importanti, presenti naturalmente, che regolano l'estensione del processo coagulativo. Queste includono l'antitrombina III (AT-III), la proteina C, la proteina S e l'inibitore della via del fattore tissutale (*Tissue Factor Pathway Inhibitor*, TFPI). L'AT-III è un inibitore delle serin-proteasi che regola prima di tutto il fattore Xa e la trombina, ma anche, in grado minore, i fattori IXa, XIa e XIIa. Quando la trombina nel sangue circolante incontra l'endotelio intatto, la trombina lega la trombomodulina, il suo recettore endoteliale. Il complesso trombina-trombomodulina in seguito attiva la proteina C in proteina C attiva. In presenza del cofattore rappresentato dalla proteina S, la proteina C attivata lisa e inattiva il fattore Va e il fattore VIIIa. Il fattore Va inattivato è infatti un anticoagulante funzionale che inibisce la coagulazione. L'inibitore finale è il TFPI, che rapidamente blocca l'attivazione del fattore X da parte del fattore VII e del fattore tissutale spostando il sito di attivazione del fattore tissutale e del fattore VII a quello del fattore IX (vedi Figg. 475-1 e 475-2).

Una volta che si è formato un tappo stabile di fibrina e piastrine, il sistema fibrinolitico limita la sua estensione e lisa anche il coagulo (fibrinolisi) per ristabilire l'integrità vascolare. La plasmina, prodotta dal plasminogeno per azione dell'attivatore del plasminogeno urochinasi simile o di tipo tissutale, scioglie il tappo di fibrina. Nel processo di dissoluzione del tappo di fibrina, vengono generati i prodotti di degradazione della fibrina. La via fibrinolitica è regolata dall'inibitore dell'attivatore del plasminogeno e dall'α_2-antiplasmina. Infine il flusso di sangue dentro e intorno al tappo è fondamentale, affinché il flusso del sangue ritorni al fegato, dove i complessi dei fattori coagulativi attivati sono rimossi e nuove proteine pro- e anticoagulanti vengono sintetizzate per mantenere l'omeostasi del sistema emostatico.

PATOLOGIA. La carenza congenita di una singola proteina procoagulante porta a patologie emorragiche, in cui il deficit di anticoagulante (inibitore di un fattore della coagulazione) predispone il paziente all'eccessiva trombosi. Nelle patologie acquisite dell'emostasi, si verificano frequentemente problemi multipli con l'emostasi, che perturbano e alterano l'emostasi. Una patologia primaria (la sepsi) e i suoi effetti secondari (shock e acidosi) attivano la coagulazione e la fibrinolisi, penalizzando la capacità dell'ospite di ripristinare le normali funzioni di emostasi. Quando la sepsi scatena la **coagulazione intravascolare disseminata**, i fattori della coagulazione procoagulanti e le proteine anticoagulanti vengono consumate, lasciando il sistema dell'emostasi squilibrato e propenso al sanguinamento o alla coagulazione. In maniera simile, i neonati e i pazienti con epatopatia grave hanno carenze di sintesi sia delle proteine procoagulanti sia di quelle anticoagulanti. Questa disregolazione fa sì che il paziente sia predisposto sia all'emorragia sia alla trombosi, a seguito di stimoli lievi o moderati che comportano alterazioni maggiori nel processo di emostasi.

Nella valutazione di laboratorio dell'emostasi, i parametri vengono manipolati per permettere la valutazione di aspetti isolati dell'emostasi e limitare la multifunzionalità di alcune delle sue componenti. Il processo di coagulazione è studiato nel plasma scoagulato con il citrato per legare il calcio, con l'aggiunta di fosfolipidi per mimare la reazione di superficie normalmente prodotta dalla membrana piastrinica e con uno stimolo che scatena la coagulazione. Il calcio viene aggiunto per far ripartire il processo coagulativo. Questo comporta anomalie come il fatto che *in vivo* la via della coagulazione fisiologica in cui il fattore VIIa attiva il fattore IX viene bypassata; invece nel tempo di protrombina (PT), il fattore VIIa attiva il fattore X. Se questa fosse la reale situazione fisiologica, ci sarebbe poi *in vivo* un meccanismo di bypass che migliorerebbe il grave deficit di fattore VIII e fattore IX, le due cause più comuni di sanguinamento abbondante.

475.1 • Valutazione clinica e laboratoristica dell'emostasi

ANAMNESI. Per la maggior parte delle patologie dell'emostasi, la storia clinica fornisce le informazioni più utili. Per una condizione emorragica, l'anamnesi dovrebbe stabilire il sito o i siti di sanguinamento, la gravità e la durata dell'emorragia e l'età all'esordio. Il sanguinamento è stato spontaneo o si è verificato dopo un trauma? C'è stata una storia precedente personale o familiare di problemi simili? I sintomi correlano con il grado di lesione o di trauma? Le ecchimosi sono comparse spontaneamente? Ci sono ematomi ed ecchimosi per traumi minimi? Se il paziente ha avuto un intervento chirurgico precedente o importanti cure odontoiatriche, c'è stato un sanguinamento abbondante? Se un bambino o un adolescente è stato sottoposto a chirurgia a carico delle superfici mucose, come una tonsillectomia o un'estrazione dentaria maggiore, l'assenza di un sanguinamento in genere permette di escludere un disordine emorragico ereditario. Guarigioni lente o ritardate di una lesione superficiale possono suggerire una patologia emorragica ereditaria. Nelle femmine in età post-puberale, è importante raccogliere un'attenta anamnesi sui flussi mestruali. Poiché alcune patologie emorragiche comuni, come la malattia di von Willebrand (*von Willebrand Disease*, VWD), presentano un'incidenza abbastanza alta, le madri e i membri della famiglia possono presentare la stessa lieve patologia di sanguinamento e possono non essere consapevoli che la storia mestruale delle figlie è anormale. Le donne con VWD lieve, che hanno una storia non grave di ecchimosi frequenti, presentano una riduzione delle ecchimosi durante la gravidanza e la somministrazione di contraccettivi orali. Alcuni farmaci, come l'acido acetilsalicilico e altri farmaci antinfiammatori non steroidei, possono inibire la funzione piastrinica, aumentando i sintomi del sanguinamento nei pazienti con una bassa conta piastrinica o emostasi anomala.

Oltre il periodo neonatale, le patologie trombotiche sono relativamente rare fino all'età adulta. Nel neonato, le carenze fisiologiche di cause procoagulanti e anticoagulanti causano la disregolazione del meccanismo dell'emostasi, ed eventi clinici possono condurre all'emorragia o alla trombosi. Se un bambino o un adolescente presenta una trombosi venosa profonda o un'embolia polmonare, deve essere ottenuta una storia familiare dettagliata per valutare la trombosi venosa profonda, l'embolia polmonare, l'infarto miocardico o l'ischemia negli altri membri della famiglia. Anche in assenza di una storia familiare, la presenza di una trombosi nel bambino o nell'adolescente dovrebbe dare luogo a una valutazione del soggetto per una predisposizione ereditaria o acquisita alla trombosi.

ESAME OBIETTIVO. L'esame obiettivo dovrebbe individuare prima di tutto se i sintomi del sanguinamento interessano le mucose o la cute (sanguinamento cutaneo-mucoso) o i muscoli e le articolazioni (sanguinamento profondo). L'esame dovrebbe determinare la presenza di petecchie, ecchimosi, ematomi, emartri o sanguinamento mucoso. I pazienti con difetti nelle interazioni tra le piastrine e la parete dei vasi sanguigni (VWD o difetti di funzione piastrinica) in genere hanno sanguinamenti cutaneomucosi, che possono includere l'epistassi, menorragia, petecchie, ecchimosi, ematomi occasionali e, meno comunemente, ematuria e sanguinamento gastrointestinale. I soggetti con una carenza dei fattori della coagulazione, come l'emofilia (carenza di fattore VIII o fattore IX), presentano sintomi di sanguinamento profondo nei muscoli e nelle articolazioni, con ecchimosi molto più estese e formazione di ematomi. I pazienti con VWD lieve o altre patologie del sanguinamento lieve possono non mostrare reperti anormali all'esame fisico. I soggetti con patologie della matrice del collagene e della parete vascolare possono presentare articolazioni eccessivamente mobili e cute lassa associate con ecchimosi facili (sindrome di Ehlers-Danlos).

I pazienti che sono sottoposti alla valutazione per patologie trombotiche dovrebbero essere interrogati su tumefazione, calore, dolore degli arti o degli organi interni (trombosi venosa), sulla dispnea inspiegabile e sulle polmoniti "persistenti" soprattutto in assenza di febbre (embolia polmonare) e varici e cambiamenti postflebitici. I trombi arteriosi in genere causano un'acuta e importante compromissione della funzione degli organi, come stroke, infarto miocardico o estremità doloranti, bianche e fredde.

TEST DI LABORATORIO. I pazienti che hanno una storia positiva di sanguinamento o che presentano emorragie in atto dovrebbero effettuare una conta piastrinica, un PT e un tempo di tromboplastina parziale (PTT). Se i risultati sono normali, dovrebbero essere considerati un tempo di trombina per valutare la funzione del fibrinogeno e i test per il VWF. Negli individui con test di screening risultati negativi, dovrebbero essere testati i singoli fattori della coagulazione. In un paziente con storia di sanguinamenti anomali e con una storia familiare positiva, test di screening normali non dovrebbero precludere successive valutazioni di laboratorio.

Non ci sono test di screening utili per le patologie ereditarie trombotiche. Se la storia familiare è positiva o la trombosi clinica non è spiegata, dovrebbero essere condotti saggi specifici per gli anticoagulanti. La trombosi è rara nel bambino e quando presente la possibilità di una predisposizione ereditaria deve essere considerata e valutata in laboratorio.

Tempo di emorragia. Il tempo di emorragia determina la funzione di piastrine e la loro interazione con la parete vascolare. Sono stati sviluppati strumenti standardizzati monouso, che permettono di controllare la lunghezza e la profondità dell'incisione cutanea. Il bracciale di uno sfigmomanometro sul braccio e gonfiato fino a 40 mmHg per bambini e adulti. Nei neonati a termine e nei bambini più giovani, è stato sviluppato uno strumento modificato che si usa a una pressione più bassa. Il tempo di emorragia è un test di laboratorio difficile da standardizzare, e ci sono molte variazioni interindividuali e tra i laboratori. Sebbene la conta piastrinica $<100\,000/mm^3$ venga associata a un tempo di emorragia prolungato, un prolungamento del tempo di emorragia sproporzionato può suggerire un difetto qualitativo delle piastrine o la VWD. Dopo aver effettuato l'incisione della cute con il dispositivo che misura il tempo di emorragia, il sangue viene raccolto dal margine dell'incisione a intervalli di 30 secondi finché il sanguinamento non cessa. Anche se ogni laboratorio stabilisce il proprio range di normalità, il sanguinamento in genere si ferma entro 4-8 minuti. Una valutazione accurata del tempo di emorragia richiede la cooperazione del paziente.

Analizzatore della funzione piastrinica. In un tentativo di valutare gli stadi precoci dell'emostasi (funzione piastrinica e interazione del VWF durante un taglio profondo), sono stati sviluppati molti analizzatori di piastrine *in vitro*. L'esperienza maggiore è stata con l'analizzatore di funzione piastrinica (PFA-100). Il PFA-100 misura l'adesione-aggregazione piastrinica nel sangue intero col taglio profondo quando esposte sia al collagene-adrenalina sia al collagene-ADP. I risultati sono riportati come tempo di chiusura misurato in secondi. Il PFA-100 ha una sensibilità variabile, in particolare nella valutazione della VWD e dei difetti di funzione piastrinica. Il PFA-100 è sensibile ad alcune varianti di VWD che sono caratterizzate da una riduzione dell'antigene VWF o della sua attività (vedi Capitolo 477). La sensibilità del PFA-100 alle patologie della funzione piastrinica meno gravi è controversa, e permangono dubbi sulla sua specificità. Sono necessari studi ulteriori per stabilire quando il PFA-100 possa essere usato come strumento di screening.

Conta piastrinica. La conta piastrinica è essenziale nella valutazione del bambino con una storia positiva di sanguinamento perché la trombocitopenia è la più comune causa acquisita di diatesi emorragica nel bambino. I pazienti con una conta piastrinica >50 000/mm^3 raramente presentano un sanguinamento clinico importante. La trombocitosi nei bambini in genere è reattiva e non viene associata a un sanguinamento o a complicanze trombotiche. Una grave trombocitosi persistente in assenza di una patologia sottostante può richiedere una valutazione per la rara presentazione pediatrica della trombocitemia isolata o della policitemia vera.

TEMPO DI PROTROMBINA E TEMPO DI TROMBOPLASTINA PARZIALE ATTIVATA. Poiché i fattori della coagulazione sono nominati in ordine di scoperta, essi non necessariamente riflettono l'ordine sequenziale di attivazione (Tab. 475-1). Infatti i fattori III, IV e VI non sono stati trovati in successione come proteine indipendenti; quindi questi termini non sono più usati. Il doppio meccanismo dell'attivazione coagulativa è stato chiamato via **intrinseca** (attivazione di superficie) ed **estrinseca** (mediata dal fattore tissutale). Lo studio del meccanismo dell'emostasi è poi complicato dal fatto che l'interazione *in vivo* può usare vie diverse da quelle studiate nei test di laboratorio. Il PT misura l'attivazione della coagulazione mediata dal fattore tissutale (tromboplastina) in presenza del calcio. L'aggiunta di fattore tissutale causa una bassa attivazione di produzione di fattore VIIa. Il complesso fattore tissutale-fattore VIIa attiva il fattore X. Quando il fattore X è attivato dalla via intrinseca o estrinseca, si genera il fattore Xa. Sulla superficie fosfolipidica piastrinica, il fattore Xa si unisce al fattore V e al calcio (il complesso "protrombinasi") per attivare la protrombina in trombina (anche detta *fattore IIa*). Una volta che si è generata la trombina, il fibrinogeno viene convertito in un coagulo di fibrina, punto terminale della reazione (vedi Fig. 475-2). Il PT non è allungato a seguito della carenza di fattore VIII, IX, XI o XII. Nella maggior parte dei laboratori, un PT normale è 10-13 secondi. Il PT è stato standardizzato utilizzando l'**International Normalized Ratio** (**INR**) così che i valori possono essere comparati tra i diversi laboratori e le dfferenti strumentazioni. Questo rapporto è usato per determinare simili livelli di anticoaugulazione con farmaci simili al warfarin.

TABELLA 475-1. Fattori della coagulazione

FATTORE COAUGULATIVO	SINONIMO	PATOLOGIA
I	Fibrinogeno	Defici congenito (afibrinogenemia) o disfunzione (disfibrinogenemia)
II	Protrombina	Deficit congenito o disfunzione
V	Fattore labile, proaccelerina	Deficit congenito (paraemofilia)
VII	Fattore stabile o proconvertina	Deficit congenito
VIII	Fattore antiemofilico	Deficit congenito, emofilia A (emofilia classica)
IX	Fattore di Christmas	Deficit congenito, emofilia B
X	Fattore di Stuart-Prower	Deficit congenito
XI	Precursori di tromboplastina plasmatica	Deficit congenito, talvolta chiamato emofilia C
XII	Fattore di Hageman	Deficit congenito non è associato a sintomi clinici
XIII	Fattore stabilizzante la fibrina	Deficit congenito

Tempo di tromboplastina parziale. La via intrinseca coinvolge l'attivazione iniziale del fattore XII, che viene accelerata da altre due proteine plasmatiche, la precallicreina e il chininogeno ad alto peso molecolare. Nel laboratorio clinico il fattore XII viene attivato utilizzando una superficie (silice o vetro) o un attivatore per contatto, come l'acido ellagico. Il fattore XIIa a sua volta attiva il fattore XI a fattore XIa, il quale poi catalizza la trasformazione del fattore IX a IXa. Sulla superficie fosfolipidica piastrinica, il fattore IXa si unisce al fattore VIII e al calcio per attivare il fattore X (complesso "tenasi").

Questo processo è accelerato dall'interazione con fosfolipidi e calcio ai livelli che coinvolgono il fattore V e VIII. Una carenza isolata di un solo fattore della coagulazione può portare all'aumento isolato del PT, del PTT o di entrambi, in base al livello del fattore nella cascata coagulativa. Questo è utile per determinare la carenza ereditaria dei fattori della coagulazione; tuttavia, nelle patologie acquisite dell'emostasi che si incontrano nella pratica clinica, in genere è carente >1 fattore, e quindi il relativo aumento del PT e PTT deve essere determinato.

Le misure del PTT come effettuate nei laboratori di analisi riguardano in genere il PTT "attivato"; tuttavia, la maggior parte si riferisce a esso come *PTT*. Questo test misura l'inizio della coagulazione a livello del fattore XII in livelli in sequenza fino al punto finale della cascata coagulativa. Esso non misura il fattore VII, XIII o gli anticoaugulanti. Il PTT utilizza un attivatore di contatto (silice, caolino o acido ellagico) in presenza di calcio e fosfolipidi. A causa della differenza dei reagenti e degli strumenti di laboratorio, il range normale per il PTT varia tra un laboratorio di un ospedale e un altro. I range normali per il PTT sono molto più variabili da laboratorio a laboratorio che quelli del PT.

Quindi, i meccanismi studiati dal PT e dal PTT permettono la valutazione della carenza dei fattori della coagulazione, anche se queste vie possono non essere le stesse di quelle che si verificano fisiologicamente. *In vivo*, il fattore VIIa attiva i fattori IX e X, ma come studiato di routine nei laboratori clinici la via attraverso cui il fattore VIIa attiva il fattore IX non è valutabile. Se il complesso fattore tissutale-fattore VIIa attivasse solo il fattore X, potrebbe essere difficile spiegare perché le patologie più severe del sanguinamento sono le carenze del fattore VIII (emofilia A) e fattore IX (emofilia B). *In vivo*, la trombina è generata e ritorna indietro ad attivare il fattore XI e accelerare il processo coagulativo. La coagulazione nel PTT può essere prolungata dalla carenza del fattore XII, della precallicreina e del chininogeno ad alto peso molecolare; queste sono condizioni asintomatiche.

Tempo di trombina. Il tempo di trombina misura il gradino finale della cascata coagulativa, in cui il fibrinogeno è convertito in fibrina. Il tempo di trombina normale varia tra i laboratori, ma è in genere 11-15 secondi. Un aumento del tempo di trombina si verifica con la riduzione dei livelli del fibrinogeno (*ipofibrinogenemia* o *apofibrinogenemia*), con la disfunzione del fibrinogeno (*disfibrinogenemia*) o con l'uso delle sostanze che interferiscono con la polimerizzazione della fibrina, come l'eparina o i prodotti di degradazione della fibrina. Se la contaminazione eparinica è una causa potenziale dell'aumento del tempo di trombina, è in genere richiesto il tempo di reptilasi.

Tempo di reptilasi. Il tempo di reptilasi utilizza il veleno di serpente per coagulare il fibrinogeno. A differenza del tempo di trombina, il tempo di reptilasi non è sensibile all'eparina ed è aumentato solo dal fibrinogeno diminuito o non funzionale e dai prodotti di degradazione della fibrina. Quindi se il tempo di trombina è aumentato ma il tempo di reptilasi è normale, l'aumento del tempo di trombina è dovuto all'eparina e non indica la presenza di prodotti di degradazione della fibrina o ridotta concentrazione o funzione del fibrinogeno.

Studi di mixing. Se è presente un inspiegato aumento del PT, del PTT o del tempo di trombina, viene praticato in genere uno studio di *mixing*. Plasma normale viene aggiunto a quello del paziente, e il PT e il PTT vengono ripetuti. La correzione del PT e del PTT attraverso il *mixing* 1:1 con plasma normale suggerisce il deficit dei fattori della coagulazione, perché un livello del 50% di proteine singole della coagulazione è sufficiente per produrre un PT e un PTT normale. Se il tempo di coagulazione non è corretto o è solo parzialmente corretto è in genere presente un inibitore. Un inibitore della coagulazione è un prodotto chimico simile all'eparina che ritarda la coagulazione o un anticorpo diretto contro uno specifico fattore coagulativo o un fosfolipide usato nei test di coagulazione. In pazienti ricoverati, la più comune causa di questo reperto è la contaminazione eparinica del campione. La presenza di eparina nel preparato può essere scoperta utilizzando il tempo di trombina e il tempo di reptilasi, come detto in precedenza. Se lo studio di *mixing* non corregge i valori o se questi si allungano, e il paziente presenta un sanguinamento clinico, un inibitore di uno specifico fattore della coagulazione (anticorpi diretti contro il fattore), soprattutto il fattore VIII, il fattore IX, il fattore X, può essere presente. Se il paziente non presenta sintomi di sanguinamento e sia il PTT che lo studio di *mixing* sono allungati, è spesso presente un anticoagulante simil-lupus (vedi Capitolo 482). Questi pazienti in genere presentano un PTT allungato, non sanguinano e possono avere una predisposizione clinica alla coagulazione eccessiva.

Analisi dei fattori della coagulazione. Ciascuno dei fattori della coagulazione può essere misurato nei laboratori clinici utilizzando il plasma con carenza di fattori singoli. Per la maggior parte dei fattori coagulativi, l'attività è misurata contro una miscela di plasmi normali o contro uno standard, in cui il 100% di attività è espresso a 100 UI/dL. Per definizione, 1 unità internazionale (UI) di ciascun fattore è definita come quella quantità presente in 1 mL di plasma normale riferito a uno standard definito dall'Organizzazione Mondiale della Sanità (OMS). In generale, un grave deficit del fattore VIII o del fattore IX è <1 UI/dL (<1% del normale), un deficit moderato è 1-4 UI/dL, mentre uno lieve è >5 UI/dL ma inferiore al range normale (Tab. 475-2). Per la maggior parte dei fattori della coagulazione, il range normale è 50-150 UI/dL (50-150%).

TABELLA 475-2. Valori di riferimento per i test coagulativi in bambini sani*

TEST	28-31 SETT. GESTAZIONALI	30-36 SETT. GESTAZIONALI	A TERMINE	1-5 ANNI	6-10 ANNI	11-18 ANNI	ADULTO
TEST DI SCREENING							
PT (sec)	15,4 (14,6-16,9)	13,0 (10,6-16,2)	13,0 (10,1-15,9)	11 (10,6-11,4)	11,1 (10,1-12,0)	11,2 (10,2-12,0)	12 (11,0-14,0)
APTT (sec)	108 (80-168)	53,6 (27,5-79,4)[§]	42,9 (31,3-54,3)[‡]	30 (24-36)	31 (26-36)	32 (26-37)	33 (27-40)
BT (min)				6 (2,5-10)[‡]	7 (2,5-13)[‡]	5 (3-8)[‡]	4 (1-7)
PROCOAGULANTI							
Fibrinogeno	256 (160-550)	243 (150-373)[§]	283 (167-399)	276 (170-405)	279 (157-400)	300 (154-448)	278 (156-40)
II	31 (19-54)	45 (20-77)[‡]	48 (26-70)[‡]	94 (71-116)[‡]	88 (67-107)[‡]	83 (61-104)[‡]	108 (70-146)
V	65 (43-80)	88 (41-144)[§]	72 (34-108)[‡]	103 (79-127)	90 (63-116)[‡]	77 (55-99)[‡]	106 (62-150)
VII	37 (24-76)	67 (21-113)[‡]	66 (28-104[‡]	82 (55-116)[‡]	86 (52-120)[‡]	83 (58-115)[‡]	105 (67-143)
VIII procoagulante	79 (37-126)	111 (5-213)	100 (50-178)	90 (59-142)	95 (58-132)	92 (53-131)	99 (50-149)
VWF	141 (83-223)	136 (78-210)	153 (50-287)	82 (60-120)	95 (44-144)	100 (46-153)	92 (50-158)
IX	18 (17-20)	35 (19-65)[‡§]	53 (15-91)[†‡]	73 (47-104)[‡]	75 (63-89)[‡]	82 (59-122)[‡]	109 (55-163)
X	36 (25-64)	41 (11-71)[‡]	40 (12-68)[‡]	88 (58-116)[‡]	75 (55-101)[‡]	79 (50-117)	106 (70-152)
XI	23 (11-33)	30 (8-52)[‡§]	38 (40-66)[‡]	30 (8-52)[‡]	38 (10-66)	74 (50-97)[‡]	97 (56-150)
XII	25 (5-35)	38 (10-66)[‡§]	53 (13-93)[‡]	93 (64-129)	92 (60-140)	81 (34-137)[‡]	108 (52-164)
PK	26 (15-32)	33 (9-89)[‡]	37 (18-69)[‡]	95 (65-130)	99 (66-131)	99 (53-145)	112 (62-162)
HMWK	32 (19-52)	49 (9-89)[‡]	54 (6-102)[‡]	98 (64-132)	93 (60-130)	91 (63-119)	92 (50-136)
XIIIa[‖]		70 (32-108)[‡]	79 (27-131)[‡]	108 (72-143)	109 (65-151)	99 (57-140)	105 (55-155)
XIIIb[‖]		81 (35-127)[‡]	76 (30-122)[‡]	113 (69-156)[‡]	116 (77-154)[‡]	102 (60-143)	98 (57-137)
ANTICOAGULANTI							
ATIII	28 (20-38)	38 (14-62)[‡§]	63 (39-87)[‡]	111 (82-139)	111 (90-131)	106 (77-132)	100 (74-126)
Proteina C		28 (12-44)[‡§]	35 (17-53)[‡]	66 (40-92)[‡]	69 (45-93)‡	83 (55-111)[‡]	96 (64-128)
Proteina S							
Totale (U/mL)		26 (14-38)[‡§]	36 (12-60)[‡]	86 (54-118)	78 (41-114)	72 (52-92)	81 (61-113)
Libera (U/mL)				45 (21-69)	42 (22-62)	38 (26-55)	45 (27-61)
Plasminogeno (U/mL)		170 (112-248)[‖]	195 (125-265)[‖]	98 (78-118)	92 (75-108)	86 (68-103)	99 (77-122)
TPA (ng/mL)		8,48 (3,00-16,70)	9,6 (5,0-18,9)	2,15 (1,0-4,5)[‡]	2,42 (1,0-5,0)[‡]	2,16 (1,0-4,0)[‡]	1,02 (0,68-1,36)
α_2AP (U/mL)		78 (40-116)	85 (55-115)	105 (93-117)	99 (89-110)	98 (78-118)	102 (68-136)
PAI-1		5,4 (0,0-12,2)[‡]	6,4 (2,0-15,1)	5,42 (1,0-10,0)	6,79 (2,0-12,0)[‡]	6,07 (2,0-10,0)[‡]	3,60 (0,0-11,0)

*Tutti i fattori tranne il fibrinogeno sono espressi in unità/mL (fibrinogeno in mg/mL), il plasma intero normale ne contiene 1 U/mL. Tutti i dati sono espressi come media seguita dai limiti superiori e inferiori che comprendono il 95% della popolazione normale.

[†]Livelli per 19-27 settimane e 28-31 settimane derivano da sorgenti multiple e non possono essere analizzate statisticamente.

[‡]Valori significativamente diversi da quelli degli adulti.

[§]Valori significativamente diversi da quelli del neonato a termine.

[‖]Valore fornito come CTA CTA unità/mL.

APTT, *Activated Partial Thromboplastin Time* (tempo di tromboplastina parziale attivato); α_2AP, α_2 antiplasmina; BT, *Bleeding Time* (tempo di emorragia); CTA, *Committee on Thrombolytic Agent* (comitato sugli agenti trombolitici [unità]); HMWK, *High Molecular Weight Kininogen* (chininogeno a elevato peso molecolare); PAI-1, *Plasminogen Activator Inibitors* (inibitori dell'attivatore del plasminogeno); PK, *Prekallikrein* (precallicreina); PT, *Prothrombin Time* (tempo di protrombina); TPA, *Tissue-Type Plasminogen Activator* (attivatore tipo tissutale plasminogeno); VWF, *von Willebrand Factor* (fattore di von Willebrand).

Dati da Andrew M, Paes B, Johnston M: Development of the hemostatic system in the neonate and young infant. *Am J Pediatr Hematol Oncol* 1990; 12:95; e Andrew M, Vegh P, Johnston M, et al: Maturation of the hemostatic system during childhood. *Blood* 1992; 80:1998.

Nei pazienti con emofilia A o B, gli inibitori dei fattori VIII o IX possono svilupparsi dopo terapia sostitutiva. Per determinare la quantità di inibitore presente, il saggio clinico standard di questi inibitori della coagulazione è il dosaggio di Bethesda. Una Unità Bethesda è definita come la quantità che inibisce il 50% del fattore coagulativo nel plasma normale.

Aggregazione piastrinica. Quando si sospetta un difetto della funzione qualitativa delle piastrine, viene in genere prescritto il test di aggregazione piastrinica. Un plasma ricco di piastrine del paziente viene attivato con uno di una serie di agonisti (ADP, adrenalina, collagene, trombina o recettore della trombina e ristocetina). Test ripetuti o effettuati in altri membri della famiglia sintomatici possono aiutare a determinare la natura ereditaria del difetto. Molti farmaci, soprattutto l'acido acetilsalicilico, altri farmaci antinfiammatori non steroidei e l'acido valproico, alterano i risultati dei test di funzione piastrinica. Alcuni aggregometri piastrinici misurano il rilascio specifico di ADP dalle piastrine, come evidenziato dalla luminescenza prodotta (lumiaggregometro) e sono più sensibili nel determinare le anomalie della reazione di rilascio delle piastrine dai granuli di deposito.

Test per la predisposizione trombotica. La predisposizione ereditaria alla trombosi si associa a una riduzione della funzione anticoaugulante (proteina C, proteina S, AT-III); la presenza di una molecola di fattore V che è resistente all'inattivazione mediata dalla proteina C (fattore V di Leiden); elevati livelli di procoagulanti (una mutazione del gene della protrombina); o un deficit della fibrinolisi (carenza di plasminogeno). Quando i pazienti sono stati sottoposti a screening per la tendenza protrombotica, test specifici sugli anticoagulanti naturali sono necessari. Anche se sono in genere disponibili test immunologici e funzionali, i saggi funzionali della proteina C, proteina S e AT-III sono in genere clinicamente utili.

Il **fattore V di Leiden** è una mutazione comune del fattore V che si associa a un elevato rischio di trombosi. Una mutazione puntiforme della molecola del fattore V previene l'inattivazione del fattore Va mediata dalla proteina C attivata e, quindi, la persistenza del fattore Va. Il difetto è anche noto come *resistenza alla proteina C attivata* e viene facilmente diagnosticato con i test sul DNA.

La **mutazione del gene della protrombina** (**G20210A**) è una mutazione della porzione non-codificante del gene della protrombina, con una G in posizione 20210 sostituita da una A. Questa mutazione aumenta la quantità di RNA messaggero per la protrombina, è associata a elevati livelli di protrombina e predispone alla trombosi. Questa anomalia è facilmente identificata attraverso i test di analisi molecolare del DNA.

Aumento dell'omocisteina. I livelli di omocisteina possono essere elevati come risultato di mutazioni genetiche, causando omocistinuria. Questi pazienti sono predisposti alla trombosi venosa e arteriosa così come a un aumento dell'aterosclerosi.

Test per il sistema fibrinolitico. Il tempo di lisi del coagulo di euglobina è un test di screening usato in alcuni laboratori per valutare la fibrinolisi. Test più specifici sono disponibili nella maggior parte dei laboratori per determinare i livelli di plasminogeno, di attivatore del plasminogeno e dell'inibitore della fibrinolisi. Un aumento nella fibrinolisi può essere associato con sintomi emorragici e un ritardo nella fibrinolisi è associato alla trombosi.

SVILUPPO DELL'EMOSTASI. Il neonato normale presenta un livello ridotto della maggior parte dei procoagulanti e degli anticoagulanti (vedi Tab. 475-1). In generale, è presente un'anomalia molto più marcata nei prematuri. Sebbene esistano differenze maggiori nei normali range tra i neonati e i prematuri, questi range variano molto tra i laboratori. Durante la gravidanza, si verifica una progressiva maturazione e un aumento dei fattori della coagulazione sintetizzati dal fegato. Il neonato molto prematuro presenterà PT e PTT aumentati, così come un'importante riduzione delle proteine anticoagulanti (proteina C, proteina S e AT-III). I livelli di fibrinogeno, i fattori V e VIII, il VWF e le piastrine sono vicine al normale durante gli ultimi periodi di gravidanza (vedi Capitolo 103.4). Poiché la proteina C e la S sono fisiologicamente ridotte, i fattori V e VIII normali non sono equilibrati dalle loro proteine regolatrici. D'altra parte, il deficit fisiologico delle proteine procoagulanti vitamina K dipendenti (fattori II, VII, IX e X) è parzialmente riequilibrata dalla fisiologica riduzione dell'AT-III. L'effetto netto è che i neonati (soprattutto i prematuri) presentano un rischio maggiore per le complicanze da sanguinamento, da trombosi o entrambi.

Chalmers EA: Neonatal coagulation problems. *Arch Dis Child Fetal Neonatal Ed* 2004;89:F475–F478.

Coller BS, Schneiderman PI: Clinical evaluation of hemorrhagic disorders: The bleeding history and differential diagnosis of purpura. In Hoffman R, Benz EJ, Shattil SJ, et al (editors): *Hematology: Basic Principles and Practice,* 4th ed. Philadelphia, Elsevier Churchill Livingstone, 2005, pp 1975–1999.

Esmon CT: Blood coagulation. In Nathan DG, Orkin SH, Ginsburg D, et al (editors): *Hematology of Infancy and Childhood,* 6th ed. Philadelphia, WB Saunders, 2003, pp 1475–1496.

Handin RI: Blood platelets and the vessel wall. In Nathan DG, Orkin SH, Ginsburg D, et al (editors): *Hematology of Infancy and Childhood,* 6th ed. Philadelphia, WB Saunders, 2003, pp 1457–1476.

Lusher JM: Clinical and laboratory approach to the bleeding patient. In Nathan DG, Orkin SH, Ginsburg D, et al (editors): *Hematology of Infancy and Childhood,* 6th ed. Philadelphia, WB Saunders, 2003, pp 1515–1526.

Monagle P, Andrew M: Acquired disorders of hemostasis. In Nathan DG, Orkin SH, Ginsburg D, et al (editors): *Hematology of Infancy and Childhood,* 6th ed. Philadelphia, WB Saunders, 2003, pp 1631–1668.

Monagle P, Andrew M: Developmental hemostasis: Relevance to newborns and infants. In Nathan DG, Orkin SH, Ginsburg D, et al (editors): *Hematology of Infancy and Childhood,* 6th ed. Philadelphia, WB Saunders, 2003, pp 121–168.

Montgomery RR, Gill JC, Scott JP: Hemophilia and von Willebrand disease. In Nathan DG, Orkin SH, Ginsburg D, et al (editors): *Hematology of Infancy and Childhood,* 6th ed. Philadelphia, WB Saunders, 2003, pp 1547–1576.

Parmar N, Albisetti M, Berry LR, Chan AK: The fibrinolytic system in newborns and children. *Clin Lab* 2006;52:115–124. Erratum in *Clin Lab* 2006;52:324.

Peyvandi F, Jayandharan G, Chandy M, et al: Genetic diagnosis of haemophilia and other inherited bleeding disorders. *Haemophilia* 2006;12:82–89.

Scott JP: Bleeding and thrombosis. In Kliegman R, Greenbaum L, Lye P (editors): *Practical Strategies in Pediatric Diagnosis and Therapy,* 2nd ed. Philadelphia, WB Saunders, 2004, pp 240–247.

Sugar NF, Taylor JA, Feldman KW: Bruises in infants and toddlers: Those who don't cruise rarely bruise. *Arch Pediatr Adolesc Med* 1999;153:399–403.

Capitolo 476 ■ Difetti ereditari dei fattori coagulativi (patologie emorragiche)

L'**emofilia A** (carenza di fattore VIII) e l'**emofilia B** (carenza di fattore IX) sono i difetti congeniti dei fattori della coagulazione più comuni e gravi. I reperti clinici nell'emofilia A e B sono virtualmente identici. L'**emofilia C** è la patologia emorragica associata a ridotti livelli del fattore XI (vedi Capitolo 476.2). Livelli ridotti del *fattore di contatto* (fattore XII, chininogeno ad alto peso molecolare e precallicreina) sono associati a un aumento significativo del tempo di tromboplastina parziale attivato (APTT; detto anche *PTT, Partial Thromboplastin Time*), ma non all'emorragia, come discusso nel Capitolo 476.3. Altre carenze dei fattori della coagulazione che sono meno comuni sono discussi in modo esaustivo nei sottocapitoli successivi.

476.1 • Deficit di fattore VIII o fattore IX (emofilia A o B)

I deficit dei fattori VIII e IX sono le patologie emorragiche ereditarie più comuni e severe. Nel 1985 sono stati clonati i geni per entrambi i fattori, VIII e IX. Successivamente, sono stati sviluppati concentrati ricombinanti di fattore VIII e IX per trattare i pazienti con emofilia, e quindi evitare il rischio di infezioni trasmesse con la trasfusione di derivati plasmatici.

FISIOPATOLOGIA. I fattori VIII e IX fanno parte di un complesso richiesto per l'attivazione del fattore X. Assieme ai fosfolipidi e al calcio, formano il complesso "tenasi" o fattore attivante il fattore X. La Figura 475-2 mostra il processo coagulativo come si verifica nei test, con il fattore X che viene attivato da entrambi i complessi del fattore VIII e IX o il complesso del fattore tissutale e del fattore VII. *In vivo*, il complesso del fattore VIIa e del fattore tissutale attiva il fattore IX per dare inizio alla coagulazione. In laboratorio, il tempo di protrombina (*Prothrombin Time*, PT) misura l'attivazione del fattore X mediata dal fattore VII ed è pertanto normale in pazienti con carenza del fattore VIII o del IX.

Dopo una lesione, l'evento emostatico iniziale è la formazione del tappo piastrinico, assieme alla produzione del coagulo di fibrina che previene una successiva emorragia. Nell'emofilia A e B, la formazione del coagulo è ritardata e non è robusta. Una produzione inadeguata di trombina compromette la formazione di un coagulo di fibrina con legami crociati stretti per supportare il tappo piastrinico. I pazienti con l'emofilia formano lentamente un coagulo soffice e friabile. Quando si verifica un sanguinamento non trattato in uno spazio chiuso, come un'articolazione, la cessazione del sanguinamento può essere la conseguenza del tamponamento. Con ferite aperte, in cui il tamponamento non può verificarsi, il sanguinamento profuso può comportare un'importante perdita di sangue. Il coagulo che si è formato può essere friabile e un nuovo sanguinamento si verifica durante la lisi fisiologica dei coaguli o con nuovi traumi minimi.

MANIFESTAZIONI CLINICHE. Né il fattore VIII né il fattore IX attraversa la placenta; i sintomi del sanguinamento possono essere presenti dalla nascita o manifestarsi nel feto. Solo circa il 2% dei neonati con emofilia va incontro a emorragia endocranica e il 30% dei neonati maschi con emofilia sanguinano con la circoncisione. Quindi, in assenza di una storia familiare positiva (l'emofilia ha un'elevata frequenza di mutazioni spontanee) l'emofilia può rimanere non diagnosticata alla nascita. Chiari sintomi di lividi facili, ematomi intramuscolari ed emartri iniziano quando il bambino "inizia ad andare in perlustrazione". Il sanguinamento da lacerazioni minori traumatiche della bocca (un frenulo torto) può persistere per ore o giorni e può portare i genitori a richiedere la valutazione medica. Anche in casi di emofilia grave, solo il 90% presenta un'evidenza di facili sanguinamenti a partire da un anno di età. Sebbene il sanguinamento possa verificarsi in ogni area del corpo, il segno distintivo dell'emofilia è l'**emartro**. Il sanguinamento intrarticolare può essere indotto da un trauma minore; molti emartri sono spontanei. L'emorragia articolare più precoce compare più comunemente a carico delle caviglie. Nel bambino più grande e nell'adolescente, l'emartro delle ginocchia e dei gomiti sono altrettanto comuni. Laddove le emorragie intrarticolari precoci del bambino sono riconosciute solo dopo una tumefazione maggiore e un accumulo di fluido nello spazio articolare, i bambini più grandi sono frequentemente in grado di riconoscere il sanguinamento prima del medico. Essi accusano una sensazione di calore, formicolio nell'articolazione come primo segno di un'emorragia intrarticolare precoce. Dopo episodi ripetuti di sanguinamento nella stessa articolazione, i pazienti con emofilia severa possono sviluppare un'articolazione "bersaglio". Il sanguinamento ricorrente può poi divenire spontaneo a causa dei cambiamenti patologici presenti nell'articolazione.

Sebbene la maggior parte delle emorragie muscolari sia clinicamente evidente perché c'è un dolore localizzato o un gonfiore, il sanguinamento nel muscolo ileopsoas richiede una specifica menzione. I pazienti possono perdere grandi volumi di sangue nel **muscolo ileopsoas** e andare incontro a shock ipovolemico, riferendo solo con un vago dolore nell'area dell'inguine. L'anca è mantenuta flessa, ruotata internamente per irritazione dell'ileopsoas. La diagnosi viene fatta clinicamente a causa dell'incapacità di estendere l'anca, ma deve essere confermata con l'ecografia o la TC (Fig. 476-1). Un sanguinamento a rischio per la vita in un paziente con emofilia è causato dall'emorragia in strutture vitali (sistema nervoso centrale, vie aeree superiori) o da sanguinamenti esterni (emorragie gastrointestinali o ileopsoas). Un pronto trattamento con concentrati dei fattori della coagulazione è imperativo per queste emorragie a rischio per la vita. Se un trauma cranico è di sufficiente gravità da suggerire la valutazione radiologica, il ripristino dei fattori dovrebbe precedere la valutazione radiologica. Le emorragie a rischio per la vita richiedono una terapia sostitutiva per ottenere un livello uguale a quello del plasma normale (100 UI/dL o 100%).

I pazienti con emofilia lieve che hanno il fattore VIII o IX a livelli >5 UI/dL in genere non presentano emorragie spontanee. Questi individui possono presentare un sanguinamento prolungato dopo cure odontoiatriche, interventi chirurgici o lesioni per traumi di modesta entità.

REPERTI DI LABORATORIO E DIAGNOSI. Il test di screening di laboratorio che è alterato dal ridotto livello di fattore VIII o fattore IX è il PTT. Nell'emofilia severa, il PTT è in genere 2-3 volte il limite superiore di normalità. I risultati degli altri test di screening del meccanismo di emostasi (conta piastrinica, tempo di emorragia, tempo di protrombina e tempo di trombina) sono normali. A meno che il paziente non possieda un inibitore per il fattore VIII o IX, il *mixing* del plasma normale con il plasma del paziente comporta la correzione del PTT. Il dosaggio specifico per il fattore VIII e IX confermerà la diagnosi di emofilia. Se la correzione non si verifica con il mixing, può essere presente un inibitore. Nel 25-30% dei pazienti con emofilia che ricevono infusioni di fattore VIII o IX si può sviluppare uno specifico anticorpo anti-fattore. Questi anticorpi sono diretti contro il sito attivo di coagulazione e sono chiamati *inibitori*. In questi pazienti il dosaggio quantitativo di Bethesda per gli inibitori dovrebbe essere eseguito per misurare il titolo anticorpale.

DIAGNOSI DIFFERENZIALE. Nei neonati con manifestazioni gravi di emorragia, la diagnosi differenziale include la trombocitopenia grave; le gravi patologie della funzione piastrinica, come la sindrome di Bernard-Soulier e la trombastenia di Glanzmann; la malattia di von Willebrand tipo 3 (grave); e la carenza di vitamina K. I test di screening sull'emostasi dovrebbero differenziare questi casi dall'emofilia.

GENETICA E CLASSIFICAZIONE. L'emofilia si verifica in circa 1:5000 maschi, con l'85% che presenta deficit del fattore VIII e il 10-15% che presenta deficit del fattore IX. L'emofilia non mostra un'apparente predilezione razziale, comparendo in tutti i gruppi etnici. La gravità dell'emofilia è classificata in base al livello di base del paziente di fattore VIII o IX, perché il livello del fattore in genere correla con la gravità dei sintomi del sanguinamento. Per definizione un'unità internazionale (UI) di ciascun fattore è definita come quella quantità presente in 1 mL di plasma normale rispetto a uno standard stabilito dall'Organizzazione Mondiale della Sanità (OMS); quindi 100 mL di plasma normale presentano 100 UI/dL (100% di attività) di ciascun fattore. Per semplificare discussione, da qui in avanti in questo capitolo verrà usato il termine *% di attività* per riferirsi alla percentuale trovata nel plasma normale (100% di attività). I concentrati dei fattori vengono anche riferiti rispetto uno standard internazionale dell'OMS, così le dosi terapeutiche sono in genere riferite a unità internazionali (UI). L'**emofilia severa** è caratterizzata dalla presenza di <1% di attività dello specifico fattore della coagulazione e il sanguinamento è spesso spontaneo. I pazienti con **emofilia moderata** presentano livelli di 1-5% e richiedono traumi lievi per indurre il sanguinamento. Individui con **emofilia lieve** presentano livelli >5%: possono trascorrere molti anni prima che la condizione venga diagnosticata ed essa richiede traumi significativi per causare emorragia. Il livello emostatico per il fattore VIII è >30-40% e per il fattore IX è

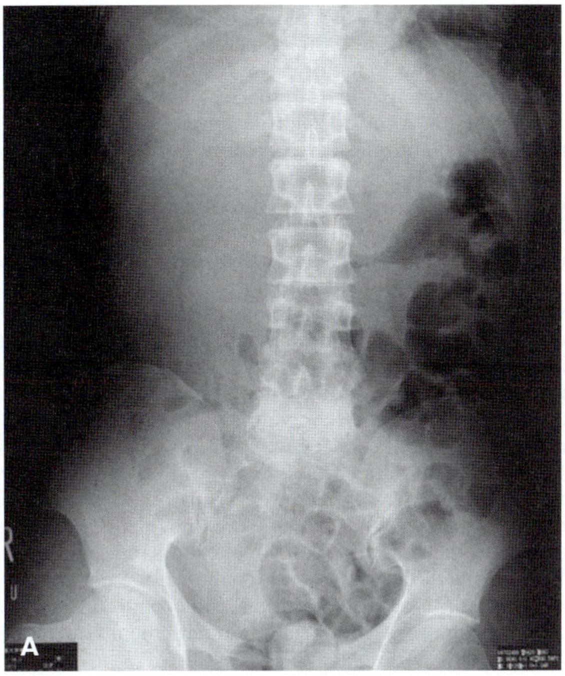

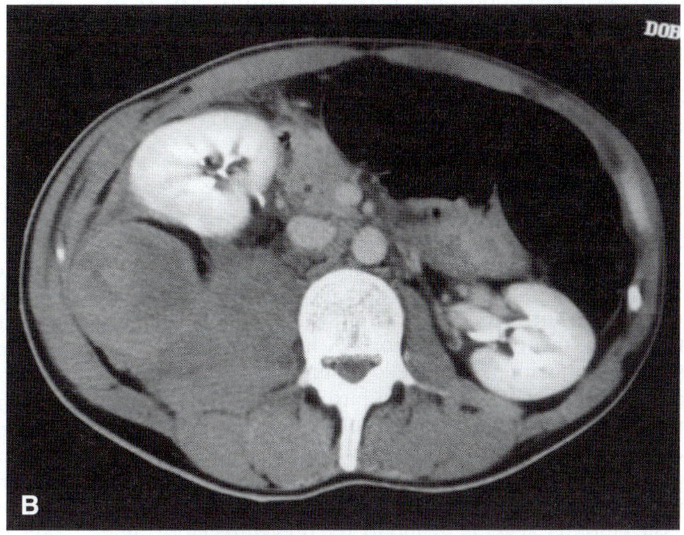

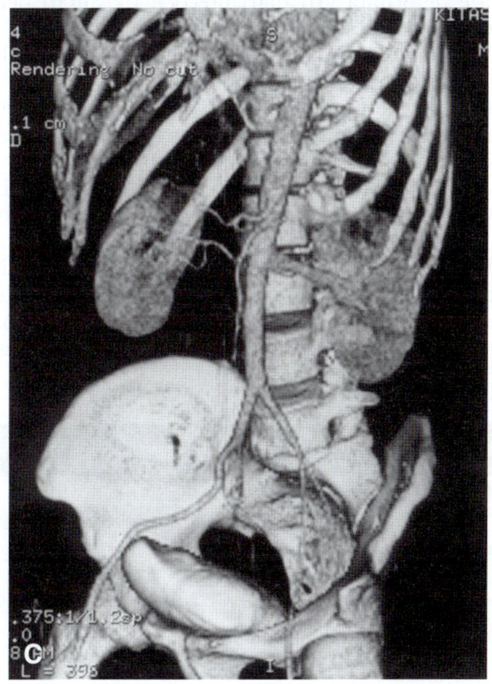

Figura 476-1. Ematoma massivo nel muscolo ileopsoas. La TC mostra un ematoma massivo nel muscolo ileopsoas destro in un paziente con emofilia B. Un maschio di 38 anni con deficit grave del fattore IX (emofilia B) è stato ricoverato per dolore addominale basso a destra di gravità progressivamente crescente e iperestesia. Inoltre, presentava un comune raffreddore con tosse severa e inappetenza da circa una settimana. *A*, Una radiografia addominale mostra un segno positivo dello psoas sul lato destro e un colon spostato a sinistra. *B*, La TC mostra un ematoma massivo del muscolo ileopsoas destro, che comporta la dislocazione anteriore del rene destro. *C*, Immagine tridimensionale ricostruita che mostra più chiaramente la dislocazione renale e i grossi vasi, stirati ma intatti. Questi sono reperti utili per le procedure diagnostiche, perché il progressivo dolore addominale basso a destra può simulare perfettamente un'appendicite acuta. L'emorragia è stata gestita con successo attraverso il ripristino del fattore IX, per una settimana senza alcuna ricaduta. Il paziente non aveva alcun inibitore del fattore IX. (Da Miyazaki K, Higashihara M: Massive hemorrhage into the iliopsoas muscle. *Intern Med* 2005;44:158.)

>25-30%. Il limite più basso dei livelli del fattore VIII e IX nei soggetti normali è circa del 50%.

I geni per i fattori VIII e IX sono localizzati vicino alla porzione terminale del braccio lungo del cromosoma X e, pertanto, sono caratteri legati alla X. La maggior parte dei pazienti presenta una riduzione quantitativa del fattore proteico della coagulazione; il 5-10% dei soggetti con emofilia A e il 40-50% di quelli con emofilia B producono una proteina malfunzionante. Circa il 45-50% dei pazienti con emofilia A grave presenta la stessa mutazione, nella quale è presente un'inversione interna nel gene del fattore VIII che comporta la mancata produzione della proteina stessa. Questa mutazione può essere individuata nel sangue dei pazienti o dei portatori e nel liquido amniotico attraverso tecniche molecolari. A causa delle molteplici cause genetiche alla base delle carenze dei fattori VIII e IX, la maggior parte dei pazienti è classificata in base alla quantità di attività coagulativa del fattore VIII o IX. Nel neonato, i livelli di fattore VIII possono essere artificialmente elevati a causa della risposta di fase acuta scatenata dal processo della nascita. Questo può causare nel paziente con forma lieve la presenza di livelli di fattore VIII normali o vicini al normale. I pazienti con emofilia grave presenteranno livelli non evidenziabili. Al contrario, i livelli del fattore IX sono fisiologicamente bassi nel neonato. Se è presente un caso di emofilia grave nella famiglia, un livello non misurabile di fattore IX è diagnostico per una grave emofilia B. In alcuni pazienti con carenza lieve di fattore IX, la presenza dell'emofilia può essere confermata solo dopo diverse settimane di vita.

Attraverso la lionizzazione del cromosoma X, alcune **donne portatrici** di emofilia A o B presentano una riduzione del fattore VIII o IX sufficiente per avere patologie emorragiche lievi. I livelli di questi fattori dovrebbero essere determinati in tutti i portatori conosciuti per determinare la necessità di trattamento in caso di chirurgia o sanguinamento clinico.

Poiché il fattore VIII è trasportato nel plasma dal fattore di von Willebrand, il rapporto tra il fattore VIII e quello di von Willebrand è talvolta usato per diagnosticare i portatori dell'emofilia. Quando possibile, le mutazioni genetiche specifiche dovrebbero essere identificate e utilizzate per testare altri membri della famiglia che sono a rischio sia di avere l'emofilia sia di esserne portatori.

TRATTAMENTO. Una terapia appropriata precoce è il segno distintivo di un eccellente trattamento dell'emofilia. Quando si verifica un sanguinamento lieve-moderato, i livelli di fattore VIII o IX devono essere portati ai livelli emostatici nel range di 35-50%. Per emorragie maggiori a rischio per la vita, la dose dovrebbe mirare a ottenere un livello del 100% di attività.

Il calcolo della dose di fattore VIII (FVIII) ricombinante o di fattore IX (FIX) ricombinante è quella che segue:

$$\text{dose di FVIII (UI)} = \text{\% desiderata (aumento del F VIII)} \times$$
$$\times \text{ peso corporeo (kg)} \times 0{,}5$$
$$\text{dose di FIX (UI)} = \text{\% desiderata (aumento del F IX nel plasma)} \times$$
$$\times \text{ peso corporeo} \times 1{,}4$$

Per il fattore VIII, la correzione è basata sul volume di distribuzione del fattore VIII, mentre per il fattore IX la correzione si basa sul volume di distribuzione e sul livello di aumento osservato del livello plasmatico dopo l'infusione del fattore IX ricombinante.

La Tabella 476-1 riassume il trattamento di alcuni comuni tipi di emorragia in un paziente con emofilia.

Con l'avvento dei prodotti sostitutivi ricombinanti, la **profilassi** è diventata lo standard terapeutico per la maggior parte dei bambini con emofilia severa, in modo da prevenire emorragie spontanee e deformità articolari precoci. I risultati della profilassi sono stati impressionanti nella prevenzione della malattia articolare cronica. Se si sviluppano articolazioni bersaglio, viene spesso iniziata una profilassi "secondaria".

Con l'emofilia lieve del fattore VIII, il fattore VIII endogeno spontaneamente dal paziente può essere rilasciato attraverso la somministrazione di desmopressina acetato. Nei pazienti con deficit di fattore VIII moderato o severo i livelli di fattore VIII immagazzinati nell'organismo sono inadeguati e il trattamento con desmopressina è inefficace. Il rischio di esposizione del paziente con emofilia lieve alle patologie trasmesse con le trasfusioni assieme al costo dei prodotti ricombinanti rendono accettabile l'uso della desmopressina, se è efficace. Una forma concentrata endonasale di desmopressina acetato può anche essere usata per trattare pazienti con emofilia A lieve. La dose è 150 μg (1 spruzzo) per bambini che pesano <50 kg e 300 μg (2 spruzzi) per bambini e giovani adulti che pesano >50 kg. La maggior parte dei centri somministra un trial di desmopressina per determinare il livello di fattore VIII ottenuto dopo la sua infusione. La desmopressina non è efficace nel trattamento dell'emofilia da carenza di fattore IX.

PROFILASSI. Molti pazienti vengono ora trattati con una profilassi a vita per prevenire emorragie articolari spontanee. In genere, i programmi vengono iniziati alla prima emorragia articolare. I bambini piccoli spesso richiedono l'inserimento di un catetere centrale per assicurare un accesso venoso. Questi programmi, anche se costosi, sono altamente efficaci nel prevenire o limitare molto il grado di patologia articolare. Il trattamento è in genere somministrato ogni 2-3 giorni per mantenere un livello plasmatico misurabile del fattore della coagulazione (1-2%) quando misurato appena prima della successiva infusione (livello più basso). Poiché la terapia genica potrà essere disponibile entro la durata di vita del paziente pediatrico, mantenere normali le articolazioni mediante la profilassi è una priorità ragionevole. Se si sviluppa un'artropatia moderata, la prevenzione di un sanguinamento futuro richiederà livelli di fattori della coagulazione plasmatici più alti. Nel bambino più grande che non sta ricevendo una profilassi primaria, una profilassi secondaria è frequentemente iniziata se si sviluppa un'articolazione bersaglio.

TRATTAMENTO DI SUPPORTO. Sebbene sia facile avvertire i genitori che il loro bambino dovrà evitare i traumi, questo consiglio è praticamente privo di utilità. I bambini nell'età del gioco sono attivi, sono curiosi di tutto e si fanno male facilmente. Misure efficaci includono l'informazione preventiva, incluso l'utilizzo di seggiolini da auto, poltrone gonfiabili, casco da bicicletta e l'evitare i comportamenti ad alto rischio. Si dovrebbe consigliare ai ragazzi più grandi di evitare sport di contatto violenti, ma questa è ancora una sfida. Ragazzi con emofilia grave spesso presentano emorragie in assenza di un trauma noto. Interventi precoci psicosociali aiutano la famiglia a ottenere un equilibrio tra l'iperprotezione e il

TABELLA 476-1. Trattamento dell'emofilia

TIPO DI EMORRAGIA	EMOFILIA A	EMOFILIA B
Emartro*	40 UI/kg concentrato di fattore VIII† al giorno 1; poi 20 UI/kg al giorno 2, 3, 5 finché la funzione articolare non ritorna normale o ai livelli di base. Considerare trattamento addizionale a giorni alterni per 7-10 giorni. Considerare la profilassi.	60-80 UI/kg al giorno 1; poi 40 UI/kg al giorno 2, 4. Considerare un trattamento addizionale a giorni alterni per 7-10 giorni. Considerare la profilassi.
Ematoma importante muscolare o sottocutaneo	20 UI/kg concentrato di fattore VIII; può richiedere il trattamento a giorni alterni fino alla completa guarigione.	40 UI/kg concentrato di fattore IX‡; può richiedere trattamento ogni 2-3 giorni fino a completa guarigione.
Bocca, denti decidui o estrazione dentaria	20 UI/kg concentrato di fattore VIII; terapia antifibrinolitica; estrazione della dentatura decidua.	40 UI/kg concentrato di fattore IX‡; terapia antifibrinolitica§; estrazione della dentatura decidua.
Epistassi	Applicare una compressione per 15-20 minuti; comprimere con una garza di vaselina; terapia antifibrinolitica; 20 UI/kg di concentrato di fattore VIII se questo trattamento si rivela inefficace.**	Applicare una compressione per 15-20 minuti; comprimere con una garza di vaselina; terapia antifibrinolitica; 30 UI/kg di concentrato di fattore IX‡ se questo trattamento si rivela inefficace.
Chirurgia maggiore, emorragia a rischio per la vita	50-75 UI/kg concentrato di fattore VIII, poi iniziare infusione continua di 2-4 UI/kg/h per mantenere il fattore VIII >100 UI/dL per 24 h, poi somministrare 2-3 UI/kg/ora in infusione continua per 5-7 giorni per mantenere la concentrazione >50 UI/dL e ulteriori 5-7 di giorni alla concentrazione di >30 UI/dL.	120 UI/kg concentrato di fattore IX‡, poi 50-60 UI/kg ogni 12-24 h per mantenere il fattore IX a >40 UI/dL per 5-7 giorni e poi >30 UI/dL per 7 giorni.
Emorragia nell'ileopsoas	50 UI/kg concentrato di fattore VIII, poi 25 UI/kg ogni 12 h fino a quando asintomatico, poi 20 UI/kg a giorni alterni per un totale di 10-14 giorni.‖	120 UI/kg concentrato di fattore IX‡; poi 50-60 UI/kg ogni 12-24 ore per mantenere il fattore IX a >40 UI/dL fino a quando asintomatico, poi 40-50 UI a giorni alterni per un totale di 10-14 giorni.‖¶
Ematuria	Riposo a letto; 11/2 × liquidi di mantenimento; se non controllata dopo 1-2 giorni, 20 UI/kg di concentrato di fattore VIII; se non controllata, somministrare prednisone (a meno che non sia HIV-positivo).	Riposo a letto; 11/2 × liquidi di mantenimento; se non controllata dopo 1-2 giorni, 40 UI/kg concentrato di fattore IX‡; se non controllata, somministrare prednisone (a meno che non sia HIV-positivo).
Profilassi	20-40 UI/kg concentrato di fattore VIII a giorni alterni per ottenere una concentrazione minima ≥1%.	30–50 UI/kg concentrato di fattore IX‡ ogni 2-3 giorni per ottenere una concentrazione minima ≥1%.

*Per l'emartrosi dell'anca, una valutazione ortopedica per possible aspirazione è consigliabile per prevenire la necrosi avascolare della testa femorale.
**OTC prodotti promuoventi la coagulazione possono essere utili.
†Per l'emofilia lieve o moderata, la desmopressina, 0,3 μg/kg, dovrebbe essere usata al posto del concentrato di fattore VIII, se si sa che il paziente risponde con un livello emostatico di fattore VIII; se vengono somministrate dosi ripetute, monitorare i livelli di fattore VIII per la tachifilassi.
‡Dosi definite applicate per il concentraro di fattore IX ricombinante; per il concentrato di fattore IX derivato dal plasma, usare il 70% della dose definita.
§Non somministrare terapia antifibrinolitica prima di 4-6 ore dopo una dose di concentrato del complesso della protrombina.
‖Valutazioni radiologiche ripetute dovrebbero essere praticate prima che la terapia venga sospesa.
¶Se sono richieste dosi ripetute di concentrato di fattore IX, usare concentrato altamente purificato specifico di fattore IX.
Adattata da Montgomery RR, Gill JC, Scott JP: Hemophilia and von Willebrand disease. In Nathan DG, Orkin SH (editors): *Nathan and Oski's Hematology of Infancy and Childhood*, 5th ed. Philadelphia, WB Saunders, 1998.

permissivismo. I pazienti con emofilia dovrebbero evitare l'acido acetilsalicilico e altri farmaci antinfiammatori non steroidei che colpiscono la funzione piastrinica. Il bambino con una patologia emorragica dovrebbe essere vaccinato contro l'epatite B, anche se i prodotti ricombinanti possono evitare l'esposizione alle patologie trasmesse dalle trasfusioni. I pazienti esposti ai plasma derivati dovrebbero essere sottoposti periodicamente a screening per l'epatite B e C, l'HIV e alterazioni della funzione epatica.

COMPLICANZE CRONICHE. Le complicanze a lungo termine dell'emofilia A e B includono l'artropatia cronica, lo sviluppo di un inibitore del fattore VIII o IX e il rischio di patologie infettive trasmesse con le trasfusioni. Sebbene l'approccio aggressivo e la profilassi abbiano ridotto i problemi dell'artropatia cronica, essi non sono stati eliminati.

Storicamente, l'artropatia cronica ha costituito la maggiore disabilità a lungo termine associata all'emofilia. La storia naturale dell'emofilia non trattata è quella di emorragie cicliche ricorrenti in specifiche articolazioni, incluse le emorragie nella stessa articolazione (bersaglio). Nei bambini piccoli, l'articolazione si distende facilmente e un grande volume di sangue può riempire l'articolazione finché non compare il tamponamento o non si interviene con una terapia. Dopo l'emorragia articolare, enzimi proteolitici sono rilasciati dai globuli bianchi nello spazio articolare e il ferro dell'eme induce la proliferazione dei macrofagi, portando a flogosi sinoviale. La sinovia si ispessisce e sviluppa nel cavo articolare proiezioni arboriformi "panno" che sono molto facili a essere stirate e che possono provocare ulteriori emorragie. La superficie cartilaginea diventa erosa e infine può anche esporre l'osso vivo, lasciando l'articolazione suscettibile all'anchilosi articolare. Nel paziente più grande con artropatia avanzata, il sanguinamento nell'articolazione bersaglio, con la sua sinovia assottigliata, causa dolore severo perché l'articolazione può avere un piccolo spazio per contenere il sangue. Una volta che si vede che si sta sviluppando un'articolazione bersaglio, al paziente viene in genere somministrata una profilassi a breve o lungo termine per prevenire la progressione dell'artropatia e ridurre l'infiammazione.

L'infusione del fattore coagulativo carente può indurre una risposta immune in pazienti con carenza sia di fattore VIII sia di fattore IX. Gli **inibitori** sono anticorpi diretti contro il fattore VIII o il fattore IX, che bloccano l'attività coagulativa. La mancata risposta di un episodio emorragico alla terapia sostitutiva è in genere il primo segno di un inibitore. Meno frequentemente, gli inibitori vengono riconosciuti durante i test di follow-up. Gli inibitori si sviluppano in circa il 25-35% dei pazienti con emofilia A; la percentuale è un po' più bassa in pazienti con emofilia B, molti dei quali producono una proteina non funzionalmente inattiva che li rende meno suscettibili alla risposta immune. Il fattore IX altamente purificato o il fattore IX ricombinante sembrano aumentare la frequenza di sviluppo dell'inibitore e alcuni inibitori anti-fattore IX inducono l'anafilassi. Molti pazienti che presentano un inibitore lo perdono a seguito di trasfusioni continue regolari. Altri presentano un elevato titolo di anticorpi con infusioni successive e possono necessitare di programmi di **desensibilizzazione**, in cui dosi elevate di fattore VIII o fattore IX vengono infuse allo scopo di saturare l'anticorpo e permettere all'organismo di sviluppare una tolleranza. I programmi di induzione della tolleranza immune per il fattore IX hanno causato la sindrome nefrosica in alcuni pazienti. È stato usato il rituximab, uso non registrato, come terapia alternativa per pazienti con un elevato titolo di inibitori che sono andati incontro a fallimento dei programmi di induzione della tolleranza immune. Se la desensibilizzazione fallisce, gli episodi di sanguinamento vengono trattati con fattore ricombinante VIIa o con concentrati del complesso protrombinico attivato. L'uso di questi prodotti bypassa l'inibitore in molti casi, ma può aumentare il rischio di trombosi. I pazienti con inibitori si devono rivolgere a centri che si occupano di molti di questi pazienti e che hanno programmi integrati per l'emofilia.

Nel passato, il trattamento con prodotti derivati dal plasma trasmetteva l'epatite B e C così come l'HIV a un grande numero di pazienti con emofilia. Nell'era dei prodotti ricombinanti, il rischio di acquisire queste infezioni dovrebbe essere minimo, ma i pazienti dovrebbero ricevere un'appropriata immunizzazione contro l'epatite B. Quelli che sono esposti ai prodotti ematici dovrebbero essere monitorati per l'epatite B e C così come per l'HIV.

TRATTAMENTO INTEGRATO. Oggi i pazienti con emofilia sono meglio gestiti nei centri integrati dell'emofilia. Questi centri sono dedicati al paziente e all'educazione della famiglia così come alla prevenzione e/o al trattamento delle complicanze dell'emofilia, inclusi l'artropatia cronica, lo sviluppo di inibitori e anche le infezioni, come l'epatite C e l'HIV. Questi centri coinvolgono una équipe di medici, infermiere, ortopedici, fisioterapisti e psicoterapeuti tra gli altri. L'educazione rimane cruciale nel trattamento dell'emofilia, perché i pazienti che stanno ricevendo la profilassi possono avere meno "esperienza" nel riconoscere gli episodi di sanguinamento in confronto ai bambini malati degli anni passati.

476.2 • Deficit di fattore XI (emofilia C)

Il deficit di fattore XI è una patologia autosomica associata a sintomi di sanguinamento lieve-moderato. È frequentemente riscontrata negli ebrei askenaziti, ma è stato trovata in molti altri gruppi etnici. In Israele, 1-3/1000 sono omozigoti per questo difetto, mentre gli ebrei sefarditi sono raramente colpiti.

La tendenza al sanguinamento non è così grave come nel deficit di fattore VIII o IX. Il sanguinamento associato alla carenza di fattore XI non è correlata con la quantità di fattore XI. Alcuni pazienti con deficit severo possono avere sintomi minimi o non averne al momento della chirurgia maggiore. A meno che il paziente non abbia precedentemente subito un intervento chirurgico senza sanguinamento abbondante, la terapia sostitutiva dovrebbe essere considerata e somministrata nel periodo preoperatorio in base alla natura della procedura chirurgica. Non esiste un concentrato di fattore XI approvato disponibile negli Stati Uniti; pertanto, il medico deve usare plasma fresco congelato (PFC).

Il sanguinamento durante la chirurgia minore può essere controllato con la compressione locale; in caso di estrazioni dentarie, i pazienti possono essere strettamente monitorati e trattati solo se si verifica l'emorragia. In un soggetto con carenza omozigote del fattore XI, il PTT è spesso più allungato rispetto ai pazienti con deficit severo sia di fattore VIII sia di IX. Il paradosso dei minori sintomi clinici assieme a un PTT più lungo è sorprendente, ma si verifica perché il fattore VIIa può attivare il fattore IX *in vivo*. La carenza di fattore XI può essere confermata da dosaggi specifici per il fattore XI. Le infusioni di plasma di 1 UI/kg in genere aumentano la concentrazione plasmatica del 2%. Pertanto, l'infusione di plasma a 10-15 mL/kg comporterà un livello plasmatico del 20-30%, in genere sufficiente a controllare un'emorragia moderata. Sarebbero necessarie infusioni di plasma più frequenti per ottenere livelli più elevati di fattore XI. Dal momento che l'emivita del fattore XI è in genere ≥48 ore, in genere non è difficile mantenere adeguati i livelli di fattore XI.

Il sanguinamento cronico nelle articolazioni è raramente un problema e, per la maggior parte dei pazienti, la carenza di fattore XI è un problema solo al momento di un intervento chirurgico maggiore, a meno che ci sia un secondo difetto dell'emostasi sottostante (per es. malattia di von Willebrand).

476.3 • Deficit del fattore di contatto (patologie non emorragiche)

Il deficit del "fattore di contatto" (fattore XII, precallicreina e chininogeno ad alto peso molecolare) causa un allungamento del PTT, ma non sintomi emorragici. Dal momento che questi fattori di contatto agiscono nella tappa iniziale della via intrinseca della coagulazione, a seconda del reagente usato per determinare il PTT, esso è marcatamente aumentato quando questi fattori sono assenti. Perciò, si presenta la situazione paradossale in cui il PTT è molto allungato ma non sono presenti segni clinici di sanguinamento. È importante che questi soggetti siano bene informati sul significato della loro carenza del fattore coagulativo, perché non necessitano di trattamento, anche in caso di chirurgia maggiore.

476.4 • Deficit di fattore VII

La carenza di fattore VII è una patologia emorragica rara che viene in genere scoperta solo allo stato omozigote. I soggetti con questa carenza possono presentare emorragia endocranica spontanea e sanguinamento mucocutaneo frequente. Questi pazienti presentano un PT marcatamente aumentato, ma un PTT normale. Il dosaggio per il fattore VII mostra una marcata riduzione del fattore VII. Dal momento che l'emivita del fattore VII è di 2-4 ore, la terapia con plasma fresco congelato è difficile ed è spesso complicata dal sovraccarico di fluidi. Un concentrato di fattore VIIa ricombinante in commercio si è rivelato talvolta efficace nel trattamento di alcuni pazienti con deficit di fattore VII, ma questo uso non è stato approvato dalla FDA.

DEFICIT NEI FATTORI DELLA VIA COMUNE (FATTORI I, II, V E X) CHE CAUSANO ALLUNGAMENTO SIA DEL PT CHE DEL PTT

476.5 • Deficit di fattore X

La carenza di fattore X è una rara patologia autosomica che comporta sanguinamento mucocutaneo e post-traumatico. Questa carenza è il risultato sia di una carenza quantitativa sia di una molecola disfunzionante. Una riduzione dei livello del fattore X si associa all'allungamento del PT e del PTT. In pazienti con difetto ereditario del fattore X, i livelli di fattore X possono essere aumentati utilizzando il plasma fresco congelato o il concentrato del complesso protrombinico. L'emivita del fattore X è di circa 30 ore e il suo volume di distribuzione è simile a quello del fattore IX. Quindi 1 U/kg aumenterà i livelli plasmatici di fattore X dell'1%.

Anche se è raramente un problema nei pazienti pediatrici, l'amiloidosi sistemica può essere associata alla carenza di fattore X a causa dell'assorbimento del fattore X sulla proteina amiloide. In caso di amiloidosi, la terapia trasfusionale spesso non si è rivelata efficace a causa della rapida clearance del fattore X.

476.6 • Deficit di protrombina (fattore II)

La carenza di protrombina è causata o da un livello marcatamente ridotto di protrombina (ipoprotrombinemia) o da una protrombina funzionalmente anomala (disprotrombinemia). I test di laboratorio nei pazienti omozigoti mostrano allungamento del PT e del PTT. I dosaggi per il fattore II, o protrombina, mostrano un livello marcatamente ridotto di protrombina. I pazienti vengono trattati con i concentrati del complesso protrombinico o con PFC. Nella carenza di protrombina, il plasma fresco congelato è utile, perché l'emivita della protrombina è di 3-5 giorni. La somministrazione di 1 UI/kg di protrombina aumenterà l'attività plasmatica dell'1%.

476.7 • Deficit di fattore V

La carenza di fattore V è una patologia emorragica lieve-moderata autosomica recessiva che è stata anche chiamata **paraemofilia.** Gli emartri si presentano raramente; il sanguinamento mucocutaneo e gli ematomi sono i sintomi più comuni. La menorragia severa è un sintomo frequente nelle donne. La valutazione di laboratorio mostra un allungamento del PT e del PTT. Dosaggi specifici per il fattore V mostrano una riduzione nei livelli di fattore V. Il plasma fresco congelato è attualmente l'unico prodotto terapeutico disponibile che contiene il fattore V. Il fattore V viene perso rapidamente dal PFC depositato. I pazienti con deficit del fattore V severo sono trattati con infusioni di PFC a 10 mL/kg ogni 12 ore. Raramente, un paziente con una storia familiare negativa di sanguinamento ha anticorpi contro il fattore V acquisiti. Spesso, questi pazienti non sanguinano perché il fattore V nelle piastrine impedisce un eccessivo sanguinamento.

476.8 • Deficit combinato di fattori V e VIII

La carenza combinata dei fattori V e VIII è secondaria all'assenza di una proteina di trasporto intracellulare, ERGIC-53, che è responsabile del trasporto dei fattori V e VIII dal reticolo endoplasmatico all'apparato di Golgi. ERGIC-53 è codificata sul cromosoma 18. La carenza di fattori V e VIII non è correlata ai geni difettivi per questa proteina, ma è secondaria a un deficit di una proteina di trasporto. Questo spiega la carenza paradossale di due fattori, uno codificato sul cromosoma 1 e l'altro sul cromosoma X.

476.9 • Deficit del fibrinogeno (fattore I)

L'**afibrinogenemia congenita** è una rara patologia autosomica recessiva in cui è presente un'assenza del fibrinogeno. Questi pazienti non sanguinano così frequentemente come i pazienti con l'emofilia e raramente presentano gli emartri. I pazienti affetti si possono presentare nel periodo neonatale con emorragia gastrointestinale o con ematomi dopo parto vaginale. Oltre a un prolungamento marcato del PT e del PTT, anche il tempo di trombina è allungato. In assenza di una coagulopatia da consumo, un livello non misurabile di fibrinogeno è diagnostico. In aggiunta alla carenza quantitativa del fibrinogeno, sono stati riportati una serie di fibrinogeni non funzionanti (**disfibrinogenemia**). Attualmente, non sono disponibili in commercio concentrati di fibrinogeno. Dal momento che l'emivita plasmatica del fibrinogeno è 2-4 giorni, il trattamento con PFC o con il crioprecipitato è efficace. Il livello emostatico del fibrinogeno è >60 mg/dL. Ogni sacca di crioprecipitato contiene 100-150 mg di fibrinogeno. Alcuni dosaggi clinici per il fibrinogeno sono inibiti da elevate dosi di eparina. Pertanto, un tempo di trombina marcatamente allungato, associato a un basso livello di fibrinogeno, dovrebbe essere valutato con la determinazione del tempo di reptilasi. Un tempo di reptilasi aumentato conferma che i livelli funzionali di fibrinogeno sono bassi e che l'eparina non è presente.

476.10 • Deficit del fattore XIII (fattore stabilizzante la fibrina o deficit della transglutaminasi)

Dal momento che il fattore XIII è responsabile dei legami crociati della fibrina per stabilizzare il coagulo di fibrina, i sintomi di un'emorragia ritardata sono secondari all'instabilità del coagulo. Tipicamente, i pazienti vanno incontro a un trauma un giorno e poi presentano ecchimosi o un ematoma il giorno seguente. I sintomi clinici includono lievi ecchimosi, ritardata caduta del moncone ombelicale dopo 4 settimane, scarsa guarigione delle ferite e aborti spontanei ricorrenti nelle donne. I risultati degli abituali test di screening per l'emostasi sono normali in pazienti con carenza di fattore XIII. I test di screening per la carenza di fattore XIII sono basati sull'osservazione che vi sia un'aumentata solubilità del coagulo a causa della marcata formazione dei legami crociati. Il coagulo normale rimane insolubile in presenza di urea 5 M, mentre in un paziente con carenza di fattore XIII il coagulo si dissolve. Dosaggi più specifici per il fattore XIII sono eseguiti con metodiche immunologiche. Poiché l'emivita del fattore XIII è 5-7 giorni e il livello di emostasi è 2-3% di attività, l'infusione di plasma fresco congelato o di crioprecipitato correggerà in questi pazienti la carenza. Il plasma contiene 1 UI/dL e il crioprecipitato contiene 75 UI/sacca. Nei pazienti con importanti manifestazioni emorragiche, la profilassi può essere ottenuta con infusione di crioprecipitato ogni 3-4 giorni.

476.11 • Deficit di antiplasmina o dell'inibitore dell'attivatore del plasminogeno

La carenza dell'antiplasmina o dell'inibitore dell'attivatore del plasminogeno, che sono proteine antifibrinolitiche, comporta un'aumentata produzione di plasmina e la lisi prematura del coagulo di fibrina. I pazienti presentano un sanguinamento mucocutaneo, ma raramente emorragie articolari. Poiché i risultati degli abituali test dell'emostasi sono normali, lo studio ulteriore per un paziente con storia di emorragie dovrebbe includere il tempo di lisi del coagulo di euglobina (se disponibile), che misura l'attività fibrinolitica ed è accorciato in presenza di questi difetti. Test specifici per l'α_2-antiplasmina e l'inibitore dell'attivatore del plasminogeno sono ora disponibili. I pazienti vengono trattati con PFC.

Abshire T: An approach to target joint bleeding in hemophilia: Prophylaxis for all or individualized treatment? *J Pediatr* 2004;145:581–583.

Bauer KA: Rare hereditary coagulation factor abnormalities. In Nathan DG, Orkin SH, Ginsburg D, et al (editors): *Hematology of Infancy and Childhood,* 6th ed. Philadelphia, WB Saunders, 2003, pp 1577–1582.

Bolton-Maggs PH: Factor XI deficiency and its management. *Haemophilia* 2000;6(Suppl 1):100–109.

Bolton-Maggs PH, Perry DJ, Chalmers EA, et al: The rare coagulation disorders: Review with guidelines for management from the United Kingdom Haemophilia Centre Doctors' Organisation. *Haemophilia* 2004;10: 593–628.

Bolton-Maggs PH, Stobart K, Smyth RL: Evidence-based treatment of haemophilia. *Haemophilia* 2004;10(Suppl 4):20–24.

Chalmers EA: Haemophilia and the newborn. *Blood Rev* 2004;18:85–92.

Dunn AL, Abshire TC: Recent advances in the management of the child who has hemophilia. *Hematol Oncol Clin North Am* 2004;18:1249–1276.

Funk M, Schmidt H, Escuriola-Ettingshausen C, et al: Radiological and orthopedic score in pediatric hemophilic patients with early and late prophylaxis. *Ann Hematol* 1998;77:171–174.

Hedner U: Recombinant factor VIIa (NovoSeven) as a hemostatic agent. *Semin Hematol* 2001;38(4 Suppl 12):43–47.

Kern M, Blanchette V, Stain AM, et al: Clinical and cost implications of target joints in Canadian boys with severe hemophilia A. *J Pediatr* 2004; 145:628–634.

Key NS: Inhibitors in congenital coagulation disorders. *Br J Haematol* 2004;127:379–391.

Manco-Johnson M: Hemophilia management: Optimizing treatment based on patient needs. *Curr Opin Pediatr* 2005;17:3–6.

Montgomery RR, Gill JC, Scott JP: Hemophilia and von Willebrand Disease. In Nathan DG, Orkin SH, Ginsburg D, et al (editors): *Hematology of Infancy and Childhood,* 6th ed. Philadelphia, WB Saunders, 2003, pp 1547–1576.

O'Connell NM: Factor XI deficiency. *Semin Hematol* 2004;41(1 Suppl 1):76–81.

Oldenburg J, Ananyeva NM, Saenko EL: Molecular basis of haemophilia A. *Haemophilia* 2004;10(Suppl 4):133–139.

Capitolo 477 ■ Malattia di von Willebrand

La più comune patologia emorragica ereditaria è la malattia di (*von Willebrand Disease*, vWD) e alcune segnalazioni suggeriscono che sia presente nell'1-2% della popolazione generale. La vWD è ereditata in modo autosomico, ma la maggior parte dei centri riporta più donne affette che uomini. Dal momento che la menorragia è il sintomo maggiore, sono soprattutto le donne a ricorrere al trattamento medico e quindi a venire diagnosticate. La vWD è classificata sulla base del fatto che la proteina sia quantitativamente ridotta ma non assente (tipo 1), qualitativamente anormale (tipo 2) o assente (tipo 3) (Fig. 477-1). Le mutazioni in loci differenti che codificano per differenti domini funzionali del fattore di von Willebrand (*von Villebrand Factor*, vWf) causano le differenti varianti della vWD.

FISIOPATOLOGIA. Il vWf è una grossa glicoproteina multimerica che viene sintetizzata nei megacariociti e nelle cellule endoteliali, depositata nei granuli α piastrinici e nei corpi di Weibel-Palade della cellula endoteliale. I multimeri a più elevato peso molecolare del vWf sono responsabili della normale interazione del vWf con la matrice subendoteliale e le piastrine. Durante la normale emostasi, il vWf aderisce alla matrice subendoteliale dopo un danno vascolare. Quando il vWf si lega alla matrice subendoteliale, la sua conformazione cambia per fare sì che le piastrine aderiscano al vWf attraverso il loro recettore glicoproteina IB (GPIB). Le piastrine sono poi attivate causando il reclutamento di altre piastrine ed esponendo la fosfatidilserina, che è un'importante tappa regolatoria per quelle dipendenti dal fattore V e dal fattore VIII nella cascata coagulativa. Il vWf serve anche come proteina di trasporto per il fattore plasmatico VIII. Una carenza grave di vWf causa una carenza secondaria nel fattore VIII, anche se il gene per il fattore VIII è normale. Questa è la causa del deficit autosomico del fattore VIII, ora conosciuto per essere un'anomalia molecolare del vWf e nota come *vWD tipo 2N.*

MANIFESTAZIONI CLINICHE. I pazienti con vWD in genere presentano sintomi di **emorragia mucocutanea**, incluse ecchimosi eccessive, epistassi, menorragia, emorragia postoperatoria, in particolare dopo una chirurgia mucosa, come la tonsillectomia o l'estrazione del dente del giudizio. Dal momento che la storia mestruale di un'adolescente è in genere inserita nel contesto negli altri membri della famiglia, un sanguinamento mestruale eccessivo non sempre viene riconosciuto come anormale, perché altre nella famiglia possono essere colpite dalla stessa patologia. Se una donna con flussi mestruali presenta una sideropenia, dovrebbe essere effettuata un'anamnesi dettagliata per ecchimosi e altri sintomi emorragici ed essa dovrebbe essere sottoposta a ulteriori valutazioni dell'emostasi.

Poiché il vWf è una proteina di fase acuta, lo stress può aumentarne i livelli. Quindi i pazienti non sanguineranno con procedure che comportano uno stress maggiore, come l'appendicectomia e il parto, ma possono sanguinare eccessivamente nel momento di interventi chirurgici estetici o alle mucose. I sintomi dovuti a traumi possono diminuire durante la gravidanza, perché i livelli di vWf possono essere doppi o tripli in quel periodo. Raramente, i pazienti con vWD possono avere teleangectasie gastrointestinali. Questa combinazione causa emorragie maggiori e un numero più elevato di ricoveri per i pazienti con una forma grave. Nei pazienti con il tipo 3, o omozigoti per la vWD, i sintomi emorragici sono molto più importanti. Questi pazienti vengono in genere diagnosticati presto durante la loro vita e possono presentare epistassi gravi o menorragia che comporta una perdita di sangue maggiore e possibilmente shock. Pazienti con la vWD di tipo 3 severo possono presentare emorragie articolari o emorragie spontanee nel sistema nervoso centrale.

REPERTI DI LABORATORIO. Anche se storicamente i pazienti con vWD sono stati descritti come portatori di un allungamento del tempo di emorragia e del tempo di tromboplastina parziale, questi reperti sono frequentemente normali nei pazienti con la vWD di tipo 1. Risultati normali ai test di screening non precludono la diagnosi di vWD. Dal momento che non esiste un singolo test che abbia dimostrato la capacità di scoprire la vWD, se la storia è suggestiva di una patologia emorragica mucocutanea, dovrebbero essere condotti i test per la vWD, inclusi un dosaggio quantitativo per l'antigene vWD, il test per l'attività del vWf (attività del cofattore della ristocetina), il test per l'attività del

	Normale	Tipo 1	Tipo 3	Tipo 2A	Tipo 2B	Tipo 2N	Tipo 2M	PT-VWD	BSS
WVF Ag	N	↓	assente	↓	↓	N o ↓	↓ o N	↓	N
WVF Rco	N	↓	assente	↓↓↓	↓	N o ↓	↓↓↓	↓	N
F VIII	N	↓ o N	1-3%	N o ↓	N o ↓	↓↓	N	N	N
RIPA	N	spesso N	assente	↓	spesso N	N	↓	N	assente
LD-RIPA	assente	assente	assente	assente	↑↑↑	assente	assente	↑↑↑	assente
PFA	N	↑	↑↑↑	↑	↑	N	↑	↑	↑↑↑
BT	N	N o ↑	↑↑↑	↑	↑	N	↑	↑	↑↑↑
Conta piastrinica	N	N	N	N	↓	N	N	↓	↓
Tx abituale		DDAVP conc. VWF	conc. VWF	conc. VWF (DDAVP)	conc. VWF (DDAVP)	conc. VWF (DDAVP)	conc. VWF (DDAVP)	piastrine	piastrine
Risposta alla DDAVP		buona	nessuna	variabile	diminuzione delle piastrine	variabile	variabile	diminuzione delle piastrine	nessuna o modesta
Risposta ai conc VWF		buona	buona	buona	buona	buona	buona	diminuzione delle piastrine	non risposta
Frequenza nella pop. generale		? (riportata 1-2%)	molto rara 1:250 000	rara	rara	rara	rara	rara	rara
Multimeri VWF	N	N ma ↓	assente	anormale	anormale	N ma ↓	N ma ↓	anormale	normale

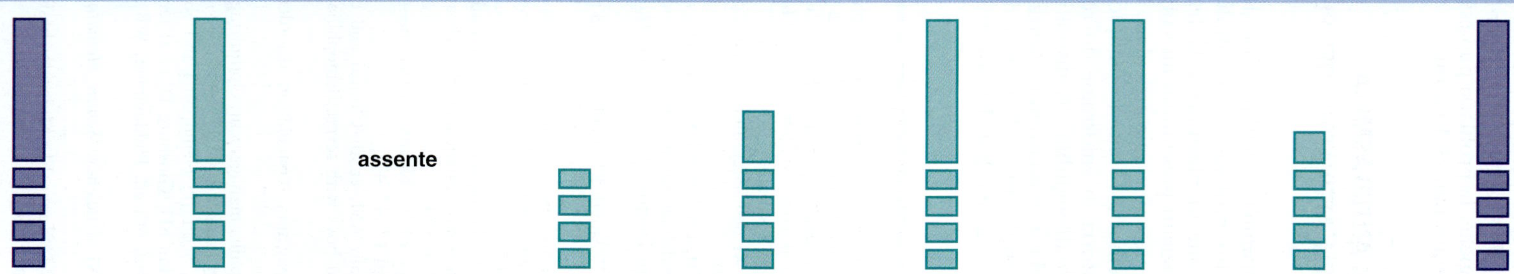

Figura 477-1. Varianti comuni di malattia di von Willebrand (vWD) e altre patologie correlate. Test di laboratorio sono elencati a *sinistra*, e i risultati più comunemente riscontrati nei pazienti con queste patologie sono mostrati. N, normale; ↑, incremento; ↓, riduzione. Una rappresentazione grafica dei multimeri del fattore di von Willebrand (vWf) viene mostrata alla base di ciascuna colonna. Un'*ombreggiatura più leggera* illustra una riduzione dell'intensità e la *lunghezza della figura* rappresenta la dimensione relativa dei multimeri. PT-vWD, pseudo-vWD di tipo piastrinico; BSS, *Bernard Soulier Syndrome* (sindrome di Bernard Soulier); FVIII, fattore VIII; vWf:Ag, antigene von Willebrand; vWf:RCo, *Ristocetin Cofactor Activity* (attività del cofattore ristocetina); BT, *Bleeding Time* (tempo di emorragia); PFA, *Platelet Function Analyzer* (analizzatore di funzione piastrinica); conc. vWf, concentrato di vWf; Tx, trattamento. RIPA, *Ristocetin Reducted Platelet Aggregation to Standard Dose Ristocetin* (ridotta aggregazione piastrinica ristocetina alla dose standard di ristocetina); DDVAP, desmopressina; LD-RIPA, *Ristocetin Induced Platelet Aggregation to Low Dose Ristocetin* (aggregazione piastrinica ristocetina indotta a bassa dose di ristocetina).

fattore plasmatico VIII, la determinazione della struttura del vWf (multimeri del vWf) e una conta piastrinica. Anche se la conta piastrinica è in genere normale nella maggior parte dei pazienti, quelli con la malattia di tipo 2B o con una patologia di tipo piastrinico (pseudo-vWD) possono presentare una trombocitopenia cronica. La Figura 477-1 elenca le varianti di vWD e riassume i loro reperti di laboratorio. I livelli del vWf variano con il gruppo sanguigno (tipo 0 <A <B <AB) che può confondere la diagnosi clinica della vWD ereditaria. Inoltre, esiste una controversia riguardo la definizione clinica della vWD "vera". La genetica molecolare può chiarire la diagnosi della vWD di tipo 1, ma possono esistere altri modificatori genetici al di fuori del gene del vWf, che sono in grado di influenzare in modo significativo la diagnosi. Più lieve è il fenotipo del paziente, maggiore è la difficoltà nella diagnosi.

GENETICA. Il cromosoma 12 contiene il gene per il vWf. In ognuna delle varianti del tipo 2 elencate nella Figura 477-1 sono colpite specifiche aree della molecola. Il fenotipo può guidare la diagnosi genetica della mutazione specifica. Alcune ricerche sono in corso per chiarire se tutti i casi di vWD di tipo 1 sono correlati a mutazioni del gene vWf sul cromosoma 12 o se ci sono dei modificatori genetici, come il gruppo sanguigno, che causa il fenotipo di vWD. I test clinici e genetici per le varianti della vWD sono disponibili solo in pochi laboratori di riferimento.

VARIANTI DELLA MALATTIA DI VON WILLEBRAND

La **vWD tipo 1** è la forma più comune e comprende l'85% dei casi. I sintomi emorragici includono epistassi, lividi e menorragia. Se il sanguinamento è eccessivo, la somministrazione di desmopressina (DDAVP) alla dose di 0,3 μg/kg endovena aumenterà il livello di vWf e di fattore VIII da 3 a 5 volte. La DDAVP endonasale è particolarmente utile per il trattamento ambulatoriale degli episodi emorragici. La dose è 150 μg (1 spruzzo) per bambini che pesano <50 kg e 300 μg (2 spruzzi) per quelli che pesano >50 kg.

La **vWD tipo 2A** è causata da un'anomala proteolisi del vWf, con la presenza solo dei multimeri più piccoli del vWf. Questo comporta la riduzione dell'antigene del vWF con una maggiore riduzione nell'attività del vWf. Anche se la DDAVP è sicura in questi pazienti non è sempre efficace, perché i multimeri normali non vengono mantenuti nel plasma. Un sanguinamento importante dovrebbe essere trattato con la terapia sostitutiva del vWf.

La **vWD tipo 2B** può essere causata da una delle centinaia mutazioni che comportano un vWf "iperattivo". Il vWf anomalo si lega spontaneamente alle piastrine, con conseguente rapida clearance delle piastrine e del vWf. I multimeri a più elevato peso molecolare vengono preferibilmente rimossi dalla circolazione, ed è comune una trombocitemia moderata-grave. La diagnosi di laboratorio è basata sul reperto che il vWf 2B iperattivo si lega alle piastrine e le agglutina a basse concentrazioni di ristocetina, una concentrazione che non agglutinerebbe le normali piastrine. Se viene somministrata a questi pazienti la DDAVP, il vWf 2B iperattivo anormale verrebbe rilasciato in circolo e potrebbe insorgere una grave trombocitopenia. I pazienti in genere rispondono all'infusione di vWf.

La **vWD tipo 2M** è causata da mutazioni che comportano la riduzione della funzione legante le piastrine del vWf. Quindi, i livelli di attività del vWf sono significativamente più bassi dei livelli dell'antigene vWf. Il legame di questa proteina al fattore VIII è normale: pertanto, i livelli di fattore VIII sono simili a quelli dell'antigene vWf. La DDAVP aumenterà i livelli del vWf e del fattore VIII, ma il rilascio di un vWf tipo 2M non ha sufficiente attività per consentire l'arresto dell'emorragia. Pertanto, può essere necessaria la terapia sostitutiva del vWf.

La **vWD tipo 2N** è causata dalla riduzione del legame del vWf al fattore VIII. Questa patologia è anche nota come **emofilia autosomica.** Con questa variante, l'interazione delle piastrine con il vWf è normale, ma il vWf tipo 2N si lega debolmente (o per niente) al fattore VIII, causando una rapida clearance del fattore VIII che viene debolmente complessato dal vWf. Quindi il livello del fattore VIII è ridotto molto più del livello del vWf. Comunemente, i pazienti che hanno un sanguinamento sintomatico sono eterozigoti composti che hanno ereditato un gene per il tipo 1 di vWD da un genitore e un gene per il tipo 2N di vWD dall'altro. Di rado, le mutazioni del tipo 2N vengono ereditate da entrambi i genitori e i livelli di vWf sono normali. In un paziente che è eterozigote composto per il tipo 1 e 2N, un allele non sintetizza la proteina e l'altro ne produce una funzionalmente anomala e, come risultato, tutto il vWf è funzionalmente anomalo. Sebbene la DDAVP provochi il rilascio del vWf tipo 2N, livelli aumentati di fattore VIII possono essere talora inadeguati per l'emostasi normale. Un trial per la DDAVP è indicato per stabilire la risposta e l'emivita del vWf e del fattore VIII dopo l'infusione. La terapia sostitutiva del vWf è in genere efficace.

La **vWD di tipo piastrinico (pseudo-vWD)** è in realtà un'anomalia del recettore GPIb delle piastrine. Questa può essere considerata l'anomalia inversa del tipo 2B, in quanto il recettore GPIb sulle piastrine è iperfunzionante e lega il vWf plasmatico spontaneamente. Questo comporta una **trombocitopenia** e la perdita di multimeri vWf ad alto peso molecolare, che sono indistinguibili da quelli visibili nella vWD tipo 2B. Test specifici, tuttavia, mostrano che questa è un'anomalia piastrinica piuttosto che un'anormalità plasmatica.

La **vWD di tipo 3** è un deficit di vWf a ereditarietà omozigote o eterozigote mista. I pazienti mostrano livelli plasmatici non misurabili di vWf e bassi, ma misurabili, livelli di fattore VIII. Questi pazienti presenteranno emorragie maggiori, ma solo raramente presentano emorragie articolari. Questa forma grave, molto rara, si verifica in circa 1:250 000 soggetti. Un'emorragia endocranica, un'epistassi maggiore e la menorragia nelle donne sono caratteristiche maggiori. Gli episodi di emorragia richiedono il trattamento con concentrati contenenti il vWf, che è una proteina sia plasmatica sia piastrinica. Dal momento che il trattamento con i concentrati contenenti il vWf correggono solo il livello plasmatico di vWf, i pazienti con emorragia grave possono avere bisogno di essere trasfusi con concentrati piastrinici per correggere la piastrinopenia. La DDAVP non è efficace nella vWD tipo 3.

DIAGNOSI E DIAGNOSI DIFFERENZIALE. La diagnosi di vWD dipende dal riscontro di bassi livelli di almeno una delle misure di laboratorio del vWf notate in Figura 477-1. La diagnosi differenziale dell'emorragia mucocutanea include anomalie del numero piastrinico, della funzione piastrinica o della parete vascolare (vedi Capitolo 484). Nell'assistere i bambini, è importante ricordare che la causa maggiore di questi reperti è il trauma, soprattutto non accidentale, ovvero l'abuso sul bambino.

COMPLICANZE. Le complicanze da sanguinamento dovute alla vWD sono rare. Nelle adolescenti, la perdita di sangue per menorragia può portare a un'anemia severa, sia acuta, con segni e sintomi di ipovolemia, sia cronica, per una carenza di ferro. I soggetti con la vWD tipo 3 possono manifestare emorragia articolare o muscolare simile ai soggetti con emofilia.

TRATTAMENTO. Il trattamento della vWD è diretto a incrementare i livelli plasmatici di vWf e fattore VIII. Dal momento che il gene per il fattore VIII è normale nei pazienti con vWD, l'aumento della concentrazione plasmatica di vWf permette un normale reintegro e la sopravvivenza del fattore VIII endogeno. La forma più comune di vWD è il tipo 1. In questi pazienti, il farmaco sintetico DDAVP induce il rilascio di vWf dalle cellule endoteliali. In alcuni pazienti con le varianti tipo 2, la DDAVP può essere egualmente efficace, ma in altre circostanze, il vWf rilasciato è funzionalmente alterato. I pazienti con la vWD possono non rispondere adeguatamente alla DDAVP perché rilasciano un vWf anomalo (soprattutto le varianti tipo 2); perché essi presentano la malattia tipo 3, in cui non c'è un vWf da rilasciare; o perché essi hanno una clearance accelerata del vWf rilasciato. Un piccolo sottogruppo di bambini e adulti, soprattutto i lattanti, non rilasciano il vWf in risposta alla DDAVP. In questi casi deve essere usata la terapia sostitutiva. Una terapia sostitutiva attuale utilizza il vWf derivato dai concentrati plasmatici che contengono anche il fattore VIII. Il vWf si distribuisce solo nello spazio intravascolare, perché è molto grande. Durante il frazionamento plasmatico, i multimeri vWf sono alterati in diverso grado. Pertanto, 1 U/kg aumenterà il livello plasmatico dell'1,5%. L'emivita plasmatica sia del fattore VIII sia del vWf è 12 ore, ma l'alterazione del vWf durante il frazionamento comporta un'emivita di 8-10 ore quando vengono infusi i concentrati. I concentrati di vWf ricombinanti o purificati (non contenenti il fattore VIII) saranno probabilmente disponibili nel prossimo futuro. Questo può essere utile per la profilassi o nella gestione prechirurgica. Quando usati per l'emorragia acuta, tuttavia, questi concentrati di vWf, che contengono una quantità bassa o nulla di fattore VIII, possono richiedere di essere supplementari con un'infusione di fattore VIII ricombinante per la prima infusione. Sia il fattore VIII sia il vWf sono necessari per la normale emostasi. Se viene ripristinato solo il vWf, la correzione endogena del livello del fattore VIII impiega 12-24 ore. Le estrazioni dentarie e talvolta le emorragie nasali possono essere controllate con DDAVP e l'agente antifibrinolitico, come l'acido ε-aminocaproico.

Favaloro EJ, Lillicrap D, Lazzari MA, et al: von Willebrand disease: Laboratory aspects of diagnosis and treatment. *Haemophilia* 2004;10:164–168.

Federici AB: Clinical diagnosis of von Willebrand disease. *Haemophilia* 2004;10(Suppl 4):169–176.

Gill JC: Diagnosis and treatment of von Willebrand disease. *Hematol Oncol Clin North Am* 2004;18:1277–1299.

Mannucci PM: Treatment of von Willebrand's disease. *N Engl J Med* 2004;351:683–694.

Mannucci PM: Desmopressin (DDAVP) in the treatment of bleeding disorders: The first 20 years. *Blood* 1997;90:2515–2521.

Montgomery RR, Gill JC, Scott JP: Hemophilia and von Willebrand disease. In Nathan DG, Orkin SH, Ginsburg D, et al (editors): *Hematology of Infancy and Childhood,* 6th ed. Philadelphia, WB Saunders, 2003, pp 1547–1576.

Sadler JE: Von Willebrand disease type 1: A diagnosis in search of a disease. *Blood* 2003;101:2089–2093.

Shankar M, Lee CA, Sabin CA, et al: von Willebrand disease in women with menorrhagia: A systematic review. *BJOG* 2004;111:734–740.

Werner EJ: von Willebrand disease in children and adolescents. *Pediatr Clin North Am* 1996;43:683–707.

White GC, Sadler EA: Von Willebrand disease: Clinical aspects and therapy. In Hoffman R, Benz EJ, Shattil SJ, et al (editors): *Hematology: Basic Principles and Practice,* 4th ed. Philadelphia, Elsevier Churchill Livingstone, 2005, pp 2121–2135.

Capitolo 478 ■ Predisposizione ereditaria alla trombosi

La trombosi nei bambini sono frequentemente associate a uno stato protrombotico acquisito o ereditario. È stato identificato un numero significativo di cause ereditarie di trombosi (Tabb. 478-1 e 478-2). Il neonato, a causa della carenza fisiologica di diverse proteine regolatrici, è particolarmente predisposto sia all'emorragia sia alla trombosi. Per entrambe le proteine anticoagulanti e per la maggior parte dei fattori procoagulanti, più il neonato è prematuro maggiore è la carenza. Il neonato piccolo è particolarmente a rischio perché gli interventi per garantirgli un supporto spesso includono il posizionamento di cateteri di grosso calibro all'interno delle vene e delle arterie maggiori. Quelli con carenze ereditarie degli anticoagulanti possono presentare sintomi più gravi. Dopo il periodo neonatale, i bambini piccoli sembrano presentare un certo grado di resistenza alla trombosi clinica, anche se presentano un deficit ereditario eterozigote di una proteina antico-

TABELLA 478-1. Stati protrombotici comuni

CONGENITI
Deficit di anticoagulanti
AT-III, proteina C o proteina S, plasminogeno
Resistenza alla proteolisi mediata dal cofattore
Fattore V Leiden
Alti livelli di procoagulanti
Mutazione 20210 dell protrombina
Elevati livelli di fattore VIII
Danno all'endotelio
Omocisteinemia
ACQUISITI
Ostruzione al flusso
Cateteri centrali
Gravidanza
Policitemia/disidratazione
Immobilizzazione
Danno
Trauma, chirurgia
Infiammazione
IBD, vasculiti, infezioni, sindrome di Behçet
Ipercoagulabilità
Gravidanza
Tumori maligni
Sindrome da anticorpi antifosfolipidi
Sindrome nefrosica
Contraccettivi orali
L-asparaginasi
Livelli elevate di fattore VIII
ALTRE CONDIZIONI RARE
Congenita
Disfibrinogenemia
Acquisita
Emoglobinuria parossistica notturna
Trombocitemia
Protesi vascolari

AT-III, antitrombina III; IBD, *Inflammatory Bowel Disease* (malattia infiammatoria cronica).

TABELLA 478-2. Patologie trombotiche ereditarie

CLASSIFICAZIONE E PATOLOGIE	EREDITARIETÀ	ASPETTI CLINICI
CARENZA O ANORMALITÀ QUALITATIVA DEGLI INIBITORI DEI FATTORI ATTIVATI DELLA COAGULAZIONE		
Deficit di AT	AD	Tromboembolia venosa (in siti abituali e non), resistenza all'eparina
Deficit di TM	AD	Tromboembolia venosa
Deficit di proteina C	AD	Tromboembolia venosa
Deficit di proteina S	AD	Tromboembolia venosa e arteriosa
Resistenza all'APC	AD	Tromboembolia venosa e arteriosa
LISI DIFETTOSA DEL COAGULO		
Disfibrinogenemia	AD	Trombosi venosa più frequente rispetto alla trombosi arteriosa
Deficit di plasminogeno	AD, AR	Tromboembolia venosa
Deficit del TPA	AD	Tromboembolia venosa
Eccesso di attività del PAI-1	AD	Tromboembolia venosa e arteriosa
DIFETTO METABOLICO		
Iperomocisteinemia	Sconosciuta	Tromboembolia venosa e precoce malattia vascolare aterosclerotica
ANOMALIA DELLO ZIMOGENO O DEL COFATTORE DELLA COAGULAZIONE		
Mutazione della protrombina	AD	Tromboembolia venosa
Livelli elevati di fattore VIII	Sconosciuta	Tromboembolia venosa
Livelli elevati di fattore IX	Sconosciuta	Tromboembolia venosa
Livelli elevati di fattore X	Sconosciuta	Tromboembolia venosa
Livelli elevati di fattore XI	Sconosciuta	Tromboembolia venosa

AD, autosomica dominante; APC, *Activate Protein C* (proteina C attivata); AR, autosomico recessivo; AT, antitrombina; PAI-1, *Plasminogen Activator Inhibitor-1* (inibitore dell'attivatore e del plasminogeno-1); TM, trombomodulina; TPA, *Tissue Plasminogen Activator* (attivatore del plasminogeno tissutale).

Da Robetorye RS, Rodgers GM: Update on selected inherited venous thrombic disorders. *Am J Hematol* 2001;68:256-268.

Modificata con il permesso da Rodgers GM, Chandler WL: Laboratory and clinical aspects of inherited thrombotic disorders. *Am J Hematol* 1992;41:113-122. Ristampata per gentile concessione di Wiley-Liss, Inc., a subsidiary of John Wiley & Sons, Inc.

agulante. Quando viene scoperto un trombo nel bambino piccolo, in particolare nel caso in cui l'anamnesi familiare sia anormale, dovrebbe essere iniziata una valutazione per una predisposizione trombotica. Nei bambini e negli adolescenti, le trombosi sono spesso scatenate da interventi medici o chirurgici maggiori.

FISIOPATOLOGIA E MANIFESTAZIONI CLINICHE. I principali anticoagulanti fisiologici sono illustrati nelle Figure 475-1 e 475-2. Una predisposizione ereditaria alla trombosi può essere causata da carenze delle proteine regolatorie proteina C, proteina S, antitrombina III e plasminogeno; la sintesi di una proteina procoagulante che non può essere inibita dalla sua proteina regolatoria, fattore V Leiden; elevati livelli di proteina procoagulante; mutazioni della protrombina (G20210A) ed elevati livelli di un acido organico tossico, l'omocisteinia.

La mutazione ereditaria del fattore V, **fattore V Leiden**, porta a una molecola di fattore V che quando viene attivata non viene successivamente inattivata dalla proteina C attivata. Questo lascia il paziente con un fattore V "attivo" e non regolato con la cosiddetta resistenza alla proteina C attivata. Inoltre, dopo la proteolisi a opera della proteina C attivata-fattore inattivato, il fattore Va (Vai) è un anticoagulante funzionale che inibisce la coagulazione. I soggetti con mutazione della protrombina (G20210A) presentano una mutazione all'estremità 3′ non tradotta dell'RNA messaggero per la protrombina che comporta livelli aumentati di sintesi della protrombina. I bambini con queste mutazioni ereditarie presentano un aumentata frequenza di trombosi venose. Le giovani donne hanno un rischio aumentato di trombosi venose in gravidanza o mentre assumono anticoncezionali per os. Esse altresì sono ad altro rischio di aborti ricorrenti. Nei giovani adulti con trombosi, il fattore V Leiden e la mutazione del gene della protrombina (G20210A) sono le anomalie più comuni associate. Il fattore V Leiden si trova in circa il 5% dei bianchi e la mutazione del gene della protrombina è presente nell'1-2% dei casi; la prevalenza di queste mutazioni in altre popolazioni etniche è minore.

Il deficit eterozigote delle proteine anticoagulanti, proteina C, proteina S o antitrombina III comporta una tendenza verso la malattia tromboembolica venosa a un'età precoce. Il caso speciale di porpora neonatale fulminante, caratterizzato da porpora necrotica della cute e trombosi dei vasi maggiori, è causato dal deficit omozigote della proteina C. Questi neonati sono stati probabilmente trascurati in passato perché i sintomi erano considerati secondari alla sepsi e alla coagulazione intravascolare disseminata. Poiché il neonato è fisiologicamente carente di proteina C, la sua assenza è difficile da determinare, tranne che in un laboratorio che abbia stabilito i range normali per i neonati a termine e pretermine. Se un soggetto presenta livelli non dosabili di proteina C, questa è per lo più una patologia ereditaria. Tuttavia la carenza fisiologica di proteina C nel neonato, associata alla sepsi vera, può pure condurre a livelli quasi indosabili di proteina C.

TEST DI LABORATORIO. Non ci sono test di screening per la predisposizione ereditaria alla trombosi; quindi sono necessari test specifici per la proteina C e S, l'antitrombina III, il fattore V Leiden e la protrombina 20210. Un'attenta anamnesi familiare può rivelare eventi tromboembolici nei membri della famiglia in età giovane, ma l'assenza di un'anamnesi positiva non permette di escludere una predisposizione ereditaria alla trombosi. Se viene sospettato il difetto ereditario di proteine anticoagulanti o regolatorie, dovrebbero essere condotti test specifici. Le tecniche che quantificano il livello e la funzione dell'antitrombina III, della proteina C e della proteina S libera sono ben stabilite. I test molecolari per il fattore V Leiden e il gene della mutazione protrombinica (G20210A) sono più specifici e sensibili rispetto ai test basati sulla coagulazione.

TRATTAMENTO. Il deificit omozigote della proteina C si presenta con una porpora fulminante nelle prime ore di vita. Il plasma fresco congelato (PFC) è l'unica fonte immediatamente disponibile di proteina C. Un miglioramento dei sintomi in genere richiede 10-15 mL/kg di PFC ogni 8-12 ore. Sono in corso trial clinici che utilizzano concentrati plasmatici di proteina C, che elimina la necessità di grandi quantità di PFC. Un concentrato di proteina C ricombinante attivata (dotrecognina-α) è stato approvato per il trattamento della sepsi dell'adulto, ma non per quello della carenza ereditaria. Ci sono pochi casi riportati in cui il concentrato della proteina C attivata è stato usato con successo per trattare la carenza di proteina C omozigote. Dopo che i sintomi del neonato sono migliorati, la quantità di PFC o di concentrato di proteina C viene regolata attraverso il monitoraggio dei livelli di proteina C. Quando il lattante è oltre il periodo neonatale, warfarin ad alte dosi (per ottenere un **International Normalized Ratio** [INR] nel range di 3-5) può prevenire la maggior parte dei problemi trombotici, ma la trombosi acuta intercorrente richiede PFC addizionale o concentrato di proteina C (vedi anche Capitolo 479).

I pazienti che presentano una trombosi associata a una predisposizione ereditaria alla coagulazione dovrebbero essere trattati con anticoagulanti (vedi Capitolo 479). La terapia sostitutiva in genere non è indicata. I soggetti con omocistinuria dovrebbero ricevere anticoagulanti assieme al trattamento della loro patologia primaria (vedi Capitolo 85.3).

Bhojwani D, Hart D: Thrombophilia in childhood. *Curr Probl Pediatr Adolesc Health Care* 2004;34:190–212.

Chalmers EA: Heritable thrombophilia and childhood thrombosis. *Blood Rev* 2001;15:181–189.

David M, Andrew M: Venous thromboembolic complications in children. *J Pediatr* 1993;123:337–346.

de Moerloose P, Alhenc-Gelas M, Boehlen F, et al: Deep venous thrombosis and thrombophilia: Indications for testing and clinical implications. *Semin Vasc Med* 2001;1:89–96.

Esmon CT: Blood coagulation. In Nathan DG, Orkin SH, Ginsburg D, et al (editors): *Hematology of Infancy and Childhood,* 6th ed. Philadelphia, WB Saunders, 2003, pp 1475–1496.

Heller C, Nowak-Gottl U: Maternal thrombophilia and neonatal thrombosis. *Best Pract Res Clin Haematol* 2003;16:333–345.

Hoppe C, Matsunaga A: Pediatric thrombosis. *Pediatr Clin North Am* 2002;49:1257–1283.

Langlois NJ, Wells PS: Risk of venous thromboembolism in relatives of symptomatic probands with thrombophilia: A systematic review. *Thromb Haemost* 2003;90:17–26.

Male C, Kuhle S, Mitchell L: Diagnosis of venous thromboembolism in children. *Semin Thromb Hemost* 2003;29:377–390.

Monagle P, Chan A, Massicotte P, et al: Antithrombotic therapy in children: The Seventh ACCP Conference on Antithrombotic and Thrombolytic Therapy. *Chest* 2004;126:645S–687S.

Monagle P, Andrew M: Acquired disorders of hemostasis. In Nathan DG, Orkin SH, Ginsburg D, et al (editors): *Hematology of Infancy and Childhood,* 6th ed. Philadelphia, WB Saunders, 2003, pp 1631–1668.

Robetorye RS, Rodgers GM: Update on selected inherited venous thrombotic disorders. *Am J Hematol* 2001;68:256–268.

Scott JP: Bleeding and thrombosis. In Kliegman R, Greenbaum L, Lye P (editors): *Practical Strategies in Pediatric Diagnosis and Therapy,* 2nd ed. Philadelphia, WB Saunders, 2004, pp 240–247.

Seligsohn U, Lubetsky A: Genetic susceptibility to venous thrombosis. *N Engl J Med* 2001;344:1222–1231.

Capitolo 479 ■ Patologie trombotiche acquisite

L'occlusione di un vaso sanguigno da parte di un tappo piastrinico o di un coagulo di fibrina può presentarsi nei vasi di qualsiasi dimensione. Un grande numero di patologie sistemiche è associato all'occlusione dei vasi arteriosi e venosi di diverso calibro, incluse le vasculiti, come il lupus eritematoso sistemico (vedi Capitolo 157) e la malattia di Kawasaki (vedi Capitolo165); difetti metabolici, come l'omocisteinemia (vedi Capitolo 85) e le emoglobinopatie, come l'anemia a cellule falciformi (vedi Capitolo 462) e la policitemia (vedi Capitolo 466 e 467). L'attivazione della coagulazione come complicanza della coagulazione intravascolare disseminata può portare alla trombosi microvascolare e macrovascolare (vedi Capitolo 483). Anche gli interventi medici possono causare la predisposizione alla trombosi, come quando i neonati malati hanno cateteri inseriti in vasi maggiori o quando i bambini con leucemia linfoblastica acuta ricevono l'agente chemioterapico L-asparaginasi, che riduce le proteine anticoagulanti. Oltre al danno vasale, i meccanismi che portano alla trombosi includono uno o più dei seguenti: *anomala aggregazione-adesione piastrinica, attivazione del meccanismo della coagulazione, sistema anticoagulante difettivo o carente, ridotta attività fibrinolitica* e *riduzione del flusso sanguigno.* La trombosi arteriosa sembra dipendere dalla lesione del vaso e dall'attivazione piastrinica in condizioni di flusso elevato, mentre la trombosi venosa in genere si presenta in condizioni di basso flusso associate ad attivazione del meccanismo coagulativo o a un difettoso sistema inibitore-fibrinolitico.

EPIDEMIOLOGIA. Anche se gli eventi trombotici acquisiti ed embolici non sono comuni nei bambini sani, la tromboembolia è una complicanza frequente nei neonati malati e nei pazienti con patologie specifiche (vedi Tab. 478-1). Negli Stati Uniti l'incidenza della malattia tromboembolica al momento del ricovero in ospedale è di circa 10/100 000 bambini/anno, ma può variare di molto in base all'età del bambino. I neonati e gli adolescenti più grandi presentano tassi maggiori.

MANIFESTAZIONI CLINICHE. Le trombosi arteriose si presentano con importante disfunzione degli organi a causa dell'ischemia (arti freddi e senza polso). Questi reperti possono essere scatenati dalla formazione di trombi nel sito di danno vasale o causati da emboli. Gli accidenti venosi in genere si presentano con organi o arti caldi, aumentati di volume o di consistenza soffice. Una trombosi venosa profonda (TVP) può essere asintomatica e si presenta solo dopo lo sviluppo di un'embolia polmonare. In generale, gli eventi occlusivi venosi nei bambini presentano un esordio acuto o improvviso.

DIAGNOSI. La diagnosi di trombosi si ottiene mediante eco Doppler o angioRM. In casi speciali (trombosi degli arti superiori), può essere necessaria l'angiografia con contrasto. Lo screening coagulativo di routine è raramente utile per diagnosticare un evento tromboembolico. Gli studi negli adulti hanno suggerito che un saggio quantitativo del **D-dimero** (che si forma quando la fibrina con legami crociati viene proteolisata dalla plasmina) è uno strumento di screening sensibile per la TVP e soprattutto per l'embolia polmonare (vedi Capitolo 406). Nella coagulazione intravascolare disseminata acuta i risultati del test di screening sono gravemente anormali, caratterizzati dalla trombocitopenia, ipofibrinogenemia, allungamento del tempo di protrombina (*Prothrombin Time*, PT) e del tempo di tromboplastina parziale (*Partial Thromboplastin Time*, PTT) e aumentati livelli di D-dimero (vedi Capitolo 483).

Le patologie comunemente associate alle trombosi sono elencate nella Tabella 478-1. La **sindrome da anticoagulante lupico** è un caso speciale in cui un inibitore apparente della coagulazione causa una predisposizione alla trombosi. In laboratorio, l'anticoagulante lupico causa allungamento del PTT che non si corregge mescolando 1:1 con plasma normale. L'anticorpo è diretto contro il fosfolipide, utilizzato come reagente nel PTT. I test specifici confermano la presenza di un anticorpo antifosfolipide. Anche se il PTT è allungato, il paziente con sindrome da anticoagulante lupico isolato in genere non presenta un rischio di emorragia aumentato. Paradossalmente il 5-20% di questi individui può sviluppare trombosi venose o arteriose. La sindrome da anticoagulante lupico, sia da solo sia come componente della sindrome antifosfolipidi, può essere primitiva (idiopatica) o associata al lupus eritematoso sistemico; all'infezione, soprattutto l'HIV; alla reazione ai farmaci o ad altre malattie autoimmuni. Caratteristiche correlate includono *livedo reticularis*, trombocitopenia, aborti ricorrenti e trombosi (arteriosa, venosa o entrambe). Alcuni bambini possono presentare un anticoagulante lupico transitorio dopo una virosi. Il trattamento della trombosi associata ad anticoagulante lupico include l'eparina e il warfarin, con o senza l'acido acetilsalicilico.

La **diagnosi differenziale** della malattia tromboembolica è dipendente dall'organo colpito e dal tipo di vaso. Per patologie arteriose, la diagnosi alternativa più comune è rappresentata da alcune forme di arterite (malattia di Kawasaki o lupus eritematoso sistemico). Per la trombosi venosa degli arti, i traumi e le infezioni possono causare reperti clinici simili. Un processo infiltrativo polmonare di qualsiasi eziologia può condurre a sintomi respiratori e altri reperti simili a quelli dell'embolia polmonare.

COMPLICANZE. L'occlusione arteriosa acuta provoca una disfunzione d'organo severa a causa dell'ischemia. Le complicanze della malattia tromboembolica venosa sono molto più spesso correlate ai cambiamenti a lungo termine della stasi venosa, con gonfiore, cambiamenti cutanei e dolore degli arti affetti. Questi reperti agli arti superiori sono stati recentemente considerati come comuni complicanze a lungo termine dei cateteri venosi centrali.

TRATTAMENTO

Trombosi venosa e tromboflebite. La tromboflebite superficiale è trattata con farmaci antinfiammatori (agenti anti-inifammatori non steroidei), compresse calde e sollevamento della parte colpita. I pazienti con TVP o tromboflebite sono trattati con anticoagulanti e raramente con agenti trombolitici. L'anticoagulante eparinico che impiega eparina standard non frazionata o a basso peso molecolare (*Low Molecular Weight*, LMW) dovrebbe essere utilizzata a dose piena per 3-5 giorni, con warfarin aggiunto per altri 6 mesi in pazienti con trombosi venosa prossimale (sopra le ginocchia). L'utilizzo della terapia trombolitica dovrebbe probabilmente essere limitato a situazioni che mettono in pericolo la vita o l'arto. È poco chiaro quale sia il miglior trattamento dei pazienti con trombosi isolata delle vene del polpaccio, ma anticoagulanti a breve durata di azione possono ritardare il ricovero e previene la progressione.

Embolia polmonare. Il paziente con embolia polmonare acuta può essere trattato con eparina o, meno frequentemente, con farmaci trombolitici (vedi Capitolo 406). La maggior parte dei pazienti dovrebbe ricevere eparina e in seguito warfarin, come descritto nella Tabella 479-1. La terapia trombolitica dovrebbe essere riservata ai casi di embolia polmonare a rischio per la vita (o "trombo a sella"), perché negli adulti produce miglioramenti clinici più rapidi della terapia eparinica, ma la sopravvivenza generale e le anomalie della funzione polmonare a lungo termine sembrano essere le stesse in entrambi i gruppi di trattamento. L'embolectomia è usata raramente quando è presente un embolo grosso e non c'è beneficio a seguito della terapia trombolitica o anticoagulante.

Trombosi arteriosa. La terapia fibrinolitica con attivatore del plasminogeno di tipo tissutale ricombinante, seguita dall'anticoagulazione eparinica, è stata usata con successo per trattare la trombosi arteriosa acuta di recente insorgenza. Raramente, viene praticata la rimozione chirurgica del coagulo se la trombolisi non ha successo o se la trombosi colpisce un organo maggiore o un arto. La trombolisi non dovrebbe essere usata in caso di recente intervento chirurgico e di trombosi o emorragia del sistema nervoso centrale.

Stroke. L'ictus ischemico comunemente si presenta con emiparesi, perdita di conoscenza o convulsioni. L'occlusione arteriosa nel cervello può verificarsi come componente di una patologia sistemica (emoglobinopatia a cellule falciformi) o dopo l'embolizzazione sia derivante da un vaso danneggiato (aneurisma carotideo dopo il trauma) o da trombi venosi che entrano nella circolazione arteriosa attraverso il forame ovale (vedi Capitolo 601). Spesso l'ictus è idiopatico. La causa di ictus più comune identificata nei bambini è l'emoglobinopatia a cellule falciformi. La trombosi venosa dei vasi cerebrali (trombosi dei seni venosi) può essere riscontrata nelle cardiopatie cianogene, nelle lesioni infiammatorie e infettive cerebrali o dei tessuti circostanti, ne-

TABELLA 479-1. Confronto tra agenti antitrombotici

	TERAPIA TROMBOLITICA	EPARINA NON FRAZIONATA*	WARFARIN	EPARINA LMW (ENOXAPARINA)
Indicazione	Esordio recente di trombi con pericolo di vita	Trombi di epoca indeterminata	Anticoaugulanti orali a lungo termine	Trombi di epoca indeterminata
Dose	rTPA 0,1-0,2 mg/kg/ora ev	75 U/kg/bolo, 20-28* U/kg/ora in infusione continua ev	0,1-0,2 mg/kg/die per os	1,0-1,5* mg/kg in 12 ore sc
Regolazione	Dose aumentata per mancanza di un effetto clinico	↑ dose di 5-10% in 6 ore fino al raggiungimento del livello adeguato del PTT	↑ dose ogni 2 giorni di 20-30% fino a INR appropriato e stabile	↑ o ↓ di 10-20%
Decorso	6-12 ore	5-14 giorni	Settimane-mesi	5 giorni-6 mesi
Monitoraggio/obiettivo	"Stato litico": FDP o D-dimero (TPA)	PTT 2-2½ tempo di controllo; tempo di trombina infinito; livello di eparina 0,3-0,7 U/mL	INR 2,0-3,0	Livello eparina LMW 4 ore dopo la 4ª dose = 0,5-1,0 U/mL
Meccanismo	Attivazione del plasminogeno in plasmina	Accelerano l'inattivazione AT-III-dipendente del trombina, F Xa	Inibisce la carbossilazione vitamina K dipendente del F II, VII, IX, X, proteina C e S	Accelerano l'inattivazione AT-III-dipendente del F Xa e della trombina
Rischio emorragico	Medio alto	Basso	Basso	Basso

*Una dose maggiore è richiesta nei neonati.
AT-III, antitrombina III; F, fattore; FDP, *Fibrin Degradation Product* (prodotti di degradazione del fibrinogeno); INR, *International Normalized Ratio;* LMW, *Low Molecular Weight* (basso peso molecolare); PTT, *Partial Thromboplastin Time* (tempo di tromboplastina parziale); rTPA, *Recombinant Tissue-Type Plasminogen Activator* (attivatore ricombinante del plasminogeno di tipo tissutale); U, unità.
L'**acido acetilsalicilico** è l'unico agente antipiastrinico comunemente usato e la dose abituale è 80 mg/die. Non c'è bisogno di monitorare la terapia con l'acido acetilsalicilico.

gli stati di iperviscosità o di trombofilia congenita. L'approccio terapeutico all'ictus arterioso o venoso è controverso. La terapia antipiastrinica con l'acido acetilsalicilico è sicura. La terapia eparinica può migliorare l'esito dell'ictus negli adulti, anche se il rischio di ictus emorragico può essere aumentato. La trombosi dei seni venosi in assenza di emorragia è di solito trattata con l'eparina. La presenza di un ictus emorragico è una **controindicazione** alla terapia anticoagulante. Non è noto se la terapia trombolitica sia efficace e sicura nei bambini con ictus non emorragici, ma, se usata, dovrebbe solo essere istituita nei pazienti entro 3 ore dall'esordio dei sintomi.

479.1 • TERAPIA TROMBOLITICA E ANTICOAGULANTE

La Tabella 479-1 fornisce un elenco degli agenti anticoagulanti comunemente utilizzati.

EPARINA NON FRAZIONATA (STANDARD). L'eparina amplifica la velocità con cui l'antitrombina III neutralizza l'attività di diverse proteine attivate della coagulazione, soprattutto il fattore Xa e la trombina. La durata dell'emivita dell'eparina somministrata per via endovenosa è di circa 60 minuti negli adulti e può essere ridotta fino a 30 minuti nel neonato. L'eparina non attraversa la placenta. L'emivita dell'eparina è dose-dipendente: più elevata è la dose più lunga è l'emivita in circolo. Nella patologia trombotica, l'emivita può essere accorciata rispetto al normale nei pazienti con una tromboembolia grave (embolia polmonare) e più lunga del normale nei pazienti con cirrosi e uremia.

L'anticoagulazione con l'eparina è **controindicata** nelle seguenti circostanze: recente emorragia nel sistema nervoso centrale; emorragia da siti inaccessibili; ipertensione maligna; endocardite batterica; precedente chirurgia dell'occhio, cervello o midollo spinale e somministrazione in corso di anestesia regionale o lombare. Un difetto della coagulazione preesistente o un'emorragia anomala sono una controindicazione relativa. Nonostante questa precauzione la frequenza dell'emorragia nei pazienti a cui viene somministrata l'eparina è 0,2-1%.

Le linee guida per la terapia che utilizzano l'eparina non frazionata sono illustrate nella Tabella 479-1. Nei neonati con bassi livelli di fattori della coagulazione, nei pazienti con inibitore lupico o in pazienti con elevati livelli di fattore VIII (come conseguenza dello stress o della chirurgia), il PTT non riflette correttamente il livello di anticoagulazione, pertanto i livelli specifici di eparina dovrebbero essere valutati in modo che il livello di eparina sia 0,35-0,7 U/mL o mediante il saggio dell'antifattore Xa o 0,2-0,4 U/mL mediante il saggio con il solfato di protamina.

L'eparina può essere neutralizzata immediatamente utilizzando il solfato di protamina. A causa della rapida clearance dell'eparina, fermare l'infusione rappresenta il trattamento adeguato per la maggior parte dei pazienti. Un milligrammo di solfato di protamina neutralizza 90-110 unità di eparina. Dal momento che l'eparina presenta un decadimento rapido *in vivo*, dovrebbe essere somministrata solo metà della dose totale di protamina. Un test di coagulazione viene effettuato per determinare se si sia verificata un'adeguata neutralizzazione; in caso contrario, può essere somministrata della protamina addizionale. La protamina da sola ha un effetto anticoagulante, quindi, se ne viene data troppa, il tempo di coagulazione può essere allungato. Anche se la protamina in eccesso ha un effetto anticoagulante, essa raramente (o mai) è causa di emorragia clinica. Una volta che l'eparina è stata neutralizzata, il paziente ritorna allo stato iniziale "protrombotico".

EPARINA A BASSO PESO MOLECOLARE. L'eparina a basso peso molecolare (*Low Molecular Weight*, LMW) rappresenta un'alternativa efficace e conveniente alla terapia eparinica standard e il suo utilizzo è descritto nella Tabella 479-1. Moltissime eparine ed eparinoidi sono attualmente impiegati in trial clinici. La maggior parte dell'esperienza pediatrica è data dall'enoxaparina. I pazienti adulti che ricevono eparina LMW raramente necessitano di monitoraggio dei loro livelli eparinici, ma nei pazienti pediatrici c'è una maggiore imprevedibilità di risposta. Il monitoraggio per assicurare che il livello terapeutico è stato raggiunto è critico. Il PTT non può essere usato per monitorare l'eparina LMW; dovrebbe essere impiegato un saggio specifico. Una volta che venga raggiunto il range terapeutico, il monitoraggio di routine non è richiesto o lo è poco frequentemente. Quando l'eparina LMW è usata per la profilassi contro la trombosi, la dose è 0,5 mg/kg nelle 12 ore per via sottocutanea, con l'obiettivo di ottenere un livello di 0,3 U/mL 4 ore dopo l'iniezione.

WARFARIN. I derivati cumarinici sono farmaci anticoagulanti che agiscono diminuendo i livelli funzionali dei fattori della coagulazione vitamina K-dipendenti: II, VII, IX e X, così come la proteina C e la proteina S (anticoagulanti vitamina K-dipendenti). Questi farmaci inibiscono la carbossilazione vitamina K-dipendente dei precursori delle proteine coinvolte nel processo della coagulazione. Il warfarin probabilmente agisce in modo competitivo inibendo il metabolismo della vitamina K. Dopo la somministrazione di warfarin, i livelli dei fattori II, VII, IX e X diminuiscono gradualmente, in base all'emivita di ciascun fattore plasmatico. Siccome il fattore VII presenta un'emivita più breve, il suo livello è il primo a diminuire, seguito dai fattori IX e X e infine dal fattore II. In genere sono richiesti 4-5 giorni per ridurre i livelli di tutti e 4 i fattori compatibili con l'anticoagulazione efficace.

Il tempo di protrombina (PT) è il test della coagulazione usato per determinare l'anticoagulazione warfarinica. Le attuali raccomandazioni sono basate sull'International Normalized Ratio

(INR), che permettono il rapporto dei valori di PT utilizzando una grande varietà di reagenti e strumenti. L'INR standard nel trattamento della trombosi è 2-3. La Tabella 479-1 presenta le linee guida per la somministrazione del warfarin ai bambini. Per pazienti con valvole cardiache meccaniche e per quelli con deficit omozigote di proteina C, l'INR dovrebbe essere 3-4.

L'effetto collaterale più serio del warfarin è l'emorragia. Questa è spesso collegata ai cambiamenti nella dose o nel metabolismo del farmaco. L'aggiunta o la rimozione di alcuni farmaci nei regimi terapeutici del paziente possono avere effetti significativi sull'anticoagulazione orale. L'effetto del warfarin può, per esempio, essere aumentato dalla somministrazione di antibiotici, salicilati, steroidi anabolizzanti, cloralio idrato, lassativi, allopurinolo, vitamina E e metilfenidato idrocloruro; il suo effetto può essere diminuito dai barbiturici, vitamina K, contraccettivi orali, fenitoina e altri agenti. L'emorragia indotta dal warfarin è trattata mediante la sospensione del farmaco e la somministrazione orale di vitamina K. Generalmente la quantità di vitamina K somministrata è uguale alla quantità giornaliera di warfarin. La vitamina K può essere somministrata per via orale, sottocutanea o endovenosa (non intramuscolare), ma le forme parenterali hanno un'emivita molto più lunga e possono superare la correzione. La correzione della coagulopatia inizia entro 6-8 ore e dovrebbe essere completata in 24-48 ore. Se il paziente sta presentando un'emorragia importante o a rischio per la vita, dovrebbe essere trasfuso plasma fresco congelato (15 mL/kg) contemporaneamente a vitamina K.

Le controindicazioni agli anticoagulanti cumarolici sono essenzialmente le stesse di quelle della terapia eparinica. Gli anticoagulanti orali sono teratogeni, attraversano la placenta e non dovrebbero essere prescritti in gravidanza, in particolare nel primo trimestre. Anche se il latte materno contiene il warfarin, la quantità è insignificante e il farmaco può essere usato per trattare la madre in allattamento senza un significativo effetto sul neonato.

TERAPIA TROMBOLITICA. Gli agenti trombolitici, come l'attivatore ricombinante di tipo tissutale del plasminogeno (*Recombinant Tissue-Type Plasminogen Activator,* rTPA), attivano il plasminogeno per lisare il coagulo ematico attraverso la digestione enzimatica; l'rTPA è più spesso usato nei pazienti pediatrici per la terapia trombolitica, come descritto nella Tabella 479-1. Perché questa terapia sia efficace, il paziente dovrebbe avere un coagulo relativamente fresco (<3-5 giorni), il coagulo deve essere accessibile all'agente litico, e ci deve essere un'adeguata quantità di plasminogeno. Una volta che si è formata la plasmina, essa si lisa la fibrina. Agenti relativamente più specifici per la fibrina rispetto ad altri agenti trombolitici urochinasi e streptochinasi, l'rTPA attiva il plasminogeno dentro o sul coagulo di fibrina. Trial clinici con l'rTPA suggeriscono che esso raramente produce uno stato iperfibrinolitico sistemico. La dose iniziale di rTPA è 0,1 mg/kg/ora. Sarebbe utile monitorare un effetto terapeutico ricercando una concentrazione aumentata del D-dimero o dei prodotti di degradazione del fibrinogeno. Dosi elevate o un decorso più prolungato della terapia trombolitica sono probabilmente associate con un aumentato rischio di complicanze emorragiche. Basse dosi di rTPA sono state efficaci nel ripristinare la pervietà dei cateteri vascolari occlusi.

PREVENZIONE

Non ci sono stati trial ufficiali di prevenzione della malattia tromboembolica venosa nei bambini. I bambini con condizioni protrombotiche conosciute che stanno per essere immobilizzati per un periodo protratto probabilmente dovrebbero ricevere un trattamento profilattico con enoxaparina 0,5 mg/kg ogni 12 ore mentre sono immobili. Più controverso è l'uso di questa terapia per i bambini che sono immobilizzati per un periodo prolungato a causa di patologie mediche severe, soprattutto se è associato a infiammazione o trauma.

Anton N, Massicotte MP: Venous thromboembolism in pediatrics. *Semin Vasc Med* 2001;1:111–122.

Bauer KA: Role of thrombophilia in deciding on the duration of anticoagulation. *Semin Thromb Hemost* 2004;30:633–637.

Chan AK, Deveber G, Monagle P, et al: Venous thrombosis in children. *J Thromb Haemost* 2003;1:1443–1455.

Christiansen SC, Cannegieter SC, Koster T, et al: Thrombophilia, clinical factors and recurrent venous thrombotic events. *JAMA* 2005;293: 2352–2361.

Di Nisio M, Middeldorp S, Buller HR: Direct thrombin inhibitors. *N Engl J Med* 2005;353:1028–1040.

Goldenberg NA, Knapp-Clevenger R, Manco-Johnson MJ: Elevated plasma factor VIII and D-dimer levels as predictors of poor outcomes of thrombosis in children. *N Engl J Med* 2004;351:1081–1088.

Jilma B, Kamath S, Lip GY: ABC of antithrombotic therapy: Antithrombotic therapy in special circumstances. II—In children, thrombophilia, and miscellaneous conditions. *BMJ* 2003;326:93–96.

Johnson MC, Parkerson N, Ward S, et al: Pediatric sinovenous thrombosis. *J Pediatr Hematol Oncol* 2003;25:312–315.

Kyrle PA, Eichinger S: Deep vein thrombosis. *Lancet* 2005;365:1163–1174.

Lim W, Crowther MA, Eikelboom JW: Management of antiphospholipid antibody syndrome. *JAMA* 2006;295:1050–1057.

Male C, Kuhle S, Mitchell L: Diagnosis of venous thromboembolism in children. *Semin Thromb Hemost* 2003;29:377–390.

Monagle P, Chan A, Massicotte P, et al: Antithrombotic therapy in children: The Seventh ACCP Conference on Antithrombotic and Thrombolytic Therapy. *Chest* 2004;126(3 Suppl):645S–687S.

Nowak-Gottl U, Straeter R, Sebire G, et al: Antithrombotic drug treatment of pediatric patients with ischemic stroke. *Paediatr Drugs* 2003;5:167–175.

Ozturk MA, Haznedaroglu IC, Turgut M, et al: Current debates in antiphospholipid syndrome: The acquired antibody-mediated thrombophilia. *Clin Appl Thromb Hemost* 2004;10:89–126.

Rieder MJ, Reiner AP, Gage BF, et al: Effect of VKORC1 haplotypes on transcriptional regulation and warfarin dose. *N Engl J Med* 2005;352: 2285–2292.

Streif W, Goebel G, Chan AKC, et al: Use of low molecular mass heparin (enoxaparin) in newborn infants: A prospective cohort study of 62 patients. *Arch Dis Child Fetal Neonatal Ed* 2003;88:F365–F370.

Sutor AH, Chan AK, Massicotte P: Low-molecular-weight heparin in pediatric patients. *Semin Thromb Hemost* 2004;30(Suppl 1):31–39.

Watson LI, Armon MP: Thrombolysis for acute deep vein thrombosis. *Cochrane Database Syst Rev* 2004; Oct 18(4):CD002783.

Wells PS, Anderson DR, Rodger M, et al: Excluding pulmonary embolism at the bedside without diagnostic imaging: Management of patients with suspected pulmonary embolism presenting to the emergency department by using a simple clinical model and D-dimer. *Ann Intern Med* 2001;135: 98–107.

Capitolo 480 ■ Deficit postneonatale di vitamina K

Anche se è stata riportata una malattia emorragica "tardiva" in bambini allattati al seno, il deficit di vitamina K che si verifica dopo il periodo neonatale è in genere secondario a un apporto orale di vitamina K insufficiente, a un'alterazione della flora intestinale dovuta all'uso prolungato di antibiotici di largo spettro o al malassorbimento di vitamina K. Il malassorbimento intestinale dei grassi può accompagnare la fibrosi cistica o l'atresia delle vie biliari e comporta un deficit di vitamine liposolubili contenute negli alimenti, con ridotta sintesi dei fattori coagulativi vitamina K-dipendente (fattori II, VII, IX e X e proteina C e S). In questi casi è indicata la somministrazione in profilassi di vitamina K idrosolubile per via orale (2-3 mg/24 h per bambini e 5-10 mg/24 h per adolescenti e adulti) oppure la vitamina K può essere somministrata a 1-2 mg per via endovenosa. In pazienti con cirrosi avanzata, la sintesi di molti fattori della coagulazione può essere ridotta a causa del danno epatocellulare. In questi pazienti, la vitamina K può rivelarsi inefficace. Le proprietà anticoagulanti del warfarin e degli anticoagulanti correlati dipendono dall'interferenza con la vitamina K, con riduzione concomitante dei fattori II, VII, IX e X. Il veleno per ratti (superwarfarin) causa deficit simili e la vitamina K è uno specifico antidoto.

Bolton-Maggs P, Brook L: The use of vitamin K for reversal of over-warfarinization in children. *Br J Haematol* 2002;118:839–840.
Monagle P, Andrew M: Acquired disorders of hemostasis. In Nathan DG, Orkin SH, Ginsburg D, et al (editors): *Hematology of Infancy and Childhood*, 6th ed. Philadelphia, WB Saunders, 2003, pp 1631–1668.

Capitolo 481 ■ Epatopatie

Dal momento che tutti i fattori della coagulazione sono prodotti esclusivamente nel fegato tranne il fattore VIII, le anomalie della coagulazione sono molto comuni nei pazienti con epatopatia. Solo il 15% di questi pazienti presenta stati emorragici clinicamente importanti. La gravità dell'anomalia coagulativa sembra essere direttamente proporzionale all'estensione del danno epatocellulare. Il meccanismo più comune che causa il difetto è la sintesi diminuita dei fattori coagulativi. I pazienti con epatopatia grave tipicamente presentano livelli di attività del fattore VIII nel plasma da normali ad aumentati (non ridotti). In alcuni casi, la coagulazione intravasale disseminata (vedi Capitolo 483) o l'iperfibrinolisi possono complicare la patologia epatica, rendendo difficile la distinzione in laboratorio tra l'epatopatia grave e coagulazione disseminata intravasale.

Il trattamento della coagulopatia della epatopatia consiste nel ripristino con plasma fresco congelato (PFC) o crioprecipitato. Il PFC (10-15 mL/kg) contiene tutti i fattori della coagulazione, ma la sostituzione del fibrinogeno per l'ipofibrinogenemia severa può richiedere il crioprecipitato alla dose di 1 sacca/5 kg di peso corporeo. Poiché una diminuzione dei fattori della coagulazione vitamina K-dipendenti è comune nei pazienti con epatopatia cronica, la terapia con vitamina K può essere data come prova. La vitamina K può essere somministrata per via orale, sottocutanea o endovenosa (non intramuscolare) alla dose di 1 mg/24 h per i neonati, 2-3 mg/24 h per i bambini e 5-10 mg/24 h per gli adolescenti e gli adulti. L'incapacità di correggere la coagulopatia con la vitamina K indica che il difetto coagulativo può essere causato da ridotti livelli di fattori coagulativi che non sono vitamina K dipendenti e/o da inadeguata sintesi delle proteine precorritrici della vitamina K. In caso di epatopatia grave, è spesso difficile raggiungere la correzione delle anomalie della coagulazione senza una terapia vigorosa con PFC o crioprecipitato. Alcuni pazienti con emorragia dovuta all'epatopatia hanno risposto alla terapia con desmopressina, mentre altri hanno risposto al trattamento con fattore VIIa ricombinante.

Frequentemente, l'epatopatia severa è associata con l'allungamento moderato del tempo di emorragia, il quale non viene corretto né dalla vitamina K né dal ripristino del plasma. Si è trovato che la desmopressina (0,3 μg/kg ev) è efficace nell'accorciare il tempo di emorragia ed è stata impiegata efficacemente per aumentare l'emostasi prima della biopsia epatica.

Atkison PR, Jardine L, Williams S, et al: Use of recombinant factor VIIa in pediatric patients with liver failure and severe coagulopathy. *Transplant Proc* 2005;37:1091–1093.
Kaul V, Munoz SJ: Coagulopathy of liver disease. *Curr Treat Options Gastroenterol* 2000;3:433–438.
Monagle P, Andrew M: Acquired disorders of hemostasis. In Nathan DG, Orkin SH, Ginsburg D, et al (editors): *Hematology of Infancy and Childhood*, 6th ed. Philadelphia, WB Saunders, 2003, pp 1631–1668.

Capitolo 482 ■ Inibitori acquisiti della coagulazione

Gli anticoagulanti (inibitori) acquisiti circolanti sono anticorpi che reagiscono o cross-reagiscono con i fattori della coagulazione o con componenti utilizzate nei test di screening coagulativi (fosfolipidi), prolungando così i test di screening, come il tempo di protrombina e il tempo di tromboplastina parziale. Alcuni di questi anticoagulanti sono autoanticorpi che reagiscono con i fosfolipidi e perciò interferiscono con la coagulazione *in vitro*, ma non *in vivo*. La forma più comune di questi anticorpi antifosfolipidi è stata chiamata *anticoagulante lupico* (vedi Capitolo 479). Questo anticoagulante si trova in pazienti con lupus eritematoso sistemico (vedi Capitolo 157) in quelli con le altre patologie vascolari del collagene e talvolta in seguito a comuni infezioni virali, incluso l'HIV. Inibitori spontanei simil-lupus si sono sviluppati transitoriamente in bambini dopo l'infezione virale incidentale. Questi inibitori transitori non sono in genere associati alla trombosi.

Anche se l'anticoagulante lupico classico è più spesso associato a una predisposizione alla trombosi piuttosto che ai sintomi emorragici, i sintomi del sanguinamento in un paziente con anticoagulante lupico possono essere causati dalla trombocitopenia, come manifestazione della sindrome antifosfolipidi o del lupus stesso, o raramente, da un coesistente anticorpo specifico contro la protrombina (fattore II). Questo anticorpo antiprotrombina non inattiva la protrombina, ma causa una clearance accelerata della proteina, con conseguenti bassi livelli di protrombina.

Raramente, gli anticorpi possono svilupparsi spontaneamente contro uno specifico fattore coagulativo, come il fattore VIII o il fattore di von Willebrand, simile a quelli più frequentemente presenti nei pazienti più anziani. Questi pazienti sono predisposti a emorragie eccessive e possono richiedere uno specifico trattamento. Nei pazienti con una carenza ereditaria di un fattore coagulativo (fattore VIII o IX), gli anticorpi possono svilupparsi dopo esposizione a concentrati di fattori trasfusi. Questi anticorpi inibitori individuabili negli emofilici sono discussi nel Capitolo 476.

REPERTI DI LABORATORIO. Gli inibitori contro i fattori coagulativi specifici in genere colpiscono i fattori VIII, IX e X o raramente la protrombina. In base al bersaglio dell'anticorpo, il tempo di protrombina, il tempo di tromboplastina parziale oppure entrambi possono essere allungati. Il meccanismo attraverso cui l'anticorpo inibitore funziona determina se il mescolare il plasma del paziente con plasma normale normalizzerà (correggerà) il tempo di coagulazione. Il plasma del paziente contenente gli anticorpi diretti contro il sito attivo del fattore della coagulazione (fattore VIII o IX) non si correggerà mescolando 1:1 con plasma normale, mentre se contiene gli anticorpi che aumentano la clearance del fattore protrombina, saranno corretti in una miscela 1:1 con plasma normale. Per stabilire quale fattore sia deficitario, si utilizzano test specifici per i singoli fattori.

TRATTAMENTO. La gestione del paziente con un inibitore contro uno specifico fattore coagulativo è la stessa che per un paziente con emofilia che presenta allo anticorpi contro il fattore VIII o il fattore IX. Le infusioni di fattore VIIa ricombinante o di concentrati del complesso attivato della protrombina possono essere necessarie per controllare un'emorragia significativa. Gli inibitori spontanei che si sviluppano dopo un'infezione virale tendono a scomparire entro poche settimane o mesi. Gli inibitori che accompagnano una patologia sottostante spesso scompaiono quando la patologia primaria viene trattata. L'anticoagulante lupico spesso scompare dopo un trattamento appropriato del lupus eritematoso sistemico.

Bernini JC, Buchanan GR, Ashcraft J: Hypoprothrombinemia and severe hemorrhage associated with lupus anticoagulant. *J Pediatr* 1993;123:937–939.

Levine JS, Branch DW, Rauch J: The antiphospholipid syndrome. *N Engl J Med* 2002;346:752–763.
Monagle P, Andrew M: Acquired disorders of hemostasis. In Nathan DG, Orkin SH, Ginsburg D, et al (editors): *Hematology of Infancy and Childhood*, 6th ed. Philadelphia, WB Saunders, 2003, pp 1631–1668.
Moraca RJ, Ragni MV: Acquired anti-FVIII inhibitors in children. *Haemophilia* 2002;8:28–32.
Roberts HR, Monroe DM, White GC: The use of recombinant factor VIIa in the treatment of bleeding disorders. *Blood* 2004;104:3858–3864. Epub 2004;Aug 24.
Savage WJ, Kickler TS, Takemoto CM: Acquired coagulation factor inhibitors in children after topical bovine thrombin exposure. *Pediatr Blood Cancer* 2006;Mar 8.

Capitolo 483 ■ Coagulazione intravascolare disseminata

La **microangiopatia trombotica** si riferisce a un gruppo eterogeneo di patologie, inclusa la coagulazione intravascolare disseminata (CID), che comportano il consumo dei fattori della coagulazione, della piastrine e delle proteine anticoagulanti. Le conseguenze di questo processo includono la deposizione intravascolare diffusa di fibrina, che portano all'ischemia tissutale e alla necrosi, a uno stato generalizzato emorragico e all'anemia emolitica.

EZIOLOGIA. Ogni processo patologico a rischio di vita associato a ipossia, acidosi, necrosi tissutale, shock e/o danno endoteliale può scatenare la CID; è stato riportato un grande numero di condizioni associate, inclusi lo shock settico (soprattutto la meningococciemia), la trasfusione di sangue incompatibile, l'infezione da rickettsie, il morso di serpente, la porpora fulminante, l'emangioma gigante e i tumori maligni, soprattutto la leucemia promielocitica acuta (Tab. 483-1). Anche se i sintomi clinici sono primariamente emorragici, l'evento scatenante è in genere l'attivazione eccessiva della coagulazione che consuma sia gli anticoagulanti fisiologici (proteina C, proteina S e antitrombina III) sia i procoagulanti, portando a una carenza di fattori V e VII, protrombina, fibrinogeno e piastrine. Comunemente il risultato clinico di questa sequenza di eventi è l'emorragia. La disregolazione dell'emostasi può anche comportare trombosi cutanee, nei reni e negli altri organi.

MANIFESTAZIONI CLINICHE. In genere la CID accompagna una malattia sistemica grave. L'emorragia si verifica frequentemente per prima dai siti di prelievo venoso o di incisione chirurgica. La cute può presentare ecchimosi e petecchie. La necrosi tissutale può coinvolgere molti organi e può essere vista maggiormente come infarto di grandi aree cutanee, del tessuto sottocutaneo o dei reni. L'anemia causata dall'emolisi può svilupparsi rapidamente a causa di un'anemia emolitica microangiopatica.

REPERTI DI LABORATORIO. Non c'è una sequenza di eventi ben definita. Alcuni fattori della coagulazione (fattori II, V e VIII e fibrinogeno) e le piastrine possono essere consumati dal processo coagulativo intravascolare in corso, con un risultante allungamento dei tempi di protrombina, di tromboplastina parziale e di trombina. La conta piastrinica può essere profondamente depressa. Lo striscio di sangue può contenere globuli rossi frammentati o a elmetto (schistociti). Inoltre, poiché il meccanismo fibrinolitico è attivato, i prodotti di degradazione del fibrinogeno (FDP, D-dimero) compaiono nel sangue circolante. Il D-dimero è formato dalla fibrinolisi del coagulo di fibrina con legami crociati. Il saggio del D-dimero è un test sensibile come gli FDP (*Fibrogen Degradation Product*) e più specifico per l'attivazione della coagulazione e della fibrinolisi.

TABELLA 483-1. Cause di coagulazione intravascolare disseminata

INFEZIONI
Meningococcemia (porpora fulminante)
Altri batteri Gram negativi (*Haemophilus, Salmonella, Escherichia coli*)
Batteri Gram positivi (streptococchi di gruppo B, stafilococchi)
Rickettsie (febbre maculosa delle Montagne Rocciose)
Virus (Cytomegalovirus, herpes simplex, febbre emorragica)
Malaria
Micosi
DANNO TISSUTALE
Trauma del sistema nervoso centrale (trauma cranico importante)
Fratture multiple con emboli grassosi
Danno da schiacciamento
Shock profondo o asfissia
Ipotermia o ipertermia
Ustioni massive
NEOPLASIE MALIGNE
Leucemia acuta promielocitica
Leucemia acuta monoblastica o mielocitica
Tumori maligni disseminati (neuroblastoma)
VELENI O TOSSINE
Morsi di serpente
Punture di insetti
MICROANGIOPATIE
Porpora trombotica trombocitopenica o sindrome uremico-emolitica "severe"
Emangioma gigante (sindrome di Kasabach-Merritt)
PATOLOGIE GASTROINTESTINALI
Epatite fulminante
Malattia infiammatoria cronica severa
Pancreatiti
PATOLOGIE TROMBOTICHE EREDITARIE
Carenze di antitrombina-III
Deficit omozigote di proteina C
NEONATI
Tossiemia materna
Infezione da streptococco di gruppo B
Abruptio placentae
Sindrome da distress respiratorio severo
Enterocolite necrotizzante
Malattia congenita virale (Cytomegalovirus, herpes simplex)
Eritrobalstosi fetale
Trasfusione fetale gemello-gemello
VARIE
Rigetto severo acuto del trapianto
Reazione acuta emolitica trasfusionale
Vasculite severa
Malattia di Kawasaki
Trombosi indotta dall'eparina
Infusione di concentrati del complesso di protrombina "attivato"
Iperpiressia/encefalopatia, sindrome da shock emorragico
Abruptio placentae

Modificata da Montgomery RR, Scott IP: Hemostasis: Diseases of the fluid phase. In Nathan DG, Oski FA (editors): *Hematology of Infancy and Childhood*, 4th ed., Vol. 2. Philadelphia, WB Saunders, 1993.

TRATTAMENTO. I primi due stadi nel trattamento della CID sono i più critici: (1) trattare i fattori scatenanti che causano la CID e (2) ripristinare l'omeostasi normale correggendo lo shock, l'acidosi e l'ipossia che in genere complicano la CID. Se il problema sottostante può essere controllato, l'emorragia cessa velocemente e c'è un miglioramento dei reperti di laboratorio anormali. Componenti derivati dal sangue sono usati per la terapia sostitutiva nei pazienti con emorragia. Questo può consistere di infusioni piastriniche (per la trombocitopenia), crioprecipitato (per l'ipofibrinogenemia) e/o plasma fresco congelato (per il ripristino degli altri fattori coagulativi e degli inibitori naturali).

Nella CID associata a sepsi, un trial controllato di drotrecogina-α (concentrato di proteina C attivata [*Activated Protein C*, APC]) in adulti con la sepsi ha migliorato la sopravvivenza in modo statisticamente significativo in quelli trattati con APC. I trial clinici che utilizzano il concentrato di proteina C nella porpora fulminante e l'APC nei bambini con sepsi non hanno mostrato un miglioramento statisticamente significativo. Il ruolo di questi prodotti nell'infanzia resta da definire.

Il ruolo dell'eparina nella CID è limitato ai pazienti che hanno una trombosi vascolare in associazione alla CID. Questi individui dovrebbero essere trattati come elencato nel Capitolo 479, con molta attenzione alla terapia sostitutiva per mantenere una conta piastrinica adeguata e quindi limitare le complicanze emorragiche.

La prognosi dei pazienti con CID è innanzi tutto dipendente dall'esito del trattamento della patologia primaria e alla prevenzione del danno d'organo irreversibile.

Bernard GR, Vincent JL, Laterre PF, et al: Efficacy and safety of recombinant human activated protein C or severe sepsis. *N Engl J Med* 2001;344: 699–709.

Fourrier F: Recombinant human activated protein C in the treatment of severe sepsis: An evidence-based review. *Crit Care Med* 2004;32(11 Suppl): S534–S541.

Franchini M, Manzato F: Update on the treatment of disseminated intravascular coagulation. *Hematology* 2004;9:81–85.

Levi M, Ten Cate H: Disseminated intravascular coagulation. *N Engl J Med* 1999;341:586–592.

Liebman HA, Weitz IC: Disseminated intravascular coagulation. In Hoffman R, Benz EJ, Shattil SJ, et al (editors): *Hematology: Basic Principles and Practice*, 4th ed. Philadelphia, Elsevier Churchill Livingstone, 2005, pp 2169–2182.

Monagle P, Andrew M: Acquired disorders of hemostasis. In Nathan DG, Orkin SH, Ginsburg D, et al (editors): *Hematology of Infancy and Childhood*, 6th ed. Philadelphia, WB Saunders, 2003, pp 1631–1668.

Sparrow A, Willis F: Management of septic shock in childhood. *Emerg Med Australas* 2004;16:125–134.

Toh CH, Dennis M: Disseminated intravascular coagulation: Old disease, new hope. *BMJ* 2003;327:974–977.

Capitolo 484 ■ Patologie delle piastrine e dei vasi sanguigni

MEGACARIOPOIESI. Le piastrine sono frammenti cellulari non nucleati prodotte dai megacariociti nel midollo osseo e in altri tessuti. I megacariociti sono cellule grandi polipoidi. Quando un megacariocita raggiunge la maturità, si verifica la frammentazione del citoplasma e viene liberato un grande numero di piastrine. Le piastrine circolano con un'emivita di 10-14 giorni. La **trombopoietina** (TPO) è il fattore di crescita primitivo che controlla la produzione piastrinica. I livelli di TPO sembrano correlare inversamente con il numero delle piastrine e la massa megacariocitaria. Pertanto, i livelli del TPO sono più elevati negli stati trombocitopenici associati a diminuita megacariopoiesi midollare e possono essere variabili negli stati di aumentata produzione piastrinica.

Le piastrine giocano ruoli emostatici multipli. La superficie piastrinica possiede un numero di importanti recettori per le proteine adesive incluso il fattore di von Willebrand (vWf) e il fibrinogeno, così come i recettori per gli agonisti che scatenano l'aggregazione piastrinica come la trombina, il collagene e l'adenosina di fosfato (ADP). In seguito a un danno alla parete vasale, il collagene sottoendoteliale si lega al vWf, il quale va incontro a un cambiamento conformazionale che induce il legame del complesso della glicoproteina piastrinica Ib (GPIb) (il recettore per il vWf). Questo processo è chiamato *adesione piastrinica*. Le piastrine subiscono quindi l'attivazione. Durante il processo di attivazione, le piastrine producono il trombossano A_2 dall'acido arachidonico attraverso la via dell'enzima ciclossigenasi. Dopo l'attivazione esse rilasciano gli agonisti come l'ADP, l'adenosina trifosfato (ATP), il Ca^{2+}, la serotonina, i fattori della coagulazione nell'ambiente circostante. Il fibrinogeno circolante si lega al suo recettore sulle piastrine attivate, il complesso della glicoproteina IIb-IIIa (GPIIb-IIIa), assemblando le piastrine in un processo detto *aggregazione*. Questa serie di eventi forma un tappo emostatico nel sito della lesione vasale. La serotonina e l'istamina che sono liberate durante l'attivazione aumentano la vasocostrizione locale. Inoltre, agendo assieme alla parete vasale per formare il tappo piastrinico le piastrine offrono la superficie catalitica in cui i fattori coagulativi si assemblano ed eventualmente generano la trombina attraverso una serie sequenziale di clivaggi enzimatici. Infine, le proteine contrattili delle piastrine e il citoscheletro mediano la retrazione del coagulo.

TROMBOCITOPENIA. La normale conta piastrinica è 150-450 × 10^9/L. La *trombocitopenia* si riferisce a una riduzione della conta piastrinica a $<150 \times 10^9$/L. Le cause di trombocitopenia includono: (1) produzione diminuita su basi congenite o acquisite; (2) sequestro di piastrine in una milza ingrandita o in altri organi; (3) aumentata distruzione di piastrine normalmente sintetizzate su basi immuni o non immuni (vedi anche Capitoli 468, 469 e 483) (Tabb. 484-1 e 484-2 e Fig. 484-1).

TABELLA 484-1. Diagnosi differenziale della trombocitopenia nel bambino e nell'adolescente

TROMBOCITOPENIE DA CONSUMO
Sindromi da consumo piastrinico primario
Trombocitopenia immune
PTI acuta e cronica
Malattie autoimmuni con PTI cronica come manifestazione
Trombocitopenia ciclica
Sindrome linfoproliferativa autoimmune e sue varianti
Lupus eritematoso sistemico
Sindrome di Evans
Sindrome da anticorpi antifosfolipidi
Trombocitopenia immune neoplasia associata
Trombocitopenia associata all'HIV
Trombocitopenia neonatale immune
Alloimmune
Autoimmune (per es. porpora trombocitopenica immune materna)
Trombocitopenia immune farmaco-indotta (inclusa la trombocitopenia indotta da eparina)
Porpora post-transfusionale
Allergia e anafilassi
Trombocitopenia post-trapianto
Trombocitopenia non immune
Trombocitopenia da infezione
Batteriemia o fungiemia
Infezione virale
Protozoaria
Patologie trombotiche microangiopatiche
Sindrome uremico-emolitica
Porpora trombotica trombocitopenica
Trapianto di midollo osseo associato a microangiopatia
Farmaco-indotta
Piastrine a contatto con un materiale esterno
Cardiopatie congenite
Effetti piastrinici farmaco-indotti per via diretta (ristocetina, protamina)
vWD tipo piastrinico o tipo 2B
Sindromi combinate da consumo piastrinico e del fibrinogeno
Coagulazione intravascolare disseminata
Sindrome di Kasabach-Merritt
Sindrome emofagocitica virus-associata
DIFETTOSA PRODUZIONE PIASTRINICA
Patologie ereditarie (vedi Capitolo 40)
Patologie acquisite
Anemia aplastica
Sindrome mielodisplasica
Processo infiltrativo midollare
Osteoporosi
Stati di deficit nutrizionale (ferro, folati, vitamina B_{12}, anoressia nervosa)
Trombocitemia indotta dai farmaci o dalle radiazioni
Ipossia neonatale o insufficienza placentare
SEQUESTRO
Ipersplenismo
Ipotermia
Ustioni

HIV, virus dell'immunodeficienza umana; vWD, malattia di von Willebrand.
Da Nathan DG, Orkin SH, Ginsburg D: *Nathan and Oskis Hematology of Infancy and Childhood*, 6th ed., Vol. 2. Philadelphia, WB Saunders, 2003, p 1598.

TABELLA 484-2. Classificazione delle trombocitopenie fetale e neonatale*

	CONDIZIONE
Fetale	**Patologia alloimmune**
	Infezione congenita (per es. CMV, toxoplasma, rosolia, HIV)
	Aneuploidia (per es. trisomia 18, 13, o 21, o triploidia)
	Patologia autoimmune (per es. PTI, LES)
	Severa malattia emolitica da Rh
	Congenita/ereditaria (per es. sindrome di Wiskott-Aldrich)
Esordio precoce neonatale (<72 ore)	**Insufficienza placentare** (per es. PET, IUGR, diabete)
	Asfissia perinatale
	Infezione perinatale (per es. *Escherichia coli*, GBS, *Haemophilus influenzae*)
	CID
	Patologia alloimmune
	Patologia autoimmune (per es. PTI, LES)
	Infezione congenita (per es. CMV, toxoplasma, rosolia, HIV)
	Trombosi (per es. aortica, vena renale)
	Sostituzione midollo osseo (per es. leucemia congenita)
	Sindrome di Kasabach-Merritt
	Malattia metabolica (per es. acidemia propionica e metilmalonica)
	Congenita/ereditaria (per es. TAR, CAMT)
Esordio tardivo neonatale (>72 ore)	**Sepsi a esordio tardivo**
	NEC
	Infezione congenita (per es. CMV, toxoplasma, rosolia, HIV)
	Autoimmuni
	Sindrome di Kasabach-Merritt
	Malattia metabolica (per es. acidemia propionica e metilmalonica)
	Congenita/ereditaria (per es. TAR, CAMT)

CAMT, *Congenital Amegakaryocytic Thrombocytopenia* (trombocitopenia amegacariocitica congenita); CMV, Cytomegalovirus; CID, coagulazione intravascolare disseminata; GBS, *Group B Streptococcus* (streptococco di gruppo B); PTI, porpora trombocitopenica immune; IUGR, *Intrauterine Growth Restriction* (ritardo di crescita intrauterino); NEC, *Necrotizing EnteroColitis* (enterocolite necrotizzante); PET, pre-eclampsia; LES, lupus eritematoso sistemico; TAR, trombocitopenia-assenza del radio.

*Le condizioni più comuni sono mostrate in neretto.

Da Roberts I, Murray NA: Neonatal thrombocytopenia: Causes and management. *Arch Dis Child Fetal Neonatal Ed* 2003;88:F359-F364.

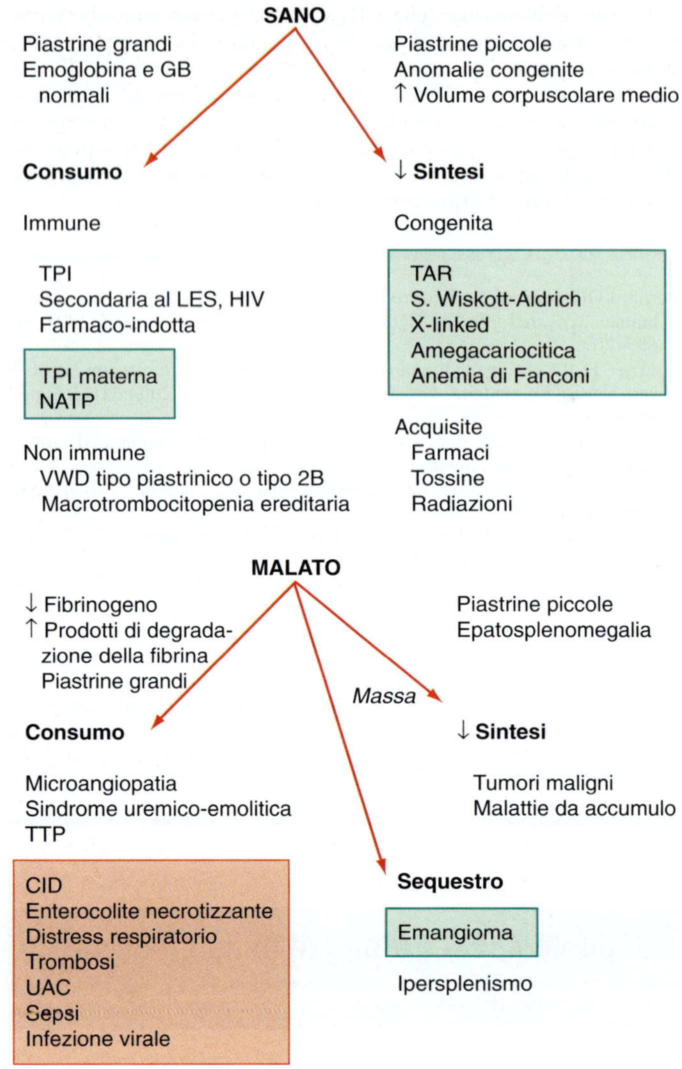

Figura 484-1. Diagnosi differenziale delle sindromi trombocitopeniche dell'infanzia. Le sindromi inizialmente sono separate in base alla loro manifestazione clinica. Le caratteristiche che portano alla diagnosi sono mostrate in *corsivo*. I meccanismi e le patologie comuni che portano a questi reperti sono mostrati nella *parte bassa* della figura. Le patologie che comunemente colpiscono i neonati sono elencate nelle *caselle ombreggiate*. GB, globuli bianchi; TPI, porpora trombocitopenica idiopatica; CID, coagulazione intravascolare disseminata; LES, lupus eritematoso sistemico; NATP, porpora trombocitopenica alloimmune neonatale; TAR, trombocitopenia-assenza del radio; vWD, malattia di von Willebrand; TTP, porpora trombotica trombocitopenica; UAC, catetere arterioso ombelicale. (Da Scott JP: Bleeding and thrombosis. In Kliegman RM [editor]: *Practical Strategies in Pediatric Diagnosis and Therapy*. Philadelphia, WB Saunders, 1996, p. 849. Da Kliegman RM, Marcdante KJ, Jenson HB, et al [editors]: *Nelson Essentials of Pediatrics*, 5th ed. Philadelphia, Elsevier/Saunders, 2006, p 716.)

484.1 • PORPORA TROMBOCITOPENICA IDIOPATICA

La più comune causa d'esordio di una trombocitopenia in un bambino per il resto sano è la porpora trombocitopenica idiopatica (autoimmune) (PTI).

EZIOLOGIA. In un esiguo numero di bambini, 1-4 settimane dopo l'esposizione a infezioni virali comuni, si sviluppa un autoanticorpo diretto contro la superficie piastrinica. Il bersaglio antigenico esatto per la maggior parte di questi anticorpi in molti casi di PTI acuta rimane sconosciuto. Dopo il legame dell'anticorpo alla superficie piastrinica, il complesso anticorpo-piastrina circolante viene riconosciuto dal recettore Fc dei macrofagi splenici e, in seguito, ingerito e distrutto. Una storia recente di patologia virale è descritta nel 50-65% dei casi di PTI dell'infanzia. Il motivo per cui alcuni bambini rispondono a infezioni comuni con una malattia autoimmune rimane sconosciuto. La maggior parte dei comuni virus infettivi è stata descritta in associazione alla PTI, incluso il virus di Epstein Barr (vedi Capitolo 251) e l'HIV (vedi Capitolo 273). La PTI correlata al virus di Epstein Barr è in genere di breve durata e segue il decorso della mononucleosi infettiva. La PTI HIV-associata è in genere cronica.

MANIFESTAZIONI CLINICHE. La presentazione tipica della PTI è quella di un bambino di 1-4 anni precedentemente sano che presenta un esordio improvviso di petecchie generalizzate e porpora. I genitori spesso riferiscono che il bambino il giorno prima stava bene e ora si è coperto con lividi e macchie purpuree. Spesso è presente un'emorragia gengivale e delle membrane mucose, in particolare con una trombocitopenia profonda (conta piastrinica $<10 \times 10^9/L$). È presente una storia di infezione virale che precede di 1-4 settimane l'esordio della trombocitopenia. L'esame obiettivo è normale, tranne che per i reperti di porpora e petecchie. La splenomegalia è rara, come la linfoadenopatia o il pallore. Un sistema di classificazione facile da usare è stato proposto dal Regno Unito per caratterizzare la gravità dell'emorragia nella PTI in base ai sintomi e ai segni, ma non alla conta piastrinica:

1. **Assenza di sintomi**
2. **Sintomi lievi: lividi e petecchie, epistassi occasionali di lieve entità, minima interferenza con le attività della vita quotidiana**
3. **Moderata: lesioni cutanee e mucose più severe, epistassi più problematica e menorragia**
4. **Grave: episodi emorragici (menorragia, epistassi, melena) che richiedono trasfusioni o ricovero in ospedale, sintomi che interferiscono seriamente con la qualità di vita**

La presenza di reperti anormali, come l'epatosplenomegalia o la linfoadenomegalia marcata, suggeriscono altre diagnosi (leucemia). Quando l'esordio è insidioso, soprattutto in un adolescente, è più probabile che la PTI cronica o la trombocitopenia sia una manifestazione di una patologia sistemica, come il lupus eritematoso sistemico (LES).

Nel 70-80% dei bambini che si presentano con una PTI acuta, la risoluzione spontanea si verifica entro 6 mesi. La terapia non sembra modificare la storia naturale della patologia. Meno dell'1% dei pazienti presenta un'emorragia endocranica. Quelli che preferiscono un trattamento attivo sostengono che l'obiettivo di una precoce terapia è di far aumentare la conta piastrinica $>20 \times 10^9/L$ prevenendo la rara insorgenza di emorragia endocranica. Circa il 20% dei bambini che si presenta con PTI acuta sviluppa in seguito una PTI cronica.

REPERTI DI LABORATORIO. La trombocitopenia grave (conta piastrinica $<20 \times 10^9/L$) è comune, le dimensioni piastriniche sono normali o aumentate, riflettendo l'aumentato ricambio piastrinico. Nella PTI acuta il valore di emoglobina, la conta dei globuli bianchi (GB) e la conta differenziale dovrebbero essere normali. L'emoglobina può essere ridotta se ci sono state epistassi o menorragia profuse. L'esame del midollo osseo mostra una normale serie granulocitica ed eritrocitaria, con un numero di megacariociti di regola normale o aumentato. Alcuni dei megacariociti possono sembrare immaturi in accordo con un turnover piastrinico aumentato. Le **indicazioni per l'aspirato midollare** includono un'anormalità nella conta di GB o un'anemia inspiegata, così come reperti suggestivi di insufficienza midollare all'anamnesi e all'esame obiettivo. Altri test di laboratorio dovrebbero essere effettuati come indicato dalla storia e dall'esame obiettivo. Negli adolescenti con una PTI di nuova insorgenza, dovrebbero essere ricercati gli anticorpi antinucleo per escludere il LES. Gli studi per l'HIV dovrebbero essere condotti nelle popolazioni a rischio, soprattutto negli adolescenti sessualmente attivi. La ricerca di anticorpi piastrinici si rivela talvolta utile nella PTI acuta. Un test di Coombs dovrebbe essere invece eseguito se è presente un'anemia inspiegata per escludere la sindrome di Evans (anemia emolitica autoimmune e trombocitopenia) (vedi Capitolo 464) o prima di iniziare la terapia con IgG-anti-D endovena.

DIAGNOSI DIFFERENZIALE. Il bambino in buone condizioni generali con trombocitopenia moderata-severa, un esame emocromocitometrico completo per altro normale e un normale esame fisico presenta una limitata diagnosi differenziale che include l'esposizione a farmaci che inducono anticorpi farmaco-dipendenti, sequestro splenico dovuto a una precedente ipertensione portale non rilevata e di rado processi aplastici precoci, come l'anemia di Fanconi (vedi Capitolo 468). Oltre a sindromi congenite, come la trombocitopenia amegacariocitica e la sindrome della trombocitopenia-assenza del radio, la maggior parte dei processi che interferiscono con la produzione di piastrine causa anche un'anomala sintesi di globuli rossi e bianchi e quindi manifestano anche diverse anomalie dell'esame emocromocitometrico completo. Patologie che causano aumentata distruzione piastrinica su base non immune sono in genere patologie sistemiche gravi con ovvi reperti clinici (per es. sindrome uremico-emolitica [*Hemolytic-Uremic Syndrome*, HUS], coagulazione intravascolare disseminata [CID]) (vedi Tab. 484-1 e Fig. 484-1). Un aumento isolato della milza suggerisce un potenziale ipersplenismo causato sia da una patologia epatica sia dalla trombosi della vena porta. La trombocitopenia autoimmune può rappresentare una manifestazione iniziale di LES, infezione da HIV o, di rado, linfoma. La sindrome di Wiskott-Aldrich (*Wiskott-Aldrich Syndrome*, WAS; vedi Capitolo 125.2) deve essere considerata in giovani maschi che presentano una ridotta conta piastrinica, in particolare se è presente una storia di eczema e di infezioni ricorrenti.

TRATTAMENTO. Non ci sono dati che mostrano che il trattamento modifichi l'esito clinico a breve e a lungo termine della PTI. Molti pazienti con PTI di nuova insorgenza presentano sintomi lievi, con reperti limitati alle petecchie e alla porpora cutanea, nonostante la severa trombocitopenia. Rispetto ai soggetti di controllo non trattati, il trattamento sembra essere in grado di indurre un aumento rapido nella conta piastrinica al livello teorico di sicurezza $>20 \times 10^9/L$, anche se non ci sono dati che indichino che la terapia precoce prevenga l'emorragia endocranica. Gli anticorpi antipiastrine si legano alle piastrine trasfuse così come alle piastrine autologhe. Quindi, la trasfusione piastrinica nella PTI è in genere controindicata a meno che l'emorragia non stia mettendo in pericolo la vita. Gli approcci iniziali della gestione della PTI includono i seguenti provvedimenti.

1. Nessuna terapia tranne che l'educazione e il counseling della famiglia e del paziente per i soggetti con sintomi minimi, lievi e moderati, come prima definito. Questo approccio enfatizza la natura benigna della PTI ed evita le montagne russe terapeutiche che si incontrano una volta iniziata la terapia. Questo approccio è molto meno costoso e gli effetti collaterali sono minimi.
2. Le immunoglobuline endovena (IVIG). L'IVIG alla dose di 0,8-1 g/kg/die per 1-2 giorni induce un aumento rapido nella conta piastrinica (in genere $>20 \times 10^9/L$) nel 95% dei pazienti entro 48 ore. L'IVIG sembra ridurre la fagocitosi Fc-mediata delle piastrine ricoperte di anticorpi. La terapia di IVIG è costosa e necessita di tempi lunghi. Inoltre, dopo l'infusione, è presente un'elevata frequenza di cefalea e vomito suggestivi di meningite asettica indotta dalla IVIG.
3. Terapia anti-D endovenosa. Per i pazienti Rh positivi, anti-D endovena alla dose di 50-75 μg/kg causa un aumento della conta piastrinica $>20 \times 10^9/L$ nell'80-90% dei pazienti in 48-72 ore. Quando somministrata a pazienti Rh positivi, gli anti-D endovena inducono una lieve anemia emolitica. I complessi anticorpo-eritrocita si legano ai recettori Fc macrofagici e interferiscono con la distruzione piastrinica, causando così un aumento nella conta piastrinica. Gli anti-D endovena sono inefficaci nei pazienti Rh negativi.
4. Prednisone. La terapia corticosteroidea è stata usata per molti anni per trattare la PTI cronica e acuta in adulti e bambini. Dosi di prednisone di 1-4 mg/kg/24 h sembrano indurre un più rapido aumento nella conta piastrinica rispetto ai pazienti non trattati con PTI. Se l'esame del midollo osseo debba essere eseguito per scoprire altre cause di trombocitopenia, soprattutto la leucemia linfoblastica acuta, prima dell'inizio della terapia con prednisone nella PTI oppure no è controverso. La terapia corticosteroidea è in genere continuata per 2-3 settimane finché la conta piastrinica $>20 \times 10^9/L$ viene raggiunta, con un rapido decremento per evitare gli effetti collaterali a lungo termine della terapia steroidea, soprattutto il ritardo di crescita, il diabete mellito e l'osteoporosi.

Ciascuno di questi farmaci può essere usato per le ricadute delle PTI, che comunemente si verificano molte settimane dopo un iniziale decorso della terapia.

Nel caso speciale dell'emorragia endocranica, possono essere utilizzate multiple modalità, inclusi la trasfusione piastrinica, l'IVIG, i corticosteroidi ad alte dosi e una tempestiva consulenza chirurgica con programmi per una splenectomia di urgenza.

Attualmente non c'è un consenso riguardo la gestione della PTI acuta dell'infanzia. L'American Society of Hematology ha pubblicato delle linee guida per il trattamento degli adulti con PTI, ma c'è un importante disaccordo in questo campo. L'unico consenso è il fatto che i pazienti che stanno sanguinando in modo significativo dovrebbero essere trattati e questi possono rappresentare solo il 5% dei bambini con PTI. Le emorragie endocraniche rimangono rare e non ci sono dati che mostrano che il trattamento attualmente riduca la sua incidenza.

Il ruolo della splenectomia nella PTI dovrebbe essere riservato a una o due situazioni. Il bambino più grande (≥4 anni) con PTI grave di durata >1 anno (PTI cronica) e i cui sintomi non sono facilmente controllati con la terapia è un candidato per la splenectomia. La splenectomia deve essere anche considerata quando un'emorragia a rischio per la vita (emorragia endocranica) complica la PTI acuta, se la conta piastrinica non può essere corretta rapidamente con la trasfusione di piastrine e la somministrazione di IVIG e corticosteroidi. La splenectomia è associata con un rischio a vita di infezioni importanti post-splenectomia causata dagli organismi capsulati.

PORPORA TROMBOCITOPENICA IDIOPATICA CRONICA. Circa il 20% dei pazienti che presentano una PTI acuta e che ha una trombocitopenia persistente da **>6 mesi** si ritiene sia affetto da una trombocitopenia cronica. A quel punto, dovrebbe essere condotta un'attenta rivalutazione per patologie associate, soprattutto per le patologie autoimmuni, come il LES; le malattie infettive croniche, come quella da HIV; le cause non immuni di trombocitopenia cronica, come la malattia di von Willebrand di tipo piastrinico e tipo 2B, la trombocitopenia legata alla X, la sindrome linfoproliferativa autoimmune, la sindrome dell'immunodeficienza comune variabile, la macrotrombocitopenia autosomica e la WAS (anche questa legata alla X). La terapia dovrebbe essere orientata al controllo dei sintomi e alla prevenzione delle emorragie gravi. Nella PTI, la milza è la sede primaria sia della sintesi di anticorpi antipiastrine sia della distruzione piastrinica. La splenectomia ha successo portando a una completa guarigione il 64-68% dei bambini con PTI cronica. Questo deve essere controbilanciato al rischio cronico di infezioni gravi post-splenectomia. Questa decisione è spesso condizionata dai problemi dello stile di vita così come dalla facilità con cui il bambino può essere gestito utilizzando la terapia medica, come l'IVIG, i corticosteroidi, gli anti-D endovena o il rituximab (vedi Capitolo 464). L'AMG 531, una proteina stimolante la trombopoiesi, ha manifestato qualche successo nel trattamento di adulti con trombocitopenia immune cronica. Prima della splenectomia, il bambino dovrebbe ricevere i vaccini antipneumoccoccici e antimeningoccici e, dopo la splenectomia, dovrebbe ricevere una profilassi penicillinica per un certo numero di anni. È controverso se la profilassi penicillinica debba durare per tutta la vita.

484.2 • Trombocitopenia farmaco-indotta

Un certo numero di farmaci è associato alla trombocitopenia immune come risultato di una reazione immune o di un danno megacariocita. Alcuni farmaci comuni usati dai pediatri che causano trombocitopenia includono l'acido valproico, la fenitoina, i sulfonamidi e il trimetoprim-sulfametoxazolo. La trombocitopenia indotta dall'eparina (e raramente la trombosi) è talvolta presente nei pazienti pediatrici, ma si verifica quando, dopo esposizione all'eparina, il paziente ha anticorpi diretti contro il complesso del fattore piastrinico 4 antieparinico.

484.3 • Distruzione piastrinica non immune

Le sindromi come la CID (vedi Capitolo 483), l'HUS (vedi Capitolo 518) e la porpora trombotica trombocitopenica (PTT) condividono il quadro ematologico di una microangiopatia trombotica in cui si verifica la distruzione dei globuli rossi e una trombocitopenia da consumo causata dal deposito di piastrine e fibrina nella microcircolazione. L'anemia emolitica microangiopatica è caratterizzata dalla presenza di frammenti eritrocitari, incluse le cellule a elmetto, gli schistociti e le cellule a sperone.

484.4 • Sindrome uremico-emolitica

Vedi anche il Capitolo 518. La sindrome uremico-emolitica (*Hemolitic Uremic Syndrome*, HUS), una patologia acuta dell'infanzia e della prima fanciullezza, in genere consegue a un episodio di gastroenterite acuta, spesso scatenata dall'*Escherichia coli* 0157:H7. In breve poi compaiono i segni e i sintomi di anemia emolitica, trombocitopenia e insufficienza renale acuta. Talvolta i sintomi neurologici sono associati a questi reperti. L'*E. coli* 0157:H7 produce una specifica tossina (verotossina) che si lega e danneggia preferenzialmente le cellule endoteliali renali.

L'anemia emolitica è caratterizzata da eritrociti morfologicamente anormali, con la presenza di cellule a elmetto, sferociti, schistociti, cellule a sperone e altre anomalie della forma. La presenza di trombocitopenia nonostante un numero normale di megacariociti midollari è indice di un'eccessiva distruzione piastrinica. I risultati dei test per la CID sono in genere normali, tranne che per i livelli elevati di D-dimero. L'esame delle urine mostra proteine, eritrociti e cilindri. L'anuria e la grave iperazotemia indicano un grave danno renale. Il trattamento della maggior parte dei casi di HUS coinvolge l'istituzione di un'attenta gestione dei fluidi e una tempestiva dialisi appropriata. Il trattamento con la plasmaferesi è in genere riservato ai pazienti con HUS associata a complicanze neurologiche maggiori.

484.5 • Porpora trombotica trombocitopenica

La porpora trombotica trombocitopenica (PTT) è una rara combinazione di **febbre, anemia emolitica microangiopatica, trombocitopenia, alterazione della funzionalità renale** e **cambiamenti del sistema nervoso centrale** che è clinicamente simile alla HUS, sebbene la PTT in genere insorga negli adulti e occasionalmente negli adolescenti. I trombi nei piccoli vasi dentro il sistema nervoso centrale causano segni neurologici sfumati e variabili che variano da cambiamenti dell'umore e dell'orientamento all'afasia, alla cecità e alle convulsioni. Le manifestazioni iniziali sono spesso aspecifiche (debolezza, dolore, vomito); un pronto riconoscimento di questa patologia è critico. I **reperti di laboratorio** danno prove importanti per la diagnosi e mostrano un'anemia emolitica microangiopatica caratterizzata da eritrociti morfologicamente anomali, con schistociti, sferociti, cellule a elmetto e un'elevata conta reticolocitaria assieme alla trombocitopenia. Gli studi coagulativi non sono in genere diagnostici. L'azotemia e la creatinemia sono di solito elevate. Il trattamento delle TPP è la plasmaferesi (*plasma exchange*), che è efficace nell'80-95% dei casi. I corticosteroidi e la splenectomia sono riservati ai casi refrattari.

La maggior parte dei casi di PTT è causata da un deficit acquisito di una metalloproteinasi (ADAMTS-13) che è responsabile del clivaggio dei multimeri di vWf ad alto peso molecolare e sembre giocare un ruolo guida nell'evoluzione della microangiopatia trombotica. Invece, i livelli della metalloproteinasi nella HUS sono di solito normali. Il deficit congenito della metalloproteinasi causa rari casi familiari di PTT, di solito manifestantesi come episodi ricorrenti di trombocitopenia e anemia emolitica, con o senza cambiamenti neurologici che spesso si presentano nell'infanzia. La carenza può essere trattata con infusioni ripetute di plasma fresco congelato.

484.6 • Sindrome di Kasabach-Merritt

Vedi anche il Capitolo 505. L'associazione di un emangioma gigante con una coagulazione intravascolare localizzata che causa la trombocitopenia e l'ipofibrinogenemia è detta *sindrome di Kasabach-Merritt*. Il sito dell'emangioma è evidente nella maggior parte dei pazienti, ma gli emangiomi retroperitoneali e intraddominali possono richiedere le indagini di imaging per essere scoperti. Le piastrine con attivazione della coagulazione sono intrappolate dentro all'emangioma, con consumo del fibrinogeno e comparsa dei suoi prodotti di degradazione. Malformazioni arterovenose interne alle lesioni possono causare insufficienza cardiaca. Alcuni Autori discutono sul fatto che la sindrome di Kasabach-Merritt è realmente un'emangioendotelioma kaposiforme piuttosto che un semplice emangioma. Lo striscio di sangue periferico mostra alterazioni microangiopatiche. Modalità multiple sono state usate per trattare la sindrome di Kasabach-Merritt, inclusa l'incisione chirurgica (se possibile), la fotocoagulazione laser, corticosteroidi ad alte dosi, terapia radiante locale e agenti antiangiogenici, come l'interferone-α_2. Nel tempo la maggior parte dei pazienti che vengono diagnosticati nell'infanzia presentano una regressione dell'emangioma. Il trattamento della coagulopatia associata può trarre beneficio dalla terapia antifibrinolitica con acido ε-aminocaproico.

484.7 • Sequestro

La trombocitopenia si sviluppa in soggetti con splenomegalia massiva dal momento che la milza si comporta come una spugna per le piastrine e ne sequestra un grande numero. La maggior parte di questi pazienti presenta anche una lieve leucopenia e anemia all'emocromo. I soggetti che hanno una trombocitopenia causata dal sequestro splenico dovrebbero essere valutati per la diagnosi eziologica della splenomegalia incluse infezioni, cause infiammatorie, infiltrative, neoplastiche, ostruttive ed emolitiche.

484.8 • Sindromi trombocitopeniche congenite

Vedi Tabella 484-2. La **trombocitopenia amegacariocitica congenita** è causata da un raro difetto nell'ematopoiesi che in genere si manifesta nei primi giorni o settimane di vita, quando il bambino presenta petecchie e porpora a causa della profonda trombocitopenia. Altri reperti oltre a quelli cutanei e mucomembranosi all'esame obiettivo sono normali. L'esame del midollo osseo mostra l'assenza di megacariociti. Questi pazienti spesso evolvono in insufficienza midollare (aplasia) nel tempo. La trombocitopenia amegacariocitaria è causata da una mutazione nel recettore TPO della cellula staminale, che è essenziale per lo sviluppo di tutte le linee cellulari ematopoietiche. Il trapianto di midollo osseo è curativo.

La sindrome della **trombocitopenia-assenza del radio** (*Thrombocytopenia-Absent Radius*, **TAR**) consiste in una trombocitopenia (assenza o ipoplasia dei megacariociti) che si presenta nella prima infanzia con anomalie bilaterali del radio di diversa gravità, che vanno da cambiamenti lievi ad arti marcatamente accorciati (Fig. 484-2). Molti di questi individui presentano anche altre anomalie scheletriche dell'ulna, del radio e degli arti inferiori. I pollici sono presenti. Un'intolleranza alle formule con latte vaccino (presente nel 50%) può complicare la gestione inducendo emorragia gastrointestinale, aumentata trombocitopenia, eosinofilia e reazione leucemoide. La trombocitopenia della sindrome TAR va frequentemente in remissione dopo i primi anni di vita. Le basi molecolari della sindrome TAR devono ancora essere definite, ma viene suggerita un'ereditarietà autosomica recessiva.

La **sindrome di Wiskott-Aldrich** (*Wiskott-Aldrich Syndrome*, **WAS**) è caratterizzata da trombocitopenia con piastrine molto piccole, eczema e infezioni ricorrenti a causa dell'immunodeficienza (vedi Capitolo 125.2). La WAS viene ereditata come una patologia correlata alla X e il gene per la WAS è stato sequenziato. La proteina WAS sembra giocare un ruolo integrante nella regolazione dell'architettura citoscheletrica delle piastrine e dei linfociti T in risposta a segnali cellulari recettore-mediati. La proteina WAS è comune a tutte le cellule della linea ematopoietica. L'analisi molecolare di famiglie con trombocitopenia correlata alla X ha mostrato che molti dei membri affetti hanno mutazioni puntiformi all'interno del gene WAS, mentre individui con la manifestazione completa della WAS presentano grandi delezioni genetiche. L'esame del midollo osseo nella WAS mostra il numero normale di megacariociti, anche se si possono presentare caratteristiche morfologiche bizzarre. Le piastrine trasfuse presentano un'emivita normale. La splenectomia spesso corregge la trombocitopenia, suggerendo che le piastrine prodotte nella WAS subiscono una distruzione accelerata. Dopo la splenectomia, questi pazienti sono a rischio aumentato di infezioni invasive e richiedono profilassi antibiotica a vita contro gli organismi capsulati. Circa il 5% dei pazienti con la WAS sviluppa tumori maligni linforeticolari. Il trapianto di midollo osseo è curativo per la WAS.

Un notevole numero di **sindromi trombocitopeniche ereditarie** conosciute come sindromi di Sebastian, Epstein, May-Hegglin e Fechtner, sono caratterizzate da macrotrombocitopenia autosomica dominante, neutrofili con corpi inclusi oltre a una varietà di patologie, incluse sordità, nefropatia e/o patologia oculare. È stato dimostrato che queste sono dovute a mutazioni differenti nella catena 9 del gene della miosina non muscolare. Alcuni soggetti con macrotrombocitopenia ereditata come carattere recessivo presentano anomalie di 22q11. La trombocitopenia è in genere lieve e non progressiva.

484.9 • Trombocitopenia neonatale

Vedi anche il Capitolo 103.4. La trombocitopenia nel neonato raramente è indicativa di una patologia primaria della megacariopoiesi, ma più spesso costituisce l'esito di patologie sistemiche e del trasferimento di anticorpi materni diretti contro le piastrine fetali. La trombocitopenia può verificarsi in diverse infezioni fetali e neonatali e può essere responsabile di severe emorragie spontanee. La trombocitopenia neonatale spesso si verifica assieme a infezioni virali congenite, soprattutto la rosolia e il Cytomegalovirus; infezioni protozoarie, come la toxoplasmosi; la sifilide e infezioni batteriche, soprattutto quelle causate da bacilli Gram-negativi. La costellazione di marcata trombocitopenia e reperti addominali anomali è comune nell'enterocolite necrotizzante e altre cause di necrosi intestinale. La piastinopenia in un bambino ammalato richiede una pronta ricerca per patogeni virali e batterici.

La trombocitopenia mediata da anticorpi nel neonato si verifica per il trasferimento placentare di anticorpi materni diretti contro le piastrine fetali. La porpora trombocitopenica alloimmune neonatale (PTAN) è causata dallo sviluppo di anticorpi materni contro antigeni presenti sulle piastrine fetali che sono condivisi con il padre e riconosciuti come estranei dal sistema immunitario materno. Questo rappresenta l'equivalente piastrinico della malattia da incompatibilità Rh del neonato. L'incidenza della PTAN è 1/4000-5000 nati vivi. Le manifestazioni cliniche della PTAN sono quelle di un bambino apparentemente sano che entro i primi giorni dal parto presenta petecchie generalizzate e porpora. Gli esami di laboratorio non mostrano una trombocitopenia materna pur con una trombocitopenia neonatale moderata o grave. Un'anamnesi attenta non deve documentare una trombocitopenia nella madre. Fino al 30% dei neonati con PTAN grave possono presentare emorragia endocranica, prenatale e perinatale. A differenza della malattia da Rh, le prime gravidanze possono essere seriamente colpite e le successive gravidanze possono essere colpite anche più seriamente delle prime.

La **diagnosi** di PTAN viene fatta mediante il controllo della presenza di alloanticorpi materni diretti contro le piastrine paterne. Studi specifici devono essere fatti per identificare l'alloantigene bersaglio. La causa più comune è l'incompatibilità nei confronti dell'alloantigene piastrinico HPA-1a. Sono stati identificati polimorfismi specifici della sequenza di DNA che permettono test informativi prenatali per identificare le gravidanze a rischio. La diagnosi differenziale della PTAN include il trasferimento transplacentare di autoanticorpi antipiastrine (PTI materna) e più comunemente un'infezione virale o batterica.

Il **trattamento** della PTAN richiede la somministrazione di IVIG alla madre durante la gestazione. La terapia in genere inizia nel secondo trimestre e viene continuata durante tutta la gravidanza. La conta piastrinica fetale può essere monitorata con prelievi percutanei dal cordone ombelicale. Il parto dovrebbe avvenire attraverso taglio cesareo. Dopo il parto, se persiste una grave trombocitopenia, la trasfusione di un'unità di piastrine che condividono gli alloantigeni materni (per es. piastrine materne lavate) causerà un rialzo della conta piastrinica per permettere un'emostasi efficace. Dopo aver avuto un bambino affetto, è importante un counseling genetico per informare i genitori dell'elevato rischio di trombocitopenia nelle gravidanze successive.

Bambini nati da madri affette da PTI (**PTI materna**) sembrano avere un rischio minore di emorragia severa rispetto ai neonati con PTAN, anche se si verifica una severa trombocitopenia. La conta piastrinica materna preesistente può presentare un qualche valore predittivo in quanto una trombocitopenia materna severa prima del parto comporta un elevato rischio di trombocitopenia fetale. Nelle madri che hanno avuto una splenectomia per PTI, la conta piastrinica materna può essere normale e non è predittiva di trombocitopenia fetale.

Il **trattamento** include la somministrazione perinatale di corticosteroidi alla madre e la somministraizione di IVIG e talvolta corticosteroidi al neonato dopo il parto. La trombocitopenia in un neonato, se dovuta a NAPT o a PTI materna, in genere si

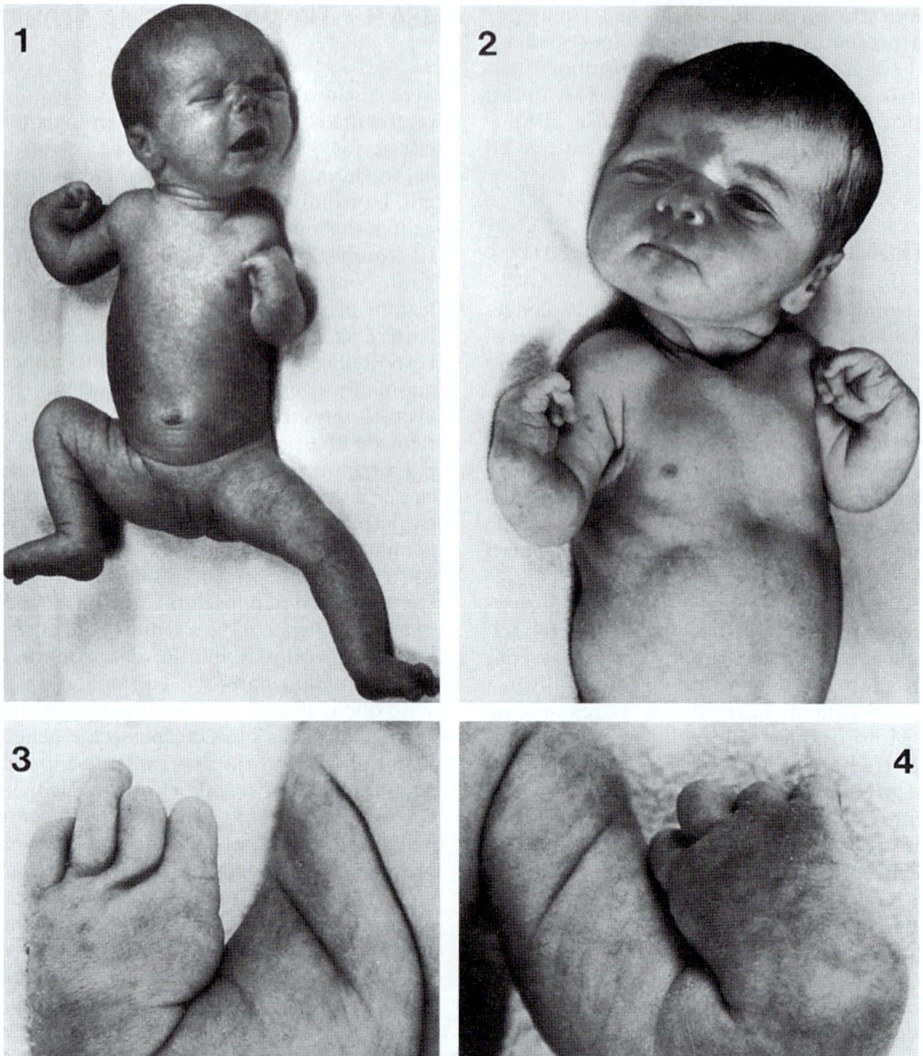

Figura 484-2. Neonato, primo figlio di genitori giovani sani, con trombocitopenia-assenza del radio pienamente espressa, incluse la trombocitopenia, l'ipereosinofilia e l'anemia. Si possono evidenziare l'ipoplasia dell'omero distale e della spalla, la displasia bilaterale dell'anca, calcagni lievemente tali e la clinodattilia di entrambi i mignoli. Questo paziente ha una pronunciata allergia al latte vaccino, con esposizione seguita da diarrea, vomito e riduzione del peso e della conta piastrinica, che lo ha obbligato a una dieta libera dal latte vaccino. Inoltre, si possono notare naso persistentemente depresso a sella e gambe incavate. (Da Wiedemann H-R, Kunze J, Grosse F-R [editors]: *Clinical Syndromes*, 3rd ed. [English translation]. London, Mosby-Wolfe, 1997, p 430.)

risolve entro i 2-4 mesi dopo il parto. Il periodo di rischio più elevato è l'immediato periodo perinatale.

Due sindromi di insufficienza congenita della produzione delle piastrine spesso si presentano nel periodo neonatale. Nella **trombocitopenia amegacariocitica**, il neonato manifesta petecchie e porpora poco dopo la nascita. I reperti all'esame fisico sono altrimenti normali. I megacariociti sono assenti dal midollo osseo. Questa sindrome è causata da una mutazione nel recettore TPO megacariocitario che è essenziale per lo sviluppo di tutte le linee cellulari ematopoietiche. In genere si sviluppa una pancitopenia e il trapianto di cellule staminali ematopoietiche è curativo. La **sindrome TAR** consiste in una piastrinopenia che si presenta nella prima infanzia, con anomalie radiali bilaterali di diversa severità, che vanno da cambiamenti lievi a marcato accorciamento degli arti. I pollici sono presenti. In molti di questi individui, ci sono anche altre anomalie scheletriche degli arti inferiori. L'intolleranza alle formule con latte vaccino è presente nel 50% dei pazienti. La sindrome TAR va frequentemente in remissione dopo i primi anni di vita (vedi Capitolo 484.8) (vedi Fig. 484-2).

484.10 • Trombocitopenia dovuta a patologie acquisite che causano una ridotta produzione

Le patologie del midollo osseo che inibiscono la megacariopoiesi in genere colpiscono la produzione di globuli rossi e bianchi. Patologie infiltrative, inclusi i tumori maligni, come la leucemia linfoblastica acuta, l'istiocitosi, i linfomi e le malattie da accumulo, in genere causano anomalie all'esame obiettivo (linfoadenopatia, epatosplenomegalia, o masse) o anomalie della conta leucocitaria o anemia. I processi aplastici possono presentarsi come trombocitopenia isolata, anche se ci sono in genere indizi nella conta cellulare ematica completa (leucopenia, neutropenia, anemia o macrocitosi). I bambini con anemia aplastica costituzionale (anemia di Fanconi) spesso presentano anomalie all'esame, incluse le anomalie radiali, altre anomalie scheletriche, bassa statura, microcefalia e iperpigmentazione. L'esame del midollo osseo dovrebbe essere condotto quando la trombocitopenia è associata a anomalie ritrovate all'esame obiettivo o all'esame delle altre linee cellulari ematiche.

484.11 • Patologie della funzione piastrinica

Il tempo di emorragia e l'analizzatore di funzione piastrinica (PFA-100™) sono i soli test comunemente disponibili per lo screening dell'anomalia di funzione piastrinica. Il tempo di emorragia misura le interazioni delle piastrine con la parete vasale e quindi viene influenzato sia dalla conta sia dalla funzione piastrinica. Il valore predittivo del tempo di emorragia è problematico perché il tempo di emorragia è dipendente da un certo numero di altri fattori, incluse l'esperienza dei tecnici e la collaborazione del paziente. Un tempo di emorragia normale non identifica un difetto lieve di funzione piastrinica in un soggetto clinicamente sintomatico. Il PFA-100™ misura l'adesione piastrinica e l'aggregazione in sangue intero a concentrazioni elevate quando il sangue viene esposto sia all'epinefrina-collagene sia al collagene-ADP. I risultati sono riportati come tempo di chiusura misurato in secondi. Il PFA-100™ sembra essere più sensibile del tempo di emorragia, pertanto molti laboratori clinici hanno sostituito il tempo di emorragia con l'uso del PFA-100™. Sebbene il valore del PFA-100™ sia prolungato nella vWD così come nei difetti congeniti e acquisiti della funzione piastrinica, l'uso del PFA-100™ come test di screening rimane controverso. Sia il tempo di emorragia sia il PFA-100™ identificano la malattia di von Willebrand moderata-severa e i difetti di funzione piastrinica. Entrambi sono variabilmente insensibili alle anomalie di funzione piastrinica lievi. Il tempo di emorragia è l'unico test comunemente disponibile per valutare l'interazione piastrinica con la parete vasale.

La funzione piastrinica nei laboratori clinici è attualmente misurata usando l'aggregometro piastrinico. Nell'aggregometro, agonisti, come il collagene, l'ADP, la ristocetina, l'acido arachidonico e la trombina vengono aggiunti al plasma ricco di piastrine e l'aggregazione delle piastrine nel tempo viene misurata da una macchina automatica. Allo stesso tempo, altri strumento misurano il rilascio del contenuto granulare, come l'ATP, dalle piastrine dopo l'attivazione. La capacità delle piastrine di aggregare e la loro attività metabolica possono essere determinate contemporaneamente.

484.12 • Patologie acquisite della funzione piastrinica

Un certo numero di patologie sistemiche è associato con disfunzione piastrinica, più comunemente un'epatopatia, una nefropatia (uremia) e patologie che liberano quantità aumentate di prodotti di degradazione del fibrinogeno. Queste patologie causano frequentemente allungamento del tempo di emorragia e sono spesso associate con altre anomalie del meccanismo coagulativo. Il più importante elemento della gestione è il trattamento della patologia primaria. Se il trattamento del processo primario non è praticabile, le infusioni di desmopressina si sono rivelate utili nel promuovere l'emostasi e correggere il tempo di emorragia. In alcuni pazienti, le trasfusioni di piastrine e/o il crioprecipitato si sono anche rivelati utili nel migliorare l'emostasi.

Molti farmaci alterano la funzione piastrinica. Il farmaco più comunemente usato negli adulti che altera la funzione piastrinica è l'acido acetilsalicilico, il quale acetila irreversibilmente l'enzima cicloossigenasi, che è critico per la formazione del trombossano A_2. L'acido acetilsalicilico in genere causa una disfunzione piastrinica moderata, che diventa più evidente se è presente un'altra anomalia del meccanismo dell'emostasi. Altri farmaci comunemente usati che colpiscono la funzione piastrinica includono i farmaci antinfiammatori non steroidei, l'acido valproico e la penicillina ad alte dosi. Quando un paziente viene valutato per una possibile disfunzione piastrinica è di importanza critica escludere la presenza di altri agenti esogeni e studiare il paziente, se possibile, previa sospensione dei farmaci per almeno 2 settimane.

484.13 • Anomalie congenite della funzione piastrinica

I difetti gravi della funzione piastrinica in genere si presentano con petecchie e porpora poco dopo la nascita, soprattutto dopo parto naturale. Difetti nel complesso piastrinico GPIb (il recettore per il vWf) o nel complesso GPIIIb-IIa (il recettore del fibrinogeno) causano una disfunzione piastrinica congenita grave.

La **sindrome di Bernard-Soulier**, una patologia severa congenita della funzione piastrinica, è causata dall'assenza o da un deficit severo del recettore per il vWf (complesso GPIb) sulla membrana piastrinica. Questa sindrome è caratterizzata da trombocitopenia, con piastrine giganti e un tempo di emorragia marcatamente aumentato (>20 minuti). I test di aggregazione piastrinica mostrano assente aggregazione piastrinica indotta da ristocetina, ma normale aggregazione con gli altri agonisti. La ristocetina induce il legame del vWf alle piastrine e agglutina le piastrine. I risultati degli studi del vWf sono normali. Il complesso GPIb interagisce con il citoscheletro piastrinico; un difetto in questa interazione si ritiene sia la causa dell'aumentata dimensione piastrinica. La sindrome di Bernard-Soulier è una patologia a eredità autosomica recessiva. Le mutazioni genetiche che causano la sindrome di Bernard-Soulier sono di solito identificate nei geni che formano il complesso GPIb delle glicoproteine IBα, IBβ e IX.

La **tromboastenia di Glanzmann** è una patologia congenita associata a grave disfunzione piastrinica, che comporta un allungamento del tempo di emorragia e una conta piastrinica normale. Le piastrine hanno dimensione e caratteristiche morfologiche normali allo striscio di sangue periferico e il tempo di emorragia è marcatamente allungato. Gli studi di aggregazione mostrano un'aggregazione anomala o assente con tutti gli agonisti usati eccetto la ristocetina, perché la ristocetina agglutina le piastrine e non richiede piastrine metabolicamente attive. Questa patologia è causata dalla carenza del recettore piastrinico per il fibrinogeno GPIIIb-IIa, un complesso di integrine sulla superficie piastrinica che va incontro a cambiamenti conformazionali quando le piastrine sono attivate. Il fibrinogeno si lega a questo complesso quando la piastrina è attivata e causa l'aggregazione piastrinica. Determinato da mutazioni identificabili nei geni per la GPIIIb o la GPIIa, questa patologia è ereditata in modo autosomico recessivo.

Il deficit ereditario dei granuli di deposito piastrinici si presenta in 2 sindromi ben caratterizzate ma rare che coinvolgono il deficit dei granuli intracitoplasmatici. Il **deficit dei granuli densi** è caratterizzato dall'assenza dei granuli che contengono ADP, ATP, Ca^{2+} e serotonina. Questa patologia viene diagnosticata dal ritrovamento che l'ATP non è rilasciato con gli studi sull'aggregazione piastrinica e idealmente è caratterizzata con studi di microscopia elettronica. La **sindrome delle piastrine grigie** è causata dall'assenza dei granuli piastrinici α, che comporta piastrine che sembrano grigie alla colorazione di Wright del sangue periferico. In questa rara sindrome, l'aggregazione e il rilascio sono assenti con la maggior parte degli agonisti diversi dalla trombina e dalla ristocetina. Gli studi al microscopio elettronico sono diagnostici.

ALTRE PATOLOGIE EREDITARIE DELLA FUNZIONE PIASTRINICA. Anomalie nella via di attivazione piastrinica e di rilascio del contenuto dei granuli causano un gruppo eterogeneo di difetti di funzione piastrinica che si manifestano, in genere, con ematomi, epistassi e/o menorragia. I sintomi possono essere subdoli e spesso si fanno più evidenti dopo un intervento ad alto rischio, come la tonsillectomia o l'adenoidectomia o con la somministrazione di farmaci anti-infiammatori non steroidei. In laboratorio, il tempo di emorragia è variabile e il tempo di chiusura misurato con PFA-100™ è frequentemente, ma non sempre, allungato. Gli studi di aggregazione piastrinica mostrano un'aggregazione carente con 1 o 2 agonisti e/o il rilascio del contenuto granulare.

La formazione del trombossano dall'acido arachidonico dopo l'attivazione della fosfolipasi è critica per la normale funzione piastrinica. La carenza o la disfunzione degli enzimi, come la cicloossigenasi e la trombossano sintasi, che metabolizzano l'acido arachidonico, causano un'anormale funzione piastrinica. Nell'aggregometro, le piastrine provenienti da questi pazienti non aggregano in risposta all'acido arachidonico.

Il difetto di funzione piastrinica più comune è quello caratterizzato da un tempo di emorragia variabile e un'anormale aggregazione con 1 o 2 agonisti, in genere ADP e/o collagene. Questi pazienti hanno un'aggregazione normale con la trombina. Alcuni di questi individui hanno solo un rilascio diminuito di ATP dai granuli intracitoplasmatici. Questo difetto di rilascio selettivo è una causa comune di lieve difetto della funzione piastrinica.

TRATTAMENTO DEI DIFETTI DI FUNZIONE PIASTRINICA. Il successo del trattamento dipende dalla gravità sia della diagnosi sia dell'evento emorragico. In tutti i difetti di funzione piastrinica gravi, la desmopressina 0,3 μg/kg endovena può essere usata per gli episodi emorragici lievi-moderati. Oltre al suo effetto di stimolazione dei livelli di vWf e fattore VIII, la desmopressina corregge il tempo di emorragia e garantisce una normale emostasi in molti soggetti con difetti di funzione piastrinica lievi-moderati. Per soggetti con la sindrome di Bernard-Soulier o la tromboastenia di Glanzmann, le trasfusioni di piastrine 1 U/5-10 kg correggono il difetto nell'emostasi e possono essere salvavita. Raramente si sviluppano anticorpi contro la proteina piastrinica carente, rendendo il paziente refrattario alle piastrine trasfuse. In questi pazienti, l'ultilizzo di fattore VIIa ricombinante è stato efficace e questo trattamento è sotto trial clinici. In entrambe le patologie, ci si attende che il trapianto di cellule staminali possa essere risolutivo.

484.14 • PATOLOGIE DEI VASI SANGUIGNI

PORPORA DI SCHÖNLEIN-HENOCH. La porpora di Schönlein-Henoch (*Henoch-Schönlein Purpura*, HSP) è caratterizzata dall'improvviso sviluppo di un rash purpurico, artriti, dolore addominale e coinvolgimento renale (vedi Capitolo 166.1). Il caratteristico rash, formato da petecchie e spesso porpora palpabile, in genere coinvolge gli arti inferiori e le natiche. I risultati degli studi sulla coagulazione sono normali. Le lesioni anatomopatologiche nella cute, nell'intestino e nella sinovia sono rappresentate da vasculite leucocitoclastica, danni infiammatori all'endotelio capillare e postcapillare delle venule mediati dai globuli bianchi e dai macrofagi. Il fattore scatenante la HSP è sconosciuto. Nel rene la lesione è la glomerulonefrite focale con deposito di immunoglobuline A. I risultati degli studi di coagulazione così come la conta piastrinica sono normali nella HSP.

SINDROME DI EHLERS-DANLOS. La sindrome di Ehlers-Danlos è un patologia comune della struttura del collagene che causa facilità di ematomi e ritardata guarigione delle ferite (vedi Capitolo 658). Reperti suggestivi all'esame fisico includono una pelle morbida, vellutata e iperelastica; lassità articolari che sono facilmente sublussabili; cicatrici inusuali. Sono state descritte più di 10 varianti della sindrome di Ehlers-Danlos. La forma più grave è stata associata a una rottura improvvisa dei visceri. I risultati dei test di screening coagulativi sono in genere normali anche se il tempo di emorragia può essere lievemente aumentato. I risultati degli studi di aggregazione piastrinica sono normali o lievemente anormali, con deficit di aggregazione con il collagene.

PATOLOGIE ACQUISITE. Lo scorbuto, la terapia corticosteroidea cronica e la malnutrizione severa sono associate a "indebolimento" della matrice del collagene che fa da supporto ai vasi sanguigni. Quindi questi fattori sono associati a facilità alle ecchimosi, in particolare in presenza dello scorbuto, emorragie gengivali o caduta dei denti. Le lesioni cutanee che inizialmente compaiono come petecchie e porpora possono essere presenti nelle sindromi vasculitiche, come il LES.

Andrews RK, Berndt MC: Platelet physiology and thrombosis. *Thromb Res* 2004;114:447–453.

Aronis S, Platokouki H, Avgeri M, et al: Retrospective evaluation of long-term efficacy and safety of splenectomy in chronic idiopathic thrombocytopenic purpura in children. *Acta Paediatr* 2004;93:638–642.

Beck CE, Nathan PC, Parkin PC, et al: Corticosteroids versus intravenous immune globulin for the treatment of acute immune thrombocytopenic purpura in children: A systematic review and meta-analysis of randomized controlled trials. *J Pediatr* 2005;147:521–527.

Bengston KL, Skinner MA, Ware RE: Successful use of anti-CD20 (rituximab) in severe, life-threatening childhood immune thrombocytopenic purpura. *J Pediatr* 2003;143:67–73.

Blanchette V: Childhood chronic immune thrombocytopenic purpura (ITP). *Blood Rev* 2002;16:23–26.

Bussel JB, Kuter DJ, George JN, et al: AMG 531, a thrombopoiesis-stimulating protein, for chronic ITP. *N Engl J Med* 2006;355:1672–1681.

Bussel JB, Zabusky MR, Berkowitz RL, et al: Fetal alloimmune thrombocytopenia. *N Engl J Med* 1997;337:22–26.

Coppo P, Bengoufa D, Veyradier A, et al: Severe ADAMTS13 deficiency in adult idiopathic thrombotic microangiopathies defines a subset of patients characterized by various autoimmune manifestations, lower platelet count, and mild renal involvement. *Medicine (Baltimore)* 2004;83:233–244.

de Alarcon PA: Immune or idiopathic thrombocytopenic purpura (ITP) in childhood: What are the risks and who should be treated? *J Pediatr* 2003;143:287–289.

de Paepe A, Malfait F: Bleeding and bruising in patients with Ehlers-Danlos syndrome and other collagen vascular disorders. *Br J Haematol* 2004;127:491–500.

Geddis AE, Kaushansky K: Inherited thrombocytopenias: Toward a molecular understanding of disorders of platelet production. *Curr Opin Pediatr* 2004;16:15–22.

Horton TM, Stone JD, Yee D, et al: Case series of thrombotic thrombocytopenic purpura in children and adolescent. *J Pediatr Hematol Oncol* 2003;25:336–339.
Iyori H, Bessho F, Ookawa H, et al: Intracranial hemorrhage in children with immune thrombocytopenic purpura: Japanese Study Group on Childhood ITP. *Ann Hematol* 2000;79:691–695.
Kokame K, Miyata T: Genetic defects leading to hereditary thrombotic thrombocytopenic purpura. *Semin Hematol* 2004;41:34–40.
Kuhne T, Buchanan GR, Zimmerman S, et al: A prospective comparative study of 2,540 infants and children with newly diagnosed idiopathic thrombocytopenic purpura (ITP) from the Intercontinental Childhood ITP Study Group. *J Pediatr* 2003;143:605–608.
Posan E, McBane RD, Grill DE, et al: Comparison of PFA-100 testing and bleeding time for detecting platelet hypofunction and von Willebrand disease in clinical practice. *Thromb Haemost* 2003;90:483–490.
Ramasamy I: Inherited bleeding disorders: Disorders of platelet adhesion and aggregation. *Crit Rev Oncol Hematol* 2004;49:1–35.
Roberts I, Murray NA: Neonatal thrombocytopenia: Causes and management. *Arch Dis Child Fetal Neonatal Ed* 2003;88:F359–F364.
Seri M, Pecci A, Di BF, et al: MYH9-related disease: May-Hegglin anomaly, Sebastian syndrome, Fechtner syndrome, and Epstein syndrome are not distinct entities but represent a variable expression of a single illness. *Medicine (Baltimore)* 2003;82:203–215.
Snapper SB, Rosen FS: A family of WASPs. *N Engl J Med* 2003;348:350–351.
Tarrantino MD, Young G, Bertolone SJ, et al: Single dose of anti-D immune globulin at 75 μg/kg is as effective as intravenous immune globulin at rapidly raising the platelet count in newly diagnosed immune thrombocytopenic purpura in children. *J Pediatr* 2006;148:489–494.
Wang J, Wiley JM, Luddy R, et al: Chronic immune thrombocytopenic purpura in children: Assessment of rituximab treatment. *J Pediatr* 2005; 146:217–221.

Sezione 8 — La milza — Bruce M. Camitta

Capitolo 485 ■ Anatomia e funzione della milza

ANATOMIA. L'abbozzo splenico è riconoscibile a partire dalle 5 settimane di gestazione. Alla nascita, la milza pesa circa 11 g. Poi in seguito aumenta di dimensioni fino alla pubertà, raggiungendo un peso di 135 g prima di diminuire di dimensioni durante l'età adulta. Le maggiori componenti spleniche sono il compartimento linfoide (*polpa bianca*) e il sistema di filtro (*polpa rossa*). La polpa bianca è formata da guaine di cellule T con centri geminativi contenenti le cellule B. La polpa rossa presenta uno scheletro di cellule reticolari fisse, macrofagi mobili, lacune endoteliali parzialmente collassate (cordoni di Billroth) e i sinusoidi splenici. Una *zona marginale* ricca in cellule dendritiche (presentanti l'antigene) separa la polpa rossa dalla polpa bianca. La capsula splenica contiene muscolo liscio e si contrae in risposta all'epinefrina.

Circa il 10% del sangue che giunge alla milza scorre rapidamente attraverso una rete vascolare chiusa. L'altro 90% scorre più lentamente attraverso un sistema aperto (i *cordoni splenici*) dove viene filtrato attraverso fessure di 1-5 μm prima di attraversare i sinusoidi splenici.

FUNZIONE. La peculiarità dell'anatomia e del flusso ematico della milza permette di svolgere funzioni di deposito, filtrazione e immunologiche. La milza riceve il 5-6% della gittata cardiaca, ma normalmente contiene solo 25 mL di sangue. Essa può contenerne molto di più quando si ingrandisce. L'emopoiesi è una funzione splenica maggiore a 3-6 mesi di vita fetale, ma poi scompare. L'emopoiesi splenica può ricomparire in pazienti affetti da mielofibrosi o anemia emolitica severa. Il fattore VIII e le piastrine sono immagazzinate nella milza e possono essere rilasciati dallo stress o dalla somministrazione di epinefrina. Trombocitosi e leucocitosi si verificano con la perdita della funzione di riserva splenica. Un'elevata conta piastrinica dopo la perdita della funzione splenica non è associata con un aumentato rischio di trombosi nei bambini.

Il lento flusso di sangue che supera i macrofagi e attraverso piccole aperture nelle pareti dei sinusoidi facilita la funzione di filtro della milza. Un eccesso di membrana viene rimosso da eritrociti giovani; la perdita di questa funzione è caratterizzata da cellule bersaglio, poichilocitosi e diminuita fragilità osmotica. La milza è la sede primitiva per la distruzione dei globuli rossi vecchi; questa funzione viene assunta dalle altre cellule del sistema reticoloendoteliale dopo splenectomia. La milza rimuove anche le cellule danneggiate e anormali, come gli sferociti e i globuli rossi ricoperti di anticorpi. Le inclusioni intracitoplasmatiche possono essere rimosse dai globuli rossi senza lisi cellulare. L'iposplenia funzionale o anatomica è caratterizzata da una persistenza in circolo di cellule contenenti inclusi nucleari (**corpi di Howell-Jolly**), emoglobina denaturata (**corpi di Heinz**) e altri residui nei globuli rossi: quest'ultimi possono comparire come "**appendici**" alla microscopia indiretta.

Le immunoglobuline, la properdina e la tuftsina sono prodotte nella milza. La milza ha un ruolo minore nella risposta anticorpale ad antigeni iniettati per via intramuscolare o sottocutanea, ma è richiesta per la produzione precoce anticorpale dopo esposizione endovenosa ad antigeni. Soggetti giovani (non immuni) o iposplenici sono a rischio aumentato di sepsi causata dai pneumococchi e altri batteri capsulati. La milza può anche utilizzare il sistema fagocitario per catturare e distruggere i parassiti intracellulari. La milza può essere un importante sito di produzione anticorpale nella porpora trombocitopenica immune.

Chadburn A: The spleen: Anatomy and anatomical function. *Semin Hematol* 2000;37(Suppl 1):13–21.
Steininger B, Barth P: Microanatomy and function of the spleen. *Adv Anat Embryol Cell Biol* 2000;151:1–101.

Capitolo 486 ■ Splenomegalia

MANIFESTAZIONI CLINICHE. Una milza soffice e sottile può essere palpabile nel 15% dei neonati, nel 10% dei bambini normali e nel 5% degli adolescenti. Nella maggior parte degli individui, la milza deve aumentare di 2-3 volte le sue dimensioni prima di essere palpabile. La milza viene esaminata meglio con il paziente supino palpando l'addome verso il margine costale sinistro da sotto quando il paziente inspira profondamente. Una milza ingrandita può scendere nella pelvi; quando vi è un sospetto di splenomegalia, l'esame addominale dovrebbe iniziare da una sede più bassa. Un reticolo venoso addominale superficiale può essere presente quando la splenomegalia è il risultato dell'ipertensione portale. La scoperta o la conferma radiologica dell'ingrandimento splenico viene fatta con l'ecografia, la TC o la scansione colloidale sulfurea con Tecnezio-99m. Quest'ultimo inoltre valuta le funzioni spleniche.

DIAGNOSI DIFFERENZIALE. Cause specifiche di splenomegalia sono elencate nella Tabella 486-1. I problemi principali sono discussi di seguito.

Pseudosplenomegalia. Connessioni mesenteriche enormemente ampie possono essere causa di una milza mobile o ptosica. Un lobo sinistro ingrandito del fegato, una massa del quadrante superiore sinistro o un ematoma splenico possono essere confusi con splenomegalia. Cisti spleniche possono contribuire o mimare la splenomegalia; queste possono essere congenite (epidermidi) o acquisite (pseudocisti) dopo un trauma o un infarto. Le cisti sono di solito asintomatiche e vengono scoperte nella valutazione radiologica. Anche la splenosi dopo rottura splenica o una milza accessoria (presente nel 10% dei soggetti normali) può mimare una splenomegalia; la maggior parte non è palpabile. La sindrome del polisplenismo congenito include difetti cardiaci, anomalie degli organi addominali localizzati a sinistra, polmoni bilobati, atresia biliare e pseudosplenomegalia (vedi Capitolo 431.11).

Ipersplenismo. Un'aumentata funzione splenica (sequestro o distruzione di cellule circolanti) comporta una citopenia nel sangue periferico, un'aumentata attività del midollo osseo e la splenomegalia. È in genere secondaria a un'altra patologia e può essere curata con il trattamento della condizione sottostante o, se assolutamente necessario, moderata attraverso la splenectomia.

Splenomegalia congestizia (sindrome di Banti). La splenomegalia può conseguire all'ostruzione delle vene epatica, portale o splenica. La malattia di Wilson (vedi Capitolo 354.2), la galattosemia (vedi Capitolo 87.2), l'atresia biliare (vedi Capitolo 353) e il deficit di α-1 antitripsina (vedi Capitolo 354.6) possono portare a un'infiammazione epatica, fibrosi e ostruzione vascolare. Le anomalie congenite delle vene portali (assenza o ipoplasia) o spleniche possono causare un'ostruzione vascolare. Onfaliti settiche o tromboflebiti possono essere spontanee o verificarsi come risultato della cateterizzazione venosa ombelicale nei neonati e possono anche comportare un'obliterazione secondaria di questi vasi. Il flusso venoso splenico può essere ostruito da masse di eritrociti falcizzati. Quando la milza è il sito di ostruzione vascolare, la splenectomia cura l'ipersplenismo. Tuttavia, l'ostruzione in genere

TABELLA 486-1. Diagnosi differenziale della splenomegalia per fisiopatologia

LESIONI ANATOMICHE
Cisti, pseudocisti
Amartomi
Sindrome polisplenica
Emangiomi e linfoangiomi
Ematoma o rottura (traumatica)
Amartoma

IPERPLASIA CAUSATA DA PATOLOGIE EMATOLOGICHE

Emolisi Acuta e Cronica*
Emoglobinopatie (malattia falciforme nell'infanzia con o senza crisi di sequestro e variante falcemica, talassemia major, emoglobina instabile)
Patologie della membrana eritrocitaria (sferocitosi ereditaria, ellissocitosi, piropoichilocitosi)
Deficit di enzimi eritrocitari (carenza grave di G6PD, deficit di piruvato chinasi)
Emolisi immune (emolisi autoimmune e isoimmune)
Emoglobinuria parossistica notturna

Deficit cronico di ferro

Ematopoiesi extramidollare
Anemie emolitiche severe
Patologie mieloproliferative: leucemia mieloide cronica (LMC), LMC giovanile, mielofibrosi con metaplasia mieloide, policitemia vera
Osteopetrosi
Pazienti che ricevono fattori stimolanti colonie granulocitarie e granulocito-macrofagiche

INFEZIONI†

Batteriche
Sepsi acuta: *Salmonella typhi*, *Streptococcus pneumoniae*, *Haemophilus influenzae* tipo b, *Staphylococcus aureus*
Infezioni croniche: endocarditi infettive, meningococciemia cronica, brucellosi, tularemia, malattia da graffio di gatto
Infezioni locali: ascesso splenico (*S. aureus*, streptococchi, meno spesso le specie di *Salmonella*, specie polimicrobiche), ascesso epatico piogenico (batteri anaerobi, batteri intestinali Gram-negativi), colangiti

Virali*
Infezioni virali acute, soprattutto nei bambini
Cytomegalovirus congenito (CMV), herpes simplex, rosolia
Epatiti, A, B, e C; CMV
Virus di Epstein-Barr (EBV)
Sindromi virali emofagocitiche: CMV, EBV, HHV-6
Virus dell'immunodeficienza umana (HIV)

Spirochete
Sifilide, soprattutto congenita
Leptospirosi

Rickettsie
Febbre maculosa delle Montagne Rocciose
Febbre Q
Tifo

Funghi/Micobatteri
Tubercolosi miliare
Istoplasmosi disseminata
Blastomicosi del Sud America
Candidosi sistemica (in pazienti immunodepressi)

Parassiti
Malaria
Toxoplasmosi, soprattutto congenita
Toxocara canis, *Toxocara cati* (larve viscerali migranti)
Leishmaniosi (kala-azar)
Schistosomiasi (coinvolgimento epatico-portale)
Tripanosomiasi
Fascioliasi

PROCESSI IMMUNOLOGICI E INFIAMMATORI*
Lupus eritematoso sistemico
Artrite reumatoide
Malattia mista dei tessuti connettivali
Vasculiti sistemiche
Malattia da siero
Ipersensibilità a farmaci, soprattutto fenitoina
Graft versus host disease
Sindrome di Sjögren
Crioglobulinemia
Amiloidosi
Sarcoidosi
Linfocitosi a grandi granuli e neutropenia
Sindrome dell'istiocitosi
Sindrome emofagocitica (non virale, familiare)

TUMORI MALIGNI
Primitivi: leucemia (acute, cronica), linfoma, angiosarcoma, malattia di Hodgkin
Metastasi

MALATTIE DA ACCUMULO
Lipidosi (malattia di Gaucher, malattia di Niemann-Pick, gangliosidosi infantile GM_1)
Mucopolisaccaridosi (Hurler, tipo Hunter)
Mucolipidosi (malattia a cellule I, sialidosi, deficit multiplo di sulfatasi, fucosidosi)
Difetti nel metabolismo dei carboidrati: galattosemia, intolleranza al fruttosio
Sindrome dell'istiocita blu mare

CONGESTIZIA*
Scompenso cardiaco
Cirrosi o fibrosi epatica
Ostruzione venosa extraepatica portale (trombosi), splenica e delle vene epatiche (trombosi, sindrome di Budd-Chiari)

*Comuni.
†Infezioni croniche o ricorrenti suggeriscono una sottostante immunodeficienza.
G6PD, glucosio-6-fosfato deidrogenasi; HHV-6, herpesvirus umano 6.
Da Kliegman RM, Greenbaum LA, Lye PS: *Practical Strategies in Pediatric Diagnosis and Therapy*, 2nd ed. Philadelphia, Elsevier, 2004, p 347.

è presente nei sistemi portale o epatico. In questi ultimi casi lo shunt porto-cavale può essere più utile, perché sia l'ipertensione portale sia la trombocitopenia contribuiscono al sanguinamento delle varici.

Aslanidou E, Fotoulaki M, Tsitouridis I, Nousia-Arvanitakis S: Partial splenic embolization: Successful treatment of hypersplenism, secondary to biliary cirrhosis and portal hypertension in cystic fibrosis. *J Cyst Fibrosis* 2006;Dec 6. E pub ahead of print.

Subhasis RC, Rajiv C, Kumar SA, et al: Surgical treatment of massive splenomegaly and severe hypersplenism secondary to extrahepatic portal venous obstruction in children. *Surg Today* 2007;37:19–23.

Capitolo 487 ■ Iposplenismo, trauma splenico e splenectomia

IPOSPLENISMO. L'assenza congenita della milza è associata a cardiopatie cianogene complesse, destrocardia, polmoni bilateralmente trilobati e organi addominali eterotopici (**sindrome di Ivemark**; vedi Capitolo 431.11). La funzione splenica è di solito normale nei bambini con **polisplenia congenita.** L'**iposplenismo congenito** può presentarsi nei neonati normali, soprattutto i prematuri. I bambini con emoglobinopatia a cellule falciformi (vedi Capitolo 462.1) possono avere un'ipofunzione splenica già al sesto mese di vita. Inizialmente questo è causato da un'ostruzione vascolare, che può essere corretta con la trasfusione di emazie. La milza alla fine va incontro ad autoinfarti e diventa fibrotica e permanentemente non funzionate. L'iposplenismo funzionale può anche presentarsi nella malaria (vedi Capitolo 285), dopo l'irradiazione del quadrante superiore sinistro, e quando la funzione reticoloendoteliale della milza è severamente colpita (come nell'anemia emolitica grave o nella malattia da accumulo metabolico). L'ipofunzione splenica è stata riportata occasionalmente in pazienti con vasculiti, nefriti, malattie infiammatorie croniche, malattia celiaca, sindrome di Pearson, anemia di Fanconi e graf versus host disease.

L'ipofunzione splenica è caratterizzata da inclusioni eritrocitarie dallo striscio di sangue periferico, **"appendici"** alla microscopia di interferenza e scarsa captazione di tecnezio alla scintigrafia della milza. I pazienti con iposplenismo funzionale o asplenia sono a rischio per la sepsi da organismi capsulati (pneumococchi).

TRAUMI. Un danno alla milza può verificarsi a seguito di traumi addominali. Piccole rotture capsulari spleniche possono causare dolore addominale o riferito alla spalla sinistra come risultato dell'irritazione peritoneale causata dal sangue. Lacerazioni maggiori comportano una perdita di sangue più severa, con dolore simile e segni di ipovolemia. Milze precedentemente ingrandite (come in pazienti con storia di mononucleosi infettiva) vanno più facilmente incontro a rottura a seguito di traumi minori. La TC con mezzo di contrasto per via endovenosa è la modalità di imaging migliore per determinare i traumi splenici.

Il **trattamento** di un piccolo danno capsulare include l'attenta osservazione, con attenzione ai cambiamenti nei segni vitali o nei reperti addominali, determinazioni seriate dell'emoglobina; inoltre la disponibilità di intervento chirurgico immediato in caso di deterioramento delle condizioni del paziente (vedi Capitolo 71). La trasfusione di emazie necessaria dovrebbe essere minima (<25 mL/kg/48 ore). Questi pazienti sono in genere ricoverati in ospedale per 10-14 giorni e devono limitare le loro attività per mesi. La laparotomia, con o senza splenectomia, è indicata nelle emorragie addominali più severe nei pazienti che hanno un'instabilità o un deterioramento clinici, o quando viene sospettato il danno di un altro organo. Una splenectomia parziale e la riparazione splenica dovrebbero essere preferite alla splenectomia quando possibile.

SPLENECTOMIA. La splenectomia dovrebbe essere limitata a indicazioni specifiche dove la terapia medica è (o è stata) inefficace. Queste includono la rottura splenica traumatica, i difetti anatomici, l'anemia emolitica severa, la citopenia immune, le malattie metaboliche da accumulo e l'ipersplenismo secondario. Il rischio maggiore a lungo termine della splenectomia è l'infezione batterica non controllabile (sepsi o meningite). Questo rischio è soprattutto elevato in bambini più piccoli di 5 anni al momento dell'intervento chirurgico. Il rischio di sepsi è minore quando la splenectomia viene eseguita per traumi, difetti di membrana eritrocitaria e trombocitopenia immune (2-4%) piuttosto che quando è presente una deficienza immune preesistente (sindrome di Wiskott-Aldrich, malattia di Hodgkin) o un blocco reticoloendoteliale (malattia da accumulo, anemia emolitica grave) (8-30%). Il ricorso alla splenectomia laparoscopica ha diminuito la morbilità e il tempo di ricovero in ospedale.

I batteri capsulati, come lo *Streptococcus pneumoniae* (>60% dei casi), *Haemophilus influenzae* e *Neisseria meningitidis* rendono conto di >80% dei casi di sepsi post-splenectomia. Dal momento che la milza è responsabile della filtrazione del sangue e delle prime risposte anticorpali, la sepsi (con o senza meningite) può progredire rapidamente, portando a morte entro 12-24 ore dall'esordio. I pazienti febbrili splenectomizzati dovrebbero essere trattati prontamente con antibiotici. Questo trattamento dovrebbe essere iniziato a casa se l'accesso alle terapie mediche definitive è ritardato. Una cefalosporina ad ampio spettro (cefotaxime 50 mg/kg ogni 8 ore) o la vancomicina (10 mg/kg ogni 6 ore) per coprire i pneumococchi penicillino-resistenti è raccomandata finché non sia nota la sensibilità allo specifico antibiotico. I pazienti splenectomizzati sono anche a rischio aumentato di contrarre infezioni protozoarie, come la malaria e la babesiosi.

La gestione **preoperatoria, intraoperatoria** e **postoperatoria** può ridurre il rischio di infezioni postsplenectomia. È importante accertarsi della necessità della splenectomia e, se possibile, posticipare l'operazione finché il paziente non compia 5 anni di età. Vaccini antipneumococchi, meningococchi e *Haemophilus influenzae* somministrati prima della splenectomia possono ridurre la sepsi post-splenectomia. Tuttavia, l'efficacia dei vaccini non coniugati è minore nei bambini più piccoli di 2 anni e nei pazienti immunodepressi. Nei pazienti con un trauma, la riparazione splenica o una parziale splenectomia dovrebbero essere considerate allo scopo di preservare la funzione splenica. Una splenectomia parziale o una parziale embolizzazione splenica possono essere sufficienti per migliorare alcune forme di anemia emolitica. Fino al 50% dei bambini la cui milza viene rimossa a causa di un trauma presentano una splenosi spontanea; la splenosi chirurgica (distribuire piccoli pezzi di milza in addome) può ridurre il rischio di sepsi nei pazienti la cui splenectomia è richiesta per un trauma. Tuttavia, in entrambi i casi, il tessuto splenico che ricresce ha frequentemente una funzione inadeguata. La profilassi con penicillina V (125 mg due volte al giorno per i bambini con meno di 5 anni; 250 mg due volte al giorno per i bambini più grandi di 5 anni) dovrebbe essere somministrata per almeno 2 anni dopo la splenectomia (almeno fino ai 6 anni di età). La profilassi può essere continuata fino all'età adulta per i pazienti ad alto rischio. La penicillina riduce il rischio di sepsi pneumococcica nei pazienti più giovani con emoglobina SS, ma altre popolazioni non sono state ancora studiate a fondo. Anche se il rischio maggiore è il periodo immediato postoperatorio, i report delle morti che si verificano molti anni dopo la splenectomia suggeriscono che il rischio (e la necessità di una profilassi) può perdurare per tutta la vita. Altre misure postoperatorie includono l'educazione del paziente e della famiglia, l'indossare un braccialetto con informazioni mediche, la tempestiva valutazione e il trattamento della febbre.

Bader-Meunier B, Gauthier F, Archambaud F, et al: Long-term evaluation of the beneficial effect of subtotal splenectomy for management of hereditary spherocytosis. *Blood* 2001;97:399–403.

Castagnola E, Fioredda F: Prevention of life-threatening infections due to encapsulated bacteria in children with hyposplenia or asplenia: A brief review of current recommendations for practical purposes. *Eur J Haematol* 2003;71:319–326.

Hansen K, Singer DB: Asplenic-hyposplenic overwhelming sepsis: Postsplenectomy sepsis revisited. *Pediatr Dev Pathol* 2001;4:105–121.

Upadhyaya P: Conservative management of splenic trauma: History and current trends. *Pediatr Surg Int* 2003;19:617–627.

Sezione 9 — Il sistema linfatico — Bruce M. Camitta

Capitolo 488 ■ Anatomia e funzione del sistema linfatico

Il sistema linfatico include i linfociti circolanti, i vasi linfatici, i linfonodi, la milza, le tonsille, le adenoidi, le placche di Peyer e il timo. La linfa, un ultrafiltrato del sangue, viene raccolta dai capillari linfatici che sono presenti in tutti gli organi eccetto il cervello e il cuore. Questi si uniscono per formare vasi progressivamente più larghi che drenano le regioni del corpo. Durante il loro decorso, i vasi linfatici portano la linfa ai linfonodi. Nei linfonodi la linfa viene filtrata attraverso cavità dove il materiale particolato e gli organismi infettivi vengono fagocitati, processati e presentati come antigeni ai linfociti circostanti. Queste azioni stimolano la produzione anticorpale, le risposte T-cellulari e la produzione di citochine (vedi Capitolo 122).

La composizione della linfa può variare con il sito di drenaggio della linfa. È di solito chiara, ma la linfa drenata dal tratto gastrointestinale può essere lattescente (chilo) per la presenza dei grassi. Il contenuto proteico è intermedio tra quello di un essudato e di un trasudato. Il livello proteico può essere aumentato con l'infiammazione e nella linfa drenata dal fegato o dall'intestino. La linfa contiene numeri variabili di linfociti.

Capitolo 489 ■ Anomalie dei vasi linfatici

Le anomalie dei vasi linfatici possono essere congenite o acquisite. I segni e sintomi possono conseguire a un aumento della massa linfatica tissutale o dalla perdita di linfa. La **linfangectasia** è la dilatazione dei vasi linfatici. La linfangectasia polmonare causa distress respiratorio (vedi Capitolo 392). Il coinvolgimento dei linfatici intestinali causa ipoproteinemia e linfocitopenia secondaria alla perdita di linfa nell'intestino (vedi Capitolo 335). Il **linfangioma** (igroma cistico) è una massa di linfatici dilatati. Alcune di queste lesioni presentano anche una componente emangiomatosa (vedi Capitolo 505). Il trattamento chirurgico viene complicato da un'elevata incidenza di ricaduta. La sclerosi intralesionale con l'OK-432, un derivato streptococcico, è stata usata con successo in pazienti selezionati. Le lesioni macrocistiche sembrano rispondere meglio rispetto al linfangioma microcistico alla scleroterapia. La **displasia linfatica** può causare problemi multisistemici. Questi includono il linfedema, l'ascite chilosa, il chilotorace e i linfangiomi dell'osso, del polmone e degli altri siti.

Il **linfedema** è causato dall'ostruzione al flusso linfatico. Il linfedema congenito si può trovare nella sindrome di Turner, di Noonan e nella malattia di Milroy ereditata in modo autosomico dominante. Molte famiglie con malattia di Milroy presentano mutazioni nel *FLT4* che codificano per il gene per il recettore-3 per il fattore di crescita vascolare endoteliale. È stata riportata anche un'ereditarietà correlata alla X e autosomica recessiva. Il **linfedema precoce** (malattia di Meige) causa un progressivo edema degli arti inferiori, in genere in femmine durante il periodo puberale o la gravidanza. Il linfedema è anche stato trovato in associazione alla linfangectasia intestinale, alla malformazione cerebrovascolare, alla ptosi, alle unghie gialle distrofiche, alla distichiasi e alla colestasi. Le mutazioni in *FOXC2* sono associate alla sindrome del linfedema-distichiasi, che presenta linfedema a esordio puberale. Un'ostruzione acquisita dei linfatici può derivare da tumori, fibrosi post-irradiazione e cicatrizzazione postinfiammatoria. La filariasi è una causa importante di linfedema in Africa, Asia, e America Latina; dei 120 milioni di persone stimate infette, circa 40 milioni (soprattutto adulti e adolescenti grandi) si ritiene che presentino linfedema e idrocele. Il danno al vaso linfatico maggiore può causare la formazione di fluido linfatico nell'addome (ascite chilosa) o nel torace (chilotorace).

La **linfangite** è un'infiammazione dei linfatici che drena un area di infezione. Strie dolenti, eritematose si estendono prossimalmente dall'area infetta. Anche i linfonodi regionali possono essere dolenti. Gli streptococchi di gruppo A e lo *Staphiloccoccus aureus* sono i patogeni più frequenti.

Addiss DG, Beach MJ, Streit TG, et al: Randomised placebo-controlled comparison of ivermectin and albendazole alone and in combination for *Wuchereria bancrofti* microfilaraemia in Haitian children. *Lancet* 1997; 350:480–484.

Banieghbal B, Davies MR: Guidelines for successful treatment of lymphangioma with OK-432. *Eur J Pediatr Surg* 2003;13:103–107.

Fischer P, Supali T, Maizels RM: Lymphatic filariasis and *Brugia timori*: Prospects for elimination. *Trends Parasitol* 2004;20:351–355.

Giguere CM, Bauman NM, Smith RJ: New treatment options for lymphangioma in infants and children. *Ann Otol Rhinol Laryngol* 2002;111: 1066–1075.

Levinson KL, Feingold E, Ferell R, et al: Age of onset in hereditary lymphedema. *J Pediatr* 2003;142:704–708.

Mulliken JB, Fishman SJ, Burrows PE: Vascular anomalies. *Curr Pediatr Surg* 2000;37:527–584.

Orvidas LJ, Kasperbauer JL: Pediatric lymphangioma of the head and neck. *Ann Otol Rhinol Laryngol* 2000;109:411–421.

Schuster T, Grantzow R, Nicolai T: Lymphangioma colli: A new classification contributing to prognosis. *Eur J Pediatr Surg* 2003;13:97–102.

Capitolo 490 ■ Linfoadenopatia

La maggior parte dei linfonodi non è in genere palpabile nel neonato. Con l'esposizione antigenica, il tessuto linfoide aumenta di volume, così che i linfonodi cervicali, ascellari e inguinali sono spesso palpabili durante l'infanzia. Non sono considerati ingranditi finché il loro diametro non supera 1 cm nei linfonodi cervicali e ascellari e 1,5 cm nei linfonodi inguinali. Altri linfonodi in genere non sono palpabili o visualizzati con le radiografie abituali.

DIAGNOSI. L'ingrandimento del linfonodo è causato dalla proliferazione di elementi linfoidi normali o dall'infiltrazione con cellule maligne e fagocitiche. Nella maggior parte dei pazienti, un'attenta anamnesi e un esame fisico completo suggeriscono la diagnosi corretta. Masse non linfoidi (costa cervicale, cisti del dotto tireoglosso, rottura di cisti dell'arco o del solco branchiale infetta, igroma cistico, gozzo, tumore del muscolo sternocleidomastoideo, tiroiditi, ascesso tiroideo e neurofibroma) si verificano frequentemente nel collo e meno frequentemente in altre aree. Linfonodi acutamente infetti sono in genere dolenti e la cute sovrastante può anche essere eritematosa e calda. Una fluttuazione suggerisce la formazione di un ascesso. I linfonodi tubercolari possono essere fusi l'un l'altro. Con infezioni croniche, molti dei segni sopraddetti possono non essere presenti. Linfonodi invasi da un tumore sono in genere fissi e duri e possono essere fusi in pacchetti o fissi alla cute o alle strutture sottostanti.

L'**adenopatia generalizzata** (accrescimento di >2 regioni linfonodali non contigue) è causata da una patologia sistemica (Tab. 490-1) ed è spesso accompagnata da reperti obiettivi anormali in altri sistemi. Al contrario, l'adenopatia regionale è più frequentemente il risultato di un'infezione nei linfonodi coinvolti e/o nell'area di drenaggio (Tab. 490-2). Quando dovuta ad agenti infettivi diversi dai batteri, l'adenopatia può essere caratterizzata da sedi anatomiche atipiche, un decorso prolungato, una fistolizzazione, assenza di un'infezione piogena precedente e dati insoliti nell'anamnesi (graffio di gatto, esposizione alla tubercolosi, malattia venerea). Un linfonodo fisso e duro dovrebbe sempre far sorgere il dubbio del tumore maligno, indipendentemente dalla presenza o dall'assenza di sintomi sistemici o altri reperti obiettivi anormali.

TRATTAMENTO. La valutazione e il trattamento della linfoadenopatia vengono guidati dal probabile agente eziologico, come determinato dall'anamnesi e dall'esame obiettivo. Molti pazienti con adenopatia cervicale hanno una storia compatibile con un'infezione virale e non necessitano di un intervento. Se si sospetta un'infezione batterica, è indicato un trattamento antibiotico di copertura per almeno gli streptococchi e gli stafilococchi. I soggetti che non rispondono agli antibiotici per via orale, come dimostrato dalla tumefazione e dalla febbre persistente, richiedono antibiotici antistafiloccoccici per via endovenosa. Se non c'è una risposta in 1-2 giorni o se ci sono segni di ostruzione delle vie aeree o uno stato settico significativo, dovrebbero essere eseguite la TC o l'ecografia al collo. Se è presente pus, può essere aspirato, sotto guida TC o ecografia, oppure se è molto esteso, può richiedere l'incisione e il drenaggio. Dovrebbe essere eseguita

TABELLA 490-1. Diagnosi differenziale delle linfoadenopatie generalizzate sistemiche

LATTANTE	BAMBINO	ADOLESCENTE
CAUSE COMUNI		
Sifilide	Infezione virale	Infezione virale
Toxoplasmosi	EBV	EBV
CMV	CMV	CMV
HIV	HIV	HIV
	Toxoplasmosi	Toxoplasmosi
		Sifilide
CAUSE RARE		
Malattia di Chagas (congenita)	Malattia da siero	Malattia da siero
Leucemia congenita	LES, JRA	LES, JRA
Tubercolosi congenita	Leucemia/linfoma	Leucemia/linfoma/malattia di Hodgkin
Reticoloendoteliosi	Tubercolosi	Malattia linfoproliferativa
Patologia linfoproliferativa	Morbillo	Tubercolosi
Malattia da accumulo metabolica	Sarcoidosi	Istoplasmosi
Patologia istiocitica	Infezione fungina	Sarcoidosi
	Lebbra	Infezione fungina
	Istiocitosi delle cellule di Langerhans	Lebbra
	Malattia granulomatosa cronica	Reazione da farmaci
	Istiocitosi dei seni	Malattia di Castleman
	Reazione da farmaci	

CMV, Cytomegalovirus; EBV, virus di Epstein-Barr; HIV, virus dell'immunodeficienza umana; JRA, *Juvenile Rheumatoid Arthritis*, (artrite reumatoide giovanile [come la malattia di Still]); LES, lupus eritematoso sistemico.

Da Kliegman RM, Greenbaum LA, Lye PS: *Practical Strategies in Pediatric Diagnosis and Therapy*, 2nd ed. Philadelphia, Elsevier, 2004, p 863.

TABELLA 490-2. Siti di linfoadenopatia locale e patologia associata

CERVICALE
Infezione orofaringea (virale o streptococco di gruppo A, stafilococcica)
Infezione del cuoio capelluto
Linfadenite da micobatteri (tubercolosi e micobatteriosi non tubercolare)
Infezione virale (EBV, CMV, HHV-6)
Malattia da graffio di gatto
Toxoplasmosi
Malattia di Kawasaki
Malattia tiroidea
Malattia di Kikuchi
Istiocitosi dei seni
Patologia linfoproliferativa autoimmune
AURICOLARE ANTERIORE
Congiuntiviti
Altre infezioni oculari
Tularemia oculoghiandolare
Cellulite facciale
Otite media
Infezione virale (soprattutto rosolia, parvovirus)
SOPRACLAVICOLARE
Tumori maligni o infezioni nel mediastino (destra)
Tumori maligni metastatici dell'addome (sinistra)
Linfoma
Tubercolosi
EPITROCLEARE
Infezioni delle mani, infezioni delle braccia*
Linfoma[†]
Sarcoidosi
Sifilide
INGUINALE
Infezione delle vie urinarie
Malattie veneree (soprattutto la sifilide o il linfogranuloma venereo)
Altre infezioni perineali
Infezione suppurativa degli arti inferiori
Lebbra
ILARI (NON PALPABILI, INDIVIDUATI ALLA RADIOGRAFIA O TC TORACICA)
Tubercolosi[†]
Istoplasmosi[†]
Blastomicosi[†]
Coccidioidomicosi[†]
Leucemia/linfoma[†]
Malattia di Hodgkin[†]
Tumori maligni metastatici*
Sarcoidosi[†]
Malattia di Castleman
ASCELLARE
Malattia da graffio di gatto
Infezione del braccio o della parete toracica
Tumori maligni della parete toracica
Leucemia/linfoma
Brucellosi
ADDOMINALE
Tumori maligni
Adeniti mesenteriche (morbillo, tubercolosi, Yersinia, streptococco di gruppo A)

*Unilaterale.
[†]Bilaterale.
CMV, Cytomegalovirus; TC, tomografia computerizzata; EBV, virus di Epstein-Barr; HHV-6, herpesvirus umano 6.
Da Kliegman RM, Greenbaum LA, Lye PS: *Practical Strategies in Pediatric Diagnosis and Therapy*, 2nd ed. Philadelphia, Elsevier 2004, p 864.

inoltre la colorazione di Gram e la coltura del pus. Il drenaggio chirurgico viene richiesto per un ascesso. Dovrebbe essere documentate prima del trattamento la dimensione dei linfonodi colpiti: un insufficiente decremento nelle dimensioni in 10-14 giorni suggerisce la necessità di ulteriori indagini. Questo può comprendere un emocromo completo con formula; sierologia per il virus di Epstein Barr, Cytomegalovirus, *Toxoplasma* e la malattia da graffio di gatto; i test sierologici per l'antistreptolisina O oppure l'antiDNAasi; il test intradermico alla tubercolina e la radiografia del torace. Se queste non sono diagnostiche, la consulenza con un infettivologo o uno specialista oncologo può essere di aiuto. La biopsia deve essere considerata se c'è una febbre persistente o inspiegata, perdita di peso, sudorazione notturna, linfonodi duri o fissi ai tessuti vicini. La biopsia può anche essere indicata se si verifica un aumento delle dimensioni sopra i valori base in 2 settimane, non diminuzione delle dimensioni in 4-6 settimane e non ritorno in 8-12 settimane, oppure se si sviluppano nuovi segni e sintomi.

Haberman TM, Steensma PA: Lymphadenopathy. *Mayo Clin Proc* 2000; 75:723–732.
Nield LS, Kamat D: Lymphadenopathy in children: When and how to evaluate. *Clin Pediatr* 2004;43:25–33.
Peters TR, Edwards KM: Cervical lymphadenopathy and adenitis. *Pediatr Rev* 2000;21:399–405.
Soldes OS, Younger JG, Hirschl RB: Predictors of malignancy in childhood peripheral lymphadenopathy. *J Pediatr Surg* 1999;34:1447–1452.
Tokuda Y, Kishaba Y, Kato J, Nakazato N: Assessing the validity of a model to identify patients for lymph node biopsy. *Medicine* 2003;82:414–418.
Twist CJ, Link MP: Assessment of lymphadenopathy in children. *Pediatr Clin North Am* 2002;49:1009–1025.

490.1 • Malattia di Kikuchi-Fujimoto (linfadenite istiocitica necrotizzante)

La malattia di Kukichi-Fujimoto è una patologia rara, autolimitantesi, che si riscontra più comunemente nei bambini rispetto agli adulti di provenienza asiatica. La presentazione può comprendere la febbre di origine sconosciuta, ma, più spesso, si verifica in bambini di 8-16 anni come adenite unilaterale cervicale posteriore, febbre, astenia e leucopenia. Il range delle dimensioni dei linfonodi è di 0,5-6 cm, sono dolenti o molli nel 50% dei casi, possono essere multipli e devono essere distinti dal linfoma.

L'eziologia è sconosciuta e la diagnosi viene fatta se le caratteristiche istologiche del linfonodo mostrano monociti plasmacitoidi a mezzaluna e assenza di neutrofili. La malattia si risolve in 6 mesi, anche se negli stessi pazienti si può sviluppare il lupus eritematoso sistemico.

490.2 • Istiocitosi dei seni con linfoadenopatia massiva (malattia di Rosai-Dorfman)

Questa malattia non frequente, benigna e autolimitantesi di eziologia sconosciuta presenta una distribuzione mondiale, ma è più comune in Africa e nei Caraibi. Bambini e adolescenti si presentano con adenopatia cervicale massiva simmetrica non dolente associata a febbre, leucocitosi, VES aumentata e aumento policlonale di immunoglobuline G. Si verifica raramente alla nascita o nei fratelli, inoltre i maschi sono più affetti delle femmine.

Talvolta, si associa con autoanticorpi contro gli eritrociti o la sinovia e si può verificare un coinvolgimento extralinfonodale. I siti includono la cute, la cavità nasale e i seni, il palato, l'orbita, l'osso e il sistema nervoso centrale. La diagnosi richiede una biopsia, che dimostra istiociti contenenti linfociti fagocitati. La diagnosi differenziale include l'istiocitosi a cellule di Langerhans e il linfoma.

La terapia è in genere non necessaria perché questa patologia è autolimitantesi, anche se una patologia extralinfonodale o persistente o esacerbazioni e remissioni possono rispondere al prednisone. I casi refrattari sono stati trattati con l'escissione chirurgica o la radiazione.

490.3 • Malattia di Castleman

Questa rara patologia linfoproliferativa, anche detta *iperplasia linfonodale angiofollicolare*, è di eziologia sconosciuta ma presenta un'associazione all'herpesvirus umano 8 e si presenta in adolescenti e giovani adulti in forme localizzate o multicentriche. L'herpesvirus 8 umano può stimolare un'eccessiva produzione di interleuchina 6 (IL-6). L'ingrandimento di un solo linfonodo, più spesso nel mediastino o nell'addome, è la presentazione localizzata più comune. Alcuni di questi pazienti possono presentare febbre, sudorazione notturna, perdita di peso e affaticamento. Il trattamento include la chirurgia e/o la terapia radiante.

La malattia di Castleman multifocale è una patologia sistemica che causa linfoadenopatia, epatosplenomegalia, febbre, anemia e ipergammaglobulinemia policlonale. La malattia di Castleman multicentrica può essere associata con l'infezione da HIV, la linfoadenopatia associata a malattia autoimmune, la sindrome POEMS (polineuropatia, organomegalia, endocrinopatia, proteine M e lesioni cutanee) e linfoma non Hodgkin. Il trattamento comprende gli steroidi, gli anticorpi monoclonali per l'IL-6 e per il recettore per l'IL-6 (tocilizumab), agenti antivirali e interferone-α. La chemioterapia per il linfoma diffuso a grandi cellule B può essere di beneficio in alcuni pazienti.

Bosch X, Guilabert A, Miquel R, et al: Enigmatic Kikuchi-Fujimoto disease. *Am J Clin Pathol* 2004;122:141–152.
Carbone A, Passannante A, Gloghini A, et al: Review of sinus histiocytosis with massive lymphadenopathy (Rosai-Dorfman disease) of head and neck. *Ann Otol Rhinol Laryngol* 1999;108:1095–1104.
Casper C: The aetiology and management of Castleman disease at 50 years: Translating pathophysiology to patient care. *Br J Haematol* 2005;129: 3–17.
Chuang CH, Yan DC, Chiu CH, et al: Clinical and laboratory manifestations of Kikuchi's disease in children and differences between patients with and without prolonged fever. *Pediatr Infect Dis J* 2005;24:551–554.
Dispenzieri A, Gertz MA: Treatment of Castleman's disease. *Curr Treat Options Oncol* 2005;6:255–266.
Guihot A, Couderc LJ, Agbalika F, et al: Pulmonary manifestations of multicentric Castleman's disease in HIV infection: A clinical, biological and radiological study. *Eur Respir J* 2005;26:118–125.
Herrada J, Cabanillas F, Rice L, et al: The clinical behavior of localized and multicentric Castleman disease. *Ann Intern Med* 1998;128:657–662.
Kojima M, Nakamura S, Nishikawa M, et al: Idiopathic multicentric Castleman's disease: A clinicopathologic and immunohistochemical study of five cases. *Pathol Res Pract* 2005;201:325–332.
Lin HC, Su CY, Huang SC: Kikuchi's disease in Asian children. *Pediatrics* 2005;115:e92–e96.
Nishimoto N: Clinical studies in patients with Castleman's disease, Crohn's disease, and rheumatoid arthritis in Japan. *Clin Rev Allergy Immunol* 2005; 28:221–229.
Parez N, Bader-Meunier B, Roy CC, et al: Paediatric Castleman disease: Report of seven cases and review of the literature. *Eur J Pediatr* 1999; 158:631–637.
Pulsoni A, Anghel G, Falcucci P, et al: Treatment of sinus histiocytosis with massive lymphadenopathy (Rosai-Dorfman disease): Report of a case and literature review. *Am J Hematol* 2002;69:67–71.
Raveenthiran V, Dhanalakshmi M, Rao PVH, et al: Rosai-Dorfman disease: Report of a 3-year-old girl with critical review of treatment options. *Eur J Pediatr Surg* 2003;13:350–354.
Scagni P, Peisino MG, Bianchi M, et al: Kikuchi-Fujimoto disease is a rare cause of lymphadenopathy and fever of unknown origin in children. *J Pediatr Hematol Oncol* 2005;27:337–340.

Parte XXI ▪ Neoplasie maligne e benigne

Capitolo 491 ▪ Epidemiologia delle neoplasie dell'infanzia e dell'adolescenza*

Nina S. Kaddan-Lottick

Le neoplasie nei soggetti di età ≤19 anni non sono frequenti; con un'incidenza annuale aggiustata per età di 16,5/100 000, rappresentano solo circa l'1% (12 400 casi/anno) di tutte le nuove occorrenze di tumore negli USA. Anche se la percentuale di sopravvivenza a 5 anni è migliorata dal 56% nel 1974 a >81% nel 2000 (Fig. 491-1), le neoplasie maligne rimangono la seconda più comune causa di morte (12,8%) tra soggetti di età compresa tra 1 e 14 anni negli USA. Studi clinici cooperativi multi-istituzionali sono tuttora in corso per ricercare nuovi trattamenti e nuove modalità per migliorare ulteriormente la sopravvivenza. Per via del crescente numero di pazienti che sopravvivono alla malattia, la ricerca clinica è anche rivolta alla qualità della vita di questi soggetti e alle conseguenze tardive della terapia affrontata dai bambini e dagli adulti colpiti da patologia tumorale durante l'infanzia. Il National Cancer Institute stima che nel 1997 c'erano 269 700 soggetti vivi (di tutte le età) colpiti da neoplasia durante l'infanzia, corrispondenti a 1/810 con <20 anni e 1/1000 con una età compresa fra i 20 e i 39 anni della popolazione degli USA.

Le neoplasie dell'età pediatrica differiscono notevolmente da quelle dell'adulto, sia per prognosi e distribuzione per istologia, sia per sede del tumore. Fra le diverse categorie di tumori pediatrici (Tab. 491-1), le neoplasie linfoematopoietiche (come la leucemia linfoblastica acuta, il linfoma) rappresentano circa il 40%, le neoplasie del sistema nervoso centrale circa il 30% e i tumori embrionali e i sarcomi circa il 10%. D'altro canto, i tumori epiteliali di organi quali i polmoni, il colon, la mammella e la prostata sono più comuni nell'età adulta. Diversamente dal pattern di incidenza in questa età, in cui la probabilità di avere una neoplasia tende ad aumentare rapidamente, in pediatria esiste un range relativamente ampio, con due picchi: nella prima infanzia e poi nell'adolescenza (Fig. 491-2). Durante il primo anno di vita, sono più comuni i **tumori embrionali** quali il neuroblastoma, il nefroblastoma (tumore di Wilms), il retinoblastoma, il rabdomiosarcoma, l'epatoblastoma e il medulloblastoma (Fig. 491-3). Questi tumori sono molto meno comuni nei bambini più grandi e nell'adulto, quando i processi di differenziazione cellulare si sono considerevolmente ridotti. I tumori embrionali, le leucemie acute, i linfomi di non-Hodgkin e i gliomi hanno un picco di incidenza tra i 2 e i 5 anni di età. Con l'aumentare dell'età dei bambini, cresce l'incidenza delle neoplasie dell'osso, della malattia di Hodgkin, delle neoplasie delle cellule germinali gonadiche (carcinomi testicolari e ovarici) e di altri carcinomi. L'adolescenza è un periodo di transizione fra le neoplasie comuni della prima infanzia e i carcinomi tipici dell'età adulta.

Le neoplasie dell'infanzia comprendono diversi generi di tumori maligni, definiti "cancro", e di tumori non maligni che derivano da alterazioni di processi genetici che coinvolgono il controllo della crescita e dello sviluppo cellulare. Sebbene molte malattie genetiche si correlino con un aumentato rischio di sviluppare neoplasie durante l'infanzia, si pensa che queste malattie siano responsabili di <5% di tutte le neoplasie (vedi Capitolo 492). Quelle più rilevanti, che conferiscono una suscettibilità a sviluppare neoplasie durante l'infanzia, sono le neurofibromatosi di tipo 1 e 2, la sindrome di Down, la sindrome di Beckwith-Wiedemann, la sclerosi tuberosa, la malattia di von Hippel-Lindau, lo xeroderma pigmentosum, la teleangectasia, la sindrome del nevo basocellulare e la sindrome di Li-Fraumeni (P53). La variabilità dei pattern di incidenza delle singole neoplasie pediatriche nel mondo implica l'influenza di fattori di rischio aggiuntivi, genetici ed epidemiologici, che rimangono da definire.

Diversamente dai tumori epiteliali dell'adulto, solo una piccola porzione di quelli pediatrici sembra essere correlata con l'esposizione a fattori ambientali noti (Tab. 491-2). Solamente un piccolo numero di neoplasie pediatriche è ricongiungibile all'esposizione a radiazioni ionizzanti e a diversi agenti chemioterapici (vedi Capitolo 706). L'associazione tra l'esposizione fetale e la neoplasia pediatrica non è chiara ed è stata dimostrata solo tra l'assunzione di dietilstilbestrolo da parte della madre durante la gravidanza e lo sviluppo di adenocarcinoma vaginale nelle figlie nell'adolescen-

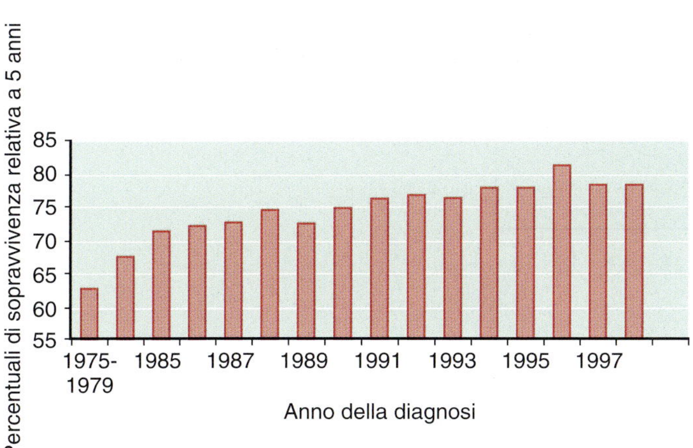

Figura 491-1. Percentuali (%) di sopravvivenza relativa a 5 anni a partire dalla diagnosi di tutti i tumori in bambini con ≤19 anni di età. Le percentuali si fondano sul follow-up di pazienti valutati nel 2003. (Da Ries LAG, Harkins D, Krapcho M, et al (editors): *SEER Cancer Statistics Review*, 1975-2003. Bethesda, MD, National Cancer Institute. http://seer.cancer.gov/csr/1975_2003/, based on November 2005 SEER data submission, posted to the SEER web site, 2006.)

*L'Autore vuole ringraziare il lavoro di James G. Gurney e Melissa L. Bondy per il Capitolo 483, "Epidemiologia delle neoplasie dell'infanzia e dell'adolescenza", della precedente edizione di questo volume.

TABELLA 491-1. Percentuali di incidenza e sopravvivenza delle neoplasie maligne per età fra i bambini degli Stati Uniti

	PERCENTUALE DI INCIDENZA ANNUALE PER MILIONE DI BAMBINI, 2000-2003							SOPRAVVIVENZA A 5 ANNI, ETÀ ≤19 ANNI ALLA DIAGNOSI, 1996-2003 (%)
	≤14 anni	≤19 anni	≤1 anno	≤4 anni	5-9 anni	10-14 anni	15-19 anni	
Tutte le neoplasie insieme	147,8	163,2	230,8	205,1	111,9	124,2	209,1	77,9
Leucemie	47,8	43,2	45,2	86,3	38,4	28,3	29,6	75,2
Linfatica acuta	37,9	32,7	19,6	79,4	31,9	19,7	17,1	81,4
Mieloide acuta	7,5	8,0	18,5	9,0	4,7	7,2	9,2	50,5
Linfomi	15,1	23,4	8,5	8,4	13,7	22,8	48,1	86,9
Malattia di Hodgkin	5,3	11,4	–	1,1	4,1	10,7	29,5	94,6
Linfomi non-Hodgkin	6,2	8,4	–	3,7	6,3	8,9	15,1	79,4
Tumori intracranici e intraspinali del sistema nervoso centrale e miscellanea	31,9	28,9	32,3	40,7	31,9	25,0	19,9	71,7
Astrocitoma	15,6	14,3	12,5	19,1	15,5	13,6	10,4	82,6
Tumori embrionali	7,5	6,6	11,3	10,4	7,5	4,6	3,8	67,3
Ependimomi e tumori del plesso corioideo	3,0	2,6	4,4	5,2	2,2	1,7	1,4	73,5
Neuroblastoma e altri tumori delle cellule nervose periferiche	9,9	7,6	50,5	19,2	3,4	1,7	–	68,9
Retinoblastoma	3,9	3,0	23,8	8,7	–	–	–	97,0
Tumori renali	7,8	6,2	17,1	18,7	4,7	1,1	1,3	87,1
Nefroblastoma	7,5	5,7	17,1	18,5	4,3	–	–	88,3
Tumori epatici	2,5	2,1	12,5	4,4	0,9	0,7	0,9	47,1
Epatoblastoma	2,1	1,6	11,8	4,3	–	–	–	59,2
Tumori dell'osso	6,3	8,5	–	1,4	5,0	12,4	15,1	65,1
Osteosarcoma	3,9	5,2	–	–	3,1	8,0	9,0	65,8
Tumore di Ewing e altri sarcomi	2,0	2,5	–	1,0	1,5	3,6	4,0	59,0
Sarcomi dei tessuti molli	10,7	12,1	17,5	10,7	7,9	12,2	16,3	69,2
Rabdomiosarcoma	5,3	4,9	5,1	8,3	4,4	3,8	3,8	61,0
Tumori delle cellule germinali	5,5	11,5	20,8	3,9	2,1	7,4	29,1	89,7
Carcinomi e melanomi	5,7	16,2	–	1,8	3,1	12,1	47,5	89,2

Basato sulla International Classification of Childhood Cancer (ICCC). Le percentuali sono per 1 000 000 di bambini e sono aggiustate per età sulla popolazione standard degli Stati Uniti del 2000. – = percentuale che non può essere calcolata per la presenza di <6 casi per intervallo di età.

Da Ries LAG, Harkins D, Krapcho M, et al (editors): *SEER Cancer Statistics Review, 1975-2003*. Bethesda, MD, National Cancer Institute. http://seer.cancer.gov/csr/1975_2003/, based on November 2005 SEER data submission, posted to the SEER web site, 2006.

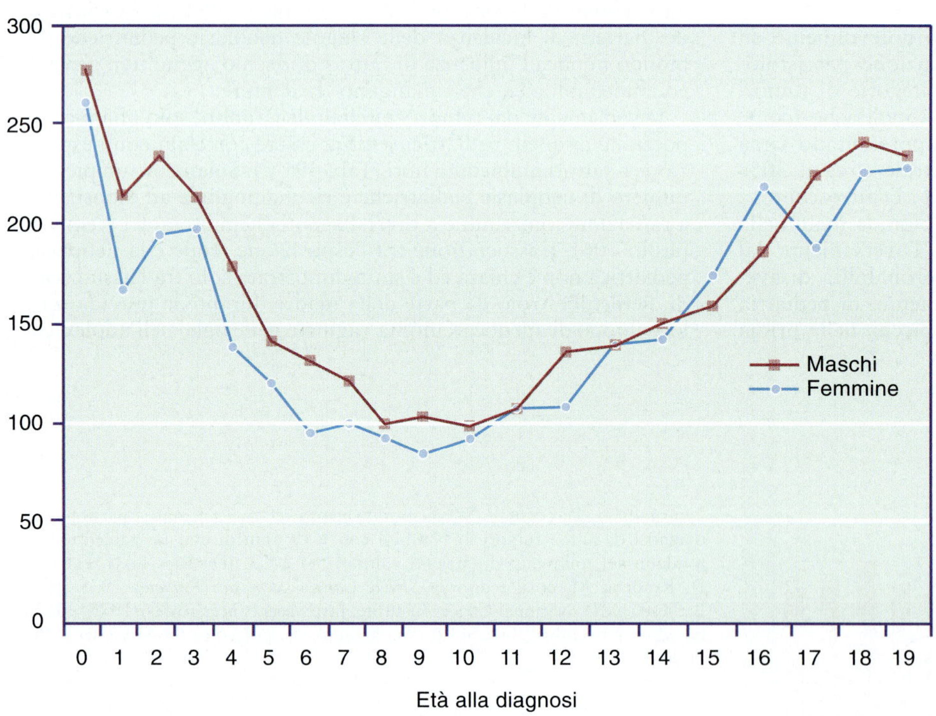

Figura 491-2. Percentuali di incidenza di neoplasie in relazione all'età e al sesso per milione di bambini negli USA. (Da Ries LAG, Smith MA, Gurney JG, et al [editors]: *Cancer Incidence and Survival Among Children and Adolescents: United States SEER Program 1975-1995*. Bethesda, MD, National Cancer Institute, SEER Program, 1999.)

za. I fattori ambientali che sono stati oggetto di studio, ma senza il ritrovamento di una convincente evidenza causale, sono i campi magnetici non ionizzanti, i pesticidi, le esposizioni lavorative a sostanze chimiche da parte dei genitori, i fattori alimentari e il fumo di sigaretta. I virus sono stati associati con determinate neoplasie pediatriche, come per esempio i poliomavirus (BK, JC, SV40) con il tumore cerebrale e il virus di Epstein-Barr con il linfoma non-Hodgkin, ma l'importanza eziologica non rimane chiara. Dal momento che l'eziologia dei tumori nei bambini è ancora, per la maggior parte, poco conosciuta, gli studi di epidemiologia hanno dimostrato che probabilmente il meccanismo è multifattoriale, risultando forse da potenziali interazioni fra tratti di predisposizione genetica ed esposizione a fattori ambientali. Sono in corso studi per valutare il ruolo dei polimorfismi dei geni che codificano per enzimi implicati nell'attivazione o nel metabolismo degli xenobiotici; la protezione delle cellule da

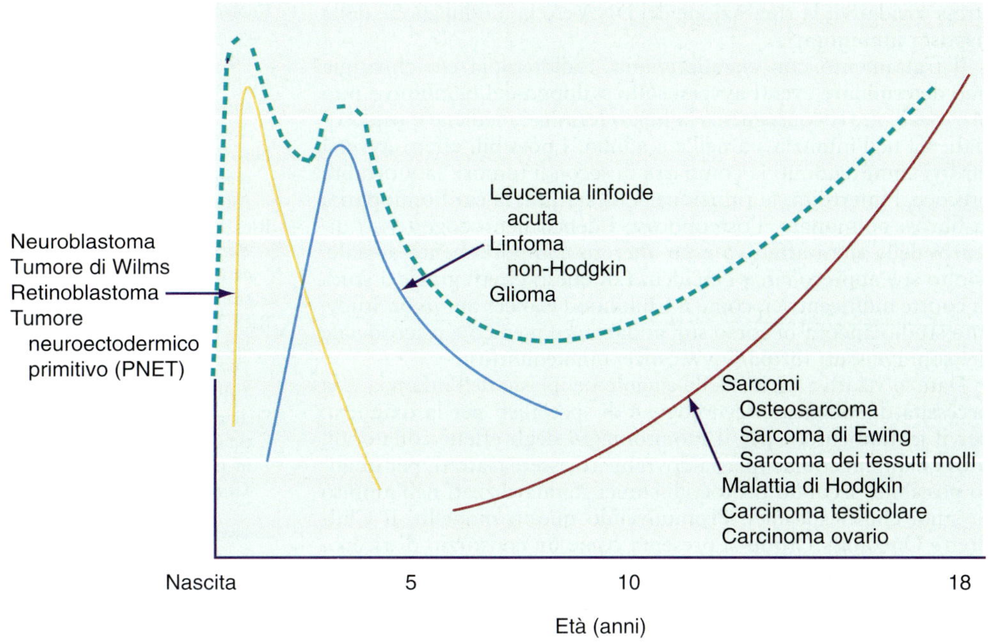

Figura 491-3. Incidenza generale, per età, dei più comuni tipi di tumore in età pediatrica. L'incidenza cumulativa di tutte le neoplasie è rappresentata dalla linea tratteggiata. (Per gentile concessione del dottor Archie Bleyer.)

TABELLA 491-2. Fattori di rischio noti per neoplasie pediatriche selezionate

TIPO DI NEOPLASIA	FATTORI DI RISCHIO	COMMENTI
Leucemia linfatica acuta	Radiazioni ionizzanti	Anche se principalmente di rilevanza anamnestica, l'esposizione prenatale ai raggi X per esami diagnostici aumenta il rischio.
		Pure la radioterapia terapeutica aumenta il rischio.
	Razza	I bambini bianchi negli USA hanno un rischio due volte maggiore rispetto ai neri.
	Fattori genetici*	La sindrome di Down ha un rischio aumentato di 10-20 volte. Anche la neurofibromatosi di tipo 1, la sindrome di Bloom, l'atassia-teleangectasia e l'istiocitosi a cellule di Langerhans, fra le altre, si associano a un rischio aumentato.
Leucemia mieloide acuta	Chemioterapici	Agenti alchilanti ed epipodofillotossine aumentano il rischio.
	Fattori genetici*	La sindrome di Down e la neurofibromatosi di tipo 1 sono strettamente correlate. La monosomia 7 familiare e diverse altre sindromi genetiche sono associate anche a un aumentato rischio.
Neoplasie cerebrali	Radiazioni ionizzanti terapeutiche della testa	A esclusione della radioterapia oncologica, un aumentato rischio da terapia radiante è essenzialmente di importanza anamnestica.
	Fattori genetici*	La neurofibromatosi di tipo 1 è strettamente correlata con i gliomi del nervo ottico e meno frequentemente con altri tumori del sistema nervoso centrale. La sclerosi tuberosa e diverse altre sindromi genetiche si associano a un aumentato rischio.
Malattia di Hodgkin	Familiarità	I gemelli monozigoti e i fratelli sono ad aumentato rischio.
	Infezioni	Il virus di Epstein-Barr si associa a un aumentato rischio.
Linfoma non-Hodgkin	Immunodeficienza	L'immunodeficienza acquisita o congenita e le terapie immunosoppressive hanno un rischio aumentato.
	Infezioni	Il virus di Epstein-Barr in Africa si associa con il linfoma di Burkitt.
Osteosarcoma	Radiazioni ionizzanti	La radioterapia e l'esposizione prolungata al radio aumenta il rischio.
	Chemioterapia	Gli agenti alchilanti aumentano il rischio.
	Fattori genetici*	Il rischio è apparentemente aumentato nella sindrome di Li-Fraumeni e nel retinoblastoma ereditario.
Sarcoma di Ewing	Razza	I bambini bianchi hanno un'incidenza circa 9 volte superiore rispetto ai bambini neri negli USA.
Neuroblastoma		Non sono dimostrati fattori di rischio.
Retinoblastoma	Fattori genetici*	Non sono dimostrati fattori di rischio.
Tumore di Wilms	Anomalie congenite	L'aniridia, la sindrome di Beckwith-Wiedemann e altre malattie congenite e genetiche si associano a un aumentato rischio.
	Razza	È stato riportato che i bambini asiatici hanno circa la metà del rischio dei bambini bianchi e neri.
Carcinoma midollare del rene	Tratto per l'anemia a cellule falciformi	Eziologia sconosciuta
Rabdomiosarcoma	Anomalie congenite e malattie genetiche	La sindrome di Li-Fraumeni e la neurofibromatosi di tipo 1 sono considerate a rischio aumentato. Vi è una qualche correlazione con l'aumentata incidenza di difetti alla nascita.
Epatoblastoma	Fattori genetici*	La sindrome di Beckwith-Wiedemann, l'emi-ipertrofia, la sindrome di Gardner e la familiarità per la poliposi adenomatosa sono associate a un aumentato rischio.
Leiomiosarcoma	Immunosoppressione e infezione da EBV	Il virus di Epstein-Barr è associato con il leiomiosarcoma in tutte le forme di immunosoppressione congenite o acquisite, ma non al leiomiosarcoma dei soggetti immunocompetenti.
Tumori maligni a cellule germinali	Criptorchidismo	Il criptorchidismo è un fattore di rischio per i tumori a cellule germinali del testicolo.

Da Gurney JG, Bondy ML: Epidemiologic research methods and childhood cancer. In Pizzo PA, Poplack DG (editors): *Principles and Practice of Pediatric Oncology*, 4th ed. Philadelphia, Lippincott Williams & Wilkins, 2001, pp 13-20.
*Vedi la Tabella 492-2.

stress ossidativi; la riparazione del DNA e/o la modulazione della risposta immunitaria.

Il trattamento con chemioterapia, radioterapia e/o chirurgia può determinare eventi avversi sullo sviluppo del bambino e può provocare gravi conseguenze a lungo termine, mediche e psicosociali, sia nell'infanzia sia nell'età adulta. I possibili **effetti avversi tardivi** comprendono la comparsa di secondi tumori, la mortalità precoce, l'infertilità, la riduzione della statura, la cardiomiopatia, la fibrosi polmonare, l'osteoporosi, i deficit neurocognitivi, i disturbi della sfera affettiva e un alterato comportamento sociale. Molto si è appreso circa l'incidenza di questi effetti grazie a studi di coorte multicentrici, come il Childhood Cancer Survivor Study, uno studio ancora in corso sull'andamento medico e psicosociale dei sopravvissuti (http://www.cancer.umn.edu/ltfu).

Date la relativa rarità delle singole neoplasie dell'infanzia e la necessità di sofisticate tecnologie e di specialisti per la diagnosi, per il trattamento e per il monitoraggio degli effetti collaterali, tutti i bambini con neoplasia dovrebbero essere trattati, per quanto possibile, secondo protocolli clinici standardizzati nell'ambito di studi clinici specifici. Promuovendo questo modello, il **Children's Oncology Group** si presenta come un consorzio di ricerca multi-istituzionale che favorisce la cooperazione di ricerca clinica, biologica ed epidemiologica in oltre 200 istituzioni affiliate in Stati Uniti, Canada e altri Paesi (http://www.curesearch.org). La partecipazione coordinata in questi trial di ricerca è stato il principale fattore ad aumentatare la sopravvivenza per molti bambini con tumore. Altri studi in corso sono fondamentali per capire meglio l'eziologia delle neoplasie pediatriche, per migliorare la sopravvivenza in neoplasie con prognosi infausta e per ottimizzare la qualità della vita dei sopravviventi.

COME INFLUENZARE L'INCIDENZA DELLE NEOPLASIE

I pediatri hanno l'opportunità di educare i bambini, gli adolescenti e i loro genitori circa il significato della prevenzione delle malattie tumorali. Ci sono solo poche cause ambientali riconosciute come predisponenti alle neoplasie dell'infanzia e possono essere evitate. Un esempio è la vaccinazione per l'epatite B, che riduce l'incidenza dell'epatoblastoma nell'adolescenza e nell'infanzia. Un obiettivo della medicina pediatrica è quello di insegnare ai bambini quali stili di vita salutari adottare per ridurre il loro rischio di sviluppare neoplasie durante l'età adulta, come evitare il fumo, l'alcol, diete ricche di grassi e obesità. Più presto queste abitudini vengono trasmesse, maggiore è il vantaggio per il resto della vita e con ogni probabilità esse continueranno a essere mantenute anche da adulti.

Ahlbom IC, Cardis E, Green A, et al: ICNIRP (International Commission for Non-Ionizing Radiation Protection) Standing Committee on Epidemiology: Review of the epidemiologic literature on EMF and Health. *Environ Health Perspect* 2001;109(Suppl 6):911–933.

Anderson RN, Smith BL: Deaths: leading causes for 2001. *National Vital Statistics Report* 2003;52(9):1–86.

Buffler PA, Kwan ML, Reynolds P, et al: Environmental and genetic risk factors for childhood leukemia: appraising the evidence. *Cancer Invest* 2005;1:60–75.

Childhood Cancer Survivorship: Improving Care and Quality of Life. Institute of Medicine, August 2003. http://www.iom.edu/CMS/28312/4931/14782.aspx

Draper G, Vincent T, Kroll ME, et al: Childhood cancer in relation to distance from high voltage power lines in England and Wales: a case-control study. *BMJ* 2005;330:1290–1292.

Gurney JG, Bondy ML: Epidemiologic research methods and childhood cancer. In Pizzo PA, Poplack DG (editors): *Principles and Practice of Pediatric Oncology,* 4th ed. Philadelphia, Lippincott Williams & Wilkins, 2002, pp 13–20.

Gurney JG, Smith MA, Olshan AF, et al: Clues to the etiology of childhood brain cancer: N-nitroso compounds, polyomaviruses and other factors of interest. *Cancer Invest* 2001;19:640–650.

Hudson MM, Mertens AC, Yasui Y, et al: Health status of adult long-term survivors of childhood cancer: A report from the Childhood Cancer Survivor Study. *JAMA* 2003;290:1583–1592.

Kaatsch P, Steliarova-Foucher E, Crocetti E, et al: Time trends of cancer incidence in European children (1978–1997): Report from the automated childhood cancer information system project. *Eur J Cancer* 2006;42:1961–1971.

Merks JHM, Caron HN, Hennekam RCM: High incidence of malformation syndromes in a series of 1,073 children with cancer. *Am J Med Genetics* 2005;134A:132–143.

Ness KK, Mertens AC, Hudson MM, et al: Limitations on physical performance and daily activities among long-term survivors of childhood cancer. *Ann Intern Med* 2005;143:639–647.

Ries LAG, Harkins D, Krapcho M, et al (editors): *SEER Cancer Statistics Review, 1975–2003.* Bethesda, MD, National Cancer Institute. http://seer.cancer.gov/csr/1975_2003/, based on November 2005 SEER data submission, posted to the SEER web site, 2006.

Ries LAG, Smith MA, Gurney JG, et al (editors): *Cancer Incidence and Survival Among Children and Adolescents: United States SEER Program 1975–1995.* Bethesda, MD, National Cancer Institute, SEER Program, 1999.

Steliarova-Foucher E, Stiller C, Kaatsch P, et al: Geographical patterns and time trends of cancer incidence and survival among children and adolescents in Europe since the 1970s (the ACCIS project): An epidemiological study. *Lancet* 2004 Dec 11;364(9451):2097–2105.

Capitolo 492 ■ Biologia molecolare e cellulare dei tumori Laura L. Worth

Le neoplasie sono un complesso di malattie che derivano da alterazioni che possono verificarsi in un vasto numero di geni. Alterazioni di normali processi cellulari come la traduzione del segnale, il controllo del ciclo cellulare, la riparazione del DNA, la crescita e la differenziazione cellulare, la regolazione translazionale, la senescenza e l'apoptosi (morte cellulare programmata) possono determinare un fenotipo maligno. Inoltre, le cellule staminali neoplastiche possono avere un ruolo in alcune neoplasie, quali CML, AML, ALL, i gliomi e il carcinoma mammario. Queste cellule che danno origine al tumore hanno capacità proprie di rigenerazione e proliferazione, simili a quelle delle cellule staminali non maligne.

GENI COINVOLTI NELL'ONCOGENESI

Nello sviluppo dei tumori sono implicate due principali classi di geni: gli oncogeni e i geni oncosoppressori. I **proto-oncogeni** sono geni cellulari importanti per le normali funzioni cellulari; essi codificano per diverse proteine, compresi i fattori trascrizionali, i fattori di crescita e i recettori per i fattori di crescita. Queste proteine sono elementi fondamentali per l'organizzazione della traduzione del segnale che regola la crescita, la moltiplicazione e la differenziazione cellulare. I proto-oncogeni possono essere alterati dando origine agli **oncogeni**, che una volta tradotti possono innescare una trasformazione maligna della cellula.

I tre principali meccanismi attraverso i quali i proto-oncogeni possono essere attivati includono: l'amplificazione, le mutazioni puntiformi e la traslocazione (Tab. 492-1). *MYC* codifica per una proteina che regola la trascrizione ed è un esempio di proto-oncogene attivato dall'amplificazione (Fig. 492-1). I pazienti affetti da un neuroblastoma in cui il gene *MYC* è amplificato 10-300 volte hanno una prognosi peggiore (Fig. 492-2). Anche le mutazioni puntiformi possono attivare i proto-oncogeni. Il proto-oncogene *NRAS* codifica per una proteina che lega il nucleotide guanina con attività di guanosina trifosfatasi, importante nel segnale di traduzione ed è mutato nel 25-30% delle leucemie acute non mieloidi, dando origine a una proteina costitutivamente attiva. Il gene *RET* codifica per un recettore transmembrana tirosinchinasi, che è importante come segnale di traduzione. Una sua mutazione puntiforme determina l'attivazione costitutiva della tirosinchinasi, come riscontrato nelle sindromi con neoplasie multiple e nelle forme familiari di carcinoma della

TABELLA 492-1. Attivatori oncogenici dei tumori pediatrici

MECCANISMO	CROMOSOMA	GENI	FUNZIONE DELLA PROTEINA	TUMORE
Traslocazione cromosomica	t(9;22)	*BCR-ABL*	Tirosinchinasi chimerica	Leucemia linfatica acuta, leucemia mieloide cronica
	t(1:19)	*E2A-PBX1*	Fattore di trascrizione chimerico	Leucemia linfatica acuta pre-B
	t(14:18)	*CMYC*	Fattore di trascrizione	Linfoma di Burkitt
	t(15;17)	*APL-RARα*	Fattore di trascrizione chimerico	Leucemia acuta promielocitica
Amplificazione genica	Amplificazione	*NMYC*	Fattore di trascrizione	Neuroblastoma
	Amplificazione	*EGFR*	Fattore di crescita, tirosinchinasi	Glioblastoma
Mutazione puntiforme	1p	*NRAS*	GTPasi	Leucemia mieloide acuta
	10q	*RET*	Tirosinchinasi	Neoplasie endocrine multiple, tipo 2

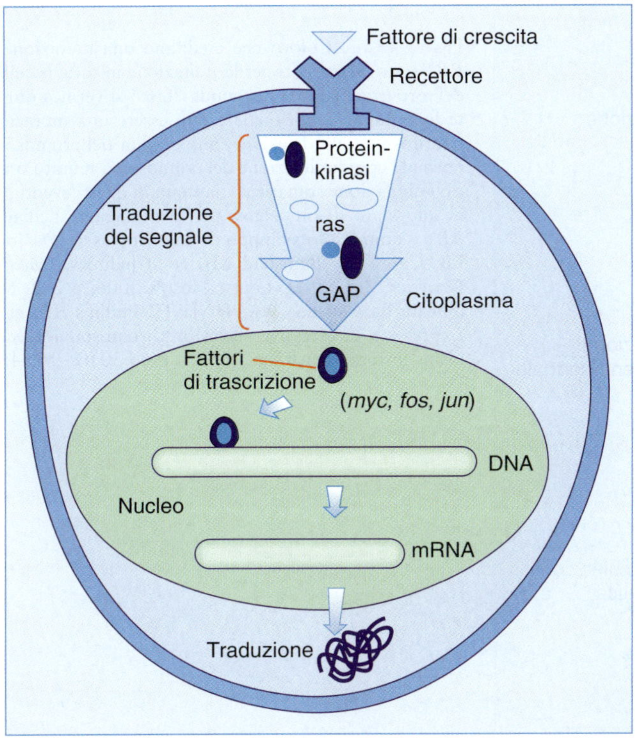

Figura 492-1. I principali meccanismi della regolazione cellulare. I *fattori di crescita* esterni (proteine e ormoni steroidei, come il fattore di crescita epidermico) si legano ai *recettori di membrana per i fattori di crescita*, attivando un *segnale di traduzione* della via che coinvolge geni come il *RAS*. I componenti della via di traduzione del segnale interagiscono con i *fattori nucleari di trascrizione*, quali il *MYC* e il *FOS*, che possono legare e regolare regioni del DNA. (Da Jorde LB, Carey JC, Bamshad MJ, et al [editors]: *Medical Genetics*, 3rd ed. St. Louis, Mosby, 2006, p. 231.)

tiroide. Il terzo meccanismo con cui i proto-oncogeni si attivano è la traslocazione cromosomica. In alcune forme di leucemia e linfomi, le sequenze che regolano il fattore di trascrizione sono collocate poco prima dei geni dei recettori per le cellule T o per le immunoglobuline, con una conseguente trascrizione di questi geni che causa la leucemia, priva di controllo. Le traslocazioni cromosomiche possono anche determinare una **fusione di geni;** la trascrizione del gene che deriva da una fusione può determinare la produzione di una proteina chimerica con attività nuove e potenzialmente oncogeniche. Le neoplasie dovute alla fusione di geni comprendono tumori solidi dell'infanzia, quali il sarcoma di Ewing [t(11;22)] e il rabdomiosarcoma alveolare [t(2;13) o t(1;13)]. Le traslocazioni determinano la produzione di nuove proteine che sono utili come marker per la diagnosi. Quella che è stata descritta meglio nelle leucemie è il **cromosoma Philadelphia t(9;22)**, che dà luogo alla proteina BCR/ABL riscontrata nella leucemia mieloide cronica e determina una tirosinchinasi costitutivamente attivata. Inoltre, la proteina è localizzata nel citoplasma in prossimità del nucleo, esponendo la chinasi a un nuovo spettro di substrati.

L'alterazione della regolazione dei geni oncosoppressori è un altro meccanismo coinvolto nell'oncogenesi. I geni oncosoppressori sono importanti nella regolazione della crescita cellulare e della morte cellulare programmata (o apoptosi). Sono stati definiti *oncogeni recessivi*, perché è necessaria l'inattivazione di entrambi gli alleli di ciascuno di essi per dare origine a un fenotipo maligno. Il modello di **sviluppo del tumore "in due fasi" di Knudson** era fondato sull'osservazione del comportamento del gene oncosoppressore *RB*. Nelle forme sporadiche di retinoblastoma entrambi i suoi alleli devono essere inattivati (Fig. 492-3), ma nelle forme familiari i bambini ereditano un allele inattivato da un genitore e quindi necessitano solo dell'inattivazione dell'allele normale. Questo spiega perché i casi familiari di retinoblastoma si manifestano più precocemente nell'infanzia rispetto alle forme sporadiche, dal momento che è richiesta una sola "fase".

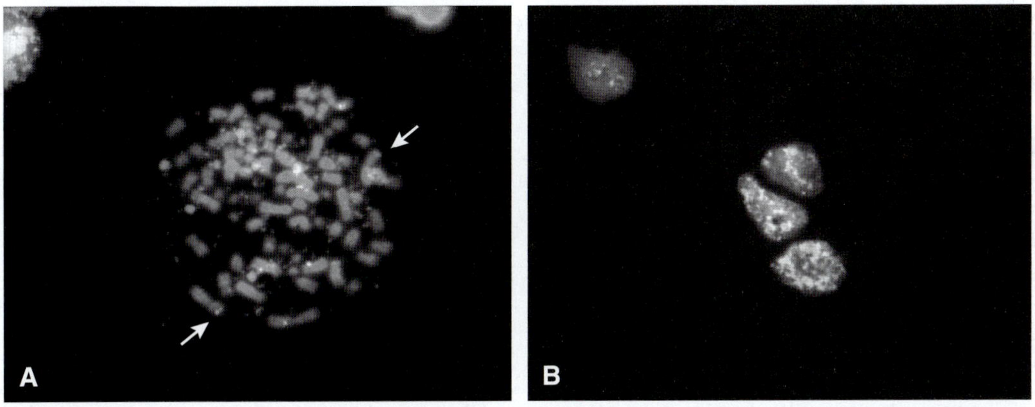

Figura 492-2. Fluorescenza di ibridazione *in situ* con sonda di *MYCN* in un neuroblastoma avanzato. *A*, Espansione in metafase di una cellula tetraploide di neuroblastoma che rivela la presenza di *double minute chromosomes*. L'intensità del segnale di fluorescenza varia a seconda delle dimensioni del *double minute chromosom* e del numero di copie di *MYCN* contenute. Le frecce bianche evidenziano il segnale fluorescente proveniente dal locus normale di *MYCN* sul tratto distale del braccio corto del cromosoma 2. *B*, Nuclei di cellule di neuroblastoma in interfase che dimostrano vari gradi di intensità di fluorescenza da parte di *double minute chromosomes*. (Immagini per gentile concessione di J. Biegel, Children's Hospital of Philadelphia. Già pubblicate in Nussbaum RL, McInnes RR, Willard HF [eds]: *Thompson and Thompson Genetics in Medicine*, 6th ed. Philadelphia, WB Saunders, 2004, p. 331.)

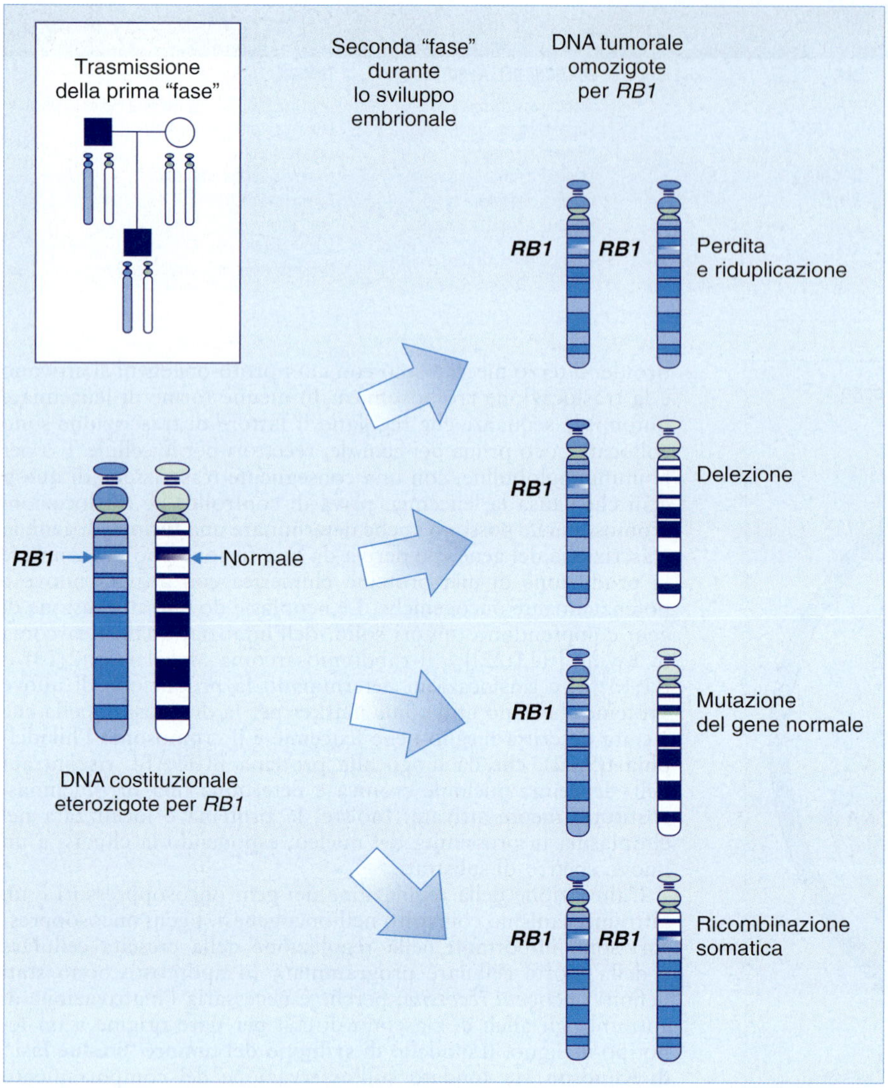

Figura 492-3. Coloro che ereditano una mutazione di *RB1* sono eterozigoti per la mutazione in tutte le cellule del loro organismo. La seconda "fase" si verifica durante lo sviluppo embrionale e può essere una mutazione puntiforme, una delezione, una perdita del cromosoma normale con duplicazione del cromosoma mutato o una ricombinazione somatica. Ciascuno di questi eventi porta allo stato di omozigosi per la mutazione dell'allele *RB1* e quindi allo sviluppo di una neoplasia. (Da Jorde LB, Carey JC, Bamshad MJ, et al [editors]: *Medical Genetics*, 3rd ed. St. Louis, Mosby, 2006, p 233. Modificata da Cavenee WK, Dryja TP, Phillips RA, et al: Expression of recessive alleles by chromosomal mechanisms in retinoblastoma. *Nature* 1983;305:779-784.)

Un'altra fondamentale proteina oncosoppressiva è la p53, nota come "guardiano del genoma" in quanto vigila sulla presenza di danni cromosomici e previene la replicazione cellulare fino a che il danno non sia riparato. Nel caso sia presente un danno che non può essere riparato, la p53 innesca l'apoptosi e la cellula muore. Oltre il 50% dei tumori ha la p53 alterata. Le mutazioni del gene *P53* sono importanti in molte neoplasie, compresi i carcinomi della mammella, del colon-retto, del polmone, dell'esofago, dello stomaco, dell'ovaio e della prostata, dei gliomi, dei sarcomi e di alcune leucemie.

SINDROMI CHE PREDISPONGONO ALLO SVILUPPO DI NEOPLASIE

Diverse sindromi, con differenti meccanismi, si associano a un aumentato rischio di sviluppare neoplasie (Tab. 492-2). Uno dei meccanismi prevede l'**inattivazione dei geni oncosoppressori**, come *RB* nel retinoblastoma familiare. È interessante il fatto che un paziente affetto da un retinoblastoma, in cui un allele è inattivato in tutte le sue cellule, ha un aumentato rischio di sviluppare anche un osteosarcoma. Nei soggetti che possono maturare sarcomi, leucemie e neoplasie a carico di mammella, osso, polmoni e cervello è stata anche descritta una forma familiare, la sindrome di Li-Fraumeni, in cui viene ereditato un allele di *P53* mutato. La neurofibromatosi è caratterizzata dalla proliferazione di cellule che originano dalla cresta neurale, determinando neurofibromi. Questi pazienti sono ad alto rischio di sviluppare schwannomi maligni e feocromocitomi. La neurofibromatosi è spesso ereditata con modalità autosomica dominante, anche se il 50% dei casi ha un'anamnesi familiare negativa e si sviluppa per un'alta percentuale di mutazioni spontanee del gene *NF1*.

Un secondo meccanismo responsabile della predisposizione ereditaria a sviluppare neoplasie è dovuto a un **deficit dei processi di riparazione del DNA**. Le sindromi che si associano a un eccessivo numero di cromosomi alterati per un difetto della riparazione comprendono la sindrome di Bloom (bassa statura, eritema teleangectasico fotosensibile), l'atassia-teleangectasia (atassia nell'infanzia con progressiva degenerazione dei motoneuroni) e l'anemia di Fanconi (bassa statura, malformazioni scheletriche e renali, pancitopenia). Per via della ridotta capacità di riparare le mutazioni cromosomiche, le cellule accumulano alterazioni del DNA che provocano un incremento significativo della probabilità di sviluppare neoplasie, soprattutto leucemie. Analogamente, lo xeroterma pigmentoso aumenta il rischio di sviluppare neoplasie cutanee, per un difetto di riparazione delle mutazioni del DNA provocate dai raggi ultravioletti. Queste malattie hanno una modalità di trasmissione autosomica recessiva.

La terza categoria di predisposizione ereditaria a sviluppare neoplasie è caratterizzata da **difetti della sorveglianza da parte del sistema immunitario**. Questo gruppo include i pazienti con la sindrome di Wiskott-Aldrich, una grave immunodeficienza combinata, varie immunodeficienze comuni e la sindrome linfoproliferativa X-linked. Le più comuni forme di neoplasia in questi soggetti sono il linfoma e la leucemia. I provvedimenti terapeutici per i bambini immunodeficienti con neoplasia sono molto meno

TABELLA 492-2. Suscettibilità familiare o genetica per le neoplasie

MALATTIA	NEOPLASIA	COMMENTO
SINDROMI CROMOSOMICHE		
Cromosoma 11p- (delezione) con sporadica aniridia	Tumore di Wilms	Si associa a malformazioni genitourinarie, ritardo mentale, gene *WT1*
Cromosoma 13q- (delezione)	Retinoblastoma Sarcoma	Si associa a ritardo mentale, malformazioni scheletriche; autosomico dominante (bilaterale) o sporadico per nuove mutazioni del gene *RB1*
Trisomia 21	Leucemia linfoide o non linfoide, soprattutto leucemia megacariocitica Reazione leucemoide transitoria	Il rischio di leucemia linfatica acuta è aumentato del 20%; il rischio di leucemia mieloide acuta è aumentato del 400%; i pazienti hanno una più elevata sensibilità alla chemioterapia
Sindrome di Klinefelter (47, XXY)	Carcinoma mammario Tumori extragonadici a cellule germinali	–
Trisomia 8	Preleucemia	–
Sindrome di Noonan	Leucemia mielomonocitica giovanile	Autosomico dominante; mutazioni del gene *PTPN11*
Monosomia 5 o 7	Sindrome mielodisplastica	Infezioni ricorrenti possono precedere la neoplasia
INSTABILITÀ CROMOSOMICA		
Xeroderma pigmentoso	Carcinoma a cellule basali e squamoso Melanoma	Autosomico recessivo; fallimento della riparazione del DNA danneggiato dai raggi UV. Mutazioni del gene *XP* sul cromosoma 3p25
Anemia di Fanconi	Leucemia Sindrome mielodisplastica Neoplasie epatiche Rari tumori di testa e collo Neoplasie gastrointestinali e genitourinarie	Autosomico recessivo; fragilità cromosomica; positività del test del diepossibutano; mutazioni della famiglia di geni *FANCX*
Sindrome di Bloom	Leucemia Linfoma Tumori solidi	Autosomico recessivo; aumento degli scambi di cromatidi; mutazioni del gene *BLM*, un componente della famiglia di geni per RecQ elicasi
Atassia-teleangectasia	Linfoma Leucemia Tumori solidi del sistema nervoso centrale e non-neurali (meno comunemente)	Autosomico recessivo; sensibilità ai raggi X, ai farmaci radiomimetici; mutazione del gene oncosoppressore *ATM*
Sindrome del nevo displastico	Melanoma	Autosomico dominante; alcuni casi si associano a mutazioni del gene *CDKN2A*
Sindrome di Rothmund-Thompson	Osteosarcoma Neoplasie cutanee	Autosomico recessivo; mutazione nella famiglia di geni per RecQ elicasi
Sindrome di Werner (invecchiamento precoce)	Sarcomi dei tessuti molli	Autosomico recessivo; mutazione del gene *WRN* (componente della famiglia di geni per RecQ elicasi)
SINDROMI DA IMMUNODEFICIENZA		
Sindrome di Wiskott-Aldrich	Linfoma, leucemia	X-linked recessivo; mutazioni del gene *WAS* (Xp11.22-23); la proteina WASp interviene nel segnale di traduzione, associata con il riarrangiamento del filamento di actina del citoscheletro
Immunodeficienza X-linked (sindrome di Duncan)	Malattia linfoproliferativa	X-linked; l'infezione da virus di Epstein-Barr può essere fatale; mutazione al locus genico *SH2D1A*
Agammaglobulinemia X-linked (malattia di Bruton)	Linfoma, leucemia	X-linked; mutazione del gene *BKT* con conseguente assenza di cellule B mature
Immunodeficienza combinata grave	Leucemia, linfoma	X-linked; mutazioni del gene *ADA*
ALTRE		
Neurofibromatosi di tipo 1	Neurofibroma Gliomi del nervo ottico Neurinoma dell'acustico Astrocitoma Meningioma Feocromocitoma Sarcoma	Autosomico dominante, mutazione dell'oncogene soppressore, *NF1*
Neurofibromatosi di tipo 2	Neurinoma dell'acustico bilaterale Meningiomi	Autosomico dominante; mutazione dell'oncogene soppressore *NF2*
Sclerosi tuberosa	Nevi fibroangiomatosi Rabdomioma miocardico	Autosomico dominante
Sindrome di Gorlin-Goltz (sindrome del carcinoma basocellulare)	Multipli carcinomi a cellule basali Medulloblastoma	Autosomico dominante; mutazione del gene *PTCH*
Sindrome di Li-Fraumeni	Osso Sarcoma dei tessuti molli Mammella	Mutazione del gene oncosoppressore *P53*, autosomico dominante
Retinoblastoma	Sarcoma	Autosomico recessivo; aumentato rischio di sviluppare secondi tumori 10-20 anno dopo, mutazione del gene oncosoppressore *RB*
Emi-ipertrofia ± sindrome di Beckwith	Tumore di Wilms Epatoblastoma Carcinoma adrenocorticale	Gene *WT1*. Il 25% sviluppa tumori, soprattutto nei primi 5 anni di vita
Malattia di von Hippel-Lindau	Emangioblastoma di cervelletto e retina Feocromocitoma Neoplasia renale	Autosomico dominante, mutazione del gene oncosoppressore *VHL*
Sindrome con neoplasie endocrine multiple, tipo 1 (sindrome di Wermer)	Neoplasie di paratiroidi, isole pancreatiche e ipofisi	Autosomico dominante; mutazione del gene oncosoppressore *PYGM*
Sindrome con neoplasie endocrine multiple, tipo 2A (sindrome di Sipple)	Carcinoma midollare della tiroide Iperparatiroidismo Feocromocitoma	Autosomico dominante; mutazioni nelle regioni ricche di Cys del gene *RET* attivano questo proto-oncogene. Il *RET* codifica per una tirosinchinasi; occorre controllare i livelli di calcitonina e calcio

Continua

TABELLA 492-2. Suscettibilità familiare o genetica per le neoplasie – *continua*

MALATTIA	NEOPLASIA	COMMENTO
Neoplasie endocrine multiple di tipo 2B (sindrome con neurinomi mucinosi multipli)	Neurinomi mucinosi Feocromocitoma Carcinoma midollare della tiroide Aspetto marfanoide Neuropatia	Autosomico dominante; la mutazione del sito catalitico (codone 883 o 914) attiva il proto-oncogene. Il *RET* codifica per una tirosin-kinasi
Poliposi adenomatosa familiare	Carcinoma colonrettale e tiroideo Carcinomi duodenali e periampollari Epatoblastoma pediatrico	Autosomico dominante; mutazione del gene *APC*
Poliposi familiare giovanile	Carcinoma colonrettale	Autosomico dominante; mutazione del gene *SMAD4*
Carcinoma del colon ereditario senza poliposi (sindrome di Lynch, NHPCC)	Carcinoma del colon	Autosomico dominante; mutazione dei geni del mismatch repair; *hMSH2, hMLH1, PMS1, PMS2, hMSH6, hMSG3*
Sindrome di Turcot	Neoplasie cerebrali in età pediatrica Aumentato rischio di carcinoma del colon e poliposi	Mutazione del gene *APC*
Poliposi adenomatosa del colon	Adenocarcinoma del colon	Autosomico dominante, gene *APC*
Sindrome di Gardner	Adenocarcinoma del colon Neoplasie del cranio e dei tessuti molli	Autosomico dominante, gene *APC*
Sindrome di Peutz-Jeghers	Carcinoma gastrointestinale Neoplasie ovariche	Autosomico dominante, il gene *LKB1* codifica per una Ser/Thr chinasi che regola il ciclo cellulare, il metabolismo, la polarità della cellula
Emocromatosi	Carcinoma epatocellulare	Autosomico dominante; neoplasie associate alla cirrosi epatica
Malattia da deposito di glicogeno 1 (malattia di von Gierke)	Carcinoma epatocellulare	Autosomico recessivo; neoplasie associate alla cirrosi epatica. Mutazione della glucosio-6-fosfatasi o del gene della glucosio-6-fosfatasi translocasi
Tirosinemia, galattosemia	Carcinoma epatocellulare	Autosomico recessivo; neoplasie associate alla cirrosi epatica
BRCA1 e BRCA2	Neoplasie di mammella e ovaio	Deficit della riparazione del DNA
Tratto della cellula falciforme	Carcinoma midollare del rene	Eziologia sconosciuta

efficaci che nei bambini non immunodeficienti con neoplasie simili, suggerendo un ruolo del sistema immunitario nel trattamento così come nella prevenzione delle neoplasie.

ALTRI FATTORI ASSOCIATI ALL'ONCOGENESI

VIRUS. Molti virus sono stati considerati come responsabili nella patogenesi delle neoplasie. La correlazione tra il **virus di Epstein-Barr** (**EBV**, *Epstein-Barr Virus*) e il linfoma di Burkitt e il carcinoma nasofaringeo è stata identificata oltre 30 anni fa, anche se l'infezione da EBV da sola non è sufficiente per la trasformazione maligna. L'EBV è associato anche alla malattia di Hodgkin con cellularità mista e linfociti-depleti, così come con alcuni linfomi a cellule T, il che è particolarmente interessante in quanto normalmente questo virus non infetta i linfociti T. L'evidenza più significativa dell'EBV nella linfogenesi è il suo ruolo causale diretto nella malattia linfoproliferativa a cellule B nelle persone immunocompromesse, soprattutto nei soggetti affetti da AIDS. L'EBV si associa inoltre al leiomiosarcoma nei soggetti immunocompromessi.

Nei bambini con infezione cronica da **epatite B** (HBsAg positivi) il rischio di sviluppare un epatocarcinoma è aumentata di oltre 200 volte. Negli adulti il periodo di latenza tra l'infezione virale e lo sviluppo dell'epatocarcinoma è di circa 20 anni, ma nei bambini che contraggono l'infezione virale per trasmissione perinatale questo periodo può essere di 6-7 anni. I fattori aggiuntivi, che sono necessari per la trasformazione maligna degli epatociti infettati dal virus, non sono ancora stati identificati. Anche l'**infezione da virus C** rappresenta un fattore di rischio per l'epatocarcinoma e si associa con il linfoma splenico.

Quasi tutti i carcinomi della cervice presentano il **papillomavirus** (**HPV**, *Human PapillomaVirus*) e specialmente quelli di tipo 16 e 18 vi sono altamente correlati, mentre i tipi 31, 33, 35, 45 e 56 hanno una minore frequenza associativa. Al contrario, i papillomavirus a basso rischio, compresi i tipi 6 e 11, che comunemente si trovano al livello delle verruche genitali, si trovano raramente collegati. Come altri virus associati alle neoplasie, la presenza isolata di HPV non è sufficiente a determinare la trasformazione neoplastica. Si pensa che il meccanismo con cui HPV 19 induce quest'ultima coinvolga i geni *P53* e *RB*, che regolano il ciclo cellulare agendo come guardiani del passaggio tra le fasi G1/S e G2/M. Interferendo con queste proteine, HPV altera la regolazione della crescita cellulare.

L'**herpes virus umano 8** (**HHV8**) si associa al sarcoma di Kaposi, un linfoma primitivo a cellule B e alla variante della malattia di Castleman a plasmacellule che colpiscono soprattutto pazienti affetti da AIDS. Il **virus umano della leucemia a cellule T di tipo 1** (**HTLV-1**) si correla con la leucemia a cellule T dell'adulto e con il linfoma.

IMPRINTING GENOMICO. Lo sviluppo di neoplasie è stato anche correlato con l'imprinting genomico, che è la selettiva inattivazione di uno dei due alleli di un determinato gene dipendente dall'eredità dalla madre o dal padre. Normalmente a essere inattivato è il gene materno *IGF2* (*Insulin-like Growth Factor receptor 2*) e si pensa che l'inattivazione sia secondaria alla metilazione di specifiche sequenze CpG davanti al promotore dell'*IGF2*, con una conseguente interferenza con la trascrizione del gene stesso. In alcuni tumori di Wilms vi è una perdita della metilazione delle sequenze che precedono il promoter del gene materno, con susseguente trascrizione ed espressione del gene *IGF2* materno. Analogamente, anche il gene *H19* (il cui ruolo non è ben chiaro), un gene materno inizialmente trascritto in modo attivo, è silenziato con la metilazione. La sindrome di Beckwith-Weidemann da crescita eccessiva, caratterizzata da macrosomia, macroglossia, emiipertrofia, onfalocele e malformazioni renali, si associa anche a un aumentato rischio di tumore di Wilms, epatoblastoma, rabdomiosarcoma, neuroblastoma e carcinoma adrenocorticale. Il rischio più elevato di sviluppare neoplasie è dovuto a modificazioni del pattern di metilazione dei geni sul cromosoma 11p15. La fertilizzazione *in vitro* è stata correlata ad alterazioni dell'imprinting e allo sviluppo di alcuni casi della sindrome di Beckwith-Weidemann associata al tumore di Wilms e al retinoblastoma.

TELOMERASI. I telomeri sono una serie di decine o centinaia di sequenze di TTAGGG ripetute al termine dei cromosomi; essi sono importanti per stabilizzare le parti terminali del cromosoma e limitare le rotture, le traslocazioni e la perdita di DNA. Con la replicazione del DNA vi è un progressivo accorciamento della lunghezza dei telomeri, che è un segno di invecchiamento della cellula e può essere un segnale di senescenza. In alcune circostanze la **telomerasi**, un enzima che aggiunge telomeri alle porzioni terminali dei cromosomi, può diventare attiva. L'aggiunta di telomeri si può osservare in linee di cellule immortalizzate e nella maggior parte di quelle neoplastiche, con un conseguente possibile vantaggio di queste cellule sulla sopravvivenza, dal momento che si permette loro di continuare a moltiplicarsi. Un trattamento mirato a inibire l'attività della telomerasi potrebbe indurre la morte della cellula.

Attiyeh EF, London WB, Mosse YP, et al: Chromosome 1p and 11q deletions and outcome in neuroblastoma. *N Engl J Med* 2005;353:2243–2253.

Blackburn E: Telomeres and telomerase; their mechanisms of action and the effects of altering their functions. *FEBS Letters* 2005;579:859–862.

Hitchens MP, Wong JJL, Suthers G, et al: Inheritance of a cancer-associated MLHI germ-line epimutation. *N Engl J Med* 2007;356:697–705.

Jordan CT, Guzman ML, Noble M: Cancer stem cells. *N Engl J Med* 2006;355:1253–1260.

Messahel B, Hing S, Nash R, et al: Clinical features of molecular pathology of solid tumours in childhood. *Lancet Oncol* 2005;6:421–430.

Mitelman F, Johansson B, Mertens F: Fusion genes and rearranged genes as a linear function of chromosome aberrations in cancer. *Nature Genetics* 2004;36:331–334.

Moll AC, Imhof SM, Cruysberg JRM, et al: Incidence of retinoblastoma in children born after in-vitro fertilization. *Lancet* 2003;361:309–310.

Prawitt D, Enklar T, Gartner-Rupprecht B, et al: Microdeletion and IGF2 loss of imprinting in a cascade causing Beckwith-Wiedemann syndrome with Wilms' tumor. *Nature Genetics* 2005;37:785–786.

Quackenbush J: Microarray analysis and tumor classification. *N Engl J Med* 2006;354:2463–2472.

Reinhart B, Chaillet JR: Genomic imprinting: cis-acting sequences and regional control. *Int Rev Cytol* 2005:243;173–213.

Schiavi F, Boedeker CC, Bausch B, et al: Predictors and prevalence of paraganglioma syndrome associated with mutations of the SDHC gene. *JAMA* 2005;294:2057–2062.

Windschwendter M, Fiegl H, Egle D, et al: Epigenetic stem cell signature in cancer. *Nat Genet* 2007;39:157–164.

Capitolo 493 ■ Principi per la diagnosi

Archie Bleyer

I sintomi e i segni clinici sono importanti per riconoscere le neoplasie maligne e per trattare i tumori benigni nei bambini e negli adolescenti. Oltre alle classiche manifestazioni, qualunque sintomo o segno persistente o difficilmente spiegabile dovrebbe essere considerato come un potenziale indicatore di una neoplasia o di una condizione preneoplastica. Oltre a porre la diagnosi, il pediatra e l'oncologo pediatra devono anche comunicarla al paziente stesso e alla sua famiglia con sensibilità e professionalità.

SEGNI E SINTOMI. Diversamente dai classici segni premonitori di neoplasia negli adulti (Tab. 493-1), non vi è un elenco riconosciuto dei sintomi e dei segni di malattia neoplastica nei bambini, per diverse ragioni. Innanzitutto, quelli di una malattia oncologica sono molto più variabili e poco specifici nei pazienti pediatrici che negli adulti. Inoltre, i tipi di neoplasie che colpiscono durante i primi 20 anni di vita variano in modo sensazionale in questo lasso di tempo più che in qualunque altro range di età comparabile (vedi Capitolo 491). Diversamente dalle neoplasie dell'adulto, le neoplasie in età pediatrica hanno origine dalle strutture viscerali più profonde e dagli organi parenchimatosi e non dagli strati epiteliali che circondano i dotti e le ghiandole e che compongono la cute. In età pediatrica le metastasi sono già presenti al momento della diagnosi nell'80% dei casi, percentuale che scende al 20% nel caso degli adulti. Nei bambini, poi, i sintomi o i segni dell'esordio della malattia sono molto più spesso provocati dalle metastasi che non dal tumore primitivo. I neonati e i bambini piccoli non possono esprimere o localizzare i loro disturbi, diversamente dagli adulti e i test diagnostici possono non avere la stessa utilità o precisione. A tutto ciò si aggiunge la variabilità della fisiologia e della biologia dell'ospite

TABELLA 493-1. Segni e sintomi più frequenti di neoplasia nei bambini e negli adulti

ADULTI*
Modificazione delle abitudini intestinali e urinarie
Sangue nelle feci
Noduli mammari o in altra sede
Abbassamento della voce o tosse fastidiosa
Difficoltà nella deglutizione
Ulcera che non guarisce
Variazione di una escrescenza o di un neo
BAMBINI†
Massa addominale
Linfoadenopatia persistente
>1 linea ematopoietica alterata
Deficit neurologico specifico
Ipertensione endocranica
Diffuso ampliamento del ponte
Proptosi
Riflesso bianco della pupilla
Dolore/edema a un ginocchio o a una spalla monolaterale
Sanguinamento o masse vaginali

*Elaborata dalla American Cancer Society nel 1950.
†Elaborata da University of Texas M.D. Anderson Cancer Center.

in relazione alla crescita e allo sviluppo dai primi mesi di vita all'adolescenza.

Per questi motivi, i segni di una malattia oncologica nei bambini sono spesso attribuiti ad altre cause, prima che venga riconosciuta la neoplasia. I ritardi nella diagnosi sono particolarmente problematici durante la tarda adolescenza e sono dovuti a diversi fattori predominanti a questa età, compresa, negli Stati Uniti, la perdita della copertura dell'assicurazione sulla salute.

Sebbene non vi sia un elenco chiaramente stabilito delle indicazioni per la presenza di una neoplasia nei giovani, le neoplasie più comuni nei bambini suggeriscono alcune linee guida che possono essere utili a riconoscere precocemente i segni e i sintomi della malattia (Tab. 493-2; vedi anche Tab. 493-1). La maggior parte di essi è tuttavia aspecifica e risulta necessario fare una diagnosi differenziale con altre patologie. Ciononostante, questi campanelli d'allarme fanno pensare ai più frequenti tumori dell'infanzia e sono particolarmente utili per una diagnosi precoce. Inoltre, vi sono alcuni segni e sintomi aggiuntivi, seppure meno comuni (Tab. 493-3).

ESAME OBIETTIVO. Le neoplasie pediatriche più comuni possono essere distinte in 5 categorie in base ai tessuti o ai sistemi interessati: il sistema linfoematopoietico, il sistema nervoso, il gruppo embrionale, il tessuto connettivo e il sistema gonadico. Pertanto, durante la visita medica è utile porre particolare attenzione alle manifestazioni di "sangue, cervello, addome e ossa" (le *quattro B* dell'inglese: "blood, brain, belly, bone") per mettere in evidenza eventuali segni di neoplasia.

Le alterazioni a carico del sistema ematopoietico si manifestano con pallore (indicativo di anemia), sanguinamenti dagli orifizi, petecchie, porpora ed ecchimosi (indicative di trombocitopenia o coagulazione intravascolare disseminata), celluliti o altri segni di infezione (rivelatori di leucopenia), noduli cutanei (sintomatici di leucocitosi) e altre alterazioni degli elementi maturi del sangue. Le alterazioni a carico del sistema linfatico comprendono la linfoadenopatia (Fig. 493-1), la sindrome della vena cava superiore o la dispnea quando il paziente è in posizione supina, che risultano suggestivi per la presenza di una massa nel mediastino superoanteriore o di un aumento del volume del timo (Fig. 493-2). Un ingrossamento dei linfonodi cervicali è frequente nei bambini con una infezione e nei pazienti con un linfoma; se poi appare persistente o progressivo, spesso senza dolore associato, è suggestivo di un linfoma e comporta la necessità di eseguire una biopsia.

Tra le manifestazioni del sistema nervoso centrale che possono suggerire una neoplasia vi sono la riduzione del livello di coscienza, la paralisi del VI nervo cranico, le crisi epilettiche, la ptosi

TABELLA 493-2. Comuni manifestazioni di malattie oncologiche dell'infanzia

SEGNI E SINTOMI	SIGNIFICATO	ESEMPIO
EMATOLOGICI		
Pallore, anemia	Infiltrazione del midollo osseo	Leucemia, neuroblastoma
Petecchie, trombocitopenia	Infiltrazione del midollo osseo	Leucemia, neuroblastoma
Febbre, faringite, neutropenia	Infiltrazione del midollo osseo	Leucemia, neuroblastoma
SISTEMICI		
Dolore osseo, zoppia, artralgia	Tumore primitivo dell'osso, metastasi ossea	Osteosarcoma, sarcoma di Ewing, leucemia, neuroblastoma
Febbre di origine sconosciuta, perdita di peso, sudorazione notturna	Neoplasia linforeticolare	Malattia di Hodgkin, linfoma non-Hodgkin
Linfoadenopatia non dolorosa	Neoplasia linforeticolare, metastasi da tumore solido	Leucemia, malattia di Hodgkin, linfoma non-Hodgkin, linfoma di Burkitt, carcinoma tiroideo
Lesione cutanea	Neoplasia primitiva o metastatica	Neuroblastoma, leucemia, istiocitosi a cellule di Langerhans, melanoma
Massa addominale	Tumore adrenorenale	Neuroblastoma, tumore di Wilms, linfoma
Ipertensione	Neoplasia del sistema nervoso simpatico	Neuroblastoma, feocromocitoma, tumore di Wilms
Diarrea	Polipeptide vasoattivo intestinale	Neuroblastoma, ganglioneuroma
Massa nei tessuti molli	Tumore locale o metastatico	Sarcoma di Ewing, osteosarcoma, neuroblastoma, carcinoma tiroideo, rabdomiosarcoma, granuloma eosinofilo
Diabete insipido, galattorrea, ridotto accrescimento	Coinvolgimento neuroendocrino di ipotalamo o ipofisi	Adenoma, craniofaringioma, prolattinoma, istiocitosi a cellule di Langerhans
Vomito, disturbi del visus, atassia, cefalea, papilledema, paralisi dei nervi cranici	Ipertensione endocranica	Neoplasia cerebrale primitiva, metastasi
SEGNI OFTALMOLOGICI		
Leucocoria	Pupilla bianca	Retinoblastoma
Ecchimosi periorbitali	Metastasi	Neuroblastoma
Miosi, ptosi, eterocromia	Sindrome di Horner: compressione dei nervi simpatici cervicali	Neuroblastoma
Opsomioclono, atassia	Neuromediato? Autoimmune?	Neuroblastoma
Esoftalmo, proptosi	Tumore dell'orbita	Rabdomiosarcoma, linfoma
MASSA TORACICA		
Mediastino anteriore	Tosse, stridore, polmonite, compressione tracheobronchiale	Tumore a cellule germinali, linfoma a cellule T, malattia di Hodgkin
Mediastino posteriore	Compressione vertebrale o delle radici nervose; disfagia	Neuroblastoma, cisti neuroenterica

Da Kliegman RM, Marcdante KJ, Jenson HB, et al (editors): *Nelson Essentials of Pediatrics*, 5th ed. Philadelphia, WB Saunders, 2006, p 729.

TABELLA 493-3. Segni e sintomi non comuni di neoplasia nei bambini

DIRETTAMENTE CORRELATI AL TUMORE
Sindrome della vena cava superiore
Noduli sottocutanei
Reazione leucemoide
Miastenia grave
Eterocromia
NON DIRETTAMENTE CORRELATI ALLA CRESCITA DEL TUMORE
Diarrea cronica
Polimioclono-opsoclono
Arresto della crescita
Sindrome di Cushing
Distrofia pseudomuscolare

Modificata da Vietti TJ, Steuber CP: Clinical assessment and differential diagnosis of the child with suspected cancer. In Pizzo PA, Poplack DG (editors): *Principles and Practice of Pediatric Oncology*, 4th ed. Philadelphia, Lippincott Williams & Wilkins, 2002, pp 149-160.

palpebrale, la riduzione dell'acuità visiva e l'aumento della pressione intracranica, che può essere diagnosticata per la presenza di papilledema (Fig. 493-3). Qualunque deficit neurologico focale sensitivo o motorio, soprattutto a carico dei nervi cranici, dovrebbe essere indagato per escludere la presenza di una neoplasia.

Le alterazioni del sistema embrionale generalmente si manifestano all'esame obiettivo con una organomegalia o con la presenza di una massa addominale. In ogni caso, qualunque massa non meglio definita in qualsiasi zona dell'organismo andrebbe considerata di natura maligna, fino a prova contraria. Un aumento diffuso del ponte è un reperto radiologico generalmente osservato con la RM (Fig. 493-4): quasi sempre indica una neoplasia e può essere considerato patognomonico; inoltre, se non localizzato, è altamente suggestivo per un astrocitoma e viene trattato di conseguenza anche senza l'esecuzione di un accertamento bioptico, sia per il rischio sia per la difficoltà della procedura chirurgica in questa zona del cervello. Il retinoblastoma generalmente si pre-

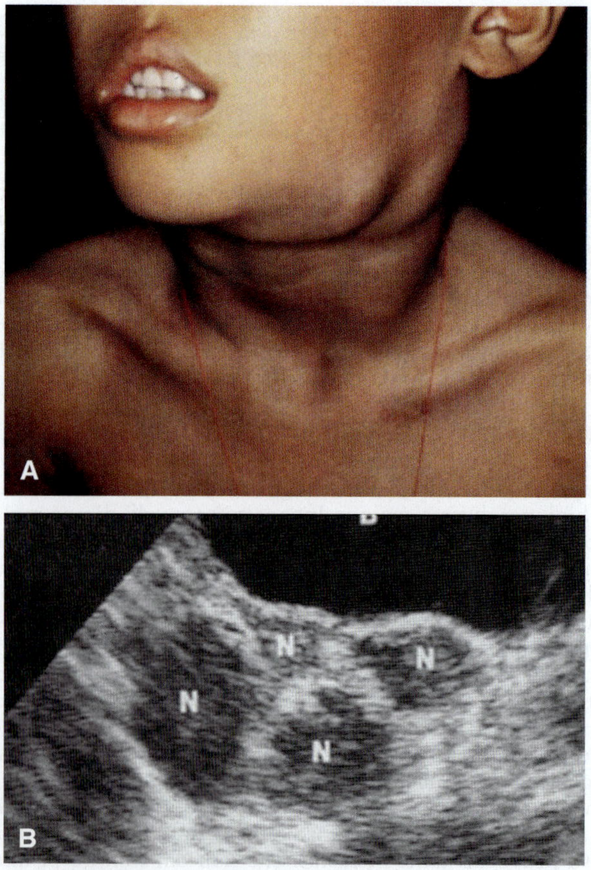

Figura 493-1. Linfoadenopatia cervicale. Come appare all'esame obiettivo (*A*) e all'ecografia (*B*). N, linfonodi di dimensioni aumentate. (Da Sinniah D, D'Angio GJ, Chatten J, et al: *Atlas of Pediatric Oncology*. London, Arnold, 1996.)

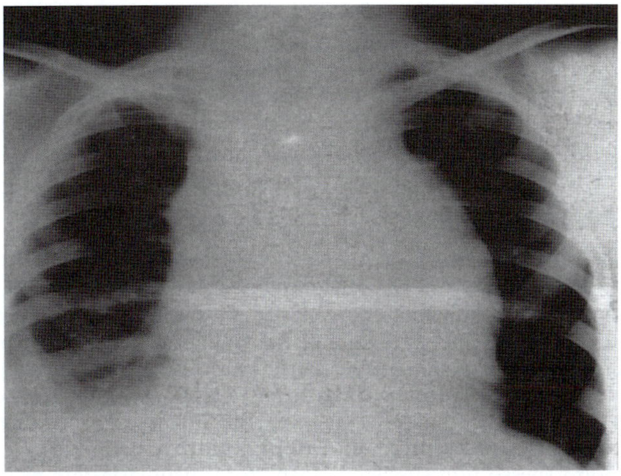

Figura 493-2. Massa del mediastino supero-anteriore da linfoma non-Hodgkin. (Da Sinniah D, D'Angio GJ, Chatten J, et al: *Atlas of Pediatric Oncology*. London, Arnold, 1996.)

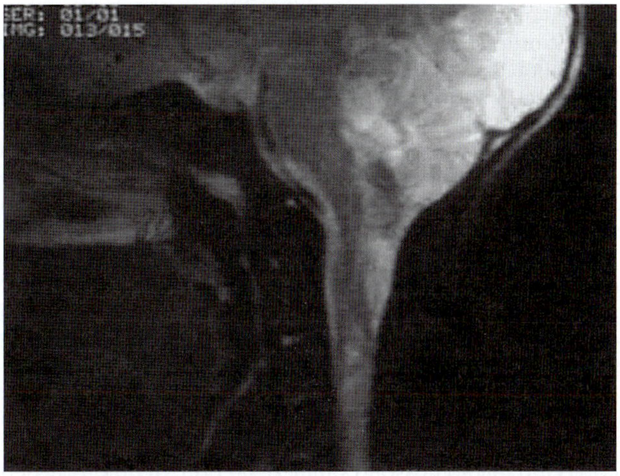

Figura 493-4. Neoplasia del tronco encefalico alla RM. (Da Sinniah D, D'Angio GJ, Chatten J, et al: *Atlas of Pediatric Oncology*. London, Arnold, 1996.)

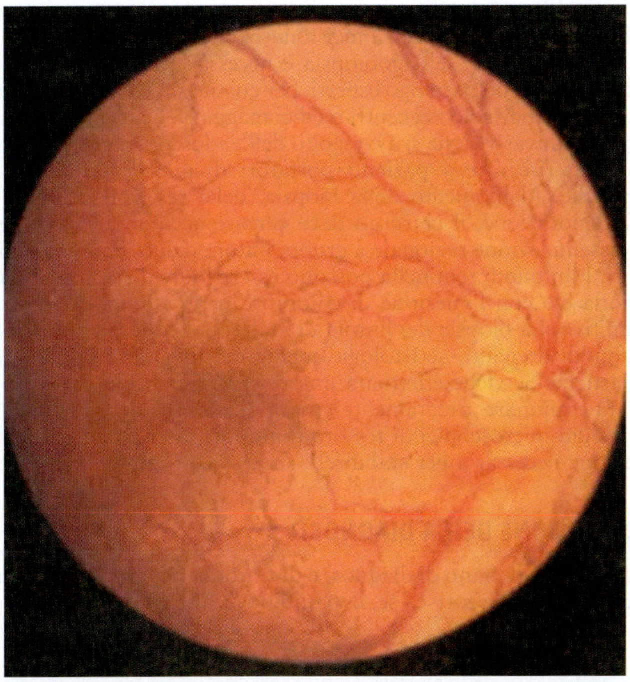

Figura 493-3. Papilledema all'esame del fundus. (Da Sinniah D, D'Angio GJ, Chatten J, et al: *Atlas of Pediatric Oncology*. London, Arnold, 1996.)

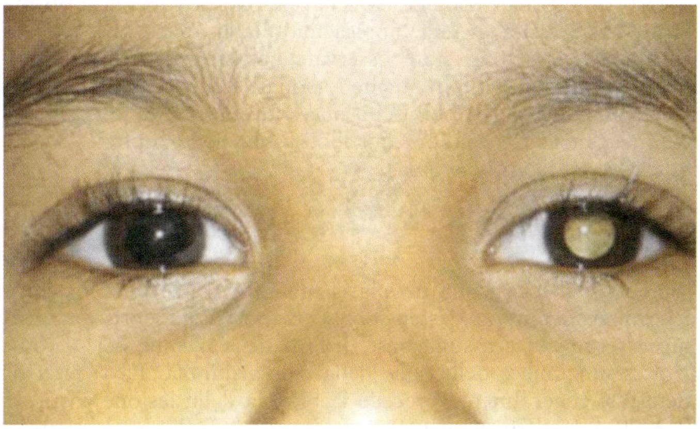

Figura 493-5. Riflesso bianco della pupilla nell'occhio di sinistra. (Da Sinniah D, D'Angio GJ, Chatten J, et al: *Atlas of Pediatric Oncology*. London, Arnold, 1996.)

senta con un riflesso bianco della pupilla (Fig. 493-5), al posto del classico riflesso rosso per la luce incidente. Questo riflesso bianco è essenzialmente patognomonico del retinoblastoma, anche se gli amartomi astrocitari, la malattia di Coats e l'ipertrofia persistente del vitreo primario possono simulare questo segno. Nei neonati, anche le macchie cutanee color "mirtillo" ("blueberry muffin") possono essere indicative di un neuroblastoma. Una massa sacrococcigea generalmente è un teratoma, che può andare incontro a una trasformazione maligna se non viene rimossa.

MANIFESTAZIONI CORRELATE CON L'ETÀ. Dal momento che nei bambini i diversi tipi di tumore si manifestano a età specifiche, il medico dovrebbe effettuare un'anamnesi e un esame obiettivo personalizzati a seconda dell'età del paziente. I tumori embrionali, compreso il neuroblastoma, generalmente si presentano durante i primi due anni di vita (vedi Fig. 491-3). Tra i 2 e i 5 anni vi è il picco di incidenza delle leucemie linfatiche acute, del linfoma non-Hodgkin e dei glomi, mentre durante l'adolescenza predominano i tumori dell'osso, la malattia di Hodgkin e i tumori delle gonadi e del tessuto connettivo. Pertanto, per i neonati e per i bambini più piccoli andrebbe portata una particolare attenzione alla possibilità di tumori embrionali e intra-addominali (per es. il tumore di Wilms, il retinoblastoma, il teratoma, il neuroblastoma e i tumori epatici). Nell'età prescolare e nei primi anni della scuola i bambini che presentano segni e sintomi compatibili dovrebbero essere attentamente valutati per escludere la leucemia, il linfoma e i tumori cerebrali. Occorre infine che gli adolescenti vengano esaminati per escludere i sarcomi e i tumori gonadici e anche per la malattia di Hodgkin.

DIAGNOSI PRECOCE

Dal momento che molte neoplasie pediatriche sono curabili, la diagnosi precoce è fondamentale. Inoltre, per alcuni tipi di tumore infantile è indicato un trattamento meno aggressivo se la malattia è diagnosticata in fase iniziale piuttosto che in fase avanzata. Infatti, la diagnosi precoce spesso permette di ridurre la dose e la durata del trattamento necessario e quindi può non solo portare a una maggiore efficacia della terapia, ma può anche evitarne al paziente una intensa e prolungata.

La prognosi per le malattie oncologiche pediatriche dipende soprattutto dal tipo di tumore, dall'estensione della malattia al momento della diagnosi e dalla rapidità di risposta al trattamento. La diagnosi precoce permette di somministrare tempestivamente il trattamento più adatto e di conseguenza di ottimizzare le possibilità di terapia. Anche se la maggior parte dei medici nella pratica quotidiana raramente incontra bambini con una neoplasia non ancora diagnosticata, essi dovrebbero ricordarsi di escludere la sua possibilità, soprattutto di fronte a un decorso atipico di un disturbo comune, a manifestazioni insolite che non si addicono a condizioni usuali e a qualunque sintomo persistente che crei dubbi diagnostici.

I ritardi nella diagnosi sono piuttosto frequenti in particolari situazioni cliniche. Il sintomo cardine sia dell'osteosarcoma sia del sarcoma di Ewing è il dolore localizzato e generalmente persistente. Considerando che questi tumori si manifestano durante la seconda decade di vita, periodo in cui normalmente vi è un incremento dell'attività fisica, i pazienti spesso ritengono che il dolore sia conseguente a un trauma. Una semplice radiografia può aiutare a confermare la diagnosi. I tumori del nasofaringe o dell'orecchio medio possono simulare un'otite. Il dolore auricolare prolungato, non altrimenti spiegabile, la suppurazione nasale, l'edema retrofaringeo e il trisma andrebbero considerati come possibili segni di neoplasia.

I sintomi precoci della leucemia possono essere costituiti da febbricola, dolore osseo e articolare. L'emocromo, soprattutto in caso di anemia normocitica o lieve trombocitopenia, può indicare la necessità di una biopsia midollare, anche se le cellule leucemiche non sono state osservate nel sangue periferico. Le neoplasie possono colpire anche i neonati e occorre prenderle in considerazione nei bambini con masse in una qualunque sede o con macchie cutanee color "mirtillo" ("blueberry muffin", segno indicativo di neuroblastoma).

STADIAZIONE

Quando si sospetta una neoplasia maligna, il primo obiettivo è determinarne il tipo e l'estensione. Una ipotesi diagnostica spesso può essere avanzata sulla base dell'età del paziente, dei sintomi di presentazione e della sede della massa dubbia. La ricerca di metastasi generalmente precede la biopsia della lesione sospetta (Tab. 493-4). Il chirurgo può decidere alla luce di più elementi se effettuare una resezione completa o se utilizzare una procedura più limitata sapendo qual è il grado di disseminazione della malattia. Gli esami preoperatori sono stabiliti in relazione all'ipotesi diagnostica. La TC e la RM sono esami non invasivi che possono essere utili per valutare la presenza di lesioni metastatiche; può anche essere necessario sottoporre il paziente all'aspirato osteomidollare, alla biopsia o a entrambi. Questi esami vengono utilizzati anche per valutare lo stadio della malattia, informazione fondamentale per la prognosi e per pianificare il piano terapeutico. Oltre alle metodologie tradizionali, l'analisi del DNA può essere utile per identificare i pattern di espressione genica di alcuni tumori, che permettono di stabilire una stadiazione più accurata e una classificazione del tumore.

ISTOPATOLOGIA

L'esame istologico è fondamentale per la diagnosi di qualsiasi tumore. Il campione di tessuto tumorale dovrebbe essere ottenuto in particolari condizioni, che permettano di effettuare un ampio spettro di valutazioni patologiche. In alcuni casi, come nel sospetto di un linfoma, potrebbe essere necessario del tessuto fresco per esami specifici. Alcuni di questi studi richiedono tempo, per cui non è possibile discutere la diagnosi con i familiari del paziente subito dopo l'intervento.

Molto spesso non sussiste il sospetto di neoplasia fino al momento dell'intervento chirurgico e il decorso dei successivi eventi prevede il reintervento per ottenere un adeguato materiale diagnostico, valutare l'estensione della malattia (stadiazione) e rimuovere il tumore residuo, trasformando l'iniziale procedura chirurgica in un intervento oncologico.

In molti casi la diagnosi può essere confermata per mezzo dell'agobiopsia, che evita l'incisione o interventi maggiori. Tuttavia, nell'utilizzo dell'agobiopsia è necessaria la presenza di un radiologo e di un patologo esperti, per cui questa tecnica è generalmente possibile solo nei centri medici maggiori. Le tecniche chirurgiche mininvasive, che si avvalgono dell'endoscopia, generalmente vengono riservate a pazienti portatori di masse addominali o toraciche. Al momento della biopsia, della resezione radicale o dell'esplorazione, il chirurgo deve cercare accuratamente i segni di disseminazione regionale a gruppi linfonodali o ad organi adiacenti. I linfonodi sentinella possono essere individuati con la scintigrafia e/o con l'iniezione di coloranti in prossimità del tumore primitivo. La biopsia dei linfonodi andrebbe limitata ai principali linfonodi drenanti, se istologicamente negativi per le cellule neoplastiche. Se viene effettuata una resezione radicale, il patologo dovrà esaminare attentamente i margini per escludere la presenza di residui microscopici di tessuto tumorale, essendo questa informazione necessaria per stabilire il successivo trattamento.

DISCUSSIONE DELLA DIAGNOSI

Occorre che il piano di diagnosi e di trattamento sia attentamente illustrato ai genitori e, se il bambino è abbastanza grande da

TABELLA 493-4. Minimo work-up (elaborazione) necessario per i comuni tumori dell'età pediatrica per valutare il tumore primitivo e le potenziali metastasi*

	MIDOLLO OSSEO ASPIRATO/BIOPSIA	RADIOGRAFIA DEL TORACE	TC	RM	SCINTIGRAFIA OSSEA	ANALISI DEL CSF	MARKER SPECIFICI	ALTRI ESAMI
Leucemia	Sì	Sì	–	–	–	Sì	–	–
Linfoma non-Hodgkin	Sì	Sì	Sì	–	Sì	Sì	–	–
Malattia di Hodgkin	Sì	Sì	Sì	–	Sì	–	–	Scintigrafia con Gallio
Tumori del SNC	–	–	ó	Sì	–	Sì	–	–
Neuroblastoma	Sì	–	Sì	–	Sì	ó	VMA, HVA	Scintigrafia con MIBG
Tumore di Wilms	–	Sì	Sì	–	–	ó	–	–
Rabdomiosarcoma	Sì	Sì	Sì	–	Sì	Sì (solo per i tumori parameningei)	–	–
Osteosarcoma	–	Sì	Sì (del torace)	Sì (per i tumori primitivi)	Sì	–	–	–
Sarcoma di Ewing	Sì	Sì	Sì (del torace)	Sì (per i tumori primitivi)	Sì	–	–	–
Tumori a cellule germinali	–	Sì	Sì	RM per l'encefalo	–	–	AFP, HCG	–
Tumori epatici	–	Sì	Sì	–	–	–	AFP	–
Retinoblastoma	±**	–	Sì, se RM non disponibile	Sì (dell'encefalo)	±	Sì	–	Analisi del gene del retinoblastoma

*Singoli casi possono necessitare di ulteriori accertamenti.

**Se si sospetta una invasione del midollo osseo.

Da Kliegman RM, Marcdante KJ, Jenson HB, et al (editors): *Nelson Essentials of Pediatrics*, 5th ed. Philadelphia, WB Saunders, 2006, p. 730.

AFP, α-fetoproteina; SNC, sistema nervoso centrale; CSF, liquido cerebrospinale (*CerebroSpinal Fluid*); HCG, gonadotropina corionica umana (*Human Chorionic Gonadotropin*); HVA, acido omovanillico (*HomoVanillic Acid*); MIBG, metaiodobenzilguanidina; VMA, acido vanilmandelico (*Vanillylmandelic Acid*).

capire, anche al paziente stesso. La migliore politica è quella di discutere onestamente. Ai bambini vanno date tutte le informazioni che essi possono comprendere e che possono essere loro necessarie, o che desiderano o vogliono conoscere. Gli effetti del trattamento, come la possibile necessità di amputare un arto, la perdita dei capelli durante la chemioterapia e l'eventuale compromissione funzionale temporanea o permanente devono essere anticipati e discussi ampiamente. Bisogna inoltre affrontare la possibilità e la probabilità del decesso per la neoplasia, in maniera adeguata a seconda dell'età del paziente. È spesso necessario ripetere le informazioni diverse volte prima che i membri della famiglia, disperati, capiscano del tutto. Durante il trattamento, i genitori, i pazienti, i fratelli e lo staff medico avranno bisogno di aiuto per esprimere le loro emozioni di ansia, frustrazione, senso di colpa e rabbia. Figure professionali esperte, compresi gli assistenti sociali per l'infanzia, gli psicologi specializzati per i bambini e gli psichiatri, gli assistenti d'infanzia e gli insegnanti con particolare esperienza con studenti affetti da malattie oncologiche dovrebbero essere contattati dal pediatra, dall'oncologo pediatra e dagli infermieri, se risultasse necessario.

Guillerman RP, Braverman RM, Parker BR: Imaging studies in the diagnosis and management of pediatric malignancies. In Pizzo PA, Poplack DG (editors): *Principles and Practice of Pediatric Oncology,* 5th ed. Philadelphia, Lippincott Williams & Wilkins, 2006; pp 256–289.

Malogolowkin M, Quinn JJ, Vietti TJ, Steuber CP: Clinical assessment and differential diagnosis of the child with suspected cancer. In Pizzo PA, Poplack DG (editors): *Principles and Practice of Pediatric Oncology,* 5th ed. Philadelphia, Lippincott Williams & Wilkins, 2006; pp 145–159.

Quackenbush J: Microarray analysis and tumor classification. *N Engl J Med* 2006;354:2463–2472.

Sinniah D, D'Angio GJ, Chatten J, et al: *Atlas of Pediatric Oncology.* London, Arnold, 1996.

Triche TJ, Sorenson PHB: Molecular pathology of pediatric malignancies. In Pizzo PA, Poplack DG (editors): *Principles and Practice of Pediatric Oncology,* 4th ed. Philadelphia, Lippincott Williams & Wilkins, 2002, pp 161–204.

Capitolo 494 ■ Principi di trattamento

Archie Bleyer

Il trattamento dei bambini con malattia neoplastica è uno dei compiti più complessi della pediatria. Prevede prima di tutto la necessità assoluta di avere una diagnosi corretta (compreso il sottotipo), per poi fare un'accurata stadiazione dell'estensione della malattia al fine di stabilire il sottogruppo prognostico; quindi è necessario programmare un'appropriata terapia a livello multidisciplinare e spesso multimodale, nonché occorrono assidui controlli per escludere recidive e per monitorare gli eventuali effetti collaterali derivanti dalla malattia e dalle terapie praticate. Tramite il programma di terapia, ogni bambino affetto da neoplasia dovrebbe avere a disposizione l'esperienza di gruppi di specialisti che si occupano della terapia delle neoplasie pediatriche, inclusi oncologi pediatri, patologi, radiologi, chirurghi, radioterapisti, infermieri e personale di supporto, tra cui nutrizionisti, assistenti sociali, psicologi, farmacisti, altri medici specialisti e insegnanti con esperienza lavorativa con bambini gravemente malati.

La migliore risposta al trattamento delle neoplasie si osserva durante le fasi iniziali della terapia; come per gli adulti, le terapie sottoposte ai pazienti con una malattia recidiva sono molto meno efficaci di quelle ai soggetti con una malattia in prima diagnosi. Tutti i pazienti con una neoplasia dovrebbero fare riferimento appena possibile a un adeguato centro specializzato, già quando vi è anche solo il sospetto di una malattia oncologica. I centri del Nord America sono riportati sul sito web del Children's Oncology Group (www.childrensoncologygroup.org), mentre sul sito del National Cancer Institute sono riportati gli studi clinici in oncologia (www.clinicaltrials.gov). I notevoli risultati ottenuti sulla terapia per le neoplasie infantili negli ultimi 30 anni non si sarebbero potuti raggiungere senza la collaborazione dei pazienti e dei loro medici curanti ai programmi di ricerca clinica presso questi centri. Negli Stati Uniti, il National Cancer Institute's Clinical Trials Cooperative Groups Program ha permesso di ridurre di oltre l'80% la mortalità per malattie oncologiche tra i bambini con meno di 15 anni, nonostante un continuo incremento dell'incidenza di neoplasie in questo stesso intervallo di tempo (Fig. 494-1). Questo importante risultato deriva da una efficace collaborazione multimodale, multicentrica e multidisciplinare.

DIAGNOSI E STADIAZIONE

Una diagnosi accurata e la stadiazione della malattia è di fondamentale importanza, soprattutto per i tumori dell'età pediatrica, che hanno alte probabilità di guarigione, in quanto il tipo di terapia dipende fortemente dalla natura della neoplasia. Inoltre, sono stati stabiliti alcuni **sottogruppi prognostici** in relazione allo stadio della malattia per la maggior parte delle neoplasie pediatriche. Di conseguenza, i bambini con prognosi migliore vengono

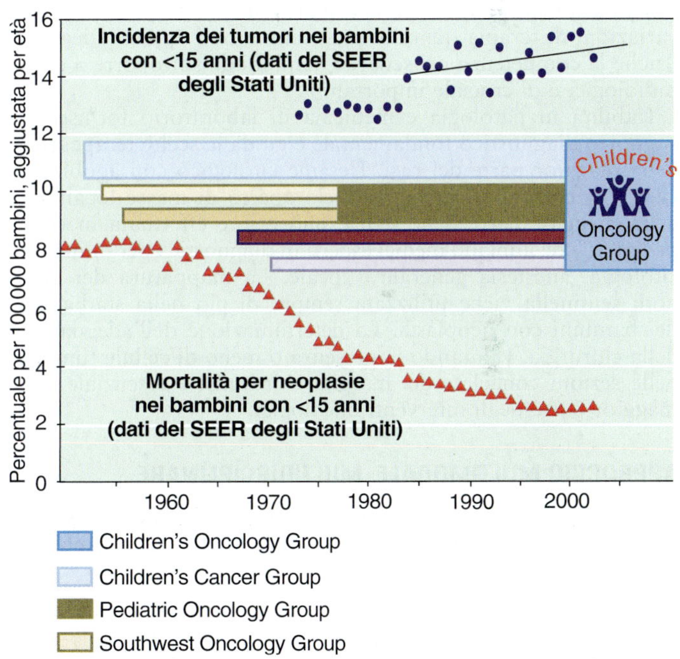

Figura 494-1. Riduzione della percentuale nazionale della mortalità tra i bambini <15 anni (triangoli) negli Stati Uniti, come diretta conseguenza del National Cooperative Group Program sponsorizzato dal National Cancer Institute e confronto con la crescente incidenza di neoplasie prima dei 15 anni di età (cerchi). Le barre orizzontali indicano il periodo di esistenza dei gruppi cooperativi oncologici nazionali pediatrici, che sono iniziati con il Children's Cancer Group (CCG) nel 1955. Gli altri gruppi sono il Pediatric Oncology Group (POG), che è derivato dalle divisioni pediatriche del Southwest Oncology Group e del Cancer and Acute Leukemia Group B, il National Wilms Tumor Study Group e l'Intergroup Rhabdomyosarcoma Study Group. Nel 2000, i quattro gruppi cooperativi pediatrici si sono fusi nel Children's Oncology Group. (I dati di incidenza e mortalità provengono da Ries LAG, Eisner MP, Kosary CL, et al [editors]: *SEER Cancer Statistics Review, 1975-2002*, National Cancer Institute, Bethesda, MD; *http://seer.cancer.gov/csr/1975_2002/*, sulla base dei dati SEER inviati nel novembre 2004 e pubblicati sul sito di SEER nel 2005. I dati sulla mortalità sono percentuali nazionali e le incidenze derivano dal programma del SEER, che rappresenta circa il 15% degli Stati Uniti.)

sottoposti a un trattamento meno aggressivo, di minore durata o con l'esclusione di almeno una modalità tra chirurgia, radioterapia e chemioterapia e in ogni caso con basse dosi di queste ultime due. Pertanto un'accurata stadiazione riduce il rischio di eventi avversi acuti importanti e di complicanze a lungo termine della terapia in pazienti la cui prognosi indica che ne risulta sufficiente una meno aggressiva. Presso un centro oncologico con esperienza limitata sulla gestione di questi trattamenti si corre il rischio che il paziente con prognosi migliore venga sottoposto a un trattamento troppo aggressivo. D'altro canto, anche un trattamento minimo è chiaramente un rischio, se la diagnosi e lo stadio di malattia non sono stabiliti correttamente, potendo compromettere una situazione che altrimenti avrebbe alte probabilità di guarigione.

Gli **esami radiologici** rappresentano una fase critica per la valutazione della maggior parte dei bambini con tumori solidi (per le neoplasie diverse dalla leucemia). RM, TC, ecografia, scintigrafia (esami di medicina nucleare), PET e spettroscopia, a seconda della situazione, hanno tutti un ruolo fondamentale nell'apprezzamento delle neoplasie pediatriche, non solo al momento della diagnosi per determinare l'estensione della malattia e l'approccio terapeutico più adeguato, ma anche durante il follow-up per verificare se la terapia è stata efficace. Inoltre, risulta sempre maggiore il numero di neoplasie infantili in cui si valutano l'entità di una risposta al trattamento e la rapidità con cui si ottiene, utilizzando tecniche diagnostiche in grado di quantificare tale risposta e che indirizzano in modo mirato le variazioni di terapia quando quest'ultima non appare adeguata. Anche la competenza nel sedare i bambini da sottoporre a esami radiologici è di cruciale importanza.

L'abilità in patologia e medicina di laboratorio fornisce un supporto diagnostico fondamentale e guida le scelte terapeutiche nella maggior parte dei casi. L'esame citologico con agobiopsia evita l'esecuzione di biopsie a cielo aperto di masse localizzate nella maggior parte delle sedi e può essere effettuata in centri pediatrici che abbiano medici esperti in diagnostica per immagini, citologia, anestesia generale e locale. La **mappatura dei linfonodi sentinella** viene utilizzata sempre di più nella stadiazione dei bambini con neoplasia. La determinazione dell'adeguatezza della chirurgia, valutando la presenza o meno di cellule tumorali nelle sezioni congelate dei margini chirurgici, è essenziale nella maggior parte degli interventi oncologici.

APPROCCIO MULTIMODALE, MULTIDISCIPLINARE

Molti ultraspecialisti pediatrici sono coinvolti nella diagnosi, nella terapia e nel trattamento dei bambini affetti da una malattia oncologica; sono altresì partecipi della fornitura delle principali modalità di trattamento e dei molteplici servizi di supporto (Fig. 494-2). Spesso sono utilizzate contemporaneamente più di due modalità principali: la chemioterapia è quella di più largo impiego, seguita, in ordine di frequenza, dalla chirurgia, dalla radioterapia e dalla terapia con agenti biologici (Fig. 494-3).

Le leucemie che colpiscono frequentemente i bambini sono trattate unicamente con la chemioterapia e solo una piccola percentuale di pazienti viene sottoposta a una radioterapia encefalica o encefalospinale come profilassi o per il trattamento di una leucemia estesa al sistema nervoso centrale. Anche il trattamento della maggior parte dei bambini con il linfoma non-Hodgkin prevede la sola chemioterapia. Le eccezioni comprendono voluminosi tumori non linfoblastici non-Hodgkin, in cui la radioterapia è spesso efficace e i tumori primitivi di Burkitt addominali operabili, in cui soltanto la chirurgia può essere risolutiva. Il trattamento locale con la chirurgia o la radioterapia, o con entrambe, è un importante elemento per la terapia della maggior parte dei tumori solidi, compresa la malattia di Hodgkin, ma la chemioterapia sistemica con più agenti risulta generalmente necessaria, perché spesso sussiste una disseminazione del tumore, anche se non dimostrabile. Molte volte la chemioterapia da sola non è sufficiente a eradicare tumori con residui voluminosi. Tuttavia, non risulta infrequente che i bambini affetti da un tumore necessitino di un trattamento che prevede tutte e tre le modalità (vedi Fig. 494-3). Purtroppo la maggior parte dei trattamenti che riescono efficaci nei bambini con una neoplasia ha un ristretto indice terapeutico (cioè una piccola finestra tra efficacia e tossicità). Gli eventi avversi acuti e cronici di questi trattamenti possono essere minimizzati, ma non eliminati completamente.

Negli ultimi 10 anni, la terapia con agenti biologici è diventata un'importante modalità di trattamento per alcuni tipi di neoplasie pediatriche (vedi Fig. 494-3). Questa strategia generalmente fa riferimento all'immunoterapia, a modulatori della risposta biologica o a molecole endogene che hanno effetti terapeutici quando somministrate a dosi sovrafisiologiche. Alcuni esempi sono l'acido retinico nella terapia della leucemia acuta promielocitica, gli anticorpi monoclonali nel trattamento di alcuni linfomi non-Hodgkin, l'imatinib mesilato per la leucemia mieloide cronica e per la leucemia positiva per il cromosoma Philadelphia e la metaiodiobenzilguanidina radioattiva per il neuroblastoma.

La chemioterapia è impiegata più largamente nei bambini che negli adulti, in quanto i bambini tollerano meglio gli eventi avversi acuti e le neoplasie che colpiscono l'infanzia sono più responsive a essa. La radioterapia invece viene usata con moderazione, perché i bambini sono più vulnerabili degli adulti agli effetti avversi tardivi.

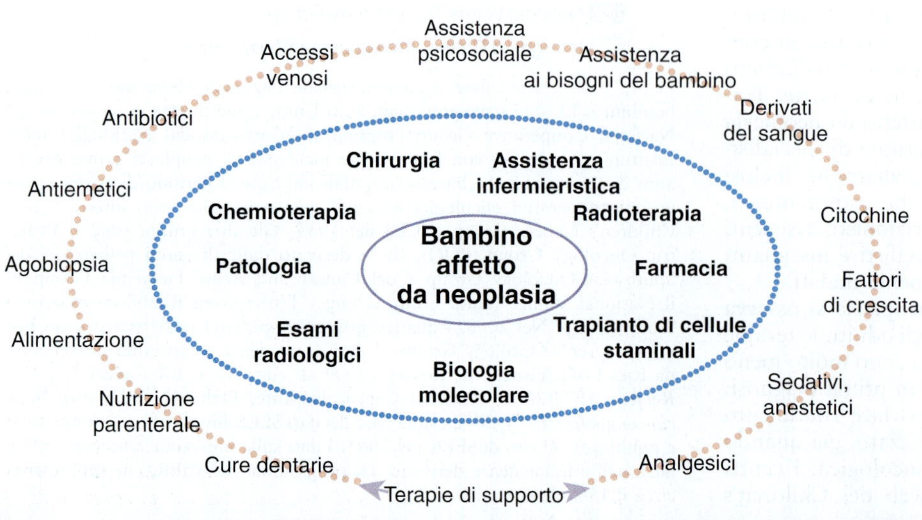

Figura 494-2. Multidisciplinarietà nella terapia dei bambini affetti da malattie oncologiche. Il cerchio più interno indica le modalità primarie e quello esterno identifica gli elementi della terapia di supporto a cui tutti i bambini con neoplasia hanno accesso.

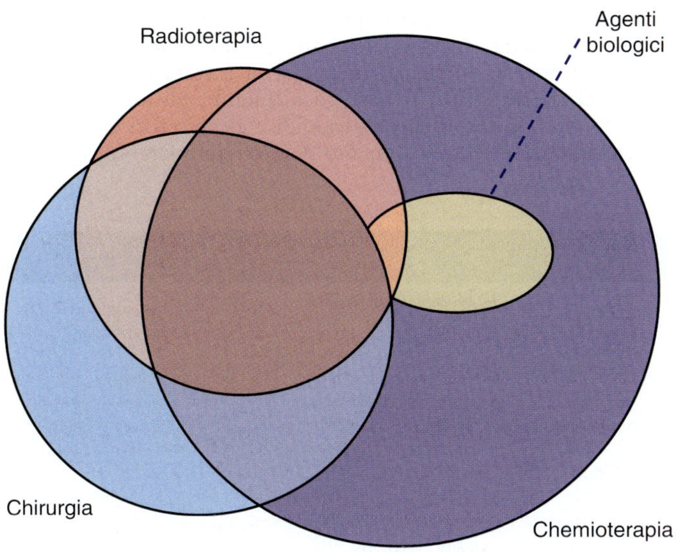

Figura 494-3. Le modalità primarie di terapia utilizzate nel trattamento dei bambini con neoplasia. Le dimensioni relative dei cerchi identificano la proporzione approssimativa del ruolo complessivo nel trattamento dei piccoli pazienti affetti da neoplasia.

Se si riesce, il trattamento andrebbe fatto a pazienti ambulatoriali. I bambini dovrebbero continuare a vivere a casa e a frequentare per quanto possibile la scuola per l'intera durata del trattamento. Sempre più spesso le terapie per le neoplasie pediatriche sono somministrate a pazienti ambulatoriali, grazie all'avvento di innovazioni quali le pompe di infusione programmabili, regimi di chemioterapia per via orale, dimissioni ospedaliere precoci con programmi di terapia di supporto intensivi e servizi domiciliari per la continuazione. Alcuni bambini perdono una considerevole parte delle lezioni scolastiche durante il primo anno dalla diagnosi per via delle terapie intense, degli effetti collaterali e delle complicanze che derivano dalla malattia di base e dalle terapie stesse. Andrebbe incoraggiato un sostegno scolastico, affinché essi non rimangano indietro con il programma; occorrerebbe fornire un supporto quando necessario. Dovrebbe inoltre esistere un servizio scolastico all'interno dell'ospedale per quei bambini che devono passare la maggior parte del loro tempo ricoverati per sottoporsi alle terapie per la loro patologia o per il trattamento degli effetti collaterali.

Lo sviluppo di terapie selettive e altamente efficaci per le neoplasie, sia dei bambini sia degli adulti, è stato ostacolato dalla scarsa conoscenza dei meccanismi molecolari che stanno alla base della trasformazione neoplastica. Le continue scoperte di meccanismi molecolari e cellulari, che spiegano il processo della cancerogenesi, hanno portato allo sviluppo crescente di tali trattamenti specifici, in genere noti come **terapie molecolari target**. La loro principale caratteristica è l'assenza di tossicità sui tessuti normali, così che l'addizionale beneficio terapeutico si correla con una minima tossicità aggiunta. Molti dei nuovi agenti biologici, come l'imatinib e il rituximab, rientrano in questa categoria (Tab. 494-1). Sono in aumento le **terapie complementari** e **alternative** somministrate dai genitori ai figli con neoplasie non sempre informando le figure mediche che seguono il piccolo paziente (vedi Capitolo 59). Molti di questi rimedi non sono mai stati valutati con studi rigorosi e la maggior parte risulta inefficace; alcuni sono tossici o interferiscono con il metabolismo di altri farmaci. La resistenza *de novo* o acquisita alla chemioterapia e alla radioterapia rimane un problema (Tab. 494-2). Importanti avanzamenti in questa disciplina hanno ridotto l'empirismo della terapia, ma rimane ancora molto da fare.

CHEMIOTERAPIA

La modalità di trattamento più ampiamente utilizzata in pediatria è la chemioterapia (vedi Fig. 494-3). La chemioterapia quasi sempre prevede la combinazione di più farmaci, come lo schema VAC (vincristina, doxorubicina [adriamicina] o dactinomicina [actinomicina D] e ciclofosfamide) e lo schema CHOP (ciclofosfamide, doxorubicina [adriamicina], vincristina e prednisone). Storicamente, l'uso sequenziale dei singoli farmaci raramente ha dato risposte complete, quelle parziali generalmente erano sporadiche e transitorie e la recidiva più rapida quando veniva

TABELLA 494-1. Inibitori della protein-tirosinchinasi e anticorpi monoclonali

AGENTE	CHINASI	NEOPLASIA
Imatinib	BCR-ABL	CML
		ALL a cellule T
	PDGFRα	Sindrome da ipereosinofilia
		Mastocitosi sistemica
	PDGFRβ	CML
	cKIT	Mastocitosi sistemica
		Tumori mesenchimali del tratto gastrointestinale (GIST)
Dasatinib	BCR-ABL	CML
		ALL con cromosoma Philadelphia
Nilotinib	BCR-ABL	CML
		ALL con cromosoma Philadelphia
Gefitinib	EGFR	Tumore polmonare non a piccole cellule
		Glioblastoma
Erlotinib	EGFR	Tumore polmonare non a piccole cellule
		Glioblastoma
Trastuzumab	ERBB2/HER-2	Tumore della mammella
Cetuximab	EGFR	Tumore polmonare non a piccole cellule
		Neoplasia a cellule squamose di testa/collo
Bevacizumab	VEGFR-1, -2	Tumore polmonare non a piccole cellule
		Tumore della mammella
		Carcinoma renale

ALL, leucemia linfatica acuta (*Acute Lymphoblastic Leukemia*); CML, leucemia mieloide cronica (*Chronic Myelogenous Leukemia*).

TABELLA 494-2. Meccanismi di farmaco-resistenza dei farmaci antineoplastici utilizzati più spesso nel trattamento dei tumori pediatrici

FARMACO	MECCANISMO D'AZIONE
AGENTI ALCHILANTI	
Ciclofosfamide/ifosfamide	↑ riparazione del DNA, ↑ degli "spazzini" dei radicali liberi, ↑ aldeide deidrogenasi (catabolismo)
Dacarbazina	↑ riparazione del DNA
Cisplatino	↓ uptake, ↑ riparazione del DNA, ↑ degli "spazzini" dei radicali liberi
Carboplatino	↓ uptake, ↑ riparazione del DNA, ↑ degli "spazzini" dei radicali liberi
ANTIMETABOLITI	
Metotrexato	↓ trasporto, ↑ DHFR (target), ↓ affinità per DHFR, ↓ poliglutammazione
Mercaptopurine	↓ attivazione, ↑ catabolismo
Citarabina	↓ desossicitidina chinasi (attivazione), ↑ dCTP, ↓ trasporto, ↑ citidina deaminasi (catabolismo)
Fluorouracile	↓ attivazione, ↑ timidilato sintasi (target), ↓ affinità per la timidilato sintasi
ANTIBIOTICI ANTITUMORALI	
Antracicline	MDR, ↓ attività della topoisomerasi II, ↑ degli "spazzini" dei radicali liberi
Dactinomicina	MDR
ALCALOIDI	
Alcaloidi della Vinca	↓ affinità per la tubulina (target), MDR
Epipodofillotossine	↑ riparazione del DNA, MDR, ↓ attività della topoisomerasi II
Paclitaxel	MDR
MISCELLANEA	
Corticosteroidi	Perdita o alterazione del recettore per i glucocorticoidi
L-Asparaginasi	↓ asparagina sintetasi nei linfoblasti

↑, aumenta; ↓, riduce; DHFR, diidrofolato reduttasi; dCTP, desossicitidina trifosfato; MDR, resistenza a più farmaci (*MultiDrug Resistance*) mediata da ↑ della glicoproteina di membrana P-170.
Da Nathan DG, Orkin SH, Ginsburg D, Look AT (eds): *Nathan & Oski's Hematology of Infancy and Childhood*, 6th ed. Philadelphia, WB Saunders, 2003, p. 1295.

utilizzato un singolo farmaco. La chemioterapia combinata è diventata standard quando la combinazione di farmaci con differenti meccanismi d'azione e tossicità non sovrapponibili (per es. POMP [mercaptopurina, vincristina, metotrexato e prednisone], VAMP [vincristina, doxorubicina (adriamicina), metotrexato e prednisone] e MOPP [mostarda azotata, vincristina, prednisone e procarbazina] è stata per la prima volta dimostrata efficace nel trattamento della leucemia nei bambini. La maggior parte dei farmaci citotossici impiegati in pediatria è stata selezionata tra diverse classi di agenti, tra cui gli alchilanti, gli antimetaboliti, gli antibiotici, gli ormoni, gli alcaloidi e gli inibitori della topoisomerasi (Tab. 494-3). L'aumento dell'attività metabolica e della

TABELLA 494-3. Comuni agenti chemioterapici utilizzati nei bambini

FARMACO	MECCANISMO D'AZIONE O CLASSIFICAZIONE	INDICAZIONI	EFFETTI AVVERSI	MONITORAGGIO DEL LIVELLO DEL FARMACO	COMMENTI
Metotrexato	Antagonista dell'acido folico; inibisce la diidrofolato reduttasi	ALL, linfoma non-Hodgkin, osteosarcoma, linfoma di Hodgkin, medulloblastoma	Mielosoppressione, mucositi, stomatiti, dermatiti, epatiti Se somministrato a lungo: osteopenia e fratture ossee patologiche Se somministrato ad alte dosi: tossicità renale e a livello del sistema nervoso centrale Se somministrato per via intratecale: aracnoiditi, leucoencefalopatia, leucomielopatia	I livelli plasmatici devono essere monitorizzati quando vengono somministrate dosi elevate e quando vengono somministrate dosi ridotte a un paziente con insufficienza renale e devono essere somministrati supplementi di analoghi dei folati	La somministrazione per via sistemica può avvenire per via orale, im o ev; può anche essere somministrato per via intratecale
6-Mercaptopurina	Analogo delle purine; inibisce la sintesi delle purine	ALL	Mielosoppressione, necrosi epatica, mucositi; l'allopurinolo aumenta la tossicità	Il monitoraggio durante il trattamento non è disponibile, né indicato	L'allopurinolo inibisce il metabolismo
Citarabina	Analogo della pirimidina; inibisce la DNA polimerasi	ALL, AML, linfoma non-Hodgkin, linfoma di Hodgkin	Nausea, vomito, mielosoppressione, congiuntiviti, mucositi, disfunzione del sistema nervoso centrale Con la somministrazione per via intratecale: aracnoiditi, leucoencefalopatia, leucomielopatia	Il monitoraggio durante il trattamento non è disponibile, né indicato	La somministrazione per via sistemica può avvenire per via orale, im o ev; può anche essere somministrato per via intratecale
Ciclofosfamide	Alchilante della guanina; inibisce la sintesi del DNA	ALL, linfoma non-Hodgkin, linfoma di Hodgkin, sarcoma dei tessuti molli, sarcoma di Ewing	Nausea, vomito, mielosoppressione, cistite emorragica, fibrosi polmonare, inappropriata secrezione di ADH, neoplasie vescicali, anafilassi	Il monitoraggio durante il trattamento non è disponibile, né indicato	Necessita di attivazione epatica e quindi è meno efficace in caso di insufficienza epatica
Ifosfamide	Alchilante della guanina; inibisce la sintesi del DNA	Linfoma non-Hodgkin, tumore di Wilms, sarcomi, germinomi e tumori testicolari	Nausea, vomito, mielosoppressione, cistite emorragica, fibrosi polmonare, inappropriata secrezione di ADH, neoplasie vescicali, disfunzione del sistema nervoso centrale, cardiotossicità, anafilassi	Il monitoraggio durante il trattamento non è disponibile, né indicato	
Doxorubicina e daunorubicina	Lega il DNA, si intercala	ALL, AML, osteosarcoma, sarcoma di Ewing, linfoma di Hodgkin, linfoma non-Hodgkin, neuroblastoma	Nausea, vomito, miocardiopatia, urine rosse, necrosi tissutale se stravasa, mielosoppressione, congiuntiviti, dermatiti da raggi, aritmie	Il monitoraggio durante il trattamento non è disponibile, né indicato	
Dactinomicina	Lega il DNA, inibisce la trascrizione	Tumore di Wilms, rabdomiosarcoma, sarcoma di Ewing	Nausea, vomito, necrosi tissutale se stravasa, mielosoppressione, radiosensibilizzazione, ulcerazioni nasali	Il monitoraggio durante il trattamento non è disponibile, né indicato	
Bleomicina	Lega il DNA, rompe le catene di DNA	Malattia di Hodgkin, linfoma non-Hodgkin, germinomi	Nausea, vomito, polmonite, stomatiti, fenomeno di Raynaud, fibrosi polmonare, dermatiti	Il monitoraggio durante il trattamento non è disponibile, né indicato	
Vincristina	Inibisce la formazione di microtubuli	ALL, linfoma non-Hodgkin, malattia di Hodgkin, tumore di Wilms, sarcoma di Ewing, neuroblastoma, rabdomiosarcoma	Cellulite nella sede di infusione, neuropatia periferica, stipsi, ileo paralitico, dolore mandibolare, inappropriata secrezione di ADH, crisi comiziali, ptosi, lieve mielosoppressione	Il monitoraggio durante il trattamento non è disponibile, né indicato	Deve essere somministrata solo ev; non deve essere fatta stravasare
Vinblastina	Inibisce la formazione dei microtubuli	Malattia di Hodgkin; istiocitosi a cellule di Langerhans	Cellulite nella sede di infusione, leucopenia	Il monitoraggio durante il trattamento non è disponibile, né indicato	Deve essere somministrata solo ev; non deve essere fatta stravasare
L-Asparaginasi	Deplezione di L-asparagina	ALL; AML, quando utilizzata in combinazione con l'asparaginasi	Pancreatiti allergiche, iperglicemia, disfunzione delle piastrine e coagulopatie, encefalopatie	Il monitoraggio durante il trattamento non è disponibile, né indicato	PEG-asparaginasi oggi è da preferirsi alla L-asparaginasi
Pegaspargasi	Polietilene glycol-coniugato di L-asparagina	ALL	Indicata per prolungate deplezioni di asparagina e per i pazienti allergici alla L-asparaginasi	Il monitoraggio durante il trattamento non è disponibile, né indicato	
Prednisone e desametasone	Lisi delle cellule linfatiche	ALL; malattia di Hodgkin, linfoma non-Hodgkin	Sindrome di Cushing, cataratta, diabete ipertensione, miopatia, osteoporosi, infezioni, ulcera peptica, psicosi	Il monitoraggio durante il trattamento non è disponibile, né indicato	
Carmustina (nitrosourea)	Carbamilazione del DNA; inibisce la sintesi di DNA	Tumori del SNC, linfoma non-Hodgkin, malattia di Hodgkin	Nausea, vomito, mielosoppressione ritardata (4-6 settimane); fibrosi polmonare, stomatiti cancerogene	Il monitoraggio durante il trattamento non è disponibile, né indicato	Aumenta il metabolismo del fenobarbital, riducendone l'attività
Carboplatino e cisplatino	Inibisce la sintesi del DNA	Tumori delle gonadi; osteosarcoma, neuroblastoma, tumori del SNC, germinomi	Nausea, vomito, insufficienza renale, mielosoppressione, ototossicità, tetania, nefrotossicità, neurotossicità, sindrome emolitica-uremica, anafilassi	Il monitoraggio durante il trattamento non è disponibile, né indicato	Gli aminoglicosidi possono aumentare la nefrotossicità
Etoposide	Inibitore della topoisomerasi	ALL, linfoma non-Hodgkin, germinomi	Nausea, vomito, mielosoppressione, leucemia secondaria	Il monitoraggio durante il trattamento non è disponibile, né indicato	
Etretinato (analogo della vitamina A) e tretinoina	Stimola la normale differenziazione	Leucemia promielocitica acuta; neuroblastoma	Secchezza delle fauci, perdita di capelli, pseudotumor cerebri, prematura saldatura delle epifisi	Il monitoraggio durante il trattamento non è disponibile, né indicato	

ADH, ormone antidiuretico (*AntiDiuretic Hormone*); ALL, leucemia linfocitica acuta; AML, leucemia mieloide acuta (*Acute Myelogenous Leukemia*); SNC, sistema nervoso centrale; IM, intramuscolare; EV, endovena.

proliferazione rende le cellule maligne più suscettibili agli effetti citotossici di questi farmaci (Fig. 494-4). Dal momento che la maggior parte dei chemioterapici agisce sul ciclo cellulare, gli effetti avversi generalmente si correlano alla cinetica della proliferazione delle singole popolazioni di cellule. Sono particolarmente suscettibili quei tessuti o organi con un elevato ricambio cellulare: midollo osseo, mucosa orale e intestinale, epidermide, fegato e spermatozoi. I più comuni eventi avversi acuti sono la mielosoppressione (neutropenia e piastrinopenia sono le situazioni più problematiche), l'immunodepressione, la nausea e il vomito, la tossicità epatica, le mucositi del tratto superiore e inferiore dell'apparato gastrointestinale, le dermatiti e l'alopecia.

Fortunatamente, i tessuti danneggiati recuperano con buona rapidità, per cui gli effetti avversi acuti sono quasi sempre reversibili. Quelli potenzialmente pericolosi per la vita dei chemioterapici sono la neutropenia grave associata a infezioni, micosi o polmoniti micotiche da immunodepressione e la setticemia, non di rado associata a un focolaio infettivo intravascolare (Tab. 494-4; vedi Capitoli 177 e 178). La miocardiopatia provocata dalle antracicline (quali la doxorubicina e la daunorubicina) e l'insufficienza renale da derivati del platino possono essere pericolose per la vita e spesso provocano disabilità.

Le cellule che non si replicano o che lo fanno lentamente, quali i neuroni, le cellule muscolari, il tessuto connettivo e l'osso, sono

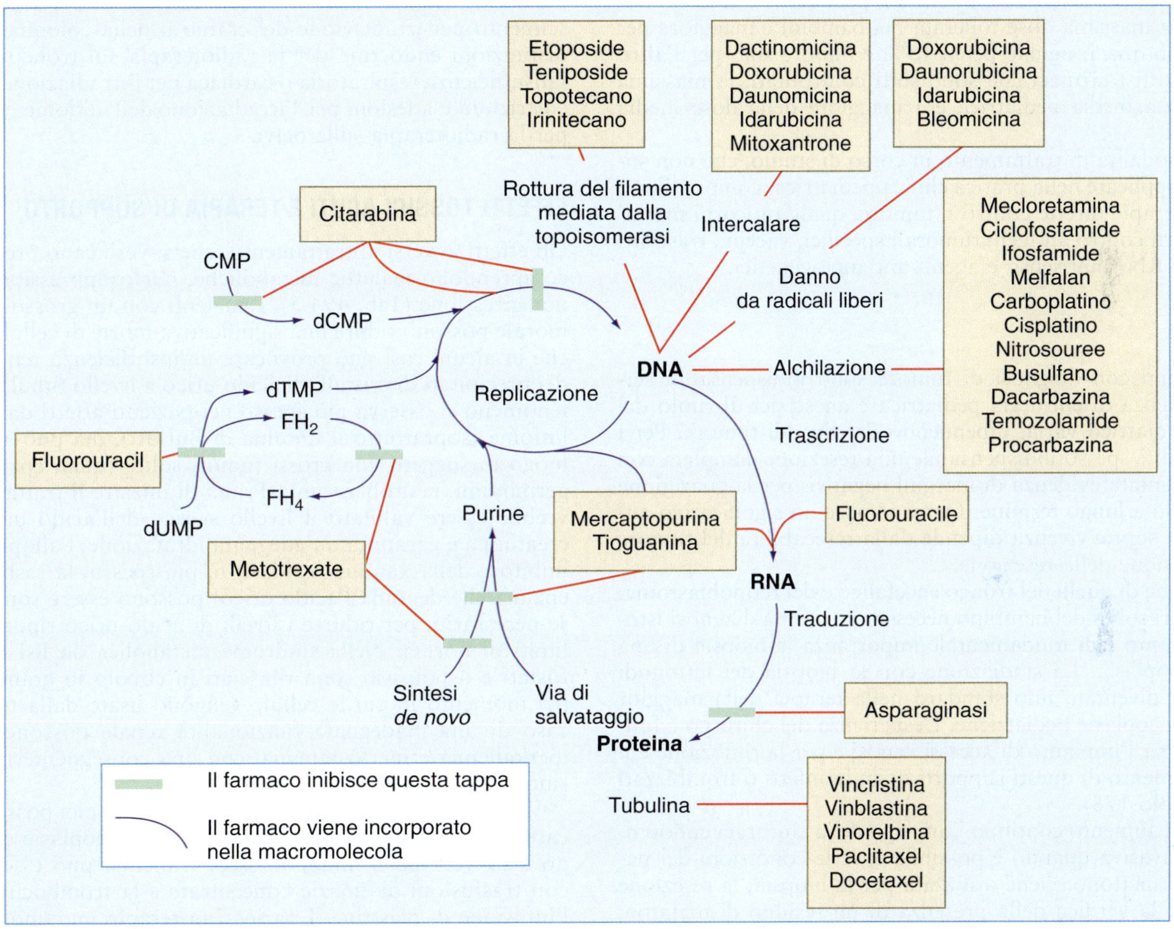

Figura 494-4. Sito d'azione dei farmaci antineoplastici più comunemente utilizzati. CMP, citidina monofosfato; dCMP, desossicitidina monofosfato; dTMP, desossitimidina monofosfato; dUMP, desossiuridina monofosfato; FH_2, diidrofolato; FH_4, tetraidrofolato. (Rielaborata da Balis FM, Holcenberg JS, Blaney SM: General principles of chemotherapy. In Pizzo PA, Poplack DG [editors]: *Principles and Practice of Pediatric Oncology*, 4th ed. Philadelphia, Lippincott Williams & Wilkins, 2002, p. 241.)

TABELLA 494-4. Complicanze infettive delle neoplasie

FATTORI PREDISPONENTI	EZIOLOGIA	SEDE DELL'INFEZIONE	AGENTE INFETTIVO
Neutropenia	Chemioterapia, infiltrazione del midollo osseo	Sepsi, shock, polmonite, tessuti molli, proctite, mucosite	*Staphylococcus aureus*, *Staphylococcus epidermidis*, *Escherichia coli*, *Pseudomonas aeruginosa*, *Candida*, *Aspergillus*, batteri anaerobi orali e rettali
Immunosoppressione, linfopenia, disfunzione linfo-monocitaria	Chemioterapia, prednisone	Polmonite, meningite, infezione virale diffusa	*Pneumocystis carinii*, *Cryptococcus neoformans*, *Mycobacterium*, *Nocardia*, *Listeria monocytogenes*, *Candida*, *Aspergillus*, *Strongyloides*, *Toxoplasma*, virus della varicella-zoster, Cytomegalovirus, herpes simplex
Splenectomia	Durante la malattia di Hodgkin	Sepsi, shock, meningite	Pneumococco, *Haemophilus influenzae*, meningococco
Catetere venoso centrale a permanenza	Nutrizione, somministrazione di chemioterapici	Sepsi, tragitto tunnellizzato del catetere, punto d'uscita	*S. epidermidis*, *S. aureus*, *Candida albicans*, *P. aeruginosa*, *Aspergillus*, *Corynebacterium JK*, *Streptococcus faecalis*, *Mycobacterium fortuitum*, *Propionibacterium acnes*

Da Kliegman RM, Marcdante KJ, Jenson HB, et al (editors): *Nelson Essentials of Pediatrics*, 5th ed. Philadelphia, WB Saunders, 2006, p. 733.

meno sensibili agli effetti della chemioterapia e della radioterapia. Tuttavia, i bambini non sono risparmiati dalla tossicità a livello di questi tessuti, probabilmente anche perché sono ancora in fase di proliferazione, pure se a una velocità inferiore rispetto ad altri tessuti, durante la crescita e lo sviluppo. Alcuni chemioterapici possono essere particolarmente tossici per questi tessuti, ma più spesso negli adulti che non nei bambini; per esempio, i bambini sono risparmiati dagli effetti neurotossici della vincristina e del metotrexato e dalla cardiotossicità da antracicline, che interessano soprattutto gli adulti.

In realtà, in molte circostanze, i bambini possono tollerare gli eventi avversi acuti della chemioterapia meglio degli adulti. La massima dose tollerata in loro, espressa in relazione alla superficie corporea o al peso, comunemente è maggiore rispetto a quella degli adulti. Dal confronto tra farmaci antineoplastici testati in trial di fase I, su pazienti sia adulti sia pediatrici, è stato dimostrato che la massima dose tollerata nei bambini è maggiore per il 70% dei farmaci, uguale per il 15% e minore solo per l'altro 15%. Per tutti i farmaci che sono stati confrontati, la massima dose tollerata media pediatrica era maggiore della dose media negli adulti.

Nuove modalità di trattamento in corso di studio, che non sono ancora applicate nella pratica clinica pediatrica, comprendono specifiche terapie dirette contro il tumore, quali anticorpi monoclonali diretti contro antigeni tumorali specifici, vaccini, trascritti di DNA ed RNA antisenso e agenti antiangiogenetici.

CHIRURGIA

Per i bambini con diagnosi di tumore sono indispensabili servizi d'eccellenza di chirurgia pediatrica e anestesici. Il ruolo del chirurgo pediatrico varia, dipendendo dal tipo di tumore. Per i tumori solidi è spesso indispensabile una resezione completa con una documentata evidenza di margini negativi, per la guarigione o il controllo a lungo termine. Quasi sempre un significativo aumento della sopravvivenza dipende dalla resecabilità del tumore e dall'estensione della resezione.

A eccezione di quelli del tronco encefalico e del retinoblastoma, tutti i tumori solidi del bambino necessitano di una diagnosi istologica; pertanto è di fondamentale importanza la biopsia di una sospetta neoplasia. La stadiazione con la biopsia dei linfonodi sentinella è diventata uno standard nella terapia della maggior parte delle neoplasie pediatriche. L'esperienza del chirurgo è fondamentale per l'impianto di accessi venosi e per la rimozione e il riposizionamento di questi supporti quando infetti o trombizzati (vedi Capitolo 178).

Risulta in aumento continuo l'impiego della chirurgia endoscopica mini-invasiva quando è possibile e, se le condizioni del paziente lo permettono, viene utilizzata per la biopsia, la resezione del tumore, la verifica della presenza di un residuo di malattia, la valutazione della risposta al trattamento, l'escissione delle aderenze e la splenectomia.

RADIOTERAPIA

La radioterapia viene utilizzata con cautela nei bambini, che sono molto più suscettibili degli adulti agli effetti avversi tardivi delle radiazioni ionizzanti. Con l'applicazione delle **radiazioni conformazionali** in oncologia pediatrica è stato fatto un fondamentale passo avanti. Questa tecnica, molto più comunemente nota come **radioterapia a intensità modulata**, risparmia il tessuto normale adattando il volume da irradiare alla forma del tumore, così da permettere la distribuzione delle dosi più alte al suo livello ed esporre di meno il tessuto normale adiacente o sulla scia del fascio di radiazioni. Un altro esempio è la terapia con radiazioni protoniche, che è stata ideata per essere utilizzata soprattutto nei bambini con una malattia oncologica. Con fasci molto più focalizzati e con migliori tecniche di sedazione e immobilizzazione, la radioterapia viene adoperata sempre più di frequente nei bambini. I suoi effetti collaterali acuti sono meno gravi di quelli della chemioterapia e dipendono dalla parte del corpo irradiata e dalla tecnica utilizzata. La dermatite è l'effetto avverso generale più comune, in quanto la cute rimane sempre nel campo di trattamento. Nausea e diarrea sono comuni eventi avversi subacuti a livello addominale. La mucosite di vari gradi quasi sempre trova luogo quando la mucosa orale o intestinale sono comprese nel volume di trattamento. La sonnolenza risulta frequente con l'irradiazione del cranio. L'alopecia si osserva quando è irradiato il cuoio capelluto.

La maggior parte dei protocolli di radioterapia prevede un trattamento per 5 giorni alla settimana per 4-7 settimane, in proporzione alla dose necessaria per controllare il tumore e in relazione alla quantità e alla natura dei tessuti normali compresi nel campo d'irradiazione. La maggior parte degli eventi avversi può avvenire mesi o anni dopo e generalmente dipende dalla dose somministrata. Il tipo di tossicità ritardata deriva anche dalla sede dell'irradiazione. Alcuni esempi sono il deficit di accrescimento per irradiazione del cranio o della colonna vertebrale, disfunzioni endocrine per la radioterapia sul tronco encefalico, l'insufficienza respiratoria o cardiaca per l'irradiazione del torace, costrizioni e adesioni per l'irradiazione dell'addome e l'infertilità per la radioterapia sulla pelvi.

EFFETTI TOSSICI ACUTI E TERAPIA DI SUPPORTO

Gli effetti avversi al trattamento, che si verificano precocemente, comprendono malattie metaboliche, mielosoppressione e immunodepressione (Tab. 494-5). I pazienti con un grosso residuo tumorale possono subire una significativa morte di cellule tumorali, che in alcuni casi può provocare un'insufficienza renale, per via dei precipitati di cristalli di acido urico a livello tubulare. Questo fenomeno si osserva più spesso nei pazienti affetti da leucemia e linfoma (soprattutto il linfoma di Burkitt), ma può anche avere luogo in soggetti con grossi tumori solidi (quali epatoblastomi, germinomi, neuroblastomi). Prima di iniziare il trattamento, dovrebbe essere valutato il livello sierico dell'acido urico e della creatinina e garantita un'adeguata idratazione; l'allopurinolo (un inibitore della xantina ossidasi) o, più spesso, la rasburicasi (un enzima che degrada l'acido urico) possono essere somministrati, se necessario, per ridurre i livelli di acido urico riportandoli nei limiti di norma. Nella **sindrome** metabolica **da lisi tumorale**, i fosfati e il potassio sono rilasciati in circolo in grandi quantità nel momento in cui le cellule vengono lisate dalla terapia. Nel caso di una inadeguata funzionalità renale possono verificarsi iperkaliemia e iperfosfatemia, con una conseguente ipocalcemia sintomatica.

Virtualmente tutti i trattamenti chemioterapici possono provocare la **mielosoppressione**, come anche le neoplasie che invadono e sovvertono il midollo osseo. L'anemia può essere corretta con trasfusioni di emazie concentrate e la trombocitopenia con l'infusione di piastrine. I pazienti in terapia immunosoppressiva dovrebbero ricevere derivati del sangue irradiati per prevenire la graft-versus-host disease. La granulocitopenia (granulociti $< 500/mm^3$) mette a rischio di contrarre infezioni pericolose per la vita. I soggetti con una granulocitopenia febbrile andrebbero ospedalizzati e trattati con antibiotici ad ampio spettro per via parenterale, nell'attesa dei risultati degli esami colturali sul sangue, sulle urine o su materiali provenienti da possibili sedi di infezione (vedi Capitolo 177). Occorre che il trattamento sia continuato fino a quando la febbre non cala e i granulociti non aumentano. Se la febbre persiste per oltre una settimana, mentre il paziente sta assumendo antibiotici ad ampio spettro, bisogna prendere in considerazione la possibilità di un'infezione micotica. Le micosi da *Candida* e *Aspergillus* sono comuni nei soggetti immunodepressi. I microrganismi opportunistici come lo *Pneumocystis carinii* possono provocare polmoniti fatali. Il trattamento profilattico con trimetoprim-sulfametoxazolo viene somministrato quando si prevede un'immunosoppressione grave o prolungata.

I **virus** a bassa patogenicità possono provocare gravi infezioni in caso di immunosoppressione secondaria alla malattia neoplastica o al suo trattamento. I pazienti non andrebbero sottoposti a vac-

TABELLA 494-5. Emergenze oncologiche

MALATTIA	MANIFESTAZIONE	EZIOLOGIA	TUMORE	TRATTAMENTO
METABOLICHE				
Iperuricemia	Nefropatia uremica; gotta	Sindrome da lisi tumorale	Linfoma, leucemia	Allopurinolo, alcalinizzazione delle urine; idratazione e diuresi, rasburicasi
Iperkaliemia	Aritmie, arresto cardiaco	Sindrome da lisi tumorale	Linfoma, leucemia	Kayexalato, bicarbonato di sodio, glucosio e insulina; ricerca di pseudoiperkaliemia da lisi delle cellule leucemiche in provetta
Iperfosfatemia	Tetania ipocalcemica; metastasi calcifiche, fotofobia, prurito	Sindrome da lisi tumorale	Linfoma, leucemia	Idratazione, diuresi forzata; arresto dell'alcalinizzazione; idrossi-alluminio per via orale per legare i fosfati
Iponatriemia	Crisi epilettiche, letargia, nessun sintomo	SIADH; perdita di sodio attraverso i liquidi e il vomito	Leucemia, tumori del SNC	Restrizione dell'assunzione di acqua per la SIADH; reintroduzione di sodio se ridotto
Ipercalcemia	Anoressia, nausea, poliuria, pancreatite, ulcera gastrica; allungamento del PR, riduzione dell'intervallo QT	Riassorbimento osseo; paratormone ectopico, vitamina D o prostaglandine	Metastasi ossee, rabdomiosarcoma	Idratazione e diuresi forzata con furosemide; corticosteroidi; mitramicina; calcitonina, difosfonati
EMATOLOGICHE				
Anemia	Pallore, debolezza, insufficienza cardiaca	Mielosoppressione o infiltrazione midollare; sanguinamenti	Qualunque chemioterapico	Trasfusione di emazie concentrate
Trombocitopenia	Petecchie, emorragie	Mielosoppressione o infiltrazione midollare	Qualunque chemioterapico	Trasfusione di piastrine
Coagulazione intravascolare disseminata	Shock, emorragie	Sepsi, ipotensione, fattori rilasciati dal tumore	Leucemia promielocitica, altre	Plasma fresco congelato; piastrine, trattamento dell'infezione
Neutropenia	Infezioni	Mielosoppressione o infiltrazione midollare	Qualunque chemioterapico	Se febbrile, somministrare antibiotici ad ampio spettro e G-CSF se indicato
Iperleucocitosi (>50 000/mm^3)	Emorragie, trombosi; infiltrati polmonari, ipossia; sindrome da lisi tumorale	Leucostasi; occlusioni vasali	Leucemia	Leucaferesi; chemioterapia
Graft-versus-host disease	Dermatiti, diarrea, epatiti	Immunosoppressione e derivati del sangue non irradiati; trapianto di midollo osseo	Tutti quando c'è immunosoppressione	Corticosteroidi; ciclosporina; immunoglobuline
PROCESSI OCCUPANTI SPAZIO				
Compressione midollare	Dolore alla schiena ± radicolopatia *Midollo al di sopra di T10*: debolezza simmetrica, aumento dei riflessi osteo-tendinei profondi; presenza di un livello di sensibilità; plantare-cutaneo in estensione *Conus medullaris (T10-L2)*: debolezza simmetrica, aumento del riflesso rotuleo; riduzione degli achillei; perdita della sensibilità a livello della sella; plantare-cutaneo in estensione o meno *Cauda equina (sotto L2)*: debolezza asimmetrica; assenza dei riflessi profondi e deficit della sensibilità; plantare-cutaneo in flessione	Metastasi vertebrali o dello spazio extramidollare	Neuroblastoma; medulloblastoma	RM o mielografia per la diagnosi; corticosteroidi; radioterapia; laminectomia; chemioterapia
Ipertensione endocranica	Confusione, coma, vomito, cefalea, ipertensione, bradicardia, crisi epilettiche, papilledema, idrocefalo; paralisi del III e del VI nervo cranico	Tumore cerebrale primitivo o metastatico	Neuroblastoma, astrocitoma; glioma	TC o RM per la diagnosi; corticosteroidi; fenitoina; ventricolostomia, derivazione; radioterapia; chemioterapia
Sindrome della vena cava superiore	Eccessiva distensione delle vene del collo, edema del capo e del collo, cianosi, proptosi, sindrome di Horner	Massa del mediastino superiore	Linfoma	Chemioterapia; radioterapia
Compressione della trachea	Insufficienza respiratoria	Massa mediastinica che comprime la trachea	Linfoma	Radiazioni, corticosteroidi

Da Kliegman RM, Marcdante KJ, Jenson HB, et al (editors): *Nelson Essentials of Pediatrics*, 5th ed.
SNC, sistema nervoso centrale; G-CSF, fattori di crescita per i granulociti (*Granulocyte Colony-Stimulating Factor*); SIADH, sindrome da inappropriata secrezione di ormone antidiuretico (*Syndrome of Inappropriate AntiDiuretic Hormone secretion*).

cinazioni con virus vivi. I bambini in trattamento chemioterapico ed esposti alla varicella dovrebbero ricevere le immunoglobuline per la varicella zoster e, se si sviluppa la malattia, andrebbero ospedalizzati e trattati con aciclovir per via endovenosa.

Il **trattamento del dolore** è di cruciale importanza. Le linee guida dell'Organizzazione Mondiale della Sanità (OMS) sono particolarmente utili nel trattamento del dolore secondario a una malattia oncologica e alle relative terapie (vedi Capitolo 77).

È comune che i soggetti oncologici in trattamento perdano >10% del peso corporeo. Talvolta i pazienti riducono l'apporto di alimenti a causa di una nausea transitoria correlata alla terapia, di stomatiti e di vomito. La perdita dell'appetito non deve allarmare. La malnutrizione è un rischio che corrono i pazienti sottoposti a un trattamento radiante che coinvolge l'addome o la testa e il collo, a una chemioterapia intensiva o a una irradiazione total body e alte dosi di chemioterapici prima del trapianto del midollo. Se la nutrizione per via orale non si dimostra adeguata, alcuni possono avere bisogno di un supporto alimentare attraverso un sondino naso-gastrico o per via parenterale.

EFFETTI COLLATERALI TARDIVI

I danni ai tessuti con un basso potenziale riparativo spesso provocano deficit tardivi o permanenti. Per esempio, una neoplasia cerebrale o midollare può esitare in una paresi permanente o in una disfunzione autonomica, la miocardiopatia indotta dalle antracicline generalmente produce una disfunzione cardiaca refrattaria ai trattamenti e la leucoencefalopatia determinata dalla somministrazione di metotrexato per via intratecale e dalla radioterapia a livello del sistema nervoso centrale spesso è solo parzialmente reversibile. I tipi potenziali di eventi avversi tardivi dipendono dall'età del bambino al momento del trattamento, dalla localizzazione del tumore e dalla terapia somministrata. Una buona risorsa per il pediatra, per il paziente e per i familiari che vogliono sapere quali possono essere questi eventi è il sito *www.survivorshipguidelines.org*.

Gli effetti avversi tardivi alla terapia possono provocare gravi morbilità (Tabb. 494-6 e 494-7). Un'ampia resezione chirurgica può determinare la perdita di importanti strutture funzionali.

TABELLA 494-6. Linee guida generali per la valutazione e il trattamento degli effetti collaterali tardivi: tossicità tardiva da radiazioni

SISTEMA	POSSIBILI EFFETTI	LINEE GUIDA PER IL MONITORAGGIO
Sistema nervoso centrale	Pubertà precoce, deficit dell'ormone della crescita e altri deficit ipofisari e ipotalamici	Monitoraggio neuroendocrino, compreso lo stato della crescita e delle gonadi
	Deficit cognitivi, leucoencefalopatia, secondi tumori del SNC (che crescono con l'aumentare della dose)	Test neurocognitivi e psicologici Visita neurologica
	Ictus, ototossicità, mielite, cecità, neuropatia periferica	Esame audiometrico e visita oculistica Visita neurologica
Occhi	Cataratta Cornea, dotto lacrimale, retina, congiuntiva, sclera, neurite ottica	Visita oculistica
Cuore	Miocardiopatia Pericardite Coronaropatia Insufficienza valvolare	ECG, ecocardiogramma, esame Holter o esame da sforzo a seconda della dose, dell'età al momento del trattamento, dei sintomi e dell'esposizione o meno alle antracicline
Polmoni	Fibrosi polmonare	Test di funzionalità respiratoria
Tiroide	Ipotiroidismo franco o compensato Noduli tiroidei o neoplasia della tiroide Ipertiroidismo	Test di funzionalità tiroidea
Gonadi	Insufficienza ovarica Oligo/azospermia Disfunzione delle cellule di Leydig	LH, FSH Estradiolo o testosterone Consulto per la fertilità o valutazione endocrinologica Visita ginecologica Esame dello sperma Stadiazione di Tanner Anamnesi mestruale
Secondi tumori	Sarcomi Tumori del SNC Tumore della mammella Melanoma Neoplasie cutanee diverse dal melanoma Tumori della tiroide Altri tumori solidi	Visite mediche complete annuali Particolare attenzione agli organi compresi nei campi della radioterapia Mammografia per escludere il carcinoma mammario nei pazienti di sesso femminile
Altro	Qualunque organo compreso nel campo della radioterapia può sviluppare una disfunzione o può essere a rischio di contrarre una seconda neoplasia	Periodici controlli della funzionalità degli organi a rischio

Da Friedman DL, Meadows AT: Late effects of childhood cancer therapy. *Pediatr Clin North Am* 2002;49, p. 1084.
SNC, sistema nervoso centrale; ECG, elettrocardiogramma; FSH, ormone follicolo-stimolante (*Follicle-Stimulating Hormone*); LH, ormone luteinizzante (*Luteinizing Hormone*).

TABELLA 494-7. Linee guida generali per la valutazione e il trattamento degli effetti collaterali tardivi: tossicità tardiva da chemioterapia

SISTEMA	AGENTI	POSSIBILI EFFETTI COLLATERALI	LINEE GUIDA DEL MONITORAGGIO
Sistema nervoso centrale	Chemioterapia intratecale	Deficit cognitivi; Leucoencefalopatia (aumento del rischio con l'aumento della dose)	Valutazione neurocognitiva
	Alte dosi di metotrexato		Valutazione neurologica
Cuore	Antracicline	Miocardiomiopatia	ECG, ecocardiogramma, esame Holter o prove da sforzo, in relazione alla dose, all'età al momento del trattamento, dei sintomi e dell'esposizione o meno a radiazioni
		Aritmie	
Udito	Derivati del platino	Perdita dell'udito	Esame audiometrico
Polmoni	Bleomicina	Pneumopatia restrittiva	Prove di funzionalità respiratoria
	Nitrosouree		
Vescica	Ciclofosfamide	Cistite emorragica cronica	Esame delle urine
	Ifosfamide	Neoplasie vescicali secondarie	
Fegato	Metotrexato	Insufficienza epatica	Esame della funzionalità epatica
	Tioguanina	Malattia da occlusione venosa (dactinomicina, busulfano, tioguanina)	Eco Doppler
	Mercaptopurine		
	Dactinomicina		
	Busulfano		
Reni	Derivati del platino	Insufficienza renale o scompenso renale	Esame delle urine
	Alte dosi di metotrexato	Riduzione/insufficienza degli elettroliti renali	Funzionalità renale
	Ifosfamide		Clearence della creatinina
Gonadi	Agenti alchilanti	Insufficienza ovarica; menopausa precoce	LH, FSH
			Estradiolo o testosterone
	Nitrosouree	Insufficienza testicolare; disfunzione delle cellule di Leydig	Consulto per la fertilità o valutazione endocrinologia
			Visita ginecologica
			Esame dello sperma
			Stadiazione di Tanner
			Anamnesi mestruale
Secondi tumori	Agenti alchilanti: mecloretamina più di altri	Leucemia	Emocromo
	Inibitori della topoisomerasi II		
	Derivati del platino		
	Ciclofosfamide	Carcinoma transizionale della vescica	Esame delle urine

Da Friedman DL, Meadows AT: Late effects of childhood cancer therapy. *Pediatr Clin North Am* 2002;49:1085.
ECG, elettrocardiogramma; FSH, ormone follicolo-stimolante; LH, ormone luteinizzante.

La radioterapia può arrecare un danno d'organo irreversibile, con sintomi e limitazioni funzionali che dipendono dall'organo coinvolto e dalla severità del danno. Molti disturbi correlati alla radioterapia non diventano evidenti fino a quando il paziente non ha completato lo sviluppo, come l'asimmetria fra le aree irradiate e quelle non irradiate o l'asimmetria delle estremità. L'irradiazione di campi che comprendono ghiandole endocrine può provocare l'ipotiroidismo, deficit ipofisari o l'infertilità. A dosi terapeutiche, la radioterapia encefalica può determinare la comparsa di deficit neurologici e l'irradiazione del rachide può dare origine a un ritardo dell'accrescimento.

Anche con la chemioterapia si può correre il rischio di danni organici a lungo termine. Di particolare interesse sono la leucoencefalopatia dopo un trattamento con il metotrexato ad alte dosi; l'infertilità nei pazienti di sesso maschile sottoposti ad agenti alchilanti (per es. la ciclofosfamide); un danno miocardio generato dalle antracicline; una fibrosi polmonare provocata dalla bleomicina; pancreatiti dall'asparaginasi; un'insufficienza renale dall'ifosfamide, dalle nitrosouree o dai derivati del platino; una riduzione dell'udito da cisplatino. Lo sviluppo di queste sequele può risultare dose-dipendente ed è generalmente irreversibile. Dovrebbero essere compiuti esami appropriati prima di iniziare con questi farmaci e periodicamente durante il trattamento, per verificare che non ci siano danni d'organo precedenti alla terapia e per monitorare gli effetti collaterali indotti dal trattamento.

Forse il più grave evento avverso tardivo è la comparsa di un **secondo tumore** in un paziente trattato con successo per un altro tumore. Il rischio sembra essere cumulativo, aumentando di circa lo 0,5% per anno, con un'incidenza di circa il 12% a 25 anni dal primo trattamento. I soggetti che sono stati trattati per una neoplasia pediatrica dovrebbero essere visitati annualmente, ponendo particolare attenzione ai possibili effetti avversi tardivi della terapia, comprese le seconde neoplasie.

TERAPIE PALLIATIVE

In tutte le fasi della presa in carico del bambino affetto da una neoplasia, i principi delle terapie palliative dovrebbero essere applicati per alleviare il dolore e la sofferenza e per migliorarne il benessere (vedi Capitolo 40). Il dolore è una grande causa di sofferenza per i pazienti oncologici. Può derivare dall'ostruzione o dalla compressione degli organi, dalle metastasi ossee o può essere di origine neuropatica. Ci si dovrebbe occupare del dolore secondo un protocollo che prevede alcune tappe, come raccomandato dall'OMS, in accordo con il principio di selezione dell'analgesico appropriato, prescritto al giusto dosaggio e somministrato in modo corretto, nonché scegliendo un appropriato schema di dosaggio per prevenire la persistenza del dolore e per alleviare quello logorante (vedi Capitolo 77). Inoltre, il dosaggio andrebbe titolato attentamente per prevenire, anticipare e gestire gli effetti collaterali. Bisognerebbe prendere in considerazione la possibilità di servirsi dei farmaci adiuvanti e di compiere ulteriori tentativi con altri antidolorifici.

Gli obiettivi principali nella terapia di chi sta morendo devono essere evitare l'angoscia per il paziente, per la famiglia e per i caregiver; portare assistenza secondo i desideri suoi e della famiglia; assecondare e difendere i modelli clinici, culturali ed etici.

Bradlyn AS: Health-related quality of life in pediatric oncology: current status and future challenges. *J Pediatr Oncol Nurs* 2004;21:137–140.

Cardous-Ubbink MC, Heinen RC, Langeveld NE, et al: Long-term cause-specific mortality among five-year survivors of childhood cancer. *Pediatr Blood Cancer* 2004;42:563–573.

Dickerman JD: The late effects of childhood cancer therapy. *Pediatrics* 2007;119:554–568.

Eshelman D, Landier W, Sweeney T, et al: Facilitating care for childhood cancer survivors: integrating children's oncology group long-term follow-up guidelines and health links in clinical practice. *J Pediatr Oncol Nurs* 2004;21:271–280.

Fallon M, Hanks G, Cherny N: Principles of control of cancer pain. *BMJ* 2006;332:1022–1024.

Harris MB: Palliative care in children with cancer: which child and when? *J Natl Cancer Inst Monogr* 2004;(32):144–149.

Hoffer FA: Interventional radiology in pediatric oncology. *Eur J Radiol* 2005;53:3–13.

Hudson MM, Mertens AC, Yasui Y, et al: Health status of adult long-term survivors of childhood cancer. *JAMA* 2003;290:1583–1592.

Joensuu A: Sunitinib for imatinib-resistant GIST. *Lancet* 2006;368:1303–1304.

Juweid ME, Cheson BD: Positron-emission tomography and assessment of cancer therapy. *N Engl J Med* 2006;354:496–507.

Kelly KM: Complementary and alternative medical therapies for children with cancer. *Eur J Cancer* 2004;40:2041–2046.

Krause DS, Van Etten RA: Tyrosine kinases as targets for cancer therapy. *N Engl J Med* 2005;353:172–187.

Lobo RA: Potential options for preservation of fertility in women. *N Engl J Med* 2005;353:64–73.

Mack JW, Grier HE. The Day One Talk. *J Clin Oncol* 2004;22:563–566.

Mocellin S, Mandruzzato S, Bronte V, et al: Part 1: Vaccines for solid tumours. *Lancet Oncol* 2004;5:681–689.

Mocellin S, Semenzato G, Mandruzzato S, et al: Part II: Vaccines for haematological malignancy disorders. *Lancet Oncol* 2004;5:727–737.

Nathan PC, Furlong W, Barr RD: Challenges to the measurement of health-related quality of life in children receiving cancer therapy. *Pediatr Blood Cancer* 2004;43:215–223.

Oeffinger KC, Mertens AC, Sklar AC, et al: Chronic health conditions in adult survivors of childhood cancer. *N Engl J Med* 2006;355:1572–1582.

Offit K, Sagi M, Hurley K: Preimplantation genetic diagnosis for cancer syndromes. *JAMA* 2006;296:2727–2730.

Patenaude AF, Kupst MJ: Psychosocial functioning in pediatric cancer. *J Pediatr Psychol* 2005;30:9–27.

Pollock BH, Knudson AG: Preventing cancer in adulthood: Advice for the pediatrician. In Pizzo PA, Poplack DG (editors): *Principles and Practice of Pediatric Oncology,* 5th ed. Philadelphia, Lippincott Williams & Wilkins, 2006;pp 1617–1628.

Prasad D, Schiff D: Malignant spinal-cord compression. *Lancet Oncol* 2005;6:15–24.

Pui CH, Relling MV: Can the genotoxicity of chemotherapy be predicted? *Lancet* 2004;364:917–918.

Reaman GH: Pediatric cancer research from past successes through collaboration to future transdisciplinary research. *J Pediatr Oncol Nurs* 2004;21:123–127.

Ross L, Johansen C, Dalton SO, et al: Psychiatric hospitalization among survivors of cancer in childhood or adolescence. *N Engl J Med* 2003;349: 650–656.

Shamberger RC, Jaksic T, Ziegler MM: General principles of surgery. In Pizzo PA, Poplack DG (editors): *Principles and Practice of Pediatric Oncology,* 5th ed. Philadelphia, Lippincott Williams & Wilkins, 2006; pp 405–420.

Sharma R, Tobin P, Clarke SJ: Management of chemotherapy-induced nausea, vomiting, oral mucositis, and diarrhoea. *Lancet Oncol* 205;6:93–102.

Spielberger R, Stiff P, Bensinger W, et al: Palifermin for oral mucositis after intensive therapy for hematologic cancers. *N Engl J Med* 2004;351: 2590–2598.

Steward AF: Hypercalcemia associated with cancer. *N Engl J Med* 2005;352: 373–378.

Tarbell NJ, Yock Kooy TH: General principles of radiation oncology. In Pizzo PA, Poplack DG (editors): *Principles and Practice of Pediatric Oncology,* 6th ed. Philadelphia, Lippincott Williams & Wilkins, 2006; pp 421–432.

Uren A, Toretsky JA: Pediatric malignancies provide unique cancer therapy targets. *Curr Opin Pediatr* 2005;17:14–19.

Capitolo 495 ■ Leucemie

David G. Tubergen e Archie Bleyer

Le leucemie sono le neoplasie più comuni dell'infanzia, rappresentando circa il 41% di tutte quelle che colpiscono i bambini con <15 anni. Nel 2002, negli Stati Uniti, sono stati diagnosticati circa 2500 casi di leucemia nei bambini con <15 anni, con una incidenza annuale di 4,5 casi per 100 000 bambini. La leucemia linfocitica acuta (ALL, *Acute Lymphoblastic Leukemia*) comprende circa il 77% dei casi di leucemia pediatrica, la leucemia mieloide acuta (AML, *Acute Myelogenous Leukemia*) l'11%, la leucemia mieloide cronica (CML, *Chronic Myelogenous Leukemia*) il 2-3% e la leucemia mieloide cronica giovanile (JCML, *Juvenile Chronic Myelogenous Leukemia*) l'1-2%. I restanti casi sono provocati da diverse forme acute e croniche che non trovano una collocazione nelle classiche definizioni di ALL, AML, CML o JCML.

Le leucemie possono essere definite come un gruppo di malattie neoplastiche in cui alterazioni genetiche a carico della cellula ematopoietica danno origine a un'abnorme proliferazione clonale. Il progenitore di queste cellule ha un vantaggio sulla crescita rispetto agli elementi cellulari normali, a causa di un aumento della percentuale di proliferazione e di una riduzione delle apoptosi spontanee. Questo fenomeno provoca un sovvertimento del normale funzionamento del midollo osseo, che con il passare del tempo porta a un quadro di insufficienza midollare. Gli elementi clinici, le indagini di laboratorio e le risposte ai trattamenti variano in relazione al tipo di leucemia.

Pizzo PA and Poplack DG (editors): *Principles and Practice of Pediatric Oncology,* 5th ed. Philadelphia, Lippincott Williams & Wilkins, 2005.

495.1 • LEUCEMIA LINFOCITICA ACUTA

L'ALL dell'infanzia è stata la prima neoplasia disseminata, che ha dimostrato di essere curabile e che pertanto ha rappresentato un modello per i principi di diagnosi, prognosi e trattamento in oncologia. In realtà si tratta di un gruppo eterogeneo di neoplasie con diverse alterazioni genetiche distinte, responsabili di altrettanti quadri clinici, con risposte differenti alle terapie.

EPIDEMIOLOGIA. Ogni anno negli Stati Uniti si diagnosticano circa 2000 casi di ALL in bambini con <15 anni. Si ha un sorprendente picco di incidenza tra 2-6 anni e sono più frequentemente colpiti i maschi delle femmine, a tutte le età. Decenni fa sembrava che questo picco correlato all'età fosse proprio dei soggetti di razza bianca nei Paesi socioeconomicamente avanzati, ma poi è stato osservato anche nelle popolazioni di razza nera negli Stati Uniti. La malattia risulta più frequente nei bambini con particolari anomalie genetiche, come la sindrome di Down, la sindrome di Bloom, l'atassia-teleangectasia e la sindrome di Fanconi. Nei gemelli omozigoti, il rischio per il secondo gemello, se il fratello è affetto da leucemia, è maggiore rispetto a quello della popolazione generale, risultando >70% se la diagnosi nel primo gemello è stata fatta durante il primo anno di vita e se i gemelli hanno condiviso la stessa placenta (monocorionici). Inoltre, indipendentemente dall'essere omo o eterozigoti, se il primo gemello sviluppa l'ALL tra 5-7 anni il rischio per il secondo è di circa il doppio rispetto a quello della popolazione generale.

EZIOLOGIA. In realtà, in tutti i casi, l'eziologia dell'ALL rimane sconosciuta, anche se diversi fattori genetici e ambientali sono stati correlati alla leucemia in età pediatrica (Tab. 495-1). L'esposizione a radiazioni per esami diagnostici sia in utero sia durante l'infanzia è stata associata a un'aumentata incidenza di ALL, che potrebbe inoltre essere in relazione a determinati fattori ambientali, secondo segnalazioni e studi di cluster geografici che sono stati pubblicati. Finora nessun altro fattore oltre alle radiazioni è stato identificato negli Stati Uniti. In alcuni Paesi in via di sviluppo è stata osservata un'associazione fra l'ALL a cellule B e l'infezione virale di Epstein-Barr.

PATOGENESI. La classificazione dell'ALL è fatta sulla base della tipizzazione delle cellule maligne nel midollo osseo, in relazione alla morfologia, alle caratteristiche fenotipiche con la valutazione dei marker di membrana e alle caratteristiche citogenetiche e genetico-molecolari. La **morfologia** da sola in genere è sufficiente a stabilire la diagnosi, ma sono indispensabili altre indagini per una corretta classificazione della malattia, che possono avere una notevole influenza sia sulla prognosi sia sulla scelta della terapia più appropriata. Il più importante elemento riconoscitivo a livello morfologico, indicativo di una leucemia a cellule B mature, è la distinzione dei 3 sottotipi (L1, L2, L3) secondo il FAB (gruppo di studio cooperativo franco-americano-britannico). Il tipo L3, noto anche come leucemia di Burkitt, è una delle neoplasie a crescita più rapida nell'uomo e che necessita di un diverso approccio terapeutico. Dal punto di vista fenotipico, i marker di superficie dimostrano che circa l'85% dei casi di ALL deriva da progenitori delle cellule B, circa il 15% dalle cellule T e circa l'1% dalle cellule B. Una piccola percentuale di bambini con diagnosi di leucemia presenta una malattia con marker di superficie di derivazione sia linfocitica sia mielocitica. Gli immunofenotipi spesso si correlano alle manifestazioni cliniche della malattia (Tab. 495-2).

Nella maggior parte dei pazienti con l'ALL sono state riscontrate **anomalie cromosomiche** (Tab. 495-3, Fig. 495-1). Le alterazioni quali le traslocazioni o le delezioni, che possono comprendere un diverso numero di cromosomi, sono indici prognostici particolarmente importanti. L'identificazione delle specifiche sequenze per la leucemia del gene alterato in campioni archiviati di sangue neonatale di alcuni bambini che hanno sviluppato l'ALL in un momento successivo indica l'importanza di eventi uterini nell'iniziazione della trasformazione maligna, ma il lungo lasso di tempo che in alcuni bambini precede l'esordio della malattia, che può essere anche di 14 anni, supporta l'ipotesi che sono necessarie anche altre mutazioni per indurre l'espressione della malattia stessa. Specifiche mutazioni cromosomiche, come la traslocazione t(9;22), che esprime la proteina di fusione BCR-ABL, suggerisco-

TABELLA 495-1. Fattori predisponenti alla leucemia nell'infanzia

MALATTIE GENETICHE
- Sindrome di Down
- Sindrome di Fanconi
- Sindrome di Bloom
- Anemia di Diamond-Blackfan
- Sindrome di Schwachman
- Sindrome di Klinefelter
- Sindrome di Turner
- Neurofibromatosi di tipo 1
- Atassia-teleangectasia
- Grave immunodeficienza combinata
- Emoglobinuria parossistica notturna
- Sindrome di Li-Fraumeni

FATTORI AMBIENTALI
- Radiazioni ionizzanti
- Farmaci
- Agenti alchilanti
- Nitrosouree
- Epipodofillotossina
- Esposizione al benzene
- Età avanzata della madre

TABELLA 495-2. Correlazione fra immunofenotipo e quadro clinico

	PRO-B, CD10$^-$	PRE-B IMMATURI, CD10$^+$	PRE-B	B MATURI	CELLULE T
N. pazienti	52	635	156	39	124
Sesso (% maschi)	39	53	50	85	75
Età (anni)					
<1 (%)	33	1	6	3	1
1–<10 (%)	50	82	80	64	62
≥ 10 (%)	17	17	14	33	37
Leucociti $<100 \times 10^9$/L					
Mediana	38	33	42	77	87
≤20 (%)	38	75	53	69	23
>50 (%)	44	11	21	5	57
Piastrine $<100 \times 10^9$ L (%)	77	75	81	56	56
Emoglobina ≤8 g/dL (%)	58	40	60	21	15
Splenomegalia (%)*	50	34	46	28	57
Epatomegalia (%)*	56	46	48	36	61
Massa mediastinica (%)	0	0	1	0	72
Linfoadenopatia	35	36	41	54	78
Interessamento del SNC	10	1	1	0	11

SNC, sistema nervoso centrale.
*>4 cm al di sotto del margine costale.
Da Nathan DG, Orkin SH, Ginsburg D, et al (editors): *Nathan & Oski's Hematology of Infancy and Childhood*, 6th ed. Philadelphia, WB Saunders, 2003, p. 1139. Dati forniti da Reiter A, Schrappe M, Ludwig WD, et al: Chemotherapy in 998 unselected childhood acute lymphoblastic leukemia patients. Results and conclusions of the multicenter trial ALL-BFM 86. *Blood* 1994;84:3122-3123.

TABELLA 495-3. Alterazioni cromosomiche comuni nelle leucemie acute dei bambini

MALATTIA	SOTTOTIPO	ALTERAZIONE CROMOSOMICA	INFLUENZA SULLA PROGNOSI
ALL	Pre-B	Trisomia 4 e 10	Favorevole
		t(12;21)	
	Pre-B	t(4;11)	Sfavorevole
	Pre-B	t(9;22)	Sfavorevole
	A cellule B	t(8;14)	Nessuna
	Generale	Iperdiploidie	Favorevole
	Generale	Iperdiploidie	Sfavorevole
AML	M1*	t(8;21)	Favorevole
	M4*	inv(16)	Favorevole
	M3*	t(5;17)	Favorevole
	Generale	del(7)	Sfavorevole
	Infantile	t(4;11)	Sfavorevole

* Secondo la classificazione franco-americano-britannica delle leucemie mielogeniche acute (vedi Tab. 495-4).
ALL, leucemia linfocitica acuta; AML, leucemia mielocitica acuta.

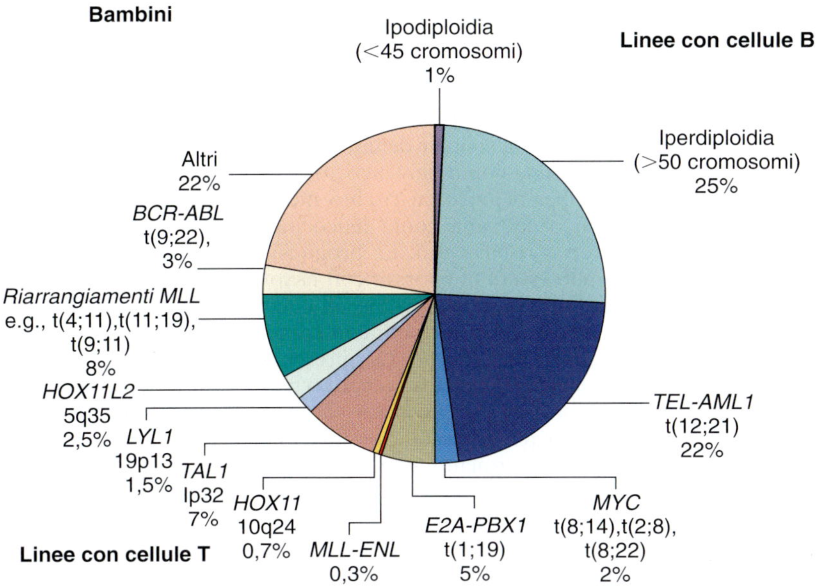

Figura 495-1. Frequenza stimata dei genotipi specifici di leucemia linfocitica acuta (ALL) nei bambini. Le lesioni genetiche che si riscontrano esclusivamente nei casi di leucemia a cellule T sono indicate in viola. Tutti gli altri sottotipi genetici si riscontrano esclusivamente o principalmente nei casi di ALL a cellule B. (Da Pui CH, Relling MV, Downing JR: Acute lymphoblastic leukemia. *N Engl J Med* 2004;350:1535-1548.)

no la necessità di ulteriori approfondimenti genetico-molecolari. Le tecniche di PCR e di fluorescenza con ibridazione *in situ*, per esempio, forniscono la possibilità d'identificare mutazioni puntiformi e di studiare anche poche cellule neoplastiche durante il follow-up; tuttavia, l'utilità clinica di questi approfondimenti deve ancora essere stabilita con chiarezza. Lo sviluppo della microanalisi del DNA permette di valutare l'espressione di centinaia di geni nella cellula leucemica. Questa tecnica permetterà di comprendere ancora meglio la biologia di base dell'ALL e procurerà importanti indicazioni circa l'approccio terapeutico.

MANIFESTAZIONI CLINICHE. La presentazione iniziale dell'ALL è generalmente aspecifica e di entità relativamente lieve. Sono quasi sempre presenti anoressia, astenia, irritabilità e una febbricola intermittente. Può aversi un dolore osseo, o meno frequentemente articolare, soprattutto agli arti inferiori. I pazienti spesso contemplano in anamnesi una recente infezione delle vie aeree superiori, nei precedenti 1-2 mesi. Meno di frequente, i sintomi possono durare da qualche mese, con dolori localizzati soprattutto a livello osseo o articolare e con presenza anche di tumefazioni alle articolazioni. Il dolore osseo è grave e può svegliare il paziente durante la notte. Quando la malattia progredisce, i segni e i sintomi da interessamento midollare diventano più evidenti con la comparsa del pallore cutaneo, di astenia, ematomi o epistassi, ma anche di febbre, che può risultare secondaria a un'infezione.

All'**esame obiettivo**, i reperti di pallore, svogliatezza, lesioni cutanee tipo porpora e petecchie, o emorragie cutanee, possono essere segni di un'insufficienza midollare (vedi Capitolo 493). La natura proliferativa della malattia può manifestarsi linfoadenopatia, splenomegalia o, meno comunemente, epatomegalia. Nei pazienti con un dolore osseo o articolare, si può trovare una specifica sensibilità in corrispondenza dell'osso oppure un edema o un versamento articolare obiettivamente evidente. Nondimeno, anche il coinvolgimento midollare si può accompagnare a un dolore osseo profondo, ma la dolorabilità non sarà evocata. Rare volte i pazienti manifestano segni d'ipertensione endocranica, indicativi di un coinvolgimento del sistema nervoso centrale (SNC) da parte della leucemia. Questi segni includono il papilledema (vedi Fig. 493-3), le emorragie retiniche e i deficit dei nervi cranici. Le difficoltà respiratorie generalmente sono conseguenti all'anemia, ma possono verificarsi anche per ostruzione delle vie aeree da parte di una massa voluminosa del mediastino anteriore (per es. per interessamento del timo o dei linfonodi). Questo disturbo si osserva più tipicamente negli adolescenti di sesso maschile affetti dall'ALL a cellule T, la quale determina altresì un aumento dei leucociti.

L'ALL a cellule pre-B immature (CD10$^+$ o CALLA$^+$) è l'immunofenotipo più comune (vedi Tab. 495-2), che esordisce tra 1-10 anni, quando la conta leucocitaria media risulta di 33 000, sebbene il 75% dei pazienti abbia <20 000 leucociti; la trombocitopenia è presente nel 75% dei casi e l'epatosplenomegalia nel 30-40%. In tutti i tipi di leucemia, i sintomi da interessamento del SNC sono presenti all'esordio nel 5% dei pazienti (10-20% hanno blasti nel liquido cerebrospinale). È possibile un interessamento dei testicoli (20%) e delle ovaie (30%), che non necessita tuttavia di un accertamento bioptico.

DIAGNOSI. L'ipotesi diagnostica viene suggerita dagli elementi riscontrati nel sangue periferico, che sono indicativi di un'alterazione midollare. L'anemia e la trombocitopenia sono presenti nella maggior parte dei pazienti. Generalmente, con i normali esami di laboratorio non si osservano cellule leucemiche nel sangue periferico. Molti pazienti con ALL hanno un numero di leucociti <10 000/μL. In alcuni casi le cellule leucemiche sono inizialmente scambiate per linfociti atipici ed è solo in successivi accertamenti che vengono invece riconosciute come parte di un clone maligno. Quando i risultati dell'emocromo suggeriscono la possibilità di una leucemia, andrebbe subito analizzato il midollo per porre una diagnosi. In genere è sufficiente il solo aspirato midollare, ma talvolta è necessaria una biopsia per prelevare un'adeguata quantità di tessuto per le analisi o per escludere altre possibili cause di alterazione.

La diagnosi di ALL è posta quando il midollo presenta una invasione da parte di una popolazione omogenea di linfociti >25%. La stadiazione dell'ALL si fonda anche sulla valutazione del liquido cerebrospinale (CSF, *CerebroSpinal Fluid*). L'aumento dei linfoblasti e dei leucociti nel CSF è infatti suggestivo di un interessamento leucemico liquorale o meningeo e risulta indicativo di uno stadio di malattia più avanzato, ponendo la necessità di terapie combinate sistemiche e per il SNC. La puntura lombare di stadiazione può essere fatta contemporaneamente alla prima somministrazione di chemioterapia intratecale, quando la diagnosi di leucemia è stata già stabilita con l'esame midollare.

DIAGNOSI DIFFERENZIALE. L'ALL deve innanzitutto essere differenziata dall'AML. Le altre patologie maligne, che invadono il midollo osseo e provocano un suo malfunzionamento, sono il neuroblastoma, il rabdomiosarcoma, il sarcoma di Ewing e il retinoblastoma; altre cause di alterazione midollare primaria sono l'anemia aplastica (congenita o acquisita) e la mielofibrosi. L'alterazione di una singola linea cellulare, come si osserva nell'anemia eritroblastica transitoria, nella trombocitopenia autoimmune e nella neutropenia congenita o acquisita, talora è difficilmente distinguibile dall'ALL e può essere necessario effettuare un esame del midollo osseo. Altre diagnosi differenziali per l'ALL riguardano la mononucleosi infettiva in pazienti con esordio acuto di febbre e linfoadenopatia e l'artrite reumatoide in soggetti con febbre ed edema articolare. Anche questi quadri possono richiedere la biopsia midollare per una diagnosi precisa.

TRATTAMENTO. Il fattore prognostico più importante nell'ALL è il trattamento: senza un'adeguata terapia, la malattia è fatale. Negli ultimi 40 anni, la sopravvivenza dei bambini con l'ALL è aumentata grazie ai trial clinici, che hanno permesso di migliorare le terapie e l'evoluzione della malattia (Fig. 495-2).

La scelta del trattamento si fonda sulla stima del rischio clinico di ricaduta nel singolo paziente, che varia in modo significativo tra i diversi sottotipi dell'ALL. I tre fattori predittivi principali sono l'età del paziente al momento della diagnosi, il numero di leucociti all'esordio e la velocità di risposta al trattamento (cioè quanto rapidamente le cellule leucemiche vengono eliminate dal midollo o dal sangue periferico). Differenti gruppi di studio utilizzano elementi diversi per definire il rischio, ma l'età compresa tra 1-10 anni e una conta dei leucociti <50 000/μL sono largamente adoperati per definire un rischio medio, mentre bambini di età >10 anni o con una conta leucocitaria iniziale >50 000 sono considerati a rischio alto. La prognosi dei pazienti a rischio più elevato può essere migliorata con la somministrazione di una terapia più intensa, anche se con un maggiore pericolo di tossicità. I bambini con l'ALL e quelli con specifiche alterazioni cromosomiche, quali t(9;22) o t(4;11), presentano un rischio di recidiva ancora maggiore, anche se vengono trattati con terapia intensiva. Trial clinici hanno dimostrato che la prognosi dei pazienti con una risposta più lenta alla terapia può migliorare con un trattamento maggiormente aggressivo rispetto a quello considerato necessario per i soggetti che rispondono in tempi più brevi.

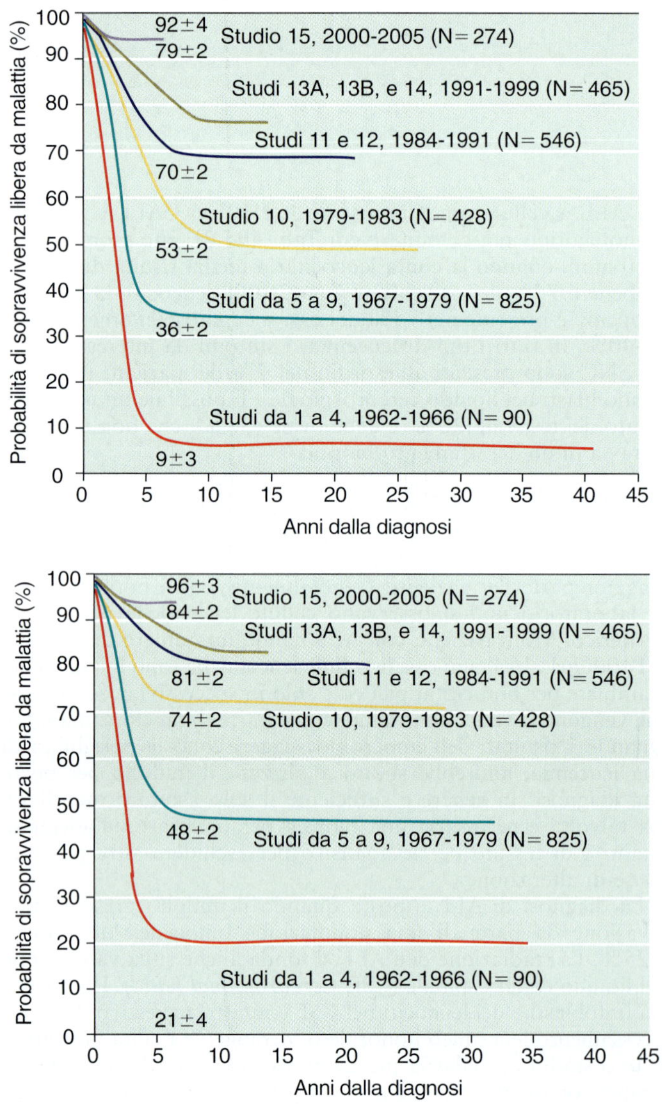

Figura 495-2. Analisi secondo Kaplan-Meier della sopravvivenza libera da malattia (*A*) e della sopravvivenza globale (*B*) su 2628 bambini con nuova diagnosi di ALL. I pazienti sono stati arruolati in 15 studi consecutivi condotti al St. Jude Children's Research Hospital dal 1962 al 2005. Sono illustrate la stima di assenza di malattia a 5 anni e quella della sopravvivenza globale (±SE, *Survival Estimate*), eccetto che per lo Studio 15, di cui sono disponibili solo i risultati preliminari a 4 anni. I risultati dimostrano un continuo miglioramento dell'andamento clinico nelle ultime 4 decadi. La differenza delle percentuali della libertà da malattia e della sopravvivenza globale si riducono nei periodi più recenti, suggerendo che le ricadute o i secondi tumori che si verificano dopo le attuali terapie sono più refrattari ai trattamenti. (Da Pui CH, Evans WE: Treatment of acute lymphoblastic leukemia. *N Engl J Med* 2006;354:166-178.)

La maggior parte dei bambini con l'ALL è trattata all'interno di trial clinici condotti da gruppi cooperativi nazionali o internazionali. Generalmente, la terapia iniziale è disegnata per estirpare le cellule leucemiche dal midollo osseo, nella fase nota come **induzione della remissione**. Durante questa fase, la terapia è solitamente somministrata per 4 settimane e consiste in vincristina settimanale, corticosteroidi quali desametazone o prednisone e dosi ripetute di L-asparaginasi o una singola dose di una preparazione a lunga durata di asparaginasi pegilata. Si possono anche utilizzare citarabina o metotrexato per via intratecale, oppure entrambi. I pazienti a rischio più alto ricevono inoltre la daunomicina a intervalli settimanali. Con questo approccio, il 98% dei pazienti va in **remissione**, definita per la presenza di <5% di blasti nel midollo e un ritorno dei leucociti e delle piastrine ai valori nell'intervallo di normalità dopo 4-5 settimane dall'inizio del trattamento. La chemioterapia intratecale si impiega in genere all'inizio della terapia e poi ancora durante l'induzione.

La seconda fase del trattamento è focalizzata sulla **terapia del SNC**, nel tentativo di prevenire le ricadute tardive. La chemioterapia intratecale è somministrata ripetutamente per mezzo di rachicentesi in concomitanza con la chemioterapia sistemica intensiva. La probabilità di ricaduta tardiva sul SNC è in questo modo ridotta a <5%. Una piccola percentuale di soggetti con caratteristiche che predicono un alto rischio di recidiva a livello del SNC può essere sottoposta a radioterapia craniospinale, cui sono specialmente candidati coloro che, al momento della diagnosi, hanno linfoblasti e un aumento dei leucociti nel CSF o segni di leucemia estesa a livello del SNC, come la presenza di paralisi dei nervi cranici.

Dopo che è stata indotta la remissione, molti regimi prevedono 14-28 settimane di politerapia con farmaci e schedule variamente combinate a seconda del gruppo di rischio del paziente. Per finire, i pazienti assumono quotidianamente la mercaptopurina e settimanalmente il metotrexato, in genere con dosi intermittenti di vincristina e corticosteroidi. Questo periodo, noto come **fase di mantenimento** della terapia, dura dai 2 ai 3 anni, a seconda del protocollo utilizzato. Molti pazienti beneficiano della somministrazione di una fase intensiva ritardata del trattamento (intensificazione ritardata), circa 5-7 mesi dopo l'inizio della terapia e dopo una fase di relativa non tossicità (durante il mantenimento), per permettere un recupero dall'inizio della terapia intensiva. Un piccolo numero di soggetti con fattori prognostici particolarmente sfavorevoli, soprattutto quelli con la traslocazione t(9;22), nota come cromosoma di Philadelphia, possono essere sottoposti a un trapianto di midollo osseo durante la prima remissione. Questo cromosoma dell'ALL è simile, ma non identico, al cromosoma di Philadelphia della leucemia mieloide cronica (CML).

Il trattamento può anche essere stratificato in relazione ai profili di espressione genica delle cellule leucemiche. In particolare, l'espressione di riarrangiamenti genici indotta dall'esposizione ad agenti chemioterapici può essere predittiva di quali pazienti hanno un'ALL resistente ai farmaci (vedi Capitolo 494). Inoltre, il **test**

farmacogenetico per il gene della tiopurina S-metiltransferasi, che converte la mercaptopurina o la tioguanina (entrambi pro-farmaci) in agenti chemioterapici attivi, permette di individuare i metabolizzatori rapidi (associati all'effetto tossico) o i metabolizzatori lenti (associati all'inefficacia del trattamento), rendendo possibile l'ottimizzazione del dosaggio dei farmaci (vedi Capitolo 56).

Il principale ostacolo alla guarigione è la recidiva della malattia, che si realizza al livello del midollo osseo nel 15-20% dei pazienti con l'ALL e si correla a gravi conseguenze, soprattutto se ha luogo durante o subito dopo il completamento della terapia. Una chemioterapia intensiva con farmaci non utilizzati in precedenza, seguita da un trapianto allogenico di cellule staminali, può aumentare la sopravvivenza a lungo termine di alcuni casi con recidiva midollare (vedi Capitolo 134).

I soggetti con una recidiva a livello del SNC generalmente presentano i segni e i sintomi di ipertensione endocranica e possono avere isolate paralisi dei nervi cranici. La diagnosi è prontamente confermata dalla dimostrazione della presenza delle cellule leucemiche nel CSF e raramente da esami radiologici. Il trattamento prevede la somministrazione di farmaci per via intratecale e l'irradiazione craniospinale. Deve essere impostata anche una chemioterapia sistemica, in quanto questi pazienti sono ad alto rischio di una recidiva anche a livello midollare. La maggior parte dei soggetti con recidiva leucemica limitata al SNC va bene, soprattutto quelli in cui essa si verifica dopo che la chemioterapia è stata completata o durante l'ultima fase del trattamento.

Una ricaduta testicolare si osserva nell'1-2% dei bambini con l'ALL, in genere dopo il completamento della terapia. Questa ricaduta si presenta con un edema non dolente di uno o entrambi i testicoli e la diagnosi è confermata con la biopsia del testicolo colpito. Il trattamento prevede una chemioterapia sistemica e una radioterapia locale. Un'alta percentuale di questi bambini può essere ritrattata con successo e la sopravvivenza è buona.

TERAPIA DI SUPPORTO. Una particolare attenzione alle terapie mediche di supporto è essenziale per gestire con successo i programmi di chemioterapia aggressiva. I pazienti con estese masse tumorali sono a rischio di sviluppare una sindrome da lisi tumorale, nel momento in cui si inizia la terapia. L'insufficienza renale associata a valori molto alti di acido urico sierico può essere prevenuta con l'urato ossidasi. La chemioterapia spesso provoca una grave mielosoppressione, che può rendere necessario trasfondere emazie e piastrine e che spesso richiede la somministrazione empirica di potenti antibiotici ad ampio spettro in caso di sepsi febbrile neutropenica. I pazienti devono ricevere un trattamento profilattico per la polmonite da *Pneumocystis carinii* durante la chemioterapia e per alcuni mesi dopo il suo completamento.

L'efficacia della terapia ha trasformato l'ALL da malattia acuta con un elevato indice di mortalità a malattia cronica. Tuttavia, il trattamento cronico può portare serie conseguenze educative, per lo sviluppo e psicosociali ai bambini con l'ALL, nonché considerevoli costi economici e stress per i loro familiari. A causa dell'intensità della terapia, si possono verificare effetti tossici tardivi e acuti. È essenziale la presenza di uno schieramento di professionisti per la terapia delle malattie neoplastiche, adeguatamente addestrati ed esperti nella gestione della moltitudine di problematiche che possono derivare, per ridurre le complicanze e ottenere risultati migliori.

PROGNOSI. Al giorno d'oggi, la maggior parte dei bambini con l'ALL può avere una lunga aspettativa di vita, con una sopravvivenza a 5 anni dalla diagnosi >80% (vedi Fig. 495-2). Il principale fattore prognostico è la scelta della terapia strettamente correlata al rischio, mentre gli altri fattori sono il genere di trattamento scelto in relazione al tipo di ALL, lo stadio della malattia, l'età del paziente e l'entità della risposta alla prima terapia (favorevole se il paziente risponde in <1 mese). Gli elementi comunemente considerati sfavorevoli sono una età <1 anno o >10 anni al momento della diagnosi, una leucocitosi >100 000/μL alla diagnosi o una risposta lenta alla prima terapia. Le alterazioni cromosomiche, quali le ipodiploidie, il cromosoma Philadelphia, i riarrangiamenti genici MLL e le traslocazioni [t(1:19) o t(4;11)], sono indici prognostici negativi. Caratteristiche più favorevoli comprendono la rapida risposta al trattamento, la iperdiploidia, la trisomia di specifici cromosomi e il riarrangiamento di TEL/AML1.

La **minima malattia residua** (**MRD**) può essere valutata con specifiche sonde molecolari per le traslocazioni e con altri marcatori del DNA contenuto nelle cellule leucemiche. La MRD può essere quantitativa e fornire una stima di quante cellule leucemiche sono ancora presenti nel midollo. Sebbene non sia noto quanta MRD possa essere eliminata dai meccanismi di difesa immunitaria del paziente, la presenza di un suo alto grado al termine dell'induzione è suggestiva per una prognosi sfavorevole e per un aumentato rischio di recidiva.

Balduzzi A, Valsecchi MG, Uderzo C, et al: Chemotherapy versus allogeneic transplantation for very-high-risk childhood acute lymphoblastic leukaemia in first complete remission: Comparison by genetic randomization in an international prospective study. *Lancet* 2005;366:635–642.

Carroll WL, Bhojwani D, Min DJ, et al: Pediatric acute lymphoblastic leukemia. *Hematology Am Soc Hematol Educ Program* 2003:102–131.

Claudio J, Rocha C, Cheng C, et al: Pharmacogenetics of outcome in children with acute lymphoblastic leukemia. *Blood* 2005;105:4752–4758.

Hijiya N, Hudson MM, Lensing S, et al: Cumulative incidence of secondary neoplasms as a first event after childhood acute lymphoblastic leukemia. *JAMA* 2007;297:1207–1215.

Holleman A, Cheok MH, den Boer ML, et al: Gene-expression patterns in drug-resistant acute lymphoblastic leukemia cells and response to treatment. *N Engl J Med* 2004;351:533–542.

Kadan-Lottick NS, Ness KK, Bhatia S, et al: Survival variability by race and ethnicity in childhood acute lymphoblastic leukemia. *JAMA* 2003;290:2008–2014.

Murray MJ, Tang T, Ryder C, et al: Childhood leukaemia masquerading as juvenile idiopathic arthritis. *BMJ* 2004;329:959–961.

Pui CH, Cheng C, Leung W, et al: Extended follow-up of long-term survivors of childhood acute lymphoblastic leukemia. *N Engl J Med* 2003;349:640–648.

Pui CH, Evans WE: Treatment of acute lymphoblastic leukemia. *N Engl J Med* 2006;354:166–178.

Pui CH, Relling MV, Downing JR: Acute lymphoblastic leukemia. *N Engl J Med* 2004;350:1535–1548.

Ravindranath Y: Down syndrome and leukemia: New insights into the epidemiology, pathogenesis, and treatment. *Pediatric Blood & Cancer* 2005;44:1–7.

Saha V: Simplifying treatment for children with ALL. *Lancet* 2007;369: 82–83.

Stanulla M, Schaeffeler E, Flohr T, et al: Thiopurine methyltransferase (TPMT) genotype and early treatment response to mercaptopurine in childhood acute lymphoblastic leukemia. *JAMA* 2005;293:1485–1489.

Stanulla M, Schünemann HJ: Thioguanine versus mercaptopurine in childhood ALL. *Lancet* 2006;368:1304–1306.

Winick NJ, Carroll WL, Hunger SP: Childhood leukemia—new advances and challenges. *N Engl J Med* 2004;351:601–604.

495.2 • Leucemia mieloide acuta

EPIDEMIOLOGIA. L'AML è responsabile dell'11% dei casi di leucemia infantile negli Stati Uniti, con circa 370 nuove diagnosi ogni anno. Un sottotipo, la leucemia acuta promielocitica, è più frequente in alcune regioni del mondo, ma la diffusione degli altri tipi è generalmente uniforme. Sono state individuate diverse alterazioni cromosomiche associate all'AML, ma nella maggior parte dei pazienti non è possibile identificare fattori genetici o ambientali predisponenti (vedi Tab. 495-3). D'altro canto, sono stati individuati numerosi fattori di rischio, tra cui le radiazioni ionizzanti, gli agenti chemioterapici (agenti alchilanti, epipodofillotossine), i solventi organici, l'emoglobinuria parossistica notturna e alcune sindromi come quella di Down, l'anemia di Fanconi, la sindrome di Bloom, la sindrome di Kostmann, la sindrome di Shwachman-Diamond, la sindrome di Diamond-Blackfan, la sindrome di Li-Fraumeni e la neurofibromatosi di tipo 1.

PATOGENESI. L'elemento distintivo dell'AML è che >30% delle cellule del midollo osseo sulla preparazione ottenuta dall'aspirato o dalla biopsia midollare rappresenta una popolazione di blasti abbastanza omogenea, con caratteristiche simili a quelle degli stati precoci di differenziazione della serie mielo-mono-megacariocitica. La più nota classificazione in sottotipi dell'LMA è il sistema FAB (Tab. 495-4), che tuttavia si basa sul solo aspetto morfologico, mentre nella pratica corrente è necessario l'uso della citometria di flusso per l'identificazione degli antigeni di superficie e delle tecniche per lo studio dei cromosomi e di genetica molecolare per fare indagini più precise e per mirare la scelta della terapia.

MANIFESTAZIONI CLINICHE. I sintomi e i segni dell'AML, come avviene nell'ALL, sono dovuti all'invasione del midollo osseo da parte di cellule maligne e alla conseguente insufficienza midollare. Sicché i pazienti con l'AML possono presentare alcuni o tutti i disturbi associati all'**insufficienza midollare** dell'ALL. In più, questi soggetti manifestano segni e sintomi non propri dell'ALL, quali i **noduli sottocutanei** o le lesioni cutanee di colore violaceo ("blueberry muffin"), gli infiltrati gengivali, segni e reperti di laboratorio di **coagulazione intravascolare disseminata** (tipica della leucemia acuta promielocitica) e masse distinte, note come **cloromi** o **sarcomi granulocitici**. Queste masse possono essere osservate in assenza di un chiaro coinvolgimento midollare e sono tipiche della sottocategoria M2 dell'ALM con la traslocazione t(8;21). I cloromi si possono anche osservare a livello dell'orbita o dello spazio epidurale. I sintomi da interessamento del SNC sono molto più comuni nell'ALM che nell'ALL.

DIAGNOSI. L'aspirato e la biopsia midollari dei pazienti con l'ALM tipicamente rivelano la presenza di un midollo ipercellulato, con presenza di cellule piuttosto simili tra loro, con caratteristiche che permettono la sottoclassificazione FAB della malattia. Speciali colorazioni consentono di identificare le cellule contenenti la mieloperossidasi, che conferma sia l'origine mielogenica della leucemia sia la diagnosi. Alcune alterazioni cromosomiche e alcuni marker genetico-molecolari sono caratteristici di specifici sottotipi (vedi Tab. 495-2).

TRATTAMENTO. Una polichemioterapia aggressiva è efficace per indurre la remissione in circa l'80% dei pazienti. Una terapia mirata verso specifici marker genetici può risultare efficace (Tab. 495-5). Oltre il 10% dei pazienti muore per infezioni o emorragie prima di ottenere la remissione. Il trapianto del midollo o di cellule staminali da parte di consanguinei dopo la remissione ha dimostrato di migliorare la sopravvivenza libera da malattia nel 60-70% dei pazienti. La chemioterapia continuativa, per i soggetti che non hanno un donatore, è meno efficace del trapianto di midollo, ma in alcuni è comunque curativa. I trapianti di midollo o di cellule staminali da non consanguinei possono costituire una terapia efficace, ma comportano un rischio significativo di graft-versus-host disease, oltre alle complicanze associate con la terapia intensiva mieloablativa. Un elemento a favore del trapianto allogenico è tuttavia che pure se l'effetto **graft-versus-leukemia** si verifica nell'ALM, è difficile dimostrare che abbia luogo quando sia di cellule staminali ematopoietiche in pazienti con l'ALL.

La leucemia acuta promielocitica, caratterizzata da un riarrangiamento genico che coinvolge il recettore per l'acido retinoico, è molto responsiva alla somministrazione di **acido retinoico** in associazione con le antracicline. L'efficacia di questa terapia rende superfluo il trapianto di midollo alla prima remissione.

La terapia di supporto per i pazienti affetti dall'ALM è sostanzialmente la stessa dei soggetti con l'ALL. Il trattamento intensivo provoca una soppressione midollare prolungata con un'alta incidenza di infezioni gravi.

TABELLA 495-4. Classificazione franco-americano-britannica (FAB) delle leucemie mielogeniche acute

SOTTOTIPO	NOME COMUNE
M1	Leucemia mieloblastica acuta senza maturazione
M2	Leucemia mieloblastica acuta con maturazione
M3	Leucemia acuta promielocitica
M4	Leucemia acuta mielomonocitica
M5	Leucemia acuta monocitica
M6	Eritroleucemia
M7	Leucemia acuta megacariocitaria

Clark JJ, Smith FO, Arceci RJ: Update in childhood acute myeloid leukemia: Recent developments in the molecular basis of disease and novel therapies. *Curr Opin Hematol* 2003;10:31–39.

Cushing T, Clericuzio C, Wilson C, et al: Risk for leukemia in infants without Down syndrome who have transient myeloproliferative disorder. *J Pediatr* 2006;148:687–689.

Kantarjian H, Giles F, Wunderle L, et al: Nilotinib in imatinib-resistant CML and Philadelphia chromosome-positive ALL. *N Engl J Med* 2006;354:2542–2550.

Kolb EA, Pan Q, Ladanyi M, et al: Imatinib mesylate in Philadelphia chromosome-positive leukemia of childhood. *Cancer* 2003;98:2643–2650.

Linabery AM, Olshan AF, Gamis AS, et al: Exposure to medical test irradiation and acute leukemia among children with Down Syndrome: A report from the children's oncology group. *Pediatrics* 2006;118:e1499–e1508.

Pui CH, Relling MV, Downing JR: Acute lymphoblastic leukemia. *N Engl J Med* 2004;350:1535–1548.

Ross ME, Mahfouz R, Onciu M et al: Gene expression profiling of pediatric acute myelogenous leukemia. *Blood* 2004;104:3679–3687.

Talpaz M, Shah NP, Kantarjian H, et al: Dasatinib in imatinib-resistant Philadelphia chromosome-positive leukemias. *N Engl J Med* 2006;354: 2531–2540.

TABELLA 495-5. Implicazioni terapeutiche delle alterazioni cromosomiche comuni nelle leucemie mielogeniche acute pediatriche e nelle sindromi mielodisplasiche

ALTERAZIONI CROMOSOMICHE	GENI ALTERATI	NORMALE MORFOLOGIA	PROGNOSI	TRATTAMENTO RACCOMANDATO
t(8;21)	*AML1-ETO*	FAB AML-M2	Favorevole	Chemioterapia intensiva, con alte dosi di citarabina
inv(16), t(16;16)	*CBFB-MYHII*	FAB AML-M4Eo	Favorevole	Chemioterapia intensiva, con alte dosi di citarabina
t(15;17)	*PML-RARA*	FAB AML-M3	Favorevole	Chemioterapia intensiva, con ATRA e antracicline
t(11;17)	*PLZF-RARA*	FAB AML-M3	Favorevole	Chemioterapia intensiva, con ATRA e antracicline
alterazioni di 11q23	riarrangiamenti *MLL*	FAB AML-M4 o AML-M5	Sfavorevole	Chemioterapia intensiva, con alte dosi di citarabina e MRD HSCT
t(3;v)	*EVI1*	MDS/AML	Sfavorevole	Chemioterapia intensiva con o senza HSCT
t(3;5)	*NPM-MLF*	MDS/AMS	Sfavorevole	Chemioterapia intensiva con o senza HSCT
del(7q), −7	Sconosciuto	MDS/FAB AML-M0	Sfavorevole	Chemioterapia intensiva con o senza HSCT
del(5q), −5	Sconosciuto	MDS/FAB AML-M0	Sfavorevole	Chemioterapia intensiva con o senza HSCT

Da Nathan DG, Orkin SH, Ginsburg D, et al (editors): *Nathan and Oski's Hematology of Infancy and Childhood*, 6th ed. Philadelphia, WB Saunders, 2003, p. 1177.
AML, leucemia mielocitica acuta; ATRA, acido trans retinoico (*All-Trans Retinoic Acid*); FAB, classificazione franco-americano-britannica; HSCT, trapianto di cellule staminali ematopoietiche (*Hematopoietic Stem Cell Transplantation*); MDS, sindromi mielodisplastiche (*Myelodysplastic Syndrome*); MRD, *Matched Related Donor*.

Woods WG, Barnard DR, Alonzo TA, et al: Prospective study of 90 children requiring treatment for juvenile myelomonocytic leukemia or myelodysplastic syndrome. *J Clin Oncol* 2002;20:434–440.

Woods WG, Neudorf S, Gold S, et al: A comparison of allogeneic bone marrow transplantation, autologous bone marrow transplantation, and aggressive chemotherapy in children with acute myeloid leukemia in remission. *Blood* 2001;97:56–62.

495.3 • Sindrome di Down, leucemia acuta e mieloproliferazione

La leucemia acuta si verifica 14 volte più di frequente nei bambini con la sindrome di Down che non nella popolazione generale (vedi Capitolo 81), mentre la proporzione fra ALL e ALM in questi bambini resta la stessa. Negli affetti dall'ALL il risultato atteso per il trattamento è identico a quello degli altri bambini, ma i pazienti con la sindrome di Down sono particolarmente sensibili al metotrexato e ad altri antimetaboliti, che possono risultare più tossici se somministrati alle dosi standard. I pazienti con la sindrome di Down e l'ALM, comunque, hanno una prognosi migliore, con >80% di lunghe sopravvivenze. Dopo la fase di induzione, questi soggetti necessitano inoltre di una terapia meno aggressiva per raggiungere i medesimi risultati.

Circa il 10% dei neonati con la sindrome di Down può sviluppare una leucemia transitoria o una sindrome **mieloproliferativa** caratterizzata da un aumento dei leucociti e dalla presenza di blasti nel sangue periferico, in associazione ad anemia, trombocitopenia ed epatosplenomegalia. Questo quadro in genere si risolve nell'arco di alcuni giorni o poche settimane dall'esordio. Anche se questi neonati possono avere bisogno di un temporaneo supporto trasfusionale, non necessitano di chemioterapia. Ciononostante, i pazienti con la sindrome di Down che sviluppano questa leucemia transitoria o una sindrome mieloproliferativa vanno sottoposti a un attento follow-up, in quanto il 20-30% di loro svilupperà una leucemia tipica (spesso acuta megacariocitica) dopo i 3 anni di vita (in media a 16 mesi). Nei blasti dei soggetti con la sindrome di Down con malattia mielolinfoproliferativa transitoria o con leucemia sono presenti mutazioni del *GATA1* (un fattore di trascrizione che controlla la megacariopoiesi). La malattia mielolinfoproliferativa transitoria può colpire anche pazienti che non hanno le caratteristiche fenotipiche della sindrome di Down, i blasti dei quali possono avere una trisomia 21, suggerendo un mosaicismo.

495.4 • Leucemia mieloide cronica

La CML è una malattia clonale del tessuto ematopoietico che rappresenta il 2-3% di tutte le leucemie dell'infanzia. In circa il 99% dei casi vi sono traslocazioni specifiche t(9;22)(q34;q11), note come **cromosoma Philadelphia**. La malattia è stata associata all'esposizione a radiazioni ionizzanti, ma in realtà solo pochi bambini con la CML hanno subito tale pregressa esposizione. La malattia è caratterizzata clinicamente da una iniziale fase cronica in cui il clone neoplastico produce un elevato numero di leucociti con prevalenza di forme mature, ma con un aumentato numero di granulociti immaturi. La **milza** è spesso ingrossata e provoca frequentemente un dolore a livello del quadrante superiore sinistro dell'addome. Oltre alla leucocitosi, sono evidenti una lieve anemia e una trombocitopenia.

Tipicamente la fase cronica dura per 3-4 anni, quindi la CML evolve verso un'accelerazione, o "crisi blastica". A questo punto, gli elementi del sangue aumentano enormemente e non è possibile controllarli con farmaci come le idrossiuree. Si possono poi osservare altre manifestazioni, quali l'iperuricemia e i sintomi neurologici, che sono correlati con l'incremento della viscosità ematica con una conseguente ridotta perfusione del SNC.

I sintomi di presentazione della CML sono aspecifici e possono comprendere febbre, astenia, perdita di peso e anoressia. Può anche aversi la splenomegalia. La diagnosi è suggerita dall'aumento del numero di cellule mieloidi differenziate in forme mature nel sangue periferico e nel midollo osseo ed è confermata dagli studi di citogenetica che dimostrano la presenza del caratteristico cromosoma Philadelphia. Le tecniche di biologia molecolare generalmente permettono di evidenziare il riarrangiamento del gene **BCR-ABL**. Questa traslocazione, anche se tipica della CML, si osserva peraltro anche in una piccola percentuale di pazienti con l'ALL o l'ALM.

L'**imatinib mesilato**, un agente specifico per l'inibizione della tirosina chinasi di BCR-ABL, è stato utilizzato negli adulti e ha dimostrato di poter dare buone risposte in oltre il 70% dei pazienti (vedi Tab. 494-1). La limitata esperienza nei bambini suggerisce che potrebbe essere impiegato tranquillamente, con risultati paragonabili a quelli osservati negli adulti. Nell'attesa di poterlo somministrare, i segni e i sintomi della CML, disabilitanti e minacciosi per la vita durante la fase cronica, possono essere controllati con le idrossouree, che determinano un graduale ritorno dei leucociti a valori normali. Si ottengono risposte morfologiche e citogenetiche protratte, ma la possibilità di ristabilimento è aumentata dal trapianto allogenico di cellule staminali o di midollo, con guarigioni superiori all'80% dei casi.

495.5 • Leucemia mieloide cronica giovanile

La JCML, nota anche come leucemia mielomonocitica giovanile, è una proliferazione clonale di cellule staminali ematopoietiche che generalmente colpisce bambini <2 anni. I pazienti affetti non hanno il cromosoma Philadelphia, tipico della CML; presentano rash cutanei, linfoadenopatia e splenomegalia. L'emocromo spesso evidenzia un aumento dei leucociti, talora trombocitopenia ed eritroblasti. Il midollo osseo possiede un pattern mielodisplastico, con i blasti che rappresentano <30% delle cellule. Non sono evidenti alterazioni citogenetiche specifiche. La JCML è rara, costituendo <2% di tutte le leucemie infantili; i pazienti con neurofibromatosi di tipo 1 hanno comunque una predisposizione a svilupparla. I trattamenti adottati sono soprattutto aneddotici. Il trapianto di cellule staminali rappresenta la migliore opportunità di guarigione, che tuttavia resta inferiore a quella della classica CML.

495.6 • Leucemia infantile

Circa il 2% dei casi di leucemia durante l'infanzia si verifica prima dell'anno di vita. Diversamente da quanto capita nei bambini più grandi, la proporzione tra l'ALL e l'ALM è di 2:1. Alcuni casi sembrano dovuti all'esposizione della madre agli inibitori della topoisomerasi II del DNA. Sono caratteristiche dell'ALL infantile alcune alterazioni biologiche isolate e una prognosi particolarmente severa. Oltre i due terzi dei casi presentano un riarrangiamento del gene MLL a livello della banda di traslocazione 11q23; questo sottogruppo di pazienti è quello con il rischio maggiore di ricaduta. Questi soggetti spesso presentano un'iperleucocitosi ed estese infiltrazioni tissutali, che provocano un'organomegalia, compreso l'interessamento del SNC. I noduli sottocutanei noti come **leucemia cutanea** e la tachipnea da diffusa infiltrazione polmonare da parte delle cellule leucemiche si osservano molto più spesso nei neonati che non nei bambini più grandi. L'aspetto morfologico delle cellule leucemiche è generalmente quello di grossi linfoblasti irregolari (FAB L2), con un fenotipo negativo per il CD10 (cALLa).

Programmi di chemioterapia particolarmente intensiva comprendenti il trapianto di cellule staminali sono stati studiati per i bambini con riarrangiamento della banda 11q23 di MLL, ma nessuno ha ancora dimostrato la sua efficacia. I neonati affetti da una leucemia senza il riarrangiamento di 11q23 hanno una prognosi simile a quella dei bambini più grandi con l'ALL. I neonati con l'ALM spesso presentano un coinvolgimento del SNC o della cute e hanno il sottotipo FAB M4, che è comunemente definito **leucemia mielomonocitica acuta**. Il trattamento è lo stesso di quello per i bambini più grandi con l'ALM. È necessaria una meticolosa terapia di supporto per via della giovane età e della necessità di una terapia aggressiva.

Bajwa RPS, Skinner R, Windebank KP, et al: Demographic study of leukaemia presenting within the first 3 months of life in the Northern Health Region of England. *J Clin Pathol* 2004;57:186–188.

Capitolo 496 ■ Linfomi

Mitchell S. Cairo e M. Brigid Bradley

Il linfoma è la terza neoplasia più comune tra i bambini degli Stati Uniti, con un'incidenza annuale di 15 casi per 1 milione di bambini di età ≤14 anni. Le due principali categorie di linfoma, linfoma o malattia di Hodgkin (HD, *Hodgkin Disease*) e il linfoma non-Hodgkin (NHL, *Non-Hodgkin Lymphoma*), hanno manifestazioni cliniche e trattamenti differenti.

496.1 • Linfoma di Hodgkin

L'HD è una neoplasia del sistema linforeticolare che rappresenta il 6% delle neoplasie infantili. Negli Stati Uniti costituisce anche circa il 5% di quelle in persone con ≤14 anni e circa il 15% tra 15-19 anni. È invece rara nei bambini con <10 anni.

EPIDEMIOLOGIA. L'incidenza dell'HD presenta un andamento bimodale, in relazione all'età. Nei Paesi industrializzati il primo picco si ha intorno ai 20 anni e il secondo dopo i 50, mentre nei Paesi in via di sviluppo il primo picco si ha prima dell'adolescenza. Tra i bambini piccoli è stata osservata una predominanza dei maschi sulle femmine, con una proporzione di 4:1 per i bambini di età compresa fra 3-7 anni, 3:1 per quelli tra 7-9 anni e 1,3:1 per quelli di età >10 anni. La maggiore diffusione in singole famiglie o razze può suggerire una predisposizione genetica o una comune esposizione a un agente eziologico. Il rischio per un gemello omozigote di un bambino affetto è di 100 volte, mentre per i gemelli eterozigoti il rischio non risulta aumentato. Studi su famiglie fanno pensare a una incrementata associazione dell'HD con specifici antigeni HLA. Diverse ricerche suggeriscono che possono essere coinvolti agenti infettivi, come l'herpes virus 6, il Cytomegalovirus e il virus di Epstein-Barr (EBV, *Epstein-Barr Virus*). Il ruolo di quest'ultimo è supportato da studi sierologici prospettici. Un vasto numero di pazienti con l'HD e con elevati titoli anticorpali per l'HBV suggerisce che l'infezione da EBV può precedere lo sviluppo dell'HD, una possibilità che è supportata anche dall'evidenza del genoma dell'EBV con l'ibridazione *in situ* nelle cellule Reed-Sternberg. Gli antigeni per l'EBV sono stati rinvenuti in tessuti dell'HD, anche se la presenza dell'EBV non costituisce un elemento prognostico. L'HD può essere il risultato finale di processi patologici multipli, compresa l'infezione virale e l'esposizione dell'ospite geneticamente predisposto a un agente sensibilizzante. Una pre-esistente immunodeficienza, sia congenita, come l'atassia-teleangectasia, sia acquisita, come l'infezione da HIV, aumenta il rischio di sviluppare l'HD.

EZIOLOGIA. La **cellula di Reed-Sternberg** (Fig. 496-1*E*) è una grossa cellula (15-45 μm di diametro) con nucleo multiplo o plurilobato. È l'elemento tipico dell'HD, anche se cellule simili si osservano nella mononucleosi infettiva, nell'NHL e in altre malattie. Ha una origine clonale e deriva dalle cellule germinali B centrali. L'HD è caratterizzata da un numero variabile di cellule circondate da un infiltrato infiammatorio di linfociti, plasmacellule ed eosinofili in proporzioni differenti, a seconda del sottotipo istologico dell'HD. Altre caratteristiche che distinguono il sottotipo istologico comprendono vari gradi di fibrosi e la presenza di bande di collagene, di necrosi o di cellule reticolari maligne.

Il **sistema di classificazione di Rye** (Tab. 496-1) definisce quattro principali sottotipi istologici: predominanza linfocitaria (**LP**, *Lymphocyte Predominant*) (Fig. 496-1*A* e *B*), sclerosi nodulare (**NS**, *Nodular Sclerosing*) (Fig. 496-1C), cellularità mista (**MC**, *Mixed Cellularity*) (Fig. 496-1*D*) e deplezione linfocitaria (**LD**, *Lymphocyte Depleted*). La LP colpisce il 10-15% dei pazienti, è più comune tra i maschi, interessa i più giovani e generalmente si presenta come malattia localizzata. La MC si osserva nel 30% dei casi, è più comune tra i bambini ≤10 anni e spesso si presenta come una malattia avanzata estesa a livello extralinfonodale. La LD è rara nei bambini, ma frequente nei pazienti con infezione da HIV. La NS, infine, è il sottotipo più comune, interessa il 40% dei pazienti più giovani e il 70% degli adolescenti con l'HD.

Il **sistema di classificazione secondo la Revised European-American Classification of Lymphoid Neoplasms** (**REAL**) (vedi Tab. 496-1) include due variazioni rispetto al più vecchio sistema Rye. Oltre alla classica malattia di Hodgkin, esso prevede la predominanza linfocitaria (LPHD) e anche il linfoma Hodgkin-like anaplastico a grandi cellule. Il sottotipo a predominanza linfocitaria è molto simile dal punto di vista clinico e per il fenotipo delle cellule di Reed-Sternberg al linfoma a cellule B di basso grado. La maggior parte dei pazienti con l'LPHD si presenta con una malattia di recente insorgenza e ha un'ottima prognosi. Il linfoma Hodgkin-like anaplastico a grandi cellule risponde poco alla chemioterapia convenzionale per l'HD ed è stato riportato che ha una risposta migliore ai regimi più aggressivi utilizzati per l'NHL. L'HD sembra originare dal tessuto linfoide e si diffonde ai linfonodi adiacenti secondo una modalità relativamente ordinata. Può manifestare una disseminazione per via ematogena, con l'interessamento di fegato, milza, osso, midollo osseo o cervello e generalmente si accompagna a sintomi sistemici. È stato dimostrato che i livelli sierici di diverse **citochine**, ottenute sia da linee cellulari coltivate sia da tessuto di HD, risultano aumentati. Le citochine possono essere responsabili dei sintomi sistemici quali la febbre e la sudorazione notturna (interleuchina 1 o 2) e della perdita di peso (fattore di necrosi tissutale), oltre a influire sulla proliferazione delle cellule di Reed-Sternberg e a indurre l'immunosoppressione (fattore di crescita trasformante-β). Possono essere identificati vari gradi di **alterazione immunitaria cellulare** nella maggior parte dei casi di nuova diagnosi di HD. La severità del deficit immunitario varia con l'estensione della malattia e persiste perfino dopo una terapia efficace, ma non è noto se questo fenomeno predispone alla malattia o se ne sia una conseguenza.

MANIFESTAZIONI CLINICHE. I pazienti presentano di frequente una linfoadenopatia cervicale o sovraclaveare non dolente, duro-elastica, fissa e palpabile. I linfonodi interessati sono più fissi di quelli infiammatori. La maggior parte dei casi possiede vari gradi di interessamento mediastinico. Una epatosplenomegalia clinicamente evidente viene osservata di rado. In relazione all'estensione e alla localizzazione della malattia linfonodale ed extralinfonodale, i pazienti possono manifestare sintomi e segni per l'ostruzione delle vie aeree (dispnea, ipossia, tosse), un versamento pleurico o pericardio, un'insufficienza epatica o una infiltrazione midollare (anemia, neutropenia o trombocitopenia). L'interessamento sottodiaframmatico è raro e si verifica in circa il 3% dei casi. I **sintomi sistemici**, classificati come **sintomi B**, importanti nella stadiazione, sono la febbre >39 °C senza una causa apparente, la perdita >10% del peso corporeo negli ultimi 3 mesi o la sudorazione notturna profusa. Alcuni soggetti hanno un esordio con febbre di origine non nota. Meno comuni e non considerati come fattori prognostici negativi sono il prurito, la letargia, l'anoressia o il dolore che peggiora con l'ingestione di alcol. I pazienti manifestano anche alterazioni a carico del sistema immunitario, che spesso persistono durante e dopo la terapia. Questi comprendono l'anergia ai test cutanei per l'ipersensibilità ritardata, un'anomala risposta dell'immunità cellulare, una lieve riduzione del rapporto CD4:CD8 e una diminuzione della cito-

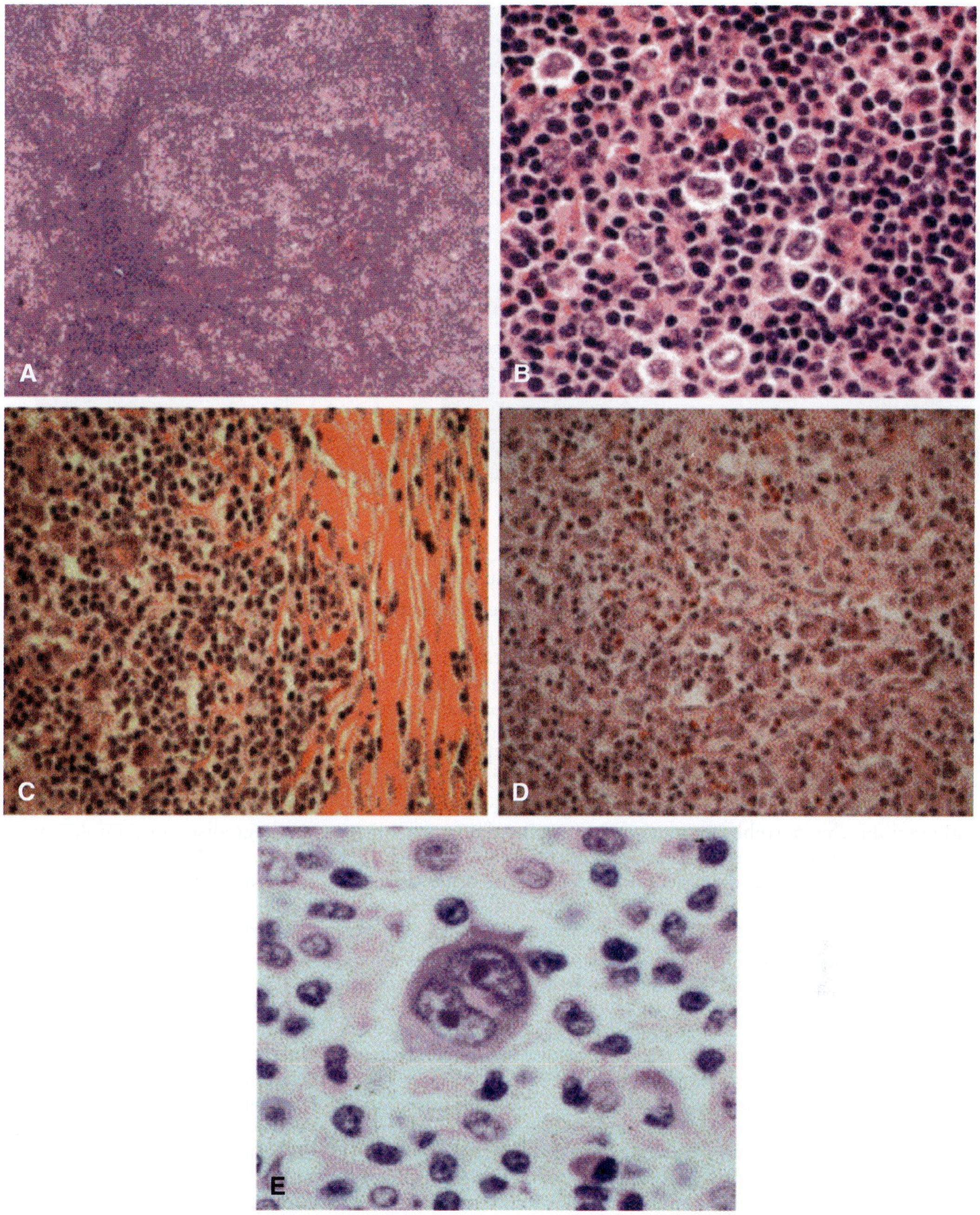

Figura 496-1. Sottotipi istologici di linfoma di Hodgkin. *A*, Colorazioni con ematossilina ed eosina di linfoma di Hodgkin a predominanza linfocitica (NLPHL), che rilevano una proliferazione nodulare con un aspetto "tarlato". *B*, Immagine ad alta risoluzione per mostrare le cellule neoplastiche L e H nell'NLPHL. *C*, Linfoma di Hodgkin classico, sottotipo con sclerosi nodulare. Tra le cellule infiammatorie si osservano grosse cellule mono- e binucleate di Reed-Sternberg. *D*, Linfoma di Hodgkin classico, sottotipo a cellularità mista, che rivela un aumentato numero di cellule di Reed-Sternberg su uno sfondo di cellule infiammatorie miste senza modificazioni sclerotiche. *E*, Immagine ad alta risoluzione di una classica cellula di Reed-Sternberg, con cellule binucleate a evidenti nucleoli eosinofili e citoplasma relativamente abbondante.

TABELLA 496-1. Sistemi di classificazione della malattia di Hodgkin

CLASSIFICAZIONE RYE
Predominanza linfocitaria
Cellularità mista
Sclerosi nodulare
Deplezione linfocitaria
NUOVA CLASSIFICAZIONE OMS/REAL
Predominanza nodulare linfocitaria
Linfoma di Hodgkin classico
Ricca di linfociti
Cellularità mista
Sclerosi nodulare
Deplezione linfocitica
Linfoma Hodgkin-like anaplastico a grandi cellule

REAL, *Revised European-American Classification of Lymphoid Neoplasms* (Classificazione rivista delle neoplasie linfoidi europea-americana); OMS, Organizzazione Mondiale della Sanità.

tossicità delle cellule natural killer. Anche l'immunità umorale può essere danneggiata dopo il trattamento.

DIAGNOSI. I pazienti con una linfoadenopatia persistente, di non chiara natura, la cui associazione a un sottostante processo infiammatorio o infettivo non risulta evidente, andrebbero sottoposti a una radiografia del torace per escludere l'esistenza di una massa mediastinica prima di procedere con una biopsia linfonodale (Fig. 496-2). Salvo che risultino segni o sintomi che facciano deporre diversamente, ulteriori esami di laboratorio possono venire rimandati fino a quando non siano disponibili gli esiti della biopsia. I soggetti con linfonodi persistentemente aumentati di volume, anche dopo che una infezione da mononucleosi sia stata dimostrata con esami ematochimici, dovrebbero essere sottoposti a una biopsia. La formale escissione bioptica è da preferire all'agobiopsia, che permette tuttavia di prelevare un'adeguata quantità di tessuto sia per gli esami di microscopia ottica, sia per i necessari esami immunocitochimici e molecolari, colturali e citogenetici, nel caso in cui gli esami di routine non siano risultati

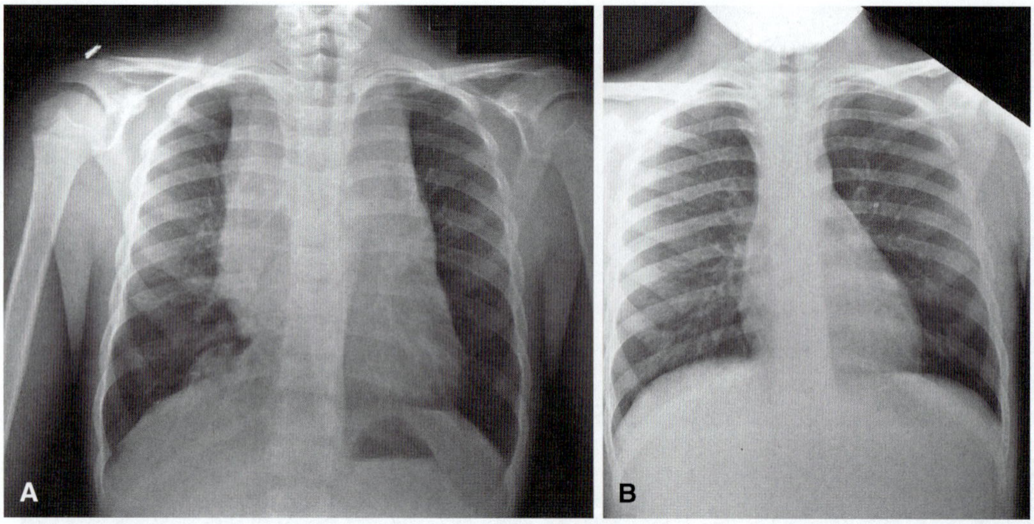

Figura 496-2. *A*, Massa mediastinica anteriore in un paziente con malattia di Hodgkin, prima della terapia. *B*, Dopo 2 mesi di chemioterapia, la massa mediastinica è scomparsa.

sufficienti a ottenere una diagnosi precisa. Avviene raramente di porre una diagnosi di HD certa su materiale congelato. L'ideale, piuttosto, consisterebbe nel congelare e conservare il materiale ottenuto con la biopsia per renderlo disponibile per eventuali ulteriori accertamenti. Una volta posta la diagnosi di HD, è necessario valutare la sua estensione (cioè fare una stadiazione) per stabilire la terapia più adeguata (Tab. 496-2). La **stadiazione prevede** l'esecuzione dell'anamnesi, dell'esame obiettivo e di esami radiologici, inclusi la radiografia del torace, la TC di torace, addome e pelvi, la scintigrafia con il gallio e la PET. Gli **esami di laboratorio** comprendono l'emocromo completo per identificare le alterazioni che potrebbero suggerire un coinvolgimento midollare, il rapporto della sedimentazione eritrocitaria, i valori di rame e ferritina sierici, che possiedono una funzione prognostica e, se alterati al momento della diagnosi, sono utili come riferimento basale per valutare l'efficacia della terapia. Gli esami per la funzionalità epatica, anche se non particolarmente sensibili a indicare un coinvolgimento del fegato, possono tornare utili per la scelta della terapia e per monitorare le relative complicanze. La radiografia del torace risulta particolarmente importante per valutare le dimensioni delle masse mediastiniche in relazione al diametro maggiore del torace. La TC del torace definisce più chiaramente l'estensione delle masse mediastiniche, quando presenti, e permette di individuare linfonodi ilari e l'eventuale coinvolgimento del parenchima polmonare, che potrebbe non risultare evidente alla sola radiografia. La TC o la RM dell'addome possono identificare il coinvolgimento di linfonodi sottodiaframmatici, l'aumento delle dimensioni e le alterazioni a carico di fegato e milza. L'aspirato e la biopsia midollari dovrebbero essere

TABELLA 496-2. Classificazione in stadi di Ann Arbor per la malattia di Hodgkin

STADIO	DEFINIZIONE
I	Coinvolgimento di un solo linfonodo (1) o di un solo organo o sito extralinfatico (I_E)
II	Coinvolgimento di due o più linfonodi dallo stesso lato del diaframma (II) o coinvolgimento localizzato di un organo o sito extralinfatico e uno o più linfonodi dallo stesso lato del diaframma (II_E)
III	Coinvolgimento di linfonodi da entrambi i lati del diaframma (III), che può essere accompagnato dal coinvolgimento della milza (III_S) o da quello localizzato di un organo o di un sito extralinfatico (III_E) o entrambi (III_{SE})
IV	Coinvolgimento diffuso o disseminato di uno o più organi o tessuti extralinfatici con o senza coinvolgimento linfonodale

L'assenza o presenza di febbre $>$38 °C per 3 giorni consecutivi, la profusa sudorazione notturna o una perdita di $\geq$10% del peso iniziale nei 6 mesi precedenti, senza causa apparente, devono essere annotati in tutti i casi rispettivamente con le lettere A o B.

Da Lister TA, Crowther D, Sutcliffe SB, et al: Report of a committee convened to discuss the evaluation and staging of patients with Hodgkin's disease: Cotswolds meeting. *J Clin Oncol* 1989;7:1630-1636.

effettuati in soggetti con malattia avanzata (stadio III o IV) o con sintomi di tipo B (febbre, perdita di peso, sudorazione notturna). Gli studi radiologici sull'osso si eseguono in pazienti con dolore osseo e/o valori elevati di fosfatasi alcalina. La linfangiografia, impiegata in passato per determinare il coinvolgimento dei linfonodi addominali, al giorno d'oggi è raramente utilizzata. Si osservano molti più falsi positivi nei bambini che negli adulti e la procedura è tecnicamente complessa. La scintigrafia con il Gallio 67 è particolarmente utile per identificare le aree ipercaptanti, che possono essere rivalutate in un secondo momento al termine del trattamento, soprattutto nei pazienti con masse mediastiniche che non regrediscono completamente alla radiografia o alla TC del torace. La PET con il fluorodesossiglucosio, rispetto alla scintigrafia con il Gallio 67, ha il vantaggio di necessitare di un solo giorno di procedura, di possedere una maggiore risoluzione, una migliore dosimetria, una minore attività intestinale e di fornire un potenziale quantitativo. Tuttavia, le percentuali di falsi positivi e falsi negativi la rendono ancora sottoutilizzata nella diagnosi dell'HD nei bambini.

Quando la radioterapia costituiva una strategia terapeutica accettabile per i pazienti con stadio precoce dell'HD, veniva effettuata una laparotomia esplorativa con splenectomia per valutare la presenza e l'estensione del coinvolgimento addominale. Tuttavia, ora non esiste più alcun ruolo per la stadiazione chirurgica nel trattamento dei pazienti pediatrici con l'HD. La classificazione per la stadiazione dell'HD correntemente utilizzata è quella adottata dalla Conferenza di Ann Arbor nel 1971, rivista nel 1989 (vedi Tab. 496-2). L'HD può essere sottoclassificata nelle categorie A o B: la *A* è utilizzata per i pazienti asintomatici e la *B* per i soggetti che manifestano sintomi di tipo B. La malattia extralinfatica, dovuta alla diretta estensione della malattia da una stazione linfonodale, è definita dalla categoria E. L'integrale risoluzione della malattia all'esame clinico e agli esami strumentali, o la riduzione di almeno il 70-80% e la negativizzazione della scintigrafia con il Gallio o della PET inizialmente positiva per via della fibrosi residua, sono considerate una risposta completa nell'HD.

TRATTAMENTO. La chemioterapia e la radioterapia sono efficaci nel trattamento dell'HD. Quello attuale, nei pazienti pediatrici, prevede pertanto l'utilizzo combinato della chemioterapia con o senza basse dosi di radioterapia a campo esteso. Il trattamento è in gran parte stabilito in relazione allo stadio della malattia, all'età alla diagnosi, alla presenza o meno dei sintomi B e della linfoadenopatia ilare o della malattia linfonodale bulky. Inizialmente si impiegava la sola radioterapia, a dosi standard di 3500-4000 Gy, con remissione prolungata e una percentuale di guarigione del 40-95% in caso di HD di basso stadio chirurgico. Questa modalità, tuttavia, ha determinato una grave morbilità tardiva, per ritardi nella crescita, disfunzione tiroidea, tossicità cardiaca e polmonare. Il regime **MOPP** (mecloretamina [mostarda azotata], vincristina, procarbazina e prednisone), introdotto nel 1964, è stato il primo regime di chemioterapia combinata adoperato nel trattamento dell'HD ed è stata la principale pietra miliare nella terapia dei suoi stadi avanzati. Determinava una risposta completa nel 70-80% dei casi e la guarigione a 10 anni nel 40-50% dei soggetti con la malattia nello stadio avanzato. Tuttavia, provocava anche una grave tossicità acuta e tardiva. Il desiderio di ridurre gli effetti collaterali ha stimolato vari tentativi di ridurre l'intensità della chemioterapia e della dose e del volume d'irradiazione.

Gli agenti chemioterapici comunemente utilizzati per trattare i bambini e gli adolescenti con l'HD sono la ciclofosfamide, la procarbazina, la vincristina o la vinblastina, il prednisone o desametasone, la doxorubicina, la bleomicina, la dacarbazina, l'etoposide, il metotrexato e la citosina arabinoside. I regimi di chemioterapia combinata attualmente in uso sono il **COPP** (ciclofosfamide, vincristina, procarbazina e prednisone) o l'**ABVD** (doxorubicina [adriamicina], bleomicina, vinblastina e dacarbazina) e il **BEACOPP** (bleomicina, etoposide, doxorubicina, ciclofosfamide, vincristina, procarbazina, prednisone), utilizzato soprattutto nei bambini con stadi avanzati della malattia (Tab. 496-3). Sono stati studiati regimi differenti per ridurre le potenziali tossicità, come per esempio il **COPP/ABV** (ciclofosfamide, vincristina, procarbazina, prednisone/doxorubicina, bleomicina e vinblastina). Inizialmente veniva somministrato un minimo di sei cicli di chemioterapia, con una significativa tossicità cumulativa, comprese le seconde neoplasie, la sterilità e l'insufficienza cardiaca e polmonare. I protocolli "adattati sul rischio" si basano sui criteri di stadiazione e sulla rapidità della risposta alla prima chemioterapia, con lo scopo di ridurre le dosi totali dei farmaci e la durata del trattamento, nonché di eliminare la radioterapia.

RECIDIVA. La maggior parte delle recidive si verifica nei primi 3 anni dalla diagnosi, ma ne sono state riportate anche dopo 10 anni. La recidiva non può essere, in effetti, prevista con precisione in questa malattia. I fattori prognostici negativi sono le dimensioni del tumore, lo stadio al momento della diagnosi e la presenza di sintomi B. I pazienti che non ottengono la remissione o che hanno una ricaduta nei primi 12 mesi dall'inizio del trattamento sono candidati a una chemioterapia mieloablativa e al **trapianto autologo di cellule staminali** con o senza la radioterapia aggiunta. Questo trattamento è più efficace nei soggetti con malattia chemoresponsiva. Il **trapianto allogenico** mieloablativo **di cellule staminali** riduce il pericolo di ricaduta nei pazienti ad alto rischio o refrattari al trattamento. Tuttavia, non ha determinato un miglioramento nella sopravvivenza globale negli studi effettuati, a causa di un'aumentata mortalità associata al trapianto. Questi risultati, comunque, suggeriscono un effetto graft-versus-HD. L'utilizzo di regimi non tossici non mieloablativi per diminuire la morbilità e la mortalità, associate al regime di trattamento con il trapianto allogenico mieloablativo di cellule staminali ma ancora dotate di effetto graft-versus-HD, è ancora poco studiato.

PROGNOSI. Con l'utilizzo degli attuali regimi terapeutici, i pazienti con fattori prognostici favorevoli e una malattia di basso grado hanno una sopravvivenza libera da malattia dell'85-90% e una sopravvivenza globale a 5 anni del 95%. Nei pazienti con una malattia di grado avanzato queste sopravvivenze si attestano invece rispettivamente all'80-85% e al 90%. La prognosi dopo la recidiva dipende dal tempo che intercorre fra il termine del trattamento e la recidiva stessa, la sua sede (linfonodale versus extralinfatica) e la presenza, in essa, di sintomi B. I soggetti con ricaduta dopo >12 mesi dal termine della sola chemioterapia o da un trattamento combinato hanno la prognosi migliore e generalmente rispondono a una nuova terapia standard, con una conseguente lunga sopravvivenza nel 60-70% dei casi. Un trapianto autologo mieloablativo di cellule staminali in pazienti con malattia refrattaria o recidiva entro i 12 mesi dal termine del trattamento porta invece a una sopravvivenza a lungo termine del 40-50%. Le complicanze tardive sono correlate alla radioterapia e alla chemioterapia; si trovano comprese le seconde neoplasie (quali la leucemia mieloide acuta, le neoplasie di mammella, polmone e tiroide e il linfoma non-Hodgkin), la sepsi (per la splenectomia o l'irradiazione della milza), la sterilità, la bassa statura, l'ipotiroidismo, la carie dentale, le disfunzioni polmonari subcliniche e la cardiopatia ischemica.

TABELLA 496-3. Regimi di chemioterapia comunemente impiegati in bambini e adulti con malattia di Hodgkin

REGIME DI CHEMIOTERAPIA	AGENTI FARMACOLOGICI
ABVD	Doxorubicina (adriamicina), bleomicina, vinblastina, dacarbazina
ABVE (DBVE)	Doxorubicina (adriamicina), bleomicina, vincristina, etoposide
VAMP	Vincristina, doxorubicina (adriamicina), metotrexato, prednisone
OPPA ± COPP (femmine)	Vincristina, prednisone, procarbazina, doxorubicina (adriamicina), ciclofosfamide, vincristina, prednisone, procarbazina
OEPA ± COPP (maschi)	Vincristina, etoposide, prednisone, doxorubicina (adriamicina), ciclofosfamide, vincristina, prednisone, procarbazina
COPP/ABV	Ciclofosfamide, vincristina, prednisone, procarbazina, doxorubicina (adriamicina), bleomicina, vinblastina
BEACOPP (stadio avanzato)	Bleomicina, etoposide, doxorubicina (adriamicina), ciclofosfamide, vincristina, prednisone, procarbazina
COPP	Ciclofosfamide, vincristina, prednisone, procarbazina
CHOP	Ciclofosfamide, doxorubicina (adriamicina), vincristina, prednisone
ABVE-PC (DBVE-PC)	Doxorubicina (adriamicina), bleomicina, vincristina, etoposide, prednisone, ciclofosfamide

Claviez A, Klingebiel T, Beyer J, et al: Allogeneic peripheral blood stem cell transplantation following fludarabine-based conditioning in six children with advanced Hodgkin disease. *Ann Hematol* 2004;83:237–241.

Hjalgrim HH, Askling J, Rostgaard K, et al: Characteristics of Hodgkin's lymphoma after infectious mononucleosis. *N Engl J Med* 2003;349:1324–1332.

Hudson MM, Donaldson SS: Hodgkin disease. In Pizzo PA, Poplack DG (editors): *Principles and Practice of Pediatric Oncology,* 4th ed. Philadelphia, Lippincott Williams & Wilkins, 2002, pp 637–660.

Hueltenschmidt B, Sautter-Bihl ML, Lang O, et al: Whole body positron emission tomography in the treatment of Hodgkin disease. *Cancer* 2001;91:302–310.

Peggs KS, Hunter A, Chopra R, et al: Clinical evidence of a graft-versus-Hodgkin's-lymphoma effect after reduced-intensity allogeneic transplantation. *Lancet* 2005;365:1934–1940.

Pileri SA, Ascani S, Leoncini L, et al: Hodgkin lymphoma: the pathologist's viewpoint. *J Clin Pathol* 2002;55:162–176.

Schwartz CL: The management of Hodgkin disease in the young child. *Curr Opin Pediatr* 2003;15:10–16.

Thomson AB, Wallace WH: Treatment of paediatric Hodgkin disease. A balance of risks. *Eur J Cancer* 2002;38:468–477.

Yung L, Linch D: Hodgkin's lymphoma. *Lancet* 2003;361:943–950.

496.2. • LINFOMA NON-HODGKIN

L'NHL rappresenta circa il 60% di tutti i linfomi nei bambini e negli adolescenti e l'8-10% di tutte le neoplasie dei bambini di età compresa tra i 5-19 anni, con una diffusione annuale negli Stati Uniti di 750-800 casi all'anno nei bambini con ≤19 anni. Anche se oltre il 70% dei pazienti è in uno stadio avanzato al momento della diagnosi, la prognosi è molto migliorata, con una sopravvivenza del 90-95% quando la malattia è circoscritta e del 60-90% quando è avanzata.

EPIDEMIOLOGIA. Benché la maggior parte dei bambini e degli adolescenti si presenti con una NHL *de novo*, un piccolo numero di essi ne sviluppa una secondaria a specifiche malattie, quali le immunodeficienze ereditarie o acquisite (varie sindromi da immunodeficienza combinata, la sindrome di Wiskott-Aldrich), le infezioni virali (HIV, EBV) o come parte di sindromi genetiche (atassia-teleangectasia, sindrome di Bloom). La gran parte dei soggetti che sviluppano l'NHL, tuttavia, non manifesta una evidente causa genetica o ambientale.

PATOGENESI. I quattro principali sottotipi patologici dell'NHL nei bambini e negli adolescenti sono: il linfoma di Burkitt (BL, *Burkitt Lymphoma*), che rappresenta il 40% degli NHL; il linfoma linfoblastico (LL), con una percentuale del 30%; il linfoma diffuso a grandi cellule B (DLBCL, *Diffuse Large B-Cell Lymphoma*), 20%; il linfoma anaplastico a grandi cellule (ALCL, *Anaplastic Large Cell Lymphoma*), 10% (Fig. 496-3). La maggior parte dei bambini e degli adolescenti con l'NHL ha neoplasie di alto grado con un andamento clinico aggressivo se confrontato con quello dell'adulto, che invece ha in genere una malattia indolente di grado medio-basso. Quasi tutti gli NHL del bambino e dell'adolescente provengono da aberrazioni nelle cellule germinali. Pressappoco tutte le forme di BL e DLBCL derivano dalle cellule di tipo B; i casi di LL sono a cellule T nell'80% delle occorrenze e a cellule B nel 20%; i casi di ALCL sono nel 70% a cellule T, nel 20% a cellule null e nel 10% a cellule B. Alcuni sottotipi patologici hanno specifiche aberrazioni citogenetiche. I bambini con il BL frequentemente (90%) presentano la traslocazione t(8;14), meno comunemente (10%) la traslocazione t(2;8) o t(8;22). I pazienti con l'ALCL hanno spesso (≥5%) una traslocazione t(2;5), mentre quelli con DLBCL e LL manifestano numerose anomalie citogenetiche differenti.

MANIFESTAZIONI CLINICHE. Le manifestazioni cliniche dell'NHL dell'infanzia e dell'adolescenza dipendono soprattutto dal sottotipo patologico e dalle sedi coinvolte primariamente e secondariamente. Gli NHL sono tumori a crescita rapida e possono provocare sintomi in relazione alle dimensioni e alla sede. Circa il 70% dei casi si presenta con una malattia avanzata in stadio III o IV (Tab. 496-4), con estensione extralinfonodale per un coinvolgimento gastrointestinale, del midollo osseo e del sistema nervoso centrale (SNC). Il **BL frequentemente si manifesta** come una malattia addominale (tipo sporadico) o del capo-collo (tipo endemico), con un'invasione midollare o del SNC. L'**LL è rappresentato comunemente** da una massa sovradiaframmatica intratoracica o mediastinica e ha una tendenza a diffondersi anche al livello del midollo osseo e del SNC. Il **DLBCL in genere è costituito** da un interessamento primario dell'addome e del mediastino e raramente si dissemina a livello del midollo o del SNC. L'**ALCL**, infine, **prevede manifestazioni** primariamente cutanee (10%) o una malattia sistemica (febbre, perdita di peso) con disseminazione al livello del fegato, della milza, dei polmoni, del mediastino o della cute; disseminazioni al livello del midollo e del SNC sono rare.

Le manifestazioni specifiche per sede comprendono un ingrossamento rapido dei linfonodi non doloroso, la tosse, la sindrome della vena cava superiore (SVC, *Superior Vena Cava*), la dispnea per l'interessamento toracico, masse addominali (di grosse dimensioni e con rapido accrescimento), l'ostruzione intestinale, sintomi da intussuscezione, l'ascite con coinvolgimento addominale, la congestione nasale, l'otodinia, la riduzione dell'udito, l'ingrossamento delle tonsille per coinvolgimento dell'anello di Waldeyer e il dolore da localizzazioni cutanee (primitive o secondarie).

TABELLA 496-4. Sistema di stadiazione di St. Jude per il linfoma non-Hodgkin infantile

STADIO	DESCRIZIONE
I	Un singolo tumore (extralinfonodale) o una singola area (linfonodale), con esclusione del mediastino o dell'addome
II	Un singolo tumore (extralinfonodale) con coinvolgimento di linfonodi regionali
	Due o più stazioni linfonodali dallo stesso lato del diaframma
	Due singoli tumori (extralinfonodali) con o senza linfonodi regionali coinvolti dallo stesso lato del diaframma
	Un tumore del tratto gastroenterico principale, generalmente a livello ileocecale, con o senza coinvolgimento dei soli linfonodi mesenterici, che devono essere grossolanamente resecati (>90%)
III	Due singoli tumori (extralinfonodali) sui lati opposti del diaframma
	Due o più stazioni linfonodali sopra e sotto il diaframma
	Qualunque tumore primario intratoracico (mediastinico, pleurico o timico)
	Qualunque malattia primariamente estesa a livello intra-addominale
IV	Tutte le precedenti, con iniziale coinvolgimento del sistema nervoso centrale o del midollo osseo al momento della diagnosi

Da Murphy SB: Classification, staging and end results of treatment of childhood non-Hodgkin's lymphomas: Dissimilarities from lymphomas in adults. *Semin Oncol* 1980;7:332-339.

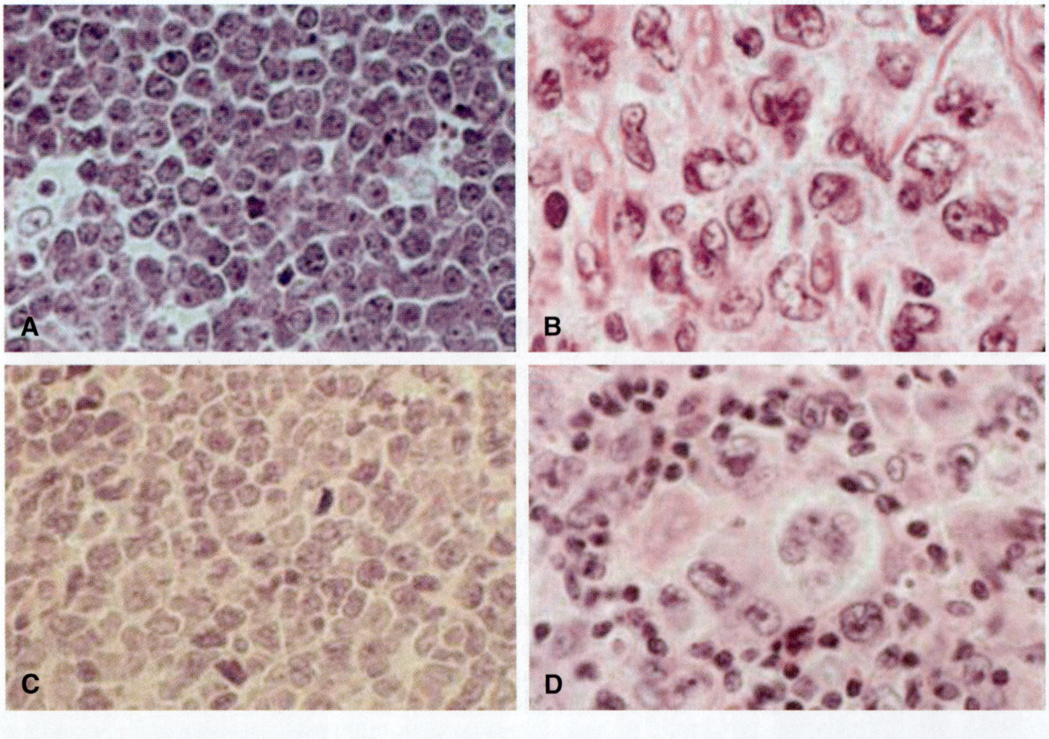

Figura 496-3. Distribuzione del linfoma non-Hodgkin nell'infanzia e nell'adolescenza. Colorazioni con ematossilina ed eosina che dimostrano la morfologia del linfoma di Burkitt (*A*, alto ingrandimento), del linfoma diffuso a grandi cellule B (*B*, alto ingrandimento), del linfoma a precursori linfoblastici T (*C*, alto ingrandimento) e del linfoma anaplastico a grandi cellule (*D*, alto ingrandimento). (Da Cairo MS, Raetz E, Lim MS, et al: Childhood and adolescent non-Hodgkin lymphoma: New insights in biology and critical challenges for the future. *Pediatr Blood Cancer* 2005;45:753-769.)

Tre manifestazioni cliniche che necessitano di particolari accorgimenti terapeutici comprendono la sindrome SVC, secondaria a una grossa massa mediastinica che ostruisce il flusso sanguigno e le vie aeree; la paraplegia acuta, secondaria a una compressione spinale o del SNC da parte di localizzazioni confinanti dell'NHL; la sindrome da lisi tumorale, secondaria a gravi alterazioni metaboliche, comprese l'iperuricemia, l'iperfosfatemia, l'iperkaliemia e l'ipocalcemia da lisi massiva di cellule neoplastiche.

REPERTI DI LABORATORIO. Gli esami di laboratorio e radiologici consigliati sono: emocromo completo, elettroliti, acido urico, calcio, fosforo, bilirubina, urea, alanina aminotransferasi e aspartato aminotransferasi, aspirato e biopsia osteomidollare bilaterale, puntura lombare con esame citologico, conta delle cellule e delle proteine su liquido cerebrospinale, radiografia del torace, TC di collo, torace, addome e pelvi, PET e radiografie ossee (opzionale) e TC al cranio (opzionale) (Tab. 496-5). Il tessuto tumorale (da biopsia, midollo osseo, liquido cerebrospinale o toracentesi/paracentesi) dovrebbe essere analizzato con un citofluorimetro per la tipizzazione immunofenotipica (T, B o null) e citogenetica (cariotipo). Esami aggiuntivi potrebbero comprendere la fluorescenza con ibridazione *in situ* o l'RT-PCR quantitativa per specifiche traslocazioni genetiche, studi di riarrangiamento genico delle cellule T e B e il profilo molecolare con i microarrangiamenti degli oligonucleotidi.

DIAGNOSI DIFFERENZIALE. La linfoadenopatia della testa e del collo dovrebbe essere differenziata dalle linfoadenopatie a eziologia infettiva; le masse mediastiniche dall'HD e dai germinomi; il coinvolgimento addominale da altre masse neoplastiche addominali quali il tumore di Wilms, il neuroblastoma e il rabdomiosarcoma; il coinvolgimento del midollo dalla leucemia linfocitica acuta a precursori delle cellule B (Pre-B) e dalla leucemia linfocitica acuta a cellule T. La TC e la PET, insieme alla flussocitometria, alla citogenetica e alla genetica molecolare su tessuto bioptico e tumorale, generalmente permettono di differenziare l'NHL da altre patologie.

TRATTAMENTO. La principale modalità di trattamento dell'NHL di bambini e adolescenti è la polichemioterapia per via sistemica e intratecale. La chirurgia viene utilizzata soprattutto per la diagnosi e/o per ottenere materiale bioptico e per la stadiazione di malattia, ma raramente si impiega per asportare masse voluminose. Della radioterapia ci si avvale raramente, se non mai, eccetto che in particolari circostanze, come nel caso di coinvolgimento del SNC nell'LL o occasionalmente nel BL, nella SVC acuta e nelle paraplegie acute. I pazienti alla diagnosi e ad alto rischio di sindrome da lisi tumorale, soprattutto con un BL avanzato/bulky o un LL, necessitano di una decisa idratazione e della somministrazione di inibitori della xantina ossidasi (allopurinolo, 10 mg/kg/die per os in tre assunzioni quotidiane) o, più spesso, di urato ossidasi ricombinante (rasburicasi, 0,2 mg/kg/die per os una volta al giorno per 1-3 giorni).

Il trattamento specifico per la malattia localizzata o avanzata è simile per il BL e il DLBCL. Le loro forme localizzate richiedono una polichemioterapia della durata variabile da 6 settimane a 6 mesi. Gli schemi comunemente usati sono COPAD (ciclofosfamide, vincristina, prednisone e doxorubicina), come dimostrato dal recente studio internazionale B-NHL (FAB/LMB 96 [franco-americano-britannico, linfoma a cellule B mature]), o COMP (ciclofosfamide, vincristina, metotrexato, 6-mercaptopurina e prednisone). La malattia avanzata in genere viene trattata per 4-6 mesi con una polichemioterapia secondo il protocollo FAB/LMB 96 o BFM (Berlino-Francoforte-Monaco) NHL 90.

L'LL localizzato e avanzato di solito richiede un trattamento di almeno 24 mesi. I migliori risultati nelle forme avanzate si ottengono servendosi del protocollo BFM NHL 90, che si avvale di un approccio terapeutico simile a quello per la leucemia acuta dell'infanzia, con un ciclo di chemioterapia d'induzione, una fase di consolidamento, una fase intermedia di mantenimento, una fase di reinduzione (solo nelle malattie avanzate) e un anno di terapia di mantenimento con la 6-mercaptopurina e il metotrexato.

L'ALCL localizzato può richiedere solo l'exeresi cutanea o una terapia più aggressiva simile a quella per le forme avanzate, che vengono comunemente trattate con il protocollo BFM NHL 90 o con il protocollo COG di APO (doxorubicina, prednisone e vincristina) con l'aggiunta di VP-16, Ara-C o vinblastina.

La chemioterapia intratecale viene adoperata per limitare la progressione della malattia in tutti i sottotipi di NHL di bambini e adolescenti e può prevedere la somministrazione di metotrexato, idrocortisone o Ara-C per via intratecale.

I pazienti con NHL che sviluppano una malattia progressiva o recidivante necessitano di una chemioterapia di reinduzione e di un trapianto allogenico o autologo di cellule staminali. La scelta tra uno schema specifico di terapia o il trapianto dipende dal sottotipo patologico, dalla precedente terapia, dalla sede della recidiva e dalla disponibilità di un donatore compatibile.

TABELLA 496-5. Esami pretrattamento per la stadiazione del linfoma non-Hodgkin pediatrico

Emocromo completo
Elettroliti sierici, acido urico, LDH, creatinina, calcio, fosforo
Funzionalità epatica (ALT, AST)
Rx torace
TC di collo, torace, addome, pelvi
Tomografia a emissione di protoni
Aspirato e biopsia ossea bilaterale
Esame liquorale con citologia, conta delle cellule e delle proteine

ALT, alanina aminotransferasi; AST, aspartato aminotransferasi.

TERAPIE DI SUPPORTO

Alcuni pazienti necessitano di profilassi con G-CSF per prevenire la febbre e la neutropenia secondarie alla chemioterapia mielosoppressiva e antibiotici profilattici per prevenire le infezioni. Di routine vengono collocati cateteri venosi centrali a permanenza, per facilitare i frequenti prelievi di sangue, la somministrazione della chemioterapia e l'esecuzione delle trasfusioni, la nutrizione parenterale per prevenire la perdita di peso e la denutrizione.

COMPLICANZE

I pazienti che ricevono polichemioterapie per malattie avanzate corrono il rischio acuto di gravi mucositi, infezioni, citopenie che richiedono la trasfusione di eritrociti e di piastrine, squilibri elettrolitici e denutrizione. Le complicanze tardive possono comprendere il ritardo nella crescita, la cardiotossicità, la tossicità gonadica con infertilità e secondi tumori.

PROGNOSI

La prognosi è ottima per la maggior parte delle forme di NHL nei bambini e negli adolescenti. I pazienti con una malattia localizzata hanno una sopravvivenza del 90-100% e quelli con una forma avanzata del 60-95%. La variabilità della sopravvivenza dipende dal sottotipo patologico, dal volume tumorale alla diagnosi espresso dal livello sierico di LDH, dall'interessamento o meno del SNC e dalla presenza di specifiche sedi coinvolte nella disseminazione della malattia. Specifici sottotipi citogenetici e geneticomolecolari possono anche risultare importanti per la prognosi e nell'influenzare specifiche strategie terapeutiche.

Cairo MS, Bishop M: Tumour lysis syndrome: new therapeutic strategies and classification. *Br J Haematol* 2004;127:3–11.

Cairo MS, Sposto R, Hoover-Regan M, et al: Childhood and adolescent large-cell lymphoma (LCL): A review of the Children's Cancer Group experience. *Am J Hematol* 2003;72:53–63.

Cairo MS, Sposto R, Perkins SL, et al: Burkitt's and Burkitt-like lymphoma in children and adolescents: A review of the Children's Cancer Group experience. *Br J Haematol* 2003;120:660–670.

Dave SS, Wright G, Tan B, et al: Prediction of survival in follicular lymphoma based on molecular features of tumor-infiltrating immune cells. *N Engl J Med* 2004;351:2159–2169.

Hummel M, Bentink S, Berger H, et al: A biologic definition of Burkitt's lymphoma from transcriptional and genomic profiling. *N Engl J Med* 2006;354:2419–2430.

Patte C, Auperin A, Michon J, et al: The Societe Francaise d'Oncologie Pediatrique LMB89 protocol: highly effective multiagent chemotherapy tailored to the tumor burden and initial response in 561 unselected children with B-cell lymphomas and L3 leukemia. *Blood* 2001;97:3370–3379.

Peniket AJ, Ruiz de Elvira MC, Taghipour G, et al: An EBMT registry matched study of allogeneic stem cell transplants for lymphoma: allogeneic transplantation is associated with a lower relapse rate but a higher procedure-related mortality rate than autologous transplantation. *Bone Marrow Transplant* 2003;31:667–678.

Reiter A, Schrappe M, Tiemann M, et al: Improved treatment results in childhood B-cell neoplasms with tailored intensification of therapy: A report of the Berlin-Frankfurt-Munster Group Trial NHL-BFM 90. *Blood* 1999;94:3294–3306.

Capitolo 497 ■ Tumori cerebrali nell'infanzia

John F. Kuttesch Jr. e Joann L. Ater

I tumori cerebrali primitivi del sistema nervoso centrale (SNC) sono un gruppo eterogeneo di malattie, che insieme rappresentano la seconda più frequente neoplasia dell'infanzia e dell'adolescenza. La mortalità complessiva per questa patologia è del 45% circa e inoltre i pazienti che la contraggono sono quelli che hanno la morbilità più alta, soprattutto neurologica, rispetto alle altre neoplasie dell'infanzia. La prognosi è migliorata nel tempo, grazie al progresso delle tecniche neurochirurgiche e radioterapiche e all'introduzione della chemioterapia come modalità di trattamento. L'approccio per la terapia di queste neoplasie è di tipo multimodale: se fattibile, la chirurgia con un'asportazione completa della lesione è fondamentale, mentre la radioterapia e la chemioterapia sono utilizzate a seconda della diagnosi, dell'età del paziente e di altri elementi.

EZIOLOGIA. L'eziologia dei tumori cerebrali pediatrici non è ben definita. È nota una predominanza nel sesso maschile dell'incidenza del medulloblastoma e dell'ependimoma. Le sindromi familiari ed ereditarie associate a un'aumentata incidenza dei tumori cerebrali rappresentano circa il 5% dei casi (Tab. 497-1). Anche l'esposizione a radiazioni ionizzanti a livello del cranio è accompagnata a una più elevata incidenza di questi tumori. Sono stati riportati casi sporadici di tumori cerebrali familiari, senza l'evidenza di una sindrome ereditaria. Gli eventi molecolari associati alla tumorigenesi dei casi pediatrici non sono noti.

EPIDEMIOLOGIA. Ogni anno vengono diagnosticati circa 2200 tumori cerebrali primitivi fra bambini e adolescenti, con un'incidenza annuale complessiva di 28 casi per milione di bambini <19 anni. L'incidenza dei tumori del SNC è maggiore nei lattanti e nei bambini ≤7 anni (≈36 casi/milione di bambini), piuttosto che nei bambini più grandi e negli adolescenti (≈21 casi/milione) (Fig. 497-1).

PATOGENESI. Fra le oltre 100 categorie istologiche e i sottotipi di tumori cerebrali primitivi descritti nella classificazione dei tumori del SNC e delle meningi dall'Organizzazione Mondiale della Sanità (OMS), 5 rappresentano l'80% di tutti i tumori pediatri-

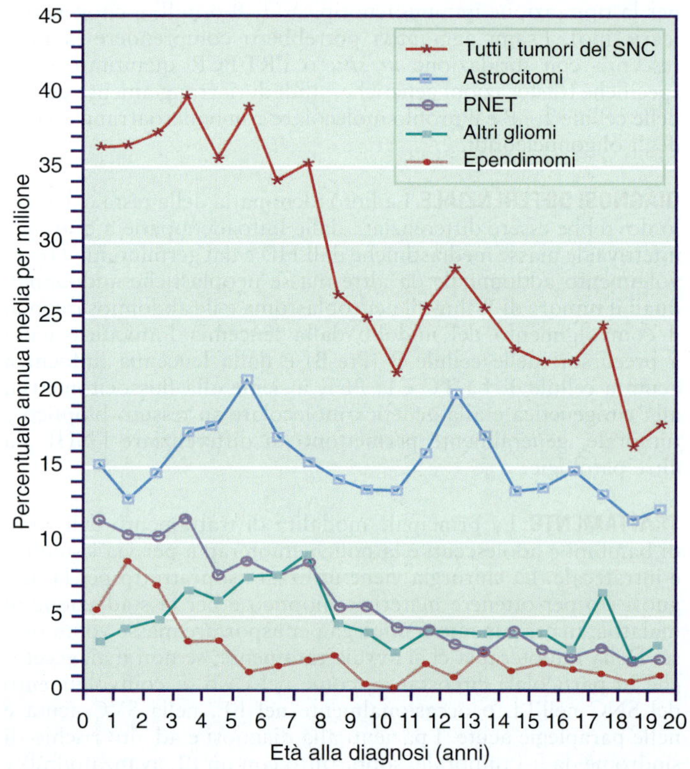

Figura 497-1. Incidenza specifica per età dei tumori cerebrali maligni dell'infanzia da SEER 1986-1994. SNC, sistema nervoso centrale; PNET, tumori primitivi neuroectodermici. (Rielaborata da Gurney JC, Smith MA, Bunin GR: *National Cancer Institute SEER Program*. NIH publication No. 99-4649. Bethesda, MD, National Cancer Institute, 1999, pp 51-63.)

TABELLA 497-1. Sindromi familiari associate con i tumori cerebrali infantili

SINDROME	MANIFESTAZIONI A CARICO DEL SNC	CROMOSOMA	GENE
Neurofibromatosi di tipo 1 (autosomica dominante)	Gliomi delle vie ottiche, astrocitomi, tumori maligni delle guaine dei nervi periferici, neurofibromi	17q11	NF1
Neurofibromatosi di tipo 2 (autosomica dominante)	Schwannomi vestibolari, meningiomi, ependimomi spinali, astrocitomi spinali, amartomi	22q12	NF2
von Hippel-Lindau (autosomica dominante)	Emangioblastoma	3p25-26	VHL
Sclerosi tuberosa (autosomica dominante)	Astrocitoma subependimale a cellule giganti, tuberi corticali	9q34	TSC1
		16q13	TSC2
Li-Fraumeni (autosomica dominante)	Astrocitoma, tumore neuroectodermico primitivo	17q13	TP53
Cowden (autosomica dominante)	Gangliocitoma displastico cerebellare (malattia di Lhermitte-Duclos)	10q23	PTEN
Turcot (autosomica dominante)	Medulloblastoma	5q21	APC
	Glioblastoma	3p21	hMLH1
		7p22	hPSM2
Carcinoma del nevo basale (autosomica dominante)	Medulloblastoma	9q31	PTCH

Modificata da Kleihues P, Cavenee WK: *World Health Organization Classification of Tumors: Pathology and Genetics of Tumors of the Nervous System*. Lyon, IARC Press, 2000.

ci: l'astrocitoma pilocitico giovanile, il medulloblastoma/tumore primitivo neuroectodermico (PNET, *Primitive NeuroEctodermal Tumor*), l'astrocitoma diffuso, l'ependimoma e il craniofaringioma (Tab. 497-2).

Il Childhood Brain Tumor Consortium ha riportato una modesta prevalenza della localizzazione sottotentoriale delle neoplasie (43,2%), seguita da quella sopratentoriale (40,9%) e dalle multiple (11%). Sussistono differenze correlate all'età, circa la localizzazione primaria del tumore (Fig. 497-2). Durante il primo anno di vita, infatti, predominano i tumori sovratentoriali, che includono, più comunemente, i tumori dei plessi corioidei e i teratomi. Tra 1-10 anni, prevalgono invece i tumori sottotentoriali, per la maggiore incidenza dell'astrocitoma pilocitico giovanile e del medulloblastoma. Dopo i 10 anni di età, tornano maggiormente numerosi i tumori sovratentoriali, tra i quali il più comune è l'astrocitoma diffuso. I tumori delle vie ottiche e della regione ipotalamica, del tronco e della regione pinealemesencefalica sono più comuni nei bambini e negli adolescenti, che non negli adulti.

MANIFESTAZIONI CLINICHE. La presentazione clinica dei pazienti con tumori cerebrali dipende dalla sede del tumore, dal suo tipo e dall'età del bambino. I segni e i sintomi sono dovuti all'ostruzione delle vie di drenaggio del liquido cerebrospinale (CSF, *CerebroSpinal Fluid*) da parte del tumore con una conseguente **ipertensione endocranica**, o a deficit neurologici focali. Lievi modificazioni della personalità, dello stato mentale e del linguaggio possono precedere questi segni e sintomi classici, che sono spesso conseguenti a lesioni sovratentoriali (corticali). Nei bambini piccoli, la diagnosi di neoplasia cerebrale può essere ritardata, perché i sintomi sono simili a quelli di malattie più comuni come le patologie gastrointestinali. I neonati con le suture craniche aperte possono presentare segni da ipertensione endocranica quali il vomito, la letargia e l'irritabilità, come pure più tardivamente una macrocefalia. La **classica triade** di cefalea, nausea e vomito e papilledema è tipica nei tumori della linea mediana o sottotentoriali, così come si associano a questi tumori le alterazioni dell'equilibrio, della deambulazione e della coordinazione e la visione offuscata, la diplopia e il nistagmo. Il **torcicollo** può essere dovuto a una erniazione delle tonsille cerebellari. I tumori del tronco possono associarsi a una paralisi dello sguardo, a paralisi multiple dei nervi cranici e a deficit del primo motoneurone (emiparesi, iperreflessia, clonie). I **tumori sovratentoriali**, più comunemente, si accompagnano invece a deficit focali come la debolezza motoria, modificazioni della sensibilità, disturbi del linguaggio, crisi epilettiche e alterazioni dei riflessi. I neonati con neoplasie sovratentoriali possono manifestare la preferenza per una mano. I tumori delle vie ottiche provocano alterazioni della vista quali una riduzione dell'acuità visiva, la pupilla di Marcus Gunn (deficit papillare afferente), il nistagmo e/o difetti del campo visivo. I tumori della regione sovrasellare e del terzo ventricolo possono presentarsi all'inizio con **deficit neuroendocrini** quali il diabete insipido, la galattorrea, una pubertà precoce o ritardata e l'ipotiroidismo. La **sindrome diencefalica** compare con un deficit dello sviluppo, il dimagrimento, l'aumento dell'appetito e l'euforia e si osserva nei neonati e nei bambini piccoli con tumori in questa sede. La **sindrome di Parinaud** è tipica dei tumori della regione pineale e comporta la paralisi dello sguardo verso l'alto, la dilatazione della pupilla durante l'accomodazione ma non dopo uno stimolo luminoso, il nistagmo convergente o retrattorio e la retrazione palpebrale. I tumori midollari e la disseminazione spinale dei tumori cerebrali possono avere luogo con deficit motori e/o sensitivi delle vie lunghe, deficit intestinali e vescicali e rachialgie o dolore radicolare. I segni e i sintomi di una disseminazione meningea da tumore cerebrale o da leucemia sono simili a quelli dei tumori sottotentoriali.

DIAGNOSI. La valutazione del paziente con un sospetto tumore cerebrale è di prioritaria importanza. Essa dovrebbe comprendere l'anamnesi completa, l'esame obiettivo completo (compre-

TABELLA 497-2. Distribuzione dei tumori cerebrali in relazione all'istologia

ISTOLOGIA	DISTRIBUZIONE (% DEL TOTALE)
Medulloblastoma/tumore neuroectodermico primitivo	20
Astrocitoma pilocitico giovanile	20
Astrocitoma di basso grado	15
Astrocitoma di alto grado	7
Ependimoma	7
Craniofaringioma	7
Tumori primitivi non classificati	7
Tumori dei plessi corioidei, germinomi, oligodendrogliomi, meningiomi, tumori misti, tumori parenchimali della pineale	1-2 (ciascun gruppo istologico)

Adattata da Fuller GN: Central nervous system tumors. In Parham DM (editor): *Pediatric Neoplasia: Morphology and Biology*. Philadelphia, Lippincott-Raven, 1996, pp 153-204.

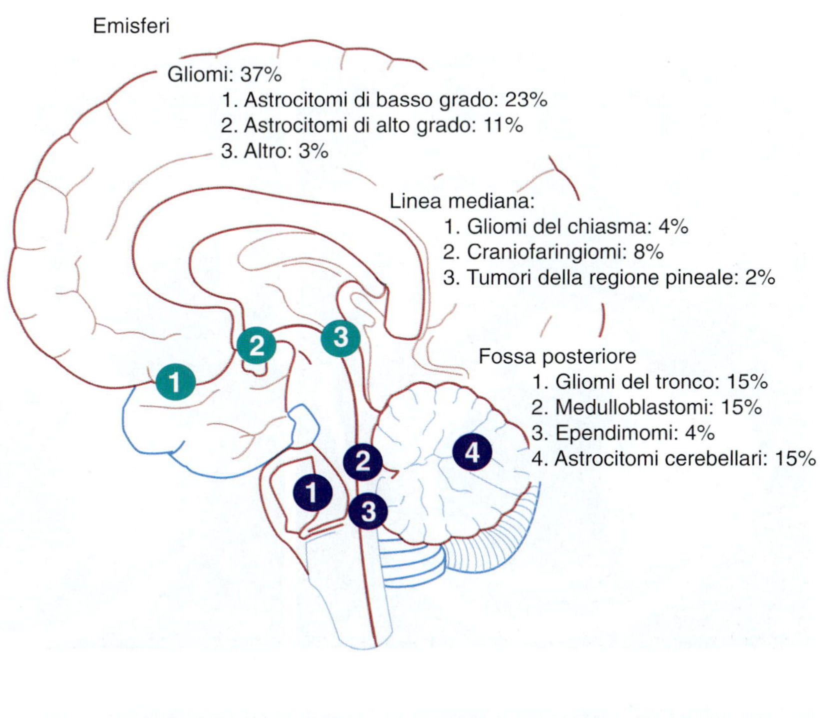

Figura 497-2. I tumori cerebrali pediatrici possono colpire qualunque sede del sistema nervoso centrale. Sono illustrate la frequenza relativa dei diversi tipi istologici di tumore cerebrale e la distribuzione anatomica. (Rielaborata da Albright AL: Pediatric brain tumors. *CA Cancer J Clin* 1993;43:272-288.)

sa la valutazione oftalmologica) e l'esame obiettivo neurologico acompagnato dagli esami neuroradiologici. Per i tumori cerebrali primitivi, la **RM** è l'esame standard. I tumori della regione pituitaria/sovrasellare, delle vie ottiche e sottotentoriali sono meglio definiti con essa che non con la TC. I pazienti con tumori della linea mediana e della regione chiasmatica di ipofisi/sovrasellare/delle vie ottiche dovrebbero essere sottoposti a una valutazione per escludere **disfunzioni neuroendocrine**. La consulenza oftalmologia risulta utile nei soggetti con tumori che interessano le vie ottiche, al fine di documentare l'impatto della malattia sull'oculomozione, sull'acuità visiva e sul campo visivo. La regione sovrasellare e pineale sono tipiche dei germinomi, per la cui diagnosi possono risultare d'aiuto la misurazione sierica e liquoreale della **β-gonadotropina corionica umana** e dell'**α-fetoproteina**. Nei tumori che hanno la tendenza a disseminare a livello delle leptomeningi, come il medulloblastoma/PNET, l'ependimoma e i germinomi, riesce utile eseguire una puntura lombare per l'analisi citologica del CSF; la rachicentesi è controindicata nei soggetti con un idrocefalo di nuova diagnosi secondario a una ostruzione del flusso del CSF oppure in soggetti con tumori sottotentoriali. La puntura lombare in questi casi può provocare un'erniazione cerebrale, con gravi conseguenze neurologiche e decesso. Pertanto, nei bambini con un tumore cerebrale di nuova diagnosi e segni da ipertensione endocranica, la rachicentesi è generalmente rinviata fino al momento dell'intervento o del posizionamento di una derivazione.

TUMORI SPECIFICI

ASTROCITOMI. Gli astrocitomi sono un gruppo eterogeneo di tumori pediatrici del SNC; essi lo possono interessare per intero e rappresentano circa il 40% di questi tumori.

Gli astrocitomi di basso grado (LGA, *Low-Grade Astrocytomas*) sono quelli più frequenti nell'infanzia e sono caratterizzati da un decorso clinico indolente. L'**astrocitoma pilocitico giovanile** (**JPA**, *Juvenile Pilocytic Astrocytoma*) è quello più comune nei bambini e rappresenta circa il 20% di tutti i tumori cerebrali (Fig. 497-3). Sulla base delle caratteristiche clinicopatologiche utilizzate nel Classification System dell'OMS, il JPA è classificato come un tumore di grado I. Anche se esso può essere localizzato in qualunque parte del SNC, la classica sede di comparsa è costituita dal **cervelletto.** Altre sedi frequenti sono la regione di ipotalamo/terzo ventricolo, il nervo ottico e la regione chiasmatica. L'aspetto neuroradiologico classico, ma non esclusivo, del JPA è costituito dalla presenza di un linfonodo assumente mezzo di contrasto sulla parete di una massa cistica (vedi Fig. 497-3). Dal punto di vista microscopico si notano due elementi caratteristici: fasci di tessuto fibrillare compatto inframmezzati da aree spongiformi microcistiche isolate. La presenza delle **fibre di Rosenthal**, che sono considerate masserelle di filamenti gliali all'interno delle aree compatte, aiuta a porre la diagnosi. Il JPA ha un basso potenziale metastatico ed è raramente invasivo. Una piccola percentuale di questi tumori può progredire e dare origine a una disseminazione leptomeningea, soprattutto nel caso dei tumori che interessano le vie ottiche. Il JPA molto di rado subisce una trasformazione maligna in un tumore più aggressivo. Quello del nervo ottico e del chiasma è relativamente frequente nei pazienti affetti da neurofibromatosi di tipo 1 (con un'incidenza del 15%). Diversamente che nel caso degli astrocitomi fibrillari diffusi, non sono evidenti nel JPA alcune tipiche alterazioni citogenetiche e non sussistono neanche alterazioni molecolari note. Altri tumori con caratteristiche clinicopatologiche simili a quelle del JPA colpiscono questa stessa fascia pediatrica di età, quali lo xantoastrocitoma pleiomorfo, l'astrocitoma desmoplastico dell'infanzia e l'astrocitoma subependimale a cellule giganti.

Il secondo più frequente è l'**astrocitoma fibrillare infiltrante**, un gruppo di tumori caratterizzato da un pattern di infiltrazione diffusa delle cellule tumorali all'interno del tessuto nervoso normale e con un potenziale di trasformazione neoplastica. Sulla base delle caratteristiche clinicopatologiche, questi tumori comprendono gli astrocitomi di basso grado (grado II, OMS), quelli maligni (astrocitomi anaplastici, grado III, OMS) e il glioblastoma multiforme (grado IV, OMS). All'interno di questo gruppo, l'LGA fibrillare rappresenta il secondo astrocitoma più comune nei bambini, costituendo il 15% dei tumori cerebrali. Istologicamente, questi tumori di basso grado dimostrano un'aumentata cellularità se confrontata con quella del parenchima cerebrale normale, con poche figure mitotiche, pleiomorfismo nucleare e microcisti. L'elemento caratteristico sulla RM è l'assenza di assunzione di mezzo di contrasto. Le alterazioni genetico-molecolari riscontrate fra gli astrocitomi diffusi di basso grado infiltranti comprendono le mutazioni di P53 e l'iperespressione della catena α del fattore di crescita di derivazione piastrinica e del recettore α di tale fattore. Questi tumori possono trasformarsi in astrocitomi maligni, uno sviluppo che si correla con l'accumulo di multiple mutazioni molecolari acquisite.

Il **trattamento clinico** degli LGA si basa su un approccio multimodale, che comprende per prima la chirurgia, come pure la radioterapia e la chemioterapia. L'andamento dei JPA è migliore rispetto a quello degli LGA fibrillari. Con una exeresi chirurgica radicale, la sopravvivenza globale raggiunge l'80-100%, mentre nei

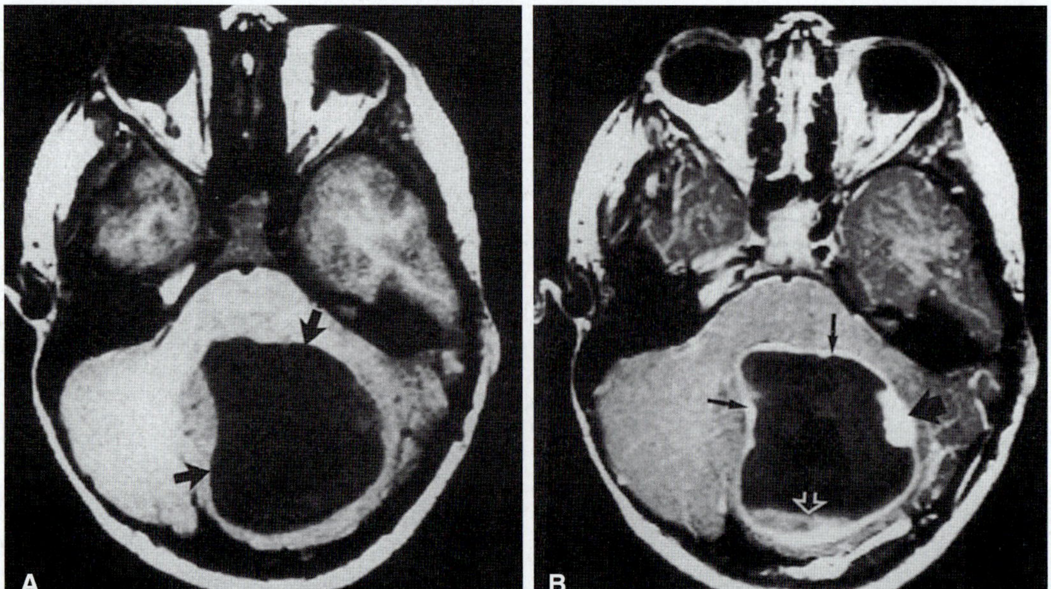

Figura 497-3. *A*, Sequenza assiale T1 pesata della RM di un paziente con un astrocitoma pilocitico cerebellare, con predominante componente cistica (ipointensa) (*frecce*), che coinvolge l'emisfero cerebellare sinistro e il verme. *B*, Sequenza T1 pesata con Gadolinio della RM dello stesso bambino, che dimostra una impregnazione di mezzo di contrasto della componente solida (*freccia spessa*) e della capsula (*freccia sottile*), con un livello di materiale assumente mezzo di contrasto sul fondo della cisti (*freccia aperta*). (Da Kuhn JP, Slovis TL, Haller JO: *Caffey's Pediatric Diagnostic Imaging*, 10th ed. Philadelphia, Mosby, 2004, p 576.)

pazienti con resezione parziale (<80%) la sopravvivenza varia dal 50 al 95%, a seconda della sede anatomica del tumore. I soggetti che hanno subito una resezione parziale e che presentano uno stato neurologico stabile secondo l'attuale strategia vanno seguiti con uno stretto follow-up clinico e radiologico. In caso di progressione, andrebbe presa in considerazione la possibilità di un reintervento. Nei pazienti in cui questa seconda chirurgia non sia stata radicale o non sia proponibile, risulterà efficace la radioterapia, che viene erogata sul letto tumorale a una dose totale cumulativa di 50-55 Gy somministrati quotidianamente per 6 settimane. In passato, i pazienti con neoplasie profonde dalla linea mediana venivano trattati empiricamente con la radioterapia senza previa chirurgia o biopsia, con una sopravvivenza variabile del 33-75%. Tuttavia, le moderne tecniche chirurgiche e le innovazioni nella radioterapia possono portare un impatto positivo sulla sopravvivenza e sul decorso clinico. Il ruolo della chemioterapia nel trattamento dell'LGA è in via di sviluppo. A causa delle conseguenze sulla morbilità causata dalla radioterapia nei bambini, sono stati valutati diversi approcci con la chemioterapia, soprattutto nei bambini <5 anni. La risposta completa a essa appare bassa; tuttavia questo approccio ha permesso di prolungare il controllo della malattia nel 70-100% dei casi. I pazienti con tumori della linea mediana al livello della regione ipotalamo/chiasmatica tendono ad andare meno bene. Considerati insieme, gli approcci chemioterapici hanno permesso di posticipare e potenzialmente di evitare la radioterapia. In un trial negli Stati Uniti ancora in corso, gli investigatori stanno confrontando l'efficacia e la tollerabilità di uno schema di chemioterapia a base di carboplatino con uno a base di lomustina (CCNU) in bambini <10 anni affetti da un LGA in progressione. Sono anche in corso trial clinici sull'utilizzo di temozolomide o vinblastina. È poi in studio l'approccio primario nel trattamento clinico di soggetti selezionati con LGA biologicamente indolenti. Un gruppo comprende pazienti con neurofibromatosi di tipo 1, che può progredire in un LGA del chiasma/vie ottiche o del tronco che viene riscontrato casualmente. Un altro gruppo include pazienti con astrocitomi del tronco che hanno avuto una risoluzione dei sintomi clinici dopo il posizionamento di una derivazione ventricolare e che non necessitano di ulteriori interventi.

Gli **astrocitomi maligni** sono molto meno comuni nei bambini e negli adolescenti che non negli adulti, rappresentando circa il 7-10% di tutti i tumori dell'infanzia. Tra questi, l'**astrocitoma anaplastico** (grado III, OMS) (Fig. 497-4) è più frequente del **glioblastoma multiforme** (grado IV, OMS). L'istopatologia degli astrocitomi anaplastici dimostra un aumento della cellularità rispetto agli atrocitomi diffusi di basso grado, atipie cellulari e nucleari, presenza di mitosi e di proliferazione microvascolare in modo variabile. I reperti istopatologici tipici del glioblastoma multiforme comprendono invece la densità cellulare, un alto indice mitotico, la proliferazione microvascolare e foci di necrosi tumorale. Sono disponibili pochi dati sulle alterazioni molecolari degli astrocitomi maligni dei bambini. Un indice prognostico sfavorevole è costituito dall'iperespressione di P53, la cui frequenza di mutazione è simile a quella osservata negli adulti, anche se nei bambini <3 anni è più bassa. Questo fatto suggerisce l'esistenza di meccanismi differenti dell'oncogenesi tra bambini di età diverse. La migliore strategia terapeutica per gli astrocitomi maligni deve ancora essere definita, per cui quella standard continua a essere costituita dalla resezione chirurgica, seguita dalla radioterapia conformazionale e quindi, generalmente, da un regime di chemioterapia a base di nitrosouree. Un trial pediatrico ha dimostrato un miglioramento della sopravvivenza nei soggetti trattati, dopo la radioterapia, con lomustina e vincristina rispetto a quelli solo radiotrattati. Allo stesso modo, uno studio sugli adulti affetti da glioblastoma ha dimostrato un significativo miglioramento della sopravvivenza in quelli sottoposti a un trattamento con temozolomide durante e dopo la radioterapia, rispetto a quest'ultima usata da sola. Questo trattamento radiante concomitante è in corso di studio anche per i gliomi di alto grado dell'infanzia.

Gli **oligodendrogliomi** sono tumori rari nei bambini. Questi tumori infiltranti si localizzano soprattutto a livello della corteccia cerebrale e originano dalla sostanza bianca. Istologicamente, sono costituiti da cellule rotondeggianti con uno scarso citoplasma e microcalcificazioni. Il riscontro di una massa corticale calcifica alla TC in un paziente con crisi epilettiche è suggestivo per un oligodendroglioma. Le strategie terapeutiche sono simili a quelle per gli astrocitomi infiltranti.

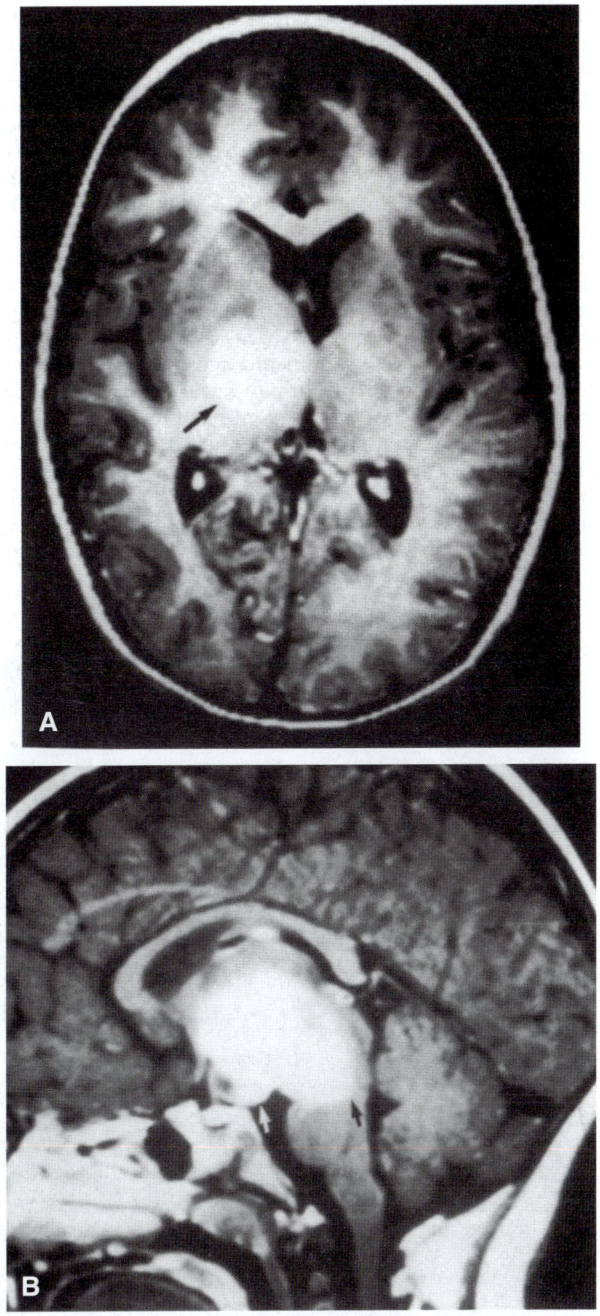

Figura 497-4. *A*, Sequenza assiale T1 pesata con Gadolinio di una RM di un astrocitoma di grado III del talamo di destra, che dimostra una diffusa assunzione di mezzo di contrasto (*freccia*). *B*, Sequenza T1 pesata sagittale di RM che dimostra l'assunzione di mezzo di contrasto di un astrocitoma di grado III del talamo con estensione al mesencefalo (*freccia nera*) e all'ipotalamo (*freccia bianca*). (Da Kuhn JP, Slovis TL, Haller JO: *Caffey's Pediatric Diagnostic Imaging*, 10th ed. Philadelphia, Mosby, 2004, p 595.)

GLIOMI MISTI. I gliomi misti sono composti da due o più tipi distinti di cellule gliali (astrocitoma, oligodendroglioma ed ependimoma) e risultano rari nei pazienti pediatrici.

TUMORI EPENDIMALI. Questi tumori originano dalle cellule ependimali che rivestono le pareti del sistema ventricolare. L'ependimoma (grado II, OMS) è il più frequente tra essi, colpisce soprattutto l'infanzia e rappresenta il 10% delle neoplasie pediatriche. Circa il 70% degli ependimomi infantili è localizzato a livello della fossa posteriore. L'età media dei pazienti è di 6 anni, con un 30% circa dei casi che si verifica prima dei 3 anni. L'incidenza della disseminazione leptomeningea è circa del 10%. La presentazione clinica dipende dalla sede del tumore. La RM ne dimostra uno ben circoscritto, con un'assunzione di mezzo di contrasto variabile e complessa, con o senza aree cistiche (Fig. 497-5). Questi tumori generalmente non sono invasivi, si estendono nel lume ventricolare e/o dislocano strutture normali. Le caratteristiche istologiche comprendono le pseudorosette perivascolari, le rosette ependimali, una morfologia nucleare monomorfa e occasionali foci di necrosi senza palizzate. La chirurgia è il trattamento di prima scelta e l'estensione della resezione è uno dei principali fattori prognostici, insieme all'età, con una prognosi peggiore per i bambini più piccoli, e alla sede del tumore, con una prognosi più infausta che viene comportata dalla localizzazione nella fossa posteriore spesso osservabile nei bambini piccoli. La chirurgia da sola raramente è sufficiente, ma una terapia multimodale, in cui si trovi in associazione con la radioterapia, ha determinato una sopravvivenza a lungo termine in circa il 40% dei casi dopo una exeresi quasi completa. La recidiva della malattia è soprattutto locale. La radioterapia conformazionale è raccomandata per la maggior parte dei bambini che abbiano l'ependimoma e l'ependimoma anaplastico. Il primo è sensibile a diversi agenti chemioterapici, sebbene il ruolo della chemioterapia nel suo trattamento multimodale non sia ancora chiaro. Alcuni trial limitati hanno dimostrato che un trattamento chemioterapico ad alte dosi con recupero di cellule staminali nel sangue periferico non risulta benefico. Studi recenti sono diretti a chiarire la dose ottimale di radiazioni, l'utilità di una seconda chirurgia dopo la chemioterapia e ulteriori valutazioni sull'utilizzo di chemioterapici classici e nuovi. Nell'ependimoma non compaiono tipiche alterazioni citogenetiche o genetico-molecolari. Tuttavia, studi preliminari suggeriscono l'esistenza di sottotipi geneticamente distinti, per esempio l'associazione tra le alterazioni del gene NF2 e l'ependimoma spinale. L'ependimoma anaplastico (grado III, OMS) è raro nell'infanzia; è contraddistinto da un alto indice mitotico e da caratteristiche istologiche di proliferazione microvascolare e necrosi con pseudopalizzate. L'ependimoma mixopapillare (grado I, OMS) è un tumore a lenta crescita, che deriva dal filum terminale e dal cono midollare.

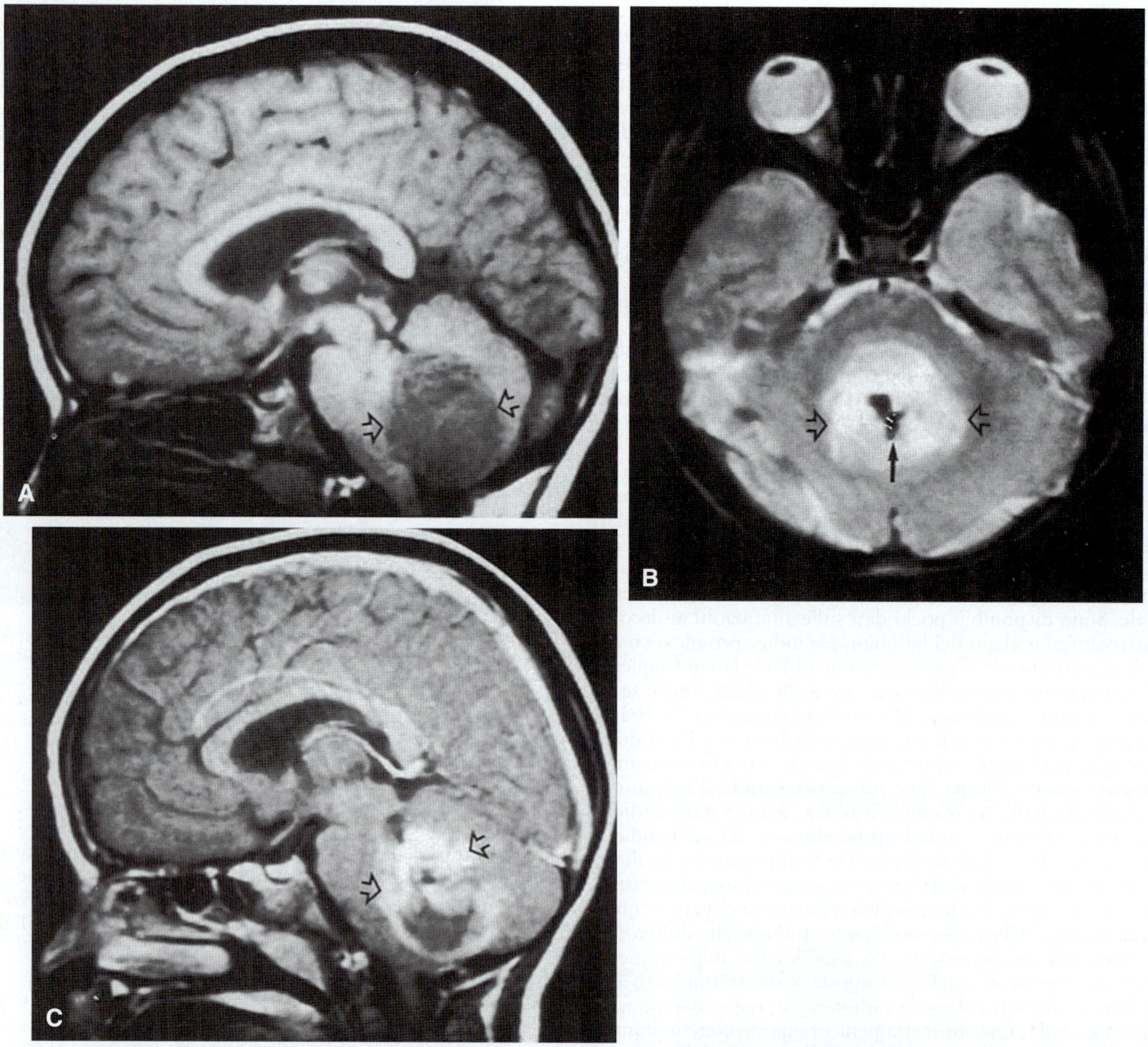

Figura 497-5. *A*, Sequenza sagittale T1 pesata di un paziente con ependimoma, che evidenzia una massa ipointensa (*frecce*) all'interno del IV ventricolo. *B*, Sequenza assiale T2 pesata di un ependimoma che dimostra una lesione iperintensa (*frecce aperte*) e un'area centrale ipointensa per le calcificazioni (*freccia chiusa*) all'interno del IV ventricolo. C, Sequenza sagittale T1 pesata con Gadolinio che dimostra un ependimoma (*frecce*). (Da Kuhn JP, Slovis TL, Haller JO: *Caffey's Pediatric Diagnostic Imaging*, 10th ed. Philadelphia, Mosby, 2004, p 579.)

TUMORI DEI PLESSI CORIOIDEI. I tumori dei plessi corioidei rappresentano il 2-4% dei tumori del SNC in età pediatrica. Sono quelli più frequenti nei bambini con <1 anno e costituiscono il 10-20% dei tumori del SNC che si manifestano durante l'infanzia. Si tratta di tumori intraventricolari epiteliali che derivano dal plesso corioideo. I bambini hanno segni e sintomi da ipertensione endocranica. Nei neonati possono comparire la macrocefalia e deficit neurologici focali, mentre nei bambini questi tumori sono soprattutto sovratentoriali a livello dei ventricoli laterali. Il **papilloma dei plessi corioidei** (grado I, OMS), la forma più comune, radiologicamente appare come una lesione ben delimitata e istologicamente assomiglia molto ai plessi corioidei normali. Il **carcinoma dei plessi corioidei** (grado III, OMS) è una neoplasia maligna potenzialmente metastatica per vie liquorali. Questa malignità è evidente a livello istologico per la presenza di pleiomorfismi nucleari, un elevato indice mitotico e un aumento della densità cellulare. L'immunopositività per la transtiretina (prealbumina) è utile per confermare la diagnosi. Queste neoplasie si associano alla **sindrome di Li-Fraumeni** e il **virus 40 della scimmia** può avere un ruolo sulla loro eziologia. Dopo una resezione chirurgica completa, la sopravvivenza per il papilloma dei plessi corioidei si avvicina al 100%, mentre quella del carcinoma al 20-40%. Alcune segnalazioni suggeriscono che la radioterapia e/o la chemioterapia possono migliorare il controllo del carcinoma.

TUMORI EMBRIONALI. I tumori embrionali, o **tumori neuroectodermici primitivi** (**PNET**), tra quelli maligni del SNC sono i più frequenti nei bambini, rappresentandone circa il 20-25%. Possono disseminare a livello del nevrasse. Il gruppo comprende il medulloblastoma, i PNET sovratentoriali, l'ependimoblastoma, il medulloepitelioblastoma e il tumore teratoide/rabdoide atipico, tutti classificati istologicamente come tumori di grado IV secondo l'OMS.

Il **medulloblastoma** rappresenta il 90% dei tumori embrionali ed è una neoplasia cerebellare che colpisce soprattutto i maschi a un'età media di 5-7 anni. La maggior parte dei medulloblastomi interessa la parte mediana del verme cerebellare, sebbene i pazienti più vecchi possano manifestare localizzazioni a livello degli emisferi cerebellari. La TC e la RM mostrano una massa solida, omogenea, assumente mezzo di contrasto al livello della fossa cranica posteriore, che provoca un'ostruzione del IV ventricolo e dell'idrocefalo. Oltre il 30% dei pazienti si presenta alla diagnosi con un interessamento radiologico delle leptomeningi. Tra i diversi tipi istologici di questo tumore, il più frequente è quello che deriva dalla lamina monomorfa, con cellule indifferenziate classicamente di piccole dimensioni, di colore blu e di forma rotondeggiante. La differenziazione neuronale è più comune tra questi tumori ed è istologicamente caratterizzata dalla presenza di rosette di Homer Wright e da una immunopositività per la sinaptosina. Una variante anaplastica può comportare una prognosi peggiore. I pazienti hanno segni e sintomi dell'ipertensione endocranica (cefalea, nausea, vomito, modificazioni dello stato mentale e ipertensione) e presentano disfunzioni cerebellari (atassia, disequilibrio, dismetria). La valutazione clinica standard di stadiazione comprende la RM encefalospinale, sia prechirurgica sia postchirurgica, così come la puntura lombare dopo la risoluzione dell'ipertensione endocranica (Fig. 497-6). Il sistema di stadiazione secondo Chang, inizialmente fondato sulla valutazione chirurgica, è stato modificato al fine di inserire i dati degli esami neuroradiologici per identificare le categorie a rischio. Le caratteristiche cliniche che hanno consistentemente dimostrato di avere un significato prognostico sono l'età al momento della diagnosi, l'estensione della malattia e quella della exeresi chirurgica. I pazienti con meno di 4 anni hanno una prognosi peggiore, in parte per l'aumentata incidenza di disseminazione della malattia alla diagnosi e in parte per le strategie terapeutiche del passato, che si avvalevano di terapie meno aggressive. I soggetti con malattia disseminata al momento della diagnosi (M >0), compresa anche la sola positività del CSF per le cellule neoplastiche (M1), hanno un andamento clinico decisamente peggiore rispetto a quelli senza disseminazione (M0). Analogamente, i pazienti con una grossa malattia residua dopo la chirurgia hanno una prognosi peggiore di quelli sottoposti a una resezione radicale.

Gli studi citogenetici e geneticomolecolari hanno dimostrato molteplici anomalie nel medulloblastoma. L'alterazione più comune comprende le delezioni del cromosoma 17p, che si osservano nel 30-40% dei casi e che non sono associate alle mutazioni della P53. Sono stati proposti due nuovi sistemi di stratificazione del rischio per il medulloblastoma, combinando i marcatori molecolari con gli elementi clinici. Un sistema si basa sull'analisi retrospettiva dei dati sulle varianti istologiche (classica, desmoplastica nodulare, anaplastica a grandi cellule), sull'espressione di TRKC, MYCC, ERBB2 e MYCC e sulle ca-

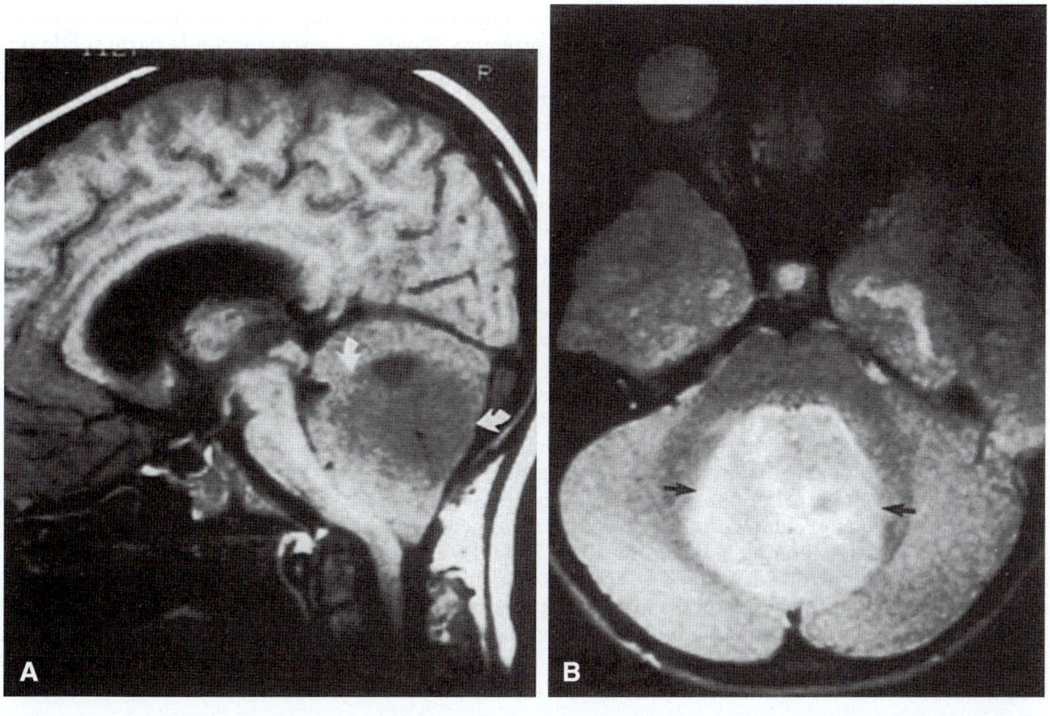

Figura 497-6. RM di un medulloblastoma. *A*, Sequenza sagittale T1 pesata che dimostra una lesione ipointensa che interessa il verme (*frecce*). *B*, Sequenza assiale T2 pesata che evidenzia una lesione iperintensa (*frecce*) con aree ipointense per la presenza di infarti emorragici acuti in un medulloblastoma del verme. (Da Kuhn JP, Slovis TL, Haller JO: *Caffey's Pediatric Diagnostic Imaging*, 10th ed. Philadelphia, Mosby, 2004, p 574.)

ratteristiche cliniche dei bambini con il medulloblastoma. Uno studio ha dimostrato che la combinazione di queste ultime e dell'espressione di ERBB2 era in grado di fornire informazioni molto accurate per discriminare il rischio legato alla malattia. Un altro studio ha indicato come il profilo dell'espressione genica sia predittivo della prognosi del medulloblastoma indipendentemente dalle variabili cliniche. Entrambi gli approcci devono ancora essere confermati su valutazioni prospettiche più ampie. Con l'evoluzione della tecnologia del riarragiamento genico, alcuni studi preliminari hanno identificato cluster di geni/espressione genica che sembrano essere associati con il medulloblastoma metastatico e con la prognosi.

Per il medulloblastoma è auspicabile un approccio terapeutico di tipo multimodale, con la chirurgia come punto di partenza. Il medulloblastoma è comunque sensibile sia alla chemioterapia sia alla radioterapia, dal momento che si sa che la chirurgia da sola non è sufficiente. L'efficacia della radioterapia è stata rilevata negli anni '40, con il miglioramento della sopravvivenza globale al 30%. Con gli avanzamenti tecnologici nella neurochirurgia, nella neuroradiologia e nella radioterapia stessa e allo stesso tempo con l'evidenza della chemioterapia come strategia terapeutica efficace, la prognosi complessiva di tutti i pazienti si avvicina al 60-70%. Il trattamento radiante standard per il medulloblastoma comprende l'irradiamento craniospinale con una dose cumulativa totale di 30-36 Gy e una sul letto tumorale di 50-55 Gy. Con queste dosi, in bambini con meno di 3 anni vengono tuttavia provocate gravi sequele neurologiche tardive, compresi la microcefalia, la difficoltà di apprendimento, il ritardo mentale, disfunzioni neuroendocrine (deficit della crescita, ipotiroidismo, ipogonadismo e pubertà assente/ritardata) e/o secondi tumori. Per altro, anche nei bambini più grandi possono verificarsi le sequele tardive, quali difficoltà di apprendimento, disfunzioni neuroendocrine e/o secondi tumori. Queste osservazioni hanno portato a stratificare gli approcci terapeutici in tre categorie: (1) pazienti <3 anni; (2) pazienti >3 anni con rischio standard, con asportazione chirurgica radicale e nessuna evidenza di disseminazione di malattia (M0); (3) pazienti >3 anni ad alto rischio, con malattia disseminata (M >0) e/o voluminoso residuo di malattia dopo la chirurgia. Con un approccio terapeutico basato sul rischio, i bambini affetti da un medulloblastoma ad alto rischio vengono sottoposti alla radioterapia craniospinale a dose piena, con chemioterapia durante e dopo.

In bambini con medulloblastoma non metastatico e una resezione ampia, la sola chemioterapia (metotrexato, ciclofosfamide, vincristina, carboplatino, etoposide) determina una sopravvivenza del 90%. La presenza di un residuo tumorale (sopravvivenza del 56%) o di metastasi (38%) determina una prognosi sfavorevole.

I **tumori neuroectodermici primitivi sovratentoriali** rappresentano il 2-3% delle neoplasie cerebrali infantili, soprattutto durante la prima decade di vita. Questi tumori sono istologicamente simili al medulloblastoma e risultano costituiti da cellule neuroepiteliali indifferenziate o scarsamente differenziate. Dal punto di vista istologico, i pazienti hanno una prognosi più sfavorevole rispetto a quelli con il medulloblastoma da quando si è cominciata a utilizzare la terapia combinata. In recenti trial clinici, i bambini con questi tumori sono considerati nel gruppo di quelli ad alto rischio e ricevono una chemioterapia ad alte dosi in associazione alla radioterapia craniospinale.

Il **tumore teratoide/rabdoide atipico** è una neoplasia embrionale particolarmente aggressiva, che colpisce soprattutto bambini <5 anni e che può trovarsi in qualunque sede del nevrasse. Dal punto di vista istologico si tratta di cellule eterogenee, comprese cellule rabdoidi, che esprimono antigeni della membrana epiteliale e antigeni dei neurofilamenti. Il tipico pattern citogenetico è la delezione parziale o completa del cromosoma 22q, che è stata associata con la mutazione del gene INI1. La relazione tra questa mutazione e la tumorigenesi non è chiara. La prognosi, anche dopo l'introduzione di una terapia multimodale con chemioterapia intensiva, è molto sfavorevole, ma sono stati riportati casi di lunga sopravvivenza.

L'**ependimoblastoma** e il **medullomioblastoma** sono rari tumori embrionali altamente maligni, che possono colpire i bambini durante i primi anni di vita.

TUMORI PARENCHIMALI DELLA PINEALE. Questi tumori sono la seconda più frequente neoplasia, dopo i germinomi, al livello della regione pineale. Comprendono il pinealoblastoma, che colpisce soprattutto durante l'infanzia, e i tumori parenchimali misti. L'approccio terapeutico a questo gruppo di malattie è multimodale. In passato si rivolgeva una particolare attenzione alla sede delle masse e alle potenziali complicanze dell'intervento chirurgico, ma con i recenti sviluppi delle tecniche neurochirurgiche e della tecnologia chirurgica, la morbilità e la mortalità associate al trattamento si sono ridotte in modo significativo. La biopsia stereotassica di questi tumori può essere un valido strumento per porre la diagnosi; tuttavia, andrebbe sempre presa in considerazione la possibilità di una resezione radicale della lesione, prima di intraprendere una terapia aggiuntiva. Il pinealoblastoma è la variante più maligna ed è considerato un sottogruppo dei PNET infantili. I regimi di chemioterapia prevedono l'utilizzo di derivati del platino, di ciclofosfamide, etoposide (VP-16) e vincristina e/o lomustina. Alcuni dati hanno dimostrato che la sopravvivenza dei PNET della regione pineale, trattati in modo combinato con la chemioterapia e la radioterapia, si avvicina al 70% a 5 anni, analogamente a quanto si è osservato per il medulloblastoma. Il pinealocitoma generalmente è trattato con la resezione chirurgica.

TUMORI NEURONALI/NEURONALI-GLIALI MISTI. I tumori neuronali e neuronali-gliali misti sono un gruppo eterogeneo di neoplasie a crescita lenta e con scarsa progressione maligna. Si accompagnano a una prognosi favorevole dopo l'asportazione chirurgica. Sono classificati come tumori di grado I o II secondo l'OMS. Le patologie di questa categoria comprendono i gangliogliomi, i tumori neuroepiteliali disembrioplastici, gli astrocitomi desmoplastici dell'infanzia e i gangliogliomi desmoplastici dell'infanzia.

CRANIOFARINGIOMA. Il craniofaringioma (grado I, OMS) è un tumore frequente nell'infanzia, rappresentando il 7-10% di tutte le neoplasie pediatriche. L'adamantinoma, una sua variante, è tipico poi di questa età. Questi tumori presentano una componente solida e una cistica e si localizzano nella regione sovrasellare. Sono poco invasivi, aderiscono al parenchima cerebrale adiacente e inglobano le normali strutture encefaliche. La RM mostra la presenza di un tumore solido con strutture cistiche contenenti un liquido di media densità, mentre la TC può indicare calcificazioni associate con la parte solida o con la parete delle aree cistiche. La chirurgia è la principale strategia terapeutica, con una resezione radicale risolutiva nel caso di piccole lesioni. Sono controversi i ruoli relativi della chirurgia e della radioterapia nel trattamento di tumori complessi e di grosse dimensioni, cui si trova associata una significativa morbilità (panipopituitarismo, deficit della crescita, deficit del visus), per via della sede anatomica. La chemioterapia non gioca nessun ruolo nei craniofaringiomi.

TUMORI MENINGEI. I meningiomi sono tumori rari nell'infanzia. Queste neoplasie derivano dal foglietto dell'aracnoide e generalmente presentano una crescita molto lenta. Nei bambini, la maggior parte di essi si associa a una predisposizione genetica, come nel caso della neurofibromatosi di tipo 2, oppure alla sindrome del nevo basale o ancora a una precedente esposizione a radiazioni (secondo tumore).

GERMINOMI. I germinomi del SNC sono un gruppo eterogeneo di tumori; colpiscono soprattutto i bambini e nascono prevalentemente a livello delle strutture della linea mediana delle regioni pineale e sovrasellare. Rappresentano l'1-2% dei tumori cerebrali pediatrici, con un picco d'incidenza a 10-12 anni. In generale si trova una predominanza nel sesso maschile, sebbene i tumori sovrasellari colpiscano più frequentemente le femmine. Queste neoplasie sono multifocali nel 5-10% dei casi; colpiscono più spesso le popolazioni asiatiche rispetto a quelle europee. Come per i germinomi periferici, l'analisi dei marcatori come l'**α-fetoproteina** e la **β-gonadotropina corionica umana** può risultare utile per porre la diagnosi e monitorare la risposta al trattamento. Anche la biopsia è raccomandata per la diagnosi, sebbene i germinomi non-germinomatosi possano venire diagnosticati solo sulla base dell'aumento dei marker proteici. Gli approcci terapeutici per i germinomi e per i tumori misti a cellule germinali sono differenti. La probabilità di sopravvivenza dei pazienti con germinomi puri supera il 90%; il loro trattamento postchirurgico è un po' controverso nel definire i relativi ruoli della chemioterapia e della radioterapia. Sono per esempio stati riportati eccellenti risultati nei soggetti che hanno ricevuto >40 Gy a livello locale e l'irradiazione craniospinale; così come uno stesso tipo di esito si è avuto quando la chemioterapia è stata introdotta nei protocolli che utilizzavano dosi ridotte di radiazioni (24 Gy solo sul letto tumorale). Più recentemente, trial clinici hanno comunque studiato l'uso della chemioterapia e della radioterapia a dosi ridotte. L'approccio terapeutico dei germinomi non-germinomatosi è invece più aggressivo, con la combinazione di regimi di chemioterapia più intensi con la radioterapia craniospinale. La sopravvivenza per questi tumori è marcatamente ridotta rispetto a quella riportata per i germinomi, essendo del 40-70% a 5 anni. Alcuni trial hanno dimostrato che alte dosi di chemioterapia con il recupero di cellule staminali nel sangue periferico risultano benefiche. Se ciò venisse confermato in studi più vasti, le future strategie potrebbero prevedere l'utilizzo di queste alte dosi insieme a una radioterapia a dosi ridotte.

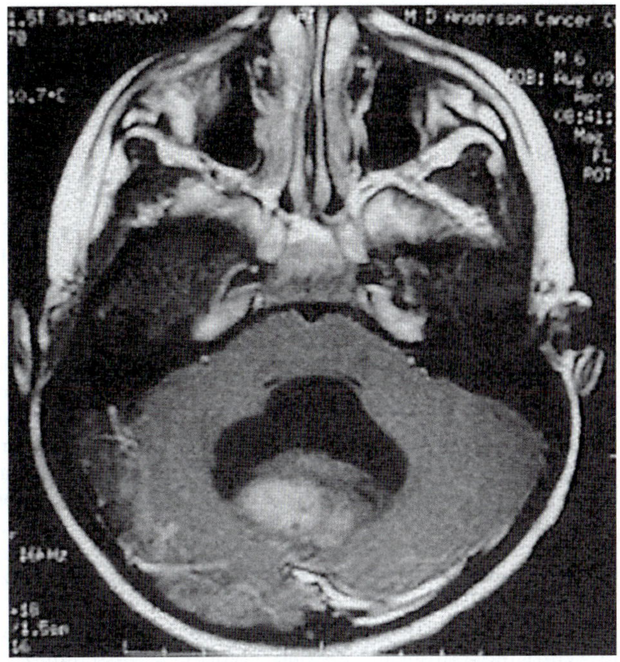

Figura 497-7. Sequenza T1 pesata dopo somministrazione di Gadolinio (sagittale) di un glioma diffuso infiltrante del tronco in una bambina di 10 anni con cefalea, paralisi dei nervi cranici e ipostenia a sinistra.

TUMORI DEL TRONCO CEREBRALE. I tumori del tronco sono un gruppo eterogeneo che rappresenta il 10-15% dei tumori primitivi del SNC nell'infanzia. La prognosi dipende dalla localizzazione del tumore, dalle caratteristiche radiologiche e dalle condizioni cliniche del paziente. I soggetti con queste neoplasie possono presentare deficit motori, dei nervi cranici, cerebellari e/o segni da ipertensione endocranica. Sulla base delle valutazioni della RM e clinica, i tumori del tronco possono essere classificati in 4 tipi: focali (5-10% dei pazienti), esofitici posteriormente (5-10%), cervicomidollari (5-10%) e intrinseci diffusi (70-85%) (Figg. 497-7 e 497-8). La resezione chirurgica è il primo approccio terapeutico per i tumori focali e quelli esofitici posteriormente e si accompagna a una prognosi favorevole. Dal punto di vista istologico, questi due gruppi generalmente comprendono gliomi di basso grado.

I tumori cervicomidollari, per via della loro sede, possono non essere aggredibili chirurgicamente, ma sono sensibili al trattamento radiante. I tumori intrinseci diffusi, caratterizzati dalla presenza di un glioma pontino diffuso infiltrante, comportano invece una prognosi sfavorevole, indipendentemente dall'istologia, e non si possono affrontare chirurgicamente. La biopsia nei bambini con un riscontro radiologico di un tumore intrinseco diffuso è controversa e non è consigliabile, a meno che non vi sia il sospetto di una patologia diversa, come un'infezione, una demielinizzazione, una malformazione vascolare, una sclerosi multipla o una lesione metastatica. Queste diagnosi sono tuttavia molto più frequenti negli adulti. L'approccio standard per il trattamento dei gliomi

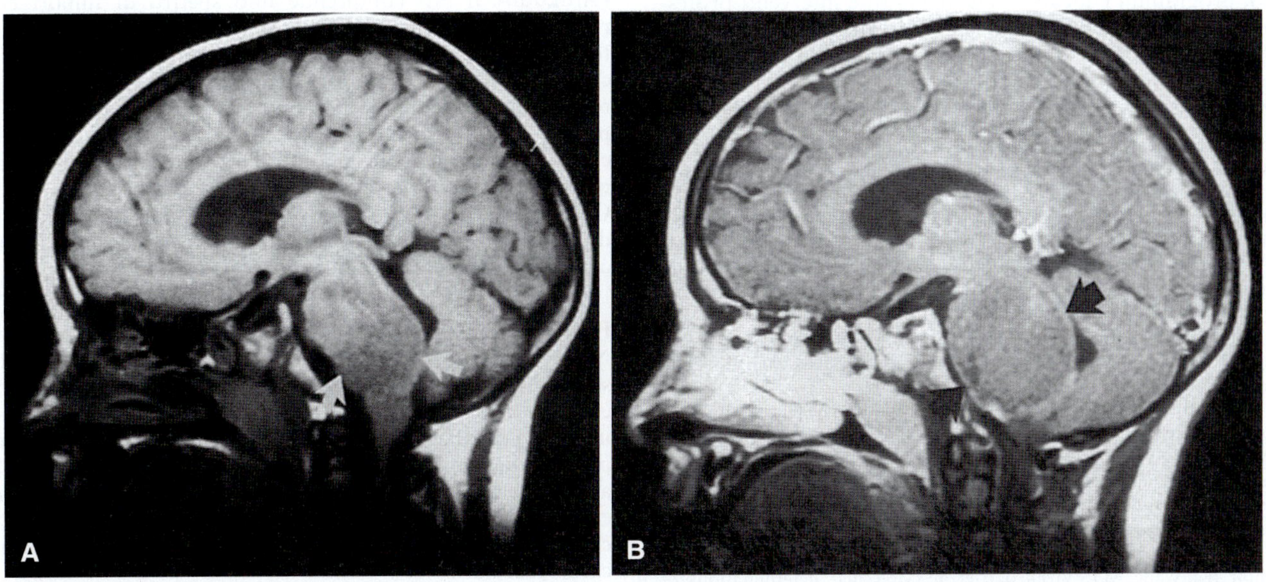

Figura 497-8. *A*, Sequenza sagittale T1 pesata di una RM che dimostra un astrocitoma del tronco che determina un allargamento del ponte per la presenza di un'area lievemente ipointensa (*frecce*). *B*, Sequenza sagittale T1 pesata dopo somministrazione di Gadolinio che dimostra un astrocitoma del tronco, con una massa (*frecce*) lievemente ipointensa, che non assume mezzo di contrasto e che determina un allargamento del ponte. (Da Kuhn JP, Slovis TL, Haller JO: *Caffey's Pediatric Diagnostic Imaging*, 10th ed. Philadelphia, Mosby, 2004, p 577.)

pontini infiltranti diffusi è la radioterapia, con una sopravvivenza mediana di 12 mesi nella migliore delle situazioni. L'utilizzo di chemioterapici, compresa la chemioterapia ad alte dosi con recupero di cellule staminali dal sangue periferico, non ha ancora portato risultati per la sopravvivenza dei pazienti. Alcune recenti strategie comprendono la valutazione di agenti investigazionali da soli o in associazione con la radioterapia, similmente agli approcci perseguiti nei pazienti con gliomi maligni.

TUMORI METASTATICI. Le metastasi cerebrali provocate da altri tumori dell'infanzia sono rare. La leucemia linfatica acuta infantile e il linfoma non-Hodgkin possono produrre metastasi leptomeningee, provocando sintomi da idrocefalo comunicante. I **cloromi**, che sono un ammasso di cellule leucemiche mieliodi, possono localizzarsi in qualunque punto del nevrasse. Raramente si hanno metastasi parenchimali cerebrali da linfoma, neuroblastoma, rabdomiosarcoma, sarcoma di Ewing, osteosarcoma e sarcoma renale a cellule chiare. L'approccio terapeutico si basa sulla diagnosi istologica specifica e può comprendere la radioterapia, la somministrazione di chemioterapici per via intratecale e/o di una chemioterapia per via sistemica. Il medulloblastoma è il tumore cerebrale infantile che più comunemente metastatizza a livello extraneurale. Meno comunemente queste metastasi si osservano da gliomi maligni, PNET ed ependimomi. Le derivazioni ventricoloperitoneali possono favorire la disseminazione extraneurale, soprattutto al livello della cavità peritoneale, ma anche a quello sistemico.

COMPLICANZE E LORO TRATTAMENTO TARDIVO

I dati del National Cancer Institute SEER Program indicano che >70% dei pazienti con tumori cerebrali durante l'infanzia avrà una lunga sopravvivenza. Almeno la metà di questi soggetti avrà tuttavia disturbi cronici, come diretta conseguenza del tumore e dei relativi trattamenti. Questi disturbi comprendono i deficit neurologici cronici come quelli focali motori e sensitivi, le crisi comiziali, i deficit neurocognitivi (ritardo nello sviluppo, difficoltà di apprendimento) e le alterazioni neuroendocrine (ipotiroidismo, deficit di accrescimento, pubertà ritardata o assente). Questi pazienti sono anche ad alto rischio di sviluppare secondi tumori. Alcuni interventi di supporto multidisciplinare per i bambini con tumori cerebrali sia durante sia dopo il trattamento aiutano a migliorare la loro sopravvivenza. L'ottimizzazione del controllo delle crisi, la fisioterapia, il supporto endocrinologico con la somministrazione dell'ormone della crescita e il supporto tiroideo, programmi educativi personalizzati e interventi professionali possono migliorare la qualità della vita dei bambini che sopravvivono alla diagnosi di tumore cerebrale.

Fernandez-Teijeiro A, Betensky RA, Sturla LM, et al: Combining gene expression profiles and clinical parameters for risk stratification in medulloblastomas. *J Clin Oncol* 2004; 22:994–998.

Freeman CR, Perilongo G: Chemotherapy for brain stem gliomas. *Childs Nerv Syst* 1999;15:545–553.

Gajjar A, Hernan R, Kocak M, et al: Clinical, histopathologic, and molecular markers of prognosis: Toward a new disease risk stratification system for medulloblastoma. *J Clin Oncol* 2004;22:984–993.

Grill J, Sainte-Rose C, Jouvet A, et al: Treatment of medulloblastoma with postoperative chemotherapy alone: An SFOP prospective trial in young children. *Lancet Oncol* 2005;6:573–580.

Gurney JC, Smith MA, Bunin GR: In Reis LAG, Smith MA, Gurney JC, et al (editors): *Cancer Survival and Incidence Among Children and Adolescents: United States SEER Program 1975–1995.* Bethesda, MD, National Cancer Institute SEER Program. NIH publication No. 99–4649, 1999, pp 51–63.

Kleihues P, Cavenee WK: *World Health Organization Classification of Tumours: Pathology and Genetics of Tumours of the Nervous System.* Lyon, IARC Press, 2000.

Mellinghoff IK, Wang MY, Vivanco I, et al: Molecular determinations of the response of glioblastomas to EGFR kinase inhibitors. *N Engl J Med* 2005;353:2012–2024.

Merchant TE, Mulhern RK, Krasin MJ, et al: Preliminary results from a phase II trial of conformal radiation therapy and evaluation of radiation-related CNS effects for pediatric patients with localized ependymoma. *J Clin Oncol* 2004;15:3156–3162.

Packer RJ, Cohen BH, Coney K: Intracranial germ cell tumors. *Oncologist* 2000;5:312–320.

Pollack IF, Finkelstein SD, Woods J, et al: Expression of p53 and prognosis in children with malignant gliomas. *N Engl J Med* 2002;346:420–426.

Rutkowski S, Bode U, Deinlein F, et al: Treatment of early childhood medulloblastoma by postoperative chemotherapy alone. *N Engl J Med* 2005;352:978–986.

Shaw EG, Wisoff JH: Prospective clinical trials of intracranial low-grade glioma in adults and children. *Neurooncol* 2003;5:153–160.

Strother DR, Pollac IF, Fisher PG, et al: Tumors of the central nervous system. In Pizzo PA, Poplack DG (editors): *Principles and Practice of Pediatric Oncology,* 5th ed. Philadelphia, Lippincott Williams & Wilkins, 2006.

Stupp R, Mason WP, van den Bent MJ, et al: Radiotherapy plus concomitant and adjuvant temozolomide for glioblastoma. *N Engl J Med* 2005;352:987–996.

Zebrack BJ, Gurney JG, Oeffinger K, et al: Psychological outcomes in long-term survivors of childhood brain cancer: A report from the Childhood Cancer Survivors Study. *J Clin Oncol* 2004;22:999–1006.

Capitolo 498 ■ Neuroblastoma

Joann L. Ater

Il neuroblastoma (NB) è una neoplasia embrionale del sistema nervoso simpatico periferico con presentazione clinica e decorso eterogenei. Lo spettro clinico del NB è variabile, andando da una regressione spontanea in alcuni casi a tumori particolarmente aggressivi non responsivi a trattamenti multimodali in altri. È attualmente accertata l'esistenza di oltre un tipo di NB.

EPIDEMIOLOGIA. Il NB è la terza più comune neoplasia in età pediatrica, rappresentando circa il l8% dei tumori dell'infanzia. Ogni anno negli Stati Uniti sono diagnosticati circa 500 nuovi casi. Il NB è anzi la neoplasia diagnosticata più di frequente nei neonati, rappresentando il 28-39% dei tumori neonatali. L'età media al momento della diagnosi è di 2 anni e il 90% dei casi è diagnosticato prima dei 5 anni. L'incidenza è leggermente più alta nei ragazzi e nei soggetti di razza bianca.

PATOLOGIA. Il NB comprende uno spettro di tumori con vari gradi di differenziazione neurale, andando da piccole cellule tondeggianti indifferenziate (neuroblastomi) a tumori contenenti cellule ganglionali mature (ganglioneuroblastomi o ganglioneuromi). Queste neoplasie possono assomigliare ad altri **tumori a piccole cellule tondeggianti**, quali il rabdomiosarcoma, il sarcoma di Ewing e il linfoma non-Hodgkin. La prognosi varia in relazione al tipo istologico (classificazione secondo Shimada). Costituiscono fattori prognostici la quantità di stroma, il grado di differenziazione delle cellule tumorali, la presenza di nucleoli ampi e prominenti e l'indice di mitosi carioressi.

PATOGENESI. L'evento genetico iniziale che scatena la nascita del NB non è noto. La patogenesi è probabilmente correlata alla successione di eventi mutageni, prenatali e perinatali, che possono essere provocati da fattori ambientali e genetici. Un'aumentata incidenza di NB è stata correlata ad alcune occupazioni materne e paterne che comportano l'esposizione ad agenti chimici, al lavoro agricolo e ai lavori che mettono a contatto con apparecchiature elettroniche. Le forme familiari di NB rappresentano l'1-2% dei casi. Il NB può anche trovarsi associato ad alcune malformazioni cardiovascolari.

Le **caratteristiche genetiche** del tessuto tumorale del NB, che possono avere un'importanza prognostica e che vengono correntemente utilizzate insieme ai fattori clinici per programmare il trattamento, sono l'amplificazione del proto-oncogene MYCN (N-myc) e l'iperdiploidia del DNA nelle cellule tumorali (Tab. 498-1). L'amplificazione del MYCN ha un ruolo prognostico importante, indipendentemente dallo stadio e dall'età, ed è strettamente associata con una fase avanzata del tumore e con una prognosi sfavorevole. L'iperdiploidia conferisce la prognosi migliore se il bambino al momento della diagnosi ha <1 anno. Le alterazioni genetiche, compresa la perdita di eterozigosi di 1p, 11q e 14q e l'acquisto di 17q, si trovano spesso al livello del tessuto tumorale del NB. Altri fattori biologici che si correlano alla prognosi comprendono poi il livello di espressione del recettore del fattore di crescita del nervo (Trk-A), della proteina associata alla resistenza ai farmaci e all'attività della telomerasi. Questi fattori sono in corso di valutazione nei trial clinici, per capire se ci si potrà servire di loro per migliorare ulteriormente l'approccio terapeutico relativo al rischio di recidiva. Pertanto, la terapia può essere ridotta nei bambini a basso rischio, che possono beneficiare di una terapia minima, mentre può essere intensificata per quelli ad alto rischio.

MANIFESTAZIONI CLINICHE. Il NB può mimare molte altre patologie e può essere difficile da diagnosticare. Si può sviluppare in qualunque sede in cui si trovi tessuto del sistema nervoso simpatico. I suoi segni e sintomi riflettono la sede del tumore e la sua estensione. La maggior parte dei casi origina nell'addome, sia a livello delle ghiandole surrenali sia a quello dei gangli simpatici retroperitoneali. Generalmente si tratta di una massa nodulare, fissa, palpabile a livello del fianco o lungo la linea mediana, che provoca dolenzia a livello addominale. Agli esami radiografici o alla TC, la massa spesso risulta calcifica e può avere emorragie focali. Il tumore di Wilms, un'altra massa localizzata nel fianco di frequente riscontro nei bambini, generalmente non calcifica. Il NB nel 30% dei casi prende origine dai gangli cervicali, toracici o pelvici. Alcune forme di malattia metastatica possono accompagnarsi a molteplici segni e sintomi, quali la febbre, l'irritabilità, un ridotto accrescimento, il dolore osseo, noduli sottocutanei bluastri, proptosi ed ecchimosi periorbitali (Fig. 498-1). Le più frequenti sedi per le metastasi sono le ossa lunghe e quelle del cranio, il midollo osseo, il fegato, i linfonodi e la cute. Le metastasi polmonari sono rare, rappresentando <3% dei casi. La diagnosi prenatale talvolta è possibile attraverso l'ecografia.

Meno comunemente si ha un esordio con segni e sintomi neurologici. La localizzazione a livello del ganglio cervicale superiore può determinare la **sindrome di Horner**. Il NB paraspinale può invadere i forami di coniugazione, dando origine a un sintomo da compressione spinale e radicolare. Il NB può altresì presentarsi come una sindrome paraneoplastica su base autoimmune, con un quadro di atassia o **opsomioclono** ("occhi e piedi danzanti"). In questi casi, il tumore primitivo è localizzato a livello toracico o addominale e il cervello non presenta segni d'interessamento. Alcuni tumori producono catecolamine, che possono provocare un aumento della sudorazione e un'ipertensione e altri rilasciano il peptide intestinale vasoattivo, responsabile di una diarrea secretoria. Bambini <1 anno possono manifestare uno stadio tipico, il 4S, spesso caratterizzato da noduli tumorali sottocutanei, coinvolgimento massivo del fegato e con un piccolo tumore primitivo e senza coinvolgimento osseo.

TABELLA 498-1. Neuroblastoma: gruppi di rischio

GRUPPO DI RISCHIO	STADIO INSS	ETÀ	STATO DI MYCN	ISTOLOGIA SECONDO SHIMADA	SOPRAVVIVENZA
Basso	1	Tutti	Qualunque	Qualunque	90-100%
	2	<1 anno	Qualunque	Qualunque	
	2	>1 anno	Qualunque	Favorevole	
	4S	<1 anno	<10 copie	Favorevole	
Medio	3	>1 anno	<10 copie	Favorevole	75-98%
	3 e 4	<1 anno	<10 copie	Qualunque	
	4S	<1 anno	<10 copie	Sfavorevole	
Alto	2	>1 anno	Qualunque	Sfavorevole	20-60%
	3	Tutti	>10 copie	Qualunque	
	4	<1 anno	>10 copie	Qualunque	
	4	>1 anno	Qualunque	Qualunque	

INSS, *International Neuroblastoma Staging System* (sistema di stadiazione internazionale del neuroblastoma).

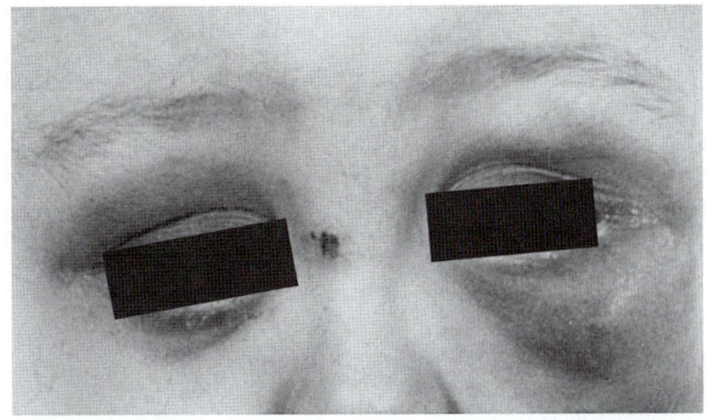

Figura 498-1. Metastasi periorbitali di neuroblastoma con proptosi ed ecchimosi.

DIAGNOSI. Il NB generalmente si manifesta come una massa o come masse multiple sulle radiografie, sulla TC o sulla RM (Fig. 498-2). I marker tumorali, l'acido omovanillico e l'acido vanilmandelico nelle urine risultano aumentati nel 95% dei casi e aiutano a confermare la diagnosi. La diagnosi patologica è fatta sul tessuto tumorale ottenuto con la biopsia. Il NB può essere diagnosticato anche senza la biopsia della massa tumorale, quando si mostra con l'apparenza tipica e il paziente presenta neuroblasti nel midollo osseo (Fig. 498-3) e un aumento dell'acido vanilmandelico o di quello omovanillico nelle urine.

La valutazione delle localizzazioni metastatiche comprende l'esecuzione di radiografie ossee per indagare il coinvolgimento dell'osso corticale e l'aspirato o la biopsia osteomidollare per studiare il midollo. In protocolli sperimentali, ci si può avvalere anche della PET e dello studio con lo iodio 131 o con lo **iodio 123 metaiodobenzilguanidina (I-123 MIBG)**, per definire meglio l'estensione della malattia. La sua estensione clinica e l'età del paziente, insieme ai marker citogenetici e molecolari effettuati su campioni di tessuto patologico, vengono utilizzati per stimare la prognosi e per guidare la scelta della terapia correlata al rischio. Sebbene in passato siano stati impiegati molti sistemi di classificazione dello stadio di malattia, al giorno d'oggi quello universalmente riconosciuto è l'**International Neuroblastoma Staging System (INSS**, Sistema di Stadiazione Internazionale del Neuroblastoma) (Tab. 498-2). In esso, lo stadio 1 comprende tumori confinati all'organo o alla struttura d'origine; nello stadio 2 i tumori si estendono oltre questa struttura, ma non attraversano la linea mediana, con (stadio 2B) o senza (stadio 2A) il coinvolgimento dei linfonodi ipsilaterali; nel 3 le neoplasie oltrepassano la linea mediana, con o senza interessamento bilaterale dei linfonodi; nello stadio 4, infine, i tumori sono disseminati in sedi distanti (osso, midollo osseo, fegato, linfonodi distanti, altri organi). Lo stadio 4S interessa poi i bambini <1 anno con malattia disseminata al fegato, alla cute o al midollo osseo, senza coinvolgimento osseo e con un tumore primitivo che diversamente sarebbe stadiato come 1 o 2.

TRATTAMENTO. I più importanti fattori prognostici clinici e biologici correntemente usati per determinare la scelta del trattamento sono l'età del paziente alla diagnosi, lo stadio di malattia, lo stato del MYCN e l'istologia secondo Shimada (vedi Tab. 498-1). La prognosi è migliorata con gli attuali regimi di trattamento. Quelli per il NB a basso rischio sono la chirurgia per gli stadi 1 e 2 e l'osservazione per lo stadio 4S. Nello stadio 2, anche con un piccolo residuo tumorale, la percentuale di guarigione è >90% senza ulteriori terapie e pure la chemioterapia o la radioterapia, per i rari casi di recidive locali, possono portare alla guarigione. I bambini con una compressione midollare alla diagnosi possono

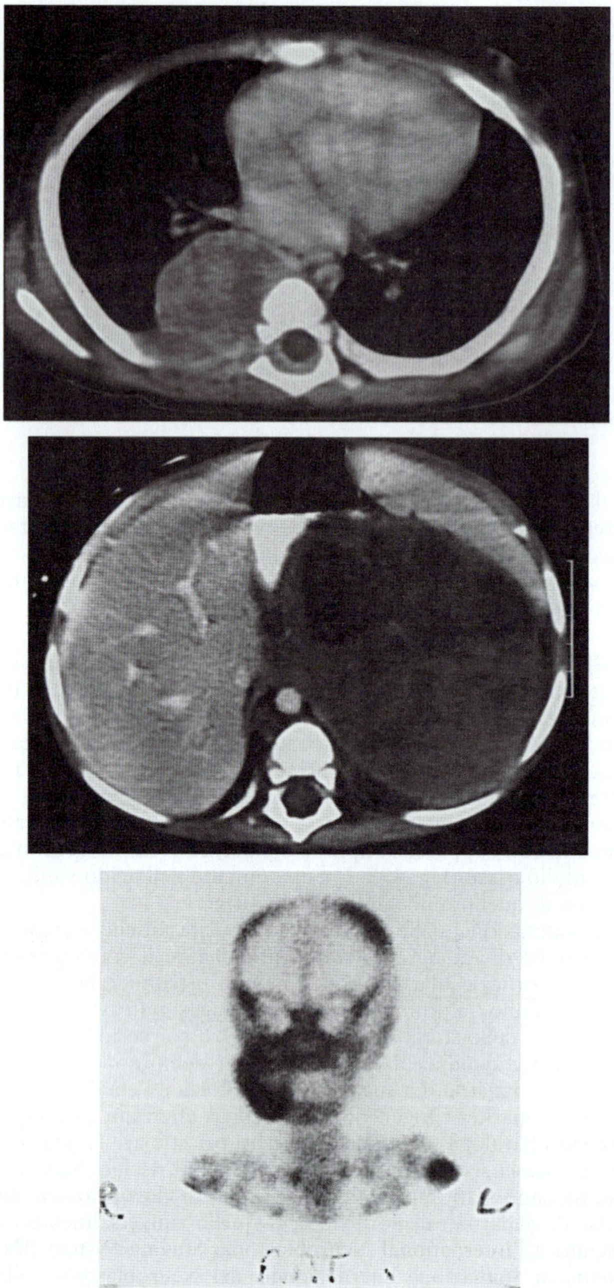

Figura 498-2. *In alto*, TC di un neuroblastoma toracico con estensione intraspinale alla diagnosi. *Al centro*, TC di una localizzazione primitiva a livello surrenale con estensione ai linfonodi. *In basso*, Scintigrafia ossea con tecnenzio difosfonato che dimostra un diffuso coinvolgimento osseo.

avere bisogno di un trattamento urgente con la chemioterapia, la chirurgia o la radioterapia al fine di evitare un danno neurologico. Lo stadio 4S ha una prognosi particolarmente favorevole, con una sopravvivenza di circa il 100% con la sola terapia di supporto, in quanto la neoplasia regredisce spontaneamente. La chemioterapia e la resezione del tumore primario non migliorano la sopravvivenza. I neonati con meno di 2 mesi con stadio 4S sono a maggiore rischio se hanno un grave coinvolgimento epatico e respiratorio. In alcuni neonati, basse dosi di ciclofosfamide o una radioterapia a basse dosi sul fegato possono essere raccomandate per alleviare i sintomi. Per i bambini con un NB di stadio 4S che necessitano di un trattamento per controllare i sintomi la sopravvivenza è dell'81%.

Il trattamento del NB a rischio intermedio prevede la chirurgia, la chemioterapia e in alcuni casi la radioterapia. La chemioterapia

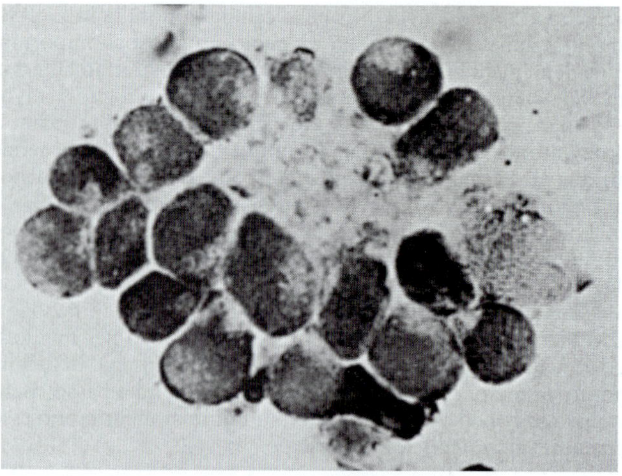

Figura 498-3. Cellule di neuroblastoma da un aspirato midollare. Aggregati cellulari che spesso contengono ≥3 cellule con o senza evidenza di formazione di rosette. Le rosette che circondano una massa centrale di materiale fibrillare sono caratteristiche del neuroblastoma.

generalmente comprende dosi medie di cisplatino o carboplatino, ciclofosfamide, etoposide e doxorubicina somministrati per diversi mesi. La radioterapia viene impiegata per i tumori con risposta incompleta alla chemioterapia. I bambini con stadio 3 di malattia e i neonati con stadio 4 e caratteristiche favorevoli hanno una prognosi eccellente, con una sopravvivenza superiore al 90% con questo trattamento moderato. In questo gruppo di rischio intermedio, è importante ottenere materiale diagnostico adeguato per operare la classificazione patologica di Shimada e per ottenere l'amplificazione del MYCN, in modo tale che i bambini con caratteristiche sfavorevoli possano ricevere un trattamento più aggressivo e quelli con caratteristiche favorevoli possano essere risparmiati da una terapia eccessivamente tossica.

Il trattamento standard per i NB ad alto rischio (vedi Tab. 498-1) prevede una chemioterapia d'induzione per ottenere una risposta completa o parziale. In questo secondo caso, è raccomandata la resezione del tumore primitivo, seguita dalla radioterapia focale sul residuo tumorale. Dopo l'induzione si prosegue quindi con una chemioterapia ad alte dosi e con il trapianto autologo di cellule staminali (SCT, *Stem Cell Transplantation*). Uno studio randomizzato nazionale ha dimostrato un miglioramento significativo della sopravvivenza grazie a questo trapianto, in confronto che con la sola chemioterapia. L'aggiunta dell'acido *cis*-retinoico dopo l'SCT per 1 anno aumenta la sopravvivenza a 5 anni, libera da recidive al 50% rispetto al 20% dei casi trattati con la sola chemioterapia senza l'SCT o l'acido *cis*-retinoico.

Sarebbe comunque necessaria una terapia migliore per la maggior parte dei pazienti con un NB ad alto rischio. Nuovi trattamenti attualmente in corso di studio comprendono nuovi agenti chemioterapici, chemioterapie ad alte dosi con liberazione di multiple cellule staminali, anticorpi monoclonali combinati con fattori di crescita e vaccini antitumorali. È anche auspicabile che gli studi biologici sul NB possano condurre all'identificazione di nuovi target genetici per la terapia stessa.

PREVENZIONE. Attualmente non si conosce nessuna possibilità di prevenire il neuroblastoma. A livello mondiale, il tentativo di migliorare la sopravvivenza con una diagnosi precoce utilizzando il dosaggio delle catecolamine nei bambini non si è dimostrato efficace.

Attiyeh EF, London WB, Mosse YP, et al: Chromosome 1p and 11q deletions and outcome in neuroblastoma. *N Engl J Med* 2005;353:2243–2253.
Blaes F, Fuhlhuber V, Korfei M, et al: Surface-binding autoantibodies to cerebellar neurons in opsoclonus syndrome. *Ann Neurol* 2005;58:313–317.

TABELLA 498-2. International Neuroblastoma Staging System

STADIO	DEFINIZIONE	INCIDENZA (%)	SOPRAVVIVENZA A 5 ANNI*
1	Tumore localizzato con asportazione ampia, con o senza residuo microscopico di malattia; linfonodi ipsilaterali negativi per la presenza di cellule tumorali (i linfonodi attaccati e rimossi con il tumore primitivo possono essere positivi)	5	≥90%
2A	Tumore localizzato con asportazione incompleta; linfonodi non aderenti ipsilaterali negativi per la presenza di cellule tumorali	10	70-80%
2B	Tumore localizzato con o senza asportazione completa, con linfonodi non aderenti ipsilaterali positivi. I linfonodi controlaterali aumentati di volume devono essere negativi per cellule neoplastiche	10	70-80%
3	Tumore unilaterale non resecabile infiltrante attraverso la linea mediana[†], con o senza coinvolgimento dei linfonodi regionali; o tumore unilaterale localizzato con coinvolgimento dei linfonodi regionali controlaterali; o tumore della linea mediana con estensione bilaterale per infiltrazione (resecabile) o per coinvolgimento dei linfonodi	25	40-70%
4	Qualunque tumore primitivo con disseminazione a livello di linfonodi distanti, osso, midollo osseo, fegato, cute e altri organi (eccetto per lo stadio 4S)	60	85-90% se l'età alla diagnosi è <18 mesi 30-40% se l'età alla diagnosi è >18 mesi
4S	Tumore primitivo localizzato (come per gli stadi 1, 2A o 2B), con disseminazione limitata alla cute, al fegato e al midollo osseo[‡] (limitatamente ai bambini con <1 anno)	5	>80%

*La sopravvivenza è influenzata da altri elementi, quali l'amplificazione di MYCN. Le percentuali sono approssimate.

[†]La linea mediana è definita in relazione alla colonna vertebrale. I tumori che originano da un lato e che attraversano la linea mediana possono infiltrare o superare il lato opposto della colonna vertebrale.

[‡]Il coinvolgimento del midollo nello stadio 4S dovrebbe essere minimo (<10% del totale delle cellule nucleate identificate come maligne alla biopsia o all'aspirato midollare). Un più estensivo coinvolgimento del midollo va considerato uno stadio 4. La scintigrafia con il MIBG (se fattibile) deve essere negativa a livello del midollo.

Da Kliegman RM, Marcdante KJ, Jenson HB, et al (editors): *Nelson Essentials of Pediatrics*, 5th ed. Philadelphia, WB Saunders, 2006, p 746. Modificata da Brodeur GM et al: Revisions of the International Criteria for Neuroblastoma Diagnosis, Staging, and Response to Treatment. *J Clin Oncol* 1993;11:1466-1477.

MIBG, metaiodobenzilguanidina.

Brodeur GM: Neuroblastoma: Biological insights into a clinical enigma. *Nature Rev Cancer* 2003;3:203–216.

De Roos AJ, Olshan AF, Teschke K, et al: Parental occupational exposures to chemicals and incidence of neuroblastoma in offspring. *Am J Epidemiol* 2001;154:106–114.

George RE, Lipshultz SE, Lipsitz SR, et al: Association between congenital cardiovascular malformations and neuroblastoma. *J Pediatr* 2004;144: 444–448.

Goldsby RE, Matthay KK: Neuroblastoma: Evolving therapies for a disease of many faces. *Paediatr Drugs* 2004;6:107–122.

Inagaki J, Yasui M, Sakata N, et al: Successful treatment of chemoresistant stage 3 neuroblastoma using irinotecan as a single agent. *J Pediatr Hematol Oncol* 2005;27:604–606.

Matthay KK, Villablanca JG, Seeger RC, et al: Treatment of high-risk neuroblastoma with intensive chemotherapy, radiotherapy, autologous bone marrow transplantation, and 13-cis-retinoic acid. *N Engl J Med* 1999;341:1165–1173.

Nickerson HJ, Matthay KK, Seeger RC, et al: Favorable biology and outcome of stage IV-S neuroblastoma with supportive care or minimal therapy: A Children's Cancer Group study. *J Clin Oncol* 2000;18:477–486.

Perez CA, Matthay KK, Atkinson JB, et al: Biological variables in the outcome of stages I and II neuroblastoma treated with surgery as primary therapy: A Children's Cancer Group Study. *J Clin Oncol* 2000;18:18–26.

Rudnick E, Khakoo Y, Antunes NL, et al: Opsoclonus-myoclonus-ataxia syndrome in neuroblastoma: Clinical outcome and antineuronal antibodies: A report from the Children's Cancer Group Study. *Med Pediatr Oncol* 2001;36:612–622.

Schmidt ML, Lukens JN, Seeger RC, et al: Biologic factors determine prognosis in infants with stage IV neuroblastoma: A prospective Children's Cancer Group Study. *J Clin Oncol* 2000;18:1260–1268.

Van Noesel MM, Versteeg R: Pediatric neuroblastomas: Genetic and epigenetic 'Danse Macabre.' *Gene* 2004; 325:1–15.

Woods WG: Screening for neuroblastoma: The final chapters. *J Pediatr Hematol Oncol* 2003;25:3–4.

Capitolo 499 ■ Neoplasie renali

Norman Jaffe e Vicki Huff

499.1 • Tumore di Wilms

EZIOLOGIA. Il tumore di Wilms, anche noto come **nefroblastoma**, è una complessa neoplasia embrionale mista dei reni composta da tre elementi: blasti, epitelio e stroma. La maggior parte dei tumori di Wilms è sporadica, anche se l'1-2% dei pazienti ha un'anamnesi familiare, con una predisposizione ereditata come un **carattere autosomico dominante.** I casi familiari si associano a un'età minore alla diagnosi e a un'aumentata frequenza di malattia bilaterale, anche se questi non sono elementi che si osservano in tutte le famiglie. Nella maggior parte di esse, inoltre, non si trovano anomalie congenite. A questo tumore si associano spesso i resti nefrogenici.

Tra le alterazioni genetiche osservate in questa neoplasia, è stato isolato un **gene**, il WT1, localizzato a livello di 11p13 (Tab. 499-1). Il WT1 codifica per un fattore di trascrizione a dita di zinco, che è fondamentale per il normale sviluppo del rene. Circa il 20% dei tumori di Wilms ha mutazioni di WT1 e la maggior parte di esse è tumore-specifica. I pazienti con questo tumore con anomalie congenite spesso sono portatori di mutazioni germinali di WT1. La predisposizione familiare generalmente non è associata alle alterazioni di WT1; in questi casi, i geni coinvolti sono localizzati a livello di 19q13 e 17q.

Nei pazienti affetti sono frequentemente riportate numerose sindromi e anomalie congenite (Tab. 499-2). La **sindrome di WAGR** è provocata dalla delezione del gene contiguo, che comporta la presenza del tumore di Wilms, dell'aniridia, di anomalie genitourinarie (criptorchidismo, ovaie sostituite da banderelle di tessuto fibroso, utero bicorne, genitali ambigui) e di un ritardo mentale. I soggetti con questa sindrome hanno una delezione costituzionale del cromosoma 11p13, dove sono localizzati il WT1 e il gene dell'aniridia, il PAX6. La **sindrome di Denys-Drash** è caratterizzata dallo pseudoermafroditismo maschile, da un'insufficienza renale precoce per sclerosi mesangiale e da un aumentato rischio di sviluppare un tumore di Wilms. Coloro che contraggono questa sindrome sono tipicamente portatori di una mutazione missense del gene WT1. La **sindrome di Beckwith-Wiedemann** è caratterizzata da emi-ipertrofia, macroglossia e visceromegalia, con un

TABELLA 499-1. Alterazioni genetiche osservate nei tumori di Wilms

GENE	CARATTERISTICHE DEL TUMORE DI WILMS	FREQUENZA	TIPO DI ALTERAZIONE
WT1	Non selezionato	~20%	Delezioni, mutazioni tronche, missense negli esoni codificanti a dita di zinco
β-catenina	Non selezionato	~15%	Mutazioni missense o delezioni interessanti i siti di fosforilazione delle proteine
	Tumori con mutazioni WT1 (~20% del totale)	~50%	-
p53	Anaplastico (~5% del totale)	~80%	Mutazioni missense e tronche

TABELLA 499-2. Sindromi associate con il tumore di Wilms e loro caratteristiche cliniche e cromosomiche

SINDROME	CARATTERISTICHE CLINICHE	CROMOSOMA O ALTRE ALTERAZIONI
WAGR	Aniridia, anomalie genitourinarie, ritardo mentale	Delezione di 11p13 (loci WT1 e PAX6)
Denys-Drash	Esordio precoce di insufficienza renale con sclerosi mesangiale, pseudoermafroditismo maschile, aumentato rischio di tumore di Wilms	Mutazioni di WT1
Beckwith-Wiedemann	Organomegalia (fegato, rene, surrene, pancreas), macroglossia, onfalocele, emi-ipertrofia	Sono state descritte la disomia uniparentale paterna, la duplicazione di 11p15.5, la perdita dell'imprinting e la mutazione di p57KIP57. Delezione di 11p15.5 (locus WT2). Possono anche essere coinvolti i geni IGF2 e/o H19.

rischio del 3-5% di sviluppare un tumore di Wilms. In alcuni casi sono state riportate diverse alterazioni a carico di 11p15.5 ed è stato ipotizzato che in questa regione sia localizzato un secondo gene del tumore di Wilms, il WT2. Anche la perdita dell'imprinting del gene del fattore di crescita 2 insuline-like, un processo epigenetico, è associato al tumore di Wilms. Altre sindromi o malattie con un incrementato rischio di questa neoplasia comprendono l'emi-ipertrofia, l'aniridia sporadica, le anomalie genitourinarie, la sindrome di Pearlman, la sindrome di Sotos, la neurofibromatosi (la malattia di von Recklinghausen) e la malattia di von Willebrand. Le anomalie genitourinarie che si trovano più spesso con il tumore di Wilms sono l'ipoplasia, la fusione e l'ectopia renali, le duplicazioni dei collettori, l'ipospadia e il criptorchidismo.

EPIDEMIOLOGIA. L'incidenza del tumore di Wilms è di circa 8 casi per milione di bambini <15 anni. Generalmente colpisce tra i 2 e i 5 anni, sebbene sia stato anche riscontrato nei neonati, negli adolescenti e negli adulti. Rappresenta circa il 6% delle neoplasie pediatriche ed è il secondo tumore addominale più frequente nell'infanzia. Può interessare uno o entrambi i reni; l'incidenza del tumore di Wilms bilaterale è del 7%. Può accompagnarsi a emi-ipertrofia, aniridia e altre anomalie congenite, soprattutto del tratto genitourinario. È anche stato descritto in associazione a numerose sindromi.

PATOGENESI. Sono state distinte due grosse categorie di tumore di Wilms: favorevole e sfavorevole. La prima forma è quella più comune e generalmente ha una buona prognosi. È caratterizzata dalla presenza di blasti, epitelio e stroma privi di ectopie e anaplasie. Una piccola porzione di elementi sarcomatosi nello stroma, in un tipo altrimenti apparentemente favorevole, non influenza comunque in maniera negativa la prognosi. Nella forma sfavorevole si trovano invece nuclei di dimensioni aumentate e ipercromici e figure mitotiche multipolari. Le aree di anaplasia possono essere focali o diffuse e sono predittive di un'alta probabilità di recidiva e di decesso. Questa forma tende a colpire soggetti più grandi e di razza non bianca. Il sarcoma a cellule chiare è un sottotipo della forma sfavorevole e metastatizza di solito al livello dell'osso. Il tumore rabdoide, che può metastatizzare nel cervello, non è più classificato come un sottotipo del tumore di Wilms.

I linfonodi o altre sedi di possibili metastasi sono in genere i luoghi migliori per identificare l'anaplasia, che è estremamente rara nei bambini con <2 anni. Se il sospetto è alto, sono indicate tecniche di campionatura più approfondite per ricercarla, soprattutto nei bambini più grandi. Il fenomeno di solito non si osserva una volta che sia stata somministrata la chemioterapia. L'anaplasia delle cellule muscolari scheletriche non sembra associata a un'aumentata incidenza di recidiva.

MANIFESTAZIONI CLINICHE. Il tumore di Wilms generalmente si presenta con una massa addominale. Viene spesso scoperto per caso e non è raro che il genitore se ne accorga facendo il bagno al bambino. Può anche essere riscontrato durante una visita medica. Queste masse renali variano per dimensioni, in genere sono omogenee e fisse e occasionalmente possono superare la linea mediana. Alcuni pazienti possono avere un dolore addominale e il vomito; l'ematuria si osserva nel 12-25% dei casi. È stata anche descritta l'ipertensione, probabilmente secondaria a una ischemia renale. Rare volte si possono osservare un rapido ingrossamento addominale e un'anemia per sanguinamento nel parenchima renale o pelvico. Quando il tumore cresce nelle vene renali o nella vena cava è possibile un'embolizzazione nel cuore o nei polmoni, con gravi conseguenze.

DIAGNOSI. Qualunque massa addominale in un bambino dovrebbe essere considerata maligna, fino a che le immagini radiologiche e gli esami di laboratorio non definiscono la sua vera natura. In caso di dubbio, al termine degli accertamenti è opportuno effettuare una biopsia o una exeresi per la verifica dell'istologia. Il tumore di Wilms va differenziato da diverse altre neoplasie addominali e pelviche (Tab. 499-3). Una volta che viene riscontrata una massa, occorre effettuare un accurato esame obiettivo, seguito da esami ematochimici come l'emocromo completo e quello della funzionalità epatica e renale e infine dalla ricerca di specifici marker secreti dal sospetto tumore. Gli esami radiologici comprendono una radiografia dell'addome, un'ecografia e una TC e/o RM.

La TC fornisce la conferma dell'origine intrarenale della massa (Fig. 499-1). Può anche procurare informazioni circa l'estensione del tumore, lo sviluppo all'interno della vena cava inferiore e l'integrità del rene controlaterale. I tumori assumono poco mezzo di contrasto, la cui somministrazione è quindi utile per determinare la funzionalità del rene non colpito in previsione di una nefrectomia. Anche la RM aiuta a definire l'estensione del tumore. L'ecografia può contribuire a identificarlo e dà informazioni sull'integrità della vena cava inferiore e circa la presenza della neoplasia nella vena renale o nella vena cava. Qualche volta può risultare necessaria l'esecuzione dell'angiografia per pianificare la

TABELLA 499-3. Diagnosi differenziale dei tumori addominali e pelvici nei neonati e nei bambini

TUMORE	ETÀ	SEGNI CLINICI	ESAMI DI LABORATORIO
Wilms	Prescolare	Massa unilaterale al fianco, aniridia, emi-ipertrofia	Ematuria; scintigrafia ossea (sarcoma a cellule chiare)
Neuroblastoma	Prescolare	Ostruzione GI/GU, occhi da procione, mioclono-opsoclono, diarrea, noduli cutanei (neonati)	Aumento di VMA; aumento di HVA; aumento della ferritina; masse con calcificazioni puntiformi Midollo osseo positivo
Linfoma non-Hodgkin	>1 anno	Intussuscezione nei bambini >2 anni	Aumento dell'acido urico; midollo osseo positivo
Rabdomiosarcoma	Qualunque	Ostruzione GI/GU, sarcoma botrioide, sanguinamento vaginale, massa paratesticolare	
Germinoma/teratoma	Prescolare, adolescenza	Ragazze: dolore addominale, sanguinamento vaginale. Ragazzi: massa testicolare, "idrocele" di recente esordio Massa/fossetta sacrococcigea	Aumento di hCG; aumento di AFP
Epatoblastoma	Dalla nascita ai 3 anni	Fegato ingrossato, fisso	Aumento di AFP
Epatoma	Scolare, adolescenza	Fegato ingrossato e fisso; epatite B, cirrosi	Aumento di AFP

AFP, α-fetoproteina; GI, gastrointestinale; GU, genitourinario; hCG, gonadotropina corionica umana (*Human Chorionic Gonadotropin*); HVA, acido omovanillico (*HomoVanillic Acid*); VMA, acido vanilmandelico (*VanillylMandelic Acid*).

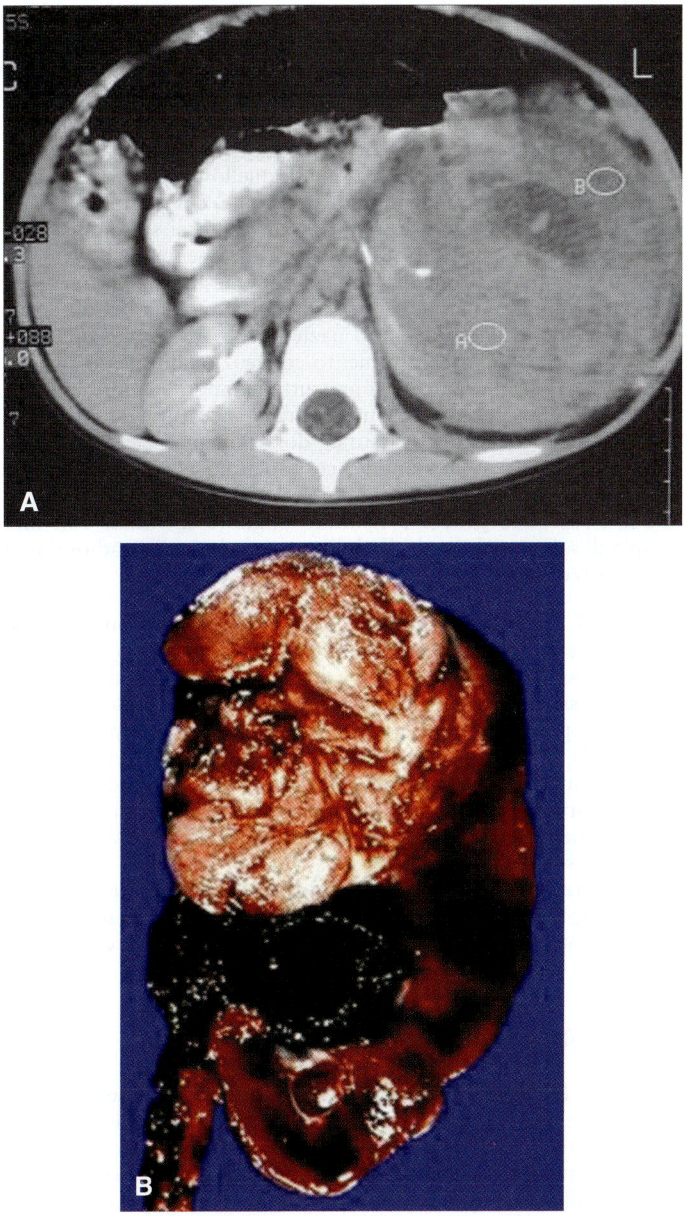

Figura 499-1. *A*, TC dell'addome che dimostra un voluminoso tumore di Wilms sinistro. *B*, Anatomia patologica del tumore resecato illustrato in *A*.

procedura dell'intervento. Le radiografie dell'osso tornano utili nel caso di un sarcoma a cellule chiare del rene e la RM o la TC dell'encefalo nel caso di un tumore rabdoide maligno.

Occorre una valutazione radiologica del torace per verificare l'esistenza di metastasi polmonari. La TC del torace non è eseguita di routine, perché le metastasi da tumore di Wilms possono essere facilmente identificate con la sola radiografia convenzionale. Occasionalmente, in soggetti con radiografie del torace normali, una TC può evidenziare noduli isolati, la cui vera natura è tuttavia incerta.

STADIAZIONE. La stadiazione sistemica più spesso utilizzata è stata sviluppata dal National Wilms Tumor Study group (gruppo di studio nazionale del tumore di Wilms) (Tab. 499-4) e lo stadio si correla con la prognosi (Tab. 499-5). Nello stadio I il tumore è confinato a un solo rene e, per definizione, è asportato completamente con la superficie della capsula intatta. Anche nello stadio II ha lo stesso confinamento, anche se la capsula può essere invasa o il tumore può essersi infiltrato nei tessuti molli perirenali. Nello stadio III è presente un residuo tumorale postchirurgico, senza estensione ematogena; la disseminazione è confinata nell'addome

TABELLA 499-4. Sistema di stadiazione sviluppato dal Third National Wilms Tumor Study (terzo studio nazionale del tumore di Wilms)

STADIO	DESCRIZIONE
Stadio I	Tumore limitato al rene e asportato completamente. Superficie capsulare intatta; assenza di erosioni tumorali; assenza di residui evidenti sui margini di resezione
Stadio II	Tumore esteso oltre il rene, ma asportato completamente. Estensione regionale del tumore; infiltrazione dei vasi; tumore biopsiato o disseminazione locale limitata al fianco. Assenza di evidenti residui tumorali sopra o vicino ai margini di resezione
Stadio III	Residuo tumorale non ematogeno confinato all'addome. Coinvolgimento dei linfonodi ilari, periaortici o limitrofi; diffusa disseminazione peritoneale da parte del tumore; impianti peritoneali del tumore, tumore esteso oltre i margini chirurgici microscopicamente o macroscopicamente; tumore non completamente asportato per un'infiltrazione locale in strutture vitali
Stadio IV	Ulteriore estensione rispetto allo stadio III (polmone, fegato, osso, cervello)
Stadio V	Coinvolgimento renale bilaterale alla diagnosi

Modificata dal National Wilms' Tumor Study Committee: Wilms' tumor: status report, 1990. *J Clin Oncol* 1991; 9: 877-887.

TABELLA 499-5. Tumore di Wilms: sopravvivenza in relazione all'istologia e allo stadio

	SOPRAVVIVENZA	
ISTOLOGIA/STADIO	2 ANNI (%)	4 ANNI (%)
Favorevole I	98	97
Favorevole II	96	94
Favorevole III	91	88
Favorevole IV	88	82
Anaplastico I	89	89
Anaplastico II-IV	56	54

Modificata dal National Wilms' Tumor Study Committee: Wilms' tumor: status report, 1990. *J Clin Oncol* 1991; 9: 877-887.

e può coinvolgere il letto perirenale, i linfonodi drenanti o i tessuti e gli organi circostanti per contiguità. Lo stadio IV è caratterizzato dalla presenza di metastasi ematogene, che generalmente interessano i polmoni e raramente il fegato. Lo stadio V vede il coinvolgimento di entrambi i reni.

TRATTAMENTO. Le controversie sul trattamento del tumore di Wilms riguardano l'uso della chemioterapia e della radioterapia preoperatorie, nonché la composizione degli agenti chemioterapici. L'intento è di ridurre l'incidenza e la natura degli effetti tardivi utilizzando la terapia più adeguata. Le indicazioni per la nefrectomia parziale devono ancora essere definite, così come il ruolo della sola chirurgia nei pazienti con tumore di Wilms a basso rischio. Non è ancora stato stabilito quale sia l'esame radiologico preoperatorio migliore per stimare la natura della malattia nel rene colpito e in quello controlaterale nelle forme di tumore di Wilms bilaterale.

Occorre operare un'asportazione chirurgica. La pervietà della vena cava inferiore dovrebbe essere valutata prima della resezione; se non è pervia, bisogna somministrare una chemioterapia preoperatoria. Durante l'intervento va esaminato anche il rene controlaterale, per escludere una malattia bilaterale. Il fegato va invece ispezionato per la possibilità di metastasi, anche se la TC, la RM e l'ecografia ne possono avere evidenziate alcune prima dell'intervento. I linfonodi retroperitoneali devono essere valutati e quelli sospetti biopsiati. Bisogna fare ogni tentativo di evitare una disseminazione del tumore.

La maggior parte dei centri effettua la chemioterapia secondo le linee guida approvate dal National Wilms Tumor Study group. Per i tumori di stadio I e II con istologia favorevole si somministrano la vincristina e l'actinomicina D; per quelli di stadio III sempre con istologia favorevole si adoperano la vincristina, l'actinomicina D e la doxorubicina, nonché si attua la radioterapia sul letto tumorale; per lo stadio IV con istologia favorevole vengono impiegate la vincristina, l'actinomicina D e la doxorubicina e la radioterapia viene somministrata in tutte le sedi note di malattia, soprattutto a livello polmonare. Se il tumore è esteso a livello epatico, va presa in considerazione la resezione chirurgica, piuttosto che la radioterapia. Anche i restanti tumori che non rispondono alla chemioterapia e alla radioterapia, o quelli che recidivano, vanno valutati per la resezione chirurgica o in alternativa per una chemioterapia sperimentale.

Per i tumori con istologia sfavorevole, si adoperano la vincristina, l'actinomicina D, la doxorubicina e il ciclofosfamide, con la radioterapia su tutti i siti di malattia noti. Il sarcoma a cellule chiare dell'osso risponde alla combinazione di cisplatino, doxorubicina e radioterapia. Può essere presa in considerazione anche una terapia aggiuntiva con ciclofosfamide o ifosfamide.

La maggior parte dei pazienti tollera molto bene il trattamento, anche se la terapia può provocare effetti collaterali sia acuti sia tardivi. La maggior parte di quelli acuti è costituita da nausea, vomito e mielosoppressione con possibili infezioni sovraimposte. Per la nausea e il vomito transitori in genere vengono somministrati antiemetici. L'actinomicina D e la doxorubicina possono provocare ulcere orali, tuttavia spesso lievi e senza conseguenze. La vincristina può invece dare luogo a stipsi e dolore addominale. Gli effetti collaterali cronici coinvolgono i sistemi gastrointestinale, epatico, cardiaco, riproduttore e scheletrico. Un'ostruzione intestinale può derivare da aderenze, fibrosi o volvoli. Accade raramente che la radioterapia provochi enteriti o malassorbimento. Una grave insufficienza epatica può derivare da una malattia veno-occlusiva, che di solito è dovuta all'assunzione di actinomicina D in concomitanza con la radioterapia sul fegato.

L'insufficienza cardiaca congestizia può avere origine da un trattamento con la doxorubicina, soprattutto se somministrata in associazione con la radioterapia polmonare. La dose cumulativa è generalmente limitata a 200-300 mg/m^2, per evitare la cardiotossicità soprattutto nei pazienti con metastasi polmonari che dovranno ricevere appunto la radioterapia.

Quella toracica, invece, può compromettere lo sviluppo mammario e il trattamento sull'utero può determinare un basso peso alla nascita dei bambini. La radioterapia sulle ovaie può provocare una menopausa precoce e una ridotta fertilità. Dopo una radioterapia sull'emiaddome con una sola parte di colonna vertebrale compresa nel campo di irradiazione si può verificare anche una cifoscoliosi, che tuttavia generalmente si può evitare con le tecniche moderne.

Le recidive del tumore e le metastasi polmonari si possono sviluppare entro i primi due anni dalla diagnosi. Sono state sviluppate diverse schedule di follow-up per la valutazione precoce e il trattamento, come la valutazione mensile con un esame clinico e con una radiografia del torace per i primi due anni. L'intervallo fra le visite di controllo nei successivi 3 anni va quindi aumentando e dal quinto anno esse divengono annuali. L'ecografia dell'addome viene eseguita annualmente dopo il completamento del trattamento, per valutare una eventuale recidiva e per verificare l'integrità del rene controlaterale. Coloro che sopravvivono a lungo devono essere sottoposti a controlli sistematici con misurazione della pressione sanguigna, della proteinuria, della creatininemia, della clearence renale e delle dimensioni renali, soprattutto dopo il trattamento per un tumore di Wilms bilaterale.

Tumore di Wilms inoperabile. La chemioterapia viene utilizzata per i tumori non operabili. In queste circostanze la diagnosi è generalmente posta con un'agobiopsia per via percutanea, con la selezione del trattamento in base al criterio istologico. Per i tumori con istologia favorevole, ci si serve della vincristina e dell'actinomicina D per gli stadi I e II, della vincristina, dell'actinomicina D e della doxorubicina per gli stadi III e IV. Per i tumori con istologia sfavorevole, il trattamento prevede invece una combinazione di vincristina, actinomicina D, doxorubicina e ciclofosfamide. Nella maggior parte dei casi si ottiene una riduzione delle dimensioni del tumore. La prognosi per le neoplasie inoperabili e sottoposte a chemioterapia, chirurgia e, se necessario, radioterapia, è generalmente favorevole, con una percentuale di sopravvivenza >50%.

Tumore di Wilms bilaterale. La chemioterapia per il tumore di Wilms bilaterale è identica a quella utilizzata per i tumori non operabili ed è somministrata per rendere il tumore suscettibile di asportazione chirurgica, che può prevedere una nefrectomia monolaterale e una parziale controlaterale oppure nefrectomie parziali bilaterali. Queste procedure permettono l'ablazione del tessuto tumorale e la conservazione di quello sano. Le procedure chirurgiche sono dipendenti dall'estensione del tumore e dalla risposta alla chemioterapia. Dopo l'intervento si somministra la chemioterapia e spesso la radioterapia. Raramente ci si avvale di quest'ultima anche prima della chirurgia. Queste strategie terapeutiche determinano una percentuale di sopravvivenza del 60-85%.

Chemioterapia di salvataggio. I pazienti che presentano una recidiva durante o dopo il trattamento convenzionale spesso rispondono a terapie alternative, soprattutto quando i tumori hanno un'istologia favorevole. In queste circostanze può essere utilizzata l'associazione di vincristina, doxorubicina, ciclofosfamide e actinomicina D o ifosfamide, carboplatino ed etoposide. Si è fatto uso anche della chemioterapia ad alte dosi con trapianto di midollo osseo. In genere il risultato migliore si ottiene con una terapia di salvataggio multidisciplinare con chirurgia, radioterapia e chemioterapia.

PROGNOSI. Vi è una notevole correlazione tra il contenuto di DNA delle cellule del tumore di Wilms, il sottotipo istologico e la risposta al trattamento. Le linee staminali sia del tumore primitivo sia delle metastasi variano da uno stato diploide a una bassa aneuploidia (iperdiploidi). I tumori a contenuto iperdiploide sono anche caratteristici delle varietà anaplastiche (sfavorevoli) e hanno numerose traslocazioni complesse. Essi rispondono poco alla chemioterapia. La prognosi è peggiore nel caso di tumori di grosse dimensioni (>500 g), di stadio avanzato (III e IV) e con un sottotipo istologico sfavorevole.

Il tumore di Wilms è un paradigma del successo del trattamento multidisciplinare e >60% dei pazienti generalmente sopravvive indipendentemente dallo stadio di malattia. Gli stadi dal I al III hanno una probabilità di guarigione >90%.

499.2 • ALTRI TUMORI RENALI DEL BAMBINO

NEFROMA MESOBLASTICO CONGENITO. Il nefroma mesoblastico congenito è una neoplasia congenita singola del rene, che raramente metastatizza. Colpisce più frequentemente i maschi e produce renina. Si presenta come una massa renale solitaria, voluminosa, fissa e infiltrante. Macroscopicamente e microscopicamente assomiglia a un leiomioma o a un leiomiosarcoma di basso grado, con nefroni intrappolati. Al microscopio si osservano fibroblasti o miofibroblasti. Questo tumore comprende la **maggior parte di quelli renali congeniti.** Il più delle volte è considerato benigno e vi sono pareri diversi circa l'utilità della chemioterapia. Una segnalazione ha messo in evidenza che la vincristina e l'actinomicina somministrate come terapia adiuvante non prevengono le metastasi. Un'altra segnalazione ha riportato che la malattia metastatica sembra rispondere alla vincristina, alla doxorubicina e al ciclofosfamide.

RESIDUI NEFROGENI. L'espressione "residui nefrogeni", o **blastomi nodulari renali,** o **nefroblastomatosi** si riferisce alla persistenza anomala di tessuto embrionale renale. La buona sopravvivenza e la percentuale di risposte del tumore di Wilms bilaterale suggeriscono una sua stretta relazione con tali residui nefrogeni. È stato suggerito che un breve trattamento con un ciclo di chemioterapia relativamente poco tossica, come la vincristina e l'actinomicina D, può essere efficace per ridurre il volume dei reni colpiti. Blastemi e alterazioni nefroblastiche sembrano rimanere nei reni di molti, se non di tutti, i soggetti trattati, indipendentemente dalla riduzione del volume renale. Il riscontro di residui nefrogeni in un rene impone un'attenta valutazione di quello controlaterale. Può essere indicato anche un follow-up radiologico con TC. Non è noto se la chemioterapia sia in grado di ridurre il rischio di sviluppare in seguito un tumore di Wilms.

NEFROBLASTOMA MULTICISTICO. I tumori renali talvolta possono contenere cisti, alcune delle quali possono essere associate al tumore di Wilms. Diverse definizioni sono state utilizzate per indicare queste neoplasie, per esempio **nefroblastoma cistico parzialmente differenziato, nefroblastoma policistico** e **nefroma multiloculare.** La maggior parte dei casi colpisce pazienti <1 anno. Questo tipo di tumore ha un aspetto biologico benigno. Tuttavia, se risulta evidente l'associazione con un tumore di Wilms, è giustificato un trattamento chemioterapico.

CARCINOMA RENALE. Il carcinoma renale è raro nella prima decade di vita, ma occasionalmente è stato riportato in bambini e adolescenti. In genere si presenta con una massa addominale e/o con ematuria. L'asportazione completa può portare alla guarigione. A volte è consigliabile un trattamento adiuvante con l'interferone e con il 5-fluorouracile.

CARCINOMA MIDOLLARE RENALE. È un tumore raro, altamente aggressivo, che si associa al tratto dell'anemia falciforme e che si manifesta con ematuria e una massa a livello del fianco. Le metastasi sono generalmente già presenti al momento della diagnosi. La prognosi è severa.

Blakely ML, Ritchey ML: Controversial issues in the maintenance of Wilms' tumor. *Semin Pediatr* 2001;10:127–131.

de Kraker J, Graf N, van Tinteren H, et al: Reduction of postoperative chemotherapy in children with stage 1 intermediate-risk and anaplastic Wilms' tumour (SIOP 93–01 trial): A randomized controlled trial. *Lancet* 2004;364:1229–1235.

Dome JS, Liu T, Krasin M, et al: Improved survival for patients with recurrent Wilms tumor: The experience at St. Jude Children's Research Hospital. *J Pediatr Hematol Oncol* 2002;24:192–198.

Firoozi F, Kogan BA: Follow-up and management of recurrent Wilms' tumor. *Urol Clin North Am* 2003;30:869–879.

Fischbach BV, Trout KL, Lewis J, et al: WAGR syndrome: A clinical review of 54 cases. *Pediatrics* 2005;116:984–988.

Fukuzawa R, Breslow NE, Morison IM, et al: Epigenetic differences between Wilms' tumours in white and east-Asian children. *Lancet* 2004;363: 446–451.

Gronskov K, Olsen JH, Sand A, et al: Population-bases risk estimates of Wilms tumor in sporadic aniridia. *Hum Genet* 2001;109:11–18.

Kalapurakal JA, Dome JS, Perlman EJ, et al: Management of Wilms' tumour: Current practice and future goals. *Lancet Oncol* 2004;5:37–46.

Malcolm AW, Jaffe N, Folkman MJ, et al: Bilateral Wilms' tumor. *Int J Radiat Oncol Biol Phys* 1980;6:167–174.

Patel K, Livni N, Macdonald D: Renal medullary carcinoma, a rare cause of haematuria in sickle cell trait. *Br J Haematol* 2006;132:1.

Pirich LM, Chou P, Walterhouse DO: Prolonged survival of a patient with sickle cell trait and metastatic renal medullary carcinoma. *J Pediatr Hematol Oncol* 1999;21:67–69.

Pritchard-Jones K, Pritchard J: Success of clinical trials in childhood Wilms' tumour around the world. *Lancet* 2004;364:1468–1470.

Ritchey ML: The role of preoperative chemotherapy for Wilms' tumor: The NWTSG perspective. Wilms' Tumor Study Group. *Semin Urol Oncol* 1999;17:21–27.

Shamberger RC: Pediatric renal tumors. *Semin Surg Oncol* 1999;16:105–120.

Capitolo 500 ■ Sarcomi dei tessuti molli

Carola A.S. Arndt

L'incidenza annuale dei sarcomi dei tessuti molli è di 8,4 casi per milione di bambini di razza bianca di età <14 anni. Il rabdomiosarcoma ne rappresenta oltre la metà. La prognosi si correla in modo molto deciso all'estensione della malattia al momento della diagnosi, alla sede del tumore primitivo e al tipo di trattamento.

RABDOMIOSARCOMA

EPIDEMIOLOGIA. Il più comune sarcoma dei tessuti molli dell'età pediatrica, il rabdomiosarcoma, rappresenta circa il 3,5% delle neoplasie infantili. In teoria può colpire qualunque sede anatomica, ma generalmente si osserva al livello della testa e del collo (25%), del tratto genitourinario (22%) degli arti (18%); il retroperitoneo e le altre sedi rappresentano i restanti siti del tumore primitivo. L'incidenza per ciascuna sede anatomica è correlata sia all'età del paziente sia al tipo di tumore. Le lesioni che colpiscono gli arti sono maggiormente frequenti nei bambini più grandi e hanno un'istologia di tipo alveolare. Il rabdomiosarcoma ha una frequenza più alta nei pazienti con neurofibromatosi ed è stato associato con il tumore mammario materno nella sindrome di Li-Fraumeni, suggerendo un'influenza genetica.

PATOGENESI. Si pensa che il rabdomiosarcoma derivi dallo stesso mesenchima embrionale del muscolo striato scheletrico. Sulla base dell'aspetto microscopico, proviene dal gruppo dei tumori a piccole cellule rotondeggianti che include il sarcoma di Ewing, il neuroblastoma e il linfoma non-Hodgkin. La diagnosi definitiva di un preparato patologico può richiedere uno studio immunoistochimico, mediante anticorpi antimuscolo scheletrico (desmina, actina muscolo-specifica, Myo-D) e la microscopia elettronica.

La determinazione dello specifico sottotipo istologico è importante per pianificare il trattamento e per stabilire la prognosi. Se ne riconoscono quattro: il **tipo embrionale**, che rappresenta circa il 60% dei casi e ha una prognosi intermedia; il **tipo botrioide**, una variante della forma embrionale in cui le cellule tumorali e uno stroma edematoso si proiettano in un organo cavitato simile a un grappolo d'uva. Questo tipo si osserva più spesso nella vagina, nell'utero, nella vescica, nel nasofaringe e nell'orecchio medio. Il **tipo alveolare** include il 15% dei casi e spesso è caratterizzato dalle traslocazioni cromosomiche 2;13 o 1;13; in esso, le cellule tumorali tendono a crescere in gruppi che spesso hanno spazi simili a fenditure, che li fanno assomigliare ad alveoli. I tumori alveolari si localizzano con maggiore frequenza nel tronco e negli arti e sono quelli con la prognosi peggiore. Il **tipo pleiomorfico** (forma adulta), infine, è raro nell'infanzia e rappresenta solo l'1% dei casi.

MANIFESTAZIONI CLINICHE. La più comune modalità di presentazione è una massa, dolente o meno. I sintomi sono provocati dalla dislocazione o dall'ostruzione di strutture normali (Tab. 500-1). L'origine a livello nasofaringeo può associarsi a una congestione nasale, alla respirazione orale, a epistassi e alla difficoltà

TABELLA 500-1. Sintomi clinici comuni del rabdomiosarcoma

REGIONE	SINTOMI
Testa e collo	Massa asintomatica, può mimare un ingrossamento linfonodale
Orbite	Proptosi, chemosi, paralisi oculare, massa palpebrale
Nasofaringe	Russamento, voce nasale, epistassi, rinorrea, dolore locale, disfagia, paralisi dei nervi cranici
Seni paranasali	Tumefazione, dolore, sinusite, ostruzione, epistassi, paralisi dei nervi cranici
Orecchio medio	Otite cronica media, otorragia, paralisi dei nervi cranici, polipi estrudenti
Laringe	Raucedine, tosse secca
Tronco	Massa asintomatica (generalmente)
Vie biliari	Epatomegalia, ittero
Retroperitoneo	Massa non dolente, ascite, ostruzione gastrointestinale o dellle vie urinarie, sintomi da compressione spinale
Vescica/prostata	Ematuria, ritenzione urinaria, massa addominale, stipsi
Genitali femminili	Estrusione polipoide vaginale di tessuto mucoso sanguinante, noduli vulvari
Genitali maschili	Massa scrotale dolente o non dolente
Arti	Massa dolente, può essere molto piccola ma con un coinvolgimento linfonodale secondario
Metastasi	Sintomi aspecifici, associati alla diagnosi di leucemia

Da McDowell HP: Update on childhood rhabdomyosarcoma. *Arch Dis Child* 2003;88:354-357.

a deglutire e masticare. L'estensione regionale intracranica può provocare la paralisi dei nervi cranici, la cecità e segni di ipertensione endocranica con cefalea e vomito. Quando il tumore si sviluppa al livello del viso o delle guance può determinare tumefazione, dolore, trisma e, man mano che si estende, la paralisi dei nervi cranici. Le neoplasie del collo possono dare luogo a una progressiva tumefazione con sintomi neurologici causati dall'estensione regionale. I tumori primitivi dell'orbita in genere sono diagnosticati precocemente durante il loro decorso, in quanto provocano la proptosi, un edema periorbitale, una ptosi, variazioni dell'acuità visiva e dolore locale. Quando la neoplasia interessa l'orecchio medio, i più comuni segni precoci sono il dolore, l'ipoacusia, l'otorrea cronica o l'evidenza di una massa nel canale auricolare; l'estensione del tumore provoca la paralisi dei nervi cranici e segni tipici di un espanso intracranico posizionato in quella sede. Una tosse persistente e un progressivo stridore possono accompagnare il rabdomiosarcoma laringeo. Dal momento che la maggior parte di questi segni e sintomi è anche associata ad altre malattie comuni dell'infanzia, i medici devono prestare attenzione alla possibilità del tumore.

Il rabdomiosarcoma del tronco o degli arti spesso viene notato per la prima volta dopo un trauma e inizialmente può essere scambiato per un ematoma, ma se l'edema non si risolve o se tende ad aumentare di volume, si deve appunto considerare la possibilità della neoplasia. Il coinvolgimento del tratto genitourinario può provocare l'ematuria, l'ostruzione del tratto urinario inferiore, infezioni ricorrenti delle vie urinarie, l'incontinenza o una massa palpabile a livello dell'addome o all'esplorazione rettale. I tumori paratesticolari generalmente si manifestano come una massa non dolente, che si accresce rapidamente al livello dello scroto. Il rabdomiosarcoma vaginale può invece presentarsi come una massa a grappolo d'uva di tessuto tumorale, noto come **sarcoma botrioide**, che protrude dall'orifizio della vagina e che può provocare sintomi a carico delle vie urinarie o dell'intestino crasso. Si possono verificare un sanguinamento vaginale o un'ostruzione dell'uretra o del retto. Quadri simili si possono osservare nelle localizzazioni primitive a livello uterino.

Tutti questi tumori possono disseminare precocemente e presentarsi con sintomi quali dolore o insufficienza respiratoria associati alle metastasi polmonari. Un esteso coinvolgimento dell'osso può determinare un'ipercalcemia sintomatica, ciò che in questi casi può rendere difficile l'identificazione della lesione primitiva.

DIAGNOSI. Per porre una diagnosi precoce del rabdomiosarcoma è necessario sospettarlo. L'aspetto microscopico è di un **tumore a piccole cellule rotondeggianti di colore blu**, come anche nel neuroblastoma, il linfoma e il sarcoma di Ewing. La diagnosi differenziale dipende dalla sede di presentazione, mentre quella definitiva si fonda sulla biopsia, sull'aspetto microscopico e sui risultati delle colorazioni immunoistochimiche. Una lesione localizzata a un arto può essere scambiata per un ematoma o un emangioma, una lesione orbitale che provoca proptosi può essere trattata come una cellulite orbitale, o possono mancare sintomi da ostruzione vescicale. Gli adolescenti possono ignorare l'esistenza di lesioni paratesticolari per lunghi periodi di tempo. Sfortunatamente, spesso possono trascorrere anche molti mesi tra i sintomi iniziali e la biopsia. Le procedure diagnostiche sono soprattutto condizionate dall'area interessata. La TC o la RM riescono necessarie per valutare la sede del tumore primitivo. Nel caso di segni e sintomi a livello della testa e del collo, occorre fare radiografie per valutare la massa del tumore e per osservare l'erosione dell'osso. La TC o la RM vanno invece eseguite per quantificare l'estensione intracranica, nonché per determinare il coinvolgimento dell'osso o l'erosione della base cranica. Per i tumori addominali e pelvici, sono utili l'ecografia, la TC con contrasto o la RM (Fig. 500-1). Una scintigrafia ossea con radionuclidi, la TC del torace e l'aspirato e la biopsia ossea bilaterale vanno effettuati per valutare il paziente e per stabilire l'esistenza di una malattia metastatica al fine di pianificare il trattamento. L'elemento più critico della fase diagnostica è costituito dall'esame del tessuto tumorale, che prevede l'utilizzo di specifiche colorazioni istochimiche e immunoistochimiche. La valutazione citogenetica e la genetica molecolare possono risultare utili per identificare specifiche traslocazioni cromosomiche di proteine di fusione presenti nel rabdomiosarcoma alveolare. Bisogna esaminare anche i linfonodi, per escludere la disseminazione della malattia soprattutto nel caso dei tumori degli arti.

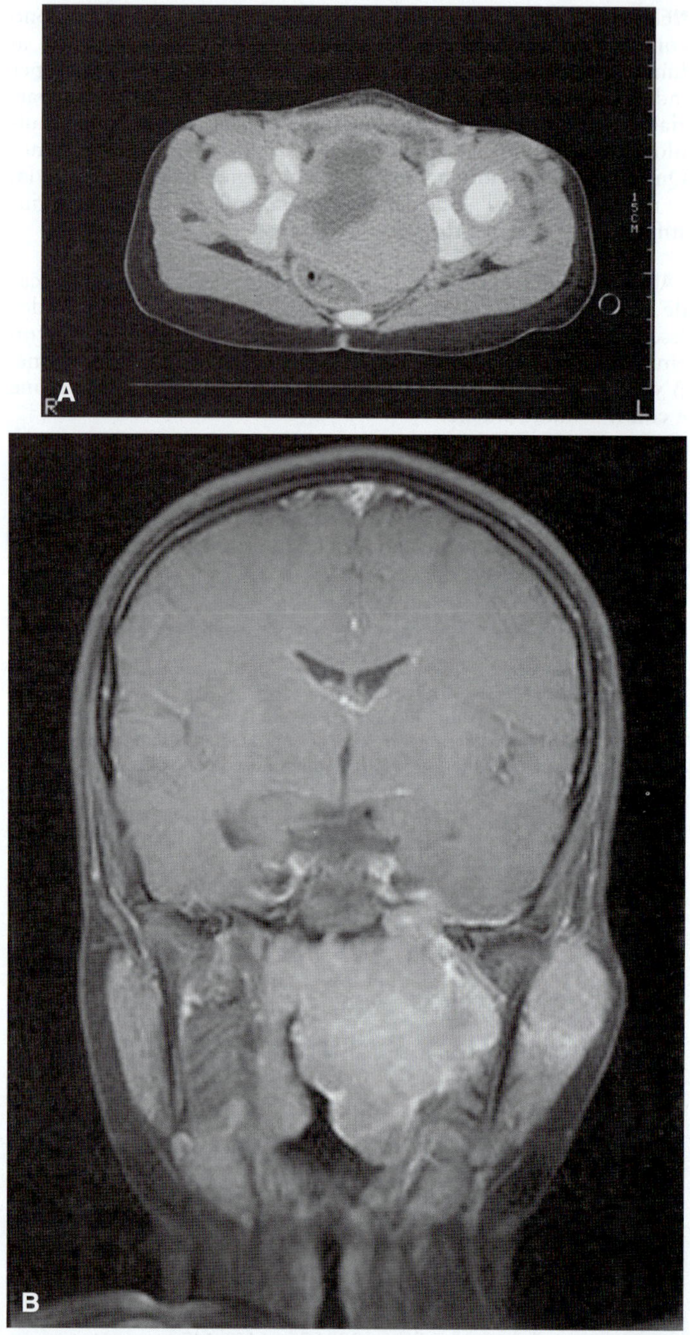

Figura 500-1. *A*, TC pelvica di un bambino con un rabdomiosarcoma vescicale. *B*, RM di un bambino con un rabdomiosarcoma parameningeo.

TRATTAMENTO. I pazienti con tumori completamente asportati hanno la prognosi migliore, ma sfortunatamente la maggior parte dei rabdomiosarcomi non è asportabile in modo radicale. Al momento della chirurgia vanno attentamente definiti i margini della neoplasia e occorre operare un'adeguata valutazione della malattia a livello regionale oppure della metastatizzazione a strutture adiacenti o ai linfonodi regionali, anche se la procedura chirurgica consiste nella sola biopsia. Il trattamento dipende dalla localizzazione del tumore primitivo e dallo stadio di malattia, che definiscono il gruppo clinico. La maggior parte dei pazienti viene sottoposta a una chemioterapia preoperatoria, con l'intento di ridurre l'estensione della chirurgia e per preservare gli organi vitali, soprattutto il tratto genitourinario. I tumori del gruppo I vengono trattati con l'exeresi locale completa seguita da una chemioterapia per ridurre la probabilità di metastasi successive. I tumori del gruppo II (residuo tumorale microscopico) sono invece trattati con la chirurgia, seguita dalla radioterapia locale e dalla chemioterapia sistemica. Dei tumori del gruppo III (voluminoso residuo tumorale) ci si occupa mediante una chemioterapia sistemica seguita dalla radioterapia e se possibile dalla chirurgia. Per il rabdomiosarcoma di gruppo IV (metastatico), infine, il trattamento consiste principalmente in una chemioterapia sistemica e nella radioterapia. Gli agenti chemioterapici standard sono la vincristina, la dactinomicina e la ciclofosfamide, mentre sono in corso di valutazione in trial terapeutici il topotecano e l'irinotecano.

PROGNOSI. I fattori prognostici sono costituiti dallo stadio, dall'istologia e dalla sede del tumore primitivo. Tra i soggetti con una neoplasia operabile, l'80-90% ha una lunga sopravvivenza libera da malattia, così come il 70% circa dei pazienti con una neoplasia asportata in modo incompleto; allo stesso modo, possiede un'alta probabilità di guarigione il tumore non operabile localizzato in particolari sedi favorevoli, come l'orbita. I casi di malattia disseminata hanno al contrario una prognosi sfavorevole; solo circa la metà dei pazienti ha una remissione e poco oltre il 50% di questi guarisce. La prognosi risulta inoltre peggiore nei bambini più grandi rispetto a quelli più piccoli. Per tutti i pazienti è comunque importante sorvegliare gli effetti tardivi del trattamento oncologico (come la ridotta crescita dell'osso secondaria alla radioterapia, la sterilità da ciclofosfamide e le seconde neoplasie).

ALTRI SARCOMI DEI TESSUTI MOLLI

I sarcomi dei tessuti molli non-rabdomiosarcomi sono un gruppo eterogeneo di tumori, che rappresenta il 3% di tutte le neoplasie dell'infanzia (Tab. 500-2). Dal momento che sono relativamente rari nei bambini, molte delle informazioni circa la loro anamnesi naturale e il trattamento derivano dagli studi su pazienti adulti. In ogni caso, nei bambini l'età media alla diagnosi è 12 anni, con un rapporto maschi:femmine di 2,3:1. Questi tumori si localizzano frequentemente nel tronco o negli arti inferiori. I tipi istologici più comuni sono il sarcoma sinoviale (42%), il fibrosarcoma (13%), l'istiocitoma fibroso maligno (12%) e i tumori neurogenici (10%). Gli studi di genetica molecolare spesso si dimostrano utili nella diagnosi, in quanto molte di queste neoplasie hanno tipiche traslocazioni cromosomiche.

La chirurgia rimane la terapia fondamentale, ma prima dell'exeresi chirurgica andrebbe effettuata un'attenta ricerca di metastasi polmonari e ossee. La disseminazione linfonodale è rara e la dissezione di routine non è raccomandata. Occorre prendere in considerazione la chemioterapia e la radioterapia per i tumori di grosse dimensioni, di alto grado e non operabili, sebbene il ruolo della chemioterapia, per queste neoplasie, non sia chiaramente definito come per il rabdomiosarcoma. I soggetti con una malattia inoperabile o metastatica sono trattati con una polichemioterapia in aggiunta alla radioterapia e/o alla chirurgia. Alla sopravvivenza si correlano la dimensione del tumore, lo stadio (gruppo clinico), l'invasività e il grado istologico.

Arndt CAS, Crist WM: Medical progress: Common musculoskeletal tumors of childhood and adolescence. *N Engl J Med* 1999;341:342–352.

Baker KS, Anderson JR, Lind MP, et al: Benefit of intensified therapy for patients with local or regional embryonal rhabdomyosarcoma: Results from the Intergroup Rhabdomyosarcoma Study IV. *J Clin Oncol* 2000;18:2427–2434.

TABELLA 500-2. Caratteristiche dei tipi più frequenti di sarcoma dei tessuti molli non-rabdomiosarcomi

TIPO DI TESSUTO	TUMORE	ANAMNESI NATURALE E BIOLOGIA
Adiposo	Liposarcoma	Un tumore molto raro. Generalmente localizzato a livello degli arti o del retroperitoneo; si associa a traslocazione non casuale t(12; 16) (q13; p11). Tende a essere localmente invasivo e raramente metastatizza; un'ampia asportazione locale è la terapia di scelta. Il ruolo della chemioterapia e della radioterapia nel trattare grossi residui o localizzazioni metastatiche non è chiaro.
Fibroso	Fibrosarcoma	Il più comune sarcoma dei tessuti molli nei bambini <1 anno. Il fibrosarcoma congenito è una neoplasia di basso grado che comunemente origina a livello degli arti o del tronco e raramente metastatizza. Il trattamento di scelta è l'asportazione chirurgica; si può osservare una importante risposta alla chemioterapia preoperatoria. Nei bambini >4 anni l'anamnesi naturale è simile a quella degli adulti (sopravvivenza a 5 anni del 60%); generalmente si utilizzano un'ampia chirurgia e una chemioterapia preoperatoria.
	Istiocitoma fibroso maligno	Frequentemente localizzato a livello del tronco o degli arti, negli strati profondi del sottocute. Istologicamente si riconoscono le varianti storiformi, a cellule giganti, mixoide e angiomatoide. Il tipo angiomatoide tende a colpire i pazienti più giovani ed è trattabile con la sola resezione chirurgica. L'ampia asportazione chirurgica è il trattamento di scelta. La chemioterapia produce regressioni obiettive della malattia.
Vascolare	Emangiopericitoma	Spesso localizzato a livello degli arti inferiori o del retroperitoneo; può presentarsi con ipoglicemia e rachitismo ipofosfatemico. L'istologia può essere sia benigna sia maligna. Sono state descritte traslocazioni non casuali t(12; 19) (q13; q13) e t(13; 22) (q22; q11). Un'ampia asportazione chirurgica è il trattamento di scelta. La chemioterapia e la radioterapia possono produrre risposte.
	Angiosarcoma	Raro nei bambini; il 33% dei casi colpisce la cute, il 25% i tessuti molli e il 25% il fegato, la mammella e l'osso. Negli adulti si associa a linfoedema cronico e all'esposizione al cloruro di vinile. La sopravvivenza è bassa (12% a 5 anni), nonostante alcune risposte alla chemio/radioterapia.
	Emangioendotelioma	Può colpire i tessuti molli, il fegato e il polmone. Le lesioni localizzate hanno un andamento favorevole; le lesioni polmonari ed epatiche spesso sono multifocali e hanno una prognosi sfavorevole.
Nervi periferici	Neurofibrosarcoma	Anche noto come tumore maligno della guaina dei nervi periferici. Si sviluppa in oltre il 16% dei pazienti con NF1 e questi pazienti sviluppano circa il 50% delle forme di questo tumore. Sono state riportate delezioni dei cromosomi 22q11-q13 o 17q11 e mutazioni della p53. Frequentemente si localizza nel tronco e negli arti ed è generalmente invasivo a livello locale. L'asportazione chirurgica completa è necessaria per garantire la sopravvivenza; la risposta alla chemioterapia è subottimale.
Sinovia	Sarcoma sinoviale	Il più comune NRSTS in molte casistiche. Spesso si manifesta nella terza decade, ma il 33% dei pazienti ha <20 anni. Tipicamente origina in prossimità del ginocchio o della coscia ed è caratterizzato da una traslocazione non casuale di t(X; 18) (p11; q11). È indispensabile un'asportazione ampia. La radioterapia è efficace per i residui microscopici di malattia e una chemioterapia a base di ifosfamide è attiva nelle malattie avanzate.
Sconosciuto	Sarcoma alveolare delle parti molli	Tumore a lenta crescita; tende a recidivare o a metastatizzare a livello polmonare ed encefalico a distanza di anni dalla diagnosi. Spesso origina a livello degli arti e della zona testa-collo. È stata ipotizzata un'origine miogenica. È raccomandata l'asportazione del tumore primitivo e delle localizzazioni metastatiche quando possibile.
Muscolo liscio	Leiomiosarcoma	È spesso localizzato a livello del tratto digerente e può associarsi alla traslocazione t(12; 14) (q14; q23). Si associa al virus di Epstein-Barr nelle sindromi da immunodeficienza (compreso l'AIDS). Il trattamento di scelta è l'asportazione chirurgica.

NF, neurofibromatosi; NRSTS, sarcomi dei tessuti molli non-rabdomiosarcomi (*NonRhabdomyoSarcoma Soft Tissue Sarcoma*).

Crist WM, Anderson JR, Meza JL, et al: Intergroup rhabdomyosarcoma study: IV. Results for patients with nonmetastatic disease. *J Clin Oncol* 2001;19:3091–3102.

McDowell HP: Update on childhood rhabdomyosarcoma. *Arch Dis Child* 2003;88:354–357.

Meyer WH, Spunt SL: Soft tissue sarcomas of childhood. *Cancer Treat Rev* 2004;30:269–280.

Spunt SL, Poquette CA, Hurt YS, et al: Prognostic factors for children and adolescents with surgically resected nonrhabdomyosarcoma soft tissue sarcoma: An analysis of 121 patients treated at St. Jude Children's Research Hospital. *J Clin Oncol* 1999;17:3697—3705.

Stevens MCG: Treatment for childhood rhabdomyosarcoma: The cost of cure. *Lancet Oncol* 2005;6:77–84.

Capitolo 501 ■ Neoplasie dell'osso

Carola A.S. Arndt

501.1 • Tumori maligni dell'osso

L'incidenza annuale dei tumori maligni dell'osso negli Stati Uniti è di circa 7 casi per milione di bambini di razza bianca con <14 anni; la diffusione è leggermente più bassa nei bambini afroamericani. L'osteosarcoma è quello più frequente tra i bambini e gli adolescenti, seguito dal sarcoma di Ewing (Tab. 501-1; Fig. 501-1). Nei bambini con <10 anni, tuttavia, quest'ultimo è più comune dell'altro. Entrambi i tipi risultano comunque in numero maggiore nella seconda decade di vita.

OSTEOSARCOMA

EPIDEMIOLOGIA. L'incidenza annuale dell'osteosarcoma negli Stati Uniti è di 5,6 casi per milione di bambini di età <15 anni. Il periodo a più elevato rischio per contrarlo è durante lo scatto della crescita nell'adolescenza, ciò che suggerisce un'associazione tra il rapido sviluppo dell'osso e la trasformazione maligna. I pazienti con osteosarcoma sono più alti rispetto ai loro coetanei.

TABELLA 501-1. Confronto delle caratteristiche dell'osteosarcoma e della famiglia dei tumori di Ewing

CARATTERISTICA	OSTEOSARCOMA	FAMIGLIA DEI TUMORI DI EWING
Età	Seconda decade	Seconda decade
Razza	Tutte le razze	Soprattutto la razza bianca
Sesso (m:f)	1,5:1	1,5:1
Cellule	Cellule fusiformi-producenti calcificazioni	Piccole cellule tondeggianti indifferenziate, probabilmente di origine neurale
Predisposizione	Retinoblastoma, sindrome di Li-Fraumeni, malattia di Paget, radioterapia	Nessuna nota
Sede	Metafisi delle ossa lunghe	Dialisi delle ossa lunghe, ossa piatte
Presentazione	Dolore locale ed edema; spesso anamnesi di un trauma	Dolore locale ed edema; febbre
Radiografia	Destrusione sclerotica (meno comunemente di aspetto litico); aspetto a sole nascente	Soprattutto litica, con reazione periosteale multilamellare ("a bulbo di cipolla")
Diagnosi differenziale	Sarcoma di Ewing, osteomielite	Osteomielite, granuloma eosinofilo, linfoma, neuroblastoma, rabdomiosarcoma
Metastasi	Polmoni, ossa	Polmoni, ossa
Trattamento	Chemioterapia, chirurgia ablativa del tumore primitivo	Chemioterapia, radioterapia e/o chirurgia del tumore primitivo
Andamento	Senza metastasi: guarigione nel 70% dei casi; con metastasi alla diagnosi, sopravvivenza ≤20%	Senza metastasi: guarigione nel 60% dei casi; con metastasi alla diagnosi, sopravvivenza del 20-30%

PATOGENESI. Anche se la causa dell'osteosarcoma è sconosciuta, alcune malattie genetiche o acquisite risultano predisponenti; i soggetti affetti da **retinoblastoma ereditario** corrono per esempio un rischio significativamente più alto. Inizialmente si pensava che le sedi di formazione di questo tumore fossero solo quelle precedentemente irradiate, ma più di recente è stato osservato che esso può originare anche in aree lontane, per cui la predisposizione in questi pazienti può essere correlata alla perdita dell'eterozigosi del gene RB. L'osteosarcoma si osserva anche nella **sindrome di Li-Fraumeni**, che è una patologia associata alla mutazione nelle cellule germinali del gene p53 con conseguenti neoplasie di tipo familiare. I parenti con la **sindrome di Li-Fraumeni** hanno diversi tipi di neoplasie nei familiari di primo grado, tra cui il carcinoma mammario, i sarcomi dei tessuti molli, i tumori cerebrali, la leucemia, il carcinoma adrenocorticale e altri. La **sindrome di Rothmund-Thomson** è una rara patologia che si associa a bassa statura, teleangectasie cutanee, mani e piedi piccoli, pollici ipoplasici o assenti e alto rischio di sviluppare un osteosarcoma. Questo può inoltre essere indotto dall'irradiazione per il sarcoma di Ewing, dalla radioterapia craniospinale per i tumori cerebrali o da alte dosi di radioterapia per altre neoplasie. Altre malattie benigne che possono associarsi a una trasformazione maligna in osteosarcoma sono la malattia di Paget, l'encondromatosi, le esostosi ereditarie multiple e la displasia fibrosa.

La diagnosi patologica di osteosarcoma è tratta con la dimostrazione di cellule neoplastiche di forma affusolata, altamente maligne, pleomorfe, associate alla formazione di osteoidi maligni e osso. Esistono quattro sottotipi patologici di osteosarcoma convenzionale di alto grado: osteoblastico, fibroblastico, condroblastico e teleangectasico. Non sussistono differenze significative sull'andamento clinico dei diversi sottotipi, anche se la componente condroblastica può non rispondere bene alla chemioterapia. Deve ancora essere valutato il ruolo prognostico di diversi geni come quelli associati alla resistenza ai farmaci, i geni oncosoppressori e quelli correlati all'apoptosi.

L'**osteosarcoma teleangectasico** può essere confuso con una cisti ossea aneurismatica, a causa del suo aspetto radiologico litico. Tipicamente l'osteosarcoma di alto grado origina a livello della diafisi delle ossa lunghe e invade la cavità midollare. Può anche trovarsi insieme a una massa nei tessuti molli. In base alle caratteristiche cliniche, si distinguono due varianti dalla sua forma convenzionale, quella parosteale e quella periosteale. Il **sarcoma parosteale** è un tumore a basso grado, ben differenziato, che non invade la cavità midollare e si osserva più frequentemente nella parte posterodistale del femore. Spesso risulta curativa la sola resezione chirurgica, per la scarsa tendenza di questo tumore metastatizzare. L'**osteosarcoma periosteale** è una rara variante, che prende origine dalla superficie dell'osso e che ha una più alta probabilità di disseminazione metastatica rispetto al tipo parosteale, con una prognosi intermedia.

MANIFESTAZIONI CLINICHE. Le più comuni manifestazioni d'esordio dell'osteosarcoma sono il dolore, la zoppia e l'edema. Dal momento che questi tumori si verificano più spesso in adolescenti fisicamente attivi, i primi disturbi possono essere attribuiti a traumi sportivi o a strappi muscolari; qualunque dolore osseo o articolare che non risponda alla terapia conservativa entro un ragionevole lasso di tempo dovrebbe quindi essere ulteriormente indagato. Segni clinici aggiuntivi possono comprendere la limitazione funzionale, il versamento articolare, la dolenzia e la sensazione di calore locale. I risultati degli esami di laboratorio di routine, come l'emocromo completo e gli esami ematochimici, generalmente sono normali, anche se la fosfatasi alcalina o la lattico deidrogenasi possono risultare aumentate.

DIAGNOSI. Bisogna sospettare una neoplasia ossea quando il paziente lamenta un dolore osseo profondo (che spesso provoca il

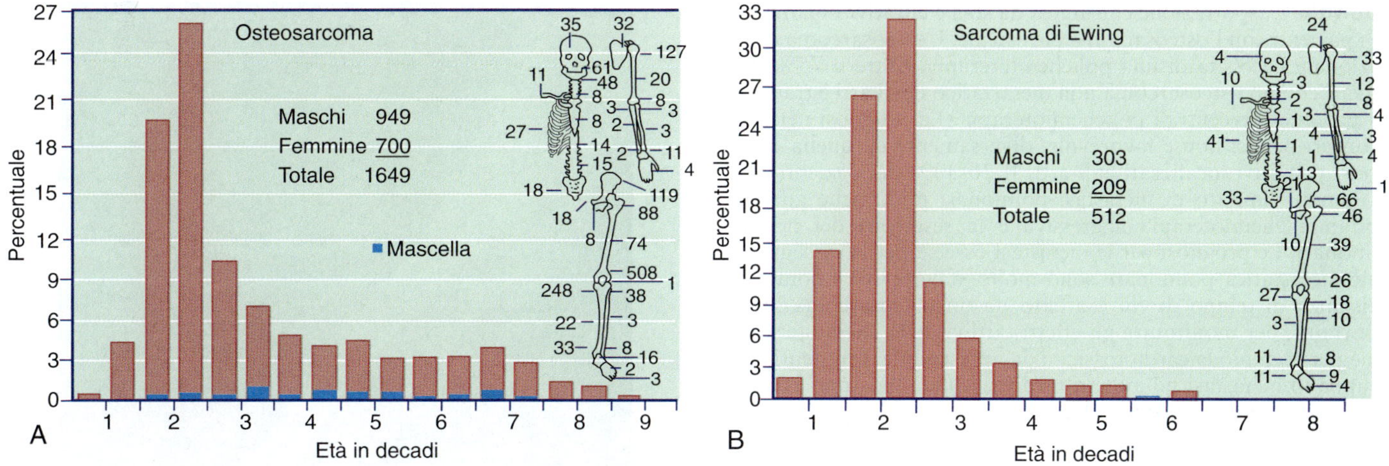

Figura 501-1. *A*, Distribuzione per età e sede di 1649 casi di osteosarcoma in una casistica della Mayo Clinic. *B*, Distribuzione per età e sede di 512 casi di sarcoma di Ewing in una casistica della Mayo Clinic. (Da Unni KK [editor]: *Dahlin's Bone Tumors: General Aspects and Data on 11,087 Cases*, 5th ed. Philadelphia, Lippincott-Raven, 1996. Ristampato su concessione della Mayo Foundation.)

risveglio durante la notte), ha una massa palpabile e l'evidenza di una lesione sulla radiografia. Questa lesione può essere mista, con un aspetto litico e blastico, ma si vede di solito la nuova formazione ossea. Il classico aspetto radiologico è quello di un **sole nascente** (Fig. 501-2). Quando si sospetta un osteosarcoma, il paziente andrebbe indirizzato presso un centro specializzato nel trattamento dei tumori ossei. La biopsia e l'asportazione chirurgica dovrebbero essere eseguite dallo stesso chirurgo, così che la sede dell'incisione bioptica possa essere scelta in maniera da non compromettere la successiva procedura di salvataggio dell'arto. Il tessuto da esaminare dai punti di vista molecolare e biologico si ottiene generalmente al momento della biopsia iniziale, prima della quale risulta opportuno effettuare la RM della lesione primaria e dell'intero osso interessato, per valutare i rapporti del tumore con i nervi e le strutture vascolari e la sua estensione ai tessuti molli e al livello delle articolazioni, nonché le lesioni saltate. Lo studio per escludere le metastasi va effettuato prima della biopsia e prevede l'esecuzione di una TC del torace e di una scintigrafia ossea per verificare, rispettivamente, la mancanza di localizzazioni polmonari e ossee. La **diagnosi differenziale** di una lesione osteolitica comprende l'istiocitosi, il sarcoma di Ewing, il linfoma e la cisti ossea.

TRATTAMENTO. Con la chemioterapia e la chirurgia, la sopravvivenza a 5 anni libera da recidive di soggetti con un osteosarcoma non metastatico degli arti è del 65-75%. L'asportazione chirurgica completa del tumore è fondamentale per la prognosi. L'attuale strategia terapeutica è quella di sottoporre il paziente a una chemioterapia preoperatoria con lo scopo di facilitare il recupero dell'arto e di trattare immediatamente la malattia micrometastatica. Dopo questa chemioterapia, oltre l'80% dei pazienti può essere sottoposto a un intervento di salvataggio dell'arto. Alcuni centri utilizzano la chemioterapia intra-arteriosa per infondere gli agenti chemioterapici direttamente nell'arteria che alimenta il tumore, anche se questa tecnica non ha dimostrato di essere migliore della chemioterapia sistemica tradizionale. È importante riprendere la chemioterapia appena possibile dopo l'intervento. Le metastasi polmonari presenti al momento della diagnosi dovrebbero essere asportante in toracotomia. I farmaci attivi attualmente impiegati nella polichemioterapia convenzionale sono la doxorubicina, il cisplatino, il metotrexato e l'ifosfamide.

Uno dei più importanti fattori prognostici è la risposta istologica alla chemioterapia. Un gruppo cooperativo internazionale sta valutando in un trial randomizzato l'aggiunta postoperatoria di alte dosi di ifosfamide ed etoposide alla terapia standard con cisplatino, doxorubicina e metotrexato, al fine di migliorare la prognosi dei casi con scarsa risposta istologica. I pazienti che quindi rispondono bene verranno randomizzati per l'ulteriore

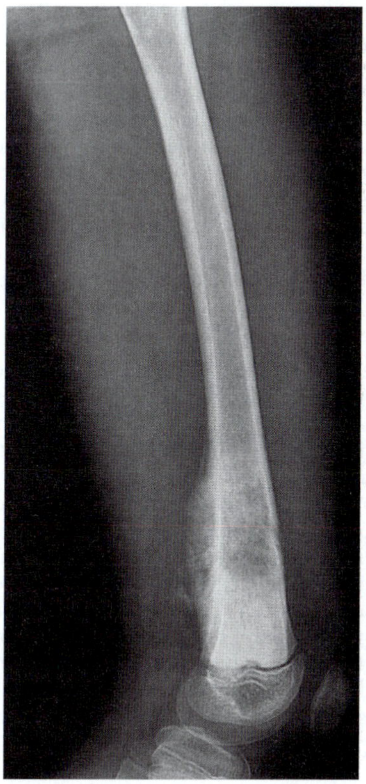

Figura 501-2. Radiografia di un osteosarcoma del femore con tipico aspetto a "sole nascente" della lesione ossea.

somministrazione di interferone α2b PEGilato. Dopo la chirurgia di salvataggio dell'arto è necessario un intenso programma di riabilitazione e di fisioterapia per recuperare la massima funzionalità possibile.

Per i soggetti che sono stati sottoposti all'amputazione di un arto, è essenziale un precoce adattamento alle protesi e una rieducazione al cammino per renderli capaci di recuperare le proprie attività nel modo più normale possibile. Prima della chirurgia definitiva, i pazienti con neoplasie localizzate su ossa portanti vanno istruiti sull'uso delle stampelle per evitare di caricare l'osso indebolito e quindi per eludere le fratture patologiche. Il ruolo della chemioterapia nei due tipi di osteosarcoma (parosteale e periosteale) non è ben definito.

PROGNOSI. L'asportazione chirurgica da sola è curativa solamente per i pazienti con l'osteosarcoma parosteale. L'osteosarcoma convenzionale necessita di una polichemioterapia. Oltre il 75% dei soggetti con un osteosarcoma non metastatico degli arti è trattato con protocolli recenti di polichemioterapia. La prognosi nei casi di tumori pelvici non è favorevole, diversamente da quella per i tumori primitivi localizzati agli arti. Il 20-30% dei pazienti con un numero limitato di metastasi polmonari può anche guarire dopo una chemioterapia aggressiva e la resezione dei noduli polmonari. Le prognosi per le metastasi ossee e per la disseminazione metastatica polmonare sono molto sfavorevoli. I controlli a distanza di tempo di chi è affetto da un osteosarcoma sono importanti, per monitorare gli effetti tardivi della chemioterapia come per esempio la cardiotossicità da antracicline. I pazienti che sviluppano metastasi polmonari tardive, isolate, possono beneficiare della sola asportazione chirurgica.

SARCOMA DI EWING

EPIDEMIOLOGIA. L'incidenza del sarcoma di Ewing negli Stati Uniti è di 2,1 casi per milione di bambini; rimane molto raro tra i bambini afroamericani. Si tratta di un sarcoma indifferenziato dell'osso che può anche originare dai tessuti molli. Il termine **famiglia dei sarcomi di Ewing** si riferisce a un gruppo di tumori indifferenziati a piccole cellule tonde che si pensa originino dalla cresta neurale, generalmente caratterizzati dalla stessa traslocazione cromosomica. Questa famiglia comprende il sarcoma di Ewing dell'osso e dei tessuti molli e il **tumore neuroectodermico primitivo** periferico. I protocolli di trattamento per queste neoplasie sono gli stessi, che abbia origine sia dall'osso sia dai tessuti molli. Le sedi anatomiche da cui si sviluppa il tumore primitivo sono soprattutto gli arti e l'asse centrale (pelvi, colonna e parete toracica); quelli che nascono dalla parete toracica sono spesso definiti **tumori Askin.**

PATOGENESI. L'immunoistochimica permette di differenziare il sarcoma di Ewing dagli altri **tumori a piccole cellule tondeggianti blu**, quali il linfoma, il rabdomiosarcoma e il neuroblastoma. Le colorazioni immunoistochimiche possono infatti dimostrare la positività per certi marcatori neurali delle cellule tumorali (enolasi neurone-specifica e S-100), soprattutto nelle neoplasie neuroectodermiche primitive periferiche. È invece assente la positività per i marcatori muscolari (per es. la desmina, l'actina). Inoltre, la glicoproteina di superficie MIC-2 è generalmente espressa. Una traslocazione cromosomica specifica, t(11;22) o una sua variante, si trova nella maggior parte dei tumori della famiglia dei sarcomi di Ewing. L'esame citogenetico per la traslocazione di routine o la PCR per la fusione chimerica dei prodotti genici EWS/FLI1 o EWS/ERG possono risultare utili per confermare la diagnosi nelle neoplasie altamente indifferenziate.

MANIFESTAZIONI CLINICHE. I sintomi sono simili a quelli dell'osteosarcoma. Dolore, edema, limitazione funzionale e alterata sensibilità al di sopra dell'osso colpito o dei tessuti molli sono i sintomi comuni alla presentazione. Voluminosi tumori primitivi della parete toracica possono determinare difficoltà respiratorie, mentre se sono paraspinali o vertebrali i pazienti possono presentare sintomi da compressione midollare. Spesso il sarcoma di Ewing si associa a **manifestazioni sistemiche** quali febbre o perdita di peso; i pazienti possono essere trattati per una presunta osteomielite. Si può anche verificare un ritardo nella diagnosi quando il dolore e l'edema vengono attribuiti a un trauma sportivo.

DIAGNOSI. La diagnosi dove essere sospettata nel caso di dolore e tumefazione, con o senza sintomi sistemici e con l'evidenza radiologica di una lesione ossea primitiva litica circondata da una reazione periostale, tipicamente **a bulbo di cipolla** (Fig. 501-3). Spesso con la RM o la TC si osserva una vasta area associata che

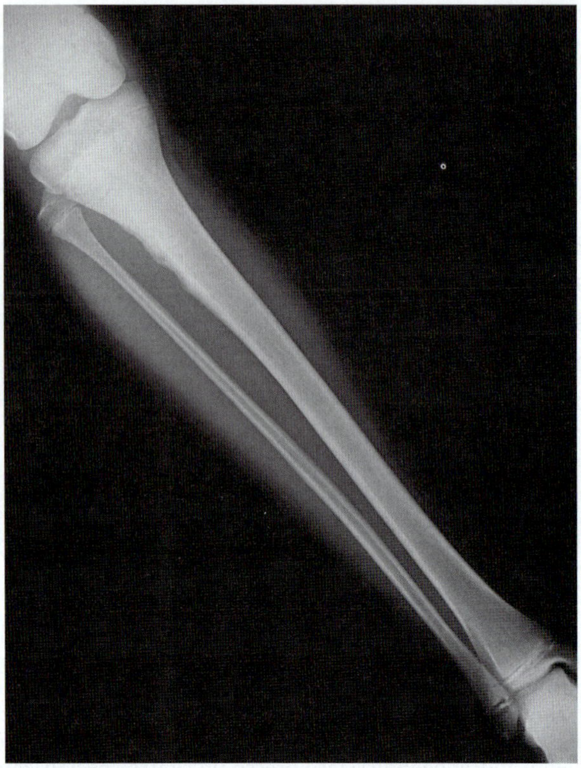

Figura 501-3. Radiografia di un sarcoma di Ewing della tibia che dimostra la protuberanza periosteale o "a bulbo di cipolla".

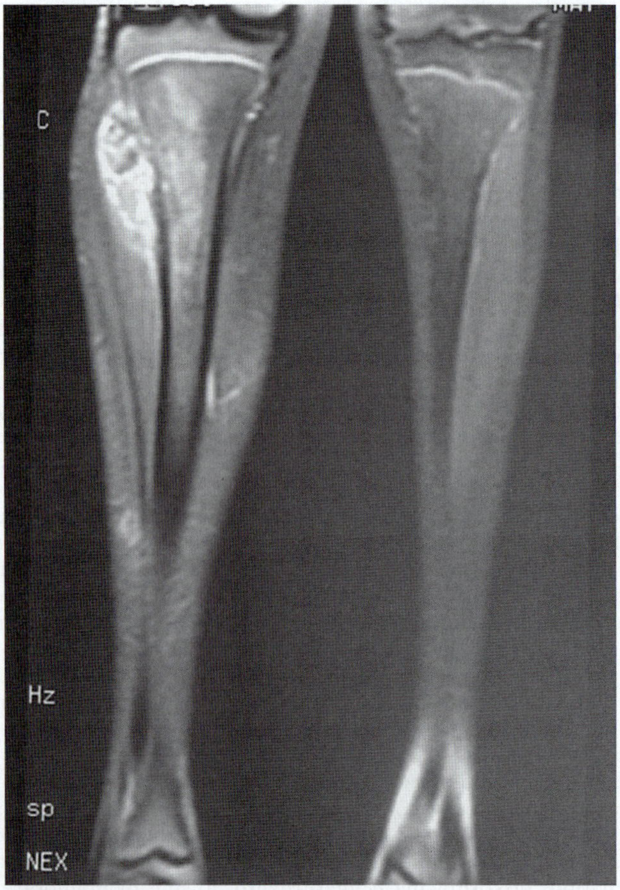

Figura 501-4. RM di un sarcoma di Ewing della tibia che evidenzia una voluminosa massa estesa ai tessuti molli.

coinvolge i tessuti molli (Fig. 501-4). La **diagnosi differenziale** va posta con l'osteosarcoma, l'osteomielite, l'istiocitosi a cellule di Langerhans, il linfoma primitivo dell'osso, il neuroblastoma metastatico e il rabdomiosarcoma nel caso di una lesione che coinvolga solo i tessuti molli. I pazienti andrebbero inviati presso un centro specializzato nel trattamento dei tumori ossei per una valutazione e per l'esecuzione della biopsia. Per l'apprezzamento della malattia metastatica è utile eseguire una TC del torace, la scintigrafia ossea e l'aspirato o biopsia midollare in almeno due sedi. La RM del tumore e dell'intera lunghezza dell'osso colpito è indicata per determinare l'esatta estensione della massa a livello dei tessuti molli e dell'osso e per valutare i rapporti del tumore con le strutture neurovascolari. Per evitare di compromettere il successivo intervento di salvataggio dell'arto con una inadeguata incisione per la biopsia, lo stesso chirurgo dovrebbe eseguire entrambi. Spesso risulta adeguata l'esecuzione della biopsia TC guidata della lesione al fine di prelevare tessuto diagnostico. È importante ottenere del tessuto adeguato per potere eseguire le colorazioni specifiche, la citogenetica e gli studi molecolari.

TRATTAMENTO. I tumori della famiglia del sarcoma di Ewing si riescono a trattare meglio con un approccio multidisciplinare, che prevede l'intervento del chirurgo, dell'oncologo e del radioterapista. La polichemioterapia è importante, perché può causare una rapida riduzione del tumore e generalmente si somministra appena possibile per avere un controllo locale della malattia. L'aggiunta di ifosfamide ed etoposide agli agenti convenzionali, quali la vincrisina, la doxorubicina e la ciclofosfamide, migliora l'andamento del sarcoma di Ewing non metastatico. La chemioterapia in genere determina un'importante riduzione della massa dei tessuti molli e un rapido e significativo miglioramento del dolore. Recenti studi randomizzati stanno inoltre valutando il ruolo della sua intensità di dose per il sarcoma di Ewing metastatico e non. Un trial di un gruppo cooperativo internazionale sta valutando se la chemioterapia mieloablativa e il recupero di cellule staminali sono superiori alla chemioterapia con irradiazione polmonare per i pazienti con metastasi polmonari. Sono in corso studi sulla chemioterapia mieloablativa anche nei soggetti con una malattia ad alto rischio (metastasi ossee e midollari), nonché sull'utilizzo di antiangiogenetici in associazione alla chemioterapia standard. Il sarcoma di Ewing è considerato un tumore radiosensibile e il controllo locale si può ottenere con la radioterapia o con la chirurgia. La prima si associa al rischio di secondi tumori radioindotti, soprattutto l'osteosarcoma, a causa di un danno sulla crescita ossea nei soggetti con uno sviluppo scheletrico ancora immaturo; molti centri le preferiscono quindi la resezione chirurgica, se possibile. È importante fornire al paziente le stampelle, se risulta interessato un osso portante, per evitare una frattura patologica prima che sia ottenuto un definitivo controllo locale. La chemioterapia va ripresa appena possibile dopo la chirurgia.

PROGNOSI. I pazienti con tumori di piccole dimensioni, non metastatici, localizzati distalmente a livello degli arti, hanno la prognosi migliore, con guarigione in oltre il 75% dei casi. La presenza di una traslocazione cromosomica può essere correlata con la prognosi. I soggetti con tumori pelvici, finora, hanno avuto una prognosi peggiore. Quelli con una malattia metastatica alla diagnosi, soprattutto se vi sono metastasi ossee o del midollo osseo, presentano una prognosi sfavorevole, con $<30\%$ di sopravvivenze a lungo termine. Nuove strategie sono in corso di studio per i casi di prognosi peggiore, come per esempio una chemioterapia particolarmente intensiva con recupero di cellule staminali dal sangue periferico.

Il follow-up a lungo termine è importante, per il rischio di effetti tardivi del trattamento come la cardiotossicità da antracicline, i secondi tumori, soprattutto nel campo d'irradiazione, e le recidive, che talvolta compaiono anche a 10 anni di distanza dalla diagnosi iniziale.

501.2 • TUMORI BENIGNI E PROCESSI SIMIL-TUMORALI DELL'OSSO

Le lesioni benigne dell'osso nei bambini sono relativamente frequenti, diversamente da quelle maligne, che sono più rare e che da queste devono essere differenziate. Alcune, anche se istologicamente benigne, possono essere minacciose per la vita. Non è sufficiente il solo elemento anamnestico o i soli esami strumentali per escludere l'origine maligna o suggerire che non si ha a che fare con un tumore. Devono essere sfruttate tutte le possibilità diagnostiche, quando ci si trova davanti una lesione ossea di natura non chiara. Le lesioni benigne possono essere non dolorose oppure dolenti, soprattutto se si trovano insieme a una frattura patologica. Il dolore notturno che risveglia il bambino è suggestivo di una lesione maligna, ma la sua scomparsa dopo l'assunzione di acido acetilsalicilico è tipica di lesioni benigne, come nel caso dell'osteoma osteoide. Le lesioni che crescono rapidamente in genere sono di natura maligna, ma diverse lesioni benigne, come la cisti ossea aneurismatica, possono ingrandirsi più velocemente della maggior parte delle neoplasie maligne. Alcune malattie, come l'osteomielite, possono simulare l'aspetto di tumori benigni dell'osso.

Molte neoplasie benigne dell'osso sono diagnosticate accidentalmente o dopo una frattura patologica, il trattamento della quale è simile a quello delle fratture non patologiche nella stessa sede. È raro che per i tumori ossei benigni vi sia un'interferenza con la normale cicatrizzazione; inoltre, le fratture raramente provocano modificazioni o la guarigione di questi tumori, che generalmente vengono trattati dopo che la frattura si è saldata.

Le radiografie di qualunque lesione ossea sospetta dovrebbero essere fatte in due proiezioni. Possono inoltre essere necessari ulteriori accertamenti per giungere alla diagnosi corretta e per guidare le scelte terapeutiche. Anche se queste lesioni si rivelano benigne, spesso vanno operate.

L'**osteocondroma** (**esostosi**) è una delle più comuni lesioni benigne ossee nei bambini. Dal momento che spesso è completamente asintomatico e che non viene riconosciuto, la sua vera incidenza non è nota. La maggior parte si sviluppa nell'infanzia, a partire dalla metafisi di un osso lungo, soprattutto sull'estremità distale del femore, su quella prossimale dell'omero e su quella prossimale della tibia. La lesione cresce poi con il bambino fino alla maturazione dello scheletro. La maggior parte è diagnosticata tra 5-15 anni, quando il bambino o i genitori notano una protuberanza non dolente dell'osso. In alcuni casi viene riconosciuta in seguito all'irritazione esercitata dalla pressione durante l'esercizio fisico o durante altre attività. Radiologicamente l'osteocondroma si presenta sottoforma di diramazioni o come proiezioni a base ampia dalla superficie dell'osso, in genere in una direzione che si allontana dell'articolazione adiacente. Invariabilmente, la lesione alla radiologia appare più piccola di quanto sembri alla palpazione, in quanto il "cappello" di cartilagine che la sovrasta non è apprezzabile, sebbene possa essere spesso anche oltre un centimetro. Sia la corticale sia lo spazio midollare dell'osso coinvolto sono in continuità con la lesione. La degenerazione maligna in un condrosarcoma è rara nei bambini, ma può verificarsi in circa l'1% degli adulti. Non sempre l'osteocondroma viene asportato chirurgicamente, a meno che non sia sufficientemente grande da provocare sintomi o non cresca rapidamente.

L'**esostosi multipla ereditaria** è una malattia decritta ma rara, caratterizzata dalla presenza di osteocondromi multipli. I bambini con forme gravi possono avere una statura ridotta, un'asimmetria della lunghezza degli arti, arresti prematuri e parziali del consolidamento dell'epifisi e deformità a livello sia degli arti superiori sia di quelli inferiori. Questi soggetti devono essere attentamente monitorati durante lo sviluppo.

L'**encondroma** è una lesione benigna di cartilagine ialina che interessa la parte centrale dell'osso; è quasi sempre asintomatica e si osserva a livello delle mani. Nella maggior parte dei casi il reperto è occasionale, anche se spesso viene diagnosticata in seguito a una frattura patologica. Dal punto di vista radiologico, le lesioni occupano il canale midollare, sono radiotrasparenti e dotate di margini netti. Al loro interno si possono trovare alcune calcificazioni puntiformi, che risultano molto più comuni negli adulti che nei bambini. Quasi tutti gli encondromi sono solitari. Nella maggior parte dei casi non è necessario un trattamento; l'asportazione e l'innesto osseo sono riservati alle lesioni sintomatiche o sufficientemente grandi da indebolire la struttura dell'osso. Il coinvolgimento multifocale configura la **malattia di Ollier** e può associarsi a una displasia ossea, a bassa statura, all'asimmetria della lunghezza degli arti e a deformità articolari, alcune delle quali possono essere corrette o prevenute con la chirurgia. Quando gli encondromi multipli si associano ad angiomi dei tessuti molli, si parla di **sindrome di Maffucci**. In entrambe queste malattie multifocali è stata riportata un'alta percentuale di trasformazione maligna.

Il **condroblastoma** è una rara lesione generalmente localizzata al livello delle epifisi delle ossa lunghe. Nella maggior parte dei pazienti si osserva nella seconda decade, con un dolore da lieve a moderato a livello dell'articolazione adiacente. Sedi frequenti sono l'anca, la spalla e la caviglia. L'atrofia muscolare e la fragilità locale possono costituire gli unici segni clinici. Alla radiologia la lesione appare radiotrasparente, con margini netti al livello delle epifisi o delle apofisi, raramente con un'estensione metafisaria attraverso la diafisi. In prossimità dell'articolazione si può osservare una deformità dell'osso subcondrale, un versamento o un'erosione dell'articolazione. È importante riconoscere queste lesioni, perché nella maggior parte dei casi possono essere trattate con l'asportazione chirurgica e l'innesto di osso prima che si verifichi la distruzione dell'articolazione.

Il **fibroma condromixoide** è un raro tumore benigno dell'infanzia, una lesione metafisaria che in genere provoca dolore e fragilità locali. A volte, tuttavia, può essere asintomatico. Alla radiologia si mostra con margini netti, sclerotici e frastagliati. L'arto inferiore è colpito più spesso. Il trattamento di solito consiste nell'asportazione chirurgica e nell'innesto osseo o nella resezione en bloc.

L'**osteoma osteoide** è un piccolo tumore benigno dell'osso che la maggior parte delle volte viene diagnosticato tra i 5 e i 20 anni di età. Il quadro clinico è caratteristico e consiste nella comparsa di un dolore non remittente e in aumento graduale, spesso più intenso durante la notte e che risponde all'assunzione di acido acetilsalicilico. I maschi sono colpiti molto più di frequente delle femmine. Può essere coinvolto qualunque osso, ma le sedi più comuni sono il femore e la tibia a livello prossimale. Lesioni vertebrali possono determinare la scoliosi o alcuni sintomi che mimano malattie neurologiche. L'esame clinico, quando viene colpito l'arto inferiore, può evidenziare zoppia, atrofia e debolezza. La palpazione e il movimento non modificano la sintomatologia. Le radiografie sono suggestive, evidenziando l'esistenza di una lesione radiotrasparente circolare o ovale a livello della metafisi o della diafisi (con un diametro di 0,5-1 cm), circondata da osso sclerotico. Il centro trasparente, o nido, dimostra un'intensa assunzione di mezzo di contrasto nelle scansioni per l'osso. Circa il 25% degli osteomi osteoidi non è visualizzabile sulle radiografie, bensì mediante la TC. A causa delle piccole dimensioni della lesione e della sua localizzazione in prossimità dello strato corticale dell'osso, anche la RM non è particolarmente sensibile nell'individuazione degli osteomi osteoidi. Il trattamento prevede la rimozione della lesione, tramite un'asportazione en bloc, un curettage o l'asportazione del nido per via percutanea sotto guida della TC. I soggetti con un dolore moderato possono essere trattati con i salicilati. Alcune lesioni si risolvono invece spontaneamente con il raggiungimento della maturità scheletrica.

L'**osteoblastoma** è una lesione localmente distruttiva che cresce in modo progressivo prediligendo le vertebre, anche se possono essere colpite quasi tutte le ossa. La maggior parte dei pazienti lamenta un esordio insidioso con un dolore sordo, che può continuare per mesi prima che venga sentito il parere di un medico. Le lesioni spinali possono provocare sintomi neurologici o deficit. L'aspetto radiologico è variabile e meno tipico rispetto ad altri tumori benigni dell'osso. Circa il 25% degli osteoblastomi presenta caratteristiche suggestive di una neoplasia maligna, rendendo necessaria in molti casi l'esecuzione di una biopsia. Le lesioni espansive spinali spesso coinvolgono gli elementi posteriori. I trattamenti prevedono il curettage e l'impianto di osso o un'asportazione en bloc, facendo attenzione a preservare le radici nervose nel caso delle lesioni spinali. A volte può risultare necessario stabilizzare la colonna.

I **fibromi** (**fibromi non calcifici, difetto fibroso corticale, difetto fibroso metafisario**) sono lesioni fibrose dell'osso che colpiscono il 40% dei bambini con >2 anni. Si presentano più spesso come un difetto di calcificazione piuttosto che come una neoplasia e sono generalmente asintomatici. Nella maggior parte dei casi vengono diagnosticati per caso, in occasione di radiografie eseguite per altri motivi, in genere per escludere una frattura dopo un trauma. Fratture patologiche occasionali possono interessare lesioni particolarmente estese. Di solito durante la visita non si osservano alterazioni. Le radiografie evidenziano una trasparenza eccentrica a margini netti sulla corticale della metafisi. Le lesioni possono essere multiloculate ed espanse, con estensione dalla corticale alla midollare e con l'asse maggiore parallelo a quello dell'osso. Nel 50% dei casi sono bilaterali o multiple. A causa dell'aspetto radiologico, la maggior parte di esse non va sottoposta a biopsia o trattamento. Dopo il raggiungimento della maturità scheletrica possono regredire spontaneamente. Il curettage e l'innesto osseo potrebbero risultare raccomandabili per lesioni che occupano >50% del diametro dell'osso, a causa del rischio di frattura patologica.

Le **cisti ossee monocamerali** possono manifestarsi in qualunque momento dell'infanzia, ma sono rare prima dei 3 anni e dopo la maturità scheletrica. La causa di queste lesioni piene di liquido è sconosciuta e alcune si risolvono spontaneamente dopo il raggiungimento della maturità scheletrica. Nella maggior parte dei casi sono asintomatiche fino al momento della diagnosi, che spesso coincide con una frattura patologica, che può essere conseguente a traumi relativamente lievi come per esempio lanciare o prendere una palla. Queste cisti, alla radiologia, appaiono lesioni solitarie, localizzate al centro della porzione midollare dell'osso. Risultano più comuni a livello del tratto prossimale di omero o femore. Spesso si estendono alla diafisi (ma non l'attraversano) e hanno margini netti. Si osservano un assottigliamento e una espansione della corteccia, ma non superano lo spessore della diafisi adiacente. Il trattamento prevede la guarigione della frattura patologica, seguita dall'aspirazione e dall'iniezione locale di metilprednisolone o midollo osseo. Iniezioni ripetute, curettage e innesto di osso riescono talvolta necessari per curare lesioni recidive.

La **cisti ossea aneurismatica** è una lesione reattiva dell'osso che si osserva in soggetti con <20 anni. La lesione è caratterizzata da spazi cavernosi pieni di sangue e aggregati solidi di tessuto. Anche se il femore, la tibia e la colonna vertebrale sono le sedi più frequentemente colpite, questa lesione espansiva, che cresce progressivamente, si sviluppa in qualsiasi punto. Dolore e tumefazione sono frequenti. Il coinvolgimento spinale può portare alla compressione midollare o delle radici nervose, con conseguenti sintomi neurologici, compresa la paralisi. Le radiografie evidenziano una distruzione litica eccentrica e un'espansione della metafisi circondata da una sottile rima sclerotica di osso. Gli elementi posteriori della colonna vertebrale sono coinvolti più comunemente rispetto al corpo vertebrale. Diversamente dalla maggior parte degli altri tumori benigni, che sono generalmente confinati a un singolo osso, le cisti ossee aneurismatiche possono interessare vertebre adiacenti. La crescita rapida è tipica e può far pensare a una neoplasia maligna. Il trattamento consiste nel curettage e nell'innesto osseo o nell'asportazione. Le lesioni spinali possono necessitare di una stabilizzazione della colonna dopo la loro asportazione. Come per altri tumori benigni, si tenta di preservare le radici e le altre strutture vitali. Le recidive dopo il trattamento chirurgico si osservano nel 20-30% dei pazienti, sono maggiormente comuni nei bambini più piccoli rispetto a quelli più grandi e generalmente si verificano nei primi 1-2 anni dopo il trattamento.

La **displasia fibrosa** è un'anomalia di sviluppo caratterizzata dalla sostituzione con tessuto fibroso dell'osso spongioso. Le lesioni possono essere solitarie o multifocali (poliostosi), relativamente stabili o progressivamente più severe. Nella maggior parte dei casi i bambini risultano asintomatici, anche se quelli con un interessamento del cranio possono avere rigonfiamenti o esoftalmo. Il dolore e la zoppia sono tipici del coinvolgimento del femore prossimale. L'asimmetria degli arti, la curvatura della tibia o del femore e le fratture patologiche possono essere segnalate già all'esordio. La triade di malattia poliostotica, pubertà precoce e pigmentazione cutanea è nota come sindrome di Albright. Le caratteristiche radiologiche della displasia fibrosa comprendono una lesione espansiva litica o a vetro smerigliato della matafisi o della diafisi. Questa lesione ha margini netti ed è spesso circondata da una densa rima di osso sclerotico. Possono aversi curvature, soprattutto del tratto prossimale del femore. In genere il trattamento prevede l'osservazione. La chirurgia è tuttavia indicata per i pazienti con deformità progressive, dolore o fratture patologiche incombenti. L'innesto di osso non è efficace come negli altri tumori benigni, perché la lesione spesso recidiva nell'osso trapiantato. Tecniche di chirurgia ricostruttiva sono spesso necessarie per migliorare la stabilità dell'osso.

La **displasia osteofibrosa** colpisce i bambini da 1 a 10 anni. Questa lesione generalmente interessa la tibia ed è clinicamente, radiologicamente e istologicamente distinta dalla displasia fibrosa. La maggior parte dei bambini presenta un edema anteriore o un aumento delle dimensioni della gamba. La progressione è rara dopo i 10 anni. Le radiografie dimostrano lesioni diafisarie radiotrasparenti solitarie o multiple, corticali, circondate da sclerosi. Si trova spesso una curvatura anteriore della tibia. L'aspetto radiologico ricorda molto quello dell'adamantimoma, una neoplasia maligna, rendendo così necessaria la biopsia più di frequente che non per altre neoplasie benigne dell'osso. Il trattamento prevede l'osservazione. Alcune lesioni regrediscono spontaneamente. L'asportazione e l'innesto osseo dovrebbero venire evitati fino a che il bambino non superi i 10 anni, a causa dell'alta percentuale di recidive prima di questa età. Le caratteristiche patologiche regrediscono con l'immobilizzazione.

Il **granuloma eosinofilo** è una malattia monostotica o poliostotica senza coinvolgimento extrascheletrico, ciò che lo distingue dalle altre forme di istiocitosi a cellule di Langerhans (le varianti di Hand-Schüller-Christian o di Letterer-Siwe), che possono avere una prognosi meno favorevole (vedi Capitolo 507). Di solito si presenta durante le prime tre decadi di vita ed è più frequente nei maschi di 5-10 anni. Il cranio è la sede più frequentemente colpita, ma può essere coinvolto qualunque osso. In genere i pazienti presentano dolore locale ed edema. Un'aumentata sensibilità e una sensazione calore si verificano spesso nell'area dell'osso coinvolto. Le lesioni spinali possono provocare dolore, rigidità e talvolta sintomi neurologici. L'aspetto radiologico delle lesioni ossee è simile a quello di tutte le forme di istiocitosi a cellule di Langerhans, ma è sufficientemente variabile da mimare molte altre lesioni ossee benigne e maligne. Le lesioni radiotrasparenti hanno margini ben definiti o irregolari con un'espansione dell'osso coinvolto e la formazione di nuovo osso periosteale. Il coinvolgimento della colonna vertebrale può provocare una compressione uniforme o un appiattimento del corpo vertebrale. È opportuna una valutazione completa dello scheletro, in quanto il coinvolgimento poliostotico e le tipiche lesioni del cranio sono altamente suggestive. La biopsia è spesso necessaria per confermare la diagnosi, a causa della presenza di numerose diagnosi differenziali radiologiche. Il trattamento prevede il curettage e l'innesto osseo, la radioterapia a basse dosi o le iniezione di steroidi. Si possono osservare lesioni sintomatiche, dal momento che la maggior parte delle lesioni ossee regredisce spontaneamente e non recidiva. I bambini con lesioni ossee dovrebbero essere valutati per escludere un coinvolgimento viscerale, perché il trattamento delle malattie di Hand-Schüller-Christian e di Letterer-Siwe risulta più complesso e spesso sistemico.

Arndt CAS, Crist WM: Common musculoskeletal tumors of childhood and adolescence. *N Engl J Med* 1999;341:342–352.

Campanacci M, Capanna R, Picci P: Unicameral and aneurysmal bone cysts. *Clin Orthop Relat Res* 1986;204:25–36.

Campanacci M, Laus M: Osteofibrous dysplasia of the tibia and fibula. *J Bone Joint Surg Am* 1981;63:367–375.

Dahlin DC, Ivins JC: Benign chondroblastoma: A study of 125 cases. *Cancer* 1972;30:401–413.

De Alava E, Gerald WL: Molecular biology of the Ewing's sarcoma/primitive neuroectodermal tumor family. *J Clin Oncol* 2000;18:204–213.

Freiberg AA, Loder RT, Heidelberger KT: Aneurysmal bone cysts in young children. *J Pediatr Orthop* 1994;14:86–91.

Ginsberg JP, Woo SY, Johnson ME, et al: Ewing's sarcoma family of tumors. In Pizzo PA, Poplack DG (editors): *Principles and Practice of Pediatric Oncology*, 4th ed. Philadelphia, Lippincott Williams & Wilkins, 2002, pp 973–1016.

Gorlick R, Anderson P, Andrulis I, et al: Biology of childhood osteogenic sarcoma and potential targets for therapeutic development: meeting summary. *Clin Cancer Res* 2003;9:5442–5453.

Grier H, Krailo M, Tarbell N, et al: Addition of ifosfamide and etoposide to standard chemotherapy for Ewing's sarcoma and primitive neuroectodermal tumor of bone. *N Engl J Med* 2003;348:694–701.

Grier RJ: Surgical options for children with osteosarcoma. *Lancet Oncol* 2005;6:85–92.

Kneisl JS, Simon MA: Medical management compared with operative treatment for osteoid osteoma. *J Bone Joint Surg Am* 1992;74:179–185.

Marina N, Gebhardt M, Teot L, et al: Biology and therapeutic advances for pediatric osteosarcoma. *Oncologist* 2004;9:422–441.

Rodriguez-Galindo C, Sount SL, Pappo AS: Treatment of Ewing sarcoma family of tumors: Current status and outlook for the future. *Med Pediatr Oncol* 2003;40:276–287.

Schmale GA, Conrad EU III, Raskind WH: The natural history of hereditary multiple exostoses. *J Bone Joint Surg Am* 1994;76:986–992.

Capitolo 502 ■ Retinoblastoma

Cynthia E. Herzog

EPIDEMIOLOGIA. Il retinoblastoma colpisce 3,7 casi per milione negli Stati Uniti, senza distinzioni di razza o sesso. Globalmente, il 60% circa dei casi è unilaterale e non ereditario, il 15% unilaterale ed ereditario e il 25% bilaterale ed ereditario. Il coinvolgimento bilaterale alla presentazione si osserva nel 42% dei pazienti con <1 anno, nel 21% dei bambini con 1 anno e meno frequentemente nei bambini più grandi.

La forma ereditaria è associata all'inattivazione del **gene del retinoblastoma (RB1)**, che è localizzato sul cromosoma 13q14 e codifica per la **proteina retinoblastoma (pRb)**, un oncosoppressore, che controlla la fase di transizione nel ciclo cellulare e interviene nell'apoptosi e nella differenziazione cellulare. Sono stati osservati diversi tipi di mutazione, fra cui le traslocazioni, le delezioni, le inserzioni, le mutazioni puntiformi e le mutazioni epigenetiche come l'ipermetilazione della regione promoter. Il tipo di mutazione predisponente influenza la penetranza e l'espressione del suo sviluppo. Le forme ereditarie generalmente risultano multifocali e bilaterali, mentre quelle non ereditarie tendono a essere unilaterali e monofocali.

In accordo con il modello delle "due tappe" dell'oncogenesi, per lo sviluppo del tumore sono necessari due eventi mutazionali (vedi Capitolo 492). Nella forma ereditaria, la prima mutazione del gene RB1 è ereditata attraverso le cellule germinali e la seconda si verifica in seguito nelle cellule somatiche della retina. Le seconde mutazioni, che portano allo sviluppo del retinoblastoma, spesso consistono nella perdita dell'allele normale e in quella concomitante dell'eterozigosi. Alcuni bambini con la forma ereditaria hanno nuove mutazioni germinali ed entrambi i genitori sono normali. I portatori delle alterazioni dell'oncogene RB1 eterozigoti presentano un'espressione fenotipica variabile. Nella forma non ereditaria le due mutazioni si verificano entrambe nelle cellule somatiche della retina.

PATOGENESI. Istologicamente, il retinoblastoma si presenta come un tumore a piccole cellule tondeggianti blu con tendenza a formare rosette. Può originare in qualunque strato di cellule nucleate della retina, presenta diversi gradi di differenziazione e tende a diventare troppo grande rispetto al supporto ematico che riceve e quindi ad avere necrosi e calcificazioni.

I tumori endofitici derivano dalla superficie interna della retina, crescono all'interno del vitreo e possono provocare una **disseminazione vitreale** verso altre sedi della retina. I tumori esofitici originano dallo strato retinico più esterno e possono determinarne un distacco della retina. Questi tumori possono disseminare per estensione diretta verso la coroide o lungo il decorso del nervo ottico in prossimità della lamina cribrosa o per via ematogena o linfatica verso sedi distanti.

MANIFESTAZIONI CLINICHE. Solo circa il 10% dei retinoblastomi è diagnosticato in occasione delle visite di screening nel contesto di un'anamnesi familiare positiva. Tipicamente il retinoblastoma si presenta con una **leucocoria**, un riflesso pupillare bianco (Fig. 502-1) che spesso è il primo segno che si osserva al posto del riflesso rosso quando si fa la valutazione di routine del neonato o durante una visita completa o nelle fotografie fatte con il flash. Lo strabismo spesso può essere una modalità di presentazione iniziale. Con l'avanzamento della malattia si osservano l'infiammazione dell'orbita, la presenza di sangue nella camera anteriore o irregolarità pupillari. Il dolore generalmente si trova quando sussiste un glaucoma secondario.

DIAGNOSI. La diagnosi si pone sulla base delle tipiche caratteristiche oftalmologiche. La biopsia è controindicata. La valutazione generalmente richiede un esame oftalmologico completo in anestesia generale, per poter visualizzare meglio entrambi gli occhi e per permettere anche di fotografare e mappare il tumore. Il distacco della retina e le emorragie vitreali possono complicare questa valutazione.

L'ecografia dell'orbita e la TC o la RM sono utilizzate per valutare l'estensione della malattia a livello oculare e per verificare quella extraoculare. Occasionalmente si osserva un tumore a livello dell'area pineale, un fenomeno noto come **retinoblastoma trilaterale**. La RM permette di visionare meglio il coinvolgimento del nervo ottico. La scintigrafia ossea, l'esame liquorale e la valutazione del midollo osseo sono necessari solo se esiste un sospetto clinico, di laboratorio o strumentale emerso da altri accertamenti.

La **diagnosi differenziale** comprende il vitreo iperplastico primario, la malattia di Coats, la cataratta, la larva viscerale migrante, il coloboma coroidale e la retinopatia del prematuro.

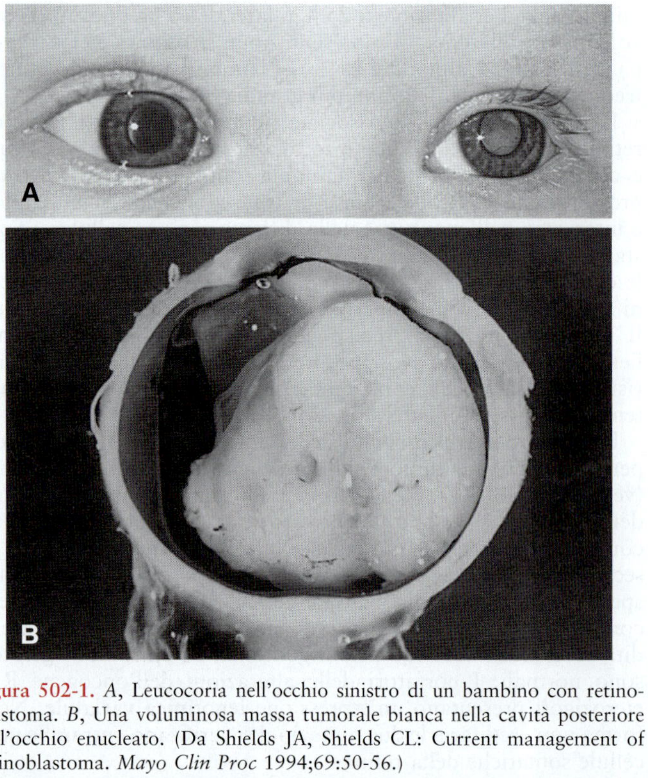

Figura 502-1. *A*, Leucocoria nell'occhio sinistro di un bambino con retinoblastoma. *B*, Una voluminosa massa tumorale bianca nella cavità posteriore dell'occhio enucleato. (Da Shields JA, Shields CL: Current management of retinoblastoma. *Mayo Clin Proc* 1994;69:50-56.)

TRATTAMENTO. Il trattamento dipende dalle dimensioni e dalla sede del tumore. L'obiettivo primario è la guarigione, quindi viene prospettata la preservazione della vista. Sono in via di sviluppo tecniche più moderne per il controllo locale del tumore endooculare e schemi di chemioterapia più efficaci; l'enucleazione primaria viene eseguita sempre di meno.

Nella maggior parte dei casi la malattia unilaterale si presenta come un tumore solitario di grosse dimensioni. L'enucleazione viene effettuata se non vi è la possibilità di salvare la vista. Quando la malattia è bilaterale, la chemioriduzione in associazione a una **terapia focale** (la fotocoagulazione con laser o la crioterapia) hanno rimpiazzato il tradizionale approccio con l'enucleazione dell'occhio più gravemente colpito e la radioterapia dell'altro occhio. Se fattibile, i tumori piccoli possono venire trattati con una terapia locale, seguita da un attento follow-up per evidenziare recidive o la crescita di nuovi tumori. I tumori più grossi spesso rispondono alla polichemioterapia con il carboplatino, la vincristina e l'etoposide. Se questo approccio fallisce, bisogna prendere in considerazione la radioterapia esterna, anche se può provocare significative deformazioni dell'orbita e un'aumentata incidenza di secondi tumori in pazienti con mutazioni della linea germinale. La brachiterapia o la radioterapia con una placca episclerale, se attuabili, rappresentano un'alternativa con meno morbilità. L'enucleazione va riservata ai casi non responsivi o ai tumori ricorrenti.

Tutti i parenti di primo grado dei bambini con un retinoblastoma dovrebbero essere visitati per escludere retinomi o cicatrici retiniche, che possono essere suggestivi per una predisposizione a questo tumore anche se la forma maligna non si è sviluppata.

PROGNOSI. Negli Stati Uniti è stato guarito circa il 95% dei retinoblastomi che raramente avevano un'estensione extraoculare. Le attuali strategie, che sfruttano la chemioterapia in combinazione con la terapia focale, mirano a preservare la vista evitando la radioterapia e l'enucleazione. Le visite oculistiche di routine dovrebbero essere effettuate fino a circa 6 anni, per escludere la comparsa di nuove lesioni. La prognosi per i pazienti con metastasi non è buona.

I bambini con mutazioni di RB1 nella linea germinale sono a rischio di sviluppare un secondo tumore, soprattutto osteosarcomi e anche sarcomi dei tessuti molli e melanomi maligni. Il rischio di neoplasie cerebrali, delle cavità nasali, dell'occhio e dell'orbita è ulteriormente aumentato dalla radioterapia. Altri effetti collaterali avversi tardivi da radioterapia sono costituiti dalla cataratta, dalle deformazioni dell'orbita, dalla disfunzione dei dotti lacrimali e dal danno vascolare tardivo sulla retina.

Abramson DH, Schefler AC: Update on retinoblastoma. *Retina* 2004;24: 828–848.

Classon M, Harlow E: The retinoblastoma tumour suppressor in development and cancer. *Nat Rev Cancer* 2002:2:910–917.

Kleinerman R, Tucker MA, Tarone RF, et al: Risk of new cancers after radiotherapy in long-term survivors of retinoblastoma: An extended follow-up. *J Clin Oncol* 2005;23:2272–2279.

Lohman DR, Gallie BL: Retinoblastoma: Revisiting the model prototype of inherited cancer. *Am J Med Genet C (Semin Med Genet)* 2004;129:23–28.

Richter S, Vandezande K, Chen N, et al: Sensitive and efficient detection of *RB1* gene mutations enhances care of families with retinoblastoma. *Am J Hum Genet* 2003;72:253–269.

Rodriguez-Galindo C, Wilson MW, Haik BG, et al: Treatment of metastatic retinoblastoma. *Ophthalmology* 2003;110:1237–1240.

Capitolo 503 ■ Neoplasie gonadiche e germinomi Cynthia E. Herzog

EPIDEMIOLOGIA. I germinomi maligni (GCT, *Germ Cell Tumor*) e i tumori delle gonadi sono rari, con un'incidenza di 12 casi per milione di persone con <20 anni; i germinomi costituiscono i tumori gonadici più maligni dell'infanzia. L'incidenza varia in relazione all'età e al sesso. I tumori sacrococcigei colpiscono soprattutto le bambine. I GCT testicolari si osservano soprattutto prima dei 4 anni e dopo la pubertà e colpiscono più spesso la razza bianca rispetto a quella nera, mentre i germinomi ovarici hanno una lieve prevalenza nella razza nera. La sindrome di Klinefelter si associa a un aumentato rischio di germinomi mediastinici; la sindrome di Down, i testicoli ritenuti, l'infertilità, l'atrofia testicolare e le ernie inguinali presentano un rischio più elevato di sviluppare neoplasie testicolari. Il rischio di GCT testicolare è aumentato nei parenti di primo grado e soprattutto nei gemelli omozigoti.

PATOGENESI. I tumori delle cellule germinali e non germinali derivano rispettivamente da cellule germinali primordiali e dall'epitelio celomico. I GCT testicolari e sacrococcigei della prima infanzia tipicamente hanno una delezione di 1p e 6q e un acquisto di 1q, nonché una mancanza dell'isocromosoma 12p, che è altamente caratteristico dei GCT maligni dell'adulto. Il GCT testicolare può anche subire la perdita dell'imprinting. Dal momento che il GCT può contenere elementi sia benigni sia maligni in aree diverse del tumore, è essenziale eseguire una valutazione estesa della lesione, per confermare una diagnosi corretta. I principali sottotipi istologici includono il teratoma (maturo e immaturo), il tumore del seno endodermico e il carcinoma embrionale (Fig. 503-1). I tumori non germinali delle ovaie comprendono le neoplasie epiteliali (sierose e mucinose) e del cordone stromale; tra quelli del testicolo si trovano i tumori del cordone stromale (a partire dalle cellule di Leyding e dalle cellule di Sertoli).

MANIFESTAZIONI CLINICHE E DIAGNOSI. La presentazione clinica dei germinomi dipende dalla loro sede. I tumori ovarici spesso risultano piuttosto voluminosi in relazione al momento in cui vengono diagnosticati. I GCT extragonadici si localizzano sulla linea mediana, come al livello della regione sovrasellare, della regione pineale, del collo, del mediastino e delle aree retroperitoneali e sacrococcigee. I sintomi sono correlati all'effetto massa, ma i GCT intracranici spesso si presentano con deficit dell'ipofisi anteriore e posteriore (vedi Capitolo 497).

Il livello di **α-fetoproteina (AFP) sierica** risulta aumentato nei tumori del seno endodermico e può esserlo lievemente anche nei teratomi. I neonati hanno livelli di AFP più elevati, che scendono a quelli tipici dell'adulto intorno agli 8 mesi; pertanto, alti valori di AFP vanno interpretati con cautela nei primi mesi di vita. Un aumento della subunità β della **gonadotropina corionica umana** si osserva nel coriocarcinoma e nei germinomi. La lattato deidrogenasi, anche se aspecifica, può essere un marcatore utile, che se risulta aumentato rappresenta un'importante conferma per la diagnosi e un valore da monitorare per la risposta del tumore o la recidiva. Nei pazienti con lesioni intracraniche questi marcatori possono venire dosati sia a livello sierico sia a livello liquorale. La diagnosi inizia con l'esame clinico e con gli esami radiologici, come le radiografie del torace e l'ecografia dell'addome. La TC e la RM possono definire meglio il tumore primitivo. Se sussiste

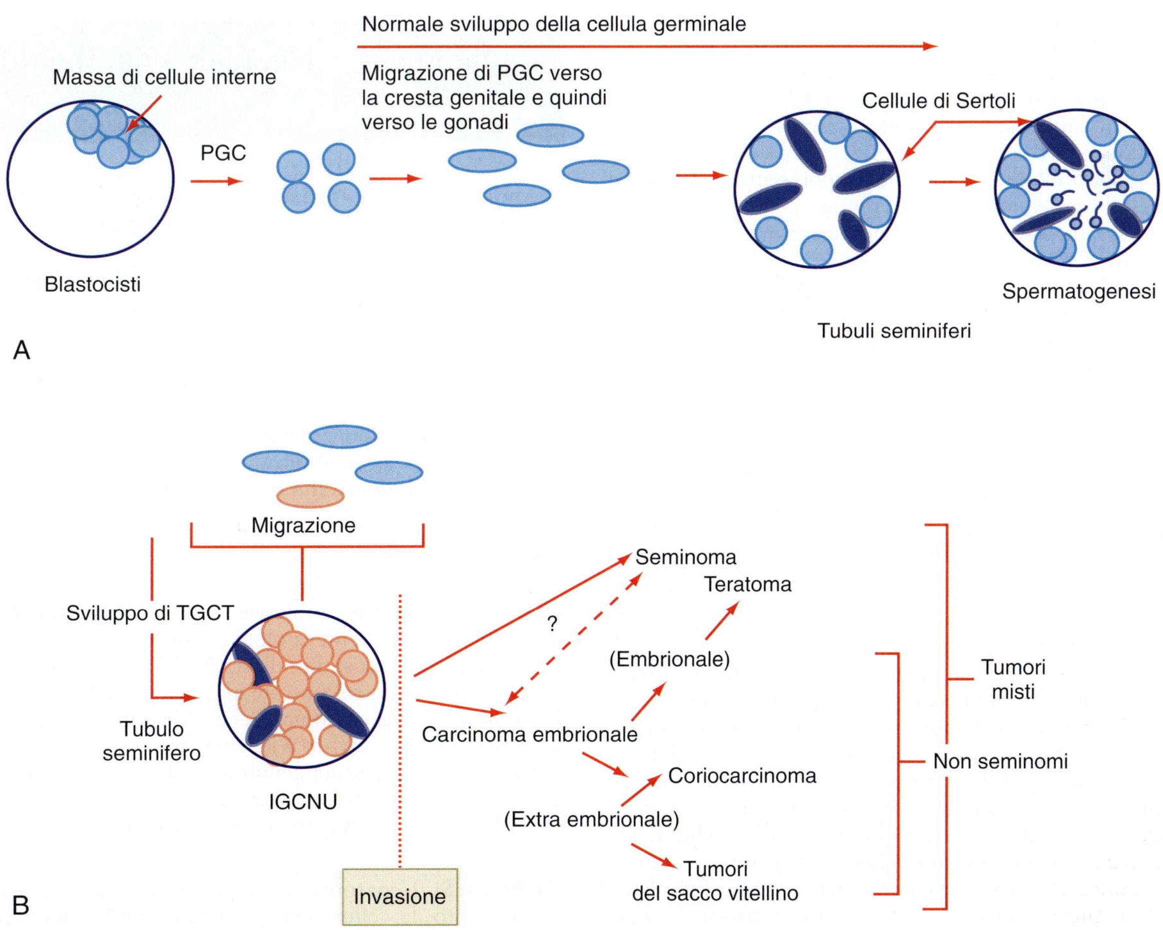

Figura 503-1. *A*, Normale sviluppo della cellula germinale. *B*, Modello per l'origine e l'istogenesi di sottotipi differenti di germinoma testicolare. IGCNU, neoplasia germinale intratubulare non classificata (*Intratubular Germ Cell Neoplasia Unclassified*); PGC, cellula germinale primaria (*Primary Germ Cell*); TGCT, germinoma testicolare (*Testicular Germ Cell Tumor*).

il forte sospetto che vi sia una neoplasia a cellule germinali, è indicata la stadiazione preoperatoria con la TC del torce e la scintigrafia ossea. La resezione chirurgica primaria è consigliabile per i tumori giudicati operabili, con l'eccezione delle lesioni intracraniche, perché la diagnosi può essere stabilita con i soli esami radiologici e con la determinazione dell'AFP o della subunità β della gonadotropina corionica umana.

I **gonadoblastomi** spesso si osservano in soggetti con disgenesie gonadiche e tutti o in parte derivano dal cromosoma Y. La disgenesia gonadica è caratterizzata da un fallimento del raggiungimento del pieno sviluppo maschile dei genitali esterni. Se viene diagnosticata, occorre esaminare l'aspetto delle gonadi con l'ecografia o con la TC e l'asportazione chirurgica del tumore è generalmente risolutiva. È raccomandata la resezione profilattica delle gonadi disgeniche al momento della diagnosi, perché i gonadoblastomi si sviluppano spesso e alcuni contengono elementi tumorali di cellule germinali maligne. I gonadoblastomi possono produrre anomale quantità di estrogeno.

I **teratomi** possono localizzarsi in diverse sedi e si presentano come masse solide. Non si associano a un aumento dei marcatori fino a che non subiscono una trasformazione in senso maligno. L'area sacrococcigea è la sede dove vengono osservati più frequentemente, soprattutto nel periodo neonatale; possono tuttavia essere diagnosticati già in utero o alla nascita e con una maggiore incidenza nel sesso femminile. La percentuale di trasformazione maligna è variabile, andando da <10% in bambini con <2 mesi a >50% in bambini con >4 mesi.

I **germinomi** si sviluppano a livello intracranico, nel mediastino e nelle gonadi. Quando sono localizzati nelle ovaie vengono chiamati **disgerminomi**, nei testicoli **seminomi**. Generalmente i marcatori sono negativi, tranne che nelle forme maligne. I tumori del seno endotermico o del sacco vitellino e i coriocarcinomi sono tumori altamente maligni dal punto di vista istologico. Entrambi possono localizzarsi nelle gonadi o in sedi extragonadiche. I carcinomi embrionali più spesso si trovano a livello testicolare.

I **tumori gonadici non germinomi** risultano molto rari in pediatria e interessano soprattutto l'ovaio. Nei bambini si osservano solo occasionalmente i carcinomi epiteliali (generalmente tumori dell'adulto), i tumori delle cellule di Sertoli-Leydig e i tumori a cellule granulose. I carcinomi rappresentano circa un terzo delle neoplasie ovariche nelle femmine con <20 anni, la maggior parte dei quali si osserva nell'adolescenza e appaiono di tipo sieroso o mucinoso. I tumori delle cellule di Sertoli-Leydig e a cellule granulose producono ormoni che possono provocare la virilizzazione, la femminizzazione o una pubertà precoce in relazione allo stato puberale e all'equilibrio tra le cellule di Sertoli (che producono estrogeni) e quelle di Leydig (che producono androgeni). La valutazione diagnostica generalmente si focalizza sul principale sintomo dell'inappropriato effetto degli ormoni sessuali e sulla misurazione degli ormoni coinvolti, che riflette la produzione gonadotropino-indipendente degli ormoni sessuali. Possono anche essere effettuati appropriati esami per escludere un tumore gonadico secernente. La chirurgia è generalmente risolutiva e al momento non esiste una terapia efficace per la malattia non chirurgica.

TRATTAMENTO. L'asportazione chirurgica completa del tumore è spesso indicata, eccetto che per quelli intracranici, il cui trattamento primario consiste nella radioterapia e nella chemioterapia. Per le neoplasie testicolari è indicato un approccio inguinale. Quando non è possibile effettuare un'asportazione completa, è consigliabile una chemioterapia preoperatoria, con successiva revisione chirurgica. Per i teratomi sia maturi sia immaturi e per i tumori maligni completamente resecati, il trattamento si limita alla chirurgia. Regimi chemioterapici a base di cisplatino risultano generalmente curativi nei GCT, che non possono essere completamente asportati, anche nel caso in cui vi siano metastasi. Eccetto che per i GCT del sistema nervoso centrale, la radioterapia ha un ruolo limitato solo ai tumori non suscettibili di asportazione completa e refrattari alla chemioterapia.

PROGNOSI. La percentuale di guarigione per i bambini con GCT è >80%. L'età è il fattore di sopravvivenza più predittivo per quelli extragonadici. I bambini con >12 anni hanno un rischio di decesso quattro volte superiore, che arriva a 6 volte se il tumore è localizzato a livello toracico. L'istologia possiede una scarsa influenza sulla prognosi. Quella dei GCT extragonadici non operati è leggermente peggiore.

Cushing B, Giller R, Cullen JW, et al: Randomized comparison of combination chemotherapy with etoposide, bleomycin, and either high-dose or standard-dose cisplatin in children and adolescents with high risk malignant germ cell tumors: A pediatric intergroup study—Pediatric Oncology Group 9049 and Children's Cancer Group 8882. *J Clin Oncol* 2004;22:2691–2700.

Horwich A, Shipley J, Huddart R: Testicular germ-cell cancer. *Lancet* 2006;367:754–764.

Marina N, London WB, Frazier L, et al: Prognostic factors in children with extragonadal malignant germ cell tumors: A pediatric intergroup study. *J Clin Oncol* 2006;24:2544–2548.

Rogers PC, Olson TA, Cullen JW, et al: Treatment of children and adolescents with stage I testicular and stages I or II ovarian malignant germ cell tumors: A pediatric intergroup study—Pediatric Oncology Group 9048 and Children's Cancer Group 8891. *J Clin Oncol* 2004;22:563–569.

Schneider DT, Schuster AE, Fritsch MK, et al: Genetic analysis of mediastinal nonseminomatous germ cell tumors in children and adolescents. *Genes Chromosomes Cancer* 2002;3:115–125.

Young JL, Wu XC, Roffers SD, et al: Ovarian cancer in children and young adults in the United States, 1992–1997. *Cancer* 2003;97:2694–2700.

Capitolo 504 ■ Neoplasie del fegato

Cynthia E. Herzog

I tumori epatici sono rari nel bambino. Quelli primitivi del fegato rappresentano circa l'1% delle neoplasie pediatriche, con un'incidenza annuale di 1,6 casi per milione di bambini negli Stati Uniti. Il 50-60% dei tumori epatici dell'infanzia è maligno, >65% di questi è un epatoblastoma e la maggior parte dei rimanenti è un carcinoma epatocellulare. Fra quelli rari rientrano l'angiosarcoma, il germinoma maligno, il rabdomiosarcoma epatico e il sarcoma indifferenziato. Anche i più frequenti tumori maligni dell'infanzia, come il neuroblastoma e il linfoma, possono metastatizzare a livello epatico. I tumori benigni del fegato, che generalmente si presentano durante i primi 6 mesi di vita, sono l'emangioma, l'amartoma e l'emangioendotelioma.

EPATOBLASTOMA

EPIDEMIOLOGIA. L'epatoblastoma colpisce soprattutto bambini con <3 anni e ha un'eziologia sconosciuta. Si associa con la poliposi adenomatosa familiare. Nella maggior parte dei tumori studiati sono state riscontrate alterazioni della via APC (Antigen Presenting Cell)/β-catenina. L'epatoblastoma si associa anche con la sindrome di Beckwith-Wiedemann e può presentare una perdita simile dell'imprinting genomico del gene del fattore di crescita 2 insulino-simile. Inoltre, minore è il peso alla nascita, maggiori, in proporzione diretta, risultano l'incidenza e il rischio.

PATOGENESI. L'epatoblastoma può essere di tipo epiteliale, accompagnato da cellule maligne fetali o embrionali (sia miste sia come elementi singoli), oppure di tipo misto, con presenza di elementi mesenchimali ed epiteliali. Un'istologia puramente fetale è predittiva di una evoluzione più favorevole.

MANIFESTAZIONI CLINICHE. L'epatoblastoma in genere si presenta come una voluminosa massa addominale asintomatica. Origina dal lobo destro 3 volte più frequentemente di quello sinistro ed è di solito una lesione singola. Con la progressione della malattia, possono verificarsi una perdita di peso, l'anoressia, il vomito e un dolore addominale. Le metastasi dell'epatoblastoma interessano più spesso i linfonodi regionali e i polmoni.

Un marcatore sierico tumorale, l'α-**fetoproteina** (**AFP**), è utilizzato per la diagnosi e il monitoraggio dei tumori epatici, in quanto il suo livello risulta aumentato in quasi tutti gli epatoblastomi. La bilirubina e gli enzimi epatici abitualmente sono normali. L'anemia è comune e la trombocitosi si osserva in circa un terzo dei pazienti. La sierologia per l'epatite B e C andrebbe fatta, ma in genere è negativa.

Gli esami radiologici dovrebbero comprendere le radiografie e l'ecografia dell'addome, per caratterizzare la massa epatica. L'ecografia può differenziare le masse epatiche maligne dalle lesioni vascolari benigne. Sia la TC sia la RM sono metodiche accurate per definire l'estensione del tumore intraepatico e per pianificare l'intervento chirurgico. La valutazione della malattia metastatica prevede l'esecuzione della TC del torace e della scintigrafia ossea.

TRATTAMENTO. In generale, la guarigione dei tumori epatici infantili dipende dalla possibilità di asportare completamente il tumore primitivo (Fig. 504-1). Può essere reciso fino all'85% del fegato, con possibilità di rigenerazione epatica entro 3-4 mesi dalla chirurgia. Il cisplatino, in associazione con la vincristina e il 5-fluorouracile o doxorubicina, risultano efficaci e aumentano le possibilità di guarigione dopo un intervento radicale. Nei tumori di basso grado si può raggiungere una percentuale di sopravvivenza >90% con il trattamento multimodale, che prevede la chi-

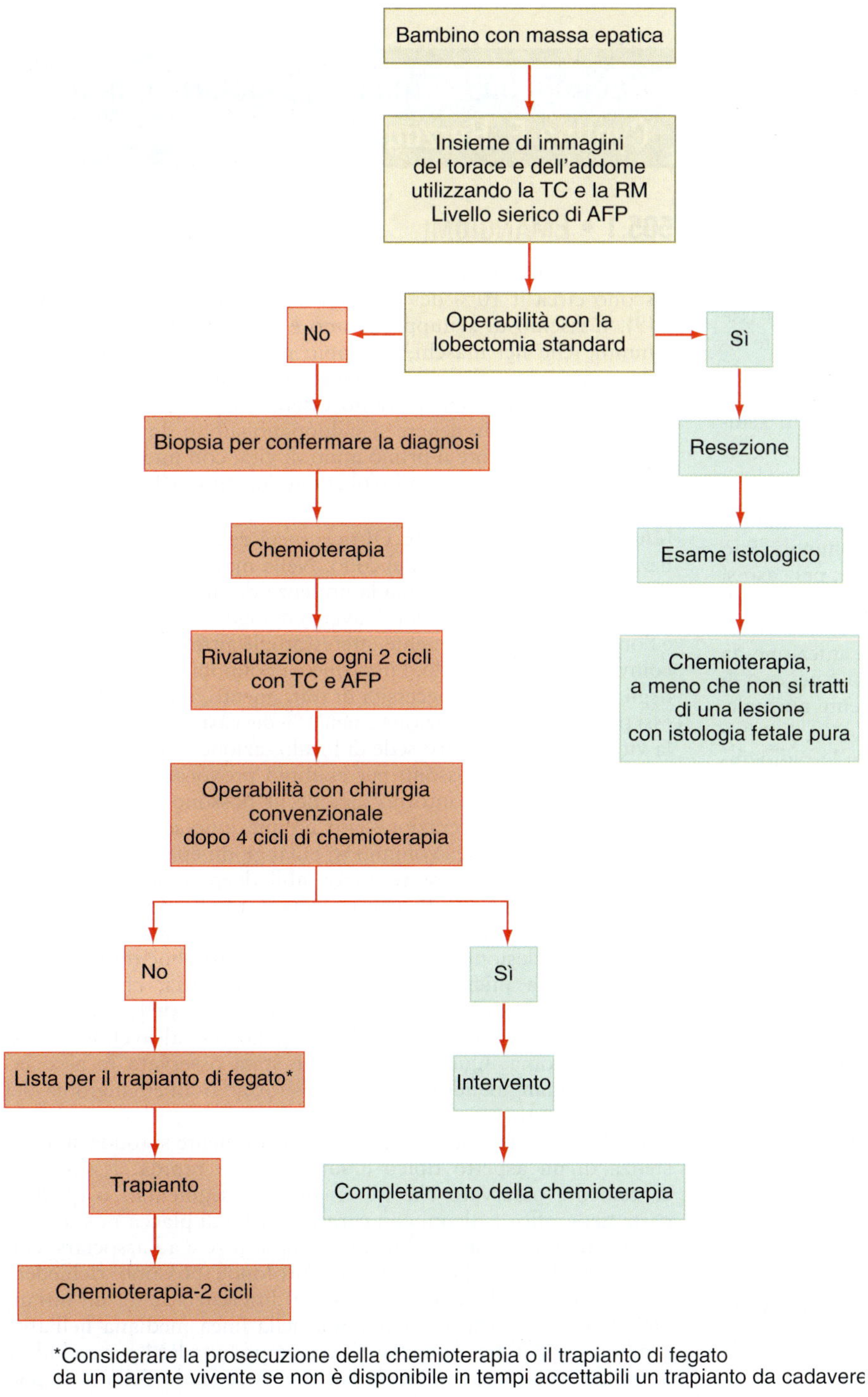

Figura 504-1. Algoritmo del trattamento del bambino con diagnosi di epatoblastoma. AFP, α-fetoproteina. (Da Tiao GM, Bobey N, Allen S, et al: The current management of hepatoblastoma: A combination of chemotherapy, conventional resection, and liver transplantation. *J Pediatr* 2005;146:204-211.)

rurgia e la chemioterapia adiuvante. Con tumori non asportabili al momento della diagnosi, la percentuale scende al 60%. Una malattia metastatica riduce ulteriormente la sopravvivenza, ma una completa regressione della malattia, con una probabilità di sopravvivenza di circa il 25%, risulta spesso ottenibile mediante la chemioterapia e l'asportazione del tumore primitivo oppure nel caso di una localizzazione polmonare isolata. Il trapianto di fegato costituisce una possibilità per i tumori epatici maligni non operabili e determina una buona sopravvivenza a lungo termine. Le condizioni cliniche precedenti il trapianto sono un importante elemento predittivo e il trapianto stesso risulta molto più efficace, come la chirurgia primaria, rispetto a una terapia di salvataggio.

CARCINOMA EPATOCELLULARE

EPIDEMIOLOGIA. Il carcinoma epatocellulare interessa più spesso gli adolescenti e di solito si associa all'infezione da virus B o C. È più frequente nell'Asia dell'Est e nelle aree in cui l'epatite da virus B è endemica ed è infatti già stata dimostrata una ridotta incidenza in seguito all'introduzione della vaccinazione per questa epatite. Nelle aree endemiche il carcinoma epatocellulare ha la tendenza a presentarsi con un andamento bimodale, con il picco dell'età più giovane che si sovrappone a quello dell'età di presentazione dell'epatoblastoma. Si osserva anche nella forma cronica della tirosinemia ereditaria, nella galattosemia, nella malattia di accumulo di glicogeno, nel deficit di α_1-antitripsina e nella cirrosi biliare. Un altro fattore di rischio è la contaminazione alimentare da aflatossina B.

PATOGENESI. Il carcinoma epatocellulare generalmente si presenta come un tumore multicentrico, invasivo, costituito da grosse cellule pleiomorfe senza un substrato cirrotico. La variante fibrolamellare si osserva più spesso negli adolescenti e nei giovani adulti. Anche se precedenti segnalazioni hanno ipotizzato che questo tipo abbia una prognosi migliore, dati più recenti sembrano smentire questo dato.

MANIFESTAZIONI CLINICHE. Il carcinoma epatocellulare di solito si manifesta con una massa epatica, una distensione addominale e sintomi quali anoressia, calo ponderale e dolore addominale. Può esordire con un episodio acuto di dolore addominale, nel caso si verifichi una rottura del tumore e dell'emoperitoneo. Il livello di AFP è aumentato in circa il 60% dei bambini. Nelle aree endemiche si osserva frequentemente una concomitante infezione da virus B e C, ciò che non avviene nei Paesi occidentali o nei casi di carcinoma fibrolamellare. La bilirubina è generalmente normale, ma gli enzimi epatici possono essere alterati.

Le indagini radiologiche dovrebbero comprendere le radiografie e l'ecografia dell'addome per caratterizzare la massa epatica. Quest'ultima può differenziare le masse maligne dalle lesioni vascolari benigne. La TC e la RM sono metodiche accurate per definire l'estensione del tumore a livello epatico e per pianificare l'intervento chirurgico. La valutazione della malattia metastatica prevede l'esecuzione di una TC del torace e di una scintigrafia ossea.

TRATTAMENTO. A causa della multifocalità del carcinoma epatocellulare, la sua asportazione completa è operabile solo nel 30-40% dei casi e tuttavia anche con essa solo il 30% dei bambini sopravvive a lungo. La chemioterapia, che prevede l'utilizzo del cisplatino, della doxorubicina, dell'etoposide e del 5-fluorouracile, ha dimostrato qualche effetto, ma è difficile ottenere un miglioramento della sopravvivenza a lungo termine. Altre tecniche di trattamento, quali la chemioembolizzazione e il trapianto di fegato, sono in corso di valutazione.

Austin MT, Leys CM, Feurer ID, et al: Liver transplantation for childhood hepatic malignancy: A review of the United Network for Organ Sharing (UNOS) database. *J Pediatr Surg* 2006;41:182–186.

Darbari A, Sabin KM, Shapiro CN, et al: Epidemiology of primary hepatic malignancies in U.S. children. *Hepatology* 2003;38:560–566.

Katzenstein HM, Krailo MD, Malogolowkin MH, et al: Hepatocellular carcinoma in children and adolescents: Results from the Pediatric Oncology Group and Children's Cancer Group Intergroup Study. *J Clin Oncol* 2002;20:2789–2797.

Katzenstein HM, Krailo MD, Malogolowkin MH, et al: Fibrolamellar hepatocellular carcinoma in children and adolescents. *Cancer* 2003;97: 2006–2012.

Llovet JM, Burroughs A, Bruix J: Hepatocellular carcinoma. *Lancet* 2003;362: 1907–1916.

Otte JB, Pritchard J, Aronson DC, et al: Liver transplantation for hepatoblastoma: Results from the International Society of Pediatric Oncology (SIOP) study SIOPEL-1 and review of the world experience. *Pediatr Blood Cancer* 2004;42:74–83.

Schnater JM, Kohler SE, Lamers WH, et al: Where do we stand with hepatoblastoma? A review. *Cancer* 2003;98:668–678.

Tiao GM, Bobey N, Allen S, et al: The current management of hepatoblastoma: A combination of chemotherapy, conventional resection, and liver transplantation. *J Pediatr* 2005;146:204–211.

Capitolo 505 ■ Tumori vascolari benigni

Cynthia E. Herzog

505.1 • EMANGIOMI

Gli emangiomi, i tumori benigni dell'infanzia più comuni, colpiscono circa il 10% dei bambini nati a termine (vedi Capitolo 649). Il rischio di svilupparne uno è 3-5 volte più elevato nelle femmine che nei maschi, è doppio nei neonati prematuri e 10 volte superiore nei figli di donne sottoposte all'esame dei villi coriali. Gli emangiomi possono essere già presenti al momento della nascita, ma in genere si sviluppano subito dopo e crescono rapidamente durante il primo anno di vita, con un rallentamento nei successivi 5 anni e un'involuzione intorno ai 10-15 anni.

MANIFESTAZIONI CLINICHE. Oltre la metà degli emangiomi si localizza a livello del capo o del collo. Nella maggior parte dei casi si tratta di lesioni solitarie, ma la presenza di oltre una lesione cutanea aumenta la probabilità di avere emangiomi viscerali. Il fegato è l'organo più comunemente interessato; le altre sedi a poter essere coinvolte sono il cervello, l'intestino e i polmoni. La maggior parte degli emangiomi non necessita di trattamento, ma il 10% circa di essi provoca una disfunzione e nell'1% dei casi sono pericolosi per la vita a causa della loro sede di localizzazione. Quelli che circondano le vie aeree possono per esempio provocare un'ostruzione delle stesse e quelli intorno agli occhi possono compromettere la vista. La loro ulcerazione con un'infezione secondaria è una complicanza comune. Voluminosi emangiomi epatici, o emangioendoteliomi, possono essere responsabili di epatomegalia, anemia, trombocitopenia e insufficienza cardiaca ad alta portata.

La **sindrome di Kasabach-Merritt** è caratterizzata dalla presenza di una lesione in rapida crescita, di trombocitopenia, anemia emolitica microangiopatica e coagulopatia, che derivano tutte dall'intrappolamento dei globuli rossi e delle piastrine e dall'attivazione del sistema della coagulazione al livello dei vasi dell'emangioma. Questa sindrome è stata osservata in associazione all'emangioendotelioma kaposiforme o all'emangioma del cuoio capelluto.

La diagnosi delle lesioni cutanee generalmente si fonda sull'esistenza di un aspetto tipico e sulla crescita rapida. È stato recentemente osservato che gli emangiomi segmentali o quelli a carta geografica e alcuni con caratteristiche di placca possiedono un'elevata tendenza a sviluppare complicanze e ad associarsi con anomalie di sviluppo. Le lesioni profonde possono richiedere uno studio radiologico per aiutare a differenziarle da un linfangioma. La presenza di emangiomi della linea mediana nell'area lombosacrale indica la necessità di eseguire una RM per escludere anomalie neurologiche asintomatiche. A seconda della sede può essere necessario sentire il parere degli oculisti o dei chirurghi. In caso di lesioni cutanee multiple è consigliabile l'esecuzione di una ecografia o di una RM del fegato.

TRATTAMENTO. La maggior parte degli emangiomi non richiede un trattamento specifico, al di là del rassicurare i genitori. Il trattamento è invece indicato per gli emangiomi pericolosi per la vita o minacciosi per le funzioni vitali, come anche per la vista. La tipica terapia iniziale è costituita dal prednisone (1-3 mg/kg/die per os); talvolta si impiegano dosi più elevate o si somministrano steroidi a livello intralesionale. Circa il 30% degli emangiomi regredisce in modo significativo con l'uso degli steroidi e la riduzione inizia precocemente, nell'arco di una settimana. Anche l'interferone (IFN)-α (1-3 MU/m^2/die) è stato utilizzato come terapia iniziale e nei pazienti che non avevano risposto agli steroidi. Anche se sono state riportate risposte superiori al 70%, il rischio di eventi avversi neurologici nel 10-20% dei casi rende comunque necessaria una certa cautela. In alcuni casi ci si è avvalsi della terapia con il laser.

Il trattamento dei pazienti con la sindrome di Kasabach-Merritt generalmente consiste in una terapia di supporto e nel contemporaneo inizio di una terapia con steroidi o con IFN-α. La somministrazione di eparina è controindicata e le trasfusioni di piastrine dovrebbero essere limitate ai casi di emorragie minacciose per la vita, perché possono scatenare esse stesse un sanguinamento. Può riuscire efficace la somministrazione di acido aminocaproico o di acido tranexanico. Il fallimento di queste terapie giustifica il ricorso a trattamenti meno convenzionali, come la radioterapia, l'embolizzazione o la resezione chirurgica.

Bruckner AL, Frieden IJ: Hemangiomas of infancy. *J Am Acad Dermatol* 2003;48:477–496.
Chiller KG, Passaro D, Frieden IJ: Hemangiomas of infancy: Clinical characteristics, morphologic subtypes, and their relationship to race, ethnicity, and sex. *Arch Dermatol* 2002;138:1567–1576.

505.2 • Linfangioma e igroma cistico

Le malformazioni linfatiche, come il linfangioma e l'igroma cistico, che originano dal sacco linfatico embrionale, rappresentano le seconde neoplasie vascolari benigne più comuni nei bambini. In circa la metà dei casi sono localizzate a livello del capo e del collo e sono presenti già alla nascita, con una maggiore evidenza dopo i 2 anni di età. Non vi è una predisposizione in relazione al sesso. Può esserci regressione spontanea, ma non è tipica.

Le malformazioni linfatiche si presentano come masse soffici e non dolenti, traslucide se superficiali. Quelle intratoraciche possono essere sintomatiche, comportandosi come masse mediastiniche o provocando un versamento pericardico o pleurico. Un rapido accrescimento si può verificare in caso di un'infezione o di sanguinamento. Le lesioni localizzate possono essere asportate chirurgicamente, ma ciò può risultare complicato, per via della loro natura infiltrante. Nel caso di lesioni asportate solo parzialmente è comune la recidiva. L'aspirazione può dare un temporaneo miglioramento in caso di emergenza, come negli eventi di dispnea, ma si verificherà di lì a poco una recidiva. L'iniezione di agenti sclerosanti, la laser terapia e la somministrazione sistemica di IFN sono terapie utilizzate. L'agente sclerosante di scelta è lo streptococco immunoterapeutico OK-432, che nella maggior parte dei casi evita il ricorso alla chirurgia e che sembra essere particolarmente efficace per i linfangiomi macrocistici del capo e del collo.

Brewis C, Pracy JP, Albert DM: Treatment of lymphangiomas of the head and neck in children by intralesional injection of OK-432 (Picibanil). *Clin Otolaryngol* 2000;25:130–134.
Giguere CM, Bauman NM, Sato Y, et al: Treatment of lymphangiomas with OK-432 (Picibanil) sclerotherapy: A prospective multi-institutional trial. *Arch Otolaryngol Head Neck Surg* 2002;128:1137–1144.

Capitolo 506 ■ Tumori rari

Cynthia E. Herzog

506.1 • Tumori della tiroide

L'incidenza dei tumori della tiroide nei pazienti con <20 anni negli Stati Uniti è di 4,9 casi per milione. La maggior parte delle neoplasie in questa fascia d'età si osserva tra gli adolescenti (vedi Capitolo 570). Il tumore della tiroide è circa 4 volte più frequente nelle femmine che nei maschi e 2,5 volte più comune nei bianchi che nei neri. Il maggiore fattore di rischio è costituito dalla precedente esposizione a radiazioni, soprattutto a livello del capo e del collo. Questo tumore rappresenta inoltre circa il 10% delle seconde neoplasie nei soggetti sopravvissuti a malattie oncologiche, soprattutto con pregressa diagnosi di linfoma di Hodgkin, non solo a causa della radioterapia, ma anche per l'utilizzo degli agenti alchilanti. Nella maggior parte dei casi si tratta di carcinomi differenziati (papillare e follicolare). Il carcinoma midollare della tiroide (MTC, *Medullary Thyroid Carcinoma*) può manifestarsi come forma familiare, soprattutto nelle **neoplasie endocrine multiple** (MEN, *Multiple Endocrine Neoplasia*, di tipo 2). Nella MEN di tipo 2a, l'MTC generalmente interessa bambini più grandi e adulti e può associarsi al feocromocitoma e all'iperplasia delle paratiroidi. La MEN di tipo 2b è invece associata a un esordio di MTC in età molto precoce. Altre caratteristiche della MEN 2b sono i neurinomi mucosi e l'habitus marfanoide. La MEN di tipo 2 si trova in relazione alla mutazione del protooncogene *RET*, mentre le traslocazioni che coinvolgono il *RET* si osservano in circa la metà delle neoplasie tiroidee differenziate dell'età pediatrica. I pazienti con un'anamnesi familiare di MTC andrebbero sottoposti a test genetici e a una tiroidectomia totale profilattica. Mutazioni particolari del *RET* si correlano a specifici fenotipi e al rischio di sviluppare precocemente l'MTC. Per questo motivo l'età in cui viene effettuata la tiroidectomia dipende dal tipo di mutazione del *RET*, ma dovrebbe essere eseguita comuqnue prima dei 2 anni nei soggetti affetti dalla MEN 2b. Il paziente necessiterà per il resto della sua vita di un trattamento sostitutivo con ormoni tiroidei.

I pazienti si presentano con una massa tiroidea e/o una linfoadenopatia cervicale; sono rari i sintomi correlati a livelli alterati degli ormoni tiroidei. Circa il 20% dei noduli tiroidei nei bambini è maligno, in confronto al 10% degli adolescenti e degli adulti. L'ago aspirato è una procedura diagnostica utilizzata spesso per valutare quelli dell'adulto, ma nella popolazione pediatrica non è ancora stato validato, soprattutto nei preadolescenti; in questi pazienti è raccomandata, piuttosto, l'asportazione chirurgica dei linfonodi. La valutazione preoperatoria comprende la determinazione del livello degli ormoni tiroidei, l'ecografia della tiroide, la radiografia e la TC del torace. La tiroidectomia totale per una malattia confinata a un solo lobo è controversa in età pediatrica, per via della buona prognosi e del rischio di complicanze come l'ipoparatiroidismo. Tuttavia, la tiroidectomia totale o subtotale riduce il rischio di recidive locali. La dissezione dei linfonodi di routine non è indicata, ma andrebbe eseguita nei casi di interessamento dei linfonodi cervicali. Per eradicare quindi la malattia residua e per trattare le metastasi polmonari, che interessano il 6-10% dei casi, si usa il trattamento a base di iodio 131. Le metastasi polmonari sono evidenziabili meglio con il radioiodio, dopo la resezione della malattia di base.

Hung W, Sarlis NJ: Current controversies in the management of pediatric patients with well-differentiated nonmedullary thyroid cancer: A review. *Thyroid* 2002;12:683–702.

Machens A, Holzhausen H-j, Thanh PN, et al: Malignant progression from C-cell hyperplasia to medullary thyroid carcinoma in 167 carriers of RET germline mutations. *Surgery* 203;134:425–31.

Sherman SI: Thyroid carcinoma. *Lancet* 2003;361:501–510.

Szinnai G, Meier C, Komminoth P, et al: Review of multiple endocrine neoplasia type 2A in children: Therapeutic results of early thyroidectomy and prognostic value of codon analysis. *Pediatrics* 203;111:e132–e139.

506.2 • Melanoma

L'incidenza del melanoma in soggetti con <20 anni negli Stati Uniti è di 4,2 casi per milione, con una maggiore prevalenza negli adolescenti (vedi Capitolo 650) specie di sesso femminile. L'incidenza nei gruppi di età più giovane negli Stati Uniti è rimasta stabile, ma è rapidamente cresciuta negli adulti. Anche se l'esposizione al sole è un fattore di rischio ben noto per gli adulti, il suo ruolo in età pediatrica è meno chiaro, ma in ogni caso i pediatri dovrebbero consigliare ai loro pazienti di evitarla, per ridurre il rischio di sviluppare un melanoma in età adulta. I soggetti con la pelle chiara e con familiarità per il melanoma sono particolarmente a rischio. Altri fattori di rischio riconosciuti per i bambini sono il nevo gigante peloso (>20 cm), la sindrome del nevo displastico e lo xeroderma pigmentoso.

Il riscontro di un nevo che cresce rapidamente, di colore scuro, che ha cambiato pigmentazione, con bordi irregolari o che sanguina facilmente deve essere considerato sospetto, anche se molti dei melanomi diagnosticati nei bambini non avevano queste caratteristiche. La diagnosi è di tipo patologico. Va in ogni caso posta particolare attenzione a quella nei bambini, perché la distinzione con altre lesioni, soprattutto con il nevo di Spitz, può essere difficile.

Le raccomandazioni sulla terapia si fondano sui dati riportati per gli adulti. Il primo trattamento per tutti i melanomi, ma soprattutto per quelli più superficiali, consiste nell'asportazione locale con la mappatura dei linfonodi e la biopsia del linfonodo sentinella. Se quest'ultimo è positivo, è raccomandata la loro dissezione formale. La somministrazione adiuvante di alte dosi di interferone si è dimostrata efficace nell'adulto, mentre la chemioterapia combinata con gli agenti biologici e con la vaccinoterapia non è risultata valida nel trattamento delle metastasi a distanza. Se la prognosi sia migliore nei bambini rispetto agli adulti non è chiaro.

Mones JM, Ackerman AB: Melanomas in prepubescent children: Review comprehensively, critique historically, criteria diagnostically, and course biologically. *Am J Dermatopathol* 2003;25:223–238.

Pappo AS: Melanoma in children and adolescents. *Eur J Cancer* 2003;39: 2651–2661.

506.3 • Carcinoma nasofaringeo

Il carcinoma nasofaringeo è raro nella popolazione pediatrica, ma è uno dei tumori nasofaringei più comuni nei bambini. Negli adulti, l'incidenza è maggiore nel sud della Cina, ma è anche frequente fra gli Inuit e nella popolazione dell'Africa del nord e del nord-est dell'India. In Cina è raro tra i bambini, ma nelle altre popolazioni citate una percentuale significativa di casi interessa l'età pediatrica, soprattutto l'adolescenza. Il rapporto maschi:femmine è di 2:1; la razza nera risulta maggiormente colpita. Nella popolazione pediatrica i carcinomi nasofaringei hanno un'istologia indifferenziata più spesso che negli adulti e si associano al virus di Epstein-Barr. Questo carcinoma è stato associato con specifici tipi di HLA.

La maggior parte dei pazienti pediatrici si presenta con una malattia locoregionale avanzata, con linfoadenopatia cervicale. Si possono riscontrare epistassi, trisma e deficit dei nervi cranici. La diagnosi è posta con la biopsia del nasofaringe o dei linfonodi cervicali. Nella maggior parte dei casi il livello di lattato deidrogenasi è aumentato, ma questo elemento è aspecifico. La TC o la RM del capo e del collo riescono necessarie per determinare l'estensione locale della malattia. La radiografia del torace, la TC, la scintigrafia ossea e l'ecografia epatica sono utilizzate per valutare la presenza di metastasi. Può tornare utile la ricerca di IgA anti virus di Epstein-Barr e della proteina ZEBRA (anticorpi anti Epstein-Barr virus Bam H1Z proteina transattivata).

Il trattamento prevede la combinazione di chemioterapia e radioterapia, con la chemioterapia a base di cisplatino che viene somministrata prima e insieme alla radioterapia. La prognosi dipende dall'estensione della malattia; i pazienti con metastasi a distanza ce l'hanno infausta. L'uso della radioterapia a intensità modulata ha migliorato il controllo locale della malattia e ha ridotto gli effetti avversi tardivi associati alla radioterapia, compresi la disfunzione ormonale, le carie dentali, la fibrosi e i secondi tumori.

Ayan I, Kaytan E, Ayan N: Childhood nasopharyngeal carcinoma: From biology to treatment. *Lancet Oncol* 2003;4:13–21.

Tsao SW, Lo KW, Huang DP: Nasopharyngeal carcinoma. In Tselis A, Jenson HB (editors): *Epstein-Barr Virus*. New York, Taylor and Francis, 2006, pp 273–295.

506.4 • Adenocarcinoma del colon e del retto

Il carcinoma colorettale è raro nella popolazione pediatrica, in cui comunque vi è una predominanza nei maschi rispetto a quella nel sesso femminile degli adulti. Anche nei soggetti con malattie predisponenti, come la poliposi adenomatosa familiare e la sindrome di Peutz-Jeghers, questa neoplasia generalmente non si manifesta fino all'età adulta, anche se sono disponibili i test genetici e lo screening può essere fatto durante l'infanzia o l'adolescenza.

Il carcinoma del colon ereditario non secondario alla poliposi, una patologia autosomica dominante, può comparire precocemente con una neoplasia del colon che ha la predisposizione a sviluppare neoplasie in altri organi (ovaie, encefalo, reni, utero). Mutazioni a livello germinale dei geni deputati alla riparazione del DNA provocano errori in questo e instabilità dei microsatelliti.

I sintomi alla presentazione comprendono sangue nelle feci o melena, dolore addominale, perdita di peso e modificazioni dell'alvo. Spesso i segni sono sfumati e portano a un ritardo nella diagnosi, che viene posta in una fase di malattia già avanzata.

I sottotipi istologici differiscono da quelli osservati negli adulti, con una prevalenza dei tumori mucinosi. Il trattamento prevede una resezione chirurgica quando possibile, con la chemioterapia per i tumori non operabili. La radioterapia è utile nel trattamento dei carcinomi del retto.

Grady WM: Genetic testing for high-risk colon cancer patients. *Gastroenterology* 2003;124:1574–1594.

Marcos I, Borrego S, Urioste M, et al: Mutations in the DNA mismatch repair gene *MLH1* associated with early onset colon cancer. *J Pediatr* 2006;148: 837–839.

506.5 • Carcinoma adrenocorticale

Il carcinoma adrenocorticale è infrequente, ma si associa alle sindromi di Li-Fraumeni e di Beckwith-Wiedemann. Per via della sua rarità nei bambini e dell'associazione con la sindrome di Li-Fraumeni, la diagnosi dovrebbe essere puntualizzata con la valutazione genetica e con l'esecuzione dei test genetici. Il tumore può manifestarsi in qualunque momento dell'infanzia, ma è più comune durante i primi dieci anni di vita ed è inoltre più frequente nel sesso femminile. In Brasile risulta 10 volte più diffuso che negli Stati Uniti. I bambini più piccoli tipicamente si presentano con un quadro di virilizzazione, mentre negli adolescenti possono mancare le disfunzioni endocrine, oppure possono sviluppare una sindrome di Cushing. La prognosi dipende dalle dimensioni del tumore, dalla sua estensione e dalla possibilità o meno di asportarlo chirurgicamente; rimane tuttavia sfavorevole per i tumori non operabili o metastatici, anche se risponde alla chemioterapia a base di mitotano e cisplatino.

Michalkiewicz E, Sandrini R, Figueiredo B, et al: Clinical and outcome characteristics of children with adrenocortical tumors: A report from the International Pediatric Adrenocortical Tumor Registry. *J Clin Oncol* 2004;5:838–845.

506.6 • TUMORE DESMOPLASTICO A PICCOLE CELLULE TONDE

Il tumore desmoplastico a piccole cellule tonde è una neoplasia di recente osservazione che colpisce soprattutto il sesso maschile durante l'adolescenza. Si associa alla traslocazione fra il gene del tumore di Ewing e quello del tumore di Wilms t(11;22)(p13;q12). I pazienti tipicamente manifestano una malattia addominale diffusa senza una chiara origine della lesione primitiva e a volte con estensione anche extra-addominale. Nonostante un trattamento aggressivo con chirurgia, chemioterapia e radioterapia, nella maggior parte dei casi la prognosi rimane infausta.

Gerald WL, Ladanyi M, de Alava E: Clinical, pathologic, and molecular spectrum of tumors associated with t(11;22)(p13;q12): Desmoplastic small round-cell tumor and its variants. *J Clin Oncol* 1998;16:3028–3036.

Capitolo 507 ■ Istiocitosi dell'infanzia

Stephan Ladisch

Le istiocitosi dell'infanzia rappresentano un gruppo di patologie diverse; anche se ognuna di esse risulta rara, possono tutte essere gravi nella loro manifestazione clinica. Queste malattie sono raggruppate insieme perché hanno in comune l'aumentata proliferazione o l'accumulo di cellule del sistema monocito-macrofagico, che origina dal midollo osseo. Anche se talvolta sono difficili da distinguere clinicamente, una diagnosi precisa è essenziale per le scelte terapeutiche. Una loro classificazione sistematica si fonda sugli aspetti istopatologici (Tab. 507-1). Una meticolosa e accurata valutazione del materiale bioptico ottenuto al momento della diagnosi risulta essenziale. Questo apprezzamento comprende la microscopia elettronica e l'immunofissazione, che possono richiedere particolari procedure.

CLASSIFICAZIONE E ANATOMIA PATOLOGICA. Sulla base delle caratteristiche istopatologiche si distinguono tre classi di istiocitosi dell'infanzia. La istiocitosi pediatrica meglio conosciuta, precedentemente nota come **istiocitosi X**, rappresenta la classe I e comprende il granuloma eosinofilo (vedi Capitolo 501), la **malattia di Hand-Schüller-Christian** e la **malattia di Letterer-Siwe**. La definizione di **istiocitosi a cellule di Langerhans (LCH,** *Langerhans' Cell Histiocytosis*) si riferisce alla classe I delle istiocitosi. La normale cellula di Langerhans è una *antigen-presenting cell* (APC) della cute. L'elemento caratteristico di tutte le forme di LCH è costituito da una proliferazione clonale delle cellule della linea monocitaria con le caratteristiche, alla microscopia elettronica, della cellula di Langerhans. Esse sono i **granuli di Birbeck**, granuli bilamellari simili a una racchetta da tennis, che risultano diagnostici quando vengono osservati nel citoplasma delle cellule di lesioni dell'LCH. I granuli di Birbeck esprimono un antigene di nuova caratterizzazione, la langerina (CD207), che è coinvolto nella presentazione degli antigeni da parte dei linfociti T. La diagnosi definitiva di LCH può anche essere fondata sulla dimostrazione della positività per il CD1a delle cellule lesionali, che può essere effettuata utilizzando tessuto fissato. Le lesioni possono contenere varie proporzioni di cellule di Langerhans, contenenti granuli, linfociti, granulociti, monociti ed eosinofili.

Diversamente da quella di classe I con predominanza di una APC (la cellula di Langerhans), le **istiocitosi di classe II** sono malattie proliferative non maligne, caratterizzate dall'accumulo di cellule che processano l'antigene (i macrofagi). Le **linfoistiocitosi emofagocitiche** sono il risultato di una emofagocitosi e di un'attivazione (up regulation) incontrollate delle citochine infiammatorie, simili alle sindromi con attivazione macrofagica (vedi Tab. 154-5). L'infiltrazione tissutale da parte dei linfociti T CD8 e di macrofagi attivati e la ipercitochinemia sono elementi caratteristici. Queste cellule fagocitiche, al microscopio ottico, appaiono morfologicamente simili ai macrofagi normali e non hanno i due elementi peculiari (i granuli di Birbeck e la positività per il CD1a) tipici delle cellule dell'LCH. Le due principali patologie classificate come istiocitosi di classe II possiedono elementi patologici indistinguibili. Una è la **linfoistiocitosi emofagocitica familiare (FHLH,** *Familial Hemophagocytic LymphoHistiocytosis*), un tempo nota come linfoistiocitosi eritrofagocitica familiare, autosomica recessiva e unica forma ereditaria; alcune sue specifiche alterazioni genetiche comprendono le mutazioni della perforina, di Munc 13-4 e della Sintassina-11. L'altra è la **sindrome emofagocitica associata alle infezioni**, detta anche linfoistiocitosi emofagocitica secondaria (Tab. 507-2). Entrambe

TABELLA 507-1. Classificazione delle istiocitosi dell'infanzia

CLASSE	PATOLOGIA	CARATTERISTICHE CELLULARI DELLE LESIONI	TRATTAMENTO
I	Istiocitosi a cellule di Langerhans	Cellule di Langerhans (CD1a-positivo) con granuli di Birbeck	Terapia locale per le lesioni isolate; chemioterapia per la malattia disseminata
II	Linfoistiocitosi eritrofagocitica familiare*	Macrofagi reattivi morfologicamente normali con prevalenza di eritrofagociti	Chemioterapia; trapianto allogenico di midollo osseo
	Sindrome emofagocitica associata alle infezioni†		
III	Istiocitosi maligna	Proliferazione neoplastica di cellule con caratteristiche di monociti/macrofagi o di loro precursori	Chemioterapia, comprese le antracicline
	Leucemia monocitica acuta		

*Detta anche linfoistiocitosi emofagocitica familiare (FHLH).
†Detta anche linfoistiocitosi emofagocitica secondaria.

TABELLA 507-2. Infezioni associate alla sindrome emofagocitica

VIRUS
Adenovirus
Cytomegalovirus
Virus dengue
Virus di Epstein-Barr
Herpes simplex virus
HIV
Parvovirus B19
Virus della varicella-zoster

BATTERI
Babesia microti
Brucella abortus
Enterobatteri Gram-negativi
Haemophilus influenzae
Mycoplasma pneumoniae
Staphylococcus aureus
Streptococcus pneumoniae

MICETI
Candida albicans
Cryptococcus neoformans
Histoplasma capsulatum

MICOBATTERI
Mycobacterium tuberculosis

RICKETTSIE
Coxiella brunetii

PARASSITI
Leishmania donovani

Da Nathan DG, Orkin SH, Ginsburg D, et al (editors): *Nathan and Oski's Hematology of Infancy and Childhood*, 6th ed. Philadelphia, WB Saunders, 2003, p. 1381.

queste patologie sono caratterizzate da una infiltrazione degli organi coinvolti da parte di macrofagi e linfociti attivati, in cui il difetto dei linfociti è considerato la principale alterazione. Queste patologie sono inoltre raggruppate insieme con la definizione di **linfoistiocitosi emofagocitiche** (**HLH**, *Hemophagocytic Lympho-Histiocytosis*) (Tab. 507-3).

Le lesioni cellulari miste delle istiocitosi di classe I e II suggeriscono che può trattarsi di patologie della regolazione immunitaria, come risultato di una inusuale e non identificata stimolazione antigenica o di una risposta cellulare immunitaria alterata e in qualche modo deficitaria. Mutazioni del gene della perforina (PRF1) o del gene Munc 13-4 provocano un ridotto funzionamento dei linfociti citotossici, la cui attività è inibita nella FHLH.

Le **istiocitosi di classe III**, d'altro canto, sono inequivocabilmente neoplasie delle cellule monocito-macrofagiche. Secondo questa definizione, la leucemia monocitica acuta e la vera istiocitosi maligna sono istiocitosi di classe III (vedi Capitolo 495). Risulta controversa l'esistenza di neoplasie delle cellule di Langerhans. In alcuni casi di LCH è stata dimostrata la presenza di cloni cellulari.

507.1 • Istiocitosi di classe I

MANIFESTAZIONI CLINICHE. Le LCH hanno una modalità di presentazione estremamente variabile. Lo scheletro è coinvolto nell'80% dei casi e può costituire l'unico organo colpito, soprattutto nei bambini con >5 anni. Le lesioni ossee possono essere singole o multiple e si localizzano soprattutto a livello del cranio (Fig. 507-1). Altre sedi interessate sono la pelvi, il femore, le vertebre, la mascella e la mandibola, che possono essere asintomatiche oppure associate a dolore o tumefazione locale. Il coinvolgimento della colonna può provocare un crollo dei corpi vertebrali, che si può osservare radiologicamente e può provocare una compressione secondaria del midollo. Nelle ossa piatte e lunghe si notano lesioni osteolitiche con bordi netti senza una manifesta formazione di nuovo osso reattivo fino a che le lesioni stesse non guariscono. Quelle che interessano le ossa lunghe portanti possono diventare responsabili di fratture patologiche. Otiti croniche purulente sono frequenti, in associazione con lesioni distruttive delle mastoidi. Le alterazioni destruenti della mandibola e della mascella possono far sembrare i denti, alla radiologia, non più ancorati. Con la risposta alla terapia, la guarigione può essere completa.

In circa il 50% dei pazienti si ha un coinvolgimento cutaneo in qualunque fase del decorso della malattia, generalmente sotto forma di una dermatite squamosa, papulare, seborroica difficile da trattare al livello del cuoio capelluto, dell'area perineale, ascellare o della regione retroauricolare. Le lesioni possono estendersi fino a coinvolgere il dorso, il palmo delle mani e la pianta dei piedi. L'esantema può essere petecchiale o emorragico, anche in assenza di trombocitopenia. Una linfoadenopatia localizzata o diffusa è presente in circa il 33% dei pazienti, mentre l'epatosplenomegalia si osserva nel 20% circa dei casi. Si possono rilevare vari gradi di insufficienza epatica, con ittero e ascite.

L'esoftalmo, quando presente, è spesso bilaterale ed è provocato da un accumulo di tessuto granulomatoso a livello retro-orbitale. Le mucose gengivali possono venire coinvolte da lesioni infiltranti, che superficialmente assomigliano a una candida. L'otite media compare nel 30-40% dei casi; le lesioni distruttive dell'orecchio medio possono portare alla sordità. Nel 10-15% dei pazienti sulle radiografie si notano infiltrati polmonari. Le lesioni possono andare da una fibrosi diffusa o infiltrati nodulari disseminati fino a cisti diffuse. Lo pneumotorace può raramente costituire una complicanza. Se i polmoni risultano gravemente coinvolti, si possono verificare tachipnea e una progressiva insufficienza respiratoria. Una insufficienza ipofisaria o un coinvolgimento ipotalamico possono provocare un ritardo nella crescita. Inoltre, i pazienti possono avere un diabete insipido; quelli con sospetto LCH devono essere indagati per la capacità di concentrare le urine, prima di essere sottoposti alla biopsia. Si può di rado osservare un panipopituitarismo. Può essere rilevabile anche un ipotiroidismo primario dovuto a una infiltrazione della tiroide.

I pazienti affetti in modo grave possono avere manifestazioni sistemiche, con la febbre, la perdita di peso, un malessere generale, l'irritabilità e un deficit dello sviluppo. Il coinvolgimento

TABELLA 507-3. Caratteristiche distintive delle linfoistiocitosi reattive

	GENETICA	INFEZIONE VIRALE	FUNZIONE CELLULARE IMMUNITARIA	MISCELLANEA
HLH, genetiche	Autosomiche recessive	Generalmente associata	↓ CMI, ↓ attività dei NK, ↓ monociti killer, ↓ CMI	Deficit di perforina, ipertrigliceridemia, mutazioni di perforina (PRF1), Munc 13-4
Secondariamente associate alle infezioni	Sporadiche	Sì	↓ CMI, NL o ↑ NK in stretta associazione con EBV, ↓ alterazioni dell'attività killer associata a EBV	Precoce coagulopatia nel decorso della malattia
XLP	X-linked sporadiche	EBV	NL o ↑ NK, NL o ↑ anomalo dell'attività killer associata a EBV	Mutazione SH2DIA, grave epatite, spesso fatale
SHML	Sporadica	EBV?	Non riportato	Fenomeni autoimmuni
LG	Sporadica	EBV	↓ CMI	Sviluppo di linfoma

Da Nathan DG, Orkin SH, Ginsburg D, et al (editors): *Nathan and Oski's Hematology of Infancy and Childhood*, 6th ed. Philadelphia, WB Saunders, 2003, p. 1387.
CMI, immunità cellulo-mediata (*Cell-Mediated Immunity*); EBV, virus di Epstein-Barr (*Epstein-Barr Virus*); HLH, linfoistiocitosi emofagocitica; LG, granulomatosi linfomatoide (*Lymphomatoid Granulomatosis*); NK, natural killer; NL, normale; SHML, istiocitosi sinusale con linfoadenopatia massiva (*Sinus Histiocytosis with Massive Lymphadenopathy*); XLP, sindrome linfoproliferativa X-linked.

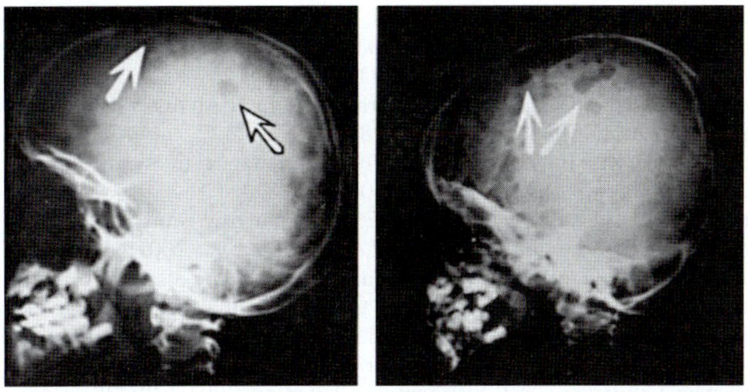

Figura 507-1. Due radiografie del cranio di pazienti con istiocitosi a cellule di Langerhans (LCH). *A sinistra*, la paziente ha >2 anni e presenta un coinvolgimento limitato alle ossa (*frecce*). Ha avuto un buon recupero. *A destra*, il paziente ha <2 anni e presenta una malattia avanzata dell'osso, febbre, anemia, gravi eruzioni cutanee, linfoadenopatia generalizzata, epatosplenomegalia, infiltrati polmonari e un'evoluzione fatale nonostante la chemioterapia. Questi due pazienti rappresentano i due estremi dello spettro clinico della LCH.

del midollo osseo può provocare l'anemia e la trombocitopenia. Due evenienze rare, ma gravi e inusuali, dell'LCH riguardano il coinvolgimento epatico (che porta a cirrosi) e il particolare interessamento del sistema nervoso centrale (SNC), caratterizzato da atassia, disartria e altri sintomi neurologici. Il coinvolgimento epatico si associa a una malattia multisistemica che spesso è già presente al momento della diagnosi, mentre quello del SNC, progressivo e istopatologicamente caratterizzato da gliosi e per cui non è nota una terapia, può essere osservato solo molti anni dopo la diagnosi iniziale di LCH, che poteva anche basarsi su una moderata malattia ossea. In nessuna di queste due manifestazioni si evidenziano le cellule di Langerhans o i granuli di Birbeck.

Dopo la biopsia, che risulta diagnostica e che si ottiene più facilmente a livello delle lesioni cutanee o ossee, è necessario sottoporre il paziente a un'attenta valutazione clinica e di laboratorio. Gli esami necessari sono: l'emocromo completo, la funzionalità epatica, la coagulazione, lo studio dell'osso, la radiografia del torace e la valutazione dell'osmolarità urinaria. Inoltre, è opportuno indagare attentamente qualunque organo o sistema che alla valutazione medica o agli esami eseguiti abbia dimostrato di essere coinvolto, al fine di stabilire l'estensione della malattia pretrattamento.

TRATTAMENTO E PROGNOSI. Il decorso clinico della malattia che interessa un singolo sistema (soprattutto l'osso, i linfonodi o la cute) è generalmente benigno, con un'elevata probabilità di remissione spontanea. Pertanto il trattamento dovrebbe essere minimo e diretto ad arrestare la progressione di una lesione ossea a rischio di provocare un danno permanente prima della sua risoluzione spontanea. Il curettage, o meno spesso una radioterapia locale a basse dosi (5-6 Gy), possono proporsi questa finalità. Una malattia multisistemica, invece, andrebbe sottoposta a una polichemioterapia sistemica. Sono stati proposti numerosi schemi differenti di terapia, ma l'elemento chiave è la presenza della vinblastina o dell'etoposide, che si sono dimostrati entrambi efficaci per l'LCH. Il trattamento multisistemico prevede invece una terapia multipla, designata a ridurre il rischio di una riattivazione della malattia e di effetti collaterali tardivi. La risposta alla terapia, contrariamente a quanto si pensava, può essere alta, soprattutto se la diagnosi è corretta e tempestiva. Le terapie sperimentali, da impiegare solo per le forme non responsive (spesso in bambini molto piccoli con forme multisistemiche e insufficienza d'organo che non hanno risposto alla terapia iniziale), comprendono quella immunosoppressiva con ciclosporina/globuline antitimociti e alcune possibilità con nuovi agenti e modalità, come l'imatinib, la 2-clorodesossiadenosina e il trapianto di cellule staminali. Gli attuali approcci terapeutici e i protocolli sperimentali per le istiocitosi di classe I e II si possono trovare sul sito web della Histiocyte Society: www.histio.org/society.

507.2 • Istiocitosi di classe II: linfoistiocitosi emofagocitica

Vedi sopra: "Classificazione e patologia".

MANIFESTAZIONI CLINICHE. Le principali forme di HLH, quella familiare (FHLH) e quella secondaria, hanno una presentazione clinica molto simile, che consiste in un processo patologico generalizzato, più spesso con febbre, rash cutaneo macropapulare e/o con petecchie, perdita di peso e irritabilità (Tab. 507-4). La FHLH è caratterizzata anche da una grave immunodeficienza. I bambini con l'FHLH hanno sempre <4 anni, mentre quelli con l'HLH secondaria possono contrarla in età più avanzata. **L'esame obiettivo** spesso permette di apprezzare un'epatosplenomegalia, una linfoadenopatia, un'insufficienza respiratoria e sintomi da coinvolgimento del SNC, ma diversamente dalla meningite asettica le cellule nel liquido cerebrospinale sono gli stessi macrofagi fagocitaci riscontrati nel sangue periferico o nel midollo osseo. La diagnosi si fonda sulle caratteristiche patologiche della biopsia della cute o del midollo osseo. Gli esami di laboratorio alterati, che si riscontrano in entrambe le forme dell'HLH, comprendono l'iperlipidemia, l'iperfibrinogenemia, l'aumento degli enzimi epatici, un grave incremento dei recettori solubili per l'interleuchina 2 rilasciati dai linfociti attivati, livelli molto elevati di ferritina sierica (spesso >10 000) e citopenia (soprattutto pancitopenia da emofagocitosi nel midollo). Non è possibile distinguere la FHLH dall'HLH secondaria sulla base delle sole manifestazioni cliniche e degli esami di laboratorio, anche se i marcatori genetici per la FHLH possono complementare l'anamnesi familiare positiva per i fratelli affetti. L'HLH può anche manifestarsi senza le mutazioni dei geni della perforina o di Munc 13-4, ma in associazione a 5 dei seguenti elementi: febbre, splenomegalia, citopenia di 2 linee cellulari, ipertrigliceridemia o iperfibrinogenemia, iperferritinemia, aumento di SCD25 (recettore dell'interleuchina 2), riduzione o assenza di NK ed evidenza di emofagocitosi a livello del midollo osseo, del liquido cerebrospinale o dei linfonodi.

TRATTAMENTO E PROGNOSI. La distinzione diagnostica tra la FHLH e la HLH secondaria talvolta si basa sull'esordio acuto dell'HLH secondaria in presenza di un'infezione documentata. In questo caso, il trattamento della sottostante infezione, in associazione alla terapia di supporto, è fondamentale. Se la diagnosi è posta in un contesto di immunodeficienza iatrogena, il trattamento immunosoppressore andrebbe interrotto e dovrebbe essere iniziata una terapia di supporto durante il trattamento specifico per la sottostante infezione. Quando la FHLH (mutazioni dei geni per la perforina o Munc 13-4) è diagnosticata o sospetta e quando non può essere documentata un'infezione, la terapia generalmente prevede l'utilizzo di etoposide, steroidi e metotrexato intratecale. Alcuni raccomandano le globuline antitimociti e la ciclosporina come terapia di mantenimento. Tuttavia, anche

TABELLA 507-4. Criteri diagnostici per la linfoistiocitosi emofagocitica

Febbre >38,5 °C e persistente per ≥7 giorni
Splenomegalia >3 cm
DUE DELLE SEGUENTI ALTERAZIONI EMATOLOGICHE:
Anemia (con emoglobina >9 g/dL)
Trombocitopenia (>100 000 cellule/μL)
Neutropenia (<1000 neutrofili/μL)
UNA DELLE SEGUENTI ALTERAZIONI:
Ipertrigliceridemia >2,0 nmol/l
Ipofibrinogenemia <150 mg/dL
e
Emofagocitosi a livello di midollo osseo, milza o linfonodi
Nessuna evidenza di iperplasia midollare o neoplasia maligna

Da Nathan DG, Orkin SH, Ginsburg D, et al (editors): *Nathan and Oski's Hematology of Infancy and Childhood*, 6th ed. Philadelphia, WB Saunders, 2003, p. 1379. Adattata da MacMahon HE, Bedizel M, Ellis CA: Familial erythrophagocytic lymphohistiocytosis. *Pediatrics* 1963; 32:868-879.

con la chemioterapia la FHLH rimane una malattia fatale, spesso dopo una recidiva. Il **trapianto allogenico di cellule staminali** è efficace in circa il 60% dei soggetti con la FHLH.

Nell'HLH secondaria, invece, quando può essere documentata una infezione e questa viene efficacemente trattata, la prognosi è buona senza altri trattamenti specifici. Quando non è possibile documentare una infezione trattabile, che è ciò che capita nella maggior parte dei casi con la HLH secondaria, la prognosi può essere infausta come per la FHLH ed è consigliato un trattamento chemioterapico identico, a base di etoposide. È stato ipotizzato che, per il suo effetto citotossico sui macrofagi, questo agente blocchi la produzione di citochine, il processo di emofagocitosi e l'accumulo di macrofagi, tutti eventi che possono contribuire alla patogenesi della sindrome emofagocitica associata alle infezioni. Un ampio spettro di agenti infettivi, quali virus (per es. Cytomegalovirus, virus di Epstein-Barr, herpes virus 6), miceti, protozoi e batteri possono scatenare l'HLH secondaria, generalmente nel contesto di uno stato di immunodeficienza (vedi Tab. 507-2). Una valutazione completa per le infezioni andrebbe fatta nei pazienti immunodeficienti con emofagocitosi. Rare volte la stessa sindrome può essere identificata in concomitanza di una patologia reumatologica (per es. il lupus eritematoso sistemico, la malattia di Kawasaki) o di una neoplasia (leucemia); in questi casi il trattamento della sottostante malattia può determinare la risoluzione dell'emofagocitosi. In alcuni soggetti si sono dimostrati efficaci l'interferone e le immunoglobuline endovena.

507.3 • Istiocitosi di classe III

La leucemia monocitica acuta e la vera istiocitosi maligna sono considerate istiocitosi di classe III (vedi Capitolo 495), perché sono inequivocabilmente neoplasie della linea monocito-macrofagica.

Arico M, Danesino C, Pende D, et al: Pathogenesis of haemophagocytic lymphohistiocytosis. *Br J Haematol* 2001;114:761–769.

Arico M, Imashuku S, Clementi R, et al: Hemophagocytic lymphohistiocytosis due to germline mutations in SH2D1A, the X-linked lymphoproliferative disease gene. *Blood* 2001;97:1131–1133.

Broadbent V, Gadner, H: Current therapy for Langerhans cell histiocytosis. *Hematol Oncol Clin North Am* 1998;12:327–328.

Domachowske JB: Infectious triggers of hemophagocytic syndrome in children. *Pediatr Infect Dis J* 2006;25:1067–1068.

Durken M, Finckenstein FG, Janka GE: Bone marrow transplantation in hemophagocytic lymphohistiocytosis. *Leuk Lymphoma* 2001;41:89–95.

Feldmann J, Callebaut I, Raposo G, et al: Munc 13–4 is essential for cytolytic granules fusion and is mutated on a form of familial hemophagocytic lymphohistiocytosis (FHL3). *Cell* 2003;115:461–473.

Gadner H, Grois N, Arico M, et al: A randomized trial of treatment for multisystem Langerhans' cell histiocytosis. *J Pediatr* 2001;138:728–734.

Hait E, Liang M, Degar B, et al: Gastrointestinal tract involvement in Langerhans cell histiocytosis: case report and literature review. *Pediatrics* 2006; 118:e1593–e1599.

Horne A, Janka G, Egeler R, et al: Hematopoietic stem cell transplantation in haemophagocytic lymphohistiocytosis. *Br J Haematol* 2005;129:622–630.

Kogawa K, Lee SM, Villanueva J, et al: Perforin expression in cytotoxic lymphocytes from patients with hemophagocytic lymphohistiocytosis and their family members. *Blood* 2002;99:61–66.

Lee SM, Sumegi J, Villanueva J, et al: Patients of African ancestry with hemophagocytic lymphohistiocytosis share a common haplotype of PRFI with a 50 delt mutation. *J Pediatr* 2006;149:134–137.

Leonidas JC, Guelfguat M, Valderrama E: Langerhans' cell histiocytosis. *Lancet* 2003;361:1293–1295.

Montella L, Insabato L, Palmieri G: Imatinib mesylate for cerebral Langerhans'-cell histiocytosis. *N Engl J Med* 2004;351:1034–1035.

Ouachee-Chardin M, Elie C, de Saint Basile G, et al: Hematopoietic stem cell transplantation in hemophagocytic lymphohistiocytosis: A single-center report of 48 patients. *Pediatrics* 2006;117:e743–e750.

Palazzi DL, McClain KL, Kaplan SL: Hemophagocytic syndrome in children: An important diagnostic consideration in fever of unknown origin. *Clin Infect Dis* 2003;36:306–312.

Valladeau J, Dezutter-Dambuyant C, Saeland S: Langerin/CD207 sheds light on formation of Birbeck granules and their possible function in Langerhans cells. *Immunol Res* 2003;28:93–107.

Writing Group of the Histiocyte Society: Histiocytosis syndromes in childhood. *Lancet* 1987;1:208–209.

Parte XXII ▪ Nefrologia

Sezione 1 — Malattia glomerulare — Ira D. Davis ed Ellis D. Avner

Capitolo 508 ▪ Introduzione alle malattie glomerulari

508.1 • Anatomia del glomerulo

I reni giacciono nello spazio retroperitoneale, leggermente sopra il livello dell'ombelico. Hanno una lunghezza e un peso variabili approssimativamente da 6 cm e 24 g in un neonato a termine a 12 cm o più e 150 g in un adulto. I reni (Fig. 508-1) hanno uno strato esterno, la corteccia, che contiene i glomeruli, i tubuli convoluti prossimali e distali e i dotti collettori e uno strato interno, la sostanza midollare, che contiene i tubuli retti, le anse di Henle, i vasa recta e i dotti collettori terminali (Fig. 508-2).

L'irrorazione a ciascun rene di solito è garantita da un'arteria renale principale che origina dall'aorta; possono essere presenti arterie renali multiple. L'arteria principale si riparte all'interno della midollare in rami segmentali, che a loro volta si dividono nelle arterie interlobari che attraversano la midollare fino alla giunzione con la corteccia. A questo punto, le arterie interlobari si diramano per formare arterie arcuate, che corrono parallele alla superficie dei reni. Le arterie interlobulari originano dalle arterie arcuate e danno vita alle arteriole afferenti dei glomeruli. Le cellule muscolari specializzate, nella parte dell'arteriola afferente e della macula densa all'interno del tubulo distale accanto al glomerulo, formano l'apparato iuxtaglomerulare che controlla la secrezione di renina. L'arteriola afferente si divide nella rete capillare glomerulare, che quindi si fonde nell'arteriola efferente (Fig. 508-3). Le arteriole efferenti dei glomeruli accanto alla midollare (glomeruli iuxtamidollari) sono più grandi di quelli nella corteccia esterna e garantiscono l'apporto ematico (vasa recta) ai tubuli e alla midollare.

Ogni rene contiene circa 1 milione di nefroni (glomeruli e tubuli associati). Negli esseri umani, la formazione dei nefroni

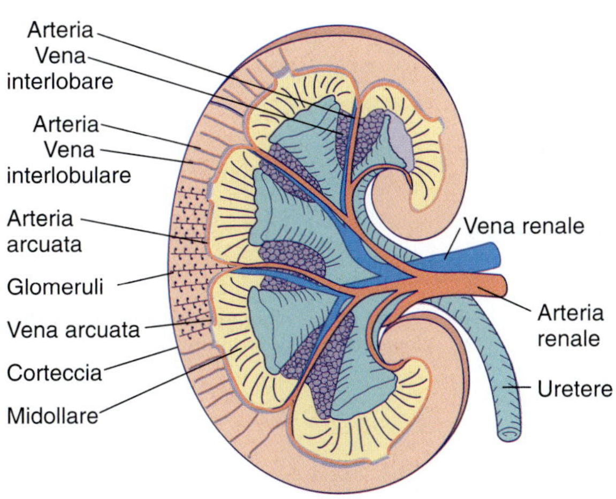

Figura 508-1. Morfologia generale della circolazione renale. (Da Pitts RF: *Physiology of the Kidney and Body Fluids*, 3rd ed. Chicago, Year Book Medical Publishers, 1974.)

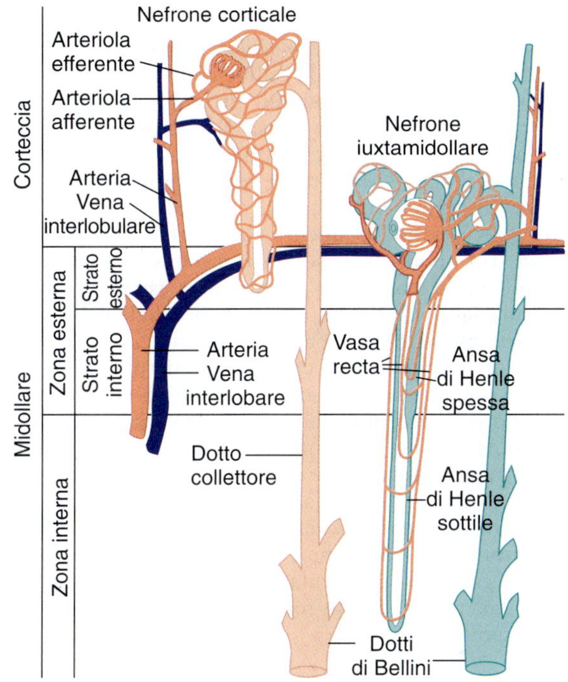

Figura 508-2. Confronto tra l'irrorazione dei nefroni corticali e iuxtamidollari. (Da Pitts RF: *Physiology of the Kidney and Body Fluids*, 3rd ed. Chicago, Year Book Medical Publishers, 1974.)

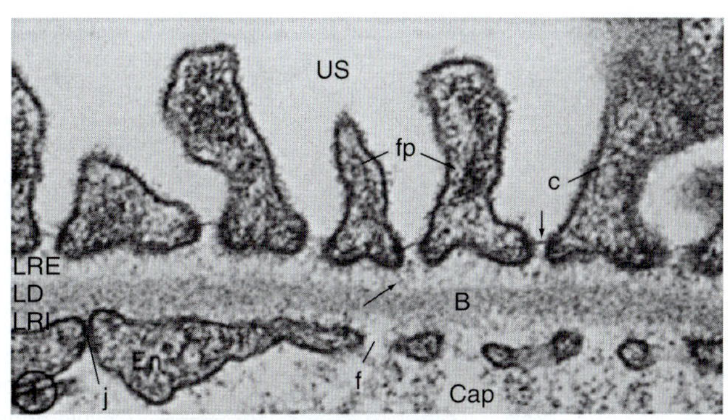

Figura 508-3. Fotografia al microscopio elettronico della parete capillare glomerulare normale (Cap) che mostra l'endotelio (En) con le sue fenestrazioni (f), la membrana basale glomerulare (B) con il suo strato denso centrale, la lamina densa (LD) e l'adiacente lamina rara, interna (LRI) ed esterna (LRE) (*freccia lunga*), nonché i podociti delle cellule epiteliali (fp) con il loro rivestimento cellulare spesso (c). Il filtrato glomerulare attraversa le finestre endoteliali, la membrana basale e le fessure di filtrazione (*freccia corta*) tra i podociti delle cellule epiteliali per raggiungere lo spazio urinario (US) (×60 000). J indica la giunzione tra due cellule endoteliali. (Da Farquhar MG, Kanwar YS: Functional organization of the glomerulus: State of the science in 1979. In Cummings NB, Michael AF, Wilson CB (editors): *Immune Mechanisms in Renal Disease*. New York, Plenum, 1982.)

è completa alla nascita, ma la maturazione, funzionale con la crescita e l'allungamento dei tubuli, continua durante i primi dieci anni di vita. Dato che dopo la nascita non possono formarsi nuovi nefroni, la loro perdita progressiva può condurre all'insufficienza renale. Un numero ridotto di nefroni alla nascita può essere associato all'ipertensione nell'età adulta, presumibilmente correlata all'iperfiltrazione e alla sclerosi "prematura" dei nefroni sovraccaricati. Questa ipotesi stimolante, se provata, potrebbe individuare un rischio maggiore di ipertensione e di complicanze cardiovascolari associate a essa nel periodo neonatale.

La rete glomerulare dei capillari specializzati funge da meccanismo di filtrazione dei reni. I capillari glomerulari sono rivestiti da cellule endoteliali (Fig. 508-4) e hanno un citoplasma molto sottile che contiene molti fori (fenestrazioni). La membrana basale glomerulare (GBM, *Glomerular Basement Membrane*) forma uno strato continuo tra le cellule endoteliali e mesangiali su un lato e le cellule epiteliali sull'altro. La membrana ha 3 strati: (1) una lamina centrale densa al microscopio elettronico; (2) la lamina rara interna, che giace tra la lamina densa e le cellule endoteliali; (3) la lamina rara esterna, tra la lamina densa e le cellule epiteliali. Le cellule epiteliali viscerali coprono il capillare e proiettano "podociti" che si attaccano alla lamina rara esterna. Tra i podociti vi sono spazi o fessure di filtrazione. Il mesangio (cellule mesangiali e matrice) si estende tra i capillari glomerulari sul lato delle cellule endoteliali della GBM e forma la parte mediale della parete capillare; esso può fungere da struttura di supporto per i capillari glomerulari e probabilmente ha un ruolo nella regolazione del flusso ematico e nella filtrazione glomerulare, nonché nell'eliminazione delle macromolecole (come gli immunocomplessi) dal glomerulo tramite la fagocitosi intracellulare oppure mediante il trasporto attraverso i canali intracellulari fino alla regione iuxtaglomerulare. La capsula di Bowman, che circonda il glomerulo, è costituita da (1) una membrana di base, che è in continuità con le membrane basali dei capillari glomerulari e dei tubuli prossimali, (2) cellule epiteliali parietali, che sono in continuità con le cellule epiteliali viscerali.

Fogo A: Renal pathology. In Avner ED, Harmon WE, Niaudet P (editors): *Pediatric Nephrology*, 5th ed. Baltimore, Lippincott Williams & Wilkins, 2004, pp 475–500.

Kon V, Ichikawa I: In Avner ED, Harmon WE, Niaudet P (editors): *Pediatric Nephrology*, 5th ed. Baltimore, Lippincott Williams & Wilkins, 2004, pp 25–44.

508.2 • Filtrazione glomerulare

Quando il sangue attraversa i capillari glomerulari, il plasma viene filtrato attraverso le loro pareti. L'ultrafiltrato, che non contiene cellule, include tutte le sostanze nel plasma (elettroliti, glucosio, fosfati, urea, creatinina, peptidi, proteine a basso peso molecolare), tranne le proteine (come l'albumina e le globuline), con un peso molecolare di ≥65 kd. Il filtrato si raccoglie nello spazio di Bowman ed entra nei tubuli, dove la sua composizione viene modificata dalla secrezione e dall'assorbimento di soluti e liquidi in base a meccanismi omeostatici tubulari rigidamente regolati, finché abbandona il rene sotto forma di urina.

La filtrazione glomerulare è il risultato netto di forze contrastanti attraverso la parete capillare. La forza per l'ultrafiltrazione (pressione idrostatica capillare glomerulare) è il risultato della pressione arteriosa sistemica, modificata dal tono delle arteriole afferenti ed efferenti. La forza principale che si oppone all'ultrafiltrazione è la pressione oncotica capillare glomerulare, che viene creata dal gradiente tra l'elevata concentrazione delle proteine plasmatiche all'interno del capillare e l'ultrafiltrato quasi privo di proteine nella capsula di Bowman. La filtrazione può essere modificata dalla velocità del flusso del plasma glomerulare, dalla pressione idrostatica all'interno della capsula di Bowman e dalla permeabilità della parete capillare glomerulare.

Benché la filtrazione glomerulare cominci attorno alla nona settimana di vita fetale, la funzione renale non è necessaria per la normale omeostasi intrauterina, perché la placenta funge da organo escretorio fetale principale. Dopo la nascita, la velocità di filtrato glomerulare (GFR, *Glomerular Filtration Rate*) aumenta fino al termine della crescita verso la fine del secondo decennio di vita. Per favorire il confronto tra i valori di GFR dei bambini e degli adulti, la GFR viene standardizzata sulla superficie corporea (1,73 m^2) di un adulto di 70 kg. Anche dopo la correzione in base all'area di superficie, la GFR di un bambino non si avvicina ai valori dell'adulto fino al terzo anno di vita (Fig. 508-5).

La GFR può essere stimata mediante la misurazione del livello di creatinina nel siero (Fig. 508-6). La creatinina deriva dal metabolismo muscolare; la sua produzione è relativamente costante e la sua escrezione avviene prevalentemente tramite la filtrazione glomerulare, benché la secrezione tubulare possa diventare importante nell'insufficienza renale. Contrariamente alla concentrazione dell'azotemia, che è influenzata dallo stato di idratazione e dal bilancio dell'azoto, il livello di creatinina nel siero è prevalentemente influenzato dal livello della funzione glomerulare. La creatinina sierica è importante solo per stimare la GFR in stato di equilibrio. Un paziente può avere un livello di creatinina normale senza un'efficace funzione renale poco dopo l'insorgenza di una insufficienza renale acuta con anuria. In questo contesto clinico,

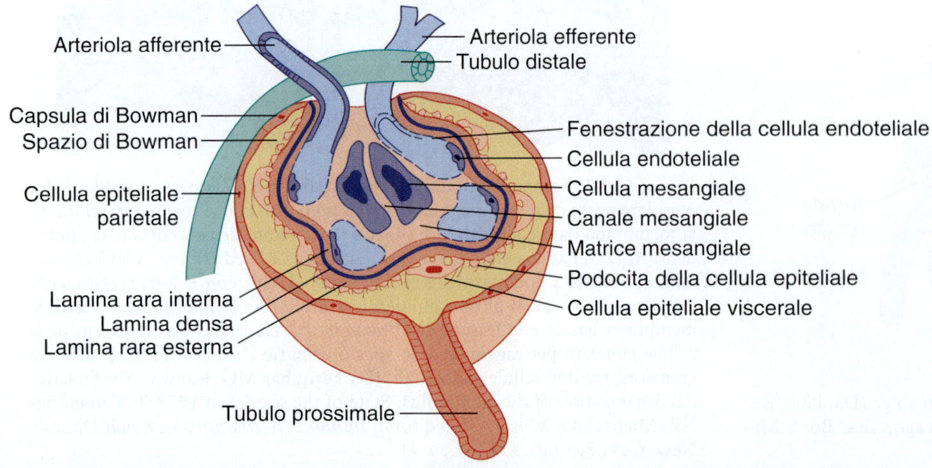

Figura 508-4. Rappresentazione schematica del glomerulo e delle strutture circostanti.

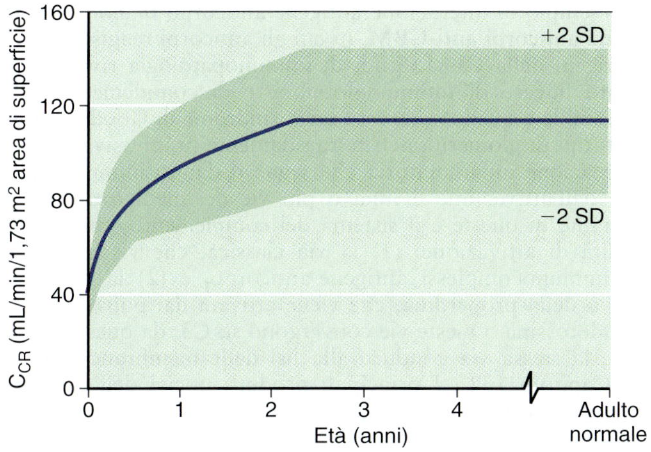

Figura 508-5. Alterazioni nel valore normale della velocità di filtrazione glomerulare misurata in base alla clearance della creatinina (CCR), quando standardizzata su mL/min/1,73 m² di superficie corporea. La *linea continua* indica la media, l'*area ombreggiata* include due deviazioni standard. (Da McCrory W: *Developmental Nephrology*. Cambridge, MA, Harvard University Press, 1972.)

la creatinina sierica può essere una misura non sensibile della funzione renale ridotta, perché il livello della stessa non aumenta oltre il valore normale finché la GFR non scende del 30-40%. La cistatina C, un inibitore della proteasi di 13,6 kd prodotto dalle cellule nucleate, è un marker endogeno che può essere più affidabile delle misurazioni della creatinina sierica nello stimare la GFR, dato che i livelli sierici non sono interessati da sesso, altezza, massa muscolare, bilirubina o emolisi.

La misurazione precisa della GFR viene effettuata quantificando la clearance di una sostanza liberamente filtrata attraverso la parete capillare e che non viene né riassorbita né secreta dai tubuli. La clearance (C_s) di questa sostanza è il volume di plasma che, quando viene completamente privato della sostanza contenuta, produce una quantità di tale sostanza uguale a quella escreta nelle urine in un periodo di tempo specificato. La clearance è rappresentata dalla seguente formula: C_s (mL/min) = U_s (mg/mL) × V (mL/min)/P_s (mg/mL), dove C_s è uguale alla clearance della sostanza s, U_s riflette la concentrazione urinaria di s, V rappresenta la velocità di flusso urinario e P_s è uguale alla concentrazione plasmatica di s. Per correggere la clearance in base all'area della superficie corporea, la formula è:

$$\text{Clearance corretta (mL/min/1,73 m}^2\text{)} = \text{Cs (mL/min)} \times \frac{1{,}73}{\text{area di superficie (m}^2\text{)}}$$

La GFR viene misurata in maniera ottimale dalla clearance di inulina, un polimero di fruttosio con un peso molecolare di circa 5 kd. Ma dato che la tecnica di clearance dell'inulina è scomoda, la GFR viene comunemente stimata dalla clearance della creatinina endogena. Quando la GFR è relativamente normale, la clearance della creatinina si avvicina molto a quella dell'inulina; man mano che la GFR si riduce, una quantità crescente della creatinina totale nell'urina viene secreta dai tubuli e questo determina una clearance della creatinina che sovrastima progressivamente la GFR effettiva. Pertanto, quando il livello di creatinina sierica supera i 2,0 mg/dL (180 μmol/L), le alterazioni della funzione renale devono essere monitorate mediante la concentrazione della creatinina sierica.

L'assenza delle proteine plasmatiche con dimensioni maggiori di quelle dell'albumina dal filtrato glomerulare conferma l'efficacia della parete capillare glomerulare come barriera di filtrazione. I fattori principali che limitano la filtrazione di queste e altre macromolecole includono le dimensioni e la carica ionica.

Studi sulla clearance delle macromolecole negli animali non hanno rilevato alcuna limitazione alla filtrazione di molecole con dimensioni fino a quelle dell'inulina, ma con l'ulteriore aumento delle dimensioni la filtrazione via via diminuisce, avvicinandosi a zero per le sostanze con dimensioni pari a quelle dell'albumina. Studi morfologici suggeriscono che la barriera di filtrazione selettiva per dimensioni è costituita dalla GBM.

La cellula endoteliale, la membrana basale e la cellula epiteliale della parete capillare glomerulare possiedono cariche ioniche negative forti, che sono una conseguenza di due frazioni caricate negativamente: i proteoglicani (eparansolfato) e le glicoproteine contenenti acido sialico. Le proteine nel sangue hanno un punto isoelettrico relativamente basso e recano una carica negativa netta, per cui vengono respinte dai siti caricati negativamente nella parte capillare glomerulare, limitando così la filtrazione.

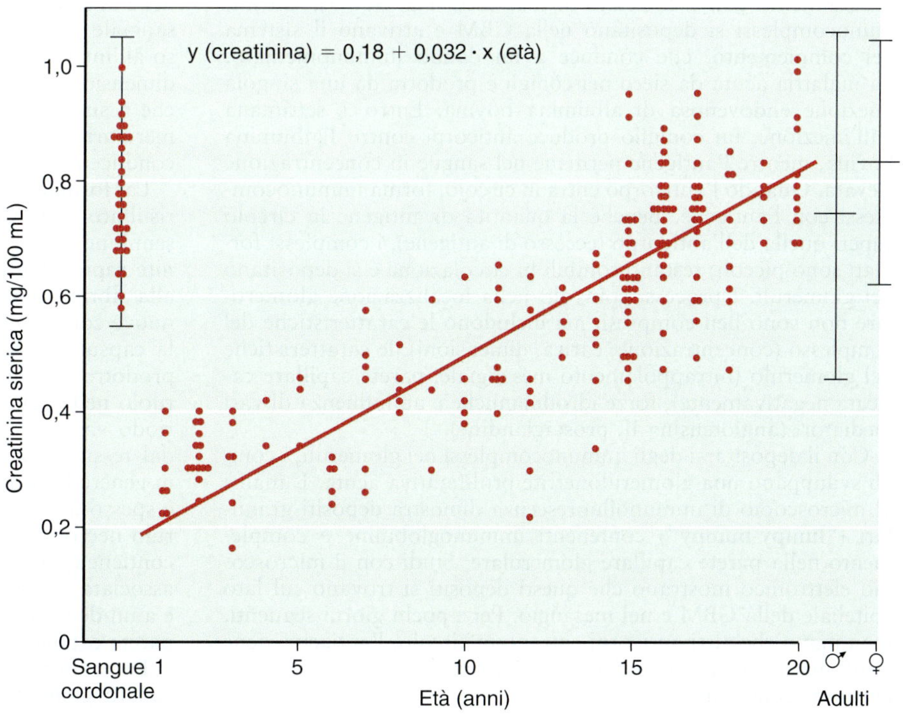

Figura 508-6. La creatinina sierica in relazione all'età. (Tratta da McCrory W: *Developmental Nephrology*. Cambridge, MA, Harvard University Press, 1972.)

Arant BS Jr: Postnatal development of renal function during the first year of life. *Pediatr Nephrol* 1987;1:308–313.
Finney H, Newman DJ, Thakkar H, et al: Reference ranges for plasma cystatin C and creatinine measurements in premature infants, neonates, and older children. *Arch Dis Child* 2000;82:71–75.
Kon V, Ichikawa I: In Avner ED, Harmon WE, Niaudet P (editors): *Pediatric Nephrology*, 5th ed. Baltimore, Lippincott Williams & Wilkins, 2004, pp 25–44.
Schwartz GJ, Haycock GB, Spitzer A: Plasma creatinine and urea concentration in children: Normal values for age and sex. *J Pediatr* 1976;88:828–837.

508.3 • Malattie glomerulari

PATOGENESI. Il danno glomerulare può essere la conseguenza di disturbi genetici, immunologici o della coagulazione. Le malattie genetiche del glomerulo derivano da: (1) mutazioni negli esoni del DNA che codificano le unità trascrizionali, le quali subiscono la traslazione nei ribosomi che formano le proteine situate all'interno del glomerulo, dell'interstizio o dell'epitelio tubulare; (2) mutazioni nei geni di regolazione che controllano la trascrizione del DNA; (3) una modifica post-trascrizionale anomala delle trascrizioni dell'RNA; (4) una modifica post-traslazionale anomala delle proteine. Il danno immunologico è la causa più comune e determina una **glomerulonefrite**, termine generico per indicare numerose malattie nonché termine istopatologico che significa infiammazione dei capillari glomerulari. L'evidenza che la glomerulonefrite deriva da danno immunologico include: (1) analogie morfologiche e immunopatologiche con la glomerulonefrite sperimentale immunomediata; (2) la dimostrazione di immunoreagenti (immunoglobuline, complemento) nei glomeruli; (3) anomalie nel complemento sierico e il riscontro di autoanticorpi (anti-GBM) in alcune di queste malattie (Fig. 508-7). Sembra che vi siano 2 meccanismi principali di danno immunologico: (1) il deposito glomerulare degli immunocomplessi antigene-anticorpo circolanti e (2) l'interazione dell'anticorpo con l'antigene locale *in situ*. Nell'ultima circostanza, l'antigene può essere un componente normale del glomerulo (il dominio non collagenoso [NC-1] del collagene di tipo IV, un antigene putativo nella nefrite anti-GBM umana) oppure un antigene che si è depositato nel glomerulo.

Nelle malattie **mediate da immunocomplessi** l'anticorpo è prodotto contro e si combina con un antigene circolante che generalmente non è correlato al rene (vedi Fig. 508-7). Gli immunocomplessi si depositano nella GBM e attivano il sistema del complemento, che conduce a un danno immunomediato. La malattia acuta da siero nei conigli è prodotta da una singola iniezione endovenosa di albumina bovina. Entro 1 settimana dall'iniezione, un coniglio produce anticorpi contro l'albumina bovina, mentre l'antigene permane nel sangue in concentrazione elevata. Quando l'anticorpo entra in circolo, forma immunocomplessi con l'antigene. Benché la quantità di antigene in circolo superi quella dell'anticorpo (eccesso di antigene), i complessi formati sono piccoli, restano solubili in circolazione e si depositano nei glomeruli. I processi coinvolti nella localizzazione glomerulare non sono ben compresi, ma includono le caratteristiche del complesso (concentrazione, carica, dimensioni), le caratteristiche del glomerulo (intrappolamento mesangiale, parete capillare caricata negativamente), forze idrodinamiche e un'influenza di vari mediatori (angiotensina II, prostaglandine).

Con il depositarsi degli immunocomplessi nei glomeruli, i conigli sviluppano una glomerulonefrite proliferativa acuta. L'analisi al microscopio di immunofluorescenza dimostra depositi granulari (**"lumpy-bumpy"**) contenenti immunoglobuline e complemento nella parete capillare glomerulare. Studi con il microscopio elettronico mostrano che questi depositi si trovano sul lato epiteliale della GBM e nel mesangio. Per i pochi giorni seguenti, man mano che altri anticorpi entrano in circolo, l'antigene viene in ultima analisi rimosso dalla circolazione e la glomerulonefrite entra in remissione.

Un esempio di interazione antigene-anticorpo *in situ* è la **malattia da anticorpi anti-GBM**, in cui gli anticorpi reagiscono con gli antigeni della GBM. Studi di immunopatologia rivelano un deposito lineare di immunoglobuline e di complemento sulla GBM, simile a quello osservato nella sindrome di Goodpasture e in certi tipi di glomerulonefrite rapidamente progressiva.

La reazione infiammatoria che segue il danno immunologico deriva dall'attivazione di una o più vie dei mediatori. La più importante di queste è il sistema del complemento, che ha due modalità di attivazione: (1) la via classica, che viene attivata dagli immunocomplessi antigene-anticorpo, e (2) la via alternativa o della properdina, che viene attivata dai polisaccaridi e dall'endotossina. Queste vie convergono su C3; da questo punto in poi, la stessa via conduce alla lisi delle membrane cellulari (vedi Capitolo 132). I principali prodotti nocivi dell'attivazione del complemento sono generati dopo l'attivazione del C3 e includono l'anafilotossina (che stimola le proteine contrattili all'interno delle pareti vascolari e aumenta la permeabilità vascolare) e fattori chemiotattici (C5a), che richiamano i neutrofili e forse i macrofagi al sito di attivazione del complemento, dove le cellule rilasciano sostanze che danneggiano le cellule vascolari e le membrane basali.

Il sistema della coagulazione può essere attivato direttamente, dopo il danno alle cellule endoteliali che espone lo strato subendoteliale trombogeno (che avvia la cascata di coagulazione), oppure indirettamente, dopo l'attivazione del complemento. Depositi di fibrina possono presentarsi all'interno dei capillari glomerulari oppure nella capsula glomerulare in formazioni a semiluna. L'attivazione del processo di coagulazione può innescare il sistema delle chinine, che produce anche fattori chemiotattici e analoghi all'anafilotossina.

ANATOMIA PATOLOGICA. Il glomerulo può essere leso da numerosi meccanismi, ma possiede solo un numero limitato di risposte istopatologiche, per cui differenti malattie possono produrre alterazioni microscopiche simili.

La proliferazione delle cellule glomerulari si verifica nella maggior parte delle forme di glomerulonefrite e può essere generalizzata, con l'interessamento di tutti i glomeruli, o focale, con l'interessamento di alcuni ma non di altri. All'interno di un singolo glomerulo, la proliferazione può essere diffusa e coinvolgere tutte le sue parti, oppure segmentale e interessare solo alcune aree ma non altre. In generale, la proliferazione riguarda le cellule endoteliali e mesangiali ed è frequentemente associata a un aumento nella matrice mesangiale (vedi Fig. 508-7). La proliferazione mesangiale può derivare da una deposizione dell'immunocomplesso all'interno del mesangio, provocando un ingrossamento nelle dimensioni e nel numero delle cellule e nella matrice mesangiale, che a sua volta può provocare l'aumento delle dimensioni glomerulari e il restringimento dei lumi dei capillari glomerulari, conducendo all'insufficienza renale.

La **formazione di semilune** nella capsula di Bowman è un risultato della proliferazione delle cellule epiteliali parietali. Le semilune si sviluppano in varie forme di glomerulonefrite (definite **rapidamente progressive**) e si pensa che siano una risposta alla fibrina depositata nella capsula di Bowman. Le semilune nuove contengono fibrina, cellule epiteliali in proliferazione della capsula di Bowman, materiale simile alla membrana basale prodotto da queste cellule e macrofagi che possono avere un ruolo nella genesi della lesione glomerulare. Nell'arco di un periodo variabile da giorni a settimane, la semiluna viene invasa dal tessuto connettivo (semiluna fibroepiteliale), determinando in genere l'obsolescenza glomerulare. La formazione di semilune è spesso associata alla morte delle cellule glomerulari. Il glomerulo necrotico ha un caratteristico aspetto eosinofilo e di solito contiene residui nucleari. La formazione di semilune è usualmente associata alla proliferazione generalizzata delle cellule mesangiali e a un deposito di immunocomplessi o anticorpi anti-GBM nella parete capillare glomerulare.

Determinate forme di glomerulonefrite acuta mostrano un essudato glomerulare di cellule ematiche, tra cui neutrofili, eosi-

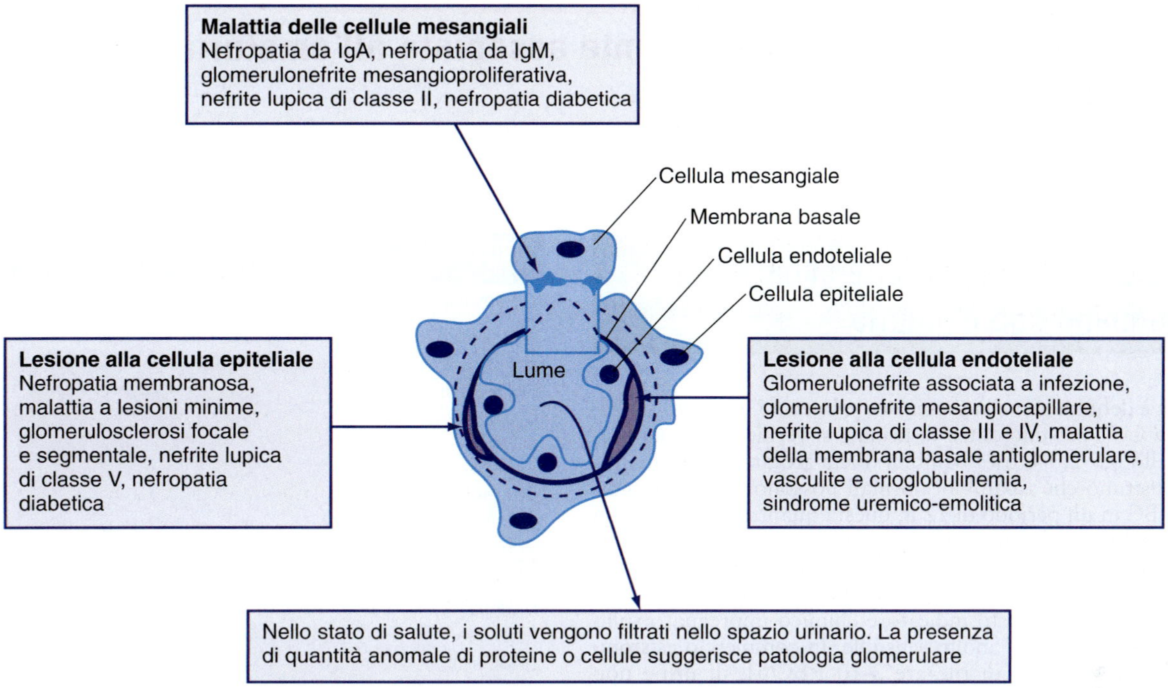

Figura 508-7. Ubicazione cellulare del danno durante la glomerulonefrite. Le cellule mesangiali sono direttamente esposte alla circolazione. Il deposito di immunocomplessi all'interno di queste cellule è tipicamente osservato nelle malattie come la nefropatia da IgA; esso causa la proliferazione e l'espansione delle cellule conducendo a ematuria, proteinuria e compromissione renale. Le cellule epiteliali, in associazione alla membrana basale, consentono la filtrazione dei soluti plasmatici ma ritardano il passaggio delle cellule e delle proteine plasmatiche. La malattia correlata a queste cellule è caratterizzata dalla presenza di depositi sottoepiteliali e dall'appiattimento dei podociti che si innestano nella membrana basale con il conseguente sconvolgimento della barriera di filtrazione e la proteinuria. La malattia delle cellule endoteliali può derivare dal deposito di immunocomplessi (come si verifica nella glomerulonefrite mesangiocapillare), dall'attacco degli anticorpi alla membrana basale (malattia di Goodpasture) oppure da un trauma e dall'attivazione della coagulazione (sindrome uremico-emolitica). La proliferazione delle cellule endoteliali e la necrosi sono accompagnate dall'accumulo di leucociti e dalla rottura della membrana basale, dalla formazione di semilune nonché dall'alterazione dell'architettura glomerulare. Ne consegue un quadro nefritico rapidamente progressivo. (Da Chadban SJ, Atkins RC: Glomerulonephritis. *Lancet* 2005;365:1797-1806.)

nofili, basofili e cellule mononucleate. L'aspetto ispessito della GBM può derivare da un aumento reale della larghezza della membrana (come si verifica nella glomerulopatia membranosa), da un deposito massivo di immunocomplessi con caratteristiche di colorazione simili alla membrana (come accade nel lupus eritematoso sistemico) oppure dall'interposizione di cellule mesangiali e di matrice nello spazio subendoteliale tra le cellule endoteliali e la GBM. Quest'ultimo caso può conferire alla membrana di base un aspetto diviso, come viene riscontrato nella glomerulonefrite membrano-proliferativa di tipo I e in altre patologie.

Il termine **sclerosi** si riferisce alla presenza di tessuto cicatriziale all'interno del glomerulo e viene occasionalmente utilizzato dai patologi per indicare un aumento nella matrice mesangiale.

La **fibrosi tubulointerstiziale** è presente in tutti i pazienti affetti da una malattia glomerulare che sviluppano un danno renale progressivo. Questa fibrosi è iniziata da una lesione ai tubuli renali e determina infiltrati di cellule mononucleate che liberano fattori solubili che a loro volta promuovono la fibrosi. Inoltre, le proteine matrici dell'interstizio renale cominciano ad accumularsi, portando infine alla distruzione dei tubuli renali e dei capillari peritubulari. La trasformazione effettiva dell'epitelio tubulare in tessuto mesenchimale può contribuire alla fibrosi tubulointerstiziale progressiva.

Chadban SJ, Atkins RC: Glomerulonephritis. *Lancet* 2005;365:1797–1806.

Fogo A: Renal pathology. In Avner ED, Harmon WE, Niaudet P (editors): *Pediatric Nephrology,* 5th ed. Baltimore, Lippincott Williams & Wilkins, 2004, pp 475–500.

Stevens LA, Coresh J, Greene T, Levey AS: Assessing kidney function-measured and estimated glomerular filtration rate. *N Engl J Med* 2006;354:2473–2483.

Sezione 2 — Malattie particolarmente associate all'ematuria — Ira D. Davis ed Ellis D. Avner

Capitolo 509 ■ Valutazione clinica del bambino con ematuria

L'ematuria è definita come la presenza di almeno 5 eritrociti (RBC, *Red Blood Cell*) per microlitro di urina e si verifica con una prevalenza dello 0,5-2,0% tra i bambini di età scolare. Studi quantitativi dimostrano che i bambini normali possono eliminare oltre 500 000 RBC in un periodo di 12 h; questa quantità aumenta con la febbre e/o lo sforzo fisico. In ambiente clinico, le stime qualitative vengono ottenute mediante strisce reattive ("stick") urinarie, che si avvalgono di una reazione chimica tra l'emoglobina (o mioglobina) e un composto indicatore chimico impregnato sullo stick "perossidasi-simile" molto sensibile. In commercio esistono strisce reattive in grado di rilevare 3-10 RBC/μL di urine non centrifugate, con ematuria significativa suggerita dalla presenza di >50 RBC/μL. Risultati falsamente negativi possono verificarsi in presenza di formalina (usata come conservante dell'urina) o di elevate concentrazioni urinarie di acido ascorbico. Risultati falsamente positivi possono invece essere osservati in bambini con febbre o successivamente a uno sforzo oppure in presenza di sangue mestruale o urine alcaline con un pH >9 o con una contaminazione con agenti ossidanti come il perossido di idrogeno usato per pulire il perineo prima di prelevare un campione. L'analisi al microscopio di 10-15 mL di urine appena centrifugate è essenziale per confermare la diagnosi di ematuria suggerita da uno stick positivo. Analisi delle urine di screening devono essere eseguite durante le visite di controllo del bambino sano a 5 anni e una volta durante il secondo decennio di vita (vedi Capitolo 5).

Urine rosse **senza** RBC vengono osservate in una serie di stati (Tab. 509-1). Le urine eme-positive senza RBC sono determinate dalla presenza dell'emoglobina o della mioglobina. L'emoglobinuria senza ematuria può verificarsi in caso di emolisi, mentre la mioglobinuria senza ematuria ha luogo in presenza della sindrome da rabdomiolisi derivante da un danno muscolare scheletrico ed è generalmente associata a un aumento di cinque volte della concentrazione della creatinchinasi nel plasma. È possibile che si riscontri una rabdomiolisi in seguito a una miosite virale, a una lesione da schiacciamento, ad anomalie gravi degli elettroliti (ipernatriemia, ipofosfatemia), a ipotensione, a coagulazione intravascolare disseminata, a tossine (farmaci e veleno) e ad attacchi convulsivi prolungati. L'urina emenegativa può apparire rossa, color cola o rosso bordeaux, a causa dell'ingestione di varie sostanze, di cibi (more, barbabietole) o di coloranti alimentari, mentre urine scure (o nere) possono essere la conseguenza di vari metaboliti urinari (vedi Tab. 509-1).

La valutazione del bambino con ematuria inizia con un'anamnesi attenta, l'esame obiettivo e l'analisi delle urine. Queste informazioni vengono utilizzate per determinare il livello dell'ematuria (tratto urinario superiore o inferiore) e per stabilire l'urgenza della valutazione in base alla sintomatologia. Considerazioni speciali vanno riservate all'anamnesi familiare, all'identificazione di anomalie anatomiche/sindromi malformative e alla presenza di una ematuria importante.

Le cause dell'ematuria sono elencate nella Tabella 509-2. Le sedi di quella del tratto urinario superiore sono all'interno del nefrone (glomerulo, tubuli convoluti/collettori e interstizio), mentre quelle del tratto urinario inferiore originano dal sistema pelvocaliceale, dall'uretere, dalla vescica o dall'uretra. L'ematuria dall'interno del glomerulo è spesso associata a urine brune, color cola o rosso bordeaux, alla proteinuria >100 mg/dL tramite stick urinario, a rilievi microscopici urinari di cilindri eritrocitari e a RBC urinari deformati (in particolare acantociti). L'ematuria che origina dai tubuli convoluti o collettori può essere associata alla presenza di leucociti o di cilindri cellulari epiteliali dei tubuli renali. Le sedi dell'ematuria del tratto urinario inferiore possono essere associate a una ematuria macroscopica, a una terminale (comparsa di ematuria macroscopica al termine del mitto urinario), a coaguli ematici, a una morfologia normale degli eritrociti urinari all'analisi microscopica e a una proteinuria minima all'esame con strisce reattive (<100 mg/dL).

TABELLA 509-1. Test di ematuria falsamente positivi

EME POSITIVI
Emoglobina
Mioglobina
EME NEGATIVI
Farmaci
Clorochina
Deferoxamina
Ibuprofene
Ferro-sorbitolo
Metronidazolo
Nitrofurantoina
Fenazopiridina (Pyridium)
Fenolftaleina
Fenotiazine
Rifampina
Salicilati
Sulfasalazina
Coloranti (verdura/frutta): bietole, more, coloranti alimentari
Metaboliti
Acido omogentisico
Melanina
Metemoglobina
Porfirina
Tirosinosi
Urati

I pazienti con ematuria possono presentarsi con una quantità di sintomi indicatori di malattie specifiche. Le urine color tè o cola, un edema facciale/corporeo, l'ipertensione e l'oliguria suggeriscono una sindrome nefritica acuta. Le malattie che comunemente si presentano come tale sindrome includono la glomerulonefrite postinfettiva, la nefropatia da IgA, la glomerulonefrite membrano-proliferativa, la porpora di Henoch-Schönlein (HSP, *Henoch-Schönlein Purpura*), la nefrite da lupus eritematoso sistemico (SLE, *Systemic Lupus Erythematosus*), la granulomatosi di Wegener, la poliarterite nodosa microscopica, la sindrome di Goodpasture e la sindrome uremico-emolitica. Un'anamnesi di recente infezione del tratto respiratorio superiore, cutanea o gastrointestinale suggerisce una glomerulonefrite acuta, la sindrome uremico-emolitica o la nefrite da HSP. Una eruzione cutanea e dolori articolari fanno pensare a una nefrite da HSP o da SLE. L'urgenza, la disuria e una febbre inspiegata indicano una infezione delle vie urinarie, mentre una colica renale suggerisce la nefrolitiasi. Una massa a livello del fianco può voler dire idronefrosi, malattia cistica, trombosi delle vene renali o tumore. L'ematuria associata a cefalea, alterazioni della vista, epistassi o insufficienza cardiaca segnalano un'ipertensione significativa. I pazienti con un'anamnesi di trauma richiedono una valutazione immediata. L'abuso deve essere sospettato in qualsiasi bambino che si presenti con escoriazioni senza spiegazione ed ematuria.

TABELLA 509-2. Cause di ematuria nei bambini

EMATURIA GLOMERULARE
Malattia renale isolata
Nefropatia da IgA (malattia di Berger)
Sindrome di Alport (nefrite ereditaria)
Nefropatia della membrana basale glomerulare sottile
GN postinfettiva (GN poststreptococcica)
Nefropatia membranosa
GN membranoproliferativa
Glomerulosclerosi segmentale focale
Malattia dell'antimembrana basale glomerulare
Malattia multisistemica
Nefrite da lupus eritematoso sistemico*
Nefrite da porpora di Henoch-Schönlein
Granulomatosi di Wegener
Poliarterite nodosa
Sindrome di Goodpasture
Sindrome emolotico-uremica
Glomerulopatia a cellule falciformi
Nefropatia da HIV
EMATURIA EXTRAGLOMERULARE
Tratto urinario superiore
Tubulointerstiziale
Pielonefrite
Nefrite interstiziale
Necrosi tubulare acuta
Necrosi papillare
Nefrocalcinosi
Vascolare
Trombosi arteriosa/venosa
Malformazioni (aneurismi, emangiomi)
Sindrome dello schiaccianoci
Cristalluria
Calcio
Ossalato
Acido urico
Emoglobinopatia (malattia/trait a cellule falciformi, emoglobina SC)
Anatomica
Idronefrosi
Malattia renale cistica
Malattia renale policistica
Displasia multicistica
Tumore (Wilms, rabdomiosarcoma, angiomiolipoma)
Trauma
Tratto urinario inferiore
Infiammazione (infettiva e non infettiva)
Cistite
Uretrite
Urolitiasi
Trauma
Coagulopatia
Sforzo intenso
Sindrome di Munchausen/Sindrome di Munchausen per procura

*Denota glomerulonefrite che si presenta con ipocomplementemia.
GN, glomerulonefrite.

Un'anamnesi familiare attenta è fondamentale nella valutazione iniziale del bambino con ematuria, date le numerose cause genetiche di patologie renali. Le malattie glomerulari ereditarie includono la nefrite ereditaria (sindrome di Alport), la malattia della membrana basale glomerulare sottile, la nefrite da SLE e la nefropatia da IgA (malattia di Berger). Altre malattie renali con ematuria con una componente ereditaria comprendono la malattia policistica renale, l'urolitiasi e la malattia/il trait a cellule falciformi.

L'esame obiettivo è fondamentale per valutare l'origine dell'ematuria. L'ipertensione, l'edema, l'epatosplenomegalia o segni di insufficienza cardiaca suggeriscono una glomerulonefrite acuta. Numerose malformazioni sono associate a una malattia renale, tra cui la sindrome di VATER (anomalie dei corpi Vertebrali, atresia Anale, fistola TracheoEsofagea e displasia Renale). Masse addominali possono essere causate da valvole uretrali posteriori, dall'ostruzione della giunzione ureteroplevica, dalla malattia del rene policistico o dal tumore di Wilms. L'ematuria osservata nei pazienti con anomalie neurologiche o cutanee può essere il risultato di una malattia cistica renale o di tumori collegati a numerose sindromi, tra cui la sclerosi tuberosa, la sindrome di von Hippel-Lindau e la sindrome di Zellweger (cerebroepatorenale). Anche le anomalie anatomiche dei genitali esterni possono essere associate a malattia renale.

I pazienti con una ematuria macroscopica presentano anche altri problemi, a causa dell'ansia che si genera nei genitori. Questa entità deve per esempio essere distinta dall'uretrorragia, che si riferisce a una emorragia uretrale (in assenza di urine) associata alla disuria e a macchie di sangue sulla biancheria dopo la minzione. Questo stato, che si verifica spesso nei ragazzi in età prepuberale a intervalli di parecchi mesi per un periodo di più anni, ha un decorso benigno e autolimitante. Le cause comuni dell'ematuria macroscopica sono elencate nella Tabella 509-3. Ciò che più di frequente la determina sono le infezioni del tratto urinario documentate o sospette. Meno del 10% dei pazienti ha una evidenza di glomerulonefrite. Episodi ricorrenti di ematuria macroscopica suggeriscono la nefropatia da IgA, la sindrome di Alport, la malattia della membrana basale glomerulare sottile, l'ipercalciuria o l'urolitiasi.

La Figura 509-1 illustra un approccio generale alla valutazione di laboratorio e radiologica del paziente con una ematuria glomerulare o extraglomerulare. I pazienti asintomatici con una ematuria microscopica isolata non devono essere sottoposti alla valutazione diagnostica prima che siano stati raccolti almeno altri 2 campioni di urina, nell'arco di un periodo di 1-2 settimane, che dimostrino un numero di eritrociti anomalo. In questo modo si riducono da 10 a 100 volte le indagini non necessarie.

Un bambino che abbia una ematuria microscopica isolata asintomatica persistente, con una durata superiore alle 2 settimane, pone un dilemma relativamente al grado di ulteriori indagini diagnostiche da eseguire (Tab. 509-4). Con questa presentazione clinica, una malattia significativa delle vie urinarie è un evento raro. La valutazione iniziale di questi bambini dovrebbe includere una urinocoltura, seguita da un esame su un campione isolato delle urine per la concentrazione di calcio e creatinina nei pazienti con coltura negativa. Nei pazienti afroamericani va inclusa una ricerca di malattia a cellule falciformi. Se questi studi risultano normali, è indicata un'analisi delle urine di tutti i parenti di primo grado. Occorre considerare l'ecografia renale e vescicale per escludere lesioni come tumori, malattia cistica, idronefrosi o urolitiasi. L'ecografia delle vie urinarie è l'indagine che fornisce più informazioni riguardo ai pazienti che si presentano con una ematuria macroscopica, dolore addominale, dolore al fianco o trauma. Se queste indagini risultano normali, si consiglia una valutazione della creatinina sierica e degli elettroliti.

L'individuazione di determinate anomalie ematologiche può restringere la diagnosi differenziale. In questo contesto, l'anemia può essere causata da (1) un'emodiluizione secondaria all'ipervolemia associata a una insufficienza renale acuta; (2) una ridotta produzione di globuli rossi nell'insufficienza renale cronica; (3) un'emolisi da sindrome emolitico-uremica o da SLE; (4) una per-

TABELLA 509-3. Cause comuni di ematuria macroscopica

Infezione del tratto urinario
Stenosi meatale
Irritazione perineale
Trauma
Urolitiasi/ipercalciuria
Coagulopatia
Tumore
Glomerulare
Nefropatia da IgA
Sindrome di Alport (nefrite ereditaria)
Malattia della membrana basale glomerulare sottile
Glomerulonefrite postinfettiva
Nefrite da porpora di Henoch-Schönlein
Nefrite da lupus eritematoso sistemico

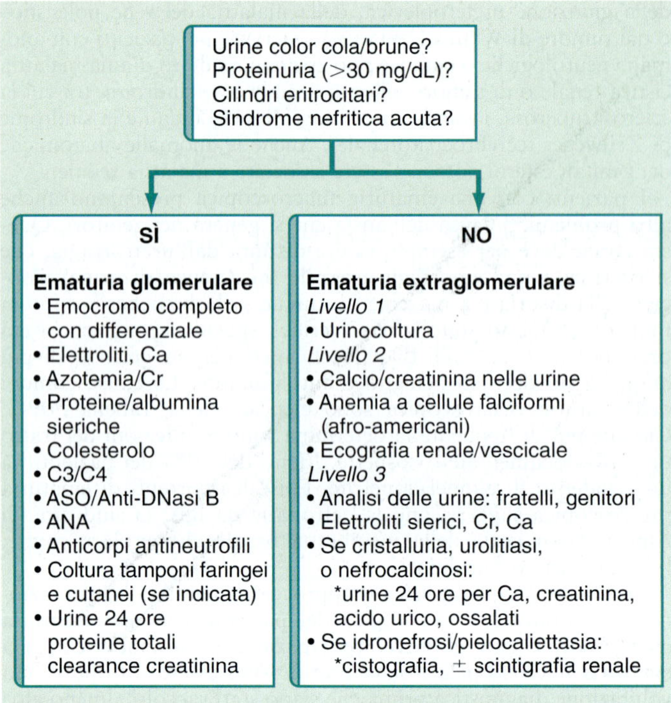

Figura 509-1. Algoritmo dell'approccio generale alla valutazione di laboratorio e radiologica del paziente con ematuria glomerulare o extraglomerulare. ANA, anticorpo antinucleare; ASO, antistreptolisina O; BUN, azoto ureico ematico (*Blood Urea Nitrogen*); C3/C4, complemento; CBC, esame del sangue completo; Cr, creatinina; RBC, eritrocita.

TABELLA 509-4. Diagnosi differenziale di ematuria sintomatica e asintomatica

CONFERMARE LA PRESENZA DI GLOBULI ROSSI
Sintomatica
Sintomi renali
Infezioni del tratto urinario
Nefrolitiasi
Uretrorragia
Sintomi sistemici
Porpora di Henoch-Schönlein
Sclerosi tuberosa
Asintomatica
Ipercalciuria
Malattia cistica
Ostruzione
Vascolare
Malformazione arterovenosa
Trombosi
Trauma
Tumore
Emoglobinopatie
Coagulopatie
Ematuria indotta da sforzo
Ematuria familiare benigna (membrana basale sottile)
Glomerulonefrite (in risoluzione)
Nefrite postinfettiva acuta
Nefropatia da IgA
Porpora di Henoch-Schönlein

Da Kliegman RM, Greenbaum LA, Lyle PS: *Practical Strategies in Pediatric Diagnosis and Therapy*, 2nd ed. Philadelphia, Elsevier, 2004.

dita di sangue per emorragia polmonare come riscontrata nella sindrome di Goodpasture o nella melena in pazienti con l'HSP o la sindrome emolitico-uremica. L'esame dello striscio del sangue periferico può rivelare un processo microangiopatico coerente con la sindrome uremico-emolitica, la trombosi delle vene renali, la vasculite o il LES. In quest'ultimo caso, la presenza di autoanticorpi può determinare un test di Coombs positivo, la presenza di anticorpi antinucleo, leucopenia e malattia multisistemica. La trombocitopenia può essere la conseguenza di una ridotta produzione di piastrine (tumori maligni) o di un loro aumentato consumo (SLE, porpora trombocitopenica idiopatica, sindrome emolitico-uremica, trombosi delle vene renali). Benché la morfologia dei globuli rossi urinari possa risultare normale con un'emorragia del tratto inferiore e dismorfica con un'emorragia glomerulare, la morfologia cellulare è correlabile in maniera affidabile al sito dell'ematuria. Il test di screening migliore per una diatesi emorragica è un'anamnesi accurata. Di norma non vengono eseguiti studi sulla coagulazione a meno che l'anamnesi familiare o personale non suggerisca una tendenza all'emorragia.

La cistouretrografia minzionale è necessaria solo nei pazienti con una infezione delle vie urinarie, cicatrici renali, idrouretere pielocaliectasia. La cistoscopia è una procedura non necessaria e costosa nei soggetti con ematuria, che comporta i rischi associati all'anestesia. Questa procedura deve essere riservata alla valutazione dei rari casi di bambini con una massa vescicale osservata all'ecografia, anomalie uretrali causate da un trauma, valvole uretrali posteriori o tumore. L'ematuria macroscopica unilaterale localizzata mediante la cistoscopia viene osservata raramente nel paziente pediatrico.

Si raccomanda di inviare a un nefrologo pediatra i pazienti con nefrite (glomerulonefrite, nefrite tubulointerstiziale), ipertensione, insufficienza renale, urolitiasi/nefrocalcinosi o un'anamnesi familiare di malattia renale come la malattia renale policistica o la nefrite ereditaria. La biopsia renale è indicata per i bambini con una ematuria microscopica persistente o una ematuria macroscopica ricorrente associata a una funzione renale ridotta, a proteinuria o a ipertensione.

I bambini con una ematuria isolata asintomatica persistente e una valutazione normale vanno sottoposti a un controllo annuale dei valori di creatinina sierica e a uno trimestrale della pressione sanguigna e delle urine fino alla risoluzione dell'ematuria. Le diagnosi da considerare in questa situazione includono la glomerulonefrite postinfettiva in risoluzione, la malattia della membrana basale sottile, la nefropatia IgA o lo sforzo/trauma pesante. Occorre considerare un invio al nefrologo pediatra per i pazienti con una ematuria asintomatica persistente con una durata superiore a 1 anno.

Bergstein J, Leiser J, Andreoli S: The clinical significance of asymptomatic gross and microscopic hematuria in children. *Arch Pediatr Adolesc Med* 2005;159:353–355.

Cohen RA, Brown RS: Microscopic hematuria. *N Engl J Med* 2003;348:2330–2338.

Feld LG, Waz WR, Perez LM, et al: Hematuria. An integrated medical and surgical approach. *Pediatr Clin North Am* 1997;44:1191–1210.

Meyers KE: Evaluation of hematuria in children. *Urol Clin North Am* 2004;3:559–573.

Capitolo 510 ■ Malattie glomerulari isolate con ematuria macroscopica ricorrente

Circa il 10% dei bambini con ematuria macroscopica ha una forma di glomerulonefrite acuta o cronica che può essere associata a una malattia sistemica. L'ematuria grave, che di solito è caratterizzata da urine brune o color cola, può essere non dolorosa o associarsi a un vago dolore al fianco o all'addome. La presentazione con un'ematuria macroscopica è comune entro 1-2 giorni dall'insorgenza di un'infezione apparentemente virale del tratto respiratorio superiore in molte forme di glomerulonefrite, come la nefropatia da IgA e tipicamente si risolve entro 5 giorni. Questo periodo relativamente breve contrasta con uno di latenza di 7-21 giorni che si verifica tra la comparsa di una faringite streptococcica o un'infezione cutanea impetiginizzata e lo sviluppo di una glomerulonefrite acuta poststreptococcica. In queste circostanze, l'ematuria macroscopica può durare fino a 4-6 settimane. Ematuria macroscopica può essere osservata anche nei bambini con malattie della membrana basale glomerulare (GBM, *Glomerular Basement Membrane*), come la nefrite ereditaria (sindrome di Alport) e la malattia della GBM sottile. Tutte queste patologie possono manifestarsi anche sotto forma di una ematuria microscopica e/o di una proteinuria senza ematuria macroscopica.

510.1 • Nefropatia da IgA (nefropatia di Berger)

La nefropatia da IgA è la malattia glomerulare cronica più comune in tutto il mondo. È caratterizzata da una predominanza di IgA all'interno dei depositi mesangiali del glomerulo in assenza di malattie sistemiche come il lupus eritematoso o la porpora di Henoch-Schönlein. Altre patologie con importanti depositi mesangiali di IgA includono l'artrite reumatoide, la spondilite anchilosante, l'artrite reattiva, la malattia infiammatoria intestinale, la malattia celiaca, la dermatite erpetiforme, l'HIV e la cirrosi epatica.

ANATOMIA PATOLOGICA E DIAGNOSI PATOLOGICA. Nel glomerulo si osservano una proliferazione mesangiale focale e segmentale e una matrice mesangiale aumentata (Fig. 510-1). Alcuni bambini mostrano una proliferazione mesangiale generalizzata, che può essere associata alla formazione di semilune e tessuto cicatriziale. L'IgA è l'immunoglobulina predominante depositata nel mesangio (Fig. 510-2), ma quantità minori di IgG, IgM, C3 e properdina sono comuni. Depositi mesangiali densi al microscopio elettronico vengono osservati nella maggior parte dei pazienti; inoltre, possono essere rilevati nelle regioni subendoteliali e subepiteliali della GBM.

La nefropatia da IgA è una malattia a immunocomplessi che sembra essere causata da anomalie nel sistema delle immunità IgA. Gruppi familiari di nefropatia da IgA indicano l'importanza dei fattori genetici e l'analisi genetica sul genoma suggerisce la sua associazione a 6q22-23 nei parenti con la stessa nefropatia IgA.

MANIFESTAZIONI CLINICHE E DI LABORATORIO. La maggior parte dei bambini con nefropatia da IgA negli Stati Uniti e in Europa si presenta con un'ematuria macroscopica, mentre quella microscopica e/o la proteinuria costituiscono la presentazione più comune in Giappone. Altri tipi di presentazione includono la sindrome nefritica acuta, la sindrome nefrosica o una sindrome nefritica-nefrosica combinata. La nefropatia da IgA viene osservata più frequentemente nei maschi che nelle femmine. L'ematuria macroscopica si verifica spesso in combinazione con un'infezione gastrointestinale o delle vie respiratorie superiori e può essere accompagnata a dolore lombare. La proteinuria è spesso inferiore a 1000 mg/24 h nei pazienti con un'ematuria microscopica asintomatica. Un'ipertensione da lieve a moderata viene frequentemente osservata nei soggetti con la sindrome nefritica o nefrosica, ma raramente è abbastanza grave da causare emergenze ipertensive. Livelli sierici normali di C3 nella nefropatia da IgA aiutano a distinguere questa malattia dalla glomerulonefrite poststreptococcica. I livelli sierici di IgA non hanno invece un valore diagnostico, in quanto risultano elevati solo nel 15% dei pazienti.

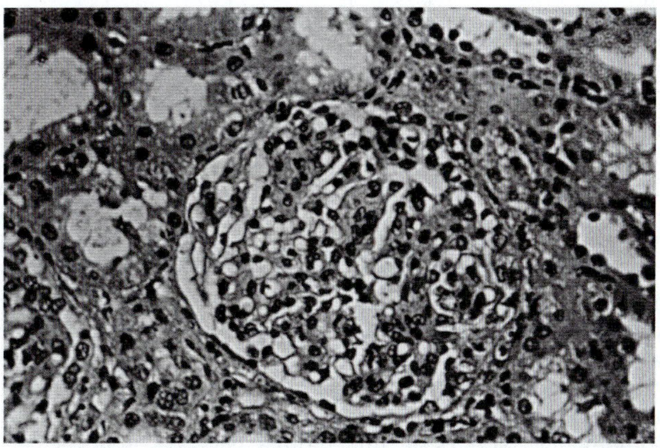

Figura 510-1. L'analisi mediante microscopia ottica della nefropatia da IgA dimostra una proliferazione mesangiale segmentale e una matrice aumentata (×180).

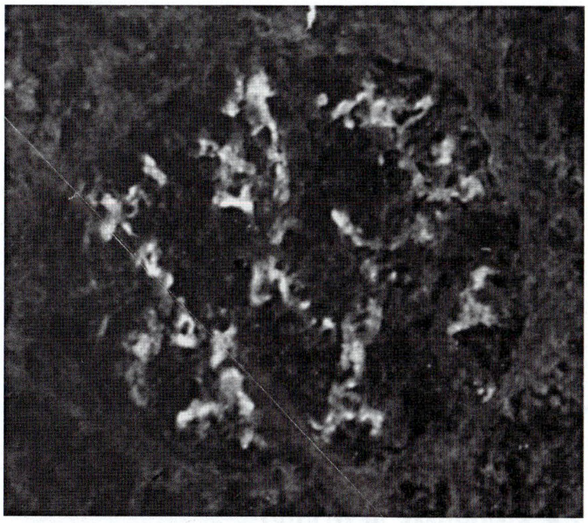

Figura 510-2. L'analisi mediante microscopio di immunofluorescenza dei campioni bioptici di un bambino con episodi di ematuria macroscopica dimostra un deposito mesangiale di immunoglobulina A (×150).

PROGNOSI E TRATTAMENTO. Benché la nefropatia da IgA non porti un danno renale significativo nella maggior parte dei bambini, nel 20-40% dei casi si sviluppa una malattia progressiva 15-20 anni dopo l'esordio. Pertanto, la maggior parte dei bambini con nefropatia da IgA non manifesta una disfunzione renale progressiva fino all'età adulta e questo pone l'esigenza di un attento follow-up a lungo termine. Gli indicatori prognostici sfavorevoli includono un'ipertensione persistente, una funzione renale diminuita e una proteinuria importante o prolungata. Una prognosi peggiore è suggerita dell'evidenza istologica di una proliferazione mesangiale diffusa, di semilune glomerulari estese, di glomerulosclerosi e di alterazioni tubulointerstiziali, tra cui l'infiammazione e la fibrosi.

Il trattamento primario della nefropatia da IgA è un controllo adeguato della pressione sanguigna. L'olio di pesce, che contiene acidi grassi polinsaturi omega 3 antinfiammatori, riduce la velocità di progressione renale negli adulti. La terapia immunosoppressiva con corticosteroidi a giorni alterni, oppure regimi farmacologici combinati e più intensi, possono risultare utili in alcuni pazienti. Gli inibitori dell'enzima di conversione dell'angiotensina e gli antagonisti dei recettori dell'angiotensina II sono efficaci nel ridurre la proteinuria e nel ritardare la velocità di progressione del danno renale, quando vengono usati come agenti singoli o in combinazione. La tonsillectomia può ridurre la frequenza dell'ematuria macroscopica e la velocità di progressione della malattia renale. I soggetti con una nefropatia da IgA possono sopportare con successo un trapianto renale. Benché la malattia ricorrente sia frequente, la perdita del trapianto causata da nefropatia da IgA si verifica solo nel 15-30% dei pazienti.

Bartosik LP, Lajoie, Sugar L, et al: Predicting progression in IgA nephropathy. *Am J Kidney Dis* 2001;38:728–735.

Delos Santos NM, Wyatt RJ: Pediatric IgA nephropathies: Clinical aspects and therapeutic approaches. *Semin Nephrol* 2004;24:269–286.

Dillon JJ: Angiotensin-converting enzyme inhibitors and angiotensin receptor blockers for IgA nephropathy. *Semin Nephrol* 2004;24:218–224.
Donadio JV, Grande JP: The role of fish oil/omega-3 fatty acids in the treatment of IgA nephropathy. *Semin Nephrol* 2004;3:225–243.
Gharavi AG, Yan Y, Scolari F, et al: IgA nephropathy, the most common cause of glomerulonephritis is linked to 6q22-23. *Nat Genet* 2000;26:354–357.
Samuels JA, Strippoli GF, Craig JC, et al: Immunosuppressive treatments for immunoglobulin A nephropathy: A meta-analysis of randomized controlled trials. *Nephrology (Carlton)* 2004;4:177–185.
Wang AY, Lai FM, Yu AW, et al: Recurrent IgA nephropathy in renal transplant allografts. *Am J Kidney Dis* 2001;38:588–596.
Wyatt RJ, Hogg RJ: Evidence-based assessment of treatment options for children with IgA nephropathies. *Pediatr Nephrol* 2001;16:156–167.
Xie Y, Chen X, Nishi S, et al: Relationship between tonsils and IgA nephropathy as well as indications of tonsillectomy. *Kidney Int* 2004;65:1135–1144.

510.2 • Sindrome di Alport

La sindrome di Alport (AS, *Alport Syndrome*), ossia la nefrite ereditaria, è una malattia geneticamente eterogenea causata da mutazioni nei geni che codificano per il collagene di tipo IV, un componente importante delle membrane basali. Queste alterazioni genetiche sono associate a una marcata variabilità nella presentazione clinica, nell'anamnesi naturale o nelle anomalie istologiche.

GENETICA. Circa l'85% dei pazienti ha una malattia legata al cromosoma X, causata da una mutazione nel gene *COL4A5*, che codifica la catena α5 del collagene di tipo IV. I soggetti con un sottotipo di AS legata al cromosoma X e una leiomiomatosi diffusa dimostrano una mutazione contigua all'interno dei geni *COL4A5* e *COL4A6*, che codificano rispettivamente le catene α5 e α6 del collagene di tipo IV. Le forme di AS autosomiche recessive sono causate da mutazioni nei geni *COL4A3* e *COL4A4* sul cromosoma 2, che codificano rispettivamente le catene α3 e α4 del collagene di tipo IV. Una forma autosomica dominante collegata al locus del gene *COL4A3-COL4A4* si presenta nel 5% dei casi.

ANATOMIA PATOLOGICA. I campioni bioptici dei reni durante il primo decennio di vita possono mostrare poche alterazioni alla microscopia ottica. Successivamente, i glomeruli possono sviluppare una proliferazione mesangiale e un ispessimento della parete capillare, con una conseguente sclerosi glomerulare progressiva. Con il progredire della malattia si sviluppano un'atrofia tubulare, un'infiammazione interstiziale e una fibrosi, nonché compaiono cellule tubulari o interstiziali contenenti lipidi, definite anche cellule schiumose. In generale, le indagini immunopatologiche non sono diagnostiche.

Nella maggior parte dei pazienti, le indagini di microscopia elettronica rivelano un ispessimento diffuso, un assottigliamento, la divisione e la stratificazione delle membrane basali dei glomeruli (Fig. 510-3) e dei tubuli. Tuttavia, nelle famiglie con le manifestazioni cliniche tipiche di AS, l'analisi ultrastrutturale della GBM può essere completamente normale, evidenziare alterazioni non specifiche oppure dimostrare solo un assottigliamento uniforme.

MANIFESTAZIONI CLINICHE. Tutti i soggetti con l'AS presentano un'ematuria microscopica asintomatica, che può risultare intermittente nelle bambine e nei maschi più giovani. Episodi singoli o ricorrenti di ematuria macroscopica, che in genere si verificano 1-2 giorni dopo un'infezione delle vie aree superiori, si osservano in circa il 50% dei pazienti. La proteinuria compare spesso nei soggetti maschi, ma può mancare del tutto, risultare lieve o intermittente nelle femmine. La presenza di una proteinuria progressiva, spesso superiore a 1 g/24 h, è frequente entro la seconda decade di vita e può essere sufficientemente grave da causare una sindrome nefrotica.

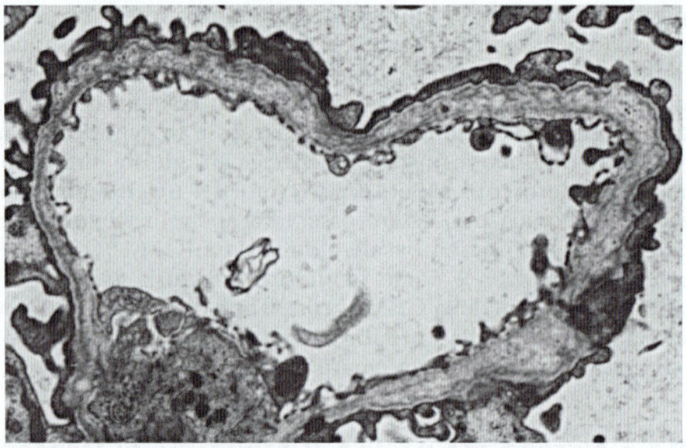

Figura 510-3. L'analisi con microscopio elettronico dei campioni bioptici di un bambino con sindrome di Alport evidenzia l'ispessimento, l'assottigliamento, la frammentazione e la stratificazione della membrana basale glomerulare (×1650). (Da Yum M, Bergstein JM: Basement membrane nephropathy. *Hum Pathol* 1983;14:996-1003.)

Le manifestazione extrarenali dell'AS includono deficit dell'udito e anomalie oculari. La perdita dell'udito neurosensoriale bilaterale, che non è mai congenita all'esordio, avviene nel 90% dei maschi emizigoti con un'AS legata al cromosoma X, nel 10% delle femmine eterozigoti con un'AS legata al cromosoma X e nel 67% dei soggetti con un'AS autosomica recessiva. Questo deficit comincia nel campo delle alte frequenze, ma progredisce fino a interessare il normale dialogo verbale, imponendo l'uso di ausili per l'udito. Le anomalie oculari, che affliggono il 30-40% dei pazienti con un'AS legata dal cromosoma X, includono il lenticono anteriore (protrusione della regione centrale del cristallino nella camera anteriore), la degenerazione maculare ed erosioni corneali. La leiomiomatosi dell'esofago, dell'albero tracheobronchiale e dei genitali femminili, nonché le anomalie piastriniche, sono eventi rari.

DIAGNOSI. Un'attenta anamnesi familiare, un'analisi di screening delle urine dei parenti di primo grado, un audiogramma e un esame oftalmologico sono fondamentali per formulare la diagnosi di AS. La presenza del lenticono anteriore è patognomonica. L'insorgenza dell'AS è molto probabile in un soggetto con ematuria e con almeno due tra le seguenti caratteristiche cliniche: degenerazione maculare, erosioni corneali ricorrenti, ispessimento e assottigliamento della GBM e sordità neurosensoriale. L'assenza di colorazione della membrana basale epidermica per la catena α5 del collagene di tipo IV negli emizigoti maschi e la colorazione della membrana basale epidermica discontinua nelle eterozigoti femmine è patognomonica dell'AS legata al cromosoma X. L'analisi mutazionale o l'analisi di linkage non sono facilmente disponibili per un impiego clinico di routine. La diagnosi prenatale è possibile per le famiglie con membri affetti da AS legata al cromosoma X che siano portatori di una mutazione identificata.

PROGNOSI E TRATTAMENTO. Il rischio di una disfunzione renale progressiva che conduca a un'insufficienza renale terminale (ESRD, *End-Stage Renal Disease*) è massimo tra gli emizigoti e gli omozigoti autosomici recessivi. Questa insufficienza ha luogo prima dei 30 anni in circa il 75% degli emizigoti con AS legata al cromosoma X, mentre il rischio negli eterozigoti per la forma legata al cromosoma X è del 12% a 40 anni e del 30% a 60. I fattori di rischio per la progressione sono un'ematuria macroscopica durante l'infanzia, una sindrome nefrosica e un ispessimento grave della GBM. Una variazione intrafamiliare dell'espressione fenotipica causa differenze significative nell'età di esordio della ESRD tra i membri della famiglia. Non esiste una terapia per l'AS, sebbene alcuni studi suggeriscano che la ciclosporina e gli ACE-inibitori possano rallentare la velocità di progressione del danno renale. Un trattamento attento delle complicanze dell'insufficienza renale, come l'ipertensione, l'anemia e lo squilibrio elettrolitico, è fondamentale. I pazienti con una ESRD vengono trattati con dialisi e trapianto di rene (vedi Capitolo 535.3). Tuttavia, circa il 5% di coloro che ricevono questo trapianto sviluppa una nefrite da anti-GBM, che si verifica prevalentemente nei soggetti maschi con AS legata al cromosoma X che sviluppano l'ESRD prima dei 30 anni.

Jais JP, Knebelmann B, Giatras I, et al: X-linked Alport syndrome: Natural history and genotype-phenotype correlations in girls and women belonging to 195 families: A "European Community Alport Syndrome Concerted Action" study. *J Am Soc Nephrol* 2003;14:2603–2610.

Kashtan CE: Familial hematuria due to type IV collagen mutations: Alport syndrome and thin basement membrane nephropathy. *Curr Opin Pediatr* 2004;16:177–181.

Proesmans W, Van Dyck M: Enalapril in children with Alport syndrome. *Pediatr Nephrol* 2004;19:271–275.

Wang YY, Rana K, Tonna S, et al: COL4A3 mutations and their clinical consequences in thin basement membrane nephropathy (TBMN). *Kidney Int* 2004;65:786–790.

510.3 • Malattia della membrana basale glomerulare sottile

La malattia della GBM sottile è definita dalla presenza di un'ematuria microscopica persistente e l'assottigliamento isolato della GBM all'analisi con microscopio elettronico. L'ematuria isolata in più membri di una famiglia, senza disfunzione renale, viene definita ematuria familiare benigna.

La malattia della GBM sottile può essere sporadica oppure trasmessa come trait autosomico dominante. Sono presenti mutazioni nei geni *COL4A3* e *COL4A4* negli eterozigoti con ematuria familiare benigna. Sono inoltre stati riferiti parenti con un assottigliamento isolato della GBM e l'assenza di mutazioni identificate all'interno dei geni del collagene di tipo IV.

In genere sussiste un'ematuria microscopica persistente, che spesso viene osservata per la prima volta durante l'infanzia. L'ematuria può esordire nell'età adulta e risultare intermittente. Può inoltre esservi un'ematuria macroscopica, in particolare dopo un'infezione respiratoria. Non esiste terapia. L'insufficienza renale progressiva, l'ipertensione, la proteinuria e le manifestazioni extrarenali sono eventi rari e suggeriscono la presenza dell'AS. L'assottigliamento della GBM è stato osservato anche nella nefropatia da IgA.

Savige J, Rana K, Tonna S, et al: Thin basement membrane nephropathy. *Kidney Int* 2003;64:1169–1178.

Capitolo 511 ■ Glomerulonefrite associata a infezioni

511.1 • Glomerulonefrite poststreptococcica acuta

Si tratta di un classico esempio di **sindrome nefritica acuta** caratterizzata dalla comparsa improvvisa di ematuria macroscopica, edema, ipertensione e insufficienza renale. La glomerulonefrite poststreptococcica acuta è una delle cause glomerulari più comuni di ematuria macroscopica nei bambini, superata solo dalla nefropatia da IgA.

EZIOLOGIA ED EPIDEMIOLOGIA. La glomerulonefrite poststreptococcica segue l'infezione faringotonsillare o cutanea causata da determinati ceppi "nefritogenici" dello streptococco β-emolitico del gruppo A. Non è chiaro quali siano i fattori che consentono solo a certi ceppi di streptococchi di essere nefritogenici. La glomerulonefrite poststreptococcica di solito compare dopo la faringite streptococcica durante i mesi freddi e le infezioni cutanee streptococciche o il pioderma durante i mesi caldi. Benché siano state descritte epidemie di nefrite in associazione a infezioni della gola (sierotipo 12) e della pelle (sierotipo 49), questa malattia è in genere sporadica.

ANATOMIA PATOLOGICA. I reni appaiono ingrossati simmetricamente. Anche tutti i glomeruli sono ingranditi e relativamente esangui e mostrano una proliferazione mesangiale diffusa con un aumento della matrice mesangiale (Fig. 511-1). La presenza di leucociti polimorfonucleati è comune nei glomeruli durante la fase precoce della malattia. Nei casi gravi possono essere osservate semilune e un'infiammazione interstiziale, alterazioni tuttavia aspecifiche della glomerulonefrite poststreptococcica. La microscopia in immunofluorescenza rivela depositi granulari (*lumpy-bumpy*) di immunoglobuline e complemento sulla membrana basale glomerulare e nel mesangio. Alla microscopia elettronica si notano depositi elettrondensi o "gibbosità" sul lato epiteliale della membrana basale glomerulare (Fig. 511-2).

PATOGENESI. Benché le indagini morfologiche e una riduzione nel livello del complemento sierico (C3) siano fortemente suggestive di glomerulonefrite poststreptococcica mediata da immunocomplessi, i meccanismi precisi mediante i quali gli streptococchi nefritogenici inducono la formazione di complessi non sono ancora stati determinati. Nonostante le somiglianze cliniche e istologiche con la malattia del siero acuta dei conigli, il riscontro di immunocomplessi circolanti nella glomerulonefrite poststreptococcica non è costante e l'attivazione del complemento avviene prevalentemente attraverso la via alternativa piuttosto che attraverso la via classica (attivata dall'immunocomplesso).

MANIFESTAZIONI CLINICHE. La glomerulonefrite poststreptococcica è più frequente nei bambini di età compresa tra i 5 e i 12 anni ed è rara prima dei 3 anni. Il paziente tipico sviluppa una sindrome nefritica acuta 1-2 settimane dopo una precedente faringite streptococcica oppure 3-6 settimane dopo un evento di pioderma streptococcico. La gravità dell'interessamento renale varia da un'ematuria microscopica asintomatica con funzione renale normale a un'insufficienza renale acuta. In base alla gravità della compromissione renale, i pazienti possono sviluppare gradi variabili di edema, ipertensione e oliguria. Inoltre, possono insorgere un'encefalopatia e/o un'insufficienza cardiaca causate da

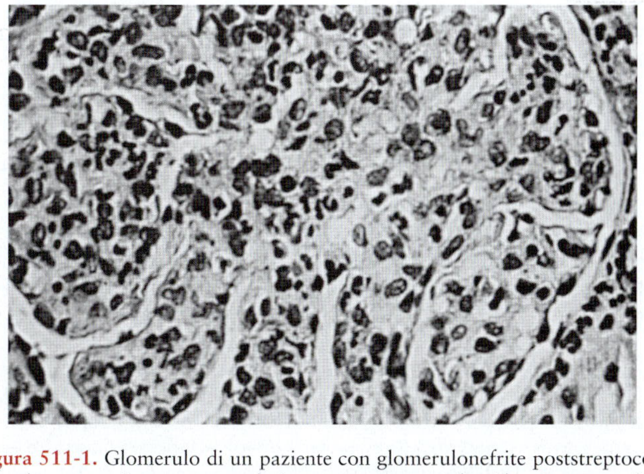

Figura 511-1. Glomerulo di un paziente con glomerulonefrite poststreptococcica che appare ingrossato e relativamente esangue ed evidenzia una proliferazione mesangiale e un'essudazione di neutrofili (×400).

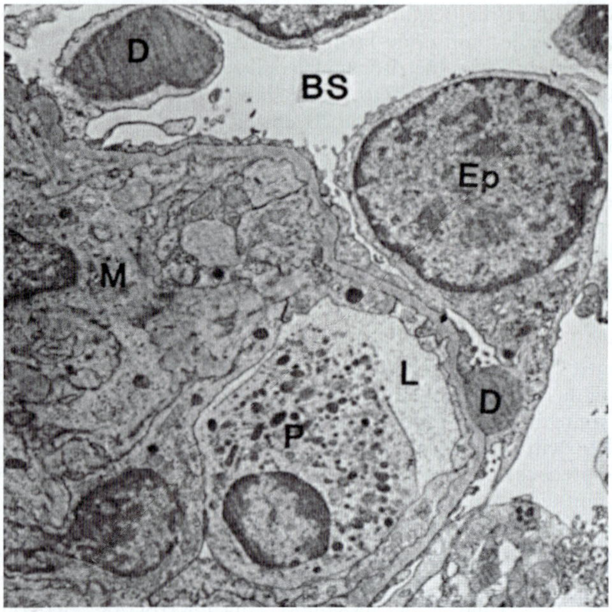

Figura 511-2. Analisi al microscopio elettronico della glomerulonefrite poststreptococcica, che dimostra depositi elettrondensi (D) sul lato delle cellule epiteliali (Ep) della membrana basale glomerulare. È presente un leucocita polimorfonucleato (P) all'interno del lume (L) del capillare. BS, capsula di Bowman (*Bowman Space*); M, mesangio.

ipertensione o ipervolemia. L'encefalopatia può essere determinata anche dagli effetti tossici diretti degli streptococchi sul sistema nervoso centrale. Tipicamente l'edema deriva dalla ritenzione d'acqua e di sali; nel 10-20% dei casi può svilupparsi una sindrome nefrosica. Sintomi aspecifici come malessere, letargia, dolore addominale o al fianco e febbre sono comuni. Sono stati riferiti anche un edema sottoglottico acuto e la compromissione delle vie aeree. In generale la fase acuta si risolve entro 6-8 settimane. Benché l'escrezione urinaria di proteine e l'ipertensione in genere si normalizzino entro 4-6 settimane dall'esordio, l'ematuria persistente può durare per 1-2 anni.

DIAGNOSI. L'analisi delle urine dimostra la presenza di eritrociti, spesso in associazione a cilindri eritrocitari, proteinuria e leucociti polimorfonucleati. Può sussistere una lieve anemia normocromica causata dall'emodiluizione e dalla modesta emolisi. Il livello di C3 nel siero è di solito diminuito nella fase acuta e torna normale 6-8 settimane dopo l'esordio.

La conferma della diagnosi richiede un'evidenza chiara di infezione streptococcica invasiva. Una coltura di tampone faringeo positiva può sostenere la diagnosi o può semplicemente rappresentare lo stato del portatore. D'altro canto, un elevato titolo anticorpale agli antigeni streptococcici conferma una recente infezione streptococcica. Un elemento importante è che il titolo anti-streptolisina O è comunemente alto dopo un'infezione faringea, ma raramente aumenta dopo le infezioni cutanee streptococciche. Il miglior titolo anticorpale singolo in grado di documentare un'infezione streptococcica cutanea è l'anti-DNasi B. Il test Streptozyme®, un test di agglutinazione su vetrino, è utile e semplice per individuare anticorpi contro streptolisina O, DNasi B, ialuronidasi, streptochinasi e nicotinamide-adenina dinucleotidasi.

La diagnosi clinica di glomerulonefrite poststreptococcica è abbastanza probabile in un bambino con una sindrome nefritica acuta, l'evidenza di una infezione streptococcica recente e un basso livello di C3. Tuttavia, è importante considerare altre diagnosi, come il lupus eritematoso sistemico e una grave esacerbazione della glomerulonefrite cronica. La biopsia renale deve essere considerata solo in presenza di un'insufficienza renale acuta, di una sindrome nefrosica, dell'assenza di un'infezione streptococcica evidente o di livelli di complemento normali. Inoltre, viene considerata l'opportunità di eseguire la biopsia quando l'ematuria e la proteinuria, la riduzione della funzione renale e/o un livello C3 basso persistono per oltre 2 mesi dall'insorgenza.

La diagnosi differenziale della glomerulonefrite poststreptococcica include molte delle cause di ematuria elencate nella Tabella 509-2 e nella Tabella 511-1. La glomerulonefrite acuta può comparire anche in seguito a un'infezione da stafilococchi coagulasi-positivi e coagulasi-negativi, *Streptococcus pneumoniae* e batteri Gram-negativi. L'endocardite batterica può determinare una glomerulonefrite ipocomplementemica con insufficienza renale. La glomerulonefrite acuta può insorgere infine per causa di talune malattie micotiche, rickettsie e virali, in particolare l'influenza.

TABELLA 511-1. Riepilogo delle principali malattie renali che si manifestano come glomerulonefrite acuta

MALATTIE	GLOMERULONEFRITE POSTSTREPTOCOCCICA	NEFROPATIA DA IGA	SINDROME DI GOODPASTURE	GLOMERULONEFRITE IDIOPATICA RAPIDAMENTE PROGRESSIVA
Manifestazioni cliniche				
Età e sesso	Tutte le età, media 7 anni, 2:1 maschi	10-35 anni, 2:1 maschi	15-30 anni, 6:1 maschi	Adulti, 2:1 maschi
Sindrome nefritica acuta	90%	50%	90%	90%
Ematuria asintomatica	Occasionalmente	50%	Rara	Rara
Sindrome nefrosica	10-20%	Rara	Rara	10-20%
Ipertensione	70%	30-50%	Rara	25%
Insufficienza renale acuta	50% (transitoria)	Molto rara	50%	60%
Altro	Periodo di latenza 1-3 settimane	Segue sindromi virali	Emorragia polmonare; anemia sideropenica	Nessuna
Reperti di laboratorio	↑ titoli ASO (70%) Streptozyme® positivo (95%) ↓ C3-C9; C1 normale, C4	↑ IgA sieriche (50%) IgA nei capillari dermici	Positività agli anticorpi anti-GBM	ANCA positiva in alcuni
Immunogenetica	HLA-B12, D"EN" (9)*	HLA-Bw 35, DR4 (4)*	HLA-DR2 (16)*	Nessuna definita
Patologia renale				
Microscopia ottica	Proliferazione diffusa	Proliferazione focale	Proliferazione focale → diffusa con semilune	GN con semilune
Immunofluorescenza	IgG granulare, C3	IgA mesangiali diffuse	IgG lineari, C3	Assenza di immunodepositi
Miscroscopio elettronico	Masse sottoepiteliali	Depositi mesangiali	Assenza di depositi	Assenza di depositi
Prognosi	95% si risolvono spontaneamente 5% RPGN o lentamente progressive	Progressione lenta nel 25-50%	75% si stabilizzano o migliorano se trattati presto	75% si stabilizzano o migliorano se trattati presto
Terapia	Di supporto	Incerta (le opzioni includono steroidi, olio di pesce e ACE-inibitori)	Sostituzione del plasma (plasma exchange), steroidi, ciclofosfamide	Terapia intermittente, o boli, con steroidi

*Rischio relativo.
ACE, enzima di conversione dell'angiotensina (*Angiotensin-Converting Enzyme*); ANCA, anticorpo anticitoplasma dei neutrofili (*AntiNeutrophil Cytoplasmatic Antibody*); ASO, anti-streptolisina O; GBM, membrana basale glomerulare; GN, glomerulonefrite; HLA, antigene leucocitario umano (*Human Leukocyte Antigen*); Ig, immunoglobulina.
Tratta da Kliegman RM, Greenbaum LA, Lye PS: *Practical Strategies in Pediatric Diagnosis and Therapy*, 2nd ed. Philadelphia, Elsevier, 2004, p 427.

COMPLICANZE. Le complicanze gravi di questa malattia derivano dall'ipertensione e dall'insufficienza renale acuta. L'ipertensione viene riscontrata nel 60% dei pazienti e può essere associata a un'encefalopatia ipertensiva nel 10% dei casi. Altre complicanze potenziali includono insufficienza cardiaca, iperpotassiemia, iperfosfatemia, ipocalcemia, acidosi, crisi convulsive e uremia.

PREVENZIONE. Una pronta terapia antibiotica sistemica delle infezioni streptococciche faringee e cutanee non elimina il rischio della glomerulonefrite. I familiari dei pazienti con glomerulonefrite acuta vanno sottoposti a coltura per lo streptococco β-emolitico del gruppo A e, in caso di positività, anche al trattamento.

TRATTAMENTO. Il trattamento è rivolto agli effetti acuti dell'insufficienza renale e dell'ipertensione (vedi Capitolo 535.1). Benché si raccomandi un ciclo di 10 giorni di terapia antibiotica sistemica con la penicillina per limitare la diffusione degli organismi nefritogenici, la terapia antibiotica non influenza il decorso naturale della glomerulonefrite. La limitazione dell'assunzione di sodio, la diuresi ridotta in genere con furosemide per via endovenosa e una terapia farmacologica con calcioantagonisti, vasodilatatori o ACE-inibitori sono le terapie standard utilizzate per l'ipertensione.

PROGNOSI. La remissione completa si verifica in oltre il 95% dei bambini. La mortalità nella fase acuta può essere evitata mediante un trattamento appropriato dell'insufficienza renale acuta, dell'insufficienza cardiaca e dell'ipertensione. La fase acuta raramente può essere grave e condurre alla ialinizzazione glomerulare e a una malattia renale cronica. Tuttavia la diagnosi di glomerulonefrite poststreptococcica acuta va messa in dubbio nei pazienti con una malattia renale cronica, perché possono sussistere altre diagnosi, come la glomerulonefrite membranoproliferativa. Le recidive sono estremamente rare.

Clark G, White RHR, Glasgow EF, et al: Poststreptococcal glomerulonephritis in children: Clinicopathological correlations and long-term prognosis. *Pediatr Nephrol* 1988; 2:381–388.
Dodge WF, Spargo BH, Travis LB, et al: Poststreptococcal glomerulonephritis in children: A prospective study. *N Engl J Med* 1972;286:273–278.
Potter EV, Lipschultz SA, Abidh S, et al: Twelve to fifteen-year follow-up of patients with poststreptococcal acute glomerulonephritis in Trinidad. *N Engl J Med* 1982;307:725–729.
White AV, Hoy WE, McCredie DA: Childhood post-streptococcal glomerulonephritis as a risk factor for chronic renal disease in later life. *Med J Aust* 2001;10:492–496.

511.2 • Altre infezioni croniche

La comparsa della glomerulonefrite è stata documentata nel corso di numerose infezioni croniche, tra cui l'endocardite batterica causata da *Streptococcus viridans* e altri organismi, shunt ventricoloatriali per l'idrocefalo infettati da *Staphylococcus epidermidis*, la sifilide, l'epatite da virus B, l'epatite da virus C e la candidosi. Le infezioni parassitarie associate alla malattia glomerulare includono la malaria, la schistosomiasi, la leishmaniosi, la filariosi, l'echinococcosi, la tripanosomiasi e la toxoplasmosi. In ognuna di esse l'organismo infettante ha una bassa virulenza e l'ospite è cronicamente contagiato da antigeni estranei. In presenza di elevati livelli di antigene circolante, la risposta anticorpale dell'ospite conduce alla formazione di immunocomplessi che si depositano nei reni e innescano l'infiammazione glomerulare.

I reperti istopatologici possono assomigliare a una glomerulonefrite poststreptococcica, membranosa o membranoproliferativa. Le manifestazioni cliniche sono generalmente quelle della nefrite acuta o della sindrome nefrotica. Il livello del fattore C3 del complemento è spesso ridotto.

L'eradicazione dell'infezione prima che si sviluppi un danno glomerulare grave in genere porta alla risoluzione della glomerulonefrite. È stata descritta la progressione a un'insufficienza renale terminale, ma si tratta di un evento raro.

Chesney RW, O'Regan S, Guyda HJ, et al: *Candida* endocrinopathy syndrome with membranoproliferative glomerulonephritis: Demonstration of glomerular *Candida* antigen. *Clin Nephrol* 1976;5:232–238.
Connor FL, Rosenberg AR, Kennedy SE, et al: HBV associated nephrotic syndrome: Resolution with oral lamivudine. *Arch Dis Child* 2003;88:446–449.
Hendrickse RG, Adeniyi A: Quartan malarial nephrotic syndrome in children. *Kidney Int* 1979;16:64–74.
Hunte W, Al-Ghraoui F, Cohen RJ: Secondary syphilis and the nephrotic syndrome. *J Am Soc Nephrol* 1993;3:1351–1355.
Meyers CM, Seeff LB, Stehman-Breen CO, et al: Hepatitis C and renal disease: An update. *Am J Kidney Dis* 2003;42:631–657.
Neugarten J, Baldwin DS: Glomerulonephritis in bacterial endocarditis. *Am J Med* 1984;77:297–304.
Ozdamar SO, Gucer S, Tinaztepe K: Hepatitis-B virus associated nephropathies: A clinicopathological study in 14 children. *Pediatr Nephrol* 2003;181:23–28.
Ray PE, Xu L, Rakusan T, Liu XH: A 20-year history of childhood HIV-associated nephropathy. *Pediatr Nephrol* 2004;10:1075–1092.
Vella J, Carmody M, Campbell E, et al: Glomerulonephritis after ventriculoatrial shunt. *Q J Med* 1995;88:911–918.
Walters S, Levin M: Infectious diseases and the kidney. In Barratt TM, Avner ED, Harmon WE (editors): *Pediatric Nephrology*, 4th ed. Baltimore, Lippincott Williams & Wilkins, 1999, pp 1079–1102.

Capitolo 512 ■ Glomerulopatia membranosa (glomerulonefrite)

Benché la glomerulopatia membranosa sia la causa più frequente di sindrome nefrosica negli adulti, di rado determina l'ematuria nei bambini. Tipicamente si presenta come una malattia renale isolata, ma può anche essere associata a malattie sistemiche, tra cui quelle autoimmuni come il lupus eritematoso sistemico o la porpora trombocitopenica autoimmune cronica, la sarcoidosi, il neuroblastoma, il gonadoblastoma, la terapia con oro o penicillamina, la sifilide e infezioni da virus dell'epatite B e C. Queste cause secondarie sono più comuni nei bambini che negli adulti e la loro identificazione risulta importante, perché il trattamento di queste malattie può condurre alla risoluzione delle lesioni glomerulari.

ANATOMIA PATOLOGICA. I glomeruli mostrano un ispessimento diffuso della membrana basale glomerulare (GMB, *Glomerular Basement Membrane*), senza alterazioni proliferative significative (Fig. 512-1). È probabile che questo ispessimento derivi dalla produzione di materiale simile alla membrana da parte delle cellule epiteliali viscerali in risposta agli immunocomplessi depositati sul lato epiteliale della membrana stessa. Questo nuovo materiale può assomigliare in certe aree a punte sul lato epiteliale della GBM. La microscopia di immunofluorescenza mostra depositi granulari di IgG e C3 situati su questo lato, quando la GBM viene esaminata mediante microscopia elettronica. All'immunofluorescenza è visibile la colorazione lineare per IgG, IgA e C3 lungo la membrana basale tubulare.

PATOGENESI. Studi morfologici suggeriscono che la glomerulopatia membranosa sia una malattia mediata da immunocomplessi. La patogenesi molecolare della nefropatia membranosa nell'uomo resta sconosciuta. Esistono alcuni fattori genetici che possono influenzare la suscettibilità alla malattia e/o la sua progressione. Quella con insorgenza neonatale è caratterizzata da anticorpi materni anti-endopeptidasi neutre (NEP, *Neutral EndoPeptidase*), che

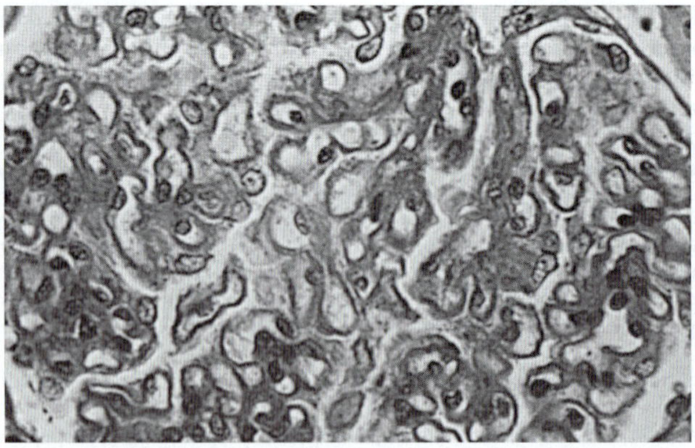

Figura 512-1. Glomerulo di un paziente con glomerulopatia membranosa che dimostra un ispessimento diffuso della membrana basale glomerulare in assenza di proliferazione cellulare (×400).

attraversano la placenta nelle madri con deficit genetico dell'antigene NEP. La NEP è una metalloendopeptidasi di membrana che nelle madri produce anticorpi. L'alloimmunizzazione mediante NEP fetali induce anticorpi materni che attraversano la placenta, avviando la glomerulopatia membranosa.

MANIFESTAZIONI CLINICHE. Nei bambini la glomerulopatia membranosa è maggiormente frequente durante la seconda decade di vita. In genere la malattia si presenta come una sindrome nefrosica ed è infatti responsabile del 2-6% dei casi di sindrome nefrosica del bambino (vedi Capitolo 527). La maggior parte dei pazienti presenta un'ematuria microscopica e talvolta macroscopica. In circa il 20% dei bambini si riscontra una ipertensione. I livelli di C3 risultano normali, tranne nei casi di lupus eritematoso sistemico, in cui possono essere ridotti.

DIAGNOSI. La diagnosi di nefropatia membranosa viene confermata solo mediante una biopsia renale, dato che non esiste un test di laboratorio diagnostico specifico. Le indicazioni consuete per la biopsia includono la presentazione della sindrome nefrosica in un bambino, di solito di età superiore ai 10 anni, oppure l'esistenza di ematuria e proteinuria inspiegate. I pazienti con glomerulopatia membranosa hanno un rischio aumentato di **trombosi delle vene renali**.

PROGNOSI E TRATTAMENTO. Il decorso clinico è variabile. I bambini che si presentano con una proteinuria asintomatica di grado ridotto possono ottenere una remissione spontanea. Studi di follow-up di 1-14 anni suggeriscono che il 20% dei bambini progredisce verso un'insufficienza cronica renale, mentre il 40% continua con la malattia attiva. Lo stato nefrosico può essere controllato limitando l'assunzione di sale e con agenti diuretici (vedi Capitolo 527). La proteinuria può essere ridotta dagli ACE-inibitori o dagli antagonisti dei recettori dell'angiotensina II (da soli o in combinazione). La terapia immunosoppressiva con il prednisone in associazione al clorambucil o alla ciclofosfamide può essere di aiuto negli adulti per rallentare la velocità di progressione della malattia renale, in particolare nei pazienti con una proteinuria grave o prolungata, insufficienza renale o ipertensione. Non esistono dati controllati sull'uso di questi agenti nei bambini. Il rituximab, un anticorpo monoclonale contro l'antigene CD20 delle cellule B, si è dimostrato una terapia efficace in un numero ridotto di pazienti adulti.

Cattran DC: Idiopathic membranous glomerulonephritis. *Kidney Int* 2000;59:1983–1994.

Debiec H, Nauta J, Coulet F, et al: Role of truncating mutations in *MME* gene in fetomaternal alloimmunization and antenatal glomerulopathies. *Lancet* 2004;364:1252–1259.

Eddy AA, Symons JM: Nephrotic syndrome in childhood. *Lancet* 2003;362:629–639.

Louis CU, Morgenstern BZ, Butani L: Thrombotic complications in childhood-onset idiopathic membranous nephropathy. *Pediatr Nephrol* 2003;18:1298–1300.

Makker SP: Treatment of membranous nephropathy in children. *Semin Nephrol* 2003;23:379–385.

Pape L, Mengel M, Offner G, et al: Cyclosporin A-induced remission of primary membranous glomerulonephritis in a child. *Nephrol Dial Transplant* 2004;19:3207.

Remuzzi G, Chiurchiu C, Abbate M, et al: Rituximab for idiopathic membranous nephropathy. *Lancet* 2002;360:923–924.

Capitolo 513 ■ Glomerulonefrite membranoproliferativa (mesangiocapillare)

Il termine **glomerulonefrite cronica** implica una lesione glomerulare continua che spesso conduce a una distruzione glomerulare e a un'insufficienza renale terminale. La glomerulonefrite membranoproliferativa (MPGN, *MembranoProliferative Glomerulo-Nephritis*) è la causa più comune di glomerulonefrite cronica nei bambini più grandi e nei giovani adulti.

ANATOMIA PATOLOGICA E PATOGENESI. Inizialmente la MPGN veniva differenziata dalle altre forme di glomerulonefrite cronica in base alla presenza di ipocomplementemia nella maggior parte dei pazienti. In alcuni l'ipocomplementemia deriva da un anticorpo, definito fattore nefritico C3, che attiva la via alternativa del complemento. Sono stati descritti tre tipi istologici di MPGN.

La **MPGN di tipo I** è la forma più comune. I glomeruli rivelano un'accentuazione dell'aspetto lobulare a causa di un aumento generalizzato della matrice e delle cellule mesangiali (Fig. 513-1). La parete capillare glomerulare appare ispessita, spesso con tratti di duplicazione o divisione dovuta all'interposizione di matrice e citoplasma mesangiale tra le cellule endoteliali e la membrana basale glomerulare (GBM, *Glomerular Basement Membrane*). Possono essere presenti semilune, che diventano indice di cattiva prognosi se si trovano in una percentuale elevata di glomeruli. La microscopia di immunofluorescenza rivela C3 e quantità minori di immunoglobuline nel mesangio e lungo le pareti dei capillari periferici con un aspetto lobulare (Fig. 513-2). La microscopia elettronica conferma l'esistenza di depositi simili a immunocomplessi nelle regioni mesangiali e subendoteliali.

Nella **malattia di tipo II** le alterazioni mesangiali sono meno evidenti rispetto al tipo I. Le pareti capillari mostrano un ispessimento irregolare a nastro dovuto all'accumulo di depositi elettrondensi. La divisione della membrana è rara, ma la presenza di semilune è comune. Alla microscopia elettronica i depositi densi vengono visti come ispessimenti della GBM in una regione distinta dalla lamina densa. Depositi vengono osservati anche nella capsula di Bowman, nel mesangio e nelle membrane basali dei tubuli. Gli studi di immunofluorescenza dimostrano C3 e immunoglobuline minime lungo il margine del materiale di deposito denso.

Nella **malattia di tipo III** i risultati della microscopia ottica e dell'immunofluorescenza assomigliano a quelli ottenuti nella malattia di tipo I. La microscopia elettronica rivela depositi subepiteliali e subendoteliali associati alla disgregazione e stratificazione della porzione della lamina densa della GBM.

MANIFESTAZIONI CLINICHE. La MPGN è più frequente nella seconda decade di vita. La maggior parte dei pazienti si presenta con una sindrome nefrosica (vedi Capitolo 527), mentre altri possono manifestare una sindrome nefritica acuta caratterizza-

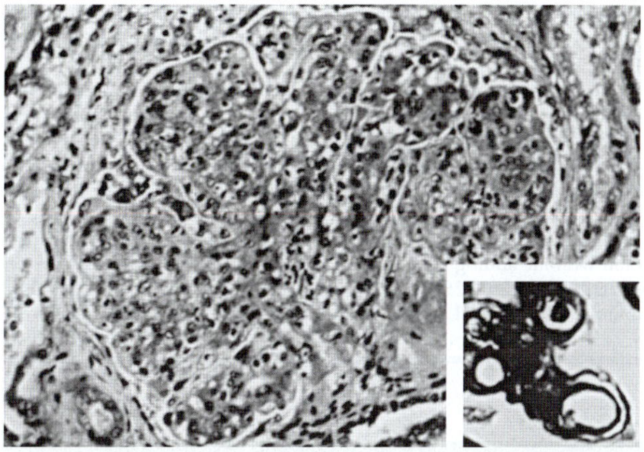

Figura 513-1. Glomerulo di un paziente con glomerulonefrite membranoproliferativa di tipo I che mostra un aspetto lobulare accentuato, un aumento generalizzato della matrice e della parete mesangiale e la "divisione" della parete capillare glomerulare (dettaglio) (×250). (Tratta da Kim Y, Michael F: Idiopathic membranoproliferative glomerulonephritis. *Annu Rev Med* 1980;31:273-288.)

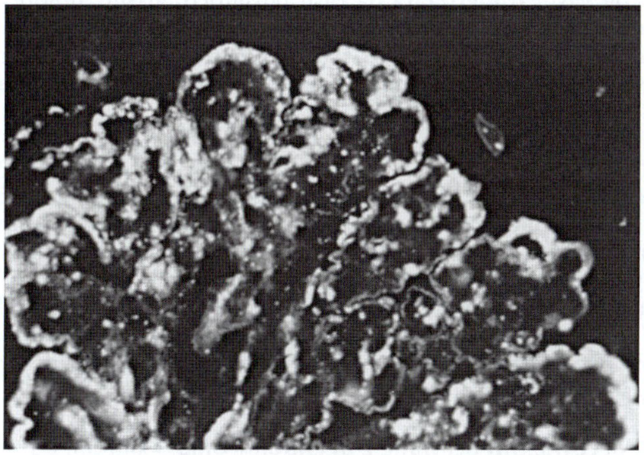

Figura 513-2. Microscopia di immunofluorescenza nella glomerulonefrite membranoproliferativa di tipo I che mostra depositi granulari di C3 lungo la membrana basale glomerulare e nel mesangio. (Tratta da Kim Y, Michael F: Idiopathic membranoproliferative glomerulonephritis. *Annu Rev Med* 1980;31:273-288.)

ta da un'ematuria macroscopica o microscopica asintomatica e proteinuria. La funzione renale può essere normale o diminuita. L'ipertensione è comune. Il livello del complemento C3 nel siero può essere ridotto.

DIAGNOSI E DIAGNOSI DIFFERENZIALE. La diagnosi di MPGN viene effettuata mediante una biopsia renale. Le indicazioni per effettuare la biopsia includono la sindrome nefrosica in un bambino di età superiore ai 10 anni, una proteinuria significativa con ematuria microscopica e un'ipocomplementemia con durata superiore alle 8 settimane in un bambino con nefrite acuta.

Sia la MPGN sia la glomerulonefrite poststreptococcica possono essere associate a ematuria macroscopica, ipertensione, livelli di C3 ridotti e titoli anticorpali antistreptococcici elevati. I pazienti con glomerulonefrite poststreptococcica migliorano entro 2 mesi dall'esordio, mentre la sindrome nefritica, la proteinuria e l'ipocomplementemia persistono nel bambino con MPGN e generalmente impongono una biopsia renale.

PROGNOSI E TRATTAMENTO. Benché alcuni pazienti si riprendano completamente, circa il 50% di quelli con MPGN progredisce a una malattia renale terminale 10 anni dopo l'esordio. I fattori associati a una prognosi infausta includono una sindrome nefrosica al momento dell'insorgenza, la presenza istologica di una MPGN di tipo II e una ridotta velocità di filtrazione glomerulare 1 anno dopo l'esordio. La recidiva dell'MPGN in un allotrapianto in seguito a un trapianto renale si verifica in circa il 30% dei soggetti con MPGN di tipo I e nel 90% di quelli con MPGN di tipo II e questo suggerisce una malattia sistemica. Non esiste una terapia definitiva, benché sia stata riferita una stabilizzazione dell'andamento clinico in molti pazienti sottoposti a 3-7 anni di prednisone a giorni alterni.

Bergstein JM, Andreoli SP: Response of type I membranoproliferative glomerulonephritis to pulse methylprednisolone and alternate-day prednisone therapy. *Pediatr Nephrol* 1995;9:268–271.
Cansick JC, Lennon R, Cummins CL, et al: Prognosis, treatment and outcome of childhood mesangiocapillary (membranoproliferative) glomerulonephritis. *Nephrol Dial Transplant* 2004;19:2769–2777.
McEnery PT: Membranoproliferative glomerulonephritis: The Cincinnati experience—cumulative renal survival from 1957 to 1989. *J Pediatr* 1990;116:S109–S114.
Tarshish P, Bernstein J, Tobin JN, et al: Treatment of mesangiocapillary glomerulonephritis with alternate-day prednisone—a report of The International Study of Kidney Disease in Children. *Pediatr Nephrol* 1992;6:123–130.
Yanagihara T, Hayakawa M, Yoshida J, et al: Long-term follow-up of diffuse membranoproliferative glomerulonephritis type I. *Pediatr Nephrol* 2005;20:585–590.

Capitolo 514 ■ Glomerulonefrite associata a lupus eritematoso sistemico

Il lupus eritematoso sistemico (LES) è caratterizzato da febbre, calo ponderale, rash, alterazioni ematologiche, artrite e coinvolgimento di cuore, polmoni, sistema nervoso centrale e reni (vedi Capitolo 157). La malattia renale, una delle caratteristiche più comuni del LES nell'infanzia, talvolta può essere l'unica manifestazione.

ANATOMIA PATOLOGICA E PATOGENESI. Le manifestazioni cliniche del LES sono mediate da immunocomplessi. Vengono osservate aberrazioni nella funzione delle cellule B e T.

La classificazione della nefrite lupica da parte dell'Organizzazione Mondiale della Sanità (OMS) si fonda su una combinazione di caratteristiche rilevate mediante la microscopia ottica, quella elettronica e l'immunofluorescenza. Nei pazienti con **nefrite di classe I secondo l'OMS** non vengono individuate anomalie istologiche. Nella **nefrite di classe II secondo l'OMS** (nefrite lupica mesangiale) i glomeruli mostrano depositi mesangiali contenenti immunoglobuline e complemento e la microscopia ottica può rivelare un'ipercellularità mesangiale lieve (**classe II-A**) o moderata e una matrice aumentata (**classe II-B**).

Nella **nefrite di classe III secondo l'OMS** (glomerulonefrite lupica segmentale focale), i depositi mesangiali si trovano in quasi tutti i glomeruli e si osservano depositi subendoteliali tra le cellule endoteliali e la membrana basale glomerulare. Oltre alla proliferazione mesangiale focale e segmentale, alcuni glomeruli mostrano la necrosi della parete capillare, la formazione di semilune e la sclerosi.

La **nefrite di classe IV secondo l'OMS** (nefrite lupica proliferativa diffusa) è la forma più comune e più grave. Tutti i glomeruli contengono significativi depositi mesangiali e subendoteliali di immunoglobuline e complemento. Ogni glomerulo mostra una proliferazione mesangiale. Le pareti capillari di solito sono ispessite secondariamente a depositi subendoteliali (creando lesioni a fil di ferro) e spesso presentano necrosi, formazione di semilune e tessuto cicatriziale.

La **nefrite di classe V secondo l'OMS** (nefrite lupica membranosa) è la meno comune. Istologicamente assomiglia alla glomerulopatia membranosa idiopatica, tranne per la presenza di una proliferazione mesangiale da lieve a moderata.

La trasformazione della lesione istologica da una classe all'altra è comune; avviene con maggiore probabilità fra i pazienti trattati in modo inadeguato e di solito causa la progressione a una lesione istologica più grave.

MANIFESTAZIONI CLINICHE. I bambini con il LES sono soprattutto adolescenti femmine. L'evidenza clinica di malattia renale si trova nel 30-70% dei casi. I referti clinici nei pazienti con le forme più lievi (tutte quelle di classe II, alcune di classe III) di nefrite lupica includono l'ematuria, una funzione renale normale e una proteinuria <1 g/24 h. Alcuni soggetti con la malattia di classe III e tutti quelli con la malattia di classe IV presentano ematuria e proteinuria, funzione renale ridotta, sindrome nefrosica o insufficienza renale acuta. In rari casi di glomerulonefrite proliferativa l'analisi delle urine può essere completamente normale. I pazienti con la nefrite di classe V in genere hanno una sindrome nefrosica.

DIAGNOSI. La diagnosi di LES viene suggerita dall'individuazione di anticorpi antinucleo circolanti ed è confermata provando che questi anticorpi che reagiscono con il DNA nativo a doppia elica. Nella maggior parte dei pazienti con malattia attiva, i livelli di C3 e C4 sono ridotti. Dal momento che manca una correlazione chiara tra le manifestazioni cliniche e la gravità del coinvolgimento renale, in tutti i pazienti con LES va eseguita una biopsia renale, i cui risultati vengono utilizzati per guidare la scelta delle terapie immunosoppressive.

TERAPIA. I bambini con LES devono essere trattati da specialisti in pediatria presso centri in cui sia possibile fornire un'assistenza medica e psicologica sia ai pazienti sia ai familiari. Nella nefrite lupica la terapia immunosoppressiva è volta a ottenere una remissione clinica e sierologica, definita come normalizzazione dei livelli di anti-DNA, C3 e C4. In tutti i pazienti la terapia viene iniziata con prednisone a 1-2 mg/kg/die in 2 o 3 dosi, seguito da una lenta riduzione degli steroidi nell'arco di 4-6 mesi a cominciare da 4-6 settimane dopo il raggiungimento della remissione sierologica. Per i pazienti con forme più gravi di nefrite (classi III e IV secondo l'OMS), 6 infusioni endovenose mensili consecutive di ciclofosfamide a 500-1 000 mg/m^2 seguite da una somministrazione ogni 3 mesi per 18 mesi sembrano ridurre il rischio di progressione del danno renale. L'azatioprina a un dosaggio quotidiano in dose singola di 1,5-2,0 mg/kg può essere usata come agente "risparmiatore di steroidi" nei pazienti con una nefrite lupica di classe I o II. Alcune segnalazioni di casi provenienti da centri singoli suggeriscono un potenziale vantaggio del mofetil micofenolato nei pazienti con nefrite lupica lieve. Il rituximab, un anticorpo monoclonale chimerico specifico per il CD20 umano, può risultare efficace nei pazienti con una nefrite lupica di tipo IV resistente alle terapie immunosoppressive convenzionali.

PROGNOSI. Una terapia immunosoppressiva aggressiva migliora la prognosi del LES nei bambini. Una sopravvivenza renale senza la necessità di dialisi viene riscontrata nell'80% dei pazienti a 10 anni dopo la diagnosi di nefrite lupica. I casi di nefrite lupica proliferativa diffusa, classe IV secondo l'OMS, mostrano il rischio massimo di progressione a un'insufficienza renale terminale. I timori riguardanti gli effetti collaterali della terapia immunosoppressiva cronica e il rischio di recidiva durano per tutta la vita. Deve essere adottata una particolare attenzione al fine di ridurre al minimo il rischio di osteoporosi, obesità, ipertensione e diabete mellito associato alla terapia steroidea cronica. Il rischio di neoplasie maligne o d'infertilità è aumentato nei pazienti che assumono una dose cumulativa di ciclofosfamide >20 g.

Baqi N, Moazami S, Singh A, et al: Lupus nephritis in children: A longitudinal study of prognostic factors and therapy. *J Am Soc Nephrol* 1996;7:924–929.
Bogdanovic R, Nikolic V, Pasic S, et al: Lupus nephritis in childhood: A review of 53 patients followed at a single center. *Pediatr Nephrol* 2004;19:36–44.
Edelbauer M, Jungraithmayr T, Zimmerhackl LB: Rituximab in childhood systemic lupus erythematosus refractory to conventional immunosuppression. *Pediatr Nephrol* 2005;20:811–813.
Hagelberg S, Lee Y, Bargman J, et al: Longterm followup of childhood lupus nephritis. *J Rheumatol* 2002;29:2635–2642.
Illei GG, Austin HA, Crane M, et al: Combination therapy with pulse cyclophosphamide plus pulse methylprednisolone improves long-term renal outcome without adding toxicity in patients with lupus nephritis. *Ann Intern Med* 2001;135:296–298.
Perfumo F, Martini A: Lupus nephritis in children. *Lupus* 2005;14:83–88.

Capitolo 515 ■ Nefrite della porpora di Henoch-Schönlein

La nefrite della porpora di Henoch-Schönlein (HSP, *Henoch-Schönlein Purpura*) (porpora anafilattoide) è una vasculite dei piccoli vasi caratterizzata da rash purpurico, artrite, dolore addominale e glomerulonefrite (vedi Capitolo 166.1). La nefrite da HSP e la nefropatia da IgA hanno reperti istopatologici renali identici, ma reperti sistemici vengono osservati solo nella nefrite da HSP.

ANATOMIA PATOLOGICA E PATOGENESI. Nella nefrite da HSP le anomalie glomerulari e tubulointerstiziali alla micoscopia ottica, di immunofluorescenza ed elettronica sono praticamente indistinguibili dai reperti patologici della nefropatia da IgA; tuttavia la formazione di semilune è più comune e più estesa. Benché la patogenesi della nefrite da HSP resti sconosciuta, questa malattia sembra mediata dalla formazione di immunocomplessi che contengono IgA1 polimeriche all'interno dei capillari di pelle, intestino e glomeruli.

MANIFESTAZIONI CLINICHE E DI LABORATORIO. I sintomi e i segni di nefrite da HSP tipicamente compaiono 1-3 settimane dopo una infezione delle vie respiratorie superiori (vedi Capitolo 166.1). La diagnosi della HSP si fonda su un insieme di risultati clinici. Benché l'ematuria macroscopica sia presente nel 20-30% dei casi, i pazienti possono anche manifestare un'ematuria microscopica isolata, ematuria e proteinuria; la sindrome nefritica acuta, la sindrome nefrosica e l'insufficienza renale acuta sono meno comuni. Manifestazioni renali di nefrite da HSP si verificano fino a 12 settimane dopo l'esordio dell'HSP. Una manifestazione urologica rara di questa malattia è l'**ureterite**, associata a dolore lombare e a colica renale. L'ureterite in genere viene osservata nei bambini di età inferiore ai 5 anni e spesso conduce a una stenosi ureterale con successiva idronefrosi, che richiede la correzione chirurgica.

PROGNOSI E TRATTAMENTO. La prognosi della nefrite da HSP è generalmente favorevole, benché il rischio di malattia renale cronica sia del 2-5%. La presentazione con la sola ematuria microscopica isolata è accompagnata dalla prognosi migliore, mentre quella con una sindrome nefrosica e/o nefritica acuta è associata al rischio massimo di sviluppare ipertensione, ipertensione associata alla gravidanza, ematuria e insufficienza renale cronica.

Non esistono dati controllati che dimostrino che gli steroidi, gli agenti citotossici o gli anticoagulanti alterino il decorso di questa malattia. Studi non controllati suggeriscono il valore potenziale della terapia con corticosteroidi ad alte dosi e di quella citotossica con la ciclofosfamide o l'azatioprina nei pazienti con la glomerulonefrite con semilune o una proteinuria significativa. L'aggiunta di dipiridamolo e/o di eparina/warfarin può portare un ulteriore beneficio nei pazienti con forme gravi di nefrite. Alcuni studi suggeriscono che le somministrazioni per brevi periodi di prednisone a basse dosi a partire dalla diagnosi riducono il rischio successivo di sviluppare segni clinici di nefrite. Non vi sono dati controllati che indichino l'esistenza di una terapia in grado di ridurre il rischio di progressione a una malattia renale grave. La tonsillectomia non sembra alterare il corso della nefrite da HSP. I bambini con le forme più gravi restano a rischio di malattia renale cronica nell'età adulta.

Algoet C, Proesmans W: Renal biopsy 2–9 years after Henoch Schonlein purpura. *Pediatr Nephrol* 2003;18:471–473.
Foster BJ, Bernard C, Drummond K, et al: Effective therapy for severe Henoch-Schönlein purpura nephritis with prednisone and azathioprine: A clinical and pathologic study. *J Pediatr* 2000;136:370–375.
Halling S, Soderberg M, Berg U: Henoch Schonlein nephritis: Clinical findings related to renal function and morphology. *Pediatr Nephrol* 2005;20:46–51.
Niaudet P, Habib R: Methylprednisolone pulse therapy in the treatment of severe forms of Henoch-Schönlein purpura nephritis. *Pediatr Nephrol* 1998;12:238–243.
Ronkainen J, Nuutinen M, Koskimies O: The adult kidney 24 years after childhood Henoch-Schonlein purpura: A retrospective cohort study. *Lancet* 2002;360:666–670.
Tarshish P, Bernstein J, Edelmann CM Jr: Henoch-Schonlein purpura nephritis: Course of disease and efficacy of cyclophosphamide. *Pediatr Nephrol* 2004;19:51–56.

Capitolo 516 ■ Glomerulonefrite rapidamente progressiva (con semilune)

L'espressione "rapidamente progressiva" descrive il decorso clinico di numerose forme di glomerulonefrite (GN), la cui anomalia comune riguarda l'osservazione istopatologica di semilune nella maggior parte dei glomeruli. L'anamnesi naturale in quasi tutte le forme è la progressione rapida a insufficienza renale terminale.

CLASSIFICAZIONE. Le semilune possono essere osservate in numerosi tipi ben definiti di GN, tra cui: (1) le forme di GN mediate da immunocomplessi (GN poststreptococcica, nefrite lupica, GN mebranoproliferativa e nefrite della porpora di Henoch-Schönlein/IgA); (2) GN mediata da anticorpi contro la membrana basale glomerulare, come la malattia di Goodpasture; (3) GN mediata da anticorpi anticitoplasma dei neutrofili (ANCA, *AntiNeutrophil Cytoplasmatic Antibody*), ossia la poliarterite nodosa microscopica e la granulomatosi di Wegener (Tab. 516-1). I reperti tipici agli esami con microscopio ottico, di immunofluorescenza e al microscopio elettronico persistono nonostante la formazione di semilune. Questi reperti istologici, unitamente alle caratteristiche cliniche e agli studi di laboratorio appropriati, rivelano la malattia sottostante. In un piccolo gruppo di pazienti, tuttavia, questa non viene identificata chiaramente e/o essi sono considerati affetti da una GN rapidamente progressiva (con semilune) "idiopatica".

ANATOMIA PATOLOGICA E PATOGENESI. Le semilune vengono osservate all'interno della capsula di Bowman e sono costituite da cellule epiteliali proliferanti della capsula, materiale simile a membrana basale, fibrina, nonché da macrofagi (Fig. 516-1). Si presume che lo stimolo alla formazione delle semilune sia il deposito di fibrina nello spazio di Bowman, probabilmente a causa della necrosi o della distruzione della parete capillare glomerulare. Molti pazienti presentano depositi di immunocomplessi sulla parete capillare o una colorazione lineare per anticorpi IgG verso la membrana basale glomerulare. Studi con microscopia in immunofluorescenza o elettronica nei pazienti con forme di GN ANCA-mediate tipicamente non mostrano alcuna evidenza di una lesione immunologica. Il livello del fattore C3 del complemento è normale.

TABELLA 516-1. Classificazione della glomerulonefrite rapidamente progressiva (con semilune) (GNRP)

TIPO DI GNRP	FREQUENZA
GNRP MEDIATA DA ANTICORPI ANTI-GBM	20%
Sindrome di Goodpasture	
Nefrite anti-GBM idiopatica	
Nefropatia membranosa con semilune	
GNRP ASSOCIATA A IMMUNODEPOSITI GRANULARI	40%
Post-infettiva	
Glomerulonefrite poststreptococcica	
Endocardite batterica	
Nefrite da shunt	
Ascessi viscerali, altre infezioni non streptococciche	
Non infettiva	
Lupus eritematoso sistemico	
Porpora di Henoch-Schönlein	
Crioglobulinemia mista	
Tumori solidi	
Malattia renale primaria	
Glomerulonefrite membranoproliferativa	
Nefropatia da IgA	
Nefrite da immunocomplessi idiopatica	
GNRP SENZA IMMUNODEPOSITI GLOMERULARI	40%
Vasculite	
Poliarterite	
Vasculite da ipersensibilità	
Granulomatosi di Wegener	
GNRP idiopatica	

GBM, mebrana basale glomerulare.
Tratta da Kliegman RM, Greenbaum LA, Lye PS: *Practical Strategies in Pediatric Diagnosis and Therapy*, 2nd ed. Philadelphia, Elsevier, 2004, p 426.

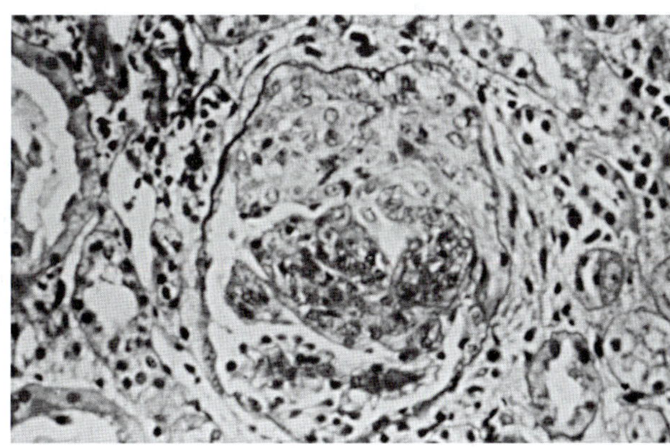

Figura 516-1. Esame al microscopio ottico di un campione bioptico di un bambino con glomerulonefrite in porpora di Henoch-Schönlein che mostra una semiluna sovrapposta al glomerulo (×180).

MANIFESTAZIONI CLINICHE. La maggior parte dei pazienti sviluppa un'insufficienza renale acuta associata alla sindrome nefritica e/o nefrosica. In genere la progressione verso l'insufficienza renale terminale si verifica entro settimane o mesi dall'esordio.

DIAGNOSI E DIAGNOSI DIFFERENZIALE. Devono essere eseguiti studi sierologici appropriati, come i titoli degli anticorpi antinucleo, C3 e antidesossiribonucleotidasi per delineare i tipi specifici della GN. Forme rare di vasculite, come la granulomatosi di Wegener e la poliarterite nodosa microscopica, possono essere suggerite dall'osservazione di anticorpi ANCA diretti contro la mieloperossidasi o la proteinasi-3 sierica del citoplasma dei neutrofili. La diagnosi è confermata dalla biopsia renale.

PROGNOSI E TRATTAMENTO. I bambini con un decorso rapidamente progressivo associato a una GN poststreptococcica di solito guariscono spontaneamente. Spesso si ha una risposta terapeutica eccellente utilizzando un terapia combinata di corticosteroidi e agenti citotossici (ciclofosfamide) nei pazienti con lupus eritematoso sistemico, nefropatia da IgA e porpora di Henoch-Schönlein. Gli esiti renali nelle altre malattie che causano la GN rapidamente progressiva sono meno favorevoli, con evoluzione in insufficienza renale terminale entro 2-3 anni. Una terapia intermittente combinata con metilprednisolone e ciclofosfamide orale può essere efficace, soprattutto nei pazienti con granulomatosi di Wegener. Segnalazioni su casi clinici indicano la validità della plasmaferesi o della linfocitasferesi.

Bacon PA: The spectrum of Wegener's granulomatosis and disease relapse. *N Engl J Med* 2005;352:330–332.
Frosch M, Foell D: Wegener granulomatosis in childhood and adolescence. *Eur J Pediatr* 2004;163:425–434.
Furuta T, Hotta O, Yusa N, et al: Lymphocytapheresis to treat rapidly progressive glomerulonephritis: A randomized comparison with steroid-pulse treatment. *Lancet* 1998;352:203–204.
Hattori M, Kurayama H, Koitabashi Y: Antineutrophil cytoplasmic autoantibody-associated glomerulonephritis in children. *J Am Soc Nephrol* 2001;12:1493–1500.
Savage J, Davies D, Falk RJ, et al: Antineutrophil cytoplasmic antibodies and associated diseases: A review of the clinical and laboratory features. *Kidney Int* 2000;57:846–862.
Valentini RP, Smoyer WE, Sedman AB, et al: Outcome of antineutrophil cytoplasmic autoantibodies-positive glomerulonephritis and vasculitis in children: A single-center experience. *J Pediatr* 1998;132:325–328.
von Vigier RO, Trummler SA, Laux-End R, et al: Pulmonary renal syndrome in childhood: A report of twenty-one cases and a review of the literature. *Pediatr Pulmonol* 2000;29:382–388.

Capitolo 517 ■ Malattia di Goodpasture

La malattia di Goodpasture è caratterizzata da emorragie polmonari e glomerulonefrite associate ad anticorpi comunemente diretti contro epitopi specifici del collagene di tipo IV all'interno della membrana basale alveolare del polmone e della membrana basale glomerulare (GBM, *Glomerular Basement Membrane*) del glomerulo. L'eziologia di questi anticorpi è sconosciuta. Questa malattia va distinta dalla **sindrome di Goodpasture**, che è invece un quadro clinico di emorragia polmonare e glomerulonefrite che può essere osservato in molte malattie, tra cui il lupus eritematoso sistemico, la porpora di Henoch-Schönlein, la poliarterite nodosa e la granulomatosi di Wegener. In alcuni pazienti la nefrite da anti-GBM si verifica senza emorragia polmonare e si presenta come una glomerulonefrite rapidamente progressiva. Anticorpi anticitoplasma dei neutrofili si trovano nel 25% dei soggetti con la sindrome di Goodpasture e possono essere una variante della vasculite.

ANATOMIA PATOLOGICA. Nella maggior parte dei casi le alterazioni alla microscopia ottica assomigliano a quelle della glomerulonefrite rapidamente progressiva. La microscopia di immunofluorescenza dimostra un deposito lineare continuo di IgG lungo la GBM (Fig. 517-1).

MANIFESTAZIONI CLINICHE. La malattia di Goodpasture è rara nell'infanzia. In genere i pazienti si presentano con un'emottisi associata a un'emorragia polmonare che possono essere pericolose per la vita. Le manifestazioni renali includono la sindrome nefritica acuta con ematuria, la proteinuria e l'ipertensione. Una disfunzione renale progressiva si verifica nell'arco di giorni o settimane. Il livello di complemento C3 nel siero è normale.

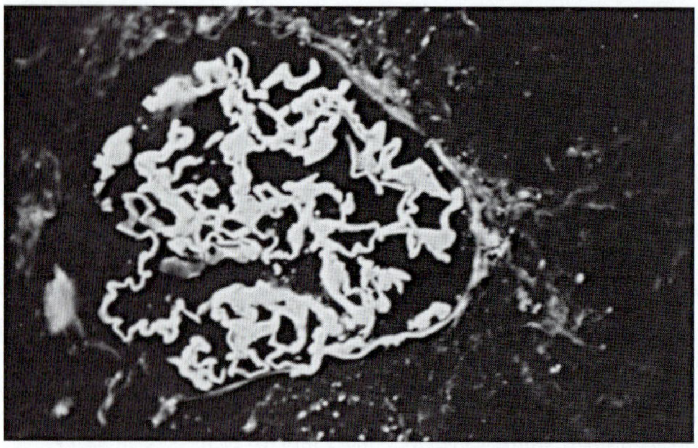

Figura 517-1. La fotografia al microscopio in immunofluorescenza mostra la colorazione lineare continua di IgG lungo la membrana basale glomerulare, come avviene nelle malattie mediate dagli anticorpi antimembrana basale glomerulare (×250).

DIAGNOSI. La diagnosi è suggerita dalla biopsia renale e viene confermata dagli anticorpi sierici diretti contro la GBM, che escludono inoltre altre malattie associate alla sindrome di Goodpasture.

PROGNOSI E TRATTAMENTO. I pazienti che sopravvivono all'emorragia polmonare in genere progrediscono fino all'insufficienza renale terminale. I tassi di sopravvivenza e recupero della funzione renale sono migliorati con la terapia intermittente con boli di metilprednisolone, ciclofosfamide orale e plasmaferesi, benché non siano disponibili dati controllati.

Gittins N, Basu A, Eyre J, et al: Cerebral vasculitis in a teenager with Goodpasture's syndrome. *Nephrol Dial Transplant* 2004;19:3168–3171.
Hudson BG: The molecular basis of Goodpasture and Alport syndromes: Beacons for the discovery of the collagen IV family. *J Am Soc Nephrol* 2004;15:2514–2527.
Levy JB, Turner N, Rees AJ, et al: Long-term outcome of anti-glomerular basement membrane antibody disease treated with plasma exchange and immunosuppression. *Ann Intern Med* 2001;134:1033–1042.
McCarthy LJ, Cotton J, Danielson C, et al: Goodpasture's syndrome in childhood: Treatment with plasmapheresis and immunosuppression. *J Clin Apher* 1994;9:116.

Capitolo 518 ■ Sindrome uremico-emolitica

La sindrome uremico-emolitica (HUS, *Hemolytic-Uremic Syndrome*) è la causa più frequente di insufficienza renale acuta nei bambini piccoli. È classicamente caratterizzata dalla triade di anemia emolitica microangiopatica, trombocitopenia e uremia. La HUS presenta tratti comuni con la porpora trombotica trombocitopenica (TTP, *Thrombotic Thrombocytopenic Purpura*), tranne per il fatto che quest'ultima tende a colpire le giovani donne adulte quale malattia recidivante con febbre, grave coinvolgimento del sistema nervoso centrale e trombocitopenia.

EZIOLOGIA. Una enterite acuta con diarrea causata dalla *Escherichia coli* 0157:H7, con produzione di una tossina Shiga-like, precede l'80% o oltre dei casi di HUS nei Paesi sviluppati. Il serbatoio di questo organismo è il tratto intestinale degli animali domestici. In genere la trasmissione avviene mediante la carne non sufficientemente cotta o il latte non pastorizzato. Alcune epidemie sono state registrate in seguito generalmente all'ingestione di hamburger non sufficientemente cotti nei fast-food. Inoltre, manifestazioni con epidemia di diarrea si verificano dopo avere nuotato in piscine, laghi o stagni contaminati, nonché dopo avere mangiato latte, formaggio, lattuga o succo di mele contaminati; la trasmissione può avvenire, mediante contatto personale, in edifici, centri di assistenza diurna, centri di terapia dei bambini, fattorie con produzione di prodotti caseari o centri di agriturismo infestati. L'organismo produce una verotossina Shiga-like che viene assorbita dall'intestino e avvia la lesione delle cellule endoteliali. La HUS è inoltre associata alla *Shigella* e, meno comunemente, ad altre infezioni batteriche (*Salmonella*, *Campylobacter*, *Streptococcus pneumoniae*, *Bartonella*) e virali (coxsackievirus, echovirus, influenza, varicella, HIV, Epstein-Barr); può svilupparsi anche con l'uso di contraccettivi orali, mitomicina o ciclosporina, oppure con l'esposizione a un copolimero di pirano, che induce la produzione d'interferone. Inoltre, è stato riferito un quadro clinico simile a quello della HUS nelle malattie che portano un danno significativo alle cellule endoteliali, come il lupus eritematoso sistemico, l'ipertensione maligna, la preeclampsia, l'insufficienza renale postpartum e la nefrite da radiazioni. Numerose segnalazioni ne descrivono la comparsa in più di un membro della stessa famiglia. Le manifestazioni familiari in genere non si trovano associate alla diarrea e possono essere malattie autosomiche recessive o dominanti. Mutazioni nel componente H del complemento (che inibisce l'attivazione della via alternativa del complemento) vengono osservate nel 10-20% dei casi familiari. Il deficit completo del fattore di von Willebrand metalloproteasi (che cliva i multimeri dei fattore di von Willebrand) e della proteina cofattore di membrana è responsabile di altri casi familiari.

ANATOMIA PATOLOGICA. Le alterazioni glomerulari iniziali, che costituiscono il risultato del deposito subendoteliale e mesangiale di un materiale granulare e amorfo di origine sconosciuta, includono l'ispessimento delle pareti capillari, il restringimento del lume dei capillari e l'allargamento del mesangio. Nei capillari e nelle arteriole glomerulari risultano osservabili anche trombi di fibrina, che possono condurre a una necrosi corticale.

I glomeruli gravemente compromessi progrediscono a una sclerosi totale o parziale. Una compromissione vascolare grave può rendere non funzionanti anche altri glomeruli a causa dell'ischemia. Nelle piccole arterie e nelle arteriole gravemente interessate la proliferazione intimale concentrica conduce a una occlusione vascolare.

PATOGENESI. L'evento primitivo nella patogenesi della sindrome è la lesione delle cellule endoteliali, che a livello capillare e arteriolare nei reni conduce a una coagulazione localizzata. Il reperto di una coagulazione intravascolare disseminata è insolito. L'anemia microangiopatica deriva da un danno meccanico ai globuli rossi (RBC, *Red Blood Cell*) quando questi attraversano i vasi alterati. La trombocitopenia è causata da un danno o da un'adesione delle piastrine alla microvascolarizzazione intrarenale o sistemica. Gli RBC danneggiati e le piastrine vengono eliminati dalla circolazione dal fegato e dalla milza. I casi familiari ricorrenti non diarroici e sporadici di HUS sono associati a livelli di complemento (C3) basso dovuti alla sua disregolazione e attivazione in seguito a una lesione scatenante alle cellule endoteliali.

MANIFESTAZIONI CLINICHE. La HUS è più frequente nei bambini di età inferiore a 4 anni. In genere la sua insorgenza è preceduta da una gastroenterite caratterizzata da febbre, vomito, dolore addominale e diarrea all'inizio acquosa e poi ematica. Meno spesso i pazienti possono presentarsi dopo un'infezione del tratto respiratorio superiore. La comparsa improvvisa di pallore, irritabilità, debolezza, letargia e oliguria in genere si verifica 5-10 giorni dopo la malattia gastrointestinale o respiratoria iniziale. L'esame obiettivo può rivelare disidratazione, edema, petecchie, epatosplenomegalia e irritabilità marcata.

DIAGNOSI E DIAGNOSI DIFFERENZIALE. La diagnosi è sostenuta dalle osservazioni dell'anemia emolitica microangiopatica, della trombocitopenia e dell'insufficienza renale acuta (Tabb. 518-1 e 518-2). In genere il valore dell'emoglobina è compreso tra 5-9 g/dL. Lo striscio del sangue periferico rivela schizociti, echinociti e RBC frammentati (vedi Capitolo 447). I livelli plasmatici di emoglobina sono alti, mentre quelli plasmatici di aptoglobina risultano diminuiti. La conta dei reticolociti è moderatamente elevata e il risultato del test di Coombs è negativo. La leucocitosi è significativa e di solito la conta dei leucociti può essere superiore a 30 000/mm^3. Inoltre il 90% dei pazienti si rileva la trombocitopenia (20 000-100 000/mm^3). I reperti dell'analisi delle urine risultano sorprendentemente lievi e di solito sono costituiti da una ematuria microscopica di grado modesto e una proteinuria. In genere il tempo di tromboplastina parziale e quello di protrombina sono normali. Normalmente il prolungamento dei parametri coagulativi è causato più da un deficit della vitamina K che da coagulazione intravascolare disseminata. Le manifestazioni renali variano da una insufficienza renale lieve a una acuta, con oliguria o anuria che richiede la dialisi. Gli studi radiografici con bario rivelano spasmi colici e difetti di riempimento precoci transitori; la colite può apparire come un'"impronta di pollice". Le stenosi intestinali sono esiti rari.

La HUS deve sempre essere considerata in un bambino con una insorgenza improvvisa d'insufficienza renale acuta. L'anamnesi tipica, il quadro clinico e i risultati di laboratorio confermano la diagnosi nella maggior parte dei casi. Vanno escluse altre cause di insufficienza renale acuta, soprattutto quelle che possono essere associate a un'anemia emolitica microangiopatica, come il lupus eritematoso sistemico e l'ipertensione maligna. Una biopsia renale è raramente indicata.

TABELLA 518-1. Definizione della sindrome uremico-emolitica postdiarroica: Centers for Disease Control and Prevention, 1996

DESCRIZIONE CLINICA

La sindrome uremico-emolitica (HUS) è caratterizzata da esordio acuto di anemia emolitica microangiopatica, lesione renale e una conta piastrinica ridotta. Anche nella porpora trombocitopenica trombotica (TTP) si trovano queste caratteristiche, ma essa può includere inoltre il coinvolgimento del sistema nervoso centrale e la febbre e può avere un esordio più graduale. La maggior parte dei casi di HUS (ma pochi di TTP) si verificano dopo una malattia gastrointestinale acuta (in genere diarroica).

CRITERI DI LABORATORIO PER LA DIAGNOSI

Quelli che seguono sono entrambi presenti in un qualche momento durante la malattia:

- anemia (esordio acuto) con alterazioni microangiopatiche (cioè schistociti, echinociti o schizociti) sullo striscio del sangue periferico;
- lesione renale (esordio acuto) evidenziata da ematuria, proteinuria o livello di creatinina elevato (cioè ≥1,0 mg/dL in un bambino di età inferiore ai 13 anni o ≥1,5 mg/dL in una persona di 13 anni o più o un aumento ≥50% rispetto al basale).

Nota: In genere, ma non sempre, nelle fasi iniziali della malattia è possibile individuare una conta piastrinica ridotta, che tuttavia in seguito può diventare normale o persino elevata. Se la conta piastrinica ottenuta entro 7 giorni dall'esordio della malattia gastrointestinale non è <150 000/mm^3, devono essere considerate altre diagnosi.

CLASSIFICAZIONE DEL CASO

Probabile

- Una malattia acuta diagnosticata come HUS o TTP che soddisfa i criteri di laboratorio in un paziente privo di un'anamnesi chiara di diarrea acuta o ematica nelle precedenti 3 settimane, oppure
- Una malattia acuta diagnosticata come HUS o TTP che (a) abbia un esordio entro 3 settimane dall'insorgenza di diarrea acuta o ematica e (b) soddisfi i criteri di laboratorio tranne per il fatto che non vengono confermate alterazioni microangiopatiche.

Confermata

Una malattia acuta diagnosticata come HUS o TTP che soddisfa i criteri di laboratorio ed è cominciata entro 3 settimane dall'inizio di un episodio di diarrea acuta o ematica.

COMMENTO

Alcuni ricercatori considerano la HUS e la TTP come parti di un continuum patologico. Pertanto non vengono indicati criteri per diagnosticare la TTP sulla base del coinvolgimento del SNC e della febbre, perché i casi diagnosticati clinicamente come TTP postdiarroica devono soddisfare i criteri per la HUS. Questi casi sono riferiti come HUS postdiarroica.

Tratta da Elliott EJ, Robins-Browne RM: Hemolytic uremic syndrome. *Curr Probl Pediatr Adolesc Health Care* 2005;35: 305-344.

TABELLA 518-2. Classificazione della sindrome uremico-emolitica (HUS)

TIPO DI HUS	EZIOLOGIA
HUS TIPICA (POSTDIARROICA)	
Infezione postgastrointestinale	Organismi che producono Shiga tossine, di solito enteroemorragici: *Escherichia coli* e *Shigella dysenteriae*
HUS ATIPICA	
Infezione del tratto urinario	*E. coli* con produzione di Shiga tossina
Postinfettiva	Infezione al di fuori del tratto gastrointestinale (per es. polmoni, sistema nervoso centrale) con organismi che producono neuraminidasi, di solito *Streptococcus pneumoniae*
Familiare (autosomica dominante o recessiva)	Regolazione anomala della via del complemento (per es. difetto genetico nel controllo della produzione del fattore H, fattore I o della proteina cofattore di membrana)
	Regolazione anomala della coagulazione (per es., difetto genetico o anticorpi che comportano una riduzione dell'attività di ADAMTS-13)
Associata all'uso di farmaci	Immunosoppressori (per es. ciclosporina, FK-506, OKT3, mitomicina C); altro (per es. ganciclovir, pillola contraccettiva orale, crack cocaine, chinino)
Associazioni rare riferite	Lupus eritematoso sistemico, sclerosi sistemica, dopo trapianto di midollo osseo, leucemia, nail-patella syndrome, dopo glomerulonefrite streptococcica

Tratta da Elliott EJ, Robins-Browne RM: Hemolytic uremic syndrome. *Curr Probl Pediatr Adolesc Health Care* 2005;35: 305-344.

I pazienti con una trombosi bilaterale delle vene renali (vedi Capitolo 519.7) possono essere difficili da distinguere da quelli con la HUS. Entrambe le malattie possono essere precedute da una patologia gastrointestinale associata a disidratazione, pallore ed evidenza di anemia emolitica microangiopatica, trombocitopenia e insufficienza renale acuta. Un ingrossamento renale marcato e l'assenza di flusso venoso renale all'ecografia renale Doppler è coerente con una trombosi venosa renale.

COMPLICANZE. Le complicanze includono anemia, acidosi, iperkaliemia, sovraccarico di liquidi, insufficienza cardiaca, ipertensione e uremia. Le manifestazioni extrarenali del sistema nervoso centrale, del tratto gastrointestinale, del cuore e dei muscoli scheletrici possono essere pericolose per la vita. Le disfunzioni del sistema nervoso centrale includono irritabilità, convulsioni, infarti dei nuclei della base e della corteccia cerebrale, cecità corticale e coma. Le manifestazioni gastrointestinali comprendono la colite ischemica e infiammatoria, la perforazione intestinale, l'invaginazione e l'epatite. La necrosi pancreatica focale può causare pancreatite acuta, intolleranza al glucosio, diabete mellito insulinodipendente e livelli di lipasi elevati. Nei casi con coinvolgimento cardiaco possono comparire pericarditi, disfunzione miocardica e aritmie. Sono state inoltre riferite altre complicanze come necrosi cutanea, parotite, disfunzione surrenale e rabdomiolisi.

PROGNOSI E TRATTAMENTO. Un trattamento di supporto con un'attenzione meticolosa ai liquidi e agli elettroliti, il controllo dell'ipertensione, una nutrizione aggressiva e l'istituzione precoce della dialisi hanno consentito di ottenere una riduzione della mortalità causata da questa malattia dall'80% a meno del 10% nel corso degli ultimi 30 anni. Gli antibiotici vanno evitati nei pazienti con una enterite acuta che si presuma secondaria all'*E. coli* 0157:H7, in quanto possono accrescere il rischio di sviluppare la HUS. La nefroprotezione nella prima fase della HUS può essere ottenuta prevenendo la disidratazione con liquidi per via endovenosa. La terapia antitrombotica non produce alcun beneficio terapeutico dimostrato. Non esistono studi prospettici controllati che valutino il valore della plasmaferesi nella HUS preceduta dalla diarrea. Tuttavia, la plasmaferesi o la somministrazione di plasma fresco congelato possono risultare utili nella porpora trombocitopenica trombotica o nella HUS non preceduta dalla diarrea, oppure nei bambini con una HUS ricorrente familiare o con un coinvolgimento grave del sistema nervoso centrale. Tuttavia, possono esacerbare la HUS causata da *S. pneumoniae* e dovrebbero quindi essere evitate in presenza di questa infezione. La dialisi peritoneale controlla le anomalie dei liquidi e degli elettroliti, mantiene un volume intravascolare normale e fornisce l'opportunità di un supporto nutrizionale aggressivo. Può inoltre contribuire alla dissoluzione dei trombi vascolari rimuovendo gli inibitori della fibrinolisi e l'inibitore-1 attivante il plasminogeno circolante, con la conseguente attivazione delle normali vie fibrinolitiche endogene. La resina legante la Shiga tossina si è rivelata inefficace nel diminuire la prevalenza degli eventi mortali o extrarenali gravi. Gli studi *in vitro* che si avvalgono di inibitori della Shiga tossina sintetici multivalenti più potenti o di batteri sottoposti a ingegneria genetica che neutralizzano grandi quantità di Shiga tossina sembrano promettenti nel ridurre l'incidenza della HUS associata a diarrea.

Con un trattamento aggressivo dell'insufficienza renale acuta, oltre il 90% dei pazienti sopravvive alla fase acuta della HUS preceduta dalla diarrea. La morte o una insufficienza renale terminale si verificano nel 12% dei casi (0-30% dei pazienti in vari studi). Ipertensione, proteinuria e velocità di filtrazione glomerulare ridotte (<80 mL/min/1,73 m^2) subentrano nel 25% dei casi. La prognosi generale della HUS è associata a esiti renali negativi nel lungo periodo, se sono presenti sintomi a carico del sistema nervoso centrale (coma, stroke, convulsioni) durante la malattia acuta ed è necessaria la dialisi. Altri fattori predittivi di gravità acuta o cronica includono una conta dei globuli bianchi >20 000, la colite ischemica e l'ipertensione. I pazienti che si riprendono dalla fase acuta richiedono un follow-up a lungo termine, perché le complicanze come ipertensione, insufficienza renale cronica e proteinuria possono comparire fino a 20 anni dopo. Il trapianto del rene può avere successo, benché possa verificarsi una recidiva di malattia, in particolare nei casi familiari e non associati a diarrea. Il trapianto combinato di fegato e reni può essere un'alternativa per i casi familiari associati a mutazioni del fattore H del complemento.

Ake JA, Jelacic S, Ciol MA, et al: Relative nephroprotection during *Escherichia coli* O157:H7 infections: Association with intravenous volume expansion. *Pediatrics* 2005;115:e673–e680.

Banatvala N, Griffin PM, Greene KD, et al: The United States national prospective hemolytic-uremic syndrome study: Microbiologic, serologic, clinical, and epidemiologic findings. *J Infect Dis* 2001;183:1063–1070.

Bonnardeaux A, Pichette V: Complement dysregulation in haemolytic uraemic syndrome. *Lancet* 2003;362:1514–1516.

Cabrera GR, Fortenberry JD, Warshaw BL, et al: Hemolytic-uremic syndrome associated with invasive *Streptococcus pneumoniae* infection. *Pediatrics* 1998;101:699–703.

Centers for Disease Control and Prevention: Laboratory-confirmed non-0157 shiga toxin–producing *escherichia coli*–Connecticut, 2000–2005. *MMWR* 2007;56:29–31.

Centers for Disease Control and Prevention: *Escherichia coli* 0157:H7 infection associated with drinking raw milk–Washington and Oregon, November–December 2005. *MMWR* 2007;56:165–167.

Coppo P, Bussel A, Charrier S, et al: High-dose plasma infusion versus plasma exchange as early treatment of thrombotic thrombocytopenic purpura/hemolytic-uremic syndrome. *Medicine* 2003;82:27–38.

Crump JA, Sulka AC, Langer AJ, et al: An outbreak of *Escherichia coli* O157:H7 infections among visitors to a dairy farm. *N Engl J Med* 2002;347:555–560.

DeCaluwe H, Harrison LM, Mariscalco MM, et al: Procalcitonin in children with *Escherichia coli* O157:H7 associated hemolytic uremic syndrome. *Pediatr Res* 2006;59:579–583.

Eliott EJ, Robins-Browne RM: Hemolytic uremic syndrome. *Curr Probl Pediatr Adolesc Health Care* 2005;35:305–344.

Garg AX, Suri RS, Barrowman N, et al: Long-term renal prognosis of diarrhea-associated hemolytic uremic syndrome. *JAMA* 2003;290:1360–1370.

Noris M, Brioschi S, Caprioli J, et al: Familial haemolytic uraemic syndrome and an *MCP* mutation. *Lancet* 2003;362:1542–1546.

Oakes RS, Siegler RL, Me Reynolds MA, et al: Predicters of fatality in post-diarrheal hemolytic uremic syndrome. *Pediatrics* 2006;117:1656–1662.
Olie KH, Florquin S, Groothoff JW, et al: Atypical relapse of hemolytic uremic syndrome after transplantation. *Pediatr Nephrol* 2004;19:1173–1176.
Remuzzi G, Ruggenenti P, Codazzi D, et al: Combined kidney and liver transplantation for familial haemolytic uraemic syndrome. *Lancet* 2002;359:1671–1672.
Spizzirri FD, Rahman RC, Bibiloni N, et al: Childhood hemolytic-uremic syndrome in Argentina: Long-term follow-up and prognostic features. *Pediatr Nephrol* 1997;11:156–160.
Tarr PI, Gordon CA, Chandler WL: Shiga-toxin-producing *Escherichia coli* and haemolytic uraemic syndrome. *Lancet* 2005;365:1073–1086.
Trachtman H, Cnaan A, Christen E, et al: Effect of an oral Shiga toxin-binding agent on diarrhea-associated hemolytic uremic syndrome in children. *JAMA* 2003;290:1337–1344.
Wong CS, Jelacic S, Habeeb RL, et al: The risk of the hemolytic-uremic syndrome after antibiotic treatment of *Escherichia coli* O157:H7 infections. *N Engl J Med* 2000; 342:1930–1936.

Capitolo 519 ■ Cause di ematuria dovute al tratto urinario superiore

519.1 • Nefrite interstiziale (vedi Capitolo 532)

519.2 • Nefropatia tossica (vedi Capitolo 533)

519.3 • Necrosi corticale (vedi Capitolo 534)

519.4 • Pielonefrite (vedi Capitolo 538)

519.5 • Nefrocalcinosi (vedi Capitolo 547)

519.6 • Anomalie vascolari

Emangiomi, angiomi e malformazioni arteriovenose dei reni e del tratto urinario inferiore sono cause rare di ematuria. In genere questa si presenta come ematuria macroscopica e passaggio di coaguli di sangue. Se viene interessato il tratto superiore è possibile che si sviluppi una colica renale. La diagnosi è confermata dall'angiografia.

L'emorragia unilaterale delle vene varicose dell'uretere sinistro, che deriva dalla compressione della vena renale sinistra fra l'aorta e l'arteria mesenterica superiore, viene definita **sindrome dello schiaccianoci**. Tipicamente i pazienti con questa sindrome manifestano un'ematuria microscopica persistente (occasionalmente un'ematuria macroscopica ricorrente), che può essere accompagnata da proteinuria, dolore addominale inferiore, dolore al fianco o ipotensione ortostatica. La diagnosi è confermata dall'ecografia Doppler, dalla TC o dall'angiografia in risonanza magnetica.

Shin JI, Park JM, Lee SM, et al: Factors affecting spontaneous resolution of hematuria in childhood nutcracker syndrome. *Pediatr Nephrol* 2005;20: 609–613.
Chang CT, Hung CC, Ng KK, et al: Nutcracker syndrome and left unilateral haematuria. *Nephrol Dial Transplant* 2005;20:460–461.

519.7 • Trombosi della vena renale

EPIDEMIOLOGIA. La trombosi della vena renale (RVT, *Renal Vein Thrombosis*) si verifica in due situazioni cliniche distinte. Nei neonati e nei lattanti è comunemente associata ad asfissia, disidratazione, shock, sepsi, stati di ipercoagulabilità congeniti; si sviluppa anche in lattanti figli di madri con diabete mellito. Nei bambini più grandi viene invece riscontrata nei casi di sindrome nefrosica, cardiopatia cianotica, stati ipercoabulabili ereditari e in seguito all'esposizione ad agenti di contrasto angiografici.

PATOGENESI. La RVT inizia nella circolazione venosa intrarenale e può diffondersi alla vena renale principale e alla vena cava inferiore. La formazione dei trombi è mediata dal danno alle cellule endoteliali che deriva da ipossia, endotossine o mezzi di contrasto. Altri fattori contribuenti includono: (1) l'ipercoagulabilità dovuta alla sindrome nefrosica o a mutazioni nei geni che codificano i fattori di coagulazione (come il gene che produce il fattore V di Leiden); (2) l'ipovolemia e la riduzione di flusso sanguigno associati a uno shock settico, alla disidratazione o alla sindrome nefrosica; (3) l'agglutinazione intravascolare dovuta alla policitemia.

MANIFESTAZIONI CLINICHE. Lo sviluppo della RVT è generalmente segnalato dall'insorgenza improvvisa di un'ematuria macroscopica e di masse unilaterali o bilaterali al fianco. I pazienti possono inoltre manifestare un'ematuria microscopica, dolore al fianco, ipertensione o oliguria. La RVT in genere è unilaterale; quella bilaterale causa un'insufficienza renale acuta.

DIAGNOSI. La diagnosi di RVT è suggerita dallo sviluppo dell'ematuria e di masse al fianco in un paziente con fattori clinici predisponenti. I pazienti possono inoltre avere un'anemia emolitica microangiopatica e una trombocitopenia. L'ecografia evidenzia un ingrossamento marcato del rene, mentre le indagini con radionuclidi rivelano una funzione renale scarsa o assente nel rene o nei reni interessati. Gli studi eco-Doppler della vena cava inferiore e della vena renale confermano la diagnosi, mentre quelli con mezzo di contrasto devono essere evitati per ridurre il rischio di un ulteriore danno vascolare.

DIAGNOSI DIFFERENZIALE. La diagnosi differenziale della RVT include altre cause di ematuria associate ad anemia emolitica microangiopatica o all'ingrossamento renale, ossia la sindrome uremico-emolitica, l'idronefrosi, la malattia del rene policistico, il tumore di Wilms, gli ascessi o l'ematoma. Tutti i pazienti vanno sottoposti a una valutazione per condizioni di ipercoagulabilità congeniti e, nei bambini più grandi, acquisiti.

TRATTAMENTO. Il trattamento primario della RVT consiste in una terapia di supporto, che include la correzione dello squilibrio dei liquidi e degli elettroliti e il trattamento dell'insufficienza renale. Il trattamento con anticoagulanti o agenti trombolitici, tra cui la streptochinasi, l'urochinasi o l'attivatore del plasminogeno tissutale ricombinante, è comune ma resta controverso. I soggetti con una trombosi della vena cava inferiore possono richiedere una trombectomia chirurgica. I bambini con un'ipertensione grave refrattaria ai farmaci antipertensivi possono venire sottoposti a un intervento di nefrectomia.

PROGNOSI. La mortalità perinatale causata dalla RVT si è ridotta in maniera significativa nel corso degli ultimi 20 anni. Tuttavia, l'atrofia renale parziale o completa è una complicanza comune nel neonato, che conduce all'insufficienza renale, a una disfunzione tubulare renale e all'ipertensione sistemica. Queste complicanze vengono osservate anche nei bambini più grandi, benché il recupero della funzione renale sia comune in quelli con RVT dovuta a una sindrome nefrosica o a una cardiopatia cianogena.

Bokenkamp A, von Kries R, Nowak-Gottl U, et al: Neonatal renal venous thrombosis in Germany between 1992 and 1994: Epidemiology, treatment and outcome. *Eur J Pediatr* 2000;159:44–48.
Kosch A, Kuwertz-Broking E, Heller C, et al: Renal venous thrombosis in neonates: Prothrombotic risk factors and long-term follow-up. *Blood* 2004;104:1356–1360.
Kuhle S, Massicotte P, Chan A, et al: Data from the 1-800-NO-CLOTS Registry. A case series of 72 neonates with renal vein thrombosis. *Thromb Haemost* 2004;92:729–733.

519.8 • Ipercalciuria idiopatica

Questa entità, che può essere ereditata con modalità autosomica dominante, può presentarsi come un'ematuria macroscopica ricorrente, un'ematuria microscopica persistente, una disuria o un dolore addominale senza la formazione di calcoli. L'ipercalciuria può essere causata da stati che provocano ipercalcemia, come l'iperparatiroidismo, l'intossicazione da vitamina D, l'immobilizzazione e la sarcoidosi. Può trovarsi associata alla sindrome di Cushing, alla terapia corticosteroidea, a una disfunzione tubulare secondaria alla sindrome di Fanconi (malattia di Wilson, sindrome oculocerebrorenale), alla sindrome di Williams, all'acidosi tubulare renale o alla sindrome di Bartter. Può inoltre essere osservata in pazienti con **malattia di Dent**, ossia una forma di nefrolitiasi legata al cromosoma X e associata al rachitismo ipofosfatemico. Benché si ritenga che la formazione di microcristalli e la conseguente irritazione tissutale inducano i sintomi, il meccanismo preciso mediante il quale l'ipercalciuria causa l'ematuria o la disuria resta sconosciuto.

DIAGNOSI. L'ipercalciuria viene diagnosticata sulla base di un'escrezione di calcio nelle urine superiore a 4 mg/kg in 24 ore. Un test di screening nei pazienti che non possono raccogliere un campione di urine delle 24 ore può essere condotto su un campione singolo misurando le concentrazioni di calcio e creatinina. Un rapporto calcio/creatinina (mg/mg) su campione singolo superiore a 0,2 suggerisce l'ipercalciuria, benché nei bambini di età inferiore ai 7 mesi possano essere normali rapporti fino a 0,8.

TRATTAMENTO. Se non trattata, l'ipercalciuria conduce alla nefrolitiasi in circa il 15% dei casi. I diuretici tiazidici orali possono normalizzare l'escrezione urinaria di calcio stimolando il suo riassorbimento nei tubuli prossimale e distale. Questa terapia può inoltre arrestare l'ematuria macroscopica o la disuria e prevenire la nefrolitiasi. Tuttavia le indicazioni precise al trattamento con tiazidici restano controverse. Nei pazienti con ematuria macroscopica o disuria viene eseguita una terapia con l'idroclorotiazide a un dosaggio di 1-2 mg/kg/24 h quale dose mattutina singola. La dose viene titolata verso l'alto fino a che l'escrezione urinaria di calcio nelle 24 ore sia <4 mg/kg e fino alla risoluzione delle manifestazioni cliniche. Dopo 1 anno di trattamento, in genere questa somministrazione viene sospesa, ma può essere ripresa in caso di recidiva di ematuria macroscopica, nefrolitiasi o disuria. Durante la terapia con l'idroclorotiazide, il livello di potassio nel siero deve essere monitorato periodicamente per evitare l'ipokaliemia. Anche il **citrato di potassio** a un dosaggio di 1 mEq/kg/24 h può risultare utile, in particolare nei pazienti con una ridotta escrezione urinaria di citrato e una disuria sintomatica. La limitazione del sodio è importante, perché l'escrezione del calcio corrisponde a quella di sodio. In particolare, non è raccomandata la limitazione dell'assunzione del calcio con la dieta (tranne nei bambini con un'anamnesi di assunzione massiva), dal momento che è un elemento indispensabile per la crescita e vista l'assenza di prove che dimostrino una relazione tra la minore assunzione e una riduzione dei suoi livelli urinari.

Bhimma R, Robbs J: Nutcracker. *Lancet* 2005;365:1280–1281.
Kari JA, Farouq M, Alshaya HO: Familial hypomagnesemia with hypercalciuria and nephrocalcinosis. *Pediatr Nephrol* 2003;18:506–510.
Knohl SJ, Scheinman SJ: Inherited hypercalciuric syndromes: Dent's disease (CLC-5) and familial hypomagnesemia with hypercalciuria (paracellin-1). *Semin Nephrol* 2004;24:55–60.
Magen D, Adler L, Mandel H, et al: Autosomal recessive renal proximal tubulopathy and hypercalciuria: A new syndrome. *Am J Kidney Dis* 2004;43:600–606.
Polito C, Iolascon G, Nappi B, et al: Growth and bone mineral density in long-lasting idiopathic hypercalciuria. *Pediatr Nephrol* 2003;18:545–547.
Polito C, LaManna A, Cioce F, et al: Clinical presentation and natural course of idiopathic hypercalciuria in children. *Pediatr Nephrol* 2000;15:211–214.
So NP, Osorio AV, Simon SD, et al: Normal urinary calcium/creatinine ratios in African-American and Caucasian children. *Pediatr Nephrol* 2001;16:133–139.
Stapleton FB: Childhood stones. *Endocrinol Metab Clin North Am* 2002;31:1001–1015.
Vachvanichsanong P, Malagon M, Moore ES: Recurrent abdominal and flank pain in children with idiopathic hypercalciuria. *Acta Paediatr* 2001;90:643–648.

Capitolo 520 ■ Malattie ematologiche che causano ematuria

520.1 • Nefropatia dell'anemia a cellule falciformi

L'ematuria macroscopica o microscopica può essere osservata nei bambini con la malattia a cellule falciformi o il trait a cellule falciformi. I segni e i sintomi si risolvono spontaneamente nella maggior parte dei pazienti (vedi Capitolo 462.1). Con ogni probabilità l'ematuria deriva da una microtrombosi secondaria alla falcizzazione in una midollare renale relativamente ipossica, acida e ipertonica, dove si trova una stasi vascolare. In questi pazienti possono inoltre essere presenti ischemia, necrosi papillare e fibrosi interstiziale. Altre manifestazioni cliniche della nefropatia da cellule falciformi includono la poliuria determinata da un difetto di concentrazione delle urine, l'acidosi tubulare renale e la proteinuria associata a una lesione glomerulare che assomiglia alla glomerulosclerosi segmentale focale o alla glomerulonefrite membranoproliferativa. Gli ACE-inibitori, come l'enalapril, sono spesso usati per ottenere una riduzione dell'escrezione di proteine con le urine nei pazienti dove questa in un giorno supera i 500 mg. Anche l'idrossiurea può aiutare a ridurla. La nefropatia da anemia a cellule falciformi può alla fine condurre all'ipertensione e all'insufficienza renale, che possono progredire a insufficienza renale terminale.

Fitzhugh CD, Wigfall DR, Ware RE: Enalapril and hydroxyurea therapy for children with sickle nephropathy. *Pediatr Blood Cancer* 2005;45:982–985.
Pham PT, Pham PC, Wilkinson AH, et al: Renal abnormalities in sickle cell disease. *Kidney Int* 2000;57:1–8.
Scheinman JI: Sickle cell disease and the kidney. *Semin Nephrol* 2003;23:66–76.

520.2 • Coagulopatie e trombocitopenia

L'ematuria macroscopica o microscopica può essere associata a malattie ereditarie o acquisite della coagulazione (emofilia, coagulazione intravascolare disseminata, trombocitopenia). In questi casi, tuttavia, in genere essa non è il sintomo iniziale ma si sviluppa dopo altre manifestazioni (vedi Parte XX, Sezione 7).

Capitolo 521 ■ Anomalie anatomiche associate a ematuria

521.1 • Anomalie congenite

L'ematuria macroscopica o microscopica può essere associata a molti tipi di diverse malformazioni del tratto urinario. L'insorgenza improvvisa dell'ematuria macroscopica dopo un trauma lieve al fianco è spesso associata all'ostruzione della giunzione ureteropelvica o a reni cistici (vedi Capitolo 537).

521.2 • Malattia del rene policistico autosomica recessiva

Nota anche come **malattia policistica infantile**, l'ARPKD (*Autosomal Recessive Polycystic Kidney Disease*) è una malattia autosomica recessiva con un'incidenza compresa tra 1:10 000 e 1:40 000. Il gene dell'ARPKD codifica per la fibrocistina, una proteina di grandi dimensioni (>4000 aminoacidi) con molteplici motivi strutturali. La sua funzione nel normale sviluppo del rene e la fisiopatologia della sua espressione anomala nell'ARPKD sono sconosciute.

ANATOMIA PATOLOGICA. Entrambi i reni sono significativamente ingrossati e mostrano in maniera evidente innumerevoli cisti nella midollare e nella corteccia. Le analisi al microscopio dimostrano microcisti che si irradiano dalla midollare alla corteccia situate prevalentemente all'interno dei tubuli e dei dotti collettori, benché siano state riferite cisti transitorie nel tubulo prossimale del feto. Lo sviluppo della fibrosi interstiziale progressiva e dell'atrofia tubulare durante le fasi avanzate della malattia conduce alla fine all'insufficienza renale. Il coinvolgimento epatico è caratterizzato da un'anomalia di base della placca duttale, che conduce alla proliferazione dei dotti biliari e all'ectasia, così come a una fibrosi epatica, ed è indistinguibile dalla fibrosi epatica congenita o malattia di Caroli.

MANIFESTAZIONI CLINICHE. Il paziente tipico presenta masse bilaterali all'altezza del fianco durante il periodo neonatale o la prima infanzia. L'ARPKD può essere associata a oligoidramnios, ipoplasia polmonare, distress respiratorio e pneumotorace spontaneo nel periodo neonatale. Possono essere presenti la facies di Potter e altri componenti del complesso dell'oligoidramnios, tra cui orecchie con impianto basso, micrognazia, naso appiattito, difetti nel posizionamento degli arti e deficit di crescita. Entro le prime settimane di vita viene generalmente riscontrata un'ipertensione, spesso grave. Normalmente la diuresi non è diminuita, benché in alcuni casi vengano riscontrate l'oliguria e un'insufficienza renale acuta. L'iponatriemia transitoria, spesso in presenza di un'insufficienza renale acuta, è comune nel periodo neonatale e spesso risponde alla diuresi. La funzione renale è generalmente compromessa, ma inizialmente, nel 20-30% dei pazienti, può risultare normale. Raramente, l'ARPKD si presenta dopo l'infanzia con insufficienza renale, ipertensione o epatosplenomegalia correlata alla fibrosi epatica.

L'evidenza clinica di una malattia epatica rilevata alle indagini di laboratorio cliniche o radiologiche è presente in circa il 45% dei neonati e si ritiene sia del 100% in caso di patologia dimostrata all'esame microscopico. I pazienti con l'ARPKD corrono il rischio di sviluppare: (1) colangite ascendente, varici, ipersplenismo correlato all'ipertensione della portale e (2) disfunzione epatica progressiva, che raramente conduce all'insufficienza epatica franca e alla cirrosi. Un sottogruppo di bambini più grandi può presentarsi con un'epatosplenomegalia e manifestare una malattia renale lieve che viene scoperta per caso durante studi di imaging dell'addome.

DIAGNOSI. La diagnosi di ARPKD è fortemente suggerita da masse palpabili e bilaterali a livello del fianco in un neonato con ipoplasia polmonare, oligoidramnios e ipertensione, nonché in assenza di cisti renali all'ecografia dei genitori. Reni significativamente ingrossati e uniformemente iperecogeni con una distinzione corticomidollare scarsa vengono comunemente osservati all'ecografia (Fig. 521-1). La diagnosi è sostenuta dai segni clinici o di laboratorio di fibrosi epatica, da reperti patologici di anomalie della placca duttale osservati alla biopsia epatica, dalla dimostrazione anatomica e istologica di ARPKD in un fratello o dalla consanguineità genitoriale. La diagnosi differenziale include altre cause di ingrossamento renale bilaterale, come la displasia multicistica, l'idronefrosi, il tumore di Wilms e la trombosi bilaterale della vena renale. Il test diagnostico prenatale mediante l'analisi di linkage o direttamente della mutazione può essere eseguito nelle famiglie in cui vi sia almeno un bambino interessato.

TRATTAMENTO. Il trattamento è di supporto. Un supporto ventilatorio aggressivo è spesso necessario nel periodo neonatale a causa dell'ipoplasia polmonare, dell'ipoventilazione e delle numerose patologie respiratorie della prematurità (che sono comuni). È fondamentale un trattamento attento dell'ipertensione, delle anomalie dei liquidi e degli elettroliti, nonché delle manifestazioni cliniche di insufficienza renale. I bambini con un'insufficienza respiratoria grave o un'intolleranza alimentare causata dai reni ingrossati possono necessitare di interventi di nefrectomia unilaterale o bilaterale, che impongono l'esigenza di una terapia di sostituzione renale.

PROGNOSI. La mortalità si è molto abbassata, nonostante circa il 30% dei pazienti muoia nel periodo neonatale per le complicanze dell'ipoplasia polmonare. Il supporto respiratorio neonatale e le terapie sostitutive renali hanno aumentato di oltre l'80% la sopravvivenza a 10 anni dei bambini che arrivano oltre il 1° anno di vita. Si stima poi che la sopravvivenza a 15 anni sia pari al 70-80%. Un'insufficienza renale terminale viene riscontrata in oltre il 50% dei bambini e in genere si verifica durante il primo decennio di vita. Di conseguenza, la dialisi e il trapianto renale sono diventati terapie standard per questi pazienti. La morbilità e la mortalità nei bambini più grandi sono correlate alle complicanze dell'insufficienza renale cronica e alla malattia epatica.

Adeva M, El-Youssef M, Rossetti S, et al: Clinical and molecular characterization defines a broadened spectrum of autosomal recessive polycystic kidney disease (ARPKD). *Medicine* 2006;85:1–21.

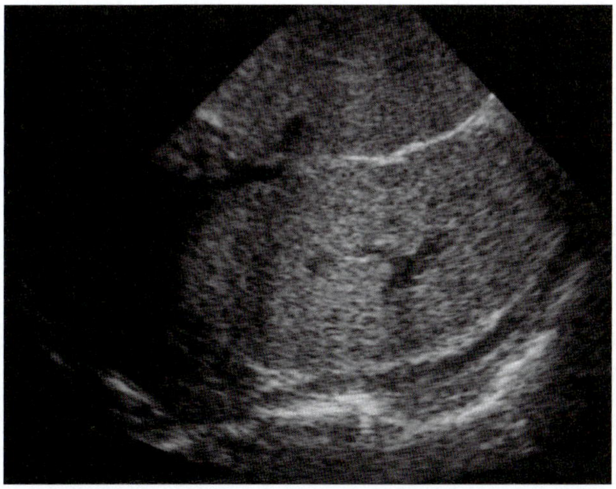

Figura 521-1. Ecografia di un neonato con malattia del rene policistico autosomica recessiva che mostra un ingrossamento renale (9 cm) e un'aumentata ecogenicità diffusa con perdita completa della differenziazione corticomidollare derivante da più interfacce cistiche piccole.

Bergmann C, Senderek J, Kupper F, et al: PKHD1 mutations in autosomal recessive polycystic kidney disease (ARPKD). *Hum Mutat* 2004;23:453–463.

Davis ID, Ho M, Hupertz V, et al: Survival of childhood polycystic kidney disease following renal transplantation: The impact of advanced hepatobiliary disease. *Pediatr Transplant* 2003;7:364–369.

Dell KM: Cystic and dysplastic disorders: Polycystic kidney diseases. In Kaplan BS, Meyers KM (editors): *Requisites in Pediatrics: Nephrology/Urology.* St. Louis, Harcourt, 2004.

Dell KM, Avner ED: Autosomal recessive polycystic kidney disease. In GeneClinics: Clinical Genetic Information Resource [database online]. University of Washington, Seattle. Available at http://www.geneclinics.org/.

Guay-Woodford LM: Autosomal recessive polycystic kidney disease (ARPKD): New insights from the identification of the ARPKD gene, PKHD1. *Pediatr Res* 2002;52:830–831.

Guay-Woodford LM, Desmond RA: Autosomal recessive polycystic kidney disease: The clinical experience in North America. *Pediatrics* 2003;111:1072–1080.

Roy S, Dillon MJ, Trompeter RS, et al: Autosomal recessive polycystic kidney disease: Long-term outcome of neonatal survivors. *Pediatr Nephrol* 1997;11:302–306.

Zerres K, Rudnik-Schoneborn S, Deget F, et al: Autosomal recessive polycystic kidney disease in 115 children: Clinical presentation, course and influence of gender. *Acta Paediatr* 1996;85:437–445.

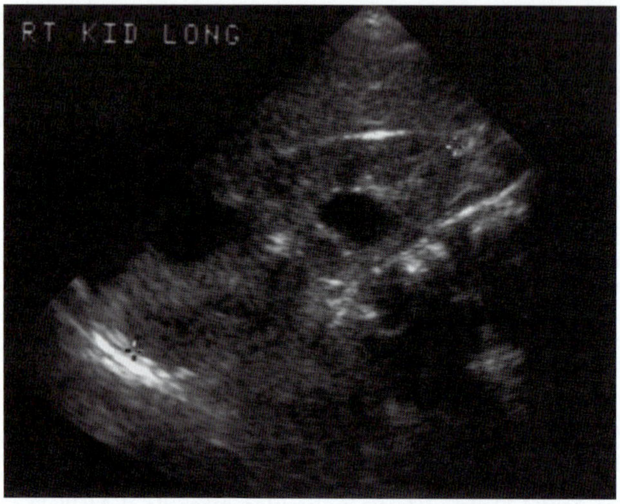

Figura 521-2. Ecografia di un bambino di 18 mesi con malattia del rene policistico autosomica dominante che mostra un ingrossamento renale (10 cm) e due grandi cisti.

521.3 • Malattia del rene policistico autosomica dominante

La malattia del rene policistico autosomica dominante (ADPKD, *Autosomal Dominant Polycystic Kidney Disease*) è la malattia renale umana ereditaria più comune. Il modello autosomico dominante di ereditarietà si verifica con un'incidenza di 1/500-1/1000. Circa l'85% dei pazienti mappa sul gene *PKD1* sul braccio corto del cromosoma 16, che codifica la policistina, una glicoproteina transmembrana. Un altro 10-15% dei casi mappa sul gene *PKD2* sul braccio lungo del cromosoma 4, che codifica la policistina 2, un canale per i cationi non selettivo. I pazienti restanti possono mappare su altri loci ancora da determinare.

ANATOMIA PATOLOGICA. Entrambi i reni sono ingrossati e mostrano cisti corticali e midollari che originano da tutte le regioni del nefrone.

PRESENTAZIONE CLINICA. Benché l'ADPKD sintomatica in genere si presenti tra i quaranta e i cinquant'anni, è possibile che i sintomi, tra cui l'ematuria macroscopica o microscopica, il dolore al fianco bilaterale, le masse addominali, l'ipertensione e l'infezione del tratto urinario, vengano osservati anche nei bambini e nei neonati. In genere l'ecografia renale dimostra macrocisti bilaterali multiple (Fig. 521-2), nonostante nella prima fase della malattia possa essere osservata anche una malattia unilaterale.

L'ADPKD è una malattia sistemica che interessa molti apparati. Possono essere presenti cisti nel fegato, nel pancreas, nella milza e nelle ovaie. Gli **aneurismi intracranici**, che sembrano raccogliersi all'interno di certe famiglie, sono una causa importante di mortalità negli adulti, ma risultano rari nei bambini. In circa il 12% di questi viene riscontrato il prolasso della valvola mitrale e possono trovarsi anche diverticoli intestinali ed ernie.

DIAGNOSI. L'ADPKD è confermata dalla presenza di reni ingrossati con macrocisti bilaterali in un paziente con un parente di primo grado interessato dalla malattia. L'assenza di un'anamnesi familiare non preclude tuttavia questa diagnosi, perché i membri della famiglia potrebbero avere una malattia silente oppure il bambino colpito può presentare una nuova mutazione, che si verifica nel 5-10% dei casi. Tra i pazienti con un'ADPKD geneticamente definita, i risultati dell'ecografia renale di screening possono risultare normali nel 20% dei casi a 20 anni, in meno del 5% a 30 anni.

La diagnosi prenatale è suggerita dalla presenza di reni ingrossati con o senza cisti all'ecografia nelle famiglie con un'ADPKD nota. Il test prenatale del DNA è disponibile per le famiglie con membri colpiti la cui malattia sia determinata da mutazioni note nei geni *PKD1* o *PKD2*.

La diagnosi differenziale include le cisti renali associate alla malattia del rene glomerulocistico, la sclerosi tuberosa e la malattia di von Hippel-Lindau, che può essere ereditata secondo un modello autosomico dominante. Le manifestazioni neonatali dell'ADPKD e dell'ARPKD possono non essere distinguibili.

TRATTAMENTO E PROGNOSI. Il trattamento è principalmente di supporto. Il controllo della pressione sanguigna è fondamentale, in quanto la velocità di progressione della malattia è correlata alla presenza di ipertensione. Gli ACE-inibitori e/o gli antagonisti dei recettori dell'angiotensina II costituiscono gli agenti di elezione.

Benché l'ADPKD neonatale possa essere letale, una sopravvivenza a lungo termine dei reni e del paziente stesso è possibile per i bambini che sopravvivono al periodo neonatale. La presentazione dell'ADPKD nei bambini più grandi ha una prognosi favorevole, con una funzione renale normale durante l'infanzia rilevata in >80% dei casi.

Davis ID, MacRae DK, Sweeney WS, et al: Can progression of autosomal dominant or autosomal recessive polycystic kidney disease be prevented? *Semin Nephrol* 2001;21:430–440.

Dell KM, McDonald R, Watkins S, et al: Polycystic kidney disease. In Avner ED, Harmon W, Niaudet P (editors): *Pediatric Nephrology,* 5th ed. Philadelphia, Lippincott Williams & Wilkins, 2004, pp 675–699.

Fick GM, Duley IT, Johnson AM, et al: The spectrum of autosomal dominant polycystic disease in children. *J Am Soc Nephrol* 1994;4:1654–1660.

Fick-Brosnahan GM, Tran ZV, Johnson AM, et al: Progression of autosomal-dominant polycystic kidney disease in children. *Kidney Int* 2001;59:1979–1980.

Kelleher CL, McFann KK, Johnson AM, et al: Characteristics of hypertension in young adults with autosomal dominant polycystic kidney disease compared with the general U.S. population. *Am J Hypertens* 2004;17:1029–1034.

Kubo S, Nakajima M, Fukuda K, et al: A 4-year-old girl with autosomal dominant polycystic kidney disease complicated by a ruptured intracranial aneurysm. *Eur J Pediatr* 2004;163:675–677.

Martinez-Vea A, Bardaj A, Gutierrez C, et al: Exercise blood pressure, cardiac structure, and diastolic function in young normotensive patients with polycystic kidney disease: A prehypertensive state. *Am J Kidney Dis* 2004;44:216–223.

Ong AC, Harris PC: Molecular pathogenesis of ADPKD: The polycystin complex gets complex. *Kidney Int* 2005;67:1234–1247.
Perrone RD: Extrarenal manifestations of ADPKD. *Kidney Int* 1997;51: 2022–2036.
Rossetti S, Chauveau D, Kubly V, et al: Association of mutation position in polycystic kidney disease 1 (PKD1) gene and development of a vascular phenotype. *Lancet* 2003;361:2196–2101.

521.4 • Traumi

I lattanti e i bambini sono più sensibili al danno renale in seguito a una contusione o a un trauma penetrante della schiena o dell'addome a causa della minore massa muscolare che "protegge" il rene. Possono verificarsi un'ematuria macroscopica o microscopica, un dolore al fianco, la rigidità addominale; possono altresì essere presenti lesioni associate. Il trauma uretrale può venire determinato da lesioni da schiacciamento, spesso associate alla frattura della pelvi o a un danno diretto. Questo tipo di lesione va sospettata in presenza di un'ematuria macroscopica sul meato uretrale esterno.

Buckley JC, McAninch JW: Pediatric renal injuries: Management guidelines from a 25-year experience. *J Urol* 2004;172:687–690.
Dreitlein DA, Suner S, Basler J: Genitourinary trauma. *Emerg Med Clin North Am* 2001;19:569–590.
Grantham JJ, Torres VE, Chapman AB, et al: Volume progression in polycystic kidney disease. *N Engl J Med* 2006;354:2122–2130.

521.5 • Tumori renali (vedi Capitoli 498 e 499)

Capitolo 522 ■ Cause di ematuria del tratto urinario inferiore

522.1 • Cause infettive di cistite e uretrite

L'ematuria macroscopica o microscopica può essere associata a infezioni batteriche, micobatteriche o virali della vescica (vedi Capitolo 538). La manifestazione di ematuria può correlarsi alla profondità e alla gravità della reazione infiammatoria all'interno della parete della vescica.

L'uretrite si può presentare con ematuria macroscopica o microscopica collegata a urgenza e piuria. Occasionalmente l'urinocoltura rivela batteri, *Ureaplasma* o *Chlamydia*, ma in genere è negativa. Deve essere ricercata un'anamnesi di trauma. Il disturbo spesso si risolve spontaneamente. Nei bambini di età superiore a 8 anni, il trattamento di elezione è una terapia di 10 giorni con la doxiciclina unitamente a un analgesico urinario come la fenazopiridina per alleviare il dolore. Se l'approccio conservativo fallisce, può essere necessaria la cistoscopia per determinare la natura di un'eventuale anomalia sottostante, come la presenza di un'ulcera o un'infiammazione.

522.2 • Cistite emorragica

La cistite emorragica (vedi anche Capitolo 259) viene definita come un'emorragia acuta o cronica della vescica. I pazienti spesso si presentano con un'ematuria macroscopica e con disuria. Nelle forme gravi l'emorragia può condurre a una riduzione dei livelli di emoglobina. La cistite emorragica può sorgere in risposta a tossine chimiche (ciclofosfamide, penicilline, busulfan, tiotepa, coloranti, insetticidi), virus (tipi di adenovirus 11 e 21, poliomavirus BK, influenza A), radiazione e amiloidosi. L'idratazione e l'uso del MESNA bisolfito (350 mg/m^2 ogni 6 h), che inattiva i metaboliti della ciclofosfamide, aiutano a proteggere la vescica dall'irritazione chimica correlata all'uso della ciclofosfamide ev per molte malattie. La somministrazione di ciclofosfamide orale al mattino seguita da una idratazione orale aggressiva per il resto della giornata è molto efficace nel ridurre al minimo il rischio della cistite emorragica. L'irrigazione della vescica con una soluzione salina, l'allume, il nitrato d'argento o l'acido aminocaproico può essere necessaria nelle forme più gravi della malattia. L'ematuria macroscopica associata alla cistite emorragica virale in genere si risolve entro 1 settimana.

DeVries CR, Freiha FS: Hemorrhagic cystitis: A review. *J Urol* 1990;143: 1–9.
Hale GA, Rochester RJ, Heslop HE, et al: Hemorrhagic cystitis after allogeneic bone marrow transplantation in children: Clinical characteristics and outcome. *Biol Blood Marrow Transplant* 2003;9:698–705.
Pahari A, Rees L: BK virus-associated renal problems—clinical implications. *Pediatr Nephrol* 2003;18:743–748.

522.3 • Sforzo intenso

L'ematuria macroscopica o microscopica può verificarsi in seguito a uno sforzo intenso. Questa forma è rara nelle femmine e può essere associata a disuria. Il colore delle urine può variare da rosso a nero e in esse si possono trovare coaguli di sangue. I risultati dell'urinocoltura, della pielografia ev, della cistouretrografia minzionale e della cistoscopia sono normali nella maggior parte dei pazienti. Sembra trattarsi di una condizione benigna e in genere l'ematuria si risolve entro 48 ore dopo la sospensione dello sforzo. L'assenza di cilindri eritrocitari o l'evidenza della malattia renale e la presenza di disuria e coaguli ematici in alcuni pazienti suggeriscono che la sorgente dell'emorragia risiede nel tratto urinario inferiore. Nella diagnosi differenziale occorre considerare la possibilità di una rabdomiolisi con mioglobinuria o emoglobinuria quando esistono sintomi associati nel contesto clinico appropriato.

Abarbanel J, Benet AE, Lask D, et al: Sports hematuria. *J Urol* 1990;143:887–890.
Gambrell RC, Blount BW: Exercise-induced hematuria. *Am Fam Physician* 1996;53:905–911.
Siegel AJ, Hennekens CH, Solomon HS, et al: Exercise-related hematuria. *JAMA* 1979;241:391–392.

522.4 • Sindrome di Münchausen per procura (vedi Capitolo 36.2)

Sezione 3 — Malattie particolarmente associate a proteinuria — Beth A. Vogt ed Ellis D. Avner

Capitolo 523 ■ Approccio al bambino con proteinuria

Ritrovare una proteinuria all'analisi delle urine di screening eseguita di routine è un evento comune; il 10% dei bambini di età compresa tra 8 e 15 anni risulta prima o poi positivo al test con strisce reattive. La difficoltà consiste nel distinguere il bambino con la proteinuria correlata a una malattia renale da quello altrimenti sano con forme transitorie o altre forme benigne.

Il test con strisce reattive (stick) offre una valutazione qualitativa dell'escrezione di proteine con le urine. Le strisce reattive rilevano in primo luogo l'albuminuria e sono meno sensibili alle altre forme di proteinuria (proteine a basso peso molecolare, proteine di Bence Jones, gamma globuline). Le alterazioni visive nel colore della striscia sono una misura semiquantitaviva della concentrazione in aumento delle proteine nelle urine. La striscia può essere negativa, con tracce (10-20 mg/dL), 1+ (30 mg/dL), 2+ (100 mg/dL), 3+ (300 mg/dL) e 4+ (1000-2000 mg/dL).

Risultati falsamente negativi possono verificarsi nei pazienti con urine diluite (peso specifico <1,005) oppure in stati patologici in cui la proteina urinaria predominante non sia l'albumina. Risultati, invece, falsamente positivi possono essere osservati in soggetti con un'ematuria macroscopica, una contaminazione con agenti antisettici (clorexidina, benzalconio cloruro), un pH urinario >7,0 o nel caso di una terapia con fenazopiridina. La striscia reattiva può diventare falsamente positiva nei pazienti con urine molto concentrate. Una striscia deve essere considerata positiva alle proteine se registra ≥1+ (30 mg/dL) in un campione di urina il cui peso specifico sia ≤1,015, mentre se questo è >1,015, la striscia deve essere ≥2+ per poter essere considerata clinicamente significativa.

Dato che la reazione della striscia offre solo una misurazione qualitativa dell'escrezione di proteine con le urine, i bambini con una proteinuria persistente vanno sottoposti a un'analisi quantitativa con un rapporto spot proteine/creatinina (UPr/UCr) nelle urine più preciso. Questo rapporto viene calcolato dividendo la concentrazione UPr (mg/dL) per quella UCr (mg/dL) e di preferenza va eseguito sul primo campione di urine del mattino, per eliminare la possibilità di una proteinuria ortostatica (posturale) (vedi Capitolo 525). Rapporti <0,5 nei bambini più giovani di 2 anni e <0,2 nei bambini di 2 anni o più grandi suggeriscono un'escrezione proteica normale, mentre un rapporto >3 indica una probabile proteinuria nell'intervallo nefrotico. I rapporti UPr/UCr possiedono una stretta correlazione con le determinazioni dell'escrezione di proteine in base a una raccolta delle urine cronometrata.

Le raccolte delle urine delle 24 h offrono informazioni più precise sull'escrezione UPr ma risultano più difficili da ottenere e molto imprecise e sono state ampiamente sostituite dal rapporto proteine/creatinina su campioni singoli. Un ragionevole limite superiore dell'escrezione di proteine normale nei bambini sani è 150 mg/24 h (0,15 g/24 h). Più specificamente, questa escrezione viene definita come ≤4 $mg/m^2/h$, mentre un'escrezione anomala si configura pari a 4-40 $mg/m^2/h$ e un intervallo nefrotico come >40 $mg/m^2/h$.

Abitbol C, Zilleruelo G, Freundlich M, et al: Quantitation of proteinuria with urinary protein/creatinine ratios and random testing with dipsticks in nephrotic syndrome. *J Pediatr* 1990;116:243–247.

D'Amico G, Bazzi C: Pathophysiology of proteinuria. *Kidney Int* 2003;63: 809–825.

Hogg R, Portman RJ, Milliner D, et al: Evaluation and management of proteinuria and nephrotic syndrome in children: Recommendations from a pediatric nephrology panel established at the National Kidney Foundation Conference of Proteinuria, Albuminuria, Risk, Assessment, Detection, and Elimination. *Pediatrics* 2000;105:1242–1249.

Tryggvason K, Patrakka J, Wartiovaara J: Hereditary proteinuria syndromes and mechanisms of proteinuria. *N Engl J Med* 2006;354:1387–1401.

Vehaskari VM, Rapola J: Isolated proteinuria: Analysis of a school-age population. *J Pediatr* 1982;101:661–668.

Capitolo 524 ■ Proteinuria transitoria

La maggior parte dei bambini con una striscia reattiva urinaria positiva alle proteine presenta valori normali di questa striscia alle misurazioni ripetute. Del 10% dei bambini che ha proteinuria secondo una singola misurazione, solo l'1% è risultato affetto da una forma persistente dopo misurazioni in 4 occasioni distinte. Questo fenomeno, definito **proteinuria transitoria**, può avere varie cause: una temperatura >38,3 °C (vedi Capitolo 174), lo sforzo (vedi Capitolo 685), la disidratazione, l'esposizione al freddo, l'insufficienza cardiaca, crisi convulsive o stress. In genere, la proteinuria non supera 2+ sulla striscia reattiva. Il meccanismo della proteinuria transitoria è sconosciuto. Non occorre alcuna valutazione o terapia per i bambini con questa condizione benigna.

Jensen H, Henriksen K: Proteinuria in non-renal infectious disease. *Acta Med Scand* 1974;196:75–82.

Marks MI, McLaine PN, Drummond KN: Proteinuria in children with febrile illnesses. *Arch Dis Child* 1970;45:250–253.

Poortmans JR: Post-exercise proteinuria in humans. *JAMA* 1985;253:236–240.

Vehaskari VM, Rapola J: Isolated proteinuria: Analysis of a school-age population. *J Pediatr* 1982;101:661–668.

Capitolo 525 ■ Proteinuria ortostatica (posturale)

La proteinuria ortostatica è la causa più comune di proteinuria persistente nei bambini in età scolare e negli adolescenti e si verifica fino nel 60% dei bambini con proteinuria persistente. I bambini con questa condizione di solito sono asintomatici ed essa viene scoperta durante un'analisi delle urine di routine. Essi eliminano quantità normali o minimamente aumentate di proteine in posizione supina, mentre in posizione eretta l'escrezione aumenta di 10 volte, fino a 1000 mg/24 h (1 g/24 h). Sono assenti ematuria, ipertensione, ipoalbuminemia, edema e disfunzione renale.

In un bambino con una proteinuria asintomatica persistente, il primo passo nella valutazione è escludere la proteinuria ortostatica, eseguendo un'analisi delle urine completa e un rapporto proteine/creatinina singolo su un campione delle urine del mattino. È importante che il bambino vuoti completamente la vescica prima di andare a letto e raccolga il campione emesso immediatamente dopo essersi alzato alla mattina. L'assenza di proteinuria in questo campione (striscia reattiva negativa o tracce di proteine e rapporto UPr/Cr <0,2) per 3 giorni consecutivi conferma la diagnosi di proteinuria ortostatica. Non occorre alcun altro esame e il paziente e la famiglia vanno rassicurati circa la natura benigna della condizione. D'altro canto, se vi sono altre anomalie nell'analisi delle urine (ematuria) o il rapporto UPr/Cr risulta >0,2, il paziente deve essere indirizzato a un nefrologo pediatra per la valutazione.

La causa della proteinuria ortostatica è sconosciuta, benché tra quelle possibili figurino l'emodinamica renale alterata e l'ostruzione parziale della vena renale in posizione eretta. Studi di follow-up a lungo termine negli adulti suggeriscono che sia un processo benigno, ma dati simili non sono disponibili per i bambini, per cui un tale follow-up in loro è prudente per monitorare una evidenza di malattia renale, tra cui ematuria, ipertensione, edema, funzione renale diminuita o proteinuria superiore a 1000 mg/24 h.

Cho BS, Choi YM, Kang MI, et al: Diagnosis of nutcracker phenomenon using renal Doppler ultrasound in orthostatic proteinuria. *Nephrol Dial Transplant* 2001;16:1620–1625.

Devarajan P: Mechanisms of orthostatic proteinuria: Lessons from a transplant donor. *J Am Soc Nephrol* 1993;4:36–39.

Springberg PD, Garrett LE Jr, Thompson AL, et al: Fixed and reproducible orthostatic proteinuria: Results of a 20-year follow-up study. *Ann Intern Med* 1982;97:516.

Capitolo 526 ■ Proteinuria persistente

I soggetti con una proteinuria significativa nel primo campione di urine del mattino per 3 giorni consecutivi (>1+ sulla striscia reattiva oppure rapporto proteine/creatinina >0,2) soffrono di proteinuria persistente. La proteinuria persistente indica una malattia renale e può essere causata da disturbi glomerulari o tubulari.

526.1 • Proteinuria glomerulare

Numerose malattie renali sono caratterizzate da un'aumentata permeabilità della parete capillare glomerulare, che conduce alla proteinuria glomerulare (Tab. 526-1). Questa può variare da <1 g a >30 g/24 h. Può essere definita *selettiva* (quando si verifica una perdita delle proteine del plasma di peso molecolare fino a quello dell'albumina compreso) o *non selettiva* (se si ha una perdita di albumina o delle proteine di peso maggiore, come le IgG). La determinazione della selettività delle proteine urinarie ha un valore clinico ridotto, a causa della considerevole sovrapposizione tra le varie forme di malattia renale. Quando è "selettiva", tuttavia, può identificare pazienti nefrotici con la massima probabilità di rispondere ai corticosteroidi (vedi Capitolo 527).

La proteinuria glomerulare deve essere sospettata in qualsiasi paziente con un rapporto proteine/creatinina delle prime urine del mattino >1,0 o con una proteinuria di qualsiasi grado accompagnata da ipertensione, ematuria, edema o disfunzione renale. Tra i disturbi caratterizzati prevalentemente dalla proteinuria figurano la glomerulosclerosi segmentale, la glomerulonefrite proliferativa mesangiale, la nefropatia membranosa, la glomerulonefrite membranoproliferativa, l'amiloidosi, la nefropatia diabetica e la glomerulonefrite correlata a obesità. Altri disturbi renali che possono avere la proteinuria come tratto prominente includono la glomerulonefrite postinfettiva, la nefropatia da IgA, la nefrite lupica, la nefrite della porpora di Henoch-Schönlein e la sindrome di Alport.

TABELLA 526-1. Cause di proteinuria

PROTEINURIA TRANSITORIA
Febbre
Esercizio fisico
Disidratazione
Esposizione al freddo
Insufficienza cardiaca congestizia
Crisi convulsive
Sforzo
PROTEINURIA ORTOSTATICA (POSTURALE)
MALATTIE GLOMERULARI CARATTERIZZATE DA PROTEINURIA ISOLATA
Glomerulosclerosi segmentale focale
Glomerulonefrite proliferativa mesangiale
Nefropatia membranosa
Glomerulonefrite membranoproliferativa
Amiloidosi
Nefropatia diabetica
Nefropatia a cellule falciformi
MALATTIE GLOMERULARI CON PROTEINURIA QUALE TRATTO DISTINTIVO
Glomerulonefrite postinfettiva acuta
Nefropatia da IgA
Nefrite della porpora di Henoch-Schönlein
Nefrite lupica
Sindrome di Alport
MALATTIE TUBULARI
Cistinosi
Malattia di Wilson
Sindrome di Lowe
Galattosemia
Nefrite tubulointerstiziale
Avvelenamento da metalli pesanti
Necrosi tubulare acuta
Displasia renale
Malattia policistica renale
Nefropatia da reflusso

La valutazione iniziale di un bambino con proteinuria persistente deve includere la misurazione della creatinina sierica e del panel di elettroliti, il rapporto proteine/creatinina nelle prime urine del mattino, il livello di albumina nel siero e il livello di C3. Questo bambino va quindi mandato da un nefrologo pediatra per un ulteriore esame e per il trattamento. La biopsia renale è spesso necessaria per definire la diagnosi e guidare la terapia.

Nei bambini asintomatici con proteinuria di grado ridotto (rapporto proteine/creatinina 0,2-1,0), in cui tutti gli altri risultati siano normali, la biopsia renale può non essere indicata, in quanto il processo sottostante può essere transitorio/in risoluzione oppure perché i tratti patologici specifici di una malattia renale cronica possono non essere ancora apparenti. Questi pazienti devono essere sottoposti a una rivalutazione periodica (ogni 4-6 mesi a meno che non diventino sintomatici), che comprenda un esame obiettivo e la determinazione della pressione sanguigna, l'analisi delle urine e la misurazione delle creatinina sierica e del rapporto proteine/creatinina nelle prime urine del mattino. Le indicazioni alla biopsia renale includono una proteinuria ingravescente (rapporto proteine/creatinina >1,0) e/o lo sviluppo dell'ematuria, un'ipertensione o una funzione renale ridotta.

Bergstein JM: A practical approach to proteinuria. *Pediatr Nephrol* 1999;13:697–700.

Mahan, JD, Turman MA, Mentser MI: Evaluation of hematuria, proteinuria, and hypertension in adolescents. *Pediatr Clin North Am* 1997; 44:1573–1589.

Roy S: Proteinuria. *Pediatr Ann* 1996;25:277–282.

Wilmer WA, Rovin BH, Hebert CJ, et al: Management of glomerular proteinuria: A commentary. *J Am Soc Nephrol* 2003;14:3217–3232.

526.2 • Proteinuria tubulare

Una serie di malattie renali che interessano principalmente il compartimento tubulointerstiziale del rene possono causare una proteinuria persistente di grado ridotto (rapporto proteine/creatinina <1,0). Nello stato sano, grandi quantità di proteine con un peso molecolare inferiore a quello dell'albumina vengono filtrate dal glomerulo e riassorbite nel tubulo prossimale. Una lesione ai tubuli prossimali può determinare una capacità di riassorbimento ridotta e la perdita di queste proteine a basso peso molecolare nelle urine.

La proteinuria tubulare (vedi Tab. 526-1) può essere osservata nei disturbi acquisiti ed ereditari e può essere associata ad altri difetti della funzione tubulare prossimale, come la glicosuria, la fosfaturia, il mancato riassorbimento del bicarbonato e l'aminoaciduria. Raramente la proteinuria tubulare rappresenta un dilemma diagnostico, perché la malattia sottostante in genere viene individuata prima che venga rilevata la proteinuria.

I pazienti asintomatici con una proteinuria persistente in genere hanno una proteinuria glomerulare e non tubulare. Nei casi occulti, queste proteinurie possono essere distinte mediante una elettroforesi delle urine: in quella tubulare viene rilevata una quantità di albumina ridotta o nulla, mentre nella glomerulare la proteina maggiore è proprio l'albumina.

Alt JM, Von der Heyde D, Assel E, et al: Characteristics of protein excretion in glomerular and tubular disease. *Contrib Nephrol* 1981;24:115–121.

Capitolo 527 ■ Sindrome nefrosica

La sindrome nefrosica è una malattia primariamente pediatrica ed è 15 volte più comune nei bambini che negli adulti. L'incidenza è di 2-3/100 000 bambini all'anno e la maggior parte di quelli interessati mostrerà una malattia con lesioni minime sensibile agli steroidi. I tratti caratteristici sono una proteinuria massiva (>3,5 g/24 h negli adulti o 40 mg/m^2/h nei bambini), l'ipoalbuminemia (<2,5 g/dL), l'edema e l'iperlipidemia.

EZIOLOGIA. La maggior parte dei bambini (90%) con la sindrome nefrosica soffre di una forma idiopatica, le cui cause includono una malattia a lesioni minime (85%), una proliferazione mesangiale (5%) e una glomerulosclerosi segmentale focale (10%). Il restante 10% presenta una sindrome nefrosica secondaria correlata a malattie sistemiche (Tab. 527-1) glomerulari, come la nefropatia membranosa o la glomerulonefrite membranoproliferativa (Tab. 527-2).

FISIOPATOLOGIA. L'anomalia sottostante alla sindrome nefrosica è un aumento della permeabilità della parete capillare glomerulare, che conduce a una proteinuria massiva e all'ipoalbuminemia. La causa della maggiore permeabilità non è ben compresa. Nella malattia a lesioni minime è possibile che la disfunzione delle cellule T conduca all'alterazione delle citochine, e ciò determina una perdita di glicoproteine caricate negativamente all'interno della parete capillare glomerulare. Nella glomerulosclerosi segmentale focale, un fattore plasmatico forse prodotto dai linfociti può essere responsabile di tale aumento della permeabilità. In alternativa, alcune mutazioni nelle proteine dei podociti (podocina, α-actinina 4) sono associate alla glomerulosclerosi segmentale focale (Tab. 527-3). La sindrome nefrosica resistente agli steroidi è invece associata a mutazioni nei geni *NPHS2* (podocina) e *WT1*.

Benché il meccanismo della formazione dell'edema nella sindrome nefrosica non sia completamente noto, sembra probabile che, nella maggior parte dei casi, una perdita massiva di proteine con le urine conduca all'ipoalbuminemia, il che determina una riduzione nella pressione oncotica plasmatica e la trasudazione di liquido dal compartimento intravascolare allo spazio interstiziale. La diminuzione del volume intravascolare riduce a sua volta la pressione di perfusione renale, attivando il sistema renina-angiotensina-aldosterone, che stimola il riassorbimento tubulare del sodio. Il volume intravascolare ridotto stimola inoltre il rilascio dell'ormone antidiuretico, che aumenta il riassorbimento dell'acqua del dotto collettore.

Questa teoria non vale per tutti i pazienti con sindrome nefrosica, perché alcuni in realtà hanno un volume intravascolare aumentato con livelli plasmatici di renina e aldosterone diminuiti. Pertanto nella formazione dell'edema, in questi casi, possono essere coinvolti anche altri fattori, tra cui un'avidità renale primitiva per il sodio e l'acqua.

Nello stato nefrosico, i livelli dei lipidi nel siero (colesterolo, trigliceridi) risultano elevati per due ragioni. Per prima cosa, l'ipoalbuminemia stimola la sintesi generalizzata delle proteine epatiche, compresa la sintesi delle lipoproteine. Inoltre, il catabolismo dei lipidi è diminuito, in conseguenza dei livelli plasmatici diminuiti della lipasi delle lipoproteine correlati alle maggiori perdite urinarie di questo enzima.

Nephrotic syndrome in children: Prediction of histopathology from clinical and laboratory characteristics at time of diagnosis. A report of the International Study of Kidney Disease in Children. *Kidney Int* 1978;13:159.
Van de Walle JGJ, Donckerwolcke RA: Pathogenesis of edema formation in the nephrotic syndrome. *Pediatr Nephrol* 2001;16:283.

527.1 • Sindrome nefrosica idiopatica

Circa il 90% dei bambini con sindrome nefrosica soffre della sindrome nefrosica idiopatica. Questa include 3 tipi istologici: la malattia a lesioni minime, la proliferazione mesangiale e la glomerulosclerosi segmentale focale. A loro volta tali disturbi possono rappresentare 3 malattie distinte, con manifestazioni cliniche simili; o altrimenti possono costituire lo spettro di una singola malattia.

ANATOMIA PATOLOGICA. Nella **sindrome nefrosica a lesioni minime** (**MCNS**, *Minimal Change Nephrotic Syndrome*), che rappresenta l'85% dei casi totali di sindrome nefrosica nei bambini, i glomeruli appaiono normali o mostrano un aumento minimo nelle cellule mesangiali e nella matrice. I risultati alla microscopia in immunofluorescenza sono tipicamente negativi e l'analisi al microscopio elettronico rivela semplicemente una scomparsa dei podociti delle cellule epiteliali. Oltre il 95% dei casi risponde alla terapia con corticosteroidi.

Alla microscopia ottica, la **proliferazione mesangiale** (5% dei casi totali) è caratterizzata da un aumento diffuso delle cellule mesangiali e della matrice. La microscopia in immunofluorescenza può mostrare da tracce IgM e/o IgA mesangiali. La microscopia elettronica rivela invece quantità aumentate di cellule mesangiali e matrice nonché la perdita dei podociti delle cellule epiteliali. Circa il 50% dei pazienti con questa lesione istologica risponde alla terapia con corticosteroidi.

Nella **glomerulosclerosi segmentale focale** (**FSGS**, *Focal Segmental GlomeruloSclerosis*) (10% di tutti i casi), i glomeruli mostrano una proliferazione mesangiale e la formazione di tessuto cicatriziale segmentale alla microscopia ottica (Fig. 527-1, Tab. 527-2). La microscopia in immunofluorescenza indica una positività per IgM e C3 nelle aree di sclerosi segmentale, mentre quella elettronica evidenzia una cicatrizzazione segmentale del glomerulo con l'obliterazione del lume capillare glomerulare. Una lesione simile può essere osservata con l'infezione da HIV, il

TABELLA 527-1. Cause di sindrome nefrosica nel bambino*

MALATTIE GENETICHE	CAUSE SECONDARIE
Sindrome nefrosica tipica	**Infezioni**
Sindrome nefrosica congenita di tipo finlandese	Epatite B, C
Glomerulosclerosi segmentale focale	HIV-1
Sclerosi mesangiale diffusa	Malaria
Sindrome di Denys-Drash	Sifilide
Displasia immuno-ossea di Schimke	Toxoplasmosi
Proteinuria con o senza sindrome nefrosica	**Farmaci**
Nail-patella syndrome	Penicillamina
Sindrome di Alport	Oro
Sindromi multisistemiche con o senza sindrome nefrosica	Farmaci antinfiammatori non steroidei
Sindrome di Galloway-Mowat	Pamidronato
Malattia di Charcot-Marie-Tooth	Interferone
Sindrome di Jeune	Mercurio
Sindrome di Cockayne	Eroina
Sindrome di Laurence-Moon-Biedl-Bardet	Litio
Malattie metaboliche con o senza sindrome nefrosica	**Malattie immunologiche o allergiche**
Sindrome di Alagille	Malattia di Castleman
Deficit di α_1 antitripsina	Malattia di Kimura
Malattia di Fabry	Puntura di ape
Acidemia glutarica	Allergeni alimentari
Malattia da accumulo del glicogeno	**Associata a malattie maligne**
Sindrome di Hurler	Linfoma
Malattie delle lipoproteine	Leucemia
Citopatie mitocondriali	**Iperfiltrazione glomerulare**
Malattia a cellule falciformi	Oligomeganefronia
SINDROME NEFROSICA IDIOPATICA	Obesità patologica
Malattia con lesioni minime	Adattamento alla riduzione dei nefroni
Glomerulosclerosi segmentale focale	
Nefropatia membranosa	

*Può anche essere la conseguenza di malattie glomerulari infiammatorie, normalmente associate a caratteristiche di nefrite, per esempio vasculite, nefrite lupica, glomerulonefrite membranoproliferativa, nefropatia da IgA.
Tratta da Eddy AA, Symons JM: Nephrotic syndrome in childhood. *Lancet* 2003; 362:629-638.

TABELLA 527-2. Riepilogo delle malattie renali che si presentano sotto forma di sindrome nefrosica idiopatica

	SINDROME NEFROSICA A LESIONI MINIME	GLOMERULOSCLEROSI FOCALE SEGMENTALE	NEFROPATIA MEMBRANOSA	GLOMERULONEFRITE MEMBRANOPROLIFERATIVA	
				Tipo I	Tipo II
FREQUENZA*					
Bambini	75%	10%	<5%	10%	10%
Adulti	15%	15%	50%	10%	10%
Manifestazioni cliniche					
Età (anni)	2-6, alcuni adulti	2-10, alcuni adulti	40-50	5-15	5-15
Sesso	2:1 maschi	1,3:1 maschi	2:1 maschi	Maschi-femmine	Maschi-femmine
Sindrome nefrosica	100%	90%	80%	60%	60%
Proteinuria asintomatica	0	10%	20%	40%	40%
Ematuria	10-20%	60-80%	60%	80%	80%
Ipertensione	10%	20% precoce	Rara	35%	35%
Velocità di progressione a insufficienza renale	Non progredisce	10 anni	50% in 10-20 anni	10-20 anni	5-15 anni
Malattie associate	Allergia? Morbo di Hodgkin, di solito nessuna	Nessuno	Trombosi vena renale, cancro, SLE, epatite B	Nessuno	Lipodistrofia parziale
Reperti di laboratorio	Manifestazioni di sindrome nefrosica	Manifestazioni di sindrome nefrosica	Manifestazioni di sindrome nefrosica		
	↑ BUN in 15-30%	↑ BUN in 20-40%		C1, C4, C3-C9 bassi	C1, C4 normali, C3-C9 bassi
Immunogenetica	HLA-B8, B12 (3,5)[†]	Mutazioni in podocina, α-actinina-4, altri geni	HLA-DRw3 (12-32)[†]	Non definita	Fattore nefritico C3 non definito
Patologia renale					
Microscopica ottica	Normale	Lesioni sclerotiche focali	GBM ispessita, spike	GBM ispessita, proliferazione	Lobulazione
Immunofluorescenza	Negativa↑	IgM, C3 nelle lesioni	IgG granulare fine, C3	IgG granulare, C3	Solo C3
Microscopia elettronica	Fusione dei podociti	Fusione dei podociti	Depositi sottoepiteliali	Depositi mesangiali e subendoteliali	Depositi densi
Risposta agli steroidi	90%	15-20%	Può esserci progressione lenta	Non definita	Non definita

*Frequenza approssimativa quale causa di sindrome nefrotica idiopatica. Circa il 10% dei casi di sindrome nefrotica nell'adulto sono dovuti a varie patologie che di solito si presentano come glomerulonefrite acuta.
[†]Rischio relativo.
BUN, azotemia (*Blood Urea Nitrogen*); C, complemento; GBM, membrana basale glomerulare (*Glomerular Basement Membrane*); HLA, antigene leucocitario umano (*Human Leukocyte Antigen*); Ig, immunoglobulina; SLE, lupus eritematoso sistemico (*Systemic Lupus Erythematosus*); epatite B, virus epatite B; ↑, elevato.
Modificata da Couser WG: Glomerular disorders. In Wyngaarden JB, Smith LH, Bennett JC (editors): *Cecil Textbook of Medicine*, 19th ed. Philadelphia, WB Saunders, 1992, p 560.

TABELLA 527-3. Sindrome nefrosica nei bambini dovuta a malattie genetiche del podocita

GENE	NOME	POSIZIONE	EREDITARIETÀ	MALATTIA RENALE
SINDROME NEFROSICA RESISTENTE AGLI STEROIDI				
NPHS1	Nefrina	19q13.1	Recessiva	Sindrome nefrosica congenita di tipo finlandese
NPHS2	Podocina	1q25	Recessiva	FSGS
FSGS1	α-actinina-4 (α*ACTN4*)	19q13	Dominante	FSGS
FSGS2	Sconosciuto	11q21-22	Dominante	FSGS
WT1	Gene soppressore del tumore di Wilms	11p13	Dominante	Sindrome di Denys-Drash con sclerosi mesangiale diffusa
				Sindrome di Frasier con FSGS
LMX1B	Omeodominio proteina LIM	9q34	Dominante	Nail-patella syndrome
SMARCAL1	Regolatore della cromatina correlato a SW1/SNF2, matrice-associato, actina-dipendente, sottofamiglia a-like 1	2q35	Recessiva	Displasia immuno-ossea di Schimke con FSGS*
SINDROME NEFROSICA CHE RISPONDE AGLI STEROIDI				
Sconosciuta	Sconosciuta	Sconosciuta	Recessiva	MCNS

*Espressione del podocita di *SMARCAL1* supposta ma non ancora definita. Mutazioni in un'altra proteina, CD2-AP o NEPH1 (proteina nuova strutturalmente correlata a nefrina), causano sindrome nefrotica congenita nei topi. Una variante mutazionale del gene *CD2AP* è stata identificata in alcuni pazienti con sindrome nefrotica resistente agli steroidi.
Da Eddy AA, Symons JM: Nephrotic syndrome in childhood. *Lancet* 2003; 362:629-638.

reflusso vescicoureterale e l'abuso di eroina per via endovenosa. Solo il 20% dei pazienti con la FSGS risponde al prednisone. La malattia è spesso progressiva: alla fine interessa tutti i glomeruli e conduce a un'insufficienza renale terminale nella maggior parte dei pazienti.

MANIFESTAZIONI CLINICHE. La sindrome nefrosica idiopatica è più comune nei maschi che nelle femmine (2:1) e in genere si manifesta tra i 2 e i 6 anni. È stata tuttavia riferita già a partire dai 6 mesi di età e per tutta l'età adulta. La MCNS colpisce l'85-90% dei pazienti di età inferiore ai 6 anni, mentre la FSGS si sviluppa nei bambini più grandi. Tra il 20 e il 30% degli adolescenti ha la MCNS. È possibile che l'incidenza della FSGS sia in aumento; può essere più frequente negli afroamericani o negli ispanici. L'episodio iniziale e le recidive possono fare seguito a infezioni lievi e occasionalmente a reazioni dovute a punture di insetto (come l'ape) o all'edera velenosa. I bambini in genere presentano un edema lieve, che inizialmente viene osservato attorno agli occhi e negli arti inferiori. Da principio la sindrome nefrosica può essere oggetto di una diagnosi errata quale disturbo allergico, a causa della tumefazione periorbitale che si riduce durante il giorno. Con il passare del tempo, tuttavia, la tumefazione diviene generalizzata, con lo sviluppo di ascite, versamenti pleurici ed edema genitale. L'anoressia, l'irritabilità, un dolore addominale e la diarrea sono comuni, mentre risultano rari l'ipertensione e l'ematuria macroscopica. La diagnosi differenziale del bambino con un edema marcato include l'enteropatia con perdita di proteine, l'insufficienza epatica, l'insufficienza cardiaca congestizia, la glomerulonefrite acuta o cronica e un insufficiente apporto di proteine. Una diagnosi diversa dalls MCNS deve essere valutata in relazione a una età <1 anno, all'anamnesi familiare, a reperti extrarenali (artrite, rash, anemia), all'ipertensione o a un edema polmonare, all'insufficienza renale acuta o cronica e all'ematuria.

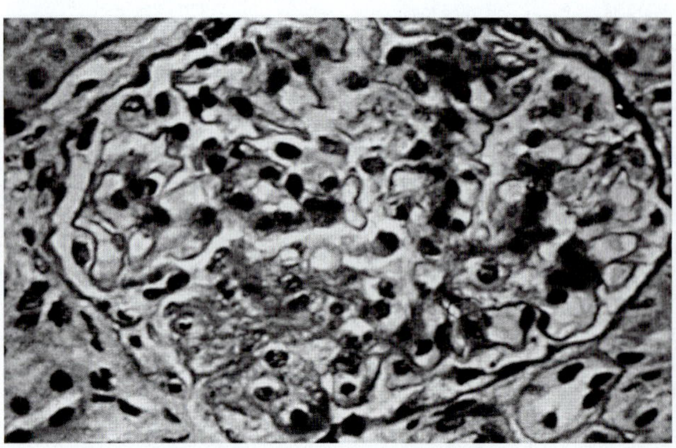

Figura 527-1. Glomerulo di un paziente con sindrome nefrotica resistente agli steroidi che mostra ipercellularità mesangiale e un'area di sclerosi nella porzione inferiore (×250).

DIAGNOSI. L'analisi delle urine rivela una proteinuria 3+ o 4+; l'ematuria microscopica può essere presente nel 20% dei bambini. Il rapporto proteine/creatinina nelle urine spot è superiore a 2,0, mentre l'escrezione di proteine con le urine è superiore a 3,5 g/24 h negli adulti e a 40 $mg/m^2/h$ nei bambini. Il valore della creatinina sierica è generalmente normale, ma può essere aumentato a causa della minore perfusione renale derivante dalla contrazione del volume intravascolare. Nel siero, il livello di albumina è generalmente <2,5 g/dL, mentre quelli di colesterolo e trigliceridi risultano elevati. I livelli di C3 e C4 appaiono normali. Nella maggior parte dei bambini una biopsia renale non è necessaria.

TRATTAMENTO. I bambini con il primo episodio da lieve a moderato di sindrome nefrosica ed edema possono essere trattati come pazienti esterni. Quelli colpiti dalla patologia possono frequentare la scuola e partecipare alle attività fisiche tollerate. La fisiopatologia e la terapia della sindrome nefrotica vanno discusse attentamente con la famiglia, per accrescere la loro comprensione della malattia del bambino. Bisogna ridurre l'assunzione di sodio, adottando una dieta iposodica che può essere normalizzata quando il bambino entra in remissione. Benché non vi siano dati a sostegno della loro sicurezza ed efficacia, molti clinici utilizzano i diuretici orali per i bambini con sindrome nefrosica, il cui uso dovrebbe comunque essere riservato ai pazienti con sintomi gravi e mantenuto sotto attento monitoraggio, data la possibilità di aumentare il rischio di complicanze tromboemboliche.

I bambini con un edema sintomatico grave, tra cui versamenti pleurici importanti, ascite o edema genitale severo, dovrebbero essere ricoverati. Oltre a una limitazione all'assunzione di sodio, se il bambino è iponatriemico può essere necessaria una restrizione dei liquidi. Uno scroto gonfio può essere sollevato con cuscini per migliorare la rimozione dei liquidi per opera della gravità. La diuresi può essere aumentata somministrando la clorotiazide (10 mg/kg/dose ev ogni 12 h) o il metolazone (0,1 mg/kg/dose per os due volte al giorno) seguita dalla furosemide a 30 min di distanza (1-2 mg/kg/dose ev ogni 12 h).

La somministrazione ev di albumina umana al 25% (0,5 g/kg/dose ogni 6-12 h somministrati in 1-2 h) seguita dalla furosemide (1-2 mg/kg/dose ev) risulta spesso necessaria quando la restrizione dei liquidi e i diuretici per via parenterale non sono efficaci. Questa terapia richiede un monitoraggio attento dello stato idroelettrolitico e della funzione renale. Il sovraccarico di volume sintomatico, con ipertensione e insufficienza cardiaca, è una complicanza potenziale della terapia parenterale con albumina, in particolare con infusioni rapide. I bambini con l'esordio della sindrome nefrosica tra 1 e 8 anni di età hanno una maggiore probabilità di avere una MCNS che risponde agli steroidi, la terapia con i quali può essere avviata senza una biopsia renale diagnostica. Per i bambini che presentano invece i tratti che rendono la MCNS meno probabile (ematuria, ipertensione, insufficienza renale, ipocomplementemia, età <1 anno o >8 anni) la biopsia renale deve essere considerata prima di avviare la terapia.

Ai bambini con MCNS presunta occorre somministrare prednisone (dopo avere verificato un test PPD negativo) a un dosaggio di 60 mg/m^2/die (massimo giornaliero: 80 mg divisa in 2-3 dosi) per almeno 4 settimane consecutive. Esistono valide prove che un trattamento iniziale di 6 settimane di terapia steroidea **quotidiana** può ridurre il tasso di recidive, benché la frequenza degli effetti collaterali indotti dagli steroidi sia superiore. Dall'80% al 90% dei bambini risponde alla terapia con steroidi (urine con tracce o assenza di proteine per 3 giorni consecutivi) per 2 settimane. La maggior parte di quelli responsivi alla terapia con prednisone ha una risposta entro le prime 4 settimane.

Dopo un ciclo iniziale di 6 settimane, il prednisone va ridotto a 40 mg/m^2/die a giorni alterni, in dose mattutina singola. Questa dose **a giorni alterni** viene quindi ridotta lentamente e interrotta nel corso dei 2-3 mesi successivi. I bambini che continuano a presentare proteinuria (2+ o superiore) dopo 8 settimane di terapia con steroidi vengono considerati resistenti a essi e devono quindi essere sottoposti a una biopsia renale diagnostica.

Molti bambini con sindrome nefrosica sperimentano almeno 1 recidiva (proteinura 3-4+ insieme all'edema). Benché in passato siano stati riferiti tassi di recidiva del 60-80%, quello nei bambini trattati con steroidi a cicli iniziali più lunghi può ridursi fino al 30-40%.

Le recidive vanno trattate con dosi giornaliere frazionate di prednisone ai dosaggi sopra indicati finché il bambino entra in remissione (urine con tracce o assenza di proteine per 3 giorni consecutivi). La dose di prednisone viene quindi passata a giorni alterni e gradualmente sospesa nell'arco di 1-2 mesi.

Un sottogruppo di pazienti va incontro alla recidiva durante la terapia con steroidi a giorni alterni oppure entro 28 giorni dalla sospensione della terapia con prednisone. Questi pazienti vengono definiti **steroido-dipendenti.** Quelli che rispondono bene alla terapia con il prednisone ma che ricadono ≥4 volte in un periodo di 12 mesi vengono invece detti pazienti con **frequenti ricadute**. I bambini, infine, che non reagiscono alla terapia con il prednisone entro 8 settimane si dicono **steroido-resistenti.** La sindrome nefrotica resistente agli steroidi generalmente si rivela una FSGS (80%), una MCNS (20%) e raramente una proliferativa mesangiale.

I pazienti steroido-dipendenti, quelli con frequenti recidive e quelli steroido-resistenti possono essere candidati per agenti alternativi, in particolare se soffrono di tossicità grave da corticosteroidi (aspetto cushingoide, ipertensione, cataratta e/o deficit di crescita). La **ciclofosfamide** prolunga la durata della remissione e riduce il numero di ricadute nei bambini con una sindrome nefrosica con **frequenti recidive** e **steroido-dipendente**. I potenziali effetti collaterali del farmaco (neutropenia, varicella disseminata, cistite emorragica, alopecia, sterilità, rischio aumentato di neoplasie maligne future) devono essere valutati con attenzione insieme alla famiglia prima di avviare il trattamento. Il quantitativo di ciclofosfamide è di 2-3 mg/kg/24 h, in una dose orale singola per una durata totale di 8-12 settimane. La terapia con il prednisone a giorni alterni viene spesso proseguita durante la somministrazione della ciclofosfamide. Durante questa terapia la conta dei globuli bianchi va monitorata settimanalmente e nel caso dovesse scendere sotto i 5000/mm^3 la terapia stessa deve essere interrotta.

Un'opzione aggiuntiva per il bambino con una sindrome nefrosica complicata è la somministrazione di **metilprednisolone a boli ad alte dosi**, in genere sotto forma di bolo di 30 mg/kg (massimo 1000 mg), con le prime 6 dosi a giorni alterni seguite da un regime a scalare per periodi fino a 18 mesi. La ciclofosfamide può essere aggiunta a questo regime in pazienti selezionati. La **ciclosporina** (3-6 mg/kg/24 h divisa ogni 12 h) o il **tacrolimus** (0,15 mg/kg/24 h ogni 12 h) sono efficaci nel mantenere remissioni prolungate nei bambini con la sindrome nefrotica e sono utili come agenti risparmiatori di steroidi. Occorre monitorare la comparsa di effetti collaterali, tra cui l'ipertensione, la nefrotossicità, l'irsutismo e l'iperplasia gengivale. Il **micofenolato** può far perdurare la remissione nei bambini con una sindrome nefrotica dipendente da steroidi e frequentemente recidivante. La maggior parte dei pazienti che risponde alla terapia con ciclosporina, tacrolimus o micofenolato tende comunque a recidivare quando il farmaco viene sospeso. Gli ACE-inibitori e i bloccanti dell'angiotensina II possono tornare utili quale terapia aggiuntiva per ridurre la proteinuria nei pazienti resistenti agli steroidi.

COMPLICANZE. L'infezione è la complicanza principale della sindrome nefrosica. I bambini in recidiva hanno una sensibilità aumentata alle infezioni batteriche a causa delle perdite urinarie di immunoglobuline e del fattore B properdinico, di una immunità cellulo-mediata deficitaria, della terapia immunosoppressiva, della malnutrizione e dell'edema/ascite che fungono da potenziale "mezzo di coltura". La **peritonite batterica spontanea** è il tipo di infezione più frequente, benché possano essere riscontrate sepsi, polmonite, cellulite e infezioni delle vie urinarie. Nonostante lo *Streptococcus pneumoniae* sia l'organismo più comune a determinare la peritonite, possono essere rilevati anche batteri come l'*Escherichia coli.* Dato che la febbre e i reperti obiettivi possono risultare minimi in presenza di una terapia corticosteroidea, diventano fondamentali un elevato indice di sospetto, una valutazione tempestiva (comprendente le colture del sangue e dei liquidi peritoneali) e l'inizio rapido di una terapia antibiotica. Il ruolo della profilassi antibiotica durante la recidiva della sindrome nefrosica è controverso.

Tutti i bambini con una sindrome nefrosica devono ricevere il vaccino pneumococcico polivalente (se non sono stati vaccinati in precedenza), possibilmente quando sono in remissione e durante la giornata senza la terapia con prednisone. I bambini con una sierologia negativa per la varicella vanno vaccinati contro di essa mentre sono in remissione oppure mentre stanno assumendo steroidi a dosi ridotte a giorni alterni. I bambini nefrosici non immuni in recidiva esposti alla varicella devono ricevere immunoglobuline antivaricella-zoster entro 72 h dall'esposizione. Il vaccino contro l'influenza va somministrato annualmente.

I bambini con una sindrome nefrosica hanno inoltre un rischio maggiore di eventi tromboembolici, con un'incidenza del 2-5%, molto minore in ogni caso rispetto al rischio registrato negli adulti. Possono essere osservate trombosi arteriose e venose, tra cui la trombosi della vena renale, l'embolia polmonare, la trombosi del seno sagittale e quella dei cateteri centrali arteriosi e venosi. Il rischio di trombosi è correlato all'aumento dei fattori protrombotici (fibrinogeno, trombocitosi, emoconcentrazione, relativa immobilizzazione) e alla diminuzione dei fattori fibrinolitici (perdite con le urine di antitrombina III, proteine C ed S). La profilassi anticoagulante non è raccomandata nei bambini, tranne nel caso in cui abbiano accusato un precedente evento trombotico. La terapia diuretica molto aggressiva deve essere evitata e l'uso di cateteri centrali va limitato, perché questi possono accrescere la probabilità di complicanze coagulative.

L'iperlipidemia, soprattutto nei pazienti con una sindrome nefrosica complicata, può essere un fattore di rischio per una malattia cardiovascolare; l'infarto miocardio è invece una complicanza rara nei bambini. È stato suggerito di considerare l'impiego di farmaci che inibiscano la 3-idrossi-3-metilglutaril coenzima A (HMG-CoA) reduttasi per trattare questa iperlipidemia.

PROGNOSI. La maggior parte dei bambini con una sindrome nefrosica che risponde agli steroidi ha recidive ripetute, che generalmente si riducono in frequenza man mano che il bambino cresce. Benché non esista un sistema provato per prevedere il decorso individuale, i pazienti che rispondono rapidamente agli steroidi e quelli che non presentano recidive durante i primi 6 mesi dopo la diagnosi probabilmente avranno un decorso con ricadute non frequenti. È importante comunicare alla famiglia che il bambino con una sindrome nefrosica che reagisce agli steroidi ha scarse probabilità di sviluppare un'insufficienza renale cronica, che in genere la malattia non è ereditaria e che il soggetto (in assenza di una terapia prolungata con la ciclofosfamide) rimarrà fertile. Per ridurre al minimo gli effetti della malattia, il medico deve sottolineare che il paziente va considerato normale quando è in remissione e può seguire una dieta e un'attività senza limitazioni e senza la necessità di verificare la proteinuria.

I bambini con una sindrome nefrosica resistente agli steroidi, per lo più causata dalla FSGS, in genere hanno una prognosi molto più sfavorevole. Essi sviluppano un'insufficienza renale progressiva, che in ultima analisi conduce a un'insufficienza renale terminale e richiede la dialisi o il trapianto. Una sindrome nefrosica ricorrente si sviluppa nel 30-50% dei riceventi di trapianto con la FSGS. La plasmaferesi, l'assorbimento di proteine plasmatiche su colonne con proteina A, la ciclosporina o il tacrolimus ad alte dosi e gli ACE-inibitori possono ridurre la proteinuria in questi pazienti.

Barletta GM, Smoyer WE, Bunchman TE, et al: Use of mycophenolate mofetil in steroid-dependent and -resistant nephrotic syndrome. *Pediatr Nephrol* 2003;18:833–837.

Cattran DC, Appel GB, Hebert LA, et al., for the North America Nephrotic Syndrome Study Group: A randomized trial of cyclosporine in patients with steroid-resistant focal segmental glomerulosclerosis. *Kidney Int* 1999; 56:2220–2226.

Constantinescu AR, Shah HB, Foote EF, et al: Predicting first-year relapses in children with nephrotic syndrome. *Pediatrics* 2000;105:492–495.

Eddy AA, Symons JM: Nephrotic syndrome in childhood. *Lancet* 2003;362:629–639.

Hinkes B, Wiggins RC, Gbadegesin R, et al: Positional cloning uncovers mutations in PLCEI responsible for a nephrotic syndrome variant that may be reversible. *Nat Genet* 2006;38:1397–1405.

Hogg R, Portman RJ, Milliner D, et al: Evaluation and management of proteinuria and nephrotic syndrome in children: Recommendations from a pediatric nephrology panel established at the National Kidney Foundation Conference of Proteinuria, Albuminuria, Risk, Assessment, Detection, and Elimination. *Pediatrics* 2000;105:1242–1249.

Leonard MB, Feldman HI, Shults J, et al: Long-term, high-dose glucocorticoids and bone mineral content in childhood glucocorticoid-sensitive nephrotic syndrome. *N Engl J Med* 2004;351:868–875.

Loeffler K, Gowrishankar M, Yiu V: Tacrolimus therapy in pediatric patients with treatment-resistant nephrotic syndrome. *Pediatr Nephrol* 2004; 19:281–287.

Mao J, Zhang Y, Du L, et al: NPHS1 and NPHS2 gene mutations in Chinese children with sporadic nephrotic syndrome. *Pediatr Res* 2007;61:117–122.

Mucha B, Ozaltin F, Hinkes BG, et al: Mutations in the Wilms' tumor 1 gene cause isolated steroid resistant nephrotic syndrome and occur in exons 8 and 9. *Pediatr Res* 2006;59:325–331.

527.2 • Sindrome nefrosica secondaria

La sindrome nefrosica secondaria può manifestarsi quale tratto secondario di molte forme di malattie glomerulari. La nefropatia membranosa, la glomerulonefrite membranoproliferativa, la glomerulonefrite postinfettiva, la nefrite lupica e la nefrite della porpora di Henoch-Schönlein possono tutte avere una componente nefrosica (vedi Tabb. 527-1 e 527-2). La sindrome nefrosica secondaria deve essere sospettata nei pazienti di età >8 anni che presentino ipertensione, ematuria, disfunzione renale, sintomatologia extrarenale (rash, artralgie, febbre) o livelli ridotti di complemento nel siero.

In certe aree del mondo, la malaria e la schistosomiasi sono le cause principali della sindrome nefrosica. Altri agenti infettivi che vi risultano associati includono il virus dell'epatite B, il virus dell'epatite C, la filaria, la lebbra e l'HIV.

La sindrome nefrosica è stata associata a neoplasie maligne, in particolare nella popolazione adulta. Nei pazienti con tumori solidi, come i carcinomi del polmone e del tratto gastrointestinale, la patologia renale spesso assomiglia alla glomerulopatia membranosa. Il coinvolgimento renale è presumibilmente mediato da immunocomplessi costituiti da antigeni tumorali e anticorpi antitumorali specifici. Nei pazienti con linfomi, in particolare il linfoma di Hodgkin, la patologia renale spesso assomiglia alla MCNS. Il meccanismo proposto per la sindrome nefrosica è che il linfoma produce una linfochina che aumenta la permeabilità della parete capillare glomerulare. La sindrome può svilupparsi prima o dopo l'individuazione della neoplasia maligna, può risolversi man mano che il tumore regredisce e può ricomparire se esso recidiva.

La sindrome nefrosica compare inoltre durante la terapia con numerosi farmaci e sostanze chimiche. Il quadro istologico può assomigliare a quello della glomerulopatia membranosa (penicillamina, captopril, oro, farmaci antinfiammatori non steroidei, composti del mercurio), della MCNS (probenecid, etosussimide, metimazolo, litio) o della glomerulonefrite proliferativa (procainamide, clorpropamide, fenitoina, trimetadione, parametadione).

Barsoum RS: Schistosomal glomerulopathies. *Kidney Int* 1993;44:1–12.

Herman ES, Klotman PE: HIV-associated nephropathy: Epidemiology, pathogenesis, and treatment. *Semin Nephrol* 2003;23:200–208.

Ronco PM: Paraneoplastic glomerulopathies: New insights into an old entity. *Kidney Int* 1999;56:355–377.

Sitprija V: Nephropathy in falciparum malaria. *Kidney Int* 1998;34:867.

527.3 • Sindrome nefrosica congenita

I neonati che sviluppano una sindrome nefrosica entro i primi 3 mesi di vita vengono considerati affetti da una forma congenita. La causa più comune è la sindrome nefrosica congenita di tipo finlandese, un disturbo autosomico recessivo più frequente nelle popolazioni di origine scandinava (incidenza 1:8000). La sindrome nefrosica congenita può essere causata da mutazioni in 1 dei 2 geni *NPHS1* e *NPHS2*, che codificano rispettivamente per le proteine nefrina e podocina. La nefrina e la podocina sono componenti chiave del diaframma fissurato della cellula epiteliale glomerulare e si pensa che svolgano un ruolo essenziale nella funzione normale della barriera di filtrazione glomerulare. Le caratteristiche patologiche maggiori del tipo finlandese sono la dilatazione dei tubuli prossimali, l'ipercellularità mesangiale e la sclerosi glomerulare.

I neonati con questa sindrome finlandese si presentano con una proteinuria massiva (individuabile in utero dalla presenza dell'alfafetoproteina aumentata), una placenta grande e un edema marcato. I tratti clinici aggiuntivi includono la prematurità, il distress respiratorio e la diastasi delle suture craniche. La storia naturale della malattia è di edema persistente, infezioni ricorrenti e insufficienza renale progressiva con morte entro i 5 anni di età. I corticosteroidi e gli agenti immunosoppressori non sono di alcuna utilità.

Gli ACE-inibitori, l'indometacina e la nefrectomia unilaterale possono diminuire la proteinuria e migliorare lo stato nefrosico. I pazienti richiedono un supporto nutrizionale aggressivo e infine una dialisi cronica e il trapianto del rene. Nelle famiglie a rischio di sindrome nefrosica congenita di tipo finlandese, la diagnosi prenatale viene suggerita da un livello di α-fetoproteina aumentato nel liquido amniotico e può essere confermata dall'analisi del DNA.

Altre cause della sindrome nefrosica congenita includono infezioni congenite come la sifilide, la toxoplasmosi, la rosolia e il Cytomegalovirus. È stato riferito che anche l'HIV e l'epatite B causano questa sindrome nel periodo neonatale (Tab. 527-4). Lo stato nefrosico, che generalmente è meno grave rispetto alla sindrome congenita di tipo finlandese, può migliorare o risolversi trattando l'infezione di base.

La **sclerosi mesangiale diffusa** è una malattia glomerulare rara osservata in una minoranza di bambini con sindrome nefrosica congenita. Il riscontro patologico caratteristico è la sclerosi progressiva del mesangio glomerulare, mentre il quadro clinico è caratterizzato dalla rapida perdita della funzione renale, con una insufficienza renale terminale che si sviluppa nell'arco di mesi o anni. La sclerosi mesangiale diffusa può verificarsi come malattia isolata o nel contesto della **sindrome di Denys-Drash**, una malattia caratterizzata dal tumore di Wilms e dallo pseudoermafroditismo maschile, determinato da una mutazione del gene del tumore di Wilms (*WT1*) sul cromosoma 11.

Holmberg C, Tryqqvason K, Kestila MK, Jalanko HJ: Congenital nephrotic syndrome. In Avner E, Harmon W, Niaudet P (editors): *Pediatric Nephrology*, 5th ed. Philadelphia, Lippincott Williams & Wilkins, 2004, pp 503–516.

Lenkkeri U, Mannikko M, McCready P, et al: Structure of the gene for congenital nephrotic syndrome of the Finnish type *(NPHS 1)* and characterization of mutations. *Am J Hum Genet* 1999;64:51–61.

Mannikko M, Kestila M, Lenkkeri U, et al: Improved prenatal diagnosis of the congenital nephrotic syndrome of the Finnish type based on DNA analysis. *Kidney Int* 1997;51:868.

McTaggart SJ, Algar E, Chow CW, et al: Clinical spectrum of Denys-Drash and Frasier syndrome. *Pediatr Nephrol* 2001;16:335–339.

Papez KE, Smoyer WE: Recent advances in congenital nephrotic syndrome. *Curr Opin Pediatr* 2004;16:165–170.

Patrakka J, Martin P, Salonen R, et al: Proteinuria and prenatal diagnosis of congenital nephrosis in fetal carriers of nephrin gene mutations. *Lancet* 2002;359:1575–1576.

TABELLA 527-4. Cause di sindrome nefrosica nei bambini di età inferiore a 1 anno

CAUSE SECONDARIE
Infezioni
Sifilide
Cytomegalovirus
Toxoplasmosi
Rosolia
Epatite B
HIV
Malaria
Reazioni a farmaci
Tossine
Mercurio
Lupus eritematoso sistemico
Sindrome con malattia renale associata
Nail-patella syndrome
Sindrome di Lowe
Nefropatia associata a malformazione cerebrale congenita
Sindrome di Drash: tumore di Wilms
Sindrome uremico-emolitica
CAUSE PRIMARIE
Sindrome nefrosica congenita
Sclerosi mesangiale diffusa
Malattia con lesioni minime
Sclerosi segmentale focale
Nefropatia membranosa

Da Kliegman RM, Greenbaum LA, Lye PS: *Practical Strategies in Pediatric Diagnosis and Therapy*, 2nd ed. Philadelphia, Elsevier, 2004, p 418.

Sezione 4 — Disordini tubulari

Capitolo 528 ■ Funzione tubulare

Katherine MacRae Dell ed Ellis D. Avner

L'acqua e gli elettroliti vengono filtrati liberamente a livello del glomerulo. Pertanto il contenuto di elettroliti dell'"ultrafiltrato" all'inizio del tubulo prossimale è simile a quello del plasma. Processi rigidamente regolati di riassorbimento tubulare e/o di secrezione tubulare determinano il contenuto finale di acqua e la composizione di elettroliti delle urine. Il movimento "sostanziale" dei soluti tende ad avere luogo nelle porzioni prossimali del nefrone, mentre le regolazioni fini in genere si verificano distalmente (vedi anche Capitolo 52).

SODIO. Il sodio è essenziale per conservare il bilancio idrico extracellulare e quindi la volemia. Il rene è in grado di mettere in atto significative alterazioni nell'escrezione del sodio, in una vasta gamma di stati normali e patologici. Esistono 4 siti principali deputati al trasporto del sodio. Circa il 60% di questo viene assorbito nel tubulo prossimale da un trasporto associato al glucosio o agli aminoacidi, il 25% nell'ansa di Henle ascendente (mediato dall'NKCC2, il trasportatore sodio-potassio-cloro sensibile alla bumetanide) e il 15% nel tubulo distale (mediato dall'NCCT, il cotrasportatore cloro-sodio sensibile al tiazide) e nel tubulo collettore (mediato dall'EnaC, il canale epiteliale del sodio). L'escrezione urinaria normalmente si avvicina a un'assunzione pari a 2-6 mEq/kg/24 h per un bambino che consumi una dieta americana tipica, tolti gli 1-2 mEq/kg/24 h richiesti per i normali processi metabolici. Tuttavia, negli stati di riduzione di volume (disidratazione, perdita di sangue) o di volemia ridotta (shock settico, stati di ipoalbuminemia, insufficienza cardiaca), può verificarsi una riduzione ingente dell'escrezione del sodio con le urine, fino a 1 mEq/L. Le alterazioni nello stato del volume vengono individuate da barorecettori negli atri, nell'arteriola afferente, nel seno carotideo e dalla macula densa, che rileva le variazioni nell'apporto di cloro. I meccanismi ormonali principali che mediano il bilancio del sodio includono l'asse renina-angiotensina-aldosterone, il fattore natriuretico atriale e la noradrenalina. L'angiotensina II e l'aldosterone aumentano rispettivamente il riassorbimento del sodio nel tubulo prossimale e nei tubuli distali. La noradrenalina, rilasciata in risposta alla riduzione di volume, non agisce direttamente sui meccanismi del trasporto tubulare, ma influisce sul bilancio del sodio riducendo l'afflusso di sangue renale e di conseguenza abbassando il carico filtrato di sodio e stimolando il rilascio di renina. In presenza di una riduzione di volume più grave, viene rilasciato anche l'ormone antidiuretico (vedi Capitolo 530). L'escrezione di sodio è promossa dal fattore natriuretico atriale e dalla soppressione di renina.

POTASSIO. L'omeostasi del potassio extracellulare è regolata, perché alterazioni minori delle concentrazioni plasmatiche del potassio determinano effetti ingenti sulla funzione cardiaca, neurale e neuromuscolare (vedi Capitolo 52.4). In particolare, tutto il potassio filtrato viene completamente riassorbito nel tubulo prossimale, cosicché l'escrezione urinaria di potassio è del tutto dipendente dalla secrezione tubulare da parte dei canali del potassio presenti nelle principali cellule del tubulo collettore. I fattori che promuovono questa escrezione del potassio includono l'aldosterone, una maggiore cessione di sodio al nefrone distale e una velocità di flusso urinario aumentata.

CALCIO. Una proporzione significativa del calcio filtrato (70%) viene riassorbita nel tubulo prossimale. Il calcio aggiuntivo viene riassorbito nell'ansa di Henle ascendente (20%), nonché nel tubulo distale e nel dotto collettore (5-10%). Il calcio viene riassorbito da un movimento passivo tra le cellule (assorbimento paracellulare) in un processo guidato dal riassorbimento del cloruro di sodio e dalla secrezione del potassio nel lume. Inoltre, la captazione del calcio è attivamente regolata dai recettori del calcio, da trasportatori specifici e dai canali del calcio. I fattori che promuovono il riassorbimento includono il paratormone (rilasciato in risposta all'ipocalcemia), la calcitonina, la vitamina D, i diuretici tiazidici e la deplezione di volume (vedi Capitolo 571). I fattori che invece agevolano l'escrezione del calcio comprendono l'espansione di volume, l'aumentata assunzione di sodio e i diuretici come il mannitolo e la furosemide.

FOSFATO. La maggior parte del fosfato filtrato viene riassorbita nel tubulo prossimale mediante il trasporto attivo. Il riassorbimento viene aumentato dalla limitazione dell'assunzione di fosforo con la dieta, dalle contrazioni di volume e dall'ormone della crescita. Il paratormone e l'espansione di volume aumentano l'escrezione di fosfato.

MAGNESIO. Circa il 25% del magnesio filtrato viene riassorbito nel tubulo prossimale. La modulazione dell'escrezione del magnesio renale si verifica principalmente nell'ansa di Henle ascendente, con un certo contributo del tubulo convoluto distale. Benché siano stati identificati trasportatori di magnesio specifici, i meccanismi precisi di regolazione non sono ancora stati compresi.

MECCANISMI DI ACIDIFICAZIONE E DI CONCENTRAZIONE. Questo tema viene affrontato nelle sezioni dedicate all'acidosi tubulare renale e al diabete insipido nefrogenico (vedi Capitoli 529 e 530).

CONSIDERAZIONI SULLO SVILUPPO. Le capacità di trasporto tubulari dei neonati (in particolare dei neonati prematuri) e dei bambini piccoli sono inferiori a quelle degli adulti. Benché la nefrogenesi (formazione di nuove unità glomerulari/tubulari) sia completa attorno alla 36ª settimana di gestazione, durante l'infanzia si verifica una maturazione tubulare significativa. L'immaturità tubulare renale, la diminuita velocità di filtrazione glomerulare, il ridotto gradiente di concentrazione e la minore reattività all'ormone antidiuretico sono caratteristici dei bambini piccoli. Questi fattori possono contribuire a una regolazione poco efficace dell'omeostasi acido-base, acqua, soluti ed elettroliti, in particolare durante le malattie acute.

Baum M, Quigley R, Satlin L: Maturational changes in renal tubular transport. *Curr Opin Nephrol Hypertens* 2003;12:521–526.

Jones DP, Chesney RW: Tubular function: In Avner ED, Harmon WE, Niaudet P (editors): *Pediatric Nephrology,* 5th ed. Philadelphia, Lippincott Williams & Wilkins, 2004, pp 45–72.

Schrier RW (editor): *Renal and Electrolyte Disorders,* 6th ed. Philadelphia, Lippincott Williams & Wilkins, 2003.

Van't Hoff WG: Molecular developments in renal tubulopathies. *Arch Dis Child* 2000;83:189–191.

Capitolo 529 ■ Acidosi tubulare renale

Katherine MacRae Dell ed Ellis D. Avner

L'acidosi tubulare renale (RTA, *Renal Tubular Acidosis*) è uno stato patologico caratterizzato da un'acidosi metabolica con gap anionico normale derivante da una compromissione del riassorbimento del bicarbonato oppure dell'escrezione di acidi (ioni idrogeno) con le urine. Esistono forme primarie e secondarie ereditarie e acquisite, di cui 3 principali: RTA prossimale (tipo II), RTA distale (tipo I) e RTA ipokaliemica (tipo IV). Le lesioni miste (quelle con elementi del tipo I e II), che interessano prevalentemente pazienti con un deficit ereditario dell'anidrasi carbonica, vengono da alcuni Autori definite RTA di tipo III.

ACIDIFICAZIONE URINARIA NORMALE. L'acidificazione urinaria comprende 2 processi: il riassorbimento del bicarbonato e l'escrezione degli ioni idrogeno. Il riassorbimento del bicarbonato avviene nel tubulo prossimale e determina il recupero del bicarbonato filtrato in una percentuale di circa l'85%. Nei neonati risulta meno efficiente e l'escrezione del bicarbonato renale può avere luogo con concentrazioni <22 mmol/L. Il bicarbonato stesso non è assorbito direttamente attraverso un trasportatore specifico, ma tramite un processo indiretto. Il riassorbimento dei bicarbonati da parte dei tubuli prossimali inizia con la secrezione di uno ione idrogeno in cambio di uno ione sodio, che nel lume tubulare si lega al bicarbonato e, sotto l'influenza dell'anidrasi carbonica, viene convertito in anidride carbonica e acqua. L'anidride carbonica si diffonde quindi nelle cellule tubulari prossimali, dove una serie di reazioni chimiche determina la creazione di una molecola di bicarbonato (che entra nei capillari peritubulari) e di uno ione idrogeno, che può partecipare alla stabilizzazione (*buffering*) del bicarbonato nel lume tubulare. Il restante 15% del bicarbonato viene riassorbito a livello distale. La secrezione della carica acida quotidiana (approssimativamente 1 mEq/kg/24 h prodotto durante i normali processi cellulari) è accompagnata dalla secrezione di ioni idrogeno (mediata dalla H^+ ATPasi presente nelle cellule intercalate del tubulo collettore), dall'ammoniogenesi e dalla formazione di acidi titolabili (quando gli ioni H^+ vengono stabilizzati dagli acidi organici come il fosfato).

529.1 • Acidosi tubulare renale prossimale (tipo II)

PATOGENESI. La RTA prossimale deriva da un riassorbimento del bicarbonato da parte del tubulo prossimale. Le forme isolate ereditate o acquisite esistono, ma sono rare. Sono state riferite forme autosomiche dominanti isolate nonché una forma autosomica recessiva associata ad anomalie oculari. La RTA prossimale in genere si manifesta come una componente della disfunzione tubulare prossimale o della **sindrome di Fanconi,** caratterizzata da una proteinuria a basso peso molecolare, glicosuria, fosfaturia, aminoaciduria e appunto RTA prossimale. Vengono rilevate entrambe le forme, autosomica e dominante, della sindrome di Fanconi primitiva, mentre quella secondaria può verificarsi quale componente di una delle numerose patologie tubulari renali ereditate oppure negli stati patologici acquisiti. Le cause della RTA e della sindrome di Fanconi, molte delle quali costituite da patologie ereditate, sono illustrate nella Tabella 529-1. In questa sezione vengono trattate due patologie, la **cistinosi** e la **sindrome di Lowe.** Altre forme ereditate includono la **galattosemia** (vedi Capitolo 87.2), l'**intolleranza al fruttosio ereditaria** (vedi Capitolo 87.3), la **tirosinemia** (vedi Capitolo 85.2) e la **malattia di Wilson** (vedi Capitolo 354.2). La **malattia di Dent**, o nefrolitiasi recessiva, viene invece discussa nel Capitolo 531.3. Nei bambini una forma grave della sindrome di Fanconi secondaria è l'esposizione alla ifosfamide, un componente di molti regimi terapeutici per il tumore di Wilms e altri tumori solidi.

La **cistinosi** è una malattia sistemica causata da un difetto nel metabolismo della cistina, che determina un accumulo di cristalli di cistina nella maggior parte degli organi principali,

TABELLA 529-1. Classificazione dell'acidosi tubulare renale

PROSSIMALE (TIPO II)
Isolata
Sporadica
Ereditaria
Sindrome di Fanconi
Primitiva
Sporadica
Ereditaria
Cistinosi
Sindrome di Lowe
Galattosemia
Tirosinemia
Intolleranza ereditaria al fruttosio
Sindrome di Fanconi-Bickel
Malattia di Wilson
Malattie mitocondriali
Malattia di Dent (nefrolitiasi recessiva)
Secondaria
Metalli pesanti (piombo, cadmio, mercurio)
Tetraciclina scaduta
Gentamicina
Ifosfamide
Ciclosporina/tacrolimo
DISTALE (TIPO I)
Primitiva
Sporadica
Ereditaria
Secondaria
Nefrite interstiziale
Uropatia ostruttiva
Reflusso vescicoureterale
Pielonefrite
Rigetto di trapianto
Nefropatia a cellule falciformi
Sindrome di Ehlers-Danlos
Nefrite lupica
Nefrocalcinosi
Malattia di Cacchi Ricci
Cirrosi epatica
Tossine/farmaci
Amfotericina B
Litio
Toluene
Cisplatino
IPERKALIEMICA (TIPO IV)
Primitiva
Sporadica
Ereditaria
Secondaria
Ipoaldosteronismo
Malattia di Addison
Iperplasia surrenale congenita
Eparinizzazione prolungata
Pseudoipoaldosteronismo (tipo I o II)
Uropatia ostruttiva
Pielonefrite
Nefrite interstiziale
Diabete mellito
Nefropatia a cellule falciformi
Trimetoprim/sulfametoxazolo
ACE-inibitori
Ciclosporina

in particolare il rene, il fegato, l'occhio e il cervello. Si verifica con una incidenza compresa tra 1:100 000-1:200 000, che in determinate popolazioni, come i Franco-Canadesi, è tuttavia molto più alta. Sono stati descritti almeno 3 modelli clinici. I bambini piccoli con la forma più grave (*cistinosi infantile* o *nefropatica*) si presentano nei primi 2 anni di vita con una disfunzione tubulare grave e un difetto di crescita. Se la malattia non viene trattata, i bambini sviluppano una malattia renale terminale entro il 10° anno di vita. Una forma più lieve interessa gli adolescenti ed è caratterizzata da anomalie tubulari meno gravi e da una progressione più lenta verso l'insufficienza renale. Esiste infine una forma benigna dell'adulto senza interessamento renale. La cistinosi è causata da mutazioni nel gene *CTNS*, che codifica per una proteina nuova, la cistinosina, che si ritiene sia un trasportatore lisosomiale per la cistina guidato dall'H^+. Studi sul genotipo fenotipici dimostrano che i pazienti con cistinosi nefropatica grave hanno mutazioni che conducono alla perdita completa della funzione della cistinosina. I soggetti con malattia clinica più lieve presentano invece mutazioni che conducono all'espressione di proteine parzialmente funzionali. I casi di cistinosi nefropatica si presentano con **manifestazioni cliniche** che riflettono la loro disfunzione tubulare pronunciata e la sindrome di Fanconi, con poliuria e polidipsia, deficit di crescita e rachitismo. La febbre, causata dalla disidratazione o da una minore produzione di sudore, è un evento comune. Tipicamente chi è coinvolto ha una pelle chiara ed è biondo per la minore pigmentazione. Si verifica fotofobia. Con la fibrosi tubulointerstiziale progressiva, l'insufficienza renale è inevitabile. Si osserva inoltre una retinopatia e la riduzione dell'acuità visiva, come anche l'ipotiroidismo, l'epatosplenomegalia e una maturazione sessuale ritardata.

La **diagnosi** di cistinosi è suggerita dall'osservazione di cristalli di cistina nella cornea ed è confermata dalla misurazione aumentata del contenuto di cistina nei leucociti che risulta aumentata. La diagnosi prenatale viene eseguita sulle famiglie a rischio.

La **terapia** è volta a correggere le anomalie metaboliche associate alla sindrome di Fanconi o all'insufficienza renale cronica. In aggiunta, è disponibile una terapia specifica con **cisteamina**, che si lega alla cistina e la converte in cisteina. Questa facilita il trasporto lisosomiale e riduce la cistina tissutale. La cisteamina orale non raggiunge livelli adeguati nei tessuti oculari, sicché risulta necessaria una terapia aggiuntiva con cisteamina in gocce. La somministrazione precoce del farmaco può prevenire o ritardare il deterioramento della funzione renale. I pazienti con un deficit della crescita che in questo modo non migliorano possono beneficiare della terapia con l'ormone della crescita. Il trapianto renale è una opzione possibile nei soggetti con insufficienza renale; con il prolungarsi della sopravvivenza possono diventare evidenti altre complicanze, tra cui anomalie del sistema nervoso centrale, debolezza muscolare, disfunzione della deglutizione e insufficienza pancreatica. Non è chiaro se la terapia con la cisteamina a lungo termine le possa ridurre.

La **sindrome di Lowe** (*sindrome di Lowe oculocerebrorenale*) è una malattia recessiva rara caratterizzata da cataratta congenita, ritardo mentale e sindrome di Fanconi. Viene causata da mutazioni nel gene *OCRL1*, che codifica per la proteina fosfatidilinositol polifosfato 5-fosfatasi. Si ritiene che le anomalie siano dovute al trasporto anomalo di vescicole all'interno dell'apparato del Golgi. I reni mostrano alterazioni tubulointerstiziali aspecifiche. Vengono inoltre osservati un ispessimento della membrana basale glomerulare e alterazioni nei mitocondri del tubulo prossimale.

I pazienti con sindrome di Lowe tipicamente si presentano nell'infanzia con cataratta, deficit di crescita progressivo, ipotonia e sindrome di Fanconi. È comune una proteinuria significativa. Spesso si sviluppano cecità e insufficienza renale. Vengono inoltre riscontrate anomalie comportamentali caratteristiche, tra cui capricci, cocciutaggine, stereotipia (comportamenti ripetitivi) e ossessioni. Non esiste una terapia specifica per la malattia renale o i deficit neurologici. In genere occorre eseguire una rimozione della cataratta.

MANIFESTAZIONI CLINICHE DELLA RTA PROSSIMALE E DELLA SINDROME DI FANCONI. I pazienti con RTA prossimale isolata, sporadica o ereditata si presentano con un deficit della crescita nel 1° anno di vita. Altri sintomi possono includere la poliuria, la disidratazione (dovuta a perdite di sodio), l'anoressia, il vomito, la costipazione e l'ipotonia. I soggetti con la sindrome di Fanconi mostrano sintomi aggiuntivi secondari alla deplezione di fosfato, come il rachitismo. Quelli con malattie sistemiche vi aggiungono i segni e i sintomi specifici della malattia sottostante. È presente un'acidosi metabolica con gap non anionico. In generale, l'analisi delle urine nei casi di RTA prossimale isolata è priva di rilevanza. Il loro pH è acido (<5,5), perché in questi pazienti i meccanismi di acidificazione distali sono intatti. Gli indici urinari nei soggetti con la sindrome di Fanconi dimostrano vari gradi di fosfaturia, aminoaciduria, glicosuria, uricosuria, nonché livelli elevati di sodio e potassio. In base alla natura della malattia sottostante, può aversi l'evidenza di un'insufficienza renale cronica, con un livello sierico di creatinina elevato.

529.2 • Acidosi tubulare renale distale (tipo I)

PATOGENESI. La RTA distale si sviluppa in seguito a un danneggiamento del meccanismo di acidificazione urinaria distale (secrezione di ioni idrogeno). Le cause primitive o secondarie possono determinare un funzionamento danneggiato o compromesso di uno o più trasportatori o proteine coinvolti nel processo di acidificazione, tra cui l'H^+/ATPasi, gli scambiatori di anioni l'HCO_3^-/Cl^- o i componenti della via dell'aldosterone. A causa dell'escrezione compromessa degli ioni idrogeno, il pH delle urine non può essere più basso di 5,5, nonostante la presenza di acidosi metabolica grave. La perdita di bicarbonato di sodio determina ipercloremia e ipokaliemia. È generalmente presente anche **ipercalciuria**, che può condurre a nefrocalcinosi o a nefrolitiasi. Anche l'acidosi metabolica cronica danneggia l'escrezione urinaria di citrato. L'**ipocitraturia** aumenta ulteriormente il rischio del deposito di calcio nei tubuli. L'osteopatia è comune e deriva dalla mobilizzazione dei componenti organici dall'osso che fungono da tampone per l'acidosi cronica. Possono verificarsi forme sia sporadiche sia ereditate. Come nella RTA prossimale, così anche nella RTA distale può presentarsi qualche complicanza delle malattie dei tubuli distali ereditate o acquisite.

MANIFESTAZIONI CLINICHE. I pazienti con la RTA distale condividono tratti comuni con quelli con la RTA prossimale, tra cui l'acidosi metabolica con gap non anionico e il ritardo di crescita. Tuttavia, i tratti distintivi della RTA distale includono la nefrocalcinosi e l'ipercalciuria. La massiva deplezione del fosfato e del bicarbonato, caratteristica della RTA prossimale, è generalmente assente.

Le cause della RTA distale primaria e secondaria sono elencate nella Tabella 529-1. Benché rare, sono state identificate 3 forme ereditarie specifiche, tra cui una autosomica recessiva associata a una sordità neurosensoriale.

La **malattia di Cacchi Ricci** è una patologia sporadica relativamente rara nei bambini, benché non sia insolita negli adulti. È caratterizzata da una dilatazione cistica delle porzioni terminali dei dotti collettori nel punto in cui questi entrano nelle piramidi renali. All'ecografia i pazienti mostrano spesso una nefrocalcinosi midollare (Fig. 529-1). Nonostante essi mantengano tipicamente una funzione renale normale per tutta l'età adulta, le complicanze includono la nefrolitiasi, la pielonefrite, l'ipostenuria (incapacità di concentrare le urine) e la RTA distale. Sono state riferite associazioni tra la malattia di Cacchi Ricci e la sindrome di Beckwith-Wiedemann (o emipertrofia).

529.3 • Necrosi tubulare renale iperkaliemica (tipo IV)

PATOGENESI. La RTA di tipo IV si verifica in conseguenza della produzione compromessa di aldosterone (ipoaldosteronismo) o da alterata risposta renale all'aldosterone ("pseudo"-ipoaldosteronismo). Dato che l'aldosterone esercita un effetto diretto sull'H^+/ATPasi responsabile della secrezione dell'idrogeno, la conseguenza è l'acidosi. Inoltre, l'aldosterone è un potente stimolante della secrezione del potassio nel tubulo collettore. La perdita del suo effetto determina quindi l'iperkaliemia. Questo influenza ulteriormente lo stato acido-base, inibendo l'ammoniogenesi e quindi l'escrezione degli ioni idrogeno. Il deficit di aldosterone tipicamente si verifica in conseguenza a disturbi della ghiandola surrenale, come la malattia di Addison o qualche forma di iperplasia surrenale congenita. Nei bambini, la mancata reattività all'aldosterone è una causa molto comune di RTA di tipo IV. Questo può avvenire in maniera transitoria, durante un episodio di pielonefrite acuta o di ostruzione acuta delle vie urinarie, oppure cronicamente, in particolare nei neonati e nei bambini con un'anamnesi di uropatia ostruttiva. Questi ultimi pazienti possono presentare un'iperkaliemia significativa, persino nei casi in cui la funzione renale è normale o solo lievemente danneggiata. Sono stati individuati esempi rari di forme ereditate di RTA di tipo IV.

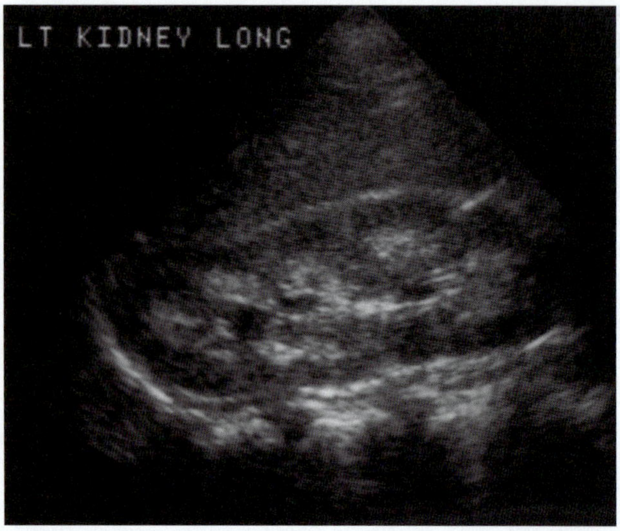

Figura 529-1. Ecografia di un bambino con acidosi tubulare renale distale che mostra nefrocalcinosi midollare.

MANIFESTAZIONI CLINICHE. I pazienti con RTA di tipo IV, analogamente a quelli con i tipi I e II, possono presentare un deficit della crescita nei primi anni di vita. Risultano comuni la poliuria e la disidratazione (da deplezione di sale). Rare volte, i pazienti (soprattutto quelli con pseudoipoaldosteronismo di tipo I) si presentano con un'iperkaliemia pericolosa per la sopravvivenza. Quelli con uropatie ostruttive possono manifestare in maniera acuta i segni e i sintomi della pielonefrite, come febbre, vomito e urine maleodoranti. Gli esami di laboratorio rivelano un'acidosi metabolica iperkaliemica con un gap non anionico. Le urine possono risultare alcaline o acide. Livelli elevati di sodio in esse, con livelli di potassio eccessivamente bassi, riflettono l'assenza dell'effetto prodotto dall'aldosterone.

APPROCCIO DIAGNOSTICO ALLA RTA

Il primo passo nella valutazione di un paziente con sospetta RTA è confermare la presenza di un'acidosi metabolica con un gap anionico normale, identificare le anomalie elettrolitiche, esaminare la funzione renale ed escludere altre cause di perdita di bicarbonato, come la diarrea (vedi Capitolo 52). L'acidosi metabolica associata alla disidratazione diarroica è estremamente comune e in generale migliora correggendo la deplezione di volume. I pazienti con una diarrea protratta possono consumare le loro riserve di bicarbonato total-body e possono avere un'acidosi persistente nonostante l'apparente ripristino dello stato del volume. Nei casi in cui un soggetto abbia un'anamnesi recente di diarrea grave, la valutazione completa per la RTA deve essere ritardata di parecchi giorni, per permettere un tempo adeguato di ricostituzione delle riserve di bicarbonato total-body. Se in questo contesto l'acidosi persiste oltre alcuni giorni, sono indicati studi aggiuntivi.

Occorre eseguire una puntura venosa per misurare gli elettroliti sierici, l'azotemia, il calcio, il fosforo, la creatinina e il pH. I prelievi traumatici (come i campioni dal calcagno), piccoli volumi di sangue in provette per la raccolta di campioni "da adulti" oppure tempi di trasporto prolungati con i campioni che restano a temperatura ambiente possono condurre a livelli di bicarbonato falsamente bassi, spesso in associazione a un valore di potassio nel siero elevato. L'acidosi iperkaliemica reale è coerente con la RTA di tipo IV, mentre il riscontro di un livello di potassio normale o ridotto suggerisce il tipo I o II. Il **gap anionico su sangue** va calcolato utilizzando la formula $[Na^+]^-$ $[Cl^- + HCO_3^-]$. Valori <12 dimostrano l'assenza del gap anionico, mentre >20 sono fortemente indicativi della sua presenza. Se viene rilevato un gap anionico di questo tipo, occorre prendere in considerazione altre diagnosi (acidosi lattica, errori congeniti del metabolismo, ingestioni). Se si nota una tachipnea, va eseguita un'analisi dei gas ematici arteriosi per escludere la possibilità di una malattia acido-base mista, che interessa prevalentemente i componenti respiratori e metabolici. Un'anamnesi dettagliata, con particolare attenzione alla crescita e allo sviluppo, malattie diarroiche recenti o ricorrenti e qualsiasi anamnesi familiare di ritardo mentale, mancato sviluppo, malattia renale terminale, morti di neonati o aborti spontanei è fondamentale. L'esame obiettivo deve determinare i parametri di crescita e lo stato del volume, nonché la presenza di tratti dismorfici che suggeriscano una sindrome sottostante.

Una volta che l'esistenza dell'acidosi metabolica con un gap non anionico è stata confermata, il pH delle urine può essere d'aiuto per distinguere le cause distali da quelle prossimali. Un pH $<5{,}5$, in questo caso, suggerisce una RTA prossimale, mentre i pazienti con una RTA distale tipicamente hanno un pH urinario $>6{,}0$. Il **gap anionico su urine** ($[Na^+$ urinario $+ K^+$ urinario$] - Cl^-$ urinario) viene talvolta calcolato per una conferma della diagnosi di RTA distale. Un gap positivo suggerisce un deficit di ammoniogenesi e, quindi, la possibilità di questa diagnosi, mentre un gap negativo è coerente con la deplezione di bicarbonato nei tubuli (deplezione di bicarbonato gastrointestinale). Va inoltre effettuata l'analisi delle urine per determinare la presenza di glicosuria, proteinuria o ematuria, che suggeriscono la possibilità di una disfunzione o di un danno tubulare più globale. Le misurazioni del calcio e della creatinina casuali o sulle 24 ore identificano l'ipercalciuria. Bisogna infine eseguire l'ecografia renale per identificare anomalie strutturali di base, come le uropatie ostruttive, nonché per determinare l'esistenza di una nefrocalcinosi.

TERAPIA E PROGNOSI DELLA RTA

In tutte le forme di RTA il caposaldo della terapia è la sostituzione del bicarbonato. I pazienti con la RTA prossimale ne richiedono spesso ingenti quantità, fino a 20 mEq/kg/24 h sotto forma di soluzione di bicarbonato o sodio citrato. Il requisito di base della RTA distale è generalmente compreso tra 2-4 mEq/kg/24 h, benché possa variare a seconda dei pazienti. Quelli con sindrome di Fanconi di solito richiedono una integrazione di fosfato. I soggetti con la RTA distale devono essere monitorati per rilevare un eventuale sviluppo di ipercalciuria; quelli con un'ipercalciuria sintomatica (episodi ricorrenti di ematuria macroscopica), con nefrocalcinosi o nefrolitiasi possono necessitare di diuretici tiazidici per ridurre l'escrezione di calcio con le urine. I pazienti con la RTA di tipo IV possono necessitare di una terapia cronica dell'iperkaliemia con una resina a scambio di sodio-potassio.

La prognosi dipende in larga misura dalla natura di qualsiasi malattia di base, se presente. I pazienti con la RTA prossimale o distale isolata in terapia mostrano generalmente un miglioramento nella crescita, a condizione che i livelli di bicarbonato nel siero vengano mantenuti nell'intervallo di normalità. I soggetti con una malattia sistemica e la sindrome di Fanconi possono accusare una morbilità costante con deficit della crescita, rachitismo e segni e sintomi correlati alla malattia di base.

529.4 • RACHITISMO ASSOCIATO AD ACIDOSI TUBULARE RENALE • Russell W. Chesney

Il rachitismo può essere presente nella RTA primitiva, in particolare in quella prossimale o di tipo II. L'ipofosfatemia e la fosfaturia sono comuni in queste sindromi, che sono anche caratterizzate da un'acidosi metabolica ipercloremica, vari gradi di bicarbonaturia e, spesso, ipercalciuria e ipercaluria. In genere, una demineralizzazione ossea senza rachitismo manifesto viene rilevata nella RTA distale e di tipo I. Questa malattia ossea metabolica può essere caratterizzata da dolore osseo, ritardo della crescita, osteopenia e, occasionalmente, fratture patologiche. Benché l'acidosi metabolica acuta negli animali con deficit di vitamina D possa danneggiare la conversione di 25-idrossivitamina D (25[OH]D) in 1,25-diidrossivitamina D ($1{,}25[OH]_2D$), con conseguenti livelli ridotti di questo metabolita attivo, i livelli circolanti di $1{,}25(OH)_2D$ nei pazienti con uno dei due tipi di RTA sono normali, mentre se i pazienti con RTA soffrono di un'insufficienza renale cronica, i livelli sierici del metabolita spesso risultano in effetti ridotti.

La demineralizzazione ossea nella RTA distale è probabilmente correlata al riassorbimento osseo, perché il calcio carbonato nell'osso serve da tampone contro l'acidosi metabolica dovuta agli ioni idrogeno trattenuti dai pazienti con la RTA.

La somministrazione del bicarbonato sufficiente per invertire l'acidosi arresta la dissoluzione ossea e l'ipercalciuria comuni nella RTA distale. La RTA prossimale viene trattata con integrazioni di bicarbonato o fosfato per via orale per guarire il rachitismo. Possono essere necessarie dosi di fosfato simili a quelle usate per l'ipofosfatemia familiare o per la sindrome di Fanconi. La vitamina D è indicata per bilanciare l'iperparatiroidismo secondario che complica la terapia con il fosfato per via orale. Con la terapia, la crescita nei pazienti con la RTA di tipo II (prossimale) è superiore a quella nei casi con sindrome di Fanconi.

Hsu SY, Tsai IJ, Tsau YK: Comparison of growth in primary Fanconi syndrome and proximal renal tubular acidosis. *Pediatr Nephrol* 2005;2 0:460.

Alper SL: Genetic diseases of acid-base transporters. *Annu Rev Physiol* 2002; 64:899–923.

Gahl WA: Early oral cysteamine therapy for nephropathic cystinosis *Eur J Pediatr* 2003;162 (Suppl 1):S38–S41.

Chan JCM, Scheinman JI, Roth KS: Renal tubular acidosis. *Pediatr Rev* 2001;22:277–286.

Izzedine H, Launay-Vacher V, Isnard-Bagnis C, et al: Drug-induced Fanconi's syndrome. *Am J Kidney Dis* 2003;41:292–309.

Kalatzis V, Antignac C: New aspects of the pathogenesis of cystinosis. *Pediatr Nephrol* 2003:18:207–215.

Nicoletta JA, Schwartz GJ: Distal renal tubular acidosis. *Curr Opin Pediatr* 2004;16:194–198.

Rodriguez-Soriano J: New insights into the pathogenesis of renal tubular acidosis—from functional to molecular studies. *Pediatr Nephrol* 2000; 14:1121–1136.

Wappner RS: Lowe syndrome. In GeneClinics: Clinical Genetic Information Resource [database online]. Seattle, University of Washington, July 2001 (updated September 2003). Available at *http://www.geneclinics.org/*.

Wuhl E, Haffner D, Offner G, et al: Long-term treatment with growth hormone in short children with nephropathic cystinosis. *J Pediatr* 2001; 138:880–887.

Capitolo 530 ■ Diabete insipido nefrogeno Katherine MacRae Dell ed Ellis D. Avner

Il diabete insipido nefrogeno (NDI, *Nephrogenic Diabetes Insipidus*) congenito è una malattia rara del metabolismo dell'acqua, caratterizzata da un'incapacità di concentrare le urine, anche in presenza dell'ormone antidiuretico (ADH, *AntiDiuretic Hormone*). Il modello di ereditarietà più comune è la malattia recessiva collegata al cromosoma X. Raramente questa malattia interessa le bambine, ciò che probabilmente avviene in seguito a una inattivazione del cromosoma X. Sono state descritte anche forme autosomiche recessive, con un interessamento equivalente di maschi e femmine. Il fenotipo clinico delle forme autosomiche recessive è simile a quello della forma collegata all'X. Forme secondarie (acquisite), parziali o complete, possono aversi nelle malattie che coinvolgono la funzione tubulare renale, tra cui le uropatie ostruttive, l'insufficienza renale acuta o cronica, le malattie cistiche renali, la nefrite interstiziale, la nefrocalcinosi o nefropatia tossica dovuta a ipokaliemia, l'ipercalcemia, il litio o l'amfotericina B.

PATOGENESI. La capacità di concentrare le urine (e pertanto di assorbire l'acqua) richiede la presenza di un gradiente di concentrazione intatto nella midollare renale e l'attitudine a modulare la permeabilità dell'acqua nel tubulo collettore. Questa permeabilità è mediata dall'ADH (chiamato anche arginina vasopressina), che viene sintetizzato nell'ipotalamo e immagazzinato nell'ipofisi posteriore. In situazioni basali il tubulo collettore è impermeabile all'acqua, ma in risposta alla maggiore osmolarità sierica (rilevata dagli osmorecettori nell'ipotalamo) e/o a una grave riduzione di volume, l'ADH viene rilasciato nella circolazione sistemica e quindi si lega ai suoi recettori, la vasopressina V2 (AVPR2), sulla membrana basolaterale delle cellule del tubulo collettore. Il legame dell'ormone al proprio recettore attiva una cascata ciclica dipendente dall'adenosina monofosfato, che determina il movimento dei canali dell'acqua preformati (aquaporina 2 [AQP2]) sulla membrana luminale del dotto collettore, rendendolo permeabile all'acqua. La presenza di difetti nel gene *AVPR2* causa la forma più comune di NDI legata al cromosoma X. Mutazioni nel gene *AQP2* sono state identificate nei pazienti con una forma autosomica recessiva più rara. Le famiglie con un rischio di NDI legato al cromosoma X possono usufruire di un test prenatale. I pazienti con forme secondarie dello NDI possono evidenziare una resistenza all'ADH dovuta a un'espressione deficitaria di aquaporina (intossicazione da litio). Una resistenza all'ADH secondaria in genere si verifica in seguito alla perdita del gradiente midollare ipertonico in seguito alla diuresi di soluti o a un danno tubulare, con conseguente incapacità di assorbire il sodio o l'urea.

MANIFESTAZIONI CLINICHE. I pazienti con uno NDI congenito tipicamente si presentano nel periodo neonatale con una poliuria massiva, una deplezione di volume, un'ipernatriemia e un'ipertermia. L'irritabilità e il pianto sono tratti comuni. Vengono inoltre osservati la costipazione e uno scarso incremento ponderale. In seguito a episodi multipli di disidratazione ipernatriemica, i bambini possono manifestare un ritardo dello sviluppo e un ritardo mentale. L'enuresi, causata da grandi volumi di urine, è comune. Data la necessità di consumare grandi quantitativi di acqua durante il giorno, i pazienti hanno spesso un appetito ridotto e assumono cibo in dosi insufficienti; per di più, anche con un'integrazione calorica adeguata, essi manifestano ancora anomalie di crescita. I soggetti con uno NDI congenito sono caratterizzati anche da disturbi comportamentali, tra cui l'iperattività e disturbi nella memoria a breve termine. Quelli che presentano la forma secondaria di solito vengono diagnosticati in una fase più avanzata della vita, soprattutto sulla base di ipernatriemia e poliuria. In questo gruppo, i sintomi associati come il ritardo dello sviluppo e le anomalie comportamentali sono meno comuni.

DIAGNOSI. In un neonato maschio la diagnosi è suggerita da poliuria, ipernatriemia e urine diluite. Devono essere eseguite misurazioni simultanee dell'osmolalità sierica e di quella urinaria. Se il valore della prima è 290 mOsm/kg o superiore e quello della seconda risulta inferiore a 290 mOsm/kg, non è necessario eseguire un test formale con deprivazione dell'acqua. Dato che la diagnosi differenziale include le cause di **diabete insipido centrale**, l'incapacità di rispondere all'ADH (e pertanto la presenza dello NDI) va confermata dalla somministrazione di vasopressina (10-20 μg per via intranasale), seguita da misurazioni seriali orarie delle osmolalità urinaria e sierica per 4 ore. Nei pazienti con un possibile diabete insipido "parziale" o secondario, in cui il valore iniziale dell'osmolalità sierica può essere <290 mOsm/kg, occorre considerare la necessità di un test di deprivazione dell'acqua. I liquidi vanno evitati e si deve procedere a una misurazione periodica delle osmolalità urinaria e sierica finché il valore di quella sierica sarà >290 mOsm/kg; si fa quindi assumere la vasopressina, come prima. I criteri per un'interruzione prematura del test di deprivazione dell'acqua includono una riduzione del peso corporeo superiore al 3%. Se lo NDI viene confermato o sospettato, è necessaria una valutazione aggiuntiva che includa un'anamnesi dettagliata per valutare possibili esposizioni ad agenti tossici, la determinazione della funzionalità renale mediante i livelli di creatinina sierica e azoto ureico nel sangue e un'ecografia renale per identificare uropatie ostruttive o una malattia cistica. Data la produzione massiva di urine, i pazienti con uno NDI congenito possono accusare una idronefrosi non ostruttiva di gravità variabile.

TRATTAMENTO E PROGNOSI. Il trattamento dello NDI include: (1) il mantenimento di un'assunzione adeguata di liquidi e l'accesso libero all'acqua; (2) la riduzione al minimo della produzione di urine, limitando il carico dei soluti con una dieta scarsamente osmolare a ridotto contenuto di sodio; (3) la somministrazione di farmaci volti a diminuire la produzione di urina. Per i neonati si deve preferire il latte umano o un latte artificiale povero di soluti. La maggior parte dei neonati con lo NDI congenito richiede una gastrostomia o un'alimentazione nasogastrica, per garantire un'assunzione di liquidi adeguata di giorno e di notte. L'apporto di sodio nei pazienti più grandi deve essere <0,7 mEq/kg/24 h. I **diuretici tiazidici** (2-3 mg/kg/24 h di idroclorotiazide) inducono effettivamente una perdita di sodio e stimolano il riassorbimento di acqua da parte dei tubuli prossimali. È spesso indicato l'uso di diuretici a risparmio di potassio, in particolare l'amiloride (0,3 mg/kg/24 h in 3 dosi divise). I pazienti con una risposta inadeguata ai soli diuretici possono trarre beneficio dall'aggiunta di **indometacina** (2 mg/kg/24 h), che ha l'effetto supplementare di ridurre l'escrezione dell'acqua in alcuni pazienti. In essi, la funzione renale deve essere monitorata attentamente, in quanto l'indometacina può causare nel tempo il deterioramento della funzione renale. I pazienti con uno NDI secondario possono non richiedere farmaci, ma devono avere libero accesso all'acqua e inoltre vanno sottoposti a un attento monitoraggio degli elettroliti nel siero e dello stato del volume, in particolare nei momenti di malattie acute sovrapposte.

La prevenzione della disidratazione ricorrente e dell'ipernatriemia nella forma congenita ha significativamente migliorato l'esito dello sviluppo neurologico. Tuttavia, i disturbi comportamentali restano un problema significativo. Inoltre, l'uso cronico di farmaci antinfiammatori non steroidei può predisporre i pazienti a un'insufficienza renale. La prognosi dei soggetti con uno NDI secondario generalmente dipende dalla natura della malattia di base.

Bonilla-Felix M: Development of water transport in the collecting duct. *Am J Physiol Renal Physiol* 2004;287:F1093-F1101.

Knoers NV: Nephrogenic diabetes insipidus. In GeneClinics: Clinical Genetic Information Resource [database online]. Seattle, University of Washington, February 2000 (updated January 2005). Available at *http://www.geneclinics.org/*.

Saborio P, Tipton GA, Chan JCM: Diabetes insipidus. *Pediatr Rev* 2000;21:122-129.

Capitolo 531 ■ Sindromi di Bartter/Gitelman e altre anomalie ereditarie del trasporto tubulare

Katherine MacRae Dell ed Ellis D. Avner

531.1 • Sindrome di Bartter

La sindrome di Bartter è una forma rara di alcalosi metabolica ipokaliemica con ipercalciuria e un modello di ereditarietà autosomico recessivo (vedi Capitolo 52). Ne esistono due sottotipi clinici distinti: la sindrome di Bartter **prenatale** (chiamata anche sindrome da iperprostaglandine E) si presenta tipicamente nell'infanzia e ha un fenotipo più grave rispetto alla sindrome "classica", comprendente polidramnios, iposodiemia e disidratazione grave. Il fenotipo più lieve, la sindrome di Bartter **classica**, si presenta anch'essa nell'infanzia, con un mancato sviluppo e un'anamnesi di episodi recidivanti di disidratazione. La sindrome di Gitelman, quale malattia correlata al fenotipo, presenta invece un difetto genetico particolare ed è illustrata nel Capitolo 531.2. È stata riferita anche una variante geneticamente distinta della sindrome di Bartter associata a sordità neurosensoriale e a un'insufficienza renale cronica.

PATOGENESI. I tratti biochimici della sindrome di Bartter, tra cui l'alcalosi metabolica ipokaliemica con ipercalciuria, assomigliano a quelli osservati con l'uso cronico di diuretici dell'ansa e riflettono un difetto nel trasporto di sodio, cloro e potassio nell'ansa di Henle ascendente. La perdita di sodio e cloro, con la conseguente contrazione del volume, stimola l'asse renina/angiotensina II/aldosterone. L'aldosterone promuove la captazione del sodio e la secrezione del potassio, esacerbando l'ipopotassiemia; inoltre, spinge distalmente alla secrezione degli ioni idrogeno, peggiorando l'alcalosi metabolica. L'ipokaliemia stimola le prostaglandine, che attivano ulteriormente l'asse renina/angiotensina II/aldosterone. La sindrome di Bartter è stata associata a 3 difetti genetici distinti nei trasportatori dell'ansa di Henle, ciascuno dei quali contribuisce, in qualche modo, allo spostamento di sodio e cloro. Le mutazioni nei geni che codificano per il trasportatore sodio potassio 2 cloro NKCC2 (il sito di azione della furosemide) o il canale del potassio ROMK a livello del lume determinano la sindrome di Bartter neonatale. I difetti nei geni che producono il canale del cloro basolaterale ClC-Kb danno origine invece alla sindrome di Bartter classica.

MANIFESTAZIONI CLINICHE. Si può avere un'anamnesi di polidramnios. All'esame obiettivo possono essere presenti tratti dismorfici, tra cui una facies triangolare, orecchie sporgenti, occhi grandi con strabismo e bocca spiovente. La consanguineità suggerisce l'esistenza di una malattia autosomica recessiva. I bambini più grandi possono avere un'anamnesi di episodi ricorrenti di disidratazione e di mancato sviluppo e possono presentare le anomalie biochimiche classiche dell'alcalosi metabolica ipokaliemica. I livelli di calcio nelle urine sono usualmente elevati, così come i livelli urinari del sodio e del potassio. I livelli sierici della renina, dell'aldosterone e della prostaglandine E sono spesso marcatamente alti, in particolare nella forma prenatale più grave. La pressione sanguigna risulta solitamente normale, benché i pazienti con la forma prenatale possano accusare iposodiemia grave, con conseguenti disidratazione e ipotensione. Di solito la funzione renale è normale. All'ecografia si può riscontrare una nefrocalcinosi derivante dall'ipercalciuria.

DIAGNOSI. Generalmente la diagnosi si fonda sulla presentazione clinica e sui risultati di laboratorio. Quella nel bambino in età neonatale è suggerita dall'ipokaliemia, di solito $<2,5$ mmol/L, con alcalosi metabolica. L'ipercalciuria è usuale, mentre l'ipomagnesiemia viene riscontrata in un minor numero di pazienti ed è più comune nella sindrome di Gitelman. Dato che i tratti della sindrome di Bartter assomigliano all'uso cronico di diuretici dell'ansa, nell'analisi differenziale occorre considerare anche l'abuso di tali diuretici, pure nei bambini piccoli. Anche il vomito cronico può generare un quadro clinico simile, che tuttavia può essere distinto mediante la **misurazione** del **cloro urinario**, che risulta elevato nella sindrome di Bartter e basso nei pazienti con tale vomito. Dal punto di vista istologico i reni mostrano un'iperplasia dell'apparato iuxtaglomerulare. Raramente vengono eseguite biopsie renali per diagnosticare questa malattia.

TRATTAMENTO E PROGNOSI. Il trattamento per la sindrome di Bartter è volto a prevenire la disidratazione, a conservare lo stato nutrizionale e a correggere l'ipokaliemia. Risulta necessaria un'integrazione di potassio, spesso a dosi molto alte. Perfino con una terapia appropriata, i valori del potassio nel siero possono non normalizzarsi, in particolare nei pazienti con la forma neonatale. I neonati e i bambini piccoli possono richiedere anche un'integrazione di sodio. L'indometacina, un inibitore delle prostaglandine, può risultare efficace. Se viene prestata una grande attenzione al bilancio elettrolitico, allo stato del volume e alla crescita, la prognosi nel lungo periodo è generalmente buona. In un ridotto numero di pazienti, l'ipokaliemia cronica, la nefrocalcinosi e la terapia cronica con l'indometacina possono portare a una nefrite interstiziale e un'insufficienza renale croniche.

531.2 • Sindrome di Gitelman

La sindrome di Gitelman (spesso considerata una variante della sindrome di Bartter) è una rara causa autosomica recessiva di alcalosi metabolica ipokaliemica, con i tratti distintivi di **ipocalciuria** e **ipomagnesiemia**. Tipicamente questa malattia si manifesta in una fase avanzata dell'infanzia o nella prima età adulta.

PATOGENESI. I tratti biochimici della sindrome di Gitelman assomigliano a quelli dell'uso cronico di diuretici tiazidici. I tiazidi agiscono sul cotrasportatore del sodio e del cloro NCCT, presente nel tubulo convoluto distale. L'analisi genetica e studi sulle mutazioni hanno consentito di individuare nei pazienti alcuni difetti nel gene che codifica per l'NCCT.

MANIFESTAZIONI CLINICHE. I pazienti tipicamente vengono colpiti dalla sindrome a un'età più avanzata rispetto a quelli con la sindrome di Bartter. Hanno spesso un'anamnesi di spasmi e crampi muscolari ricorrenti, presumibilmente causati da ridotti livelli sierici di magnesio. In genere non possiedono un'anamnesi di episodi di disidratazione ricorrente. Le anomalie biochimiche includono l'ipokaliemia, l'alcalosi metabolica e l'ipomagnesiemia. Il livello di calcio nelle urine è generalmente molto basso (al contrario che nella sindrome di Bartter, dove invece spesso risulta elevato) e quello di magnesio è alto. Di solito i livelli della renina e dell'aldosterone sono normali e la secrezione di prostaglandine E non è elevata. Il deficit della crescita è meno evidente che nella sindrome di Bartter, ma comunque può sussistere.

DIAGNOSI. La diagnosi viene suggerita in un adolescente o in un adulto che si presenti con un'alcalosi metabolica ipokaliemica, con ipomagnesiemia e ipocalciuria.

TRATTAMENTO. La terapia è volta a correggere l'ipokaliemia e l'ipomagnesiemia mediante integrazioni di potassio e magnesio. Il supplemento di sodio o la terapia con gli inibitori delle prostaglandine in genere non sono necessari, in quanto i pazienti in genere non mostrano episodi di deplezione di volume o una escrezione elevata di prostaglandine E.

531.3 • ALTRE ANOMALIE EREDITARIE DEL TRASPORTO TUBULARE

Sono state identificate anomalie ereditarie nei diversi trasportatori di ciascun segmento del nefrone e ne sono stati caratterizzati i difetti molecolari. L'acidosi tubulare renale e il diabete insipido nefrogeno sono discussi in maniera dettagliata rispettivamente nei Capitoli 529 e 530. La **cistinuria** è una malattia autosomica recessiva osservata prevalentemente nei pazienti con origini mediorientali ed è caratterizzata dalla formazione ricorrente di calcoli. Viene causata da un difetto nel trasportatore ad alta affinità della L-cistina e degli aminoacidi dibasici presenti nel tubulo prossimale.

La **nefrolitiasi collegata all'X** (**Malattia di Dent**) è contraddistinta dalla formazione ricorrente di calcoli e dalla progressione verso la sindrome di Fanconi. Coerentemente con l'ereditarietà collegata all'X, viene riscontrata quasi esclusivamente nei soggetti di sesso maschile. È determinata da mutazioni nel gene che codifica per il canale del cloro voltaggio-dipendente CLN5, presente in tutto il nefrone. Nell'ansa di Henle, alcune mutazioni dell'attivazione e disattivazione nel gene del recettore del calcio, che media la sua captazione indotta dall'ormone paratiroideo, ingenerano rispettivamente ipoparatiroidismo o iperparatiroidismo gravi.

Nel dotto collettore, l'acquisizione di mutazioni della funzione del gene che codifica il canale del sodio epiteliale causa una forma di ipertensione ereditata chiamata **sindrome di Liddle**. I pazienti con questa malattia hanno una captazione del sodio costitutiva nel dotto collettore, con ipokaliemia e con l'aldosterone soppresso. Al contrario, le mutazioni con perdita della funzione comportano pseudoipoaldosteronismo, caratterizzato da una grave deplezione di sodio e da iperkaliemia. Una variante di quest'ultima malattia è associata ad anomalie sistemiche, tra cui difetti nel cloro del sudore, e può assomigliare alla fibrosi cistica.

Hebert SC: Bartter syndrome. *Curr Opin Nephrol Hypertens* 2003;12:527-532.

Jeck N, Reinalter SC, Henne T, et al: Hypokalemic salt-losing tubulopathy with chronic renal failure and sensorineural deafness. *Pediatrics* 2001;108:E5.

Kleta R, Bockenhauer D: Bartter syndrome and other salt-losing tubulopathies. *Nephron Physiol* 2006;104:73-80.

Thakker RV: Pathogenesis of Dent's disease and related syndromes of X-linked nephrolithiasis. *Kidney Int* 2000;57:787-793.

Vehaskari VM: Inherited Na transport disorders: The taming of the syndromes. *Curr Opin Pediatr* 2004;16:182-187.

Capitolo 532 ■ Nefrite tubulointerstiziale

Katherine MacRae Dell ed Ellis D. Avner

Nefrite tubulointerstiziale (TIN, *TubuloInterstitial Nephritis*, nota anche come nefrite interstiziale) è il termine utilizzato per indicare gli stati caratterizzati da un'infiammazione tubulointerstiziale e un danno con risparmio relativo dei glomeruli e dei vasi. Esistono forme primitive acute e croniche. La nefrite interstiziale può trovarsi anche con le malattie glomerulari primitive, nonché con le malattie sistemiche che interessano il rene.

NEFRITE TUBULOINTERSTIZIALE ACUTA

ANATOMIA PATOLOGICA E PATOGENESI. I tratti distintivi della TIN acuta sono un'infiltrazione linfocitica dello spazio tubulointerstiziale, un edema tubulare e gradi variabili di danno tubulare. Possono essere presenti eosinofili, soprattutto nella TIN indotta da farmaci; occasionalmente si verificano granulomi. La patogenesi non è totalmente compresa, ma è stato postulato un meccanismo immunomediato dalle cellule T. Numerosi farmaci, in particolare antimicrobici, anticonvulsivi e analgesici, sono stati implicati quali agenti eziologici (Tab. 532-1). Altre cause includono infezioni, malattie glomerulari primitive e malattie sistemiche come il lupus eritematoso (SLE, *Systemic Lupus Erythematosus*).

MANIFESTAZIONI CLINICHE. La presentazione classica della TIN acuta è costituita da febbre, rash e artralgia nel contesto di un valore della creatinina sierica in aumento. Benché nella TIN indotta dai farmaci sia possibile notare la "triade" completa, molti pazienti con la forma acuta non evidenziano tutti i tratti tipici. Il rash, se presente, può variare da maculopapulare a urticarioide ed è spesso transitorio. I pazienti manifestano frequentemente i sintomi costituzionali aspecifici di nausea, vomito, astenia e perdita di peso. Può aversi un dolore al fianco dovuto alla distensione della capsula renale in seguito a un ingrossamento renale acuto di tipo infiammatorio. Se la TIN è determinata da una malattia sistemica come lo SLE, la presentazione clinica sarà coerente con i suoi segni e sintomi specifici. Contrariamente alla presentazione tipica dell'insufficienza renale acuta osservata con la malattia glomerulare, il 30-40% dei pazienti con la TIN acuta non è oligurico. Può sussistere un'eosinofilia periferica, soprattutto nella TIN indotta dai farmaci. Qualche grado di ematuria microscopica è sempre presente, ma l'ematuria e la proteinuria significative sono rare. Un'eccezione è tuttavia rappresentata dai pazienti con una TIN causata dai farmaci antinfiammatori non steroidei (FANS), che possono dare luogo a una sindrome nefrotica. L'analisi delle urine può rivelare globuli bianchi e cilindri granulari o ialini, ma solo raramente vengono riscontrati cilindri eritrocitari, tipici di una malattia glomerulare. La presenza di eosinofili nelle urine non è né sensibile né specifica.

DIAGNOSI. Generalmente la diagnosi si fonda sulla presentazione clinica e sui risultati di laboratorio. Un'anamnesi attenta del momento di esordio della malattia in relazione all'esposizione ai farmaci è fondamentale qualora si sospetti una TIN indotta dai farmaci. Data la natura immunomediata della TIN, in generale i segni o i sintomi compaiono 1-2 settimane dopo l'esposizione. Nei bambini gli antimicrobici sono un agente stimolante comune e i FANS costituiscono una causa importante della forma acuta della malattia. È necessario monitorare l'analisi delle urine ed eseguire misurazioni seriali della creatinina sierica e degli elettroliti. L'ecografia renale non è diagnostica, ma può dimostrare reni ingrossati ed iperecogeni. La rimozione di un sospetto agente causante seguita da un miglioramento spontaneo della funzione renale è fortemente suggestiva della diagnosi e in genere non vengono eseguiti ulteriori esami. Nei casi più gravi, in cui la causa non sia chiara o in cui la funzione renale del paziente peggiori rapidamente, può essere indicata una biopsia renale.

TRATTAMENTO E PROGNOSI. In generale il trattamento è di supporto ed è volto a risolvere le complicanze dell'insufficienza renale acuta, come l'iperkaliemia e il sovraccarico volemico. Numerosi studi non controllati suggeriscono che i pazienti con una compromissione renale significativa possano trarre beneficio da un trattamento con corticosteroidi, sebbene altri studi, sempre non controllati, non siano riusciti a dimostrare esiti simili. Nei pazienti con un miglioramento rapido della funzione renale senza terapia la prognosi risulta eccellente, ma quando l'insufficienza renale diventa prolungata la prognosi deve essere cauta. La TIN acuta grave dovuta a una qualsiasi causa che non si risolva può progredire a una forma cronica.

NEFRITE TUBULOINTERSTIZIALE CRONICA

Nei bambini, in genere, la TIN cronica è determinata da una malattia renale congenita di base, come un'uropatia ostruttiva o un reflusso vescicoureterale (vedi Tab. 532-1). Questa TIN può verificarsi sotto forma di una malattia idiopatica, benché sia più frequente negli adulti. Il **complesso nefronoftisi giovanile (JN,** *Juvenile Nephronophthisis*)/**malattia midollare cistica renale** è un

TABELLA 532-1. Eziologia della nefrite interstiziale

ACUTA
Farmaci
Antimicrobici
Derivati della penicillina
Cefalosporine
Sulfamidici
Trimetoprim-sulfametoxazolo
Ciprofloxacina
Tetracicline
Derivati dell'eritromicina
Amfotericina B
Anticonvulsivi
Carbamazepina
Fenobarbital
Fenitoina
Valproato sodico
Altri farmaci
Diuretici
Allopurinolo
Cimetidina
Ciclosporina
Farmaci antinfiammatori non steroidei
Inibitori della proteasi
Inibitori della pompa protonica
Infezioni
Batteri associati a pielonefrite acuta
Specie di streptococco
Cytomegalovirus
Virus di Epstein-Barr
Virus dell'epatite B
Istoplasmosi
Virus dell'immunodeficienza umana
Hantavirus
Adenovirus
Toxoplasma gondii
Associata a malattia
Glomerulonefrite (per es. lupus eritematoso sistemico)
Rigetto di allo trapianto acuto
Nefrite tubulointerstiziale e sindrome da uveite
Sarcoidosi
Idiopatica
CRONICA
Farmaci e tossine
Analgesici
Ciclosporina
Litio
Metalli pesanti
Infezioni (vedi Acuta)
Associata a malattia
Metaboliche/ereditarie
Cistinosi
Ossalosi
Malattia di Fabry
Malattia di Wilson
Nefropatia a cellule falciformi
Sindrome di Alport
Nefronoftisi giovanile/malattia midollare cistica
Malattia renale policistica
Immunologica
Lupus eritematoso sistemico
Rigetto di allotrapianto cronico
Nefrite tubulointerstiziale e sindrome da uveite
Urologica
Valvole uretrali posteriori
Sindrome di Eagle-Barrett
Ostruzione della giunzione ureteropelvica
Reflusso vescicoureterale
Varie
Nefropatia balcanica
Nefropatia da erbe cinesi
Irradiazione
Sarcoidosi
Neoplasia
Idiopatica

gruppo di malattie cistiche renali ereditate che condividono un fenotipo istologico comune della TIN cronica. La JN è generalmente ereditata come tratto autosomico recessivo. Benché risulti rara negli Stati Uniti, è alla base del 10-20% dei casi di malattia renale terminale in Europa. I pazienti tipicamente si presentano con poliuria, deficit di crescita, anemia "inspiegata" e insufficienza renale cronica nella tarda infanzia o nell'adolescenza. Le varianti con un coinvolgimento extrarenale includono la **sindrome di Senior-Løken** (retinite pigmentosa), la **sindrome di Joubert** e l'**aprassia oculomotoria del tipo di Cogan**. La **malattia midollare cistica renale** è invece autosomica dominante e si presenta tipicamente nell'età adulta. La **nefrite tubulointerstiziale con uveite** è una sindrome autoimmune rara di TIN cronica, con una uveite anteriore e granulomi del midollo osseo, che si verifica prevalentemente nelle adolescenti. Una TIN cronica viene osservata in tutte le forme di malattia renale progressiva, indipendentemente dalla causa di base e la gravità della malattia interstiziale è il fattore singolo più importante per predire la progressione a una malattia renale terminale.

ANATOMIA PATOLOGICA E PATOGENESI. La fisiopatologia della TIN cronica è indefinita, ma i dati suggeriscono che è immunomediata. Dal punto di vista macroscopico, i reni possono apparire pallidi e piccoli per l'età, mentre sul piano microscopico vengono rilevati un'atrofia tubulare e un "dropout" con fibrosi interstiziale e un'infiammazione interstiziale linfocitaria a chiazze. I pazienti con JN presentano spesso piccole cisti caratteristiche nella regione corticomidollare. Nella TIN cronica primitiva i glomeruli vengono in parte risparmiati, fino alla fase avanzata della malattia. I soggetti con una TIN cronica secondaria a una malattia glomerulare primitiva mostrano l'evidenza istologica di quest'ultima.

MANIFESTAZIONI CLINICHE. I tratti clinici della TIN cronica risultano spesso aspecifici e possono riflettere i segni e i sintomi dell'insufficienza renale cronica (vedi Capitolo 535). Si hanno spesso astenia, ritardo di crescita, poliuria, polidipsia ed enuresi. L'anemia è frequente ed è un tratto particolarmente pronunciato della nefronoftisi giovanile. Dato che il danno tubulare conduce di frequente alla deplezione di sale renale, l'ipertensione significativa costituisce un evento insolito.

DIAGNOSI. La diagnosi è suggerita dai segni e dai sintomi di un danno tubulare renale, come la poliuria e un valore di creatinina sierico elevato, associati a un'anamnesi indicativa di una malattia cronica, come un'enuresi di vecchia data o la presenza di un'anemia resistente alla terapia con il ferro. Studi radiografici, in particolare l'ecografia, possono fornire una prova ulteriore di cronicità, come reni piccoli ed ecogeni, cisti corticomidollare suggestiva di JN o reperti di uropatia ostruttiva. Una cistouretrografia minzionale può dimostrare un reflusso vescicoureterale o anomalie della vescica. Se si sospetta la JN, è disponibile la diagnosi molecolare. Nei casi in cui l'origine non sia chiara può essere eseguita una biopsia renale, che tuttavia può non risultare diagnostica quando la malattia è avanzata. Molte patologie renali allo stato terminale hanno un aspetto istologico comune di infiammazione e fibrosi tubulare.

TRATTAMENTO E PROGNOSI. La terapia è volta a mantenere il bilancio di liquidi ed elettroliti e a evitare un'ulteriore esposizione ad agenti nefrotossici. I pazienti con uropatie ostruttive possono richiedere una integrazione di sale e una terapia con resina legante il potassio. La prevenzione delle infezioni mediante una profilassi antibiotica è importante per rallentare la progressione del danno renale in questi pazienti. La prognosi nei soggetti con la TIN cronica è dipendente, in larga misura, dalla natura della malattia di base. Quelli che hanno un'uropatia ostruttiva o un reflusso vescicoureterale possono presentare un grado diverso di danno renale e pertanto un decorso variabile. La malattia renale terminale, se si verifica, può svilupparsi nel corso di un periodo variabile da mesi ad anni e costituisce comunque il risultato della progressione uniforme della JN entro l'adolescenza.

Alon U: Tubulointerstitial nephritis. In Avner ED, Harmon WE, Niaudet P (editors): *Pediatric Nephrology,* 5th ed. Philadelphia, Lippincott Williams & Wilkins, 2004, pp 817-831.

Clarkson MR, Giblin L, O'Connell FP, et al: Acute interstitial nephritis: Clinical features and response to corticosteroid therapy. *Nephrol Dial Transplant* 2004;19:2778-2883.

Harris DC: Tubulointerstitial nephritis. *Curr Opin Nephrol Hypertens* 2001;10:303–313.

Hildebrandt F, Omram H: New insights: Nephronophthisis—medullary cystic kidney disease. *Pediatr Nephrol* 2001;16:168-176.

Rossert J: Drug-induced acute interstitial nephritis. *Kidney Int* 2001; 60:804-817.

Sezione 5 — Nefropatie tossiche – insufficienza renale

Capitolo 533 ■ Nefropatia tossica

Beth A. Vogt ed Ellis D. Avner

I farmaci, gli agenti diagnostici (i mezzi di contrasto radiografici iodati) e le sostanze chimiche possono alterare i reni in maniera diretta (attraverso la riduzione del flusso di sangue renale, la necrosi tubulare acuta, l'ostruzione intratubulare) o indiretta (tramite l'induzione di una reazione allergica o da ipersensibilità nei vasi o nell'interstizio). Inoltre, gli animali marini, i rettili e gli insetti producono numerose nefrotossine biologiche che causano un'insufficienza renale acuta spesso attraverso l'induzione della rabdomiolisi (veleno di serpenti). Gli agenti nefrotossici comuni e le loro manifestazioni cliniche sono elencati nella Tabella 533-1.

TABELLA 533-1. Sindromi renali prodotte dalle nefrotossine

SINDROME NEFROSICA
ACE-inibitori
Composti del mercurio
Farmaci antinfiammatori non steroidei
Interferone
Penicillamina
Sali d'oro

DIABETE INSIPIDO NEFROGENO
Amfotericina B
Colchicina
Demeclociclina
Litio
Metossiflurano
Propossifene
Vinblastina

VASCULITE RENALE
Idralazina
Isoniazide
Numerosi altri farmaci che possono causare una reazione di ipersensibilità
Propiltiouracile
Sulfamidici

NEFROCALCINOSI O NEFROLITIASI
Allopurinolo
Bumetanide
Etilenglicole
Furosemide
Metossiflurano
Topiramato
Vitamina D

INSUFFICIENZA RENALE ACUTA
ACE-inibitori
Aciclovir
Alotano
Amfotericina B
Aminoglicosidici
Ciclosporina
Cisplatino
Etilenglicole
Farmaci antinfiammatori non steroidei
Ifosfamide
Litio
Metalli pesanti
Metossiflurano
Mezzi di contrasto
Paracetamolo
Tacrolimus
Tossine biologiche (serpente, ragno, ape, vespa)
Vancomicina

SINDROME DI FANCONI
Aminoglicosidici
Cisplatino
Erbe cinesi (aristolochico)
Ifosfamide
Lisolo
Metalli pesanti (cadmio, piombo, mercurio e uranio)
Tetraciclina scaduta

ACIDOSI TUBULARE RENALE
Amfotericina B
Litio
Toluene

NEFRITE INTERSTIZIALE
Agenti di radiocontrasto
Amidopirine
p-Aminosalicilati
Canamicina
Cefalosporine
Ciclosporina
Cimetidina
Cisplatino
Colistina
Etilenglicole
Farmaci antinfiammatori non steroidei
Fenacetina
Fenilbutazone
Ferro
Foscarnet
Funghi velenosi
Gentamicina
Indometacina
Interferone-a
Litio
Mannitolo
Mitomicina C
Neomicina
Penicilline (soprattutto meticillina)
Pentamidina
Polimixina B
Rame
Rifampina
Sali d'oro
Sali di mercurio
Salicilato
Streptomicina
Sulfamidici
Tacrolimus
Tetracloroetilene
Tetracloruro di carbonio
Trimetoprim-sulfametoxazolo

La nefrotossicità risulta spesso reversibile, se l'agente nocivo viene prontamente rimosso.

Anche se le sostanze utili non devono essere evitate a causa della loro potenziale nefrotossicità, le seguenti misure preventive possono comunque ridurre i rischi: (1) l'utilizzo dell'ecografia, della RM o di scansioni con radionuclidi al posto degli studi con mezzi di contrasto nei pazienti con una malattia renale preesistente; (2) l'adozione di agenti non nefrotossici al posto di quelli nefrotossici; (3) l'uso della dose efficace minore possibile dell'agente in combinazione a un monitoraggio del suo livello nel sangue; (4) la riduzione appropriata di tutti i dosaggi farmacologici nei soggetti con insufficienza renale, guidata da nomogrammi ben sviluppati; (5) l'astensione dall'impiego simultaneo di numerosi agenti nefrotossici. Quando possibile, i soggetti a rischio vanno idratati bene prima di una procedura o di una terapia farmacologica; l'acetilcisteina prima e durante una procedura con radiocontrasto, per esempio, previene il deterioramento della funzione renale se i pazienti risultano ben idratati.

Aronoff GR, Berns JS, Brier ME, et al (editors): *Drug Prescribing in Renal Failure,* 4th ed. Philadelphia, American College of Physicians, 1999.

Chesney RW, Jones DW: Nephrotoxins. In Avner E, Harmon W, Niaudet P (editors): *Pediatric Nephrology,* 5th ed. Philadelphia, Lippincott Williams & Wilkins, 2004, pp 987-1004.

Kay J, Chow WH, Chan TM, et al: Acetylcysteine for prevention of acute deterioration of renal function following elective coronary angiography and intervention. *JAMA* 2003;289:553-558.

O'Brien KL, Selanikio JD, Hecdivert C, et al: Epidemic of pediatric deaths from acute renal failure caused by diethylene glycol poisoning. *JAMA* 1998;279:1175-1180.

Perazella MA: Crystal-induced acute renal failure. *Am J Med* 1999;106: 459-465.

Schwartz A, Perez-Canto A: Nephrotoxicity of antiinfective drugs. *Int J Clin Pharmacol Ther* 1998;35:164-167.

Sturmer T, Elseviers MM, De Broe ME: Nonsteroidal anti-inflammatory drugs and the kidney. *Curr Opin Nephrol Hypertens* 2001;10:161–163.

Timmer RH, Sands JM: Lithium intoxication. *J Am Soc Nephrol* 1999;10: 666-674.

Capitolo 534 ■ Necrosi corticale

Beth A. Vogt ed Ellis D. Avner

La necrosi corticale renale rappresenta un comune risultato finale di diversi tipi di lesione ai reni. In genere li interessa entrambi e può essere a chiazze o coinvolgere l'intera corteccia.

EZIOLOGIA. Nei neonati la necrosi corticale è più comunemente associata a insulti ipossici/ischemici determinati da un'asfissia perinatale, un distacco della placenta e una trasfusione gemello-gemello o fetale-materna. Altre cause includono la trombosi vascolare renale e la cardiopatia congenita grave. Dopo il periodo neonatale, la necrosi corticale viene riscontrata soprattutto nei bambini con shock settico o sindrome uremico-emolitica grave, nonché nelle adolescenti con un'insufficienza renale acuta correlata a gravidanza. Ciò che meno di frequente porta alla necrosi corticale sono i morsi di serpente, l'endocardite infettiva e la terapia con farmaci antifibrinolitici (acido tranexamico).

ANATOMIA PATOLOGICA. Le porzioni di corteccia renale interessate evidenziano infarti con la congestione dei glomeruli, la trombosi delle arteriole e la necrosi dei tubuli.

PATOGENESI. La necrosi corticale ha luogo quando la lesione delle cellule endoteliali progredisce in associazione a un diminuito flusso sanguigno corticale renale. Le tossine o altri mediatori che presumibilmente si sviluppano durante lo shock, la sindrome uremico-emolitica o la sepsi possono danneggiare le cellule endoteliali e instaurare una coagulazione intrarenale, causando trombosi e necrosi corticale.

MANIFESTAZIONI CLINICHE. La necrosi corticale si presenta sotto forma di un'insufficienza renale acuta, che si verifica nei soggetti con le cause predisponenti menzionate in precedenza. La produzione di urina risulta diminuita e può esservi un'ematuria macroscopica e/o microscopica. L'ipertensione è comune e può trovarsi una trombocitopenia in conseguenza della lesione microvascolare renale.

DIAGNOSI. All'inizio della malattia la diagnosi è sostenuta dall'osservazione ecografica di reni di dimensioni normali o ingrossati, non ostruiti. Le valutazioni ecografiche sequenziali mostrano una riduzione progressiva delle loro dimensioni, indicativa di un'atrofia renale. Le scansioni dei reni con radionuclidi indicano una ridotta o assente perfusione renale con una funzione che ritarda o manca. La diagnosi differenziale include altre cause di insufficienza renale acuta (vedi Tab. 535-1).

TRATTAMENTO E PROGNOSI. La terapia è di supporto e comprende il ripristino del volume, la correzione dell'ipossia e il trattamento della sepsi. Possono essere necessari un trattamento medico delle complicanze dell'insufficienza renale acuta e una dialisi di supporto. I bambini con necrosi corticale possono avere un recupero renale parziale o non averlo affatto e la prognosi dipende dalla quantità di corteccia renale sopravvissuta. I bambini con un recupero parziale corrono un rischio maggiore di sviluppare una malattia renale cronica.

Agraharkar M, Fahlen M, Siddiqui M, et al: Waterhouse-Friderichsen syndrome and bilateral renal cortical necrosis in meningococcal sepsis. *Am J Kidney Dis* 2000;36:396-400.

Lerner GR, Kurnetz R, Bernstein J, et al: Renal cortical and renal medullary necrosis in the first 3 months of life. *Pediatr Nephrol* 1992;6:516-518.

Manley HJ, Bailie GR, Eisele G: Bilateral renal cortical necrosis associated with cefuroxime axetil. *Clin Nephrol* 1998;49:268-270.

Palapattu GS, Barbaris Z, Raijfer J: Acute bilateral renal cortical necrosis as a cause of postoperative renal failure. *Urology* 2001;58:281.

Capitolo 535 ■ Insufficienza renale

Beth A. Vogt ed Ellis D. Avner

535.1 • INSUFFICIENZA RENALE ACUTA

L'insufficienza renale acuta (ARF, *Acute Renal Failure*) è una sindrome clinica in cui un improvviso deterioramento della funzione renale causa l'incapacità dei reni di conservare l'omeostasi di liquidi ed elettroliti. L'ARF si verifica nel 2-3% dei bambini ricoverati presso i centri pediatrici di terzo livello e nell'8% dei neonati presso le unità di terapia intensiva neonatali.

PATOGENESI. Per convenzione, l'ARF è stata classificata in 3 categorie: prerenale, renale intrinseca e postrenale (Tab. 535-1).

L'**ARF prerenale**, chiamata anche azotemia prerenale, è caratterizzata dalla diminuzione del volume arterioso circolante effettivo, che conduce a una perfusione renale inadeguata e a una minore velocità di filtrazione glomerulare (GFR, *Glomerular Filtration Rate*). È assente un'evidenza di danno renale. Le cause comuni di questa ARF includono la disidratazione, la sepsi, l'emorragia, l'ipoalbuminemia grave e l'insufficienza cardiaca. Se la causa sottostante dell'ipoperfusione renale viene pronta-

TABELLA 535-1. Cause comuni di insufficienza renale acuta

PRERENALI
Disidratazione
Emorragia
Sepsi
Ipoalbuminemia
Insufficienza cardiaca
RENALI INTRINSECHE
Glomerulonefrite
Postinfettive/poststreptococciche
Lupus eritematoso
Porpora di Henoch-Schönlein
Membranoproliferative
Antimembrana basale glomerulare
Sindrome emolitico-uremica
Necrosi tubulare acuta
Necrosi corticale
Trombosi della vena renale
Rabdomiolisi
Nefrite interstiziale acuta
Infiltrazione tumorale
Sindrome da lisi tumorale
POSTRENALI
Valvole uretrali posteriori
Ostruzione della giunzione ureteropelvica
Ostruzione della giunzione ureterovescicale
Ureterocele
Tumore
Urolitiasi
Cistite emorragica
Vescica neurogena

mente invertita, la funzione dei reni torna normale, mentre se l'ipoperfusione è sostenuta può svilupparsi un danno intrinseco del parenchima renale.

L'**ARF renale intrinseca** include una varietà di disturbi caratterizzati dal danno del parenchima renale, tra cui l'ipoperfusione/ischemia sostenuta. Molte forme di **glomerulonefrite** possono causare l'ARF, come per esempio la glomerulonefrite postinfettiva, la nefrite lupica, la nefrite da porpora di Henoch-Schönlein, la glomerulonefrite membranoproliferativa e la nefrite della membrana basale antiglomerulare.

La **sindrome uremico-emolitica** (HUS, *Hemolytic-Uremic Syndrome*) è stata descritta come la causa più comune dell'ARF intrinseca negli Stati Uniti (vedi Capitolo 518). I suoi tratti cardinali includono l'ARF, l'anemia emolitica microangiopatica e la trombocitopenia. Benché sia stata collegata a numerosi fattori, l'origine più frequente nei Paesi sottosviluppati è costituita dal danno alle cellule endoteliali indotto dalla tossina *Shigella*, mentre negli altri Paesi essa viene più spesso determinata dall'*Escherichia coli* (OI57:H7).

La **necrosi tubulare acuta** (**ATN**, *Acute Tubular Necrosis*) si sviluppa soprattutto nei neonati e nei bambini in stato critico che sono stati esposti a insulti nefrotossici e/o ischemici. Il processo patologico tipico è costituito dalla necrosi delle cellule tubulari, sebbene nei pazienti con l'ATN clinica non vengano sempre riscontrate alterazioni istologiche significative. I meccanismi di lesione possono includere le alterazioni dell'emodinamica intrarenale, l'ostruzione tubulare e il reflusso passivo del filtrato glomerulare attraverso le cellule tubulari danneggiate nei capillari peritubulari.

La **sindrome da lisi tumorale** è una forma specifica di ARF correlata alla lisi cellulare spontanea o indotta dalla chemioterapia nei pazienti con neoplasie maligne linfoproliferative. Questa sindrome è prevalentemente determinata dall'ostruzione dei tubuli da parte di cristalli di acido urico (vedi Capitoli 495 e 499).

La **nefrite interstiziale acuta** è una causa sempre più comune di ARF e generalmente rappresenta una conseguenza di una reazione da ipersensibilità a un agente terapeutico o a vari agenti infettivi (vedi Capitolo 532).

L'**ARF postrenale** include una varietà di disturbi caratterizzati dall'ostruzione del tratto urinario. Nei neonati e nei lattanti, gli stati congeniti come le valvole uretrali posteriori e l'occlusione della giunzione ureteropelvica bilaterale sono responsabili della maggior parte dei casi di ARF. Altre malattie come l'urolitiasi, un tumore (intra-addominale o entro il tratto urinario), la cistite emorragica e la vescica neurogena possono dare origine a un'ARF nei bambini più grandi e negli adolescenti. In un soggetto che abbia entrambi i reni funzionanti, l'ostruzione deve essere bilaterale, per causare l'ARF. La risoluzione dell'ostruzione di solito determina un ripristino della funzione renale, eccetto che nei pazienti con una displasia renale associata o un'occlusione prolungata del tratto urinario.

MANIFESTAZIONI CLINICHE E DIAGNOSI. Un'anamnesi attenta è fondamentale per definire l'origine dell'ARF. Un neonato con un'anamnesi di 3 giorni di vomito e diarrea molto probabilmente ha un'ARF prerenale causata dalla deplezione del volume. Un bambino di 6 anni con una faringite recente che presenti un edema periorbitale, l'ipertensione e un'ematuria macroscopica molto probabilmente soffre di un'ARF intrinseca correlata a una glomerulonefrite postinfettiva acuta. Un bambino in condizioni critiche con un'anamnesi di ipotensione protratta ed esposizione a farmaci nefrotossici molto facilmente soffre di ATN. Un neonato che abbia un'anamnesi di idronefrosi all'ecografia prenatale e una vescica o una prostata palpabili assai presumibilmente patisce un'ostruzione congenita del tratto urinario, possibilmente correlata a valvole uretrali posteriori.

L'esame obiettivo deve essere accurato e occorre prestare attenzione allo stato del volume. La tachicardia, membrane mucose secche e una perfusione periferica insufficiente suggeriscono un volume circolante inadeguato e l'eventualità di un'ARF prerenale (vedi Capitoli 54 e 55). Un edema periferico, il verificarsi di rantoli e un ritmo di galoppo cardiaco presuppongono un sovraccarico del volume e la possibilità di un'ARF intrinseca da glomerulonefrite o un'ATN. La presenza di un rash e di artrite può indicare il lupus eritematoso sistemico (SLE, *Systemic Lupus Erythematosus*) o una nefrite da porpora di Henoch-Schönlein. Masse palpabili sul fianco sono suggestive di una trombosi della vena renale, di tumori, di una malattia cistica o di un'ostruzione del tratto urinario.

REPERTI DI LABORATORIO. Le anomalie di laboratorio possono includere l'anemia (in genere da diluizione o emolitica, come nel caso di SLE, di trombosi della vena renale, di HUS); la leucopenia (SLE); la trombocitopenia (SLE, trombosi della vena renale, HUS); l'iponatriemia (da diluizione); l'acidosi metabolica; concentrazioni sieriche elevate di azoto ureico nel sangue, di creatinina, di acido urico, di potassio e di fosfato (funzione renale diminuita) e l'ipocalcemia (iperfosfatemia).

Il livello sierico di C3 può essere ridotto (glomerulonefrite postinfettiva, SLE o glomerulonefrite membranoproliferativa) ed è possibile che nel siero vengano individuati anticorpi ad agenti streptococcici (glomerulonefrite poststreptococcica), nucleari (SLE), citoplasmatici neutrofili (granulomatosi di Wegener, poliarterite microscopica) o della membrana glomerulare basale (malattia di Goodpasture).

La presenza di ematuria, proteinuria e cilindri eritrocitari o granulari suggerisce un'ARF intrinseca e in particolare una malattia glomerulare. Se si rilevano leucociti e cilindri leucocitari con un'ematuria e una proteinuria di grado ridotto, è possibile l'esistenza di una malattia tubulointerstiziale. Eosinofili urinari possono trovarsi nei bambini con nefrite tubulointerstiziale causata da farmaci.

Gli indici urinari possono tornare utili per differenziare l'ARF prerenale da quella intrinseca (Tab. 535-2). I pazienti con urine di peso specifico elevato ($>$1,020), un'osmolalità urinaria alta (UOsm $>$500 mOsm/kg), sodio nelle urine ridotto (UNa $>$20 mEq/L) e una sua frazione di escrezione (FENa) $<$1% ($>$2,5% nei neonati) molto probabilmente soffrono di un'ARF prerenale. I soggetti in cui il peso specifico è $<$1,010, l'osmolalità urinaria

TABELLA 535-2. Analisi delle urine, analisi chimica delle urine e osmolalità nell'insufficienza renale acuta

	IPOVOLEMIA	NECROSI TUBULARE ACUTA	NEFRITE INTERSTIZIALE ACUTA	GLOMERULONEFRITE	OSTRUZIONE
Sedimento	Scarso	Cilindri granulari ampi, brunastri	Leucociti, eosinofili, cilindri cellulari	Eritrociti, cilindri eritrocitari	Scarso o ematico
Proteine	Assenti o scarse	Assenti o scarse	Minime ma possono aumentare con i FANS	Aumentate, >100 mg/dL	Basse
Sodio nelle urine, mEq/L*	>20	>30	>30	<20	<20 (acuta) >40 (pochi giorni)
Osmolalità nelle urine mOsm/kg	>400	<350	<350	>400	<350
Escrezione frazionaria di sodio% †	<1	>1	Varie	<1	<1 (acuta) >1 (pochi giorni)

*La sensibilità e la specificità del sodio nelle urine <20 nel differenziare l'azotemia prerenale dalla necrosi tubulare sono rispettivamente pari al 90 e all'82%.
†L'escrezione frazionaria del sodio è data dal rapporto urine/plasma (U/P) del sodio diviso per il rapporto U/P della creatinina × 100. La sensibilità e la specificità dell'escrezione frazionaria di sodio <1% nella differenziazione dell'azotemia prerenale dalla necrosi tubulare acuta sono rispettivamente pari al 96 e al 95%.
FANS, farmaci antinfiammatori non steroidei.
Tratta da Singri N, Ahya SN, Levin ML: Acute renal failure. *JAMA* 2003;289:747-751.

ridotta (UOsm <350 mOsm/kg), il sodio nelle urine elevato (UNa >40 mEq/L) e una FENa maggiore del 2% (>10% nei neonati) hanno verosimilmente un'ARF intrinseca.

$$\text{FENa}\ (\%) = \frac{\text{UNa} \times \text{PCr}}{\text{PNa} \times \text{UCr}} \times 100$$

La radiografia del torace può presentare cardiomegalia e congestione polmonare (sovraccarico di liquidi). L'ecografia renale può rivelare idronefrosi e/o idrouretere, indicativi di un'ostruzione del tratto urinario. La biopsia renale può in ultima analisi essere necessaria per determinare la causa dell'ARF nei pazienti che non presentano una forma prerenale o postrenale chiaramente definita.

Nei soggetti ad alto rischio (trauma, intervento chirurgico), l'individuazione precoce dell'insufficienza renale (prima di un aumento dei livelli dell'azoto ureico nel sangue o della creatinina) può essere determinata misurando la lipocalina associata alla gelatinasi neutrofila nel siero o nelle urine, che si accumula nei reni dopo una lesione renale ischemica acuta.

TRATTAMENTO

GESTIONE MEDICA. Nei lattanti e nei bambini con ostruzione del tratto urinario, come un neonato con un sospetto di valvole ureterali posteriori, è necessario inserire immediatamente un catetere vescicale per garantire un drenaggio adeguato del tratto urinario. Il suo posizionamento può inoltre essere considerato nei bambini più grandi e negli adolescenti non deambulanti per monitorare accuratamente la produzione di urine durante l'ARF.

La determinazione dello stato del volume è di fondamentale importanza durante la valutazione iniziale di un paziente con l'ARF. Se non esiste un'evidenza di sovraccarico del volume o d'insufficienza cardiaca, il volume intravascolare deve essere espanso mediante la somministrazione endovenosa di una soluzione salina isotonica a 20 mL/kg nell'arco di 30 min. In assenza di perdita di sangue o d'ipoproteinemia, per l'espansione del volume non sono necessarie soluzioni contenenti colloide. L'ipovolemia grave può richiedere boli di liquidi aggiuntivi (vedi Capitoli 53 e 68). La determinazione della pressione venosa centrale può tornare utile se sussistono dubbi sull'adeguatezza del volume di sangue. Dopo il suo ripristino, in genere i pazienti ipovolemici urinano entro 2 h; una mancata minzione indica che si è in presenza di un'ARF intrinseca o postrenale.

La terapia con diuretici va considerata solo dopo avere verificato l'adeguatezza del volume di sangue circolante. Il mannitolo (0,5 g/kg) e la furosemide (2-4 mg/kg, o in alternativa il bumetanide a 0,1 mg/kg) possono essere fatti assumere in una singola dose ev. Se la produzione di urina non migliora, è possibile considerare un'infusione continua di diuretici. Per ridurre il flusso sanguigno corticale renale, molti medici somministrano la dopamina (2-3 μg/kg/min) in associazione a una terapia diuretica, benché non vi siano dati controllati a sostegno di questa pratica. Esistono evidenze scarse che i diuretici o la dopamina possano prevenire l'ARF o accelerare il recupero. Il mannitolo può essere efficace nell'insufficienza renale indotta dai pigmenti (mioglobina, emoglobina).

In assenza di una risposta alla stimolazione con diuretici, la loro somministrazione deve essere interrotta; sicché la restrizione dei liquidi diviene fondamentale. I pazienti con un volume intravascolare normale vanno inizialmente sottoposti a una limitazione di 400 mL/m^2/24 h (perdite insensibili), più una quantità di liquidi uguale alla produzione di urine nella giornata. Le perdite di liquidi extrarenali (sangue, tratto gastrointestinale) devono essere sostituite, millilitro per millilitro, con altri liquidi appropriati. I pazienti marcatamente ipovolemici possono richiedere un'ulteriore limitazione, che prevede l'omissione della sostituzione delle perdite insensibili, della produzione di urine e delle perdite extrarenali per ridurre il volume intravascolare espanso. L'assunzione di liquidi, la produzione di urine e di feci, il peso corporeo e gli esami chimici sierici devono essere monitorati su base quotidiana.

Nell'ARF, il rapido sviluppo di **iperkaliemia** (livello di potassio nel siero >6 mEq/L) può condurre ad aritmia e arresto cardiaci e morte. La prima alterazione elettrocardiografica riscontrata nei pazienti con un'iperkaliemia in sviluppo è la comparsa di onde T con picchi. Questa manifestazione può essere quindi seguita da un ampliamento degli intervalli QRS, la depressione del segmento ST, aritmie ventricolari e arresto cardiaco (vedi Capitolo 52.4). Quando il potassio nel siero sale oltre 6,0 mEq/L occorre avviare le procedure volte a ridurre le sue scorte corporali. Le sue fonti esogene (dieta, liquidi endovenosi, nutrizione parenterale totale) vanno eliminate. Occorre inoltre somministrare la resina sodio polistirene sulfonato, 1 g/kg per os o tramite un clistere di ritenzione, la quale scambia il sodio con il potassio impiegando possibilmente diverse ore ad agire. Una dose singola di 1 g/kg può abbassare il livello del potassio nel siero di circa 1 mEq/L. Questa terapia può quindi essere ripetuta ogni 2 h, con limitazioni nella frequenza date prevalentemente dal rischio di sovraccarico di sodio.

Gli incrementi più gravi del potassio nel siero (>7 mEq/L), soprattutto se sono accompagnati da alterazioni elettrocardiografiche, richiedono alcune misure di emergenza in aggiunta alla resina. Per la precisione, occorre far assumere i seguenti agenti:

- **gluconato di calcio in soluzione al 10%, 1,0 mL/kg ev, in 3-5 min**
- **bicarbonato di sodio, 1-2 mEq/kg ev, in 5-10 min**
- **insulina regolare, 0,1 U/kg, con soluzione di glucosio al 50%, 1 mL/kg, in 1 h**

Il gluconato di calcio contrasta l'aumento dell'irritabilità miocardica indotto dal potassio, ma non abbassa il livello di potassio nel siero. La somministrazione del bicarbonato di sodio, dell'insulina e del glucosio abbassa il livello di potassio nel siero, spostandolo dal compartimento extracellulare a quello intracellulare. Un effetto simile è stato riferito con l'impiego intenso degli antagonisti β-adrenergici negli adulti, ma non esistono dati controllati per i pazienti pediatrici. Dal momento che la durata dell'azione di queste misure di emergenza è di poche ore, l'iperkaliemia va gestita mediante dialisi.

L'**acidosi metabolica** lieve è comune nell'ARF, a motivo della ritenzione di ioni idrogeno, fosfato e solfato, ma raramente richiede un intervento terapeutico. Se l'acidosi è grave (pH arterioso <7,15, bicarbonato sierico <8 mEq/L) o contribuisce all'iperkaliemia, risulta necessaria una terapia. Bisogna correggere parzialmente l'acidosi per via endovenosa, generalmente facendo assumere una quantità di bicarbonato sufficiente per aumentare il pH arterioso a 7,20 (valore che si avvicina a un livello di bicarbonato nel siero di 12 mEq/L). Il resto della correzione può essere condotto mediante la somministrazione orale di bicarbonato di sodio dopo la normalizzazione dei livelli sierici di calcio e fosfato. La citata correzione per via endovenosa può precipitare la tetania nei pazienti con un'insufficienza renale, perché la sua rapidità riduce la concentrazione di calcio ionizzata (vedi anche Capitolo 52).

L'**ipocalcemia** viene trattata principalmente abbassando il livello di fosforo nel siero. Il calcio non deve essere somministrato per via endovenosa, tranne nei casi di tetania, per evitare il deposito dei suoi sali nei tessuti. I pazienti vanno istruiti al rispetto di una dieta a basso contenuto di fosforo ed è necessario fare loro assumere per via orale i leganti del fosfato, allo scopo di legare gli eventuali fosfati ingeriti e di aumentare la loro escrezione per via gastrointestinale. Gli agenti comuni includono il sevelamer, il calcio carbonato e il calcio acetato. I leganti a base alluminio, comunemente impiegati in passato, vanno evitati, per l'evidente rischio di tossicità dell'alluminio.

L'**iponatriemia** è in genere un disturbo della diluizione che deve essere corretto mediante la limitazione dei liquidi piuttosto che con l'assunzione di sodio cloruro. La somministrazione di soluzione salina ipertonica (3%) va limitata ai pazienti con un'iponatriemia sintomatica (convulsioni, letargia) o a quelli con un livello di sodio nel siero <120 mEq/L. La correzione acuta del sodio sierico a 125 mEq/L (mmol/L) deve essere ottenuta utilizzando la seguente formula:

$$\text{mEq NaCl necessari} = 0{,}6 \times \text{peso (kg)} \times [125 - \text{sodio nel siero (mEq/L)}]$$

I pazienti con l'ARF sono predisposti a **emorragia gastrointestinale**, a causa della disfunzione piastrinica uremica, dell'aumentato stress e dell'esposizione all'eparina se è stata attivata l'emodialisi o la terapia sostitutiva renale continua. Gli H_2-bloccanti orali o endovenosi come la ranitidina vengono comunemente impiegati per prevenire questa complicanza.

È possibile che si sviluppi un'**ipertensione** dall'iperreninemia associata al processo patologico primitivo e/o all'espansione del volume extracellulare di liquidi e questo evento è massimamente frequente nei pazienti con l'ARF accompagnata dalla glomerulonefrite o dalla HUS. La limitazione dell'assunzione di sale e acqua è fondamentale e la somministrazione di diuretici può risultare utile (vedi Capitolo 445). Per una riduzione relativamente rapida della pressione sanguigna è possibile utilizzare l'isradipina (0,05-0,15 mg/kg per dose, dose massima 5 mg quattro volte al giorno). Gli agenti ad azione prolungata come i calcioantagonisti (amlodipina, 0,1-0,6 mg/kg/24 h ogni giorno o divisa per due volte al giorno) o β-bloccanti (propranololo, 0,5-8 mg/kg/24 h divisi per due o tre volte al giorno; labetalolo, 4-40 mg/kg/24 h divisi per due o tre volte al giorno) può essere utile per conservare il controllo della pressione sanguigna. I bambini con un'ipertensione sintomatica grave (urgenza/emergenza ipertensiva) devono essere trattati con infusioni continue di nitroprussiato di sodio (0,5-10 μg/kg/min), labetalolo (0,25-3,0 mg/kg/h) o esmololo (150-300 μg/kg/min) e convertiti agli antipertensivi a dosaggio intermittente quando divengono più stabili.

I **sintomi neurologici** nell'ARF possono includere cefalea, crisi convulsive, letargia e confusione. I potenziali fattori eziologici comprendono l'iponatriemia, l'ipocalcemia, l'ipertensione, l'emorragia cerebrale, la vasculite cerebrale e lo stato uremico. Il diazepam è l'agente più efficace per controllare le crisi convulsive e occorre mirare la terapia alla causa precipitante.

L'**anemia** dell'ARF è generalmente lieve (emoglobina 9-10 g/dL) e deriva principalmente dall'espansione del volume (emodiluizione). I bambini con HUS, SLE, emorragia attiva o ARF prolungata possono richiedere una trasfusione di emazie concentrate, se il loro livello di emoglobina scende al di sotto di 7 g/dL. Nei pazienti ipervolemici, la trasfusione di sangue comporta il rischio di un'ulteriore espansione del volume, che può precipitare l'ipertensione, l'insufficienza cardiaca e l'edema polmonare. Una trasfusione lenta (4-6 h) con emazie concentrate (10 mL/kg) riduce il rischio di ipervolemia. L'uso di globuli rossi freschi, lavati, riduce il rischio di iperpotassiemia. In presenza di ipervolemia o iperpotassiemia grave il sistema più sicuro per eseguire le trasfusioni di sangue è rappresentato dalla dialisi/ultrafiltrazione.

La **nutrizione** è fondamentale nei pazienti che sviluppano l'ARF. Nella maggior parte dei casi occorre limitare l'assunzione di sodio, potassio e fosforo e quella di proteine va moderatamente limitata, mentre bisogna massimizzare quella di calorie per ridurre al minimo l'accumulo di scorie azotate. Nei pazienti con un'ARF in condizioni critiche deve essere considerata un'iperalimentazione parenterale con aminoacidi essenziali.

DIALISI. Le indicazioni alla dialisi nell'ARF includono:

- **sovraccarico di volume con evidenza di ipertensione e/o edema polmonare refrattario alla terapia con diuretici**
- **iperpotassiemia persistente**
- **grave acidosi metabolica che non risponde al trattamento medico**
- **sintomi neurologici (stato mentale alterato, crisi convulsive)**
- **azotemia superiore a 100-150 mg/dL (o inferiore se in aumento rapido)**
- **squilibrio calcio/fosforo, con tetania ipocalcemica**

La dialisi trova un'altra indicazione nell'incapacità di garantire un apporto nutrizionale adeguato a causa del bisogno di una severa limitazione dei liquidi. Nei pazienti con un'ARF, la dialisi può essere necessaria per alcuni giorni o fino a 12 settimane; molti la richiedono per 1-3 settimane. I vantaggi e gli svantaggi dei 3 tipi di dialisi sono presentati nella Tabella 535-3.

TABELLA 535-3. Dialisi peritoneale (PD) a confronto con emodialisi intermittente (IHD) a confronto con terapia sostitutiva renale continua (CRRT)

	PD	IHC	CRRT
BENEFICI			
Rimozione di liquidi	+	++	++
Clearance di urea e creatinina	+	++	+
Clearance del potassio	++	++	+
Clearance delle tossine	+	++	+
COMPLICANZE			
Dolore addominale	+	–	–
Emorragia	–	+	+
Disequilibrio	–	+	–
Sbilancio elettrolitico	+	+	+
Necessità di eparinizzazione	–	+	+
Iperglicemia	+	–	–
Ipotensione	+	++	+
Ipotermia	–	–	+
Infezione dell'accesso centrale	–	+	+
Ernia inguinale/addominale	+	–	–
Peritonite	+	–	–
Perdita di proteine	+	–	–
Compromissione respiratoria	+	–	–
Trombosi vascolare	–	+	+

Adattata da Rogers MC: *Textbook of Pediatric Intensive Care*. Baltimore, Williams & Wilkins, 1992.

L'**emodialisi intermittente** è utile nei soggetti con uno stato emodinamico relativamente stabile. Questo processo molto efficace consente una rimozione dei liquidi e degli elettroliti in sedute di 3-4 ore, mediante l'uso di un circuito extracorporeo azionato da una pompa e di un grande catetere venoso centrale. L'emodialiasi intermittente può essere eseguita 3-7 volte alla settimana, in base al bilancio dei liquidi e degli elettroliti.

La **dialisi peritoneale** viene utilizzata soprattutto nei neonati e nei bambini piccoli, sebbene possa trovare impiego nei bambini più grandi e negli adolescenti di tutte le età. Il dialisato iperosmolare viene infuso nella cavità peritoneale attraverso un catetere per dialisi peritoneale posizionato mediante un intervento chirurgico o per via percutanea. Il liquido viene lasciato riposare per 45-60 min e quindi viene drenato dal paziente per gravità (manualmente o con l'uso di un variatore), ottenendo in questo modo una rimozione dei liquidi e degli elettroliti. In base all'equilibrio di questi ultimi, i cicli vengono ripetuti per 8-24 h/giorno. Non è necessaria una terapia anticoagulante; questa dialisi è controindicata nei pazienti con una patologia addominale significativa.

La **terapia di sostituzione renale continua** (CRRT, *Continuous Renal Replacement Therapy*) è indicata per i pazienti con uno stato emodinamico instabile, una sepsi concomitante o un'insufficienza multiorgano in un contesto di terapie intensive. Si tratta di una terapia extracorporea in cui liquidi, elettroliti e soluti di piccole e medie dimensioni vengono continuamente rimossi dal sangue (24 h/die) tramite una macchina specializzata azionata da una pompa. Di solito si inserisce un catetere a doppio lume nella succlavia, nella giugulare interna o nella vena femorale. Il paziente viene quindi connesso al circuito della CRRT azionato dalla pompa, la quale passa continuamente il suo sangue attraverso un filtro ad alta permeabilità.

La CRRT può essere eseguita in 3 modalità di base. Nell'emofiltrazione venovenosa continua, una grande quantità di liquido passa per pressione attraverso un filtro, portando con sé per convezione altre molecole come l'urea, la creatinina, il fosforo e l'acido urico. Il volume di sangue viene ricostituito mediante infusione ev di un liquido di sostituzione con una composizione desiderata di elettroliti simile a quella del sangue. La dialisi di emofiltrazione venovenosa continua utilizza il principio della diffusione, facendo circolare il dialisato in direzione controcorrente sul lato ultrafiltrato della membrana. Non viene utilizzato il liquido di sostituzione. L'emofiltrazione continua si serve invece sia del liquido di sostituzione sia del dialisato e offre la più efficace eliminazione dei soluti tra tutte le forme di CRRT.

PROGNOSI. Il tasso di mortalità nei bambini con ARF è variabile e dipende interamente dalla natura del processo patologico di base, piuttosto che dall'insufficienza renale stessa. I bambini con un'ARF causata da una malattia limitata ai reni, come la glomerulonefrite postinfettiva, hanno un tasso di mortalità molto basso (<1%), mentre quelli in cui essa sia collegata a una insufficienza multiorgano presentano un tasso molto alto (>90%).

La prognosi di recupero della funzione renale dipende dalla malattia che ha precipitato l'ARF. Questo recupero risulta probabile in seguito a un'ARF dovuta a cause prerenali, all'HUS, all'ATN, alla nefrite interstiziale acuta o alla sindrome da lisi tumorale; al contrario, si configura come raro quando l'ARF deriva dalla maggior parte dei tipi di glomerulonefrite rapidamente progressivi, da una trombosi bilaterale della vena renale o da una necrosi corticale bilaterale. Per trattare le sequele dell'ARF, che includono l'insufficienza renale cronica, l'ipertensione, l'acidosi tubulare renale e il difetto di concentrazione delle urine, può essere necessaria una terapia medica prolungata.

Andreoli SP: Acute renal failure in the newborn. *Semin Perinatol* 2004;28: 112–123.

Bellomo R, Chapman M, Finfer S, et al: Low-dose dopamine in patients with early renal dysfunction: A placebo-controlled randomized trial. Australian and New Zealand Intensive Care Society (ANZICS) Clinical Trials Group. *Lancet* 2000;356:2139–2143.

Bunchman TE, McBryde KD, Mottes TE, et al: Pediatric acute renal failure: Outcome by modality and disease. *Pediatr Nephrol* 2001;16:1067–1071.

Chan JCM, Williams DM, Roth KS: Kidney failure in infants and children. *Pediatr Rev* 2002;23:47–59.

Herget-Rosenthal S: One step forward in the early detection of acute renal failure. *Lancet* 2005;365:1205–1206.

Lamiere N, Van Biesen W, Vanholder R: Acute renal failure. *Lancet* 2005;365:417–430.

Lamiere N, Vanholder R, Vab Biesen W: Loop diuretics for patients with acute renal failure. *JAMA* 2002;288:2599–2600.

Manns M, Sigler MH, Teehan BP: Continuous renal replacement therapies: An update. *Am J Kidney Dis* 1998;32:185–207.

Singri N, Ahya SN, Levin ML: Acute renal failure. *JAMA* 2003;289: 747–751.

Williams DM, Sreedhar SS, Mickell JJ, Chan JCM: Acute kidney failure. *Arch Pediatr Adolesc Med* 2002;156:893–900.

535.2 • MALATTIA RENALE CRONICA

La malattia renale cronica (CKD, *Chronic Kidney Disease*) è definita come una compromissione renale (proteinuria) e/o una velocità di filtrazione glomerulare <60 mL/min/1,73 m^2 per >3 mesi. La diffusione nella popolazione pediatrica è di circa 18 per 1 milione. La prognosi per il neonato, il bambino o l'adolescente è migliorata notevolmente nel corso degli ultimi 4 decenni, grazie ai progressi compiuti nel trattamento medico (supporto nutrizionale aggressivo, eritropoietina ricombinante, ormone della crescita ricombinante), alle tecniche di dialisi e al trapianto renale.

EZIOLOGIA. Nei bambini la CKD può essere la conseguenza di una malattia renale congenita, acquisita, ereditata o metabolica e la causa sottostante è strettamente correlata all'età al momento della prima individuazione. Nei pazienti di età inferiore ai 5 anni, la CKD costituisce spesso il risultato di anomalie congenite come l'ipoplasia renale, la displasia e/o l'uropatia ostruttiva. Altre origini includono la sindrome nefrosica congenita, la sindrome da deficit della muscolatura addominale (*prune belly*), la necrosi corticale, la glomerulosclerosi segmentale focale, la malattia del rene policistico, la trombosi della vena renale e la sindrome uremico-emolitica.

Dopo il quinto anno di età, predominano invece le malattie acquisite (varie forme di glomerulonefrite, tra cui la nefrite lupica) ed ereditate (nefronoftisi giovaline familiare, sindrome di Alport). Una CKD correlata a malattie metaboliche (cistinosi, iperossaluria) e a determinate patologie ereditate (malattia del rene policistico) può manifestarsi durante tutti gli anni dell'infanzia.

PATOGENESI. Oltre alla compromissione crescente con malattie genetiche strutturali/metaboliche continue, il danno renale può progredire nonostante l'eliminazione dell'insulto originario.

La **compromissione dell'iperfiltrazione** può costituire un'importante via comune finale di distruzione glomerulare, indipendentemente dalla causa di base della malattia renale. Man mano che si perdono nefroni, quelli residui vanno incontro a una ipertrofia strutturale e funzionale caratterizzata da un aumento del flusso di sangue glomerulare. Nei nefroni che sopravvivono la forza di propulsione per la filtrazione glomerulare è aumentata. Sebbene questa iperfiltrazione compensatoria conservi temporaneamente la funzione renale totale, essa può determinare un danno progressivo ai glomeruli sopravvissuti, per esempio tramite l'effetto diretto della pressione idrostatica elevata sull'integrità della parete capillare e/o l'effetto tossico del maggior traffico di proteine attraverso la parete capillare stessa. Con il passare del tempo, man mano che la popolazione dei nefroni sclerosati aumenta, quelli sopravvissuti vengono sottoposti a un carico escretorio aumentato, che dà origine a un circolo vizioso di flusso ematico glomerulare in aumento e a una compromissione dell'iperfiltrazione.

La **proteinuria** stessa può contribuire al declino della funzione renale, come è stato evidenziato da alcuni studi che hanno dimostrato un effetto positivo della sua riduzione. Le proteine che attraversano la parete capillare glomerulare possono esercitare un effetto tossico diretto e reclutare monociti/macrofagi, accrescendo il processo di sclerosi glomerulare e di fibrosi tubulointerstiziale. L'**ipertensione** non controllata può esacerbare la progressione della malattia, generando una nefrosclerosi arteriolare e incrementando la lesione da iperfiltrazione precedentemente descritta.

Anche l'**iperfosfatemia** può aumentare la progressione della malattia, causando un deposito di calcio-fosfato nell'interstizio renale e nei vasi sanguigni. L'iperlipidemia, uno stato comune nei pazienti con una CKD, può influenzare negativamente la funzione glomerulare mediante un danno mediato dagli ossidanti.

La CKD può essere considerata un continuum della malattia, con manifestazioni biochimiche e cliniche che si estendono con la progressione del deterioramento della funzione renale. Le manifestazioni fisiopatologiche sono illustrate nella Tabella 535-4. La terminologia per descrivere gli stadi della malattia renale cronica è standardizzata (Tab. 535-5).

Malattia renale terminale (ESRD, *End-Stage Renal Disease*) è per esempio un termine amministrativo che negli Stati Uniti viene usato per indicare tutti i pazienti trattati con dialisi o trapianto renale. Questi soggetti costituiscono un sottogruppo di quelli con una CKD di stadio 5.

TABELLA 535-4. Fisiopatologia della malattia renale cronica

MANIFESTAZIONE	MECCANISMI
Accumulo di prodotti di scarto azotati	Riduzione della velocità di filtrazione glomerulare
Acidosi	Sintesi ridotta dell'ammoniaca Riassorbimento compromesso del bicarbonato Escrezione di acido netta ridotta
Ritenzione di sodio	Eccessiva produzione di renina Oliguria
Deplezione di sodio	Diuresi di soluto Danno tubulare
Difetto di concentrazione delle urine	Diuresi di soluto Danno tubulare
Iperpotassiemia	Riduzione della velocità di filtrazione glomerulare Acidosi metabolica Eccessiva assunzione di potassio Ipoaldosteronismo iporeninemico
Osteodistrofia renale	Produzione renale di 1,25-diidrossicolecalciferolo compromessa Iperfosfatemia Ipocalcemia Iperparatiroidismo secondario
Ritardo di crescita	Apporto calorico insufficiente Osteodistrofia renale Acidosi metabolica Anemia Resistenza all'ormone della crescita
Anemia	Produzione di eritropoietina ridotta Deficit di ferro Deficit di folati Deficit di vitamina B_{12} Sopravvivenza ridotta degli eritrociti
Tendenza all'emorragia	Funzione piastrinica difettosa
Infezione	Funzione granulocitaria difettosa Funzioni immunitarie cellulari compromesse Cateteri per dialisi residenti
Sintomi neurologici (astenia, difficoltà di concentrazione, cefalea, sonnolenza, perdita di memoria, crisi convulsive, neuropatia periferica)	Fattori uremici Tossicità dovuta all'alluminio Ipertensione
Sintomi gastrointestinali (intolleranza all'alimentazione, dolore addominale)	Reflusso gastroesofageo Motilità gastrointestinale ridotta
Ipertensione	Sovraccarico di volume Eccessiva produzione di renina
Iperlipidemia	Attività di lipasi delle lipoproteine plasmatiche ridotta
Pericardite/miocardiopatia	Fattori uremici Ipertensione Sovraccarico di liquidi
Intolleranza al glucosio	Resistenza all'insulina tissutale

TABELLA 535-5. Terminologia standardizzata per gli stadi della malattia renale cronica

STADIO	DESCRIZIONE	GFR (mL/min/1,73 m²)
Stadio 1	Danno renale con GFR normale o aumentata	>90
Stadio 2	Danno renale con una lieve riduzione della GFR	60-89
Stadio 3	Riduzione moderata della GFR	30-59
Stadio 4	Riduzione grave della GFR	5-29
Stadio 5	Insufficienza renale	<15 o in dialisi

GFR, velocità di filtrazione glomerulare.

MANIFESTAZIONI CLINICHE. La presentazione clinica della CKD è piuttosto varia e dipende dalla malattia renale di base. I bambini e gli adolescenti con una CKD causata da glomerulonefrite cronica (glomerulonefrite membranoproliferativa) possono presentarsi con edema, ipertensione, ematuria e proteinuria. I neonati e i bambini con malattie congenite come la displasia renale e l'uropatia ostruttiva possono manifestare un mancato sviluppo nel periodo neonatale, una disidratazione da poliuria, un'infezione del tratto urinario o un'insufficienza renale manifesta. Molti neonati con la CKD vengono identificati all'ecografia prenatale e questo consente un intervento diagnostico e terapeutico precoce. I bambini con la nefronoftisi giovanile familiare possono avere una presentazione molto tenue, con disturbi aspecifici come la cefalea, l'astenia, la letargia, l'anoressia, il vomito, la polidipsia, la poliuria e un deficit della crescita nel corso di più anni.

L'esame obiettivo può rivelare pallore e colorito giallognolo. I pazienti con una CKD non trattata di lunga durata possono rivelare una statura ridotta e alcune anomalie ossee tipiche dell'osteodistrofia renale (vedi anche Capitoli 529.3 e 529.4). Nei bambini con una CKD dovuta alla glomerulonefrite cronica (o in quelli con un'insufficienza renale avanzata originata da altre cause) si possono trovare edema, ipertensione e altri segni di sovraccarico del volume di liquido extracellulare.

I reperti di laboratorio includono aumenti dell'azotemia e della creatinina sierica. Nei bambini il grado di disfunzione renale può venire determinato applicando la seguente formula, che fornisce una stima della velocità di filtrazione glomerulare:

$$\text{GFR (mL/min/1,73 m}^2\text{)} = \frac{\text{k peso (cm)}}{\text{creatinina sierica (mg/dL)}}$$

dove k è 0,33 per i neonati di età inferiore a 1 anno con un ridotto peso alla nascita, 0,45 per quelli della stessa età con un peso appropriato per l'età gestazionale a termine, 0,55 per i bambini e le adolescenti e 0,70 per gli adolescenti.

I **reperti di laboratorio** possono inoltre rivelare iperkaliemia, iponatriemia (se sussiste un sovraccarico del volume), acidosi, ipocalcemia, iperfosfatemia e un aumento dell'acido urico. I pazienti con una forte proteinuria possono maturare un'ipoalbuminemia. In genere un esame emocromocitometrico evidenzia un'anemia normocromica, normocitica. I livelli del colesterolo e dei trigliceridi nel siero sono solitamente elevati. Le analisi delle urine, nei bambini con una CKD originata dalla glomerulonefrite, mostrano ematuria e proteinuria, mentre in quelli in cui essa è dovuta a lesioni congenite come la displasia renale, di solito rivelano un peso specifico ridotto e anomalie minime.

TRATTAMENTO

Il trattamento della CKD è volto a: (1) sostituire le funzioni renali assenti/diminuite, che si deteriorano progressivamente in parallelo con la progressiva perdita di GFR; (2) rallentare l'evolversi della disfunzione renale. I bambini con CKD devono essere trattati presso un centro medico in grado di fornire servizi multidisciplinari, tra cui l'assistenza medica, infermieristica, sociale, nutrizionale e psicologica.

La gestione richiede un attento monitoraggio dello stato clinico e di laboratorio del paziente. I controlli ematici da eseguire di routine includono i livelli degli elettroliti sierici, dell'azotemia, della creatinina, del calcio, del fosforo, dell'albumina, della fosfatasi alcalina e dell'emoglobina. Una misurazione periodica dei livelli dell'ormone paratiroideo (PTH, *ParaThyroid Hormone*) intatto e studi radiologici dell'osso possono tornare utili per individuare un'evidenza precoce di osteodistrofia renale. Occorre eseguire periodicamente l'ecografia al fine di identificare un'ipertrofia ventricolare sinistra e una disfunzione cardiaca che possono verificarsi quali conseguenze delle complicanze della CKD.

GESTIONE DEI LIQUIDI E DEGLI ELETTROLITI. La maggior parte dei bambini con CKD mantiene un equilibrio normale tra sodio e acqua grazie all'assunzione di sodio da una dieta appropriata. I neonati e i bambini con una CKD dovuta a displasia renale possono essere poliurici, con ingenti perdite di sodio con le urine. Questi bambini possono trarre beneficio da un'alimentazione a bassa densità calorica e a elevato volume, con l'integrazione del sodio. I bambini con ipertensione, edema o insufficienza cardiaca possono necessitare di una limitazione del sodio e di una terapia diuretica. La riduzione dei liquidi raramente appare necessaria, finché lo sviluppo di una malattia renale terminale non richiede l'avvio della dialisi.

Nella maggior parte dei bambini con CKD, il bilancio di potassio viene mantenuto fino a quando la funzione renale non si deteriora così tanto da richiedere l'inizio della dialisi. Tuttavia, nei pazienti con un'insufficienza renale moderata e un'eccessiva assunzione di potassio con la dieta è possibile che si sviluppi l'iperkaliemia, un'acidosi grave o un ipoaldosteronismo iporeninemico (correlato alla distruzione dell'apparato iuxtaglomereulare che secerne la renina). L'iperkaliemia può venire trattata limitando l'assunzione del potassio, somministrando agenti alcalinizzanti orali e/o mediante una terapia con la resina sodio polistirene sulfonato.

ACIDOSI. Un'acidosi metabolica si sviluppa in quasi tutti i bambini con CKD in conseguenza della ridotta escrezione netta di acidi dai reni compromessi. Per conservare il livello del bicarbonato di sodio >22 mEq/L è possibile somministrarlo in compresse (650 mg corrispondono a 8 mEq di base) o utilizzare un preparato con 1 mEq sodio citrato/mL).

NUTRIZIONE. In genere i pazienti con una CKD necessitano di una limitazione progressiva di vari componenti dietetici man mano che la funzione renale diminuisce. L'assunzione, con la dieta, di fosforo, potassio e sodio va definita in base agli esami di laboratorio e al bilancio idrico del paziente. Nei neonati vengono normalmente impiegati tipi artificiali di latte, che contengono una quantità ridotta di fosfato.

L'apporto calorico ottimale è sconosciuto, ma si raccomanda di fornire almeno quello indicato per l'età. L'apporto proteico, invece, deve essere pari a 2,5 g/kg/24 h e occorre sia costituito da proteine ad alto valore biologico, che vengono metabolizzate prevalentemente in aminoacidi instabili piuttosto che in scorie azotate. Le proteine con il valore biologico massimo sono quelle delle uova e del latte e quindi della carne, del pesce e del pollame.

L'assunzione alimentare va corretta in base alla risposta, se possibile consultando un dietista esperto nella CKD infantile. L'apporto calorico può essere aumentato nei bambini integrando il latte artificiale con componenti modulari di carboidrati, grassi (olio di trigliceridi a catena media) e proteine secondo la tolleranza mostrata. Nei bambini più grandi e negli adolescenti possono essere utili prodotti enterali disponibili in commercio. Se l'apporto calorico resta inadeguato e/o l'aumento ponderale e la velocità di crescita non risultano ottimali, occorre considerare l'alimentazione con un sondino enterale. Le integrazioni possono venire apportate mediante un sondino nasogastrico, la gastrostomia o un sondino gastrodigiunale. In genere vengono fatte assumere infusioni notturne continue con o senza la somministrazione di boli diurni.

I bambini possono andare incontro a un deficit delle vitamine solubili in acqua, per l'inadeguato apporto alimentare o per le perdite causate dalla dialisi. Queste vitamine devono essere garantite di routine, utilizzando preparazioni come il Nephrocaps®. Le integrazioni di zinco e ferro vanno effettuate solo se i deficit vengono confermati e in genere quella delle vitamine liposolubili A, E e K non è necessaria.

CRESCITA. La statura ridotta è una conseguenza a lungo termine significativa della CKD infantile. I bambini affetti hanno uno stato resistente all'ormone della crescita (GH, *Growth Hormone*): i suoi livelli sono elevati, ma quelli del fattore della crescita 1 insulino-simile risultano ridotti e sussistono gravi anomalie delle proteine leganti il fattore della crescita insulino-simile.

I bambini con CKD con un'altezza inferiore −2 SD, nonostante un'assistenza medica ottimale (apporto calorico adeguato e trattamento effettivo dell'osteodistrofia renale, dell'anemia e dell'acidosi metabolica) possono trarre giovamento da dosaggi farmacologici di GH ricombinante umano (rHuGH, *Recombinant Human GH*). Il trattamento può essere avviato con 0,05 mg/kg/24 h per via sottocutanea, con correzioni periodiche del dosaggio per raggiungere l'obiettivo di una velocità di crescita normale per l'età.

La terapia con rHuGH continua finché il paziente: (1) raggiunge il 50° percentile dell'altezza media dei genitori; (2) arriva a un'altezza adulta finale; (3) viene sottoposto a un trapianto renale. Il trattamento a lungo termine eleva in maniera significativa l'altezza adulta finale, che per alcuni pazienti arriva a essere quella normale e induce un recupero persistente della crescita.

OSTEODISTROFIA RENALE. L'espressione osteodistrofia renale viene usata per indicare uno spettro di disturbi ossei osservati nei pazienti con CKD. La malattia più comune che riguarda i bambini è quella da elevato turn-over osseo, che viene causata dall'iperparatiroidismo secondario. Il reperto patologico scheletrico è in questo caso costituito da un'osteite fibrosa cistica.

La **fisiopatologia** dell'osteodistrofia renale è complessa. Nella fase iniziale della CKD, quando la GFR si riduce a circa il 50% del normale, la diminuzione della massa renale funzionale conduce a un declino dell'attività della 1α-idrossilasi renale, con una produzione ridimensionata di vitamina D (1,25-diidrossicolecalciferolo). Questo deficit della vitamina D attivata causa un ridotto assorbimento di calcio intestinale, un'ipocalcemia e un aumento dell'attività della ghiandola paratiroide. Una secrezione eccessiva di ormone paratoroideo (PTH, *ParaThyroid Hormone*) tenta di correggere l'ipocalcemia mettendo in atto un incremento del riassorbimento osseo. Più avanti nel corso della CKD, quando la GFR si riduce al 20-25% del normale, i meccanismi di compensazione per accrescere l'escrezione del fosfato diventano inadeguati e causano un'iperfosfoatemia, che promuove ulteriormente l'ipocalcemia e un'aumentata secrezione di PTH.

Le **manifestazioni cliniche** dell'osteodistrofia renale includono debolezza muscolare, dolore osseo e fratture in seguito a un trauma minimo. Nei bambini in crescita possono essere riscontrate alterazioni rachitiche, deformità vare e valghe delle ossa lunghe e scivolamento della testa del femore. Gli esami di laboratorio possono dimostrare un livello di calcio sierico ridotto, uno di fosforo sierico aumentato, un innalzamento della fosfatasi alcalina e un livello di PTH normale. Nelle radiografie delle mani, dei palmi e delle ginocchia si nota un riassorbimento sottoperiosteo dell'osso con l'ampliamento delle metafisi.

Gli obiettivi del **trattamento** sono di prevenire la deformità ossea e di normalizzare la velocità di crescita adottando interventi dietetici e farmacologici. Occorre che i bambini e gli adolescenti seguano una dieta a basso contenuto di fosforo e che i neonati siano alimentati con latte artificiale con la medesima caratteristica. Dato che è impossibile limitare completamente l'assunzione del fosforo, vengono impiegati alcuni leganti del fosfato per accrescere l'escrezione di quest'ultimo con le feci. Sebbene anamnesticamente il calcio carbonato e il calcio acetato siano stati i leganti più usati, sta affermandosi l'impiego di alcuni più nuovi, non basati sul calcio, come il savelamer, in particolare nei pazienti predisposti all'ipercalcemia. Considerato inoltre che l'alluminio può essere assorbito dal tratto gastrointestinale e può condurre a tossicità, i leganti con base alluminio devono essere evitati.

Il fondamento della terapia dell'osteodistrofia renale è la somministrazione di vitamina D. La **terapia con vitamina D** è indicata nei pazienti con: (1) livelli di 25-idrossi-vitamina D al di sotto dell'intervallo stabilito per lo stadio particolare di CKD; (2) livelli di PTH superiori all'intervallo fissato per lo stadio di CKD. I pazienti con livelli bassi di 25-idrossi-vitamina D vanno trattati con l'ergocalciferolo, mentre quelli il cui livello di 25-idrossi-vitamina D risulti normale ma che ne hanno uno elevato di PTH devono essere trattati con 0,01-0,05 μg/kg/24 h di calcitriolo (0,25 μg in capsule o 1 μg/mL in sospensione). Nuovi analoghi della vitamina D attivata, come il paracalcitolo e il doxecalciferolo, vengono adottati sempre più spesso, soprattutto nei pazienti predisposti all'ipercalcemia. I leganti del fosfato e la vitamina D vanno regolati in modo da mantenere il livello del PTH entro l'intervallo stabilito e i livelli sierici di calcio e fosfato entro l'intervallo normale per l'età. Molti nefrologi tentano di conservare il prodotto calcio/fosforo ($Ca \times PO_4$) <55 per ridurre al minimo la possibilità del deposito tissutale di sali di calcio-fosforo.

MALATTIA ADINAMICA DELL'OSSO. La malattia adinamica dell'osso (malattia da scarso turn-over osseo) è stata individuata sia in bambini sia in adulti con CKD. Il reperto patologico è l'osteomalacia ed è associato a una soppressione del PTH, forse correlata all'utilizzo diffuso dei leganti del fosfato contenti calcio e degli analoghi della vitamina D.

ANEMIA. Nei pazienti con CKD l'anemia appare principalmente il risultato di una produzione inadeguata di eritropoietina da parte dei reni compromessi e di solito diviene manifesta negli stadi 3-4 della malattia.

Altri possibili fattori contribuenti includono il deficit di ferro, quello di acido folico o di vitamina B_{12} e la ridotta sopravvivenza degli eritrociti. La terapia con l'eritropoietina umana ricombinante (rHuEPO, *Recombinant Human ErythroPoietin*) ha ridotto la necessità di una trasfusione. La somministrazione dell'eritropoietina di solito viene avviata quando la concentrazione dell'emoglobina scende sotto 10 g/dL, a un dosaggio di 50-150 mg/kg/dose per via sottocutanea 1-3 volte alla settimana. La dose viene quindi corretta per conservare la concentrazione di emoglobina tra i 12 e i 13 g/dL. Tutti i pazienti in cui viene utilizzata una terapia con rHuEPO devono ricevere un'integrazione di ferro per via orale o endovenosa. Quelli che sembrano resistenti alla rHuEPO vanno sottoposti a un controllo per appurare deficit di ferro, perdita di sangue occulto, infezione/stato infiammatorio cronico, deficit di vitamina B_{12} o folati e fibrosi del midollo osseo correlata a un iperparatiroidismo secondario. I meriti della terapia con eritropoietina sono riassunti nella Tabella 535-6. Un'opzione alternativa è la darbopoeitina alfa, un agente ad azione prolungata somministrato a un dosaggio di 0,45 mcg/kg/settimana, il cui vantaggio principale è costituito dal fatto che può essere dosato da una volta alla settimana a una volta al mese per la sua durata di azione prolungata.

TABELLA 535-6. Meriti della terapia con eritropoietina umana ricombinante o con darbopoietina

BENEFICI
Mancata necessità/riduzione al minimo della necessità di trasfusioni di sangue
Ridotta sensibilizzazione agli antigeni di istocompatibilità
Ridotta esposizione alle malattie infettive
Minori probabilità di sovraccarico cronico di ferro
Miglioramento dell'appetito
Maggiore tolleranza allo sforzo
Miglioramento del sonno
Miglioramento del benessere fisico
POTENZIALI COMPLICANZE
Deficit di ferro
Ipertensione
Crisi convulsive
Coagulazione dell'accesso vascolare
Aplasia eritrocitaria pura (riferita negli adulti a causa degli anticorpi all'eritropoietina umana ricombinante)

IPERTENSIONE. I bambini con la CKD possono presentare un'ipertensione sostenuta correlata a un sovraccarico del volume e/o a una eccessiva produzione di renina collegata alla malattia glomerulare. I bambini ipertesi con un sospetto sovraccarico del volume devono seguire una dieta iposodica (2-3 g/24 h) e possono trarre giovamento da una terapia con diuretici. I diuretici tiazidici (idroclorotiazide 2 mg/kg/24 h due volte al giorno) sono la prima classe di scelta per i bambini con una disfunzione renale lieve (CKD stadi 1-3). Tuttavia, quando la GFR stimata scende a CKD di fase 4, i tiazidi risultano meno efficaci e occorre passare ai diuretici dell'ansa (furosemide 1-2 mg/kg/dose due o tre volte al giorno). Gli **ACE-inibitori** (enalapril, lisinopril) e i bloccanti dell'angiotensina II (losartan) sono gli antipertensivi di elezione in tutti i bambini con una malattia renale proteinurica, a causa della loro potenziale capacità di rallentare la progressione a una ESRD. Tuttavia deve essere posta estrema attenzione nell'utilizzo di questi agenti, monitorando la funzione renale e il bilancio degli elettroliti, in particolare nei bambini con una CKD avanzata. I calcioantagonisti (amlodipina), i β-bloccanti (propranololo, atenololo) e gli agenti ad azione centrale (clonidina) possono essere utili quali agenti aggiuntivi nei bambini con una CKD in cui sia impossibile controllare la pressione sanguigna limitando l'assunzione di sodio con la dieta o somministrando diuretici e ACE-inibitori.

VACCINAZIONI. I bambini con la CKD devono ricevere tutte le vaccinazioni standard secondo il programma previsto per i bambini sani. Vanno invece evitati i vaccini vivi per i bambini con una CKD correlata a glomerulonefrite durante il trattamento con farmaci immunosoppressori. È tuttavia fondamentale adoperarsi in ogni modo per fare assumere vaccini virali vivi (parotite, morbillo, rosolia, varicella) prima del trapianto renale, perché il loro uso è sconsigliato nei pazienti immunosoppressi. Tutti i bambini con CKD devono sottoporsi all'annuale vaccinazione antinfluenzale. I dati indicano tuttavia che questi bambini possono rispondere in maniera non ottimale alle vaccinazioni.

REGOLAZIONE DEL DOSAGGIO DEI FARMACI. Dato che molti farmaci vengono escreti dai reni, è possibile che il loro dosaggio debba essere regolato nei pazienti con la CKD, per ottimizzarne l'efficacia e ridurre al minimo il rischio di tossicità (vedi Capitolo 716). Le strategie di correzione includono l'allungamento dell'intervallo tra le dosi, la riduzione del dosaggio assoluto o entrambe queste misure.

PROGRESSIONE DELLA MALATTIA. Sebbene non esistano terapie definitive per migliorare la funzione renale nei bambini o negli adulti con la CKD, vi sono numerose strategie che possono risultare efficaci per rallentare la velocità di progressione della disfunzione renale. Un controllo ottimale dell'ipertensione (ossia il mantenimento della pressione sanguigna al di sotto del 75° percentile e se possibile anche meno) è fondamentale in tutti i pazienti. Gli ACE-inibitori o i bloccanti dei recettori dell'angiotensina II devono essere i farmaci antipertensivi di elezione nei bambini ipertesi con una malattia renale proteinurica cronica. Questi agenti inoltre vanno fortemente considerati nei bambini con la CKD che presentino una proteinuria significativa, anche in assenza dell'ipertensione. Occorre mantenere il fosforo sierico entro l'intervallo di normalità per l'età e il prodotto calcio-fosforo deve essere <55, per ridurre al minimo il deposito renale di calcio-fosforo. Un trattamento sollecito delle complicanze infettive e degli episodi di disidratazione può minimizzare la perdita aggiuntiva del parenchima renale.

Altre raccomandazioni potenzialmente utili includono la correzione dell'anemia con l'eritropoietina o la darbopoietina alfa, il controllo dell'iperlipidemia, l'astensione dal fumo di sigaretta, la prevenzione dell'obesità e la riduzione al minimo dell'impiego di farmaci antinfiammatori non steroidei. Benché la limitazione di proteine con la dieta si sia rivelata utile negli adulti, in generale non viene suggerita per i bambini, per il timore di effetti collaterali sulla crescita e sullo sviluppo.

535.3 • MALATTIA RENALE TERMINALE

L'ESRD rappresenta lo stato in cui la disfunzione renale di un paziente è giunta al punto in cui l'omeostasi e la sopravvivenza non possono più essere sostenuti con la funzione renale nativa e una gestione medica massima. A partire da qui, diviene necessaria la terapia di sostituzione renale (dialisi o trapianto). L'obiettivo finale per i bambini con l'ESRD è costituito appunto da un trapianto renale riuscito (vedi Capitolo 536), perché consente lo stile di vita più normale e la possibilità di riabilitazione per loro e per la famiglia.

Il 75% dei bambini statunitensi con l'ESRD richiedono un periodo di dialisi prima che possa essere eseguito il trapianto. Si raccomanda di avviare i piani di sostituzione renale quando il bambino raggiunge la CKD di stadio 4. Il momento ottimale per cominciare la dialisi, tuttavia, si fonda su una combinazione di caratteristiche biochimiche e cliniche del paziente, tra cui un sovraccarico di liquidi refrattario, uno squilibrio elettrolitico, un'acidosi, un deficit della crescita oppure sintomi uremici, compresi l'astenia, la nausea e un rendimento scolastico compromesso. In generale, la maggior parte dei nefrologi tenta di iniziare la dialisi sufficientemente presto, per prevenire lo sviluppo di gravi anomalie idriche ed elettrolitiche, la malnutrizione e i sintomi uremici. Il trapianto preventivo prima dell'avvio della dialisi viene utilizzato sempre più spesso.

La scelta della modalità di dialisi deve essere personalizzata per adattarla alle esigenze di ciascun bambino. Negli Stati Uniti, due terzi dei bambini con l'ESRD vengono trattati con la dialisi peritoneale, mentre un terzo con l'emodialisi. L'età è un fattore importante nella selezione della modalità di dialisi: l'88% dei neonati e dei bambini, dalla nascita ai 5 anni, viene trattato con la dialisi peritoneale, mentre il 54% di quelli di età superiore ai 12 anni con l'emodialisi.

La **dialisi peritoneale** è una tecnica che utilizza la membrana peritoneale del paziente quale dializzatore. L'acqua corporea in eccesso viene rimossa da un gradiente osmotico creato dall'elevata concentrazione del destrosio nel dialisato; le scorie vengono eliminate mediante la diffusione dai capillari peritoneali nel dialisato. L'accesso alla cavità peritoneale si ottiene da un catetere di Tenckhoff tunnellizzato inserito chirurgicamente.

La dialisi peritoneale può essere eseguita in modalità ambulatoriale continua oppure come qualsiasi altra forma di terapia automatizzata con un variatore (ciclica continua, intermittente o intermittente notturna). La maggior parte dei bambini statunitensi che vengono sottoposti alla dialisi peritoneale utilizza una terapia guidata da un variatore, che consente al paziente e alla famiglia di essere liberi dalle esigenze della dialisi durante le ore diurne, dal momento che gli scambi vengono eseguiti automaticamente dalla macchina durante il sonno. Questo permette un'attività diurna ininterrotta, una riduzione del numero di connessioni e disconnessioni del catetere (con conseguente riduzione del rischio di peritonite) e una diminuzione del tempo richiesto dai pazienti e dai genitori per eseguire la dialisi, con abbassamento del rischio di spossatezza e stanchezza estrema. Dato che la dialisi peritoneale non ha la stessa efficienza dell'emodialisi, deve essere eseguita quotidianamente invece che 3 volte alla settimana; i suoi vantaggi sono elencati nella Tabella 535-7.

L'**emodialisi**, contrariamente alla dialisi peritoneale, è generalmente eseguita in un contesto ospedaliero. Tipicamente, i bambini e gli adolescenti vengono sottoposti a tre sedute di 3 o 4 ore alla settimana, durante le quali vengono rimosse le scorie di liquido e soluto. L'accesso alla circolazione del bambino viene ottenuto mediante una fistola arteriovenosa creata chirurgicamente, un innesto o un catetere residente nella succlavia o nella giugulare interna.

TABELLA 535-7. Meriti della dialisi peritoneale nei pazienti pediatrici con malattia renale terminale

VANTAGGI
Possibilità di eseguire la dialisi a casa
Tecnicamente più semplice dell'emodialisi, soprattutto nei neonati
Possibilità di vivere a una distanza maggiore dall'istituto ospedaliero
Libertà di frequentare la scuola e le attività postscolastiche
Dieta meno restrittiva
Meno costosa dell'emodialisi
Indipendenza (adolescenti)
SVANTAGGI
Cattivo funzionamento del catetere
Infezioni correlate al catetere (peritonite, sito di uscita)
Compromissione dell'appetito (per la cavità peritoneale piena)
Imaging corporeo negativo
Esaurimento della persona che fornisce assistenza

Brouhard BH, Donaldson LA, Lawry KW, et al: Cognitive functioning in children on dialysis and post-transplantation. *Pediatr Transplant* 2000;4:261-267.

Coulthard MG, Crosier J: Outcome of reaching end stage renal failure in children under 2 years of age. *Arch Dis Child* 2002;87:511-517.

El Nahas AM, Bello AK: Chronic kidney disease: The global challenge. *Lancet* 2005;365:331-340.

Neu AM, Fivush BA: Immunizations for pediatric dialysis patients. *Adv Ren Replace Ther* 2000;7:239-246.

Goodman WG, Goldin J, Kuizon BD, et al: Coronary artery calcification in young adults with end-stage renal disease who are undergoing dialysis. *N Engl J Med* 2000;342:1478-1483.

Haffner D, Schaefer F, Nissel R, et al: Effect of growth hormone treatment on the adult height of children with chronic renal failure. *N Engl J Med* 2000;343:923-930.

Hebert LA, Wilmer WA, Falkenhain ME, et al: Renoprotection: One or many therapies? *Kidney Int* 2001;59:1211-1226.

Hogg RJ, Furth S, Lemley KV, et al: National Kidney Foundation's Kidney Disease Outcomes Quality Initiative clinical practice guidelines for chronic kidney disease in children and adolescents: Evaluation, classification, and stratification. *Pediatrics* 2003;111:1416-1421.

Hingorani S, Watkins SL: Dialysis for end-stage renal disease. *Curr Opin Pediatr* 2000;12:140-145.

Lewis EJ, Hunsicker LG, Clarke WR, et al: Renoprotective effect of the angiotensin-receptor antagonist irbesartan in patients with nephropathy due to type 2 diabetes. *N Engl J Med* 2001;345:851-860.

Martin KJ, Olgaard K, Coburn JW, et al: Diagnosis, assessment, and treatment of bone turnover abnormalities in renal osteodystrophy. *Am J Kidney Dis* 2004;43:558-565.

McDonald SP, Craig JC: Long-term survival of children with end-stage renal disease. *N Engl J Med* 2004;350:2654-2662.

Parekh RS, Carroll CE, Wolfe RA, et al: Cardiovascular mortality in children and young adults with end-stage kidney disease. *J Pediatr* 2002; 141:197-207.

Parekh RS, Flynn JT, Smoyer WE, et al: Improved growth in young children with severe chronic renal insufficiency who use specified nutritional therapy. *J Am Soc Nephrol* 2001;12:2418-2426.

Sanchez CP: Prevention and treatment of renal osteodystrophy in children with chronic renal insufficiency and end-stage renal disease. *Semin Nephrol* 2001;21:441-450.

Seikaly MG, Ho PL, Emmett L, et al: Chronic renal insufficiency in children: The 2001 Annual Report of the NAPRTCS. *Pediatr Nephrol* 2003; 18:796-804.

Warady BA, Alexander SR, Watkins S, et al: Optimal care of the pediatric end-stage renal disease patient on dialysis. *Am J Kidney Dis* 1999; 33:567-583.

Warady BA, Belden B, Kohaut E: Neurodevelopmental outcome of children initiating peritoneal dialysis in early infancy. *Pediatr Nephrol* 1999; 13:759-765.

Capitolo 536 ■ Trapianto renale

Rodrigo E. Urizar

Il trattamento ottimale dei bambini con una malattia renale terminale (ESRD, *End-Stage Renal Disorder*) è un trapianto renale (RT, *Renal Transplantation*) precoce da un donatore consanguineo vivente (LRD-RT, *Living Related Donor-Renal Transplantation*). I vantaggi tecnici, le strategie di supporto e in particolare l'uso di sostanze immunosoppressive efficaci consentono inoltre un tasso elevato di successo nei trapianti renali da donatore non consanguineo vivente o cadavere (CAD)-RT (*Cadaveric-Renal Transplantation*).

EPIDEMIOLOGIA. Lo U.S. Renal Data System documenta 20 nuovi casi di ESRD per milione di bambini all'anno, con un picco tra gli 11 e i 15 anni di età. Precedentemente al 1° anno di età, l'incidenza è di 0,2 pazienti/milione all'anno. Il North American Pediatric Renal Transplant Cooperative Study (NAPRTCS) ha riportato la registrazione e il successivo follow-up, dal gennaio 2003, di oltre l'80% dei bambini americani e canadesi con un'insufficienza renale cronica, dialisi, trapianto ed eventi post-trapianto. Dei 13 341 bambini registrati, 7651 (57,3%) hanno ricevuto il loro primo trapianto (indice); 1713 degli 8399 trapianti primari (24%) sono stati eseguiti su base precauzionale (ossia senza una precedente dialisi). Tra gli altri, 3646 presentavano un'insufficienza renale cronica (27,3%), mentre 1519 (11,5%) dei 13 341 restanti sono in dialisi in attesa di trapianto. L'81% degli allotrapianti è stato eseguito da un donatore vivente, pochi riceventi hanno meno di 6 anni di età e pochi donatori hanno meno di 10 anni di età.

Un trapianto ben funzionante (LRD o CAD) può riabilitare completamente un paziente. Il candidato a ricevere il trapianto e i parenti devono comprendere, in ogni caso, che l'RT non rappresenta una soluzione permanente per la ESRD. Inoltre, un rene trapiantato che funzioni in maniera inadeguata (rigetto progressivo incontrollabile) è associato a una grave morbilità, a mortalità e ad un potenziale ritorno alla dialisi a lungo termine. Il carattere transitorio dei trapianti renali ha costretto i programmi di trapianto a considerarne molti per paziente, un obiettivo fortemente ostacolato dalla limitata disponibilità di reni CAD. Questa carenza può riflettere la reticenza del pubblico generale, del personale infermieristico e dei medici, nei confronti della donazione di organi. Data la forte sproporzione tra l'incremento annuo nella necessità di un RT (22%) e il numero di quelli eseguiti nello stesso periodo (8%), si stima che 100 000 reni dovranno essere distribuiti tra 180 000 pazienti in dialisi nei soli Stati Uniti. Allo stato attuale dell'approvvigionamento di organi, il gap tra la disponibilità di reni e i trapianti andrà via via ampliandosi, se non aumenteranno le donazioni da consanguinei viventi e da cadavere; altri reni, negli Stati Uniti, vengono ottenuti da donatori di età inferiore a 15 anni cerebralmente morti; inoltre, negli Stati Uniti stanno diventando sempre più accettabili altre misure, come lo xenotrapianto (ossia un trapianto tra specie diverse, oggi sporadicamente usato in campi diversi dall'RT quale misura temporanea). I criteri per l'RT sono elencati nella Tabella 536-1.

Le cause di ESRD variano con l'età del paziente e includono bambini da molto piccoli a più grandi con una frequenza decrescente, comprendendo: malattie renali congenite (53%), glomerulonefriti (20%), glomerulosclerosi segmentale focale (12%), malattie metaboliche (10%) e cause varie (5%) (Tab. 536-2). Benché le glomerulopatie interessino una proporzione significativa di questa popolazione (in particolare i soggetti fra i 13 e i 17 anni), nei bambini molto piccoli (<5 anni) predominano i processi congeniti e ostruttivi (vedi Capitolo 535.2).

TRATTAMENTO. I bambini con peso compreso tra <15-20 kg vanno sottoposti a un trapianto transperitoneale eseguendo un'incisione lungo la linea mediana; nei soggetti con peso >20 kg il rene viene invece trapiantato in posizione retroperitoneale, nella fossa iliaca destra. I vasi renali vengono anastomizzati ai vasi iliaci del ricevente e l'uretere viene reimpiantato nella vescica (ureteroneocistostomia). Il rene extraperitoneale facilita l'accesso per le future biopsie percutanee. Le valutazioni cliniche del donatore e del ricevente prima dell'RT sono riassunte nella Tabella 536-3. Una età molto giovane del ricevente può costituire un ostacolo all'RT: per i riceventi di trapianti sia LRD sia CAD, un'età inferiore ai 24 mesi è associata a una minore sopravvivenza del trapianto; risultati analoghi sono stati inoltre documentati nei bambini trapiantati con reni piccoli da donatori molto giovani.

Sebbene in generale i trapianti LRD diano esiti migliori di quelli CAD, con il tempo tra questi ultimi è stato osservato un miglioramento significativo (Tab. 536-4). Tuttavia, circa l'80% dei trapianti LRD restano funzionanti dopo 5 anni, mentre questo avviene solo nel 65% dei casi dei CAD-RT.

TABELLA 536-1. Criteri per l'esecuzione di un trapianto renale da donatore vivente o cadavere nei pazienti pediatrici

Insufficienza renale, malattia renale cronica o terminale con qualsiasi eziologia
Età, dipendente dal peso per ricevere un rene adulto
Stato nutrizionale buono
Assenza di
- Infezione attiva
- Ritardo mentale grave
- Tratto urinario ostruito (anse ileali, deviazioni del colon e procedure di aumento della vescica possono essere utili in molti casi)
- Malattia gastrointestinale, epatica, pancreatica o cardiovascolare
- Gravi disturbi psicosociali o comportamentali nonché mancata compliance nei regimi farmacologici e dietetici
- Sensibilizzazione nel ricevente
- Obesità massiva

Da Mauer SM, Nevins TE, Ascher N: Renal transplantation in children. In Edelman CM Jr (editor): *Pediatric Kidney Disease*. Boston, Little, Brown, 1992, pp 941-981.

TABELLA 536-2. Distribuzione degli stati più frequenti che conducono a una malattia renale terminale nei bambini

	N	%
GRUPPO 1		
Congeniti, metabolici, genetici		
Uropatia ostruttiva (PUV)		
Aplasia/displasia/ipoplasia	4113 (insieme)	53,9 (insieme)
Nefropatia da reflusso		
Malattie genetiche e metaboliche (cistinosi, ossalosi, PCKD, nail-patella syndrome, sindrome di Alport, complesso malattia midollare cistica, nefronoftisi)		
GRUPPO 2		
Glomerulonefriti (tutti i processi acuti e cronici immunologicamente mediati)	1015	13,3
GRUPPO 3		
FSGS	873	11,4
GRUPPO 4		
Stati rari		
Tumore di Wilms	43	0,6
Altri processi immunologici	30	0,4
HUS	206	2,7
Nefropatia da IDDM	8	0,1
Nefropatia pielo/interstiziale	146	1,9
Infarto renale	119	1,6
Nefropatia membranosa	36	0,5
GRUPPO 5		
Altro	596	7,8
Sconosciute	466	6,1
Totale	7651	100

FSGS, sclerosi glomerulare segmentale focale (*Focal Segmantal Glomerular Sclerosis*); HUS, sindrome uremico-emolitica; IDDM, diabete mellito dipendente da insulina (*Insulin-Dependent Diabetes Mellitus*); PCKD, malattia del rene policistico (tipo infantile e adulto) (*PolyCystic Kidney Disease*); PUV, valvole uretrali posteriori (*Posterior Urethral Valves*).
Nefriti IgA postinfettive (porpora di Henoch-Schönlein e nefrite di Berger), nefrite da lupus sistemico; tutti i tipi di nefrite membranoproliferativa (tipi I-II e III), sindrome di Goodpasture e varianti (nessun coinvolgimento polmonare), vasculiti (poliarterite nodosa, Wegener).
Modificata da North American Pediatric Renal Transplant Cooperative Study, 2003 Annual Report; sezione 1:1-5.

TABELLA 536-3. Valutazione clinica e di laboratorio del potenziale donatore di rene consanguineo vivente e del ricevente

RICEVENTE
Anamnesi completa ed esame obiettivo: vaccinazioni aggiornate tra cui pneumococco ed epatite B
Seduta di orientamento al trapianto: paziente (se sufficientemente grande), genitori, potenziali donatori, chirurgo che eseguirà il trapianto o suo rappresentante, nefrologo o suo rappresentante, assistente sociale
Dati di laboratorio
- Gruppo sanguigno (ABO)
- Tipizzazione tissutale (HLA-A, B, C, D/DR), MLC
- Pannello epatite, Cytomegalovirus, varicella, virus di Epstein-Barr
- Esame emocromocitometrico, complemento (C3, C4), ANA, derminazione quantitativa Ig
- Creatinina sierica, elettroliti, colesterolo, test di funzionalità epatica, profilo di coagulazione, glicemia
- Analisi delle urine, urinocoltura e colture faringee
- Radiografia del torace (due posizioni), radiografia per l'età ossea (se non disponibile precedentemente)
- Consulto neurologico e analisi EEG e CT del cervello (per i neonati)
- Valutazione odontoiatrica
- Colture: punto di uscita di tutti i cateteri e del liquido peritoneale nei pazienti sottoposti a CAPD
- Valutazione urologica completa dei soggetti con disturbi del tratto urinario ostruttivi o congeniti
- Escrezione di proteine nelle 24 ore

DONATORE
Anamnesi completa ed esame obiettivo
Radiografie del torace
Elettrocardiogramma
Ecografia renale (se necessaria IVP)
Laboratorio
- Esame emocromocitometrico, VES, gruppo sanguigno ABO, HLA e MLC
- Profilo di coagulazione
- Creatinina sierica ed elettroliti, test di funzionalità epatica, glicemia
- Analisi delle urine, urinocoltura, escrezione di proteine e creatinina nelle 24 ore
- Titoli anticorpali per epatite, Cytomegalovirus, herpes, virus di Epstein-Barr

Angiografia renale

CAPD, dialisi peritoneale ambulatoriale continua (*Continuous Ambulatory Peritoneal Dialysis*); EEG, elettroencefalogramma; VES, velocità di eritrosedimentazione; HLA, antigene leucocitario umano; IVP, pielografia endovenosa (*IntraVenous Pyelogram*).
Da Mauer SM, Nevins TE, Ascher N: Renal transplantation in children. In Edelman CM Jr (editor): *Pediatric Kidney Disease*. Boston, Little, Brown, 1992, pp 941-981.

TABELLA 536-4. Sopravvivenza a un anno dopo trapianto renale per tipo di donatore e coorti raggruppate per anni

ANNI	DONATORE VIVENTE (%)	CADAVERE (%)
1987-1990	89,3	75,2
1991-1994	91,8	85,0
1995-1998	93,9	90,3
1999-2002	95,6	91,8

Modificata da North American Pediatric Renal Transplant Cooperative Study, 2003 Annual Report; Graft Function, 5-3.

Circa il 50% degli eventi di mancato attecchimento è dovuto al rigetto, che è acuto nel 14% e cronico nel 33% dei casi. La recidiva della malattia originale si è mantenuta stabile attorno al 6,3% (Tab. 536-5). Un mancato attecchimento correlato a trombosi si verifica in circa l'11% dei pazienti, più spesso nel trapianto renale da cadavere, indipendentemente dall'età del ricevente. In quelli molto giovani, gli episodi trombotici sono correlati agli sbilanci di volume e idrici generati dalle esigenze imposte da organi normalmente grandi. Nei bambini di età più elevata, il mancato attecchimento acuto è spesso determinato da una necrosi tubulare acuta (ATN). I rischi di perdita del trapianto includono un'età del ricevente inferiore a 1 anno, un donatore cadavere di età inferiore ai 6 anni, un RT precedente, un funzionamento del trapianto ritardato (ATN) e una mancanza di terapia con gammaglobuline antilinfocitarie (ATGAM) o con OKT3.

TABELLA 536-5. Frequenza di recidiva delle glomerulopatie negli allotrapianti e perdita del trapianto

GLOMERULOPATIA	% RECIDIVA	% DANNO/PERDITA DEL TRAPIANTO
FSGS (con NS)	20-40	25
IgA	50	510
HSP	30-80	10
MN	20	5-10
MPGN I	25	5-10
MPGN II	90	20
HUS	10-50	10-50
WG	5-20	5-20
AGBM	<10 (rara nei bambini)	<1 (incerto)
SLEGN	5-10	<5
HYPEROX	Alta	Perdite elevate
Cistinosi	Il trapianto gestisce il carico di cistina	Perdita per rigetto
IGN (MPGN de novo)	Incerta	Incerta

AGBM, nefrite della membrana basale antiglomerulare (*Anti-Glomerular Basement Membrane*); FSGS, glomerulosclerosi segmentale focale; HSP, porpora di Henoch-Schönlein (*Henoch-Schönlein Purpura*); HUS, sindrome uremico-emolitica; HYPEROX, iperossalosi/ossaluria; IgA, nefrite da immunoglobuline A; IGN, glomerulonefrite idiopatica (*Idiopatic GlomeruloNephritis*); MN, nefropatia membranosa (*Membranous Nephropathy*); MPGN I e II, glomerulonefrite membranoproliferativa tipo I e tipo II; SLEGN, glomerulonefrite da lupus eritematoso sistemico (*Systemic Lupus Erythematosus GlomeruloNephritis*); WG, granulomatosi di Wegener (*Wegener Granulomatosis*).
Modificata da Denton MC, Singh AK: Recurrent and de novo glomerulonephritis in the renal allograft. *Semin Nephrol* 2000; 20:164-75; e Mauer SM, Nevins TE, Ascher N: Renal transplantation in children. In Edelman CM Jr (editor): *Pediatric Kidney Disease*. Boston, Little Brown, 1992, pp 941-981.

ISTOCOMPATIBILITÀ. I geni del complesso d'istocompatibilità maggiore (MHC, *Major Histocompatibility Complex*), presenti sul braccio corto del cromosoma 6, codificano per gli antigeni leucocitari umani (HLA; *Human Leukocyte Antigen*) (Fig. 536-1). Questi sono costituiti da proteine di classe I (antigeni tissutali al trapianto) e da immunotossicità cellulo-mediata; da proteine di classe II che controllano l'induzione della risposta immunitaria e da proteine di classe III che includono il fattore di necrosi tumorale e i componenti del complemento (C2 e C4). Ogni cromosoma 6 contiene tutte e 3 le classi di proteine: HLA-A, B e C per la classe I; HLA-DP, DQ e DR per la II e C2, C4 e fattore di necrosi tumorale per la III. Per ogni proteina esistono alleli multipli e codominanti (polimorfismo), mentre A, B e DR sono considerati i più importanti nel trapianto clinico. Gli aplotipi, ossia l'area del cromosoma

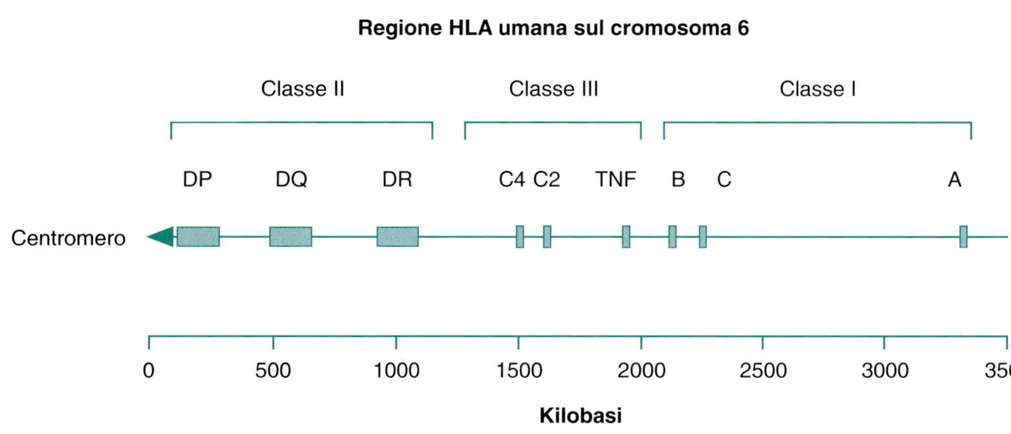

Figura 536-1. Organizzazione della regione HLA (antigene leucocitario umano) del cromosoma 6. I loci per HLA-A, B e C si trovano nella regione di classe I. Quelli che codificano per HLA-DR, DQ e DP si trovano nella regione di classe II, centromera rispetto alla classe I. Tra le classi I e II vi sono i cosiddetti geni di classe III, che codificano per alcune delle proteine del complemento, nonché per alcune citochine. (Da Grimm PC, Laufer J, Ettenger RB: The immunobiology of renal transplantation. In Edelman CM Jr (editor): *Pediatric Kidney Disease*. Boston, Little, Brown, 1992.)

6 su cui risiedono i geni HLA, vengono ereditati in gruppo, per cui ogni individuo riceve da ciascun genitore simultaneamente un aplotipo, che in questo modo determina il profilo HLA della prole. Il donatore genitore e il ricevente figlio condividono il 50% di tutti gli aplotipi, per cui il bambino avrà un antigene rappresentante dei loci di classe I, II e III di ciascun genitore; tra i gemelli, invece, è possibile che vi sia una condivisione di tutti, alcuni o nessun aplotipo (corrispondenza di 2 aplotipi, 1 aplotipo o 0 aplotipi). Un bambino ha la corrispondenza di 1 aplotipo con ciascun genitore e l'ereditarietà degli aplotipi segue modelli mendeliani codominanti (Fig. 536-2). Nella coppia donatore/ricevente geneticamente affine, la probabilità di una buona corrispondenza negli HLA aumenta e il mancato attecchimento del trapianto dovuto a una reazione di rigetto (RR) diminuisce.

REAZIONE DI RIGETTO. Nella RR acuta e cronica, entrambi i meccanismi, cellulari e umorali, danneggiano il trapianto. Gli anticorpi preformati o indotti dalle cellule T mediano una RR accelerata (iperacuta), uno stato osservato raramente al giorno d'oggi (Fig. 536-3).

La RR si manifesta con un'ipersensibilità dolorifica e una tumefazione dell'organo trapiantato, febbre, oliguria, ipertensione e aumento progressivo del livello di creatinina. L'ecografia renale può rivelare un organo ingrossato con un'iperecogenicità corticale e una scansione renale dimostra un ridotto flusso sanguigno. Il materiale bioptico prelevato dal trapianto indica i segni di rigetto con glomeruli relativamente intatti, una patologia ultrastrutturale lieve e un'immunofluorescenza glomerulare negativa. La differenziazione tra RR, necrosi tubulare acuta, tossicità da ciclosporina o da altri farmaci e ricomparsa della malattia renale originale nel trapianto richiede una biopsia renale. Dato che la corrispondenza incrociata pretrapianto rileva anticorpi anti-HLA preesistenti, la RR iperacuta è un evento molto raro. In questo stato, gli anticorpi anti-HLA si legano all'endotelio, causando una coagulazione intravascolare con la conseguente necrosi capillare glomerulare e peritubulare. Per converso, la RR cronica ispessisce e ostruisce le arteriole del trapianto, che evidenziano depositi di immunoglobuline parietali mentre i glomeruli subiscono la ialinizzazione. Nel contempo l'interstizio si riempie di cellule mononucleari attivate, alcune delle quali possono essere individuate nelle urine.

Il test di istocompatibilità è di fondamentale importanza per prolungare la sopravvivenza di trapianti renali LRD e CAD. La presenza di HLA-A, B, C e D/DR identici a quelli di un donatore fratello con MCH non stimolante offre i risultati migliori di sopravvivenza del trapianto. La seconda opzione più vantaggiosa è il donatore fratello o genitore che abbia almeno una corrispondenza di 1 aplotipo.

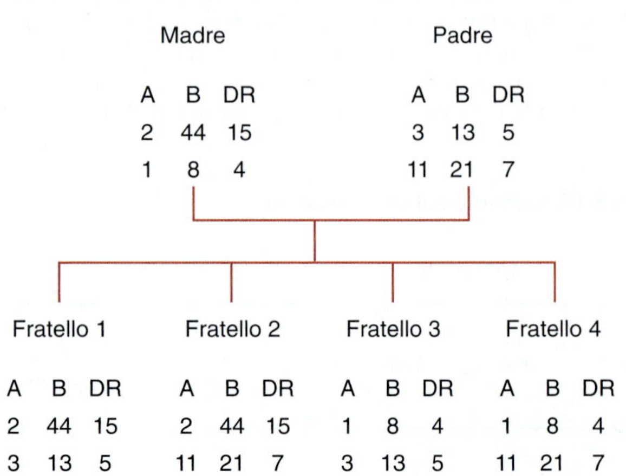

Figura 536-2. Ereditarietà degli aplotipi e profilo HLA in quattro fratelli teorici. Il fratello 1 ha una corrispondenza di 1 aplotipo con i fratelli 2 e 3 e una corrispondenza di 0 aplotipi con il fratello 4. (Da Terasaki PI, Park MA, Danovitch GM: Histocompatibility testing, crossmatching and allocation of cadaveric kidney transplants. In Danovitch GM (editor): *Handbook of Kidney Transplantation*. Boston, Little, Brown, 1992.)

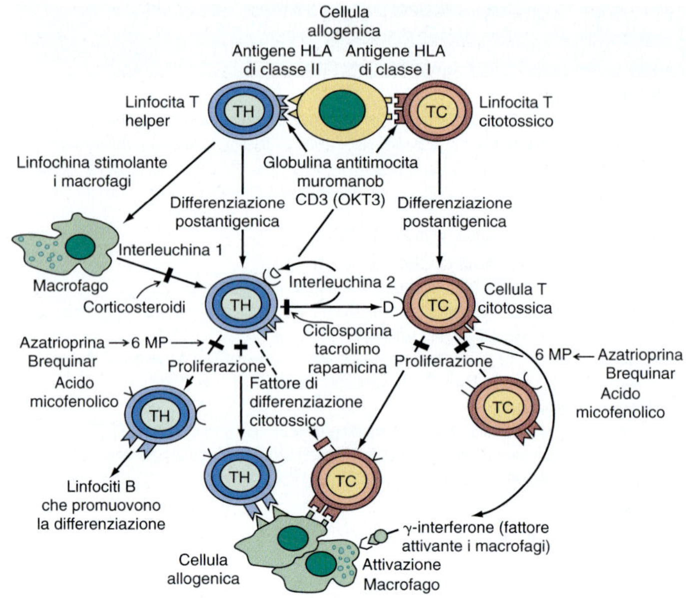

Figura 536-3. Rappresentazione di un rigetto di allotrapianto e siti di azione proposti per i farmaci immunosoppressori. (Da Shaefer MA, Collier DS: Immunosuppression for solid organ transplantation. *Dial Transplant* 1993;22:542.)

PRINCIPI DI IMMUNOSOPPRESSIONE E TERAPIA DELLA REAZIONE DI RIGETTO. La stimolazione del sistema immunitario da parte di una proteina estranea (trapianto renale) causa l'attivazione dell'infiammazione immunitaria cellulo-mediata e umorale-mediata con la distruzione delle cellule o l'RR (vedi Fig. 536-3; vedi anche Capitolo 135). Per reprimere o controllare questo processo, sono necessari farmaci immunosoppressori che evitino la perdita del trapianto. Gli immunosoppressori utilizzati clinicamente al momento e quelli sottoposti a trial clinici sono elencati nella Tabella 536-6 e nella Figura 536-3. L'immunosoppressione sequenziale con azatioprina, ciclosporina e corticosteroidi a basse dosi ha rappresentato il protocollo antirigetto utilizzato con maggiore frequenza. Tuttavia, sono stati concepiti nuovi protocolli con il risparmio dei corticosteroidi e dell'inibitore della calcineurina, con l'obiettivo di evitare il deficit della crescita e gli altri effetti negativi del prednisone, nonché la nefrotossicità della ciclosporina A (ipertensione, danno renale, aumento della creatinina sierica). Una RR acuta si è verificata nel 52,5% di tutti gli 8398 pazienti che hanno partecipato allo studio NAPRTCS, mentre non è stata documentata in 4004 (47,8%) casi di RT. La RR acuta è reversibile in oltre il 60% dei casi, mentre solo il 30% può essere invertito quando si sono verificate 4 o più crisi. Al contrario, la RR cronica è inesorabile e non risponde alla terapia; dato allora che quella immunosoppressiva rende il paziente più sensibile alle infezioni, i bambini interessati corrono un elevato rischio di perdita del trapianto, di decesso o di entrambi.

COMPLICANZE (TAB. 536-7). L'infezione è la causa più comune di morte durante il primo anno dopo un RT. Le infezioni causate da virus di Epstein-Barr (EBV, *Epstein-Barr Virus*) e Cytomegalovirus (CMV) sono particolarmente frequenti; i titoli anticorpali a entrambi vengono verificati di routine nel donatore e nel ricevente. Il CMV può essere primitivo, trasmesso dal trapianto o da trasfusioni di sangue, oppure può essere riattivato entro 1-3 mesi dai farmaci immunosoppressori in un paziente sieropositivo (Tab. 536-8). L'85-90% dei casi può essere asintomatico e autolimitarsi ma il 5-10% conduce a morte; il CMV causa un danno tissutale diretto e può scatenare una RR e una perdita del trapianto. Dosi minori di immunosoppressori, una terapia ev con ganciclovir e infusioni di immunoglobuline anti-CMV possono controllare l'infezione. Inoltre, la somministrazione

TABELLA 536-6. Sostanze immunosoppressive utilizzate con la massima frequenza nel trapianto renale pediatrico

FARMACO	MECCANISMI D'AZIONE	DOSAGGIO	TOSSICITÀ
GLUCOCORTICOIDI			
(prednisone e derivati)	Reazione antinfiammatoria di blocco immunitario: TNF-alfa e deplezione di IL-2/IL-6; deplezione anche delle cellule T (arresta il ciclo riproduttivo cellulare): riduce l'immunità cellulare	1-2 mg/kg/24 h (o 60 mg/m²/24 h) per os o ev possono equivalere a 30 mg/kg quando somministrati sotto forma di bolo ev di emergenza	Sbilancio elettrolitico, crescita stentata, IDDM, ipertensione arteriosa, cataratta, pancreatite
FARMACI A MICROMOLECOLE			
Ciclosporina A* e derivati ISA (TX) 247	Leganti immunofillina/ciclofillina; inibiscono la fosfatasi calcineurina	4-6 mg/kg/24 h	Irsutismo, ipertensione, arteriolite, RTID, danno al SNC, insufficienza renale acuta
TK506 (tacrolimus)	Leganti immunofillina/ciclofillina; inibiscono la fosfatasi calcineurina (antibiotico macrolide)	0,15-0,2 mg/kg/24 h	Insufficienza renale
Mofetil micofenolato*	Blocca la sintesi delle purine; arresta l'attivazione delle cellule T e B; altera la glicosilazione della membrana cellulare	1-3 g/24 h (o 600 mg/m²; max 2 g/24 h)	Insufficienza renale acuta post-trapianto IDDM; HTN; gastrite, diarrea, PTLD
Azatioprina	Antimetabolita, blocca la sintesi delle proteine (6-tioguanina incorporata nel DNA quale base fraudolenta)	2-3 mg/kg/24 h per os, da solo; combinato: 1-2 mg/kg/24 h	Soppressione midollo osseo, danno epatico, PTLD
Bersaglio degli inibitori della rapamicina: sirolimo* ed everolimo	Blocca la proliferazione e la maturazione delle cellule guidata dalle citochine	7,5 mg/m²/5 giorni; 5 mg/m² quando combinati	Trombocitopenia, iperlipidemia
FARMACI PROTEICI			
Deplezione degli anticorpi contro le cellule B e T o entrambe: Ig equine e di coniglio	Lega i recettori opsonizzanti sulla superficie cellulare, inibendo fagocitosi e lisi mediata dal complemento	Atgam: 1,5 mg/kg/24 h, solo ev centrale con filtro per 4-6 h; timoglobuline: ev periferica o centrale per 6 h, 1,5 mg/kg; entrambi 14-21 giorni	Conta linfociti T periferici profondi (<150-<50/mm³), brividi, febbre, artralgie, trombocitopenia, leucopenia generale, CMVI, PTLD e altri tumori
Anticorpi monoclonali murini anti-CD3 (muromonab CD3 o OKT3 ortoclone)	Lega i recettori opsonizzanti sulla superficie cellulare, inibendo fagocitosi e lisi mediata dal complemento	Solo ev; <30 kg, 2,5 mg/24 h; >30 kg, 5 mg; in bolo quotidianamente per 10-14 giorni (per ridurre la conta cellulare CD3 a < 25/mm³)	Conta linfociti T periferici profondi (<150-<50/mm³), brividi, febbre, artralgie, trombocitopenia, leucopenia generale, CMVI, PTLD e altri tumori
Nessuna deplezione anticorpi e proteine di fusione: anti-CD25 monoclonale umanizzato/chimerico Anticorpi: daclizumab, basiliximab	Anticorpo monoclonale al recettore IL-2 previene l'attivazione cellulare; nessuna sindrome da rilascio di citochine; nessun anticorpo neutralizzante	Dose 1: 1 mg/kg ev periferica/centrale, per 15 min, 24 h prima del trapianto; uguale 4 dose rimanenti a intervalli di 14 giorni; <35 kg, 2 dosi di 10 mg ciascuno, 1ª dose 2 h prima del trapianto; 2ª dose 4 giorni dopo; >35 kg, 2 dosi di 20 mg ciascuna, come sopra	Dolore addominale, diarrea, arti inferiori, edema, tremore, vertigine, IDDM, scarsa guarigione delle ferite, rash, prurito, irsutismo, visione sfocata, iperkaliemia, dispnea, ipertensione, aritmie, artralgie, neuropatie, parestesie, proteinuria

*Necessarie attente misurazioni del livello ematico per regolare la dose. Sono disponibili molti altri farmaci immunosoppressori, che tuttavia non sono ancora comunemente utilizzati in pediatria oppure al momento sono sottoposti a trial clinici: FK778, mizoribina, leflunomide, FTY720, alemtuzumab e rituximab (anticorpi monoclonali rispettivamente alle cellule CD52 e CD20) e proteine di infusione con proprietà di legame naturali: CTLA-4-Ig (LEA29).
CMV, Cytomegalovirus; SNC, sistema nervoso centrale; HTN, nefropatia ipertensiva (*HyperTensive Nephropathy*); IDDM, diabete mellito dipendente da insulina; IL, interleuchina; PTLD, malattia linfoproliferativa post-transpianto; RTID, malattia tubulo-interstiziale renale (*Renal Tubular-Interstitial Disease*); TNF, fattore di necrosi tumorale.

TABELLA 536-7. Complicanze post-trapianto nei pazienti pediatrici

Necrosi tubulare acuta
Reazione di rigetto
Tecniche: vascolari, urologiche
Recidiva della malattia renale originale
Tossicità farmacologica (immunosoppressori, antibiotici)
Infezione (particolarmente virale, sistemica); infezione di ferite o del tratto urinario
Emorragia
Pancreatite
Linfocele
Urinoma
Ostruzione intestinale

Da Mauer SM, Nevins TE, Ascher N: Renal transplantation in children. In Edelman CM Jr (editor): *Pediatric Kidney Disease*. Boston, Little, Brown, 1992, pp 941-981.

continuativa del ganciclovir per 3-5 mesi viene adottata di routine dopo il trapianto presso la maggior parte dei centri. In molti centri americani vengono utilizzate biopsie percutanee del trapianto secondo protocollo, insieme a dati clinici per diagnosticare infezioni e una RR precoce. L'assunzione di immunosoppressori va interrotta nel caso di un CMV con coinvolgimento sistemico, multiorgano (polmone, fegato, cervello oltre al rene) e la perdita del rene se la RR non risponde. Altre infezioni virali, il poliovirus BK (BKV), il virus della varicella-zoster, l'herpes simplex e l'epatite sono associati alla nefropatia del trapianto. Nei bambini l'acquisizione del BKV è con ogni probabilità una infezione primaria, in contrasto con l'attivazione del virus latente nei tubuli renali. Questa infezione può manifestarsi con febbre lieve, mialgie e gastroenterite, prima della disfunzione dell'allotrapianto. Il BKV può anche presentarsi con una forte RR acuta oppure con sindromi simili alla nefrite interstiziale e all'uropatia ostruttiva, con perdite del trapianto che variano dal 45 all'80%. La terapia dell'infezione da BKV segue gli stessi principi adottati per l'EBV e per il CMV: riduzione o interruzione degli immunosoppressori, possibilità di proseguire con gli steroidi e terapia antivirale (ganciclovir, cidofovir, leflunomide, immunoglobuline ev).

L'infezione da *Pneumocystis carinii* è meno comune, se viene somministrato il trimetoprim-sulfametoxazolo a scopo preventivo. Nel 2003, il North American Pediatric Renal Transplant Cooperative Study (NAPRTCS) ha riferito il decesso documentato di 463 pazienti su un totale di 7651 LRD-RT e CAD-RT (6,1%). Di questi decessi, 141 (30,5%) sono stati causati da una infezione, mentre il 30% è avvenuto in seguito a una malattia virale. La sopravvivenza a 5 anni dopo il trapianto per l'LRD è del 95,9%, mentre per il CAD è del 95,5%.

TABELLA 536-8. Tipi di Cytomegalovirus nel ricevente di trapianto renale pediatrico

TIPO DI INFEZIONE	TIPO DI PAZIENTE	SINTOMATICA	PREVENZIONE
Primaria	Sieronegativo con rene sieropositivo, trasfusione di leucociti, trasfusione di prodotti ematici	60%	Evitare l'infezione da CMV o impiegare una vaccinazione attiva (vaccino vivo attenuato: ceppo Towne; non molto efficace)
Riattivazione	Sieropositivo prima del trapianto	<20%	Elevato titolo di globulina anti-CMV iperimmune umana (CytoGam)
Superinfezione	Paziente sieropositivo trapiantato con rene CMV	40%	Concentrati di IgG umane (Gammagard o Polygam aspecifici per CMV)

CMV, Cytomegalovirus.
Da Snydman DR: Prevention of cytomegalovirus-associated diseases with immunoglobulin. *Transplant Proc*. 1991; 23:131.

TUMORI MALIGNI. Benché l'immunosoppressione resti un requisito essenziale per il trapianto, può tuttavia causare un aumento della replicazione dell'EBV, con una conseguente malattia linfoproliferativa post-trapianto (PTLD, *Post-Transplantation Lymphoproliferative Disorder*) aggressiva e potenzialmente letale nell'1-2% degli RT. Nel 2003 il NAPRTCS ha riferito 203 tumori maligni su 7898 RT (2,6%, con i trapianti che funzionavano per un periodo pari o superiore ai 30 giorni). Di questi 203 tumori maligni, 150 erano PTLD (73%), con un tempo medio intercorrente tra il trapianto e la formazione maligna (con diagnosi confermata) di 14 mesi (intervallo 1-20 mesi). La PTLD, che è uno stato premaligno e maligno raro, costituisce ancora, tuttavia, una causa grave di morbilità e mortalità nei bambini dopo il 1° anno successivo al trapianto. Questa malattia deve essere diagnosticata il più presto possibile in un trapiantato febbrile con linfoadenopatia, manifestazioni gastrointestinali (massa addominale, emorragia, dolore, ostruzione, perforazione, ascite), crisi convulsive o altre anomalie del sistema nervoso centrale e masse toraciche e/o mediastiniche asintomatiche. La diagnosi definitiva di PTLD, come malattia causata da EBV-CMV, deve essere formulata sulla base di un campionamento tissutale e con altri mezzi di laboratorio. Le conseguenze cliniche della crescita del virus di Epstein-Barr e gli elevati rischi di sviluppare una PTLD nel paziente immunosoppresso sono elencati nella Tabella 536-9. I pazienti con una PTLD con trapianto eseguito meno di 1 anno prima hanno una prognosi più favorevole e possono regredire semplicemente riducendo il farmaco immunosoppressore. L'adozione, nei casi più gravi, di una terapia antitumorale completa (ciclofosfamide, doxorubicina, vincristina e prednisone) non ha evidenziato una nefrotossicità e un'evidenza di RR in un numero significativo di pazienti mentre questi erano sottoposti a una terapia immunosoppressiva ridotta o non ne seguivano alcuna (immunosoppressiva) specifica.

TRAPIANTO RENALE NEI PAZIENTI HIV POSITIVI. Con lo sviluppo di una terapia antiretrovirale efficace, la prognosi del bambino HIV positivo è migliorata così tanto da poter considerare, in questi casi, l'RT su base individuale. Le condizioni per eseguire un RT o un ritrapianto nei pazienti HIV positivi richiedono che il candidato non presenti infezioni opportunistiche da 2 anni e stia seguendo un regime anti-HIV/*Pneumocystis* stabile e ben tollerato. Sono fondamentali una buona compliance, una carica virale non rilevabile (mediante reazione a catena della polimerasi), una conta dei linfociti CD4 accettabile e l'assenza di malattie complicanti.

RECIDIVA DI MALATTIA GLOMERULARE NEL TRAPIANTO. Praticamente tutte le glomerulopatie possono risvilupparsi nel trapianto e il 5-10% di tutti i trapianti viene perso attraverso questo meccanismo. Di queste, la glomerulopatia membranoproliferativa di tipo II e la glomerulosclerosi segmentale sono alcune tra le più frequenti e più difficili da trattare (vedi Tabb. 536-5 e 536-10).

La sindrome uremico-emolitica (HUS, *Hemolytic-Uremic Syndrome*) postinfettiva non recidiva; tuttavia, varietà geneticamente trasmesse non diarroiche possono svilupparsi *de novo* nell'1-3% dei casi. Inoltre, la HUS può manifestarsi in associazione alla terapia con inibitori della calcineurina (ciclosporina e altri), benché questo accada più frequentemente nel trapianto di midollo osseo che non nei trapianti di rene. Tra gli indicatori importanti dello sviluppo di una HUS non correlata a un'infezione nel trapianto renale vi sono una malattia familiare (autosomica recessiva o dominante), un trapianto eseguito prima di un periodo di 6-12 mesi dalla completa remissione della malattia primaria e l'uso di elevate dosi di ciclosporina. Nei casi familiari di LRD-RT, la terapia con contraccettivi orali e l'impiego di ATGAM e OKT3 sono controversi e forse non dovrebbero essere raccomandati nelle forme genetiche di HUS. Il trapianto combinato di fegato e rene può essere un approccio più appropriato nei soggetti con la HUS familiare (vedi Capitolo 518).

CRESCITA E TRAPIANTO RENALE. Una crescita stentata o una malnutrizione franca sono eventi frequenti nei pazienti con l'ESRD, nonostante la dialisi (vedi Capitolo 535). Una terapia di supporto (dialisi e farmaci appropriati) migliora la capacità di resistenza e induce un senso di benessere. Un trapianto renale riuscito corregge le anomalie e riabilita i pazienti.

TABELLA 536-9. Conseguenze dello sviluppo di EBV e fattori ad alto rischio per lo sviluppo di PTLD nei pazienti immunosoppressi

SINDROMI CLINICHE
Mononucleosi
Meningoencefalite
Leucoplachia capelluta o orale
Tumori costituiti da cellule muscolari lisce
Linfomi a cellule T
Malattia linfoproliferativa post-trapianto (PTLD, proliferazione incontrollata di cellule B infettate da EBV e trasformate, secondo una modalità policlonale, oligoclonale e monoclonale)
Linfoma non-Hodgkin
ALTO RISCHIO DI PTLD
Elevata carica di EBV
Infezione da EBV primaria
Immunosoppressione ad alte dosi (ciclosporina A, tacrolimus, anticorpi antilinfocitari e boli di steroidi da soli o in combinazione)
La terapia cardiaca è comunemente interessata

EBV, virus di Epstein-Barr.

TABELLA 536-10. FSGS: Caratteristiche cliniche ed effetti sull'allotrapianto

EFFETTI SUL RENE NATIVO	EFFETTI SULL'ALLOTRAPIANTO	FORME DI TERAPIA
FSGS progressiva grave e ipercellularità; clinicamente, sindrome nefrotica, insufficienza renale cronica con progressione a ESRD nel 60% dei casi	Recidiva istologica di FSGS nel trapianto 20-40%; sindrome nefrosica recidivante, cronica, ESRD in 25%	Evitare donatore consanguineo vivente e alte dosi di ciclosporina A; per terapia impiegare scambio plasmaferesi e immunoassorbimento, ciclofosfamide e OKT3; eseguire nefrectomia bilaterale pretrapianto; le forme di terapia sembrano puramente palliative
Necessari dialisi e trapianto	Favoriscono recidiva: <6 anni, insufficienza renale rapidamente progressiva, ipercellularità glomerulare, precedente recidiva, donatore consanguineo vivente con corrispondenza stretta, distribuzione familiare di FSGS, presenza di livelli alti dimostrabili di fattore di permeabilità nel sangue del ricevente	

ESRD, malattia renale terminale; FSGS, glomerulosclerosi segmentale focale.

Nella maggior parte dei bambini di età inferiore ai 5 anni in attesa del loro RT indice o in quelli con oltre 1 RT, il ritardo di crescita raggiunge rispettivamente −2,8 e −3,2 SD. Un'accelerazione della crescita dopo un trapianto renale con una durata di 6-12 mesi viene osservata nei bambini più piccoli; negli adolescenti, la terapia con l'ormone della crescita (*rh*GH) induce uno sviluppo puberale approssimativamente uguale a quello dei bambini non trattati. L'altezza finale dei bambini trattati con *rh*GH è significativamente aumentata.

L'uso quotidiano di corticosteroidi è generalmente la norma nei protocolli di trattamento per l'RT. La terapia quotidiana con prednisone ritarda la crescita, anche se lo steroide viene assunto a dosaggi relativamente bassi; pertanto, è necessario ridurre al minimo questo effetto sfavorevole molto frequente. Una terapia con prednisone a giorni alterni può ottimizzare il potenziale di crescita. La completa astensione dagli steroidi tenta di ridurre significativamente o di eliminarli, ma può aumentare il rischio di RR. Un uso giudizioso dell'ormone della crescita *rh*GH prima e dopo il trapianto del rene, unitamente a una terapia con steroidi a giorni alterni o priva di steroidi ma con somministrazione di immunosoppressori (daclizumab, tacrolimus, micofenolato), può offrire un vantaggio significativo ai bambini che necessitano di un RT.

Abouna GM: The use of marginal-suboptimal donor organs: A practical solution for organ shortage. *Adv Transpl* 2004;9:62–66.

Acott PD, Pernica JM: Growth hormone therapy before and after pediatric renal transplant. *Pediatr Transplant* 2003;7:426–440.

Ahsan N: Induction immunotherapy with IL-2Ra monoclonal antibody in kidney transplantation. *Min Urol Nefrol* 2003;55:67–79.

Benfield MR: Current status of kidney transplant: Update 2003. *Pediatr Clin North Am* 2003;50:1301–1334.

Bennett WM, Vella JP: Transplantation. In Glassock RJ (editor): Nephrology Self Assessment Program (Neph sap) 2005;4:1–63.

Charpenter B: Tacrolimus in renal transplantation: A review of recent data. *Min Urol Nefrol* 2003;55:25–32.

Dharnidharka V, Sullivan EK, Stablein DM, et al: Risk factors for post-transplant lymphoproliferative disorder (PTLD) in pediatric kidney transplantation: A report of the North American Pediatric Transplant Cooperative Study (NAPRTCS). *Transplantation* 2001;71:1065–1068.

Doyle AM, Lechler RI, Turka LA: Organ transplantation: Halfway through the first century. *J Am Soc Nephrol* 2004;15:2965–2971.

El Sayegh S, Keller MJ, Shrish H, et al: Solid organ transplantation in HIV-infected recipients. *Pediatr Transplant* 2004;8:214–221.

Fine RN, Alonso EM, Fischel JE, et al: Pediatric transplantation of the kidney, liver, and heart: Summary report. *Pediatr Transplant* 2004;8:75–86.

Halloran PF: Immunosuppressive drugs for kidney transplantation. *N Engl J Med* 2004;351:2715–2729.

Kaplan B, Herwic-Ulf MK: Renal transplantation: A half century of success and the long road ahead. *J Am Soc Nephrol* 2004;15:3270–3271.

Quist E, Jalanko H, Holmberg C: Psychosocial adaptation after solid organ transplantation in children. *Pediatr Clin North Am* 2003;50:1505–1519.

Ramos EL, Drachenberg CB: BK virus: Life cycle and interactions with host cells. *Transplant Immunol Lett* 2004;20:4–13.

Samsonov D, Briscoe DM: Long-term care of pediatric renal transplant patients: From bench to beside. *Curr Opin Pediatr* 2002;14:205–210.

Sarwal MM, Yorgin PD, Alexander S, et al: Promising early outcomes with a novel complete steroid avoidance immunosuppression protocol in pediatric renal transplantation. *Transplantation* 2001;72:13–21.

Seikali MG: Recurrence of primary disease on children after renal transplantation: An evidence based update. *Pediatr Transplant* 2004;8:113–119.

Swiatecka-Urban A: Anti-interleukin-2 receptor antibodies for prevention of rejection in pediatric renal transplant patients. Current status. *Pediatr Drugs* 2003;5:699–716.

Tsuzuki K: Role of mizoribine in renal transplantation. *Pediatr Int* 2002; 44:224–231.

United States Renal Data System: *Atlas of End Stage Renal Disease in the United States. 16th Annual Report 2004. Pediatric ESRD.* Bethesda, MD, National Institutes of Health-National Institute of Diabetes & Digestive & Kidney Diseases—Division of Kidney, Urologic & Hematologic Diseases, 2004, pp 154–166.

Vats A, Randhawa PS, Shapiro R: BK virus-associated transplant nephropathy: Diagnosis and treatment. *Transplant Immunol Lett* 2004;20:5–12.

Vitko S, Margreiter R, Weimar W, et al: Everolimus (certican) 12 month safety and efficacy versus mycophenolate mofetil in de novo renal transplant recipients. *Transplantation* 2004;78:1532–1540.

Weber LT, Hocker B, Mehl O, et al: Mycophenolate mofetil in pediatric renal transplantation. *Min Urol Nefrol* 2003;55:91–99.

Parte XXIII ■ Disordini urologici della prima e seconda infanzia

Capitolo 537 ■ Anomalie congenite e disgenesia del rene Jack S. Elder

SVILUPPO EMBRIONALE

Il rene deriva dal bottone ureterale e dal blastema metanefrico. Durante la 5ª settimana di gestazione, il dotto mesonefrico (di Wolff) dà origine al bottone ureterale che penetra nel blastema metanefrico, un'area di mesenchima indifferenziato sulla cresta nefrogenica. Il bottone ureterale va incontro a una serie di circa 15 generazioni di divisioni e dalla 20ª settimana di gestazione forma l'intero sistema collettore: uretere, pelvi renale, calici, dotti papillari e tubuli collettori. Segnali provenienti dalle cellule mesenchimali inducono la formazione dei bottoni ureterali dal dotto di Wolff come anche la ramificazione dei bottoni ureterali. Segnali reciproci provenienti dal bottone ureterico e, in seguito, dalle estremità delle sue ramificazioni inducono la condensazione e la proliferazione delle cellule mesenchimali, quindi la loro trasformazione in cellule epiteliali. Sotto l'influenza induttiva del bottone ureterale, la differenziazione del nefrone ha inizio nel corso della 7ª settimana di gestazione. A partire dalla 20ª settimana, quando il sistema collettore si è sviluppato, è presente circa il 30% dei nefroni. La nefrogenesi continua a velocità pressoché esponenziale ed è completa dalla 36ª settimana di gestazione. Attualmente, sono stati identificati almeno 16 agenti di segnalazione che regolano lo sviluppo renale. Un deficit di una qualsiasi delle attività di segnale potrebbe causare la mancata formazione del rene (**agenesia renale**), una differenziazione anormale (**disgenesia renale**) o lo sviluppo di **cisti**.

Il rene fetale ha un ruolo minore nel bilancio dei sali e nell'omeostasi idrica fetale. La velocità di produzione di urina aumenta nel corso della gestazione e, a termine, sono stati riportati volumi di 25 mL/min/1,73 m^2 a termine e di 3 volte superiori a 3 mesi di vita. L'aumento della velocità di filtrazione glomerulare è provocato da una riduzione della resistenza vascolare intrarenale e della ridistribuzione del flusso ematico intrarenale alla corticale, dove si trova un maggior numero di nefroni.

Le disgenesie renali comprendono aplasia, displasia, ipoplasia e malattia cistica.

AGENESIA RENALE. L'*agenesia renale*, o assenza di sviluppo renale, si può verificare secondariamente a un difetto del dotto di Wolff, del bottone ureterale o del blastema metanefrico. L'agenesia renale unilaterale ha un'incidenza di 1/450-1000 nati vivi. L'agenesia renale unilaterale viene spesso diagnosticata nel corso della valutazione per altre anomalie congenite (vedi Sindrome VATER, Capitolo 108) e la sua incidenza è aumentata nei neonati con arteria ombelicale unica. Nell'agenesia vera, l'uretere e l'emitrigono vescicale ipsilaterale sono assenti. Il rene controlaterale va incontro a ipertrofia compensatoria, in qualche misura già a livello prenatale ma soprattutto dopo la nascita e circa il 15% di questi bambini presenta un reflusso vescicoureterale controlaterale. La maggior parte dei maschi presenta un'assenza del vas deferens ipsilaterale a causa dell'assenza del dotto di Wolff, mentre, dal momento che il dotto di Wolff e quello di Müller sono contigui, nelle femmine sono comuni anche le anomalie del dotto di Müller. La **sindrome di Mayer-Rokitansky-Kuster-Hauser** si riferisce a un gruppo di anomalie associate che comprendono agenesia o ectopia renale unilaterale, difetti unilaterali del dotto di Müller e agenesia vaginale.

L'agenesia renale è distinta dall'aplasia in cui si osserva un nubbin di tessuto non funzionale che incappuccia un uretere, il quale può essere normale o anomalo. Clinicamente, tale distinzione può essere difficile. In alcuni soggetti la diagnosi di agenesia renale unilaterale viene posta in base al riscontro dell'assenza di un rene all'ecografia o all'urografia escretoria. Tuttavia, alcuni di questi pazienti avevano in realtà un rene ipoplasico o un rene displasico multicistico alla nascita che successivamente è andato incontro a regressione completa. Anche se la diagnosi specifica non è critica e il riscontro dell'assenza di un rene si basa sull'ecografia, è necessario uno studio di imaging funzionale come un'urografia escretoria o una scintigrafia renale, in quanto alcuni di questi pazienti potrebbero avere un rene ectopico. Se è presente un rene normale controlaterale, la funzione renale dovrebbe rimanere normale nel tempo.

L'**agenesia renale bilaterale** è incompatibile con la vita extrauterina ed è denominata **sindrome di Potter**. La morte si verifica poco dopo la nascita per ipoplasia polmonare. Il neonato ha una facies caratteristica, denominata *facies di Potter* (Fig. 537-1). Gli occhi sono ampiamente spaziati e presentano epicanto, l'impianto delle orecchie è basso, il naso è largo e piatto, il mento è sfuggente e sono presenti anomalie degli arti. Occorre sospettare un'agenesia renale bilaterale quando l'ecografia materna

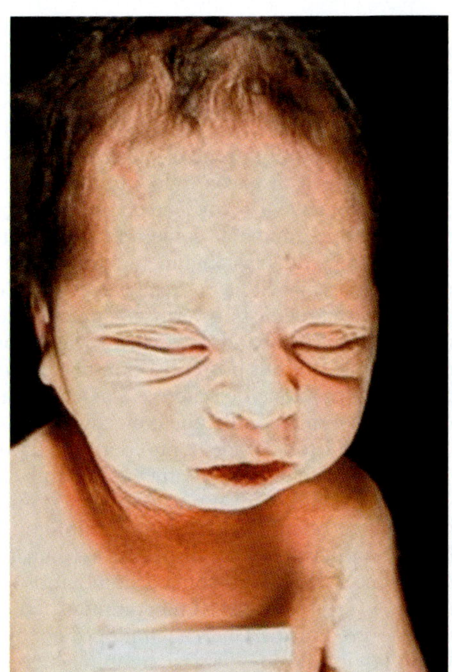

Figura 537-1. Bambino nato morto con agenesia renale che mostra la caratteristica facies di Potter.

dimostra **oligoidramnios**, mancata visualizzazione della vescica e assenza dei reni. L'incidenza di questa sindrome è di 1/3000 nati vivi, con predominanza maschile, e rappresenta il 20% dei neonati con fenotipo di Potter. Altre cause comuni di insufficienza renale neonatale associata a fenotipo di Potter comprendono la displasia renale cistica e l'uropatia ostruttiva. Cause meno comuni sono la nefropatia policistica autosomico-recessiva (infantile), l'ipoplasia renale e la displasia midollare. I neonati con agenesia renale bilaterale muoiono per insufficienza polmonare da ipoplasia polmonare piuttosto che per insufficienza renale (vedi Capitolo 101).

Il termine **adisplasia renale familiare** descrive una situazione in cui agenesia renale, displasia renale, rene multicistico (displasia) o una combinazione di queste anomalie si presentano in una singola famiglia. Questo disordine ha una modalità ereditaria autosomico-dominante con una penetranza del 50-90% e un'espressione variabile. A causa di tale associazione, alcuni clinici consigliano lo screening dei parenti di primo grado dei soggetti con diagnosi di agenesia o displasia renale, ma questa non è una pratica standardizzata.

Non è ancora chiaro se i soggetti con rene unico debbano evitare gli sport da contatto come football o karate. A favore della partecipazione c'è il fatto che vi sono altri organi unici (per esempio milza, fegato e cervello) che non impediscono il praticare sport da contatto; inoltre, sono stati segnalati pochi casi di individui che hanno perso un rene per un trauma sportivo. Contro la partecipazione sta il fatto che il rene normale controlaterale è ipertrofico e quindi non adeguatamente protetto dalle coste, per cui un trauma renale severo potrebbe avere conseguenze estremamente serie per il resto della vita. L'American Academy of Pediatrics raccomanda una "valutazione individuale per gli sport da contatto, collisione e contatto limitato".

DISGENESIA, DISPLASIA, IPOPLASIA RENALE E ANOMALIE CISTICHE DEL RENE. La *disgenesia renale* si riferisce allo sviluppo anomalo del rene, che interessa dimensioni, forma o struttura. I tre tipi principali di disgenesia sono il tipo displasico, quello ipoplasico e quello cistico. Anche se la displasia è sempre accompagnata da un ridotto numero di nefroni (ipoplasia), non è vero il contrario, in quanto l'ipoplasia può essere isolata. Quando sono presenti entrambe le condizioni si preferisce il termine **ipodisplasia**. Il termine **displasia** è tecnicamente una diagnosi istologica e si riferisce a strutture primitive disposte in modo segmentario, diffuso o focale, e nello specifico a strutture duttali primitive derivanti da un'anomala differenziazione metanefrica. Possono essere presenti anche elementi non renali, come la cartilagine. La condizione può interessare il rene intero o una parte. Se sono presenti cisti, la condizione è denominata displasia cistica. Se tutto il rene è displasico con una preponderanza di cisti, si parla di **rene displasico multicistico** (Fig. 537-2). La patogenesi della displasia è dovuta a molti fattori. La teoria del "bottone" (*bud theory*) sostiene che se il bottone ureterale si forma in posizione anomala, come un uretere ectopico, la penetrazione e l'induzione del blastema metanefrico sono anormali, con un'anomala differenziazione del rene che in seguito porta a una displasia. La displasia renale può verificarsi precocemente nella gestazione anche con una uropatia ostruttiva severa, come con i casi più severi di valvole uretrali posteriori o in un rene displasico multicistico in cui una porzione dell'uretere è assente o atresica.

Un rene multicistico è una condizione congenita in cui il rene è sostituito da cisti e non è funzionale, e può derivare da un'atresia ureterale. Le dimensioni renali sono altamente variabili. L'incidenza è di circa 1/2 000. Alcuni studi usano non correttamente i termini *rene multicistico* e *rene policistico* come sinonimi. Tuttavia, la malattia del rene policistico è un disordine ereditario che può essere autosomico recessivo o autosomico dominante e interessa entrambi i reni (vedi Capitolo 521). Il rene multicistico è di solito unilaterale e non è ereditario. Un rene multicistico bilaterale è incompatibile con la vita. Il rene displasico multicistico è la causa più comune di massa addominale nel neonato e nella maggior parte dei casi viene diagnosticato incidentalmente nel corso di un'ecografia prenatale: in alcuni individui, le cisti vengono diagnosticate

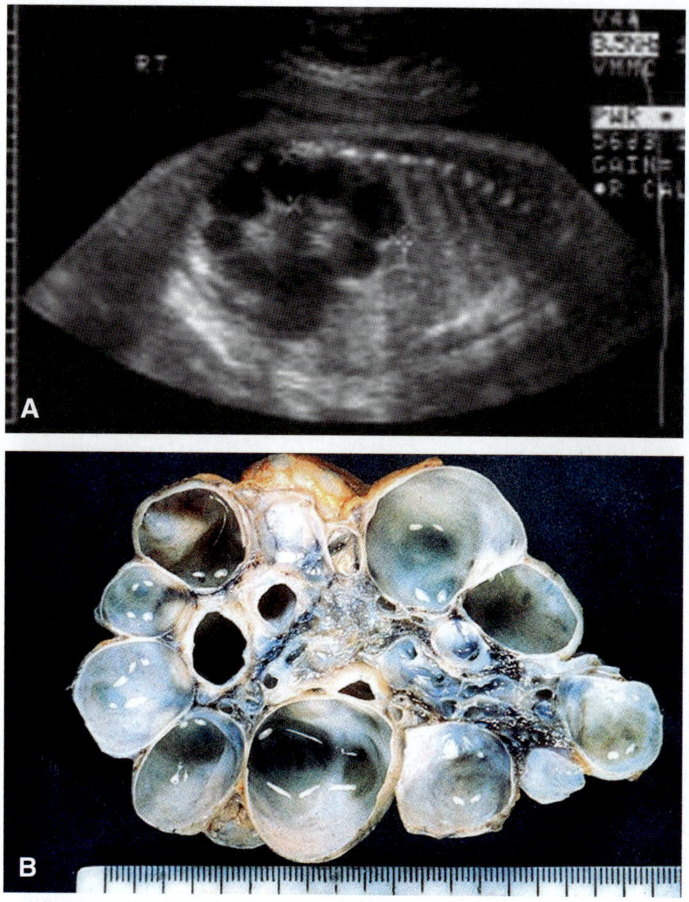

Figura 537-2. *A*, Ecografia prenatale che dimostra la presenza di un rene displasico multicistico. *B*, Campione chirurgico.

in epoca prenatale o postatale, ma non viene identificato tessuto renale a causa della regressione delle cisti in utero. Un'idronefrosi controlaterale è presente nel 5-10% dei pazienti. L'ecografia è in grado di mostrare l'aspetto caratteristico del rene sostituito da cisti multiple di dimensioni variabili che non comunicano tra loro e che non è presente parenchima identificabile; la diagnosi deve perciò essere confermata con una scintigrafia renale, la quale deve dimostrare l'assenza di funzionalità renale. È preferibile anche eseguire una cistouretrografia minzionale, poiché il 15% dei pazienti presenta un reflusso vescicoureterale controlaterale. Il trattamento è controverso, poiché vi sono state alcune segnalazioni di ipertensione renino-mediata e di tumore di Wilms insorti in questo tipo di rene. Dal momento che le neoplasie insorgono dalla componente stromale più che da quella cistica (anche se le cisti regrediscono completamente) la probabilità che il rene possa dare origine a una neoplasia non cambia e il rischio di ipertensione è dello 0,2-1,2%, mentre il rischio di tumore di Wilms è di 1/333. A causa della natura occulta di queste potenziali complicanze, molti Autori raccomandano un follow-up annuale con ecografia e determinazione della pressione arteriosa. La nefrectomia è consigliata se è presente una massa addominale, se le cisti aumentano di volume, se aumentano le dimensioni del nucleo stromale o se si sviluppa un'ipertensione. Può essere eseguita una nefrectomia laparoscopica in luogo dello screening di follow-up.

L'**ipoplasia renale** è costituita da un piccolo rene non displasico che presenta un numero di calici e nefroni inferiore al normale. Il termine comprende un gruppo di condizioni caratterizzate da un rene anormalmente piccolo e deve essere distinto dall'aplasia, in cui il rene è rudimentale. Se la condizione è unilaterale, la diagnosi di solito è posta incidentalmente durante la valutazione per un altro problema delle vie urinarie o per un'ipertensione. L'ipoplasia bilaterale di solito si presenta con le manifestazioni dell'insufficienza renale cronica ed è la causa principale di insufficienza renale terminale nel primo decennio di vita. Una storia di poliuria e polidipsia è comune. L'esame delle urine può essere normale. In una rara forma di ipoplasia bilaterale nota come **oligomeganefronia**, il numero di nefroni è severamente ridotto e quelli presenti sono fortemente ipertrofici. Il **rene di Ask-Upmark**, noto anche come **ipoplasia segmentale**, si riferisce a un rene piccolo, di solito con peso non superiore a 35 mg, con uno o più solchi profondi sulla convessità laterale, al di sotto della quale il parenchima renale consiste di tubuli simili a quelli della ghiandola tiroide. Non è chiaro se la condizione sia congenita oppure acquisita. La maggior parte dei pazienti ha 10 anni o più alla diagnosi e presenta un'ipertensione severa. Di solito la nefrectomia controlla l'ipertensione.

ANOMALIE DI FORMA E DI POSIZIONE. Durante lo sviluppo renale in genere il rene risale dalla pelvi nella sua posizione normale dietro le coste. Il normale processo di risalita e rotazione del rene può essere incompleto, risultando in ectopia renale o mancata rotazione. Il rene ectopico può trovarsi in una sede pelvica, iliaca, toracica o controlaterale. Se l'ectopia è controlaterale, nel 90% degli individui è presente una fusione dei due reni. L'incidenza di ectopia renale è di circa 1 su 900.

Le anomalie di fusione renale sono comuni. I poli inferiori dei reni possono fondersi sulla linea mediana, con la formazione di un rene a ferro di cavallo (Fig. 537-3); la porzione fusa è denominata *istmo* e può essere costituita da parenchima spesso o da una sottile banda fibrosa. Un rene a ferro di cavallo si osserva in 1/400-500 nati vivi ma è presente nel 7% delle pazienti con sindrome di Turner. Il rene a ferro di cavallo è una delle molte anomalie renali che si manifestano nel 30% delle pazienti con sindrome di Turner (vedi Capitolo 587). Il tumore di Wilms è 4 volte più frequente nel bambino con rene a ferro di cavallo che nella popolazione generale. La litiasi renale e l'idronefrosi secondaria a ostruzione della giunzione ureteropelvica sono altre potenziali complicanze tardive. L'aumentata incidenza di rene displasico multicistico che interessa uno dei due lati di un rene a ferro di cavallo sembra anch'essa essere aumentata. Nell'ectopia con fusione crociata, un rene migra sull'altro lato e il parenchima dei due reni si fonde. La funzionalità renale è di solito normale e, nel caso più comune, il rene sinistro migra sull'altro lato fondendosi con il polo inferiore del rene destro. L'inserzione dell'uretere sulla vescica non cambia e le ghiandole surrenali rimangono nella loro posizione normale. Il significato clinico di questa anomalia è che se è necessario un intervento sul rene, la vascolarizzazione renale è variabile e può rendere difficoltosa una nefrectomia parziale.

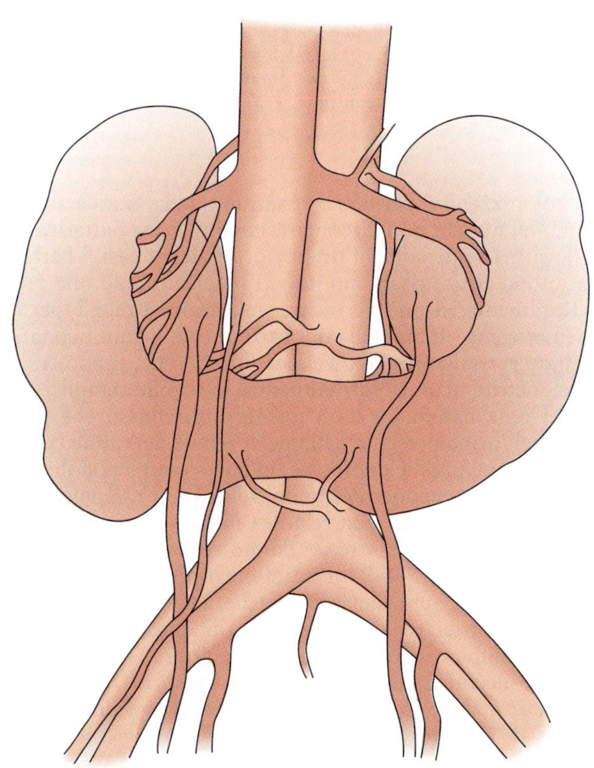

Figura 537-3. Rene a ferro di cavallo.

ANOMALIE ASSOCIATE. Le anomalie delle vie urinarie superiori sono più comuni nei bambini che presentano determinate caratteristiche fisiche. L'incidenza di anomalie renali è aumentata in presenza di arteria ombelicale unica e di anomalie di altri sistemi d'organo (cardiopatia congenita). Anomalie dell'orecchio esterno (particolarmente se il bambino presenta anomalie congenite multiple), imperforazione dell'ano e scoliosi sono associate ad anomalie renali e i neonati che le manifestano devono essere sottoposti a ecografia renale.

Aslam M, Watson AR: Unilateral multicystic dysplastic kidney: long term outcomes. *Arch Dis Child* 2006;91:820–823.

Cheng AM, Phan V, Geary DF, et al: Outcome of isolated antenatal hydronephrosis. *Arch Pediatr Adolesc Med* 2004;158:38–40.

Coplen DE, Austin PF: Outcome analysis of prenatally detected ureteroceles associated with multicystic dysplasia. *J Urol* 2004;172:1637–1639.

Damen-Elias HA, Stoutenbeek PH, Visser GH, et al: Concomitant anomalies in 100 children with unilateral multicystic kidney. *Ultrasound Obstet Gynecol* 2005;25:384–388.

Elder JS: Sports recommendations for children with solitary kidneys and other genitourinary abnormalities. In Baskin LS, Kogan BA (editors), *Handbook of Pediatric Urology*, 2nd ed. Philadelphia, Lippincott Williams & Wilkins, 2005, pp 271–277.

Grinsell MM, Showalter S, Gordon KA, Norwood VF: Single kidney and sports participation: perception versus reality. *Pediatrics* 2006;118(3): 1019–1027.

Guarino N, Cassamassima MG, Tadini B, et al: Natural history of vesicoureteral reflux associated with kidney anomalies. *Urology* 2005;65: 1208–1211.

Guarino N, Tadini B, Camardi P, et al: The incidence of associated urological abnormalities in children with renal ectopia. *J Urol* 2004;172:1757–1759.

Ismaili K, Avni FE, Alexander M, et al: Routine voiding cystourethrography is of no value in neonates with unilateral multicystic dysplastic kidney. *J Pediatr* 2005;146:759–763.

Merrot T, Lumenta CB, Tercier S, et al: Multicystic dysplastic kidney with ipsilateral abnormalities of genitourinary tract: Experience in children. *Urology* 2006;67:603–607.

Miller DC, Rumohr JA, Dunn RL, et al: What is the fate of the refluxing contralateral kidney in children with multicystic dysplastic kidney? *J Urol* 2004;172:1630–1634.

Narchi H: Risk of hypertension with multicystic kidney disease: A systematic review. *Arch Dis Child* 2005;90:921–924.

Narchi H: Risk of Wilms' tumour with multicystic kidney disease: A systematic review. *Arch Dis Child* 2005;90:147–149.

Rabelo EA, Oliveira EA, Gilva GS, et al: Predictive factors of ultrasonographic involution of prenatally detected multicystic dysplastic kidney. *BJU Int* 2005;95:868–871.

Welch TR, Wacksman J: The changing approach to multicystic dysplastic kidney in children. *J Pediatr* 2005;146:723–725.

Yamatake A, Satake S, Kaneko K, et al: Outcome and cost analysis of laparoscopic or open surgery versus conservative management for multicystic dysplastic kidney. *J Laparoendosc Adv Surg Tech A* 2005;15:190–193.

Capitolo 538 ■ Infezioni delle vie urinarie

Jack S. Elder

Vedi anche Capitolo 519.4

PREVALENZA ED EZIOLOGIA. Le infezioni delle vie urinarie (IVU o in inglese UTI, *N.d.C.*) si verificano nel 3-5% delle femmine e nell'1% dei maschi. Nelle bambine, la prima IVU di solito si verifica entro i 5 anni di età con un picco durante la prima infanzia e il periodo dell'educazione degli sfinteri (*toilet training*). Dopo la prima IVU, il 60-80% delle bambine presenta una seconda IVU entro 18 mesi. Nei bambini, la maggior parte delle IVU si verifica nel corso del primo anno di vita e sono molto più comuni nei maschi non circoncisi. La prevalenza di IVU varia con l'età. Durante il primo anno di vita il rapporto maschio:femmina è di 2,8-5,4:1, mentre oltre gli 1-2 anni di vita compare una marcata prevalenza femminile, con un rapporto maschio:femmina di 1:10.

Le IVU sono causate soprattutto da batteri del colon. Nelle femmine, il 75-90% delle infezioni è causato dall'*Escherichia coli*, seguita da *Klebsiella* spp. e *Proteus* spp. Alcune casistiche riportano che nei maschi con più di 1 anno di età, *Proteus* è una causa comune quanto l'*E. coli*; altri riportano una preponderanza di microrganismi Gram-positivi nei maschi. Lo *Staphylococcus saprophyticus* e gli enterococchi sono patogeni in entrambi i sessi. Possono verificarsi anche infezioni virali, particolarmente da adenovirus, specialmente come causa di cistite. Le IVU sono considerate un importante fattore di rischio per lo sviluppo di insufficienza renale o di nefropatia terminale nel bambino. Alcuni Autori hanno messo in discussione l'importanza delle IVU come fattore di rischio, in quanto solo il 2% dei bambini con insufficienza renale riporta un'anamnesi di IVU. Questo paradosso può essere secondario a migliori conoscenze dei rischi delle IVU e a una maggiore immediatezza della diagnosi e della terapia.

MANIFESTAZIONI CLINICHE E CLASSIFICAZIONE. Le tre forme principali di IVU sono la pielonefrite, la cistite e la batteriuria asintomatica.

La **pielonefrite** clinica è caratterizzata da uno o più dei seguenti sintomi: dolore addominale o del fianco, febbre, malessere, nausea, vomito e, occasionalmente, diarrea. I neonati possono presentare sintomi non specifici come difficoltà ad alimentarsi, irritabilità e calo ponderale. La pielonefrite è la più comune infezione batterica severa dei bambini di <24 mesi di età con febbre senza infezione focale (vedi Capitolo 175). Tali sintomi rappresentano un'indicazione della presenza di un'infezione batterica delle vie urinarie superiori. L'interessamento del parenchima renale è denominato *pielonefrite acuta*, mentre se non è presente interessamento parenchimale la condizione può essere definita *pielite*. La pielonefrite acuta può portare a un danno renale, definito come cicatrice (*scar*) pielonefritica.

La **nefrite lobare acuta** è un'infezione batterica renale localizzata che interessa >1 lobo e che rappresenta una complicanza della pielonefrite o una fase precoce dello sviluppo di un ascesso renale. Le manifestazioni sono simili a quelle della pielonefrite; l'imaging renale dimostra l'anomalia (Fig. 538-1). Un **ascesso renale** può verificarsi in seguito a una pielonefrite o può essere secondario a una batteriemia primitiva (*S. aureus*). L'**ascesso perinefrico** può essere secondario a un'infezione contigua dell'area perirenale (per esempio, osteomielite vertebrale, ascesso dello psoas) o a una pielonefrite che disseca nella capsula renale.

Il termine **cistite** definisce un interessamento vescicale; i sintomi comprendono disuria, minzione imperiosa, pollachiuria, dolore sovrapubico, incontinenza e urine maleodoranti. La cistite non provoca febbre e non causa danno renale, tuttavia la presenza di urine maleodoranti non è specifica di un'IVU.

Il termine **batteriuria asintomatica** si riferisce a una condizione che risulta in un'urinocoltura positiva senza altre manifestazioni infettive ed è più frequente nelle femmine. L'incidenza è dell'1-2% nelle bambine in età prescolare e in età scolare, e dello 0,03% nei bambini, ma l'incidenza si riduce con l'aumentare dell'età. Questa condizione è benigna e non causa danno renale, eccetto che nelle donne gravide, in cui una batteriuria asintomatica, se non trattata, può portare a un'IVU sintomatica. In alcune bambine viene diagnosticata erroneamente una batteriuria asintomatica, mentre in realtà esse sono sintomatiche, con incontinenza diurna o notturna o con bruciore perineale.

PATOGENESI E ANATOMIA PATOLOGICA. Virtualmente tutte le IVU sono infezioni ascendenti. I batteri prendono origine dalla flora fecale, colonizzano il perineo e penetrano nella vescica attraverso l'uretra. Nei maschi non circoncisi, la patogenesi batterica deriva dalla flora residente sotto il prepuzio. In alcuni casi, i batteri che provocano la cistite risalgono fino al rene causando una pielonefrite. Raramente, si può verificare un'infezione renale per diffusione ematogena, come nell'endocardite o in alcuni neonati.

Se i batteri risalgono dalla vescica fino al rene, si può verificare una pielonefrite acuta. Normalmente, le papille semplici e composte del rene hanno un meccanismo antireflusso che previene l'entrata dell'urina presente nella pelvi renale nei tubuli collettori. Tuttavia, alcune papille composte, in particolare nei poli superiore e inferiore del rene, permettono il reflusso intrarenale. Le urine infette stimolano quindi una risposta immunologica e infiammatoria e il risultato può essere un danno renale e la formazione di cicatrici renali (Fig. 538-2). I bambini di qualsiasi età con IVU febbrile possono avere una pielonefrite acuta e successivamente sviluppare cicatrici renali. L'eccezione a questa osservazione è che se un bambino con IVU ha una scintigrafia con acido 2,3-dimercaptosuccinico (DMSA) normale entro i 4 anni di età, il rischio di *scar* da pielonefrite da future IVU è ridotto. I fattori di rischio dell'ospite per un'IVU sono evidenziati nella Tabella 538-1. Il reflusso vescicoureterale è discusso nel Capitolo 539. Nelle bambine, le IVU si verificano spesso nelle fasi iniziali del

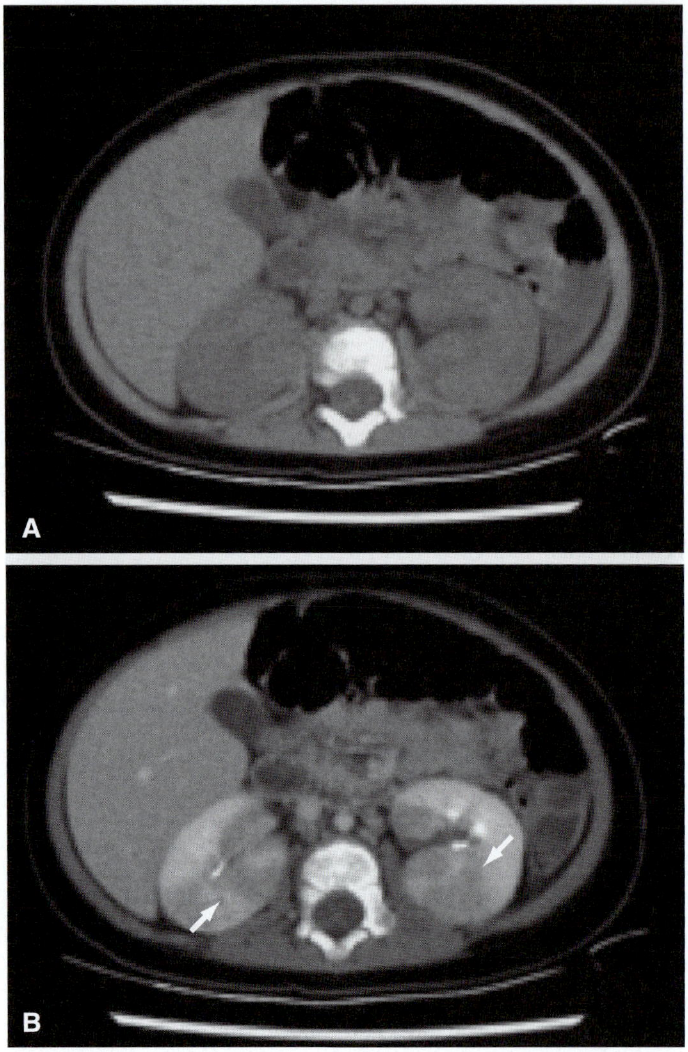

Figura 538-1. Tipiche immagini TC pre-contrasto (*A*) e con contrasto (*B*) di un paziente di 8 mesi con nefrite lobare acuta che si è presentato con nefromegalia bilaterale severa ma senza una massa focale all'ecografia. Non si osserva un'area di attenuazione nel rene prima dell'*enhancement* con il contrasto. (Da Cheng CH, Tsau YK, Lin TY: Effective duration of antimicrobial therapy for the treatment of acute lobar nephronia. *Pediatrics* 2006;117: e84-e89.)

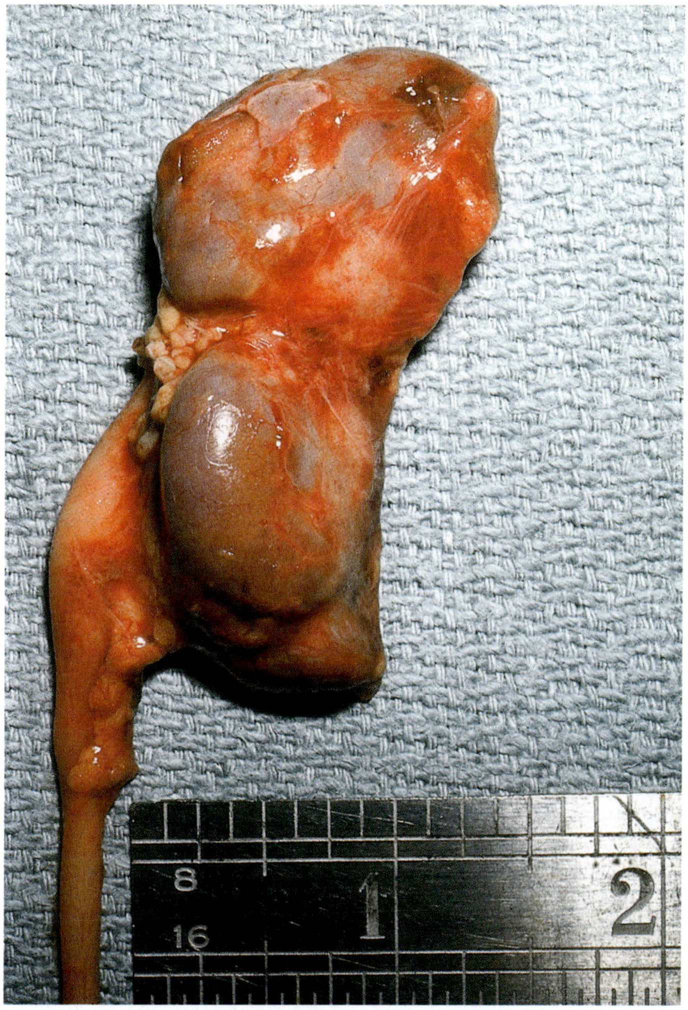

Figura 538-2. Rene con *scar* da pielonefrite recidivante.

TABELLA 538-1. Fattori di rischio per le infezioni delle vie urinarie

Sesso femminile
Maschio non circonciso
Reflusso vescicoureterale*
Toilet training
Disfunzione minzionale
Uropatia ostruttiva
Strumentazione uretrale
Pulizia perineale retro-fronte nelle femmine
Uso di bagnoschiuma?
Vestiti stretti (biancheria intima)
Infestazione da ossiuri
Stipsi
Batteri con fimbrie P
Anomalie anatomiche (aderenze labiali)
Vescica neurogena
Attività sessuale
Gravidanza

*Rischio aumentato di pielonefrite clinica, non di cistite.

toilet training a causa della disfunzione minzionale che si verifica in tale età. Il bambino o la bambina tenta di trattenere le urine per non bagnarsi, ma la vescica può avere contrazioni non inibite che ne provocano la fuoriuscita forzata: il risultato può essere un flusso urinario turbolento e ad alta pressione o un incompleto svuotamento vescicale ed entrambe le cose aumentano la probabilità di batteriuria. La disfunzione minzionale può verificarsi nel bambino che ha già raggiunto il controllo degli sfinteri e che urina infrequentemente. Problemi simili possono insorgere nei bambini in età scolare che rifiutano l'uso delle toilette della scuola. Un'uropatia ostruttiva risultante in un'idronefrosi aumenta il rischio di IVU a causa della stasi urinaria. La strumentazione uretrale nel corso di una cistografia minzionale o di un cateterismo non sterile può infettare la vescica con un microrganismo patogeno. La stipsi può aumentare il rischio di IVU in quanto può causare disfunzione minzionale.

La patogenesi delle IVU si basa in parte sulla presenza di pili o fimbrie batteriche sulla superficie dei batteri. Esistono due tipi di fimbrie, tipo I e II. Le fimbrie di tipo I si trovano nella maggior parte dei ceppi di *E. coli*. Dal momento che l'aderenza alle cellule bersaglio può essere bloccata dal d-mannosio, queste fimbrie sono denominate "mannosio-sensibili", che non hanno alcun ruolo nella pielonefrite. L'adesione delle fimbrie di tipo II non è inibita dal mannosio e sono quindi note come "mannosio-resistenti". Queste fimbrie sono espresse solo da alcuni ceppi di *E. coli*. Il recettore delle fimbrie di tipo II è un glicosfingolipide che è presente sia sulla membrana cellulare uroepiteliale sia sugli eritrociti. La frazione oligosaccaridica Gal 1-4 Gal è il recettore specifico. Dal momento che queste fimbrie possono essere agglutinate dagli eritrociti appartenenti al gruppo P, esse sono note come fimbrie P. I batteri con fimbrie P hanno una maggiore probabilità di causare una pielonefrite. Circa il 76-94% dei ceppi pielonefritogeni di *E. coli* ha fimbrie P rispetto al 19-23% dei ceppi che causano cistite.

Altri fattori dell'ospite per le IVU comprendono anomalie anatomiche che impediscono la minzione normale, come le aderenze labiali. Questa anomalia agisce da barriera e provoca minzione vaginale. Una vescica neurogena può provocare IVU se si accompagna a svuotamento vescicale incompleto o a dissinergia detrusore-sfintere, oppure a entrambe le cose. L'attività sessuale è associata a IVU nelle ragazze, in parte a causa di uno svuotamento vescicale incompleto. Il 4-7% delle donne gravide presenta batteriuria asintomatica, che può evolvere in un'IVU sintomatica. L'incidenza di IVU nei neonati allattati al seno è inferiore a quella nei lattanti che ricevono latte formulato.

La **pielonefrite xantogranulomatosa** è un raro tipo di infezione renale caratterizzato da infiammazione granulomatosa con cellule giganti e istiociti schiumosi. Si può presentare clinicamente come una massa renale o un'infezione acuta o cronica. Litiasi renale, ostruzione e infezione da *Proteus* spp. o *E. coli* contribuiscono allo sviluppo di questa lesione, che di solito impone una nefrectomia parziale o totale.

DIAGNOSI. Una IVU può essere sospettata in base ai sintomi o alle caratteristiche dell'esame delle urine oppure a entrambe, ma è necessaria un'urinocoltura per la conferma e per una terapia appropriata. La diagnosi corretta di un'IVU dipende dal prelievo di un appropriato campione di urine. Esistono diversi modi per ottenere un corretto campione di urine e alcuni sono più accurati di altri.

Nei bambini che hanno raggiunto il controllo degli sfinteri, di solito è sufficiente un campione di urine del mitto intermedio. La maggior parte degli studi non ha dimostrato alcun beneficio della pulizia formale dell'introitus prima del prelievo delle urine. Se la coltura evidenzia >100 000 colonie di un singolo patogeno, o se vi sono 10 000 colonie e il bambino è sintomatico, il bambino è considerato affetto da IVU. Nei maschi non circoncisi, il prepuzio deve essere retratto, ma se il prepuzio non è detraibile questo metodo di prelievo delle urine potrebbe essere inaffidabile. Nei lattanti, può essere utile l'applicazione di un sacchetto sterile sigillato per la raccolta delle urine dopo disinfezione della cute o dei genitali, particolarmente se la coltura è negativa. Una coltura positiva può riflettere un contaminante, particolarmente nelle bambine e nei bambini non circoncisi. In tali casi, se l'esame delle urine è positivo, il paziente è sintomatico e vi è un singolo microrganismo in coltura con una conta delle colonie >100 000, è presente una presunta IVU. Se uno qualsiasi di questi criteri non è soddisfatto, è raccomandata la conferma dell'infezione con un campione di urine prelevato con catetere.

Quando è necessaria una maggiore accuratezza rispetto alla possibilità di un'infezione, occorre un campione prelevato con catetere. Sono importanti un'appropriata preparazione della cute e una buona tecnica di cateterizzazione. L'uso di un sondino nasogastrico in polietilene 5 F o di un sondino 8 F con appropriata lubrificazione nei bambini più grandi minimizza la possibilità di trauma e contaminazione uretrale. Occorre aspirare solo pochi mL con una siringa per ottenere il campione di urine. Il cateterismo subito dopo la minzione spontanea fornisce una misura del residuo urinario vescicale e aiuta a risolvere i problemi correlati allo svuotamento vescicale.

È importante l'immediata messa in coltura del campione di urine, in quanto, se l'urina resta a temperatura ambiente per più di 60 minuti, la crescita di un contaminante minore può suggerire un'IVU quando in effetti le urine possono non essere infette. La refrigerazione è un metodo affidabile di conservare le urine fino a quando non è possibile l'urinocoltura. L'esame delle urine deve essere eseguito dallo stesso campione che è servito per l'urinocoltura. La presenza di **piuria** (leucociti nelle urine) suggerisce infezione, ma un'infezione può verificarsi in assenza di piuria; conseguentemente, una piuria può essere presente senza IVU. Nitriti ed esterasi leucocitaria di solito sono positivi in caso di urine infette. Nella cistite acuta è comune un'ematuria microscopica. La presenza di cilindri leucocitari nel sedimento urinario suggerisce l'interessamento renale, ma nella pratica si osserva raramente. Se il bambino è asintomatico e l'esame delle urine è normale, è improbabile che sia presente un'IVU. Tuttavia, se il bambino è sintomatico è possibile che si manifesti un'IVU, anche se l'esame delle urine è negativo.

In un'infezione renale acuta sono frequenti leucocitosi, neutrofilia e aumento della VES e della proteina C-reattiva. Gli ultimi due sono marker non specifici di infezione batterica e il loro aumento non significa che il bambino abbia una pielonefrite acuta. Con un ascesso renale, la conta leucocitaria è marcatamente elevata a >20 000-25 000/mm^3. Poiché nella pielonefrite è comune la sepsi, particolarmente nei lattanti e in tutti i bambini con uropatia ostruttiva, deve essere presa in considerazione un'emocoltura.

La **cistite emorragica acuta** è spesso causata dall'*E. coli*; è stata attribuita anche agli adenovirus di tipo 11 e 21. La cistite da adenovirus è molto più comune nel maschio ed è autolimitante, con un'ematuria che dura almeno 4 giorni.

La **cistite eosinofila** è una rara forma di cistite di origine oscura che occasionalmente si incontra anche nel bambino. I sintomi usuali sono quelli della cistite con ematuria, dilatazione ureterale con occasionale idronefrosi e difetti di riempimento della vescica causati da masse, le quali consistono istologicamente di infiltrati infiammatori con eosinofili. I bambini con cistite eosinofila possono essere stati esposti a un allergene. Per escludere un processo neoplastico è spesso necessaria la biopsia vescicale. Il trattamento di solito comprende antistaminici e FANS, ma in alcuni casi è necessaria l'instillazione intravescicale di dimetil-sulfossido.

La **cistite interstiziale** è caratterizzata da sintomi irritativi alla minzione come urgenza, pollachiuria e disuria, e dolore vescicale e pelvico alleviato dalla minzione con urinocoltura negativa. Il disordine interessa più frequentemente le adolescenti ed è idiopatico (vedi Capitolo 519.1). La diagnosi si pone mediante l'osservazione cistoscopica di ulcere mucose con distensione vescicale. Il trattamento comprende l'idrodistensione della vescica e l'ablazione laser delle aree ulcerate, ma nessun trattamento è risolutivo nel lungo periodo.

TRATTAMENTO. La cistite acuta deve essere trattata immediatamente per prevenire una possibile progressione a pielonefrite. Se i sintomi sono severi occorre prelevare un campione di urine vescicale per l'urinocoltura quindi iniziare immediatamente il trattamento. Se i sintomi sono lievi o la diagnosi è dubbia, il trattamento può essere ritardato fino a quando non sono noti i risultati dell'urinocoltura, mentre quest'ultima può essere ripetuta se i risultati sono incerti. Se, per esempio, in una coltura di urine del mitto intermedio crescono tra 10^4 e 10^5 colonie di un microrganismo Gram-negativo, è possibile eseguire una seconda coltura mediante cateterismo prima di iniziare il trattamento. Se il trattamento viene iniziato prima di conoscere i risultati dell'urinocoltura e l'antibiogramma, un ciclo di 3-5 giorni di terapia con trimetoprim-sulfametoxazolo è efficace nei confronti di molti ceppi di *E. coli*. Anche la nitrofurantoina (5-7 mg/kg/24 ore suddivisi in 3-4 dosi) è efficace e ha il vantaggio di essere attiva nei confronti di *Klebsiella-Enterobacter*. L'amoxicillina (50 mg/kg/24 ore) è anch'essa efficace come trattamento iniziale ma non possiede un evidente vantaggio rispetto ai sulfamidici o alla nitrofurantoina. Nelle infezioni febbrili acute suggestive di **pielonefrite**, è preferibile un ciclo di 10-14 giorni di un antibiotico ad ampio spettro in grado di raggiungere concentrazioni tessutali significative. I bambini disidratati, che vomitano o che non sono in grado di bere liquidi, con ≤1 mese di vita o in cui è possibile una sepsi urinaria, devono essere ricoverati in ospedale per la reidratazione ev e una terapia antibiotica ev. È preferibile il trattamento parenterale con ceftriaxone (50-75 mg/kg/24 ore, non superando i 2 g) o ampicillina (100 mg/kg/24 ore) con un aminoglicoside come la gentamicina (3-5 mg/kg/24 ore suddivisi in 1-3 dosi). Deve essere presa in considerazione la potenziale ototossicità e nefrotossicità e, prima di iniziare il trattamento, occorre valutare i livelli sierici di creatinina e i livelli sierici minimi di gentamicina tutti i giorni e per tutta la durata della terapia. Il trattamento con aminoglicosidi è particolarmente efficace nei confronti di *Pseudomonas* spp. e l'alcalinizzazione delle urine con bicarbonato di sodio ne aumenta l'efficacia nelle vie urinarie. Le cefalosporine orali di 3^a generazione come cefixima sono altrettanto efficaci del ceftriaxone per via parenterale contro vari microrganismi Gram-negativi diversi da *Pseudomonas*, e questi antibiotici sono ora considerati da alcuni Autori il trattamento di scelta per la terapia orale. La nitrofurantoina non deve essere usata di routine nei bambini con IVU febbrile in quanto non raggiunge concentrazioni significative nei tessuti renali. La ciprofloxacina, un fluorochinolone orale, è un agente alternativo per i microrganismi resistenti, particolarmente *Pseudomonas*, per i pazienti con più di 17 anni. È stato utilizzato anche in bambini più piccoli con fibrosi cistica e infezione polmonare secondaria a *Pseudomonas* e viene occasionalmente impiegato per terapie brevi nei bambini con IVU da *Pseudomonas*. Tuttavia, l'uso clinico dei fluorochinoloni nel bambino deve essere limitato a causa del potenziale danno per le cartilagini che è stato osservato negli studi su animali immaturi. La sicurezza e l'efficacia della ciprofloxacina orale nel bambino è in corso di studio. In alcuni bambini con IVU febbrile, è efficace l'iniezione im di una dose di carico di ceftriaxone seguita da una terapia orale con una cefalosporina di 3ª generazione. Un'urinocoltura una settimana dopo la fine del trattamento di un'IVU assicura la sterilità delle urine; nella maggior parte dei bambini ciò non è necessario, in quanto le culture sono spesso negative. I bambini con ascesso renale o perirenale o con infezioni a livello di vie urinarie ostruite spesso richiedono un drenaggio percutaneo chirurgico oltre alla terapia antibiotica e altre misure di sostegno.

In un bambino con IVU ricorrenti, l'identificazione dei fattori predisponesti è estremamente utile. Molte bambine in età scolare hanno una **disfunzione minzionale**; il trattamento di questa condizione spesso riduce la probabilità di IVU ricorrenti. Alcuni bambini con infezioni delle vie urinarie urinano infrequentemente e possono avere anche una stipsi severa. Per controllare le recidive può essere utile un counseling di genitori e pazienti per cercare di stabilire modalità più normali di minzione e defecazione. La profilassi nei confronti delle reinfezioni, per mezzo di trimetoprim-sulfametoxazolo, trimetoprim o nitrofurantoina a 1/3 della normale dosa terapeutica una volta al giorno, è spesso efficace. Anche la profilassi con amoxicillina o cefalexina può essere efficace, ma il rischio di sviluppare un'IVU può essere più elevato in quanto può essere indotta una resistenza batterica. Altre indicazioni alla profilassi a lungo termine (per es. vescica neurogena, stasi e ostruzione delle vie urinarie, reflusso, litiasi) sono discusse in altri capitoli. Attualmente vi è interesse per la terapia con probiotici, che sostituiscono la normale flora vaginale, e con succo di mirtillo, che previene l'adesione batterica e la formazione del biofilm, ma questi agenti non si sono dimostrati efficaci nel prevenire le IVU.

Le principali conseguenze del danno renale cronico causato dalla pielonefrite sono l'ipertensione arteriosa e l'insufficienza renale; quando queste condizioni vengono diagnosticate devono essere trattate appropriatamente (vedi Capitoli 445 e 535).

STUDI DI IMAGING. Lo scopo degli studi di imaging nei bambini con IVU è l'identificazione di anomalie anatomiche che predispongono all'infezione. Nei bambini con pielonefrite clinica (IVU febbrile), occorre eseguire un'ecografia renale per escludere un'idronefrosi e anomalie strutturali delle vie urinarie; l'ecografia può suggerire anche la presenza di una pielonefrite evidenziando un ingrandimento del rene. L'ecografia Power Doppler si è dimostrata leggermente più sensibile ma è inaffidabile nell'identificare tutti i casi. L'ecografia dimostra molte delle cicatrici renali ma non tutte. Normalmente, la differenza di lunghezza tra i due reni è inferiore a 1 cm e una differenza maggiore può essere un'indicazione di deficit della crescita renale. Occorre ricordare che in un bambino con pielonefrite acuta, un rene piccolo può essere ingrandito a causa dell'infezione, dando l'impressione erronea di uguali dimensioni dei due reni. L'ecografia renale è sensibile anche per l'identificazione di una nefrite lobare acuta e di una pionefrosi, una condizione che può richiedere l'immediato drenaggio del sistema collettore mediante nefrotomia percutanea. Le indicazioni alla cistouretrografia minzionale (VCUG) sono controverse e sono attualmente in corso di cambiamento. La maggior parte dei clinici la raccomanda nelle bambine che hanno avuto due o tre IVU in un periodo di 6 mesi, e nei bambini con più di una IVU. Occorre eseguire una VCUG anche se l'ecografia renale ha evidenziato qualsiasi anomalia significativa, come idronefrosi, disparità di lunghezza tra i due reni o ispessimento della parete vescicale. Il riscontro più comune è il reflusso vescicoureterale, che viene identificato in circa il 40% dei pazienti (Fig. 538-3). Il timing della VCUG è controverso. Anche se in alcuni centri lo studio viene rimandato per 2-6 settimane per permettere la risoluzione dell'infiammazione vescicale, l'incidenza di reflusso è identica, indipendentemente se la VCUG viene eseguita durante il trattamento dell'IVU o dopo 6 settimane. Di conseguenza, l'esecuzione della VCUG prima che il bambino sia dimesso dall'ospedale è appropriata e assicura la completezza della valutazione. Se disponibile, può essere effettuata nelle bambine una VCUG con radioisotopi piuttosto che una VCUG con contrasto, poiché questa tecnica provoca meno esposizione alle radiazioni delle gonadi rispetto al metodo con contrasto. Tuttavia, la VCUG con radioisotopi non fornisce una definizione anatomica della vescica, non permette una precisa gradazione del reflusso, non dimostra un diverticolo paraureterale o se il reflusso avvenga in un sistema collettore doppio o in un uretere ectopico. Nei maschi è importante la definizione radiografica dell'uretra; conseguentemente si raccomanda la VCUG con contrasto per la valutazione iniziale.

A causa della preoccupazione per il fatto che la VCUG possa essere traumatica per il bambino, alcuni genitori mettono in discussione la necessità di una VCUG se l'ecografia è normale. L'ecografia non è sensibile nell'individuare un reflusso e soltanto il 40% dei bambini con reflusso presenta qualche anomalia all'ecografia. La VCUG non deve essere effettuata di routine in anestesia generale, in quanto lo studio è incompleto senza una fase minzionale e assoggetta inutilmente il bambino ai rischi e ai costi di un'anestesia. In casi selezionati, può essere utilizzato midazolam per os (fino a 0,5 mg/kg per os, 0,2 mg/kg per via nasale), che provoca amnesia anterograda e ansiolisi: si monitorano i segni vitali e l'ossimetria pulsata e non è presente l'anestesista.

Quando la diagnosi di pielonefrite acuta è incerta, è utile la **scintigrafia renale** con DMSA marcato con tecnezio o con glucoeptonato. La presenza di aree di ipocaptazione conferma la diagnosi di pielonefrite e un radiologo esperto può distinguere un processo acuto da uno cronico. In circa il 50% dei bambini con IVU febbrile, indipendentemente dall'età, la scintigrafia con DMSA dimostra un interessamento parenchimale. Nei bambini con reflusso di grado III, IV o V e una IVU febbrile, l'80-90% mostra una pielonefrite acuta. Se la scintigrafia con DMSA evidenzia una pielonefrite acuta, il 50% circa dei bambini svilupperà una cicatrice in quella sede nei successivi 5 mesi. Tuttavia, se la scintigrafia con DMSA è normale in corso di un'IVU febbrile, non deriverà alcuna cicatrice da quella particolare infezione. La TC è un altro strumento diagnostico che può diagnosticare una pielonefrite acuta, ma l'esperienza clinica con la scintigrafia con DMSA è molto maggiore. Un algoritmo di imaging alternativo e razionale è stato proposto per i bambini con IVU febbrile: ecografia renale e scintigrafia renale con DMSA, eseguendo una VCUG se la scintigrafia evidenzia una pielonefrite acuta. L'utilità di questo approccio deve essere confermata da trial prospettici. Una scintigrafia con DMSA (Fig. 538-4) viene spesso eseguita in presenza di reflusso vescicoureterale per valutare la presenza di cicatrici renali. La scintigrafia con DMSA è lo studio più accurato e sensibile per dimostrare le cicatrici renali. L'urografia escretoria non è altrettanto sensibile rispetto alla scintigrafia con DMSA nel dimostrare le cicatrici renali; inoltre, la visualizzazione del sistema collettore nel lattante e nel bambino più piccolo è spesso subottimale, esiste un piccolo rischio di allergia al contrasto e possono essere necessari 1-2 anni perché una cicatrice renale divenga visibile all'urografia. Anche la TC è stata utilizzata per valutare le vie urinarie superiori, in quanto è efficace nel dimostrare le cicatrici renali (Fig. 538-5).

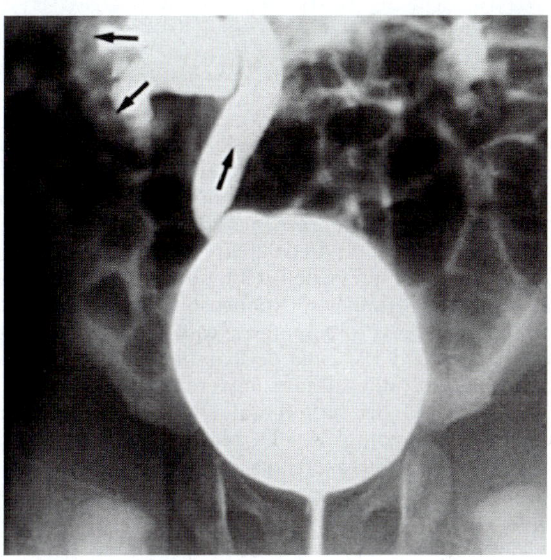

Figura 538-3. Reflusso intrarenale. Cistouretrografia minzionale in un lattante con anamnesi di infezione delle vie urinarie. Si noti il reflusso vescicoureterale destro con dilatazione ureterale, con opacificazione del parenchima renale che rappresenta il reflusso intrarenale.

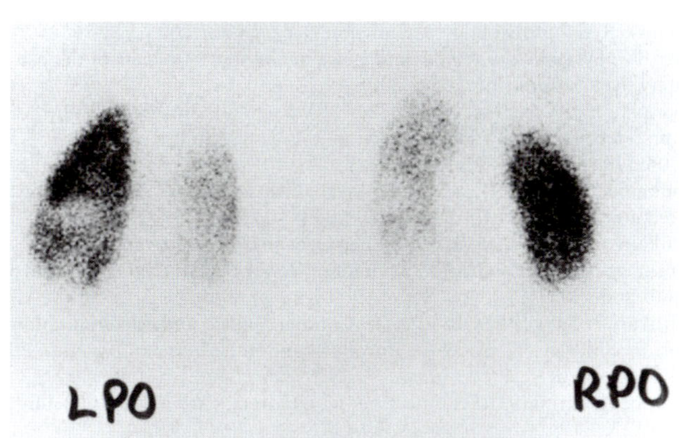

Figura 538-4. Scintigrafia renale con DMSA che evidenzia aree di ipocaptazione bilaterali indicative di pielonefrite acuta e cicatrizzazione renale.

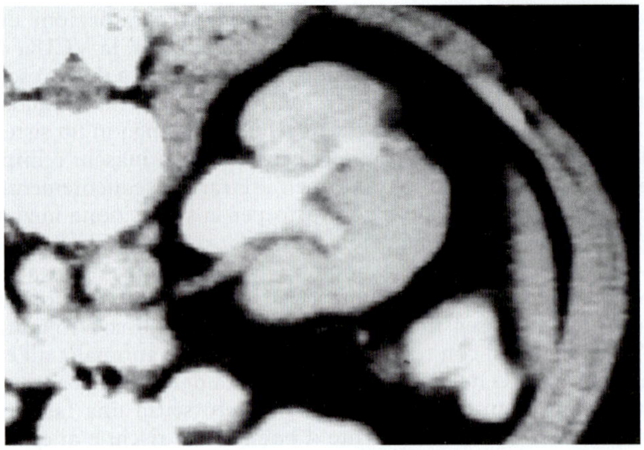

Figura 538-5. TC che evidenzia un'area di assottigliamento parenchimale corrispondente a un calice sottostante, caratteristico della cicatrizzazione (*scarring*) pielonefritica della nefropatia da reflusso.

In passato, venivano spesso eseguite la cistoscopia e la misurazione del calibro uretrale nelle bambine con IVU, ma questi studi non contribuiscono alle decisioni terapeutiche da prendere per i bambini con IVU e sono controindicati. Un tempo è stato ipotizzato che la stenosi dell'uretra femminile fosse un fattore che potesse contribuire allo sviluppo di IVU, ma è stato riscontrato che l'uretra delle bambine con IVU ricorrenti non è più stretta di quella delle bambine senza infezione.

Beattie TJ: Imaging guidelines for urinary tract infection in childhood; time for change? *Arch Dis Child* 2004; 89:398–399.

Beetz R: May we go on with antibacterial prophylaxis for urinary tract infections? *Pediatr Nephrol* 2006;21:5–13.

Bloomfield P, Hodson EM, Craig J: Antibiotics for acute pyelonephritis in children. *Cochrane Database Syst Rev* 2005;25:CD003772.

Bratalavsky G, Feustel PJ, Aslan AR, et al: Recurrence risk in infants with urinary tract infections and a negative radiographic evaluation. *J Urol* 2004;172:1610–1613.

Chen L, Hasio AL, Moore CL, et al: Utility of bedside bladder ultrasound before urethral catheterization in young children. *Pediatrics* 2005;115: 108–111.

Cheng CH, Tsau YK, Lin TY: Effective duration of antimicrobial therapy for the treatment of acute lobar nephronia. *Pediatrics* 2006;117:e84–e89.

Craig JC, Hodson EM: Treatment of acute pyelonephritis in children. *BMJ* 2004;328:179–180.

Currie ML, Mitz L, Raasch CS, et al: Follow-up urine cultures and fever in children with urinary tract infection. *Arch Pediatr Adolesc Med* 2003;157:1237–1240.

Freedman AL: Urologic diseases in North America Project: Trends in resource utilization for urinary tract infections in children. *J Urol* 2005; 173:949–954.

Giorgi LJ Jr, Bratalavsky G, Kogan BA: Febrile urinary tract infections in infants: Renal ultrasound remains necessary. *J Urol* 2005;173:568–570.

Grady RW: Systemic quinolone antibiotics in children: A review of the use and safety. *Expert Opin Drug Saf* 2005;4:623–630.

Hoberman A, Charron M, Hickey RW, et al: Imaging studies after a first febrile urinary tract infection in young children. *N Engl J Med* 2003;348:195–202.

Jahnukainen T, Chen M, Celsi G: Mechanisms of renal damage owing to infection. *Pediatr Nephrol* 2005;20:1043–1053.

Jahnukainen T, Honkinen O, Ruuskanen O, et al: Ultrasonography after the first febrile urinary tract infection in children. *Eur J Pediatr* 2006;165:556–559. Epub 2006 Mar 25.

Kontiokari T, Salo J, Eerola E, et al: Cranberry juice and bacterial colonization in children—A placebo-controlled randomized trial. *Clin Nutr* 2005; 24:1065–1072.

Larcombe J: Urinary tract infection in children. *Clin Evid* 2004;Jun(11): 509–523.

Lutter SA, Currie ML, Mitz LB, et al: Antibiotic resistance patterns in children hospitalized for urinary tract infections. *Arch Pediatr Adolesc Med* 2005;159:924–928.

McGillivray D, Mok E, Mulroney E, et al: A head-to-head comparison: "Clean-void" bag versus catheter urinalysis in the diagnosis of urinary tract infection in young children. *J Pediatr* 2005;147:451–456.

Michael M, Hodson EM, Craig JC, et al: Short compared with standard duration of antibiotic treatment for urinary tract infections: A systematic review of randomized controlled trials. *Arch Dis Child* 2002;87:118–123.

Modgil G, Baverstock A: Should bubble baths be avoided in children with urinary tract infections? *Arch Dis Child* 2006;91:863–865.

Peratoner L, Pennesi M, Bordugo A, et al: Kidney length and scarring in children with urinary tract infection: Importance of ultrasound scans. *Abdom Imaging* 2005;30:780–785.

Polito C, Rambaldi PF, Signoriello G, et al: Permanent renal parenchymal defects after febrile UTI are closely associated with vesicoureteric reflux. *Pediatr Nephrol* 2006;21:521–526.

Shah G, Upadhyay J: Controversies in the diagnosis and management of urinary tract infections in children. *Paediatr Drugs* 2005;7:339–346.

Shaikh N, Abedin S, Docimo SG: Can ultrasonography or uroflowmetry predict which children with voiding dysfunction will have recurrent urinary tract infections? *J Urol* 2005;174:1620–1622.

Singh-Grewal D, Macdessi J, Craig J: Circumcision for the prevention of urinary tract infection in boys: A systematic review of randomised trials and observational studies. *Arch Dis Child* 2005;90:853–858.

Siomou E, Papadopoulou F, Kollios KD, et al: Duplex collecting system diagnosed during the first 6 years of life after a first urinary tract infection: A study of 63 children. *J Urol* 2006;175:678–681.

Struthers S, Scanlon J, Parker K, et al: Parental reporting of smelly urine and urinary tract infection. *Arch Dis Child* 2003;88:250–252.

Thompson RH, Dicks D, Kramer SA: Clinical manifestations and functional outcomes in children with eosinophilic cystitis. *J Urol* 2005;174: 2347–2349.

Tseng MH, Lin WJ, Lo WT, et al: Does a normal DMSA obviate the performance of voiding cystourethrography in evaluation of young children after their first urinary tract infection? *J Pediatr* 2007;150:96–99.

Westwood ME, Whiting PF, Cooper J, et al: Further investigation of confirmed urinary tract infection (UTI) in children under five years: A systematic review. *BMC Pediatr* 2005;5:2.

Zamir G, Sakran W, Horowitz Y, et al: Urinary tract infection: Is there a need for routine renal ultrasonography? *Arch Dis Child* 2004;89:466–468.

Zhanel GG, Hisanaga TL, Laing NM, et al: Antibiotic resistance in outpatient urinary isolates: Final results from the North American Urinary Tract Infection Collaborative Alliance (NAUTICA). *Int J Antimicrob Agents* 2005; 26:380–388.

Zorc JJ, Levine DA, Platt SL, et al: Clinical and demographic factors associated with urinary tract infection in young febrile infants. *Pediatrics* 2005;116:644–648.

Capitolo 539 ■ Reflusso vescicoureterale

Jack S. Elder

Il flusso retrogrado di urina dalla vescica nell'uretere e nella pelvi renale è definito **reflusso vescicoureterale**. L'uretere normalmente si connette alla vescica in direzione obliqua, perforando il muscolo detrusore lateralmente e proseguendo tra la mucosa vescicale e il muscolo detrusore, in modo da creare un meccanismo a valvola (lembo valvolare) che previene il reflusso (Fig. 539-1). Il reflusso si verifica quando il tunnel sottomucoso tra la mucosa e il muscolo detrusore è breve o assente ed esso è di solito congenito, familiare e interessa l'1% circa dei bambini.

Il reflusso predispone all'infezione renale (pielonefrite) facilitando il trasporto dei batteri dalla vescica alle vie urinarie superiori (vedi Capitolo 538). La reazione infiammatoria causata da un'infezione pielonefritica può portare a un danno renale (*scarring*), denominato anche **nefropatia da reflusso**. Uno *scarring* renale esteso altera la funzione renale e può condurre a ipertensione renino-mediata (vedi Capitolo 445), insufficienza renale o nefropatia terminale (vedi Capitolo 535), ridotto accrescimento staturoponderale e morbilità durante la gravidanza. La nefropatia da reflusso un tempo era responsabile di almeno il 15-20% dei casi di nefropatia terminale nei bambini e

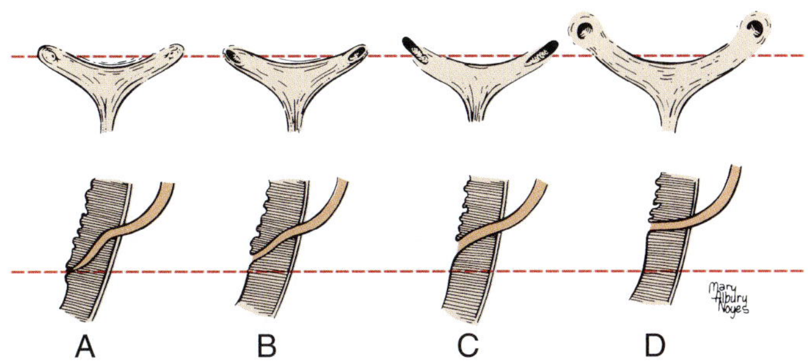

Figura 539-1. Configurazione normale e anomala degli orifizi ureterali. Da sinistra a destra, si osserva un progressivo spostamento laterale degli orifizi ureterali e l'accorciamento del tunnel intramurale. In alto, aspetto endoscopico. In basso, immagine sagittale attraverso l'uretere intramurale.

nei giovani adulti. Con una maggiore attenzione al trattamento delle infezioni delle vie urinarie (IVU) e il miglioramento delle conoscenze del reflusso, la nefropatia terminale secondaria a nefropatia da reflusso è divenuta rara. La nefropatia da reflusso resta una della cause più comuni di ipertensione nel bambino. Il reflusso in assenza di infezione o di elevata pressione vescicale non causa danno renale.

CLASSIFICAZIONE. La gravità del reflusso è classificata utilizzando la Classificazione Internazionale di Studio in gradi da I a V e si basa sull'aspetto delle vie urinarie alla cistouretrografia minzionale con contrasto (VCUG, *Voiding CystoUrethroGram*) (Figg. 539-2 e 539-3). Maggiore è il grado di reflusso, più alta è la probabilità di un danno renale. La serietà del reflusso è un'indicazione indiretta del grado dell'anomalia della giunzione ureterovescicale. Il reflusso può essere primario o secondario (Tab. 539-1). Il reflusso vescicoureterale primario deriva da una deformità anatomica della giunzione ureterovescicale (vedi Fig. 539-1). Un'instabilità vescicale può accelerare il reflusso o peggiorarne uno preesistente, se è presente una giunzione ureterovescicale solo marginalmente competente. Nei casi più gravi, si manifesta un reflusso talmente massivo nelle alte vie urinarie da sviluppare una sovradistensione della vescica. Questa condizione, la **sindrome megacisti-megauretere**, si verifica primariamente nel maschio e può essere unilaterale o bilaterale (Fig. 539-4). Il reimpianto degli ureteri nella vescica per correggere il reflusso risolve la situazione.

Circa un bambino su 125 presenta una **duplicazione** del tratto urinario superiore in cui il rene è drenato da due ureteri anziché da uno. La duplicazione può essere parziale o completa: nella duplicazione parziale, gli ureteri si uniscono al di sopra della vescica ed è presente un solo orifizio ureterale, mentre nella duplicazione completa, l'inserimento dell'uretere del polo inferiore alla vescica è superolaterale rispetto all'uretere del polo superiore. Il meccanismo a valvola dell'uretere del polo inferiore spesso è scarsamente interessato, e in almeno il 50% dei casi si verifica un reflusso nell'uretere inferiore. In alcuni individui si verifica un reflusso sia nel sistema inferiore sia in quello superiore (Fig. 539-5). Nelle anomalie di duplicazione, alcuni pazienti hanno un uretere ectopico, in cui l'uretere del polo superiore drena al di fuori della vescica (vedi Capitolo 540). Se l'uretere ectopico drena nel collo vescicale, in genere esso è ostruito ed è sede di reflusso. Le anomalie di duplicazione sono comuni anche nei bambini con ureterocele (una dilatazione cistica della porzione intramurale dell'uretere distale) e in questi pazienti è spesso presente un reflusso nell'uretere associato del polo inferiore o nell'uretere controlaterale. Il reflusso è di solito presente anche quando l'uretere sbocca in un diverticolo vescicale (Fig. 539-6).

Un reflusso è presente alla nascita nel 25% dei bambini con **vescica neurologica**, come avviene nel mielomeningocele, nell'agenesia sacrale e in molti bambini con ano imperforato alto. Un reflusso si osserva anche nel 50% dei maschi con valvole uretrali posteriori. Clinicamente, un reflusso con aumento della pressione intravescicale (come nella dissinergia sfintero-detrusoriale o

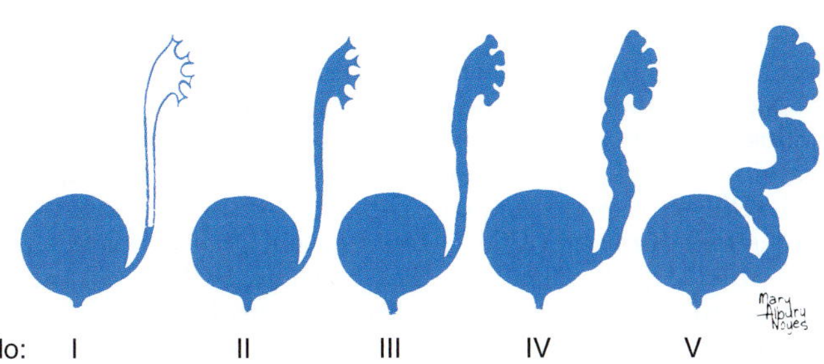

Figura 539-2. Gradi del reflusso vescicoureterale. Grado I: reflusso in uretere non dilatato. Grado II: reflusso nel sistema collettore superiore senza dilatazione. Grado III: reflusso in uretere dilatato e/o appiattimento dei fornici caliciali. Grado IV: reflusso in uretere grossolanamente dilatato. Grado V: reflusso massivo, con significativa dilatazione ureterale e tortuosità e perdita dell'impressione papillare.

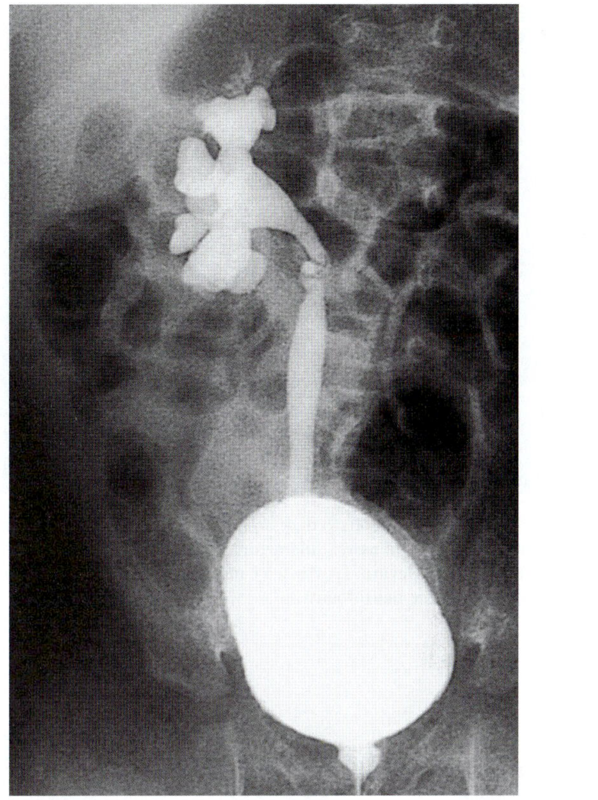

Figura 539-3. Cistouretrografia minzionale (VCUG) che evidenzia un reflusso vescicoureterale destro di IV grado con reflusso intrarenale.

TABELLA 539-1. Classificazione del reflusso vescicoureterale

TIPO	CAUSA
Primario	Incompetenza congenita del meccanismo valvolare della giunzione vescicoureterale
Primario associato ad altre malformazioni della giunzione ureterovescicale	Duplicazione ureterale
	Ureterocele con duplicazione
	Ectopia ureterale
	Diverticoli paraureterali
Secondario ad aumento della pressione vescicale	Vescica neurologica
Disfunzione vescicale non neurologica	Cistite batterica severa
Ostruzione dell'efflusso vescicale	Chirurgia della giunzione ureterovescicale
Secondario a processi infiammatori	
Corpi estranei	
Litiasi vescicale	
Cistite clinica	
Secondario a procedure chirurgiche	

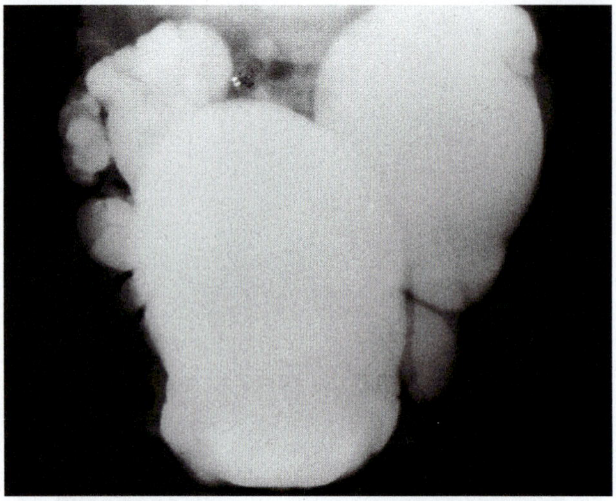

Figura 539-4. VCUG in neonato di sesso maschile con sindrome del megacisti-megauretere. Si noti la massiva dilatazione ureterale dovuta al reflusso vescicoureterale di grado elevato. La vescica è molto distesa e non vi era ostruzione uretrale o disfunzione neurologica.

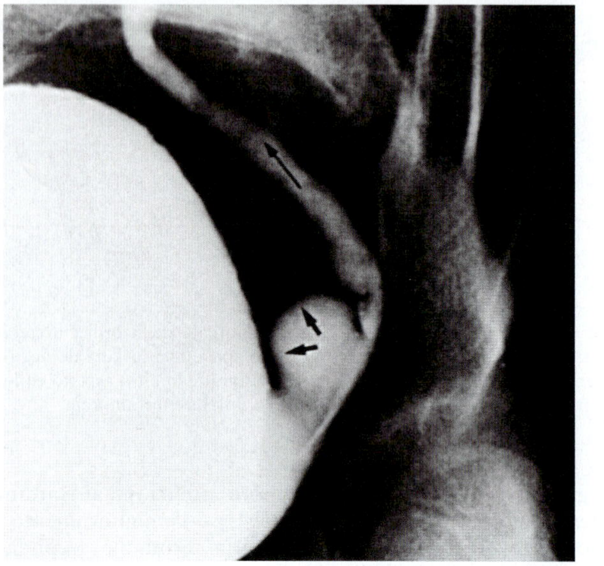

Figura 539-6. Reflusso e diverticolo vescicale. La cistouretrografia minzionale dimostra un reflusso vescicoureterale sinistro e un diverticolo paraureterale.

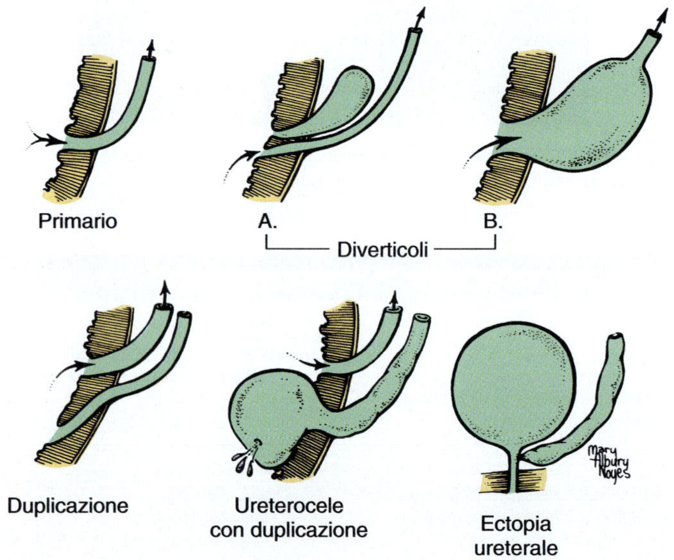

Figura 539-5. Differenti anomalie anatomiche della giunzione ureterovescicale associata a reflusso vescicoureterale.

ostruzione dell'efflusso vescicale) può portare a un danno renale, anche in assenza di infezione.

Il reflusso primario si verifica in associazione a diverse anomalie congenite delle vie urinarie: per esempio, il 15% dei bambini con rene displasico multicistico o con agenesia renale mostra un reflusso nel rene controlaterale, mentre il 10-15% dei bambini con ostruzione della giunzione ureteropelvica presenta un reflusso nel rene idronefrosico oppure nel rene controlaterale.

Il reflusso sembra essere un disordine ereditario autosomico dominante. Circa il 35% dei fratelli o sorelle dei bambini affetti da reflusso ne manifesta uno, inoltre un reflusso è presente in circa la metà dei fratelli o delle sorelle neonati. La probabilità che un fratello o una sorella abbia un reflusso è indipendente dal grado del reflusso o dal sesso del caso indice. Circa il 12% dei fratelli o sorelle con reflusso asintomatici presenta evidenze di *scarring* renale. Di conseguenza, molti ritengono che i fratelli o le sorelle di bambini con reflusso debbano essere sottoposti a screening anche se non hanno avuto un'IVU. Inoltre, anche il 50% dei bambini nati da donne con un'anamnesi di reflusso ne manifesta uno. È appropriato lo screening con una scinticistografia di tutti i fratelli o sorelle di 3 anni o meno e di qualsiasi fratello o sorella con un'IVU. Tuttavia, non vi sono linee guida generali per quanto riguarda i figli o i fratelli. I fratelli o sorelle più grandi possono essere sottoposti a ecografia renale e, se viene diagnosticata un'anomalia come un'idronefrosi o una differenza nella lunghezza dei reni, si raccomanda l'esecuzione di una VCUG. Il reflusso primitivo è meno comune negli afromericani.

MANIFESTAZIONI CLINICHE. Il reflusso viene di solito diagnosticato nel corso di una valutazione per un'IVU (vedi Capitolo 538). Tra bambini con reflusso, l'80% è di sesso femminile la cui età media alla diagnosi è di 2-3 anni. In altri bambini, si esegue una VCUG nel corso di una valutazione per disfunzione minzionale, insufficienza renale, ipertensione o altri sospetti processi patologici delle vie urinarie. Un reflusso primario può essere scoperto anche durante la valutazione per un'idronefrosi prenatale. In questo campione selezionato, l'80% dei bambini affetti è di sesso maschile, inoltre il grado di reflusso di solito è più elevato che nelle femmine in cui la diagnosi è stata posta in seguito a un'IVU. Il reflusso si risolve dopo la nascita nella maggior parte dei pazienti in cui la diagnosi è stata prenatale. Tuttavia, sono indicati ripetuti esami ecografici dopo la nascita per dimostrare la risoluzione dell'idronefrosi.

DIAGNOSI. La diagnosi di reflusso di solito richiede il cateterismo vescicale, l'instillazione di una soluzione contenente mezzo di contrasto iodato o un radiofarmaco e l'imaging radiologico del tratto urinario superiore e inferiore, rispettivamente una VCUG con contrasto o una VCUG con radionuclidi. La vescica e le vie urinarie superiori vengono visualizzate nel corso del riempimento vescicale e della minzione. Un reflusso che si verifica nel corso del riempimento vescicale è definito reflusso *a bassa pressione* o *passivo*; un reflusso durante la minzione è chiamato invece reflusso *ad alta pressione* o *attivo*. I bambini con reflusso passivo hanno una minore probabilità di avere una risoluzione spontanea del reflusso rispetto a quelli con uno attivo. L'esposizione alle radiazioni durante la VCUG con radionuclidi è significativamente inferiore a quella che si verifica con una VCUG con mezzo di contrasto. Tuttavia, gli studi con contrasto forniscono maggiori informazioni anatomiche, come la dimostrazione di un sistema collettore duplice, di un uretere ectopico, di un diverticolo paraureterale (vescicale), di un'ostruzione dell'efflusso vescicale nei maschi, di una stasi del tratto urinario superiore e di segni di disfunzione minzionale come un'uretra a "spinning top" nelle femmine. Il sistema di classificazione del reflusso per gradi si basa sull'aspetto alla VCUG. Di conseguenza, in molti centri la VCUG viene usata come studio iniziale. Per il follow-up, si preferisce spesso la cistografia con radionuclidi a causa della bassa esposizione alle radiazioni (Fig. 539-7), anche se può essere difficile determinare se la gravità del reflusso sia cambiata.

I bambini sottoposti a cistografia possono essere traumatizzati psicologicamente dal cateterismo. Una preparazione accurata da parte dei genitori o la somministrazione di midazolam per os o per via nasale (per sedazione e amnesia) o di propofol prima dell'esame possono risultare in un'esperienza meno stressante.

La **cistografia indiretta** è una tecnica diagnostica per il reflusso senza cateterismo che comprende l'iniezione iv di un radiofarmaco, il quale, essendo eliminato a livello renale, passa nella vescica. Ciò permette di visualizzare il tratto urinario inferiore mentre il paziente urina; tuttavia, questa tecnica identifica soltanto il 75% dei casi di reflusso. Un'altra tecnica che evita l'esposizione alle radiazioni comprende l'instillazione di mezzo di contrasto ecografico attraverso un catetere uretrale: i reni vengono visualizzati ecograficamente e il vantaggio risiede nell'assenza di radiazioni, benché essa sia meno accurata della VCUG con contrasto e non sia possibile la classificazione del grado del reflusso.

Dopo la diagnosi del reflusso e la sua classificazione come grado e se primario o secondario, è importante analizzare le vie urinarie superiori. Lo scopo dell'imaging delle vie urinarie superiori è di valutare la presenza di *scarring* renale e di anomalie associate delle vie urinarie. L'imaging renale può essere eseguito attraverso un'ecografia renale, una scintigrafia renale, un'urografia escretoria (pielografia intravenosa [IVP, *IntraVenous Pielogram*]) o una TC. La scintigrafia renale può mostrare se è presente uno *scarring* renale significativo o se è presente una condizione anatomica che predisponga a IVU, come un'ostruzione della giunzione ureteropelvica o della giunzione ureterovescicale, o un'anomalia di duplicazione renale con un'ostruzione ureterale; inoltre l'ecografia permette al medico di monitorare la crescita renale nel tempo. La scintigrafia renale viene di solito eseguita con acido dimercaptosuccinico (DMSA), che consente di evidenziare i dettagli della corticale renale e che è affidabile nel dimostrare virtualmente tutte le cicatrici renali come anche un'infezione acuta del parenchima renale; tuttavia, non è affidabile per quanto riguarda la dimostrazione di un'idronefrosi. La IVP comprende l'iniezione di mezzo di contrasto iodato e fornisce buoni dettagli anatomici del rene, ma questo esame viene eseguito raramente nei bambini, in quanto difficilmente fornisce altre informazioni. Solo occasionalmente si esegue una TC durante la valutazione per una IVU. Questo esame fornisce informazioni simili a quelle degli esami discussi in precedenza, ma comprende una significativa esposizione alle radiazioni.

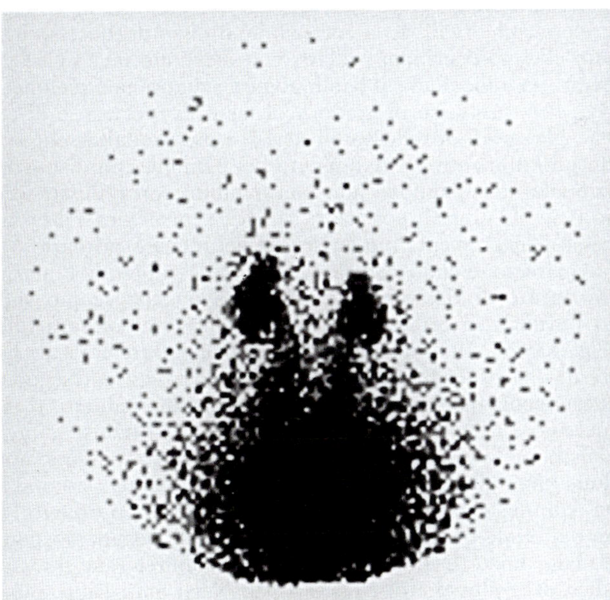

Figura 539-7. Cistografia con radionuclidi che evidenzia un reflusso bilaterale.

Il bambino deve essere valutato per una disfunzione minzionale, comprese urgenza, pollachiuria, incontinenza diurna, minzione infrequente o un'associazione di queste. Devono essere valutate le caratteristiche dell'alvo. I bambini con instabilità vescicale spesso vengono sottoposti a un regime di training vescicale (minzione a intervalli regolari) e, occasionalmente, a terapia anticolinergici oltre a profilassi antibiotica.

Dopo la diagnosi, devono essere determinate e monitorate altezza, peso e pressione arteriosa del bambino. Se l'imaging delle vie urinarie superiori evidenzia la presenza di cicatrici renali, occorre determinare la creatinina sierica. Occorre ricercare nelle urine un'infezione o una proteinuria. La cistoscopia non è utile ai fini prognostici o nella scelta del trattamento, come non è vantaggiosa la dilatazione uretrale.

STORIA NATURALE. L'incidenza di cicatrici renali o di nefropatia da reflusso aumenta con il grado del reflusso e, con la crescita e la maturazione vescicale, vi è una tendenza alla risoluzione di esso o al miglioramento nel tempo. Il reflusso di basso grado ha una maggiore probabilità di risoluzione del reflusso di grado elevato. Per i gradi I e II, la probabilità di risoluzione è simile indipendentemente dall'età alla diagnosi e dal fatto che sia unilaterale o bilaterale. Per il grado III, un'età più bassa alla diagnosi e un reflusso unilaterale sono di solito associati a tasso più elevato di risoluzione spontanea (Fig. 539-8). Il reflusso bilaterale di grado IV ha una probabilità molto minore di risolversi rispetto a un

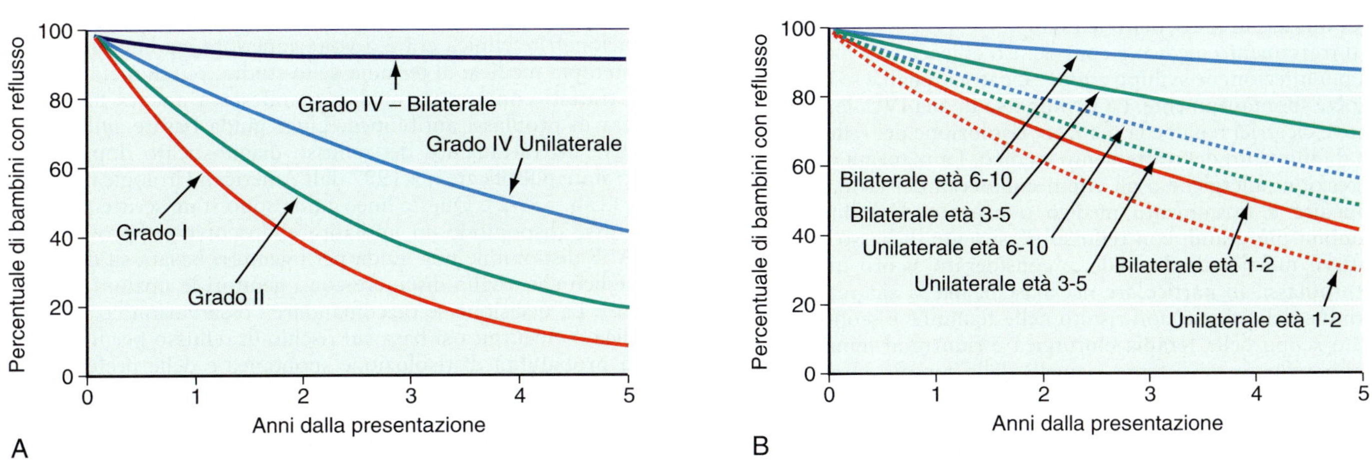

Figura 539-8. *A*, Probabilità percentuale di persistenza del reflusso, gradi I, II e IV, per 1-5 anni dopo la presentazione. *B*, Probabilità percentuale di persistenza del reflusso per età di presentazione, grado III, per 1-5 anni dopo la presentazione. (Da Elder JS, Peters CA, Arant BS Jr, et al: Pediatric Vesicoureteral Reflux Guidelines Panel Summary Report on the management of primary vesicoureteral reflux in children. *J Urol* 1997;157:1846-1851.)

medesimo grado di reflusso unilaterale. Il reflusso di grado V raramente va incontro a risoluzione. L'età media alla risoluzione del reflusso è 6 anni. Anche se non è probabile che il reflusso causi un danno renale in assenza di infezione, nelle situazioni con reflusso ad alta pressione, come nei bambini con valvole uretrali posteriori, vescica neurologica e vescica neurogena non neurogena (sindrome di Hinman), un reflusso sterile può provocare un danno renale significativo. I bambini con reflusso di grado elevato che sviluppano un'IVU hanno un rischio significativo di pielonefrite e di *scarring* renale.

TRATTAMENTO. Gli obiettivi del trattamento sono la prevenzione della pielonefrite, del danno renale e di altre complicanze del reflusso. La terapia medica si basa sul principio che il reflusso spesso si risolve nel tempo e che la morbilità o le complicanze possono essere prevenute senza ricorrere alla chirurgia. La base della terapia chirurgica risiede nel fatto che, in bambini selezionati, un reflusso persistente ha provocato o possiede la potenzialità di causare un danno renale o altre complicanze correlate al reflusso, oltre al fatto che l'eliminazione del reflusso minimizza la probabilità di tali complicanze.

In base ad alcuni studi preliminari che dimostrano l'efficacia della profilassi antibiotica nel ridurre il rischio delle complicanze del reflusso, la profilassi giornaliera continua è stata la pietra angolare del trattamento iniziale dei bambini con reflusso. I farmaci comunemente usati per la profilassi comprendono sulfametoxazolo-trimetoprim, trimetoprim e nitrofurantoina, generalmente somministrati a 1/4-1/3 della dose necessaria per trattare un'infezione acuta. La profilassi viene di solito continuata finché il reflusso non si risolve o fino a quando il rischio di reflusso per il paziente non è considerato minimo. Devono essere valutate le abitudini del bambino rispetto alla minzione e all'evacuazione, e occorre trattare la stipsi nonché qualsiasi disfunzione della minzione (vedi Capitolo 543). Se sono presenti segni o sintomi di IVU occorre eseguire un'urinocultura. Ogni 12-18 mesi si esegue una VCUG (con contrasto o radionuclidi). Per monitorare lo status delle vie urinarie superiori si deve effettuare periodicamente un imaging delle vie urinarie superiori. Una valutazione clinica di follow-up deve essere eseguita almeno annualmente, e nella stessa occasione si registrano peso, altezza e pressione arteriosa del bambino.

Sono state sollevate obiezioni sui rischi e sull'efficacia della profilassi antibiotica rispetto alla terapia intermittente (accurato monitoraggio e pronta terapia antibiotica per le IVU). Che la terapia intermittente sia sicura non è provato; attualmente sono in corso trial clinici prospettici coordinati dal NIH, come anche in Svezia. Studi retrospettivi non randomizzati hanno dimostrato che l'interruzione della terapia antibiotica nei bambini con reflusso persistente di basso grado e con funzione vescicale normale di solito è sicura nel breve termine, ma non sono stati effettuati studi longitudinali che abbiano preso in considerazione anche l'età adulta, in particolare le donne.

Il trattamento medico è considerato efficace se il bambino non ha più infezioni né sviluppa nuove cicatrici renali e se il reflusso si risolve spontaneamente. La ricomparsa di una IVU, lo sviluppo di nuove cicatrici renali e la mancata risoluzione del reflusso indicano il fallimento del trattamento medico. La mancata compliance, le reazioni allergiche o gli effetti collaterali dei farmaci possono impedire il trattamento medico o causarne il fallimento. Nei bambini più grandi con reflusso persistente di basso grado e un pattern minzionale normale, è considerato sicuro interrompere la profilassi, in particolare nei maschi, ma la sicurezza a lungo termine del reflusso non risolto nelle femmine è sconosciuta.

Lo scopo della terapia chirurgica è ridurre al minimo i rischi di un reflusso persistente e quelli della terapia non chirurgica (profilassi ed esami di follow-up). La terapia chirurgica è riservata ai bambini per i quali la terapia medica è inefficace. La correzione del reflusso può essere ottenuta sia mediante un'incisione addominale bassa o inguinale, sia laparoscopicamente o cistoscopicamente. Il trattamento chirurgico aperto comprende la modifica della normale inserzione ureterovescicale per creare un rapporto tra lunghezza dell'uretere intramurale e diametro ureterale di 4:1-5:1. Le tecniche comprendono l'apertura della vescica (intervento di Politano-Leadbetter, transtrigonale di Cohen, Glenn-Anderson), mentre altri eseguono la correzione del reflusso mediante un approccio extravescicale (detrusorrafia di Lich-Gregoir). Se è presente una semplice anomalia di duplicazione, si reimpiantano insieme entrambi gli ureteri con un impianto noto come *reimpianto con guaina comune*. Quando si corregge un reflusso associato a dilatazione ureterale severa (cioè un megauretere), l'uretere deve essere adattato o ristretto a dimensioni più normali per ottenere un normale rapporto lunghezza:ampiezza per il tunnel intramurale e un angolo vescicale viene connesso al tendine dello psoas formando uno *psoas hitch*. Se il rene con reflusso ha una funzionalità scarsa, è indicata la nefrectomia o la nefroureterectomia. È in corso di valutazione la correzione laparoscopica del reflusso sia attraverso la vescica (*vescicoscopica*) sia con approccio extravescicale.

L'intervento chirurgico aperto viene eseguito nei bambini in cui il trattamento medico non è efficace, compresi quelli con IVU in corso di trattamento, reflusso persistente e reflusso di grado IV o V. Le perdite ematiche sono minime e la degenza ospedaliera è in media di 1-2 giorni. Il tasso di successo nei bambini con reflusso primario è superiore al 95-98% per i gradi da I a IV, nel 2% è presente un reflusso persistente e nell'1% è presente un'ostruzione ureterale che richiede la correzione. Il tasso di successo è così elevato che molti urologi pediatri non eseguono una VCUG postoperatoria a meno che il bambino non sviluppi una pielonefrite clinica. Per il reflusso di grado V, il tasso di successo è di circa l'80%. Nei gradi di reflusso più bassi, è più probabile che si verifichi un fallimento del reimpianto nei bambini con disfunzione minzionale non diagnosticata. Nei bambini con reflusso secondario (valvole uretrali posteriori, vescica neurologica), il tasso di successo è leggermente più basso che nel reflusso primario.

La riparazione endoscopica del reflusso comprende l'iniezione di un agente di riempimento attraverso un cistoscopio subito sotto l'orifizio ureterale, creando un lembo valvolare artificiale (Fig. 539-9). Il vantaggio dell'iniezione subureterale è che si tratta di una procedura ambulatoriale non invasiva (eseguita in anestesia generale) senza necessità di tempo di recupero. Il tasso di successo è del 70-80% ed è più elevato per i reflussi di grado più basso. Se la prima iniezione non ha successo, possono essere eseguite una o due altre iniezioni. Nell'ottobre 2001, la Food and Drug Administration (FDA) degli Stati Uniti ha approvato l'uso di un materiale biodegradabile, microsfere di destano sospese in acido ialuronico (Deflux), per l'iniezione subureterale. Il tasso di recidiva del reflusso è di circa il 10%. Negli Stati Uniti, più del 40% degli interventi antireflusso viene eseguito con questo tipo di procedura (Fig. 539-10).

L'International Reflux Study ha dimostrato che nei bambini con reflusso di grado da III a IV, dopo 5 anni di terapia medica o chirurgica, si sono avuti risultati simili rispetto alla formazione di nuove cicatrici renali e della funzione renale. Tuttavia, l'incidenza di pielonefrite clinica era 2,5 volte superiore nei bambini trattati con terapia medica; al termine dello studio, più di metà dei bambini trattati con terapia medica manifestava ancora un reflusso ed era in profilassi antibiotica. Linee guida basate sull'evidenza relative al trattamento del reflusso diagnosticato dopo un'IVU sono state pubblicate nel 1997 dall'American Urological Association (Tab. 539-2). Queste linee guida sono state scritte prima che divenisse disponibile un impianto endoscopico approvato dalla FDA. È disponibile una guida per i genitori basata su di esse per il medico che voglia discutere con i genitori le opzioni di trattamento. La decisione se raccomandare l'osservazione o la terapia medica o chirurgica si basa sul rischio di reflusso per il paziente, sulla probabilità di risoluzione spontanea e delle preferenze dei genitori del paziente.

Afshar K, Papanikolaou F, Malek R, et al: Vesicoureteral reflux and complete ureteral duplication. Conservative or surgical management? *J Urol* 2005;173:1725–1727.

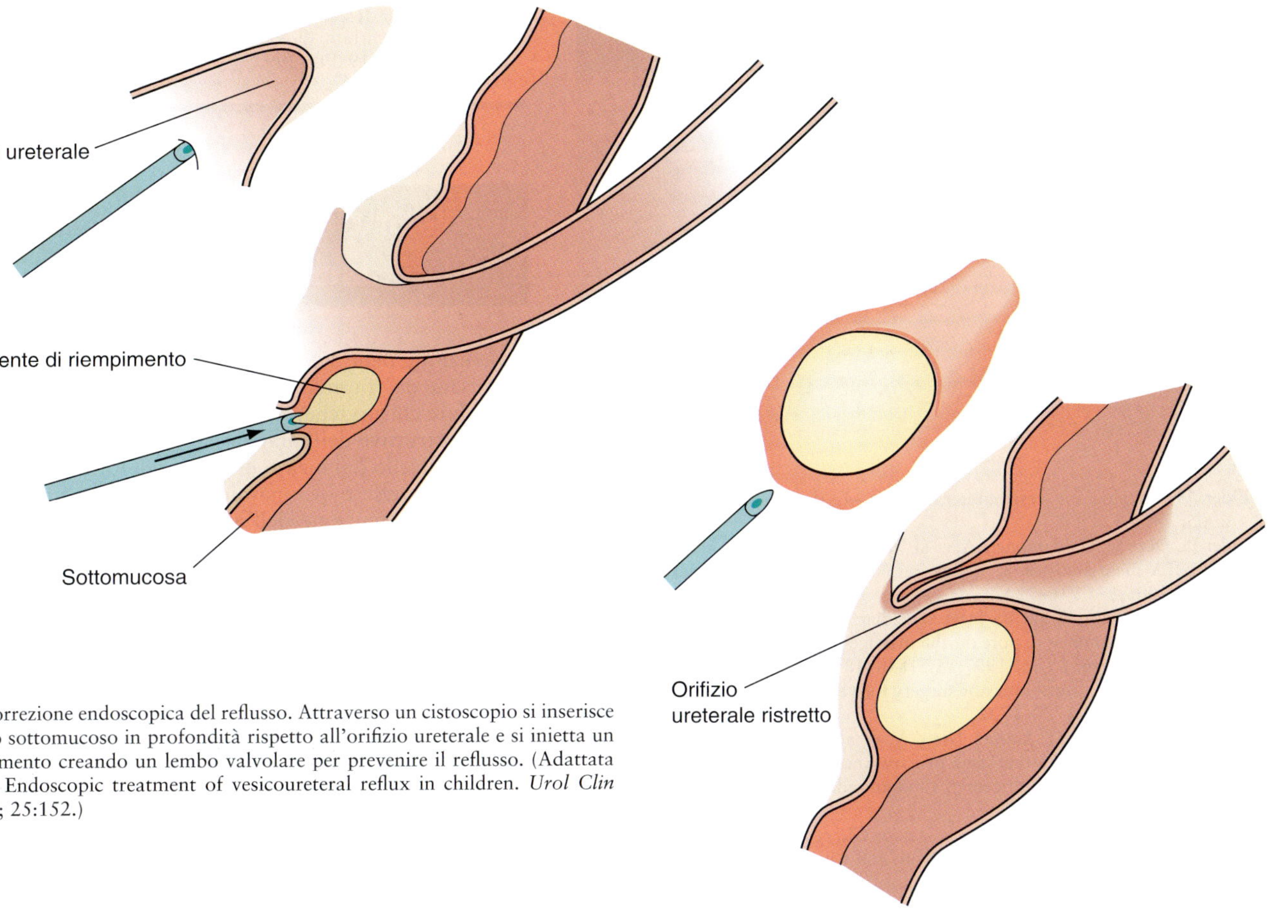

Figura 539-9. Correzione endoscopica del reflusso. Attraverso un cistoscopio si inserisce un ago nel piano sottomucoso in profondità rispetto all'orifizio ureterale e si inietta un agente di riempimento creando un lembo valvolare per prevenire il reflusso. (Adattata da Ortenberg J: Endoscopic treatment of vesicoureteral reflux in children. *Urol Clin North Am* 1998; 25:152.)

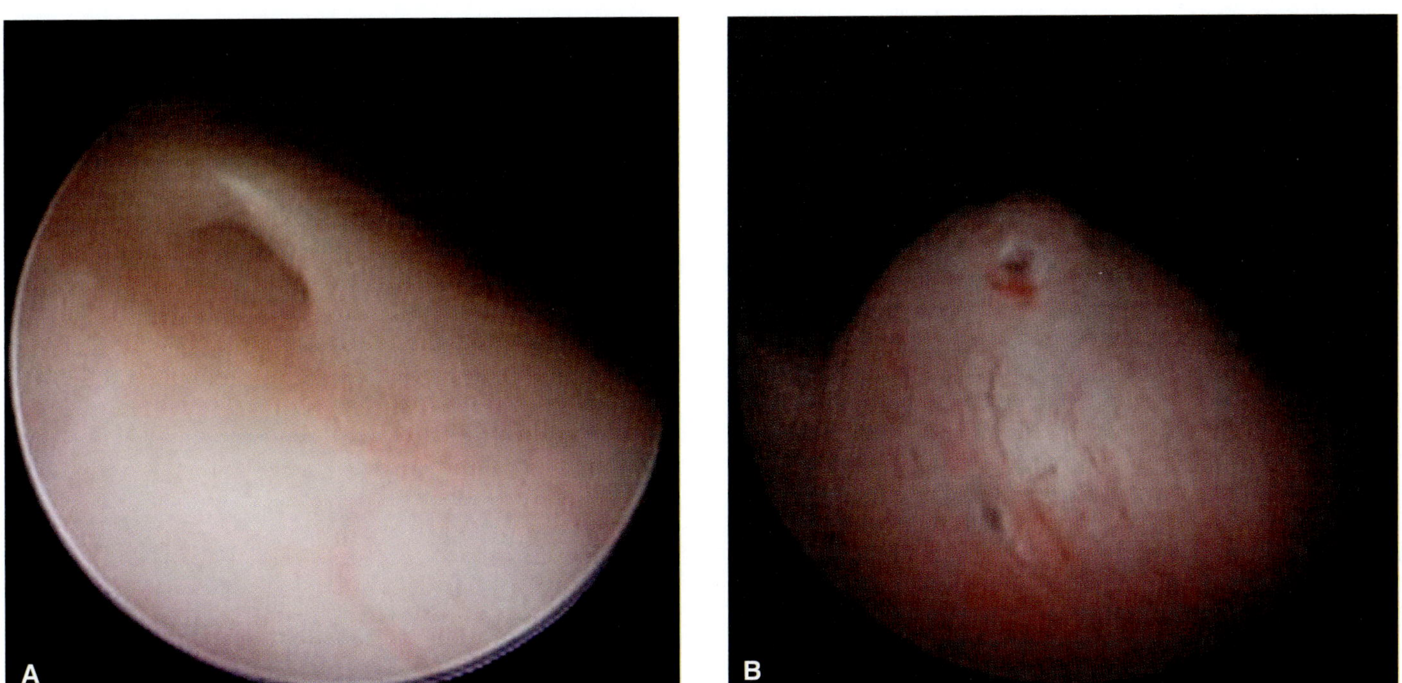

Figura 539-10. *A*, Immagine endoscopica di un uretere destro con reflusso. *B*, Lo stesso uretere dopo iniezione subureterale di microsfere di dextranomero.

Al-Sayyad AJ, Pike JG, Leonard MP: Can prophylactic antibiotics safely be discontinued in children with vesicoureteral reflux? *J Urol* 2005; 174:1587–1589.

Charbonneau SG, Tackett LD, Gray EH, et al: Is long-term sonographic follow-up necessary after uncomplicated ureteral reimplantation in children? *J Urol* 2005;174:1429–1431.

Chen HW, Yuan SSF, Lin CJ: Ureteral reimplantation for vesicoureteral reflux: Comparison of minimally invasive extravesical with transvesical and conventional extravesical techniques. *Urology* 2004;63:364–368.

Edmondson JD, Maizels M, Alpert SA, et al: Multi-institutional experience with PIC cystography—Incidence of occult vesicoureteral reflux in Children with febrile urinary tract infections. *Urology* 2006;67:608–611.

TABELLA 539-2. Trattamento consigliato del reflusso vescicoureterale diagnosticato dopo un'infezione delle vie urinarie*

GRADO	ETÀ (ANNI)	SCARRING	TRATTAMENTO INIZIALE	FOLLOW-UP
I-II	Qualsiasi	Sì/No	Profilassi antibiotica	Assenza di consenso
III-IV	0-5	Sì/No	Profilassi antibiotica	Chirurgia
III-IV	6-10	Sì/No	Unilaterale: profilassi antibiotica Bilaterale: chirurgia	Chirurgia
V	<1	Sì/No	Profilassi antibiotica	Chirurgia
V	1-5	No	Unilaterale: profilassi antibiotica	Chirurgia
V	1-5	No	Bilaterale: chirurgia	
V	1-5	Sì		Chirurgia
V	6-10	Sì/No		Chirurgia

*Riassunto delle linee guida sviluppate dalla American Urological Association; l'età si riferisce all'età al momento della diagnosi.

Elder JS: Imaging for vesicoureteral reflux—Is there a better way? *J Urol* 2005; 74:7–8.
Elder JS, Diaz M, Caldamone AA, et al: Endoscopic therapy for vesicoureteral reflux: A meta-analysis. I. Reflux resolution and urinary tract infection. *J Urol* 2006;175:716–722.
Elder JS, Peters CA, Arant BS Jr, et al: Pediatric Vesicoureteral Reflux Guidelines Panel Summary Report on the management of primary vesicoureteral reflux in children. *J Urol* 1997;157:1846–1851.
Fanos V, Cataldi L: Antibiotics or surgery for vesicoureteric reflux in children. *Lancet* 2004;364:1720–1722.
Garin EH, Olavarria F, Garcia Nieto V, et al: Clinical significance of primary vesicoureteral reflux and urinary antibiotic prophylaxis after acute pyelonephritis: A multicenter, randomized, controlled study. *Pediatrics* 2006;117:626–632.
Georgaki-Angelaki H, Kostaridou S, Daikos GL, et al: Long-term follow-up of children with vesicoureteral reflux with and without antibiotic prophylaxis. *Scand J Infect Dis* 2005;37:842–845.
Giel DW, Noe HN, Williams MA: Ultrasound screening of asymptomatic siblings of children with vesicoureteral reflux: A long-term follow-up study. *J Urol* 2005;174:1602–1604.
Hollowell JG: Screening siblings for vesicoureteral reflux. *J Urol* 2002; 168:2138–2141.
Ismaili K, Hall M, Piepsz A, et al: Primary vesicoureteral reflux detached in neonates with a history of fetal renal pelvis dilation: A prospective clinical and imaging study. *J Pediatr* 2006;148:222–227.
Jodal U, Smellie JM, Lax H, et al: Ten-year results of randomized treatment of children with severe vesicoureteral reflux. Final report of the International Reflux Study in Children. *Pediatr Nephrol* 2006;2006:785–792.
Kajbafzadeh AM, Habibi Z, Tajik P, et al: Endoscopic subureteral Urocol injection for the treatment of vesicoureteral reflux. *J Urol* 2006;175: 1480–1483.
Leroy S, Marc E, Adamsbaum C, et al: Prediction of vesicoureteral reflux after a first febrile urinary tract infection in children: Validation of a clinical decision rule. *Arch Dis Child* 2006;91:241–244.
Moorthy I, Easty M, McHigh K, et al: The presence of vesicoureteric reflux does not identify a population at risk for renal scarring following a first urinary tract infection. *Arch Dis Child* 2005;90:733–736.
Putman S, Wicher C, Wayment R, et al: Unilateral extravesical ureteral reimplantation in children performed on an outpatient basis. *J Urol* 2005;174:1987–1989.
Routh JC, Vandersteen DR, Pfefferle H, et al: Single center experience with endoscopic management of vesicoureteral reflux in children. *J Urol* 2006;175:1889–1892.
Thompson M, Simon SD, Sharma V, et al: Timing of follow-up voiding cystourethrogram in children with primary vesicoureteral reflux: Development and application of a clinical algorithm. *Pediatrics* 2005;115:426–434.
Tombesi M, Ferrari CM, Bertolotti JJ: Renal damage in refluxing and nonrefluxing siblings of index children with vesicoureteral reflux. *Pediatr Nephrol* 2005;20:1201–1202.
Van Capelle JW, De Haan T, El Sayed W, et al: The long-term outcome of the endoscopic subureteric implantation of polydimethylsiloxane for treating vesico-ureteric reflux in children: A retrospective analysis of the first 195 consecutive patients in two European centres. *BUJ Int* 2004;94:1348–1351.
Venhola M, Huttunen MP, Uhari M: Meta-analysis of vesicoureteral reflux and urinary tract infection in children. *Scand J Urol Nephrol* 2006; 40:98–102.
Wheeler D, Vimalachandra D, Hodson EM, et al: Antibiotics and surgery for vesicoureteric reflux: A meta-analysis of randomized controlled trials. *Arch Dis Child* 2003;88:688–694.
Yeung CK, Sihoe JD, Borzi PA: Endoscopic cross-trigonal ureteral reimplantation under carbon dioxide bladder insufflation: A novel technique. *J Endourol* 2005;19:295–299.

Capitolo 540 ■ Ostruzione delle vie urinarie Jack S. Elder

L'ostruzione delle vie urinarie può essere congenita (anatomica) o causata da traumi, neoplasie, litiasi, processi infiammatori o procedure chirurgiche, anche se è congenita la maggior parte delle lesioni ostruttive dell'infanzia. Le lesioni ostruttive si verificano a qualsiasi livello dal meato uretrale agli infundibuli dei calici (Tab. 540-1). Gli effetti fisiopatologici dell'ostruzione dipendono da livello, dall'estensione dell'interessamento, dall'età del bambino all'esordio e se essa è acuta o cronica.

EZIOLOGIA. Un'ostruzione ureterale che si verifica precocemente nella vita fetale dà esito a una displasia renale, che può variare

TABELLA 540-1. Tipi e cause di ostruzione delle vie urinarie

SEDE	CAUSA
Infundibuli	Congenita Litiasi Infiammatoria (tubercolosi) Traumatica Postchirurgica Neoplastica
Pelvi renale	Congenita (stenosi infundibolo-pelvica) Infiammatoria (tubercolosi) Litiasi Postchirurgica Traumatica Neoplastica (tumore di Wilms, neuroblastoma)
Giunzione ureteropelvica	Stenosi congenita Litiasi Neoplastica Infiammatoria Postchirurgica Traumatica
Uretere	Megauretere ostruttivo congenito Stenosi medioureterale Ectopia ureterale Ureterocele Uretere retrocavale Polipi fibroepiteliali ureterali Valvole ureterali Litiasi Postchirurgica Compressione estrinseca Neoplastica (neuroblastoma, linfoma e altri tumori retroperitoneali o pelvici) Infiammatoria (morbo di Crohn, malattia granulomatosa cronica) Ematoma, rinoma Linfocele Fibrosi retroperitoneale
Efflusso vescicale e uretra	Disfunzione neurologica della vescica (ostruzione funzionale) Valvole uretrali posteriori Valvole uretrali anteriori Diverticoli Stenosi uretrali (congenite, traumatiche o iatrogene) Atresia uretrale Ureterocele ectopico Stenosi meatale (maschi) Litiasi Corpi estranei Fimosi Compressione estrinseca tumorale Anomalie congenite del seno urogenitale

dal rene multicistico, associato ad atresia ureterale o pelvica (vedi Fig. 537-2), alla displasia corticale renale istologica di grado variabile nelle ostruzioni meno gravi. L'ostruzione ureterale cronica nelle ultime fasi della vita fetale (o dopo la nascita) porta a una dilatazione dell'uretere, della pelvi renale e dei calici, con anomalie del parenchima renale che variano da alterazioni tubulari minime alla dilatazione dello spazio di Bowman, dalla fibrosi glomerulare alla fibrosi interstiziale. Dopo la nascita, le infezioni possono complicare l'ostruzione e peggiorare il danno renale.

MANIFESTAZIONI CLINICHE. Un'ostruzione delle vie urinarie provoca generalmente un'**idronefrosi**, che di solito è asintomatica nelle sue fasi precoci. Un rene ostruito in seguito a un'ostruzione della giunzione ureteropelvica (UPJ) o della giunzione ureterovescicale può presentarsi come una massa oppure causare un dolore all'addome superiore o al fianco dal lato affetto. Può manifestarsi una pielonefrite in seguito alla stasi urinaria oppure una litiasi delle vie urinarie superiori, che causa dolore addominale o al fianco ed ematuria. Nell'ostruzione dell'efflusso vescicale, il mitto può essere debole e le infezioni delle vie urinarie (IVU) sono comuni. Molte di queste anomalie sono identificate mediante l'ecografia prenatale e si sospetta un'anomalia delle vie urinarie in 1 feto su 100.

Un'insufficienza renale ostruttiva può presentarsi con scarso accrescimento staturoponderale, vomito, diarrea o altri segni e sintomi non specifici. Nei bambini più grandi, un'ostruzione infravescicale può essere associata a incontinenza urinaria da sovrafflusso o a un mitto insufficiente. L'ostruzione uretrale acuta provoca dolore all'addome o al fianco, mentre l'ostruzione uretrale cronica può essere silente oppure causare un dolore addominale vago o un tipico dolore al fianco in seguito a un aumento di assunzione di liquidi.

DIAGNOSI. L'ostruzione delle vie urinarie viene spesso diagnosticata prima della nascita mediante un'ecografia, che di solito mostra un'idronefrosi. In questi bambini occorre eseguire nel periodo neonatale una valutazione più completa, che comprende gli studi di imaging. L'ostruzione delle vie urinarie è in genere silente e, nel neonato, una massa addominale palpabile è più spesso un rene displasico idronefrosico o multicistico. In caso di valvole uretrali posteriori, una lesione ostruttiva infravescicale (in particolare dei maschi) è palpabile una massa delle dimensioni di una noce che rappresenta la vescica subito sopra la sinfisi pubica. Anche la pervietà dell'uraco con drenaggio è suggestiva di ostruzione uretrale. L'ascite urinario del neonato è di solito causato da uno stravaso urinario renale o vescicale in seguito alla presenza di valvole uretrali posteriori. L'infezione e la sepsi possono essere le prime indicazioni di una lesione ostruttiva delle vie urinarie.

L'associazione di infezione e ostruzione costituisce una seria minaccia per la salute nei lattanti e nei bambini e richiede la somministrazione parenterale di antibiotici nonché il drenaggio del rene sede di ostruzione. Un'ecografia renale deve essere eseguita in tutti i bambini durante la fase acuta delle infezioni febbrili delle vie urinarie.

STUDI DI IMAGING

ECOGRAFIA RENALE. La presenza di una dilatazione del tratto renale è la caratteristica più comune dell'ostruzione e l'idronefrosi è il reperto ecografico più frequente (Fig. 540-1). La dilatazione non è sempre indicativa di ostruzione e può persistere dopo correzione chirurgica di una lesione ostruttiva. Una dilatazione può derivare da un reflusso vescicoureterale oppure può essere una manifestazione di un anormale sviluppo delle vie urinarie, anche in assenza di ostruzione. Occorre valutare la lunghezza del rene, il grado di pielectasia e lo spessore parenchimale, oltre alla presenza o meno di dilatazione ureterale. La gravità dell'idronefrosi dovrebbe essere idealmente classificata in gradi da 1 a 4 utilizzando la scala della Society for Fetal Urology (Tab. 540-2).

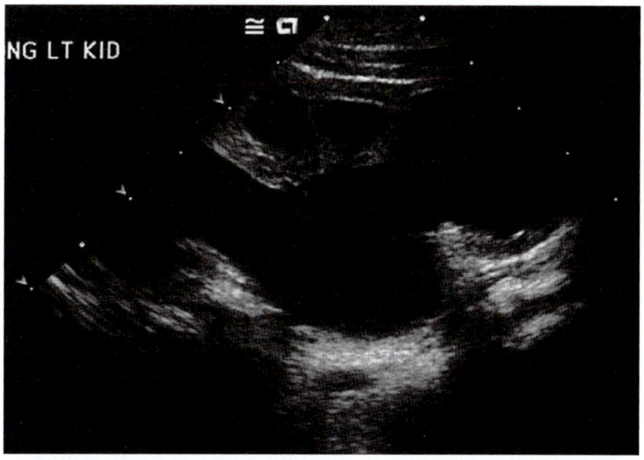

Figura 540-1. Immagine ecografica del rene sinistro con marcata dilatazione pelvica e dei calici (idronefrosi di grado 4) in un bambino con ostruzione della giunzione ureteropelvica.

TABELLA 540-2. Society for Fetal Urology Grading System for Hydronephrosis

GRADO DI IDRONEFROSI	IMMAGINE RENALE	
	COMPLESSO RENALE CENTRALE	SPESSORE PARENCHIMALE RENALE
0	Intatto	Normale
1	Splitting lieve	Normale
2	Splitting evidente, complesso confinato entro i contorni renali	Normale
3	Ampio splitting, pelvi dilatata al di fuori dei contorni renali, calici uniformemente dilatati	Normale
4	Ulteriore dilatazione di pelvi e calici (i calici possono apparire convessi)	Sottile

Da Maizels M, Mitchell B, Kass E, et al: Outcome of non specific hydronephrosis in the infant: A report from the registry of the Society for Fetal Urology. *J Urol* 1994; 152:2324.

Si deve accertare la normalità del rene controlaterale e occorre anche visualizzare la vescica per osservare un'eventuale dilatazione della parete vescicale, una dilatazione dell'uretere inferiore e se lo svuotamento vescicale è completo. Nell'ostruzione acuta o intermittente, la dilatazione del sistema collettore può essere minima e l'ecografia fuorviante.

CISTOURETROGRAFIA MINZIONALE. In tutti i casi di idronefrosi congenita e in tutti i bambini con dilatazione ureterale, occorre eseguire una cistouretrografia minzionale (VCUG), poiché la dilatazione è secondaria a reflusso vescicoureterale nel 15% dei casi. Nei maschi, la VCUG è necessaria anche per escludere un'ostruzione uretrale, particolarmente nel sospetto di valvole uretrali posteriori. Nell'ostruzione infravescicale dei lattanti, la vescica può essere palpabile a causa della distensione cronica e dell'incompleto svuotamento. Nei bambini più grandi, l'entità del flusso urinario può essere misurata in modo non invasivo con un misuratore di flusso urinario; una riduzione del flusso con una normale contrattilità vescicale è indicativa di un'ostruzione infravescicale. Quando non è possibile eseguire il cateterismo uretrale per la VCUG, si deve sospettare una stenosi uretrale o una lesione uretrale ostruttiva. L'uretrografia retrograda con mezzo di contrasto iniettato nel meato uretrale permette di delineare l'anatomia dell'ostruzione uretrale.

STUDI CON RADIOISOTOPI. La **scintigrafia renale** è utilizzata per la valutazione della funzionalità e dell'anatomia renale. I due isotopi (radiofarmaceutici) più comunemente usati sono la mercaptoacetil-triglicina (MAG-3) e l'acido dimercaptosuccinico marcato con tecnezio 99 m (DMSA). Il MAG-3, che si elimina dal tubulo renale, è utilizzato per la valutazione della funzionalità renale differenziale e, assieme alla somministrazione di furosemide, è possibile misurare anche il drenaggio urinario. Un'alternativa al MAG-3 è l'acido dietilen-tetrapenta-acetico (DTPA) che viene eliminato mediante filtrazione glomerulare. L'attività di fondo del DTPA è molto più elevata di quella del MAG-3. Il DMSA è un agente di imaging per la corticale renale e viene usato per la valutazione della funzionalità differenziale renale e per dimostrare la presenza di cicatrici renali e si usa raramente nei bambini con uropatia ostruttiva. In una scintigrafia diuretica con MAG-3, si inietta per via ev una piccola dose di MAG-3 marcato con tecnezio (Figg. 540-2 e 540-3). Durante i primi 2-3 minuti, si analizza e confronta la captazione del parenchima renale, permettendo il calcolo della funzionalità renale differenziale e successivamente si valuta l'escrezione. Dopo 20-30 minuti si inietta furosemide per via ev e si analizza la rapidità e il pattern di drenaggio dai reni alla vescica. Se non è presente ostruzione, metà dose di radionuclidi dovrebbe essere eliminata dal rene entro 10-15 minuti, periodo noto come *emivita* (t1/2). Se è presente un'ostruzione significativa del tratto superiore, la t1/2 è di solito >20 minuti. Una t1/2 di 15-20 minuti è indeterminata e le immagini generate forniscono in genere una valutazione adeguata della sede di ostruzione. Numerose variabili influenzano l'esito della scintigrafia diuretica, poiché il rene neonatale è funzionalmente immaturo e, in alcuni casi, il rene normale può non dimostrare un drenaggio normale dopo la somministrazione di diuretici, inoltre la disidratazione prolunga il transito parenchimale e può attenuare la risposta diuretica. La somministrazione di una dose insufficiente di furosemide può portare a un drenaggio inadeguato. Se è presente reflusso vescicoureterale, è obbligatorio un drenaggio continuo con catetere per prevenire il reflusso di radionuclide dalla vescica nel tratto superiore dilatato, cosa che prolungherebbe la fase di washout. A causa delle numerose variabili, la Society for Fetal Urology e il Pediatric Nuclear Medicine Club hanno sviluppato congiuntamente un metodo standardizzato per l'esecuzione della scintigrafia renale nel lattante e nel bambino, denominato la *scintigrafia ben temperata*.

La scintigrafia diuretica con MAG-3 è considerata superiore all'urografia escretoria nel lattante e nel bambino con idronefrosi, per il fatto che la presenza di meteorismo e di immaturità della

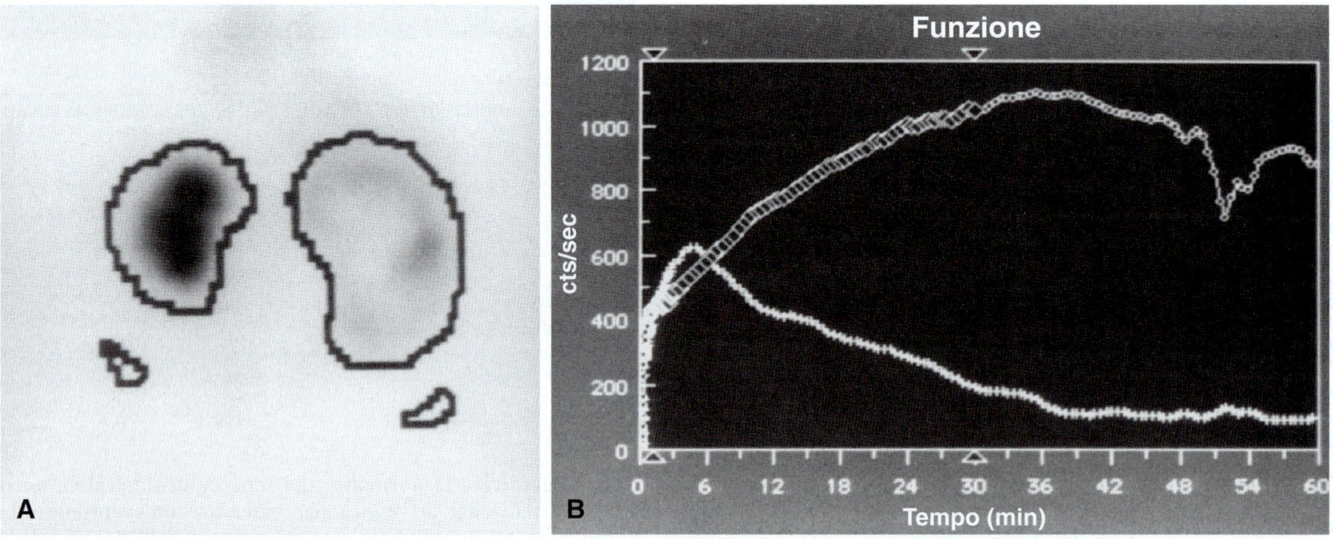

Figura 540-2. Scintigrafia renale diuretica con MAG-3 in un lattante di 6 settimane con idronefrosi destra diagnosticata con l'ecografia prenatale. Il rene destro è sul lato destro dell'immagine. *A*, Funzione renale differenziale: rene sinistro 70%, rene destro 30%. *B*, Dopo la somministrazione di furosemide, il drenaggio del rene sinistro era normale mentre il drenaggio del rene destro era rallentato, reperto compatibile con un'ostruzione del giunto ureteropelvico destro. Il rene destro è stato sottoposto a pieloplastica.

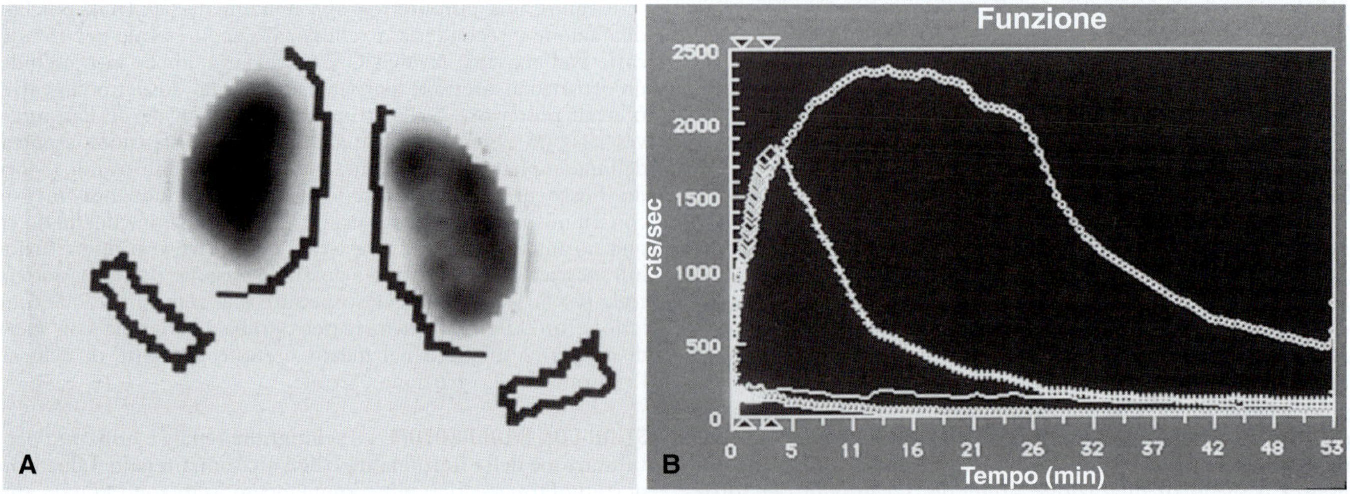

Figura 540-3. Stesso paziente della Figura 540-2. *A*, La scintigrafia diuretica con MAG-3 a 14 mesi evidenzia un'uguale funzione dei due reni e *B*, un rapido drenaggio dopo somministrazione di furosemide.

funzionalità renale spesso sono causa di una qualità subottimale delle immagini della pielografia ev (IVP). La scintigrafia diuretica fornisce inoltre una valutazione oggettiva della funzionalità relativa di ciascun rene.

UROGRAFIA ESCRETORIA. Anche se usata raramente per l'imaging delle vie urinarie nei bambini, l'IVP è utile in casi selezionati (Fig. 540-4). Occorre ricercare con una radiografia addominale in bianco la presenza di litiasi, di anomalie spinali e di un pattern anormale di meteorismo intestinale o di una grave stipsi. Nell'ostruzione infravescicale, la parete vescicale è irregolare o trabecolata a causa dell'ipertrofia del detrusore. Una radiografia eseguita dopo la minzione può evidenziare un residuo minzionale. Nell'ostruzione ureterale, il sistema collettore è dilatato al di sopra dell'ostruzione e i calici sono appiattiti. La concentrazione del mezzo di contrasto è ridotta dal lato ostruito e la comparsa del mezzo di contrasto nel sistema collettore può venire ritardata, con un aumento progressivo della concentrazione nel punto dell'ostruzione quando si eseguono le radiografie ritardate. Nell'ostruzione di grado elevato, il mezzo di contrasto può restare nel sistema collettore anche dopo 24 ore.

Uno stravaso urinario può essere diagnosticato nelle radiografie iniziali o in quelle ritardate di uno studio urografico e anche con la scintigrafia con MAG-3. Quando si sospetta un'ostruzione intermittente, l'urografia ev nel corso di un episodio doloroso acuto è spesso lo studio diagnostico più utile.

UROGRAFIA RMN. Lo studio più recente per valutare una sospetta patologia delle vie urinarie superiori è l'urografia RMN. Si idrata il bambino e si somministra ev furosemide. Successivamente, si inietta gadolinio-DTPA e si esegue una RMN di routine pesata in T1 e pesata in T2 con fast spin-echo e soppressione del tessuto adiposo con sezioni attraverso reni, ureteri e vescica. Questa metodica fornisce ottime immagini del processo patologico ed è in corso di sviluppo una metodica per la valutazione della funzionalità renale differenziale.

TOMOGRAFIA COMPUTERIZZATA. Nei bambini con sospetta litiasi ureterale, la TC spirale senza contrasto dell'addome e della pelvi è un metodo standard per dimostrare la presenza di uno o più calcoli e la loro sede nonché l'eventuale presenza di una idronefrosi prossimale significativa. Questa tecnica costituisce l'esame iniziale di scelta in questi pazienti.

ALTRI ESAMI DIAGNOSTICI. In rari casi, si può eseguire una **pielografia anterograda** (inserimento di un sondino nefrostomico percutaneo e iniezione di mezzo di contrasto) per valutare l'anatomia delle vie urinarie superiori. Tale procedura richiede di solito l'anestesia generale. Inoltre, può essere eseguito uno **studio di flusso pressione-perfusione anterogrado** (test di Whitaker), in cui si infonde liquido a una velocità determinata, di solito 10 mL/min. Si monitorano le pressioni a livello della pelvi renale e della vescica durante l'infusione e le differenze di pressione eccedenti i 20 cm H_2O sono indicative di ostruzione. In altri casi, la pielografia retrograda con cistoscopia fornisce eccellenti immagini delle vie urinarie superiori (Fig. 540-5).

TIPI SPECIFICI DI OSTRUZIONE DELLE VIE URINARIE E RELATIVO TRATTAMENTO

IDROCALICOSI. Il termine *idrocalicosi* si riferisce a una dilatazione localizzata del calice causata dall'ostruzione del suo infundibulo, denominata *stenosi infundibolare*. Tale ostruzione può essere originata durante lo sviluppo oppure secondaria a processi infiammatori come per esempio un'IVU. Quando l'anomalia non viene individuata all'ecografia prenatale oppure casualmente, viene di solito determinata durante una valutazione diagnostica

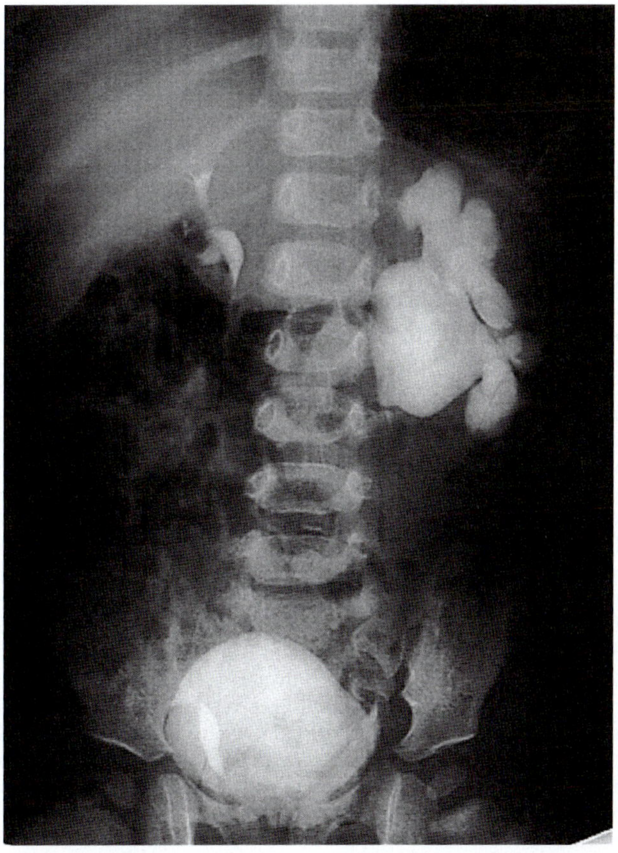

Figura 540-4. Urografia escretoria in un bambino di sesso maschile che evidenzia una dilatazione della pelvi renale sinistra e un appiattimento dei calici caratteristici di un'ostruzione della giunzione ureteropelvica.

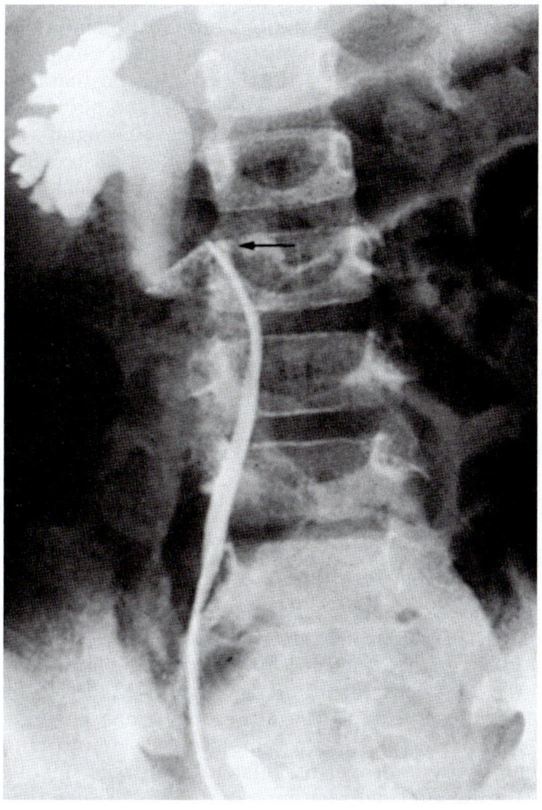

Figura 540-5. Pielografia retrograda che evidenzia una deviazione mediale di un uretere dilatato superiormente a livello della 3° vertebra lombare, caratteristico di un uretere retrocavale.

per la presenza di dolore o per una IVU. La diagnosi di stenosi infundibolare viene generalmente stabilita mediante IVP o TC con contrasto.

OSTRUZIONE DELLA GIUNZIONE URETEROPELVICA. L'ostruzione della giunzione ureteropelvica è la più comune lesione ostruttiva dell'età pediatrica, di solito causata da una stenosi intrinseca (vedi Figg. da 540-1 a 540-4). Anche un'arteria accessoria situata a livello del polo renale inferiore può essere causa di ostruzione estrinseca. L'aspetto tipico all'ecografia è un'idronefrosi di grado 3 o 4 senza dilatazione ureterale. L'ostruzione della giunzione ureteropelvica si presenta più comunemente come (1) un'idronefrosi fetale a un'ecografia materna; (2) una massa renale palpabile in un neonato o in un lattante; (3) un dolore addominale, del fianco o lombare; (4) un'IVU febbrile; o (5) un'ematuria successiva a un trauma di minima entità. Circa il 60% dei casi si verifica a sinistra e il rapporto maschio femmina è di 2:1, mentre nel 10% dei casi l'ostruzione della giunzione ureteropelvica è bilaterale. In un rene con ostruzione della giunzione ureteropelvica, la funzione renale può essere significativamente alterata dall'atrofia da pressione, ma circa metà dei reni affetti ha una funzione relativamente normale. L'anomalia viene corretta mediante una pieloplastica in cui il segmento stenotico viene escisso con la riconnessione tra uretere e pelvi renale normali. Il tasso di successo dell'intervento è del 91-98%. In molti centri, si esegue la pieloplastica per via laparoscopica, spesso con assistenza robotizzata.

Gradi minori di ostruzione della giunzione ureteropelvica possono provocare un'idronefrosi lieve, di solito non ostruttiva, e in genere questi reni hanno una funzione normale. Lo spettro delle anomalie a tipo ostruzione della giunzione ureteropelvica è stato definito come *giunzione ureteropelvica anomala*. Un'altra causa di idronefrosi lieve è rappresentata dalle pliche fetali dell'uretere superiore, che sono non ostruttive.

La diagnosi può essere difficile da porre in un lattante asintomatico in cui la dilatazione della pelvi renale è osservata casualmente all'ecografia prenatale. Dopo la nascita, si ripete lo studio ecografico per confermare la diagnosi prenatale. È necessaria una VCUG in quanto il 10-15% dei pazienti presenta un reflusso vescicoureterale ipsilaterale. Dal momento che l'oliguria neonatale può causare una decompressione temporanea di una pelvi renale dilatata, l'ideale è eseguire la prima ecografia postnatale dopo il 3° giorno di vita. Tuttavia, ritardare l'ecografia può essere poco pratico. Se non si trova una dilatazione all'ecografia iniziale, occorre eseguire un'altra ecografia a 1 mese di età. Se il rene presenta un'idronefrosi di grado 1 o 2 e il parenchima renale ha un aspetto normale, di solito è appropriato un periodo di osservazione, con ecografie renali sequenziali per monitorare la gravità dell'idronefrosi, la quale in genere scompare. Il bambino deve ricevere una **profilassi antibiotica**, di solito trimetoprim-sulfametoxazolo o trimetoprim, anche se prima dei 2 mesi di vita si preferisce l'amoxicillina. Se l'idronefrosi è di grado 3 o 4, la risoluzione spontanea è meno probabile vi è una minore probabilità di ostruzione, particolarmente se il diametro della pelvi renale è 2 cm. Si esegue una scintigrafia diuretica con MAG-3 a 4-6 settimane di vita. Se il drenaggio del tratto urinario superiore è insufficiente o la funzione differenziale renale è alterata, è consigliata una pieloplastica. Dopo la pieloplastica, la funzione differenziale renale spesso migliora ed è atteso un miglioramento del drenaggio con la stimolazione con furosemide.

Se la funzione differenziale alla scintigrafia è normale, e il drenaggio è soddisfacente, il bambino può essere seguito con ecografie seriate, anche nel caso di una idronefrosi di grado 4. Se l'idronefrosi rimane di grado elevato senza miglioramento, può essere utile una scintigrafia diuretica dopo 6-12 mesi ai fini della decisione tra osservazione continua e riparazione chirurgica. Una pronta riparazione chirurgica è indicata nei lattanti con massa addominale, grave idronefrosi bilaterale, un rene singolo o una ridotta funzionalità del rene interessato. In casi poco frequenti in cui la funzionalità renale differenziale è inferiore al 10% ma il rene comunque conserva una certa funzionalità, l'inserimento di un tubo nefrostomico per cutaneo consente il drenaggio del rene idronefrosico per alcune settimane per permettere la rivalutazione della funzione renale. In bambini più grandi che si presentano con sintomi, la diagnosi di ostruzione della giunzione ureteropelvica viene di solito posta con l'ecografia e la scintigrafia diuretica.

Nella **diagnosi differenziale** occorre considerare le seguenti entità: (1) megacalicosi, una dilatazione congenita non ostruttiva dei calici senza dilatazione della pelvi o degli ureteri; (2) reflusso vescicoureterale con marcata dilatazione e angolatura dell'uretere; e (3) ostruzione medioureterale o distale quando l'uretere non è bene visualizzabile all'urografia.

OSTRUZIONE MEDIOURETERALE. La stenosi ureterale congenita o una valvola ureterale dell'uretere medio sono anomalie rare. L'anomalia si corregge mediante escissione del segmento stenotico e la rianastomosi dei segmenti ureterali normali superiore e inferiore. L'uretere retrocavale è un'anomalia in cui l'uretere destro superiore decorre posteriormente alla vena cava inferiore. In questa anomalia, la vena cava può causare compressione estrinseca e ostruzione. Una IVP evidenzia la deviazione mediale dell'uretere destro a livello della 3ª vertebra lombare. La diagnosi può essere confermata dalla pielografia retrograda (vedi Fig. 540-5). Il trattamento chirurgico consiste nella resezione dell'uretere superiore, spostandolo davanti alla vena cava, e nella successiva rianastomosi dei segmenti superiore e inferiore. La riparazione è necessaria solo quando è presente un'ostruzione. I tumori retroperitoneali, la fibrosi causata dalle procedure chirurgiche, i processi infiammatori (come nella malattia granulomatosa cronica) e la radioterapia possono provocare un'ostruzione medioureterale acquisita.

ECTOPIA URETERALE. Un uretere che drena al di fuori della vescica è definito **uretere ectopico**. Questa anomalia è tre volte più comune nelle femmine che nei maschi e di solito viene diagnosticata prima della nascita. In genere, l'uretere ectopico drena il polo superiore di un sistema collettore doppio (due ureteri). Nelle femmine, circa il 35% di questi ureteri sbocca nella vescica a livello del collo vescicale, il 35% sbocca nel setto uretrovaginale, il 25% nella vagina e in pochi casi nella cervice uterina, nell'utero, nel dotto di Gartner o in un diverticolo uretrale. Spesso la parte terminale dell'uretere è stenotica, cosa che porta a idroureteronefrosi. Con l'eccezione dell'uretere ectopico che sbocca nel collo vescicale, nelle femmine un uretere ectopico provoca una continua incontinenza urinaria dalla parte del rene interessata dall'anomalia. Sono frequenti le IVU a causa della stasi urinaria. Nei maschi, l'uretere ectopico penetra nell'uretra posteriore (al di sopra dello sfintere esterno) nel 47% dei casi, nell'utricolo prostatico nel 10% dei casi, nella vescicola seminale nel 33% dei casi, nel dotto eiaculatore nel 5% dei casi e nel dotto deferente nel 5% dei casi. Di conseguenza, nei maschi, un uretere ectopico non provoca incontinenza e la maggior parte dei pazienti si presenta con un'IVU o un'epididimite. La valutazione comprende un'ecografia renale, una VCUG e una scintigrafia renale, che dimostra se il segmento interessato possiede una funzione significativa. L'ecografia evidenzia il rene idronefrosico affetto o una dilatazione del polo superiore e dell'uretere fino alla vescica (Fig. 540-6). Se l'uretere ectopico drena nel collo vescicale (femmine), una VCUG di solito evidenzia un reflusso nell'uretere. Altrimenti, non vi è reflusso nell'uretere ectopico, ma vi può essere reflusso nell'uretere del polo inferiore ipsilaterale o nel sistema collettore controlaterale.

Il **trattamento** dipende dallo stato dell'unità renale drenata dall'uretere ectopico. Se è presente una funzionalità renale soddisfacente, è indicato il reimpianto ureterale nella vescica o l'ureteroureterostomia (anastomosi dell'uretere ectopico del polo superiore nell'uretere del polo inferiore che ha un'inserzione normale). Se la funzionalità renale è deficitaria, è indicata la nefrectomia parziale o totale. In molti centri questa procedura viene eseguita laparascopicamente.

URETEROCELE. L'ureterocele è una dilatazione cistica dell'uretere terminale ed è ostruttivo a causa di un orifizio ureterale puntiforme. L'ureterocele è più comune nelle femmine rispetto ai maschi.

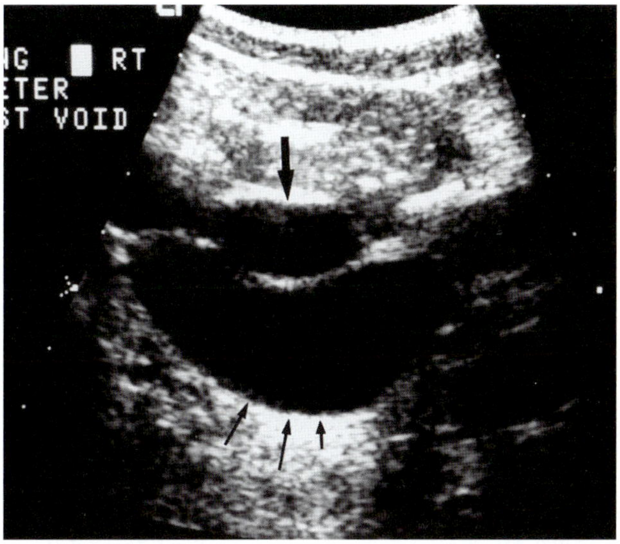

Figura 540-6. Immagine ecografia dell'uretere destro dilatato (*frecce sottili*) che si estende dietro e caudalmente rispetto a una vescica pressoché vuota (*freccia*) in una bambina con incontinenza urinaria e uretere ectopico che drena in vagina.

Nei bambini affetti di solito la diagnosi viene posta all'ecografia prenatale, ma alcuni si presentano con un'IVU. L'ureterocele può essere ectopico, nel qual caso il rigonfiamento cistico si può estendere attraverso il collo vescicale nell'uretra, o ortotopico, nel qual caso l'uretere è interamente all'interno della vescica. Sia l'ureterocele ectopico sia quello ortotopico possono essere bilaterali.

Nelle femmine, l'ureterocele è quasi sempre associato a duplicazione ureterale (Fig. 540-7), mentre nel 50% dei maschi affetti è presente un solo uretere. Se associato a duplicazione, l'ureterocele drena la metà renale superiore, che di solito ha una funzione deficitaria o è displasia a causa dell'ostruzione congenita. L'uretere del polo inferiore drena nella vescica superiormente e lateralmente all'uretere del polo superiore e presenta frequentemente reflusso.

Un **ureterocele ectopico** si estende sotto la mucosa nell'uretra. Raramente, gli ureteri ectopici di grandi dimensioni possono causare un'ostruzione dell'efflusso vescicale e ritenzione urinaria con idronefrosi bilaterale; nelle femmine, l'ureterocele può prolassare dal meato uretrale. L'ecografia è efficace nell'evidenziare l'ureterocele e se il sistema associato ostruito è duplicato o singolo. La VCUG di solito mostra un difetto di riempimento della vescica, talvolta ampio, corrispondente all'ureterocele e spesso evidenzia un reflusso nel sistema collettore del polo inferiore adiacente, dal tipico aspetto "a giglio cadente". La scintigrafia renale è l'esame che più accuratamente dimostra se il rene affetto ha una funzione significativa.

Il **trattamento** dell'ureterocele ectopico è diverso a seconda dei differenti centri e dipende dalla funzionalità del polo superiore alla scintigrafia renale e dalla presenza o meno di reflusso nell'uretere del polo inferiore. Se il polo superiore non è funzionale o se vi è un reflusso significativo nell'uretere del polo inferiore, o se il paziente è settico in seguito a un'infezione del rene idronefrosico, una terapia iniziale appropriata è l'incisione transuretrale con cauterio o laser olmio:YAG per decomprimere l'ureterocele. Tuttavia, il reflusso nell'ureterocele inciso è comune ed è necessaria la successiva escissione dell'ureterocele e il reimpianto ureterale.

L'**ureterocele ortotopico** è associato a un sistema collettore singolo o duplicato, e l'orifizio si trova nella sede attesa nella vescica (Fig. 540-8). Queste anomalie vengono di solito scoperte nel corso di una valutazione per un'idronefrosi prenatale o una IVU. L'ecografia è una metodica sensibile per l'identificazione dell'ureterocele a livello vescicale e dell'idroureteronefrosi. L'IVP rivela vari gradi di dilatazione ureterale e caliciale e nella vescica si osserva un difetto di riempimento di forma circolare. Nelle radiografie ritardate può essere chiaramente visibile la dilatazione cistica dell'uretere, ricolma di mezzo di contrasto. L'incisione transuretrale dell'ureterocele migliora efficacemente l'ostruzione, ma può causare reflusso vescicoureterale con necessità di un successivo reimpianto ureterale. Alcuni preferiscono l'escissione aperta dell'ureterocele il reimpianto come trattamento iniziale. Gli ureteroceli semplici e di piccole dimensioni scoperti accidentalmente e che non si associano a dilatazione delle vie urinarie superiori non richiedono trattamento.

MEGAURETERE. La Tabella 540-3 presenta una classificazione del megauretere. Numerosi disordini sono causa di dilatazione ureterale e molti sono non ostruttivi.

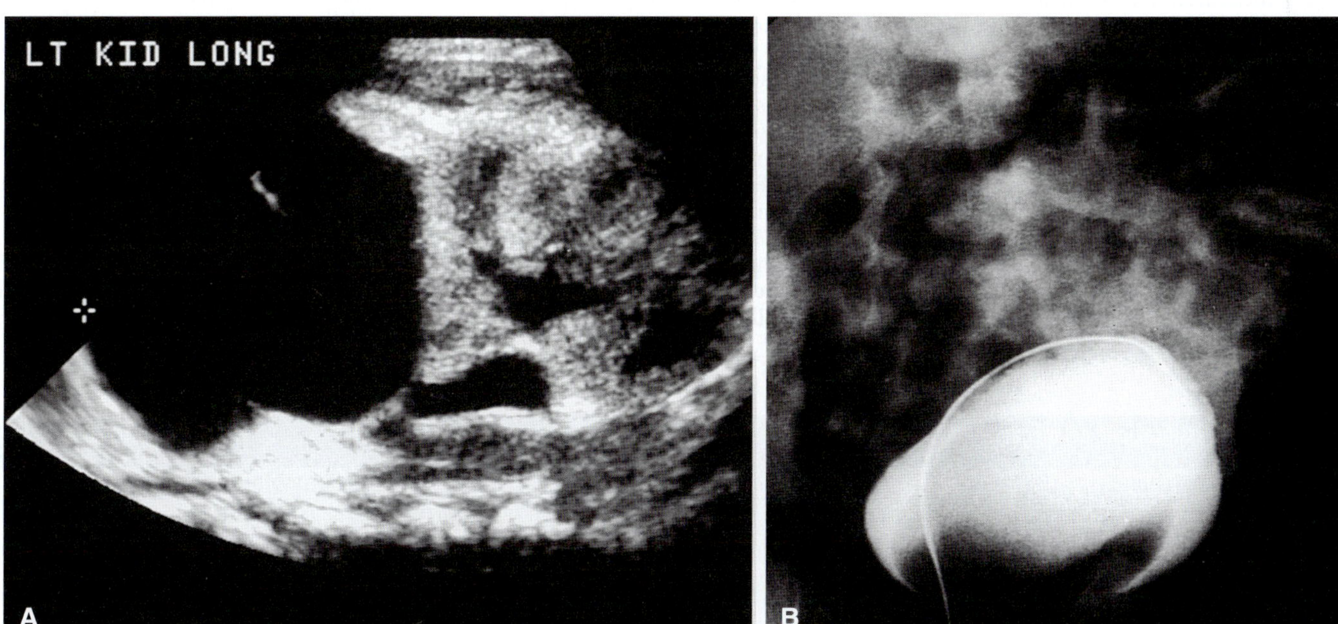

Figura 540-7. *A*, Lattante con ureterocele ectopico. L'ecografia del rene sinistro evidenzia una massiva dilatazione del polo superiore e un polo inferiore normale. *B*, la VCUG evidenzia un grosso ureterocele, che drena il polo superiore, a livello vescicale. Non è presente reflusso.

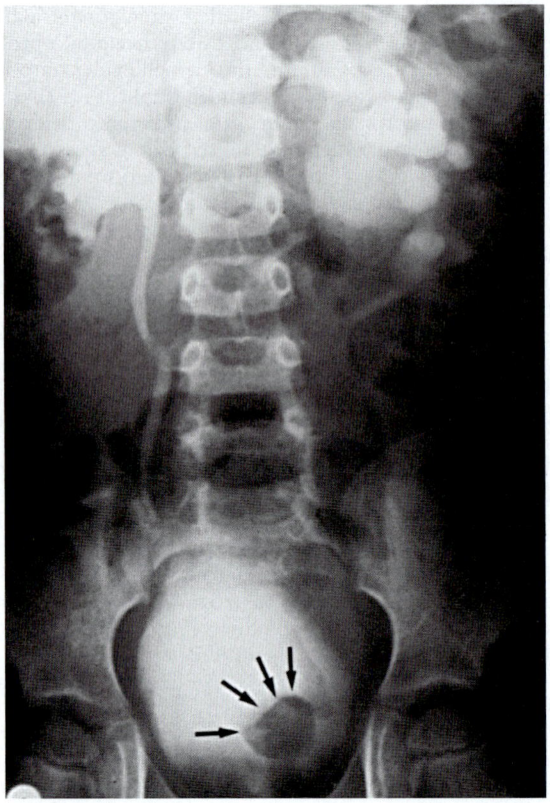

Figura 540-8. Ureterocele intravescicale semplice. L'urografia escretoria evidenzia un'idronefrosi sinistra e un difetto di riempimento circolare sul lato sinistro della vescica corrispondente a un ureterocele semplice che provoca ostruzione ureterale sinistra. Questa lesione è stata trattata mediante incisione transuretrale e drenaggio dell'ureterocele.

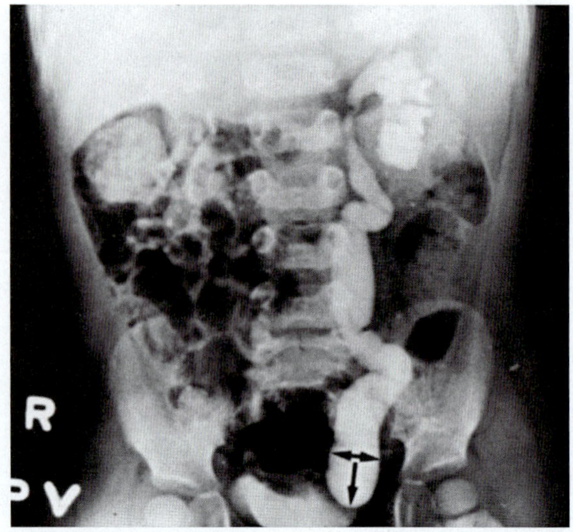

Figura 540-9. Megauretere senza reflusso con ostruzione. Urografia escretoria in una bambina con storia di infezione febbrile delle vie urinarie. Il lato destro è normale. Il lato sinistro rivela un'idroureteronefrosi con predominante dilatazione dell'uretere distale. Si noti l'aspetto caratteristico dell'uretere distale. Non era presente reflusso vescicoureterale. La diagnosi di ostruzione è stata confermata mediante scintigrafia diuretica.

Il megauretere di solito viene individuto con l'ecografia renale e vescicale di screening in seguito alla diagnosi prenatale di idronefrosi o nel periodo postnatale per un'IVU, per un'ematuria o per dolore addominale. Anamnesi ed esame obiettivo accurato, assieme alla VCUG, permettono di identificare i megaureteri secondari e i megaureteri con reflusso, come anche la sindrome "prune belly". I megaureteri con ostruzione e quelli senza ostruzione primari rappresentano probabilmente gradi variabili di gravità della stessa anomalia.

Il megauretere primario con ostruzione e senza reflusso deriva da un anomalo sviluppo dell'uretere distale, con lo strato muscolare sostituito da tessuto a base di collagene. La normale peristalsi ureterale è alterata e si verifica un allargamento dell'uretere prossimale. Non è presente di solito una vera e propria stenosi. All'IVP, l'uretere distale è più dilatato nel segmento distale e si restringe bruscamente a livello o al di sopra della giunzione vescicale (Fig. 540-9). La lesione può essere unilaterale o bilaterale e la dilatazione del sistema collettore superiore e l'appiattimento dei calici sono suggestivi di ostruzione. Il megauretere predispone alle IVU, alla litiasi urinaria, all'ematuria o al dolore del fianco a causa della stasi urinaria. Nella maggior parte dei casi, la scintigrafia diuretica e l'ecografia sequenziale possono distinguere in modo affidabile tra un megauretere con ostruzione e uno senza ostruzione. Nella maggior parte dei megaureteri senza ostruzione, l'idroureteronefrosi si riduce gradualmente (Fig. 540-10), mentre i megaureteri con ostruzione reale richiedono un trattamento chirurgico, con escissione del segmento stenotico, tapering e reimpianto dell'uretere. I risultati della ricostruzione chirurgica di solito sono buoni, ma la prognosi dipende dalla funzione renale preesistente e dall'eventuale sviluppo di complicanze.

Se la funzionalità renale differenziale è normale (>45%) e il bambino è asintomatico, sembra sicuro seguire il paziente con ecografie e scintigrafie diuretiche seriate per monitorare la funzione e il drenaggio renale. Questi bambini dovrebbero ricevere una terapia antibiotica profilattica fino a quando esiste una stasi urinaria a livello del rene e dell'uretere superiore. Se la funzione renale si deteriora, se il drenaggio del tratto urinario superiore rallenta o se si verifica un'IVU, è consigliato il reimpianto ureterale. Dal 20 al 30% dei bambini con megauretere con reflusso viene sottoposto a reimpianto ureterale.

SINDROME "PRUNE BELLY". La sindrome "prune belly", chiamata anche **sindrome della triade** o **sindrome di Eagle-Barrett**, si presenta in circa 1:40 000 nati vivi; il 95% degli individui affetti è di sesso maschile. La caratteristica associazione di assenza dei muscoli addominali, mancata discesa dei testicoli e anomalie delle vie urinarie deriva probabilmente da una grave ostruzione uretra-

TABELLA 540-3. Classificazione del megauretere

CON REFLUSSO		CON OSTRUZIONE		SENZA REFLUSSO E SENZA OSTRUZIONE	
PRIMITIVO	**SECONDARIO**	**PRIMITIVO**	**SECONDARIO**	**PRIMITIVO**	**SECONDARIO**
Reflusso primitivo	Vescica neurogena	Intriseco (megauretere primitivo con ostruzione)	Vescica neurogena	Senza reflusso, senza ostruzione	Diabete insipido
Sindrome della megacisti-megauretere	Sindrome di Hinman		Sindrome di Hinman		Infezione
Uretere ectopico	Valvole uretrali posteriori	Valvola ureterale	Valvole uretrali posteriori		Persistente dopo eliminazione dell'ostruzione
Sindrome "prune belly"	Diverticolo vescicale	Uretere ectopico	Calcolo ureterale		
	Postoperatorio	Ureterocele ectopico	Estrinseco		
			Postoperatorio		

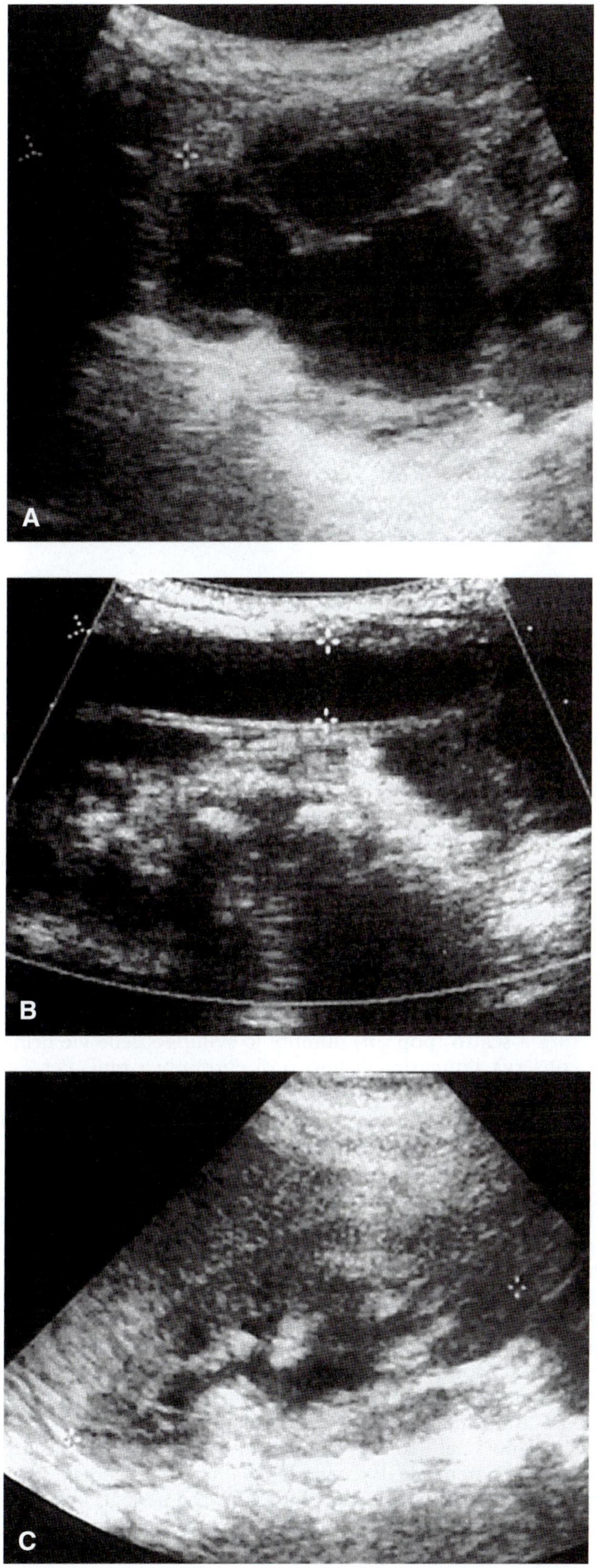

Figura 540-10. Neonato con megauretere primitivo senza reflusso. *A*, L'ecografia renale evidenzia un'idronefrosi di grado 4. *B*, Uretere dilatato. La scintigrafia renale ha dimostrato una funzione renale uguale rispetto al rene controlaterale e un drenaggio soddisfacente con la stimolazione della diuresi. *C*, Ecografia di follow-up a 10 mesi che evidenzia la completa risoluzione dell'idronefrosi.

le nella vita fetale (Fig. 540-11). Oligoidramnios e ipoplasia polmonare sono complicanze comuni nel periodo perinatale e molti dei bambini affetti sono nati morti. Le anomalie delle vie urinarie

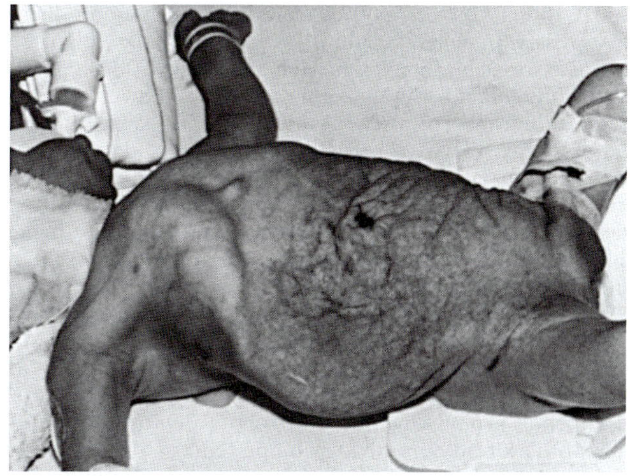

Figura 540-11. Immagine di un neonato di 1600 g con sindrome "prune belly". Si noti la mancanza di tonicità della parete addominale e l'aspetto grinzoso della cute.

comprendono una dilatazione massiva degli ureteri e delle vie urinarie superiori e una vescica di grandi dimensioni con pervietà dell'uraco o un diverticolo uracale e la maggior parte dei pazienti manifesta un reflusso vescicoureterale. L'uretra prostatica di solito è dilatata e la prostata ipoplasica, mentre l'uretra anteriore può essere dilatata, dando esito a megalouretra. Raramente è presente stenosi o atresia uretrale. I reni di solito presentano una displasia di grado variabile e i testicoli intra-addominali. Spesso è presente una malrotazione intestinale. Anomalie cardiache sono presenti nel 10% dei casi; più del 50% manifesta anomalie del sistema muscoloscheletrico, comprese anomalie degli arti e scoliosi. Nelle femmine, sono di solito presenti anomalie dell'uretra, dell'utero e della vagina.

Molti neonati con sindrome "prune belly" mostrano difficoltà a svuotare efficacemente la vescica, essendo la muscolatura vescicale poco sviluppata e l'uretra stenotica. Quando non è presente un'ostruzione, lo scopo del trattamento è la prevenzione delle infezioni delle vie urinarie mediante profilassi antibiotica. Quando è presente un'ostruzione dell'uretere o dell'uretra, misure di drenaggio temporanee, come la vescicostomia, possono favorire la conservazione della funzione renale fino a quando il bambino non è sufficientemente cresciuto per la chirurgia. In alcuni bambini con sindrome "prune belly" sono state riscontrate valvole uretrali posteriori classiche o atipiche. Le infezioni delle vie urinarie sono frequenti e devono essere prontamente trattate. La correzione del criptorchidismo mediante orchidopessi può essere difficile in questi bambini, poiché i testicoli sono situati in alto nell'addome ed è preferibile che sia eseguita nei primi 6 mesi di vita. La ricostruzione della parete addominale offre benefici estetici e funzionali.

La prognosi dipende in definitiva dal grado di ipoplasia polmonare e di displasia renale. Un terzo dei bambini con sindrome "prune belly" è nato morto o muore nei primi mesi di vita a causa di complicanze polmonari. Almeno il 30% dei sopravviventi a lungo termine sviluppa una nefropatia terminale per la displasia a causa delle complicanze delle infezioni o del reflusso e necessita infine del trapianto di rene, che, in questi bambini, offre buoni risultati.

OSTRUZIONE DEL COLLO VESCICALE. L'ostruzione del collo vescicale di solito è secondaria a ureterocele ectopico, a calcoli vescicali o a una neoplasia prostatica (rabdomiosarcoma). Le manifestazioni comprendono difficoltà di svuotamento vescicale, ritenzione urinaria, infezioni delle vie urinarie e distensione vescicale con incontinenza da sovraflusso. Un'evidente ostruzione del collo vescicale è comune nei casi di valvole uretrali posteriori, ma raramente ha un qualche significato funzionale. L'ostruzione primitiva del collo vescicale è estremamente rara.

VALVOLE URETRALI POSTERIORI. La causa più comune di grave uropatia ostruttiva nei bambini è costituita dalle valvole uretrali posteriori, che interessano 1 maschio su 8 000. le valvole uretrali sono lembi tessutali che si estendono in direzione distale rispetto all'uretra prostatica, in direzione dello sfintere urinario esterno. I lembi valvolari sono di solito separati da un'apertura a fessura. Le valvole hanno un'origine embriologica non chiara e provocano un'ostruzione di grado variabile. Circa il 30% dei pazienti sviluppa una nefropatia terminale o un'insufficienza renale cronica. L'uretra prostatica si dilata e la muscolatura vescicale si ipertrofizza. Un reflusso vescicoureterale è presente nel 50% dei pazienti e si può avere ostruzione ureterale distale a causa della distensione vescicale cronica o dell'ipertrofia della muscolatura vescicale. Le alterazioni renali variano da un'idronefrosi di grado lieve a una grave displasia renale; la loro serietà dipende probabilmente dalla gravità dell'ostruzione e dal momento d'esordio durante lo sviluppo fetale. Come in altri casi di ostruzione o displasia renale, vi può essere oligoindramnios e ipoplasia polmonare.

I bambini affetti da valvole uretrali posteriori vengono diagnosticati in epoca prenatale quando l'ecografia materna rivela un'idronefrosi bilaterale, una distensione vescicale e, se l'ostruzione è grave, oligoidramnios. Sono stati riportati interventi di decompressione vescicale prenatale con shunt vescicoamniotico per cutaneo o chirurgia fetale aperta. Mancano evidenze cliniche e sperimentali dei possibili benefici dell'intervento fetale e pochi feti affetti sono candidati a questo tipo di interventi. Le valvole uretrali posteriori diagnosticate in epoca prenatale, particolarmente quelle diagnosticate nel 2° trimestre, hanno una prognosi più sfavorevole rispetto a quelle diagnosticate dopo la nascita. Nel neonato maschio, si sospetta la presenza di valvole uretrali posteriori se è presente una **distensione vescicale** palpabile e se **il mitto è debole**. Se l'ostruzione è grave e non viene diagnosticata nel periodo neonatale, i lattanti possono avere una presentazione tardiva con crescita insufficiente da uremia o da sepsi causata dall'infezione del tratto urinario ostruito. Nei gradi minori di ostruzione, i bambini possono avere una presentazione ancora più tardiva con difficoltà a raggiungere la continenza urinaria diurna o con un'IVU. La diagnosi viene posta con una VCUG (Fig. 540-12) o con l'ecografia perineale.

Dopo aver posto la diagnosi, occorre un'accurata valutazione della funzione renale e dell'anatomia del tratto urinario superiore. Nel neonato sano, un piccolo sondino nasogastrico in polietilene (da 5 o 8 F) viene inserito in vescica e lasciato in sede per diversi giorni. L'inserimento del sondino può essere difficile, poiché la punta può arrotolarsi nell'uretra prostatica. Un segno di questo problema è che l'urina drena intorno al catetere piuttosto che attraverso di esso. Non si deve usare il catetere di Foley (con palloncino) poiché il palloncino può creare un grave spasmo della vescica, che a sua volta può causare una seria ostruzione ureterale.

Se i livelli di creatinina sierica rimangono normali o ritornano normali, il trattamento consiste nell'ablazione transuretrale dei lembi valvolari, eseguita endoscopicamente in anestesia generale. Se l'uretra è troppo piccola per l'ablazione transuretrale, si preferisce eseguire una vescicostomia temporanea, in cui la cupola vescicale viene esteriorizzata sulla parte inferiore della parete addominale. Nei bambini più grandi, le valvole possono essere eliminate e la vescicostomia chiusa.

Se i livelli di creatinina sierica rimangono elevati o aumentano nonostante il drenaggio vescicale mediante un piccolo catetere, si deve sospettare un'ostruzione ureterale secondaria, un danno renale irreversibile o una displasia renale. In tali casi, si deve eseguire una vescicostomia. La pielostomia cutanea raramente consente un miglior drenaggio rispetto alla vescicostomia cutanea e quest'ultima permette anche una crescita continuativa e regolare della vescica e un graduale miglioramento della compliance della parete vescicale.

Nel lattante con sepsi e uremia, le misure salvavita possono comprendere l'immediata correzione dello squilibrio elettrolitico e il controllo dell'infezione mediante antibiotici appropriati e

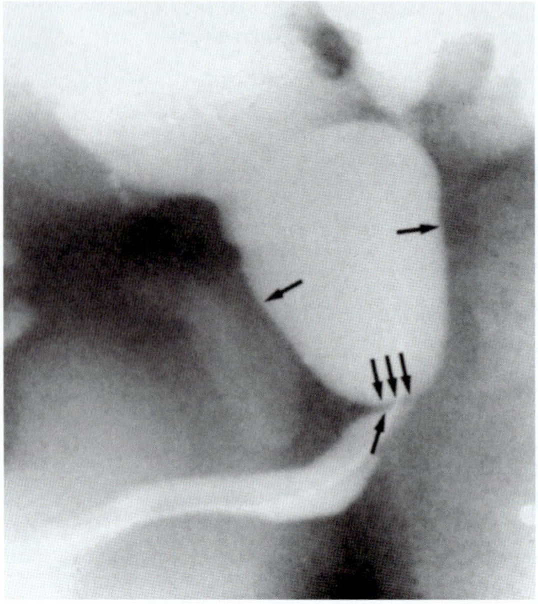

Figura 540-12. Cistouretrografia minzionale in un lattante con valvole uretrali posteriori. Si noti la dilatazione dell'uretra prostatica e il difetto di riempimento lineare trasversale corrispondente alle valvole.

può essere necessario il drenaggio dei tratti superiori mediante nefrotomia per cutanea ed emodialisi. Una volta stabilizzate le condizioni del paziente, si possono iniziare la valutazione e il trattamento. In alcuni bambini più grandi la diagnosi viene posta in seguito a debolezza del mitto, incontinenza diurna o un'IVU; questi bambini di solito vengono trattati con la rimozione primaria delle valvole.

I **fattori prognostici favorevoli** comprendono un'ecografia prenatale normale tra le 18 e le 24 settimane di gestazione, una creatinina sierica $<$0,8-1,0 mg/dL dopo decompressione vescicale e la visualizzazione della giunzione corticomidollare all'ecografia renale. In diverse situazioni, si può sviluppare una valvola con apertura a scatto (pop off) durante lo sviluppo delle vie urinarie che conserva l'integrità di uno o di entrambi i reni. Per esempio, il 15% dei bambini con valvole uretrali posteriori hanno un reflusso unilaterale in un rene displasico non funzionante, fenomeno denominato **sindrome VURD** (valvole, reflusso unilaterale, displasia). In questi bambini, l'elevata pressione vescicale viene dispersa nel rene non funzionante, permettendo un normale sviluppo del rene controlaterale. Nei neonati maschi con ascite urinario, l'urina generalmente stravasa dal sistema collettore ostruito attraverso i fornici renali, permettendo un normale sviluppo renale. I fattori prognostici sfavorevoli comprendono la presenza di oligoidramnios in utero, la diagnosi di idronefrosi prima della 24ª settimana di gestazione, una creatinina sierica $>$1,0 mg/dL dopo decompressione vescicale, la diagnosi di cisti corticali in entrambi i reni e la persistenza di incontinenza diurna oltre i 5 anni di età.

La prognosi nel neonato è correlata al grado di ipoplasia polmonare e al potenziale di recupero della funzione renale. I neonati gravemente affetti spesso nascono morti. Dei neonati che sopravvivono al periodo neonatale, il 30% circa conserva un certo grado di insufficienza renale e infine possono richiedere il trapianto di rene. In alcune casistiche, il trapianto di rene nei bambini con valvole uretrali posteriori possiede un basso tasso di successo rispetto ai bambini con vescica normale, presumibilmente a causa dell'influenza avversa dell'alterazione della funzione vescicale sulla funzione e sulla sopravvivenza del rene trapiantato.

Dopo l'ablazione delle valvole, la profilassi antibiotica è utile per la prevenzione delle IVU, in quanto l'idronefrosi spesso persiste in varia misura per molti anni. Questi bambini devono essere valutati tutti gli anni con un'ecografia renale, un esame obiettivo comprendente la valutazione della crescita somatica e della pressione arteriosa, l'esame delle urine e la determinazione dei livelli sierici degli elettroliti. Molti bambini hanno una poliuria significativa derivante da un difetto di concentrazione secondario a un'uropatia ostruttiva prolungata. Se essi acquisiscono una malattia sistemica con vomito o diarrea, o entrambe, non può essere utilizzata la diuresi per valutarne lo stato di idratazione. Questi bambini possono disidratarsi rapidamente e la soglia per il ricovero in ospedale per la reidratazione intravenosa deve essere molto bassa. Alcuni di questi pazienti hanno un'acidosi tubulare renale con la necessità di assumere bicarbonato per os. Se è presente un qualsiasi grado significativo di disfunzione renale, un deficit di crescita o ipertensione, essi devono essere seguiti da un neurologo pediatra. Se è presente un reflusso vescicoureterale, è consigliabile una strategia di attesa con profilassi antibiotica, se invece si verifica un'IVU, è necessario effettuare la correzione chirurgica.

Dopo il trattamento, i bambini con valvole uretrali spesso non raggiungono la continenza urinaria notturna precocemente come gli altri bambini. L'incontinenza può derivare da un'associazione di fattori, tra cui contrazioni vescicali non inibite, scarsa compliance vescicale, atonia vescicale, dissinergia del collo vescicale o poliuria. Spesso questi bambini richiedono una valutazione urodinamica con esami urodinamici o videourodinamici per pianificare la terapia. I bambini che non mostrano compliance hanno un rischio significativo di danno renale, anche in assenza di infezione. Il drenaggio notturno con catetere si è dimostrato utile nei bambini con poliuria e può contribuire a preservare la funzione renale. L'incontinenza urinaria di solito migliora con l'età, particolarmente dopo la pubertà. Una meticolosa attenzione alla compliance vescicale, allo svuotamento e alle infezioni può migliorare i risultati nel futuro.

ATRESIA URETRALE. La forma più grave di uropatia ostruttiva nei maschi è l'atresia uretrale. In utero è presente una vescica distesa, idroureteronefrosi bilaterale e oligoidramnios. Nella maggior parte dei casi, questi bambini nascono morti decedendo per ipoplasia polmonare. Alcuni bambini con sindrome "prune belly" presentano anche un'atresia uretrale. Se l'uraco è pervio, è improbabile un oligoidramnios e il bambino di solito sopravvive. La ricostruzione uretrale è difficile e la maggior parte dei pazienti viene trattata con una diversione urinaria continente.

IPOPLASIA URETRALE. L'ipoplasia uretrale è una rara forma di uropatia ostruttiva dei maschi meno grave dell'atresia uretrale. Nell'ipoplasia uretrale, il lume uretrale è estremamente piccolo. I neonati con ipoplasia uretrale presentano generalmente un'idronefrosi bilaterale e una distensione vescicale. L'inserimento di un piccolo sondino nasogastrico pediatrico attraverso l'uretra è difficoltoso o impossibile. Di solito si deve eseguire una vescicostomia percutanea per eliminare l'ostruzione del tratto urinario superiore e la gravità dell'insufficienza renale è variabile. I bambini più gravemente affetti sviluppano una nefropatia terminale. Il trattamento comprende la ricostruzione uretrale, la dilatazione uretrale graduale o la diversione urinaria continente.

STENOSI URETRALI. Le stenosi uretrali nei maschi di solito derivano da un trauma uretrale, sia iatrogeno (cateterismo, procedure endoscopiche, pregressa ricostruzione uretrale) sia accidentale (traumi dell'area perineale-genitale [*straddle injuries*], fratture pelviche). Dal momento che queste lesioni possono svilupparsi gradualmente, la diminuzione della forza del mitto urinario viene notata raramente dal bambino o dai genitori. Più frequentemente, l'ostruzione provoca sintomi di instabilità vescicale, ematuria o disuria. Il cateterismo vescicale è di solito impossibile. La diagnosi viene stabilita con una radiografia durante la minzione eseguita nel corso di un'orografia intravenosa o di un'uretrografia retrograda. Anche l'ecografia è stata utilizzata per la diagnosi delle stenosi uretrali e l'endoscopia conferma la diagnosi. Il trattamento endoscopico delle stenosi brevi mediante uretrotomia in visione diretta è spesso efficace e dà esito a un rilevante miglioramento del mitto urinario. Le stenosi più lunghe circondate da fibrosi periuretrale spesso richiedono un'uretroplastica. In genere devono essere evitate le procedure endoscopiche ripetute, in quanto possono causare ulteriori lesioni uretrali. La determinazione non invasiva della velocità e del pattern del flusso urinario è utile per la diagnosi e il follow-up.

Nelle femmine, le stenosi uretrali vere sono eccezionali, dal momento che l'uretra femminile è protetta dai traumi particolarmente nell'infanzia. In passato si riteneva che un anello uretrale distale fosse una causa comune di ostruzione dell'uretra femminile e che le bambine affette beneficiassero della dilatazione uretrale. La diagnosi veniva sospettata quando si osservava alla VCUG una deformità a "spinning top" dell'uretra (vedi Fig. 543-4) e quindi confermata dalla misurazione del diametro uretrale. Non vi è una correlazione tra aspetto radiografico dell'uretra alla VCUG e diametro uretrale e non vi sono differenze significative nel diametro uretrale tra bambine con cisiti ricorrenti e controlli normali simili per età. Questo aspetto radiografico è di solito secondario a una dissinergia detrusore-sfintere, di conseguenza la dilatazione uretrale nelle bambine viene raramente rilevata.

VALVOLE URETRALI ANTERIORI E DIVERTICOLI URETRALI NEL MASCHIO. Le valvole uretrali anteriori sono rare. L'ostruzione non è costituita da lembi valvolari come avviene nell'uretra posteriore, ma si tratta piuttosto di un diverticolo uretrale nell'uretra peniena che si espande durante la minzione. L'estensione distale del diverticolo provoca una compressione estrinseca dell'uretra peniena distale, causando così un'ostruzione uretrale. In genere, è presente una massa di consistenza molle sulla superficie ventrale del pene a livello della giunzione peno-scrotale; inoltre, il mitto è debole e spesso sono presenti i segni fisici associati alle valvole uretrali posteriori. Il diverticolo può essere piccolo e minimamente ostruttivo o, in altri casi, può essere altamente ostruttivo e causare insufficienza renale. Il sospetto diagnostico si pone all'esame obiettivo ed è confermato dalla VCUG. Il trattamento comprende l'escissione aperta del diverticolo o l'escissione transuretrale della cuspide uretrale distale. Diverticoli uretrali possono presentarsi occasionalmente dopo un intervento estensivo di correzione di un'ipospadia.

Una dilatazione fusiforme dell'uretra o **megalouretra** può derivare dall'iposviluppo del corpus spongiosum e delle strutture di sostegno dell'uretra. Questa condizione è di solito associata a sindrome "prune belly".

STENOSI MEATALE URETRALE NEL MASCHIO. Vedi Capitolo 544 per informazioni sulla stenosi meatale uretrale nel maschio.

Ashmead GG, Mercer B, Herbst M, et al: Fetal bladder outlet obstruction due to ureterocele: In utero "colander" therapy. *J Ultrasound Med* 2004;23:565–568.

Biard JM, Johnson MP, Carr MC, et al: Long-term outcomes in children treated by prenatal vesicoamniotic shunting for lower urinary tract obstruction. *Obstet Gynecol* 2005;106:503–508.

Capello SA, Kogan BA, Giorgi LJ Jr, et al: Prenatal ultrasound has led to earlier detection and repair of ureteropelvic junction obstruction. *J Urol* 2005; 74:1425–1428.

Chertin B, Pollack A, Koulikov D, et al: Conservative treatment of ureteropelvic junction obstruction in children with antenatal diagnosis of hydronephrosis: Lessons learned after 16 years of follow-up. *Eur Urol* 2006; 49:734–739.

DeFoor W, Minevich E, Reddy P, et al: Results of tapered ureteral reimplantation for primary megaureter: Extravesical versus intravesical approach. *J Urol* 2004;172:1640–1643.

Direnna T, Leonard MP: Watchful waiting for prenatally detected ureteroceles. *J Urol* 2006;175:1493–1495.

Fefer S, Ellsworth P: Prenatal hydronephrosis. *Pediatr Clin North Am* 2006;53: 429–447.

Gundeti MS, Ransley PG, Duffy PG, et al: Renal outcome following heminephrectomy for duplex kidney. *J Urol* 2005;173:1743–1744.

Holmdahl G, Sillen U: Boys with posterior urethral valves: Outcome concerning renal function, bladder function and paternity at ages 31 to 44 years. *J Urol* 2005;174:1031–1034.

Hwang AH, McAleer IM, Shapiro E, et al: Congenital mid ureteral strictures. *J Urol* 2005;174:1999–2002.
Hwang WY, Peters CA, Zurakowski D, et al: Renal biopsy in congenital ureteropelvic junction obstruction: Evidence for parenchymal maldevelopment. *Kidney Int* 2006;69:137–143.
Krishnan A, deSouza A, Konijeti R, et al: The anatomy and embryology of posterior urethral valves. *J Urol* 2006;175:1214–1220.
Lee RS, Retik AB, Borer JG, et al: Pediatric robot assisted laparoscopic dismembered pyeloplasty: Comparison with a cohort of open surgery. *J Urol* 2006;175:683–687.
McDaniel BB, Jones RA, Scherz H, et al: Dynamic contrast-enhanced MR urography in the evaluation of pediatric hydronephrosis: Part 2, anatomic and functional assessment of ureteropelvic junction obstruction. *AJR Am J Roentgenol* 2005;185:1608–1614.
Narasimhan KL, Mahajan JK, Kaur B, et al: The vesicoureteral reflux dysplasia syndrome in patients with posterior urethral valves. *J Urol* 2005;174:1433–1435.
Nguyen MT, Pavlock CL, Zderic SA, et al: Overnight catheter drainage in children with poorly compliant bladders improves post-obstructive diuresis and urinary incontinence. *J Urol* 2005;174:1633–1636.
Perez-Brayfield MR, Baseman A, Kirsch AJ: Adolescent urology. *Adolesc Med Clin* 2005;16:215–227.
Piaggio L, Franc-Guimond J, Figueroa TE, et al: Comparison of laparoscopic and open partial nephrectomy for duplication anomalies in children. *J Urol* 2006;175:2269–2273.
Shukla AR, Cooper J, Patel RP, et al: Prenatally detected primary megaureter: A role for extended follow-up. *J Urol* 2005;173:1353–1356.
Sty JR, Pan CG: Genitourinary imaging techniques. *Pediatr Clin North Am* 2006;53 339–361.
Tsai JD, Huang FY, Lin CC, et al: Intermittent hydronephrosis secondary to ureteropelvic junction obstruction: Clinical and imaging features. *Pediatrics* 2006;117:139–146.
Yee DS, Shanberg AM, Duel BP, et al: Initial comparison of robotic-assisted laparoscopic versus open pyeloplasty in children. *Urology* 2006;67:599–602.

Capitolo 541 ■ Anomalie della vescica

Jack S. Elder

ESTROFIA VESCICALE

L'estrofia della vescica urinaria si presenta in 1 ogni 35 000-40 000 nati vivi. Il rapporto tra maschio e femmina è di 2:1. La gravità varia da una semplice epispadia a un'estrofia completa della cloaca, la quale comprende l'esposizione di tutto l'intestino posteriore e della vescica.

MANIFESTAZIONI CLINICHE. Si ipotizza che le anomalie della vescica derivino dalla mancata penetrazione del mesoderma nell'estensione cefalica della membrana cloacale; l'estensione di questa mancata penetrazione determina il grado dell'anomalia. Nella classica estrofia vescicale (Fig. 541-1), la vescica protrude dalla parete addominale con la mucosa esposta; inoltre, l'ombelico è spostato verso il basso, i rami del pube sono ampiamente separati sulla linea mediana e i muscoli del retto sono separati. Nei **maschi**, è presente un'epispadia completa con chordee dorsale e la lunghezza complessiva del pene è circa la metà di quella dei bambini non affetti. In genere, lo scroto è appena separato dal pene ed è ampio e incavato, come sono inoltre frequenti criptorchidismo ed ernia inguinale. Le **femmine** invece presentano anche epispadia, con separazione delle due metà del clitoride e un'ampia separazione delle labbra. L'ano è spostato anteriormente in entrambi i sessi e vi può essere prolasso rettale. Anche i rami pubici sono ampiamente separati e i pazienti con estrofia tendono a essere più bassi del normale. Le conseguenze di un'estrofia vescicale non trattata sono l'incontinenza urinaria totale e un aumento dell'incidenza di cancro della vescica, di solito un adenocarcinoma. Le deformità genitali possono produrre disabilità sessuale in entrambi i sessi, in particolare nei maschi. L'ampia separazione dei rami pubici provoca un'andatura a base allargata caratteristica ma non una disabilità significativa. Nell'estrofia vescicale classica, le vie urinarie superiori sono di solito normali.

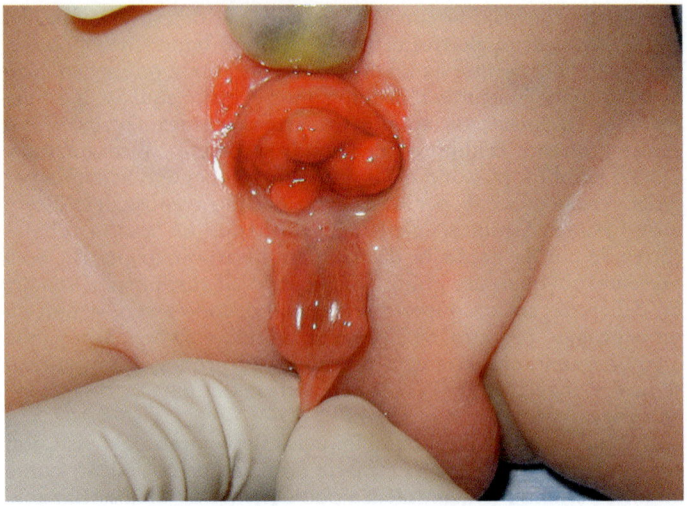

Figura 541-1. Classica estrofia vescicale in un neonato maschio. La vescica è esposta sulla linea mediana; il cordone ombelicale è spostato in direzione caudale; il pene presenta epispadia e lo scroto appare largo.

TRATTAMENTO. Il trattamento dell'estrofia vescicale deve iniziare alla nascita. La vescica deve essere ricoperta da un involucro in materiale plastico per mantenere umida la mucosa vescicale. *L'applicazione di garze o garze alla vaselina sulla mucosa vescicale deve essere evitata, poiché causa un'irritazione significativa.* Il bambino deve essere subito trasferito presso un centro specializzato nel trattamento di queste anomalie. La terapia convenzionale comprende una serie di procedure ricostruttive in diversi tempi, ma si è diffusa anche una procedura ricostruttiva in un tempo singolo. Questi pazienti tendono a manifestare **allergia al lattice**, per cui occorre prendere precauzioni relativamente a esso.

Il trattamento da preferire è un'immediata chiusura della vescica estrofica. Durante tale procedura si mobilizza la parete addominale e si congiungono i rami pubici lungo la linea mediana. Se la chiusura della vescica viene eseguita nelle prime 48 ore di vita, spesso è presente una mobilità dei rami pubici sufficiente da consentire l'approssimazione della sinfisi pubica. Se la procedura viene rimandata, occorre eseguire un'osteotomia pelvica per congiungere i rami e quindi creare una sinfisi pubica per sostenere la chiusura vescicale. La chiusura vescicale precoce può essere applicata a quasi tutti i neonati con estrofia vescicale classica. Il trattamento deve essere differito in situazioni selezionate quando si ritiene che l'intervento sia eccessivamente rischioso o complesso, come in un neonato prematuro, o se dovesse essere eseguito da un chirurgo inesperto.

La ricostruzione totale comprende la chiusura della vescica e della parete addominale e, nei maschi, la correzione dell'epispadia utilizzando la tecnica del dissemblaggio penieno, in cui i due corpi cavernosi e l'uretra vengono mobilizzati separatamente in tre parti. Dopo l'intervento, il tratto urinario superiore del bambino viene attentamente monitorato per il possibile sviluppo di idronefrosi e di infezioni. La maggior parte dei bambini con estrofia vescicale presenta un reflusso vescicoureterale e deve ricevere una profilassi antibiotica. Nei maschi, se l'epispadia non è corretta alla nascita, si può eseguirne la riparazione di solito a 1-2 anni di età, periodo in cui il bambino mostra un'incontinenza urinaria totale poiché non esiste uno sfintere urinario esterno.

Lo stadio finale della ricostruzione comprende la creazione di uno sfintere per il controllo vescicale e la correzione del reflusso vescicoureterale. Quando il bambino ha 3-6 anni, la capacità vescicale dovrebbe essere di almeno 80-90 mL e l'individuo deve avere raggiunto il controllo rettale. Di solito, la capacità vescicale viene monitorata ogni 12-24 mesi mediante cistoscopia in anestesia.

Alla pubertà, il pelo pubico è spesso distribuito ai lati dei genitali esterni. Per garantire un aspetto più normale del pube si può eseguire una plastica del mons pubis.

PROGNOSI. Questo piano di trattamento ha permesso, in alcuni centri, di raggiungere un tasso di continenza del 60-70%, con un deterioramento del tratto urinario superiore inferiore al 15%. Tale tasso di continenza riflette non soltanto una ricostruzione efficace, ma anche la qualità e le dimensioni della vescica. Le vescica ricostruita non si rilassa durante lo svuotamento come in un bambino normale; al contrario, il paziente deve svuotarla mediante una manovra di Valsalva. I bambini sottoposti a intervento ricostruttivo da neonati hanno una maggiore probabilità di avere una vescica normalmente funzionante. I bambini che rimangono incontinenti per più di un anno dopo la ricostruzione del collo vescicale o quelli che non sono eleggibili per la ricostruzione di esso a causa di una ridotta capacità vescicale sono candidati a una procedura ricostruttiva alternativa per ottenere la continenza. In casi selezionati, l'iniezione cistoscopica di microsfere di destranomero o polidimetilsiloxano nel collo vescicale può fornire una coaptazione sufficiente da permettere la continenza. In alternativa, se il bambino non è un candidato alla terapia endoscopica, le possibilità comprendono (1) cistoplastica di aumento, in cui la vescica viene allargata con un patch di colon o di intestino tenue per aumentarne la capacità; (2) creazione di una neovescica utilizzando il colon o l'intestino tenue inserendo una stomia addominale continente attraverso la quale può essere eseguito un cateterismo intermittente pulito; (3) inserimento di uno sfintere urinario artificiale, con possibile cistoplastica di aumento; (4) ureterosigmoidostomia, in cui gli ureteri vengono distaccati dalla vescica e suturati al colon sigma; i pazienti eliminano le urine e le feci dal retto e per la continenza di basano sullo sfintere anale; e (5) procedura di Mainz II, in cui il colon sigma viene riconfigurato in una "vescica" alla quale vengono connessi gli ureteri e il paziente elimina le urine 3-6 volte al giorno attraverso il retto (in questo caso, le feci tendono a essere più solide). L'ureterosigmoidostomia si associa a un rischio significativo di pielonefrite cronica, danno del tratto urinario superiore, acidosi metabolica da assorbimento di ione idrogeno e cloro nell'intestino e un rischio di almeno il 15% a lungo termine di carcinoma del colon. I pazienti dei Paesi sottosviluppati spesso vengono sottoposti a intervento di Mainz II perché il tasso di continenza è elevato e perché la pielonefrite e le alterazioni del tratto urinario superiore non sono frequenti.

Il follow-up a distanza ha dimostrato che, anche se i maschi con estrofia hanno un pene che è la metà della lunghezza normale, essi di solito hanno una funzione sessuale soddisfacente. La fertilità è invece ridotta, forse a causa delle lesioni iatrogene degli organi sessuali secondari durante la ricostruzione. Grazie ai metodi di riproduzione artificiale, pressoché tutti gli uomini possono essere fertili. Nelle donne la fertilità non è ridotta, ma il prolasso uterino durante la gravidanza rappresenta un problema. Inoltre, nelle donne che sono state sottoposte a una diversione urinaria continente, può essere necessario il parto cesareo.

ALTRE ANOMALIE CON ESTROFIA

I bambini con i casi più complessi di **estrofia cloacale**, che ha un'incidenza di 1 su 400 000, mostrano un onfalocele, gravi anomalie di colon e retto e spesso una sindrome dell'intestino corto, l'anomalia più grave trattata dagli urologhi pediatri. Circa il 50% dei pazienti presenta un'anomalia del tratto urinario superiore e il 50% una spina bifida. Nessun bambino con estrofia cloacale ha mai raggiunto una normale continenza urinaria o fecale. Le correnti tecniche ricostruttive portano a un esito soddisfacente nella maggior parte dei pazienti con diversione urinaria permanente (sia un condotto ileale sia una diversione urinaria continente) e colostomia. Dal momento che il pene nei bambini con estrofia cloacale di solito è di dimensioni ridotte, la ricostruzione genitale nei maschi con estrofia cloacale si è dimostrata insoddisfacente. In passato, la maggior parte degli specialisti prescriveva l'assegnazione del sesso femminile a questi bambini, ma attualmente si è dibattuto se essi, che hanno un cariotipo 46,XY e un imprinting androgenico in utero, possano avere una soddisfacente identità di genere femminile. Le decisioni riguardanti l'assegnamento del genere devono essere prese unitamente dai medici che si occupano del bambino (team chirurgico, endocrinologo pediatra, neuropsichiatria infantile ed esperto in etica) e dalla famiglia.

L'**epispadia** rientra nello spettro delle anomalie associate a estrofia, e interessa circa 1 su 117 000 maschi e 1 su 480 000 femmine. Nei maschi, la diagnosi è ovvia in quanto il prepuzio è distribuito primariamente sull'aspetto ventrale dell'asta e il meato uretrale si trova sul dorso del pene. L'epispadia distale nel maschio è di solito associata a normale controllo urinario e a un tratto urinario superiore normale e deve essere riparata a 6-12 mesi di età. Nelle femmine, il clitoride è bifido e l'uretra divisa dorsalmente. Nei maschi con forme più gravi e in tutte le femmine con epispadia è presente un'incontinenza urinaria totale poiché lo sfintere è formato in modo incompleto e vi è un'ampia separazione dei rami pubici. Questi bambini richiedono procedure di ricostruzione chirurgica analoghe a quelle della 2ª e 3ª fase del trattamento dei pazienti con estrofia vescicale classica.

DIVERTICOLI VESCICALI

I diverticoli vescicali di solito si manifestano a livello della giunzione ureterovescicale e sono associati a reflusso vescicoureterale (Fig. 541-2), poiché il diverticolo interferisce con la normale inserzione del lembo valvolare tra uretere e vescica. Diverticoli congeniti possono manifestarsi anche in altre sedi. I diverticoli vescicali sono inoltre comunemente associati a ostruzione uretrale distale come le valvole uretrali posteriori o una disfunzione vescicale neurologica. I piccoli diverticoli non richiedono altro trattamento che quello della malattia primitiva, mentre quelli di grandi dimensioni possono contribuire a uno svuotamento inefficiente, a residuo e stasi urinaria e a infezioni delle vie urinarie e devono perciò essere rimossi.

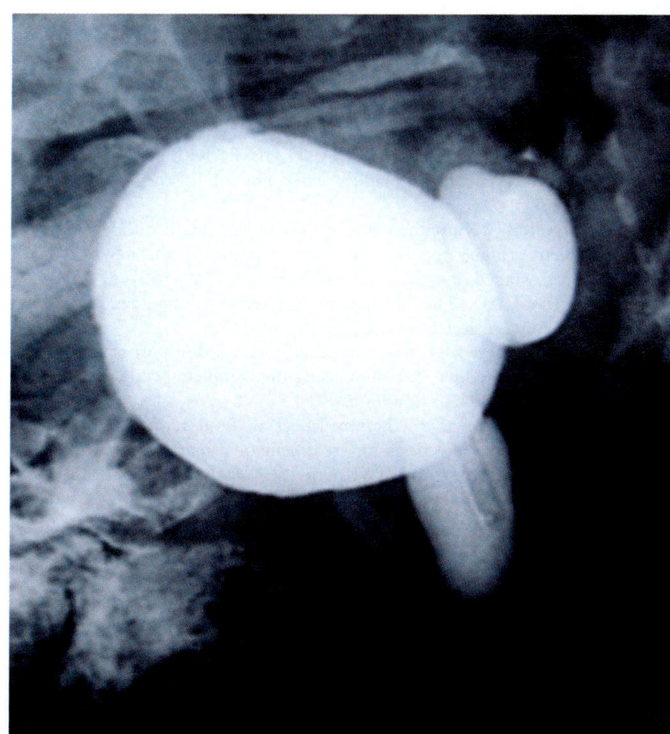

Figura 541-2. Diverticolo vescicale evidenziato alla cistouretrografia minzionale in un neonato con valvole uretrali posteriori.

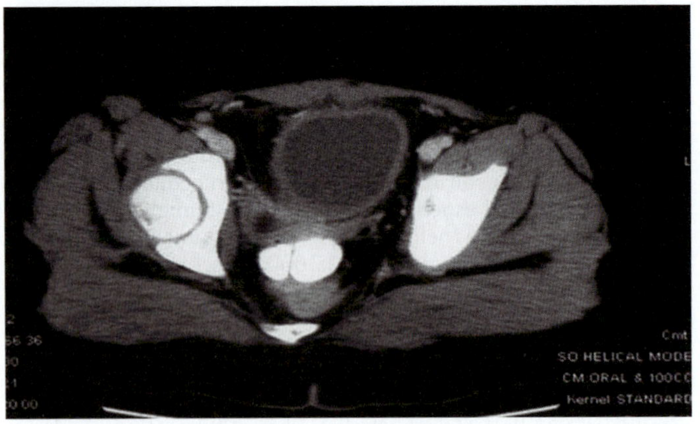

Figura 541-3. TC che evidenzia un ascesso dell'uraco in una bambina di 8 anni. La condizione è stata trattata con drenaggio ed escissione.

ANOMALIE DELL'URACO

Le anomalie dell'uraco sono più comuni nei maschi che nelle femmine. La pervietà dell'uraco può manifestarsi come anomalia isolata; può essere associata a sindrome "prune belly" o a valvole uretrali posteriori. In questa condizione è presente un drenaggio urinario continuo dall'ombelico. Il tratto deve essere escisso chirurgicamente. Un'altra anomalia dell'uraco è la cisti uracale, che può infettarsi. I segni e sintomi comuni comprendono dolore sovrapubico, sintomi irritativi durante lo svuotamento e una massa infraombelicale, che può essere eritematosa. La diagnosi viene stabilita con l'ecografia o la TC (Fig. 541-3) e il trattamento comprende la terapia antibiotica intravenosa, il drenaggio e l'escissione. Altre anomalie dell'uraco comprendono il diverticolo uracale, che è un diverticolo della cupola vescicale, e il seno uracale sterno, una fistola a fondo cieco che si apre in corrispondenza dell'ombelico. Tali lesioni devono essere rimosse.

Allen JW, Song J, Velcek FT: Acute presentation of infected urachal cysts: Case report and review of diagnosis and therapeutic interventions. *Pediatr Emerg Care* 2004;20:108–111.

Borer JG, Gargollo PC, Hendren WH, et al: Early outcome following complete primary repair of bladder exstrophy in the newborn. *J Urol* 2005;174:1674–1678.

Borer JG, Gargollo PC, Kinnamon DD, et al: Bladder growth and development after complete primary repair of bladder exstrophy in the newborn with comparison to staged approach. *J Urol* 2005;174:1553–1557.

Gearhart JP, Baird AD: The failed complete repair of bladder exstrophy: Insights and outcomes. *J Urol* 2005;174:1669–1672.

Husmann DA, Gearhart JP: Loss of the penile glans and/or corpora following primary repair of bladder exstrophy using the complete penile disassembly technique. *J Urol* 2004;172:1696–1700.

Lottmann HB, Margarayan M, Bernuy M, et al: Long-term effects of dextranomer endoscopic injections for treatment of urinary incontinence: An update of a prospective study of 31 patients. *J Urol* 2006;175:1485–1489.

Meyer-Bahlburg HF: Gender identity outcome in female-raised 46,XY persons with penile agenesis, cloacal exstrophy of the bladder, or penile ablation. *Arch Sex Behav* 2005;34:423–438.

Mitchell ME: Bladder exstrophy repair: Complete primary repair of exstrophy. *Urology* 2005;65:5–8.

Nelson CP, Dunn RL, Wei JT, et al: Surgical repair of bladder exstrophy in the modern era: Contemporary practice patterns and the role of hospital case volume. *J Urol* 2005;174:1099–1102.

Pahernik S, Beetz R, Schede J, et al: Rectosigmoid pouch (Mainz pouch II) in children. *J Urol* 2006;175:284–287.

Reiner WG, Kropp BP: A 7-year experience of genetic males with severe phallic inadequacy assigned female. *J Urol* 2004;172:2395–2398.

Capitolo 542 ■ Vescica neurologica

Jack S. Elder

La disfunzione vescicale neurologica nei bambini è di solito congenita e può derivare da difetti del tubo neurale o altre anomalie del midollo spinale (vedi Capitolo 592). Sono invece meno comuni le malattie acquisite e le lesioni traumatiche del midollo spinale. Anche i tumori del sistema nervoso centrale, il teratoma sacrococcigeo e le anomalie del midollo spinale associate ad ano imperforato (vedi Capitolo 341) possono dare esito a un'anomala innervazione della vescica o dello sfintere o di entrambi.

DIFETTI DEL TUBO NEURALE. I difetti del tubo neurale costituiscono un gruppo di diverse anomalie della colonna vertebrale che interessano la funzione del midollo spinale, tra cui il mielomeningocele e il meningocele (vedi Capitolo 592). In seguito alla supplementazione con acido folico e allo screening prenatale, l'incidenza di difetti del tubo neurale è in diminuzione negli USA e in molti altri Paesi. In Terranova (Canada), l'incidenza è diminuita da 4,67 per 1 000 nati vivi nel 1992-1996 all'1,01 per 1000 nati vivi nel 1998-2002. Rimane tuttora elevata in molte parti del mondo; nella provincia di Shanxi (Cina), per esempio, l'incidenza è di 13,87 per 1 000 nati vivi. Pochi centri medici negli Stati Uniti eseguono la chiusura prenatale del mielomeningocele, ma gli studi di follow-up del tratto urinario non hanno dimostrato un definito miglioramento della funzione del tratto urinario inferiore. Per chiarire questo problema sono in corso trial di randomizzazione delle madri alla chiusura del mielomeningocele prenatale in rapporto alla chiusura postatale per valutare gli esiti urologici, neurologici e relativi alla qualità della vita.

MANIFESTAZIONI CLINICHE E DIAGNOSI. Le conseguenze urologiche più importanti della disfunzione vescicale neurologica associata a difetti del tubo neurale sono l'incontinenza urinaria (vedi Capitolo 543), le infezioni delle vie urinarie (IVU; vedi Capitolo 538) e l'idronefrosi da reflusso vescicoureterale o dissinergia detrusore-sfintere. La pielonefrite (vedi Capitolo 519.4) e il deterioramento della funzione renale (vedi Capitolo 535) sono cause frequenti di morte prematura degli individui affetti.

Nel neonato, si eseguono l'ecografia renale, la valutazione del residuo minzionale e la cistouretrografia minzionale dopo la chiusura del mielomeningocele. Il 10-15% dei pazienti presenta un'idronefrosi e il 25% un reflusso vescicoureterale. Deve essere inoltre eseguito uno studio urodinamico, il quale comprende il riempimento della vescica con soluzione fisiologica, la determinazione del volume e della pressione vescicale e la valutazione del tono sfinteriale. Durante il riempimento vescicale, la vescica può presentare contrazioni non inibite (premature) ai bassi volumi, un volume vescicale normale con contrazione al volume appropriato o atonia (mancanza di contrazione vescicale). Anche la compliance o l'elasticità vescicale può essere ridotta. Lo sfintere può evidenziare un tono normale con rilassamento durante la contrazione vescicale, un tono ridotto o assente oppure un tono normale o elevato che aumenta durante la contrazione vescicale (denominato dissinergia detrusore-sfintere) (Fig. 542-1).

DANNO RENALE. Il danno renale di solito deriva dall'incapacità dello sfintere di rilassarsi durante una contrazione vescicale. Tale dissinergia causa un'ostruzione funzionale dell'efflusso vescicale, il quale a sua volta porta a elevata pressione intravescicale, ipertrofia e trabecolazione della muscolatura vescicale e trasmissione dell'elevata pressione alle vie urinarie superiori con idronefrosi (Fig. 542-2). Il reflusso vescicoureterale e le IVU complicano il problema. Il trattamento comprende la riduzione della pressione vescicale con farmaci anticolinergici (oxibutinina, 0,2 mg/kg/24 ore suddivisi in 2-3 dosi) e cateterismo sterile intermittente ogni 3-4 ore. Se è presente un reflusso vescicoureterale o

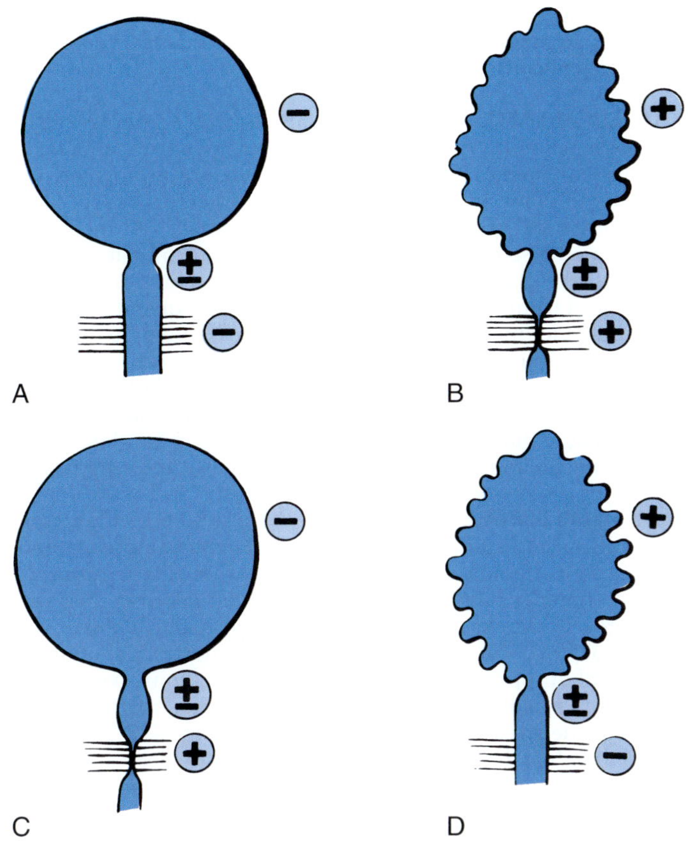

Figura 542-1. Classificazione della disfunzione vescicale neurologica in base all'innervazione, la tonicità e alla coordinazione del detrusore e degli sfinteri descritta da Guzman. Questa classificazione si basa su dati provenienti da studi di imaging, cistometrografia ed elettromiografia degli sfinteri. I pazienti del gruppo B sono a rischio di sviluppo di reflusso e idronefrosi. Per una guida nel trattamento dell'incontinenza, il gruppo A trae beneficio da procedure che aumentano la resistenza dell'efflusso, il gruppo B da anticolinergici o procedure di aumento vescicale, il gruppo C dal cateterismo intermittente, e il gruppo D sia dall'aumento della resistenza dell'efflusso che dall'aumento vescicale sia farmacologico sia chirurgico. La maggior parte dei pazienti richiede il cateterismo intermittente per svuotare la vescica (Modificata da Gonzalez R: Urinary incontinence. In Kelalis PK, King LR, Belman AB (editors): *Clinical Pediatric Urology.* Philadelphia, WB Saunders, 1992, p 387.)

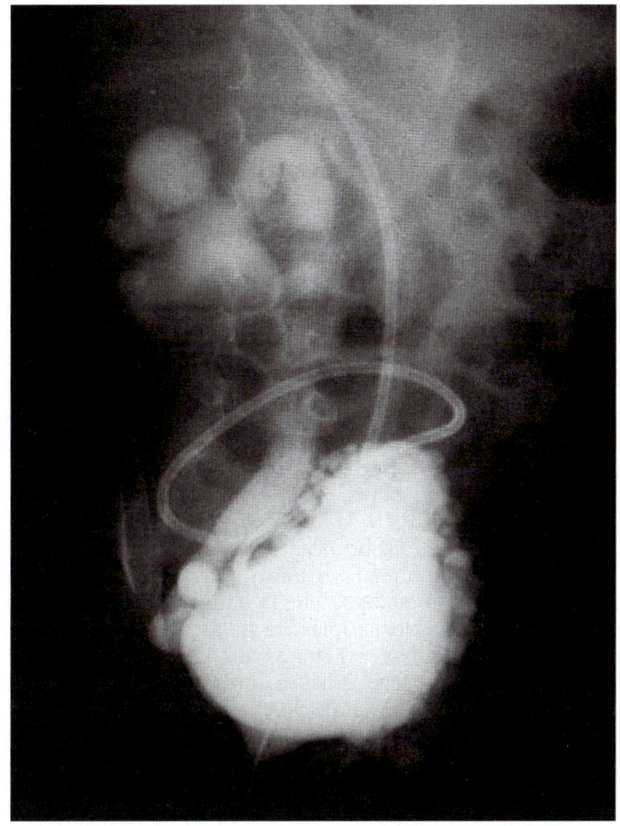

Figura 542-2. Cistouretrografia minzionale in un lattante con mielodisplasia che evidenzia una grave trabecolatura vescicale con diverticoli multipli e reflusso vescicoureterale di 5° grado. La valutazione ha evidenziato una severa dissinergia detrusore-sfintere.

si manifestano IVU, è invece indicata la profilassi antibiotica. Nel neonato o nel lattante con reflusso grave, nei casi in cui il cateterismo intermittente è difficoltoso o i farmaci anticolinergici non sono tollerati, un'alternativa consiste nella diversione urinaria temporanea mediante vescicostomia per cutanea. Altre possibilità per il soggetto con grave dissinergia detrusore-sfintere sono la sovradilatazione uretrale o l'iniezione transuretrale di tossina botulinica (Botox) nello sfintere. Quest'ultima procedura richiede l'anestesia generale e causa incompetenza dello sfintere per 4-6 mesi. Il cateterismo sterile intermittente e la terapia anticolinergica guariscono il reflusso anche nell'80% dei bambini con reflusso di 1° o 2° grado. Nei bambini con alterazioni del tratto urinario superiore, il cateterismo notturno continuo permette un significativo rilassamento vescicale e può ridurre l'ispessimento della parete vescicale. Quelli con reflusso più grave, invece, richiedono spesso la correzione endoscopica del reflusso o l'intervento aperto antireflusso seguito da cateterismo intermittente e farmaci anticolinergici, mentre nei bambini più grandi con mielomeningocele e reflusso di grado elevato, con IVU e con idronefrosi, può essere necessaria l'enterocistoplastica di aumento con cateterismo intermittente.

INCONTINENZA URINARIA. L'incontinenza nel bambino con vescica neurologica può derivare da denervazione parziale o totale dello sfintere, da iper-reflessia vescicale, scarsa compliance vescicale, ritenzione urinaria cronica o una combinazione di questi fattori. L'incontinenza viene spesso affrontata intorno ai 4 anni e l'intervento viene adattato alle necessità del singolo individuo. Quasi tutti i bambini richiedono il cateterismo sterile intermittente per non bagnarsi. Questa tecnica permette un efficiente svuotamento vescicale con un rischio minimo di IVU sintomatica. Il tratto urinario deve essere rivalutato mediante un'ecografia renale, una cistouretrografia menzionale e uno studio urodinamico, compreso lo studio della capacità vescicale. Se il tono dello sfintere è sufficiente e la vescica ha una compliance adeguata, il cateterismo intermittente ogni 3-4 ore è di solito efficace nel mantenere il bambino asciutto. Se sono presenti contrazioni da instabilità vescicale si prescrive un farmaco anticolinergico come ossibutinina cloruro, iosciamina o tolterodina per aumentare la capacità vescicale. Se è presente incompetenza sfinterica, si prescrivono farmaci α-adrenergici per migliorare la resistenza dell'efflusso. Con l'autocateterismo intermittente si osserva batteriuria nel 50% dei bambini, ma raramente essa è asintomatica. In assenza di reflusso non sembrano esservi motivi di preoccupazione. La profilassi antibatterica è spesso efficace nel mantenere le urine sterili quando si usa il cateterismo intermittente. Anche l'esecuzione del cateterismo intermittente con un catetere nuovo ogni volta (silicone idrofilo o standard) è abbastanza efficace nella prevenzione della batteriuria ed evita la necessità di profilassi antibiotica. Con questo piano di trattamento, il 40-85% dei pazienti è asciutto a seconda della loro definizione di incontinenza. Alcuni bambini indossano un pannolino o un tampone nella biancheria intima, ma riferiscono di essere asciutti.

Se l'incontinenza persiste nonostante tali misure, la chirurgia ricostruttiva del tratto urinario può assicurare quasi sempre una continenza completa o soddisfacente. Se la resistenza uretrale è bassa, l'impianto di uno sfintere artificiale è di solito una misura efficace. Tale sfintere consiste in un manicotto gonfiabile che viene posizionato intorno al collo vescicale, un palloncino di regolazione della pressione impiantato nello spazio retroperitoneale e un meccanismo a pompa impiantato nello scroto (nei maschi) e nelle grandi labbra (nelle femmine). In alternativa, sono spesso efficaci le procedure di ricostruzione del collo vescicale come uno *sling* periruretrale. Se la capacità vescicale o la sua compliance sono basse, o se sono presenti contrazioni non inibite persistenti nonostante la terapia anticolinergica, è efficace l'ingrandimento della vescica con un *patch* di intestino tenue o di colon, intervento denominato **cistoplastica di aumento** o **enterocistoplastica.** Questi pazienti necessitano ancora di cateterismo sterile intermittente. Se il cateterismo uretrale è difficoltoso, può essere incorporato una stomia continente nella ricostruzione del tratto urinario. Una metodica comune è la **procedura di Mitronoff**, in cui l'appendice viene isolata dal ceco sul suo peduncolo vascolare e quindi interposta tra vescica e parete addominale per permettere il cateterismo intermittente attraverso una stomia asciutta.

Complicanze. Con l'enterocistoplastica possono insorgere diverse potenziali complicanze.

INFEZIONI DELLE VIE URINARIE. Le urine sono di solito colonizzate da batteri Gram-negativi e il tentativo di renderle sterili per periodi prolungati di solito è destinato al fallimento. Tuttavia, non vi sono evidenze che la batteriuria cronica nei pazienti sottoposti a enterocistoplastica sia associata a danno renale e devono pertanto essere trattate solo le IVU sintomatiche.

ACIDOSI. La superficie mucosa intestinale in contatto con le urine assorbe ioni ammonio, cloro e idrogeno e perde potassio. Ne può derivare acidosi metabolica ipercloremica, che può eventualmente richiedere il trattamento medico (vedi Capitolo 52). L'acidosi cronica può compromettere la crescita scheletrica e tale complicanza è maggiormente frequente nei pazienti con compromissione della funzione renale e in quelli in cui è stato usato il colon per ingrandire la vescica. Per superare le limitazioni dell'enterocistoplastica nei pazienti con insufficienza renale cronica, può essere usato un segmento gastrico invece di un segmento del colon o dell'intestino tenue. Lo stomaco secerne ioni cloro e idrogeno; pertanto, l'acidosi metabolica preesistente rimane stabile o migliora. Tuttavia, la possibilità di un'alcalosi metabolica intrattabile e di ulcera peptica dell'aumento vescicale ha ridotto l'entusiasmo per questa procedura. Un aumento composito che utilizza lo stomaco e l'intestino tenue o il colon è associato a poche complicanze metaboliche.

PERFORAZIONE. La perforazione della vescica aumentata è una complicanza potenzialmente fatale che deriva più spesso dalla sovradistensione acuta o cronica della vescica aumentata. I pazienti con questa complicanza di solito si presentano con serio dolore addominale e segni di peritonite. Sono necessari diagnosi e trattamento immediati con laparotomia esploratoria, nonché chiusura della vescica. È importante una stretta aderenza al programma di cateterismo intermittente prescritto per evitare la sovradistensione vescicale.

LITIASI VESCICALE. Una litiasi vescicale si è sviluppata in almeno il 70% dei bambini seguiti per 10 anni dopo l'enterocistoplastica. I calcoli si sviluppano in risposta al muco che si accumula nella vescica e agisce da nido per la formazione dei calcoli. Questa complicanza può essere prevenuta mediante irrigazione giornaliera della vescica con soluzione fisiologica sterile.

CARCINOMA A CELLULE TRANSIZIONALI INVASIVO. Un carcinoma a cellule transizionali invasivo è stato rilevato in circa il 2% dei pazienti sottoposti a enterocistoplastica. La patogenesi è incerta, ma si ipotizza che essa sia correlata alla batteriuria e al contatto intestino-vescica. È prudente consigliare esami endoscopici annuali o studi citologici urinari a cominciare dal 10° anno dopo l'intervento.

STIPSI. Molti pazienti con spina bifida presentano anche problemi intestinali con stipsi e alcuni traggono beneficio da una tecnica nota come procedura con clisma a continenza anterograda di Malone (*Malone antegrade continence enema procedure*), in cui l'appendice viene esternalizzata sulla cute per consentire l'inserzione di un catetere nel cieco per clismi anterogradi. La stomia è continente e tutti i giorni può essere eseguito un clisma anterogrado con acqua corrente. Questa forma di trattamento permette al paziente di essere continente per quanto riguarda le feci e maggiormente autosufficiente.

ALLERGIA AL LATTICE. L'allergia al lattice (vedi Capitolo 148) è un problema molto rilevante che si osserva in almeno la metà dei pazienti con spina bifida e con altre condizioni urologiche, che necessitano di un cateterismo sterile intermittente e di procedure ricostruttive del tratto urinario. Questa allergia IgE mediata è acquisita ed è secondaria a ripetuta esposizione all'allergene del lattice. L'allergia al lattice può manifestarsi con congiuntivite allergica, starnuti, prurito, orticaria o anafilassi quando si gonfia un palloncino oppure se l'esaminatore indossa un paio di guanti in lattice. Durante un intervento, un individuo sensibilizzato può presentare shock anafilattico. Un ambiente senza lattice deve essere assicurato a tutti i bambini con spina bifida in ambulatorio, in ospedale e durante le procedure operatorie. I bambini affetti devono anche indossare un braccialetto medico informativo.

DISRAFISMO SPINALE OCCULTO. Circa 1 su 4000 pazienti presenta un disrafismo spinale occulto, categoria che comprende lipomeningocele, lipoma intradurale, diastematomielia, tensione del filum terminale, cisti-fistola dermoide, radici nervose aberranti, meningocele sacrale anteriore e i tumori della cauda equina (vedi Capitolo 592). Più del 90% dei pazienti mostra un'anomalia cutanea al di sopra della parte inferiore della colonna vertebrale, tra cui una piccola fossetta, un ciuffo di peli, una malformazione vascolare dermica o un lipo sottocutaneo (Fig. 542-3). Spesso questi bambini hanno piedi cavi, discrepanza delle dimensioni muscolari e della forza tra gli arti inferiori e un'andatura anormale. I neonati e i lattanti spesso presentano un'obiettività neurologica normale, mentre i bambini più grandi non hanno sensibilità perineale e presentano lombalgia. La funzione delle vie urinarie inferiori è anormale nel 40% dei pazienti, comprendendo incontinenza, IVU ricorrenti e imbrattamento fecale (*soiling*). La probabilità di un esame normale è inversamente correlata all'età del bambino al momento della correzione chirurgia della lesione spinale. Dei bambini con urodinamica anormale, il 60% ritorna alla norma; mentre dei bambini più grandi, solo il 27% ritorna alla norma. La gestione del tratto urinario negli altri bambini è simile a quella descritta in precedenza per i difetti del tubo neurale.

AGENESIA SACRALE. L'agenesia sacrale si definisce come assenza di una sola parte o di entrambe le parti o di tutti i corpi vertebrali inferiori. Tale condizione è più comune nei figli di donne diabetiche. Questi bambini hanno una natica appiattita e un solco intergluteo breve e basso, ma di solito non mostrano deformità ortopediche, anche se qualcuno presenta piedi cavi. La palpazione dell'area coccigea permette di identificare le vertebre assenti. Circa il 20% dei casi non è individuato fino all'età di 3-4 anni; molti sono diagnosticati dopo il fallimento dell'educazione degli sfinteri. Gli studi urodinamici in questi bambini evidenziano diversi pattern e la maggior parte di essi necessita di cateterismo sterile intermittente e farmacoterapia per rimanere asciutti.

ANO IMPERFORATO. Tra il 30 e il 45% dei bambini con ano imperforato alto presenta una vescica neurologica, spesso a causa di agenesia sacrale. I neonati con ano imperforato devono essere sottoposti a ecografia spinale durante la valutazione iniziale; se essi hanno difficoltà all'educazione degli sfinteri, deve essere eseguita una valutazione urologia completa con imaging del tratto urinario superiore e inferiore ed esami urodinamici. Per ulteriori dettagli vedi il Capitolo 341.

PARALISI CEREBRALE. I bambini con paralisi cerebrale (vedi Capitolo 598.1) hanno un ragionevole controllo della vescica. Tuttavia, essi raggiungono la continenza in un'età successiva a quella degli altri bambini non affetti. In generale, il 25-50% di questi pazienti è incontinente e il rischio è direttamente correlato alla serietà del deficit fisico e le vie urinarie superiori sono di solito

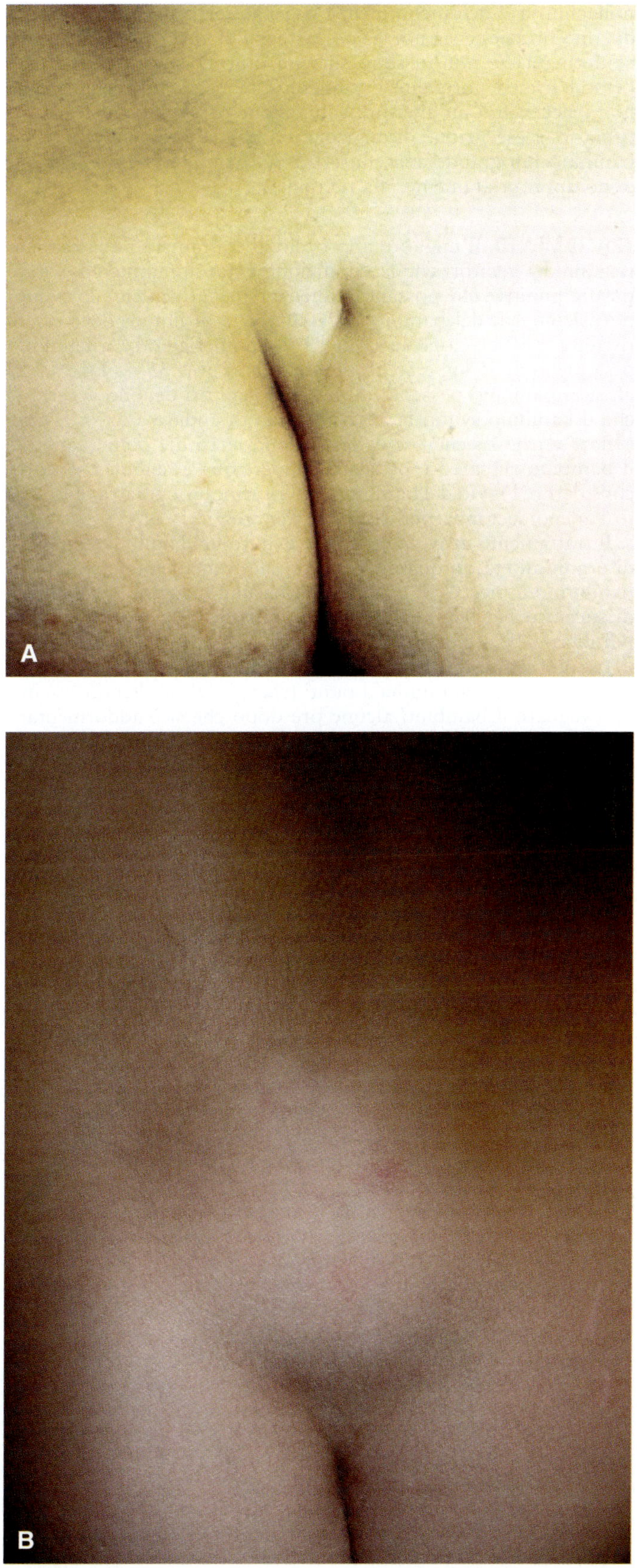

Figura 542-3. *A,* Aspetto delle natiche di un adolescente con *tethered cord* secondario a lipomeningocele. Si noti la fossetta sacrale e la deviazione del solco intergluteo a sinistra. *B,* Deposito di tessuto adiposo sul sacro in una bambina con *tethered cord* secondario a lipomeningocele.

normali. Gli studi urodinamici hanno dimostrato che la maggior parte di questi pazienti presenta contrazioni vescicali non inibite. Di solito si rivelano efficaci lo svuotamento vescicale programmato e la terapia anticolinergica, mentre solo raramente è necessario il cateterismo sterile intermittente.

Alpert SA, Cheng EY, Zebold KF, et al: Clean intermittent catheterization in genitally sensate children: Patient experience and health related quality of life. *J Urol* 2005;174:1616–1619.
Altaweel W, Jednack R, Bilodeau C, et al: Repeated intradetrusor botulinum toxin type A in children with neurogenic bladder due to myelomeningocele. *J Urol* 2006;175:1102–1105.
Elder JS: Latex allergy: Time for a change. *J Urol* 2006;175:1193–1194.
Gilbert SM, Hensle TW: Metabolic consequences and long-term complications of enterocystoplasty. *J Urol* 2005;173:1080–1086.
Joseph DB: Bladder rehabilitation in children with spina bifida: State of the art. *J Urol* 2005;173:1850–1851.
Kaufman BA: Neural tube defects. *Pediatr Clin North Am* 2004;51: 389–419.
Lottmann HB, Margaryan M, Bernuy M, et al: Long-term effects of dextranomer endoscopic injections for treatment of urinary incontinence: An update of a prospective study of 31 patients. *J Urol* 2006;175:1485–1489.
Metcalfe PD, Casale AJ, Kiefer MA, et al: Spontaneous bladder perforations: A report of 500 augmentations in children and analysis of risk. *J Urol* 2006;175:1466–1471.
Nguyen MT, Pavlock CL, Zderic, SA, et al: Overnight catheter drainage in children with poorly compliant bladders improves post-obstructive diuresis and urinary incontinence. *J Urol* 2005;174:1633–1636.
Nogueira M, Greenfield SP, Wan J, et al: Tethered cord in children: A clinical classification with urodynamic correlation. *J Urol* 2004;172:1677–1680.
Ozkan KU, Bauer SB, Khoshbin S, et al: Neurogenic bladder dysfunction after sacrococcygeal teratoma resection. *J Urol* 2006;175:292–296.
Snodgrass WT, Adams R: Initial urologic management of myelomeningocele. *Urol Clin North Am* 2004;31:427–434.
Soergel TM, Cain MP, Misseri R, et al: Transitional cell carcinoma of the bladder following augmentation cystoplasty for the neuropathic bladder. *J Urol* 2004;172:1649–1651.
Tanaka ST, Stone AR, Kurzrock EA: Transverse myelitis in children: Long-term urological outcomes. *J Urol* 2006;175:1865–1868.
Thomas J, Elder JS: Neuropathic bladder in children. *AUA Update Series,* 2007.

Capitolo 543 ■ Disfunzione minzionale

Jack S. Elder

MINZIONE NORMALE ED EDUCAZIONE DEGLI SFINTERI

Il feto svuota la vescica mediante una contrazione riflessa della vescica associata a una simultanea e a un rilassamento dello sfintere. La ritenzione delle urine consiste nell'inibizione dell'attività contrattile del detrusore mediata dai nervi simpatici e pudendi, accompagnata dalla chiusura del collo vescicale e dell'uretra prossimale con aumento dell'attività dello sfintere esterno.

Il neonato ha un riflesso di svuotamento vescicale coordinato anche 15-20 volte al giorno. Nel tempo, la capacità della vescica aumenta. Nei bambini fino ai 14 anni di età, la capacità vescicale media in once è uguale all'età più 2.

A 2-4 anni, il bambino è pronto dal punto di vista dello sviluppo a iniziare l'educazione degli sfinteri. Per raggiungere il controllo cosciente della vescica, devono essere presenti diverse condizioni: consapevolezza del riempimento vescicale, inibizione corticale (modulazione soprapontina) delle contrazioni vescicale riflesse (instabili), capacità di contrarre coscientemente lo sfintere esterno per prevenire l'incontinenza, normale crescita vescicale e motivazione del bambino a rimanere asciutto. La fase di transizione dello svuotamento si riferisce al periodo in cui il bambino sta acquisendo il controllo vescicale: le bambine assumono tipicamente il controllo vescicale prima dei bambini, e normalmente il controllo delle feci viene raggiunto prima di quello delle urine.

ENURESI NOTTURNA

Dall'età di 5 anni, il 90-95% dei bambini è quasi completamente continente durante il giorno, mentre l'80-85% è continente la notte. Si definisce enuresi notturna (vedi Capitolo 22.3) lo svuotamento vescicale durante la notte dopo i 5 anni, età in cui è previsto il controllo volontario della minzione. L'enuresi può essere primitiva (la percentuale stimata, 75-90%, dei bambini con enuresi; controllo notturno delle urine mai raggiunto) o secondaria (10-25%; il bambino è rimasto asciutto la notte per almeno alcuni mesi e quindi si è sviluppata l'enuresi). Inoltre, il 75% dei bambini con enuresi si bagna solo la notte, mentre il 25% si bagna sia il giorno sia la notte. Questa distinzione è importante perché i bambini con entrambe le forme hanno una maggiore probabilità di avere anomalie del tratto urinario.

EPIDEMIOLOGIA. Circa il 60% dei bambini con enuresi notturna è di sesso maschile, con un'anamnesi familiare positiva nel 50% dei casi. Anche se l'enuresi notturna primitiva può essere poligenica, sono stati localizzati geni candidati sui cromosomi 12 e 13. Se un genitore era enuretico, ciascun figlio ha il 44% di rischio di enuresi; se entrambi i genitori erano enuretici ciascun figlio ha una probabilità del 77%. L'enuresi notturna senza evidenti sintomi relativi allo svuotamento durante il giorno interessa anche il 20% dei bambini all'età di 5 anni; essa scompare spontaneamente nel 15% circa dei bambini interessati ogni anno successivo. La sua frequenza negli adulti è inferiore all'1%.

PATOGENESI. La patogenesi dell'enuresi notturna (normali abitudini menzionali durante il giorno) è multifattoriale (Tab. 543-1).

MANIFESTAZIONI CLINICHE E DIAGNOSI. Occorre eseguire un'accurata anamnesi, specialmente rispetto all'assunzione di liquidi di notte e al pattern dell'enuresi notturna. I bambini con diabete insipido (vedi Capitolo 559), diabete mellito (vedi Capitolo 590) e con nefropatie croniche (vedi Capitolo 559) possono avere un'elevata diuresi obbligata e una polidipsia compensatoria. Occorre informarsi dai familiari se il bambino russa durante la notte. Un esame obiettivo completo dovrebbe comprendere la palpazione dell'addome e l'esame rettale dopo svuotamento vescicale per valutare la possibilità di una distensione vescicale cronica. Il bambino con enuresi notturna deve essere esaminato accuratamente per la ricerca di anomalie neurologiche e spinali. Esiste un aumento dell'incidenza di batteriuria nelle bambine enuretiche e, in tal caso, deve essere studiata e trattata (vedi Capitolo 538), anche se ciò non sempre porta a una risoluzione dell'enuresi. Occorre eseguire un esame delle urine dopo digiuno notturno per la valutazione del peso specifico o dell'osmolarità o di entrambi, per escludere che una poliuria sia la causa della pollachiuria e dell'incontinenza e per accertarsi che la capacità di concentrazione sia normale. L'assenza di glicosuria deve essere confermata. Se non vi sono sintomi diurni, l'esame obiettivo e l'esame urine è normale e l'urinocultura è negativa, generalmente non è necessaria un'ulteriore valutazione per patologie del tratto urinario. L'esecuzione di un'ecografia renale è ragionevole in un bambino più grande con enuresi o nei bambini che non rispondono appropriatamente alla terapia.

TABELLA 543.1. Cause di enuresi notturna

Ritardo maturativo dei meccanismi corticali che consentono il controllo volontario del riflesso minzionale
Disordini del sonno
"Sonno profondo" (nessun pattern specifico del sonno identificato)
L'enuresi può verificarsi in qualunque fase del sonno
Tutti i bambini hanno la maggiore difficoltà a svegliarsi nel primo terzo della notte, la minore difficoltà nell'ultimo terzo, ma i bambini enuretici hanno maggiore difficoltà a svegliarsi di quelli con controllo vescicale normale
Ridotta produzione di ormone antipiretico durante la notte, con aumento della diuresi
I bambini enuretici spesso vengono descritti come quelli che "bagnano il letto"
Fattori genetici; i cromosomi 12 e 13q sono i siti probabili del gene dell'enuresi
Anamnesi familiare dei bambini enuretici spesso positiva per enuresi
Fattori organici, come IVU o uropatia ostruttiva
Fattori psicologici più spesso coinvolti nell'enuresi secondaria
Apnea del sonno (russamento) secondaria a ipertrofia adenoidea

TRATTAMENTO. Il migliore approccio al trattamento è la rassicurazione dei genitori che la condizione è autolimitante ed evitare misure punitive che possano influenzare negativamente lo sviluppo psicologico del bambino. L'assunzione di liquidi deve essere ristretta a 60 cL dopo le 18 o 19 del pomeriggio se il bambino pesa meno di 35 kg, a 85 cL se il bambino pesa 35-45 kg e a 110 cL se il bambino pesa più di 45 kg. I genitori devono accertarsi che il bambino svuoti la vescica prima di andare a letto. È utile evitare anche zucchero e caffeina dopo le 16 del pomeriggio. Se il bambino russa ed è presente un'ipertrofia adenoidea, occorre considerare l'invio del bambino dall'otorinolaringoiatra, in quanto l'adenoidectomia può risolvere l'enuresi.

Il trattamento attivo deve essere evitato nei bambini con meno di 6 anni di età, in quanto l'enuresi è estremamente comune nei bambini più piccoli. Il trattamento ha una maggiore probabilità di successo nei bambini vicini alla pubertà rispetto ai bambini più piccoli.

La più semplice misura iniziale è la **terapia motivazionale** e comprende un diagramma a punti (*star chart*) per le notti asciutte. Svegliare il bambino alcune ore dopo che si è addormentato per farlo urinare spesso consente un risveglio asciutto, anche se questa misura non è curativa. Alcuni studi hanno consigliato che i bambini trattengano le urine per periodi progressivamente crescenti durante il giorno, ma non vi sono evidenze che questo approccio sia efficace.

La terapia di condizionamento comprende l'uso di un sistema di allarme sonoro o vibratorio connesso a un sensore di umidità posto nella biancheria intima. L'allarme suona quando si verifica lo svuotamento e ha lo scopo di svegliare il bambino e spingerlo a urinare. Questa forma di terapia è considerata curativa ed è stato riportato un successo del 30-60%. Spesso, l'allarme sonoro sveglia altri componenti della famiglia e non il bambino enuretico; spesso è necessario l'uso continuativo per diversi mesi. La **terapia di condizionamento** tende a essere efficace soprattutto nei bambini più grandi. Un'altra forma di terapia alla quale rispondono alcuni bambini è l'autoipnosi. Il ruolo principale della terapia psicologica è di aiutare il bambino ad affrontare psicologicamente l'enuresi e di motivarlo a urinare durante la notte se si sveglia con la vescica piena.

La **terapia farmacologica** ha lo scopo di trattare sintomatologicamente l'enuresi e pertanto è considerata di seconda linea e non curativa. Come sottolineato nel Capitolo 22.3, i confronti diretti tra sistemi di allarme e terapia farmacologia sono a favore dei primi a causa di un minor tasso di recidive, anche se i tassi di risposta iniziali sono equivalenti. Una forma di trattamento è la desmopressina acetato, un analogo sintetico dell'ormone antidiuretico che riduce la produzione di urine nel corso della notte. È disponibile sotto forma di compressa, con un dosaggio di 0,2-0,6 mg prima di andare a letto. Nel passato è stato usato come spray nasale al dosaggio da 10 μg (1 spray) a 40 μg (4 spray in totale) prima di andare a letto. Si deve utilizzare la minore dose efficace. Nei bambini con rinorrea, lo spray nasale non viene assorbito e quindi è inefficace. La restrizione dei fluidi durante la notte è importante e il farmaco non dovrebbe essere usato se il bambino ha una malattia sistemica con vomito o diarrea. È stata riportata una iponatremia in alcuni bambini con lo spray nasale, prima di tutto in soggetti che non usavano il farmaco appropriatamente. L'iponatremia non è stata riportata i bambini che usavano le compresse. La desmopressina acetato è efficace in almeno il 40% dei bambini. Se efficace, deve essere usata per 3-6 mesi e quindi deve essere fatto un tentativo di ridurre il dosaggio. Se la riduzione del dosaggio risulta in una recidiva dell'enuresi, il bambino deve ritornare alla dose più alta. Non sono stati riportati eventi avversi con l'uso a lungo termine della desmopressina acetato. Un altro agente farmacologico è l'imipramina, un antidepressivo triciclico. Questo farmaco possiede un leggero effetto anticolinergico e α-adrenergico, riduce leggermente la diuresi e può anche alterare il ritmo del sonno. La dose di imipramina è di 25 mg nei bambini di 6-8 anni di età, 50 mg nei bambini di 9-12 anni di età e di 75 mg negli adolescenti. I tassi di successo riportati sono del 30-60%. Gli effetti collaterali comprendono ansia, insonnia e secchezza del cavo orale, e disturbi del ritmo cardiaco. Il farmaco inoltre è una della cause più comuni di avvelenamento da farmaci soggetti a ricetta medica nei bambini più piccoli. L'ossibutinina cloruro, un farmaco anticolinergico puro, è stato usato in alcuni bambini con enuresi notturna primitiva, ma il tasso di risposta è basso, in parte a causa della durata di azione che è soltanto di 6 ore.

Nei casi che non rispondono alla terapia, l'associazione di più terapie spesso è efficace. Per esempio, l'uso dell'allarme associato alla desmopressina è più efficace di entrambi i trattamenti da soli. Inoltre, l'associazione di ossibutinina cloruro e desmopressina è più efficace di entrambi i farmaci somministrati singolarmente. Desmopressina e imipramina non devono essere associati.

INCONTINENZA DIURNA

L'incontinenza diurna non secondaria ad anomalie neurologiche è comune nei bambini. All'età di 5 anni, il 95% dei bambini è rimasto asciutto durante la notte in un determinato momento e il 92% è continente. A 7 anni, il 96% dei bambini è continente, anche se il 15% presenta saltuariamente urgenza minzionale significativa. A 12 anni, il 99% dei bambini è continente durante il giorno. La causa più comune di incontinenza diurna è **un'instabilità vescicale pediatrica** (definita anche come vescica iperattiva o non inibita oppure come spasmi vescicali). La Tabella 543-2 elenca le cause di incontinenza diurna nei bambini. Aspetti importanti dell'anamnesi comprendono il pattern dell'incontinenza (cioè la frequenza), il volume di urine perso durante gli episodi di incontinenza, se l'incontinenza è associata a urgenza o ad atti come il ridere ecc., se si verifica anche dopo lo svuotamento e se è continua. Devono essere valutate la frequenza di svuotamento e se sia presente enuresi notturna, un mitto forte e continuo, oppure una sensazione di svuotamento vescicale incompleto. È utile un diario minzionale che registri quando il bambino è asciutto o bagnato. Devono essere ricercati altri problemi urologici come infezioni delle vie urinarie (IVU), reflusso, disordini neurologici o un'anamnesi familiare di anomalie di duplicazione. Occorre valutare anche le abitudini dell'alvo, poiché l'incontinenza è comune nei bambini con stipsi o encopresi, o entrambe le cose. Incontinenza diurna può essere presente in bambine con una storia di abuso sessuale. L'esame obiettivo è diretto all'identificazione dei segni e sintomi delle cause organiche di incontinenza: bassa statura, ipertensione, aumento di volume di reni o vescica ed entrambi, stipsi, aderenze labiali, ectopia ureterale (dalla Fig. 543-1 alla Fig. 543-3), anomalie sacrali o del dorso (vedi Fig. 542-3) e anomalie neurologiche. Devono essere eseguiti un esame delle urine o un'urinocultura o entrambi per la ricerca di eventuali infezioni. In alcuni casi, è appropriato il controllo del volume urinario residuo postminzionale o della velocità del flusso urinario. Le metodiche di imaging sono riservate ai bambini con segni e sintomi fisici significativi, un'anamnesi familiare di anomale delle vie urinarie, IVU o ai pazienti che non rispondono appropriatamente alla terapia. È indicata un'ecografia renale con o senza cistouretrografia menzionale. Devono essere eseguiti studi urodinamici se vi sono evidenze di malattia neurologica e può essere utile se la terapia empirica non è efficace.

TABELLA 543-2. Cause di incontinenza urinaria nell'infanzia

Vescica instabile pediatrica (vescica non inibita)
Minzione infrequente
Dissinergia detrusore-sfintere
Vescica neurologica non neurologica (sindrome di Hinman)
Minzione vaginale
Incontinenza da aumento della pressione addominale (riso)
Cistite
Ostruzione dell'efflusso vescicale (valvole uretrali posteriori)
Uretere ectopico e fistola
Anomalie dello sfintere (epispadia, estrofia, anomalie del seno urogenitale)
Neurologica
Incontinenza da sovrafflusso
Traumatica
Iatrogena
Comportamentale
Combinata

VESCICA INSTABILE (IPERATTIVA) PEDIATRICA

I bambini con vescica iperattiva di solito presentano frequenza urinaria, urgenza e incontinenza da urgenza. Spesso le bambine si accovacciano per cercare di impedire l'incontinenza (atteggiamento denominato **riverenza di Vincent**). La vescica in questi bambini è più piccola del normale e presenta forti contrazioni non inibite. Circa il 25% dei bambini con enuresi notturna presentano anche sintomi di iperattività vescicale. Molti bambini indicano che non percepiscono lo stimolo a urinare, anche prima della dell'incontinenza. Nelle femmine, è comune una storia di IVU ricorrenti, ma l'incontinenza può persistere a lungo anche dopo che le infezioni sono state messe sotto controllo.

Non è chiaro se in questi casi la disfunzione minzionale è una sequela delle IVU o se è la disfunzione minzionale a predisporre alle IVU ricorrenti. Nelle bambine, l'uretrocistografia minzionale evidenzia spesso una dilatazione uretrale (*spinning top deformity*; Fig. 543-4) e un restringimento del collo vescicale con ipertrofia della parte vescicale. L'aspetto dell'uretra deriva da un inadeguato rilassamento dello sfintere urinario esterno e la stipsi è comune.

La vescica iperattiva va quasi sempre incontro a risoluzione, ma il tempo per la risoluzione è altamente variabile, talvolta fino agli anni dell'adolescenza. La terapia iniziale consiste nella minzione programmata, ogni 1,5-2 ore. Inoltre, è importante il trattamento della stipsi e delle IVU. Un altro trattamento è il biofeedback, in cui si insegna ai bambini esercizi per i muscoli del pavimento pelvico (**esercizi di Kegel**), in quanto vi sono evidenze che l'esecuzione giornaliera di questi esercizi può ridurre o eliminare le contrazioni della vescica instabile. Il biofeedback può inoltre comprendere studi di flusso con elettromiografia dello

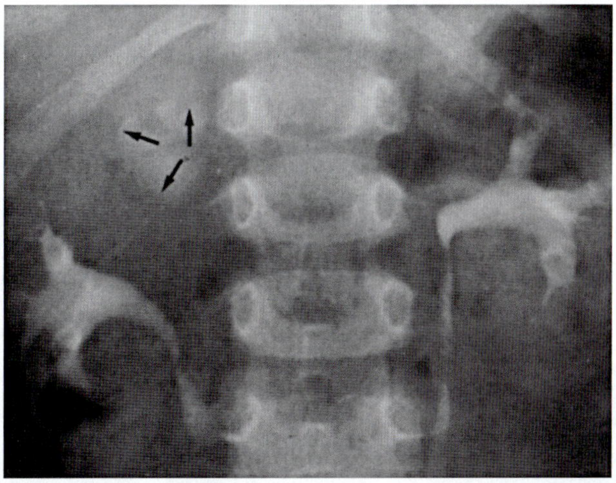

Figura 543-1. Duplicazione del sistema collettore destro con uretere ectopico. L'urografia escretoria in una bambina con pattern minzionale normale e "sgocciolamento" urinario costante. Il rene sinistro è normale, mentre sul lato destro, ben visualizzato, si osserva il sistema collettore inferiore di un rene duplicato. Sul polo superiore, di fronte al primo e al secondo corpo vertebrale, si noti l'accumulo di mezzo di contrasto corrispondente a un polo superiore scarsamente funzionale drenato da un uretere che sbocca nel vestibolo.

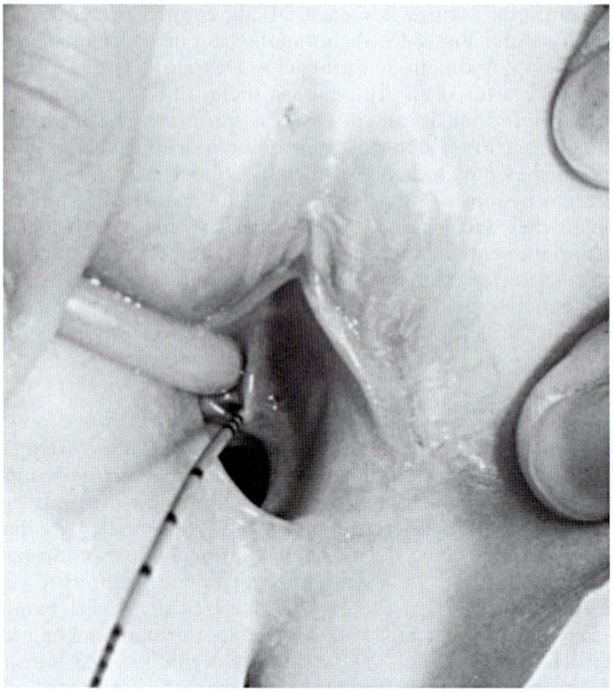

Figura 543-2. L'immagine mostra un uretere ectopico che sbocca nel vestibolo in prossimità del meato uretrale. Il sottile catetere ureterale con tacche trasversali è stato introdotto nell'uretere ectopico. Questa bambina aveva un pattern minzionale normale e "sgocciolamento" urinario costante.

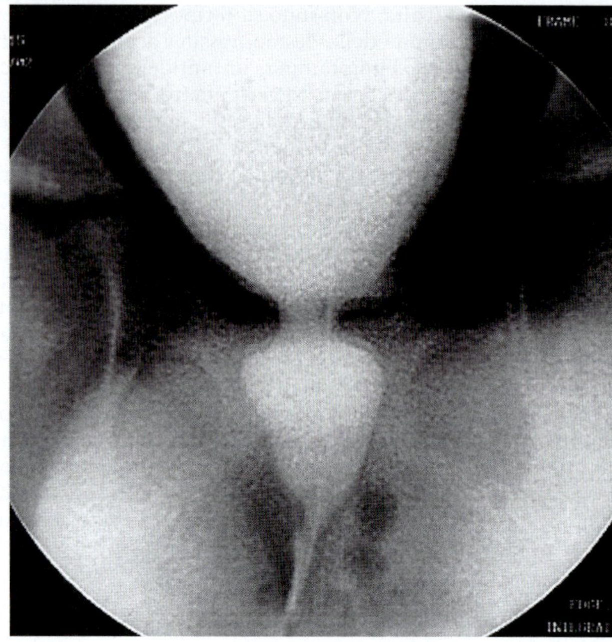

Figura 543-4. Deformità a "spinning top". La cistouretrografia dimostra una dilatazione uretrale con stenosi uretrale distale e contrazione del collo vescicale.

sfintere per accertare che il pavimento pelvico si rilassi durante la minzione e anche un'ecografia per la valutazione del residuo urinario postminzionale. La terapia anticolinergica con ossibutinina cloruro, iosciamina o tolterodina riduce l'iperattività vescicale e può favorire il raggiungimento della continenza. Il trattamento con un α-bloccante come la terazosina o la doxazina può facilitare lo svuotamento vescicale favorendo il rilassamento del collo vescicale; gli α-bloccanti hanno lievi proprietà anticolinergiche. Se la terapia farmacologia è efficace, occorre ridurre periodicamente il dosaggio per determinare la necessità di continuare la terapia. I bambini che non rispondono alla terapia devono essere valutati urodinamicamente per escludere altre possibili forme di disfunzione vescicale o sfinteriale. Nei casi refrattari, la neuromodulazione sacrale è una nuova tecnica che si è dimostrata promettente.

VESCICA NEUROLOGICA NON NEUROLOGICA (SINDROME DI HINMAN)

La sindrome di Hinman è una malattia più grave ma meno comune che comprende il mancato rilassamento dello sfintere esterno durante lo svuotamento in bambini senza anomalie neurologiche. I bambini con questa sindrome, chiamata anche **dissinergia detrusore-sfintere**, presentano di solito un mitto irregolare (a getti improvvisi), IVU ricorrenti, stipsi, encopresi, oltre a bagnarsi di giorno e di notte. La valutazione dei bambini affetti rivela spesso reflusso vescicoureterale, vescica con trabecolatura parietale e

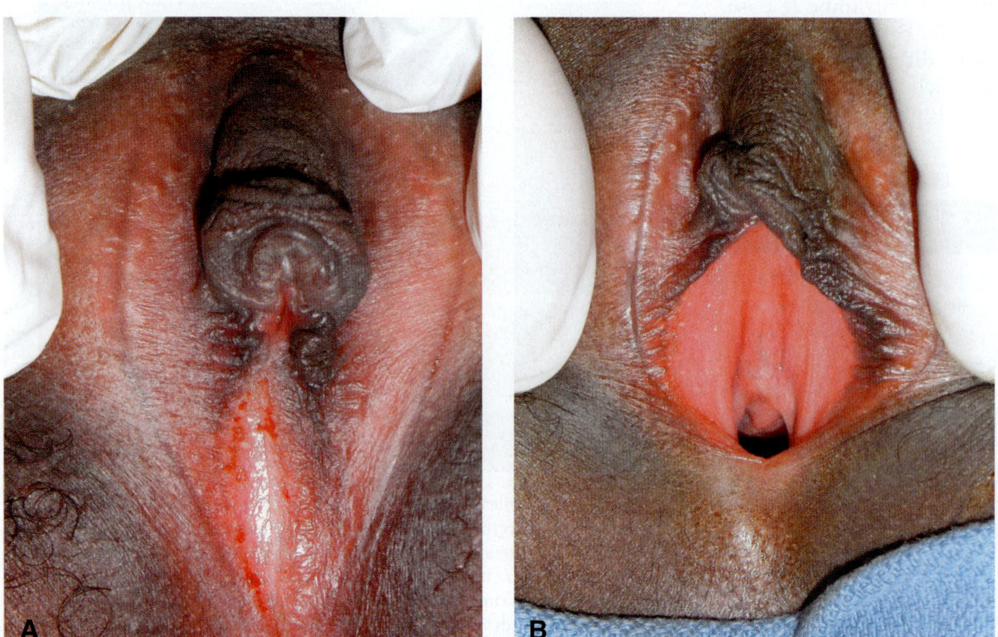

Figura 543-3. *A*, Aderenze labiali. Si noti l'impossibilità di visualizzare il meato uretrale e la vagina. *B*, Aspetto normale dei genitali femminili esterni dopo lisi delle aderenze labiali.

un ridotto tasso di flusso urinario con pattern intermittente. Nei casi gravi si possono verificare idronefrosi, insufficienza renale e anche nefropatia terminale. Si ritiene che la patogenesi di questa sindrome comprenda l'acquisizione di abitudini minzionali anormali durante la fase di educazione degli sfinteri; la sindrome si osserva raramente nei bambini più piccoli. Sono indicati studi urodinamici e RMN della colonna vertebrale per escludere una causa neurologica della disfunzione vescicale. Il trattamento di solito è complesso e può comprendere una terapia anticolinergica e α-bloccante, la programmazione della minzione, il trattamento della stipsi, le modifiche comportamentali e l'incoraggiamento al rilassamento durante la minzione. Anche il biofeedback è stato usato con successo nei bambini più grandi per insegnare il rilassamento dello sfintere esterno. In alcuni casi, l'iniezione di tossina botulinica nello sfintere esterno può assicurare una sua paralisi temporanea, riducendo quindi la resistenza all'efflusso e, nei casi gravi, è necessario il cateterismo intermittente per assicurare lo svuotamento vescicale. In pazienti selezionati, è necessaria la diversione urinaria esterna per protegge le vie urinarie superiori. Questi bambini richiedono un trattamento a lungo termine e un attento follow-up.

MINZIONE INFREQUENTE

La minzione infrequente è un comune disordine della minzione, di solito associato infezioni delle vie urinarie. I bambini affetti (in genere bambine) urinano solo 2 volte al giorno invece delle normali 4-7 volte. Con la sovradistensione vescicale e la ritenzione prolungata delle urine, la crescita batterica può portare a IVU ricorrenti. Alcuni di questi bambini sono affetti da stipsi. Alcuni presentano anche occasionali episodi di incontinenza dovuti a urgenza da sovrafflusso. Il disordine è comportamentale. Se il bambino ha IVU frequenti, il trattamento comprende la profilassi antibatterica e l'incoraggiamento a uno svuotamento vescicale frequente e completo mediante una doppia minzione fino a quando viene ristabilito un normale pattern minzionale.

MINZIONE VAGINALE

Nelle bambine con minzione vaginale, si verifica di solito un'incontinenza dopo la minzione una volta che la bambina si alza in piedi. Di solito il volume di urine è di 5-10 mL. Una delle cause più comuni è costituita dalle aderenze labiali (vedi Fig. 543-3). Questa lesione si osserva nelle bambine più piccole e può essere trattata topicamente con l'applicazione sulle aderenze di una crema contenente estrogeni o mediante una lisi ambulatoriale delle aderenze. Alcune bambine hanno una minzione vaginale perché non aprono a sufficienza le gambe durante la minzione. Queste bambine di solito sono sovrappeso o non abbassano la biancheria intima fino alle caviglie al momento di urinare. Il trattamento comprende il consiglio di aprire le gambe a sufficienza durante la minzione. Il modo più efficace a questo scopo è di far sedere la bambina sul sanitario con il viso rivolto verso il muro.

ALTRE CAUSE DI INCONTINENZA NELLE BAMBINE

L'**ectopia ureterale**, di solito associata a una duplicazione del sistema collettore nelle bambine, si riferisce a una situazione in cui l'urina drena al di fuori della vescica, spesso in vagina o nell'uretra distale. Può produrre un'incontinenza urinaria caratterizzata da un costante sgocciolamento urinario per tutto il giorno, anche se il bambino urina regolarmente. Talvolta la produzione di urina dal segmento renale drenato dall'uretere ectopico è ridotta e il drenaggio urinario viene confuso con perdite vaginali acquose. Le bambine con un'anamnesi di perdite vaginali o incontinenza e un pattern minzionale anormale richiedono una valutazione accurata. L'orifizio ectopico di solito è di difficile localizzazione. All'ecografia o all'urografia intravenosa è possibile sospettare una duplicazione del sistema collettore (Fig. 543-1), ma il sistema collettore superiore drenato dall'uretere ectopico di solito ha una funzionalità scarsa o ritardata. La TC renale contribuisce a escludere le duplicazioni meno evidenti che possono non essere diagnosticate con l'urografia intravenosa. Può essere necessario l'esame in anestesia dell'orifizio ureterale ectopico nel vestibolo o nella vagina. In questi casi, il trattamento è rappresentato dalla nefrectomia parziale, con rimozione del segmento del polo superiore del rene duplicato e del suo uretere fino al margine pelvico o dalla ureteroureterostomia ipsilaterale in cui l'uretere ectopico del polo superiore viene anastomizzato all'uretere del polo inferiore normalmente posizionato.

La ***giggle incontinence*** interessa tipicamente le bambine tra i 7 e i 15 anni di età. L'incontinenza si presenta improvvisamente durante l'atto del ridere e lo svuotamento vescicale è completo. Si ritiene che la causa risieda nell'improvviso rilassamento dello sfintere urinario. I farmaci anticolinergici e la minzione programmata sono raramente efficaci. Il trattamento più efficace è il metilfenidato a basso dosaggio.

L'incontinenza totale nelle bambine può essere secondaria a epispadia. Questa condizione, che interessa soltanto 1 bambina su 480 000, è caratterizzata dalla separazione della sinfisi pubica, separazione del lato sinistro e destro del clitoride e da pervietà uretrale. Il trattamento consiste nella ricostruzione del collo uretrale o nell'inserimento di uno sfintere urinario artificiale per la riparazione dell'uretra non competente. A certe malformazioni del seno urogenitale può essere associata un'uretra breve e non competente. La diagnosi di tali malformazioni richiede un elevato indice di sospetto e un attento esame obiettivo di tutte le bambine incontinenti. In questi casi, la ricostruzione uretrale e vaginale spesso permette di ripristinare la continenza.

DISORDINI MINZIONALI SENZA INCONTINENZA

Alcuni bambini presentano un esordio improvviso di pollachiuria grave, urinando anche ogni 10-15 minuti durante il giorno, senza disuria, IVU, incontinenza diurna o nicturia. L'età in cui più comunemente si presentano questi sintomi è tra i 4 e i 6 anni, dopo l'educazione degli sfinteri, e la grande maggioranza degli individui affetti è di sesso maschile. Questa condizione è denominata **sindrome della pollachiuria diurna**. La condizione è funzionale e non vi sono problemi anatomici. Spesso la sindrome si presenta subito prima che il bambino inizi la scuola materna o se ha problemi emozionali legati a situazioni di stress familiare. Questi bambini devono essere controllati per le IVU e il medico deve accertare che il bambino svuoti la vescica in modo soddisfacente. Occasionalmente, può essere implicata un'ossiuriasi. La condizione è autolimitata e i sintomi generalmente si risolvono entro 2-3 mesi. La terapia anticolinergica raramente è efficace. Alcuni bambini manifestano la **sindrome della disuria-ematuria**, in cui il bambino presenta una disuria senza IVU e un'ematuria microscopica o macroscopica. Tale condizione interessa i bambini che hanno raggiunto il controllo degli sfinteri ed è spesso secondaria a ipercalciuria. Occorre valutare l'eliminazione di calcio e creatinina nelle urine delle 24 ore. Un'eliminazione di calcio nelle 24 ore di più di 4 mg/kg non è normale e deve essere trattata con tiazidi, poiché alcuni di questi bambini possono essere a rischio di urolitiasi.

Akbal C, Genc Y, Burbu B, et al: Dysfunctional voiding and incontinence scoring system: Quantitative evaluation of incontinence symptoms in pediatric population. *J Urol* 2005;173:969–973.

Ayan S, Kaya K, Topsakal K, et al: Efficacy of tolterodine as a first-line treatment for non-neurogenic voiding dysfunction in children. *BJU Int* 2005;96:411–414.

Bower WF, Yip SK, Yeung CK: Dysfunctional elimination symptoms in childhood and adulthood. *J Urol* 2005;174:1623–1627.

Feldman AS, Bauer SB: Diagnosis and management of dysfunctional voiding. *Curr Opin Pediatr* 2006;18:139–147.

Firoozi F, Batniji R, Aslan AR, et al: Resolution of diurnal incontinence and nocturnal enuresis after adenotonsillectomy in children. *J Urol* 2006; 175:1885–1888.

Fitzgerald MP, Thom DH, Wassel-Fyr C, et al: Childhood urinary symptoms predict adult overactive bladder symptoms. *J Urol* 2006;175:989–993.
Glazener CM, Evans JH, Cheuk DK: Complementary and miscellaneous interventions for nocturnal enuresis in children. *Cochrane Database Syst Rev* 2005 Apr 18:CD005230.
Glazener CM, Evans JH, Peto RE: Alarm interventions for nocturnal enuresis in children. *Cochrane Database Syst Rev* 2005 Apr 18:CD002911.
Hjalmas K, Arnold T, Bower W, et al: Nocturnal enuresis: An international evidence based management strategy. *J Urol* 2004;171:2545–2561.
Humphreys MR, Reinberg YE: Contemporary and emerging drug treatments for urinary incontinence in children. *Paediatr Drugs* 2005;7:151–162.
Joinson C, Heron J, Butler U, et al: Psychological differences between children with and without soiling problems. *Pediatrics* 2006;117:1575–1583.
Kilic N, Balkan E, Akgoz S, et al: Comparison of the effectiveness and side-effects of tolterodine and oxybutynin in children with detrusor instability. *Int J Urol* 2006;13:105–108.
Klijn AJ, Asselman M, Vijverberg MA, et al: The diameter of the rectum on ultrasonography as a diagnostic tool for constipation in children with dysfunctional voiding. *J Urol* 2004;172:1986–1988.
Kramer SA, Rathbun SR, Elkins D, et al: Double-blind placebo controlled study of alpha-adrenergic receptor antagonists (doxazosin) for treatment of voiding dysfunction in the pediatric population. *J Urol* 2005;173: 2121–2124.
Neveus T, von Gontard A, Hoebeke P, et al: The standardisation of terminology of lower urinary tract function in children and adolescents: Report from the Standardisation Committee of the International Children's Continence Society (ICCS). *J Urol* 2006;176:314–324.
Nguyen MT, Pavlock CL, Zderic SA, et al: Overnight catheter drainage in children with poorly compliant bladders improves post-obstructive diuresis and urinary incontinence. *J Urol* 2005;174:1633–1636.
Robson WL, Leung AK, Van Howe R: Primary and secondary nocturnal enuresis: Similarities in presentation. *Pediatrics* 2005;115:956–959.
Sommer BR, O'Hara R, Askari N, et al: The effect of oxybutynin treatment on cognition in children with diurnal incontinence. *J Urol* 2005;173: 2125–2127.
Thumfart J, Roehr CC, Kapelari K, et al: Desmopressin associated symptomatic hyponatremic hypervolemia in children. Are there predictive factors? *J Urol* 2005;174:294–298.
Van de Walle JG, Bogaert GA, Mattsson S, et al: A new fast-melting oral formulation of desmopressin: A pharmacodynamic study in children with primary nocturnal enuresis. *BJU Int* 2006;97:603–609.
Yagci F, Kibar Y, Akay O, et al: The effect of biofeedback treatment on voiding and urodynamic parameters in children with voiding dysfunction. *J Urol* 2005;174:1994–1997.

Capitolo 544 ■ Anomalie del pene e dell'uretra Jack S. Elder

IPOSPADIA

Il termine **ipospadia** si riferisce a un orifizio uretrale che si trova sulla superficie ventrale dell'asta, condizione che interessa 1 neonato maschio su 250. È presente uno sviluppo incompleto del prepuzio, noto come **cappuccio dorsale**, in cui il prepuzio si trova sugli aspetti dorsale e laterale dell'asta ed è assente centralmente. Alcuni bambini con ipospadia, particolarmente quelli con ipospadia prossimale, presentano una **chordee**, condizione per cui il pene è incurvato centralmente durante l'erezione. È stato ipotizzato che l'incidenza di ipospadia sia in aumento, forse a causa dell'esposizione in utero a sostanze chimiche di tipo estrogenico o a *endocrine disruptor* di tipo antiandrogenico (per es. policlorobifenili, fitoestrogeni).

MANIFESTAZIONI CLINICHE. L'ipospadia è classificata in base alla posizione del meato uretrale dopo aver valutato la presenza o no di chordee (Fig. 544-1). La deformità viene descritta come balanica (del glande), coronale, sottocoronale, mediopeniena, penoscrotale, scrotale o perineale. Circa il 60% dei casi appare distale, il 25% sottocornale o mediopeniene, mentre il 15% prossimale. Nei casi più gravi, lo scroto è bifido e talvolta si estende sulla base dorsale del pene (*engulfment* scrotale). Esiste anche una variante megameatale, in cui il prepuzio è normale, ma è presente ipospadia distale o sottocoronale, con meato a "bocca di pesce". Questi casi possono non essere diagnosticati fino a quando non viene eseguita una circoncisione.

L'ipospadia è di solito un'anomalia isolata, ma è anche comune nei maschi con anomalie congenite multiple. Circa il 10% dei maschi con ipospadia presenta un testicolo criptorchide; come sono comuni anche le ernie inguinali. Nel neonato, la diagnosi differenziale dell'ipospadia prossimale associata a testicolo criptorchide deve comprendere forme di genitali ambigui, in particolare una virilizzazione femminile (iperplasia surrenalica congenita) e disgenesia gonadica mista. Occorre eseguire un cariotipo nei pazienti con ipospadia prossimale o mediopeniena e criptorchidismo (vedi Capitolo 584). Nei bambini con ipospadia penoscrotale, occorre prendere in considerazione una cistouretrografia minzionale, poiché il 5-10% di questi bambini presenta un utricolo prostatico dilatato, che rappresenta un residuo del sistema di Mueller (vedi Capitolo 554). L'incidenza di altre anomalie del tratto genitorurinario nei bambini con ipospadia è basso.

Le complicanze dell'ipospadia non trattata comprendono (1) sia anomalie della morfologia del mitto, sia deflessione centrale o allargamento marcato; (2) disfunzione sessuale secondaria alla curvatura del pene; (3) infertilità se il meato uretrale è prossimale; e (4) stenosi meatale (congenita), che è rara. Lo scopo della terapia dell'ipospadia è quello di correggere le deformità funzionali ed estetiche. Mentre la riparazione dell'ipospadia è raccomandata per i bambini con ipospadia mediopeniena e prossimale, alcuni bambini con ipospadia distale non evidenziano anomalie funzionali e non richiedono una correzione chirurgica.

TRATTAMENTO. Il trattamento inizia nel periodo neonatale. Occorre evitare la circoncisione poiché il prepuzio spesso viene utilizzato nell'intervento di correzione. L'età ideale per la correzione in un bambino sano sono i 6-12 mesi, poiché non vi sono più rischi derivanti dall'anestesia generale a questa età rispetto a 2-3 anni, la crescita del pene negli anni successivi è lenta, il bambino non ricorda la procedura chirurgica e la necessità di analgesici dopo l'intervento è minore che nei bambini più grandi. Con l'eccezione dell'ipospadia prossimale, in teoria tutti i casi vengono corretti in un singolo intervento su base ambulatoriale. L'intervento più comune consiste nella tubularizzazione della lamina uretrale distale al meato uretrale, che viene ricoperta con un lembo dal peduncolo al prepuzio, denominato *intervento con lamina incisa e tubularizzata* (TIP). I casi più prossimali richiedono una correzione in due tempi. Il tasso di complicanze è basso: 5% per le ipospadia distali, 10% per le ipospadie mediopeniene e 15-20% per le ipospadie prossimali. Le complicanze più comuni comprendono la fistola uretrocutanea e la stenosi meatale. Altre complicanze comprendono un mitto deformato e deformità uretrali. Il trattamento di queste complicanze di solito è immediato. La correzione dell'ipospadia è un intervento tecnicamente impegnativo e deve essere eseguito da un chirurgo esperto e specialista in urologia pediatrica.

CHORDEE SENZA IPOSPADIA

In alcuni bambini è presente una curvatura ventrale del pene (**chordee**) e uno sviluppo incompleto del prepuzio (**cappuccio dorsale**), ma il meato uretrale si trova sulla punta del glande (Fig. 544-2). Nella maggior parte di questi bambini, l'uretra è normale ma vi è scarsità di cute ventrale del pene oppure bande ventrali inelastiche e sporgenti di fascia del dartos che impediscono un'erezione corretta. Tuttavia, in alcuni casi, l'uretra è breve e ipoplasica ed è necessaria un'uretroplastica formale per la riparazione. L'unico segno di questa anomalia nel neonato può essere un prepuzio a cappuccio ed è consigliata la correzione in anestesia generale a 6 mesi di età.

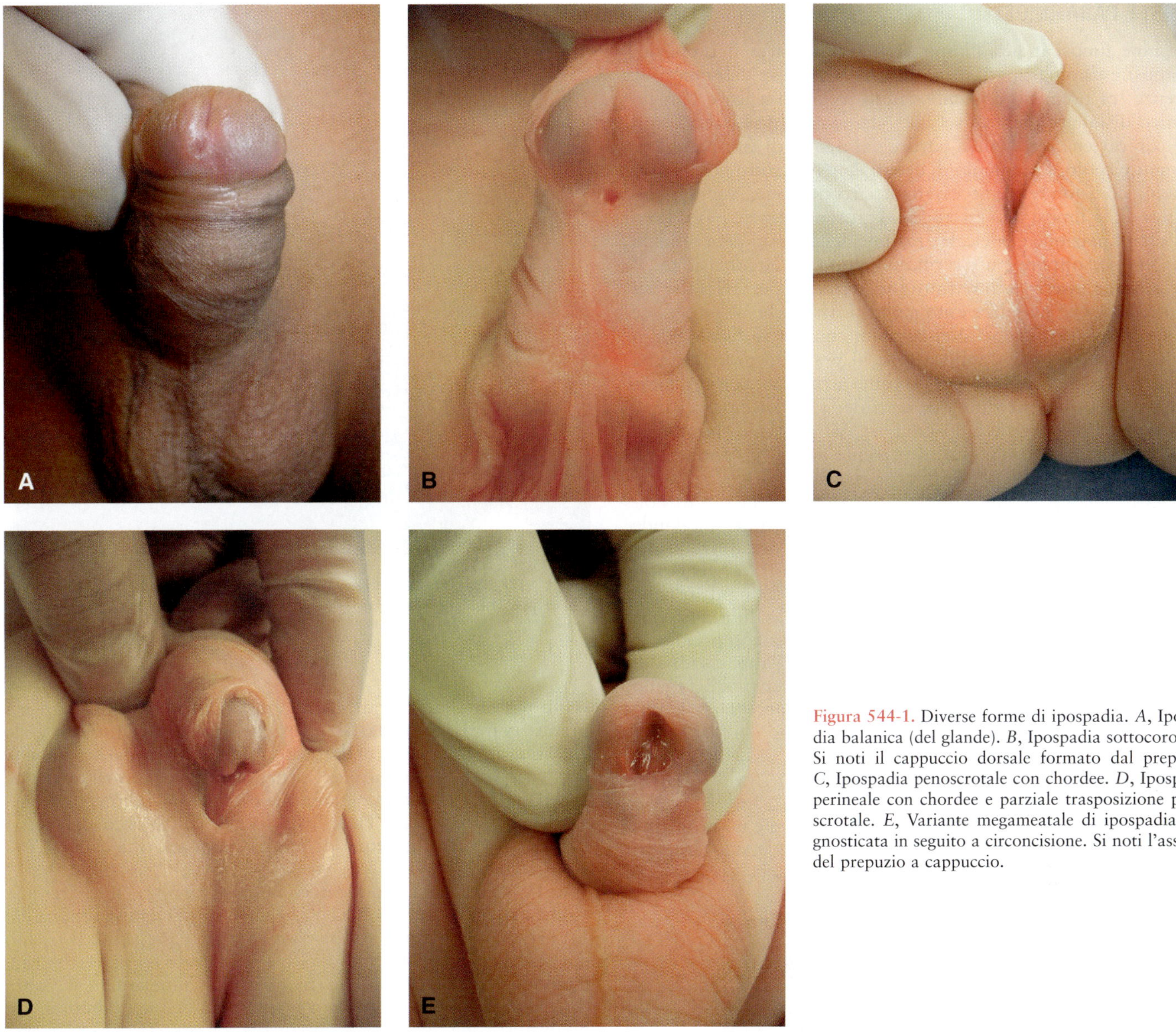

Figura 544-1. Diverse forme di ipospadia. *A*, Ipospadia balanica (del glande). *B*, Ipospadia sottocoronale. Si noti il cappuccio dorsale formato dal prepuzio. *C*, Ipospadia penoscrotale con chordee. *D*, Ipospadia perineale con chordee e parziale trasposizione penoscrotale. *E*, Variante megameatale di ipospadia diagnosticata in seguito a circoncisione. Si noti l'assenza del prepuzio a cappuccio.

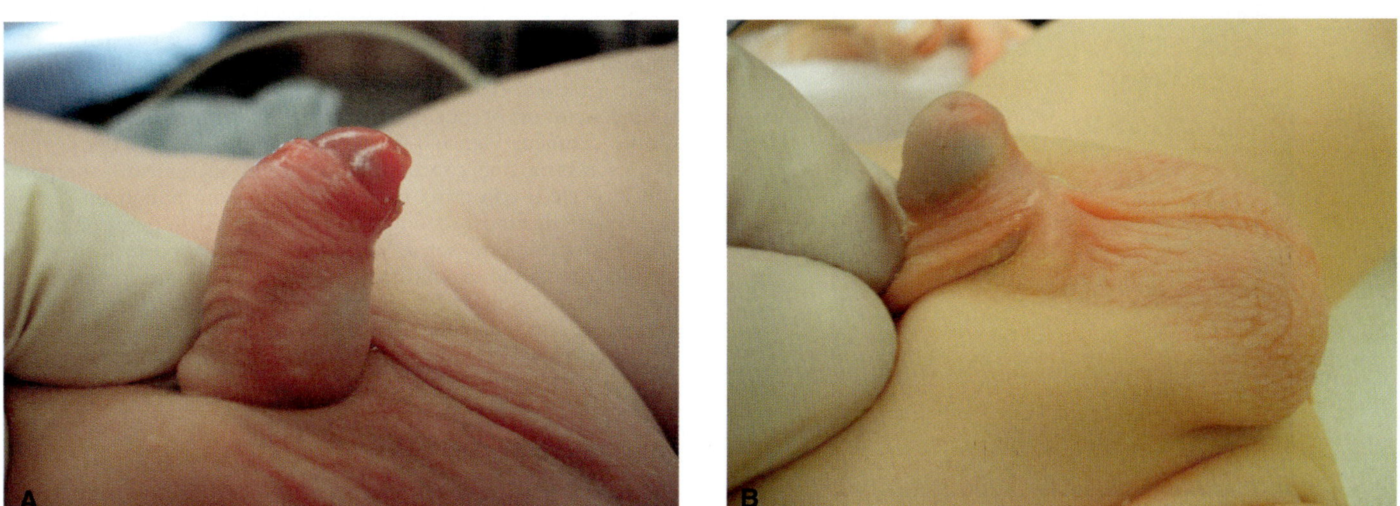

Figura 544-2. *A* e *B*, Due esempi di chordee con ipospadia. Si noti il prepuzio a cappuccio e la sede normale del meato uretrale.

FIMOSI E PARAFIMOSI

Il termine **fimosi** indica l'impossibilità di retrarre il prepuzio. La fimosi è fisiologica alla nascita. Con il passare del tempo, le aderenze tra prepuzio e glande vanno incontro a lisi e l'anello fimotico distale si allenta. Nel 90% dei maschi non circoncisi il prepuzio diviene retraibile a partire dai 3 anni di età. Nel bambino più piccolo, l'accumulo di detriti epiteliali sotto il prepuzio è fisiologico e non rende necessaria la circoncisione. Nei bambini più grandi, la fimosi può essere fisiologica, può essere patologica per l'infiammazione e la cicatrizzazione della punta del prepuzio (Fig. 544-3), oppure può verificarsi dopo la circoncisione. Il prepuzio può essere stato retratto forzatamente per 2-3 volte nel passato, cosa che può dare esito a una cicatrice che ne impedisce una successiva retrazione. Nei bambini con fimosi fisiologica o patologica persistente, l'applicazione al prepuzio di una crema contenente corticosteroidi per 3 volte al giorno per un mese allenta l'anello fimotico nei due terzi dei casi. La circoncisione è consigliata se si verifica un gonfiore del prepuzio durante la minzione o se la fimosi è ancora presente dopo i 10 anni di età e la terapia corticosteroidea topica si rivela inefficace.

Si verifica una **parafimosi** quando il prepuzio viene retratto oltre il solco coronale e quindi non può essere riportato sul glande (Fig. 544-4). Si verifica una stasi venosa dolorosa a livello del prepuzio retratto con edema che a sua volta porta al peggioramento del dolore e all'impossibilità di retrarre il prepuzio nella posizione iniziale. Il trattamento comprende la lubrificazione del glande e del prepuzio e quindi una manovra comprendente simultaneamente la compressione del glande e l'applicazione di una trazione distale sul prepuzio per tentare di spingere l'anello fimotico oltre il solco coronale. In rari casi è necessaria la circoncisione in anestesia generale.

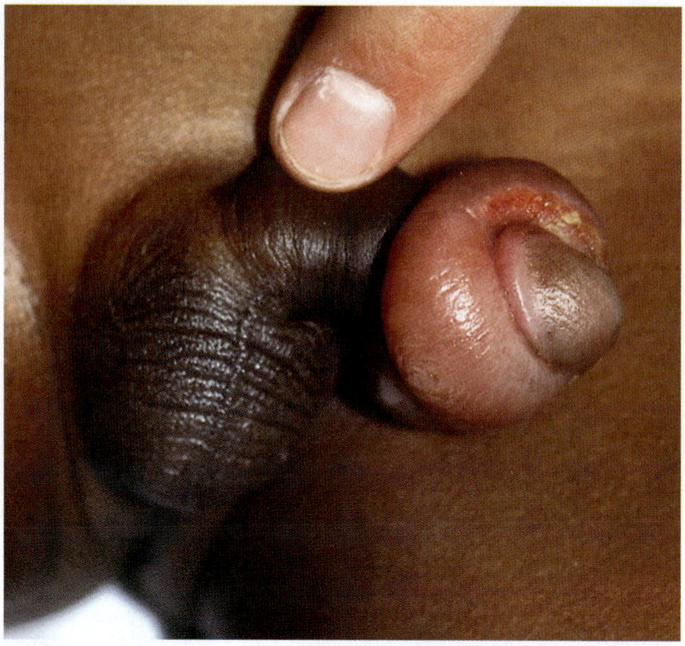

Figura 544-4. Parafimosi. Il prepuzio è stato retratto prossimalmente al glande e si è notevolmente rigonfiato secondariamente all'edema alla congestione venosa.

CIRCONCISIONE

Se effettuare la circoncisione dei bambini o meno è un problema controverso. Negli Stati Uniti, la circoncisione viene eseguita di solito per motivi culturali. Le ragioni addotte a favore di questa pratica comprendono la riduzione del rischio di infezioni delle vie urinarie (IVU) e di malattie sessualmente trasmesse, nonché la prevenzione del tumore del pene, della fimosi e dell'infezione da HIV e della balanite. Quando si esegue una circoncisione nel neonato, è consigliata l'anestesia locale, con blocco del nervo dorsale o con applicazione di EMLA in crema (lidocaina 2,5% e prilocaina 2,5%).

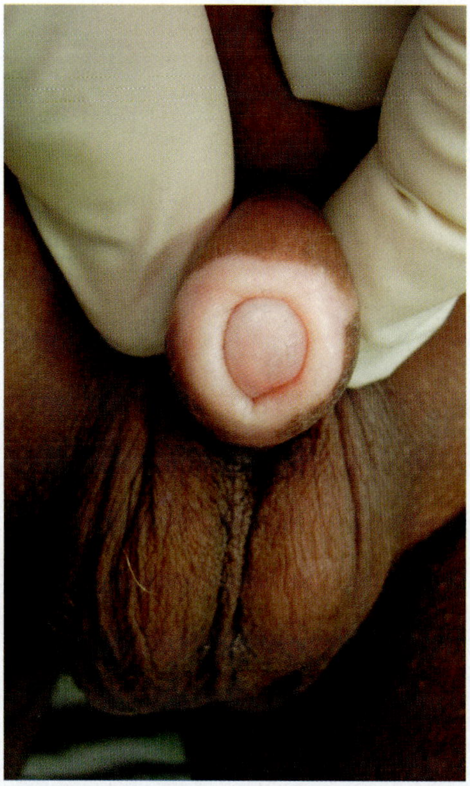

Figura 544-3. Balanite xerotica obliterante. Si noti la placca cicatriziale biancastra.

Le IVU sono 10-15 volte più comuni nel bambino non circonciso che in quello circonciso e i patogeni originari hanno origine dai batteri che colonizzano lo spazio tra glande e prepuzio. Il rischio di IVU febbrili (vedi Capitolo 538) è più elevato tra la nascita e i 6 mesi, ma vi è un aumento del rischio di IVU almeno fino ai 5 anni di età. Molti studi consigliano la circoncisione nei bambini con predisposizione alle IVU, come quelli con idronefrosi congenita e con reflusso vescicoureterale. La circoncisione riduce il rischio di infezioni sessualmente trasmesse negli adulti (vedi Capitolo 119), in particolare l'AIDS (vedi Capitolo 273). Vi sono stati soltanto pochi casi di uomini adulti circoncisi alla nascita che in seguito hanno sviluppato un carcinoma del pene, ma nei Paesi scandinavi, dove pochi maschi vengono circoncisi e il livello di igiene è buono, l'incidenza di tumore del pene è bassa. Le complicanze dopo la circoncisione neonatale comprendono emorragia, infezione della ferita, stenosi meatale, fimosi secondaria, rimozione di un prepuzio insufficiente e aderenze peniene serrate (ponte cutaneo; Fig. 544-5); mentre nello 0,2-3,0% dei pazienti è necessaria una procedura operatoria successiva. I bambini con idrocele o con ernia di grosse dimensioni hanno un rischio particolare di fimosi secondaria. Le complicanze potenzialmente gravi comprendono sepsi, amputazione della parte distale del glande, rimozione di una quantità eccessiva di cute prepuziale e fistola uretrocutanea. La circoncisione non deve essere eseguita in neonati con ipospadia, chordee senza ipospadia o deformità a cappuccio dorsale (controindicazione relativa) o nei bambini con pene di piccole dimensioni.

TORSIONE DEL PENE

La torsione del pene è un difetto di rotazione dell'asta peniena. Di solito ha un andamento antiorario, cioè verso il lato sinistro (vedi Fig. 544-6). Nella maggior parte dei casi, lo sviluppo del pene è

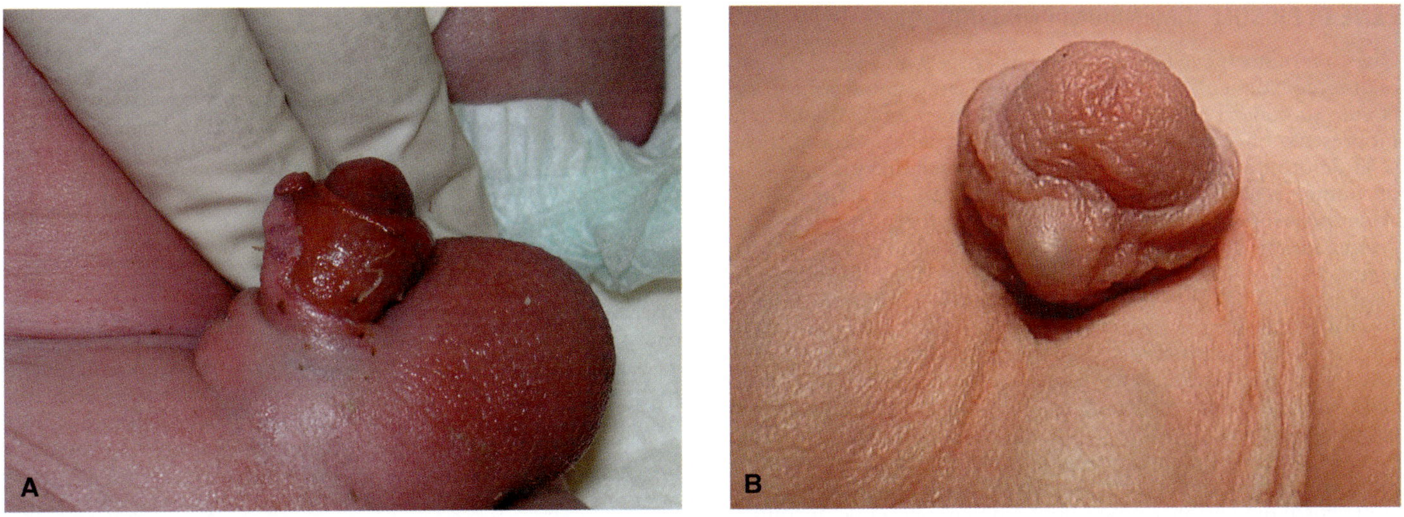

Figura 544-5. Complicanze della circoncisione. *A*, Asta peniena denudata. Con le terapie locali, il pene è guarito e presentava un aspetto normale. *B*, Cisti da incisione epiteliale mediana.

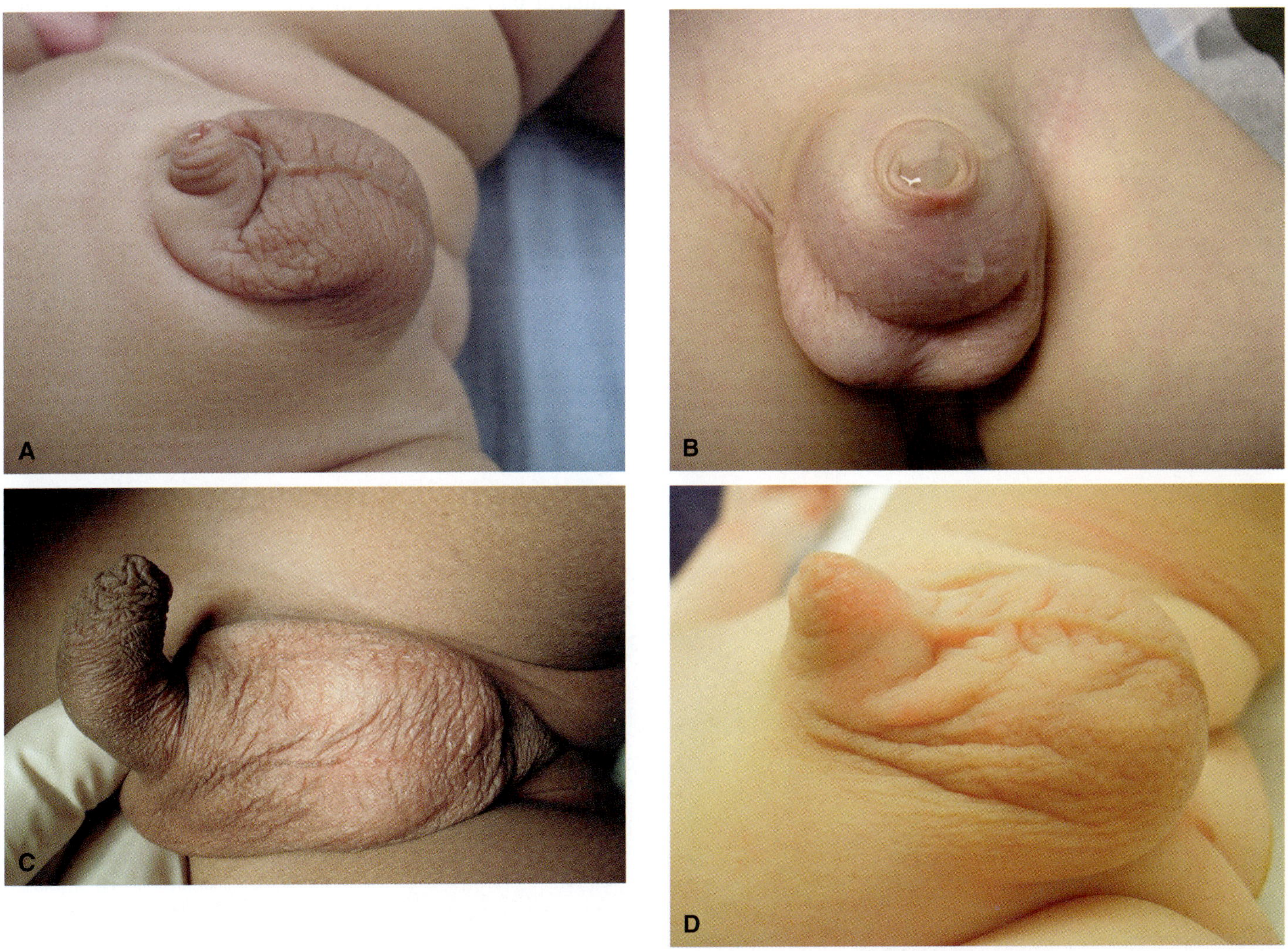

Figura 544-6. Esempi di deformità in cui la circoncisione neonatale è controindicata. *A*, pene nascosto. *B*, Megaprepuzio. *C*, Torsione del pene a sinistra. *D*, Pene palmato; si noti la connessione dello scroto con l'asta.

normale e la condizione non viene riconosciuta fino all'esecuzione della circoncisione o fino a quando il prepuzio non diviene detraibile. La torsione del pene si verifica anche in alcuni bambini con ipospadia. Il difetto ha principalmente un significato estetico e la correzione della rotazione non è necessaria se questa è inferiore a 60 gradi rispetto alla linea mediana.

PENE DI PICCOLE DIMENSIONI (INCOSPICUO)

Questo termine (*pene inconspicuo*) si riferisce a un pene che appare di piccole dimensioni. Un **pene palmato** è una condizione in cui la cute scrotale si estende sul ventre del pene e questa deformità rappresenta un'anomalia della giunzione tra pene e scroto. Anche se la deformità può apparire lieve, se si esegue una circoncisione di routine, il pene può ritrarsi nello scroto con una fimosi secondaria (**pene intrappolato**). Il **pene nascosto** è un pene normalmente sviluppato che appare coperto dal cuscinetto adiposo sovrapubico (Fig. 544-7). Questa anomalia può essere congenita, iatrogena dopo la circoncisione o derivare da obesità. La correzione chirurgica è indicata per motivi estetici o se è presente un'anomalia funzionale se il mitto tende ad allargarsi. Un **pene intrappolato** è una forma acquisita di pene inconspicuo e si riferisce a un fallo che rimane affondato nel cuscinetto adiposo sovrapubico dopo la circoncisione (Fig. 544-8). Questa deformità può verificarsi dopo una circoncisione neonatale in un neonato che ha un significativo ingrossamento dello scroto per un idrocele o per un ernia inguinale di grosse dimensioni oppure dopo una circoncisione di routine in un lattante con pene palmato. Questa complicanza può predisporre alle IVU e può causare ritenzione urinaria. Il trattamento iniziale di un pene intrappolato deve comprendere l'uso topico di un corticosteroide in crema, che spesso allenta l'anello fimotico. In alcuni casi, è necessaria una riparazione secondaria a 6-9 mesi.

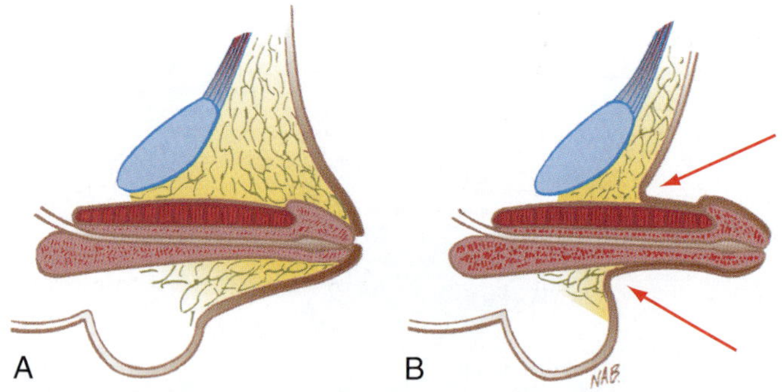

Figura 544-7. Pene nascosto (*A*), che può essere visualizzato con la retrazione della cute lateralmente all'asta (*B*) (Da Wein AJ, Kavoussi LR, Novick AC, et al [editors]: *Campbell-Walsh Urology*, Chapter 126, Fig. 126-4, p. 2339.)

MICROPENE

Si definisce micropene un pene normalmente formato che è almeno 2,5 DS al di sotto delle dimensioni medie (Fig. 544-9). Di solito, il rapporto tra lunghezza dell'asta e la sua circonferenza è normale. La misura corretta è quella della **lunghezza con stiramento del pene**, che si misura stirandolo e misurando la distanza dalla base del pene sotto la sinfisi pubica fino alla punta del glande. La lunghezza media del pene del neonato a termine è di 3,5 ±0,7 cm e il diametro è di 1,1 ±0,2 cm. La diagnosi di micropene si pone se la lunghezza con stiramento è inferiore a 1,9 cm. Il micropene deriva da un'anomalia ormonale che si verifica dopo la 14ª settimana di gestazione. Cause comuni comprendono ipogonadismo ipogonadotropo, ipogonadismo ipergonadotropico (insufficienza testicolare primitiva) e il micropene idiopatico. Se è presente anche un deficit di ormone della crescita può verificarsi un'ipoglicemia. La causa più frequente di micropene è l'incapacità dell'ipotalamo di produrre un'adeguata quantità di ormone rilasciante le gonadotropine (GnRH), come avviene in genere nella sindrome di Kallmann (vedi Capitolo 584), nella sindrome di Prader-Willi (vedi Capitolo 108) e nella sindrome di Lawrence-Moon-Biedl. In alcuni casi è presente un deficit di ormone della crescita. L'insufficienza testicolare primitiva può derivare da disgenesia gonadale o da sindrome dei testicoli rudimentali e si verifica anche nella **sindrome di Robinow** (caratterizzata da ipoplasia dei genitali, avambracci corti, bozze frontali, ipertelorismo, fessure palpebrali ampie, naso corto e largo, filtro lungo, mento piccolo, brachidattilia e cariotipo normale). Tutti i bambini con queste sindromi devono essere valutati dal punto di vista endocrinologico e urologico. La **valutazione** comprende l'esecuzione del cariotipo, una valutazione della funzione ipofisaria anteriore e della funzione testicolare, e una RMN per determinare l'integrità anatomica dell'ipotalamo e dell'ipofisi anteriore come anche delle strutture cerebrali mediane. Uno dei problemi più complessi è valutare se sia essenziale una terapia con androgeni durante l'infanzia, poiché la stimolazione androgenica della crescita del pene in un bambino prepubere può limitare la crescita potenziale del pene durante la pubertà. Studi su piccoli gruppi di uomini con micropene evidenziano che molti, anche se non tutti, hanno una funzione sessuale soddisfacente. Di conseguenza, una decisione di riassegnazione di genere viene presa raramente.

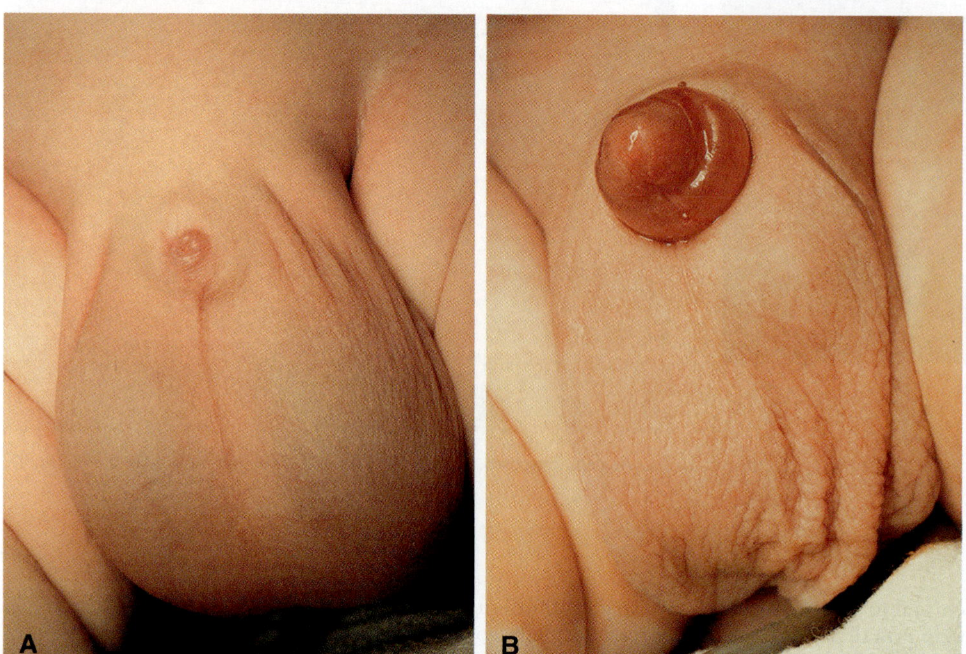

Figura 544-8. *A*, Pene intrappolato (nascosto) derivante da circoncisione. *B*, Lo stesso paziente dopo revisione della circoncisione. (Da Wein AJ, Kavoussi LR, Novick AC, et al [editors]: *Campbell-Walsh Urology*, Fig. 126-2a e b, p. 2340.)

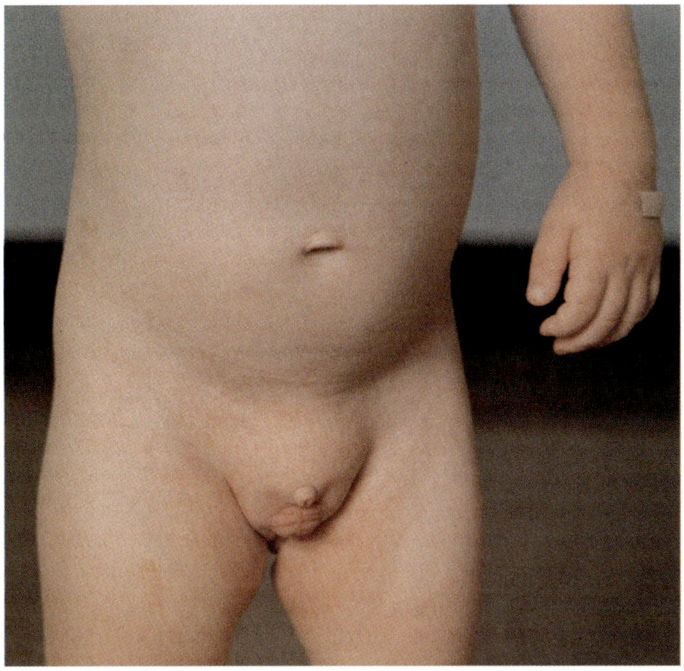

Figura 544-9. Micropene secondario a ipopituitarismo in bambino di 8 anni. (Da Wein AJ, Kavoussi LR, Novick AC, et al [editors]: *Campbell-Walsh Urology* color photo Fig. 126-5A, p. 2341.)

ALTRE ANOMALIE DEL PENE

L'**agenesia del pene** interessa circa 1 bambino su 10 milioni. Il cariotipo è quasi sempre 46XY e l'aspetto comune è quello di uno scroto ben sviluppato con testicoli in sede e assenza dell'asta del pene. Sono comuni le anomalie delle vie urinarie superiori. Nella maggior parte dei casi, è consigliata la riassegnazione di genere nel periodo neonatale. La **difallia** può variare da un piccolo pene accessorio alla duplicazione completa. La **curvatura laterale del pene** è di solito causata da una crescita eccessiva o da un'ipoplasia del corpo cavernoso e di solito è congenita. La riparazione chirurgica è consigliata all'età di 6-12 mesi.

STENOSI MEATALE

La stenosi meatale è una condizione che quasi sempre è acquisita e che si verifica dopo la circoncisione neonatale. Essa probabilmente deriva da una grave infiammazione del glande denudato. Se il meato è puntiforme, il bambino svuota la vescica con un mitto fine e forzato che arriva a grande distanza. Questi pazienti possono presentare disuria, pollachiuria o ematuria, o un'associazione di queste condizioni, senza IVU, tra i 3 e gli 8 anni di età. Altri bambini presentano una deflessione dorsale del mitto. Anche se il meato può essere piccolo, l'idronefrosi o la difficoltà a svuotare la vescica sono estremamente rare a meno che non vi sia una **balanite xerotica obliterante** (dermatite cronica di eziologia sconosciuta, che interessa generalmente glande e prepuzio e che si estende solo talvolta nell'uretra). Il **trattamento** consiste nella meatoplastica, in cui il meato uretrale viene aperto chirurgicamente, procedura che può essere eseguita in anestesia a livello ambulatoriale oppure in anestesia locale (EMLA) con o senza sedazione. Non è necessaria la cistoscopia di routine.

ALTRE ANOMALIE DELL'URETRA MASCHILE

La **cisti uretrale parameatale** si presenta come una piccola cisti asintomatica su un lato del meato uretrale. Il trattamento consiste nell'escissione in anestesia. La **fistola uretrale congenita** è una rara deformità in cui è presente una fistola a partire dall'uretra peniena e di solito è un'anomalia isolata. Il trattamento consiste nella chiusura della fistola. La **megalouretra** è un'uretra di grandi dimensioni che di solito si associa a uno sviluppo anormale del *corpus spongiusum*. Questa condizione è più comunemente nota come sindrome "prune belly" (vedi Cap. 540). La **duplicazione uretrale** è una rara condizione in cui due canali uretrali si trovano sullo stesso piano sagittale e l'uretra più normale è quella posizionata più ventralmente. Alcuni bambini presentano un'uropatia ostruttiva significativa e richiedono un intervento maggiore di chirurgia ricostruttiva. L'**ipoplasia uretrale** è una rara condizione in cui l'uretra è estremamente piccola ma pervia. In alcuni casi, è necessaria una vescicostomia cutanea temporanea per un drenaggio urinario soddisfacente. È necessario un ingrandimento graduale dell'uretra oppure un intervento maggiore di uretroplastica. L'**atresia uretrale** si riferisce al mancato sviluppo dell'uretra e quasi sempre è fatale, a meno che l'uraco non rimanga pervio durante la gravidanza.

PROLASSO URETRALE (FEMMINA)

Il prolasso uretrale si osserva soprattutto nelle bambine nere tra 1 e 9 anni di età. I segni più comuni sono rappresentati da perdite ematiche sulla biancheria intima o sul pannolino, anche se possono essere presenti disuria o fastidio a livello perineale (Fig. 544-10). Un esaminatore inesperto potrebbe scambiare questi sintomi per abuso sessuale. La terapia usuale consiste nell'applicazione di estrogeni in crema da 2 a 3 volte al giorno per 3-4 settimane e in semicupi. L'escissione chirurgica e la riapposizione dei margini della mucosa sono curative.

ALTRE LESIONI DELL'URETRA FEMMINILE

La **cisti parauretrale** deriva dalla ritenzione di secrezioni nelle ghiandole di Skene secondariamente a ostruzione duttale (Fig. 544-11). Queste lesioni sono presenti alla nascita e la maggior parte regredisce durante le prime 4-8 settimane, anche se occasionalmente sono necessari incisione e drenaggio. Un **prolasso di ureterocele ectopico** appare come una massa cistica che protrude dall'uretra ed è un sintomo di presentazione nel 10% delle bambine con ureterocele, che è una dilatazione cistica della parte terminale dell'uretere (Fig. 544-12). Occorre eseguire un'ecografia per

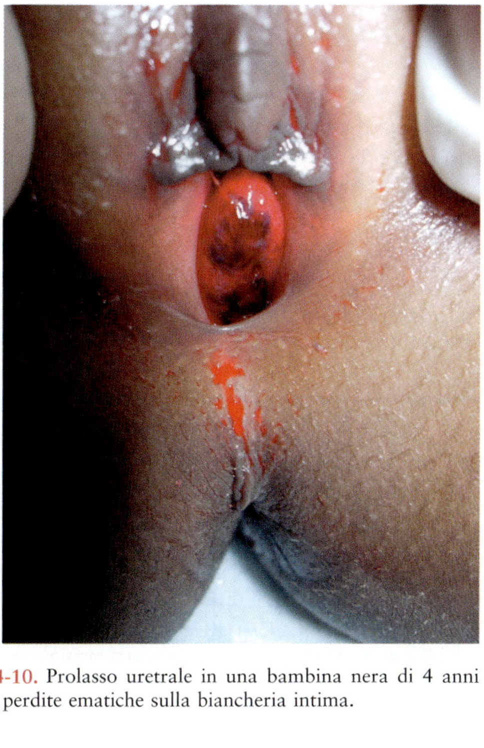

Figura 544-10. Prolasso uretrale in una bambina nera di 4 anni che aveva presentato perdite ematiche sulla biancheria intima.

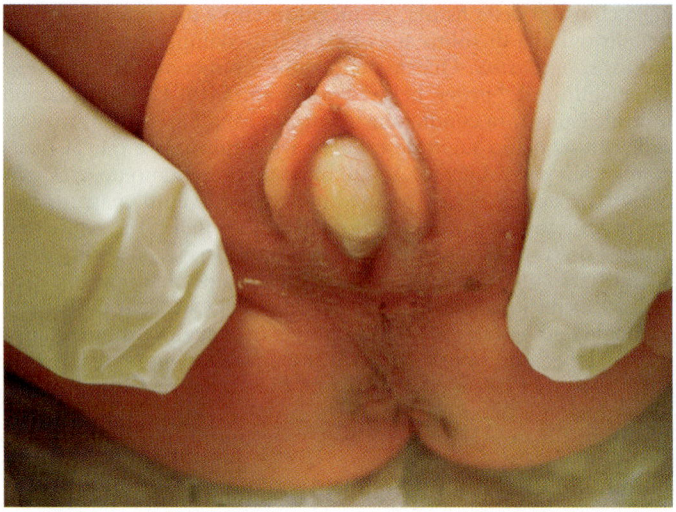

Figura 544-11. Cisti parauretrale in una neonata.

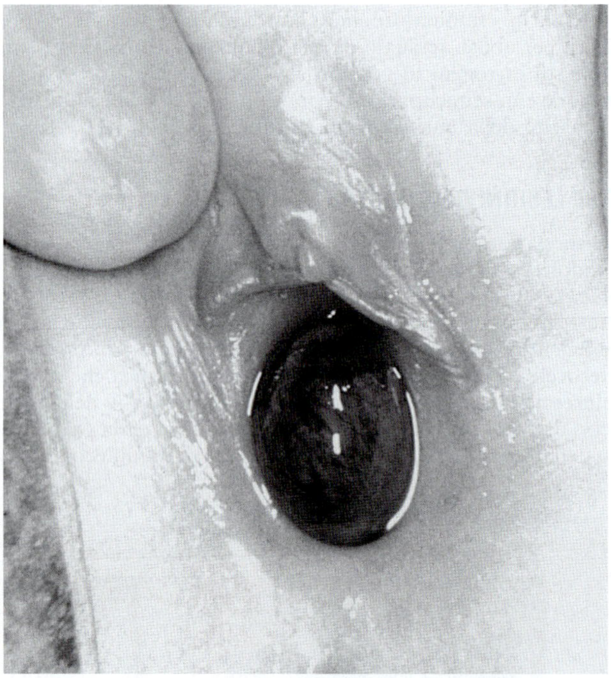

Figura 544-12. Prolasso di ureterocele ectopico in una neonata. La bambina aveva un sistema collettore del polo superiore non funzionale connesso all'ureterocele.

visualizzare le vie urinarie superiori per la conferma diagnostica. Di solito, può essere inciso l'ureterocele oppure può essere necessaria una procedura ricostruttiva delle vie urinarie superiori.

American Academy of Pediatrics, Task Force on Circumcision: Circumcision policy statement. *Pediatrics* 1999;103:686–693.

Auvert B, Taljaard D, Lagarde E, et al: Randomized, controlled intervention trial of male circumcision for reduction of HIV infection risk: The ANRS 1265 Trial. *PLoS Med* 2005;2:e298. Epub 2005 Oct 25.

Baskin LS, Ebbers MB: Hypospadias: Anatomy, etiology, and technique. *J Pediatr Surg* 2006;41:463–472.

Carmichael SL, Shaw GM, Laurent C, et al: Maternal progestin intake and risk of hypospadias. *Arch Pediatr Adolesc Med* 2005;159:957–962.

Castellsague X, Bosch X, Munoz N, et al: Male circumcision, penile human papillomavirus infection, and cervical cancer in female partners. *N Engl J Med* 2002;346:1105–1112.

Elder JS: Abnormalities of the genitalia in boys and their surgical management. In Wein AJ, Kavoussi LR, Novick AC, et al (editors): *Campbell-Walsh Urology,* 9th ed. Philadelphia, Elsevier, in press.

Gargollo PC, Kozakewich HP, Bauer SB, et al: Balanitis xerotica obliterans in boys. *J Urol* 2005;174:1409–1412.

Horowitz M, Sulzhauer E: The "learning curve" in hypospadias surgery. *BJU Int* 2006;97:593–596.

Husmann DA: The androgen insensitive micropenis: Long-term follow-up into adulthood. *J Pediatr Endocrinol Metab* 2004;17:1037–1041.

Kurzrock EA, Karpman E: Hypospadias: Pathophysiology and etiologic theories. *Pediatr Endocrinol Rev* 2004;1:288–295.

Lee PA, Houk CP: Outcome studies among men with micropenis. *J Pediatr Endocrinol Metab* 2004;17:1043–1053.

Lund L, Wai KH, Mui LM, et al: An 18-month follow-up study after randomized treatment of phimosis in boys with topical steroid versus placebo. *Scand J Urol Nephrol* 2005;39:78–81.

Meau-Petit V, Marcou V, Trivin C, et al: Idiopathic male pseudohermaphroditism: Variations in presentation and management. *J Pediatr Endocrinol Metab* 2005;18:569–575.

Misra M, Maclaughlin DT, Donahoe PK, et al: Measurement of Müllerian inhibiting substance facilitates management of boys with microphallus and cryptorchidism. *J Clin Endocrinol Metab* 2002;87:3598–3602.

Nelson CP, Bloom DA, Kinast R, et al: Patient-reported sexual function after oral mucosa graft urethroplasty for hypospadias. *Urology* 2005;66: 1086–1089.

Nelson CP, Dunn R, Wan J, et al: The increasing incidence of newborn circumcision: Data from the nationwide inpatient sample. *J Urol* 2005; 173:978–981.

Nelson CP, Park JM, Wan J, et al: The increasing incidence of congenital penile anomalies in the United States. *J Urol* 2005;174:1573–1576.

Palmer JS, Elder JS, Palmer LS: The use of betamethasone to manage the trapped penis following neonatal circumcision. *J Urol* 2005;174: 1577–1578.

Schoen EJ, Colby CJ, To TT: Cost analysis of neonatal circumcision in a large health maintenance organization. *J Urol* 2006;175:1111–1115.

Wilcox D, Snodgrass W: Long-term outcome following hypospadias repair. *World J Urol* 2006;24:248–253.

Zorc JJ, Levine DA, Platt SL, et al: Clinical and demographic factors associated with urinary tract infection in young febrile infants. *Pediatrics* 2005;116:644–648.

Capitolo 545 ■ Disordini e anomalie dei contenuti scrotali Jack S. Elder

CRIPTORCHIDISMO

La mancata discesa di un testicolo nello scroto indica che il testicolo non è disceso, assente o retrattile.

EPIDEMIOLOGIA. Un testicolo non disceso (**criptorchidismo**) è il disordine più comune della differenziazione sessuale nei maschi. Alla nascita, il 4,5% circa dei maschi ha un testicolo non disceso. Dal momento che la discesa testicolare si verifica in gravidanza, il 30% dei neonati maschi prematuri ha un testicolo non disceso; l'incidenza è del 3,4% a termine. La maggior parte dei testicoli non discesi discende spontaneamente durante i primi 3 mesi di vita ed entro i 6 mesi l'incidenza si riduce allo 0,8%. Se il testicolo non è disceso entro 4 mesi, esso rimarrà nella stessa condizione. Il criptorchidismo è bilaterale nel 10% dei casi. Vi sono alcune evidenze che l'incidenza di criptorchidismo è in aumento. Anche se il criptorchidismo è di solito considerato una condizione congenita, un numero sempre crescente di bambini più grandi riceve una diagnosi di criptorchidismo. In genere, questi bambini hanno un testicolo scrotale che "risale" in posizione inguinale bassa e quindi necessita di orchidopessi. Alcuni bambini hanno un criptorchidismo secondario successivo a intervento per ernia inguinale. Questa complicanza è particolarmente comune nei neonati e nei lattanti e interessa l'1-2% dei pazienti sottoposti a intervento di riparazione di ernia inguinale.

PATOGENESI. Il processo di discesa testicolare è regolato da un'interazione tra fattori ormonali e meccanici, tra cui testosterone, diidrotestosterone, fattore inibente mülleriano, gubernaculum, pressione intra-addominale e nervo genitofemorale. Il testicolo si sviluppa alla 7-8ª settimana di gestazione. Alla 10-11ª settimana, le cellule di Leydig producono testosterone, che stimola la differenziazione del dotto di Wolff (mesonefrico) in epididimo, vaso deferente, vescicola seminale e dotto eiaculatorio. A 32-36 settimane il testicolo, che è ancora ancorato all'anello inguinale interno mediante il gubernaculum, inizia il processo di discesa. Il gubernaculum distende il canale inguinale e guida il testicolo nello scroto. Dopo la discesa testicolare, il processo vaginale che è pervio di solito va incontro a involuzione.

MANIFESTAZIONI CLINICHE. Un testicolo non disceso può essere classificato come **addominale** (non palpabile), **affacciato sul canale inguinale** (addominale ma che può essere spinto nella parte superiore del canale inguinale), **inguinale**, **"in ascensore"** (può essere spinto nello scroto ma si ritrae immediatamente sul tubercolo pubico) ed **ectopico** (tasca inguinale superficiale o, raramente, perineale). La maggior parte dei testicoli non discesi si trova nel canale inguinale o appena distalmente al canale inguinale. Circa il 10% dei bambini criptorchidi manifesta un testicolo non palpabile; in questi bambini il testicolo è presente ed è addominale o inguinale nel 50% dei casi, mentre è assente secondariamente a una torsione testicolare perinatale nel 50% dei casi. In un neonato con fenotipo maschile con testicoli non palpabili bilateralmente, si dovrebbe considerare la possibilità che l'individuo sia una femmina virilizzata con iperplasia surrenalica congenita (vedi Capitolo 577). In un bambino con testicolo non disceso e ipospadia mediopeniena o prossimale, deve essere invece considerata la possibilità di una condizione intersesso.

Le **conseguenze del criptorchidismo** comprendono infertilità, neoplasia maligna testicolare, ernia associata, torsione del testicolo criptorchide e i possibili effetti psicologici di uno scroto vuoto.

Il testicolo non disceso è istologicamente normale alla nascita, ma alterazioni patologiche possono essere evidenziate dai 6-12 mesi di vita. Ritardo della maturazione delle cellule germinali, riduzione delle cellule germinali, ialinizzazione dei tubuli seminiferi e riduzione del numero delle cellule di Leydig: queste sono alterazioni progressive nel tempo se il testicolo rimane non disceso. Allo stesso modo, anche se meno gravi, si osservano alterazioni nel testicolo controlaterale non disceso dopo 4-7 anni. Dopo il trattamento per un testicolo non disceso unilaterale, l'85% dei pazienti è fertile, una percentuale leggermente inferiore al tasso di fertilità del 90% che si osserva in una popolazione non selezionata di adulti maschi. Al contrario, in seguito a orchidopessi bilaterale, soltanto il 50-60% dei pazienti è fertile.

Il rischio di una **neoplasia maligna delle cellule germinali** (vedi Capitolo 503) che si sviluppa in un testicolo non disceso è da 4 a 10 volte più elevato che nella popolazione generale ed è circa di 1 su 80 in un testicolo non disceso unilaterale e da 1 su 40 a 1 su 50 in caso di testicoli non discesi bilateralmente. Il picco d'età per lo sviluppo di una neoplasia del testicolo è 15-45 anni. Il tumore più frequente che si sviluppa in un testicolo non disceso è il **seminoma** (65%); al contrario, dopo orchidopessi, i seminomi rappresentano soltanto il 30% dei tumori del testicolo. Se l'orchidopessi riduca il rischio di sviluppare un cancro del testicolo è controverso, ma non è frequente che i tumori del testicolo si verifichino dopo un orchidopessi eseguita prima dei 2 anni di età.

I testicoli non discesi sono di solito accompagnati da ernie inguinali indirette che però sono raramente sintomatiche. Sono rari anche la torsione e l'infarto del testicolo non disceso, ma possono comunque verificarsi a causa dell'eccessiva mobilità di questi testicoli. Di conseguenza, dolore e/o edema inguinale in un bambino con testicolo non disceso devono suscitare il sospetto di un'ernia incarcerata o di una torsione testicolare del testicolo non disceso.

I **testicoli non discesi ascendenti** o "acquisiti" sono diagnosticati sempre più spesso. I bambini affetti hanno un testicolo disceso alla nascita, ma durante l'infanzia, di solito tra i 4 e i 10 anni di età, il testicolo non rimane nello scroto. In tali bambini spesso si riscontra un'anamnesi di testicolo retrattile. Con la salita testicolare, all'esame obiettivo il testicolo può spesso essere riportato nello scroto, ma è presente un'evidente tensione sul funicolo spermatico. Questa condizione si ritiene derivi dall'involuzione incompleta del processo vaginale con restrizione dell'allungamento del funicolo spermatico, il quale provoca uno spostamento graduale del testicolo dalla sua posizione scrotale.

I **testicoli retrattili** possono essere erroneamente diagnosticati come testicoli non discesi. I bambini con più di un anno di età hanno frequentemente un riflesso cremasterico molto vivace, e se il bambino è ansioso o *ticklish* durante l'esame scrotale, può essere difficile riportare il testicolo nello scroto. I bambini devono essere esaminati con le gambe rilassate in posizione a rana e, se il testicolo può essere riportato nello scroto senza difficoltà, esso è probabilmente retrattile. Il testicolo deve essere monitorato ogni 6-12 mesi con successivi esami obiettivi, perché potrebbe essere un testicolo non disceso acquisito. In generale, almeno un terzo dei bambini con testicolo retrattile svilupperà un testicolo non disceso acquisito e i bambini <7 anni di età alla diagnosi di un testicolo retrattile sono quelli a maggior rischio. La maggior parte degli Autori ritiene che i bambini con un testicolo retrattile non abbiano un rischio aumentato di infertilità o di neoplasia maligna.

All'**esame obiettivo** dello scroto, è importante che il bambino sia completamente svestito per aiutarlo a rilassarsi. Se è difficile palpare il testicolo, spesso è utile il "test del sapone"; si applica sapone sul canale inguinale e sulla mano dell'esaminatore, riducendo l'attrito in modo significativo e facilitando l'identificazione di testicolo in sede inguinale. Un sintomo "leggero" che un testicolo è assente è l'ipertrofia del testicolo controlaterale, ma questo reperto non è diagnostico al 100%.

TRATTAMENTO. Il testicolo non disceso congenito deve essere trattato chirurgicamente non oltre i 9-15 mesi. Mediante un'anestesia somministrata da un anestesista pediatra, è indicata la correzione chirurgica a 6 mesi, poiché la discesa spontanea del testicolo non si verifica oltre i 4 mesi di vita. La maggior parte dei testicoli può essere riportata nello scroto mediante una orchidopessi che comprende un'incisione inguinale, la mobilizzazione del testicolo e del funicolo spermatico e la correzione dell'ernia inguinale indiretta: tale procedura viene generalmente eseguita a livello ambulatoriale e ha un tasso di successo del 98%. In alcuni bambini con un testicolo in prossimità dello scroto, può essere eseguito un intervento di Bianchi o orchidopessi prescrotale. In questa procedura, l'intero intervento viene eseguito attraverso un'incisione lungo il margine dello scroto. Spesso anche l'ernia inguinale associata può essere corretta mediante questa incisione. I vantaggi di questo approccio rispetto a quello inguinale comprendono un minore tempo operatorio e un minore dolore postoperatorio.

Il **trattamento ormonale** è usato raramente. La teoria è che, dal momento che la discesa testicolare è regolata dagli androgeni, la gonadotropina corionica umana (che stimola la produzione di testosterone da parte delle cellule di Leydig) o l'ormone rilasciante l'ormone luteinizzante (LHRH) possono stimolare la discesa testicolare. Anche se il trattamento ormonale è stato utilizzato in Europa, i trial randomizzati e controllati non hanno dimostrato l'efficacia di nessuna di queste due preparazioni ormonali nello stimolare la discesa testicolare. Vi sono alcune evidenze preliminari che la buserelina, un analogo dell'LHRH, può essere utile nell'aumentare il numero delle cellule germinali e nel normalizzare l'istologia testicolare.

In circa il 50% dei bambini in cui il testicolo non è palpabile, esso è intra-addominale o in posizione alta nel canale inguinale; nel restante 50%, il testicolo è assente (atrofico) secondariamente a torsione testicolare perinatale e questa situazione è definita ***vanishing testis.*** È stato proposto l'utilizzo dell'imaging per determinare se è presente il testicolo. L'ecografia si è dimostrata inefficace nel localizzare il testicolo non palpabile. Al contrario, la TC è relativamente accurata nel dimostrare la presenza del testicolo. La RMN è ancora più accurata, ma lo svantaggio è che nella maggior parte dei bambini è necessaria una forte sedazione. Dal momento che l'imaging non si è dimostrato affidabile al 100% nell'evidenziare la presenza del testicolo, nella maggior parte dei centri si esegue una laparoscopia diagnostica. Questa procedura permette una valutazione rapida e sicura se il testicolo sia intra-addominale. Nella maggior parte dei casi, l'orchidopessi del testicolo intra-addominale localizzato subito all'interno dell'anello inguinale interno ha successo, ma nei casi più difficili, o quando il testicolo sembra essere atrofico, occorre prendere in considerazione l'orchiectomia. Una orchidopessi in due stadi è talvolta necessaria in bambini con testicolo addominale alto e tali pazienti vengono trattati con tecniche laparoscopiche presso molti centri. Sono disponibili protesi testicolari per i bambini più grandi e gli adolescenti quando l'assenza della gonade nello scroto può avere un effetto psicologico indesiderabile. La FDA ha approvato un impianto testicolare contenente soluzione fisiologica ed è attualmente in corso di valutazione un impianto solido in silicone "da modellare". L'inserimento precoce nell'infanzia di protesi testicolari è consigliato nei bambini con anarchia (assenza di entrambi i testicoli).

EDEMA DELLO SCROTO

L'aumento di volume dello scroto può essere acuto o cronico, doloroso o non doloroso. L'insorgenza improvvisa di edema dello scroto richiede una pronta valutazione, poiché alcune condizioni, come la torsione testicolare e l'ernia inguinale incarcerata, richiedono un trattamento chirurgico d'emergenza. La diagnosi differenziale è evidenziata nelle Tabelle 545-1 e 545-2.

MANIFESTAZIONI CLINICHE. È utile un'anamnesi dettagliata nel determinare la causa dell'edema, che deve comprendere (1) l'insorgenza del dolore (con la torsione testicolare il dolore ha spesso un esordio improvviso e può essere associato all'attività fisica o a un trauma genitale minore); (2) la durata del dolore; (3) l'irradiazione del dolore (il dolore inguinale è comune nella torsione testicolare, nell'ernia inguinale o nell'epididimite, e può essere presente un dolore associato al fianco in caso di espulsione di un calcolo ureterale); (4) pregressi episodi di dolore simile, che sono comuni nei bambini con torsione testicolare intermittente o ernia inguinale; (5) nausea e vomito, che sono associati a torsione testicolare ed ernia inguinale; e (6) sintomi urinari irritativi, come disuria, urgenza e pollachiuria, che sono indicativi di un'infezione delle vie urinarie che può causare epididimite. I bambini con patologia delle vie urinarie inferiori come stenosi uretrale o vescica neurologica possono avere una tendenza all'epididimite.

L'**esame obiettivo** può essere difficile nei bambini con scroto doloroso. Alcuni hanno consigliato l'esecuzione di un blocco del funicolo spermatico o la somministrazione di un'analgesia intravenosa per facilitare l'esame obiettivo, ma tale misura di solito non è necessaria. L'eritema della parete scrotale è comune nella torsione testicolare, nell'epididimite, nella torsione appendicolare e nell'ernia incarcerata. Nei bambini con normale riflesso cremasterico, la torsione testicolare è improbabile. L'assenza di riflesso cremasterico, tuttavia, non è diagnostica.

TABELLA 545-1. Diagnosi differenziale delle masse scrotali nei bambini e negli adolescenti

DOLOROSA	NON DOLOROSA
Torsione testicolare	Idrocele
Torsione appendicolare	Ernia inguinale*
Epididimite	Varicocele*
Trauma: rottura del testicolo, ematocele	Spermatocele*
Ernia inguinale (incarcerata)	Tumore testicolare*
Parotite, orchite	Porpora di Henoch-Schönlein*
	Edema scrotale idiopatico

*Può essere associato a dolore.

TABELLA 545-2. Diagnosi differenziale dell'ingrossamento scrotale nel neonato

Idrocele
Ernia inguinale (riducibile)
Ernia inguinale (incarcerata)*
Torsione testicolare*
Ematoma scrotale
Tumore testicolare
Peritonite da meconio
Epididimite*

*Può essere associata a dolore.

ESAMI DI LABORATORIO E DIAGNOSI. Gli esami di laboratorio pertinenti comprendono un esame delle urine e un'urinocoltura. Un esame delle urine positivo è indicativo di epididimite. Gli esami del sangue non sono utili per la diagnosi, a meno che non si sospetti un tumore del testicolo. Dopo la valutazione iniziale, gli studi di imaging possono essere utili nel porre la diagnosi, poiché permettono di stabilire la normalità del flusso ematico, oppure se è ridotto o aumentato. Gli studi di imaging comprendono l'ecografia Doppler a colori e una scintigrafia del flusso ematico testicolare. Inoltre, se è presente un idrocele e il testicolo non è palpabile, oppure se viene riscontrata un'anomalia del testicolo, può essere utile l'ecografia. Gli studi di imaging non sono accurati al 100%; essi non devono essere utilizzati per decidere se un bambino con dolore testicolare deve essere inviato a consulenza urologica. L'ecografia Doppler a colori è lo studio di imaging più utilizzato e permette la valutazione del flusso ematico testicolare e delle caratteristiche morfologiche testicolari. L'accuratezza è del 95%, se l'operatore è esperto. Si può avere un'ecografia Doppler falsa negativa (che evidenzia un normale flusso ematico testicolare) in un bambino con torsione testicolare se il grado di torsione è inferiore a 360 gradi e la durata della torsione è breve, in quanto vi può essere la continuazione della perfusione testicolare. Inoltre, nei bambini prepuberi il flusso sanguigno può essere difficile da dimostrare in almeno il 30% dei testicoli normali. La scintigrafia del flusso testicolare con ^{99m}Tc-pertecnetato può dimostrare se è presente flusso ematico al testicolo. Dopo iniezione intravenosa del radionuclide, si eseguono scansioni statiche e di flusso. La torsione testicolare spesso appare come una "macchia fredda" di assenza di flusso nel testicolo interessato. Le condizioni infiammatorie di solito causano iperemia. L'accuratezza nel dimostrare il flusso ematico è di circa il 95%. Una scintigrafia falsa positiva può verificarsi in un bambino con torsione testicolare se il grado di torsione è inferiore a 360 gradi. L'esame spesso può essere eseguito in emergenza durante il giorno, ma durante la notte possono essere necessarie 2-3 ore per eseguirlo e interpretarlo.

TORSIONE DEL TESTICOLO (FUNICOLO SPERMATICO)

EZIOLOGIA. La torsione del testicolo richiede una diagnosi e un trattamento immediati per salvare il testicolo. La torsione è la causa più comune di dolore testicolare nei bambini di 12 anni o più ed è poco frequente nei bambini con meno di 10 anni. È causata da inadeguata fissazione del testicolo nello scroto, il quale dà esito a una ridondanza della tunica vaginale, permettendo quindi un'eccessiva mobilità del testicolo. l'attaccamento anormale è stata denominato *deformità a batacchio di campana* e spesso è bilaterale. Subito dopo che si è verificata la torsione inizia la congestione venosa; successivamente si interrompe il flusso arterioso. La probabilità di sopravvivenza del testicolo dipende dalla durata e dalla gravità della torsione. Entro 4-6 ore di assenza del flusso ematico al testicolo, si può verificare una perdita irreversibile della spermatogenesi.

DIAGNOSI. La torsione testicolare causa acutamente dolore ed edema dello scroto. All'esame obiettivo, lo scroto appare ingrossato e il testicolo è di solito dolente e spesso difficile da esaminare. Il riflesso cremasterico quasi sempre è assente. La condizione può essere distinta da un'ernia incarcerata in quanto è assente la tumefazione in area inguinale. Se il dolore è durato meno di 4-6 ore, si può tentare la detorsione manuale. Nei 2/3 dei casi il testicolo andato incontro a torsione può essere ruotato all'interno, per cui la detorsione può essere tentata nella direzione opposta (per es. il testicolo sinistro è ruotato in senso orario). Una detorsione manuale efficace può portare a un drammatico sollievo dal dolore.

TRATTAMENTO. Il trattamento consiste nell'immediata esplorazione chirurgica seguita dalla detorsione. Se il testicolo viene esplorato entro 6 ore dalla torsione, almeno il 90% delle gonadi sopravvive. La sopravvivenza diminuisce rapidamente con un ritardo superiore alle 6 ore. Se il grado di torsione è di 360 gradi o meno, il testicolo può avere sufficiente flusso arterioso per consentire la sopravvivenza della gonade, anche dopo 24-48 ore. Il testicolo viene quindi fissato nello scroto con suture riassorbibili, intervento denominato *orchidopessi scrotale*, per prevenire una torsione futura. Anche il testicolo controlaterale deve essere fissato nello scroto, poiché la condizione anatomica predisponente spesso è bilaterale. Se il testicolo appare non vitale si esegue un'orchiectomia (Fig. 545-1). Una torsione testicolare può verificarsi anche nel feto o nel neonato. Essa deriva dall'incompleto attaccamento della tunica vaginale alla parete scrotale ed è "extravaginale". Quando la torsione si verifica in utero, il bambino di solito nasce con un testicolo di grandi dimensioni, duro e non dolente. Di solito, l'emiscroto ipsilaterale è ecchimotico (Fig. 545-2). In questi casi, il testicolo raramente è vitale in quanto la torsione raramente è stata un evento remoto. Tuttavia, il testicolo controlaterale ha un aumento del rischio di torsione fino a un mese dopo il termine. Molti urologi pediatri consigliano l'esplorazione per porre la diagnosi, rimuovere il testicolo necrotico e fissare il testicolo controlaterale. In altri casi, l'esame iniziale è normale e l'edema scrotale acuto viene riconosciuto solo in seguito e, in tali casi, occasionalmente il testicolo può essere salvato.

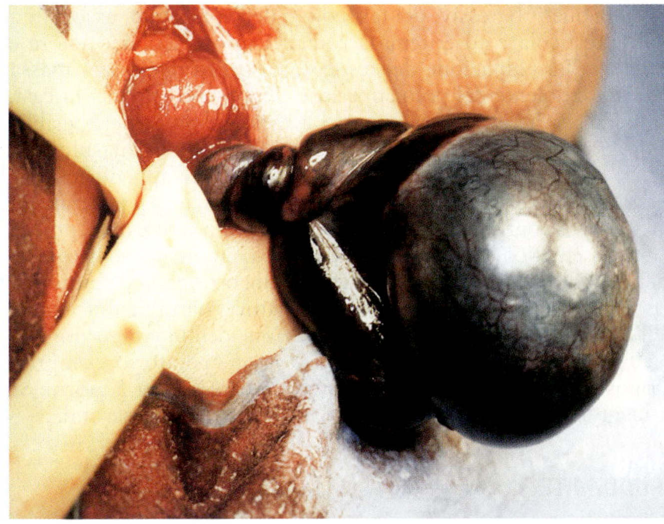

Figura 545-1. Torsione testicolare sinistra in un adolescente; il testicolo è necrotico.

TORSIONE DELL'APPENDICE DEL TESTICOLO (IDATIDE DI MORGAGNI)

La torsione dell'appendice del testicolo o idatide di Morgagni è la causa più comune di dolore testicolare nei bambini tra i 2 e 10 anni di età ma è rara negli adolescenti. L'appendice del testicolo è una struttura a peduncolo che rappresenta il residuo vestigiale embrionale del sistema duttale di Müller (paramesonefrico) che è connesso al polo superiore del testicolo. Quando va incontro a torsione, si verificano un'infiammazione e una

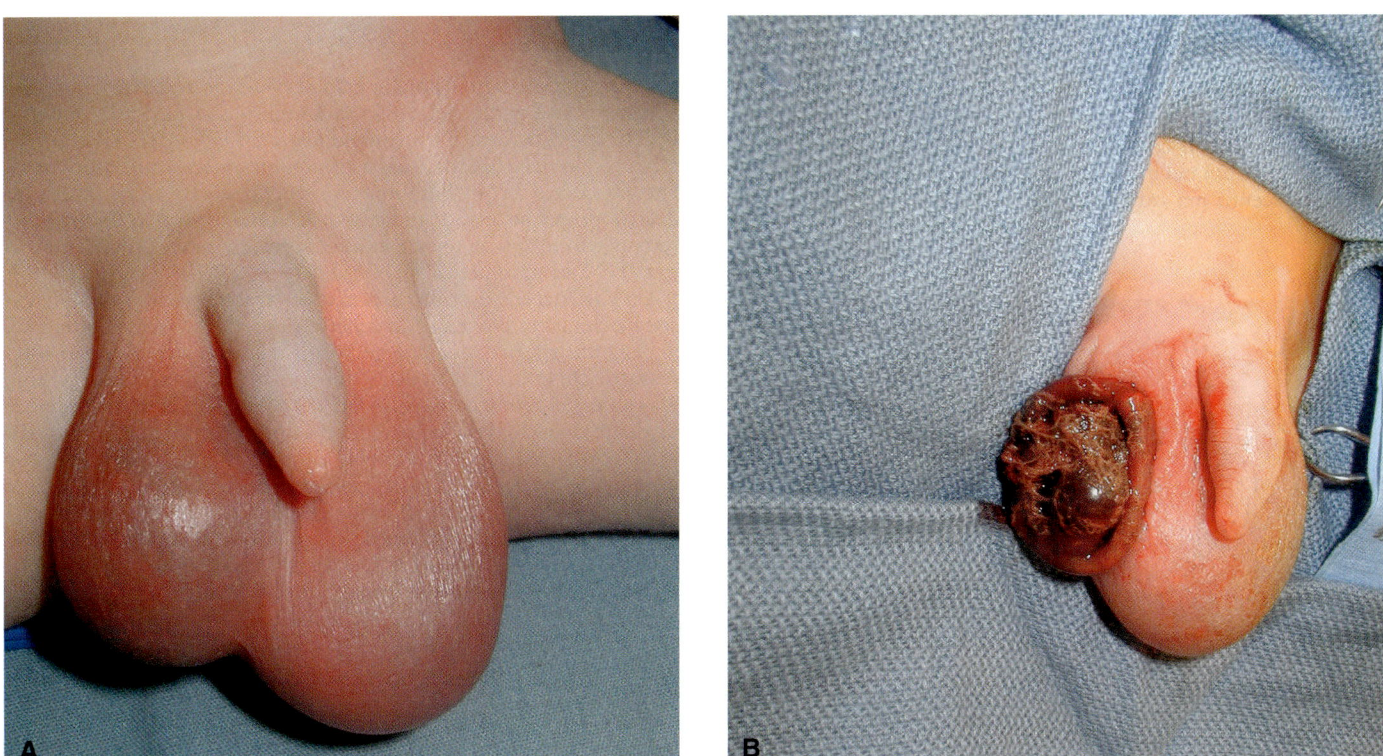

Figura 545-2. Torsione testicolare destra in un neonato. L'emiscroto destro è più scuro e il testicolo appare indurito e ingrandito.

tumefazione progressivi del testicolo e dell'epididimo, associati a dolore testicolare ed eritema scrotale. L'insorgenza del dolore è graduale. La palpazione del testicolo di solito rivela una massa indurita e dolente del polo superiore (Fig. 545-3). In alcuni casi, l'appendice che è andata incontro a torsione può essere visibile attraverso la cute scrotale, con il segno della "macchia blu". In alcuni bambini, la distinzione della torsione dell'appendice dalla torsione testicolare è difficoltosa. In questi casi, una scintigrafia di flusso o un'ecografia Doppler a colori possono essere utili, poiché il flusso ematico testicolare è normale o aumentato. In questi casi, il radiologo spesso identifica la tumefazione dell'epididimo e pone una diagnosi di epididimite. La storia naturale di torsione dell'appendice del testicolo è la risoluzione dell'infiammazione in 3-10 giorni. Si consiglia un trattamento non operatorio, compresi il riposo a letto e l'analgesia con steroidi e FANS per 5 giorni. Se la diagnosi è incerta, è raccomandata l'esplorazione scrotale.

EPIDIDIMITE

L'infiammazione acuta dell'epididimo è un'infezione ascendente retrograda dall'uretra attraverso il vaso deferente nell'epididimo. Questa condizione causa dolore, eritema e tumefazione acuta dello scroto. È rara prima della pubertà e deve sollevare il dubbio di un'anomalia congenita del dotto di Wolff, come un uretere ectopico che sbocca nel vaso deferente. Nei bambini più piccoli, il microrganismo responsabile è spesso l'*Escherichia coli*. Dopo la pubertà, l'epididimite diviene progressivamente più frequente ed è la causa principale di tumefazione scrotale dolorosa acuta nei maschi giovani e sessualmente attivi. L'esame delle urine di solito rivela una piuria. L'epididimite può essere infettiva (di solito gonococco o **clamidia**), ma spesso il microrganismo resta indeterminato. Altre cause comprendono la porpora di Henoch-Schönlein, la febbre mediterranea familiare e le infezioni da enterovirus e adenovirus. Il trattamento consiste nel riposo a letto e in una terapia antibiotica (vedi Capitolo 119). La diagnosi differenziale con la torsione può essere difficile e nei bambini è di solito necessaria l'esplorazione chirurgica.

VARICOCELE

Un varicocele è una condizione congenita in cui vi è un'anormale dilatazione del plesso pampiniforme nello scroto (Fig. 545-4). La dilatazione del plesso venoso pampiniforme deriva da incompetenza valvolare della vena spermatica. Circa il 15% dei maschi adulti presenta un varicocele; di questi, il 15% circa è subfertile. Il varicocele è la più comune causa correggibile (e, in teoria, la sola) su subfertilità nel maschio. Un varicocele si trova nel 5-15% degli adolescenti, ma raramente viene diagnosticato in bambini con meno di 10 anni, poiché esso si distende solo dopo che si è verificato l'aumento del flusso sanguigno associato alla pubertà. Il varicocele si verifica prevalentemente a livello del lato sinistro, è bilaterale nel 10% dei casi e raramente interessa il lato destro. Un varicocele in un bambino con meno di 10 anni o sul lato destro potrebbe essere indicativo di una massa addominale o retroperitoneale; in questi casi occorre eseguire un'ecografia o una TC addominale.

Un varicocele è di solito una massa paratesticolare non dolente, spesso descritta come un "sacchetto di vermi". Occasionalmente, il paziente riferisce un dolore sordo a livello del testicolo interessato. Di solito il varicocele non è evidente quando il paziente è supino perché decompresso; al contrario, il varicocele diviene evidente quando il paziente è in posizione eretta e aumenta di volume con la manovra di Valsala. Gli studi hanno dimostrato che la maggior parte dei pediatri non ricerca di routine il varicocele negli adolescenti maschi. Il varicocele è in genere classificato in 3 gradi: il **grado 1** è palpabile solo con la manovra di Valsalva; il **grado 2** è palpabile senza manovra di Valsalva ma non è visibile all'ispezione e il **grado 3** è visibile all'ispezione. I bambini con varicocele di grado 3 hanno il massimo rischio di arresto della crescita testicolare. Le dimensioni testicolari devono essere documentate con un calibro, un orchimetro o un'ecografia scrotale, perché se il testicolo sinistro interessato è significativamente più piccolo del testicolo destro, probabilmente la spermatogenesi è stata influenzata negativamente.

Lo scopo della varicocelectomia è quello di massimizzare le probabilità di fertilità. Il trattamento chirurgico del varicocele

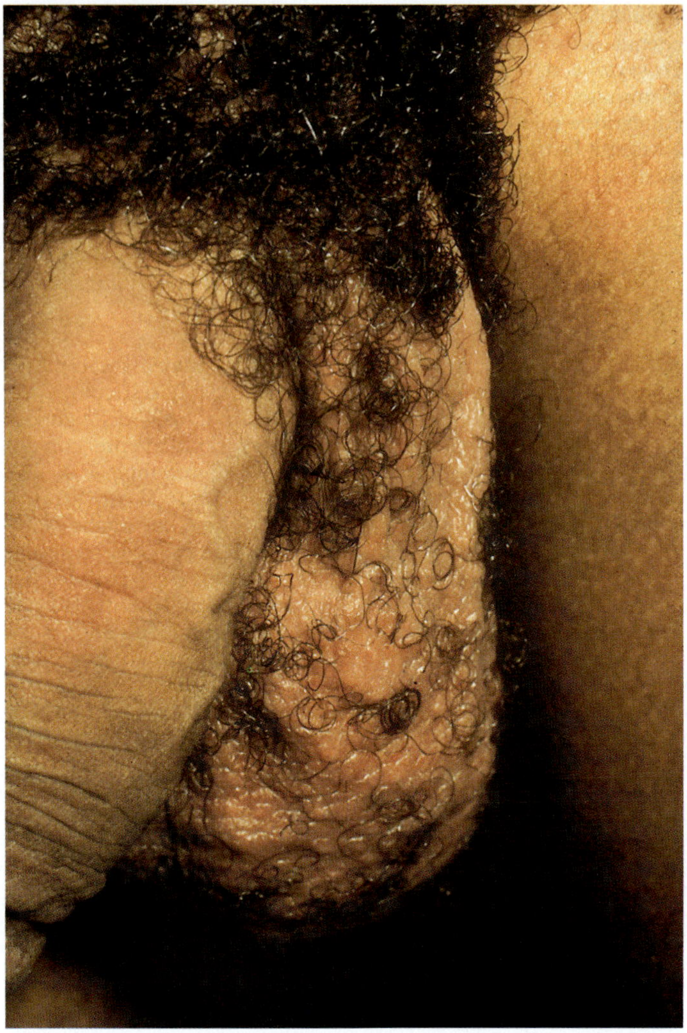

Figura 545-4. Varicocele sinistro in un ragazzo adolescente.

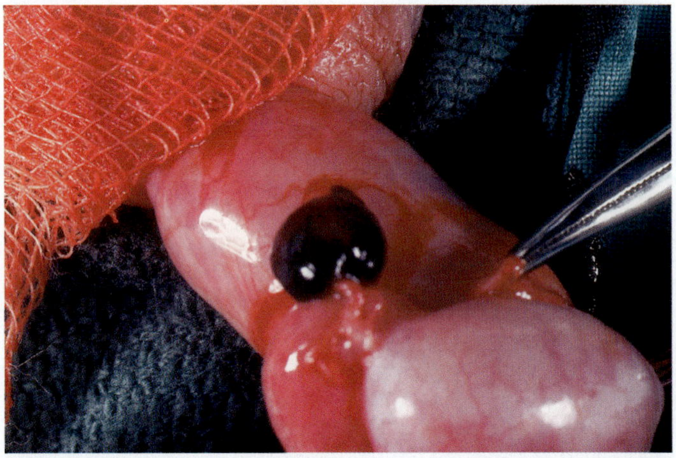

Figura 545-3. Torsione dell'appendice del testicolo; il testicolo è necrotico (freccia).

nei bambini e negli adolescenti è indicato nei soggetti con significativa disparità nelle dimensioni testicolari o dolore del testicolo interessato, oppure se il testicolo controlaterale è patologico o assente. Il testicolo interessato di solito si ingrandisce e raggiunge le dimensioni del testicolo normale nei successivi 1-2 anni. La varicocelectomia deve essere presa in considerazione anche nei bambini con un grosso varicocele di grado 3, anche senza disparità nelle dimensioni testicolari. L'intervento prevede diverse tecniche con la legatura delle vene del plesso pampiniforme mediante un'incisione inguinale o sottoinguinale (con o senza microscopia operatoria) o con la legatura della vena spermatica interna nel retroperitoneo. Si sta diffondendo anche l'intervento in laparoscopia. L'intervento si esegue su base ambulatoriale.

SPERMATOCELE

Uno spermatocele è una lesione cistica contenente sperma che è connessa al polo superiore del testicolo sessualmente maturo. Lo spermatocele di solito non è dolente e rappresenta un riscontro accidentale nel corso dell'esame obiettivo. Un ingrandimento dello spermatocele o la comparsa di dolore sono indicazioni alla rimozione.

IDROCELE

EZIOLOGIA. Un idrocele è un accumulo di liquido nella tunica vaginale (Fig. 545-5). L'1-2% dei neonati maschi presenta un idrocele. Nella maggior parte dei casi, l'idrocele è non-comunicante (il processo vaginale è stato obliterato durante lo sviluppo) e, in tali casi, il liquido dell'idrocele scompare entro 1 anno di età. Se è presente un processo vaginale persistentemente pervio, l'idrocele persiste, si ingrandisce progressivamente durante il giorno, mentre è più piccolo al mattino. Una rara variante di idrocele è l'idrocele addominoscrotale in cui è presente un grosso idrocele teso che si estende nella cavità addominale inferiore. In alcuni bambini più grandi, un idrocele non comunicante può derivare da una condizione infiammatoria all'interno dello scroto, come una torsione testicolare, una torsione dell'appendice del testicolo, un'epididimite o un tumore testicolare. Il rischio a lungo termine di un idrocele comunicante è lo sviluppo di un'ernia inguinale. Anche alcuni bambini più grandi e alcuni adolescenti maschi possono sviluppare un idrocele. In alcuni casi in questo gruppo d'età compare un idrocele dopo un episodio di trauma scrotale e di orchiepididimite, mentre in altri lo sviluppo è più insidioso.

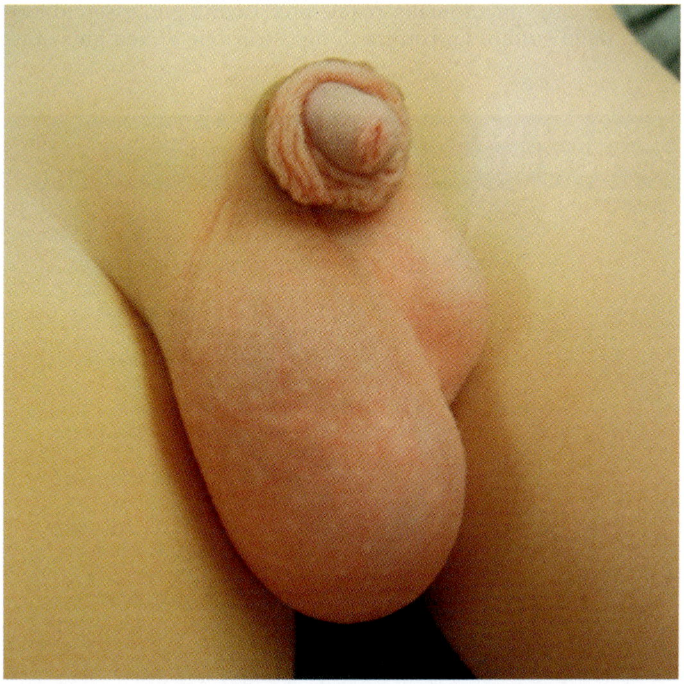

Figura 545-5. Neonato con idrocele destro di grandi dimensioni.

DIAGNOSI. All'esame obiettivo, l'idrocele è liscio e non dolente. La transilluminazione dello scroto conferma la natura della massa piena di liquido. È importante palpare il testicolo, poiché alcuni giovani uomini possono sviluppare un idrocele in associazione a un tumore del testicolo. Se la compressione della massa piena di liquido riduce completamente l'idrocele, la diagnosi probabile è quella di ernia inguinale/idrocele.

TRATTAMENTO. La maggior parte degli idroceli congeniti si risolve entro i 12 mesi di età in seguito a riassorbimento del liquido. Tuttavia, se l'idrocele è di grandi dimensioni e teso deve essere presa in considerazione la correzione chirurgica precoce, perché è difficile verificare che il bambino non abbia un'ernia e gli idroceli di grandi dimensioni di rado scompaiono spontaneamente. Un idrocele che persiste oltre i 12-18 mesi è di solito comunicante e deve essere operato. La correzione chirurgica è simile a un'erniorrafia (vedi Capitolo 343). Attraverso un'incisione inguinale, si identifica il funicolo spermatico, si drena il liquido dell'idrocele e si esegue una legatura alta del processo vaginale. Se un bambino più grande presenta un idrocele di grandi dimensioni, spesso occorre eseguire una laparoscopia diagnostica per determinare se sia presente un processo vaginale pervio e, se l'anello inguinale interno è chiuso, l'idrocele può essere corretto con un'incisione scrotale.

ERNIA INGUINALE

L'ernia inguinale è discussa nel Capitolo 343.

TUMORI DEL TESTICOLO

I tumori testicolari e paratesticolari possono presentarsi a qualsiasi età, anche nel neonato. Circa il 35% dei tumori testicolari prepuberi è maligno; più spesso sono tumori del sacco vitellino, anche se in questo gruppo d'età possono manifestarsi rabdomiosarcoma e leucemia. Negli adolescenti maschi, il 98% delle masse testicolari solide non dolenti è maligno (vedi Capitolo 503). La maggior parte di questi tumori si presenta come una massa testicolare di consistenza dura che non transillumina. Occorre eseguire un'ecografia scrotale per confermare la presenza di una massa testicolare; l'ecografia può inoltre contribuire a evidenziare il tipo di tumore testicolare. Devono essere dosati i marker tumorali sierici, comprese **α-fetoproteina** e **β-gonadotropina corionica umana**. La terapia definitiva comprende l'esplorazione chirurgica attraverso un'incisione inguinale: nella maggior parte dei casi si esegue un'orchiectomia radicale, che consiste nella rimozione dell'intero testicolo e del funicolo spermatico. In un bambino prepubere, se l'ecografia o l'esplorazione chirurgica evidenziano che il tumore è localizzato e benigno (come un teratoma o una cisti epidermoide) può essere appropriato un intervento conservativo con rimozione della sola massa.

Agarwal PK, Diaz M, Elder JS: Retractile testis—Is it really a normal variant? *J Urol* 2006;175:1496–1499.

Alukal JP, Zurakowski D, Atala A, et al: Testicular hypotrophy does not correlate with grade of adolescent varicocele. *J Urol* 2005;174:2367–2370.

Barthold JS: Is adjuvant hormonal therapy indicated in cryptorchidism? *Nat Clin Pract Urol* 2005;2:366–367.

Barthold JS, Gonzalez R. The epidemiology of congenital cryptorchidism, testicular ascent and orchiopexy. *J Urol* 2003;170:2396.

Caroppo E, Niederberger C, Elhanby C, et al: Effect of cryptorchidism and retractile testes on male factor infertility: A multicenter, retrospective, chart review. *Fertil Steril* 2005;83:1581–1584.

Cayan S, Acar D, Ulger S, et al: Adolescent varicocele repair: Long-term results and comparison of surgical techniques according to optical magnification use in 100 cases at a single university hospital. *J Urol* 2005;174:2003–2006.

De Kretser DM: Differences in the prevalence of cryptorchidism. *Lancet* 2004;363:1250–1252.

Eaton SH, Cendron MA, Estrada CA, et al: Intermittent testicular torsion: Diagnostic features and management outcomes. *J Urol* 2005;174: 1532–1535.

Eggener SE, Lotan Y, Cheng EY: Magnetic resonance angiography for the nonpalpable testis: A cost and cancer risk analysis. *J Urol* 2005;173:1745–1749.

Hack WW, Meijer RW, van der Voort-Doedens LM, et al: Natural course of acquired undescended testis in boys. *Br J Surg* 2003;90:728–731.

Husmann DA: Cryptorchidism and its relationship to testicular neoplasia and microlithiasis. *Urology* 2005;66:424–426.

Hutson JM, Hasthorpe S: Testicular descent and cryptorchidism: The state of the art in 2004. *J Pediatr Surg* 2005;40:297–302.

Kollin C, Hesser U, Ritzen EM, et al: Testicular growth from birth to two years of age, and the effect of orchiopexy at age nine months: A randomized, controlled study. *Acta Paediatr* 2006;95:318–324.

Lam WW, Yap TL, Jacobsen AS, et al: Colour Doppler ultrasonography replacing surgical exploration for acute scrotum: Myth or reality? *Pediatr Radiol* 2005;35:597–600.

Lee PA: Fertility after cryptorchidism: Epidemiology and other outcome studies. *Urology* 2005;66:427–431.

Livne PM, Sivan B, Karmazyn B, et al: Testicular torsion in the pediatric age group: Diagnosis and treatment. *Pediatr Endocrinol Rev* 2003;1:128–133.

Mansbach JM, Forbes P, Peters C: Testicular torsion and risk factors for orchiectomy. *Arch Pediatr Adolesc Med* 2005;159:1167–1171.

Mouriquand P: The normal testis. *Arch Dis Child* 2007;92:3.

Pierik FH, Burdorf A, de Muinck Keizer-Schrama SM, et al: The cryptorchidism prevalence among infants in the general population of Rotterdam, the Netherlands. *Int J Androl* 2005;28:248–252.

Rajimwale A, Brant WO, Koyle MA: High scrotal (Bianchi) single-incision orchiopexy: A "tailored" approach to the palpable undescended testis. *Pediatr Surg Int* 2004;20:618–622.

Salzhauer EW, Sokol A, Glassberg KI: Paternity after adolescent varicocele repair. *Pediatrics* 2004;114:1631–1633.

Sandlow J: Pathogenesis and treatment of varicoceles. *BMJ* 2004;328: 967–968.

Schwentner C, Oswald L, Kreczy A, et al: Neoadjuvant gonadotropin-releasing hormone therapy before surgery may improve the fertility index in undescended testes: A prospective randomized trial. *J Urol* 2005;173: 974–977.

Skakkebaek NE, Jorgensen N, Main KM, et al: Is human fecundity declining? *Int J Androl* 2006;29:2–11.

Somekh E, Gorenstein A, Serour F: Acute epididymitis in boys: Evidence of a post-infectious etiology. *J Urol* 2004;171:391–394.

Yang DM, Lim JW, Kim JE, et al: Torsed appendix testis: Gray scale and color Doppler sonographic findings compared with normal appendix testis. *J Ultrasound Med* 2005;24:87–91.

Yerkes EB, Robertson FM, Gitlin J, et al: Management of perinatal torsion: Today, tomorrow or never? *J Urol* 2005;174:1579–1582.

Capitolo 546 ■ Traumi del tratto genitourinario Jack S. Elder

EZIOLOGIA. I traumi del tratto genitourinario nel bambino di solito derivano da traumi chiusi durante cadute, attività sportive o incidenti con veicoli a motore (vedi Capitolo 71). In più di metà dei casi, sono presenti anche lesioni maggiori del cervello, del midollo spinale, dello scheletro, dei polmoni o di organi addominali. I bambini hanno un rischio più elevato di trauma renale chiuso rispetto agli adulti perché hanno meno grasso corporeo e perché i reni non si trovano direttamente dietro le coste. Anche i bambini con un'anomalia renale preesistente (come un'idronefrosi secondaria a ostruzione della giunzione ureteropelvica, un rene a ferro di cavallo o un'ectopia renale) hanno un rischio più elevato di trauma renale. Un trauma chiuso dell'addome o del fianco causa spesso un danno renale. Una caduta può causare una lesione da decelerazione che dà esito a una lesione del peduncolo renale, interrompendo il flusso ematico al rene. Se la vescica è piena, un trauma chiuso dell'addome inferiore può causare una rottura della vescica. La rottura dell'uretra membranosa si verifica nel 5% delle fratture di bacino. I traumi perineali sono di solito associati a trauma del bulbo uretrale. I segni e i sintomi di trauma delle vie urinarie comprendono microematuria o macroematuria, emorragia dal meato uretrale, dolore dell'addome o del fianco, massa del fianco, frattura delle coste inferiori o dei processi trasversi lombari ed ematoma perineale o scrotale.

DIAGNOSI. La valutazione del paziente ha inizio dopo lo stabilimento di vie aeree adeguate e la stabilizzazione emodinamica (vedi Capitolo 66). In caso di trauma addominale significativo, macroematuria o >50 eritrociti per campo ad alto ingrandimento, o sospetta lesione renale (trauma da decelerazione, dolore del fianco o ecchimosi a livello del fianco), è indicato l'imaging renale. Inoltre, la vescica deve essere cateterizzata, a meno che non vi sia fuoriuscita di sangue dal meato uretrale, cosa che costituisce un'indicazione di una potenziale lesione uretrale. L'inserimento del catetere in presenza di una lesione uretrale può aumentare l'estensione del danno e convertire una lacerazione parziale dell'uretra membranosa in una rottura totale. In questi pazienti, deve essere eseguita un'uretrografia retrograda iniettando un mezzo di contrasto radiopaco nel meato uretrale sotto guida fluoscopica. Le radiografie in proiezione obliqua dimostrano l'estensione della lesione e se la continuità uretrale è conservata o è stata interrotta.

Occorre eseguire una TC **spirale trifasica** per valutare reni, ureteri e vescica. Le immagini ritardate sono importanti per identificare un eventuale stravaso renale di sangue o di urina. Un'efficiente funzionalità di entrambi i reni senza stravaso di solito esclude una lesione renale significativa. Le lesioni renali sono classificate in base alla scala in gradi presentata nella Tabella 546-1. Le lesioni renali minori sono le più comuni e comprendono le contusioni del parenchima renale e le lacerazioni corticali poco profonde che non coinvolgono il sistema collettore. Le lesioni renali maggiori includono invece le lacerazioni profonde che interessano il sistema collettore, la rottura del rene e le lesioni del peduncolo renale (Fig. 546-1). La completa assenza di funzionalità di un rene senza ipertrofia compensatoria controlaterale (indicativa di assenza congenita) deve essere considerata come un'indicazione di una lesione maggiore del peduncolo renale. L'angiografia renale, un tempo usata per l'ulteriore valutazione delle lesioni renali (in particolare in caso di sospetta lesione di un peduncolo renale) viene ora utilizzata di rado perché questi pazienti sono spesso emodinamicamente instabili e il trattamento non è significativamente influenzato dai risultati dell'angiografia. In alcuni casi, un'anomalia renale preesistente può essere dimostrata dallo studio. La rottura di un'ostruzione di una giunzione

TABELLA 546-1. Scala di gravità del trauma renale dell'American Association for the Surgery of Trauma Organ

GRADO*	TIPO	DESCRIZIONE
I	Contusione	Micro- o macroematuria, studi urologici normali
	Ematoma	Sottocapsulare, non in espansione e senza lacerazione parenchimale
II	Ematoma	Ematoma perirenale non in espansione confinato al retroperitoneo renale
	Lacerazione	Spessore parenchimale della corticale renale senza stravaso urinario <1 cm
III	Lacerazione	Spessore parenchimale della corticale renale senza lacerazione del sistema collettore e senza stravaso urinario >1 cm
IV	Lacerazione	Lacerazione parenchimale che si estende attraverso la corticale renale, la midollare e il sistema collettore
	Vascolare	Lesione dell'arteria o della vena renale principale con emorragia contenuta dalla strutture circostanti
V	Lacerazione	Rene con rottura completa
	Vascolare	Avulsione dell'ilo renale, devascolarizzazione del rene

*Avanzare di 1 grado per le lesioni bilaterali fino al grado III.

Adattata da Moore EE, Shackford SR, Pachter HL, et al: Organ injury scaling: Spleen, liver, and kidney. *J Trauma* 1989;29:1664-1666.

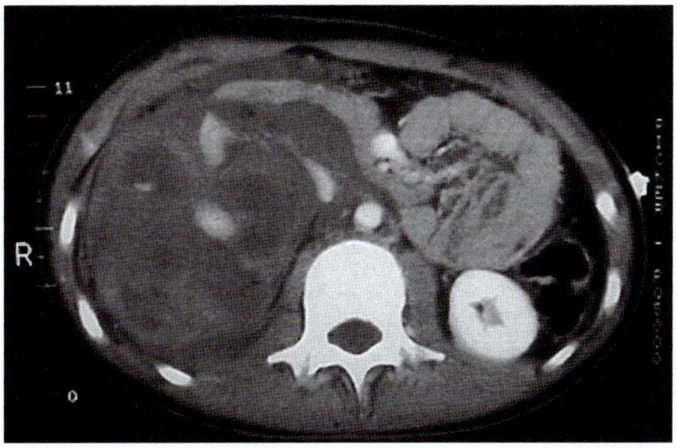

Figura 546-1. TC di una bambina con trauma renale maggiore in seguito a caduta dalla bicicletta. La TC dimostra una rottura del rene destro con stravaso urinario.

ureteropelvica può essere evidente se il rene è intatto ma l'uretere distale non è visualizzabile.

TRATTAMENTO. Le lesioni renali minori, come le contusioni, vengono trattate con il riposo a letto e il monitoraggio dei segni vitali, fino alla risoluzione del dolore dell'addome e del fianco e della macroematuria. I bambini con una lesione renale maggiore di solito vengono ricoverati in unità intensiva per il monitoraggio continuo dei segni vitali e della diuresi. Si somministrano anche antibiotici per via ev. Queste lesioni devono essere gestite in modo conservativo, perché la fascia di Gerota causa spesso un tamponamento dell'emorragia dal rene e una guarigione del parenchima lesionato si può osservare anche in presenza di uno stravaso urinario significativo. Circa il 10% dei bambini con una lesione renale maggiore va incontro a esplorazione chirurgica a causa di instabilità dinamica, stravaso persistente o ematuria persistente, oppure per la correzione di un'anomalia renale congenita. Può essere difficile identificare il parenchima normale e quello devitalizzato, come è significativa la probabilità di dovere eseguire una nefrectomia. Se il bambino viene sottoposto a esplorazione chirurgica per altre lesioni addominali, occorre esaminare anche il rene traumatizzato. Se è presente uno stravaso persistente a causa di un'ostruzione ureterale intermittente provocata da un coagulo, il problema può essere risolto inserendo endoscopicamente uno stent a doppia J temporaneo tra vescica e rene. Se è presente una lesione del peduncolo renale, è necessaria invece la nefrectomia. Il rene può essere salvato con una rivascolarizzazione renale d'emergenza soltanto se l'esplorazione chirurgica del rene avviene entro 2-3 ore dal trauma. L'esplorazione chirurgica occorre in tutti i casi di trauma penetrante del rene. Oltre alla perdita della funzione renale, la complicanza a lungo termine dei traumi renali è l'ipertensione renino-mediata. I bambini con lesioni renali devono essere sottoposti a determinazione periodica della pressione arteriosa. Le lesioni ureterali sono di solito iatrogene e le lesioni ureterali da trauma chiuso o da trauma penetrante richiedono l'immediata attenzione chirurgica. Quando è possibile il cateterismo vescicale, occorre eseguire una cistografia statica mediante l'infusione del mezzo di contrasto attraverso il catetere per gravità, idealmente per mezzo della fluoroscopia. Si possono eseguire proiezioni in antero-posteriore e oblique, inoltre deve essere eseguita una radiografia dopo minzione perché, in alcuni casi, la presenza di uno stravaso può essere occultata dalla vescica piena. La rottura vescicale può essere intraperitoneale o extraperitoneale. Tutte le rotture intraperitoneali richiedono la riparazione chirurgica. Le quasi-rotture extraperitoneali minori possono essere invece trattate con drenaggio mediante catetere, ma in generale è necessario il trattamento chirurgico.

Il trattamento delle lesioni dell'uretra membranosa è controverso. Disfunzione erettile, stenosi uretrale e incontinenza urinaria sono le principali complicanze tardive della rottura dell'uretra membranosa e la terapia ha lo scopo di ridurne il rischio. Spesso è presente un grosso ematoma pelvico con tamponamento spesso e un tentativo immediato di riparare la lesione può essere tecnicamente difficile e risultare in un'emorragia significativa. Molte di queste lesioni sono trattate inizialmente mediante cistotomia sovrapubica temporanea con drenaggio vescicale continuo per 3-6 mesi. Successivamente, può essere eseguita un'uretroplastica aperta o endoscopica. In alternativa, alcuni tentano di ottenere la continuità uretrale in anestesia e lasciano un catetere uretrale in sede per diversi mesi. Questi pazienti di solito richiedono una successiva uretroplastica aperta o endoscopica.

Le lesioni del pene sono rare. Alcuni bambini che stanno apprendendo il controllo degli sfinteri possono subire un trauma del glande se il coperchio del sanitario cade loro addosso mentre stanno urinando. Questi bambini spesso presentano un ematoma che ricopre la metà distale del glande e, in genere, non hanno difficoltà a urinare né necessitano di una valutazione approfondita. Alcuni bambini possono inavvertitamente sviluppare una lesione da strangolamento causata da un capello attorcigliato intorno al pene; in genere si osserva una costrizione molto stretta con grave edema distale e dolore e l'identificazione e l'incisione del capello permettono l'immediata risoluzione dell'edema. Dopo l'eliminazione del capello occorre valutare la vascolarizzazione dell'uretra e del pene. Gli adolescenti che hanno rapporti sessuali molto intensi possono sperimentare una rottura di uno dei corpi cavernosi. Questi soggetti presentano un edema severo dell'asta e richiedono un'esplorazione e un intervento d'emergenza. Anche i bambini con traumi penetranti del pene richiedono lo sbrigliamento e l'intervento d'emergenza.

Le lesioni testicolari sono relativamente poco frequenti nei bambini, a causa delle piccole dimensioni dei testicoli e della loro mobilità all'interno dello scroto. Tali lesioni derivano di solito da un trauma chiuso nel corso di un'attività sportiva. Di solito, questi pazienti presentano una significativa tumefazione scrotale, dolore testicolare e dolorabilità locale. L'ecografia dimostra la rottura della tunica albuginea (la capsula del testicolo) e un'emorragia circostante. L'immediato trattamento chirurgico delle lesioni testicolari aumenta il tasso di salvataggio del testicolo. Una lesione rara è il trauma da cerniera lampo, che può interessare sia lo scroto sia il prepuzio. Questo problema generalmente si verifica in bambini che non indossano biancheria intima. La cerniera può essere tagliata con un cutter da osso o da metallo. Generalmente non è necessaria la sedazione.

American Academy of Pediatrics, Committee on Sports Medicine and Fitness: Medical conditions affecting sports participation. *Pediatrics* 2001;107:1205–1209.

Buckley JC, McAninch JW: The diagnosis, management, and outcomes of pediatric renal injuries. *Urol Clin North Am* 2006;33:33–40.

Buckner BJ, Parousis V, Tarry W, et al: Strangulation injuries of the glans penis: A case series. *W V Med J* 2004;100:187–188.

Holmes JH 4th, Wiebe DJ, Tataria M, et al: The failure of nonoperative management in pediatric solid organ injury: A multi-institutional experience. *J Trauma* 2005;59:1309–1313.

Inoue N, Crook SC, Yamamoto LG: Comparing 2 methods of emergent zipper release. *Am J Emerg Med* 2005;23:480–482.

Johnson B, Christensen C, Dirusso S, et al: A need for reevaluation of sports participation recommendations for children with a solitary kidney. *J Urol* 2005;17:686–689.

Mohr AM, Pham AM, Lavery RF, et al: Management of trauma to the male external genitalia: The usefulness of American Association for the Surgery of Trauma organ injury scales. *J Urol* 2003;170:2311–2315.

Muram D, Levitt CJ, Frasier LD, et al: Genital injuries. *J Pediatr Adolesc Gynecol* 2003;16:149–155.

Nance ML, Lutz N, Carr MC, et al: Blunt renal injuries in children can be managed nonoperatively: Outcome in a consecutive series of patients. *J Trauma* 2004;57:474–478.

Onen A, Ozturk H, Yayla M, et al: Genital trauma in children: Classification and management. *Urology* 2005;65:986–990.

Onen A, Subasi M, Arslan H, et al: Long-term urologic, orthopedic, and psychological outcome of posterior urethral rupture in children. *Urology* 2005;66:174–179.

Otgun I, Karnak I, Senocak ME, et al: Late urodynamic findings after treating traumatic rupture of the posterior urethra in boys. *BJU Int* 2006;97:367–370.
Rogers CG, Knight V, MacUra KJ, et al: High-grade renal injuries in children—Is conservative management possible? *Urology* 2004;64: 574–579.
Wan J, Corvino TF, Greenfield SP, et al: Kidney and testicle injuries in team and individual sports: Data from the national pediatric trauma registry. *J Urol* 2003;170:1528–1523.

Capitolo 547 ■ Litiasi urinaria

Jack S. Elder

La litiasi urinaria in età pediatrica è meno comune negli Stati Uniti che in altri Paesi del mondo. L'ampia variabilità geografica nell'incidenza di litiasi in età pediatrica è correlata a fattori climatici, dietetici e socioeconomici. Circa il 7% dei calcoli urinari si verifica in bambini con meno di 16 anni di età. Negli Stati Uniti, molti bambini con litiasi hanno un'anomalia metabolica. Le eccezioni sono rappresentate dai pazienti con vescica neurologica (vedi Capitolo 542) che hanno una tendenza alla litiasi renale successiva alle infezioni e dai pazienti con ricostruzione delle vie urinarie con un tratto intestinale, che predispone alla litiasi vescicale. I calcoli metabolici sono due volte più frequenti nei maschi rispetto alle femmine e sono rari negli afroamericani. Nel Sud-Est asiatico, i calcoli urinari sono endemici e sono correlati a fattori dietetici.

FORMAZIONE DEI CALCOLI. La composizione e il sito dei calcoli urinari variano a seconda della patogenesi. La maggior parte dei "calcoli" spontanei è composta da cristalli di calcio ossalato o fosfato; altri sono dovuti a cristalli di acido urico, cistina o ammonio, o a cristalli di fosfato, oppure a un'associazione di queste sostanze (Tab. 547-1). Il rischio di formazione di calcoli aumenta in presenza di concentrazioni crescenti di questi cristalli e si riduce in presenza di concentrazioni crescenti di inibitori. I calcoli renali si sviluppano da cristalli che si formano sul calice e si aggregano per formare un calcolo. I calcoli vescicali possono essersi formati nel rene e quindi sono migrati lungo l'uretere oppure possono essersi formati primitivamente in vescica. La formazione dei calcoli dipende da 4 fattori: matrice, precipitazione-cristallizzazione, epitassi e assenza di inibitori della formazione dei calcoli nelle urine. La **matrice** è una mistura di proteine, zuccheri non amminici, glucosamina, acqua e residui organici che compongono fino al 2-9% del peso secco dei calcoli urinari ed è disposta all'interno dei calcoli in lamine concentriche. La **precipitazione-cristalizzazione** si riferisce alla supersaturazione delle urine da ioni specifici che formano i cristalli. I cristalli si aggregano per forze chimiche ed elettriche. Aumentando la saturazione delle urine rispetto agli ioni aumenta il tasso di enucleazione, la crescita e l'aggregazione dei cristalli e aumenta la probabilità di formazione e crescita dei calcoli. L'**epitassi** fa riferimento all'aggregazione di cristalli di differente composizione ma con struttura spaziale simile: si formano così cristalli di natura eterogenea. Le strutture spaziali dei calcoli di ossalato di calcio e di urato monopodico sono simili, e i cristalli di ossalato di calcio possono aggregarsi su un nucleo di cristalli di urato monopodico. L'urina contiene anche **inibitori della formazione di calcoli**, compresi ioni citrato, difosfonato e magnesio.

MANIFESTAZIONI CLINICHE. I bambini con urolitiasi di solito presentano microematuria o macroematuria. Se il calcolo si trova nella pelvi renale, nel calice o nell'uretere e provoca ostruzione, si verifica un severo dolore all'addome o al fianco (colica renale). In genere, il dolore è irradiato anteriormente allo scroto o alle grandi labbra. Spesso il dolore è intermittente, corrispondendo a periodi di ostruzione del flusso urinario, che aumenta la pressione nel sistema collettore. Se il calcolo si trova nell'uretere distale, il bambino può presentare sintomi irritativi di disuria, urgenza e pollachiuria; se invece il calcolo trasmigra nella vescica, il bambino di solito è asintomatico; infine, se il calcolo si trova nell'uretra, possono verificarsi disuria e difficoltà dello svuotamento. Alcuni bambini eliminano piccole quantità di materiale simile a sabbia.

TABELLA 547-1. Classificazione dell'urolitiasi

CALCOLI DI CALCIO (OSSALATO DI CALCIO E FOSFATO DI CALCIO)*
Ipercalciuria
Da assorbimento
Stravaso renale
Da riassorbimento
Acidosi tubulare distale, tipo 1 (fosfato di calcio)
Iperparatiroidismo
Sarcoidosi
Somministrazione di furosemide
Eccesso di vitamina D
Immobilizzazione
Somministrazione di corticosteroidi
Morbo di Cushing
Iperuricosuria
Cistinuria eterozigote
Iperossaluria (ossalato di calcio)
Iperossaluria primitiva, tipi 1 e 2
Iperossaluria secondaria
Iperossaluria enterica
Ipocitruria
Acidosi tubulare renale
CALCOLI DI CISTINA
Cistinuria
CALCOLI DI STRUVITE (MAGNESIO, AMMONIO, FOSFATO)
Infezioni delle vie urinarie (microrganismi produttori di ureasi)
Corpo estraneo
Stasi urinaria
CALCOLI DI ACIDO URICO
Iperuricosuria
Sindrome di Lesch-Nyhan
Disordini mieloproliferativi
Da chemioterapia
Malattia intestinale infiammatoria
CALCOLI DA INDINAVIR
NEFROCALCINOSI

*Più comuni.

DIAGNOSI. Il 90% circa dei calcoli urinari presenta qualche grado di calcificazione e, conseguentemente, risulta radiopaco alla radiografia addominale senza mezzo di contrasto. Alcuni calcoli hanno un diametro di pochi millimetri e possono non essere evidenti, in particolare se si trovano nell'uretere. I calcoli di struvite (fosfato, ammonio, magnesio) sono radiopachi. I calcoli di cistina, di xantina e di acido urico possono essere radiotrasparenti, ma di solito sono leggermente opachi. Alcuni bambini presentano una **nefrocalcinosi**, cioè la calcificazione del tessuto renale in sé, la quale si osserva più comunemente nei neonati prematuri trattati con furosemide (che provoca ipercalciuria) e nei bambini con rene a spugna midollare.

In un bambino con sospetta colica renale, si esegue una **TC spirale senza contrasto** dell'addome e della pelvi (Fig. 547-1). Questo studio richiede solo pochi minuti, è accurato nel delineare il numero e la sede dei calcoli e dimostra se il rene interessato è affetto da idronefrosi. Meno frequentemente si esegue un'urografia escretoria. Questo studio dimostra un ritardo della visualizzazione del sistema collettore rispetto al lato normale; e se è presente un calcolo ureterale vi è una disposizione a colonna del mezzo di contrasto fino al calcolo. Se il calcolo è radiotrasparente o di piccole dimensioni, l'urografia può non evidenziare il calcolo. Di conseguenza, si preferisce una TC spirale senza contrasto.

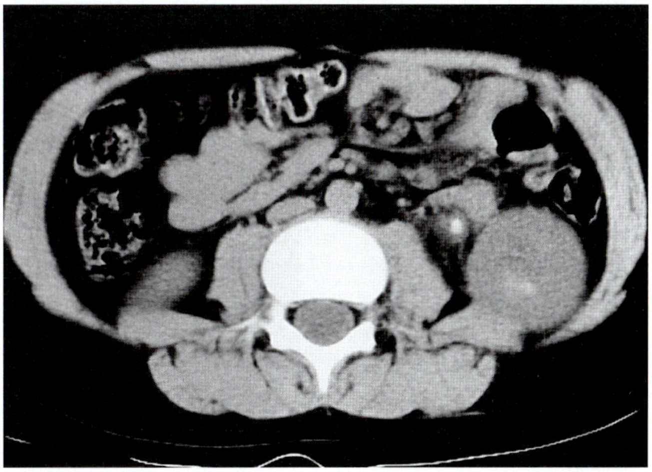

Figura 547-1. TC senza contrasto della parte media dell'addome che evidenzia un rene destro ingrandito con leggere calcificazioni nella pelvi renale e un uretere inspessito con un piccolo calcolo di ossalato di calcio impattato. (Da Kuhn JP, Slovis T, Haller J [editors]: *Caffey's Pediatric Diagnostic Imaging*, 10th ed. Philadelphia, Mosby, 2003, p 1799.)

TABELLA 547-2. Test di laboratorio per la valutazione dell'urolitiasi

SIERO
Calcio
Fosforo
Acido urico
Elettroliti e gap anionico
Creatinina
Fosfatasi alcalina
URINE
Esame delle urine
Urinocultura
Rapporto calcio:creatinina
Spot test per la cistinuria
Raccolta delle urine delle 24 ore per:
Clearance della creatinina
Calcio
Fosfato
Ossalato
Acido urico
Aminoacidi di basici (se il risultato dello spot test per la cistinuria è positivo)

Un'altra alternativa consiste nell'eseguire una radiografia senza contrasto dell'addome e della pelvi associato a un'ecografia renale. Se, però, è presente un piccolo calcolo nell'uretere, potrebbe non essere dimostrato da questi due esami; e se il calcolo non causa una riduzione del flusso urinario al momento dello studio, l'ecografia renale può non evidenziare l'idronefrosi. In un bambino che ha ricevuto la diagnosi di litiasi, si possono usare una serie di radiografie serieate o l'ecografia renale per seguire lo stato del calcolo, se esso è aumentato o diminuito di volume o se si è spostato. Se un bambino ha un calcolo nella pelvi renale, si deve sospettare un'ostruzione della giunzione ureteropelvica. In alcuni casi, può essere difficile determinare se in questo bambino l'idronefrosi è secondaria a un calcolo ostruente o all'ostruzione della giunzione ureteropelvica o a entrambe le cose.

Qualsiasi materiale che somigli a un calcolo deve essere inviato a un laboratorio specializzato nell'analisi chimica dei calcoli.

VALUTAZIONE METABOLICA. Occorre eseguire una valutazione metabolica per i più comuni fattori predisponenti in tutti i bambini con urolitiasi, ricordando che spesso coesistono fattori strutturali, infettivi e metabolici. Tale valutazione non deve essere eseguita in un bambino nella fase di espulsione di un calcolo, perché l'alterazione della dieta e dell'idratazione, come anche l'effetto dell'ostruzione sul rene, può alterare i risultati dello studio. Gli esami di laboratorio di base necessari sono elencati nella Tabella 547-2 e i valori normali per la raccolta delle urine delle 24 ore sono elencati nella Tabella 547-3. Nei bambini con ipercalciuria, sono necessari ulteriori studi dell'eliminazione del calcio con restrizione del calcio dietetico e carico di calcio se necessario.

PATOGENESI DI SPECIFICI CALCOLI RENALI

CALCOLI DI OSSALATO DI CALCIO E DI FOSFATO DI CALCIO. La maggior parte dei calcoli urinari nei bambini negli Stati Uniti è composta da ossalato di calcio o da fosfato di calcio, o da entrambi. Il più comune disordine metabolico in questi individui è l'**ipercalciuria normocalcemica**. Il 30-60% dei bambini con calcoli di calcio ha un'ipercalciuria senza ipercalcemia. Altre anomalie metaboliche che predispongono alla litiasi comprendono iperossaluria, iperuricosuria, ipocitruria, cistinuria eterozigote, ipomagnesuria, iperparatiroidismo e acidosi tubulare renale (vedi Capitolo 529).

L'**ipercalciuria** può essere renale da assorbimento o da riassorbimento. Nell'ipercalciuria da assorbimento il disturbo primitivo è l'iperassorbimento intestinale di calcio. In alcuni bambini, un aumento della 1,25 diidrossivitamina D è associato a un aumento dell'assorbimento di calcio, mentre in altri il processo è indipendente dalla vitamina D. L'**ipercalciuria renale** si riferisce a un'alterazione del riassorbimento tubulare renale del calcio (vedi Capitolo 519.8). La perdita renale di calcio causa una lieve ipocalcemia che a sua volta provoca un aumento della produzione di paratormone, con aumento dell'assorbimento intestinale del calcio e un aumento della mobilizzazione dei depositi di calcio. L'ipercalciuria da riassorbimento non è comune e si osserva nei pazienti con iperparatiroidismo primitivo. L'eccesso di paratormone stimola l'assorbimento intestinale del calcio e la mobilizzazione dei depositi di calcio. Un breve sommario della valutazione metabolica dei bambini si trova nella Tabella 547-4.

L'**iperossaluria** è un'altra potenziale causa importante di urolitiasi. L'ossalato aumenta il prodotto di solubilità della cristallizzazione del calcio ossalato di 7-10 volte più del calcio. Di conseguenza, l'iperossaluria aumenta in modo significativo la probabilità di precipitazione dell'ossalato di calcio. L'ossalato si trova in concentrazioni elevate nel tè, negli spinaci e nel rabarbaro. L'iperossaluria primitiva è un raro disordine autosomico recessivo che può essere ulteriormente classificato in aciduria glicolica e in aciduria L-glicerica. La maggior parte dei pazienti con iperossaluria primitiva ha un'aciduria glicolica; nelle urine degli individui affetti è presente un aumento degli acidi ossalico e glicolico. Entrambi i difetti causano un aumento della produzione endogena di ossalato, con ipo-ossaluria, urolitiasi, nefrocalcinosi e danno renale. Nei pazienti non trattati si verifica il decesso per insufficienza renale entro i 20 anni di età. L'**ossalosi**, definita come deposizione extrarenale di ossalato di calcio, si verifica quando è presente insufficienza renale con aumento dell'ossalato plasmatico. I depositi di ossalato di calcio compaiono dapprima nei vasi sanguigni e nel midollo osseo e quindi nel resto dell'organismo. L'iperossaluria secondaria è più comune e può verificarsi in pazienti con aumento dell'assunzione di ossalato e di precursori dell'ossalato come la vitamina C, in quelli con deficit di piridossina e nei bambini con malassorbimento intestinale.

L'**iperossaluria enterica** si riferisce a disturbi come la malattia intestinale infiammatoria (vedi Capitolo 333), l'insufficienza pancreatica (vedi Capitolo 347) e le malattie biliari, in cui è presente malassorbimento gastrointestinale degli acidi grassi, che legano il calcio endoluminale e formano sali che vengono eliminati nelle feci. Normalmente, il calcio forma un complesso con l'ossalato per ridurre l'assorbimento di ossalato, ma se il calcio non è disponibile, vi è un aumento dell'assorbimento di ossalato non legato.

L'**ipocitruria** si riferisce a una ridotta eliminazione di citrato, che è un inibitore della formazione di calcoli di calcio. Il citrato

TABELLA 547-3. Biochimica delle urine: valori normali

COSTITUENTE URINARIO	ETÀ	VALORE SINGOLO (CASUALE)	24 ORE	COMMENTI
Calcio	0-6 mesi	<0,8 mg/mg creatinina	<4 mg/kg/24 ore	Variazione prandiale
	7-12 mesi	<0,6 mg/mg creatinina		Sodio-dipendente
	≥2 anni	<0,21 mg/mg creatinina		
Ossalato*	<1 anno	0,15-0,26 mmol/mmol creatinina	≥2 anni; <0,5 mmol/1,73 m^2/24 ore	Valore singolo (casuale) mmol/mmol altamente età-dipendente
	1-≤5 anni	0,11-0,12 mmol/mmol creatinina		Tasso di escrezione/1,73 m^2 costante nel corso dell'infanzia e dell'età adulta
	5-12 anni	0,006-0,15 mmol/mmol creatinina		
	>12 anni	0,002-0,083 mmol/mmol creatinina		
Acido urico	Neonato a termine	3,3 mg/dL GFR†	<815 mg/1,73 m^2/24 ore	Tasso di escrezione/1,73 m^2 da >1 anno di età costante per tutta l'infanzia
	>3 anni	<0,53 mg/dL GFR		
Magnesio	>2 anni	<0,12 mg/mg creatinina	<88 mg/1,73 m^2/24 ore	Tasso di escrezione/1,73 m^2 costante nel corso dell'infanzia
Citrato		>400 mg/g creatinina		Dati limitati per l'infanzia
Cistina		<75 mg/g creatinina	<60 mg/1,73 m^2/24 ore	Cistina >250 mg/g creatinina suggerisce cistinuria omozigote

* Dosaggio dell'ossalato ossidasi.
† (mg/dL acido urico) (concentrazione di creatinina sierica/concentrazione di creatinina urinaria).
GFR, velocità di filtrazione glomerulare.
Da Milliner DS: Urolithiasis. In Avner ED, Harmon WE, Naiudet P (editors): *Pediatric Nephrology*, 5th ed. Philadelphia, Lippincott Williams & Wilkins, 2004, p. 1103, per gentile concessione.

TABELLA 547-4. Valutazione metabolica dei bambini con ipercalciuria

	CALCIO SIERICO	RESTRIZIONE DEL CALCIO (URINE)	CALCIO A DIGIUNO (URINE)	CARICO DI CALCIO (URINE)	PARATORMONE
Ipercalciuria da assorbimento	N	N o A	N	A	A
Ipercalciuria renale	N	A	A	A	N
Ipercalciuria da riassorbimento	A	A	A	A	A

A, aumentato; N, normale.

agisce come un inibitore dell'urolitiasi calcica formando complessi con il calcio, aumentando la solubilità del calcio nelle urine e inibendo l'aggregazione dei cristalli di fosfato di calcio e di ossalato di calcio. Disordini come la diarrea cronica, il malassorbimento intestinale e l'acidosi tubulare renale possono causare ipocitruria. Il disturbo può inoltre essere idiopatico.

L'**acidosi tubulare renale** (RTA) è una sindrome che coinvolge un disturbo dell'equilibrio acido-base a livello renale che può essere classificato in tre tipi, uno dei quali predispone ai calcoli renali che di solito sono di fosfato di calcio (vedi Capitolo 529). Nel tipo 1, il neurone distale non secerne idrogenioni nel tubulo distale. Il pH urinario non è mai inferiore a 5,8 e ne deriva un'acidosi ipokaliemica ipercloremica. I pazienti sviluppano nefrolitiasi, nefrocalcinosi, perdita di forza muscolare e osteomalacia. La RTA di tipo 1 può essere un disordine autosomico dominante ma più spesso è acquisito e associato a malattie sistemiche come la sindrome di Sjögren, la malattia di Wilson, la cirrosi biliare primitiva e la tiroidite linfocitaria, come pure può derivare dall'assunzione di amfotericina B, litio o toluene (un solvente organico associato all'abitudine di annusare colla).

Il 5-8% dei pazienti con **fibrosi cistica** (vedi Capitolo 400) presenta urolitiasi. In genere, i calcoli sono di calcio e spesso si manifestano nell'adolescenza o nella prima età adulta. Una nefrocalcinosi microscopica si verifica anche nei bambini più piccoli con questa malattia. Questi pazienti non hanno un'ipercalciuria e la tendenza all'urolitiasi è stata attribuita a un'incapacità di eliminare un carico di cloruro di sodio o al malassorbimento intestinale.

Altri disturbi possono avere un ruolo nel causare calcoli di calcio. L'**iperuricosuria** può essere correlata alla crescita epitattica dei cristalli di ossalato di calcio intorno a un nucleo di acido urico o all'azione dell'acido urico come controinibitore dei mucopolisaccaridi urinari, che inibiscono la cristallizzazione dell'ossalato di calcio. La **cistinuria eterozigote** si osserva in alcuni pazienti con calcoli di calcio. Il meccanismo è sconosciuto ma può essere simile a quello dell'acido urico. La sarcoidosi può causare un aumento della sensibilità alla vitamina D_3 (colecalciferolo) e quindi un elevato assorbimento di calcio dal tratto gastrointestinale. Nella sindrome di Lesch-Nyhan è presente un eccesso di sintesi di acido urico. Tali pazienti hanno una maggiore probabilità di formare calcoli di acido urico, ma alcuni di questi calcoli possono essere calcificati. L'**immobilità** può causare ipercalciuria da mobilizzazione dei depositi di calcio. I corticosteroidi ad alte dosi possono causare ipercalciuria e precipitazione di ossalato di calcio. Anche la furosemide, somministrata in unità intensiva neonatale, può causare ipercalciuria, urolitiasi e nefrocalcinosi gravi.

In alcuni bambini, i calcoli di calcio sono idiopatici. Prima di porre questa diagnosi è necessaria una valutazione metabolica completa.

CALCOLI DI CISTINA. La cistinuria comprende l'1% dei calcoli renali nei bambini. La condizione è un raro disturbo autosomico recessivo delle cellule epiteliali del tubulo renale che previene l'assorbimento dei 4 aminoacidi dibasici (cistina, ornitina, arginina e lisina) con eccesso di eliminazione renale di queste sostanze. L'unica complicanza nota di questa malattia familiare è la formazione di calcoli a causa della ridotta solubilità della cistina. I pazienti hanno di solito urine acide, cosa che provoca un tasso più elevato di precipitazione. Nel paziente omozigote, l'eliminazione giornaliera di cistina supera di solito i 500 mg e la formazione dei calcoli si verifica in età precoce. Gli eterozigoti eliminano 100-300 mg/die e, di solito, non presentano urolitiasi clinica. Il contenuto di zolfo della cistina conferisce ai calcoli il loro debole aspetto radiopaco.

CALCOLI DI STRUVITE. Le infezioni delle vie urinarie (vedi Capitolo 538) causate dai batteri produttori di ureasi (più spesso *Proteus* spp. e occasionalmente *Klebsiella* spp., *Escherichia coli*, *Pseudomonas* spp. e altri) risultano nell'alcalinizzazione e nell'eccessiva produzione di ammonio che può portare alla precipitazione di fosfato di ammonio e magnesio (struvite) e di fosfato di calcio. Nel rene, i calcoli hanno spesso una configurazione ramificata (a corna di cervo) e riempiono i calici. I calcoli agiscono da corpi estranei causando ostruzione, perpetuando le infezioni e causando un danno renale graduale. I pazienti con calcoli di struvite possono anche presentare anomalie metaboliche che predispongono alla formazione di calcoli. Questi calcoli si osservano spesso nei bambini con vescica neurogena, particolarmente in quelli sottoposti a procedura di ricostruzione con condotto ileale (vedi Capitolo 542). Calcoli di struvite possono formarsi nella vescica ricostruita dei bambini che sono stati sottoposti a ricostruzione del tratto urinario con cistoplastica di aumento o diversione continente o a entrambe le procedure.

CALCOLI DI ACIDO URICO. I calcoli che contengono acido urico rappresentano meno del 5% di tutti i casi di litiasi nei bambini negli Stati Uniti, ma sono più comuni nei Paesi meno sviluppati. Iperuricosuria con o senza iperuricemia è il fattore sottostante più comune nella maggior parte dei casi. I calcoli sono radiotrasparenti e la diagnosi deve essere sospettata quando è presente un'urina persistentemente acida e una cristalluria di urati.

Un'iperuricosuria può derivare da diversi errori congeniti del metabolismo della purina, che porta a un'eccessiva produzione di acido urico, il prodotto finale del metabolismo della purina negli esseri umani. Anche i bambini con sindrome di Lesch-Nyhan e i pazienti con deficit di glucosio-6-fosfatasi formano calcoli di urati. Nei bambini con sindrome dell'intestino corto, e particolarmente in quelli con ileostomia, la disidratazione e l'acidosi croniche sono talvolta complicate dalla litiasi da acido urico.

Una della cause più comuni di litiasi da acido urico è il rapido turnover della purina che si osserva in certi tumori e malattie mieloproliferative. Il rischio di litiasi da acido urico è particolarmente elevato quando il trattamento di queste malattie causa la rapida degradazione delle nucleoproteine. Calcoli o *sludge* di acido urico possono riempire l'intero sistema collettore superiore e causare insufficienza renale e perfino anuria. Anche gli urati sono presenti nei calcoli contenenti calcio. In questi casi, può essere presente più di un fattore predisponente alla formazione di calcoli. Un disordine correlato è la litiasi da 2,8-diidrossiadenina che deriva da un deficit di adenina fosforibosiltransferasi. I calcoli sono radiotrasparenti e possono essere differenziati dai calcoli di acido urico con la spettrofotometria di massa ma non con le analisi chimiche di routine. A differenza dell'acido urico, che è solubile nelle urine alcaline, la solubilità della 2,8 diidrossiadenina varia di poco negli intervalli fisiologici di pH.

CALCOLI DI INDINAVIR. L'indinavir solfato è un inibitore delle proteasi approvato per il trattamento dell'infezione da HIV. Almeno il 4% dei pazienti sviluppa una nefrolitiasi sintomatica. La maggior parte dei calcoli è radiotrasparente e composta di indinavir monoidrato, anche se in alcuni casi è stato evidenziato ossalato di calcio o fosfato di calcio o entrambi. Dopo ciascuna dose, il 12% del farmaco viene eliminato immodificato nelle urine. Le urine di questi pazienti spesso contengono cristalli di caratteristici rettangoli e cristalli a ventaglio o a stella. L'indinavir è solubile a un pH inferiore a 5,5; di conseguenza, si deve prendere in considerazione la terapia di dissoluzione mediante acidificazione urinaria con cloruro di ammonio o acido ascorbico.

NEFROCALCINOSI. Il termine nefrocalcinosi si riferisce alla deposizione di calcio nel tessuto renale. Spesso la nefrocalcinosi è associata a urolitiasi. Le cause più comuni sono terapia con furosemide (somministrata ai neonati prematuri), RTA distale, iperparatiroidismo, rene a spugna midollare, rachitismo ipofosfatemico, sarcoidosi, necrosi corticale, iperossaluria, immobilizzazione prolungata, sindrome di Cushing, iperuricosuria e candidasi renale.

TRATTAMENTO

In un bambino con un calcolo renale o ureterale, la decisione di rimuovere il calcolo dipende dalla sede, dalle dimensioni e dalla composizione (se nota), e dalla presenza o meno di infezione. Piccoli calcoli ureterali spesso vengono eliminati spontaneamente, anche se il bambino può presentare una grave colica renale. Le parti più strette dell'uretere comprendono la giunzione ureteropelvica e la parte media dell'uretere, dove interseca l'arteria iliaca comune; il segmento più stretto è la giunzione ureterovescicale. I **bloccanti α-adrenergici**, come tamsulosina, terazosina e doxazosina, si sono dimostrati in grado di facilitare l'eliminazione dei calcoli negli adulti diminuendo la pressione ureterale al di sotto del calcolo e riducendo la frequenza delle contrazioni peristaltiche dell'uretere ostruito. Effetti positivi simili sono stati notati con i calcioantagonisti con o senza corticosteroidi. Anche se questi farmaci sono stati usati in bambini con calcoli ureterali, la loro sicurezza ed efficacia non sono state dimostrate. In alcuni casi, l'inserimento endoscopico di uno **stent ureterale** dopo il calcolo permette di alleviare il dolore e dilata l'uretere sufficientemente da permettere il passaggio del calcolo. Nei casi di bambini con un calcolo di acido urico o di un lattante con calcolo da furosemide, può essere efficace la terapia di dissoluzione.

Se il calcolo non viene eliminato, o sembra improbabile che possa essere eliminato, oppure se è presente un'infezione delle vie urinarie associata, è necessaria la rimozione (Tab. 547-5). La **litotrissia** dei calcoli vescicali, ureterali e dei piccoli calcoli della pelvi renale per mezzo del laser all'olmio (attraverso un ureteroscopio flessibile o rigido) è abbastanza efficace. La litotrissia con onde shock extracorporee è stata utilizzata con successo nei bambini con calcoli renali e ureterali, con un tasso di successo superiore al 75%. Nei bambini con urolitiasi, deve essere trattato il disordine metabolico di base (Tab. 547-6). Dal momento che la litiasi deriva dall'eccessiva concentrazione di sostanze specifiche nelle urine, il mantenimento di una diuresi elevata per mezzo di un'elevata assunzione di liquidi è spesso un metodo efficace per prevenire altri calcoli. Un'elevata assunzione di liquidi deve essere continuata durante la notte e di solito è necessario che il bambino si alzi almeno una volta per notte per urinare e bere altra acqua.

Nei bambini con ipercalciuria, è necessaria una certa riduzione dell'assunzione di calcio e di sodio, ma occorre attenzione in un bambino che cresce. Anche i diuretici tiazidici riducono l'elimi-

TABELLA 547-5. Opzioni per il trattamento chirurgico primario rispetto alle dimensioni e alla sede

CALCOLI	LITOTRISSIA CON ONDE D'URTO	URETEROSCOPIA	NEFROLITOTOMIA PERCUTANEA
RENALE			
<1 cm	Più comune	Opzionale	Opzionale
1-2 cm	Più comune	Opzionale	Opzionale
>2 cm	Opzionale	Rara	Più comune
POLO INFERIORE			
<1 cm	Più comune	Opzionale	Opzionale
>1 cm	Opzionale	Opzionale	Più comune
URETERALE			
Prossimale	Più comune	Opzionale	Occasionale
Distale	Opzionale	Più comune	Rara

Da Durkee CT, Balcom A: Surgical management of urolithiasis. *Pediatr Clin North Am* 2006; 53: 465-477, per gentile concessione.

TABELLA 547-6. Terapia indicata per l'urolitiasi causata da anomalie metaboliche

ANOMALIA METABOLICA	TRATTAMENTO INIZIALE	TRATTAMENTO DI SECONDA SCELTA
Ipercalciuria	Riduzione del sodio della dieta	Citrato di potassio
	Calcio della dieta secondo RDA	Fosfato neutro
	Diuretici tiazidici	
Iperossaluria	Correzione dell'ossalato della dieta	Fosfato neutro*
	Citrato di potassio	Magnesio
		Piridossina*
Aciduria ipocitrica	Citrato di potassio	
	Bicarbonato	
Iperuricosuria	Alcalinizzazione	Allopurinolo
Cistinuria	Alcalinizzazione	Tiopronina
	Riduzione del sodio della dieta	D-penicillamina
		Captopril

*Terapia iniziale nell'iperossaluria primitiva.
RDA, quota giornaliera raccomandata.
Da Milliner DS: Urolithiasis. In Avner ED, Harmon WE, Niaudet P (editors): *Pediatric Nephrology,* 5th ed. Philadelphia, Lippincott Williams & Wilkins, 2004, p 1104, per gentile concessione.

nazione renale del calcio. È utile l'aggiunta di potassio citrato, un inibitore dei calcoli di calcio, con un dosaggio di 1-2 mEq/kg/24 ore. Un'ottima fonte di citrato è la limonata, in quanto 120 g di succo di limone contengono 84 mEq di acido citrico. Una miscela giornaliera di 120 g di succo di limone ricostituito in 2 l d'acqua e addolcito dovrebbe aumentare significativamente i livelli urinari di citrato. Nei casi difficili, occorre somministrare anche ortofosfato neutro, anche se è scarsamente tollerato.

Nei pazienti con calcoli di acido urico, è utile l'allopurinolo, un inibitore della xantina ossidasi efficace nel ridurre la produzione sia di acido urico sia di 2,8-diidrossiadenina e che può servire a controllare le recidive di entrambi i tipi di calcoli. Inoltre, è utile l'alcalinizzazione urinaria con bicarbonato di sodio o citrato di sodio. Il pH urinario dovrebbe essere almeno 6,5 e può essere monitorato a domicilio dalla famiglia.

Anche il mantenimento di un elevato pH urinario può prevenire la recidiva dei calcoli di cistina. La cistina è molto più solubile quando il pH urinario è superiore a 7,5 e l'alcalinizzazione delle urine con bicarbonato di sodio o citrato di sodio è efficace. Un altro farmaco importante è la D-penicillamina, un agente chelante che si lega alla cisteina o all'omocisteina, aumentando la solubilità del prodotto.

Anche se poco tollerata da molti pazienti, ne è stata segnalata l'efficacia nel dissolvere i calcoli di cistina e nel prevenire le recidive quando non sono utili l'idratazione e l'alcalinizzazione urinaria. L'N-acetilcisteina sembra avere una bassa tossicità e può essere efficace nel controllare la cistinuria, ma manca un'esperienza a lungo termine.

Il trattamento della RTA di tipo 1 comprende la correzione dell'acidosi metabolica e la compensazione delle perdite di sodio e di potassio. È necessaria la terapia con citrato di sodio o citrato di potassio oppure con entrambi. Quando si corregge l'acidosi metabolica, l'eliminazione del citrato urinario ritorna normale.

Il trattamento dell'iperossaluria primitiva comprende il trapianto epatico in quanto gli enzimi difettivi sono epatici. Idealmente, il trapianto dovrebbe essere effettuato prima della comparsa di insufficienza renale. Nei casi più gravi, è necessario anche il trapianto di rene.

Afshar K, McLorie G, Papanikolaou F, et al: Outcome of small residual stone fragments following shock wave lithotripsy in children. *J Urol* 2004;172:1600–1603.

Borghi L, Schianchi T, Meschi T, et al: Comparison of two diets for the prevention of recurrent stones in idiopathic hypercalciuria. *N Engl J Med* 2002;346:77–84.

Cameron MA, Sakhaee K, Moe OW: Nephrolithiasis in children. *Pediatr Nephrol* 2005;20:1587–1592.

DeFoor W, Dharamsi N, Smith P, et al: Use of mobile extracorporeal shock wave lithotripter: Experience in a pediatric institution. *Urology* 2005;65:778–781.

Durkee CT, Balcom A: Surgical management of urolithiasis. *Pediatr Clin North Am* 2006;53:465–477.

Holdgate A, Pollock T: Systematic review of the relative efficacy of non-steroidal anti-inflammatory drugs and opioids in the treatment of acute renal colic. *BMJ* 2004;328:1401–1404.

Hollingsworth JM, Rogers MAM, Kaufman SR, et al: Medical therapy to facilitate urinary stone passage: a meta-analysis. *Lancet* 2006;368:1171–1179.

Lande MB, Varade W, Erkan E, et al.: Role of urinary supersaturation in the evaluation of children with urolithiasis. *Pediatr Nephrol* 2005;20:491–494.

Minevich E, DeFoor W, Reddy P, et al: Ureteroscopy is safe and effective in prepubertal children. *J Urol* 2005;174:276–279.

Moe OW: Kidney stones: Pathophysiology and medical management. *Lancet* 2006;367:333–334.

Nicoletta JA, Lande MB: Medical evaluation and treatment of urolithiasis. *Pediatr Clin North Am* 2006;53:479–491.

Palmer JS, Donaher ER, O'Riordan MA, et al: Diagnosis of pediatric urolithiasis: Role of ultrasound and computerized tomography. *J Urol* 2005;174:1413–1416.

Parmar MS: Kidney stones. *BMJ* 2004;328:1420–1424.

Preminger GM, Assimos DG, Lingeman JE, et al: Chapter 1: AUA guideline on management of staghorn calculi: Diagnosis and treatment recommendations. *J Urol* 2005;173:1991–2000.

Prie D, Huart V, Bakouh N, et al: Nephrolothiasis and osteoporosis associated with hypophosphatemia caused by mutations in the type 2a sodium-phosphate cotransporter. *N Engl J Med* 2002;347:983–991.

Yilmaz E, Batislam E, Basar MM, et al: The comparison and efficacy of 3 different (alpha) 1-adrenergic blockers for distal ureteral stones. *J Urol* 2005;173:2010–2012.

Parte XXIV ▪ Disturbi ginecologici dell'infanzia

Capitolo 548 ▪ Anamnesi ed esame obiettivo Joseph S. Sanfilippo

PERIODO NEONATALE. Dopo l'esame obiettivo generale, la valutazione ginecologica iniziale della neonata inizia con l'esame delle mammelle. Comunemente, in seguito alla produzione di estrogeni endogeni da parte della madre, il tessuto mammario aumenta temporaneamente di dimensioni nel periodo neonatale; si può anche osservare una secrezione simil-lattea dal capezzolo. L'ingrandimento monolaterale persistente associato a dolorabilità e febbre dovrebbe suggerire una mastite o, raramente, un ascesso mammario. Occorre palpare delicatamente l'addome alla ricerca di segni di organomegalia e valutare se i genitali esterni presentano segni di ambiguità. Le labbra dovrebbero essere separate con delicatezza, consentendo l'ispezione dell'area dell'introito-imene. L'abduzione delle anche con le labbra delicatamente retratte frequentemente facilita l'ispezione dell'area dell'introito. Spesso si può percepire un imene normale protuberante associato a una perdita vaginale mucoide bianca acquosa. Nelle primissime settimane di vita può verificarsi un sanguinamento vaginale di modesta entità, che riflette la diminuzione dei livelli circolanti di estrogeni materni. A completamento della fase ispettiva, si effettua l'esplorazione rettale. Spesso è palpabile una struttura sulla linea mediana, indicativa dell'utero, mentre gli annessi non dovrebbero risultare palpabili a questa età.

ETÀ PREPUBERALE. Una paziente pediatrica o adolescente che si sottopone alla sua prima visita ginecologica andrebbe trattata con un'attenzione particolare, perché l'incontro iniziale può preparare adeguatamente il terreno a tutte le visite future. Se l'esame è doloroso o spiacevole oppure se si verifica una significativa mancanza di rapporto tra la paziente e l'esaminatore, la bambina può subire conseguenze psicologiche durature. Un atteggiamento gentile e dolce da parte del medico riuscirà a fare sì che la paziente si rilassi.

L'anamnesi viene ottenuta primariamente dai genitori, che andrebbero coinvolti in modo integrale nell'esame obiettivo di una figlia di questo gruppo di età. Sarebbe necessario che le pazienti abbiano la sensazione di poter controllare l'esame, siano a loro volta coinvolte e non sperimentino fastidio. Il raggiungimento di questi obiettivi viene facilitato da un'adeguata spiegazione prima dell'esame.

Molte informazioni si possono ottenere attraverso l'ispezione dell'area vulvovaginale. Idealmente la paziente viene collocata in posizione a gambe di rana (*frog-leg*), seguita dalla posizione genupettorale con manovra di Valsalva, che consente l'adeguata valutazione del terzo inferiore dell'area vaginale introitale. Spesso si può ricorrere all'ingrandimento utilizzando un colposcopio o una lente di ingrandimento manuale; è importante anche un'adeguata documentazione. La visualizzazione del vestibolo permette di esaminare la possibile presenza di perdite. L'aspirazione di eventuali liquidi nella vagina e il lavaggio dovrebbero essere realizzati con una tecnica asettica. S'introduce un tubo endovenoso (butterfly) in un catetere vescicale numero 12 e il tutto viene collegato a una siringa da tubercolina da 1 mL, potendo ricavare ed esaminare in questo modo campioni umidi. Si dovrebbero ottenere colture per la valutazione della vulvovaginite. Altri strumenti utilizzati per l'esame genitale sono l'otoscopio o il vaginoscopio di Cameron-Myers. La delicata trazione sulle labbra verso l'alto e l'esterno espone ulteriormente l'introito vaginale per la valutazione. Anche i tamponi di alginato di calcio sono utili, specialmente per ottenere colture dalla vagina. Esistono numerose varianti dell'imene normale e occorre fare attenzione a determinare se una paziente presenta un imene imperforato, microperforato o settato. Se si effettua un esame inadeguato nel contesto di un ambulatorio ospedaliero, occorrerebbe prendere in considerazione la sedazione o l'esame in anestesia.

ADOLESCENZA. In questo gruppo di età l'anamnesi può inizialmente essere ottenuta in presenza dei genitori della paziente. Tuttavia si dovrebbe mettere al corrente l'adolescente del concetto di riservatezza, offrendole l'opportunità di fornire il proprio racconto faccia a faccia, senza i genitori. Ciò può essere realizzato nella stanza di visita prima dell'esame obiettivo. Bisognerebbe considerare le preoccupazioni relative alla presenza di perdite vaginali, al rischio di infezioni sessualmente trasmesse, alla gravidanza o alle alterazioni mestruali. I medici dovrebbero ottenere la fiducia dell'adolescente, garantire un'atmosfera rilassata per l'esame e comunicare la propria disponibilità alla consulenza. Le indicazioni alla prima visita pelvica sono presentate nella Tabella 548-1.

Se l'adolescente non presenta uno dei criteri elencati nella Tabella 548-1, l'American College of Obstetrician and Gynecologists raccomanda che il "primo incontro ginecologico" sia realizzato a una età compresa fra i 13 e i 15 anni (Tab. 548-2). Questo incontro non rende obbligatorio l'esame pelvico ma rappresenta un'opportunità per il medico di fornire un'educazione all'adolescente.

Un suggerimento per il colloquio è l'utilizzo del metodo mnemonico *HEADSS is VG* (vedi Capitolo 111) illustrato di seguito:

TABELLA 548-1. Indicazioni proposte per l'esame pelvico nelle adolescenti

Età 21 anni, sessualmente non attiva
Sessualmente attiva entro 3 anni dall'inizio dei rapporti sessuali
Irregolarità mestruali, fase acuta
Grave dismenorrea
Dolore addominale inspiegabile
Disuria inspiegabile
Perdite vaginali anomale

Modificata da The adolescent obstetric-gynecologic patient. *ACOG Technical Bull* 1990;145:3.

TABELLA 548-2. Raccomandazioni per la prima visita ginecologica

Età compresa fra 13 e 15 anni
Il "primo incontro ginecologico" non comporta necessariamente una visita pelvica
Prima visita pelvica in caso di Pap test nei primi 3 anni dall'inizio dei rapporti sessuali (coitarca) o all'età di 21 anni

American College of Obstetricians and Gynecologists Teen Tool Kit, 2003.

Home (casa): ambiente domestico, dinamiche e relazioni familiari, condizioni di vita.

Education (educazione): frequenza della scuola, perdita di anni scolastici, voti attuali rispetto a quelli dell'anno precedente, atteggiamento nei confronti della scuola, argomenti più ostici e più graditi, obiettivi: università, carriera.

Activities (attività): attività fisica, sport, esercizio, hobby, amicizie, tempo extrascolastico, fine settimana.

Drugs (droghe): sigarette/tabacco senza fumo, alcol e/o altre droghe: uso a scuola o alle feste; utilizzo da parte di amici e proprio; frequenza e quantità assunta.

Sexuality (sessualità): attrazione sessuale: per il sesso opposto o per lo stesso; rapporti sessuali: età del primo, numero di partner totale e attuale, recente cambio del partner, contraccezione, infezioni sessualmente trasmesse, gravidanze pregresse, aborti.

Suicide/depression (suicidio/depressione): sentimenti nei propri confronti, esperienza di depressione o di altri disturbi di salute mentale, pregressi pensieri suicidi, pregressi tentativi di suicidio, problemi del sonno.

Violence (violenza): gestione dei conflitti domestici (ossia, ritorno a casa tardi la sera), a scuola, al lavoro, armi in casa, porto d'armi, sesso non consensuale, contatto fisico.

Gangs (bande): fa parte o ha amici che fanno parte di una banda, numero di bande nella scuola superiore, notare eventuali segni sulla pelle che segnalano l'appartenenza a una banda.

Il fattore più importante per quanto riguarda il colloquio è quello di stabilire il rapporto, sottolineando alla paziente il principio della riservatezza. È necessario dedicare un tempo sufficiente alla visita ambulatoriale e questa parte del colloquio (anamnesi) dovrebbe avvenire direttamente tra la paziente e il medico.

ESAME PELVICO. La paziente adolescente con un problema specifico per cui è necessario l'esame pelvico (sanguinamento uterino anomalo, vulvovaginite, primo Pap test dopo 3 anni dall'inizio dei rapporti sessuali vaginali), andrebbe coinvolta nel processo dell'esame stesso, che viene realizzato preferibilmente senza i genitori, ma con una accompagnatrice che può aiutare ad affrontare gli eventuali aspetti psicosociali avversi della situazione. Il medico e la paziente dovrebbero comunicare durante tutta la durata dell'esame. Questo andrebbe effettuato in posizione litotomica dorsale, cercando di mantenere il contatto oculare. Occorrerebbe la disponibilità di speculum di dimensioni appropriate, inclusi i Pedersen piccoli (profondità di 8 cm). Meglio evitare lo speculum da 4-5 cm, perché solitamente non consente una visualizzazione ottimale; può tuttavia essere appropriato l'uso dello speculum pediatrico di Huffman.

L'ispezione della vulva è seguito dalla palpazione delle ghiandole uretrali di Bartolini e di Skene. Si valuta quindi il clitoride, che normalmente è largo 2-4 mm. Un clitoride di larghezza superiore a 10 mm, specialmente in presenza di altri segni di virilizzazione, risulta anormale. Sarebbe necessario valutare anche la configurazione dell'imene. Prima dell'introduzione dello speculum bisognerebbe subito dire alla paziente che avvertirà una sensazione di pressione e prima di toccare l'introito vaginale è utile toccare la coscia interna con lo speculum stesso. Si dovrebbe evitare di traumatizzare l'uretra; lo spostamento posteriore della forchetta facilita ulteriormente l'appropriato posizionamento dello speculum. Spesso è utile discutere con l'adolescente riguardo alle tecniche per rilassare la muscolatura perineale.

Dopo avere completato la parte di esame con lo speculum, si procede con l'esame bimanuale. Nella ragazza vergine l'esame monodigitale con un dito guantato e ben lubrificato consente di palpare adeguatamente le pareti vaginali e la cervice e di valutare in maniera bimanuale l'utero e gli annessi. Si apprezza anche il cul-de-sac.

Negli Stati Uniti sono disponibili numerose risorse educative per le adolescenti che si sottopongono alla loro prima visita pelvica. Tra queste vi sono:

North American Society for Pediatric and Adolescent Gynecology (http://www.naspag.org)

The Society for Adolescent Medicine (http://www.adolescent.health.org)

Association of Reproductive Health Professionals (http://www.arhp.org)

GYN101 (http://www.gyn101.com)

L'American College of Obstetricians and Gynecologists ha reso disponibile un "tool kit", che comprende informazioni su come stabilire un ambiente favorevole per la valutazione ginecologica dell'adolescente, strumenti per la valutazione stessa, suggerimenti su come parlare con gli adolescenti, volantini per loro e tutta una serie di risorse per i professionisti sanitari (indirizzo: 409 12th Street, SW, PO Box 96920, Washington, DC 20090-6920).

Cavanaugh R: Obtaining a personal and confidential history from adolescents. An opportunity for prevention. *J Adolesc Health Care* 1986;72:118–122.

Elford K, Spence J: The forgotten female: Pediatric and adolescent gynecological concerns and their reproductive consequences. *J Pediatr Adolesc Gynecol* 2002;15:65–77.

Farrington PF: Pediatric vulvo-vaginitis. *Clin Obstet Gynecol* 1997;40:135–140.

Kass-Wolff JH, Wilson EE: Pediatric gynecology: Assessment strategies and common problems. *Semin Reprod Med* 2003;21:329–338.

Phillips S, Bohannon W, Heald F: Teenagers' choices regarding the presence of family members during the examination of genitalia. *J Adolesc Health Care* 1986;7:245–249.

Pokorny SF, Stormer J: Atraumatic removal of secretions from the prepubertal vagina. *Am J Obstet Gynecol* 1987;156:581–582.

Ricciardi R: First pelvic examination in the adolescent. *Nurse Pract Forum* 2000;11:161–169.

Saipik R: Adolescent contraception. In Sanfilippo JS, Muram D, Dewhurst J, et al. (editors): *Pediatric Adolescent Gynecology,* 2nd ed. Philadelphia, WB Saunders, 2001, pp 305–317.

Sanders JM Jr, DuRant RH, Chastain DO: Pediatricians' use of chaperones when performing gynecologic examinations on adolescent females. *J Adolesc Health Care* 1989;10:110–114.

Talbot CW: The gynecologic examination of the pediatric patient. *Pediatr Ann* 1986;15:501–505, 508.

Capitolo 549 ■ Vulvovaginite

Joseph S. Sanfilippo

La vulvovaginite è il problema ginecologico più comune nell'infanzia e nell'adolescenza. Tra le principali manifestazioni cliniche, in ordine di frequenza, vi sono le perdite vaginali, l'eritema, la dolorabilità e il prurito. Possono comparire anche la disuria e il sanguinamento, ma sono meno comuni. L'irritazione vulvovaginale è dovuta all'assenza di cuscinetti adiposi labiali e di peli pubici per la protezione dei genitali esterni. Le piccole labbra tendono ad aprirsi quando la bambina si accovaccia; ciò, a sua volta, provoca l'esposizione dei tessuti sensibili all'interno dell'anello imenale. La stretta vicinanza dell'orifizio anale alla vagina consente il trasferimento dei batteri fecali all'area vulvovaginale. Anche la masturbazione può essere un fattore contribuente.

Nel periodo prepuberale, con livelli di estrogeni relativamente bassi, il sottile epitelio vaginale atrofico è suscettibile all'invasione batterica. La vulvovaginite ricorrente, specialmente quella aspecifica, di solito cessa quando la bambina raggiunge la pubertà, gli estrogeni aumentano e il pH vaginale diventa più acido. Tale modificazione è dovuta in parte all'aumentata produzione di acido acetico e acido lattico, un fenomeno accompagnato dall'incremento della proliferazione delle cellule superficiali e del glicogeno, così come dall'arricchimento della normale flora batterica (Tab. 549-1).

L'esame colturale e citologico vaginale e la vaginoscopia possono essere indicati per la valutazione delle pazienti pediatriche

TABELLA 549-1. Vulvovaginite specifica

MICRORGANISMO	PRESENTAZIONE	DIAGNOSI	TRATTAMENTO
Enterobiasi (ossiuri)	Prurito perineale (notturno); sintomi gastrointestinali; contaminazione vulvovaginale variabile da parte delle feci	Vermi adulti nelle feci o uova sulla cute perianale	Mebendazolo; da ripetere dopo 3 settimane se necessario
Giardiasi	Contaminante fecale asintomatico, perdite vaginali, diarrea, sindrome da malassorbimento	Protozoi flagellati (cisti o trofozoiti) nelle feci	Metronidazolo o quinacrina
Mollusco contagioso	Lesioni vulvari, noduli con area ombelicata; nucleo bianco di materiale similcaseoso	Isolamento del poxvirus	Curettage dermico della papula
Phthirus pubis (pediculosi del pube)	Prurito, escoriazione, macule cutanee blu; interno coscia o addome inferiore	Lendini sugli steli piliferi, pidocchi sulla cute o sugli indumenti	Lozione di lindane; vedi anche Capitolo 667
Sarcoptes scabiei (scabbia)	Prurito notturno, vescicole pruriginose, pustole in linee	Acari; uova scure, punti delle feci (microscopici)	Lindane 1%
Shigella species (shigellosi)	Febbre, malessere, contaminazione fecale, diarrea; sangue e muco, crampi, pus nelle feci	Feci; leucociti ed eritrociti, positività alla *Shigella*	Trimetoprim-sulfametoxazolo, ampicillina o tetraciclina
Staphylococcus e *Streptococcus*	Perdite vaginali nell'area vulvovaginale; diffusione dalla lesione primaria	Risultati colturali positivi per il microrganismo appropriato	Penicillina, una cefalosporina o clindamicina

Da Sanfilippo JS: Adolescent girls with vaginal discharge. *Pediatr Ann* 1986;15:509-512, 516-519.

con una vulvovaginite. Lo stick per l'esterasi leucocitaria è un test di screening rapido per la vaginite e la cervicite. La tecnica è stata utilizzata per l'identificazione della tricomoniasi, della *Candida* e della vaginosi batterica e anche per valutare le secrezioni cervicali allo scopo d'identificare le infezioni gonococciche e da clamidie.

LEUCORREA FISIOLOGICA. Si tratta di perdite che riflettono i livelli circolanti di estrogeni. Il trattamento consiste nel rassicurare la paziente che si tratta di un processo normale e autolimitato.

PERDITE VAGINALI PATOLOGICHE. Le perdite vaginali sono un comune sintomo di presentazione nelle pazienti pediatriche. Spesso rappresentano il sintomo primario della vulvite, della vaginite o della vulvovaginite. Possibili segni e sintomi associati sono il prurito, la minzione frequente, la disuria e l'enuresi. La vulvite si manifesta primariamente con disuria e prurito ed è associata a eritema della vulva; ha comunemente un decorso più protratto rispetto alla vaginite, che è invece caratterizzata da perdite senza disuria e da prurito o eritema associati. La vulvovaginite comporta una combinazione di tali manifestazioni. Si dovrebbero notare il colore, l'odore e la durata delle perdite. Sebbene vi siano numerose cause di vulvovaginite nelle pazienti pediatriche, tra le cause più comuni vi sono la scarsa igiene perineale, l'infezione da *Candida* e i corpi estranei.

VULVOVAGINITE ASPECIFICA. Le pazienti con scarsa igiene perineale spesso sviluppano una malattia nota come vulvovaginite aspecifica, la quale rappresenta il 70% di tutti i casi di vulvovaginite pediatrica. Le perdite sono caratteristicamente marroni o verdi, di odore fetido e associate a pH vaginale di 4,7-6,0. Nel 68% dei casi riportati, questa vaginite è associata a batteri coliformi secondari a contaminazione fecale. Gli altri microrganismi batterici che più comunemente si associano sono lo streptococco emolitico e lo stafilococco coagulasi-positivo, che vengono spesso trasmessi manualmente dal nasofaringe. Anche indumenti, prodotti chimici, cosmetici e saponi o detergenti utilizzati per il bagno o per la lavatrice possono causare un'irritazione che porta alla vulvovaginite aspecifica. Sono chiamati in causa gli indumenti troppo aderenti come i jeans, i body, le calzamaglie, i collant e le mutandine sintetiche o i pannolini di carta rivestiti di plastica. Occasionalmente questa malattia può risultare in una infezione cronica, che può provocare significative conseguenze psicologiche per la bambina e per i genitori. L'esame obiettivo dovrebbe sottolineare l'importanza di evitare la "fissazione vaginale", promuovendo un'appropriata igiene perineale.

Un trattamento efficace dovrebbe dunque comprendere istruzioni per tale igiene, l'evitare indumenti intimi aderenti, praticare semicupi con sapone neutro e lasciare asciugare la vulva all'aria. Si dovrebbero istruire le pazienti ad avere abitudini appropriate per quanto riguarda l'evacuazione dell'intestino e della vescica urinaria, sottolineando la necessità di rimuovere il materiale fecale dall'area vulvovaginale. La vulvovaginite ricorrente andrebbe trattata con antibiotici sistemici come l'amoxicillina o una cefalosporina. Gli estrogeni topici in crema o l'unguento di polimixina spesso si rivelano utili.

VULVOVAGINITE SPECIFICA. La *Gardnerella vaginalis* è il microrganismo più comunemente coltivato nelle pazienti pediatriche o adolescenti con vulvovaginite, seguita dalla *Candida*. Tra gli altri microrganismi identificati vi sono enterococchi e batteri anaerobi come il *Peptococcus*, il *Peptostreptococcus*, la *Veillonella parvula*, l'*Eubacterium*, il *Propionibacterium* e la *Bacteroides* species. Occorrerebbe prendere in considerazione anche i protozoi, gli elminti e i virus, quali agenti eziologici. Il trattamento dipende dal microrganismo responsabile (vedi Tab. 549-1).

CISTI VAGINALI. Si tratta di cisti rare, frequentemente riscontrate come reperto occasionale. Rappresentano residui del dotto wolffiano o mülleriano oppure cisti da inclusione epiteliale. Il trattamento dipende dalla loro localizzazione e dal loro aspetto; di solito vengono sottoposte a osservazione, ma la resezione è raccomandata se diventano sintomatiche.

CISTI DEL DOTTO DI GARTNER. Rappresentano una porzione rudimentale del dotto wolffiano. Nelle ragazze di solito il dotto regredisce completamente, ma possono rimanere residui lungo le pareti anterolaterali della vagina. Le cisti sono state associate a dispareunia nelle adolescenti sessualmente attive, sintomatologia che giustifica la resezione chirurgica.

SINECHIE CLITORIDEE. Spesso si trovano associate a un prurito che interessa l'area clitoridea e possono essere dovute allo sfregamento dell'area genitale anteriore durante la deambulazione. L'eritema è variabile. Se il cappuccio clitorideo sembra essere agglutinato al glande clitorideo la valutazione può essere dolorosa. Il trattamento consiste nell'applicazione quotidiana di creme estrogeniche nell'area periclitoridea per un periodo di 1-2 settimane. Di solito questo si rivela sufficiente; raramente diventa necessario l'intervento chirurgico.

ADERENZE LABIALI. In questa malattia, le piccole labbra presentano una linea centrale di aderenza che si estende da un'area immediatamente inferiore al clitoride e quindi alla forchetta (Fig. 549-1). Le aderenze labiali sono comunemente osservate nelle pazienti di età inferiore a 6 anni e spesso sono asintomatiche. Di solito le lesioni sono associate a un'infiammazione locale e allo stato ipoestrogenico dell'adolescenza. L'accumulo di urine in vagina e la vulvovaginite ricorrente forniscono un habitat continuo favorevole alle infezioni ricorrenti delle vie urinarie. Questi sintomi urinari compaiono nel 20-40% delle pazienti e andrebbero trattati.

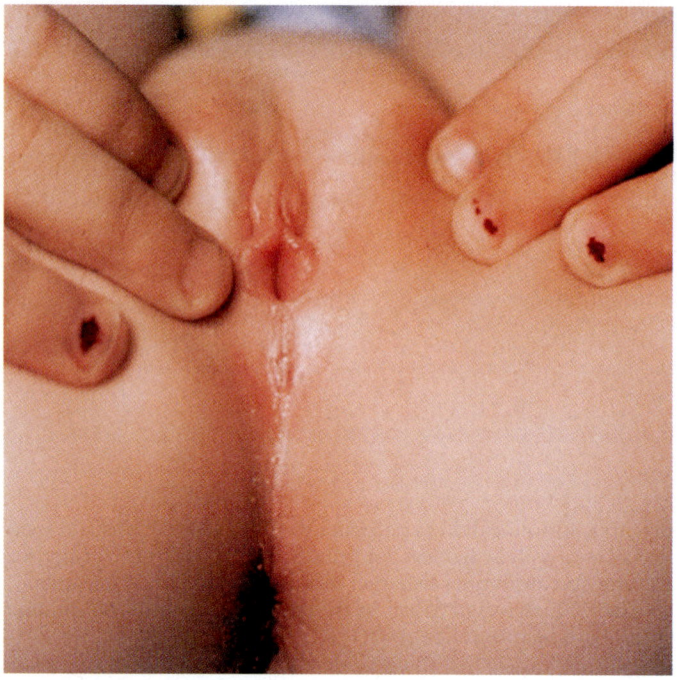

Figura 549-1. Aderenze labiali.

Le creme a base di estrogeni topici applicate ogni sera per 1 settimana rappresentano il trattamento di scelta e risultano efficaci in oltre il 90% dei casi. La detersione seguita dall'applicazione periodica di un unguento blando come il petrolato o l'ossido di zinco dovrebbe proseguire per 1-2 mesi dopo la separazione delle aderenze, al fine di prevenire la recidiva. La separazione meccanica è consigliabile solo se le aderenze sembrano rispondere facilmente e se non provoca un trauma significativo. Dopo l'intervento si dovrebbe riconsiderare se la paziente presenta cause predisponenti, come la presenza di un setto vaginale.

CANDIDIASI. L'infezione da *Candida* è spesso associata a un eritema da pannolino. La vulvovaginite da *Candida*, sebbene rara in epoca infantile, deve essere presa in considerazione specialmente nelle pazienti con candidiasi mucocutanea cronica. La presenza di tessuto infettato da *Candida* può essere indicativo di un'immunosoppressione significativa. Si dovrebbero escludere fattori sottostanti come il diabete mellito. Il trattamento con una crema a base di imidazoli (clotrimazolo) è frequentemente efficace, tranne nei casi di candidiasi mucocutanea cronica.

MOLLUSCO CONTAGIOSO. Si tratta di una comune infezione della cute causata dal virus del mollusco contagioso, o poxvirus. Il mollusco contagioso si presenta come una papula ombelicata, cupoliforme, in cui l'ombelicatura centrale è solitamente associata a un core polposo. Le lesioni vulvari sembrano dovute a un'autoinoculazione o a un contatto ravvicinato (sessuale o non sessuale) con un individuo infetto. Il periodo di incubazione è di 2-7 settimane. La diagnosi viene confermata dalla visualizzazione al microscopio ottico delle inclusioni virali (corpi del mollusco) nel core centrale. Il trattamento consiste nell'attesa; se le lesioni persistono, possono essere eliminate mediante un delicato curettage. Tra gli altri metodi di terapia vi sono la criochirurgia e l'elettrocauterizzazione (vedi Capitolo 666).

INTERTRIGINE. L'intertrigine può apparire nelle aree genitocrurali insieme a frizione, obesità e umidità in queste zone. Si può associare anche alla miliaria e a un'infezione secondaria. Le aree interessate appaiono rosse e macerate. L'igiene scrupolosa, accompagnata con blandi emollienti e talvolta corticosteroidi leggeri, risulta un trattamento efficace.

IMPETIGINE. Questa entità viene comunemente identificata durante le primissime settimane di vita. Di solito è causata dallo *Staphylococcus aureus*, spesso dal fago gruppo II, tipo 71, che può essere acquisito dalla madre, da altri parenti o dal personale. L'impetigine tende a interessare la vulva e le aree periombelicali, provocando lesioni o pustole che successivamente diventano crostose e che possono estendersi diffusamente e complicarsi se non viene istituito prontamente il trattamento con antibiotici.

MALASSEZIA FURFUR. Questa malattia viene scatenata dal *Pityrosporum orbicolare* e si manifesta con macule squamose sul tronco nei pazienti in età postpuberale, ma sono state riportate anche lesioni al volto e all'area genitale. La diagnosi viene confermata mediante la visualizzazione delle ife e delle spore su preparato umido con idrossido di potassio al 10%. Il trattamento richiede l'applicazione di imidazoli topici (clotrimazolo).

HERPES SIMPLEX. Il virus dell'herpes simplex di tipo 1 e 2 interessa l'area vulvare. Sebbene i due tipi non siano esclusivamente sito-specifici, il 2 è comunemente responsabile delle lesioni genitali, mentre l'1, in generale, delle lesioni orofacciali. L'infezione è caratterizzata da papule che si trasformano in vescicole e dal fatto che il virus interessa i gangli delle radici dorsali. Nella diagnosi differenziale sono comprese tutte le lesioni erose o pustolose, così come l'herpes zoster. La diagnosi definitiva viene confermata dalla coltura o dalla visualizzazione del virus al microscopio elettronico. Il trattamento con aciclovir topico riduce la sua diffusione e accelera la guarigione (vedi Capitolo 249).

PAPILLOMAVIRUS UMANO. Questo virus è associato a numerosi sierotipi, tra cui quelli 6, 11, 16 e 18 vengono solitamente riscontrati nella regione anogenitale. I tipi 16 e 18 si associano particolarmente a lesioni maligne e premaligne della vulva e della cervice. La diagnosi differenziale comprende il mollusco contagioso, il condiloma acuminato e la neoplasia vulvare intraepiteliale. La possibilità di abuso sessuale deve essere fortemente presa in considerazione quando tali lesioni vengono identificate. Il trattamento si basa sui sintomi e sui segni di presentazione.

LICHEN SCLEROSO. Si tratta di una malattia cutanea atrofica cronica caratterizzata da piccole papule appiattite, di colore da rosa ad avorio e con un diametro di diversi millimetri. Le papule sembrano confluire in placche che diventano rugose e atrofiche. Le lesioni anogenitali assumono frequentemente un aspetto "a clessidra" o "a 8" (Fig. 549-2). Le vescicole e le bolle possono

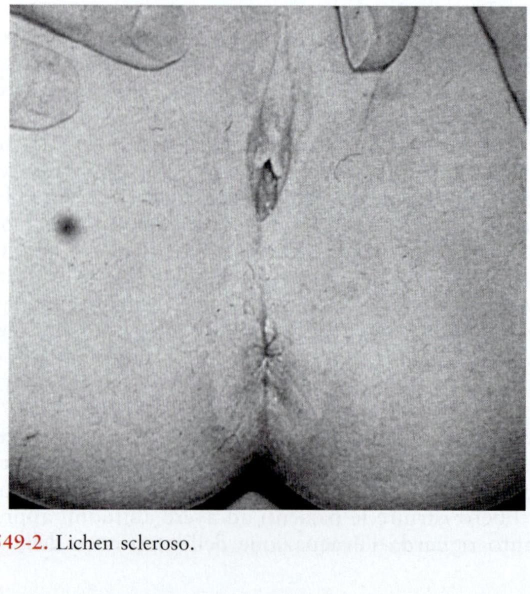

Figura 549-2. Lichen scleroso.

diffondersi alla vulva con un'emorragia associata. Il lichen scleroso si presenta spesso in età prepuberale; il 10-15% dei casi compare nei bambini.

L'esordio nella maggior parte dei bambini solitamente avviene prima dell'età di 7 anni. Il paziente più giovane riportato in letteratura medica era un neonato di alcune settimane di vita. La comparsa del menarca spesso porta al miglioramento spontaneo delle lesioni, ma solitamente il processo continua. Le pazienti sono spesso sintomatiche in modo intermittente e non esiste una relazione diretta tra il menarca e il miglioramento dei sintomi o la risoluzione della malattia. Si possono verificare l'atrofia delle piccole labbra e la fimosi del clitoride, così come la contrattura dell'introito.

La causa del lichen scleroso è sconosciuta, ma si ritiene che sia correlato a una malattia autoimmune. Vi è un'associazione tra alcuni tipi HLA. Non sono documentati raggruppamenti familiari. Ci può essere una relazione tra il lichen scleroso e la morfea (sclerodermia localizzata). La diminuzione dell'attività della 5-α-reduttasi è stata proposta come una possibile causa determinante. Nel 75% dei pazienti è stata dimostrata l'immunofluorescenza positiva per la fibrina, per il complemento sierico (C3) e per l'immunoglobulina M (IgM) nell'area interessata.

Il trattamento è sintomatico; di solito gli emollienti e i corticosteroidi topici forniscono sollievo. I corticosteroidi costituiscono la prima scelta negli adulti e sono risultati efficaci anche nei bambini. Inizialmente viene impiegata una crema di idrocortisone all'1-2%. In caso di mancata risposta, è raccomandato un breve ciclo con betametasone dipropionato allo 0,05% o con clotrimazolo. A questo trattamento sono associati minimi effetti collaterali. Dopo la risposta iniziale, si può utilizzate un corticosteroide topico più leggero per prevenire la recidiva. Sono stati proposti anche gli estrogeni e gli androgeni topici, che però possono provocare perdite vaginali e altri disturbi secondari, come la ginecomastia e l'ingrandimento del clitoride. Le infezioni secondarie andrebbero trattate con antibiotici. Alcuni individui affetti mostrano il fenomeno di Koebner, sicché dovrebbero evitare gli indumenti troppo aderenti e i traumi genitali. È stata proposta anche la laserterapia.

LICHEN PLANUS. Il lichen planus vulvare è spesso associato a lesioni mucose orali e sottocutanee. Le lesioni vulvari sono caratterizzate da papule appiattite, violacee, angolari e possono simulare la leucoplachia. Le lesioni orali sono invece costituite da papule bianche minute che formano un aspetto merlettato e di solito sono localizzate nella mucosa buccale. Le lesioni sono intensamente pruriginose e possono diventare escoriate e macerate; nei casi gravi possono comparire erosioni e ulcerazioni. Per la diagnosi è necessaria la biopsia. La riacutizzazione o la recidiva è comune.

Il trattamento consiste in corticosteroidi intralesionali topici e antistaminici per controllare il prurito. In caso di lichen planus vulvare ipertrofico di lunga data può comparire un carcinoma squamocellulare, per cui sono raccomandabili il follow-up a lungo termine e la valutazione istologica di eventuali alterazioni o aree altrimenti sospette.

LICHEN SIMPLEX CRONICO (NEURODERMATITE). Si tratta di una placca lichenificata, cronica, che provoca prurito. È dovuta a uno sfregamento e un grattamento persistenti della cute vulvare; compaiono escoriazioni e fissurazioni. Le labbra assumono l'aspetto di lesioni edematose, ipertrofiche, bianche. Le alterazioni possono comparire sul monte del pube e sulle grandi labbra e provocano grattamento e infiammazione, instaurando un circolo vizioso. La malattia è rara nei bambini. È raccomandato il trattamento con antistaminici e corticosteroidi topici o intralesionali. Il triamcinolone (5-10 mg/mL) è stato utilizzato per l'iniezione intralesionale.

DERMATITE SEBORROICA. Si presenta sotto forma di chiazze eritematose, oleose, circoscritte, che possono essere riscontrate sul volto, sul cuoio capelluto e sul torace, così come sulle aree intertriginose del corpo. Possono anche esservi associate fissurazioni e infezione secondaria perivulvari; l'infezione secondaria batterica o da candida è piuttosto comune e provoca dolore, prurito, disuria ed emorragia vaginale. Gli episodi acuti vengono trattati preferibilmente con semicupi o con una soluzione topica di acetato di alluminio (soluzione di Burow). Si dovrebbero eliminare i fattori esacerbanti, come gli indumenti aderenti o i calzoni sintetici. In caso di infezione secondaria andrebbero somministrati antibiotici sistemici con un appropriato farmaco antimicotico topico.

DERMATITE ATOPICA (ECZEMA). Interessa il 3% di tutti i bambini. I pazienti si presentano con febbre da fieno e/o asma e in genere hanno una familiarità positiva. La lesione vulvare è caratteristicamente una malattia cronica accompagnata da prurito intenso, eritema, papule e vescicole, con essudazione e formazione di croste nelle aree interessate. Sull'area vulvare si possono associare chiazze squamose lichenificate, circoscritte. Spesso il prurito provoca il grattamento, che porta all'escoriazione delle lesioni. L'infezione secondaria batterica o da candida è comune.

Gli antistaminici sono necessari per il controllo del prurito. I semicupi con sapone leggero e lubrificanti risultano utili e anche i corticosteroidi topici come l'idrocortisone all'1% appaiono efficaci. Le infezioni secondarie batteriche, virali o da candida richiedono un trattamento specifico (vedi Capitolo 144).

DERMATITE. Nella dermatite allergica o irritativa da contatto, la vulva può essere interessata da lesioni edematose, eritematose ed essudative, che talvolta sono accompagnate da vescicole o pustole. La dermatite cronica da contatto è spesso associata a lesioni ispessite e lichenificate. L'indizio per la diagnosi corretta di questa malattia è la limitazione della dermatite all'area di contatto con l'agente eziologico. Può anche sussistere un'infezione secondaria batterica o da candida. Alcuni comuni agenti eziologici sono i saponi, le polveri, le bolle di sapone, i deodoranti femminili spray, i farmaci topici, la carta igienica, la gomma e alcuni tipi di indumenti.

Il trattamento dovrebbe comprendere l'evitare gli agenti implicati, l'uso di semicupi e l'applicazione di garze con soluzione topica di acetato di alluminio (soluzione di Burow) durante gli episodi acuti. I corticosteroidi topici leggeri, come l'idrocortisone 0,5-1% in crema, applicati diverse volte al giorno possono favorire ulteriormente la guarigione e alleviare l'irritazione vulvare. La recidiva si può prevenire con la rimozione dell'agente eziologico responsabile.

FOLLICOLITE. Può insorgere spontaneamente oppure in seguito alla rasatura o ad altri metodi depilatori come la ceretta. Porta alla formazione di un'eruzione papulopustolosa secondaria all'infiammazione del follicolo pilifero. Può comparire in qualunque regione cutanea in cui sono presenti peli. All'esame obiettivo si identificano pustole di dimensioni comprese tra 2 e 10 mm, che possono essere perforate nel centro da un pelo visibile e che vengono in seguito sostituite da papule rosse. L'agente più comune è lo *S. aureus*, ma può verificarsi anche la *Pseudomonas aeruginosa*, associata alla "follicolite da bagno caldo". Il trattamento comprende semicupi e detersione con una soluzione di iodopovidone una o due volte al giorno. Quando le infezioni stafilococciche non rispondono, il trattamento diventa con la clindamicina, una cefalosporina o l'eritromicina.

PSORIASI VULVARE. È frequentemente associata a lesioni in altre parti del corpo ed è caratterizzata da papule o placche violacee con una crosta argentea, aderente, spessa (Fig. 549-3). Le aree intertriginose possono mostrare psoriasi "invertita", una variante che non interessa gli arti. Le lesioni vulvari risultano mal delimitate e possono presentarsi come chiazze squamose, più comunemente sul monte del pube; spesso resistono alla terapia. Si dovrebbe utilizzare una crema a base di corticosteroidi (idrocortisone 1%), in associazione al controllo dell'infezione secondaria e del prurito.

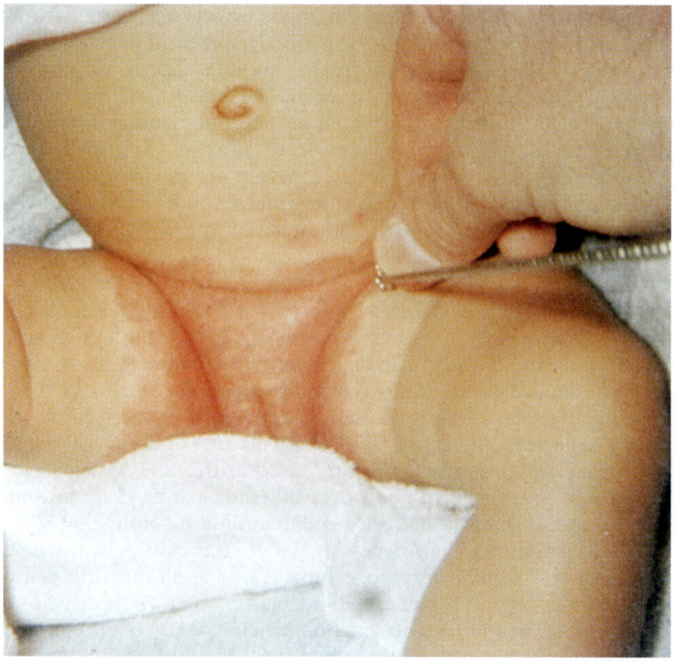

Figura 549-3. Psoriasi vulvare.

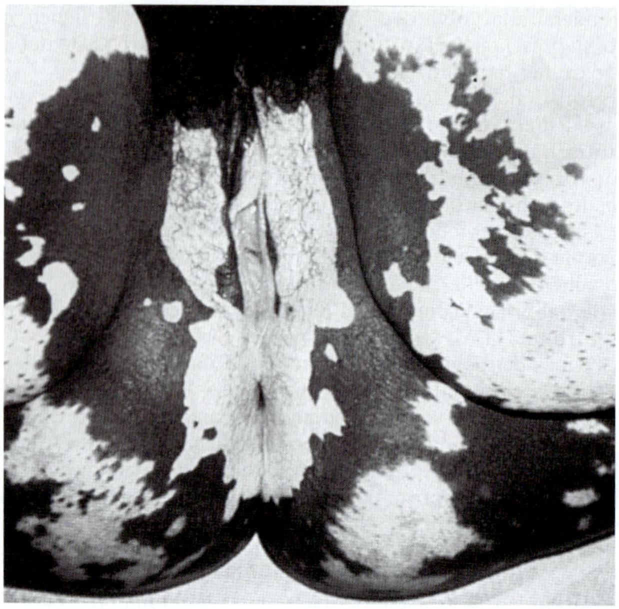

Figura 549-4. Vitiligine.

ENTEROBIASI. Gli ossiuri (*Enterobius vermicularis*) sono elminti che possono trasportare batteri del colon al perineo, provocando una vulvovaginite ricorrente. Quelli di sesso femminile emergono dall'ano e depositano le uova, causando la vulvovaginite in circa il 20% delle donne infettate. Il test del nastro adesivo dovrebbe essere utilizzato per ricercare il microrganismo quando viene sospettato o nei casi di una vulvovaginite ricorrente non diagnosticata. Le pazienti presentano tipicamente prurito ed episodi notturni di grattamento. Il trattamento consiste nel pirantel pantoato (vedi Tab. 549-1).

SHIGELLOSI. La *Shigella flexneri* e la *Shigella sonni* provocano vari sintomi gastrointestinali, in associazione alla vaginite. Il 47% delle pazienti si presenta con perdite vaginali emorragiche e il 2% con diarrea. Gli antibiotici sistemici sono il trattamento di scelta. La colonizzazione dell'intestino da parte della shigella può portare a sintomi gastrointestinali subclinici nel 10% dei membri familiari.

VITILIGINE. Si presenta sotto forma di chiazze ben delimitate di colore da rosa ad avorio, che tendono a diffondersi e a confluire (Fig. 549-4). La cute al di sopra della chiazza è liscia e non mostra alterazioni palpabili. Può essere differenziata dal lichen scleroso perché le chiazze iperpigmentate sono asintomatiche. Non è necessario alcun trattamento a meno che non compaiano problemi estetici.

ULCERE AFTOSE. Le ulcere aftose della regione genitale e quelle della mucosa orale hanno dimensioni comprese tra 1 e 10 mm e presentano un fondo giallo-grigiastro; possono recidivare e durare almeno 7-10 giorni. L'eziologia rimane sconosciuta. Le lesioni della vulva possono essere trattate con corticosteroidi topici e, se necessario, con anestetici topici.

REAZIONI A FARMACI ASSOCIATE A LESIONI VULVARI. L'eritema multiforme si può presentare con ulcere genitali che accompagnano lesioni dei palmi delle mani, delle piante dei piedi e di altre parti del corpo, che di solito persistono per circa 1 settimana e che possono rappresentare una reazione allergica a un farmaco oppure precedere l'eruzione dell'herpes simplex.

SINDROME DI STEVENS-JOHNSON. Si tratta di una variante dell'eritema multiforme, con un interessamento più grave delle membrane mucose. Tra i farmaci che provocano questa sindrome vi sono gli antinfiammatori non steroidei, i sulfamidici e alcuni anticonvulsivanti. Anche il *Mycoplasma pneumoniae* può causarla. In generale, il periodo prodromico è di 1-14 giorni ed è caratterizzato da febbre, cefalea, mal di gola e malessere. Possono essere presenti vomito e diarrea. La mucosa orale e gli occhi possono venire colpiti simultaneamente (vedi Capitolo 653).

NECROLISI EPIDERMICA TOSSICA. Queste lesioni sono secondarie a numerosi farmaci; il 20-30% dei pazienti muore. La cute sembra ustionata; l'erosione e l'ulcerazione vulvare possono essere estese. Le sinechie e l'atrofia vulvari risultanti possono provocare dispareunia.

IPERTROFIA LABIALE. L'ipertrofia delle piccole labbra è rara, ma può essere monolaterale o bilaterale. Occasionalmente è sintomatica, con la paziente che lamenta irritazione o fastidio quando cammina, quando va in bicicletta o in moto o durante il rapporto sessuale. Nella paziente asintomatica il trattamento comprende la rassicurazione, mentre in quella sintomatica il tessuto in eccesso può essere asportato riavvicinando la cute con punti staccati o con una chiusura sottocuticolare. Può essere necessario posizionare un catetere di Foley nel periodo postoperatorio immediato.

MORBO DI CROHN. Si tratta di una malattia granulomatosa non caseosa che interessa il tratto gastrointestinale. Si verificano disturbi ginecologici fin nel 24% delle donne, tra cui l'eritema, l'edema e la successiva formazione di un'ulcera. Le ulcere cutanee della vulva sono a fessura, profonde e multiple. Può comparire un'infezione secondaria. La diagnosi, confermata dalla biopsia, deve essere distinta da altri difetti, come la sarcoidosi, i condilomi acuminati, i condilomi lati e l'idrosadenite suppurativa. Il trattamento del disturbo gastrointestinale con steroidi e antibiotici è l'obiettivo primario della terapia. Le lesioni vulvari vengono trattate con l'applicazione locale di steroidi e antibiotici sistemici per le infezioni secondarie.

MALATTIA DI BEHÇET. Si tratta di una rara malattia cronica multisistemica associata a una vasculite occlusiva; una malattia sistemica multiorgano caratterizzata da ulcere aftose orali o genitali ricorrenti e uveite, vasculite cutanea, sinovite e meningoencefalite. Ulcere genitali compaiono nel 58-78% dei pazienti come lesioni maculari, rosse, dolorose. Il trattamento sintomatico comprende anestetici topici come la lidocaina gel. Gli steroidi intralesionali possono risultare necessari per le ulcere sintomatiche. Nelle forme gravi della malattia il trattamento ha compreso la colchicina o il metotrexato.

Brown MR, Cartwright PC, Snow BW: Common office problems in pediatric urology and gynecology. *Pediatr Clin North Am* 1997;44:1091–1115.
Fisher G, Rogers M: Treatment of childhood vulvar lichen sclerosus with potent topical corticosteroid. *Pediatr Dermatol* 1997;14:235–238.
Fivozinsky KB, Laufer MR: Vulvar disorders in adolescence. A literature review. *J Reprod Med* 1998;43:763–773.
Joishy M, Ashtekar CS, Jain A, et al: Do we need to treat vulvovaginitis in prepubertal girls? *Br Med J* 2005;330:186–188.
Kokotos F: Vulvovaginitis. *Pediatr Rev* 2006;27:116–117.
Koumantakis EE, Hassan EA, Deligeoroglou EK, et al: Vulvovaginitis during childhood and adolescence. *J Pediatr Adolesc Gynecol* 1997;10:39–43.
Leung AK, Robson WL, Tay-Uyboco J: The incidence of labial fusion in children. *J Paediatr Child Health* 1993;29:235–236.
Powell J, Wojnarowska F. Childhood vulvar lichen sclerosus: an increasingly common problem. *J Am Acad Dermatol* 2001;44:803–806.
Quint EH, Smith YR: Vulvar disorders in adolescent patients. *Pediatr Clin North Am* 1999;46:593–606, ix.
Rau F, Muram D: Vulvovaginitis in children. In Sanfilippo JS, Muram D, Dewhurst J, et al. (editors): *Pediatric Adolescent Gynecology,* 2nd ed. Philadelphia, WB Saunders, 2001, p 199.
Ridley C: Dermatologic conditions of the vulva. In Sanfilippo JS, Muram D, Dewhurst J, et al. (editors): *Pediatric Adolescent Gynecology,* 2nd ed. Philadelphia, WB Saunders 2001, p 216.
Schroeder B: Vulvar disorders in adolescents. *Obstet Gynecol Clin North Am* 2000;27:35–48.
Styed TS, Braverman P: Vaginitis in adolescents. *Adolesc Med Clin* 2004; 15:235–251.
Stricker T, Navratil F, Sennhauser FH: Vulvovaginitis in prepubertal girls. *Arch Dis Child* 2003;88:324–326.

Capitolo 550 ■ Emorragia

Joseph S. Sanfilippo

Tra le entità responsabili del sanguinamento vaginale isolato nella paziente pediatrica vi sono l'esposizione a steroidi sessuali esogeni, i corpi estranei, la cistite emorragica, l'ipotiroidismo, la pubertà precoce, le cisti ovariche, i traumi che possono essere associati o meno ad abuso sessuale, il prolasso uretrale, la vulvovaginite, le neoplasie e altre cause meno comuni. Vedi il Capitolo 115 per una discussione sui disturbi mestruali.

CORPO ESTRANEO. Un corpo estraneo è comunemente responsabile del sanguinamento vaginale nelle pazienti pediatriche; la sua presenza può essere suggerita da una perdita di odore sgradevole che si riscontra assieme all'emorragia. Quello più comunemente identificato è costituito da tamponi di carta igienica. La radiografia diretta o l'ecografia della pelvi spesso si rivelano utili. Un corpo estraneo vaginale è stato riscontrato nel 18% delle preadolescenti con un sanguinamento vaginale associato o meno a perdita e nel 50% di quelle in cui il sanguinamento non includeva perdite.

PROLASSO URETRALE. Il sanguinamento vulvare può essere associato a un prolasso uretrale. Questa rara malattia è caratterizzata dal fatto che la mucosa uretrale protrude attraverso il meato e forma una massa vulvare sensibile, separata dalla vagina, che sanguina facilmente. Le pazienti possono avere difficoltà a urinare, a seconda delle dimensioni della massa e che questa ostruisca o meno il meato uretrale. L'entità risponde all'applicazione topica di estrogeni, perché l'uretra distale è sensibile a essi. Spesso il prolasso uretrale sfugge alla diagnosi in presenza di sanguinamento urogenitale.

TRAUMA GENITALE. Sebbene la maggior parte delle lesioni in quest'area sia accidentale, si deve prendere in considerazione la possibilità dell'abuso fisico o sessuale. Le lesioni contusive possono provocare la rottura dei vasi sanguigni sottostanti alla cute perineale. Il sangue che si accumula sotto la cute forma un ematoma, che può presentarsi come una massa rotonda, tesa e dolorabile. La contusione della vulva di solito non richiede alcun trattamento. Spesso un piccolo ematoma vulvare può essere controllato mediante la pressione con un pacchetto di ghiaccio. Possono essere necessari analgesici.

Le lesioni penetranti nell'area vaginale giustificano una ulteriore e attenta valutazione, che comprenda la seria presa in considerazione della possibilità di un abuso sessuale (vedi Capitolo 36). È necessario un esame dettagliato, specialmente in presenza di sanguinamento attivo. Occorre anche considerare la possibilità di un trauma intestinale o della vescica urinaria.

TUMORI GENITALI. In presenza di un sanguinamento vaginale nelle pazienti pediatriche si dovrebbero prendere in considerazione i tumori benigni e maligni della vulva. Un ampio spettro di entità, che va dagli emangiomi capillari a tumori maligni come il rabdomiosarcoma, richiede una diagnosi istologica e un trattamento appropriati. Tra i tumori maligni più comuni vi sono il carcinoma endodermico, che si verifica più spesso nei bambini più piccoli; il carcinoma mesonefrico, che origina dal residuo di un dotto mesonefrico e si riscontra più spesso nelle bambine dai 3 anni in su; e l'adenocarcinoma a cellule chiare, che è spesso associato a un'anamnesi di esposizione prenatale al dietilstilbestrolo.

MALFORMAZIONE VENOSA CAPILLARE DELLE GRANDI LABBRA. La malformazione venosa capillare è stata descritta come una causa del sanguinamento vaginale nelle pazienti pediatriche, con espansione nel volume vaginale in risposta alle alterazioni ormonali della pubertà. La diagnosi differenziale comprende l'emangioma e altre malformazioni vascolari. La diagnosi si basa su una valutazione che includa l'ecografia, la RM e l'arteriografia addominale. La malformazione può essere asportata localmente.

Anveden-Hertzberg L, Gauderer MW, Elder JS: Urethral prolapse: An often misdiagnosed cause of urogenital bleeding in girls. *Pediatr Emerg Care* 1995;11:212–214.
Hickey M, Balen A: Menstrual disorders in adolescence: investigation and management. *Hum Reprod Update* 2003;9:493–504.
Imai A, Horibe S, Tamaya T: Genital bleeding in premenarcheal children. *Int J Gynaecol Obstet* 1995;49:41–45.
Kanbur N, Derman O, Kutluk T, et al: Coagulation disorders as the cause of menorrhagia in adolescents. *J Adolesc Med Health* 2004;16:183–185.
Kempinaire A, De Raeve L, Roseeuw D, et al: Capillary-venous malformation in the labia majora of a 12-year-old girl. *Dermatology* 1997;194:405–407.
Lavin C: Dysfunctional uterine bleeding in adolescents. *Curr Opin Pediatr* 1996;8:328–332.
Minjarez D: Abnormal bleeding in adolescents. *Semin Reprod Med* 2003;21:363–373.
Strickland JL, Wall J: Abnormal uterine bleeding in adolescents. *Obstet Gynecol Clin North Am* 2003;30:321–335.
Strickland JL: Management of abnormal bleeding in adolescents. *Mo Med* 2004;101:38–41.
Templeman C, Hertweck SP, Muram D, et al: Vaginal bleeding in childhood and menstrual disorders in adolescence. In Sanfilippo JS, Muram D, Dewhurst J, et al. (editors): *Pediatric and Adolescent Gynecology,* 2nd ed. Philadelphia, WB Saunders, 2001, pp 237–247.

Capitolo 551 ■ Malattie della mammella

Joseph S. Sanfilippo

Iniziando a circa 6 settimane di gestazione, le cellule epidermiche migrano al mesenchima e formano le creste mammarie. Alla fine si formano le gemme mammarie, i dotti lattiferi e le ghiandole mammarie pienamente sviluppate. Lo sviluppo mammario normalmente ha luogo nel sesso femminile tra gli 8,5 e i 13 anni di vita. La velocità della crescita è variabile e la formazione risulta spesso asimmetrica. Lo sviluppo può non completarsi finché la donna non ha raggiunto i 20 anni.

AUTOESAME DELLE MAMMELLE. La diagnosi precoce è fondamentale per migliorare la terapia delle anomalie mammarie, tra cui il carcinoma. Sebbene vi siano controversie, le istruzioni all'autoesame delle mammelle vanno prese in considerazione nelle adolescenti (Tab. 551-1). Questo autoesame è comunque indicato specialmente nelle ragazze a partire dall'età di 20 anni, quando sono positive per i geni *BRCA1* e/o *BRCA2*.

ANOMALIE CONGENITE. L'assenza completa della mammella, o amastia, è rara; essa è solitamente unilaterale e spesso associata ad altre anomalie come la sindrome di Poland (aplasia dei muscoli pettorali, deformità delle coste, dita palmate e aplasia del nervo radiale). L'amastia può essere iatrogena, a seguito dell'accidentale asportazione di una gemma mammaria. L'atelia consiste invece nell'assenza di uno o di entrambi i capezzoli. Anche tale anomalia è rara e può non trovarsi associata a un'assenza del tessuto mammario. Entrambe richiedono la correzione chirurgica.

Le mammelle soprannumerarie (polimastia) e i capezzoli soprannumerari (politelia) sono relativamente comuni (Fig. 551-1); tali strutture compaiono lungo le linee del latte e di solito sono asintomatiche. Esiste un'associazione tra la politelia e alcune anomalie dell'apparato urinario e cardiovascolare. In generale, l'asportazione chirurgica delle mammelle o dei capezzoli in soprannumero non è necessaria, ma se diventano sintomatici può essere indicata.

L'ipoplasia delle mammelle è di grado variabile, andando da un'assenza quasi totale di tessuto mammario a mammelle ben formate che vengono tuttavia considerate troppo piccole dalla paziente. Esistono tre cause generali di sviluppo scarso o assente: (1) l'inizio può essere ritardato e le mammelle si formano lentamente, ma sono normali per quanto riguarda tutti gli altri aspetti; (2) l'anamnesi familiare della paziente può comprendere uno sviluppo tardivo; (3) la funzione ovarica può essere inefficace o soppressa. Il trattamento dipende dalla causa sottostante.

L'atrofia è osservata occasionalmente nelle adolescenti ed è quasi costantemente secondaria ad alterazioni alimentari come quelle che si verificano in caso di anoressia nervosa. La correzione del disturbo sottostante permette di ripristinare il tessuto mammario.

TABELLA 551-1. Come effettuare l'autoesame delle mammelle

1. Sdraiarsi. Per spianare la mammella destra collocare un cuscino al di sotto della spalla destra. Se le mammelle sono voluminose, usare la mano destra per tenere la mammella destra mentre questa viene palpata con la sinistra.
2. Usare i cuscinetti sensibili delle tre dita centrali della mano sinistra. Cercare eventuali noduli con un movimento di sfregamento.
3. Esercitare una certa pressione per percepire le differenze nel tessuto mammario.
4. Palpare completamente tutta la mammella e l'area del torace per comprendere il tessuto mammario che si estende verso la spalla. Dedicare un tempo sufficiente per effettuare l'esame in modo completo. Nelle donne con mammelle piccole sono necessari almeno 2 minuti per esaminare ciascuna mammella. Le mammelle più voluminose richiedono più tempo.
5. Utilizzare la stessa modalità per palpare ogni parte del tessuto mammario. Scegliere il metodo che si ritiene più comodo. I tre metodi preferiti dalle donne e dai loro medici sono quello circolare, a orologio o ovale; verticale; a cuneo.
6. Dopo avere esaminato completamente la mammella destra, esaminare la sinistra utilizzando lo stesso metodo. Confrontare ciò che si è palpato in una mammella con l'altra.
7. Si possono esaminare anche le mammelle durante il bagno, quando la pelle è umida e può essere più facile palpare i noduli.
8. Si possono controllare le mammelle allo specchio; osservare eventuali alterazioni delle dimensioni o del profilo, fossette sulla cute o secrezioni spontanee dal capezzolo.

Riprodotta per gentile concessione dell'American Cancer Society.

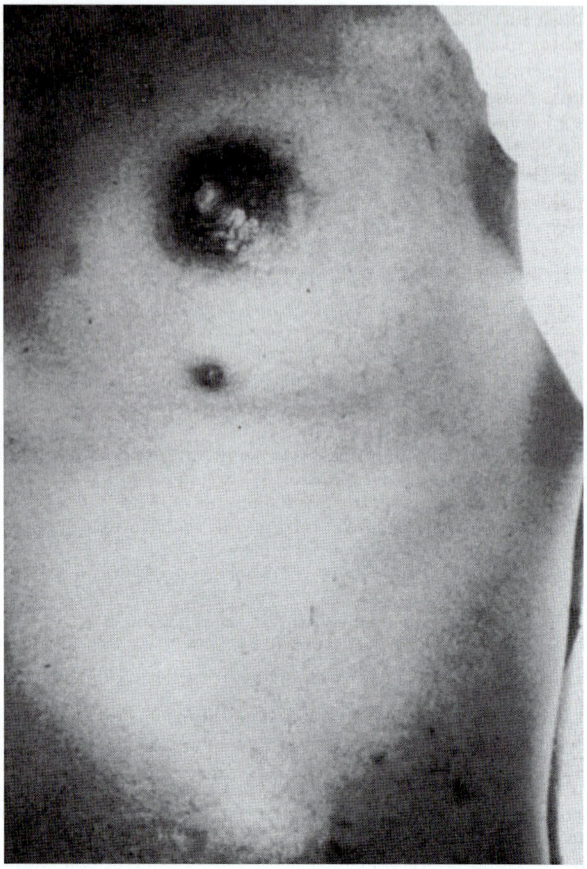

Figura 551-1. Politelia.

ANOMALIE MAMMARIE NEONATALI. L'ipertrofia mammaria bilaterale può insorgere in seguito all'aumento degli ormoni steroidi materni endogeni circolanti nell'ultimo periodo della gestazione. Essa può essere associata a perdite dai capezzoli note come "latte della strega". La ripetuta manipolazione della mammella può riacutizzare la malattia. Talvolta l'ipertrofia si trova associata a una mastite causata da una infezione stafilococcica o streptococcica; andrebbero somministrati antibiotici.

MASTODINIA. L'ingorgo mammario doloroso (mastodinia) è solitamente associato ai cicli ovulatori; è raro nelle adolescenti fino a circa 18 mesi dopo il menarca, ossia il tempo che può essere necessario per la stabilizzazione dei cicli. Frequentemente il dolore mammario si presenta in maniera ciclica. Gli analgesici come i farmaci antinfiammatori non steroidei, tra cui l'ibuprofene, e l'uso di un reggiseno di adeguato sostegno sono spesso utili per alleviare il disagio.

MASSE MAMMARIE. Un'indagine retrospettiva sulla malattia mammaria nelle adolescenti ha evidenziato che circa il 54% di esse ha fibroadenomi e il 13% un'ipertrofia verginale. La malattia mammaria fibrocistica o proliferativa si verifica in circa il 24%. Il rabdomiosarcoma primario, il rabdomiosarcoma metastatico, il neuroblastoma metastatico e il linfoma non-Hodgkin compaiono nel 2-3% di tutti i casi di masse mammarie in questo gruppo di età. Tra le altre diagnosi vi sono la politelia, il tessuto mammario accessorio, la mastite, l'emangioma, la necrosi adiposa e i linfonodi intramammari. Le masse mammarie durante l'adolescenza possono essere dovute a diverse cause:

- fibroadenoma
- malattia fibrocistica
- cisti mammaria
- ascesso/mastite
- papilloma intraduttale
- necrosi adiposa/lipoma
- cistosarcoma filloide
- iperplasia adenomatosa
- lesioni rare (emangiomi, linfangiomi, linfoma)
- tessuto mammario normale
- tumore

Un'anamnesi e un esame obiettivo esaustivi sono raccomandati per ogni paziente pediatrica o adolescente che presenti una massa mammaria. Il disturbo clinico dovrebbe essere esaminato con un radiologo prima di intraprendere ogni valutazione radiologica. L'agoaspirato e l'agobiopsia risultano spesso fondamentali per l'apprezzamento delle anomalie mammarie palpabili. In età adolescenziale possono comparire anche tumori di grosse dimensioni. Sebbene spesso si sospetti un tumore maligno a causa della rapida crescita della massa e dell'ulcerazione cutanea, l'incidenza è comunque molto bassa. I tumori mammari possono manifestarsi in varie modalità. Il fibroadenoma gigante nell'adolescenza può essere trattato mediante l'enucleazione semplice.

TUMORI MALIGNI. Sebbene rari, <1% di essi si verifica in donne di età inferiore ai 30 anni e il tumore della mammella colpisce le adolescenti. Il menarca precoce, in associazione a cicli anovulatori, è un fattore di rischio. Il rapporto estrogeni/androgeni sembra essere critico e gli androgeni hanno un effetto protettivo.

Il *cistosarcoma filloide*, un raro tumore mammario negli adulti, può comparire nell'adolescenza. È caratterizzato da un ingrandimento mammario asimmetrico accompagnato da una massa circoscritta, solida e mobile. Può simulare un fibroadenoma gigante. Spesso il tumore aumenta rapidamente di dimensioni e può diventare piuttosto voluminoso. La sua fissazione alla cute o alla parete toracica è rara. La maggior parte di questi tumori è benigna, ma sono stati riportati cistosarcomi filloidi maligni con metastasi. L'asportazione è la terapia iniziale preferita nelle adolescenti, indipendentemente dalla classificazione istologica della lesione. Il *cistosarcoma maligno* ha una maggiore probabilità di recidivare rispetto a una lesione benigna. In un'adolescente è stato riportato un cistosarcoma filloide metastatico fatale.

I tumori mammari possono costituire anche la prima manifestazione di recidiva (extramidollare) nella leucemia linfoblastica acuta. In letteratura è riportato un caso di sarcoma mammario indotto da radiazioni in un'adolescente e un caso di liposarcoma in una ragazza nera di 17 anni che precedentemente era stata sottoposta a mastectomia totale.

MACROMASTIA (IPERTROFIA VERGINALE). La causa dell'ingrandimento mammario massivo durante la pubertà e la prima adolescenza è sconosciuta, ma l'anomalia probabilmente rappresenta un'aumentata sensibilità dell'organo bersaglio agli estrogeni circolanti. È bilaterale, spesso si verifica nel corso di un breve periodo di tempo e più comunemente interessa le ragazze di 13-17 anni. Nelle adolescenti con macromastia possono comparire disturbi fisici e psicologici; spesso avvengono disturbi di postura e disagio. La mastoplastica riduttiva è il trattamento di scelta, ma dovrebbe essere rimandata all'adolescenza tardiva, per consentire un completo sviluppo della mammella. L'intervento chirurgico spesso comporta la rilocalizzazione del capezzolo, che può portare a una sensibilità ridotta e ad alterazioni dell'allattamento. Inoltre, si dovrebbe fornire un intenso supporto emotivo.

MAMMELLE TUBEROSE. Si tratta di una deformità che porta alla formazione di mammelle che ricordano una pianta a radice tuberosa. Può fare seguito all'uso di steroidi esogeni, specialmente con l'induzione dello sviluppo puberale. L'intervento chirurgico è necessario per la correzione.

MASTITE E ASCESSO. Per la mastite e l'ascesso mammario possono essere necessari l'antibioticoterapia così come l'incisione e il drenaggio. Si stima che la mastite si verifichi frequentemente dopo un piercing mammario, con tassi di infezione stimati del 10-20%. È inoltre comune nel periodo postpartum.

TRAUMI E INFIAMMAZIONI. I traumi mammari nelle adolescenti sono diventati più comuni, a causa del maggiore numero di donne giovani che partecipano a sport di contatto. Di solito il trauma comporta una contusione o un ematoma e si risolve con alterazioni cistiche tardive o fibrosi con retrazione della cute o del capezzolo al di sopra dell'area lesionata. Queste alterazioni tardive possono simulare quelle associate ai tumori maligni; la biopsia può essere l'unico metodo per differenziare le due situazioni.

DISPLASIA MAMMARIA. Si tratta di una lesione comune caratterizzata da alterazioni associate al ciclo mestruale. Lo squilibrio ormonale può causare risposte esagerate nel tessuto mammario, specialmente nei quadranti superiore ed esterno durante la fase premestruale del ciclo. L'estensione del trattamento dipende dal grado dei sintomi; spesso è utile l'ibuprofene. Inoltre, andrebbero eliminate le metilxantine e la caffeina (caffè, tè, bevande con aggiunta di carbonati) dalla dieta.

PERDITE DAL CAPEZZOLO. Queste perdite devono essere valutate attentamente, distinguendo tra la presenza di galattorrea (fuoriuscita spontanea di latte), sangue o altre secrezioni (Tab. 551-2). La valutazione della galattorrea nei bambini è simile a quella per gli adulti. I livelli di prolattina vengono dosati per escludere un prolattinoma ipofisario. Se si sospetta un tumore o un adenoma ipofisario in base a elevati livelli sierici di prolattina, è necessario procedere agli appropriati accertamenti radiologici (TC, RM). Un'altra causa di galattorrea è l'ipotiroidismo in associazione ad alti livelli di ormone tireostimolante, che stimola inoltre il rilascio di prolattina. Anche i farmaci possono provocare galattorrea (Tab. 551-3). Il trattamento della galattorrea (non correlata alla tiroide) si basa primariamente sui dopaminoagonisti come la bromocriptina o la cabergolina. L'intervento chirurgico, di solito

TABELLA 551-2. Diagnosi differenziale delle perdite dal capezzolo

TIPO	DIAGNOSI DIFFERENZIALE (IN ORDINE DI FREQUENZA)
Lattea	Galattorrea
Multicolore/viscosa	Ectasia duttale
Purulenta	Mastite
Acquosa	Papilloma Carcinoma
Sierosa/sieroematica	Papilloma intraduttale Alterazioni fibrocistiche Carcinoma Ectasia duttale

Da Neinstein LS: Breast masses in adolescents. *Adolesc Pediatr Gynecol* 1994;7:119.

TABELLA 551-3. Farmaci che causano galattorrea

Aloperidolo	Domperidone	Narcotici
Amfetamine	Estrogeni	Prostaglandine
Amitriptilina	Flufenazina	Reserpina
Androgeni	Inibitori della monoamino ossidasi	Sulpiride
Anestetici	Meprobamato	Trifluoperazina
Cimetidina	Metildopa	
Clorpromazina	Metoclopramide	

Adattata da Yazigi RA, Quintero CH, Salameh WA: Prolactin disorders. *Fertil Steril* 1997;67:215-225, riprodotta per gentile concessione dell'American Society for Reproductive Medicine.

l'ipofisectomia transfenoidale, è raramente necessario. È stata riportata anche una galattorrea secondaria a un intervento chirurgico della parete toracica in un'adolescente, che si verificò per 2 mesi in associazione a un'amenorrea transitoria.

La secrezione ematica dal capezzolo può essere indicativa di ectasia duttale. Sono necessarie la valutazione citologica e la consulenza chirurgica. Sono state riportate anche perdite dal capezzolo in associazione ai tubercoli di Montgomery. Queste secrezioni possono risultare episodiche e presentare un colore variabile da chiaro a marrone, ma di solito non sono lattee. Le perdite evolvono nell'arco di 3-5 settimane, possono associarsi a noduli mammari e costituiscono un disturbo benigno, autolimitato. Papillomi mammari intraduttali sono stati descritti nelle adolescenti.

ASIMMETRIA MAMMARIA. A partire dall'età neonatale, lo sviluppo mammario può essere unilaterale. Nelle adolescenti, non è raro per circa il 25% delle pazienti che sussista un elemento di asimmetria mammaria, che persiste dopo i 18 anni. L'asimmetria è comune specialmente negli stadi di Tanner 2 e 4.

Dufos C, Plo-Bureau G, Thibaud E, et al: Breast diseases in adolescents. *Endocr Dev* 2004;7:183–196.
Faden H: Mastitis in children from birth to 17 years. *Pediatr Infect Dis J* 2005;24:1113.
Jacobs VR, Golombeck K, Jonat W, et al: Mastitis nonpuerperalis after nipple piercing: Time to act. *J Fertil Womens Med* 2003;48:226–231.
Michels KB, Willett WC: Breast cancer—early life matters. *N Engl J Med* 2004;351:1679–1681.
Neinstein L: Breast disease in adolescents and young women. *Pediatr Clin North Am* 1999;46:607–629.
Ogletree RJ, Hammig B, Drolet JC, et al: Knowledge and intentions of ninth-grade girls after a breast self examination program. *J Sch Health* 2004;74:365–369.
Quint E, Simmons P: Breast masses in a teenage patient: *J Pediatr Adolesc Gynecol* 2001;14:47–48.
Shannon C, Smith IE: Breast cancer in adolescents and young women. *Eur J Cancer* 2003;39:2632–2642.
Templeman C, Hertweck SP: Breast disorders in the pediatric and adolescent patient. *Obstet Gynecol Clin North Am* 2000;27:19–34.

TABELLA 552-1. Cause di irsutismo

PERIFERICHE
Idiopatico
Insensibilità parziale agli androgeni (deficit di 5α-reduttasi)
Sindrome HAIR-AN (*Hirsutism, Androgenization, Insulin Resistance, and Acanthosis Nigricans*; irsutismo, androgenizzazione, insulinoresistenza e acanthosis nigricans)
Iperprolattinemia
OVARICHE
Sindrome dell'ovaio policistico (ovaie policistiche, anovulazione cronica)
Neoplasia ovarica (cellula di Sertoli-Leydig, cellule della granulosa, tecoma, ginandroblastoma, cellule lipoidi, luteoma, ipernefroma, tumore di Brenner)
Disgenesia ovarica (mosaicismo di Turner con antigene XY o H-Y positivo)
SURRENALICHE
Sindrome di Cushing
Iper-responsività surrenalica
Iperplasia surrenalica congenita (classica, criptica, a esordio adulto)
Deficit di 21-idrossilasi
Deficit di 11-idrossilasi
Deficit di 3β-idrossisteroide
Deficit di 17α-idrossilasi
Neoplasia surrenalica (adenoma carcinoma corticale)
ESOGENE
Minoxidil
Fenitoina
Ciclosporina
Steroidi anabolizzanti
Acetazolamide
Penicillamina
Contraccettivi orali con progestinici androgeni
Danazolo
Psoraleni
Idroclorotiazide
Fenotiazine
ANOMALIE CONGENITE
Trisomia 18 (sindrome di Edwards)
Sindrome di Cornelia de Lange
Sindrome di Hurler
Ipotiroidismo giovanile

Adattata da Bailey-Pridham DD, Sanfilippo JS: Hirsutism in the adolescent female. *Pediatr Clin North Am* 1989;36:581-599.

Capitolo 552 ■ Irsutismo e sindrome dell'ovaio policistico Joseph S. Sanfilippo

L'**irsutismo** (eccessiva crescita pilifera) deve essere distinto dalla virilizzazione, che oltre all'aumento dei peli corporei comporta anche l'acne, l'approfondimento della voce, la modificazione dell'habitus corporeo dovuta alla crescita della massa muscolare e la clitoromegalia. Il pubarca prematuro è definito come la comparsa dei peli genitali e/o ascellari prima dell'età di 8 anni. L'adrenarca, ossia l'aumentata produzione di androgeni dalle ghiandole surrenali, di solito si verifica tra i 12 e i 18 anni ed è discusso nel Capitolo 575.3.

Si ritiene che la **sindrome dell'ovaio policistico** (POC, *Polycystic Ovarian Syndrome*) abbia le sue origini nella pubertà. Di solito le adolescenti si presentano con disturbi mestruali associati o meno a irsutismo (Tab. 552-1). Tra le altre caratteristiche vi sono un'acne grave, la perdita dei capelli e l'obesità. Le donne adulte possono essere infertili e hanno un rischio aumentato di diabete mellito di tipo 2 e di complicanze cardiovascolari. Spesso la valutazione ecografica identifica ovaie multicistiche, con un caratteristico aspetto "a collana di perle". La prevalenza delle ovaie policistiche aumenta durante tutta la pubertà e può arrivare al 26% entro l'età di 15 anni.

La PCOS (*Polycystic ovaries, Chronic anovulation, and Stein-Leventhal syndrome*, ovaie policistiche, anovulazione cronica e sindrome di Stein-Leventhal) è la causa ovarica di irsutismo più comunemente diagnosticata; è controverso se il difetto di base sia centrale (regolazione ipotalamica o ipofisaria delle gonadotropine), ovarico (deficit di un ormone peptidico, probabilmente l'inibina, con conseguente anomalo feedback all'ipofisi) o l'insulinoresistenza. Il quadro ormonale abituale della PCOS inizia con il rilascio alterato di ormone luteinizzante (LH, *Luteinizing Hormone*) (un rapporto tra esso e l'ormone follicolo-stimolante di 2:1 o 3:1, una riduzione della frequenza pulsata e un lieve aumento dell'ampiezza pulsatile dell'LH); inoltre, si osservano maggiori livelli circolanti di testosterone e androstenedione. Le adolescenti con iperandrogenismo mostrano una pulsatilità esagerata dell'LH, simile a quella riscontrata nelle donne adulte con la PCOS. L'incidenza di quest'ultima nelle donne di età compresa tra 18 e 25 anni è dell'8-26%, a seconda dei criteri diagnostici, tra i quali compaiono l'oligomenorrea, livelli clinici e/o sierici indicativi di iperandrogenismo e segni ecografici di follicoli multipli (di diametro 9-10 mm).

L'anamnesi familiare è importante, perché la PCOS è più comune nei parenti di primo grado delle donne con questa malattia. Le indagini dovrebbero comprendere: gli androgeni sierici (testosterone, androstenedione e deidroepiandrosterone), l'ormone tireostimolante, la tiroxina, la prolattina, la glicemia e l'insulina a digiuno e il 17-idrossiprogesterone (17OHP).

Le pazienti con la PCOS dovrebbero essere distinte da quelle con l'AOCAH (*Adult-Onset Congenital Adrenal Hyperplasia*, iperplasia surrenalica congenita a esordio nell'adulto), che presentano livelli estremamente elevati di 17OHP a digiuno (vedi oltre).

La PCOS è associata a una resistenza periferica all'insulina e a elevati livelli dell'LH, con un conseguente aumento della produzione ovarica di androgeni. L'iperinsulinemia è associata a una maggiore biodisponibilità del fattore di crescita insulino simile-1 (IGF-1, *Insulin-like Growth Factor-1*) e a una depressione della produzione di IGF-1 carrier protein (IGFBP-1). Anche l'attivazione del recettore dell'IGF-1 può essere coinvolta nell'aumento della produzione di androgeni. La conversione periferica dell'androstenedione ovarico in testosterone contribuisce all'incremento comunemente identificato dei livelli di testosterone totale, che fanno parte integrante del quadro ormonale della PCOS. Oltre allo stato iperinsulinemico, queste pazienti hanno elevati rischi cardiovascolari a lungo termine d'ipertensione e coronaropatia e spesso presentano anche un aumento dei livelli totali di trigliceridi.

L'insulinoresistenza fa parte integrante della **sindrome HAIR-AN**, nella quale si verificano la mutazione del recettore dell'insulina, così come la presenza di anticorpi circolanti diretti contro di esso e difetti postrecettoriali. I difetti del trasporto di glucosio, nonché elevati livelli di insulina stimolano l'attività del citocromo P450c 17β, un enzima attivamente coinvolto nella produzione di androgeni da parte dell'ovaio. Nella PCOS vi è anche un'alterata regolazione del sistema enzimatico del citocromo P450c 17β.

L'irsutismo nell'adolescenza può anche essere dovuto a una forma eterozigote del deficit di 21-idrossilasi, denominata AOCAH. Diverse altre forme di iperplasia surrenalica congenita e anomalie congenite si trovano inoltre associate all'irsutismo. Dal punto di vista clinico, può essere difficile distinguere tra la PCOS e l'AOCAH.

L'**ipertricosi ovarica**, che può essere familiare, è una variante della PCOS e viene definita come la presenza di isole separate di cellule luteinizzate all'interno dell'ovaio che contribuiscono all'aumentata produzione di androgeni. La produzione di androgeni ovarici e i suoi effetti periferici sono simili a quelli associati alla PCOS.

Anche i farmaci, l'irradiazione e l'irritazione cronica (posizionamento di un gesso) possono dare origine a una crescita pilifera localizzata, non endocrinologica.

TRATTAMENTO DELLE PAZIENTI CON IRSUTISMO. Il migliore trattamento per l'irsutismo secondario a iperprolattinemia è costituito dalla bromocriptina. Nelle pazienti con ovaie multicistiche (policistiche) e ipotiroidismo primario, la policistosi ovarica si risolve rapidamente con adeguate dosi di terapia sostitutiva tiroidea. Se l'irsutismo è generato da una causa esogena, come un farmaco, tale agente andrebbe eliminato. Anche quando il più elevato effetto androgeno tissutale risulta invertito dal trattamento appropriato, i follicoli piliferi convertiti in follicoli terminali possono ancora produrre quel tipo di peli. L'elettrolisi può fornire un migliore aspetto estetico, con la garanzia che, se l'anomalia sottostante viene controllata, non si dovrebbe verificare alcuna crescita di nuovi peli. La sindrome o la malattia di Cushing, i tumori producenti androgeni e l'iperplasia surrenalica congenita sono discussi nei Capitoli 577 e 578. La metformina, una sostanza insulino-sensibilizzante, è raccomandata per le pazienti iperinsulinemiche con PCOS. L'obiettivo è di avere livelli circolanti d'insulina più efficaci, insieme a una riduzione dell'LH e del testosterone sierici con la PCOS, entro 4-8 settimane. È essenziale

TABELLA 552-2. Trattamenti farmacologici*

SOSTANZA	MECCANISMO D'AZIONE	VANTAGGI E SVANTAGGI	ESEMPI	UTILIZZI: IRSUTISMO, ACNE	UTILIZZI: OLIGOMENORREA O AMENORREA	UTILIZZI: INDUZIONE DELL'OVULAZIONE	UTILIZZI: RIDUZIONE DELL'INSULINA
Combinazioni di estrogeni e progestinici	Aumentano la SHBG, sopprimono l'LH e l'FSH, sopprimono la produzione ovarica di androgeni; il progestinico può agire da antiandrogeno	Esposizione ciclica dell'endometrio a estrogeni e progestinici; efficaci per l'irsutismo e per l'acne; possono aumentare il rischio di trombosi e anomalie metaboliche; effetti antiandrogeni vantaggiosi del drospirenone	Etinilestradiolo e norgestimato; etinilestradiolo e desogestrel; etinilestradiolo e drospirenone	X	X		
Antiandrogeni	Inibiscono il legame degli androgeni al recettore per gli androgeni	Efficaci per l'irsutismo e l'acne; rischio di iperkaliemia (spironolattone) o di epatite (flutamide)	Ciproterone acetato, spironolattone, flutamide	X			
Glucocorticoidi	Sopprimono la corticotropina e quindi la produzione surrenalica di androgeni	Attenuano la componente surrenalica dell'eccesso di androgeni; rischi a lungo termine di intolleranza al glucosio, insulinoresistenza, osteopenia, aumento ponderale	Prednisone, desametasone	X	X	X	
Inibitori della 5α-reduttasi	Inibiscono la 5α-reduttasi	Non sono mirati in modo specifico all'isoenzima della 5α-reduttasi nell'unità pilosebacea	Finasteride	X			
Inibitori dell'ornitina decarbossilasi	Inibiscono l'ornitina decarbossilasi	Minima efficacia documentata; utilizzati topicamente	Eflornitina idrocloruro	X			
Antiestrogeno	Induce l'aumento di FSH, LH	Moderatamente efficace in monoterapia, meno efficace nei pazienti obesi; può essere utile in associazione a terapie insulinoriducenti	Clomifene citrato			X	
Biguanide	Diminuisce la produzione epatica di glucosio, riducendo secondariamente i livelli di insulina; può avere effetti diretti sulla steroidogenesi ovarica	Notevole efficacia nel ristabilire la ciclicità mestruale, meno valido per l'irsutismo; di solito associata a calo ponderale iniziale; può avere effetti indesiderati gastrointestinali	Metformina	X	X	X	X
Tiazolidinedioni	Aumentano l'azione dell'insulina a livello dei tessuti bersaglio (adipocita, muscolo); possono avere effetti diretti sulla steroidogenesi ovarica	Estremamente efficaci nel ridurre i livelli di insulina e androgeni, modesti effetti sull'irsutismo; associati ad aumento ponderale	Pioglitazone	X	X	X	X

*FSH, ormone follicolo-stimolante (*Follicle-Stimulating Hormone*); LH, ormone luteinizzante; SHBG, *Sex Hormone-Binding Globulin*.
Da Ehrmann DA: Polycystic ovary syndrome. *N Engl J Med* 2005; 352: 1223-1236.

che le pazienti trattate siano sottoposte a una preterapia e alla valutazione periodica della funzionalità epatica.

La metformina funziona al meglio con un calo ponderale nei pazienti obesi. Tra le altre terapie vi sono la pillola contraccettiva estrogeno-dominante (non androgenica) oppure, se questa non è ben tollerata, i GNRH agonisti. L'irsutismo è trattato con un antiandrogeno (spironolattone, ciproterone) più un contraccettivo orale (Tab. 552-2).

Tra gli effetti indesiderati a lungo termine della PCOS vi sono l'aumentata incidenza di diabete mellito di tipo 2, l'iperlipidemia e la malattia cardiovascolare.

Cedars M: Polycystic ovarian syndrome: What is it and how should we treat it? *J Pediatr* 2004;144:4–6.

Driscoll D: Polycystic ovarian syndrome in adolescence *Ann N Y Acad Sci* 2003;997:49–55.

Ehrmann DA: Polycystic ovary syndrome. *N Engl J Med* 2005;352:1223–1236.

Elmer KB, George RM: HAIR-AN syndrome: A multisystem challenge. *Am Fam Physician* 2001;15:2385–2390.

Fraser IS, Kovacs G: Current recommendations for the diagnostic evaluation and follow-up of patients presenting with symptomatic polycystic ovary syndrome. *Best Pract Res Clin Obstet Gynaecol* 2004;18:813–823.

Homburg R, Lambalk CB: Polycystic ovary syndrome in adolescence—a therapeutic conundrum. *Hum Reprod* 2004;19:1039–1042.

Legro R: Detection of insulin resistance and its prognosis in adolescent polycystic ovarian syndrome. *J Pediatr Endocrinol Metab* 2002;15 Suppl 5:1367–1378.

Mulchahey K: In support of metformin use in adolescent polycystic ovarian syndrome. *J Pediatr Adolesc Gynecol* 2002;15:109–111.

Ploufee L Jr: Disorders of excessive hair growth in the adolescent. *Obstet Gynecol Clin North Am* 2000;27:79–99.

Salmi DJ, Zisser HC, Jovanovic L: Screening for and treatment of polycystic ovary syndrome in teenagers. *Exp Biol Med* 2004;229:369–377.

Capitolo 553 ■ Trattamento delle neoplasie e delle anomalie del Pap test

Joseph S. Sanfilippo

La neoplasia ginecologica più comune riscontrata nell'infanzia è di origine ovarica e di solito si presenta sotto forma di una massa addominale. Le neoplasie ovariche costituiscono l'1% di tutte le neoplasie infantili e l'8% di tutti i tumori maligni e addominali è di origine ovarica (vedi Capitolo 503). Inoltre, il 10-30% delle neoplasie ovariche operate durante l'infanzia e l'adolescenza è maligno. Vi sono poi i tumori paraovarici, che sono i secondi in ordine di frequenza, seguiti dalle neoplasie uterine. Anche la vagina e la vulva possono essere sedi di lesione benigna o maligna nell'infanzia, mentre la displasia cervicale può verificarsi nell'adolescenza. Le masse mammarie sono discusse nel Capitolo 551.

La chemioterapia per qualsiasi tumore, specialmente mediante agenti alchilanti (ciclofosfamide, busulfan, clorambucil e mostarda azotata), porta un danno alla cellula germinale nell'ovaio postpuberale, mentre l'ovaio prepuberale, dall'altra parte, è estremamente resistente al danneggiamento chemioterapico delle cellule germinali. L'effetto della terapia contraccettiva orale combinata per proteggere l'ovaio durante la chemioterapia nelle adolescenti rimane controverso.

Le sopravvissute a tumore infantile che sono state precedentemente sottoposte a una irradiazione addominale o ovarica presentano un aumentato tasso di aborti spontanei. Tuttavia, l'incidenza di malformazioni congenite non è più alta rispetto alla popolazione generale. Le pazienti con segni di insufficienza ovarica prematura possono essere candidate alla tecnologia di riproduzione assistita con l'uso di ovociti da donatrice.

OVAIE

CISTI OVARICHE NEONATALI E PEDIATRICHE. La maggior parte delle volte le manifestazioni cliniche dei tumori ovarici sono il dolore e/o una massa addominale. Le cisti ovariche funzionali persistono raramente oltre il periodo neonatale. Nelle adolescenti la neoplasia più comune è il teratoma, che è solitamente benigno, anche se possono verificarsene di maligni. Spesso una calcificazione alla radiografia addominale è il segno caratteristico di un teratoma benigno. Durante l'intervento chirurgico andrebbe esaminato l'ovaio opposto e, in caso di dubbi sull'eventualità di una neoplasia, si dovrebbe ottenere un campione bioptico. Gli adenomi ovarici sono il secondo tumore benigno più comune.

I carcinomi ovarici sono estremamente rari nell'infanzia, responsabili di 1:500 tumori maligni (Tab. 553-1); colpiscono il 4% delle donne. I tumori della cellula germinale sono i più comuni. Le cellule germinali primordiali possono trasformarsi in disgerminoma, teratomi maligni, tumori del seno endodermico, carcinomi embrionali, neoplasie a cellule miste e gonadoblastomi. I teratomi immaturi e i tumori del seno endodermico sono tumori maligni più aggressivi dei disgerminomi e compaiono in una percentuale significativamente più alta di ragazze giovani (età <10 anni). In questo gruppo di età, sono stati riportati tassi di sopravvivenza a 10 anni del 73% per i carcinomi epiteliali, del 44% per i tumori stromali del cordone sessuale, del 73% per i disgerminomi, del 33% per i teratomi maligni, del 39% per i tumori del seno endodermico, del 25% per i carcinomi embrionali, del 30% per altre neoplasie della cellula germinale e del 100% per i gonadoblastomi. Di solito i disgerminomi sono associati alla disgenesia gonadica XY; per la loro diagnosi sono importanti le sonde Y-DNA. Anche i marker tumorali come l'α-fetoproteina (AFP), l'antigene carcinoembrionario e l'antigene CA 125 sono utilizzati per valutare i tumori maligni ovarici (vedi Tabb. 553-1 e 553-2). I tumori della cellula germinale sono associati a positività all'AFP, alla gonadotropina corionica umana (HCG, *Human Chorionic Gonadotropin*) e all'antigene carcinoembrionario.

Il trattamento consiste nell'asportazione chirurgica, seguita dalla chemioterapia postoperatoria; la radioterapia è spesso necessaria. La stadiazione all'inizio della terapia è di massima importanza. In molti casi è indicata una procedura di second-look per decidere sul successivo trattamento di tali neoplasie.

CARCINOMA EMBRIONALE. Questo tumore maligno rappresenta il 6% delle neoplasie ovariche pediatriche e l'8% dei tumori della cellula germinale. La paziente manifesta dolore e distensione addominali in progressivo aumento. Il carcinoma della cellula embrionale è estremamente maligno e l'età media di identificazione è compresa fra 13 e 15 anni. Complessivamente, il 60% delle pazienti presenta segni e sintomi endocrinologici, tra i quali vi possono essere una pseudopubertà precoce, un sanguinamento vaginale anomalo e l'irsutismo. Il carcinoma embrionale produce l'HCG e l'AFP. Il trattamento comporta la salpingo-ooforectomia per la malattia in stadio I.

TABELLA 553-1. Tumori maligni ovarici nelle adolescenti

CELLULA GERMINALE (PIÙ COMUNI)
Disgerminoma
Teratoma immaturo
Tumore del seno endodermico
Coriocarcinoma
Carcinoma embrionale
TUMORI STROMALI DEL CORDONE SESSUALE
Tumore della cellula stromale della granulosa
Tumore della cellula di Sertoli-Leydig
Tumore della cellula lipoide
Ginandroblastoma
TUMORI EPITELIALI

TABELLA 553-2. Marker tumorali nel siero

MARKER	TUMORE ASSOCIATO
CA 125	Tumori epiteliali (specialmente sierosi)
	Teratoma immaturo (raro)
α-fetoproteina	Tumori del seno endodermico
	Carcinomi embrionali
	Tumori misti della cellula germinale
	Teratoma immaturo (raro)
Gonadotropina corionica umana	Coriocarcinoma
	Carcinomi embrionali
	Tumori misti della cellula germinale
	Poliembrioma
Lattato deidrogenasi	Disgerminoma
	Tumori misti della cellula germinale
Estradiolo	Tesomi
	Tumori della cellula della granulosa dell'adulto
Testosterone	Tumori della cellula di Sertoli
	Tumori della cellula di Leydig (dell'ilo)
F9 embrioglicano	Carcinoma embrionale
	Tumore del sacco vitellino
	Coriocarcinoma
	Teratoma immaturo
Inibina	Tumore della cellula della granulosa-teca
Sostanza inibente mülleriana	Tumore della cellula della granulosa-teca

TUMORE DEL SENO ENDODERMICO. Questi tumori sono i più letali di tutti quelli ovarici. L'età media all'esordio è di 19 anni. Il tumore del seno endodermico produce AFP come marker tumorale utile. Sono tumori radiosensibili. Possono essere trattati chirurgicamente se nello stadio I, mediante una salpingo-ooforectomia unilaterale, ma la chemioterapia può essere necessaria indipendentemente dallo stadio.

CORIOCARCINOMA. Il coriocarcinoma primario dell'ovaio è estremamente raro e spesso fatale; lo 0,6% dei tumori della cellula germinale è rappresentato da coriocarcinomi.

TUMORE MISTO DELLA CELLULA GERMINALE. La frequenza dei tumori misti della cellula germinale rispetto a tutte le neoplasie ovariche dell'infanzia è del 4%.

TUMORE STROMALE DEL CORDONE SESSUALE. I tumori stromali del cordone sessuale costituiscono il 5% delle neoplasie ovariche e tra essi il più comune è il tumore della cellula della granulosa. Nella variante giovanile si possono osservare una precocità isosessuale e occasionalmente la virilizzazione. Le caratteristiche istologiche tipiche comprendono un'architettura nodulare, la formazione di follicolo, microcisti, la necrosi cellulare e un'aumentata attività mitotica.

TUMORE DELLA CELLULA DI SERTOLI-LEYDIG. Viene anche definito come tumore stromale del cordone sessuale e rappresenta il 2% dei tumori ovarici pediatrici, benché sia raro nelle ragazze in età prepuberale. La paziente presenta segni di virilizzazione. Il trattamento comprende la salpingo-ooforectomia unilaterale per la malattia in stadio I.

CISTI FOLLICOLARI OVARICHE. Queste cisti si verificano dalla nascita alla pubertà e di solito scompaiono spontaneamente. All'esame ecografico, la cisti si presenta come un'area anecogena, frequentemente con un diametro massimo >20 mm; si osservano anche un edema del parenchima ovarico e un ingrandimento follicolare della zona corticale.

SINDROME DELL'OVAIO POLICISTICO (PCOS). Questa sindrome si presenta con una disfunzione mestruale e con segni e sintomi di un eccesso di androgeni, spesso all'epoca della pubertà. L'irregolarità mestruale può andare dall'amenorrea all'oligomenorrea (vedi Capitolo 552).

CISTI OVARICHE FUNZIONALI ED EMORRAGICHE. Queste cisti costituiscono una parte integrante dello sviluppo follicolare durante il ciclo mestruale, ma occasionalmente una di esse può persistere e aumentare di diametro. Dopo l'ovulazione, viene denominata corpo emorragico. Le cisti sono spesso sintomatiche e vengono meglio valutate all'ecografia. La terapia di attesa per una presunta cisti funzionale è appropriata, con un follow-up ecografico e i contraccettivi orali monofasici possono facilitare la sua soppressione.

TORSIONE OVARICA. La torsione di un annesso è una complicanza che dovrebbe sempre essere presa in considerazione nella diagnosi differenziale dei tumori ovarici o nel dolore addominale in una paziente; è necessario un intervento chirurgico tempestivo. Spesso la torsione si presenta con un dolore addominale penetrante intermittente che, in molti casi, si irradia inferiormente all'arto ipsilaterale. Nell'infanzia si può verificare anche la torsione ovarica bilaterale. Quando viene diagnostica la torsione unilaterale, può essere indicata l'ooforopessi (plicatura) degli annessi controlaterali.

L'incidenza della torsione ovarica in uno studio era del 25% (16 masse ovariche benigne su 63). La diagnosi può essere facilitata dall'ecografia con Color Doppler. La torsione degli annessi spesso può essere valutata e trattata con l'uso degli studi Doppler flow e con la laparoscopia. Di solito la causa sottostante è una cisti o una neoplasia ovarica associata. La ripresa della funzione ovarica dopo la detorsione laparoscopica è stata riportata con l'identificazione del normale sviluppo follicolare all'ecografia, per cui si raccomanda che la torsione degli annessi venga trattata in modo conservativo.

AUTOAMPUTAZIONE DELL'OVAIO. Questa entità si presenta come una piccola massa calcifica che fluttua liberamente associata all'assenza degli annessi. Il soggetto può essere asintomatico e l'ecografia è spesso utile per confermare la diagnosi. Si è ipotizzato che la torsione prenatale o subclinica porti alla necrosi, alla calcificazione e alla separazione degli annessi dal loro peduncolo vascolare.

TUMORI OVARICI GIOVANILI DELLA CELLULA DELLA GRANULOSA. Questi tumori rappresentano l'1-2% di tutti i tumori ovarici. L'età media all'esordio è di 7,6 anni, con un intervallo tra 6 mesi e 17,5 anni. La maggior parte delle pazienti manifesta una distensione addominale e una precocità sessuale. Con l'avvento della chemioterapia multifarmacologica, tra cui gli schemi a base di cisplatino, la prognosi appare sempre più favorevole. Tuttavia, la neurotossicità, in particolare l'ototossicità e la depressione del midollo osseo, costituiscono complicanze gravi.

INSUFFICIENZA OVARICA PREMATURA IN ASSOCIAZIONE A CHEMIOTERAPIA E/O RADIOTERAPIA. L'incidenza dell'insufficienza ovarica prematura è cresciuta con l'aumento della sopravvivenza dei bambini e degli adolescenti con neoplasie. La terapia ormonale sostitutiva in un approccio simile a quello per la menopausa, ossia una terapia sostitutiva degli estrogeni fisiologici con l'aggiunta di progestinici, garantisce lo sviluppo dei caratteri sessuali secondari e la regolarità dei cicli mestruali.

CERVICE

La diffusione della displasia e del carcinoma *in situ* è di 18,8/1000 per l'età di 15-19 anni, mentre quella della neoplasia intraepiteliale cervicale (CIN, *Cervical Intraepithelial Neoplasia*) di qualunque grado, dimostrata alla biopsia, nella popolazione adolescente è di 13,3/1000. Il Sistema di Classificazione di Bethesda del Pap test è largamente utilizzato per la diagnosi (Tab. 553-3).

R 28/10/2011 Caso Cottardi V.

TABELLA 553-3. Classificazione di Bethesda 2001 dei Pap test

TIPO DI CAMPIONE
Indicare se striscio convenzionale (Pap test) o su liquido o altro

ADEGUATEZZA DEL CAMPIONE
Soddisfacente per la valutazione (descrivere la presenza o l'assenza della componente endocervicale/zona di trasformazione e di altri eventuali indicatori di qualità, per esempio sangue parzialmente oscurante, infiammazione)
Non soddisfacente per la valutazione... (specificare il motivo)
  Campione rifiutato/non processato (specificare il motivo)
  Campione processato ed esaminato, ma non soddisfacente per la valutazione di anomalie epiteliali a causa di (specificare il motivo)

CLASSIFICAZIONE GENERALE (FACOLTATIVA)
Negativo per lesioni intraepiteliali o malignità
Anomalie delle cellule epiteliali: vedi "Interpretazione/risultato" (specificare squamoso o ghiandolare come appropriato)
Altro: vedi "Interpretazione/risultato" (per es. cellule endometriali in una donna di 40 anni o più)

ANALISI AUTOMATICA
Se lo striscio è stato esaminato da un dispositivo automatico, specificare il dispositivo e il risultato

TEST ANCILLARI
Fornire una breve descrizione dei metodi del test e riportare il risultato in modo che sia facilmente compreso dal medico

INTERPRETAZIONE/RISULTATO
Negativo per lesioni intraepiteliali o malignità (in assenza di segni cellulari di neoplasia, ciò va specificato nella parte "Classificazione generale" sopra e/o nella sezione "Interpretazione/risultato" del referto, se sono presenti o meno microrganismi o altri reperti aspecifici)
Microrganismi
Trichomonas vaginalis
Microrganismi fungini morfologicamente compatibili con *Candida* spp.
Modificazione della flora suggestiva di vaginosi batterica
Batteri morfologicamente compatibili con *Actinomyces* spp.
Alterazioni cellulari compatibili con virus dell'herpes simplex
Altri reperti aspecifici (referto facoltativo; elenco non esaustivo)
Alterazioni cellulari reattive associate a
  Infiammazione (include la riparazione tipica)
  Radiazione
  Dispositivo contraccettivo intrauterino
Presenza di cellule ghiandolari postisterectomia
Atrofia

ALTRO
Cellule endometriali (in una donna di 40 anni o più)
(Specificare se negativo per lesione squamosa intraepiteliale)

ANOMALIE DELLE CELLULE EPITELIALI
Cellule squamose
Cellule squamose atipiche
  Di significato indeterminato (ASC-US)
  Non si può escludere una lesione intraepiteliale squamosa di alto grado (ASC-H)
  Lesione intraepiteliale squamosa di basso grado che comprende papillomavirus umano/displasia lieve/neoplasia intraepiteliale cervicale 1
  Lesione intraepiteliale squamosa di alto grado che comprende displasia moderata e grave, CIS/neoplasia intraepiteliale cervicale 2 e neoplasia intraepiteliale cervicale 3
  con caratteristiche sospette di invasione (se si sospetta l'invasione)
  Carcinoma squamocellulare
Cellule ghiandolari
Atipiche
  Cellule endocervicali (non altrimenti specificato o specificare nei commenti)
  Cellule endometriali (non altrimenti specificato o specificare nei commenti)
  Cellule ghiandolari (non altrimenti specificato o specificare nei commenti)
Atipiche
  Cellule endocervicali, suggestive di neoplasia
  Cellule ghiandolari, suggestive di neoplasia
Adenocarcinoma endocervicale in situ
Adenocarcinoma
  Endocervicale
  Endometriale
  Extrauterino
  Non altrimenti specificato

ALTRE NEOPLASIE MALIGNE (SPECIFICARE)

NOTE EDUCATIVE E SUGGERIMENTI (FACOLTATIVO)
I suggerimenti dovrebbero essere sintetici e compatibili con le linee guida di follow-up clinico pubblicate dalle organizzazioni professionali (possono essere inclusi riferimenti a pubblicazioni rilevanti)

Da http://www.bethesda2001.cancer.gov/terminology.html.
CIS, carcinoma in situ.

La frequenza globale di risultati anomali del Pap test nella popolazione adolescente è del 3,8 e l'1% di tutti i Pap test anormali è associato alla CIN. L'infezione da papillomavirus (vedi Capitolo 263) e l'alterazione della flora vaginale sono reperti compatibili nei pazienti con la CIN. I risultati anormali del Pap test nelle adolescenti sono correlati a una CIN significativa e dovrebbero essere seguiti in caso di una lesione di basso grado (Fig. 553-1), mentre qualora ci sia una lesione più avanzata (lesione intraepiteliale squamosa di alto grado [ASC-H]), la paziente andrebbe inviata allo specialista per ulteriori approfondimenti. Sembra che il vaccino contro il papillomavirus umano riduca l'incidenza della CIN. Tra le altre anomalie patologiche della cervice vi sono i polipi cervicali e i tumori mesodermici misti: questi ultimi possono rappresentare un sarcoma misto, eterologo o omologo, della cervice uterina.

UTERO (TUMORI BENIGNI E MALIGNI DEL CORPO DELL'UTERO)

L'*adenocarcinoma* del corpo è raro nell'infanzia e nell'adolescenza, ma può presentarsi con il sintomo frequente di un sanguinamento vaginale non associato a precocità sessuale. Il trattamento consiste nell'isterectomia con l'asportazione delle ovaie, seguita da una radioterapia e/o chemioterapia adiuvanti, a seconda dei reperti operatori. I tumori mesodermici misti e i leiomiomi in un'adolescente dovrebbero essere inclusi nella diagnosi differenziale di una massa pelvica. Anche il leiomiosarcoma, sebbene molto raro, è stato osservato in questo gruppo di età; la presentazione è variabile, ma di solito compare un sanguinamento vaginale anomalo.

VAGINA

La cisti del dotto di Gartner (mesonefrico) è una comune anomalia della parete vaginale. Di solito costituisce un reperto accidentale e non necessita di alcuna terapia specifica, ma nelle pazienti sessualmente attive, se si trova associata a dispareunia, l'asportazione può essere necessaria. Le cisti del dotto paramesonefrico (di Müller) spesso diventano sintomatiche al menarca quando la cavità si riempie di sangue mestruale.

Il sarcoma botrioide, un carcinoma vaginale che si verifica primariamente nelle pazienti pediatriche, viene trattato preferibilmente mediante l'asportazione chirurgica, seguita solitamente dalla chemioterapia. Ogni lesione vulvare dubbia dovrebbe essere sottoposta a un esame istologico. Il liposarcoma della vulva è stato riportato in una ragazza di 15 anni ed è stato anche descritto il melanoma maligno della vulva in una paziente di 14 anni.

Calaminus G, Wessalowski R, Harms D, et al: Juvenile granulosa cell-tumors of the ovary in children and adolescents: Results from 33 patients registered in a prospective cooperative study. *Gynecol Oncol* 1997;64:447–452.
Falcone T, Bedaiwy MA: Fertility preservation and pregnancy outcome after malignancy. *Curr Opin Obstet Gynecol* 2005;17:21–26.
Fields KR, Neinstein LS: Uterine myomas in adolescents: Case reports and a review of the literature. *J Pediatr Adolesc Gynecol* 1996;9:195–198.
Guido R: Guidelines for screening and treatment of cervical disease in the adolescent. *J Pediatr Adolesc Gynecol* 2004;17:301–311.
Guido R, Schiffman M, Solomon D, et al, ASCUS LSIL Triage Study (ALTS) Group: Postcolposcopy management strategies for women referred with low-grade squamous intraepithelial lesions or human papillomavirus DNA-positive atypical squamous cells of undetermined significance: A two-year prospective study. *Am J Obstet Gynecol* 2003;188:1401–1405.
Kozlowski K: Ovarian masses. *Adolesc Med* 1999;10:337–350, vii.
Owens K, Honebrink A: Gynecologic care of medically complicated adolescents. *Pediatr Clin North Am* 1999;46:631–642, ix.
Ozcan C, Celik A, Ozok G, et al: Adnexal torsion in children may have a catastrophic sequel: Asynchronous bilateral torsion. *J Pediatr Surg* 2002;37:1617–1620.
Parker-Jones K: Gynecologic issues in pediatric oncology. Clin Obstet Gynecol 1997;40:200–209.
Pienkowski C, Baunin C, Gayrard M, et al: Ovarian masses in adolescent girls. *Endocr Dev* 2004;7:163–182.

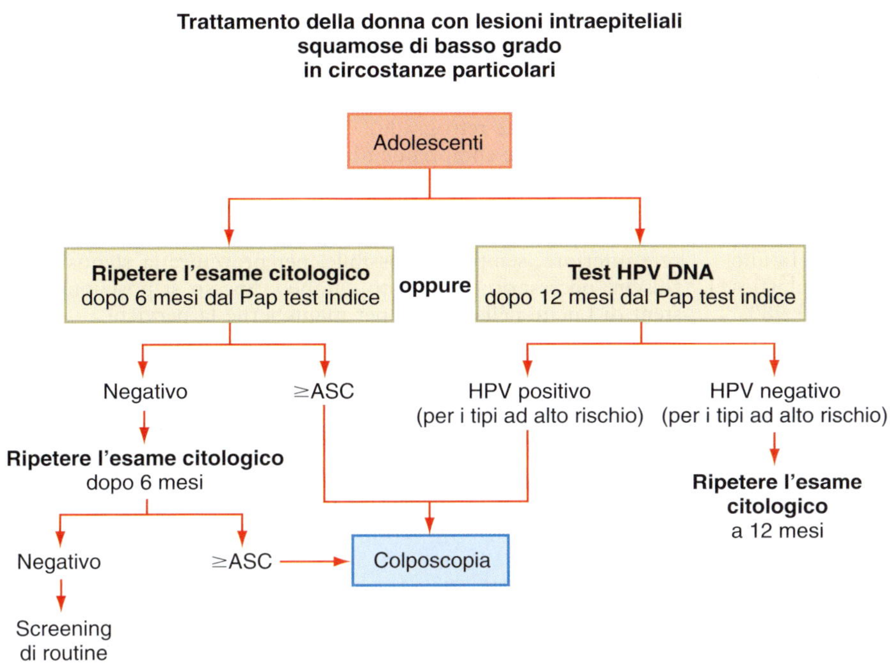

Figura 553-1. Trattamento della lesione intraepiteliale squamosa di basso grado nella paziente adolescente. A causa dell'elevato tasso di papillomavirus umano (HPV, *Human PapillomaVirus*) in questa popolazione e dell'assenza di screening per il tumore cervicale, la colposcopia può essere ritardata. Accettabili alternative a essa sono la ripetizione del Pap test dopo 6 mesi da quello iniziale o un test per l'HPV da solo a distanza di 12 mesi dal Pap test incidente. Se il risultato è normale per 2 Pap test successivi, l'adolescente potrà tornare per lo screening annuale. Si dovrebbe notare che il test per l'HPV eseguito a 12 mesi viene effettuato senza Pap test; la sua aggiunta non aumenta la sensibilità d'identificare una lesione di alto grado, ma aumenta il numero di pazienti in cui è necessaria la colposcopia. Il test per l'HPV viene prorogato a 12 mesi in modo da lasciare un periodo di tempo sufficiente per la risoluzione dell'infezione. (Da Guido R. Guidelines for screening and treatment of cervical disease in the adolescent. *J Pediatr Adolesc Gynecol* 2004;17:303-311. © 2004 The North American Society for Pediatric & Adolescent Gynecology.)

Piippo S, Mustaniemi L, Lenko H, et al: Surgery for ovarian masses during childhood and adolescence: A report of 79 cases. *J Pediatr Adolesc Gynecol* 1999;12:223–227.

Pomeranz A, Sabnis S: Misdiagnosis of ovarian masses in children and adolescents. *Pediatr Emerg Care* 2004;20:172–174.

Capitolo 554 ■ Anomalie vulvovaginali e mülleriane Joseph S. Sanfilippo

EMBRIOLOGIA. L'utero si forma attraverso la fusione degli elementi caudali dei dotti mülleriani, un processo che si verifica a 8 settimane di gestazione. La fusione inizia dall'estremità caudale (tubercolo di Müller) e si completa al livello superiore del fondo. È presente un setto mediano fino alla fine del primo trimestre di gestazione.

La vagina si forma dalla porzione terminale del canale uterovaginale (tubercolo di Müller). Il tessuto origina in modo combinato dal dotto urogenitale e dal dotto di Müller ed è noto come placca epiteliale vaginale. Estroflessioni bilaterali della lamina epiteliale vaginale circondano la porzione caudale del canale uterino. La canalizzazione della lamina vaginale inizia e procede in direzione caudale per formare la vagina. Il processo allunga la struttura vaginale, lasciando che i 2/3 craniali restino di origine mülleriana e l'1/3 caudale di origine urogenitale.

Il sistema paramesonefrico è responsabile dello sviluppo del tratto mülleriano. L'insufficiente fusione laterale o il mancato riassorbimento del setto verticale mediano portano alla comparsa di un'anomalia mülleriana. A causa dell'intimo sviluppo anatomico ed embrionale dei sistemi urinario e genitale, spesso anche le vie urinarie sono interessate; si possono verificare anche difetti dello scheletro, come una spina bifida occulta. Nelle Tabelle 554-1 e 554-2 sono presentate le comuni anomalie del dotto di Müller e le malattie ereditarie associate.

IMENE IMPERFORATO. La paziente si presenta con un'amenorrea primaria; le caratteristiche sessuali secondarie sono normali. Per l'imene imperforato è necessario l'intervento chirurgico. Dopo la risoluzione dell'ostruzione del tratto di efflusso, si dovrebbe valutare il canale vaginale alla ricerca di altri eventuali difetti.

TABELLA 554-1. Comuni anomalie mülleriane

Idrocolpo	Accumulo di muco o di liquido non ematico nella vagina
Emiematometro	Segmento atresico della vagina con accumulo di liquido mestruale
Idrosalpinge	Accumulo di liquido sieroso nella tuba di Falloppio, spesso conseguenza finale della piosalpinge
Utero didelfo	Due cervici, ciascuna delle quali è associata a un corno uterino
Utero bicorne	Una cervice associata a due corni uterini
Utero unicorne	Conseguente alla mancata discesa di uno dei due dotti di Müller

TABELLA 554-2. Malattie ereditarie associate ad anomalie mülleriane

MODALITÀ DI EREDITARIETÀ	MALATTIA	DIFETTO MÜLLERIANO ASSOCIATO
Autosomica dominante	Camptobrachidattilia	Setti vaginali longitudinali
	Mani-piedi-genitali	Incompleta fusione mülleriana
Autosomica recessiva	Kaufan-McCusick	Setti vaginali trasversi
	Johanson-Blizzard	Setti vaginali longitudinali
	Anomalie renali-genitali-orecchio medio	Atresia vaginale
	Sindrome di Fraser	Incompleta fusione mülleriana
	Sindrome dell'ernia uterina	Residui persistenti del dotto di Müller
Poligenica/multifattoriale	Sindrome di Mayer-Rokitansky-Küster-Hauser	Aplasia di Müller
X-linked	Sindrome dell'ernia uterina	Residui persistenti del dotto di Müller

Da Shulman L, Elias S: Developmental abnormalities of the female reproductive tract: Pathogenesis and nosology. *Adolesc Pediatr Gynecol* 1988;1:232.

ASSENZA CONGENITA DELLA VAGINA (SINDROME DI MAYER-ROKITANSKY-KÜSTER-HAUSER). L'incidenza riportata è di 1/4 000-5 000 nati. La causa è sconosciuta. L'agenesia vaginale è caratterizzata da amenorrea primaria, vulva normale, anomalie dell'utero, assottigliamento delle tube di Falloppio, ovaie normali, cariotipo e fenotipo femminili normali e anomalie associate (più frequentemente renali e scheletriche). L'anomalia è spesso scoperta nell'adolescenza e ha significative implicazioni anatomiche, fisiologiche e psicologiche per la paziente e la famiglia.

Di solito il **trattamento** viene rimandato finché la paziente non sia pronta per essere sessualmente attiva. L'approccio non chirurgico per creare una vagina funzionale comprende l'uso di dilatatori di dimensioni progressivamente maggiori, che richiedono l'impegno da parte della paziente a rispettarne l'utilizzo quotidiano. Quando si raggiunge la dimensione massima che consente il coito, la paziente deve utilizzare quotidianamente il dilatatore oppure avere rapporti sessuali con una frequenza tale da mantenere la lunghezza adeguata. Vi è anche una procedura laparoscopica vulvare (vaginoplastica vulvare) in cui una cannula con punta a oliva collegata al filo di sutura viene collocata nell'area dell'introito e i fili di sutura vengono tirati in alto attraverso lo spazio di Retzius. Il progressivo aumento di tensione dei fili di sutura introdotti attraverso un dispositivo collocato sull'addome per "tirarli" porta allo sviluppo di una vagina funzionale. In uno studio su 52 pazienti con agenesia vaginale, la vaginoplastica laparoscopica ha portato a un "successo funzionale" del 98%. In alternativa, si è rivelato efficace l'intervento chirurgico con procedura di McIndoe, che comporta un innesto cutaneo split-thickness nell'area vaginale.

A questa sindrome si associano alcune lesioni che interessano altri apparati. Le più comuni sono le anomalie delle vie urinarie, che comportano principalmente l'assenza unilaterale di un rene o di un uretere (27%) e le anomalie scheletriche (12%), che riguardano principalmente lo sviluppo vertebrale.

INCOMPLETA FUSIONE VERTICALE DELLA VAGINA. I setti vaginali trasverso e longitudinale rappresentano l'incompleta canalizzazione della vagina. Comunemente la paziente si presenta con amenorrea e dolore ciclico, che è dovuto a criptomenorrea. L'agenesia di Müller deve essere differenziata dall'insensibilità agli androgeni (femminilizzazione testicolare), nella quale di solito i livelli di testosterone si trovano entro quelli che si osservano nel maschio. L'agenesia mülleriana risulta più comune, con un'incidenza riportata di 1/50 000-20 000, seconda per frequenza alla disgenesia gonadica fra le cause di amenorrea primaria.

Sono osservate anomalie renali nel 34% e scheletriche nel 12% delle pazienti con anomalie mülleriane: l'agenesia renale unilaterale si verifica nel 15% delle pazienti, mentre le anomalie scheletriche più frequenti sono quelle vertebrali. La sindrome di Klippel-Feil è stata associata all'agenesia mülleriana. Di solito le pazienti presentano un cariotipo femminile normale (46 XX), ma si verifica anche la traslocazione autosomica dei cromosomi 12q e 14q. Sono stati riportati casi di fratelli e di famiglie con un'espressione variabile di difetti nei sistemi mülleriano, renale e scheletrico.

L'ecografia pelvica è utile per definire l'anomalia e la TC e la RM forniscono ulteriori dettagli, mentre di solito la laparoscopia è riservata alla valutazione di una massa pelvica e delle anomalie che vi si trovano insieme. La valutazione radiologica ed ecografica è indicata per identificare anomalie associate. Si dovrebbe ottenere un cariotipo.

È meglio rinviare la vaginoplastica finché la paziente non abbia raggiunto la maturità e occorre in ogni caso che venga accompagnata da un counseling per la paziente e per la famiglia. La procedura di McIndoe comporta l'uso di un innesto cutaneo, di solito dalle natiche, per creare una vagina dopo l'appropriata dissezione dell'area vulvovaginale. L'epitelio vaginale artificiale si trasforma citologicamente in una mucosa vaginale di aspetto quasi normale. Altre procedure ricostruttive hanno compreso l'uso di lembi fasciocutanei. Vari sistemi di dilatazione possono anche portare all'aumento delle dimensioni vaginali, fino a rendere possibile il rapporto sessuale. È stato riportato il carcinoma squamocellulare della vagina ricostruita, che sembra essere correlato al tipo di tessuto trapiantato. In questo caso, di solito la radioterapia è il principale metodo di trattamento.

SETTI VAGINALI TRASVERSI. L'incidenza di tale lesione è circa di 1/80 000 femmine. In genere la paziente presenta un'amenorrea che può essere associata a dolore pelvico ciclico, a una massa pelvica e a criptomenorrea. Sebbene di solito restino asintomatici fino alla pubertà, gli idrometrocolpi possono insorgere nell'infanzia. I setti vaginali trasversi possono trovarsi insieme ad altre anomalie congenite, sebbene ciò si verifichi meno spesso che con l'agenesia mülleriana. La sede più comune per il setto è tra il terzo medio e il terzo superiore della vagina. Le pazienti presentano un utero funzionale, benché la loro fertilità sia spesso compromessa; il 47%, in uno studio retrospettivo, aveva avuto un aborto spontaneo. La prognosi è peggiore per le ostruzioni più alte. Vi è anche un'aumentata incidenza dell'endometriosi secondaria a una mestruazione retrograda.

La valutazione comprende un esame pelvico attento spesso accompagnato dall'imaging per descrivere le anomalie anatomiche. Il **trattamento** consiste nella resezione chirurgica dell'ostruzione dal basso. Si dovrebbe tentare l'anastomosi dei segmenti superiore e inferiore, sempre se possibile, per prevenire la stenosi. Può riuscire necessario un innesto cutaneo. Spesso si posiziona uno stent di Lucite nella vagina per mantenerne la pervietà.

ALTERAZIONI DELLA FUSIONE LATERALE. Comprendono tutta una serie di varianti anatomiche del setto longitudinale non ostruttivo, così come l'emivagina ostruita. Quest'ultima può essere associata a utero didelfo e spesso a una massa pelvica, che rappresenta la mestruazione retrograda associata all'emivagina occlusa. Le mestruazioni, spesso cicliche, indicano un tratto di efflusso non ostruito da uno dei due corni uterini.

ANOMALIE UTERINE. L'incidenza delle anomalie uterine è compresa tra 1/100 e 1/1 000. L'anomalo sviluppo della cavità uterina può avere varie manifestazioni cliniche. Le pazienti possono presentarsi con amenorrea primaria o con mestruazioni irregolari o anche regolari. Ci può essere una massa pelvica asintomatica o la dismenorrea. Nelle adolescenti e nelle donne adulte, una gravidanza andata male e l'infertilità possono sollevare il primo sospetto di un'anomalia uterina.

La diagnosi dovrebbe comprendere un esame ecografico, la valutazione del tratto renale e l'esame dello scheletro alla ricerca di eventuali anomalie. La cariotipizzazione e la laparoscopia diagnostica possono risultare necessarie, a seconda della presentazione e degli esami di laboratorio.

Il **trattamento** dipende dall'anomalia specifica e la riparazione chirurgica fino a oggi ha compreso la resezione isteroscopica. Dal punto di vista storico, sono state proposte vari tipi di metroplastica: di Strassman, "a cuneo" di Jones, di Tompkins. Si deve altresì risolvere l'ostruzione al tratto di efflusso, per la quale può essere necessario creare una finestra vaginale o asportare un'emivagina. Occorre inoltre valutare la mestruazione retrograda in un corno uterino, che se presente va corretta chirurgicamente in modo appropriato.

ATRESIA CONGENITA DELLA CERVICE UTERINA. Questa anomalia estremamente rara, definita con l'aiuto dell'imaging pelvico, spesso si presenta alla pubertà con criptomenorrea, amenorrea e dolore pelvico. È associata ad anomalie renali significative nel 5-10% delle pazienti. All'esame obiettivo si riscontra la completa assenza della cervice in un utero comunque palpabile. Può essere necessaria l'isterectomia. Tra le altre anomalie associate vi sono le cisti mesonefriche, che sono residui dei dotti di Wolff, la reduplicazione incompleta dei genitali interni (per es. l'utero didelfo) e l'aplasia renale unilaterale. Inoltre, sono state riportate anomalie gastrointestinali (42,9%), respiratorie (47,6%), del sistema nervoso centrale (28,6%), cardiovascolari (38,1%) e muscoloscheletriche (33,3%).

DUPLICAZIONE VULVARE COMPLETA. Questa rara anomalia congenita si presenta nell'infanzia ed è costituita da due vulve, due vagine e due vesciche urinarie, un utero didelfo, un singolo retto e ano e due apparati renali.

IPERTROFIA LABIALE. L'allungamento delle piccole labbra può comparire alla nascita. Di solito non ha conseguenze, ma può essere indicata la revisione chirurgica in presenza di sintomi fastidiosi o di una sporgenza quando si indossano indumenti aderenti.

ANOMALIE CLITORIDEE. L'agenesia del clitoride è rara. La sua duplicazione è stata riportata spesso in associazione ad anomalie degli organi pelvici, tra cui l'agenesia delle strutture delle vie genitali e l'esotropia vescicale.

ANOMALIE DELL'IMENE. L'imene imperforato può trovarsi nelle pazienti pediatriche ed è spesso associato a mucocolpo; si può anche osservare idrometrocolpo. Tra le altre anomalie vi sono l'imene cribriforme e l'imene stenotico.

ANOMALIE CLOACALI. Queste lesioni sono costituite da un seno urogenitale comune in cui sboccano l'orifizio uretrale e quello anale. L'apertura singola (cloaca) richiede la correzione chirurgica.

TRATTAMENTO DELLE EMERGENZE ASSOCIATE ALLE MALFORMAZIONI CONGENITE DELLE VIE GENITALI FEMMINILI

Le manifestazioni cliniche delle anomalie mülleriane sono varie. Può riscontrarsi una massa pelvica, associata o meno a sintomi; una massa vaginale prominente o un'emivagina sono indicative di un'ostruzione completa o parziale del tratto di efflusso. Un'adolescente può presentarsi con un dolore pelvico legato ad amenorrea primaria oppure diversi mesi dopo l'inizio del menarca. Le pazienti possono anche essere asintomatiche finché non si osservano aborti ripetuti. Quando la presentazione è invece acutamente sintomatica, può rendersi necessario il trattamento di emergenza.

OSTRUZIONE DEL TRATTO DI EFFLUSSO. L'ostruzione può essere dovuta a numerose anomalie distinte, tra cui l'imene imperforato, il setto vaginale trasverso e un corno rudimentale non comunicante. Con il progressivo accumulo di liquido prossimalmente all'ostruzione, l'ematocolpo, l'ematometro o l'ematometrocolpo che ne risultano provocano il dolore ciclico o una massa pelvica. Queste ostruzioni vengono valutate meglio tenendo conto della loro localizzazione.

VAGINA DISTALE/IMENE IMPERFORATO. Si tratta dell'anomalia ostruttiva più comune e di cui sono riportati casi familiari. Nel periodo neonatale e nella prima infanzia può essere diagnosticata per la presenza di una membrana sporgente dovuta a un mucocolpo da stimolazione estrogenica materna. Se non viene identificata a quest'epoca, spesso rimane inosservata fino alla pubertà, quando si accumula liquido mestruale. Le manifestazioni cliniche spesso sono costituite da una membrana prominente di colore blu-nero, dolore, amenorrea primaria e caratteristiche sessuali secondarie normali. A seconda della circostanza, le pazienti possono avere un dolore addominale ciclico o una massa pelvica.

Il **trattamento** richiede l'incisione/resezione della membrana, risolvendo così l'ostruzione alla via di efflusso. L'intervento dovrebbe essere effettuato all'epoca della diagnosi, se la paziente è sintomatica. Inoltre, sebbene la lesione possa venire riparata in qualunque momento durante il periodo neonatale, l'infanzia o l'adolescenza, l'intervento chirurgico è facilitato dalla stimolazione estrogenica e quindi idealmente andrebbe operato nell'adolescenza.

SETTO TRASVERSO PROSSIMALE O MEDIOVAGINALE. I difetti di fusione verticale possono portare a setto trasverso, che può essere imperforato e associato a ematocolpo o ematometro nelle adolescenti o mucocolpo nelle bambine. Con un'apertura puntiforme, il liquido si accumula in vagina. Può essere presente una massa, come nel caso dell'imene imperforato. La vagina appare breve o a fondo cieco. L'approccio alla resezione del setto dipende dalla presenza o dall'assenza di un'apertura: nel primo caso, si dovrebbe tentare la cannulazione con resezione del setto, con successivo possibile stent vaginale.

CORNA RUDIMENTALI. Questa emergenza deriva dalla presenza di un corno con un endometrio funzionale e un'ostruzione al tratto di efflusso. Come avviene in altri tipi di tale ostruzione, la manifestazione clinica primaria è costituita dal dolore addominale inferiore grave con una massa pelvica. Tuttavia, a differenza delle altre forme, di solito non si ha un'amenorrea primaria, perché è improbabile che anche il corno opposto sia ostruito. È stata riportata la rottura asintomatica di un corno rudimentale in un'adulta.

L'ecografia è indicata per la visualizzazione del corno rudimentale. Si dovrebbe ottenere anche un pielogramma endovenoso o una scansione ecografica renale, a causa delle anomalie associate. Se si riscontrano i segni di un endometrio funzionale, è raccomandata l'asportazione chirurgica.

GRAVIDANZA IN UN CORNO RUDIMENTALE. Si verifica in 1/40 000 gravidanze e in 1/5 000-15 000 gravidanze ectopiche. Può essere dovuta a una banda fibrosa o fibromuscolare che collega l'utero unicorne e il corno rudimentale, ma l'80-85% dei casi è di tipo non comunicante, probabilmente a motivo della migrazione transperitoneale degli spermatozoi o dell'uovo fecondato. A differenza delle gravidanze tubariche, quelle in un corno rudimentale spesso non sono identificate prima del secondo trimestre e dal momento che la maggior parte dei corni ha una muscolatura più spessa, tipicamente la rottura si verifica più tardi.

Nella maggior parte dei casi la diagnosi viene posta soltanto dopo la rottura, quando le pazienti manifestano un dolore addominale acuto e segni peritoneali e sono spesso in condizioni di shock. Quando avviene la rottura, l'emorragia peritoneale può essere massiva e minacciosa per la vita e richiede un intervento chirurgico immediato. La mortalità materna è circa del 5% e nel 90% dei casi si verifica entro 10-15 minuti dopo la rottura, mentre la morte del feto avviene il 98% delle volte.

Prima della rottura, la diagnosi può essere difficile. Andrebbe sospettata in ogni donna gravida con un corno rudimentale noto e tali pazienti dovrebbero essere strettamente monitorate fino a che non venga documentata una gravidanza intrauterina. Nelle donne in cui precedentemente non è stato identificato tale corno, i reperti all'esame pelvico iniziale sono simili a quelli della gravidanza ectopica tubarica e comprendono la deviazione della cervice da un lato con una massa annessiale sul lato opposto. I reperti ecografici includono invece un sacco gestazionale extrauterino e una placenta all'interno del corno in prossimità di un utero leggermente ingrandito.

Il **trattamento** consiste nella resezione chirurgica del corno rudimentale.

RITENZIONE URINARIA ACUTA. L'ostruzione della via di efflusso che porta all'accumulo di liquido nella vagina o nell'utero può provocare la ritenzione urinaria in seguito al mucocolpo nei primi anni di vita o all'ematocolpo, all'ematometro o all'ematometrocolpo durante gli anni puberali. Il liquido ritenuto comprime l'uretra e ciò si aggrava quando l'utero pieno esercita pressione sulla parete posteriore della vescica e altera l'angolo dell'uretra. La pressione sul plesso sacrale esercitata dalla vagina distesa può essere un fattore contribuente.

Le manifestazioni cliniche abituali nelle adolescenti sono il dolore addominale inferiore e l'incapacità di svuotare la vescica. Possono sussistere anche l'esitazione e uno svuotamento incompleto della vescica per diversi giorni, prima della presentazione. In genere le adolescenti manifestano un'amenorrea primaria, un'anamnesi di dolore addominale inferiore ciclico e una massa pelvica. Tuttavia, se l'ostruzione è unilaterale, come nel caso del corno rudimentale non comunicante o nell'emivagina ostruita, la paziente può avere cicli mestruali regolari.

La cateterizzazione uretrale può fornire un sollievo temporaneo ma immediato. In caso di resistenza entro un catetere di gomma di dimensioni appropriate, si può utilizzare un sondino pediatrico da nutrizione o, se necessario, si può introdurre un ago spinale per via soprapubica per svuotare la vescica. Le urine andrebbero inviate per essere sottoposte a esame e coltura, in quanto la stasi urinaria favorisce l'infezione. Dopo avere trattato la malattia acuta, i disturbi sottostanti e la massa ostruente dovrebbero essere valutati in modo appropriato. Le infezioni delle vie urinarie sono state associate anche ad anomalie mülleriane. Ciò può essere dovuto ad anomalie renali con reflusso vescicoureterale oppure può precedere la ritenzione in seguito all'ostruzione della via di efflusso vaginale. È indicato il trattamento antibiotico.

TRAUMA GENITALE ACUTO PRIMA DEL MENARCA. Il trauma genitale acuto durante l'infanzia può manifestarsi sotto forma di lacerazioni e abrasioni genitali superficiali che non presentano sanguinamento attivo e possono essere semplicemente tenute sotto osservazione. Il sanguinamento attivo in seguito a un trauma nell'area genitale merita invece una valutazione appropriata, che di solito comprende l'esame in anestesia con riparazione chirurgica. Le indagini medico-legali possono essere indicate in caso di sospetto abuso sessuale. L'applicazione di estrogeni topici in crema sembra facilitare il processo di guarigione nell'area vulvovaginale e andrebbe presa in considerazione dopo l'intervento.

American College of Obstetrics and Gynecology. Nonsurgical diagnosis and management of vaginal agenesis. *Int J Gynaecol Obstet* 2002;79:167–170.
Folch M, Pigem I, Konge J: Müllerian agenesis: Etiology, diagnosis and management. *Obstet Gynecol Surv* 2000;55:644–649.
Gell J: Mullerian anomalies. *Semin Reprod Med* 2003;21:375–388.
Lin P, Bhatnagar K, Nettleton G, et al: Female genital anomalies affecting reproduction. *Fertil Steril* 2002;78:899–915.
Merit D: Evaluating and managing acute genital trauma pre-menarche girls. *J Pediatr Adolesc Gynecol* 1999;12:237–238.
Nagele F, Langle R, Stolzlechner J, et al: Noncommunicating rudimentary horn-obstetric and gynecologic implications. *Acta Obstet Gynecol Scand* 1995;74:566–568.
Porcu E: Imaging in pediatric and adolescent gynecology. *Endocr Dev* 2004;7:9–22.
Scarsbrook AF, Moore NR: MRI appearances of mullerian duct abnormalities. *Clin Radiol* 2003;58:747–754.
Siegel MJ: Magnetic resonance imaging of the adolescent female pelvis. *Magn Reson Imaging Clin N Am* 2002;10:303–324.
Stallion A: Vaginal obstruction. *Semin Pediatr Surg* 2000;9:128–134.
Troiano RN, McCarthy SM: Mullerian duct anomalies: Imaging and clinical issues. *Radiology* 2004;233:19–34.
Yamada G, Satoh Y, Baskin LS, et al: Cellular and molecular mechanisms of development of the external genitalia. *Differentiation* 2003;71:445–460.
Yu TJ, Lin MC: Acute urinary retention in two patients with imperforate hymen. *Scand J Urol ,Nephrol* 1993;27:543–544.

Capitolo 555 ■ Esigenze ginecologiche particolari Joseph S. Sanfilippo

SOGGETTI CON RITARDO MENTALE. Le bambine con ritardo mentale si trovano di fronte a diverse problematiche ginecologiche, che comprendono livelli variabili di conoscenza della riproduzione, della sessualità e della contraccezione. È stato dimostrato che programmi di counseling specificamente rivolti a tale questione risultano utili, specialmente per chi vive nella comunità. Anche l'igiene perineale è un motivo di preoccupazione. Spesso le giovani donne con ritardo mentale grave non sono in grado di essere istruite dalle loro madri a gestire l'igiene intima durante le mestruazioni; la maggior parte delle donne con un livello di funzionamento più alto è alla fine in grado di essere istruita, in particolare quelle che sono state educate all'uso della toilette. Modificazioni comportamentali cicliche (pianto, autolesionismo e capricci) prima della mestruazione sono comuni, dovute suppostamente a dolore o a crampi, in quanto il 65% delle pazienti risponde ai farmaci antinfiammatori non steroidei (FANS). Se il trattamento con questi non è efficace, la pillola contraccettiva e il depo-medrossi-progesterone acetato hanno migliorato il comportamento nel 40-66% dei casi. Anche gli inibitori selettivi del re-uptake della serotonina sono risultati validi.

L'abuso sessuale è uno dei principali motivi di preoccupazione; fino al 25% delle donne con ritardo mentale ne ha subito uno.

Si possono prendere in considerazione numerosi tipi di approccio per sopprimere i cicli mestruali. Il depo-medrossi-progesterone acetato, di solito prescritto alla dose di 150 mg, può essere somministrato ogni 3 mesi. In alternativa, i contraccettivi orali o sotto forma di cerotto non producono amenorrea, ma determinano una diminuzione del flusso mestruale. Negli Stati Uniti, prima di prendere qualsiasi decisione sulla sterilizzazione di queste pazienti si dovrebbe affrontare una discussione approfondita con i genitori o i tutori e, idealmente, una consulenza con un comitato etico. Negli Stati Uniti, i genitori di bambine con una grave disabilità dello sviluppo possono scegliere la sterilizzazione associata a una terapia estrogenica ad alte dosi (prima dell'inizio della pubertà), per attenuare la crescita della figlia.

Chamberlain A, Rauth J, Passer A, et al: Issues in fertility control for mentally retarded female adolescents: 1. Sexual activity, sexual abuse, and contraception. *Pediatrics* 1984;73:445–450.
Elkins TE, Gafford LS, Wilks CS, et al: A model clinic approach to the reproductive health concerns of the mentally handicapped. *Obstet Gynecol* 1986;68:185–188.
Elkins TE, Kope S, Ghaziuddin M, et al: Integration of a sexuality counseling service into a reproductive health program for persons with mental retardation. *J Pediatr Adolesc Gynecol* 1997;10:24–27.
Gunther DF, Dickema DS: Attenuating growth in children with profound developmental disability. *Arch Pediatr Adolesc Med* 2006;160:1013–1017.
Owens K, Honebrink A: Gynecologic care of mentally complicated adolescents. *Pediatr Clin North Am* 1999;46:631–642, ix.
Paransky OI, Zurawin RK: Management of menstrual problems and contraception in adolescents with mental retardation: A medical, legal, and ethical review with new suggested guidelines. *J Pediatr Adolesc Gynecol* 2003;16:223–235.
Quint EH, Elkins TE, Sorg CA, et al: The treatment of cyclical behavioral changes in women with mental disabilities. *J Pediatr Adolesc Gynecol* 1999;12:139–142.
Tharinger D, Horton CB, Millea S: Sexual abuse and exploitation of children and adults with mental retardation and other handicaps. *Child Abuse Negl* 1999;14:301–312.

Capitolo 556 ■ Tecniche di imaging ginecologico Joseph S. Sanfilippo

L'approccio ecografico transaddominale è il più attuabile nelle pazienti pediatriche e adolescenti. È necessaria una vescica distesa, che funge da finestra di visualizzazione e facilita l'identificazione dell'utero e delle ovaie; la distensione della vescica da parte delle urine allontana dalla pelvi le anse intestinali piene di gas e migliora l'imaging. Di solito si utilizza un trasduttore da 7,5 o 5,0 MHz, specialmente nelle bambine di taglia più grande e nelle adolescenti. L'ecografia è uno strumento di screening fondamentale, che consente una diagnosi appropriata nelle pazienti che si presentano con genitali ambigui, masse ovariche o uterine, amenorrea primaria e dolore addominale o pelvico (Tab. 556-1).

Masse pelviche possono essere identificate a qualunque età. Le cisti ovariche e l'idrocolpo o l'idrometrocolpo sono le anomalie più comunemente riscontrate nelle neonate. L'idrocolpo è definito come una dilatazione della vagina di solito associata a un accumulo di liquido sieroso o di urine (in presenza di una fistola urogenitale). L'idrometrocolpo provoca la dilatazione dell'utero e della vagina e può essere associato a un'atresia vaginale o cervicale, a una stenosi o a un imene imperforato. La maggior parte delle cisti ovariche (cisti semplici) di grosse dimensioni nell'infanzia può essere semplicemente sottoposta a un'osservazione con esami ecografici seriali e tende a diminuire di dimensioni o a risolversi completamente. Di fronte a una massa solida è necessaria una diagnosi istologica.

TABELLA 556-1. Normali dimensioni ovariche e uterine

OVAIO

Alla nascita

Lunghezza 15 mm, larghezza 3 mm, spessore 2,5 mm

Volume ovarico 0,7 cm^3*

Dopo la pubertà

Lunghezza 22,5-50,0 mm

Larghezza 1,5-3,0 cm; spessore 0,6-1,5 cm

Volume ovarico 1,8-5,7 cm^3*

UTERO

Alla nascita

Lunghezza 2,3-4,6 cm

Diametro anteroposteriore 0,8-2,2 cm

Fino ai 7 anni

Lunghezza 2,5-3,3 cm

Diametro anteroposteriore 0,4-1,0 cm

Dopo la pubertà

Lunghezza 6 cm

*Il volume ovarico può essere determinato mediante la seguente formula: lunghezza × altezza × larghezza = 0,523.

Da Sanfilippo JS, Lavery JP: The spectrum of ultrasound: Antenatal to adolescent years. *Semin Reprod Endocrinol* 1988;6:45-53.

La RM risulta utile per la valutazione delle anomalie del dotto di Müller. Andrebbe utilizzata assieme alla valutazione ecografica e, se necessario, a tecniche come la genitografia. Per la valutazione delle anomalie ovariche sono state impiegate l'ecografia tridimensionale e il Doppler. L'ecografia tridimensionale permette di differenziare in modo più chiaro le lesioni ovariche benigne da quelle maligne e riduce i falsi positivi.

Kurjak A, Jupesic S, Sparac V, et al: Three-dimensional ultrasonographic and power Doppler characterization of ovarian lesions. *Ultrasound Obstet Gynecol* 2000;16:365–371.

Lang IM, Babyn P, Oliver GD: MR imaging of pediatric uterovaginal anomalies. *Pediatr Radiol* 1999;29:163–170.

Porcu E: Imaging in pediatric and adolescent gynecology. *Endocr Dev* 2004;7:9–22.

Siegel MJ: Magnetic resonance imaging of the adolescent female pelvis. *Magn Reson Imaging Clin N Am* 2002;10:303–324, vi.

Warner BW, Kuhn JC, Barr LL: Conservative management of large ovarian cysts in children: The value of serial pelvic ultrasonography. *Surgery* 1992;112:749–755.

Parte XXV ▪ Il sistema endocrino

Sezione 1 — Alterazioni della funzione ipotalamica e dell'ipofisi

Capitolo 557 ▪ Ormoni dell'ipotalamo e dell'ipofisi John S. Parks ed Eric I. Felner

L'IPOFISI: LA GHIANDOLA MAESTRA

L'ipofisi è la ghiandola che più di ogni altra regola il sistema ormonale. Essa riceve segnali dall'ipotalamo e risponde inviando ormoni ipofisarici alle ghiandole bersaglio. Queste producono a loro volta ormoni che forniscono un feedback negativo a livello ipotalamico e ipofisario. Questo meccanismo di feedback consente all'ipofisi di regolare la quantità di ormoni rilasciati all'interno del flusso sanguigno dalle ghiandole bersaglio. Il ruolo centrale dell'ipofisi in questo sistema ormonale e la sua proprietà di interpretare e rispondere a una grande quantità di segnali hanno portato a definire l'ipofisi la "ghiandola maestra".

ANATOMIA DELL'IPOFISI. L'ipofisi si trova alla base del cranio nella cavità a forma di sella dell'osso sfenoide: la sella turcica. La struttura ossea protegge e circonda l'ipofisi bilateralmente e inferiormente. La dura, uno spesso strato di tessuto connettivo, forma il tetto della sella. Uno strato esterno della dura continua all'interno della sella formando un rivestimento. L'ipofisi è extradurale e normalmente non è in contatto con il liquido cerebrospinale. L'ipofisi è collegata all'ipotalamo dal peduncolo ipofisario. Esso è composto da un lobo anteriore (**adenoipofisi**) e uno posteriore (**neuroipofisi**). Il lobo anteriore costituisce circa l'80% del peduncolo.

EMBRIOLOGIA DELL'IPOFISI. L'ipofisi anteriore ha origine dalla tasca di Rathke come invaginazione dell'ectoderma orale (Fig. 557-1). Essa poi si distacca dall'epitelio orale e diventa una struttura indipendente di cellule rapidamente proliferanti. Alla sesta settimana di gestazione, non si ha più la connessione tra la tasca di Rathke e l'orofaringe e la tasca stabilisce un collegamento diretto con l'estensione inferiore dell'ipotalamo, che genera il peduncolo ipofisario, o infundibolo. Frammenti persistenti della connessione originale tra la tasca di Rathke e la cavità orale possono svilupparsi in **craniofaringiomi**, il tipo di tumore più comune in quest'area.

VASCOLARIZZAZIONE DELL'IPOFISI. La vascolarizzazione dell'ipofisi ha origine dalla carotide interna tramite le arterie ipofisiarie inferiore, media e superiore. Questa rete di vasi forma una circolazione portale unica che collega l'ipotalamo e l'ipofisi. I rami delle arterie ipofisiarie superiori penetrano nel peduncolo e formano una rete di vasi che attraversano il peduncolo stesso e terminano in una rete di capillari all'interno del lobo anteriore. È attraverso questo sistema venoso portale che gli ormoni ipotalamici vengono trasportati nell'ipofisi anteriore. Gli ormoni dell'ipofisi anteriore, a loro volta, vengono secreti in un plesso secondario di vene portali che defluiscono nei seni venosi durali.

TIPOLOGIA CELLULARE DELL'IPOFISI ANTERIORE. Una serie di fattori di attivazione trascrizionale espressi sequenzialmente regola la differenziazione e la proliferazione delle cellule dell'ipofisi anteriore (Fig. 557-1). Queste proteine sono membri di una grande famiglia di proteine leganti il DNA che assomigliano ai **geni omeobox**. Le conseguenze delle mutazioni in molti di questi geni sono evidenti nelle forme di deficit dell'ormone ipofisario nell'uomo. Cinque tipi di cellule dell'ipofisi anteriore producono 6 ormoni peptidici. Le cellule somatotrope producono l'ormone della crescita (*Growth Hormone*, GH); le cellule lattotrope producono la prolattina (PRL); le cellule tireotrope generano l'ormone stimolante la tiroide (*Thyroid-Stimulating Hormone*, TSH); le cellule corticotrope esprimono la proopiomelanocortina (POMC), il precursore dell'ormone adrenocorticotropo (*Adrenocorticotropic Hormone*, ACTH); e le cellule gonadotrope esprimono sia l'ormone luteinizzante (*Luteinizing Hormone*, LH) sia l'ormone follico-stimolante (*Follicle-Stimulating Hormone*, FSH).

Ormone della crescita. Il GH dell'uomo è una catena polipeptidica singola di 191 aminoacidi sintetizzata, depositata e secreta dalle cellule somatotrope dell'ipofisi. Il suo gene (*GH1*) è il primo di un gruppo di 5 geni strettamente correlati sul braccio lungo del cromosoma 17 (q22-24). Gli altri 4 geni (*CS1*, *CS2*, *GH2*, *CSP*) hanno un'identità di sequenza con *GH1* superiore al 90%.

Il GH viene secreto in modo pulsatile sotto la regolazione degli ormoni ipotalamici. La secrezione alternata dell'ormone di rilascio dell'ormone della crescita (*Growth-Hormone-Releasing-Hormone*, GHRH), che stimola il rilascio di GH, e della somatostatina, che inibisce il rilascio di GH, regolano la secrezione ritmica del GH. I picchi di GH si verificano quando i picchi di GHRH coincidono con le depressioni di somatostatina. Anche la grelina, un peptide prodotto nel nucleo arcuato dell'ipotalamo e in quantità molto maggiori dallo stomaco, stimola la secrezione di GH. I fattori fisiologici hanno un ruolo nella stimolazione e nell'inibizione di GH. Il sonno, l'esercizio fisico, lo stress, i traumi, patologie acute, la pubertà, il digiuno e l'ipoglicemia stimolano il rilascio di GH, mentre l'iperglicemia, l'ipotiroidismo e i glucocorticoidi inibiscono il rilascio di GH.

Il GH si lega alle molecole recettoriali sulla superficie delle cellule bersaglio. Il recettore del GH è una catena singola di 620 aminoacidi con un dominio extracellulare, un dominio a membrana singola e un dominio citoplasmico. I frammenti scissi proteoliticamente del dominio extracellulare circolano nel plasma e agiscono come una proteina legante il GH. Il dominio citoplasmico del recettore del GH è privo di attività chinasica intrinseca; invece, il legame del GH induce alla dimerizzazione del recettore e all'attivazione di una chinasi associata al recettore (*Janus Kinase*, Jak2). La fosforilazione della chinasi e di altri substrati proteici avvia una serie di eventi che porta ad alterazioni nella trascrizione del gene nucleare. Il trasduttore di segnale e l'attivatore di trascrizione 5b (*Signal Transducer and Activator of Transcription*, STAT5b) svolgono un ruolo fondamentale nell'attivazione del recettore di legame nel cambio della trascrizione del gene.

Gli effetti biologici del GH comprendono aumenti lineari della crescita, ispessimento osseo, crescita del tessuto morbido, sintesi proteica, rilascio di acidi grassi dal tessuto adiposo, insulino-resistenza e controllo della glicemia. Le azioni mitogene del GH vengono mediate tramite l'incremento della sintesi del fattore

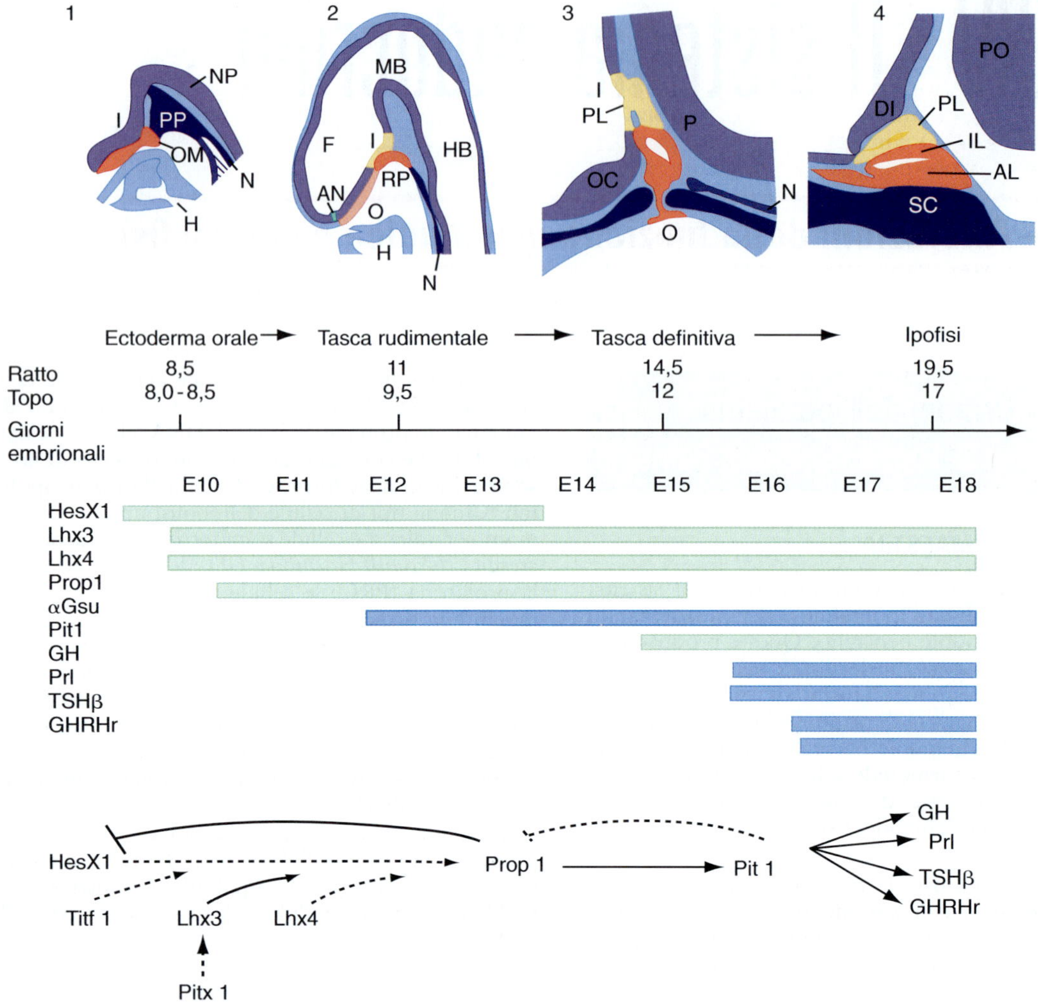

Figura 557-1. Sviluppo dell'ipofisi. *A,* figure della sezione mediosagittale o parasagittale dell'embrione di un ratto, che mostra lo sviluppo dell'ipofisi: (1) crescita della porzione preinfundibulare della piastra neurale e definizione dell'area della tasca di Rathke presunta; (2) formazione di una tasca rudimentale, con assenza del mesoderma tra la tasca e il pavimento del diencefalo; (3) formazione della tasca definitiva e del lobo posteriore con invasione della cresta neurale e del tessuto mesenchinale e separazione delle cavità cerebrale e orale; (4) ipofisi nascente. Fasi corrispondenti nello sviluppo del topo. AL, lobo anteriore; AN, poro neurale anteriore; F, prosencefalo, cervello anteriore; H, cuore; HB, romboencefalo; I, infundibolo; IL, lobo intermedio; MB, mesencefalo; N, notocorda; NP, piastra neurale; O, cavità orale; OC, chiasma ottico; OM, membrana orale; P, flessura pontina; PL, lobo posteriore; PO, ponte; PP, piastra precordale; RP, tasca di Rathke; SC, cartilagine sfenoidale. *B,* Cascata dei fattori di trascrizione che regolano lo sviluppo dell'ipofisi anteriore. Viene indicato il tempo approssimativo dell'espressione dell'mRNA nel topo per i fattori di trascrizione (barra verde) e per altri geni marcatori (barre blu). Le frecce rappresentano l'attivazione; le linee interrotte rappresentano la repressione. Le frecce nere intere indicano gli effetti supportati dall'analisi dei mutanti ipofisarici. Le frecce spezzate rappresentano le ipotetiche interazioni che possono essere rivelate dall'analisi dell'espressione in altri mutanti ipofisarici. E, giorno embrionale. (Da Dattani M, Preece M: Growth hormone deficiency and related disorders: Insights into causation, diagnosis, and treatment. *Lancet* 2004;363:1997.)

di crescita insulino-simile (*Insulin-Like Growth Factor*, IGF-I), in precedenza definito somatomedina C, una catena peptidica singola di 70 aminoacidi codificata da un gene sul braccio lungo del cromosoma 12. L'IGF-I ha una considerevole analogia con l'insulina. L'IGF-I circolante viene sintetizzato principalmente nel fegato e formato localmente nelle cellule del mesoderma e dell'ectoderma, soprattutto nella placca di accrescimento dei bambini, dove il suo effetto è esercitato dal meccanismo paracrino o autocrino. I livelli circolatori dell'IGF-I sono correlati ai livelli sanguigni del GH e allo stato nutrizionale. L'IGF-I circola legato a diverse proteine. La principale di queste è un complesso di 150-kd (*Insulin-Like Growth Factor-Binding Protein*, IGF-BP3), di cui vi è carenza nei bambini con deficit di GH. L'IGF-I ricombinante nell'uomo può avere un potenziale terapeutico in condizioni caratterizzate dalla resistenza dell'organo bersaglio al GH come la sindrome di Laron e lo sviluppo di anticorpi al GH somministrato. L'IGF-II è una catena proteica singola di 67 aminoacidi codificata da un gene sul braccio corto del cromosoma 11. Presenta delle omologie con l'IGF-I. Le conoscenze riguardo il suo ruolo fisiologico sono scarse, ma sembra essere un importante mitogeno nell'osteocita, dove è presente in concentrazioni assai superiori rispetto a quelle dell'IGF-I.

Prolattina. La PRL è una catena peptidica di 199 aminoacidi sintetizzata dalle cellule lattotrope dell'ipofisi. La regolazione della PRL è unica perché la PRL è secreta in modo costante a meno che non sia attivamente inibita dalla dopamina, prodotta dai neuroni nell'ipotalamo. Un'affezione dell'ipotalamo o del peduncolo ipofisario può determinare livelli elevati di PRL. Elevati livelli sierici di PRL comportano un'antagonizzazione della dopamina, stati di ipotiroidismo primitivo, somministrazione dell'ormone di rilascio della tireotropina (*Thyrotropin-Releasing Hormone*, TRH), stress fisiologico (shock) e tumori dell'ipofisi. Gli antagonisti della dopamina e i processi che causano alterazioni dell'ipofisi riducono i livelli di PRL.

Il ruolo fisiologico primario della PRL è l'iniziazione e il mantenimento dell'allattamento. La PRL prepara le mammelle per l'allattamento e stimola la produzione di latte dopo il parto. Durante la gravidanza, la PRL stimola comunque lo sviluppo delle cellule secretorie del latte, ma non si ha produzione di latte a causa degli alti livelli di estrogeno e di progesterone. Dopo il parto, i livelli di estrogeno e progesterone si riducono e stimoli fisiologici, quali quello all'allattamento e la stimolazione dei capezzoli, inducono il rilascio di PRL e danno inizio all'allattamento.

Ormone stimolante la tiroide. Il TSH è costituito da 2 catene glicoproteiche (α e β) unite da legami di idrogeno; la subunità α è composta da 89 aminoacidi ed è identica alle altre glicoproteine (FSH, LH, gonadotropina corionica [*Chorionic Gonadotropin*, hCG]), mentre la subunità β, composta da 112 aminoacidi, è specifica per il TSH.

Il TSH viene immagazzinato nei granuli secretori e messo in circolazione principalmente in risposta al TRH, prodotto dall'ipotalamo. Il TRH viene liberato dall'ipotalamo nel sistema portale ipofisario, stimolando infine il rilascio di TSH dalle cellule tireotrope. Il TSH stimola il rilascio della tiroxina (T_4) e della triiodotironina (T_3) dalla tiroide tramite la formazione di adenosina monofosfato ciclico (cAMP) e del sistema del secondo messaggero, la proteina G. Oltre all'inibizione del feedback negativo da parte di T_3, il rilascio di TRH e TSH viene inibito anche dalla dopamina, dalla somatostatina e dai glucocorticoidi.

Il deficit di TSH causa l'inattività e l'atrofia della tiroide, mentre un eccesso di TSH causa ipertrofia e iperplasia tiroidea.

Ormone adrenocorticotropo. L'ACTH è una catena peptidica di 39 aminoacidi derivata dal clivaggio proteolitico della **POMC**, un precursore glicoproteico di 240 aminoacidi dell'ipofisi. La POMC contiene anche le sequenze per le lipotropine (LPH), gli ormoni melanocito-stimolanti (*Melanocyte-Stimulating Hormones*, MSH) e le β-endorfine (β-END).

La secrezione di ACTH è regolata dall'ormone di rilascio della corticotropina (*Corticotropin-Releasing Hormone*, CRH), un peptide di 41 aminoacidi che si trova prevalentemente nell'eminenza mediana ma anche in altre aree intra- ed extracerebrali. L'ACTH viene secreto in modalità diurna. Esso agisce sulla corteccia surrenalica per stimolare la sintesi e la secrezione del cortisolo. I livelli di ACTH e di cortisolo sono più elevati la mattina al momento del risveglio, sono bassi nel tardo pomeriggio e la sera e raggiungono il loro punto più basso 1 o 2 ore dopo l'inizio del sonno. L'ACTH sembra anche essere il principale ormone pigmentario dell'uomo. Simili al TRH e al TSH, il CRH e l'ACTH funzionano tramite la formazione del cAMP e del sistema del secondo messaggero della proteina G. Benché il CRH sia il principale regolatore della secrezione di ACTH, sono implicati anche altri ormoni. L'arginina vasopressina (AVP), l'ossitocina, l'angiotensina II e la colecistochinina stimolano il rilascio di CRH e ACTH, mentre il peptide natriuretico atriale (*Atrial Natriuretic Peptide*, ANP) e gli oppioidi ne inibiscono il rilascio. Il cortisolo inibisce il CRH e l'ACTH. Anche condizioni fisiologiche come lo stress, il digiuno e l'ipoglicemia stimolano il rilascio di CRH e ACTH.

Ormone luteinizzante e ormone follico-stimolante. Gli ormoni gonadotropi comprendono due glicoproteine: l'LH e l'FSH. Esse contengono la stessa subunità α, come il TSH e l'hCG ma diverse subunità β. I recettori per l'FSH sulle cellule della granulosa ovarica e sulle cellule testicolari del Sertoli mediano la stimolazione di FSH per lo sviluppo follicolare nell'ovaio e per la gametogenesi nei testicoli. Legandosi a recettori specifici sulle cellule della teca ovarica e sulle cellule testicolari del Leydig, l'LH stimola la luteinizzazione dell'ovaio e la funzione delle cellule testicolari del Leydig. I recettori per l'LH e l'FSH appartengono a una classe di recettori con 7 domini proteici di membrana. L'occupazione del recettore attiva l'adenilil-ciclasi tramite la mediazione della proteina G.

L'ormone di rilascio dell'ormone luteinizzante, un decapeptide, è stato isolato, sintetizzato e utilizzato a fini terapeutici. Poiché porta al rilascio di LH e FSH dalle stesse cellule gonadotrope, sembra esserci un solo ormone di liberazione della gonadotropina.

La secrezione di LH è inibita dagli androgeni e dagli estrogeni, mentre la secrezione di FSH è soppressa dalla produzione gonadica dell'inibina, una glicoproteina di 31 kd prodotta dalle cellule del Sertoli. L'**inibina** è costituita dalle subunità α e β unite da legami disolfuro. Si genera anche il dimero β-β (**activina**); il suo effetto biologico è di stimolare la secrezione di FSH. Le caratteristiche biologiche dell'inibina e dell'activina sono oggetto di ricerca. Oltre al suo effetto endocrino, l'activina ha effetti paracrini nel testicolo. Essa facilita la produzione di testosterone LH-indotto, indicando un effetto diretto delle cellule del Sertoli sulle cellule di Leydig.

TIPOLOGIA DELLE CELLULE DELL'IPOFISI POSTERIORE. Il lobo posteriore dell'ipofisi è parte di un'unità funzionale, la neuroipofisi, costituita dai neuroni dei nuclei supraottico e paraventricolare dell'ipotalamo; gli assoni neuronali, che formano il peduncolo ipofisario, o infundibolo; e le terminazioni assoniche dell'eminenza mediana o del lobo posteriore. L'arginina vasopressina (AVP; ormone antidiuretico [*Antidiuretic Hormone*, ADH]) e l'ossitocina sono i due ormoni prodotti dalla neurosecrezione nei nuclei ipotalamici e liberati dall'ipofisi posteriore. Sono octapeptidi e differiscono solo per due aminoacidi.

Ormone antidiuretico. L'ADH regola la conservazione dell'acqua a livello del rene aumentando la permeabilità all'acqua del dotto collettore. L'ADH stimola la traslocazione dei canali dell'acqua tramite la sua interazione con i recettori della vasopressina 2 (V2) nel dotto collettore, che agisce tramite le proteine G per aumentare l'attività dell'adenilil ciclasi e aumentare la permeabilità all'acqua. I recettori V2 mediano anche il fattore di von Willebrand e l'attivatore del plasminogeno tissutale. Ad alte concentrazioni, l'ADH attiva i recettori V1 nelle cellule del muscolo liscio e negli epatociti ed esercita effetti pressori e glicogenolitici tramite la mobilizzazione delle riserve di calcio intracellulare. Recettori V3 separati mediano la stimolazione della secrezione di ACTH. Questi effetti producono l'idrolisi di fosfatidilinositolo piuttosto che la produzione di AMP ciclico.

L'ADH e la sua proteina accompagnatrice, la neurofisina II, sono codificate dallo stesse gene. Un singolo preproormone viene scisso e le due parti vengono trasportate nelle vescicole neurosecretorie dell'ipofisi posteriore e vengono rilasciate in quantità equimolare.

L'ADH ha un'emivita breve e risponde rapidamente ai cambiamenti di idratazione. Gli stimoli per il suo rilascio sono l'aumentata osmolalità del plasma, percepita dagli osmorecettori ipotalamici e la riduzione del volume plasmatico, percepita dai barorecettori del seno carotideo dell'arco aortico.

Ossitocina. L'ossitocina stimola le contrazioni uterine al momento del travaglio e del parto in risposta alla distensione del tratto riproduttivo e stimola la contrazione delle cellule mammarie preposte all'allattamento con conseguente fuoriuscita del latte.

Capitolo 558 ■ Ipopituitarismo

John S. Parks ed Eric I. Felner

Il termine ipopituitarismo indica una riduzione della produzione di ormone della crescita (GH, *Growth Hormone*) isolata o associata a deficit di altri ormoni ipofisari. I bambini colpiti mostrano un'alterazione della crescita post-natale, corretta da specifica terapia sostitutiva con GH. L'incidenza di ipopituitarismo è compresa tra 1 su 4000 e 1 su 10 000 nati. Con la conoscenza dei geni che indirizzano lo sviluppo ipofisario (vedi Fig. 557-1) o la produzione ormonale, si può attribuire un sempre maggior numero di casi a specifiche patologie genetiche (Tab. 558-1). Nel 13% dei casi di carenza isolata di ormone della crescita (IGHD, *Isolated Growth Hormone Deficiency*) e nel 20% dei casi di carenze ormonali ipofisarie multiple (MPHD, *Multiple Pituitary Hormone Deficiency*) si riscontrano mutazioni di tali geni. Un'anamnesi familiare positiva aumenta la probabilità di trovare mutazioni, mentre la carenza di ACTH la diminuisce.

TABELLA 558-1. Classificazione eziologica dei deficit ormonali ipofisari multipli

GENE O POSIZIONE	FENOTIPO	EREDITARIETÀ
FORME GENETICHE		
POU1F1 (PIT1)	GH, TSH, PRL	R, D
PROP1	GH, TSH, PRL, LH, FSH, ± ACTH, variabile AP	R
LHX3	GH, TSH, PRL, LH, FSH, variabile IA, ± collo corto	R
LHX4	GH, TSH, ACTH, piccola IA, IPE, ± sindrome di Arnold Chiari	D
TPIT	ACTH, grave forma neonatale	R
HESX1	GH, variabile per altri, piccola IA, IPE	R, D
SOX3	Deficit variabili, ± MR, IPE; piccola IA e peduncolo	AX
PTX2	Sindrome di Rieger	D
GLI2	Oloprosencefalia, difetti mediali	D
GLI3	Sindrome di Hall-Pallister	D
Sonic hedgehog	Deficit di GH con singolo incisivo centrale	D
FORME ACQUISITE		
Idiopatica		
Irradiazione	Deficit di GH precede gli altri deficit	
Infiammazione/Infiltrazione	Istiocitosi, sarcoisdosi, meningite, encefalite, tubercolosi	
Autoimmune	Ipofisite	
Postchirurgica	Sezione del peduncolo, compromissione vascolare	
Tumore	Craniofaringioma, glioma, pinealoma, adenoma, germinoma, glioma ottico	
Trauma	Maltrattamento, sindrome del bambino battuto, veicoli a motore, incidente, perinatale	
Ipotiroidismo	Primario o acquisito	
EZIOLOGIA INCERTA		
Idiopatica		
Assenza congenita dell'ipofisi		
Displasia setto-ottica		
Trauma alla nascita		
Encefalocele		
Idrocefalo		

ACTH, *Adrenocorticotropic Hormone* (ormone corticotropo); IA, ipofisi anteriore; D, dominante; IPE, ipofisi posteriore ectopica; FSH, *Follicle-Stimulating Hormone* (ormone follicolostimolante); GH, *Growth Hormone* (ormone della crescita); LH, *Luteinizing Hormone* (ormone luteinizzante); PRL, *Prolactin* (prolattina); R, recessivo; TSH, *Thyroid-Stimulating Hormone* (ormone tiroide-stimolante); AX, associato a X.

CARENZA MULTIPLA DI ORMONI IPOFISARI

FORME GENETICHE. I fattori di attivazione trascrizionale espressi sequenzialmente orientano la differenziazione e la proliferazione dei vari tipi cellulari dell'ipofisi anteriore (vedi Fig. 557-1). Queste proteine appartengono a un'ampia famiglia di proteine di trasporto del DNA simili ai geni homeobox. Le mutazioni producono forme diverse di carenza multipla di ormoni ipofisari. I geni *HESX1*, *LHX3*, *LHX4* e *PTX2*, presenti in stadi precoci dello sviluppo ipofisario, possono essere espressi anche in altri organi e loro eventuali mutazioni tendono a produrre fenotipi che, oltre all'ipopituitarismo, comprendono anomalie di altri organi.

HESX1. Il gene *HESX1* è espresso nei precursori di tutti e cinque i tipi cellulari dell'ipofisi anteriore, precocemente durante lo sviluppo embrionale. Le sue mutazioni comportano un fenotipo complesso, con difetti nello sviluppo del nervo ottico. Gli eterozigoti per mutazioni con perdita di funzione manifestano deficit isolato di GH associato a ipoplasia del nervo ottico. Negli omozigoti si può avere espressione completa della **displasia setto-ottica** (DSO), caratterizzata da incompleto sviluppo del setto pellucido con ipoplasia del nervo ottico e altre anomalie mediali. Nei bambini, l'osservazione clinica di nistagmo e di disturbi visivi indirizza alla scoperta di anomalie cerebrali e del nervo ottico. Nel 25% dei pazienti la DSO è associata a deficit di ormoni ante o post-ipofisari. I pazienti presentano spesso la triade caratterizzata da: ipoplasia dell'ipofisi anteriore, assottigliamento del peduncolo ipofisario e macchia brillante costituita dall'ipofisi posteriore ectopica. La maggior parte dei casi di DSO non presenta però mutazioni *HESX1*.

LHX3. L'*LHX3* attiva il promoter α-GSU e agisce sinergicamente a POU1F1 per aumentare la trascrizione di PRL, β-TSH e promotori di POU1F1. Il fenotipo ormonale prodotto da mutazioni recessive con perdita di funzione di questo gene assomiglia a quello prodotto da mutazioni di *PROP1*. Sono presenti deficit multipli di GH, PRL, TSH, LH e FSH, ma non di ACTH. Non è chiaro se i deficit siano presenti sin dalla nascita o se compaiano nel bambino successivamente. Alcuni individui affetti mostrano un ingrandimento dell'ipofisi anteriore. Nei primi pazienti descritti, si evidenziavano inusuale brevità del collo e rigidità della colonna cervicale che consentiva la rotazione del collo solo di 90 gradi, rispetto ai 150-180 di una rotazione normale.

LHX4. Mutazioni del gene *LHX4* a ereditarietà dominante producono un consistente deficit di GH, associato in modo variabile a deficit di TSH e ACTH. Si possono associare inoltre piccola fossa ipofisaria, con forma a V, malformazione di Chiari 1, ectopia dell'ipofisi posteriore.

PYX2. La sindrome di Rieger si manifesta in un fenotipo complesso, causato da mutazioni del gene del fattore di trascrizione *PTX2*. Questo gene è riferito anche a *RIEG1*. Si esprime in vari tessuti, compresa l'ipofisi anteriore. I bambini con sindrome di Rieger, oltre a gradi diversi di deficit degli ormoni anteipofisari, presentano colobomi dell'iride e anomalo sviluppo di reni, del tratto gastrointestinale e dell'ombelico.

PROP1. *PROP1* è stato trovato nei nuclei delle cellule produttrici di somatotropo, prolattina e tireotropina. Fra i suoi ruoli vi è anche la deviazione verso l'espressione POU1F1, per cui è stato chiamato "profeta di PIT1". Mutazioni di PROP1 sono la causa più comune di MPHD recessivo. Tali mutazioni sono 10 volte più frequenti delle combinazioni totali di mutazioni in altri geni di fattori di trascrizione ipofisari. Le più comuni sono delezioni di uno o due paia di basi nell'esone 2, seguite da missense, nonsense e mutazioni di *splice site*. Deficit di ormoni anteipofisari sono raramente evidenti nel periodo neonatale. La crescita durante il primo anno di vita è migliore che con difetti di POU1F1. Mediamente verso i 6 anni si arriva alla diagnosi di deficit di GH e il riconoscimento di un deficit di TSH è tardivo rispetto a quello di GH. I livelli di PRL basale e dopo stimolazione con TRH tendono a essere più alti che nelle mutazioni POUF1. La maggior parte dei bambini con mutazioni *PROP1* sviluppa un deficit di LH e FSH. Alcuni iniziano spontaneamente la pubertà, che in seguito si blocca. Le ragazze presentano amenorrea secondaria, mentre i ragazzi regressione del volume testicolare e delle caratteristiche sessuali secondarie. Nel 30% dei pazienti con difetti *PROP1* si evidenzia nel tempo una parziale carenza di ACTH. Nella maggior parte dei pazienti le dimensioni dell'ipofisi sono ridotte, ma in alcuni si manifesta invece un progressivo ingrossamento della ghiandola. All'interno della sella turcica si sviluppa inizialmente una massa centrale, che può espandersi superiormente e il cui contenuto cellulare durante la fase di ingrandimento non è noto. Con il tempo, il contenuto della massa appare in degenerazione, con aree cistiche multiple. La massa può persistere come struttura stabile o può scomparire completamente, lasciando una "sella vuota". La RM può evidenziare, in stadi diversi, microadenoma, macroadenoma, craniofaringioma o cisti della tasca di Ratke.

POU1F1 (PIT1). POU1F1 (originariamente PIT1) era identificata come una proteina nucleare che lega i promoter di GH e PRL e risulta necessaria per l'origine e la funzione matura degli ormoni somatotropo, lattotropo e tireotropo. Mutazioni dominanti e recessive in POU1F1 sono responsabili di deficit completo di GH e PRL e variabile di TSH. Individui affetti presentano una crescita fetale quasi normale ma, nel primo anno di vita, un grave deficit di sviluppo. Con una normale produzione di LH e di FSH, la pubertà inizia spontaneamente, ma più tardivamente rispetto alla norma. Questi pazienti non sono a rischio di sviluppare deficit di ACTH e le dimensioni ipofisarie sono normali o piccole.

Altre forme congenite di MPHD. Una grave MPHD a insorgenza precoce, compreso il deficit di ACTH, è spesso associata alla triade: ipoplasia dell'ipofisi anteriore, assenza o assottigliamento del peduncolo ipofisario ed ectopia dell'ipofisi posteriore, che appare come macchia brillante alla RM. La maggior parte dei casi è sporadica; più frequente nel sesso maschile. Alcuni presentano anomalie del gene *SOX3*, localizzato sul cromosoma X, ma non è chiara la situazione genetica nella maggior parte dei casi.

L'**ipoplasia ipofisaria** può manifestarsi come fenomeno isolato o in associazione a più estese anomalie di sviluppo, come l'anencefalia o l'oloprosencefalia. Anomalie della porzione mediale del volto (fessurazione del labbro, del palato) o la scoperta di un incisivo centrale mascellare solitario indicano, con elevata probabilità, un deficit di GH o di un altro ormone antero o postero-ipofisario. Nella **sindrome di Hall-Pallister**, l'assenza dell'ipofisi si associa ad amartoblastoma ipotalamico, polidactilia postassiale, displasia ungueale, epiglottide bifida, ano imperforato e anomalie di cuore, polmoni e reni.

Forme acquisite. Qualsiasi lesione che danneggi l'ipotalamo, il peduncolo ipofisario o l'ipofisi anteriore può provocare deficit ormonale ipofisario. Data la non selettività delle lesioni, si osservano solitamente deficit ormonali multipli. La lesione più comune è il craniofaringioma (vedi Capitolo 497). Il germinoma del sistema nervoso centrale, il granuloma eosinofilo (istiocitosi), la tubercolosi, la sarcoidosi, la toxoplasmosi, la meningite e gli aneurismi possono provocare una distruzione ipotalamo-ipofisaria. Traumi, compresa la sindrome del bambino sbattuto, incidenti automobilistici, trazione da parto, anossia e infarto emorragico possono danneggiare l'ipofisi, il suo peduncolo o l'ipotalamo.

DEFICIT ISOLATO E INSENSIBILITÀ AL GH

FORME GENETICHE DI DEFICIT DI ORMONE DELLA CRESCITA. Il deficit isolato di GH (IGHD) è causato da anomalie del recettore del GHRH, dei geni dell'ormone della crescita e dei geni localizzati sul cromosoma X (Tab. 558-2).

Recettore del GHRH. Mutazioni recessive della perdita di funzione nel recettore del GHRH interferiscono con la proliferazione di cellule somatotrope durante lo sviluppo ipofisario e interrompono i segnali più importanti per il rilascio di GH. L'ipofisi anteriore si presenta piccola, in accordo con l'osservazione che le cellule somatotrope normalmente rappresentano più del 50% del volume ipofisario. La crescita fetale, diminuita, è seguita da grave deficit dello sviluppo postnatale.

GH1. Il gene GH1 è uno del gruppo di 5 geni sul cromosoma 17q22-24. Questo gruppo derivava da successive duplicazioni di un gene capostipite del GH. Un *crossing-over* diseguale durante la meiosi produce una varietà di delezioni del gene. Piccole delezioni (<10 kb) rimuovono solo il gene *GH1*, mentre quelle ampie (45kb) rimuovono uno o più geni adiacenti (*CSL*, *CS1*, *GH2*, *CS2*). Il fenotipo di crescita è identico con sola delezione *GH1* o delezioni multiple di uno o più geni adiacenti. La perdita di *CS1*, *GH2* e *CS2* senza perdita di *GH1* provoca deficit di somatomammotropina corionica e di GH placentare nella circolazione materna ma non comporta ritardo della crescita fetale o postnatale. Bambini omozigoti per delezioni del gene *GH1* rispondono bene alla terapia con GH.

TABELLA 558-2. Classificazione eziologica della carenza o dell'insensibilità isolata al GH

GENE O POSIZIONE	FENOTIPO		EREDITARIETÀ
DEFICIT DI GH			
Recettore del GHRH	IGHD, piccola IA	Basso GH, Basso IGF-I	R
GH1	IGHD, piccola o normale IA	Basso GH, Basso IGF-I	R, D
GH1	GH biologicamente inattivo	Alto GH, Basso IGF-I	D
BTK (Xq21.3-q22)	IGHD, ipogammaglobulinemia	Basso GH, Basso IGF-I	AX
SOX3 (Xq27.1)	IGHD, RM	Basso GH, Basso IGF-I	AX
INSENSIBILITÀ AL GH			
Recettore del GH	Variabile GHBP	Alto GH, Basso IGF-I	R, D
STAT5b	Immunodeficienza	Alto GH, basso IGF-I	R
IGF-I	IUGR, RM, sordità	Alto GH, Basso IGF-I	R
Subunità acido-labile	Statura lievemente inferiore alla norma	GH Normale, Basso IGF-I	R
Recettore dell'IGF-I	IUGR	Alto GH, Alto IGF-I	

IA, ipofisi anteriore; D, dominante; IPE, ipofisi posteriore ectopica; IGHD, *Isolated Growth Hormone Deficiency* (carenza isolata di ormone della crescita); IUGR, *Intrauterine Growth Retadation* (ritardo di crescita intrauterina); RM, ritardo mentale; R, recessivo; AX, associato a X.

Mutazioni nel gene *GH1* trasmesse con ereditarietà recessiva producono un fenotipo simile. Sono descritte mutazioni missense, nonsense e frameshit. La più comune coinvolge il quarto e l'ultimo introne del gene. Queste mutazioni eliminano il normale *splice donor site* e promuovono l'uso di un sito alternativo. L'mRNA abnorme codifica una proteina più lunga di quella normale, priva di attività biologica.

Anche la IGHD autosomica dominante è dovuta a mutazioni di *GH1*. Le mutazioni normalmente coinvolgono errori di *splice site* nell'introne 3. Si verifica iperproduzione di una proteina 20-kd, priva degli aminoacidi normalmente codificati a livello dell'esone 3. L'accumulo di questa proteina interferisce con l'elaborazione, l'immagazzinamento e la secrezione della normale proteina GH 22-kd. Sono noti ulteriori deficit di TSH e/o ACTH come complicanze tardive in pazienti con mutazioni dominanti in *GH1*.

La bassa statura da GH biologicamente inattivo è caratterizzata da livelli di GH circolante da normali ad alti, se si utilizza un dosaggio immunologico, ma da livelli di GH più bassi se si utilizza l'analisi della proliferazione cellulare, del legame col recettore o dell'attivazione del recettore. Un esempio ben documentato presenta un bambino omozigote per mutazione missense del gene *GH1*. La sostituzione della glicina al posto della normale serina in posizione 53 previene la formazione di un ponte disolfuro tra il residuo 53 e quello 165. La molecola mutante possiede un'attività subnormale nella funzione immunitaria, di legame con il recettore e di attivazione della via di segnalazione Jak2/Stat5. Il trattamento con ormone della crescita produce un aumento dei livelli di IGF-I e del ritmo di crescita, con raggiungimento di una statura adulta normale.

IGHD associata a X. Due loci sul cromosoma X sono stati associati a ipopituitarismo. Il primo si trova a livello di Xq21.3-q22 nella regione del gene della timidina chinasi di Bruton (*BTK*). Mutazioni di questa regione producono **ipogammaglobulinemia** e IGHD. Il secondo locus si trova più lontano sul braccio lungo, a livello Xq24-q27.1, una regione che contiene il gene del fattore di trascrizione SOX2. Anomalie in questo locus sono state associate a IGHD con ritardo mentale e a MPHD con la triade costituita da ipolplasia ipofisaria, mancanza del peduncolo ipofisario, ed ectopia dell'ipofisi posteriore.

Forme acquisite. L'asse del GH è più suscettibile a patologie acquisite rispetto agli altri assi ipotalamo-ipofisari. Fra le cause di deficit acquisito di GH si ricordano: radioterapia in caso di tumore, meningite, istiocitosi e trauma.

Bambini sottoposti a radioterapia per tumori del SNC o per prevenire infiltrazione del SNC (leucemia) corrono il rischio di sviluppare un deficit di GH. L'irradiazione della colonna contribuisce a una crescita scarsa e sproporzionata del tronco, indipendentemente dalla situazione del GH. La crescita rallenta tipicamente durante la radioterapia o la chemioterapia, migliora per 1-2 anni e in seguito declina con il manifestarsi del deficit di GH. La dose e la frequenza della radioterapia sono importanti fattori determinanti dell'ipopituitarismo. Il deficit di GH è quasi universale 5 anni dopo la terapia con una dose totale ≥35 Gy. Dosi intorno ai 20 Gy comportano difetti più lievi. Il deficit di GH è il difetto più comune, ma si può verificare anche carenza di TSH e ACTH. Diversamente da altre forme di ipopituitarismo, la pubertà tende a essere precoce piuttosto che ritardata. I medici in genere incontrano questi bambini verso gli 8-10 anni, mentre stanno crescendo a una velocità normale per età cronologica ma subnormale per lo stadio di sviluppo puberale.

INSENSIBILITÀ ALL'ORMONE DELLA CRESCITA

ANOMALIE DEL RECETTORE DELL'ORMONE DELLA CRESCITA. L'insensibilità all'ormone della crescita è causata da un'alterazione distale alla via di produzione del GH. La sindrome di Laron implica mutazioni del recettore del GH. I bambini con questa malattia assomigliano, da un punto di vista clinico, a quelli con CIGH grave. Alla nascita la lunghezza tende a essere 1 DS inferiore rispetto alla media e, a un anno di età, si evidenzia una grave bassa statura con altezza inferiore di più di 4 DS alla media. I livelli basali e dopo stimolo di GH tendono a essere elevati, mentre sono bassi quelli di IGF-I. Il recettore del GH possiede un dominio extracellulare che lega il GH, un dominio transmembrana, e un dominio di segnalazione intracellulare. Mutazioni nel dominio extracellulare interferiscono con il legame del GH. L'attività della proteina legante l'ormone della crescita (GHBP) sierico, che rappresenta la forma circolante del recettore di membrana del GH, è generalmente bassa. Mutazioni nel dominio transmembrana possono interferire con la fissazione del recettore alla membrana plasmatica. In questi casi l'attività della GHBP circolante è normale o aumentata. Mutazioni nel dominio intracellulare interferiscono con la segnalazione JAK/STAT.

FORME POST-RECETTORIALI DI INSENSIBILITÀ AL GH. Alcuni bambini con grave deficit di crescita, alti livelli di GH e bassi di IGF-I e con normali valori di GHBP presentano anomalie distali al legame e all'attivazione del recettore del GH. In diversi casi si sono trovate mutazioni nel trasduttore del segnale della codificazione del gene e nell'attivatore della trascrizione 5b (STAT5b). L'alterazione di questa chiave intermedia che comunica l'attivazione del recettore per la trascrizione genica comporta un deficit di crescita analogo a quello della sindrome di Laron. Questi pazienti inoltre soffrono di infezioni polmonari croniche, dato il ruolo importante di STAT5b nella segnalazione di interleuchine e citochine.

ANOMALIE DEL GENE IGF-I. Anomalie del gene IGF-I producono un grave deficit di crescita sia prenatale sia postnatale. In pazienti con delezione dell'esone e mutazione missense sono presenti microcefalia, ritardo mentale e sordità. È probabile che questi pazienti rispondano al trattamento con IGF-I ricombinante.

ANOMALIE DELLA PROTEINA LEGANTE-IGF. Una mutazione del gene che codifica la subunità acido-labile del 165-kdIGF-I circolante e il complesso della subunità acido-labile IGF-BP3 si associa a bassa statura. I livelli di IGF-I totale sono molto bassi. Nel caso di omozigosi per mutazione ALS, non si evidenzia incremento dei livelli di IGF-I o incremento della velocità di crescita durante il trattamento con GH.

ANOMALIE DEL GENE DEL RECETTORE IGF-I. Anche mutazioni del recettore IGF-I compromettono la crescita prenatale e postnatale. Il fenotipo è meno grave rispetto a quello da assenza di IGF-I. L'altezza in età adulta è più vicina al range di normalità e gli individui affetti non manifestano ritardo mentale o sordità.

MANIFESTAZIONI CLINICHE

IPOPITUITARISMO CONGENITO. Il bambino ipopituitarico è normalmente di dimensioni e peso normali alla nascita, sebbene quelli con MPHD e difetti genetici del gene *GH1* o *GHR* abbiano una lunghezza alla nascita di 1 DS inferiore alla media. A 1 anno di età, bambini con gravi difetti della produzione o dell'azione del GH sono inferiori di 4 DS alla media. Quelli con deficit meno gravi crescono a una velocità inferiore del 25% per l'età e gradualmente si allontanano dai normali percentili di altezza. La chiusura ritardata delle epifisi permette la crescita oltre l'età in cui normalmente è ultimata.

I neonati con difetti congeniti dell'ipofisi o dell'ipotalamo manifestano normalmente emergenze neonatali, come apnea, cianosi o **grave ipoglicemia** con o senza crisi epilettiche. Nei ragazzi, la presenza di **micropene** costituisce ulteriore indizio diagnostico. La carenza di GH può accompagnarsi a ipotiroidismo e iposurrenalismo. È frequente un ittero prolungato, dovuto a incremento della bilirubina coniugata e non coniugata, che può essere confuso con un'**epatite neonatale**.

Nel bambino molto piccolo la testa è rotonda e la faccia corta e larga; l'osso frontale è prominente e la radice del naso, depressa, presenta una tipica forma a sella. Il naso è piccolo e le pieghe nasolabiali appaiono ben sviluppate; gli occhi sono un po' sporgenti; la mandibola e il mento sono iposviluppati e i denti, a iruzione tardiva, sono frequentemente stipati. Si evidenziano inoltre brevità del collo e ipoplasia laringea. Il tono della voce è alto e rimane tale dopo la pubertà. Gli arti sono ben proporzionati, con mani e piedi piccoli. Il peso solitamente è normale in rapporto all'altezza, ma si ha nel complesso un aspetto sovrappeso per eccesso di tessuto adiposo e carenza di massa muscolare. I genitali sono di solito piccoli per l'età e la maturazione sessuale può essere ritardata o assente. I peli facciali, ascellari e pubici normalmente sono scarsi e i capelli fini. È compromessa soprattutto l'altezza, che conferisce a questi bambini un aspetto grassottello. Nel 10-15% dei bambini con panipopituitarismo e in quelli con IGHD compare ipoglicemia sintomatica, in genere postprandiale. L'intelligenza è di solito normale.

IPOPITUITARISMO ACQUISITO. Il bambino è inizialmente normale. Gradatamente compaiono manifestazioni simili a quelle dell'ipopituitarismo idiopatico, che via via progrediscono. Nei casi di distruzione completa o quasi dell'ipofisi, sono presenti segni di insufficienza pituitarica. L'atrofia di surrene, tiroide e gonadi è responsabile di perdita di peso, astenia, sensibilità al freddo, torpore mentale e assenza di sudorazione. Si evidenzia la mancata comparsa della maturazione sessuale o la sua regressione, se già presente. Ci può essere atrofia delle gonadi e del tratto genitale, con amenorrea e perdita dei peli pubici e ascellari. Si manifesta tendenza all'ipoglicemia. La crescita diminuisce drammaticamente. Può essere presente precocemente un diabete insipido, che tende però a migliorare spontaneamente in rapporto alla progressiva distruzione dell'anteipofisi.

Se la lesione è rappresentata da un **tumore in espansione**, si possono verificare sintomi come cefalea, vomito, disturbi visivi, modificazioni patologiche del sonno, calo della performance scolastica, crisi epilettiche, poliuria e deficit di crescita. Il rallentamento della crescita può anticipare i segni neurologici e i vari sintomi, specialmente in caso di craniofaringiomi, ma i sintomi da deficit ormonale ammontano solo a un 10% dei disturbi presenti. Dopo un intervento chirurgico si evidenziano per primi i segni di insufficienza ipofisaria. Nei bambini con craniofaringiomi sono comuni difetti del campo visivo, atrofia ottica, papilledema e paralisi di nervi cranici.

REPERTI DI LABORATORIO. Si sospetta una carenza di GH in bambini con deficit di crescita postnatale da moderato a grave. I criteri per l'insufficienza di crescita includono un'altezza inferiore dell'1% per età e sesso, o un'altezza più di 2 DS inferiore all'altezza media dei genitori, aggiustata in base al sesso. La carenza acquisita di GH si può verificare a qualsiasi età; nei casi a esordio acuto, l'altezza può essere nel range della normalità. Per la diagnosi ha grande importanza il sospetto clinico, perché le valutazioni di laboratorio, nel caso del GH, mancano di sufficiente specificità. Possono essere indicativi bassi livelli sierici di IGF-I e di IGF-BP3 GH-dipendente; i livelli di IGF-1 e di IGF-BP3 devono essere confrontati con i valori normali per età scheletrica piuttosto che cronologica. Si può effettivamente escludere una carenza di GH, in presenza di valori al limite superiore del range di normalità per età. I valori di IGF-I nei bambini con crescita normale e in quelli con ipopituitarismo si sovrappongono durante la prima infanzia e l'infanzia.

La **diagnosi definitiva** di deficit di GH richiede tradizionalmente la dimostrazione di una risposta scarsa o assente del GH ai test di stimolo. Ne sono utilizzabili vari, in grado di determinare un rapido incremento dei livelli di GH nei bambini normali, fra cui la somministrazione di insulina, arginina, clonidina o glucagone. Nei quadri da carenza cronica di GH, la dimostrazione di una crescita scarsa e lineare, l'età scheletrica ritardata e un picco dei livelli di GH (<10 ng/mL) in 2 successivi test di stimolo, sono compatibili con diagnosi di deficit di GH. Nelle forme acute, un forte sospetto clinico, e un basso picco dei livelli di GH (<10 ng/mL) in due successivi test di stimolo, indirizzano alla diagnosi di deficit di GH. Questo limite abbastanza arbitrario, è maggiore di 3 o 5 ng/mL rispetto a quello valido per la diagnosi di carenza di GH nell'adulto. La frequenza di risposte negative del GH a un singolo test standard, in bambini con crescita normale, è valutato intorno al 20%. Generalmente le analisi con anticorpi monoclonali sottostimano la concentrazione di GH rispetto a quelle con più precoci anticorpi policlonali. Non tutti gli Autori sono d'accordo su quali criteri adottare, tenendo conto dell'età, del genere e delle caratteristiche del dosaggio del GH. La stimolazione con GHRH di solito produce una risposta maggiore nei bambini con carenza di GH da disordini ipotalamici e non produce risposta in quelli con recettore GHRH, *GH1*, *POU1F1*, *PROP1* e mutazioni *LHX3*. La maggior parte dei bambini normali in fase prepubere non raggiunge valori di GH <10 ng/mL con 2 test farmacologici. Può essere necessario un carico estrogenico per 3 giorni prima che il test per il GH raggiunga una maggiore specificità diagnostica.

Nei trent'anni in cui l'HGH è stato ottenuto in sede autoptica dall'estrazione da cellule ipofisarie umane, le scorte erano nettamente limitate e si trattavano solo i pazienti con carenza classica di GH. Con l'avvento di scorte illimitate di GH ricombinante, si sono ridefiniti i criteri di carenza di GH, per includere anche bambini con deficit minori. Si valutava normalmente la secrezione spontanea di GH, misurando i suoi livelli ogni 20 minuti nell'arco di 24 o 12 ore (dalle 20.00 alle 8.00) Alcuni bambini di bassa statura con normali livelli basali di GH, se sottoposti a test di stimolo, mostrano una scarsa secrezione spontanea di GH. Si ritiene che questi bambini abbiano una **disfunzione della neurosecrezione di GH.** Tuttavia i frequenti dosaggi di GH mancano di specificità diagnostica. Il range di secrezione spontanea di GH in bambini con normale crescita prepubere è molto ampio, con notevole sovrapposizione dei valori rispetto a quelli osservati in bambini con classica carenza di GH. Mentre nei pazienti con ipopituitarismo grave (classico), sono ben chiari i criteri clinici e di laboratorio, per quelli di bassa statura, con deficit minori di GH, i criteri diagnostici sono invece incerti.

Oltre a stabilire la diagnosi di carenza di GH, è necessario esaminare le altre funzioni ipofisarie. Con il dosaggio dei livelli di TSH, tiroxina (T4), ACTH, cortisolo, gonadotropine e steroidi gonadici si possono evidenziare altri deficit ormonali ipofisari. In presenza di normale risposta alla somministrazione dei realising ipotalamici per TSH, ACTH, o gonadotropina, il difetto è localizzato a livello ipotalamico. In presenza di deficit di TSH, i livelli sierici di TSH e di T4 sono bassi. Un normale incremento di TSH e PRL dopo stimolazione con TRH depone per un danno ipotalamico, mentre l'assenza di risposta per uno ipofisario. Elevati livelli plasmatici di PRL in un paziente ipopituitarico sono significativi di un difetto ipotalamico piuttosto che ipofisario. Alcuni bambini con craniofaringiomi hanno alti livelli prechirurgici di PRL, ma, dopo l'intervento chirurgico, si instaura un deficit di PRL per danno ipofisario. Con adeguate valutazioni, può essere evidenziato un deficit di ormone antidiuretico.

REPERTI RADIOLOGICI. L'RX standard del cranio è stato sostituito dalla tomografia computerizzata e, in misura crescente, dalla risonanza magnetica. La TC è utile per valutare le calcificazioni soprasellari associate a craniofaringiomi e le erosioni ossee che accompagnano l'istiocitosi. La RM fornisce una proiezione più dettagliata dell'anatomia ipotalamica e ipofisaria. In molti casi di grave MPHD a esordio precoce, si evidenzia la triade: piccola ipofisi anteriore, peduncolo ipofisario assente o assottigliato e macchia brillante da ipofisi posteriore ectopica alla base dell'ipotalamo (Fig. 558-1). Nelle forme idiopatiche e genetiche di IGHD è frequente un'altezza dell'ipofisi anteriore inferiore alla norma, che indica una piccola adenoipofisi. Nei bambini con ipopituitarismo i craniofaringiomi sono frequenti, mentre sono rari gli adenomi ipofisari. In pazienti con mutazioni *PROP1* o *LHX3* sono frequenti sia l'ipoplasia sia il marcato ingrossamento dell'ipofisi anteriore.

La maturazione scheletrica è ritardata nei pazienti con IGHD e lo può essere ancora di più in presenza di deficit di GH associato a quello di TSH. L'assorbimetria a doppio raggio fotonico evidenzia carenza di mineralizzazione ossea, deficit di massa corporea magra e corrispondente incremento di tessuto adiposo.

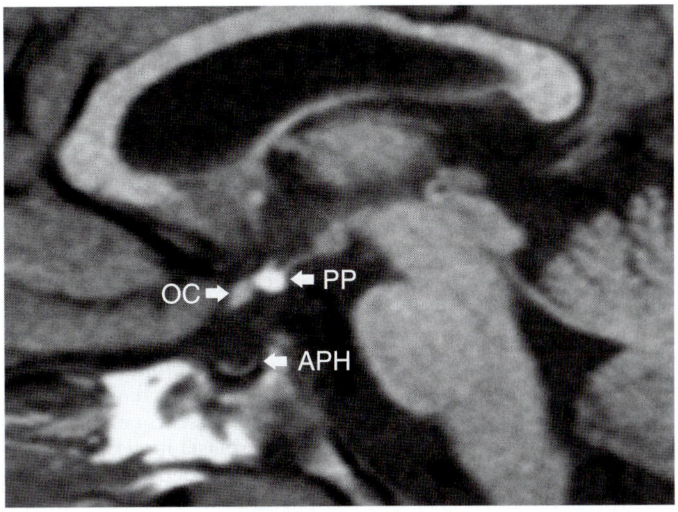

Figura 558-1. Una scansione sagittale RM mostra ipoplasia dell'ipofisi anteriore. APH, ipoplasia dell'ipofisi anteriore; OC, chiasma ottico (qui normale); PP, ipofisi posteriore (qui ectopica). Il peduncolo che connette l'ipofisi all'ipotalamo non è visibile. (Da Dattani MT, Prece M: Growth hormone deficiency and related disordes: Insights into causation, diagnosis, and treatment. *Lancet* 2004;363:1977-1986.)

DIAGNOSI DIFFERENZIALE. Numerose sono le cause di alterazioni della crescita (vedi Capitolo 37). Vanno prese in considerazione patologie sistemiche, come malattie infiammatorie intestinali, malattia celiaca, malattie renali occulte, e anemia. Pazienti con patologie sistemiche mostrano spesso un deficit del peso corporeo più marcato di quello dell'altezza. D'altronde, non pochi bambini normali presentano bassa statura (>3 DS rispetto alla media per età) e crescita annua uguale o inferiore a 5 cm, pur in presenza di normali livelli di GH dopo test di stimolo e normale secrezione episodica spontanea. La maggior parte di questi bambini mostra un aumento della velocità di crescita in corso di trattamento con GH a dosaggi paragonabili a quelli usati nella terapia dei bambini ipopituitarici. In questi pazienti i livelli plasmatici di IGF-I sono normali o bassi. Parecchi gruppi di bambini trattati hanno raggiunto un'altezza adulta normale o quasi. Studi diversi hanno evidenziato delle modificazioni nell'altezza definitiva comprese fra −2,5 e +7,5 cm, se confrontate con le previsioni pretrattamento. Non c'è la possibilità di predire correttamente quali fra questi bambini diventeranno più alti da adulti dopo trattamento con GH e quali invece presentano una compromissione dell'altezza definitiva.

Le strategie diagnostiche per differenziare una carenza permanente di GH da altre cause di alterazione della crescita sono incomplete. Bambini con una combinazione di bassa statura genetica e ritardo costituzionale della crescita presentano bassa statura, velocità di crescita inferiore alla media ed età ossea ritardata. Numerosi di questi individui evidenziano minime risposte secretorie di GH ai test di stimolazione. Bambini con diagnosi di carenza di GH idiopatica o acquisita, trattati con hGH e rivalutati da adulti, mostrano, nella maggioranza dei casi, un picco di livelli di GH nel range di normalità.

RITARDO COSTITUZIONALE DELLA CRESCITA. Il ritardo costituzionale della crescita è una variante comune della crescita normale. Le misurazioni di peso e altezza dei bambini colpiti sono normali alla nascita e la crescita risulta nella norma per i primi 4-12 mesi. L'altezza si mantiene a un percentile più basso durante l'infanzia. Lo *spurt* di crescita puberale è ritardato, così che la loro velocità di crescita continua a diminuire, mentre quella dei loro compagni di classe comincia ad accelerare. Un'anamnesi dettagliata spesso rivela altri familiari (frequentemente uno o entrambi i genitori) con problemi di bassa statura nell'infanzia, pubertà ritardata e statura finale normale. I livelli di IGF-I tendono a essere bassi per età cronologica ma nel range di normalità per età ossea. Le risposte dell'ormone della crescita ai test di stimolazione tendono a essere più basse rispetto ai bambini con un più tipico timing puberale. La prognosi circa la possibilità di normale statura da adulti, in questi bambini, richiede prudenza. Le previsioni basate sull'altezza e sull'età ossea tendono a sovrastimare l'eventuale altezza in misura maggiore nei maschi che nelle femmine. Ragazzi con ritardo puberale che supera i due anni beneficiano di un breve periodo di terapia con testosterone, per accelerare la pubertà dopo i 14 anni di età. Si ritiene che la causa di questa variante della normale crescita sia la persistenza di un relativo stato ipogonadotropo tipico dell'infanzia (vedi Capitolo 12).

IPOTIROIDISMO PRIMARIO. L'ipotiroidismo primario è più frequente della carenza di GH. La diagnosi viene stabilita sulla base dei bassi livelli di T4 totale o libero e degli alti livelli di TSH. La risposta al test di stimolo per il GH può essere scarsa e può essere presente un ampliamento della sella. L'iperplasia ipofisaria recede durante la terapia sostitutiva con ormoni tiroidei. Dato che l'ormone tiroideo costituisce un prerequisito necessario alla normale sintesi di GH, è sempre meglio valutarlo prima di dosare il GH.

DWARFISMO PSICOSOCIALE. La deprivazione emotiva è causa importante di ritardo della crescita e può mimare l'ipopituitarismo. Tale condizione è nota come dwarfismo psicosociale, dwarfismo da deprivazione materna o bassa statura iperfagica. Il meccanismo con cui la deprivazione sensoriale ed emotiva interferisce con la crescita non è completamente chiaro. La presenza di un ipopituitarismo funzionale è indicata da bassi livelli di IGF-I e da inadeguata risposta del GH ai test di stimolazione. La pubertà può essere normale o anche comparire precocemente. Un'anamnesi accurata e un'osservazione attenta rivelano il disturbo della relazione madre-figlio o di quella familiare e consentono la diagnosi (vedi Capitolo 37). Può risultare difficile avere le prove, perché i genitori, o comunque chi si occupa del bambino, spesso dissimulano la reale situazione familiare e di rado i bambini parlano della loro situazione. I bambini con deprivazione emotiva spesso manifestano appetito perverso o vorace, enuresi, encopresi, insonnia, accessi palesi, collere improvvise. Il sottogruppo di bambini con iperfagia e normale indice di massa corporea tende a recuperare il difetto di crescita se collocato in un ambiente meno stressante.

TRATTAMENTO. La Lawson Wilkins Pediatric Endocrine Society, l'Academy of Pediatrics e la GH Research Society hanno tutte pubblicato linee guida per il trattamento con hGH. Nei bambini con classica carenza di GH, il trattamento deve essere iniziato il prima possibile, per colmare il gap in altezza dei pazienti rispetto ai coetanei durante l'infanzia e per ottenere i risultati migliori in età adulta. Le dosi raccomandate di hGH sono, durante l'infanzia, di 0,18-0,3 mg/kg/settimana, mentre nella pubertà si utilizzano dosaggi maggiori. Si somministra GH ricombinante per via sottocutanea in 6-7 dosi refratte. La massima risposta al GH si ottiene nel primo anno di trattamento. La velocità di crescita in questo primo anno è tipicamente intorno al 95° percentile, ma tende a diminuire nei successivi anni di trattamento. Se la velocità di crescita scende al 25° percentile, prima di aumentare la dose, si deve valutare la sua compliance. Si utilizzano trattamenti combinati con GH e agonisti dell'LHRH nella speranza di interrompere la pubertà e, ritardando la chiusura epifisaria, prolungare la crescita. Questa strategia può incrementare la statura definitiva, ma anche la discrepanza tra la maturità fisica dei bambini con carenza di GH rispetto ai coetanei, e inoltre compromettere la mineralizzazione ossea. Si cerca di prevenire la chiusura epifisaria nei ragazzi utilizzando farmaci che inibiscono l'aromatasi, enzima responsabile della conversione degli androgeni in estrogeni. La terapia con ormone della crescita deve essere continuata fino in prossimità della statura finale. I criteri per sospendere la terapia comprendono la decisione del paziente, qualora si ritenga soddisfatto dell'altezza raggiunta, una velocità di crescita inferiore a 2,54 cm/anno e un'età ossea >14 anni nelle femmine e >16 nei maschi.

Alcuni pazienti, durante la terapia con GH, sviluppano anche un ipotiroidismo primario o centrale. Analogamente c'è il rischio di insufficienza surrenalica che, se non riconosciuta, può risultare fatale. Valutazioni periodiche della funzionalità tiroidea e surrenalica sono quindi raccomandate in tutti i pazienti in terapia con GH. Negli Stati Uniti l'IGF-I ricombinante è stato approvato per uso terapeutico. Si somministra per via sottocutanea 2 volte/die. Per ridurre il rischio di ipoglicemia si pratica l'iniezione in concomitanza del pasto o di uno spuntino. In certe situazioni, è risultato più efficace del GH in pazienti con anomalie del recettore del GH e dei geni *STAT5b*, e anche in pazienti con grave carenza di GH che abbiano sviluppato anticorpi antiGH. Si sta valutando la sua utilità nel migliorare la velocità di crescita e la statura finale in categorie più ampie di bambini con bassa statura.

Le dosi di GH usate per trattare bambini con classica carenza di GH migliorano normalmente la crescita anche di bambini privi di deficit di GH. Sono in corso vari studi per determinare la gamma completa di bambini che possono beneficiare del trattamento con GH. Negli Stati Uniti il GH è normalmente approvato per il trattamento del deficit di crescita in bambini con sindrome di Turner, stadio finale pretrapianto dell'insufficienza renale, sindrome di Prader Willi, deficit di crescita intrauterina e bassa statura idiopatica. Le ultime indicazioni riguardano un'altezza inferiore dell'1,2% (−2,25 DS) per età e sesso, un'altezza prevista inferiore al 5° percentile ed epifisi ancora aperte. Studi sugli effetti del trattamento con GH sull'altezza dell'adulto, suggeriscono un aumento medio di 5,08-7,62 cm, in base alla dose e alla durata del trattamento.

Nei bambini con MPHD, la terapia sostitutiva deve comprendere anche le altre carenze ormonali. Nei soggetti con deficit di TSH, si somministrano ormoni tiroidei a dosaggio sostitutivo completo. In quelli con carenza di ACTH, la dose ottimale di idrocortisone non deve superare i 10 mg/m^2/die. Si aumenta la dose in caso di malattie o nella preparazione a intervento chirurgico. In pazienti con carenza di gonadotropine, si somministrano steroidi gonadici se l'età ossea corrisponde a quella in cui normalmente inizia la pubertà. Per i neonati con microfallo, una terapia con cicli di 1-2-3 mesi di iniezioni intramuscolari mensili di 25 mg di testosterone cipionato o di testosterone enantato può portare a una normale dimensione del pene senza effetti indesiderati sulla maturazione ossea.

COMPLICANZE ED EFFETTI COLLATERALI DEL TRATTAMENTO CON HGH. Alcuni pazienti trattati con GH hanno sviluppato una leucemia. L'incremento del rischio è attribuibile ai bambini con fattori di rischio aggiuntivi, come irradiazione cranica. Il trattamento con ormone della crescita non aumenta il rischio di recidiva di tumori cerebrali o leucemia. Altri riportano effetti secondari tra cui *pseudotumor cerebri*, slittamento dell'epifisi capitale femorale, ginecomastia e peggioramento della scoliosi. Si verifica un aumento dell'acqua corporea totale durante le prime due settimane di terapia. I livelli prandiali e postprandiali di insulina sono caratteristicamente bassi prima del trattamento e si normalizzano durante la terapia sostitutiva con GH. La terapia non aumenta il rischio di diabete mellito di tipo 1, ma quello di tipo 2.

All'epoca del trattamento con GH di estrazione ipofisaria, c'era il rischio di comparsa della malattia di **Creutzfeldt-Jakob** (CK) per almeno 10-20 anni dopo la terapia e di anticorpi anti-GH: i pazienti che sviluppavano tali anticorpi diventavano resistenti al trattamento. L'utilizzo di GH ricombinante negli ultimi 20 anni ha eliminato il rischio di malattia CK e ha ridotto la formazione di anticorpi durante il trattamento.

Abuzzahabab MJ, Schneider A, Goddard A, et al: IGF-I receptor mutations resulting in intrauterine and postnatal growth retardation. *N Engl J Med* 2003;349:2211–2222.

Allen DB, Fost N: hGH for short stature: ethical issues raised by expanded access. *J Pediatr* 2004;144:648–652.

Amar AP, Weiss MH: Pituitary anatomy and physiology. *Neurosurg Clin North Am* 2003;14(1):11–23.

Badaru A, Wilson DM: Alternatives to growth hormone stimulation testing in children. *Trends Endocrinol Metab* 2004;15(6):252–258.
Besson A, Salemi S, Deladoey J, et al: Short stature caused by a biologically inactive mutant growth hormone. *J Clin Endocrinol Metab* 2005;90:2493–2499.
Carel JC, Ecosse E, Nicolino M, et al: Adult height after long term treatment with recombinant growth hormone for idiopathic isolated growth hormone deficiency: Observational follow up of the French population based registry. *Br Med J* 2002;25:70–73.
Committee on Drugs and Committee on Bioethics: Considerations related to the use of recombinant human growth hormone in children. *Pediatrics* 1997;99:122–129.
Dattani MT: Growth hormone deficiency and combined pituitary hormone deficiency: Does the genotype matter? *Clin Endocrinol* 2005;63:121–130.
Dattani MT, Preece M: Growth hormone deficiency and related disorders: Insights into causation, diagnosis, and treatment. *Lancet* 2004;363: 1977–1986.
Domene HM, Bengolea SV, Martinez AS, et al: Deficiency of the circulating insulin-like growth factor system associated with inactivation of the acid-labile subunit gene. *N Engl J Med* 2004;350:570–577.
Finkelstein BS, Imperiale TF, Speroff T, et al: Effect of growth hormone therapy on height in children with idiopathic short stature. *Arch Pediatr Adolesc Med* 2002;156:230–240.
Growth Hormone Research Society: Consensus guidelines for the diagnosis and treatment of growth hormone (GH) deficiency in childhood and adolescence: Summary statement of the GH Research Society. *J Clin Endocrinol Metab* 2000;85:3990–3993.
Hwa V, Little B, Adiyaman P, et al: Severe growth hormone insensitivity resulting from total absence of signal transducer and activator of transcription 5b. *J Clin Endocrinol Metab* 2005;90:4260–4266.
Kofoed EM, Hwa V, Little B, et al: Growth hormone insensitivity associated with a *STAT5b* mutation. *N Engl J Med* 2003;349:1139–1147.
Kojima M, Hosoda H, Date Y, et al: Grhelin is a growth-hormone releasing acylated peptide from stomach. *Nature* 1999;402:656–660.
Leschek EW, Rose SR, Yanovski JA, et al: Effect of growth hormone treatment on adult height in peripubertal children with idiopathic short stature: A randomized, double-blind, placebo-controlled trial. *J Clin Endocrinol Metab* 2004;89:3140–3148.
Rosenfeld RG, Rosenbloom AL, Guevara-Aguirre J: Growth hormone (GH) insensitivity due to primary GH receptor deficiency. *Endocrinol Rev* 1994;15:369–390.
Schmiegelow M, Lassen S, Weber L, et al: Dosimetry and growth hormone deficiency following cranial irradiation of childhood brain tumors. *Med Pediatr Oncol* 1999;33:564–571.
Traggiai C, Stanhope R: Endocrinopathies associated with midline cerebral and cranial malformations. *J Pediatr* 2002;140:252–255.
Woods KA, Camacho-Hubner C, Savage MO, et al: Intrauterine growth retardation and postnatal growth failure associated with deletion of the insulin-like growth factor gene. *N Engl J Med* 1996;35:1363–1367.
Yanovski JA, Rose SR, Municchi G, et al: Treatment with luteinizing hormone-releasing hormone agonist in adolescents with short stature. *N Engl J Med* 2003;348:908–917.

Capitolo 559 ■ Diabete insipido

David T. Breault e Joseph A. Majzoub

Il diabete insipido (DI) si manifesta clinicamente con poliuria e polidipsia e può essere provocato da carenza di vasopressina (DI centrale) o da insensibilità renale alla vasopressina (DI nefrogenico). Entrambi i tipi di DI, centrale e nefrogenico, possono derivare da difetti ereditari congeniti o a esordio neonatale oppure essere secondari a varie cause (Tab. 559-1).

FISIOLOGIA DEL BILANCIO IDRICO

Il controllo della tonicità extracellulare (osmolalità) e del volume all'interno di un range ristretto è fondamentale per una normale struttura e funzionalità cellulari (vedi Capitolo 52). La tonicità del liquido extracellulare viene regolata quasi esclusivamente dall'introduzione e dall'escrezione di acqua, mentre il volume extracellulare dipende dall'assunzione e dall'escrezione di sodio. Il controllo della tonicità plasmatica e del volume intravascolare richiede una completa integrazione di vari sistemi: endocrino, nervoso, comportamentale e paracrino (Fig. 559-1). La vasopressina, principale regolatore della tonicità, viene secreta dall'ipofisi posteriore in risposta a un aumento della tonicità plasmatica. L'omeostasi del volume è in gran parte regolata dal sistema renina-angiotensina-aldosterone, con il contributo della vasopressina e del peptide natriuretico.

La vasopressina, un peptide di 9 aminoacidi, che possiede attività antidiuretica e pressoria, è sintetizzata nei nuclei ipotalamici paraventricolare e sopraottico. Viene quindi trasportata per via assonica all'ipofisi posteriore, dove è immagazzinata in attesa del suo rilascio nella circolazione sistemica. L'emivita della vasopressina circolante è di 5 minuti. La vasopressina viene secreta, oltre che in risposta allo stimolo osmotico, anche per una significativa diminuzione del volume e della pressione intravascolari (per un decremento minimo dell'8%) tramite le vie afferenti dei barocettori dell'arco aortico (seno carotideo) e

TABELLA 559-1. Diagnosi differenziale di poliuria e polidipsia

DIABETE INSIPIDO (DI)
DI centrale
Genetico (autosomico dominante)
Acquisito
Trauma (chirurgico o accidentale)
Malformazioni congenite
Tumori
Patologie infiltrative, autoimmuni, infettive
Farmaci
DI nefrogenico
Genetico (collegato ad X, autosomico recessivo, autosomico dominante)
Acquisito
Ipercalcemia, ipocaliemia
Farmaci
Patologie renali
POLIDIPSIA PRIMARIA
DIABETE MELLITO

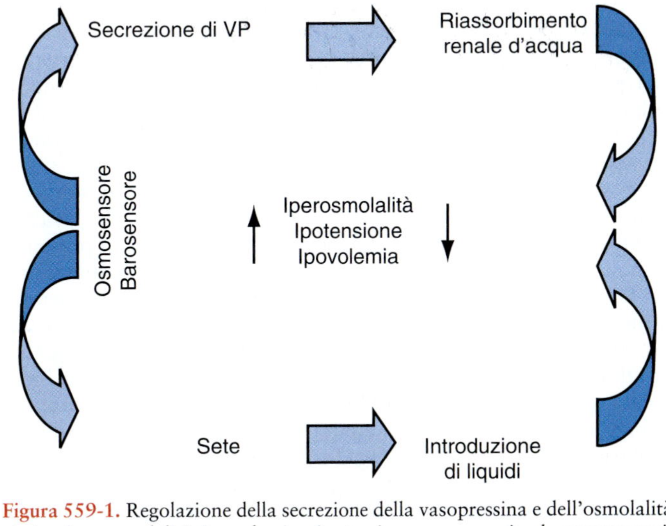

Figura 559-1. Regolazione della secrezione della vasopressina e dell'osmolalità sierica. Iperosmolalità, ipovolemia e ipotensione sono recepite da osmosensori, recettori di volume e barocettori, rispettivamente. Questi stimolano contemporaneamente la secrezione di vasopressina (VP) e la sete. La vasopressina, agendo a livello renale, provoca un aumento del riassorbimento di acqua (antidiuresi). La sete comporta un incremento dell'ingestione di acqua. I risultati di questi cicli a doppio feedback negativo provocano riduzione dell'iperosmolalità o ipotensione/ipovolemia. Stimoli ulteriori per la secrezione di vasopressina sono rappresentati da nausea, ipoglicemia e dolore. (Da Muglia LJ, Majzoub JA: Disorders of the posterior pituitary. In Sperling MA [editor] *Pediatric Endocrinology*, 2nd ed. Philadelphia, WB Saunders, 2002.)

dei recettori di volume situati a livello atriale e nelle vene polmonari. Le stimolazioni osmotiche ed emodinamiche agiscono quindi sinergicamente.

La sensazione della sete è regolata da neuroni corticali e ipotalamici. La soglia della sete è approssimativamente di 10 mOsm/kg (circa 293 mOsm/kg) maggiore di quella per il rilascio della vasopressina. Perciò, in condizioni di iperosmolalità, il rilascio della vasopressina precede l'inizio della sete, consentendo la ritenzione dell'acqua ingerita. I chemorecettori presenti nell'orofaringe agiscono rapidamente controregolando il rilascio di vasopressina dopo ingestione di acqua.

La vasopressina esercita i suoi effetti principali a livello renale, attraverso i recettori V2 localizzati principalmente nel tubulo collettore, il braccio ascendente dell'ansa di Henle a parete spessa, e nei tubuli periglomerulari. Il gene umano del recettore V2 è localizzato nel braccio lungo del cromosoma X (Xq28) a livello del locus associato a **diabete insipido congenito, vasopressina-resistente, collegato a X.** L'attivazione del recettore V2 comporta un incremento intracellulare di adenosina monofosfato ciclica, con conseguente introduzione del canale per l'acqua aquaporina-2 nella membrana apicale (luminale). Ciò permette il movimento dell'acqua lungo il suo gradiente osmotico dal lume tubulare all'interno dell'interstizio midollare ipertonico, con escrezione di urina concentrata. Al contrario dell'aquaporina-2, le aquaporine -3 e -4 sono espresse a livello della membrana basolaterale delle cellule del dotto collettore mentre l'aquaporina-1 nel tubulo prossimale. Questi canali contribuiscono inoltre alla capacità di concentrazione dell'urina.

Il **peptide natriuretico atriale** (PNA), inizialmente isolato dal muscolo cardiaco atriale, ha numerosi importanti effetti sull'equilibrio dell'acqua e dei sali, comprese la stimolazione della natriuresi, l'inibizione del riassorbimento del sodio e l'inibizione della secrezione di vasopressina. Il PNA viene espresso nelle cellule endoteliali e muscolari lisce vascolari, dove regola la vasodilatazione delle arterie. Il PNA viene inoltre espresso nel cervello, insieme ad altri composti della famiglia natriuretica, il cui ruolo non è stato ancora ben definito.

APPROCCIO AL PAZIENTE CON POLIURIA, POLIDIPSIA E IPERNATRIEMIA

Nei bambini può essere difficile stabilire la causa di poliuria e polidipsia patologiche (oltre i 2 L/m^2/24 ore). I bambini possono presentare irritabilità, deficit di sviluppo e febbre intermittente. Nei pazienti con sospetto DI è necessaria un'attenta anamnesi volta a quantificare l'introduzione e l'escrezione giornaliera di liquidi nel bambino e a stabilire il quadro minzionale, nicturia ed enuresi primaria o secondaria. Tramite un esame obbiettivo completo si deve verificare lo stato di idratazione del paziente, cercando inoltre segni di alterazioni visive e disfunzioni del sistema nervoso centrale o di carenza di altri ormoni ipofisari. In presenza di poliuria o polidipsia patologiche, è necessaria la valutazione dei seguenti parametri: osmolalità sierica, sodiemia, potassiemia, azoto ureico, glicemia, creatininemia e calcemia; mentre, a livello urinario, osmolalità, peso specifico e glicosuria. Si pone diagnosi di DI se l'osmolalità sierica risulta maggiore di 300 mOsm/kg e quella urinaria inferiore a 300 mOsm/kg. Un DI è invece improbabile se l'osmolalità sierica è inferiore a 300 mOsm/kg o quella urinaria supera 600 mOsm/kg. In presenza di osmolalità sierica minore di 300 mOsm/kg (ma maggiore di 270 mOsm/kg) e di poliuria e polidipsia patologiche, per porre diagnosi di DI e per differenziare la forma centrale da quella nefrogenica, è opportuno sottoporre il paziente al test da deprivazione di acqua.

Nel paziente postneurochirurgico, è probabile un DI qualora l'iperosmolalità (osmolalità sierica >300 mOsm/kg) sia associata a osmolalità urinaria minore di quella sierica. È molto importante differenziare una poliuria postchirurgica dovuta a DI centrale da una normale eliminazione di liquidi somministrati intraoperatoriamente. In entrambi i casi, può essere associato un notevole volume (>200 mL/m^2/ora) di urina diluita, nonostante in pazienti con DI l'osmolalità sierica sia alta in rapporto a quella di pazienti sottoposti a diuresi postoperatoria.

559.1 • CAUSE DI IPERNATRIEMIA (VEDI CAPITOLO 52.3)

DIABETE INSIPIDO CENTRALE

Il diabete insipido centrale può derivare da cause diverse: mutazioni genetiche del gene della vasopressina, trauma (accidentale o chirurgico) dei neuroni produttori di vasopressina, malformazioni congenite ipotalamiche o ipofisarie, tumori, patologie infiltrative, autoimmuni e infettive dei neuroni produttori di vasopressina o del peduncolo e un incremento del metabolismo della vasopressina. In circa il 10% dei bambini con DI centrale, l'eziologia rimane idiopatica. Possono essere presenti deficit di altri ormoni ipofisari (vedi Capitolo 558).

Il DI centrale autosomico dominante si presenta normalmente entro i primi 5 anni di vita e dipende da mutazioni del gene della vasopressina. Numerose mutazioni possono essere responsabili di difetti del processing del gene nel gruppo di neuroni per l'espressione della vasopressina. Anche la **sindrome di Wolfram** (che comprende DI, diabete mellito, atrofia ottica e sordità) deriva da deficit di vasopressina. Si è identificato il gene di questo disturbo, ma la sua funzione è ancora sconosciuta. Varie anomalie cerebrali congenite, come la **displasia setto-ottica** con agenesia del corpo calloso, la sindrome di Kabuki, l'oloprosencefalia e l'ipoplasia ipofisaria familiare con assenza del peduncolo, possono essere associate a DI centrale e a difetti nella percezione della sete. Anche la sindrome da "sella vuota", forse da infarto ipofisario non riconosciuto, nei bambini si può associare a DI.

Cause comuni di DI centrale sono un trauma (della base del cervello) e un intervento neurochirurgico (nella regione ipotalamica o ipofisaria). La **risposta postchirurgica** ha un tipico andamento **trifasico** che comprende una fase iniziale di DI transitorio, della durata variabile dalle 12 alle 48 ore, seguita da una seconda fase con sindrome da inappropriata secrezione di ormone antidiuretico, che si protrae fino al decimo giorno, la quale può quindi essere seguita da DI permanente. La fase iniziale può dipendere da edema locale che interferisce con la normale secrezione di vasopressina; la seconda fase risulta da un rilascio incontrollato di vasopressina da parte dei neuroni necrotici, mentre nella terza fase si verifica DI permanente qualora sia distrutto più del 90% dei neuroni.

Data la particolare distribuzione anatomica dei neuroni secernenti vasopressina in una vasta area ipotalamica, i tumori responsabili di DI devono essere molto voluminosi e infiltrati o essere localizzati strategicamente in prossimità della base dell'ipotalamo, dove convergono gli assoni contenenti vasopressina prima dell'ingresso nell'ipofisi posteriore. Tipici di questa regione sono germinomi e pinealomi, tra i più comuni tumori cerebrali primitivi associati a DI. I germinomi possono essere molto piccoli e non identificabili con RM per parecchi anni dopo l'inizio della poliuria. Nei bambini con DI idiopatico o non spiegabile, in aggiunta alle indagini seriali di RM, si può effettuare il dosaggio della subunità β della gonadotropina corionica umana, spesso secreta da germinomi e pinealomi. I craniofaringiomi e i gliomi ottici, se molto voluminosi, possono provocare DI centrale, sebbene quest'ultimo sia più frequente come loro complicanza postchirurgica. Neoplasie ematologiche, come la leucemia mielocitica acuta, possono provocare DI attraverso un'infiltrazione del peduncolo ipofisario e della sella.

L'istiocitosi a cellule di Langherans e l'ipofisite linfocitica sono due tipi comuni di patologie infiltrative responsabili di DI centrale. L'**ipofisite** è causa del 50% dei casi di DI centrale "idiopatico". Le infezioni che interessano la base del cervello, compresa la meningite (meningococcica, criptococcica, da listeria, da toxoplasma), l'infezione congenita da Cytomegalovirus e la patologia infiammatoria cerebrale non specifica possono provocare DI centrale, spesso transitorio. Le sostanze in grado di inibire il rilascio della vasopressina comprendono l'etanolo, la fentoina, gli antagonisti degli oppiacei, l'alotano e agenti α-adrenergici.

DIABETE INSIPIDO NEFROGENICO

Il DI nefrogenico (vasopressina-insensibile) (DIN) insorge per cause genetiche o acquisite. Le cause genetiche sono meno comuni, ma più gravi rispetto a quelle acquisite. Nel DIN genetico, la poliuria e la polidipsia compaiono di solito entro le prime settimane di vita, ma diventano evidenti dopo lo svezzamento o quando si instaurano lunghi periodi di sonno notturno. Molti neonati manifestano inizialmente febbre, vomito e disidratazione. Il deficit di sviluppo può essere secondario all'ingestione di notevoli quantità di acqua, che comportano malnutrizione calorica. L'ingestione e l'escrezione protratte di notevoli volumi di acqua può portare a idronefrosi non ostruttiva, idrouretere e megavescica.

Il **DIN congenito associato a X** deriva da mutazioni inattivanti del recettore V2 della vasopressina. Il **DIN congenito autosomico recessivo** dipende da difetti del gene dell'aquaporina-2. Una **forma autosomica dominante di DIN** è associata a mutazioni del processing del gene dell'aquaporina-2.

Il DI nefrogenico può dipendere da ipercalcemia o ipocaliemia o dall'utilizzo dei seguenti farmaci: litio, demeclociclina, foscarnet, clozapina, amfotericina, meticillina, rifampicina. Si osserva compromissione della capacità renale di concentrare l'urina anche in presenza di ostruzione ureterale, insufficienza renale cronica, malattia policistica del rene, malattia midollare cistica, sindrome di Sjogren e anemia a cellule falciformi. Una diminuzione dell'ingestione proteica o sodica oppure un'eccessiva introduzione di acqua, come nella polidipsia primaria, possono comportare decremento della tonicità dell'interstizio midollare renale e DI nefrogenico.

TRATTAMENTO DEL DIABETE INSIPIDO CENTRALE

TERAPIA CON LIQUIDI. In presenza di integrità del meccanismo della sete e di libero accesso all'introduzione orale di liquidi, un paziente con DI completo può riuscire a mantenere l'osmolalità e il sodio plasmatici ai limiti alti del range della normalità, nonostante notevoli fastidi. Nei neonati e nei bambini molto piccoli si preferisce spesso una terapia esclusivamente liquida, data la loro necessità di notevoli quantità di liquidi nutritivi (3 L/m^2/24 ore). L'utilizzo di analoghi della vasopressina è in questi casi controindicato, per il rischio di grave iponatremia.

Analoghi della vasopressina. Nei bambini più grandi, per il trattamento del DI centrale, è preferibile l'uso di analoghi della vasopressina a lunga durata, come la dDAVP (desmopressina). La dDAVP è disponibile in una preparazione per uso endonasale (inizio 5-10 min) e in compresse (inizio 15-30 min). La preparazione endonasale di dDAVP (10 μg/0,1 mL) può essere somministrata con un sondino nasale (permettendo la titolazione della dose) o con uno spray. La dose appropriata viene stabilita empiricamente in base alla durata desiderata dell'azione antidiuretica. Lo spray nasale eroga 10 μg (0,1 mL) e rappresenta la preparazione standard nel trattamento dell'enuresi primaria dei bambini più grandi. La terapia dell'enuresi con dDAVP costituisce un provvedimento transitorio, in quanto non incide sulla condizione sottostante e deve perciò essere utilizzato con cautela. Per prevenire l'intossicazione da acqua, il paziente dovrebbe avere almeno un'ora di pausa urinaria tra una dose e l'altra nell'arco della giornata. Sono disponibili anche le compresse di dDAVP, ma richiedono una dose almeno dieci volte maggiore rispetto a quella utilizzata per la somministrazione per via endonasale. Dosaggi orali compresi fra 25 e 300 μg ogni 8-12 ore sono sicuri ed efficaci nei bambini.

Vasopressina in soluzione acquosa. Si preferisce trattare il DI centrale postchirurgico a insorgenza acuta, con la somministrazione continua di vasopressina sintetica in soluzione acquosa (pitressina). Nella maggior parte dei casi, l'introduzione complessiva di liquidi durante l'azione antidiuretica si dovrebbe limitare a 1 L/m^2/24 ore. Un tipico dosaggio della terapia con vasopressina per via endovenosa è 1,5 mU/kg/ora, che corrisponde a una concentrazione di circa 10 pg/mL. In certi casi, per un DI acuto conseguente a intervento di chirurgia ipotalamica (ma non transfenoidale), possono essere necessarie concentrazioni iniziali maggiori per il rilascio di una sostanza che inibisce la secrezione di vasopressina. Si devono evitare concentrazioni di vasopressina superiori a 1000 pg/mL per il rischio di necrosi cutanea, rabdomiolisi e disturbi del ritmo cardiaco. In pazienti postchirurgici trattati con infusioni di vasopressina, si deve passare dalla somministrazione endovenosa a quella orale di liquidi il prima possibile, per consentire la ripresa della sensazione della sete, se intatta, allo scopo di favorire la regolazione dell'osmolalità.

TRATTAMENTO DEL DIABETE INSIPIDO NEFROGENICO

Il trattamento del DIN acquisito si focalizza, se possibile, sull'eliminazione del disordine di base, come sostanze dannose, ipercalcemia, ipocaliemia o ostruzione ureterale, mentre è più complesso trattare un diabete insipido nefrogenico congenito. L'obiettivo principale è garantire l'introduzione di una quantità adeguata di calorie necessarie alla crescita e di evitare una grave disidratazione. Si devono preferire gli alimenti a più alto contenuto calorico per carico osmotico (Na <1 mmol/kg/24 ore), per massimizzare la crescita e minimizzare la quantità di urina necessaria a eliminare il carico di soluti. Tuttavia, anche instaurando precocemente la terapia, sono comuni deficit di crescita e ritardo mentale.

L'approccio farmacologico al trattamento del DIN comprende l'utilizzo dei diuretici tiazidici, che tendono a diminuire la diuresi complessiva. Sembra che i tiazidici inducano una modesta deplezione del volume urinario per un aumento dell'eliminazione sodica a spese dell'acqua e un decremento della percentuale di filtrazione glomerulare, che comporta riassorbimento tubulare prossimale di acqua e di sodio. Indometacina e amiloride si possono utilizzare in associazione ai tiazidici per diminuire più rapidamente la poliuria. In alcuni soggetti con DIN si sono usate alte dosi di dDAVP, in associazione a indometacina, utili in pazienti con difetti genetici nel recettore V2, associati a ridotta affinità di trasporto per la vasopressina.

Knoers N, Monnens LH: Nephrogenic diabetes insipidus: Clinical symptoms, pathogenesis, genetics and treatment. *Pediatr Nephrol* 1992; 6:476–482.

Maghnie M, Cosi G, Genovese E, et al: Central diabetes insipidus in children and young adults. *N Engl J Med* 2000; 343:988–1007.

Muglia LJ, Majzoub JA: Disorders of the posterior pituitary. In Sperling MA (editor): *Pediatric Endocrinology*, 2nd ed. Philadelphia, WB Saunders, 2002.

Capitolo 560 ■ Altre anomalie del metabolismo e dell'azione dell'arginina-vasopressina

David T. Breault e Joseph A. Majzoub

Nei bambini l'iposodiemia (sodio plasmatico <130 mEq/L) è normalmente associata a gravi malattie sistemiche ed è più frequentemente dovuta a (1) deplezione del volume intravascolare, (2) eccessiva perdita di sali o (3) sovraccarico di liquidi ipotonici, specialmente nei lattanti (vedi Capitolo 52). La sindrome da inappropriata secrezione di ormone antidiuretico (SIADH, *Syndrome of Inappropriate Antidiuretic Hormone*) è raramente causa di iposodiemia nei bambini.

L'approccio iniziale al paziente iposodiemico prevede la valutazione del volume plasmatico. Un'attenta revisione anamnestica, comprese variazioni di peso corporeo, un esame obiettivo e segni vitali aiutano a determinare se il paziente è ipo o ipervolemico. Ulteriori indagini comprendono gli esami di laboratorio con elettroliti sierici, azotemia, creatininemia, uricemia, sodiuria, peso specifico e osmolalità urinari (vedi Capitolo 52.3) (Tabb. 560-1 e 560-2).

CAUSE DI IPOSODIEMIA

SINDROME DI INAPPROPRIATA SECREZIONE DI ORMONE ANTIDIURETICO. La SIADH è caratterizzata da iposodiemia, inappropriata concentrazione urinaria (>100 mOsm/kg), volume plasmatico normale o modicamente aumentato, da normo a ipersodiuria e ipouricemia. La SIADH non è frequente nei bambini, in cui la maggior parte dei casi è dovuta a eccessiva somministrazione di vasopressina per il trattamento del diabete insipido centrale. Si può accompagnare anche a encefalite, tumori cerebrali, trauma cranico, patologia psichiatrica, periodo postictale dopo crisi epilettiche generalizzate, dopo nausea prolungata, polmonite, meningite tubercolare e AIDS. La SIADH è causa della seconda fase iposodiemica della risposta trifasica dopo intervento ipotalamo-ipofisario (vedi Capitolo 559). In più del 35% dei pazienti, a circa una settimana dall'intervento chirurgico, si può verificare una degenerazione neuronale con necrosi cellulare e conseguente rilascio di vasopressina. Farmaci comuni possono incrementare la secrezione di vasopressina o mimarne l'azione, con conseguente iposodiemia, e fra di essi oxcarbazepina, carbamazepina, clorpropamide, vinblastina, vincristina e antidepressivi triciclici.

SINDROME NEFROGENICA DA INAPPROPRIATA ANTIDIURESI (NSIAD, *NEPHROGENIC SYNDROME OF INAPPROPRIATE ANTIDIURESIS*). Sono state descritte mutazioni con aumento di funzione nel gene del recettore V2 della vasopressina, in due neonati maschi con quadro clinico simile a quello della SIADH e livelli indosabili di vasopressina. Anche mutazioni attivanti nel gene aquaporina-2 possono portare allo stesso risultato, anche se, per ora, non sono ancora ben descritte.

DISIDRATAZIONE SISTEMICA. Le manifestazioni iniziali di disidratazione sistemica sono rappresentate spesso da ipersodiemia e iperosmolalità, che successivamente stimolano la secrezione di vasopressina e diminuiscono l'eliminazione di acqua. Mano a mano che la disidratazione progredisce, l'ipovolemia e/o l'ipotensione diventano stimolo maggiore per il rilascio di vasopressina, ma in seguito diminuisce la clearance dell'acqua libera. L'escrezione urinaria del sodio è bassa (normalmente <10 mEq/L) a causa del basso tasso di filtrazione glomerulare e concomitante attivazione del sistema renina-angiotensina-aldosterone, eccetto che nella patologia renale primaria o in pazienti sottoposti a terapia diuretica.

PERDITA DI SALI. L'iposodiemia può essere dovuta a perdita primaria di cloruro di sodio, come in specifiche malattie renali (malattia policistica renale congenita, nefrite acuta interstiziale, insufficienza renale cronica), del tratto gastrointestinale, (gastroenterite) e delle ghiandole sudoripare (fibrosi cistica). L'iposodiemia non è dovuta solamente alla perdita di sali, perché quest'ultima provoca anche ipovolemia, con conseguente incremento della vasopressina. La carenza di mineralcorticoidi, lo pseudoipoaldosteronismo (talvolta in bambini con ostruzione o infezione delle vie urinarie) e i diuretici possono portare a deplezione di cloruro di sodio.

DIMINUZIONE DEL VOLUME PLASMATICO EFFETTIVO. L'iposodiemia può derivare da diminuzione effettiva del volume plasmatico, come nell'insufficienza cardiaca congestizia, nella cirrosi, nella sindrome nefrotica, nella ventilazione meccanica a pressione positiva, nelle ustioni gravi, nella displasia broncopolmonare dei neonati, nella fibrosi cistica con ostruzione e nell'asma di grado severo. Il conseguente decremento della gittata cardiaca comporta una diminuzione dell'escrezione di acqua e sali, come nella disidratazione sistemica, e un aumento della secrezione di vasopressina. Nei pazienti con alterazione della gittata cardiaca e ipertrofia atriale (insufficienza cardiaca congestizia, patologia polmonare), le concentrazioni di peptide natriuretico atriale sono più elevate, con conseguente iposodiemia da ipersodiuria. Questi pazienti normalmente presentano un'eliminazione urinaria di sodio molto scarsa. Diversamente dai pazienti disidratati, queste persone possono presentare un eccesso di sodio corporeo totale, per attivazione del sistema renina-angiotensina-aldosterone, ed edemi periferici.

POLIDIPSIA PRIMARIA (AUMENTATA INGESTIONE DI ACQUA). In pazienti con funzione renale normale, il rene è in grado di eliminare urina diluita con osmolalità pari a 50 mOsm/kg. Per espellere un carico giornaliero di soluti di 500 mOsm/m^2, il rene deve produrre 10 L/m^2/die di urina. Tuttavia, per evitare l'iposodiemia, il consumo giornaliero massimo di acqua, per un individuo con normale funzionalità renale, è di 10 L/m^2. I neonati, però, non sono in grado di diluire le urine fino a questo punto, correndo il rischio di un'intossicazione da acqua se l'assunzione della stessa supera i 4 L/m^2/die (approssimativamente 60 mL/ora in un neonato). Molti neonati sviluppano crisi epilettiche iposodiemiche transitorie ma sintomatiche se alimentati con acqua pura priva di elettroliti, piuttosto che con latte materno o in polvere.

DIMINUZIONE DELLA CLEARANCE DELL'ACQUA LIBERA. L'iposodiemia dovuta a diminuzione della clearance renale dell'acqua libera, anche in assenza di un incremento della secrezione di vasopressina, può dipendere da insufficienza surrenalica, ipotiroidismo, o dall'effetto diretto di alcuni farmaci sul rene. Per una normale clearance dell'acqua libera sono necessari, indipendentemente dalla vasopressina, sia i mineralcorticoidi sia i

TABELLA 560-1. Diagnosi differenziale dell'iposodiemia

MALATTIA	STATO DEL VOLUME INTRAVASCOLARE	SODIO URINARIO
Disidratazione sistemica	Basso	Basso
Diminuzione significativa del volume plasmatico	Basso	Basso
Perdita di sali primaria	Basso	Basso
Perdita di sali cerebrale	Basso	Molto alto
SIADH	Alto	Alto
Diminuzione della clearance dell'acqua libera	Normale o alto	Normale o alto
Polidipsia primaria	Normale o alto	Normale
Iponatremia dei corridori	Basso	Basso
NSIAD	Alto	Alto
Pseudoiposodiemia	Normale	Normale
Iposodiemia fittizia	Normale	Normale

NSIAD, *Nephrogenic Syndrome of Inappropriate Antidiuresis* (sindrome da inappropriata antidiuresi); SIADH, *Syndrome of Inappropriate Antidiuretic Hormone Secretion* (inappropriata secrezione di ormone antidiuretico).

TABELLA 560-2. Parametri clinici per differenziare SIADH, sindrome da perdita di sali per cause cerebrali e diabete insipido centrale

PARAMETRI CLINICI	SIADH	PERDITA DI SALI CEREBRALE	DI CENTRALE
Sodio sierico	Basso	Basso	Alto
Eliminazione urinaria	Normale o bassa	Alta	Alta
Sodio urinario	Alto	Molto alto	Basso
Stato del volume intravascolare	Normale o alto	Basso	Basso
Acido urico sierico	Basso	Normale o alto	Alto
Livello di vasopressina	Alto	Basso	Basso

glicocorticoidi. In pazienti con iposodiemia idiopatica si devono quindi ricercare un'insufficienza surrenalica o tiroidea. Inoltre pazienti con insufficienza surrenalica e diabete insipido possono non avere sintomi di quest'ultimo fino a che la terapia con glicocorticoidi smaschera la necessità di una sostituzione con vasopressina. Certi farmaci possono inibire l'escrezione dell'acqua attraverso un'azione diretta sul nefrone, con conseguente iponatremia; questi farmaci comprendono alte dosi di ciclofosfamide, vinblastina, cisplatino e carbamazepina.

SINDROME DA PERDITA DI SALI DI ORIGINE CEREBRALE. La sindrome da perdita di sali di origine cerebrale è il risultato di una ipersecrezione del peptide natriuretico atriale e si verifica principalmente nelle malattie del sistema nervoso centrale, compresi tumori cerebrali, trauma cranico, idrocefalo, neurochirurgia, accidenti vascolari cerebrali e morte encefalica. L'iposodiemia si accompagna a elevata sodiuria (spesso >150 mEq/L), poliuria, ipovolemia, iper o normouricemia, soppressione della vasopressina ed elevate concentrazioni di peptide natriuretico atriale (>20 pmol/L). Si distingue in questo modo dalla SIADH, caratterizzata da diuresi normale o diminuita, normovolemia, ipouricemia, modesta ipersodiuria ed elevati livelli di vasopressina. La distinzione tra sindrome da perdita di sali di origine cerebrale e SIADH è importante, dal momento che il trattamento, nelle due patologie, è completamente diverso.

IPOSODIEMIA DEI CORRIDORI. Un eccesso di ingestione di liquidi durante le corse su lunghe distanze (maratoneti) può portare a grave iposodiemia da attivazione, ipovolemia-indotta, della secrezione di AVP, unita a eccessiva ingestione di acqua, ed è correlata a una competizione di lunga durata, aumento di peso e variazioni estreme dell'indice di massa corporea.

PSEUDOIPOSODIEMIA E ALTRE CAUSE DI IPOSODIEMIA. La pseudoiposodiemia può essere dovuta a ipertrigliceridemia (vedi Capitolo 52). Elevati livelli lipidici comportano una relativa diminuzione del contenuto sierico di acqua. Poiché gli elettroliti sono disciolti nella fase acquosa del siero, essi sembrano bassi se espressi come frazione del volume sierico totale. Il contenuto elettrolitico è tuttavia normale, se espresso come frazione dell'acqua sierica. Un'iposodiemia fittizia si può verificare qualora si prelevi sangue da una sede prossimale al punto di infusione endovenosa di liquido ipotonico.

L'iposodiemia si associa anche a iperglicemia, che provoca ingresso di acqua nello spazio intravascolare. Il sodio sierico diminuisce di 1,6 mEq/L per ogni 100 mg/dL di aumento della glicemia oltre i 100 mg/dL. Il glucosio di solito non è un agente osmoticamente attivo e non stimola il rilascio di vasopressina, probabilmente perché si riequilibra spontaneamente attraverso le membrane plasmatiche. In presenza di carenza insulinica e iperglicemia, tuttavia, il glucosio si comporta come agente osmotico, presumibilmente perché il suo normale accesso intracellulare è prevenuto da siti osmosensori. In queste circostanze si viene a creare un gradiente osmotico che stimola il rilascio di vasopressina.

TRATTAMENTO DELL'IPOSODIEMIA

Pazienti con disidratazione sistemica e ipovolemia possono essere reidratati con liquidi e sali, come una normale soluzione fisiologica o la soluzione Ringer lattato. In virtù dell'attivazione del sistema renina-angiotensina-aldosterone, si verifica una ritenzione di sodio con diuresi acquosa, non appena si ripristina il volume e diminuiscono le concentrazioni di vasopressina. In queste condizioni, si deve usare una certa cautela per prevenire una correzione troppo rapida dell'iposodiemia, che può essere responsabile di mielinosi pontina centrale, caratterizzata da demielinizzazione assonica in ampie regioni, con potenziale danno cerebrale irreversibile.

L'iposodiemia da effettiva ipovolemia per problemi cardiaci, epatici, renali o polmonari è più difficile da trattare. Il trattamento della patologia di base è la terapia più efficace, anche se quella meno facilmente applicabile. Per esempio, pazienti cui è stata sospesa la ventilazione a pressione positiva, rapidamente mostrano diuresi acquosa e risoluzione dell'iposodiemia, cioè non appena si ripristina la gettata cardiaca e diminuiscono le concentrazioni di vasopressina.

Pazienti con iponatremia da perdita primaria di sali richiedono una terapia supplementare con cloruro di sodio e liquidi. Inizialmente, può essere necessario il ripristino per via endovenosa del volume perso con le urine, con liquidi contenenti cloruro di sodio, alla dose di 150-450 mEq/L, a seconda dell'entità della perdita di sali; successivamente si passa a una supplementazione per via orale. Questo trattamento contrasta con quello della SIADH, che si basa sulla restrizione di acqua senza supplementazione di sodio.

TRATTAMENTO DI EMERGENZA DELL'IPOSODIEMIA. L'evoluzione dell' iposodiemia acuta (esordio <12 ore) o della sodiemia inferiore a 120 mEq/L, si può associare a letargia, psicosi, coma o crisi epilettiche generalizzate, specialmente nei bambini più piccoli. L'iposodiemia acuta può provocare un aumento del volume cellulare e disfunzioni neuronali o ernia cerebrale. Il trattamento di emergenza dell'alterazione cerebrale da iponatremia acuta prevede la restrizione di acqua e può richiedere correzione rapida con infusione di soluzione salina ipertonica al 3%. Dopo l'inizio della terapia, la sodiemia dovrà aumentare solo fino al livello necessario a migliorare la situazione psichica, e mai più di 0,5 mEq/L/ora o 12 mEq/L/24 ore.

TRATTAMENTO DELLA SIADH. La SIADH cronica viene trattata nel modo migliore con la restrizione orale di liquidi. Con antidiuresi completa (osmolalità urinaria di 1000 mOsm/kg) un normale carico renale giornaliero obbligato di soluti di 500 mL/m^2 dovrà essere escreto in 500 mL/m^2 di acqua. Questo, più la perdita extrarenale di liquidi di 500 mL/m^2, richiede una limitazione dell'ingestione orale di liquidi a 1 L/m^2/24 ore, per evitare iponatremia. Nei bambini piccoli, l'entità della restrizione orale di liquidi può non consentire l'introduzione di un numero di calorie adeguato per la crescita. In questi casi può essere indicata la creazione di un diabete insipido nefrogenico utilizzando la demeclociclina, in modo da consentire un introito di liquidi sufficiente per la crescita. Il conivaptan, un antagonista del recettore V2, diminuisce la permeabilità del dotto collettore all'acqua, producendo un'adeguata *aquaresis* (aumento di volume delle urine senza perdita di sodio). Esso è efficace nel trattamento della SIADH dell'adulto.

TRATTAMENTO DELLA PERDITA DI SALI DI ORIGINE CEREBRALE. Il trattamento dei pazienti con perdita di sali cerebrale consiste nel ripristinare il volume intravascolare con acqua e cloruro di sodio, come nelle altre condizioni di disidratazione sistemica. Si devono trattare, se possibile, anche le cause alla base del problema, normalmente dovuto a lesione cerebrale acuta. La terapia richiede la continua sostituzione delle perdite di sodio urinarie (volume per volume).

Albanese A, Hindmarsh P, Stanhope R: Management of hyponatremia in patients with acute cerebral insults. *Arch Dis Child* 2001;85:246–251.

Almond CS, Shin AY, Fortescue EB, et al: Hyponatremia among runners in the Boston Marathon. *N Engl J Med* 2005;352:1550–1556.

Feldman BJ, Rosenthal SM, Vargas GA, et al: Nephrogenic syndrome of inappropriate antidiuresis. *N Engl J Med* 2005; 352:1884–1890.

The Medical Letter: Conivaptan (Vaprisol) for hyponatremia. *Med Lett* 2006;48:51–52.

Muglia LJ, Majzoub JA: Disorders of the posterior pituitary. In Sperling MA (editor): *Pediatric Endocrinology,* 2nd ed. Philadelphia, WB Saunders, 2002.

Capitolo 561 ■ Iperpituitarismo, alta statura e sindromi da crescita eccessiva

Pinchas Cohen e Melanine Shim

IPERPITUARISMO

L'**ipersecrezione primaria** di ormoni ipofisari, rara nei bambini, è di solito la conseguenza di un adenoma ipofisario. L'iperpituitarismo primario non deve essere confuso con l'iperpituitarismo **secondario**, che è una conseguenza di diminuito feedback per specifiche carenze ormonali, come nell'ipogonadismo, nell'iposurrenalismo o nell'ipotiroidismo. In alcuni casi, l'ipersecrezione ormonale di lunga durata è accompagnata da iperplasia ipofisaria con ampliamento, erosione sellare e, raramente, ipertensione endocranica. Gli elevati livelli di ormoni ipofisari inibiscono prontamente la normale successiva sostituzione degli ormoni degli organi bersaglio. L'iperplasia ipofisaria può essere secondaria a stimolazione ectopica di ormoni ipotalamici, come si è visto nel caso di un paziente con sindrome di Cushing secondaria a ipersecrezione dell'ormone di rilascio della corticotropina, o in bambini con acromegalia secondaria alla stimolazione da parte dell'ormone di rilascio del GH (GHRH), prodotto da vari tumori sistemici.

L'adenoma più frequente durante l'infanzia è il prolattinoma, seguito dal corticotropinoma e infine dal somatotropinoma, che producono rispettivamente prolattina, corticotropina e ormone della crescita. Nei bambini sono noti numerosi casi di tireotropinoma, mentre non esistono dati pediatrici riguardo al gonadotropinoma. Per la natura monoclonale della maggior parte degli adenomi ipofisari, è implicito che quasi tutti originano da un evento clonale in una singola cellula. Si ritiene che alcuni tumori ipofisari possano dipendere da stimolazione con ormoni di rilascio ipotalamici, e in altri casi, come nella sindrome di McCune-Albright, il tumore sia causato da una mutazione attivante costitutiva del gene $G_S\alpha$ della proteina-G. La presentazione clinica dipende tipicamente dall'ormone ipofisario ipersecreto. Sono comuni alterazioni della crescita e/o della maturazione sessuale, come risultato dell'ipersecrezione di entrambi gli ormoni, o di compressione locale da parte del tumore.

ALTA STATURA

La normale distribuzione dell'altezza comporta che il 2,5% della popolazione diventi più alto di 2 DS (97,5%) rispetto alla media. Tuttavia, l'accettazione sociale e anche il desiderio di essere alti (gigantismo) rendono l'alta statura un disagio non comune. Nel Nord America è decisamente inusuale, per i maschi, la richiesta di aiuto in relazione a una statura eccessiva, mentre in Europa è più frequente. Per le femmine l'alta statura è diventata più accettabile da un punto di vista sociale, nonostante ragazze molto alte possano, ancora oggi, desiderare di limitare il loro tasso di crescita.

DIAGNOSI DIFFERENZIALE DELL'ALTA STATURA. La Tabella 561-1 elenca le cause di alta statura nell'infanzia e nell'adolescenza. Fra queste, la variante normale, l'alta statura familiare o costituzionale, è di gran lunga la causa più comune. Quasi invariabilmente è presente un'anamnesi familiare positiva per alta statura, in assenza di patologie organiche. Il bambino è spesso alto per tutta l'infanzia e gode di salute eccellente. I genitori di un adolescente costituzionalmente alto possono riflettere il loro disagio in quanto ragazzi alti ai tempi dell'adolescenza. Non presentano anomalie all'esame obiettivo e anche gli esami di laboratorio, quando presenti, sono sempre negativi.

La **sindrome di Klinefelter (sindrome XXY)** è una patologia comune (1:500-1000 nati maschi) associata ad alta statura, lieve ritardo mentale, ginecomastia e basso rapporto tra il segmento superiore e inferiore del corpo. I testicoli sono costantemente piccoli nonostante la produzione androgenica da parte delle cellule di Leidyg sia spesso ai livelli bassi del range di normalità. Sono alterate la spermatogenesi e la funzionalità delle cellule del Sertoli, con conseguente sterilità. La **sindrome XYY** è associata ad alta statura e a possibili problemi comportamentali e mentali. La **sindrome di Marfan** è una patologia del tessuto connettivo autosomica dominante, caratterizzata da alta statura, aumento dell'estensione delle braccia e diminuzione del rapporto tra segmento superiore e inferiore del corpo (vedi Capitolo 700). Possono essere presenti inoltre aracnodactilia, problemi oculari e alterazioni cardiache. L'**omocistinuria** è un errore congenito, autosomico recessivo, del metabolismo degli aminoacidi, che provoca, se non trattata, ritardo mentale. Parecchie delle sue caratteristiche assomigliano a quelle della sindrome di Marfan, soprattutto le manifestazioni oculari (vedi Capitolo 85). L'ipertiroidismo negli adolescenti è associato a rapida crescita, ma normale statura da adulto. È quasi sempre causato dalla malattia di Graves ed è molto più comune nelle femmine (vedi Capitolo 569). L'obesità esogena è una condizione comune negli adolescenti e può essere associata a rapida crescita lineare con maturazione precoce; l'altezza da adulti però è tipicamente normale.

TABELLA 561-1. Diagnosi differenziale dell'alta statura e delle sindromi da crescita eccessiva

ECCESSIVA CRESCITA FETALE
Diabete mellito materno
Gigantismo cerebrale (sindrome di Sotos)
Sindrome di Weaver
Sindrome di Beckwith-Wiedemann
Altre sindromi da eccesso di IGF-II
ECCESSIVA CRESCITA POSTNATALE CON ALTA STATURA NELL'INFANZIA
Alta statura familiare (costituzionale)
Gigantismo cerebrale
Sindrome di Beckwith-Wiedemann
Obesità esogena
Ipersecrezione di GH (gigantismo ipofisario)
Sindrome di McCune-Albright o MEN associata a ipersecrezione di GH
Pubertà precoce
Sindrome di Marfan
Sindrome di Klinefelter (XXY)
Sindromi da eccesso di SHOX
Sindrome di Weaver
Sindrome dell'X fragile
Omocistinuria
XYY
Ipertiroidismo
ECCESSIVA CRESCITA POSTNATALE CON ALTA STATURA NELL'ADULTO
Alta statura familiare (costituzionale)
Carenza di androgeni o estrogeni/resistenza agli estrogeni (nei maschi)
Femminilizzazione testicolare
Carenza/resistenza di ACTH/cortisolo
Ipersecrezione di GH (gigantismo ipofisario)
Sindrome di Marfan
Sindrome di Klinefelter (XXY)
XYY

ACTH, *Adrenocorticotropic Hormone* (ormone corticotropo); GH, *Growth Hormone* (ormone della crescita); IGF, *Insulin-like Growth Factor* (fattore di crescita insulino-simile).

Lo scopo della valutazione diagnostica dell'alta statura è quello di distinguere le diverse e frequenti varianti costituzionali normali dalle rare condizioni patologiche. Spesso, quando l'anamnesi è suggestiva per alta statura familiare e l'esame obiettivo è completamente normale, non sono necessari ulteriori esami di laboratorio. È importante disporre di una radiografia per l'età ossea, che serve per prevedere l'altezza da adulti e come base per la discussione con la famiglia e per eventuali decisioni circa la gestione del caso. Se, tuttavia, l'anamnesi è indicativa di qualcuna delle patologie sopra menzionate o se l'esame obiettivo rivela delle anomalie, si devono eseguire ulteriori test di laboratorio. Per l'ipersecrezione di GH, sono esami di screening eccellenti il fattore-I di crescita insulino-simile (IGF-I) e la proteina-3 che lega IGF (IGFBP-3), valutabili con un test di soppressione al glucosio. L'evidenza laboratoristica di un eccesso di GH autorizza la valutazione dell'ipofisi con RM. L'analisi cromosomica viene utilizzata nei maschi, specialmente in presenza di una diminuzione del rapporto tra segmento superiore e inferiore del tronco o di ritardo mentale. Se l'esame obiettivo pone il sospetto di sindrome di Marfan o di omocistinuria, può essere richiesta una consulenza cardiologia e oculistica. Quando si sospetta un ipertiroidismo, l'esecuzione dei test di funzionalità tiroidea possono confermare o meno la diagnosi.

La **pubertà precoce**, sia centrale (aumento della secrezione di gonadotropine) sia periferica (aumentata secrezione di androgeni, estrogeni, o di entrambi), porta inizialmente a una accelerazione lineare della crescita durante l'infanzia, che mima lo *spurt* puberale. Poiché è accelerata anche la maturazione scheletrica, l'altezza da adulto è solitamente compromessa. La valutazione diagnostica e il trattamento della pubertà precoce sono discussi altrove in questo testo.

Sebbene la pubertà ritardata possa essere associata nell'infanzia a bassa statura, come con il ritardo costituzionale, il ritardo della pubertà e della completa maturazione sessuale può comportare un proseguimento della crescita durante l'età adulta, con alta statura finale. Il dato di alta statura con epifisi aperte, dovuto a mutazione del recettore estrogenico in un maschio con normale maturazione sessuale di tipo maschile, sottolinea il ruolo fondamentale degli estrogeni nel promuovere la chiusura epifisaria, ponendo fine alla normale crescita scheletrica. Una carenza di aromatasi porta ad alta statura con analogo meccanismo. Inoltre, l'insensibilità agli androgeni è associata, nelle femmine, ad alta statura, dimostrando un ruolo degli androgeni in questo processo.

TRATTAMENTO DELL'ALTA STATURA. La rassicurazione della famiglia e dei pazienti è la chiave del trattamento dell'alta statura come variabile normale. L'utilizzo dell'età ossea per prevedere l'altezza da adulto può dare un certo conforto, così come la rassicurazione sull'accettazione sociale di questa condizione. Il trattamento di ragazze e ragazzi con crescita eccessiva deve essere ristretto ai pazienti con (1) altezza prevista da adulto maggiore di 3 DS rispetto alla media (198,12 cm nei maschi, 180,34 cm nelle femmine) e (2) significativo disagio psicosociale. Se la famiglia è molto motivata al trattamento, si può considerare un trial con ormoni steroidei. La terapia si propone di accelerare la pubertà e la chiusura epifisaria ed è quindi di scarso aiuto in caso di pubertà ritardata; inoltre, essa va iniziata possibilmente in epoca prepubere o in caso di pubertà precoce. Nei ragazzi, il trattamento deve iniziare prima che l'età ossea raggiunga i 14 anni; si utilizza il testosterone enantato alla dose di 500 mg im ogni 2 settimane per 6 mesi. Nelle femmine gli estrogeni per via orale a dosaggi vari sono efficaci nel ridurre l'altezza prevista in media di 5-10 cm. Questo è un risultato diretto dei noti effetti degli steroidi sessuali nel promuovere la chiusura epifisaria; la terapia deve iniziare, tuttavia, prima che l'età ossea raggiunga i 12 anni. Nelle ragazze si usa con successo l'etinil-estradiolo orale alla dose di 0,15-0,5 mg/die fino alla fine della crescita. Se necessario, si può aggiungere un progestinico dopo un anno di sola terapia estrogenica. Gli effetti collaterali a breve termine del trattamento con estrogeni per l'alta statura comprendono: irregolarità mestruali, aumento di peso, nausea, dolore agli arti, galattorrea, patologia mammaria benigna, colelitiasi, ipertensione e trombosi. Come potenziale complicanza a lungo termine, in fasi successive della vita, si può presentare una riduzione della fertilità. La mancanza di vasta esperienza con questo tipo di terapia e i rischi connessi, richiede, prima di cominciare, un'attenta valutazione e la discussione con la famiglia.

Il meccanismo dell'azione estrogenica comprende effetti sulla produzione di GH e di IGF e a livello epifisario. Gli estrogeni mediano la chiusura epifisaria sia nei maschi sia nelle femmine. Se si comincia la terapia in ragazze prepuberi, si nota che l'altezza da adulte è inferiore di 5-6 cm rispetto alle previsioni pretrattamento. Quando la terapia invece viene iniziata dopo l'avvio della pubertà, il decremento nell'altezza definitiva non è così notevole.

Nei ragazzi con alta statura la terapia è meno problematica. Gli estrogeni sono probabilmente i più efficaci nell'accelerare la chiusura epifisaria, ma non sono ovviamente utilizzabili nei maschi. Anche gli androgeni accelerano la maturazione scheletrica, presumibilmente attraverso l'aromatizzazione in estrogeni, ma si associano a virilizzazione.

PROLATTINOMA

Gli adenomi ipofisari prolattina-secernenti sono i tumori più comuni dell'ipofisi durante l'adolescenza (vedi Capitolo 497). Con l'avvento della RM, si riescono a identificare molti di questi tumori, soprattutto i microadenomi (<1cm). I segni con cui si manifestano più frequentemente sono cefalea, amenorrea e galattorrea. La malattia colpisce le femmine con frequenza doppia rispetto ai maschi; la maggior parte delle pazienti ha avuto una normale pubertà prima di diventare sintomatica. Solo poche presentano pubertà ritardata. In alcuni congiunti con neoplasia endocrina multipla di tipo I (*Multiple Endocrine Neoplasia,* MEN), i prolattinomi sono una caratteristica tipica dell'adolescenza.

I livelli di prolattina possono essere moderatamente (40-50 ng/mL) o marcatamente (10 000-15 000 ng/mL) aumentati. La maggior parte dei prolattinomi nei bambini è voluminosa (macroadenomi) e provoca un ampliamento sellare e in alcuni casi difetti del campo visivo. Circa 1/3 dei pazienti con macroadenomi sviluppa ipopituitarismo, in particolare deficit di GH. In alternativa, gli adenomi prolattina-secernenti possono anche mostrare un'ipersecrezione di GH e/o di TSH.

I prolattinomi non devono essere confusi con l'iperprolattinemia e con l'iperplasia ipofisaria, che si verificano in pazienti con ipotiroidismo primario, facilmente trattato con ormone tiroideo (vedi Capitolo 556). Un aumento moderato di prolattina (<200 ng/mL) si può associare all'assunzione di vari farmaci, a disfunzione del peduncolo ipofisario, a craniofaringioma e ad altre condizioni benigne. Il trattamento della maggior parte dei bambini consiste nella resezione chirurgica per via transfrontale o transfenoidale. Nella maggior parte dei pazienti il prolattinoma può essere trattato efficacemente anche da un punto di vista medico con bromocriptina o cabergolina a lunga durata d'azione. Circa l'80% dei pazienti adulti risponde con una diminuzione del tumore e un marcato decremento dei livelli sierici di prolattina.

CORTICOTROPINOMA

In ambito pediatrico i corticotropinomi sono gli adenomi più comuni prima della pubertà, sebbene facciano la loro comparsa a tutte le età. La **malattia di Cushing** configura specificamente un adenoma ipofisario ACTH-secernente, che stimola l'ipersecrezione di cortisolo. Al momento della diagnosi, gli adenomi responsabili della malattia di Cushing sono significativamente più piccoli degli altri tipi di adenomi. L'indicatore più sensibile dell'ipersecrezione di glicocorticoidi nei bambini è il deficit di crescita, che generalmente precede le altre manifestazioni. I pazienti presentano un aumento del peso corporeo, più spesso centripeto che generalizzato, e sono comuni, inoltre, arresto della pubertà, astenia e depressione.

La chirurgia transfenoidale è il trattamento di elezione per la malattia di Cushing nei bambini. Si riportano remissioni iniziali nel 70-98% dei pazienti e successi a lungo termine nel 50-98% dei casi. Si osserva spesso, dopo l'intervento, un iposurrenalismo transitorio residuo, che può persistere fino a 30 mesi.

IPERSECREZIONE DI ORMONE DELLA CRESCITA E GIGANTISMO IPOFISARIO

Nei giovani con epifisi aperte, l'iperproduzione di GH comporta **gigantismo**, mentre in pazienti con epifisi chiuse acromegalia. Spesso alcune caratteristiche dell'**acromegalia** sono presenti nel gigantismo, anche nei bambini e negli adolescenti. Dopo la chiusura epifisaria le caratteristiche acromegaliche diventano più evidenti.

Il gigantismo ipofisario è raro, più spesso provocato da un adenoma ipofisario, ma è noto un caso di gigantismo in un bambino di 2 anni e mezzo con tumore ipotalamico, presumibilmente GHRH-secernente. Altri tumori, per esempio quelli nell'ambito della MEN, soprattutto a livello pancreatico, provocano acromegalia per ipersecrezione di GHRH con conseguente iperplasia delle cellule somatotrope. La caratteristica clinica principale del gigantismo è l'accelerazione della crescita staturale per l'ipersecrezione di GH. Il quadro clinico comprende lineamenti facciali grossolani con ingrandimento di mani e piedi. Nei bambini piccoli, la rapida crescita della testa può precedere quella staturale. Alcuni pazienti presentano problemi comportamentali e visivi. Nella maggior parte dei casi riportati, la crescita anomala diventa evidente alla pubertà, ma si riporta il caso di un bambino con esordio precoce nel periodo neonatale e di un altro al ventunesimo mese di età. Raramente si riporta nel gigantismo una crescita in altezza superiore a 243,48 cm. Le **caratteristiche acromegaliche** consistono principalmente in un allargamento delle porzioni distali del corpo, anche se altre parti possono essere coinvolte nella crescita abnorme: aumenta la circonferenza del cranio, il naso diventa largo e la lingua è spesso ingrossata, con alterazione dei lineamenti del viso. Anche la crescita mandibolare è eccessiva e i denti si distanziano. Sono comuni alterazioni del campo visivo e anomalie neurologiche, più tardivamente compaiono segni di ipertensione endocranica. Le dita delle mani e dei piedi aumentano soprattutto in larghezza, ci può essere cifosi dorsale e sintomi precoci sono rappresentati da astenia e debolezza. I livelli di GH sono elevati e possono occasionalmente superare i 100 ng/mL. Normalmente non si ottiene soppressione dei livelli di GH con iperglicemia o con il test da carico di glucosio. I livelli di IGF-I e di IGFBP-3 sono molto elevati nell'acromegalia, mentre non altrettanto lo sono altri fattori di crescita.

Il gigantismo è raro, con solo un centinaio di casi riportati. L'esordio del gigantismo è di solito drammatico, diversamente dall'esordio insidioso dell'acromegalia nell'adulto. La stessa massa tumorale può essere responsabile di cefalea, modificazioni visive da compressione del nervo ottico e ipopituitarismo. Circa la metà dei pazienti presenta anche una marcata iperprolattinemia come risultato di adenomi plurisecernenti, che producono GH e prolattina. Ciò è dovuto al fatto che le cellule mammosomatotrope sono il più comune tipo di cellule GH-secernenti coinvolte nel gigantismo infantile. I tumori ipofisari GH-secernenti sono di solito adenomi eosinofili o cromofobi. Gli adenomi possono compromettere altre funzioni dell'ipofisi anteriore per espansione o per degenerazione cistica. Si può verificare una diminuzione della secrezione di gonadotropine, tireotropina o corticotropina. Ci può essere ritardo della maturazione sessuale o ipogonadismo. Quando l'ipersecrezione di GH si accompagna a deficit gonadotropinico, una crescita accelerata in altezza può persistere per decadi. In alcuni casi, il tumore si espande in sede sovrasellare, coinvolgendo lo sfenoide, il nervo ottico e il cervello. In pediatria, i tumori GH-secernenti sono più localmente invasivi o aggressivi che nell'adulto.

L'eziologia è incerta, sebbene studi sugli acromegalici suggeriscano, in molti casi, mutazioni che comportano la presenza di proteine-G attivate, con riduzione dell'attività della GTPasi. La conseguenza è un aumento dell'adenosina monofosfato ciclica intracellulare ipofisaria e incremento della secrezione di GH. La **sindrome di McCune-Albright** (MAS), causata da mutazioni con conseguenti proteine-G attivate, può comprendere anche tumori a cellule somatotrope con ipersecrezione di GH. Circa il 20% dei pazienti con gigantismo presenta MAS (che consiste comunemente nella triade: pubertà precoce, macchie caffellatte, displasia fibrosa). I tumori GH-secernenti sono stati descritti nelle adenomatosi endocrine multiple e in associazione a neurofibromatosi, sclerosi tuberosa e complesso di Carney.

Mutazioni attivanti delle proteine stimolanti $G_s\alpha$ sono state trovate in lesioni ipofisarie nell'ambito della MAS, e si ritengono responsabili di altri adenomi ghiandolari osservati in questa condizione. Mutazioni somatiche puntiformi della proteina $G_s\alpha$ sono state identificate nelle cellule somatotrope di più del 40% degli adenomi ipofisari sporadici GH-secernenti.

DIAGNOSI DI ECCESSO DI ORMONE SOMATOTROPO. L'elemento diagnostico chiave nell'eccesso di GH è la mancata soppressione dei livelli sierici di GH a valori inferiori a 5 ng/dL dopo somministrazione orale di glucosio alla dose di 1,75 g/kg (fino a un massimo di 75 g). Questo test valuta la capacità dell'IGF-I di sopprimere la secrezione di GH in quanto il glucosio stimola la secrezione di insulina, con conseguente soppressione di IGFBP-I e incremento acuto dei livelli di IGF-I libero. L'aumento di IGF-I libero inibisce la secrezione di GH entro 30-90 minuti. Questo test può essere alterato in pazienti diabetici. Una singola misurazione di GH risulta inadeguata, perché viene secreto in modo pulsatile e può dare esito a risultati falsamente positivi o falsamente negativi. La valutazione della concentrazione sierica di IGF-I è un test di screening sensibile per eccesso di GH, in quanto è stata dimostrata un'ottima correlazione lineare dose-risposta tra i livelli sierici di IGF-I e la secrezione media di GH nelle 24 ore. Un elevato livello di IGF-I in un paziente con sospetto clinico è solitamente indicativo di eccesso di GH. Può sorgere potenziale confusione nella valutazione di adolescenti normali, dato che durante la pubertà si hanno livelli più elevati di IGF-I rispetto all'adulto; il livello di IGF-I deve essere rapportato quindi all'età e al sesso. I livelli sierici di IGFBP-3 sono marker sensibili di eccesso di GH e possono essere elevati nonostante normali livelli di IGF-I. Se i reperti di laboratorio suggeriscono un eccesso di GH, è necessario confermare la presenza di adenoma ipofisario con una RM. Nei rari casi in cui non si identifica alcuna massa ipofisaria, si può trattare di un microadenoma ipofisario occulto o di un tumore ectopico. Si esegue una TC quando la RM non fornisce alcuna indicazione.

TRATTAMENTO DELL'IPERSECREZIONE DI ORMONE DELLA CRESCITA. Gli obiettivi della terapia consistono nella rimozione o nella diminuzione della massa ipofisaria, per ripristinare una normale secrezione di GH, normali livelli di IGF-I e di IGFBP-3, normale secrezione degli altri ormoni ipofisari e per prevenire eventuali recidive.

Per gli adenomi ben circoscritti il trattamento elettivo è rappresentato dall'intervento chirurgico per via transfenoidale, che può essere risolutivo. Il tumore deve essere rimosso completamente. La probabilità di riuscita dell'intervento dipende notevolmente dall'esperienza del chirurgo, dalla dimensione e dall'estensione della massa. Dosaggi intraoperatori di GH possono migliorare i risultati della resezione tumorale. La chirurgia transfenoidale è sicura sia nei bambini sia negli adulti. In passato, era necessario un approccio per via transcranica. L'obiettivo fondamentale del trattamento è normalizzare i livelli di GH. I livelli di GH (<1 ng/mL entro due ore dal carico di glucosio) e i livelli sierici di IGF-I (range normale aggiustato per età) sono i test migliori per definire una terapia biochimica.

Se la secrezione di GH non si è normalizzata dopo l'intervento chirurgico, le ulteriori possibilità terapeutiche comprendono l'irradiazione dell'ipofisi e la terapia medica. Si raccomanda la radioterapia qualora l'ipersecrezione di GH non si sia regolarizzata dopo l'intervento. In più del 99% dei pazienti la terapia radiante previene l'ulteriore crescita del tumore, ma comporta un ritardo nella diminuzione dei livelli di GH. Esso si riduce a circa il 50% dei valori iniziali dopo 2 anni, al 75% a 5 anni e circa al 90% a 15 anni. L'ipopituitarismo è un esito prevedibile e si manifesta nel 40-50% dei pazienti dopo 10 anni dalla terapia radiante.

La chirurgia non è risolutiva in un numero significativo di pazienti e quindi, in questi casi, la terapia medica ha un ruolo importante. La terapia con analoghi della somatostatina a lunga durata d'azione, con agonisti della dopamina e anche con i nuovi antagonisti del GH, è efficace e ben tollerata.

Gli **analoghi della somatostatina** sono molto efficaci nel trattamento di pazienti con eccesso di GH. L'octreotide sopprime il GH a valori inferiori a 2,5 ng/mL nel 65% dei pazienti con acromegalia e normalizza i livelli di IGF-I nel 70% dei casi. Gli effetti dell'octreotide sono prolungati nel tempo; esso comporta pure una diminuzione del tumore, ma generalmente modesta. In un ragazzo pubere con gigantismo ipofisario, si è ottenuta una consistente soppressione del GH utilizzando una pompa sc a infusione continua di octreotide. Formulazioni a lunga durata d'azione, compresi l'octreotide e il lanreotide a lunga durata, producono una significativa soppressione di GH e di IGF-I in pazienti acromegalici, utilizzando iniezioni im di formulazioni depot mensilmente o bisettimanalmente. Le preparazioni a rilascio sostenuto non sono state formalmente testate nei bambini. L'iniezione di octreotide nella popolazione pediatrica è stata utilizzata alla dose di 1-40 μg/kg/die.

Per i pazienti con ipersecrezione sia di GH sia di prolattina, si utilizzano gli agonisti della dopamina e la **bromocriptina**, che legano i recettori della dopamina ipofisaria di tipo 2 (D_2) e sopprimono la secrezione di GH, nonostante il loro preciso meccanismo d'azione non sia chiaro. Con questo tipo di trattamento i livelli di prolattina vengono spesso soppressi in modo adeguato; raramente, invece, si normalizzano i livelli di GH e di IGF-I. Meno del 20% dei pazienti raggiunge livelli di GH inferiori a 5 ng/mL e meno del 10% ottiene una normalizzazione dei livelli di IGF-I. In una minoranza di pazienti si verifica inoltre una riduzione delle dimensioni del tumore. La bromocriptina viene utilizzata come coadiuvante nel trattamento medico dell'eccesso di GH e il suo effetto si somma a quello dell'octreotide. Maggiore efficacia, testimoniata da normali livelli di IGF-I e dalla riduzione delle dimensioni del tumore, si ottiene con altri agonisti della dopamina (pergolide, cabergolina). Il dosaggio della bromocriptina è compreso tra 10-60 mg/die per os diviso in quattro somministrazioni. Tuttavia solo una minima parte di pazienti beneficia di dosi maggiori di 20 mg/die. Il suo utilizzo è sicuro nei bambini per lungo tempo, ma gli effetti collaterali comprendono nausea, vomito, dolore addominale, aritmie, ostruzione nasale, ipotensione ortostatica, disturbi del sonno e astenia. La dose di cabergolina è di 0,25-1 mg per os 1-2 volte la settimana, ma non è stata ben definita una dose pediatrica.

Gli antagonisti del recettore del GH bloccano specificamente l'attività del GH a livello dei suoi siti effettori. Il **pegvisomant** è un analogo del GH che compete con il GH endogeno per il legame con il suo recettore. Esso sopprime efficacemente i livelli di GH e di IGF-I sia in pazienti acromegalici con tumori ipofisari sia in quelli con iperproduzione ectopica di GHRH. I livelli di IGF-I vengono normalizzati nel 90% dei pazienti trattati giornalmente con questo farmaco per 3 mesi o più. Non è stato testato sui bambini, mentre la dose per l'adulto è di 10-30 mg per iniezione sottocutanea una volta al giorno. È efficace anche la terapia settimanale combinata con analoghi della somatostatina e pegvisomant.

SINDROME DI SOTOS (GIGANTISMO CEREBRALE)

I bambini con gigantismo cerebrale (sindrome di Sotos) si presentano alla nascita oltre il 90° percentile sia in lunghezza sia in peso; può essere presente anche macrocefalia. La sindrome di Sotos è causata da aploinsufficienza del gene NSD1 (recettore nucleare contenente il dominio SET gene-1). Nonostante sia caratterizzata da rapido accrescimento, non c'è alcuna evidenza che si tratti di una patologia endocrina. Si è ipotizzato un difetto ipotalamico, ma nessuno lo ha dimostrato da un punto di vista funzionale o all'indagine autoptica. La crescita è rapida e all'età di un anno i bambini malati hanno un'altezza che supera il 97° percentile. Questo accrescimento accelerato continua nei primi 4-5 anni per ritornare poi entro i limiti di norma (Fig. 561-1). La pubertà inizia di solito in epoca normale o lievemente anticipata. La statura da adulto si situa al limite superiore del range di normalità. Le mani e i piedi sono larghi, con notevole spessore del tessuto sottocutaneo. Sono evidenti macrocefalia e dolicocefalia, prognatismo, ipertelorismo, taglio obliquo antimongoloide degli occhi. Sono caratteristiche una certa goffaggine e andatura impacciata, e i bambini affetti mostrano una notevole difficoltà negli sport, nell'imparare ad andare in bicicletta e in altre attività che richiedono coordinazione. La maggior parte dei pazienti presenta gradi diversi di ritardo mentale; in alcuni bambini possono essere predominanti carenze percettive. La maturazione ossea è compatibile con l'altezza. I livelli di GH e di IGF-I, nonché la valutazione di altri parametri endocrini, risultano nella norma; in questa sindrome non ci sono marker laboratoristici o radiologici. Sono comuni alterazioni elettroencefalografiche; altri studi hanno rivelato frequentemente una dilatazione del sistema ventricolare. I pazienti hanno un maggior rischio di neoplasie; sono stati riportati casi di carcinoma epatico e di tumore di Wilms, carcinoma ovarico e neoplasie parotidee.

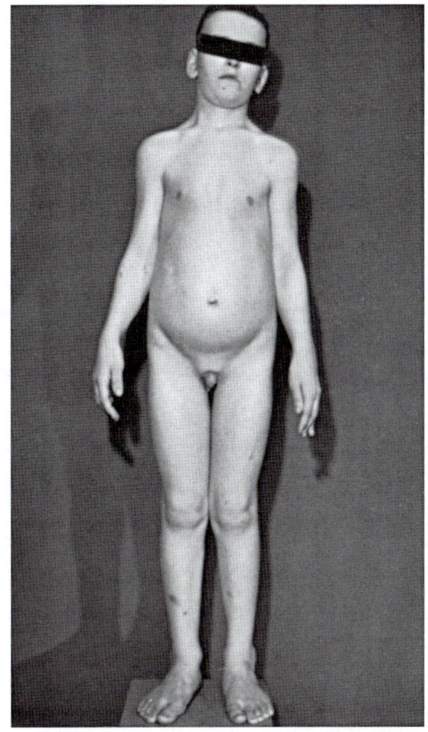

Figura 561-1. Gigantismo cerebrale in un ragazzo di 8 anni. L'altezza corrispondeva a un'età di 12 anni, così come l'età ossea. Il QI era di 60. Erano presenti anomalie elettroencefalografiche. Si noti la prominenza delle bozze frontali e della mandibola, e la grandezza di mani e piedi. Lo sviluppo sessuale era adeguato all'età cronologica. Le valutazioni ormonali erano normali. L'altezza da adulto era di 208 cm, con normale sviluppo sessuale. Il numero delle scarpe era 51.

ECCESSIVA CRESCITA FETALE

Il diabete materno è la causa più frequente di neonati grandi per età gestazionale (*Large for Gestational Age*, LGA). Anche in assenza di sintomi clinici o di anamnesi familiare positiva, la nascita di un neonato eccessivamente grosso deve indurre alla valutazione di un eventuale diabete materno (o gestazionale).

È stato descritto un gruppo di malattie associate a eccessiva crescita somatica e crescita di specifici organi, definite, nel loro complesso, come sindromi da crescita eccessiva. Sembra che queste malattie siano causate da eccessiva disponibilità di un fattore-II di crescita insulino-simile (IGF-II) codificato dal gene *Igf2*. Tra queste patologie la meglio descritta è la **sindrome di Beckwith-Wiedemann** (BWS), che è una sindrome malformativa iperaccrescitiva con incidenza di 1:13 700 nati. Si manifesta come eccessiva crescita fetale in cui il quadro clinico è dominato dall'ipertrofia. Tipicamente alla nascita sono evidenti macroglossia, epatosplenomegalia, nefromegalia e ipoglicemia con iperinsulinemia da iperplasia delle cellule pancreatiche β in un neonato LGA. Questi bambini sono predisposti a essere affetti da specifici tumori infantili, compresi il tumore di Wilms e il carcinoma adrenocorticale. La superespressione di IGF-II nella BWS può essere dovuta a un certo numero di alterazioni genetiche, comprese duplicazione del gene, perdita dell'eterozigosi e perdita o diminuzione dell'imprinting del gene *Igf2*. Vari studi hanno localizzato i geni *imprinted* coinvolti nella BWS e associati a tumori infantili sul cromosoma 11p. Questi comprendono, oltre a *Igf2*, il gene *H19*, che è coinvolto nella soppressione di *Igf2*, e *WT-1* (il gene del tumore di Wilms). Mutazioni in GPC3, gene Glypican 3 (che codifica per un recettore di membrana neutralizzante di IGF-II), provocano una patologia correlata, la **sindrome da crescita eccessiva di Simpson-Golabi-Behmel**.

Cannavo S, Venturino M, Curto L, et al: Clinical presentation and outcome of pituitary adenomas in teenagers. *Clin Endocrinol (Oxf)* 2003;58: 519–527.

Cecconi M, Forzano F, Milani D, et al: Mutation analysis of the NSD1 gene in a group of 59 patients with congenital overgrowth. *Am J Med Genet* 2005;134:247–253.

Clemmons DR: Role of insulin-like growth factor-I in diagnosis and management of acromegaly. *Endocr Pract* 2004;10:362–371.

Colao A, Di Sarno A, Landi ML, et al: Long-term and low-dose treatment with cabergoline induces macroprolactinoma shrinkage. *J Clin Endocrinol Metab* 1997;82:3574–3579.

Colao A, Loche S, Cappabianca P, et al: Pituitary adenomas in children and adolescents: Clinical presentation, diagnosis, and therapeutic strategies. *Endocrinologist* 2000;10:314–327.

Daughaday WH: Pituitary gigantism. *Endocrinol Metab Clin North Am* 1992;21:633–647.

Feensta J, de Herder WW, Van der Beld AW, et al: Combined therapy with somatostatin analogues and weekly pegvisomant in active acromegaly. *Lancet* 2005;365:1644–1646.

Freda PU, Katznelson LO, Van der Lely AJ, et al: Long-acting somatostatin analog therapy of acromegaly: a meta-analysis. *J Clin Endocrinol Metab* 2005;90:4465–4473.

Kane LA, Leinung MC, Scheithaver BW, et al: Pituitary adenomas in childhood and adolescence. *J Clin Endocrinol Metab* 1994;79:1135–1140.

Lee JM, Howell JD: Tall girls: the social shaping of a medical therapy. *Arch Pediatr Adolesc Med* 2006;160:1035–1039.

Melmed S: Acromegaly. *N Engl J Med* 2006;355:2558–2572.

Morison IM, Becroft DM, Taniguchi T, et al: Somatic overgrowth associated with overexpression of insulin-like growth factor II. *Nature Med* 1996;2:311–316.

Rajasoorya C, Holdaway IM, Wrightson P, et al: Determinants of clinical outcome and survival in acromegaly. *Clin Endocrinol (Oxf)* 1994;41: 95–102.

Serri O: Progress in management of hyperprolactinoma. *N Engl J Med* 1994;331:942–944.

Sorgo W, Scholler K, Heinze E, et al: Critical analysis of height reduction in estrogen treated tall girls. *Eur J Pediatr* 1984;142:260–265.

Sotos JF: Overgrowth: Genetic syndromes and other disorders associated with overgrowth. *Clin Pediatr* 1997;36:157–170.

Vance ML, Laws ER: Role of medical therapy in the management of acromegaly. *Neurosurgery* 2005;56:877–885.

Venn A, Bruinsma F, Werther G, et al: Oestrogen treatment to reduce the adult height of tall girls: Long-term effects on fertility. *Lancet* 2004;364: 1513–1518.

Capitolo 562 ■ Fisiologia della pubertà

Luigi Garibaldi

Tra la prima infanzia e l'età di 8-9 anni circa (stadio prepuberale), l'asse ipotalamo-ipofisi-gonadi è quiescente, come dimostra l'assenza di concentrazioni sieriche dosabili di ormone luteinizzante (LH) e di ormoni sessuali (estradiolo nelle femmine, testosterone nei maschi). In questa fase, l'attività dell'ipotalamo e dell'ipofisi può essere soppressa da vie di controllo neuronale scarsamente rappresentate.

Da 1 a 3 anni prima dell'inizio della pubertà clinicamente manifesta, cominciano a diventare evidenti durante il sonno bassi livelli sierici di LH (periodo peripuberale). Tale secrezione notturna di LH si verifica in modo pulsatile e probabilmente riflette le scariche episodiche endogene di ormone ipotalamico di rilascio delle gonadotropine (GnRH). La pulsatilità notturna dell'LH continua ad aumentare in ampiezza e, in minor misura, in frequenza, via via che ci si avvicina alla pubertà clinica. Questa secrezione pulsatile di gonadotropine è responsabile di iperplasia e di maturazione delle gonadi nonché della secrezione di ormoni sessuali. La comparsa delle caratteristiche sessuali secondarie nella fase precoce della pubertà rappresenta l'apice visibile della prolungata attiva interazione tra ipotalamo, ipofisi e gonadi nel periodo peripuberale. In corrispondenza della fase intermedia della pubertà, la pulsatilità dell'LH diventa evidente anche durante il giorno e si verifica a intervalli di circa 90-120 min.

Un secondo evento critico si verifica nella media o tarda adolescenza nelle ragazze, con la comparsa del ciclo mestruale e dell'ovulazione. Si sviluppa un meccanismo di feedback positivo che incrementa i livelli di estrogeni a metà del ciclo per uno specifico aumento dell'LH.

I fattori che normalmente attivano o inibiscono i neuroni ipotalamici responsabili della secrezione di GnRH (un'unità neurosecretoria conosciuta come generatore pulsatile di GnRH) sono sconosciuti. Negli altri primati, una diminuzione del tono GABA-ergico nei neuroni ipotalamici (acido γ-aminobutirrico) con conseguente incremento di quello glutaminergico attiva il generatore pulsatile del GnRH. Sono probabilmente numerosi i neurotrasmettitori coinvolti sia nell'uomo sia negli altri primati.

È chiaro che il GnRH è il principale, ma non il solo, ormone responsabile dell'inizio e della progressione della pubertà, dal momento che lo sviluppo puberale può essere riprodotto nell'uomo e in animali sessualmente immaturi o con deficit gonadotropinico tramite la somministrazione pulsatile di GnRH. Mutazioni del gene *GPR54* (un gene del recettore della proteina G-accoppiata) provocano una forma autosomica recessiva di ipogonadismo ipogonadotropo. Difetti di questo sistema receptor-ligand non riguardano la migrazione neuronale di GnRH, in contrasto con l'ipogonadismo ipogonadotropo associato a X della sindrome di Kallmann, ma ripristinano l'attività dei neuroni ipotalamici secernenti GnRH.

L'interpretazione delle modificazioni ormonali della pubertà è complessa per diversi motivi. In primo luogo, le gonadotropine ipofisarie sono eterogenee e si trovano in circolo in varie isoforme: più isoforme di LH biologicamente attive possono essere preponderanti durante la pubertà. In secondo luogo, l'immunoreattività dell'LH è variabile nei diversi dosaggi immunologici e i risultati delle misurazioni dell'LH possono cambiare ampiamente a seconda dei laboratori. In terzo luogo, la secrezione pulsatile di gonadotropine e il sinergismo tra ormone follicolo-stimolante (FSH) e LH nel promuovere la maturazione gonadica rendono difficile l'interpretazione di un singolo dosaggio di gonadotropine sieriche. È decisamente più significativa la valutazione delle gonadotropine in campioni sierici ottenuti da prelievi seriali (ogni 10-20 min per 12-24 ore) o in campioni di urina raccolti in un certo periodo. Esistono, inoltre, importanti differenze sessuali nella maturazione dell'ipotalamo e dell'ipofisi e le concentrazioni sieriche di LH aumentano più precocemente durante la pubertà nei maschi rispetto alle femmine.

Gli effetti degli steroidi gonadici (testosterone nei maschi, estradiolo nelle femmine) sulla crescita e sulla maturazione dell'osso sono fondamentali. Nei ragazzi, sia un deficit di aromatasi sia i difetti dei recettori estrogenici comportano un ritardo nella fusione epifisaria e alta statura. Queste osservazioni indicano che sono gli estrogeni, più che gli androgeni, i responsabili del processo di maturazione ossea che si conclude con fusione epifisaria e cessazione della crescita. Gli estrogeni mediano anche l'incremento della produzione di ormone della crescita, il quale soltanto in presenza di un effetto diretto degli steroidi sessuali sulla crescita dell'osso è responsabile dello spurt di crescita puberale.

L'età di inizio della pubertà è variabile ed è più strettamente correlata con la maturazione ossea che con l'età cronologica (vedi Capitolo 12). Nelle femmine, il **bottone mammario** è normalmente il primo segno di pubertà (10-11 anni), seguito dalla comparsa di **peli pubici** 6-12 mesi dopo. Il menarca compare di solito dopo un intervallo di 2-2,5 anni, ma che può anche diventare di 6 anni. Negli Stati Uniti, almeno un segno di pubertà è presente in circa il 95% delle ragazze all'età di 12 anni e nel 99% delle femmine a 13 anni. Il picco della velocità di crescita in altezza si verifica precocemente (allo stadio mammario II-III, tipicamente tra gli 11 e i 12 anni) nelle ragazze e precede sempre il menarca. L'età media di comparsa del menarca è di 12 anni e 3/4. Ci sono, tuttavia, notevoli variazioni nella sequenza dei cambiamenti che riguardano lo spurt accrescitivo, il bottone mammario, i peli pubici e la maturazione dei genitali esterni e interni.

Nei maschi, la **crescita dei testicoli** (>3 mL in volume o 2,5 cm nel diametro maggiore) e l'ispessimento dello scroto, rappresentano il primo segno di pubertà. Sono seguiti dalla pigmentazione dello scroto e dalla crescita del pene (vedi Capitolo 12) e per ultimi compaiono i **peli pubici**. La comparsa di **peli ascellari** normalmente si ha nella fase intermedia della pubertà. Nei maschi, a differenza delle femmine, l'accelerazione della crescita inizia dopo la pubertà, prosegue bene ed è massima in corrispondenza dello stadio genitale IV-V (tipicamente tra i 13 e i 14 anni). Nei maschi, lo spurt accrescitivo si verifica circa 2 anni dopo le femmine e la crescita può continuare fino al 18° anno d'età.

Fattori genetici e ambientali possono modificare l'inizio della pubertà. Dopo un abbassamento dell'età del menarca verificatosi nel secolo scorso (probabilmente in rapporto a una maggiore nutrizione e a un miglioramento della salute in generale) negli ultimi 30-40 anni essa si è stabilizzata. Le femmine afroamericane possono essere più avanzate nello sviluppo delle caratteristiche sessuali secondari per età, rispetto alle coetanee bianche. È nota una correlazione positiva tra il grado di adiposità e la precocità dello sviluppo puberale nelle femmine. Al contrario, danzatrici, ginnaste, atlete impegnate nella corsa e in altri sport in cui coesistono magrezza e attività fisica forzata fin dall'infanzia frequentemente evidenziano un ritardo notevole della pubertà o del menarca e di solito da adulte presentano oligomenorrea o amenorrea (vedi Capitolo 689). Il ritardo puberale è comune anche nei maschi che praticano attività fisica molto intensa. Tali osservazioni supportano la tesi che il bilancio energetico sia strettamente correlato all'attività del generatore pulsatile del GnRH e dei meccanismi che danno inizio e sostengono la pubertà, probabilmente attraverso segnali ormonali, comprese le adipochine.

Anche gli androgeni corticosurrenalici ricoprono un ruolo nella maturazione sessuale. I livelli sierici di deidroepiandrosterone (DHEA) e del suo solfato (DHEAS) cominciano ad aumentare circa verso i 6-8 anni, prima di un qualunque incremento dell'LH o degli ormoni sessuali e prima che compaiano le più precoci modificazioni cliniche della pubertà: tale processo è stato chiamato adrenarca. Il DHEAS è lo steroide surrenalico a 19 atomi di carbonio circolante più abbondante e la sua concentrazione sierica rimane abbastanza stabile nelle 24 ore. Di solito si utilizza una singola misurazione di quest'ormone come marker di secrezione androgenica surrenalica. Nonostante l'adrenarca tipicamente preceda di pochi anni l'inizio dell'attività gonadica (gonadarca), i due processi non hanno rapporti di causa-effetto, perché l'adrenarca e il gonadarca si presentano dissociati in condizioni quali la pubertà precoce centrale e l'insufficienza corticosurrenalica.

Capitolo 563 ■ Disordini dello sviluppo puberale Luigi Garibaldi

Si definisce pubertà precoce la comparsa delle caratteristiche sessuali secondarie prima degli 8 anni nelle femmine e dei 9 anni nei maschi. Questa definizione è in parte arbitraria, perché esistono variazioni molto notevoli dell'età in cui inizia la pubertà nei bambini normali a seconda dei differenti gruppi etnici.

Lo sviluppo puberale precoce può essere classificato come **gonadotropino-dipendente**, definito anche pubertà precoce **centrale** o vera, oppure **gonadotropino-indipendente**, definito pubertà precoce **periferica** o pseudopubertà precoce (Tab. 563-1). La pubertà precoce vera è sempre isosessuale e dipende dall'attivazione dell'asse ipotalamo-ipofisi-gonadi. L'incremento, gonadotropino-mediato, delle dimensioni e dell'attività delle gonadi porta a un aumento della secrezione di ormoni sessuali e a una progressiva maturazione sessuale. Nella pseudopubertà precoce, compaiono alcune delle caratteristiche sessuali secondarie, ma non esiste attivazione della normale interazione ipotalamo-ipofisi-gonadica. In quest'ultimo gruppo le caratteristiche sessuali possono essere isosessuali o eterosessuali (o "controsessuali") (vedi Capitoli 584-589).

La pseudopubertà precoce può indurre maturazione dell'asse ipotalamo-ipofisi-gonadico ed eventualmente innescare una precocità sessuale vera. Questa forma mista di pubertà precoce si verifica comunemente nell'iperplasia surrenalica congenita, nella

TABELLA 563-1. Condizioni che provocano pubertà precoce

PUBERTÀ GONADOTROPINO-DIPENDENTE (PUBERTÀ PRECOCE VERA)
Idiopatica
Lesioni organiche cerebrali
Amartoma ipotalamico
Tumori cerebrali, idrocefalo, grave trauma cranico, mielomeningocele
Ipotiroidismo, prolungato e non trattato
PUBERTÀ COMBINATA GONADOTROPINO-DIPENDENTE E GONADOTROPINO-INDIPENDENTE
Iperplasia surrenalica congenita trattata
Sindrome di McCune-Albright, tardiva
Pubertà precoce maschile familiare, tardiva
PUBERTÀ GONADOTROPINO-INDIPENDENTE (PSEUDOPUBERTÀ PRECOCE)
Femmine
Condizioni isosessuali (femminilizzanti)
Sindrome di McCune-Albright
Cisti ovariche autonome
Tumori ovarici
Tumore a cellule della granulosa-teca associato a malattia di Ollier
Teratoma, corionepitelioma
Tumore del cordone sessuale con tubuli anulari (SCTAT) associata a sindrome di Peutz-Jeghers
Tumore surrenalico femminilizzante
Estrogeni esogeni
Condizioni eterosessuali (mascolinizzanti)
Iperplasia surrenalica congenita
Tumore surrenalico
Tumori ovarici
Difetto dei recettori dei glucocorticoidi
Androgeni esogeni
Maschi
Condizioni isosessuali (mascolinizzanti)
Iperplasia surrenalica congenita
Tumore surrenalico
Tumore a cellule di Leydig
Pubertà precoce maschile familiare
Isolata
Associata a pseudoipoparatiroidismo
Tumori hCG secernenti
Sistema nervoso centrale
Epatoblastoma
Tumore mediastinico associato a sindrome di Klinefelter
Teratoma
Difetto del recettore dei glicocorticoidi
Androgeni esogeni
Condizioni eterosessuali (femminilizzanti)
Tumori surrenalici femminilizzanti
SCTAT associata alla sindrome di Peutz-Jeghers
Estrogeni esogeni
PUBERTÀ PRECOCE INCOMPLETA (PARZIALE)
Telarca precoce
Adrenarca precoce
Menarca precoce

sindrome di McCune-Albright e nella pubertà precoce familiare limitata ai maschi, quando l'età ossea raggiunge il range puberale (10,5-12,5 anni).

563.1 • Pubertà precoce gonadotropino-dipendente

La condizione si verifica almeno 5-10 volte più frequentemente nelle femmine che nei maschi ed è di solito sporadica, sebbene esistano alcuni casi familiari. Circa il 90% dei casi di precocità sessuale nelle femmine è idiopatica. Tuttavia, nel 25-75% dei maschi e nell'8-10% delle ragazze con pubertà precoce centrale, può essere rilevata un'anomalia strutturale del SNC. Inoltre, è stata riportata un'alta prevalenza di precocità sessuale idiopatica nelle ragazze adottate da nazioni in via di sviluppo, con la limitazione che la data esatta di nascita può essere incerta.

MANIFESTAZIONI CLINICHE. Lo sviluppo sessuale può cominciare a una qualsiasi età e generalmente segue la sequenza osservata nella pubertà normale. Nelle ragazze, il primo segno è lo sviluppo delle mammelle, mentre i peli pubici possono apparire simultaneamente, ma spesso compaiono più tardi. Seguono la maturazione dei genitali esterni, la comparsa dei peli ascellari e la comparsa delle mestruazioni. I primi cicli mestruali possono essere più irregolari di quelli della pubertà normale; inoltre, sono solitamente anovulatori, ma è stato riportato un caso di gravidanza in una bambina di 5 anni e mezzo (Fig. 563-1).

Nei ragazzi, l'ingrossamento dei testicoli è seguito dall'aumento del pene, dalla comparsa dei peli pubici e dall'acne. Sono comuni le erezioni e si possono verificare eiaculazioni notturne, inoltre la voce si abbassa e si accelera la crescita in altezza. Biopsie testicolari hanno mostrato la stimolazione di tutti gli elementi testicolari e si è osservata la spermatogenesi, anche precocemente, verso i 5-6 anni. Sia nei maschi sia nelle femmine sono avanzati l'altezza, il peso e la maturazione ossea. L'aumento della velocità di maturazione ossea comporta una precoce chiusura epifisaria e la statura finale è inferiore a quella che si sarebbe raggiunta altrimenti. Senza trattamento, circa un terzo delle ragazze e una percentuale anche più ampia di ragazzi arriva, da adulti, a un'altezza inferiore al 5° percentile. Lo sviluppo mentale è solitamente compatibile con l'età cronologica e sono comuni comportamento emotivo e oscillazioni del tono dell'umore, ma problemi psicologici più seri sono rari.

Nonostante il decorso clinico sia variabile, sono tre i pattern principali di progressione puberale che si possono identificare. La maggior parte delle bambine (particolarmente quelle che all'inizio hanno meno di 6 anni) e dei bambini mostra rapidamente una progressiva precocità sessuale, caratterizzata da veloce maturazione fisica e ossea, con perdita del potenziale di crescita. Molte bambine (generalmente quelle che iniziano dopo il sesto anno di età) mostrano una variante della precocità sessuale centrale a progressione più lenta, caratterizzata da un avanzamento parallelo della maturazione ossea e della crescita lineare, con potenziale di crescita preservato. Una variante a progressione lenta della precocità sessuale centrale si verifica anche nei maschi, ma è meno comune che nelle femmine. Una piccola percentuale di bambine presenta una forma di pubertà precoce centrale spontaneamente regressiva o non sostenuta. Tale variabilità nel decorso naturale della precocità sessuale sottolinea la necessità di tenere sotto osservazione longitudinale i bambini alla comparsa dello sviluppo sessuale, prima di prendere in considerazione un trattamento.

REPERTI DI LABORATORIO. Le concentrazioni di ormoni sessuali sono solitamente appropriate allo stadio della pubertà in entrambi i sessi. Le concentrazioni sieriche di estradiolo nelle bambine sono basse o indosabili nella fase iniziale della precocità sessuale, come nella pubertà normale. Nei bambini, i livelli sierici di testosterone sono misurabili o nettamente elevati nel momento in cui i genitori si rivolgono al medico, soprattutto se si fanno prelievi di sangue al mattino presto. I dosaggi sensibili immunometrici (compresi quelli immunoradiometrici, immunofluorimetrici e chemiluminescenti) per LH hanno sostituito il tradizionale dosaggio radioimmunologico dell'LH e offrono una maggiore sensibilità diagnostica utilizzando campioni di sangue randomiz-

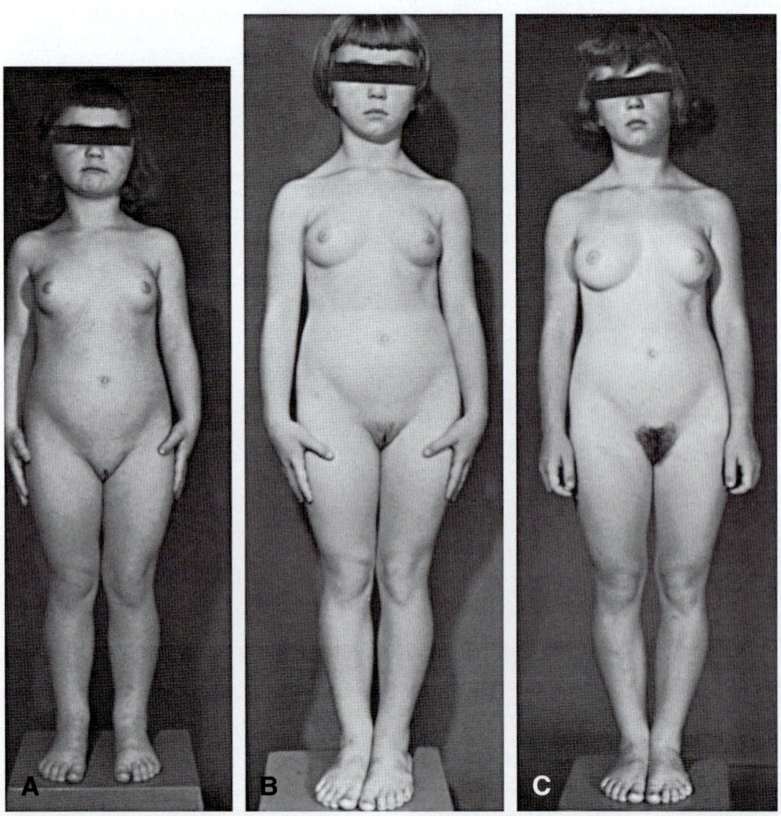

Figura 563-1. Decorso naturale della pubertà precoce idiopatica centrale. Il paziente *(A)* a 3 anni e 11 mesi, *(B)* a 5 anni e 8 mesi, e *(C)* a 8 anni e mezzo di età. Lo sviluppo mammario e il sanguinamento vaginale erano iniziati a 2 anni e mezzo. L'età ossea era di 7 anni e mezzo a 3 anni e 11 mesi e di 14 anni a 8 anni di età. L'intelligenza e l'età dentaria erano normali per l'età cronologica. La crescita era completata a 10 anni; l'altezza definitiva era di 142 cm. Al tempo in cui il paziente si era presentato all'osservazione medica, non era disponibile alcuna terapia efficace.

zati. Con i dosaggi sensibili, nei bambini in età prepubere non sono rilevabili concentrazioni sieriche di LH, che però diventano dosabili nel 60-75% delle bambine e in percentuale più alta in bambini con precocità sessuale centrale. Misurazioni dell'LH in campioni ematici seriali ottenuti durante il sonno hanno maggiore significato diagnostico di un singolo campione casuale e mostrano tipicamente una ben definita secrezione pulsatile di LH. La somministrazione endovenosa di ormone di rilascio delle gonadotropine (test di stimolazione al GnRH) o di un suo agonista (test di stimolazione con leuprolide) è di notevole aiuto diagnostico, particolarmente per i maschi, in cui, nella fase iniziale della pubertà precoce, si verifica una vivace risposta dell'LH (picco di LH >5-10 UI/L) con prevalenza dell'LH sull'ormone follicolo-stimolante (FSH). Nelle femmine con precocità sessuale, tuttavia, al II stadio mammario, la secrezione notturna di LH e la risposta dell'LH al test con GnRH può essere abbastanza bassa, fino all'inizio dello stadio III (picco di LH-immunometrico, spesso <5 UI/L) e il rapporto tra LH e FSH può rimanere basso fino allo stadio intermedio della pubertà. Nelle ragazze con "bassa" risposta dell'LH, la natura centrale della precocità sessuale può essere provata valutando i livelli puberali di estradiolo (>50 pg/mL), 20-24 ore dopo la stimolazione con leuprolide.

La maturazione ossea è variabilmente avanzata, spesso più di 2-3 DS. Nelle ragazze, l'ecografia pelvica evidenzia un progressivo ingrandimento delle ovaie, seguito dall'incremento dell'utero, fino a dimensioni tipiche della pubertà. L'RM normalmente dimostra il fisiologico aumento dell'ipofisi, come si verifica nella pubertà normale; può anche rivelare una patologia del SNC (vedi Capitolo 563-2).

DIAGNOSI DIFFERENZIALE. Cause organiche di precocità sessuale che riguardano il SNC possono essere determinate con una RM, particolarmente nelle femmine con rapido sviluppo mammario, in quelle con estradiolo >30 pg/mL, nelle bambine con meno di 6 anni e in tutti i maschi. Tuttavia, nei bambini che non hanno segni o sintomi neurologici, le lesioni del SNC che provocano pubertà precoce sono raramente maligne e di rado sono necessari un intervento neurochirurgico o una terapia radiante. Alcuni esperti raccomandano l'esecuzione di RM in tutti i bambini con pubertà precoce centrale.

Nella diagnosi differenziale vanno prese in considerazione cause **gonadotropino-indipendenti** di pubertà precoce isosessuale (vedi Tab. 563-1). Per le femmine, queste comprendono tumori ovarici, cisti ovariche funzionalmente autonome, tumori surrenalici femminilizzanti, sindrome di McCune-Albright e sorgenti esogene di estrogeni. Per i maschi, l'iperplasia surrenalica congenita, tumori surrenalici, tumori a cellule di Leydig, neoplasie che producono gonadotropina corionica e pubertà precoce familiare maschile.

TRATTAMENTO. L'osservazione che le cellule ipofisarie gonadotrope richiedono una stimolazione da parte del GnRH di tipo pulsatile, piuttosto che continua, per mantenere un rilascio continuo di gonadotropine, fornisce la ragione per l'utilizzo degli agonisti del GnRH nel trattamento della pubertà precoce centrale. Per il vantaggio di essere più potenti e di avere una più lunga durata di azione rispetto al GnRH nativo, questi agonisti del GnRH (dopo un breve periodo di stimolazione) "desensibilizzano" le cellule gonadotrope dell'ipofisi dall'effetto stimolatorio del GnRH endogeno e bloccano effettivamente la progressione della precocità sessuale centrale.

Virtualmente tutti i maschi e un largo sottogruppo di femmine con pubertà precoce a progressione rapida sono candidati per questo trattamento, mentre le bambine con pubertà precoce a progressione lenta non ottengono benefici in termini di prognosi di altezza dalla terapia con agonisti del GnRH. I neonati con basso peso alla nascita possono presentare un alto rischio di bassa statura definitiva e richiedere perciò un trattamento della pubertà precoce più aggressivo. Pochi pazienti necessitano di trattamento unicamente per ragioni psicologiche o sociali, compresa la notevole ansia dei genitori. Formulazioni depot degli agonisti del GnRH a lunga durata di azione, che mantengono pressoché costante la concentrazione sierica del farmaco per settimane, costituiscono la preparazione di elezione per il trattamento della pubertà precoce centrale. Il leuprolide acetato, la sola preparazione depot approvata negli Stati Uniti per questo uso, si somministra alla dose di 0,25-0,3 mg/kg (per un minimo di 7,5 mg) per via im una volta ogni 4 settimane. Altre preparazioni a lunga durata di azione (D-Trp6-GnRH, goserelin acetato) sono approvate per il trattamento della pubertà precoce in altre nazioni. L'effetto collaterale più fastidioso è una frequente raccolta liquida sterile nella sede di iniezione e si verifica in meno del 3-5% dei pazienti trattati. Nei bambini con queste reazioni locali, si deve cambiare il trattamento, utilizzando iniezioni sottocutanee di leuprolide in soluzione acquosa, una o due volte al giorno (dose totale di 60 mg/kg/die) o somministrazione endonasale dell'agonista del GnRH nafarelin, 800 mg in 2 somministrazioni/die. Il potenziale per la compliance irregolare con la somministrazione giornaliera, assieme al variabile assorbimento per via endonasale del nafarelin, può limitare il beneficio a lungo termine delle ultime preparazioni sull'altezza definitiva. Preparazioni depot di leuprolide con più lunga durata di azione (90 giorni) non sono attualmente approvate dalla FDA per il trattamento della precocità sessuale, ma appaiono promettenti. Impianti sottocute (effetto di rilascio fino a 12-18 mesi) di agonisti del GnRH (histrelin) si sono dimostrati efficaci nei trial preliminari. Gli antagonisti del GnRH sono relativamente nuovi e non sono stati sufficientemente studiati per il trattamento della pubertà precoce; inoltre, si stanno valutando anche degli antagonisti del GnRH per via orale.

Il trattamento comporta una diminuzione della velocità di crescita, generalmente a valori idonei all'età e ancor più della velocità di maturazione ossea. Alcuni bambini, particolarmente quelli con maggiore incremento (puberale) dell'età ossea, possono mostrare una marcata decelerazione della velocità di crescita e un arresto completo della maturazione ossea. Il trattamento porta a un miglioramento dell'altezza prevista, sebbene l'altezza finale dei pazienti, seguita dalla chiusura epifisaria, sia di circa 1 DS minore dell'altezza media dei genitori. Nelle femmine, lo sviluppo mammario può regredire allo stadio II-III di Tanner. Più comunemente, la dimensione delle mammelle rimane immodificata nelle ragazze allo stadio III-V o può anche aumentare lievemente per progressiva deposizione di tessuto adiposo. Diminuisce però la quantità di tessuto ghiandolare. I peli pubici solitamente rimangono stabili nelle bambine o possono anche aumentare leggermente durante il trattamento, in rapporto al graduale incremento degli androgeni surrenalici. Il ciclo, se presente, cessa. L'ecografia pelvica dimostra una diminuzione delle dimensioni di ovaie e utero. Nei maschi, si verifica una diminuzione delle dimensioni testicolari, una regressione variabile dei peli pubici e della frequenza delle erezioni. Eccetto che per un decremento reversibile della densità ossea (di incerto significato clinico), non si sono registrati effetti collaterali seri degli analoghi del GnRH nei bambini trattati per pubertà precoce. Se il trattamento è efficace, le concentrazioni sieriche dell'ormone sessuale diminuiscono a livelli prepuberi (testosterone, <10-20 ng/dL nei maschi; estradiolo, <5-10 pg/mL nelle femmine). Le concentrazioni sieriche di LH e FSH, valutate con metodiche sensibili immunometriche, diminuiscono a valori inferiori a 1 UI/L nella maggior parte dei pazienti, sebbene quasi mai i livelli di LH ritornino davvero a valori prepuberi (<0,1 UI/L). Inoltre, le risposte incrementali di FSH e LH alla stimolazione con GnRH diminuiscono a meno di 1-2 UI/L. I livelli sierici di LH e di ormoni sessuali rimangono soppressi finché si continua la terapia, ma la pubertà riprende prontamente non appena essa si interrompe, tipicamente a un'età cronologica "puberale". Nelle femmine, il menarca e i cicli ovulatori di solito compaiono in media dopo 18 mesi (range 6-24 mesi) dalla sospensione della terapia. L'aggiunta di ormone della crescita umano (hGH) agli agonisti del GnRH è stata utilizzata nei bambini con pubertà precoce, età ossea notevolmente avanzata e con previsione di bassa statura. I dati disponibili, sebbene limitati, indicano che la terapia combinata può aumentare l'altezza da adulti.

563.2 • PUBERTÀ PRECOCE DA LESIONI CEREBRALI ORGANICHE

EZIOLOGIA. Gli amartomi ipotalamici rappresentano la più comune lesione cerebrale responsabile di pubertà precoce vera (Fig. 563-2). Questa malformazione congenita consiste nella presenza, in sedi ectopiche, di tessuto nervoso contenente neuroni GnRH-secernenti, che può anche fungere da generatore pulsatile accessorio di GnRH. Alla RM appare come una piccola massa peduncolata attaccata al *tuber cinereum* o al pavimento del terzo ventricolo oppure, meno di frequente, come una massa sessile (Fig. 563-3) che rimane di dimensioni stabili con il passare degli anni. Questa lesione può anche essere associata a crisi gelastiche o psicomotorie. Un'ampia varietà di lesioni del SNC, che coinvolgono solitamente l'ipotalamo, come cicatrizzazione, invasione o pressione, sono state associate a precocità sessuale gonadotropino-dipendente. Queste lesioni probabilmente inducono una maturazione sessuale attraverso l'interruzione di vie di controllo puberale scarsamente caratterizzate. Si può trattare di cicatrici postenecefalitiche, di meningite tubercolare, di sclerosi tuberosa, di grave trauma cranico e di idrocefalo, isolati o associati a mielomeningocele. Le neoplasie che provocano pubertà precoce comprendono astrocitomi, ependimomi e tumori del tratto ottico, mentre quelle dell'ultimo tipo (tipicamente gliomi ottici a lenta progressione o indolenti) sono le più frequenti (15-20%) nei bambini con neurofibromatosi di tipo 1 (NF-1); costituiscono, inoltre, il principale fattore eziologico della precocità sessuale centrale, presenti in un piccolo sottogruppo (circa il 3%) di bambini con NF-1.

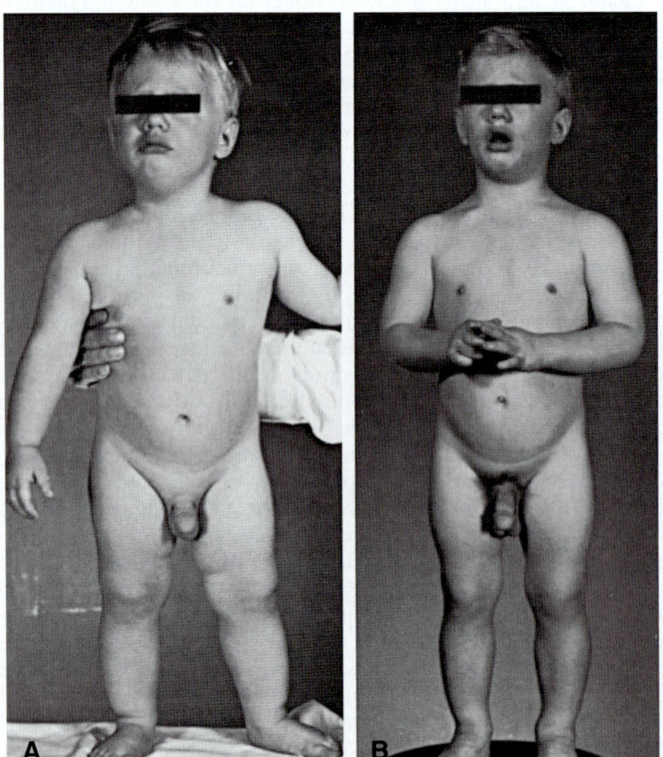

Figura 563-2. Decorso naturale della pubertà precoce con lesione del sistema nervoso centrale. Fotografie a 1 anno e mezzo *(A)* e a 2 anni e mezzo *(B)* di età. L'accelerazione della crescita, lo sviluppo muscolare, la maturazione ossea erano in rapporto alla maturazione dei caratteri sessuali secondari. All'età di 1 anno e mezzo, il paziente cominciava ad avere frequenti episodi di movimenti rapidi, non finalizzati; più tardi nel corso degli anni comparvero crisi di riso incontrollabili con movimenti oculari. A 7 anni mostrava labilità emotiva, comportamento aggressivo e tendenze distruttive. Sebbene fosse sospettato un amartoma ipotalamico, esso non è stato comprovato fino a che si è resa disponibile la TC, quando il paziente aveva ormai 23 anni. Le epifisi erano fuse all'età di 9 anni; la statura definitiva era di 142 cm. All'età di 24 anni, ha sviluppato un carcinoma a cellule embrionali retroperitoneale.

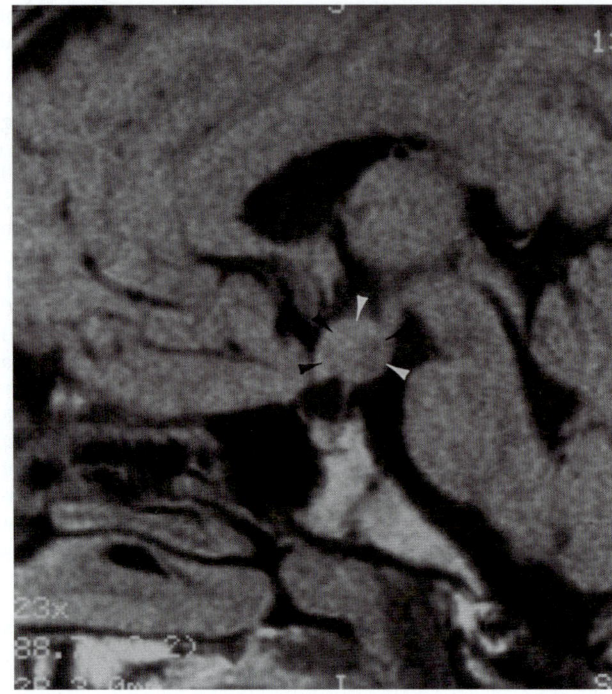

Figura 563-3. RM di una lesione del sistema nervoso centrale in una bambina con pubertà precoce centrale. A 6 anni la bambina si trovava a uno stadio IV di sviluppo mammario e di accelerazione della crescita. Le concentrazioni sieriche di ormone luteinizzante e di estradiolo erano nel range dell'adulto. L'immagine in proiezione mediosagittale T1 mostra una massa ipotalamica isointensa (*punta di freccia*), tipica dell'amartoma. (Da Sharafuddin M, Luisiri A, Garibaldi LR, et al: MR imaging diagnosis of central precocious puberty: Importance of changes in the shape and size of the pituitary gland. *Am J Roengenol* 1994; 162:1167.)

Circa la metà dei tumori della regione epifisaria è rappresentata da germinomi o astrocitomi; il rimanente comprende una notevole varietà di tipi tumorali istologicamente distinti. Questi tumori provocano pubertà precoce attraverso l'interruzione di vie inibitorie dal SNC verso l'ipotalamo o, solo nei maschi, tramite la secrezione di gonadotropina umana corionica (hCG), che stimola le cellule di Leydig dei testicoli. I germinomi intracranici hCG-secernenti di solito non provocano pubertà precoce nelle femmine, presumibilmente perché senza la stimolazione di FSH non si può realizzare la completa funzionalità ovarica.

MANIFESTAZIONI CLINICHE. Alcuni di questi tumori o malformazioni (amartomi ipotalamici) mantengono dimensioni stabili o crescono lentamente, senza produrre segni, se non la pubertà precoce. Per le lesioni responsabili di sintomi neurologici, le manifestazioni neuroendocrine possono essere presenti 1-2 anni prima che il tumore possa essere evidenziato radiologicamente. I segni o sintomi ipotalamici, come il diabete insipido, adipsia, ipertermia, strane grida o risa (crisi gelastiche), obesità e cachessia, devono suggerire la possibilità di una lesione intracranica. Segni visivi (proptosi, diminuzione dell'acuità visiva, difetti del campo visivo) possono essere le prime manifestazioni di un glioma ottico.

La precocità sessuale è sempre isosessuale e il pattern endocrino è generalmente quello di bambini senza lesioni organiche dimostrabili. Una precocità sessuale rapidamente progressiva in bambini molto piccoli suggerisce la possibilità di un amartoma ipotalamico. In condizioni diverse dall'amartoma ipotalamico, si può verificare deficit dell'ormone della crescita, che può essere mascherato dall'effetto di incremento della crescita dovuto agli aumentati livelli di ormoni sessuali.

TRATTAMENTO. Indipendentemente dalla causa, la terapia con agonisti del GnRH è efficace sia nei bambini con lesioni cerebrali organiche responsabili di pubertà precoce centrale, sia in quelli con precocità sessuale idiopatica, e questi analoghi rappresentano la terapia di elezione per arrestare lo sviluppo sessuale precoce. Questo include pazienti con amartoma ipotalamico, se la pubertà precoce è la sola manifestazione. Nei pazienti con amartoma ipotalamico in associazione a crisi gelastiche o psicomotorie intrattabili, tuttavia, la terapia radiante stereotattica (chirurgia a raggi gamma) è efficace e meno rischiosa dell'intervento neurochirurgico. Per altre lesioni neurologiche, la terapia dipende dalla natura e dalla sede del processo patologico. Per i pazienti con associata carenza di ormone della crescita, si deve prendere in considerazione la terapia combinata con ormone della crescita.

563.3 • PUBERTÀ PRECOCE DOPO IRRADIAZIONE DEL CERVELLO

La terapia radiante, generalmente per leucemia o tumori intracranici, accresce considerevolmente il rischio di pubertà precoce, sia che l'irradiazione venga diretta all'area ipotalamica, sia ad aree del cervello anatomicamente distanti dall'ipotalamo. Una bassa dose di radiazioni (18-24 Gy) accelera l'inizio della pubertà quasi esclusivamente nelle femmine. Un'alta dose di radiazioni (25-47 Gy), al contrario, sembra essere l'innesco dello sviluppo sessuale precoce in entrambi i sessi e il rischio di precocità sessuale è inversamente proporzionale all'età del bambino al momento in cui è stato sottoposto a terapia radiante.

Questo tipo di precocità sessuale spesso si verifica con deficit di ormone della crescita e può essere associata ad altre condizioni (irradiazione spinale, ipotiroidismo), che peggiorano la prognosi di un'altezza accettabile da adulto. A meno di una notevole attenzione ai primi i segni di sviluppo puberale in questi bambini, la combinazione di deficit di ormone della crescita ed effetti degli steroidi sessuali nel promuovere la crescita spesso porta a una "normale" velocità di crescita, a spese di un rapido avanzamento dell'età ossea, con problemi per quanto riguarda il potenziale dell'altezza da adulti.

TRATTAMENTO. Gli analoghi del GnRH sono efficaci nell'arrestare la progressione puberale in questo gruppo di pazienti. Tuttavia, è necessario diagnosticare e trattare prontamente un concomitante deficit di GH (e/o deficit di ormone tiroideo) per migliorare la prognosi dell'altezza da adulti.

Paradossalmente, è possibile che si sviluppi successivamente un ipopituitarismo con carenza di gonadotropine, come effetto tardivo di un'alta dose di radiazioni al SNC in pazienti con o senza un'anamnesi di pubertà precoce e può risultare necessaria terapia sostitutiva con steroidi sessuali.

563.4 • SINDROME DA PUBERTÀ PRECOCE E IPOTIROIDISMO

Nei bambini con ipotiroidismo non trattato, l'inizio della pubertà è normalmente ritardato, fino a che la maturazione epifisaria non raggiunge i 12-13 anni di età. In un bambino con ipotiroidismo non trattato, l'associazione di pubertà precoce ed età ossea prepubere non è di certo fisiologica, seppure comune, e si può verificare in un 50% di bambini con severo ipotiroidismo di lunga durata. Questi bambini presentano le comuni manifestazioni di ipotiroidismo, compreso il ritardo della crescita e della maturazione ossea (vedi Capitolo 566). La causa dell'ipotiroidismo è spesso una tiroidite linfocitica non diagnosticata e raramente una tiroidectomia o una terapia con dosi eccessive di farmaci antitiroidei. Lo sviluppo sessuale nelle femmine consiste essenzialmente in un ingrossamento mammario e nella comparsa di mestruazioni; queste ultime possono comparire anche in bambine con un incremento mammario minimo. L'ecografia pelvica può rivelare ovaie ingrandite e multicistiche, invece i maschi hanno uno sviluppo testicolare associato o meno a modesto aumento del pene in assenza di peli pubici. L'ingrandimento sellare, tipico dell'ipotiroidismo primario di lunga data, può essere dimostrato con un RX del cranio o con RM. I livelli plasmatici di TSH sono notevolmente elevati, spesso oltre i 500 μU/mL, mentre quelli della prolattina moderatamente. Sebbene l'FSH sierico sia basso e l'LH indosabile, se misurati con specifici dosaggi, le altissime concentrazioni di TSH sembrerebbero interagire con il recettore dell'FSH (o "specificità spillover"), provocando sulle gonadi effetti FSH-simili, in assenza di effetti dell'LH. Come conseguenza, nei maschi affetti, a differenza della pubertà precoce vera si verifica ingrossamento testicolare senza sostanziale stimolazione delle cellule di Leydig e senza secrezione di testosterone. Nelle femmine, la produzione di estrogeni ovarici avviene senza il concomitante aumento degli androgeni e, di conseguenza, la pubertà precoce associata a ipotiroidismo si comporta come una forma incompleta di pubertà gonadotropino-dipendente. Il trattamento dell'ipotiroidismo riporta rapidamente nella norma le manifestazioni cliniche e biochimiche. Spesso nei mesi seguenti l'inizio della terapia sostitutiva con ormone tiroideo si verificano rapido avanzamento dell'età ossea e progressione della pubertà centrale. La terapia con analoghi del GnRH deve essere iniziata rapidamente in questi pazienti, per prevenire un grave difetto di statura nell'adulto. Il macrorchidismo (volume testicolare >30 mL) può persistere nel maschio adulto nonostante adeguata terapia con tiroxina.

563.5 • TUMORI GONADOTROPINO-SECERNENTI

TUMORI EPATICI. La pubertà precoce isosessuale può essere non comunemente associata a epatoblastoma. Tutti i casi riportati erano di sesso maschile, con un'età di inizio variabile dai 4 mesi agli 8 anni (in media 2 anni). La diagnosi può essere suggerita da un'epatomegalia o da una massa nel quadrante superiore. Le cellule tumorali producono hCG, che stimola i recettori dell'LH a livello delle cellule di Leydig dei testicoli. Questi ultimi sono solo minimamente ingranditi e l'istologia testicolare rivela un'iperplasia interstiziale in assenza di spermatogenesi. I livelli plasmatici di hCG e α-fetoproteina sono di solito notevolmente elevati; vengono utilizzati come marker per seguire nel tempo gli effetti della terapia. I livelli plasmatici di testosterone sono elevati e quelli di FSH e LH, con dosaggi specifici, immunometrici, sono bassi; in passato i livelli di LH apparivano falsamente elevati per una reazione crociata con l'hCG al dosaggio radioimmunologico.

Il trattamento di questi tumori è analogo a quello degli altri carcinomi epatici; la prognosi di sopravvivenza a 1-2 anni dal momento della diagnosi è negativa.

ALTRI TUMORI. Corioncarcinomi gonadotropina corionica-secernenti, teratocarcinomi o teratomi (anche chiamati pinealomi ectopici o teratomi atipici), localizzati nel SNC, nel mediastino, nelle gonadi o anche nelle ghiandole surrenali, possono provocare pubertà precoce, più comunemente (da 10 a 20 volte) nei maschi che nelle femmine. I pazienti spesso presentano livelli molto elevati di hCG e α-fetoproteina. I tumori mediastinici, ma non quelli gonadici, possono essere causa di pubertà precoce nei maschi con sindrome di Klinefelter.

PSEUDOPUBERTÀ PRECOCE. Le cause surrenaliche di pseudopubertà sono discusse nel Capitolo 577 e quelle gonadiche nei Capitoli 585 e 588.

563.6 • Sindrome di McCune-Albright (pubertà precoce con displasia fibrosa poliostotica e anormale pigmentazione)

Questa disfunzione endocrina è associata a disomogenea pigmentazione cutanea e a displasia fibrosa del sistema scheletrico. Sebbene la precocità sessuale nelle femmine fosse in passato la principale endocrinopatia riconosciuta, erano presenti anche alterazioni dell'ipofisi, della tiroide e del surrene. La malattia è caratterizzata da iperfunzione autonoma di molte ghiandole ed è causata da una mutazione missense nel gene che codifica la α-subunità di GS, la proteina G che stimola la formazione di adenosina monofosfato (cAMP), con conseguente formazione di proteina oncogena putativa gsp. Ne deriva un'attivazione dei recettori (recettori della corticotropina [ACTH], del TSH, dell'FSH e dell'LH), che opera tramite un meccanismo cAMP-dipendente, e proliferazione cellulare. Poiché la mutazione è più somatica che genomica, si esprime in modo diverso nelle diverse ghiandole e nei diversi tessuti, da cui notevole variabilità dell'espressione clinica nei vari pazienti. La pubertà precoce è stata descritta soprattutto nelle femmine (Fig. 563-4). L'età media di inizio è di circa 3 anni, ma si è verificato sanguinamento vaginale molto precocemente, al quarto mese di età, e caratteristiche sessuali secondarie sono comparse al sesto mese. Le bambine piccole hanno livelli di LH e di FSH soppressi, che non rispondono alla stimolazione con GnRH. I livelli di estradiolo possono variare da valori normali a notevolmente elevati (>900 pg/mL), sono spesso ciclici e possono venire correlati alla dimensione delle cisti. Nei maschi, la pubertà precoce è meno comune, ma sono stati individuati diversi casi. Al contrario dell'incremento ovarico nelle bambine, nei maschi l'ingrossamento testicolare è abbastanza simmetrico. È seguito da aumento del pene e da comparsa di peli pubici, come avviena nella pubertà normale. L'istologia testicolare ha dimostrato ampi tubuli seminiferi e una minima o assente iperplasia delle cellule di Leydig: tali reperti possono semplicemente riflettere il fatto che il prelievo bioptico era stato ottenuto in uno stadio precoce dello sviluppo puberale. Tanto nelle bambine quanto nei bambini, se l'età ossea raggiunge il normale range puberale, allora inizia la secrezione di gonadotropine e la risposta al GnRH acquista connotazioni puberali. La pubertà precoce vera (gonadotropino-dipendente) sostituisce la precedente pseudo-pubertà precoce (gonadotropino-indipendente). Nelle femmine, i cicli mestruali cominciano a regolarizzarsi, ma spesso non completamente, e si è documentata fertilità.

La progressione puberale è variabile in questi pazienti. Le cisti ovariche funzionanti spesso scompaiono spontaneamente; raramente si consiglia l'aspirazione o l'exeresi chirurgica delle cisti. Per le femmine con persistente secrezione di estradiolo, agenti che interferiscono con le fasi finali della biosintesi estrogenica, per esempio inibitori dell'aromatasi come il testolactone o il letrozolo (1,25-2,5 mg/die per os) o l'anastrozolo (1 mg/die per os), o antiestrogeni (come il tamoxifene) possono limitare, in modo variabile, gli effetti estrogenici sulla maturazione puberale e ossea. Gli stessi composti si utilizzano nei maschi, in associazione ad antiandrogeni (come lo spironolattone 50-100 mg/2 volte al giorno, o flutamide 125-250 mg/2 volte al giorno). Tali composti non sono approvati dalla FDA per questa indicazione; il tamoxifene e la flutamide possono essere epatotossici e alte dosi di spironolattone possono di rado provocare iperkaliemia. Una terapia associata con analoghi del GnRH a lunga durata di azione è indicata solo per i pazienti in cui la pubertà si sposti da una forma gonadotropino-indipendente a una in cui predomina il meccanismo gonadotropino-dipendente.

MANIFESTAZIONI EXTRAGONADICHE. L'ipertiroidismo che si verifica in questa condizione differisce da quello caratteristico della malattia di Graves. C'è un'uguale distribuzione nei maschi e nelle femmine; i gozzi sono multinodulari. L'ipertiroidismo clinico non è comune nei bambini, ma sono riportati gozzi, livelli modicamente elevati di triiodotironina, livelli soppressi di TSH e anomalie ecografiche. Solo raramente è necessaria una tiroidectomia.

In pazienti con associata sindrome di Cushing, nella prima infanzia compare iperplasia surrenalica bilaterale, antecedente alla precocità sessuale. I livelli di ACTH sono bassi, ma la funzionalità surrenalica non è soppressa da alte dosi di desametazone. Il trattamento consiste nella surrenalectomia bilaterale.

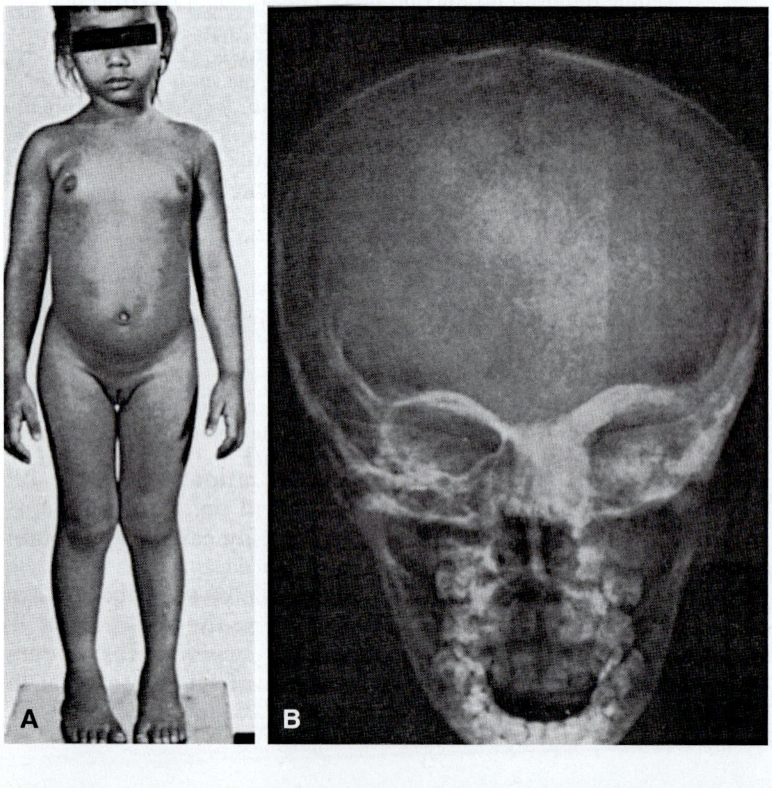

Figura 563-4. Pubertà precoce associata a displasia fibrosa poliostotica (sindrome di McCune-Albright) in una bambina di 4 anni e mezzo; in questo momento erano normali l'età staturale e quella ossea. Menarca a 4 anni. *A*, Notare lo sviluppo mammario bilaterale, le macchie iperpigmentate sull'addome e la prominenza della parte sinistra del volto. *B*, L'indagine radiologica rivelò una displasia fibrosa nell'estremità distale dell'ulna sinistra e un ispessimento delle ossa intorno all'orbita sinistra e nella porzione mascellare delle ossa frontali.

L'ipersecrezione di ormone della crescita si verifica di rado e si manifesta clinicamente con gigantismo o acromegalia oppure con aumento della velocità di crescita anche in assenza di pubertà precoce e maschi e femmine sono colpiti in uguale misura. I livelli sierici di ormone della crescita sono elevati e aumentano durante il sonno; sono incrementati dalla tireotropina (TRH) e scarsamente inibiti dal carico orale di glucosio. I livelli sierici di prolattina nella maggior parte dei pazienti sono aumentati, ma in meno della metà è dimostrabile un tumore ipofisario. L'octreotide, un analogo della somatostatina a lunga durata di azione, è stato utilizzato per trattare l'ipersomatotropinismo. La prognosi *quod vitam* è favorevole, ma le lesioni ossee possono comportare deformità, fratture ripetute, dolore e occasionale compressione dei nervi cranici.

Fra le manifestazioni extraghiandolari, la fosfaturia, con rachitismo o con osteomalacia, è la più comune. Sono rari i problemi cardiovascolari o epatici, ma possono essere pericolosi per la vita (grave colestasi neonatale).

563.7 • Pubertà precoce maschile familiare gonadotropino-indipendente

Questa rara forma, autosomica dominante, di precocità sessuale si trasmette da un maschio affetto e una femmina non affetta portatrice del gene, che passa alla prole di sesso maschile. Verso i 2-3 anni compaiono i segni della pubertà e i testicoli sono solo modestamente aumentati. Le biopsie testicolari mostrano maturazione delle cellule di Leydig, talvolta marcata ipoplasia. Può essere presente maturazione dei tubuli seminiferi. I livelli di testosterone sono molto alti come nella pubertà precoce vera; tuttavia, i livelli basali di LH sono prepuberi, è assente la secrezione pulsatile di LH, la quale, inoltre, non risponde alla stimolazione con GnRH. La causa dell'attivazione delle cellule di Leidyg indipendentemente dalla stimolazione con LH è una mutazione missense del recettore del'LH, che porta all'attivazione costitutiva della produzione di cAMP. La maturazione ossea può essere notevolmente avanzata; se essa raggiunge il range di età puberale, la maturazione ipotalamica sposta il meccanismo dello sviluppo puberale verso una forma gonadotropino-dipendente. Questa sequenza di eventi è simile a quella che si verifica nei bambini con sindrome di McCune-Albright (vedi paragrafo precedente) o in quelli con iperplasia surrenalica congenita (vedi Capitolo 577.1).

La pubertà precoce gonadotropino-indipendente è stata diagnosticata in pochi bambini, senza legami di parentela, con pseudoipoparatiroidismo di tipo IA, che avevano una singola mutazione della proteina $G_S\alpha$, la quale è inattivante alla normale temperatura corporea e provoca pseudoipoparatiroidismo, ma alla temperatura più bassa dei testicoli, è costituzionalmente attivante e comporta stimolazione dell'adenilciclasi oltre a produzione di testosterone. Sebbene questa mutazione differisca da quella costitutiva del recettore dell'LH, che normalmente provoca pubertà precoce maschile familiare gonadortopino-indipendente, l'esito finale è lo stesso.

TRATTAMENTO. Bambini piccoli sono stati trattati con successo con ketoconazolo (600 mg/die in dosi refratte ogni 8 ore), un antimicotico che inibisce la C-17,20-liasi e la sintesi del testosterone. Altri Autori utilizzano una combinazione di antiandrogeni (come lo spironolattone 50-100 mg/2 volte al giorno o flutamide 125-250 mg/2 volte al giorno) e inibitori dell'aromatasi (letrozolo 2,5 mg/2 o anastrozolo 1 mg/die), perché gli estrogeni derivati dagli androgeni stimolano la maturazione ossea. Questi farmaci non sono in grado di riportare il testosterone a concentrazioni normali (prepuberi) o di compensare completamente gli effetti sfavorevoli degli elevati livelli di ormoni sessuali. Essi rallentano, ma non arrestano, la progressione della pubertà e non migliorano la prognosi circa l'altezza. I maschi con maturazione del generatore pulsatile di GnRH necessitano di una terapia combinata con agonisti del GnRH.

563.8 • Sviluppo precoce incompleto (parziale)

Isolate manifestazioni di precocità senza sviluppo di altri segni di pubertà non sono infrequenti; le due forme più comuni sono rappresentate dal telarca nelle femmine e dalla crescita di peli sessuali in entrambi i sessi.

TELARCA PRECOCE. Questo termine si riferisce a una condizione transitoria di isolato sviluppo mammario, che più spesso compare nei primi 2 anni di vita; in alcune bambine, è presente fino dalla nascita e persiste. Lo sviluppo mammario può essere asimmetrico e spesso di grado diverso. La crescita e la maturazione ossea sono normali o lievemente avanzate, mentre i genitali non mostrano segni di stimolazione estrogenica. Di solito questa condizione è sporadica e raramente familiare. Lo sviluppo mammario può regredire dopo 2 anni, in genere persiste per 3-5 anni ed è raramente progressivo. Il menarca compare all'età giusta, come normale è la riproduzione. I livelli sierici basali di FSH e la risposta dell'FSH alla stimolazione con GnRH possono essere maggiori dei controlli normali. I livelli plasmatici di LH e di estradiolo sono consistentemente minori dei limiti di dosabilità. L'indagine ecografia delle ovaie dimostra normali dimensioni, ma non sono rare piccole cisti (<9 mm).

In alcune bambine di alcune fasce di età, lo sviluppo mammario può essere associato a manifestazioni definite, dovute agli effetti sistemici degli estrogeni, come accelerazione della crescita e progressione dell'età ossea. L'ecografia pelvica può evidenziare un ingrandimento ovarico o uterino. Questa condizione, definita **telarca esagerato o atipico**, differisce dalle forme centrali di pubertà precoce in quanto regredisce spontaneamente. La stimolazione con GnRH o leuprolide provoca una risposta significativa dell'FSH, bassa dell'LH, e (dopo solo leupride) un moderato incremento dell'estradiolo a 24 ore (mediamente 60-90 pg/mL). La patogenesi della forma di telarca tipico o esagerato non è chiara, sebbene un ritardo nel passaggio da un asse ipofiso-ovarico attivato (neonatale-infantile) a uno inattivo (prepubere) possa sottendere a entrambe le condizioni. Il telarca precoce è una condizione benigna, ma può essere il primo segno di una pubertà precoce vera o di una pseudopubertà precoce, o può essere dovuto a esposizione a estrogeni esogeni. Oltre a un'anamnesi dettagliata, può essere necessario stabilire un'età ossea. Le concentrazioni sieriche di FSH, LH ed estradiolo generalmente sono basse e non diagnostiche e raramente l'ecografia pelvica è indicativa. È importante la continua osservazione, perché la condizione non è facilmente distinguibile dalla pubertà precoce vera. La regressione e la recidiva suggeriscono cisti follicolari funzionanti. La presenza di telarca in bambine con più di 3 anni più spesso è provocata da una condizione diversa rispetto al telarca precoce.

PUBARCA PRECOCE (ADRENARCA). Si applica questo termine alla comparsa di peli sessuali prima dell'ottavo anno nelle femmine e del nono nei maschi, senza altre evidenze di maturazione. È molto più frequente nelle femmine rispetto ai maschi e si verifica più spesso nelle bambine di razza nera che non nelle altre. I peli appaiono sul monte di Venere e sulle grandi labbra nelle femmine, nella zona perineale e scrotale nei maschi, mentre i peli ascellari solitamente sono più tardivi. È comune un odore ascellare di tipo adulto. I bambini mostrano un'altezza e un'età ossea leggermente avanzate. L'adrenarca precoce è un evento maturativo precoce, legato alla produzione surrenalica di androgeni e questo fatto coincide con la precoce maturazione della zona reticolare, con associato decremento nell'attività della 3 β-idrossisteroido deidrogenasi e incremento dell'attività della C-17,20-liasi. Queste modificazioni enzimatiche comportano un aumento delle concentrazioni sieriche basali e dopo stimolazione con ACTH, di Δ^5-steroidi (17-idrossipregnenolone e DHEA) e, in minor misura, di Δ^4-steroidi (particolarmente androstenedione), rispetto a coetanei di controllo. I livelli di questi steroidi e di DHEAS sono normalmente paragonabili a quelli di altri bambini in stadi precoci della normale pubertà.

L'adrenarca precoce è una condizione a progressione lenta che non richiede terapia. Tuttavia, un sottogruppo di pazienti con pubarca precoce presenta una o più caratteristiche di effetti sistemici degli androgeni, come una marcata accelerazione della crescita, aumento del clitoride (nelle femmine) o del pene (nei maschi), acne cistica o età ossea avanzata (>2 DS rispetto alla media per età). In questi pazienti con **adrenarca precoce atipico**, è indicato un test di stimolazione con ACTH, che misuri gli steroidi intermedi (soprattutto le concentrazioni sieriche di 17-idrossiprogesterone), per escludere un'iperplasia surrenalica congenita non classica da carenza di 21-idrossilasi. Studi epidemiologici e genetici molecolari hanno mostrato che la frequenza di deficit non classica di 21-idrossilasi è approssimativamente intorno al 3-6% di bambini non selezionati con pubarca precoce; la frequenza di altri difetti enzimatici (per es. carenza di 3 β-idrossisteroido deidrogenasi o 11 β-idrossilasi) è molto bassa. Sebbene l'adrenarca precoce idiopatico sia considerato una forma benigna, osservazioni longitudinali suggeriscono che circa il 50% delle femmine con adrenarca precoce presenti da adulto un rischio maggiore di **iperandrogenismo** e di **sindrome dell'ovaio policistico**, da solo, o più spesso in combinazione con altri componenti di questa sindrome metabolica (insulino-resistenza con possibilità di un progressivo diabete di tipo 2, dislipidemia, ipertensione, aumento del grasso addominale). Anche se la sfavorevole progressione dell'iperandrogenismo puberale può essere prevenuta con agenti insulino-sensibilizzanti (metformina 850-1000 mg/die) o con interventi sullo stile di vita (dieta, esercizio fisico), questo deve ancora essere provato da ampi studi. Si è ben documentato invece un aumento del rischio di adrenarca precoce e di sindrome metabolica in bambini nati piccoli per età gestazionale; sembra che venga associato a insulino-resistenza e decremento della riserva delle cellule β, probabilmente come conseguenza di iponutrizione fetale.

MENARCA PRECOCE. Si tratta di un evento raro, molto meno frequente del telarca precoce o dell'adrenarca precoce e costituisce una diagnosi di esclusione. In bambine con sanguinamento vaginale isolato in assenza di altre caratteristiche sessuali secondarie, devono essere attentamente escluse le cause più comuni come vulvovaginite, corpo estraneo o abuso sessuale, nonché quelle meno comuni, come prolasso uretrale e sarcoma botrioide. La maggior parte delle bambine con menarca precoce idiopatico mostra solo da uno a tre episodi di sanguinamento; la pubertà si verifica in tempi giusti e i cicli mestruali sono normali. Anche i livelli plasmatici di gonadotropine sono normali, ma quelli di estradiolo possono essere elevati, probabilmente per secrezione estrogenica episodica da parte dell'ovaio. L'indagine ecografica ha evidenziato occasionalmente cisti ovariche follicolari.

563.9 • Precocità indotta da farmaci

Numerosi farmaci possono indurre la comparsa di caratteristiche sessuali secondarie, le quali possono essere confuse con la pubertà precoce. È importante un'anamnesi attenta, focalizzata sulle possibilità di esposizione accidentale per ingestione di ormoni sessuali. Casi di pseudopubertà precoce si sono verificati sia nei maschi sia nelle femmine per ingestione accidentale di estrogeni (compresa la pillola contraccettiva) e per somministrazione di steroidi anabolizzanti. Cosmetici a base di estrogeni, creme per i capelli e creme per aumentare il seno hanno causato sviluppo mammario nelle femmine e ginecomastia nei maschi, poiché gli estrogeni sono facilmente assorbiti attraverso la cute. La notevole frequenza di telarca precoce e di pseudopubertà precoce a Porto Rico è stata attribuita alla contaminazione di carne, particolarmente di pollo, con estrogeni usati negli animali da allevamento, ma non ne esistono prove. Estrogeni esogeni possono produrre un'intensa colorazione marrone scuro dell'areola mammaria, solitamente non presente nelle forme endogene di precocità. Le modificazioni precoci scompaiono dopo la cessazione dell'esposizione agli ormoni. L'utilizzo di testosterone in gel o creme da applicare sulla cute per il trattamento dell'ipogonadismo maschile comporta una virilizzazione dei bambini e delle bambine, in seguito al contatto cutaneo, e assorbimento sistemico, a livello dell'area dove il gel o la crema è stato applicato da un membro della famiglia.

Antoniazzi F, Zamboni G, Bertoldo F: Bone development during GH and GnRH analog treatment. *Eur J Endocrinol* 2004;151:S47–54.

Carel JC, Lahlou N, Jaramillo O, et al: Treatment of central precocious puberty by subcutaneous injections of leuprorelin 3-month depot (11.25 mg). *J Clin Endocrinol Metab* 2002;87:4111–4116.

Carel JC, Lahlou N, Roger M, et al: Precocious puberty and statural growth. *Hum Reprod Update* 2004;10:135–147.

Chalumeau M, Chemaitilly W, Trivin C, et al: Central precocious puberty in girls: An evidence-based diagnosis tree to predict central nervous system abnormalities. *Pediatrics* 2002;109:61–67.

Chalumeau M, Hadjiathanasiou CG, Ng SM, et al: Selecting girls with precocious puberty for brain imaging: Validation of European evidence-based diagnosis rule. *J Pediatr* 2003;143:445–450.

Hirsch HJ, Gillis D, Strich D, et al: The histrelin implant: A novel treatment for central precocious puberty. *Pediatrics* 2005;116:e798–e802.

Ibanez L, Dimartino-Nardi J, Potau N, et al: Premature adrenarche–normal variant or forerunner of adult disease? *Endocr Rev* 2000;21:671–696.

Ibanez L, Ferrer A, Marcos MV, et al: Early puberty: Rapid progression and reduced final height in girls with low birth weight. *Pediatrics* 2000;106:E72.

Ibanez L, Ferrer A, Ong K, et al: Insulin sensitization early after menarche prevents progression from precocious pubarche to polycystic ovary syndrome. *J Pediatr* 2004;144:4–6.

Ibanez L, Potau N, Marcos MV, et al: Adrenal hyperandrogenism in adolescent girls with a history of low birthweight and precocious pubarche. *Clin Endocrinol (Oxf)* 2000;53:523–527.

Ibanez L, Potau N, Zampolli M, et al: Use of leuprolide acetate response patterns in the early diagnosis of pubertal disorders: Comparison with the gonadotropin-releasing hormone test. *J Clin Endocrinol Metab* 1994;78:30–35.

Kaplowitz PB, Slora EJ, Wasserman RC, et al: Earlier onset of puberty in girls: Relation to increased body mass and race. *Pediatrics* 2001;108:347–353.

Klein K, Barnes KM, Jones JV, et al: Increase in final height in precocious puberty after long-term treatment with LHRH agonists: The National Institutes of Health experience. *J Clin Endocrinol Metab* 2001;86: 4711–4716.

Latronico AC, Lins TS, Brito VN, et al: The effect of distinct activating mutations of the luteinizing hormone receptor gene on the pituitary-gonadal axis in both sexes. *Clin Endocrinol (Oxf)* 2000;53:609–613.

Leger J, Reynaud R, Czernichow P: Do all girls with apparent idiopathic precocious puberty require gonadotropin-releasing hormone agonist treatment? *J Pediatr* 2000;137:819–825.

Lumbroso S, Paris F, Sultan C: McCune-Albright syndrome: Molecular genetics. *J Pediatr Endocrinol Metab* 2002;15(Suppl 3):875–882.

Mul D, Oostdijk W, Drop SL: Early puberty in adopted children. *Horm Res* 2002;57:1–9.

Neville KA, Walker JL: Precocious pubarche is associated with SGA, prematurity, weight gain, and obesity. *Arch Dis Child* 2005:90:258–261.

Ng SM, Kumar Y, Cody D, et al: Cranial MRI scans are indicated in all girls with central precocious puberty. *Arch Dis Child* 2003;88:414–418.

Palmert MR, Boepple PA: Variation in the timing of puberty: Clinical spectrum and genetic investigation. *J Clin Endocrinol Metab* 2001;86:2364–2368.

Pucarelli I, Segni M, Ortore M, et al: Combined therapy with GnRH analog plus growth hormone in central precocious puberty. *J Pediatr Endocrinol Metab* 2000;13:811–820.

Ritzen EM: Early puberty: What is normal and when is treatment indicated? *Horm Res* 2003;60:31–34.

Saenger P, Rincon M: Precocious puberty: McCune-Albright syndrome and beyond. *J Pediatr* 2003;143:9–10.

Seminara SB, Messager S, Chatzidaki EE, et al: The GPR54 gene as a regulator of puberty. *N Engl J Med* 2003;349:1614–1626.

Stanhope R: Gonadotropin-dependent precocious puberty and occult intracranial tumors: Which girls should have neuro-imaging? *J Pediatr* 2003;143:426–427.

Tanaka T, Niimi H, Matsuo N, et al: Results of long-term follow-up after treatment of central precocious puberty with leuprorelin acetate: Evaluation of effectiveness of treatment and recovery of gonadal function. *J Clin Endocrinol Metab* 2005;90:1371–1376.

Teilmann G, Pedersen CB, Kold Jensen T, et al: Prevalence and incidence of precocious pubertal development in Denmark: An epidemiologic study based on national registries. *Pediatrics* 2005;116:1323–1328.

Terasawa E, Fernandez DL: Neurobiological mechanisms of the onset of puberty in primates. *Endocr Rev* 2001;22:111–151.

Tuvemo T, Gustafsson J, Proos LA, et al: Suppression of puberty in girls with short acting intranasal versus subcutaneous depot GnRH agonist. *Horm Res* 2002;57:27–31.
Tuvemo T, Jonsson B, Gustafsson J, et al: Final height after combined growth hormone and GnRH analogue treatment in adopted girls with early puberty. *Acta Paediatr* 2004;93:1456–1462.
Van Beek JT, Sharafuddin MJ, Kao SC, et al: Prospective evaluation of pituitary size and shape on MR imaging after suppressive hormonal therapy in central precocious puberty. *Pediatr Radiol* 2000;30:444–446.
Virdis R, Street ME, Bandello MA, et al: Growth and pubertal disorders in neurofibromatosis type 1. *J Pediatr Endocrinol Metab* 2003;16: 289–292.
Walvoord EC, Pescovitz OH: Combined use of growth hormone and gonadotropin-releasing hormone analogues in precocious puberty: Theoretic and practical considerations. *Pediatrics* 1999;104: 1010–1014.

Sezione 2 — Malattie della tiroide — Stephen LaFranchi

Capitolo 564 ■ Sviluppo e fisiologia della tiroide

SVILUPPO FETALE

La forma bilobata della tiroide fetale si riconosce già alla settima settimana di gestazione e alla decima sono visibili i caratteristici follicoli tiroidei oltre alla formazione di colloide. La sintesi di tireoglobulina ha inizio dalla quarta settimana, la captazione di iodio nell'ottava-decima, mentre la sintesi e la secrezione di tiroxina (T_4) e, in minor misura, di triiodotironina (T_3), cominciano a partire dalla dodicesima settimana di gestazione. Quattro fattori di trascrizione, TTF-1, PAX8, Foxe1 e Hhex, sono importanti per la morfogenesi e per la differenziazione della tiroide, nonché per la sua migrazione caudale fino alla sede definitiva. Questi fattori legano anche i promotori dei geni della tireoglobulina e della perossidasi, influenzando così la produzione di ormoni tiroidei. I neuroni ipotalamici sintetizzano l'ormone di rilascio della tireotropina (TRH) alla sesta-ottava settimana, mentre il sistema vascolare portale dell'ipofisi inizia a svilupparsi all'ottava-decima settimana e la secrezione di ormone stimolante la tiroide (TSH) comincia a essere evidente alla dodicesima settimana di gestazione. La maturazione dell'asse ipotalamo-ipofiso-tiroideo si verifica dopo il secondo mese e mezzo di gestazione, ma la maturazione dei normali rapporti di feedback non si attua fino a circa il terzo mese postnatale. Un altro fattore trascrizionale, il Pit-1, è importante per la differenziazione e la crescita delle cellule tireotrope, somatotrope e lattotrope.

FISIOLOGIA DELLA TIROIDE

La principale funzione della ghiandola tiroidea consiste nella sintesi di T_4 e di T_3. Il solo ruolo fisiologico dello iodio conosciuto è quello della sintesi di tali ormoni; la quantità raccomandata di iodio nella dieta è di 30 μg/kg/die per i lattanti, di 90-120 μg/die per i bambini e di 150 μg/die per gli adolescenti e gli adulti. L'apporto medio di iodio negli Stati Uniti è diminuito di circa il 50% tra il 1970 (320 μg/L) e il 1990 (145 μg/L), sebbene attualmente pare si sia stabilizzato. Qualsiasi sia la forma chimica con cui viene ingerito, lo iodio raggiunge con molta probabilità la tiroide sotto forma di ioduro. Il tessuto tiroideo presenta una particolare avidità per lo iodio ed è in grado di captarlo (con un gradiente di 100:1), trasportarlo e concentrarlo nel lume follicolare per la sintesi dell'ormone tiroideo. Il trasporto dello iodio è effettuato dal symporter della pompa sodio/ioduro.

Prima che lo iodio assunto possa reagire con la tiroxina, esso deve essere ossidato e tale reazione è catalizzata dalla **perossidasi tiroidea.** Le cellule tiroidee elaborano anche una specifica tireoproteina, una globulina con circa 120 unità tirosiniche (**tireoglobulina**). La iodinazione della tiroxina porta alla formazione di monoiodotirosina e diiodotirosina; due molecole di diiodotirosina si uniscono a formare una molecola di T_4, oppure una molecola di diiodotirosina e una di monoiodotirosina si legano a formare il T_3. Appena sintetizzati, gli ormoni vengono accumulati sotto forma di tireoglobulina nel lume follicolare (colloide) fino a quando non sono pronti per rifornire le cellule dell'organismo. La tireoglobulina è una grande glicoproteina globulare con peso molecolare di circa 660 000. Il T_4 e il T_3 vengono liberati dalla tireoglobulina per l'attivazione di proteasi e peptidasi.

La potenza metabolica del T_3 è 3-4 volte maggiore di quella del T_4. Negli adulti, la tiroide produce ogni giorno circa 100 μg di T4 e 20 μg di T_3. Solo il 20% del T_3 circolante è secreto dalla tiroide e il rimanente si forma dalla deiodinazione del T_4 a livello epatico, renale, tiroideo e di altri tessuti periferici, a opera di una 5′-deiodinasi di tipo I. La seleniocisteina è il centro attivo della iodotironina-deiodinasi. Perciò, il selenio indirettamente gioca un ruolo nella crescita e nello sviluppo normali. Nell'ipofisi e nel cervello, circa l'80% del T_3 richiesto viene prodotto localmente dal T_4 a opera di un enzima diverso, cioè la 5′-deiodinasi di tipo II. I livelli ematici di T_3 sono circa la metà di quelli di T_4, ma il T_3 è l'ormone tiroideo fisiologicamente attivo.

Gli ormoni tiroidei aumentano il consumo di ossigeno, stimolano la sintesi proteica, influenzano la crescita e la differenziazione e influiscono sul metabolismo di carboidrati, di lipidi e di vitamine. Gli ormoni liberi entrano nelle cellule, dove il T_4 può essere convertito in T_3 tramite deiodinazione. Il trasportatore 8 monocarbossilato è un trasportatore attivo specifico per l'ormone tiroideo, che facilita l'ingresso di T_4 nella cellula. Mutazioni di *MCT8* sono associate ad alti livelli di T_3, a resistenza all'ormone tiroideo e a grave ritardo psicomotorio associato a X. Il T_3 intracellulare entra successivamente nel nucleo, dove si lega al recettore per l'ormone tiroideo, il quale appartiene a una superfamiglia di recettori di ormoni steroidei che comprendono i glicocorticoidi, gli estrogeni, il progesterone, la vitamina D e i retinoidi. Sono espresse quattro diverse isoforme del recettore dell'ormone tiroideo (α_1, α_2, β_1, β_2) nei diversi tessuti; la proteina prodotta da quello che in passato era chiamato proto-oncogene c-*erb* A (ora *THRA2*) è stata identificata come il recettore α_2 dell'ormone tiroideo nel cervello e nell'ipotalamo. I recettori dell'ormone tiroideo sono formati da un dominio ligand-binding (che lega il T_3), regione cardine, e da un dominio DNA-binding (*zinc finger*). Il legame di T_3 attiva gli elementi di risposta del recettore dell'ormone tiroideo, con conseguente produzione di mRNA codificato, sintesi proteica e secrezione specifica per le cellule bersaglio. In questo modo un singolo ormone, il T_4, agendo attraverso isoforme del recettore dell'ormone tiroideo tessuto-specifiche ed elementi di risposta tiroidea gene-specifici, può produrre effetti multipli nei vari tessuti.

Circa il 70% del T_4 circolante è saldamente legato alla TBG, il 50% all'albumina; lo 0,3% del T_3 circola non legato o libero. Dato che la concentrazione di TBG è alterata in molte circostanze cliniche, essa va valutata per potere interpretare i livelli di T_4 o di T_3.

REGOLAZIONE DELLA TIROIDE

La tiroide è regolata dal TSH, una glicoproteina prodotta e secreta dall'ipofisi anteriore. Quest'ormone attiva l'adenil ciclasi tiroidea ed è importante in tutte le fasi della biosintesi dell'ormone tiroideo, dalla captazione dello iodio al rilascio degli ormoni tiroidei. Il TSH è composto da due subunità (catene), legate in modo non-covalente: α e β. La subunità α è comune anche all'ormone luteinizzante, follicolo-stimolante e alla gonadotropina corionica; la specificità di ogni ormone è quindi conferita dalla subunità beta. La sintesi e il rilascio di TSH sono stimolati dall'ormone di rilascio del TSH (TRH), sintetizzato nell'ipotalamo e secreto nell'ipofisi. Il TRH è stato trovato in altre sedi del cervello oltre all'ipotalamo e in molti altri organi; a prescindere dalla sua funzione endocrina, può essere un neurotrasmettitore. Il TRH è un semplice tripeptide. In condizioni di diminuita produzione di ormone tiroideo, il TSH e il TRH aumentano. L'introduzione esogena o l'aumento della sintesi di ormone tiroideo comportano invece un'inibizione della produzione di TSH e di TRH. Tranne nel neonato, i livelli sierici di TRH sono molto bassi.

Un ulteriore controllo del livello degli ormoni tiroidei circolanti si verifica in periferia. In molte malattie non tiroidee, diminuisce la produzione di T_3 extratiroideo; i fattori che inibiscono la 5′-deiodinasi tipo I della tiroxina comprendono il digiuno, la malnutrizione cronica, le malattie acute e certi farmaci. In queste condizioni i livelli di T_3 possono essere significativamente diminuiti, mentre quelli di T_4 libero e di TSH rimangono normali. Presumibilmente, la diminuzione dei livelli di T_3 porta a un decremento del tasso di produzione di ossigeno, dell'uso del substrato e di altri processi catabolici.

Cavalieri RD: Iodine metabolism and thyroid physiology: Current concepts. [Review.] *Thyroid* 1997;7:177–181.

De Felice M, Di Lauro F: The development of the thyroid gland: What we know and what we would like to know. *Curr Opin Endocrinol Metab* 2005;12:4.

Fisher DA, Brown RS: Thyroid physiology in the perinatal period and during childhood. In Braverman LE, Utiger RD (editors): *Werner & Ingbar's The Thyroid: A Fundamental and Clinical Text,* 8th ed. Philadelphia, Lippincott Williams & Wilkins, 2000, p 959.

Friesema ECH, Grueters A, Biebermann H, et al: Association between mutations in a thyroid hormone transporter and severe X-linked psychomotor retardation. *Lancet* 2004;364:1435–1437.

Hollowell JG, Staehling NW, Hannon WH, et al: Iodine nutrition in the United States – Trends and public health implications: Iodine excretion data from National Health and Nutrition Examination Surveys I and III (1971–1974 and 1988–1994). *J Clin Endocrinol Metab* 1998;83:3401–3408.

564.1 • STUDI SULL'ORMONE TIROIDEO

ORMONI TIROIDEI SIERICI. Sono disponibili vari metodi per misurare tutti gli ormoni tiroidei nel siero: T_4, T_4 libero, T_3, e T_3 libero. È presente nel siero anche un T_3 metabolicamente inerte (3,5′,3′-triiodotironina), chiamato T_3 *reverse.* Nell'interpretazione dei dati, si deve tener conto dell'età, particolarmente nei neonati.

La tireoglobulina è un dimero glicoproteico secreto attraverso la superficie apicale del tireocita all'interno della colloide. Piccole quantità circolanti possono essere misurate nel siero. I livelli aumentano dopo stimolazione con TSH (detta anche tireotropina) e diminuiscono invece con la sua soppressione. I livelli sono più elevati nel neonato, in pazienti con malattia di Graves e altre forme di patologia tiroidea autoimmune e in quelle con gozzo endemico. Gli incrementi maggiori di tireoglobulina si verificano in pazienti con carcinoma differenziato della tiroide, mentre neonati con aplasia tiroidea possono avere livelli sierici molto bassi di tireoglobulina.

I livelli sierici di TSH sono degli indicatori estremamente sensibili dell'ipotiroidismo primario. Ormai si utilizzano correntemente dei nuovi dosaggi di terza generazione (dosaggi chemiluminescenti), in grado di misurare anche un TSH completamente soppresso, con valori inferiori al range di normalità. Questi dosaggi sensibili del TSH ovviano alla necessità del test di stimolazione con TRH per la diagnosi della maggior parte dei pazienti con patologie tiroidee.

TIROIDE NEL FETO E NEL NEONATO. Il T_4 sierico fetale aumenta progressivamente, dalla metà della gestazione fino al termine, raggiungendo valori di circa 11,5 μg/dL. I livelli fetali di T_3 sono bassi prima della ventesima settimana e poi aumentano gradualmente fino a circa 45 ng/dL al termine. I livelli di T_3 *reverse* (la forma inattiva del T_3), tuttavia, sono alti nel feto (250 ng/dL alla trentesima settimana) e diminuiscono a 150 ng/dL al termine. I livelli sierici di TSH aumentano gradualmente fino al termine a 10 mU/L. Circa un terzo del T_4 materno passa dalla madre al feto, attraverso la placenta. Il T_4 materno può giocare un ruolo nello sviluppo fetale, soprattutto del cervello, prima che inizi la sintesi fetale di ormoni tiroidei. Il feto di una madre ipotiroidea può essere a rischio per danno neurologico e un feto ipotiroideo può essere parzialmente protetto fino al parto dal T_4 materno. La quantità di T_4 che passa attraverso la placenta non è sufficiente a interferire con la diagnosi di ipotiroidismo congenito nel neonato.

Alla nascita, si verifica un rilascio acuto di TSH; il picco delle concentrazioni sieriche raggiunge le 60 mU/L in 30 min nei neonati a termine. Nelle successive 24 ore si verifica un rapido declino, che continua più gradualmente nei successivi 5 giorni, fino a raggiungere valori inferiori a 10 μU/mL. L'aumento acuto di TSH produce, in 4 ore, un drammatico incremento dei livelli di T_4 fino a circa 16 μg/dL e di T_3 a circa 300 ng/dL. Questo T_3 deriva ampiamente dall'aumento della conversione periferica del T_4 in T_3. I livelli di T_4 gradualmente diminuiscono durante la prima-seconda settimana di vita, a valori di 12 μg/dL. I livelli di T_3 diminuiscono poi durante la prima settimana di vita a valori inferiori a 200 ng/mL. Nei lattanti i livelli sierici di T_4 libero sono compresi tra 0,9-2,3 ng/dL e diminuiscono nell'infanzia a 0,7-1,8 ng/dL. Le concentrazioni sieriche di T_3 libero sono di circa 540 pg/dL nei lattanti, e declinano a 210-440 pg/dL durante l'infanzia. I livelli di T_3 *reverse* si mantengono per 2 settimane (200 ng/dL) e decrescono alla quarta settimana intorno ai 50 ng/dL. Nei neonati pretermine, le modificazioni della funzionalità tiroidea dopo la nascita sono simili da un punto di vista qualitativo, ma inferiori quantitativamente, a quelli dei neonati a termine. I livelli sierici di T_4 e di T_3 sono proporzionali all'età gestazionale e al peso alla nascita.

GLOBULINA SIERICA CHE LEGA LA TIROXINA. Gli ormoni tiroidei sono trasportati nel plasma legati alla TBG, una glicoproteina sintetizzata dal fegato. Talvolta è necessaria la valutazione dei livelli di TBG, perché aumentano o diminuiscono in molte situazioni cliniche, con conseguenze sul livello della tiroxina totale. La TBG lega circa il 70% del T_4 e il 50% del T_3. I livelli di TBG aumentano in gravidanza, nel periodo neonatale e con la somministrazione di estrogeni (contraccettivi orali), perfenazina o eroina, e diminuiscono con gli androgeni, gli steroidi anabolizzanti, i glicocorticoidi e l'L-asparaginasi. Questi effetti sono il risultato della modulazione della sintesi epatica di TBG. La fentoina (difenilidantoina) è un'altra causa di alterazione dei test di funzionalità tiroidea indotta da farmaci. La fentoina, un induttore degli enzimi epatici, stimola la degradazione epatica di T_4 e ne accelera il trasporto nei tessuti. Il fenobarbital e la carbamazepina hanno un effetto simile. Alcuni farmaci, particolarmente la fentoina, inibiscono anche il legame del T_4 e del T_3 con la TBG. Un aumento o una diminuzione dei livelli di TBG si verifica anche in alcuni profili genetici (vedi Capitolo 565). I livelli di TBG possono diminuire notevolmente per un calo della produzione, in presenza di malattie epatiche, oppure per perdita (intestinale da enteropatia proteino-disperdente o urinaria) come nella sindrome nefrotica congenita.

STUDI IN VIVO CON RADIONUCLIDE. I test diretti di funzionalità tiroidea, notevolmente migliorati, hanno reso meno utili gli studi sulla captazione del radioiodio. Il meccanismo di captazione e concentrazione dello iodio da parte della tiroide può essere valutato mediante la misurazione della captazione dell'isotopo radioattivo ^{123}I (emivita di 13 ore). La tecnologia consente ora di utilizzare dosi di radioiodio (0,1-0,5 mCi) che sono solo una piccola parte di quelle che si utilizzavano per lo ^{131}I. Il tecnezio (^{99m}Tc) è un isotopo particolarmente utilizzato per i bambini, perché, contrariamente allo iodio, possiede un'emivita di sole 6 ore. Lo studio della tiroide può essere indicato nell'agenesia ghiandolare, per valutare la presenza di tessuto tiroideo, e per trovare tessuto tiroideo ectopico; inoltre la captazione tiroidea può essere indicata per la valutazione di eventuali noduli "caldi". Tali studi dovrebbero utilizzare il ^{99m}Tc pertecnato o lo ^{123}I, che hanno il vantaggio di una bassa esposizione a radiazioni e un'alta qualità dello scintigramma. L'uso di ^{131}I nei bambini dovrebbe essere limitato a quelli con tumore tiroideo.

STUDI ECOGRAFICI DELLA TIROIDE. Le indagini tiroidee con ultrasuoni sono in grado di determinare la sede, le dimensioni e la forma della ghiandola, nonché di valutare la natura solida o cistica dei noduli. L'ecografia non è affidabile come le indagini con radionuclidi, nella valutazione dei neonati in cui si sospetti una disgenesia tiroidea, particolarmente un'ectopia ghiandolare. Le indagini ultrasonografiche sono utilizzate per l'identificazione della posizione della tiroide normale nei bambini con sospetto di cisti del dotto tireoglosso. Nei bambini con tiroidite autoimmune, gli ultrasuoni rivelano un'ipoecogenicità cicatriziale. Gli esami ecografici sono più accurati dell'esame obiettivo nella valutazione delle dimensioni di un gozzo e di noduli tiroidei.

Fisher DA: Physiological variations in thyroid hormones: Physiological and pathophysiological considerations. *Clin Chem* 1996;42:135–139.
Haddow JE, Palomaki GE, Allan WC, et al: Maternal thyroid deficiency during pregnancy and subsequent neuropsychological development of the child. *N Engl J Med* 1999;341:549–555.
Murphy N, Hume R, van Toor H, et al: The hypothalamic-pituitary-thyroid axis in preterm infants: Changes in the first 24 hours of postnatal life. *J Clin Endocrinol Metab* 2004;89:2824–2831.
O'Reilly DS: Thyroid function tests–Time for a reassessment. *Br Med J* 2000;320: 1332–1334.
Pop VJ, Brouwers EP, Vader HL, et al: Maternal hypothyroxinaemia during early pregnancy and subsequent child development: A 3-year follow-up study. *Clin Endocrinol (Oxf)* 2003;59:282–288.
Xu F, Sullivan K, Houston R, et al: Thyroid volumes in US and Bangladeshi schoolchildren: Comparison with European schoolchildren. *Eur J Endocrinol* 1999;140:498–504.

Capitolo 565 ■ Difetti della globulina che lega la tiroxina

Le alterazioni dei livelli della globulina che lega la tiroxina (TBG) non sono associate a malattie cliniche e non richiedono trattamento. Di solito sono scoperte in occasione della ricerca di diminuzione o di aumento dei livelli di tiroxina (T_4) e possono essere motivo di confusione nella diagnosi dell'ipo o dell'ipertiroidismo.

Il deficit di TBG si verifica in una malattia dominante associata a X. La carenza congenita di TBG è più spesso scoperta attraverso i programmi di screening per l'ipotiroidismo neonatale che utilizzano, come esame principale, il dosaggio dei livelli di T_4. I pazienti presentano bassi livelli di T_4 ed elevata captazione su resina di triiodotironina (RT_3U), ma normali livelli di T_4 libero e di ormone stimolante la tiroide (TSH). La diagnosi è confermata dall'assenza o da bassi livelli di TBG. Il deficit di TBG si verifica in 1 su 2400 neonati maschi, il 36% dei quali mostra livelli di TBG inferiori a 1 mg/dL. Forme più lievi di carenza di TBG si verificano in circa uno su 4200 neonate femmine eterozigoti, mentre un deficit completo di TBG (<5 μg/dL) si riscontra molto meno frequentemente. Tre delle nove famiglie in cui si è documentata carenza completa di TBG presentano la mutazione di un codone (da leucina a prolina); altri pazienti con ridotta affinità della TBG per il T_4 hanno mutazioni in altri punti, che alterano la struttura terziaria della proteina. Il deficit acquisito di TBG compare in corso di terapia con androgeni e glicocorticoidi, insufficienza epatica (non epatite), patologia renale e proteinuria e nefropatie proteino-disperdenti.

L'eccesso di TBG è un'anomalia benigna dominante associata a X, che si verifica in circa 1 su 25 000 persone e che è stata riscontrata principalmente negli adulti, sebbene programmi di screening neonatale ne hanno rivelato la presenza anche nel neonato. Il livello di T_4 è elevato, il T_3 è variabilmente elevato, il TSH e il T_4 libero sono normali, con RT_3U diminuita. Sono i livelli elevati di TBG che confermano la diagnosi. Nei neonati, si sono trovati livelli di T_4 fino a 95 μg/dL, che scendono a 20-30 μg/dL dopo 2-3 settimane. Livelli così alti di T_4 possono essere in parte correlati, nei neonati, a valori normalmente elevati di TBG durante il primo mese di vita, presumibilmente come effetto degli estrogeni materni. I pazienti sono eutiroidei. Studi familiari hanno indicato che altri individui possono esserne affetti. L'aumento acquisito di TBG si verifica durante la gravidanza, trattamento con estrogeni, epatite e con certi farmaci (clofibrato, metadone, perfenazina).

L'**ipertirosinemia disalbuminemica familiare** è una malattia autosomica dominante che può essere confusa con l'ipertiroidismo. Il legame notevolmente aumentato del T_4 a una variante anomala dell'albumina porta a una aumento delle concentrazioni sieriche di T_4. Tuttavia, i livelli di T_4 libero, T_3 libero e TSH sono normali, mentre quelli di T_3 sono normali o solo lievemente elevati. I pazienti colpiti sono eutiroidei.

LaFranchi SH, Snyder DB, Sesser DE, et al: Follow-up of newborns with elevated screening T_4 concentrations. *J Pediatr* 2003;143:296–301.
Mandel SH, Hanna CE, Boston BA, et al: Thyroxine binding globulin deficiency detected by newborn screening. *J Pediatr* 1993; 122:227–230.
Refetoff S, Murata Y, Mori Y, et al: Thyroxine-binding globulin: Organization of the gene and variants. *Horm Res* 1996;45:128–138.

Capitolo 566 ■ Ipotiroidismo

L'ipotiroidismo è dovuto a una diminuzione della produzione di ormone tiroideo o da un difetto dell'attività del recettore dell'ormone stesso (Tab. 566-1). La malattia può essere presente sin dalla nascita oppure venire acquisita. Se i sintomi appaiono dopo un periodo di apparente normalità funzionale tiroidea, il quadro può essere veramente "acquisito" o semplicemente sembrarlo, poiché esistono diversi difetti congeniti in cui le manifestazioni della carenza sono ritardate. È preferibile evitare il termine cretinismo, sebbene spesso sia usato come sinonimo di carenza iodica endemica e ipotiroidismo congenito.

IPOTIROIDISMO CONGENITO

La maggior parte dei casi di ipotiroidismo congenito non è ereditaria e deriva da una disgenesia tiroidea. Alcuni possono essere familiari, normalmente provocati da errori congeniti della sintesi di ormone tiroideo, altri invece associati a gozzo. In molti casi, la carenza di ormone tiroideo è grave e i sintomi si sviluppano nelle prime settimane di vita. In altri, si evidenziano deficit di minore entità e le manifestazioni possono essere ritardate per mesi.

TABELLA 566-1. Classificazione eziologica dell'ipotiroidismo congenito

IPOTIROIDISMO CENTRALE (IPOFISARIO)
Mutazioni PIT-1
Carenza di tireotropina (TSH), ormone della crescita, e prolattina
Mutazioni PROP-1
Carenza di TSH, ormone della crescita, prolattina, LH, FSH, ±ACTH
Carenza di ormone di rilascio della tireotropina (TRH)
È isolata?
Carenze ipotalamiche multiple (per es. displasia setto-ottica)
Mancata responsività al TRH
Mutazioni del recettore del TRH
Carenza di TSH
Mutazioni della catena β
Carenze ipofisarie multiple (per es. craniofaringioma)
Mancata responsività al TSH
Mutazione $G_s\alpha$ (per es. pseudoipoparatiroidismo di tipo IA)
Mutazioni del recettore del TSH
IPOTIROIDISMO PRIMARIO
Difetto dello sviluppo fetale della tiroide
Aplasia, Ipoplasia, Ectopia (disgenia)
Difetti della sintesi dell'ormone tiroideo (per es. ipotiroidismo con gozzo)
Difetto del trasporto iodico
Difetti della perossidasi tiroidea
Mutazioni dell'ossidasi tiroidea: omozigote, permanente; eterozigote, transitoria
Difetti della sintesi di tireoglobulina
Difetti della deiodinazione
Difetti nel trasporto dell'ormone tiroideo
Carenza di iodio (gozzo endemico)
Tipo neurologico
Tipo mixedematoso
Anticorpi materni
Anticorpi bloccanti i recettori della tireotropina (TRBAb, detti anche immunoglobulina inibitrice del legame della tireotropina)
Farmaci materni
Radioiodio, ioduro
Propiltiouracile, metimazolo
Amiodarone

ACTH, *Adrenocorticotropic Hormone* (ormone adrenocorticotropo); FSH, *Follicle-Stimulating Hormone* (ormone follicolo-stimolante); LH, *Luteinizing Hormone* (ormone luteinizzante).

EPIDEMIOLOGIA. La frequenza dell'ipotiroidismo congenito desumibile dai programmi di screening su scala nazionale è di 1 su 4000 nati in tutto il mondo; la frequenza è minore negli afroamericani (1/32 000) e più alta negli ispanici e nei nativi americani (1/2000). La frequenza è doppia nelle femmine rispetto ai maschi.

EZIOLOGIA

Disgenesia tiroidea. Alcune forme di disgenesia tiroidea (aplasia, ipoplasia o ectopia ghiandolare) sono le cause più comuni di ipotiroidismo congenito, in circa l'85% dei casi; il 10% è dovuto a un errore congenito nella sintesi di tiroxina, mentre un 5% è il risultato di anticorpi materni transplacentari che bloccano il recettore della tireotropina (TRBAb). In circa un terzo dei casi di disgenesia, anche un'indagine sensibile come la scintigrafia può non trovare residui di tessuto tiroideo (aplasia tiroidea). Negli altri due terzi si ritrovano residui di tessuto tiroideo in sedi ectopiche, dalla base della lingua (tiroide linguale) fino alla normale posizione nel collo (ipoplasia tiroidea).

La precisa causa della disgenesia tiroidea non è conosciuta nella maggior parte dei casi: essa è un evento sporadico, ma occasionalmente sono stati riportati anche casi familiari. Anomalie di sviluppo della tiroide, come la cisti del dotto tireoglosso e l'emiagenesia, sono presenti nell'8-10% dei parenti di primo grado dei bambini con disgenesia tiroidea e tale dato supporta l'ipotesi di una sottostante componente genetica.

Tre fattori di trascrizione, il TTF-1, il FOXE1 e il PAX-8, sono importanti per la differenziazione e la morfogenesi della tiroide e mutazioni in questi geni si associano a disgenesia tiroidea: inoltre, sono stati descritti difetti genetici che comportano assenza o inefficacia della tireotropina.

Un altro fattore di trascrizione, l'NKX2.1, è espresso sia nella tiroide sia nel sistema nervoso centrale. Nell'ipotiroidismo congenito con problemi neurologici persistenti, compresa l'atassia, nonostante un precoce trattamento con ormone tiroideo, sono state rilevate mutazioni di NKX2.1.

Il frequente reperto di disgenesia tiroidea in uno solo di due gemelli monozigoti suggerisce l'intervento di un fattore nocivo durante la vita intrauterina, il quale potrebbe essere rappresentato da anticorpi antitiroidei materni. Sebbene gli anticorpi antiperossidasi tiroidea (*Thyroid PerOxidase*, TPO) siano stati trovati in alcune coppie madre-neonato, è stata evidenziata solo una modesta patogenicità. La dimostrazione in alcuni neonati con disgenesia tiroidea di anticorpi citotossici e bloccanti la crescita della tiroide, come nelle loro madri, indica un più probabile meccanismo patogenetico.

La più comune forma di disgenesia tiroidea è l'ectopia ghiandolare, che può essere dimostrata da un'indagine ecografica. Nella maggior parte dei casi viene rivelata durante gli screening neonatali, ma in alcuni bambini il tessuto tiroideo ectopico (linguale, sublinguale, subioideo) può essere in grado di produrre per molti anni un'adeguata quantità di ormone tiroideo, oppure può smettere nella prima infanzia. I bambini arrivano all'osservazione clinica per la crescita di una massa alla base della lingua o nel collo, in corrispondenza della linea mediana, di solito a livello dell'osso ioide. Occasionalmente, l'ectopia si associa a cisti del dotto tireoglosso e si può verificare nei fratelli. La rimozione chirurgica del tessuto tiroideo in presenza di eutiroidismo porta di norma a ipotiroidismo, perché la maggior parte dei pazienti non possiede altro tessuto tiroideo.

Deficit della sintesi di tiroxina (disormonogenesi). Vari difetti nella biosintesi dell'ormone tiroideo possono essere responsabili di ipotiroidismo congenito; la frequenza nei programmi di screening neonatale è di 1/30 000-50 000 nati. Questi difetti sono trasmessi in modo autosomico recessivo. Quasi sempre è presente **gozzo**. Se il difetto è incompleto si ha una compensazione e il suo esordio dell'ipotiroidismo può essere ritardato per anni.

Difetto del trasporto dello iodio. Questo raro difetto coinvolge mutazioni nel symporter della pompa sodio-iodio. Tra i diversi casi attualmente riportati, si è individuato in 9 bambini imparentati fra loro della setta Hutterite e in circa nella metà dei casi giapponesi. È presente consanguineità in circa un terzo delle famiglie.

In passato, l'ipotiroidismo clinico con o senza gozzo spesso si sviluppava nei primi mesi di vita e tale condizione è stata rilevata con i programmi di screening neonatale. In Giappone, tuttavia, pazienti non trattati ritardano la comparsa di gozzo e ipotiroidismo dopo il decimo anno di età, probabilmente per l'alto contenuto iodico (spesso 19 mg/die) della dieta giapponese.

I meccanismi energia-dipendenti per la concentrazione dello iodio sono carenti nella tiroide e nelle ghiandole salivari. In contrasto con altri difetti della sintesi dell'ormone tiroideo, la captazione del radioiodio e del pertecnato è bassa; per la diagnosi può essere utile richiedere il rapporto di ^{123}I saliva-siero. Questa condizione risponde al trattamento con alte dosi di ioduro di potassio, ma è preferibile quello con tiroxina (T_4).

Difetti della perossidasi tiroidea nell'organificazione e coniugazione. È il più comune tra i difetti della sintesi di T_4. Dopo che lo ioduro viene captato dalla tiroide, è rapidamente ossidato a ioduro reattivo, che viene poi incorporato nelle unità tirosiniche della tireoglobulina. Questo processo richiede la formazione di H_2O_2, perossidasi tiroidea ed ematina (un cofattore enzimatico); si possono evidenziare difetti di ciascuna di queste componenti ed esiste una notevole eterogeneità clinica e biochimica. Nel programma di screening neonatale olandese, in 23 bambini si è trovato un difetto completo dell'organificazione (1/60 000), ma la frequenza in altre zone non è nota. Un reperto caratteristico in tutti i pazienti con questo difetto è rappresentato dalla marcata diminuzione della radioattività tiroidea dopo assunzione di perclorato e di tiocianato, somministrati due ore dopo l'assunzione di una dose di radioiodio per l'esame. In questi pazienti, il perclorato emette il 40-90% del radioiodio rispetto a meno del 10%

degli individui normali. Sono state riportate parecchie mutazioni del gene TPO in bambini con ipotiroidismo congenito. Anche pazienti con la **sindrome di Pendred**, una malattia che comprende sordità neurosensoriale e gozzo, mostrano una positiva eliminazione di perclorato. La sindrome di Prended è dovuta al difetto di una proteina di trasporto del solfato, presente sia nella ghiandola tiroidea sia nella coclea.

L'ossidasi tiroidea 2 aiuta la formazione di H_2O_2. Mutazioni inattivanti bi-alleliche producono un ipotiroidismo congenito permanente, mentre lesioni di un singolo gene provocano ipotiroidismo transitorio.

Difetti della sintesi di tireoglobulina. Questo eterogeneo gruppo di alterazioni, caratterizzato da gozzo, elevati livelli di ormone stimolante la tiroide (TSH), bassi livelli di T_4 e bassi o assenti livelli di tireoglobulina (TG), è stato riportato in circa un centinaio di pazienti. Difetti molecolari, soprattutto mutazioni puntiformi, sono stati descritti in parecchi pazienti.

Difetti di deiodinasi. La monoiodotirosina e la diiodotirosina rilasciate dalla tireoglobulina sono deiodate in condizioni normali nella tiroide o nei tessuti periferici a opera di una deiodinasi. Lo iodio liberato viene riciclato per la sintesi degli ormoni tiroidei. Pazienti con deficit di questo enzima presentano una grave carenza di iodio, per la costante perdita urinaria di tiroxine non deiodate, con conseguente deficit ormonale e gozzo. Il difetto di deiodinazione può essere limitato alla sola tiroide o ai soli tessuti periferici, oppure può riguardare tutte le sedi.

Difetti del trasporto dell'ormone tiroideo. Il passaggio dell'ormone tiroideo nella cellula è facilitato da trasportatori di membrana. In cinque maschi con ritardo mentale associato a X, si è trovata una mutazione in questo gene trasportatore, transporter monocarbossilato 8 (MCT8), localizzato sul cromosoma X. Il deficit di trasportatore comporta un impedimento al passaggio di T_3 all'interno dei neuroni; questa sindrome è caratterizzata da elevati livelli sierici di T_3 e ritardo psicomotorio.

Anticorpi antirecettore della tireotropina. Una causa poco frequente di ipotiroidismo congenito transitorio è rappresentata da un anticorpo materno antirecettore della tireotropina (TRBAb), spesso misurato come immunoglobulina inibitrice del legame della tireotropina. Il passaggio transplacentare di TRBAb materno inibisce, nel neonato, il legame del TSH con il suo recettore. La frequenza è di circa 1 su 50 000-100 000 neonati. Il sospetto deve nascere in presenza di un'anamnesi positiva per patologia tiroidea materna di natura immunitaria, compresa la tiroidite di Hashimoto, la malattia di Graves, l'ipotiroidismo anche in presenza di terapia sostitutiva, oppure per ipotiroidismo congenito ricorrente di natura transitoria in un fratello o sorella. In questi casi, è necessario controllare i livelli materni di TRBAb durante la gravidanza. I neonati affetti e le loro mamme possono anche presentare anticorpi stimolanti il recettore della tireotropina (TRSAbs) e anticorpi TPO. Il pertecnato di tecnezio e lo ^{125}I possono anche non evidenziare tessuto tiroideo, mimando l'agenesia tiroidea, ma l'indagine ecografia è in grado di dimostrare la presenza della ghiandola. Al miglioramento della situazione, le indagini evidenziano una tiroide normale, dopo l'interruzione della terapia sostitutiva. L'emivita degli anticorpi è di 21 giorni e la remissione dell'ipotiroidismo si verifica in circa 3-6 mesi. La corretta diagnosi di questa causa di ipotiroidismo congenito evita trattamenti protratti non necessari, richiama l'attenzione dei medici sulla possibilità che si ripeta in una futura gravidanza e permette una prognosi favorevole.

Somministrazione di radioiodio. Si può verificare ipotiroidismo come conseguenza di involontaria assunzione di radioiodio durante la gravidanza per il trattamento della malattia di Graves o di un tumore tiroideo. La tiroide fetale è in grado di captare lo ioduro verso i 70-75 giorni. Se si somministra radioiodio a una donna in età fertile, è sempre necessario un preventivo test di gravidanza prima di assumere la dose di ^{131}I, senza tenere conto dell'anamnesi mestruale o dell'uso di contraccettivi. È controindicata inoltre la somministrazione di radioiodio a donne che allattano, dal momento che viene escreto nel latte materno.

Deficit di tireotropina. Il deficit di tireotropina si può verificare in una qualunque delle condizioni associate a difetti dello sviluppo dell'ipofisi o dell'ipotalamo (vedi Capitolo 558). Più spesso in queste condizioni il deficit di TSH è secondario a carenza di ormone di rilascio della tireotropina (*Thyrotropin-Realising Hormone*, TRH). L'ipotiroidismo da deficit di TSH si trova in 1 su 30 000-50 000 neonati; gran parte dei programmi di screening è volta a scoprire l'ipotiroidismo primario, senza essere in grado di individuare numerosi casi di ipotiroidismo centrale. La maggior parte dei neonati affetti ha carenze ipofisarie multiple e presenta ipoglicemia, ittero persistente, micropene in associazione a displasia setto-ottica, labbro leporino, ipoplasia di un'emifaccia e altre anomalie mediali del volto. Mutazioni Pit-1 sono una causa recessiva di ipotiroidismo centrale secondario a deficit di TSH. I bambini possono presentare anche deficit dell'ormone della crescita e di prolattina. Pit-1, un fattore di trascrizione genetica, è essenziale per la differenziazione, il mantenimento e la proliferazione delle cellule somatotrope, lattotrope e tireotrope. La valutazione della prolattina e della risposta del TSH alla stimolazione con TRH può consentire di formulare una diagnosi. Un deficit della risposta prolattinemica al test con TRH deve indurre alla valutazione del gene Pit-1.

PROP-1 è un altro importante fattore di trascrizione nello sviluppo ipofisario e nella produzione ormonale. Neonati con mutazione del gene PROP-1 ("profeta" di Pit-1) non presentano solo una carenza di TSH, di GH e di prolattina, ma anche di LH e di FSH e in modo variabile anche di ACTH.

La carenza isolata di TSH è una rara malattia autosomica recessiva riportata in alcuni pazienti imparentati. Studi sul DNA su due bambini giapponesi e su tre bambini in due famiglie greche imparentate hanno rivelato diversi punti di mutazione nel gene della subunità β del TSH; in due fratelli tedeschi una mutazione che provoca un codone stop dovuto a frameshift, infine mutazioni *splice site* in due famiglie turche.

Mancata responsività alla tireotropina. Una mutazione del gene del recettore del TSH è stata riportata in tre fratelli con livelli elevati di TSH e normali di T_4; due di loro erano stati scoperti nell'ambito di uno screening neonatale e, nonostante la persistente resistenza al TSH per tutta l'infanzia, sono rimasti eutiroidei senza alcun trattamento. Pazienti descritti in tre altre ricerche, con presunte mutazioni del gene del recettore del TSH, presentavano invece un grave ipotiroidismo con necessità di terapia. La malattia, congenita, si trasmette in modo autosomico recessivo e sono state documentate mutazioni omo- ed eterozigotiche composte del gene del recettore del TSH.

Si è trovato un ipotiroidismo congenito di modesta entità in neonati che successivamente hanno sviluppato uno **pseudoipoparatiroidismo di tipo I_a**. La causa molecolare della resistenza al TSH in questi pazienti è l'alterazione generalizzata dell'attivazione dell'adenosina ciclica monofosfato, dovuta a deficit genetico della subunità α della proteina G_S di regolazione della guanina nucleotidica (vedi Capitolo 573).

Anomalie del recettore dell'ormone di rilascio della tireotropina. È stato riportato il caso di un paziente con anomalie del recettore del TRH, deficit isolato di TSH e ipotiroidismo. Si era sospettata questa condizione a causa della carenza simultanea di TSH e di prolattina al test di stimolazione con TRH. Le indagini hanno rivelato una mutazione composta eterozigote del gene che codifica per il recettore del TRH, con conseguente incapacità del recettore di legare il TRH.

NON RESPONSIVITÀ ALL'ORMONE TIROIDEO. Questa patologia autosomica dominante è dovuta a mutazioni del recettore dell'ormone tiroideo. La maggior parte dei pazienti presenta gozzo e livelli elevati di T_4, T_3, T_4 libero e T_3 libero. Questi reperti spesso hanno portato all'erronea diagnosi di malattia di Graves, nonostante la maggior parte dei pazienti fosse clinicamente eutiroidea. La non responsività può essere presente in modo variabile nei tessuti. Possono essere presenti sfumate caratteristiche di ipotiroidismo, compreso un ritardo mentale, della crescita e della maturazione scheletrica. D'altra parte, possono comparire caratteristiche compatibili con l'ipertiroidismo, come tachicardia e iperreflessia. Si presume che questi pazienti mostrino diverse resistenze all'ormone tiroideo nei vari tessuti. Da un punto di vista neurologico i pazienti possono presentare, con probabilità aumentata, un deficit di attenzione con iperattività; tuttavia non è vero il contrario, perché individui con disturbo da deficit dell'attenzione e con iperattività non hanno un aumento del rischio di resistenza all'ormone tiroideo.

I livelli di TSH misurati con dosaggio sensibile sono diagnostici, dal momento che non appaiono soppressi come nella malattia di Graves, pur essendo tuttavia moderatamente elevati o normali, ma comunque inappropriati per i livelli di T_4 e di T_3. La mancata soppressione del TSH indica che la resistenza è generalizzata e colpisce sia l'ipofisi sia i tessuti periferici. Sono state individuate mutazioni in più di 40 punti distinti nel dominio del legame dell'ormone del β-recettore tiroideo. Fenotipi diversi non sono in correlazione con i genotipi e si è osservata la stessa mutazione in soggetti con resistenza generalizzata o ipofisaria isolata, anche in persone non appartenenti alla medesima famiglia. Inoltre, un bambino omozigote per mutazione del recettore ha evidenziato una grave, insolita resistenza. Questi casi confermano l'effetto negativo dominante dei recettori mutanti, in cui la proteina recettoriale mutante inibisce la normale azione del recettore negli eterozigoti. Il reperto di elevati livelli di T_4 in corso di screening neonatale dovrebbe suggerire la possibilità di questa diagnosi. Normalmente non è necessario alcun trattamento, a meno che non siano presenti ritardo della crescita e della maturazione scheletrica.

Due bambini nati da unione fra consanguinei presentano una forma di resistenza tiroidea autosomica recessiva. Questi neonati hanno evidenziato ipotiroidismo solo tardivamente nel corso della vita e studi genetici hanno rivelato una delezione del recettore tiroideo β in un individuo: la resistenza, in questa forma, appare molto più grave.

Raramente, la resistenza all'ormone tiroideo può selettivamente colpire l'ipofisi. Dal momento che i tessuti periferici non sono resistenti all'ormone, i pazienti avevano gozzo e manifestazioni di ipertiroidismo. I reperti di laboratorio erano gli stessi della resistenza generalizzata. Questa condizione deve essere differenziata da un tumore ipofisario TSH-secernente. In un certo numero di pazienti è stato riportato successo terapeutico con vari farmaci compresi D-tiroxina, TRIAC (acido triiodotiroacetico), e TETRAC (acido tetraiodiotiroacetico). La somministrazione di bromocriptina, che interferisce con la secrezione di TSH, in altri ha ottenuto buoni risultati.

Esposizione allo iodio. Un ipotiroidismo congenito può dipendere da un'eccessiva esposizione fetale allo iodio. L'esposizione perinatale si può verificare per l'uso di antisettici a base di iodio applicati sulla cute in preparazione al taglio cesareo o anche in sede cervicale per il parto. Alcuni studi riportano casi in neonati di madri giapponesi che consumano notevoli quantità di un'alga marina ricca di iodio. Queste condizioni sono transitorie e non devono essere confuse con altre forme di ipotiroidismo. Nel neonato, anche antisettici a contenuto iodico per uso topico usati nelle nursery e dai chirurghi possono provocare ipotiroidismo congenito transitorio, specialmente nei neonati di scarso peso alla nascita e possono condurre ad alterazioni dei test di screening neonatale. In altri bambini, le fonti di iodio sono rappresentate da alcune preparazioni usate nel trattamento dell'asma. In pochi casi, la causa dell'ipotiroidismo era l'amiodarone, un farmaco antiaritmico ad alto contenuto iodico e, nella maggior parte di questi, è presente gozzo (vedi Capitolo 568.3).

Gozzo endemico da carenza iodica. Praticamente sconosciuto negli Stati Uniti, il gozzo endemico da carenza di iodio è la causa più comune di ipotiroidismo congenito nel resto del mondo. La carenza iodica borderline provoca più facilmente problemi nel neonato pretermine, che dipende dalla madre per l'approvvigionamento di iodio per la normale produzione di ormone tiroideo.

FUNZIONE TIROIDEA NEI NEONATI PRETERMINE. La funzione postnatale tiroidea nei bambini pretermine è qualitativamente simile, ma quantitativamente ridotta, in rapporto a quella di neonati a termine. Il T_4 sierico del cordone diminuisce in rapporto all'età gestazionale e al peso alla nascita. La scarica postnatale di TSH è ridotta e i neonati con complicanze inerenti alla prematurità, come la sindrome da distress respiratorio, evidenziano un decremento del T_4 sierico nella prima settimana di vita. Quando le complicanze si risolvono, gradualmente aumenta anche il T_4 sierico, tanto che generalmente alla sesta settimana di vita si colloca nel range dei bambini nati a termine. Le concentrazioni sieriche di T_4 libero sono meno coinvolte, e spesso si rivelano normali se misurate con metodiche di *equilibrium dialysis*. Anche neonati pretermine mostrano, con alta frequenza, un'elevazione transitoria del TSH e un apparente ipotiroidismo primario transitorio. I bambini prematuri, nati prima della ventottesima settimana di gestazione, possono incorrere in problemi dovuti alla combinazione di immaturità dell'asse ipotalamo-ipofiso-tiroideo e perdita del contributo materno di ormone tiroideo, diventando possibili candidati per una terapia sostitutiva temporanea; sono necessari studi ulteriori.

MANIFESTAZIONI CLINICHE. La maggior parte dei bambini con ipotiroidismo congenito è asintomatica alla nascita, anche in presenza di agenesia completa della tiroide. Questo fatto è attribuito al passaggio transplacentare di una modesta quantità di T_4 materno, che determina livelli fetali che sono circa il 33% dei normali alla nascita. Questi bassi livelli sierici di T_4 e i concomitanti alti livelli di TSH rendono possibile l'identificazione dei neonati ipotiroidei.

Per la diagnosi di ipotiroidismo congenito, i medici si basano sui dati dello screening neonatale. Tuttavia si verificano errori di laboratorio e per questo deve essere sempre ricercata la presenza di segni e di sintomi precoci. L'ipotiroidismo congenito è due volte più comune nelle femmine che nei maschi. Prima dei programmi di screening neonatale, l'ipotiroidismo congenito raramente veniva individuato nei neonati, perché i segni e i sintomi non erano sufficientemente evidenti. Anche nelle prime settimane di vita si può sospettare e diagnosticare un ipotiroidismo, ma si trovano manifestazioni meno caratteristiche. Il peso e la lunghezza alla nascita sono normali, ma le dimensioni craniche possono essere leggermente aumentate per la presenza di mixedema cerebrale. Un prolungamento dell'ittero fisiologico, causato da ritardata maturazione della glicuro-coniugazione, può rappresentare il segno più precoce. Difficoltà nell'alimentazione (in particolare lentezza, apatia, sonnolenza e crisi di soffocamento durante l'allattamento) sono spesso presenti durante il primo mese di vita. Le difficoltà respiratorie, dovute in parte a macroglossia, comprendono episodi apneici, respirazione rumorosa e ostruzione nasale. Si può verificare anche la tipica sindrome da distress respiratorio. I bambini affetti piangono poco, dormono molto, hanno scarso appetito e sono generalmente indolenti, inoltre ci può essere stipsi, che normalmente non risponde al trattamento. L'addome è espanso e di solito è presente ernia ombelicale. La temperatura corporea è subnormale, spesso inferiore a 35 °C, e la cute, particolarmente quella degli arti, è fredda e a chiazze. Può essere presente edema ai genitali e agli arti. C'è inoltre bradicardia e sono comuni soffi cardiaci, cardiomegalia e versamento pericardico asintomatico, come anche è spesso presente anemia macrocitica refrattaria al trattamento con ematinici. Dato che la comparsa dei sintomi è graduale, la diagnosi clinica spesso è ritardata.

Circa il 10% dei bambini con ipotiroidismo congenito presenta associazione ad altre anomalie congenite; le più comuni sono quelle cardiache, ma sono riportate anche anomalie oculari e quelle del sistema nervoso centrale.

Se l'ipotiroidismo congenito rimane insospettato e non trattato, tali manifestazioni evolvono. Gradatamente, nei mesi seguenti, si rende più evidente un ritardo dello sviluppo psicofisico, e al 3°-6° mese di età il quadro clinico è completamente sviluppato (Fig. 566-1). In presenza di una carenza parziale di ormone tiroideo, i sintomi possono essere modesti, la sindrome incompleta e l'esordio ritardato. Sebbene il latte materno contenga notevoli quantità di ormoni tiroidei, in particolare di T_3, esso non è sufficiente a proteggere il bambino allattato al seno materno dall'ipotiroidismo congenito e non ha effetti sullo screening neonatale.

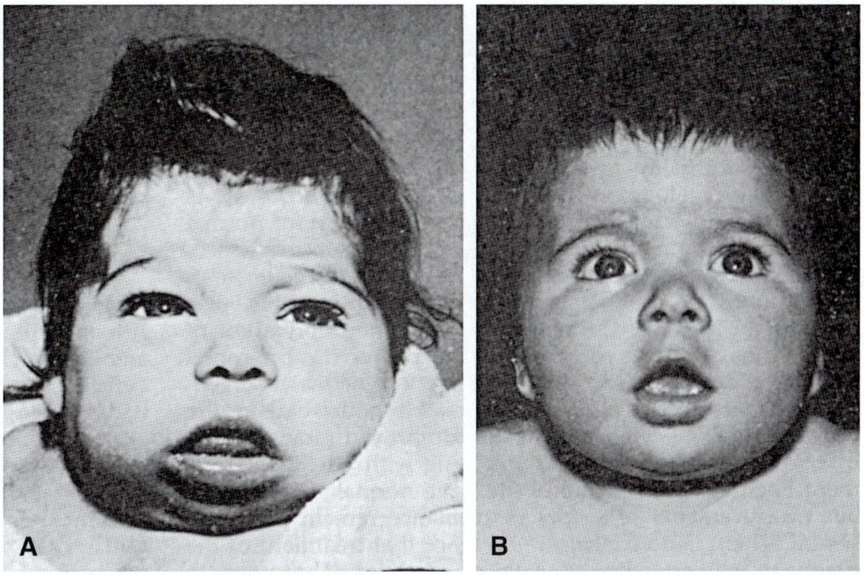

Figura 566-1. Ipotiroidismo congenito in una bambina di 6 mesi. In epoca neonatale mangiava poco ed era stitica. Presentava rinorrea persistente e macroglossia; era sempre assonnata, non sorrideva e non riusciva a sorreggere il capo. *A*, Notare il viso paffuto, l'espressione ottusa e l'impianto basso dei capelli sulla fronte. Le indagini rivelavano una trascurabile captazione iodica. Lo sviluppo osseo corrispondeva a quello di un neonato. *B*, Dopo quattro mesi di trattamento, notare il viso meno paffuto, la riduzione dei capelli sulla fronte e l'espressione vivace e attenta.

La crescita del bambino è ritardata, gli arti sono corti e le dimensioni craniche normali o aumentate. Le fontanelle, anteriore e posteriore, sono generalmente aperte; l'osservazione di questi segni alla nascita può servire come indizio per una ricerca precoce dell'ipotiroidismo congenito. Solo il 3% dei neonati normali presenta una fontanella posteriore più ampia di 0,5 cm. Gli occhi appaiono distanziati e la radice del naso, che appare largo, è infossata. Le fessure palpebrali sono ristrette e le palpebre edematose. La bocca è mantenuta aperta e protrude una lingua voluminosa, inoltre la dentizione è ritardata. Il collo è corto e tozzo, e ci può essere deposizione di cuscinetti adiposi in sede clavicolare e tra il collo e le spalle. Le mani sono larghe e le dita corte. La cute è secca e squamosa, con scarsa perspirazione. È evidente il mixedema, particolarmente nella cute delle palpebre, del dorso delle mani e dei genitali esterni. La pelle è pallida, con un colorito verdastro. La carotenemia può essere responsabile di una colorazione giallastra della cute, ma le sclere rimangono bianche. Il cuoio capelluto è ispessito e i capelli ruvidi, fragili e scarsi. La linea di inserzione dei capelli è molto bassa sulla fronte, che appare rugosa, soprattutto se il bambino piange.

Lo sviluppo è normalmente ritardato. I neonati ipotiroidei appaiono letargici e acquisiscono in ritardo la capacità di stare seduti e in piedi, hanno inoltre la voce rauca e non imparano a parlare. Il grado di ritardo fisico e mentale aumenta con l'età, mentre la maturazione sessuale può essere ritardata o non verificarsi affatto.

La muscolatura è solitamente ipotonica, ma in rari casi si verifica una pseudoipertrofia muscolare generalizzata (**sindrome di Kocher-Debré-Sémélaigne**). I bambini più grandi presentano un aspetto atletico proprio a causa dell'ipertrofia, particolarmente nella muscolatura del polpaccio. La sua patogenesi è sconosciuta; eventuali modificazioni istochimiche e ultrastrutturali non specifiche osservate all'indagine bioptica dei muscoli tornano nella norma dopo il trattamento. I maschi sviluppano più facilmente questa sindrome, che è stata osservata in fratelli nati da consanguinei. I pazienti presentano un ipotiroidismo grave e di lunga durata.

REPERTI DI LABORATORIO. La maggior parte dei programmi di screening neonatale nel Nord America misura i livelli di T_4 e solo successivamente quelli del TSH se esso è basso. Questo approccio è in grado di identificare i neonati con ipotiroidismo primario, alcuni con ipotiroidismo ipotalamico e ipofisario, e i bambini con un ritardo nell'incremento dei livelli di TSH. Gli screening europei e giapponesi, invece, sono basati sulla misurazione primaria del TSH; alcuni programmi nordamericani hanno adottato lo screening primario del TSH. Questo approccio è in grado di rilevare i neonati con ipotiroidismo primario, e anche bambini con ipotiroidismo subclinico (T_4 normale e TSH elevato), ma non conosce neonati con ritardo dell'elevazione del TSH e con ipotiroidismo ipotalamico o ipofisario. In tutti i test, si deve fare molta attenzione al range normale dei valori in base all'età del paziente, particolarmente nella prima settimana di vita (Tab. 566-2). Qualunque sia l'approccio utilizzato per lo screening, alcuni neonati non vengono diagnosticati a causa di errori tecnici o umani; i medici dovrebbero quindi essere molto attenti alla manifestazioni cliniche di ipotiroidismo.

I livelli sierici di T_4 o di T_4 libero sono bassi, mentre quelli di T_3 possono essere normali e non aiutare per niente la diagnosi. Se il difetto è primariamente nella tiroide, i livelli di TSH sono elevati, spesso maggiori di 100 mU/L. I livelli sierici di prolattina sono elevati se rapportati a quelli del TSH, invece i livelli sierici di tireoglobulina sono solitamente bassi nei neonati con agenesia tiroidea o con difetti della sintesi o della secrezione della tireoglobulina, mentre possono essere elevati in presenza di tessuto ghiandolare ectopico e di altri errori congeniti della sintesi della tiroxina.

Speciale attenzione va posta nella valutazione dei gemelli identici; in alcuni casi riportati, lo screening neonatale non è in grado di trovare il gemello discordante con ipotiroidismo, e perciò è assente la diagnosi, fino al 4°-5° mese di età. Apparentemente, la trasfusione di sangue eutiroideo prelevato dal gemello non affetto normalizza i livelli sierici di T_4 e di TSH nel gemello ipotiroideo nello screening iniziale.

Il ritardo dello sviluppo osseo può essere dimostrato radiologicamente alla nascita in circa il 60% dei neonati con ipotiroidismo congenito e indica una certa deprivazione di ormone tiroideo durante la vita intrauterina. L'epifisi femorale distale, normalmente presente alla nascita, è spesso assente (Fig. 566-2*A*). In pazienti non diagnosticati e non trattati, la discrepanza tra l'età cronologica e lo sviluppo osseo aumenta. Le epifisi spesso presentano foci multipli di ossificazione (disgenesia epifisaria) (Fig. 566-2*B*), sono comuni deformazioni (o "a rostro"), della dodicesima vertebra toracica o della prima o della seconda lombare. L'RX del cranio mostra fontanelle e suture ampie; è comune la presenza di ossa tra le suture (wormiane). La sella turcica è spesso allargata e tondeggiante; in rari casi può presentare erosioni o ispessimento; inoltre si può verificare un ritardo nella formazione ed eruzione dei denti. Può essere presente una cardiomegalia o un versamento pericardico.

La scintigrafia può aiutare a individuare le cause sottostanti nei bambini con ipotiroidismo congenito, ma non bisogna ritardare troppo il trattamento per eseguire questi studi. A questo scopo lo ^{123}I ioduro di sodio è superiore al ^{99m}Tc pertecnato sodico. L'eco-

TABELLA 566-2. Test di funzionalità tiroidea

ANALITA O PROCEDURA	CAMPIONE	VALORI RI RIFERIMENTO (USA)		FATTORE DI CONVERSIONE	VALORI DI RIFERIMENTO (SI)
Tireoglobulina tiroidea	S	Sangue del cordone ombelicale	14,7-101,1 ng/mL	× 1	14,7-101,1 μg/L
			10,6-92,0		
		Nascita-35° mese	5,6-41,9		10,6-92,0
		3-11 anni	2,7-21,9		5,6-41,9
		12-17 anni			2,7-21,9
Ormone stimolante la tiroide	S	Prematuro (28-36 settimane)			
		Prima settimana di vita	0,7-27,0 mUI/L	× 1	0,7-27,0 mUI/L
		Neonato a termine			
		Nascita-4 giorni	1,0-38,9		1,0-28,9
		2-20 settimane	1,7-9,1		1,7-9,1
		5 mesi-20 anni	0,7-6,4		0,7-6,4
Globulina legante la tiroxina (*Thyroxine Blinding Globulin*, TBG)	S		ng/dL		ng/dL
		Sangue del cordone ombelicale	1,4-94	× 10	14-94
		1-4 settimane	1,0-9,0		10-90
		1-12 mesi	2,0-7,6		20-76
		1-5 anni	2,9-5,4		29-54
		5-10 anni	2,5-5,0		25-50
		10-15 anni	2,1-4,6		21-46
		Adulto	1,5-3,4		15-34
Tiroxina	S	Neonati a termine		× 12,9	Neonati a termine
		1-3 giorni	8,2-19,9 μg/dL		1-3 giorni 106-256 nmol/L
		1 settimana	6,0-15-9		1 settimana 77-205
		1-12 mesi	6,1-14,9		1-12 mesi 79-192
		Bambini prepuberi			Bambini prepuberi
		1-3 anni	6,8-13,5 μg/dL		1-3 anni 88-174 nmol/L
		3-10 anni	5,5-12,8		3-10 anni 71-175
		Ragazzi puberi e adulti			Ragazzi puberi e adulti
			4,2-13,0 μg/dL		54-167 nmol/L
Tiroxina, libera	S	Neonati		× 12,9	Neonati a termine
		3 giorni	2,0-4,9 ng/dL		3 giorni 26-631 pmol/L
		Lattanti			Lattanti
			0,9-2,6 ng/dL		12-33 pmol/L
		Bambini prepuberi			Bambini prepuberi
			0,8-2,2 ng/dL		10-28 pmol/L
		Ragazzi puberi e adulti			Ragazzi puberi e adulti
			0,8-2,3 ng/dL		10-30 pmol/L
Tiroxina, totale	W	Esame neonatale (carta da filtro)	6,2-22 μg/dL	× 12.9	80-283 nmol/L
Triiodotironina, libera	S		pg/dL		pmol/L
		Sangue del cordone ombelicale	20-240	× 0,01536	0,3-0,7
		1-3 giorni	200-610		3,1-9,4
		6 settimane	240-560		3,7-8,6
		Adulto (20-50 anni)	230-660		3,5-10,0
Test di captazione su resina della triiodotironina	S				Captazione frazionata
		Neonato 26-36%		× 0,01	0,26-0,36
		Successivamente 26-35%			0,26-0,35
Triiodotironina, totale	S		ng/dL		nmol/L
		Sangue del cordone ombelicale	30-70	× 0,0154	0,46-1,08
		Neonato	75-260		1,16-4,00
		1-5 anni	100-260		1,54-4,00
		5-10 anni	90-240		1,39-3,70
		10-15 anni	80-210		1,23-3,23
		Successivamente	115-190		1,77-2,93

S, siero; W, *Whole Blood* (sangue intero).
Adattata da Nicholson JF, Pesce MA: Reference Ranges for Laboratory Tests and Procedures. In Beherman RE, Kliegman RM, JensonHB (eds.) *Nelson textbook of Pediatrics*, 17th ed. Philadelphia, Elsevier Science, 2004, pp 2412-2413.

grafia della tiroide è un'indagine utile, ma vari studi dimostrano che non è in grado di rivelare tessuto ghiandolare ectopico, evidenziato invece dalla scintigrafia. I livelli sierici di tireoglobulina sono bassi nell'agenesia ed elevati nell'ectopia ghiandolare e nel gozzo, ma c'è un'ampia sovrapposizione dei range. La dimostrazione di tessuto ghiandolare ectopico è diagnostica di disgenesia tiroidea e definisce la necessità di un trattamento con T_4 per tutta la vita. La mancata dimostrazione di tessuto tiroideo indica invece l'aplasia tiroidea, ma questo dato si presenta anche in neonati con TRBAb e in quelli con deficit di captazione dello iodio. Una ghiandola in sede normale con una normale capacità di captare il radionuclide suggerisce un difetto nella biosintesi dell'ormone tiroideo. In passato, pazienti con ipotiroidismo e gozzo hanno richiesto notevoli indagini, compresi studi con radiodiodio, test di eliminazione del perclorato, studi cinetici, cromatografia e studi del tessuto tiroideo, per determinare la natura biochimica del difetto. La maggior parte viene ora valutata con test genetici mirati per difetti delle varie fasi della via biosintetica della tiroxina.

L'elettrocardiogramma può mostrare onde P e T a basso voltaggio, con diminuita ampiezza del complesso QRS e suggerisce una diminuzione della funzionalità del ventricolo sinistro e versamento pericardico. L'elettroencefalogramma frequentemente

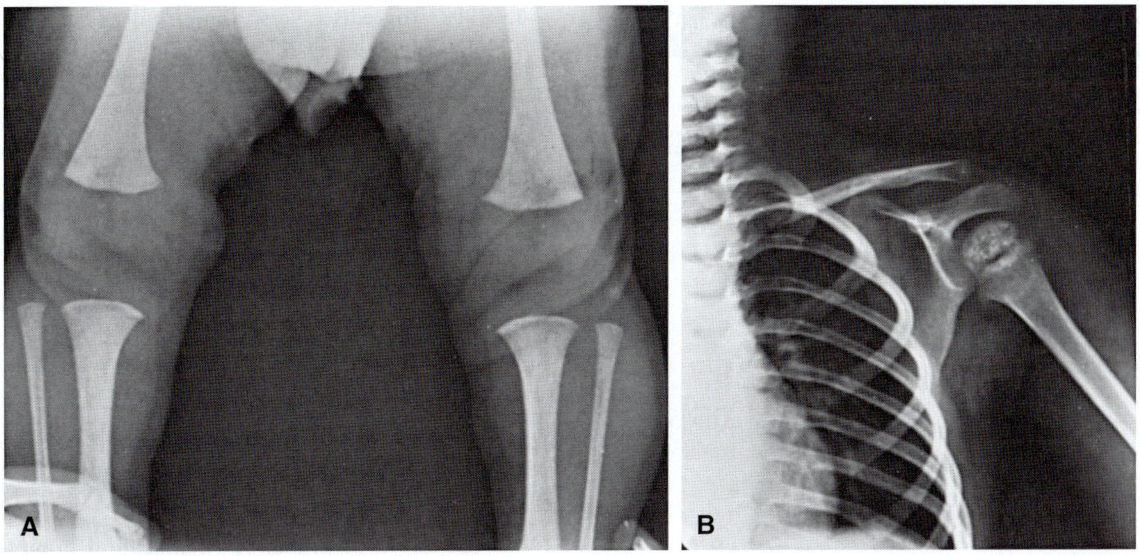

Figura 566-2. Ipotiroidismo congenito. *A*, Assenza dell'epifisi femorale distale in un neonato di 3 mesi nato a termine. Ciò depone per l'insorgenza dell'ipotiroidismo durante la vita fetale. *B*, Disgenesia epifisaria della testa dell'omero in una bambina di 9 anni inadeguatamente trattata con ormone tiroideo.

evidenzia basso voltaggio. Nei bambini con più di 2 anni di età, il colesterolo sierico è di solito aumentato. La RM cerebrale prima del trattamento è normale, sebbene la spettroscopica protonica in risonanza magnetica dimostri alti livelli di composti contenenti colina, possibile indice di blocco della maturazione mielinica.

TRATTAMENTO. Il trattamento di elezione è raprresentato dalla levotiroxina somministrata per via orale. Dato che l'80% del T_3 circolante si forma dalla monodeiodinazione del T_4, i livelli sierici di T_4 e di T_3 ritornano normali nei bambini trattati. Questo è vero anche nel cervello, dove l'80% del T_3 necessario è prodotto localmente dal T_4. Nei neonati, la dose iniziale raccomandata è di 10-15 μg/kg (da 37,5 a 50 μg/die). Neonati con ipotiroidismo più grave, con T_4 sierico <3 μg/dL, devono iniziare con quantità maggiori, ai valori alti del range del dosaggio. Le compresse di tiroxina non devono essere mescolate con latte contenente proteine della soia o ferro, perché possono legarsi al T_4 e inibirne l'assorbimento. I livelli di T_4 o T_4 libero e di TSH devono essere monitorati a intervalli regolari (circa ogni mese nei primi sei mesi di vita, poi ogni 2-3 mesi dal sesto mese al secondo anno) e mantenuti nel range di normalità per età. Bambini con ipotiroidismo richiedono circa 4 μg/kg/die e gli adulti solo 2 μg/kg/die.

Più tardi, per alcuni bambini, può essere necessario confermare la diagnosi, per escludere la possibilità di ipotiroidismo transitorio. Questo non è necessario invece in bambini con ectopia tiroidea provata o in quelli con elevati livelli di TSH dopo il 6°-12° mese di terapia per scarsa compliance o dosaggio inadeguato di T_4. L'interruzione della terapia al terzo anno di età per 3-4 settimane provoca un marcato aumento dei livelli di TSH nei bambini con ipotiroidismo permanente.

Il solo effetto negativo dell'L-tiroxina-sodica è dose-dipendente. Una dose eccessiva può provocare craniosinostosi e problemi comportamentali. Un bambino più grande (8-13 anni) con ipotiroidismo acquisito può presentare *pseudotumor cerebri* nei primi 4 mesi di trattamento. In bambini più grandi, dopo che il recupero della crescita è completo, la velocità di crescita fornisce un buon indice dell'adeguatezza della terapia. I genitori devono essere avvertiti circa le modificazioni del comportamento e dell'attività che si possono presentare con la terapia e si deve fare particolare attenzione a eventuali deficit neurologici o comportamentali.

PROGNOSI. Con l'avvento dei programmi di screening neonatale per l'individuazione dell'ipotiroidismo congenito, la prognosi per i neonati colpiti è notevolmente migliorata. La diagnosi precoce e un adeguato trattamento dalle prime settimane di vita portano a una normale crescita della statura e dell'intelligenza, analoga a quella di fratelli o sorelle non malati. Alcuni programmi di screening riportano che la maggior parte dei neonati colpiti gravemente, come quelli con i più bassi livelli di T_4 e ritardo della maturazione scheletrica, ha un QI ridotto (5-10 punti) e altre sequele neuropsicologiche, come scoordinazione, ipotonia, ipertonia, scarsa capacità di attenzione e problemi di linguaggio. Circa il 20% dei bambini presenta un deficit neurosensoriale dell'udito. Senza trattamento, i bambini colpiti hanno un grave ritardo di crescita e un marcato deficit mentale. L'ormone tiroideo è fondamentale per il normale sviluppo cerebrale nei primi mesi postnatali; la diagnosi biochimica può essere formulata subito dopo la nascita e si deve iniziare rapidamente un trattamento efficace, per prevenire un danno cerebrale irreversibile. Un ritardo nella diagnosi, la non correzione rapida dell'iniziale ipotiroidismo, un trattamento inadeguato e una scarsa compliance nei primi 2-3 anni di vita comportano gradi variabili di danno cerebrale. Quando l'esordio dell'ipotiroidismo si verifica dopo i 2 anni di età, migliora molto la previsione di un normale sviluppo, anche se la diagnosi e il trattamento sono ritardati, indicando così come l'ormone tiroideo sia molto importante per una rapida crescita cerebrale del neonato.

IPOTIROIDISMO ACQUISITO

EPIDEMIOLOGIA. Studi in bambini in età scolare riportano che l'ipotiroidismo compare in circa lo 0,3% (1/333). L'ipotiroidismo acquisito è più comunemente il risultato di una tiroidine linfocitica cronica; il 6% dei ragazzi tra i 12-19 anni presenta una patologia tiroidea autoimmune, che si verifica nelle femmine con frequenza doppia rispetto ai maschi.

EZIOLOGIA. La causa più comune di ipotiroidismo acquisito (Tab. 566-3) è la tiroidine linfocitica cronica (vedi Capitolo 567). La **patologia tiroidea autoimmune** può far parte di sindromi polighiandolari; bambini con sindrome di Down, di Turner e di Klinefelter, con malattia celiaca o diabete, presentano un rischio maggiore di presentare patologia tiroidea autoimmune (vedi Capitolo 567). Altre malattie autoimmuni con aumentato rischio di ipotiroidismo, comprendono la sindrome di Sjoegren, la sclerosi multipla, l'anemia perniciosa, la malattia di Addison e l'insufficienza ovarica. Nonostante compaia tipicamente nell'adolescente, si può verificare anche precocemente, nel primo anno di vita.

TABELLA 566.3. Classificazione eziologica dell'ipotiroidismo acquisito

AUTOIMMUNE (IPOTIROIDISMO ACQUISITO)
Tiroidite di Hashimoto
Sindrome autoimmune polighiandolare, tipo I e II
IATROGENICO
Propiltiouracile, metimazolo, ioduro, litio, amiodarone
Irradiazione
Radioiodio
Tiroidectomia
MALATTIE SISTEMICHE
Cistinosi
Istiocitosi a cellule di Langerhans
EMANGIOMI (VOLUMINOSI) DEL FEGATO (IODIOTIRONINA DEIODINASI DI TIPO 3)
RESISTENZA ALL'ORMONE DELLA TIROIDE (SOLO OCCASIONALI MANIFESTAZIONI CLINICHE DI IPOTIROIDISMO)

Alcuni pazienti con disgenesia tiroidea congenita o con difetti genetici incompleti nella sintesi dell'ormone tiroideo, possono non mostrare manifestazioni cliniche fino all'infanzia, come se avessero un ipotiroidismo acquisito; attualmente questi casi vengono di norma scoperti con gli screening neonatali. La tiroidectomia subtotale per tireotossicosi o per tumore, può esitare in ipotiroidismo, come la rimozione di tessuto tiroideo ectopico. Il tessuto tiroideo in una cisti del dotto tireoglosso normalmente costituisce la sola sorgente di ormone tiroideo, e la sua escissione comporta un ipotiroidismo. Dal momento che le ghiandole subioidee di solito simulano la cisti del dotto tireoglosso, in questi pazienti, prima dell'intervento, è indicata un'indagine ecografia o una scintigrafia.

Bambini con **cistinosi nefropatica**, una malattia caratterizzata da accumulo lisosomiale di cistina nei tessuti dell'organismo, sviluppano una ridotta funzionalità tiroidea. L'ipotiroidismo può essere manifesto, ma sono comuni delle forme subcliniche, ed è indicato un controllo periodico dei livelli di TSH. All'età di 13 anni, 2/3 di questi pazienti richiedono una terapia sostitutiva con T_4.

L'infiltrazione istiocitica della tiroide in bambini con istiocitosi a cellule di Langerhans può portare a ipotiroidismo.

L'**irradiazione** incidentale della zona tiroidea durante il trattamento della malattia di Hodgkin, o di altre patologie maligne della testa e del collo, oppure prima di un trapianto di midollo osseo, spesso portano a danno tiroideo. Circa un terzo di questi bambini sviluppa elevati livelli di TSH a un anno dalla terapia e il 15-20% progredisce verso l'ipotiroidismo in 5-7 anni. Alcuni medici raccomandano controlli periodici del TSH, ma altri consigliano di trattare tutti i pazienti esposti con dosi di T_4 soppressive del TSH.

Un'ingestione protratta di **farmaci** contenenti iodio può causare ipotiroidismo, normalmente accompagnato da gozzo (vedi Capitolo 568). L'amiodarone, un farmaco antiaritmico con il 37% di peso molecolare fornito da iodio, ha provocato ipotiroidismo in circa il 20% dei bambini trattati. Per il suo elevato contenuto di iodio, esso lede direttamente la funzionalità tiroidea inibendo la 5'-deiodinasi, che converte il T_4 in T_3. Bambini trattati con questo farmaco vanno monitorati con dosaggi seriali di T_4, T_3 e TSH. Altri farmaci possono indurre ipotiroidismo, come carbonato di litio, interferone α, talidomide, stavudina e aminoglutetimide.

Ipotiroidismo può comparire in bambini con voluminosi **emangiomi** epatici, per incremento dell'attività della deiodinasi di tipo 3, che catalizza la conversione di T_4 in rT_3 e di T_3 in T_2. La secrezione tiroidea è aumentata, ma non è sufficiente a compensare il notevole aumento della degradazione di T_4 a rT_3.

MANIFESTAZIONI CLINICHE. Normalmente il primo segno è rappresentato dalla decelerazione della crescita, segno che spesso, però, non viene riconosciuto (Figg. 566-3 e 566-4). Il gozzo, che può essere presente, tipicamente non è né molle né duro, ma con una consistenza gommosa e una superficie irregolare. Si sviluppano in modo insidioso modificazioni mixedematose della cute, stipsi, intolleranza al freddo e astenia, e aumenta la necessità di dormire. Sorprendentemente, il lavoro scolastico e la sua qualità di solito non ne risentono, anche nelle forme di ipotiroidismo grave. La maturazione ossea è ritardata, spesso di molto, e dà un'indicazione della durata dell'ipotiroidismo. Gli adolescenti hanno tipicamente una pubertà ritardata, mentre i bambini più piccoli possono manifestare una pseudopubertà precoce con galattorrea. Quest'ultima è il risultato di un aumento della secrezione di prolattina da stimolazione del TRH. La pubertà precoce, caratterizzata da sviluppo mammario nelle femmine e macrorchidismo nei maschi, sembra essere il risultato di concentrazioni di TSH elevate in modo abnorme, che si legano al recettore dell'ormone follicolo-stimolante con conseguente stimolazione.

Alcuni bambini presentano cefalea e problemi visivi; essi di solito hanno un ingrossamento iperplastico dell'ipofisi, talvolta con espansione soprasellare, nell'ipotiroidismo di lunga durata; si ritiene che questa condizione sia il risultato di iperplasia delle cellule tireotrope, ma può essere scambiata per un tumore ipofisario (vedi Capitolo 558). Altre caratteristiche comprendono compressione nervosa, atassia, debolezza muscolare o crampi, disturbi mestruali, bradicardia, aumento di peso e anomalie dei

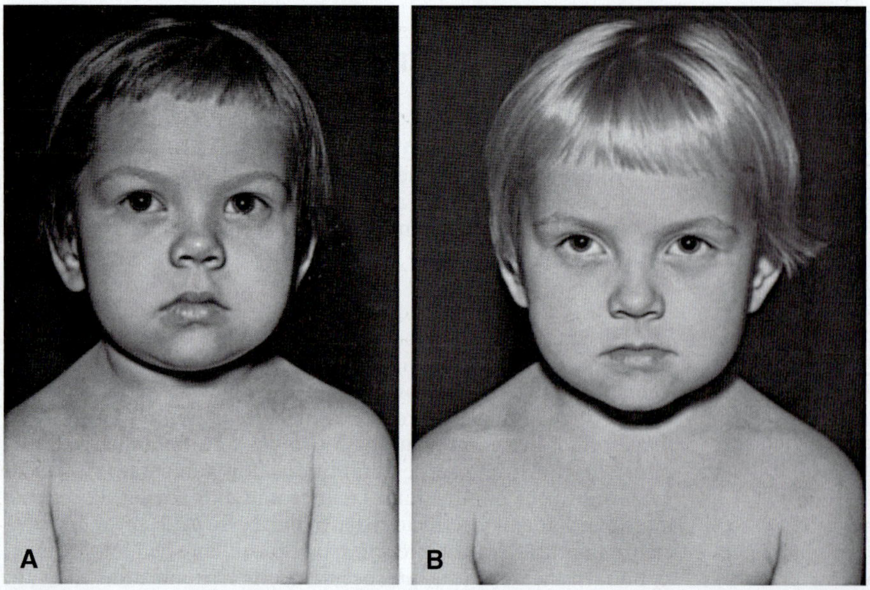

Figura 566-3. *A*, Ipotiroidismo acquisito in una bambina di 6 anni. È stata trattata per 3 anni con vari farmaci ematinici, per la presenza di anemia refrattaria. Ha presentato inoltre un arresto quasi completo della crescita, stipsi e indolenza per 3 anni. L'età staturale era di 3 anni, mentre quella ossea di 4. Presentava un colorito giallastro e un aspetto infantile, con scarso sviluppo della radice del naso. Colesterolo sierico, 501 mg/dL; captazione del radioiodio, 7% a 24 ore; PBI, 2,8 mg/dL. *B*, Dopo 18 mesi di terapia, notare lo sviluppo del naso, l'aumento della lucentezza e la diminuzione della pigmentazione dei capelli, e un aspetto più maturo del viso. L'età staturale era di 5 anni e mezzo, mentre quella ossea di 7 anni. C'era stato un deciso miglioramento delle condizioni generali. Il menarca è comparso all'età di 14 anni. L'altezza definitiva è stata di 155 cm. Ha acquisito il diploma di scuola secondaria. La malattia è stata efficacemente controllata con somministrazione giornaliera di L-tiroxina sodica.

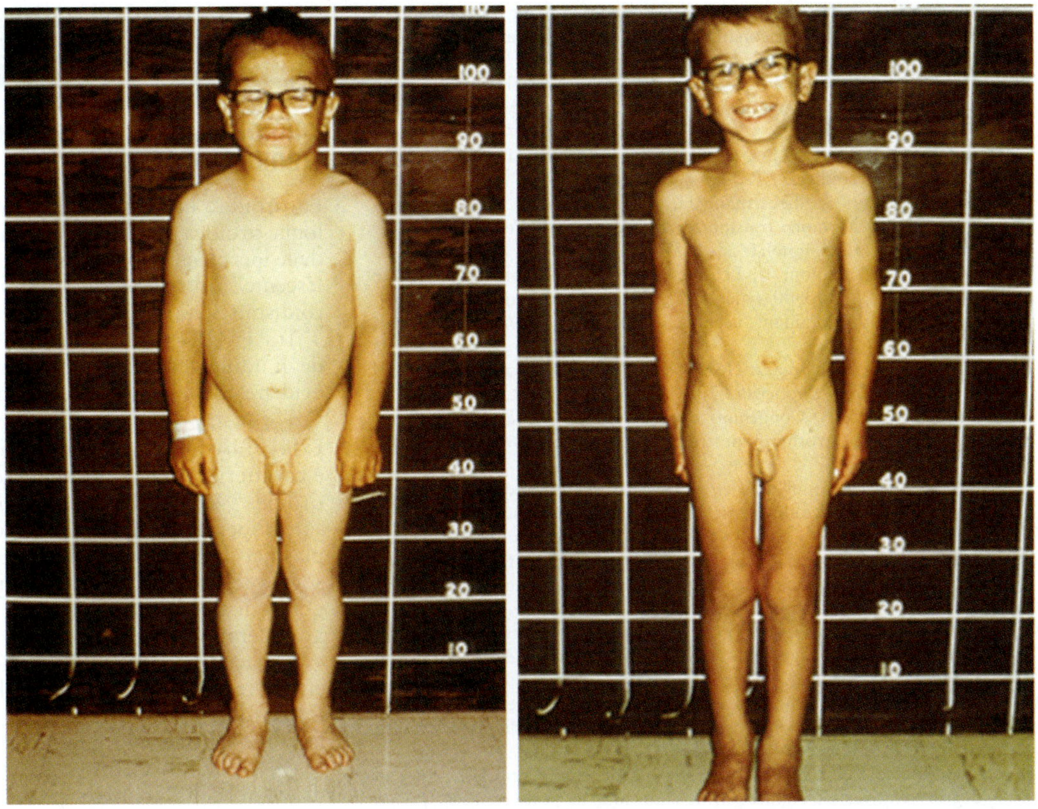

Figura 566-4. *A*, Bassa statura (108 cm, <3° percentile), mixedema generalizzato, espressione sonnolente, addome voluminoso e capelli secchi sono i segni di ipotiroidismo in questo ragazzo di 12 anni. Le proporzioni corporee sono immature per la sua età (1.25:1). *B*, Stesso ragazzo dopo 4 mesi di trattamento. L'altezza è aumentata di 4 cm; notare la notevole modificazione dell'habitus corporeo dovuto a scomparsa del mixedema generalizzato, miglioramento del tono muscolare e una vivace espressione del volto. (Da LaFranchi SH: Hypotiroidism. *Pediatr Clin North Am* 1979; 26:44.)

dati di laboratorio (iponatremia, anemia macrocitica, ipercolesterolemia, aumento delle CPK, iperprolattinemia). Le complicazioni dell'ipotiroidismo grave sono indicate nella Tabella 566-4.

Tutte queste modificazioni ritornano nella norma con una adeguata terapia sostitutiva con T_4, ma nei bambini con ipotiroidismo di lunga durata, il recupero della crescita può essere incompleto (vedi Fig. 566-4). Durante i primi 18 mesi di trattamento, la maturazione scheletrica spesso supera le aspettative di crescita in altezza, con conseguente perdita di circa 7 cm rispetto all'altezza prevista da adulti; le cause non sono note.

STUDI DIAGNOSTICI E TRATTAMENTO. Il trattamento e gli studi diagnostici sono gli stessi descritti per l'ipotiroidismo congenito. La misurazione degli anticorpi antitireoglobulina e antiperossidasi (definiti precedentemente antimicrosomiali) può indicare come causa un tiroidite autoimmune. Generalmente, non c'è indicazione per indagini morfologiche. Nei casi con gozzo da patologia autoimmune, se si esegue un'indagine ecografica essa dimostrerà tipicamente un ingrossamento diffuso con ipoecogenicità cicatriziale. Durante il primo anno di trattamento, possono presentarsi: peggioramento del rendimento scolastico, sonnolenza, irrequietezza, scarsa capacità di attenzione e problemi comportamentali, ma sono transitori; se la famiglia viene avvertita di queste manifestazioni, si può migliorare la gestione del caso. I sintomi riportati beneficiano di una terapia con T_4 sottodosata, che va aumentata lentamente.

TABELLA 566-4. Patogenesi delle complicanze generali nel trattamento dell'ipotiroidismo complicato

COMPLICANZA	PATOGENESI
Insufficienza cardiaca	Alterazioni della funzione ventricolare sistolica e diastolica e aumento delle resistenze vascolari periferiche
Insufficienza ventilatoria	Diminuzione del drive ventilatorio ipercapnico e ipossico
Iponatremia	Alterazione renale dell'escrezione dell'acqua libera e sindrome da inappropriata secrezione di ormone antidiuretico (SIADH)
Ileo	Ipomobilità intestinale
Sensibilità ai farmaci	Riduzione della percentuale di filtrazione e aumento della sensibilità ai sedativi e agli analgesici
Ipotermia e assenza di febbre alla sepsi	Diminuzione della risposta termogenetica
Delirio, demenza, crisi epilettiche, encefalopatia da stupor e coma	Diminuzione dell'azione dell'ormone tiroideo sul SNC e iponatremia e ipercapnia
Insufficienza surrenalica	Associata malattia surrenalica o ipofisaria, o alterazione reversibile dell'asse ipotalamo-ipo- fiso-surrenalico da stress
Coagulopatia	Sindrome acquisita di von Willebrand (tipo I), e decremento dei fattori VIII, VII, V, IX e X

Da Roberts CG, Landerson PW: Hypotiroidism. *Lancet* 2004;363:793-803.

Adams A, Matthews C, Collingwood TH, et al: Genetic analysis of 29 kindreds with generalized and pituitary resistance to thyroid hormone. *J Clin Invest* 1994;94:506–515.

American Academy of Pediatrics; Rose SR; Section on Endocrinology and Committee on Genetics, American Thyroid Association; Brown RS; Public Health Committee, Lawson Wilkins Pediatric Endocrine Society; Foley T, Kaplowitz PB, Kaye CI, Sundararajan S, Varma SK: Update of newborn screening and therapy for congenital hypothyroidism. *Pediatrics* 2006; 117:2290–2303.

Asajura Y, Tachibana K, Adachi M, et al: Hypothalamic-pituitary hypothyroidism detected by neonatal screening for congenital hypothyroidism using measurement of thyroid-stimulating hormone and thyroxine. *Acta Paediatr* 2002;91:172–177.

Bilimoria KY, Pescovitz OH, DiMeglio LA: Autoimmune thyroid dysfunction in children with type 1 diabetes mellitus: Screening guidelines based on a retrospective analysis. *J Pediatr Endocrinol Metab* 2003;16:1111–1117.

Borck G, Topaloglu AK, Korsch E, et al: Four new cases of congenital secondary hypothyroidism due to a splice site mutation in the thyrotropin-beta gene: Phenotypic variability and founder effect. *J Clin Endocrinol Metab* 2004;89:4136–4141.

Castanet M, Park SM, Smith A, et al: A novel loss-of-function mutation in TTF-2 is associated with congenital hypothyroidism, thyroid agenesis and cleft palate. *Hum Mol Genet* 2002;11:2051–2059.

Conrad SC, Chiu H, Silverman BI: Soy formula complicates management of congenital hypothyroidism. *Arch Dis Child* 2004;89:37–40.

De Vijlder JJ: Primary congenital hypothyroidism: defects in iodine pathways. *Eur J Endocrinol* 2003;149:247–256.

Doyle DA, Gonzalez I, Thomas B, et al: Autosomal dominant transmission of congenital hypothyroidism, neonatal respiratory distress, and ataxia caused by a mutation of NKX2-1. *J Pediatr* 2004;145:190–193.
Eugene D, Djemli A, VanVliet G: Sexual dimorphism of thyroid function in newborns with congenital hypothyroidism. *J Clin Endocrinol Metab* 2005;90:2696–2700.
Eugster EA, LeMay D, Xerin JM, et al: Definitive diagnosis in children with congenital hypothyroidism. *J Pediatr* 2004;144:643–647.
Friesema EC, Grueters A, Biebermann H, et al: Association between mutations in a thyroid hormone transporter and severe X-linked psychomotor retardation. *Lancet* 2004;364:1435–1437.
Grasberger H, Ringkananont U, Lefrancois P, et al. Thyroid transcription factor 1 rescues PAX8/p300 synergism impaired by a natural PAX8 paired mutation with dominant negative activity. *Mol Endocrinol* 2005; 19:1779–1791.
Gruters A, Krude H, Biebermann H. Molecular genetic defects in congenital hypothyroidism. *Eur J Endocrinol* 2004;151(Suppl 3):U39.
Heyerdahl S, Oerbeck B: Congenital hypothyroidism: Developmental outcome in relation to levothyroxine treatment variables. *Thyroid* 2003;13: 1029–1038.
Huang SA, Tu HM, Harney JW, et al: Severe hypothyroidism caused by type 3 iodothyronine deiodinase in infantile hemangiomas. *N Engl J Med* 2000;343: 185–189.
Ishiguro H, Yasuda Y, Tomita Y, et al: Long-term follow-up of thyroid function in patients who receive bone marrow transplantation during childhood and adolescence. *J Clin Endocrinol Metab* 2004;89:5981–5986.
Karlson B, Gustafsson J, Hedov G, et al: Thyroid dysfunction in Down's syndrome: Relation to age and thyroid autoimmunity. *Arch Dis Child* 1998;79:242–245.
Kaspers S, Kordonouri O, Schober F, et al: Anthropometry, metabolic control, and thyroid autoimmunity in type 1 diabetes with celiac disease: A multicenter survey. *J Pediatr* 2004;145:790–795.
Leger J, Marinovic D, Garel C, et al: Thyroid developmental anomalies in first degree relatives of children with congenital hypothyroidism. *J Clin Endocrinol Metab* 2002;87:575–580.
Madison LD, LaFranchi S: Screening for congenital hypothyroidism: current controversies. *Curr Opin Endocrinol Metab* 2005;12:36.
Mandel SJ, Hermos RJ, Larson CA, et al: Atypical hypothyroidism and the very low birthweight infant. *Thyroid* 2000;10:693–695.
Moreno JC, Bikker H, Kempers MJE, et al: Inactivating mutations in the gene for thyroid oxidase 2 (THOX2) and congenital hypothyroidism. *N Engl J Med* 2002;347:95–102.
Murphy N, Jume R, van Toor H, et al: The hypothalamic-pituitary-thyroid axis in preterm infants: Changes in the first 24 hours of postnatal life. *J Clin Endocrinol Metab* 2004;89:2824–2831.
Nishiyama S, Mikeda T, Okada T, et al: Transient hypothyroidism or persistent hyperthyrotropinemia in neonates born to mothers with excessive iodine intake. *Thyroid* 2004;14:1077–1083.
Oerbeck B, Sundet K, Kase BF, et al: Congenital hypothyroidism: Influence of disease severity and L-thyroxine treatment on intellectual, motor, and school-associated outcomes in young adults. *Pediatrics* 2003;112:923–930.
Oerbeck B, Sundet K, Kase BF, et al: Congenital hypothyroidism: No adverse effects of high dose thyroxine treatment on adult memory, attention, and behavior. *Arch Dis Child* 2005;90:132–137.
Olivieri A, Stazi A, Mastroiacovo P, et al. A population-based study on the frequency of additional congenital malformations in infants with congenital hypothyroidism: Data from the Italian registry for congenital hypothyroidism (1991–1998). *J Clin Endocrinol Metab* 2002;87:557–562.
Roberts CG, Landenson PW: Hypothyroidism. *Lancet* 2004;363:793–803.
Rovet J: Congenital hypothyroidism: Treatment and outcome. *Curr Opin Endocrinol Diabetes* 2005;12:42.
Rovet J: Children with congenital hypothyroidism and their siblings: Do they really differ? *Pediatrics* 2005;115:e52–57.
Schoen EJ, Clapp W, To TT, et al: The key role of newborn thyroid scintigraphy with isotopic iodine (123I) in defining and managing congenital hypothyroidism. *J Pediatr* 2004;114:e683–688.
Scott DA, Wang R, Kreman VC, et al: The Pendred syndrome is caused by mutations in a putative sulphate transporter gene (PDS). *Nat Genet* 1999;17:411.
Selva KA, Harper A, Downs A, et al: Neurodevelopmental outcomes in congenital hypothyroidism: Comparison of initial T_4 dose and time to reach target T_4 and TSH. *J Pediatr* 2005;147:775–780.
Teng W, Shan Z, Teng X, et al: Effect of iodine in take on thyroid diseases in China. *N Engl J Med* 2006;354:2783–2792.
Trueba SS, Auge J, Mattei G, et al. PAX8, TITF1, and FOXE1 gene expression patterns during human development: new insight into human thyroid development and thyroid dysgenesis-associated malformations. *J Clin Endocrinol Metab* 2005;90:455–462.

Capitolo 567 ■ Tiroidite

TIROIDITE LINFOCITICA (TIROIDE DI HASHIMOTO, TIROIDE AUTOIMMUNE)

La tiroidite linfocitica rappresenta la causa più comune di patologia tiroidea nei bambini e negli adolescenti e giustifica molte delle iperplasie tiroidee precedentemente definite gozzo "dell'adolescente" o "semplice". È inoltre la causa più frequente di ipotiroidismo acquisito, con o senza gozzo.

Tra l'1-2% dei bambini di età scolare più piccoli e il 4-6% degli adolescenti risulta positivo agli anticorpi antitiroidei come evidenza della tiroide autoimmune.

EZIOLOGIA. Questa tipica patologia autoimmune organo-specifica è caratterizzata istologicamente da infiltrazione linfocitaria della tiroide. Nelle fasi precoci della malattia, può essere presente solo l'iperplasia; questa è seguita da infiltrazione di linfociti e plasmacellule tra i follicoli e da aplasia follicolare. Quasi sempre sono presenti anche follicoli linfoidi con centri germinativi e il grado di atrofia e di fibrosi dei follicoli è variabile, da forme lievi a moderate.

Gli accumuli di linfociti intratiroidei differiscono da quelli ematici. Circa il 60% delle cellule linfoidi infiltrate è costituito da linfociti T e circa il 30% esprime marker delle cellule B; la popolazione cellulare T è rappresentata da cellule helper ($CD4^+$) e cellule citotossiche ($CD8^+$). È chiara la partecipazione di eventi cellulari nella patogenesi. Certi aplotipi HLA (HLA-DR4, HLA-DR5) sono associati ad aumentato rischio di gozzo e di tiroiditi, mentre altri (HLA-DR3) a una variante atrofica della tiroidite.

Sono coinvolti anche una grande varietà di autoanticorpi contro diversi antigeni tiroidei. Anticorpi antiperossidasi tiroidea (TPOAb) (in precedenza definiti "anticorpi antimicrosomiali") e anticorpi contro la tireoglobulina sono rintracciabili nel siero del 90% dei bambini con tiroidite linfocitica e in molti pazienti con malattia di Graves. I TPOAb inibiscono l'attività enzimatica e stimolano la citotossicità delle cellule killer naturali. Non sembra che gli anticorpi antitireoglobulina giochino un ruolo nella distruzione autoimmune della ghiandola. Spesso sono presenti anticorpi bloccanti il recettore della tireotropina, specialmente in pazienti con ipotiroidismo, e attualmente pare che siano correlati allo sviluppo di ipotiroidismo e di atrofia ghiandolare in pazienti con tiroidite autoimmune.

MANIFESTAZIONI CLINICHE. La malattia è due volte più frequente nelle femmine che nei maschi. Può comparire durante i primi tre anni di vita, ma diventa nettamente più frequente dopo il sesto anno di età, raggiungendo un picco di incidenza durante l'adolescenza. Le più comuni manifestazioni cliniche sono il gozzo e il ritardo della crescita. Il gozzo può manifestarsi insidiosamente, essere di piccole dimensioni o voluminoso. Nella maggior parte dei pazienti, la tiroide è diffusamente aumentata di volume, di consistenza dura e non molle. In circa il 30% dei pazienti, la ghiandola appare globulare o nodulare. La maggior parte dei bambini colpiti è asintomatica e clinicamente eutiroidea; alcuni possono riportare sintomi di pressione a livello del collo. Alcuni bambini manifestano segni clinici di ipotiroidismo, ma altri, clinicamente eutiroidei, hanno indici bioumorali tipici dell'ipotiroidismo. Una minoranza di pazienti presenta manifestazioni tipiche dell'ipertiroidismo, come nervosismo, irritabilità, aumento della sudorazione e iperattività, ma i risultati delle indagini di laboratorio non corrispondono necessariamente a ipertiroidismo. Occasionalmente, la patologia può coesistere con la malattia di Graves. Nella tiroidite linfocitica può comparire oftalmopatia, in assenza di malattia di Graves.

Il decorso clinico è variabile. Il gozzo può diminuire o addirittura scomparire spontaneamente oppure persistere inalterato per anni, sebbene il paziente rimanga eutiroideo. La maggior parte dei bambini che all'esordio sono eutiroidei rimane tale, nonostante una certa percentuale gradualmente sviluppi ipotiroidismo, in mesi o anni. Nel corso di alcuni anni, la metà dei bambini con ipotiroidismo subclinico ritorna eutiroidea, mentre l'altra metà sviluppa un ipotiroidismo manifesto. La tiroidite rappresenta la causa della maggior parte dei casi di ipotiroidismo senza gozzo (atrofico).

Comunemente la tiroidite colpisce più individui della stessa famiglia; l'incidenza nei fratelli o nei genitori di bambini colpiti è intorno al 25%. In queste famiglie la presenza di autoanticorpi antitireoglobulina e antiperossidasi tiroidea è ereditaria e la malattia si trasmette con modalità autosomica dominante, a ridotta penetranza nei maschi. La concomitanza, nei familiari di pazienti, di tiroidite linfocitica, ipotiroidismo "idiopatico" e malattia di Graves rende convincente l'evidenza di un rapporto di base tra queste tre condizioni patologiche. La malattia è stata associata a molte altre patologie autoimmuni. La tiroidite autoimmune si verifica nel 10% di pazienti con sindrome autoimmune polighiandolare di tipo I (APS-1), caratterizzata dall'acronimo APECED, cioè poliendocrinopatia autoimmune-candidosi-displasia ectodermica. L'APS-1 consiste di due elementi della triade dell'ipoparatiroidismo, malattia di Addison e candidosi mucocutanea (sindrome "HAM"). Questa relativamente rara malattia autosomica recessiva presente nell'infanzia è causata da mutazioni del gene regolatore autoimmune (*AIRE*) sul cromosoma 21q22.3. La tiroidite autoimmune si verifica nel 70% dei pazienti con APS-2 (sindrome di Schmidt), che consiste nell'associazione fra malattia di Addison e diabete mellito insulino-dipendente o patologia tiroidea autoimmune. L'eziologia è sconosciuta ed è tipicamente presente nei giovani adulti. La patologia tiroidea autoimmune tende a essere associata ad anemia perniciosa, a vitiligine o ad alopecia. TPOAb sono stati trovati in circa il 20% dei bambini bianchi e nel 4% di quelli neri con diabete mellito. La patologia tiroidea autoimmune ha un'aumentata incidenza in bambini con rosolia congenita. La tiroidite linfocitica è associata anche a certe patologie cromosomiche, in particolare la sindrome di Turner e la sindrome di Down. Nei bambini con sindrome di Down, uno studio riporta che il 28% presenta anticorpi antitiroidei (soprattutto anti-TPO), il 7% evidenzia ipotiroidismo subclinico, il 7% ipotiroidismo conclamato e il 5% ipertiroidismo. In un lavoro che riguardava bambine con sindrome di Turner, il 41% delle pazienti aveva anticorpi antitiroidei (ancora soprattutto anti-TPO), il 18% gozzo e l'8% ipotiroidismo subclinico o manifesto. Un altro studio su 75 bambine con sindrome di Turner evidenzia che la patologia tiroidea autoimmune aumenta dalla prima (15%) alla terza (30%) decade di vita. Anche i maschi con sindrome di Klinefelter sono a rischio di patologia tiroidea autoimmune. La diagnosi differenziale è riportata nella Tabella 567-1.

REPERTI DI LABORATORIO. I test di funzionalità tiroidea sono spesso normali, sebbene il livello dell'ormone stimolante la tiroide (TSH) possa essere lievemente o anche moderatamente elevato in alcuni individui, con cosiddetto ipotiroidismo subclinico. Il fatto che molti bambini con tiroidite linfocitica non presentino elevati livelli di TSH indica che il gozzo può essere provocato dalla infiltrazione linfocitica o da immunoglobuline stimolanti la crescita. Bambini piccoli con tiroidite linfocitica presentano anticorpi sierici anti-TPO, ma il test per titolare gli anticorpi tiroidei antitireoglobulina è positivo in meno del 50% dei casi. Anticorpi anti-TPO e antitireoglobulina sono stati individuati in quantità analoghe in adolescenti con tiroidite linfocitica. Quando si utilizzano i test ematologici, si scopre circa il 95% dei pazienti con tiroidite autoimmune. I livelli nei bambini e negli adolescenti sono inferiori a quelli dell'adulto con tiroidite linfocitica, e, nei casi dubbi, sono consigliate valutazioni ripetute, perché le concentrazioni possono aumentare tardivamente nel corso della malattia. L'RM e l'ecografia tiroidea non sono normalmente necessarie. L'RM tiroidea mostra, nel 50% dei bambini, una distribuzione irregolare e disuniforme del radioisotopo e in circa il 60% o più la somministrazione di perclorato porta a una eliminazione di iodio dalla tiroide maggiore del 10%. L'ecografia tiroidea mostra ipoecogenicità cicatriziale nella maggior parte dei pazienti. La diagnosi definitiva è stabilita dalla biopsia della tiroide; questa procedura è di rado clinicamente indicata.

Anticorpi antitiroidei possono essere individuati anche in quasi la metà dei fratelli di pazienti colpiti e in una percentuale significativa di mamme di bambini con sindrome di Down o sindrome di Turner, in assenza di dimostrabile patologia tiroidea. Si sono individuati anche nel 20% dei bambini con diabete mellito e nel 23% di quelli con sindrome da rosolia congenita.

TRATTAMENTO. In presenza di ipotiroidismo, è indicato il trattamento sostitutivo con levotiroxina (50-150 μg/die). Il gozzo spesso tende a decrescere, ma persiste per anni. Un gozzo voluminoso in un paziente eutiroideo dovrebbe regredire con dosi soppressive di levotiroxina. I livelli anticorpali fluttuano, sia nei pazienti trattati sia in quelli non trattati, e persistono per anni. Dato che, in un certo numero di casi, la malattia è autolimitante, con periodiche rivalutazioni è possibile stabilire la necessità o meno di continuare la terapia. Anche i pazienti non trattati devono periodicamente essere controllati. Sebbene il trattamento di pazienti con ipotiroidismo subclinico (T_4 e T_4 libero normali, TSH elevato) sia controverso, si preferisce trattare questi bambini fino al completamento della crescita e della pubertà, per poi rivalutarne la funzionalità tiroidea. Noduli voluminosi persistenti nonostante la terapia soppressiva devono essere valutati dal punto di vista istologico dato che, in pazienti con tiroidite linfocitica, si possono sviluppare sia il linfoma sia il carcinoma tiroideo.

TABELLA 567-1. Caratteristiche delle sindromi tiroiditiche

CARATTERISTICHE	TIROIDITE DI HASHIMOTO	TIROIDITE *POST PARTUM* INDOLORE	TIROIDITE SPORADICA INDOLORE	TIROIDITE SUBACUTA INDOLORE	TIROIDITE SUPPURATIVA	TIROIDITE DI RIEDEL
Rapporto fra i sessi (F:M)	8-9:1	–	2:1	5:1	1:1	3-4:1
Cause	Autoimmune	Autoimmnune	Autoimmune	Sconosciute	Infettive	Sconosciute
Reperti patologici	Infiltrazione linfocitica, centri germinali, fibrosi	Infiltrazione linfocitica	Infiltrazione linfocitica	Cellule giganti, granulomi	Formazione di ascesso	Fibrosi densa
Funzionalità tiroidea	Ipotiroidismo	Tireotossicosi, ipotiroidismo o entrambi	Tireotossicosi, ipotiroidismo o entrambi	Tireotossicosi, ipotiroidismo o entrambi	Di solito eutiroidismo	Di solito eutiroidismo
Anticorpi anti-TPO	Alto titolo, persistente	Alto titolo, persistente	Alto titolo, persistente	Basso titolo, o assente o transitorio	Assente	Normalmente presenti
VES	Normale	Normale	Normale	Alto	Alto	Normale
Captazione dello ^{123}I dopo 24 ore	Variabile	<5%	<5%	<5%	Normale	Basso o normale

VES, velocità di eritrosedimentazione; ^{123}I, iodio 123; TPO, perossidasi tiroidea
Da Pearce EN, Farwell AP, Braverman LE: Thyroiditis. N Engl J Med 2003; 348: 2646--2654

ALTRE CAUSE DI TIROIDITE

Condizioni specifiche come la tubercolosi, la sarcoidosi, la parotite e la malattia da graffio di gatto possono essere cause rare di tiroidite (vedi Tab. 567-1).

La **tiroidite acuta suppurativa** non è frequente e di solito è preceduta da infezione respiratoria. È colpita soprattutto la porzione inferiore del lobo sinistro. Si può formare un ascesso. Tipicamente gli agenti infettivi sono rappresentati da microrganismi anaerobi, con o senza aerobi. Il microrganismo più comune è lo *Streptococcus viridans*, seguito dallo *Staphylococcus aureus* e dallo *Pneumococcus*. Episodi ricorrenti, o reperti di flora batterica mista, suggeriscono che l'infezione provenga da residui del **dotto tireoglosso**, o, più spesso, dalla **fistola del seno piriforme**. La notevole sensibilità ghiandolare, la tumefazione, l'eritema, la disfagia e la limitazione funzionale nei movimenti sono segni caratteristici. Sono comuni febbre, brividi e mal di gola ed è presente leucocitosi. Gli scintigrammi della tiroide spesso rivelano una diminuzione della captazione nelle aree colpite e l'ecografia può evidenziare una massa ecogenicamente complessa. La funzionalità tiroidea è solitamente normale, ma si è verificata tireotossicosi da dismissione di ormone tiroideo in un bambino con tiroidite suppurativa da *Aspergillus*. Se si forma un ascesso, sono indicati l'incisione e il drenaggio, con successiva somministrazione parenterale di antibiotici. Dopo la risoluzione dell'infezione, è consigliato un esofagogramma con bario o una TC con contrasto per cercare eventuali fistole: se se ne trova una, è indicato il trattamento chirurgico.

La **tiroidite subacuta granulomatosa** (malattia di De Quervain) è rara nei bambini. Si ritiene abbia un'eziologia virale e una remissione spontanea. La malattia diventa manifesta dopo unínfezione delle vie aeree superiori, con vaga dolorabilità in corrispondenza della tiroide e febbre modesta, seguite da un dolore intenso nella regione della ghiandola tiroidea. L'infiammazione comporta immissione in circolo di ormone tiroideo preformato. I livelli sierici di T_4 e T_3 sono elevati e possono essere presenti modesti segni di ipertiroidismo, ma la captazione del radioiodio è depressa. La velocità di eritrosedimentazione è aumentata. Il decorso è variabile e normalmente passa da una fase di eutiroidismo a una con ipotiroidismo; in qualche mese normalmente si ha la remissione. Occasionalmente questa condizione si sovrappone a una tiroidite linfocitica.

Dittmar M, Kahaly GJ: Immunoregulatory and susceptibility genes in thyroid and polyglandular autoimmunity. *Thyroid* 2005;15:239–250.

Gruneiro de Papendieck L, Iorcansky S, Coco R: High incidence of thyroid disturbances in 49 children with Turner syndrome. *J Pediatr* 1987;111:258–261.

Hollowell JG, Staehling NW, Flanders D, et al: Serum TSH, T4, and thyroid antibodies in the United States Population (1988 to 1994): National Health and Nutrition Examination Survey (NHANES III). *J Clin Endocrinol Metab* 2002;87:489–499.

Jaruratanasirikul S, Leethanaporn K, Khuntigij P, et al: The clinical course of Hashimoto's thyroiditis in children and adolescents: 6 years longitudinal follow-up. *J Pediatr Endocrinol Metab* 2001;14:177–184.

Marwaha RK, Sen S, Tandon H, et al: Familial aggregation of autoimmune thyroiditis in first-degree relatives of patients with juvenile autoimmune thyroid disease. *Thyroid* 2003;13:297–300.

Nabhan ZM, Kreher NC, Eugster EA: Hashitoxicosis in children: Clinical features and natural history. *J Pediatr* 2005;146:533–536.

Pearce EN, Farwell AP, Braverman LE: Thyroiditis. *N Engl J Med* 2003;348:2646–2654.

Rallison ML, Dobyns BM, Meikle AW, et al: Natural history of thyroid abnormalities: Prevalence, incidence, and regression of thyroid diseases in adolescents and young adults. *Am J Med* 1991;91:363–370.

Rich EJ, Mendelman PM: Acute suppurative thyroiditis in pediatric patients. *Pediatr Infect Dis J* 1987;6:936–940.

Tuzsuz B, Beker DB: Thyroid dysfunction in children with Down's syndrome. *Acta Paediatr* 2001;90:1389–1393.

Capitolo 568 ■ Gozzo

Il gozzo consiste in un aumento di volume della tiroide. Pazienti con ingrossamento tiroideo possono presentare una funzionalità ghiandolare normale (**eutiroidismo**), diminuita (**ipotiroidismo**) o aumentata (**ipertiroidismo**). Il gozzo può essere congenito o acquisito, endemico o sporadico.

Spesso il gozzo è dovuto a un aumento della secrezione ipofisaria dell'ormone stimolante la tiroide (TSH), in risposta a un decremento dei livelli circolanti di ormoni tiroidei. L'aumento di volume tiroideo può dipendere anche da processi infiltrativi, di natura infiammatoria o neoplastica. Il gozzo dei pazienti con malattia di Graves e tireotossicosi è causato da anticorpi stimolanti il recettore della tireotropina (TRSAb).

568.1 • Gozzo congenito

Il gozzo congenito è di norma sporadico e può essere dovuto a un difetto della sintesi della tiroxina fetale (T_4) o alla somministrazione di ioduro o di farmaci antitiroidei durante la gravidanza, per il trattamento di una tireotossicosi materna. Lo ioduro e i farmaci gozzigeni attraversano la placenta e, ad alte dosi, possono interferire con la sintesi dell'ormone tiroideo, causando gozzo e ipotiroidismo nel feto. La concomitante somministrazione di ormone tiroideo e farmaci gozzigeni, non è in grado di prevenire questo effetto, perché il T_4 attraversa la placenta in quantità insufficiente. Gli ioduri si trovano in molti antitussigeni utilizzati nella terapia dell'asma; queste preparazioni devono essere evitate durante la gravidanza, visto che spesso sono risultate responsabili di gozzo congenito. Anche l'amiodarone, un farmaco antiaritmico contenente il 37% di iodio, è responsabile di gozzo congenito con ipotiroidismo. Anche quando il bambino è clinicamente eutiroideo, può manifestarsi ritardo della maturazione ossea, con bassi livelli di T_4, elevati livelli di TSH. In donne gravide con malattia di Graves in terapia antitiroidea, questi effetti sul feto si possono verificare per assunzione di propiltiouracile alla dose di solo 100-200 mg/die; per questo tutti i bambini vanno sottoposti, alla nascita, a una valutazione della tiroide. Può essere indicata la somministrazione di ormone tiroideo ai neonati colpiti, sia per trattare l'ipotiroidismo clinico sia per accelerare la scomparsa del gozzo e prevenire un danno cerebrale. Dato che raramente questa condizione è permanente, il trattamento può essere sospeso quando i farmaci antitiroidei siano stati eliminati dal neonato, di solito dopo 1-2 settimane.

L'aumento di volume della tiroide alla nascita talvolta è sufficiente a provocare un distress respiratorio tale da interferire con l'allattamento e può portare anche alla morte. Il capo deve essere mantenuto in accentuata iperestensione. Se l'ostruzione respiratoria è grave, più che la tracheotomia è indicata una tiroidectomia parziale (Fig. 568-1).

Quasi sempre è presente gozzo nei bambini con ipertiroidismo congenito. Questi gozzi di solito non sono voluminosi; i neonati manifestano sintomi clinici di ipertiroidismo. Le madri spesso hanno un'anamnesi positiva per malattia di Graves; in questi casi il gozzo deriva dal passaggio transplacentare di immunoglobulina materna stimolante la tiroide (vedi Capitolo 569.1). Anche mutazioni attivanti il recettore del TSH sono riconosciute causa di gozzo congenito.

Qualora non sia evidenziabile alcun fattore causale, si deve sospettare la presenza di un **difetto della sintesi** di ormone tiroideo. I programmi di screening neonatale sono in grado di rivelare ipotiroidismo congenito causato da questo tipo di difetti in uno su 30 000-50 000 nati. In presenza di ipotiroidismo neonatale, è opportuno iniziare immediatamente la terapia con ormone tiroideo, rimandando altri studi a momenti successivi. Se si sospetta un difetto specifico, si possono eseguire test genetici per l'identificazione di una mutazione (vedi Capitolo 566). Dato che questi

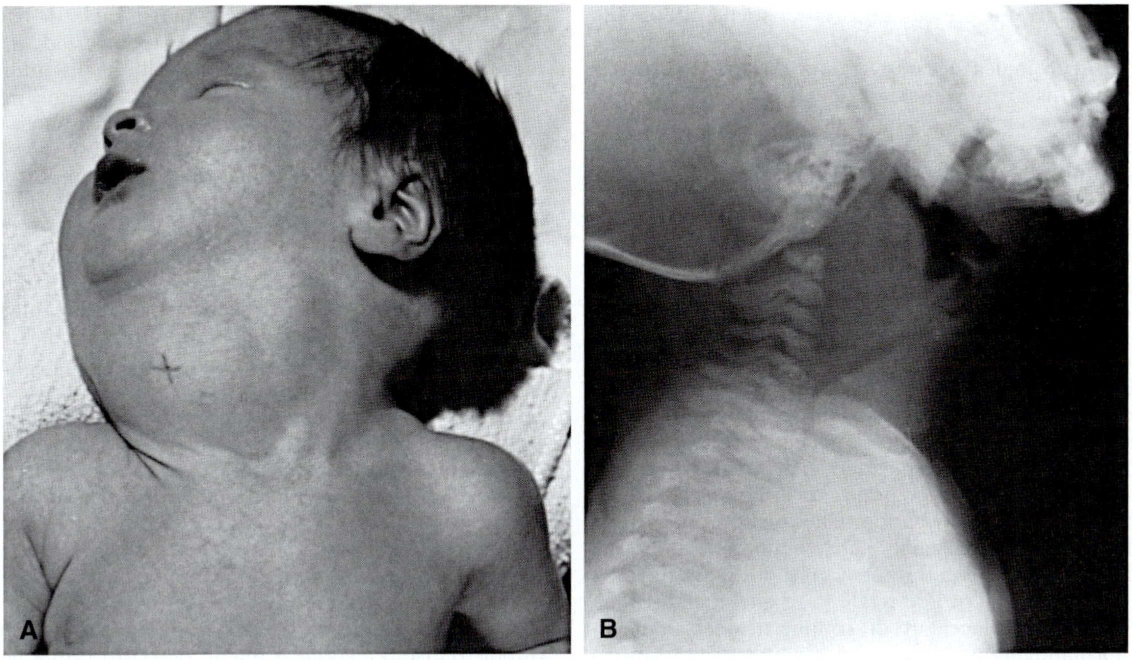

Figura 568-1. Gozzo congenito in neonato. *A*, Voluminoso gozzo congenito in un bambino nato da madre con tireotossicosi, trattata durante la gravidanza con ioduro e metimazolo. *B*, Un neonato di 6 settimane (non lo stesso di *A*) con distress respiratorio e massa cervicale sin dalla nascita. L'intervento ha rivelato un voluminoso gozzo che circondava quasi completamente la trachea. Una tiroidectomia parziale ha alleviato completamente i sintomi. Risulta evidente come in questi bambini non sia opportuna una tracheotomia. Non è stata individuata la causa del gozzo.

difetti si trasmettono tramite dei geni recessivi, la consulenza genetica può aiutare la diagnosi. Il monitoraggio ecografico ripetuto in gravidanza può essere utile per scoprire gozzi già in epoca fetale (vedi Capitolo 96).

La carenza iodica responsabile di gozzo congenito è rara nei Paesi sviluppati, ma persiste in isolate aeree endemiche (vedi oltre). Più importante è il riconoscimento di una grave carenza iodica in gravidanza, che può essere responsabile di danno neurologico durante lo sviluppo fetale, anche in assenza di gozzo. La carenza iodica può portare a ipotiroidismo fetale e materno, che ostacola il trasferimento, parzialmente protettivo, di ormoni tiroidei materni.

Se il "gozzo" è lobulato, asimmetrico, duro o molto voluminoso, nella diagnosi differenziale va preso in considerazione un teratoma della tiroide o di una sede vicina (vedi Capitolo 570).

568.2 • Gozzo endemico e cretinismo

EZIOLOGIA

CARENZA IODICA. È chiara l'associazione tra carenza dietetica di iodio e incidenza di gozzo o cretinismo. Un deficit moderato di iodio può essere compensato da un aumento dell'efficienza della sintesi di ormone tiroideo. Lo iodio liberato a livello tissutale ritorna rapidamente nella tiroide, che risintetizza prevalentemente triiodotironina (T_3) in quantità maggiore della norma. Questa aumentata attività è possibile grazie a ipertrofia e iperplasia compensatorie (gozzo), in grado di soddisfare la domanda tissutale di ormone tiroideo. In certe aree geografiche la carenza iodica è notevole, con conseguente scompenso e ipotiroidismo. Si stima che un miliardo di individui nei Paesi in via di sviluppo viva in zone con carenza iodica.

L'acqua marina è ricca di iodio; il contenuto iodico del pesce e dei crostacei è alto. Il gozzo endemico è quindi raro nelle popolazioni che vivono in vicinanza del mare. Lo iodio è carente nell'acqua e nei prodotti provenienti dal Pacifico occidentale e dalla zona dei Grandi Laghi statunitensi. Si ha una carenza iodica anche più grave in certe vallate delle Alpi, dell'Himalaya, delle Ande, del Congo e in regioni montuose della Papua Nuova Guinea. In Paesi come gli Stati Uniti, dove lo iodio è fornito da alimenti provenienti da altre aree e dal sale iodato, il gozzo endemico è scomparso. Negli Stati Uniti il sale iodato contiene ioduro di potassio (100 μg/g), che garantisce un'ottima profilassi. In questo Paese un ulteriore introito iodico è costituito da iodati usati nella produzione del pane, dai coloranti contenenti iodio e dai disinfettanti iodati usati nell'industria casearia. La dose giornaliera di iodio raccomandata per i neonati è maggiore di 90 μg/die; questa quantità, negli Stati Uniti, è superata nei neonati allattati al seno e di 4 volte nei neonati allattati con latte di mucca.

Manifestazioni cliniche. Se la carenza iodica è lieve, non compare aumento di volume della tiroide, se non nei momenti in cui aumenta la domanda di ormone tiroideo, come durante i periodi di crescita rapida, nell'adolescente o in gravidanza. In regioni a moderata carenza iodica, il gozzo presente in bambini in età scolare può scomparire con la maturità, e ricomparire durante la gravidanza o l'allattamento. I gozzi da carenza iodica sono molto più comuni nelle femmine che nei maschi. In aree con grave carenza iodica, come nelle zone montuose iperendemiche della Papua Nuova Guinea, quasi la metà della popolazione presenta gozzi voluminosi e il cretinismo endemico è comune.

I livelli sierici di T_4 sono spesso bassi nelle persone con gozzo endemico, sebbene l'ipotiroidismo clinico sia raro. Questo è vero in Nuova Guinea, in Congo, nell'Himalaya, e nel Sud America. Nonostante i bassi livelli sierici degli ormoni tiroidei, le concentrazioni di TSH sono spesso normali o solo moderatamente aumentate. Inoltre, anche i livelli di T_3 sono aumentati in pazienti con normali valori di T_4, indicando, in questa malattia, una secrezione tiroidea preferenziale di T_3.

Il **cretinismo endemico** è la conseguenza più grave della carenza iodica; si verifica solo in associazione geografica a gozzo endemico. Il termine cretinismo endemico comprende due sindromi diverse ma sovrapponibili: una **forma neurologica** e una **mixedematosa.** La frequenza di queste due forme varia nelle diverse popolazioni. In Papua Nuova Guinea, si verifica quasi solo la forma neurologica, mentre nello Zaire, predomina quella mixedematosa. In tutte le aree endemiche si sono trovate entrambe le forme e alcuni individui presentano caratteristiche intermedie o miste.

La **sindrome neurologica** è caratterizzata da ritardo mentale, sordomutismo, disturbi della stazione eretta e dell'andatura, segni piramidali come cloni ai piedi, segno di Babinski e iperreflessia patellare. I pazienti presentano gozzo eutiroideo, hanno un normale sviluppo puberale e una normale statura da adulti, con lieve o assente alterazione della funzionalità tiroidea. Anche i pazienti con la **forma mixedematosa** presentano ritardo mentale, sordità e sintomi neurologici, ma, al contrario della forma neurologica, hanno una crescita e uno sviluppo sessuale ritardati, mixedema e assenza di gozzo. I livelli sierici di T_4 sono bassi e il TSH marcatamente elevato. Il ritardo della maturazione scheletrica può oltrepassare la terza decade di vita e oltre. L'ecografia tiroidea dimostra atrofia ghiandolare.

Patogenesi. La patogenesi della **sindrome neurologica** è stata attribuita a carenza iodica e a ipotiroxinemia durante la gravidanza, con ipotiroidismo fetale e postnatale. Sebbene alcuni Autori abbiano attribuito il danno cerebrale a un effetto diretto della carenza iodica fetale, la maggior parte ritiene che i sintomi neurologici siano dovuti a ipotiroxinemia fetale e materna. È noto che nel cervello umano sono presenti recettori per l'ormone tiroideo prima dello sviluppo della tiroide fetale ed è anche chiaro che esiste un passaggio transplacentare di ormone tiroideo materno nel feto, che normalmente può migliorare gli effetti dell'ipotiroidismo fetale sul sistema nervoso in via di sviluppo. L'introduzione di iodio dopo la nascita di solito è sufficiente a garantire una funzionalità tiroidea normale o solo lievemente alterata. La patogenesi della forma mixedematosa con atrofia tiroidea è invece più sconcertante. Ricerche di ulteriori fattori ambientali che possano provocare un ipotiroidismo permanente postnatale hanno condotto a incriminare la carenza di selenio, alimenti gozzigeni, tiocianati e *Yersinia*. Studi nella Cina occidentale suggeriscono che l'autoimmunità tiroidea possa giocare un ruolo. I soggetti affetti da cretinismo mixedematoso con atrofia tiroidea, ma non quelli eutiroidei, presentano delle immunoglobuline bloccanti la crescita della tiroide, del tipo di quelle riscontrate in neonati con ipotiroidismo congenito sporadico. In riferimento a questi dati, altri Autori sono scettici sull'eventuale ruolo patogenetico delle immunoglobuline bloccanti la crescita tiroidea.

Trattamento. In molti Paesi in via di sviluppo la somministrazione intramuscolare, alle femmine, di una singola dose di olio di seme di papavero iodato previene la carenza iodica durante future gravidanze, per circa 5 anni. Questa forma di terapia, somministrata a bambini con cretinismo mixedematoso con meno di 4 anni, porta a eutiroidismo in 5 mesi. Tuttavia, i bambini più grandi rispondono scarsamente e gli adulti non rispondono alle iniezioni di olio iodato, dimostrando l'incapacità della tiroide a sintetizzare l'ormone; questi pazienti richiedono una terapia con T_4. Mediante gli sforzi dell'Organizzazione Mondiale della Sanità e i suoi programmi di iodinazione del sale in tutti i Paesi del mondo, la carenza iodica endemica mondiale è stata ridotta di circa il 50%. Nella provincia cinese dello Xinjiang, dove sono falliti i metodi usuali, la iodinazione dell'acqua per le irrigazioni ha aumentato i livelli iodici del terreno, degli animali e degli uomini.

568.3 • Gozzo acquisito

La maggior parte dei gozzi acquisiti è sporadica e dipende da varie cause; i pazienti sono normalmente eutiroidei ma possono essere ipotiroidei. La causa più comune di gozzo acquisito è rappresentata dalla tiroidite linfocitica (vedi Capitolo 567). Altre cause comprendono l'eccessiva ingestione di iodio e certi farmaci, compresi l'amiodarone e il litio. I difetti biochimici intrinseci sono quasi sempre associati a gozzo; possono essere lievi e manifestarsi più tardivamente durante l'infanzia. La comparsa dell'alterazione in un fratello, l'esordio precoce e la possibile associazione con ipotiroidismo (ipotiroidismo con gozzo) costituiscono indizi importanti per la diagnosi.

GOZZO DA IODURO. Una piccola percentuale di pazienti trattati con preparazioni contenenti ioduro per periodi prolungati manifesta un gozzo. Gli ioduri sono solitamente addizionati, per i loro effetti espettoranti, nei farmaci per la tosse e in preparazioni per l'asma. I gozzi da ioduro sono di consistenza dura, con un aumento diffuso del volume, e in alcuni casi si può sviluppare ipotiroidismo. Negli individui normali, la somministrazione acuta di una notevole quantità di ioduri inibisce l'organificazione dello iodio e la sintesi dell'ormone tiroideo (effetto Wolff-Chaikoff). Questo effetto ha una durata limitata e non comporta ipotiroidismo permanente. Se però la somministrazione di ioduro continua, nelle persone normali un meccanismo autoregolatore limita la captazione iodica consentendo la diminuzione del livello di ioduri intratiroidei e una normale organificazione. In pazienti con gozzo da ioduro, questo meccanismo non si verifica, per la presenza di una preesistente anomalia della biosintesi dell'ormone tiroideo. I pazienti più suscettibili alla comparsa di gozzo da ioduro sono quelli con tiroidite linfocitica, o con un errore congenito subclinico della sintesi dell'ormone tiroideo, e quelli parzialmente tiroidectomizzati.

Anche il **carbonato di litio**, normalmente utilizzato nel trattamento delle forme maniaco-depressive, può causare gozzo. Il litio compete con lo iodio e ne consegue una diminuzione della sintesi e del rilascio di T_4 e T_3; il meccanismo che porta a gozzo o ipotiroidismo è simile a quello descritto prima per il gozzo da ioduro. Litio e iodio agiscono anche sinergicamente nella genesi del gozzo; si dovrebbe quindi evitare di utilizzarli insieme.

L'**amiodarone**, un farmaco usato nel trattamento delle aritmie cardiache, può provocare disfunzione tiroidea con gozzo, in quanto è ricco di iodio. È inoltre un potente inibitore della 5′-deiodinasi, impedendo la conversione del T_4 in T_3. Può causare ipotiroidismo, particolarmente in pazienti con sottostanti patologie immunitarie; in altri pazienti provoca ipertiroidismo.

GOZZO SEMPLICE (GOZZO COLLOIDALE). Una minoranza di bambini con gozzo eutiroideo ha un gozzo semplice, condizione a eziologia ignota, non associata a ipotiroidismo o ipertiroidismo, che non è provocata da infiammazione o neoplasia. Questo quadro è più frequente nelle femmine e ha un picco di incidenza prima e durante la pubertà. L'indagine istologica della ghiandola rivela un quadro normale o dimensioni follicolari variabili, colloide densa ed epitelio appiattito. Il gozzo può essere piccolo o voluminoso. Ha una consistenza dura nella metà dei casi e occasionalmente è asimmetrico o nodulare. I livelli di TSH sono normali o bassi, lo scintigramma è normale e gli anticorpi antitiroidei sono assenti. Senza una biopsia, può non essere distinguibile da una tiroidite linfocitica; di norma però la biopsia non è indicata. La terapia con ormone tiroideo può aiutare a evitare la progressione verso un voluminoso gozzo multinodulare, sebbene sia difficile separare l'effetto del trattamento dalla storia naturale, che comunque tende a una riduzione delle dimensioni. I pazienti devono essere rivalutati periodicamente; sia perché alcuni possono avere una tiroidite linfocitica priva di anticorpi, sia per il rischio di modificazioni della funzionalità tiroidea (vedi Capitolo 567).

GOZZO MULTINODULARE. È raro il riscontro di un gozzo di consistenza dura, con superficie lobulata e singoli o multipli noduli palpabili. Possono essere presenti aree di modificazione cistica, emorragia e fibrosi. L'incidenza di questa condizione è notevolmente diminuita con l'utilizzo del sale iodato a scopo preventivo. Si pensa che la causa sia uno stimolo gozzigeno modesto, ma di lunga durata. L'indagine ecografica può rivelare multiple lesioni anecogene ed ecogene, che corrispondono nello scintigramma ad aree non funzionanti. Le indagini della tiroide sono di solito normali. Alcuni bambini con tiroidite linfocitica cronica sviluppano un gozzo multinodulare; il TSH può essere elevato e possono essere presenti anticorpi antitiroidei. Raramente i bambini presentano un "gozzo tossico multinodulare", caratterizzato da soppressione del TSH e ipertiroidismo. La patologia si verifica in bambini con la **sindrome di McCune-Albright** (normalmente associata a ipertiroidismo) e sono stati descritti i casi di tre bambini (che comprendono due fratelli) con anomalie digitali e malattia cistica renale. Noduli evidenti nel contesto di un gozzo multinodulare, particolarmente quelli che non rispondono alla terapia sostitutiva con T_4, devono essere valutati con un ago-aspirato con ago sottile, in quanto non è facile escludere una patologia maligna.

GOZZO TOSSICO (IPERTIROIDISMO). Vedi Capitolo 569.

568.4 • Gozzo intratracheale

Una delle molte localizzazioni ectopiche del tessuto tiroideo è nel contesto tracheale. La tiroide intraluminale si trova al di sotto della mucosa tracheale ed è frequentemente in continuità con la tiroide normalmente situata in sede extratracheale. Il tessuto tiroideo è suscettibile di aumento di volume, che coinvolge sia la tiroide in sede normale sia quella ectopica. In presenza di ostruzione delle vie aeree associata a gozzo, è necessario chiarire se l'ostruzione è extra o endotracheale. Se le manifestazioni ostruttive sono lievi, la somministrazione di levotiroxina sodica normalmente comporta un diminuzione del volume del gozzo. Se i sintomi sono gravi, è invece indicata l'exeresi chirurgica del gozzo endotracheale (vedi Capitolo 568.1).

Gozzo congenito

Bikker H, den Hartog MT, Baas F, et al: A 20-base pair duplication in the human thyroid peroxidase gene results in a total iodide organification defect and congenital hypothyroidism. *J Clin Endocrinol Metab* 1994;79:248–252.

Caron P, Moya CM, Malet D, et al: Compound heterozygous mutations in the thyroglobulin gene (1143delC and 6725G → A [R2223H]) resulting in fetal goitrous hypothyroidism. *J Clin Endocrinol Metab* 2003;88: 3546–3453.

Vade A, Gottschalk ME, Yetter EM, et al: Sonographic measurements of the neonatal thyroid gland. *J Ultrasound Med* 1997;16:395–399.

Vicens-Calvet E, Potau N, Carreras E, et al: Diagnosis and treatment in utero of goiter with hypothyroidism caused by iodine overload. *J Pediatr* 1998;133:147–148.

Gozzo endemico e cretinismo

Aghini-Lombardi F, Antonangeli L, Pinchera A, et al: Effect of iodized salt on thyroid volume of children living in an area previously characterized by moderate iodine deficiency. *J Clin Endocrinol Metab* 1997;82:1136–1139.

Benmiloud M, Chaouki ML, Gutekunst R, et al: Oral iodized oil for correcting iodine deficiency: Optimal dosing and outcome indicator selection. *J Clin Endocrinol Metab* 1994;79:20–24.

Boyages SC, Halpern JP, Maberly GF, et al: A comparative study of neurological and myxedematous endemic cretinism in western China. *J Clin Endocrinol Metab* 1988;67:1262–1271.

Boyages SC, Halpern JP, Maberly GF, et al: Endemic cretinism: Possible role for thyroid autoimmunity. *Lancet* 1989;2:529–532.

Boyages SC, Halpern JP, Maberly GF, et al: Supplementary iodine fails to reverse hypothyroidism in adolescents and adults with endemic cretinism. *J Clin Endocrinol Metab* 1990;70:336–341.

DeLange F: Iodine deficiency as a cause of brain damage. *Postgrad Med J* 2001;77:217–220.

Delange F, de Benoist B, Pretell E, et al: Iodine deficiency in the world: Where do we stand at the turn of the century? *Thyroid* 2001;11:437–447.

WHO, UNICEF, and ICCIDD: Assessment of the iodine deficiency disorders and monitoring their elimination. Geneva,WHO publ.WHO/NHD/01.1, 2001;1–107.

Gozzo acquisito

Brix TH, Kyvik KO, Hegedus L: Major role of genes in the etiology of simple goiter in females: A population-based twin study. *J Clin Endocrinol Metab* 1999;84:3071–3075.

Daneman D, Davy T, Mancer K, et al: Association of multinodular goiter, cystic renal disease, and digital anomalies. *J Pediatr* 1985;107:270–272.

Feuillan PP, Shawker T, Rose SR, et al: Thyroid abnormalities in the McCune-Albright syndrome: Ultrasonography and hormonal studies. *J Clin Endocrinol Metab* 1990;71:1596–1601.

Jaruratanasirkul S, Leethanaporn K, Suchat K: The natural clinical course of children with an initial diagnosis of simple goiter: A 5-year longitudinal follow-up. *J Pediatr Endocrinol Metab* 2000;13:1109–1113.

Lisboa HR, Gross JL, Orsolin A, et al: Clinical examination is not an accurate method of defining the presence of goiter in schoolchildren. *Clin Endocrinol* 1996;45:471–475.

Capitolo 569 ■ Ipertiroidismo

L'ipertiroidismo deriva da un'eccessiva secrezione di ormone tiroideo e, durante l'infanzia, con poche eccezioni, è dovuto alla malattia di Graves (Tab. 569-1). La **malattia di Graves** è un patologia autoimmunitaria; la produzione di un'immunoglobulina stimolante la tiroide (*Thyroid-Stimulating Immunoglobulin*, TSI) comporta un gozzo tossico diffuso. Sia nei casi familiari (autosomici dominanti) sia in quelli sporadici di ipertiroidismo non autoimmunitario, sono state trovate mutazioni della linea germinale del **recettore dell'ormone stimolante la tiroide** (*Thyroid-Stimulating Hormone*, **TSH**), con conseguenti mutazioni attivanti (aumento di funzione). Questi pazienti, in cui la malattia si presenta nel periodo neonatale o successivamente durante l'infanzia, evidenziano un'iperplasia tiroidea con gozzo e soppressione del TSH. In alcuni casi di adenomi tiroidei sono state identificate diverse mutazioni attivanti. Compare ipertiroidismo in alcuni pazienti con la **sindrome di McCune-Albright**, come conseguenza di mutazione attivante della subunità α della proteina G; questi pazienti tendono ad avere un gozzo multinodulare. Altre rare cause di ipertiroidismo nei bambini includono il gozzo uninodulare tossico (malattia di Plummer), il carcinoma iperfunzionante della tiroide, la tireotossicosi factitia, la tiroidite subacuta e la tiroidite acuta suppurativa. La soppressione del TSH plasmatico indica che l'origine dell'ipertiroidismo non è ipofisaria. L'ipertiroidismo da eccesso di tireotropina è raro e, nella maggior parte dei casi, è dovuto a resistenza ipofisaria all'ormone tiroideo. I tumori ipofisari TSH-secernenti sono stati riportati solo nell'adulto. Nei neonati di madri con malattia di Graves, l'ipertiroidismo è quasi sempre un fenomeno transitorio; la malattia di Graves classica, durante il periodo neonatale, è rara. Coriocarcinoma, mola idatiforme e struma ovarico sono altre possibili cause di ipertiroidismo nell'adulto, ma non nel bambino.

569.1 • Malattia di Graves

EPIDEMIOLOGIA. La malattia di Graves compare in circa lo 0,02% dei bambini (1:5000). Ha un picco di incidenza nel periodo che va dagli 11 ai 15 anni; il rapporto femmine/maschi è di 5:1. La maggior parte dei bambini con malattia di Graves presenta un'anamnesi familiare positiva per alcune forme di patologia tiroidea autoimmunitaria. In Giappone, la malattia di Graves familiare, definita come malattia di Graves in un parente di 1° grado, si verifica nel 2-3% dei casi.

EZIOLOGIA. Ingrossamento del timo, splenomegalia, linfoadenopatia, infiltrazione linfocitica e plasmacellulare della tiroide e dei tessuti retro-orbitali, linfocitosi periferica, sono reperti tipici della malattia di Graves. Nella ghiandola tiroidea, prevalgono le cellule helper (CD4+), in densi aggregati linfoidi; in zone invece di minore densità cellulare, predominano le cellule T citotossiche. La percentuale di linfociti B attivati infiltranti la tiroide è maggiore che nel sangue periferico. Un presupposto deficit di linfociti T soppressori consente l'espressione delle cellule T helper, sensibilizzate all'antigene del TSH, che interagiscono con le cellule B. Queste cellule si differenziano in plasmacellule, che producono anticorpi stimolanti il recettore della tireotropina (TRSAb). I

TABELLA 569-1. Cause di ipertiroidismo

CAUSE DI IPERTIROIDISMO	CARATTERISTICHE FISIOPATOLOGICHE	FREQUENZA
STIMOLATORI CIRCOLANTI DELLA TIROIDE		
Malattia di Graves	Immunoglobuline stimolanti la tiroide	Comune
Malattia di Graves neonatale	Immunoglobuline stimolanti la tiroide	Molto rara
Tumore tireotropino secernente	Adenoma ipofisario	Rara
Iperemesi gravidica	Secrezione di gonadotropina corionica umana	Non comune
Coriocarcinoma	Secrezione di gonadotropina corionica umana	Rara
Anomalie del recettore della tireotropina	Secrezione di gonadotropina corionica umana	Molto rara
AUTONOMIA TIROIDEA		
Gozzo multinodulare tossico	Mutazioni attivanti del recettore della tireotropina o della proteina G	Comune
Adenoma tossico solitario	Mutazioni attivanti del recettore della tireotropina o della proteina G	Comune
Ipertiroidismo congenito	Mutazioni attivanti del recettore della tireotropina	Molto rara
Ipertiroidismo da iodio (*Jod-basedow*)	Sconosciuta; eccesso iodico con produzione sregolata di ormone tiroideo	Non comune negli Stati Uniti e in altre zone con sufficiente presenza di iodio
DISTRUZIONE DEI FOLLICOLI TIROIDEI		
Tiroidite subacuta	Probabile infezione virale	Non comune
Tiroidite indolore o postpartum	Autoimmune	Comune
Tiroidite da amiodarone	Effetto tossico diretto del farmaco	Non comune
Tiroidite acuta (infettiva)	Infezione tiroidea (batterica, micotica ecc.)	Non comune
ORMONE TIROIDEO ESOGENO		
Iatrogenico	Eccessiva ingestione di ormone tiroideo	Comune
Factitia	Eccessiva introduzione di ormone tiroideo	Rara
Tireotossicosi da hamburger	Ghiandola tiroidea incorporata nel macinato di manzo	Probabilmente rara
TESSUTO TIROIDEO ECTOPICO		
Struma ovarico	Teratoma ovarico contenete tessuto tiroideo	Rara
Carcinoma tiroideo follicolare metastatico	Grande massa tumorale secernente autonomamente ormone tiroideo	Rara
Resistenza ipofisaria all'ormone tiroideo	Mutazione del recettore dell'ormone tiroideo con maggiore espressione ipofisaria rispetto ai tessuti periferici	Rara

Da Cooper DS: Hypertiroidism. *Lancet* 2003; 362:459-468.

TRSAb legano il recettore del TSH e stimolano l'adenosina ciclica monofosfato, come il TSH. Oltre ai TRSAb, possono essere prodotti degli anticorpi che bloccano il recettore della tireotropina (TRBAb) e il decorso clinico della malattia è solitamente correlato al rapporto fra questi due tipi di anticorpi.

L'oftalmopatia della malattia di Graves è dovuta ad anticorpi diretti contro antigeni comuni alla tiroide e ai muscoli oculari. I recettori del TSH sono stati identificati negli adipociti retro-orbitali e possono rappresentare un bersaglio per gli anticorpi. Gli anticorpi antimuscoli extraoculari e antifibroblasti orbitali stimolano la sintesi di glucosaminoglicani da parte dei fibroblasti stessi e producono effetti citotossici sulle cellule muscolari.

La malattia di Graves è associata a HLA-B8 e HLA-DR3; il secondo tipo corre un rischio 7 volte maggiore di malattia di Graves. La malattia di Graves è associata anche ad altre patologie connesse con HLA-D3, come la malattia di Addison, il diabete mellito insulino-dipendente, la miastenia grave e la malattia celiaca. Nei bambini con malattia di Graves sono stati descritti: lupus eritematoso sistemico, artrite reumatoide, vitiligine, porpora trombocitopenica idiopatica, anemia perniciosa. Nei familiari, le condizioni più frequentemente associate a malattia di Graves sono la tiroidite linfocitica autoimmunitaria e l'ipotiroidismo. Nei bambini giapponesi, la malattia di Graves è associata a diversi aplotipi HLA: HLA-DRB1*0405 e HLA-DQB1*0401.

MANIFESTAZIONI CLINICHE. Circa il 5% dei pazienti con ipertiroidismo ha meno di 15 anni; il picco di incidenza in questi bambini si ha nell'adolescenza. In bambini nati da madri con una storia di ipertiroidismo, la malattia di Graves comincia tra la sesta settimana e il secondo anno di età. L'incidenza è circa 5 volte maggiore nelle femmine che nei maschi.

Il decorso clinico, nei bambini, è notevolmente variabile, ma di solito non è fulminante come in molti adulti (Tab. 569-2). I sintomi si sviluppano lentamente; l'intervallo tra l'esordio e la diagnosi è normalmente di 6-12 mesi, e può essere maggiore nei bambini prepuberi rispetto agli adolescenti. I primissimi segni nei bambini possono essere disturbi emotivi con iperattività motoria. I bambini diventano irritabili, eccitabili e piangono facilmente per una certa labilità emotiva. Hanno un sonno agitato e tendono ad allontanare le coperte. Il rendimento scolastico peggiora per scarsa capacità di attenzione e per lo scarso sonno. L'estensione delle braccia può rivelare un certo tremore delle dita. Può essere presente un appetito vorace, accompagnato da perdita di peso o comunque da un mancato incremento. Le dimensioni della tiroide sono variabili. Può essere così minimamente ingrandita, da sfuggire inizialmente alla valutazione, ma, con un esame attento, in quasi tutti i pazienti è possibile trovare un gozzo diffuso, a consistenza molle, con superficie liscia. Nella maggior parte dei pazienti e rilevabile esoftalmo, solitamente di lieve entità. Possono essere presenti mancanza dell'abbassamento della palpebra superiore quando lo sguardo è rivolto in basso, difetti di convergenza e retrazione della palpebra superiore con rarità dell'ammiccamento (Figg. 569-1 e 569-2). Le manifestazioni oculari possono essere dolorose e produrre eritema palpebrale, chemosi, diminuzione della funzione della muscolatura extraoculare e decremento dell'acuità visiva (coinvolgimento del nervo corneale o ottico). La cute è liscia e arrossata, con eccessiva sudorazione. L'astenia muscolare non è frequente, ma può essere abbastanza intensa da portare a indebolimento. Tachicardia, palpitazioni, dispnea, cardiomegalia e insufficienza cardiaca danno al paziente un senso di malessere, ma raramente mettono in pericolo la sua vita. Una rara complicanza è rappresentata dalla fibrillazione atriale. Il reflusso mitralico, probabilmente da disfunzione dei muscoli papillari, è la causa del soffio sistolico apicale presente in alcuni pazienti. La pressione arteriosa sistolica e l'ampiezza del polso sono aumentate. Molti dei reperti della malattia di Graves dipendono da un'iperattività del sistema nervoso simpatico.

La **"crisi", o "tempesta" tiroidea**, è una forma di ipertiroidismo che si manifesta con esordio acuto, ipertermia, grave tachicardia, insufficienza cardiaca e irrequietezza. Il quadro può progredire

TABELLA 569-2. Sintomi maggiori e segni di ipertiroidismo e di malattia di Graves e condizioni associate alla malattia di Graves

MANIFESTAZIONI DI IPERTIROIDISMO
Sintomi
Iperattività, irritabilità, alterazione del tono dell'umore, insonnia, ansia
Intolleranza al caldo, aumento della sudorazione
Palpitazioni
Astenia, debolezza
Dispnea
Perdita di peso con aumento dell'appetito (aumento di peso nel 10% dei pazienti)
Prurito
Defecazioni più frequenti
Sete e poliuria
Oligomenorrea o amenorrea, perdita della libido
Segni
Tachicardia sinusale, fibrillazione atriale (rara nei bambini), tachicardia sopraventricolare
Tremori fini, ipercinesi, iperreflessia
Cute calda, umida
Eritema palmare, onicolisi
Perdita di capelli
Osteoporosi
Ipercalcemia
Debolezza muscolare e debilitazione
Insufficienza cardiaca ad alta gittata
Corea
Paralisi periodica (ipokaliemica) (soprattutto nei maschi asiatici)
Psicosi (rara)
MANIFESTAZIONI DI MALATTIA DI GRAVES
Gozzo diffuso
Oftalmopatia
Sensazione di sabbia e disagio agli occhi
Pressione o dolore retrobulbare
Occhi distanziati e retrazione
Edema periorbitale, cremosi, iniezione sclerale
Esoftalmo (proposi)
Disfunzione dei muscoli extraoculari
Cheratite da esposizione
Neuropatia ottica
Dermopatia localizzata (rara nei bambini)
Iperplasia linfoidi
Acropachia tiroidea (rara nei bambini)
CONDIZIONI ASSOCIATE A MALATTIA DI GRAVES
Diabete mellito di tipo I
Malattia di Addison
Vitiligine
Anemia perniciosa
Alopecia areata
Miastenia grave
Malattia celiaca

Adattamento da Weetman AP: Graves diseases. *N Engl J Med* 2000;343:1236-1248.

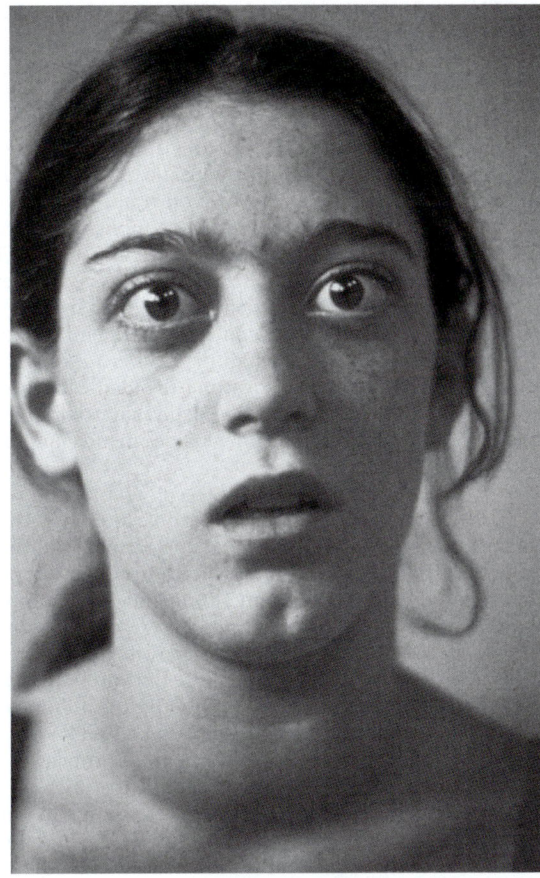

Figura 569-1. Ragazza di 15 anni con la malattia di Graves classica. Il quadro clinico comprende gozzo ed esoftalmo. È stata trattata con farmaci antitiroidei, con buona risposta.

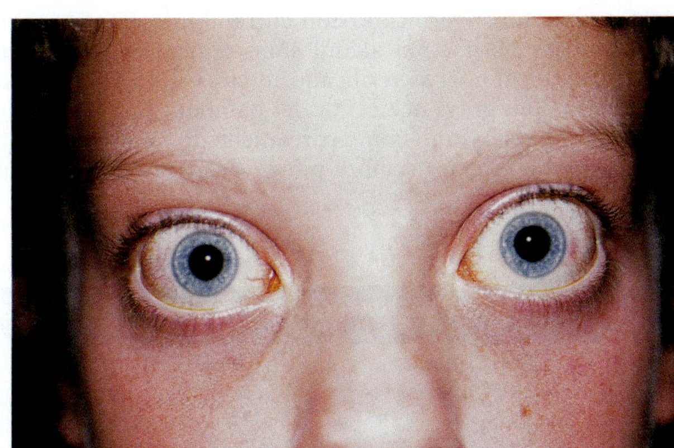

Figura 569-2. Retrazione delle palpebre superiori e fissità (segno di Dalrymple). (Da Kanski JJ: *Systemic Diseases and the Eye: Signs and Differential Diagnosis*. London, Mosby, 2001, Fig. 2.230.)

rapidamente verso il delirio, il coma e la morte. Eventi precipitanti comprendono un trauma, il parto, infezioni o un intervento chirurgico. L'**ipertiroidismo "apatico" o "mascherato"** è un'altra forma di ipertiroidismo, caratterizzata da estrema indolenza, apatia e cachessia. Si può verificare anche una combinazione di entrambe le forme. Questi sintomi sono comunque complessivamente rari nei bambini.

REPERTI DI LABORATORIO. I livelli sierici di tiroxina (T_4), triiodotironina (T_3), T_4 libero, T_3 libero sono elevati. In alcuni pazienti, i livelli di T_3 possono essere più alti di quelli di T_4. I valori del TSH sono soppressi a livelli inferiori di quelli normali. Sono spesso presenti anticorpi antitiroidei, compresi quelli antiperossidasi tiroidea. La maggior parte dei pazienti con diagnosi recente di malattia di Graves presenta TRSAb misurabili; la loro scomparsa è indice di remissione della malattia. Fra i bambini affetti da malattia di Graves congenita, quelli molto piccoli spesso presentano una maturazione scheletrica avanzata e craniostenosi. La densità ossea può essere ridotta al momento della diagnosi, ma torna normale con il trattamento.

DIAGNOSI DIFFERENZIALE. Raramente la diagnosi pone delle difficoltà, una volta preso in considerazione l'ipertiroidismo. Livelli elevati di T_4 o di T_4 libero e di T_3, in associazione a livelli soppressi di TSH sono di solito diagnostici (vedi Tab. 569-1). La presenza di TRSAb stabilisce la causa di malattia di Graves.

Altre cause di ipertiroidismo non sono frequenti. Se è apprezzabile un nodulo tiroideo, o se è elevato soprattutto il T_3, si deve considerare la possibilità di un nodulo tiroideo funzionale. L'indagine scintigrafia è diagnostica, se dimostra una captazione nodulare in assenza di captazione nella restante ghiandola (o "nodulo caldo"). Se sono presenti pubertà precoce, displasia fibrosa poliostotica, pigmentazione con macchie caffellatte, è verosimile un disturbo autonomo della tiroide, nella sindrome di McCune-Albright. Pazienti con resistenza generalizzata all'ormone tiroideo hanno elevati livelli di T_4 libero, ma valori di TSH inaspettatamente alti o normali. I pazienti con resistenza ipofisaria isolata all'ormone della tiroide presentano un ipertiroidismo clinico, ma i loro livelli di TSH sono elevati o normali e devono essere differenziati dai pazienti con tumori ipofisari secernenti TSH, che hanno elevati livelli sierici della catena α del TSH. La maggior parte delle altre cause di ipertiroidismo non è frequente e può portare a diagnosi erronea. Pazienti con elevati livelli di globulina che lega la tiroide (TBG) o con ipertiroxinemia familiare disalbuminemica hanno livelli normali di T_4 libero e di TSH.

Se l'ipertiroxinemia è dovuta a **ormone tiroideo esogeno**, i livelli di T_4 libero e di TSH sono gli stessi della malattia di Graves, ma il livello della tireoglobulina è molto basso, mentre in pazienti con malattia di Graves è elevato.

TRATTAMENTO. La maggior parte degli endocrinologi pediatrici raccomanda di iniziare la terapia medica con farmaci antitiroidei piuttosto che con radioiodio o tiroidectomia subtotale, sebbene il radioiodio sia accettato come trattamento iniziale in bambini con più di 10 anni. Tutte le opzioni terapeutiche presentano vantaggi e svantaggi (Tab. 569-3). I due farmaci antitiroidei più usati sono il propiltiouracile (PTU) e il metimazolo. Entrambi inibiscono l'incorporazione dello ioduro inorganico captato, all'interno di composti organici, e sopprimono inoltre i livelli di TRSAb, interessando così l'immunità tiroidea direttamente. Tuttavia, ci sono importanti differenze fra questi due farmaci. Il metimazolo è almeno 10 volte più potente del PTU in base al peso e ha un'emivita sierica più lunga (6-8 ore rispetto a 0,5 ore); il PTU generalmente si somministra tre volte al giorno, il metimazolo una sola volta. A differenza del metimazolo, il PTU presenta un alto legame proteico e ha maggiori difficoltà ad attraversare la placenta e a passare nel latte materno; teoricamente, quindi, il PTU è il farmaco di elezione durante la gravidanza e l'allattamento. Il PTU, più del metimazolo, inibisce la conversione extratiroidea del T_4 in T_3; questo può essere vantaggioso nel trattamento della tireotossicosi neonatale.

Effetti collaterali si verificano con entrambi; la maggior parte di essi è di lieve entità, ma alcuni sono pericolosi per la vita. Effetti collaterali minori si verificano in circa il 10-20% dei casi, mentre altri più gravi nel 2-5% dei bambini. Tali effetti non sono prevedibili e possono comparire anche dopo una terapia di una certa durata. Appare sempre più evidente che questi effetti sono minori nei pazienti trattati con metimazolo. È frequente una granulocitopenia transitoria (<2000/mm^3), asintomatica e non prodromica di agranulocitosi, tale da non dover di solito sospendere la terapia. Sono comuni anche rash cutanei di tipo orticarioide. Possono essere affrontati con una breve sospensione della terapia, che può essere successivamente ripresa alternando i farmaci antitiroidei. L'effetto collaterale più grave è rappresentato da reazioni di ipersensibilità e comprende l'agranulocitosi (0,1-0,5%), l'epatite (0,2-1%), l'insufficienza epatica, una sindrome poliartritica simile al lupus, la glomerulonefrite e una vasculite ANCA-positiva che coinvolge la cute e altri organi. Queste reazioni sono state riportate con entrambi i farmaci, sebbene l'epatite si verifichi quasi esclusivamente con PTU. Pazienti che presentano effetti collaterali gravi ai farmaci devono essere trattati con radioiodio o tiroidectomia. Sono stati riportati casi di difetti congeniti della cute (aplasia cutis) in neonati esposti, durante la vita fetale, al metimazolo, ma questa associazione non sembra essere forte.

Il dosaggio iniziale di PTU è 5-10 mg/kg/die suddiviso in 3 dosi giornaliere, invece quello del metimazolo è 0,25-1,0 mg/kg/die in una sola o in due dosi giornaliere. Nei bambini molto piccoli devono essere utilizzati dei dosaggi iniziali più bassi. Dopo l'inizio del trattamento è necessaria un'attenta sorveglianza. Un incremento dei livelli sierici di TSH oltre i valori normali indica un sovradosaggio e comporta un incremento volumetrico del gozzo. La risposta clinica alla terapia si evidenzia in 3-6 settimane e di solito in 3-4 mesi si raggiunge un adeguato controllo. A questo punto si diminuisce la dose al valore minimo richiesto per mantenere uno stato di eutiroidismo.

La terapia farmacologica deve necessariamente durare 5 anni o più, perché a 2 anni esiste una percentuale di remissione del 25%. In caso di recidiva, questa solitamente si verifica nel terzo o quasi sempre entro il sesto mese dalla sospensione. In caso di ricaduta va ripresa la terapia. Pazienti con più di 13 anni, di sesso maschile, con un più alto indice di massa corporea, e quelli con gozzi più piccoli e livelli di T_3 modestamente elevati hanno remissioni più precoci.

Agenti bloccanti β-adrenergici come il propanololo (0,5-2,0 mg/kg/die per os, in tre somministrazioni quotidiane) è un adiuvante utilizzato nella gestione dei pazienti con grave tireotossicosi. Ulteriori terapie per la **tempesta tiroidea** sono indicate nella Tabella 569-4. Gli ormoni tiroidei potenziano l'azione delle catecolamine, compresi tachicardia, tremore, eccessiva sudorazione, retrazione e fissità palpebrale. Questi sintomi si riducono con l'uso del propanololo, che non incide, tuttavia, sulla funzione tiroidea e sull'esoftalmo.

TABELLA 569-3. Trattamenti per l'ipertiroidismo causato da malattia di Graves

TRATTAMENTI	VANTAGGI	SVANTAGGI	COMMENTO
Farmaci antitiroidei	Non invasivo Costo iniziale inferiore	Percentuale di guarigione (30-80%; media 40-50%)	Trattamento di prima scelta nei bambini, negli adolescenti e durante la gravidanza
		Effetti collaterali ai farmaci	Trattamento iniziale dei casi gravi o come preparazione preoperatoria
	Basso rischio di ipotiroidismo permanente Possibili remissioni da effetti immunitari	Richiesta compliance farmacologica	
Iodio radioattivo ^{131}I	Guarigione dell'ipertiroidismo	Ipotiroidismo permanente quasi inevitabile	Non c'è evidenza di infertilità, difetti alla nascita, tumori
	Maggior costo effettivo	Possibile peggioramento dell'oftalmopatia Una eventuale gravidanza deve essere rinviata di 6-12 mesi, la madre non può allattare al seno; modesto rischio potenziale di esacerbazione dell'ipertiroidismo	Miglior trattamento per i noduli tossici e per il gozzo multinodulare tossico
Chirurgia	Trattamento rapido, efficace specialmente in pazienti con gozzo voluminoso	Terapia più invasiva	Potenziale uso in gravidanza in presenza di effetti collaterali maggiori dei farmaci antitiroidei Utile quando vi sia il sospetto della presenza di un nodulo
		Potenziali complicanze (danno al nervo laringeo ricorrente, ipoparatiroidismo) Maggior costo della terapia Ipotiroidismo permanente; dolore; cicatrice	Opzione per i pazienti che rifiutano il radioiodio

Da Cooper DS: Hyperthyroidsm. *Lancet* 2003; 362:459-468.

TABELLA 569-4. Trattamento della tempesta tiroidea negli adolescenti

OBIETTIVO	TRATTAMENTO
Inibizione dell'ormone tiroideo formazione e secrezione	Propiltiouracile (PTU), 400 mg ogni 8 ore per os o con sondino nasogastrico Ioduro di sodio, 1 g per via endovenosa in 24 ore, o soluzione satura di KI, 5 gocce ogni 8 ore
Blocco del simpatico	Propanololo, 20-40 mg ogni 4-6 ore, o 1 mg per via endovenosa lentamente (ripetere la dose fino al rallentamento della frequenza cardiaca); non indicato in pazienti con asma o insufficienza cardiaca che non sia correlata alla frequenza
Terapia con glicocorticoidi	Idrocortisone, 50-100 mg per via endovenosa ogni 6 ore
Terapia di supporto	Liquidi per via endovenosa (a seconda dell'indicazione: glucosio, elettroliti, vitamine) Controllo della temperatura (coperte refrigeranti, paracetamolo; evitare i salicilati) Ossigeno se richiesto Digitale per l'insufficienza cardiaca e per rallentare la risposta ventricolare; pentobarbital per la sedazione Trattamento di eventi precipitanti (per es. infezione)

Da Goldman L, Ausiello D: *Cecil Textbook of Medicine*, 22nd ed, Philadelphia, WB Saunders, 2004, p 1401.

Il trattamento chirurgico, o con radioiodio, è indicato quando, nell'ambito della gestione medica, non sia possibile un'adeguata cooperazione, quando un'adeguata terapia non sia in grado di mantenere una remissione permanente o quando gravi effetti collaterali precludano l'utilizzo ulteriore di farmaci antitiroidei. La tiroidectomia subtotale, che risulta essere più sicura se eseguita da un team esperto, si può eseguire solo dopo che il paziente ha raggiunto, in 2-3 mesi, una situazione di eutiroidismo, con metimazolo o PTU. Dopo che si è ottenuto l'eutiroidismo, si aggiunge alla terapia una soluzione satura di ioduro di potassio, alla dose di 5 gocce/die, per le due settimane prima dell'intervento, allo scopo di diminuire la vascolarizzazione ghiandolare. Le complicanze dell'intervento chirurgico sono rare, e comprendono l'ipoparatiroidismo (transitorio o permanente) e la paralisi delle corde vocali. L'incidenza di iper o ipotiroidismo residuale dipende dall'entità dell'intervento. La più utilizzata è la tiroidectomia subtotale. L'incidenza di recidiva è bassa ma l'ipotiroidismo può superare il 50% dei casi.

Il radioiodio è una terapia per la malattia di Graves, efficace, relativamente sicura, di prima scelta o alternativa nei bambini con più di 10 anni. Non è necessario il pretrattamento con farmaci antitiroidei; in caso di assunzione pregressa, il paziente deve sospendere la terapia una settimana prima la somministrazione di radioiodio. Molti endocrinologi pediatrici preferiscono scegliere una dose di radioiodio che garantisca una completa ablazione del tessuto tiroideo. Questo obiettivo può essere raggiunto con una dose di 300 μCi/g di tessuto tiroideo, o una dose totale di circa 15 μCi. Essenzialmente tutti i pazienti trattati con questa dose diventano ipotiroidei; il tempo di comparsa dell'ipotiroidismo è in media di 11 settimane, con un range da 9 a 28. Poiché gli effetti totali del trattamento possono non essere completi per 1-6 mesi, si raccomanda una terapia suppletiva con un antagonista β-adrenergico e dosi più basse di farmaci antitiroidei. Nonostante le preoccupazioni circa un'eventuale oncogenesi da radiazione o un danno genetico, il follow-up eseguito dopo un cinquantina di anni, in pazienti trattati da bambini, non ha evidenziato ciò che si temeva. Il rischio di adenoma benigno può aumentare (0,6-1,9% in uno studio). Con dosi più basse di radioiodio, l'ipotiroidismo si verifica nel 10-20% dei pazienti dopo il primo anno e in circa il 3% negli anni successivi.

L'**oftalmopatia** ha una remissione graduale e normalmente indipendente dall'ipertiroidismo. Un forma grave può richiedere un trattamento con alte dosi di prednisone, radioterapia orbitale (di valore dubbio), o decompressione chirurgica orbitale. Il fumo di sigaretta è un fattore di rischio per la patologia oculare tiroidea e deve essere evitato o comunque sospeso per impedire la progressione del coinvolgimento oculare.

569.2 • Ipertiroidismo congenito

EZIOLOGIA E PATOGENESI. La malattia di Graves neonatale è causata dal passaggio transplacentare di TRSAb, ma l'esordio clinico, la severità e il decorso possono essere modificati dalla contemporanea presenza di TRBAb e dal passaggio transplacentare di farmaci antitiroidei assunti dalla madre. In presenza di livelli molto alti di TRSAb, di norma si verifica un ipertiroidismo neonatale classico, ma se il neonato è stato esposto a farmaci antitiroidei, l'esordio dei sintomi è ritardato di 3-4 giorni, tempo necessario alla degradazione dei farmaci antitiroidei di provenienza materna. Se sono presenti anche TRBAb, l'esordio dei sintomi ipertiroidei può essere ritardato anche di alcune settimane. Le mamme di questi bambini presentano una malattia di Graves in forma attiva, o in remissione, o raramente un ipotiroidismo con anamnesi positiva per tiroidite linfocitica.

L'ipertiroidismo neonatale si verifica solo in circa il 2% dei neonati di madri con anamnesi di malattia di Graves. Il reperto di livelli molto alti di TRSAb in queste mamme di solito fa prevedere la comparsa di patologia neonatale. La tachicardia fetale e il gozzo possono consentire una diagnosi prenatale. A differenza della malattia di Graves e di tutti gli altri agenti, l'ipertiroidismo neonatale colpisce i maschi più frequentemente delle femmine. La malattia di solito presenta una remissione spontanea in 6-12 settimane, ma può persistere più a lungo, a seconda dei livelli di TRSAb. Si può anche verificare un'ipertiroxinemia asintomatica. Raramente, la malattia di Graves neonatale classica non presenta remissione, ma persiste per alcuni anni o più. Questi bambini mostrano una notevole anamnesi familiare di malattia di Graves. In questi bambini, il passaggio di TRSAb dalla madre apparentemente si confonde con l'esordio infantile di una malattia di Graves autonoma.

MANIFESTAZIONI CLINICHE. Molti neonati sono prematuri, con un difetto della crescita intrauterina. La maggior parte presenta gozzo. Il bambino è estremamente irrequieto, irritabile e iperattivo, ansioso e insolitamente vigile. Possono essere presenti microcefalia e dilatazione ventricolare. Gli occhi sono molto aperti e ci può essere esoftalmo (Fig. 569-3). Si manifestano inoltre tachicardia e

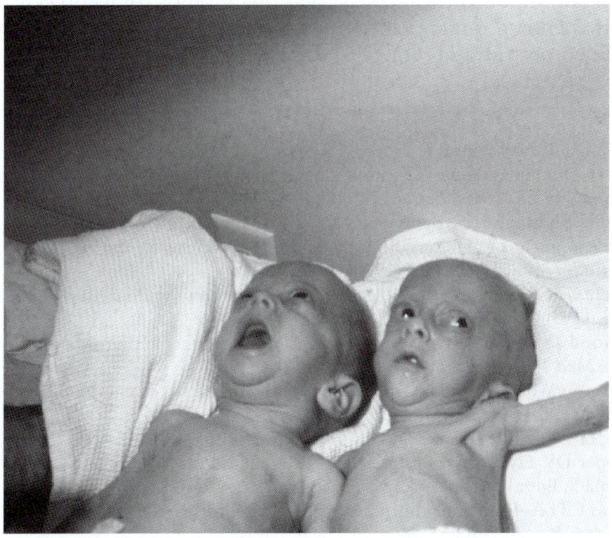

Figura 569-3. Gemelli maschi con ipertiroidismo neonatale confermato dall'alterazione dei test di funzionalità tiroidea. Il quadro clinico comprende perdita del tessuto sottocutaneo per ipermetabolismo, occhi distanziati e sguardo fisso ansioso. È stata fatta diagnosi di malattia di Graves neonatale, in assenza di analoga patologia materna; essi manifestavano invece un ipertiroidismo persistente, non transitorio. All'età di 8 anni, sono stati trattati con radioiodio. Si ritiene che abbiano avuto una qualche altra forma di ipertiroidismo neonatale, come un'attivazione costitutiva del recettore del TSH.

tachipnea, con ipertermia. Nei neonati più gravi, si verifica una progressione della sintomatologia; compare una perdita di peso nonostante l'appetito vorace, aumenta l'epatosplenomegalia e si manifesta ittero. Possono esserci inoltre una grave ipertensione e scompenso cardiaco. Il neonato può anche morire se non si instaura prontamente un'adeguata terapia. I livelli sierici di T_4 sono notevolmente aumentati, con TSH soppresso. Sono comuni un'aumentata età ossea, prominenza frontale con faccia triangolare e sinostosi cranica, specialmente nei neonati con persistenti manifestazioni cliniche di ipertiroidismo.

TRATTAMENTO. Il trattamento del neonato consiste nella somministrazione orale di propanololo (1-2 mg/kg/die, per os in tre somministrazioni giornaliere) e PTU (5-10 mg/kg/die, in tre somministrazioni giornaliere distanziate di 8 ore), o metimazolo (0,25-1,0 mg/kg/die, con una somministrazione ogni 12 ore); si può aggiungere ioduro di potassio (1 goccia ogni 8 ore). Se durante la gravidanza si utilizza il propanololo per trattare la tireotossicosi materna, questo attraversando la placenta, può causare depressione respiratoria nel neonato. Se lo stato di tireotossicosi è severo, può essere indicata la somministrazione parenterale di liquidi e corticosteroidi. Se si verifica insufficienza cardiaca, può essere indicata la digitalizzazione. Una volta raggiunta una condizione di eutiroidismo, rimane necessario solo il trattamento con antitiroidei. Il dosaggio deve essere ridotto gradualmente, per mantenere eutiroideo il neonato. La maggior parte dei casi presenta una remissione verso il terzo-quarto anno di età.

Occasionalmente l'ipertiroidismo neonatale non va in remissione, ma persiste nell'infanzia. Questi pazienti possono avere un'anamnesi di notevole ipertiroidismo familiare. L'ipertiroidismo neonatale, senza evidenza di patologia autoimmunitaria nella mamma o nel bambino, è dovuto a mutazione del gene TSHR che produce l'attivazione costitutiva del recettore. Quando si sospendono i farmaci antitiroidei, ricompare ipertiroidismo; questi bambini devono essere trattati con radioiodio o con la chirurgia.

PROGNOSI. Se si ritarda il trattamento, progredisce la maturazione ossea e compaiono microcefalia e ritardo mentale. Lo sviluppo intellettivo è normale nella maggior parte dei neonati con malattia di Graves trattati, anche se alcuni possono mostrare lesioni da ipertiroidismo fetale. In alcuni bambini, l'ipertiroidismo in epoca intrauterina sopprime il meccanismo di feedback ipotalamo-ipofiso-tiroideo e si sviluppa un ipotiroidismo centrale permanente, il quale richiede una terapia sostitutiva con ormone tiroideo per tutta la vita.

Akamizu T, Nakamura Y, Tamaoki A, et al: Prevalence and clinico-epidemiology of familial Graves' disease in Japan based on nationwide epidemiologic survey in 2001. *Endocrinol J* 2003;50:429–436.

Azizi F, Khamseh ME, Bahreynian M, et al: Thyroid function and intellectual development of children of mothers taking methimazole during pregnancy. *J Endocrinol Invest* 2002;25:586–589.

Birrell G, Cheetham T: Juvenile thyrotoxicosis; Can we do better? *Arch Dis Child* 204;89:745–750.

Cawood T, Moriarty P, O'Shea D: Recent developments in thyroid eye disease. *Br Med J* 2004;329:385–390.

Chan W, Wong GW, Fan DS, et al: Ophthalmopathy in childhood Graves' disease. *Br J Ophthalmol* 2002;86:740–742.

Cooper DS: Antithyroid drugs. *N Engl J Med* 2005;352:905–917.

Cooper DS: Hyperthyroidism. *Lancet* 2003;362:459–468.

Iwama S, Ikezaki A, Kikuoka N, et al: Association of HLA-DR, DQ genotypes and CTLA-4 gene polymorphism with Graves' disease in Japanese children. *Horm Res* 2005;63:55–60.

Kempers MJ, van Tijn DA, van Trotsenburg AS, et al: Central congenital hypothyroidism due to gestational hyperthyroidism: Detection where prevention failed. *J Clin Endocrinol Metab* 2003;88:5851–5857.

Kopp P, van Sande J, Parma J, et al: Brief report: Congenital hyperthyroidism caused by a mutation in the thyrotropin-receptor gene. *N Engl J Med* 1995;332:150–154.

Mastorakos G, Mitsiades NS, Doufas AG, et al: Hyperthyroidism in McCune-Albright syndrome with a review of thyroid abnormalities sixty years after the first report. *Thyroid* 1997;7:433–439.

Milham S Jr: Scalp defects in infants of mothers treated for hyperthyroidism with methimazole or carbimazole during pregnancy. *Teratology* 1985;32:321.

Nabhan Z, Kreher NC, Eugster EA: Hashitoxicosis in children: Clinical features and natural history. *J Pediatr* 2005;146:533–536.

Nesbesio TD, Siddiqui AR, Pescovitz OH, et al: Time course to hypothyroidism after fixed-dose radioablation therapy of Graves' disease in children. *J Pediatr* 2002;141:99–103.

Pearce EN: Diagnosis and management of thyrotoxicosis. *BMJ* 2006;332: 1369–1373.

Polak M: Hyperthyroidism in early infancy: Pathogenesis, clinical features and diagnosis with a focus on neonatal hyperthyroidism. *Thyroid* 1998;8:1171–1177.

Read CH, Tansey MJ, Menda Y: A 36-year retrospective analysis of the efficacy and safety of radioactive iodine in treating young Graves' patients. *J Clin Endocrinol Metab* 2004;89:4229–4233.

Rivkees SA, Cornelius EA: Influence of iodine-131 dose on the outcome of hyperthyroidism in children. *J Pediatr* 2003;111:745–749.

Skuza KA, Sills IN, Stene M, et al: Prediction of neonatal hyperthyroidism in infants born to mothers with Graves' disease. *J Pediatr* 1996;128:264–268.

Sugino K, Ito K, Mimura T, et al: Surgical treatment of Graves' disease in children. *Thyroid* 2004;14:447–452.

Weber G, Ielo V, Vigone MC, et al: Neonatal hyperthyroidism: report of eight cases. *Ital J Pediatr* 2001;27:757.

Zimmerman D, Lteif AN: Thyrotoxicosis in children. *Endocrinol Metab Clin North Am* 1998;27:109–126.

Capitolo 570 ■ Carcinoma della tiroide

EPIDEMIOLOGIA. Il carcinoma della tiroide è raro nell'infanzia; l'incidenza annuale nei bambini di età inferiore a 15 anni è approssimativamente di due casi su 100 000. Diversamente da altre patologie maligne dei bambini, il carcinoma della tiroide normalmente ha un decorso lento, anche dopo lo sviluppo di metastasi polmonari.

PATOGENESI. I fattori genetici e l'esposizione a radiazioni sono due fattori importanti nella patogenesi del carcinoma tiroideo. Nel 3-33% dei carcinomi papillari e nel 68-80% di quelli post-radiazioni, si è trovata una modificazione del proto-oncogeno *RET*, come nei bambini bielorussi esposti a radiazioni dopo la catastrofe nucleare di Chernobyl o in quelli sottoposti a irradiazione terapeutica esterna durante l'infanzia. Mutazioni puntiformi inattivanti del gene soppressore del tumore *p53* sono rare in pazienti con carcinoma tiroideo differenziato, ma comuni in quelli con carcinoma tiroideo anaplastico. Complessivamente, il 5-10% dei casi di carcinoma papillare della tiroide è familiare e di norma ereditario, con modalità autosomica dominante.

La ghiandola tiroidea, nei bambini, è particolarmente sensibile all'esposizione a radiazioni esterne, probabilmente senza che vi sia una dose-soglia; 1 Gy comporta un rischio relativo 7,7 di carcinoma tiroideo. In passato, circa l'80% dei bambini con tumore tiroideo aveva ricevuto, durante l'infanzia, una dose inappropriata di radiazioni al collo e nelle zone circostanti, per la presenza di patologie benigne come iperplasia timica, ipertrofia tonsillare e adenoidea, emangiomi, nevi, eczema, tinea capitis e "adenite cervicale". Dopo che si è interrotto l'utilizzo delle radiazioni per queste patologie benigne, è scomparsa anche questa causa di carcinoma tiroideo. Tuttavia, la sopravvivenza a lungo termine di bambini che, per patologia neoplastica, sono stati curati con appropriata terapia radiante nella zona del collo ha reso questa causa di carcinoma e di noduli tiroidei progressivamente prevalente. Dosi più alte, precocità del trattamento e appartenenza al sesso femminile sono fattori che aumentano il rischio di carcinoma tiroideo. I dati che si riferiscono al rischio a lungo termine per tumore sono scarsi, ma il 15-20% dei bambini che ha ricevuto terapia radiante e chemioterapia per malattia di Hodgkin, leucemia, trapianto di midollo osseo, tumori cerebrali e altre patologie maligne del capo e del collo presenta livelli elevati di ormone stimolante la tiroide (TSH) nel primo anno di terapia, mentre il 5-20% progredisce verso un ipotiroidismo nei 5-7 anni successivi. La maggior parte di ampi gruppi di bambini trattati presenta un'incidenza del 10-30% di noduli tiroidei benigni e un aumento della frequenza di tumore tiroideo. Quest'ultimo fa la sua comparsa nell'arco di 3-5 anni dall'irradiazione, raggiungendo un picco in 15-25 anni. Non si conosce il motivo per cui c'è un periodo dopo il quale non si sviluppano più tumori tiroidei. La somministrazione di ^{131}I a scopo terapeutico o diagnostico non aumenta il rischio di tumore tiroideo.

In pazienti con tiroidite linfocitica cronica è stato riportato un carcinoma tiroideo differenziato; non è chiaro se vi sia un aumento del rischio di carcinoma tiroideo nei bambini con patologia tiroidea autoimmune. Al contrario, l'infiltrazione linfocitica nel carcinoma tiroideo comporta una prognosi più favorevole, rappresentando forse un segno di risposta immunitaria al tumore.

Istologicamente, i carcinomi si suddividono in papillari (80%), follicolari (17%), midollari (2%) o misti differenziati. Di norma questi tumori crescono lentamente e possono rimanere silenti per anni. Il tipo di tumore e il decorso naturale della malattia è analogo in pazienti irradiati o no, con la sola eccezione della multicentricità, più frequente in quelli conseguenti a radiazioni. I tumori tiroidei indifferenziati (anaplastici) sono rari nei bambini e di norma presentano un decorso rapidamente fatale. Nei residui del dotto tireoglosso, durante l'infanzia, sono riportati casi di carcinoma tiroideo, più frequentemente il carcinoma papillare. Nei bambini sono stati riportati anche linfomi e teratomi della tiroide.

MANIFESTAZIONI CLINICHE. Le bambine sono colpite con frequenza doppia rispetto ai maschi. L'età media al momento della diagnosi è di 9 anni, ma l'esordio può anche essere più precoce, nel primo anno di vita. Un singolo nodulo indolore della tiroide o nel collo è solitamente il primo segno della malattia. Rappresentano fattori di rischio per carcinoma le dimensioni notevoli, la durezza, la fissità rispetto ai tessuti adiacenti e la paralisi delle corde vocali. Spesso, al momento della diagnosi, è presente un coinvolgimento dei linfonodi cervicali. Un qualunque ingrossamento di un linfonodo cervicale richiede l'esame della tiroide, che può talora presentare un tumore primitivo troppo piccolo per essere percepito mediante palpazione; la diagnosi si basa perciò sull'indagine bioptica del linfonodo. I polmoni rappresentano la sede più frequente di metastasi al di fuori del collo, anche in assenza di manifestazioni cliniche a esse riferibili; radiologicamente appaiono come infiltrazione miliare diffusa o con aspetto nodulare, soprattutto nelle regioni basali. Possono essere confuse con tubercolosi, istoplasmosi o sarcoidosi. Altre sedi di metastasi comprendono il mediastino, le ossa lunghe, il cranio e l'ascella. Quasi tutti i bambini sono eutiroidei, ma raramente il carcinoma può essere funzionante e produrre sintomi di ipertiroidismo.

DIAGNOSI. Il test più importante per la diagnosi in presenza di nodulo solitario, è l'agoaspirazione con ago sottile (*Fine-Needle Aspiration*, FNA). L'indagine ecografica della tiroide può fornire informazioni sulle caratteristiche del nodulo (solido o cistico) e sull'eventuale presenza di altri noduli non palpabili. Una scintigrafia che utilizzi preferibilmente ^{123}I o ^{99m}T-pertecnato offre indicazioni sulla capacità di captazione e sul fatto che il nodulo sia "caldo", "caldissimo" o "freddo". La maggior parte dei noduli freddi è benigna. Né l'ecografia né la scintigrafia è in grado di differenziare una lesione benigna da una maligna. Un campione ottenuto con FNA può essere interpretato come tumore benigno, maligno, indeterminato oppure come un campione inadeguato. L'esperienza di FNA nei bambini comporta un 5-10% di falsi negativi, un 1-2% di falsi positivi, con un'accuratezza diagnostica complessiva del 90-95%. I test di funzionalità tiroidea sono normali, ma la tiroidite di Hashimoto è stata associata a carcinoma tiroideo.

TRATTAMENTO. Dal momento che il carcinoma tiroideo differenziato è un patologia cronica con lunga sopravvivenza, la terapia ottimale è ancora in evoluzione. Il carcinoma papillare di piccole dimensioni (<1 cm), il tipo meno aggressivo, può essere efficacemente trattato con tiroidectomia subtotale e dosi soppressive di ormone tiroideo. Tuttavia, è sempre più evidente che la maggior parte dei pazienti è gestita meglio con una tiroidectomia totale o quasi totale. I carcinomi papillari tendono a essere multicentrici e diversi studi dimostrano che la metà di questi bambini, all'esordio, mostra già un coinvolgimento dei linfonodi regionali. Per i carcinomi papillari di più ampie dimensioni, i carcinomi follicolari o con coinvolgimento dei linfonodi regionali, il trattamento di elezione è la tiroidectomia totale con escissione dei linfonodi regionali. Non c'è ragione per una dissezione radicale del collo. La tiroidectomia è di solito seguita da una dose ablativa di ^{131}I (30-100 mCi). Solo i pazienti sottoposti a tiroidectomia totale devono essere monitorati con scintigrafia total body con radioiodio e dosaggio della tireoglobulina sierica.

Dopo l'intervento, tutti i pazienti devono essere trattati con L-tiroxina sodica a dosi sufficienti a sopprimere il TSH a livelli inferiori alla norma. La tireoglobulina sierica (Tg) rappresenta un marker eccellente di recidiva tumorale e si deve eseguire una determinazione periodica dei suoi livelli che, in presenza di terapia soppressiva con L-tiroxina (T_4), devono essere inferiori a 3 ng/mL. Pazienti con livelli sierici di Tg elevati devono essere sottoposti a una scintigrafia total body con radioiodio e a una scintigrafia ed ecografia della tiroide, per localizzare la sorgente di Tg e approntare un adeguato piano terapeutico.

PROGNOSI. Per qualsiasi tipo di terapia, la sopravvivenza o la recidiva non appaiono diverse nei pazienti con o senza coinvolgimento dei linfonodi cervicali. Tutti i pazienti con metastasi cervicali o polmonari hanno una sopravvivenza di parecchi anni. Più del 95% dei pazienti è in vita dopo 25 anni dal trattamento iniziale, se il tumore era intratiroideo, inferiore a 2 cm di diametro e classificato di grado 1. Tumori più voluminosi, con metastasi a distanza, e con gradi maggiori di atipia sono associati a un aumento cumulativo della mortalità. I carcinomi tiroidei che esprimono telomerasi e recettore IGF-1 mostrano manifestazioni cliniche più aggressive, mentre quelli che esprimono symporter sodio-ioduro sono associati a minore rischio di recidiva.

570.1 • Nodulo solitario della tiroide

I noduli solitari della tiroide sono frequenti nei bambini. Sono percepibili mediante palpazione in circa il 2% dei ragazzi di età compresa fra gli 11 e i 18 anni; l'indagine ecografica permette di evidenziare verosimilmente una maggiore frequenza, come negli adulti. I fattori genetici giocano un ruolo eziologico. La maggior parte dei noduli tiroidei nei bambini è benigna. La malignità si verifica nel 15% dei casi, forse per decremento dell'esposizione a radiazioni nei bambini (Tab. 570-1). I bambini esposti a radiazione evidenziano un'elevata incidenza di adenoma benigno e di carcinoma della tiroide.

Le patologie benigne che possono presentarsi sotto forma di nodulo solitario comprendono adenomi benigni (follicolare, embrionale, a cellule di Hurthle), nodulo colloidale (adenomatosi), cisti semplice, tiroidite linfocitica, ascesso tiroideo e anomalie di sviluppo come la cisti del dotto tireoglosso o l'emiagenesia. Una massa tiroidea che compaia improvvisamente o che si ingrandisca rapidamente indica un'emorragia intracistica o un adenoma benigno. Nella maggior parte dei casi, il bambino è eutiroideo e gli studi di funzionalità tiroidea sono normali. Se la causa del nodulo è rappresentata dalla tiroidite linfocitica, il T_4 può essere basso, il TSH elevato e sono in genere presenti anticorpi antitiroidei. Se si esegue una scintigrafia, essa può rivelare un difetto della classica forma a farfalla. Raramente, la tiroidite linfocitica può essere associata a carcinoma. L'ecografia è particolarmente utilizzata per individuare lesioni cistiche.

TABELLA 570-1. Classificazione eziologica dei noduli solitari della tiroide

Follicolo linfoide, come parte della tiroidite linfocitica cronica
Anomalie dello sviluppo della tiroide
Emiagenesia
Cisti intratiroidea del dotto tireoglosso
Ascesso tiroideo (tiroidite acuta suppurativa)
Cisti semplice
Neoplasie
Benigne
Nodulo colloidale (adenomatoso)
Adenoma follicolare
Adenoma tossico
Non tiroidee (per es. linfoemangioma)
Maligne
Carcinoma papillare
Carcinoma follicolare
Carcinoma misto papillare-follicolare
Indifferenziato (anaplastico)
Carcinoma midollare
Non tiroidee
Linfoma
Teratoma

Gli studi diagnostici per determinare le cause sottostanti comprendono i test di funzionalità tiroidea, la determinazione degli anticorpi antitiroide, l'indagine ecografica della tiroide e l'FNA. La scintigrafia e lo studio della captazione sono utili se si trovano livelli soppressi di TSH, che suggeriscono un nodulo "caldo". La risposta alla prova di soppressione con T_4 per vedere un'eventuale riduzione delle dimensioni del nodulo non è realizzabile. Sebbene i carcinomi tiroidei generalmente si presentino come noduli solidi, noduli "freddi", la maggior parte dei noduli freddi è rappresentata da lesioni benigne. L'FNA è utilizzato per evitare la chirurgia in caso di nodulo benigno. Tuttavia, si deve rapidamente ricorrere al trattamento chirurgico se il nodulo è duro o cresce rapidamente, se ci sono segni di coinvolgimento tracheale o delle corde vocali e in presenza di ingrossamento dei linfonodi adiacenti. Tutte le persone con un'anamnesi positiva per irradiazione del collo e del capo devono essere sottoposte a un'attenta valutazione della tiroide, almeno ogni due anni, per tutta la vita.

Raramente, i noduli tiroidei possono essere funzionanti, con ipertiroidismo (**malattia di Plummer**). La captazione del radionuclide è concentrata nel nodulo ("caldissimo" o "caldo") e gli studi di funzionalità tiroidea indicano che il nodulo è autonomamente funzionante. Questi noduli sono di solito benigni, ma è stata riportata una piccola percentuale di malignità. I livelli di T_4 sono normali, ma i livelli di triiodotironina (T_3) sono elevati (T_3 tossicosi) e quelli di TSH soppressi. Il trattamento consiste nella rimozione chirurgica del nodulo.

570.2 • Carcinoma midollare

Il carcinoma midollare della tiroide deriva dalle cellule parafollicolari (cellule C) della tiroide e ha un'incidenza del 2% di tutte le patologie maligne. Il sintomo più comune è il gozzo o un nodulo tiroideo palpabile. L'indagine radiografica può evidenziare una densa, conglomerata, omogenea calcificazione della tiroide. Sono comuni le metastasi ai linfonodi regionali e al fegato; anche queste possono calcificare. Può portare a morte, ma è frequente una lunga sopravvivenza.

I tumori si possono presentare come patologia sporadica, come malattia familiare autosomica dominante e come componente di due distinte sindromi autosomiche dominanti. La predisposizione a tutte queste forme è stata associata a mutazioni della linea germinale del proto-oncogeno *RET* sul cromosoma 10q11.2. Se il tumore compare sporadicamente, è di solito unicentrico, ma nelle forme familiari è normalmente multicentrico e ha inizio come iperplasia delle cellule parafollicolari. I tumori sono spesso troppo piccoli per essere percepiti palpatorialmente, scintigraficamente ed ecograficamente nei pazienti a rischio di tali famiglie. La diagnosi di carcinoma midollare deve portare alla ricerca accurata di tumori associati, particolarmente il feocromocitoma. Non ci sono manifestazioni clinicamente rilevabili degli alti livelli sierici di calcitonina o del peptide gene-correlato a essa. Ciononostante, questi test sono utili per lo screening e il monitoraggio della terapia.

NEOPLASIA ENDOCRINA MULTIPLA, TIPO IIA. Quando l'iperplasia o il carcinoma a cellule C è associato a iperplasia surrenalica o feocromocitoma e iperplasia paratiroidea, si parla di neoplasia endocrina multipla (*Multiple Endocrine Neoplasia*, MEN) di tipo IIA. La modalità di trasmissione per la MEN-IIA è autosomica dominante, con alto grado di penetranza ed espressività variabile. Per la MEN-IIA e per i casi familiari di carcinoma midollare della tiroide sono state descritte almeno 19 diverse specifiche mutazioni missense dell'esone 10 o 11 del dominio extracellulare del gene *RET*. L'analisi del DNA permette una precisa identificazione dei trasportatori del proto-oncogeno *RET*. L'iperplasia delle cellule C o i tumori appaiono di solito più precocemente rispetto al feocromocitoma. I feocromocitomi sono frequentemente bilaterali e possono essere multipli. È noto che l'iperplasia surrenalica midollare precede il feocromocitoma, ma il periodo latente è breve. L'ipercalcemia è una manifestazione tardiva e indica iperparatiroidismo. Le ghiandole paratiroidi possono mostrare iperplasia delle cellule principali o solo ipercellularità.

NEOPLASIA ENDOCRINA MULTIPLA, TIPO IIB. Gli aspetti distintivi della MEN tipo IIB, anche chiamata **sindrome dei neurinomi mucosi**, consistono in neurinomi multipli associati a un tipico fenotipo con carcinoma midollare e feocromocitoma. Anche questa malattia è autosomica dominante e il 93% dei familiari presenta mutazione missense del proto-oncogeno *RET*. Tuttavia, la mutazione si verifica nell'esone 16, il dominio catalitico tirosina di *RET*; tutti i pazienti hanno gli stessi punti di mutazione.

Molto spesso i neurinomi compaiono sulla lingua, sulla mucosa orale, delle labbra e sulla congiuntiva. Possono essere presenti neurofibromi periferici e macchie caffellatte ed è frequente la ganglioneuromatosi intestinale. È presente una diffusa proliferazione dei nervi e delle cellule gangliari nella mucosa, nella sottomucosa, nello strato muscolare e in quello sottosieroso a livello dell'intestino tenue e crasso e dell'esofago. Il paziente può avere alta statura, con aracnodactilia e habitus marfanoide. Sono comuni scoliosi, *pectus excavatum*, piede cavo e ipotonia muscolare. Le palpebre possono essere ispessite e rovesciate, le labbra aperte e tumide e ci può essere prognatismo. Difficoltà dell'alimentazione, scarso succhiamento, diarrea, stipsi e deficit di crescita possono cominciare nelle fasi più precoci o nell'infanzia, molti anni prima del manifestarsi dei neurinomi o dei sintomi endocrini.

TRATTAMENTO. Per tutti i bambini in cui studi del DNA abbiano dimostrato mutazioni genetiche, è indicata la tiroidectomia totale. L'individuazione di forme familiari di questo tumore è critica per la diagnosi precoce nei bambini a rischio. I dati suggeriscono che la tiroidectomia deve essere precoce, perché il carcinoma midollare è stato trovato anche in un bambino di 6 mesi con MEN-IIB e in uno di 3 anni con MEN-IIA. Nella MEN-IIA, esiste una correlazione tra la specifica mutazione e l'esordio dell'iperplasia a cellule C o del carcinoma midollare. Mutazioni del codone 634 si verificano in età precoce, mentre quelle dei codoni 618, 620 e 804 tendono a essere più tardive. In tutti questi bambini, prima di ricorrere alla terapia chirurgica, deve essere ricercato un feocromocitoma. Il monitoraggio dei livelli di calcitonina è utile per seguire il decorso della malattia dopo l'intervento e per la ricerca di lesioni metastatiche. Sono consigliati screening periodici per la scoperta di eventuali feocromocitoma e iperparatiroidismo.

Acharya S, Sarafoglou K, LaQuaglia M, et al: Thyroid neoplasms after therapeutic radiation for malignancies during childhood or adolescence. *Cancer* 2003;97:2397–2403.

Amrikachi M, Ponder TB, Wheeler TM, et al: Thyroid fine-needle aspiration biopsy in children and adolescents: Experience with 218 aspirates. *Diagn Cytopath* 2005;32:189–192.
Antonelli A, Miccoli P, Fallahi P, et al: Role of neck ultrasonography in the follow-up of children operated on for thyroid papillary cancer. *Thyroid* 2003;13:479–484.
Borson-Chazot F, Causeret S, Lifante JC, et al: Predictive factors for recurrence from a series of 74 children and adolescents with differentiated thyroid cancer. *World J Surg* 2004;28:1088–1092.
Collins BJ, Chiappetta G, Schneider AB, et al: RET expression in papillary thyroid cancer from patients irradiated in childhood for benign conditions. *J Clin Endocrinol Metab* 2002;87:3941–3946.
Degnan BM, McClellan DR, Francis GL: An analysis of fine-needle aspiration biopsy of the thyroid in children and adolescents. *J Pediatr Surg* 1996;31:903–907.
Grigsby PW, Gal-or A, Michalski JM, Doherty GM: Childhood and adolescent thyroid cancer. Cancer 2002;95:724–732.
Hansen PS, Brix TH, Bennedbaek FN, et al: The relative importance of genetic and environmental factors in the aetiology of thyroid nodularity: A study of healthy Danish twins. *Clin Endocrinol* 2005;62:380–386.
Hegedüs L: The thyroid nodule. *N Engl J Med* 2004;351:1764–1771.
Hung W, Sarlis NJ. Current controversies in the management of pediatric thyroid patients with well-differentiated nonmedullary thyroid cancer: A review. *Thyroid* 2002;8:683–702.
Lafferty AR, Batch JA: Thyroid nodules in childhood and adolescence–Thirty years of experience. *J Pediatr Endocrinol Metab* 1997;10:479–486.
Lando A, Holm K, Nysom K, et al: Serum thyroglobulin as a marker of thyroid neoplasms after childhood cancer. *Acta Paediatr* 2003;92: 1284–1290.
Peretz A, Leibermann E, Kapelushnik J, et al: Thyroglossal duct carcinoma in children: Case presentation and review of the literature. *Thyroid* 2004;14:777–785.
Ries LAG, Eisner MP, Kosary CL, et al: SEER Cancer Statistics Review, 1975–2000. Bethesda, MD, National Cancer Institute, 2003. Available at *seer.cancer.gov/csr/1975_2000.*
Svensson J, Nilsson PE, Olsson C, et al: Interpretation of normative thyroid volumes in children and adolescents: Is there a need for a multivariate model? *Thyroid* 2004;14:536–543.
Szinnai G, Meier C, Komminoth P, Zumsteg UW: Review of multiple endocrine neoplasia type 2A in children: Therapeutic results of early thyroidectomy and prognostic value of codon analysis. *Pediatrics* 2003;111: E132–139.
Utiger RD: The multiplicity of thyroid nodules and carcinomas. *N Engl J Med* 2005;352:2376–2378.
Zimmerman D: Thyroid neoplasia in children. *Curr Opin Pediatr* 1997;9: 413–418.

Sezione 3 — Malattie delle ghiandole paratiroidi — Daniel A. Doyle e Angelo M. DiGeorge

Capitolo 571 ■ Ormoni e peptidi dell'omeostasi del calcio e del metabolismo osseo

L'ormone paratiroideo (PTH) e la vitamina D sono i principali regolatori dell'omeostasi del calcio (vedi Capitoli 48 e 701). La calcitonina e il peptide PTH-correlato (*Peptide PTH-Related*, PTHrP) sono importanti soprattutto nel feto.

ORMONE PARATIROIDEO. Il PTH è un peptide di 84 aminoacidi (9500 Da), ma la sua attività biologica risiede nei primi 34. Le paratiroidi sintetizzano un pre-pro-PTH (catena di 115 aminoacidi) e un ormone proparatiroideo (90 aminoacidi). Il pre-pro-PTH si trasforma in pro-PTH e quest'ultimo in PTH. Il PTH (1-84) è il maggior prodotto della secrezione ghiandolare, ma viene rapidamente metabolizzato nel fegato e nel rene in frammenti più piccoli COOH-terminali, regione media, NH_2-terminali.

La presenza di questi frammenti nel siero ha portato alla messa a punto di vari sistemi di dosaggio. I frammenti 1-34 amino-terminali (N-terminali) sono dotati di attività biologica, ma sono presenti, a livello circolatorio, in basse quantità; il dosaggio di questi frammenti è il più utilizzato per verificare modificazioni acute della secrezione. I frammenti carbossi-terminali (C-terminali) e le porzioni intermedie, sebbene biologicamente inerti, rimangono più a lungo in circolo e rappresentano l'80% del PTH plasmatico immunoreattivo; i valori del frammento C-terminale sono 50-500 volte i livelli dell'ormone attivo. I dosaggi del frammento C-terminale sono utili per la diagnosi di iperparatiroidismo, ma, dal momento che tali frammenti vengono rimossi dalla circolazione per opera della filtrazione glomerulare, sono meno utili per la valutazione dell'iperparatiroidismo secondario caratteristico della patologia renale. Solo certi radioimmunodosaggi sensibili per il PTH sono in grado di differenziare le basse concentrazioni dell'ipoparatiroidismo dai livelli normali. Un dosaggio sensibile immunochemiluminometrico della durata di 15 minuti, messo a punto per un utilizzo intraoperatorio, può essere di aiuto al chirurgo, perché fornisce informazioni utili.

In condizioni di ipocalcemia, il segnale viene trasferito tramite un recettore calcio-sensibile, con incremento della secrezione di PTH (Fig. 571-1). Il PTH stimola l'attività dell'1 α-idrossilasi renale, aumentando la produzione di 1,25-diidrossicolecalciferolo (1,25-$[OH]_2D_3$). L'aumento dei livelli di 1,25-$[OH]_2D_3$ induce la sintesi di una proteina legante il calcio (calbindina-D) nella mucosa intestinale, con conseguente assorbimento di calcio. Il PTH mobilizza anche il calcio attraverso un incremento del riassorbimento osseo, mediato dall'1,25-$[OH]_2D_3$. Gli effetti del PTH sull'osso e sul rene sono mediati dal legame con specifici recettori sulle membrane delle cellule bersaglio e dall'attivazione di una via di trasduzione che coinvolge la proteina G associata al sistema dell'adenilciclasi (vedi anche Capitolo 573).

Il recettore di rilevazione del calcio regola la secrezione di PTH e il riassorbimento di calcio dai tubuli renali, in risposta ad alterazione delle concentrazioni sieriche del calcio. Il gene per il recettore è localizzato sul cromosoma 3q13.3-q21 e codifica una proteina della superficie cellulare composta da 1078 aminoacidi, espressa nelle paratiroidi e nel rene e appartenente alla famiglia dei recettori associati alla proteina G. In presenza di un recettore per il calcio normalmente funzionante, l'ipocalcemia induce la secrezione di PTH e l'ipercalcemia la deprime. Mutazioni con perdita di funzione provocano un incremento del set-point per il calcio sierico, con conseguente **ipercalcemia ipercalciurica familiare** e iperparatiroidismo neonatale grave. L'ipercalcemia ipercalciurica acquisita può essere dovuta agli autoanticorpi contro il recettore per il calcio e si manifesta assieme a ipercalcemia e iperparatiroidismo. Mutazioni con aumento di funzione comportano una diminuzione della secrezione di PTH in risposta all'ipocalcemia, responsabile della sindrome dell'ipocalcemia ipercalciurica familiare (vedi Fig. 571-1).

PEPTIDE CORRELATO ALL'ORMONE PARATIROIDEO. Il PTHrP è un omologo del PTH solo nei primi 13 aminoacidi del suo amino-terminale, 8 dei quali sono identici al PTH. Il suo gene si trova sul braccio corto del cromosoma 12 e quello del PTH sul braccio corto del cromosoma 11.

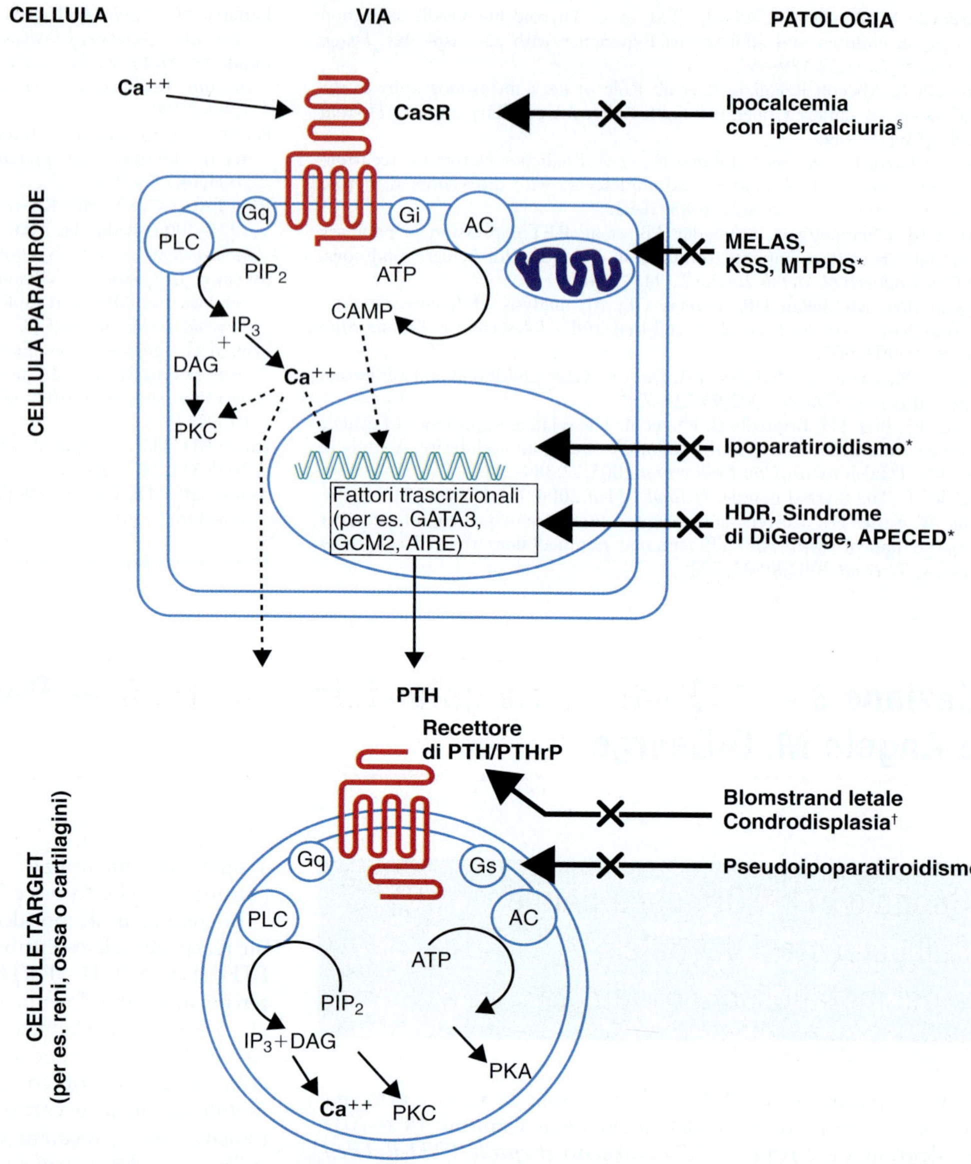

Figura 571-1. Alcuni degli agenti coinvolti nell'omeostasi del calcio. I recettori di CaSR e PTH/PTHrP mediano i loro effetti attraverso vie di segnalazione associate alla proteina G, che a turno attivano i sistemi dell'adenilciclasi (AC) e della fosfolipasi C (PLC). APECED (*Autoimmune Poliendocrinopathy-Candidosis-Ectodermal Dystrophy*), poliendocrinopatia autoimmune-candidosi-distrofia ectodermica; DAG (*Diacylglycerol*) diacilglicerolo; Gi (*G Inhibitory protein*), proteina inibitrice G; Gq (*G-Pertussis-Toxin-Insensitive-Protein*), proteina G insensibile alla tossina della pertosse; HDR (*Hypoparathyroidism, Deafness, and Renal Anomalies*), ipoparatiroidismo, sordità e anomalie renali; IP_3 (*Inositol* 1,45-*triphosphate*), inositolo 1,45 trifosfato; KSS (*Kearns-Sayre Syndrome*), sindrome di Kearns-Sayre (oftalmoplegia esterna progressiva, retinopatia pigmentata, blocco cardiaco, e cardiomiopatia); MELAS (*Mitochondrial Encephalopathy, Stroke-like Episodes, and Lactic Acidosis*), encefalopatia mitocondriale, episodi ictus-simili e acidosi lattica; MTPDS (*Mitochondrial Trifunctional Protein Deficiency Syndrome*), sindrome da deficit della proteina trifunzionale mitocondriale; PIP_2 (*Phosphatidyl Inositol* 4,5-*bisphosphate*), fosfatidil inositolo 4,5-bifosfato; PKC (*Protein Kinase* C), proteinchinasi C.
* Patologie da carenza di PTH.
† Deficit da difetto del recettore di PTH/PTHrP.
‡ Deficit da insensibilità al PTH per difetti a valle del recettore di PTH/PTHrP.
§ Deficit da alterato set point nell'asse Ca^{++}/PTH, associato a mutazione con aumento di funzione di CaSR.
(Da Thakker RV: Genetic Development in Hypoparathyroidism. *Lancet* 2001;357:974-976, per gentile concessione.)

Il PTHrP, come il PTH, attiva i recettori specifici nelle cellule del rene e dell'osso, e aumenta l'adenosina monofosfato ciclica urinaria e la produzione renale di 1,25-$[OH]_2D_3$. Esso viene prodotto in quasi tutti i tipi cellulari dell'organismo, compresi tutti i tessuti dello stadio embrionale e somatico dello sviluppo. Il PTHrP è importante per il normale sviluppo fetale. Mutazioni inattivanti del recettore per PTH/PTHrP comportano una patologia ossea letale, caratterizzata da arti corti e maturazione ossea notevolmente avanzata, conosciuta col nome di condrodisplasia di Blomstrand (vedi Fig. 571-1). Il PTHrP ha un ruolo paracrino o autocrino, perché i livelli sierici sono bassi, eccetto poche situazioni cliniche. Il sangue del cordone ombelicale contiene livelli di PTHrP tre volte superiori a quelli sierici dell'adulto; è prodotto dalle paratiroidi fetali e rappresenta il principale agente stimolante il passaggio materno-fetale di calcio. Il PTHrP è essenziale per una normale maturazione scheletrica del feto, che richiede 30 g di calcio. Durante la gravidanza, l'assorbimento materno di calcio aumenta da circa 150 mg/die a 400 mg durante il secondo trimestre.

Come nel sangue del cordone ombelicale, i livelli di PTHrP sono aumentati durante la lattazione e in pazienti con ipertrofia mammaria benigna. Il latte materno e quello bovino pastorizzato hanno livelli di PTHrP 10 000 volte superiori a quelli del plasma normale. La maggior parte dei casi di malignità della sindrome da ipercalcemia ormonale è causata da elevate concentrazioni di PTHrP.

VITAMINA D. Vedi Capitolo 48.

CALCITONINA. La calcitonina (CT) è un polipeptide di 32 aminoacidi. Il suo gene si trova sul cromosoma 11p ed è strettamente associato a quello del PTH. Il gene per CT codifica tre peptidi: CT, un peptide carbossiterminale di 21 aminoacidi (catacalcina) e un peptide correlato al gene di CT. La catacalcina e la CT sono secrete assieme in quantità equimolari dalle cellule parafollicolari (cellule C) della ghiandola tiroidea. La CT pare essere di poca importanza nei bambini e negli adulti, perché anche livelli molto alti in pazienti con carcinoma midollare della tiroide (un tumore che deriva dalle cellule C) non provocano ipercalcemia. Nel feto, tuttavia, i livelli circolanti sono alti e sembra che aumentino il metabolismo osseo e la crescita scheletrica. Mentre nel cordone ombelicale e nei bambini più piccoli le concentrazioni circolanti sono elevate, i livelli nei bambini più grandi e nell'adulto sono bassi. I lattanti e i bambini con ipotiroidismo congenito (e presunto deficit di cellule C) hanno livelli di CT inferiori rispetto a quelli di bambini normali.

La sua azione pare essere indipendente da quella del PTH e della vitamina D. Si ritiene che il suo principale effetto biologico sia l'inibizione del riassorbimento osseo, attraverso una diminuzione del numero e dell'attività degli osteoclasti che riassorbono l'osso. Questa azione della CT viene sfruttata nel trattamento della malattia di Paget. La CT viene sintetizzata anche in altri organi, come il tratto gastrointestinale, il pancreas, il cervello e l'ipofisi. Si ritiene che in questi organi, la CT si comporti come un neurotrasmettitore a effetto inibitorio locale sulla funzionalità cellulare.

Capitolo 572 ■ Ipoparatiroidismo

EZIOLOGIA (TAB. 572-1). L'ipocalcemia è un evento frequente tra la dodicesima e la settantaduesima ora di vita, soprattutto nei neonati prematuri, con asfissia, e in quelli nati da madri diabetiche (ipocalcemia neonatale precoce) (vedi Capitolo 106). Dopo i primi 2-3 giorni e per la prima settimana di vita, anche il tipo di alimentazione è un fattore determinante per il livello sierico del calcio (ipocalcemia neonatale tardiva). Il ruolo giocato dalle ghiandole paratiroidi in questi neonati ipocalcemici rimane da chiarire, sebbene, come fattore patogenetico, sia considerata un'immaturità delle paratiroidi. In un gruppo di neonati con ipocalcemia idiopatica transitoria (1-8 settimane di vita), i livelli sierici dell'ormone paratiroideo (*Parathyroid Hormone*, PTH) sono significativamente inferiori a quelli di neonati normali. È possibile che l'immaturità funzionale sia una manifestazione del ritardo nello sviluppo degli enzimi che convertono il PTH ghiandolare in PTH secreto; sono possibili però altri meccanismi.

TABELLA 572-1. Classificazione eziologica dell'ipocalcemia

DEFICIT DI ORMONE PARATIROIDEO (PTH)
- Aplasia o ipoplasia delle paratiroidi
  - Con delezione 22q11
    - Sindrome di DiGeorge
    - Sindrome velocardiofacciale
    - Sindrome conotronco-facciale
  - Con delezione 10p13
  - Con diabete mellito materno o embriopatia da acido retinoico
  - Con ipoparatiroidismo isolato correlato a X
  - Con mutazione di *GCMB* (missing B della cellula gliale), autosomica recessiva
  - Con ritardo e dimorfismo (sindrome di Sanjad-Sakati), autosomica recessiva
  - Con sordità e displasia renale (mutazione di *GATA3*)
  - Con osteosclerosi (sindrome di Kenny-Caffey), mutazione di *TBCE*
- Soppressione della secrezione neonatale da iperparatiroidismo materno
- Mutazione del gene dell'ormone preproparatiroideo
  - Autosomica dominante
- Mutazione attivante del recettore per il Ca^{2+}
  - Sporadica
  - Autosomica dominante
- Paratiroidite autoimmune
  - Isolata
  - Con poliendocrinopatia autoimmune tipo I, APECED
    - Mutazione del gene *AIRE*
- Lesioni infiltrative
  - Emosiderosi (trattamento della talassemia)
  - Depositi di rame (malattia di Wilson)

DIFETTI DEL RECETTORE DEL PARATORMONE (PSEUDOIPOPARATIROIDISMO)
- Tipo IA (mutazione inattivante di $G_s\alpha$)
  - Con pubertà precoce gonadotropino-indipendente
- Tipo IB (imprinting paterno di *GNAS1*)
- Tipo II (normale risposta del cAMP)

MUTAZIONI DEL DNA MITOCONDRIALE
- Sindrome di Kearns-Sayre
- Sindrome midollo pancreas di Pearson
- Mutazione della catena lunga del 3-idrossiacilcoenzima A deidrogenasi

CARENZA DI MAGNESIO
- Perdita renale di magnesio (autosomica dominante)
- Malassorbimento di magnesio (autosomica recessiva)
- Terapia con aminoglicosidi

ECCESSO DI FOSFATI INORGANICI ESOGENI
- Lassativi
- Bevande dolci con acido fosforico

CARENZA DI VITAMINA D
- Nutrizionale
- Vitamina D-dipendente (rachitismo)
  - Mutazione dell'1α-(OH)asi (P450)

APLASIA O IPOPLASIA DELLE GHIANDOLE PARATIROIDI. Spesso è associata alla **sindrome di DiGeorge/velocardiofacciale** (vedi Fig. 571-1). Questa sindrome compare in uno su 4000 neonati. Nel 90% dei pazienti, la malattia è dovuta a una delezione del cromosoma 22q11.2. Circa il 25% di questi pazienti eredita l'anomalia cromosomica da un genitore. L'ipocalcemia neonatale si verifica nel 60% dei pazienti colpiti, ma nella maggior parte è transitoria; l'ipocalcemia può recidivare o può esordire successivamente nel corso della vita. È frequente l'associazione con anomalie della terza e quarta tasca faringea; esse comprendono difetti conotroncali del cuore nel 25% dei casi, insufficienza velofaringea nel 32%, fissurazione del palato nel 9%, anomalie renali nel 35% e aplasia timica con grave immunodeficienza nell'1%. Questa sindrome è stata riportata anche in un piccolo numero di pazienti con delezione del cromosoma 10p13, in neonati di madri diabetiche e in bambini nati da madri trattate, nelle fasi precoci della gravidanza, con acido retinoico per acne.

IPOPARATIROIDISMO RECESSIVO CORRELATO A X. Sono stati descritte varie tipologie familiari di ipoparatiroidismo con modalità diverse di trasmissione. In due numerosi gruppi familiari del Nord America, questa malattia viene trasmessa con un gene recessivo correlato a X localizzato su Xq26-q27. In queste famiglie, l'esordio di crisi apiretiche si verifica in modo caratteristico nei neonati dalla seconda settimana al sesto mese di vita. L'assenza di tessuto paratiroideo dopo esame dettagliato di un bambino con questa condizione suggerisce un difetto dell'embriogenesi.

IPOPARATIROIDISMO AUTOSOMICO RECESSIVO CON CARATTERISTICHE DISMORFICHE. Questa sindrome è stata descritta in bambini mediorientali. Per quasi tutte le numerose decine di pazienti affetti, è presente consanguineità tra i genitori. Si instaura precocemente una notevole ipocalcemia e le caratteristiche dismorfiche comprendono microcefalia, occhi infossati, naso a becco, micrognatismo e orecchie grandi e flosce. Il ritardo di crescita è grave, sia nella fase intrauterina sia in quella postnatale, ed è frequente il ritardo mentale. Il gene responsabile si trova sul cromosoma 1q42-43. La forma autosomica recessiva di ipoparatiroidismo, che compare con la patologia autoimmunitaria polighiandolare tipo I è descritta oltre. In pochi pazienti con ipoparatiroidismo isolato a ereditarietà autosomica recessiva sono state trovate mutazioni del gene del PTH.

SINDROME HDR. Mutazioni del gene *GATA3* provocano ipoparatiroidismo, sordità neurosensoriale, anomalie renali. La proteina codificata da questo gene è essenziale per lo sviluppo delle paratiroidi, dell'apparato uditivo e dei reni. Il gene *GATA3* è localizzato sul cromosoma 10p14 e non c'è sovrapposizione con la regione critica della sindrome di DiGeorge, a livello 10p13 (vedi Fig. 571-1).

SOPPRESSIONE DELLA SECREZIONE NEONATALE DI PTH DA IPERPARATIROIDISMO MATERNO. Questo può comportare una transitoria ipocalcemia del neonato. Sembra che l'ipocalcemia neonatale derivi da soppressione delle ghiandole paratiroidee fetali conseguente all'esposizione a elevati livelli di calcio nel siero materno e fetale. Di solito entro le prime tre settimane di vita si sviluppa tetania, ma può ritardare al primo mese o anche oltre se il bambino è allattato al seno. L'ipocalcemia può persistere per settimane o mesi. Se la causa dell'ipocalcemia in un neonato è sconosciuta, vanno eseguite valutazioni della calcemia, fosforemia e del PTH anche nella madre. La maggior parte delle madri affette è asintomatica e la causa del loro iperparatiroidismo di solito è rappresentata da un adenoma paratiroideo.

IPOPARATIRPOIDISMO AUTOSOMICO DOMINANTE. Questi pazienti hanno una mutazione attivante (aumento di funzione) del recettore per il Ca^{2+}, che conferisce al recettore stesso uno stato "attivato", con conseguente inibizione della secrezione di PTH anche in presenza di ipocalcemia. Questi pazienti presentano ipercalciuria.

L'ipocalcemia è solitamente di modesta entità e può anche non richiedere ulteriore trattamento nell'infanzia (vedi Fig. 571-1).

IPOPARATIROIDISMO ASSOCIATO A PATOLOGIE MITOCONDRIALI. Mutazioni del DNA mitocondriale nella sindrome di Kearns-Sayre e della proteina mitocondriale trifunzionale sono associate a ipoparatiroidismo. Si deve prendere in considerazione la diagnosi di citopatia mitocondriale in pazienti con sintomi non spiegabili, come oftalmoplegia, perdita dell'udito neurosensoriale, disturbi della conduzione cardiaca e tetania (vedi Fig. 571-1).

IPOPARATIROIDISMO CHIRURGICO. La tiroidectomia può essere complicata dalla rimozione o dal danno alle ghiandole paratiroidi. Si può sviluppare ipoparatiroidismo anche se le paratiroidi, una volta identificate, sono lasciate intatte al momento dell'intervento. Questo può dipendere da un'interferenza con il flusso ematico o da un edema o fibrosi postoperatoria. I sintomi tipici di tetania possono comparire bruscamente nel periodo postoperatorio e possono essere temporanei o permanenti. In alcuni casi, i sintomi si possono sviluppare insidiosamente e non venire scoperti fino a mesi dopo la tiroidectomia. Occasionalmente, il primo segno di ipoparatiroidismo chirurgico può essere lo sviluppo di una cataratta. È necessario monitorare attentamente la funzionalità paratiroidea in tutti i pazienti sottoposti a tiroidectomia.

La deposizione di pigmenti a base di ferro o di rame nelle ghiandole paratiroidee (talassemia, malattia di Wilson) può portare a ipoparatiroidismo.

IPOPARATIROIDISMO AUTOIMMUNE. Il reperto di anticorpi antiparatiroide indica un meccanismo autoimmunitario nella genesi l'ipoparatiroidismo ed è frequente l'associazione con altre patologie autoimmunitarie o anticorpi organo-specifici. L'ipoparatiroidismo autoimmune è spesso associato alla malattia di Addison e alla candidosi mucocutanea cronica. L'associazione di almeno due di queste tre condizioni è stata provvisoriamente classificata come **malattia autoimmune polighiandolare tipo I.** È nota inoltre come poliendocrinopatia autoimmune/candidosi/distrofia ectodermica. Questa sindrome ereditaria si trasmette con modalità autosomica recessiva e non è correlata a un qualche singolo aplotipo HLA. Un terzo dei pazienti con questa sindrome presenta tutte e tre le componenti, mentre due terzi ne ha invece solo due. La candidosi quasi sempre precede le altre patologie (il 70% dei casi si verifica in bambini con meno di 5 anni di età); l'ipoparatiroidismo (90% dopo i 3 anni) di solito compare prima della malattia di Addison (90% dopo i 6 anni di età). Molte altre patologie compaiono in momenti diversi, come alopecia areata o totale, malassorbimento, anemia perniciosa, insufficienza gonadica, epatite attiva cronica, vitiligine e diabete insulino-dipendente. Alcune di queste associazioni possono non manifestarsi fino all'età adulta. Una patologia autoimmune della tiroide costituisce un reperto raro.

Fratelli affetti possono mostrare la stessa varietà di patologie, o quadri diversi (ipoparatiroidismo, malattia di Addison). La malattia è molto frequente nella popolazione finlandese e iraniana. Il gene di questa malattia è denominato *AIRE* (*Autoimmune Regulator*, regolatore autoimmunitario) ed è localizzato sul cromosoma 21q22. Esiste un fattore di trascrizione che gioca un ruolo essenziale nello sviluppo della tolleranza immunitaria. Pazienti con la malattia di Addison come parte della sindrome poliendocrinopatia tipo I rivelano una reattività autoanticorpale specifica per il surrene, diretta contro l'enzima di separazione della catena laterale.

IPOPARATIROIDISMO IDIOPATICO. Questo termine deve essere riservato a quell'esiguo numero di bambini con ipoparatiroidismo in cui non si sia definito alcun meccanismo causale. La maggior parte dei bambini in cui l'esordio dell'ipoparatiroidismo si verifica dopo i primi anni di vita presenta una **patologia autoimmunitaria.** In alcuni pazienti con ipoparatiroidismo acquisito sono stati identificati autoanticorpi contro i domini cellulari del recettore del calcio. Si dovrebbero sempre prendere in considerazione, nella diagnosi differenziale, forme incomplete di sindrome di DiGeorge o una mutazione attivante del recettore del calcio.

Manifestazioni cliniche. Esiste una serie di deficit paratiroidei con manifestazioni cliniche diverse, che spaziano dall'assenza di sintomatologia a forme complete di deficit di lunga durata. La carenza modesta può essere rilevata solo con appropriate indagini di laboratorio. Dolore muscolare e crampi sono manifestazioni precoci; l'evoluzione porta a intorpidimento, rigidità e parestesie a mani e piedi. Ci può essere solo una positività ai segni di Chvostek o di Trousseau, o spasmi laringei o carpopedali. A intervalli di giorni, settimane o mesi possono manifestarsi convulsioni con o senza perdita di coscienza. Questi episodi possono iniziare con dolore addominale, seguito da rigidità tonica, retrazione del capo e cianosi. L'ipoparatiroidismo è frequentemente confuso con l'epilessia; cefalea, vomito, ipertensione endocranica e papilledema possono essere associati alle convulsioni e indicare la presenza di un tumore cerebrale.

In pazienti con ipocalcemia di lunga durata, l'eruzione dentaria è tardiva e irregolare. La formazione dello smalto è irregolare e i denti possono essere particolarmente teneri. La cute può presentarsi secca e squamosa e le unghie delle dita delle mani e dei piedi possono evidenziare delle linee orizzontali. Quando presente, la candidosi mucocutanea precede lo sviluppo dell'ipoparatiroidismo; l'infezione da candida più spesso coinvolge le unghie, la mucosa orale, gli angoli della bocca e, meno spesso, la cute; essa è difficile da trattare.

Le cataratte presenti nei pazienti con malattia di lunga durata non trattata sono una diretta conseguenza dell'ipoparatiroidismo; si possono manifestare altre patologie oculari autoimmunitarie, come la cheratocongiuntivite. Le manifestazioni legate alla malattia di Addison, alla tiroidite linfocitica, all'anemia perniciosa, all'alopecia areata o totale, all'epatite e alla insufficienza gonadica primitiva possono essere associate a quelle dell'ipoparatiroidismo.

Se si inizia il trattamento con notevole ritardo può manifestarsi una compromissione psicofisica permanente.

Reperti di laboratorio. La calcemia è bassa (5-7 mg/dL) e la fosfatemia elevata (7-12 mg/dL). I livelli ematici di calcio ionizzato (di solito circa il 45% del totale) riflettono meglio l'adeguatezza fisiologica, ma sono anch'essi bassi. Il livello sierico della fosfatasi alcalina è normale o basso e quello di 1,25-$[OH]_2D3$ è solitamente basso, ma, in alcuni bambini con grave ipocalcemia, è stato trovato elevato. La magnesiemia è normale, ma deve sempre essere indagata in pazienti ipocalcemici. I livelli di PTH sono bassi se misurati con metodiche immunometriche. La somministrazione del frammento 1-34 umano di PTH (teriparatide acetato) comporta un incremento dei livelli urinari di adenosina ciclica monofosfato e fosfato. Questa risposta è in grado di differenziare l'ipoparatiroidismo dallo pseudoipoparatiroidismo. Con l'avvento di dosaggi del PTH molto sensibili, normalmente questo test non è necessario. L'indagine radiografica delle ossa occasionalmente rivela un aumento della densità limitato alle metafisi, indicativo di intossicazione da metalli pesanti o un aumento della densità della lamina dura. L'indagine radiografica o la TC del cranio possono evidenziare calcificazioni dei gangli basali. All'elettrocardiogramma è presente un prolungamento dell'intervallo QT, che scompare con la correzione dell'ipocalcemia. L'elettroencefalogramma rivela di norma segni diffusi di attività rallentata; il tracciato ritorna normale dopo che la concentrazione sierica del calcio è stata riportata nel range della normalità da qualche settimana, a meno che non si sia verificato un danno cerebrale irreversibile o che l'insufficienza paratiroidea non si associ a epilessia. Se l'ipoparatiroidismo compare in un soggetto affetto da malattia di Addison, la calcemia può essere inizialmente normale, ma, dopo che l'insufficienza surrenalica è stata efficacemente trattata, si evidenzia l'ipocalcemia.

Trattamento. Il trattamento di urgenza della tetania neonatale consiste nell'iniezione per via endovenosa di 5-10 mL di una soluzione al 10% di calcio gluconato, alla velocità di 0,5-1 mL/min, con contemporaneo monitoraggio della frequenza cardiaca. In aggiunta, si deve somministrare 1,25-diidrocolecalciferolo (calcitriolo). Il dosaggio iniziale è di 0,25 μg/die; il dosaggio va mantenuto in un range compreso tra 0,01 e 0,10 μg/kg/die, fino a un massimo di 1-2 μg/die. Il calcitriolo ha una breve emivita e deve essere somministrato in due dosi equivalenti; ha il vantaggio di effetti rapidi (1-4 giorni) e anche di un rapido ritorno all'ipocalcemia dopo sospensione in caso di sovradosaggio (livelli di calcio cominciano a diminuire in 3-4 giorni). Il calcitriolo è fornito in soluzione per os.

È necessario assicurare un adeguato apporto di calcio. Può essere attuata una supplementazione di calcio con la somministrazione di calcio gluconato o di calcio glubionato, in modo da garantire 800 mg/die di calcio, ma raramente è essenziale. Devono essere diminuiti nella dieta tutti gli alimenti ad alto contenuto di fosforo, come il latte, le uova e il formaggio.

Nelle fasi precoci del trattamento sono indicate sia la valutazione clinica del paziente che frequenti determinazioni della calcemia, per determinare la dose più idonea di calcitriolo o vitamina D_2. In caso di ipercalcemia, si deve interrompere la terapia e, al ripristino di una condizione di normocalcemia, si deve riprendere, ma a dosaggi inferiori. Nei casi di lunga durata è improbabile la remissione di eventuali modificazioni cerebrali o dentarie. Pigmentazione, diminuzione della pressione arteriosa o calo ponderale possono indicare un'insufficienza surrenalica, che richiede uno specifico trattamento. Pazienti con ipercalciuria ipocalcemica autosomica dominante, possono andare incontro a nefrocalcinosi e danno renale se trattati con vitamina D.

Diagnosi differenziale. Deve essere presa in considerazione l'ipomagnesiemia in pazienti con ipocalcemia di natura sconosciuta. Concentrazioni sieriche di magnesio inferiori a 1,5 mg/dL (1,2 mEq/L) sono di solito anomale. L'ipomagnesiemia familiare con ipocalcemia secondaria è stata riportata in 50 pazienti, la maggior parte dei quali aveva sviluppato tetania e crisi epilettiche all'età di 2-6 settimane. La somministrazione di calcio è inefficace, mentre quella di magnesio corregge prontamente sia i livelli di calcio sia quelli di magnesio. La supplementazione orale di magnesio è necessaria per mantenere i livelli di quest'ultimo nel range della normalità. Sono state descritte due forme genetiche. Una è causata da un gene autosomico recessivo situato sul cromosoma 9, che comporta uno specifico difetto dell'assorbimento del magnesio. L'altro è dovuto a un gene autosomico dominante sul cromosoma 11q23, con perdita renale di magnesio.

Ipomagnesiemia si verifica anche nelle sindromi da malassorbimento, come il morbo di Crohn e la fibrosi cistica. Pazienti con malattia polighiandolare autoimmune di tipo I e ipoparatiroidismo possono presentare anche una concomitante steatorrea e bassi livelli di magnesio. La terapia con aminoglicosidi provoca ipomagnesiemia con aumento delle perdite urinarie. Non è chiaro come i bassi livelli di magnesio portino a ipocalcemia. I dati suggeriscono che l'ipomagnesiemia comprometta il rilascio di PTH e induca resistenza agli effetti dell'ormone, ma possono essere operativi anche altri meccanismi.

L'intossicazione con fosfati inorganici porta a ipocalcemia e tetania. Neonati a cui sono somministrate alte dosi di fosfati inorganici, sia come lassativi sia come enemi di fosfato sodico, hanno manifestato una tetania a esordio improvviso, con calcemia inferiore a 5 mg/dL e livelli notevolmente elevati di fosfati. I sintomi sono scomparsi rapidamente con la somministrazione endovenosa di calcio. Il meccanismo dell'ipocalcemia non è chiaro (vedi Capitolo 52.6).

Ipocalcemia può comparire precocemente durante il trattamento della leucemia acuta linfoblastica. Normalmente è associata a iperfosfatemia, con conseguente distruzione dei linfoblasti.

Ipocalcemia episodica sintomatica si verifica nella **sindrome di Kenny-Caffey**, caratterizzata da stenosi midollare delle ossa lunghe, bassa statura, ritardo della chiusura delle fontanelle e dell'età ossea, e anomalie oculari. Sono state riportate modalità di trasmissione ereditaria autosomica dominante e autosomica recessiva. Mutazioni del gene *TBCE* (1q43-44) alterano l'organizzazione microtubulare delle cellule malate.

Capitolo 573 ■ Pseudoipoparatiroidismo (osteodistrofia ereditaria di Albright)

Al contrario dell'ipoparatiroidismo, nello pseudoipoparatiroidismo (PHP) le ghiandole paratiroidi sono normali o iperplastiche e sono in grado di sintetizzare e secernere l'ormone paratiroideo (PTH). I livelli sierici di PTH immunoreattivo sono elevati, anche se il paziente è ipocalcemico, e possono essere alti anche in presenza di normocalcemia. Né il PTH esogeno né quello endogeno è in grado di aumentare i livelli sierici di calcio o di diminuire quelli di fosforo. I difetti genetici del **sistema dell'AMPciclico connesso al recettore dell'ormone** sono classificati in diversi tipi, a seconda del fenotipo e dei reperti biochimici.

TIPO IA. Il tipo IA accoglie la maggior parte dei pazienti con PHP. Essi presentano un difetto genetico della subunità α della proteina stimolante che lega la guanosina ($G_S\alpha$). Questo fattore di associazione è necessario affinché il PTH, dopo il legame con i recettori della superficie cellulare, possa attivare l'adenosina monofosfato ciclica (AMP). Sono state documentate mutazioni eterogenee del gene di $G_S\alpha$, localizzato sul cromosoma 20q13.2. Il deficit di una subunità in $G_S\alpha$ rappresenta un difetto cellulare generalizzato e giustifica l'associazione del PHP di tipo Ia ad altre malattie endocrine. Il difetto, ereditario, si trasmette con modalità autosomica dominante e si pensa che la rarità della trasmissione padre-figlio sia dovuta a una diminuzione della fertilità maschile.

La tetania è spesso il segno d'esordio. I bambini colpiti hanno una corporatura bassa, tozza e un viso tondeggiante. Normalmente è presente brachidattilia con retrazione cutanea del dorso della mano. Meno frequentemente è colpito il secondo metacarpale, così che il dito indice può occasionalmente essere più lungo del medio. Analogamente, di rado è colpito il secondo metatarsale. Si possono associare altre anomalie scheletriche, come falangi corte e larghe, curvatura, esostosi e ispessimento del cranio. Questi pazienti frequentemente presentano depositi di calcio e metaplasia ossea a livello del tessuto sottocutaneo. In pazienti che ricevono una diagnosi tardiva, sono frequenti: ritardo mentale di grado modesto, calcificazione dei gangli basali e cataratta lenticolare.

Alcuni parenti di bambini colpiti possono presentare le stesse stigmate anatomiche del PHP, ma avere livelli sierici di calcio e di fosforo normali, nonostante la riduzione dell'attività della proteina $G_S\alpha$; tuttavia, i livelli di PTH possono essere lievemente elevati. Questa condizione è stata denominata **pseudopseudoipoparatiroidismo.** Spesso, con l'aumentare dell'età, si passa da una condizione di normocalcemia a una di ipocalcemia. Questi pazienti, fenotipicamente simili ma metabolicamente diversi, possono appartenere alla stessa famiglia e presentare le stesse mutazioni della proteina $G_S\alpha$. Non si conosce il motivo per cui i fattori provochino un'ipocalcemia clinicamente manifesta in certi pazienti e non in altri. Si pensa che la mutazione di $G_S\alpha$ sia trasmessa dal padre nello pseudopseudoipoparatiroidismo e dalla madre nei pazienti con la malattia di tipo Ia. Il gene può subire un imprinting tessuto-specifico.

Oltre alla resistenza al PTH, anche la resistenza ad altri recettori associati a proteina G per l'ormone stimolante la tiroide (TSH), per le gonadotropine e per il glucagone può portare a effetti metabolici diversi. L'ipotiroidismo clinico non è frequente, ma sono elevati i livelli basali di TSH ed è esagerata la risposta del TSH all'ormone di rilascio della tireotropina. Nell'ambito di programmi di screening neonatale, la scoperta di livelli di tiroxina moderatamente diminuiti, con TSH aumentato, ha portato alla scoperta del PHP tipo Ia nell'infanzia. Negli adulti, è frequente l'alterazione gonadica, che si manifesta con immaturità sessuale, amenorrea, oligomenorrea e infertilità. Ciascuna di queste anomalie può essere correlata al deficit della sintesi di AMP ciclico secondario alla carenza di $G_S\alpha$, ma non è chiaro per quale motivo la resistenza ad altri ormoni proteina G-dipendenti (corticotropina, vasopressina) sia molto più rara.

I livelli sierici di calcio sono bassi e quelli di fosforo e di fosfatasi alcalina elevati. La diagnosi clinica può essere confermata dalla dimostrazione di una risposta notevolmente diminuita, riguardante l'eliminazione urinaria di fosfati e AMP ciclico, dopo infusione endovenosa del frammento sintetico umano del PTH 1-34 (teriparatide acetato). La diagnosi definitiva è stabilita dalla dimostrazione di una proteina G mutata.

Tipo Ia con pubertà precoce. È stato riportato il caso di due bambini con PHP tipo Ia e pubertà precoce gonadotropino-indipendente (vedi Capitolo 563.6). Avevano una mutazione termosensibile della proteina G_S. Questa, alla normale temperatura corporea (37 °C), va incontro a degradazione con conseguente PHP, ma, alla temperatura inferiore dei testicoli (33 °C), porta a un'attivazione costitutiva del recettore dell'ormone luteinizzante e a pubertà precoce.

TIPO IB. I pazienti colpiti hanno normali livelli di attività della proteina G e un normale fenotipo. Presentano una resistenza tessuto-specifica al PTH, ma non ad altri ormoni. I livelli sierici di calcio, fosforo e di PTH immunoreattivo sono analoghi a quelli di pazienti con PHP di tipo Ia. Questi pazienti, però, non presentano un aumento dell'AMPciclico in risposta alla somministrazione esogena di PTH. Il PTH biologicamente attivo non è aumentato. La fisiopatologia dell'alterazione in questo gruppo di pazienti è legata a un'isodisomia uniparentale, paterna, del cromosoma 20q e comporta una metilazione di *GNAS1*. Questo, solo con la perdita del gene *GNAS1* materno, porta a resistenza al PTH nei tubuli prossimali renali, con conseguente alterazione dell'omeostasi minerale ionica.

TIPO II. Il tipo II è stato scoperto solo in pochi pazienti e si differenzia dalla forma I in quanto l'escrezione urinaria di AMPciclico è elevata, sia in condizioni basali sia dopo stimolazione con PTH, mentre la fosfaturia non aumenta. Da un punto di vista fenotipico, i pazienti sono normali ed è presente ipocalcemia. Il difetto è distale all'AMPciclico, perché quest'ultimo è normalmente attivato, ma la cellula non è in grado di rispondere al suo segnale.

Capitolo 574 ■ Iperparatiroidismo

La causa di un'eccessiva produzione di ormone paratiroideo (PTH) può essere rappresentata da un difetto primario delle ghiandole paratiroidi, come un adenoma o un'iperplasia (iperparatiroidismo primario).

Più spesso, l'incremento della produzione di PTH è compensatorio, solitamente volto a correggere uno stato di ipocalcemia che può avere origini diverse (iperaparatiroidismo secondario). Nel rachitismo da deficit di vitamina D e nelle sindromi da malassorbimento, è scarso l'assorbimento intestinale del calcio, ma l'ipocalcemia e la tetania possono essere prevenute da un aumento dell'attività delle paratiroidi. Nello **pseudoipoparatiroidismo**, i livelli di PTH sono elevati perché una mutazione della proteina $G_S\alpha$ interferisce con la risposta al PTH stesso. Nelle fasi precoci delle patologie renali croniche, l'iperfosfatemia si accompagna a un parallelo decremento della concentrazione del calcio, con conseguente aumento del PTH, ma, negli stadi avanzati di insufficienza renale, diminuisce anche la produzione di 1,25-$[OH]_2D_3$, con peggioramento dell'ipocalcemia e ulteriore stimolazione del PTH. In alcuni casi, se la stimolazione delle paratiroidi è sufficientemente intensa e protratta, le ghiandole possono continuare a secernere alti livelli di PTH per mesi o per anni dopo un trapianto renale, con conseguente ipercalcemia.

EZIOLOGIA. L'iperparatiroidismo infantile è una patologia rara. L'esordio durante l'infanzia depone a favore di un singolo adenoma benigno, che di solito si manifesta dopo il decimo anno di età. È noto un gruppo di famiglie in cui parecchi membri presentano iperparatiroidismo a trasmissione autosomica dominante. La maggior parte dei soggetti affetti è adulta, ma circa un terzo degli ascendenti è stato colpito da bambino. In queste famiglie alcuni pazienti sono asintomatici e sono stati individuati solo con attente valutazioni. In altri parenti compare un iperparatiroidismo nell'ambito di una serie di altre patologie, quadro noto come sindrome da **neoplasia endocrina multipla** (MEN) o sindrome iperparatiroidismo-tumore della mandibola.

L'iperparatiroidismo grave neonatale è una patologia rara. I sintomi si sviluppano rapidamente dopo la nascita e consistono in anoressia, irritabilità, letargia, stipsi e mancanza di sviluppo. L'indagine radiografica rivela riassorbimento osseo subperiostale, osteoporosi e fratture patologiche. I sintomi possono essere lievi e risolversi senza trattamento; oppure possono presentare rapidamente un decorso fatale, se la diagnosi e il trattamento vengono ritardati. Istologicamente, le paratiroidi mostrano iperplasia diffusa. In alcune famiglie sono stati colpiti dei fratelli e in parecchi nuclei è stata riportata consanguineità fra i genitori. La maggior parte dei casi si è verificata in famiglie con caratteristiche cliniche e biochimiche di **ipercalcemia ipocalciurica familiare**. Bambini con iperparatiroidismo grave neonatale possono essere omo o eterozigoti per mutazione del gene del recettore sensibile al Ca^{2+}, mentre la maggior parte degli individui con una copia di questa mutazione evidenzia un'ipercalcemia ipocalciurica familiare autosomica dominante.

La **MEN tipo I** è una patologia autosomica dominante caratterizzata da iperplasia o neoplasia del pancreas endocrino (che secerne gastrina, insulina, polipeptide pancreatico e occasionalmente glucagone), dell'ipofisi anteriore (che di solito secerne prolattina) e delle ghiandole paratiroidee. Nella maggior parte delle famiglie, l'iperparatiroidismo rappresenta in genere la manifestazione d'esordio, con una diffusione vicina al 100% a 50 anni di età, mentre si verifica solo di rado nei ragazzi con meno di 18 anni. Con adeguate indagini sul DNA, è possibile scoprire alla nascita, con un'accuratezza del 99%, i portatori del gene, evitando così inutili programmi di screening biochimico.

Il gene per la MEN tipo I si trova sul cromosoma 11q13; funziona come un gene oncosoppressore e segue le due ipotesi prevalenti dello sviluppo del tumore. La prima mutazione (germinale) è ereditaria e recessiva per l'allele dominante e non comporta sviluppo tumorale. Per eliminare l'allele normale è necessaria una seconda mutazione (somatica), che dà successivamente origine al tumore.

La **sindrome iperparatiroidismo-tumore della mandibola** è una patologia autosomica dominante caratterizzata da adenomi paratiroidei e tumori fibro-ossei della mandibola. Possono essere presenti anche: malattia policistica renale, amartomi renali e tumore di Wilms. Sebbene questa patologia colpisca principalmente gli adulti, si è riscontrata anche più precocemente, in bambini di 10 anni.

La **MEN tipo II** può essere associata a iperparatiroidismo (vedi Capitolo 570.2).

L'**iperparatiroidismo neonatale transitorio** è un patologia poco frequente, riscontrata in bambini nati da madri ipoparatiroidee (ipoparatiroidismo idiopatico o chirurgico) o pseudoipoparatiroidee. In tutti questi casi la patologia materna non era stata diagnosticata o era stata inadeguatamente trattata durante la gravidanza. La causa della malattia è rappresentata dall'esposizione cronica, durante la vita intrauterina, all'ipocalcemia, con conseguente iperplasia delle paratiroidi fetali. Nel neonato le manifestazioni coinvolgono principalmente le ossa e la guarigione si completa tra il quarto e il settimo mese di età.

MANIFESTAZIONI CLINICHE. A tutte le età, le manifestazioni cliniche di ipercalcemia, qualunque sia la causa, comprendono astenia muscolare, affaticamento, cefalea, anoressia, dolore addominale, nausea, vomito, stipsi, polidipsia, poliuria, perdita di peso e febbre. Se l'ipercalcemia è di lunga durata, il calcio si può depositare nel parenchima renale (nefrocalcinosi), con progressiva diminuzione della funzionalità renale. Si possono formare calcoli renali con coliche ed ematuria. Le modificazioni ossee possono provocare dolore alla schiena o agli arti, alterazioni dell'andatura, ginocchio valgo, fratture e tumori. Si può verificare diminuzione dell'altezza, per compressione vertebrale; il paziente può essere costretto a letto. Con l'avvento di dosaggi a pannello automatico, che includono la determinazione della calcemia, è aumentato il numero di diagnosi di pazienti completamente asintomatici.

Il dolore addominale talvolta è molto rilevante e può accompagnare una **pancreatite acuta**. Si può verificare una crisi paratiroidea, che si manifesta con livelli ematici di calcio maggiori di 15 mg/dL e progressiva oliguria, iperazotemia, *stupor* e coma. Nei neonati sono comuni mancanza di sviluppo, iponutrizione e ipotonia. Come postumi di una ipercalcemia di lunga durata possono comparire ritardo mentale, convulsioni e cecità.

REPERTI DI LABORATORIO. Il livello sierico del calcio è elevato; 39 dei 45 bambini con adenoma presentavano valori superiori a 12 mg/dL. L'ipercalcemia è più severa nei neonati con iperplasia paratiroidea; sono frequenti concentrazioni variabili da 15 a 20 mg/dL, fino a valori di 30 mg/dL. Anche se la calcemia totale è borderline o solo lievemente aumentata, i livelli del calcio ionizzato sono spesso aumentati. La fosforemia è ridotta a circa 3 mg/dL o meno e la magnesiemia è bassa. Le urine possono presentare un peso specifico basso e non modificabile e l'azotemia e l'uricemia possono essere elevate. In pazienti con adenomi e lesioni scheletriche sono presenti elevati livelli di fosfatasi, ma nei neonati con iperplasia, la fosfatasi alcalina può essere normale anche in presenza di compromissione ossea diffusa.

I livelli sierici di PTH, misurati con sieri immunizzanti carbossiterminali, sono elevati, specialmente in rapporto alla calcemia. I risultati possono essere molto diversi da un laboratorio all'altro, a seconda dell'anticorpo usato. I livelli di calcitonina sono normali. Un'ipercalcemia acuta può stimolare il rilascio di calcitonina; ma con una ipercalcemia cronica non si verifica ipercalcitoninemia.

La maggior parte dei reperti radiografici caratteristici e di un certo rilievo sono rappresentati da riassorbimento osseo subperiostale, meglio visibile lungo i margini delle falangi delle mani. Nel cranio, si può evidenziare una notevole trabecolatura o un aspetto granulare per rarefazione focale; la lamina dura può essere assente. Nelle forme più avanzate, si possono evidenziare rarefazione generalizzata, cisti, tumori, fratture e deformità. Circa il 10% dei pazienti mostra segni radiografici di rachitismo. L'indagine radiografica dell'addome può rivelare calcoli renali o nefrocalcinosi.

DIAGNOSI DIFFERENZIALE. Altre cause di ipercalcemia possono manifestarsi con un quadro simile e vanno differenziate dall'iperparatiroidismo (Tab. 574-1). L'ipofosfatemia con l'ipercalcemia sono caratteristiche dell'iperparatiroidismo primario; anche elevati livelli di PTH hanno significato diagnostico. Nelle altre forme di ipercalcemia, eccetto l'iperparatiroidismo e l'ipercalcemia ipocalciurica familiare, i livelli di PTH sono soppressi. Dosi farmacologiche di corticosteroidi abbassano la calcemia a valori normali in pazienti con ipercalcemia dovuta ad altre cause, ma generalmente non incidono sui valori calcemici degli iperparatioridei.

TRATTAMENTO. In tutte le forme è indicata l'esplorazione chirurgica. È necessario ispezionare molto attentamente tutte le paratiroidi; un eventuale adenoma deve essere rimosso; nei bambini si sono trovati pochissimi carcinomi. La maggior parte dei neonati con ipercalcemia severa richiede una paratiroidectomia totale; forme meno gravi invece possono avere una remissione spontanea. Una parte della ghiandola paratiroidea può essere autoinnestata nell'avambraccio. Nel postoperatorio il paziente deve essere controllato attentamente per la possibilità che si sviluppi ipocalcemia e tetania; può essere necessaria per qualche giorno la somministrazione endovenosa di gluconato di calcio. La calcemia torna poi gradualmente nella norma ed è opportuno mantenere, solo per qualche mese dopo l'intervento, una dieta ad alto contenuto di calcio e fosforo.

TABELLA 574-1. Classificazione eziologica dell'ipercalcemia

ECCESSO DI ORMONE PARATIROIDEO (PTH)
Iperparatiroidismo primario
Adenoma
Sporadico
Autosomico dominante
Sindrome da iperparatiroidismo/tumore della mandibola
Iperplasia o adenoma
Neoplasia endocrina multipla tipo I
Mutazione del gene di MEN I (11q13)
Iperplasia paratiroidea dell'infanzia
Mutazione inattivante del recettore sensibile al Ca^{2+}
Secondaria a ipoparatiroidismo materno
Produzione ectopica di PTH
Tumori non endocrini
ECCESSO DI PEPTIDE CORRELATO ALL'ORMONE PARATIROIDEO (PTHrP)
Tumori non endocrini
Ipertrofia mammaria benigna
MUTAZIONE INATTIVANTE DEL RECETTORE SENSIBILE AL Ca^{2+}
Ipercalcemia ipocalciurica familiare eterozigote
Iperparatiroidismo grave neonatale
MUTAZIONE ATTIVANTE DEL RECETTORE DI PTH/PTHrP
Autosomica dominante
Condrodisplasia metafisaria tipo Jansen
MUTAZIONE INATTIVANTEDEL RECETTORE DI PTH/PTHrP
Autosomica recessiva
Condrodisplasia di Blomstrand
ECCESSO DI VITAMINA D
Iatrogenico
Da produzione ectopica
Sarcoidosi, tubercolosi, lesioni granulomatosa, necrosi adiposa sottocutanea
Latte addizionato in modo eccessivo
CAUSA SCONOSCIUTA
Sindrome di Williams (delezione 7q11.23)
ALTRI
Ipofosfatasia
Mutazione del gene della fosfatasi alcalina non tessuto-specifica
Immobilizzazione prolungata
Tireotossicosi
Ipervitaminosi A
Leucemia
Ipercalcemia ipocalciurica acquisita (autoanticorpi contro il recettore sensibile al calcio)

Nel 50-90% degli adulti è possibile una diagnosi differenziale tra un singolo adenoma e l'iperplasia diffusa, utilizzando TC, ecografia real-time, scintigrafia a sottrazione di immagini con Tc-sestamibi e Tc-pertecnetato da soli o in combinazione. Chirurghi esperti raramente richiedono queste procedure, poiché attualmente, per localizzare e rimuovere la sorgente dell'aumentata secrezione di PTH, ci si basa spesso sul prelievo di campioni venosi selettivi per il dosaggio intraoperatorio del PTH stesso.

PROGNOSI. La prognosi è buona se la malattia viene riconosciuta precocemente e trattata chirurgicamente. In presenza di lesioni ossee diffuse, le difformità possono essere permanenti. È consigliata l'estensione delle indagini ad altri familiari.

574.1 • Altre cause di ipercalcemia

IPERCALCEMIA IPOCALCIURICA FAMILIARE (IPERCALCEMIA FAMILIARE BENIGNA). Questi pazienti di solito sono asintomatici e l'ipercalcemia è un reperto casuale, durante le indagini di routine eseguite per altre condizioni. Le paratiroidi sono normali, i livelli di PTH sono inappropriatamente normali e la paratiroidectomia non è in grado di correggere l'ipercalcemia. La magnesiemia è alta, normale o moderatamente elevata. Il rapporto calcio/clearance della creatinina è di solito diminuito, nonostante l'ipercalcemia. La malattia è ereditaria con modalità autosomica dominante ed è causata dalla mutazione di un gene sul cromosoma 3q2. La penetranza è vicina al 100% e i pazienti possono essere riconosciuti precocemente nell'infanzia tramite la valutazione delle concentrazioni sieriche e urinarie di calcio. È importante indagare per scoprire altri familiari affetti, onde evitare inutili interventi chirurgici sulle paratiroidi. Il difetto di base in questa malattia è legato a una mutazione inattivante del gene del recettore sensibile al Ca^{2+}. Questo recettore associato alla proteina G, è sensibile ai livelli del Ca^{2+} libero nel sangue e innesca l'insieme di reazioni volte ad aumentare il Ca^{2+} extracellulare in presenza di ipocalcemia. Questo recettore per l'omeostasi calcica è funzionante nelle paratiroidi e nel rene; mutazioni inattivanti portano a un innalzamento del set-point del Ca^{2+} sierico, con conseguente ipercalcemia da lieve a moderata negli eterozigoti.

MALATTIE GRANULOMATOSE. Nel 30-50% di bambini con sarcoidosi, e meno spesso in quelli con altre patologie granulomatose, come la tubercolosi, si verifica ipercalcemia. I livelli di PTH sono soppressi e quelli di 1,25-$[OH]_2D_3$ elevati. La sorgente **ectopica di 1,25-$[OH]_2D_3$** è il macrofago attivato, attraverso la stimolazione dell'interferone α dai linfociti T, presenti in abbondanza nelle lesioni granulomatose. Contrariamente a quella delle cellule tubulari renali, l'1α-idrossilasi macrofagica non risponde alla regolazione omeostatica. La somministrazione orale di prednisone (2 mg/kg/die) abbassa i livelli sierici di 1,25-$[OH]_2D_3$ a valori normali e corregge l'ipercalcemia.

IPERCALCEMIA DELLE NEOPLASIE. L'ipercalcemia si verifica frequentemente negli adulti colpiti da una serie di tumori solidi, ma meno spesso nei bambini. È stata riportata in neonati con tumori rabdoidi maligni del rene o con nefroma mesoblastico congenito e in bambini con neuroblastoma, medulloblastoma, leucemia, linfoma di Burkitt, disgerminoma e rabdomiosarcoma. I livelli sierici di PTH raramente sono elevati. Nella maggior parte dei pazienti, l'ipercalcemia associata a neoplasia è dovuta agli elevati livelli di peptide correlato all'ormone paratiroideo (PTHrP) e non al PTH. Raramente i tumori producono 1,25-$[OH]_2D_3$ o PTH ectopico.

CAUSE VARIE DI IPERCALCEMIA. Si può verificare ipercalcemia nei bambini con **necrosi adiposa sottocutanea**. I livelli di PTH sono normali. Per esempio, in un neonato erano alti i livelli di 1,25-$[OH]_2D_3$ e la biopsia della lesione cutanea rivelava infiltrazione granulomatosa, facendo supporre che il meccanismo dell'ipercalcemia non fosse simile a quello di pazienti con altre patologie granulomatose. In un altro neonato, sebbene i livelli di 1,25-$[OH]_2D_3$ fossero normali, il PTH era soppresso, dimostrando come l'ipercalcemia non fosse correlata al PTH. Il trattamento con prednisone è efficace.

L'**ipofosfatasia**, specialmente la forma severa infantile, è normalmente associata a ipercalcemia da lieve a moderata (vedi Capitolo 703). I livelli sierici di fosforo sono normali e bassi quelli della fosfatasi alcalina. All'indagine radiografica, le ossa mostrano lesioni simil-rachitiche. I livelli urinari di fosfoetanolamina, di pirofosfato inorganico, e di piridossal 5′-fosfato sono elevati; ciascuno di essi è un substrato naturale dell'enzima fosfatasi alcalina non tessuto-specifica (fegato, osso, rene). Mutazioni missense del gene della fosfatasi alcalina non tessuto-specifica, portano, in questa patologia autosomica recessiva, all'inattivazione dell'enzima.

L'**ipercalcemia idiopatica dell'infanzia** si manifesta con mancanza di sviluppo e ipercalcemia durante il primo anno di vita, seguito da remissione spontanea. I livelli sierici di fosforo e PTH sono normali. L'ipercalcemia è dovuta a un aumento dell'assorbimento di calcio. Nella patogenesi può essere coinvolta la vitamina D. Sono stati riportati livelli di 1,25-$[OH]_2D_3$ sia normali sia elevati. Un eccessivo aumento dei livelli di 1,25-$[OH]_2D_3$ in risposta alla somministrazione di PTH, alcuni anni dopo la fase ipercalcemica, suggerisce che la vitamina D abbia un ruolo nella patogenesi. È stata riportata anche una scarsa risposta della calcitonina all'iniezione endovenosa di calcio.

Il 10% dei pazienti con **sindrome di Williams** presenta anche un'ipercalcemia infantile. Il fenotipo comprende difficoltà nell'alimentazione, crescita rallentata, viso da elfo (mandibola piccola, mascella prominente, naso rivolto all'insù), patologie nefrovascolari e personalità socievole "cocktail party". Le lesioni cardiache sono rappresentate da stenosi aortica sopravalvolare, stenosi polmonare periferica, ipoplasia aortica, stenosi dell'arteria coronaria e difetto settale, atriale o ventricolare. Se l'ipercalcemia persiste, si può sviluppare nefrocalcinosi. Il QI è 50-70 ed è curiosamente accompagnato da un aumento della quantità e della qualità dei vocaboli utilizzati, della memoria uditiva e dell'uso sociale del linguaggio. Nel 90% dei pazienti si verifica una delezione submicroscopica del cromosoma 7q11.23, che include delezione di un allele dell'elastina: tale difetto sembra responsabile dei problemi vascolari. La diagnosi definitiva può essere stabilita da una fluorescenza specifica nel sito dell'ibridazione. L'ipercalcemia e i sintomi inerenti al SNC possono essere dovuti a delezione di geni adiacenti. L'ipercalcemia può essere controllata efficacemente sia con prednisone sia con calcitonina.

È stata riportata un'**ipervitaminosi D** con ipercalcemia, per assunzione di bevande a base di latte addizionato non correttamente con vitamina D. Non tutti i pazienti con ipervitaminosi D sviluppano ipercalcemia. I neonati colpiti possono manifestare mancanza di accrescimento, nefrolitiasi, diminuzione della funzionalità renale e osteosclerosi. I livelli sierici di 25[OH]D sono i migliori indicatori di ipervitaminosi D, più dei livelli di 1,25-$[OH]_2D_3$, perché il 25[OH]D ha un'emivita più lunga.

L'**immobilizzazione prolungata** può portare a ipercalcemia e occasionalmente a diminuzione della funzionalità renale, ipertensione ed encefalopatia. I bambini con rachitismo ipofosfatemico sottoposti a intervento chirurgico con conseguente immobilizzazione per un lungo periodo di tempo sono a rischio di ipercalcemia: pertanto, è necessario diminuire o sospendere la supplementazione con vitamina D.

La **condrodisplasia metafisaria tipo Jansen** è una rara malattia genetica caratterizzata da dwarfismo con arti corti e ipercalcemia severa ma asintomatica (vedi Capitolo 702). I livelli circolanti di PTH e di PTHrP sono indosabili. Questi pazienti presentano una mutazione attivante del recettore PTH-PTHrP, che comporta un'alterata omeostasi calcica e anomalie della crescita della placca.

Ahonen P, Myllarniemi S, Sipla I, et al: Clinical variation of autoimmune polyendocrinopathy-candidiasis-ectodermal dystrophy (APECED) in a series of 68 patients. *N Engl J Med* 1990;322:1829–1836.

Brown EM: The calcium-sensing receptor (CaR) and its disorders. *Hormones* 2002;1:10–21.

Cook JS, Stone MS, Hansen JR: Hypercalcemia in association with subcutaneous fat necrosis of the newborn: Studies of calcium-regulating hormones. *Pediatrics* 1992;90:93–96.

Cooper L, Wertheimer J, Levey R, et al: Severe primary hyperparathyroidism in a neonate with two hypercalcemic parents: Management with parathyroidectomy and heterotopic autotransplantation. *Pediatrics* 1986;78: 263–268.

Ding C, Buckingham B, Levine M: Familial isolated hypoparathyroidism caused by a mutation in the gene for the transcription factor GCMB. *J Clin Invest* 2001;108:1215–1220.

Ewart AK, Morris CA, Atkinson D, et al: Hemizygosity at the elastin locus in a developmental disorder, Williams syndrome. *Nat Genet* 1993;5:11–16.

Fedde KN, Michell MP, Whyte MP, et al: Aberrant properties of alkaline phosphatase in patients with clinical expressivity in severe forms of hypophosphatasia. *J Clin Endocrinol Metab* 1996;81:2587–2594.

Gillis D, Hirsch HJ, Peylan-Ramu N, et al: Parathyroid adenoma after radiation in an 8-year old boy. *J Pediatr* 1998;132:892–893.

Hobbs MR, Pole AR, Pidisirng GN, et al: Hyperparathyroidism-jaw tumor syndrome: The HRPT2 locus is within a 0.7-cM region on chromosome 1q. *Am J Hum Genet* 1999;64:518–525.

Irvin GL, Carneiro DM: Management changes in primary hyperparathyroidism. *JAMA* 2000;284:934–936.

Jacabus CH, Holick MF, Shao G, et al: Hypervitaminosis D associated with drinking milk. *N Engl J Med* 1992;326:1173–1177.

Kahn KT, Uma R, Farag TI, et al: Kenny-Caffey syndrome in six Bedouin sibships: Autosomal recessive inheritance is confirmed. *Am J Med Genet* 1997;69:126–132.

Key LL, Thorne M, Pitzer B, et al: Management of neonatal hyperparathyroidism with parathyroidectomy and autotransplantation. *J Pediatr* 1990;116:923–926.
Kollars J, Zarroug AE, van Heerden J, et al: Primary hyperparathyroidism in pediatric patients. *Pediatrics* 2005;115:974–980.
Kovacs CS, Kronenberg HM: Maternal-fetal calcium and bone metabolism during pregnancy, puerperium and lactation. *Endocr Rev* 1997;18:832–872.
Learoyd DL, Twigg SM, Robinson BG, et al: The practical management of multiple endocrine neoplasia. *Trends Endocrinol Metab* 1995;6:273.
Levitt M, Gessert C, Finberg L: Inorganic phosphate (laxative) poisoning resulting in tetany in an infant. *J Pediatr* 1973;82:479–481.
Li Y, Song Y-H, Muir A, et al: Autoantibodies to the extracellular domain of the calcium-sensing receptor in patients with acquired hypoparathyroidism. *J Clin Invest* 1996;97:910–914.
Liu J, Litman D, Weinstein LS, et al: A GNAS1 imprinting defect in pseudohypoparathyroidism type 1B. *J Clin Invest* 2000;107:793.
Marx SJ: Hyperparathyroid and hypoparathyroid disorders. *N Engl J Med* 2000;343:1863–1875.
McKay C, Furman WL: Hypercalcemia complicating childhood malignancies. *Cancer* 1993;72:256–260.
Miric A, Vechio JD, Levine MA: Heterogeneous mutations in the gene encoding the α-subunit of the stimulatory G protein of adenylyl cyclase in Albright hereditary osteodystrophy. *J Clin Endocrinol Metab* 1993;76:1560–1568.
Nakamoto JM, Sandstrom AT, Van Dop C, et al: Pseudohypoparathyroidism type Ia from maternal but not paternal transmission of a $G_s\alpha$ gene mutation. *Am J Med Genet* 1998;77:261–267.
Pallais JC, Kifor O, Chen YB, et al: Acquired hypocalciuric hypercalcemia due to autoantibodies against the calcium-sensing receptor. *N Engl J Med* 2004;351:362–368.
Parvari R, Hershkovitz F, Grossman N, et al: Mutation of TBCE causes hypoparathyroidism-retardation-dysmorphism and autosomal recessive Kenny-Caffey syndrome. *Nat Genet* 2002;32:448–452.
Pearce SH: Multiple endocrine neoplasia type I (MEN 1): Recent advances (commentary). *Clin Endocrinol* 1997;47:513–514.
Pearce SH, Williamson C, Thaker RV, et al: A familial syndrome of hypocalcemia with hypercalciuria due to mutations in the calcium-sensing receptor. *N Engl J Med* 1996;335:1115–1122.
Pollak MR, WuChou YH, Marx SJ, et al: Familial hypocalciuric hypercalcemia and neonatal severe hyperparathyroidism: Effects of mutant gene dosage on phenotype. *J Clin Invest* 1994;93:1108–1112.
Ryan AK, Goodship JA, Wilson DI, et al: Spectrum of clinical features associated with interstitial chromosome 22q11 deletions: A European collaborative study. *J Med Genet* 1997;34:708–804.
Schipani E, Langman CB, Juppner H, et al: Constitutively activated receptors for parathyroid hormone and parathyroid hormone-related peptide in Jansen's metaphyseal chondrodysplasia. *N Engl J Med* 1996;335:708–714.
Shalev H, Phillip M, Landau D, et al: Clinical presentation and outcome in primary familial hypomagnesaemia. *Arch Dis Child* 1998;78:127–130.
Stewart AF: Translational implications of the parathyroid calcium receptor. *N Engl J Med* 2004;351:324–326.
Tean BT, Farnebo F, Larson C, et al: Familial isolated hyperparathyroidism maps to the hyperparathyroidism-jaw tumor locus in 1q21-q32 in a subset of families. *J Clin Endocrinol Metab* 1998;83:2114–2120.
Tengan CH, Kiyomoto BH, Moraes CT, et al: Mitochondrial encephalomyopathy and hypoparathyroidism associated with a duplication and a deletion of mitochondrial deoxyribonucleic acid. *J Clin Endocrinol Metab* 1998;83:125–129.
Thakker RV: Genetic developments in hypoparathyroidism. *Lancet* 2001;357:974–976.
Thomas BR, Bennett JD: Symptomatic hypocalcemia and hypoparathyroidism in two infants of mothers with hyperparathyroidism and familial benign hypercalcemia. *J Perinatol* 1995;15:23–26.
Toft AD: Surgery for primary hyperparathyroidism—sooner rather than later. *Lancet* 2000;355:1478–1479.
Trump D, Dixon PH, Mumm S, et al: Localization of X-linked idiopathic hypoparathyroidism to a 1.5 Mb region on Xq26-q27. *J Med Genet* 1998;35:905–909.
Van Esch H, Groenen P, Devriendt K, et al: GATA3 haplo-insufficiency causes human HDR syndrome. *Nature* 2000;406:419–422.
Walder RY, Shalev H, Sheffield VC, et al: Familial hypomagnesiemia maps to chromosome 9q not to the X chromosome: Genetic linkage mapping and analysis of a balanced translocation breakpoint. *Hum Mol Genet* 1997;6:1491–1497.
Watanabe T, Bai M, Yasuda T, et al: Familial hypoparathyroidism: Identification of a novel gain of function mutation in transmembrane domain 5 of the calcium-sensing receptor. *J Clin Endocrinol Metab* 1998;83:2497–2502.
Weinstein LS, Yu S: The role of genomic imprinting of $G_s\alpha$ in the pathogenesis of Albright hereditary osteodystrophy. *Trends Endocrinol Metab* 1999;10:81–85.

Sezione 4 — Malattie delle ghiandole surrenali — Perrin C. White

Capitolo 575 ■ Fisiologia delle ghiandole surrenali

575.1 • Istologia ed embriologia

La ghiandola surrenale è composta da due tessuti endocrini: midollare e corticale. Le cellule cromaffini della midollare surrenalica derivano dal neuroectoderma, mentre quelle della corteccia surrenalica derivano dal mesoderma. Le cellule mesodermiche contribuiscono anche allo sviluppo delle gonadi. Le ghiandole surrenali e le gonadi possiedono in comune alcuni enzimi coinvolti nella sintesi degli steroidi; un errore congenito della steroidogenesi in un tessuto può essere presente anche nell'altro.

La corteccia surrenalica consiste di tre zone: la zona glomerulare, la più esterna, localizzata immediatamente sotto la capsula; la zona fascicolata, cioè quella intermedia; e infine la zona reticolare, la più interna, adiacente alla midollare. La zona fascicolata è la più ampia, e costituisce i 2/3 della corteccia; la zona glomerulare rappresenta circa il 15% e quella reticolare circa il 10%. Le cellule della glomerulare sono piccole, con un basso rapporto citoplasma/nucleo, un numero intermedio di inclusioni lipiche e nuclei più piccoli contenenti cromatina più condensata rispetto alle cellule delle altre due zone. Le cellule della zona fascicolata sono voluminose, con un alto rapporto citoplasma/nucleo e molte inclusioni lipidiche, che conferuiscono al citoplasma un aspetto spumoso, vacuolare. Le cellule sono disposte in cordoni radiali. Le cellule della zona reticolare formano invece dei cordoni irregolarmente anastomizzati. Il rapporto citoplasma/nucleo è intermedio e il citoplasma compatto ha un contenuto relativamente basso di lipidi.

La zona glomerulare sintetizza aldosterone, il più potente mineralcorticoide naturale nell'uomo. La zona fascicolata produce cortisolo, il più potente glicocorticoide naturale dell'uomo, e la zona fascicolata e quella reticolare sintetizzano gli androgeni surrenalici.

La midollare surrenalica è formata principalmente da cellule neuroendocrine (cromaffini) e da cellule gliali (sustentacolari) inframmezzate a tessuto connettivo e cellule vascolari. Le cellule neuroendocrine sono poliedriche, con citoplasma abbondante e nucleo piccolo, di colore chiaro. Al microscopio elettronico il citoplasma rivela numerosi grossi granuli di secrezione, contenenti catecolamine. Le cellule gliali hanno citoplasma scarso e nuclei più basofili.

Il primo abbozzo della ghiandola surrenale può essere fatto risalire alla terza-quarta settimana di gestazione, appena cefalico al mesonefro in via di sviluppo. Alla quinta-sesta settimana, la cresta gonadica si sviluppa all'interno delle cellule steroidogenetiche delle gonadi e della corteccia surrenalica; le cellule gonadiche e surrenaliche si separano: quelle surrenaliche migrano in sede retroperitoneale, mentre quelle gonadiche si spostano caudalmente. Alla sesta-ottava settimana di gestazione, le ghiandole aumentano rapidamente di volume, le cellule della parte più interna della corteccia si differenziano nella forma della zona fetale e la rima subcapsulare esterna rimane come zona definitiva. L'abbozzo della ghiandola surrenale è invaso a questo punto da elementi nervosi simpatici che si differenziano in cellule cromaffini, capaci di sintetizzare e accumulare catecolamine. La catecol-O-metiltransferasi, che converte la noradrenalina in adrenalina, è espressa successivamente durante la gravidanza. Alla fine dell'ottava settimana di gestazione, la ghiandola surrenalica con la sua capsula si colloca al polo superiore del rene. Alla nona-dodicesima settimana, le cellule della zona fetale sono in grado di sintetizzare attivamente steroidi. Nel feto al secondo mese, le ghiandole surrenaliche appaiono più voluminose dei reni, ma a partire dal quarto mese i reni crescono rapidamente diventando, alla fine del sesto, il doppio rispetto ai surreni. Nel neonato a termine, le ghiandole surrenaliche sono circa un terzo del rene e il loro peso complessivo è di 7-9 g. Alla nascita, la corteccia fetale interna occupa circa l'80% della ghiandola, e la "vera" corteccia esterna il 20%. In pochi giorni la corteccia fetale comincia a involversi, riducendosi del 50% verso il primo mese di vita. Al contrario, la midollare surrenalica è relativamente scarsa alla nascita e subisce un progressivo proporzionale incremento anche oltre il sesto mese di vita postnatale. A un anno, le ghiandole surrenali pesano insieme meno di 1 g. La crescita surrenalica tuttavia comporta il raggiungimento di un peso complessivo, da adulti, di 8 g. Le zona fascicolata e quella glomerulare sono completamente differenziate verso circa il terzo anno di età. La zona reticolare si sviluppa completamente alla pubertà.

Una crescita precoce del surrene fetale sembra indipendente dall'ormone adrenocorticotropo (ACTH), ma, almeno dalla metà fino alla fine della gestazione, l'ACTH risulta essenziale per la crescita e la maturazione dei surreni. Non è ancora chiaro a quale stadio delle sviluppo fetale si stabilisca il meccanismo di feedback nella regolazione dell'ACTH da parte del cortisolo, ma l'esperienza clinica suggerisce che i normali rapporti di feedback ipofiso-surrenalici siano operativi nel primo trimestre.

Altri fattori importanti per la crescita fetale e per la steroidogenesi comprendono la gonadotropina corionica fetale e una serie di fattori peptidici di crescita prodotti dalla placenta e dal feto.

Due fattori di trascrizione sono critici per lo sviluppo delle ghiandole surrenaliche: il fattore steroidogenetico 1 (SF-1; NR5A1) e DAX-1 (inversione sessuale dosaggio-sensibile, ipoplasia surrenalica congenita, cromosoma X; NR0B1). SF-1 è importante anche nella regolazione trascrizionale di parecchi geni che codificano per gli enzimi coinvolti nella steroidogenesi. Alterazioni di SF-1, codificato sul cromosoma 9q33, comportano agenesia surrenalica e gonadica, assenza delle cellule gonadotrope ipofisarie e iposviluppo dell'ipotalamo ventrale mediale. Mutazioni del gene DAX1, codificato su Xp21, portano a ipoplasia surrenalica congenita e ipogonadismo ipogonadotropo. DAX1 gioca un ruolo importante nella regolazione della steroidogenesi.

575.2 • Biosintesi degli steroidi surrenalici

Il colesterolo rappresenta il substrato iniziale per la biosintesi di tutti gli steroidi (Fig. 575-1). Sebbene le cellule della corteccia surrenalica siano in grado di sintetizzare colesterolo ex novo a partire dall'acetato, le lipoproteine plasmatiche circolanti provvedono per l'80% al rifornimento di colesterolo per la sintesi degli ormoni corticali. Specifici recettori della superficie cellulare per le lipoproteine a bassa densità (LDL) legano le LDL circolanti e le internalizzano con un processo di endocitosi recettore-mediato. Il colesterolo viene accumulato in vescicole sotto forma di esteri e successivamente idrolizzato da un'idrolasi per gli esteri del colesterolo, quando sia necessario rendere disponibile del colesterolo libero per la sintesi degli steroidi.

Il limite di velocità della steroidogenesi surrenalica è il passaggio del colesterolo attraverso la membrana mitocondriale esterna e interna. Questo richiede parecchie proteine, compreso il recettore periferico per le benzodiazepine e la proteina regolatrice acuta steroidogenetica (StAR). La proteina StAR ha un'emivita molto breve e la sua sintesi viene indotta rapidamente da fattori trofici (corticotropina); in questo modo, il meccanismo di regolazione della biosintesi degli steroidi è più rapido (inferiore all'ora).

A livello della membrana mitocondriale interna, viene accorciata la catena laterale del colesterolo, per la produzione di pregnenolone. Questa reazione è catalizzata da un enzima che rompe la catena laterale del colesterolo (colesterolo desmolasi, P450scc, CYP11A1), un enzima citocromo P450 (CYP). Come gli altri P450, questa è un'emoproteina legata alla membrana, con massa molecolare di circa 50 kDa. Essa cattura elettroni da un sistema mitocondriale di trasporto di elettroni NADPH-dipendente, che consiste di due proteine accessorie, l'adrenoxina reduttasi (una flavoproteina) e l'adrenoxina (una piccola proteina contenente ferro non eme). Gli enzimi P450 utilizzano elettroni e ossigeno per idrossilare il substrato, con la formazione di H_2O. In questo passaggio per la rottura della catena laterale del colesterolo, si verificano tre successive reazioni ossidative per rompere il legame del carbonio C20,22. Il pregnenolone diffonde poi fuori dal mitocondrio ed entra nel reticolo endoplasmatico. Le reazioni successive variano a seconda della zona della corteccia surrenalica.

ZONA GLOMERULARE. Nella zona glomerulare, il pregnenolone è convertito in progesterone da una 3β-idrossi-steroidodeidrogenasi (HSD3B2), un enzima NAD^+-dipendente del tipo "deidrogenasi a catena corta". Il progesterone si trasforma in 11-desossicorticosterone per mezzo di una 21-idrossilasi (P450c21, CYP21), che è un altro citocromo P450. Come gli altri P450 del reticolo endoplasmatico, esso utilizza un sistema di trasporto degli elettroni con solo una proteina accessoria, il citocromo P450 ossidoreduttasi.

Il desossicorticosterone rientra poi nei mitocondri e viene convertito in aldosterone da un'aldosterone sintasi (P450aldo, CYP11B2), un enzima P450 strutturalmente correlato alla desmolasi del colesterolo. Anche l'aldosterone sintasi effettua tre successive ossidazioni: l'11β-idrossilazione, la 18-idrossilazione e un'ulteriore ossidazione del gruppo metilico sul carbonio 18 con formazione di un gruppo aldeidico.

ZONA FASCICOLATA. Nel reticolo endoplasmatico della zona fascicolata, il pregnenolone e il progesterone vengono convertiti da un 17α-idrossilasi (P450c17, CYP17) a 17idrossi pregnenolone e 17idrossi progesterone, rispettivamente. Questo enzima non viene espresso nella zona glomerulare, che quindi non è in grado di sintetizzare steroidi idrossilati in posizione 17. Il 17idrossipregnenolone è trasformato in 17idrossi progesterone e in 11desossicortisolo dagli stessi enzimi 3β-idrossisteroido e 21-idrossilasi rispettivamente, attivi nella zona glomerulare. Così, anomalie ereditarie di questi enzimi compromettono la sintesi sia dell'aldosterone sia del cortisolo (vedi Capitolo 577). Infine l'11-desossicortisolo rientra nei mitocondri ed è convertito a cortisolo da una steroido 11β-idrossilasi (P450c11, CYP11B1). Questo enzima è strettamente correlato con l'aldosterone sintasi, ma ha bassa attività 18-idrossilasica e non ha attività 18-ossidasica. Pertanto, in circostanze normali, la zona fascicolata non è in grado di produrre aldosterone.

ZONA RETICOLARE. Nella zona reticolare e per la stessa estensione della zona fascicolata, l'enzima 17-idrossilasi possiede un'ulteriore capacità, cioè quella di rompere il legame tra il carbonio 17 e il carbonio 20. Questo converte il 17-idrossipregnenolone a deidroepiandrosterone (DHEA). Il deidroepiandrosterone viene trasformato in androstenedione da una 3β-idrossi-steroidodeidrogenasi. Questo può essere ulteriormente convertito, in altri tessuti, in testosterone e in estrogeni.

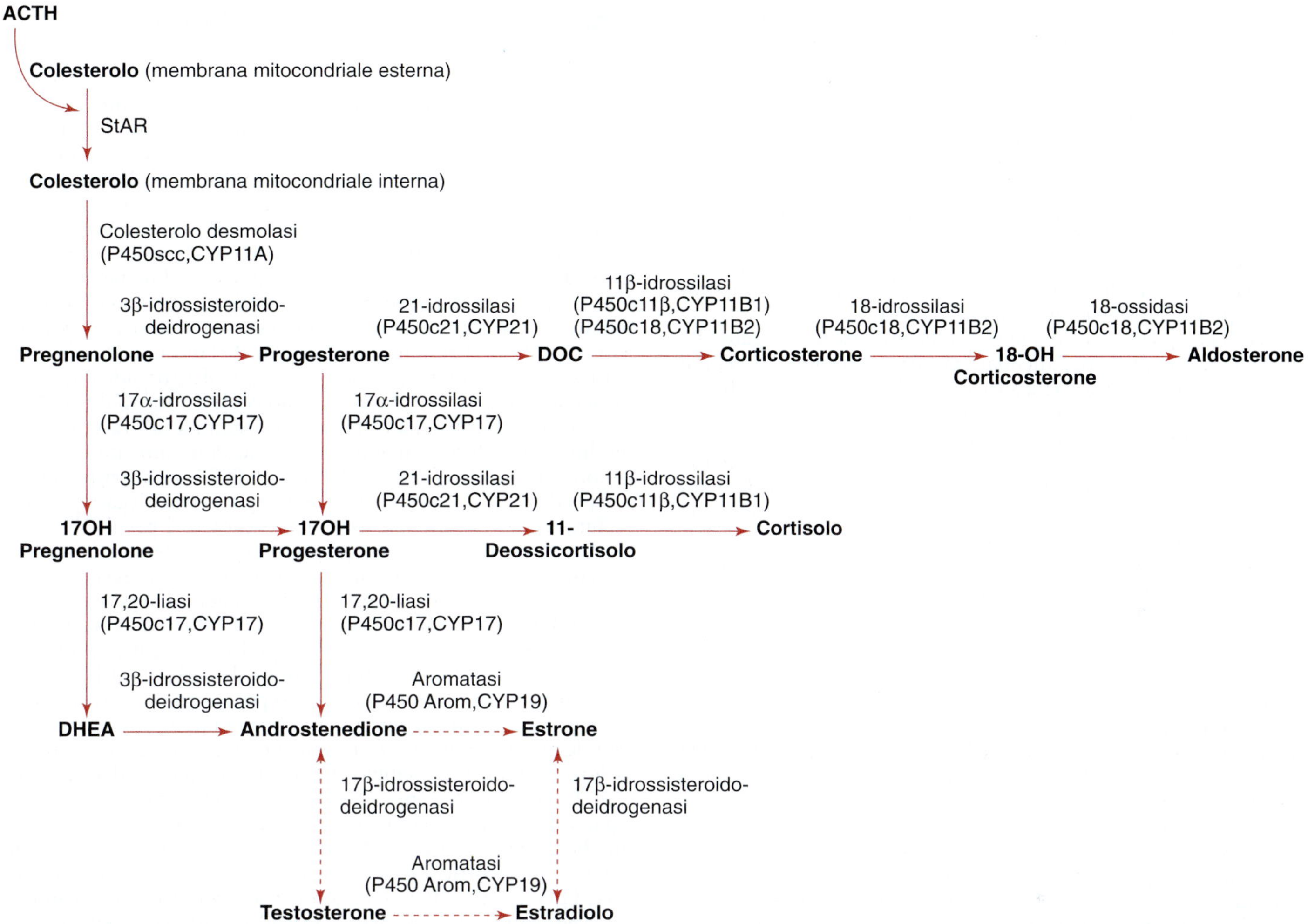

Figura 575-1. Via biosintetica degli steroidi. La via per la sintesi surrenalica di mineralcorticoidi (aldosterone), glicocorticoidi (cortisolo) e androgeni (DHEA, androstenedione) è indicata verticalmente. Per ogni bioconversione è indicata l'attività enzimatica. Il nome sistematico per le attività mediate da specifici citocromi P450, viene indicato tra parentesi. Le reazioni indicate dalla freccia si verificano principalmente nelle gonadi, non nei surreni. Il P450c11β media l'attività dell'11β-idrossilasi nella zona fascicolata, per convertire l'11-desossicorticosterone (DOC) in corticosterone, e l'11-desossicortisolo in cortisolo. Il P450c18 media l'attività della 11β-idrossilasi, della 18-idrossilasi e della 18-ossidasi nella zona glomerulare per la conversione del DOC ad aldosterone.

UNITÀ FETOPLACENTARE. La sintesi di steroidi nel surrene fetale è diversa da quella che si realizza nella ghiandola nel periodo postnatale. Il colesterolo LDL sintetizzato dal fegato fetale rappresenta la maggiore sorgente di colesterolo per la sintesi di steroidi nel surrene fetale. La ghiandola fetale ha una bassa attività 3β-idrossi-steroidodeidrogenasica e un'alta attività steroidosulfochinasica. In questo modo, il surrene fetale produce soprattutto DHEA e DHEA solfato (DHEAS) e, con una 16α-idrossilazione epatica, 16α-idrossiDHEAS. La placenta, che ha attività steroidosolfatasica, utilizza il DHEA e il DHEAS come substrati per l'estrone e l'estradiolo e il 16α-OH DHEAS come substrato per l'estriolo. L'estrone placentare e l'estradiolo derivano in uguale misura da precursori sia materni sia fetali; l'estriolo è quasi esclusivamente prodotto da substrati di origine fetale. Oltre a provvedere substrati per la sintesi placentare di estrogeni, il surrene fetale produce una quantità significativa di cortisolo, molto del quale è convertito in cortisone dall'enzima 11β-idrossi-steroidodeidrogenasi. Mano a mano che ci si avvicina al termine della gravidanza, la concentrazione di cortisolo fetale aumenta per aumento della secrezione di cortisolo e per diminuzione della conversione del cortisolo in cortisone. Nella fase intermedia della gestazione sono prodotti bassi livelli di aldosterone, ma la capacità di secrezione di questo ormone aumenta verso il termine.

575.3 • Regolazione della corteccia surrenalica

REGOLAZIONE DELLA SECREZIONE DI CORTISOLO. La secrezione di glicocorticoidi è regolata principalmente dall'ormone adrenocorticotropo (corticotropina, ACTH), un peptide di 39 aminoacidi prodotto dall'ipofisi anteriore. Esso viene sintetizzato come parte di un peptide precursore ad alto peso molecolare, noto come pro-opiomelanocortina (POMC). Questo precursore rappresenta anche la sorgente di β-lipotropina (β-LPH). ACTH e β-LPH sono separati ulteriormente per la produzione di un ormone α e β-melanocita-stimolante, di un peptide del lobo intermedio corticotropina-simile (CLIP), di γ-LPH, di β e γ-endorfina e di encefalina (vedi Capitolo 557).

L'ACTH viene rilasciato con secrezione pulsatile di ampiezza variabile fra il giorno e la notte, da cui dipende il normale ritmo diurno della secrezione di cortisolo. La pulsatilità del cortisolo e dell'ACTH si verifica ogni 30-120 min, è più alta durante lo stato di veglia e cala durante il tardo pomeriggio e la sera, raggiungendo il minimo una o due ore dopo l'addormentamento.

L'ormone di rilascio della corticotropina (CRH), sintetizzato dai neuroni della divisione parvicellulare del nucleo ipotalamico paraventricolare, è il più importante stimolatore della secrezione di ACTH. L'arginin-vasopressina (AVP) aumenta l'azione del

CRH. Stimoli nervosi di origine cerebrale provocano il rilascio di CRH e di AVP (vedi Capitolo 557). L'AVP e il CRH sono secreti nella circolazione portale ipofisaria in modo pulsatile. Questa secrezione pulsatile è a sua volta responsabile del rilascio pulsatile (ultradiano) dell'ACTH. Il ritmo circadiano del rilascio della corticotropina è probabilmente indotto da un corrispondente ritmo circadiano della secrezione ipoatalamica di CRH, regolato dai nuclei soprachiasmatici con impulsi provenienti da altre aree cerebrali. Il cortisolo esercita un feedback negativo sulla sintesi e sulla secrezione di ACTH, CRH e AVP. L'ACTH inibisce la sua stessa secrezione, con un feedback mediato a livello ipotalamico. Così la secrezione di cortisolo dipende dall'interazione di ipotalamo, ipofisi, surrene e altri stimoli nervosi.

L'ACTH agisce attraverso uno specifico recettore collegato alla proteina G, per attivare l'adenilato ciclasi e aumentare i livelli di adenosina monofosfato ciclica (AMP). L'AMP ciclico ha effetti a breve termine (minuti o ore) sul trasporto del colesterolo nel mitocondrio, aumentando l'espressività della proteina regolatoria acuta (StAR) della steroidogenesi. Gli effetti a lungo termine (da ore a giorni) della stimolazione dell'ACTH consistono nell'aumento della captazione del colesterolo LDL e dell'espressività dei geni che codificano gli enzimi necessari alla sintesi del cortisolo. Questi effetti trascrizionali si verificano almeno in parte attraverso un aumento dell'attività della proteinchinasi A, che fosforila diversi fattori trascrizionali di regolazione.

REGOLAZIONE DELLA SECREZIONE DI ALDOSTERONE. L'entità della sintesi di aldosterone, che normalmente è da 100 a 1000 volte inferiore a quella del cortisolo, è regolata principalmente dal sistema renina-angiotensina e dai livelli di potassio, mentre l'ACTH ha solo un effetto a breve termine. In risposta al decremento del volume intravascolare, l'apparato juxta-glomerulare del rene secerne la renina. La renina è un enzima proteolitico che converte l'angiotensinogeno (substrato della renina), una α 2-globulina prodotta dal fegato, in un decapeptide inattivo, l'angiotensina I. L'enzima convertitore dell'angiotensina del polmone e di altri tessuti rapidamente trasforma l'angiotensina I nell'octapeptide biologicamente attivo angiotensina II. Dalla trasformazione dell'angiotensina II si ottiene l'angiotensina III, un eptapeptide. L'angiotensina II e III sono potenti stimolatori della secrezione di aldosterone; l'angiotensina II è il più potente agente vasopressore. L'angiotensina II e III occupano un recettore correlato alla proteina G che attiva la fosfolipasi C. Quest'ultima proteina idrolizza il fosfatidilinositolo bifosfato in inositolo trifosfato e diacilglicerolo, che aumenta i livelli intracellulari del calcio e attiva la proteinchinasi C e le chinasi calmodulina-attivate (CaM). Allo stesso modo, l'aumento dei livelli extracellulari di potassio depolarizza la membrana cellulare e aumenta il flusso di calcio attraverso i canali del calcio di tipo L "voltage-gate". La fosforilazione dei fattori di regolazione trascrizionale da parte delle CaM chinasi aumenta la trascrizione dell'aldosterone sintasi (CYP11B2), necessaria alla sintesi di aldosterone.

REGOLAZIONE DELLA SECREZIONE DI ANDROGENI SURRENALICI. Il meccanismo di regolazione degli androgeni surrenalici, deidroepiandrosterone e androstenedione, non è completamente chiarito. L'adrenarca è quel processo di maturazione delle ghiandole surrenaliche che comporta un aumento della secrezione surrenalica di androgeni tra i 5 e i 20 anni.

Il processo comincia prima dei più precoci segni di pubertà e continua negli anni, quando si verifica la pubertà. Istologicamente, sembra essere legato alla zona reticolare. Mentre l'ACTH stimola acutamente la produzione di androgeni surrenalici e rappresenta chiaramente lo stimolo principale per il rilascio del cortisolo (vedi oltre), altri fattori sono implicati nella stimolazione degli androgeni surrenalici. Questi includono un relativo decremento dell'espressione della 3β-idrossi-steroidodeidrogenasi nella zona reticolare e possibilmente un aumento dell'attività della 17,20-liasi per la fosforilazione di CYP17 o un aumento dell'espressione del citocromo b5.

575.4 • AZIONE DEGLI ORMONI STEROIDEI SURRENALICI

Gli ormoni steroidei agiscono tramite alcuni distinti recettori che corrispondono alle attività biologiche ormonali conosciute: glicocorticoide, mineralcorticoide, progestinica, estrogenica e androgenica. Questi recettori appartengono ad una grande famiglia di fattori trascrizionali nucleari che comprende, fra gli altri, i recettori dell'ormone tiroideo e dell'acido retinoico. Essi possiedono una struttura comune, con un dominio ligand-binding carbossiterminale e un dominio DNA-binding nella regione intermedia. Quest'ultimo dominio contiene due "zinc fingers", ognuno dei quali è formato da un anello di aminoacidi stabilizzati a livello di 4 residui cisteinici che chelano uno ione zinco.

I recettori per i glicocorticoidi e i mineralcorticoidi si trovano principalmente nel citoplasma. Le molecole ormonali diffondono attraverso la membrana cellulare e si legano a tali recettori, che modificano la loro configurazione e successivamente si trasferiscono nel nucleo, dove si legano al DNA in corrispondenza di specifici siti di risposta ormonale. I recettori legati possono reclutare altri fattori trascrizionali coregolatori per il DNA.

Mentre steroidi differenti possono avere le stesse attività biologiche, per la loro capacità di legare lo stesso recettore, un certo steroide può esercitare effetti biologici diversi nei diversi tessuti. La varietà delle risposte ormonali è dovuta ai diversi geni regolati dall'ormone nei vari tessuti. Oltre a ciò, nei vari tessuti sono espresse differenti combinazioni di coregolatori e questo comporta che ogni ormone steroideo possa produrre molti effetti diversi. Inoltre, gli enzimi possono aumentare o diminuire l'affinità degli steroidi per i loro recettori e modulare in questo modo la loro attività. Per esempio, l'11β-idrossi-steroidodeidrogenasi tipo 1 (HSD11B1) converte il cortisone, che non è in grado di legarsi al recettore dei glicocorticoidi, in cortisolo, che invece è un glicocorticoide attivo. Questo fa aumentare le concentrazioni locali di glicocorticoidi nei vari tessuti, specialmente nel fegato, dove i glicocorticoidi mantengono la secrezione epatica di glucosio (vedi sotto). Al contrario, l'11β-idrossi-steroidodeidrogenasi tipo 2 (HSD11B2) ossida, particolarmente a livello renale, il cortisolo a cortisone e ciò impedisce che i recettori dei mineralcorticoidi siano occupati da alti livelli di cortisolo (vedi sotto).

AZIONI DEI GLICOCORTICOIDI. I glicocorticoidi sono essenziali per la vita. Il termine glicocorticoidi si riferisce alla capacità di questi ormoni di regolare il metabolismo del glucosio. I glicocorticoidi hanno inoltre effetti multipli sul metabolismo di carboidrati, lipidi e proteine. Essi regolano anche le funzioni immunitaria, circolatoria e renale. Influenzano la crescita, lo sviluppo, il metabolismo osseo e l'attività del sistema nervoso centrale.

In situazioni di stress, la secrezione di glicocorticoidi può aumentare fino a 10 volte. Questo comporta un aumento della capacità di sopravvivenza attraverso un incremento delle contrattilità cardiaca, della gittata cardiaca, della sensibilità agli effetti pressori delle catecolamine e di altri ormoni pressori, la capacità di lavoro dei muscoli scheletrici e la capacità di mobilizzare energia dai depositi.

Effetti metabolici. L'azione primaria dei glicocorticoidi sul metabolismo dei carboidrati consiste nell'aumento della produzione di glucosio attraverso una stimolazione della gluconeogenesi epatica. I glicocorticoidi aumentano anche la resistenza cellulare all'insulina, facendo così diminuire l'ingresso del glucosio nelle cellule. Questa inibizione della captazione di glucosio si attua negli adipociti, nelle cellule muscolari e nei fibroblasti. Oltre a questa attività anti-insulinica, i glicocorticoidi possono avere anche un'azione sinergica con l'insulina nella protezione contro il digiuno di lunga durata, tramite la stimolazione della produzione e dell'accumulo di glicogeno nel fegato. Entrambi gli ormoni stimolano l'attività della glicogeno-sintetasi e diminuiscono la glicogenolisi. L'eccesso di glicocorticoidi può causare iperglicemia, invece un deficit può portare a ipoglicemia.

I glicocorticoidi aumentano i livelli di acidi grassi liberi stimolando la lipolisi, diminuendo la captazione cellulare del glucosio e la produzione di glicerolo, necessario per la riesterificazione degli acidi grassi. La lipolisi è stimolata anche per un effetto permissivo nei confronti di altri fattori lipolitici, come l'adrenalina. Questa azione si ripercuote sugli adipociti in modo diverso a seconda della loro localizzazione anatomica. In pazienti con eccesso di glicocorticoidi, il tessuto adiposo è scarso alle estremità, ma aumenta in tronco (obesità centripeta), collo e viso (facies lunaris). Questo può implicare effetti sulla differenziazione degli adipociti.

I glicocorticoidi generalmente esercitano un'azione catatilica/antianabolica sul metabolismo proteico. La proteolisi a livello di tessuto adiposo, muscolo scheletrico, osso, tessuto linfoide e connettivo, aumenta i substrati aminoacidici che possono essere poi utilizzati nella gluconeogenesi. Il muscolo cardiaco e il diaframma sono quasi completamente risparmiati da questo effetto catabolico.

Effetti circolatori e renali. I glicocorticoidi hanno un effetto inotropo positivo sul cuore, aumentando l'indice di lavoro del ventricolo sinistro. Inoltre, essi hanno un effetto permissivo sull'azione dell'adrenalina e della noradrenalina sia sul cuore sia sui vasi. In assenza di glicocorticoidi, diminuisce la gettata cardiaca e può comparire shock; in condizioni di eccesso ormonale frequentemente si sviluppa ipertensione. Questa può essere dovuta all'attivazione del recettore dei mineralcorticoidi (vedi oltre), che si verifica quando la 11β-idrossi-steroidodeidrogenasi è saturata da eccessivi livelli di glicocorticoidi.

Crescita. L'eccesso di glicocorticoidi inibisce la crescita in altezza e la maturazione scheletrica nei bambini. Questo effetto è dovuto principalmente alla loro azione inibitoria a livello epifisario. Può però essere in parte mediato dal decremento dei livelli dell'ormone della crescita e del fattore 1 di crescita insulino-simile (IGF-1) e dall'aumento della proteina 1 che lega IGF (IGFBP-1), che inibisce la crescita somatica diminuendo i livelli di IGF-1 libero circolante.

Nonostante l'eccesso di glicocorticoidi comprometta nettamente la crescita, essi sono necessari, per altro, alla crescita e allo sviluppo normali. Nel feto e nel neonato, accelerano la differenziazione e lo sviluppo dei vari tessuti. Queste azioni includono lo sviluppo sei sistemi epatico e gastrointestinale e anche la produzione di surfattante da parte del polmone fetale. I glicocorticoidi sono spesso somministrati a donne in gravidanza con rischio di parto prematuro, allo lo scopo di accelerare questi processi di maturazione (vedi Capitolo 96.8).

Effetti immunologici. I glicocorticoidi giocano un ruolo importante nella regolazione immunitaria. Inibiscono la sintesi dei precursori di glicolipidi e prostaglandine e le azioni della bradichinina. Bloccano anche l'istamina e la sintesi e gli effetti delle citochine protoinfiammatorie (fattore tumorale-α di necrosi, interleuchina-1, interleuchina-6). Queste azioni fanno diminuire il processo infiammatorio. Alte dosi di glicocorticoidi provocano una riduzione di monociti, eosinofili e linfociti, specialmente le cellule T. Essi agiscono inducendo almeno in parte l'arresto del ciclo cellulare alla fase G1 e attivando l'apoptosi, con effetti mediati dal recettore per i glicocorticoidi. Gli effetti sui linfociti si esercitano principalmente sulle cellule T helper 1 e da qui sull'immunità cellulare, mentre le cellule T helper 2 sono sparite, lasciando una risposta soprattutto umorale. Dosi farmacologiche di glicocorticoidi possono anche diminuire la quantità di tessuto immunologicamente attivo (milza, timo e linfonodi).

I glicocorticoidi aumentano il numero delle cellule polimorfonucleate circolanti. Inoltre diminuiscono la diapedesi, la chemiotassi e la fagocitosi da parte delle cellule polimorfonucleate. Di conseguenza la mobilità di queste cellule è alterata a tal punto che non sono in grado di arrivare nella sede della infiammazione per organizzare un'appropriata risposta immunitaria. Alti livelli di glicocorticoidi diminuiscono le risposte cellulari infiammatoria e immunitaria, ed aumentano la sensibilità a certe infezioni batteriche, virali, micotiche e parassitarie.

Effetti sulla cute, osso e sul calcio. I glicocorticoidi inibiscono i fibroblasti, con conseguente aumento delle ecchimosi e scarsa guarigione delle ferite per atrofia cutanea. Questo effetto spiega l'assottigliamento della cute e le strie che compaiono nei pazienti con sindrome di Cushing.

I glicocorticoidi hanno l'effetto complessivo di diminuire la calcemia e sono utilizzati nella terapia di urgenza per certi tipi di ipercalcemia. Questo effetto ipocalcemizzante probabilmente dipende da una diminuzione dell'assorbimento intestinale del calcio e del riassorbimento renale di calcio e fosforo. La calcemia, tuttavia, generalmente non scende sotto i livelli normali, per un aumento secondario della secrezione dell'ormone paratiroideo.

L'effetto a lungo termine più significativo di un eccesso di glicocorticoidi sul metabolismo del calcio e dell'osso è rappresentato dall'**osteoporosi**. I glicocorticoidi inibiscono l'attività osteoblastica diminuendo il numero e l'attività degli osteoblasti. Diminuiscono inoltre l'attività osteoclastica, ma in minor grado, con conseguente basso turn over osseo e bilancio complessivamente negativo. La tendenza dei glicocorticoidi a provocare ipocalcemia e ipofosfatemia, provoca un iperparatiroidismo secondario. Queste azioni diminuiscono l'apposizione di osso e provocano una perdita netta della quota minerale dell'osso.

Effetti sul sistema nervoso centrale. I glicocorticoidi penetrano senza difficoltà attraverso la barriera emato-encefalica ed esplicano effetti diretti sul metabolismo cerebrale. Diminuiscono certi tipi di edema del SNC e sono frequentemente utilizzati per trattare l'ipertensione endocranica. Stimolano l'appetito e provocano insonnia, con una riduzione delle fasi del sonno caratterizzate da movimenti oculari rapidi. Aumentano inoltre l'irritabilità e la labilità emotiva, con un'alterazione della memoria e della capacità di concentrazione. Un aumento lieve-moderato di glicocorticoidi per un periodo di tempo limitato spesso causa una sensazione di euforia o di benessere, ma un eccesso o un deficit possono associarsi a depressione clinica. L'eccesso di glicocorticoidi può portare a **psicosi** in alcuni pazienti.

Gli effetti dei glicocorticoidi a livello cerebrale sono mediati in larga misura dall'interazione con i recettori dei mineralcorticoidi e anche dei glicocorticoidi (talvolta definiti in questo caso recettori di tipo I e di tipo II rispettivamente). L'attivazione dei recettori di tipo II aumenta la sensibilità dei neuroni ippocampali al neurotrasmettitore serotonina, che può aiutare a spiegare l'euforia associata ad alte dosi di glicocorticoidi. I glicocorticoidi inibiscono la secrezione di ormone di rilascio della corticotropina (CRH) nell'ipotalamo anteriore, ma lo stimolano nei nuclei centrali dell'amigdala e nei nuclei laterali della stria terminalis, dove può mediare sensazioni di paura e ansia. I glicocorticoidi, inoltre, e anche altre steroidi, possono avere effetti non gnomici a livello di attività di modulazione dei recettori dell'acido gamma-aminobutirrico (GABA) e dell'N-metil-D-aspartato (NMDA).

AZIONI DEI MINERALCORTICOIDI. Il più importante mineralcorticoide è l'aldosterone e, in minor misura, l'11-desossicorticosterone; il corticosterone e il cortisolo non sono normalmente importanti come mineralcorticoidi, se non quando sono secreti in eccesso. I mineralcorticoidi hanno azioni più limitate rispetto ai glicocorticoidi. La loro funzione maggiore consiste nella regolazione del volume intravascolare con ritenzione di sodio ed eliminazione di potassio e di ioni idrogeno. Esercitano quest'azione a livello renale, intestinale, salivare e delle ghiandole sudoripare. L'aldosterone può avere effetti distinti in altri tessuti. I recettori per i mineralcorticoidi sono stati trovati nel cuore e nell'endotelio vascolare e l'aldosterone aumenta la fibrosi miocardica nell'insufficienza cardiaca.

I mineralcorticoidi esplicano la loro azione principale nei tubuli contorti distali e nei dotti collettori corticali del rene, dove inducono il riassorbimento di sodio e la secrezione di potassio. Nei dotti collettori della midollare agiscono in modo permissivo nei confronti della vasopressina, con aumento del flusso osmotico di acqua. Pertanto, pazienti con deficit di mineralcorticoidi possono manifestare perdita di peso, ipotensione, iponatremia e iperkaliemia, mentre pazienti con eccesso di mineralcorticoidi sviluppano ipertensione, ipokaliemia e alcalosi metabolica (vedi Capitoli 576-579).

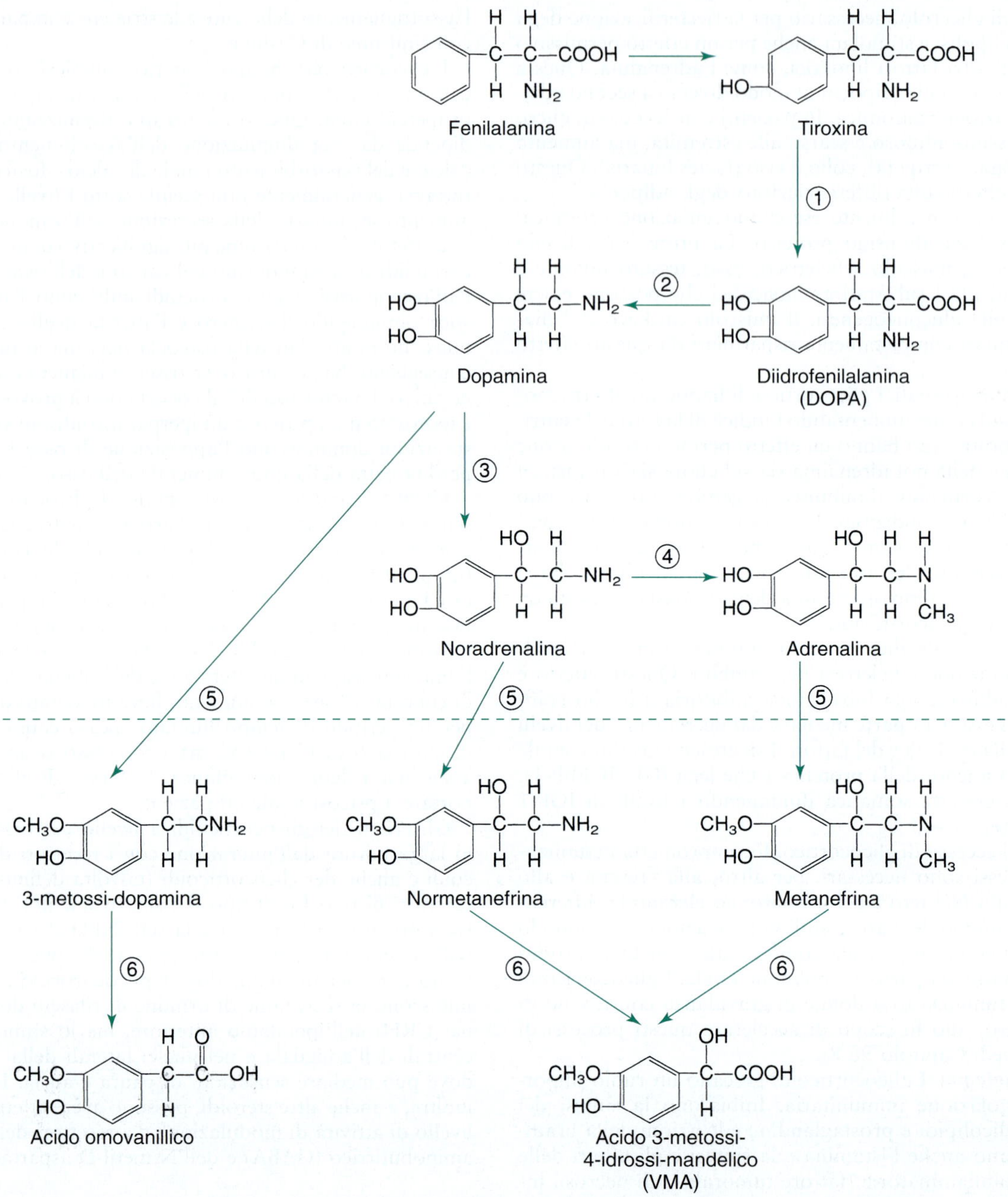

Figura 575-2. Biosintesi (sopra la linea) e metabolismo (sotto la linea) delle catecolamine noradrenalina e adrenalina. Enzimi: 1, tiroxina idrossilasi; 2, dopa decarbossilasi; 3, dopamina betaossidasi; 4, feniletanolamina-N-metiltansferasi; 5, catecol-*O*-metiltransferasi; 6, monoaminoossidasi.

Il meccanismo con cui l'aldosterone interviene nell'escrezione sodica non è chiarito. La maggior parte degli effetti dell'aldosterone è probabilmente dovuta a modificazioni dell'espressione genica mediata dal recettore dei mineralcorticoidi e infatti, in risposta all'aldosterone, aumentano i livelli di subunità sia di Na^+ e K^+-ATPasi sia del canale epiteliale del sodio (*Epithelial Sodium Channel*, ENaC).

Il recettore dei mineralcorticoidi mostra in vitro analoga affinità per il cortisolo e l'aldosterone, tuttavia, in vivo, il cortisolo ha una attività mineralcorticoide debole. Questa discrepanza dipende dall'azione dell'11β-idrossi-steroidodeidrogenasi di tipo 2, che converte il cortisolo in cortisone. Il cortisone non è in grado di legare il recettore, mentre l'aldosterone non costituisce un substrato dell'enzima. L'inibizione farmacologica o genetica di questo enzima consente al cortisolo il legame con il recettore dei mineralcorticoidi e provoca ipertensione e ritenzione sodica.

AZIONE DEGLI ANDROGENI SURRENALICI. Molte delle azioni degli androgeni surrenalici sono esercitate tramite la loro conversione in androgeni ed estrogeni attivi, come il testosterone, il diidrotestosterone, l'estrone e l'estradiolo. Nel maschio adulto, meno del 2% degli androgeni biologicamente importanti deriva dalla produzione surrenalica, mentre nella donna circa il 50% degli androgeni ha un'origine surrenalica. Il contributo del surrene al livello degli estrogeni circolanti è importante soprattutto in condizioni patologiche, come nei tumori surrenalici femminilizzanti. Gli androgeni surrenalici contribuiscono al fisiologico sviluppo dei peli pubici e ascellari durante la normale pubertà. Giocano inoltre un ruolo importante nella fisiopatologia dell'iperplasia surrenalica congenita, dell'adrenarca prematuro, di tumori surrenalici e della sindrome di Cushing (vedi Capitoli 577 e 578).

Nell'uomo, i livelli circolanti di DHEA e DHEAS, i principali androgeni surrenalici, raggiungono il massimo nel giovane adulto, per poi diminuire. Da ciò si ritiene che le modificazioni fisiologiche correlate all'età possano essere invertite con la somministrazione di DHEA e sono stati suggeriti (ma non provati) effetti benefici sull'insulino-resistenza, densità minerale ossea, massa muscolare, rischio cardiovascolare, obesità, rischio di cancro, autoimmunità e sistema nervoso centrale.

Corticosteroidi di sintesi. Sono stati ottenuti molti analoghi sintetici del cortisone e dell'idrocortisone. Il prednisone e il prednisolone sono derivati con un ulteriore doppio legame nell'anello A. Simile al cortisone, il prednisone non è uno steroide attivo, ma è convertito a prednisolone per opera di un 11β-idrossisteroidodeidrogenasi epatica. Prednisone e prednisolone sono 4-5 volte più potenti per quanto riguarda l'azione antinfiammatoria e sul metabolismo dei carboidrati, ma possiedono effetti lievemente inferiori sulla ritenzione di acqua e sodio rispetto al cortisolo. I derivati alogenati hanno effetti diversi. Il betametasone e il desametasone mostrano una potenza glicocorticoide 40-50 volte maggiore di quella del cortisolo, ma con effetti mineralcorticoidi scarsi. Questi analoghi sono utilizzati solitamente a dosi farmacologiche per le loro proprietà antinfiammatorie e immunosoppressive. Il fludrocortisone possiede un'attività antinfiammatoria 15 volte più potente rispetto all'idrocortisone, ma, essendo 125 volte più attivo dei mineralcorticoidi, viene utilizzato nel trattamento del deficit di aldosterone.

575.5 • MIDOLLARE SURRENALICA

Gli ormoni principali della midollare sono le catecolamine fisiologicamente attive: dopamina, noradrenalina e adrenalina (Fig. 575-2). La sintesi di catecolamine si attua anche a livello cerebrale, nelle terminazioni nervose simpatiche, e nel tessuto cromaffine extramidollare. I metaboliti delle catecolamine sono escreti con le urine, principalmente l'acido 3-metossi-4-idrossimandelico (VMA), la metanefrina, e la normetanefrina. Quando si sospetta un feocromocitoma della midollare e del sistema nervoso simpatico, si ricorre al dosaggio delle metanefrine urinarie e delle catecolamine (vedi Capitolo 581).

Il rapporto tra adrenalina e noradrenalina nella ghiandola surrenalica varia con l'età. Nelle fasi fetali precoci, l'adrenalina è praticamente assente; alla nascita è predominante la noradrenalina. Nell'adulto, la noradrenalina raggiunge solo il 10-30% delle amine pressorie midollari.

Gli effetti delle catecolamine sono mediati da una serie di recettori adrenergici correlati alla proteina G. Sia la noradrenalina sia l'adrenalina aumenta la pressione arteriosa media, ma solo l'adrenalina aumenta la gittata cardiaca. Con l'aumento delle resistenze vascolari periferiche, la noradrenalina aumenta anche la pressione arteriosa sistolica e diastolica, con una lieve riduzione della frequenza cardiaca. L'adrenalina aumenta la frequenza cardiaca e, diminuendo le resistenze vascolari periferiche, provoca un decremento della pressione diastolica. Gli effetti iperglicemico e calorigeno della noradrenalina sono molto meno pronunciati di quelli dell'adrenalina.

Aguilera G, Rabadan-Diehl C: Vasopressinergic regulation of the hypothalamic-pituitary-adrenal axis: Implications for stress adaptation. *Regul Pept* 2000;96: 23–29.

Allen DB: Growth suppression by glucocorticoid therapy. *Endocrinol Metab Clin North Am* 1996;25:699–717.

Ashwell JD, Lu FW, Vacchio MS: Glucocorticoids in T cell development and function. *Annu Rev Immunol* 2000;18:309–345.

Bamberger CM, Schulte HM, Chrousos GP: Molecular determinants of glucocorticoid receptor function and tissue sensitivity to glucocorticoids. *Endocr Rev* 1996;17:245–261.

de Kloet ER, Vreugdenhil E, Oitzl MS, et al: Brain corticosteroid receptor balance in health and disease. *Endocr Rev* 1998;19:269–301.

Itoi K, Seasholtz AF, Watson SJ: Cellular and extracellular regulatory mechanisms of hypothalamic corticotropin-releasing hormone neurons. *Endocr J* 1998;45:13–33.

Jenkins BD, Pullen CB, Darimont BD: Novel glucocorticoid receptor coactivator effector mechanisms. *Trends Endocrinol Metab* 2001;12:122–126.

Lamberts SW, Bruining HA, de Jong FH: Corticosteroid therapy in severe illness. *N Engl J Med* 1997;337:1285–1292.

Lane NE, Lukert B: The science and therapy of glucocorticoid-induced bone loss. *Endocrinol Metab Clin North Am* 1998;27:465–483.

Lupien SJ, McEwen BS: The acute effects of corticosteroids on cognition: Integration of animal and human model studies. *Brain Res Brain Res Rev* 1997;24:1–27.

Manelli F, Giustina A: Glucocorticoid-induced osteoporosis. *Trends Endocrinol Metab* 2000;11:79–85.

Matsusaka T, Ichikawa I: Biological functions of angiotensin and its receptors. *Annu Rev Physiol* 1997;59:395–412.

Miller WL: Early steps in androgen biosynthesis: From cholesterol to DHEA. *Baillieres Clin Endocrinol Metab* 1998;12:67–81.

Peter M, Dubuis JM: Transcription factors as regulators of steroidogenic P-450 enzymes. *Eur J Clin Invest* 2000;30(Suppl 3):14–20.

Rainey WE, White PC: Functional adrenal zonation and regulation of aldosterone biosynthesis. *Curr Opin Endocrinol Diabet* 1998;5:175–182.

Stocco DM: StAR protein and the regulation of steroid hormone biosynthesis. *Annu Rev Physiol* 2001;63:193–213.

Tomlinson JW, Walker EA, Bujalska IJ, et al: 11β-Hydroxysteroid dehydrogenase type 1: A tissue-specific regulator of glucocorticoid response. *Endocr Rev* 2004;25:831–866.

Wallberg AE, Wright A, Gustafsson JA: Chromatin-remodeling complexes involved in gene activation by the glucocorticoid receptor. *Vitam Horm* 2000;60:75–122.

White PC: Genetic diseases of steroid metabolism. *Vitam Horm* 1994;49: 131–195.

White PC: Abnormalities of aldosterone synthesis and action in children. *Curr Opin Pediatr* 1997;9:424–430.

White PC, Mune T, Agarwal AK: 11β-Hydroxysteroid dehydrogenase and the syndrome of apparent mineralocorticoid excess. *Endocr Rev* 1997;18: 135–156.

Yanovski JA, Cutler GBJ: Glucocorticoid action and the clinical features of Cushing's syndrome. *Endocrinol Metab Clin North Am* 1994;23:487–509

Capitolo 576 ■ Insufficienza surrenalica

Nell'insufficienza surrenalica primaria, lesioni congenite o acquisite della corticale impediscono la produzione di cortisolo e spesso di aldosterone (Tab. 576-1). L'insufficienza surrenalica primaria acquisita viene definita morbo di Addison. Alterazioni dell'ipotalamo o dell'ipofisi anteriore possono provocare un deficit di corticotropina (ACTH), con conseguente ipofunzione surrenalica corticale; in questo caso si parla di insufficienza surrenalica secondaria (Tab. 576-2).

576.1 • INSUFFICIENZA SURRENALICA PRIMARIA

L'insufficienza surrenalica può essere causata da alterazioni genetiche che non sempre si manifestano nell'infanzia e da patologie acquisite, come quelle autoimmunitarie. Tuttavia, spesso la suscettibilità a certe patologie autoimmunitarie riconosce una base genetica, perciò la precedente distinzione non ha valore assoluto.

EZIOLOGIA EREDITARIA

DIFETTI CONGENITI DELLA STEROIDOGENESI. La causa più comune di insufficienza surrenalica nell'infanzia è rappresentata dall'iperplasia surrenalica congenita nelle forme con perdita di sali (vedi Capitolo 577). Circa il 75% dei neonati con deficit della 21-idrossilasi, quasi tutti i neonati con iperplasia surrenalica lipoidea e la maggior parte di quelli con deficit di 3β-idrossi-steroidodeidrogenasi manifestano, nel periodo neonatale, sintomi da perdita di sali perché non sono in grado di sintetizzare cortisolo e aldosterone.

IPOPLASIA SURRENALICA CONGENITA. Di solito l'iposurrenalismo si manifesta acutamente nel periodo neonatale, ma può comparire

TABELLA 576-1. Cause di insufficienza surrenalica primaria

DIAGNOSI	CARATTERISTICHE CLINICHE ASSOCIATE ALL'INSUFFICIENZA SURRENALICA	PATOGENESI O GENETICA
SURRENALITE AUTOIMMUNE		
Surrenalite autoimmune isolata	Non altre caratteristiche	Associazione con *HLA-DR*, *CTLA4*
Surrenalite autoimmune come parte di APS		
APS tipo 1 (APECED)	Ipoparatiroidismo, candidosi mucocutanea cronica, altre patologie autoimmuni	Mutazioni del gene *AIRE* (21q22.3)
APS tipo 2	Patologia tiroidea, diabete mellito, altre patologie autoimmuni (raro nei bambini)	Associazione con *HLA-DR*, *CTLA-4*
APS tipo 4	Altre patologie autoimmuni, escluse quelle tiroidee o diabete (raro nei bambini)	Associazione con *HLA-DR*, *CTLA-4*
SURRENALITE INFETTIVA		
Surrenalite tubercolare	Altre manifestazioni d'organo della tubercolosi	Tubercolosi
AIDS	Altre patologie associate all'AIDS	HIV-1, Cytomegalovirus
Surrenalite micotica	Soprattutto in pazienti immunosoppressi	Criptococcosi, istoplasmosi, coccidioidomicosi
DISORDINI GENETICI CON INSUFFICIENZA SURRENALICA		
Adrenoleucodistrofia, adrenomieloneuropatia	Demielinizzazione del SNC (adrenoleucodistrofia cerebrale), del midollo spinale o dei nervi periferici (adrenomieloneuropatia)	Mutazione del gene *ABCD1* che codifica per la proteina perossisomiale della adrenoleucodistrofia
Iperplasia surrenalica congenita		
Deficit di 21-idrossilasi	Genitali ambigui nelle femmine	Mutazione di *CYP21*
Deficit di 11β-idrossilasi	Genitali ambigui nelle femmine e ipertensione	Mutazione di *CYP11B1*
Deficit di 3β-HSD tipo 2	Genitali ambigui nei maschi, virilizzazione postnatale nelle femmine	Mutazione di *HSD3B2*
Deficit di 17α-idrossilasi	Genitali ambigui nei maschi, mancanza di pubertà in entrambi i sessi, ipertensione	Mutazione di *CYP17*
Ipoplasia surrenalica congenita lipoidea	Inversione sessuale XY	Mutazioni del gene (*STAR*) della proteina regolatoria acuta steroidogenica; mutazioni di *CYP11A* (che codifica P450scc), mutazione di PDR
Deficit di piro-ossidoreduttasi	Sindrome di Antler-Bixler	
Sindrome di Smith-Lemli-Opitz	Ritardo mentale, malformazioni craniofacciali, deficit di crescita	Mutazioni del gene *DHCR7* della 7-didrocolesteroloreduttasi
Ipoplasia surrenalica congenita		
Correlata all'X	Ipogonadismo ipogonadotropo	Mutazioni di *NROB1* (*DAX1*)
Sindrome del gene contiguo Xp21	Distrofia muscolare di Duchenne e deficit di glielo-chinasi (ritardo psicomotorio)	Delezione della distrofia muscolare di Duchenne, glicerolochinasi, e geni *NROB1* (*DAX1*)
Correlata a SF-1	Inversione sessuale XY	Mutazione di *NR5A1* (*SF1*)
Sindrome IMAGe	Ritardo della crescita intrauterina, displasia metafisaria, insufficienza surrenalica e anomalie genitali (IMAGe)	Sconosciuta
Sindrome di Kearms-Sayre	Oftalmoplegia esterna, degenerazione retinica, difetti della conduzione cardiaca; altre endocrinopatie	Delezioni del Dna mitocondriale
Sindromi da insensibilità all'ACTH (deficit di glicocorticoidi familiare)	Deficit di glicocorticoidi, ma non laterazioni della sintesi dei mineralcorticoidi	
Tipo 1	Alta statura	Mutazioni del recettore ACTH (*MC2R*)
Tipo 2	Non ci sono altre caratteristiche	Sconosciuta
Sindrome della tripla A (sindrome di Allgrove)	Alacrimia, acalasia; sintomi addizionali, compresi disturbi neurologici, sordità, ritardo mentale, ipercheratosi	Mutazioni del gene tripla A (*AAAS*) che codifica per la proteina WD-repeat
EMORRAGIA SURRENALICA BILATERALE	Sintomi della patologia sottostante	Shock settico, specificamente sepsi meningococcica (sindrome di Waterhouse-Friderichsen); sindrome antifosfolipide primaria
INFILTRAZIONE SURRENALICA	Sintomi della patologia sottostante	Metastasi surrenaliche, linfoma surrenalico primario, sarcoidosi, amiloidosi, emocromatosi
SURRENALECTOMIA BILATERALE	Sintomi della patologia sottostante	Sindrome di Cushing non risolta
INSUFFICIENZA SURRENALICA DA FARMACI	Non ci sono altri sintomi	Trattamento con mitotano, aminoglutetimide, etomidate, ketoconazolo, suramin, mifepristone

HSD, 3β-idrossi-steroidodeidrogenasi.
Da Arlt W, Allolio B: Adrenal insufficiency. *Lancet* 2003;361:1881-1892.

tardivamente durante l'infanzia o anche nell'età adulta, ma con un esordio più insidioso. L'indagine istologica della corticale surrenalica ipoplasica rivela un quadro di disorganizzazione e citomegalia. La malattia colpisce principalmente i maschi ed è causata da una mutazione del gene *DAX1* (*NR0B1*), che fa parte della famiglia dei recettori ormonali nucleari, localizzato su Xp21. Bambini con ipoplasia surrenalica congenita (*Adrenal Hypoplasia Congenital*, AHC) non hanno pubertà, per la presenza di ipogonadismo ipogonadotropo; sia l'AHC sia l'ipogonadismo ipogonadotropo sono dovuti alla stessa mutazione del gene *DAX1*. Il **criptorchidismo**, spesso presente in questi bambini, è probabilmente la manifestazione precoce dell'ipogonadismo ipogonadotropo.

L'AHC è presente anche in una sindrome da **delezione di un gene contiguo**, assieme alla distrofia muscolare di Duchenne, al deficit della glicerolo chinasi, a ritardo mentale o a una combinazione di queste patologie.

DEFICIT DI SF-1. Il fattore di trascrizione SF-1 è essenziale per lo sviluppo surrenalico e gonadico (vedi Capitolo 575). Rari pazienti eterozigoti per mutazione di SF-1 (*NR5A1*) manifestano insufficienza surrenalica nonostante la presenza di una normale copia del gene sull'altro cromosoma. I maschi evidenziano un'alterazione dello sviluppo testicolare e possono avere un fenotipo femminile, analogamente ai pazienti con iperplasia surrenalica lipoidea (vedi Capitolo 577).

ADRENOLEUCODISTROFIA (ALD). In questa malattia, il deficit surrenalico si associa a demielinizzazione del sistema nervoso centrale (vedi Capitoli 86 e 599.3). Nei tessuti e nei liquidi corporei, sono presenti elevati livelli di acidi grassi a catena molto lunga, per alterata ossidazione a livello dei perossisomi.

La forma più frequente di ALD è una malattia legata all'X che può presentarsi in modo diverso. Il quadro clinico più frequente comprende un disturbo neurologico degenerativo che compare nell'infanzia o nell'adolescenza ed evolve fino a una grave demenza e a un deterioramento della vista, dell'udito, del linguaggio e dell'andatura, con esito fatale in pochi anni. Una forma più lieve

TABELLA 576-2. Cause dell'insufficienza surrenalica secondaria

DIAGNOSI	COMMENTO
Tumori ipofisari	Insufficienza surrenalica secondaria soprattutto nell'ambito di panipopituitarismo; sintomi ulteriori (alterazioni del campo visivo): generalmente adenomi, il carcinoma è raro; conseguenza della crescita tumorale, del trattamento chirurgico o di entrambi
Altri tumori della regione ipotalamo-ipofisaria	Craniofaringioma, meningioma, ependimoma e metastasi intra o soprasellari
Irradiazione ipofisaria	Irradiazione craniospinale nella leucemia, irradiazione per tumori esterni all'asse ipotalamo-ipofisi, irradiazione di tumori ipofisari
Ipofisite linfocitica	
Isolata	Ipofisite autoimmune; più frequente in gravidanza (80%); soprattutto ipopituitarismo, ma anche deficit isolato di ormone adrenocorticotropo
Come parte di APS	Associata a patologia tiroidea autoimmune e, meno frequentemente, a vitiligine, a insufficienza gonadica primaria, a diabete tipo 1 e ad anemia perniciosa
Isolata congenita	È un deficit dell'enzima che scinde la pro-opiomelanocortina?
Deficit di ACTH	
Sindrome da deficit di pro-opiomelanocortina	Mutazioni del gene della pro-opiomelanocortina; triade clinica di insufficienza surrenalica, obesità a esordio precoce e capelli rossi
Deficit combinato di ormoni ipofisari	Mutazioni del gene che codifica il fattore ipofisario di trascrizione di Pit1 (*PROP1*), progressivo sviluppo di panipopituitarismo nel seguente ordine: GH, PRL, TSH, LH/FSH, (ACTH). Mutazioni nell'homeobox gene *HESX1*, deficit combinato di ormoni ipofisari, ipoplasia del nervo ottico, difetti cerebrali mediali (displasia setto-ottica)
Apoplessia ipofisaria	Esordisce principalmente con improvvisa e severa cefalea, disturbi visivi, nausea o vomito
(Sindrome di Sheehan)	Sindrome da istiocitosi, apoplessia surrenalica o necrosi con esordio nel periodo postpartum per notevole perdita ematica o ipotensione
Infiltrazione o granuloma ipofisario	Tubercolosi, actinomicosi, sarcoidosi, granulomatosa di Wegener
Trauma cranico	Per esempio lesioni del peduncolo ipofisario
Precedente eccesso cronico di glicocorticoidi	Somministrazione esogena di glicocorticoidi per più di 4 settimane, ipersecrezione endogena di glicocorticoidi da sindrome di Cushing

FSH, ormone follicolo stimolante; GH, ormone della crescita; LH, ormone luteinizzante; PRL, prolattina; TSH, tireotropina.
Da Arlt W, Allolio B: Adrenal insufficiency. *Lancet* 2003;361:1881-1892.

di ALD correlata a X è la adrenomieoloneuropatia (ALM), che inizia nella tarda adolescenza o nelle prime fasi dell'età adulta. Molti pazienti presentano insufficienza surrenalica al momento dell'esordio delle manifestazioni neurologiche, ma la malattia di Addison può essere presente anche in assenza di sintomi neurologici, o può precederli di molti anni. L'adrenoleucodistrofia legata all'X (X-ALD) è dovuta a mutazioni del gene *ABCD1* localizzato su Xq28. Il gene codifica un trasportatore di membrana coinvolto nel trasporto di acidi grassi a catena molto lunga all'interno dei perossisomi. In pazienti con X-ALD sono state descritte più di 400 mutazioni; la maggior parte delle famiglie con X-ALD presenta un'unica mutazione. I quadri clinici possono variare anche all'interno di una stessa famiglia, forse a causa di un gene modificante o per altri fattori sconosciuti. Non c'è un rapporto tra grado di lesione neurologica e gravità dell'insufficienza surrenalica. È auspicabile la diagnosi prenatale mediante studio del DNA e screening familiare, con dosaggio di acidi grassi a catena molto lunga e analisi della mutazione. Femmine eterozigoti per trasportatori del gene X-ALD possono sviluppare sintomi nella mezza età o successivamente. L'insufficienza surrenalica è rara.

L'ALD neonatale è una rara malattia autosomica recessiva. I neonati presentano un deterioramento neurologico e hanno o acquisiscono segni di insufficienza surrenalica. La maggior parte dei pazienti manifesta un grave ritardo mentale e muore prima del quinto anno di età. Questa malattia fa parte della sindrome di Zellweger (cerebro-epato-renale), in cui non si sviluppano i perossisomi a causa di mutazioni in qualcuno dei vari geni che controllano lo sviluppo di questi organuli.

DEFICIT FAMILIARE DI GLICOCORTICOIDI. Questa forma di insufficienza surrenalica cronica è caratterizzata da un deficit isolato di glicocorticoidi, elevati livelli di ACTH e normale produzione di aldosterone. Non compaiono qui manifestazioni da perdita di sali, presenti nella maggior parte delle altre forme di insufficienza surrenalica; i pazienti manifestano invece principalmente ipoglicemia, crisi epilettiche e aumento della pigmentazione durante la prima decade di vita. La malattia colpisce entrambi i sessi in uguale misura ed è ereditaria con modalità autosomica recessiva. È presente una marcata atrofia corticale, con relativo risparmio della zona glomerulare. In circa il 40% di questi pazienti sono state descritte numerose mutazioni del gene per il recettore dell'ACTH.

Un'altra sindrome da resistenza all'ACTH si verifica in associazione ad **acalasia** cardiale gastrica e ad **alacrimia** (**sindrome di Allgrove** o **della tripla A**). Questi pazienti spesso manifestano un progressivo deterioramento neurologico, che comprende alterazioni del sistema autonomo, ritardo mentale, sordità e neuropatia motoria. Questa sindrome è ereditaria con trasmissione autosomica recessiva e il gene AAAS è stato mappato sul cromosoma 12q13. La proteina codificata, l'aladina, partecipa alla regolazione del trasporto nucleocitoplasmatico di altre proteine.

POLIENDOCRINOPATIA AUTOIMMUNE TIPO I (APS-1)

Nonostante il morbo di Addison autoimmunitario compaia molto spesso in modo sporadico (vedi oltre), può appartenere a due sindromi, che consistono entrambe di una serie di patologie autoimmuni. La **poliendocrinopatia autoimmune tipo I** (**APS-1**), conosciuta anche come sindrome da poliendocrinopatia autoimmune/candidosi/distrofia ectodermica (*Autoimmune Polyendicrinopathy/Candidiasis/Ectodermal Dystrophy*, APECED), è ereditaria con trasmissione mendeliana autosomica recessiva, mentre la APS-2 (vedi oltre) ha una ereditarietà complessa. La **candidosi mucocutanea cronica** è molto spesso la prima manifestazione della APS-1, seguita da ipoparatiroidismo e poi da morbo di Addison, che si sviluppa tipicamente nelle fasi precoci dell'adolescenza. Altre patologie autoimmunitarie strettamente associate comprendono insufficienza gonadica, alopecia, vitiligine, cheratopatia, ipoplasia dello smalto, distrofia ungueale, malassorbimento intestinale ed epatite cronica attiva. Nel 10% dei pazienti compaiono anche ipotiroidismo e diabete mellito tipo 1. Alcune componenti di questa sindrome continuano a progredire fino alla quinta decade di vita. La presenza in questi pazienti di autoanticorpi antisurrene e anticellule a secrezione steroidea indica normalmente un'alta probabilità di sviluppare il morbo di Addison o, nelle femmine, insufficienza gonadica. L'insufficienza surrenalica nella APS-1 può evolvere rapidamente; sono stati riportati casi di esito fatale in pazienti precedentemente diagnosticati e di morte inspiegabile in fratelli di pazienti con questa patologia. Ne deriva la necessità di monitorare strettamente i pazienti con APS-1 e di valutare accuratamente i fratelli apparentemente sani di pazienti con questa malattia.

In pazienti con APS-1 sono stati descritti autoanticorpi contro gli enzimi CYP21, CYP17 e CYP11A1. Il gene responsabile della APS-1 viene detto regolatore autoimmune-1 (*AIRE1*); è localizzato sul cromosoma 21q22.3. Il gene *AIRE1* codifica una proteina che funge da fattore trascrizionale, con un ruolo importante nella riposta immunitaria. In pazienti con APS-1 sono state descritte circa 40 diverse mutazioni del gene *AIRE1*, di cui due (R257X e delezione 3-bp) sono più frequenti. In una famiglia è stata documentata una trasmissione autosomica dominante, per una specifica mutazione missense (G228W).

ALTERAZIONI DELLA SINTESI/METABOLISMO DEL COLESTEROLO. Pazienti con alterazioni della sintesi o del metabolismo del colesterolo, che comprendono la abetalipoproteinemia con deficit di lipoproteine contenenti lipoproteina B e l'ipercolesterolemia familiare, con diminuzione o alterazione dei recettori delle LDL, mostrano una limitazione della funzionalità surrenalica. Insufficienza surrenalica è stata descritta in pazienti con la **sindrome di Smith-Lemli-Opitz** (SLOS), una malattia autosomica recessiva che si presenta con anomalie facciali, microcefalia, anomalie degli arti, e ritardo dello sviluppo. Nella patogenesi della SLOS sono implicate mutazioni del gene che codifica per la sterolDELTA7-reduttasi, sul cromosoma 11q12-q13, con conseguente alterazione delle fasi finali della sintesi del colesterolo e notevole aumento del 7-deidrocolesterolo, notevole diminuzione del colesterolo e insufficienza surrenalica. La **malattia di Wolman** è una rara patologia autosomica recessiva, dovuta a mutazioni del gene che codifica l'acido-lipasi lisosomiale umana. Gli esteri del colesterolo si accumulano a livello lisosomiale nella maggior parte degli organi, con conseguente insufficienza funzionale dell'organo stesso. Neonati nel primo o secondo mese di vita presentano epatosplenomegalia, steatorrea, distensione addominale e arresto della crescita. Sono presenti insufficienza surrenalica e calcificazioni surrenaliche bilaterali; la morte sopravviene di solito nei primi anni di vita. Il gene per l'acido-lipasi lisosomiale è stato mappato sul cromosoma 10q23.2-23.3; sono stati chiariti i difetti genetici dei pazienti con malattia di Wolman.

CARENZA DELLA GLOBULINA CHE LEGA I CORTICOSTEROIDI (*CORTICOSTEROID-BINDING GLOBULIN*, CBG) E DIMINUZIONE DELL'AFFINITÀ DI LEGAME PER IL CORTISOLO. Queste alterazioni portano a una diminuzione dei livelli plasmatici del cortisolo, ma con normale cortisolo libero urinario e normali livelli plasmatici di ACTH. In adulti con alterazioni della CBG è stata descritta una notevole frequenza di ipotensione e astenia.

EZIOLOGIA ACQUISITA

MORBO DI ADDISON AUTOIMMUNE. La causa più frequente di morbo di Addison è la distruzione autoimmune della ghiandola. I surreni possono essere così piccoli da non risultare visibili all'autopsia e nelle sezioni microscopiche si possono trovare solo frammenti di tessuto. Solitamente la midollare non viene colpita e presenta una marcata infiltrazione linfocitaria nell'area occupata precedentemente dalla corticale. Nei quadri avanzati di malattia, vengono annullate tutte le funzioni surrenaliche, ma nelle fasi precoci si può avere un deficit isolato di cortisolo. Nel plasma della maggior parte dei pazienti sono dosabili anticorpi anticitoplasma surrenalico; il più frequente autoantigene è rappresentato dalla 21-idrossilasi (CYP21).

La malattia di Addison può far parte di due sindromi poliendocrine autoimmuni. Il tipo I (APS-1) è stato discusso precedentemente. La **poliendocrinopatia autoimmune tipo II** (**APS-2**), consiste nel morbo di Addison associato a patologia autoimmune tiroidea (sindrome di Schmidt) o a diabete di tipo 1 (sindrome di Carpenter). Possono essere presenti anche insufficienza gonadica, vitiligine, alopecia e gastrite atrofica cronica, con o senza anemia perniciosa. In questi pazienti sono aumentati l'HLA-D3 e l'HLA-D4, ai quali pare correlato un incremento del rischio di contrarre la malattia; a questa patologia sono stati inoltre associati alleli al complesso di istocompatibilità maggiore di classe I dei geni A e B catena-correlati (MICA e MICB). La malattia è più frequente nelle femmine di mezza età e si può presentare in molte generazioni della stessa famiglia. In questi pazienti si sono trovati anche autoanticorpi antisurrene, in particolare quelli contro gli enzimi CYP21 e CYP17 e CYP11A1.

INFEZIONI. In passato la tubercolosi è stata una causa frequente di distruzione surrenalica, ma ora lo è molto meno. L'eziologia infettiva più frequente dell'insufficienza surrenalica è quella meningococcica (vedi Capitolo 190); nella sindrome di Waterhouse-Friderichsen si verifica una crisi surrenalica dovuta a questo agente. Pazienti con AIDS possono manifestare una serie di anomalie subcliniche dell'asse ipotalamo-ipofiso-surrenalico, ma è rara una vera insufficienza surrenalica. Tuttavia, farmaci utilizzati nel trattamento dell'AIDS possono alterare l'omeostasi degli ormoni surrenalici.

FARMACI. Il ketoconazolo, un farmaco antimicotico, può provocare insufficienza surrenalica tramite l'inibizione degli enzimi surrenalici. La rifampicina e i farmaci anticonvulsivanti come la fentoina e il fenobarbital riducono l'efficacia e la biodisponibilità della terapia sostitutiva con ormoni corticosteroidi, mediante l'induzione a livello epatico di enzimi che metabolizzano gli steroidi stessi. Il mitotane (o,p′-DDD), usato nel trattamento del carcinoma surrenalico e della sindrome di Cushing refrattaria (vedi Capitoli 578 e 581), è citotossico per la corticale surrenalica e può alterare anche il metabolismo extrasurrenalico del cortisolo. In una notevole percentuale di pazienti trattati con mitotano compaiono segni di insufficienza surrenalica.

EMORRAGIA INTRASURRENALICA. Si può verificare nel periodo neonatale come conseguenza di un travaglio difficoltoso (soprattutto nella presentazione podalica) o per causa sconosciuta. Si valuta un'incidenza percentuale di 3 per 100 000 nati vivi. L'emorragia può essere sufficientemente estesa da portare a morte per ipovolemia o iposurrenalismo. I segni di presentazione possono essere una massa addominale, anemia, ittero inspiegabile o ematoma scrotale. Spesso inizialmente l'emorragia è asintomatica e viene identificata solo in un secondo momento per la presenza di calcificazioni dei surreni. È stata descritta anche un'emorragia surrenalica in periodo fetale. Dopo la nascita, l'emorragia surrenalica compare più frequentemente in pazienti trattati con anticoagulanti. Può anche essere la conseguenza di un abuso infantile.

MANIFESTAZIONI CLINICHE. L'insufficienza surrenalica primaria porta a deficit di cortisolo e aldosterone. Tenendo conto delle normali azioni di questi ormoni, già discusse nel Capitolo 575, si possono comprendere molto più facilmente i segni e i sintomi dell'insufficienza surrenalica.

L'ipoglicemia è una caratteristica importante ed è spesso accompagnata da chetosi, poiché l'organismo tenta di utilizzare gli acidi grassi come sorgente energetica alternativa. La chetosi è aggravata dall'anoressia, dalla nausea e dal vomito, che compaiono frequentemente.

La carenza di cortisolo comporta un decremento della gittata cardiaca e del tono vascolare; inoltre le catecolamine come l'adrenalina hanno, in assenza di cortisolo, minori effetti inotropi e pressori. Questi problemi si manifestano inizialmente come ipotensione ortostatica nei bambini più grandi e possono progredire fino allo shock in pazienti di qualsiasi età. Sono aumentati dalla carenza di aldosterone, responsabile di ipovolemia da diminuzione del riassorbimento del sodio nel nefrone distale.

Ipotensione e diminuzione della gittata cardiaca provocano un decremento della filtrazione glomerulare con conseguente diminuzione della capacità renale di eliminare acqua libera. In risposta all'ipotensione, anche per mancanza di inibizione da parte del cortisolo, l'ipofisi posteriore secerne vasopressina (AVP). Questi fattori diminuiscono l'osmolalità plasmatica e in particolare portano a iponatremia. L'iponatremia è dovuta anche alla carenza di aldosterone è può essere molto severa in caso di deficit combinato sia di cortisolo sia di aldosterone.

Oltre all'ipovolemia e all'iponatremia, il deficit di aldosterone provoca iperkaliemia per diminuzione dell'escrezione di potassio nel nefrone distale. Il deficit di solo cortisolo non provoca iperkaliemia.

La carenza di cortisolo decresce il feedback ipotalamo-ipofisario, con conseguente incremento della secrezione di ACTH. L'iperpigmentazione è dovuta all'ACTH e ad altri ormoni peptidici (ormone stimolante i γ-melanociti), derivati dal precursore dell'ACTH pro-opiomelanocortina. In pazienti con carnagione chiara, la cute può assumere un colorito bronzeo. La pigmentazione può essere più evidente nelle pieghe cutanee, nelle mucose e in corrispondenza delle cicatrici. In pazienti di pelle scura, può essere visibile più facilmente nella mucosa gengivale e orale.

La presentazione clinica dell'insufficienza surrenalica dipende dall'età del paziente, in caso di coinvolgimento contemporaneo di cortisolo e aldosterone e dall'entità dell'eziologia. Nella prima infanzia le cause più comuni sono rappresentate da errori congeniti della biosintesi degli steroidi, sepsi, ipoplasia surrenalica congenita ed emorragia surrenalica. I neonati, rispetto ai bambini più grandi, hanno una richiesta relativamente maggiore di aldosterone, per immaturità renale e anche per il basso contenuto sodico del latte umano e di quello in polvere. Nel neonato, i segni principali di esordio dell'insufficienza surrenalica sono rappresentati da iperkaliemia, iponatremia, ipoglicemia. La chetosi è presente raramente, perché i neonati generano meno chetoni dei bambini più grandi. Di solito non è rilevabile la melanodermia, che si sviluppa in settimane e mesi, e l'ipotensione ortostatica è ovviamente difficile da dimostrare nel neonato.

La malattia nei neonati ha un andamento acuto. Dopo solo pochi giorni di diminuita attività, anoressia e vomito, si possono già sviluppare gravi alterazioni elettrolitiche.

Nei bambini più grandi con morbo di Addison, l'esordio è solitamente più graduale ed è caratterizzato da astenia muscolare, malessere, anoressia, vomito, perdita di peso e ipotensione ortostatica. Spesso la melanodermia è assente. Sono frequenti l'ipoglicemia, la chetosi, l'iponatremia. Nei bambini più grandi l'iperkaliemia tende a manifestarsi più tardivamente rispetto ai neonati, perciò la presentazione clinica può essere facilmente confusa con una gastroenterite o altre infezioni acute. La cronicità dei sintomi può fare sospettare la possibilità del morbo di Addison, ma questa diagnosi va presa in considerazione in tutti i bambini con ipotensione ortostatica, iponatremia, ipoglicemia e chetosi.

Nell'insufficienza surrenalica primaria con deficit di mineralcorticoidi, si manifesta un bisogno di sali. Astenia, mialgia, febbre, eosinofilia, linfocitosi, ipercalcemia e anemia possono essere presenti nel deficit di glicocorticoidi.

REPERTI DI LABORATORIO. L'iponatremia, l'ipoglicemia, la chetosi e l'iperkaliemia sono già state discusse. In un bambino in condizioni critiche, l'elettrocardiogramma è utile per rilevare rapidamente l'iperkaliemia. Frequentemente è presente acidosi e, se il paziente è disidratato, sono elevati i livelli plasmatici di azoto ureico.

I livelli di cortisolo possono talvolta situarsi al limite inferiore del range di normalità, ma risultano invariabilmente bassi in rapporto al grado di malattia del paziente. I livelli di ACTH sono elevati nell'insufficienza surrenalica primaria, ma possono richiedere tempo prima di essere pronti. Similmente, i livelli di aldosterone possono situarsi nel range della normalità, ma essere inappropriatamente bassi in rapporto all'iponatremia, all'iperkaliemia e all'ipovolemia del paziente. L'attività retinica plasmatica è elevata. Gli eosinofili ematici possono essere aumentati, ma questo raramente ha valore diagnostico.

L'escrezione urinaria di sodio e cloruro è aumentata, mentre è diminuita quella di potassio; questi dati però sono di difficile valutazione in singoli campioni di urina. Un'interpretazione accurata degli elettroliti urinari richiede una raccolta delle urine più prolungata (24 ore) e la conoscenza dell'introito di sodio e potassio del paziente.

Il **test più accurato** per la diagnosi di insufficienza surrenalica è la misurazione dei livelli sierici di cortisolo prima e dopo somministrazione di ACTH; i livelli basali sono bassi e non aumentano, come di norma, dopo la somministrazione di ACTH. Occasionalmente, livelli basali normali che non aumentano dopo somministrazione di ACTH possono indicare l'assenza di riserva surrenalica. Una basso livello iniziale, seguito da una significativa risposta all'ACTH, può indicare un'insufficienza surrenalica secondaria. Tradizionalmente, questo test è stato studiato per misurare i livelli di cortisolo prima e 30 o 60 minuti dopo la somministrazione di 0,250 mg di cosintropina (ACTH 1-24) per rapida infusione endovenosa. Anche l'aldosterone può transitoriamente aumentare in risposta a questa dose di ACTH e può quindi essere valutato. Un test con bassa dose (0,5-1 μg di ACTH 1-24/1,73 m^2) è più sensibile per la valutazione della riserva ipofiso-surrenalica, ma ha minore specificità (più falsi positivi).

DIAGNOSI DIFFERENZIALE. All'inizio, spesso è necessario distinguere il morbo di Addison da patologie più acute, come la gastroenterite con disidratazione o la sepsi. Ulteriori test hanno lo scopo di identificare le cause specifiche dell'insufficienza surrenalica. Se si sospetta un'iperplasia surrenalica congenita, si devono misurare i livelli dei precursori del cortisolo (17-idrossiprogesterone) ed eseguire un test di stimolazione con ACTH (vedi Capitolo 577). Elevati livelli di acidi grassi a catena molto lunga sono diagnostici di adrenoleucodistrofia. La presenza di anticorpi antisurrene suggerisce una patogenesi autoimmune. Pazienti con morbo di Addison autoimmune devono essere monitorati con attenzione, per la possibilità che si sviluppino altre patologie autoimmuni. Nei bambini, la malattia che si associa più frequentemente è l'ipoparatioridismo, sospettata in presenza di ipocalcemia ed elevati livelli di fosfati.

Ecografia, TC o RM possono essere di aiuto per definire le dimensioni delle ghiandole surrenaliche.

TRATTAMENTO. Il trattamento dell'insufficienza surrenalica acuta deve essere immediato e deciso. Se la diagnosi di insufficienza surrenalica non è ancora stabilita, si deve prelevare un campione di sangue prima di iniziare la terapia, per la determinazione di elettroliti, glucosio, ACTH, cortisolo, aldosterone e attività retinica plasmatica. Se le condizioni del paziente lo permettono, mentre si sta iniziando rianimazione con liquidi, si può eseguire un test di stimolazione con ACTH. Per correggere ipoglicemia, ipovolemia e iponatremia, è necessaria la somministrazione endovenosa di glucosio al 5% in soluzione salina allo 0,9%. Se l'iperkaliemia è severa, può richiedere trattamento per via endovenosa con calcio e/o bicarbonato, per via rettale con resina legante il potassio, o per via endovenosa con infusione di glucosio e insulina. Un derivato idrosolubile dell'idrocortisone, l'idrocortisone sodio succinato, va somministrato per via endovenosa. Deve essere dato a intervalli di 6 ore per le prime 24 ore, al dosaggio di 10 mg per i neonati, 25 mg per i bambini piccoli, 50 mg per quelli un po' più grandi e 100 mg per gli adolescenti. Se l'andamento è soddisfacente, queste dosi devono essere ridotte durante le successive 24 ore. Con la somministrazione di soluzione salina, coadiuvata dall'effetto mineralcorticoide di alte dosi di idrocortisone, si ottiene un adeguato apporto di liquidi e di sodio.

Si deve fare particolare attenzione a quei rari pazienti che presentano insufficienza surrenalica e contemporaneamente ipotiroidismo, perché la tiroxina può aumentare la clearance del cortisolo. In tal modo, se l'ipotiroidismo viene trattato senza prima aver provveduto a una adeguata terapia sostitutiva con glicocorticoidi, si può provocare una **crisi surrenalica**.

Quando le manifestazioni acute sono sotto controllo, la maggior parte dei pazienti richiede una terapia sostitutiva cronica per il deficit di cortisolo e aldosterone. L'idrocortisone può essere assunto per via orale alla dose di 10 mg/m^2/die in tre somministrazioni; alcuni pazienti richiedono 15 mg/m^2/die per combattere l'astenia, specialmente durante il giorno. Possono essere utilizzate dosi equivalenti (20-25% della dose dell'idrocortisone) di prednisone o prednisolone, in due somministrazioni giornaliere. Nell'insufficienza surrenalica primaria, per monitorare l'adeguatezza della terapia sostitutiva con glicocorticoidi, ci si basa sui livelli di ACTH; nell'iperplasia surrenalica congenita si utilizzano invece i livelli del precursore ormonale (vedi Capitolo 577). In situazioni di stress, come nei periodi di infezione o di procedure chirurgiche minori, la dose di idrocortisone deve essere aumentata di 2-3 volte. Interventi chirurgici maggiori in anestesia generale richiedono la somministrazione endovenosa di alte dosi di idrocortisone, analoghe a quelle utilizzate per l'insufficienza surrenalica acuta. In presenza di deficit di aldosterone, si somministra fludrocortisone per via orale (un mineralcorticoide), alla dose di 0,05-0,3 mg/die. Misurazioni dell'attività retinica plasmatica sono utili per monitorare l'adeguatezza della terapia sostitutiva con fludrocortisone. Il sovradosaggio cronico di glicocorticoidi porta a obesità, bassa statura e osteoporosi, mentre quello di fludrocortisone comporta tachiacardia, ipertensione e occasionalmente ipokaliemia.

La terapia sostitutiva con deidroepiandrosterone (DHEA) nell'adulto rimane controversa; bambini prepuberi non producono normalmente grosse quantità di DHEA. Molti adulti con morbo di Addison lamentano un calo dell'energia e la terapia con DHEA può risolvere questo problema, particolarmente in donne in cui gli androgeni surrenalici rappresentino circa la metà della secrezione androgenica complessiva. Tuttavia, mancano studi ampi e ben controllati in proposito.

Può essere necessaria un'ulteriore terapia, diretta contro la causa sottostante dell'insufficienza surrenalica, in caso di infezioni e di certi difetti metabolici. L'approccio terapeutico della adrenoleucodistrofia comprende la somministrazione di glicerolo trioleato e glicerolo trierucato (olio di Lorenzo), trapianto di midollo osseo e lovastatina (vedi Capitolo 599.3).

576.2 • INSUFFICIENZA SURRENALICA SECONDARIA

EZIOLOGIA

BRUSCA INTERRUZIONE DELLA SOMMINISTRAZIONE DI GLICOCORTICOIDI. L'insufficienza surrenalica secondaria si verifica più frequentemente in presenza di soppressione dell'asse ipotalamo-ipofiso-surrenalico, per prolungata somministrazione di alte dosi di un potente glicocorticoidi, qualora l'agente sia improvvisamente sospeso o la dose sia diminuita troppo velocemente. I pazienti a rischio per questo problema comprendono quelli con leucemia, asma (particolarmente se il paziente è passato dalla somministrazione di corticosteroidi per via orale a quella per via inalatoria), collagenopatie vascolari o altre condizioni autoimmuni e quelli sottoposti a trapianto tissutale o a interventi neurochirurgici. Non è nota la durata massima e la dose di glicocorticoidi che porta a questo problema, ma si suppone che possano essere somministrate alte dosi di glicocorticoidi (l'equivalente di più di 10 volte la secrezione fisiologica di cortisolo) per almeno una settimana, senza la necessità di una diminuzione del dosaggio. D'altra parte, quando si somministrano alte dosi di desametasone a bambini leucemici, possono essere necessari due mesi o più dopo la cessazione della terapia, prima che i test di funzionalità surrenalica ritornino nella norma. Segni e sintomi di insufficienza surrenalica sono molto più probabili in pazienti che abbiano subito stress come gravi infezioni o interventi chirurgici.

DEFICIT DI CORTICOTROPINA (ACTH). Una patologia ipotalamica o ipofisaria può provocare un deficit di corticotropina (vedi Capitolo 558), di solito associato a carenza di altri ormoni, come l'ormone della crescita e la tireotropina. Lesioni che colpiscono la zona ipofisaria, come il craniofaringioma e il germinoma, sono le cause più comuni di deficit di corticotropina. In molti casi l'ipofisi o l'ipotalamo sono danneggiati durante la rimozione chirurgica o la radioterapia di tumori della parte mediale del cervello. Raramente la causa del deficit corticotropinico è rappresentata da un'ipofisite autoimmune.

Si possono verificare anche lesioni ipofisarie congenite. Può essere colpita la sola ipofisi, o altre strutture mediali, come il nervo ottico o il setto pellucido. Il secondo tipo di anomalia viene definita **displasia setto-ottica**, o sindrome di de Morsier. Anomalie dello sviluppo cerebrale più gravi, come l'anencefalia e l'oloprosencefalia, possono coinvolgere anche l'ipofisi. Queste patologie sono solitamente sporadiche, sebbene si siano verificati pochi casi a eredità autosomica recessiva. È stato riportato anche il deficit isolato di corticotropina in diversi casi riguardanti fratelli. Sono descritti casi di pazienti con deficit ipofisari multipli per mutazioni del gene *PROP1*, con deficit progressivo di ACTH/cortisolo. La carenza isolata di ormone di rilascio della corticotropina è stata documentata in famiglie arabe, con caratteristiche autosomiche recessive.

PRESENTAZIONE CLINICA. La secrezione di aldosterone non viene coinvolta nell'insufficienza surrenalica secondaria, perché il surrene è, per definizione, intatto, e il sistema renina-angiotensina non viene coinvolto. Così, i segni e i sintomi sono quelli del deficit di cortisolo. I neonati spesso presentano ipoglicemia. Bambini più grandi hanno ipotensione ortostatica o astenia. Gli elettroliti sono di solito normali.

Se l'insufficienza surrenalica è dovuta a difetti anatomici congeniti o acquisisti che coinvolgono l'ipofisi, possono essere associati segni di carenza di altri ormoni ipofisari. In caso di deficit gonadotropinico, il pene può avere dimensioni ridotte nei neonati maschi. Neonati con ipotiroidismo secondario spesso manifestano ittero. I bambini con deficit dell'ormone della crescita, crescono poco dopo il primo anno di vita.

Alcuni bambini con anomalie ipofisarie presentano ipoplasia di un'emifaccia. Bambini con ipoplasia del nervo ottico possono manifestare una severa riduzione del visus. Di solito hanno un caratteristico nistagmo errante, che però spesso si rende evidente solo dopo diversi mesi di età.

TRATTAMENTO. Si può evitare l'insufficienza surrenalica secondaria iatrogenica (causata da somministrazione cronica di glicocorticoidi), utilizzando dosi inferiori di glicocorticoidi per via sistemica per più brevi periodi di tempo. Se si ritiene che un paziente possa essere a rischio, riducendo rapidamente la dose a un livello equivalente o lievemente inferiore alla sostituzione fisiologica (circa 10 mg/m^2/die di idrocortisone) e poi scendendo ulteriormente in qualche settimana, si consente alla corticale surrenalica di riprendersi senza sviluppare segni di insufficienza. Pazienti con lesioni anatomiche dell'ipofisi devono essere trattati con glicocorticoidi per il resto della loro vita. La sostituzione con mineralcorticoidi non è necessaria. In pazienti con panipopituitarismo il trattamento del deficit cortisolemico può causare escrezione di acqua libera che rivela un diabete insipido centrale. Quando si inizia la terapia con cortisolo in pazienti panipopituitarici, è necessario monitorare attentamente gli elettroliti.

Abdu TAM, Clayton RN: The low-dose synanthem test for the assessment of secondary adrenal insufficiency. *Curr Opin Endocrinol* 2000;7:116–121.

Arlt W, Allolio B: Adrenal insufficiency. *Lancet* 2003;361:1881–1893.

Anderson RA, Bryson GM, Parks JS: Lysosomal acid lipase mutations that determine phenotype in Wolman and cholesterol ester storage disease. *Mol Genet Metab* 1999;68:333–345.

Berberogly M, Aycan Z, Oeal G, et al: Syndrome of congenital adrenocortical unresponsiveness to ACTH: Report of six patients. *J Pediatr Endocrinol Metab* 2001;14:1113–1118.

Boles RG, Roe T, Senadheera D, et al: Mitochondrial DNA deletion with Kearns-Sayre syndrome in a child with Addison disease. *Eur J Pediatr* 1998;157:643–647.

Clark AJL, Metherell L, Swords FM, et al: The molecular pathogenesis of ACTH insensitivity syndromes. *Ann Endocrinol* 2001;62:207–211.

Cooper MS, Stewart PM: Corticosteroid insufficiency in acutely ill patients. *N Engl J Med* 2003;348:727–734.

Coursin DB, Wood KE: Corticosteroid supplementation for adrenal insufficiency. *JAMA* 2002;287:236–240.

Dickstein G: Hypothalamo-pituitary-adrenal axis testing: Nothing is sacred and caution in interpretation is needed. *Clin Endocrinol* 2001;54:15–16.

Drake AJ, Howells RJ, Shield PH, et al: Symptomatic adrenal insufficiency presenting with hypoglycaemia in asthmatic children with asthma receiving high dose inhaled fluticasone propionate. *Br Med J* 2002;324:1081–1082.

Eledrisi MS, Verghese AC: Adrenal insufficiency in HIV infection: A review and recommendations. *Am J Med Sci* 2001;321:137–144.

Fujieda K, Tajima T: Molecular basis of adrenal insufficiency. *Pediatr Res* 2005;57(5 pt 2):62R–69R.

Heino M, Peterson P, Kudoh J, et al: APECED mutations in the autoimmune regulator (AIRE) gene. *Hum Mutat* 2001;18:205–211.

Huysman MWA, Hokken-Koelega ACS, De Ridder MAJ, et al: Adrenal function in sick very preterm infants. *Pediatr Res* 2000;48:629–633.

Kemp S, Pujol A, Waterham HR, et al: ABCD1 mutations and the X-linked adrenoleukodystrophy mutation database: Role in diagnosis and clinical correlations. *Hum Mutat* 2001;18:499–515.
Krivit W, Peters C, Dusenbery K, et al: Case report: Wolman disease successfully treated by bone marrow transplantation. *Bone Marrow Transplant* 2000;26:567–570.
Moser H, Dubey P, Fatemi A: Progress in X-linked adrenoleukodystrophy. *Curr Opin Neurol* 2004;17:263–269.
Myhre AG, Undlien DE, Lovas K, et al: Autoimmune adrenocortical failure in Norway autoantibodies and human leukocyte antigen class II associations related to clinical features. *J Clin Endocrinol Metab* 2002;87:618–623.
Pearce SHS, Cheetham TD: Autoimmune polyendocrinopathy syndrome type 1: Treat with kid gloves. *Clin Endocrinol* 2001;54:433–435.
Peters C, Charnas LR, Tan Y, et al: Cerebral X-linked adrenoleukodystrophy: The international hematopoietic cell transplantation experience from 1982 to 1999. *Blood* 2004;104:881–888.
Ronghe MD, Barton J, Jardine PE, et al: The importance of testing for adrenoleukodystrophy in males with idiopathic Addison's disease. *Arch Dis Child* 2002;86:185–189.
Salvatori R: Adrenal insufficiency. *JAMA* 2005;294:2481–2488.
Sandrini F, Farmakidis C, Kirschner LS, et al: Spectrum of mutations of the AAAS gene in Allgrove syndrome: Lack of mutations in six kindreds with isolated resistance to corticotropin. *J Clin Endocrinol Metab* 2001;86:5433–5437.
Vaidya B, Pearce S, Kendall-Taylor P: Recent advances in the molecular genetics of congenital and acquired primary adrenocortical failure. *Clin Endocrinol* 2000;53:403–418.
Velaphi SC, Perlman JM: Neonatal adrenal hemorrhage: Clinical and abdominal sonographic findings. *Clin Pediatr* 2001;40:545–548.

Capitolo 577 ■ Iperplasia surrenale congenita e patologie correlate

L'iperplasia surrenale congenita (CAH, *Congenital Adrenal Hyperplasia*) è un'alterazione familiare autosomica recessiva della biosintesi del cortisolo (la steroidogenesi normale viene discussa nel Capitolo 575). Il deficit di cortisolo comporta un aumento della secrezione di corticotropina (ACTH), che a sua volta provoca iperplasia surrenale e iperproduzione di metaboliti intermedi. In base al livello del deficit enzimatico, ci possono essere segni, sintomi e reperti di laboratorio di carenza o eccesso di mineralcorticoidi; virilizzazione incompleta o pubertà prematura nei maschi; virilizzazione o infantilismo sessuale nelle femmine (Fig. 577-1 e 577-2 e Tab. 577-1).

577.1 • Iperplasia surrenale congenita da deficit della 21-idrossilasi

EZIOLOGIA. Oltre il 90% dei casi di CAH è dovuto a deficit di 21-idrossilasi. Questo enzima P450 (CYP21, P450c21) idrossila il progesterone e il 17-idrossiprogesterone (17-OHP), rispettivamente a 11-desossicorticosterone (DOC) e 11-desossicortisolo (vedi Fig. 575-1). Queste conversioni sono a loro volta necessarie per la sintesi di aldosterone e di cortisolo. Nelle forme più gravi di questa malattia, vi è quindi una carenza di entrambi gli ormoni, associata a perdita di sali. I pazienti con deficit un po' meno grave sono invece in grado di sintetizzare una quantità adeguata di aldosterone, ma presentano livelli elevati di androgeni surrenalici; questa patologia configura un quadro di virilizzazione semplice. Queste due forme sono definite nel loro complesso come deficit classico di 21-idrossilasi. Pazienti con malattia non classica presentano livelli di androgeni moderatamente elevati e possono manifestare, dopo la nascita, segni di eccesso androgenico.

EPIDEMIOLOGIA. Il classico deficit di 21-idrossilasi compare, nella maggior parte delle popolazioni, in circa 1 su 15 000-20 000 nati. Circa il 70% dei neonati colpiti ha la forma con perdita di sali, mentre il 30% quella con virilizzazione semplice. Le popolazioni yupik ed eschimesi dell'Alaska hanno un'incidenza di 1:280; una frequenza elevata è stata riportata anche nelle isole Reunion francesi (1:2100), in Brasile (1:7500) e nelle Filippine (1:7000). Negli Stati Uniti, la CAH è meno frequente fra i bambini afroamericani rispetto ai bianchi (1:42 000 rispetto a 1:15 500). La malattia non classica ha un'incidenza di circa 1 su 1000 nella popolazione generale, ma si verifica più frequentemente in specifici gruppi etnici, come gli ebrei ashkenaziti, gli ispanici e gli slavi.

GENETICA. Sono due i geni per la steroido 21-idrossilasi, *CYP21P* (*CYP21A1P*, *CYP21A*) e *CYP21* (*CYP21A2*, *CYP21B*) che si

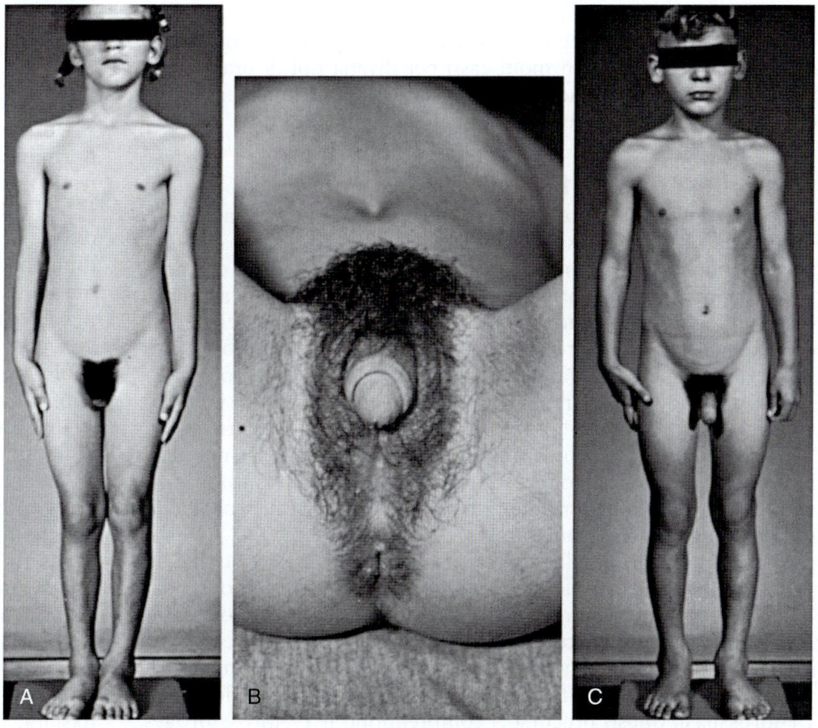

Figura 577-1. *A*, Bambina di 6 anni con iperplasia surrenale congenita virilizzante. L'età staturale era di 8 anni e mezzo, e quella ossea di 13. *B*, Notare l'ingrossamento clitorideo e la fusione delle grandi labbra. C, Fratello maschio di 5 anni, considerato normale dai genitori. L'età staturale era di 8 anni e quella ossea di 12 e mezzo.

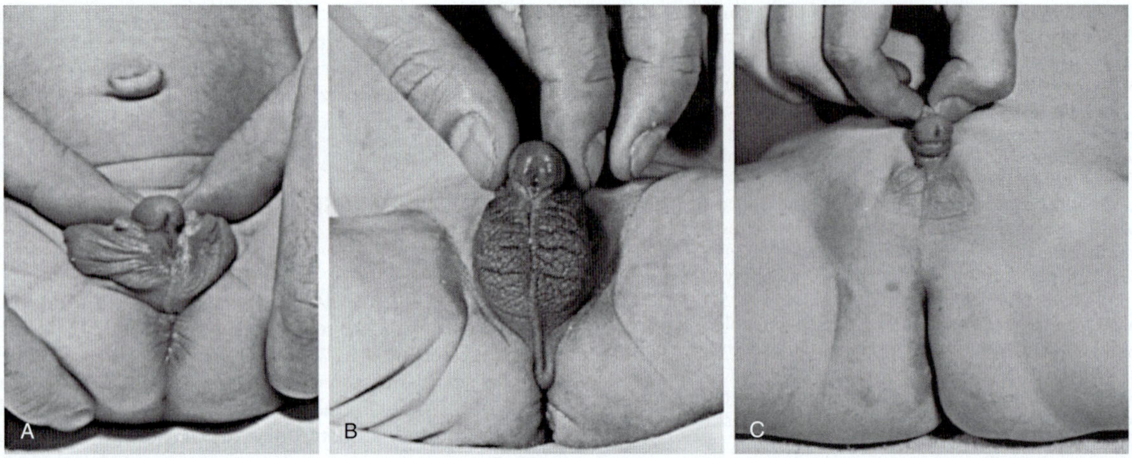

Figura 577-2. Tre casi di pseudoermafroditismo femminile con iperplasia surrenale congenita non trattata. A tutte e tre alla nascita è stato erroneamente attribuito un sesso maschile e ciascuna possiede normali cromosomi sessuali. I neonati A e B presentavano una forma con perdita di sali. Il neonato C è stato visitato a un anno per criptorchidismo. Notare l'uretra completamente peniena; un grado così completo di virilizzazione è raro nelle femmine con iperplasia surrenale; la maggior parte di questi bambini manifesta perdita di sali.

alternano in tandem con due geni per il quarto componente del complemento (C4A e C4B) nell'antigene leucocitario umano del complesso di istocompatibilità maggiore (HLA) sul cromosoma 6p21.3, tra il locus HLA-B e HLA-DR. In questa sede sono localizzati molti altri geni. *CYP21* è un gene attivo; *CYP21P* è identico per il 98% nella sequenza del DNA a *CYP21*, ma è uno pseudogene per 9 diverse mutazioni. Oltre il 90% delle mutazioni che provocano deficit di 21-idrossilasi è rappresentato da ricombinazioni tra *CYP21* e *CYP21P*. Nel 20% dei casi si tratta invece di delezioni generate da ineguale *crossing-over* meiotico tra *CYP21* e *CYP21P*, mentre le rimanenti sono rappresentate da transfer non reciproci di mutazioni nocive da *CYP21P* a *CYP21*, fenomeno denominato conversione genetica.

Le mutazioni nocive di *CYP21P* hanno vari effetti sull'attività enzimatica qualora siano trasferite su *CYP21*. Parecchie mutazioni impediscono completamente la sintesi di una proteina funzionale, mentre altre sono mutazioni missense (con sostituzioni aminoacidiche) che producono enzimi dotati dell'1-50% della normale attività. La gravità della malattia è correlata alle mutazioni veicolate da individui affetti; per esempio, pazienti con malattia con perdita di sali normalmente portano mutazioni su entrambi gli alleli, che azzerano completamente l'attività enzimatica. Se invece i pazienti sono eterozigoti (come si verifica in molti casi) per diversi tipi di mutazioni, la gravità dell'espressione della malattia è largamente determinata dall'attività dell'allele meno severamente colpito fra i due.

PATOGENESI E MANIFESTAZIONI CLINICHE

Deficit di aldosterone e cortisolo. Poiché la 21-idrossilazione è necessaria sia alla sintesi di cortisolo sia a quella di aldosterone, nella forma della malattia con perdita di sali sono carenti entrambi gli ormoni. Questa forma costituisce circa il 70% dei casi della carenza classica di 21-idrossilasi. I segni e i sintomi del deficit cortisolemico e aldosteronemico, assieme alla fisiopatologia che li sottende, sono essenzialmente quelli descritti nel Capitolo 576. Essi comprendono progressiva perdita di peso, anoressia, vomito, disidratazione, astenia, ipotensione, ipoglicemia, iponatremia e iperkaliemia. Questi problemi si sviluppano tipicamente nei neonati colpiti verso la seconda settimana di vita. Se i bambini non vengono trattati, si possono manifestare shock, aritmie cardiache e morte in giorni o settimane.

La CAH differisce da altre cause di insufficienza surrenale primaria, per l'accumulo del precursore steroideo a monte del blocco enzimatico. Dal momento che il cortisolo non viene sintetizzato in modo efficiente, i livelli di ACTH sono elevati, con conseguente iperplasia della corticale surrenale e livelli di precursori steroidei anche 100 volte quelli normali. Nel caso del deficit di 21-idrossilasi, questi precursori comprendono il 17-idrossiprogesterone e il progesterone. Il progesterone e forse altri metabolici agiscono come antagonisti per il recettore dei mineralcorticoidi e questo può aggravare gli effetti del deficit di aldosterone nei pazienti non trattati.

Eccesso prenatale di androgeni. Il problema più importante legato all'accumulo di precursori steroidei è che il 17-idrossiprogestreone viene indirizzato nella via biosintetica degli androgeni, con conseguente aumento dei livelli di androstenedione, convertito in sede extrasurrenale in testosterone. Questo problema in epoca fetale comincia verso l'ottava-decima settimana di gestazione e porta, nelle femmine, a un anomalo sviluppo genitale (vedi Fig. 577-1 e 577-2).

I genitali esterni di maschi e femmine solitamente appaiono identici nelle fasi precoci della gestazione (vedi Capitolo 583). Le femmine colpite, esposte in utero ad alti livelli di androgeni surrenalici, presentano genitali esterni mascolinizzati (vedi Fig. 577-1 e 577-2): si verifica cioè un ingrossamento clitorideo con fusione parziale o completa delle grandi labbra. Normalmente la vagina ha un'apertura in comune con l'uretra (seno urogenitale). Il clitoride può essere così aumentato di volume da assomigliare a un pene; dal momento che l'uretra si apre al di sotto di questo organo, molte di queste femmine sono scambiate per maschi con ipospadia e criptorchidismo. Il grado di virilizzazione normalmente è maggiore nelle femmine con la forma di deficit di 21-idrossilasi con perdita di sali. Gli organi genitali interni sono normali, perché le femmine colpite hanno ovaie normali e non testicoli e questi non secernono ormone anti-müelleriano.

Nelle femmine, l'esposizione cerebrale prenatale ad alte dosi di androgeni può influenzare successivi comportamenti sessuali dimorfi. Le ragazze tendono a essere interessate a giochi di tipo maschile, come macchinine e trenini, spesso diminuisce l'interesse per le bambole e mostrano, durante il gioco, una certa aggressività. Da adulte possono manifestare uno scarso interesse per il ruolo materno e c'è un aumento nella frequenza di omosessualità. Ciò nonostante, la maggior parte ha un atteggiamento eterosessuale e non presenta confusione di genere o disforia. È raro che le femmine ricoprano un ruolo maschile.

I neonati maschi appaiono normali alla nascita e per questo nei bambini la diagnosi può essere ritardata fino a che non si sviluppano segni di insufficienza surrenale. Dato che il peggioramento può essere molto rapido, i neonati maschi sono molto più a rischio per esito fatale rispetto alle femmine. Per questa ragione, molti Stati hanno istituito screening neonatali per questa patologia (vedi Screening neonatale, oltre).

Eccesso postnatale di androgeni. Bambini di entrambi i sessi non trattati, o trattati in modo inadeguato, sviluppano, dopo la nascita, ulteriori segni di iperproduzione androgenica. I maschi

TABELLA 577-1. Diagnosi e trattamento dell'iperplasia surrenale congenita

MALATTIA	GENE RESPONSABILE E CROMOSOMA	SEGNI E SINTOMI	REPERTI DI LABORATORIO	MISURE TERAPEUTICHE
Deficit di 21-idrossilasi Forma classica	CYP21 6p21.3	Deficit di glicocorticoidi	↓Cortisolo, ↑ACTH ↑↑17-idrossiprogestreone basale e dopo stimolazione con ACTH Iponatremia, iperkaliemia ↑Renina plasmatica	Sostituzione con glicocorticoidi (idrocortisone)
		Deficit di mineralcorticoidi (crisi da perdita di sali)	↑Androgeni sierici	Sostituzione con mineralcorticoidi (fludrocortisone)
		Pseudoermafroditismo femminile Virilizzazione postnatale in maschi e femmine	↑Androgeni sierici	Vaginoplastica e riduzione clitoridea Soppressione con glicocorticoidi
Deficit di 21 idrossilasi Forma non classica	CYP21 6p21.3	Adrenarca precoce, irregolarità mestruali, irsutismo, acne, infertilità	↑17-idrossiprogesterone basale e dopo stimolazione con ACTH ↑Androgeni sierici	Soppressione con glicocorticoidi
Deficit di 11β-idrossilasi	CYP11B1 8q24.3	Deficit di glicocorticoidi	↓Cortisolo, ↑ACTH ↑↑11-desossicortisolo e desossicorticosterone basali e dopo stimolo con ACTH	Somministrazione di glicocorticoidi (idrocortisone)
		Pseudoermafroditismo femminile	↑Androgeni sierici	Vaginoplastica e riduzione clitoridea
		Virilizzazione postnatale in maschi e femmine	↑Androgeni sierici	Soppressione con glicocorticoidi
		Ipertensione	↓Renina plasmatica, ipokaliemia	Soppressione con glicocorticoidi
Deficit di 3β-idrossisteroido-deidrogenasi, forma classica	HSD3B2 1p13.1	Deficit di glicocorticoidi	↓Cortisolo, ↑ACTH ↑↑Δ5 steroidi (pregnenolone, 17-idrossi pregnenolone, DHEA) basali e dopo stimolazione con ACTH	Sostituzione con glicocorticoidi (idrocortisone)
		Deficit di mineralcorticoidi (crisi da perdita di sali)	Iponatremia, iperkaliemia ↑Renina plasmatica	Sostituzione con mineralcorticoidi (fludrocortisone), supplementazione con cloruro di sodio
		Pseudoermafroditismo maschile e femminile	↑DHEA, ↓androstenedione, testosterone, estradiolo	Correzione chirurgica dei genitali e sostituzione con ormoni sessuali al momento opportuno, in accordo con il sesso con cui sono cresciuti
		Adrenarca precoce, alterazioni della pubertà	↑DHEA, ↓androstenedione, testosterone e estradiolo	Soppressione con glicocorticoidi
Deficit di 17α-idrossilasi/17,20-liasi	CYP17 10q24.3	Carenza di cortisolo(il corticosterone è un adeguato glicocorticoidi)	↓Cortisolo, ↑ACTH ↑DOC, corticosterone Bassi gli steroidi 17α-idrossilati; scarsa risposta all'ACTH	Somministrazione di glicocorticoidi (idrocortisone)
		Pseudoermafroditismo maschile	↓Androgeni sierici; scarsa risposta all'hCG	Orchidopessi o rimozione dei testicoli intra-addominali; sostituzione con ormoni sessuali, compatibili con il sesso con cui sono stati cresciuti
		Infantilismo sessuale	↓Androgeni o estrogeni sierici	Sostituzione con ormoni sessuali compatibili con il sesso con cui sono stati cresciuti
		Ipertensione	↓Renina plasmatica; ipokaliemia	Soppressione con glicocorticoidi
Iperplasia surrenale congenita lipoidea	StAR 8p11.2	Deficit di glicocorticoidi	↑ACTH Bassi livelli di tutti gli ormoni steroidei, con diminuzione o assenza di risposta all'ACTH	Sostituzione con glicocorticoidi (idrocortisone)
		Deficit di mineralcorticoidi (crisi da perdita di sali)	Iponatremia, iperkaliemia ↓Aldosterone, ↑renina plasmatica	Sostituzione con mineralcorticoidi (fludrocortisone); supplementazione con cloruro di sodio
		Pseudoermafroditismo maschile	Assenza o diminuzione della risposta all'hCG nello pseudoermafroditismo maschile	Orchidopessi o rimozione dei testicolo intra-addominali; terapia sostitutiva con ormoni sessuali compatibili con il sesso con cui sono stati cresciuti
		Scarso sviluppo puberale o insufficienza ovarica prematura nelle femmine	↑FSH, ↑LH, ↓estradiolo (postpuberale)	Sostituzione con estrogeni
Deficit di P450 ossidoreduttasi	POR 7q11.3	Deficit di glicocorticoidi	↓Cortisolo, ↑ACTH ↑Pregnenolone, ↑progesterone	Sostituzione con glicocorticoidi (idrocortisone) Correzione chirurgica dei genitali e sostituzione con ormoni sessuali compatibili con il sesso con cui sono stati cresciuti
		Pseudoermafroditismo maschile e femminile	↑Androgeni prenatali sierici, ↓androgeni e estrogeni alla pubertà	
		Virilizzazione materna	Diminuito rapporto tra androgeni ed estrogeni	
		Sindrome di Antley-Bixler		

con la forma di virilizzazione semplice del deficit di 21-idrossilasi spesso hanno una diagnosi ritardata, perché appaiono normali e raramente sviluppano insufficienza surrenale.

I segni di eccesso androgenico comprendono una rapida crescita somatica e un'accelerazione della maturazione scheletrica. Per questo i pazienti durante l'infanzia sono alti, ma la prematura chiusura epifisaria causa una cessazione relativamente precoce della crescita e una statura da adulti scarsa (vedi Fig. 577-1). Può essere eccessivo anche lo sviluppo muscolare. Possono comparire peli pubici e ascellari, acne e abbassamento del tono della voce. Il pene, lo scroto e la prostata possono cominciare ad aumentare, mentre **i testicoli hanno di solito dimensioni prepuberi**, tanto da apparire relativamente piccoli in rapporto all'aumento del pene. Occasionalmente, anche delle cellule corticosurrenali ectopiche presenti in sede testicolare, possono andare incontro a iperplasia, analogamente a quelle surrenaliche, producendo neoplasie dei residui surrenalici in sede testicolare (vedi Capitolo 585). Nelle femmine il clitoride può cominciare a ingrossarsi (vedi Fig. 577-1). Sebbene i genitali interni siano di tipo femminile, le mammelle e le mestruazioni non compaiono fino a che si instaura un'adeguata terapia che sopprime l'iperproduzione androgenica.

Nel **deficit non classico di 21-idrossilasi** possono comparire segni simili, ma più lievi, di eccesso androgenico. In questa forma attenuata, i livelli di cortisolo e aldosterone sono normali; le femmine presentano alla nascita genitali esterni nella norma. Maschi e femmine possono manifestare pubarca precoce e precoce sviluppo dei peli pubici e ascellari. Successivamente possono comparire irsutismo, acne, disordini mestruali e infertilità. Tuttavia, molte femmine e molti maschi sono asintomatici.

REPERTI DI LABORATORIO (VEDI TAB. 577-1). Pazienti con malattia con perdita di sali presentano reperti di laboratorio legati all'insufficienza di cortisolo e aldosterone, fra cui iponatremia, iperkaliemia, acidosi metabolica e spesso ipoglicemia; queste anomalie si possono però sviluppare anche dopo 1-2 settimane dalla nascita. I livelli ematici di **17-idrossiprogesterone** sono notevolmente elevati; sono alti, nei primi 2-3 giorni di vita, anche in bambini sani, e soprattutto in quelli ammalati o prematuri. Dopo l'infanzia, quando compare il ritmo circadiano del cortisolo, anche i livelli di 17-idrossiprogesterone variano nell'arco della giornata, presentandosi più alti al mattino e più bassi la notte. Nei pazienti con la forma da perdita di sali, i livelli ematici di cortisolo di solito sono bassi, mentre in pazienti con virilizzazione semplice sono spesso normali, ma inappropriatamente bassi in rapporto ai livelli di ACTH e di 17-idrossiprogesterone. Oltre al 17-idrossiprogesterone, nelle femmine sono elevati anche i livelli di androstenedione e testosterone; quest'ultimo invece non è incrementato nei maschi, perché anche i neonati maschi normali hanno elevati livelli testosteronemici, se confrontati con quelli successivi durante l'infanzia. I livelli urinari di 17-chetosteroidi e di pregnantriolo sono alti, ma attualmente vengono utilizzati di rado, perché è più semplice ottenere campioni di sangue rispetto a una raccolta di urina nelle 24 ore. I livelli di corticotropina (ACTH) sono elevati, ma non hanno maggiore utilità diagnostica del 17-idrossiprogesterone. I livelli plasmatici di renina sono alti, e l'aldosterone sierico è inappropriatamente basso in rapporto a essi. Tuttavia, nei primi giorni di vita, la renina è alta anche in condizioni normali.

La diagnosi di deficit di 21-idrossilasi si basa soprattutto sulla determinazione dei valori di 17-idrossiprogesterone prima e 30 e 60 minuti dopo la somministrazione endovenosa di un bolo di 0,125-0,25 mg di cosintropina (ACTH 1-24). Esiste un nomogramma che permette di distinguere facilmente pazienti normali da quelli con deficit di 21-idrossilasi classico o non classico. I portatori eterozigoti di questa anomalia autosomica recessiva tendono ad avere livelli di 17-idrossiprogesterone più alti dopo stimolazione con ACTH rispetto ai soggetti sani, ma in queste due categorie di persone si registra una certa sovrapposizione dei risultati.

DIAGNOSI DIFFERENZIALE. Le condizioni intersessuali sono discusse nel Capitolo 589. La tappa iniziale nella valutazione di un neonato con genitali ambigui è rappresentata da un accurato esame fisico, per definire l'anatomia dei genitali, localizzare il meato uretrale, palpare lo scroto o le labbra e le regioni inguinali alla ricerca dei testicoli (gonadi palpabili indicano quasi sempre la presenza di tessuto testicolare, a testimonianza che il neonato sia geneticamente maschio) e per ricercare altre eventuali anomalie anatomiche. L'ecografia può essere utilizzata per dimostrare la presenza o l'assenza dell'utero e spesso è in grado di localizzare le gonadi. Una rapida analisi del cariotipo (come l'ibridazione fluorescente *in situ* o i nuclei in interfase per i cromosomi X e Y), è in grado di determinare rapidamente il sesso genetico del neonato. Tutti questi dati sono facilmente ottenibili prima dei risultati dei test ormonali e permettono quindi ai medici di dare informazioni ai genitori sia sul sesso genetico del bambino sia sull'anatomia delle strutture riproduttive interne. Nelle femmine ermafrodite, l'iniezione di mezzo di contrasto nel seno urogenitale consente di dimostrare la presenza di vagina e di utero; pertanto, la maggior parte dei chirurghi utilizza questa informazione per formulare un piano di intervento chirurgico.

DIAGNOSI PRENATALE. La diagnosi prenatale di deficit della 21-idrossilasi è possibile nel terzo trimestre tramite analisi del DNA, ottenuto da campioni di villi coriali o nel secondo trimestre con l'amniocentesi. Normalmente si ricorre a questa indagine perché i genitori hanno già un altro bambino affetto. Più spesso si analizza il gene *CYP21* per mutazioni frequenti ma strettamente associate, però possono essere utilizzati dei marker microsatelliti altamente polimorfi, se è disponibile per un confronto genetico un bambino malato (per es. caso indice).

SCREENING NEONATALE. Dato che il deficit di 21-idrossilasi spesso non viene diagnosticato nei maschi colpiti fino a quando non si manifesta una grave insufficienza surrenale, molti Stati hanno istituito programmi di screening neonatale. Questi programmi valutano i livelli di **17-idrossiprogesterone** in campioni di sangue essiccato, ottenuti dal calcagno e assorbito su filtro di carta; gli stessi filtri sono analizzati contemporaneamente per altre condizioni genetiche, come l'ipotiroidismo e la fenilchetonuria. I neonati sospetti sono richiamati rapidamente per ulteriori indagini (dosaggio degli elettroliti e ripetizione del 17-idrossiprogesterone) a circa due settimane di età. Neonati con malattia da perdita di sali spesso, a questa età, presentano alterazioni elettrolitiche, ma di solito non sono gravi. I programmi di screening sono pertanto efficaci nel prevenire molti casi di crisi surrenale in bambini malati. La forma non classica della malattia non è facilmente rilevabile dallo screening neonatale, ma ciò è di scarso interesse clinico perché, comunque, in questo tipo di deficit di 21-idrossilasi l'insufficienza surrenale non si verifica.

La difficoltà maggiore con gli odierni programmi di screening neonatale è rappresentata dal fatto che, una volta trovati tutti i neonati affetti, il livello limite del 17-idrossiprogesterone per la ripetizione dell'indagine è così basso, che sono molto frequenti i falsi positivi (per es. il test ha basso valore predittivo positivo). Questo problema è maggiore nei neonati prematuri. Il genotyping per *CYP21* potrebbe migliorare la specificità, ma non è disponibile di routine.

TRATTAMENTO

Terapia sostitutiva con glicocorticoidi. Il deficit di cortisolo è trattato con glicocorticoidi. Il trattamento sopprime inoltre l'iperproduzione corticale di androgeni, riducendo i problemi inerenti alla crescita eccessiva, alla maturazione scheletrica e alla virilizzazione. Questo obiettivo spesso richiede dosi maggiori di glicocorticoidi rispetto a quelle necessarie in altre forme di insufficienza surrenale, tipicamente 15-20 mg/m^2/die di idrocortisone somministrato per os in tre dosi giornaliere. I neonati di solito necessitano di dosaggi al limite superiore di questo range. Dosi doppie o triple sono indicate durante i **periodi di stress**, come un'infezione o un intervento chirurgico. Il trattamento con glicocorticoidi deve essere continuato indefinitamente in tutti i pazienti con deficit classico di 21-idrossilasi, ma non è necessario in pazienti con la forma non classica, almeno fino a che compaiono segni di iperproduzione androgenica. La terapia deve essere individualizzata. È opportuno mantenere uno standard di crescita lineare che segua le linee percentili; l'incrocio con una linea percentile più alta presuppone un sottodosaggio terapeutico, mentre la perdita di altezza percentile spesso è indice di un sovradosaggio di glicocorticoidi. Anche un eccessivo aumento di peso può essere la spia di un sovradosaggio. È necessario monitorare con esami periodici lo sviluppo puberale e la maturazione scheletrica con radiografie seriali della mano e del polso per età ossea. I livelli ormonali, in particolare quelli del 17-idrossiprogesterone e dell'androstenedione, devono essere misurati di primo mattino, prima dell'assunzione della terapia giornaliera, o a una distanza di tempo adeguata alla somministrazione dei farmaci. In genere, i livelli desiderabili di 17-idrossiprogesterone si situano nel range alto della normalità o molte volte appaiono normali; di solito si ottengono livelli bassi-normali solo utilizzando alte dosi di glicocorticoidi.

Nella maggior parte delle ragazze con un buon controllo della malattia, il menarca compare all'età adeguata, ma può essere ritardato in quelle con un controllo non ottimale.

Bambini con virilizzazione semplice, soprattutto maschi, non ricevono diagnosi fino ai 3-7 anni, quando la maturazione scheletrica può essere avanzata di 5 o più anni rispetto all'età cronologica. In parecchi bambini, specialmente se l'età ossea è uguale o maggiore a 12 anni, quando si inizia il trattamento, si può verificare una **pubertà spontanea gonadotropino-dipendente**, perché la terapia con idrocortisone, sopprimendo la produzione di androgeni surrenalici, stimola, in presenza di un adeguato livello di maturazione ipotalamica, il rilascio di gonadotropine ipofisarie. Questa forma di pubertà precoce vera forzata può essere trattata con un analogo dell'ormone di rilascio delle gonadotropine, come leuprolide.

Maschi con deficit di 21-idrossilasi sottoposti a terapia inadeguata possono sviluppare neoplasie dei residui di tessuto surrenale in sede testicolare, che normalmente regrediscono con l'aumentare del dosaggio dei glicocorticoidi. RM testicolare, ecografia e color Doppler aiutano a definire il carattere e l'estensione della malattia. È descritto, per i tumori che non rispondono alla terapia, un approccio chirurgico con salvaguardia dei testicoli.

Terapia sostitutiva con mineralcorticoidi. Pazienti con malattia con perdita di sali (per es. deficit di aldosterone) richiedono una sostituzione con **fludrocortisone**. Nei primi mesi di vita, i neonati possono avere bisogno di dosi molto alte di mineralcorticoidi, solitamente 0,1-0,3 mg/die suddivisi in due somministrazioni, ma possono arrivare anche a 0,4 mg/die e spesso richiedono una supplementazione di sodio (cloruro di sodio, 1-3 g) in aggiunta a essi. Per i neonati un po' più grandi e i bambini piccoli è indicata una dose di mantenimento di 0,05-0,1 mg/die di fludrocortisone. In molti pazienti, la virilizzazione semplice può essere controllata più facilmente con basse dosi di fludrocortisone in aggiunta all'idrocortisone, anche qualora i livelli di aldosterone siano normali, pur in assenza di terapia sostituiva con mineralcorticoidi. La terapia va valutata monitorando i segni vitali; tachicardia e ipertensione sono segni di sovradosaggio di mineralcorticoidi. Nella prima infanzia, a ogni aggiustamento terapeutico, vanno controllati gli elettroliti plasmatici. L'attività retinica plasmatica è utile per valutare l'adeguatezza della terapia; deve essere mantenuta nel range della normalità o vicino a esso, ma non soppressa.

Possono essere utilizzati anche antiandrogeni, con un inibitore dell'aromatasi (blocco della conversione degli androgeni in estrogeni), ormone della crescita con o senza agonisti dell'LH-RH e si può ricorrere alla surrenectomia in caso di scarso controllo medico del paziente.

Trattamento chirurgico dei genitali ambigui. Tra il secondo e il sesto mese di vita, le femmine con notevoli segni di virilizzazione vengono solitamente sottoposte a intervento chirurgico. Se vi è una notevole ipertrofia clitoridea, vengono ridotte le dimensioni del clitoride, con escissione parziale dei corpi cavernosi e mantenimento dei fasci neurovascolari; tuttavia, un'ipertrofia moderata può diventare molto meno visibile, anche senza chirurgia, mano a mano che la bambina cresce. Al momento dell'intervento clitorideo, si eseguono solitamente anche la vaginoplastica e la correzione del seno urogenitale; spesso è necessaria una revisione successiva, durante l'adolescenza.

È necessario discutere a fondo i rischi e i benefici della terapia chirurgica con i genitori delle bambine. Non sono molti i follow-up a lungo termine disponibili per valutare gli esiti funzionali in pazienti sottoposte alle **moderne** tecniche chirurgiche. L'assegnazione sessuale dei neonati con una **situazione di intersessualità** (compresa la CAH) si basa solitamente sulle aspettative di funzionalità e fertilità nell'età adulta, ottenibili con la correzione chirurgica precoce dei genitali esterni, conformemente all'assegnazione del sesso. Nell'ambito della CAH è rara una identità psicosessuale confusa. Tuttavia, oppositori profani e medici di questa pratica per altre condizioni di intersessualità dichiarano che, così facendo, si ignora una qualsiasi predisposizione al ruolo corrispondente al genere prenatale parziale e si preclude al paziente la possibilità di decidere la propria identità sessuale, femminile o maschile, e il tipo di correzione chirurgica. Questi individui e gruppi sostengono che il trattamento dovrebbe essere volto principalmente a educare i pazienti, la famiglia e gli altri circa la situazione medica, la terapia e su come affrontare una condizione di intersessualità. Essi propongono di ritardare il trattamento chirurgico fino a che lo stesso paziente non sia in grado di decidere se si debba praticare una correzione, e quale. Per fare decollare questa pratica, sarebbero necessari studi di follow-up a lungo termine.

Negli adolescenti e nelle femmine adulte con scarso controllo del deficit di 21-idrossilasi (irsutismo, obesità, amenorrea), la surrenectomia bilaterale laparoscopica (con successiva sostituzione ormonale) può essere più efficace della terapia medica.

Trattamento prenatale. Oltre alla consulenza genetica, l'obiettivo principale della diagnosi prenatale è quello di facilitare un appropriato trattamento prenatale delle femmine affette. Le precauzioni per le gravidanze a rischio consistono nella somministrazione di desametasone, uno steroide che attraversa facilmente la placenta, al dosaggio di 20 μg/kg/die di peso della donna gravida, in due o tre dosi giornaliere. Il desametasone sopprime la secrezione di steroidi del surrene fetale, compresa quella di androgeni. Se si inizia alla sesta settimana di gestazione si registra, nelle femmine, un miglioramento della virilizzazione dei genitali esterni. Si esegue poi la biopsia dei villi coriali per determinare il sesso e il genotipo del feto. Si continua la terapia solo se il feto è femmina ed è colpito. L'analisi del DNA delle cellule fetali isolate dal plasma materno per la determinazione del sesso e per l'analisi del gene *CYP21* permette l'identificazione precoce del feto femmina affetto. Nei bambini esposti a questa terapia, non sono stati descritti specifici effetti negativi, ma i dati attualmente disponibili sono insufficienti per determinare se vi siano rischi a lungo termine, in particolare nei maschi e nelle femmine non colpite che non ricavano benefici dal trattamento. Gli effetti collaterali materni comprendono edema, eccessivo aumento di peso, ipertensione, intolleranza al glucosio, caratteristiche facciali di tipo cushingoide, e notevoli striae rubrae. In certe sedi, si effettua la terapia prenatale seguendo attentamente un protocollo istituzionale, ma spesso, in altre, viene praticata dai ginecologi come opzione di routine.

577.2 • Iperplasia surrenale congenita da deficit della 11β-idrossilasi

EZIOLOGIA. Il deficit di 11β-idrossilasi è dovuto a una mutazione del gene *CYP11B1*, localizzato sul cromosoma 8q24. *CYP11B1* media la 11-idrossilazione dell'11-desossicortisolo in cortisolo. Dal momento che l'11-desossicortisolo non viene convertito in cortisolo, aumentano i livelli di corticotropina. Di conseguenza, si accumulano precursori, particolarmente l'11-desossicortisolo e il desossicorticosterone, che, come nel deficit di 21-idrossilasi, vengono indirizzati verso la biosintesi di androgeni. Tuttavia, dato che il gene adiacente *CYP11B2*, che codifica l'aldosterone sintasi, non viene coinvolto in questa malattia, l'aldosterone viene prodotto normalmente.

EPIDEMIOLOGIA. Il deficit di 11β-idrossilasi copre circa il 5% dei casi di ipoplasia surrenale, con un'incidenza di 1/250 000 fino a 1/100 000. Sono state identificate più di 30 mutazioni di *CYP11B1*. La malattia compare con relativa frequenza nelle popolazioni ebree di origine nordafricana (1 su 15 000-17 000 nati vivi); in questo gruppo etnico quasi tutti gli alleli portano una mutazione da Arg448 a His (R448H). Questa malattia si manifesta in una forma classica, severa, e molto raramente in una forma non classica, più lieve.

MANIFESTAZIONI CLINCHE. Nonostante la sintesi del cortisolo non sia efficiente, la capacità sintetica dell'aldosterone è normale e l'enzima aldosterone sintasi consente la sintesi anche di corticosterone a partire dal progesterone, che rimane inalterato. Di conseguenza, raramente i pazienti manifestano segni di insufficienza surrenale come ipotensione, ipoglicemia, iponatremia e iperkaliemia. Circa i due terzi dei pazienti diventano **ipertesi**, anche se in tempi molto lunghi. L'ipertensione è una probabile conseguenza degli elevati livelli di desossicorticosterone, che possiede attività mineralcorticoide. I neonati, una volta iniziato il trattamento con idrocortisone, possono transitoriamente sviluppare segni di deficit aldosteronemico. Probabilmente ciò è dovuto alla brusca soppressione della secrezione del desossicorticosterone in un paziente con atrofia della zona glomerulare dovuta a cronica soppressione dell'attività reninica.

Tutti i segni e i sintomi di eccesso androgenico presenti nel deficit di 21-idrossilasi compaiono anche in quello di 11-idrossilasi.

REPERTI DI LABORATORIO. I livelli plasmatici di 11-desossicortisolo e desossicorticosterone sono elevati. Dato che il desossicorticosterone e i metaboliti hanno un'attività mineralcorticoide, la reninica plasmatica risulta soppressa. Di conseguenza, i livelli di aldosterone sono bassi anche se la capacità di sintetizzare aldosterone è intatta. Occasionalmente si manifesta alcalosi ipokaliemica.

TRATTAMENTO. I pazienti vengono trattati con idrocortisone a dosi analoghe a quelle utilizzate per il deficit di 21-idrossilasi. Talvolta nei bambini è necessaria una terapia sostitutiva transitoria con mineralcorticoidi, ma raramente va proseguita oltre. L'ipertensione spesso regredisce con il trattamento glicocorticoide, ma se è di lunga durata, può anche essere necessaria un'ulteriore terapia.

In queste circostanze si possono utilizzare i calcioantagonisti.

577.3 • Iperplasia surrenale congenita da deficit di 3β-idrossisteroido-deidrogenasi

EZIOLOGIA. Il deficit di 3β-idrossisteroido-deidrogenasi (3β-HSD) si verifica in meno del 2% dei pazienti con iperplasia surrenale. Questo enzima è necessario alla conversione dei Δ5 steroidi (pregnenolone, 17-idrossiprogesterone, deidroepiandrosterone [DHEA],) in Δ4 steroidi (progesterone, 17-idrossiprogesterone e androstenedione). Questa carenza enzimatica comporta una diminuzione della sintesi di cortisolo, aldosterone e androstenedione, ma un aumento della produzione di DHEA (vedi Fig. 575-1). L'enzima 3β-HSD espresso nella corticale del surrene viene codificato dal gene *HSD3B2*, localizzato sul cromosoma 1p13.1. Sono state descritte più di 30 mutazioni del gene *HSD-D3B2* in pazienti con deficit di 3β-HSD.

MANIFESTAZIONI CLINICHE. Poiché nei pazienti con la forma classica di questa malattia non vengono sintetizzati né il cortisolo né l'aldosterone, i neonati sono soggetti a **crisi da perdita di sali**. Dal momento che non vengono sintetizzati nemmeno testosterone e androstenedione, i maschi presentano un quadro di virilizzazione incompleta. Si può verificare ipospadia di varia entità, con o senza scroto bifido o criptorchisdismo. Poiché i livelli di DHEA sono elevati e questo ormone è un debole androgeno, le femmine sono moderatamente virilizzate, con ingrossamento clitorideo da lieve a moderato. Dopo la nascita, la continua ipersecrezione di DHEA può provocare adrenarca precoce. Durante l'adolescenza e l'età adulta, compaiono nelle femmine irsutismo, irregolarità mestruali e ovaio policistico. I maschi manifestano gradi diversi di ipogonadismo, sebbene possa essere presente adeguato sviluppo dei caratteri sessuali secondari. Si è dimostrato, tuttavia, un difetto persistente della 3β-HSD testicolare, con un alto rapporto tra Δ5 e Δ4 steroidi nel sangue refluo dai testicoli.

REPERTI DI LABORATORIO. Il segno distintivo di questa malattia è la notevole elevazione dei Δ5 steroidi (come il 17-idrossipregnenolone, e il DHEA), a monte del blocco enzimatico. I pazienti possono avere anche livelli elevati di 17-idrossiprogesterone, per l'attività della 3β-HSD nei tessuti periferici extrasurrenalici; questi pazienti possono essere confusi con quelli con deficit di 21-idrossilasi. Tuttavia il rapporto tra 17-idrossipregnenolone e 17-idrossiprogesterone è notevolmente alto nel deficit di 3β-HSD, mentre è basso in quello di 21-idrossilasi. L'attività reninica plasmatica è elevata nelle forme con perdita di sali.

DIAGNOSI DIFFERENZIALE. Raramente bambine con adrenarca prematuro (o donne con segni di eccesso androgenico) presentano livelli da modesti a moderati di DHEA. Si ritiene che queste pazienti manifestino una forma "non classica di deficit di 3β-HSD". Tuttavia, non sono state trovate in queste pazienti mutazioni del gene *HSD3B2*, pertanto la forma non classica di questo deficit è attualmente molto rara. L'attività della 3β-HSD della zona fascicolata e reticolare della corticale surrenale, corrispondenti all'attività di CYP17 (17-idrossilasi/17,20-liasi), normalmente diminuisce durante l'adrenarca, per facilitare la sintesi di DHEA, ed elevazioni così modeste del DHEA in bambine prepuberi o donne di solito rappresentano un normale variante.

TRATTAMENTO. È necessaria sia la sostituzione glicorticoide che quella mineralcorticoide con idrocortisone e fludrocortisone, rispettivamente, come nel deficit di 21-idrossilasi. I maschi genetici incompletamente virilizzati, cresciuti come maschi, possono beneficiare nella prima infanzia di diverse iniezione di un preparato depot del testosterone, per aumentare le dimensioni del pene. Alla pubertà è necessaria la terapia sostitutiva con testosterone.

577.4 • Iperplasia surrenale congenita da deficit della 17-idrossilasi

EZIOLOGIA. Meno dell'1% dei casi di CAH è dovuto a deficit della 17-idrossilasi. Un singolo polipeptide, il CYP17, catalizza due distinte reazioni: la 17-idrossilazione del pregnenolone e del progesterone, rispettivamente a 17-idrossipregnenolone e 17-idrossiprogesterone, e la reazione della 17,20-liasi che trasforma il 17-idrossipregnenolone in DHEA e, in misura minore, il 17-idrossiprogesterone in Δ4-androstenedione. Il DHEA e l'androstenedione sono steroidi precursori del testosterone e degli estrogeni (vedi Fig. 575-1). L'enzima viene espresso sia nella corticale surrenale sia nelle gonadi ed è codificato da un gene sul cromosoma 10q24.3. La maggior parte delle mutazioni interferisce sia con l'attività dell'idrossilasi sia con quella della liasi, ma rare mutazioni possono inibire una sola delle due attività.

MANIFESTAZIONI CLINICHE E REPERTI DI LABORATORIO. Pazienti con deficit di 17-idrossilasi non sono in grado di sintetizzare cortisolo, ma possono produrre corticosterone. Poiché il corticosterone è un glicocorticoide attivo, i pazienti non sviluppano insufficienza surrenale. È presente un'iperproduzione di desossicorticosterone, l'immediato precursore del corticosterone, con conseguenti **ipertensione**, **ipokaliemia** e soppressione della secrezione della renina e dell'aldosterone, come si verifica nel deficit di 11-idrossilasi. Tuttavia, in contrasto con quanto succede in quest'ultima patologia, i pazienti con deficit di 17-idrossilasi non sono in grado di sintetizzare gli ormoni sessuali. Pertanto, i maschi manifestano una **virilizzazione incompleta** con fenotipo femminile (ma le gonadi sono di solito palpabili nella regione inguinale o delle labbra) o con ambiguità sessuale (pseudoermafroditismo maschile). Le femmine in genere presentano un'**insufficienza dello sviluppo sessuale** al momento in cui si dovrebbe verificare la **pubertà**. Il deficit di 17-idrossilasi nelle femmine deve essere preso in considerazione nella diagnosi differenziale con l'ipogonadismo primario (vedi Capitolo 587). Oltre all'aumento del DOC, alla soppressione della renina e dell'aldosterone e al decremento degli steroidi 17-idrossilati, il cortisolo e gli steroidi sessuali non rispondono rispettivamente alla stimolazione con ACTH umano e con gonadotropina corionica.

TRATTAMENTO. I pazienti con deficit di 17-idrossilasi richiedono terapia sostitutiva con cortisolo per sopprimere la secrezione di desossicorticosterone e controllare quindi l'ipertensione. Possono rendersi necessari altri farmaci antipertensivi. Alle femmine si devono aggiungere estrogeni al momento delle pubertà. I pazienti geneticamente maschi richiedono un supplementazione con estrogeni o androgeni a seconda dell'indirizzo sessuale. Analogamente alla sindrome da insensibilità agli androgeni (vedi Capitolo 584), i soggetti geneticamente maschi con deficit grave di 17-idrossilasi cresciuti come femmine richiedono una gonadectomia al momento o prima della pubertà, per la possibilità di degenerazione neoplastica dei testicoli ritenuti in sede addominale.

577.5 • Iperplasia surrenale lipoidea

EZIOLOGIA E PATOGENESI. L'iperplasia surrenale lipoidea è una patologia rara, riportata in meno di 100 pazienti, prevalentemente giapponesi. Si verifica un notevole accumulo di colesterolo e di lipidi nella corticale surrenale e nelle gonadi, associato a gravi alterazioni della steroidogenesi. L'iperplasia surrenale lipoidea è normalmente causata da mutazioni del gene per la proteina regolatoria acuta della steroidogenesi (StAR), una proteina mitocondriale che promuove il passaggio del colesterolo all'interno della membrana mitocondriale. Sono state descritte mutazioni del gene *CYP114* (*P450 scc*) in due pazienti con iperplasia surrenale lipoidea.

Una parte del colesterolo è in grado di entrare nei mitocondri anche in assenza di StAR, tanto che si potrebbe supporre che questa alterazione non modifichi completamente la biosintesi steroidea. Tuttavia, l'accumulo di colesterolo nel citoplasma ha un effetto citotossico, che provoca la necrosi di tutte le cellule steroidogenetiche in cui normalmente è espressa StAR. Questo si verifica prima della nascita nel surrene e nei testicoli. Di norma, però, le ovaie non sintetizzano steroidi prima della pubertà, così che in questa sede non si accumula colesterolo e le ovaie possono mantenere la capacità di sintetizzare estrogeni fino all'adolescenza.

MANIFESTAZIONI CLINICHE. I pazienti con iperplasia surrenale lipoidea normalmente non sono in grado di sintetizzare steroidi surrenalici. Sono frequenti le manifestazioni da **perdita di sali** e molti neonati muoiono precocemente nell'infanzia. I soggetti geneticamente maschi incapaci di sintetizzare androgeni manifestano un **fenotipo femminile**, pur in presenza di gonadi maschili. I soggetti geneticamente femmine appaiono normali alla nascita e alla pubertà possono presentare femminilizzazione con comparsa del ciclo mestruale. Esse tuttavia evolvono verso un quadro di **ipogonadismo ipergonadotropo**, con accumulo di colesterolo che provoca la necrosi delle cellule della granulosa (steroidosintetiche) nell'ovaio.

REPERTI DI LABORATORIO. Nell'iperplasia surrenale lipoidea gli steroidi surrenalici e ovarici sono bassi, con scarsa o assente risposta alla stimolazione (ACTH, gonadotropina corionica umana). I livelli plasmatici di renina sono aumentati.

Indagini morfologiche dei surreni mostrano una massiccia ipertrofia ghiandolare che nel neonato aiuta a indirizzarsi verso la diagnosi di iperplasia lipoidea.

TRATTAMENTO. I pazienti richiedono terapia sostitutiva con glicocorticoidi e mineralcorticoidi. Ai soggetti geneticamente maschi viene di solito assegnato il sesso femminile; così, sia i maschi sia le femmine ricevono una terapia con estrogeni all'età della pubertà.

577.6 • Deficit di P450 ossidoreduttasi (sindrome di Antley-Bixler)

EZIOLOGIA, PATOGENESI E MANIFESTAZIONI CLINICHE. Il P450 ossidoreduttasi (POR, gene localizzato sul cromosoma 7q11.3) è necessario per l'attività di tutti gli enzimi del sistema del citocromo P450 microsomiale (vedi Capitolo 575), compresi gli enzimi surrenalici CYP17 e CYP21. Di conseguenza, un deficit completo di POR rende inattive tutte le attività microsomiali P450. Questo fatto nel topo provoca la morte già in fase embrionale e presumibilmente anche nell'uomo. Pazienti con mutazioni che diminuiscono, ma non sopprimono, l'attività di POR, presentando un deficit parziale di 17-idrossilasi e 21-idrossilasi surrenaliche. Il deficit di 17-idrossilasi porta a mascolinizzazione incompleta nei maschi, mentre quello di 21-idrossilasi è responsabile di virilizzazione femminile. Inoltre è diminuita l'attività dell'aromatasi (*CYP19*) placentare, con azione incontrastata degli androgeni prodotti dal surrene fetale. Ciò peggiora la virilizzazione dei feti femmina e può comportare anche virilizzazione della madre. Sebbene sia strana la virilizzazione femminile nonostante un deficit parziale di *CYP17* (necessario per la biosintesi androgenica), può essere utilizzata una via sintetica alternativa, in cui il 17-idrossiprogesterone è trasformato in 5α-pregano-3α, 17α-diol-20-one, un metabolita che rappresenta un substrato decisamente migliore per l'attività 17,20-liasica di *CYP1* rispetto al solito substrato, il 17-idrossipregnenolone (vedi Capitolo 575). Il metabolita è poi convertito, attraverso diverse tappe enzimatiche, in diiidrotestosterone, un potente androgeno.

Poiché sono alterati altri enzimi P450, spesso i pazienti (ma non sempre) hanno varie anomalie congenite, definite nel loro complesso **sindrome di Antley-Bixler**. Esse comprendono carniosinostosi, brachicefalia, ipertrofia delle bozze frontali, grave ipoplasia di un'emifaccia con proptosi e stenosi o atresia coanale, sinostosi omeroradiale, curvatura mediale dell'ulna, dita delle mani lunghe, magre con camptodattilia, ali iliache strette, curvatura anteriore del femore e malformazioni cardiache e renali. I precisi difetti metabolici responsabili di questa malattia sono ancora incerti, ma coinvolgono alterazioni del metabolismo dell'acido retinoico o di un teratogeno correlato oppure un deficit di lanosterolo14-demetilasi (*CYP51*). Il dato che simili anomalie possano dipendere dall'esposizione materna al ketoconazolo, un farmaco antimicotico che inibisce *CYP51*, supporta la seconda possibilità.

EPIDEMIOLOGIA. L'incidenza precisa non è nota. Raramente si manifesta con il deficit della 21-idrossilasi, ma si può verificare con analoga frequenza in altre forme di CAH.

REPERTI DI LABORATORIO. Gli steroidi sierici, esclusi quelli 17- o 21-idrossilati, sono per la maggior parte aumentati, compresi il pregnenolone e il progesterone. Anche i 17-idrossi e i 21-desossisteroidi sono aumentati, compresi il 17-idrossipregnenolone, il 17-idrossiprogesterone e il 21-desossicortisolo. I metaboliti steroidei urinari possono essere determinati con spettrometria quantitativa di massa. I metaboliti i cui livelli sono aumentati comprendono: pregnandiolo, pregnantriolo, pregnantriolone e metaboliti del corticosterone. I metaboliti urinari del cortisolo sono diminuiti. L'analisi genetica dimostra mutazioni del gene POR.

DIAGNOSI DIFFERENZIALE. Questa malattia deve essere distinta da altre forme di iperplasia surrenale congenita, particolarmente il deficit di 21-idrossilasi nelle femmine, che è altrettanto comune e ha dati di laboratorio similari. Si pone il sospetto di deficit di *POR* se la madre presenta virilizzazione o se si associano anomalie proprie della sindrome di Antley-Bixler. Al contrario, la virilizzazione sia della madre sia del figlio può essere dovuta a un luteoma gravidico, ma in questo caso non si osservano anomalie postnatali della biosintesi corticosteroidea. La sindrome di Antley-Bixler si può verificare anche in assenza di alterazioni della biosintesi steroidea, per mutazioni del recettore del fattore di crescita fibroblastica, FGRF2.

577.7 • Deficit dell'aldosterone sintasi

EZIOLOGIA. Si tratta di una rara patologia autosomica recessiva in cui è alterata la sintesi di corticosterone e aldosterone. È stato accuratamente studiato un gruppo di pazienti ebrei iraniani. La maggioranza dei casi dipende da mutazioni del gene *CYP11B2*, che codifica per l'aldosterone sintasi; tuttavia, in altre famiglie è stato escluso il linkage di *CYP11B2*. In assenza di mutazioni di *CYP11B2*, la malattia è stata chiamata ipoaldosteronismo familiare iper-reninemico di tipo 2; il gene o i geni responsabili non sono ancora stati determinati.

L'aldosterone sintasi media le tre reazioni finali della sintesi dell'aldosterone dal desossicorticosterone (11-idrossilazione, 18-idrossilazione, 18-ossidazione). Benché l'11-idrossilazione richieda la conversione del desossicorticosterone a corticosterone, questa reazione può essere catalizzata anche da un altro enzima correlato, il CYP11B1, localizzato nella zona fascicolata, che non è colpita dalla malattia. Per la stessa ragione, questi pazienti presentano una normale biosintesi del cortisolo.

La malattia è stata classificata in due tipi, definiti deficit di corticosterone metilossidasi di tipo I e di tipo II. Essi differiscono solo per i livelli dell'immediato precursore dell'aldosterone, il 18-idrossicorticosterone; i livelli sono bassi nel tipo I ed elevati nel tipo II. Queste differenze non corrispondono a una semplice via di particolari mutazioni e sono di scarsa importanza clinica.

MANIFESTAZIONI CLINICHE. I neonati con deficit di aldosterone sintasi possono avere gravi alterazioni elettrolitiche, con **iponatremia, iperkaliemia** e **acidosi metabolica**. Tuttavia, dal momento che la sintesi del cortisolo non viene intaccata, i neonati raramente presentano quadri analoghi a quelli dei bambini non trattati con forme da perdita di sali dell'iperplasia surrenale congenita, come il deficit della 21-idrossilasi. È per questo motivo che parecchi neonati sfuggono alla diagnosi. Successivamente, durante l'infanzia o nella prima fanciullezza, si possono manifestare mancanza di sviluppo e crescita scarsa. Gli adulti spesso sono asintomatici; sebbene possano sviluppare alterazioni elettrolitiche in caso di deplezione sodica conseguente a varie procedure, per esempio per preparazione intestinale per un enema al bario.

REPERTI DI LABORATORIO. I neonati presentano un'elevata attività reninica plasmatica. I livelli di aldosterone sono diminuiti; possono situarsi ai limiti inferiori del range di normalità ma sono comunque sempre inappropriatamente bassi in rapporto al grado di iperkaliemia o iper-reninemia. I livelli di corticosterone sono spesso elevati. Alcuni pazienti, ma non tutti, mostrano un notevole aumento dei livelli di 18-idrossicorticosterone, ma bassi valori di questo steroide non escludono la diagnosi. Nelle famiglie in cui il 18-idrossicorticosterone è elevato negli individui colpiti, questa anomalia biochimica persiste nell'adulto, anche in assenza di alterazioni elettrolitiche.

DIAGNOSI DIFFERENZIALE. È importante distinguere il deficit di aldosterone sintasi dall'insufficienza surrenale primaria, in cui sono interessati sia il cortisolo sia l'aldosterone (comprese le forme con perdita di sali dell'iperplasia surrenale congenita), perché la seconda condizione è usualmente associata a un rischio molto maggiore di shock e iponatremia. La distinzione risulta chiara dopo appropriate indagini di laboratorio. Lo pseudoipoaldosteronismo (vedi Capitolo 52) può avere alterazioni elettrolitiche analoghe e iper-reninemia, ma i livelli di aldosterone sono elevati e questa condizione solitamente non risponde al fludrocortisone.

TRATTAMENTO. Il trattamento consiste nella somministrazione di fludrocortisone (0,05-0,3 mg/die), cloruro di sodio o entrambi, che riportano nella norma i livelli plasmatici di renina. Con l'aumentare dell'età, i segni da carenza di sali di solito migliorano e spesso è possibile interrompere la terapia.

577.8 • IPERALDOSTERONISMO GLICOCORTICOIDO-SOPPRIMIBILE

EZIOLOGIA. L'iperaldosteronismo glicocorticoido-sopprimibile (aldosteronismo trattabile con glicocorticoidi, iperaldosteronismo familiare tipo I) è una forma autosomica dominante di **ipertensione a bassa renina**, in cui l'iperaldosteronismo è rapidamente soppresso dalla somministrazione con glicocorticoidi. Questo effetto inusuale dei glicocorticoidi suggerisce che la malattia è regolata dalla secrezione di ACTH e aldosterone e non dal sistema renina-angiotensina. In aggiunta alla secrezione di aldosterone regolata in modo abnorme dall'ACTH, vi è una notevole iperproduzione di 18-idrossicortisolo e 18-ossicortisolo. La sintesi di questi steroidi richiede l'attività della 17-idrossilasi (CYP17), che è normalmente espressa solo nella zona fascicolata, e l'attività dell'aldosterone sintasi (CYP11B2), normalmente espressa solo nella zona glomerulare. Inoltre, queste caratteristiche implicano che l'aldosterone sintasi sia espressa in modo simile all'enzima 11-idrossilasi (*CYP11B1*), strettamente correlato. La malattia è causata da un ineguale *crossing-over* meiotico tra i geni *CYP11B1* e *CYP11B2*, che sono strettamente associati sul cromosoma 8q24. Si produce un ulteriore gene "ibrido", che possiede sequenze regolatrici di *CYP11B1* giustapposte alle sequenze di *CYP11B2*. Come conseguenza si ha una inappropriata espressione dell'enzima *CYP11B2*-simile con l'attività dell'aldosterone sintasi nella zona fascicolata del surrene.

MANIFESTAZIONI CLINICHE. Alcuni bambini colpiti non hanno sintomi e la diagnosi viene stabilita dopo la scoperta incidentale di un'ipertensione moderata, tipicamente di 30 mmHg superiore rispetto ai membri coetanei della famiglia non affetti. Altri presentano una più evidente ipertensione sintomatica con cefalea, vertigini e disturbi visivi. Un'anamnesi familiare positiva per ipertensione a insorgenza precoce o precoci ictus può insospettire il medico e orientarlo nella diagnosi. Alcuni pazienti manifestano ipokaliemia cronica (ma questo non è un reperto consistente) che di solito è modesta.

REPERTI DI LABORATORIO. I pazienti hanno elevati livelli plasmatici e urinari di aldosterone e un'attività reninica plasmatica soppressa. Non sempre è presente ipokaliemia. I livelli plasmatici e urinari di 18-ossicortisolo e 18-idrossicortisolo sono notevolmente aumentati. Il gene ibrido *CYP11B1/CYP11B2* può essere trovato facilmente con metodiche di genetica molecolare. Tuttavia, questi dosaggi non sono utilizzabili di routine.

DIAGNOSI DIFFERENZIALE. Questa malattia deve essere distinta dall'aldosteronismo primario da iperplasia bilaterale o da adenoma aldosterone-secernente (vedi Capitolo 579). La maggior parte dei casi di aldosteronismo primario è sporadica, sebbene siano state descritte rare famiglie colpite.

I pazienti con aldosteronismo primario possono anche avere elevati livelli di 18-idrossicortisolo e 18-ossicortisolo e questi dati dovrebbero essere usati con cautela per distinguere un aldosteronismo primario da uno sopprimibile con glicocorticoidi. Può essere utile una prova terapeutica con desametasone, se la secrezione di aldosterone è soppressa, e se si sono approntati i test genetici per identificare l'eventuale presenza del gene ibrido dell'iperaldosteronismo sopprimibile con glicocorticoidi.

TRATTAMENTO. L'iperaldosteronismo che risponde ai glicocorticoidi viene trattato quotidianamente con tali sostanze, in genere il desametasone, alla dose di 25 μg/kg/die in due somministrazioni. Se necessario, gli effetti dell'aldosterone possono essere bloccati con un diuretico risparmiatore di potassio, come lo spironolattone, l'eplerenone o l'amiloride. L'ipertensione si risolve in pazienti in cui non sia grave o di vecchia data. Se l'ipertensione è presente da lungo tempo, può essere necessario aggiungere altri farmaci antipertensivi, come i calcioantagonisti.

CONSULENZA GENETICA. Vista la modalità di trasmissione ereditaria autosomica dominante, i membri delle famiglie a rischio devono essere valutati per scoprire questa causa di ipertensione, facilmente trattabile.

Arlt W, Walker EA, Draper N, et al: Congenital adrenal hyperplasia caused by mutant P450 oxidoreductase and human androgen synthesis: Analytical study. *Lancet* 2004;363:2128–2135.
Auchus RJ: The genetics, pathophysiology, and management of human deficiencies of P450c17. *Endocrinol Metab Clin North Am* 2001;30:101–119.
Bose HS, Sato S, Aisenberg J, et al: Mutations in the steroidogenic acute regulatory protein (StAR) in six patients with congenital lipoid adrenal hyperplasia. *J Clin Endocrinol Metab* 2000;85:3636–3639.
Consensus statement on 21-hydroxylase deficiency from the Lawson Wilkins Pediatric Endocrine Society and the European Society for Paediatric Endocrinology. *J Clin Endocrinol Metab* 2002;87:4048–4053.
Dluhy RG: Glucocorticoid-remediable aldosteronism. *Endocrinologist* 2001; 11:263–268.
Fluck CE, Tajima T, Pandey AV, et al: Mutant P450 oxidoreductase causes disordered steroidogenesis with and without Antley-Bixler syndrome. *Nat Genet* 2004;36:228–230.
Giacaglia LR, Mendonca BB, Madureira G, et al: Adrenal nodules in patients with congenital adrenal hyperplasia due to 21-hydroxylase deficiency: Regression after adequate hormonal control. *J Pediatr Endocrinol Metab* 2001;14:415–419.
Gmyrek GA, New MI, Sosa RE, et al: Bilateral laparoscopic adrenalectomy as a treatment for classic congenital adrenal hyperplasia attributable to 21-hydroxylase deficiency. *Pediatrics* 2002;109:E28.
Hughes IA, Houk C, Ahmed SF, Lee PA: Consensus statement on management of intersex disorders. *Arch Dis Child* 2006;91:554–562.
Katsumata N, Ohtake M, Hojo T, et al: Compound heterozygous mutations in the cholesterol side chain cleaving enzyme (CYP11A) causing congenital adrenal insufficiency in humans. *J Clin Endocrinol Metab* 2002;87: 3808–3813.
Krege S, Walz KH, Hauffa BP, et al: Long-term follow-up of female patients with congenital adrenal hyperplasia from 21-hydroxylase deficiency, with special emphasis on the results of vaginoplasty. *BJU Int* 2000;86:253–259.
Lajic S, Nordenstrom A, Ritzen EM, et al: Prenatal treatment of congenital adrenal hyperplasia. *Eur J Endocrinol* 2004;151(Suppl 3): U63–69.
Merke DP, Bornstein SR: Congenital adrenal hyperplasia. *Lancet* 2005; 365:2125–2136.
Meyer-Bahlburg HF: Gender and sexuality in classic congenital adrenal hyperplasia. *Endocrinol Metab Clin North Am* 2001;30:155–171.
Morgan JF, Murphy H, Lacey JH, Conway G: Long term psychosocial outcome for women with congenital adrenal hyperplasia: Cross sectional survey. *Br Med J* 2005;330:340–341.
New MI: Prenatal treatment of congenital adrenal hyperplasia: The United States experience. *Endocrinol Metab Clin North Am* 2001;30:1–13.
Nordenstrom A, Wedell A, Hagenfeldt L, et al: Neonatal screening for congenital adrenal hyperplasia: 17-Hydroxyprogesterone levels and CYP21 genotypes in preterm infants. *Pediatrics* 2001;108:E68.
Pang S: Congenital adrenal hyperplasia owing to 3 beta-hydroxysteroid dehydrogenase deficiency. *Endocrinol Metab Clin North Am* 2001;30:81–99.
Rangecroft L: Surgical management of ambiguous genitalia. *Arch Dis Child* 2003;88:799–801.
Schnitzer JJ, Donahoe PK: Surgical treatment of congenital adrenal hyperplasia. *Endocrinol Metab Clin North Am* 2001;30:137–154.
Speiser PW, White PC: Congenital adrenal hyperplasia. *N Engl J Med* 2003; 349:776–788.
Tajima T, Fujieda K, Kouda N, et al: Heterozygous mutation in the cholesterol side chain cleavage enzyme (P450scc) gene in a patient with 46,XY sex reversal and adrenal insufficiency. *J Clin Endocrinol Metab* 2001;86: 3820–3825.
Therrell BL: Newborn screening for congenital adrenal hyperplasia. *Endocrinol Metab Clin North Am* 2001;30:15–30.
White PC: Steroid 11-beta-hydroxylase deficiency and related disorders. *Endocrinol Metab Clin North Am* 2001;30:61–79.

Capitolo 578 ■ Sindrome di Cushing

La sindrome di Cushing è il risultato di livelli ematici molto elevati di cortisolo o di altri glicocorticoidi, per causa iatrogena o per secrezione endogena di cortisolo, dovuta a neoplasia surrenalica o a ipersecrezione di corticotropina (ormone adrenocorticotropo [ACTH]) da tumore ipofisario (malattia di Cushing) (Tab. 578-1).

TABELLA 578-1. Classificazione eziologica dell'iperfunzione surrenalica

ECCESSO DI ANDROGENI
Iperplasia surrenalica congenita
Deficit di 21-idrossilasi (P450c21)
Deficit di 11β-idrossilasi (P450c11)
Difetto della 3β-idrossisteroido deidrogenasi
Tumore
Carcinoma
Adenoma
ECCESSO DI CORTISOLO (SINDROME DI CUSHING)
Iperplasia surrenalica bilaterale
Ipersecrezione di corticotropina (malattia di Cushing)
Secrezione ectopica di corticotropina
Corticotropina esogena
Displasia corticosurrenale nodulare
Malattia corticosurrenale nodulare pigmentata (complesso di Carney)
Tumore
Carcinoma
Adenoma
ECCESSO DI MINERALCORTICOIDI (SINDROME IPERTENSIVA IPOKALIEMICA)
Iperaldosteronismo primario
Adenoma secernente aldosterone
Iperplasia corticosurrenale micronodulare bilaterale
Aldosteronismo sopprimibile con glicocorticoidi
Tumore
Adenoma
Carcinoma
Eccesso di desossicorticosterone
Iperplasia surrenalica congenita
11β-idrossilasi (P450c11)
17α-idrossilasi (P450c17)
Tumore (carcinoma)
Apparente eccesso di mineralcorticoidi
Deficit di 11β-idrossisteroidodeidrogenasi
ECCESSO DI ESTROGENI (SINDROME SURRENALICA FEMMINILIZZANTE)
Carcinoma
Adenoma
Ipercorticismo misto e tumore

EZIOLOGIA. La causa più comune di sindrome di Cushing è rappresentata da una prolungata somministrazione esogena di glicocorticoidi, specialmente alle alte dosi utilizzate nel trattamento delle patologie linfoproliferative. Non ci sono di solito problemi diagnostici, ma il trattamento di iperglicemia, ipertensione, aumento di peso, ritardo della crescita in altezza e osteoporosi spesso complica la terapia con glicocorticoidi.

La **sindrome di Cushing endogena** nei neonati è più frequentemente causata da un tumore surrenalico secernente, di solito un carcinoma maligno, ma occasionalmente anche un adenoma benigno (vedi Capitolo 580). Pazienti con questi tumori spesso mostrano segni di ipercortisolismo assieme a segni di ipersecrezione di altri steroidi, come gli androgeni, gli estrogeni e l'aldosterone.

Sebbene estremamente rara nell'infanzia, la causa più frequente di sindrome di Cushing endogena in bambini maggiori di 7 anni è la **malattia di Cushing**, in cui l'eccessiva secrezione di ACTH da parte di un adenoma ipofisario causa un'iperplasia surrenalica bilaterale. Tali adenomi, spesso troppo piccoli per essere identificati con le tecniche diagnostiche morfologiche, vengono definiti microadenomi. Si tratta principalmente di cellule cromofobe, che mostrano spesso una immunocolorazione positiva per l'ACTH e il suo precursore, la pro-opiomelanocortina (POMC).

La sindrome di Cushing ACTH-dipendente può anche essere dovuta a produzione ectopica di ACTH, sebbene questa forma sia rara nei bambini. La secrezione ectopica di ACTH nei bambini si associa al carcinoma pancreatico a cellule insulari, al neuroblastoma o al ganglioneuroblastoma, all'emangiopericitoma, al tumore di Wilm e al carcinoide timico. L'ipertensione è più frequente nella sindrome da ACTH ectopico rispetto alle altre forme di sindrome di Cushing, poiché livelli molto elevati di cortisolo possono sopraffare l'11β-idrossisteroido deidrogenasi renale (vedi Capitolo 575), con aumento dell'effetto dei mineralcorticoidi (ritenzione di sali).

La **malattia surrenalica primaria pigmentata nodulare** (*Primary Pigmented Nodular Adrenocortical Disease*, PPNAD) è una forma particolare di sindrome di Cushing ACTH-indipendente, che normalmente si presenta prima del ventesimo anno di età. Si può verificare come evento isolato o, più comunemente, come un disordine familiare associato ad altre manifestazioni. Le ghiandole surrenali sono piccole e con caratteristici noduli multipli, piccoli (<4 mm di diametro), pigmentati (neri), contenenti ampie cellule con citoplasma ricco di lipofuscina; tra i noduli vi è atrofia corticale.

Questa patologia surrenalica compare come una delle manifestazioni del **complesso di Carney**, una malattia autosomica dominante che comprende anche lentiggini delle zone mediali del volto e nevi blu, mixomi cardiaci e cutanei, tumori ipofisari, tiroidei e testicolari, e schwannomi melanotici pigmentati. Il complesso di Carney è ereditario con modalità autosomica dominante, sebbene siano noti casi sporadici. I loci genetici del complesso di Carney sono stati localizzati sul cromosoma 2p16 e il gene per la subunità regolatoria tipo 1α della proteinchinasi A (PRKAR1A) sul cromosoma 17q22-24.

La sindrome di Cushing ACTH-indipendente con iperplasia nodulare o adenoma si verifica raramente, nei casi di **sindrome di McCune-Albright**, con sintomi che iniziano nella primissima infanzia o nell'infanzia. La sindrome di McCune-Albright è dovuta a una mutazione somatica della proteina G, $G_S\alpha$, con conseguente inibizione dell'attività della guanosina trifosfatasi e attivazione costitutiva dell'adenilato ciclasi. Quando la mutazione è presente nel tessuto surrenalico, l'ACTH stimola in modo indipendente il cortisolo e la divisione cellulare. Altri tessuti in cui compaiono mutazioni attivanti sono l'osso (con conseguente displasia fibrosa), gonadi, tiroide e ipofisi. Le manifestazioni cliniche dipendono da quali tessuti sono coinvolti.

Le lesioni surrenaliche comprendono iperplasia diffusa, iperplasia nodulare, adenoma e raramente carcinoma, come parte della neoplasia endocrina multipla tipo 1, una patologia autosomica dominante, in cui si verifica una in attivazione eterozigote del gene soppressore del tumore menin (**MEN1**) sul cromosoma 11q13 (vedi Capitolo 574).

MANIFESTAZIONI CLINICHE. Segni di sindrome di Cushing sono stati trovati in bambini con meno di 1 anno. Nei neonati la malattia è più grave e i dati clinici sono più evidenti rispetto ai bambini più grandi. La faccia è rotondeggiante, con guance prominenti e carnagione arrossata (facies lunaris). Nei bambini più piccoli è frequente l'obesità generalizzata. Nei pazienti con neoplasie surrenaliche, spesso sono presenti segni di virilizzazione; può comparire irsutismo del viso e del tronco, peli pubici, acne, abbassamento del tono della voce, ingrossamento del clitoride nelle femmine. Si ha un'alterazione della crescita, con l'altezza che scende sotto al 3° percentile, eccetto i casi in cui la notevole virilizzazione produca una crescita normale o anche accelerata. È frequente l'ipertensione, che può essere responsabile di insufficienza cardiaca. Un aumento della suscettibilità alle infezioni può portare a sepsi fatale.

Nei bambini più grandi, oltre all'obesità, è comune la bassa statura. Le sole manifestazioni precoci possono essere rappresentate dallo sviluppo graduale di obesità e dalla decelerazione o dall'arresto della crescita. I bambini più grandi più spesso hanno un'obesità più grave a livello del viso e del tronco, rispetto agli arti. Sono comuni striae rubrae sui fianchi, sull'addome e sulle cosce. Lo sviluppo puberale può essere ritardato o può comparire amenorrea in ragazze in età postmenarcale. Astenia, cefalea e labilità emotiva possono essere rilevanti. Spesso sono presenti ipertensione e iperglicemia; quest'ultima può evolvere verso un diabete franco. È frequente l'osteoporosi, con possibili fratture patologiche.

REPERTI DI LABORATORIO. I livelli ematici di cortisolo sono solitamente elevati alle 8.00 e diminuiscono almeno del 50% a mezzanotte, eccetto che nei neonati e nei bambini piccoli in cui non si è ancora stabilito un ritmo diurno. I pazienti con sindrome di Cushing perdono il ritmo circadiano, e i livelli di cortisolo sono analoghi sia a mezzanotte sia alle 8.00. Ottenere dei campioni di sangue durante il giorno presenta delle difficoltà logistiche per la valutazione di un paziente esterno, ma il cortisolo può essere misurato anche in campioni di saliva, ottenibili a domicilio e ad appropriate ore del giorno. Livelli notturni elevati di cortisolo salivare, fanno sospettare la sindrome di Cushing.

L'escrezione urinaria di cortisolo libero è aumentata. È preferibile ricavare questo dato da campioni di urina delle 24 ore ed esprimerlo come rapporto fra microgrammi di cortisolo escreto per grammi di creatinina. Questo rapporto è indipendente dalle dimensioni corporee e dalla completezza della raccolta urinaria.

Spesso risulta utile una singola dose del test di soppressione con desametasone; nei soggetti normali una dose di 25-30 μg/kg (al massimo 2 mg) alle 23.00 porta a un decremento dei livelli di cortisolo a meno di 5 μg/dL alle 8.00 del giorno successivo, ma non nei pazienti con sindrome di Cushing.

Il test di tolleranza glicidica è spesso alterato, nonostante gli alti livelli insulinemici. Gli elettroliti sierici sono spesso normali, ma il potassio può essere diminuito, specialmente in pazienti con tumori secernenti ACTH ectopico.

Dopo aver stabilito la diagnosi di sindrome di Cushing, è necessario determinare se sia dovuta a un adenoma ipofisario, a un tumore secernente ACTH ectopico o a un tumore surrenalico che produce cortisolo. Le concentrazioni di ACTH sono normalmente soppresse in pazienti con tumori cortisolo-secernenti, sono molto alte in quelli con tumori secernenti ACTH ectopico, ma possono anche essere normali in pazienti con adenomi ipofisari ACTH-secernenti. Dopo un bolo endovenoso di ormone di rilascio della corticotropina (CRH), i pazienti con sindrome di Cushing ACTH-dipendente hanno una risposta esagerata di ACTH e cortisolo, mentre quelli con neoplasie surrenaliche non presentano alcun incremento né di ACTH né di cortisolo. La seconda fase del test di soppressione al desametasone consiste nella somministrazione di desametasone, da 30 a 120 μg/kg/die in 4 dosi, nei giorni successivi. In bambini con sindrome di Cushing ipofisaria, la dose maggiore, ma non la minore, è in grado di sopprimere i livelli sierici di cortisolo. Tipicamente, pazienti con sindrome di Cushing ACTH-dipendente non mostrano soppressione dei livelli di cortisolo dopo desametasone.

La TC virtualmente è in grado di trovare tutti i tumori surrenalici maggiori di 1,5 cm. La RM evidenzia gli adenomi ipofisari ACTH-secernenti, ma molti di essi sono troppo piccoli per essere scoperti; l'utilizzo di un mezzo di contrasto, come il gadolinio, aumenta la sensibilità dell'indagine. Qualora non si riesca a visualizzare l'adenoma ipofisario, per localizzare la neoplasia può essere necessario prelevare bilateralmente dei campioni ematici dai seni petrosi inferiori, per misurare le concentrazioni di ACTH prima e dopo somministrazione di CRH.

DIAGNOSI DIFFERENZIALE. La sindrome di Cushing è sospettata frequentemente nei bambini con obesità, particolarmente quando siano presenti striae rubrae e ipertensione. I bambini con obesità semplice sono solitamente alti, mentre quelli con sindrome di Cushing sono bassi o hanno una decelerazione della velocità di crescita. Sebbene l'escrezione urinaria di cortisolo sia spesso elevata nell'obesità semplice, i livelli notturni salivari di cortisolo sono normali e la secrezione è normalmente soppressa dalla somministrazione orale di basse dosi di desametasone.

Nei pazienti con resistenza generalizzata ai glicocorticoidi, si hanno elevati livelli di cortisolo e ACTH, in assenza di evidenza clinica di sindrome di Cushing. I pazienti possono essere asintomatici o presentare ipertensione, ipokaliemia e pseudopubertà precoce; queste manifestazioni sono causate da un aumento dei mineralcorticoidi e degli androgeni surrenalici in risposta agli elevati livelli di ACTH. Sono state identificate mutazioni del recettore dei glicocorticoidi. È stato riportato il caso di un paziente con assenza di fenotipo cushingoide nonostante la presenza di adenoma ipofisario e malattia di Cushing biochimicamente comprovata. In questo paziente, il deficit della conversione del cortisone a cortisolo comporta un aumento della clearance del cortisolo, che protegge il paziente dall'eccesso dell'ormone.

TRATTAMENTO. Il trattamento di elezione della malattia di Cushing ipofisaria nei bambini è l'intervento di microchirurgia ipofisaria per via transfenoidale. La percentuale complessiva di successi a un follow-up inferiore ai 10 anni è del 60-80%. Basse concentrazioni sieriche o urinarie postoperatorie di cortisolo costituiscono un elemento predittivo favorevole di remissione a lungo termine nella maggior parte dei casi. Le recidive vengono trattate con il reintervento o con irradiazione ipofisaria.

La ciproeptadina, un antagonista serotoninergico ad azione centrale che blocca il rilascio di ACTH, è stato utilizzato per trattare la malattia di Cushing negli adulti; non si hanno remissioni dopo l'interruzione della terapia. Questo composto raramente è utilizzato nei bambini. Nel periodo preoperatorio, per normalizzare i livelli circolanti di cortisolo e ridurre la morbilità e la mortalità perioperatorie, si utilizzano degli inibitori della steroidogenesi surrenalica (metirapone, ketoconazolo, aminoglutetimide).

Se l'adenoma ipofisario non risponde al trattamento o se l'ACTH viene secreto da un tumore metastatico ectopico, si deve ricorrere alla surrenectomia. Questo intervento spesso può essere eseguito in laparoscopia. La permanenza dell'adenoma ipofisario dopo la surrenectomia può provocare un aumento della secrezione di ACTH, evidenziato principalmente da un marker caratteristico, l'iperpigmentazione cutanea. Questa condizione viene chiamata **sindrome di Nelson**.

Gli adenomi corticali benigni sono trattati con surrenectomia unilaterale. Talvolta si tratta di adenomi bilaterali; in questi casi il trattamento elettivo è costituito dalla surrenectomia subtotale. In altre situazioni, si può ottenere un risultato eccellente con la rimozione del solo tumore. I carcinomi surrenalici metastatizzano frequentemente, soprattutto nel fegato e nel polmone, e non hanno prognosi favorevole, nonostante la rimozione della lesione primitiva. Raramente queste neoplasie sono bilaterali e richiedono la surrenectomia totale. Spesso è impossibile differenziare forme maligne da altre benigne, attraverso il solo reperto istologico.

La gestione dei pazienti sottoposti a surrenectomia necessita di un'adeguata preparazione preoperatoria e di una terapia sostitutiva postoperatoria con un corticosterioide. Le noeoplasie che producono corticosteroidi di norma provocano l'atrofia del tessuto surrenalico normale, ed è necessaria la terapia sostitutiva con cortisolo (10 mg/m^2/die in tre somministrazioni, da iniziare nell'immediato periodo postoperatorio), fino a che non si ristabilisce l'asse ipotalamo-ipofiso-surrenalico. Le complicanze postoperatorie comprendono: sepsi, pancreatite, trombosi, ritardo nella chiusura della ferita e collasso improvviso, soprattutto nei neonati con sindrome di Cushing. Si verifica un sostanziale recupero della crescita, della progressione puberale e un aumento della densità ossea, che rimane però alterata, e l'altezza in età adulta spesso è compromessa.

Bourdeau I, D'amour P, Hamet P, et al: Aberrant membrane hormone receptors in incidentally discovered bilateral macronodular adrenal hyperplasia with subclinical Cushing's syndrome. *J Clin Endocrinol Metab* 2001;86:5534–5540.

Devoe DJ, Miller WL, Conte FA, et al: Long-term outcome in children and adolescents after transsphenoidal surgery for Cushing's disease. *J Clin Endocrinol Metab* 1997;82:3196–3202.

Gafni RI, Papanicolaou DA, Nieman LK: Nighttime salivary cortisol measurement as a simple, noninvasive, outpatient screening test for Cushing's syndrome in children and adolescents. *J Pediatr* 2000;137:30–35.

Hiroi N, Chrousos GP, Kohn B, et al: Clinical Case Seminar: Adrenocortical-pituitary hybrid tumor causing Cushing's syndrome. *J Clin Endocrinol Metab* 2001;86:2631–2637.

Kirk JMW, Brain CE, Carson DJ, et al: Cushing's syndrome caused by nodular adrenal hyperplasia in children with McCune-Albright syndrome. *J Pediatr* 1999;134:789–792.

Lacroix A, N'Diaye N, Tremblay J, et al: Ectopic and abnormal hormone receptors in adrenal Cushing's syndrome. *Endocr Rev* 2001;22:75–110.

Lienhardt A, Grossman AB, Dacie JE, et al: Relative contributions of inferior petrosal sinus sampling and pituitary imaging in the investigation of children and adolescents with ACTH-dependent Cushing's syndrome. *J Clin Endocrinol Metab* 2001;86:5711–5714.

Newell-Price J, Bertagna X, Grossman AB, et al: Cushing's syndrome. *Lancet* 2006;367:1605–1617.

Raff H, Findling JW: A physiologic approach to diagnosis of the Cushing syndrome. *Ann Intern Med* 2003;138:980–991.

Raffin-Sanson ML, de Keyzer Y, Bertagna X: Syndromes of ectopic ACTH secretion: Recent pathophysiological progresses and their clinical implications. *Endocrinologist* 2000;10:97–106.

Stratakis CA, Kirschner LS, Carney JA: Clinical and molecular features of the Carney complex: Diagnostic criteria and recommendations for patient evaluation. *J Clin Endocrinol Metab* 2001;86:4041–4046.

Stratakis CA: Genetics of adrenocortical tumors: Gatekeepers, landscapers and conductors in symphony. *Trends Endocrinol Metab* 2003;14:404–410.

Capitolo 579 ■ Iperaldosteronismo primario

L'iperaldosteronismo primario comprende patologie causate dall'ipersecrezione di aldosterone, indipendentemente dal sistema renina-angiotensina. Queste condizioni sono caratterizzate da **ipertensione**, **ipokaliemia** e soppressione del sistema renina-angiotensina.

EZIOLOGIA. Gli adenomi aldosterone-secernenti sono unilaterali e sono stati descritti anche in bambini di 3 anni e mezzo e colpiscono soprattutto le femmine. Nei bambini più grandi, più frequentemente maschi, tende a verificarsi invece un'iperplasia corticosurrenale bilaterale micronodulare. Può manifestarsi anche un iperaldosteronismo primario da iperplasia surrenale unilaterale. L'iperaldosteronismo sopprimibile con glicocorticoidi è discusso nel Capitolo 577.

EPIDEMIOLOGIA. Queste condizioni sono abbastanza rare nei bambini, ma possono rappresentare il 5-10% dei casi di ipertensione nell'adulto. Nonostante si tratti di una patologia solitamente sporadica, sono stati riportati casi di famiglie con diversi membri colpiti.

MANIFESTAZIONI CLINICHE. Una parte dei bambini colpiti è asintomatica e la diagnosi viene posta dopo la scoperta casuale di un'ipertensione moderata. Altri presentano invece un'ipertensione grave (fino a 240/150 mmHg), con cefalea, vertigini, nicturia, enuresi e polidipsia. I bambini con grave ipokaliemia manifestano astenia e malessere, tetania, paralisi intermittente, affaticamento e crescita insufficiente.

REPERTI DI LABORATORIO. Spesso è presente ipokaliemia. Il pH sierico e le concentrazioni di anidride carbonica e di sodio sono elevati, mentre sono diminuiti i livelli di cloro e di magnesio. La calcemia è normale, anche in bambini con tetania manifesta. Il pH urinario è neutro o alcalino ed è elevata l'escrezione urinaria di potassio. I livelli plasmatici di aldosterone possono essere normali o aumentati. Anche la concentrazione di aldosterone nelle urine delle 24 ore è aumentata. I livelli plasmatici di renina sono persistentemente bassi.

È controverso quale sia l'indagine elettiva per la diagnosi di iperaldosteronismo primario. Sia i livelli di aldosterone sia quelli di renina possono variare a seconda dei giorni, della postura, dell'introito di sodio, rendendo difficile stabilire un range di riferimento costante. Sarebbe opportuno redigere un protocollo che codifichi una procedura di prelievo costante, per esempio a metà giornata, dopo che il paziente è rimasto seduto per 15 minuti. Se possibile, alcune settimane prima dell'esame sarebbe opportuno sospendere la terapia farmacologica antipertensiva, come anche altri farmaci che possano interferire con la secrezione di renina o aldosterone, compresi i diuretici, i β-bloccanti, gli inibitori dell'enzima di conversione dell'angiotensina, i bloccanti i recettori dell'angiotensina, la clonidina e gli agenti antinfiammatori non steroidei. Nei pazienti che assumono tutti questi farmaci, può essere necessaria la sostituzione con bloccanti α-adrenergici o calcioantagonisti, che hanno minori effetti sui valori dell'esame. Il rapporto tra le concentrazioni plasmatiche di aldosterone e l'attività reninica è sempre alto e rappresenta un efficace test di screening per l'iperaldosteronismo primario. L'aldosterone non diminuisce con la somministrazione di soluzione salina o fludrocortisone e la renina non risponde alla restrizione di sali e di liquidi. I livelli urinari di 18-ossicortisolo e 18-idrossicortisolo possono essere aumentati, ma non tanto quanto nella forma di iperaldosteronismo sopprimibile con glicocorticoidi.

DIAGNOSI DIFFERENZIALE. L'iperaldosteronismo primario deve essere differenziato da quello glicocorticoido-sopprimibile (vedi Capitolo 577.7), che è trattato specificamente assieme ai glicorticoidi. In presenza di un'ereditarietà autosomica dominante, il sospetto si indirizza verso il secondo disturbo. La diagnosi di iperaldosteronismo glicocorticoido-sopprimibile si basa sul test di soppressione con desametasone o su specifiche ricerche genetiche. Più in generale, con le indagini precedentemente descritte, l'iperaldosteronismo primario deve essere distinto da altre forme di ipertensione.

TRATTAMENTO. Il trattamento dell'adenoma aldosterone-secernente consiste nella rimozione chirurgica; inizialmente era eseguita con laparotomia e surrenectomia; successivamente sono state messe a punto tecniche laparoscopiche di enucleazione di adenomi aldosterone-secernenti e di surrenectomia. Nell'iperaldosteronismo da iperplasia surrenalica bilaterale si attua una terapia medica con antagonisti dei mineralcorticoidi, come lo spironolattone o l'eplerenone, che spesso sono in grado di normalizzare la pressione arteriosa e la potassiemia. I dati sono più numerosi per lo spironolattone, ma questo farmaco possiede anche proprietà antiandrogeniche e può essere sconsigliato per i maschi adolescenti. L'eplerenone è un antimineralcorticoide più specifico, ma si ha meno esperienza nel suo utilizzo pediatrico. Come alternativa, può essere utilizzato un bloccante i canali epiteliali del sodio, come l'amiloride, con l'aggiunta di altri antipertensivi. Nei pazienti in cui sia difficile il controllo con la terapia medica, si deve prendere in considerazione la surrenectomia unilaterale.

Gordon RD: The challenge of more robust and reproducible methodology in screening for primary aldosteronism. *J Hypertens* 2004;22:251–255.

Grim CE: Evolution of diagnostic criteria for primary aldosteronism: Why is it more common in "drug-resistant" hypertension today? *Curr Hypertens Rep* 2004;6:485–492.

Kaplan NM: The current epidemic of primary aldosteronism: Causes and consequences. *J Hypertens* 2004;22:863–869.

Capitolo 580 ■ Tumori surrenalici

EPIDEMIOLOGIA. I tumori surrenalici sono rari nell'infanzia. Possono comparire a tutte le età, ma più frequentemente in bambini con meno di 10 anni. Nel 2-10% dei casi, il tumore è bilaterale e in oltre il 90% dei bambini colpiti sono presenti sintomi di iperfunzione endocrina (vedi Tab. 578-1). I tumori possono essere associati a emi-ipertrofia, di solito nei primi anni di vita. Possono essere associati anche la **sindrome di Beckwith-Wiedemann** e altri difetti congeniti, in particolare anomalie del tratto genitourinario, del sistema nervoso centrale e di tipo amartomatoso.

EZIOLOGIA. In pazienti con carcinoma surrenalico isolato e anche in altri appartenenti a famiglie con neoplasie rare, sono state trovate mutazioni germiline in p53 (sul cromosoma 17p13.1). In casi di carcinoma surrenalico sporadico è stata riportata perdita di eterozigosi che coinvolge i cromosomi 2, 4, 1, e 18 e di sovraespressione del gene *IGF2* (cromosoma 11p15.5).

580.1 • Tumori corticosurrenalici virilizzanti

MANIFESTAZIONI CLINICHE. Il sintomo di esordio più comune nei bambini con tumori corticosurrenalici è rappresentato dalla virilizzazione. Nei maschi, il quadro clinico è simile a quello della virilizzazione semplice dell'iperplasia surrenalica congenita: accelerazione della velocità di crescita e dello sviluppo muscolare, acne, ingrossamento del pene e sviluppo precoce dei peli pubici e ascellari. Nelle femmine, i tumori surrenalici virilizzanti causano una mascolinizzazione di bambine in precedenza normali, con ingrossamento clitorideo, accelerazione della crescita, modificazioni della voce e sviluppo prematuro dei peli pubici e ascellari.

In aggiunta alla virilizzazione, il 20-40% dei bambini con tumori surrenalici presenta anche la sindrome di Cushing (vedi Capitolo 578). Mentre nei bambini con tumori surrenalici la virilizzazione si può manifestare anche da sola (50-80%), di solito ciò non accade nel caso della sindrome di Cushing.

REPERTI DI LABORATORIO. I livelli sierici di deidroepiandrosterone (DHEA), il DHEA solfato e l'androstenedione sono usualmente elevati, spesso in modo notevole. Frequentemente sono aumentati anche i livelli di testosterone, in seguito alla conversione periferica dell'androstenedione, ma sono stati riportati casi di bambini con tumori surrenalici a prevalente secrezione testosteronemica. Anche i 17-ketosteroidi urinari (metaboliti degli steroidi sessuali) sono aumentati. Molti tumori surrenalici manifestano un deficit relativo dell'attività 11β-idrossilasica e secernono un'aumentata quantità di desossicorticosterone; questi pazienti sono ipertesi e i tumori sono maligni.

Lo studio delle neoplasie può essere eseguito con indagini ecografiche, TC o RM. È necessaria la valutazione preoperatoria di eventuali metastasi al torace, addome e pelvi. Spesso non è possibile differenziare istologicamente le forme benigne da quelle maligne.

TRATTAMENTO. Il trattamento è chirurgico. Si raccomanda solitamente un approccio transperitoneale, ma è possibile la rimozione laparoscopica. Molti di questi tumori sono altamente maligni e metastatizzano ampiamente, ma in caso di tumori meno maligni, incapsulati, è possibile la guarigione con regressione delle manifestazioni di virilizzazione dopo la rimozione chirurgica. La resezione incompleta, con residui tissutali maggiori di 100 g, tumori più ampi di 200 cm^3, l'età superiore a 3 anni e mezzo al momento della diagnosi, la presenza di sintomi per più di 6 mesi e un marcato incremento dei livelli urinari dei 17-ketosteroidi e dei 17-idrossisteroidi, sono tutti fattori associati a prognosi infausta. Dopo l'intervento, i pazienti devono essere strettamente monitorati da un punto di vista biochimico, con frequenti valutazioni dei livelli degli androgeni surrenalici e da un punto di vista morfologico. La recidiva dei sintomi o anomalie biochimiche devono indirizzare prontamente alla ricerca di metastasi. Queste coinvolgono primariamente fegato, polmone e linfonodi regionali. La maggior parte delle recidive metastatiche appare entro un anno dalla resezione tumorale. Se possibile, si interviene chirurgicamente di nuovo per la rimozione delle metastasi e si instaura un'adeguata terapia. La terapia radiante non è in genere utile. Nei bambini, i farmaci chemioterapici come cisplatino, etoposide, ifosfamide e carboplatino, 5-fluorouracile e leucovorina hanno un utilizzo limitato e la loro efficacia non è stabilita. La terapia con o,p′-DDD (mitotano), un agente adrenolitico, può migliorare i sintomi d'ipercortisolismo o di virilizzazione nelle forme recidivanti, ma non migliora la sopravvivenza. Anche altri farmaci che interferiscono con la sintesi degli steroidi surrenalici come il ketoconazolo, l'aminoglutetimide e il metirapone, possono migliorare i sintomi da eccesso steroideo, ma non la sopravvivenza.

La neoplasia di una sola ghiandola surrenale può produrre atrofia nella controlaterale, per eccessiva produzione di cortisolo, che inibisce la normale stimolazione da parte dell'ormone adrenocorticotropo sulla ghiandola normale. Di conseguenza, dopo la rimozione chirurgica della neoplasia, si può evidenziare un'insufficienza surrenalica. Questa evenienza va prevenuta con la somministrazione di 10-25 mg di idrocortisone ogni 6 ore, iniziando il giorno stesso dell'intervento e continuando per 3-4 giorni. È necessaria inoltre una terapia con quantità adeguate di liquidi, cloruro di sodio e glucosio.

580.2 • Tumori surrenalici femminilizzanti

Tumori surrenalici femminilizzanti possono essere rappresentati sia da adenomi sia da carcinomi. Possono produrre solo estrogeni oppure anche androgeni, cortisolo o mineralcorticoidi (vedi Fig. 575-1). In questi tumori sono stati trovati alti livelli di attività aromatasica e di espressione del gene *CYP19* (*P450arom*), assenti nel normale tessuto surrenalico.

MANIFESTAZIONI CLINICHE. I tumori possono diventare sintomatici a qualsiasi età dopo il sesto mese. Spesso la prima manifestazione è rappresentata dalla ginecomastia nel maschio o da telarca prematuro nella femmina. La crescita e lo sviluppo possono essere normali oppure può comparire una concomitante virilizzazione con acne, abbassamento della voce, ingrossamento del pene o del clitoride e accelerazione della maturazione scheletrica. Negli adulti è frequente l'ipertensione, che non si osserva però nei bambini.

REPERTI DI LABORATORIO. Oltre agli elevati livelli plasmatici e urinari di estrogeni, sono spesso presenti anche elevati livelli plasmatici di androgeni (per es. il deidroepiandrosterone e il suo derivato solfato) e urinari di 17-ketosteroidi. Le concentrazioni plasmatiche di gonadotropine sono soppresse e non rispondono alla stimolazione con ormone di rilascio delle gonadotropine. L'indagine radiografica può evidenziare delle calcificazioni tumorali, ma la localizzazione di solito viene fatta con la TC.

TRATTAMENTO. Se è possibile la resezione, la ginecomastia regredisce e i valori ormonali ritornano nella norma.

Koch CA, Pacak K, Chrousos GP: The molecular pathogenesis of hereditary and sporadic adrenocortical and adrenomedullary tumors. *J Clin Endocrinol Metab* 2002;87:5367–5384.

Ribeiro RC, Figueiredo B: Childhood adrenocortical tumours. *Eur J Cancer* 2004;40:1117–1126.

Stratakis CA: Genetics of adrenocortical tumors: Gatekeepers, landscapers and conductors in symphony. *Trends Endocrinol Metab* 2003;14:404–410.

Capitolo 581 ■ Feocromocitoma

I feocromocitomi, tumori secernenti catecolamine, derivano dalle cellule cromaffini. La sede di origine più frequente (circa il 90%) è la midollare surrenale; tuttavia, si possono sviluppare in qualunque luogo lungo la catena simpatica addominale e spesso in prossimità dell'aorta a livello dell'arteria mesenterica inferiore o della sua biforcazione. Possono comparire anche nella zona perisurrenalica, nella parete vescicale o ureterale, nella cavità toracica e nella regione cervicale. Il 10% si verifica nei bambini, con una maggiore frequenza tra i 6 e i 14 anni di età. Le dimensioni tumorali variano da 1 a 10 cm di diametro e più spesso si localizzano a destra. In più del 20% dei bambini affetti il tumore è bilaterale; nel 30-40% dei bambini il tumore è bilaterale e presente anche in aree extrasurrenaliche o solo in zone extrasurrenaliche.

Il feocromocitoma può essere ereditato come un carattere autosomico dominante. Nelle famiglie interessate, nei soggetti colpiti la diagnosi avviene tra la prima e la quinta decade di vita e più della metà di essi presenta tumori multipli.

Il feocromocitoma può essere associato ad altre sindromi, come la **neurofibromatosi** e la **malattia di von Hippel-Lindau**, e fare parte della sindrome da **neoplasia endocrina multipla** (*Multiple Endocrine Neoplasia*, MEN) di tipo 2A e 2B. Il gene *NF1* della neurofibromatosi è un gene tumore-soppressore sul cromosoma 17q11.2. In famiglie con MEN-2A e MEN-2B, sono state trovate mutazioni nella linea germinale del proto-oncogeno *RET* sul cromosoma 10 (10q11.2) e, nella sindrome di von Hippel-Lindau, mutazioni nella linea germinale in un gene tumore-soppressore sul cromosoma 3p25-26. Il feocromocitoma può essere associato anche alla sclerosi tuberosa, alla sindrome di Sture-Weber e all'atassia-teleangectasia. Mutazioni somatiche dei geni associati a sindromi tumorali familiari sono stati trovati in forme non familiari di feocromocitoma.

MANIFESTAZIONI CLINICHE. Le caratteristiche cliniche del feocromocitoma dipendono da un'eccessiva produzione di adrenalina e noradrenalina. Tutti i pazienti prima o poi manifestano ipertensione. È soprattutto un'ipertensione parossisitica a dovere indicare un feocromocitoma. A differenza dell'adulto, l'ipertensione nel bambino è molto più spesso costante, piuttosto che parossistica. In caso di forme parossistiche, di solito gli attacchi all'inizio sono rari, ma diventano più frequenti ed eventualmente evolvono verso uno stato ipertensivo costante. Tra gli attacchi di ipertensione, i pazienti possono essere asintomatici. Durante gli attacchi, il paziente riferisce cefalea, palpitazioni, dolore addominale e vertigini; possono comparire anche pallore, vomito, sudorazione e rendersi evidenti convulsioni o altre manifestazioni di encefalopatia ipertensiva. Nei casi gravi, si sviluppa un dolore precordiale con irradiazione alle braccia; edema polmonare e cardio ed epatomegalia. I sintomi sono esacerbati dall'attività fisica. Il bambino ha un buon appetito ma, dato l'ipermetabolismo, non aumenta di peso e può anzi sviluppare una cachessia grave. Poliuria e polidipsia possono essere tali da far sospettare un diabete insipido. Il deficit di crescita può essere grave. La pressione arteriosa sistolica si aggira tra i 180 e i 260 mmHg, quella diastolica tra i 120 e i 210 mmHg, con eventuale cardiomegalia. L'indagine oftalmoscopica può rivelare papilledema, emorragie, essudati e vasocostrizione arteriolare.

REPERTI DI LABORATORIO. A livello urinario possono essere presenti proteinuria, qualche cilindro e occasionalmente glicosuria. Una ematuria macroscopica può indicare la localizzazione del tumore nella parete vescicale. Talvolta è presente policitemia. La diagnosi prevede la dimostrazione di elevati livelli ematici ed urinari di catecolamine e dei loro metaboliti.

Il feocromocitoma produce adrenalina e noradrenalina. Normalmente, la noradrenalina plasmatica deriva dalla produzione surrenalica e dalle terminazioni nervose adrenergiche, mentre l'adrenalina proviene principalmente dal surrene. Al contrario di quanto succede nell'adulto con feocromocitoma, in cui sono elevate sia l'adrenalina sia la noradrenalina, nei bambini il feocromocitoma produce principalmente noradrenalina. L'escrezione urinaria totale di catecolamine di solito supera i 300 µ/die. L'escrezione urinaria di acido vanillmandelico (VMA, acido 3-metossi-4-idrossimandelico), il maggiore metabolita dell'adrenalina e della noradrenalina, è aumentato come anche l'escrezione di metanefrina (vedi Fig. 575-2). I livelli di catecolamine possono essere misurati con metodiche radioimmunologiche e con metodiche di cromatografia liquida ad alta prestazione. L'escrezione di metaboliti catecolaminergici può essere simile nei bambini con feocromocitoma o con neuroblastoma, sebbene il neuroblastoma di solito non provochi ipertensione. I livelli urinari della maggior parte delle catecolamine sono però più alti nel feocromocitoma, anche se le concentrazioni di dopamina e acido omovanillico sono di solito maggiori nel neuroblastoma. L'escrezione urinaria giornaliera di questi composti aumenta con l'età e alimenti contenenti vaniglia e frutta possono essere responsabili di falsi positivi per VMA. Certi farmaci interferiscono con il dosaggio fluorometrico delle catecolamine.

L'ecografia, la TC o la RM sono in grado di localizzare facilmente la maggior parte dei tumori nell'area surrenalica; non si deve dimenticare che frequentemente sono bilaterali. I tumori extrasurrenalici possono invece porre dei problemi. Si utilizza la ^{131}I-metaiodobenzil-guanidina (MBIG), per localizzare nell'organismo eventuale tessuto cromaffine o tumori molto piccoli. Raramente oggi è necessario, per la localizzazione della neoplasia, la cateterizzazione venosa con prelievo di sangue a vari livelli per la determinazione delle catecolamine.

DIAGNOSI DIFFERENZIALE. Devono essere prese in considerazione le varie cause di ipertensione nei bambini, come patologie renali o nefrovascolari, la coartazione dell'aorta, l'ipertiroidismo, la sindrome di Cushing, il deficit di 11β-idrossilasi, 17α-idrossilasi, o 11β-idrossisteroido deidrogenasi (isoenzima tipo 2), iperaldosteronismo primario, tumori corticosurrenalici e ipertensione essenziale (vedi Capitolo 445). L'eventualità di un'ipofunzione renale monolaterale può dipendere dalla compressione dell'uretere o dell'arteria renale da parte del feocromocitoma. L'ipertensione parossistica può essere associata a porfiria o disautonomia familiare. L'escrezione urinaria di VMA è bassa nella disautonomia familiare per la presenza di un deficit di rilascio più che di sintesi delle catecolamine. Nella diagnosi differenziale vanno considerati anche patologie cerebrali, diabete insipido, diabete mellito e ipertiroidismo. Nei pazienti con neurofibromatosi l'ipertensione può essere causata da un coinvolgimento nefrovascolare o da un concomitante feocromocitoma.

Anche il neuroblastoma, il ganglioneuroblastoma e il ganglioneuroma producono frequentemente catecolamine. I tumori neurogeni secernenti comunemente sono responsabili di ipertensione, eccessiva sudorazione, rossore, pallore, rash, poliuria e polidipsia. La diarrea cronica può essere sufficientemente persistente da far sospettare una malattia celiaca.

TRATTAMENTO. La terapia consiste nella rimozione chirurgica del tumore, ma si tratta di un intervento altamente rischioso. È essenziale un'attenta gestione pre, intra e postoperatoria. È necessaria la somministrazione preoperatoria di un carico di liquidi e di α- e β-bloccanti. Poiché nei bambini spesso questi tumori sono multipli, un'approfondita esplorazione transaddominale per tutte le eventuali sedi offre le migliori opportunità di trovarli tutti. La scelta dell'anestesia più appropriata e l'incremento del volume plasmatico con introduzione di adeguate quantità di liquidi durante l'intervento chirurgico sono fondamentali per evitare una precipitosa caduta della pressione arteriosa intraoperatoria o nell'arco delle prime 48 ore postoperatorie. La manipolazione e la rimozione di questi tumori provoca un marcato incremento della secrezione di catecolamine, con conseguente aumento della pressione arteriosa e della frequenza cardiaca. La sorveglianza postoperatoria deve essere continua.

Sebbene questi tumori spesso siano istologicamente maligni, il solo indice sicuro di malignità è la comparsa di metastasi, di invasività locale, che preclude la resezione chirurgica o ematica. Circa il 10% di tutti i feocromocitomi surrenalici è maligno. Questi tumori sono rari nell'infanzia; i feocromocitomi pediatrici maligni si localizzano molto più frequentemente in sede extrasurrenalica. È opportuno un follow-up prolungato, perché nel corso degli anni si possono manifestare tumori funzionanti in altre sedi. L'esame dei parenti del paziente può evidenziare la presenza, in altri individui, di tumori insospettati, anche asintomatici.

Capitolo 582 ■ Masse surrenaliche

582.1 • INCIDENTALOMA SURRENALICO

Sempre più frequentemente si scoprono masse surrenaliche in pazienti sottoposti a TC o RM addominale, per motivi che non riguardano i surreni. La frequenza della scoperta di singole masse surrenaliche varia da meno dell'1% a oltre il 4% delle TC addominali negli adulti. La scoperta incidentale di queste masse pone ai medici un dilemma sia per quanto riguarda le fasi diagnostiche da intraprendere sia per quanto riguarda il trattamento. La diagnosi differenziale dell'incidentaloma surrenalico comprende lesioni benigne come cisti, cisti emorragiche, ematomi e mielolipomi. Queste lesioni possono essere visualizzate con la TC o con la RM. Se la natura della lesione non è chiara, è necessaria un'ulteriore valutazione per escludere adenomi benigni, feocromocitomi, carcinoma surrenalico e metastasi carcinomi primitivi in altre sedi. Gli adenomi corticosurrenalici benigni, non funzionanti, rappresentano la maggior parte degli incidentalomi. Sono necessari: anamnesi attenta, esame fisico, valutazione endocrina e ricerca di secrezione autonoma di cortisolo, androgeni, mineralcorticoidi o catecolamine. I tumori funzionanti vanno rimossi chirurgicamente. Anche se la massa surrenalica non è funzionante e ha dimensioni di 4-6 cm, si consiglia l'intervento chirurgico. Lesioni uguali o inferiori a 3 cm devono essere seguite clinicamente con periodiche ripetizioni della TC o della RM. Il trattamento deve essere individualizzato; gli incidentalomi surrenalici non funzionanti possono aumentare di volume e cominciare a secernere. Indagini morfologiche e talvolta l'aspirazione con ago sottile possono essere d'aiuto nella definizione della massa.

582.2 • CALCIFICAZIONI SURRENALICHE

Calcificazioni surrenaliche si possono verificare in varie situazioni, alcune gravi e altre senza particolari conseguenze. Le calcificazioni surrenaliche sono spesso scoperte incidentalmente durante indagini radiologiche dell'addome sia di neonati sia di bambini. Può essere presente un'anamnesi di anossia o di trauma alla nascita. L'emorragia surrenalica al momento o subito dopo la nascita costituisce probabilmente il fattore più frequente che determina la successiva calcificazione. Sebbene sia consigliabile verificare la riserva corticosurrenalica di questi pazienti, raramente si evidenziano alterazioni funzionali.

Neuroblastomi, ganglioneuromi, carcinomi corticali, feocromocitomi, cisti surrenaliche possono essere responsabili di calcificazioni, particolarmente se l'emorragia si è verificata all'interno della neoplasia. Quasi sempre in queste patologie la calcificazione è monolaterale.

In passato, la tubercolosi era una causa frequente di calcificazioni surrenaliche e di morbo di Addison. Si possono sviluppare calcificazioni anche nei surreni di bambini che hanno sofferto di sindrome di Waterhouse-Friderichsen; di solito sono asintomatici. Neonati con la sindrome di Wolman, un raro disturbo da accumulo lipidico per deficit dell'acido lipasi lisosomiale, presentano estese calcificazioni bilaterali dei surreni (vedi Capitolo 86.2).

Agrons GA, Lonergan GJ, Dickey GE, et al: Adrenocortical neoplasms in children: Radiologic-pathologic correlation. *Radiographics* 1999;19:989–1008.
Barzon L, Boscaro M: Diagnosis and management of adrenal incidentalomas. *J Urol* 2000;163:398–407.
Bravo EL: Evolving concepts in the pathophysiology, diagnosis and treatment of pheochromocytoma. *Endocr Rev* 1994;15:356–368.
Brunt LM, Moley JF: Adrenal incidentaloma. *World J Surg* 2001;25:905–913.
Ciftci AO, Senocak ME, Tanyel FC, et al: Adrenocortical tumors in children. *J Pediatr Surg* 2001;36:549–554.
Ein SH, Weitzman S, Thorner P, et al: Pediatric malignant pheochromocytoma. *J Pediatr Surg* 1994;29:1197–1201.

Eisenhoffer G, Lenders JWM, Linehan WM, et al: Plasma normetanephrine and metanephrine for detecting pheochromocytoma in von Hippel-Lindau disease and multiple endocrine neoplasia type 2. *N Engl J Med* 1999; 340:1872–1879.

Ghazi AAM, Mofid D, Rahimi F, et al: Oestrogen and cortisol producing adrenal tumour. *Arch Dis Child* 1994;71:358–359.

Kjellman M, Roshani L, Teh BT, et al: Genotyping of adrenocortical tumors: Very frequent deletions of the MEN1 locus in 11q13 and of a 1-centimorgan region in 2p16. *J Clin Endocrinol Metab* 1999;84:730–735.

Koch CA, Vortmeyer AO, Huang SC, et al: Genetic aspects of pheochromocytoma. *Endocr Regul* 2001;35:43–52.

LaFranchi SH, Hanna CE, Mandel SH: Feminizing adrenal adenoma secreting estrone presenting as prepubertal gynecomastia. *J Pediatr Endocrinol* 1989;3:261–265.

Latronico AC, Pinto EM, Domenice S, et al: An inherited mutation outside the highly conserved DNA-binding domain of the p53 tumor suppressor protein in children and adults with sporadic adrenocortical tumors. *J Clin Endocrinol Metab* 2001;86:4970–4973.

Magill SB, Raff H, Shaker JL, et al: Comparison of adrenal vein sampling and computed tomography in the differentiation of primary aldosteronism. *J Clin Endocrinol Metab* 2001;86:1066–1071.

Mayer SK, Oligny LL, Deal C, et al: Childhood adrenocortical tumors: Case series and reevaluation of prognosis–a 24-year experience. *J Pediatr Surg* 1997;32:911–915.

Mendonca BB, Lucon AM, Menezes CAV, et al: Clinical, hormonal and pathological findings in a comparative study of adrenocortical neoplasms in childhood and adulthood. *J Urol* 1995;154:2004–2009.

Moneva MH, Gomez-Sanchez CE: Establishing a diagnosis of primary hyperaldosteronism. *Curr Opin Endocrinol Diabet* 2001;8:124–129.

Phornphutkul C, Okubo T, Wu K, et al: Aromatase P450 expression in a feminizing adrenal adenoma presenting as isosexual precocious puberty. *J Clin Endocrinol Metab* 2001;86:649–652.

Prys-Roberts C: Phaeochromocytoma–recent progress in its management. *Br J Anaesth* 2000;85:44–57.

Reincke M, Beuschlein F, Slawik M, et al: Molecular adrenocortical tumourigenesis. *Eur J Clin Invest* 2000;30:63–68.

Ross JH: Pheochromocytoma: Special considerations in children. *Urol Clin North Am* 2000;27:393–402.

Siren J, Tervahartiala P, Sivula A, et al: Natural course of adrenal incidentalomas: Seven-year follow-up study. *World J Surg* 2000;24:579–582.

Wajchenberg BL, Albergaria Pereira MA, Medonca BB, et al: Adrenocortical carcinoma: Clinical and laboratory observations. *Cancer* 2000;88:711–736.

Wilkin F, Gagne N, Paquette J, et al: Pediatric adrenocortical tumors: Molecular events leading to insulin-like growth factor II gene overexpression. *J Clin Endocrinol Metab* 2000;85:2048–2056.

Young J, Bulun SE, Agarwal V, et al: Aromatase expression in a feminizing adrenocortical tumor. *J Clin Endocrinol Metab* 1996;81:3173–3176.

Sezione 5 — Patologie delle gonadi — Robert Rapaport

Capitolo 583 ■ Sviluppo e funzione delle gonadi

DIFFERENZIAZIONE EMBRIONALE DELLE GONADI. La gonade fetale indifferenziata, bipotenziale, prende origine da un ingrossamento della cresta urogenitale, vicino alla regione che darà origine ai reni e alla corticale surrenalica. Alla 6ª settimana di gestazione, le gonadi contengono cellule germinali, cellule stromali, che diventeranno cellule di Leydig nei testicoli, o cellule della teca, interstiziali o ilari nelle ovaie, e cellule di supporto che diventeranno cellule del Sertoli nei testicoli o cellule della granulosa nelle ovaie. In assenza di un fattore di determinazione testicolare, che si ritiene essere SRY (*Sex-determining Region on the Y chromosome*, cioè regione determinante il sesso sul cromosoma Y), lo sviluppo gonadico evolve in senso ovarico. Si pensa che SRY sia normalmente soppresso da un fattore putativo 2 (non ancora identificato) che funziona come repressore dello sviluppo in senso maschile.

Per lo sviluppo di **ovaie normali** è necessario un complemento cromosomico 46,XX. Sia il braccio corto sia quello lungo del cromosoma X possiede geni per il normale sviluppo ovarico. Il locus DSS (*Dosage Sensitive/Sex Reversal*) associato al gene *DAX1* responsabile dell'iperplasia surrenale congenita correlata a X e dell'ipogonadismo ipogonadotropo, membro della superfamiglia dei recettori nucleari, agisce come repressore dell'espressione genetica in senso maschile. *DAX1* esplica la sua azione tramite il legame con un recettore nucleare SF-1 correlato (fattore-1 steroidogenetico). Il gene del *signaling WNT4 in vitro* sovraregola *DAX1*, con conseguente soppressione della sintesi androgenica nelle femmine XX. I WNT sono *secret ligand* che attivano il segnale recettore mediato per la via di trasduzione e sono coinvolti nella modulazione dell'espressione genetica e del comportamento, adesione e polarità cellulari. In una diciottenne 46,XX, con assenza delle strutture di derivazione mülleriana (utero e tube), agenesia renale unilaterale e segni clinici di iperandrogenismo è stata trovata una mutazione con perdita di funzione del gene *WNT4*. Nella differenziazione sessuale può anche essere coinvolto uno *splicing* alternativo del gene del tumore di Wilms. Mutazioni WT1 sono associate alla sindrome di Denys-Drash (insufficienza renale a insorgenza precoce con anomalie dei genitali esterni e tumore di Wilms). Aploinsufficienza della forma di un 3-aminoacido [KTS] di *WT1* è stata implicata nella disgenesia gonadica di pazienti con sindrome di Fraser (glomerulopatia progressiva a esordio tardivo e disgenesia gonadica 46,XY). Mutazioni del gene *FOXL2* sono associate a insufficienza ovarica. Anche geni autosomici giocano un ruolo nella normale organogenesi ovarica e nello sviluppo testicolare. Alcune condizioni di disgenesia gonadica sono associate ad anomalie cromosomiche. Una delezione del braccio corto del cromosoma X produce le tipiche alterazioni somatiche della sindrome di Turner (vedi Capitolo 81).

Lo **sviluppo dei testicoli** richiede il braccio corto del cromosoma Y; in questa sede è stato identificato un fattore di determinazione testicolare ed è stato clonato il suo gene, denominato *SRY*. Durante la meiosi maschile, il cromosoma Y si dovrebbe separare dal cromosoma X in modo che entrambi non entrino nello stesso spermatozoo. La porzione maggiore del cromosoma Y è composta da sequenze Y-specifiche che non si appaiano con il cromosoma X. Tuttavia, una porzione minore del cromosoma Y condivide delle sequenze con il cromosoma X e in questa regione si può verificare un appaiamento. I geni e le sequenze in questa area si ricombinano tra i cromosomi sessuali, che si comportano come geni autosomici. Si usa il termine pseudoautosomico per descrivere il comportamento genetico di questi geni. Il gene *SRY* è localizzato sulla porzione prossimale 35-kb di questo appaiamento e la regione di scambio (pseudoautosomica) del cromosoma Y. Essa contiene una proteina non istone del gruppo ad alta mobilità (HMG box), lasciando supporre che *SRY* possa essere un regolatore trascrizionale di altri geni coinvolti nella differenziazione sessuale. La cresta gonadica si forma intorno al 33° giorno di gestazione. *SRY* compare al 41° giorno, con un picco al 44°, quando i cordoni testicolari diventano visibili per la prima volta e persiste nell'età adulta. Questi geni comprendono SOX9, un gene *SRY*-correlato, contenente un motivo omologo comune con il gruppo box 9 ad alta mobilità (HMG box 9) di *SRY*, localizzato sul cromosoma 17, che risulta in una inversione sessuale e displasia camptomelica, il fattore 1 steroidogenetico (SF-1) sul cromosoma 9q33 e i geni del tumore di Wilms (*WT1*), specialmente la forma KSTiso sul cromosoma 11p13, necessaria per lo sviluppo precoce di gonadi, surrene, rene, fattore 9 di crescita fibroblastica (FGF-9), GATA-4 e XH-2. Anche SOY9 interagisce con la heat shock protein 70 (HSP) nei testicoli. Quando gli eventi della ricombinazione si estendono oltre la regione pseudoautosomica, può avvenire un trasferimento di specifico DNA di X e Y tra i due cromosomi. Si verificano in questo modo delle ricombinazioni aberranti nei cromosomi X con *SRY*, che danno origine a un maschio XX, oppure nei cromosomi Y che hanno perso *SRY*, portando a **femmine XY**. *SRY* agisce come un regolatore trascrizionale per aumentare la proliferazione cellulare, attira nella cresta genitale cellule interstiziali dai mesonefri adiacenti e stimola la differenziazione delle cellule del Sertoli. Le cellule del Sertoli agiscono come un organizzatore delle linee cellulari steroidogenetiche e germinali e producono l'**ormone antimülleriano** (AMH), che provoca la regressione del sistema duttale femminile. Essi esprimono bassi livelli di *SRY* (per ulteriori geni coinvolti nello sviluppo sessuale, Tab. 583-1).

FUNZIONE DEI TESTICOLI. Nel primo trimestre di gravidanza, i livelli di gonadotropina corionica placentare raggiungono un picco (8-12 settimane) e stimolano le cellule di Leydig fetali a secernere testosterone, il maggior prodotto ormonale del testicolo. Questo periodo è fondamentale per la normale virilizzazione del feto XY. Difetti in questo processo portano a diverse forme di sviluppo maschile atipico (vedi Capitolo 589.2). Dopo la virilizzazione, i livelli fetali di testosterone diminuiscono, ma sono mantenuti a bassi livelli nella seconda metà della gravidanza dall'ormone luteinizzante (LH), secreto dall'ipofisi fetale, per consentire la crescita del pene.

Nell'ambito della normale transizione dalla vita intra- a quella extrauterina, probabilmente come risultato dell'improvvisa mancanza degli ormoni placentari e materni, il neonato subisce un transitorio incremento postnatale di gonadotropine e di steroidi sessuali. Nel maschio, l'LH e il testosterone raggiungono il picco al primo-secondo mese di vita e raggiungono livelli prepuberi al quarto-sesto mese. L'ormone follicolostimolante (FSH) e l'inibina B, hanno un picco al terzo mese e diminuiscono a livelli prepuberi al nono e al 15° mese, rispettivamente. L'innalzamento dell'LH è maggiore. Nelle femmine, invece, predomina l'incremento dell'FSH. Si ha il picco dell'FSH intorno al terzo, sesto mese, poi

TABELLA 583-1. Geni noti coinvolti nelle malattie dello sviluppo sessuale (dsd)

GENE 46,XY DSD	PROTEINA	N. OMIM DATA BASE	LOCUS	EREDITARIETÀ	GONADE	STRUTTURE MÜLLERIANE	GENITALI ESTERNI	CARATTERISTICHE ASSOCIATE/VARIANTI FENOTIPICHE
MALATTIE DELLO SVILUPPO GONADICO (TESTICOLARE): ALTERAZIONI DI SINGOLI GENI								
WT1	TF	607102	11p13	AD	Testicolo disgenetico	±	Femminili o ambigui	Tumore di Wilm, anomalie renali, tumori gonadici (WAGRm, sindrome di Denys-Drash e di Frasier)
SF1 (*NR5A1*)	Recettore nucleare TF	184757	9q33	AD/AR	Testicolo disgenetico	±	Femminili o ambigui	I fenotipi più gravi comprendono insufficienza surrenalica primaria; quelli più lievi disgenesia gonadica parziale isolata
SRY	TF	480000	Yp11.3	Y	Testicolo disgenetico o ovotestis	±	Femminili o ambigui	
SOX9	TF	608160	17q24-25	AD	Testicolo disgenetico o ovotestis	±	Femminili o ambigui	Displasia camptomelica (riarrangiamenti di 17q24 Fenotipo più lieve rispetto a mutazioni puntiformi
DHH	Molecola *signaling*	605423	12q13.1	AR	Testicolo disgenetico	±	Femminili	Il grave fenotipo di un paziente includeva neuropatia minifascicolare, altri pazienti presentavano disgenesia gonadica isolata
ATRX	Elicasi (? Ristrutturazione della cromatina)	300032	Xq13.3	X	Testicolo disgenetico	–	Femminili, ambigui o maschili	α-talassemia, ritardo mentale
ARX	TF	3003382	Xp22.13	X	Testicolo disgenetico	–	Ambigui	Lissencefalia associata a X, epilessia, instabilità della temperatura
MALATTIE DELLO SVILUPPO GONADICO (TESTICOLARE): MODIFICAZIONI CROMOSOMICHE DEI GENI CANDIDATI CHIAVE COINVOLTI								
DMRT1	TF	602424	9p24.3	Delezione monosomica	Testicolo disgenetico	±	Femminili o ambigui	Ritardo mentale
DAX1 (*NROB1*)	Recettore nucleare di TF	300018	Xp21.3	DupXp21	Testicolo disgenetico ovaio	±	Femmnili o ambigui	
WNT4	Molecola *signaling*	603490	1p35	Dup1p35	Testicolo disgnetico	+	Ambigui	Ritardo mentale
ALTERAZIONI DELLA SINTESI O DELL'AZIONE ORMONALE								
LHGCR	Recettore della proteina G	152790	2p21	AR	Testicolo	–	Femminili, ambigui, o micropene	Ipoplasia delle cellule di Leydig
DHCR7	Enzima	602858	11q12-13	AR	Testicolo	–	Variabili	Sindrome di Schimidt-Lemli-Opitz: lineamenti grossolano del volto, sindattilia del secondo e terzo dito, crescita insufficiente, ritardo dello sviluppo, anomalie cardiache e viscerali
StAR	Proteina di membrana mitocondriale	600617	8p11.2	AR	Testicolo	–	Femminili	Iperplasia surrenalica congenita lipoidea (insufficienza surrenalica primaria), insufficienza puberale
CYP11A1	Enzima	118485	15q23-24	AR	Testicolo	–	Femminili o ambigui	Iperplasia surrenalica congenita (insufficienza surrenalica primaria), insufficienza puberale
HSD3B2	Enzima	201810	1p13.1	AR	Testicolo	–	Ambigui	CAH, insufficienza surrenalica primaria, androgenizzazioone parziale per aumento del DHEA
CYP17	Enzima	202110	10q24.3	AR	Testicolo	–	Femminili, ambigui o micropene	CAH, ipertensione da aumento del corticosterone e 11-desossicorticosterone (eccetto il deficit isolato di 17,20-liasi)
POR (P450 ossidoreduttasi)	Enzima CYP donatore di elettroni	124015	7q11.2	AR	Testicolo	–	Maschili o ambigui	Caratteristiche miste di deficit di 21-idrossilasi, deficit di 17α-idrossilasi/17,20-liasi, deficit di aromatasi, talvolta associato a craniosinostosi di Antley-Bixler
HSD17B3	Enzima	605573	9q22	AR	Testicolo	–	Femminili o ambigui	Androgenizzazione parziale alla pubertà, aumento del rapporto androstenedione: testosterone

TABELLA 583-1. Geni noti coinvolti nelle malattie dello sviluppo sessuale (dsd) – *continua*

GENE	PROTEINA	N. OMIM DATA BASE	LOCUS	EREDITARIETÀ	GONADE	STRUTTURE MÜLLERIANE	GENITALI ESTERNI	CARATTERISTICHE ASSOCIATE/VARIANTI FENOTIPICHE
46,XY DSD								
SRD5A2	Enzima	607306	2p23	AR	Testicolo	–	Ambigui o micropene	Androgenizzazione parziale alla pubertà, aumento del rapporto testosterone: DHT
AMH	Molecola *signaling*	600957	19p13.3-13.2	AR	Testicolo	+	Maschili normali	Sindrome da persistenza dei dotti mülleriani; genitali esterni maschili, criptorchidismo bilaterale
AMH-recettore	Recettore transmembrana di serina-treonina chinasi	600956	12q13	AR	Testicolo	–	Maschili normali	
Recettore androgenico	Recettore nucleare TF	3130700	Xq11-12	X	Testicolo	–	Femminili, ambigui, micropene, o maschili normali	Spettro fenotipico variabile da sindrome da insensibilità androgenica (genitali esterni femminili) completa e insensibilità androgenica parziale (ambigui), a genitali maschili normali/infertilità
46, XX DSD								
MALATTIE DELLO SVILUPPO GONADICO (OVARICO)								
SRY	TF	480000	Yp11.3	Traslocazione	Testicolo o ovotestis	–	Maschili o ambigui	
SOX9	TF	608160	17q24	Dup17q24	ND	–	Maschili o ambigui	
ECCESSO ANDROGENICO								
HSD3B2	Enzima	201810	1p13	AR	Ovaio	+	Clitoridomegalia	CAH, insufficienza surrenalica primaria, parziale androgenizzazione per aumento di DHEA
CYP21A2	Enzima	201910	6p21-23	AR	Ovaio	+	Ambigui	CAH, spettro fenotipico variabile da forme gravi con perdita di Sali associate a insufficienza surrenalica, a forme di virilizzazione semplice con funzionalità surrenalica compensata, aumento del 17-OHprogesterone
CYP11B1	Enzima	20210	8q21-22	AR	Ovaio	+	Ambigui	CAH, ipertensione per aumento dell'11-desossicortisolo e 11-desossicorticosterone
POR (P450 ossidoreduttasi)	Enzima CYP donatore di elettroni	124015	7q11.2	AR	Ovaio	+	Ambigui	Caratteristiche miste di deficit di 21-idrossilasi, deficit di 17α-idrossilasi/17,20 liasi e deficit di aromatasi; associata a craniosinostosi di Antley-Bixler
CYP19	Enzima	107910	15q21	AR	Ovaio	+	Ambigui	Androgenizzazione materna durante la gravidanza, sviluppo mammario alla pubertà, tranne in casi parziali
Recettore dei glicocorticoidi	Recettore nucleare TF	138040	5q31	AR	Ovaio	+	Ambigui	Aumento dell'ACTH, del 17-idrossiprogesterone, e del cortisolo; insufficiente soppressione del desametasone (paziente eterozigotico per mutazione di CYP21)

ACTH, adrenocorticotropina; AD, autosomico dominante (spesso da mutazione ex novo); AR, autosomico recessivo; CAH, *Congenital Adrenal Hyperplasia* (iperplasia surrenalica congenita); ND, non determinato; TF, *Transcription Factor* (fattore di trascrizione); WAGR, *Wilms, Aniridia, Genital Anomalies, and Retardation* (Wilms, aniridia, anomalie genitali e ritardo); X, cromosoma X; Y, cromosoma Y. Sono compresi riarrangiamenti cromosomici suscettibili di includere geni chiave.

Lee PA, Houk CP, Ahmed SF, Hughes IA: International Consensus Conference on Intersex organized by the Lawson Wilkins Pediatric Endocrine Society and the European Society for Paediatric Endocrinology. Consensus statement on management of intersex disorders. International Consensus Conference on Intersex. *Pediatrics* 2006 Aug; 118(2):e488-500.

diminuisce verso il dodicesimo, ma rimane dosabile per 24 mesi. Sotto l'influenza dell'LH l'estradiolo aumenta con un massimo al secondo-sesto mese. La risposta dell'inibina B è variabile, con un picco tra il secondo e il dodicesimo mese, e rimane a livelli pressappoco puberali fino al 24° mese. L'impennata neonatale è importante per la maturazione postnatale delle gonadi, la stabilizzazione dei genitali esterni maschili e probabilmente anche per l'identità di genere e il comportamento sessuale. L'incremento postnatale dell'LH e del testosterone è assente o scarso nei neonati con ipopituitarismo, criptorchidismo e sindrome da insensibilità completa agli androgeni (*Complete Androgen Insensivity Syndrome*, CAIS). Lo sviluppo della secrezione pulsatile notturna dell'LH è un marker dell'inizio della pubertà (vedi Capitolo 562).

In assenza di specifiche cellule bersaglio, il 6-8% del testosterone è convertito da una 5α-reduttasi in diidrotestosterone, un altro potente androgeno (Fig. 583-1), e circa lo 0,3% è trasformato da un'aromatasi in estradiolo (vedi Fig. 575-1). Circa la metà del testosterone circolante è legato alla globulina di trasporto degli ormoni sessuali (SHBG) e metà all'albumina; solo il 2% circola in forma libera. I livelli plasmatici di SHBG sono bassi alla nascita, aumentano rapidamente durante i primi 10 giorni di vita e in seguito rimangono stabili fino all'inizio della pubertà. L'ormone tiroideo gioca un ruolo in questo incremento fisiologico, perché neonati con atireosi presentano livelli molto bassi di SHBG.

L'ormone antimülleriano (AMH; precedentemente riferito alla sostanza inibitrice mülleriana [MIS]), l'inibina e l'attivina fanno parte del fattore di crescita β di trasformazione (TGF-β) che appartiene alla superfamiglia dei fattori di crescita, che comprende 45 membri, tra cui le proteine ossee morfogenetiche (BMP). I membri della superfamiglia di TGF-β sono coinvolti nella regolazione dei processi di sviluppo e in varie patologie umane, comprese la condrodisplasia e il tumore.

L'AMH, un ormone glicoproteico omodimerico di 140-kd, è il prodotto più precoce delle cellule del Sertoli del testicolo fetale. Sintetizzato come pro-ormone, per diventare attivo sul recettore di membrana, necessita della rimozione del suo frammento carbossi-terminale. Il gene per AMH si trova sul cromosoma 19. La sua trascrizione viene iniziata da *SOX9* che agisce attraverso il box HMG, sebbene la sua espressione sia sovraregolata da SF-1 che lega il suo promoter e che in seguito interagisce con *SOX9*, *WTI* e *GATA4*. Sono stati identificati due distinti recettori serina/treonina con un singolo dominio transmembrana. Il recettore attivato di tipo 1 segnala alla famiglia SMAD dei mediatori intracellulari.

Il gene del recettore di AMH (sul cromosoma 12) è espresso nelle cellule del Sertoli e anche nel dotto mülleriano fetale, e nelle cellule della granulosa postnatali. Durante la differenziazione sessuale, AMH provoca l'involuzione dei precursori embriologici della cervice, dell'utero e, assieme a SFI, delle tube di Falloppio (dotti mülleriani).

L'AMH viene secreto nei maschi dalle cellule del Sertoli durante sia la vita fetale sia quella postnatale. Nelle femmine, è prodotto dalle cellule della granulosa a partire dalla 36ª settimana di gestazione fino alla menopausa, ma a livelli inferiori. La concentrazione sierica di AMH nei maschi è maggiore alla nascita, mentre

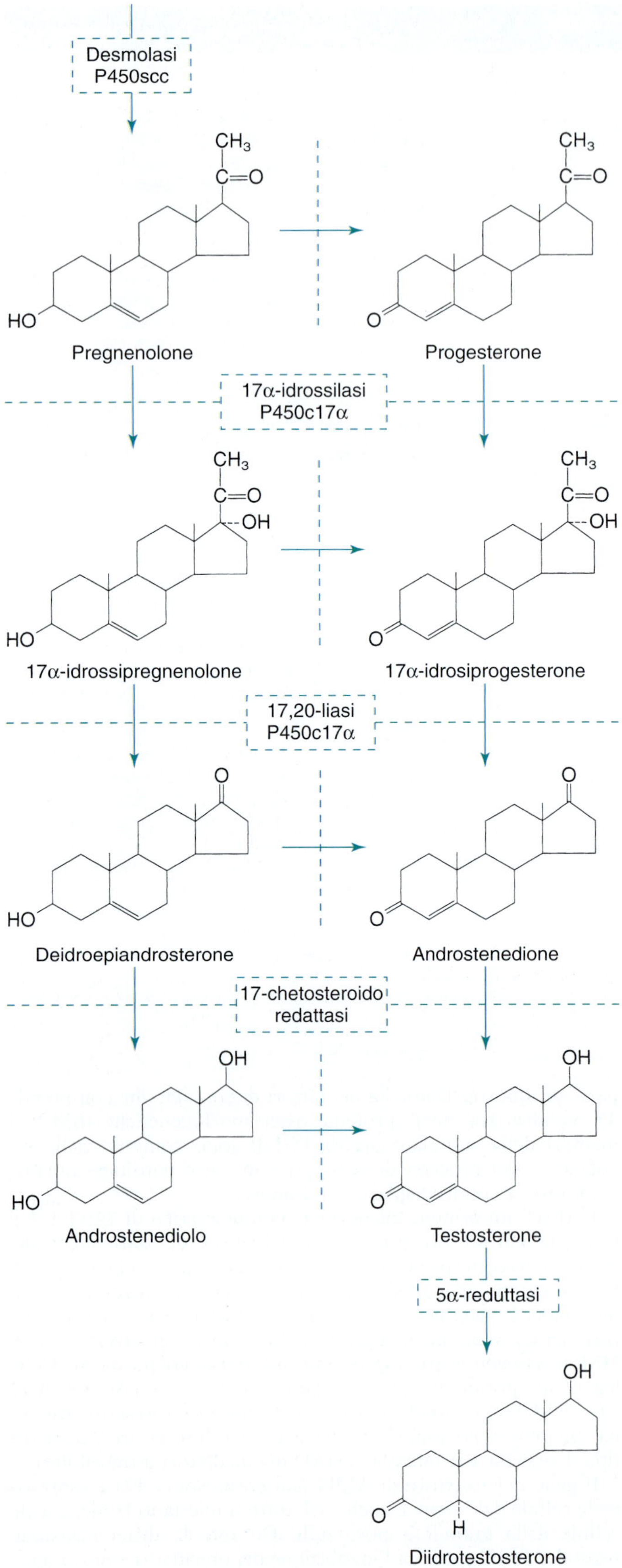

Figura 583-1. Biosintesi degli androgeni. La linea tratteggiata indica i difetti enzimatici associati ad alterazioni 46XY della differenziazione sessuale. La linea tratteggiata verticale indica un difetto della 3β-idrossisteroido deidrogenasi. Un singolo polipeptide, P450c17, catalizza sia l'attività della 17α-idrossilasi che quella della 17,20-liasi.

nelle femmine è più alta alla pubertà. Dopo la pubertà, entrambi i sessi hanno concentrazioni sieriche simili di AMH.

L'inibina è un altro ormone glicoproteico secreto dalle cellule del Sertoli dei testicoli e dalle cellule della granulosa e della teca delle ovaie. L'inibina A consiste di una subunità α disolfuro associata a una subunità β, mentre l'inibina B è formata dalla stessa subunità α associata alla subunità β-B.

Le attivine sono dimeri delle subunità B, entrambe omodimeri (BA/BA, BB/BB) o eterodimeri (BA/BB). Le inibine selettivamente inibiscono, e invece le attivine stimolano, la secrezione ipofisaria di FSH. Con l'utilizzo di immunodosaggi specifici per l'inibina A o B, è stato mostrato che l'inibina A è assente nei maschi ed è presente soprattutto nella fase luteale nelle donne. L'inibina B è la forma principale di inibina nei maschi e nelle femmine durante la fase follicolare. L'inibina B può essere utilizzata come marker della funzione delle cellule del Sertoli nel maschio. L'FSH stimola la secrezione di inibina B nei maschi e nelle femmine, ma solo nei primi è evidente una via regolatoria gonadotropino-indipendente. I livelli di inibina B sono attualmente studiati in bambini con varie forma di alterazioni gonadiche e puberali. La follistatina, simile all'attivina e all'inibina (una proteina glicosilata a catena singola), è prodotta dalle gonadi e da altri tessuti come l'ipotalamo, i reni, i surreni e la placenta. La follistatina inibisce la secrezione di FSH principalmente attraverso il legame con le attivine, con conseguente blocco degli effetti delle attivine a livello ovarico e ipofisario.

Sono conosciuti numerosi altri ormoni peptidici coinvolti come mediatori dello sviluppo e della funzione dei testicoli. Questi comprendono neuroormoni, come l'ormone di rilascio dell'ormone della crescita, l'ormone di rilascio delle gonadotropine (GnRH), l'ormone di rilascio della corticotropina, l'ossitocina, l'arginin-vasopressina, la somatostatina, la sostanza P e il neuropeptide Y; fattori di crescita come i fattori di crescita insulino-simili (*Insulin-Like Growth Factors*, IGF) e le proteine che legano IGF, TGF-β, fibroblasto-, piastrine-derivati e fattori di crescita nervosa; peptidi vasoattivi; inoltre, citochine immunoderivate come il fattore di necrosi tumorale e le interleuchine IL-1, IL-2, IL-4 e IL-6.

I pattern clinici delle modificazioni puberali variano notevolmente (vedi Capitoli 12 e 562). Nel 95% dei maschi, lo sviluppo dei genitali comincia tra i 9 anni e mezzo e i 13 anni e mezzo, raggiungendo la maturità a 13-17 anni. In una minoranza di ragazzi normali, la pubertà inizia dopo i 15 anni. In alcuni, lo sviluppo puberale si completa in meno di 2 anni, ma in altri richiede un tempo maggiore, di 4 anni e mezzo. Lo *spurt* accrescitivo puberale si verifica più tardi nei maschi rispetto alle femminine, in rapporto a certi livelli di maturazione sessuale; per esempio, il picco di velocità della crescita in altezza non si realizza nel maschio fino a che non siano ben sviluppati i genitali, ma nelle femmine la velocità di crescita raggiunge solitamente il massimo quando si sono sviluppati il capezzolo e l'areola, ma prima di un significativo incremento mammario.

L'età media della produzione di spermatozoi (spermarca) è 14 anni. Questo evento si verifica nella fase intermedia della pubertà, come attestato dai peli pubici, dalle dimensioni testicolari, dallo scatto di crescita e dai livelli di testosterone. I livelli notturni di FSH si collocano nel range dell'adulto al momento dello spermarca; la prima eiaculazione consapevole si verifica in questo periodo.

FUNZIONE DELLE OVAIE. In assenza del gene *SRY*, la gonade indifferenziata può essere identificata istologicamente come ovaio alla decima-undicesima settimana di gestazione. Gli ovociti sono presenti dal quarto mese di gestazione e raggiungono il picco di 7 milioni al quinto mese di gestazione. Per un normale mantenimento, gli ovociti necessitano delle cellule della granulosa per formare i follicoli primordiali. I recettori funzionali dell'FSH (ma non dell'LH) sono presenti negli ovociti dei follicoli primari durante lo sviluppo follicolare. I normali cromosomi X sono necessari per mantenere gli ovociti. Al contrario delle cellule somatiche, in cui è attivo solo un cromosoma X, nelle cellule germinali sono attivi entrambi. Alla nascita, le ovaie contengono circa un milione di follicoli attivi, che diminuiscono di mezzo milione all'epoca del menarca. Successivamente, essi diminuiscono alla velocità di 1000/mese e a una velocità anche maggiore dopo i 35 anni di età.

Gli ormoni dell'ovaio fetale derivano per la maggior parte dall'unità fetoplacentare. Come nei maschi, si verifica in epoca fetale un picco di gonadotropine e in seguito anche al secondo-terzo mese di vita, arrivando ai livelli minimi a circa 6 anni. Sia nella primissima infanzia sia nell'infanzia, i livelli di gonadotropine sono maggiori nelle femmine che nei maschi.

I più importanti estrogeni prodotti dall'ovaio sono l'estradiolo-17 (E2) e l'estrone (E1); l'estriolo è un metabolita dei due precedenti e tutti e tre possono essere trovati nelle urine di donne mature. Gli estrogeni derivano anche dagli androgeni del surrene e del testicolo (vedi Fig. 575-1). Questa conversione spiega come in certi tipi di disordini della differenziazione sessuale nei maschi, si verifichi alla pubertà una femminilizzazione; nel deficit di 17-chetosteroido-reduttasi, per esempio, il blocco enzimatico comporta un notevole incremento della produzione di androstenedione, che nei tessuti periferici viene convertito in estradiolo ed estrone; questi estrogeni, in aggiunta a quelli direttamente sintetizzati dal testicolo, causano ginecomastia. Gli estrogeni regolano una serie di attività funzionali diverse in molti tessuti. Esistono due distinti recettori per gli estrogeni, con diversi pattern di espressione. Le ovaie sintetizzano anche progesterone, uno steroide progestazionale; la corticale surrenalica e il testicolo sintetizzano progesterone come precursore di altri ormoni surrenalici e testicolari.

Nell'ovaio è stata identificata una serie di altri ormoni con effetti autocrini, paracrini e intracrini. Essi comprendono inibine, attivine, relaxina e fattori IGF-1, TGF-α e TGF-β e citochine.

I livelli plasmatici di estradiolo aumentano lentamente ma regolarmente con il progredire della maturazione sessuale e sono correlati alle manifestazioni cliniche dello sviluppo puberale, all'età ossea e all'incremento dei livelli di FSH. I livelli di LH non aumentano fino a quando non sono ben sviluppate le caratteristiche sessuali secondarie. Gli estrogeni, similmente agli androgeni, inibiscono la secrezione sia di LH sia di FSH (feedback negativo). Nelle femmine, gli estrogeni provocano anche l'incremento dell'LH che si verifica alla metà del ciclo mestruale. L'acquisizione di questo feedback positivo è un'altra tappa fondamentale della pubertà.

L'età media del menarca nelle ragazze americane è 12,5-13,5 anni, ma il range di "normalità" è ampio, e l'1-2% delle femmine "normali" non sono ancora mestruate a 16 anni. Può variare anche l'età di comparsa dei segni puberali, che secondo studi recenti sono molto più precoci dei tempi passati, specialmente negli afroamericani degli Stati Uniti (vedi Capitolo 12). Il menarca è generalmente in stretto rapporto con l'età scheletrica (vedi Capitoli 12 e 562). La maturazione e la chiusura epifisarie sono almeno in parte estrogeno-dipendenti, come dimostrato in un maschio di 28 anni, normalmente virilizzato, con incompleta chiusura epifisaria per completa insensibilità agli estrogeni da difetto del recettore estrogenico.

SUSSIDI DIAGNOSTICI. Il miglioramento della sensibilità e della specificità dei dosaggi degli ormoni ipofisari e gonadici, misurabili anche in piccole quantità di sangue, ha contribuito al rapido progresso della comprensione delle relazioni normali e patologiche fra ipotalamo, ipofisi e gonadi. Per esempio nei maschi, le misurazioni di LH, di FSH e di testosterone possono rivelare difetti ipofiso-testicolari. L'integrità delle cellule di Leydig nell'infanzia può essere valutata con la determinazione della risposta del testosterone alla somministrazione di gonadotropina corionica umana (5000 UI/die per 3 giorni). L'integrità e la maturazione dell'asse ipotalamo-ipofiso-gonadico nei maschi e nelle femmine può essere studiata con la somministrazione di ormone di rilascio delle gonadotropine (GnRH) o di un analogo del GnRH. Un dosaggio ultrasensibile dell'LH è in grado di differenziare tra maschi con pubertà ritardata e quelli con ipogonadismo ipogonadotropo completo, ma non parziale.

Nei neonati sono stati documentati normali livelli di inibina B; la inibina B può essere un marker di spermatogenesi e anche di neoplasia, come il tumore delle cellule della granulosa. L'inibina può essere coinvolta nella soppressione tumorale. Il dosaggio dei recettori estrogenici può essere clinicamente utile nella gestione dei vari tipi di neoplasia ovarica. La misurazione di AMH serve alla valutazione di bambini con gonadi non apprezzabili clinicamente e alterazioni dello sviluppo sessuale.

SUSSIDI TERAPEUTICI. Gli effetti estrogenici di un idrocarburo aromatico polialogenato (PHAH) possono in parte essere dovuti all'inibizione della solfatazione dell'estradiolo per opera della estrogeno solfotransferasi (SULT1E1), un'importante via di inattivazione estrogenica. In condizioni naturali gli estrogeni somministrati per via orale vengono rapidamente metabolizzati dagli enzimi gastrointestinali ed epatici; per questo vengono somministrati coniugati o sotto forma di esteri. La preparazione orale più ampiamente utilizzata è quella che contiene estrogeni coniugati di derivazione equina ed etinilestradiolo. Sono utilizzati anche cerotti cutanei a contenuto estrogenico, con assorbimento transdermico. Con il miglioramento della comprensione degli estrogeni e delle loro interazioni con i recettori, è stata sintetizzata una nuova classe di composti, definiti modulatori selettivi del complesso estrogeno-recettore. Per esempio, il raloxifene, un derivato benzotiofenico non steroideo, agisce come un agonista estrogenico nell'osso e nel fegato e come antagonista estrogenico nell'utero e nella mammella. Gli androgeni come il testosterone, sono generalmente iniettati per via intramuscolare come esteri a lunga durata di azione (enantato o cipionato, i più comuni), per la loro potenza e la risposta costante. Sono stati utilizzati anche cerotti transdermici di testosterone applicati in sede scrotale o non scrotale e un gel cutaneo, soprattutto negli ipogonadici adulti, per la difficoltà di titolare le dosi necessarie durante l'infanzia e l'adolescenza. Preparazioni orali, come il metiltestosterone e il fluossimesterone, non provocano una potente risposta androgenica e possono essere epatotossiche. Il testosterone undecanoato, un'altra preparazione orale, è utilizzato in Europa ma non negli Stati Uniti. Sono in fase di studio preparazioni sublinguali (microsfere o compresse) e buccali (assorbimento attraverso la mucosa orale) di testosterone.

Bergada I, Bergada C, Campo S: Role of inhibins in childhood and puberty. *J Pediatr Endocrinol Metab* 2001;14:343–353.

Biason-Lauber A, Konrad D, Navratil F, et al: A WNT4 mutation associated with Müllerian-duct regression and virilization in a 46,XX woman. *N Engl J Med* 2005;351:792–798.

Bouvattier C, Carel JC, Lecointre C, et al: Postnatal changes of T, LH, and FSH in 46,XY infants with mutations in the AR gene. *J Pediatr Endocrinol Metab* 2002;87:29–32.

Habert R, Lejeune H, Saez J: Origin, differentiation and regulation of fetal and adult Leydig cells. *Mol Cell Endocrinol* 2001;179:47–74.

Hughes IA: Female development–all by default? *N Engl J Med* 2004;351: 748–750.

Josso N, diClemente N, Gouedard L: Anti-müllerian hormone and its receptors. *Mol Cell Endocrinol* 2001;179:25–32.

Koopman P: The genetics and biology of vertebrate sex determination. *Cell* 2001;105:843–847.

Ostrer H: Sex determination: Lessons from families and embryos. *Clin Genet* 2001;59:207–215.

Pierik FH, Vreeburg JTM, Stijnen T, et al: Serum inhibin B as a marker of spermatogenesis. *J Clin Endocrinol Metab* 1998;83:3110–3114.

Quigley CA: The postnatal gonadotropin and sex steroid surge: Insights from the androgen insensitivity syndrome. (Editorial.) *J Clin Endocrinol Metab* 2002;87:24–28.

Rajpert-De Meyts E: Expression of anti-müllerian hormone during normal and pathological gonadal development: Association with differentiation of Sertoli and granulosa cells. *J Clin Endocrinol Metab* 1999;84:3836–3844.

Rey RA, Belville C, Nihoul-Fékété C, et al: Evaluation of gonadal function in 107 intersex patients by means of serum anti-müllerian hormone measurements. *J Clin Endocrinol Metab* 1999;84:627–631.

Sequera AM, Fideleff HL, Boquete HR, et al: Basal ultra sensitive LH assay: A useful tool in the early diagnosis of male pubertal delay? *J Pediatr Endocrinol Metab* 2002;15:589–596.

Swerdloff RS, Wang C, Cunningham G, et al: Long-term pharmacokinetics of transdermal testosterone gel in hypogonadal men. *J Clin Endocrinol Metab* 2000;85:4500–4510.

Teixeira J, Maheswaran S, Donahue PK: Müllerian inhibiting substance: An instructive development hormone with diagnostic and possible therapeutic applications. *Endocr Rev* 2001;22:657–674.

Capitolo 584 ■ Ipofunzione del testicolo

L'ipofunzione testicolare può essere primaria nel testicolo (ipogonadismo primario) o secondaria a deficit di gonadotropine ipofisarie (ipogonadismo secondario). I pazienti con ipogonadismo primario presentano elevati livelli di gonadotropine (ipergonadotropo); quelli con ipogonadismo secondario mostrano invece livelli gonadotropinici bassi o assenti (ipogonadotropo).

584.1 • Ipogonadismo ipergonadotropo nel maschio (ipogonadismo primario)

I difetti della produzione androgenica che coinvolgono il testicolo fetale e comportano un'alterata virilizzazione maschile sono discussi nel Capitolo 589.2.

EZIOLOGIA. L'anorchia congenita si verifica nello 0,6% dei maschi con testicoli non palpabili (1/20 000 maschi). Questi bambini hanno genitali esterni nella norma, a significare che una noxa patogena ha danneggiato il testicolo del feto geneticamente maschio, in un momento successivo alla differenziazione sessuale (14ª settimana di vita fetale). Alcuni definiscono questa condizione come **sindrome del "vanishing testis"**. La malattia è stata riportata in gemelli monozigoti. L'andamento familiare della patologia suggerisce un'eziologia genetica. Pertanto un termine più appropriato potrebbe essere **sindrome da regressione testicolare embrionale**. Nei primi mesi dopo la nascita si sono trovati livelli bassi di testosterone (<10 ng/dL) e notevolmente elevati di ormone luteinizzante (LH) e follicolo-stimolante (FSH); successivamente il livelli gonado-tropinemici tendono a scendere anche in bambini agonadici, risalendo a valori molto alti durante la pubertà. La stimolazione con gonadotropina corionica umana (hCG) non evoca un aumento dei livelli di testosterone. Le concentrazioni sieriche di ormone anti-mülleriano (AMH) sono basse o indosabili.

È stata descritta una sindrome del **testicolo rudimentale**, in cui i testicoli sono molto piccoli; si tratta di una forma congenita con eredità autosomica recessiva o correlata a X. La causa è sconosciuta. L'atrofia testicolare può essere la conseguenza di un danno vascolare, come si può verificare per esempio per maldestra manipolazione testicolare durante procedure chirurgiche per la correzione di criptorchidismo o come conseguenza di torsione testicolare bilaterale. Nella pubertà o nell'età adulta, talvolta un'orchite parotitica acuta può danneggiare i testicoli, ma di solito è compromessa solo la funzione riproduttiva del testicolo. La vaccinazione di routine di tutti i bambini in età prepubere dovrebbe prevenire questa complicanza.

Un danno testicolare è una conseguenza frequente di **chemioterapia** o **radioterapia** per neoplasia. La frequenza e l'estensione del danno dipendono dall'agente patogeno, dalla dose totale, dalla durata della terapia e dall'intervallo di osservazione post-terapia. Un'altra variabile importante è l'età in cui si effettua la terapia; le cellule germinali sono più vulnerabili nei maschi prepuberi che in quelli puberi e post-puberi. La chemioterapia provoca danni maggiori se vengono utilizzati più farmaci. L'uso di agenti alchilanti come la ciclofosfamide nei bambini prepuberi non danneggia lo sviluppo puberale, anche in presenza di danno istologico alle cellule germinali. Alte dosi di ciclofosfamide e ifosfamide sono associate a infertilità. La maggior parte dei farmaci chemioterapici provoca più frequentemente azoospermia e infertilità piuttosto che lesioni delle cellule di Leydig. Anche il cisplatino provoca azoospermia transitoria o oligospermia. L'interleuchina-2 può danneggiare le funzione delle cellule di Leydig, mentre l'interferone-α non incide sulla funzionalità gonadica.

Il **danno da radiazioni** è dose-dipendente (vedi Capitolo 706). Con una dose maggiore di 0,1 Gy si può osservare azoospermia temporanea e con dosi maggiori di 0,2 Gy azoospermia permanente. Le cellule di Leydig sono le più resistenti all'irradiazione. Con dosi fino a 6 Gy si possono verificare danni di lieve entità, come da alti livelli di LH; dosi più elevate di 30 Gy nella maggior parte dei casi provocano ipogonadismo. Se possibile, i testicoli dovrebbero essere protetti dall'irradiazione. Negli adolescenti, dopo trattamento infantile multimodale per tumore, la funzione testicolare deve essere valutata con attenzione. Possono essere indicate una terapia sostitutiva con testosterone e una valutazione della fertilità.

Il termine ipogonadismo è stato ampiamente utilizzato per descrivere degli aspetti presenti in bambini con una serie di sindromi da malformazioni multiple. La parola si riferisce spesso al criptorchidismo, a un pene di piccole dimensioni o a un'anomalia scrotale. In molte di queste sindromi, poco si sa circa la funzionalità testicolare; l'ipogonadismo ipogonadotropo o ipergonadotropo è stato dimostrato in varie circostanze.

In pazienti con la **sindrome di Prader-Willi** è stato riportato sia un ipogonadismo ipogonadotropo che uno ipergonadotropo, probabilmente secondario a criptorchidismo e al suo trattamento (vedi Capitoli 80 e 81). In questi pazienti, la terapia con ormone della crescita porta a un miglioramento della composizione corporea, della funzionalità psicomotoria e della crescita. Dato che sono stati riportati casi di morte in pochi pazienti con sindrome di Prader-Willi trattati con ormone della crescita, è indispensabile porre estrema cautela prima di intraprendere questa terapia. In pazienti con la sindrome da sole cellule di Sertoli, sono documentati testicoli piccoli e azoospermia (aplasia delle cellule germinali, o **sindrome di Del Castillo**).

Vari gradi di ipogonadismo compaiono anche in una significativa percentuale di pazienti con aberrazioni cromosomiche, come nella **sindrome di Klinefelter** o nei **maschi XX**.

MANIFESTAZIONI CLINICHE. Alla nascita si sospetta un ipogonadismo primario se i testicoli e il pene sono piccoli. I parametri volumetrici di riferimento sono variabili a seconda della popolazione. La situazione spesso non è apprezzabile fino alla pubertà, quando dovrebbero svilupparsi le caratteristiche sessuali secondarie. I peli facciali, pubici e ascellari sono scarsi o assenti; non si manifesta né acne né stempiatura dei capelli e la voce rimane sui toni alti. Il pene e lo scroto mantengono un aspetto infantile e possono essere quasi nascosti dal tessuto adiposo pubico; i testicoli sono piccoli o assenti. Il tessuto adiposo si accumula nella regione delle anche e delle natiche e talvolta in sede mammaria e addominale. La chiusura epifisaria è ritardata; di conseguenza gli arti sono lunghi. L'apertura delle braccia e di parecchi centimetri superiore all'altezza e la distanza fra la sinfisi pubica e la punta del piede è maggiore di quella tra la sinfisi e il vertice. Le proporzioni del corpo configurano un aspetto di tipo **eunucoide**. Il rapporto tra segmento superiore e inferiore è molto inferiore a 0,9. Molti individui con gradi leggeri di ipogonadismo possono essere scoperti solo con studi particolari dell'asse ipotalamo-ipofiso-gonadico. L'esame dei testicoli deve essere eseguito di routine dai pediatri; il volume testicolare deve essere comparato con quello dell'orchidometro standard.

DIAGNOSI. I livelli sierici di FSH e in misura minore di LH sono elevati oltre il range di normalità per l'età. Questi alti valori indicano che anche nel bambino prepubere è attivo un feedback ipotalamo-gonadico. Dopo gli 11 anni, l'LH e l'FSH aumentano notevolmente, raggiungendo il range degli individui castrati. Non è utile la valutazione del testosterone in epoca prepubere, perché i valori sono normalmente bassi a quest'età e poi aumentano durante la pubertà fino ad attestarsi su valori propri dell'adulto. Durante la pubertà, questi livelli si correlano meglio con le dimensioni testicolari, lo stadio della maturazione sessuale e l'età ossea, più che con l'età cronologica. In pazienti con ipogonadismo primario, i livelli di testosterone rimangono bassi a tutte le età. Si verifica un aumento modesto o nessun aumento dopo somministrazione di hCG, contrariamente a quanto succede nei maschi normali in cui esso provoca un significativo incremento dei livelli plasmatici di testosterone in qualsiasi stadio. La valutazione delle concentrazioni sieriche di AMH e di inibina possono dare un'idea della presenza delle gonadi e della loro funzione.

SINDROME DI NOONAN

EZIOLOGIA. Il termine sindrome di Noonan è stato applicato a maschi e femmine con cariotipo normale che presentano certe caratteristiche fenotipiche presenti anche in femmine con la sindrome di Turner (vedi Capitolo 81). La sindrome di Noonan si verifica in 1:1000-2500 nati vivi. La malattia è autosomica dominante con espressione variabile. Sono stati riportati casi autosomici recessivi e sporadici. Nella maggior parte dei pazienti studiati sono state trovate mutazioni missense in *PTPN11*, un gene sul cromosoma 12q24.1 che codifica la proteina non recettoriale tirosina fosfatasi SHP-2. Anche mutazioni del gene *KRAS* possono provocare la sindrome di Noonan.

MANIFESTAZIONI CLINICHE. Le anomalie più frequenti sono rappresentate da bassa statura, pterigio del collo, petto carenato o torace a imbuto, cubito valgo, cardiopatia congenita destra e facies caratteristica. Sono comuni anche ipertelorismo, epicanto, piega palpebrale antimongoloide, ptosi, micrognazia e anomalie auricolari. Altre anomalie, come clinodattilia, ernie e malformazioni vertebrali sono più rare. Il QI medio in età scolare di bambini affetti è di 86, con un range di variabilità da 53 a 127. Il QI verbale tende a essere migliore del precedente. È frequente la perdita dell'udito neurosensoriale ad alta frequenza. Il difetto cardiaco è rappresentato più spesso da stenosi valvolare polmonare, miocardiopatia ipertrofica o difetto atriale settale. Sono state descritte epatosplenomegalia, gravi malattie ematologiche, compreso il deficit dei fattori XI e XII, leucemia linfoblastica acuta, leucemia mieolomonocitica cronica. Sono state riportate caratteristiche sia della sindrome di Noonan sia della neurofibromatosi di tipo 1, ma è stata esclusa l'evenienza di linkage. Caratteristiche simili a quelle della sindrome di Noonan possono presentarsi in varianti fenotipiche della mutazione del gene NF1, facendo supporre l'esistenza di un locus per la sindrome di Noonan anche nel cromosoma 17q. Pochi pazienti con *NF1* e caratteristiche della sindrome di Noonan sono poi stati descritti come sindrome di Turner. I maschi frequentemente manifestano criptorchidismo e testicoli piccoli; possono essere ipogonadici o normali. La pubertà è ritardata di due anni; l'altezza adulti viene di solito raggiunta alla fine della seconda decade di vita e si mantiene al limite inferiore del range di normalità. La diagnosi prenatale si basa sull'osservazione, in feti con cariotipo normale, edema o idropi e femore corto.

TRATTAMENTO. La somministrazione di ormone della crescita umano migliora la velocità di crescita analogamente a quanto osservato in pazienti con sindrome di Turner, senza effetti collaterali sullo spessore della parete ventricolare. In pochi pazienti però si è osservato un miglioramento dell'altezza da adulti. I pazienti con sindrome di Noonan e dimostrabili mutazioni di *PTNP11*, crescono meno e sono meno responsivi al trattamento con ormone della crescita di quelli senza mutazioni. Presentano livelli più bassi di IGF1 e più alti di GH, forse per resistenza parziale al GH dovuta a difetti del segnale postrecettoriale.

SINDROME DI KLINEFELTER

Vedi anche Capitoli 81 e 561.

EZIOLOGIA. Circa 1 su 500 nati maschi presenta un complemento cromosomico 47,XXY, che rappresenta la più frequente aneuploidia dei cromosomi sessuali nei maschi. Nell'ambito dei ritardi mentali, l'incidenza è circa dell'1%, compreso tra pazienti con QI maggiore di 50 e bambini ricoverati in ospedali psichiatrici o che si sono rivolti a cliniche psichiatriche. Nei maschi sterili, l'incidenza è del 3% e in quelli con oligospermia o azoospermia è del 5-10%. L'aberrazione cromosomica più frequente dipende da una non disgiunzione meiotica del cromosoma X durante la gametogenesi dei genitori; il cromosoma X aggiuntivo è di origine materna nel 54% e paterna nel 46% dei pazienti. Un'età della madre elevata predispone alla non disgiunzione meiotica e a questa sindrome, ma nella maggior parte dei casi l'età materna non è avanzata. Uno studio nazionale in Danimarca ha rivelato un'incidenza prenatale di 213 per 100 000 feti maschili e, standardizzata in base all'età materna, di 153/100 000. Nel maschio adulto, l'incidenza era invece solo di 40/100 000, perché solo 1 su 4 adulti maschi con sindrome di Klinefelter viene diagnosticato.

Il complemento 47,XXY è il più comune nei pazienti con sindrome di Klinefelter (80%); alcuni presentano dei mosaici: 46,XY/47,XXY, 46,XY/48,XXYY, 45,X/46,XY/47,XXY o 46,XX/47,XXY. Raramente la presenza di più di 2 cromosomi X dà origine a delle varianti della sindrome di Klinefelter: 48,XXXY, 49,XXXYY, 49,XXXXY, 50,XXXXYY, 47,XXY/48,XXXY, 47,XXY/49,XXXXY o 48,XXYY. Anche in presenza di molti cromosomi X, per esempio 4, il cromosoma Y determina un fenotipo maschile. Nella maggior parte dei pazienti con 4 o 5 cromosomi X, tutti i cromosomi aggiuntivi derivano dallo stesso genitore e non sono associati a una età avanzata dei genitori.

MANIFESTAZIONI CLINICHE. Raramente la diagnosi viene posta prima della pubertà, perché durante l'infanzia le manifestazioni cliniche sono poche e modeste. Dal momento che prima della comparsa delle alterazioni dello sviluppo puberale, spesso si manifestano disturbi comportamentali o psichiatrici, è necessario sospettare questa malattia in tutti i bambini con ritardo mentale e in quelli con problemi psicosociali, di apprendimento o scolastici. I bambini colpiti possono mostrarsi ansiosi, immaturi, eccessivamente timidi o aggressivi, con possibilità di atti antisociali. In alcuni di questi bambini è stato osservato un comportamento incendiario. In uno studio prospettico, un gruppo di bambini con cariotipo 47,XXY identificato alla nascita ha manifestato deviazioni relativamente modeste durante i primi 5 anni di vita. Nove presentavano una maggiore disabilità fisica, intellettiva o emotiva; alcuni erano inattivi, con funzioni motorie scarsamente organizzate e lieve ritardo nell'acquisizione del linguaggio. Spesso i problemi cominciano a diventare evidenti dopo l'inizio della scuola. I punteggi del QI totale possono essere normali, con QI verbale talvolta diminuito. Sono frequenti difetti cognitivi e verbali, mancato conseguimento di risultati adeguati in lettura, linguaggio e in matematica. Nelle fasi tardive dell'adolescenza, la maggior parte dei ragazzi con sindrome di Klinefelter ha deficit generalizzati dell'apprendimento, la maggior parte dei quali inerenti al linguaggio e sono in ritardo di 4 o 5 livelli. Nonostante queste difficoltà, la maggior parte completa la scuola superiore. La RM ad alta risoluzione ha dimostrato la riduzione nel lobo temporale sinistro del volume della materia grigia (in misura minore nei soggetti trattati con testosterone).

I pazienti tendono a essere alti, snelli e con scarso tessuto adiposo e presentano arti inferiori relativamente lunghi, ma l'habitus corporeo può cambiare notevolmente. I testicoli sono piccoli per l'età, ma questo segno può diventare evidente solo dopo la pubertà, quando non si verifica la normale crescita testicolare. Il pene è di dimensioni inferiori alla media e in qualche paziente possono esserci criptorchidismo e ipospadia.

Lo sviluppo puberale può essere ritardato, sebbene alcuni ragazzi presentino una normale virilizzazione. Lo studio riguardante il caso di un ragazzo finlandese di 14 anni 47,XXY senza mosaicismo ha evidenziato una pubertà con esordio e progressione nella norma, con normale aumento dei livelli sierici di testosterone e PSA, e decremento delle concentrazioni di leptina e SHBG. Nonostante i normali livelli testosteronemici, le concentrazioni sieriche di LH e di FSH e la loro risposta al test di stimolazione con GnRH erano elevate, a partire dai 13 anni. Circa l'80% degli adulti evidenzia **ginecomastia** e presenta peli facciali più radi, che non richiedono rasature quotidiane. Le lesioni testicolari più frequenti sono rappresentate dall'arresto spermatogenetico e dalla predominanza delle cellule del Sertoli. Negli spermatozoi è presente un'alta incidenza di aneuploidia dei cromosomi sessuali. Sono frequenti azoospermia e infertilità, sebbene siano noti rari casi di fertilità. Tecniche di fecondazione artificiale con prelievo di spermatozoi testicolari e successiva iniezione intracitoplasmatica possono portare alla nascita di bambini sani. Sono stati ritrovati anticorpi antispermatozoi in un quarto dei campioni testicolari. In pazienti con sindrome di Klinefelter senza mosaicismi, la maggior parte degli spermatozoi testicolari (94%) presenta un normale pattern di segregazione cromosomica.

I pazienti con sindrome di Klinefelter tendono a essere alti. Presentano con maggiore frequenza malattie polmonari, varici venose, tumori alle mammelle. Tra 93 **pazienti maschi con tumore mammario** non selezionati, il 7,5% presentava la sindrome di Klinefelter. Sono stati descritti anche tumori mediastinici a cellule germinali; alcuni di essi producono hCG e provocano pubertà precoce. Possono essere inoltre associati a leucemia, linfoma e altre neoplasie ematologiche. Il maggior rischio di tumore (rischio relativo 2,7) si verifica tra i 15 e i 30 anni. Un ampio studio su un gruppo di pazienti britannici ha dimostrato una frequenza standardizzata di mortalità significativamente aumentata (1,5) con particolare incremento dei decessi per diabete, epilessia, patologie vascolari periferiche e intestinali, embolia polmonare e malattie renali. È in diminuzione la mortalità per cardiopatia ischemica. Negli adulti, anomalie cerebrali strutturali sono correlate a deficit cognitivi.

In adulti con mosaicismo XY/XXY, diminuisce sia la frequenza sia la gravità delle caratteristiche tipiche della sindrome di Klinefelter. I bambini con mosaicismo presentano una prognosi migliore per virilizzazione, fertilità e adattamento psicosociale.

Varianti della sindrome di Klinefelter. Quando i cromosomi X sono più di due, le manifestazioni cliniche, compreso il ritardo mentale e le alterazioni della virilizzazione, sono molto più gravi. La variante XXYY è la più frequente (1/50 000 nati). Nella maggior parte di questi bambini compare un ritardo mentale con punteggi QI tra 60 e 80, anche se il 10% evidenzia un QI superiore a 110. Il fenotipo maschile XXYY non è sostanzialmente diverso da quello XXY, se non per il fatto che gli adulti XXYY tendono a essere più alti. La variante 49,XXXXY è sufficientemente caratteristica da essere diagnosticata nell'infanzia. L'incidenza stimata è di 1/80 000-1/100 000 nati. La malattia deriva da non-disgiunzioni sequenziali durante la meiosi. I pazienti manifestano un grave ritardo mentale, collo corto e facies tipica, con lineamenti grossolani, ipertelorismo, lieve piega mongoloide, epicanto, strabismo, naso largo e rivolto verso l'alto, bocca ampia e aperta, malformazioni auricolari. I testicoli sono piccoli e possono essere criptorchidi, lo scroto è ipoplasico e il pene di dimensioni molto scarse. Sono frequenti anche alterazioni tipiche della sindrome di Down (quinto dito con falangi curve e brevi, pieghe palmari uniche e ipotonia) e altre anomalie scheletriche (compresi difetti nella flessione dei gomiti e ridotta supinazione). Le più comuni alterazioni radiografiche sono rappresentate da sinostosi o dislocazione radioulnare, radio allungato, pseudoepifisi, scoliosi o cifosi, anca valga ed età ossea ritardata. La maggior parte dei pazienti con tali modificazioni ha un cariotipo 49,XXXXY; sono stati osservati anche diversi mosaicismi: 48,XXXY/49,XXXXY (Fig. 584-1), 48,XXXY/49,XXXXY/50,XXXXXY e 48,XXXY/49, XXXXY/50,XXXXYY. È stato riportato il caso di un neonato con diagnosi prenatale 49,XXXXY. Il feto presenta ritardo della crescita intrauterina, edema e igroma cistico del collo.

La variante 48,XXXY è relativamente rara. Le caratteristiche tipiche sono generalmente meno severe di quelle dei pazienti con 49,XXXXY e più gravi di quelle con 47,XXY. A questa condizione sono associati: lieve ritardo mentale, ritardo nell'acquisizione del linguaggio e nello sviluppo motorio, comportamento immaturo ma passivo e affabile.

In pochissimi pazienti si riportano i cariotipi 49,XYYY e 49,XXYYY. In entrambi sono comuni ritardo mentale e alterazioni dismorfiche.

REPERTI DI LABORATORIO. La maggior parte dei maschi con questa condizione rimane non diagnosticata. In tutti i pazienti con sospetta sindrome di Klinefelter, in particolare in quelli che si occupano di bambini, che lavorano in cliniche con pazienti psichiatrici e con ritardo mentale, devono essere compiute indagini cromosomiche. Durante l'infanzia, i livelli di inibina B e di AMH sono normali, ma quelli di testosterone sono inferiori ai controlli. Prima del decimo anno di età, i maschi con Klinefelter 47,XXY hanno normali livelli basali di FSH e LH. Anche la risposta al GnRH e all'hCG è normale. La crescita dei testicoli è normale nelle fasi precoci

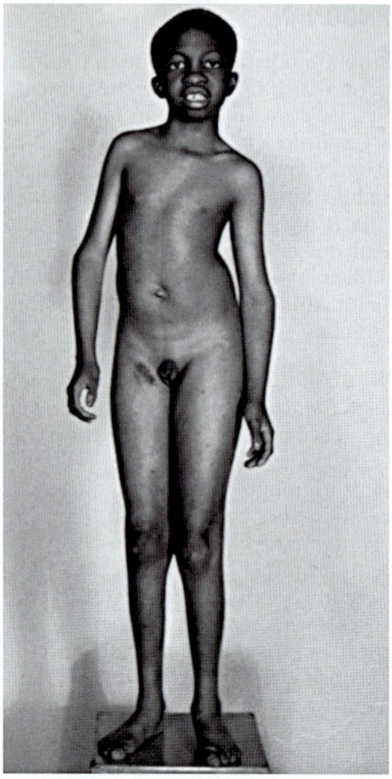

Figura 584-1. Un ragazzo di 12 anni con mosaicismo 48,XXXY/49,XXXXY con prognatismo, epicanto, scoliosi, testicoli piccoli, grave ritardo mentale, clinodattilia e sinostosi radioulnare.

della pubertà, ma nelle fasi intermedie si arresta, le gonadotropine aumentano e il testosterone rimane persistentemente basso. I livelli di inibina B sono normali nelle prime fasi della pubertà, poi diminuiscono e diventano basse nell'adulto. Elevati livelli di estradiolo, con alto rapporto estradiolo:testosterone, giustificano lo sviluppo di ginecomastia durante la pubertà. Nonostante l'ipogonadismo, la maggior parte presenta normali masse ossee. L'espansione di lunghi tratti di poliglutamina (CAG) del recettore androgenico è associata a un fenotipo più severo, che comprende ginecomastia, testicoli e pene piccoli.

La biopsia testicolare prima della pubertà può rivelare solo il deficit o l'assenza delle cellule germinali. Dopo la pubertà, le membrane dei tubuli seminiferi appaiono ialinizzate e sono presenti ammassi adenomatosi di cellule di Leydig. Predominano le cellule del Sertoli: inoltre, è caratteristica l'azoospermia e l'infertilità è comune.

TRATTAMENTO. La terapia sostitutiva con preparazioni a base di testosterone a lunga durata dipende dall'età del paziente. È opportuno iniziare verso gli 11-12 anni. Si può cominciare con una dose di estere enantato da 25-50 mg per via intramuscolare ogni 3-4 settimane, aumentando di 50 mg ogni 6-9 mesi, fino al raggiungimento della quantità necessaria nell'adulto, che è di 200-250 mg ogni 3-4 settimane. A questo punto, le iniezioni possono essere sostituite da cerotti o da gel a base di testosterone. Nei ragazzi più grandi, dosi iniziali maggiori e più cospicui incrementi possono consentire una virilizzazione più rapida. Il trattamento con testosterone provoca un aumento del volume prostatico e dei livelli degli antigeni prostata-specifici. Tecniche di fecondazione con prelievo testicolare di spermatozoi e successiva iniezione intracitoplasmatica possono portare alla nascita di bambini sani. In pazienti Klinefelter privi di mosaicismi, la maggior parte degli spermatozoi testicolari (94%) presenta un normale assetto di segregazione cromosomica. In un centro, le percentuali di recupero degli spermatozoi sono maggiori del 70% e quasi il 70% dei pazienti ha spermatozoi adeguati, di cui quasi la metà porta alla nascita di bambini normali.

MASCHI XX

Si ritiene che la malattia si verifichi in 1 su 20 000 nati maschi. Gli individui affetti hanno un fenotipo maschile, testicoli piccoli, pene piccolo, e assenza di ovaie e tessuti di origine mülleriana; questa forma è quindi ben distinta dalla malattia ovotesticolare dello sviluppo sessuale (vedi Capitolo 589.3). Questa patologia assomiglia alla sindrome di Klinefelter, ma la statura è meno alta. In una minoranza di pazienti sono presenti criptorchidismo e ipospadia. Le caratteristiche istologiche dei testicoli sono essenzialmente le stesse della sindrome di Klinefelter. I pazienti di solito arrivano all'osservazione medica in età adulta, per ipogonadismo, ginecomastia o infertilità. Si verifica ipogonadismo ipergonadotropo secondario al deficit testicolare. Pochi casi sono stati diagnosticati in epoca perinatale, per una discrepanza tra l'ecografia prenatale e il cariotipo.

Nell'80% dei maschi XX con normali genitali esterni, uno dei cromosomi X porta il gene *SRY*. Lo scambio tra Y e X si verifica nella meiosi paterna, quando si appaiano le braccia corte dei cromosomi X e Y. I maschi XX ereditano un cromosoma X materno e un cromosoma X paterno, contenente il gene traslocato che determina il sesso maschile. Questi scambi si verificano per la vicinanza del gene *SRY* con la regione pseudoautosomica quando normalmente avviene la ricombinazione tra X e Y durante la meiosi. In pochi casi di maschi 46,XX sono state identificate traslocazioni 9P. La maggior parte dei maschi XX identificati prima della pubertà presenta ipospadia o micropene; questo gruppo di pazienti di solito perde specifiche sequenze Y, facendo ipotizzare altri meccanismi di virilizzazione (vedi Capitolo 576). Per identificare piccoli segmenti di DNA con *SRY*, sono state utilizzate l'ibridazione fluorescente *in situ* e tecniche di citologia molecolare (o *Primed In Situ Labeling*, PRINS). Anomalie del frammento Yp possono comportare fenotipi sessuali ambigui.

MASCHI 45,X

Vedi anche Capitolo 583.

Nei pochi pazienti con cariotipo 45,X, sequenze Yp sono state traslocate su un cromosoma autosomico. In un caso, il braccio corto terminale del cromosoma Y è stato traslocato sul cromosoma X. In un altro, è stata ipotizzata una traslocazione *SRY/autosomica*. In un maschio con cariotipo 45,X e discondrosteosi di Leri-Weill è stata descritta anche perdita del gene *SHOX* e traslocazione di *SRY* su Xp.

MASCHI 47,XXX

Un maschio giapponese con scarso sviluppo dei peli pubici, ipoplasia scroto-testicolare (4 mL), pene normale e altezza regolare, ginecomastia e grave ritardo mentale presentava cariotipo 47,XXX per anomalo interscambio X-Y durante la meiosi paterna e non-disgiunzione X-X durante la mieosi materna.

584.2 • IPOGONADISMO IPOGONADOTROPO NEL MASCHIO (IPOGONADISMO SECONDARIO)

Nell'ipogonadismo ipogonadotropo, esiste un deficit di FSH, di LH o di entrambi. Il difetto primario può risiedere nell'ipofisi anteriore o nell'ipotalamo, come il deficit di GnRH. I testicoli sono normali, ma rimangono allo stadio prepubere per la mancanza di stimolazione gonadotropinica. La malattia può essere scoperta durante l'infanzia, verso la pubertà o, raramente, nell'età adulta. Sono state descritte varie alterazioni genetiche nei pazienti con ipogonadismo ipogonadotropo.

EZIOLOGIA

Ipopituitarismo. La maggior parte delle cause di ipopituitarismo è associata a deficit di gonadotropine e ipogonadismo ipogonadotropo (vedi Capitolo 558). In pazienti con lesioni organiche dell'ipofisi o di sedi vicine, congenite o acquisite, il deficit di gonadotropine è originariamente ipofisaroa. Nella maggior parte dei pazienti con ipopituitarismo "idiopatico", il difetto è a livello ipotalamico, per deficit di GnRH. In pazienti con deficit ormonali multipli, sono state descritte alterazioni dei fattori di trascrizione ipofisari, come PROP-1, HESX-1 e LHX-3. La presenza in un neonato maschio di micropene (<2,5 cm) con deficit dell'ormone della crescita indirizza verso la diagnosi di carenza gonadotropinica.

Deficit isolato di gonadotropine. Normalmente questa patologia riguarda più l'ipotalamo dell'ipofisi. Colpisce 1/10 000 maschi e 1/50 000 femmine e comprende un gruppo eterogeneo di entità diverse. Il deficit di GnRH può essere completo o parziale, sporadico o familiare. È stato identificato un locus per una forma autosomica recessiva di ipogonadismo ipogonadotropo idiopatico sul cromosoma 19p13.3.

La **sindrome di Kallmann**, una delle più frequenti forme genetiche di ipogonadismo ipogonadotropo, è caratterizzata dall'associazione con **anosmia** o **iposmia.** La malattia, legata a X (KAL1), è causata da mutazioni del gene *KAL* su Xp22.3. L'associazione riflette la non avvenuta migrazione di assoni olfattivi e di neuroni che esprimono GnRH, dalla loro origine comune nella placca olfattiva, all'interno del cervello. Il gene *KAL* produce anosmina-1, una glicoproteina della matrice extracellulare di 95 kDa, che facilita la crescita e la migrazione neuronali. Il gene *KAL* è espresso anche in altre diverse parti del cervello, del mesenchima facciale, dei mesonefri e metanefri, che spiegano alcune delle altre associazioni della sindrome di Kalmann con sincinesia, difetti della zona mediale del volto e agenesia renale.

Alcune famiglie presentano soggetti anosmici con o senza ipogonadismo; altre, individui ipogonadici con anosmia. In alcuni pazienti ricorrono altre manifestazioni, quali labbro e palato leporino, ipotelorismo, fessurazione mediali del volto, perdita dell'udito neurosensoriale, aplasia renale monolaterale, deficit neurologici e altre. Quando la sindrome di Kallmann è causata da delezioni terminali o interstiziali della regione Xp22.3, si associa a sindromi inerenti ai geni contigui, come deficit di steroido solfatasi, condrodisplasia punctata, ictiosi correlata a X, albinismo oculare. Nei pazienti in cui le mutazioni riguardano solo il locus KAL1, non sono descritte alterazioni mentali.

Esistono forme autosomiche dominanti e autosomiche recessive della sindrome di Kallmann.

La forma autosomica dominante (KAL2) si verifica nel 10% dei pazienti, per una mutazione con perdita di funzione del gene del recettore 1 per il fattore di crescita fibroblastica (FGFR1). A KAL2, ma non a KAL1, si associano labbro e palato leporino; mentre in entrambe le malattie possono verificarsi oligodentia e perdita dell'udito. Esiste anche una forma meno nota, autosomica recessiva, di questa malattia (KAL3).

Bambini con **ipoplasia surrenalica congenita correlata a X** presentano anche un ipogonadismo ipogonadotropo (*Hypogonadotropic HypoGonadism*, HHG) dovuto ad alterazione della secrezione di GnRH. In questi pazienti è presente una mutazione del gene *DAX1* su Xp21.2-21.3. Occasionalmente si associano, per la **sindrome del gene contiguo**, altre condizioni che comprendono deficit di glicerolo chinasi, distrofia muscolare di Duchenne, deficit di ornitina transcarbamil-transferasi. La maggior parte dei maschi con mutazioni *DAX1* sviluppa HHG durante l'adolescenza, sebbene siano stati descritti i casi di un paziente con insufficienza surrenalica a esordio nell'età adulta e parziale HHG e di due femmine con HHG e pubertà ritardata, queste ultime come parte di estese famiglie con maschi con classico HHG. Il difetto del gene *DAX1* è, tuttavia, raro in pazienti con pubertà ritardata o HHG senza almeno un'anamnesi familiare di insufficienza surrenalica.

Sono stati identificati parecchi dei difetti genetici dell'asse ipotalamo-ipofiso-gonadico. Essi coinvolgono la funzione di altri ormoni o dei loro recettori. A seconda del livello e della natura della mutazione, possono svilupparsi ipogonadismo, pubertà precoce o ambiguità sessuale. A tutt'oggi sono state identificate, come causa di HHG, otto diverse mutazioni del gene del recettore per il GnRH, la maggior parte eterozigoti. Il fenotipo, tuttavia, varia da una forma parziale a una completa di ipogonadismo. Una mutazione del gene per la subunità β dell'LH a livello ipofisario provoca HHG. A livello gonadico, difetti del recettore dell'LH portano a ipoplasia delle cellule di Leydig e alterata virilizzazione nei maschi. È stato riportato il caso di un maschio con micropene e normali testicoli, che non produceva testosterone anche dopo ripetute somministrazioni di hCG. Si è ritenuto che si potesse trattare della sindrome delle "cellule di Leydig vanishing" (in analogia con la sindrome del "vanishing testis"). Nel primo trimestre di gravidanza devono essere presenti cellule di Leydig normalmente funzionanti ma, a causa di un difetto del recettore dell'LH, l'inadeguata produzione di testosterone nel secondo e nel terzo trimestre porta a uno sviluppo insufficiente del pene alla nascita. È stata descritta, come causa di ipogonadismo in un ragazzo di 18 anni valutato per pubertà ritardata e in tre donne con pubertà ritardata e amenorrea primaria (Tab. 584-1) una nuova mutazione della subunità β dell'FSH. Sono state associate a HHG mutazioni della leptina, del recettore della leptina e dell'endopeptidasi proormonale convertasi-1 (PC-1).

Altre patologie. Si è osservato HHG in pochi pazienti con sindrome polighiandolare autoimmune, in alcuni con elevati livelli di melatonina e in quelli con una serie di altre sindromi come quella di Bardet-Biedl, quella di Prader-Willi, la sindrome con lentiggini multiple e con varie forme di atassia.

DIAGNOSI. I livelli di gonadotropine e di steroidi gonadici rimangono nel range prepubere e non compare la tipica secrezione pulsatile notturna dell'LH. La risposta gonadotropinica alla stimolazione con GnRH o con un più potente analogo del GnRH è notevolmente diminuita. Questi reperti sono però compatibili anche con quelli trovati in adolescenti normali con la nota variante di pubertà ritardata costituzionale; è quindi difficile distinguere tra le due condizioni. Molti test diversi, compresi il test di stimolazione con GnRH, TRH, metoclopramide e domperidone, hanno dato risultati non decisivi. Una singola misurazione dei livelli di testosterone alle 8.00 può essere un buon indicatore di pubertà imminente. In maschi che presentavano tutti un incremento del volume testicolare maggiore di 4 mL al 15° mese e del 77% al 12°, è stato trovato un valore maggiore di 0,7 nmol/L (20 mg/dL). Al contrario, fra i maschi con livelli di testosterone inferiori a 0,7 nmol/L, solo il 25% ha iniziato la pubertà all'età di 15 anni. L'utilizzo di un analogo del GnRH o del test con GnRH dopo 36 ore dal "priming" dell'asse ipotalamo-ipofiso-gonadico con somministrazione pulsatile di GnRH può essere in grado di differenziare gli adolescenti con ipogonadismo da quelli con pubertà ritardata.

È ipotizzabile un deficit di gonadotropine, se il paziente presenta altri deficit ipofisari, come quello dell'ormone della crescita, particolarmente se associato a quello di corticotropina (ormone adrenocorticotropo [ACTH]). La presenza di **anosmia** solitamente indica un deficit permanente di gonadotropine, ma in soggetti anosmici sono stati osservati quadri occasionali di notevole ritardo puberale (18-20 anni d'età). Nonostante l'anosmia possa essere presente nella famiglia o nel paziente sin dalla prima infanzia, raramente i pazienti la dichiarano spontaneamente, perciò si rende necessaria un'indagine approfondita e specifica in questo senso in tutti i pazienti con pubertà ritardata. Alla RM in alcuni pazienti possono evidenziarsi anomalie dei lobi olfattivi e dei solchi. Come causa di pubertà ritardata, con sempre maggiore frequenza si trovano i **prolattinomi** e per escluderli è necessaria la determinazione dei livelli plasmatici di prolattina.

Sono disponibili varie indagini per stabilire la diagnosi negli eterozigoti e in neonati con la forma associata a X della sindrome di Kallmann. Durante i primi 3-4 mesi di vita, i bambini sani evidenziano il normale incremento delle gonatropine e degli steroidi gonadici e la risposta al GnRH supera quella dei bambini prepuberi. Il maschio adulto con mutazioni KAL1 documentate presenta una perdita completa della pulsatilità dell'LH.

TRATTAMENTO. Prima di fare diagnosi di deficit isolato di GnRH e di iniziare il trattamento deve essere escluso il ritardo costituzionale della crescita. Circa il 3% dei maschi ha un volume testicolare inferiore a 4 mL a 14 anni, ma il vero ipogonadismo ipogonadotropo è raro. Anche ritardi relativamente modesti dello sviluppo sessuale e della crescita possono portare a un significativo stress psicologico e richiedere attenzione. Inizialmente, per la maggior parte dei ragazzi, sono sufficienti una spiegazione delle variabilità della pubertà e una rassicurazione. Se a 15 anni ancora non sono iniziate le manifestazioni cliniche di pubertà e i livelli di testosterone sono inferiori a 50 ng/dL, è indicata la somministrazione di testosterone per un breve periodo. Il testosterone enantato, 100 mg intramuscolo una volta al mese per 4-6 mesi, di solito porta a un aumento delle caratteristiche sessuali secondarie e della velocità di crescita; può dare l'avvio alla pubertà e può differenziare il ritardo costituzionale dalle forme di deficit isolato di gonadotropine. L'età di inizio della terapia deve essere individualizzata.

Pazienti con diagnosi di deficit di gonadotropine devono essere curati con lo stesso trattamento con testosterone usato per quelli con deficit testicolare primario (vedi Capitolo 584.1): con questa terapia, però, i testicoli rimangono piccoli. Il trattamento con hCG, somministrato per via sottocutanea o intramuscolare, alla dose di 500-1000 UI, tre volte la settimana, stimola la crescita testicolare e la spermatogenesi. Se, dopo 6-12 mesi di terapia, non si è ancora raggiunta una crescita testicolare sufficiente, si può aggiungere la gonadotropina umana menopausale alla dose di 37,5-150 UI, tre volte la settimana. Per ottenere un'adeguata spermatogenesi nell'adulto, possono essere necessari anche più di due anni di terapia. Le gonadotropine ricombinanti sono in grado di stimolare la crescita e la funzione gonadica.

Una forma di trattamento più fisiologica, ma scomoda, consiste in somministrazioni episodiche (sottocutanee o endovenose) di GnRH. È possibile la terapia a lungo termine con una pompa a infusione peristaltica programmabile. La maggior parte dei pazienti richiede circa due anni di terapia per massimizzare la crescita testicolare e ottenere la spermatogenesi.

TABELLA 584-1. Difetti genetici conosciuti che provocano ipogonadismo

DIFETTO	CONDIZIONE CLINICA	GENERE COLPITO
ORMONE DI RILASCIO DELLE GONADOTROPINE		
KAL-1	Sindrome di Kallmann	Entrambi
DAX-1	Ipoplasia surrenalica associata a X e ipogonadismo ipogonadotropo	Maschi
Recettore	Ipogonadismo ipogonadotropo familiare	Femmine
ORMONE LUTEINIZZANTE		
Subunità β	Pubertà ritardata, ipoplasia delle cellule di Leydig, infertilità	Maschi
Recettore	Pseudoermafroditismo maschile, ipoplasia delle cellule di Leydig, micropene Amenorrea	Entrambi
ORMONE FOLLICOLO-STIMOLANTE		
Subunità β	Pubertà ritardata Amenorrea	Entrambi
Recettore	Insufficienza ovarica Tumori ovarici a cellule germinali	Femmine

Acierno SA, Shagoury JK, Bo-Abbas Y, et al: A locus for autosomal recessive idiopathic hypogonadotropic hypogonadism on chromosome 19p13.3. *J Clin Endocrinol Metab* 2003;88:2730–2737.

Bahuau M, Houdayer C, Assouline B, et al: Novel recurrent nonsense mutation causing neurofibromatosis type 1 (NF1) in a family segregating both NF1 and Noonan syndrome. *Am J Med Genet* 1998;75:265–272.

Carrel AL, Myers SE, Whitman BY, et al: Growth hormone improves body composition, fat utilization, physical strength and agility, and growth in Prader-Willi syndrome: A controlled study. *J Pediatr* 2000;134:215–221.

Cotterill AM, McKenna WJ, Brady AF, et al: The short-term effects of growth hormone therapy on height velocity and cardiac ventricular wall thickness in children with Noonan syndrome. *J Clin Endocrinol Metab* 1996;81: 2291–2297.

DeRoux N, Young J, Misrahi M, et al: A family with hypogonadotropic hypogonadism and mutations in the gonadotropin-releasing hormone receptor. *N Engl J Med* 1997;337:1597–1602.
Dobs AS, Hoover DR, Chen MC, et al: Pharmacokinetic characteristics, efficacy, and safety of buccal testosterone in hypogonadal males: A pilot study. *J Clin Endocrinol Metab* 1998;83:33–39.
Geschwind DH, Boone KB, Miller BL, et al: Neurobehavioral phenotype of Klinefelter syndrome. *Ment Retard Dev Disabil Res Rev* 2000;6:107–116.
Goodfellow PN, Camerino G: DAX-1, an "antitestis" gene. *EXS* 2001; 91:57–69.
Hardelin J: Kallmann syndrome: Towards molecular pathogenesis. *Mol Cell Endocrinol* 2001;179:75–81.
Hultborn R, Hanson C, Kopf I, et al: Prevalence of Klinefelter's syndrome in male breast cancer patients. *Anticancer Res* 1997;17:4293–1497.
Itti E, Gaw Gonzalo IT, Pawlikowska-Haddal A, et al: The structural brain correlates of cognitive deficits in adults with Klinefelter's syndrome. *J Clin Endocrinol Metab* 2006;91:1423–1427.
Kadandale JS, Wachtel SS, Tunca Y, et al: Localization of SRY by primed in situ labeling in XX and XY sex reversal. *Am J Med Genet* 2000;95:71–74.
Khorram O, Patrizio P, Wang C, et al: Reproductive technologies for male infertility. *J Clin Endocrinol Metab* 2001;86:2373–2379.
Latronico AC, Anasti J, Arnhold IJ, et al: Brief report: Testicular and ovarian resistance to luteinizing hormone caused by inactivating mutations of the luteinizing hormone-receptor gene. *N Engl J Med* 1996;334:507–512.
Layman LC, Lee EJ, Peak DB, et al: Delayed puberty and hypogonadism caused by mutations in the follicle stimulating hormone β-subunit gene. *N Engl J Med* 1997;337:607–611.
Lee MM, Donahoe PK, Silverman BL, et al: Measurements of serum müllerian inhibiting substance in the evaluation of children with nonpalpable gonads. *N Engl J Med* 1997;336:1480–1486.
Limal J, Parfait B, Cabrol S, et al: Noonan Syndrome: Relationships between genotype, growth, and growth factors. *J Clin Endocrinol Metab* 2006;91: 300–306.
Matthews CH, Borgato S, Beck-Peccoz, et al: Primary amenorrhea and infertility due to a mutation in the β-subunit of follicle-stimulating hormone. *Nat Genet* 1993;5:83–86.
McCabe ERB: Vulnerability within a robust complex system-DAX1 mutations and steroidogenic axis development. *J Clin Endocrinol Metab* 2002;87: 41–43.
Merke DP, Tajima T, Baron J, et al: Hypogonadotropic hypogonadism in a female caused by an X-linked recessive mutation in the DAX1 gene. *N Engl J Med* 1999;340:1248–1252.
Meyer J, Sudbeck P, Held M, et al: Mutational analysis of the SOX9 gene in campomelic dysplasia and autosomal sex reversal: Lack of genotype/phenotype correlations. *Hum Mol Genet* 1997;6:91–98.
Muller J: Hypogonadism and endocrine metabolic disorders in Prader-Willi syndrome. *Acta Paediatr Suppl* 1997;423:58–59.
Nisbet DL, Griffin DR, Chitty LS: Prenatal features of Noonan syndrome. *Prenat Diagn* 1999;19:642–647.
Noonan JA: Noonan syndrome revisited. *J Pediatr* 1999;135:667–668.
Ogata T, Matsuo M, Muroya K, et al: 47,XXX male: A clinical and molecular study. *Am J Med Genet* 2001;98:353–356.
Patwardhan AJ, Eliez S, Bender B, et al: Brain morphology in Klinefelter syndrome: Extra X chromosome and testosterone supplementation. *Neurology* 2000;54:2218–2223.
Phillip M, Arbelle JE, Segev Y, et al: Male hypogonadism due to a mutation in the gene for the β-subunit of follicle-stimulating hormone. *N Engl J Med* 1998;338:1729–1732.
Romano AA, Blethen SL, Dana K, et al: Growth hormone treatment in Noonan syndrome: The National Cooperative Growth Study experience. *J Pediatr* 1996;128:S18–21.
Rovet J, Netley C, Keenan M, et al: The psychoeducational profile of boys with Klinefelter syndrome. *J Learn Disabil* 1996;29:180–196.
Sato N, Katsumata N, Kagami M, et al: Clinical assessment of mutation analysis of Kallman Syndrome 1 (KAL1) and fibroblast growth factor receptor 1 (FGFR1, or KAL2) in five families and 18 sporadic patients. *J Clin Endocrinol Metab* 2004;89:1079–1088.
Schiff JD, Palermo GD, Veeck LL, et al: Success of testicular sperm injection and intracytoplasmic sperm injection in men with Klinefelter Syndrome. *J Clin Endocrinol Metab* 2005;90:6263–6267.
Schubbert S, Zenker M, Rowe SL, et al: Germline KRAS mutations cause Noonan syndrome. *Nat Genet* 2006;38:331–336.
Smals AGH, Hermus ARM, Boers GHJ, et al: Predictive value of luteinizing hormone releasing hormone (LHRH) bolus testing before and after 36-hour pulsatile LHRH administration in the differential diagnosis of constitutional delay of puberty and male hypogonadotropic hypogonadism. *J Clin Endocrinol Metab* 1994;78:602–608.
Stuppia L, Calabrese G, Borrelli P, et al: Loss of the SHOX gene associated with Leri-Weill dyschondrosteosis in a 45,X male. *J Med Genet* 1999;36: 711–713.
Swerdlow AJ, Higgins CD, Schoemaker MJ, et al: Mortality in patients with Klinefelter Syndrome in Britain: A cohort study. *J Clin Endocrinol Metab* 2005;90:6516–6522.
Toledo SPA, Brunner HG, Kraaij R, et al: An inactivating mutation of the luteinizing hormone receptor causes amenorrhea in a 46,XX female. *J Clin Endocrinol Metab* 1996;81:3850–3854.
VanDop C, Burstein S, Conte FA, et al: Isolated gonadotropin deficiency in boys: Clinical characteristics and growth. *J Pediatr* 1987;111:684–692.
Wu FC, Brown DC, Butler GE, et al: Early morning plasma testosterone is an accurate predictor of imminent pubertal development in prepubertal boys. *J Clin Endocrinol Metab* 1993;76:26–31.

Capitolo 585 ■ Pseudopubertà precoce da tumori testicolari

I tumori testicolari a cellule di Leydig rappresentano una causa rara di pseudopubertà precoce e provocano un aumento di volume asimmetrico del testicolo. Essi rappresentano circa il 3% di tutti i tumori testicolari.

Le cellule di Leydig sono scarse prima della pubertà; i tumori che ne derivano sono quindi più frequenti nell'età adulta. I casi riportati nei bambini comprendono due pazienti, ciascuno appartenente a una coppia di gemelli identici. Questi tumori solitamente sono monolaterali e benigni; il 10% può diventare maligno. Caratteristico è il reperto microscopico di cristalloidi di Reinke, presente però in meno del 50% dei tumori a cellule di Leydig. In un tumore testicolare a cellule di Leydig è stata descritta una mutazione *gsp*. Nei testicoli adulti, i tumori a cellule germinali, ma non quelli a cellule del Sertoli o a cellule di Leydig, esibiscono espressione biallelica del gene umano *H19*.

Le **manifestazioni cliniche** sono quelle della pubertà nel maschio; l'esordio si colloca di solito fra i 5 e i 9 anni. È stata descritta ginecomastia. Il tumore testicolare è di solito facilmente apprezzabile e il testicolo sano controlaterale presenta dimensioni normali in rapporto all'età del paziente.

I livelli plasmatici di testosterone sono marcatamente elevati. L'ormone follicolo-stimolante e l'ormone luteinizzante sono soppressi e risulta assente la risposta alla somministrazione di ormone di rilascio delle gonadotropine (GnRH). L'indagine ecografica è in grado di rilevare tumori molto piccoli, non percepibili palpatorialmente. Anche l'agobiopsia del testicolo con ago sottile può aiutare a definire la diagnosi.

Il **trattamento** consiste nella rimozione chirurgica del testicolo malato. Dopo l'intervento, cessa la progressione della virilizzazione e possono anche scomparire alcuni dei segni di precocità presenti.

All'interno del tumore si possono sviluppare dei residui di tessuto surrenalico che simulano le neoplasie a cellule del Leydig; in assenza dei cristalloidi di Reinke, questi due tumori non sono istologicamente differenziabili. I tumori dei residui surrenalici di solito sono bilaterali e compaiono in pazienti con iperplasia surrenalica congenita, specialmente nella forma con perdita di sali, durante l'adolescenza e nei giovani adulti. Lo stimolo per la crescita dei residui di tessuto surrenalico è rappresentato da un'inadeguata terapia soppressiva con corticosteroidi, mentre il trattamento con dosi appropriate quasi sempre comporta una loro regressione. La dimostrazione della loro attività 21-idrossilasica ha fornito informazioni definitive sull'origine di tali tumori. La diagnosi errata di questo tipo di tumori in portatori di iperplasia surrenalica congenita ha comportato orchidectomie non necessarie.

La **sindrome dell'X fragile** è una causa comune di ritardo mentale ereditario, con una frequenza di 1/2000 nati. È dovuta all'amplificazione di una sequenza ripetuta di CGG nella regione 5′ non tradotta del gene *FMR1* su Xp17.3 (vedi Capitolo 81). Una caratteristica fondamentale di questa condizione è l'aumento del volume testicolare (**macrorchidismo**), che raggiunge i 40-50 mL dopo la pubertà. Sebbene questa patologia sia stata riconosciuta in un bambino molto piccolo, di soli 5 mesi, i bambini con meno di 6 anni raramente presentano ipertrofia testicolare; a 8-10 anni, la maggior parte ha un volume testicolare maggiore di 3 mL. I testicoli sono aumentati bilateralmente, non sono nodulari e sono istologicamente normali. Lo studio dell'assetto ormonale è normale. Analisi dirette del DNA volte a ricercare sequenze ripetute di CGG permettono la diagnosi definitiva (vedi Capitolo 81).

I tumori del cordone sessuale con tubuli anulari del testicolo possono provocare sviluppo mammario in giovani ragazzi. Questi tumori di solito sono associati alla malattia di Peutz-Jeghers; sono bilaterali, multifocali ed ecograficamente rilevabili. In questi maschi, l'iperproduzione di aromatasi ($P450_{arom}$) provoca femminilizzazione.

Nei maschi con criptorchidismo unilaterale, il testicolo controlaterale, nel 25% dei casi, ha dimensioni maggiori dell'altro. Si è notato un aumento del volume testicolare anche in un maschio con porpora di Schönlein Henoch e linfangiectasia. Raramente sono stati riportati casi di cisti epidermoidi e dermoidi del testicolo.

Assi A, Sironi M, Bacchioni AM, et al: Leydig cell tumor of the testis: A cytohistological, immunohistochemical, and ultrastructural case study. *Diagn Cytopathol* 1997;16:262–266.

Clark RV, Albertson BD, Monabi A, et al: Steroidogenic enzyme activities, morphology and receptor studies of a testicular rest in a patient with congenital adrenal hyperplasia. *J Clin Endocrinol Metab* 1990;70:1408–1413.

Coen P, Kulin H, Ballantine T, et al: An aromatase-producing sex-cord tumor resulting in prepubertal gynecomastia. *N Engl J Med* 1991;324:317–322.

Combes-Moukousky ME, Kottler ML, Valensi P, et al: Gonadal and adrenal catheterization during adrenal suppression and gonadal stimulation in a patient with bilateral testicular tumors and congenital adrenal hyperplasia. *J Clin Endocrinol Metab* 1994;79:1390–1394.

Fragoso MCBV, Latronico AC, Carvalho FM, et al: Activating mutation of the stimulatory G protein (gsp) as a putative cause of ovarian and testicular human stromal Leydig cell tumors. *J Clin Endocrinol Metab* 1998;83:2074–2078.

Nisula BC, Loriaux DL, Sherins RJ, et al: Benign bilateral testicular enlargement. *J Clin Endocrinol Metab* 1974;38:440–445.

Rosenberg T, Gilboa Y, Golik A, et al: Pseudoprecocious puberty in a young boy due to interstitial cell adenomas of the testis. *Helv Paediatr Acta* 1984;39:79–87.

Capitolo 586 ■ Ginecomastia

La ginecomastia, cioè la comparsa di tessuto mammario nel maschio, è una condizione frequente. È necessario distinguere la ginecomastia vera (presenza di tessuto ghiandolare mammario) dalla pseudoginecomastia (che consiste esclusivamente di tessuto adiposo), tipica dei maschi in sovrappeso. La ginecomastia è di solito un segno di squilibrio tra androgeni ed estrogeni; spesso la sua causa è ignota. È presente in molti neonati maschi, come conseguenza della normale stimolazione da parte degli ormoni materni, e gli effetti si esauriscono in poche settimane.

In un periodo che va dagli inizi della pubertà fino alla sua fase intermedia, circa due terzi dei maschi sviluppa gradi variabili di iperplasia mammaria subareolare. La ginecomastia puberale fisiologica può essere monolaterale, ma anche frequentemente bilaterale, con ingrossamento rapido o in tempi diversi. Spesso le mammelle presentano una certa sensibilità, che però è transitoria. In pochi mesi si può assistere a una regressione spontanea; raramente persiste per più di due anni. Le concentrazioni medie di ormone follicolo-stimolante, ormone luteinizzante, prolattina, testosterone, estrone ed estradiolo sono identiche a quelle presenti nei coetanei senza ginecomastia. La coltura *in vitro* di fibroblasti cutanei di derivazione pubica di maschi con ginecomastia evidenzia un eccesso di attività aromatasica. Il trattamento consiste nel rassicurare il ragazzo e la sua famiglia sulla natura fisiologica e transitoria del fenomeno. Quando l'ipertrofia è notevole, persiste e provoca seri disturbi psicologici al paziente, può essere giustificata una terapia. Il **trattamento medico** è volto generalmente alla diminuzione del rapporto estrogeni/androgeni. Il danazolo ha attività antiestrogenica, ma anche numerosi effetti collaterali. L'anastrozolo, un inibitore dell'aromatasi, alla dose di 1,0 mg per os per 6 mesi non presenta effetti diversi dal placebo nel provocare un decremento del volume mammario totale in oltre il 50% dei ragazzi con ginecomastia puberale.

Occasionalmente, lo sviluppo mammario può simulare quello femminile (fino agli stadi di Tanner 3-5) e non regredire. In questi casi, può essere indicata la rimozione **chirurgica** del tessuto mammario in eccesso e una tecnica prevede la rimozione transascellare endoscopicamente assistita del tessuto ghiandolare.

È stata descritta una ginecomastia benigna, autolimitantesi e solitamente transitoria in bambini prepuberi all'inizio della terapia con ormone della crescita umano.

La **ginecomastia familiare**, presente in parecchie famiglie, è una caratteristica correlata a X o autosomica dominante limitata al sesso. I livelli di gonadotropine, testosterone, prolattina e globulina di trasporto degli steroidi sono normali. In casi familiari e sporadici di ginecomastia è stato trovato un aumento della conversione periferica dei 19-steroidi in estrogeni (aumentata aromatizzazione) e ciò è utile a spiegare alcune situazioni.

Per esempio, la presenza in un maschio adulto, in suo figlio e in sua figlia di una sindrome con eccesso di aromatasi, ha fatto ipotizzare un'ereditarietà autosomica dominante. Nel bambino di 9 anni era presente ginecomastia e in sua sorella di 7 anni e mezzo macromastia e precocità isosessuale. Nei fibroblasti cutanei e nei linfociti trasformati *in vitro*, è stato dimostrato l'eccesso di attività aromatasica, associato a polimorfismo di $P450_{arom}$, che suggeriva una modificazione della sequenza nella regione del promoter $P450_{arom}$. In una vasta famiglia con mutazione simile del gene dell'aromatasi P450, è stata descritta una ginecomastia prepubere a trasmissione dominante, in presenza di elevati livelli sierici di estrone ma non di 17β-estradiolo. Nel topo, la rottura del gene *DAX1* provoca un aumento dell'espressione aromatasica.

In bambini prepuberi con ginecomastia, va ricercata una **fonte esogena di estrogeni**. L'esposizione accidentale o terapeutica a piccole quantità di estrogeni esogeni per inalazioni, per via transcutanea o per ingestione può provocare ginecomastia. Tre maschi hanno sviluppato ginecomastia dopo esposizione indiretta, dovuta a utilizzo di creme delle loro madri, per uso topico, contenenti estrogeni. In questi casi si può manifestare iperpigmentazione del capezzolo e dell'areola. L'esposizione a farmaci che diminuiscono i livelli di androgeni, soprattutto di quelli liberi, e aumentano quelli di estradiolo o sostituiscono gli androgeni in corrispondenza dei loro recettori mammari può provocare ginecomastia. La lavanda e certi oli essenziali di tea tree possono essere causa di ginecomastia prepubere.

Numerose altre condizioni patologiche possono provocare ginecomastia. È stata osservata in bambini con iperplasia surrenalica congenita virilizzante (**deficit di 11b-idrossilasi**) e può essere associata a tumori del testicolo a cellule di Leydig o a tumori femminilizzanti del surrene. Molti maschi con la sindrome di Peutz-Jeghers e ginecomastia presentano tumori dei cordoni sessuali con tubuli anulari dei testicoli. I testicoli possono non essere aumentati e il tumore di solito è bilaterale e multifocale. L'eccessiva produzione di aromatasi spiega la presenza di ginecomastia. Questa condizione si verifica nei pazienti con **sindrome di Klinefelter** e con altri tipi di insufficienza testicolare (stati ipergonadotropinemici). È un reperto frequente in maschi con certe forme di scarsa virilizzazione (particolarmente la **sindrome di Reifenstein**), nella sindrome con insensibilità agli androgeni e nel deficit di 17-chetosteroido reduttasi. Quando la ginecomastia si associa a galattorrea, si deve ricercare un **prolattinoma**. Per esempio, in un maschio pubere con **carcinoma fibrolamellare** del fegato, la ginecomastia e gli elevati livelli estrogenici erano attribuibili all'aumento dell'aromatizzazione degli androgeni circolanti da parte del tumore. In un bambino di 8 anni con tumore calcificante a cellule di Sertoli, la ginecomastia era dovuta ad aromatizzazione periferica degli androgeni prodotti dalle cellule di Leydig differenziatesi dalle cellule interstiziali stimolate dal tumore. L'**ipertiroidismo** altera il rapporto androgeni/estrogeni, per un aumento degli androgeni legati e una diminuzione del testosterone libero e può portare a ginecomastia.

Negli adulti, si verifica ginecomastia nella cirrosi epatica, durante la terapia digitalica per insufficienza cardiaca congestizia, nel carcinoma broncogeno, durante la somministrazione di vari farmaci non steroidei e nei fumatori di marijuana. Il ketoconazolo, un farmaco antimicotico, provoca ginecomastia per diretta inibizione della sintesi di testosterone. Vari farmaci come spironolattone, metil-dopa, fenotiazine, antidepressivi, warfarin, digitale ed eroina possono portare a ginecomastia.

Binder G, Iliev DI, Dufke A, et al: Dominant transmission of prepubertal gynecomastia due to serum estrone excess: Hormonal, biochemical, and genetic analysis in a large kindred. *J Clin Endocrinol Metab* 2005;90:484–492.

Braunstein GD: Gynecomastia. *N Engl J Med* 1993;328:490–495.

Felner EI, White PC: Prepubertal gynecomastia: Indirect exposure to estrogen cream. *Pediatrics* 2000;105:1–3.

Henley DV, Lipson N, Korach KS, Bloch CA: Prepubertal gynecomastia linked to lavender and tea tree oils. *N Engl J Med* 2007;356:479–485.

Lazala C, Saenger P: Pubertal gynecomastia. *J Pediatr Endocrinol Metab* 2002;15:553–560.

Maclaren NK, Migeon CJ, Raiti S: Gynecomastia with congenital virilizing adrenal hyperplasia (11β-hydroxylase deficiency). *J Pediatr* 1975;86:579–581.

Malozowski S, Stadel BV: Prepubertal gynecomastia during growth hormone therapy. *J Pediatr* 1995;126:659–661.

Ohyama T, Takada A, Fujikawa M, et al: Endoscope-assisted transaxillary removal of glandular tissue in gynecomastia. *Ann Plast Surg* 1998;40:62–64.

Plourde PV, Reiter EO, Jou H, et al: Safety and efficacy of anastrozole for the treatment of pubertal gynecomastia: A randomized, double-blind, placebo-controlled trial. *J Clin Endocrinol Metab* 2004;89:4428–4433.

Stratakis CA, Vottero A, Brodies A, et al: The aromatase excess syndrome is associated with feminization of both sexes and autosomal dominant transmission of aberrant P450 aromatase gene transcription. *J Clin Endocrinol Metab* 1998;83:1348–1357.

Capitolo 587 ■ Ipofunzione delle ovaie

L'ipofunzione delle ovaie può essere causata da insufficienza congenita dello sviluppo, da distruzione postnatale (ipogonadismo primario o ipergonadotropo) o da mancata stimolazione da parte dell'ipofisi e/o dell'ipotalamo (ipogonadismo secondario e terziario). Molte malattie croniche possono provocare un ipogonadismo ipogonadotropo.

587.1 • Ipogonadismo ipergonadotropo nella femmina (ipogonadismo primario)

Prima della pubertà la diagnosi di ipogonadismo ipergonadotropo è difficile. Eccetto il caso della sindrome di Turner, la maggior parte delle pazienti non presenta manifestazioni cliniche prima della pubertà.

SINDROME DI TURNER

Turner descrisse, nelle femmine adulte, una sindrome che consiste in infantilismo sessuale, pterigio del collo e gomito valgo (vedi anche Capitolo 81). Ullrich ha descritto una bambina di 8 anni con bassa statura e molte delle medesime caratteristiche fenotipiche. Il termine di sindrome di Turner-Ullrich è utilizzato spesso in Europa, ma raramente negli Stati Uniti. La malattia è definita come la combinazione di aspetti fenotipici caratteristici, con assenza completa o parziale del secondo cromosoma X, con o senza mosaicismo.

PATOGENESI. La metà dei pazienti con sindrome di Turner ha un assetto cromosomico 45,X. Circa il 15% delle pazienti presenta un mosaicismo, con 45,X e una normale linea cellulare (45,X/46,XX). Meno frequentemente si trovano altri mosaici con isocromosomi, come 45,X/46,X,i(Xq), con anelli, 45,X/46,X,r(X), o con frammenti, 45,X/46fra. È tanto più frequente trovare un mosaicismo, quanti più tessuti vengono esaminati. Il singolo cromosoma X è di origine materna in circa l'80% delle pazienti con 45,X. Il meccanismo di perdita cromosomica è sconosciuto e il rischio di questa sindrome non aumenta con l'età materna. I geni coinvolti nella sindrome di Turner sono geni correlati a X che sfuggono all'inattivazione. Un locus maggiore coinvolto nel controllo della crescita lineare è stato mappato nella regione pseudoautosomica del cromosoma X (PAR1). Si ritiene che *SHOX*, un gene contenente homeobox di 170 kb di DNA in PAR1, sia importante per il controllo della crescita nelle bambine con sindrome di Turner, in pazienti con bassa statura idiopatica e nella sindrome di Leri-Weill. Si ritiene che i geni per il controllo della normale funzione ovarica siano su Xp e forse due "supergeni" su Xq.

La sindrome di Turner si verifica in circa uno su 1500-2500 nate femmine. La frequenza del cariotipo 45,X al momento del concepimento è di circa il 3,0%, ma il 99% di questi viene spontaneamente abortito, rappresentando circa il 5-10% di tutti gli aborti. Il mosaicismo (45,X/46,XX) compare in proporzione maggiore di quanto si verifichi in altri stati di aneuploidia, ma raramente nei feti abortiti; questo dato indica una preferenziale sopravvivenza dei feti con mosaicismo.

L'ovaio fetale normale contiene circa 7 milioni di ovociti, che cominciano rapidamente a scomparire dopo il quinto mese di gestazione. Alla nascita, ce ne sono solo 2 milioni (un milione di follicoli attivi); all'epoca del menarca, sono circa 400 000-500 000 e in menopausa ne rimangono 10 000. In assenza di un cromosoma X, questo processo viene accelerato e quasi tutti gli ovociti scompaiono al secondo anno di età. In feti abortiti 45,X, il numero delle cellule germinali primordiali nella cresta gonadica appare normale, suggerendo che, nelle pazienti con sindrome di Turner, vi sia un'accelerazione del normale processo. Alla fine, le ovaie appaiono "nastriformi" e consistono esclusivamente di tessuto connettivo, ma possono persistere poche cellule germinali.

MANIFESTAZIONI CLINICHE. In molte pazienti la diagnosi di sindrome di Turner viene posta alla nascita, per la presenza di un caratteristico edema del dorso delle mani e dei piedi e ampie pieghe cutanee della nuca e del collo. Sono frequenti basso peso alla nascita e scarsa lunghezza (vedi Capitolo 81). Nell'infanzia le manifestazioni cliniche comprendono pterigio del collo, bassa attaccatura posteriore dei capelli, ipoplasia mandibolare, orecchie prominenti, epicanto, alto arco palatale, torace ampio con capezzoli notevolmente distanziati, gomito valgo e unghie a notevole convessità. La diagnosi è sospettata per la prima volta alla pubertà, quando non compare maturazione sessuale.

La bassa statura, segno fondamentale presente in tutte le bambine con sindrome di Turner, può accompagnarsi ad altre minime manifestazioni cliniche. La decelerazione della crescita comincia nella primissima e nella prima infanzia, diventa progressivamente più marcata nelle fasi successive e nell'adolescenza e porta a una statura adulta molto bassa. Al momento opportuno non compare maturazione sessuale. L'altezza media da adulte è di 143-144 cm negli Stati Uniti e nella maggior parte degli Stati del nord d'Europa, ma di 140 cm in Argentina e di 147 in Scandinavia (Fig. 587-1). L'altezza è in rapporto con l'altezza media dei genitori (media delle altezze dei genitori). Per le bambine con sindrome di Turner sono state compilate specifiche curve di crescita.

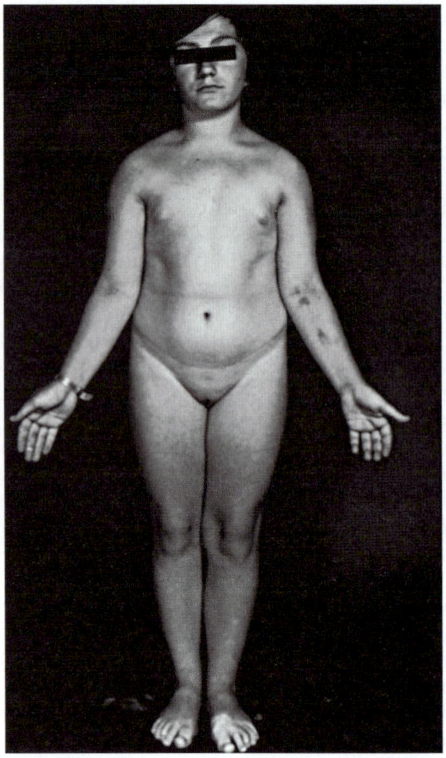

Figura 587-1. Sindrome di Turner in un ragazza di 15 anni che mostra un deficit della maturazione sessuale, bassa statura, cubito valgo e gozzo. È assente lo pterigio del collo. Il cariotipo è 45,X/46,XX.

È frequente l'associazione con altre patologie. Una valutazione cardiologica completa, compresa l'ecocardiografia, rivela in un terzo o nella metà delle pazienti isolate valvole aortiche bicuspidi non stenotiche. Nelle fasi tardive della vita, la patologia valvolare aortica può progredire verso la dilatazione dell'origine dell'aorta. Difetti meno frequenti comprendono coartazione aortica (20%), stenosi aortica, prolasso della mitrale e anomalo drenaggio venoso polmonare. In uno studio danese di 170/393 femmine con sindrome di Turner, il 38% delle pazienti 45,X presentava malformazioni cardiovascolari, rispetto all'11% di quelle con mosaicismi; l'anomalia più comune era rappresentata da alterazioni della valvola aortica e coartazione aortica. Lo pterigio del collo, in pazienti con o senza sindromi riconosciute, è associato a difetti cardiaci correlati o meno al flusso. Tra le pazienti con sindrome di Turner, quelle con pterigio del collo hanno maggiori probabilità di avere coartazione aortica rispetto a quelle senza tale malformazione. Durante l'adolescenza è necessario ripetere la valutazione cardiaca anche in pazienti senza precedenti reperti di anomalie cardiache e senza dubbio prima di affrontare una gravidanza. È necessario monitorare routinariamente la pressione arteriosa, anche in assenza di lesioni cardiache o renali, specialmente in pazienti con possibilità di dilatazione aortica. La RM può essere d'aiuto per diagnosticare e monitorare la dilatazione dell'origine aortica.

Da un quarto a un terzo delle pazienti presenta malformazioni renali (50% di quelle con cariotipo 45,X) ecograficamente rilevabili. Le alterazioni più gravi comprendono reni ectopici pelvici, rene a ferro di cavallo, doppio sistema collettore, agenesia renale monolaterale e ostruzione della giunzione ureteropelvica. È frequente anche ipertensione idiopatica. Gli studi più datati riportavano la difficoltà di evidenziare ecograficamente le ovaie negli stadi più precoci fino alle fasi più tardive dell'infanzia. Uno studio successivo, incrociato e longitudinale, condotto in Italia, non confermava tali differenze in rapporto all'età; il 27-46% delle pazienti aveva ovaie dimostrabili nelle varie età; il 76% di quelle con mosaicismo X e il 26% di quelle con il cariotipo 45,X avevano ovaie dimostrabili.

Solitamente non si verifica maturazione sessuale, ma il 10-20% delle ragazze ha uno sviluppo mammario spontaneo, mentre una piccola percentuale può avere qualche mestruazione. L'insufficienza ovarica primaria è associata a esordio precoce dell'adrenarca (aumento del DHEA solfato), ma a ritardo del pubarca (sviluppo dei peli pubici). Sono stati riportati, in donne con sindrome di Turner, casi di gravidanze, per la comparsa di mestruazioni spontanee. In alcune di queste donne sono state riportate menopausa precoce, aumento del rischio di aborto e figli con aumentato rischio di trisomia 21. Una donna con cariotipo 45,X/46,X,r(X), trattata con terapia ormonale sostitutiva, ha avuto tre gravidanze, una conclusasi con la nascita di un maschio normale 46,XY, una con una femmina con sindrome di Turner 45,X/46,Xr(X) e un aborto spontaneo.

Nel 30-50% delle pazienti si trovano anticorpi antitiroidei, antiperossidasi o antitireoglobulina. L'incidenza aumenta con l'aumentare dell'età. Dal 10 al 30% presenta **patologia tiroidea autoimmune**, con o senza gozzo. In pazienti con sindrome di Turner possono manifestarsi alterazioni, età-dipendenti, del metabolismo dei carboidrati, caratterizzate da anomala tolleranza glicidica e insulino-resistenza e, solo raramente, un diabete franco di tipo 2. In una donna 45,X è stata descritta un'alterata secrezione insulinica. I livelli di colesterolo sono elevati nell'adolescenza, in base al peso corporeo e al cariotipo.

Sono stati riportati casi di patologia infiammatoria intestinale, morbo di Crohn e colite ulcerativa, sanguinamento gastrointestinale da alterazioni vascolari mesenteriche nonché ritardato svuotamento gastrico.

Con l'RX in proiezione laterale è possibile valutare eventuali malformazioni sternali. Di solito un aumento del *carrying angle* del gomito non riveste alcun significato clinico. In circa il 10% delle adolescenti è presente scoliosi. Molto più frequentemente che nella popolazione generale, si verifica displasia congenita dell'anca. Le manifestazioni oculari comprendono disgenesia del segmento anteriore e cheratocono. Con l'età aumentano i nevi pigmentati; sono comuni i nevi melanocitici. Iperidrosi essenziale, toro mandibolare e alopecia areata compaiono raramente.

In circa il 75% delle pazienti si sviluppa un'**otite media bilaterale ricorrente**. Sono frequenti i deficit dell'udito neurosensoriale e sempre più con il passare dell'età. Problemi inerenti l'integrazione senso-motoria fine e grossolana, ritardo nella deambulazione fino al 15° mese e precoci alterazioni del linguaggio spesso pongono problemi circa un ritardo dello sviluppo, ma nella maggior parte delle pazienti l'intelligenza è normale. Tuttavia, in soggetti 45,X/46,X,r(X) si può verificare ritardo mentale, poiché la mancata inattivazione del cromosoma ad anello porta a due cromosomi X funzionali. Nelle donne adulte i deficit delle capacità percettive spaziali sono più frequenti rispetto alla popolazione generale. Alcuni dati non confermati suggeriscono l'esistenza di un locus associato a X che riguarda la funzione cognitiva, le capacità verbali e altre funzioni esecutive più alte (meglio quando l'X è di origine paterna).

La prevalenza di mosaicismo dipende in larga parte dalle tecniche usate per lo studio del pattern cromosomico. L'uso dell'ibridazione fluorescente *in situ* e della reazione a catena della polimerasi-trascrizione inversa (*Polymerase Chain Reaction*, PRC) ha aumentato la frequenza di mosaicismi fino al 60-74% dei casi.

Il mosaicismo del cromosoma Y si verifica nel 5% dei casi. Uno studio sulla popolazione femminile danese, utilizzando PCR con 5 diversi primer set, ha trovato materiale cromosomico Y nel 12,2% delle pazienti. Il gonadoblastoma era presente nel 7-10% delle pazienti Y-positive. Tuttavia, l'attuale impostazione che consiglia l'ovariectomia profilattica anche in assenza di evidenza di tumore alla RM e all'ecografia potrà necessitare in futuro di una rivalutazione. Il locus del gonadoblastoma sul cromosoma Y (GBY) è mappato vicino al centromero di Y. La presenza del solo locus SRY (regione determinante il sesso sul cromosoma Y) non è sufficiente per conferire un aumento della suscettibilità di sviluppare gonadoblastoma. Un accurato studio di 53 pazienti con sindrome di Turner eseguito utilizzando PCR nested escludeva bassi livelli di mosaicismo Y in quasi tutti i casi.

Una seconda indagine con PCR rivelava SRY nella parte distale del braccio corto del cromosoma Y in solo due soggetti. Non è tuttavia consigliato l'utilizzo routinario della PCR per trovare il cromosoma Y, allo scopo di assegnare un certo rischio di gonadoblastoma. La genotipizzazione quantitativa ad alto rendimento può fornire un metodo efficace ed economico per l'identificazione delle anomalie del cromosoma X e l'identificazione del materiale del cromosoma Y.

In pazienti con mosaicismo 45,X/46,XX, le anomalie sono poche e attenuate; la bassa statura è frequente come nelle pazienti 45,X e può essere la sola manifestazione della condizione, oltre all'insufficienza ovarica (vedi Fig. 587-1).

REPERTI DI LABORATORIO. In tutte le bambine con bassa statura è necessaria l'analisi cromosomica. In una ricerca sistematica, utilizzando l'analisi della macchia del sud del DNA leucocitario, la sindrome di Turner era presente nel 4,8% delle ragazze che si erano rivolte a un endocrinologo per bassa statura. Pazienti con un marker cromosomico in alcune o in tutte le cellule devono essere sottoposte ad analisi per lo studio delle sequenze di DNA a livello o vicine al centromero di Y.

Dopo la diagnosi è indicata un'indagine ecografica di cuore, reni e ovaie. Le più frequenti alterazioni scheletriche sono l'accorciamento del quarto osso metatarsale e metacarpale, la disgenesia epifisaria nelle articolazioni del ginocchio e del gomito, la deformità di Madelung, la scoliosi e, nelle pazienti più anziane, un'inadeguata mineralizzazione ossea.

Nella prima infanzia, i livelli plasmatici di gonadotropine, particolarmente di ormone follicolo-stimolante (FSH), sono marcatamente elevati, più di quelli dei controlli di pari età; a 2-3 anni si verifica un progressivo decremento dei livelli fino a che raggiungono un minimo a 6-8 anni, mentre a 10-11 risalgono a livelli analoghi a quelli di un adulto castrato.

Periodicamente è necessaria la valutazione degli anticorpi tiroidei antiperossidasi e, in caso di positività, la misurazione dei livelli di tiroxina e di ormone stimolante la tiroide. Studi molto ampi non sono riusciti a stabilire un ruolo primario del deficit di ormone somatotropo nella patogenesi del disturbo della crescita. Nelle adolescenti con sindrome di Turner sono state descritte alterazioni del normale pattern di secrezione dell'ormone della crescita, ma non in bambine più piccole. In vitro, monociti e linfociti risultano meno sensibili al fattore 1 di crescita insulino-simile (IGF-1).

L'American Academy of Pediatrics ha pubblicato un guida dettagliata per la sorveglianza della salute delle bambine con sindrome di Turner. Una guida per la terapia delle bambine e delle donne con sindrome di Turner è stata pubblicata nel 2007.

TRATTAMENTO. Il trattamento con **ormone della crescita** ricombinante umano aumenta la velocità di crescita e la statura definitiva nella maggior parte, ma non in tutte le bambine. Se il trattamento viene iniziato precocemente, molte ragazze superano i 150 cm. In un trial clinico negli Stati Uniti, ampio, multicentrico, controllato con placebo, 99 pazienti con sindrome di Turner, che hanno cominciato a ricevere ormone della crescita a un'età media di 10,9 anni, a dosaggi compresi tra 0,27 e 0,36 mg/kg/settimana, hanno raggiunto una statura media di 149 cm, mentre solo un terzo è arrivata a una statura adulta maggiore di 152,4 cm. In Olanda, dosi maggiori di ormone della crescita (oltre 0,6 mg/kg/settimana nel terzo anno di trattamento) hanno fatto raggiungere all'85% delle pazienti una statura adulta compresa nel range di riferimento della popolazione tedesca. Il trattamento con ormone della crescita deve essere iniziato precocemente e/o quando vi sia evidenza di una diminuzione della velocità di crescita rispetto alle curve di crescita specifiche per la sindrome di Turner. La dose iniziale di ormone della crescita è di 0,375 mg/kg/settimana. La terapia con ormone della crescita non peggiora in modo significativo la tolleranza glucidica e non provoca particolari effetti collaterali nelle pazienti con sindrome di Turner. Durante il trattamento con ormone della crescita vanno monitorati routinariamente i livelli sierici di IGF-1.

È indicata anche la terapia sostitutiva con **estrogeni**, sebbene se non vi sia accordo circa l'età d'inizio. È necessaria una preparazione psicologica delle pazienti per l'accettazione della terapia. Il miglioramento della crescita ottenuto con ormone della crescita durante l'infanzia permette di proseguire con la terapia sostitutiva con estrogeni verso i 12-13 anni. Per un maggior aumento della statura, specialmente per quelle pazienti in cui il trattamento con ormone della crescita sia iniziato solo nella tarda infanzia o nell'adolescenza, gli estrogeni possono essere ritardati fino ai 14-15 anni. È necessaria un'attenta valutazione dei conflitti psicologici conseguenti a una posticipazione della terapia estrogenica, per ottenere i migliori risultati sulla statura, e vanno considerati gli effetti sull'accrescimento osseo. La disponibilità di terapie estrogeniche a dosaggi molto bassi potrà ovviare in un prossimo futuro alla necessità di scegliere tra un'adeguata sostituzione puberale e l'ottimizzazione della statura potenziale. Dati preliminari suggeriscono che dosi mensili molto basse per via parenterale di preparati estrogenici depot, iniziate insieme al GH a 12 anni, possono migliorare la statura da adulte. La terapia estrogenica migliora la memoria verbale e non verbale in femmine con sindrome di Turner. Nelle giovani donne con sviluppo puberale adeguato all'età in cui raggiungono una normale statura definitiva, i questionari sulla salute correlata alla qualità di vita hanno ottenuto normali risultati.

Un estrogeno coniugato, alla dose di 0,3-0,625 mg, o estradiolo micronizzato, alla dose di 0,5 mg, somministrati giornalmente per 3-6 mesi, sono solitamente efficaci nell'indurre la pubertà. Successivamente gli estrogeni si somministrano in modo ciclico (ogni giorno dal primo al 23° giorno) e si aggiunge un progestinico (ogni giorno dal 10° al 23° giorno), alla dose di 5-10 g/die. Nei giorni in cui il trattamento viene sospeso, normalmente si verifica una perdita ematica da sospensione. I dati in nostro possesso riguardo all'uso di preparazioni estrogeniche transdermiche e depot nella sindrome di Turner non sono sufficienti.

L'analisi cromosomica prenatale per età materna avanzata ha rivelato una frequenza di 45,X/46,XX 10 volte maggiore di quella diagnosticata dopo la nascita. La maggior parte di queste pazienti non ha manifestazioni cliniche tipiche della sindrome di Turner e i livelli di gonadotropine sono normali. La consapevolezza di questo fenotipo lieve è importante per la consulenza alle pazienti.

Il supporto psicologico, per queste ragazze, è parte integrante del trattamento e La Turner Sindrome Society, che ha sedi locali negli Stati Uniti, e gruppi similari in Canada e in altri Paesi, provvede a un sistema di supporto molto utile alle pazienti e alle loro famiglie, in aggiunta a quello fornito dal team medico.

Sono state portate a termine gravidanze utilizzando la donazione di ovociti e la fertilizzazione *in vitro*. In donne adulte con sindrome di Turner, esiste un'alta percentuale di alterazioni non diagnosticate, che riguardano la densità minerale ossea, i lipidi e la tiroide. Sono frequenti intolleranza al glucosio, diminuzione della risposta insulinica nella prima fase, ipertensione arteriosa e diminuzione delle masse grasse libere. Con la terapia sostitutiva estrogenica peggiora la tolleranza al glucosio, ma migliorano la massa grassa libera, la pressione arteriosa e lo stato fisico generale. Il profilo neurocognitivo della donna adulta non dipende dallo stato estrogenico.

DISGENESIA GONADICA XX

Alcune femmine normali da un punto di vista genetico e fenotipico presentano lesioni ovariche identiche a quelle delle pazienti 45,X, ma senza le caratteristiche somatiche della sindrome di Turner; questa situazione viene definita disgenesia gonadica pura o disgenesia ovarica pura.

La malattia è diagnosticata raramente in età infantile, perché i genitali esterni sono normali, non sono visibili altre anomalie e la crescita è normale. Alla pubertà, non comincia la normale maturazione sessuale. I livelli plasmatici di gonadotropine sono elevati. Il ritardo della fusione epifisaria comporta un habitus di tipo **eunucoide**. L'ecografia pelvica dimostra ovaie nastriformi.

La presenza di sorelle affette, la consanguineità fra i genitori e l'assenza di mosaicismo indicano un'ereditarietà autosomica recessiva limitata al sesso femminile. La malattia è particolarmente frequente in Finlandia (1/8300 nati femmina). In questa popolazione, si è dimostrato che parecchie mutazioni nel gene del recettore per l'FSH (sul cromosoma 2p) sono la causa di questa condizione. Tali mutazioni non sono state trovate invece in donne messicane con disgenesia gonadica 46,XX. In alcune pazienti, la disgenesia gonadica XX è stata associata a sordità neurosensoriale (sindrome di Perrault). È stato riportato il caso di una paziente con questa malattia e concomitante deficit di ormone della crescita e virilizzazione. Esistono forme genetiche distinte di questa malattia. L'**agenesia mülleriana**, o sindrome di **Mayer-Rokitansky-Küster-Hauser**, che è seconda alla disgenesia gonadica come causa di amenorrea primaria, si verifica in 1:4000-1:5000 femmine ed è stata riportata in associazione a disgenesia gonadica 46,XX in un'adolescente di 17 anni con amenorrea primaria e mancanza di sviluppo mammario. È stato riportato un caso di disgerminoma con sinciziotrofoblasto a cellule giganti. Una ragazza di 18 anni con amenorrea primaria e assenza delle strutture di derivazione mülleriana, agenesia renale monolaterale e segni clinici di iperandrogenismo (fenotipo questo che assomiglia a quello della sindrome di Mayer-Rokitanky-Küster-Hauser) aveva una mutazione con perdita di funzione del gene *WNT4*. Il trattamento consiste nella terapia sostitutiva con estrogeni.

DISGENESIA GONADICA 45,X/46,XY

La disgenesia gonadica 45,X/46,XY, denominata anche **disgenesia gonadica mista**, presenta una notevole variabilità fenotipica postnatale, che può andare da un aspetto Turner-simile, fino a un fenotipo maschile con uretra peniena; è possibile comunque delineare tre quadri clinici maggiori. La bassa statura è il segno clinico principale in tutti i pazienti affetti. Il 90% dei casi diagnosticati in epoca prenatale ha un normale fenotipo maschile.

Alcuni pazienti non presentano virilizzazione; hanno un fenotipo femminile e spesso segni fisici della sindrome di Turner. Questa condizione viene di solito scoperta prima della pubertà quando, a causa della bassa statura, vengono eseguite analisi cromosomiche in una bambina, o successivamente, per mancanza di maturazione sessuale. Sono presenti le tube di Falloppio e l'utero. Le gonadi consistono in formazioni nastriformi indifferenziate intra-addominali; lo studio cromosomico delle ovaie spesso rivela una linea cellulare XY. Le gonadi nastriformi differiscono da quelle della sindrome di Turner; in aggiunta al tessuto connettivo, presentano spesso strutture tubulari cordoniformi, occasionali ammassi di cellule della granulosa e, frequentemente, cellule mesonefriche o ilari.

Alcuni bambini manifestano una virilizzazione di medio grado, rappresentata solo da clitoridomegalia prepubere. Sono presenti normali strutture mülleriane, ma alla pubertà compare virilizzazione. Queste pazienti solitamente posseggono un testicolo intra-addominale, un ovaio nastriforme controlaterale e tube di Falloppio bilaterali.

La maggior parte dei bambini presenta una **chiara ambiguità** genitale durante l'infanzia. Ci sono casi caratterizzati dalla presenza di un testicolo e un deferente in ambito labioscrotale, con gonade nastriforme controlaterale. Nonostante il testicolo, le tube di Falloppio spesso erano presenti bilateralmente. Quasi sempre si trova un utero infantile o rudimentale.

Sono stati descritti altri genotipi e fenotipi. Circa il 25% di 200 pazienti analizzati aveva un cromosoma Y dicentrico (45,X/46,X,dic Y). In alcuni pazienti il cromosoma Y può essere rappresentato solo da un frammento (45,X/45,X +fra); l'applicazione di specifiche prove per Y può stabilirne l'origine. Non è chiaro come lo stesso genotipo (45,X/46,XY) possa essere responsabile di fenotipi diversi: in alcuni pazienti sono state descritte mutazioni del gene *SRY*.

I bambini con un fenotipo femminile di solito vengono cresciuti senza problemi. Pazienti solo modestamente virilizzati sono di solito stati cresciuti come femmine, prima di arrivare alla diagnosi. Pazienti con ambiguità dei genitali vengono facilmente confusi con vari tipi di alterazioni dello sviluppo sessuale maschile. In molti casi, ma non in tutti, questi bambini sono cresciuti più facilmente come femmine; la bassa statura, la facilità della ricostruzione dei genitali e la predisposizione della gonade allo sviluppo di neoplasia favoriscono questa scelta. In alcuni pazienti seguiti fino all'età adulta, il normale testicolo putativo dimostra di essere disgenetico, con eventuale perdita della funzione delle cellule di Leydig e del Sertoli (vedi anche Capitolo 584). In uno studio su 22 pazienti australiani con disgenesia gonadica mista, non sono state trovate significative correlazioni o associazioni tra fenotipi interni ed esterni o funzione endocrina e caratteristiche morfologiche gonadiche. La scelta di crescere un bambino come maschio o femmine è stata determinata dall'aspetto dei genitali esterni. In 11 pazienti, i livelli di testosterone basale e dopo stimolazione con gonadotropina corionica umana erano inferiori rispetto ai soggetti di controllo.

Tumori gonadici, di solito **gonadoblastomi**, si verificano in circa il 25% di questi bambini. Un locus per il gonadoblastoma è stato localizzato in una regione vicina al centromero del cromosoma Y (GBY). Questi tumori a cellule germinali sono preceduti da modificazioni del carcinoma *in situ*. Di conseguenza, devono essere rimosse entrambe le gonadi in tutti i pazienti allevati come femmine e la gonade indifferenziata in quelli cresciuti come maschi.

Non c'è rapporto tra la proporzione di linee cellulari 45,X/46,XY nel sangue e nei fibroblasti e il fenotipo. In passato, tutti i pazienti arrivavano all'osservazione clinica per le loro anomalie fenotipiche. Tuttavia, mosaicismo 45,X/46,XY è stato trovato in circa il 7% dei feti con vero mosaicismo cromosomico incontrato prima della nascita. Di 76 neonati con mosaicismo 45,X/46,XY diagnosticato prima della nascita, 72 avevano un normale fenotipo maschile, 1 aveva fenotipo femminile, e solo 3 maschi presentavano ipospadia. Di 12 maschi in cui sono state esaminate le gonadi, solo 3 erano anormali. Questi dati vanno tenuti in considerazione durante la consulenza a una famiglia in cui sia fatta diagnosi prenatale del feto 45,X/46,XY.

FEMMINE XXX, XXXX E XXXXX

FEMMINE XXX. L'assetto cromosomico 47,XXX (trisomia) è la più frequente anomalia cromosomica nel sesso femminile, che si verifica in circa 1 su 1000 femmine nate vive. Nel 68% dei casi questa condizione è causata da una non disgiunzione meiotica materna, ma la maggior parte dei 45,X e la metà dei 47,XXY sono causate da errori dei cromosomi sessuali paterni. Il fenotipo è quello di una femmina normale; non vengono riconosciuti neonati o bambini affetti.

Lo sviluppo sessuale e il menarca compaiono regolarmente. La maggior parte delle donne che affrontano una gravidanza partorisce neonati normali. A 2 anni si rendono evidenti ritardo dell'uso di parole e del linguaggio e in alcuni casi si evidenziano perdita della coordinazione, scarsi risultati scolastici e comportamento immaturo. Queste bambine tendono a essere alte e magre, manifestano disturbi comportamentali e sono assegnate a classi speciali. Con la RM ad alta risoluzione, 10 soggetti 47,XXX mostravano un minore volume dell'amigdala rispetto a 20 soggetti euploidi di controllo; anche 10 47,XXY avevano una riduzione del volume dell'amigdala. In un'analisi di 155 femmine, il 62% era psichicamente normale. In questa sindrome è presente una spiccata variabilità e una piccola percentuale di femmine colpite è coordinata, socievole e con un'istruzione superiore.

FEMMINE XXXX E XXXXX. La grande maggioranza delle femmine con questi rari cariotipi presenta ritardo mentale. Frequentemente si associano epicanto, ipertelorismo, clinodattilia, pieghe palmari traverse, sinostosi radioulnare e patologia cardiaca congenita. La maturazione sessuale è spesso incompleta e in alcune può mancare. Tre donne con la sindrome da tetra-X hanno partorito, ma non sono riportate gravidanze in donne 49,XXXXX. La maggior parte delle donne 48,XXXX tendono a essere alte, con un'altezza media di 169 cm, mentre la bassa statura è caratteristica del fenotipo 49,XXXXX.

SINDROME DI NOONAN

Femmine con la sindrome di Noonan mostrano certe anomalie presenti anche in bambine 45,X con sindrome di Turner, ma hanno normali cromosomi 46,XX. Le anomalie più comuni sono le stesse di quelle di maschi con sindrome di Noonan (vedi Capitolo 584.1). Il fenotipo differisce dalla sindrome di Turner per diversi aspetti. Spesso è presente ritardo mentale; più spesso la patologia cardiaca è rappresentata da stenosi valvolare polmonare o da difetto settale atriale, piuttosto che da alterazioni aortiche; di solito compare normale maturazione sessuale, ma con un ritardo in media di 2 anni, ed è stata riportata insufficienza ovarica precoce.

ALTRI DIFETTI OVARICI

Alcune giovani donne senza anomalie cromosomiche hanno gonadi nastriformi che possono occasionalmente contenere o meno cellule germinali. Le gonadotropine sono elevate. Farmaci citotossici, specialmente agenti alchilanti come ciclofosfamide e busulfan, procarbazina, etoposide, e l'esposizione ovarica a irradiazione per il trattamento di neoplasie sono cause frequenti di insufficienza ovarica. Giovani donne con la malattia di Hodgkin dimostrano che la combinazione di chemioterapia e irradiazione pelvica può essere più nociva delle due terapie eseguite singolarmente. Dopo irradiazione o chemioterapia combinata, le adolescenti mantengono o recuperano la funzionalità ovarica con più facilità rispetto alle donne più anziane; dopo il trattamento sono possibili gravidanze normali.

L'attuale regime terapeutico comporta alcuni danni ovarici nella maggior parte delle ragazze trattate per neoplasia. La LD50 per l'ovocita umano è circa 4 Gy; dosi basse di 6 Gy hanno prodotto amenorrea primaria. La trasposizione ovarica nelle bambine prima dell'irradiazione pelvica e addominale può essere in grado di preservare la funzione dell'ovaio, diminuendo la sua esposizione a meno di 4-7 Gy.

L'**insufficienza ovarica autoimmune** si verifica nel 60% delle ragazze con più di di 13 anni con poliendocrinopatia autoimmune di tipo I (malattia di Addison, ipoparatiroidismo, candidosi). Questa patologia, conosciuta anche come sindrome polighiandolare autoimmune (*PolyGlandural Autoimmune Disease*, PGAD) di tipo I, è rara in tutto il mondo, ma non in Finlandia, dove si verifica in 1 su 25 000 persone, come risultato dell'effetto di un gene fondatore. Il gene per questa malattia è localizzato sul cromosoma 21 ed è associato a HLA-DR5. In pazienti con PGAD-1 e insufficienza ovarica, è stata descritta un'associazione a HLA-A3. Le bambine non presentano sviluppo sessuale o, nelle giovani donne, compare amenorrea secondaria. Le ovaie possono evidenziare infiltrazione linfocitica o presentarsi nastriformi. La maggior parte delle pazienti presenta anticorpi circolanti contro le cellule steroidee e autoanticorpi contro la 21-idrossilasi. Fra le pazienti con sindromi polighiandolare autoimmuni, il 5% manifesta ipogonadismo.

La malattia si verifica anche in giovani donne come evento isolato o in associazione ad altre patologie autoimmuni, con amenorrea secondaria (cioè insufficienza ovarica precoce, *Premature Ovarian Failure*, POF). Si verifica nello 0,2-0,9% delle giovani donne con meno di 40 anni. L'insufficienza ovarica precoce è una patologia eterogenea con cause diverse: cromosomiche, genetiche, enzimatiche, infettive e iatrogeniche. Quando si associa a patologia surrenalica autoimmunitaria, sono presenti anticorpi diretti contro le cellule a secrezione steroidea. Questi anticorpi reagiscono con P450scc e enzimi 17α-OH, o 21-OH. Quando si associa con altre patologie endocrine e non endocrine, ma non con forme surrenaliche autoimmuni, raramente si ritrovano anticorpi anticellule steroidee. Una seconda patologia autoimmune, spesso subclinica, è stata trovata nel 10-39% delle pazienti adulte con POF. Una diciassettenne con porpora idiopatica trombocitopenica e 47,XXX aveva POF autoimmune. Pazienti con POF non presentano i deficit neurocognitivi presenti nella sindrome di Turner.

La **galattosemia**, particolarmente la forma classica della malattia, di solito comporta danno ovarico, che comincia durante la vita intrauterina. I livelli di FSH e di ormone luteinizzante (LH) sono precocemente elevati. Il danno ovarico può essere dovuto a deficit di UDP-galattosio (vedi Capitolo 87). La **sindrome di Denys-Drash**, causata da mutazione WT1, può manifestare disgenesia gonadica.

L'**atassia-teleangectasia** può essere associata a ipoplasia ovarica e gonadotropine elevate e la causa è sconosciuta. In poche bambine sono comparsi gonadoblastomi e disgerminomi.

Si ritiene che l'ipergonadismo ipogonadotropo si verifichi anche per resistenza da parte delle ovaie a gonadotropine endogene ed esogene (sindrome di Savage). Si verifica anche in donne con POF. Questa condizione può essere causata da anticorpi antiovaio o anomalie del recettore per l'FSH. Sono state descritte mutazioni del gene del recettore dell'FSH a trasmissione autosomica recessiva (vedi anche "Disgenesia gonadica"). In poche femmine 46,XX con amenorrea primaria e ipergonadotropinemia, esistono mutazioni inattivanti del gene del recettore dell'LH. Questo lascia ipotizzare che l'azione dell'LH sia necessaria per il normale sviluppo follicolare e la normale ovulazione. Altri difetti genetici associati a insufficienza ovarica comprendono mutazioni di *FOXL2*, *GNAS*, *CYP17* e *CYP19*.

587.2 • IPOGONADISMO IPOGONADOTROPO NELLA FEMMINA (IPOGONADISMO SECONDARIO)

L'ipofunzione ovarica può essere provocata da un deficit di secrezione delle gonadotropine. Il difetto può risiedere nell'ipofisi anteriore o, più frequentemente, nell'ipotalamo.

EZIOLOGIA

Ipopituitarismo (vedi anche Capitolo 558). Lesioni congenite o acquisite dell'ipofisi o di zone a essa adiacenti quasi sempre comportano un'alterazione della secrezione delle gonadotropine e di altri ormoni ipofisari. In bambini con deficit multipli degli ormoni ipofisari, compreso il deficit di gonadotropine, sono stati descritti difetti del fattore di trascrizione ipofisario come di PROP-1.

In bambini con ipopituitarismo idiopatico, il difetto è normalmente a livello ipotalamico. In questi pazienti, la somministrazione di ormone di rilascio delle gonadotropine (GnRH) porta a un aumento dei livelli di FSH e LH, dimostrando l'integrità dell'ipofisi.

Deficit isolato di gonadotropine. È stato possibile definire questo gruppo eterogeneo di patologie con l'aiuto del test al GnRH. Nella maggior parte dei bambini, l'ipofisi è normale e il difetto è localizzato a livelli ipotalamico.

Sono stati riportati parecchi casi sporadici di **anosmia** con ipogonadismo ipogonadotropo. Le femmine ipogonadiche con anosmia sono state descritte in famiglie con sindrome di Kallmann, ma l'ipogonadismo colpisce più frequentemente i maschi di queste famiglie. Sono descritte mutazioni del gene per la subunità β dell'FSH e dell'LH.

Alcune patologie autosomiche recessive come la sindrome di Laurence-Moon-Biedl, la sindrome da lentiggini multiple e la sindrome di Carpenter, compaiono in vari casi comprendenti deficit gonadotropinico. Bambine con sindrome di Prader-Willi hanno ipogonadismo ipogonadotropo. Bambine con talassemia grave presentano deficit da danno ipofisario causato da cronico aumento del ferro, secondario a trasfusioni multiple. L'anoressia nervosa frequentemente si associa a ipogonadismo ipogonadotropo (vedi Capitolo 27).

DIAGNOSI. La diagnosi può essere semplice in pazienti con altri deficit di ormoni ipofisari, ma nei maschi è difficile differenziare un ipogonadismo ipogonadotropo isolato da una forma psicologica di pubertà ritardata. La ripetizione delle misurazioni di FSH e LH, particolarmente durante il sonno, può rivelare un iniziale incremento dei livelli gonadotropinici, che annuncia le prime fasi della pubertà. Il test di stimolazione con GnRH o con uno dei suoi analoghi può aiutare la diagnosi.

SINDROME DELL'OVAIO POLICISTICO (SINDROME DI STEIN-LEVENTHAL)

La sindrome classica dell'ovaio policistico (*Classical Polycystic Ovary Syndrome*, PCOS) è caratterizzata da obesità, irsutismo e amenorrea secondaria, con ipertrofia bilaterale delle ovaie, ma queste manifestazioni possono non essere tutte presenti (vedi anche Capitolo 552). L'esordio di solito si verifica alla pubertà o poco dopo; i segni più frequenti sono irregolarità mestruali e irsutismo. Negli anni riproduttivi, questa malattia è la causa più comune di infertilità anovulatoria. Si sono utilizzati molti termini per descrivere questa patologia: iperandrogenismo ovarico funzionale e, soprattutto nelle donne adulte, anovulazione cronica iperandrogenica. C'è un rapporto molto stretto tra l'adrenarca prematuro e il successivo sviluppo di PCOS. L'ipertrofia ovarica spesso può essere apprezzata con la palpazione combinata rettale e addominale e quasi sempre risulta evidente all'indagine ecografica (vedi Capitolo 552).

La causa della malattia, nella maggior parte delle pazienti, è incerta nonostante le indagini accurate. La PCOS è una patologia eterogenea che può associarsi a parecchie entità distinte, come il deficit di 21-idrossilasi, il deficit di 3β-idrossistroido deidrogenasi e il deficit di 17-chetoreduttasi ovarica, l'enzima che converte l'androstenedione in testosterone e l'estrone in estradiolo. La conversione del colesterolo in pregnenolone da parte dell'enzima P450scc per la scissione della catena laterale del colesterolo, codificato dal gene *CYP11A*, si verifica dopo che il colesterolo entra nel mitocondrio aiutato da una proteina regolatoria acuta steroidogenetica (*Steroidogenic Acute Regulatory Protein*, StAR). DAX1 può reprimere l'espressione del gene StAR, e SF-1 regola SF-1. Anomalie di *CYP11A* o di *DAX1* sono state trovate in donne irsute iperandrogeniche con o senza disturbi mestruali. Nella maggior parte delle pazienti con PCOS, gli elevati livelli plasmatici di testosterone libero o androstenedione non vengono soppressi dal desametasone, escludendo una patogenesi surrenalica. In alcune pazienti, i livelli sierici di testosterone totale possono non essere elevati, ma lo sono quelli di testosterone libero, con marcata diminuzione delle globuline di trasporto. Circa il 75% delle pazienti presenta un aumento del rapporto LH/FSH, un aumento dell'ampiezza e della frequenza dei livelli plasmatici di LH e una esagerata risposta al GnRH. I livelli di inibina B sono basalmente elevati e perdono la normale pulsatilità. Le ragazze in età premenarcale possono avere un rialzo diurno precoce dell'LH, maggiore di quello caratteristico notturno. Si ritiene che le alterazioni della secrezione di LH determinino iperplasia delle cellule tecali, arresto dello sviluppo follicolare e diminuzione della produzione di estradiolo. L'anormale sviluppo follicolare, uno dei segni distintivi della PCOS, può essere correlato alla disregolazione del fattore 9 di differenziazione e crescita dell'ovocita (GDF-9), ma non al fattore-15 morfogenetico osseo (BMP-15), entrambi noti come fattori di crescita ovocitaria. Questi effetti portano a iperandrogenismo e cicli irregolari o amenorrea. In bambine con sindromi virilizzanti congenite, l'asse ipotalamo-ipofisario appare programmato per un'ipersecrezione di LH al momento della pubertà, con conseguente iperandrogenismo anche quando si pensa che gli androgeni surrenalici siano adeguatamente soppressi. Molti comuni polimorfismi nel promoter del gene dell'interleuchina 6 sono associati a iperandrogenismo.

Esiste un'associazione tra **iperandrogenismo e insulino-resistenza.** Specialmente nelle pazienti obese, la PCOS può essere associata a iperinsulinismo, insulino-resistenza e acanthosis nigricans. In ragione dell'alta frequenza di PCOS, è necessario elencare almeno le condizioni più comuni associate a intolleranza glicidica e a diabete mellito di tipo 2. Adolescenti con PCOS tendono a manifestare una notevole incidenza di alterata tolleranza glucidica. L'insulino-resistenza è correlata a eccessiva fosforilazione della serina del recettore insulinico. Lo stesso processo, cioè la fosforilazione serinica, è importante nel regolare l'attività di P450c17, un enzima maggiore coinvolto nella biosintesi androgenica. Tuttavia, alcuni hanno ipotizzato che questo difetto sia l'unica anomalia nella PCOS, responsabile sia di insulino-resistenza sia di iperandrogenismo. Variazioni del gene che codifica la calpaina 10 cisteina proteasi, possono associarsi ad aumentata suscettibilità al diabete tipo 2. L'alotipo 112/121 è associato a livelli di insulina e rischio due volte maggiore di PCOS in donne afroamericane e bianche.

Per la **diagnosi** di PCOS è utile la misurazione dei livelli plasmatici di LH, FSH, prolattina, testosterone libero, globulina di trasporto degli ormoni sessuali, deidroepiandrosterone solfato (DHEAs). Fratelli di donne con PCOS hanno elevati livelli di DHEAS, mentre nelle sorelle di pazienti con PCOS, i marker dell'insulino-resistenza (iperinsulinemia a digiuno e diminuzione del rapporto tra glucosio e insulina durante il digiuno) sono associati a iperandrogenismo, ma non a irregolarità mestruali. La valutazione dell'insulino-resistenza, tuttavia, può subire delle significative variazioni personali in donne con PCOS. Per distinguere un iperandrogenismo di origine surrenalica da uno di origine ovarica, si sono utilizzate una stimolazione complessa e una inibizione farmacologica. I livelli basali e dopo stimolazione con ormone adrenocorticotropo di steroidi surrenalici possono rivelare lievi difetti della steroidogenesi surrenalica.

Si ipotizza un deficit di 17-chetoreduttasi quando sono ammalate anche le sorelle o quando sono aumentati i rapporti estrone:estradiolo e androstenedione:testosterone. Donne trattate con valproato per epilessia prima dell'età di 20 anni presentano spesso PCOS e ipertestosteronemia, ma normali livelli di LH.

In pazienti con PCOS sono stati studiati i geni candidati alla regolazione, biosintesi, trasporto e azione degli androgeni e comprendono *SF1*, *DAX1*, proteina *StAR*, *CYP17*, *CYP11B2*, *CYP21*, *CYP19*, *HSD3B2*, *HSD17B*, *LHβ*, *FSHβ*, recettore dell'FSH, recettori del GnRH, dopamina, glicocorticoidi e androgeni e SHBG.

La **base della terapia** è la soppressione ovarica con contraccettivi orali contenenti un progestinico non androgenico, come il desogestrel. Lo spironolattone, in aggiunta ai contraccettivi orali, ha rappresentato il pilastro farmacologico negli Stati Uniti per diminuire l'irsutismo. La soppressione può essere ottenuta anche con testolattone, un composto con proprietà antiandrogeniche e debolmente progestiniche. L'elettrolisi e la laser terapia sono la base del trattamento non farmacologico dell'irsutismo. È importante fare attenzione all'eventuale presenza di obesità, perché la sua correzione spesso porta al miglioramento dell'insulino-resistenza. Si sono cominciati a usare antidiabetici utilizzati nel diabete di tipo 2, per migliorare l'insulino-resistenza in donne con PCOS. I farmaci insulino-sensibilizzanti come la metformina e il troglitazone diminuiscono l'iperinsulinemia e l'iperandrogenismo ovarico. Tre mesi di terapia con metformina migliorano l'insulino-resistenza e l'esagerata risposta androgenica alla somministrazione di ACTH. Il trattamento con D-chiro-inositolo nelle donne con PCOS migliora l'azione insulinica, migliorando così anche l'azione ovarica, e diminuisce i livelli androgenici. Questo approccio stimola l'azione postrecettoriale dell'insulina. Il naltrexone, un antagonista degli oppioidi, diminuisce la secrezione insulinica nelle pazienti iperinsulinemiche con PCOS.

Aittomaki K, Lucena JLD, Pakarinen P, et al: Mutation in the follicle-stimulating hormone receptor gene causes hereditary hypergonadotropic ovarian failure. *Cell* 1995;82:959–968.

Arslanian SA, Lewy V, Danadian K, et al: Metformin therapy in obese adolescents with polycystic ovary syndrome and impaired glucose tolerance: Amelioration of exaggerated adrenal response to adrenocorticotropin with

reduction of insulinemia/insulin resistance. *J Clin Endocrinol Metab* 2002; 87:1555–1559.
Berdahl LD, Wenstrom KD, Hanson JW: Web neck anomaly and its association with congenital heart disease. *Am J Med Genet* 1995;56:304–307.
Betterle C, Volpato M: Adrenal and ovarian autoimmunity. *Eur J Endocrinol* 1998;138:16–25.
Binder G, Kock A, Wajs E, et al: Nested polymerase chain reaction study of 53 cases with Turner syndrome: Is cytogenetically undetected Y mosaicism common? *J Clin Endocrinol Metab* 1995;80:3532–3536.
Bondy CA: Care of girls and women with Turner Syndrome: A guideline of the Turner syndrome study group. *J Clin Endo Metab* 2007;92:10–25.
Calvo RM, Asuncion M, Telleria D, et al: Screening for mutations in the steroidogenic acute regulatory protein and steroidogenic factor-1 genes, and in CYP11A and dosage-sensitive sex reversal-adrenal hypoplasia gene on the X chromosome, gene-1 (DAX-1), in hyperandrogenic hirsute women. *J Clin Endocrinol Metab* 2001;86:1746–1749.
Carel JC, Mathivon L, Gendrel C, et al: Near normalization of final height with adapted doses of growth hormone in Turner syndrome. *J Clin Endocrinol Metab* 1998;83:1462–1466.
Chang HJ, Clark RD, Bachman H: The phenotype of 45,X/46,XY mosaicism: An analysis of 92 prenatally diagnosed cases. *Am J Hum Genet* 1990; 46:156–167.
De la Chesnayae E, Canto P, Ulloa-Aguirre A, et al: No evidence of mutations in the follicle-stimulating hormone receptor gene in Mexican women with 46,XX pure gonadal dysgenesis. *Am J Med Genet* 2001;98:125–128.
Doherty E, Pakarinen P, Tiitinen A, et al: A novel mutation in the FSH receptor inhibiting signal transduction and causing primary ovarian failure. *J Clin Endocrinol Metab* 2002;87:1151–1155.
Dunaif A: Insulin resistance and the polycystic ovary syndrome: Mechanism and implications for pathogenesis. *Endocr Rev* 1997;18:774–800.
Ehrmann DA, Schwarz PEH, Hara M, et al: Relationship of calpain-10 genotype to phenotype features of polycystic ovary syndrome. *J Clin Endocrinol Metab* 2002;87:1669–1673.
Escobar-Morreale HF, Luque-Ramírez M, San Millán JL: The molecular-genetic basis of functional hyperandrogenism and the polycystic ovary syndrome. *Endocr Rev* 2005;26:251–282.
Gicquel C, Gaston V, Cabrol S, et al: Assessment of Turner syndrome by molecular analysis of the X chromosome in growth-retarded girls. *J Clin Endocrinol Metab* 1998;83:1472–1476.
Gravholt CH, Fedder J, Naeraa RW, et al: Occurrence of gonadoblastoma in females with Turner syndrome and Y chromosome material: A population study. *J Clin Endocrinol Metab* 2000;85:3199–3202.
Hoek A, Schoemaker J, Drexhage HA: Premature ovarian failure and ovarian autoimmunity. *Endocr Rev* 1997;18:107–134.
Holland CM: 47,XXX in an adolescent with premature ovarian failure and autoimmune disease. *J Pediatr Adolesc Gynecol* 2001;14:77–80.
Iezzoni JC, Kap-Herr CV, Golden W, et al: Gonadoblastomas in 45,X/46,XY mosaicism. *Am J Clin Pathol* 1997;108:197–203.
Jayagopal V, Kilpatrick ES, Holding S, et al: The biological variation of insulin resistance in polycystic ovarian syndrome. *J Clin Endocrinol Metab* 2002;87:1560–1562.
Lin AE, Lippe B, Rosenfeld RD: Further delineation of aortic dilation, dissection, and rupture in patients with Turner syndrome. *Pediatrics* 1998;102: e12.
Linssen WH, van den Bent MJ, Brunner HG, et al: Deafness, sensory neuropathy, and ovarian dysgenesis: A new syndrome or a broader spectrum of Perrault syndrome? *Am J Med Genet* 1994;51:81–82.
Mazzanti L, Cacciari E, Bergamaschi R, et al: Pelvic ultrasonography in patients with Turner syndrome: Age-related findings in different karyotypes. *J Pediatr* 1997;131:135–140.
Melner MH, Feltus FA: Autoimmune premature ovarian failure–endocrine aspects of a T-cell disease: Review. *Endocrinology* 1999;140:3401–3403.
Merke DP, Tajima T, Baron J, et al: Hypogonadotropic hypogonadism in a female caused by an X-linked recessive mutation in the Dax1 gene. *N Engl J Med* 1999;340:1248–1252.
Migeon BR, Luo S, Jani M, et al: The severe phenotype of females with tiny ring X chromosomes are associated with inability of these chromosomes to undergo X inactivation. *Am J Med Genet* 1994;55:497–504.
Nester J, Jakubowicz D, Reamer P, et al: Ovulatory and metabolic effects of D-chiro-inositol in polycystic ovary syndrome. *N Engl J Med* 1999;340: 1314–1320.
Palmert MR, Gordon CM, Kartashov AI, et al: Screening for abnormal glucose tolerance in adolescent with polycystic ovary syndrome. *J Clin Endocrinol Metab* 2002;87:1017–1023.
Pasquino AM, Passeri F, Pucarelli I, et al: Spontaneous pubertal development in Turner syndrome. *J Clin Endocrinol Metab* 1997;82:1810–1813.
Patwardham AJ, Brown WE, Bender BG, et al: Reduced size of the amygdala in individuals with 47,XXY and 47,XXX karyotypes. *Am J Med Genet* 2002;114:93–98.
Quigley CA, Crowe BJ, Anglin DG, et al: Growth hormone and low dose estrogen in Turner syndrome: Results of a United States multi-center trial to near-final height. *J Clin Endocrinol Metab* 2002;87:2033–2041.
Rongen-Westerlaken C, Corel K, van den Broeck J, et al: Reference values for height, height velocity and weight in Turner syndrome. *Acta Paediatr* 1997; 86:937–942.
Rosenfeld R, Devine N, Julius Hunold J, et al: Treatment of girls with Turner syndrome (TS) with very low doses of estrogen beginning at 12 years enhances the growth-promoting effect of GH. *J Clin Endocrinol Metab* 2005;90:6424–6430.
Ross JL, Roeltgen D, Feuillan P, et al: Use of estrogen in young girls with Turner syndrome. *Neurology* 2000;54:164–170.
Schorry EK, Lovell AM, Milatovich A, et al: Ullrich-Turner syndrome and neurofibromatosis-1. *Am J Med Genet* 1996;66:423–425.
Seashore MR, Cho S, Desposito F, et al, American Academy of Pediatrics Committee on Genetics: Health supervision for children with Turner syndrome. *Pediatrics* 1995;96:1166–1173.
Sempe M, Hansson Bodallaz C, Limoni C: Growth curves in untreated Ullrich-Turner syndrome: French reference standards 1–22 years. *Eur J Pediatr* 1996;155:862–869.
Sybert VP: Cardiovascular malformations and complications in Turner syndrome. *Pediatrics* 1998;101:E11.
Telvi L, Lebar A, DelPino O, et al: 45,X/46,XY mosaicism: Report of 27 cases. *Pediatrics* 1999;104:304–308.
Thibaud E, Ramirez M, Brauner R, et al: Preservation of ovarian function by ovarian transposition performed before pelvic irradiation during childhood. *J Pediatr* 1992;121:880–884.

Capitolo 588 ■ Pseudoprecocità da lesioni dell'ovaio

I tumori ovarici sono rari in ambito pediatrico, con una frequenza di 2,6/100 000. La maggior parte delle masse ovariche è di origine benigna, ma il 10-30% può essere maligno. Le neoplasie ovariche maligne, che rappresentano i più comuni tumori genitali dell'adolescenza, ammontano all'1% delle neoplasie dell'infanzia. Più del 60% è rappresentato da neoplasie a cellule germinali, soprattutto disgerminomi, che possono secernere marker tumorali e ormoni (vedi Capitolo 503). Il 5-10% di questi si verifica in fenotipi femminili con anomalie gonadiche associate alla presenza del cromosoma sessuale Y. Il secondo gruppo più comune è rappresentato dai tumori delle cellule epiteliali (circa il 20%) e subito dopo (10%) si trovano i tumori dei cordoni sessuali/stromali (a cellule della granulosa, cellule del Sertoli e tumori mesenchimali). Nelle neoplasie ovariche si trovano molti marker, compresi α-fetoproteina, gonadotropina corionica umana hCG, antigene carcinoembrionale, oncoproteine, p105, p53, mutazioni di *KRAS*, ciclina D1, proteine e recettori epidermici correlati col fattore di crescita, catepsina B e altri. Nei tumori ovarici si sono trovati livelli variabili di espressione del gene della subunità inibina-attivina.

Lesioni funzionanti dell'ovaio consistono in cisti benigne o tumori maligni. La maggior parte sintetizza estrogeni; una piccola minoranza produce androgeni.

LESIONI ESTROGENE DELL'OVAIO. Queste lesioni provocano precocità isosessuale, ma costituiscono solo una piccola percentuale di tutti i casi di precocità. Le cisti ovariche follicolari benigne sono i tumori più frequenti associati a pubertà precoce isosessuale nelle femmine; raramente sono gonadotropino-dipendenti.

Tumore giovanile delle cellule della granulosa. Nell'infanzia, il più comune tumore ovarico con manifestazioni estrogeniche è il tumore a cellule della granulosa, sebbene esso costituisca l'1-10% di tutte le neoplasie ovariche. Queste neoplasie hanno caratteristiche istologiche distintive che li differenziano da quelle delle età successive (tumori delle cellule della granulosa dell'adulto). Le cellule presentano elevata attività mitotica, i follicoli sono spesso irregolari, sono rari i corpi di Call-Exner ed è frequente la luteinizzazione. Questo tumore può essere solido o cistico o avere caratteristiche di entrambi. Di solito è benigno. In pochi casi può essere associato a encondromi multipli (**malattia di Ollier**) e a emangiomi sottocutanei multipli (**sindrome di Maffucci**).

Manifestazioni cliniche e diagnosi. Questo tumore, osservato anche in neonati, può manifestarsi a 2 anni o anche a meno, con un quadro di precocità sessuale; circa la metà di questi tumori compare prima dei 10 anni. L'età media al momento della diagnosi è di 7,5 anni. I tumori sono quasi sempre monolaterali. Le mammelle cominciano ad aumentare di volume, diventano tondeggianti e sode, con capezzoli prominenti. I genitali esterni assomigliano a quelli di una ragazza normale alla pubertà, inoltre anche l'utero aumenta di volume. Una perdita vaginale biancastra è seguita da una mestruazione irregolare o ciclica. Non si verifica però l'ovulazione. La manifestazione di esordio può essere rappresentata da dolore o tumefazione addominale. I peli pubici sono solitamente assenti, eccetto i casi con modesta virilizzazione.

Nella maggior parte delle bambine, quando si rende evidente il quadro di precocità sessuale, risulta palpabile una massa nella regione addominale inferiore. Il tumore, però, può essere anche piccolo e sfuggire alla palpazione pur eseguendo un attento esame addominale e rettale. Si ricorre in questi casi all'indagine ecografica, anche se è più sensibile la TC multidetector. La maggior parte di questi tumori (90%) è diagnosticata a stadi di malignità molto precoci (stadio I FIGO [International Federation of Gynecology and Obstetrics]).

I livelli plasmatici di estradiolo sono notevolmente elevati. Quelli di gonadotropine sono soppressi e non rispondono alla stimolazione con GnRH. I livelli di ormone antimülleriano (AMH), inibina e α-fetoproteina sono elevati. Nel 30% dei casi si sono trovate mutazioni attivanti di Gsα e nei tumori più aggressivi è contenuta l'espressione GATA-4, mentre i livelli di AMH sono inversamente proporzionali alle dimensioni del tumore. Lo sviluppo osseo è moderatamente avanzato.

Trattamento e prognosi. Una volta stabilita la diagnosi, il tumore deve essere asportato al più presto. La prognosi è eccellente, poiché nei bambini meno del 5% di questi tumori è maligno. Tuttavia, tumori scoperti in stadi avanzati si comportano in modo aggressivo e richiedono difficili decisioni circa l'approccio chirurgico, l'utilizzo di radioterapia e chemioterapia. Negli adulti con tumori delle cellule della granulosa, l'espressione p53 si associa a prognosi sfavorevole. Immediatamente dopo l'asportazione chirurgica della neoplasia, è frequente il sanguinamento vaginale. I segni di pubertà precoce si riducono e possono scomparire in pochi mesi dopo l'intervento. La secrezione estrogenica ritorna normale.

Il tumore del cordone sessuale con tubuli anulari è una forma distinta, derivata dalle cellule della granulosa, che si verifica principalmente in pazienti con la sindrome di Peutz-Jeghers. Si tratta di neoplasie multifocali, bilaterali e solitamente benigne. La presenza di calcificazioni è ecograficamente utile. In questi tumori, l'incremento della produzione di aromatasi comporta una pubertà precoce gonadotropino-indipendente. I livelli di inibina A e B sono elevati e diminuiscono dopo l'asportazione chirurgica. In uno studio, 9 dei 13 tumori dei cordoni sessuali/stromali presentavano mutazioni dei recettori dell'ormone follicolo-stimolante (FSH), facendo ipotizzare un ruolo di questa mutazione nello sviluppo della neoplasia.

Il **corionepitelioma** è un tumore raro. Questa neoplasia ad alta malignità deriva da un preesistente teratoma. Il tumore, di solito monolaterale, produce grandi quantità di hCG, che stimola l'ovaio controlaterale a secernere estrogeni e progesterone. Elevati livelli di hCG sono diagnostici.

Cisti follicolare. Piccole cisti ovariche (<0,7 cm di diametro) sono comuni nelle bambine in epoca prepubere. Alla pubertà e in bambine con pubertà precoce isosessuale vera spesso si manifestano cisti di dimensioni maggiori (1-6 cm), secondarie a stimolazione gonadotropinica. Tuttavia, occasionalmente, simili cisti voluminose si evidenziano anche in giovani donne con pubertà precoce, in assenza di FSH e di LH. Dato che la rimozione chirurgica o l'involuzione spontanea delle cisti comporta la regressione delle modificazioni puberali, si dubita che esse possano esserne la causa. Il meccanismo di produzione di queste cisti funzionanti in modo autonomo è sconosciuto. Le cisti si possono formare una sola volta, oppure scomparire e recidivare con conseguente "va' e vieni" dei segni di pubertà precoce. Possono essere mono o bilaterali. La precocità sessuale in giovani femmine con la **sindrome di McCune-Albright** è di solito associata a cisti follicolari autonome, dovute a mutazione attivante della proteina G negli stadi precoci delle sviluppo (vedi Capitolo 563.6) Le gonadotropine sono soppresse e i livelli di estradiolo sono di solito notevolmente elevati, ma possono fluttuare ampiamente e anche ritornare normali. La stimolazione con GnRH non provoca alcun incremento gonadotropinico. Dato che in queste bambine le gonadotropine sono soppresse, il meccanismo della stimolazione ovarica è sconosciuto. L'indagine ecografica costituisce l'esame elettivo per rilevare e monitorare queste cisti. Prima di un intervento di aspirazione della cisti o di cistectomia è preferibile un breve periodo di osservazione, per verificare la risoluzione spontanea o meno della patologia. Nella diagnosi differenziale vanno tenute in considerazione le neoplasie cistiche.

LESIONI ANDROGENE DELL'OVAIO. I tumori ovarici virilizzanti sono rari a tutte le età, ma particolarmente nelle bambine in età prepubere. In una neonata di 14 giorni è stato riportato un caso di **arrenoblastoma**, ma in letteratura ci sono pochi casi di bambine colpite a un'età inferiore ai 16 anni.

Il **gonadoblastoma** compare esclusivamente in gonadi disgenetiche, particolarmente nei fenotipi femminili con un cromosoma Y (46,XY; 45,X/46,XY; 45,X/46,X-fra). Il tumore è bilaterale. In certi casi, ma non sempre, compare virilizzazione. Le caratteristiche cliniche sono simili a quelle descritte nei tumori surrenalici virilizzanti e comprendono accelerazione della crescita, acne, ipertrofia clitoridea e crescita dei peli sessuali. Solo nel 50% delle pazienti è palpabile una massa addominale. I livelli plasmatici di testosterone e androstenedione sono elevati, mentre sono soppressi quelli delle gonadotropine. Ecografia, TC, RM sono in grado di localizzare la lesione. La gonade disgenetica del fenotipo femminile con cromosoma Y va rimossa a scopo precauzionale. Quando viene asportato un tumore monolaterale, va rimossa anche la gonade disgenetica controlaterale. In uno studio immuno-istochimico di due gonadoblastomi, si è dimostrata espressione di WT1, p53, MIS e anche di inibina.

Manifestazioni di virilizzazione si verificano occasionalmente in femmine con **tumori giovanili delle cellule della granulosa**. Residui surrenalici e tumori delle cellule ilari raramente sono virilizzanti. Nei tumori ovarici (e testicolari) sono state descritte mutazioni attivanti dei geni della proteina G. Mutazioni di *GSP*, presenti di solito in tumori gonadici associati a **sindrome di McCune-Albright**, sono state osservate anche in 4 di 6 neoplasie a cellule di Leydig (tre ovarici e uno testicolare). Di dieci tumori studiati, solo in due a cellule della granulosa e in un tecoma sono state trovate mutazioni *GIP-2*.

I **tumori delle cellule di Sertoli-Leydig**, rare neoplasie del cordone sessuale/stroma, costituiscono meno dell'1% dei tumori ovarici. L'età media alla diagnosi è 25 anni; meno del 5% di questi tumori compare prima della pubertà. I livelli di AFP possono essere modicamente elevati. In un bambino di 12 mesi con tumore a cellule di Sertoli-Leydig, che manifestava precocità isosessuale, il solo marker tumorale rilevabile era rappresentato dai livelli sierici di inibina, con aumento delle subnità A e B. La sopravvivenza a 5 anni è del 70-90%.

In 102 pazienti consecutivi sottoposti ad intervento chirurgico per masse ovariche in un periodo di 15 anni, i sintomi di presentazione erano dolore addominale acuto nel 56% e massa pelvica o addominale nel 22%. Di 9 bambini operati per malignità, 3 avevano un disgerminoma, 2 un teratoma, 2 un tumore a cellule della granulosa, 1 un tumore a cellule di Sertoli-Leydig e infine 1 un tumore del sacco vitellino.

Anttonen M, Unkila-Kallio L, Leminen A, et al: High GATA-4 expression associates with aggressive behavior, whereas low anti-Müllerian hormone expression associates with growth potential of ovarian granulosa cell tumors. *J Clin Endocrinol Metab* 2005;90:6529–6535.
Calaminus G, Wessalowski R, Harms D, et al: Juvenile granulosa cell tumors of the ovary in children and adolescents: Results from 33 patients registered in a prospective cooperative study. *Gynecol Oncol* 1997;65:447–452.
Cass DL, Hawkins E, Brandt ML, et al: Surgery for ovarian masses in infants, children, and adolescents: 102 Consecutive patients treated in a 15-year period. *J Pediatr Surg* 2001;36:693–699.
Choong CS, Fuller PJ, Chu S, et al: Sertoli-Leydig cell tumor of the ovary, a rare cause of precocious puberty in a 12 month-old infant. *J Clin Endocrinol Metab* 2002;87:49–56.
Fink D, Kubik-Huch RA, Wildermuth S: Juvenile granulosa cell tumor. *Abdom Imaging* 2001;26:550–552.
Fotiou SK: Ovarian malignancies in adolescence. *Ann NY Acad Sci* 1997;816:338–346.
Kalfa, N, Ecochard A, Patte C, et al: Activating mutations of the stimulatory G protein in juvenile ovarian granulosa cell tumors: A new prognostic factor? *J Clin Endocrinol Metab* 2006;91:1842–1847.
Lazar EL, Stolar CJ: Evaluation and management of pediatric solid ovarian tumors. *Semin Pediatr Surg* 1998;7:29–34.
Powell JL, Connor GP, Henderson GS: Management of recurrent juvenile granulosa cell tumor of the ovary. *Gynecol Oncol* 2001;81:113–116.
Silverman LA, Gitelman SE: Immunoreactive inhibin, müllerian inhibitory substance, and activin as biochemical markers for juvenile granulosa cell tumors. *J Pediatr* 1996;129:918–921.
Stepanian M, Cohn D: Gynecologic malignancies in adolescents. *Adolesc Med* 2004;15:549–568.

Capitolo 589 ■ Disturbi dello sviluppo sessuale (intersessualità)

DIFFERENZIAZIONE SESSUALE (VEDI ANCHE CAPITOLO 583). Nel normale processo di differenziazione, la forma definitiva delle strutture sessuali dipende dalla presenza di normali cromosomi sessuali (o XX o XY). Per lo sviluppo di ovaie normali, sono necessari un complemento cromosomico 46,XX e fattori genetici come DAX1 e la molecola di segnalazione WNT-4. Lo sviluppo del fenotipo maschile è ancora più complesso e richiede la presenza del cromosoma Y e, specificamente, di un gene *SRY* intatto che, in associazione a geni quali *SOX9*, *SF1* e *WT1* e altri (vedi Capitolo 583), indirizzano la gonade indifferenziata verso una trasformazione testicolare. Ricombinazioni aberranti possono provocare la presenza, sui cromosomi X, del gene *SRY*, con formazione di maschi XX, oppure la perdita, sui cromosomi Y, di *SRY*, con formazione di femmine XY.

L'ormone antimülleriano (*Antimüllerian Hormone*, AMH), conosciuto anche come sostanza inibitrice mülleriana, il principale ormone testicolare prodotto nella sesta-settima settimana di gestazione, provoca la regressione dei dotti mülleriani; in sua assenza, essi persistono. L'attivazione di AMH nel testicolo richiede il gene *SF1*. Verso l'ottava settimana di gestazione, le cellule testicolari di Leydig cominciano a produrre testosterone. Durante questo periodo critico della differenziazione sessuale maschile, la secrezione di testosterone è stimolata dalla gonadotropina corionica umana placentare (hCG), che ha un picco a 8-12 settimane. Nella seconda metà della gravidanza, il testosterone viene mantenuto a livelli più bassi dall'ormone luteinizzante secreto dall'ipofisi fetale. Il testosterone dà l'avvio alla virilizzazione del dotto wolffiano in epididimo, vasi deferenti e vescicole seminali. Anche lo sviluppo dei genitali esterni richiede diidrotestosterone (DHT), un metabolita attivo del testosterone. Il DHT è necessario per la fusione delle pieghe genitali e per formare lo scroto e il pene. Perché il testosterone e il DHT producano queste modificazioni virilizzanti, è necessaria la presenza di un recettore funzionale degli androgeni, controllato da un gene correlato a X.

Nel feto XX con normale braccio lungo e corto del cromosoma X, lo sviluppo della gonade bipotenziale in senso ovarico avviene circa verso la decima-undicesima settimana. Ciò si verifica solo in assenza di *SRY*, testosterone e AMH e richiede un normale gene DAX1 nel locus DSS e la molecola WNT-4. Il fenotipo femminile si sviluppa indipendentemente dalla gonade fetale, ma la mascolinizzazione su una base potenzialmente femminile è dovuta all'azione degli ormoni prodotti dal testicolo fetale. Gli estrogeni non sono necessari per la normale differenziazione sessuale prenatale, come dimostrano pazienti 46,XX con deficit di aromatasi e topi senza recettori per l'estradiolo.

L'**intersessualità** implica una discrepanza tra la morfologia delle gonadi e quella dei genitali esterni. Aberrazioni cromosomiche possono provocare ambiguità dei genitali esterni (vedi Capitoli 584 e 587). Su un genotipo XX o XY, si possono sviluppare condizioni di differenziazione sessuale aberrante. Il nuovo, adeguato termine proposto per la condizione che un tempo era definita intersessualità, è **disturbi dello sviluppo sessuale** (*Disorders of Sex Development*, DSD). Questo termine definisce una "condizione in cui si verifica uno sviluppo atipico di cromosomi, gonadi o sesso anatomico". È preferibile usare il termine "genitali atipici" piuttosto che "ambigui". Nelle Tabelle 589-1 e 589-2 si trova il confronto tra terminologia precedente e la nuova classificazione eziologica. Alcuni dei geni coinvolti nelle disturbi dello sviluppo sessuale sono indicati nella Tabella 583-1. Inizialmente lo sviluppo dei genitali esterni ha in sé potenzialità in senso maschile e femminile (Fig. 589-1). La virilizzazione della femmina, la più comune forma di DSD, può portare a diversi fenotipi (Fig. 589-2), che iniziano dall'aspetto genitale di base dell'embrione (vedi Fig. 589-1).

589.1 • DSD 46,XX

In questa condizione, il genotipo è XX e le gonadi sono ovaie, ma i genitali esterni sono virilizzati. Dal momento che non c'è AMH (sono presenti ovaie e non testicoli), si sviluppano l'utero, le tube e le ovaie. Le varietà e le cause di questa condizione sono relativamente scarse. La maggior parte dei casi dipende dall'esposizione del feto femmina, durante la vita intrauterina, a una quantità eccessiva di androgeni endogeni o esogeni. Le modificazioni consistono principalmente in virilizzazione dei genitali esterni (ipertrofia clitoridea e fusione labioscrotale).

IPERPLASIA SURRENALICA CONGENITA (VEDI CAPITOLO 577.1). Questa è la causa più comune di ambiguità genitale e DSD 46,XX. Le femmine con deficit di 21-idrossilasi e 11-idrossilasi sono le più virilizzate, sebbene una virilizzazione minima si verifichi

TABELLA 589-1. Proposta di revisione della nomenclatura

PRECEDENTE	PROPOSTA
Intersessualità*	Disturbi dello sviluppo sessuale (DSD)
Pseudoermafroditismo maschile	DSD 46,XY
Incompleta virilizzazione di un maschio XY	
Incompleta mascolinizzazione di un maschio XY	
*Intersessualità 46,XY	
Pseudoermafroditismo femminile	DSD 46,XX
Eccessiva virilizzazione di una femmina XX	
Mascolinizzazione di una femmina XX	
*Intersessualità 46,XX	
Ermafroditismo vero	DSD ovotesticolare
*Gonadi intersessuali	
Maschio XX o Inversione sessuale XX	DSD testicolare 46,XX
Inversione sessuale XY	Disgenesia gonadica completa 46,XY

*Termine utilizzato nella precedente edizione di questo capitolo.
Da Lee PA, Houk CP, Ahmed SF, et al: Consensus statement on management of intersex disorders. *Pediatrics* 2006;118:e 448-500.

TABELLA 589-2. Classificazione eziologica dei disturbi dello sviluppo sessuale (DSD)

46,XX-DSD
Esposizione agli androgeni
Sorgente fetale/feto-placentare
Deficit di 21-idrossilasi (P450 c21)
Deficit di 11β-idrossilasi (P450 c11)
Deficit di 3β-idrossisteroido deidrogenasi II (3β-HSD II)
Citocromo p450 ossidoreduttasi (POR)
Deficit di aromatasi ($P450_{arom}$)
Mutazione del gene del recettore dei glicocorticoidi
Sorgente materna
Tumore ovarico virilizzante
Tumore surrenale virilizzante
Farmaci androgenici
Disturbi dello sviluppo ovarico
Disgenesia gonadica XX
DSD testicolare (SRY+, SOX9Dup)
Origine sconosciuta
Associato a difetti del tratto genitourinario e gastrointestinale
46,XY-DSD
Difetti dello sviluppo testicolare
Sindrome di Denys-Drash (mutazione del gene WT1)
Sindrome WAGR (tumore di Wilms, aniridia, malformazione genitourinaria, ritardo)
Elezione di 11p13
Sindrome camptomelica (gene autosomico su 17q24.3-q25.1) e mutazione di SOX9
Disgenesia gonadica pura XY (sindrome di Swyer)
Mutazione del gene SRY
Agenesia gonadica XY
Causa sconosciuta
Deficit di ormoni testicolari
Aplasia delle cellule di Leydig
Mutazione del recettore dell'LH
Iperplasia surrenalica lipoidea (P450scc); mutazione di StAR (proteina regolatrice acuta steroidogenica)
Deficit di 3β-HSD II
Deficit di 17-idrossilasi/17,20-liasi (P450c17)
Sindrome da persistenza del dotto mülleriano
Mutazioni del gene, ormone antimülleriano
Difetti del recettore dell'ormone antimülleriano
Difetto dell'azione androgenica
Mutazioni della 5α-reduttasi II
Difetti del recettore androgenico
Sindrome da completa insensibilità agli androgeni
Sindrome da parziale insensibilità agli androgeni
(Reifenstein e altre sindromi)
Sindrome di Smith-Lemli-Opitz (difetto della conversione del 7-deidrocolesterolo in colesterolo, DHCR7)
DSD ovotesticolare
XX
XY
Chimere XX/XY

Da Lee PA, Houk CP, Ahmed SF, e altri: Consensus statement on management of intersex disoerders. *Pediatrics* 2006;118;e488-500.

anche nel deficit di 3β-idrossisteroido deidrogenasi tipo II (vedi Fig. 589-1). Le forme con perdita di sali tendono ad avere gradi maggiori di virilizzazione rispetto alle altre forme. La mascolinizzazione può essere così intensa da portare a un'uretra peniena completa, e la condizione può essere assimilabile a quella di un maschio criptorchide (vedi Capitolo 577.1).

DEFICIT DI AROMATASI. In pazienti genotipicamente femmine, il deficit di aromatasi durante la vita fetale porta a DSD 46,XX con ipogonadismo ipergonadotropo alla pubertà, per insufficienza della sintesi estrogenica ovarica (vedi Fig. 575-1).

Due neonate 46,XX presentavano, alla nascita, ipertrofia clitoridea e fusione labiale posteriore. In un caso, i livelli materni plasmatici e urinari di estrogeni erano molto bassi, mentre quelli di androgeni molto alti. Anche i livelli di estrogeni nel sangue del cordone ombelicale erano molto bassi e invece elevati quelli di androgeni. Anche la seconda paziente presentava virilizzazione sin dalla nascita, per causa sconosciuta, ma il deficit di aromatasi non è stato diagnosticato fino all'età di 14 anni, quando si è ulteriormente virilizzata e non è cominciata la pubertà. A quel tempo, presentava livelli elevati di gonadotropine e di androgeni ma bassi di estrogeni, e l'indagine ecografica aveva evidenziato voluminose cisti ovariche bilaterali. Queste due pazienti dimostrano il ruolo importante dell'aromatasi nella conversione degli androgeni in estrogeni. Sono noti altri pazienti femmine e maschi con deficit di aromatasi dovuto a mutazioni del gene $P450_{arom}$ (*CYP19*). È stato descritto il caso di due fratelli; uno di essi, di 28 anni, XY, aveva raggiunto la statura di 177,6 cm (+2,5 DS) dopo aver ricevuto terapia ormonale sostitutiva; l'altro, di 24 anni, era alto 204 cm (+3,7 DS) e aveva un'età ossea di 14 anni. Per le femmine, anche in epoca prepubere, è indicata una terapia con bassi dosaggi di estradiolo, attentamente calibrati per mantenere livelli adeguati all'età ossea.

MUTAZIONE DEL GENE DEL RECETTORE DEI GLICOCORTICOIDI. Una bambina di 9 anni 46,XX con disordine dello sviluppo sessuale, che si pensava dovuto a deficit di 21-OHasi (iperplasia surrenalica congenita) fin dall'età di 5 anni, aveva elevati livelli di cortisolo basale e dopo desametasone, ipertensione, ipokaliemia, tutti elementi suggestivi per la diagnosi di resistenza generalizzata ai glicocorticoidi. È stata dimostrata una nuova mutazione eterozigote nell'esone 5 del recettore dei glicocorticoidi. In questa famiglia brasiliana, la condizione era autosomica recessiva.

Il POR, citocromo P450 ossidoreduttasi, codificato da un gene su 7q11.2, è un cofattore implicato nei difetti steroidogenetici combinati P450C17 e P3450C21. Le femmine nascono con genitali ambigui, ma la virilizzazione non prosegue dopo la nascita e i livelli androgenici sono normali o bassi. I maschi possono nascere scarsamente virilizzati. Entrambi possono presentare delle anomalie ossee come nella **sindrome di Antley-Bixler** (*Antley-Bixler Syndrome*, ABS). Al contrario, in una serie di pazienti ABS, quelli con genitali ambigui e alterazioni steroidogenetiche avevano un deficit di POR, mentre quelli senza ambiguità e normale steroidogenesi presentavano mutazioni *FGFR2*. Le caratteristiche principali di ABS comprendono craniosinostosi, grave ipoplasia di un'emifaccia, proptosi, atresia/stenosi coanale, bozze frontali, orecchie displasiche, depressione della radice del naso, sinostosi radio-omerale, fratture delle ossa lunghe e incurvamento femorale, con anomalie urogenitali.

TUMORI MATERNI VIRILIZZANTI. Raramente la causa della virilizzazione di un feto femmina durante la vita fetale è dovuta alla presenza di un tumore materno che secerne androgeni. In pochi casi, era presente un adenoma surrenalico benigno, ma in tutti gli altri si trattava di neoplasie ovariche, particolarmente androblastomi, luteomi e tumori di Krukenberg. La **virilizzazione materna** può manifestarsi con ipertrofia clitoridea, acne, abbassamento della voce, diminuzione della secrezione lattea, irsutismo e iperandrogenismo. Nel neonato, è presente ipertrofia clitoridea di varia entità, spesso con fusione labiale. Madri e bambine con DSD 46,XX inspiegato devono essere sottoposte a determinazioni dei livelli plasmatici di testosterone, deidroepiandrosterone solfato e androstenedione.

SOMMINISTRAZIONE DI FARMACI ANDROGENICI ALLA MADRE DURANTE LA GRAVIDANZA. Il testosterone e il 17-metiltestosterone possono provocare in alcuni casi condizioni intersessuali 46,XX. Il maggior numero di casi dipende dall'uso di certi composti progestinici per il trattamento delle minacce di aborto. Questi progestinici sono stati sostituiti da altri non virilizzanti.

Sono state descritte neonate con virilizzazione, assetto cromosomico 46,XX e anomalie caudali per le quali non è stato identificato alcun agente virilizzante. In questi casi, la condizione è solitamente associata ad altri difetti congeniti, particolarmente del tratto urinario e gastrointestinale. Specifiche sequenze Y del DNA, compreso *SRY*, sono assenti. In un caso, sono stati trovati rafe scrotale ed elevati livelli di testosterone, ma la causa rimane ignota.

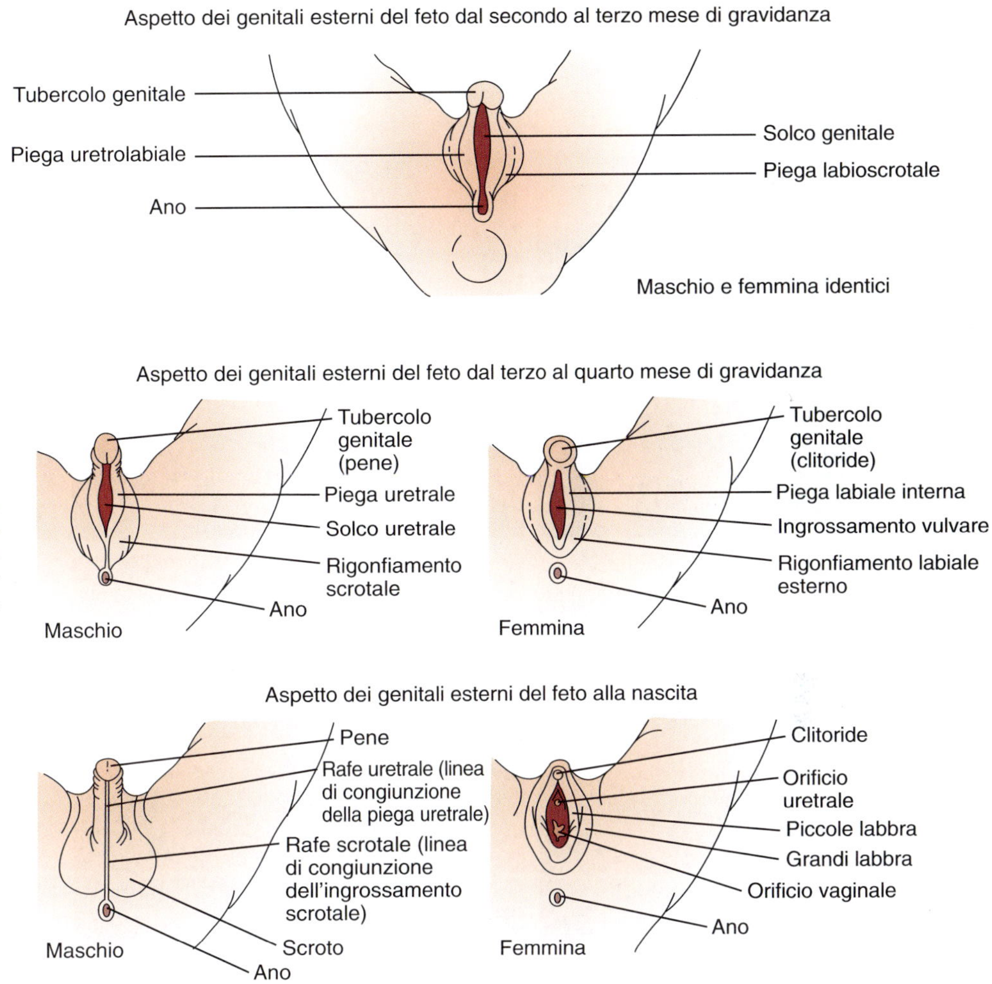

Figura 589-1. Illustrazione schematica della normale differenziazione dei genitali maschili e femminili durante l'embriogenesi. (Da Zitelli BJ, Davis HW: *Atlas of Pediatric Physical Diagnosis*, 4th edition. St. Louis, Mosby, 2002, p 328.)

589.2 • DSD 46,XY

In questa condizione, il genotipo è XY, ma i genitali esterni sono incompletamente virilizzati, ambigui o completamente femminili. Quando si trovano le gonadi, sono invariabilmente dei testicoli, variamente sviluppati, da rudimentali a normali. Dato che il processo di normale virilizzazione nel feto è molto complesso, non è una sorpresa che ci siano molte tipologie di individui XY con inadeguata virilizzazione.

DIFETTI DELLA DIFFERENZIAZIONE TESTICOLARE

La prima fase della differenziazione maschile è la conversione della gonade indifferenziata in testicolo. Nel feto XY, se si verifica una delezione del braccio corto del cromosoma Y o del gene *SRY*, non compare differenziazione in senso maschile. Il fenotipo è femminile; i dotti mülleriani sono sviluppati per assenza di AMH, ma le gonadi consistono di formazioni nastriformi indifferenziate. Al contrario, con delezioni estreme del braccio lungo del cromosoma Y (Yq-), si sono trovati maschi normalmente sviluppati, molti dei quali azoospermici e di bassa statura, indice del fatto che il braccio lungo del cromosoma Y possiede normalmente dei geni che prevengono queste manifestazioni. In altre sindromi in cui non si verifica una normale differenziazione testicolare, i cromosomi Y sono morfologicamente normali.

SINDROME DI DENIS-DRASH. L'insieme di nefropatia, genitali ambigui e **tumore di Wilms bilaterale** costituisce la caratteristica maggiore di questa sindrome (vedi Capitolo 499). La maggior parte dei casi riportati era 46,XY. Spesso erano presenti i dotti mülleriani, indice di un deficit globale della funzione testicolare fetale. I pazienti con cariotipo 46,XX hanno genitali esterni normali. La proteinuria d'esordio nell'infanzia evolve verso una **sindrome nefrotica** e insufficienza renale, nello stadio terminale, verso i 3 anni. Il più importante reperto istopatologico è rappresentato da sclerosi mesangiale focale o diffusa. Il tumore di Wilms solitamente si sviluppa in bambini con meno di 2 anni ed è frequentemente bilaterale. Sono stati riportati anche casi di gonadoblastoma.

Si sono trovate parecchie mutazioni del gene del tumore di Wilms (*WT1*), localizzato sul cromosoma 11p13. *WT1* funziona come un gene tumore-soppressore e fattore trascrizionale ed è espresso nella cresta genitale e nelle gonadi fetali. Quasi tutte le mutazioni riportate sono nella regione codificante il "dito di zinco" o vicino a essa. In un caso si è trovata una mutazione del dominio del "dito di zinco" negli alleli *WT1* di un paziente privo di anomalie genitourinarie, suggerendo che alcuni casi di tumore di Wilms sporadico possano portare la mutazione *WT1*. Nella **sindrome di Fraser**, una condizione caratterizzata da glomerulosclerosi aspecifica focale e segmentale, disgenesia gonadica 46,XY e frequente gonadoblastoma, ma senza tumore di Wilms, sono state descritte diverse mutazioni del gene *WT1* e mutazioni costituzionali eterozigoti a livello dell'introne 9.

SINDROME WAGR. Questa sindrome da geni contigui (acronimo per *Wilms tumor, Aniridia, Genitourinary malformation and Retardation*) consiste in tumore di Wilms, aniridia, malformazioni genitourinarie e ritardo mentale (vedi Capitolo 499). Questi bambini hanno la delezione di una coppia del cromosoma 11p13, evidenziabile con l'analisi del cariotipo. La regione cancellata

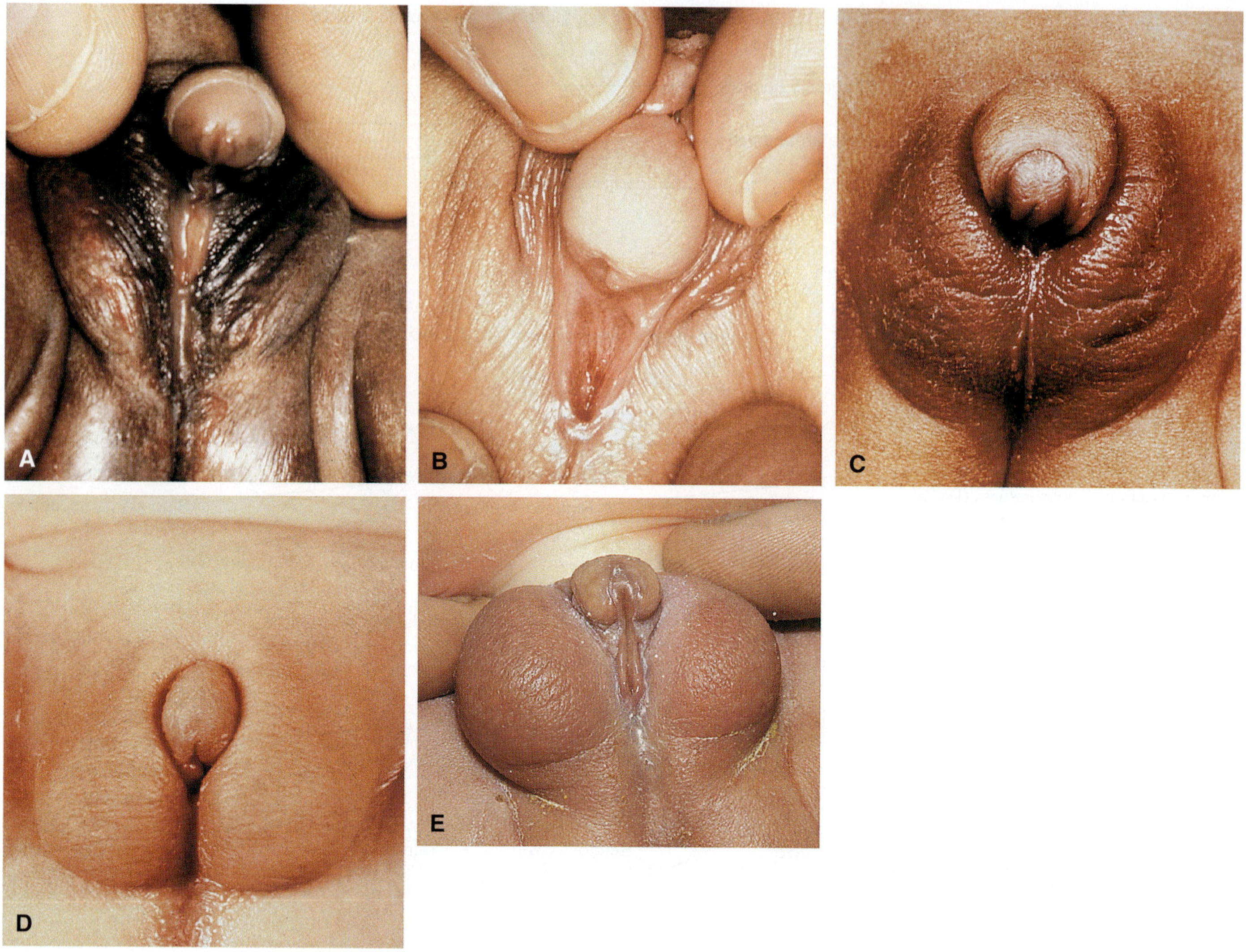

Figura 589-2. Esempi di genitali atipici. Questi casi comprendono la malattia ovotesticolare dello sviluppo sessuale *(A)* e l'iperplasia surrenalica congenita virilizzante *(B-E)*. (*B-D*, per gentile concessione di D. Becker, MD, Pittsburgh.) (Da Zitelli BJ, Davis HW: *Atlas of pediatric Physical Diagnosis*, 4th edition. St. Louis, Mosby, 2002, p. 329.)

contiene il gene dell'aniridia (*PAX6*) e il gene soppressore del tumore di Wilms (*WT1*). Solo i maschi 46,XY presentano anomalie genitali, che vanno dal criptorchidismo a grave deficit di virilizzazione. Nelle gonadi disgenetiche si sviluppano gonadoblastomi. Il tumore di Wilms solitamente si verifica verso i 2 anni di età. Alcuni casi presentano obesità di cui non è chiara l'origine, sollevando la questione della presenza in questa regione del cromosoma 11, di un gene associato a obesità e facendo definire la sindrome come **WAGRO**.

SINDROME CAMPTOMELICA (VEDI CAPITOLO 702). Questa forma di **displasia con arti corti** è caratterizzata da incurvamento anteriore di femore e tibia, scapole piccole, cavità toracica piccola e 11 paia di costole, assieme a malformazioni di altri organi. Solitamente porta a morte nella prima infanzia. Circa il 75% dei pazienti 46,XY riportati presenta un fenotipo completamente femminile; i genitali esterni e interni sono femminili. Alcuni pazienti 46,XY presentano invece genitali ambigui. Le gonadi appaiono come ovaie, ma istologicamente possono contenere elementi sia ovarici sia testicolari.

Il gene responsabile della condizione è *SOX9* (gene HMG-box SRY-correlato) e si trova su 17q24-q25. Questo gene è strutturalmente correlato con SRY e regola anche direttamente lo sviluppo del gene del collagene di tipo II (*COL2A1*). Le stesse mutazioni possono essere responsabili di diversi fenotipi gonadici. In un paziente con questa condizione è stato riportato un gonadoblastoma. L'ereditarietà è autosomica dominante. In un paziente con mutazione del gene SF1 è stata descritta insufficienza surrenalica e disgenesia gonadica 46,XY.

In pazienti con delezioni di parti di loci autosomici sul cromosoma 2q, 9p, e 10q, è stata descritta un'inversione sessuale 46,XY.

DISGENESIA GONADICA PURA XY (SINDROME DI SWYER). Il termine "pura" distingue questa forma da altre di disgenesia gonadica di origine cromosomica e associate ad anomalie somatiche. I pazienti presentano statura normale e **fenotipo femminile**, compresi vagina, utero e tube di Falloppio, ma in epoca puberale non si sviluppano le mammelle e non compare il menarca. Non è presente nessun difetto associato a 45,X. In epoca puberale i pazienti manifestano un'amenorrea primaria ipergonadotropa. I casi familiari suggeriscono una trasmissione associata a X o autosomica dominante limitata al sesso. La maggior parte dei pazienti esaminati presentava mutazioni del gene *SRY*. Nessuno aveva una mutazione di *SOX9*. Le gonadi consistono di residui nastriformi quasi completamente indifferenziati, nonostante la presenza di un cromosoma Y citogeneticamente normale. La gonade primitiva può compiere una qualche funzione testicolare, compresa la soppressione dei dotti mülleriani. Nella gonade possono essere presenti cellule dell'ilo in grado di produrre alcuni androgeni;

pertanto, in epoca puberale si possono manifestare alcuni segni di virilizzazione, come l'ipertrofia clitoridea. Le gonadi nastriformi possono subire modificazioni neoplastiche, con la comparsa di gonadoblastoma e disgerminoma, e devono essere rimosse rapidamente dopo la diagnosi, in base all'età.

La disgenesia gonadica pura si verifica anche in individui XX (vedi Capitolo 587).

SINDROME DA AGENESIA GONADICA XY (SINDROME DA REGRESSIONE TESTICOLARE EMBRIONALE). In questa rara sindrome, i genitali esterni sono lievemente ambigui ma più simili a quelli **femminili**. Sono presenti ipoplasia labiale, gradi diversi di fusione labioscrotale, microfallo simile a clitoride, orifizio uretrale perineale. Mancano utero, tessuto gonadico e di solito anche vagina. In epoca puberale, non compare sviluppo sessuale ed è presente ipergonadotropinemia. La maggior parte dei bambini viene allevata come femmina. In parecchi pazienti con agenesia gonadica XY in cui, all'esplorazione, non sono reperibili le gonadi, si documenta un incremento significativo del testosterone dopo stimolazione con hCG, che dimostra una qualche funzione delle cellule di Leydig. Sono noti fratelli con la stessa patologia.

Si ritiene che del tessuto testicolare sia attivo durante la vita fetale abbastanza a lungo da consentire all'AMH di inibire lo sviluppo dei dotti mülleriani, ma non abbastanza da consentire la virilizzazione per la produzione di testosterone In un paziente, per mezzo di prove sul DNA Y-specifiche, non si è trovata delezione del cromosoma Y. La degenerazione testicolare si verifica tra l'ottava e la dodicesima settimana di vita fetale. La regressione del testicolo prima dell'ottava settimana porta alla sindrome di Swyer; tra la quattordicesima e la ventesima settimana alla sindrome del testicolo rudimentale; dopo la ventesima settimana all'anorchia.

Nell'**anorchia bilaterale**, i testicoli sono assenti, ma in presenza di un **fenotipo maschile** completo; si presume che il tessuto con funzione testicolare fetale fosse attivo durante il periodo critico della differenziazione genitale, ma che abbia subito un danno successivamente. La presenza di anorchia bilaterale in gemelli identici e di anorchia monolaterale in gemelli identici e in fratelli suggerisce una predisposizione genetica. La coesistenza in fratelli di anorchia e della sindrome da agenesia gonadica fa presupporre una relazione tra le malattie. Nei pazienti con anorchia non sono stati descritti difetti di *SRY*.

Una revisione retrospettiva di indagini urologiche ha rivelato l'assenza di testicoli nel 21% di 691 esami. Di questi, il 73% aveva strutture cordoniformi a fondo cieco con il testicolo "vanishing" a livello del canale inguinale (59%), dell'addome (21%), dell'anello inguinale superficiale (18%) e dello scroto (2%). Si ritiene che la presenza di strutture cordoniformi in sede laparoscopica debba indurre all'esplorazione inguinale, dato che, in 4 di questi bambini, si è trovato del tessuto testicolare vitale. Non sono stati riportati i dati ormonali (test di stimolazione con hCG, livelli di AMH).

DIFETTI DEGLI ORMONI TESTICOLARI

Sono stati delineati 5 difetti genetici nella sintesi enzimatica del testosterone da parte del testicolo fetale e un difetto nella differenziazione delle cellule di Leydig. Questi difetti producono maschi 46,XY con inadeguata mascolinizzazione (vedi Fig. 583-1). Dato che i livelli di testosterone sono normalmente bassi prima della pubertà, per stabilire la capacità dei testicoli di sintetizzare testosterone nei bambini si deve eseguire il test di stimolazione con hCG.

APLASIA DELLE CELLULE DI LEYDIG. Pazienti con aplasia delle cellule di Leydig di solito presentano un **fenotipo femminile**, ma possono manifestare gradi lievi di mascolinizzazione. Sono presenti testicoli, epididimo e deferenti. Sono assenti l'utero e le tube. Alla pubertà non si verificano modificazioni con comparsa dei caratteri sessuali secondari; i peli pubici possono essere normali. L'ipotestosteronemia non risponde allo stimolo con hCG; i livelli di LH sono elevati. Le cellule di Leydig dei testicoli sono assenti o notevolmente diminuite. Il difetto può coinvolgere la mancanza dei recettori per l'LH. Nei bambini, è necessaria la stimolazione con hCG per differenziare questa condizione dalle sindromi da insensibilità agli androgeni (*Autosomal Insensivity Syndrome*, AIS). L'ereditarietà è autosomica recessiva limitata al sesso maschile. Il recettore umano dell'LH fa parte della superfamiglia legata alla proteina G, dei recettori che contengono 7 domini transmembrana. In maschi con ipogonadismo sospettati di ipoplasia o aplasia delle cellule di Leydig, sono state descritte numerose mutazioni inattivanti del recettore dell'LH.

In un maschio con ipogonadismo dovuto a mutazione del gene per la subunità β dell'FSH, si sono trovati alti livelli di LH e bassi di FSH (vedi Tab. 584-1).

IPERPLASIA SURRENALICA LIPOIDEA (VEDI ANCHE CAPITOLO 577). La forma più grave di iperplasia surrenalica congenita prende il suo nome dall'aspetto delle ghiandole surrenali ipertrofiche, dovuto all'accumulo di colesterolo e di suoi esteri. Il processo limitante la velocità della steroidogenesi è il trasporto del colesterolo libero attraverso il citoplasma, fino all'interno della membrana mitocondriale, dove agisce p450scc. Il trasporto del colesterolo all'interno dei mitocondri è mediato da una proteina regolatrice acuta steroidogenica (StAR), la cui sintesi si verifica via cAMP, attraverso una proteina che lega l'elemento di risposta AMP ciclico (CREB). StAR è una proteina di 30kDa essenziale per la steroidogenesi ed è codificata da un gene sul cromosoma 8p11.2. Il contenuto mitocondriale di StAR aumenta tra la prima e la quinta ora dopo la stimolazione con ACTH, a lungo dopo l'aumento acuto ACTH-indotto della steroidogenesi. Questo aveva portato alcuni a ritenere che anche la StAR extramitocondriale possa essere coinvolta nella risposta acuta all'ACTH.

Il livello di tutti gli steroidi sierici è basso o indosabile, mentre la corticotropina e la renina plasmatica sono elevate. Il fenotipo è femminile sia in soggetti geneticamente maschi sia in femmine; i soggetti geneticamente maschi non hanno strutture mülleriane perché i testicoli possono produrre normale AMH, ma non steroidi. Questi bambini presentano nell'infanzia crisi surrenali acute e da perdita di sali. La maggior parte dei pazienti è 46,XY. In pochi pazienti è presente alla pubertà una steroidogenesi ovarica.

Il ruolo regolatore della steroidogenesi StAR-indipendente è illustrato da due gemelle di 4 mesi 46,XX con ipoplasia surrenalica lipoidea. Una è morta al quindicesimo mese per complicanze cardiache correlate alla coartazione aortica. I surreni avevano caratteristici depositi lipidici. La gemella sopravissuta presentava un pubertà spontanea con femminilizzazione a 11 anni e mezzo, con menarca a 13,8 anni. Valutata nuovamente all'età di 15 anni, è stata scoperta una mutazione omozigote frameshift-inattivante del gene StAR. Questa scoperta e il fatto che fosse sopravvissuta fino al quarto mese con livelli dosabili di aldosterone e senza terapia sostitutiva, supporta l'ipotesi che la steroidogenesi StAR-indipendente sia in grado di continuare fino ad accumulare abbastanza lipidi intracellulari da distruggere l'attività steroidogenetica. Sono stati descritti casi di difetti parziali in maschi solo parzialmente virilizzati, e ritardato esordio della perdita di sali. Difetti completi di P450scc possono essere incompatibili con la vita, perché solo quest'enzima è in grado di convertire il colesterolo in pregnenolone, che poi diventa progesterone, un ormone essenziale per il mantenimento della normale gravidanza nei mammiferi. È stata descritta una mutazione eterozigote in P450scc in un bambino di 4 anni con inversione sessuale 46,XY, ed esordio tardivo della forma di iperplasia surrenalica lipoidea. Alla sesta-settima settimana di gestazione, quando cessa la produzione di progesterone da parte del corpo luteo materno, la placenta, che non esprime StAR, produce progesterone attraverso una steroidogenesi StAR-indipendente, utilizzando il sistema enzimatico P450scc.

DEFICIT DI 3β-IDROSSISTEROIDO DEIDROGENASI. Maschi con questa forma di iperplasia surrenalica congenita (vedi Capitolo 577) presentano gradi variabili di **ipospadia**, con o senza scroto bifido e criptorchidismo e, raramente, fenotipo completamente femminile. I neonati di solito manifestano, subito dopo la nascita, segni da perdita di sali. Sono stati riportati casi di difetti incompleti, in maschi con pubarca prematuro e come forme non classiche a esordio tardivo. Questi bambini avevano mutazioni puntiformi del gene per l'enzima 3β-idrossisteroido di tipo II, con conseguente alterazione della steroidogenesi surrenalica e gonadica; l'alterazione può essere diversa tra surreni e gonadi. La comparsa in alcuni maschi di normali modificazioni puberali, potrebbe essere spiegata con l'attività della 3β-idrossisteroido deidrogenasi di tipo I, normalmente presente in molti tessuti periferici. L'infertilità non è frequente e sono state descritte più di 31 mutazioni. Non esiste un rapporto tra il grado della perdita di sali e quello delle anomalie fenotipiche.

DEFICIT DI 17-IDROSSILASI/17,20 LIASI. Un singolo enzima (P450c17), codificato da un singolo gene sul cromosoma 10q24.3, aveva sia l'attività 17-idrossilasica sia quella 17,20 liasica nel surrene e nelle gonadi (vedi Capitolo 577). Sono state descritte molte diverse lesioni genetiche. Soggetti geneticamente maschi presentavano un fenotipo completamente femminile o, meno spesso, vari gradi di ipovirilizzazione, dalla fusione labioscrotale all'ipospadia perineale e al criptorchidismo. In entrambi i sessi genetici non compare sviluppo sessuale alla pubertà.

Nella patologia classica, è presenta una diminuzione della sintesi surrenale di cortisolo e della sintesi di steroidi sessuali di origine surrenale e ovarica (vedi Figg. 583-1 e 575-1). I livelli di desossicorticosterone (DOC) e corticosterone sono notevolmente aumentati, con conseguenti ipertensione e ipokaliemia, caratteristiche di questa forma di DSD maschile. Sebbene i livelli di cortisolo siano bassi, l'aumento dei livelli di corticotropina e corticosterone mantiene uno stato eucorticoide. L'asse renina-aldosterone è soppresso per il potente effetto mineralcorticoide degli elevati livelli di DOC. Alla pubertà non compare virilizzazione; i livelli di testosterone sono bassi e aumentati quelli di gonadotropine. Dato che la produzione fetale di AMH è normale, non sono presenti residui dei dotti mülleriani. Gonadectomia e successiva terapia sostitutiva con idrocortisone e steroidi sessuali sono indicate negli individui XY fenotipicamente femmine.

L'eredità è di tipo autosomico recessivo. Le femmine XX, di solito non sono scoperte prima di aver raggiunto un'età giovane-adulta, quando non compaiono le normali modificazioni puberali e si scoprono ipertensione e ipokaliemia. Si deve sospettare questa condizione in tutte le pazienti con amenorrea primaria e ipertensione, in cui l'assetto cromosomico sia 46,XX o 46,XY.

DEFICIT DI 17-CHETOSTEROIDO REDUTTASI. Questo enzima, definito anche 17β-idrossisteroido deidrogenasi (17β-HSD), è l'ultimo nella catena biosintetica del testosterone; è necessario per convertire l'androstenedione in testosterone, il deidroepiandrosterone in androstenediolo e l'estrone in estradiolo. Difetti enzimatici del testicolo fetale comportano un incremento di maschi 46,XY con fenotipo femminile completo o quasi. I dotti mülleriani sono assenti ed è presente una piccola vagina. La diagnosi si basa sul rapporto tra testosterone e androstenedione; in bambini prepuberi è necessaria la preventiva stimolazione con hCG.

Il difetto è ereditario con trasmissione autosomica recessiva. Sono noti almeno 4 tipi diversi di 17β-HSD, ciascuno codificato da un gene diverso o da diversi cromosomi. Il difetto enzimatico di tipo III è quello più frequente in un ampio gruppo di consanguinei della popolazione araba di Gaza. Il gene per questa patologia si trova su 9q22, ed è espresso solo nei testicoli, dove converte l'androstenedione in testosterone. La maggior parte dei pazienti viene diagnosticata alla pubertà, per la mancata comparsa di virilizzazione o di menarca. Alla pubertà i livelli di testosterone possono mostrarsi normali, presumibilmente per la conversione periferica dell'androstenedione in testosterone; in questo periodo, alcuni pazienti spontaneamente assumono un ruolo di genere maschile.

La 17β-HSD di tipo I, codificata da un gene sul cromosoma 17q21, converte l'estrone in estradiolo e si trova in placenta, ovaio, testicolo, fegato, prostata, tessuto adiposo ed endometrio. Il tipo II, il cui gene si trova sul cromosoma 16q24, ha un'attività opposta a quella dei tipi I e III (converte il testosterone in androstenedione e l'estrone in estradiolo). Il tipo IV ha un'azione simile a quella del tipo II. Una forma di deficit di 17-chetosteroido reduttasi a esordio tardivo presenta ginecomastia in maschi giovani adulti.

SINDROME DA PERSISTENZA DEI DOTTI MÜLLERIANI. In questa patologia, persistono, in maschi per il resto completamente virilizzati, dei derivati del dotto mülleriano. Sono stati riportati casi in fratelli e in gemelli identici. Il **criptorchidismo** è presente nell'80% dei maschi colpiti; e durante l'intervento per questo motivo o per ernia inguinale, si scoprono casualmente tube di Falloppio o utero. Il grado dello sviluppo mülleriano è variabile e può essere asimmetrico. Nella maggior parte la funzione testicolare è normale, ma sono riportati esempi di degenerazione testicolare. Alcuni maschi colpiti manifestano tumori testicolari dopo la pubertà. In uno studio di 38 famiglie, 16 avevano difetti del gene AMH, localizzato su braccio corto del cromosoma 19. Presentavano bassi livelli di AMH. In 16 famiglie con alti livelli di AMH, il difetto era nel gene del recettore di tipo II dell'AMH, e i 10/16 avevano identiche delezioni 27bp sull'esone 10 in almeno un allele.

Il **trattamento** consiste nella rimozione della maggior parte possibile di strutture mülleriane senza provocare danni testicolari, epididimali o dei vasi deferenti.

DIFETTI NELL'AZIONE ANDROGENICA

Nel seguente gruppo di patologie, la sintesi fetale di testosterone è normale e la difettosa virilizzazione dipende da anomalie ereditarie dell'azione androgenica.

DEFICIT DI 5α-REDUTTASI. La diminuzione, durante la vita intrauterina, della produzione di diidrotestosterone comporta, nel feto maschio, una grave ambiguità dei genitali esterni. La biosintesi e l'azione periferica del testosterone sono normali.

Il fenotipo più frequentemente associato a questa condizione è rappresentato da maschi con pene piccolo, scroto bifido, seno urogenitale con ipospadia perineale e una struttura vaginale a fondo cieco (Fig. 589-3). I testicoli si trovano nel canale inguinale

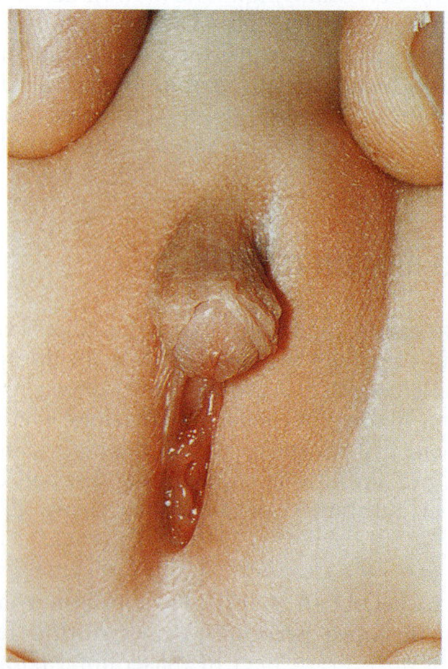

Figura 589-3. Deficit di 5α-reduttasi. (Da Wales JKH, Wit JM, Rogol AD: *Pediatric Endocrinology and Growth*, 2nd edition. Philadelphia, Elsevier/Saunders, 2003, p 165.)

o nella piega labioscrotale e sono normali da un punto di vista istologico. Non sono presenti strutture mülleriane, mentre sono presenti quelle wolffiane: vasi deferenti, epididimo e vescichette seminali. La maggior parte dei pazienti viene identificata come femmina. Alla pubertà, compare virilizzazione; aumentano le dimensioni del pene, i testicoli discendono e crescono regolarmente e si verifica spermatogenesi. Non si manifesta ginecomastia. La barba cresce in modo scarso, è assente l'acne, la prostata è piccola, e non compare recessione dell'inserzione dei capelli a livello temporale. La virilizzazione del dotto wolffiano è dovuta all'azione dello stesso testosterone, sebbene la mascolinizzazione del seno urogenitale e dei genitali esterni dipenda dall'azione del DHT durante il periodo critico della mascolinizzazione fetale. Anche la crescita dei peli facciali e della prostata dipende dal DHT.

L'altezza adulta raggiunta è vicina a quella del fratello o di altri familiari maschi. È presente, tuttavia, una significativa eterogeneità fenotipica. Si sono pertanto classificati i pazienti in 5 diversi tipi di deficit di 5α-reduttasi (SRD), che vanno da quello completamente femminile (tipo 5), parzialmente femminile (tipo 4), ambiguo (tipo 3), prevalentemente maschile con micropene (tipo 2), a quello completamente maschile senza apparenti difetti della virilizzazione (tipo 1).

In pazienti di tutto il mondo, parecchi diversi difetti del gene che porta a SRD sono stati identificati nel gene della 5α-reduttasi di tipo 2, localizzato sul braccio corto del cromosoma 2. Sono stati descritti gruppi familiari in Repubblica Dominicana, Turchia, Papua Nuova Guinea, Brasile, Messico e Medio Oriente. Non esiste una correlazione tra la severità del difetto genetico e il fenotipo.

La patologia è ereditaria con trasmissione autosomica recessiva, ma limitata al sesso maschile. Femmine omozigoti normali, con normale fertilità, stanno a dimostrare che nel sesso femminile il DHT non ha un ruolo nella differenziazione sessuale o nella funzionalità ovarica nelle fasi successive della vita. La diagnosi clinica deve essere posta nei bambini il più precocemente possibile; è necessario distinguere questa patologia dalla sindrome da insensibilità agli androgeni. La diagnosi biochimica si basa sul reperto di livelli normali di testosterone, livelli di DHT normali o bassi, con marcato incremento del rapporto tra testosterone:diidrotestosterone (>17) basale, ma soprattutto dopo stimolo con hCG, ed elevato rapporto urinario tra eziocolanolone:androsterone e tra 5α:metaboliti 5α. I bambini con insensibilità agli androgeni, presentano una normale attività della 5α reduttasi epatica e un normale rapporto tra tetraidrocortisolo:5α-tetraidrocortisolo, al contrario di quanto si verifica nella SRD.

La maggior parte ma, cosa importante, non la totalità dei bambini allevati come femmine durante l'infanzia presenta dei cambiamenti in senso maschile alla pubertà. Pare che l'esposizione al testosterone in utero, in epoca neonatale e alla pubertà, contribuisca alla formazione di un'identità di genere maschile. Nel determinare l'identità e il comportamento di genere, più spesso è necessario conoscere oltre alle influenze ormonali, come quelle androgeniche, anche quelle culturali, sociali, psicologiche, genetiche e inerenti ad altri fattori biologici. Neonati con questa condizione dovrebbero essere allevati come maschi tutte le volte che ciò sia possibile. Il **trattamento** dei neonati maschi con DHT comporta un aumento di volume del pene.

SINDROMI DA INSENSIBILITÀ AGLI ANDROGENI (AIS). Le AIS rappresentano le forme più comuni di DSD maschile e hanno un frequenza presunta di 1/20 000 maschi geneticamente tali. Questo gruppo di eterogenee patologie correlate a X è dovuto a più di 150 diverse mutazioni del gene del recettore androgenico, localizzato su Xq11-12: singole mutazioni puntiformi comportano sostituzioni aminoacidiche o codoni di stop prematuro, frameshift e interruzione prematura, delezioni del gene e mutazioni *splice site*.

Manifestazioni cliniche. La variabilità clinica dei pazienti con AIS, aventi tutti un assetto cromosomico 46,XY, spazia da un fenotipo femminile (AIS completa) a uno maschile con varie forme di ambiguità sessuale dei genitali e aspetto ipovirilizzato (AIS parziale, o sindromi cliniche come la **sindrome di Reifenstein**), a un fenotipo maschile apparentemente normale con infertilità. In tutti questi bambini, oltre ai normali cromosomi 46,XY, si trovano i testicoli e livelli normali o elevati di testosterone (Figg. 589-4 e 589-5).

Nell'**AIS completa**, una forma estrema di insufficiente virilizzazione, i maschi geneticamente tali alla nascita vengono scambiati per femmine e sono invariabilmente cresciuti come tali. I genitali esterni sono femminili. La vagina termina a fondo cieco e manca l'utero. In circa un terzo dei pazienti, si trovano residui tubarici mono o bilaterali. I testicoli sono di solito intraddominali, ma possono scendere nel canale inguinale; consistono in gran parte di tubuli seminiferi. Sono descritti casi di femmine gemelle con ernia inguinale contenente i testicoli. Alla pubertà, compare un normale sviluppo mammario e l'aspetto è femminile, ma non si presentano le mestruazioni e sono assenti i peli pubici. L'altezza di queste donne da adulte è simile a quella di maschi normali, nonostante il notevole deficit congenito di effetti androgenici.

I testicoli dei pazienti adulti producono normali livelli maschili di testosterone e DHT. Il deficit della normale virilizzazione maschile in epoca fetale riflette il difetto di risposta agli androgeni in quel periodo, ma l'assenza dei dotti mülleriani indica un'anormale produzione testicolare fetale di AMH. L'assenza degli effetti

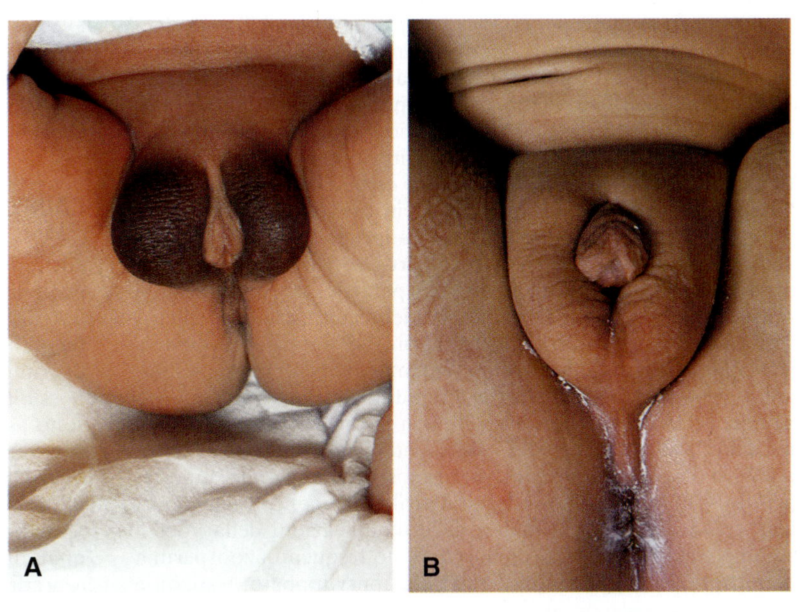

Figura 589-4. *A*, parziale insensibilità agli androgeni con discesa testicolare in una formazione labioscrotale bifida. *B*, Insensibilità agli androgeni parziale meno grave, con severa ipospadia e testicoli mal discesi. (Da Wales JKH, Woit JM, Rogol AD: *Pediatric Endocrinology and Growth*, 2nd edition. Philadephia, Elsevier/Saunders, 2003, p. 165)

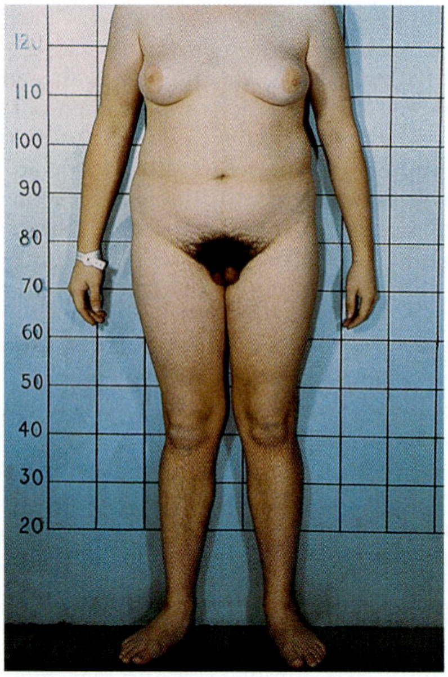

Figura 589-5. Sindrome da parziale insensibilità agli androgeni al momento dell'adolescenza, in un soggetto cresciuto come maschio. Notare la ginecomastia per aromatasi periferica del testosterone in estrogeno. L'abbondanza di peli pubici indica un'insensibilità solo parziale (Da Wales JKH, Wit JM, Rogolo AD: *Pediatric Endocrinology and Growth*, 2nd edition. Philadeplhia, Elsevier/Saunders, 2003, p. 165.)

androgenici è dovuta a una straordinaria resistenza all'azione del testosterone esogeno o endogeno a livello cellulare.

Questa patologia viene spesso diagnosticata in bambini prepuberi, quando si scopre che delle masse inguinali sono in realtà testicoli o quando in un paziente con fenotipo femminile, durante un intervento di correzione di un'ernia, si trova inaspettatamente un testicolo. Circa l'1-2% delle femmine con ernia inguinale manifesta questa patologia. Nei neonati, la diagnosi viene suggerita da un quadro di ipergonadotropinemia. Negli adulti, un sintomo frequente di presentazione è rappresentato dall'**amenorrea**. Nei bambini in epoca prepubere, è necessaria la diagnosi differenziale con altre forme di ipovirilizzazione maschile, in cui esiste completa femminilizzazione. Queste forme comprendono la disgenesia gonadica XY (sindrome di Swyer), l'agonadismo vero, l'aplasia delle cellule di Leydig compresi i difetti dei recettori dell'LH, e il deficit di 17-chetosteroido reduttasi; tutte queste condizioni, a differenza della AIS completa, sono caratterizzate da **bassi livelli di testosterone** nel neonato e nell'adulto e insufficiente risposta all'hCG negli anni prepuberi. Mentre pazienti con AIS completa hanno alla nascita genitali esterni femminili senza alcuna ambiguità, quelli con **AIS parziale** presentano una ampia varietà di aspetti fenotipici, che vanno dall'**ipospadia perineoscrotale** allo scroto bifido e al criptorchidismo, fino a una grave ipovirilizzazione caratterizzata da ipertrofia clitoridea e fusione labiale. Alcune forme di AIS parziale sono note come sindromi specifiche. Pazienti con la **sindrome di Reifenstein** presentano incompleta virilizzazione con ipogonadismo, severa ipospadia e ginecomastia (vedi Fig. 589-5). Le **sindromi di Gilbert-Dreyfuss** e di **Lubs** sono ulteriori quadri classificati come AIS parziale. In tutti i casi, si sono identificate alterazioni del gene del recettore androgenico.

Diagnosi. La diagnosi di pazienti con AIS parziale può essere particolarmente difficile durante l'infanzia. L'incremento postnatale di testosterone e di LH è diminuito nei pazienti con AIS completa (CAIS), ma non in quelli con la forma parziale (PAIS). In alcuni, specialmente quelli sufficientemente virilizzati nell'infanzia, la diagnosi non viene neppure sospettata fino alla pubertà, quando si manifesta un'inadeguata virilizzazione, con mancanza della crescita dei peli facciali e delle modificazioni della voce e la comparsa invece di ginecomastia. Sono frequenti azoospermia e infertilità. In soggetti adulti con pene iposviluppato, testicoli e infertilità, sempre più si trovano difetti del recettore androgenico. Nei recettori androgenici di una ampia famiglia cinese in cui alcuni membri affetti erano fertili, mentre altri avevano ipospadia e/o ginecomastia, è stata descritta una singola sostituzione aminoacidica. La produzione di IGF2 e di IGFBP2, ma non di IGFBP3, da parte dei fibroblasti della cute dei genitali è diminuita nella CCAIS rispetto ai normali fibroblasti cutanei, suggerendo un possibile ruolo del sistema IGF nella modulazione dell'azione androgenica.

Trattamento e prognosi. In pazienti con CAIS in cui l'orientamento sessuale sia indiscutibilmente femminile, i testicoli devono essere rimossi quanto prima dopo la loro scoperta. La rimozione laparoscopica delle gonadi contenenti il cromosoma Y è stata eseguita in pazienti con AIS e in quelli con disgenesia gonadica. In un terzo dei pazienti, verso l'età di 50 anni, si sviluppano neoplasie maligne, di solito seminomi. Molte ragazze adolescenti hanno manifestato seminomi. La terapia sostitutiva con estrogeni è indicata all'epoca della pubertà.

Le ragazze in cui non siano stati rimossi i testicoli, alla pubertà presentano un normale sviluppo mammario. In queste pazienti, la produzione di estradiolo deriva dall'attività aromatasica. Anche l'assenza dell'attività androgenica contribuisce alla femminilizzazione di queste donne.

La gestione psicosessuale e il trattamento chirurgico di pazienti con AIS parziale sono molto complessi e dipendono in larga parte dal fenotipo presente. L'osteopenia rappresenta una caratteristica dell'AIS.

Analisi molecolari hanno suggerito che il fenotipo possa dipendere da un mosaicismo somatico del gene del recettore androgenico. L'ipotesi si basa sul caso di un paziente 46,XY che presentava un codone di stop prematuro nell'esone 1 del gene AR, ma che manifestava anche virilizzazione (peli pubici e ipertrofia clitoridea), spiegata, a un esame accurato del gel di sequenziamento, dalla scoperta di alleli di tipo selvaggio. La presenza di mosaicismo modifica il fenotipo nel senso di un maggior grado di virilizzazione rispetto a quello previsto dal genotipo del solo allele mutante.

La consulenza genetica è difficile in famiglie con mutazione del gene del recettore androgenico. In aggiunta alla mancanza di correlazione tra genotipo e fenotipo, nelle famiglie esiste un'alta percentuale (27%) di mutazioni *ex novo*.

La riduzione della globulina di trasporto degli ormoni sessuali dopo somministrazione di androgeni esogeni (stanatolo), è correlata alla gravità del difetto recettoriale e può diventare un utile strumento clinico. In pazienti con AIS parziale e mutazioni varie del recettore androgenico nel dominio di legame DNA e in quello di legame alle ligandine, la terapia con androgeni ha avuto successo.

Anche in pazienti con atrofia muscolare spinale e bulbare, in cui le manifestazioni cliniche comprendevano atrofia testicolare, infertilità, ginecomastia ed elevati livelli di LH, FSH ed estradiolo verso la terza e quinta decade di vita, sono stati trovati dei recettori androgenici mutati. Mutazioni del recettore androgenico sono state descritte anche in pazienti con tumori prostatici.

CAUSE INDETERMINATE

Altri maschi XY ipovirilizzati dimostrano notevole variabilità dei genitali esterni e interni e gradi diversi di sviluppo fallico e mülleriano. I testicoli possono essere istologicamente normali o rudimentali o può esserne presente uno solo. In un notevole numero di bambini, anche con le tecniche più aggiornate, può non essere possibile trovare le cause di DSD. Alcune ambiguità dei genitali sono associate a un'ampia varietà di aberrazioni cromosomiche, che vanno sempre considerate nella diagnosi differenziale e di queste la più frequente è la sindrome 45,X/46,XY (vedi Capitolo 587.1). Per stabilire il mosaicismo, può essere necessario esaminare molti tessuti. Altre complesse sindromi genetiche, molte delle quali dipendono da mutazioni di un singolo gene, sono associate a gradi variabili di ambiguità genitale, particolarmente nel maschio. Queste forme si identificano sulla base delle malformazioni extragenitali associate.

La **sindrome di Smith-Lemli-Opitz** è una malattia autosomica recessiva causata da mutazioni del gene della sterolo δ7-reduttasi, localizzato sul cromosoma 11q12-q13. È caratterizzata da ritardo della crescita pre e post- natale, microcefalia, ptosi, narici anteverse, ampi solchi alveolari, sindattilia del secondo e terzo dito, e severo ritardo mentale (vedi Capitolo 86.3). La sua incidenza varia da 1/20 000 a 1/60 000; il 70% è rappresentato da maschi. Gli individui genotipicamente maschi solitamente presentano ambiguità genitale e, occasionalmente, completa inversione sessuale, con ambiguità genitale femminile o inversione sessuale completa con genitali esterni di tipo femminile. I derivati del dotto mülleriano sono normalmente assenti. I pazienti 46,XX hanno genitali normali. Sono state identificate due forme di sindrome di Smith-Lemli-Opitz: una **forma classica** (tipo I), descritta prima, e la sindrome acrodisgenitale, di solito letale nel primo anno, associata a severe malformazioni, polidattilia post-assiale e genitali esterni molto anomali (tipo II). La stenosi pilorica si associa alla sindrome di Smith-Lemli-Opitz tipo I e la malattia di Hirschsprung al tipo II. Nella **forma di tipo II** sono stati descritti schisi palatale, anomalie scheletriche e un caso di lipoma ipofisario. Alcuni Autori riportano uno spettro di gravità della malattia maggiore rispetto alla precedente classificazione. Nel tipo I e II sono stati trovati bassi livelli di colesterolo con aumento del suo precursore, il 7-deidrocolesterolo, in assenza di una correlazione con la gravità della malattia. I valori di apolipoproteina E materna sono invece in rapporto con la gravità. L'espressione prenatale più frequente della sindrome di Smith-Lemli-Opitz è il ritardo della crescita intrauterina (per il trattamento vedi Capitolo 86.3).

Soggetti 46,XY con DSD sono stati descritti nei fratelli con la sindrome α talassemia/ritardo mentale.

589.3 • DSD OVOTESTICOLARE

Nella DSD ovotesticolare, sono presenti tessuti sia ovarici sia testicolari, nella stessa gonade o in quella controlaterale. I pazienti presentano ambiguità genitale, che varia da un normale fenotipo femminile con solo una modesta ipertrofia clitoridea, a un fenotipo maschile con genitali esterni quasi normali (vedi Fig. 589-2A).

Circa il 70% di tutti i pazienti presenta un cariotipo 46,XX; il 97% degli africani neri è 46,XX. Meno del 10% delle persone con DSD ovotesticolare è 46,XY. Circa il 20% ha un mosaicismo 46,XX/46,XY. La metà di questi deriva da più di uno zigote e si tratta di chimere (chi 46,XX/46,XY). È dimostrata la presenza di alleli materni e paterni per alcuni gruppi sanguigni. È riportato il caso di una DSD ovotesticolare chimera, 46,XX/46,XY, derivante da mescolanza embrionale dopo fertilizzazione *in vitro*. Ciascun embrione derivava da una cellula uovo indipendente, separatamente fertilizzato.

L'esame di pazienti DSD ovotesticolari 46,XX, con indagini specifiche per Y, ha evidenziato che meno del 10% possiede una porzione del cromosoma Y compresa nel gene *SRY*. La DSD ovotesticolare è in genere sporadica, ma sono riportati casi in fratelli. La causa della maggior parte delle situazioni è sconosciuta.

La gonade rappresentata più frequentemente nella DSD ovotesticolare è l'ovotestis, anche bilaterale; se unilaterale, l'altra gonade di solito è un ovaio, talvolta un testicolo. Il tessuto ovarico è normale, ma quello testicolare è disgenetico. È possibile verificare la presenza e la funzione di tessuto testicolare misurando i livelli di testosterone basali e dopo stimolazione con hCG o i livelli di AMH. I pazienti molto virilizzati presentano una buona funzione testicolare, non hanno utero e di solito vengono cresciuti come maschi. Se esiste l'utero, la virilizzazione è modesta e minima la funzione testicolare; in questi casi può essere indicata l'assegnazione al sesso femminile e la rimozione selettiva del tessuto gonadico incoerente al sesso di assegnazione. In poche famiglie, sono stati descritti, nella stessa prole, soggetti 46,XY con DSD ovotesticolare e maschi 44,XX.

In alcuni individui 46,XX con DSD ovotesticolare allevati come femmine, sono state descritte gravidanze con prole viva, ma solo pochissimi maschi con DSD ovotesticolare sono diventati padre. Circa il 5% dei pazienti evidenzia gonadoblastomi, disgerminomi o seminomi.

DIAGNOSI E TRATTAMENTO. Nel neonato, l'ambiguità dei genitali richiede un'immediata attenzione per decidere, il più precocemente possibile, il sesso con cui il bambino dovrà essere cresciuto. La famiglia deve essere informata al più presto della situazione del bambino, in modo completo, onesto e partecipato. È necessaria una certa cautela per evitare sentimenti di colpa, vergogna e disagio. È indispensabile un'assistenza per alleviare i problemi a breve e lungo termine e per consentire al bambino di crescere in un ambiente completamente accogliente. La terapia iniziale prevede l'intervento di un team di specialisti, tra cui l'endocrinologo, il radiologo, l'urologo, lo psicologo e il genetista, che si concentrino prima di tutto sulle necessità del bambino. Il trattamento del potenziale disagio psicologico che queste patologie possono generare nel bambino o nella famiglia è di primaria importanza e richiede l'intervento dei medici e di altre figure professionali con particolare sensibilità, specializzazione ed esperienza in questo settore.

Mentre si attendono i risultati delle analisi cromosomiche, è indicata l'esecuzione di un'ecografia, per determinare la presenza di utero e ovaie. La presenza dell'utero e l'assenza di gonadi palpabili suggerisce una femmina XX virilizzata. Si deve quindi intraprendere la ricerca della sorgente della virilizzazione, compresa la determinazione degli ormoni surrenali, per escludere le forme di iperplasia surrenalica congenita, mentre occasionalmente possono essere necessari studi degli androgeni e degli estrogeni, per escludere il deficit di aromatasi. Le femmine XX virilizzate sono generalmente (ma non sempre) cresciute come femmine, anche se notevolmente virilizzate.

L'assenza dell'utero, con o senza gonadi palpabili, quasi sempre indica un'ipovirilizzazione maschile e un cariotipo XY. Sono necessarie misurazioni dei livelli di gonadotropine, testosterone, AMH e DHT, per determinare se la produzione testicolare di androgeni è normale. Maschi ipovirilizzati, totalmente femminilizzati possono essere cresciuti come femmine. Tuttavia, certi neonati di aspetto tipicamente femminile, come quelli con deficit di 5α-reduttasi, possono anche essere cresciuti come maschi, perché alla pubertà questi bambini si virilizzano normalmente. Il 6% dei bambini cresciuti come femmine durante l'infanzia vive in seguito come maschio. Un neonato con un grado analogo di femminilizzazione dovuto a un difetto del recettore androgenico, come nella CAIS, è cresciuto meglio come femmina. Neonati con cariotipo 45,XX/46,XY, in cui i fenotipi sono variabili da uno quasi completamente maschile, a uno completamente femminile, sono di solito allevati come femmine, perché sono di bassa statura e presentano l'utero; in questi casi è necessaria la gonadectomia.

Nel sospetto, in un maschio XY con micropene, di alterazioni recettoriali, la somministrazione intramuscolo di testosterone enantato (25-50 mg) può aiutare nella diagnosi differenziale e nel trattamento.

In alcuni mammiferi, le femmine esposte agli androgeni prima della nascita o nelle fasi immediatamente postnatali, nella vita adulta manifestano un comportamento sessuale non tradizionale. La maggior parte, ma non la totalità, delle ragazze sottoposte a mascolinizzazione fetale per iperplasia surrenalica congenita o per terapia progestinica materna non hanno problemi di identità sessuale, nonostante durante l'infanzia possano preferire attività e compagni di gioco maschili piuttosto che compagne di gioco femmine e giochi femminili con bambole, in ruoli materni.

Poiché si riteneva più semplice ricostruire i genitali esterni per creare una femmina sessualmente funzionante, soprattutto se già in presenza di vagina, più che creare un pene funzionante, in assenza di ragionevoli prospettive di un pene maschile ben funzionante, i neonati DSD, negli Stati Uniti, sono stati in passato quasi sempre assegnati al genere femminile. Attualmente esistono notevoli controversie circa queste decisioni. Non è detto che un sistema genitale esterno di tipo femminile scarsamente funzionante sia migliore di un pene maschile scarsamente funzionante. Inoltre, il funzionamento sessuale è in larga parte dipendente da altri fattori, neuro-ormonali e comportamentali, piuttosto che dall'aspetto fisico e dalla capacità funzionale dei genitali. Questo concetto è stato di aiuto nel caso di un individuo 46,XY in cui era stato accidentalmente ablato il pene ed era stato di conseguenza cresciuto come femmina. Alla pubertà, l'individuo è diventato maschio e ha continuato a vivere come tale con successo la sua vita.

Allo stesso modo, esistono controversie circa il momento più opportuno per praticare interventi chirurgici, invasivi e definitivi. È opportuno che il team multidisciplinare di esperti consideri la possibilità di rinviare, quando possibile e senza danneggiare la salute fisica o psicologica del bambino, la riparazione chirurgica e la gonadectomia fino a che il bambino stesso possa partecipare, con un consenso informato, alla procedura. Sono necessari studi scientifici retrospettivi e prospettici a lungo termine e in un sufficiente numero di individui con DSD, per valutare il loro stato anatomico, psicosessuale, sociale e funzionale. I risultati di questi studi potrebbero essere utilizzati per tracciare linee guida riguardanti tutti gli aspetti della gestione di neonati e bambini con DSD.

I pediatri e gli endocrinologi pediatrici, in collaborazione con altri specialisti, dovrebbero fornire una terapia di supporto continua e partecipata al paziente e alla sua famiglia per tutta l'infanzia, l'adolescenza e l'età adulta. Sono disponibili gruppi di sostegno per le famiglie e i pazienti che presentano molte delle condizioni discusse.

Bose HS, Pescovitz OH, Miller WL: Spontaneous feminization in a 46,XX female patient with congenital lipoid adrenal hyperplasia due to a homozygous frameshift mutation in the steroidogenic acute regulatory protein. *J Clin Endocrinol Metab* 1997;82:1511–1515.

Brinkmann AO: Molecular basis of androgen insensitivity. *Mol Cell Endocrinol* 2001;179:105–1099.

Cameron FJ, Montalto J, Byrt E, et al: Gonadal dysgenesis: Associations between clinical features and sex of rearing. *Endocr J* 1997;44:95–104.

Canto P, Vilchis F, Chavez B, et al: Mutations of the 5α-reductase type 2 gene in eight Mexican patients from six different pedigrees with 5α-reductase-2 deficiency. *Clin Endocrinol* 1997;46:155–160.

Chu J, Zhang R, Zhao Z, et al: Male fertility is compatible with an Arg840 Cys substitution in the AR in a large Chinese family affected with divergent phenotypes of AR insensitivity syndrome. *J Clin Endocrinol Metab* 2002;87:347–351.

Creighton S, Minto C: Managing intersex. *Br Med J* 2001;323:1264–1265.

Daaboul J, Frader J: Ethics and the management of the patient with intersex: A middle way. *J Pediatr Endocrinol Metab* 2001;14:1575–1583.

Damiani D, Fellous M, McElreavey K, et al: True hermaphroditism: Clinical aspects and molecular studies in 16 cases. *Eur J Endocrinol* 1997;136: 201–204.

Diamond DA, Mitchell C, Lamb K, et al: Sex assignment for newborns with ambiguous genitalia and exposure to fetal testosterone: Attitudes and practices of pediatric urologists. *J Pediatr* 2006;148:445–449.

Diamond M, Sigmundson K: Sex reassignment at birth. *Arch Pediatr Adolesc Med* 1997;151:298–304.

Frade Costa EM, Bilharinho Mendonca B, Inacio M, et al: Management of ambiguous genitalia in pseudohermaphrodites: New perspectives on vaginal dilation. *Fertil Steril* 1997;67:229–232.

Geissler WM, Davis DL, Wu L, et al: Male pseudohermaphroditism caused by mutation of testicular 17β-hydroxysteroid dehydrogenase 3. *Nat Genet* 1994;7:34–39.

Gul D: Third case of WAGR syndrome with severe obesity and constitutional deletion of chromosome (11)(p12p14). *Am J Med Genet* 2002;107:70–71.

Hiort O, Sinnecker GHG, Holterbus PM, et al: Inherited and de novo androgen receptor gene mutations: Investigation of single-case families. *J Pediatr* 1998;132:939–943.

Hochberg Z, Chayen R, Reiss N, et al: Clinical, biochemical and genetic findings in a large pedigree of male and female patients with 5α-reductase 2 deficiency. *J Clin Endocrinol Metab* 1996;81:2821–2827.

Kremer H, Karaaij R, Toledo SPA, et al: Male pseudohermaphroditism due to a homozygous missense mutation of the luteinizing hormone receptor gene. *Nat Genet* 1995;9:160–164.

Krob G, Braun A, Kuhnle U: True hermaphroditism: Geographical distribution, clinical findings, chromosomes and gonadal histology. *Eur J Pediatr* 1994;153:2–10.

Lee PA, Houk CP, Ahmed SF, et al: Consensus statement on management of intersex disorders. *Pediatrics* 2006;118:e488–500.

MacLaughlin DT, Donahoe PK: Sex determination and differentiation. *N Engl J Med* 2004;350:367–378.

McPherson EW, Clemens MM, Gibbons RJ, et al: X-linked α-thalassemia/mental retardation (ATR-X) syndrome: A new kindred with severe genital anomalies and mild hematologic expression. *Am J Med Genet* 1995; 55:302–306.

Mebarki F, Sanchez R, Rheaumes E, et al: Non-salt-losing male pseudohermaphroditism due to the novel homozygous N100S mutation in the type II 3 β-hydroxysteroid dehydrogenase gene. *J Clin Endocrinol Metab* 1995;80:2127–2134.

Mendonca BB, Inacio M, Costa EMF, et al: Male pseudohermaphroditism due to steroid 5α-reductase 2 deficiency. *Medicine* 1996;75:64–76.

Mendonca BB, Leite MV, DeCastro M, et al: Female pseudohermaphroditism caused by a novel homozygous mutation of the GR gene. *J Clin Endocrinol Metab* 2002;87:1805–1809.

Moisan AM, Ricketts ML, Tardy V, et al: New insight into the molecular basis of 3β-hydroxysteroid dehydrogenase deficiency: Identification of eight mutations in the HSD3 gene in eleven patients from seven new families and comparison of the functional properties of twenty-five mutant enzymes. *J Clin Endocrinol Metab* 1999;84:4410–4425.

Mongan NP, Jaaskelainen J, Green K, et al: Two de novo mutations in the AR gene cause the complete androgen insensitivity syndrome in a pair of monozygotic twins. *J Clin Endocrinol Metab* 2002;87:1057–1061.

Morishima A, Grumbach MM, Simpson ER, et al: Aromatase deficiency in male and female siblings caused by a novel mutation and the physiological role of estrogens. *J Clin Endocrinol Metab* 1995;80:3689–3698.

Mueller RF: The Denys-Drash syndrome. *J Med Genet* 1994;31:471–477.

Mullis PE, Yoshimura N, Kuhlmann B, et al: Aromatase deficiency in a female who is compound heterozygote for two new point mutations in the $P450_{arom}$ gene: Impact of estrogens on hypergonadotropic hypogonadism, multicystic ovaries, and bone densitometry in childhood. *J Clin Endocrinol Metab* 1997;82:1739–1745.

Quigley CA, French FS: Androgen insensitivity syndromes. *Curr Ther Endocrinol Metab* 1994;5:342–351.

Reardon W, Gibbons RJ, Winter RM, et al: Male pseudohermaphroditism in sibs with the α-thalassemia/mental retardation (ATR-X) syndrome. *Am J Med Genet* 1995;55:285–287.

Saenger P: New developments in congenital lipoid adrenal hyperplasia and steroidogenic acute regulatory protein. *Pediatr Clin North Am* 1997; 44:397–421.

Sarafoglou K, Ostrer H: Clinical Review 111–Familial sex reversal: A review. *J Clin Endocrinol Metab* 2000;85:483–493.

Smith EP, Boyd J, Frank GR, et al: Estrogen resistance caused by a mutation in the estrogen-receptor gene in a man. *N Engl J Med* 1994;331: 1056–1061.

Tajima T, Fujieda K, Kouda N, et al: Heterozygous mutation in the cholesterol side chain cleavage enzyme (P450scc) gene in a patient with 46,XY sex reversal and adrenal insufficiency. *J Clin Endocrinol Metab* 2001;86: 3820–3825.

Weidemann W, Peters B, Romalo G, et al: Response to androgen treatment in a patient with partial androgen insensitivity and a mutation in the deoxyribonucleic acid-binding domain of the androgen receptor. *J Clin Endocrinol Metab* 1998;83:1173–1176.

Sezione 6 — Diabete mellito nei bambini — Ramin Alemzadeh e David T. Wyatt

Capitolo 590 ■ Diabete mellito

590.1 • Introduzione e classificazione

Il diabete mellito (DM) è una frequente sindrome metabolica cronica, in cui l'iperglicemia rappresenta la caratteristica biochimica fondamentale. Le forme principali di diabete sono classificate a seconda che siano dovute a un deficit di secrezione insulinica per danno pancreatico delle cellule β (DM di tipo 1, o T1DM) o siano la conseguenza di una resistenza insulinica a livello del muscolo scheletrico, del fegato e del tessuto adiposo, con vari gradi di alterazione della cellula β (DM di tipo 2, o T2DM). T1DM è la più frequente malattia endocrino-metabolica dell'infanzia e dell'adolescenza, con importanti conseguenze per lo sviluppo fisico ed emotivo. Pazienti con T1DM devono affrontare notevoli cambiamenti del loro stile di vita, che comprendono l'inderogabile richiesta quotidiana di insulina esogena, la necessità di monitorare la glicemia e di porre attenzione all'intake dietetico. La morbilità e la mortalità derivano da squilibri metabolici acuti e da **complicanze** a lungo termine (di solito nella vita adulta) che colpiscono i piccoli e i grandi vasi con conseguenti retinopatia, nefropatia, neuropatia, cardiopatia ischemica e ostruzione arteriosa con gangrena degli arti. Le manifestazioni cliniche acute sono dovute a chetoacidosi iperglicemica ipoinsulinemica. Nella genesi del T1DM rientrano meccanismi autoimmunitari; le complicanze a lungo termine sono correlate a disturbi metabolici in cui si distinguono aspetti genetici e altri meccanismi eziologici e fisiopatologici, che portano a una alterazione della tolleranza glicidica. Una classificazione del diabete e di altri tipi di intolleranza glicidica viene illustrata nella Tabella 590-1. Sono indicate tre forme principali di diabete e alcune forme di intolleranza ai carboidrati.

DIABETE MELLITO DI TIPO 1. Definito anche diabete mellito insulino-dipendente (*Insulin-Dependent Diabetes Mellitus*, IDDM) o diabete giovanile, il T1DM è caratterizzato da livelli di insulina endogena bassi o assenti e dalla dipendenza da insulina esogena, per prevenire lo sviluppo di chetoacidosi, una complicanza acuta del T1DM pericolosa per la vita. La storia naturale della malattia comprende quattro fasi distinte: (1) autoimmunità preclinica contro le cellule β, con progressivo deficit di secrezione insulinica, (2) esordio clinico del diabete, (3) remissione transitoria, o "periodo luna di miele", e (4) diabete stabilizzato associato a complicanze acute e croniche e diminuzione della spettanza di vita. L'esordio si verifica prevalentemente nell'infanzia, a un'età media che va dai 7 ai 15 anni, ma può presentarsi a qualsiasi età. Il T1DM è caratterizzato da una distruzione autoimmunitaria delle cellule β delle insule pancreatiche. Alla patogensi contribuiscono fattori sia genetici sia ambientali. La suscettibilità al T1DM è geneticamente controllata dagli alleli dei geni del maggior complesso di istocompatibilità (*Major Histocompatibility Complex*, MHC) di classe II, che esprimono antigeni leucocitari umani (*Human Leukocyte Antigens*, HLA). È associato anche ad autoanticorpi anticitoplasma delle cellule delle insule pancreatiche (*Islet Cell Cytoplasm Autoantibodies*, ICA), anti-insulina (*Insulin*, IAA) e anti-acido glutammico decarbossilasi (*Antibodies to Glutamic Acid Decarboxylase*, GADA o GAD65), e ICA512 (IA2). Il T1DM è associato ad altre patologie **autoimmuni** come tiroidite, malattia celiaca, sclerosi multipla e malattia di Addison. In alcuni bambini e adolescenti con T1DM apparente, la distruzione delle cellule β non è mediata dall'immunità. Questo sottotipo di diabete si verifica in pazienti di origine africana o asiatica e dipende da cause note di distruzione β-insulare, come farmaci o sostanze chimiche, virus, difetti genetici mitocondriali, pancreatectomia e radiazioni ionizzanti. Questi individui possono presentare chetoacidosi, ma hanno lunghi periodi di remissione con deficit variabili di insulina, analogamente ai pazienti con T2DM.

DIABETE MELLITO DI TIPO 2. I bambini e gli adolescenti con questo tipo di diabete sono di solito obesi, ma non insulino-dipendenti, e raramente sviluppano chetoacidosi. Alcuni possono presentare chetosi durante gravi infezioni o altri stress e possono manifestare la necessità di insulina per correggere l'iperglicemia sintomatica. Questa categoria comprende la forma di diabete prevalente nell'adulto, caratterizzata da insulino-resistenza e spesso da progressivo difetto della secrezione insulinica. Questo tipo di diabete è noto come diabete mellito a esordio nell'adulto, diabete mellito non insulino-dipendente (*Non-Insulin-Dependent Diabetes Mellitus*, NIDDM) o diabete giovanile a esordio nell'età matura (*Maturity-Onset Diabetes of the Young*, MODY).

La presentazione del T2DM è tipicamente più insidiosa di quella del T1DM. Al contrario dei pazienti con T1DM, in cui la malattia è presente al momento della diagnosi, i bambini con T2DM spesso arrivano all'attenzione medica per eccesso di peso corporeo e affaticamento, come conseguenza dell'insulino-resistenza, e/o per il reperto accidentale, durante indagini di routine, di glicosuria. In questi pazienti è relativamente rara un'anamnesi positiva per poliuria e polidipsia. In molti centri diabetici, l'incidenza del T2DM nei bambini è aumentata più di 10 volte, in parte come risultato dell'obesità epidemica nei bambini (vedi Capitolo 44). Il T2DM di interesse pediatrico raggiunge quasi il 30% dei nuovi casi di diabete, specialmente in adolescenti obesi africani e messicani. L'**acanthosis nigricans** (pigmentazione scura della pelle delle pieghe e delle flessure), segno di insulino-resistenza, è presente nella maggior parte dei pazienti con T2DM ed è accompagnata da iperinsulinemia relativa al momento della diagnosi (vedi Capitolo 651). Tuttavia, l'incremento dei livelli sierici di insulina è di solito inferiore a quello di bambini e adolescenti non diabetici di uguale peso, età e sesso, suggerendo una situazione di insufficienza insulinica. In alcuni individui, è possibile una lenta evoluzione verso il T1DM.

In alcuni bambini con anamnesi familiare positiva per T2DM, l'alterata tolleranza glicidica si può manifestare nell'ambito di un'ereditarietà dominante. Questo tipo di diabete è stato definito **diabete giovanile a esordio nell'età matura** (MODY), e può richiedere trattamento insulinico. Nel MODY, non c'è evidenza di distruzione immunitaria delle cellule β e non esiste associazione con HLA. Questa sottoclasse di T2DM consiste di specifiche patologie genetiche, che coinvolgono mutazioni del gene che codifica la glucochinasi (*Glucokinase*, GK) delle cellule β pancreatiche ed epatiche o del fattore nucleare epatocitario (*Hepatocyte Nuclear Factor*, HNF) dei fattori di trascrizione nucleare (1α, 4α o 1β). Un difetto del gene che regola il trasporto del glucosio all'interno delle cellule β pancreatiche, il transporter GLUT2, può essere responsabile di altre forme di T2DM. La base genetica del T2DM comprende anche difetti della glicogeno sintasi, dei recettori insulinici, del Rad (Ras associato a diabete) e anche della apolipoproteina C-III.

ALTRI TIPI SPECIFICI DI DIABETE SECONDARIO. Gli esempi comprendono il diabete secondario a patologie pancreatiche esocrine (fibrosi cistica), ad altre patologie endocrine (sindrome di Cushing) e all'ingestione di certi farmaci o veleni (certi topicidi). Rientrano

TABELLA 590-1. Classificazione eziologica del diabete mellito

Diabete di tipo 1* (Distruzione β-cellulare, che di solito porta a deficit assoluto di insulina)
Immunomediato
Idiopatico
Diabete di tipo 2* (può variare da una forma con prevalenza di resistenza insulinica e deficit relativo di insulina, a una forma con difetto prevalentemente secretorio con insulino resistenza)
Tipo 2 dominante per mutazione del recettore 1 della sulfonilurea
Altri tipi specifici
Difetti genetici della funzione β-cellulare
Cromosoma 12, HFN-1α (MODY3)
Cromosoma 7, glucochinasi (MODY2)
Cromosoma 20, HNF-4α (MODY1)
Fattore-1 promotore dell'insulina (MODY4)
HNF-1β(MODY5)
NUROD1 (MODY6)
DNA mitocondriale
Altri
Difetti genetici dell'azione insulinica
Insulino-resistenza di tipo A
Leprecaunismo
Sindrome di Rabson-Mendenhall
Diabete lipoatrofico
Altri
Malattie del pancreas esocrino
Pancreatite
Trauma, pancreatectomia
Neoplasia
Fibrosi cistica
Emocromatosi
Pancreopatia fibrocalcolotica
Resezione pancreatica
Altri
Endocrinopatie
Acromegalia
Malattia di Cushing
Glucagonoma
Feocromocitoma
Ipertiroidismo
Somatostatinoma
Aldosteronoma
Altri
Indotto da farmaci o sostanze chimiche
Vacor
Pentamidina
Acido nicotinico
Glicocorticoidi
Ormone tiroideo
Diazzosido
Agonisti β-adrenergici
Tiazide
Dilantina
Interferone-β
Altri, ciclosporina, tacrolimus
Infezioni
Rosolia congenita
Cytomegalovirus
Altri
Altre sindromi genetiche talvolta associate a diabete
Sindrome di Down
Sindrome di Klinefelter
Sindrome di Turner
Sindrome di Wolfram
Atassia di Friedreich
Corea di Huntington
Sindrome di Lawrence-Moon-Biedl
Distrofia miotonica
Porfiria
Sindrome di Prader-Willi
Altri
Diabete mellito gestazionale
Diabete mellito neonatale
Transitorio, senza recidiva
Transitorio, con recidiva 7-20 anni dopo
Permanente dall'esordio

*Pazienti con qualsiasi forma di diabete possono richiedere il trattamento insulinico in alcuni stadi della malattia. Pertanto i pazienti non vanno classificati in base all'uso di insulina.

in questo gruppo anche certe sindromi genetiche, comprese quelle con anomalie del recettore insulinico. Non esiste associazione con HLA, autoimmunità o anticorpi anti-cellule insulari.

La Tabella 590-2 riporta in dettaglio i criteri attuali per la diagnosi di DM. Si noti che il criterio accettato per la diagnosi di diabete consiste in una glicemia a digiuno superiore a 125 mg/dL (6,9 mmol/L).

ALTERATA TOLLERANZA AL GLUCOSIO. Il termine di alterata tolleranza al glucosio (*Impaired Glucose Tolerance*, IGT) si riferisce a una fase metabolica intermedia tra la normale omeostasi glucidica e il diabete. Una glicemia a digiuno di 99 mg/dL (5,5 mmol/L) rappresenta il limite massimo dei valori "normali". Questo valore è vicino a quello oltre il quale, in risposta alla somministrazione endovenosa di glucosio, manca la secrezione insulinica della fase acuta ed è associato a un rischio progressivamente maggiore di sviluppare complicanze micro- e macro-vascolari.

Molti individui con IGT (glicemia a digiuno di 100-125 mg/dL) sono solitamente normoglicemici e possono avere livelli normali o quasi di emoglobina glicosilata. Individui con IGT spesso manifestano iperglicemia solo quando sono sottoposti a carico orale di glucosio durante il test di tolleranza glicidica.

Al di fuori della gravidanza, la IGT non è un'entità clinica, ma più che altro un fattore di rischio per diabete e patologie cardiovascolari. Si osserva come stadio intermedio in ciascuno dei processi patologici indicati nella Tabella 590-1. La IGT è spesso associata alla **sindrome da insulino-resistenza** (nota anche con il nome di sindrome X o sindrome metabolica), che consiste in insulino-resistenza, iperinsulinemia secondaria per mantenere la normale omeostasi glicidica, obesità (specialmente addominale o viscerale), dislipidemia da trigliceridi alti o da aumento delle lipoproteine ad alta o bassa densità, o di entrambe, e ipertensione (vedi Capitolo 44). L'insulino-resistenza è direttamente coinvolta nella patogenesi del T2DM. L'IGT appare come un marker di rischio caratteristico di questo tipo di diabete, almeno in parte, per la correlazione all'insulino-resistenza. I criteri diagnostici per IGT sono illustrati nella Tabella 590-2.

590.2 • Diabete mellito di tipo 1 (immuno-mediato)

EPIDEMIOLOGIA: GENETICA E AMBIENTE. Il T1DM presenta un'incidenza in rapido aumento in specifiche regioni e tende a esordire in età più precoce. Il T1DM rappresenta circa il 10% di tutti i tipi di diabete, colpendo 1,4 milioni di persone negli Stati Uniti e circa 15 milioni nel mondo. È una delle malattie croniche infantili gravi più frequenti; il 40% degli individui con diabete di tipo 1 ha meno di 20 anni. L'incidenza del T1DM è molto variabile nei diversi gruppi etnici. L'incidenza complessiva regolata per età del DM di tipo 1 varia da 0,7/100 000 per anno a Karachi (Pakistan) a circa 40/100 000 per anno in Finlandia (Fig. 590-1).

TABELLA 590-2. Criteri diagnostici di alterata tolleranza glicidica e diabete mellito

ALTERATA TOLLERANZA GLICIDICA (IGT)	DIABETE MELLITO (DM)
Glicemia a digiuno 110-125 mg/dL (6,1-7,0 mmol/L)	Sintomi* di DM più glicemia >200 mg/dL (11,1 mmol/L)
Glucosio plasmatico dopo 2 ore dal carico orale di glucosio dell'OGTT <200 mg/dL (11,1 mmol/L) ma ≥140 mg/dL	*o*
	Glicemia a digiuno ≥126 mg/dL (7 mmol/L)
	o
	Glucosio plasmatico dopo 2 ore dal carico orale di glucosio ≥200 mg/dL

*Sintomi comprendono: poliuria, polidipsia e inspiegata perdita di peso con glicosuria e chetonuria.
OGTT, *Oral Glucose Tolerance Test* (test di tolleranza orale al glucosio).
Dal Report of the Export Committee on the Diagnosis and Classification of Diabetes mellitus. *Diabetes Care* 1999;20 (Suppl 1):S5.

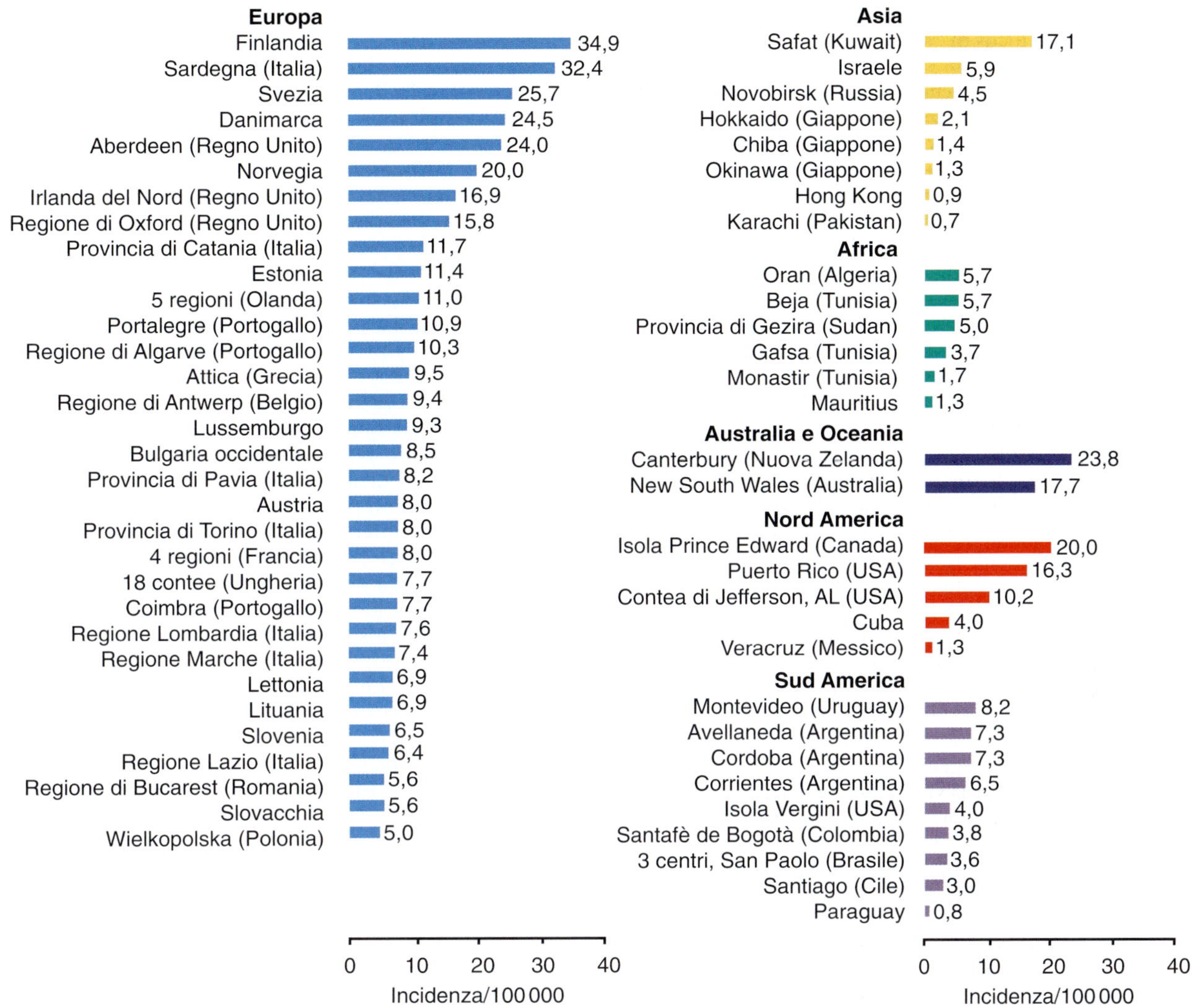

Figura 590-1. Incidenza percentuale del diabete mellito tipo 1 in varie regioni e Paesi. (Da Karvonen M, Viik-Kajander M, Moltchanova E e altri: Incidence of type I diabetes worldwide. Diabetes Mondiale (DiaMond) Project Group. *Diabetes Care* 2000;23(10):1516-1526.)

Il dato dimostra che c'è una variabilità nell'incidenza di più di 400 volte in 100 diverse popolazioni. Spesso si nota un aumento dell'incidenza in nazioni con una frequenza precedentemente bassa di diabete autoimmune; l'incidenza di T1DM in Thailandia è aumentata notevolmente da 0,2/100 000 nel periodo 1984-1985, fino a 1,65/100 000 10 anni dopo. Si prevede che l'incidenza complessiva di T1DM sarà nel 2010 maggiore del 40% rispetto a quella del 1997.

I dati provenienti dai centri diabetologici dell'Europa occidentale suggeriscono che la percentuale di incremento annuo nell'incidenza di T1DM sia del 3-4%, mentre alcuni Paesi dell'Europa centrale e orientale mostrano un aumento ancora più rapido. Questa percentuale di incremento è maggiore nei bambini più piccoli; la percentuale di incremento in funzione dell'età è di 6,3%, 3,1% e 2,4% in gruppi di bambini, rispettivamente, di 0-4 anni, 5-9 anni e 12-14 anni. Negli Stati Uniti, la prevalenza complessiva del diabete nei bambini in età scolare è di circa 1,9/1000. La frequenza, tuttavia, è più alta all'aumentare dell'età; il range è 1/1,43 bambini a 5 anni a 1/360 ragazzi a 16 anni. Tra gli afroamericani, l'incidenza di T1DM è del 30-60% rispetto a quella degli americani bianchi. L'incidenza annuale di nuovi casi negli Stati Uniti è di circa 14,9/100 000 bambini. Negli Stati Uniti si sono stimati 30 000 nuovi casi all'anno, che colpiscono 1 su 300 bambini e 1 su 100 adulti, durante l'arco della vita. Femmine e maschi sono colpiti in uguale misura; non esiste una correlazione apparente con lo stato socioeconomico. Il picco di incidenza si verifica in due gruppi di età: a 5-7 anni e al momento della pubertà. Un numero crescente di casi si manifesta tra il primo e il secondo anno di vita. Il primo picco può corrispondere al momento in cui aumenta l'esposizione agli agenti infettivi, per l'inizio della scuola; il secondo picco può corrispondere allo *spurt* di crescita puberale indotto dagli steroidi gonadici e dalla aumentata secrezione puberale di ormone della crescita (che antagonizza l'insulina). Questi possibili rapporti causa-effetto sono ancora da testare.

Geni. I geni del T1DM possono essere responsabili della suscettibilità o della protezione dalla malattia. Nonostante siano stati localizzati molti loci cromosomici associati a queste attività, sono stati identificati pochi veri geni. La genetica del T1DM non può essere classificata secondo un modello specifico di trasmissione ereditaria. I geni più importanti sono localizzati nella regione MHC HLA di classe II, sul cromosoma 6p21, denominato formalmente (IDDM1), che rappresenta circa il 60% della suscettibilità genetica a questa malattia. Il suo specifico contributo alla patogenesi di T1DM rimane sconosciuto. L'importanza degli aplotipi di classe II non dipende solo da un ben noto rischio per patologie associate a HLA-DR3 e HLA-DR4, ma anche da un'ulteriore suscettibilità associata alla catena DQα e alla catena DQβ. L'ereditarietà degli antigeni HLA-DR3 o DR4 sembra conferisca un rischio 2-3 volte maggiore di sviluppare T1DM. Quando si eredita sia DR3 sia DR4, il rischio relativo di sviluppare diabete aumenta di 7-10 volte. L'analisi del polimorfismo del DNA dopo digestione con specifiche endonucleasi di restrizione ha rivelato un'ulteriore eterogeneità della regione HLA-DR tra individui con e senza diabete, nonostante il possesso di entrambi i marker DR3 e DR4, suggerendo un locus di "suscettibilità" ancora da definire in questi marker.

Nei caucasici almeno un locus maggiore di suscettibilità può risiedere nel gene DQβ$_1$. L'assenza omozigote dell'acido aspartico in posizione 57 della catena HLA DQβ (non-Asp/non-Asp) conferisce un rischio circa 100 volte superiore di sviluppare diabete di tipo 1. Gli eterozigoti con un singolo acido aspartico in posizione 57 (non-Asp/Asp) si ammalano molto meno facilmente di diabete e sono solo marginalmente più suscettibili degli individui che hanno l'acido aspartico su entrambe le catene DQβ e che sono omozigoti Asp/Asp. Pertanto, la presenza di acido aspartico su uno o entrambi gli alleli della catena DQβ protegge contro lo sviluppo di diabete autoimmune, ma, a dire il vero, l'incidenza del DM di tipo 1 in una data popolazione è proporzionale alla frequenza degli alleli non-Asp di quella popolazione. Inoltre, l'arginina in posizione 52 della catena DQβ conferisce una marcata suscettibilità al diabete di tipo 1. Le posizioni 57 e 52 della DQβ sono critiche della molecola di HLA, che permettono o prevengono la presentazione antigenica dei recettori delle cellule T e attivano la cascata autoimmunitaria. Tuttavia, il DM di tipo 1 è unico nell'ambito delle patologie autoimmuni, nelle quali, oltre alla suscettibilità, certi aplotipi MHC provvedono a una protezione significativa. Gli alleli HLA-DRB1*0301, HLA-DRb1*0401, HLA-DQB1*0302 e HLA-DQA1*0301 di MHC (IDDM1) conferiscono suscettibilità a un rischio elevato nell'uomo, mentre altri alleli come HLA-DRB1*0403, HLA-DQB1*0602 e HLA-DQA1*0301 sono associati negativamente al DM di tipo 1 e possono conferire resistenza. L'osservazione che il 20% degli europei o degli statunitensi sono portatori di aplotipo protettivo HLA-DR2 e che ancora meno dell'1% dei bambini con DM di tipo 1 è DR2 (DQB1*0602) positivo evidenzia questa importante componente genetica.

Il T1DM rappresenta una patologia eterogenea e poligenica. Sono stati identificati circa 20 loci non HLA che contribuiscono alla suscettibilità alla patologia. È conosciuta la funzione di solo 2 loci non HLA. IDDM2 sul cromosoma 11p5.5 è una regione polimorfica che mappa minisatelliti, cioè ripetizioni in tandem di numero variabile (*Variable Number of Tandem Minisatellite Repeats*, VNTR), con alleli VNTR brevi di classe I che predispongono al DM di tipo 1 e alleli più lunghi di classe III che rivestono un effetto protettivo dominante. Questo locus contribuisce a circa il 10% della suscettibilità alla malattia. Un altro locus associato al DM di tipo 1 in alcune popolazioni è IDDM12, sul cromosoma 2q33, che mappa vicino ai 2 marker delle cellule T coinvolti nell'attivazione delle cellule T: la proteina 4 associata al linfocita citotossico T (CTLA-4) e CD28. Studi su famiglie italiane e spagnole hanno dimostrato che il polimorfismo a livello del gene di CTL4 (transizione A-G in posizione 49 dell'esone 1), detto allele G, è trasmesso preferenzialmente ai fratelli affetti.

Nella determinazione del diabete sono coinvolti anche fattori diversi dall'ereditarietà pura dei marker HLA o di altri geni. Per esempio, si trovano HLA-DR3 o HLA-DR4 in circa il 50% della popolazione generale e (non-Asp/non-Asp) in circa il 20% dei bianchi non diabetici degli Stati Uniti; tuttavia, in questi soggetti, il rischio per DM di tipo 1 è solo un decimo di quello in un fratello HLA-identico di un caso indice che possiede questi marker. Anche fratelli che condividono solo un aplotipo hanno un rischio da 6 a 10 volte maggiore di sviluppare DM di tipo 1 rispetto alla popolazione normale. Inoltre, circa il 10% dei pazienti con T1DM non possiede né HLA-DR3 né -DR4, sebbene la maggior parte dei diabetici bianchi perda almeno un acido aspartico in posizione 57 della catena DQβ. La percentuale di concordanza fra gemelli identici è solo del 30-50%, dato che suggerisce sia la partecipazione di fattori scatenanti ambientali o di altri fattori genetici, sia la selezione post-natale di certi cloni di cellule T autoreattive che portano i recettori che riconoscono il "self". Questo processo post-natale si verifica nel timo e implica che gemelli identici non siano identici riguardo al repertorio recettoriale delle cellule T in loro possesso.

Il T1DM tra gli afroamericani è associato agli stessi geni HLA dei bianchi. Se un fratello condivide entrambi gli aplotipi HLA-D con un caso indice, il rischio di diabete di tipo 1 in questo individuo è del 12-20%; per un fratello che condivide un aplotipo, il rischio è del 5-7%; se non ci sono aplotipi in comune, il rischio è solo dell'1-2%. Si può affermare che nei bianchi, il rischio complessivo per i fratelli è di circa il 6% se il probando ha meno di 10 anni e del 3% se è più grande al momento della diagnosi. Il rischio della prole di un genitore diabetico è del 2-5%, che aumenta se è diabetico il padre. Negli afroamericani, questi rischi variano da solo la metà a due terzi rispetto a quelli dei bianchi.

Ambiente. Nella prima metà del XX secolo il T1DM infantile era raro, ma la sua incidenza è rapidamente aumentata negli ultimi 50 anni. La proporzione complessiva delle nuove diagnosi in soggetti portatori di uno o entrambi gli aplotipi di suscettibilità DR4-DQ8 e DR3-DQ2 non è cambiata; ora è diminuito il numero di quelli con genotipo a rischio maggiore DR4-DQ8/DR3-DQ2, bilanciato da un aumento del numero di quelli con genotipi a rischio minore DR4-DQ8/X e DR3-DQ2/X. La proporzione complessiva dei genotipi DR3-DQ2/DR4-DQ8 è diminuita, nei bambini di età compresa tra 0 e 15 anni, dal 47% al 35% e, nei bambini di età inferiore ai 5 anni, dal 63% al 42%. L'aumento dell'incidenza del T1DM nei bambini piccoli, tuttavia, dipende dalla suscettibilità genetica di un sottogruppo della popolazione. Si noti che il rischio di sviluppare T1DM con il genotipo DR3-DQ2/DR4-DQ8 è solo del 4% e questo dato rende lo screening per questo genotipo uno strumento scadente per i soggetti a rischio. Inoltre, l'incidenza di T1DM è aumentata molto più rapidamente rispetto a quanto ci si potrebbe aspettare dai soli cambiamenti genetici nella popolazione.

L'accresciuta incidenza degli aplotipi a rischio minore e il decremento dell'età media di esordio della malattia in questo sottogruppo sono in rapporto con un **maggior effetto dell'ambiente** sullo sviluppo del diabete. Le cause comprendono l'aumento della frequenza di un fattore nocivo di vecchia data ancora indeterminato e la diminuzione della frequenza di un fattore protettivo, come allattamento al seno, infezioni lievi della prima infanzia (teoria dell'igiene) o immunità di massa contro i virus, che può essere trasmessa al feto attraverso la placenta. Possibili agenti ambientali che scatenano l'autoimmunità contro le insule comprendono cereali ed elementi dietetici, come le tossine che provengono dai tuberi, ed Enterovirus.

Si è sospettato che fattori come infezioni e composti chimici, fattori ambientali quali la stagionalità e la localizzazione geografica, possano contribuire alle differenze di incidenza e prevalenza del T1DM in varie etnie. Non sono stati individuati agenti ambientali dominanti o agenti responsabili di innescare il T1DM. I determinanti del rischio ambientale, molto studiati, possono essere classificati in: infezioni virali, alimentazione dei primi mesi e composti chimici.

INFEZIONI VIRALI E VACCINAZIONI. Nonostante il ruolo eziologico delle infezioni virali nel T1DM umano sia controverso, il virus Coxsackie B3, il virus Coxsackie B4, il Cytomegalovirus, il virus della rosolia e della parotite possono infettare le cellule β umane. Solo la rosolia congenita è associata a diabete nelle fasi successive della vita. Si stima che il 10-12% dei pazienti colpiti da rosolia congenita sviluppi T1DM e che oltre il 40% sviluppi un'alterata tolleranza glicidica. Il diabete da rosolia assomiglia al T1DM, poiché è associato a HLA-DR3 e HLA-DR4 ed è mediato da una risposta immune contro gli antigeni β-cellulari. Non esistono correlazioni convincenti tra vaccinazioni infantili e rischio di T1DM.

ASSOCIAZIONI STAGIONALI. L'incidenza di IDDM presenta variazioni stagionali e ciclicità a lungo termine. Casi di recente diagnosi si manifestano con maggiore frequenza nei mesi autunnali e invernali, rispettivamente nell'emisfero settentrionale e in quello meridionale. Le variazioni stagionali sono molto evidenti durante l'adolescenza. Il tentativo di associare una ciclicità a lungo termine con l'incidenza della parotite o di altre infezioni virali non ha avuto successo. La stagionalità nel DM di tipo 1 in pazienti belgi di età superiore a 10 anni appare ristretta a maschi HLA-DQ2/DQ8-negativi.

PUBERTÀ. Il picco puberale di esordio del diabete di tipo 1 si verifica più precocemente nelle femmine rispetto ai maschi. Questa differenza in base al sesso può essere mediata in parte dagli estrogeni oppure da geni regolati dagli estrogeni, come il gene dell'interleuchina-6 (IL6), e suggerisce che le modificazioni puberali possono contribuire ad accelerare l'esordio del DM di tipo 1 in femmine geneticamente suscettibili.

FATTORI DIETETICI. I fattori dietetici sono stati implicati nella patogenesi del T1DM, ma il loro ruolo nell'induzione dell'autoimmunità insulare rimane controverso. L'alimentazione con latte di mucca somministrata a modelli animali di T1DM è stata associata allo sviluppo di diabete in questi animali. Il probabile meccanismo consiste nel mimetismo molecolare tra un peptide a 17 aminoacidi dell'albumina sierica bovina e l'antigene insulare 69. Anche se si ritiene che ci sia una relazione stretta tra il consumo di latte di mucca e l'incidenza nazionale di diabete nei bambini, il ruolo del latte di mucca nel diabete umano è controverso. Anche composti nitrosi, derivati dalla conversione a livello intestinale dei nitrati dei vegetali e della carne introdotti con la dieta, sono stati coinvolti nello sviluppo di diabete. Il ruolo di questi composti come fattore significativo di rischio nella patogenesi del diabete rimane controverso. Un'iniziale esposizione dei neonati ai cereali prima del quarto mese, o dopo il sesto, sembra accrescere il rischio di autoimmunità insulare indipendentemente dal genotipo HLA, dall'anamnesi familiare per T1DM, dal gruppo etnico e dall'età materna. Il rischio di autoimmunità insulare in entrambi i gruppi di età è aumentato maggiormente nei bambini positivi per genotipo HLA-DRB1*03/04,DQB8.

INDICE DI MASSA CORPOREA. Gli individui in sovrappeso nella prima infanzia possono avere un rischio maggiore di T1DM. L'**ipotesi dell'acceleratore** prevede un esordio più precoce nelle persone più pesanti, senza necessariamente una modificazione del rischio, e considera il tipo 1 e il T2DM come lo stesso disordine da resistenza all'insulina, nonostante differenti substrati genetici. L'insulino-resistenza è una funzione della massa grassa e, dal momento che all'aumentare del peso corporeo nel mondo industrializzato corrisponde una più precoce presentazione (accelerazione) del T2DM, i sostenitori dell'ipotesi dell'acceleratore suggeriscono che l'età di presentazione del T1DM sia associata anche alla quantità del tessuto adiposo. Pertanto, limitare l'eccessivo aumento di peso può essere importante sia per i bambini suscettibili di T1DM sia per quelli a rischio genetico di T2DM.

FATTORI CHIMICI. Farmaci come l'allossano, la streptozotocina (STZ), la pentamidina e il Vacor® sono direttamente citotossici per le cellule β e provocano diabete mellito negli animali da esperimento e negli uomini. Negli animali suscettibili, multiple dosi sub-diabetogene di STZ inducono un danno primario alla cellula β e, successivamente, risposte immuni contro le cellule stesse, evidenziando che un danno β-cellulare può evocare una specifica autoimmnunità. Si è dimostrata autoimmunità contro le cellule β anche in soggetti dopo intossicazione con il ratticida Vacor®.

La Figura 590-2 elenca le ipotesi eziologiche correnti del T1DM come malattia autoimmune, con una componente genetica trasmessa attraverso il sistema HLA, in cui la distruzione autoimmune delle cellule β è innescata da un agente non ancora identificato. La curva di declino dell'insulina è variabile e al momento della comparsa delle caratteristiche cliniche corrisponde a una distruzione di circa l'80% della riserva secretoria insulinica. Questo processo nell'adolescente e nei pazienti più anziani può richiedere da mesi a anni, e settimane in quelli molto giovani. I titoli maggiori di anticorpi spontanei anti-insulina e anti-insule sono caratteristici della distruzione delle cellule insulari più attive, tipica dei pazienti più giovani, e può essere utile nel prevedere l'ulteriore evoluzione del diabete.

Agenti ambientali possono intervenire fungendo da modificatori della patogenesi delle malattia piuttosto che da scatenatori. Infezioni multiple durante il primo anno di vita sono associate a una diminuzione del rischio di T1DM. Un aumento del rischio si associa invece a infezioni perinatali, accoppiate a effetto protettivo di asili nido prescolari con una possibile associazione a effetti di modificazione età-dipendenti delle infezioni sullo sviluppo del sistema immune. Durante i diversi stadi di sviluppo, fattori ambientali potrebbero promuovere e attenuare la malattia, con effetti che dipendono sia dal tempo sia dalla quantità degli incontri.

PATOGENESI

Lesione autoimmunitaria. Il T1DM è una patologia cronica, autoimmune, mediata dalle cellule T, dovuta a distruzione delle insule pancreatiche. Predisposizione genetica e fattori ambientali danno l'avvio al processo autoimmunitario contro le insule pancreatiche. Si ritiene inoltre che la risposta autoimmune contro le diverse proteine bersaglio (dette epitopi) debba essere sostenuta e diversificata per periodi prolungati, in modo da superare i meccanismi protettivi. L'attacco autoimmune alle insule pancreatiche porta a una graduale e progressiva distruzione delle cellule β, con deficit della secrezione insulinica. Si stima che, all'esordio del diabete clinico, sia già distrutto l'80-90% delle insule pancreatiche. Nelle fasi iniziali del T1DM si sono ricercati segni di rigenerazione di nuove isole e si ritiene che questo fatto possa essere responsabile del "periodo luna di miele" (transitoria diminuzione della richiesta insulinica, associata a miglioramento della funzione β-cellulare). In bambini diabetici piccoli, specialmente in quelli con aplotipi DR3/DR4, la distruzione delle cellule β è

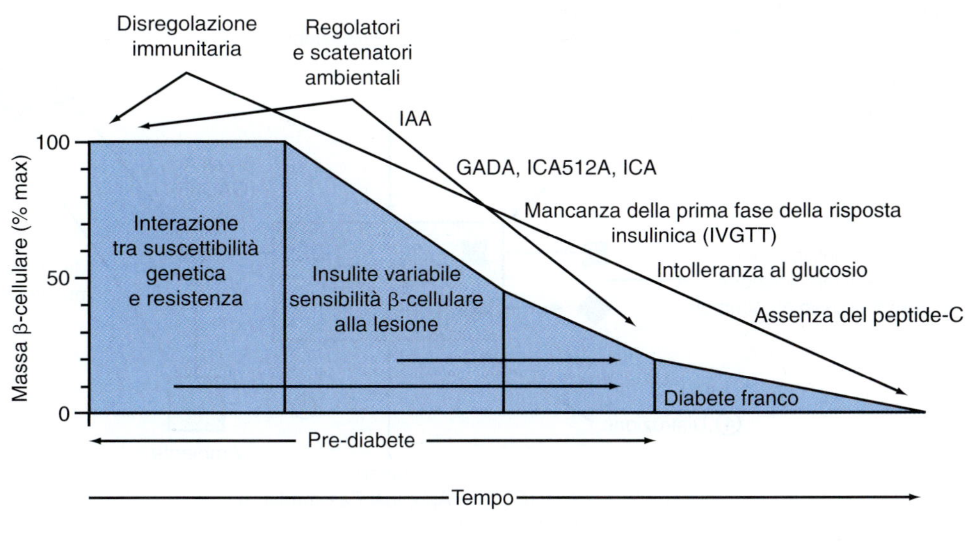

Figura 590-2. Modello di patogenesi e storia naturale di DM di tipo 1. IAA, *Insulin AutoAntibodies* (autoanticorpi anti-insulina); GADA, *Glutamic Acid Decarboxylase Antibody* (anticorpi anti-acido glutammico decarbossilasi); ICA, *Islet Cell Antibody* (anticorpi anti-insule); IVGTT, *Intravenous Glucose Tolerance Test* (test di tolleranza al carico di glucosio per via endovenosa). (Adattata da Aktinson MA, Eisenbarth GS: Type 1 diabetes: New perspective on desease pathogenesis and treatment. *Lancet* 2001;358:221-229.)

quasi completa nei primi 3 anni dopo l'esordio dell'iperglicemia, mentre, nei pazienti più grandi, una distruzione β-cellulare completa si può realizzare anche in 10 anni. Queste osservazioni indicano che l'alterazione della funzione β-cellulare all'esordio dell'iperglicemia è la conseguenza sia della distruzione delle cellule β sia dell'inibizione della secrezione insulinica mediata dalle citochine. È importante la distinzione fra distruzione delle cellule β e inibizione della secrezione insulinica, poiché una frazione di cellule β può essere recuperata, se si interviene in modo terapeuticamente efficace all'inizio di questa malattia. Una volta avviata l'autoimmunità insulare, la progressione della distruzione cellulare insulare è abbastanza variabile; alcuni pazienti mostrano una rapida progressione verso il diabete clinico, mentre altri non progrediscono. La diffusione antigene/epitope della risposta autoanticorpale è un marker importante dell'imminente progressione; quelli con un singolo autoanticorpo progrediscono lentamente, mentre quelli con autoanticorpi multipli più spesso progrediscono rapidamente. La maggior parte degli individui che vanno incontro a un diabete manifesto esprime multipli anticorpi anti-cellule insulari (GAD65, ICA512/IA-2 e IAA) prima dell'inizio del diabete. Si ritiene che la risposta autoimmune contro le cellule β pancreatiche consista di 4 fasi: (1) insulto ambientale, (2) attivazione delle cellule T, (3) differenziazione delle cellule T e (4) distruzione delle cellule β (Fig. 590-3).

Ambiente. Agenti patogeni possono dare l'avvio o precipitare il processo di autoreazione con tre meccanismi. Il primo è rappresentato dal mimetismo molecolare tra le proteine virali e proteine proprie, espresse dalle cellule β (proteina PC2 dei virus Coxsackie e GAD65, proteina capsulare del virus della rosolia e proteina insulare a 52-kd, proteina del Cytomegalovirus e proteina insulare 38-kd). Il secondo si realizza dopo un'infezione acuta delle cellule β o un danno delle stesse cellule indotto dalle citochine durante le risposte infiammatorie contro vari agenti patogeni, quando le proteine rilasciate possono essere riprese dalle cellule che presentano l'antigene (*Antigen-Presenting Cells*, APC), le quali evidenziano i propri peptidi alle cellule T. Il terzo meccanismo si realizza quando le citochine secrete durante un'infezione virale possono sovraregolare l'espressione del costimolatore e delle molecole MHC sulla superficie delle cellule APC facoltative o non facoltative, permettendo loro di presentare in forma immunogenica i propri peptidi alle cellule T. L'induzione della citochina interferone (IFN)-α che segue l'infezione enterovirale è stata implicata nella patogenesi del T1DM. L'attivazione dei recettori toll da parte dell'RNA a doppio filamento o del poli-IC (imitatore virale) attraverso l'induzione dell'IFN-α può attivare o accelerare la distruzione β-cellulare immuno-mediata. Molti studi clinici riportano che la terapia con IFN-α può essere associata a patologie autoimmunitarie, e che elevati livelli sierici di IFN-α sono associati a T1DM. L'esposizione durante le fasi precoci della vita ad agenti patogeni batterici e virali può anche essere protettiva contro lo sviluppo di T1DM.

Anche lo **stress psicosociale** che deriva da eventi gravi può contribuire a innescare il meccanismo del T1DM o il processo autoimmune alla base della malattia. Si è dimostrato che lo stress psicosociale, misurato come tensione psicosociale in famiglia, è coinvolto nell'induzione o nella progressione del diabete correlato all'immunità in bambini durante il primo anno di vita, indipendentemente dall'anamnesi familiare per diabete. È verosimile che lo stress psicosociale familiare possa interferire negativamente nei bambini, a causa dell'associazione tra livelli ormonali e segnali nervosi che a turno influenzano sia la sensibilità all'insulina/richiesta di insulina sia il sistema immunitario.

ATTIVAZIONE DELLE CELLULE T. La presentazione di autoantigeni specifici delle cellule β da parte dei macrofagi APC o delle cellule dendritiche (*Dendritic Cells*, DC) nei confronti delle cellule CD4 T helper (Th), in associazione a molecole MHC di classe II, è considerata la prima tappa delle fasi inizili del processo patologico (vedi Fig. 590-3). I macrofagi producono interleuchina (IL)-12, che stimola le cellule T CD4 a secernere interferone (IFN-γ e IL-2. IFN-γ stimola altri macrofagi a riposo a rilasciare, a turno, altre citochine, come IL-1β, il fattore di necrosi tumorale (TNF)-α, e radicali liberi ($NO_2^{\bullet}$, $O_2^{\bullet-}$), che sono tossici per le cellule β pancreatiche. Durante questo processo, le citochine inducono la migrazione di cellule citotossiche CD8 specifiche per autoantigeni delle cellule β. Su autoantigeni di riconoscimento specifici sulle

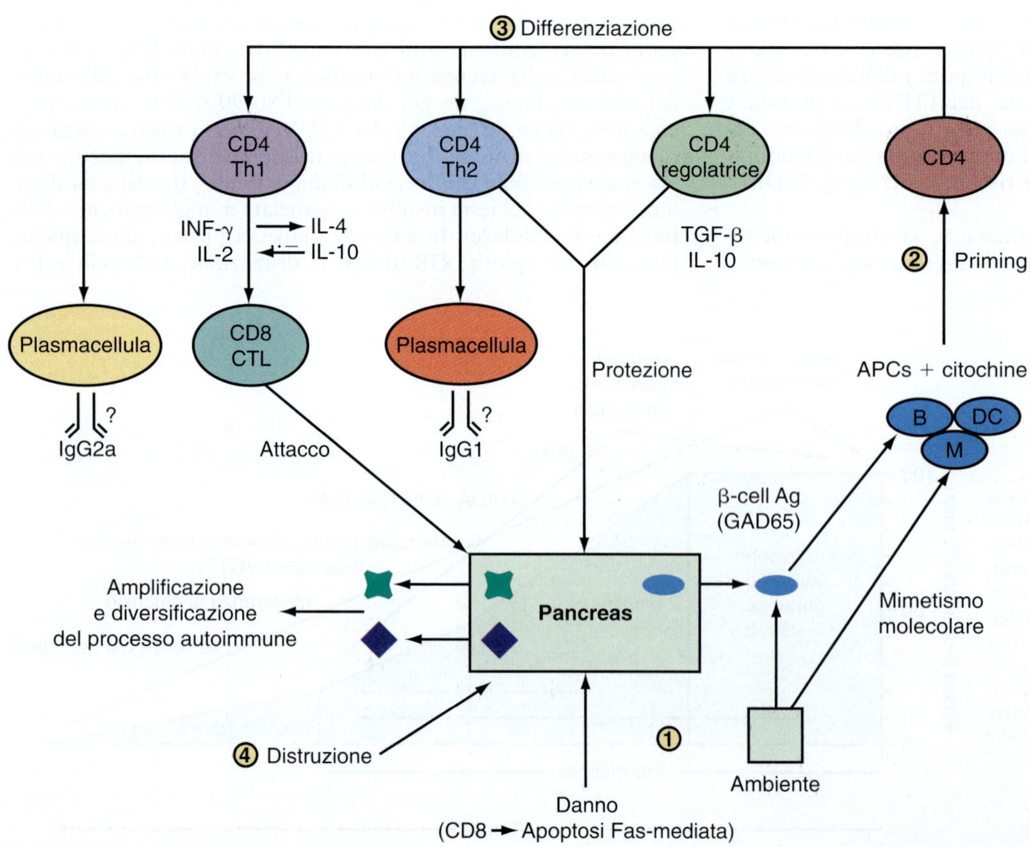

Figura 590-3. Rappresentazione schematica della risposta autoimmune contro le cellule β pancreatiche. Un danno pancreatico porta al rilascio di antigeni β-cellulari (GAD65), che sono assunti dalle cellule di presentazione antigenica (*Antigen-Presenting Cells*, APC) in modo che gli epitomi siano presentati alle cellule T CD4. Il tipo e le fasi dell'attivazione delle cellule APC, così come l'ambiente di citochine, in cui ha luogo per prima l'attivazione delle cellule T CD4, dettano la differenziazione delle cellule T autoreattive in cellule T-helper-1 diabetogene (Th1), in cellule Th2, o in cellule T regolatrici antigene-specifiche. Una risposta autoimmune con predominanza di Th1 porta al reclutamento e alla differenziazione di cellule CD (citotossiche, che attaccano le cellule β pancreatiche, portando a un rilascio massiccio di antigeni β-cellulari (Ag), con diffusione di epitomi e distruzione delle insule pancreatiche. B, linfocita B; DC, *Dendritic Cell* (cellula dendritica); M, macrofago; CTL, *Cytotoxic Cell* (cellula citotossica); TGF β, fattore di crescita-β; INF-γ, interferone-γ; IL, interleuchina. (Adattata da Casares, Brumeanu TD: Insights into the pathogenesis of T1DM: A hint for novel immunospecific therapies. *Curr Molec Med* 2001;1:357-378).

cellule β in associazione a molecole di classe 1, queste cellule T citotossiche CD8 provocano un danno β-cellulare tramite il rilascio di perforina e granzima e tramite apoptosi β-cellulare Fas-mediata.

DIFFERENZIAZIONE DELLE CELLULE T. Il diabete immuno-mediato è associato a popolazioni policlonali di cellule T, reattive contro antigeni multipli delle cellule β. Infatti, in pazienti con T1DM sono stati trovate cellule T reattive contro: acido glutammico decarbossilasi 65 (GAD65), proinsulina, tirosina fosfatasi (ICA512/IA-2), proteina-60 da shock termico (hsp60), antigene insulare 60 (ICA 69). Tra questi antigeni, GAD65 rappresenta un bersaglio precoce delle cellule T. Dal momento che GAD65 è una proteina intracellulare, può essere richiesta la lesione della cellula β, che espone l'antigene, per cominciare il processo autoimmunitario. L'associazione tra MHC di classe II e T1DM suggerisce fortemente il ruolo patogenetico delle cellule T CD4, in quanto le molecole MHC di classe II sono necessarie per l'istruzione timica dei precursori e per la restrizione delle risposte della cellula T CD4. Esiste una correlazione tra l'affinità del legame del peptide all'MHC di classe II e l'antigenicità. Mentre le molecole protettive per T1DM di classe II legano peptidi propri con alta affinità e cancellano i precursori timici, molecole di suscettibilità a T1DM di classe II legano peptidi propri con bassa affinità, oltre a provocare un'insufficiente tolleranza centrale e una fuga verso la periferia di cellule T autoreattive. Le cellule T si differenziano in cellule effettrici Th1 e Th2. Le cellule Th1 proteggono contro i batteri e i parassiti intracellulari e mediano l'ipersensibilità di tipo ritardato e il rigetto allografico acuto, mentre le cellule Th2 regolano la risposta umorale (IgE e IgG 1), mediano le reazioni allergiche e proteggono contro patologie autoimmuni organo-specifiche, come il T1DM, la sclerosi multipla, la tiroidite e il morbo di Crohn. Le cellule Th1 CD4 secernono IL-2 e IFN-α e sono associate a immunità cellulo-mediata. Le cellule Th2 secernono IL-4 e IL-10 e sono associate a risposte umorali e antinfiammatorie. Un sottogruppo di cellule T regolatrici, conosciuto come cellule T killer naturali (NKT), previene il diabete tramite la secrezione di IL-4 e/o IL-10. Anche le cellule regolatrici Th3 (CD4) tendono a esercitare un effetto antidiabetogeno tramite la secrezione del fattore β di crescita tumorale citochina soppressivo. Anomalie funzionali in queste cellule regolatrici possono anche giocare un ruolo nella patogenesi del T1DM. Un difetto funzionale relativo di una popolazione di cellule T regolatrici, conosciute come cellule $CD4^+CD25^+$, potrebbe contribuire alla mancanza di autotolleranza immunitaria nel T1DM e influenzare la sua patogenesi.

DISTRUZIONE DELLE CELLULE β. L'infiltrazione di cellule mononucleari nelle insule pancreatiche (insulite) e la riduzione delle cellule β che producono insulina rappresentano la caratteristica patologica chiave del T1DM. Campioni bioptici insulari ottenuti da pazienti prediabetici e da quelli con T1DM di recente esordio hanno dimostrato, in tutti i pazienti, vari gradi di riduzione di volume delle cellule β, non essendo ancora presente una vera insulite in circa il 50%. In presenza di insulite, l'infiltrato è composto da cellule T CD8 e CD4, cellule B e macrofagi, con una predominanza di cellule T CD8. Le cellule delle isole sede di infiammazione mostrano iperespressione di molecole MHC di classe I. Il grado di insulite e di iperespressione di molecole MHC di classe I si correla con il deterioramento del controllo glicemico e con i livelli di anticorpi GAD65. All'interno delle cellule β infiammate si trova Fas, mentre le cellule mononuclate che infiltrano le insule esprimono il ligando di Fas. Un'interazione tra Fas sulle cellule β e ligando di Fas sulle cellule infiltranti potrebbe innescare una selettiva morte apoptotica delle cellule β infiammate, portando a T1DM.

PREVISIONE E PREVENZIONE. L'autoimmunità precede il T1DM clinico e si possono utilizzare indicatori di progressione autoimmune come marker per la previsione di malattia. È possibile identificare individui a rischio per T1DM valutando una combinazione di marker genetici, immunologici e metabolici. Il locus genetico che dà maggiori informazioni, HLA di classe II, conferisce circa la metà del rischio genetico totale, ma ha un basso valore predittivo positivo (*Positive Predictive Value*, PPV), se utilizzato nella popolazione generale. Gli autoanticorpi consentono un pratica lettura dell'autoimmunità contro la cellula β sono facilmente dosabili in campioni di sangue venoso e sono diventati la base per le previsioni del T1DM. Inizialmente descritti in termini di dosaggio immunofluorescente di anticorpi anti-cellule insulari (*Islet Cell Antibody*, ICA) su sezioni pancreatiche, si valutano gli autoanticorpi nei confronti di definiti antigeni del bersaglio ICA, come l'insulina (IAA), l'acido glutamico deidrogenasi (GAD65) e l'omologo ICA512/IA-2 della tiroxina fosfatasi.

Nei parenti stretti di pazienti diabetici, il cui rischio di diabete è di circa 3,5-5%, per trovare un T1DM in via di sviluppo vengono utilizzati gli autoanticorpi. Tuttavia, la maggior parte dei casi è sporadica e non familiare e richiede uno screening della popolazione generale. Questo è stato difficile, in parte perché la percentuale di autoanticorpi osservata eccede notevolmente la bassa incidenza nei non parenti, con alti tassi di falsi positivi. La positività a un singolo definito autoanticorpo (d-aab) può dipendere da memoria persistente delle cellule B nei linfonodi o nel midollo osseo dopo breve e transitoria insulite, che non evolve in diabete clinico. Poiché durante il prediabete appare successivamente un diverso d-aab, si pensa che la presenza di multipli d-aab possa indicare un'insulite più persistente e un maggior rischio di diabete. Nei parenti di primo grado di un paziente con T1DM, il numero dei d-aab positivi può aiutare a stimare il rischio di sviluppare T1DM: basso rischio (d-aab singolo: PPV di 2-6%), rischio moderato (2 d-aab: PPV di 21-40%), e alto rischio (>2 d-aab: PPV di 59-80%), in un periodo di 5 anni. In bambini che portano un genotipo ad alto rischio di T1DM (HLA-DQB1*0201-DQA1*05/DQB1*0302-DQA1*03), l'insulite è almeno 10 volte più frequente (PPV 21%) rispetto a bambini con altri genotipi (PPV 2,2%). Inoltre, nella popolazione generale dei bambini, un numero consistente di studi ha suggerito una PPV complessiva molto bassa per un singolo d-aab (0-0,5%), mentre la PPV complessiva per multipli (≥2) d-aab è alta, fino al 19-50% (alto rischio) in un periodo di 2-8 anni. Bambini a rischio per T1DM sviluppano precocemente IAA, che possono essere seguiti da multipli anticorpi anti-insulari, basati sul grado dell'affinità di IAA all'insulina. Un'alta affinità di IAA è associata a HLADRB1*04, a giovane età di comparsa di IAA e a successiva progressione a multipli anticorpi anti-insule o T1DM.

Non si conosce un agente in grado di prevenire il T1DM. Esistono molti ostacoli a una plausibile strategia di prevenzione. Questi comprendono: (1) problemi etici di previsione, (2) dilemma del trattamento, (3) selezione della popolazione a rischio e strategie di trattamento e (4) ricerca di nuovi agenti preventivi. La capacità di prevedere futuri casi di T1DM in assenza di un agente preventivo, nonostante un maggior beneficio che può derivare dalla conoscenza della storia naturale di questa malattia, aumenta i conflitti etici correlati all'induzione di stress, cambiamenti dello stile di vita e potenziali effetti sulla possibilità di assicurare il bambino sano e la sua famiglia.

Si è riconosciuto che gli interventi più efficaci sono quelli che iniziano nelle prime fasi del processo autoimmune. Tuttavia, la predizione di malattia utilizzando marker immunologici, genetici e metabolici è molto più accurata nel periodo vicino all'esordio del diabete manifesto. Di conseguenza, molti medici e ricercatori sono di fronte a conflitti etici e clinici, in cui le forme più efficaci di terapia potrebbero coinvolgere il trattamento di individui in un periodo in cui la predizione di malattia è meno accurata. È molto difficile trovare forme di terapia efficaci e sicure da poter impiegare per gli individui che potrebbero non sviluppare mai il T1DM.

Immunoterapia del DM di tipo 1 di nuovo esordio. Il DM di tipo 1 è una patologia autoimmune mediata dalle cellule T che ha inizio, in molti casi, 3-5 anni prima dell'inizio dei sintomi clinici, continua dopo la diagnosi e può recidivare dopo trapianto insulare. Il meccanismo effettore responsabile della distruzione delle cellule β coinvolge le cellule T citotossiche e i prodotti solubili delle cellule T, come IFN-γ e TNF-α. Tali osservazioni indirizzano verso trial clinici con farmaci immunomodulatori come la ciclosporina, l'azatioprina, il prednisone e la globulina antitimocita. Questi agenti provocano un transitorio peggioramento delle valutazioni cliniche della funzione β-cellulare. Sfortunatamente, gli effetti tossici di questi farmaci, la preoccupazione per il rischio associato all'immunosoppressione e la necessità di trattamento continuo in una popolazione altrimenti sana e giovane limitano notevolmente l'uso di questi agenti.

L'immunoterapia che utilizza **anticorpi monoclonali modificati contro CD3 hOKT3γ1** si è mostrata efficace in pazienti con rigetto di allotrapianto renale ed è stata utilizzata in trial limitati in soggetti con T1DM. Il trattamento con infusioni di hOKT3β1 mitiga il deterioramento della produzione insulinica, migliorando il controllo metabolico durante il primo anno di T1DM nella maggior parte dei pazienti. Gli effetti collaterali comprendono febbre transitoria, sintomi gastrointestinali e rash con prurito, senza effetti tossici a lungo termine fino a 2 anni. Il meccanismo di azione degli anticorpi monoclonali CD3 può coinvolgere effetti diretti sulle cellule patogenetiche T e/o l'induzione di popolazioni di cellule regolatrici. La terapia per breve periodo (6 giorni) con anticorpi IgG1 umani monoclonali CD3 (ChAglyCD3), in pazienti di età compresa tra 12 e 39 anni con T1DM di nuova comparsa, preserva la funzione residua delle cellule β per almeno 18 mesi. È stata associata a una sindrome moderata "simil influenzale" e a sintomi transitori della mononucleosi virale di Epstein-Barr.

FISIOPATOLOGIA. L'insulina riveste un ruolo critico nell'accumulo e nel recupero del carburante cellulare. La sua secrezione in risposta all'alimentazione è tipicamente modulata da meccanismi intercorrelati di tipo nervoso, ormonale e dipendenti dal substrato, per consentire che gli alimenti ingeriti siano a disposizione controllata e ottenere quindi energia per uso immediato o futuro. I livelli insulinici in seguito decrescono per poi mobilizzare, durante il digiuno, l'energia accumulata. Così, nel metabolismo normale, esiste una regolare oscillazione tra lo stato iperinsulinemico anabolico post-prandiale e lo stato ipoinsulinemico catabolico del digiuno, a livello epatico, muscolare e del tessuto adiposo (Tab. 590-3). Il T1DM consiste in una condizione ipoinsulinemica catabolica progressiva, in cui l'alimentazione non inverte, bensì esaspera tali processi catabolici. In presenza di insulinopenia moderata, diminuisce l'utilizzazione del glucosio da parte del muscolo e del tessuto adiposo e compare iperglicemia post-prandiale. A valori ancora più bassi di insulina, il fegato produce una quantità eccessiva di glucosio per glicogenolisi e gluconeogenesi e ha inizio l'iperglicemia a digiuno. L'iperglicemia produce una diuresi osmotica (glicosuria) quando viene superata la soglia renale (180 mg/dL; 10 mmol/L). La conseguente perdita di calorie ed elettroliti, come avviene nella disidratazione permanente, produce uno stress fisiologico con ipersecrezione degli ormoni dello stress (adrenalina, cortisolo, ormone della crescita e glucagone). Questi ormoni, a turno, contribuiscono allo scompenso metabolico attraverso un'ulteriore alterazione della secrezione insulinica (adrenalina), antagonizzando la sua azione (adrenalina, cortisolo, ormone della crescita), promuovendo glicogenolisi, gluconeogenesi, lipolisi e chetogenesi (glucagone, adrenalina, ormone della crescita e cortisolo) e diminuendo l'utilizzazione del glucosio e la sua clearance (adrenalina, ormone della crescita, cortisolo).

La combinazione di deficit insulinico e incremento dei livelli plasmatici di ormoni controregolatori è responsabile anche dell'accelerazione della lipolisi e dell'alterazione della sintesi lipidica, con conseguente aumento della concentrazione plasmatica totale di lipidi, colesterolo, trigliceridi e acidi grassi liberi. Le interrelazioni ormonali del deficit insulinico e l'eccesso di glucagone indirizzano gli acidi grassi liberi verso la formazione di corpi chetonici; la velocità di formazione di questi composti, principalmente β-idrossibutirrato e acetoacetato, eccede la capacità di utilizzazione periferica e di escrezione renale. Quindi, l'accumulo di questi chetoacidi comporta un'acidosi metabolica o chetoacidosi diabetica (*Diabetic Ketoacidosis*, DKA) e atti respiratori compensatori rapidi, profondi, per eliminare l'eccesso di CO_2 (respiro di Kussmaul). L'acetone, formato dalla conversione non enzimatica dell'acetoacetato, è responsabile del caratteristico odore fruttato dell'alito. I chetoni sono escreti con le urine assieme ai cationi e così aumenta ulteriormente la perdita di acqua ed elettroliti. Con la progressione di disidratazione, acidosi, iperosmolalità e con la diminuzione della utilizzazione cerebrale di ossigeno, compare un'alterazione dello stato di coscienza e il paziente alla fine diventa comatoso.

TABELLA 590-3. Influenza dell'alimentazione (alta insulina) o del digiuno (bassa insulina) su alcuni processi metabolici nel fegato, muscolo e tessuto adiposo*

	INSULINA PLASMATICA ELEVATA (STATO POST-PRANDIALE)	INSULINA PLASMATICA BASSA (STATO DI DIGIUNO)
Fegato	Captazione del glucosio Sintesi di glicogeno Assenza di gluconeogenesi Litogenesi Assenza di chetogenesi	Produzione di glucosio Glicogenolisi Gluconeogenesi Assenza di litogenesi Chetogenesi
Muscolo	Captazione del glucosio Ossidazione del glucosio Sintesi di glicogeno Sintesi proteica	Assenza di capatazione del glucosio Ossidazione di acidi grassi e di chetoni Glicogenolisi Proteolisi e rilascio di aminoacidi
Tessuto adiposo	Captazione del glucosio Sintesi lipidica Captazione dei trigliceridi	Assenza di captazione del glucosio Lipolisi e rilascio di acidi grassi Assenza di captazione dei trigliceridi

*L'insulina è ritenuto il fattore che più di ogni altro regola questi processi metabolici. Il diabete mellito può essere considerato come uno stato di permanente ipoinsulinismo che, se non trattato, porta a uno stato esagerato analogo al digiuno.

MANIFESTAZIONI CLINICHE. A mano a mano che sviluppa il diabete, aumentano progressivamente i sintomi, in rapporto alla diminuzione della massa delle cellule β, al peggioramento del deficit insulinico, all'iperglicemia progressiva e all'eventuale chetoacidosi. Inizialmente, quando la glicemia aumenta oltre la soglia renale, cominciano **poliuria** intermittente o **nicturia**. Con l'ulteriore perdita di cellule β, l'iperglicemia cronica provoca una diuresi più persistente, spesso con **enuresi** notturna, e comincia a manifestarsi **polidipsia.** Le pazienti femmine possono presentare vaginite da monilia, per glicosuria cronica. Con le urine si perdono calorie (glicosuria) e ciò innesca un'**iperfagia** compensatoria. Se questa iperfagia non sta al passo con la glicosuria, si instaura una perdita del grasso corporeo, con **dimagrimento** clinico e diminuzione delle riserve di tessuto adiposo sottocutaneo. In media, un bambino sano di 10 anni introduce circa il 50% di 2000 calorie giornaliere sotto forma di carboidrati. Se il bambino diventa diabetico, le perdite giornaliere di acqua e glucosio possono ammontare a 5 L e 250 g rispettivamente, che corrispondono a 1000 calorie o al 50% dell'intake calorico giornaliero medio. Nonostante l'aumento dell'intake alimentare compensatorio, il bambino dimagrisce, perché le calorie non utilizzate vengono perse attraverso le urine.

Quando si raggiungono livelli insulinemici molto bassi, **si accumulano chetoacidi**. A questo punto, il bambino peggiora rapidamente. I chetoacidi producono dolori addominali, nausea e vomito, impedendo l'introduzione orale dei liquidi persi con le urine. La disidratazione accelera, provocando astenia e ipotensione ortostatica, ma persiste la poliuria. Come in una condizione iperosmotica, il grado di disidratazione può essere clinicamente sottostimato, perché il volume intravascolare si conserva a spese di quello intracellulare. La chetoacidosi esacerba i sintomi precedenti e porta al respiro di Kussmaul (respiri rapidi, profondi, accelerati), a un tipico odore fruttato dell'alito (acetone), alla diminuzione delle funzioni neurocognitive e anche al coma. Circa il 20-40% dei bambini con diabete di recente esordio progredisce fino a DKA prima di ricevere diagnosi.

Tutta questa progressione si verifica molto più rapidamente (in poche settimane) nei bambini più piccoli, probabilmente a causa di una più aggressiva distruzione immunitaria delle cellule β. Nei neonati, la maggior parte della perdita di peso si realizza per perdita acuta di acqua perché, al momento della diagnosi, essi non hanno avuto una prolungata perdita calorica con le urine e l'incidenza di DKA può essere maggiore. Negli adolescenti, il decorso è in genere più prolungato (vari mesi) e la maggior parte della perdita di peso è dovuta a perdita di tessuto adiposo per carenza prolungata. Un'ulteriore perdita di peso da disidratazione acuta può avvenire subito prima della diagnosi. In ogni bambino, la progressione dei sintomi può essere accelerata dallo stress per una malattia o per un trauma intercorrenti, quando gli ormoni controregolatori (dello stress) sopraffanno la limitata capacità di secrezione insulinica.

DIAGNOSI. La diagnosi di T1DM è di solito semplice. Nonostante la maggior parte dei sintomi non sia specifica, l'indizio più importante è rappresentato da una poliuria inadeguata in un bambino disidratato, dimagrito o influenzato. Iperglicemia, glicosuria e chetonuria possono essere determinate rapidamente. Una glicemia non a digiuno maggiore di 200 mg/dL (11,1 mmol/L) con sintomi tipici è diagnostica, con o senza chetonuria. Nel bambino obeso, si deve considerare la possibilità di T2DM (vedi "Diabete mellito di tipo 2", oltre). Quando l'iperglicemia è confermata, è prudente verificare se è presente DKA (specialmente se si trova chetonuria) e valutare eventuali anomalie elettrolitiche, anche se i segni di disidratazione sono minimi. Il dosaggio dell'emoglobina A_{1C} (HbA_{1C}) basale permette di stimare la durata dell'iperglicemia e servirà di confronto per valutare l'efficacia della terapia successiva.

Nel bambino non obeso, non sono necessarie valutazioni dell'autoimmunità anti-cellule β. Si possono indagare altre patologie autoimmunitarie associate a diabete di tipo 1, quali la **malattia celiaca** (attraverso la IgA transglutaminasi tissutale o le IgA totali) e la **tiroidite** (attraverso gli anticorpi antiperossidasi e antitireoglobulina). Dato che stress fisiologici di una certa entità possono alterare l'asse ipofiso-tiroideo, dopo qualche settimana, quando il bambino si è stabilizzato, si devono valutare anche la tiroxina libera (T4) e il TSH.

Raramente un bambino presenta iperglicemia transitoria con glicosuria durante uno stress fisico notevole. Questa di solito si risolve in modo permanente quando il bambino si riprende dai fattori stressanti. Tuttavia, l'iperglicemia da stress può riflettere una riserva limitata di insulina, temporaneamente evidenzata dagli ormoni controregolatori. Pertanto, un bambino con iperglicemia transitoria deve comunque essere monitorato, per verificare se si sviluppano sintomi da iperglicemia persistente, e in tal caso deve essere studiato attentamente. Non sono necessarie valutazioni particolari in un bambino che rimane clinicamente asintomatico.

Le procedure routinarie di screening, come la determinazione della glicemia post-prandiale o il test di tolleranza al carico orale di glucosio, hanno fornito scarsi risultati in bambini sani, asintomatici, anche tra quelli considerati a rischio, come i fratelli o le sorelle di bambini diabetici. Pertanto le procedure di screening non sono raccomandate nei bambini.

Chetoacidosi diabetica. La DKA è il risultato finale di anomalie metaboliche che derivano da un grave deficit insulinico o della efficacia insulinica. Il secondo caso si verifica durante lo stress, quando gli ormoni controregolatori bloccano l'azione insulinica. La DKA si verifica nel 20-40% dei bambini con diabete di nuova diagnosi e in bambini con diabete noto che non abbiano assunto le dosi di insulina o che non siano stati trattati adeguatamente in concomitanza a una patologia intercorrente. La DKA può essere arbitrariamente classificata come lieve, moderata o severa (Tab. 590-4) e il range dei sintomi dipende dalla gravità della chetoacidosi. Sono presenti: notevole chetonuria, perdita ionica, decremento dei bicarbonato sierici (o della CO_2 totale) e del pH ed elevazione dell'osmolalità sierica, che indica una disidratazione ipertonica.

TABELLA 590-4. Classificazione della chetoacidosi diabetica

	NORMALE	LIEVE	MODERATA	SEVERA[†]
CO_2 (mEq/L, venosa)*	20-28	16-20	10-15	<10
pH (venoso)	7,35-7,45	7,25-7,35	7,15-7,25	<7,5
Clinica	Assenza di modificazioni	Orientato, vivace ma affaticato	Respiro di Kussmaul; orientato ma sonnolento; eccitabile	Respiro di Kussmaul o depressa; sonnolento fino a un sensorio depresso e coma

*Le misurazioni di CO_2 e pH sono metodi dipendenti; il range di normalità può variare.
[†]Una severa ipernatriemia (Na corretto >150 mEq/L) potrebbe essere classificata come DKA severa.

TRATTAMENTO. La terapia è adattata al grado di insulinopenia al momento della comparsa. La maggior parte dei bambini con nuovo diabete (60-80%) ha sintomi da lievi a moderati, disidratazione minima senza anamnesi di vomito e non presenta chetoacidosi progressiva. Dal momento che la DKA in un bambino con nuovo diabete viene risolta, la terapia diventa identica a quella prescritta per i bambini non chetoacidosici. Bambini con diabete precedentemente diagnosticato e che hanno sviluppato DKA sono in genere riportati al loro precedente regime insulinico.

Diabete di nuova diagnosi senza chetoacidosi. Un eccellente controllo del diabete deve rispondere a molti obiettivi: mantenere un equilibrio tra stretto controllo glicemico e assenza di ipoglicemia, eliminare la poliuria e la nicturia, prevenire la chetoacidosi e permettere normale crescita e sviluppo, con effetti minimi sullo stile di vita. La terapia comprende l'inizio e la regolazione dell'insulina, l'educazione approfondita del bambino e di chi si occupa di lui e il ripristino della normale routine di vita. Nella terapia complessiva, ogni aspetto deve essere affrontato precocemente. Idealmente, la terapia può cominciare in regime ambulatoriale, per opera di un team completo comprendente endocrinologo pediatrico, personale infermieristico esperto, dietista con training come educatore per i diabetici e assistente sociale. Vanno assicurati stretti contatti tra il team medico e la famiglia. Inoltre, la terapia iniziale deve essere eseguita in ambito ospedaliero.

Terapia insulinica. Molti fattori influenzano la dose giornaliera iniziale di insulina per chilogrammo di peso corporeo. Nei ragazzi puberi di solito il dosaggio è più alto. È più alto anche in quelli in cui è necessario ripristinare un maggior deficit di glicogeno, proteine e tessuto adiposo, come anche in quelli che hanno una maggiore capacità calorica iniziale. D'altra parte, la maggior parte dei bambini con diabete di nuova diagnosi, possiede una certa funzione β-insulare residua ("periodo luna di miele"), che riduce la richiesta di insulina esogena. Bambini con diabete di lunga data e privi di riserva insulinica richiedono circa 0,7 U/kg/die se prepuberi, 1,0 U/kg/die nelle fasi intermedie della pubertà e 1,2 U/kg/die alla fine della pubertà. Una dose ragionevole nei bambini di **nuova diagnosi**, poi, rappresenta circa il 60-70% della dose sostituiva totale in base allo stato della pubertà. La dose ottimale di insulina può essere determinata solo empiricamente, con frequente automonitoraggio della glicemia e regolazioni dell'insulina da parte del diabetologo. La funzione β-cellulare residua svanisce di solito in pochi mesi e si riflette in un incremento della richiesta insulinica e in maggiori escursioni della glicemia.

La dose insulinica iniziale deve essere diretta a un grado ottimale di controllo glicemico, nel tentativo di imitare l'attività delle cellule β. Questo è limitato dalla nostra capacità di simulare l'attività β-cellulare. L'insulina esogena non ha un primo passaggio a livello epatico, mentre il 50% dell'insulina pancreatica portale è captata dal fegato, organo chiave per lo smaltimento del glucosio; l'assorbimento di una dose esogena continua nonostante l'ipoglicemia, mentre, in presenza di una clearance rapida, il rilascio endogeno di insulina cessa e i suoi livelli sierici si abbassano rapidamente; la percentuale di assorbimento di una dose iniettata varia a seconda della sede di iniezione e del livello di attività del paziente, mentre l'insulina endogena viene secreta direttamente nella circolazione portale. Nonostante queste fondamentali differenze fisiologiche, si può ottenere un controllo glicemico accettabile con i nuovi analoghi dell'insulina, usati in un regime a bolo basale, che preveda, con inizio lento, una base di insulina a lunga durata per il controllo della glicemia tra i pasti e un insulina ad azione rapida a ogni pasto.

Tutti gli analoghi insulinici sono disponibili in forma di esameri, che devono dissociarsi in monomeri a livello sottocutaneo prima di essere assorbiti nella circolazione. Così, un effetto rilevabile per l'insulina regolare (R) è ritardato di 30-60 minuti dopo l'iniezione. Questo, a turno, richiede che si ritardi il pasto di 30-60 minuti dopo l'iniezione, per un effetto ottimale, un ritardo raramente realizzabile nella vita programmata del bambino. R ha un ampio picco e una coda lunga per il bolo insulinico (Figg. 590-4 e 590-5). Questo profilo limita il controllo glicemico post-prandiale, produce picchi prolungati con eccessivi effetti ipoglicemici tra i pasti e aumenta il rischio di ipoglicemia notturna. Gli effetti indesiderati tra i pasti spesso necessitano di "alimentare l'insulina" con spuntini e di limitare il grado complessivo di controllo glicemico. Anche l'insulina NPH e la lenta hanno limiti intrinseci, perché non creano un livello di base costante di insulina, privo di picchi (vedi Fig. 590-5*C*-*E*). Questo comporta un

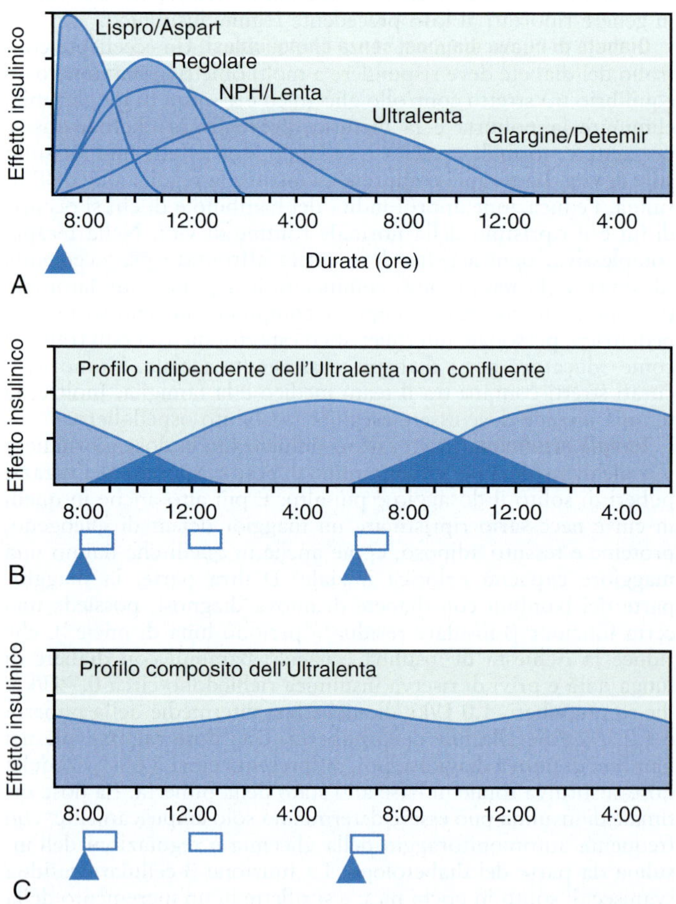

Figura 590-4. Profili indicativi dell'effetto insulinico. I pasti sono visualizzati come rettangolini sull'asse del tempo. *A*, Sono utilizzati l'effetto del picco relativo seguente e le unità di durata: Lispro® o Aspart®, picco 20 per 4 ore; regolare, picco 15 per 7 ore; NPH/lenta, picco 12 per 12 ore; ultralenta, picco 9 per 18 ore; Glargine®, picco 5 per 24 ore. Sebbene la lenta e l'ultralenta non siano più prodotte, vengono confrontate con i nuovi analoghi dell'insulina. S, Tempo di iniezione. *B*, Due iniezioni di ultralenta somministrate a colazione e a cena. Notare la sovrapposizione dei profili. *C*, Curva composita che dimostra l'effetto insulinico cumulativo per le due iniezioni di ultralenta. Per il paziente, i genitori e il personale medico si utilizza più spesso questa curva composita, perché mostra importanti effetti combinati di iniezioni multiple di insulina con la sovrapposizione delle caratteristiche variabili di assorbimento e durata.

significativo effetto ipoglicemico durante il range medio della loro durata. Pertanto, è spesso difficile predire la loro interazione con le insuline ad azione rapida. Quando R si combina con l'insulina NPH o con la lenta (vedi Fig. 590-5*E*), il profilo insulinico risultante mima in modo inadeguato la normale secrezione insulinica endogena. Vi sono ampie aree di effetto insulinico eccessivo, alternate ad altre con effetto insufficiente durante il giorno e la notte. Le insuline lente e le ultralente sono state sospese e non sono più utilizzabili.

Gli analoghi insulinici Lispro® (L) e Aspart® (A) vengono assorbiti più rapidamente perché non formano esameri. Essi consentono una discreta pulsatilità con scarsa se non nulla sovrapposizione o un breve effetto coda. Questo consente un miglior controllo dell'incremento glicemico post-prandiale e riduce l'ipoglicemia tra i pasti e notturna (vedi Fig. 590-5*A*). L'analogo Glargine® a lunga durata (G) crea un profilo più piatto nelle 24 ore, rendendo più facilmente prevedibile l'effetto combinato di un bolo rapido (L o A) sull'insulina basale, producendo un andamento dell'effetto insulinico più fisiologico (vedi Fig. 590-5*A*). Si controlla meglio l'aumento post-prandiale della glicemia e si riduce l'ipoglicemia notturna e tra i pasti.

L'ultralenta (UL), somministrata due volte al giorno, ha un accettabile profilo basale (vedi Fig. 590-4*C*) e si è mostrata del tutto efficace quando usata con Lispro® o Aspart® (vedi Fig. 590 5-*B*). Da quando UL non è più utilizzabile, nei bambini piccoli si può somministrare G ogni 12 ore, se una singola dose giornaliera non produce una completa copertura basale nelle 24 ore. Nei bambini piccoli l'insulina Glargine® basale deve rappresentare il 25-30% della dose totale e in quelli più grandi il 40-50%. La porzione rimanente della dose giornaliera totale va divisa equamente in 3 iniezioni ai tre pasti principali. Si inizia con un semplice programma di 3 o 4 dosi, basandosi sulla glicemia (Tab. 590-5). È necessario insegnare al bambino e ai suoi familiari a calcolare il contenuto carboidratico dei cibi ai pasti e a dosare più accuratamente il bolo insulinico in rapporto sia al contenuto carboidratico del pasto sia alla glicemia (vedi Tab. 590-5).

Sono necessari frequenti monitoraggi della glicemia e regolazioni dell'insulina durante le prime settimane, quando il bambino ritorna alle sue normali attività e si adatta a un nuovo programma nutrizionale, in modo da determinare le richieste giornaliere complessive di insulina. Il maggior limite fisiologico a un controllo stretto è rappresentato dall'ipoglicemia. Controlli ripetuti abbassano notevolmente il rischio di complicanze vascolari a lungo termine; sono associati a un aumento di 3 volte di ipoglicemia severa. L'uso di analoghi dell'insulina diminuisce, ma non elimina, il problema.

Alcune famiglie possono non essere in grado di praticare 4 iniezioni giornaliere. In questi casi, si deve cercare un compromesso. Un regime a 3 iniezioni che combini NHP con un analogo rapido a colazione, un analogo ad azione rapida a cena e NHP al mo-

TABELLA 590-5. Dosi dell'insulina per via sottocutanea

ETÀ (ANNI)	LIVELLO DI GLUCOSIO DI RIFERIMENTO (MG/DL)	INSULINA TOTALE GIORNALIERA (U/KG/DIE)*	INSULINA BASALE, % DELLA DOSE GIORNALIERA TOTALE	BOLO† DI INSULINA	
				Unità aggiunte per ogni 100 mg/dL oltre il livello di riferimento	Unità aggiunte per 15 g a pasto
0-5	100-200	0,6-0,7	25-30	0,50	0,50
5-12	80-150	0,7-1	40-50	0,75	0,75
12-18	80-150	1,0-1,2	40-50	1,0-2‡	1,0-2,0

*Bambini con nuova diagnosi nel "periodo luna di miele" possono richiedere solo il 60-70% della dose complessiva. La dose totale giornaliera per kg aumenta alla pubertà.

†Bambini con nuova diagnosi che non hanno l'abitudine di dosare i carboidrati dovrebbero dividere la quota non basale dell'insulina giornaliera in dosi uguali a ogni pasto. Una scala di somministrazione viene poi addizionata a ogni dose. **Per esempio**: un bambino di 6 anni che pesa 20 kg necessita di circa (0,7 U/kg/die × 20 kg = 14 U/24 h con 7 unità (50%) come quota basale e 7 unità come bolo giornaliero totale. Somministrare di base Glargine® all'ora Somministrare 2 unità di Lispro® o Aspart® prima di ogni pasto se la glicemia è nei riferimenti; sottrarre 1 unità se è inferiore e aggiungere 0,75 unità per ogni 100 mg/dL oltre il riferimento (arrotondare la dose alle 0,5 unità più vicine).

‡Per un miglior controllo, può essere aggiunta dell'insulina extra con incrementi di 50 mg/dL.

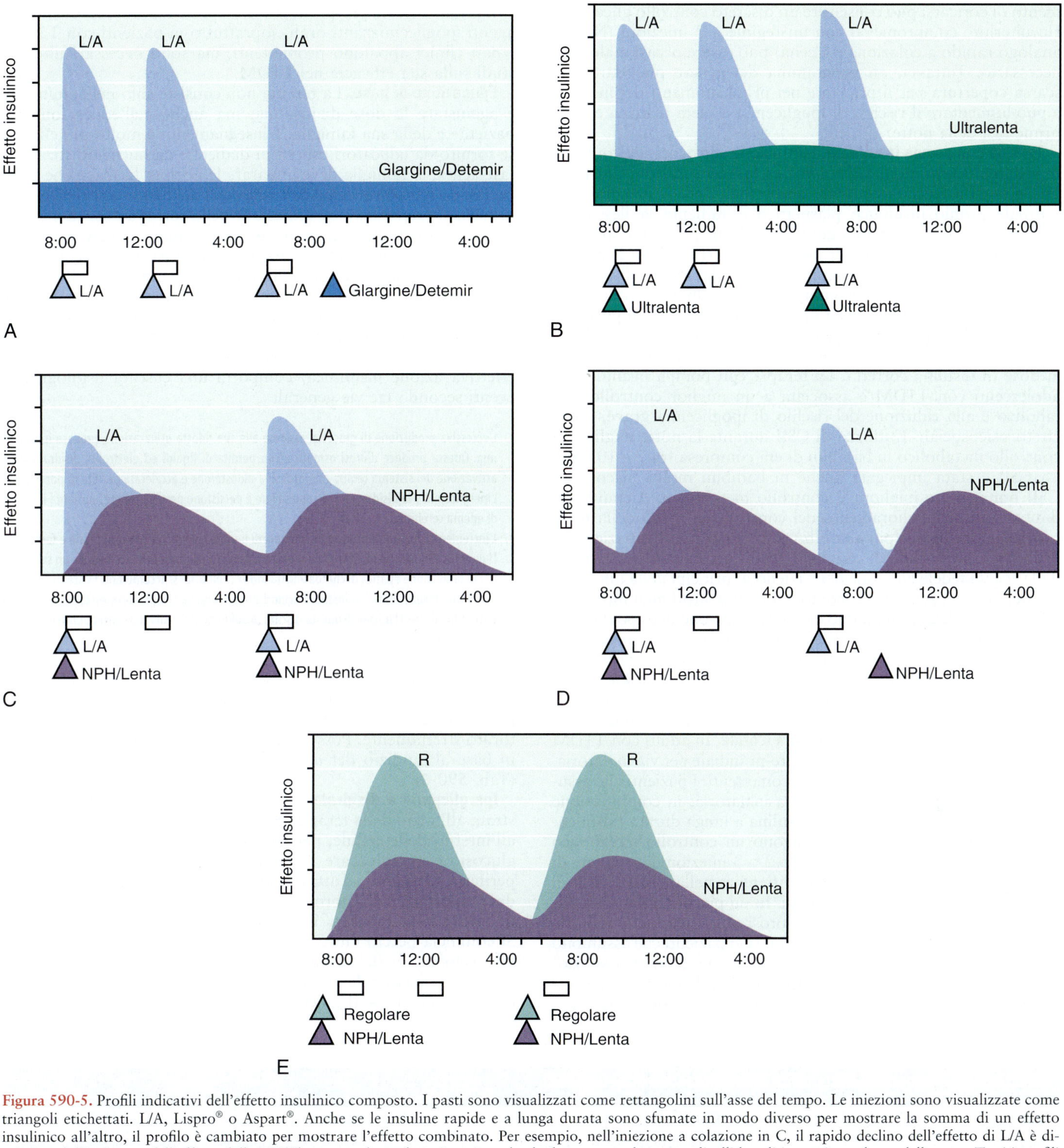

Figura 590-5. Profili indicativi dell'effetto insulinico composto. I pasti sono visualizzati come rettangolini sull'asse del tempo. Le iniezioni sono visualizzate come triangoli etichettati. L/A, Lispro® o Aspart®. Anche se le insuline rapide e a lunga durata sono sfumate in modo diverso per mostrare la somma di un effetto insulinico all'altro, il profilo è cambiato per mostrare l'effetto combinato. Per esempio, nell'iniezione a colazione in C, il rapido declino dell'effetto di L/A è diminuito dall'aumento dell'effetto della NPH/lenta, producendo un'ampia coda che lentamente decresce a livelli basali in corrispondenza della cena. Tutti i profili sono idealizzati usando l'assorbimento e la velocità di clearance medi. Ogni paziente ha velocità di assorbimento variabili, che dipendono dalla sede di iniezione, dall'attività fisica e da altre variabili. *A*, L o A pre-pasto; Glargine® al momento di coricarsi. Il rapido esordio e la breve durata di L o A riducono la sovrapposizione tra le iniezioni pre-pasto e manca un'azione durante la notte. Questo riduce il rischio di ipoglicemia. Glargine® comporta un profilo basale regolare, che agevola la previsione dell'effetto del bolo insulinico. *B*, L o A pre-pasto; ultralenta a colazione e a cena. L'ultralenta comporta un profilo basale simile a quello di Glargine®. Tuttavia, si nota un eccessivo effetto insulinico prima di cena e durante la notte. C, L o A pre-pasto; NPH o lenta a colazione e a cena. L'ampio picco di NPH o della lenta produce un rischio sostanziale di ipoglicemia prima di pranzo e durante le prime ore della notte. L'effetto insulinico in calo prima di cena e di colazione può anche permettere una svolta iperglicemia. *D*, L o A pre-pasto; NPH o lenta a colazione e al momento di coricarsi. Cambiando l'insulina a lunga azione della sera, si coprono le ore prima di colazione, ma permane il rischio di ipoglicemia durante al notte. *E*, Regolare e NPH o lenta a colazione e cena. Questo comporta il profilo meno fisiologico, con notevole eccesso prima di pranzo e durante le prime ore della notte e scarsa copertura prima di cena e colazione. Sebbene la lenta e l'ultralenta non siano più prodotte, esse vengono utilizzate per un confronto con i nuovi analoghi dell'insulina.

mento di coricarsi può consentire un discreto controllo glicemico. Un ulteriore compromesso con un regime a 2 iniezioni (NHP e analogo rapido a colazione e a cena) può essere occasionalmente necessario. Tuttavia, un programma del genere può dare una scarsa copertura per il pranzo e nei primi momenti del mattino e può aumentare il rischio di ipoglicemia a metà mattina e nelle prime fasi della notte.

Terapia con pompa insulinica. L'infusione sottocutanea continua di insulina (*Continuous Subcutaneous Insulin Infusion*, CSII) con una pompa a batteria consente una buona approssimazione del normale profilo insulinico plasmatico e aumenta la flessibilità per quanto riguarda i tempi dei pasti e degli spuntini, rispetto al programma convenzionale di iniezioni. I vari modelli di pompa insulinica possono essere programmati con algoritmi della dose di insulina personalizzata, che comprende l'insulina necessaria alla quota di carboidrati e la scala di correzione per i livelli glicemici pre-prandiali. Il paziente deve registrare la sua glicemia e il contenuto carboidratico dei cibi e il computer della pompa calcola la dose di insulina corretta. La terapia con pompa insulinica in adolescenti con T1DM è associata a un miglior controllo metabolico e alla riduzione del rischio di ipoglicemia grave, senza effetti psicosociali. L'utilizzo di CSII durante la notte migliora il controllo metabolico in bambini di età compresa fra 7 e 10 anni. La CSII è stata impiegata anche in bambini molto piccoli. La CSII non sempre migliora il controllo metabolico. Alcuni studi dimostrano un miglioramento del controllo in meno della metà e un peggioramento (più alta HbA_{1C}) in un quinto dei pazienti. È probabile che il grado di controllo glicemico dipenda soprattutto dalla scarsa fedele adesione dei pazienti ai principi della autoterapia del diabete, senza tener conto del regime insulinico intensivo. Un beneficio della pompa può essere la riduzione dell'ipoglicemia grave e di eventuali crisi epilettiche associate. Trial randomizzati che confrontano, in bambini con T1DM, somministrazioni giornaliere multiple di insulina (*Multiple Daily Insulin*, MDI) con insulina Glargine® e CSII dimostrano un analogo controllo metabolico e un'analoga frequenza di episodi ipoglicemici.

Terapie insuliniche per via inalatoria e orale. In adulti con T1DM e T2DM è stata valutata l'insulina pre-prandiale per via inalatoria. I dati metabolici preliminari sono promettenti. I pazienti che assumono insulina pre-prandiale per via inalatoria, in combinazione con una iniezione giornaliera di insulina a lunga durata (ultralenta) al momento di coricarsi ottengono un controllo metabolico simile a quello di pazienti che fanno 2 o 3 iniezioni giornaliere di insulina. Non ci sono significative differenze nella frequenza degli episodi ipoglicemici tra i due gruppi. In un piccolo numero di pazienti, sono stati riportati casi di fibrosi polmonare, che richiede un ulteriore monitoraggio e valutazione dei pazienti che assumono insulina per via inalatoria, prima che questa modalità di assunzione sia considerata sicura. La biodisponibilità dell'insulina per via inalatoria è aumentata dal fumo e ridotta in pazienti asmatici.

L'insulina orale pre-prandiale è stata valutata in confronto ad agenti ipoglicemizzanti orali, soprattutto in pazienti con T2DM. I dati clinici appaiono promettenti, ma sono necessari ulteriori studi sulla sua efficacia nel T1DM.

Educazione di base. La terapia non consiste solo nel cominciare e aggiustare la dose di insulina, ma anche nell'educazione del paziente e della sua famiglia. L'insegnamento è molto più efficace se fornito da educatori esperti in diabete e da nutrizionisti. Nella fase acuta, la famiglia deve imparare le nozioni basilari, che comprendono il monitoraggio della glicemia del bambino e dei chetoni urinari, la preparazione e l'iniezione della corretta dose di insulina per via sottocutanea al momento opportuno, trovare e trattare l'ipoglicemia, avere uno schema dietetico di base. La maggior parte delle famiglie prova ad adattarsi psicologicamente alla nuova diagnosi di diabete del loro bambino, di conseguenza mostra una limitata capacità di recepire nuove informazioni. Opuscoli informativi possono aiutare la famiglia durante i primi giorni.

Chetoacidosi. Una severa insulinopenia (o la mancanza di una effettiva azione insulinica) comporta una cascata fisiologica di eventi secondo tre vie generali.

1. **L'eccessiva produzione di glucosio, assieme alla sua ridotta utilizzazione, provoca iperglicemia. Questa produce diuresi osmotica, con perdita di liquidi ed elettroliti, disidratazione, attivazione del sistema renina-angiotensina-aldosterone e accelerata perdita di potassio. Se l'iperglicemia e la disidratazione sono severe e persistono per diverse ore, aumenta il rischio di edema cerebrale.**
2. **L'incremento dei processi catabolici comporta perdite cellulari di sodio, potassio e fosfati**
3. **L'aumento del rilascio di acidi grassi liberi dai depositi adiposi periferici fornisce un substrato per la produzione epatica di chetoacidi. Quando i chetoacidi si accumulano, i sistemi tampone diventano insufficienti e si instaura acidosi metabolica. La terapia deve essere indirizzata a entrambi gli eventi iniziali di questa cascata (insulinopenia) e alla sua conseguente fisiologica interruzione.**

L'inversione della DKA è associata a rischi inerenti, che comprendono ipoglicemia, ipokaliemia ed edema cerebrale. Qualsiasi protocollo deve essere utilizzato con cautela e il paziente va monitorato strettamente. Possono essere necessari degli aggiustamenti in base al giudizio del medico per un qualsiasi livello di DKA (Tab. 590-6).

Iperglicemia e disidratazione. L'insulina deve essere somministrata all'inizio della terapia per accelerare l'ingresso del glucosio all'interno delle cellule, per controllare la produzione epatica di glucosio e per bloccare il trasferimento degli acidi grassi dalla periferia al fegato. Tuttavia, un bolo iniziale di insulina non deve riportare nella norma la situazione troppo rapidamente, in quanto può aumentare il rischio di ipokaliemia e ipoglicemia. Si comincia perciò l'infusione di insulina **senza** un bolo iniziale, alla velocità di 0,1 U/kg/h. Questo si avvicina alla secrezione insulinica massimale in un soggetto normale durante un test orale di tolleranza al glucosio. Anche la reidratazione stessa ab-

TABELLA 590-6. Protocollo di trattamento della chetoacidosi diabetica (DKA)

TEMPO	TERAPIA	COMMENTI
Prima ora	10-20 mL/kg bolo endovenoso di NaCl 0,9% o LR Insulina a gocce a 0,05 fino a 0,10 µg/kg/ora	Rapida espansione del volume; può essere ripetuto. NPO. Monitoraggio I/O, stato neurologico. Usare il flow sheet. Tenere a portata di mano il mannitolo; 1 g/kg endovena per l'edema cerebrale.
Seconda ora fino alla risoluzione	NaCl 0,45%; più continuare insulina a gocce 20 mEq/L Kphos e 20 mEq/L KAc glucosio 5% di glucosio se la glicemia supera i 250 mg/dL (14 mmol/L)	$\text{tasso ev} = \frac{85\ \text{mL/kg} + \text{mantenimento} - \text{bolo}}{23\ \text{ore}}$
Variabile	Liquidi per via orale con insulina sottocutanea	Se K <3 mEq/L, somministrare da 0,5 a 1,0 mEq/kg come soluzione orale di K oppure aumentare il K endovena a 80 mEq/L No vomito; $CO_2 \geq 16$ mEq/L; elettroliti normali.

Notare che l'iniziale bolo endovenoso è considerato a parte dei liquidi complessivi permessi nelle prime 24 ore ed è sottratto prima di calcolare la percentuale endovenosa.
Mantenimento (24 ore) = 100 mL/kg (per i primi 10 kg) + 50 mL/kg (per i secondi 10 kg) + 25 mL/kg (per tutti i kg rimanenti)
Calcolo di un campione per un bambino di 30 kg:
prima ora = 300 mL di bolo endovenoso di NaCl 0,9% o LR

$$\text{seconda ora e successive} = \frac{(85\ \text{mL x } 30) + 1750\ \text{mL} - 300\ \text{mL}}{23\ \text{ore}} = \frac{175\ \text{mL}}{\text{ora}}\ (0{,}45\%\ \text{NaCl con 20 mEq/L KPhos e 20 mEq/L KAC})$$

I/O, dentro e fuori (urine, emesi); KAc, acetato di potassio; Kphos, fosfato di potassio; LR, soluzione Ringer lattato; NaCl, cloruro di sodio.

bassa i livelli di glucosio, migliorando la perfusione renale e aumentandone l'escrezione. La combinazione di queste terapie si solito provoca un iniziale rapido declino della glicemia. Quando la glicemia scende sotto i 180 mg/dL (10 mmol/L), si arresta la diuresi osmotica, diventando più rapida la reidratazione, senza aumentare ulteriormente la velocità di infusione.

La risoluzione dell'iperglicemia si verifica prima della correzione dell'acidosi. Per questo motivo, dopo che si sono raggiunti normali livelli glicemici, l'insulina è ancora necessaria per controllare il rilascio degli acidi grassi. Per continuare l'infusione di insulina senza provocare ipoglicemia, si deve aggiungere del glucosio all'infusione, di solito in soluzione al 5%. Il glucosio va aggiunto quando la glicemia scende a circa 250 mg/dL (14 mmol/L) per un tempo sufficiente ad adattare l'infusione prima che la glicemia scenda ulteriormente. Una volta risolta l'iperglicemia, si può ridurre la velocità massima iniziale dell'infusione di insulina.

Il ripristino del deficit di liquidi deve essere moderato, per il potenziale rischio di **edema cerebrale**. In tutti i bambini qualunque sia lo stato iperosmotico, è prudente una reidratazione cauta. L'effettiva osmolalità sierica ($E_{osm} = 2 \times [Na_{non\ corretto}] +$ [glucosio]) rappresenta un indice accurato della tonicità dei liquidi corporei e riflette l'idratazione intra ed extracellulare meglio della misurazione della osmolalità plasmatica. Si calcola con sodio e glucosio in mmol/L. Questo valore è di solito elevato all'inizio della terapia e deve progressivamente normalizzarsi. Un calo rapido o un declino lento al di sotto del range di normalità può indicare un eccesso di acqua libera nello spazio vascolare e un aumento del rischio di edema cerebrale. Perciò, al paziente non deve essere consentito introdurre liquidi per via orale, fino a che la reidratazione sia avanzata e non siano ulteriormente probabili modificazioni elettrolitiche significative. Si può dare un piccolo cubetto di ghiaccio per un apporto orale minimo. Tutti i liquidi introdotti ed eliminati devono essere monitorati con precisione.

Il calcolo del deficit di liquidi che si basa sull'osservazione di segni clinici ed è difficile nei bambini con DKA perché, nello stato ipertonico, il volume intravascolare si mantiene meglio. Per ogni grado di tachicardia, ritardato riempimento capillare, diminuzione della temperatura corporea o modificazioni ortostatiche della pressione arteriosa, il bambino con DKA deve essere più idratato rispetto al bambino con un deficit normotonico di liquidi. Il protocollo della Tabella 583-6 corregge un deficit di 85 mL/kg (disidratazione dell'8,5%) per tutti i pazienti nelle prime 24 ore. Bambini con DKA lieve si reidratano più precocemente e possono passare all'introduzione per via orale, mentre quelli con DKA severa e maggior deficit del volume richiedono 30-60 ore con questo protocollo. Questa reidratazione del bambino con DKA severa più graduale è una modalità di sicurezza. L'iniziale bolo endovenoso (20 mL/kg di soluzione Ringer lattato isotonica di sali di sodio priva di glucosio o una soluzione allo 0,9% di cloruro di sodio), valido per tutti i pazienti, assicura una rapida espansione del volume e può essere ripetuto in assenza di un miglioramento clinico in poco tempo. Questo bolo è somministrato come soluzione salina isotonica, perché il paziente è inevitabilmente ipertonico, in quanto la maggior parte dell'infusione iniziale rimane nello spazio intravascolare. I liquidi successivi sono ipotonici, per riparare il deficit di acqua libera, per consentire la reidratazione intracellulare e per permettere una più appropriata sostituzione delle continue perdite urinarie ipotoniche.

La sodiemia iniziale è di solito normale o bassa, per la diluizione osmolare dell'iperglicemia e l'effetto di un'elevata frazione lipidica priva di sodio. Una valutazione del sodio sierico ricostituito, o "vero", per ogni livello di glucosio oltre i 100 mg/dL (5,6 mmol/L), è calcolata come segue:

$$\frac{[Na^+]+\text{glucosio}-\mathit{100}\times 1{,}6}{100}$$

se il glucosio è in mg/dL, o

$$\frac{[Na^+]+\text{glucosio}-\mathit{5{,}6}\times 1{,}6}{5{,}6}$$

se il glucosio è in mmol/L.

Il sodio deve aumentare di circa 1,6 mmol/L per ogni 100 mg/dL di diminuzione del glucosio. Il sodio corretto è di solito normale o lievemente elevato e indica una moderata disidratazione ipernatremica. Se il valore corretto è maggiore di 150 mmol/L, può essere presenta una grave disidratazione ipernatriemia che necessita di una più lenta infusione di liquidi. Il sodio deve aumentare progressivamente con la terapia. La sua diminuzione può indicare un eccessivo accumulo di acqua libera e il rischio di edema cerebrale.

Perdite cataboliche. I cambiamenti metabolici in senso prevalentemente catabolico e l'acidosi provocano il movimento di potassio e fosfati dalla cellula al siero. La diuresi osmotica, l'effetto kaliuretico dell'iperaldosteronismo e la chetonuria accelerano in seguito le perdite renali di potassio e fosfati. Il sodio viene eliminato anche con la diuresi, ma le perdite di acqua libera sono maggiori di quelle isotoniche. Con malattie prolungate e con la DKA di grado severo, le perdite corporee totali possono arrivare a 10-13 mEq/kg di sodio, 5-6 mEq/kg di potassio e 4-5 mEq/kg di fosfati. Queste perdite continuano per parecchie ore durante la terapia, fino a che si inverte lo stato catabolico e la diuresi è sotto controllo. Per esempio, il 50% del sodio infuso può essere perso per via urinaria durante la terapia per via endovenosa. Anche se il deficit di sodio può essere ripristinato in 24 ore, le concentrazioni intracellulari di potassio e fosfati ritornano completamente nella norma solo in un numero consistente di giorni.

Sebbene i pazienti con DKA abbiano un deficit del potassio corporeo totale, i livelli sierici iniziali spesso sono normali o elevati. Questo è dovuto al movimento di potassio dallo spazio intracellulare al siero, in parte come tampone contro i chetoacidi e in parte per un cambiamento in senso catabolico. Questi effetti sono reversibili con la terapia e il potassio ritorna all'interno della cellula. Il miglioramento dell'idratazione aumenta il flusso ematico renale, tenendo conto di un'aumentata escrezione di potassio nell'iperaldosteronismo. Il risultato netto è spesso rappresentato da un drammatico declino dei livelli sierici di potassio, specialmente nella DKA di grado severo, che può precipitare modificazioni della conduzione cardiaca, appiattimento dell'onda T e prolungamento del complesso QRS, provocando inoltre debolezza o paralisi dei muscoli scheletrici. Il rischio di alterazioni miocardiche è aumentato in caso di shock e acidosi. I livelli di potassio devono essere seguiti attentamente e, con il monitoraggio elettrocardiografico, continuati fino a che la DKA sia sostanzialmente risolta. Se necessario, la somministrazione parenterale di potassio può essere aumentata a 80 mEq/L o, in assenza di vomito, può essere somministrato un supplemento orale. Raramente, l'insulina per via endovenosa deve essere temporaneamente sospesa.

Non è chiaro se il deficit di potassio contribuisca ai sintomi di DKA così come alla debolezza muscolare generalizzata. Nei pazienti pediatrici, non si è dimostrato che il deficit comprometta la distribuzione dell'ossigeno attraverso un deficit di 2,3-difosfoglicerato (2,3-DPG). Poiché il paziente riceve un eccesso di cloruro, che può aggravare l'acidosi, è prudente utilizzare, come fonte di potassio, il fosfato di potassio invece del cloruro di potassio. È utilizzato anche l'acetato di potassio, poiché funziona da ulteriore tampone.

In concomitanza della DKA, si è osservata occasionalmente pancreatite, specialmente in presenza di distress addominale prolungato; le amilasi sieriche possono essere elevate. Se le lipasi sieriche non sono aumentate, le amilasi sono probabilmente non specifiche o di origine salivare. La creatinina sierica, dosata per età, può essere falsamente elevata, a causa dell'interferenza da parte dei chetoni nel metodo autoanalitico. Raramente un valore iniziale elevato indica insufficienza renale e deve essere ricontrollato quando il bambino è meno chetonemico. L'azoto ureico ematico (*Blood Urea Nitrogen*, BUN) può essere elevato, con azotemia prerenale, e deve essere ricontrollato quando il bambino viene reidratato. Un lieve aumento della creatina o del BUN non è una ragione per non eseguire la terapia con potassio, in presenza di una buona escrezione urinaria.

Accumulo di chetoacidi. L'infusione insulinica a bassa velocità (0,02-0,05 U/kg/h) di solito è sufficiente a bloccare il rilascio periferico di acidi grassi, eliminando così il flusso di substrati utilizzati per la chetogenesi. Perciò, se la glicemia scende sotto i 150 mg/dL (8 mmol/L), la velocità iniziale di infusione può essere diminuita, nonostante l'aggiunta di glucosio all'infusione. La chetogenesi continua fino a che il substrato, costituito dagli acidi grassi, non sia già terminato a livello epatico, ma questa produzione diminuisce molto più rapidamente senza l'arrivo di un nuovo substrato. I tamponi bicarbonato, rigenerati a livello del tubulo renale distale e dal metabolismo dei corpi chetonici, riparano progressivamente l'acidosi, dopo che è sotto controllo la produzione di chetoacidi. La terapia con bicarbonato è raramente necessaria e può anche aumentare il rischio di ipokaliemia e di edema cerebrale.

A mano a mano che la terapia continua, si deve verificare un progressivo aumento del pH e dei bicarbonato sierici. Il respiro di Kussmaul deve cessare, come deve scomparire il dolore addominale. Un'acidosi persistente può indicare un'inadeguata terapia con insulina o liquidi, infezione o raramente acidosi lattica. I chetoni urinari possono essere positivi a lungo dopo la risoluzione della chetoacidosi, perché la reazione alla nitroprusside usata di routine per misurare i chetoni urinari con dipstick misura solo l'acetoacetato. Durante la DKA, la maggior parte dell'eccesso chetonico è rappresentato dal β-idrossibutirrato, che aumenta il normale rapporto con l'acetoacetato da 3:1 a 8:1. Con la risoluzione dell'acidosi, il β-idrossibutirrato si converte in aceotoacetato, escreto nelle urine e rilevato dal dipstick. Perciò, una persistente chetonuria non riflette accuratamente il grado di miglioramento clinico, quindi non deve essere considerata un indicatore di insuccesso terapeutico. Tutti i pazienti con DKA devono essere valutati per **eventi iniziali** che possano innescare uno scompenso metabolico.

Protocollo per DKA (vedi Tab. 590-6). Anche se la gravità della DKA è molto variabile, un approccio comune a tutti i pazienti semplifica il regime terapeutico e può essere utilizzato con tranquillità nella maggior parte dei bambini. I liquidi sono calcolati in base al peso, e non alla superficie corporea (m^2), perché raramente si può utilizzare l'altezza per il calcolo. Il protocollo Milwaukee è stato usato per più di 20 anni, e nei bambini trattati inizialmente in questo modo non si sono verificati casi di morte o di sequele neurologiche. Può essere utilizzato per bambini di tutte le età e con tutti i gradi di DKA. Nel bambino mediamente grave, in circa 24 ore è in grado di ripristinare la maggior parte dei deficit elettrolitici, di risolvere l'acidosi e di reidratare. Si considera un deficit di acqua standard (85 mL/kg), che, aggiunto al mantenimento, reintegra circa 4 L/m^2 in bambini di tutte le taglie. Bambini con DKA più lieve recuperano in 10-20 ore (e necessitano di meno liquido totale per via endovenosa, prima di passare all'assunzione orale), mentre quelli con DKA più severa richiedono l'utilizzo di questo protocollo per 30-36 ore. Quando la DKA è essenzialmente risolta (CO_2 totale >15 mEq/L; pH >7,30; sodio stabile tra 135 e 145 mEq/L; assenza di vomito), ogni bambino può facilmente passare all'assunzione orale e all'insulina per via sottocutanea. Si sospende quindi la terapia endovenosa e si somministra la prima dose di insulina sottocutanea con un pasto. Bambini con DKA di lieve entità spesso possono essere dimessi dal reparto di emergenza dopo poche ore di terapia, se si provvede a un adeguato follow-up.

Per un accurato monitoraggio dei cambiamenti di acidosi, elettroliti, bilancio idrico e stato clinico, è obbligatorio il flow-sheet, specialmente se il paziente è trasferito da un reparto di urgenza in un altro, con nuovi medici curanti. Un sistema computerizzato centrale fornisce un più completo flow-sheet, che permette un rapido aggiornamento e un'ampia disponibilità di risultati e che evidenzia il ruolo di valori critici. È invece sufficiente un flow-sheet cartaceo se si rimane con il paziente; esso va aggiornato e rivisto frequentemente. Ogni flow-sheet deve includere colonne per i dosaggi seriali di elettroliti, pH, glicemia e bilancio idrico. Nei bambini con DKA severa, si eseguono dei prelievi di sangue ogni 1-2 ore e ogni 3-4 per forme lievi e moderate.

Anche se questo protocollo vanta un lungo record di sicurezza, ogni paziente deve essere monitorato strettamente. Per tutti i casi di media entità, il monitoraggio prevede frequenti controlli neurologici, attenti a valutare ogni eventuale segno di **aumentata pressione endocranica**, o di alterazione dello stato di coscienza, depressione della respirazione, peggioramento della cefalea, bradicardia, apnea, modificazioni pupillari, papilledema e crisi epilettiche. Il mannitolo dovrebbe essere facilmente disponibile per la terapia dei primi segni di edema cerebrale. È necessario anche essere sempre informati sulle modificazioni dei parametri di laboratorio; ipokaliemia o ipoglicemia si possono instaurare rapidamente. Bambini con DKA da severa a moderata hanno un rischio maggiore e dovrebbero essere trattati in un centro di terapia intensiva. Infine, questo protocollo può non essere appropriato per alcuni pazienti, come quelli più gravemente ipernatriemici (sodio corretto >150 mEq/L), in cui può essere necessaria una reidratazione più lenta, con un'infusione di liquidi isotonici di durata maggiore.

Anche in bambini con DKA grave si è osservata una certa attività residua β-cellulare. Questa funzione può migliorare non appena il bambino si rimette dall'effetto dell'iperglicemia e degli elevati ormoni controregolatori. La secrezione residua può richiedere una riduzione della dose sottocutanea di insulina utilizzata nei primi giorni di terapia.

Coma iperosmolare non chetosico. Questa sindrome è caratterizzata da severa iperglicemia (glicemia >800 mg/dL), assenza di chetosi o chetosi lieve, acidosi non chetosica, grave disidratazione, sensorio depresso o vero e proprio coma e vari segni neurologici che possono comprendere crisi epilettiche di grande male, ipertermia, emiparesi e positività dei segni di Babinski. La respirazione è superficiale, ma può evidenziarsi, con la comparsa del respiro di Kussmaul, una coesistente acidosi metabolica (lattica). L'osmolarità sierica è comunemente di 350 mOsm/kg o maggiore. Questa condizione non è frequente nei bambini; negli adulti, la percentuale di mortalità è elevata, anche per il ritardo nel riconoscimento della patologia e quindi dell'instaurazione di un adeguata terapia. Nei bambini, sono molto frequenti danni neurologici preesistenti. Si può sviluppare un'iperglicemia notevole nell'arco di alcuni giorni e, inizialmente, la poliuria osmotica obbligata e la disidratazione possono esser parzialmente compensate da un incremento dell'introduzione di liquidi. Con il progredire della malattia, la sensazione della sete viene compromessa, per alterazione del centro ipotalamico della sete a causa dell'iperosmolarità e, in alcuni casi, di un preesistente difetto nel meccanismo ipotalamico di osmoregolazione.

La bassa produzione di chetoni è attribuita soprattutto all'iperosmolarità, che *in vitro* attenua l'effetto lipolitico dell'adrenalina e quello antilipolitico dell'insulina residua; la diminuzione della lipolisi per l'utilizzo terapeutico di bloccanti β-adrenergici può contribuire a questa sindrome. La depressione della coscienza è strettamente correlata al grado di iperosmolarità sia in questa condizione sia nella DKA. L'emoconcentrazione può predisporre anche a trombosi dell'arteria cerebrale e trombosi venose.

Il **trattamento** del coma iperosmolare non chetosico è diretto a reintegrare rapidamente il deficit del volume vascolare e a correggere invece molto lentamente lo stato iperosmolare. Si somministra una soluzione salina con tonicità dimezzata (NaCl allo 0,45%; alcuni utilizzano una soluzione salina normale) a una velocità tale da ripristinare il 50% del deficit di volume nelle prime 12 ore e il rimanente durante le successive 24. La velocità di infusione e la concentrazione salina sono titolate in modo da determinare una discesa lenta dell'osmolarità sierica. Quando la glicemia si avvicina ai 300 mg/dL, si sostituiscono i liquidi da infusione, con destrosio al 5% in un soluzione salina 0,2 normale (N). A ognuno di questi liquidi si devono aggiungere circa 20 mEq/L di cloruro di potassio, per prevenire l'ipokaliemia. La glicemia e la kaliemia vanno monitorate a intervalli di 2 ore per le prime 12 ore e a intervalli di 4 ore per le successive 24, per consentire appropriati aggiustamenti della somministrazione di potassio e insulina.

L'insulina può essere somministrata in infusione endovenosa continua, cominciando dalla seconda ora di terapia liquida. La glicemia può diminuire drasticamente con la sola terapia liquida.

Il dosaggio dell'insulina per via endovenosa deve essere 0,05 U/kg/h di regolare (a rapida-azione) invece che 0,1 U/kg/h come nei pazienti con DKA.

Trattamento dietetico. La nutrizione gioca un ruolo essenziale nel trattamento del paziente con T1DM ed è di importanza fondamentale durante l'infanzia e l'adolescenza, quando è richiesto un adeguato *intake* (apporto) calorico per affrontare le necessità energetiche, di crescita e di sviluppo puberale. Il trattamento dietetico da solo o in combinazione con una terapia insulinica appropriata previene o attenua i sintomi di iperglicemia nei pazienti diabetici. Inoltre, il tipo di alimentazione può influenzare lo sviluppo a lungo termine delle complicanze del diabete (nefropatia diabetica). Il bambino diabetico non ha particolari esigenze nutrizionali, se non quelle legate a una crescita e uno sviluppo ottimali. Nel delineare le esigenze nutrizionali del bambino si devono tenere in considerazione età, sesso, peso, attività, preferenze per certi cibi, comprese quelle culturali ed etniche.

L'intake calorico complessivo raccomandato si basa sull'entità della superficie corporea e può essere desunto da tabelle standardizzate (Tabb. 590-7 e 590-8). Le calorie complessive sono suddivise in: circa 55% di carboidrati, 30% di lipidi e 15% di proteine. Circa il 70% del contenuto carboidratico deve derivare da carboidrati complessi come l'amido, mentre deve essere limitata l'assunzione di zuccheri a elevata raffinazione. I carboidrati complessi richiedono una digestione prolungata e un assorbimento tali per cui i livelli plasmatici di glucosio salgono lentamente, mentre il glucosio che deriva da zuccheri raffinati, comprese le bibite gassate, è assorbito rapidamente e può provocare ampie oscillazioni del quadro metabolico; le bevande gassate dovrebbero quindi essere prive di zucchero. È fondamentale calcolare le calorie totali e del consumo complessivo di carboidrati piuttosto che esaminare la loro origine. Il calcolo dei carboidrati è diventato un cardine dell'educazione nutrizionale e del trattamento di pazienti con DM. Ogni unità di scambio di carboidrati ammonta a 1,5 g. Il paziente e la sua famiglia vengono informati circa il contenuto in carboidrati dei diversi alimenti e istruiti sulla lettura delle etichette dei cibi. Questo consente al paziente di modificare la sua dose di insulina in base al contenuto carboidratico del pasto. L'utilizzo del conteggio dei carboidrati e dei rapporti tra carboidrati e insulina assieme all'uso di analoghi dell'insulina a lunga durata di azione e di insulina basale a lunga durata (Detemir® e Glargine®) rende l'organizzazione dei pasti meno rigida per molti bambini. La flessibilità nell'uso dell'insulina in rapporto al contenuto di carboidrati degli alimenti migliora la qualità della vita.

Sebbene esista preoccupazione circa il potenziale effetto cumulativo della saccarina nei bambini, i dati disponibili non sostengono un rapporto fra dosi moderate e cancro della vescica. In vari prodotti sono utilizzati altri dolcificanti privi di calorie, come l'aspartame. È preferibile non utilizzare come dolcificanti artificiali come sorbitolo e xilitolo, poiché sono prodotti derivati dalla via dei polioli e sono implicati in alcune delle complicanze del diabete.

Per migliorare il controllo glicemico si utilizzano diete ad alto contenuto di fibre. Una quantità moderata di zucchero, consumata con alimenti ricchi di fibre come il pane integrale a pasto, può non avere un effetto glicemico maggiore rispetto ai suoi equivalenti privi di zucchero e a basso contenuto di fibre. Il concetto di equivalenza biologica o di "indice glicemico" degli alimenti è in fase di studio.

L'assunzione di grassi è regolata in modo tale che il rapporto tra polinsaturi:saturi aumenti a circa 1,2:1, al contrario della media stimata, per esempio, per un americano, che è di 0,3:1. Sono ridotti i grassi alimentari derivanti da fonti animali e sostituiti da grassi polinsaturi di origine vegetale. Nella cottura è opportuno sostituire il burro con la margarina e l'olio di origine animale con gli oli vegetali, così come scegliere carne magra, pollame e pesce al posto di carni grasse come il bacon. In questo modo, oltre a diminuire il numero di tuorli di uovo, si riduce anche l'assunzione di colesterolo. Queste semplici misure riducono il colesterolo-LDL, un fattore predisponente alla patologia aterosclerotica. Meno del 10% delle calorie deve derivare da grassi saturi, oltre il 10% da grassi polinsaturi e la quota rimanente da grassi monoinsaturi. La Tabella 590-8 riassume le linee guida attuali.

L'intake calorico complessivo giornaliero viene diviso come segue: 20% a colazione, 20% a pranzo, 30% a cena, lasciando un 10% per ciascuno degli spuntini a metà mattina, metà pomeriggio e alla sera, se il paziente lo desidera. Nei bambini più grandi, si può evitare lo spuntino di metà mattina e aggiungere l'equivalente calorico a pranzo. Negli Stati Uniti le associazioni regionali di diabetici in genere forniscono speciali opuscoli e libretti che descrivono semplici esempi di pasto per i bambini; il

TABELLA 590-7. Necessità caloriche per i bambini e i giovani adulti

ETÀ	KCAL RICHIESTE/KG PESO CORPOREO*
Bambini	
0-12 mesi	120
1-10 anni	100-75
Giovani donne	
11-15 anni	35
≥16 anni	30
Giovani uomini	
11-15 anni	80-55 (65)
16-20 anni	
Attività media	40
Attività fisica intensa	50
Sedentarietà	30

I numeri tra parentesi rappresentano la media.
*Graduale declino nelle calorie per unità di peso all'aumentare dell'età.
Da *Nutrition Guide for Professionals: Diabetes education and meal Planning*. Alexandria, VA, and Chicago, IL, The American Diabetes Association and The American Dietetic Association, 1988.

TABELLA 590-8. Riassunto delle linee guida dietetiche per bambini e/o adolescenti con diabete mellito di tipo 1

Piano di terapia dietetica

Promozione di una compliance ottimale

Comprendere gli obiettivi del trattamento: normale crescita e sviluppo, controllo della glicemia, mantenimento di un ottimale stato nutrizionale e prevenzione delle complicanze. Usare un approccio graduale.

Consigli e distribuzione dei nutrienti

NUTRIENTE	(%) DI CALORIE	ASSUNZIONE GIORNALIERA RACCOMANDATA
Carboidrati	Varia	
Fibre	>20 g/die	Mole fibre, specialmente solubili, quota ottimale sconosciuta
Proteine	12-20	
Grassi	<30	
Saturi	<10	
Polinsaturi	6-8	
Monoinsaturi	Il rimanente della quota lipidica	
Colesterolo		300 mg
Sodio		Evitare l'eccesso; limitare a 3000-4000 mg in caso di ipertensione

Ulteriori raccomandazioni

Energia: se si utilizza una dieta misurata, rivalutare l'energia prescritta almeno ogni 3 mesi.

Proteine: un apporto proteico elevato può contribuire alla nefropatia diabetica. Intake bassi possono far recedere una nefropatia preclinica. Tuttavia, si raccomanda il 12-20% delle calorie; è preferibile il livello inferiore del range. È necessario un approccio graduale per raggiungere il limite inferiore del range.

Alcol: nelle scuole superiori, nell'ambito di una prevenzione precoce di routine, va sottolineata l'importanza di un uso prudente di dosi moderate di alcol.

Spuntini: gli spuntini variano a seconda delle necessità individuali (generalmente 3 spuntini al giorno per i bambini, uno spuntino a metà pomeriggio e all'ora di coricarsi per i bambini più grandi e gli adolescenti).

Dolcificanti alternativi: si consiglia di usare vari dolcificanti.

Tecniche educative: non esiste una tecnica migliore delle altre. La scelta di un metodo educativo si deve basare sulle necessità del paziente. La conoscenza delle varie tecniche è importante. Si richiede un supporto e un follow-up educativo.

Disturbi alimentari: il miglior trattamento è la prevenzione. Uno scarso controllo inspiegabile o una ipoglicemia severa possono indicare un potenziale disturbo alimentare.

Esercizio fisico: l'educazione è vitale per prevenire ipoglicemia ritardata o immediata e un peggioramento dell'iperglicemia e chetosi.

Da Connell JE, Thomas-Doberson D: Nutitional Management of children and adolescent with insulin-dependent diabetes mellitus: A review by the Diabetes care and Education Dietetic Practice Group: *J Am Diet Assoc* 1991;91:1556 loro utilizzo va incoraggiato come parte del processo educativo. Lo schema del pasto spesso è basato su gruppi di alimenti scambiabili; in ognuna delle liste di scambio degli alimenti che sono principali fonti di carboidrati, proteine e grassi esiste un'ampia varietà di alimenti di sostituzione o scambio. Ci sono poche restrizioni, in modo che, con l'aiuto del medico o del dietista (o di entrambi), ogni bambino possa scegliere una dieta basata sulle proprie preferenze. È necessario sottolineare l'importanza della regolarità dell'assunzione dei cibi e della costanza dell'apporto di carboidrati. Un eccesso occasionale durante un compleanno o un'altra festa è permesso e tollerato e non incoraggia la ribellione o l'assunzione di nascosto del cibo desiderato. In occasioni speciali sono concessi torte e dolciumi, in modo che il valore dell'alimento scambiato e il contenuto di carboidrati venga modificato nello schema del pasto. È necessario fare continue modifiche agli schemi dei pasti, per venire incontro alla necessità e ai desideri di ogni bambino, sebbene per il controllo metabolico sia importante un atteggiamento alimentare regolare, con appropriati supplementi per lo sport, la crescita puberale e la gravidanza nelle adolescenti diabetiche.

Negli ultimi 20 anni, è triplicata l'incidenza di bambini e adolescenti con T1DM in sovrappeso, in rapporto all'aumento della frequenza di obesità nella popolazione generale. Alcuni Autori hanno osservato che tra i loro pazienti con T1DM, i bambini in età prescolare normopeso hanno un miglior controllo glicemico dei coetanei sovrappeso. Questo può significare che, in questo gruppo di pazienti, l'eccesso di peso corporeo impedisce di raggiungere gli obiettivi terapeutici. Vi è inoltre un aumento della frequenza di disordini alimentari tra le giovani donne con diabete. È necessario quindi che le aspettative e i consigli educativi riguardo alla nutrizione siano forniti in modo sensibile e attento, specialmente agli adolescenti.

Monitoraggio. Il successo del trattamento giornaliero del bambino diabetico può essere misurato dalla competenza acquisita dalla famiglia, e di conseguenza anche dal bambino, nell'assumersi la responsabilità della "terapia giornaliera del diabete". L'educazione iniziale e continua e la supervisione possono portare al raggiungimento di una certa confidenza nel modificare saltuariamente il dosaggio insulinico per eventuali trasgressioni dietetiche, per un esercizio fisico non abituale o anche per alcune patologie intercorrenti minori, come per ripetute reazioni ipoglicemiche non spiegabili in altro modo, e per eccessiva glicosuria. Pertanto, l'assunzione di responsabilità deve rendere relativamente indipendente dal medico per la gestione ordinaria. Il medico dovrebbe mantenere una continua supervisione interessata, condividendo la responsabilità con la famiglia e con il bambino.

L'automonitoraggio della glicemia (*Self-Monitoring of Blood Glucose*, SMBG) è una componente essenziale del trattamento del diabete. Il monitoraggio spesso deve tenere conto della dose di insulina, di un'attività fisica non abituale, di cambiamenti dietetici, ipoglicemia, patologie intercorrenti e altri fattori che possano influenzare la glicemia. Se esiste una discrepanza fra SMBG e altre misure del controllo glicemico (come la HbA_{1C}), il medico dovrebbe chiarire la situazione in modo da non minare la fiducia reciproca.

Il monitoraggio giornaliero della glicemia è stato molto incrementato per la disponibilità di strisce impregnate di glucosio ossidasi, che permette la misurazione del glucosio ematico da una goccia di sangue. Uno strumento portatile calibrato a riflettenza è in grado di fornire misurazioni accurate della glicemia. Molti strumenti contengono un chip di memoria che favorisce il richiamo di ogni misurazione, la sua media in un dato intervallo e sono in grado di evidenziare il quadro sullo schermo di un computer. Tale informazione è un utile strumento educativo per verificare il grado di controllo e modificare il regime in atto prescritto. È disponibile sul mercato un piccolo apparecchio a molla che preleva automaticamente sangue capillare in modo relativamente indolore. I genitori e il paziente devono imparare a usare l'apparecchio e a misurare il glucosio nel sangue almeno 4 volte al giorno, prima di colazione, pranzo e cena e prima di coricarsi. Non appena si inizia la terapia insulinica e quando si apportano delle modifiche che possono influenzare i livelli notturni di glucosio, si dovrebbe eseguire una SMBG a mezzanotte e alle 3.00 per cercare un'eventuale ipoglicemia notturna. Idealmente, la concentrazione ematica di glucosio dovrebbe aggirarsi dagli 80 mg/dL a digiuno fino ai 140 mg/dL dopo il pasto. In pratica, tuttavia, è accettabile un range di 60-220 mg/dL, in base all'età del paziente (Tab. 590-9). Livelli glicemici costantemente oltre questi limiti, in assenza di una causa identificabile, come l'esercizio o una modificazione alimentare, costituiscono un'indicazione per modificare il dosaggio insulinico. Se la glicemia a digiuno è elevata, si aumenta del 10-15% la dose serale di insulina a lunga durata di azione e/o si può aggiungere un'insulina ad azione rapida (Lispror® o Aspartr®) come copertura per lo spuntino serale. Se la glicemia notturna supera i limiti, si aumenta del 10-15% l'insulina giornaliera ad azione rapida (Lispror® o Aspartr®). Se la glicemia prima di coricarsi è alta, si aumenta del 10-15% la dose di insulina prima di cena. Analogamente, riduzioni di un tipo di insulina e della sua dose vanno attuate solo se le misurazioni della glicemia sono notevolmente inferiori ai limiti desiderabili.

È necessario eseguire un minimo di 4 misurazioni giornaliere della glicemia, anche se alcuni bambini e adolescenti possono avere bisogno di un monitoraggio più frequente, in base al livello della loro attività fisica e all'anamnesi di frequenti reazioni ipoglicemiche. Si devono incoraggiare le famiglie a documentarsi sufficientemente sulla gestione del diabete. Con l'automonitoraggio dei livelli glicemici prima e due ore dopo i pasti e con multiple iniezioni giornaliere di insulina, regolata come necessario, si può mantenere una glicemia vicina ai valori normali per periodi prolungati.

Un sistema continuo di monitoraggio della glicemia (*Continuous Glucose Monitoring System*, CGMS) registra i dati ottenuti da un sensore sottocutaneo ogni 5 minuti per 72 ore e fornisce ai medici un profilo continuo dei livelli di glucosio tissutale. I livelli di glucosio interstiziale sono sfasati di 13 minuti rispetto ai valori del glucosio ematico, a un qualsiasi livello dato. I valori del CGMS hanno un alto coefficiente di correlazione con quelli della glicemia in un range compreso tra 40 e 400 mg/dL. Il CGMS è minimamente invasivo e comporta la sistemazione di un piccolo catetere sottocutaneo che può essere facilmente asportato sia da adulti sia da bambini. Il sistema fornisce informazioni che permettono al paziente e al team terapeutico di regolare il regime insulinico e lo schema dietetico per migliorare il controllo glicemico. Il CGMS può essere di aiuto per trovare un'ipoglicemia notturna asintomatica e per abbassare i livelli di HbA_{1C} senza aumento del rischio di grave ipoglicemia. Nonostante potenziali inconvenienti nell'uso del CGMS, compresi compliance subottimale, errore umano, tecnica non corretta e alterazione del sensore, l'avvio del CGMS nella gestione ambulatoriale del diabete permette ai medici di diagnosticare in modo più preciso un anomalo pattern glicemico.

Il Glucowatch Biographer® usa la iontoforesi inversa per analizzare il contenuto glicidico dei liquidi interstiziali, estratti attraverso una membrana sul polso del paziente sotto all'apparecchio Glucowatch®. Il Glucowatch® fornisce in tempo reale il valore del glucosio dei liquidi interstiziali, in un range compreso tra 40 e 400 mg/dL, che rappresenta la media dei valori glicemici dei precedenti 20 minuti. Valori di glucosio compresi tra 70 e 280

TABELLA 590-9. Glicemia di riferimento pre-pasto e range medio della glicemia di 30 giorni e corrispondente HbA_{1C} per ogni gruppo di età

GRUPPI DI ETÀ	RANGE DELLA GLICEMIA DI RIFERIMENTO PRE-PASTO (mg/dL)	RANGE DELLA GLICEMIA MEDIA IN 30 GIORNI (mg/dL)	HbA_{1C} DI RIFERIMENTO (%)
<5	100-200	180-250	7,5-9,0
5-11	80-150	150-200	6,5-8,0
12-15	80-130	120-180	6,0-7,5
16-18	70-120	100-150	5,5-7,0

Nel nostro laboratorio il range di riferimento per HbA_{1C} è 4,5-5,7% (95% di intervallo di confidenza).
HBA_{1C}, emoglobina A_{1C}.

mg/dL hanno il più alto coefficiente di correlazione con i valori ematici. Oltre a ciò, l'allarme del Glucowatch® può essere utilizzato per monitorare, se necessario, l'ipoglicemia notturna. La nuova generazione di strumenti per la monitorizzazione continua del glucosio non solo fornisce i dati relativi al glucosio in tempo reale, ma consente anche l'inserimento di un allarme sopra o sotto la soglia di predeterminati livelli glicemici. Questa seconda caratteristica di sicurezza può aiutare i genitori di bambini piccoli nei confronti dell'ipoglicemia notturna.

Un indice affidabile di controllo glicemico a lungo termine è fornito dalla misurazione dell'emoglobina glicosilata. HbA_{1C} rappresenta la frazione emoglobinica a cui il glucosio e legato in circolo in modo non enzimatico. La formazione di HbA_{1C} è una reazione lenta, che dipende dalla concentrazione prevalente del glucosio ematico. Essa continua irreversibilmente per tutto il periodo di vita dei globuli rossi, di circa 120 giorni. Più alta è la concentrazione di glucosio ematico e più lunga è l'esposizione a esso dei globuli rossi, maggiore è la frazione di HbA_{1C}, espressa come percentuale di emoglobina totale. Dato che in un qualsiasi momento un campione di sangue contiene una miscela di globuli rossi di varie epoche, esposte per tempi diversi a diverse concentrazioni ematiche di glucosio, una misurazione della HbA_{1C} riflette la concentrazione media del glucosio dei 2-3 mesi precedenti. Quando misurata con metodi standardizzati per rimuovere le forme labili, la frazione di HbA_{1C} non è influenzata da un episodio isolato di iperglicemia. Di conseguenza, una misurazione di HbA_{1C} è superiore come indice di controllo glicemico di lunga durata, alle misurazioni della glicosuria o anche a multiple determinazioni della glicemia (quest'ultima può rivelare importanti fluttuazioni ma può non riflettere accuratamente la media del controllo glicemico complessivo). Si raccomanda di misurare la HbA_{1C} 3 o 4 volte all'anno per avere un profilo del controllo glicemico a lungo termine. Più basso è il livello di HbA_{1C}, e quindi migliore è il controllo glicemico, più probabile è che complicanze microvascolari come la retinopatia e la nefropatia siano meno severe, compaiano tardivamente o siano anche completamente assenti. A seconda del metodo usato per la determinazione, i valori di HbA_{1C} possono essere falsamente elevati nella talassemia (o in altre condizioni con elevata emoglobina F) e falsamente bassi nella emoglobinopatia a cellule falciformi (o altre condizioni con elevato turnover dei globuli rossi). Sebbene i valori di HbA_{1C} possano variare a seconda del metodo usato per la misurazione, in individui non diabetici, la frazione HbA_{1C} è di solito inferiore al 6%; nei diabetici, valori del 6-7,9% rappresentano un buon controllo metabolico, valori dell'8,0-9,9% un controllo adeguato e valori del 10% o maggiori un controllo scarso. Nei bambini più piccoli sono necessarie modifiche nel target di HbA_{1c} (vedi Tab. 590-9).

Esercizio. Nessun tipo di esercizio, compresi gli sport competitivi, deve essere proibito al bambino diabetico. Una complicanza importante dell'esercizio fisico nei pazienti diabetici è la presenza di una reazione ipoglicemica durante l'esercizio stesso o nelle ore successive. Se con il movimento non si verifica ipoglicemia, non sono necessarie modificazioni della dieta o della terapia insulinica, ed è probabile che la regolazione del metabolismo glicidico venga migliorata dall'aumento dell'utilizzazione muscolare di glucosio. Il fattore che maggiormente contribuisce all'ipoglicemia durante l'esercizio fisico è l'aumento della percentuale di assorbimento dell'insulina dalla sua sede di iniezione. Più alti livelli insulinici diminuiscono la produzione epatica di glucosio, che risulta quindi inadeguata per compensare l'aumentata utilizzazione di glucosio del muscolo sotto sforzo. L'esercizio regolare migliora anche la glicoregolazione attraverso un aumento del numero dei recettori insulinici. In pazienti con scarso controllo metabolico, l'esercizio intenso può precipitare una chetoacidosi, per l'aumento, indotto dall'esercizio, degli ormoni contro-regolatori.

In previsione di un esercizio intenso, prima dell'attività si può assumere una quantità di carboidrati addizionale e, prima e dopo l'attività, dovrebbe essere disponibile del glucosio sotto forma di succo di arancia, bevanda gassata non dietetica o un dolce. Con l'esperienza, per prove e per errori, ciascun paziente, sotto la guida del medico, dovrebbe sviluppare un regime appropriato per un'attività fisica regolare e pianificata, che è frequentemente associata a ipoglicemia; in questi casi, la dose totale di insulina deve essere ridotta di circa il 10-15% il giorno programmato per l'esercizio. Un esercizio prolungato, come la corsa su lunga distanza, può richiedere una riduzione delle solite dosi di insulina anche del 50% o più. È importante anche porre attenzione all'ipoglicemia ritardata parecchie ore dopo l'esercizio.

Benefici del miglioramento del controllo glicemico. Il Diabetes Control and Complication Trial (DCCT) stabiliva in conclusione un'associazione tra più alti livelli glicidici e complicanze microvascolari a lungo termine. Il trattamento intensivo produce una drammatica riduzione di retinopatia, nefropatia e neuropatia del 47-76%. I dati della popolazione di adolescenti dimostrano lo stesso grado di miglioramento e lo stesso rapporto tra misure degli esiti delle complicanze microvascolari. Gli adolescenti aumentano maggiormente di peso e sperimentano molto più frequentemente episodi ipoglicemici severi e chetoacidosi rispetto agli adulti. Altri studi di bambini e adolescenti non hanno documentato un aumento della frequenza della severità dell'ipoglicemia.

L'effetto benefico di un trattamento intensivo è stato determinato attraverso il grado di normalizzazione della glicemia, indipendentemente dal tipo di trattamento intensivo utilizzato. Il frequente monitoraggio della glicemia è stato considerato un fattore importante per ottenere un miglior controllo glicemico per gli adolescenti e gli adulti trattati con terapia intensiva. Pazienti trattati intensivamente hanno personalizzato l'obiettivo sul glucosio, frequenti modifiche basate sul monitoraggio continuo della glicemia del sangue capillare e un approccio in team che si focalizza sulla persona con diabete come prima fase della terapia ambulatoriale. La terapia era regolata costantemente per raggiungere l'obiettivo di una glicemia normale o quasi, evitando o riducendo al minimo gravi episodi di ipoglicemia. È da notare un approccio preventivo per le fluttuazioni della glicemia, con costanti modifiche che facciano da contrappeso a ogni referto di iper- o ipoglicemia.

La durata totale del diabete contribuisce allo sviluppo e alla gravità delle complicanze. Nonostante ciò, molti medici hanno delle difficoltà ad applicare il risultato della DCCT ai bambini in età prescolare, che spesso hanno un'ipoglicemia misconosciuta con unico problema di sicurezza, e ai bambini prepuberi in età scolare che non sono inclusi nella DCCT.

Regimi attuali di sostituzione insulinica intensiva. L'obiettivo di una sostituzione fisiologica dell'insulina nel T1DM si realizza con insuline a breve durata di azione, che mimano più fedelmente il brusco aumento e la breve durata dell'insulina pancreatica secreta in risposta all'introduzione di nutrienti. L'analogo insulinico Lispro® ad azione rapida ha proprietà farmacocinetiche superiori per il controllo della glicemia post-prandiale. Con due iniezioni giornaliere come l'insulina convenzionale (*Conventional Insuline*, CI), multiple iniezioni giornaliere (*Multiple Daily Injection*, MDI) o CSII, si verifica un miglioramento delle risposte alla glicemia post-prandiale. L'uso di insulina Lispro® o Aspart® riduce la frequenza dell'ipoglicemia tra i pasti, specialmente quando è attentamente bilanciato con il contenuto carboidratico dei pasti. Questo ha migliorato la modalità di somministrazione dell'insulina ai lattanti e la gestione di uno schema flessibile dei pasti.

Il contenuto carboidratico degli alimenti non influenza il controllo glicemico se si adatta l'insulina rapida pre-pasto (bolo) al contenuto di carboidrati del cibo. Ampie variazioni nell'assunzione di carboidrati non modificano le richieste di insulina basale o a lunga durata di azione (Detemir® o Glargine®). Le strategie terapeutiche insuliniche sottolineano l'importanza di somministrare dosi minori di insulina durante il giorno. Questo approccio permette di modificare le dosi di insulina per correggere l'iperglicemia, di aumentarle per l'assunzione addizionale di carboidrati o di diminuirle in caso di attività fisica. In realtà, il trattamento con bolo basale a iniezioni multiple si adatta meglio all'andamento fisiologico dell'insulina e del glucosio e può consentire inoltre un miglior controllo glicemico, rispetto al regime convenzionale con 2-3 iniezioni. Si sono sviluppati algoritmi di regolazione dell'insulina, in base all'età e alle razioni di carboidrati, per normalizzare gli elevati livelli glicemici e per compensare le alterazioni dell'introduzione di carboidrati. L'uso di iniezioni multiple flessibili (*Flexible Multiple Daily Injection*, FMDI) e di CSII in bambini con T1DM migliora il controllo glicemico senza aumento dell'incidenza di ipoglicemia severa.

Reazioni ipoglicemiche. L'ipoglicemia è la limitazione più importante a un controllo stretto dei livelli glicemici. Dopo l'iniezione, l'assorbimento e l'azione insulinica sono indipendenti dal livello di glucosio, creando così un unico rischio di ipoglicemia da un effetto insulinico non bilanciato. Gli analoghi dell'insulina possono aiutare a ridurre tale rischio, ma non sono in grado di eliminarlo. La maggior parte dei bambini con T1DM può avere una lieve ipoglicemia ogni settimana, una glicemia moderata qualche volta all'anno e un'ipoglicemia severa una volta ogni qualche anno. Questi episodi non sono di solito prevedibili, sebbene l'attività fisica, l'introduzione ritardata di un pasto o uno spuntino e ampie oscillazioni dei livelli di glucosio contribuiscano ad aumentare il rischio. Nei neonati e nei lattanti c'è un rischio maggiore, perché hanno pasti più variabili e più variabile attività fisica, non sono in grado di riconoscere precocemente i segni di ipoglicemia, e sono limitati nella loro capacità di trovare una sorgente di glucosio orale per invertire l'ipoglicemia. Il bambino molto piccolo ha un aumento del rischio di riduzione permenente della funzione cognitiva, come sequela a lungo termine di ipoglicemia severa. Per questa ragione, è necessario un grado più tranquillo di controllo glicemico, fino a quando il bambino non è cresciuto (vedi Tab. 590-9).

L'ipoglicemia si può verificare in qualsiasi momento del giorno o della notte. I sintomi precoci (ipoglicemia lieve) possono manifestarsi con un improvviso decremento della glicemia che non soddisfa i criteri standard per l'ipoglicemia in bambini non diabetici (vedi Capitolo 92). Il bambino può mostrare pallore, sudorazione, ansia o enfasi, fame, tremore e tachicardia, tutti dovuti all'aumento delle catecolamine compensatorie all'eccessivo effetto insulinico. Alterazioni comportamentali come pianto, irritabilità, aggressività e disobbedienza sono molto frequenti nei bambini. Se la glicemia scende ulteriormente, si verifica glicopenia cerebrale con sonnolenza, alterazioni della personalità, confusione mentale e alterato giudizio (ipoglicemia moderata), progressivamente fino all'incapacità di chiedere aiuto e crisi epilettiche o coma (ipoglicemia severa). Un'ipoglicemia severa prolungata può portare a una depressione del sensorio o a deficit motori focali simili a quelli dell'ictus, che persistono anche dopo che l'ipoglicemia si è risolta. Nonostante le sequele permanenti siano rare, l'ipoglicemia severa spaventa il bambino e la famiglia e può portare successivamente a una certa riluttanza ad affrontare anche un controllo glicemico moderato.

Nel bambino importanti ormoni controregolatori sono rappresentati dall'ormone della crescita, cortisolo, adrenalina e glucagone. Gli ultimi due sono fondamentali nei bambini più grandi. Molti pazienti più grandi con T1DM di lunga data perdono la loro capacità di secernere glucagone in risposta all'ipoglicemia. Nel giovane adulto, il deficit di adrenalina può svilupparsi anche come parte di una neuropatia autonoma generalizzata. Questo aumenta sostanzialmente il rischio di ipoglicemia, perché i segnali di avvertimento precoci della diminuzione dei livelli del glucosio sono dovuti al rilascio di catecolamine. Episodi ricorrenti di ipoglicemia, associati a stretto controllo metabolico, possono aggravare il deficit parziale di ormoni controregolatori, con la comparsa di una sindrome da inconsapevolezza dell'ipoglicemia e ridotta capacità di ripristinare un normale livello glicemico (ipoglicemia associata a insufficienza autonoma). Evitare l'ipoglicemia consente di guarire questa sindrome.

I fattori più importanti nel trattamento dell'ipoglicemia sono la comprensione da parte del paziente e della sua famiglia dei sintomi e dei segni della reazione e l'anticipazione dei fattori precipitanti noti, come la ginnastica e le attività sportive. Un più stretto controllo glicemico ne aumenta il rischio. È necessario insegnare alla famiglia a cogliere i tipici segni ipoglicemici o l'andamento delle registrazioni domiciliari del glucosio, per potere regolare la dose insulinica ed evitare episodi prevedibili. Sempre e ovunque dovrebbe essere disponibile una sorgente di emergenza di glucosio, anche a scuola o durante una visita agli amici. Se possibile, all'inizio, prima del trattamento, è importante documentare l'ipoglicemia, perché parecchi sintomi possono anche non essere causati dall'ipoglicemia. La maggior parte delle famiglie e dei bambini sviluppa una buona sensibilità per l'ipoglicemia vera ed è in grado di iniziare il trattamento prima del test. Anche ogni bambino con sospetta ipoglicemia da moderata a severa deve essere trattato prima del test. È importante non dare troppo glucosio; si dovrebbero somministrare 5-10 g sotto forma di succo di frutta o di bibita gassata contenente zucchero oppure un dolce e determinare la glicemia 15-20 minuti più tardi. I pazienti, i genitori e le insegnanti dovrebbero essere istruiti circa la somministrazione di glucagone, quando il bambino non sia in grado di assumere glucosio per bocca. Un kit di iniezione dovrebbe essere portato a casa e a scuola. La dose intramuscolare è di 0,5 mg se il bambino pesa meno di 20 kg, e di 1,0 mg se pesa più di 20 kg. Questo produce un breve rilascio di glucosio dal fegato. Il glucagone spesso provoca vomito, che preclude una supplementazione orale, nel caso in cui la glicemia diminuisca dopo che è terminato l'effetto del glucagone. Chi si occupa del bambino deve quindi essere preparato a portare il bambino all'ospedale, se necessario, per una somministrazione di glucosio per via endovenosa. Dosaggi minimi di glucagone (10 μg per anno di età fino a un massimo di 150 μg per via sottocutanea) sono efficaci nel trattare l'ipoglicemia nei bambini con glicemia inferiore a 60 mg/dL, quando non rispondono al glucosio per via orale e rimangono sintomatici.

Fenomeno di Somogyi, "effetto alba" e diabete instabile. Esistono moltissime ragioni per spiegare l'incremento della glicemia nelle prime ore del mattino, prima di colazione. La più comune è un semplice calo dei livelli di insulina e si nota in molti bambini che usano l'NPH o la lenta come insulina di base al pasto serale o al momento di coricarsi. Questo di solito comporta livelli mattutini routinariamente elevati di glucosio. Si ritiene che l'"**effetto alba**" sia dovuto principalmente alla secrezione notturna di ormone della crescita e a un aumento della clearance insulinica. È un processo normale, fisiologico, osservato nella maggior parte degli adolescenti non diabetici, che viene compensato con una maggiore secrezione insulinica. Un bambino con T1DM non è in grado di compensare e può avere una diminuzione dei livelli di insulina se utilizza in serata l'NPH o la lenta. L'"effetto alba" di solito è ricorrente ed eleva modestamente la maggior parte dei livelli mattutini di glucosio.

Raramente, un'iperglicemia mattutina è dovuta al **fenomeno di Somogyi**, un teorico *rebound* per ipoglicemia delle ultime fasi della notte o del mattino presto, si pensa per esagerata risposta controregolatoria. Non rappresenta una causa comune, in quanto la maggior parte dei bambini rimane ipoglicemica (assenza di rebound) dopo la diminuzione dei livelli notturni di glucosio. Sistemi di monitoraggio glicemico continuo possono aiutare a chiarire un'iperglicemia mattutina ambigua.

Il termine **diabete instabile** è stato utilizzato per descrivere il bambino, in genere una femmina adolescente, con inspiegabili e ampie fluttuazioni della glicemia, spesso con DKA ricorrente, in cui si somministrano ampie dosi di insulina. Raramente è presente un'anomalia fisiologica intrinseca, perché questi bambini di solito in ambiente ospedaliero mostrano una normale risposta insulinica. Sono generalmente presenti problemi psicosociali o psichiatrici, compresi disturbi del comportamento alimentare, e alterate dinamiche familiari, che precludono un'efficace terapia del diabete. Il ricovero in ospedale è di solito necessario per confermare l'effetto ambientale ed è essenziale la valutazione psicosociale o psichiatrica. Inoltre, i medici dovrebbero astenersi dall'usare il termine di "diabete instabile" come termine diagnostico.

Aspetti comportamentali/psicologici e disturbi dell'alimentazione. Il diabete di un bambino modifica lo stile di vita e i rapporti interpersonali dell'intera famiglia. Nei genitori sono comuni sentimenti di ansia e di colpa. Sentimenti analoghi, assieme al rifiuto, sono altrettanto frequenti nei bambini, particolarmente durante gli anni dell'adolescenza. Il conflitto familiare si associa a una scarsa adesione al trattamento e a scadente controllo metabolico tra i giovani con T1DM. Non sono caratteristici di diabete né specifiche alterazioni della personalità né disturbi psicopatologici e sono stati osservati sentimenti analoghi in famiglie in cui sono presenti altre malattie croniche.

COMPORTAMENTI ADATTATIVI. Bambini e adolescenti con T1DM devono affrontare una serie complessa di modificazioni dello sviluppo e i mutevoli fardelli della malattia. Problemi di adattamento possono ripercuotersi sul benessere psicologico e sul decorso della malattia, contribuendo a un'autogestione scadente e a uno scarso controllo metabolico. I comportamenti adattativi si riferiscono alle modalità abituali con cui si approcciano i problemi e possono essere considerati come strategie che le persone generalmente utilizzano per sopravvivere a un'ampia varietà di stress. L'adattamento a uno specifico problema si riferisce agli sforzi messi in atto per la razionale gestione del problema stesso ed è rivolto al cambiamento della situazione che provoca tensione. D'altra parte, l'adattamento alle emozioni implica sforzi per ridurre la tensione emotiva causata dall'evento stressante e per gestire o controllare emozioni che possono accompagnare o dipendere da fattori stressanti. Negli adolescenti diabetici, evitare l'adattamento e sfogare le emozioni costituiscono elementi predittivi di un'inadeguata attitudine autoterapeutica e di uno scarso controllo metabolico. È molto più probabile che aderiscano al loro regime terapeutico i pazienti che usano difese più mature e che mostrano una maggiore capacità adattativa. Le strategie di adattamento sembra che dipendano dall'età e gli adolescenti usano maggiormente un atteggiamento di evitamento rispetto ai bambini diabetici più piccoli.

NON ADESIONE. Conflitto familiare, rifiuto e sentimenti di ansia si esprimono in una mancata adesione alle istruzioni riguardanti l'alimentazione e la terapia insulinica e in una mancata compliance nell'automonitoraggio. Iperdosaggi insulinici intenzionali, con conseguente ipoglicemia, o al contrario omissione dell'insulina, spesso in associazione a eccessi dell'intake calorico e conseguente chetoacidosi, possono mascherare richieste di aiuto psicologico o tentativi manipolatori per evadere da un ambiente sentito come indesiderabile e intollerabile; occasionalmente, si possono manifestare intenti suicidi. Frequenti ricoveri in ospedale per chetoacidosi o ipoglicemia devono fare insospettire sulla presenza di un conflitto emotivo sottostante. I genitori sono spesso iperprotettivi e la maggior parte delle volte non nell'interesse del paziente. Sono comuni sentimenti di diversità o solitudine, o entrambi, giustificati dagli schemi restrittivi imposti dagli esami di urine e di sangue, dalla somministrazione di insulina e dalle limitazioni alimentari. Inoltre, la preoccupazione circa la possibilità di complicanze e la diminuzione della durata di vita dei pazienti con diabete favoriscono l'ansia. Sfortunatamente, abbonda la disinformazione circa il rischio di sviluppare diabete in fratelli o figli e di gravidanza in giovani donne diabetiche. Anche adeguate informazioni possono provocare ulteriore ansia.

La maggior parte di questi problemi può essere prevenuta attraverso una continua consulenza empatica, basata su una corretta informazione e il tentativo di infondere, nel paziente, atteggiamenti di normalità e la senzazione di essere un membro produttivo della società. Il riconoscimento del potenziale impatto di questi problemi ha indotto a organizzare in molti luoghi gruppi di discussione tra coetanei; attraverso la condivisione di problemi comuni, i sentimenti di isolamento e di frustrazione tendono a scomparire. Negli Stati Uniti i campi estivi per bambini diabetici offrono un'eccellente opportunità per l'apprendimento e la condivisione, sotto la supervisione di esperti. L'educazione circa la fisiopatologia del diabete, le dosi di insulina, la tecnica di somministrazione, l'alimentazione, l'esercizio fisico e le reazioni ipoglicemiche può essere rinforzata da personale medico e paramedico. La presenza di numerosi coetanei con problemi analoghi offre nuove idee al bambino diabetico. Il trattamento residenziale per bambini e adolescenti con difficoltà nella gestione del T1DM è un'opzione possibile solo in alcuni centri.

ANSIA E DEPRESSIONE. Si è dimostrato che esistono correlazioni significative tra scarso controllo e sintomi depressivi, alto livello di ansietà o precedente diagnosi psichiatrica. In tal senso, uno scarso controllo metabolico è correlato a maggiori livelli di disadattamento personale, sociale, scolastico o di insoddisfazione dell'ambiente familiare. Si stima che il 20-26% dei pazienti adolescenti possa sviluppare un disordine depressivo maggiore (*Major Depressive Disorder*, MDD), che è simile alla percentuale di comparsa di MDD in adolescenti non diabetici. Il decorso caratteristico del MDD in giovani soggetti diabetici e soggetti psichiatrici di controllo appare simile; tuttavia è maggiore, nel giovane diabetico, la propensione a una depressione più protratta nel tempo ed è presente un rischio più alto di recidiva tra le giovani donne diabetiche. Chi si occupa dell'assistenza di un bambino o di un adolescente con diabete deve, infatti, essere consapevole del suo ruolo fondamentale come consulente e consigliere e deve monitorare strettamente la salute mentale del paziente.

PAURA DELL'AUTOINIEZIONE E DELL'AUTOANALISI. Un'eccessiva paura dell'autoiniezione (*Fear of Self-Injecting*, FSI) di insulina (fobia dell'iniezione) può compromettere il controllo glicemico tanto quanto un atteggiamento emotivo. Allo stesso modo, la paura delle punture alle dita può essere motivo di disagio e può seriamente ostacolare l'autogestione. Può capitare che i bambini e gli adolescenti non assumano la dose di insulina o rifiutino di fare la rotazione delle sedi di iniezione, necessaria perché iniezioni ripetute nella stessa zona portano alla formazione di cicatrici sottocutanee (lipoipertrofia). L'iniezione di insulina nella cute lipoipertrofica è di solito associata a scarso assorbimento insulinico e/o perdita di insulina, con conseguente controllo glicemico subottimale.

DISTURBI ALIMENTARI. Il trattamento del T1DM richiede un costante monitoraggio dell'intake dietetico. Oltre a ciò, un peggioramento del controllo glicemico è comunemente associato a un aumento del peso corporeo. Nelle ragazze adolescenti, questi due fattori, assieme a fattori individuali, familiari e socioeconomici, possono portare a un aumento dell'incidenza di disturbi alimentari specifici e non specifici, che possono alterare il controllo glicemico e incrementare il rischio di complicanze a lungo termine. I disturbi alimentari e le condotte alimentari disfunzionali sottosoglia sono almeno due volte più frequenti nelle adolescenti con T1DM rispetto alle loro coetanee non diabetiche. La frequenza di specifici disturbi alimentari (anoressia o bulimia nervosa) varia dall'1% al 6,9% delle giovani pazienti con T1DM. L'incidenza di disturbi alimentari non specifici e di condotte alimentari disfunzionali sottosoglia è del 9% e del 14% rispettivamente. Circa l'11% delle ragazze adolescenti con T1DM assume meno insulina di quanto prescritto per perdere peso. Tra le femmine adolescenti con un disturbo alimentare, circa il 42% delle pazienti fa un uso scorretto dell'insulina, mentre l'incidenza stimata di uso scorretto nei gruppi con condotte alimentari disfunzionali sottosoglia e in quelli privi di disturbi è, rispettivamente, del 18% e del 6%. Sebbene ci sia poca informazione circa l'incidenza di disturbi alimentari tra i maschi adolescenti con T1DM, i dati disponibili suggeriscono, nella **maggior parte**, normali abitudini alimentari. Tra gli adolescenti maschi sani che partecipano al wrestling, tuttavia, il desiderio di perdere peso ha portato allo sviluppo transitorio e stagionale di anomale abitudini alimentari e comportamenti, che possono condurre all'omissione di dosi di insulina per perdere peso.

Quando problemi comportamentali/psicologici e/o disturbi alimentari sono ritenuti responsabili di scarsa compliance con il regime medico, è indicata la richiesta di consulenza per una valutazione psicologica e un eventuale trattamento. Bambini e adolescenti con fobia delle iniezioni e paura dell'autoanalisi possono essere inviati a un terapista comportamentale e beneficiare delle tecniche di desensibilizzazione e di biofeedback, per attenuare la sensazione di dolore e il disagio psicologico associato a queste procedure. Nella maggior parte dei centri americani, di norma il terapista comportamentale e gli psicologi fanno parte del team che si occupa del diabete dei bambini e possono aiutare a valutare e trattare i disturbi emotivi e comportamentali nei bambini diabetici.

Trattamento durante le infezioni. Sebbene le infezioni non siano più frequenti nei bambini diabetici rispetto ai non diabetici, esse possono spesso alterare il controllo glicemico e precipitare una DKA. Inoltre, il bambino diabetico ha un rischio maggiore di disidratazione per diuresi osmotica da iperglicemia o per vomito da chetosi. Gli ormoni controregolatori associati allo stress diminuiscono l'azione insulinica e aumentano i livelli di glucosio; tuttavia, se si verifica anoressia, la perdita dell'intake calorico aumenta il rischio di ipoglicemia. Anche se i bambini con meno di 3 anni tendono a diventare ipoglicemici e quelli più grandi sono invece portati a essere iperglicemici, l'effetto complessivo non è prevedibile. Pertanto, frequenti monitoraggi della glicemia e regolazioni della dose di insulina sono elementi essenziali delle linee guida giornaliere del bambino malato (Tab. 590-10).

Gli obiettivi complessivi sono mantenere l'idratazione, controllare i livelli glicemici ed evitare la chetoacidosi. Questo solitamente è realizzabile a domicilio, se vengono seguite le linee guida giornaliere in caso di malattia, mantenendo un contatto telefonico con lo specialista. La famiglia dovrebbe richiedere aiuto se il trattamento domiciliare non controlla chetonuria, iperglicemia o ipoglicemia o se il bambino mostra segni di disidratazione. Un bambino con notevole chetonuria e vomito deve essere ricoverato in un reparto di urgenza per un controllo generale, che ne valuti lo stato di idratazione e determini se è presente chetoacidosi, attraverso la determinazione degli elettroliti, del glucosio del pH e della CO_2 totale. Un bambino con una diminuzione della glicemia sotto i 50-60 mg/dL (2,8-3,3 mmol/L), o che non riesce a mantenere un adeguato intake alimentare orale, può richiedere la somministrazione di glucosio per via endovenosa, specialmente se è necessaria ulteriore insulina per controllare la chetonemia.

Trattamento durante gli interventi chirurgici. Gli interventi chirurgici possono alterare il controllo glicemico con le stesse modalità delle infezioni intercorrenti. Gli ormoni dello stress associati sia alla condizione di base sia alla chirurgia diminuiscono la sensibilità all'insulina. Questo aumenta i livelli di glucosio, esacerba la perdita di liquidi e può dare l'avvio alla DKA. D'altra parte, l'apporto calorico è di solito ridotto, con conseguente diminuzione dei livelli di glucosio. L'effetto netto è difficile da prevedere, proprio come durante un'infezione. Un vigile monitoraggio e frequenti regolazioni dell'insulina sono necessarie per mantenere l'euglicemia ed evitare la chetosi.

TABELLA 590-10. Linee guida per la gestione quotidiana del paziente

CHETONURIA	ANALISI DEL GLUCOSIO E INSULINA EXTRA	DOSI * CORRETTIVE DI INSULINA AD AZIONE RAPIDA	COMMENTO
Negativa o lieve[†]	ogni 2 ore	ogni 2 ore per glucosio >250 mg/dL	Cercare i chetoni a minzioni alternate
Da moderata a notevole[‡]	ogni ora	ogni ora per glucosio >250 mg/dL	Cercare i chetoni ogni minzione. Recarsi in ospedale in caso di vomito

Insulina basale: l'insulina basale Glargine® o Detemir® deve essere somministrata alla dose e al tempo abituali. L'NPH e la lenta devono essere ridotte della metà se la glicemia <150 mg/dL e l'assunzione orale è limitata.

Liquidi per via orale: privi di zucchero se la glicemia >250 mg/dL (14 mmol/L); con zucchero se la glicemia è <250 mg/dL.

Chiamare il medico o l'infermiere se la glicemia rimane elevata dopo 3 dosi extra; se la glicemia rimane inferiore a 70 mg/dL e il bambino non assume un supplemento orale; se compare disidratazione.

*Somministrare insulina in base agli schemi di dosaggio individualizzato. Somministrare anche una dose per l'introduzione di carboidrati se la glicemia >150 mg/dL.

†Per chetoni sierici misurati a domicilio <1,5 mmol/L per kit commerciale.

‡Per chetoni sierici misurati a domicilio >1,5 mmol/L.

Con l'insulina per via endovenosa e l'aggiunta di liquidi si ottiene il mantenimento del controllo glicidico e si evita la DKA. Nella maggior parte dei casi può essere utilizzata una semplice scala di regolazione dell'insulina, basata sul peso del paziente e sui livelli glicemici (Tab. 590-11). Dopo l'intervento chirurgico si continua l'insulina per via endovenosa, fino a che il bambino non inizia a introdurre liquidi per via orale; i liquidi per via endovenosa possono essere diminuiti progressivamente mano a mano che cresce l'introduzione di quelli orali. Quando si raggiunge un intake orale totale, si sospende la somministrazione per via endovenosa e si passa a quella per via sottocutanea. Quando l'intervento è elettivo, è meglio eseguirlo nelle prime ore del giorno, permettendo al paziente il massimo tempo di recupero per riprendere l'assunzione orale di liquidi e la somministrazione di insulina sottocutanea. Quando l'intervento elettivo è breve (meno di un'ora) e subito dopo viene ripreso l'intake orale totale, si può semplicemente monitorare la glicemia ogni ora e somministrare una dose di un analogo insulinico utilizzando la scala di correzione del glucosio per uso domiciliare. Se come insulina di base si utilizzano Glarginer® e Detemirr®, si somministra una dose complessiva la sera prima dell'intervento. Il bambino non deve essere dimesso fino a che la glicemia sia stabile e sia possibile un'alimentazione per via orale.

COMPLICANZE A LUNGO TERMINE: RELAZIONE CON IL CONTROLLO GLICEMICO. Il prolungamento della sopravvivenza dei diabetici si associa all'aumento dell'incidenza di complicanze. Le complicanze del DM possono essere divise in 3 categorie maggiori: (1) complicanze microvascolari, specificamente retinopatia e nefropatia; (2) complicanze macrovascolari, particolarmente accelerazione della patologia arteriosa coronarica, patologia cerebrovascolare e patologia vascolare periferica, e (3) neuropatie, periferiche e autonome che colpiscono vari organi e sistemi (Tab. 590-12). Inoltre, può comparire con maggiore frequenza cataratta.

La **retinopatia diabetica** è la principale causa di cecità negli Stati Uniti nei soggetti tra i 20 e i 65 anni. Il rischio di retinopatia diabetica dopo 15 anni di patologia diabetica è del 98% per soggetti con T1DM e del 78% per quelli con T2DM. Le opacità del cristallino (dovute a glicazione delle proteine tissutali e ad attivazione della via dei polioli) sono presenti in almeno il 5% dei soggetti con meno di 19 anni. Sebbene il controllo metabolico abbia un impatto sullo sviluppo di questa complicanza, anche i fattori genetici hanno un ruolo, dal momento che il 50% dei pazienti sviluppa retinopatia proliferativa. Le manifestazioni più precoci clinicamente evidenti della retinopatia diabetica sono classificate come retinopatia non proliferativa o background diabetico, caratterizzato da microaneurismi, emorragie puntiformi e a macchia, essudati duri e molli, dilatazione venosa e perliforme e anomalie microvascolari intraretiniche. Queste alterazioni non compromettono la visione. La forma più severa è la retinopatia diabetica proliferativa, caratterizzata da neovascolarizzazione, proliferazione fibrosa ed emorragie preretiniche e vitree. La retinopatia proliferativa, se non trattata, è inesorabilmente progressiva e compromette le visione, portando a cecità. La base del trattamento è la fotocoagulazione laser panretinica. Nelle patologie oculari diabetiche avanzate, caratterizzate da severa

TABELLA 590-11. Linee guida per la copertura insulinica endovenosa durante interventi chirurgici

GLICEMIA (mg/dL)	INFUSIONE DI INSULINA (U/kg/ora)	MONITORAGGIO DELLA GLICEMIA
<120	0,00	1 ora
121-200	0,03	2 ore
200-300	0,06	2 ore
300-400	0,08	1 ora[†]
400	0,10	1 ora[†]

Si somministra un'infusione di glucosio al 5% e una soluzione salina allo 0,45% con 20 mEq/L di potassio acetato a una velocità di mantenimento di 1,5 volte.

†Ricercare i chetoni nelle urine.

TABELLA 590-12. Linee guida di screening

	QUANDO SI DEVE INIZIARE LO SCREENING	FREQUENZA	METODO PREFERENZIALE DI SCREENING	ALTRI METODI DI SCREENING	POTENZIALE INTERVENTO
Retinopatia	In bambini prepuberi dopo una durata di 5 anni, in ragazzi puberi dopo una durata di 2 anni	1-2 all'anno	Fotografia del fundus	Angiografia con fluoresceina, oftalmoscopia midriatica	Migliorato controllo glicemico, laser terapia
Nefropatia	In bambini prepuberi dopo una durata di 5 anni, in ragazzi puberi dopo una durata di 2 anni	Annualmente	Escrezione urinaria di albumina nell'arco di una notte	Escrezione di albumina nelle 24 ore	Migliorato controllo glicemico, controllo della pressione arteriosa, ACE-inibitori
Neuropatia	Non definito	Non definita	Esame fisico	Conduzione nervosa, soglia termica e di vibrazione, pupillometria, riflessi cardiovascolari	Migliorato controllo glicemico
Patologia macrovascolare	Al momento della diagnosi	Ogni 5 anni	Lipidi	Pressione arteriosa	Statine per l'iperlipidemia Controllo della pressione arteriosa
Patologia tiroidea	Al momento della diagnosi	Ogni 2-3 anni	TSH	Anticorpi anti-perossidasi tiroidea	Tiroxina
Malattia celiaca	Al momento della diagnosi	Ogni 2-3 anni	Transglutaminasi tissutale, anticorpi anti-endomisio	Anticorpi anti-gliadina	Dieta priva di glutine

Da Glastras SJ, Moshin F, Donaghue KC: Complication of diabetes mellitus in childhood. *Pediatr Clin North Am* 2005;52:1735-1753.

emorragia vitrea o da fibrosi, spesso con distacco retinico, la vitrectomia è un'importante modalità terapeutica. Alla fine, la patologia oculare diventa quiescente, uno stadio definito come retinopatia involutiva. Un sottotipo separato di retinopatia è la maculopatia diabetica, che si manifesta con grave edema maculare che compromette la visione centrale, per cui può essere efficace la fotocoagulazione laser focale.

Le linee guida suggeriscono che i pazienti diabetici siano sottoposti a un ampio e completo esame oculistico subito dopo la diagnosi di diabete di tipo T2DM, e nei primi 3-5 anni dopo l'esordio del T1DM (ma non prima dei 10 anni di età). Ogni paziente con anomalie o sintomi visivi deve essere sottoposto a indagini oculistiche. Ogni anno, presso un oculista esperto nella diagnosi di retinopatia diabetica e del suo trattamento, andrebbero ripetute successive valutazioni per entrambi i tipi di diabete (vedi Tab. 590-12).

La **nefropatia diabetica** è la causa principale di malattia renale allo stadio terminale (*End-Stage Renal Disease*, ESRD) negli Stati Uniti. La maggior parte delle ESRD derivanti dalla nefropatia diabetica si può prevenire. La nefropatia diabetica colpisce il 20-30% dei pazienti con T1DM e il 15-20% dei pazienti con T2DM 20 anni dopo l'esordio. La speranza media di vita a 5 anni per i pazienti con ESRD correlata al diabete è inferiore al 20%. L'aumento del rischio di mortalità del T1DM può essere dovuto a nefropatia, che può ammontare al 50% dei decessi. Il rischio di nefropatia aumenta con la durata del diabete (fino ai 25-30 anni di durata, dopo i quali raramente comincia questa complicanza), il grado del controllo metabolico e la predisposizione genetica all'ipertensione essenziale. Solo il 30-40% dei pazienti con T1DM presenta ESRD. La glicazione delle proteine tissutali comporta un ispessimento della membrana basale glomerulare. Il decorso della nefropatia diabetica è lento. Si può trovare un aumento della percentuale di escrezione urinaria dell'albumina (*Albumin Excretion Rate*, AER) di 30-300 mg/24 h (20-200 µg/min), la cosiddetta microalbuminuria, che costituisce uno stadio precoce della nefropatia, da intermittente a persistente (incipiente), comunemente associata a iperfiltrazione glomerulare e ipertensione. Dal momento che la nefropatia evolve verso uno stadio precoce manifesto con proteinuria (AER >300 mg/24 h o >200 µg/min), essa si accompagna a ipertensione. Gli stadi avanzati della nefropatia sono definiti da un progressivo declino della funzione renale (diminuzione della filtrazione glomerulare ed elevazione dell'urea e della creatinina sieriche), proteinuria progressiva e ipertensione. Si riconosce la progressione della ESRD dalla comparsa di uremia, sindrome nefritica e dalla necessità di una sostituzione renale (trapianto o dialisi).

Lo screening per nefropatia diabetica è un aspetto routinario della terapia del diabete (vedi Tab. 590-12). L'American Diabetes Association (ADA) raccomanda uno screening precoce per i soggetti con T2DM e per quelli con T1DM, dopo 5 anni di durata della malattia (ma non prima della pubertà). La determinazione della AER nelle 24 ore (albumina urinaria e creatinina) e quella urinaria in un dato periodo (notturno) sono tecniche accettabili. I risultati positivi devono essere confermati da una seconda misurazione della AER, per l'alta variabilità dell'escrezione di albumina nei pazienti diabetici. Iperglicemia di breve durata, attività fisica, infezioni delle vie urinarie, ipertensione notevole, insufficienza cardiaca e patologie acute febbrili possono dare luogo ad albuminuria transitoria. È necessario tenere sotto controllo, giorno dopo giorno, la variabilità della secrezione alluminica e per questo dal terzo al sesto periodo almeno 2 o 3 raccolte urinarie devono mostrare elevati livelli, prima che sia diagnosticata la microalbuminuria e si cominci il trattamento. Dal momento della diagnosi di albuminuria, vari fattori attenuano l'effetto dell'iperfiltrazione sui reni: (1) meticoloso controllo dell'iperglicemia, (2) controllo aggressivo dell'ipertensione arteriosa, (3) controllo selettivo della dilatazione arteriolare utilizzando inibitori dell'enzima di conversione (ACE) (che diminuiscono la pressione capillare transglomerulare) e (4) restrizione proteica dietetica (perché un apporto calorico elevato di proteine aumenta la percentuale di perfusione renale). Lo stretto controllo glicemico ritarda la progressione della microalbuminuria e rallenta la progressione della nefropatia diabetica. La precedente considerevole terapia del diabete ha un persistente beneficio per 7-8 anni e può ritardare o prevenire lo sviluppo della nefropatia diabetica.

NEUROPATIA DIABETICA. Possono essere coinvolti sia il sistema nervoso autonomo sia quello periferico e gli adolescenti con diabete possono mostrare più precoci manifestazioni di neuropatia. Questa complicanza può essere fatta risalire agli effetti dell'iperglicemia e/o altri effetti del deficit insulinico sui vari costituenti dei nervi periferici. Appare probabile che abbiano un ruolo favorente la via dei polioli, la glicazione non enzimatica e/o disturbi del metabolismo del mioinositolo, che colpiscono uno o più tipi cellulari nei costituenti multicellulari dei nervi periferici. Sembra essere importante il ruolo di altri fattori, così come un possibile effetto diretto neurotrofico dell'insulina, fattori di crescita correlati all'insulina, l'ossido nitrico e proteine dello stress. La neuropatia periferica può presentarsi soprattutto in adolescenti con una lunga storia di diabete. Utilizzando test sensitivi di tipo quantitativo (*Quantitative Sensory Testing*, QST), si trova frequentemente in pazienti diabetici neurologicamente asintomatici un'anomala percezione termica cutanea negli arti sia superiori sia inferiori. La soglia del dolore termico nella mano è correlata alla durata del diabete. Non esiste una correlazione tra i punteggi QST e controllo metabolico. In circa il 10% degli adolescenti, durante le fasi tardive della pubertà e dopo la pubertà, possono essere trovate alterazioni subcliniche dei nervi motori, come la ridotta velocità di conduzione dei nervi sensitivi e l'ampiezza del potenziale di azione del nervo sensitivo. Lo scarso controllo metabolico durante la pubertà sembra indurre il deterioramento della funzione nervosa periferica nei giovani pazienti. Un segno precoce di neuropatia autonoma, quale la diminuzione della variabilità della frequenza cardiaca, può essere presente negli adolescenti con una storia di malattia di lunga durata e scarso controllo metabolico. Si possono mettere in atto varie strategie, con risultati variabili. Queste modalità di trattamento comprendono (1) miglioramento del controllo metabolico, (2) utilizzo di inibitori dell'aldoso reduttasi per diminuire la bioproduzione della via dei polioli, (3) utilizzo dell'acido α-lipoico (un antiossidante) che aumenta l'ossido nitrico tissutale e i suoi metaboliti e di anticonvulsivanti (per es. lorazepam, valproato, carbamazepina, tiagabina e topiramato) per il trattamento del dolore neurologico.

Altre complicanze nei bambini diabetici includono il dwarfismo associato a ipertrofia epatica da accumulo di glicogeno (**sindrome di Mauriac**), osteopenia e una sindrome da limitata mobilità articolare associata a cute spessa, cerea; difficoltà di crescita e ritardo di maturazione. La sindrome di Mauriac è correlata a ridotta somministrazione insulinica; essa è molto meno comune da quando si sono cominciate a utilizzare le insuline a lunga durata di azione. Le caratteristiche cliniche della sindrome di Mauriac comprendono facies lunaris, addome protuberante, debolezza dei muscoli prossimali e epatomegalia per infiltrazione di lipidi e glicogeno. La sindrome di limitata mobilità articolare è frequentemente associata a sviluppo precoce di complicanze diabetiche microvascolari, come la retinopatia e la nefropatia, che possono comparire prima dei 18 anni di età.

PROGNOSI. Il T1DM è una patologia seria, cronica. Si è valutato che la vita media di individui con diabete sia di circa 10 anni inferiore rispetto ai non diabetici. Sebbene i bambini diabetici alla fine raggiungano un'altezza adulta nel range di normalità, la pubertà può essere ritardata e la statura finale può essere inferiore a quella genetica potenziale. Da studi eseguiti su gemelli identici è chiaro che, nonostante un controllo apparentemente soddisfacente, il gemello diabetico manifesta pubertà ritardata e una sostanziale riduzione dell'altezza se l'esordio del diabete si verifica prima della pubertà. Queste osservazioni indicano che in passato i criteri convenzionali per giudicare il controllo erano inadeguati e che non veniva mai ottenuto un adeguato controllo del T1DM attraverso mezzi di routine.

L'introduzione di strumenti portatili (pompe insuliniche) che possono essere programmati per fornire CSII in modo pulsatile in rapporto ai pasti costituisce un approccio valido per la risoluzione di questi problemi di vecchia data. In individui selezionati, sono stati mantenuti per parecchi anni livelli quasi normali di glicemia e altri indici di controllo metabolico, compreso la HbA_{1C}. Questo approccio, tuttavia, deve essere riservato a persone fortemente motivate, impegnate a un rigoroso automonitoraggio della glicemia che sono consapevoli delle complicanze potenziali, come un blocco meccanico dell'apparecchio per l'infusione di insulina che provoca iperglicemia o ipoglicemia e un'infezione del sito di inserimento del catetere.

La variabilità del quadro di controllo metabolico ha una profonda influenza sulla riduzione dell'incidenza e della severità di certe complicanze. Per esempio, dopo 20 anni di diabete, si verifica un calo dell'incidenza della nefropatia tra i bambini svedesi con T1DM in cui la malattia era stata diagnosticata negli anni 1971-1975, rispetto invece ai decenni precedenti. In aggiunta, nella maggior parte dei pazienti con microalbuminuria in cui sia possibile ottenere un buon controllo, la microalbuminuria svanisce. Questo miglioramento della prognosi è direttamente correlato al controllo metabolico.

TRAPIANTO E RIGENERAZIONE DEL PANCREAS E DELLE INSULE. Nel tentativo di curare il T1DM, si è ricorsi al trapianto di un segmento di pancreas o di insule isolate. Queste procedure sono entrambe tecnicamente impegnative e associate al rischio di recidiva della malattia e di complicanze inerenti al rigetto o al suo trattamento con immunosoppressori. Le complicanze dell'immunosoppressione comprendono lo sviluppo di neoplasie. Alcuni farmaci antirigetto, particolarmente la ciclosporina e il tacrolimus, sono tossici per le insule di Langerhans, alterando la secrezione di insulina e anche causando diabete. Per cui, si esegue generalmente il trapianto segmentale di pancreas solo in associazione al trapianto di un rene, in un paziente con ESRD da nefropatia diabetica in cui il regime immunosoppressivo sia comunque indicato per il trapianto renale. Negli adulti sono stati eseguiti alcune migliaia di trapianti. Con l'esperienza e farmaci immunosoppressori di nuova generazione, il pancreas trapiantato può sopravvivere funzionalmente per più di parecchi anni, durante i quali il paziente può godere di un controllo metabolico senza, o con un minimo, di insulina esogena e manifestare la reversibilità di alcune complicanze microvascolari. Tuttavia, dato che i bambini e gli adolescenti con DM non presentano di solito ESRD, il trapianto di pancreas è un trattamento primario non raccomandato nei bambini.

Anche i tentativi di trapiantare insule isolate sono stati analogamente modificati per il problema del rigetto. Si eseguono ricerche continue per migliorare le tecniche per la produzione, la fattibilità e la riduzione dell'immunogenicità delle insule di Langerhans, nell'ottica del trapianto. Una metodo di **trapianto di insule** (**protocollo di Edmonton**) prevede l'infusione di insule pancereatiche isolate nella vena porta di un gruppo di adulti con T1DM. Questa strategia terapeutica implica l'uso di una nuova generazione di farmaci immunosoppressori, che apparentemente hanno meno effetti collaterali rispetto ad altri farmaci. Di 36 pazienti consecutivi con almeno 2 anni di follow-up dopo l'iniziale trapianto, 5 (14%) erano insulino indipendenti a 2 anni. Sebbene i pazienti abbiano sperimentato effetti collaterali minimi a seguito della terapia immunosoppressiva, sono state osservate alcune complicanze associate alle procedure di trapianto insulare che comprendono: trombosi della vena porta, sanguinamento correlato all'accesso percutaneo alla vena porta, emorragie intraepatica e subcapsulare per la terapia anticoagulante (che richiedevano trasfusione e intervento chirurgico). Nel 46% dei soggetti si sono trovati elevati livelli dei test di funzionalità epatica, ma tutti risoltisi. Inoltre, solo la metà dei pazienti è rimasta priva di insulina a 2 anni. Si ritiene che esiti positivi a lungo termine dipendano dalla composizione del trapianto insulare, specialmente dalla presenza di un alto numero di cellule insulari progenitrici (epitelio duttale). Esiste la possibilità di migliorare l'innesto di insule con la somministrazione peritrapianto di immunosoppressori, globulina antitimocita e di etanecept. È necessario un monitoraggio a lungo termine prima che si possa valutare il successo di queste tecniche.

La rigenerazione delle insule è un approccio che potrebbe in teoria curare il T1DM. Si classifica in 3 categorie:

1. Terapia in vitro utilizzando cellule coltivate trapiantate, comprese cellule embrionali staminali, cellule pancreatiche staminali e linee β-cellulari, assieme a terapia immnusoppressiva o immunoisolamento.
2. Terapia di rigenerazione ex vivo, in cui i pazienti forniscono le cellule, come cellule staminali del midollo osseo, che sono transitoriamente rimosse e indotte in vitro alla differenziazione in cellule β. Sebbene alcuni studiosi abbiano riportato successo nella transdifferenziazione di cellule embrionali staminali in cellule β pancreatiche dopo trapianto di cellule di midollo osseo in roditori, altri non hanno ottenuto questi effetti. Inoltre, a tutt'oggi, non è possibile rigenerare ripetutamente cellule produttrici di insulina partendo da cellule staminali del midollo osseo.
3. Terapia di rigenerazione in vivo, in cui i tessuti danneggiati si rigenerano da cellule del paziente stesso in vivo. È stata considerata la neogenesi di cellule β da cellule non β e la proliferazione di cellule β in vivo, particolarmente come terapia rigenerativa per il T2DM.

La terapia di rigenerazione delle cellule β pancreatiche può essere combinata con varie altre strategie terapeutiche, compresi il trapianto di insule, la terapia cellulare, la terapia genica e la terapia farmacologica, per promuovere la proliferazione e la neogenesi delle cellule β, ed esiste la speranza che queste strategie possano, in futuro, costituire un terapia per il diabete.

590.3 • Diabete mellito di tipo 2

Il T2DM è considerato una patologia poligenica aggravata da fattori ambientali, quali una bassa attività fisica o una dieta ipercalorica, ricca di lipidi. I pazienti obesi con T2DM mostrano resistenza del muscolo scheletrico all'insulina, aumentata produzione epatica di glucosio e diminuzione della secrezione insulinica indotta dal glucosio. Con il tempo, l'iperglicemia peggiora, fenomeno questo attribuito all'effetto nocivo della iperglicemia cronica (glicotossicità) o dell'iperlipidemia cronica sulla funzione β-cellulare ed è spesso accompagnato da un aumento del contenuto di trigliceridi e dalla diminuzione dell'espressione del gene dell'insulina. Numerosi studi hanno descritto il T2DM nei giovani indioamericani, negli afroamericani, negli ispanici e nei coetanei bianchi. Il T2DM pediatrico rappresenta negli adolescenti una delle forme di diabete più rapidamente in crescita. L'incidenza del T2DM tra i bambini con diabete in un centro medico è aumentata dal 4% prima del 1992 al 16% nel 1994. Tra i ragazzi di età compresa tra i 10 e i 19 anni, il T2DM ammonta a un terzo di tutti i casi di diabete pediatrico di nuova diagnosi nel corso del 1994. Complessivamente, l'incidenza del T2DM degli adolescenti è aumentata di 10 volte, dallo 0,7 al 7,2/100 000 per anno nell'area metropolitana del Midwest. L'età media di presentazione era 13,8 anni; la maggior parte dei ragazzi era notevolmente obesa. Al Children's Hospital of Wisconsis (Milwaukee), si è osservato un aumento dell'incidenza di più di 10 volte del T2DM (da meno del 2% a circa il 22% di nuovi casi di DM) in ragazzi di età compresa tra 10 e 18 anni nel decennio scorso. Erano in genere colpiti gli afroamericani (quasi il 70% dei casi), gli ispanici e le adolescenti bianche.

La comparsa epidemica di T2DM in bambini e adolescenti procede di pari passo con l'emergenza di obesità epidemica (vedi Capitolo 44). Sebbene l'obesità stessa si associ a resistenza insulinica, non si sviluppa diabete fino a che è presente qualche grado di insufficienza della secrezione di insulina. In questo modo, quando si valuta la secrezione insulinica in risposta al glucosio o a altri stimoli, la si trova sempre più bassa in persone con T2DM rispetto a controlli di pari età, sesso, peso ed analoga glicemia. Nonostante generalmente si sostenga che la distruzione autoimmune delle cellule β non si verifica nel diabete di tipo 2, marker autoimmuni del T1DM, quali GAD65, ICA512 e IAA, possono essere positivi in oltre un terzo dei casi di adolescenti con T2DM. Questi reperti riflettono un ampio spettro di anomalie pancreatiche e periferiche, che potrebbero portare a T2DM, e la presenza di questi marker autoimmuni non esclude il DM tipo 2 in bambini e adolescenti.

Nel DM di tipo 2, il deficit insulinico raramente è assoluto, così che i pazienti usualmente non hanno necessità di insulina per la sopravvivenza. Nondimeno, il controllo glicemico può essere migliorato dall'insulina esogena. La DKA, quando si verifica, è associata a stress per altre patologie, come severe infezioni, e si può risolvere quando si risolve la patologia stressante. La DKA tende a essere più frequente negli afroamericani che negli altri gruppi etnici. La maggior parte dei pazienti con T2DM rimane asintomatica per mesi o anni, poiché l'iperglicemia è così moderata che i sintomi non sono drammatici come la poliuria e la perdita di peso che accompagnano il T1DM. Può anche continuare l'aumento di peso. L'iperglicemia prolungata può essere accompagnata, nel tempo, dallo sviluppo di complicanze micro- e macro-vascolari.

Il T2DM si verifica più frequentemente in certi gruppi etnici o razziali, come negli abitanti delle isole del Pacifico, gli indiani di Pima e gli afroamericani. Si verifica anche in soggetti con ipertensione e dislipidemia. Il T2DM ha una maggiore componente genetica rispetto al T1DM. La percentuale di concordanza fra gemelli identici è virtualmente del 100% per il tipo 2 e solo del 30-50% per il tipo 1 di DM. La base genetica per il DM di tipo 2 è complessa e definita in modo incompleto; non esiste la predominanza di un singolo difetto identificato, come per l'associazione con HLA del diabete tipo 1. L'acanthosis nigricans può essere un marker di resistenza insulinica, iperinsulinemia ed eventualmente diabete di tipo 2. L'irsutismo, associato alla sindrome dell'ovaio policistico, adrenarca prematuro o a modeste mutazioni degli enzimi steroidogenetici, è associato di frequente a insulino-resistenza in bambini e adolescenti e può essere un indizio di futuro sviluppo di DM di tipo 2 (vedi Capitolo 587).

La resistenza insulinica di tipo A con **acanthosis nigricans** è caratterizzata da severa resistenza insulinica e acanthosis nigricans in assenza di obesità o lipoatrofia; le femmine colpite hanno anche iperandrogenismo, possibilmente come manifestazione secondaria dell'iperinsulinemia con stimolazione della sintesi di androgeni da parte delle cellule ovariche tecali (vedi Capitolo 587). L'intolleranza al glucosio è variabile e comprende il diabete sintomatico. L'iperandrogenismo si presenta con reperti clinici e biochimici suggestivi di sindrome dell'ovaio policistico. Alcuni casi, soprattutto nelle femmine afroamericane con obesità, acanthosis nigricans e accelerata crescita suggestiva di gigantismo possono rappresentare insulino-resistenza dovuta a obesità con down regulation del recettore insulinico. Il gigantismo può rappresentare un effetto "spillover" dell'insulina, che agisce attraverso il recettore del fattore 1 di crescita piuttosto che attraverso il recettore dell'insulina.

TRATTAMENTO. Educazione nutrizionale e **maggior esercizio fisico** sono i pilastri della terapia per bambini e adolescenti con T2DM. Questi bambini spesso provengono da un ambiente familiare con scarsa conoscenza delle corrette abitudini alimentari. I comportamenti di comune osservazione comprendono: salto dei pasti, spuntini pesanti e visione della tv per periodi eccessivi, gioco con videogame e uso del computer. Gli adolescenti si alimentano non in base al loro appetito (per es. alimentazione emotiva, associata alla visione della tv, da noia) e seguono diete cicliche (alimentazione "yo-yo"). L'approccio iniziale per il trattamento del T2DM deve mirare alla perdita di peso e all'aumento dell'attività fisica. Questo, tuttavia, spesso non ha successo.

Al momento della diagnosi, può essere necessaria la terapia insulinica, specialmente se i livelli di glucosio sono elevati o sono presenti chetoni. Con uno stretto follow-up medico, le dosi insuliniche spesso possono essere ridotte, sostituite o anche sospese, di solito in poche settimane dopo aver ottenuto il controllo della glicemia. Una terapia iniziale efficace deve includere anche la metformina (una biguanide), che diminuisce la produzione epatica di glucosio. La dose di partenza della metformina è solitamente di 500 mg due volte al giorno ai pasti. La metformina è controindicata in presenza di significative alterazioni renali o epatiche; una corretta valutazione della funzionalità epatica e renale è quindi essenziale prima di cominciare la terapia (Tab. 590-13). Una classe di farmaci, i tiazolidinedioni, aumenta l'azione dell'insulina diminuendo la produzione epatica di glucosio e facilitando l'utilizzazione di glucosio nel muscolo e nel tessuto adiposo. Dato che agiscono aumentando l'azione insulinica, possono essere utilizzati in associazione a insulina esogena e metformina. Tuttavia, i tiazolidinedioni negli Stati Uniti non sono stati approvati per uso pediatrico, e possono essere eccessivamente tossici per il fegato. L'analogo del peptide-1 glucagone-simile (GLP-1) e l'amilina sono attualmente disponibili per il trattamento del T2DM. Il GPL-1 è secreto dalle cellule L dell'intestino tenue nelle fasi post-prandiali e stimola la secrezione di insulina, mentre inibisce la risposta del glucagone. L'amilina invece inibisce per prima cosa la secrezione di glucagone. Entrambi i farmaci diminuiscono lo svuotamento gastrico e l'appetito. Gli stimolatori dell'incretina, una classe di GPL-1, conosciuta anche come dipeptidilpeptidasi-4 (DPP-4 o sitagliptina), sono efficaci nel trattamento del T2DM negli adulti. Studi in pazienti adulti con T2DM hanno dimostrato che l'analogo GPL-1, agonista del recettore del GPL-1 (sitagliptina), e l'amilina migliorano il controllo glicemico quando utilizzati in aggiunta all'insulina e alla metformina. Non sono noti dati clinici in bambini e adolescenti.

PREVENZIONE. La difficoltà di ottenere un buon controllo glicemico e di prevenire le complicanze del diabete fanno della prevenzione una strategia importante. Questo è particolarmente

TABELLA 590-13. Ipoglicemizzanti orali

FARMACO	MECCANISMO DI AZIONE	DURATA DELL'EFFETTO BIOLOGICO	DOSE GIORNALIERA ABITUALE (mg)	DOSI/DIE	EFFETTI COLLATERALI	AVVERTENZE
Biguanide	Sensibilizzazione all'insulina				Disturbi gastrointestinali, acidosi lattica	Evitare in presenza di alterazioni epatiche e renali
Metformina			1500-2500	2-3		
Sulfoniluree						
Prima generazione						
Acetoesamide		12-18	500-750	1 o divisa		
Clorpropamide		27-72	250-500	1 o divisa		
Tolbutamide		14-16	1000-2000			
Seconda generazione						
Glipizide		14-16	2,5-10	1 o divisa		
			XL:5-10	1		
Gliburide		20-24+	2,5-10	1 o divisa		
Glimepride		24+	2-4	1		
Glitinidi	Promuove la secrezione insulinica					Dosare attentamente in caso di alterazioni epatiche o renali
Repaglinide		≤24	2-16	3		
Nateglinide		4	360	3		
Inibitori dell'α-glicosidasi	Lenta idrolisi e assorbimento dei carboidrati complessi		150-300	3 (ai pasti)	Disturbi intestinali transitori	
Acarbosio						
Miglitolo			150-300	3 (ai pasti)		
Tiazolidinedioni	Sensibilizzazione periferica all'insulina				Infezioni delle vie aeree superiori, cefalea, edema, aumento di peso	
Rosiglitazone			4-8	1 o divisa		
Pioglitazone			15-45	1		
Sitagliptina	Agonista recettoriali GLP-1	24	50-100	1	Infezioni delle vie aeree superiori, angina, diarrea	Non ci sono dati per i bambini e gli adolescenti

Da Jacobson-Dickman E, Levistky L: Oral agents in managing diabetes mellitus in children and adolescent. *Pediatric Clin North Am* 2005;52:1689-1703.

vero per il T2DM, che è chiaramente associato a fattori di rischio modificabili (obesità, stile di vita sedentario). Il Diabetes Prevention Program (DPP) era concepito per prevenire o ritardare lo sviluppo di T2DM in soggetti adulti ad alto rischio per la presenza di alterata tolleranza glucidica (*Impaired Glucose Tolerance*, IGT). Il DPP ha dimostrato che uno stile di vita più intenso o l'intervento farmacologico in soggetti con IGT previene o ritarda l'esordio del T2DM. I risultati sono davvero notevoli. Gli interventi sullo stile di vita riducono l'incidenza di diabete del 58%; la metformina riduce l'incidenza del 31% se comparata con placebo. Gli effetti sono simili per l'uomo e per la donna e per tutte le razze e i gruppi etnici. Si ritiene che gli interventi sullo stile di vita abbiano analoghi effetti benefici negli adolescenti obesi con IGT. Lo screening è indicato per pazienti a rischio (Tab. 590-14). Le complicanze associate a T2DM sono indicate nella Tabella 590-15.

ALTERATA TOLLERANZA GLICIDICA. Il termine alterata tolleranza glicidica (IGT) sostituisce i termini diabete asintomatico, diabete chimico, diabete subclinico, diabete borderline e diabete latente, per evitare il marchio associato al termine diabete mellito. Etichette diagnostiche possono, infatti, influenzare la scelta di un'attività, diritto di salute o assicurazione sulla vita, e l'immagine di sé. Sebbene l'IGT rappresenti un intermediario biochimico tra il normale metabolismo glucidico e il diabete, l'esperienza ha dimostrato che pochi bambini con IGT evolvono o acquisiscono un diabete; il range stimato va dallo 0 al 10%. Esiste disaccordo se il grado di intolleranza glicidica sia utile come indice prognostico della possibilità di progressione, ma è chiaro che tra i pochi casi che progrediscono, la risposta dell'insulina durante il test di tolleranza glicidica è notevolmente alterata. Nei pazienti che sviluppano diabete clinico si trovano frequentemente sia autoanticorpi anti-cellule insulari sia anti-insulina, sia l'aplotipo HLA-DR3 o -DR4. Nella maggior parte dei bambini obesi con IGT, le risposte insuliniche durante il carico orale di glucosio sono più alte di quelle della media dei controlli dosata per età, ma non regolata per peso; questi individui hanno notevole resistenza agli effetti dell'insulina più che una totale inabilità a produrla.

In bambini sani non diabetici, la risposta glicidica durante il test di tolleranza da carico orale di glucosio è simile a tutte le età. Al contrario, le risposte dell'insulina durante il test aumentano progressivamente nella fascia di età dai 3-15 anni e sono signifi-

TABELLA 590-14. Test per il diabete tipo 2 nei bambini

Criteri*
- Sovrappeso (BMI >85° percentile per età e sesso, peso per altezza >85° percentile, o peso >120% del peso ideale per altezza)

Più

Ciascuno dei due seguenti fattori di rischio:
- Anamnesi familiare di diabete di tipo 2 in parenti di primo e secondo grado
- Razza, etnia (indioamericani, afroamericani, ispanici, abitanti delle isole asiatiche e del Pacifico)

Segni di insulino-resistenza o condizioni associate a insulino-resistenza (acanthosis nigricans, ipertensione, dislipidemia, sindrome dell'ovaio policistico)

Età di inizio: 10 anni o all'esordio della pubertà se la pubertà si verifica a un'età inferiore

Frequenza: ogni 2 anni

Test: preferibile FPG

*È necessaria una valutazione clinica per i test per il diabete in pazienti ad alto rischio in cui questi criteri non sono appropriati.

Da American Diabetes Association. Type 2 diabetes in children and adolescents. *Diabetes Care* 200;23:386. Per gentile concessione.

TABELLA 590-15. Monitoraggio per complicanze e comorbilità

CONDIZIONE	TEST DI SCREENING	COMMENTO
Ipertensione	Pressione arteriosa	
Steatosi epatica	AST, ALT, possibile ecografia epatica	
Sindrome dell'ovaio policistico	Anamnesi mestruale, valutazione dell'eccesso androgenico con testosterone libero/totale, DHEA	
Microalbuminuria	Concentrazione albuminica urinaria e rapporto albumina/creatinina	
Dislipidemia	Profilo lipidico a digiuno (colesterolo totale, LDL, HDL, trigliceridi)	Alla diagnosi e ogni 2 anni
Apnea da sonno	Studio del sonno per verificare la saturazione di ossigeno durante la notte	

Da Liu L, Hironaka K, Pihoker C: Typr 2 diabetes in youth. *Curr Probl Pediatr Adolesc Health Care* 2004;34:249-280.

cativamente più alte durante la pubertà, così che l'interpretazione di queste risposte richiede il confronto con le risposte regolate per età e pubertà.

L'interpretazione del test di tolleranza glicidica deve essere standardizzata secondo gli attuali criteri. Questi comprendono almeno 3 giorni di dieta bilanciata contenente circa il 50% di calorie dai carboidrati, il digiuno dalla mezzanotte fino al tempo del test la mattina successiva e la dose di glucosio per il test di 1,75 g/kg, ma non più di 75 g. Si prelevano campioni ematici prima dell'ingestione di glucosio 1, 2 e 3 ore dopo. La risposta arbitrariamente designata al test che identifica IGT è rappresentata da glicemia a digiuno inferiore a 126 mg/dL e un valore a 2 ore maggiore di 140 mg/dL, ma inferiore a 200 mg/dL (vedi Tab. 590-2). La determinazione delle risposte insuliniche durante il test di tolleranza glucidica non costituisce un prerequisito per giungere a una diagnosi; l'ampiezza della risposta, tuttavia, può avere un valore prognostico.

In bambini con IGT ma senza iperglicemia a digiuno, non è opportuna la ripetizione del test di tolleranza glicidica. Studi nei bambini indicano che il grado dell'alterazione della tolleranza glicidica tende a rimanere stabile o può migliorare dopo un periodo di anni, tranne nei pazienti con risposte insuliniche notevolmente alterate. Di conseguenza, nei bambini obesi non è indicata alcuna terapia, se non la diminuzione di peso. In particolare, l'uso degli ipoglicemizzanti orali deve essere riservato agli studi di ricerca. Se si sviluppano iperglicemia a digiuno o sintomi caratteristici di diabete, il bambino presenta un classico T2DM, precedentemente noto come NIDDM (vedi Tab. 590-1).

590.4 • ALTRI TIPI SPECIFICI DI DIABETE

DIFETTI GENETICI DELLA FUNZIONE DELLE CELLULE β

Diabete del giovane a esordio nella maturità. Questo sottotipo di DM comprende un gruppo di entità cliniche e genetiche eterogenee, caratterizzate da esordio precoce tra i 9 e i 25 anni, ereditarietà autosomica dominante (AD) e difetto primario della secrezione insulinica (Tab. 590-16). Criteri ristretti per la diagnosi di MODY comprendono diabete in almeno tre generazioni con trasmissione AD e diagnosi prima dei 25 anni in almeno un soggetto affetto.

Mutazioni del gene della glicochinasi responsabile di MODY2 determinano una lieve, cronica iperglicemia dovuta a modesta riduzione della risposta β-cellulare al glucosio. Il risultato di solito è rappresentato, nella maggior parte dei pazienti, da una forma relativamente lieve di diabete, con modesta iperglicemia a digiuno e IGT, che può essere trattato con basse dosi di insulina esogena.

TABELLA 590-16. Riassunto dei tipi MODY e caratteristiche cliniche speciali

	GENE MUTATO	FUNZIONE	CARATTERISTICA SPECIALE
MODY1	HNF-4α	Fattore di trascrizione	Diminuzione dei livelli di trigliceridi, apolipoproteine apoAII e apoCIII
MODY2	Glucochinasi (GCK)	Enzima, sensore del glucosio	Iperglicemia a esordio precoce ma lieve e non progressiva
MODY3	HFN-1α	Fattore di trascrizione	Diminuzione dell'assorbimento renale di glucosio e conseguente glicosuria
MODY4	IPF-1	Necessario per lo sviluppo pancreatico	
MODY5	HNF-1β	Fattore di trascrizione	Malattia renale non iperglicemica, associata ad anomalie uterine, ipospadia, lassità articolare e difficoltà di apprendimento
MODY6	NEUROD1	Fattore di differenziazione nello sviluppo delle insule pancreatiche	

Da Nakhla M, Polychronakos C: Monogenic and other unusual causes of diabetes mellitus. *Pediatric Clin North Am* 2005;52:1637-1650.

Pazienti colpiti con mutazioni di HNF-4α o di -1α mostrano anomalie più severe del metabolismo dei carboidrati, che variano da un'alterata tolleranza glicidica a diabete grave e che spesso col tempo progrediscono da una forma lieve a una severa. Circa un terzo di questi pazienti richiede insulina ed è soggetto allo sviluppo di complicanze vascolari. Pazienti con MODY2 e difetti del gene della glicochinasi possono presentare normale risposta insulinica al glucosio per via endovenosa, quando le concentrazioni ematiche di glucosio si mantengono a un livello superiore alle 7 mmol/L. Si è associato il deficit dell'attività della glicochinasi al deficit del recettore del glucosio della cellula β pancreatica. In contrasto, pazienti con MODY1 e MODY3 hanno un'alterazione più severa della secrezione insulinica e questo difetto non può essere controllato dal carico con infusione di glucosio.

Per definizione, l'assenza di una anamnesi familiare suggestiva di ereditarietà AD preclude la diagnosi di MODY. In queste circostanze, la comparsa di diabete in una persona relativamente giovane potrebbe rappresentare un T1DM in evoluzione e quindi è raccomandata la valutazione dei marker autoimmnunitari. Un DM tipo 1 più lieve, a evoluzione lenta, potrebbe essere confuso con un T2DM.

La distinzione tra le varie forme di MODY ha rilevanza clinica per la minore frequenza di complicanze vascolari nel MODY2 e, inoltre, per la necessità di trattare appropriatamente con insulina i pazienti con MODY1 e MODY3, se necessario. L'analisi molecolare per mutazioni del gene attualmente noto sui cromosomi 20, 7 e 12 sono attualmente disponibili per un uso clinico routinario che può facilitare la diagnosi e il trattamento. È stata anche descritta una forma ulteriore di MODY, dovuta a mutazione eterozigote di un fattore di trascrizione homeobox denominato fattore-1 (IPF-1) di promozione dell'insulina o MODY4, ma per ora non è disponibile un esame molecolare di routine. Altre forme meno comuni di MODY dipendono da mutazioni in altri fattori di trascrizione, compresi HNF-1β (MODY5) e NeuroD1 (MODY6).

Difetti primari o secondari nel tipo GLUT1 dei trasportatori del glucosio, una forma insulino-indipendente, possono anche essere associati a diabete. GLUT2 trasporta rapidamente il glucosio all'interno delle cellule β per la successiva fosforilazione per opera della glicochinasi, che alla fine porta alla secrezione di insulina. Il fenomeno della tossicità del glucosio può dipendere da una secondaria down-regulation dei trasportatori GLUT2.

MODY può anche essere la manifestazione di un polimorfismo del gene della glicogeno sintasi. Questo enzima è cruciale per l'accumulo del glucosio sotto forma di glicogeno a livello muscolare. Pazienti con questo difetto presentano una marcata resistenza all'insulina, ipertensione e un'anamnesi familiare significativa per diabete.

Difetti del gene mitocondriale. Mutazioni puntiformi del DNA mitocondriale sono talvolta associate a DM e sordità. Una mutazione è identica alla mutazione della MELAS *(Myopathy, Encephalopathy, Lactic Acidosis and Stroke-like syndrome* [sindrome con miopatia, encefalopatia, acidosi lattica e simil-ictus]), ma questa sindrome non è associata a diabete, così che muta l'espressione fenotipica dello stesso difetto. Un'altra forma di IDDM, talvolta associata a mutazioni mitocondriali, è la sindrome di Wolfram.

La sindrome di Wolfram è caratterizzata da diabete insipido, DM, atrofia ottica e sordità, sintomi che costituiscono l'acronimo DIDMOAD. La sindrome di Wolfram è causata da un'alterazione mitocondriale a livello di un gene nucleare mappato sul braccio corto del cromosoma 4. Sembra che alcuni pazienti con diabete abbiano insulinopenia, mentre altri presentano una secrezione significativa di insulina, come stimato dal peptide-C. In due pazienti esaminati, non si sono trovati anticorpi anti-cellule insulari, mentre la tipizzazione HLA ha rivelato DR2, che generalmente è considerato protettivo per diabete. In parecchi pazienti con diabete e sordità si è trovata una mutazione del tRNA mitocondriale; in altri questa mutazione è assente. La incidenza complessiva è di 1/770 000. La sequenza di comparsa dei segni è la seguente: IDDM non autoimmune nella prima decade, diabete insipido centrale e sordità neurosensoriale nei due terzi fino ai tre-quarti dei pazienti nella seconda decade, anomalie renali in circa la metà dei pazienti nella terza decade e complicanze neurologiche, come atassia cerebellare e miocloni nella metà fino ai due terzi dei pazienti nella quarta decade. Altre caratteristiche comprendono atrofia gonadica primaria nella maggioranza dei maschi e progressiva neurodegenerazione con morte neurorespiratoria a un'età media di 30 anni. L'assenza di diabete materno o sordità e di precedenti casi di difetto del gene mitocondriale suggeriscono un'ereditarietà di tipo autosomico recessivo.

DIABETE MELLITO DEL NEONATO

Transitorio. Il diabete mellito neonatale è raro, con un'incidenza stimata di 1 per 100 000 nati. L'esordio di T1DM persistente prima del sesto mese è raro. La sindrome del DM transitorio del neonato vede il suo esordio nella prima settimana di vita e persiste solo da alcune settimane a mesi, prima di una spontanea risoluzione. Si verifica più spesso in neonati piccoli per età gestazionale ed è caratterizzata da iperglicemia e pronunciata glicosuria, con severa disidratazione e, al tempo, acidosi metabolica ma con solo minima o assente chetonuria o chetonemia. La risposta insulinica al glucosio o alla tolbutamide è scarsa o assente; le concentrazioni plasmatiche basali di insulina sono normali. Dopo la risoluzione spontanea, la risposta insulinica agli stessi stimoli è vivace e normale, suggerendo un ritardo funzionale della maturazione della cellula β, a risoluzione spontanea. È stata riportata la comparsa della sindrome in fratelli consecutivi. Nel DM neonatale transitorio **sono comuni le anomalie del cromosoma 6**. Sono riportati dei casi di pazienti con T1DM classico che precedentemente avevano avuto un diabete transitorio del neonato. È ancora da verificare se questa associazione tra diabete transitorio del neonato seguito in momenti successivi della vita da T1DM classico sia una possibilità di comparsa o una correlazione casuale. Si deve distinguere questa sindrome dall'iperglicemia severa che si può verificare nella disidratazione ipertonica; questa condizione di solito si verifica in lattanti nel periodo perinatale, quando rispondono immediatamente alla reidratazione, con una richiesta minima di insulina.

La somministrazione di insulina è obbligatoria durante la fase attiva del DM nel neonato. Da 1 a 2 U/kg/24 h di insulina ad azione intermedia suddivisa in 2 dos di solito comportano un drammatico miglioramento e un'accelerazione della crescita e della ripresa del peso. È necessario porre molta attenzione alla riduzione della dose di insulina non appena si manifesta ipoglicemia recidiva o dopo il secondo mese di vita.

Permanente. Il DM nel periodo neonatale può essere permanente se associato a una rara sindrome di agenesia pancreatica. Il follow-up a lungo termine di una popolazione di pazienti con diabete neonatale ha rivelato che almeno una metà presentava diabete permanente, un terzo diabete transitorio e circa un quarto diabete transitorio che recidiva all'età di 7-20 anni. La maggior parte di questi neonati era piccola alla nascita. Sono stati descritti casi di gemelli affetti e di famiglie con più di un neonato affetto. Alcuni neonati con DM neonatale permanente sono inizialmente euglicemici e la malattia si presenta nel primo mese di vita.

Nei neonati sono state descritte mutazioni attivanti del gene *ABCC8* che codifica la subunità Kir6.2 del canale del potassio ATP-sensibile che produce diabete neonatale permanente. La sequenza genica di 29 pazienti con diabete neonatale permanente dimostrava che 10 pazienti avevano una delle 6 mutazioni eterozigoti nel gene KCNJ11, che codifica la subunità Kir6.2 dei canali del potassio ATP-sensibili trovata nelle cellule β pancreatiche. Mutazioni dominanti in *ABCC8* ammontano al 12% dei casi di diabete neonatale. Il diabete dipende da un meccanismo attraverso cui l'azione basale stimolatoria magnesio-nucleotide-dipendente del recettore della sulfanilurea (SUR)-1 sui pori kir è aumentata, ma è preservato il blocco da parte delle sulfoniluree. I pazienti identificati avevano severo diabete che necessitava di terapia insulinica e non producevano insulina quando stimolati con glucosio o glucagone, sebbene fossero in grado di produrla se stimolati con tolbutamide, una sulfonilurea. Perciò la terapia con sulfonilurea è più efficace dell'insulina nel diabete dovuto a mutazioni ABCC8 o KCNJII. Le patologie associate comprendono paresi e ritardo dello sviluppo in 4 pazienti, 3 dei quali mostravano anche crisi epilettiche e lieve dismorfismo.

Anomalie del gene dell'insulina. Diabete di grado variabile può dipendere da difetti del gene dell'insulina, dal difettoso passaggio da proinsulina a insulina, un difetto autosomico dominante, a varie sostituzioni aminoacidiche che alterano l'efficacia dell'insulina a livello recettoriale. Inoltre, questi difetti sono evidenti per l'alta concentrazione di insulina misurata con dosaggio radioimmunologico, mentre difetti della glicochinasi, MODY1, MODY3 e GLUT2, sono caratterizzati da deficit relativo o assoluto di secrezione insulinica per le comuni concentrazioni di glucosio.

DIFETTI GENETICI DELL'AZIONE INSULINICA. Due mutazioni del gene del recettore dell'insulina con rilevanza nei bambini sono il leprecaunismo e la sindrome di Rabson-Mendenhall.

Leprecaunismo. Questa sindrome è caratterizzata da ritardo della crescita intrauterina, ipoglicemia a digiuno e iperglicemia post-prandiale in associazione a profonda resistenza insulinica; durante il test orale di tolleranza glucidica, le concentrazioni sieriche di insulina possono essere 100 volte quelle di neonati normali di pari età. Sono stati descritti vari difetti del recettore dell'insulina, attestando così il ruolo importante dell'insulina e del suo recettore nella crescita fetale e nella morfogenesi. Inoltre, anche nella probabile completa assenza di recettori funzionali insulinici per ereditarietà omozigote di una mutazione *missense* del gene del recettore dell'insulina, con normale organogenesi e neonati nati vivi, si manifestava una forma severa di leprecaunismo. La maggior parte dei pazienti muore nel primo anno di vita.

Sindrome di Rabson-Mendenhall. Questa entità è definita da manifestazioni cliniche intermedie tra l'acanthosis nigricans con insulino-resistenza tipo A e il leprecaunismo. Le caratteristiche comprendono estrema resistenza insulinica, acanthosis nigricans, anomalie dei denti e delle unghie e iperplasia epifisaria. Non è chiaro se questa sindrome sia interamente distinta dal leprecaunismo; tuttavia, i pazienti con Rabson Mendenhall tendono a sopravvivere oltre il primo anno di vita. In questa sindrome sono stati descritti difetti del gene del recettore insulinica.

DIABETE CORRELATO ALLA FIBROSI CISTICA. Dati i miglioramenti della terapia medica di bambini con fibrosi cistica (*Cystic Fibrosis*, CF), molti sopravvivono fino alla tarda adolescenza e alle prime fasi dell'età adulta. D'altra parte, da quando lo screening annuale per il diabete è diventato routinaria nei pazienti con CF, il numero dei casi di diabete correlato a CF (*CF-Related Diabetes*, CFRD) è per lo meno duplicato. Si stima che più del 25% degli adolescenti con CF abbia il diabete. La terapia di questi pazienti è molto diversa da quella di pazienti con DM di tipo 1 o 2, perché i pazienti con CFRD presentano una fisiopatologia ben distinta e problemi nutrizionali e medici complessi.

I pazienti con CFRD sono magri e presentano deficit insulinico. La presentazione clinica è simile a quella del DM di tipo 2 nel fatto che l'esordio della malattia è insidioso ed è rara la comparsa di chetoacidosi. Sono negativi gli anticorpi anti-insulari. Non è ben definita l'incidenza di complicanze microvascolari nel CFRD, in rapporto alla durata del diabete, al controllo glicemico e alla malattia polmonare. Le complicanze macrovascolari non compaiono nel CFRD, forse per la breve durata di vita di questi pazienti. Parecchi fattori legati alla CF influenzano l'esordio e il decorso del diabete: (1) frequenti infezioni acute o croniche sono associate allo sviluppo e al declino di insulino-resistenza; (2) è necessario un incremento energetico per le infezioni e la patologia polmonare; (3) la malnutrizione si associa a scarsa sopravvivenza; (4) il malassorbimento è dovuto a insufficienza pancreatica esocrina, nonostante la supplementazione enzimatica; (5) l'alterazione dell'assorbimento dei nutrienti è causato da un anomalo tempo di transito intestinale; (6) è presente patologia epatica; (7) malattie, reflusso gastroesofageo, ritardato svuotamento gastrico, ostruzione intestinale, aumento del lavoro respiratorio e fattori psicosociali provocano comunemente anoressia e nausea; (8)

esiste un'ampia variabilità dell'intake alimentare quotidiano in rapporto allo stato di salute del paziente; (9) esiste un'alterazione della secrezione di insulina e glucagone.

Nel pancreas, il tessuto esocrino è sostituito da tessuto fibroso e adiposo; molte delle insule pancreatiche sono distrutte. Le insule rimanenti dimostrano una diminuzione del numero delle cellule β e α pancreatiche e di quelle che secernono il polipeptide pancreatico. La secrezione degli ormoni insulari insulina, glucagone e polipeptide pancreatico, in risposta a una serie di agenti stimolanti, è alterata in pazienti con CF. È possibile che l'insulino-resistenza possa giocare un ruolo anche nello sviluppo di CFRD, specialmente in concomitanza di infezioni acute.

In Danimarca, lo screening con il test da carico orale di glucosio in tutti i pazienti con CF ha dimostrato l'assenza di diabete in pazienti con meno di 10 anni, il 12% di diabete in pazienti dai 10 ai 19 anni e un 48% di diabete in adulti di 20 anni o più. In un centro del Midwest, dove si esegue uno screening annuale con il test di tolleranza glicidica, solo la metà dei bambini e un quarto degli adulti presentano una normale tolleranza glicidica. Si trova diabete nel 9% dei bambini con CF, nel 26% degli adolescenti e nel 35% degli adulti tra i 20 e i 29 anni. Circa un terzo dei pazienti con CFRD presenta iperglicemia a digiuno e due terzi CFRD senza iperglicemia a digiuno. L'iperglicemia a digiuno è esacerbata cronicamente, o in modo intermittente, dalle infezioni o dalla terapia con glicocorticoidi nel 3% dei bambini, nell'11% degli adolescenti e nel 15% degli adulti.

Quando si sviluppa iperglicemia, gli squilibri metabolici di accompagnamento sono solitamente lievi e, se la terapia insulinica diventa necessaria, sono sufficienti dosi relativamente basse a mantenere un adeguato controllo. La chetoacidosi è rara, ma si può verificare con il progressivo deterioramento della funzione delle insule pancreatiche. Il trattamento con insulina è stato descritto per il T1DM, ma il trattamento dietetico deve essere limitato per la presenza del disturbo primario.

PATOLOGIE AUTOIMMUNI. La **tiroidite linfocitica cronica (tiroidite di Hashimoto)** è frequentemente associata a T1DM nei bambini (vedi Capitolo 567). Un paziente diabetico insulino-dipendente su 5 può avere anticorpi antitiroide nel suo siero; l'incidenza è di 2-20 volte maggiore rispetto alla popolazione di controllo. Solo una piccola percentuale di questi pazienti, tuttavia, manifesta ipotiroidismo clinico; l'intervallo tra diagnosi di diabete e comparsa di patologia tiroidea è in media di 5 anni. Una periodica palpazione della tiroide è indicata in tutti i bambini diabetici; se la ghiandola appare dura o ingrandita, è necessaria la determinazione dei livelli sierici degli anticorpi anti-tiroidei e del TSH. Un livello di TSH confermato maggiore di 10 μU/mL indica l'esistenza o l'incipienza di una disfunzione tiroidea che richiede una terapia sostitutiva con ormone tiroideo. Anche una decelerazione nella velocità di crescita può essere dovuta a insufficienza tiroidea ed è, essa stessa, una ragione per valutare le concentrazioni sieriche di tiroxina e TSH.

Quando coesistono diabete e patologia tiroidea, deve essere presa in considerazione la possibilità di insufficienza surrenalica autoimmune. Si può preannunciare attraverso un decremento della richiesta insulinica, un aumento della pigmentazione della cute e della mucosa orale, desiderio di assumere sale, astenia, debolezza e ipotensione posturale o anche vere e proprie crisi addisoniane. Questa sindrome non è abituale soprattutto nella prima decade di vita, ma può manifestarsi nella seconda oppure oltre.

La **malattia celiaca**, nota come sprue non tropicale, è un altra patologia autoimmune, dovuta all'ipersensibilità al glutine presente nella dieta, che si verifica con frequenza significativa nei bambini con DM di tipo 1 (vedi Capitolo 335.2). Si stima che circa il 7,0% del bambini con DM di tipo 1 sviluppi malattia celiaca nei primi sei anni dalla diagnosi. Inoltre, l'incidenza della malattia celiaca è significativamente più alta nei bambini con meno di 4 anni e nel sesso femminile. Bambini piccoli con DM di tipo 1 e malattia celiaca presentano di norma sintomi gastrointestinali (crampi addominali, diarrea e reflusso gastroesofageo), deficit di crescita per peso inferiore al limite e inspiegate reazioni ipoglicemiche dovute a malassorbimento dei nutrienti; gli adolescenti possono rimanere asintomatici. La diagnosi di malattia celiaca va considerata se il titolo di anticorpi sierici anti-endomisio e/o anti-transglutaminasi tissutale è positivo in presenza di un normale livello sierico totale di IgA. La diagnosi è confermata dalla valutazione endoscopica e dalla biopsia dell'intestino tenue, che rivela caratteristica atrofia dei villi intestinali. La terapia consiste nella dieta priva di glutine, che è in grado di alleviare i sintomi gastrointestinali e di ridurre le escursioni glicemiche.

Gli anticorpi circolanti contro le cellule parietali gastriche e contro il fattore intrinseco sono 2-3 volte più comuni in pazienti con T1DM rispetto ai soggetti di controllo. Esistono buone correlazioni tra gli anticorpi anti-cellule parietali gastriche e gastrite atrofica e fra anticorpi contro il fattore intrinseco e malassorbimento di vitamina B_{12}. Tuttavia, l'anemia megaloblastica è rara in bambini con T1DM.

Una variante della sindrome da deficit endocrino multiplo è caratterizzata da diabete di tipo 1, atrofia idiopatica della mucosa intestinale con associata infiammazione e severo malassorbimento, deficit di IgA e anticorpi circolanti contro organi endocrini multipli, compresi tiroide, surrene, pancreas, paratiroidi e gonadi. Inoltre, membri di famiglie non diabetiche hanno una frequenza aumentata di vitiligine, malattia di Graves e sclerosi multipla, oltre a bassi livelli di complemento e anticorpi contro tessuti endocrini.

ENDOCRINOPATIE. Le endocrinopatie elencate nella Tabella 590-1 sono solo raramente causa di diabete nell'infanzia. Possono accelerare le manifestazioni di diabete in quelli con difetti congeniti o acquisiti della secrezione o dell'azione dell'insulina.

FARMACI. Alte dosi orali o parenterali di steroidi normalmente comportano una significativa resistenza insulinica che porta a intolleranza glucidica e diabete franco. I farmaci immunosoppressori come la ciclosporina e il tacrolimus sono tossici per le cellule β, e provocano IDDM in una percentuale significativa di pazienti trattati. La loto tossicità sulle cellule β pancreatiche è stato un fattore che ha contribuito a limitarne l'uso per arrestare la continua distruzione autoimmune delle cellule β. Anche la streptozotocina e il topicida Vacor® sono tossici per le cellule β, provocando diabete.

SINDROMI GENETICHE ASSOCIATE A DIABETE MELLITO. È stato descritto un certo numero di rare sindromi genetiche associate a IDDM o a intolleranza carboidratica (vedi Tab. 590-1). Queste sindromi rappresentano un ampio spettro di malattie che vanno dalla prematurità cellulare, come nelle sindromi di Werner e di Cockayne (vedi Capitolo 90), a eccessiva obesità con iperinsulinismo, resistenza all'azione insulinica e intolleranza ai carboidrati, come nella sindrome di Prader-Willi (vedi Capitolo 80). Alcune di queste sindromi sono caratterizzate da disturbi primari del recettore insulinico o da anticorpi anti-recettore in assenza di alterata secrezione insulinica. Sebbene rare, queste sindromi rappresentano modelli unici per comprendere le cause multiple di disturbi del metabolismo dei carboidrati da alterata secrezione insulinica o da alterata azione insulinica a livello recettoriali o post-recettoriale.

Epidemiologia, eziologia, patologia, classificazione e prevenzione

Atkinson MA, Eisenbarth GS: Type 1 diabetes: New perspectives on disease pathogenesis and treatment. *Lancet* 2001;358:221–229.

Atkinson MA, Ellis TM: Infants' diets and insulin-dependent diabetes: Evaluating the "cows' milk hypothesis" and a role for anti-bovine serum albumin immunity. *J Am Coll Nutr* 1997;16:334–340.

Casares S, Brumeanu TD: Insights into the pathogenesis of type 1 diabetes: A hint for novel immunospecific therapies. *Curr Molec Med* 2001;1: 357–378.

Daneman D: Type 1 diabetes. *Lancet* 2006;367:847–858.

Ferner RE: Drug-induced diabetes. *Baillieres Clin Endocrinol Metab* 1992;6: 849–866.

Hoppu S, Ronkainen MS, Kimpimäki T, et al: Insulin autoantibody isotypes during the prediabetic process in young children with increased genetic risk of type I diabetes. *Pediatr Res* 2004;55:236–242.

Hummel M, Bonifacio E, Schmid S, et al: Brief communication: Early appearance of islet autoantibodies predicts childhood type 1 diabetes in offspring of diabetic parents. *Ann Intern Med* 2004;140:882–886.

Lindley S, Dayan CM, Bishop A, et al: Defective suppressor function in CD4+CD25+ T-cells from patients with type diabetes. *Diabetes* 2005; 54:92–99.

Quinn M, Fleishman A, Rosner B, et al: Characteristics at diagnosis of type 1 diabetes in children younger than 6 years. *J Pediatr* 2006;148:366–371.

Rewers M, Norris J and Dabelea D: Epidemiology of type 1 diabetes mellitus. In Eisenbarth GS (editor): *Immunology of Type 1 Diabetes Mellitus*, 2nd edition. Boston, MA, Kluwer Acadamic Publishing Group, 2004.

Schatz DA, Maclaren NK: Cow's milk and insulin-dependent diabetes mellitus. *JAMA* 1996;276:647–648.

Solimena M, De Camilli P: Coxsackieviruses and diabetes. *Nat Med* 1995; 1:25–26.

Weill J, Vanderbecken S, Froguel P: Understanding the rising incidence of type 2 diabetes in adolescence. *Arch Dis Child* 2004;89:502–505.

Weir GC: A defective β-cell glucose sensor as a cause of diabetes. *N Engl J Med* 1993;328:729–731.

Yoon JW: The role of viruses and environmental factors in the induction of diabetes. *Curr Top Microbiol Immunol* 1990;164:95–123.

Genetica

Faas S, Trucco M: The genes influencing the susceptibility to IDDM in humans. *J Endocrinol Invest* 1994;17:477–495.

Ghosh S, Schork NJ: Genetic analysis of NIDDM: The study of quantitative traits. *Diabetes* 1996;45:1–14.

Johns DR: Mitochondrial DNA and disease. *N Engl J Med* 1995;333: 638–644.

Gillespie K, Bain SC, Barnett AH et al: The rising incidence of childhood type 1 diabetes and reduced contribution of high-risk HLA haplotypes. *Lancet* 2004;364:1699–1700.

Guo D, Li M, Zhang Y, et al: A functional variant of SUMO4, a new IκBα modifier, is associated with type 1 diabetes. *Nat Genet* 2004;36:837–841.

Huopio H, Otonkoski T, Vauhkonen I, et al: A new subtype of autosomal dominant diabetes attributable to a mutation in the gene for sulfonylurea receptor 1. *Lancet* 2003;361:301–307.

Velho G, Froguel P: Genetic, metabolic and clinical characteristics of maturity onset diabetes of the young. *Eur J Endocrinol* 1998;138:233–239.

Zamani M, Cassiman JJ: Reevaluation of the importance of polymorphic HLA class II alleles and amino acids in the susceptibility of individuals of different populations to type 1 diabetes. *Am J Med Genet* 1998;76:183–194.

Chetoacidosi diabetica

Amiel SA, Alberti KGMM: Inhaled insulin. *Br Med J* 2004;228:1215–1216.

DeWitt DE, Dugdale DC: Using new insulin strategies in the outpatient treatment of diabetes. *JAMA* 2003;289:2265–2269.

Duck SC, Wyatt DT: Factors associated with brain herniation in the treatment of diabetic ketoacidosis. *J Pediatr* 1988;113:10–14.

Dunger DB, Sperling MA, Acerini CL, et al: European Society for Pediatric Endocrinology/Lawson Wilkins Pediatric Endocrine Society consensus statement on diabetic ketoacidosis in children and adolescents. *Pediatrics* 2004;113:e133–e140.

Felner EI, White PC: Improving management of diabetic ketoacidosis in children. *Pediatrics* 2001;108:735–740.

Glaser NS, Wootton-Gorges SL, Marcin JP, et al: Mechanism of cerebral edema in children with diabetic ketoacidosis. *J Pediatr* 2004;145:164–171.

Green SM, Rothrock SG, Ho JD, et al: Failure of adjunctive bicarbonate to improve outcome in severe pediatric diabetic ketoacidosis. *Ann Emerg Med* 1998;31:41–48.

Hirsch IB: Insulin analogues. *N Engl J Med* 2005;352:174–183.

Lawrence SE, Cummings EA, Gaboury I, et al: Population-based study of incidence and risk factors for cerebral edema in pediatric diabetic ketoacidosis. *J Pediatr* 2005;146;688–692.

Medical Letter: Insulin glulisine (Apidra): a new rapid-acting insulin. *Med Lett* 2006;48:33–34.

Okuda Y, Adrogue J, Field JB, et al: Counterproductive effects of sodium bicarbonate in diabetic ketoacidosis. *J Clin Endocrinol Metab* 1996;81: 314–320.

Rosenbloom AL, Hanas R: Diabetic ketoacidosis treatment guidelines. *Clin Pediatr* 1996;261–266.

Tattersall RB: Brittle diabetes revisited: The Third Arnold Bloom Memorial Lecture. *Diabet Med* 1997;14:99–110.

Trattamento del diabete di tipo 1 nei bambini

Alemzadeh R, Ellis JN, Holzum MK, et al: Beneficial effects of continuous subcutaneous insulin infusion and flexible multiple daily insulin regimen using insulin glargine in type 1 diabetes mellitus. *Pediatrics* 2004;114: e91–e95.

Arslanian S, Ohki Y, Becker DJ, et al: The dawn phenomenon: comparison between normal and insulin-dependent diabetic adolescents. *Pediatr Res* 1992;31:203–206.

Berhe T, Postellon D, Wilson B, Stone R: Feasibility and safety of insulin pump therapy in children aged 2 to 7 years with type I diabetes: a retrospective study. *Pediatrics* 2006;117:2132–2137.

Bolli GB, Gerich JE: The "dawn phenomenon"—A common occurrence in both non-insulin and insulin-dependent diabetes mellitus. *N Engl J Med* 1984;310:746–750.

Bolli GB, Gottesman IS, Campbell PJ, et al: Glucose counter regulation and waning of insulin in the Somogyi phenomenon (posthypoglycemic hyperglycemia). *N Engl J Med* 1984;311:1214–1219.

Litton J, Rice A, Friedman N, et al: Insulin pump therapy in toddlers and preschool children with type 1 diabetes mellitus. *J Pediatr* 2002;141: 490–495.

Maniatis AK, Klingensmith GJ, Slover RH, et al: Continuous subcutaneous insulin infusion therapy in children and adolescents: An option for routine diabetes care. *Pediatrics* 2001;107: 351–356.

Rami B, Schober E: Postprandial glycaemia after regular and lispro insulin in children and adolescents with diabetes. *Eur J Pediatr* 1997;156:838–840.

Regan FM, Dunger DB: Use of new insulins in children. *Arch Dis Child* 2006;91:ep47–ep53.

Rutledge KS, Chase HP, Klingensmith GJ, et al: Effectiveness of postprandial Humalog in toddlers with diabetes. *Pediatrics* 1997;100:968–972.

Weinzimer S, Ahern JH, Doyle EA, et al: Persistence of benefits of continuous subcutaneous insulin infusion in very young children with type 1 diabetes: A follow-up report. *Pediatrics* 2004;114:1601–1605.

Wilson D, Buckingham B, Kunselman EL, et al: A two-center randomized controlled feasibility trial of insulin pump therapy in young children with diabetes. *Diabetes Care* 2005;28;15–19.

Zinman B: The physiologic replacement of insulin. *N Engl J Med* 1989; 321:363–370.

Esiti a lungo termine del diabete infantile: relazione del controllo dello sviluppo delle complicanze

The absence of a glycemic threshold for the development of long-term complications: The perspective of the Diabetes Control and Complications Trial. *Diabetes* 1996;45:1289–1298.

Bojestig M, Arnqvist HJ, Karlberg BE: Glycemic control and prognosis in type 1 diabetic patients with microalbuminuria. *Diabetes Care* 1996;19: 313–317.

Leslie ND, Sperling MA: Relation of metabolic control to complications in diabetes mellitus. *J Pediatr* 1986;108:491–497.

Nathan DM: Long-term complications of diabetes mellitus. *N Engl J Med* 1993;328:1676–1685.

Reichard P, Nilsson BY, Rosenqvist U: The effect of long-term intensified insulin treatment on the development of microvascular complications of diabetes mellitus. *N Engl J Med* 1993;329:304–309.

Rosenbloom AL: Skeletal and joint manifestations of childhood diabetes. *Pediatr Clin North Am* 1984;31:569–589.

Sandman DD, Shore AC, Tooke JE: Relation of skin capillary pressure in patients with insulin-dependent diabetes mellitus to complications and metabolic control. *N Engl J Med* 1992;327:760–764.

Wang PH: Tight glucose control and diabetic complications. *Lancet* 1993; 342:129.

Malattie e sindromi associate a diabete

Barrett TG, Bundey SE: Wolfram (DIAMOAD) syndrome. *J Med Genet* 1997;34:838–841.

Jones KL: Non-insulin dependent diabetes in children and adolescents: The therapeutic challenge. *Clin Pediatr* 1998;37:103–110.

Krook A, Brueton L, O'Rahilly S: Homozygous nonsense mutation in the insulin receptor gene in an infant with leprechaunism. *Lancet* 1993;342: 277–278.

Low L, Chernausek SD, Sperling MA: Acromegaloid patients with type-A insulin resistance: Parallel defects in insulin and insulin-like growth factor-I receptors and biological responses in cultured fibroblasts. *J Clin Endocrinol Metab* 1989;69:329–337.

Morrison EY, McKenzie K: The Mauriac syndrome. *West Indian Med J* 1989;38:180–182.

Pinhas-Hamiel O, Dolan LM, Daniels SR: Increased incidence of non-insulin-dependent diabetes mellitus among adolescents. *J Pediatr* 1996;128:608–615.
Rotig A, Cormier V, Chatelain P, et al: Deletion of mitochondrial DNA in a case of early-onset diabetes mellitus, optic atrophy, and deafness. *J Clin Invest* 1993;91:1095–1098.
Sullivan MM, Denning CR: Diabetic microangiopathy in patients with cystic fibrosis. *Pediatrics* 1989;84:642–647.
Taylor SI, Cama A, Accili D, et al: Mutations in the insulin receptor gene. *Endocr Rev* 1992;13:566–595.
Watkins PB, Whitcomb RW: Hepatic dysfunction associated with troglitazone. *N Engl J Med* 1998;338:916–917.
Winter WE, Maclaren NK, Riley WJ, et al: Congenital pancreatic hypoplasia: A syndrome of exocrine and endocrine pancreatic insufficiency. *J Pediatr* 1986;109:465–468.
Winter WE, Maclaren NK, Riley WJ, et al: Maturity-onset diabetes of youth in black Americans. *N Engl J Med* 1987;316:285–291.

Diabete del neonato

Alcolado JC, Thomas AW: Maternally inherited diabetes mellitus: The role of mitochondrial DNA defects. *Diabet Med* 1995;12:102–108.
Babenko AP, Polak M, Cavé H, et al: Activating mutations in the ABCC8 gene in neonatal diabetes mellitus. *N Engl J Med* 2006;355:456–466.
Geffner ME, Clare-Salzler M, Kaufman DL, et al: Permanent diabetes developing after transient neonatal diabetes. *Lancet* 1993;341:1095.
Gloyn AL, Pearson ER, Antcliff AF, et al: Activating mutations in the gene encoding the ATP-sensitive potassium channel subunit Kir6.2 and permanent neonatal disease. *N Engl J Med* 2004;350:1838–1849.
Metz C, Cavé H, Bertrand AM, et al: Neonatal diabetes mellitus: Chromosomal analysis in transient and permanent cases. *J Pediatr* 2002;141:483–489.
Pagliara AS, Karl IE, Kipnis DB: Transient neonatal diabetes: Delayed maturation of the pancreatic beta cell. *J Pediatr* 1973;82:97–101.
Pearson ER, Flechtner I, Njølstad PR, et al: Switching from insulin to oral sulfonylureas in patients with diabetes due to Kir6.2 mutations. *N Engl J Med* 2006;355:467–477.
von Muhlendahl KR, Herkenhoff H: Long-term course of neonatal diabetes. *N Engl J Med* 1995;333:704–708.

Ipoglicemia e diabete

Amiel SA, Tamborlane WV, Simonson DC, et al: Defective glucose counter regulation after strict glycemic control of insulin-dependent diabetes mellitus. *N Engl J Med* 1987;316:1376–1383.
Bolli GB, Fanelli CG: Unawareness of hypoglycemia. *N Engl J Med* 1995;333:1771–1772.
Cryer PE, Fisher JN, Shamoon H: Hypoglycemia. *Diabetes Care* 1994;17:734–755.
Diabetes Control and Complications Trial Research Group: Hypoglycemia in the diabetes control and complications trial. *Diabetes* 1997;46:271–286.
Gschwend S, Ryan C, Atchinson J, et al: Effects of acute hyperglycemia on mental efficiency and counterregulatory hormones in adolescents with insulin-dependent diabetes mellitus. *J Pediatr* 1995;126:178–184.
McCrimmon RJ, Gold AE, Deary IJ, et al: Symptoms of hypoglycemia in children with IDDM. *Diabetes Care* 1995;18:858–861.
Porter PA, Keating B, Byrne G, et al: Incidence and predictive criteria of nocturnal hypoglycemia in young children with insulin-dependent diabetes mellitus. *J Pediatr* 1997;130:366–372.
Silverstein JH, Gordon G, Pollock BH, et al: Long-term glycemic control influences the onset of limited joint mobility in type I diabetes. *J Pediatr* 1998;132:944–947.
Wayne EA, Dean HJ, Booth F, et al: Focal neurologic deficits associated with hypoglycemia in children with diabetes. *J Pediatr* 1990;117:575–577.

Trapianto di pancreas e di insule

Alejandro R, Lehmann R, Ricordi C, et al: Long-term function (6 years) of islet allografts in type 1 diabetes. *Diabetes* 1997;46:1983–1989.
Hering BJ, Kandaswamy R, Ansite JD, et al: Single-donor, marginal-dose islet transplantation in patients with type 1 diabetes. *JAMA* 2005;293:830–835.
Larsen JL, Stratta RJ: Consequences of pancreas transplantation. *J Investig Med* 1994;42:622–631.
Mitanchez D, Doiron B, Chen R, et al: Glucose-stimulated genes and prospects of gene therapy for type 1 diabetes. *Endocr Rev* 1997;18:520–540.
Robertson RP: Islet transplantation as a treatment for diabetes—a work in progress. *N Engl J Med* 2004;350:694–705.
Ryan EA, Lakey JR, Paty BW, et al: Successful islet transplantation: Continued insulin reserve provides long-term glycemic control. *Diabetes* 2002;51:2148–2157.
Shapiro AMJ, Ricordi C, Hering BJ, et al: International trial of the edmonton protocol for islet transplantation. *N Engl J Med* 2006;355:1318–1330.

Parte XXVI ■ Il sistema nervoso

Capitolo 591 ■ Valutazione neurologica*

Robert H.A. Haslam

L'obiettivo dell'esame neurologico è di valutare l'integrità del sistema nervoso centrale (SNC) mediante un'anamnesi dettagliata, l'esame fisico e indagini volte a determinare la localizzazione e le cause di eventuali anomalie.

ANAMNESI

L'anamnesi è fondamentale nella valutazione di un bambino con sospetti disturbi neurologici. Oltre a elencare i sintomi, in ordine cronologico di comparsa, è opportuno descriverne accuratamente la frequenza, la durata e le caratteristiche associate. I bambini con più di 3-4 anni sono solitamente in grado di contribuire alla loro storia clinica, in particolare riguardo agli aspetti collegati ai sintomi attuali. È essenziale ottenere un quadro completo della funzione e delle interazioni tra i diversi apparati, poiché le anomalie del sistema nervoso possono **inizialmente** presentarsi con manifestazioni cliniche (vomito, dolore, costipazione, disturbi del sistema urinario). Un'anamnesi dettagliata può contribuire, per esempio, ad attribuire il vomito del bambino a un aumento della pressione intracranica (*IntraCranial Pressure*, ICP), il dolore retro-orbitale alla cefalea o alla sclerosi multipla, la costipazione e la perdita di urina a un tumore del midollo spinale.

È importante iniziare l'anamnesi con una concisa descrizione dei principali sintomi, inserendoli nel contesto evolutivo. I genitori sono spesso preoccupati del ritardo di linguaggio manifestato dal figlio. La gravità di questo disturbo dipende da molti fattori, inclusi l'età del paziente paragonata all'età media di acquisizione del linguaggio, l'interazione genitori-bambino, l'integrità del sistema uditivo e il livello intellettivo. Un'approfondita conoscenza delle principali tappe evolutive è essenziale per valutare la rilevanza delle osservazioni dei genitori (vedi Capitoli 7-15).

Dopo il resoconto dei disturbi presentati dal bambino, si passa alla descrizione della gravidanza, del travaglio e del parto, in particolare se si sospetta una malattia congenita (vedi Capitoli 93-109). È opportuno indagare l'eventuale esposizione della madre, durante la gravidanza, a malattie virali e il suo status immunologico riguardo a varicella, HIV e sifilide. La presenza di ipertensione indotta dalla gravidanza o diabete gestazionale deve essere investigata. L'anamnesi dovrebbe determinare anche il numero e i risultati di ecografie e amniocentesi, oltre a includere informazioni sulla quantità di alcol consumata, il numero di sigarette fumate, l'esposizione a tossine e l'uso di farmaci e sostanze stupefacenti (legali e non) con potenziali effetti collaterali sullo sviluppo fetale. La riduzione o l'assenza di attività fetale può essere associata a una miopatia congenita o ad altri disturbi neuromuscolari. **Convulsioni** in utero possono verificarsi occasionalmente e suggeriscono un'insufficienza placentare o la presenza di uno dei rari disturbi congeniti del metabolismo, come una dipendenza da piridossina. L'attività convulsiva in utero è difficile da valutare, in particolare in una primipara. Spesso la presenza di convulsioni già in utero è accertata retrospettivamente, soltanto dopo che la madre ha avuto l'opportunità di osservare una crisi.

Le condizioni di salute postpartum della madre possono fornire utili indicazioni sulla causa dei disturbi neurologici del figlio. Gli aspetti da indagare includono presenza di febbre, dipendenza da stupefacenti, vescicole della cervice o vaginali (herpes simplex), emorragia o petecchie, anomalie della placenta.

Informazioni particolarmente importanti sono il peso alla nascita, la lunghezza e la circonferenza cranica. Per quest'ultimo dato può essere necessario richiedere la cartella clinica del bambino nell'ospedale di nascita, in particolare se si sospetta una microcefalia congenita. Il punteggio di Apgar consente invece di escludere un'asfissia perinatale. L'anamnesi fornisce diversi indicatori affidabili di disfunzione neurologica nel periodo neonatale. L'**incapacità** di un neonato a termine di **respirare spontaneamente**, tale da richiedere il riscorso alla ventilazione assistita, suggerisce un'anomalia del SNC. Mancanza di coordinazione o difficoltà della suzione, in un neonato che richiede un tempo eccessivo per alimentarsi, indicano un disturbo neurologico che è particolarmente grave se le difficoltà sono tali da richiedere l'alimentazione per gavage. Tutte le anomalie menzionate sono comuni in un neonato prematuro, in particolare in caso di peso molto basso alla nascita, ma non sono indicative necessariamente di sequele neurologiche. Un'altra informazione importante nel periodo neonatale consiste nella presenza, nella gravità e nel trattamento dell'**ittero**. L'anamnesi consente inoltre al medico di raccogliere informazioni sul benessere complessivo del bambino, sulle attività, sulle modalità del sonno e sul tipo di pianto.

La componente principale dell'anamnesi neurologica consiste nella **valutazione dello sviluppo** (vedi Capitoli 6 e 15). Per distinguere un ritardo evolutivo globale da un ritardo circoscritto a competenze specifiche (per es. quelle motorie) è necessaria una attenta valutazione del linguaggio, delle abilità sociali e motorie (motricità fine e grossolana). Un'anomalia evolutiva presente fin dalla nascita suggerisce una causa intrauterina o perinatale. Un rallentamento successivo nell'acquisizione delle competenze evolutive può implicare un'anomalia acquisita del sistema nervoso. Una perdita di competenze (**regressione**) nel corso del tempo è indicativa della **malattia degenerativa** del SNC, come un errore congenito del metabolismo. L'abilità dei genitori nel ricordare con precisione le tappe del processo di acquisizione delle diverse competenze del loro bambino è estremamente variabile. Alcuni genitori sono molto affidabili, mentre altri appaiono incerti e titubanti, in particolare se il paziente presenta un disturbo neu-

TABELLA 591-1. Screening del ritardo dello sviluppo: range superiore

ETÀ (IN MESI)	MOTRICITÀ GROSSOLANA	MOTRICITÀ FINE	ABILITÀ SOCIALI	LINGUAGGIO
3	Sostiene il peso sugli avambracci	Apre le mani spontaneamente	Sorride contestualmente	Ride e sorride
6	Si siede momentaneamente	Sposta gli oggetti	Mostra preferenze	Balbetta
9	Riesce ad alzarsi	Presa a pinza (con opposizione pollice-indice)	Gioca a nascondino e battimani	Imita i suoni
12	Cammina reggendosi con una mano	Consegna un oggetto su richiesta	Accorre quando viene chiamato	Pronuncia una o due parole significative
18	Sale le scale con aiuto	Mangia usando il cucchiaio	Mima le azioni degli altri	Pronuncia almeno sei parole
24	Corre	Costruisce una torre con sei blocchi	Gioca con gli altri	Pronuncia frasi composte da due-tre parole

*Ringrazio i Dr. Michael Esser, Hannah Glass e Adam Kirton per il loro contributo alla revisione del Capitolo 591.

roevolutivo significativo. La Tabella 591-1 fornisce alcune linee guida circa il range superiore delle capacità normali solitamente ricordate dai genitori; l'assenza di tali abilità dovrebbe allarmare il pediatra. Il Capitolo 15 include un elenco completo dei test evolutivi di screening e illustra nei dettagli le modalità di interpretazione. È utile domandare ai genitori di poter guardare le fotografie del bambino scattate a diverse età, perché talvolta forniscono informazioni precise sull'acquisizione delle diverse competenze. È inoltre importante ascoltare con attenzione il racconto dei genitori, in particolare delle madri, spesso consapevoli della presenza di un disturbo evolutivo nel figlio. Un altro elemento da non trascurare è l'eventuale ricorso a metodi terapeutici alternativi, talvolta confessato con riluttanza al medico.

L'**anamnesi familiare** è molto importante nella valutazione neurologica di un bambino, benché alcuni genitori siano poco propensi a parlare di membri familiari con disturbi neurologici debilitanti. Se il parente è istituzionalizzato, è possibile che non dispongano di molte informazioni a riguardo. La maggior parte dei genitori non esita a fornire un resoconto clinico dettagliato degli altri membri della famiglia, specialmente se lo ritengono rilevante per il loro bambino. La storia familiare dovrebbe documentare l'età e le condizioni di salute dei familiari di primo grado e la presenza di eventuali malattie neurologiche, come epilessia, cefalea, accidenti cerebrovascolari, ritardo evolutivo e disturbi ereditari. È importante segnalare il sesso e l'età alla morte di aborti o di fratelli, includendo i risultati dell'esame *post mortem*, poiché queste informazioni possono essere collegate al disturbo attuale del paziente. Deve inoltre essere ricercata la possibile **consanguineità** tra i genitori, perché in tal caso l'incidenza di malattie metaboliche e degenerative a carico del SNC aumenta significativamente.

L'indagine deve includere anche un approfondimento delle caratteristiche di personalità e comportamentali del bambino. Le informazioni sul rendimento scolastico e sulle modalità di socializzazione (che possono essere richieste direttamente alla scuola) contribuiscono spesso a chiarire la diagnosi, in particolare se gli insegnanti segnalano un brusco cambiamento. Un bambino che non è in grado di nominare almeno tre amichetti del cuore o compagni di giochi presenta uno sviluppo sociale anomalo. In caso di significativo calo della performance scolastica, è utile ottenere una descrizione del bambino prima e dopo l'esordio dei sintomi. Il colloquio con gli insegnanti può fornire informazioni preziose che completano il quadro esposto dai genitori.

ESAME NEUROLOGICO

L'esame neurologico ha inizio subito dopo la raccolta delle informazioni anamnestiche. L'**osservazione** del bambino durante l'interazione con i genitori, mentre gioca e nei momenti in cui non gli viene prestata attenzione, può fornire dati utili (vedi Capitoli 6 e 15). Le osservazioni più evidenti includono la presenza di una facies caratteristica, di una postura insolita o di un'anomalia motoria, che si manifesta con un disturbo della deambulazione o un'emiparesi. È particolarmente importante osservare il **comportamento** del paziente durante il colloquio. Un bambino alla 1ª o 2ª infanzia normalmente curioso gioca da solo per un certo periodo di tempo, ma ben presto manifesta il desiderio di essere coinvolto nel dialogo. Un bambino con un disturbo dell'attenzione può manifestare un comportamento anomalo nello studio medico, mentre un bambino con un disturbo neurologico appare letargico, disinteressato o totalmente inconsapevole di ciò che accade nell'ambiente esterno. Anche le modalità di interazione genitore-bambino devono essere osservate. L'esame neurologico di un neonato o di un bambino nato prematuro richiede un approccio modificato rispetto a un bambino più grande; le differenze nelle modalità di esame per entrambi i gruppi sono indicate nei Capitoli 7 e 94.

L'**esame** deve essere condotto in un ambiente appropriato, rassicurante e non minaccioso per il bambino. Per garantirsi la sua cooperazione, è utile presentare la visita come un gioco. Talvolta il bambino si sente maggiormente a suo agio in braccio al genitore o interagendo sul pavimento dello studio. Non è consigliabile forzare il paziente a sedersi alla scrivania, né è opportuno farlo svestire all'inizio della visita. Ottenere la cooperazione del bambino è fondamentale per poter condurre un esame neurologico completo. Il livello di partecipazione del bambino è direttamente collegato all'instaurazione di un rapporto di fiducia con il medico. Per valutare lo **status mentale**, la **funzione cognitiva** e il **livello di allerta** è possibile utilizzare diversi strumenti, a seconda dell'età del bambino. Semplici puzzle possono essere molto utili. La capacità del bambino di raccontare una storia o di disegnare contribuisce a valutare la funzione cognitiva e a determinare il livello evolutivo. Le modalità di gioco o di esplorazione della funzione di un oggetto nuovo costituiscono un eccellente indicatore della curiosità intellettiva. Il livello di allerta di un neonato dipende da molti fattori, tra i quali l'intervallo trascorso dall'ultima poppata, la temperatura della stanza e l'età gestazionale. Valutazioni sequenziali del bambino sono utili per evidenziare eventuali modifiche della funzione neurologica. Neonati prematuri (<28 settimane di gestazione) non sempre manifestano fasi di allerta, mentre una lieve stimolazione fisica in bambini più grandi è di solito sufficiente a svegliarli, determinando un breve periodo di allerta. Nei nati a termine, le modalità del sonno e la deambulazione risultano solitamente normali. Si raccomanda di prestare attenzione alla presenza di un **odore** particolare emanato dal bambino, o notato dai genitori, che può indicare un disturbo metabolico (come l'odore di rancido nella fenichetonuria o l'odore di piedi nell'acidemia isovalerica). È importante determinare se questo odore è persistente o transitorio, presentatosi solo con le malattie.

L'esaminatore deve approfittare delle occasioni offerte dal paziente e, se le circostanze lo consentono, può effettuare una valutazione preliminare della funzione cerebellare, della forza e del tono muscolare, prima di procedere all'esame dei nervi cranici. Se l'anamnesi suggerisce l'opportunità di misurare la funzione acustica, è fondamentale concentrarsi su questo aspetto quando l'attenzione e l'interesse del bambino sono ancora vivi.

TESTA. Le dimensioni e la forma della testa devono essere registrate accuratamente. La presenza di turricefalia o di oxicefalia è indice di una prematura chiusura delle suture, associata a varie forme di craniosinostosi ereditaria (vedi Capitolo 592.12). La fronte ampia può indicare idrocefalo, mentre un cranio piccolo è tipico della microcefalia. L'osservazione di un cranio squadrato indica un ematoma subdurale cronico, perché la presenza di liquido nello spazio subdurale causa un allargamento della fossa cranica media. L'esame del cuoio capelluto include l'osservazione della circolazione venosa, perché l'aumento della ICP e la trombosi del seno sagittale superiore possono causare una marcata distensione venosa. Deve essere notata la presenza di eventuali anomalie cutanee, come "aplasia cutis" o capelli torti, che indicano un disturbo genetico. Per escludere la presenza di un'aberrazione neuroevolutiva, è utile una valutazione complessiva degli aspetti antropomorfici del volto (occhi, orecchie, naso, labbra, dentizione e palato).

Alla nascita, tutti i neonati presentano due **fontanelle**: la fontanella anteriore è situata lunga la linea mediana, a livello della giunzione tra le suture coronale e sagittale; quella posteriore, delle dimensioni di un polpastrello, si trova all'intersezione tra le ossa occipitale e parietale. La fontanella posteriore, più difficile da palpare, si chiude tra le 6 e le 8 settimane di vita (ma talvolta risulta già chiusa alla nascita); la sua persistenza suggerisce la presenza di idrocefalo o di ipotiroidismo congenito. La fontanella anteriore misura approssimativamente 2 × 2 cm, ma si osserva un'estrema variabilità individuale. L'età media di chiusura è 18 mesi, ma talvolta può essere anticipata fino a 9. Una fontanella anteriore molto piccola o assente alla nascita può indicare la **prematura fusione** delle suture o **microcefalia**, mentre una fontanella particolarmente grande può indicare un'ampia gamma di problemi. Normalmente leggermente depressa e pulsatile, la fontanella è esaminabile al meglio con il lattante in posizione eretta, mentre dorme o viene allattato. Una fontanella sporgente è un indicatore affidabile dell'aumento della ICP, ma anche il pianto vigoroso può causarne la protrusione in un neonato sano.

La **palpazione** del cranio rivela tipicamente la sovrapposizione delle suture craniche nei primi giorni di vita del neonato, risultato della pressione esercitata sul cranio durante la sua discesa attraverso la pelvi. La palpazione consente di osservare la presenza di difetti cranici o di **craniotabe**, un assottigliamento dell'osso parietale che, in seguito a leggere pressione, rivela una consistenza elastica e cedevole come una pallina da ping pong. La craniotabe è spesso associata a prematurità.

L'**auscultazione** completa l'esame del cranio. I **rumori cranici** sono più intensi nell'area della fontanella anteriore, nella regione temporale o sulle orbite; la maniera migliore per ascoltarli è attraverso il diaframma dello stetoscopio. Fino ai 4 anni, lievi rumori simmetrici si rivelano anche nei bambini normali in associazione a stati febbrili. Le malformazioni arteriovenose dell'arteria cerebrale centrale, o vena di Galeno, producono un rumore sordo. Rumori che si originano dal cuore o dai grossi vasi possono essere trasmessi al cranio. In presenza di grave anemia, si riscontra spesso un rumore cranico, che scompare in seguito alla correzione dell'anemia. Anche l'aumento dell'ICP, causato da idrocefalo, tumore, effusioni subdurali o meningite purulenta, può produrre rumori cranici percepibili. Il riscontro di un rumore localizzato o intenso suggerisce l'opportunità di eseguire esami di approfondimento.

La **corretta misura della circonferenza cranica** è importante e deve essere eseguita durante ciascuna visita, annottando i valori su di un apposito diagramma. Si consiglia di utilizzare un metro di plastica non estendibile, collocandolo sulle bozze frontali, e procedendo circonferenzialmente in modo da includere la porzione più prominente dell'occipite e misurare il volume cranico maggiore. Se si riscontrano anomalie, è opportuno procedere alla misura della circonferenza cranica di genitori e fratelli del paziente. Gli errori nella misura del cranio del neonato, particolarmente frequenti, sono attribuibili a edema del cuoio capelluto, sovrapposizione delle suture, stravaso di fluido endovenoso o cefaloematoma. La velocità media di crescita del cranio in un neonato prematuro sano è di 0,5 cm nelle prime due settimane di vita, 0,75 cm nella terza settimana, e 1 cm nella quarta (e fino alla quarantesima). La circonferenza cranica di un neonato a termine misura 34-35 cm, 44 cm entro i 6 mesi, e 47 cm entro il primo anno (vedi Capitoli 7 e 8).

NERVI CRANICI

Nervo olfattivo (1). L'**anosmia**, cioè la perdita della capacità di percepire gli odori, si riscontra comunemente in associazione a infezioni del tratto respiratorio superiore nei bambini e costituisce dunque un'anomalia transitoria. Anche una frattura alla base del cranio e della lamina cribroide può causare anosmia. Occasionalmente, un bambino in fase di guarigione dalla meningite purulenta può manifestare una riduzione dell'olfatto. In rari casi, l'anosmia è congenita. Benché non si tratti di una componente di routine dell'esame neurologico, l'olfatto può essere testato già durante la 32ª settimana di gestazione, utilizzando stimoli come il caffè, la menta e altre sostanze familiari al bambino; si consiglia invece di evitare le sostanze aromatiche.

Nervo ottico (2). L'esame del disco ottico e della retina costituisce una componente importante dell'esame neurologico. Per visualizzare una porzione di retina adeguata, è necessario dilatare la pupilla. La somministrazione, ripetuta tre volte a intervalli di 15 minuti, di una goccia di una combinazione di ciclopentolato cloridato all'1%, fenilefrina idrocloride al 2,5% e tropicamide all'1% è sufficiente a produrre midriasi. I midriatici sono controindicati se la reazione della pupilla è necessaria per valutare il livello della coscienza o in presenza di cataratta. L'esame della retina è eseguito al meglio mentre il lattante succhia un capezzolo o un ciuccio, con la testa posizionata su un lato. Il medico esamina l'occhio più vicino, stimolando delicatamente il neonato per mantenerlo sveglio. Il bambino più grande può essere esaminato in braccio al genitore, distraendolo con giocattoli e oggetti luminosi. Il nervo ottico è di colore rosa salmone nel bambino e grigio-bianco nel neonato (ancora più chiaro in chi ha i capelli biondi). Questo reperto normale può essere fonte di confusione, conducendo all'erronea diagnosi di atrofia ottica.

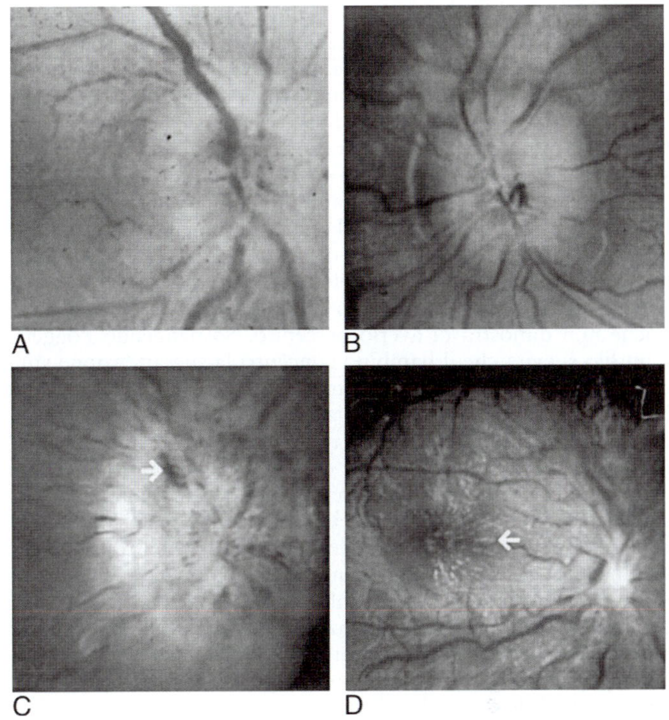

Figura 591-1. *A.* Papilledema lieve. Margini del disco indefiniti e congestione venosa. *B,* Papilledema moderato. Disco edematoso e rilevato. Vasi coperti da tessuto nervoso. *C,* Papilledema grave. Evidenti emorragie all'interno del disco (*freccia*), microinfarti (essudati molli) nello strato delle fibre nervose. *D,* Stella maculare (*freccia*), con residui edematosi distribuiti all'interno dello strato di Henle della macula.

Il **papilledema** è un rigonfiamento del disco ottico originato da un aumento della pressione intracranica. Si verifica raramente nell'infanzia, perché le suture craniche sono in grado di adattarsi all'espansione cerebrale. Nel bambino più grande, il papilledema può essere riconosciuto dalle seguenti alterazioni progressive del nervo ottico e del tessuto retinico circostante (Fig. 591-1).

1. Il nervo ottico diviene iperemico.
2. I piccoli capillari che normalmente attraversano il nervo ottico si restringono al punto da non essere più visibili.
3. Le vene più grandi si dilatano, mentre le arteriole a esse associate si restringono.
4. Il bordo del nervo ottico è difficile da distinguere dalla retina circostante, in particolare lungo il margine temporale.
5. Nella retina, si nota la comparsa di emorragie subialoidee a fiamma, che circondano il nervo ottico.
6. In alcuni casi, si sviluppa una stella maculare, provocata da un edema retinico nella regione della macula. Il papilledema deve essere differenziato dalla **papillite**, dovuta a una infiammazione del nervo ottico (neurite ottica). Il papilledema non altera l'acuità visiva, né la visione dei colori, mentre nella neurite ottica si riscontra una perdita visiva; in entrambi i disturbi, le dimensioni della macchia cieca risultano aumentate.

Le emorragie retiniche si verificano nel 30-40% dei neonati a termine. Sono più comuni in caso di parto vaginale rispetto al cesareo e non risultano associate a lesioni perinatali o complicanze neurologiche. Scompaiono spontaneamente entro una o due settimane.

VISTA (VEDI ANCHE PARTE XXVIII). A 28 settimane, bambini prematuri normali ammiccano quando una luce intensa è diretta verso i loro occhi; entro la 32ª settimana, tengono gli occhi chiusi finché la sorgente luminosa non viene rimossa. Alla 37ª settimana, i pretermine normali rivolgono la testa e gli occhi in direzione di una luce soffusa; entro questa età, si sviluppano la fissazione visiva e la capacità di seguire un target luminoso. Durante i periodi di allerta, nel neonato è possibile dimostrare il **nistagmo optocinetico**. Nei neonati a termine, l'**acuità visiva** è di circa 20/150, ma raggiunge il livello dell'adulto (20/20) entro i 6 mesi di età. I bambini troppo piccoli per essere sottoposti all'esame della vista standard (carta ottica di Snellen) sono esaminati mediante il "gioco della E". A 2,5-3 anni, un bambino con capacità visiva nella norma identifica gli oggetti della carta di Allen a una distanza di 4-5 metri. L'esame del **campo visivo** nel lattante è condotto avvicinando lentamente un oggetto di colore rosso vivo da dietro il capo del bambino, attraverso il suo campo visivo periferico, finché non dimostra di averlo percepito. Sospendendo l'oggetto a un filo si evita che il bambino concentri la sua attenzione sulla mano e il braccio dell'esaminatore. È inoltre importante avere la certezza che il bambino abbia effettivamente visto l'oggetto, escludendo la possibilità che la risposta visiva sia stata determinata piuttosto da un rumore.

La **pupilla** è difficile da esaminare nei neonati prematuri, a causa della scarsa pigmentazione dell'iride e della resistenza all'apertura della palpebra. La pupilla reagisce alla luce entro la 29ª-32ª settimana di gestazione. La simmetria delle pupille, le dimensioni e la reattività possono essere influenzate da farmaci, da lesioni cerebrali che occupano uno spazio, da disturbi metabolici e da anomalie del mesencefalo o dei nervi ottici. Nella valutazione della pupilla, è importante notare la presenza di eterocromia o di macchie di Brushfield sull'iride.

La **sindrome di Horner** è caratterizzata da miosi, ptosi, endoftalmo e anidrosi omolaterale del volto. Può essere congenita o il risultato di una lesione che coinvolge il sistema nervoso simpatico a livello del tronco cerebrale, della colonna vertebrale cervicale o del plesso simpatico (in giustapposizione all'arteria carotide). La risposta pupillare a una serie di farmaci topici (cocaina, adrenalina, idrossiamfetamina e fenilefrina) contribuisce alla localizzazione della lesione nel sistema nervoso simpatico.

Nervi oculomotore (3), trocleare (4) e abducente (6). L'occhio si muove grazie ai muscoli extraoculari, innervati dai nervi oculomotore, trocleare e abducente. Il nervo oculomotore innerva i muscoli retto superiore, mediale e inferiore, l'obliquo inferiore e i muscoli elevatori della palpebra superiore. La completa **paralisi del nervo oculomotore** causa ptosi, dilatazione pupillare, deviazione dell'occhio verso l'esterno e in basso, compromissione dei movimenti di adduzione ed elevazione. Il **nervo trocleare** innerva il muscolo obliquo superiore, perciò la sua paralisi isolata provoca una deviazione verso l'alto o verso l'esterno dell'occhio, spesso associata all'inclinazione del capo, per compensare lo spostamento verticale delle immagini. Il **nervo abducente** innerva il muscolo retto laterale, perciò la sua paralisi isolata determina una deviazione mediale dell'occhio, con conseguente incapacità di abdurre oltre la linea mediana. Nel bambino più grande, il **test del vetro rosso** è utile per diagnosticare eventuali paralisi extraoculari. Coprendo uno degli occhi con il vetro colorato, si domanda al bambino di seguire una luce bianca che si sposta in varie direzioni nel campo visivo. Il paziente vede una sola luce rosso/bianca nella direzione della funzione muscolare normale, mentre percepisce una separazione tra le immagini rossa e bianca sul piano del muscolo danneggiato. L'**oftalmoplegia internucleare** è il risultato di una lesione del fascicolo longitudinale mediale del tronco cerebrale, responsabile di una paralisi della funzione del retto mediale dell'occhio adducente, con nistagmo limitato all'occhio abducente. Nell'**oftalmoplegia interna**, la pupilla è dilatata e non risponde alla luce né all'accomodazione, ma la funzione extraoculare è normale. Al contrario, l'**oftalmoplegia esterna** è associata a ptosi e paralisi di tutti i muscoli oculari, mentre la risposta pupillare è preservata. Il **nistagmo** consiste in un rapido movimento oculare, in direzione orizzontale, verticale, rotatoria, pendolare o mista. La scossa di nistagmo comprende una fase rapida e una fase lenta ed è di solito normale quando sia presente solo nello sguardo di estrema lateralità. Come regola generale, il nistagmo orizzontale si verifica in presenza di un'anomalia del labirinto periferico, di una lesione del sistema vestibolare a livello del tronco cerebrale o del cervelletto, oppure in seguito all'assunzione di alcuni farmaci (in particolare, la fenitoina). Il nistagmo verticale indica una disfunzione del tronco cerebrale o un'anomalia strutturale.

L'esame completo dei movimenti oculari può essere effettuato già durante la 25ª settimana di gestazione, utilizzando la **manovra dell'occhio di bambola**. Questa tecnica consente di verificare i movimenti oculari orizzontali e verticali in un lattante, in un bambino non collaborante o comatoso. Se la testa viene improvvisamente ruotata verso destra, gli occhi guardano a sinistra, in maniera simmetrica. Il movimento oculare nella direzione opposta è testato ruotando la testa verso sinistra. Analogamente, una rapida flessione ed estensione del capo consente di valutare il movimento in verticale. Lattanti e bambini sani seguono un oggetto interessante o un giocattolo in tutte le direzioni. Il test della luce intermittente consente di verificare tale abilità in un soggetto non cooperativo. L'esaminatore osserva la competenza e il flusso dei movimenti oculari e determina la presenza di nistagmo, diplopia, opsoclono (oscillazioni caotiche brusche degli occhi, spesso associate a neuroblastoma o infezioni virali), bobbing oculare brusco, spontaneo movimento degli occhi verso il basso con lento ritorno alle posizioni di riposo (associato a lesioni pontine) o altre anomalie della posizione oculare. Nei bambini prematuri, si nota spesso una mancanza di coordinazione oculare a riposo, con un occhio spostato orizzontalmente di 1-2 mm rispetto all'altro. Le deviazioni degli occhi sul piano verticale richiedono ulteriori indagini di approfondimento. Lo strabismo è discusso nel Capitolo 622.

Nervo trigemino (5). La distribuzione sensoriale del volto è suddivisa in tre aree: l'area oftalmica, l'area mascellare e quella mandibolare. Ciascuna regione può essere esaminata mediante il tatto o una leggera puntura e confrontata con il lato opposto. La risposta corneale di chiusura della palpebra si può ottenere toccando la cornea con un tampone di ovatta. Nei bambini prematuri, la tecnica ideale per esaminare la funzione del nervo trigemino consiste nell'osservare le smorfie del bambino in risposta alla stimolazione del viso con una leggera puntura (lontano dall'occhio) o delle narici con un cotton-fioc. L'assenza del riflesso può essere dovuta a un difetto sensoriale (nervo trigemino) o motorio (nervo facciale). Per valutare la funzione motoria, si procede all'esame dei muscoli massetere, pterigoide e temporale durante la masticazione e alla verifica del riflesso mandibolare.

Nervo facciale (7). La riduzione dei movimenti volontari della parte inferiore del volto, con appiattimento dell'angolo nasolabiale sul lato ipsilaterale, indica una lesione del motoneurone superiore o corticospinale sopranucleare. Una lesione del motoneurone inferiore tende piuttosto a coinvolgere in uguale misura i muscoli facciali superiori e inferiori. La paralisi del nervo facciale può essere congenita o secondaria a trauma, infezione (come la malattia di Lyme), tumore intracranico, leucemia, istiocitosi, malattia granulomatosa, ipertensione, esposizione a tossine o miastenia grave. Nel bambino cooperativo, è possibile esaminare il gusto nei tre quarti anteriori della lingua, collocando una soluzione salina o glucosio a lato della lingua protrusa. I bambini sani sono in grado di identificare la sostanza senza difficoltà.

Nervo acustico (8). L'esame uditivo costituisce una componente importante della valutazione neurologica, perché difficilmente i genitori si rendono conto della presenza di un deficit nel bambino (vedi Capitolo 636). I neonati normali interrompono brevemente la suzione quando l'esaminatore suona una campanella, ma la ripetizione dello stimolo non determina l'interruzione perché il lattante si abitua. In presenza di anomalie neurologiche, tale adattamento non si verifica. I bambini con udito nella norma ruotano il capo in direzione del suono di una campanella, di un sonaglio o di un foglio accartocciato e, entro i 3 mesi di età, guardano verso la sorgente del suono. I bambini con intelligenza normale e deficit uditivo manifestano allerta visiva e rispondono in maniera appropriata a stimoli fisici. I disturbi del linguaggio e la tendenza a fare i capricci costituiscono sintomi comuni in un bambino con deficit uditivo. In caso di sospetta perdita uditiva, è indispensabile procedere all'esame audiometrico o dei potenziali evocati uditivi nel tronco encefalico (vedi Capitolo 636). I fattori di rischio che suggeriscono l'opportunità di una valutazione della funzione uditiva nei primi mesi di vita includono: una storia familiare di sordità, prematurità, grave asfissia, l'uso di farmaci ototossici nel periodo neonatale, iperbilirubinemia, anomalie congenite della testa o del collo, meningite batterica e infezioni congenite dovute a rosolia, toxoplasmosi, herpes e Cytomegalovirus. I timori dei genitori costituiscono spesso un indicatore affidabile della compromissione acustica e suggeriscono perciò l'opportunità di procedere a una valutazione completa della funzione.

La funzione vestibolare può essere valutata mediante il **test calorico**, che prevede l'irrigazione (con una siringa) di 5 mL di acqua fredda nel canale uditivo esterno, mantenendo la testa del bambino elevata di 30° rispetto alla posizione orizzontale. Nei pazienti comatosi o in stato di ottundimento, ma con il tronco encefalico integro, si osserva una deviazione degli occhi verso il lato dello stimolo. Nei soggetti svegli e in stato di allerta, si inietta una quantità di acqua inferiore (0,5 mL). Nel bambino sano, l'introduzione del liquido provoca nistagmo, con la componente veloce in direzione opposta rispetto al labirinto stimolato. L'assenza di risposta implica una grave disfunzione del tronco encefalico e del fascicolo longitudinale mediale. Se l'esame otoscopico rivela la rottura della membrana del timpano, il test calorico non può essere eseguito.

Nervo glossofaringeo (9). Il nervo glossofaringeo innerva il muscolo stilofaringeo. Lesioni isolate di questo nervo craniale si riscontrano raramente. La sua funzione può essere esaminata osservando il riflesso di apertura della bocca in risposta alla stimolazione tattile della parete faringea posteriore. Il senso del gusto nel terzo posteriore della lingua è garantito dalla porzione sensoriale del nervo glossofaringeo.

Nervo vago (10). Una lesione unilaterale del nervo vago causa debolezza e asimmetria del palato molle ipsilaterale e una voce rauca dovuta alla paralisi di una corda vocale. Lesioni bilaterali possono provocare distress respiratorio, conseguente alla paralisi delle corde vocali, come pure rigurgito nasale di liquidi, accumulo di secrezioni e immobilità del palato molle. Una lesione isolata del nervo vago può subentrare nel postoperatorio di un intervento di tracheotomia, in seguito alla resezione del nervo laringeo ricorrente; tale lesione è comune nel periodo neonatale, in bambini affetti dalla malformazione di Chiari di tipo II. Se si sospetta una lesione che coinvolge il nervo vago, è necessario procedere alla visualizzazione delle corde vocali. Per testare il riflesso della tosse nel neonato/lattante, l'esaminatore applica una leggera pressione sulla trachea, a livello della fossetta soprasternale.

Nervo accessorio (11). La lesione del nervo accessorio provoca una paralisi e atrofia dei muscoli sternomastoideo e trapezio. Il muscolo sternomastoideo ha due origini (sternale e clavicolare) e può essere testato ruotando vigorosamente capo e collo contro la mano dell'esaminatore. Le più comuni condizioni patologiche responsabili della debolezza e atrofia di questi muscoli sono: la malattia dei motoneuroni, la distrofia miotonica e la miastenia grave.

Nervo ipoglosso (12). Il nervo ipoglosso innerva la lingua. L'esame della lingua include una valutazione della motilità, delle dimensioni e della forma, nonché una verifica della presenza di atrofia o di fascicolazione. Anomalie del nucleo ipoglosso o del nervo provocano ipotrofia, debolezza e fascicolazione della lingua. Se la lesione è bilaterale, la protrusione della lingua è impossibile e può riscontarsi disfagia. La malattia di Werdnig-Hoffmann (atrofia muscolare spinale infantile, o SMA di tipo 1) e anomalie congenite nella regione del forame magno costituiscono la principale causa di lesione del nervo ipoglosso.

ESAME MOTORIO. L'esame motorio implica la valutazione dell'integrità del sistema muscoloscheletrico e la verifica della presenza di movimenti anomali, che suggeriscono un disturbo del sistema nervoso periferico o del SNC. Gli aspetti da testare sono la forza e la massa muscolare, il tono, la postura, la locomozione e la motilità, i riflessi tendinei profondi e la presenza di riflessi arcaici.

Forza. La verifica della forza muscolare è piuttosto semplice nel bambino collaborativo, al quale si domanda di stringere le dita dell'esaminatore, flettere ed estendere polso e gomito, addurre e abdurre la spalla contro resistenza. La forza dei muscoli del cingolo scapolare è valutata reggendo il neonato/lattante sotto le ascelle; in presenza di debolezza, il bambino non riesce a sostenere il peso del corpo e scivola tra le mani dell'esaminatore. La forza distale è esaminata valutando la presa palmare e la capacità di manipolare oggetti. Tra i 3 e i 4 anni, il bambino sano è in grado di collaborare attivamente con l'esaminatore, estendendo e flettendo i muscoli del piede, del ginocchio e dell'anca. L'esame del cingolo pelvico e dei muscoli prossimali degli arti inferiori è eseguito osservando in bambino mentre sale le scale o si solleva dalla posizione prona. In presenza di debolezza, il bambino si aiuta con le mani per assumere la posizione eretta (*segno di Gowers*, Fig. 591-2). In caso di debolezza degli arti inferiori, si osserva una riduzione dell'attività spontanea e un'incapacità di sostenere il peso del corpo quando l'esaminatore lo solleva per le ascelle. Oltre a esaminare individualmente ciascun gruppo muscolare, è importante confrontare la forza tra arti superiori e inferiori, e fra lato destro e sinistro. Nel bambino collaborativo, la **forza muscolare** è classificata su di una scala da 0 a 5, nei termini seguenti: 0 = assenza di contrazione; 1 = traccia di contrazione; 2 = movimento attivo se si elimina la gravità; 3 = movimento attivo contro gravità; 4 = movimento attivo contro gravità e resistenza; 5 = potenza normale. L'esame della forza muscolare include la valutazione dei muscoli respiratori, mediante osservazione dell'azione dei muscoli intercostali, del movimento del diaframma e dell'uso dei muscoli accessori. È importante inoltre valutare la massa muscolare e la nutrizione. La debolezza può essere associata a atrofia muscolare e fascicolazioni. Poiché in molti bambini piccoli si riscontra un eccesso di grasso corporeo, la presenza di atrofia o fascicolazioni in questo gruppo di età è evidenziata più facilmente nella lingua denervata.

Tono. Il tono muscolare è valutato misurando il grado di resistenza opposta quando ciascuna articolazione è mobilizzata passivamente. Il tono si modifica nel corso della crescita. Il neonato o il prematuro appaiono relativamente ipotonici rispetto a un bambino. Il tono in questo gruppo di età può essere valutato con varie manovre (vedi Capitoli 94 e 97). Quando l'arto superiore del neonato a termine è spinto delicatamente verso il torace, il gomito normalmente non raggiunge il centro dello sterno (**segno della sciarpa**). Il gomito di un neonato ipotonico si estende facilmente oltre la linea mediana dello sterno. La misura dell'angolo popliteo è un utile metodo per documentare il tono degli arti inferiori nel neonato. L'esaminatore flette l'arto inferiore del bambino sull'addome ed estende il ginocchio. Nei neonati normali a termine, l'estensione massima del ginocchio è di circa 80°. Analogamente, il tono può essere testato flettendo anca e ginocchio a 90° e ruotando l'arto inferiore verso l'interno. Nei lattanti normali, il tallone non dovrebbe superare l'ombelico. Le più comuni anomalie del tono sono spasticità, rigidità e ipotonia.

La **spasticità** è caratterizzata da un'iniziale resistenza al movimento passivo, seguita da un improvviso rilascio, che determina un bloccaggio in estensione definito "fenomeno del **coltello a serramanico**". La spasticità è più evidente nei muscoli flessori degli arti superiori e negli estensori degli arti inferiori. È associata a iperreflessia tendinea, riflesso estensore plantare, clono, riduzione dei movimenti attivi e atrofia da non-uso. La presenza di **clono** può essere dimostrata negli arti inferiori, mediante improvvisa dorsiflessione del piede, con il ginocchio parzialmente flesso. Nel neonato, 5-10 contrazioni costituiscono un riscontro normale, a meno che le contratture non siano asimmetriche. La spasticità è il risultato di una lesione che coinvolge i motoneuroni superiori, può essere unilaterale o bilaterale. La **rigidità**, dovuta a una lesione dei gangli basali, è caratterizzata da una costante resistenza al movimento passivo dei muscoli estensori e flessori. Se gli arti sono sottoposti a movimento passivo, si riscontra il tipico fenomeno della **ruota dentata**, causato dalla sovrapposizione di un tremore extrapiramidale alla rigidità. Al contrario di quanto avviene nella spasticità, la rigidità persiste nonostante la ripetizione di estensione e flessione e non si riscontra alcun rilascio della tensione. I bambini con spasticità degli arti inferiori tendono a trascinare le gambe quando gattonano oppure camminano sulle punte. I pazienti con marcata spasticità o rigidità manifestano una postura

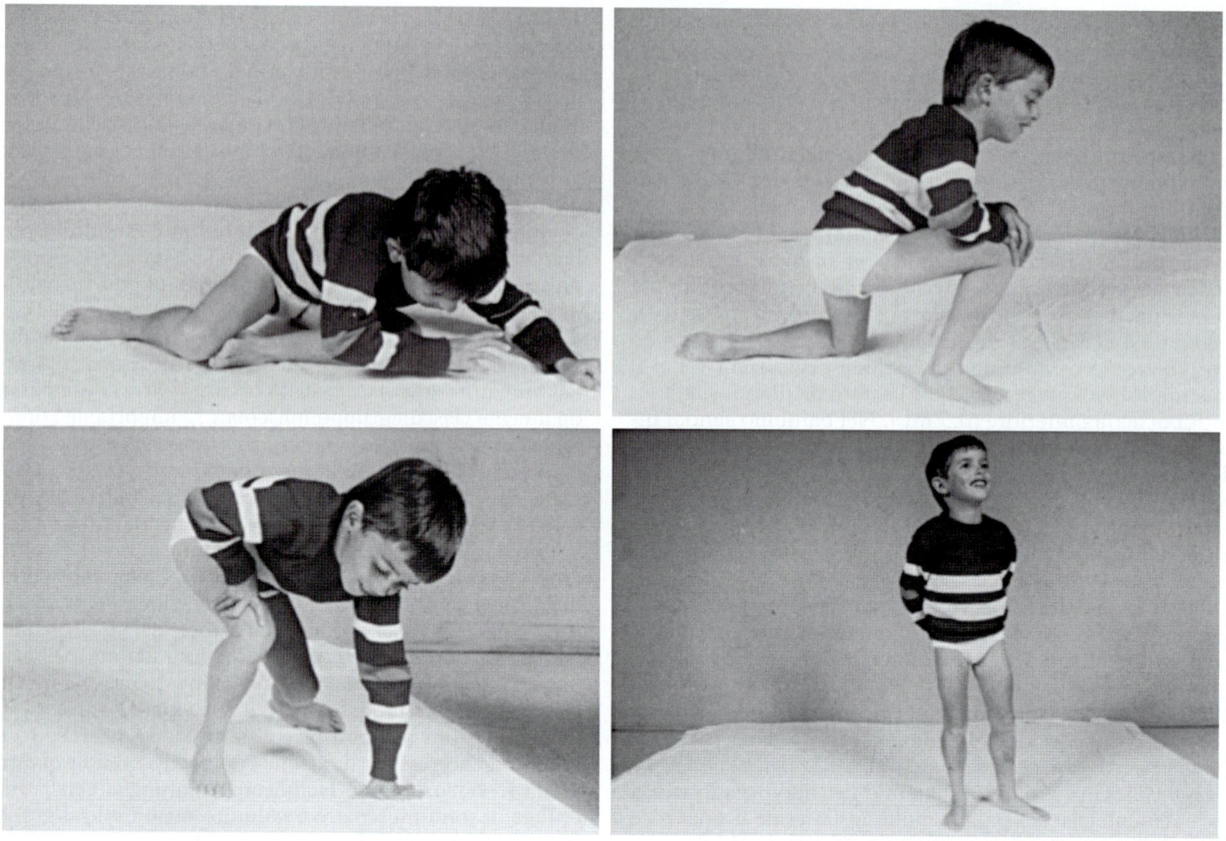

Figura 591-2. Segno di Gowers. Bambino con debolezza del cingolo pelvico dovuto alla distrofia muscolare di Duchenne.

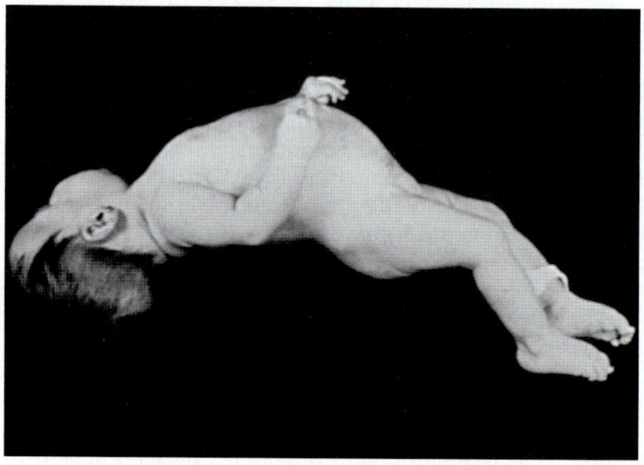

Figura 591-3. Opistotono in un lattante con lesioni cerebrali.

in **opistotono**, con dorsiflessione di capo e piedi e anteroflessione del tronco (Fig. 591-3). La **rigidità decerebrata** è caratterizzata da una marcata estensione degli arti, causata da una disfunzione o lesione del tronco encefalico a livello dei collicoli superiori. L'**ipotonia**, cioè la riduzione patologica del tono, costituisce la più comune anomalia del tono nei neonati prematuri o a termine che presentano una compromissione neurologica. La presenza di ipotonia può riflettere una patologia degli emisferi cerebrali, del cervelletto, del midollo spinale, delle cellule della cornea anteriori, dei nervi periferici, delle giunzioni mioneurali o dei muscoli. Una postura insolita è il risultato di un'anomalia del tono. Il lattante ipotonico appare **flaccido** e, quando è seduto, fatica a sostenere la testa e a mantenere la schiena eretta. In posizione supina, assume la tipica posizione "a rana", e durante la trazione si nota un significativo ritardo della testa. A 28 settimane, i neonati prematuri tendono a estendere gli arti a riposo, ma entro la 32ª settimana si osserva una flessione, in particolare degli arti inferiori. La postura normale di un neonato a termine è caratterizzata dalla flessione di tutti e quattro gli arti.

Motilità e locomozione. I bambini prematuri (<32ª settimana di gestazione) manifestano movimenti casuali, lenti e contorti, alternati ad attività rapide di tipo mioclonico degli arti. Oltre la 32ª settimana, l'attività motoria è prevalentemente flessoria. L'osservazione dei bambini più grandi nell'atto di gattonare, camminare e correre può rivelare la presenza di disturbi del movimento, che nella maggior parte dei casi tendono a scomparire a riposo o durante il sonno. L'**atassia** consiste in una mancanza di coordinazione dei movimenti o in disturbo dell'equilibrio. Può essere limitata agli altri o coinvolgere prevalentemente il tronco. L'atassia del tronco, causata dal coinvolgimento del verme cerebellare, è caratterizzata da instabilità nella posizione eretta o seduta. Anomalie degli emisferi cerebellari provocano tipicamente tremore intenzionale, non alterato dall'attenzione visiva. La presenza di atassia può essere dimostrata mediante i test indicenaso e tallone-tibia, verificando la capacità di camminare in tandem e punta-tacco, oppure, nei lattanti, osservando la capacità di raggiungere e afferrare un giocattolo. Anomalie addizionali associate alle lesioni cerebellari includono la dismetria (errori nella capacità di valutare le distanze), il rebound (incapacità di inibire un'azione muscolare, come quando l'esaminatore lascia andare improvvisamente il braccio flesso, e il paziente si colpisce il volto inavvertitamente) e l'adiadococinesia (ridotta efficacia dei movimenti alternati rapidi). Ipotonia, disartria, nistagmo e iperreflessia tendinea sono di comune riscontro in presenza di anomalie cerebellari. L'atassia sensoriale è associata a malattie del midollo spinale e dei nervi periferici. In questi disturbi il **segno di Romberg** è positivo (instabilità a occhi chiusi, ma non a occhi aperti) e vi sono spesso associate anomalie della posizione delle articolazioni e del senso della vibrazione.

La **corea** è caratterizzata da movimenti irregolari, rapidi e involontari delle principali articolazioni, del tronco e del volto. I bambini affetti sono incapaci di estendere le braccia senza produrre movimenti anomali. Manifestano la tendenza alla pronazione delle braccia sollevate al di sopra del capo. Contraggono e rilassano incessantemente il pugno (**segno della mungitrice**) e presentano un linguaggio confuso e inarticolato; si osserva una perdita dei riflessi tendinei profondi patellari e una difficoltà a mantenere in protrusione la lingua. L'**atetosi** consiste in movimenti lenti e contorti, spesso associati ad anomalie del tono muscolare. È più evidente a livello distale degli arti ed è aggravata dall'attività volontaria o dallo stress emotivo. Può coinvolgere anche il linguaggio e la deglutizione. Corea e atetosi sono il risultato di lesioni dei gangli basali e risultano piuttosto difficili da distinguere sul piano clinico. I due disturbi possono coesistere in uno stesso paziente. La **distonia** consiste in lente contorsioni involontarie che coinvolgono principalmente i muscoli prossimali degli arti, il tronco e il collo. I **tic motori** sono caratterizzati da brevi e improvvisi movimenti, solitamente sopprimibili e preceduti da una sensazione premonitrice di disagio o di tensione. I tic più comuni includono ammiccamenti, torsioni del collo, rapide alzate di spalle, smorfie.

Riflessi tendinei profondi e risposta plantare. I riflessi tendinei profondi sono facilmente evocati nella maggior parte dei lattanti e bambini. Nei nati a termine e prematuri, i riflessi più attendibili sono dati dai bicipiti, dai patellari e dall'achilleo. Sono valutati in una scala da 0 (assenza del riflesso) a 4 (marcata iperattività), con il punteggio 2 indicativo della normalità. Il riflesso tendineo achilleo, più difficile da dimostrare, è sollecitato percuotendo con il martelletto il tallone di Achille, con il piede in dorsiflessione. La stimolazione del riflesso patellare del ginocchio può provocare una **risposta crociata degli adduttori**, causando la contrazione dell'arto opposto; se presente, tale risposta non deve essere considerata anomala fino ai 6-7 mesi di età. I riflessi tendinei profondi risultano assenti o ridotti nei disturbi primari dei muscoli (miopatia), dei nervi (neuropatia), della giunzione mioneurale e nelle anomalie cerebellari. Nelle lesioni dei motoneuroni superiori si osserva tipicamente iperreflessia. L'asimmetria di questi riflessi suggerisce una lesione lateralizzata. La risposta plantare è ottenuta mediante stimolazione della porzione esterna della pianta del piede, partendo dal tallone e procedendo verso la base delle dita. Un metodo utile per ottenere la risposta consiste nell'esercitare una ferma pressione con il pollice. Il **riflesso di Babinski**, che indica una lesione dei motoneuroni superiori, è caratterizzato dall'estensione dell'alluce, con contemporaneo allargamento a ventaglio delle altre dita. Una stimolazione eccessivamente vigorosa può causare una reazione di fuga, erroneamente diagnosticabile come segno di Babinski. La maggior parte dei neonati mostra una iniziale flessione dell'alluce in seguito a stimolazione plantare. Come negli adulti, l'asimmetria della risposta plantare tra gli arti costituisce un utile segno di lateralizzazione.

Riflessi arcaici. I riflessi arcaici compaiono e scompaiono in sequenza durante fasi specifiche dello sviluppo (Tab. 591-2). La loro assenza o persistenza oltre un dato periodo segnala una disfunzione del SNC. Alcuni riflessi arcaici, come il **"rooting"** o **riflesso di ricerca** (se si stimola la pelle intorno alla bocca, il neonato gira il viso per trovare il capezzolo), ricompaiono nella vecchiaia o in presenza di specifiche malattie degenerative che coinvolgono la corteccia cerebrale. I più importanti riflessi arcaici sono quello di Moro, il riflesso di prensione palmare, il riflesso tonico del collo e quello del paracadute. Il **riflesso di Moro** è suscitato con il neonato in posizione semieretta; il capo viene lasciato ricadere all'indietro per un istante, per poi essere prontamente sostenuto con la mano dall'esaminatore; il bambino abduce ed estende simmetricamente le braccia e flette i pollici; segue un movimento di flessione e adduzione delle braccia. Una risposta asimmetrica può indicare una frattura della clavicola, una lesione del plesso brachiale o un'emiparesi. L'assenza del riflesso di Moro in un neonato a termine è un segno infausto, che segnala una seria disfunzione del SNC. Il **riflesso di prensione palmare** è suscitato collocando un dito o un oggetto nel palmo aperto di ciascuna mano. Il neonato normale afferra l'oggetto e stringe il pugno quando l'esaminatore tenta di rimuoverlo. Il **riflesso tonico del collo** è prodotto ruotando manualmente la testa da un lato, con il bambino in posizione supina. Nel lato del corpo corrispondente alla direzione del volto si osserva l'estensione dell'arto, mentre gli arti controlaterali si flettono. Una risposta tonica obbligatoria, che blocca il bambino nella posizione dello schermitore, segnala invariabilmente un disturbo del SNC. Il **riflesso del paracadute** è dimostrato sospendendo il neonato per il tronco e mimando un'improvvisa flessione in avanti, come se stesse per cadere. Il bambino reagisce spontaneamente estendendo gli arti superiori come per un meccanismo protettivo. Questo meccanismo protettivo compare prima che il bambino cominci a camminare.

TABELLA 591-2. Durata dei riflessi arcaici

RIFLESSO	ESORDIO	PIENO SVILUPPO	DURATA
Presa palmare	28ª settimana	32ª settimana	2-3 mesi
Rooting	32ª settimana	36ª settimana	Meno marcato dopo il primo mese
Moro	28ª-32ª settimana	37ª settimana	5-6 mesi
Tonico del collo	35ª settimana	1 mese	6-7 mesi
Paracadute	7-8 mesi	10-11 mesi	Resta per sempre

ESAME DELLA SENSIBILITÀ. L'esame della sensibilità è difficile da eseguire sul lattante o su un bambino non collaborativo. Ma anche i bambini disposti a cooperare si stancano presto di prove che prevedono una mutevole attenzione per compiti ripetitivi e monotoni. L'abilità del medico nel trasformare questa parte dell'esame in un gioco favorisce dunque la cooperazione. I disturbi a carico del sistema sensoriale sono meno comuni nella popolazione pediatrica rispetto agli adulti. Mentre il lattante è distratto dal genitore o da un giocattolo, l'esaminatore lo tocca con un cotton-fioc o un abbassalingua. I bambini sani dimostrano una consapevolezza dello stimolo, interrompendo per un attimo il gioco, ritirando gli arti, piangendo o guardando e toccando l'area stimolata. Purtroppo, il lattante si stanca facilmente e si disinteressa dell'esaminatore molto in fretta. Per studiare accuratamente un'area critica, può essere perciò necessario ripetere la prova a distanza di tempo.

L'identificazione del livello sensoriale associato a una **lesione del midollo spinale** può risultare molto difficile nel lattante. Talvolta l'osservazione suggerisce una differenza di colore, temperatura o perspirazione, con cute più fredda, o asciutta, al di sotto del livello della lesione spinale. Toccando delicatamente la cute al di sopra del livello della lesione spinale, viene suscitata una risposta, solitamente una contorsione o un movimento di fuga. I **riflessi addominali superficiali** possono essere assenti. In caso di lesione del midollo spinale, può manifestarsi incontinenza dello sfintere e ano beante, che si manifesta con assenza di contrazione dello sfintere anale in seguito a stimolazione della cute perianale con un oggetto appuntito, assenza di contrazione anale durante l'esame rettale. Nei maschi, è utile verificare la presenza del riflesso cremasterico. I bambini tra i 4 e i 5 anni sono in grado di partecipare attivamente all'esame della sensibilità, che prevede la verifica delle seguenti sensazioni: posizione articolare, vibrazione, temperatura, stereognosi, discriminazione tra due punti, estinzione doppia simultanea, tocco leggero e dolore. Il buon esito dell'esame dipende in gran parte dall'abilità e pazienza dell'esaminatore.

ANDATURA E POSTURA ERETTA. L'osservazione dell'andatura del bambino costituisce una componente importante dell'esame neurologico. L'andatura **spastica** è caratterizzata da rigidità; il bambino cammina a grandi falcate, come un soldatino di latta, oppure cammina sulle punte a causa di contratture del tendine di Achille. L'**emiparesi** è associata a una riduzione dell'ampiezza del movimento dell'arto superiore del lato colpito e da un movimento circolare laterale della gamba (circonduzione). I movimenti extrapiramidali, come la distonia o la corea, possono evidenziarsi quando il bambino cammina o corre. L'**atassia cerebellare** causa un'andatura instabile e a base allargata; nei casi più gravi, il bambino ha bisogno di un sostegno per non cadere. I pazienti con compromissione cerebellare presentano una ridotta capacità di camminare in tandem e punta-tacco. La debolezza del cingolo pelvico prossimale determina un'andatura ondeggiante (o anserina). I bambini colpiti tendono a sviluppare una lordosi compensatoria e fanno fatica a salire le scale. La debolezza o ipotonia degli arti inferiori può causare *genu recurvatum* e piedi piatti, con conseguente andatura goffa e incerta. Anche la scoliosi, risultato di un disturbo muscolare o del midollo spinale, può determinare un'andatura anomala.

ESAME GENERALE

L'esame fisico di altri sistemi di organi è una componente essenziale della valutazione neurologica. Lesioni cutanee suggeriscono una sindrome neuromuscolare (vedi Capitolo 596); l'epatosplenomegalia indica un errore congenito del metabolismo, una glicogenosi, l'HIV o un tumore maligno; caratteristiche dismorfiche indicano varie sindromi (vedi Capitolo 108). La presenza di soffio cardiaco può indicare febbre reumatica (corea), sclerosi tuberosa (rabdomioma cardiaco), ascesso cerebrale o trombosi (malattia cardiaca cianotica) o occlusione vascolare cerebrale (endocardite). È inoltre opportuno verificare, mediante palpazione, la presenza di linfoadenopatie o anomalie della tiroide.

SEGNI NEUROLOGICI MINORI. Questi segni devono essere interpretati con cautela, perché si evidenziano anche nei bambini normali in vari stadi dello sviluppo. I segni neurologici minori, detti anche "soft", sono suggeriti da risultati che si discostano dalla norma in alcuni specifici test motori o sensoriali. Verificarne la presenza richiede l'osservazione della performance del bambino in una serie di compiti motori a tempo, confrontando poi la qualità e precisione del movimento con il rendimento di controlli normali dello stesso sesso ed età. L'esame deve includere test di verifica della capacità di eseguire movimenti ripetitivi con le dita in rapida successione, di battere le mani e i piedi, di compiere movimenti di supinazione e di pronazione, di saltare e di camminare in tandem. A seconda dell'età, del sesso e della maturazione del sistema nervoso, si riscontra una grande variabilità nell'espressione di questi segni. Movimenti coreoatetosici minimi delle dita, con il braccio in estensione, sono normali a 4 anni, ma scompaiono entro i 7-8 anni. Lo sviluppo neurologico delle femmine risulta accelerato rispetto a quello dei maschi per la maggior parte dei compiti motori come saltellare, saltare la corda o eseguire manovre che richiedono equilibrio. Bambini con un livello intellettivo nella norma possono manifestare un segno neurologico minimo, ma la presenza di due o più segni persistenti è correlata significativamente alla presenza di una disfunzione neurologica (come un deficit di attenzione, un disturbo dell'apprendimento o una paralisi cerebrale). Poiché i segni neurologici minimi non vengono di solito associati a particolari disabilità, ma possono riscontrarsi anche nel bambino normale, non è opportuno etichettare con diagnosi improprie un paziente che manifesta alcuni di tali segni. Si raccomanda piuttosto di monitorare lo sviluppo del bambino, verificando l'eventuale insorgenza di un disturbo evolutivo.

PROCEDURE DIAGNOSTICHE PARTICOLARI

PUNTURA LOMBARE ED ESAME DEL LIQUIDO CEREBROSPINALE. L'esame della composizione del liquido cerebrospinale (LCS) è essenziale per confermare la diagnosi di meningite, encefalite ed emorragia subaracnoidea; contribuisce inoltre alla valutazione della presenza di malattie demielinizzanti, degenerative o connettiviti/vasculiti, cellule tumorali nello spazio subaracnoideo. Costituisce infine il test di elezione per la diagnosi di "pseudotumor cerebri". Per portare a termine con successo la procedura, la preparazione del paziente è fondamentale. Un infermiere esperto svolge un ruolo essenziale nel posizionare, immobilizzare e confortare il paziente. Dopo aver preparato la cute con un disinfettante, il soggetto è collocato in posizione di decubito laterale e coperto con teli sterili. Il medico indossa camice, mascherina e guanti. L'assistente provvede a flettere collo e gambe del paziente, in modo da allargare gli spazi intervertebrali. Gli spazi ideali per la puntura lombare (PL) sono L3-L4 oppure L4-L5, determinati tracciando una linea orizzontale immaginaria tra una spina iliaca anteriore superiore e l'altra. La cute e il tessuto sottocutaneo sono anestetizzati con un anestetico locale o applicando sulla pelle, 30 minuti prima della procedura, una mistura eutettica di anestetici locali composta da lidocaina e prilocaina (EMLA). Si introduce sul piano mediosagittale un ago spinale a punta smussa da 22 G con mandrino, orientandolo leggermente in direzione cefalica. Il mandrino è rimosso di frequente a mano a mano che l'ago avanza lentamente, per determinare la presenza dell'LCS. Quando l'ago penetra nella dura ed entra nello spazio subaracnoideo, si percepisce uno schiocco. Per ottenere la pressione di apertura, si utilizza un manometro e un rubinetto a tre vie. La pressione di apertura in posizione di decubito e rilassata è di circa 100 mm di acqua; in decubito laterale in flessione, il range è di 60-180 mm. La pressione di apertura è molto più elevata in un bambino non cooperativo, che piange e si dimena. La pressione è misurata con il bambino in posizione confortevole, con il capo e le gambe in estensione. È opportuno che i neonati gravemente malati rimangano in posizione eretta, perché la riduzione della ventilazione e le anomalie della perfusione responsabili di arresto cardiaco sono più comuni nella posizione di decubito laterale in questo gruppo di età.

Le **controindicazioni** per l'esecuzione della PL includono: (1) aumento dell'ICP dovuto a una sospetta lesione con presenza di una massa cerebrale o nel midollo spinale; (2) sintomi e segni di imminente erniazione cerebrale in un bambino con probabile meningite; (3) malattia grave in condizioni critiche (in rari casi); (4) infezione cutanea nel sito della PL; (5) trombocitopenia.

1. Nel primo caso, la procedura rischia di determinare un'erniazione transtentorale o delle tonsille cerebellari. L'ispezione del fondo oculare per ricerca di papilledema e una TC cerebrale sono indispensabili prima di procedere alla PL.
2. Nel secondo caso, i sintomi e segni includono una postura decerebrata o decorticata, convulsioni toniche generalizzate, anomalie nelle dimensioni e reattività pupillare, con assenza di risposta oculocefalica e deviazione oculomotoria fissa. L'imminente erniazione è associata anche ad anomalie respiratorie, tra cui iperventilazione, respiro di Cheyne-Stokes, respiro atassico, apnea e arresto respiratorio. In questi casi, il bambino deve essere trattato immediatamente con antibiotici per via endovenosa e misure atte a ridurre l'ICP. Prima di poter procedere alla PL, è opportuno il ricovero in terapia intensiva, per la stabilizzazione e per effettuare studi di imaging. La PL costituisce la procedura diagnostica di elezione nei casi di sospetta meningite batterica, in assenza di sepsi galoppante o shock o di segni e sintomi di erniazione cerebrale.
3. Nel terzo caso, la procedura è temporaneamente sospesa, perché le condizioni particolarmente critiche del paziente comportano un elevato rischio di arresto cardiorespiratorio. In tali circostanze, si preferisce effettuare un prelievo per emocoltura e sottoporre il paziente a terapia antibiotica, procedendo alla PL solo successivamente alla stabilizzazione clinica.
4. Nel quarto caso, se l'esame dell'LCS è urgente malgrado l'infezione nel sito della PL, un medico esperto può eseguire una puntura ventricolare o della cisterna magna.
5. Nel quinto caso, una trombocitopenia con conta piastrinica $<20 \times 10^9$/L può causare un'emorragia incontrollata negli spazi subaracoideo o subdurale. Dunque, la PL non è indicata fino al miglioramento dei valori, mediante infusione piastrinica.

L'LCS normale è incolore come l'acqua e contiene fino a 5 globuli bianchi/mm^3 (che sale a 5 globuli bianchi/mm^3 nel neonato). Un'elevata concentrazione di globuli bianchi o rossi determina un aspetto torbido. La presenza di polimorfonucleati (PMN) nel bambino è sempre anomala e alimenta il sospetto di un processo patologico in atto, mentre nel neonato possono raggiungere la concentrazione di 1-2/mm^3. Un'elevata conta delle PMN può indicare una meningite batterica o la fase iniziale della meningite asettica (vedi Capitolo 602). La linfocitosi dell'LCS indica: una meningite fungina, asettica o tubercolare; una malattia demielinizzante; un tumore cerebrale o midollare; un disturbo immunologico, compresa una connettivite/vasculite; un'irritazione chimica (causata da mielografia o da metotrexato intratecale).

La colorazione Gram dell'LCS è fondamentale in caso di sospetta meningite batterica, mentre per confermare la diagnosi di meningite fungina o tubercolare si utilizzano colorazioni acido-resistenti o inchiostro d'India. Il liquor è posto in un apposito mezzo di coltura, stabilito sulla base dei reperti clinici e delle analisi dell'LCS. Se l'anamnesi e l'esame clinico ne indicano l'opportunità, una porzione dell'LCS è sottoposta a esami virali (PCR o ricerca di anticorpi specifici), per l'individuazione di HSV1 e 2, West Nile Virus ed enterovirus.

L'LCS normale non contiene globuli rossi. La loro presenza suggerisce una puntura traumatica o un'emorragia subaracnoidea. In presenza di sangue, l'LCS deve essere immediatamente centrifugato. Il supernatante è solitamente limpido, ma risulta xantocromico in presenza di emorragia subaracnoidea. In caso di puntura traumatica, si nota un progressivo schiarimento del liquido durante la raccolta. La presenza di schistociti crenati non consente la differenziazione tra una puntura traumatica e un'emorragia subaracnoidea. La xantocromia può essere causata anche da iperbilirubinemia, carotenemia e da un marcato aumento della concentrazione di proteine.

In condizioni normali, il livello proteico nell'LCS del bambino è compreso tra 10 e 40 mg/dL, mentre può raggiungere i 120 mg/dL nel neonato. Il calo si verifica entro i 3 mesi di età. La concentrazione di proteine può risultare elevata in presenza di diversi processi patologici, come infezioni, malattie immunologiche, vascolari o degenerative, tumori cerebrali e midollari. In seguito a puntura traumatica, il livello di proteine sale fino a circa 1 mg/dL ogni 1000 RBCs/mm^3. L'aumento delle immunoglobuline G (IgG), che normalmente rappresentano circa il 10% delle proteine totali, si osserva nella panencefalite sclerosante subacuta, nell'encefalomielite postinfettiva e in alcuni casi di sclerosi multipla. Se si sospetta la diagnosi di sclerosi multipla, è opportuno ricercare la presenza di bande oligoclonali nell'LCS.

Nel bambino sano, la glicorrachia è pari a circa il 60% della glicemia. In caso di sospetta meningite, per prevenire un falso aumento del rapporto tra glucosio nel sangue e nell'LCS, si raccomanda di effettuare il prelievo di sangue prima della PL, quando il bambino è relativamente calmo. L'ipoglicorrachia si riscontra in associazione a malattia meningitica, in particolare batterica o tubercolare. L'aumento della glicemia può essere determinato anche da un diffuso coinvolgimento neoplastico delle meningi, un'emorragia subaracnoidea, una meningite fungina e, in alcuni casi, una meningite asettica.

È possibile inoltre ricercare nell'LCS antigeni specifici (test di agglutinazione al lattice per sospetta meningite) e metaboliti (lattato, amminoacidi, enolasi), per escludere una serie di malattie metaboliche.

PUNTURA SUBDURALE. Questa procedura, indicata per stabilire la diagnosi di versamento subdurale o ematoma, prevede l'utilizzo di un ago da 20 G con mandrino a punta smussa. Lo spazio subdurale è raggiunto dal bordo laterale della fontanella anteriore, oppure lungo il margine superiore della sutura coronale, mantenendosi almeno a 2-3 cm dalla linea mediana, per evitare lesioni del sottostante seno sagittale. Dopo un'adeguata preparazione della cute del sito chirurgico (che include la rasatura), il paziente è sistemato in posizione supina e trattenuto con fermezza dall'assistente. Dopo l'applicazione di un anestetico locale, si procede all'inserimento di ago e mandrino, fatti avanzare lentamente attraverso la cute e il tessuto sottocutaneo con un movimento "a zig zag", finché non si percepisce uno schiocco che segnala l'ingresso nella dura. Si raccomanda un'estrema cautela nell'evitare di perforare con l'ago la corteccia cerebrale, che nel lattante si trova a circa 1,5 cm dalla superficie cutanea. Per aumentare il margine di sicurezza, è opportuno applicare un perno a 5-7 mm dalla punta smussa dell'ago. Il liquido subdurale, che sotto pressione può schizzare fuori, è raccolto e inviato per l'analisi delle proteine, la conta cellulare e la coltura. La colorazione del liquido può essere xantocromica, rosso brillante o marrone-oleosa (a seconda dell'età delle raccolte subdurali). Può essere indicata una puntura bilaterale. La quantità di liquidi prelevata con le punture non dovrebbe superare un totale di 15-20 mL per ciascun lato, per evitare il sanguinamento dovuto a un improvviso spostamento del contenuto intracranico. Al termine della procedura, si applica una medicazione sterile e il bambino è sistemato in posizione seduta, per prevenire la perdita di liquido dal sito della puntura (vedi il Capitolo 602 per i dettagli del liquido subdurale associato a meningite).

PUNTURA VENTRICOLARE. La puntura ventricolare è una procedura utilizzata per la rimozione di LCS in caso di aumento potenzialmente fatale dell'ICP, associato a idrocefalo, successivamente al fallimento delle misure conservative. Il pediatra è autorizzato a ricorrere a questa procedura soltanto se non è disponibile un neurochirurgo e in presenza di un rischio immediato per il paziente. Nel neonato, la procedura è analoga alla puntura subdurale. Un ago ventricolare da 20 G con mandrino è inserito nel bordo laterale della fontanella anteriore, e orientato in direzione del canto interno dell'occhio ipsilaterale. L'ago è fatto avanzare lentamente e il mandrino è rimosso frequentemente, per determinare la presenza dell'LCS. Solitamente il ventricolo si incontra circa 4 cm dalla superficie cutanea.

PROCEDURE NEURORADIOLOGICHE. La radiografia del cranio può essere utile in alcuni casi, dimostrando la presenza di fratture, calcificazioni intracraniche, craniosinostosi, anomalie congenite, difetti ossei o un aumento dell'ICP. Un aumento acuto dell'ICP è caratterizzato da diastasi delle suture, mentre la presenza di ipertensione intracranica di vecchia data è segnalata dall'erosione dei processi clinoidei posteriori, allargamento della sella turcica e aumento dei solchi delle circonvoluzioni.

La **tomografia computerizzata (TC)** è un'importante procedura diagnostica, rapida e non invasiva, che utilizza i raggi X. Nei lattanti e bambini piccoli è necessario ricorrere alla sedazione, perché è fondamentale mantenere la testa ben ferma durante l'esame. La somministrazione per via intramuscolare di 4 mg/kg di pentobarbital 30 minuti prima della procedura (e, se necessario, di una dose supplementare di 2 mg/kg 1-1½ dopo) è solitamente efficace. Un metodo alternativo consiste nella somministrazione orale, 45 minuti prima della procedura, di 50-75 mg/kg di cloralio idrato. La TC è utile per dimostrare la presenza di malformazioni cerebrali congenite, idrocefalo e cisti porencefaliche, raccolte subdurali, atrofia cerebrale, calcificazioni intracraniche, ematoma intracerebrale, tumori e aree edematose, infarto e demielinizzazione (Tab. 591-3). L'iniezione per via endovenosa di un mezzo di contrasto esalta le aree di aumentata permeabilità vascolare dovute ad anomalie della barriera ematoencefalica (come ascessi o tumori) ed evidenzia la presenza di vasi sanguigni anomali nei casi di malformazione arteriovenosa.

La **risonanza magnetica (RM)** è una procedura non invasiva, particolarmente utile per lo studio di neoplasie, edema cerebrale, ictus acuto (RM pesata in diffusione), demielinizzazione, malattie degenerative e anomalie congenite, in particolare a carico della fossa posteriore e del midollo spinale (vedi Tab. 591-3). La RM riesce a rilevare la presenza di piccole placche in pazienti con sclerosi multipla e di aree di gliosi localizzata nei bambini con convulsioni incontrollate. Tale tecnica è utilizzata di routine nella valutazione dei candidati per la terapia chirurgica dell'epilessia. La RM non riesce a individuare la presenza di calcificazioni intracerebrali. L'utilizzo dell'agente di contrasto gadolinio-DTPA è utile per evidenziare lesioni associate a difetti della barriera ematoencefalica. **L'angio-RM** e **la flebografia-RM** forniscono immagini dettagliate delle principali strutture vascolari intracraniche e contribuiscono alla diagnosi di ictus, malformazioni vascolari o trombosi del seno venoso cerebrale. La **RM funzionale (f-RM)** consente di visualizzare ad alta risoluzione i cambiamenti

TABELLA 591-3. Procedure di imaging nelle malattie neurologiche

MALATTIA NEUROLOGICA	PROCEDURA DI IMAGING
Infarto ischemico cerebrale o cerebellare	TC nelle prime 12-24 ore; RM dopo 12-24 ore (la RM pesata in diffusione e perfusione aumenta i reperti, in particolare dopo le prime 24 ore, ma anche prima di 8 ore)
Emorragia cerebrale o cerebellare	TC nelle prime 24 ore; RM dopo 24 ore; RM e angiografia endovascolare per sospetta malformazione arterovenosa
Attacco ischemico transitorio	RM per identificare lesioni lacunari o piccole lesioni di altro tipo; ecografia delle arterie carotidi; angio-RM
Malformazione arteriovenosa	TC per emorragia acuta; RM e angiografia endovascolare il prima possibile
Aneurisma cerebrale	TC per emorragia acuta subaracnoidea; angiografia TC o endovascolare per identificare l'aneurisma; TCD per evidenziare vasospasmo
Tumore cerebrale	RM con e senza iniezione di mezzo di contrasto
Trauma craniocerebrale	TC; RM dopo l'iniziale valutazione e trattamento
Sclerosi multipla	RM con e senza iniezione di mezzo di contrasto
Meningite o encefalite	TC con e senza iniezione di mezzo di contrasto; RM dopo l'iniziale valutazione e trattamento
Ascesso cerebrale o cerebellare	TC con e senza iniezione di mezzo di contrasto per la diagnosi iniziale; se il paziente è stabile, RM invece della TC; in seguito, RM con e senza iniezione di mezzo di contrasto
Granuloma	RM con e senza iniezione di mezzo di contrasto
Demenza	RM; PET; SPECT
Disturbi motori	RM; PET
Disturbi neonatali e dello sviluppo	Ecografia nei neonati prematuri instabili; altrimenti RM
Epilessia	RM; PET; SPECT
Mal di testa	TC in pazienti con sospetto disturbo organico

PET, *Positron Emission Tomography* (tomografia a emissione di positroni); SPECT, *Single-Photon Emission Computed Tomography* (tomografia computerizzata a emissione di un fotone singolo); TCD, *TransCranial Doppler Ultrasonography* (eco Doppler transcranica).
Tratta da Gilman S: Imaging the brain. *N Engl J Med* 1998;338:812-820.

emodinamici prodotti dall'attività cerebrale localizzata durante specifiche funzioni cognitive o sensomotorie; questa tecnica è particolarmente promettente per l'indagine dello sviluppo della plasticità di tali funzioni.

L'**imaging con radionuclidi** prevede l'utilizzo di un materiale radioattivo (come ^{99}Tc) che si concentra nelle regioni dove la barriera ematoencefalica risulta danneggiata. È utile per la diagnosi di encefalite erpetica e ascesso cerebrale. La **tomografia a emissione di positroni** (*Position Emission Tomography*, PET) fornisce preziose informazioni sul metabolismo cerebrale e la perfusione, misurando il flusso sanguigno, l'uptake di ossigeno e il consumo di glucosio. Questa tecnica, molto costosa, in passato riservata agli adulti, è utilizzata sempre più spesso in centri pediatrici, in particolare se dispongono di programmi per la terapia chirurgica dell'epilessia. La **tomografia computerizzata a emissione di un fotone singolo** (*Single-Photon Emission Computed Tomography*, SPECT), che utilizza ^{99m}Tc esametil-propilene-amino-ossima (^{99m}Tc-HMPAO), costituisce una tecnica affidabile e poco costosa per esaminare il flusso cerebrale regionale. È particolarmente utile nell'indagine delle malattie vascolari nei bambini (come il lupus eritematoso sistemico), nella diagnosi dell'encefalite erpetica e nella localizzazione di scariche epilettiformi focali e tumori cerebrali ricorrenti. L'**angiografia cerebrale** è riservata allo studio dei disturbi vascolari. Nella maggior parte dei bambini, questa procedura richiede la somministrazione di un anestetico sistemico. L'uso delle tecniche a sottrazione è particolarmente utile per l'esame di malformazioni arteriovenose, aneurismi, occlusioni arteriose e trombosi venose. In molti casi, si realizza un'angiografia dei quattro vasi (carotidi interne e arterie vertebrali). L'utilizzo dell'angio-MR riduce la necessità di ricorrere all'invasiva angiografia. L'**ecografia cranica** per la diagnosi di leucomalacia periventricolare, emorragia intracranica, idrocefalo e tumori intracranici è riservata ai lattanti con fontanella aperta. Nei bambini più grandi, questa procedura è usata intraoperatoriamente per il posizionamento di shunt, la localizzazione di piccoli tumori e per dirigere l'ago in caso di biopsia. La **mielografia**, usata in passato per dimostrare la presenza di anomalie congenite, tumori e malformazioni vascolari a carico del midollo spinale, è stata ormai soppiantata dalla RM, perché consente una maggiore sensibilità e non è associata al rischio di aracnoidite (una possibile complicanza dell'iniezione del mezzo di contrasto nello spazio subaracnoide).

ELETTROENCEFALOGRAFIA. L'elettroencefalogramma (EEG) fornisce una registrazione continua dell'attività elettrica tra elettrodi di riferimento collocati sul cranio. La genesi dell'attività elettrica non è stata ancora chiarita con certezza, ma è probabile che origini dai potenziali post-sinaptici nei dendriti dei neuroni corticali. Malgrado l'amplificazione dell'attività elettrica, non tutti i potenziali sono registrabili, a causa dell'effetto tampone di cranio, muscoli, ossa, vasi sanguigni e liquido subaracnoideo. Le onde EEG sono classificate, sulla base della loro frequenza, in onde delta (1-3/s), teta (4-7/s), alfa (8-12/s) e beta (13-20/s). La frequenza di tali onde può essere alterata da vari fattori, tra cui l'età, lo stato di allerta, la chiusura degli occhi, l'assunzione di farmaci e la presenza di condizioni patologiche. Nell'EEG normale, onde lente ad alto voltaggio (complessi K) e fusi (ogni 12-14 secondi) sono confinati alle regioni cerebrali centrali durante il sonno. Le anomalie del tracciato includono punte e onde lente. Le punte, tipicamente parossistiche e ad alto voltaggio, sono seguite da onde lente. Punte e onde lente sono associate all'epilessia, ma talvolta si riscontrano anche in soggetti normali. Le punte focali sono spesso associate a lesioni irritative, incluse cisti, tumori a crescita lenta e presenza di tessuto cicatriziale gliale. L'attività epilettiforme può essere aggravata da procedure attivanti, come l'iperventilazione, la stimolazione luminosa e la deprivazione di sonno. In caso di riscontro di onde lente focali, si sospetta la presenza di una lesione circoscritta, come un ematoma, un tumore, un infarto o un processo infettivo localizzato; onde lente generalizzate suggeriscono un più diffuso processo, metabolico o infiammatorio.

Il **monitoraggio video-EEG-poligrafico** fornisce una precisa descrizione della tipologia delle convulsioni, contribuendo alla definizione della terapia. Consente inoltre la diagnosi differenziale tra convulsioni epilettiche ed eventi parossistici che mimano l'epilessia, come le pseudoconvulsioni. Tale tecnica di monitoraggio permette la misurazione dell'intensità delle convulsioni e contribuisce alla verifica dell'efficacia delle varie modalità terapeutiche. Infine, consente di registrare simultaneamente le alterazioni EEG e fisiologiche, agevolando la diagnosi nei neonati, nei quali la caratterizzazione delle convulsioni è particolarmente difficile.

Magnetoencefalografia (MEG) è utilizzata per la registrazione dei campi magnetici generati dal flusso di corrente all'interno dei neuroni. L'**imaging di sorgenti magnetiche** (*Magnetic Source Imaging*, **MSI**) costituisce una tecnica neurofisiologica avanzata che combina la MEG e la RM, per misurare i campi magnetici generati da una serie di neuroni. È particolarmente utile per l'esame dei candidati alla terapia chirurgica dell'epilessia.

POTENZIALI EVOCATI. Il potenziale evocato è la risposta elettrica che segue la stimolazione del SNC da parte di uno specifico stimolo visivo, uditivo o sensoriale. L'applicazione clinica dei potenziali evocati in età pediatrica è notevolmente aumentata negli ultimi anni. La stimolazione del sistema visivo mediante un flash o un pattern particolare (come una scacchiera bianca e nera) produce dei **potenziali evocati visivi** (VEP, *Visual Evoked Potentials*), registrati sopra l'occipite ed elaborati al computer. Lesioni che coinvolgono il sistema visivo, dalla retina alla corteccia visiva, risultano in VEP anomali. Patologie degenerative, come le malattie di Tay-Sachs, Krabbe e Pelizaeus-Merzbacher, e la lipofuscinosi neuronale ceroide mostrano anomalie VEP caratteristiche. Anche lesioni del nervo e del chiasma ottico determinano anomalie della risposta VEP. L'utilizzo di pattern come stimoli è particolarmente utile nella verifica della funzione visiva nei neonati a rischio. I VEP da flash contribuiscono alla determinazione delle sequele di asfissia in neonati a termine. I **potenziali evocati acustici troncoencefalici** (*Brainstem Auditory-Evoked Potential*, BAEP) consentono di ottenere una misurazione oggettiva dell'acuità uditiva, in particolare nei neonati o nei bambini non collaborativi, in seguito al fallimento delle tecniche di indagine standard. I BAEP risultano anomali in diverse malattie neurodegenerative infantili e sono particolarmente utili nella valutazione di pazienti con sospetto tumore dell'angolo pontocerebrale. Contribuiscono inoltre alla valutazione della funzione troncoencefalica nei pazienti comatosi, perché le onde non sono alterate né dai farmaci né dal livello di coscienza. I BAEP non costituiscono un indice accurato nel predire il recupero neurologico e le sequele. I **potenziali evocati somatosensoriali** (*SomatoSensory Evoked Potential*, SSEP) sono ottenuti stimolando un nervo periferico (peroneale o mediano) e registrando la risposta elettrica sopra la regione cervicale e la corteccia parietale somatosensoriale controlaterale. Sono utili per valutare l'integrità funzionale del sistema lemniscale dorsale e per monitorare la funzione del midollo spinale durante procedure chirurgiche in caso di scoliosi, di riparazione della coartazione dell'aorta e di mielomeningocele. I SSEP risultano anomali in molti disturbi neurodegenerativi infantili e consentono una accurata previsione dell'esito di gravi insulti al SNC.

Ellis R: Lumbar cerebrospinal fluid opening pressure measured in a flexed lateral decubitus position in children. *Pediatrics* 1994;93:622–623.

Gilman S: Imaging the brain. Parts I and II. *N Engl J Med* 1998;338:812–820, 889–896.

Haslam RH: Role of computed tomography in the early management of bacterial meningitis. *J Pediatr* 1991;119:157–159.

Mizrahi EM: Electroencephalographic/polygraphic/video monitoring in childhood epilepsy. *J Pediatr* 1984;105:1–9.

Otsubo H, Snead C: Magnetoencephalography and magnetic source imaging in children. *J Child Neurol* 2001;16:227–235.

Packer RJ, Zimmerman RA, Sutton LN, et al: Magnetic resonance imaging of spinal cord disease of childhood. *Pediatrics* 1986;78:251–256.

Piatt JH: Recognizing neurosurgical conditions in the pediatrician's office. *Pediatr Clin North Am* 2004;51:237–270.

Portnoy JM, Olson LC: Normal cerebrospinal fluid values in children: Another look. *Pediatrics* 1985;75:484–487.

Taylor MJ: Evoked potentials in paediatrics. In Halliday AM (editor): *Evoked Potentials in Clinical Testing,* 2nd ed. Edinburgh, Churchill Livingstone, 1993, p 489.

Capitolo 592 ■ Anomalie congenite del sistema nervoso centrale

Stephen L. Kinsman e Michael V. Johnston

592.1 • Difetti del tubo neurale (disrafismo)

I difetti del tubo neurale costituiscono l'anomalia congenita del sistema nervoso centrale più frequente e sono il risultato di una mancata chiusura del tubo neurale, che normalmente avviene spontaneamente tra la terza e quarta settimana dello sviluppo endouterino. La causa precisa di questi difetti non è nota, ma è ipotizzabile che i seguenti fattori influenzino negativamente lo sviluppo del SNC fin dal concepimento: ipertermia, assunzione di farmaci, malnutrizione, esposizione a sostanze chimiche, obesità o diabete materno, determinanti genetiche (come mutazioni delle vie folato-responsive o folato-dipendente). In alcuni casi, fattori nutrizionali o l'esposizione a radiazioni prima del concepimento possono aumentare la probabilità di una malformazione congenita del SNC. I principali difetti del tubo neurale includono: spina bifida occulta, meningocele, mielomeningocele, encefalocele, anencefalia, sinus dermico, midollo ancorato ("tethered cord": si tratta di una vera e propria sindrome costituita da un cono midollare ancorato in posizione estremamente bassa a causa di un filum terminale corto ed ispessito, di aderenze fibrose, o di un lipoma intradurale che fissa gli elementi neurali alla parte più

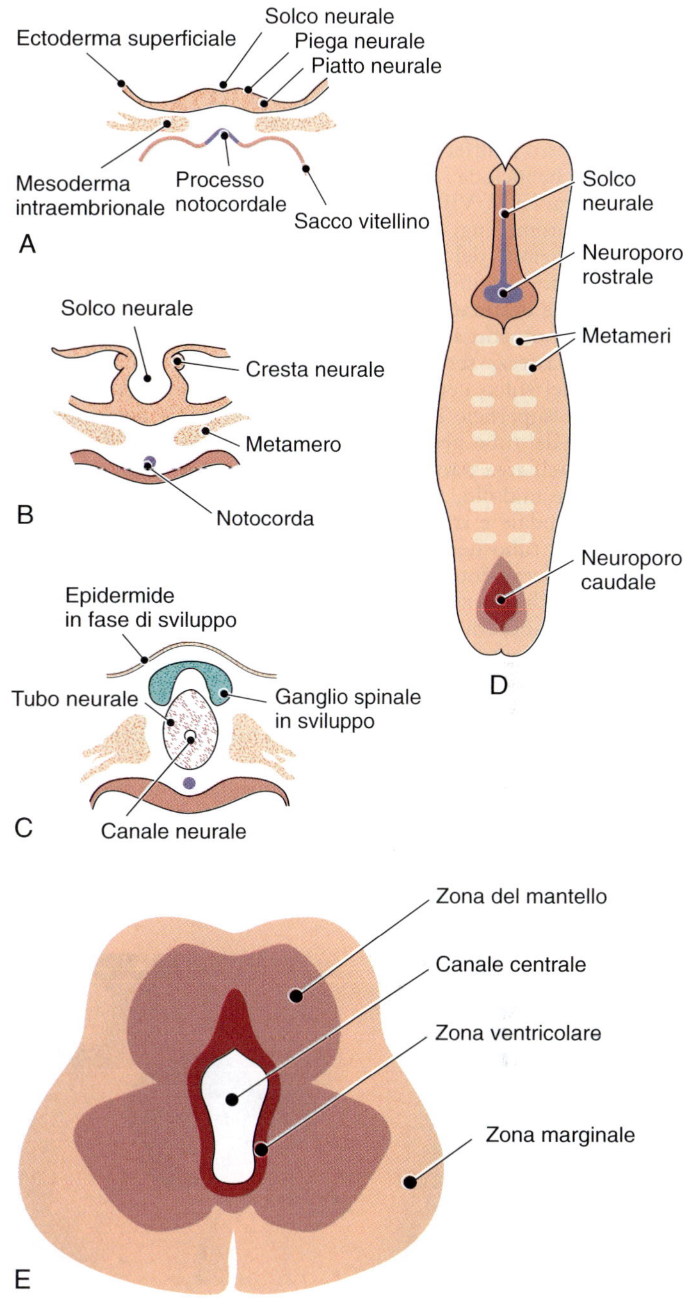

Figura 592-1. Illustrazione schematica dello sviluppo del sistema nervoso. *A*, Sezioni trasversali del piatto neurale durante la 3ª settimana. *B*, Formazione del solco e della cresta neurale. *C*, Lo sviluppo del tubo neurale è completato. *D*, Immagine longitudinale che mostra la chiusura iniziale del tubo neurale nella regione centrale. *E*, Sezione trasversale del tubo neurale dell'embrione (midollo spinale primitivo).

caudale del sacco durale, *N.d.C.*), siringomielia, diastematomielia e lipoma a livello del cono midollare e/o del filum terminale.

Il sistema nervoso umano ha origine dall'ectoderma primitivo, da cui si sviluppa anche l'epidermide. Ectoderma, endoderma e mesoderma costituiscono i tre foglietti germinali che si sviluppano entro la terza settimana. L'endoderma, in particolare il piatto notocordale e il mesoderma intraembrionale, inducono l'ectoderma sovrastante a sviluppare il piatto neurale durante la terza settimana di gestazione (Fig. 592-1*A*). L'assenza di tale induzione è responsabile della maggior parte dei difetti del tubo neurale. La rapida proliferazione cellulare all'interno del piatto neurale causa una ulteriore invaginazione del solco neurale e la differenziazione di un conglomerato di cellule, la cresta neurale, che migra lateralmente sulla superficie del tubo neurale (Fig. 592-1*B*). Il processo notocordale si trasforma nella notocorda centrale, che costituisce il fondamento intorno al quale si sviluppa la colonna vertebrale. In seguito alla formazione della colonna vertebrale, la notocorda subisce un'involuzione e si trasforma nel nucleo polposo dei dischi intervertebrali. Le cellule della cresta neurale vanno incontro a differenziazione, per formare il sistema nervoso periferico, che include i gangli spinali e autonomi, nonché i gangli dei nervi cranici V, VII, VIII, IX e X. Le creste neurali formano anche le leptomeningi e le cellule di Schwann, responsabili della mielinizzazione del sistema nervoso periferico. Si ritiene che la dura madre origini dal mesoderma parassiale. Nella regione dell'embrione destinata a divenire la testa, si osserva un pattern analogo (la notocorda è sostituita dal mesoderma precordale).

Durante la terza settimana dello sviluppo embrionale, l'invaginazione del solco neurale è completata e la separazione della sovrastante superficie ectodermica (Fig. 592-1C) determina la formazione del tubo neurale. L'iniziale chiusura del tubo neurale si realizza nell'area corrispondente alla futura giunzione tra spina dorsale e midollo; tale chiusura si completa rapidamente in direzione caudale e rostrale. Per un breve periodo, entrambe le estremità del tubo neurale rimangono aperte e il canale neurale comunica liberamente con la cavità amniotica (Fig. 592-1*D*). La mancata chiusura del tubo neurale consente l'escrezione nel liquido amniotico di sostanze fetali (α-fetoproteina [AFP], acetilcolinesterasi), utilizzate come marker biochimici dei difetti del tubo neurale. Lo screening prenatale del siero materno per AFP tra la 16ª e la 18ª settimana di gestazione è un metodo efficace per l'identificazione delle gravidanze a rischio. Normalmente, l'estremo rostrale del tubo neurale si chiude durante il 23° giorno, mentre il neuroporo caudale si chiude mediante un processo di neurulazione secondaria entro il 27° giorno, quando la maggior parte delle donne non si è ancora accorta di essere incinta.

592.2 • Spina bifida occulta

Questa anomalia comune consiste in un difetto della linea mediana dei corpi vertebrali, senza protrusione del midollo spinale o delle meningi. La maggior parte degli individui è asintomatica e non presenta segni neurologici. La presenza di ciuffi di peli, lipomi, discolorazione della cute o di un sinus dermico sulla linea mediana della parte bassa della schiena suggerisce una malformazione del midollo spinale più grave (Fig. 592-2). Nei casi di spina bifida occulta semplice, la radiografia spinale mostra un difetto di chiusura degli archi e delle lamine vertebrali posteriori, che tipicamente coinvolge L5 e S1; non si riscontrano invece anomalie delle meningi, del midollo spinale e delle radici nervose. La spina bifida occulta è occasionalmente associata a più significative anomalie evolutive del midollo spinale, che includono siringomielia, distematomielia e "tethered cord". La tecnica diagnostica di elezione per l'identificazione di tali difetti è la RM (Fig. 592-3). Alcuni utilizzano l'espressione *spina bifida occulta* per indicare semplicemente un difetto di fusione dei corpi vertebrali posteriori, non associato a una malformazione del midollo spinale. Le forme clinicamente più gravi sono definite, in maniera più corretta, **disrafismo spinale occulto**. Nella maggior parte dei casi, si tratta di manifestazioni cutanee come emangiomi, fossette, noduli o ciuffi di peli (vedi Fig. 592-2). Il **sinus dermoide** generalmente determina la formazione di una piccola apertura cutanea, collegata a un dotto, talvolta indicato da un ciuffo di peli o da un nevo vascolare. Tali seni dermoidi si sviluppano sulla linea mediana, nelle regioni lombosacrale e occipitale, dove possono comparire meningocele ed encefalocele. I tragitti dei seni dermoidi possono passare attraverso la dura madre, agendo come condotti per la diffusione di infezioni. Ri-

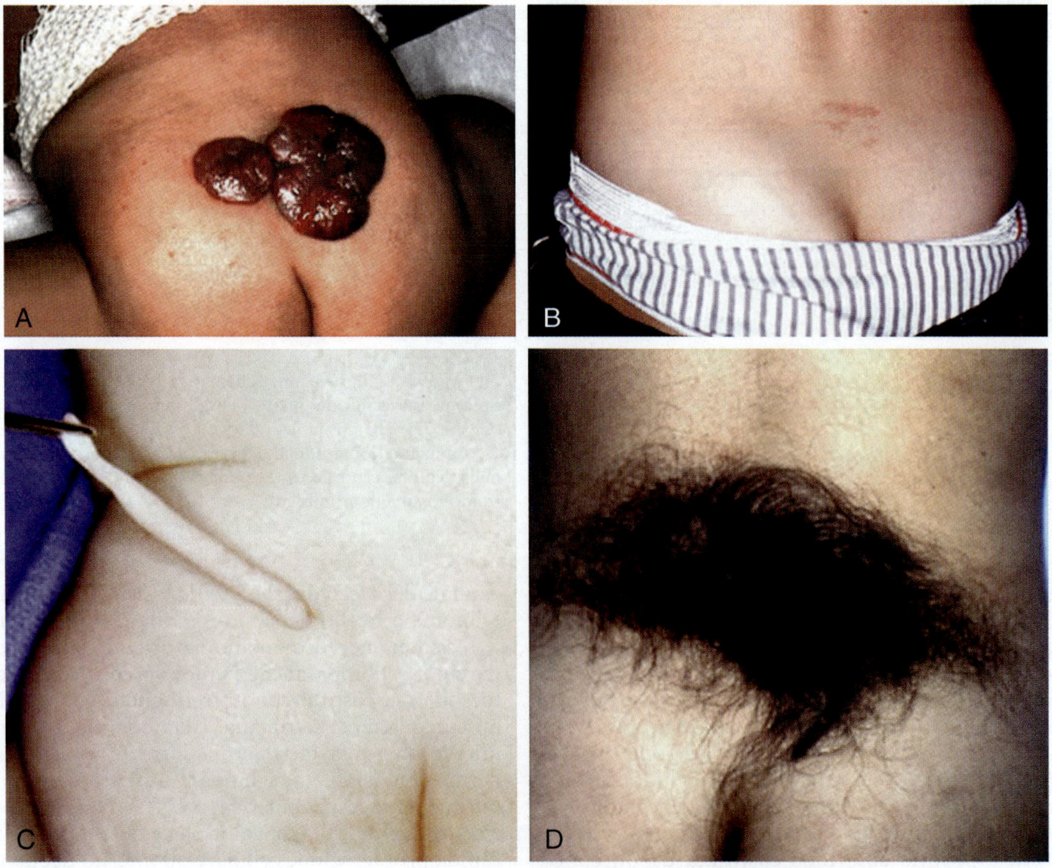

Figura 592-2. Aspetto clinico di lesioni cutanee lombosacrali congenite, combinate o isolate. *A*, Emangioma ulcerato centrato sul sinus dermico e deviazione del solco gluteo. *B*, Macchia vinacea isolata. *C*, Coda umana. *D*, Coda di fauno. (Tratta da Guggisberg D, Hadj-Rabia S, Viney C, et al: Skin markers of occult spinal dysraphism. *Arch Dermatol* 2004;140:1109-1115.)

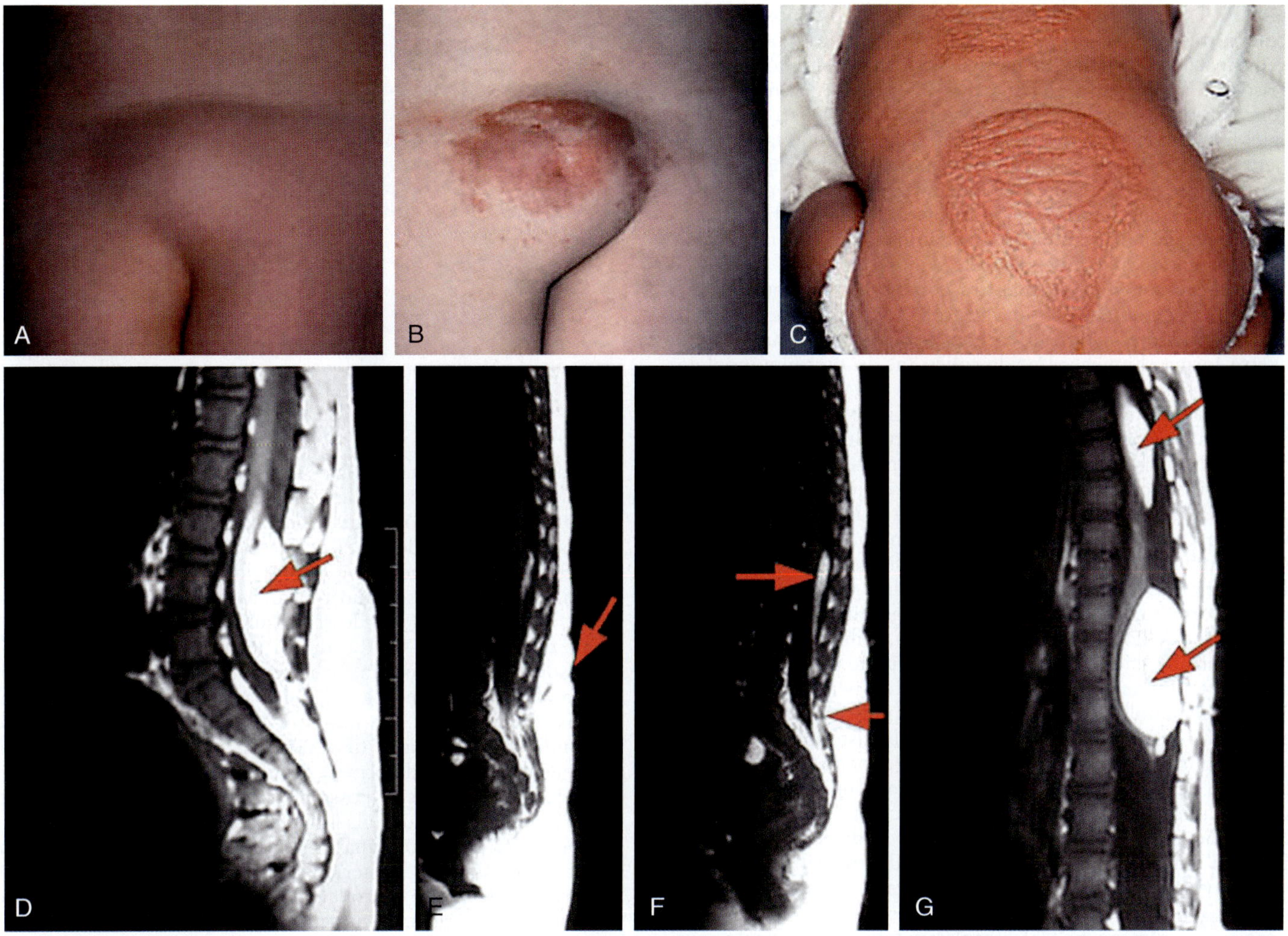

Figura 592-3. Caratteristiche cliniche (A-C) e corrispondente disrafismo spinale occulto evidenziate dalla RM sagittale e pesata in T1 del midollo spinale (D-G). *A*, Lipoma sacrale e deviazione del solco gluteo. *B*, Macchia vinacea lombare, lipoma, seno dermico e deviazione del solco gluteo. *C*, Amartomi dorsali e lombari non classificati. *D*, Lipoma del cono (*freccia*). *E*, Sinus dermico (*freccia*). *F*, Parte superiore del lipoma del filum terminale (*freccia in alto*) e fistola (*freccia in basso*). *G*, Lipomi multipli della colonna toracica (*freccia in alto*) e del cono posteriore (*freccia in basso*). (Tratta da Guggisberg D, Hadj-Rabia S, Viney C, et al: Skin markers of occult spinal dysraphism. *Arch Dermatol* 2004;140:1109-1115.)

correnti meningiti di origine occulta suggeriscono di verificare accuratamente la presenza di un piccolo tragitto di seno nella regione mediana posteriore, compresa la nuca. I seni nella parte bassa della schiena si trovano solitamente al di sopra della piega glutea, in direzione cefalica. La sindrome del "tethered cord" può essere associata.

592.3 • MENINGOCELE

Il meningocele si forma in seguito all'erniazione delle meningi dovuta a un difetto degli archi vertebrali posteriori. Il midollo spinale è solitamente normale e assume una posizione corretta nel canale spinale, benché sia possibile riscontrare tethering, siringomielia o diastematomielia. Una massa fluttuante sulla linea mediana, transilluminabile, può svilupparsi lungo la colonna vertebrale, solitamente nella parte bassa della schiena. Nella maggior parte dei casi, il meningocele è ben coperto dalla cute e non costituisce una minaccia, ma un accurato esame neurologico è obbligatorio. Nei bambini asintomatici con reperti neurologici nella norma e spessore cutaneo adeguato, l'intervento chirurgico per la rimozione del meningocele può essere rimandato. Prima della correzione chirurgica del difetto, è opportuno sottoporre il paziente a un esame accurato, che includa una radiografia diretta, l'ecografia e la RM, per determinare l'estensione del coinvolgimento del tessuto neurale ed eventuali anomalie associate (come diastematomielia, tethered cord o lipoma). La valutazione urologica, che solitamente include il cistometrogramma (CMG), consente di identificare i pazienti con vescica neurogena a rischio di compromissione renale. In presenza di una perdita di liquido cerebrospinale o di insufficiente copertura cutanea, si raccomanda l'immediato intervento chirurgico, per scongiurare il rischio di meningite. Nei bambini con meningocele è opportuno eseguire una TC craniale, per verificare l'associazione con idrocefalo. Il **meningocele anteriore** si proietta nella pelvi attraverso un difetto del sacro. I sintomi di costipazione e di disfunzione vescicale si sviluppano in seguito all'aumento delle dimensioni della lesione. I pazienti di sesso femminile possono manifestare anomalie associate del tratto genitale, come una fistola rettovaginale o setto vaginale. Le radiografie dirette dimostrano la presenza di un difetto a livello del sacro, mentre la TC o la RM evidenziano l'estensione del meningocele.

592.4 • MIELOMENINGOCELE

Il mielomeningocele, la più grave forma di disrafismo, coinvolge la colonna vertebrale e si verifica con un'incidenza di circa 1 su 4000 nati vivi.

EZIOLOGIA. La causa del mielomeningocele è sconosciuta ma, come in tutti i difetti di chiusura del tubo neurale, si osserva una predisposizione genetica; se un figlio presenta la malformazione, il rischio di ricorrenza aumenta fino al 3-4%, mentre sale fino a circa il 10% dopo due gravidanze anomale. I dati epidemiologici e la presenza di una sostanziale aggregazione familiare di anencefalia, mielomeningocele e craniorachischisi suggeriscono il contributo determinante dell'ereditarietà (su base poligenica) nell'eziologia dei difetti del tubo neurale. Senza dubbio anche i fattori nutrizionali e ambientali svolgono un ruolo importante nell'eziologia del mielomeningocele.

Il folato è coinvolto in maniera complessa nella prevenzione ed eziologia dei difetti del tubo neurale. Oltre a funzionare nelle reazioni di trasferimento di carbonio singolo, il folato esiste in diverse forme chimiche. L'acido folico (acido pteroilmonoglutarico), che costituisce la forma di folato più stabile e maggiormente ossidata, è presente raramente nei cibi, ma è contenuto in tutti i supplementi vitaminici e prodotti alimentari fortificati. I folati che si riscontrano più comunemente in natura (folati alimentari) sono i pteroilpoliglutammati, che contengono da una a sei molecole addizionali di glutammato, unite in un legame peptidico con il γ-carbossil del glutammato. I coenzimi folato sono coinvolti nei seguenti processi: (1) sintesi dell'acido deossiribonucleico (DNA); (2) sintesi delle purine; (3) generazione del pool di formato; (4) interconversione degli amminoacidi, con la conversione dell'omocisteina in metionina, utilizzata per la sintesi di S-adenosil-metionina (un agente importante per la metilazione in vivo). Le mutazioni del gene che codifica per gli enzimi coinvolti nel metabolismo dell'omocisteina colpiscono la 5,10 metilenetetraidrofolato reduttasi (MTHFR), la cistationina β-sintasi e la metionina sintasi. È probabile che in almeno il 15% dei casi di difetto del tubo neurale possa riscontrarsi un'associazione tra una variante termolabile di MTHFR e caratteristiche materne. La somministrazione periconcezionale di acido folico alle madri riduce di almeno il 50% l'incidenza del difetto del tubo neurale nelle gravidanze a rischio. Per essere efficace, la supplementazione di acido folico deve essere avviata prima del concepimento e proseguita almeno fino al completamento della neurulazione, durante la 12ª settimana di gestazione.

PREVENZIONE. L'U.S. Public Health Service raccomanda l'assunzione di 0,4 mg di acido folico al giorno a tutte le donne in età fertile. In caso di pianificazione di una gravidanza in una donna a elevato rischio (per la presenza del difetto in un precedente figlio), la terapia dovrebbe cominciare un mese prima del tentativo di concepimento, alla dose di 4 mg/die. La dieta attuale fornisce circa il 50% dell'apporto giornaliero necessario di acido folico. Per aumentarne l'assorbimento, in Canada e Stati Uniti è stata disposta nel 1988 l'aggiunta di 0,15 mg di acido folico per ogni 100 g di farina, pasta, riso e farina di mais. La quantità di acido folico aggiunto è insufficiente a massimizzare la prevenzione dei difetti del tubo neurale prevedibili. Pertanto, rimangono indispensabili programmi educativi diretti a tutte le donne che pianificano una gravidanza e possibilmente a tutte le donne in età fertile, per informarle sull'importanza di una dieta variata e sulla necessità di assumere supplementazioni di acido folico. Alcuni farmaci antagonisti dell'acido folico (come il trimetoprim e gli anticonvulsivanti carbamazepina, fenitoina, fenobarbital e primidone) aumentano il rischio di mielomeningocele. Se somministrato durante la gravidanza, l'anticonvulsivante acido valproico causa un difetto del tubo neurale in circa l'1-2% dei casi. Alcuni medici specialisti raccomandano la prescrizione di supplementi di acido folico a tutte le donne in età fertile che assumono regolarmente farmaci anticonvulsivanti.

MANIFESTAZIONI CLINICHE. Oltre a danneggiare il sistema nervoso periferico e centrale, il difetto causa disfunzioni a carico di diversi organi e strutture, incluso lo scheletro, la cute e i tratti gastrointestinale e genito-urinario. Il mielomeningocele può svilupparsi a qualsiasi livello lungo il neurasse, ma almeno il 75% dei casi è localizzato nella regione lombosacrale. L'estensione e il grado del deficit neurologico dipendono dalla localizzazione del mielomeningocele e delle lesioni associate. Una lesione nella regione sacrale inferiore causa incontinenza urinaria e fecale associata ad anestesia dell'area perineale, ma non compromette la funzione motoria. I neonati portatori di un difetto nella regione lombare centrale presentano tipicamente una struttura cistica a sacco, coperta da un sottile strato di tessuto parzialmente epitelializzato (Fig. 592-4). Residui di tessuto neurale sono visibili al di sotto della membrana, che tende a rompersi, provocando perdite di liquido cerebrospinale. L'esame del neonato rivela una paralisi flaccida degli arti inferiori, l'assenza dei riflessi tendinei profondi, una mancanza di risposta al tocco e al dolore e una elevata incidenza di deformità degli arti inferiori (piede equino, sublussazione dell'anca). Possono riscontrarsi anche una perdita urinaria continua e un rilassamento dello sfintere anale. Altri bambini non perdono urina e hanno una vescica con pressione elevata e dissinergia sfinterica. Dunque, un mielomeningocele nella regione lombare centrale tende a produrre segni a carico dei motoneuroni inferiori, dovuti ad anomalie del cono midollare. Tipicamente, il deficit neurologico si aggrava con l'estensione verso l'alto nella regione toracica del mielomeningocele. I pazienti con mielomeningocele nella parte superiore del torace o nella regione cervicale presentano solitamente un deficit neurologico minimo, nella maggior parte dei casi non associato a idrocefalo.

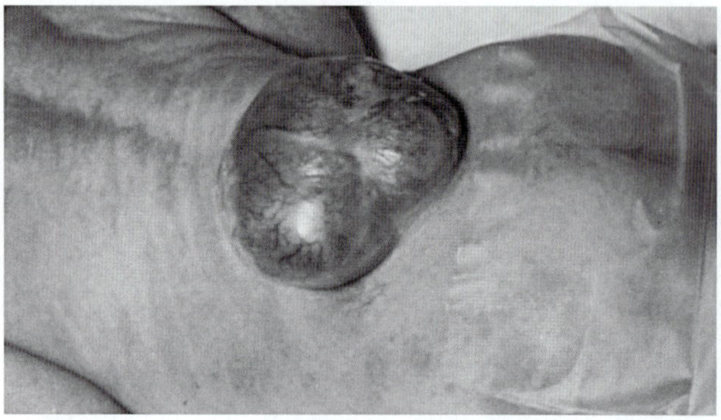

Figura 592-4. Mielomeningocele lombare coperto da un sottile strato cutaneo.

L'**idrocefalo** in associazione a **malformazione di Chiari di tipo II** si sviluppa in almeno l'80% dei pazienti con mielomeningocele. Generalmente, più la deformità è collocata in basso lungo il neurasse (sacro), meno elevato è il rischio di idrocefalo. Tuttavia, a prescindere dal livello spinale, la possibilità che si sviluppi idrocefalo deve essere sempre presa in considerazione. La dilatazione ventricolare può risultare indolente e a progressione lenta, oppure può crescere rapidamente, causando un aumento della circonferenza cranica associato a fontanella anteriore sporgente, vene della volta cranica dilatate, occhi a sole calante, irritabilità e vomito. Circa il 15% dei lattanti con idrocefalo e malformazione di Chiari di tipo II sviluppa sintomi di disfunzione romboencefalica, come difficoltà di allattamento e deglutizione, stridore respiratorio, apnea, paralisi delle corde vocali, accumulo di secrezioni e spasticità degli arti superiori. Se non trattati, questi sintomi possono risultare fatali. La cosiddetta **crisi di Chiari** è dovuta all'erniazione verso il basso del midollo e delle tonsille cerebellari attraverso il forame magno.

TRATTAMENTO. La gestione e supervisione di un bambino con mielomeningocele richiede un approccio multidisciplinare. Il pediatra si occupa solitamente della coordinazione degli interventi di un team composto da chirurghi, specialisti e terapisti della riabilitazione. La scoperta delle presenza nel neonato di una malattia devastante come il mielomeningocele causa nei genitori una reazione di disperazione e rabbia. Il medico deve informarli sull'handicap in un setting non minaccioso, dando loro il tempo di assorbire le informazioni sulla malattia, sulle complicanze associate e sulle varie procedure e programmi di trattamento. Se possibile, il confronto con altri genitori di bambini con difetti del tubo neurale può contribuire a chiarire i dubbi e le questioni più pressanti.

Solitamente, il neonato è sottoposto a **intervento chirurgico** nei primi giorni di vita. In assenza di perdite di liquido cerebrospinale, l'intervento può essere ritardato di qualche giorno, in modo da concedere ai genitori il tempo di abituarsi allo shock e di prepararsi agli inevitabili problemi che saranno chiamati ad affrontare. La valutazione delle altre anomalie congenite e della funzione renale può essere cominciata prima dell'intervento. Nella maggior parte dei centri specialistici, il mielomeningocele è trattato aggressivamente. Dopo la riparazione chirurgica, molti lattanti richiedono l'applicazione di uno shunt per il trattamento dell'idrocefalo. Se compaiono sintomi e segni di disfunzione romboencefalica, è indicata la decompressione chirurgica di midollo allungato e cervicale. Il piede equino può richiedere un'ingessatura, mentre una lussazione dell'anca deve talvolta essere corretta chirurgicamente.

La componente principale della valutazione consiste nell'attento esame del **sistema genito-urinario**. Per mantenere un volume residuo ridotto e una pressione vescicale che prevenga le infezioni del tratto urinario e il reflusso (con conseguente pielonefrite, idronefrosi e danno vescicale), è fondamentale insegnare ai genitori, e in seguito al bambino, a cateterizzare regolarmente una vescica neurogena. Per evitare lo sviluppo di allergie, è opportuno evitare l'uso di cateteri e guanti di lattice. Sulla base dei progressi del paziente e dei risultati dell'esame fisico, si effettuano periodiche urinocolture e valutazioni della funzione renale, comprendendo elettroliti sierici e creatinina, cisturetrogramma (VCUG), ecografia e cistometrografia. Tale approccio preventivo ha enormemente ridotto la necessità di ricorrere a procedure di diversione urinaria e ha contribuito al calo della morbilità e mortalità associate alla malattia renale progressiva. In alcuni casi, l'incontinenza può essere corretta mediante impianto chirurgico di uno sfintere urinario artificiale oppure (in età più avanzata) mediante ampliamento della vescica. L'**incontinenza fecale**, malgrado ponga rilevanti difficoltà (soprattutto in età scolare), non rischia di danneggiare organi vitali come la disfunzione urinaria, ma occasionalmente può svilupparsi occlusione da feci e/o megacolon. Utilizzando clisteri e supposte, è possibile abituare i bambini a evacuare in orari prestabiliti una o due volte al giorno. Un'appendicostomia per clisteri anterogradi può pure essere utile (vedi anche il Capitolo 22.4).

La possibilità di **deambulazione** funzionale, maggiore aspirazione di bambini e genitori, dipende dal livello della lesione e dall'integrità dei muscoli ileopsoas. Tale deambulazione è realizzabile nella quasi totalità dei pazienti con lesione sacrale o lombosacrale; circa il 50% dei bambini con difetti più alti deambulano con tutore. Con l'avvicinarsi dell'adolescenza e del conseguente aumento della massa corporea, la deambulazione diviene più difficile.

In alcuni centri specializzati, è stata tentata con successo la correzione chirurgica di lesioni spinali in utero. Resoconti preliminari indicano la possibile preservazione della funzione motoria e una ridotta incidenza di anomalie romboencefaliche e idrocefalia. Questi dati suggeriscono la natura progressiva del difetto in utero, dimostrando che la chirurgia prenatale può prevenire la perdita di funzione. La diagnosi in utero è facilitata dallo screening della α-fetoproteina nel siero materno e dall'ecografia fetale (vedi Capitolo 96).

PROGNOSI. Malgrado il trattamento aggressivo del mielomeningocele, il tasso di mortalità è di circa il 10-15%. Complicanze fatali possono insorgere a qualsiasi età, ma la maggior parte dei decessi si verifica prima dei 4 anni. In almeno il 70% dei sopravvissuti, si riscontra un livello intellettivo nella norma, ma i disturbi dell'apprendimento e i disturbi convulsivi sono più frequenti rispetto alla popolazione generale. Episodi di meningite o ventricolite incidono negativamente sul quoziente intellettivo definitivo. Poiché il mielomeningocele costituisce una patologia invalidante cronica, il paziente deve essere sottoposto per tutta la vita a periodici follow-up multidisciplinari. La disfunzione renale costituisce la principale causa di mortalità.

592.5 • ENCEFALOCELE

Le due principali forme di disrafismo che colpiscono la volta cranica provocano una protrusione di tessuto attraverso un difetto osseo della linea mediana, chiamato **cranio bifido**. Il **meningocele cranico** è costituito da un sacco meningeo contenente liquido cerebrospinale, mentre l'**encefalocele cranico** contiene, oltre al sacco, corteccia cerebrale, cervelletto o porzioni del tronco encefalico. L'esame al microscopio del tessuto neurale all'interno dell'encefalocele rivela spesso la presenza di anomalie. Nella maggior parte dei casi, il difetto cranico è localizzato nella regione occipitale o al di sotto dell'inion, ma in alcuni Paesi l'encefalocele frontale o nasofrontale è il più comune. L'incidenza di questa anomalia è di un decimo rispetto a quella dei difetti di chiusura del tubo neurale che coinvolgono la colonna. L'eziologia è simile a quella dell'anencefalia e del mielomeningocele. Sono stati segnalati casi di presenza contemporanea di più di una delle patologie menzionate nella stessa famiglia.

Nei lattanti con encefalocele cranico, aumenta il rischio di sviluppo di idrocefalo dovuto a stenosi dell'acquedotto, malformazione di Chiari o sindrome di Dandy-Walker. L'esame mostra un piccolo sacco dotato di un peduncolo o di una struttura cistica talmente voluminosa da eccedere le dimensioni del cranio. La lesione è completamente coperta da cute, ma possono riscontrarsi aree denudate, che richiedono l'intervento chirurgico urgente. La transilluminazione del sacco può indicare la presenza di tessuto neurale. La radiografia diretta della volta cranica e della colonna cervicale è indicata per definire l'anatomia delle vertebre. L'ecografia contribuisce a determinare il contenuto del sacco, mentre la RM o la TC consentono di definire lo spettro della lesione. La prognosi del meningocele cranico è in genere buona, mentre i pazienti con encefalocele rischiano di sviluppare disturbi visivi, microcefalia, ritardo mentale e convulsioni. In linea generale, i bambini con tessuto neurale all'interno del sacco e idrocefalo associato hanno la prognosi peggiore. La **sindrome di Meckel-Gruber** è una rara malattia autosomica recessiva caratterizzata da un encefalocele occipitale, labbra o palato fissurato, microcefalia, microftalmia, anomalie dei genitali, rene policistico e polidattilia. La diagnosi dell'encefalocele in utero è realizzabile mediante determinazione dei livelli della α-fetoproteina nel siero materno, misura del diametro biparietale utilizzando gli ultrasuoni, o identificazione dell'encefalocele stesso.

592.6 • ANENCEFALIA

I bambini anencefalici presentano una facies caratteristica, con un evidente difetto di calvario, meningi e scalpo, associato a un cervello rudimentale, risultato della mancata chiusura del neuroporo rostrale, apertura anteriore del tubo neurale. Il cervello primitivo è costituito da porzioni di tessuto connettivo, vasi e neuroglia. Gli emisferi cerebrali e cerebellari sono solitamente assenti ed è possibile identificare soltanto un residuo di tronco encefalico. L'ipofisi è ipoplasica e non si riscontrano i tratti spinali piramidali, a causa dell'assenza di corteccia cerebrale. Anomalie supplementari includono malformazioni delle orecchie, palatoschisi e difetti cardiaci congeniti (dal 10 al 20% dei casi). Nella maggior parte dei casi, il decesso avviene entro qualche giorno dalla nascita. L'incidenza dell'anencefalia è di circa 1 su 1000 nati vivi; la frequenza maggiore di riscontra in Irlanda, Galles e nel nord della Cina. Il rischio di ricorrenza è di circa il 4%, ma aumenta fino al 10% nelle donne che hanno già avuto due figli affetti da tale patologia. Oltre ai fattori genetici, sono state ipotizzate diverse cause implicate nell'anencefalia, tra le quali un basso status socioeconomico, deficit vitaminici e carenze nutrizionali, nonché un'ampia gamma di fattori ambientali e tossici. È molto probabile che l'anencefalia sia il risultato dell'interazione tra una serie di stimoli nocivi, che agiscono su di un soggetto geneticamente predisposto. Negli ultimi vent'anni, la frequenza della patologia si è progressivamente ridotta. In circa il 50% dei casi si osserva l'associazione di polidramnios. Nelle madri che hanno già partorito un figlio anencefalico, è opportuno un attento monitoraggio delle nuove gravidanze, che includa l'amniocentesi, la determinazione dei livelli di AFP e l'ecografia tra la 14ª e la 16ª settimana di gestazione.

Beeker T, Scheers M, Faber J, et al: Prediction of independence and intelligence at birth on meningomyelocele. *Childs New Syst* 2006;22:33–37.

Berry RJ, Li Z, Erickson JD, et al for the China-U.S. Collaborative Project for Neural Tube Defect Prevention: Prevention of neural-tube defects with folic acid in China. *N Engl J Med* 1999;341:1485–1490.

Fernandes ET, Reinberg Y, Vernier R, et al: Neurogenic bladder dysfunction in children: Review of pathophysiology and current management. *J Pediatr* 1994;124:1–7.

Guggisberg D, Hadj-Rabia S, Viney C, et al: Skin markers of occult spinal dysraphism in children. *Arch Dermatol* 2004;140:1109–1115.

Hernandez-Diaz S, Werler MM, Walker AM, et al: Folic acid antagonists during pregnancy and the risk of birth defects. *N Engl J Med* 2000;343:1608–1614.

Ickowicz V, Ewin D, Maugay-Laulom B, et al: Meckel-Gruber syndrome, sonography and pathology. *Ultrasound Obstet Gynecol* 2006;27:296–300.

Kibar Z, Torban E, McDearmid JR, et al: Mutations in VANGLI associated with neural-tube defects. *N Engl J Med* 2007;356:1432–1437.

Mazzola CA, Albright AL, Sutton LN, et al: Dermoid inclusion cysts and early spinal cord tethering after fetal surgery for myelomeningocele. *N Engl J Med* 2002;347:256–259.

Mitchell LE, Adzick NS, Melchionne J, et al: Spina bifida. *Lancet* 2004;364:1885–1895.

592.7 • Patologie della migrazione neuronale

Le patologie della migrazione neuronale possono provocare anomalie minori con conseguenze cliniche minime (lieve eterotopia neuronale) o devastanti (ritardo mentale, convulsioni, lissencefalia o schizencefalia, in particolare la forma a labbra aperte [Fig. 592-5]). Uno dei principali meccanismi del controllo della migrazione neuronale è il sistema delle fibre gliali radiali che indirizzano e guidano i neuroni alla sede corretta. Legati alle fibre gliali, i neuroni migrano verso siti predeterminati, dove sono liberati, per formare i sei strati della corteccia cerebrale. Nelle cavie, il prodotto di un gene, chiamato *reelin*, dirige il neurone verso la sua destinazione finale nel cervello. Un altro gene (*mdab1*), attivato da *reelin*, agisce come segnalatore. Mutazioni di questi geni causano rilevanti anomalie della migrazione neuronale. La gravità e l'estensione della patologia sono collegate a diversi fattori di natura genetica e ambientale, nonché all'epoca di insorgenza dell'insulto.

Il tubo neurale è costituito da tre zone: la zona ventricolare, quella marginale e il mantello (vedi Fig. 592-1*E*). Lo strato ependimale è composto da cellule neuroepiteliali colonnari, pseudostratificate e pluripotenti. Specifiche cellule neuroepiteliali si differenziano in neuroni primitivi o neuroblasti, che formano lo strato del mantello. La zona marginale origina da cellule dello strato esterno del neuroepitelio, destinate a trasformarsi nella sostanza bianca. Anche i glioblasti, importanti cellule di supporto primitive del SNC, derivano dalle cellule neuroepiteliali della zona ependimale, che migrano verso le zone del mantello e marginale, trasformandosi in astrociti e oligodendrociti. È probabile che la microglia origini dalle cellule mesenchimali in uno stadio successivo dello sviluppo fetale, quando i vasi sanguigni cominciano a penetrare nel sistema nervoso in crescita. I continui progressi nella comprensione delle basi molecolari dello sviluppo corticale condurranno a nuove classificazioni delle malformazioni corticali.

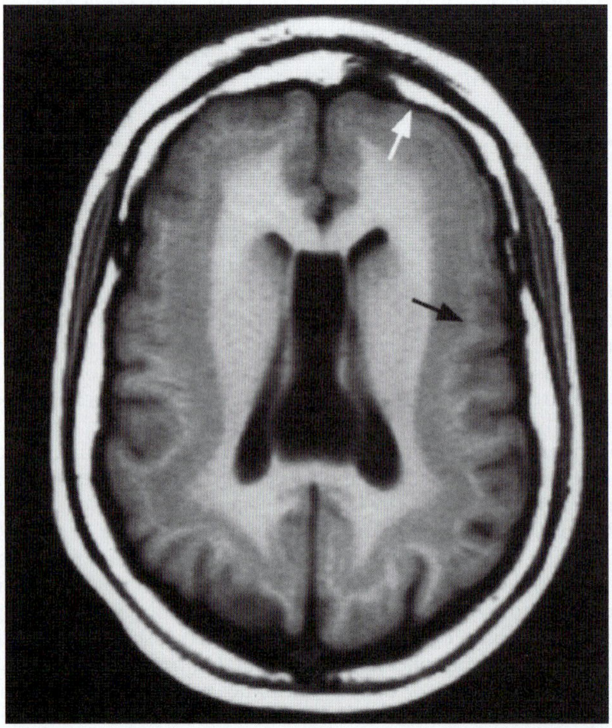

Figura 592-5. RM pesata in T1 che dimostra la presenza di eterotopia a banda. Tra la banda di sostanza grigia eterotopica e la superficie corticale si osserva un sottile strato di sostanza bianca (*freccia nera*). La lissencefalia, con assenza di organizzazione corticale, è presente in entrambi i lobi frontali (*freccia bianca*).

LISSENCEFALIA. La lissencefalia, o **agiria**, è una rara patologia caratterizzata dall'assenza di circonvoluzioni cerebrali e da una scissura silviana scarsamente sviluppata, tipica di un feto al terzo o quarto mese. Questa condizione patologica, solitamente associata ad allargamento dei ventricoli laterali ed eterotopia nella sostanza bianca, è probabilmente dovuta a un difetto nella migrazione dei neuroblasti durante le prime fasi dello sviluppo embrionale. In alcune forme, si riscontra una corteccia a 4 strati (invece di 6), con un sottile margine di sostanza bianca periventricolare ed eterotopie della sostanza grigia visibili al microscopio. I bambini con lissencefalia manifestano deficit staturo-ponderale, microcefalia, marcato ritardo dello sviluppo e gravi disturbi convulsivi. Le anomalie oculari sono comuni e includono ipoplasia del nervo

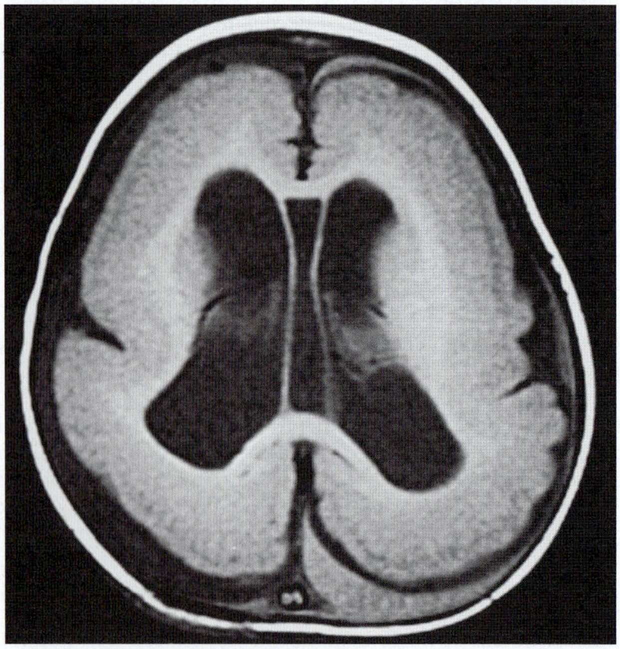

Figura 592-6. RM di un neonato con lissencefalia. Notare l'assenza di solchi cerebrali e la malformazione della scissura silviana, associata a dilatazione ventricolare.

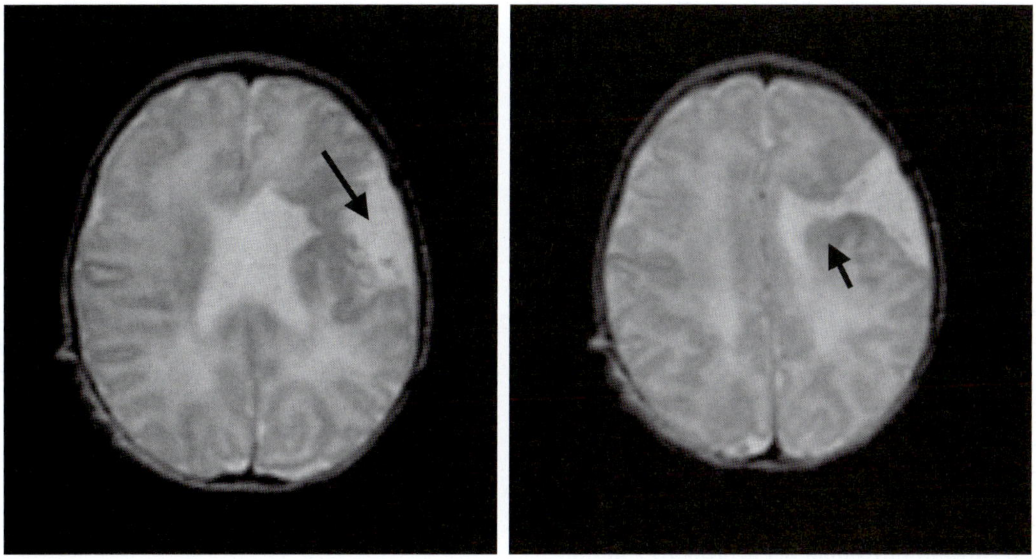

Figura 592-7. Schizencefalia unilaterale mostrata in RM assiale. Esempio di una schizencefalia a labbra chiuse con una fessura comunicante tra ventricolo e spazio extracranico (*freccia* nell'immagine a sinistra). Molte di queste fessure sono rivestite da sostanza grigia anomala (*freccia* nell'immagine a destra).

ottico e microftalmia. In circa il 15% dei casi, la lissencefalia è associata alla **sindrome di Miller-Diecker** (*Miller-Dieker Syndrome*, MDS), che determina una facies caratteristica: fronte prominente, restringimento bitemporale, narici anteverse, labbro superiore prominente e micrognazia. In circa il 90% dei bambini con MDS si riscontrano delezioni cromosomiche di 17p13.3 (visibili o submicroscopiche). Tali delezioni coinvolgono il gene LIS-1 (lissencefalia 1), mappato nella regione 17p13.3. TC e RM mostrano tipicamente un cervello liscio privo di solchi (Fig. 592-6).

SCHIZENCEFALIA. Questa patologia consiste nella presenza di **fessure** unilaterali o bilaterali all'interno degli emisferi cerebrali, dovute ad anomalie della morfogenesi (Fig. 592-7). Le fessure possono fondersi e, se ampie e unilaterali, sono facilmente confondibili con una cisti porencefalica. I bordi della fessura sono spesso circondati da tessuto cerebrale anomalo, in particolare microgiria. La TC consente di formulare la diagnosi, documentando le dimensioni e l'estensione della fessura. Il riconoscimento delle forme più lievi può richiedere la RM. Molti pazienti presentano ritardo mentale grave, convulsioni difficili da controllare e microcefalia (con tetraparesi spastica quando le fessure sono bilaterali). La schizencefalia unilaterale costituisce una causa frequente di **emiparesi congenita.**

PORENCEFALIA. Consiste nella presenza di cisti e cavità all'interno del cervello, originate da difetti dello sviluppo o lesioni acquisite (come infarti del tessuto). Le cisti porencefaliche vere sono localizzate nella regione della scissura silviana e tipicamente comunicano con lo spazio subaracnoideo e/o il sistema ventricolare. Tali cisti costituiscono anomalie evolutive della migrazione cellulare e sono spesso associate ad altre malformazioni cerebrali, come microcefalia, pattern anomalo di giri adiacenti ed encefalocele. I bambini colpiti manifestano ritardo mentale, emi o tetraparesi spastica, atrofia ottica e convulsioni. Le cisti pseudoporencefaliche si sviluppano tipicamente durante il periodo perinatale o postnatale e sono il risultato di anomalie della circolazione venosa o arteriosa (come infarti o emorragie). Tali cisti unilaterali non comunicano con una cavità piena di liquido, né sono associate ad anomalie della migrazione cellulare o a malformazioni del SNC. Le cisti pseudoporencefaliche si manifestano con emiparesi e convulsioni focali nel primo anno di vita.

OLOPROSENCEFALIA. Questo disturbo dello sviluppo cerebrale è il risultato di un difettoso clivaggio del proencefalo e dell'inadeguata induzione delle strutture encefaliche anteriori. Le anomalie, di gravità variabile, sono classificate in tre gruppi: alobari, semilobari e lobari (Fig. 592-8). Un quarto tipo, detto sintelencefalia o fusione interemisferica mediana (*Middle InterHemispheric Fusion*, MIHF), coinvolge un'area segmentale di non clivaggio dei lobi frontale posteriore e parietale. **Anomalie facciali** come ciclopia, cebocefalia, dente incisivo centrale singolo e agenesia premascellare sono comuni nei casi più gravi, perché il mesoderma precordale che induce il prosencefalo ventrale è responsabile anche dell'induzione delle strutture facciali mediane. La oloprosencefalia lobare è caratterizzata da un ventricolo unico, assenza di falce e gangli basali fusi. Il riscontro di anomalie ventricolari non è sufficiente per la formulazione della diagnosi, che richiede la dimostrazione dell'assenza di clivaggio delle strutture cerebrali della linea mediana.

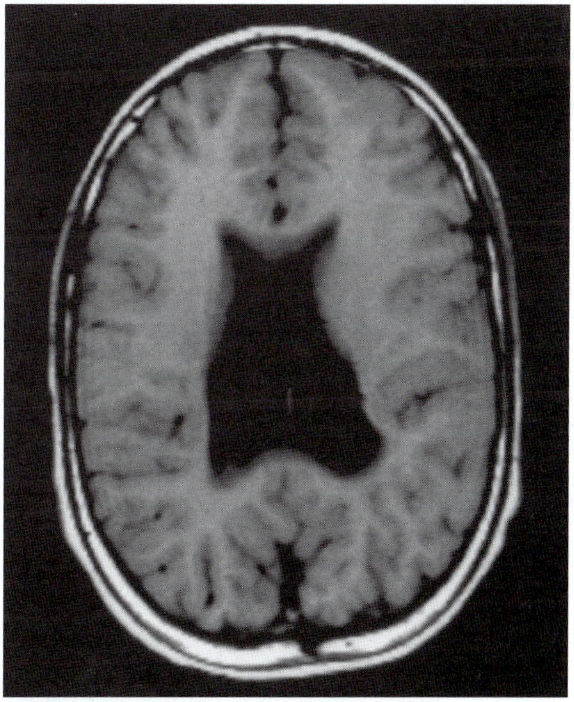

Figura 592-8. Oloprosencefalia lobare. La RM pesata in T1 mostra l'assenza di separazione tra gli emisferi e la fusione ventricolare.

Il tasso di mortalità è estremamente elevato, ma alcuni pazienti vivono per anni. Nelle forme lievi la morbilità è meno grave, ma è opportuno evitare qualsiasi prognosi. L'incidenza dell'oloprosencefalia è compresa tra 1 su 5000 e 1 su 16 000. La diagnosi prenatale può essere confermata mediante ecografia dopo la decima settimana di gestazione (nei casi più gravi). Solitamente non è possibile identificare la causa della patologia, ma è ipotizzabile un'associazione con il diabete materno. In circa il 50% dei casi, si riscontrano anomalie cromosomiche, come delezioni dei cromosomi 7q e 3p, 21q, 2p, 18p e13q, trisomia 13 e 18. È stato dimostrato che anche le mutazioni del gene "sonic hedgehog" a livello del cromosoma 7q causano oloprosencefalia.

592.8 • Agenesia del corpo calloso

L'agenesia del corpo calloso consiste in un eterogeneo gruppo di patologie con espressione variabile, dal grave ritardo mentale e deficit neurologico a soggetti asintomatici con livello intellettivo nella norma (Fig. 592-9). Il corpo calloso si sviluppa a partire dal piatto commissurale, che si trova in prossimità del neuroporo anteriore. Il danneggiamento di tale piatto durante le fasi precoci dell'embriogenesi provoca l'agenesia del corpo calloso. Se l'agenesia resta un fenomeno isolato, il paziente può risultare asintomatico. Gli individui che, oltre all'assenza del corpo calloso, presentano anomalie dovute a difetti della migrazione cellulare, come eterotopia, microgiria e pachigiria (circonvoluzioni aumentate e ampie), manifestano sintomi neurologici, tra cui ritardo mentale, microcefalia, emiparesi, diplegia e convulsioni. La TC e la RM consentono di evidenziare le caratteristiche anatomiche del disturbo, mostrando l'ampia separazione tra i corni anteriori e l'anomala posizione elevata del terzo ventricolo tra i ventricoli laterali. La RM delinea con precisione l'estensione del difetto del corpo calloso. L'assenza del corpo calloso può essere ereditata con modalità autosomica dominante. La patologia è talvolta associata a specifiche anomalie cromosomiche, in particolare la trisomia 8 e 18.

La **sindrome di Aicardi** è una patologia complessa che colpisce diversi sistemi, tipicamente associata ad agenesia del corpo calloso. Il fatto che nella quasi totalità dei casi i pazienti siano di sesso femminile suggerisce un'anomalia genetica del cromosoma X (può essere letale nei feti maschi). Le convulsioni esordiscono durante i primi mesi di vita e non rispondono agli anticonvulsivanti. L'elettroencefalogramma (EEG) registra l'attività indipendente dei due emisferi, risultato dell'assenza del corpo calloso. Tutte le pazienti manifestano ritardo mentale grave e anomalie delle vertebre, fuse o solo parzialmente sviluppate (emivertebre). I reperti tipici della sindrome di Aicardi sono le anomalie retiniche, come lacune circoscritte e coloboma del disco ottico.

592.9 • Agenesia dei nervi cranici

L'assenza dei nervi cranici o dei corrispondenti nuclei centrali, descritta in diverse malattie, può coinvolgere i nervi ottico, trigemino e uditivo, e i nervi cranici IX, X, XI, e XII. I disturbi causati includono la ptosi congenita e il fenomeno di Marcus Gunn (movimenti di suzione della mandibola causano la simultanea chiusura delle palpebre; questa sincinesia congenita è dovuta a una anomala innervazione dei nervi trigemino e oculomotorio). La **sindrome di Möbius** è caratterizzata da debolezza facciale bilaterale, spesso associata a paralisi del nervo abducente. Sono stati segnalati casi di ipoplasia o agenesia dei nuclei troncoencefalici e di assenza o riduzione del numero di fibre muscolari. La malattia si presenta nel periodo neonatale con debolezza facciale e conseguenti difficoltà di allattamento. La facies immobile e inespressiva può erroneamente suggerire la presenza di ritardo mentale. La prognosi è eccellente in molti casi e lo sviluppo procede nella norma. L'aspetto del volto può essere migliorato chirurgicamente.

592.10 • Microcefalia

La microcefalia è definita come una circonferenza cranica che misura più di tre deviazioni standard al di sotto della media per sesso ed età. Questa condizione patologica è relativamente comune, in particolare nei bambini con ritardo dello sviluppo. Può essere causata da diversi fattori, ma in molti casi si riscontra un'anomalia della migrazione neuronale durante lo sviluppo fetale (come l'eterotopia delle cellule neuronali e le atipie citoarchitetturali). Esistono due forme principali: la microcefalia primaria (genetica) e la microcefalia secondaria (non genetica). La formulazione di una diagnosi precisa è fondamentale per il counseling genetico e per la previsione dei rischi in caso di gravidanze future.

EZIOLOGIA. La microcefalia primaria comprende un gruppo di condizioni patologiche ereditate con modalità mendeliana, nelle quali non si riscontrano altre malformazioni, o associate a una specifica sindrome genetica. I neonati colpiti sono solitamente identificati alla nascita in seguito al riscontro di una circonferenza cranica inferiore alla media. I tipi più comuni includono la microcefalia familiare autosomica dominante e una serie di sindromi cromosomiche riassunte nella Tabella 592-1. La microcefalia **secondaria** è il risultato dell'esposizione a un'ampia gamma di agenti tossici che possono danneggiare il feto in utero o il lattante (in particolare nei periodi di rapida crescita cerebrale nei primi due anni di vita).

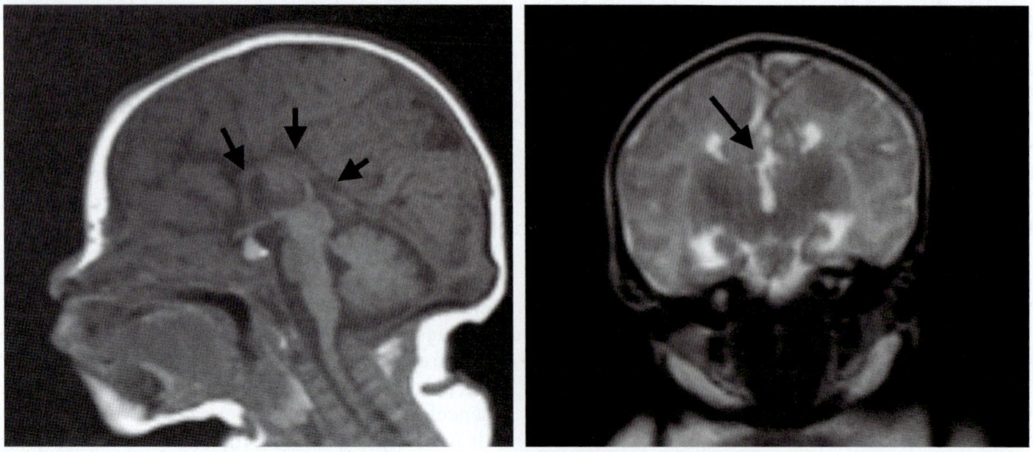

Figura 592-9. Agenesia del corpo calloso mostrata dalla RM. La scansione sul piano sagittale (a sinistra) e coronale (a destra) mostra la totale assenza di una struttura mediosagittale di sostanza bianca (*frecce* nell'immagine a sinistra). L'immagine coronale (a destra) mostra, malgrado l'artefatto da movimento, l'assenza di una struttura di collegamento tra i due emisferi (area al di sotto della *freccia*).

TABELLA 592-1. Cause della microcefalia

CAUSE	REPERTI TIPICI
PRIMARIA (GENETICA)	
1. Familiare (autosomica recessiva)	• Incidenza 1 su 40 000 nascite • Facies tipica, con fronte obliqua, naso e orecchie prominenti; grave ritardo mentale e convulsioni; scarsa differenziazione delle circonvoluzioni e citoarchitettura disorganizzata
2. Autosomica dominante	• Assenza di una facies tipica, palpebre e fronte oblique, orecchie prominenti • Crescita lineare normale, convulsioni facilmente controllabili, ritardo mentale lieve o borderline
3. Sindromi	
di Down (trisomia 21)	• Incidenza 1 su 800 • Anomalo arrotondamento dei lobi frontale e occipitale, cervelletto piccolo; giro temporale superiore stretto, tendenza a sviluppare alterazioni neurofibrillari dell'Alzheimer, anomalie ultrastrutturali della corteccia cerebrale
di Edward (trisomia 18)	• Incidenza 1 su 6500 • Basso peso alla nascita, microstomia, micrognazia, orecchie a impianto basso, occipite prominente, piede rocker-bottom, deformità in flessione delle dita, cardiopatia congenita, aumento dei giri, eterotopia dei neuroni
Cri-du-chat (5p-)	• Incidenza 1 su 50 000 • Volto ovale, epicanto prominente, orecchie a impianto basso, ipertelorismo e pianto caratteristico • Assenza di una specifica neuropatia
di Cornelia de Lange	• Ritardo di crescita pre e postnatale, sinofria, labbro superiore sottile e rivolto verso il basso • Pollice in posizione prossimale
di Rubinstein-Taybi	• Naso a becco, palpebre oblique e rivolte verso il basso, epicanto, bassa statura, pollici e alluci grandi
di Smith-Lemli-Opitz	• Ptosi, scafocefalia, epicanto, anteversione delle narici • Basso peso alla nascita, gravi disturbi dell'allattamento
SECONDARIA (NON GENETICA)	
1. Radiazioni	• Microcefalia e ritardo mentale, più grave se l'esposizione avviene nelle prime 15 settimane di gestazione
2. Infezioni congenite	
Cytomegalovirus	• Piccole dimensioni rispetto alla media, eruzione petecchiale, epato-splenomegalia, corioretinite, sordità, ritardo mentale e convulsioni • Calcificazione del SNC e microgiria
Rosolia	• Ritardo di crescita, porpora, trombocitopenia, epato-splenomegalia, cardiopatia congenita, corioretinite, cataratta e sordità • Aree perivascolari necrotiche, polimicrogiria, eterotopia, cavitazioni subependimali
Toxoplasmosi	• Porpora, epato-splenomegalia, ittero, convulsioni, idrocefalo, corioretinite e calcificazione cerebrale
3. Farmaci e abuso di sostanze	
Sindrome feto-alcolica	• Ritardo di crescita, ptosi, assenza di filtro e labbro superiore ipoplastico, cardiopatia congenita, disturbi dell'allattamento, eterotopia della neuroglia, disorganizzazione neuronale
Sindrome fetale da idantoina	• Ritardo di crescita, ipoplasia delle falangi distali, epicanto, radice nasale ampia e narici anteverse
4. Meningite/encefalite	• Infarti cerebrali, cavitazione cistica, diffusa perdita neuronale
5. Malnutrizione	• La causa di microcefalia è controversa
6. Malattie metaboliche	• Diabete mellito materno e iperfenilalaninemia materna
7. Ipertermia	• Febbre elevata durante le prime 4-6 settimane può causare microcefalia, convulsioni e anomalie facciali • Studi anatomopatologici rivelano eterotopia neuronale • Altri studi non sono riusciti a stabilire alcun collegamento tra febbre materna e anomalie fetali
8. Encefalopatia ipossica-ischemica	• Edema cerebrale diffuso iniziale; atrofia cerebrale negli stadi avanzati

MANIFESTAZIONI CLINICHE E DIAGNOSI. L'anamnesi dettagliata deve indagare in particolare la presenza di altri casi di microcefalia nella famiglia o di disturbi a carico del sistema nervoso. È importante misurare la circonferenza del paziente alla nascita. Una circonferenza molto ridotta implica infatti un processo iniziato precocemente durante lo sviluppo embrionale o fetale. Un insulto cerebrale più tardivo (in particolare dopo i due anni) determina raramente una grave microcefalia. Misure seriali sono più utili di una singola misurazione, soprattutto se l'anomalia è minima. È opportuno misurare anche la circonferenza cranica di genitori e fratelli.

La scelta degli esami di laboratorio è determinata dall'anamnesi e dall'esame fisico. Se la causa della microcefalia non è nota, è utile determinare il livello sierico materno di fenilalanina. Una concentrazione elevata in una madre asintomatica può causare un grave danno cerebrale in un bambino non fenilchetonurico. Se si sospetta una sindrome cromosomica o in presenza di facies anomala, bassa statura o anomalie congenite addizionali è utile ottenere il cariotipo. La RM consente di identificare anomalie strutturali del cervello, mentre la TC è la tecnica ideale per evidenziare calcificazioni intracerebrali. Studi supplementari includono: il dosaggio degli amminoacidi nel plasma a digiuno e nelle urine; la determinazione dell'ammoniaca nel siero; esami del gruppo TORCH, per la ricerca di toxoplasmosi, rosolia, Cytomegalovirus, herpes simplex; esame HIV di madre e bambino; prelievo di un campione urinario per la coltura del Cytomegalovirus.

TRATTAMENTO. Una volta stabilita la causa della microcefalia, è opportuno fornire alla famiglia un accurato counseling genetico e di supporto. Poiché la microcefalia è spesso associata a ritardo mentale, il medico è chiamato ad assistere i genitori nella scelta del programma più appropriato per favorire lo sviluppo del bambino (vedi Capitolo 38.2).

Barkovich AJ, Kuzniecky RI, Jackson MD, et al: Classification system for malformations of cortical development. *Neurology* 2001;57:2168–2178.

Barr M, Cohen MM: Holoprosencephaly survival and performance. *Am J Med Genet* 1999;89:116–120.

Clark GD: The classification of cortical dysplasias through molecular genetics. *Brain Dev* 2004;26:351–362.

Denis D, Chateil JF, Brun M, et al: Schizencephaly: Clinical and imaging features in 30 infantile cases. *Brain Dev* 2000;22:475–483.

Donkelaar HJ, Lammens M, Wesseling P, et al: Development and developmental disorders of the human cerebellum. *J Neurol* 2003;250:1025–1036.

d'Orsi G, Tinuper P, Bisulli F, et al: Clinical features and long term outcome of epilepsy in periventricular nodular heterotopia. Simple compared with plus forms. *J Neurol Neurosurg Psychiatry* 2004;75:873–878.

Hayashi N, Tsutsumi Y, Barkovich AJ: Morphological features and associated anomalies of schizencephaly in the clinical population: Detailed analysis of MR images. *Neuroradiology* 2002;44:418–427.

Hayashi N, Tsutsumi Y, Barkovich AJ: Polymicrogyria without porencephaly/schizencephaly. MRI analysis of the spectrum and the prevalence of macroscopic findings in the clinical population. *Neuroradiology* 2002;44:647–655.

Kinsman SL, Plawner LL, Hahn JS: Holoprosencephaly: Recent advances and insights. *Curr Opin Neurol* 2000;13:127–132.
Miller SP, Shevell MI, Patenaude Y, et al: Septo-optic dysplasia plus: A spectrum of malformations of cortical development. *Neurology* 2000;54: 1701–1703.
Nerdich JA, Nussbaum RL, Packer TC, et al: Heterogeneity of clinical severity and molecular lesions in Aicardi syndrome. *J Paediatr* 1990;116: 911–917.
Parrish ML, Roessmann U, Levinsohn MW: Agenesis of the corpus callosum: A study of the frequency of associated malformations. *Ann Neurol* 1979;6:349–354.
Richards LJ, Plachez C, Ren T: Mechanisms regulating the development of the corpus callosum and its agenesis in mouse and human. *Clin Genet* 2004;66:276–289.
Sudarshan A, Goldie WD: The spectrum of congenital facial diplegia (Moebius syndrome). *Pediatr Neurol* 1985;1:180–184.
Sztriha L: Spectrum of corpus callosum agenesis. *Pediatr Neurol* 2005;32: 94–101.

592.11 • Idrocefalo

L'idrocefalo non è una malattia specifica, ma rappresenta un gruppo eterogeneo di condizioni risultato della compromissione della circolazione e dell'assorbimento di liquido cerebrospinale o, in rari casi, dall'aumento della sua produzione causato da un papilloma del plesso coroideo (Tab. 592-2).

FISIOLOGIA. Il liquido cerebrospinale (LCS) è formato prevalentemente nel sistema ventricolare da plessi coroidei, situati nei ventricoli laterali, 3° e 4°. La quantità maggiore è prodotta nei ventricoli laterali, mentre il restante 25% circa origina da fonti extracoroidee, come l'endotelio capillare all'interno del parenchima cerebrale. L'innervazione adrenergica e colinergica del plesso coroideo garantisce il controllo neurogeno attivo della formazione di LCS. La stimolazione del sistema adrenergico riduce la produzione, mentre l'eccitazione dei nervi colinergici può raddoppiarla. Nel bambino normale, vengono prodotti circa 20 mL di LCS l'ora. Il volume totale di LCS è approssimativamente di 50 mL nel lattante e 150 mL nell'adulto. La maggior parte dell'LCS è extraventricolare. La sua produzione da parte dei plessi coroidei avviene in diversi stadi; attraverso una complessa serie di intricati passaggi, il plasma ultrafiltrato è processato in una secrezione, l'LCS.

Il flusso dell'LCS è il risultato del gradiente pressorio tra il sistema ventricolare e i canali venosi. In condizioni normali, la pressione intraventricolare può salire fino a 180 mmH_2O, mentre la pressione nel seno sagittale superiore si colloca intorno a 90 mmH_2O. L'LSC scorre dai ventricoli laterali al terzo ventricolo, passando per il forame di Monro. Attraversa poi l'acquedotto del Silvio (lungo circa 3 mm e largo 2 mm nel bambino) ed entra nel 4° ventricolo. Attraverso i forami laterali di Luschka e il forame centrale di Magendie, l'LCS lascia il 4° ventricolo ed entra nelle cisterne alla base del cervello. L'idrocefalo causato dal un'ostruzione nell'ambito del sistema ventricolare è definito **idrocefalo ostruttivo** o **non comunicante**. Dalle cisterne basali, l'LCS fluisce posteriormente, attraverso il sistema delle cisterne e al di sopra delle convessità degli emisferi cerebrali. È assorbito prevalentemente dai villi aracnoidei, attraverso le giunzioni strette del loro endotelio, grazie ai gradienti pressori descritti in precedenza. In grado minore, l'LCS è assorbito anche dai canali linfatici diretti ai seni paranasali, lungo il rivestimento delle radici nervose, e dai plessi coroidei stessi. L'idrocefalo risultato dell'obliterazione delle cisterne subaracnoidee o del malfunzionamento dei villi aracnoidi è definito **idrocefalo non ostruttivo** o **comunicante**.

TABELLA 592-2. Cause di idrocefalo

COMUNICANTE
Acondroplasia
Impronta basilare
Allargamento benigno dello spazio subaracnoideo
Papilloma del plesso coroideo
Tumore meningeale maligno
Meningite
Emorragia
NON COMUNICANTE
Stenosi acqueduttale
infettiva*
correlata alla X
Malformazione di Chiari
Malformazione di Dandy-Walker
Sindrome di Klippel-Feil
Lesioni da massa
ascesso
ematoma
tumori e disturbi neurocutanei
malformazione della vena di Galeno
sindrome di Walker-Warburg
IDRANENCEFALIA
Oloprosencefalia
Idrocefalo
Porencefalia

* Toxoplasmosi, parotite, neurocisticercosi.
Tratta da Fenichel GM: *Clinical Pediatric Neurology*, 5th ed. Philadelphia, Elsevier, 2005, p 354.

FISIOPATOLOGIA ED EZIOLOGIA. Nei bambini, l'idrocefalo ostruttivo o non comunicante si sviluppa prevalentemente a causa di una anomalia dell'acquedotto o di una lesione a carico del 4° ventricolo. La **stenosi acqueduttale** è il risultato di un anomalo restringimento dell'acquedotto del Silvio, spesso associato a ramificazione o biforcazione. In una piccola percentuale di casi, la stenosi è ereditata come tratto recessivo legato al sesso. Occasionalmente, tali pazienti presentano un difetto minore della chiusura del tubo neurale, inclusa la spina bifida occulta. In rari casi, la stenosi acqueduttale è associata a neurofibromatosi. Anche la **gliosi acqueduttale** può dare origine a idrocefalo. In seguito a meningite neonatale o emorragia subaracnoidea in un neonato prematuro, il rivestimento ependimale dell'acquedotto è interrotto e la conseguente risposta gliale determina una completa ostruzione. Sono stati segnalati casi di infezioni virali intrauterine responsabili di stesosi acqueduttale seguita da idrocefalo (e un caso di meningoencefalite parotitica). La malformazione della vena di Galeno, con conseguente espansione, può determinare un'ostruzione del flusso di LCS, a causa della sua posizione centrale. Lesioni o malformazioni della fossa cerebrale posteriore (come tumori, malformazione di Chiari e sindrome di Dandy-Walker) costituiscono un'altra rilevante causa di idrocefalo.

Nella maggior parte dei casi, l'idrocefalo non ostruttivo o comunicante è il risultato di un'emorragia subaracnoidea, solitamente conseguenza di una emorragia intraventricolare in un neonato prematuro. La presenza di sangue negli spazi subaracnoidei può causare obliterazione delle cisterne o dei villi aracnoidei o ostruzione del flusso di LCS. La meningite tubercolotica o pneumococcica tende a produrre un essudato denso e tenace, che ostruisce le cisterne basali. Anche le infezioni intrauterine possono distruggere le vie di scorrimento dell'LCS. Infine, la presenza di infiltrati leucemici nello spazio subaracnoideo rischia di produrre idrocefalo comunicante.

MANIFESTAZIONI CLINICHE. La presentazione clinica dell'idrocefalo è estremamente variabile e dipende da molti fattori, inclusa l'età di esordio, la natura delle lesione responsabile dell'ostruzione, la durata e l'entità dell'aumento della pressione intracranica (*IntraCranial Pressure*, ICP). Nel lattante, il segno principale è costituito da un accelerato aumento delle dimensioni del cranio. La fontanella anteriore appare rilevata e ampia, e le vene della volta cranica risultano dilatate. La fronte è ampia e gli occhi tendono a deviare verso il basso a causa della pressione esercitata dal recesso soprapineale dilatato sul tectum, che determina i caratteristici occhi a sole calante. Lo stiramento e la lesione delle fibre corticospinali della corteccia motoria determina segni delle vie lunghe, come iperreflessia tendinea, spasticità, clono (in particolare a livello degli arti inferiori) e segno di Babinski. Nel bambino più grande, le suture craniche sono parzialmente chiuse, perciò i segni di idrocefalo risultano più sfumati e includono: irritabilità, letargia, scarso appetito, vomito e mal di testa. Una graduale modifica della personalità e un deterioramento delle prestazioni scolastiche suggeriscono una forma di idrocefalo a lenta progressione. Misure seriali della circonferenza cranica indicano l'incremento della velocità di crescita. La percussione del cranio produce un tipico suono di "pentola fessa" (segno di Macewen), che indica la separazione delle suture. Un accorciamento dell'occipite suggerisce la malformazione di Chiari, mentre un occipite pronunciato suggerisce la malformazione di Dandy-Walker. Nella maggior parte dei casi si osservano papilledema, paralisi del nervo abducente e segni piramidali, più evidenti a livello degli arti inferiori.

Le **malformazioni di Chiari** sono classificate in due sottogruppi principali. Il **tipo I**, che produce tipicamente sintomi durante l'adolescenza e l'età adulta, solitamente non è associato a idrocefalo. I pazienti lamentano cefalee ricorrenti, cervicalgia, minzione frequente e progressiva spasticità degli arti inferiori. La deformità consiste nello spostamento delle tonsille cerebellari nel canale cervicale (Fig. 592-10). La patogenesi è sconosciuta, ma la teoria prevalente suggerisce un'ostruzione della porzione caudale del 4° ventricolo durante lo sviluppo fetale. È stato ipotizzato anche un cord tethering o anomalie addizionali (siringe). La **malformazione di Chiari di tipo II** è caratterizzata da idrocefalo progressivo associato a mielomeningocele. La lesione è il risultato di un'anomalia romboencefalica, probabilmente dovuta alla mancata formazione della curvatura pontina durante l'embriogenesi, con conseguente allungamento del 4° ventricolo e deformazione del tronco (spostamento di verme inferiore, ponte e midollo allungato nel canale cervicale; Fig. 592-11). In circa il 10% dei casi, la malformazione determina sintomi durante l'infanzia, che includono stridore respiratorio, pianto debole e apnea (alleviabile mediante shunt o decompressione della fossa posteriore). Una forma più indolente causa anomalie della deambulazione, spasticità e progressiva perdita della coordinazione durante l'infanzia. Le radiografie dirette mostrano una fossa posteriore piccola e un allargamento del canale cervicale. La TC con mezzo di contrasto e la RM mostrano la protrusione verso il canale cervicale delle tonsille cerebellari e le anomalie romboencefaliche. La malformazione è trattata mediante decompressione chirurgica.

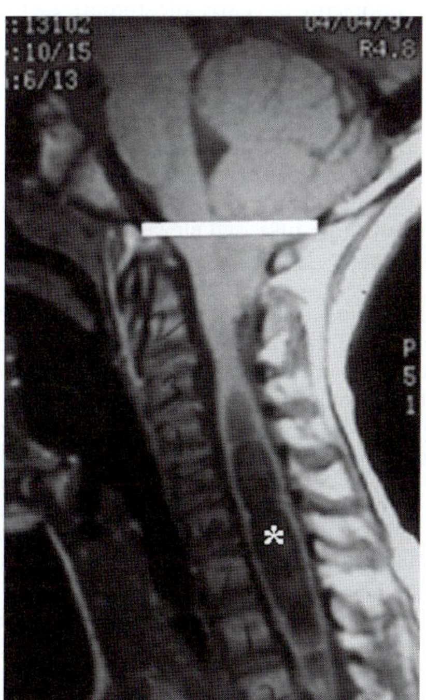

Figura 592-10. La RM sagittale di un paziente con malformazione di Chiari di tipo I. Le tonsille cerebellari risultano spostate attraverso il forame magno (*linea bianca*) nell'aspetto inferiore di C2. L'ingombro del forame è evidente. È visibile una cavità siringomielica, che si estende da C3 a T2. (Tratta da Yassari R, Frim D: Evaluation and management of the Chiari malformation type 1 for the primary care pediatrician. *Pediatr Clin North Am* 2004;51:477-490.)

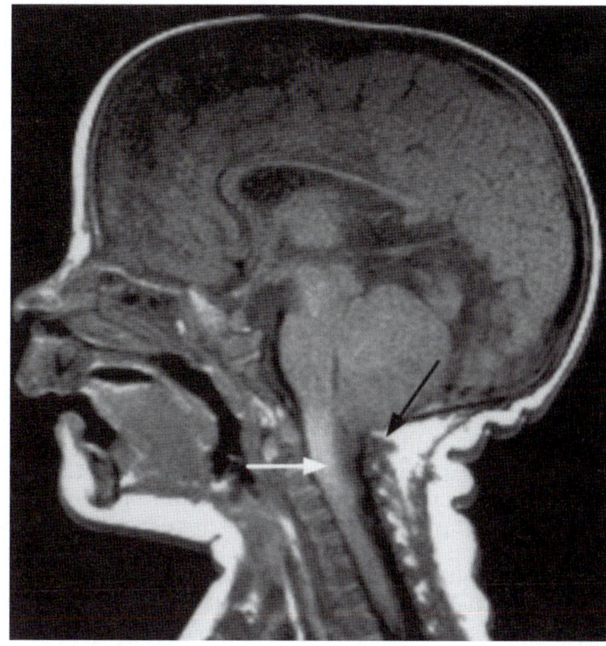

Figura 592-11. La RM mediosagittale pesata in T1 di un paziente con malformazione di Chiari. Le tonsille cerebellari (*freccia bianca*) sono discese al di sotto del forame magno (*freccia nera*). Notare l'aspetto del 4°, che appare come una piccola fessura verticale.

La **malformazione di Dandy-Walker** consiste in un'espansione cistica del 4° ventricolo nella fossa posteriore e in un'ipoplasia cerebellare della linea mediana, conseguenza del mancato sviluppo del tetto del 4° ventricolo durante l'embriogenesi (Fig. 592-12). Circa il 90% dei pazienti ha idrocefalo e un numero significativo di bambini presenta anomalie associate, come agenesia del verme cerebellare posteriore e del corpo calloso. Nel lattante, la

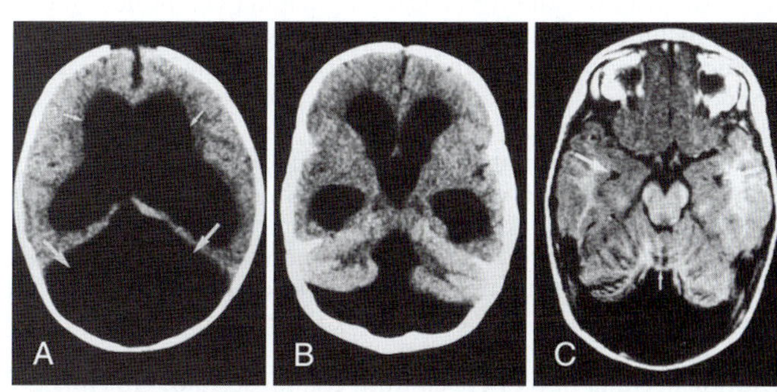

Figura 592-12. Cisti di Dandy-Walker. *A*, Immagine TC assiale (preoperatoria) che mostra un'ampia cisti nella fossa posteriore (cisti di Dandy-Walker, *freccia grande*) e la dilatazione dei ventricoli laterali (*frecce piccole*), una complicazione secondaria all'ostruzione dei canali dell'LCS all'uscita del 4° ventricolo. *B*, Nello stesso paziente, un'immagine TC assiale più bassa mostra la distensione degli emisferi cerebellari dovuta alla dilatazione del 4° ventricolo (cisti di Dandy-Walker). I ventricoli dilatati prossimali al 4° ventricolo mostrano l'ostruzione del flusso di LCS dovuta alla cisti di Dandy-Walker. *C*, RM dello stesso paziente, che mostra la riduzione delle dimensioni della cisti di Dandy-Walker e dei corni temporali (*frecce*) in seguito all'impianto di uno shunt. Il verme incompleto (*freccia piccola*) è ora riconoscibile.

malformazione si presenta con un rapido aumento della circonferenza del cranio e occipite prominente. La transilluminazione della volta cranica può risultare positiva. La maggior parte dei pazienti presenta segni delle vie lunghe, atassia cerebellare e ritardo nelle acquisizione motorie e cognitive, probabilmente dovuti alle anomalie strutturali associate. In presenza di idrocefalo, il trattamento prevede l'impianto di uno shunt nella cavità cistica (e occasionalmente anche nei ventricoli).

DIAGNOSI E DIAGNOSI DIFFERENZIALE. L'esame di un bambino con idrocefalo comincia con la raccolta dell'anamnesi. Il riscontro di una storia familiare positiva suggerisce un idrocefalo legato all'X secondario a stenosi acqueduttale. È importante verificare la presenza di una storia clinica di prematurità con emorragia intracranica, meningite o encefalite parotitica. Chiazze caffellatte multiple e altre caratteristiche cliniche della neurofibromatosi sono suggestive di un idrocefalo da stenosi acqueduttale. L'esame include una accurata ispezione, palpazione e auscultazione della volta cranica e della colonna. La circonferenza occipitofrontale è registrata e paragonata a misurazioni precedenti. Si osservano le dimensioni e la configurazione della fontanella anteriore. Il dorso deve venire ispezionato, per verificare la presenza di lesioni cutanee della linea mediana, come ciuffi di peli, lipomi o angiomi, che suggeriscono disrafismo spinale. La presenza di una fonte prominente o di anomalie della forma dell'occipite contribuiscono a chiarire la patogenesi dell'idrocefalo. La malformazione della vena di Galeno causa spesso un rumore cranico auscultabile. La transilluminazione del cranio è positiva in caso di rilevante dilatazione del sistema ventricolare o nella sindrome di Dandy-Walker. L'esame del fondo oculare è indispensabile, perché il riscontro di corioretinite suggerisce la responsabilità di un'infezione intrauterina, come la toxoplasmosi, nella genesi dell'idrocefalo. Il papilledema è osservato nei bambini più grandi, ma è raramente presente nei lattanti, perché l'incremento della pressione determina una separazione delle suture. Le radiografie dirette mostrano tipicamente separazione delle suture, erosioni dei processi clinoidei posteriori nel bambino più grande e un allargamento dei solchi delle circonvoluzioni ("segno dell'argento battuto") se l'aumento dell'ICP si protrae a lungo. La TC e/o la RM e l'ecografia costituiscono le tecniche di elezione per identificare le cause specifiche dell'idrocefalo nel neonato e per valutarne la gravità.

L'aumento della circonferenza cranica può essere confuso con l'idrocefalo secondario all'ispessimento cranico dovuto a anemia cronica, rachitismo, osteogenesi imperfetta e displasia epifisaria. Raccolte subdurali croniche possono causare una prominenza parietale ossea bilaterale. Vari disturbi metabolici e degenerativi del SNC determinano encefalomegalia, dovuta all'anomalo accumulo di sostanze all'interno del parenchima cerebrale. Questi disturbi includono malattie lisosomiali (Tay-Sachs, gangliosidosi e mucopolisaccaridosi), aminoacidurie (malattia delle urine a sciroppo d'acero) e leucodistrofie (metacromatica, malattie di Alexander e Canavan).

Anche la neurofibromatosi e il gigantismo cerebrale sono caratterizzati da un aumento della massa cerebrale. L'encefalomegalia familiare, ereditata con modalità autosomica dominante, è caratterizzata da un ritardo nelle acquisizioni motorie, ma il livello intellettivo è solitamente nella norma o lievemente inferiore. Per formulare la diagnosi è necessario procedere alla misura della circonferenza cranica dei genitori.

L'**idranencefalia** può essere confusa con idrocefalo. Gli emisferi cerebrali sono assenti o costituiti da un sacco membranoso che contiene residui di corteccia frontale, temporale o occipitale, dispersi sulla membrana. Il mesencefalo e il tronco sono relativamente integri (Fig. 592-13). La causa dell'idranencefalia è sconosciuta, ma l'occlusione bilaterale delle arterie carotidi interne durante le fasi precoci dello sviluppo fetale spiegherebbe gran parte delle anomalie. Nei lattanti colpiti, la circonferenza cranica, normale o aumentata alla nascita, aumenta troppo rapidamente nel postnatale. La transilluminazione rivela l'assenza degli emisferi cerebrali. Il bambino è irritabile, manifesta disturbi

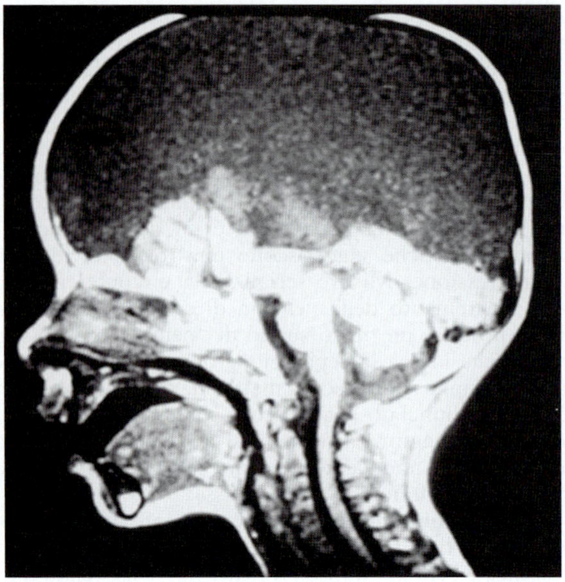

Figura 592-13. Idranencefalia. RM che mostra il tronco e il midollo spinale con residui di cervelletto e corteccia cerebrale. Il resto del cranio è riempito con LCS.

dell'allattamento e sviluppa convulsioni e tetraparesi spastica. Lo sviluppo cognitivo è minimo o del tutto assente. L'impianto di uno shunt ventricolo-peritoneale impedisce un allargamento incontrollato del cranio.

TRATTAMENTO. La terapia dell'idrocefalo dipende dalla causa. La somministrazione di acetazolamide e furosemide può fornire un sollievo temporaneo, riducendo la produzione di LCS, ma i risultati a lungo termine di questa terapia si sono rivelati deludenti. La maggior dei casi di idrocefalo richiede l'impianto di uno shunt extracranico, in particolare ventricolo-peritoneale (ma talvolta è sufficiente la ventricolostomia). Le principali complicanze dell'applicazione di shunt sono l'occlusione (con mal di testa, papilledema, emesi e alterazioni dello stato mentale) e le infezioni batteriche (con febbre, mal di testa e meningismo), solitamente dovute a *Staphylococcus epidermidis* (vedi Capitolo 180). Grazie a una meticolosa preparazione, il tasso di infezioni da shunt può essere ridotto fino a <5%. La correzione chirurgica intrauterina dell'idrocefalo fetale non ha ottenuto risultati incoraggianti, forse a causa dell'elevato tasso di malformazioni cerebrali associate.

PROGNOSI. La prognosi dipende dalla causa della dilazione ventricolare e non dalle dimensioni del mantello corticale all'epoca dell'intervento, fatta eccezione per i casi di grave compressione o stiramento del mantello. I bambini con idrocefalo presentano un rischio più elevato di presentare varie disabilità dello sviluppo. Il quoziente intellettivo medio è più basso rispetto alla popolazione generale, in particolare nelle abilità di performance (mentre nelle abilità verbali il ritardo è meno marcato). Si riscontrano spesso anomalie della funzione mnemonica. Sono comuni anche i disturbi visivi, come strabismo, anomalie visuospaziali, difetti del campo visivo e atrofia ottica, con riduzione dell'acuità visiva secondaria all'aumento dell'ICP. Le latenze dei potenziali evocati visivi sono ritardate e continuano a esserlo per un certo periodo anche dopo la correzione chirurgica dell'idrocefalo. Alcuni pazienti manifestano un comportamento aggressivo e delinquenziale. Nei soggetti con idrocefalo corretto da shunt o mielomeningocele, si riscontra spesso un'accelerazione dello sviluppo puberale, forse causata dall'aumento della secrezione di gonadotropina in risposta all'incremento della ICP. È indispensabile sottoporre i bambini con idrocefalo a follow-up multidisciplinare a lungo termine.

Chumas P, Tyagi A, Livingston J: Hydrocephalus—What's new? *Arch Dis Child Fetal Neonatal Ed* 2001;85:F149–F154.
Cochrane DD, Myles ST, Nimrod C, et al: Intrauterine hydrocephalus and ventriculomegaly: Associated abnormalities and fetal outcome. *Can J Neurol Sci* 1985;12:51–59.
Fitzsimmons JS: Laryngeal stridor and respiratory obstruction in association with myelomeningocele. *Dev Med Child Neurol* 1973;15:553–556.
Greene M, Benacerraf B, Crawford J: Hydranencephaly: US appearance during in utero evolution. *Radiology* 1985;156:779–780.
Hirsch JF, Pierre-Kahn A, Renier D, et al: The Dandy-Walker malformation. *J Neurosurg* 1984;61:515–522.
Hoffman HJ, Hendrick EB, Humphreys RP: Manifestations and management of Arnold-Chiari malformations in patients with myelomeningocele. *Childs Brain* 1975;1:255–259.
Löppönen T, Saukkonen A-L, Serlo W, et al: Accelerated pubertal development in patients with shunted hydrocephalus. *Arch Dis Child* 1996;74:490–496.
Parisi MA, Dobyns WB: Human malformations of the midbrain and hindbrain: Review and proposed classification scheme. *Mol Genet Metab* 2003;80:36–53.

TABELLA 592.3. Classificazioni clinico-genetiche delle craniosinostosi usate comunemente

CATEGORIA DIAGNOSTICA	NOME DELLA SINDROME	CAUSA
Craniosinostosi isolata	Sulla base della morfologia	Sconosciuta, costrizione uterina o mutazione di *FGFR*$_3$
Craniosinostosi sindromica	Sindrome di Antler-Bixler	Sconosciuta
	Sindrome di Apert	Solitamente una delle due mutazioni di *FGFR*$_2$
	Sindrome di Baere-Stevenson	Mutazione di *GFGR*$_2$ o *FGFR*$_3$
	Sindrome di Bailler-Gerold	Mutazione eterogenea di *TWIST*
	Sindrome di Carpenter	Sconosciuta
	Displasia craniofrontale	Gene sconosciuto in Xp22
	Sindrome di Crouzon	Numerose mutazioni di *FGFR*$_2$
	Sindrome di Crouzon mesodermo-scheletrica	Mutazione di *FGFR*$_3$
	Sindrome di Jackson-Weiss	Mutazione di *FGFR*$_2$
	Sindrome di Muenke	Mutazione di *FGFR*$_3$
	Sindrome di Pfeiffer	Mutazione di *FGFR*$_1$ o più mutazioni di *FGFR*$_2$
	Sindrome di Saethre-Chotzen	Mutazione di *TWIST*
	Sindrome di Shprintzen-Goldberg	Mutazione di *FBEN*$_1$

Tratta da Ridgway EB, Weiner HL: Skull deformities. *Pediatr Clin North Am* 2004;51:359-387.

592.12 • Craniosinostosi

La craniosinostosi è definita come la chiusura prematura delle suture craniche ed è classificata in primaria e secondaria. La **craniosinostosi primaria** consiste nella chiusura di una o più suture, dovuta ad anomalie dello sviluppo cranico. La **craniosinostosi secondaria**, che non verrà discussa in questa sede, è il risultato di un disturbo della crescita e dell'espansione cerebrale. L'incidenza della craniosinostosi è di circa 1 su 2000 nascite. Nella maggior parte dei casi, la causa è sconosciuta, ma nel 10-20% si ipotizza un'origine genetica.

SVILUPPO ED EZIOLOGIA. Durante le fasi precoci dello sviluppo, il cervello è avvolto da una guaina mesenchimale. Entro il 2° mese, nella porzione di mesenchima corrispondente al cranio comincia a evidenziarsi il tessuto osseo, mentre alla base del cranio si forma tessuto cartilagineo. Entro il 5° mese di gestazione, le ossa craniche (frontali, parietali, temporali e occipitali) appaiono ben sviluppate e separate da suture e fontanelle. Il cervello cresce rapidamente nei primi anni di vita e, in condizioni normali, tale sviluppo non incontra ostacoli grazie all'equivalente crescita lungo le linee di sutura. La causa della craniosinostosi non è nota, ma l'ipotesi prevalente suggerisce che uno sviluppo anomalo della base del cranio determini una pressione eccessiva sulla dura madre, alterando il normale sviluppo delle suture. Sono stati identificati fattori genetici in alcune cause isolate e in molte cause sindromiche di craniosinostosi (Tab. 592-3).

MANIFESTAZIONI CLINICHE E TRATTAMENTO. La maggior parte dei casi di craniosinostosi è evidente già alla nascita ed è caratterizzata dalla deformità del cranio, diretta conseguenza della prematura fusione delle suture. La palpazione delle suture rivela un margine osseo prominente. La fusione delle suture può essere confermata dalla radiografia diretta del cranio o da scansione ossea nei casi dubbi (Tab. 592-4). La chiusura prematura della sutura sagittale produce un cranio stretto e allungato (**scafocefalia**), che costituisce la forma più comune di craniosinostosi. La scafocefalia è associata a occipite prominente, fronte larga e fontanella anteriore piccola o assente. Questa malformazione è sporadica, più comune nei maschi e spesso causa difficoltà durante il travaglio, a causa della sproporzione cefalopelvica. La scafocefalia non determina né un aumento dell'ICP né idrocefalo. I risultati degli esami neurologici sono nella norma.

La **plagiocefalia frontale** è la seconda più comune forma di craniosinostosi. È caratterizzata da un appiattimento unilaterale della fronte, un'elevazione dell'orbita omolaterale e del sopracciglio e orecchio prominente sul lato opposto. La malformazione, più comune nelle femmine, è il risultato della prematura fusione della sutura coronale e sfenofrontale. L'intervento di chirurgia plastica consente di ottenere un buon risultato estetico.

La **plagiocefalia occipitale** ha spesso un'origine posturale ed è più comune nei bambini con handicap grave o incapaci di muoversi. Ma anche la fusione o sclerosi della sutura lamdoidea può causare appiattimento occipitale unilaterale associata a prominenza frontale omolaterale. La **trigonocefalia** è una rara forma

TABELLA 592-4. Epidemiologia e caratteristiche cliniche delle più comuni craniosinostosi

TIPO	EPIDEMIOLOGIA	DEFORMTÀ DEL CRANIO	PRESENTAZIONE CLINICA
Sagittale	Forma più comune che coinvolge una sola sutura, 80% maschi	Dolicocefalia o scafocefalia	Protuberanze frontali, occipite prominente, margine della sutura metopica palpabile, OFC normale e diametro biparietale ridotto
Coronale	18% delle craniosinostosi, più comune nelle femmine Associata a sindrome di Apert (con sindattilia) e con la sindrome di Crouzon (anomalie ossa sfenoidi, orbitali e facciali)	Unilaterale: plagiocefalia Bilaterale: brachicefalia, acrocefalia	Unilaterale: appiattimento della fronte sul lato colpito, guance piatte, deviazione del naso verso il lato normale, margine sopraorbitale più alto che determina il segno di Arlecchino nelle radiografie, rotazione verso l'esterno dell'orbita, che può causare ambliopia Bilaterale: fronte ampia e schiacciata. Sindattilia in presenza di sindrome di Apert, ipoplasia della parte centrale del volto e proptosi progressiva nella sindrome di Crouzon
Lambdoide	10-20% delle craniosinostosi; rapporto M:F 4:1	Plagiocefalia lambdoide/occipitale; lato destro colpito nel 70% dei casi	Appiattimento unilaterale dell'occipite, indentazione lungo la sutura sinostotica, protrusione della fronte omolaterale che determina cranio romboide, orecchio omolaterale in posizione anteriore e inferiore Bilaterale: brachicefalia con spostamento in posizione anteriore e inferiore delle orecchie
Metopica	Associazione con anomalie del cromosoma 19p	Trigoncefalia	Fronte a punta e sporgente lungo la linea mediana, ipotelorismo
Multiple		Ossicefalia	Turricefalia con seni poco sviluppati e orbite poco profonde, elevata ICP

OFC, *Occipital-Frontal Circumference* (circonferenza occipitale-frontale).
Tratta da Ridgway EB, Weiner HL: Skull deformities. *Pediatr Clin North Am* 2004;51:359-387.

di craniosinostosi dovuta alla prematura fusione della sutura metopica, che causa ipotelorismo e una fronte stretta e appuntita. I pazienti presentano un elevato rischio di sviluppare anomalie evolutive del proencefalo. La **turricefalia** è caratterizzata da un cranio a cono, causato dalla prematura fusione della sutura coronale e spesso anche delle suture sfenofrontale e frontoetmoidale. La **deformità Kleeblattschädel** determina un cranio a forma di trifoglio, con le ossa temporali molto prominenti e il resto del cranio compresso. L'idrocefalo è una complicanza comune.

La prematura fusione di una sola sutura causa raramente un deficit neurologico. In tali casi, l'unica indicazione per l'intervento chirurgico è di tipo estetico. La prognosi dipende dalla sutura coinvolta e dalla gravità della deformazione. Le probabilità di insorgenza di complicanze neurologiche, incluso l'idrocefalo e l'aumento della ICP, è più elevata in caso di fusione prematura di due o più suture. In tali casi l'intervento chirurgico è essenziale.

I principali disturbi genetici associati alla craniosinostosi includono le sindromi di Crouzon, Apert, Carpenter, Chotzen e Pfeiffer. La **sindrome di Crouzon** è caratterizzata da craniosinostosi prematura e si trasmette con modalità autosomica dominante. La forma della testa dipende dall'epoca e dall'ordine della fusione delle suture, ma la maggior parte dei bambini presenta una compressione in direzione retro-frontale del diametro del cranio o brachicefalia dovuta alla chiusura bilaterale delle suture coronali. Le orbite sono poco sviluppate e la proptosi oculare è prominente. L'ipoplasia mascellare e l'ipertelorismo orbitale completano la facies tipica.

La **sindrome di Apert** presenta molte caratteristiche in comune con la sindrome di Crouzon. Si tratta solitamente di una condizione sporadica, ma può riscontrarsi anche un'ereditarietà di tipo autosomico dominante. È associata alla prematura fusione di molteplici suture, tra cui la coronale, la sagittale, la squamosa e la lambdoidea. La facies tende a essere asimmetrica e la proptosi oculare è meno marcata rispetto alla sindrome di Crouzon. La sindrome di Apert è caratterizzata da sindattilia del 2°, 3° e 4° dito, che possono essere fuse al pollice e al 5° dito. Anomalie analoghe si riscontrano anche nel piede. Tutti i pazienti vanno incontro a una progressiva calcificazione e fusione delle ossa di mani, piedi e colonna cervicale.

La **sindrome di Carpenter** è una malattia a trasmissione autosomica recessiva determinata dalla fusione di varie suture, che tende a produrre la deformità del cranio a forma di trifoglio. La sindattilia del tessuto molle di mani e piedi è sempre presente e anche il ritardo mentale è comune. Anomalie meno comuni includono la cardiopatia congenita, opacità corneali, coxa valga e genu valgum.

La **sindrome di Chotzen** è caratterizzata da craniosinostosi asimmetrica e plagiocefalia. Si tratta della sindrome genetica più frequente, ereditata con modalità autosomica dominante. È associata ad asimmetria facciale, ptosi palpebrale, accorciamento delle dita e sindattilia del tessuto molle del 2° e 3° dito.

La **sindrome di Pfeiffer** è spesso associata a turricefalia. Gli occhi sono prominenti e distanziati, pollice e alluce sono corti e larghi. Può evidenziarsi una parziale sindattilia del tessuto molle. La maggior parte dei casi sembra sporadica, ma è stata segnalata una modalità di trasmissione autosomica dominante.

È stata dimostrata l'associazione tra mutazioni della famiglia genetica del recettore del fattore di crescita dei fibroblasti (*Fibroblast Growth Factor Receptor*, FGFR) e specifici fenotipi della craniosinostosi. Mutazioni del gene *FGFR1* localizzato sul cromosoma 8 causano la sindrome di Pfeiffer; una mutazione simile del gene *FGFR2* causa la sindrome di Apert. Mutazioni identiche del gene *FGFR2* possono determinare sia il fenotipo di Pfeiffer sia quello di Crouzon. In tutte le sindromi genetiche si riscontra un elevato rischio di insorgenza di anomalie associate, incluso idrocefalo, aumento dell'ICP, papilledema, atrofia ottica dovuta a anomalie del forame ottico, problemi respiratori secondari a deviazioni del setto nasale o atresia delle coane, disturbi del linguaggio e sordità. Il trattamento dell'aumento dell'IPC richiede una craniectomia. La gestione a lungo termine dei pazienti prevede regolari follow-up multidisciplinari. La correzione chirurgica della craniosinostosi consente di ottenere buoni risultati, con una morbilità e mortalità minime, in particolare nei neonati non sindromici.

Losee JE, Mason AC: Deformational plagiocephaly: Diagnosis, prevention, and treatment. *Clin Plast Surg* 2005;32:53–64.

Ridgway EB, Weiner HL: Skull deformities. *Pediatr Clin North Am* 2004;51:359–387.

Rutland P, Pulleyn LJ, Reardon W, et al: Identical mutations in the $FGFR_2$ gene cause both Pfeiffer and Crouzon syndrome phenotypes. *Nat Genet* 1995;9:173–176.

Sloan GM, Wells KC, Raffel C, et al: Surgical treatment of craniosynostosis: Outcome analysis of 250 consecutive patients. *Pediatrics* 1997;100:E2.

Speltz ML, Kapp-Simon KA, Cunningham M, et al: Single-suture craniosynostosis: A review of neurobehavioral research and theory. *J Pediatr Psychol* 2004;29(8):651–668.

Yassari R, Frim D: Evaluation and management of the Chiari malformation type 1 for the primary care pediatrician. *Pediatr Clin North Am* 2004;51: 477–490.

Capitolo 593 ■ Convulsioni nell'infanzia

Michael V. Johnston

Le convulsioni, o crisi epilettiche, sono definite come un cambiamento parossistico limitato nel tempo dell'attività motoria e/o comportamentale, risultato di un'attività elettrica cerebrale anomala. In età pediatrica le convulsioni sono comuni e si riscontrano il circa il 10% dei bambini. Nella maggior parte dei casi, sono provocate da disturbi somatici originati all'esterno del cervello, come febbre molto alta, infezioni, sincope, trauma cranico, ipossia, tossine o aritmia cardiaca. Spasmi affettivi e reflusso gastroesofageo possono causare eventi che simulano le convulsioni (vedi Capitolo 594). Alcuni bambini manifestano pseudoconvulsioni di natura psichiatrica. Meno di un terzo delle convulsioni in età pediatrica è causato dall'**epilessia**, una condizione patologica caratterizzata da convulsioni ricorrenti originate all'interno del cervello. In base alla classificazione epidemiologica, si pone diagnosi di epilessia in presenza di due o più attacchi convulsivi non provocati, a distanza di più di 24 ore. La prevalenza cumulativa dell'epilessia è del 3%; mentre in oltre il 50% dei casi la malattia esordisce nell'infanzia. L'incidenza annuale è inferiore (0,5-0,8%) perché molti bambini crescendo guariscono. La prognosi delle convulsioni sintomatiche o associate all'epilessia è generalmente buona, ma in alcuni casi tale sintomo segnala una grave malattia sistemica o a carico del SNC, che richiede ulteriori approfondimenti diagnostici. Il 10-20% dei bambini con epilessia presenta convulsioni ricorrenti refrattarie al trattamento farmacologico. Tali casi costituiscono spesso una sfida diagnostica e terapeutica.

VALUTAZIONE DEL PRIMO ATTACCO. La valutazione iniziale del lattante o bambino durante o poco dopo un sospetto episodio convulsivo deve includere una valutazione delle vie respiratorie, della ventilazione e della funzione cardiaca, nonché la misura di temperatura, pressione sanguigna e glicemia. In seguito al primo episodio, è importante escludere la presenza di malattie potenzialmente fatali responsabili di convulsioni, come meningite, sepsi, trauma cranico intenzionale e non, ingestione di farmaci o abuso di sostanze tossiche. Nell'anamnesi è opportuno tentare di definire i fattori che possono aver provocato l'attacco, fornendo anche una dettagliata descrizione del tipo di convulsione e dello stato postictale. Solitamente i genitori ricordano nei minimi particolari il primo attacco del figlio e sono in grado di fornire un resoconto accurato.

Il primo passo della valutazione consiste nel determinare se la convulsione ha un esordio focale o è invece piuttosto generalizzata. Le **convulsioni focali** sono caratterizzate da sintomi motori o sensoriali, che includono la rotazione forzata verso un lato di occhi e testa, movimenti clonici unilaterali che partono dal volto o dagli arti, disturbi sensoriali come parestesie o dolore localizzato in aree specifiche. Negli adolescenti o adulti, le convulsioni focali indicano solitamente una lesione localizzata, più difficile da diagnosticare nel bambino. Nel neonato, si riscontrano convulsioni focali in seguito a ictus perinatale. Le convulsioni motorie possono essere focali o generalizzate, tonico-cloniche, toniche, cloniche o atoniche. Le **convulsioni toniche** sono caratterizzate da un aumento del tono e da rigidità, mentre in quelle **atoniche** si riscontra flaccidità o assenza di movimento. Le **convulsioni cloniche** consistono nell'alternanza ritmica di contrazione e rilassamento muscolare. Il **mioclono** è definito come una contrazione muscolare improvvisa e brusca. È importante documentare la durata dell'attacco e la conservazione dello stato di coscienza. Nel corso dell'anamnesi, è opportuno determinare se l'attacco è stato preceduto da un'**aura** e indagare il comportamento del bambino nelle fasi immediatamente precedenti. L'aura più comunemente sperimentata nel periodo infantile consiste in un malessere o dolore epigastrico e in una sensazione di paura. Altri elementi da notare includono la postura, la presenza e distribuzione della cianosi, le vocalizzazioni, la perdita del controllo sfinterico (in particolare vescicale) e lo stato postictale (presenza di sonnolenza, mal di testa e emiparesi).

Oltre alla valutazione dello stato cardiorespiratorio e metabolico, l'esame deve ricercare una eventuale causa organica del disturbo convulsivo. I valori della circonferenza cranica, il peso e l'altezza del bambino sono confrontati alla media per l'età e a misurazioni precedenti. Si procede poi a un accurato esame neurologico generale. L'esame del **fondo oculare** consente di escludere al presenza di papilledema, emorragie retiniche, corioretinite, coloboma, alterazioni maculari e facoma retinico. Una facies anomala o il riscontro di segni fisici come l'epatosplenomegalia suggerisce la presenza di una malattia metabolica o di una malattia da accumulo. Il riscontro di vitiligine utilizzando una fonte di luce ultravioletta orienta verso la sclerosi tuberosa, mentre la presenza di adenomi sebacei, chiazze zigrinate, macchie caffellatte, nevo flammeo e facoma retinico suggeriscono una sindrome **neurocutanea**.

La localizzazione dei segni neurologici, come una lieve **emiparesi** con iperreflessia, un segno di Babinski dubbio e una caduta verso il basso di un arto superiore esteso quando il bambino tiene gli occhi chiusi, può indicare una lesione emisferica strutturale controlaterale, come un glioma del lobo temporale a lenta crescita. Un arresto unilaterale della crescita di unghie, mani o arti in un bambino con convulsioni focali induce a sospettare una condizione cronica, come una cisti porencefalica, una malformazione arteriovenosa o un'atrofia corticale dell'emisfero opposto.

593.1 • Convulsioni febbrili

Le convulsioni febbrili costituiscono la forma più comune di convulsioni in età pediatrica e generalmente hanno una prognosi ottima, ma in alcuni casi segnalano la presenza di una grave malattia infettiva acuta, come la sepsi o la meningite batterica. Di conseguenza, l'associazione di febbre e convulsioni richiede un approfondito esame del bambino, per determinare la causa della febbre (vedi Capitolo 175), in particolare se si tratta del primo attacco. Le convulsioni febbrili sono collegate all'età e sono rare prima dei 9 mesi e dopo i 5 anni. Il picco di esordio si riscontra tra i 14 e i 18 mesi, con un'incidenza che si avvicina al 3-4%. Una storia clinica positiva per convulsioni febbrili in fratelli e genitori suggerisce una predisposizione genetica. Studi di linkage in diverse famiglie numerose hanno consentito di mappare il gene della convulsione febbrile sui cromosomi 19p e 8q13-21. In alcune famiglie è stata dimostrata una modalità di trasmissione autosomica dominante.

MANIFESTAZIONI CLINICHE. La convulsione febbrile semplice è solitamente associata a un rapido aumento della temperatura corporea ≥39 °C. È inizialmente generalizzata e tonico-clonica, dura pochi secondi (raramente fino a 15 minuti), è seguita da un breve periodo postictale di sonnolenza e non si ripete per almeno 24 ore. La convulsione febbrile è definita complessa quando la durata è >15 minuti, quando si ripete nell'arco di 24 ore o in presenza di attività convulsiva focale o di reperti focali nel periodo postictale. Alcuni bambini con disturbo convulsivo cronico manifestano un maggior numero di attacchi quando hanno la febbre: in questi casi, non si parla di convulsioni febbrili, ma di convulsioni associate a febbre. Lo stato convulsivo epilettico (una singola convulsione che si protrae per 30 minuti o convulsioni multiple che si ripetono per almeno 30 minuti senza che il soggetto riprenda coscienza) è spesso dovuto a un'infezione del sistema nervoso centrale (come meningite batterica o virale).

Circa il 30-50% dei bambini presenta **convulsioni ricorrenti** durante successivi episodi di febbre e una minoranza di casi manifesta numerose convulsioni febbrili ricorrenti. I fattori associati al rischio di ricorrenza sono l'età <12 mesi, una temperatura non particolarmente elevata all'esordio della convulsione, una storia familiare positiva e la natura complessa dell'attacco. Le convulsioni febbrili non sono associate a una riduzione della futura performance intellettuale e, nella maggior parte dei casi, si riscontra un aumento soltanto minimo del rischio di sviluppare in seguito epilessia rispetto alla popolazione generale. I fattori associati a un drastico aumento del rischio di epilessia includono la presenza di caratteristiche complesse durante la convulsione o il periodo postictale, una storia clinica positiva per l'epilessia, un episodio iniziale di convulsione febbrile prima dei 12 mesi di età, il ritardo nelle acquisizioni evolutive o un preesistente disturbo neurologico. Il rischio di epilessia è particolarmente elevato nei bambini che hanno sperimentato uno o più episodi di convulsioni febbrili complesse, in particolare in caso di convulsioni focali in un paziente affetto da un disturbo neurologico. In presenza dei fattori di rischio elencati, l'incidenza dell'epilessia è >9%, mentre scende all'1% nei bambini con convulsioni febbrili, ma privi di fattori di rischio addizionali.

Durante la valutazione, la principale responsabilità del medico è di determinare la causa della febbre ed escludere la presenza di meningite o encefalite. *In caso di dubbi sulla possibilità di meningite, è opportuno procedere a esame del liquor (LCS) mediante puntura lombare.* In particolare, tale esame è raccomandato nei bambini al di sotto dei 12 mesi e deve essere preso in considerazione nei soggetti tra i 12-18 mesi che manifestano convulsioni complesse o che non recuperano completamente lo stato di coscienza dopo un breve periodo postictale.

Le anomalie del LCS indotte dalle convulsioni sono rare nei bambini, perciò la loro presenza deve allarmare il medico. Va considerata la possibilità di una meningoencefalite virale, causata in particolare da herpes simplex. Altre cause frequenti di convulsioni febbrili sono le infezioni virali delle prime vie aeree, la rosolia (e le infezioni da herpes 6 e 7) e l'otite media acuta.

Oltre alla glicemia, test di laboratorio addizionali, come il dosaggio sierico degli elettroliti e lo screening tossicologico, sono prescritti sulla base delle circostanze cliniche individuali (per es. un'evidente disidratazione). L'EEG non è di norma effettuato dopo una condizione febbrile semplice, ma può risultare utile per la valutazione di pazienti con caratteristiche atipiche o complesse o che presentano altri fattori di rischio per lo sviluppo di epilessia. Analogamente, le tecniche di neuroimaging sono prese in considerazione nei pazienti con aspetti atipici, come segni neurologici focali o deficit neurologici preesistenti.

TRATTAMENTO. Il trattamento di routine di un bambino con brevi convulsioni febbrili semplici include un'accurata ricerca della causa della febbre e la rassicurazione dei genitori. Benché gli antipiretici non si siano dimostrati efficaci nel prevenire la ricorrenza delle convulsioni, misure attive per il controllo della febbre (inclusa l'assunzione di antipiretici) possono contribuire a ridurre il malessere del paziente e hanno un effetto rassicurante. In un ambiente in cui è possibile ricorrere alla ventilazione assistita, può essere presa in considerazione la somministrazione di benzodiazepina come terapia di prima linea per il trattamento di convulsioni della durata superiore a 5 minuti (come descritto nel Capitolo 593.8).

L'utilità di una prolungata profilassi per la prevenzione delle convulsioni febbrili ricorrenti è oggetto di controversie e attualmente non è più raccomandata. Gli antiepilettici come la fenitoina e la carbamazepina non prevengono le convulsioni febbrili. Il fenobarbital previene la ricorrenza, ma può influire negativamente sulla funzione cognitiva. Anche il valproato di sodio è efficace, ma i potenziali rischi di questo farmaco non ne giustificano l'utilizzo in un disturbo con una prognosi eccellente a prescindere dal trattamento. L'incidenza di epatotossicità fatale indotta dal valproato è più elevata nei bambini <2 anni di età. Se i genitori sono particolarmente ansiosi, la somministrazione orale di diazepam costituisce un metodo efficace e sicuro di ridurre il rischio di ricorrenza delle convulsioni febbrili. All'esordio di ciascun episodio febbrile, il paziente assume 0,3 mg/kg di diazepam, e poi ogni 8 ore per tutta la durata della malattia (1 mg/kg/24 h per 2-3 giorni). Gli effetti collaterali (letargia, irritabilità e atassia) sono solitamente minimi e possono essere ulteriormente ridotti adeguando la dose. Una modalità terapeutica alternativa nei pazienti con convulsioni febbrili ricorrenti consiste nel prescrivere diazepam in forma di un gel, da somministrare per via rettale all'esordio dell'attacco, alla dose di 0,5 mg/kg per bambini di 2-5 anni. Questo trattamento solitamente interrompe l'attacco e riesce a prevenire la ricorrenza per 12 ore. Il trattamento preventivo o dopo l'attacco con anticonvulsivanti non si è dimostrato efficace nel ridurre il rischio di insorgenza di epilessia nei pazienti a rischio.

593.2 • Convulsioni non provocate

PRIMO ATTACCO. L'insorgenza di convulsioni non provocate da alcuno stimolo (come la febbre) talvolta annuncia lo sviluppo di un disturbo convulsivo cronico o dell'epilessia, ma soltanto una percentuale inferiore al 50% di questi bambini è destinata a presentare un secondo attacco. L'obiettivo principale dell'anamnesi è di verificare la presenza di una storia clinica positiva per l'epilessia, di un disturbo neurologico preesistente o di precedenti di convulsioni con febbre. Le circostanze cliniche individuali dovrebbero orientare la scelta dei test di laboratorio, tra il dosaggio degli elettroliti sierici, lo screening tossicologico e gli esami metabolici in urine e siero. La glicemia va effettuata dopo la prima convulsione afebbrile. La puntura lombare va riservata ai casi di sospetta meningite, encefalite, sepsi, emorragia subaracnoidea o disturbo demielinizzante. L'EEG è raccomandato nella valutazione neurodiagnostica del bambino con una prima convulsione apparentemente non provocata, perché può contribuire alla diagnosi, alla previsione del rischio di ricorrenza e all'identificazione di specifiche anomalie focali e/o sindromi epilettiche. Le tecniche di **neuroimaging** non sono raccomandate dopo la prima convulsione non provocata, a meno che l'esame neurologico non ne suggerisca l'opportunità (presenza di deficit neurologici focali). In tal caso, la RM è preferibile alla TC. Una singola convulsione non è sufficiente a giustificare la prescrizione di farmaci anticonvulsivanti. La RM può essere indicata anche in neonati e adolescenti alla prima convulsione.

CONVULSIONI RICORRENTI. L'insorgenza di almeno due convulsioni non provocate nell'arco delle 24 ore suggerisce la presenza di un disturbo epilettico responsabile della ricorrenza. Oltre all'identificazione della causa degli attacchi, l'obiettivo principale della valutazione è di stabilire la necessità di un trattamento con antiepilettici e di stimare il potenziale di risposta al trattamento e di remissione del disturbo.

L'**anamnesi** fornisce informazioni preziose sul tipo di convulsione. I genitori sono spesso in grado di descrivere nei dettagli e "simulare" l'attacco. In molti casi, i bambini con predisposizione allo sviluppo dell'epilessia sperimentano la prima crisi in associazione con una malattia virale o una febbre non molto alta. Nell'epilessia infantile sono comuni le convulsioni nelle prime ore del mattino o associate alla sonnolenza, in particolare durante la prima fase del sonno. Irritabilità, sbalzi di umore, mal di testa e sottili cambiamenti della personalità possono precedere di diversi giorni la convulsione e sono segnalati retrospettivamente dai genitori. Sulla base dei cambiamenti nell'atteggiamento del bambino, alcuni genitori sono in grado di prevedere con precisione l'insorgenza degli attacchi. La rappresentazione della convulsione da parte di genitori o di *caregiver* è spesso sorprendentemente simile all'attacco reale ed è molto più attendibile della descrizione verbale. Oltre alla natura della convulsione, è importante determinarne la frequenza, l'orario, gli eventuali fattori scatenanti e l'alternanza tra pattern diversi. Le convulsioni tonico-cloniche generalizzate sono facilmente documentabili, ma la frequenza degli episodi di assenza è spesso sottostimata dai genitori. Un prolungato cambiamento di personalità o un deterioramento intellettuale suggeriscono una **malattia degenerativa** del SNC, mentre sintomi costituzionali, come

TABELLA 593-1. Geni dell'epilessia identificati

	FUNZIONE	LOCUS	SINDROME EPILETTICA	TIPO DI CONVULSIONE
GABRA1 recettore della subunità α1 $GABA_A$	Inibizione parziale delle correnti attivate dal GABA	5q34	AD JME	TCS, miocloniche, assenze
GABRG2 recettore della subunità $GABA_A$ γ2	Rapida inibizione dei neuroni GABA-ergici	5q31	FS, CAE, $GEFS^+$	Febbrili, assenze, TCS, miocloniche, parziali
GABRD recettore della subunità GABAA δ2	Riduzione ampiezze corrente dei recettori $GABA_A$	1p36	$GEFS^-$	Convulsioni febbrili e afebbrili
SCN2A subunità α1 del canale del sodio	Rapida apertura di flusso del sodio e propagazione potenziali di azione	1q24	$GEFS^-$ BFNIC	Convulsioni febbrili e afebbrili toniche generalizzate e TCS
SCN1A subunità α1 del canale del sodio	Influsso somatodendritico di sodio	2q24	$GEFS^-$ SMEI	Febbrili, assenze, miocloniche, TCS, parziali
SCN1B subunità β21 del canale del sodio	Coadiuvare e modulare la subunità 1	19q13	$GEFS^-$	Febbrili, assenze, tonico-cloniche, miocloniche
KCNQ2 canale del potassio	Corrente M interagisce con KCNQ3	20q13	BFNC	Convulsioni neonatali
KCNQ3 canale del potassio	Corrente M interagisce con KCNQ2	8q24	BFNC	Convulsioni neonatali
ATP1A2 pompa Na^1, K^1-ATPasi	Disfunzione del trasporto ionico	1q23	BFNIC e cefalea emiplegica familiare	Convulsioni infantili
CHRNA4 recettore dell'acetilcolina della subunità α4	Modulazione della corrente nicotinica, interazione con subunità β2	20q13	ADNFLE	Convulsioni focali collegate al sonno
CHRNB recettore dell'acetilcolina della subunità β2	Modulazione della corrente nicotinica, interazione con subunità α4	1p21	ADNFLE	Convulsioni focali collegate al sonno
LGI1 ricco di leucina, attivato da glioma	Alterazione dell'omeostasi, interazione tra neuroni e glia?	10q24	ADPEAF	Convulsioni parziali con allucinazioni visive e uditive
CLCN2 canali del cloro voltaggio-dipendenti	Efflusso neuronale di cloro	3q26	IGE	TCS, miocloniche, assenze
EFHC1 proteina con motivo EF	Riduce l'apoptosi ippocampale indotta nel topo	6p12-p11	JME	TCS, miocloniche
BRD2 (RING3) Regolatore della trascrizione nucleare	?	6p21	JME	TCS, miocloniche

AD, autosomica dominante; ADNFLE, *Autosomal Dominant Nocturnal Frontal Lobe Epilepsy* (epilessia notturna del lobo frontale autosomica dominante); ADPEAF, *Autosomal Dominant Partial Epilepsy with Auditory Features* (epilessia parziale autosomica dominante con sintomi uditivi); BFNC, *Benign Familiar Neonatal Convulsions* (convulsioni neonatali familiari benigne); BFNIC, *Benign Familiar Neonatal-infantile Convulsion* (convulsioni neonatali-infantili familiari benigne); $GEFS^+$, *Generalized Epilepsy with Febrile Seizures Plus* (epilessia generalizzata con convulsioni febbrili); JME, *Juvenile Myoclonic Epilepsy* (epilessia mioclonica giovanile); SMEI, *Severe Myoclonic Epilepsy of Infancy* (grave epilessia mioclonica infantile); TCS, *Tonic-Clonic Seizures* (convulsioni tonico-cloniche); XL, *X-Linked* (correlata a X).

Tratta da Guerrini R: Epilepsy in children. *Lancet* 2006; 367:499-524.

vomito o deficit staturo-ponderale, possono indicare un disturbo metabolico primario o una lesione strutturale. Oltre a indagare su precedenti terapie con farmaci anticonvulsivanti e sulla risposta del bambino, è essenziale verificare l'eventuale assunzione di farmaci in grado di potenziare le convulsioni, come la clorpromazina e il metilfenidato. La descrizione dell'attacco e la storia familiare possono evidenziare la presenza di una sindrome epilettica genetica (Tab. 593-1), come l'epilessia notturna del lobo frontale autosomica dominante, le convulsioni neonatali familiari benigne, le convulsioni febbrili autosomiche dominanti, l'epilessia parziale con sintomi uditivi, l'epilessia del lobo frontale autosomica dominante con ritardo mentale, le assenze epilettiche e le convulsioni febbrili con successive convulsioni parzialmente complesse.

Gli esami obiettivo, oftalmologico e neurologico forniscono informazioni sulla presenza di un aumento della pressione intracranica, sindromi neurocutanee e anomalie cerebrali strutturali, come malformazioni, lesioni, infezioni o tumori.

L'EEG, indicato in tutti i casi di epilessia, è utile per determinare la natura della patologia e per valutarne la prognosi futura. Il dosaggio sierico degli elettroliti, incluso calcio e magnesio, non è raccomandato come procedura di routine. Soltanto in presenza di circostanze cliniche indicative è opportuno procedere a esami metabolici di approfondimento, come la somministrazione di piridossina e piridossalfosfato per sospette convulsioni indotte da piridossina, il dosaggio sierico di lattato e piruvato, la misura degli acidi organici nelle urine. La puntura lombare deve essere presa in considerazione nei bambini con convulsioni ripetute associate a disabilità neuroevolutiva, per verificare la presenza di una riduzione della glicorrachia causata da un disturbo del trasporto, di alterazioni dei livelli di amminoacidi, neurotrasmettitori o cofattori tipici delle malattie metaboliche o per evidenziare un'infezione cronica. Le tecniche di neuroimaging (come la RM) sono indicate nella valutazione di bambini ai quali è stata appena diagnosticata l'epilessia, in particolare se presentano deficit neurologici, convulsioni parziali o anomalie EEG focali che non rientrano nella sindrome epilettica idiopatica. In alcuni casi, è necessario l'elettrocardiogramma per escludere una sindrome QT lungo, che in rari casi provoca convulsioni e sincope (vedi Capitolo 594).

CLASSIFICAZIONE DELLE CONVULSIONI. La classificazione del tipo di convulsione (Tab. 593-2) è importante per identificare la causa del disturbo. Una precisa descrizione della tipologia costituisce la base della prognosi e contribuisce alla scelta del trattamento più adeguato. Gli anticonvulsivanti consentono di controllare rapidamente l'epilessia tonico-clonica generalizzata, ma sono meno efficaci nei pazienti con convulsioni parziali o di tipo diverso.

L'epilessia mioclonica benigna ha un esito più favorevole rispetto agli spasmi infantili. Un bambino in età scolare con epilessia parziale benigna e punte centrotemporali (epilessia rolandica) ha una prognosi eccellente e non richiede una prolungata terapia con anticonvulsivanti. La classificazione delle convulsioni può risultare complessa, perché le manifestazioni di tipi differenti sono talvolta molto simili. Le caratteristiche cliniche di un bambino con assenze possono risultare pressoché identiche a quelle di un paziente con epilessia parziale complessa. L'EEG è utile per chiarire eventuali dubbi dati dalla variabilità dell'espressione delle convulsioni in questo gruppo di età.

L'epilessia infantile è stata classificata anche secondo diverse sindromi (Tab. 593-3). Sulla base dell'età di esordio, dello sviluppo cognitivo e dei risultati dell'esame neurologico, della descrizione della tipologia, dei dati EEG (incluso il ritmo di fondo), è stato possibile classificare circa il 50% delle convulsioni in sindromi specifiche. Tale classificazione sindromica garantisce indiscutibili vantaggi rispetto alla classificazioni precedenti, orientando la scelta dell'anticonvulsivante più adatto, contribuendo all'identificazione dei potenziali candidati per la terapia chirurgica e fornendo a pazienti e familiari una prognosi accurata e affidabile. Le sindromi epilettiche definite includono gli spasmi infantili (sindrome di West), l'epilessia mioclonica benigna dell'infanzia,

TABELLA 593-2. Classificazione internazionale delle convulsioni epilettiche

CONVULSIONI PARZIALI
Parziali semplici (senza compromissione della coscienza)
- Motorie
- Sensoriali
- Autonomiche
- Psichiche

Parziali complesse (compromissione della coscienza)
- Parziali semplici, seguite da compromissione della coscienza
- Compromissione della coscienza fin dall'esordio

Convulsioni parziali con generalizzazione secondaria

CONVULSIONI GENERALIZZATE
Assenze
- Tipiche
- Atipiche

Tonico-cloniche generalizzate
Toniche
Cloniche
Miocloniche
Atoniche
Spasmi infantili

CONVULSIONI NON CLASSIFICATE

TABELLA 593-3. Classificazione delle epilessie e sindromi epilettiche

EPILESSIE COLLEGATE A UNA LOCALIZZAZIONE (FOCALI, PARZIALI)
Idiopatiche
- Epilessia infantile benigna con punte centrotemporali
- Epilessia infantile con parossismi rolandici

Sintomatiche
- La classificazione è determinata dalla localizzazione anatomica suggerita dalla storia clinica, dal tipo predominante di convulsioni, dall'EEG intercritale e ictale e dagli esami di imaging; CPS, CPC o convulsioni a generalizzazione secondaria che originano dai lobi frontali, parietali, temporali, occipitali e da localizzazioni multiple o sconosciute

Localizzate, ma la natura sintomatica o idiopatica è incerta

EPILESSIE GENERALIZZATE
Idiopatiche
- Convulsioni neonatali familiari benigne
- Convulsioni neonatali benigne
- Epilessia mioclonica infantile benigna
- Assenze infantili (picnoepilessia)
- Assenze giovanili
- Epilessia mioclonica giovanile (petit mal impulsivo)
- Epilessia grand mal al risveglio
- Altre epilessie idiopatiche generalizzate che non rientrano nelle sindromi descritte

Epilessia criptogenetica o sintomatica generalizzata
- Sindrome di West (spasmi infantili)
- Sindrome di Lennox-Gastaut
- Epilessia con convulsioni miocloniche astatiche
- Epilessia con assenze miocloniche
- Epilessia sintomatica
- Cause non specifiche
  - Encefalopatia mioclonica precoce
- Malattie specifiche che si manifestano con convulsioni

EPILESSIE E SINDROMI INDETERMINATE COME FOCALI O GENERALIZZATE
Con convulsioni generalizzate e focali
- Convulsioni neonatali
- Grave epilessia mioclonica infantile
- Epilessia con pattern punte-onda continuo durante il sonno a onde lente
- Afasia epilettica acquisita (sindrome di Landau-Kleffner)
- In assenza di convulsioni sicuramente generalizzate o focali
- Tutte le cause con GTCS in cui i reperti EEG non consentono la precisa classificazione come sicuramente generalizzate o da localizzazione (per es. GTCS durante il sonno)

SINDROMI SPECIALI
Convulsioni collegate alla situazione
- Convulsioni febbrili
- Convulsioni isolate o status epilettico isolato

Convulsioni sintomatiche acute, per esempio da astinenza da alcol, eclampsia, uremia

CPC, convulsioni parziali complesse; CPS, convulsioni parziali semplici.
Tratta da Kliegman RM, Greenbaum LA, Lye PS: *Practical Strategies in Pediatric Diagnosis and Therapy*, 2nd ed. Philadelphia, Elsevier, 2004, p. 680.

la sindrome di Lennox-Gastaut, le convulsioni febbrili, la sindrome di Landau-Kleffner, l'epilessia infantile benigna con punte centrotemporali (epilessia rolandica), l'encefalite di Rasmussen, l'epilessia mioclonica giovanile (sindrome di Janz) e la malattia di Lafora (epilessia mioclonica progressiva). Alcune di queste sindromi hanno un esito più favorevole (Tab. 593-4).

593.3 • Convulsioni parziali

Secondo alcune casistiche, il 40% delle convulsioni infantili è di tipo parziale. Sulla base della conservazione della coscienza o meno, le convulsioni parziali sono ulteriormente classificabili in semplici o complesse.

CONVULSIONI PARZIALI SEMPLICI (CPS). Il più comune sintomo di questo tipo di convulsioni è l'attività motoria. I movimenti sono asincroni clonici o tonici e tendono a coinvolgere il volto, il collo e gli arti. Le crisi versive, che consistono nella rotazione di testa e occhi, sono particolarmente comuni. Gli automatismi non si verificano, ma alcuni pazienti lamentano un'aura (mal di testa, fastidio al torace), che può costituire l'unica manifestazione della convulsione. I bambini fanno fatica a descrivere l'aura e riferiscono spesso di "sentirsi strani", come se avessero "qualcosa che striscia dentro". In media, la convulsione si protrae per 10-20 secondi. La caratteristica distintiva delle convulsioni parziali semplici è la preservazione della coscienza e della capacità di parlare durante la crisi. L'evento non è seguito da alcun fenomeno postictale. Tali convulsioni sono spesso scambiate per tic (come alzate di spalle, ammiccamenti, smorfie facciali; vedi Capitolo 23). I tic coinvolgono prevalentemente volto e spalle e possono essere facilmente soppressi, mentre le convulsioni parziali non sono controllabili. L'EEG mostra onde punta o puntute, sia unilaterali che bilaterali, o un pattern di punte multifocali.

CONVULSIONI PARZIALI COMPLESSE (CPC). Le CPC possono esordire con una crisi parziale semplice, con o senza aura, seguita da perdita dello stato di coscienza; oppure l'esordio della CPC, può coincidere con uno stato di coscienza alterato. L'aura, che si riscontra in circa un terzo dei bambini con CPS e CPC, consiste in una sensazione di malessere vago, di fastidio epigastrico o in una sensazione di paura. La presenza dell'aura è sempre indicativa di un esordio focale della crisi. Poiché le convulsioni parziali sono difficili da documentare in lattanti e bambini, la frequenza della loro associazione con le crisi parziali complesse può essere sottostimata. La perdita di coscienza può manifestarsi con un breve sguardo vacuo o una pausa improvvisa nell'attività, difficilmente osservabili dai genitori. Inoltre, nella maggior parte dei casi il bambino non è in grado di comunicare o descrivere i periodi di perdita di coscienza. Se brevi e infrequenti, tali eventi anomali sono rilevabili solo da un osservatore esperto o sono documentabili dall'EEG.

Gli **automatismi** si verificano nel 50-75% delle CPC di lattanti e bambini. La frequenza è direttamente proporzionale all'aumento dell'età del bambino. Gli automatismi compaiono dopo la perdita di coscienza e possono persistere anche nella fase postictale; il bambino non riesce a ricordarli. Nei lattanti, i comportamenti di comune riscontro sono gli automatismi alimentari (schiocco delle labbra, movimenti di masticazione e deglutizione, eccessiva salivazione). Tali movimenti rientrano nel comportamento normale dei lattanti e sono molto difficili da notare. Prolungati e ripetitivi automatismi alimentari associati a sguardo vacuo o assenza di risposta indicano quasi sempre la presenza di CPC in un neonato. Nei bambini più grandi, i movimenti più comuni consistono in automatismi gestuali semi-intenzionali, scoordinati e non pianificati, che includono toccarsi i vestiti, tirare le lenzuola, accarezzare o strofinare oggetti, camminare o correre senza direzione.

La diffusione della scarica epilettiforme durante le CPC può risultare in una **generalizzazione secondaria**, con crisi tonico-clonica. Durante la diffusione della scarica ictale attraverso l'emisfero, è possibile notare la rotazione controlaterale della testa, una postura distonica e movimenti tonici o clonici di arti e volto (come ammiccamenti). La durata media di una CPC è di 1-2 minuti, considerevolmente superiore alla durata delle CPS e delle assenze.

L'EEG intercritale delle CPC rivela onde puntute o punte-onda focali e punte multifocali. In circa il 20% dei lattanti e bambini con CPC, l'EEG intercritale risulta normale. In questi pazienti, l'identificazione delle punte e onde puntute può richiedere un EEG con deprivazione di sonno, l'applicazione di elettrodi zigomatici, tempi di registrazioni prolungati o il ricorso a video-EEG del paziente ospedalizzato (con sospensione degli anticonvulsivanti) (Fig. 593-1*A*). Alcuni bambini con CPC manifestano onde puntute o punte intercritali che originano dai lobi frontali, parietali o occipitali. La TC e la RM consentono di rivelare la presenza di un'anomalia del lobo temporale nel bambino con CPC. Tali lesioni includono sclerosi temporale mesiale, amartoma, gliosi postencefalitica, cisti subaracnoidea, infarto, malformazioni arteriovenose e glioma a lenta evoluzione (Fig. 593-2).

EPILESSIA PARZIALE BENIGNA CON PUNTE CENTROTEMPORALI. Comune nell'infanzia, l'epilessia parziale benigna con punte centrotemporali (*Benign Partial Epilepsy with Centrotemporal Spikes*, BPEC) ha una prognosi eccellente. Le caratteristiche cliniche, i reperti EEG (focolai rolandici) e l'assenza di lesioni neuropatologiche consentono una rapida diagnosi differenziale tra BPEC e CPC. La BPEC insorge prevalentemente tra i 2 e i 14 anni, con un picco di esordio tra i 9 e i 10 anni. Il disturbo colpisce bambini altrimenti sani, privi di anamnesi clinica significativa e con esame neurologico nella norma, ma si riscontra spesso una storia familiare positiva per l'epilessia. Le convulsioni sono solitamente parziali e i segni motori e somatosensoriali restano confinati al volto. I **sintomi orofaringei** includono contrazioni toniche e parestesie della lingua, insensibilità unilaterale della guancia (in particolare lungo la gengiva), suoni gutturali, disfagia e salivazione eccessiva. I sintomi orofaringei sono spesso accompagnati da contratture tonico-cloniche unilaterali

TABELLA 593-4. Sindromi epilettiche infantili con prognosi generalmente buona

SINDROME	COMMENTO
Convulsioni neonatali familiari benigne	Dominante, può risultare grave e resistente per qualche giorno. In una minoranza di pazienti si riscontrano successive convulsioni benigne febbrili e non febbrili
Convulsioni familiari infantili	Dominante, spesso in cluster (sovrapposizione con l'epilessia benigna parziale complessa dell'infanzia)
Convulsioni febbrili	Convulsioni in più membri di una stessa famiglia (epilessia generalizzata con convulsioni febbrili); la vecchia dicotomia tra convulsioni febbrili ed epilessia non è sempre applicabile
Epilessia mioclonica benigna dell'infanzia	Spesso convulsioni durante il sonno; in una rara variante, convulsioni miocloniche (toccamenti, rumori)
Epilessia idiopatica parziale con punte rolandiche	Convulsioni in coincidenza con addormentamento o risveglio; punte focali a localizzazione EEG centrotemporale; genetica
Epilessia idiopatica occipitale parziale	Forma della prima infanzia, convulsioni durante il sonno e vomito ictale, possibile esordio come status epilettico; forme tardive con sintomi della cefalea; non sempre benigna
Assenze (petit mal)	Casi con solo assenze o alcuni hanno convulsioni generalizzate; piena remissione nel 60-80%; nella maggior parte dei casi, le assenze scompaiono con la terapia, ma si riscontrano casi resistenti (non prevedibili)
Epilessia mioclonica giovanile	Esordio nell'adolescenza con convulsioni miocloniche nel primo mattino e convulsioni generalizzate durante il sonno; spesso storia clinica di assenze nell'infanzia

Tratta da Deonna T: Management of epilepsy. *Arch Dis Child* 2005;90:5-9.

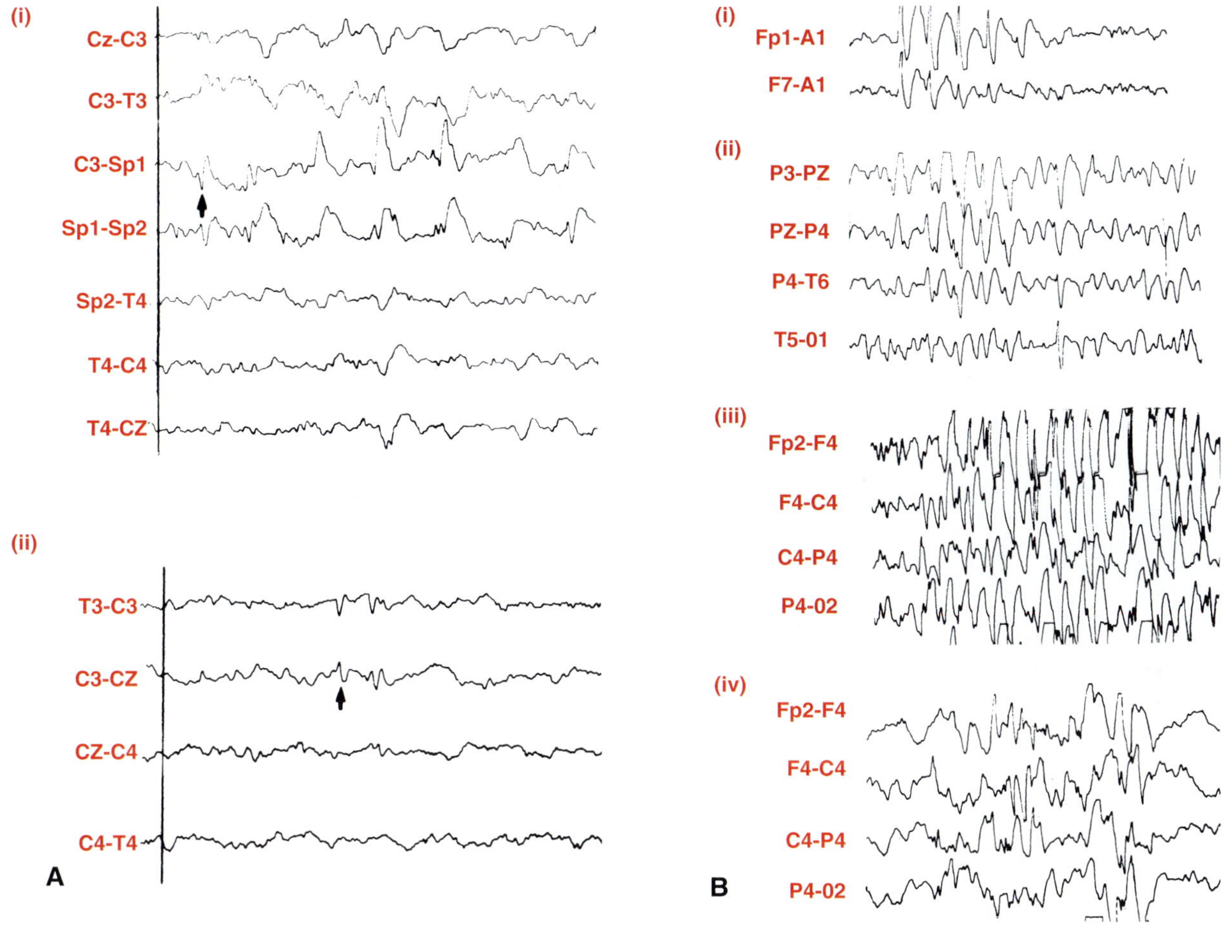

Figura 593-1. *A*, EEG di una convulsione parziale: (i) scariche a punta dal lobo temporale (*freccia*) in un paziente con CPC, (ii) punte centrali parietali sinistre (*freccia*) caratteristiche della BPEC. *B*, EEG di convulsioni generalizzate: (i) scarica punta e onda di 3/s in un paziente con assenza, con attività di fondo normale, (ii) epilessia mioclonica complessa (sindrome di Lennox-Gastaut) con punte onda lente interictali, (iii) epilessia mioclonica giovanile con punte e onda di 6/s, potenziate dalla stimolazione luminosa, e (iv) ipsaritmia con attività punte e onda irregolare e ad alto voltaggio. BPEC, epilessia parziale benigna con punte centrotemporali; CPC, convulsioni parziali complesse; EEG, elettroencefalogramma.

della parte inferiore del volto e da movimenti clonici o parestesie degli arti omolaterali. È possibile riscontrare perdita di coscienza e generalizzazione secondaria della convulsione parziale.

Circa il 20% dei bambini sperimenta una sola crisi, la maggior parte ha convulsioni sporadiche e circa un quarto presenta ripetuti cluster di convulsioni. Nel 75% dei pazienti, la BPEC si verifica durante il sonno, mentre le CPC vengono solitamente osservate durante le ore di veglia. Il pattern EEG diagnostico della BPEC è caratterizzato ripetuti da focolai di punte localizzati nell'area centrotemporale o rolandica, con attività di fondo normale (vedi Fig. 593-1*A*). Gli anticonvulsivanti sono necessari nei pazienti che sperimentano attacchi ripetuti, ma non è opportuna la loro prescrizione di routine dopo la prima crisi. Il **farmaco di elezione** è la **carbamazepina**, da somministrare per almeno 2 anni, o fino ai 14-16 anni, età in cui solitamente si verifica la remissione spontanea.

ENCEFALITE DI RASMUSSEN. Questa forma di encefalite infiammatoria subacuta è una delle cause dell'**epilessia parziale continua**. Una malattia non specifica febbrile può precedere l'esordio delle crisi focali, frequenti o continue. La malattia insorge solitamente prima dei 10 anni. Le sequele includono emiplegia, emianopsia e afasia. L'EEG rivela una diffusa attività parossistica con ritmo di fondo lento. La malattia è progressiva e potenzialmente letale, ma spesso si trasforma in autolimitante, con significativi deficit neurologici. Può essere causata da anticorpi che si legano ai recettori del glutammato, stimolandoli. Il Cytomegalovirus è stato identificato in diversi campioni chirurgici di pazienti con encefalite di Rasmussen.

593.4 • Convulsioni generalizzate

ASSENZE. Le assenze semplici o tipiche (petit mal) sono caratterizzate da un'improvvisa cessazione dell'attività motoria o dell'eloquio, accompagnata da un'espressione facciale vacua e da scosse delle palpebre. Più comuni prima dei 5 anni e nel sesso femminile, queste convulsioni non sono mai associate ad aura, raramente persistono più di 30 secondi e non sono seguite da uno stato postictale. Queste caratteristiche consentono la diagnosi differenziale con le CPC. Il bambino può sperimentare innumerevoli crisi di assenza durante il giorno, mentre le CPC sono meno frequenti. Il tono posturale è conservato, ma la testa può cadere leggermente in avanti. Immediatamente dopo la crisi, il paziente riprende l'attività interrotta, senza manifestazioni postictali. Le assenze semplici sono spesso accompagnate da automatismi comportamentali. L'iperventilazione per 3-4 minuti produce un'assenza. L'EEG mostra tipicamente una punta di 3/s seguita da una scarica generalizzata (vedi Fig. 593-1*B*). Nelle assenze complesse (atipiche) si riscontra l'associazione di componenti motorie, che consistono in movimenti mioclonici di volto, dita o arti, talvolta accompagnati da una perdita del tono posturale. Queste crisi producono un EEG tipico, con punta e onda lenta ogni 2-2,5/s.

CONVULSIONI TONICO-CLONICHE GENERALIZZATE. Tali convulsioni, piuttosto comuni, possono seguire una convulsione parziale con esordio focale (generalizzazione secondaria) oppure si verificano *de novo*. La frequente presenza di un'**aura** suggerisce un'origine focale della scarica epilettica. È importante stabilire

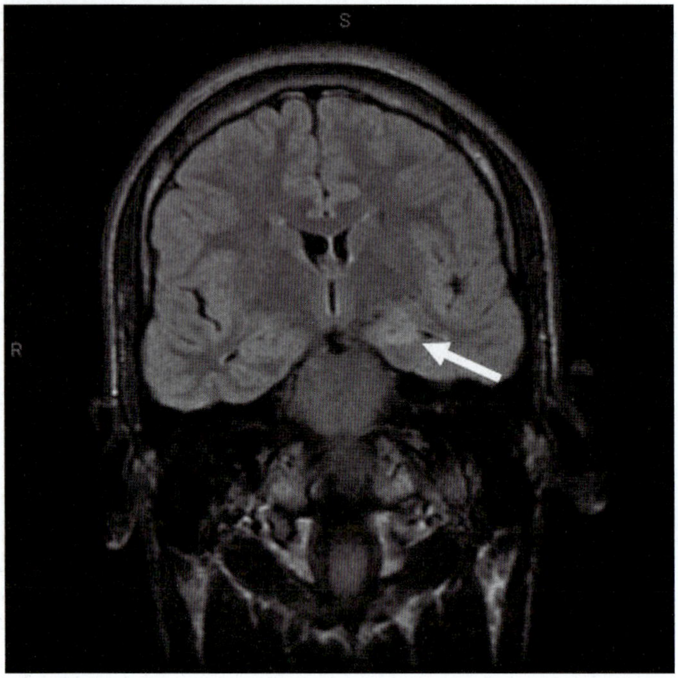

Figura 593-2. RM FLAIR coronale di un ragazzo di 13 anni con convulsioni intrattabili e sclerosi temporale mesiale (MTS). La *freccia* indica la presenza di un caratteristico segnale ad alta intensità nell'ippocampo (Tratta da Lee JYK, Adelson PD: Neurosurgical management of pediatric epilepsy. *Pediatr Clin North Am* 2004;51:441-456.)

l'area di origine dell'aura, perché può indicare la localizzazione della patologia. Il paziente perde improvvisamente conoscenza e, in alcuni casi, emette un grido stridulo. Gli occhi si rovesciano all'indietro e l'intera muscolatura somatica va incontro a contrazioni toniche. In seguito all'apnea, il paziente diviene rapidamente cianotico. La fase clonica della crisi è preannunciata da contrazioni cloniche ritmiche, alternate al rilassamento di tutti i gruppi muscolari. Tale fase clonica si presenta verso la fine dell'attacco, che solitamente si protrae per alcuni minuti. In coincidenza con la brusca conclusione della crisi, il paziente spesso emette un singhiozzo. Durante la convulsione, capita che il bambino si morda la lingua, ma raramente vomita. La perdita del controllo sfinterico, soprattutto vescicale, è frequente.

Durante la crisi, è opportuno allentare colletti o collane che stringono il collo, adagiare il paziente sul fianco e collocare con delicatezza collo e mandibola in iperestensione, per favorire la respirazione. La bocca non deve essere aperta con la forza, né con le dita, né usando un oggetto, per evitare di danneggiare i denti serrati del paziente o la cavità orofaringea. Nella fase postictale, il paziente è inizialmente semicomatoso e il sonno profondo dura da 30 minuti a 2 ore. L'esame durante la crisi o postictale rivela atassia del tronco, iperreflessia dei tendini profondi, clono e riflesso di Babinski. La fase postictale è spesso associata a vomito e a un'intensa cefalea bifrontale.

L'espressione **convulsione idiopatica** è utilizzata nei casi in cui non si riesce a identificare la causa della crisi. Diversi fattori possono scatenare convulsioni tonico-cloniche generalizzate nei bambini, tra cui febbre di lieve entità associata a infezioni del sistema nervoso non centrale, eccessivo affaticamento, stress emotivo e l'assunzione di farmaci psicotropi, teofillina e metilfenidato (in particolare se le convulsioni non sono ben controllate dai farmaci anticonvulsivanti).

EPILESSIA MIOCLONICA INFANTILE. Questo disturbo è caratterizzato da crisi ripetute di contrazioni muscolari brevi e simmetriche, con perdita del tono posturale e tendenza a cadere o accasciarsi in avanti, con il rischio di provocarsi ferite al volto e alla bocca. La diagnosi di epilessia mioclonica include un gruppo eterogeneo di disturbi con cause ed esito variabili. Nella popolazione pediatrica sono stati identificati almeno cinque sottogruppi differenti.

Mioclono infantile benigno. Il mioclono benigno esordisce durante l'infanzia e consiste in cluster di movimenti mioclonici confinati a collo, tronco e arti. L'attività mioclonica può essere confusa con spasmi infantili, ma nel primo caso l'EEG risulta normale. La prognosi è buona, con sviluppo normale e cessazione del mioclono entro i 2 anni. Il trattamento con anticonvulsivanti non è indicato.

Epilessia mioclonica tipica della prima infanzia. Questo disturbo colpisce bambini precedentemente sani, nei quali non si segnalano né anomalie della gestazione, del travaglio o del parto, né ritardi delle tappe evolutive. L'età media di esordio è intorno ai 2 anni, ma il range va dai 6 mesi ai 4 anni. La frequenza delle convulsioni miocloniche è variabile; alcuni bambini sperimentano varie crisi al giorno, altri non manifestano alcun sintomo per settimane. Un ridotto numero di pazienti ha convulsioni febbrili o crisi afebbrili tonico-cloniche generalizzate che precedono l'esordio dell'epilessia mioclonica. Circa il 50% dei pazienti sperimenta occasionalmente convulsioni tonico-cloniche oltre all'epilessia mioclonica. Nella maggior parte dei casi, l'EEG mostra rapidi complessi onda punta $\geq$2,5 Hz e un ritmo di fondo normale. Almeno un terzo dei bambini presenta una storia familiare positiva per l'epilessia, che indica un'eziologia genetica. L'esito a lungo termine è relativamente favorevole. Soltanto una minoranza dei pazienti manifesta ritardo mentale e in una percentuale >50% si verifica una remissione spontanea. In un numero significativo di bambini si riscontrano disturbi del linguaggio e dell'apprendimento, nonché problemi emotivi e comportamentali, che richiedono un follow-up multidisciplinare a lungo termine.

Epilessie miocloniche complesse. Questa diagnosi include un gruppo eterogeneo di disturbi, accomunati da una diagnosi sfavorevole. Convulsioni tonico-cloniche focali o generalizzate esordiscono nel primo anno di vita, anticipando lo sviluppo dell'epilessia mioclonica. La crisi generalizzata, spesso associata a un'infezione delle vie respiratorie superiori e a febbre non elevata, tende a trasformarsi in uno stato epilettico. Circa un terzo dei pazienti manifesta un ritardo nell'acquisizione delle tappe evolutive. Sono di comune riscontro una storia clinica di encefalopatia ipossica-ischemica nel periodo perinatale e la presenza di segni extrapiramidali e a carico dei motoneuroni superiori associati a microcefalia. Rispetto ai pazienti con epilessia mioclonica tipica, in questo gruppo si segnala più spesso una storia familiare di epilessia.

Alcuni bambini manifestano una combinazione di convulsioni miocloniche frequenti e crisi toniche. Quando l'EEG interictale rivela punte-onda lente, il disturbo è classificato come **sindrome di Lennox-Gastaut**. Tale sindrome è caratterizzata da una triade di convulsioni non trattabili di vario tipo, un EEG che rivela onde-punte lente durante lo stato di veglia e ritardo mentale. I pazienti con epilessia mioclonica complessa presentano punte-onda lente nella fase interictale e sono refrattari agli anticonvulsivanti (vedi Fig. 593-1*B*). Le crisi sono persistenti e la frequenza del ritardo mentale e dei problemi comportamentali è di circa il 75%. Il trattamento con acido valproico o benzodiazepine riduce la frequenza e l'intensità delle convulsioni. Nei pazienti refrattari agli anticonvulsivanti è opportuno considerare una dieta chetogenica.

Epilessia miocolonica giovanile (sindrome di Janz). L'epilessia mioclonica giovanile, responsabile di circa il 5% dei casi, solitamente esordisce tra i 12 e i 16 anni. È stato identificato un locus genetico sul cromosoma 6p21. I pazienti segnalano frequenti spasmi mioclonici al risveglio e lamentano una difficoltà a lavarsi i denti e pettinarsi. Poiché il mioclono si attenua nel corso della mattinata, molti pazienti non consultano il medico in questo stadio e tendono a negare il fenomeno. A qualche anno di distanza, al mattino presto insorgono convulsioni tonico-cloniche generalizzate, associate a mioclono. L'EEG mostra punte-onde irregolari ogni 4-6/s, aumentate dalla stimolazione luminosa (vedi Fig. 593-1*B*). L'esame neurologico è normale e la maggior parte dei pazienti risponde in maniera eccellente al valproato, la cui somministrazione deve proseguire per tutta la vita. L'interruzione del trattamento causa un elevato tasso di recidiva.

Epilessia mioclonica progressiva. Questo eterogeneo gruppo di disturbi genetici rari, accomunati da una prognosi infausta, include la malattia di Lafora, l'epilessia mioclonica con fibre rosse sfilacciate (*Myoclonic Epilepsy with Ragged-Red Fibers*, MERRF) (vedi Capitolo 598.2), la sialidosi di tipo II (vedi Capitolo 599.4), la lipofuscinosi ceroide (vedi Capitolo 599.2), la malattia neuropatica giovanile di Gaucher e la distrofia neuroassonale giovanile.

La **malattia di Lafora** si presenta in bambini e adolescenti tra i 10 e i 18 anni con convulsioni tonico-cloniche generalizzate. Successivamente compaiono spasmi mioclonici, sempre più evidenti e costanti con il progredire della malattia. Il deterioramento mentale caratteristico della malattia si evidenzia entro il primo anno dall'esordio delle crisi. Si riscontrano marcate anomalie neurologiche, in particolare segni cerebellari ed extrapiramidali. L'EEG mostra scariche polipunta-onda, soprattutto nella regione occipitale, con progressivo rallentamento e disorganizzazione del ritmo di fondo. Gli spasmi mioclonici sono difficili da controllare, ma una combinazione di acido valproico e una benzodiazepina (clonazepam) è efficace contro le convulsioni generalizzate. La malattia di Lafora si trasmette con modalità autosomica recessiva; la diagnosi può essere confermata, tramite biopsia cutanea, ricercando le inclusioni Shiff-positive, presenti in particolare nelle cellule duttali delle ghiandole sudoripare eccrine. Il gene per la malattia di Lafora, localizzato sul cromosoma 6p24, codifica per la proteina tirosina fosfatasi.

SPASMI INFANTILI. Gli spasmi infantili solitamente esordiscono tra i 4 e gli 8 mesi di età e sono caratterizzati da brevi contrazioni simmetriche di collo, tronco e arti. Si riscontrano almeno tre tipi di spasmi: flessori, estensori e misti. Gli spasmi flessori si verificano in scariche o cluster e consistono in improvvise flessioni del collo, delle braccia e delle gambe verso il tronco. Gli spasmi estensori, meno comuni, determinano invece l'estensione del tronco e degli arti, mentre gli spasmi misti, la forma più comune, consistono in scariche di estensione alternate a scariche di flessione. La crisi si protrae per alcuni minuti, con brevi intervalli tra ciascuno spasmo. Il pianto può precedere o seguire lo spasmo e in alcuni casi può essere confusa con una colica. Gli spasmi possono verificarsi sia durante il sonno che la veglia, ma sono più frequenti immediatamente dopo il risveglio o in momenti di sonnolenza. L'EEG più comunemente associato al disturbo, definito ipsaritmia, consiste in un pattern caotico di attività a onda lenta ad alto voltaggio, bilateralmente asincrona (vedi Fig. 593-1*B*) o in una pattern di ipsaritmia modificato.

Gli spasmi infantili sono comunemente classificati in due gruppi: gli spasmi **criptogenetici** e quelli **sintomatici**. Nel primo caso, non si segnalano né anomalie della storia clinica, della gestazione e del parto, né ritardi dello sviluppo. L'esame neurologico, la TC e la RM della testa risultano normali e non si riscontrano fattori di rischio per l'epilessia. Circa il 10-20% degli spasmi infantili è classificato come criptogenetico. Gli spasmi sintomatici sono direttamente collegati a fattori prenatali, perinatali e postnatali. I fattori prenatali e perinatali includono encefalopatia ipossica-ischemica con leucomalacia periventricolare, infezioni congenite, errori congeniti del metabolismo, sindromi neurocutanee come la sclerosi tuberosa, anomalie citoarchitetturali come la lissencefalia e la schizencefalia e la prematurità. Le condizioni postnatali includono infezioni del SNC, traumi cranici (in particolare ematoma subdurale e emorragia intraventricolare) ed encefalopatia ipossica-ischemica. Il fatto che l'esordio degli spasmi infantili e le vaccinazioni si verifichino simultaneamente, intorno ai 6 mesi, è da considerarsi una coincidenza piuttosto che un effetto degli antigeni immunizzanti.

La prognosi degli spasmi criptogenetici è buona, mentre i bambini con il tipo sintomatico presentano un rischio dell'80-90% di sviluppare ritardo mentale. I soggiacenti disturbi del SNC incidono in maniera significativa sull'esito neurologico. Sono state proposte diverse teorie sulla patogenesi degli spasmi infantili, che includono la disfunzione del sistema monoaminergico di neurotrasmissione nel tronco encefalico, la lesione delle strutture neuronali del tronco e anomalie del sistema immunitario. Un'ipotesi chiama in causa l'ormone di rilascio della corticotropina (CRH), un neurotrasmettitore putativo, metabolizzato nell'oliva inferiore. Il CRH agisce sulla ghiandola pituitaria, stimolando il rilascio dell'ormone adrenocorticotropico (ACTH); l'ACTH e i glucocorticoidi sopprimono il metabolismo e la secrezione di CRH mediante un meccanismo di feedback. Specifici stress o lesioni durante un periodo critico nello sviluppo del bambino possono causare un'eccessiva produzione di CRH, con conseguente ipereccitabilità e tendenza a sviluppare convulsioni. Il fatto che il numero dei recettori di CRH, dopo aver raggiunto il massimo, vada incontro a riduzione spontanea spiega la tendenza alla risoluzione degli spasmi infantili, anche in assenza di terapia.

SINDROME DI LANDAU-KLEFFNER. Questa rara malattia dalla causa sconosciuta è più comune nei maschi ed esordisce in media a 5 anni e mezzo. La sindrome di Landau-Kleffner (*Landau-Kleffner Syndrome*, LKS) è spesso confusa con l'autismo, perché in entrambe le patologie si riscontra una compromissione della funzione linguistica. La caratteristica principale della LKS è dunque la perdita del linguaggio in un bambino precedentemente normale. Almeno il 70% dei casi presenta un disturbo convulsivo associato. La regressione del linguaggio può essere improvvisa o graduale. L'**afasia** può essere prevalentemente recettiva o espressiva e l'agnosia uditiva è talvolta talmente grave da impedire al bambino di percepire i suoni quotidiani. La funzione uditiva è normale, ma i problemi comportamentali, come irritabilità e disturbi dell'attenzione, sono particolarmente comuni. Malgrado i disturbi di linguaggio, i bambini ottengono spesso risultati nella norma ai test di performance e visivo-spaziali. Le convulsioni sono di diverso tipo: focali o tonico-cloniche generalizzate, assenze atipiche, parziali complesse e, talvolta, miocloniche. Le scariche punte-onda di grande ampiezza predominano, soprattutto bitemporali ma anche multifocali o generalizzate. Nelle fasi iniziali della malattia, l'EEG può risultare normale. Le scariche di punte sono più evidenti durante il sonno non-REM (*Non-Rapid Eye Movement*), perciò in caso di sospetto, malgrado il tracciato della veglia risulti normale, è opportuno effettuare l'EEG durante il sonno. In presenza di un elevato indice di sospetto, nonostante tracciati della veglia e del sonno normali, si consiglia il ricovero del bambino in un centro specializzato, per essere sottoposto a una prolungata registrazione EEG e a specifici esami di neuroimaging. TC e RM solitamente non rivelano alcuna anomalia, mentre la tomografia a emissione di positroni (*Positron Emission Tomography*, PET) segnala la presenza di ipometabolismo o ipermetabolismo unilaterale o bilaterale. L'esame dei campioni chirurgici mostra una gliosi minima, ma non evidenzia alcun segno di encefalite.

L'acido valproico è l'anticonvulsivante di elezione. Alcuni pazienti richiedono una combinazione di acido valproico e clobazam per il controllo delle convulsioni. Se gli attacchi e l'afasia persistono, è opportuno considerare un trial con steroidi; il prednisone è somministrato oralmente alla dose di 2 mg/kg/24 h per il primo mese, ridotta poi a 1 mg/kg/24 h per il secondo mese. In caso di miglioramento clinico, la terapia è proseguita per altri 6-12 mesi, alla dose di 0,5 mg/kg/24 h. È fondamentale avviare al più presto la logoterapia, da proseguire per diversi anni, perché i miglioramenti della funzione linguistica richiedono tempi prolungati. In alcuni centri si raccomanda una procedura chirurgica di transezione subpiale in caso di fallimento della terapia farmacologica. La somministrazione di metilfenidato deve essere presa in considerazione nei pazienti con grave iperattività e con deficit dell'attenzione. Tuttavia, le convulsioni, se scarsamente controllate dagli anticonvulsivanti, possono essere potenziate dal metilfenidato. Anche la somministrazione per via endovenosa di immunoglobuline può essere utile nella LKS. Alcuni bambini sperimentano una recidiva dell'afasia e delle convulsioni dopo un'apparente guarigione. La maggior parte dei pazienti manifesta un significativo deficit del linguaggio in età adulta. L'esordio precoce della malattia (<2 anni) è associato a una prognosi peggiore riguardo al recupero della funzione linguistica.

593.5 • MECCANISMO DELLE CONVULSIONI

Il meccanismo preciso delle convulsioni non è noto, ma di certo sono implicati diversi fattori fisiologici. L'attacco è scatenato da un gruppo di neuroni in grado di generare una scarica, disattivando il sistema inibitorio GABA-ergico (acido γ-aminobutirrico). La trasmissione della scarica dipende da sinapsi eccitatorie glutamatergiche. È probabile che neurotrasmettitori eccitatori (glutammato, aspartato) determinino l'eccitazione neuronale agendo su specifici recettori. Si ipotizza che le convulsioni originino in aree cerebrali di morte neuronale, che promuovono lo sviluppo di nuove sinapsi ipereccitabili, responsabili delle convulsioni. Lesioni del lobo temporale (come gliomi a lenta crescita, amartomi, gliosi, sclerosi ippocampale e malformazioni arteriovenose) causano convulsioni, che cessano quando il tessuto anomalo è rimosso chirurgicamente. Sono state avanzate due ipotesi per spiegare l'origine delle convulsioni causate da lesioni cerebrali. La prima suggerisce un danneggiamento selettivo dei neuroni inibitori, con conseguente ipereccitabilità dei restanti neuroni eccitatori. La seconda ipotesi postula che i circuiti eccitatori aberranti siano una conseguenza della riorganizzazione cerebrale successiva alla lesione. Le convulsioni possono essere riprodotte in un setting sperimentale mediante il fenomeno del **kindling**. In questo modello, stimolazioni subliminali consecutive dell'amigdala provocano una convulsione generalizzata, conseguenza di un cambiamento delle sinapsi. È possibile che tale meccanismo sinaptico agisca anche nell'essere umano.

Le convulsioni sono più comuni nei lattanti e negli animali sperimentali immaturi. Nella popolazione pediatrica, alcuni tipi di convulsioni sono età-specifiche (come gli spasmi infantili); questa osservazione suggerisce che l'immaturità cerebrale aumenti la suscettibilità ad alcuni tipi di convulsioni. Ciò è confermato anche dai dati scientifici che segnalano la maggiore eccitabilità del cervello immaturo, conseguenza dell'influenza eccitatoria dei circuiti contenenti glutammato. Paradossalmente GABA, il principale neurotrasmettitore inibitorio, esercita spesso un'azione eccitatoria sul cervello immaturo. È ipotizzabile che l'aumento dell'attività eccitatoria contribuisca a conferire maggiore plasticità al cervello in sviluppo.

I fattori genetici sono responsabili di almeno il 20% dei casi di epilessia (vedi Tab. 593-1). Gli studi di linkage hanno consentito di localizzare diverse epilessie familiari, incluse le convulsioni neonatali benigne (20q e 8q), l'epilessia mioclonica giovanile (6p) e l'epilessia mioclonica progressiva (21q22.3). Il difetto genetico delle convulsioni neonatali familiari benigne è stato caratterizzato mediante l'identificazione di una delezione submicroscopica del cromosoma 20q13.3. Studi della regione della delezione hanno condotto all'identificazione di un cDNA che codifica per un nuovo canale del potassio voltaggio-dipendente: $KCNQ_2$. Anche la substantia nigra svolge un ruolo importante nello sviluppo delle convulsioni generalizzate. L'attività elettrica convulsiva si diffonde all'interno della substantia nigra, causando un aumento dell'uptake di 2-desossigluscosio negli animali adulti, mentre negli animali immaturi si riscontra un'attività metabolica minima o nulla durante la convulsione. È stato ipotizzato che l'immaturità funzionale della substantia nigra abbia un ruolo nell'aumento della suscettibilità alle convulsioni del cervello immaturo. I neuroni GABA-sensibili della pars reticulata della substantia nigra contribuiscono a prevenire le convulsioni. È probabile che le vie efferenti della substantia nigra agiscano modulando e regolando le convulsioni, ma non siano responsabili del loro esordio.

UTILIZZO DELL'EEG PER LA DIAGNOSI DI EPILESSIA. L'indagine di un attacco convulsivo dipende da molti fattori, tra cui l'età del paziente, il tipo e la frequenza delle crisi e la presenza di reperti neurologici e sintomi costituzionali. Un tracciato EEG con scariche parossistiche durante la crisi consente di formulare la diagnosi di epilessia, ma raramente le convulsioni si verificano in laboratorio. Un EEG normale non esclude la diagnosi di epilessia, perché il tracciato intercritale non presenta anomalie in circa il 40% dei pazienti. Può essere utile ricorrere a procedure di attivazione, come l'iperventilazione e l'applicazione di elettrodi zigomatici. È più facile registrare le scariche in lattanti e bambini rispetto ad adolescenti e adulti. Non è opportuno sospendere l'assunzione degli anticonvulsivanti prima di un esame EEG di routine, per il rischio di insorgenza di status epilettico.

Il monitoraggio EEG prolungato mediante video registrazione simultanea a circuito chiuso è riservato ai casi di convulsioni protratte che non rispondono alla terapia. Tale tecnica consente di registrare eventi ictali raramente evidenziabili durante gli EEG di routine e contribuisce alla classificazione della convulsione, determinandone la localizzazione e la frequenza e segnalando le alterazioni del livello di coscienza e la presenza di segni clinici. L'EEG consente una rapida diagnosi differenziale tra i pazienti con pseudoconvulsioni e quelli con epilessia vera e propria e contribuisce alla classificazione del tipo di crisi (parziale complessa piuttosto che generalizzata). La determinazione del tipo di convulsione è fondamentale per l'identificazione dei candidati alla terapia chirurgica dell'epilessia.

593.6 • TRATTAMENTO DELL'EPILESSIA

Il primo passo nella gestione dell'epilessia consiste nell'assicurarsi che il paziente presenti effettivamente un disturbo convulsivo e non una condizione che mima l'epilessia (vedi Capitolo 594). Nel bambino normale è talvolta complicato risalire alla causa dell'evento parossistico. Un risultato negativo dell'EEG suggerisce di attendere prima di procedere alla somministrazione di un anticonvulsivante, proseguendo la ricerca della causa del disturbo parossistico. Malgrado le differenze di opinione a riguardo, la maggior parte degli esperti concorda nell'evitare la prescrizione di un antiepilettico in un bambino precedentemente sano dopo la prima crisi afebbrile nelle seguenti circostanze: storia familiare negativa, risultati dell'esame obiettivo e dell'EEG nella norma, presenza di una famiglia disposta a collaborare. Il 70% circa di questi bambini non sperimenta una seconda crisi. Circa il 75% dei bambini che hanno già sperimentato due o tre crisi non provocate è destinato ad avere nuovi attacchi. La ricorrenza della convulsione, in particolare se a breve distanza dalla prima, costituisce un'indicazione per intraprendere la terapia con anticonvulsivanti. La Figura 593-3 suggerisce l'approccio ideale a un bambino con sospetto disturbo convulsivo.

Il secondo passo consiste nella scelta dell'**anticonvulsivante** più indicato. Il farmaco di elezione dipende dalla classificazione della convulsione, determinata dall'anamnesi e dall'EEG. Per ogni paziente, l'obiettivo è di controllare le crisi utilizzando un solo farmaco, con il minor numero possibile di effetti collaterali. La dose del farmaco scelto è aumentata gradualmente, fino a ottenere il controllo della convulsione o finché non compaiono effetti collaterali indesiderati. Durante questa fase, è opportuno monitorare il livello sierico dell'anticonvulsivante, modificando la dose di conseguenza. Nella Tabella 593-5 sono elencati i più comuni farmaci antiepilettici usati in età pediatrica, specificando la dose quotidiana raccomandata, i livelli sierici terapeutici e i potenziali effetti collaterali. È indicata anche la dose di carico consigliata dei farmaci utili per il trattamento dello status epilettico. Il medico dovrebbe conoscere a fondo la farmacocinetica degli anticonvulsivanti e la loro azione tossica e sottoporre il paziente a controlli regolari, in modo da ottenere il controllo delle convulsioni senza incorrere in effetti collaterali indesiderati.

Il monitoraggio sierico dei livelli degli anticonvulsivanti non è raccomandato di routine a causa dei costi elevati, ma è indispensabile nelle seguenti circostanze: (1) all'inizio della terapia, per verificare se il livello rientra nel range terapeutico; (2) in caso di scarsa compliance da parte del paziente o della famiglia; (3) in presenza di status epilettico; (4) durante le fasi di crescita accelerata; (5) nei pazienti in politerapia, in particolare per verificare le interazioni tra acido valproico, fenobarbital e lamotrigina; (6) in caso di convulsioni incontrollate o di modifica della tipologia della crisi; (7) in presenza di sintomi e segni di tossicità (dovuta al

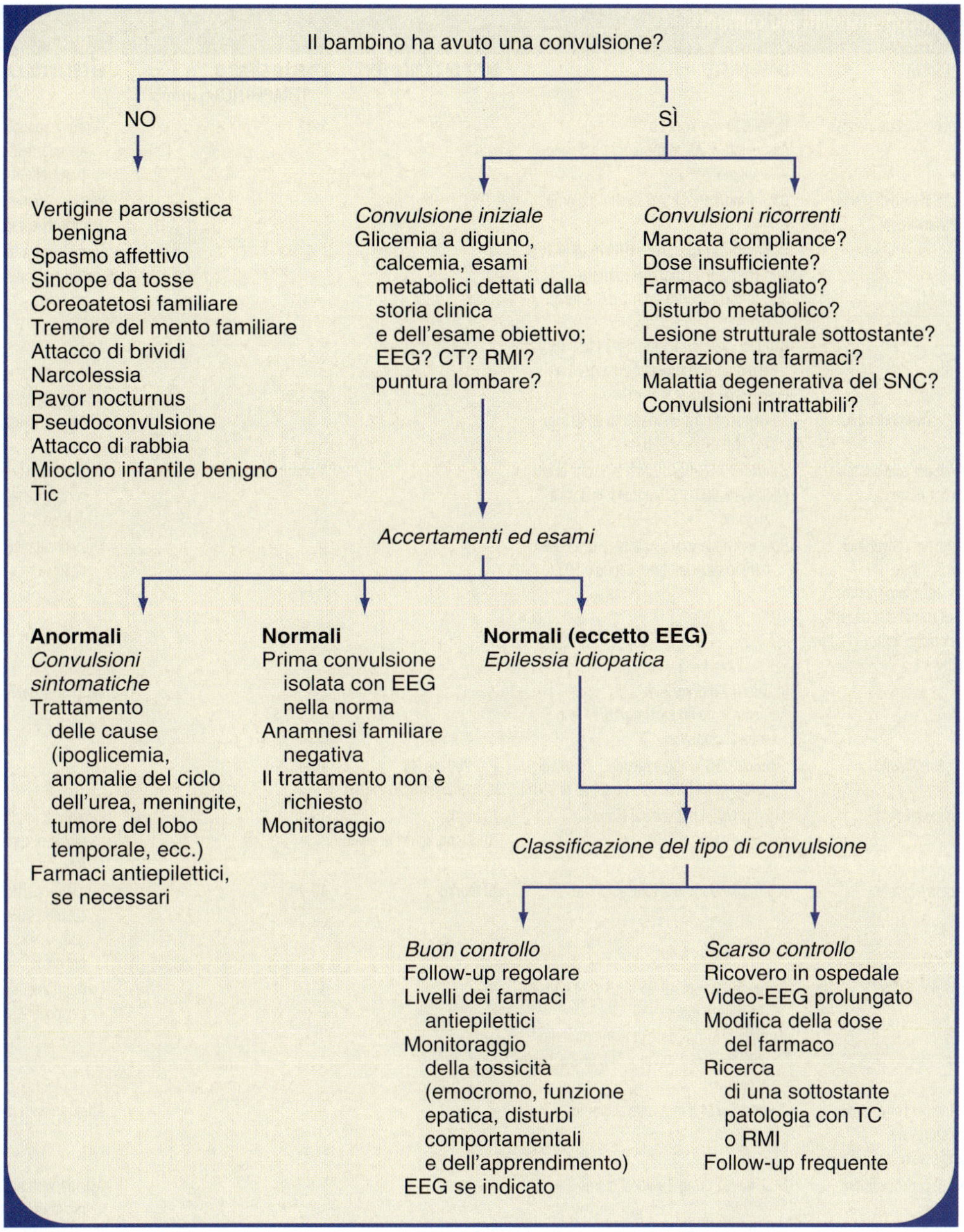

Figura 593-3. Approccio al bambino con sospetto disturbo convulsivo.

metabolita della carbamazepina, carbamazepina-10,11-eposside); (8) nei pazienti con malattia epatica o renale; (9) nei bambini con disturbi cognitivi o fisici, in particolare se assumono fenitoina, la cui tossicità è più difficile da valutare. Per ottenere il controllo delle convulsioni, il giudizio clinico del medico esperto è più affidabile di un prolungato monitoraggio. Le forme di epilessia resistenti i farmaci, talvolta associate a polimorfismi genetici dei meccanismi di trasporto del farmaco, richiedono trial di anticonvulsivanti differenti.

È oggetto di controversie anche l'opportunità di sottoporre il paziente a periodici esami del sangue (emocromo completo ed esame della funzione epatica) durante la terapia anticonvulsivante. Poiché le reazioni più gravi si sviluppano nei primi mesi di terapia, il controllo ematico mensile è raccomandato per almeno 3 mesi. Successivamente, gli esami del sangue sono prescritti solo in presenza di indicazioni cliniche.

In alcuni casi, gli anticonvulsivanti introdotti durante l'infanzia continuano a essere assunti anche nell'adolescenza, quando il paziente è in età fertile. Alcuni di essi, come la fenitoina, l'acido valproico, la carbamazepina e il primidone, sono associati a specifici **difetti congeniti** (anomalie facciali e degli arti, disrafismo spinale). Il pediatra è tenuto a informare i pazienti su questi rischi. La prescrizione di un anticonvulsivante a pazienti in stato di gravidanza è opportuna solo in caso di assoluta necessità.

Se il completo controllo delle crisi è ottenuto con un solo farmaco, in un paziente che non presenta fattori di rischio il trattamento può essere sospeso dopo almeno due anni di assenza di sintomi. I principali fattori di rischio includono: un'età di esordio inferiore a 12 anni, la presenza di disfunzioni neurologiche (come handicap motori o ritardo mentale), un'anamnesi di convulsioni neonatali e una difficoltà iniziale nell'ottenere il controllo delle crisi. In un bambino privo di fattori di rischio rilevanti che non presenta crisi per un periodo minimo di 2 anni, il rischio di recidiva è di circa il 20-25% e risulta particolarmente elevato nei primi sei mesi dopo la sospensione della terapia. I pazienti affetti da epilessia benigna con punte rolandiche o da convulsioni idiopatiche generalizzate presentano una prognosi migliore dopo la sospensione della terapia. Le recidive sono più frequenti nei casi di CPS e convulsioni miocloniche giovanili. Poiché la brusca interruzione dell'assunzione di un farmaco può causare status epilettico, la sospensione della terapia deve avvenire gradualmente, nel corso di 3-6 mesi.

TABELLA 593-5. Farmaci anticonvulsivanti più comuni

FARMACO	TIPO DI CONVULSIONI	DOSE ORALE	DOSE DI CARICO (EV)	LIVELLO SIERICO TERAPEUTICO (μg/mL)	EFFETTI COLLATERALI E TOSSICITÀ
Carbamazepina	Tonico-cloniche generalizzate, parziali	Iniziale: 10 mg/kg/24 h Aumentata a: 20-30 mg/kg/24 h 3 volte al giorno	—	8-12	Vertigini, sonnolenza, diplopia, disfunzione epatica, anemia, neutropenia, SIADH, discrasie ematiche (rare), effetti epatotossici
Clobazam	Terapia potenziante in caso di scarso controllo delle convulsioni	0,25-1 mg/kg/24 h 2 o 3 volte al giorno	—	—	Vertigini, affaticamento, aumento di peso, atassia e disturbi comportamentali
Clonazepam	Assenze Miocloniche Spasmi infantili Parziali Lennox-Gastaut Acinetiche	Bambini <30 kg: Iniziale: 0,05 mg/kg/24 h Aumento di 0,05 mg/kg/settimana Massimo: 0,2 mg/kg/24 h 2 o 3 volte al giorno Bambini >30 kg: 1,5 mg/kg/24 h 2 o 3 volte al giorno, non superare 20 mg/24 h	—	>0,013	Sonnolenza, irritabilità, agitazione, disturbi comportamentali, depressione, salivazione eccessiva
Etosuccimide	Assenze Può aumentare le convulsioni tonico-cloniche	Iniziale: 20 mg/kg/24 h Aumentare fino a un massimo di 40 mg/kg/24 h o 1,5 g/24 h	—	40-100	Fastidio addominale, eruzioni cutanee, disfunzione epatica, leucopenia
Gabapentina	Terapia potenziante per convulsioni scarsamente controllate	Bambini: 20-50 mg/kg/24 h in 3 volte al giorno Adolescenti: 900-3600 mg/24 h in 3 volte al giorno	—	Monitoraggio non necessario	Sonnolenza, vertigini, atassia, mal di testa, tremori, vomito, nistagmo, affaticamento e aumento di peso
Lamotrigina	Terapia potenziante per convulsioni scarsamente controllate Anticonvulsivante ad ampio spettro per crisi parziali complesse, assenze, miocloniche, cloniche, tonico-cloniche, Lennox-Gastaut	Dose individualizzata sulla base dell'età e dei farmaci associati (vedi Capitolo 593.6)	—	—	Eruzioni cutanee, vertigini, atassia, sonnolenza, diplopia, mal di testa, nausea, vomito
Nitrazepam	Assenze Miocloniche Spasmi infantili	Iniziale: 0,2 mg/kg/24 h Aumento lento fino a 1 mg/kg/24 h in 3 volte al giorno	—	—	Simili al clonazepam, allucinazioni
Paraldeide	Status epilettico generalizzato	Soluzione al 5% aggiungendo 1,75 mL di paraldeide a D5W, volume totale di 35 mL	150-200 mg/kg Mantenimento: 20 mg/kg	10-40	
Fenobarbital	Tonico-cloniche generalizzate Parziali	3-5 mg/kg/24 h 2 volte al giorno	20 mg/kg 20-30 mg/kg nel neonato	15-40	Iperattività, irritabilità, disturbi dell'attenzione, crisi di rabbia, disturbi del sonno, sindrome di Stevens-Johnson, depressione della funzione cognitiva
Fenitoina	Tonico-cloniche generalizzate Parziali Status epilettico	3-9 mg/kg/24 h in 2 volte al giorno	20 mg/kg	10-20	Irsutismo, ipertrofia gengivale, atassia, eruzioni cutanee, sindrome di Stevens-Johnson, nistagmo, nausea, vomito, sonnolenza, tratti somatici grossolani, discrasie ematiche
Primidone	Tonico-cloniche generalizzate Parziali	Bambini <8 anni: 10-25 mg/kg/24 h in 2 o 3 volte al giorno Bambini >8 anni: dose di mantenimento abituale, 750-1500 mg/24 h in 2 o 3 volte al giorno	—	5-12	Comportamento aggressivo, cambiamenti di personalità, simili al fenobarbital
Topiramato	Terapia potenziante per convulsioni scarsamente controllate Crisi parziali complesse refrattarie	1-9 mg/kg/24 h in 2 volte al giorno	—	—	Affaticamento, depressione cognitiva
Tiagabina	Terapia potenziante per convulsioni parziali complesse	Dose media, 6 mg 2 volte al giorno	—	—	Astenia, vertigini, disturbi dell'attenzione, nervosismo, tremori
Acido valproico	Tonico-cloniche generalizzate Assenze Miocloniche Parziali Acinetiche	Iniziale: 10 mg/kg/24 h Aumento di 5-10 mg/kg/settimana Dose usuale 30-60 mg/kg/24 h in 3-4 somministrazioni	Disponibile preparato per somministrazione endovenosa Nei bambini, in fase di sperimentazione	50-100	Nausea, vomito, anoressia, amenorrea, sedazione, tremori, aumento di peso, alopecia, epatotossicità
Vigabatrin	Spasmi infantili Terapia potenziante per convulsioni scarsamente controllate	Iniziale: 30 mg/kg/24 h 1 o 2 volte al giorno Dose di mantenimento: 30-100 mg/kg/24 h 1 o 2 volte al giorno	—	—	Iperattività, agitazione, eccitazione, sonnolenza, aumento di peso Sono stati segnalati anche riduzione del campo visivo, pallore o atrofia del nervo ottico, nevrite ottica

SIADH, *Syndrome of Inappropriate Secretion of Antidiuretic Hormone* (sindrome da inappropriata secrezione dell'ormone antidiuretico).
D5W = glucosata 5%.

Le modalità di azione, le dosi e gli effetti collaterali dei principali anticonvulsivanti sono riassunti nella Figura 593-4 e nella Tabella 593-5.

BENZODIAZEPINE. Le benzodiazepine esercitano un'azione anticonvulsivante legandosi a specifici siti GABA che stimolano la frequenza di apertura dei canali del cloro, senza incidere sulla durata della crisi (vedi Fig. 593-4). Il diazepam e il lorazepam via ev vengono utilizzati per la gestione iniziale dello status epilettico. Il diazepam in gel somministrato per via rettale (alla dose di 2,5, 5 e 10 mg) si è dimostrato un metodo efficace e sicuro per interrompere gli episodi convulsivi acuti nei bambini. Anche il midazolam per via orale o nasale è efficace negli episodi acuti. Il clonazepam è utile per il trattamento della sindrome di Lennox-Gastaut, delle convulsioni miocloniche, acinetiche e delle assenze. L'emivita di eliminazione è di 18-50 ore. L'associazione del clonazepam con la fenitoina può determinare un incremento della concentrazione sierica di quest'ultima, mentre la combinazione di clonazepam con altri farmaci depressori del SNC rischia di causare un effetto depressore eccessivo. Il clonazepam è disponibile in compresse da 0,5 e 2 mg. Il nitrazepam è efficace per il controllo delle convulsioni miocloniche. La sua emivita di eliminazione è di 18-57

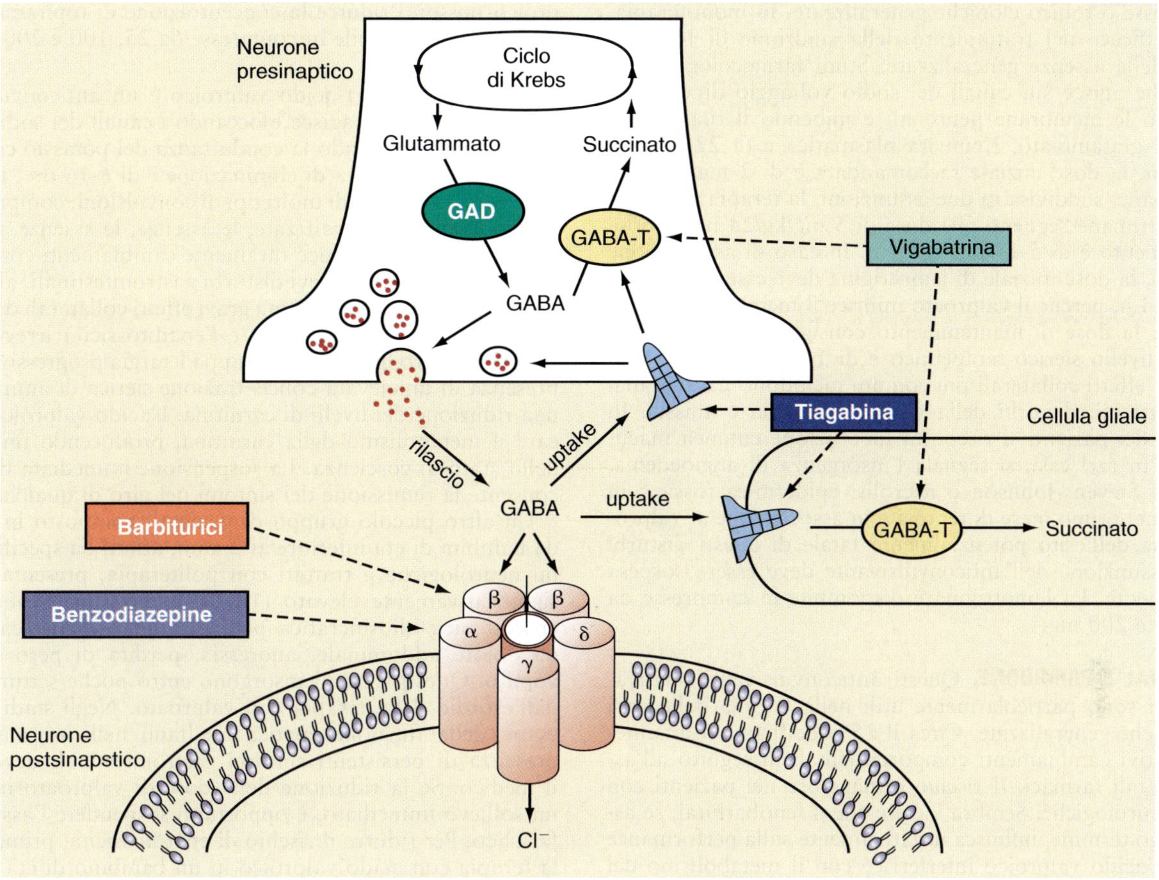

Figura 593-4. Effetti farmacologici dei farmaci antiepilettici a livello del recettore $GABA_A$. I barbiturici si legano alla subunità β di $GABA_A$, potenziando l'azione dell'agonista endogeno GABA e prolungando il tempo di apertura dei canali del cloro. Le benzodiazepine si legano alla subunità α di $GABA_A$, potenziando l'azione di GABA e incrementando la frequenza di apertura dei canali del cloro. Il vigabatrin si lega irreversibilmente a GABA-T, inibendo la degradazione del neurotrasmettitore inibitorio GABA. La tiagabina blocca l'uptake del GABA rilasciato dalle sinapsi nei neuroni presinaptici e nelle cellule gliali, permettendo a GABA di restare nel sito di azione per periodi più prolungati. GABA, acido γ-aminobutirrico; $GABA_A$, GABA di tipo A; GABA-T, GABA transaminasi; GAD, *Glutamic Acid Decarboxylase*, acido glutammico decarbossilasi. (Tratta da Leach JP, Brodie MJ: Tiagabine. *Lancet* 1998;351:203-207.)

ore. Questo farmaco, disponibile in compresse da 5 e 10 mg, può aumentare la depressione del SNC se usato in combinazione con un farmaco depressore. Il clobazam è indicato come farmaco aggiuntivo nella terapia delle convulsioni parziali complesse. La sua emivita è di 10-30 ore. Usato in associazione, il clobazam può aumentare i livelli sierici di carbamazepina, fenitoina, fenobarbital e acido valproico. È disponibile in compresse da 10 mg.

CARBAMAZEPINA. Questo farmaco è efficace nel trattamento delle convulsioni tonico-cloniche generalizzate e parziali. Analogamente alla fenitoina, agisce riducendo le ripetute scariche neuronali, bloccando i canali sodio-dipendenti e limitando l'uptake di calcio dipendente dalla depolarizzazione. In rari casi, può causare una significativa leucopenia (<1000 neutrofili/mL^3) ed epatotossicità, in particolare nei primi 3-4 mesi di terapia. Di conseguenza, in questa fase si raccomanda un esame emocromocitometrico con formula mensile e la determinazione di AST e ALT (ma una seria reazione idiosincrasica può insorgere anche in presenza di risultati dei test epatici ed ematici nella norma). L'opportunità dei test di laboratorio nelle fasi successive della terapia è stabilita sulla base della presenza di sintomi e segni preoccupanti. I parenti devono essere informati dei potenziali effetti collaterali ed esortati a riferirli tempestivamente al medico. L'eritromicina deve essere somministrata con cautela in associazione alla carbamazepina, perché i due farmaci sono in competizione metabolica nel fegato. La concentrazione plasmatica di carbamazepina è ridotta da fenitoina, fenobarbital e acido valproico. Il metabolita attivo della carbamazepina (carbamazepina-10,11-eposside) può causare tossicità anche quando i livelli del farmaco rientrano nel range terapeutico, in particolare in caso di associazione con l'acido valproico. L'iponatremia è un altro effetto collaterale segnalato di questo farmaco. La carbamazepina è disponibile in sospensione (20 mg/mL), compresse masticabili, compresse da 200 mg e compresse a rilascio controllato da 200 e 400 mg. L'emivita è di 8-20 ore. La dose quotidiana andrebbe suddivisa in 2 o 3 somministrazioni.

ETOSUCCIMIDE. L'etosuccimide esercita la sua azione anticonvulsivante bloccando i canali del calcio associati al circuito talamocorticale. È efficace nel controllo delle assenze tipiche e ha un'emivita di 60 ore. Utilizzato in associazione a fenobarbital o primidone, l'etosuccimide può ridurre i livelli sierici di questi anticonvulsivanti ed è disponibile in sciroppo (50 mg/mL) e in capsule da 250 mg.

GABAPENTIN. Questo anticonvulsivante è utilizzato come farmaco potenziante in pazienti affetti da convulsioni parziali complesse o tonico cloniche a generalizzazione secondaria. Il suo meccanismo di azione è il risultato del legame con le membrane neuronali (sinapsi eccitate dal glutammato) e dell'incremento del turnover cerebrale di GABA. L'emivita plasmatica del gabapentin è di 5-7 ore. Il farmaco è rapidamente assorbito dal tratto gastrointestinale, non si lega alle proteine plasmatiche e non viene metabolizzato. Non presenta significative interazioni con altri farmaci e risulta relativamente privo di effetti collaterali legati alla dose. Disponibile in capsule da 100, 300 e 400 mg, è raccomandato nei bambini con età minima di 12 anni.

LAMOTRIGINA. La lamotrigina è un composto feniltriazinico usata come farmaco potenziante per il controllo delle convulsioni parziali complesse o tonico cloniche generalizzate. In monoterapia, è talvolta efficace nel trattamento della sindrome di Lennox-Gastaut e delle assenze generalizzate. Studi farmacologici suggeriscono che agisce sui canali del sodio voltaggio dipendenti, stabilizzando le membrane neuronali e inibendo il rilascio soprattutto di glutammato. L'emivita plasmatica è di 22-37 ore. Nei bambini, la dose iniziale raccomandata è di 2 mg/kg/24 h per 2 settimane, suddivisa in due assunzioni; la terapia prosegue nelle due settimane seguenti alla dose di 5 mg/kg/24 h. La dose di mantenimento è di 5-15 mg/kg/24 h. In caso di associazione al valproato, la dose iniziale di lamotrigina deve essere ridotta a 0,5 mg/kg/24 h, perché il valproato inibisce il metabolismo della lamotrigina; la dose di mantenimento consigliata è di 1-5 mg/kg/24 h. Il livello sierico terapeutico è di 1-4 mg/L o 3,9-15,6 μmol/L. Gli effetti collaterali più comuni includono nausea, mal di testa, vertigini, disturbi della visione, diplopia e atassia. In circa il 3% dei pazienti si riscontra un'eruzione cutanea maculopapulare. In rari casi, si segnala l'insorgenza di angioedema, sindrome di Stevens-Johnson o necrolisi epidermica tossica, in particolare nel primo mese di terapia e in associazione al valproato. A causa dell'esito potenzialmente fatale di questi disturbi cutanei, l'assunzione dell'anticonvulsivante deve essere sospesa immediatamente. La lamotrigina è disponibile in compresse da 25, 50, 100 e 200 mg.

FENOBARBITAL E PRIMIDONE. Questi anticonvulsivanti relativamente sicuri sono particolarmente utili nella terapia delle crisi tonico-cloniche generalizzate. Circa il 25% dei bambini manifesta significativi cambiamenti comportamentali in seguito all'assunzione di tali farmaci. Il rischio è maggiore nei pazienti con anomalie neurologiche. Sembra inoltre che il fenobarbital, se assunto a lungo termine, influisca negativamente sulla performance cognitiva. L'acido valproico interferisce con il metabolismo del fenobarbital, causandone un aumento dei livelli plasmatici e della tossicità. Il fenobarbital agisce sui recettori GABA, prolungando la durata dell'apertura dei canali del cloro (vedi Fig. 593-4). L'emivita plasmatica è di 48-150 ore. Il fenobarbital è disponibile in forma di sciroppo (4 mg/mL), di compresse da 15, 30, 60 e 100 mg e in soluzione iniettabile da 30 e 120 mg/mL. Il primidone è disponibile in sospensione da 50 mg/mL e in compresse da 125 e 250 mg. L'emivita plasmatica del primidone è di 10-21 ore. Il fenobarbital è assunto in due dosi quotidiane, mentre il primidone è suddiviso in tre assunzioni. Gli esami del sangue di routine non sono indicati per questi anticonvulsivanti.

FENITOINA. La fenitoina agisce riducendo le scariche ripetitive di neuroni singoli, bloccando i canali sodio-dipendenti e riducendo l'uptake di calcio dipendente dalla depolarizzazione. È usata per il trattamento delle convulsioni tonico-cloniche a generalizzazione primaria o secondaria, delle convulsioni parziali e dello status epilettico. L'emivita plasmatica è di 7-42 ore. Diverse interazioni farmacologiche possono aumentare o ridurre l'effetto degli anticonvulsivanti associati (vedi Tab. 593-5). La fenitoina è disponibile in sospensione da 6 e 25 mg/mL, compresse masticabili da 50 mg, capsule da 100 mg e soluzione iniettabile da 100 mg/2 mL e 250 mg/5 mL. La fosfenitoina, un profarmaco della fenitoina solubile in acqua, somministrabile per via intramuscolare o endovenosa, è disponibile in concentrazione da 75 mg/mL, equivalente a 50 mg/mL di fenitoina.

TIAGABINA. La tiagabina inibisce l'attività convulsiva bloccando il reuptake del neurotrasmettitore inibitorio GABA nelle cellule neuronali e gliali (vedi Fig. 593-4). Questo farmaco, disponibile in compresse da 4, 12, 16 e 20 mg, è efficace nel trattamento nelle convulsioni parziali complesse e come farmaco potenziante.

TOPIRAMATO. Il topiramato esercita la sua azione anticonvulsivante bloccando i canali del sodio voltaggio dipendenti. È usato come farmaco potenziante per il controllo della convulsioni complesse refrattarie, con o senza generalizzazione secondaria. L'emivita di eliminazione è di 21 ore. Fenitoina, carbamazepina e acido valproico possono ridurre la concentrazione di topiramato. Questo farmaco è disponibile in compresse da 25, 100 e 200 mg.

ACIDO VALPROICO. L'acido valproico è un anticonvulsivante ad ampio spettro, che agisce bloccando i canali del sodio voltaggio dipendenti e riducendo la conduttanza del potassio calcio-dipendente. La sua emivita di eliminazione è di 6-16 ore. Il farmaco è utile per il controllo di molti tipi di convulsioni, comprende quelle tonico-cloniche generalizzate, le assenze, le assenze atipiche e le crisi miocloniche. Induce raramente cambiamenti comportamentali, ma è associato a lievi disturbi gastrointestinali, alopecia, tremore e iperfagia. Due rari ma gravi effetti collaterali del valproato sono la sindrome simil-Reye e l'epatotossicità irreversibile. Un ridotto numero di pazienti sviluppa letargia progressiva e coma in presenza di un'elevata concentrazione sierica di ammoniaca e di una riduzione dei livelli di carnitina. L'acido valproico può bloccare il metabolismo della carnitina, producendo un'alterazione dello stato di coscienza. La sospensione immediata della terapia consente la remissione dei sintomi nel giro di qualche giorno.

Un altro piccolo gruppo di pazienti, composto in particolare da bambini di età inferiore ai 2 anni, affetti da specifiche sindromi neurologiche e trattati con politerapia, presenta un rischio significativamente elevato (1:800) di sviluppare una sindrome epatotossica idiosincratica potenzialmente fatale, caratterizzata da dolore addominale, anoressia, perdita di peso e conati di vomito. Questi sintomi insorgono entro poche settimane o mesi dall'esordio della terapia con valproato. Negli stadi iniziali, gli esami della funzione epatica risultano nella norma, perciò la presenza di persistenti sintomi gastrointestinali deve allarmare il medico. Se la riduzione della dose di valproato non fornisce un sollievo immediato, è opportuno sospendere l'assunzione del farmaco. Per ridurre il rischio di epatotossicità, prima di iniziare la terapia con acido valproico in un bambino di età inferiore ai 2 anni affetto da convulsioni la cui causa è sconosciuta, è utile effettuare una serie di test di screening per la ricerca di una malattia metabolica. Tali test includono il dosaggio dei livelli sierici di ammoniaca, di amminoacidi, dei gas ematici e del rapporto lattato/piruvato, il dosaggio degli acidi organici nelle urine e della carnitina totale e libera nel siero. L'incidenza di epatotossicità potenzialmente fatale indotta dall'acido valproico si è ridotta drasticamente negli ultimi anni, grazie al minor utilizzo del farmaco nei bambini con meno due anni e alla consapevolezza dei rischi minori della monoterapia.

L'acido valproico può causare anche una riduzione dei livelli sierici di carnitina libera, inibendo l'uptake della carnitina nel plasmalemma. Alcuni studi suggeriscono che il deficit di carnitina costituisca la principale causa di epatotossicità del valproato; per prevenire questa complicanza fatale, suggeriscono perciò l'assunzione di supplementi di L-carnitina, alla dose di 50-100 mg/kg/24 h. Finché non saranno disponibili nuovi dati, si raccomanda la prescrizione di supplementi di L-carnitina nei bambini maggiormente a rischio di epatotossicità (vedi sopra). Nei bambini più grandi in terapia con acido valproico, la L-carnitina andrebbe somministrata in presenza di sintomi clinici suggestivi di deficit di carnitina (debolezza, letargia, ipotonia) oppure in caso di significativo calo dei livelli sierici di carnitina libera. L'acido valproico è disponibile in sciroppo (50 mg/mL), capsule da 250 e 500 mg, compresse da 125, 250 e 500 mg. Capsule a base di divalproex sodico, un composto di coordinazione stabile del valproato di sodio e dell'acido valproico, sono utili nei bambini che non tollerano valproato in sospensione, compresse o capsule. Il contenuto di queste capsule (da 125 mg) viene spruzzato su cibi molli che non devono essere masticati.

VIGABATRIN. Questo farmaco agisce legandosi al recettore dell'enzima di degradazione GABA transaminasi, causando un incremento dei livelli di GABA e un'inibizione della neurotrasmissione (vedi Fig. 593-4). Il vigabatrin è efficace nel controllo degli spasmi infantili, in particolare nei bambini con sclerosi tuberosa. È utile anche come terapia potenziante in presenza di convulsioni refrattarie. La sua emivita plasmatica è di 5-8 ore. Questo farmaco può causare una riduzione dei livelli plasmatici di fenobarbital e fenitoina. Sono stati segnalati anche casi di riduzione del campo visivo. Il vigabatrin è disponibile in compresse da 500 mg e bustine da 500 mg.

LEVIRACTAM. Questo farmaco dal meccanismo di azione sconosciuto è indicato come potenziante nel trattamento delle convulsioni parziali. La sua emivita plasmatica è di circa 8 ore. È disponibile in compresse da 250, 500 e 750 mg.

OXCARBAZEPINA. Questo farmaco ha un'azione simile alla carbamazepina ed è utile come potenziante nel trattamento delle convulsioni parziali in adulti e bambini. La sua emivita è di 2 ore, mentre quella del suo metabolita principale, 10-mono-idrossi oxcarbazepina (MHD), è di 9 ore. Il 30% dei pazienti con reazioni allergiche alla carbamazepina reagisce anche all'oxcarbazepina. L'iponatremia si verifica nel 2,5% dei pazienti. L'oxcarbazepina è disponibile in compresse da 150, 300 e 600 mg e in sospensione da 300 mg/5 mL.

ZONISAMIDE. Questo farmaco è utile come potenziante nel trattamento delle convulsioni parziali e delle sindromi miocloniche, ma il suo meccanismo d'azione non è stato ancora chiarito. In monoterapia, la sua emivita è di 60 ore, mentre si riduce a 30 ore in associazione a farmaci metabolizzati dal fegato. Lo zonisamide è stato associato allo sviluppo di calcoli renali. È disponibile in compresse da 100 mg.

ACTH. L'ACTH è il **farmaco di elezione** nel trattamento degli **spasmi infantili**, ma la dose e la durata della terapia variano a seconda dei casi. Anche il prednisone è efficace. Una pratica comune consiste nel somministrare per via intramuscolare 20 U/die di ACTH per due settimane; in assenza di risposta, la dose è aumentata a 30 e 40 U/die per altre 4 settimane. Se il controllo delle crisi non è completo, l'ACTH è sostituito con prednisone orale, alla dose di 2 mg/kg/die per due settimane (da proseguire per altre 4 in caso di mancata risposta). Gli effetti collaterali di ACTH includono iperglicemia, ipertensione, anomalie elettrolitiche, disturbi gastrointestinali, infezioni (come la polmonite da *Pneumocystic carinii*) e una riduzione cerebrale transitoria osservabile mediante TC. L'ACTH e il prednisone sono ugualmente efficaci nel trattamento delle convulsioni criptogenetiche e sintomatiche, consentendo di ottenere il controllo delle crisi in circa il 70% dei casi. Non si riscontra alcuna relazione tra la facilità e il grado di controllo delle convulsioni e l'esito cognitivo e neurologico finale. La risposta al farmaco è solitamente evidente nel giro di qualche settimana di terapia, ma un terzo dei pazienti che rispondono va incontro a una recidiva successivamente alla sospensione del farmaco.

DIETA CHETOGENICA. Questo trattamento andrebbe preso in considerazione nei casi di convulsioni resistenti, in particolare nei bambini con epilessia mioclonica complessa con convulsioni tonicocloniche associate. La dieta appare sicura ed efficace nei bambini di meno di 2 anni e costituisce anche la terapia di elezione nei lattanti con deficit di piruvato deidrogenasi e della proteina di trasporto del glucosio. La dieta prevede una limitazione dell'assunzione di carboidrati e proteine e un utilizzo dei grassi come principale fonte di calorie. Dopo i 2 o 3 anni, alcuni bambini non riescono a tollerare tale dieta grassa e poco appetitosa. Anche le famiglie fanno fatica ad attenersi a una dieta che richiede la precisa misurazione delle quantità di cibo ed elaborate procedure di preparazione. In alcuni casi, è utile introdurre una dieta chetogenica libera, che prevede la sostituzione dei trigliceridi a catena media con i cibi ad alto contenuto di grassi della dieta precedente. Questa dieta, benché il suo meccanismo di azione non sia noto, sembra esercitare un effetto anticonvulsivante, secondario agli elevati livelli di β-idrossibutirato e acetoacetato (risultato della chetosi). L'uso di acido valproico in associazione alla dieta chetogenica è controindicato, a causa del potenziamento del rischio di epatotossicità.

TRATTAMENTO CHIRURGICO DELL'EPILESSIA. La chirurgia andrebbe presa in considerazione nei bambini con convulsioni refrattarie, in particolare se focali, che non rispondono agli anticonvulsivanti. L'esordio focale della convulsione può risultare evidente già dall'anamnesi e dall'esame neurologico, ma l'EEG è necessario per documentare l'esatta localizzazione ed estensione delle scariche epilettogene nei candidati alla chirurgia. In molti casi è indispensabile ricorrere alla registrazione video-EEG prolungata per definire l'area epilettogena con assoluta precisione. Nei pazienti ospedalizzati, è spesso utile ridurre o sospendere l'assunzione dell'anticonvulsivante, per aumentare la probabilità di registrare l'attività epilettogena ictale e interictale. Se l'EEG con elettrodi sfenoidali non consente un'adeguata localizzazione del focolaio, l'applicazione di elettrodi subdurali può fornire informazioni preziose. In particolare, gli elettrodi subdurali sono utili nell'investigazione di focolai epilettogeni in aree diverse dal lobo temporale. I risultati dell'EEG sono integrati dai test neuropsicologici, dal test WADA (iniezione intracarotidea di amobarbital, per stabilire l'emisfero dominante), da SPECT (*Single-Photon Emission CT*, TC a emissione di fotone singolo) e PET, dalle procedure di neuroimaging, incluse TC e RM funzionale. Alcuni centri specialistici utilizzano MSI (*Magnetic Source Imaging*, fonte magnetica di imaging) e MEG (*Magnetoelectroencephalograms*, magneto-elettroencefalografia) per localizzare con maggior precisione la scarica convulsiva. I risultati dell'intervento chirurgico in bambini con un focolaio di attività epilettogena ben definito e una lesione strutturale corrispondente dimostrata da TC o RM sono molto favorevoli.

STIMOLAZIONE DEL NERVO VAGO. La sperimentazione animale ha suggerito la possibilità di interrompere o di prevenire la convulsione mediante stimolazione elettrica del nervo vago. In trial a doppio cieco condotti su 60 bambini (16 dei quali con un'età inferiore ai 12 anni), la stimolazione del nervo vago sinistro prodotta da un elettrodo impiantato riduceva le convulsioni del 31-42% entro 18 mesi. Questi risultati suggeriscono la possibilità di utilizzare tale tecnica come terapia potenziante nei pazienti refrattari alle altre forme di trattamento.

COUNSELING AI GENITORI. La maggior parte dei genitori reagisce con angoscia alla diagnosi di epilessia e richiede perciò un adeguato supporto e informazioni accurate. Il medico dovrebbe essere in grado di anticipare le domande dei genitori relative alla durata del disturbo convulsivo, agli effetti collaterali dei farmaci e delle convulsioni stesse, all'eziologia, alle ripercussioni sociali e scolastiche. Anche il senso di colpa dei genitori deve essere affrontato nel *counseling*. Una delle prime questioni spesso sollevata riguarda le restrizioni alla vita del bambino e l'opportunità o meno di informare gli insegnanti della malattia. I genitori si interrogano anche sulle implicazioni genetiche e sui rischi per eventuali future gravidanze. È importante incoraggiare i genitori a trattare il proprio figlio nella maniera più normale possibile. Nella maggior parte dei casi, le restrizioni all'attività fisica non sono necessarie; l'unico obbligo consiste nella supervisione da parte di un adulto responsabile quando il bambino nuota o fa il bagno. Durante il counseling, è opportuno spiegare il meccanismo delle convulsioni e il significato dell'epilessia nonché illustrare gli scopi e gli effetti collaterali degli anticonvulsivanti prescelti. I genitori che capiscono l'azione fondamentale e lo scopo degli anticonvulsivanti e la necessità di un trattamento con un farmaco specifico gradualmente mostrano buona compliance. Il counseling dovrebbe includere anche nozioni di pronto soccorso da mettere in pratica in caso di ricorrenza delle convulsioni. Nella maggior parte dei casi, bambini e genitori si adeguano rapidamente alle esigenze di una malattia che richiede una terapia a lungo termine. In genere, le epilessie infantili sono ben controllate dal trattamento farmacologico; i pazienti mostrano un'intelligenza nella norma e conducono una vita normale. È tuttavia importante monitorare il loro rendimento scolastico, perché i disturbi dell'apprendimento sono più comuni per loro rispetto alla popolazione generale. La cooperazione tra genitori, medici, insegnanti e bambino migliora la prognosi.

Allen JE, Ferrie CD, Livingston JH, Feltbower RG: Recovery of consciousness after epileptic seizures in children. *Arch Dis Child* 2007;91:39–41.
Baumann RJ, Duffner PK: Treatment of children with simple febrile seizures: The AAP practice parameter. *Pediatr Neurol* 2000;23:11–17.
Berg AT, Testa FM, Levy SR, et al: Neuroimaging in children with newly diagnosed epilepsy: A community-based study. *Pediatrics* 2000;196: 527–532.
Chang BS, Lowenstein DH: Epilepsy. *N Engl J Med* 2003;349:1257–1266.
Clusmann H, Kral T, Gleissner U, et al: Analysis of different types of resection for pediatric patients with temporal lobe epilepsy. *Neurosurgery* 2004;54:847–860.
Deonna T: Management of epilepsy. *Arch Dis Child* 2005;90:5–9.
French JA: First-choice drug for newly diagnosed epilepsy. *Lancet* 2007;369: 970–971.
Guerrini R: Epilepsy in children. *Lancet* 2006;367:499–524.
Hamano SI, Yamashita S, Tanaka M, et al: Therapeutic efficacy and adverse effects of adrenocorticotropic hormone therapy in West syndrome: differences in dosage of adrenocorticotropic hormone, onset of age, and cause. *J Pediatr* 2006;148:485–488.
Hamano SI, Yoshinari S, Higurashi N, et al: Developmental outcomes of cryptogenic West syndrome. *J Pediatr* 2007;150:295–299.
Hirtz D, Ashwal MD, Berg A, et al: Practice parameter: Evaluating a first nonfebrile seizure in children. *Neurology* 2000;55:616–623.
Hirtz D, Berg A, Bettis D, et al: Practice parameter: Treatment of the child with a first unprovoked seizure. *Neurology* 2003;60:166–175.
Kneen R, Appleton R: Status epilepticus with fever: How common is meningitis? *Arch Dis Child* 2005;90:3–4.
LaRoche SM, Helmers SL: The new antiepileptic drugs: Scientific review. *JAMA* 2004;291:605–614.
LaRoche SM, Helmers SL: The new antiepileptic drugs: Clinical applications. *JAMA* 2004;291:615–620.
Lee JYK, Adelson PD: Neurosurgical management of pediatric epilepsy. *Pediatr Clin North Am* 2004;51:441–456.
Lux AL, Edwards SW, Hancock E, et al: The United Kingdom infantile spasms study comparing vigabatrin with prednisolone or tetracosactide at 14 days: A multicentre, randomized controlled trial. *Lancet* 2004;364:1773–1778.
Marson A, Jacoby A, Johnson A, et al: Immediate versus deferred antiepileptic drug treatment for early epilepsy and single seizures: A randomized controlled trial. *Lancet* 2005;365:2007–2012.
Murphy JV, et al: Left vagal nerve stimulation in children with medically refractory epilepsy. *J Pediatr* 1994;134:563–566.
Nordli DR, Kuroda MM, Carroll J, et al: Experience with the ketogenic diet in infants. *Pediatrics* 2001;198:129–133.
Pohlmann-Eden B, Beghi E, Camfield C, Camfield P: The first seizure and its management in adults and children. *BMJ* 2006;332:339–342.
Romanelli P, Verdecchia M, Rodas R, et al: Epilepsy surgery for tuberous sclerosis. *Pediatr Neurol* 2004;31:239–247.
Sadleir LG, Scheffer IE: Febrile seizures. *BMJ* 2007;334:307–311.
Sankar R: Initial treatment of epilepsy with antileptic drugs: Pediatric issues. *Neurology* 2004;63:S30–S39.
Shinnar S, Pellock JM: Update on the epidemiology and prognosis of pediatric epilepsy. *J Child Neurol* 2002;17:S4–S17.
Siddiqui A, Kerb R, Weale ME, et al: Association of multidrug resistance in epilepsy with a polymorphism in the drug-transporter gene *ABCB1*. *N Engl J Med* 2003;348:1442–1448.
Wang HS, Kuo MF, Chou ML, et al: Pyridoxal phosphate is better than pyridoxine for controlling idiopathic intractable epilepsy. *Arch Dis Child* 2005;90:512–515.
Warden CR, Zibulewsky J, Mace S, et al: Evaluation and management of febrile seizures in the out-of hospital and emergency department settings. *Ann Emerg Med* 2003;41:215–222.
Wiebe S, Blume WT, Girvin JP, et al: A randomized, controlled trial of surgery for temporal-lobe epilepsy. *N Engl J Med* 2001;345:311–318.
Wong M, Schlaggar BL, Landt M: Postictal cerebrospinal fluid abnormalities in children. *J Pediatr* 2001;138:373–377.

593.7 • CONVULSIONI NEONATALI (vedi Capitoli 97-100)

I neonati sono particolarmente a rischio per lo sviluppo di convulsioni, perché in questa fase tendono a manifestarsi malattie metaboliche, tossiche, strutturali e infettive. Le crisi neonatali differiscono da quelle del bambino e dell'adulto, perché le convulsioni tonico-cloniche generalizzate non si verificano nel primo mese di vita. A causa dell'incompletezza dell'arborizzazione dei processi assonali e dendritici e della mielinizzazione, la scarica epilettica non può propagarsi nel cervello neonatale, dunque non è generalizzata.

MANIFESTAZIONI CLINICHE E CLASSIFICAZIONE. Le **convulsioni focali** consistono in contrazioni ritmiche di gruppi muscolari, in particolare degli arti e del volto. Queste crisi sono spesso associate a lesioni strutturali localizzate, a infezioni o emorragia subaracnoidea. Le convulsioni **multifocali cloniche** sono simili a quelle focali cloniche, ma implicano il coinvolgimento, spesso simultaneo, di diversi gruppi muscolari. Le **crisi toniche** sono caratterizzate da rigidità degli arti e del tronco e sono talvolta associate a deviazione fissa degli occhi. Le **crisi miocloniche** sono spasmi brevi, focali o generalizzati, degli arti o del corpo, che tendono a coinvolgere gruppi muscolari distali. Le **convulsioni minori** consistono in movimenti di masticazione, salivazione eccessiva e alterazioni del ritmo respiratorio; includono apnea, ammiccamenti, nistagmo, movimenti degli arti (per es. pedalare) cambiamenti del colorito.

Le convulsioni neonatali sono talvolta difficili da riconoscere sul piano clinico e in alcuni casi il tracciato EEG non conferma la natura parossistica di comportamenti considerati convulsivi (Tab. 593-6). Ciò nonostante, diverse caratteristiche cliniche aiutano a distinguere le convulsioni dall'attività non epilettica. Alterazioni autonomiche come tachicardia e aumento della pressione sanguigna sono comuni nelle crisi convulsive, ma non negli eventi non epilettici. I movimenti non epilettici, a differenza delle convulsioni, possono essere bloccati da una delicata costrizione. Stimoli sensoriali sono in grado di potenziare i fenomeni non epilettici, mentre non esercitano alcuna influenza sulle convulsioni. La corretta classificazione delle convulsioni neonatali è importante per selezionare l'anticonvulsivante più indicato. Le registrazioni video-EEG poligrafiche hanno contribuito alla caratterizzazione delle convulsioni neonatali e al trattamento farmacologico.

CLASSIFICAZIONE EEG DELLE CONVULSIONI NEONATALI

CONVULSIONI CLINICHE ASSOCIATE A EVENTI EEG. Le convulsioni incluse in questa categoria, di tipo focale clonico, focale tonico o mioclonico, sono registrate sul tracciato EEG. Sono dunque chiaramente epilettiche e tendono a rispondere agli anticonvulsivanti.

TABELLA 593-6. Disturbi parossistici del periodo neonatale

DISTURBI PAROSSISTICI NON EPILETTIFORMI
Nervosismo
Mioclono neonatale benigno del sonno
CONVULSIONI SINTOMATICHE ACUTE E OCCASIONALI*
Encefalopatia ipossica-ischemica
Emorragia intraventricolare
Disturbi metabolici acuti†
Sepsi-meningite
SINDROMI EPILETTICHE
Convulsioni idiopatiche neonatali benigne
Familiari
Non familiari
Epilessia focale sintomatica
Tumore cerebrale
Malformazioni dello sviluppo corticale
Malattia metabolica ereditaria; malattie mitocondriali
Sindromi epilettiche generalizzate a esordio precoce, con encefalopatia
Encefalopatia mioclonica precoce
Epilessia encefalopatica infantile precoce

*Vedi Tabella 593-7
†Ipoglicemia, ipocalcemia, ipomagnesiemia, iponatremia, ipernatremia.
Tratta da Kliegman RM, Greenbaum LA, Lye PS: *Practical Strategies in Pediatric Diagnosis and Therapy*, 2nd ed. Philadelphia, Elsevier, 2004, p. 680.

CONVULSIONI CLINICHE NON CORRELATE A EVENTI EEG. Nei neonati è possibile riscontrare convulsioni (toniche generalizzate, minori e miocloniche) in assenza di corrispondente scarica registrabile dall'EEG. Questi bambini risultano neurologicamente depressi o comatosi, a causa dell'encefalopatia ipossica-ischemica. Le convulsioni incluse in questa categoria hanno probabilmente un'origine non epilettica e non rispondono agli anticonvulsivanti.

CONVULSIONI ELETTRICHE IN ASSENZA DI CONVULSIONI CLINICHE. Convulsioni elettriche associate ad attività di fondo EEG marcatamente anomala possono svilupparsi in neonati comatosi che non assumono anticonvulsivanti. Le convulsioni elettriche possono persistere in pazienti con convulsioni focali toniche o cloniche, in assenza di segni clinici, dopo l'introduzione di un anticonvulsivante.

DIAGNOSI EZIOLOGICA. La più comune causa di convulsioni neonatali, l'encefalopatia ipossica-ischemica, è discussa nel Capitolo 99.5. Molte altre malattie possono causare gli attacchi, tra cui i disturbi metabolici, infettivi, traumatici, strutturali, emorragici, embolici e materni (Tab. 593-7). Un approccio diagnostico tempestivo e organizzato riveste un'importanza fondamentale in età neonatale, perché i sintomi convulsivi possono indicare la presenza di una malattia grave, talvolta fatale, come di una condizione potenzialmente reversibile.

Un accurato esame neurologico può contribuire a rivelare la causa del disturbo convulsivo. L'esame della **retina** può mostrare la presenza di corioretinite, che può indicare un'infezione congenita, nel qual caso è indicata nella madre e nel neonato la sierologia per il TORCH (*TO*xoplasmosi, *R*osolia, *C*ytomegalovirus e *H*erpes simplex). La **sindrome di Aicardi**, che colpisce esclusivamente le bambine, è associata a coloboma dell'iride e lacune retiniche, convulsioni refrattarie e assenza del corpo calloso. L'ispezione della **cute** può rivelare lesioni ipopigmentate caratteristiche della sclerosi tuberosa o le tipiche lesioni vescicolari dell'incontinentia pigmenti; entrambe le sindromi neurocutanee sono associate a precoci convulsioni miocloniche generalizzate. Un odore insolito emanato dal corpo del bambino suggerisce la presenza di un errore congenito del metabolismo.

Deve essere prelevato un campione di sangue per la determinazione dei livelli di glucosio, calcio, magnesio, azoto ureico e degli elettroliti. In caso di sospetta ipoglicemia, si raccomanda un test sierico ad hoc in modo da attuare un inizio tempestivo della terapia. Per un approfondimento della diagnosi e del trattamento dell'ipoglicemia, vedi il Capitolo 107. L'ipocalcemia può verificarsi isolatamente o in associazione all'ipomagnesiemia. Una calcemia ridotta è spesso collegata a un trauma da parto o a un insulto a carico del SNC nel periodo perinatale. Altre cause includono il diabete materno, la prematurità, la sindrome di DiGeorge e una dieta ricca di fosfati. L'ipomagnesiemia ($<1{,}5$ mg/dL) è spesso associata a ipocalcemia e si verifica in modo particolare in presenza di malnutrizione materna. In tali casi, le convulsioni sono resistenti alla terapia con calcio, ma rispondono alla somministrazione intramuscolare di magnesio (alla dose di 0,2 mL/kg di una soluzione di $MgSO_4$ al 50%). Per la diagnosi e il trattamento dell'ipomagnesiemia, vedi il Capitolo 106. La misura degli elettroliti sierici può segnalare una significativa iponatremia (sodio sierico <135 mEq/L) o ipernatremia (sodio sierico >150 mEq/L) come causa del disturbo convulsivo.

La **puntura lombare** è indicata virtualmente in tutti i neonati con convulsioni, a meno che la causa non sia chiaramente collegata a un disturbo metabolico come l'ipoglicemia o l'ipocalcemia, secondari a una dieta ricca di fosfati. In questo secondo caso, i neonati appaiono vigili nella fase intercritale e solitamente rispondono prontamente alla terapia. L'esame del LCS può indicare una meningite batterica o encefalite asettica (vedi Capitoli 109 e 602). La diagnosi tempestiva e una corretta terapia consentono di migliorare la prognosi in questi casi. La presenza di sangue nel LCS indica una puntura traumatica o un'emorragia subaracnoidea/intraventricolare. L'immediata centrifugazione del campione contribuisce alla differenziazione tra i due disturbi. Un supernatante trasparente suggerisce una puntura traumatica, mentre la presenza di xantocromia indica un'emorragia subaracnoidea. Nei bambini con lieve ittero, la colorazione giallastra del LCS rende meno attendibile l'esame del supernatante nel periodo neonatale.

Diversi **errori congeniti del metabolismo** causano convulsioni generalizzate nel periodo neonatale. Poiché queste condizioni sono spesso ereditate con modalità autosomica recessiva o correlata alla X, è necessario ottenere un'anamnesi familiare dettagliata, per determinare l'eventuale presenza di fratelli o di parenti con disturbi convulsivi o deceduti prematuramente. La determinazione dell'ammoniemia è utile per lo screening delle anomalie del ciclo dell'urea, come i deficit di ornitina transcarbamilasi, argininsuccinico liasi e carbamilfosfato sintetasi. Nei primi giorni di vita questi bambini, oltre a presentare convulsioni tonico-cloniche generalizzate, manifestano una letargia progressiva (fino al coma), anoressia e vomito; l'esame obiettivo rivela una fontanella sporgente. Se l'emogasanalisi rivela un gap anionico e acidosi metabolica con iperammoniemia, è opportuno procedere immediatamente

TABELLA 593-7. Cause di convulsioni neonatali

ETÀ 1-4 GIORNI
Encefalopatia ipossica-ischemica
Astinenza da farmaci, abuso materno di narcotici o barbiturici
Tossicità dei farmaci: lidocaina, penicillina
Emorragia intraventricolare
Disturbi metabolici acuti
Ipocalcemia
Asfissia perinatale, neonato piccolo per l'età gestazionale
Sepsi
Diabete materno, ipertiroidismo, ipoparatiroidismo
Ipoglicemia
Insulti perinatali, prematurità, neonato piccolo per l'età gestazionale
Diabete materno
Ipoglicemia iperinsulinemica
Sepsi
Ipomagnesiemia
Iponatremia o ipernatremia
Secrezione dell'ormone antidiuretico inappropriata o iatrogena
Errori congeniti del metabolismo
Galattosemia
Iperglicinemia
Disturbi del ciclo dell'urea
Deficit di piridossina (da considerare a qualsiasi età)
ETÀ 4-14 GIORNI
Infezione
Meningite (batterica), encefalite (enterovirale, herpes simplex)
Disturbi metabolici
Ipocalcemia
Fattori dietetici
Ipoglicemia persistente
Disturbi ereditari del metabolismo: galattosemia, fruttosemia, sensibilità alla leucina
Ipoglicemia iperinsulinemica
Preesistente ipoplasia pituitaria, tumore delle cellule insulari pancreatiche
Sindrome di Beckwith
Astinenza da farmaci, abuso materno di narcotici e barbiturici
Convulsioni neonatali benigne, familiari e non familiari
Chernictero, iperbilirubinemia
ETÀ 2-8 SETTIMANE
Infezioni
Herpes simplex o encefalite enterovirale, meningite batterica
Traumi cranici
Ematoma subdurale, maltrattamento
Disturbo metabolico ereditario
Aminoaciduria, difetti del ciclo dell'urea, acidurie organiche
Adrenoleucodstrofia neonatale
Malformazioni dello sviluppo corticale
Lissencefalia
Displasia corticale focale
Sclerosi tuberosa
Sindrome di Sturge-Weber

Tratta da Kliegman RM, Greenbaum LA, Lye PS: *Practical Strategies in Pediatric Diagnosis and Therapy*, 2nd ed. Philadelphia, Elsevier, 2004, p. 681.

al dosaggio degli acidi organici nelle urine, per verificare la possibile presenza di acidemia metilmalonica o propionica. La malattia delle urine a sciroppo d'acero (*Maple Syrup Urine Disease*, MSUD) deve essere sospettata quando, nella prima settimana di vita, l'acidosi metabolica è associata a convulsioni cloniche generalizzate, vomito e rigidità muscolare. La presenza di MSUD è segnalata da un risultato positivo al test di screening che utilizza 2,4-dinitrofenilidrazina per identificare i chetoderivati nelle urine. Altre cause metaboliche di convulsioni neonatali includono: l'iperglicinemia non chetotica, una malattia letale caratterizzata dal marcato aumento dei livelli di glicina in plasma e LCS, convulsioni generalizzate persistenti e letargia che progredisce rapidamente verso il coma; l'iperglicinemia chetotica, in cui le convulsioni sono associate a vomito, alterazioni dell'equilibrio idroelettrolitico e acidosi metabolica; la malattia di Leigh, suggerita da elevati livelli di lattato nel siero e nel LCS o da un aumento del rapporto lattato/piruvato. Anche il deficit di biotinidasi deve essere preso in considerazione. La Parte X include una dettagliata descrizione della diagnosi e del trattamento delle malattie metaboliche.

L'**iniezione non intenzionale di anestetico** locale nel feto durante il travaglio può causare intense convulsioni toniche. La flaccidità alla nascita, riflessi troncoencefalici alterati e i segni di depressione respiratoria (tali da richiedere talvolta una ventilazione assistita) sono inizialmente attribuiti al parto traumatico. Il successivo esame del neonato può mostrare una puntura d'ago sulla cute o una perforazione o lacerazione dello scalpo. La diagnosi è confermata dal riscontro un livello sierico di anestetico elevato. Il trattamento prevede misure di supporto e la promozione del flusso urinario mediante somministrazione endovenosa di liquidi (ma evitando il sovraccarico).

Le **convulsioni neonatali familiari benigne**, a trasmissione autosomica dominante, esordiscono nei primi 2-3 giorni di vita, a una frequenza di 10-20 al giorno. Tra una crisi è l'altra i pazienti appaiono normali. Le convulsioni scompaiono entro 1-6 mesi. Le **crisi del quinto giorno**, di tipo multifocale, si verificano in neonati al 5° giorno (4-6 giorni) apparentemente sani e si protraggono per meno di 24 ore. La diagnosi richiede l'esclusione delle altre cause di disturbi convulsivi. La prognosi è buona.

La **dipendenza da piridossina** è un raro disturbo da prendere in considerazione in caso di convulsioni cloniche generalizzate che esordiscono poco dopo la nascita, con segni di distress fetale in utero. Queste convulsioni sono particolarmente resistenti agli anticonvulsivanti tradizionali, come il fenobarbital o la fenitoina. La storia clinica può suggerire l'insorgenza di crisi analoghe già in utero. Si segnalano casi di dipendenza da piridossina a esordio tardivo (nella prima e seconda infanzia). Questo disturbo è ereditato con modalità autosomica recessiva. Il meccanismo biochimico preciso del difetto non è stato ancora chiarito, ma la piridossina è essenziale per la sintesi della acido glutammico decarbossilasi, a sua volta richiesta per la sintesi di GABA. Nei bambini portatori del difetto, sono necessarie grandi quantità di piridossina per mantenere la produzione di GABA a un livello adeguato. In caso di sospette convulsioni piridossina-dipendenti, è opportuno procedere alla somministrazione per via endovenosa di 10-200 mg di piridossina o di piridossalfosfato durante la registrazione EEG che deve essere prontamente eseguito qualora si sospetti la diagnosi. Se la diagnosi è confermata, le convulsioni si interrompono bruscamente e il tracciato EEG si normalizza nel giro di qualche ora. Tuttavia, non tutti i casi di dipendenza da piridossina rispondono prontamente all'iniziale bolo di piridossina per via ev. In presenza di un elevato indice di sospetto malgrado la risposta negativa alla somministrazione di piridossina, è opportuno tentare un trial di 6 settimane di piridossina orale (10-20 mg/die) o di piridossalfosfato. È probabile che in futuro la misura del livello di piridossale-5′ fosfato in plasma e LCS si dimostrerà il metodo più attendibile per confermare la diagnosi di dipendenza da piridossina. I bambini con questo difetto richiedono l'assunzione di piridossina per tutta la vita, alla dose di 10 mg/die. La diagnosi tempestiva garantisce una prognosi favorevole. I bambini non trattati presentano convulsioni persistenti e sviluppano invariabilmente un grave ritardo mentale.

Le **convulsioni da astinenza da farmaci e stupefacenti** possono presentarsi subito dopo la nascita, ma solitamente richiedono diverse settimane per svilupparsi, a causa della prolungata escrezione del farmaco da parte del neonato. I farmaci e gli stupefacenti incriminati sono: barbiturici, benzodiazepine, eroina e metadone. Il neonato appare irritabile, itterico, letargico, e può sviluppare mioclono o franche convulsioni cloniche. Se la madre nega l'utilizzo di una di queste sostanze, l'analisi del siero o delle urine consente di identificare l'agente responsabile (vedi Capitolo 106).

I neonati con convulsioni focali, sospetto ictus o emorragia intracranica e gravi **anomalie della citoarchitettura** cerebrale (come lissencefalia e schizencefalia), che appaiono normali o microcefalici, devono essere sottoposti a RM o TC. Molti medici raccomandano questi esami in tutti i neonati con convulsioni non spiegate da ipoglicemia, ipocalcemia e diselettrolitemia. Anche i neonati con anomalie cromosomiche e adrenoleucodistrofia presentano un elevato rischio di sviluppare convulsioni e devono essere sottoposti ad analisi del cariotipo (nel primo caso) e a dosaggio sierico degli acidi grassi a catena lunga (nel secondo).

TRATTAMENTO. L'utilizzo degli anticonvulsivanti è opportuno nel trattamento di neonati con convulsioni secondarie a encefalopatia ipossica-ischemica o a emorragia intracranica acuta (vedi Capitoli 99.2 e 99.5). Le dosi di fenobarbital, diazepam e degli altri farmaci sono specificate nel Capitolo 99.5. Fenitoina e fenobarbital risultano egualmente efficaci come anticonvulsionanti nel neonato, ma controllano le crisi in meno del 50% dei casi. Il diffuso utilizzo della registrazione EEG nei neonati con convulsioni minori ha consentito l'identificazione di un certo numero di pazienti con movimenti anomali non collegati alle scariche epilettiche.

PROGNOSI. La prognosi è direttamente collegata alla causa primaria del disturbo e alla gravità dell'insulto. Nei bambini ipoglicemici figli di madri diabetiche e nei casi di ipocalcemia associata a eccessiva assunzione di fosfati, la prognosi è eccellente. Al contrario, un bambino con convulsioni intrattabili dovute a grave encefalopatia ipossica-ischemica o ad anomalie citoarchitettoniche cerebrali solitamente non risponde agli anticonvulsivanti e rischia di andare incontro a status epilettico e morte precoce. Il compito del medico è di identificare tempestivamente i casi in cui il trattamento adeguato consente la remissione, evitando ritardi diagnostici che possono causare danni neurologici irreversibili.

Baxter P: Pyridoxine or pyridoxal phosphate for intractable seizures? *Arch Dis Child* 2005;90:441–442.

Gilman JT, Gal P, Duchowny MS, et al: Rapid sequential phenobarbital treatment of neonatal seizures. *Pediatrics* 1989;83:674–678.

Hillman L, Hillman R, Dodson WE: Diagnosis, treatment and follow-up of neonatal mepivacaine intoxication secondary to paracervical and pudendal blocks during labor. *J Pediatr* 1979;95:472–477.

Legido A, Clancy RR, Berman P: Neurologic outcome after electroencephalographically proven neonatal seizures. *Pediatrics* 1991;88:583–596.

Painter MJ, Scher MS, Stein AD, et al: Phenobarbital compared with phenytoin for treatment of neonatal seizures. *N Engl J Med* 1999;341:485–489.

Sankar R, Painter MJ: Neonatal seizures, after all these years we still love what doesn't work. *Neurology* 2005;64:776–777.

Sillanpää M, Jalava M, Kaleva O, et al: Long-term prognosis of seizures with onset in childhood. *N Engl J Med* 1998;338:1715–1722.

Volpe JJ: Neonatal seizures: Current concepts and revised classification. *Pediatrics* 1989;84:422–428.

593.8 • Status epilettico

Lo status epilettico è definito come una **convulsione continua**, che si prolunga più di 20-30 minuti, oppure l'insorgenza di **convulsioni in serie**, senza recupero della coscienza tra una crisi e l'altra. Lo status epilettico è classificato in generalizzato (tonico-clonico, assenze) o parziale (semplice, complesso o a generalizzazione secondaria). Le convulsioni tonico-cloniche generalizzate predominano. Tale status costituisce un'emergenza medica che richiede un immediato intervento specialistico per minimizzare l'associata mortalità e morbilità.

EZIOLOGIA. Nei bambini si riscontrano tre sottogruppi principali di status epilettico: le convulsioni febbrili prolungate; lo status epilettico idiopatico, in cui l'attacco si sviluppa in assenza di una lesione o insulto del SNC; e lo status epilettico sintomatico, risultato di un disturbo neurologico o di un'anomalia metabolica. La più comune causa di status epilettico è una convulsione febbrile che si protrae oltre 30 minuti, in particolare in un bambino con meno di 3 anni. Il gruppo idiopatico include pazienti epilettici nei quali lo status epilettico segue la sospensione improvvisa di un anticonvulsivante (in particolare benzodiazepine e barbiturici). Il rischio è più elevato nei bambini epilettici ai quali vengono somministrati antiepilettici in forma sporadica o in caso di mancata compliance. Lo status epilettico può costituire anche la presentazione iniziale dell'epilessia. La deprivazione di sonno e un'infezione intercorrente rendono il paziente epilettico maggiormente suscettibile a sviluppare status epilettico. La mortalità e la morbilità nei pazienti con status epilettico idiopatico o da convulsioni febbrili prolungate sono basse.

Lo status epilettico dovuto ad altre cause ha, invece, un tasso di mortalità molto più elevato. Solitamente la causa della morte è direttamente attribuibile all'anomalia sottostante. A differenza dei bambini con status epilettico idiopatico, molti di questi pazienti non hanno mai presentato convulsioni in precedenza. Lo status epilettico prolungato è stato associato a grave danno dell'ippocampo (**sclerosi ippocampale**). Una convulsione prolungata può costituire la manifestazione iniziale di **encefalite** e l'epilessia può rappresentare una complicanza a lungo termine di una **meningite**. I bambini con malformazioni cerebrali congenite (lissencefalia o schizencefalia) possono andare incontro a ricorrenti episodi di status epilettico, spesso refrattario agli anticonvulsivanti. Anche gli errori congeniti del metabolismo talvolta si presentano con status epilettico; i neonati manifestano una progressiva perdita di coscienza associata a deficit staturo-ponderale e vomito eccessivo. Ulteriori cause di status epilettico includono diselettrolitiemie, ipocalcemia, ipoglicemia, intossicazione da farmaci, sindrome di Reye, intossicazione da piombo, iperpiressia estrema e tumori cerebrali, in particolare nel lobo frontale.

FISIOPATOLOGIA. La relazione tra esiti neurologici e durata dello status epilettico in bambini e adulti non è stata ancora chiarita. I bambini sembrano maggiormente resistenti alle lesioni neurologiche rispetto agli adulti. Nei primati, le alterazioni patologiche si verificano nel cervello di animali ventilati dopo 60 minuti di costante attività convulsiva, se è mantenuta l'omeostasi metabolica. La morte cellulare può essere il risultato di un processo definito di "eccitotossicità", conseguenza dell'eccessivo rilascio del neurotrasmettitore eccitatorio glutammato e dell'eccessiva stimolazione dei recettori del glutammato. Le aree cerebrali più vulnerabili includono l'ippocampo, l'amigdala, il cervelletto, l'area corticale centrale e il talamo. Le alterazioni patologiche caratteristiche includono congestione venosa, piccole emorragie petecchiali e edema. I cambiamenti ischemici cellulari costituiscono il primo riscontro istologico, seguito da neuronofagia, proliferazione microgliale, perdita cellulare e aumento del numero di astrociti reattivi. Le concentrazioni neuronali di calcio, acido arachidonico e prostaglandine aumentano, promuovendo la morte cellulare. L'attività convulsiva generalizzata e prolungata può causare la disfunzione del sistema nervoso autonomo, con ipotensione e shock, acidosi lattica, mioglobinuria e necrosi tubulare acuta.

Diversi studi condotti sugli animali hanno dimostrato che la crisi diviene più difficile da interrompere e il rischio di lesione neuronale aumenta quando la convulsione persiste oltre un *periodo transizionale*, della durata compresa tra 20 e 60 minuti. Il trattamento dei bambini dovrebbe essere diretto a supportare le funzioni vitali e controllare le convulsioni il più velocemente possibile, perché la durata del periodo transizionale negli esseri umani non è nota.

TRATTAMENTO. Il trattamento iniziale prevede la valutazione dei sistemi respiratorio e cardiovascolare. I bambini devono essere trasferiti in un reparto di rianimazione. Dopo aver verificato la pervietà delle vie respiratorie, si procede alla registrazione di polso, temperatura, respiro e pressione sanguigna. Secrezioni orali eccessive sono rimosse mediante delicata aspirazione e al paziente è applicata una maschera di dimensioni adatte collegata all'ossigeno. In caso di difficoltà a ventilare con pallone Ambu, il paziente può richiedere intubazione e ventilazione assistita. Vengono inseriti un sondino nasogastrico e immediatamente un catetere ev. Se l'ipoglicemia è confermata da un test specifico, si infondono rapidamente 5 mL/kg di una soluzione di destrosio al 10%. Il prelievo di sangue consente di effettuare la conta ematica e il dosaggio di elettroliti (incluso calcio, fosforo e magnesio), glucosio, creatinina, lattato e, se indicato, del livello dell'anticonvulsivante. Sangue e urine sono ottenuti anche per gli esami metabolici e tossicologici, tenendo presente che alcuni farmaci e stupefacenti sono in grado di potenziare o scatenare lo status epilettico (anfetamine, cocaina, fenotiazine, teofillina a livelli tossici, antidepressivi triciclici). È necessario eseguire un'emogasanalisi arteriosa e monitorare la saturazione di ossigeno (SaO_2) con un ossimetro. L'esame del LCS è imperativo in caso di sospetta meningite o encefalite, verificando tuttavia l'assenza di controindicazioni alla procedura. In questo secondo caso, **prima** di poter procedere alla puntura lombare è opportuno somministrare al paziente antibiotici adeguati ed effettuare esami di imaging. Se le convulsioni sono refrattarie agli anticonvulsivanti di prima linea o il paziente è paralizzato, il monitoraggio EEG è importante per valutare la frequenza delle scariche, la loro localizzazione e la risposta alla terapia anticonvulsivante.

L'**esame obiettivo e neurologico** ricerca la presenza di traumi, papilledema, una fontanella anteriore sporgente o segni neurologici localizzati di lateralizzazione che suggeriscono un aumento della pressione intracranica (*IntraCranial Pressure*, ICP), manifestazioni di sepsi e meningite, emorragie retiniche indicative di un ematoma subdurale, respiro di Kussmaul e disidratazione, che possono indicare un'acidosi metabolica, irregolarità respiratorie provocate da disfunzioni troncoencefaliche, deficit staturo-ponderale, un odore anomalo emanato dal corpo, una pigmentazione dei capelli insolita che suggerisce un errore congenito del metabolismo, la costrizione o dilatazione pupillare causata da tossine o farmaci. Un esame ancor più approfondito deve essere effettuato dopo aver ottenuto il controllo delle convulsioni. L'opportunità di ricorrere a ulteriori esami neuroradiologici è stabilita sulla base dei reperti obiettivi e neurologici e di una precisa definizione del tipo e della frequenza delle convulsioni.

Nello status epilettico si raccomanda la somministrazione dei **farmaci** per via endovenosa; la via im è inaffidabile, per il rischio di sequestro da parte dei muscoli. Una dei problemi principali nella gestione dello status epilettico consiste nell'inappropriato utilizzo di anticonvulsivanti. Troppo spesso il primo farmaco è somministrato a una dose insufficiente e, in seguito all'assenza di risposta, si procede immediatamente all'introduzione di un farmaco diverso, senza prestare attenzione alle modalità di somministrazione. Per esempio, la fenitoina in soluzione di glucosio forma un precipitato, che la rende inefficace. È essenziale avere a disposizione vicino al letto del paziente le attrezzature per la rianimazione, in modo da poter intubare e ventilare il paziente se la depressione respiratoria si verifica.

Inizialmente, è opportuno somministrare una **benzodiazepina** (diazepam, lorazepam o midazolam), perché questi farmaci sono efficaci nell'ottenere un immediato controllo delle convulsioni tonico-cloniche prolungate nella maggior parte dei bambini. Il diazepam deve essere introdotto per via ev direttamente (non attraverso la via di infusione) in vena, alla dose di 0,1-0,3 mg/kg, a una velocità non superiore a 2 mg al minuto, per un massimo di tre dosi. In ambiente non ospedaliero o se l'accesso ev non è immediatamente disponibile, è possibile somministrare il diazepam in forma di gel rettale, alla dose di 0,2-0,5 mg/kg.

Un'altra opzione è costituita dal midazolam per via orale o nasale (0,5 mg/kg) quando l'accesso ev non è disponibile, somministrabile in sicurezza dal personale paramedico prima dell'arrivo in ospedale. Può provocare depressione respiratoria e ipotensione, soprattutto se somministrato con barbiturici. Le benzodiazepine sono altrettanto efficaci del pentobarbital, con meno effetti collaterali. Il diazepam è utile nella gestione dello status tonico-clonico, ma ha un'emivita breve, responsabile di ricorrenza della crisi in assenza di contemporanea somministrazione di un altro anticonvulsivante ad azione prolungata. Anche il lorazepam è un anticonvulsivante efficace a breve termine, con una durata di azione più lunga e una minor probabilità di causare ipotensione e arresto respiratorio. La dose raccomandata è di 0,05-0,1 mg/kg, da somministrare lentamente per via ev. La dose ideale di midazolam è di 0,15-0,3 mg/kg per via ev. In assenza di un accesso ev o in ambiente non ospedaliero, diazepam e lorazepam sono somministrabili per via rettale. Il diazepam diluito in 3 mL di NaCl allo 0,9% è inserito nel retto utilizzando una siringa e un tubo flessibile, alla dose di 0,3-0,5 mg/kg. La dose efficace di lorazepam rettale è di 0,05-0,1 mg/kg. Il livello sierico terapeutico è ottenuto entro 5-10 minuti. Il lorazepam sublinguale è utilizzabile nei bambini con convulsioni seriali che tendono a sviluppare status epilettico quando si trovano a casa. La dose sublinguale raccomandata è di 0,05-0,1 mg/kg. Collocata sotto la lingua del paziente, la compressa si scioglie in pochi secondi. Un'alternativa è costituita dal diazepam in gel rettale (dosi pediatriche di 2,5, 5 o 10 mg).

Dopo la somministrazione iniziale di diazepam o lorazepam, sono disponibili diverse opzioni per la gestione successiva. Se l'attività convulsiva si interrompe dopo la terapia con diazepam o lorazepam, o se la crisi persiste, si procede alla somministrazione di **fenitoina**. La dose di carico di fenitoina è compresa tra 15 e 30 mg/kg per via ev (aumentandola di 10 mg/kg alla volta), a una velocità di 1 mg/kg/min. Il profarmaco **fosfenitoina** ha il vantaggio di essere solubile in acqua, meno irritante dopo l'iniezione ev e facilmente assorbito dopo l'iniezione per via intramuscolare. La fosfenitoina parenterale è formulata in unità di equivalente della fenitoina (*Phenytoin Equivalent*, PE), per consentire la somministrazione della stessa quantità di fenitoina malgrado il suo peso molecolare più elevato (150 mg di fosfenitoina equivalgono a 100 mg di fenitoina). Il dosaggio in unità PE è identico alla precedente formulazione. Quest'ultima può essere diluita in soluzione fisiologica intera o diluita al 50%, ma non in soluzioni di glucosio; il farmaco non diluito può causare dolore, irritazione e flebite venosa. L'elettrocardiogramma è raccomandato durante la fase di carico, per identificare eventuali aritmie e bradicardia (complicanze rare nei bambini). L'ipotensione sistemica può essere aggravata dalla fenitoina. Se le convulsioni non ricorrono, la somministrazione di una dose di mantenimento di 3-9 mg/kg, suddivisa in due dosi quotidiane uguali, è iniziata 12-24 ore dopo. È opportuno monitorare i livelli sierici di fenitoina, perché la dose di mantenimento varia considerevolmente a seconda dell'età. Se la fenitoina non riesce a controllare lo status epilettico tonico-clonico, è necessario ricorrere a un anticonvulsivante diverso. In un alcuni centri, il **fenobarbital** è utilizzato ancor prima della fenitoina, somministrato ev in 10-30 minuti, alla dose di carico di 15-20 mg/kg o di 20-30 mg/kg nei neonati. La dose di mantenimento è di 3-5 mg/kg/24 h, suddivisa in due dosi quotidiane uguali.

Se lo status epilettico non è controllato dalle strategia descritte, il medico è chiamato a prendere decisioni terapeutiche impegnative, perché è probabile che il *periodo transizionale* sia ormai trascorso. Il trattamento successivo prevede la scelta tra l'infusione di diazepam, l'induzione di coma da barbiturici, la somministrazione di paraldeide o l'anestesia generale. In questo stadio, il paziente è solitamente sedato e può mostrare segni di depressione respiratoria, che richiedono l'intubazione e la ventilazione assistita.

La costante infusione per via ev di **midazolam** (0,20 mg/kg in bolo, 20-400 µg/kg h in infusione) o di **propofol** (1-2 mg/kg, 2-10 mg/kg h in infusione) è efficace nel controllo delle convulsioni durante uno status epilettico che non risponde agli altri anticonvulsivanti. Se la crisi continua, è opportuno prendere seriamente in considerazione la possibilità di indurre un coma da barbiturici. In un reparto di rianimazione, il paziente è intubato sotto ventilatore e sottoposto a monitoraggio EEG continuo. La dose di carico iniziale di tiopental è di 2-4 mg/kg, successivamente ridotta per ottenere la burst suppression dell'EEG. Il coma è mantenuto per almeno 48 ore, al termine delle quali il tiopental è sospeso, con conseguente calo del livello di fenobarbital fino al range terapeutico. Tale coma richiede un attento monitoraggio, perché l'ipotensione dovuta alla depressione miocardica richiede spesso una terapia pressoria.

L'**acido valproico** è un efficace anticonvulsivante nella terapia di diversi tipi di convulsioni. È disponibile in forma iniettabile ev. Studi preliminari raccomandano una dose ev di carico di 10-15 mg/kg. L'acido valproico ev può diventare un farmaco utile per lo status epilettico.

La **paraldeide** è un farmaco relativamente sicuro in età pediatrica. Una soluzione al 5% è preparata aggiungendo 1,75 mL di paraldeide (1 g/mL) a glucosata al 5%, ottenendo un volume totale di 35 mL. La dose di carico è di 150-200 mg/kg h, iniettati lentamente in 15-20 minuti; la dose di mantenimento è di 20 mg/kg/h, in infusione di una concentrazione al 5% (in bottiglia di vetro perché il farmaco è incompatibile con la plastica). La velocità di infusione può essere ridotta in caso di miglioramento. È importante utilizzare confezioni aperte al momento e verificare la data di scadenza del farmaco, perché con il tempo la paraldeide si deteriora in acetilaldeide e acido acetico.

L'anestesia generale costituisce un'alternativa nella gestione dello status epilettico successivamente al fallimento della terapia farmacologica convenzionale. È possibile utilizzare diversi agenti, come l'alotano e l'isoflurano. È probabile che l'anestesia generale agisca correggendo l'anossia cerebrale e le concomitanti anomalie metaboliche, consentendo ai farmaci precedentemente somministrati di esercitare i loro effetti. Il principale svantaggio dell'anestesia generale consiste nel fatto che deve essere somministrata da personale esperto con la disponibilità di attrezzature per lo smaltimento dei gas anestetici per lunghi periodi di tempo.

L'opportunità di proseguire la terapia anticonvulsivante successivamente allo status epilettico è oggetto di controversie. La terapia antiepilettica a lungo termine è certamente necessaria nei bambini con una malattia neurologica progressiva o con storia clinica di convulsioni ricorrenti prima dell'esordio dello status epilettico. Dopo un iniziale attacco di status epilettico idiopatico, il trattamento anticonvulsivante a lungo termine è raramente utile, in particolare se la causa è attribuibile a convulsioni febbrili prolungate. In quest'ultimo caso, la terapia anticonvulsivante è proseguita arbitrariamente per 3 mesi e poi sospesa (se il bambino resta asintomatico).

PROGNOSI. La status epilettico causa disturbi delle funzioni fisiologiche potenzialmente fatali. Il tasso di mortalità è di circa il 5% e risulta più elevato nel gruppo sintomatico (per la presenza di gravi disturbi del SNC già noti prima dell'esordio dello status epilettico). In assenza di danno neurologico progressivo (come encefalite erpetica) o di disturbi metabolici, la morbilità è poco elevata. Il riscontro di sequele neurologiche come emiplegia, sindromi extrapiramidali, ritardo mentale ed epilessia nei bambini che sperimentano status epilettico prima di aver compito l'anno è attribuibile al fatto che in questo gruppo di età aumenta la probabilità della presenza di un preesistente disturbo del SNC. Tuttavia, il rischio di danno cerebrale da status epilettico prolungato costituisce un tema ancora dibattuto. È importante notare che lo status epilettico febbrile in un bambino con disturbo neurologico rappresenta un fattore di rischio per successive convulsioni febbrili e non, mentre lo stesso status in un bambino altrimenti normale non aumenta il rischio di convulsioni. La RM eseguita su diversi lattanti ha dimostrato l'occasionale associazione tra convulsioni febbrili complesse e lesione ippocampale acuta, responsabile di atrofia. In questi bambini, l'esame anatomopatologico e le tecniche di imaging hanno rivelato la presenza di disgenesia cerebrale preesistente. Questi casi suggeriscono che la sclerosi ippocampale associata a status epilettico rifletta l'interazione tra processi preesistenti e acquisiti.

Claassen J, Hirsch LJ, Emerson RG, et al: Treatment of refractory status epilepticus with pentobarbitol, propofol, or midazolam: A systemic review. *Epilepsia* 2002;43:146–153.
Hanhan UA, Fiallos MR, Orlowski JP: Status epilepticus. *Pediatr Clin North Am* 2001;48:683.
Lowenstein DH, Alldredge BK: Status epilepticus. *N Engl J Med* 1998; 338:970–976.
Maytal J, Shinnar S, Moshe SL, et al: Low morbidity and mortality of status epilepticus in children. *Pediatrics* 1989;83:323–331.
Perez ER, Maeder P, Villemure KM, et al: Acquired hippocampal damage after temporal lobe seizures in 2 infants. *Ann Neurol* 2000;48:384–387.
Riikonen R: Childhood convulsive status epilepticus. *Lancet* 2006;368:184–185.
Riviello JJ Jr., Ashwal S, Hirtz D, et al: Practice parameter: diagnostic assessment of the child with status epilepticus (an evidence-based review). *Neurology* 2006;67:1542–1550.
Sahin M, Menache CC, Holmes GL, et al: Outcome of severe refractory status epilepticus in children. *Epilepsia* 2001;42:1461–1467.
Shinnar S, Pellock JM, Berg AT, et al: Short-term outcomes of children with febrile status epilepticus. *Epilepsia* 2001;42:47S–53S.
VanLandingham KE, Heinz ER, Cavazos JE, et al: Magnetic resonance imaging evidence of hippocampal injury after prolonged focal febrile convulsions. *Ann Neurol* 1998;43:413–426.
Wiznitzer M: Buccal midazolam for seizures. *Lancet* 2005;366:182–184.

Capitolo 594 ■ Condizioni che simulano le crisi epilettiche Michael V. Johnston

Diverse condizioni patologiche presentano caratteristiche comuni all'epilessia. Poiché questi disturbi sono spesso associati ad alterazione del livello di coscienza, a movimenti tonici o clonici e a cianosi essi tendono a essere confusi con l'epilessia. In questi casi, la somministrazione di anticonvulsivanti è inutile e rischiosa, perché i disturbi che simulano l'epilessia sono refrattari agli antiepilettici e richiedono un trattamento specifico. La diagnosi differenziale è spesso collegata all'età del paziente (Tab. 594-1).

VERTIGINI PAROSSISTICHE BENIGNE. Le vertigini parossistiche benigne (*Benign Paroxysmal Vertigo*, BPV) si sviluppano tipicamente nella prima infanzia e sono relativamente rare dopo i 3 anni. Gli attacchi, a esordio improvviso, sono associati ad atassia, responsabile della tendenza del bambino a cadere o del suo rifiuto di camminare o sedere. Il **nistagmo orizzontale** può risultare evidente durante tutta la durata dell'attacco. Il bambino appare spaventato e pallido e talvolta sono presenti nausea e vomito. La coscienza e la capacità di esprimersi non sono compromesse e l'episodio non è seguito da letargia o da sonnolenza. Gli attacchi risultano molto variabili in termini di durata (secondi o minuti), frequenza (quotidiana o mensile) e intensità. I bambini più grandi riferiscono una sensazione di vertigine (rotatoria). Anni dopo, questi pazienti tendono a sviluppare cinetosi e cefalea suggerendo un rapporto tra BPV e cefalea. La valutazione neurologica è solitamente negativa, fatta eccezione per il riscontro di un'anomalia della funzione vestibolare evidenziata dal test calorico con acqua e ghiaccio. I pazienti con cluster di attacchi normalmente rispondono alla somministrazione orale, per via ev o rettale di difenidramina, alla dose di 5 mg/kg/24 h, fino a un massimo di 300 mg/24 h.

PAVOR NOCTURNUS O TERRORE NOTTURNO. Il terrore notturno è un disturbo comune, in particolare nei bambini di età compresa tra i 5 e i 7 anni (vedi Capitolo 18). È sperimentato dall'1-3% dei bambini, ma solitamente ha una breve durata. È caratterizzato da un esordio improvviso, nella maggior parte dei casi tra mezzanotte e le due, durante gli stadi 3 o 4 del sonno a onde lente. Il bambino urla, ha le pupille dilatate e appare terrorizzato,

TABELLA 594-1. Disturbi parossistici non epilettici

PERIODO NEONATALE
Nervosismo*
Mioclono neonatale benigno del sonno*
PRIMA INFANZIA
Sincope infantile*
Spasimi affettivi
Sincope pallida
Attacchi di brividi
Torcicollo parossistico
Reazioni extrapiramidali da farmaci, distonia
Reflusso gastroesofageo con distonia
Ruminazione
Stereotipie, autismo, sindrome di Rett, sordità e cecità coesistenti
Costipazione, ritenzione delle feci
Masturbazione
Spasmo nutans
Opsoclono
Vertigini parossistiche benigne
Mioclono
Disturbi non epilettici; ansia, eccitazione, encefalopatia acuta metabolica
Mioclono benigno della prima infanzia
Iperreflessia
Emiplegia alternante infantile
Disturbi del sonno
Jactatio capitis
SECONDA INFANZIA
Spasmi affettivi*
Sincope
Emicrania e equivalenti emicranici, dolore addominale ricorrente, vomito ciclico*
Tic*
Torcicollo spasmodico
Reazione da farmaci, distonia
Coreoatetosi parossistica
Reflusso gastroesofageo
Vertigini parossistiche benigne
Mioclono non epilettico; ansia, eccitazione, encefalopatia metabolica acuta
Iperreflessia
Masturbazione
Costipazione, ritenzione delle feci*
Sogni a occhi aperti, sguardo fisso*
Stereotipie; autismo, sordità e cecità coesistenti
Sindrome di Münchausen per procura
Iperventilazione
Convulsioni psicogeniche
Amnesia globale transitoria
Disturbi del sonno*
Jactatio capitis
Terrore notturno – Pavor nocturnus
Sonnambulismo, sonniloquio
ADOLESCENZA
Sincope*
Emicrania*
Convulsioni psicogeniche
Stati dissociativi, disturbi di conversione, attacchi di panico, iperventilazione
Sogni a occhi aperti*
Disturbi del sonno*
Mioclono notturno, spasmi ipnici
Narcolessia
Sonnambulismo
Sonniloquio
Rabbia episodica
Fingersi malato
Coreoatetosi parossistica
Tremori
Tic
Reazione da farmaci, distonia
Amnesia transitoria globale

*Comune.

presenta inoltre tachicardia e iperventilazione. Di solito il bambino non parla, ma si dimena con violenza; inconsapevole della presenza dei genitori, non può essere consolato: dopo qualche minuto si addormenta e il mattino dopo non conserva alcun ricordo dell'episodio. Circa un terzo dei bambini che soffrono di terrori notturni sperimenta sonnambulismo. Nei bambini con terrori notturni persistenti e prolungati è opportuno indagare la presenza di un disturbo emotivo. Contemporaneamente alla valutazione delle dinamiche familiari, dovrebbe essere considerata la possibilità di ricorrere a una breve terapia con diazepam.

SPASMI AFFETTIVI. Gli spasmi affettivi costituiscono spesso un'esperienza drammatica per i genitori, che assistono con terrore alla perdita di coscienza del figlio, dovuta all'anossia cerebrale al picco dell'attacco. Si riscontrano due tipi principali di spasmi: la forma cianotica (i più comuni) e la forma pallida (vedi anche Capitolo 28).

Forma cianotica. Tali spasmi, solitamente prevedibili, sono espressione della rabbia o del malessere di un bambino rimproverato o innervosito. L'episodio è introdotto da un pianto breve e acuto, seguito dall'espirazione o apnea forzata. La cianosi generalizzata insorge rapidamente, con conseguente perdita di coscienza, talvolta associata a spasmi clonici ripetuti e generalizzati, opistotono e bradicardia. I risultati dell'EEG intercritale sono normali. Gli spasmi affettivi possono essere sporadici oppure ripetersi nel giro di qualche ora, ma appaiono sempre stereotipati. Rari prima dei 6 mesi, presentano un picco di insorgenza intorno ai 2 anni, mentre calano drasticamente dopo i 5 anni. La gestione degli spasmi affettivi si concentra sul supporto e sulla riassicurazione dei familiari. Tuttavia alcuni genitori, ignorando i consigli del pediatra, non possono fare a meno di gettare acqua gelata sul viso del bambino, rovesciarlo a testa in giù, tentare la respirazione bocca a bocca o persino la rianimazione cardiopolmonare. Un esame accurato, assieme alla spiegazione del meccanismo dello spasmo, ha un effetto rassicurante su molti genitori. Durante il *counseling*, è importante sottolineare la necessità che essi adottino un atteggiamento coerente ed evitino di rinforzare il comportamento del figlio. Al termine della crisi, il genitore dovrebbe mettere a letto il bambino, evitando di coccolarlo, di giocare o di tenerlo in braccio.

Forma pallida. Questi spasmi, molto meno comuni della forma cianotica, sono scatenati tipicamente da un'esperienza dolorosa o terrificante, come una caduta o uno spavento improvviso. Il bambino smette di respirare, perde rapidamente coscienza, diviene pallido e ipotonico e può sperimentare una convulsione tonica. È possibile registrare bradicardia con periodi di asistolia >2 secondi, mentre l'EEG intercritale è normale. In alcuni casi, gli spasmi possono essere indotti spontaneamente, in laboratorio, mediante compressione oculare, che produce il riflesso oculocardiaco tramite la stimolazione afferente del nervo trigemino e l'inibizione efferente del cuore per mezzo del nervo vago. Questa procedura non deve essere tentata da medici inesperti o se non si dispone di attrezzatura per la rianimazione. Nella maggior parte dei casi, il bambino risponde a misure conservative (già descritte per lo spasmo cianotico). Nei casi refrattari, si consiglia un trial di anticolinergici, con somministrazione orale di 0,01 mg/kg/24 h di atropina solfato, in dosi suddivise. Tale farmaco, che alla dose massima giornaliera di 0,4 mg, determina un aumento della frequenza cardiaca, bloccando il nervo vago, può essere usato nei casi refrattari. L'atropina è controindicata in presenza di una temperatura esterna molto elevata, perché rischia di scatenare un episodio di iperpiressia.

SINCOPE

SINCOPE SEMPLICE. La sincope è il risultato di un'alterazione del metabolismo cerebrale, conseguenza di una riduzione del flusso sanguigno cerebrale, solitamente secondaria a ipotensione sistemica. Tale riduzione del flusso causa perdita di coscienza e, assieme alla concomitante ischemia, stimola i centri corticali superiori a esercitare una funzione di inibizione sulla formazione reticolare troncoencefalica. In circa il 50% dei pazienti con sincope, la scarica neurale che parte dalla formazione reticolare determina brevi contrazioni toniche della muscolatura di volto, tronco e arti. Durante l'episodio, la deviazione fissa verso l'alto degli occhi può indurre a sospettare erroneamente la presenza di epilessia. La sincope semplice è provocata dalla stimolazione vasovagale ed è scatenata da dolore, paura, eccitazione, immobilità per periodi protratti, in particolare in un ambiente caldo. L'EEG mostra un rallentamento transitorio durante l'attacco, in assenza di scariche convulsive. Rara prima dei 10-12 anni, la sincope è prevalente nelle ragazze adolescenti. Il tilt-table test è un metodo efficace per riprodurre i sintomi di sincope, inclusa l'ipotensione, in pazienti con svenimenti inspiegabili. Se la sincope vasovagale è ricorrente, si consiglia la somministrazione orale di agenti β-bloccanti adrenergici. Di solito, la sincope si può facilmente distinguere dalla crisi epilettica per la sua breve durata, per i sintomi associati di nausea e di perspirazione e per il recupero completo della capacità di orientamento subito dopo l'evento.

SINCOPE DA TOSSE. Comune nei bambini asmatici, questo tipo di sincope tende a verificarsi poco dopo l'addormentamento. La crisi di tosse parossistica risveglia bruscamente il bambino, che ha il volto pletorico, suda molto, appare agitato e spaventato. La perdita di coscienza è associata a ipotonia muscolare generalizzata, occhi rovesciati verso l'alto e contrazioni muscolari cloniche che si protraggono per diversi secondi. L'incontinenza urinaria è frequente. Il bambino comincia a riprendersi dopo qualche secondo e recupera la coscienza nell'arco di qualche minuto. Non conserva alcun ricordo dell'episodio, fatta eccezione per gli eventi collegati alla tosse parossistica. La tosse determina un marcato aumento della pressione intrapleurica, in seguito una riduzione del ritorno venoso verso il lato destro del cuore e infine un'associata riduzione dell'efflusso ventricolare destro. Il successivo calo del riempimento ventricolare sinistro determina una rapida diminuzione del flusso sanguigno in uscita, con conseguente alterazione del flusso cerebrale, ipossia cerebrale e perdita di coscienza. La gestione dei bambini asmatici con sincope da tosse prevede un approccio aggressivo alla prevenzione della broncocostrizione.

SINDROME DEL QT LUNGO. La sindrome del QT lungo ha un'incidenza di 1/10 000-1/15 000 ed è caratterizzata da un'improvvisa perdita di coscienza durante l'esercizio fisico o un'esperienza emotivamente stressante (vedi Capitolo 435.5). L'epilessia è raramente in causa nei casi di associazione tra perdita di coscienza e sforzo o stress, mentre l'origine cardiaca deve sempre essere considerata. Il disturbo si instaura tipicamente nella tarda infanzia o nell'adolescenza; l'esordio nella prima infanzia può simulare una sindrome da morte improvvisa del lattante. Durante la sincope si riscontrano varie aritmie cardiache, in particolare fibrillazione ventricolare. Il bambino può ristabilirsi entro pochi minuti o andare incontro al decesso. L'ECG mostra un anomalo allungamento dell'intervallo QT, in particolare sotto sforzo monitorato. Un intervallo QT corretto per la frequenza cardiaca ≥0,46 msec conferma la diagnosi. Esistono almeno due varianti della sindrome: la forma dovuta a cardiopatia acquisita (miocardite, prolasso della valvola mitralica, diselettrolitemie, disturbi indotti da farmaci) e la forma congenita. La sindrome del QT lungo è ereditabile con modalità autosomica recessiva associata a sordità (sindrome di Jervell e Lange-Nielsen), oppure con modalità autosomica dominante (sindrome di Romano-Ward). Mutazioni del gene che codifica per il canale cardiaco del potassio (*KvLQT1*), legato al cromosoma 11p15.5, sono responsabili di circa il 50% dei casi di sindrome del QT lungo autosomica dominante (tipo 1 o LQT1). LQT2 è il risultato di una mutazione di un secondo gene che codifica per il canale del potassio (*HERG*), legato al cromosoma 7q35-36. La sindrome del QT lungo di tipo 3 deriva da una mutazione del gene che codifica per il canale cardiaco del sodio (*SCN5A*), legato al cromosoma 3p21-24. Una quarta variante della malattia è legata al cromosoma 4q25-27, ma il gene per LQT4 non è stato ancora identificato. Tutti i membri della famiglia di un paziente che presenta il disturbo devono sottoporsi a elettrocardiogramma a 12 derivazioni. Esami supplementari includono un test da sforzo o il monitoraggio Holter. I farmaci antagonisti β-adrenergici sono solitamente efficaci e in alcuni casi possono salvare la vita del paziente. Se la terapia farmacologica è inefficace, è possibile considerare l'impianto permanente di defibrillatori cardiaci o l'esecuzione di una simpatectomia cervicotoracica sul lato sinistro. I genitori dovrebbero apprendere le tecniche di rianimazione cardiopolmonare, perché in alcuni pazienti la ridotta attività fisica e la terapia farmacologica non ottengono il completo controllo delle crisi.

COREOATETOSI PAROSSISTICA CHINESIGENICA. Questo disturbo è caratterizzato da un improvviso esordio di coreoatetosi, unilaterale o talvolta bilaterale, oppure dall'assunzione di una posizione distonica di una gamba o un braccio, associata a disartria e a smorfie facciali. Il disturbo è scatenato da movimenti improvvisi, in particolare l'alzarsi da una posizione seduta, o da eccitazione e stress emotivo. Raramente gli attacchi persistono per oltre un minuto e non sono mai associati a perdita di coscienza. L'età di esordio tipica è compresa tra 8 e 14 anni, ma si riscontrano casi precoci (2 anni). Il bambino può presentare diversi attacchi quotidiani oppure crisi intermittenti una o due volte al mese. I risultati dell'esame neurologico, dell'EEG e degli esami di neuroimaging sono normali. Gli studi neuropatologici eseguiti in alcuni casi non hanno rivelato alcuna anomalia. La maggior parte dei casi segnalati è di tipo familiare; ciò suggerisce una trasmissione autosomica recessiva del disturbo. Gli attacchi possono essere prevenuti con l'uso di anticonvulsivanti, in particolare fenitoina. In età adulta, quando la frequenza delle crisi tende a diminuire, il farmaco può essere gradualmente sospeso.

ATTACCHI DI BRIVIDI. Gli attacchi di brividi esordiscono tra i 4 e i 6 mesi di età e possono persistere fino ai 6-7 anni. Producono una postura caratteristica, con improvvisa flessione del capo e del tronco e tremori simili a quelli prodotti versando senza preavviso acqua gelata sulla schiena di un individuo. I pazienti hanno fino a 100 attacchi al giorno, seguiti da settimane prive di sintomi. Tali brividi possono costituire il precursore infantile del tremore essenziale benigno, perché l'esame di genitori e parenti rivela un'elevata incidenza del disturbo.

TORCICOLLO PAROSSISTICO BENIGNO DELL'INFANZIA. I bambini con torcicollo parossistico benigno manifestano ricorrenti attacchi di torsione del capo, associati a pallore, agitazione e vomito, con esordio tra i 2 e gli 8 mesi. Durante l'attacco, il bambino resiste al movimento passivo della testa. Non si riscontra perdita di coscienza e la remissione spontanea si verifica entro i 2-3 anni. Come per le vertigini parossistiche benigne, in questi pazienti sono state documentate anomalie della funzione vestibolare. In presenza di torcicollo persistente, è opportuno ricercare eventuali anomalie delle vertebre cervicali, incluse dislocazioni o fratture, oppure un tumore localizzato nella fossa posteriore. Alcuni pazienti tendono a sviluppare cefalea nella tarda infanzia. Sono stati inoltre segnalati casi di bambini con cefalea familiare legata a una mutazione del canale del calcio.

TREMORE EREDITARIO DEL MENTO. Il tremore ereditario del mento provoca fremiti rapidi e ripetuti (ogni 3 secondi), facilmente confondibili con l'epilessia. Tali brevi attacchi, ereditati con modalità autosomica dominante, sono scatenati da stress, rabbia e frustrazione. I risultati dell'esame neurologico e dell'EEG sono normali.

NARCOLESSIA E CATAPLESSIA. (Vedi anche Capitolo 18.) La narcolessia esordisce raramente prima dell'adolescenza ed è caratterizzata da attacchi parossistici e incontrollabili di sonno diurno, talvolta associati a perdita transitoria del tono muscolare (**cataplessia**). L'incidenza della narcolessia è di 1 su 2000. L'EEG mostra che gli attacchi consistono in sonno REM (*Rapid Eye Movement*, cioè rapidi movimenti oculari). I pazienti narcolettici possono essere svegliati senza difficoltà e recuperano spontaneamente l'allerta, mentre le convulsioni sono seguite da sonno profondo, sonnolenza postictale, letargia e spesso cefalea. La somministrazione orale di modafinil acetamide, alla dose di 200 mg/die, ha un'efficacia superiore ai farmaci stimolanti nel controllo della narcolessia e presenta scarsi effetti collaterali. Anche la cataplessia è talvolta confusa con l'epilessia. In seguito a una crisi di riso, a stress emotivo o esperienze terrorizzanti, i pazienti sperimentano un'improvvisa perdita del tono muscolare e si accasciano al suolo. I pazienti cataplettici non perdono coscienza, ma giacciono immobili per qualche minuto, finché non recuperano il tono muscolare normale. Il trattamento prevede sonno programmato e la somministrazione di amfetamine, metilfenidato, antidepressivi triciclici. Il counseling deve approfondire gli aspetti relativi alla sicurezza, affrontando temi come la possibilità di guidare e le scelte professionali. I farmaci stimolanti e antidepressivi causano comunemente effetti collaterali che includono ansia, euforia, ipersonnolenza e sviluppo di tolleranza.

CRISI DI RABBIA O SINDROME DELLA PERDITA DI CONTROLLO EPISODICO. La sindrome della perdita di controllo episodico è una condizione non epilettica spesso confusa con gli attacchi convulsivi parziali complessi. I pazienti presentano improvvisi e ricorrenti attacchi di comportamento fisico violento, scatenato da provocazioni minime. Tali comportamenti includono calci, graffi, morsi e grida (talvolta insulti e parolacce). Il bambino o l'adolescente non sembra in grado di controllarsi e può apparite momentaneamente psicotico. L'episodio è seguito da affaticamento, amnesia e da sincero rimorso. L'EEG può rivelare anomalie non specifiche, ma durante l'attacco non si modifica. Tale riscontro consente di distinguere il disturbo dalle crisi epilettiche parziali complesse, sempre caratterizzate da anomalie nell'EEG durante la crisi.

MASTURBAZIONE. La masturbazione o i comportamenti di autostimolazione possono riscontrarsi nelle bambine tra 2 mesi e 3 anni. Episodi stereotipati di assunzione di una postura tonica sono associati a movimenti copulatori, ma non a stimolazione manuale dei genitali. La bambina appare congestionata, suda abbondantemente, emette suoni gutturali e respira in maniera irregolare, ma non perde conoscenza. L'attività masturbatoria ha un esordio improvviso, solitamente persiste per alcuni minuti (raramente ore) e tende a verificarsi in momenti di stress o noia. L'esame dovrebbe includere la verifica di un eventuale abuso o di anomalie del perineo, ma nella maggior parte dei casi non è possibile risalire ad alcuna causa. Il trattamento prevede la rassicurazione dei genitori sul fatto che il comportamento è destinato a regredire entro i 3 anni, in assenza di terapia farmacologica.

PSEUDOCONVULSIONI. La diagnosi di pseudoconvulsioni può essere formulata solo dopo un'approfondita anamnesi, un accurato esame fisico e l'esclusione della presenza di convulsioni "vere" mediante prolungata registrazione EEG. Le pseudoconvulsioni si verificano tipicamente tra i 10 e i 18 anni di età e sono più comuni nelle ragazze. Possono insorgere in pazienti con una passata anamnesi di epilessia e in soggetti che presentano anche convulsioni epilettiche. La pseudoconvulsione è talvolta piuttosto realistica, ma nella maggior parte dei casi appare bizzarra, associata a una postura insolita, verbalizzazioni e movimenti tonici o clonici insoliti. Le caratteristiche distintive della pseudoconvulsione includono assenza di cianosi, reazione pupillare alla luce normale, assenza di perdita del controllo sfinterico, risposte plantari normali, assenza di lesioni durante l'attacco (come morsicarsi la lingua). Alcuni pazienti gemono o piangono prima dell'attacco e in alcuni casi possono essere persuasi dal medico ad averne uno. L'esame psicologico rivela spesso una personalità nevrotica. Non è insolito che questi pazienti assumano 3 o 4 anticonvulsivanti, ovviamente del tutto inefficaci. Il metodo più attendibile per formulare la diagnosi differenziale consiste nel registrare l'attacco. L'EEG mostra un eccesso di artefatti muscolari durante la pseudoconvulsione, ma un ritmo di fondo privo di scariche convulsive. Inoltre, successivamente a una crisi convulsiva vera si riscontra un significativo aumento del livello sierico di prolattina, assente nei casi di pseuduconvulsione.

Ackerman MJ, Clapham DE: Ion channels-basic science and clinical disease. *N Engl J Med* 1997;336:1575–1586.
Britton JW: Syncope and seizures—Differential diagnosis and evaluation. *Clin Auton Res* 2004;14:148–159.
Broughton RJ, Fleming JA, George CF, et al: Randomized double-blind placebo-controlled crossover trial of modafinil in the treatment of excessive daytime sleepiness in narcolepsy. *Neurology* 1997;49:444–451.
Fleisher DR, Morrison A: Masturbation mimicking abdominal pain or seizures in young girls. *J Pediatr* 1990;116:810–814.
Giffin NJ, Benton S, Goadsby PJ: Benign paroxysmal torticollis of infancy: Four new cases and linkage to CACNA1A mutation. *Dev Med Child Neurol* 44:490–493.
Haslam RH, Freigang B: Cough syncope mimicking epilepsy in asthmatic children. *Can J Neurol Sci* 1985;12:45–47.
Lotz T, Jankovic J: Paroxysmal kinesigenic dyskinesias. *Semin Pediatr Neurol* 2003;10:68–79.
Macleod S, Ferrie C, Zuberi SM: Symptoms of narcolepsy in children misinterpreted as epilepsy. *Epileptic Disord* 2005;7:13–17.

Capitolo 595 ■ Cefalee

Robert H.A. Haslam

La cefalea è un disturbo comune in età pediatrica, i cui effetti sul rendimento e sulla frequenza scolastica, sulla memoria, sulla personalità e sulle relazioni interpersonali dipendono dall'eziologia, dalla frequenza e dall'intensità dei sintomi. In alcuni casi, una cefalea segnala la presenza di un disturbo grave (come un tumore cerebrale), perciò è indispensabile sottoporre ad accurata valutazione tutti i soggetti che presentano mal di testa ricorrente, grave, progressivo o non convenzionale. I bambini reagiscono alla cefalea in maniera imprevedibile. Se molto piccoli, non riescono a comunicare le caratteristiche del loro disturbo, ma possono apparire irritabili e capricciosi; talvolta manifestano vomito, preferiscono una stanza buia a causa della fotofobia oppure si strofinano con insistenza gli occhi e il capo. Nella quasi totalità dei casi, i bambini fanno fatica a descrivere i loro sintomi. Le principali cause della cefalea nell'infanzia includono: emicrania, fattori psicogeni o stress, aumento della pressione intracranica (*IntraCranial Pressure*, ICP). Cause meno comuni comprendono: errori refrattivi, strabismo, sinusite e malocclusione dentale. La cefalea è spesso la manifestazione di un'infezione a livello della testa o del collo.

595.1 • Emicrania

L'emicrania è il tipo di cefalea più frequente nella popolazione pediatrica. Nella maggior parte dei casi, il disturbo non è grave e può essere trattato con misure conservative, senza dover ricorrere all'intervento del medico. Secondo un recente studio svedese, la prevalenza dell'emicrania nella popolazione scolare tra i 7 e i 15 anni è del 4%, mentre sale dall'8 al 23% nell'adolescenza. La probabilità di sviluppare emicrania è maggiore nelle adolescenti di sesso femminile, mentre al di sotto dei 10 anni i maschi costituiscono la maggioranza. Più del 50% dei bambini va incontro a remissione spontanea dopo i 10 anni. Da adulti, il 5-10% degli uomini e il 15-20% delle donne soffre di emicrania.

La ***Cortical Spreading Depression*** (CSD), un fenomeno ritenuto responsabile dell'aura emicranica, è associata ad aumento degli ioni idrogeno e potassio nel SNC con rilascio di glutammato e di ossido nitrico. Questi cambiamenti risultano in un'oligoemia corticale regionale e nell'attivazione della porzione caudale del ganglio trigeminale. L'eccitazione del sistema vascolare trigeminale induce il rilascio di polipeptidi intestinali vasoattivi, che causano vasodilatazione, seguita da fuoriuscita di proteine plasmatiche dai vasi durali, con conseguente infiammazione localizzata di tali vasi. L'infiammazione vascolare neurogena causa l'eccitazione dei recettori sensibili al dolore. La CSD è considerata una risposta fisiologica ereditaria a una varietà di stimoli, che scatenano la crisi emicranica.

CLASSIFICAZIONE E MANIFESTAZIONI CLINICHE. Nella Tabella 595-1 sono elencati i vari tipi di emicrania.

Emicrania senza aura. Questo tipo di emicrania costituisce la forma prevalente in età pediatrica. Di tipo pulsante e martellante, tende a essere **unilaterale**, ma talvolta ha una localizzazione bifrontale o a livello delle regioni temporali. Nei bambini è solitamente meno intensa rispetto all'adulto. Il dolore persiste per 1-3 ore, ma sono stati segnalati casi che si protraggono fino a 72 ore. Poiché le attività fisiche aggravano il dolore, il bambino non è in grado di svolgere le sue attività quotidiane. Una caratteristica peculiare dell'emicrania infantile è nausea e vomito intensi, sintomi spesso più fastidiosi del dolore vero e proprio. Il vomito può essere associato a dolore addominale e febbre. Condizioni come appendicite o infezioni sistemiche sono talvolta erroneamente considerate la diagnosi primaria. Sintomi addizionali includono un estremo pallore, fotofobia, sensazione di testa vuota, fonofobia, osmofobia (avversione per gli odori) e parestesie di mani e piedi. In circa il 90% dei casi si riscontra una storia familiare positiva, in particolare dal lato materno. In assenza di tale anamnesi, la diagnosi di emicrania senza aura deve essere formulata con estrema cautela.

Altre caratteristiche dell'emicrania includono la sincronicità con la fase perimestruale o con l'ovulazione, l'insorgenza graduale in seguito a esercizio fisico intenso, l'attenuazione dei sintomi con il sonno, prodromi stereotipati (ipersonnia, iperfagia, irritabilità, sbalzi dell'umore), avversione per particolari cibi o odori e l'esordio dopo una delusione o un periodo di stress. Le manifestazioni suggestive di un disturbo più serio includono l'insorgenza improvvisa di una cefalea molto intensa, un cambiamento nelle caratteristiche della cefalea, un'emicrania progressiva che si protrae per giorni, l'associazione con la manovra di Valsava, segni sistemici cronici (come perdita di peso o febbre), manifestazioni neurologiche focali persistenti, convulsioni, perdita di coscienza, rigidità cervicale, rumori cranici, anomalie del campo visivo o papilledema (Tab. 595-2).

Emicrania con aura. In questo disturbo, l'esordio della cefalea è preceduto da un'aura, solitamente di tipo visivo raramente descritta dai bambini piccoli, che si manifesta con visione offuscata, scotoma (area di depressione all'interno del campo visivo), spettro di fortificazione (linee bianche luminose a zig zag) o distor-

TABELLA 595-1. Classificazione internazionale delle cefalee (2004)*

EMICRANIA
Emicrania senza aura
Emicrania con aura
Aura tipica con emicrania
Emicrania tipica con cefalea non-emicranica
Aura tipica senza cefalea
Emicrania emiplegica familiare
Emicrania emiplegica sporadica
Emicrania basilare
Sindromi periodiche infantili, precursori comuni dell'emicrania
Vomito ciclico
Emicrania addominale
Vertigini parossistiche benigne dell'infanzia
Emicrania retinica
Complicanze dell'emicrania
Emicrania cronica
Stato di male emicranico
Aura persistente senza infarto
Infarto emicranico
Probabile emicrania

*Headache Classification Subcommittee of the International Headache Society: *The International Classification of Headache Disorders*, 2nd Edition. Cephalalgia 2004;24(Suppl 1):9-160.

TABELLA 595-2. Indicazioni per neuroimaging in un bambino con cefalea

Segni neurologici anomali
Recente calo del rendimento scolastico, cambiamento comportamentale, ritardo di crescita
Il mal di testa sveglia il bambino durante il sonno; mal di testa nelle prime ore del mattino, con frequenza e gravità crescente
Cefalee periodiche coincidenti con convulsioni, in particolare se a esordio focale
Coincidenza di emicrania e di convulsioni in uno stesso episodio e sintomi vascolari che precedono la convulsione (20-50% di rischio di tumore o malformazione arteriovenosa)
Cefalea a grappolo nel bambino; qualsiasi bambino di età <5-6 anni che lamenta principalmente cefalea
Comparsa di sintomi o segni neurologici focali durante la cefalea (emicrania complicata)
Comparsa di segni o sintomi neurologici focali durante l'aura (eccetto i sintomi visivi tipici dell'emicrania), con lateralità fissa; segni focali dell'aura persistenti o ricorrenti nella fase della cefalea
Offuscamento visivo al picco della cefalea (invece dell'aura)
Mal di testa da breve tosse in un bambino o adolescente

Modificata da Barlow CF: *Headaches and Migraine in Childhood*. Philadelphia, JB Lippincott, 1984, p 205.

sioni irregolari degli oggetti. Alcuni pazienti sperimentano anche vertigini e sensazione di testa vuota durante questo stadio della cefalea. I sintomi sensoriali includono parestesie e insensibilità di mani e piedi. Le distorsioni dell'immagine corporea (sindrome di "Alice nel paese delle meraviglie") possono predominare come preludio di un'emicrania classica. Dopo l'esordio dell'aura, il paziente sviluppa i tipici sintomi descritti in precedenza.

L'**emicrania emiplegica**, considerata un equivalente dell'aura, è caratterizzata dall'esordio unilaterale di segni motori o sensoriali durante un episodio di emicrania. Le emisindromi, più comuni nei bambini rispetto agli adulti, sono caratterizzate da: insensibilità e torpore a livello di volto, mani e gambe; debolezza unilaterale e afasia. In età pediatrica è raro che si verifichi più di un attacco. I segni neurologici possono essere transitori o persistere per giorni. È raro che un bambino vada incontro a deficit neurologico dopo un singolo episodio. L'emicrania emiplegica nei bambini più grandi e negli adolescenti ha una prognosi relativamente favorevole; in questi casi si riscontra spesso un'anamnesi familiare positiva per eventi emiplegici analoghi. L'emicrania emiplegica familiare (*Familiar Hemiplegic Migraine*, FHM) è un disturbo autosomico dominante caratterizzato da emiplegia durante la cefalea e, in alcune famiglie, da atrofia cerebellare progressiva. In circa due terzi dei pazienti con FHM1 si riscontra una mutazione del gene *CACNA1A*, localizzato sul cromosoma 19p3. Il gene *CACNA1A* codifica per la subunità $\alpha 1$ del canale del calcio voltaggio-dipendente. FHM2 è causata da mutazioni del gene *ATP1A2*, mentre FHM3 è il risultato di una mutazione del gene *SCN1A*, che codifica per il canale del sodio voltaggio-dipendente.

L'**emicrania di tipo basilare** è considerata un precursore di quella infantile. In questi pazienti predominano i sintomi troncoencefalici, causati dalla vasocostrizione delle arterie cerebrali basilare e posteriore. I sintomi principali includono vertigini, ronzio auricolare, diplopia, visione offuscata, scotoma, atassia e cefalea occipitale. Le pupille sono talvolta dilatate e la ptosi può risultare evidente. Possono seguire alterazioni della coscienza e convulsioni generalizzate. Dopo l'attacco, si osserva una risoluzione completa dei sintomi e segni neurologici. Nella maggior parte dei casi, si riscontra un'anamnesi positiva per emicrania. Molti pazienti sviluppano emicrania con aura da adolescenti o adulti. Traumi cranici minori possono scatenare un episodio di emicrania basilare. Il disturbo è stato descritto in bambini di entrambi i sessi, ma le femmine di età inferiore ai 4 anni risultano particolarmente a rischio.

Sindromi periodiche infantili, precursori comuni dell'emicrania. Queste varianti includono il vomito ciclico (vedi Capitolo 303), l'emicrania addominale e le vertigini parossistiche benigne (vedi Capitolo 594). Il **vomito ciclico** è caratterizzato da attacchi ricorrenti, talvolta mensili, di grave vomito, talmente intenso da causare disidratazione e diselettrolitiemie, in particolare nei lattanti. Le manifestazioni sistemiche, come febbre, dolore addominale e diarrea sono inizialmente assenti, ma divengono prominenti in seguito all'eccessiva perdita di liquidi secondaria al vomito. L'attacco può protrarsi per 1-5 giorni, ma tra un attacco e l'altro la remissione dei sintomi è completa. In ciascun attacco, gli accessi di vomito si verificano almeno 5 volte all'ora, per almeno un'ora, e vi è una completa risoluzione dei sintomi tra gli attacchi. Il bambino appare pallido e preoccupato, ma non perde conoscenza. Dopo un periodo di sonno profondo, si sveglia, riprende le attività abituali e ricomincia a mangiare come se il vomito non si fosse mai verificato. Molti di questi pazienti presentano un'anamnesi positiva per emicrania e, crescendo, sono in grado di descrivere con precisione i sintomi di un tipico attacco di emicrania. Ciò lascia pochi dubbi alla diagnosi e all'associazione tra vomito ciclico ed emicrania. Il disturbo è trattato con somministrazione per via rettale o iniettiva di antiemetici, come dimenidrinato o ondansetron, e reidratazione attenta in caso di eccessiva perdita di liquidi. Il vomito ciclico dell'emicrania deve essere differenziato da disturbi gastrointestinali come l'ostruzione intestinale (malrotazione, volvolo intermittente, diaframma duodenale, cisti da duplicazione, compressione dell'arteria mesenterica superiore, ernia interna), ulcera peptica, gastrite, giardiasi, pancreatite cronica e morbo di Crohn. Anche le anomalie della motilità gastrointestinale e un'ostruzione della giunzione pelviureterica possono causare vomito ciclico. Le cause metaboliche includono disturbi del metabolismo degli amminoacidi (deficit eterozigote di ornitina trascarbamilasi), difetti di ossidazione degli acidi grassi (deficit di acil-CoA deidrogenasi a catena media), disturbi del metabolismo dei carboidrati (intolleranza ereditaria al fruttosio), porfiria intermittente acuta e lesioni del sistema nervoso centrale (tumori della fossa posteriore, ematomi o effusioni subdurali).

L'**emicrania addominale** è un disturbo ricorrente caratterizzato da dolore all'addome, mesogastrio, con periodi privi di sintomi tra un attacco e l'altro. Il dolore, solitamente descritto come sordo, da moderato a severo, può persistere da 1 a 72 ore. Benché solitamente localizzato sulla linea mediana dell'addome, nel bambino può risultare periombelicale o scarsamente localizzato. Per soddisfare i criteri dell'emicrania addominale, il bambino deve presentare almeno due dei seguenti sintomi: anoressia, nausea, vomito o pallore. Come per il vomito ciclico, un'accurata anamnesi, l'esame obiettivo e i test di laboratorio devono escludere eventuali malattie gastrointestinali sottostanti.

Due disturbi in passato elencati tra le complicanze dell'emicrania sono stati recentemente riclassificati. L'**emiplegia alternante** dell'infanzia può essere causata da un disturbo metabolico o mitocondriale, oppure da una canalopatia. L'**emicrania oftalmoplegica** è definita attualmente nevralgia cranica.

DIAGNOSI E DIAGNOSI DIFFERENZIALE. Nella maggior parte dei casi, un'approfondita anamnesi e l'esame obiettivo sono sufficienti per la formulazione della diagnosi (Tab. 595-3). L'emicrania basilare può essere confusa con diversi disturbi, come malformazioni congenite del cranio e delle vertebre cervicali, tumori della fossa posteriore, effetti di tossine e di farmaci e anomalie metaboliche, inclusa la malattia di Leigh e il deficit di piruvato decarbossilasi. Nei bambini con emicrania emiplegica, la diagnosi differenziale è con malformazioni arterovenose, MELAS (*Mitochondrial myopathy Encephalopathy Lactic Acidosis, and Strokes*, cioè miopatia mitocondriale, encefalopatia, acidosi lattica e ictus), tumori cerebrali, paralisi di Todd, disturbi della coagulazione, emoglobinopatie come l'anemia a cellule falciformi e disturbi metabolici come l'omocistinuria. Il profilo lipidico deve essere ottenuto nei bambini con emicrania e un'anamnesi familiare positiva per infarto miocardico prematuro o accidente cerebrovascolare. L'emicrania può verificarsi anche in bambini con lupus eritematoso sistemico e in caso di abuso di cocaina. La scelta degli esami di laboratorio e dei test radiologici dipende dalla costellazione dei sintomi e dai reperti dell'esame neurologico. L'elettroencefalogramma (EEG) e gli esami di imaging (TC e RM) sono raramente indicati nei bambini, a meno che la cefalea non risulti associata a una costellazione di sintomi e segni anomala o se si sospetta un aumento dell'ICP (vedi Tab. 595-2).

TRATTAMENTO. L'American Academy of Neurology ha stabilito le seguenti linee guida pratiche per il trattamento dell'emicrania:

TABELLA 595-3. Criteri diagnostici dell'emicrania

SENZA AURA	
A	Almeno 5 attacchi
B	La cefalea dura 4-72 ore (in caso di trattamento inefficace o assente)
C	La cefalea presenta almeno due delle seguenti caratteristiche: Localizzazione unilaterale Qualità pulsatile Intensità moderata o grave Aggravata dalle attività fisiche quotidiane (come camminare o salire le scale)
D	Durante la cefalea sono presenti almeno uno dei sintomi seguenti: Nausea e/o vomito Fotofobia e fonofobia
E	I sintomi non sono attribuibili ad altri disturbi
CON AURA (EMICRANIA CLASSICA)	
A	Almeno due attacchi
B	Il disturbo soddisfa i criteri per aura tipica, aura emiplegica o aura di tipo basilare
C	I sintomi non sono attribuibili ad altri disturbi
AURA TIPICA	
1	Sintomi sensoriali, visivi o di linguaggio reversibili (o una combinazione) ma assenza di debolezza motoria
2	Sintomi visivi uni o bilaterali positivi (punti o linee luminose) o negativi (perdita di campo visivo oppure sintomi sensoriali unilaterali positivi (sensazione di puntura) e/o negativi (insensibilità) o qualsiasi combinazione
3	Almeno uno dei seguenti sintomi: a) Un sintomo che si sviluppa gradualmente nel corso di un minimo di 5 minuti e/o differenti sintomi in successione o entrambi b) Ciascun sintomo dura almeno 5 minuti e non si protrae per più di 60 minuti
4	La cefalea che soddisfa i criteri per l'emicrania senza aura esordisce durante l'aura o la segue entro 60 minuti

Tratta da Silberstein SD: Migraine. *Lancet* 2004;363:381-391.

1. Riduzione della frequenza, della gravità, della durata della cefalea e dei suoi effetti disabilitanti.
2. Riduzione dell'assunzione di farmaci inefficaci e mal tollerati; sospensione di farmacoterapie inutili.
3. Miglioramento della qualità della vita.
4. Controllo del rischio di escalation nell'uso di farmaci.
5. Sostegno alla capacità del paziente di controllare la malattia.
6. Riduzione dei sintomi psicologici e dello stress collegati alla cefalea.

L'emicrania può essere prevenuta o migliorata evitando certi stimoli scatenanti. Alcuni bambini sono in grado di specificare particolari fattori che invariabilmente provocano la cefalea. I più comuni sono lo stress, la stanchezza e l'ansia. Difficoltà scolastiche o nell'ambiente familiare possono indurre uno stato di tensione nel bambino, in particolare se sottoposto a pressioni o richieste irrealistiche. Bambini che sperimentano emicrania ricorrente durante i mesi scolastici possono presentare un disturbo dell'apprendimento o possono essere stati assegnati a una classe troppo competitiva. Talvolta un cambiamento di scuola o una rivalutazione delle abilità scolastiche del bambino può costituire il passo principale nella gestione delle cefalee. Alcuni studi hanno segnalato un collegamento tra emicrania e cibi specifici, in particolare noci, cioccolato, bevande gassate contenenti caffeina, agrumi, fritti, formaggio, yogurt, cibi piccanti, carne in scatola, aringhe affumicate e cibo cinese (cefalea da glutammato monosodico). Per verificare il ruolo dei fattori dietetici, i genitori sono incoraggiati a tenere un diario o un calendario della cefalea, registrando il collegamento tra l'esordio dei sintomi e il consumo di particolari cibi. L'eliminazione del cibo incriminato è opportuna se emerge una chiara relazione con lo scatenamento della cefalea. In caso di anamnesi suggestiva, è indicato anche evitare luci lampeggianti, esposizione al sole, sforzi fisici eccessivi, traumi cranici anche lievi, rumori forti, periodi di digiuno prolungato, affaticamento, attività che causano cinetosi e assunzione di alcol e di farmaci (inclusi i contraccettivi orali). Durante l'anamnesi, è opportuno indagare il possibile collegamento tra l'emicrania e un disturbo del sonno molto comune. La frequenza e la gravità dei sintomi sono ridotte significativamente in almeno il 50% di pazienti pediatrici sottoposti ad anamnesi ed esame neurologico accurati, seguiti dalla rassicurazione da parte del medico.

La **gestione di un attacco acuto** di emicrania prevede il ricorso a un analgesico e antiemetico (Tab. 595-4). L'uso prudente di *paracetamolo* (15 mg/kg) o *ibuprofene* (7,5-10 mg/kg) *in compresse dispersibili* consente di trattare la maggior parte degli attacchi, in particolare se lievi, non frequenti e di breve durata. In molti casi, il bambino non è consapevole dell'aura o non la comunica ai genitori. Un antiemetico come il *dimenidrinato in supposte rettali* (5 mg/kg/24 h suddivisi in 4 dosi) è il farmaco di elezione se il vomito costituisce il sintomo principale. Anche la metoclopramide per via parenterale è molto efficace. Solitamente il bambino preferisce riposare in un luogo tranquillo e buio. Al risveglio, dopo alcune ore di sonno profondo, i sintomi sono scomparsi. Se gli analgesici convenzionali non sono sufficienti, i *triptani* (per es. il *sumatriptan*), agonisti specifici e selettivi dei recettori della 5-idrossitriptamina, costituiscono efficaci farmaci bloccanti nel trattamento della fase acuta dell'emicrania. Il sumatriptan è somministrabile per via sottocutanea, nasale o orale. La formulazione in spray nasale è la preferita in età pediatrica, alla dose di 5 mg nei bambini <25 kg, 10 mg (due spruzzi) nei bambini di 25-50 kg e 20 mg se ≥50 kg. La somministrazione può essere ripetuta a due ore di distanza dalla dose iniziale, evitando di superare le due dosi al giorno. Gli effetti collaterali più comuni, solitamente minori e transitori, includono vampate di calore, nausea, vomito, affaticamento e sonnolenza. I triptani sono controindicati nel trattamento di emicrania basilare e emiplegica. La Food and Drug Administration non ha approvato il loro utilizzo per pazienti di età inferiore ai 18 anni, benché numerosi studi in doppio cieco ne abbiano dimostrato l'efficacia e sicurezza in età pediatrica.

I bambini possono sviluppare gravi attacchi di emicrania o stato di male emicranico (cefalea persistente che si protrae oltre i 3 giorni), che non rispondono ai farmaci tradizionali. In tali casi, la *proclorperazina* per via endovenosa, alla dose di 0,15 mg/kg (per un massimo di 10 mg), costituisce un farmaco efficace nell'interrompere l'accesso.

La decisione di prescrivere una *terapia farmacologica continua* (**trattamento profilattico**) si basa sulla gravità e frequenza dei sintomi e sul livello di compromissione delle attività del bambino, inclusa la frequenza scolastica, il rendimento e la possibilità di partecipare alle attività ricreative. La profilassi può essere presa in considerazione se il paziente sperimenta almeno 2-4 gravi episodi al mese, che gli impediscono di frequentare la scuola con regolarità. Soltanto due farmaci sono stati sottoposti a rigorosi studi controllati, per verificarne l'efficacia e la tollerabilità in età pediatrica: il propranololo (un β-bloccante) e la flunarizina (calcioantagonista). Nei bambini con età minima di 7-8 anni, la dose di propanololo è di 10-20 mg tre volte al giorno (partendo da una dose iniziale di 10 mg/24 h e incrementandola gradualmente fino alla dose massima o all'ottenimento l'effetto terapeutico desiderato). Un errore comune consiste nel sospendere prematuramente la terapia, perché talvolta sono necessarie settimane o mesi prima che il farmaco risulti efficace. Anche la flunarizina (non disponibile negli Stati Uniti) si è dimostrata utile nella profilassi dell'emicrania pediatrica. La dose iniziale è di 5 mg prima di coricarsi, aumentabile se necessario fino a 10 mg. L'effetto collaterale più frequente è la sonnolenza. Altri farmaci in via di sperimentazione includono valproato di sodio, topiramato, levetiracetam, gabapentin, ciproeptadina e amitriptilina.

Il *trattamento comportamentale* si è rivelato efficace in bambini e adolescenti. In alcuni centri specializzati, le tecniche di biofeedback e di autoipnosi stanno gradualmente sostituendo la terapia farmacologica, a causa degli effetti collaterali di quest'ultima e del rischio di dipendenza chimica. Il biofeedback, utilizzabile nella maggior parte dei bambini con più di 8 anni, si è dimostrato efficace in diversi trial clinici. Parecchi studi mostrano una significativa riduzione nella frequenza della cefalea nei bambini trattati con autoipnosi rispetto a quelli che assumono propanololo o un placebo. Diversi centri specializzati impiegano assistenti sociali e

TABELLA 595-4. Farmaci utilizzati nel trattamento dell'emicrania nei bambini

FARMACO	DOSE	MECCANISMO	EFFETTI COLLATERALI	COMMENTI
EMICRANIA ACUTA				
Analgesici				
Paracetamolo	15 mg/kg/dose	Inibisce la sintesi delle prostraglandine	Overdose, necrosi epatica fatale, dolore addominale, nausea, emorragia gastrointestinale	
Ibuprofene	7,5-10 mg/kg/dose	Inibisce la sintesi delle prostraglandine		Preferibile nella formulazione in capsule gelatinose
Triptani (non approvati dalla FDA per bambini e adolescenti)				
Sumatriptan Spray nasale raccomandato (disponibile anche orale e sottocutaneo)	<25 kg: 5 mg 25-50 kg: 10 mg >50 kg: 20 mg	Selettivo, agonista di 5-idrossitriptamina	Seri eventi cardiaci non sono stati segnalati nei bambini	Controindicato nell'emicrania basilare ed emiplegica
PROFILASSI				
Calcioantagonisti				
Flunarizina*	5 mg prima di coricarsi	Calcioantagonista	Cefalea, letargia, vertigini	↑ Fino a 10 mg prima di coricarsi
Antipertensivi				
Propanololo (controindicato nell'asma)	10-20 mg tre volte al giorno	Agente β-bloccante adrenergico non selettivo	Vertigini, letargia	Iniziare con 10 mg/24 h ↑10 mg/settimana
Anticonvulsivanti				
Valproato di sodio	5-20 mg/kg/24 h (iniziare con 5 mg/kg/24 h)	↑GABA cerebrale	Nausea, pancreatite, epatotossicità fatale	↑5 mg/kg/settimana
Topiramato	3-9 mg/kg/24 h	↑Attività di GABA	Affaticamento, nervosismo	Iniziare con 1-3 mg/kg/24 h
Gabapentina	900-1200 mg/24 h	Sconosciuto	Sonnolenza, affaticamento, aggressività, aumento di peso	Iniziare con 300 mg ↑ 300 mg/settimana
Antistaminici				
Ciproeptadina	0,2-0,4 mg/kg prima di coricarsi	Agonista recettore H_1 e serotonina	Sonnolenza, secrezioni bronchiali dense	Massimo 0,5 mg/kg/24 h
Antidepressivi				
Amitriptilina	Bambini: 0,1 mg/kg prima di coricarsi, massimo 2 mg/kg prima di coricarsi Adolescenti: 25 mg prima di coricarsi, massimo 200 mg/24 h	Serotonina e noradrenalina nel SNC	Anomalie della conduzione cardiaca, bocca secca, costipazione, sonnolenza, confusione	Sconsigliata la sospensione brusca
GRAVE, INTRATTABILE				
Proclorperazina	0,15 mg/kg/ev (massimo 10 mg)		Agitazione, rigidità muscolare	

*Non disponibile negli Stati Uniti.
GABA, acido γ-aminobutirrico.

psicologi esperti nella gestione del dolore. In molti casi, i bambini rispondono favorevolmente all'apprendimento di tecniche di immaginazione guidata e imparano spesso a controllare il dolore associato all'emicrania senza dover ricorrere al farmaco.

595.2 • Cefalee da cause organiche

La cefalea può costituire il sintomo di esordio di un aumento dell'ICP. La tensione e trazione dei vasi sanguigni cerebrali e della dura madre si verificano inizialmente in forma sporadica, prevalentemente nelle prime ore del mattino o poco dopo il risveglio. La cefalea, di tipo diffuso e generalizzato, è più intensa a livello delle regioni occipitali e frontali. L'esordio può essere insidioso e il dolore è aggravato da qualsiasi attività che eleva l'ICP (tosse, starnuti, tensione da motilità intestinale). All'aumentare dell'ICP, il bambino diviene sempre più letargico e irritabile e sperimenta una cefalea costante. Episodi di vomito nelle prime ore del mattino sono spesso associati all'aumento dell'ICP. Le cause organiche delle cefaee in età pediatrica includono tumori cerebrali, in particolare se localizzati nella fossa posteriore, idrocefalo, meningite ed encefalite, ascesso cerebrale, ematoma subdurale, avvelenamento da piombo cronico e pseudotumor cerebri. Altre cause, non sempre associate a un aumento dell'ICP, includono malformazioni arteriovenose, aneurisma di Berry, connettiviti/vasculiti a carico del SNC, encefalopatia ipertensiva, emorragia subaracnoidea acuta e ictus. Il trattamento di questo tipo di cefalea dipende dalla causa. Il primo passo prevede una approfondita anamnesi e un accurato esame obiettivo, che deve includere la registrazione della pressione sanguigna e l'esame del fondo oculare (per la ricerca di papilledema). Gli esami di laboratorio e i test radiologici sono stabiliti sulla base dei risultati di anamnesi e esame obiettivo.

595.3 • Cefalee tensive o da stress

La cefalea tensiva o da stress è comune in età pediatrica, in particolare dopo l'esordio della pubertà, ed è molto difficile da distinguere dall'emicrania. Le due forme sono spesso associate in uno stesso paziente. La cefalea tensiva insorge raramente nelle prime ore del mattino, mentre è più frequente durante l'orario scolastico, in particolare in coincidenza con esami e compiti in classe. Benché si riscontrino casi di mal di testa continuo e persistente per settimane, solitamente il dolore, dopo aver raggiunto un picco di intensità, tende a calare durante il giorno. La cefalea è descritta come urente e bruciante, ma raramente è percepita come pulsante. Nella maggior parte dei casi, il dolore è distribuito nella regione frontale, ma può risultare localizzato sul vertice o nell'area occipitale. A differenza dell'emicrania o della cefalea da aumento dell'ICP, la cefalea da tensione non è, di regola, associata a nausea e vomito.

La **diagnosi** è formulata per esclusione, dopo il completamento dell'anamnesi e dell'esame obiettivo. Esami come l'EEG e la TC sono raramente necessari. Il trattamento prevede la ricerca dei fattori emotivi stressanti sottostanti. La capacità di comprensione del bambino dell'origine della propria cefalea è spesso sorprendente. Quando ne ha la possibilità, il bambino è spesso ansioso di condividere con il medico i suoi conflitti e le sue preoccupazioni, collegati a una scarsa autostima, alla paura del fallimento scolastico e alla mancanza di fiducia nelle proprie capacità. Talvolta la depressione infantile si esprime attraverso il sintomo del cefalea. Questi pazienti lamentano anche improvvisi cambiamenti di umore, perdita di peso, anoressia, disturbi del sonno, affaticamento e una scarsa partecipazione alle attività sociali. Un eccessivo consumo di caffeina o l'astinenza acuta da caffeina possono essere associati alla cefalea. Anche il consumo quotidiano di cola o di caffè può causare cefalea. La graduale eliminazione di queste sostanze consente la remissione dei sintomi.

Il **trattamento** della cefalea tensiva prevede la rassicurazione del paziente e la spiegazione delle modalità attraverso le quali lo stress causa il disturbo. L'ansia può determinare una costante contrazione isometrica dei muscoli temporale, massetere e trapezio, responsabili del caratteristico dolore sordo e bruciante. È opportuno favorire l'eliminazione delle situazioni ansiogene più ovvie. In alcuni casi, è possibile ricorrere alla somministrazione di paracetamolo o altri analgesici blandi, mentre sedativi e antidepressivi sono raramente necessari. I pazienti che soffrono di cefalee gravi possono trarre beneficio da un breve ricovero in ospedale, in particolare se il disturbo depressivo sottostante viene riconosciuto e affrontato. L'ambiente ospedaliero fornisce l'opportunità allo staff medico di osservare l'interazione del bambino con gli altri e le dinamiche familiari prima di formulare un piano per il counseling o l'intervento psichiatrico. Nella maggior parte dei casi, durante l'osservazione i sintomi si attenuano. Come per l'emicrania, le tecniche di biofeedback e di autoipnosi sono efficaci nel trattamento della cefalea da tensione in alcuni pazienti.

Brandes JL, Kudrow D, Stark SR, et al: Sumatriptan-naproxen for acute treatment of migraine. *JAMA* 2007;297:1443–1454.
Brousseau DC, Duffy SJ, Anderson AC, et al: Treatment of pediatric migraine headaches: A randomized, double-blind trial of prochlorperazine versus ketorolac. *Ann Emerg Med* 2004;43:256–262.
Colman I, Brown MD, Innes GD, et al: Parenteral metoclopramide for acute migraine: Meta-analysis of randomized controlled trials. *Br Med J* 2004;329:1369–1372.
Fuller G, Kaye C: Headaches. *BMJ* 2007;334:254–256.
Goadsby PJ, Kullmann DM: Another migraine gene. *Lancet* 2005;366: S345–S346.
Goadsby PJ, Lipton RB, Ferrari MD: Migraine—Current understanding and treatment. *N Engl J Med* 2002;346:257–270.
Hämäläinen ML, Hoppu K, Santavuouri P: Sumatriptan for migraine attacks in children: A randomized placebo-controlled study. *Neurology* 1997;48:1100–1103.
Hämäläinen ML, Hoppu K, Valkeila E, et al: Ibuprofen and acetaminophen for the acute treatment of migraine in children: A double-blind, randomized, placebo controlled, crossover study. *Neurology* 1997;48:103–107.
Hering-Hanit R, Gadoth N: Caffeine-induced headache in children and adolescents. *Cephalalgia* 2003;23:332–335.
Lewis D: Practice parameter: Pharmacological treatment of migraine headache in children and adolescents. *Neurology* 2004;63:2215–2224.
Lewis DW: Toward the definition of childhood migraine. *Curr Opin Pediatr* 2004;16:628–636.
Mack KJ: What incites new daily persistent headache in children? *Pediatr Neurol* 2004;31:122–125.
Medical Letter: Topiramate (Topamax) for prevention of migraine. *Med Lett Drugs Ther* 2005;47:9–10.
Olness H, MacDonald JT, Uden DL: Comparison of self-hypnosis and propranolol in the treatment of juvenile classic migraine. *Pediatrics* 1987;79:593–597.
Silberstein SD: Migraine. *Lancet* 2004;363:381–391.
Victor S, Ryan SW: Drugs for preventing migraine headaches in children. *Cochrane Database Syst Rev* 2003;4:CD002761.
Winner P, Rothner AD, Saper J, et al: A randomized double-blind placebo-controlled study of sumatriptan nasal spray in the treatment of acute migraine in adolescents. *Pediatrics* 2000;106:989–997.

Capitolo 596 ■ Sindromi neurocutanee

Robert H.A. Haslam

Le sindromi neurocutanee includono un gruppo eterogeneo di malattie, caratterizzate da anomalie a carico del sistema nervoso centrale (SNC) e della cute. La maggior parte dei disturbi è di tipo familiare e si ritiene derivi da un difetto nella differenziazione dell'ectoderma primitivo. Il gruppo comprende le neurofibromatosi, la sclerosi tuberosa, la sindrome di Sturge-Weber, la malattia di von Hippel-Lindau, la sindrome PHACE, l'atassia-teleangiectasia, la sindrome del nevo lineare, l'ipomelanosi di Ito (vedi Capitolo 652) e l'incontinentia pigmenti (vedi Capitolo 651).

596.1 • Neurofibromatosi

La neurofibromatosi (NF), o malattia di von Recklinghausen, è un disturbo comune autosomico dominante. La malattia è proteiforme, dal momento che può colpire virtualmente tutti i sistemi e gli organi, e progressiva perché, sebbene alcune caratteristiche distintive siano presenti dalla nascita, lo sviluppo delle complicanze è ritardato per decadi. La NF è il risultato di un'anomalia della differenziazione e migrazione della cresta neurale durante le fasi precoci dell'embriogenesi (vedi anche Capitolo 651).

MANIFESTAZIONI CLINICHE E DIAGNOSI. Si riscontrano due forme distinte di NF. La **NF-1** è il tipo prevalente, con un'incidenza di 1/4000. È diagnosticata in presenza di almeno due dei sette segni seguenti. (1) Sei o più macchie caffellatte dal diametro superiore di 5 mm nei soggetti prepuberi e di 15 mm negli individui postpuberi. Tali segni costituiscono il tratto distintivo della malattia e sono presenti nel 100% dei casi. Presenti fin dalla nascita, le macchie aumentano di numero e dimensioni nel corso del tempo, in particolare nel primo anno di vita, assumendo una differente pigmentazione. Sono distribuite su tutta la superficie del corpo, ma si concentrano soprattutto sul tronco e sugli arti, risparmiando spesso il volto. (2) Efelidi nella regione ascellare o inguinale, costituite da aree di iperpigmentazione del diametro di 2-3 mm. (3) Due o più noduli di Lisch, amartomi dell'iride identificabili mediante esame con lampada a fessura (Fig. 596-1), presenti nel 75% dei pazienti con NF-1 (ma non in quelli con NF-2). La prevalenza dei noduli di Lisch aumenta con l'età, dal

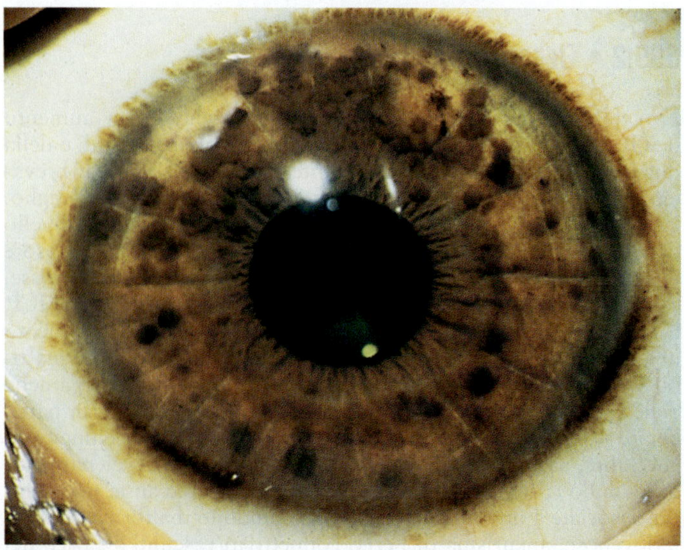

Figura 596-1. Neurofibromatosi 1 (NF-1). Amartoma pigmentato dell'iride (noduli di Lish). (Tratta da Zitelli BJ, Davis HW: *Atlas of Pediatric Physical Diagnosis*, 4th ed. St. Louis, Mosby, 2002, p 507.)

5% nei bambini con meno di 3 anni al 42% nei pazienti con 3-4 anni, fino al 100% degli adulti. (4) Due o più neurofibromi o un neurofibroma plessiforme. Tipicamente, i neurofibromi colpiscono la cute, ma possono essere localizzati anche lungo i nervi periferici, i vasi sanguigni e all'interno dei visceri (incluso il tratto gastrointestinale). Il fatto che queste lesioni compaiano solitamente durante l'adolescenza o la gravidanza suggerisce un'influenza ormonale. Piccole e di aspetto gommoso, le lesioni causano una leggera discromia violacea della cute. I neurofibromi plessiformi, solitamente evidenti fin dalla nascita, sono il risultato del diffuso ispessimento di tronchi nervosi e tipicamente sono localizzati nelle regioni orbitali e temporali del volto. La cute che li ricopre può risultare ancor più iperpigmentata delle macchie caffellatte. Tali neurofibromi possono causare un'ipertrofia e una conseguente deformità dell'osso corrispondente. (5) Una lesione ossea caratteristica come una displasia dello sfenoide (che può provocare esoftalmo pulsante) o un assottigliamento corticale delle ossa lunghe, con o senza pseudoartrosi. La scoliosi è la manifestazione ortopedica più comune della NF-1, ma non è sufficientemente specifica da essere inclusa nei criteri diagnostici. (6) Gliomi ottici, tumori relativamente benigni composti da cellule gliali e materiale mucinoso, sono presenti in circa il 15% dei casi. La maggior parte dei pazienti con glioma ottico è asintomatica e ha una visione normale o pressoché normale; circa il 20% presenta disturbi visivi o manifesta un precoce sviluppo sessuale secondario all'invasione tumorale dell'ipotalamo. I tumori del nervo ottico sintomatici tipicamente producono sintomi prima dei 6 anni di età. I bambini sono raramente consapevoli della perdita unilaterale della vista e ciò può ritardarne la diagnosi. I pazienti con glioma ottico unilaterale tipicamente mostrano un difetto pupillare afferente, diagnosticabile stimolando alternativamente ciascun occhio con una sorgente luminosa. La pupilla colpita si dilata invece di costringersi, mentre la luce diretta verso l'occhio sano causa un'identica costrizione di entrambe le pupille. La NF-1 e il neuroma plessiforme della palpebra presentano un elevato rischio di associazione con un glioma ottico omolaterale. I reperti di RM del glioma ottico includono diffuso ispessimento, allargamento localizzato o una massa focale originata dal nervo ottico o dal chiasma. (7) Un parente di primo grado con NF-1, la cui diagnosi è stata formulata sulla base dei criteri sopramenzionati. La maggior parte delle mutazioni di NF-1 si verifica nella linea germinale paterna. Il gene per NF-1, localizzato nella regione del cromosoma 17q11.2, codifica tutti gli mRNA di 11-13kb contenenti almeno 59 esoni che producono la proteina neurofibromina. Sono state finora segnalate più di 300 mutazioni indipendenti del gene per NF-1.

I bambini con NF-1 presentano un rischio elevato di sviluppare **complicanze neurologiche**. Studi effettuati con RM su bambini selezionati hanno dimostrato la presenza di anomali segnali pesati in T_2 in tratti ottici, tronco encefalico, globo pallido, talamo, capsula interna e cervelletto. Tali segnali, detti **UBO** (***Unidentified Bright Object***), tendono a scomparire con l'età; nella maggior parte dei casi non sono più percepibili dopo i 30 anni. È ipotizzabile che gli UBO, non rilevabili con la TC, costituiscano aree di demielinizzazione o aree focali di aumento del contenuto d'acqua (Fig. 596-2). Si registrano differenze di opinione riguardo alla presenza e al numero di UBO e al loro collegamento con i disturbi dell'apprendimento, con i deficit dell'attenzione, con i disturbi del linguaggio e con le difficoltà comportamentali e psicosociali che si riscontrano nel 40-60% dei bambini affetti da NF-1. Un'altra complicanza frequente è costituita dalle convulsioni cloniche parziali complesse o generalizzate. L'idrocefalo è una manifestazione rara, secondaria a stenosi acqueduttale, mentre la macrocefalia (con ventricoli di dimensioni normali) è di comune riscontro. I vasi sanguigni possono sviluppare aneurismi o una stenosi responsabile della sindrome di Moyamoya (vedi Fig. 601-2). Le sequele neurologiche di queste anomalie vascolari includono attacchi ischemici cerebrovascolari transitori, emiparesi e deficit cognitivi. I disturbi psicologici sono prevalenti, a causa della gravità e della incertezza proprie della malattia. La pubertà precoce può risultare evidente sia in presenza sia in assenza di lesioni di chiasma ottico e ipotalamo. Anche le neoplasie maligne costituiscono un problema significativo nei pazienti con NF-1. Occasionalmente, un neurofibroma può trasformarsi in neurofibrosarcoma o in schwannoma maligno. I pazienti con NF-1 rischiano di sviluppare ipertensione, causata da una stenosi vascolare renale o da un feocromocitoma. L'incidenza di feocromocitomi, rabdomiosarcomi, leucemie e tumori di Wilson è più elevata rispetto alla popolazione generale. Si riscontra inoltre un'insolita associazione tra NF-1 e leucemia mieloide, come tra NF-1 e xantogranuloma giovanile. Le patologie associate maggiormente responsabili di morbilità e mortalità sono i tumori del SNC, che includono gliomi ottici, meningiomi cerebrali e midollari, neurofibromi, astrocitomi e neurilemmomi a causa della loro aumentata incidenza nel paziente con NF-1.

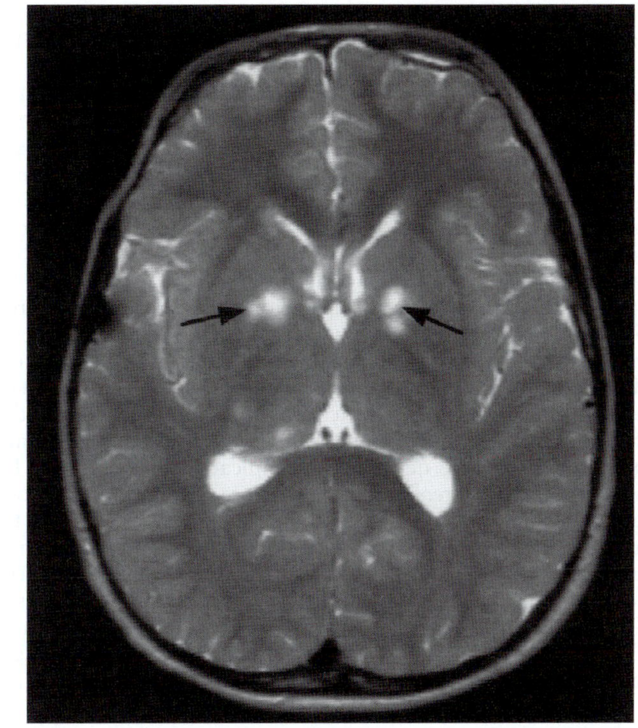

Figura 596-2. RM pesata in T_2 di un paziente con neurofibromatosi. Notare la presenza di segnali iperintensi (UBO) in un'area dei gangli basali (*frecce*).

Con un'incidenza di 1/50 000, la **NF-2** è responsabile del 10% di tutti i casi di NF. È diagnosticata in presenza di uno dei due criteri seguenti: (1) *masse bilaterali sull'ottavo nervo cranico*, compatibili con una diagnosi di neurinoma acustico (dimostrabile mediante TC o RM). (2) *Un genitore, un fratello o un figlio con NF-2* e la presenza di masse unilaterali sull'ottavo nervo o due dei disturbi seguenti: neurofibroma, meningioma, glioma, schwannoma o opacità lenticolare subcapsulare posteriore giovanile. I **neurinomi acustici bilaterali** costituiscono la caratteristica distintiva della NF-2. I sintomi di perdita uditiva, debolezza facciale, mal di testa o instabilità possono comparire già durante l'infanzia, mentre i segni di una massa a livello dell'angolo cerebellopontino si presentano più comunemente nella seconda e terza decade. Gli studi di linkage hanno dimostrato che il gene per NF-2 è localizzato vicino al centro del braccio lungo del cromosoma 22q1.11.

TRATTAMENTO. In assenza di un trattamento specifico per la NF, la gestione include il *counseling* genetico e la diagnosi precoce di complicanze curabili. Il National Institutes of Health (NIH) suggerisce di basare la scelta degli esami di laboratorio sui risultati della valutazione clinica. Nei pazienti asintomatici, gli esami di laboratorio, in particolare i potenziali evocati, l'EEG, la TC e la RM sono raramente utili. Le indicazione per gli esami di neuroimaging sono controverse, mentre si riscontra un generale consenso sull'opportunità di sottoporre tempestivamente a esame tutti i casi sintomatici (con perdita o disturbi visivi, proptosi, sintomi e segni di aumento della pressione intracranica). La NIH Consensus Development Conference ha criticato l'abitudine di effettuare di routine esami di imaging cerebrale e dei tratti ottici nei bambini NF-1 asintomatici, che richiedono raramente il trattamento. Si raccomandano piuttosto un'anamnesi dettagliata e un esame obiettivo approfondito, seguiti da un esame oftalmologico, da ripetersi a cadenza annuale fino ai 10 anni. In seguito, è sufficiente che il paziente si sottoponga a periodiche valutazioni visive di routine. Un genitore con NF presenta il 50% di rischio di trasmettere la malattia ai figli. Il tipo di NF (NF-1 o NF-2) "si riproduce direttamente" nelle generazioni successive. Poiché circa il 50% dei casi di NF è il risultato di mutazioni *de novo*, ciascun genitore dovrebbe essere esaminato attentamente (senza trascurare la ricerca dei noduli di Lisch) prima del *counseling* sui rischi di trasmissione. L'analisi diagnostica del DNA standard non è utile per lo screening prenatale del gene per NF-1, a causa delle grandi dimensioni del gene e del numero significativo di mutazioni. La diagnosi prenatale è realizzabile soltanto se la mutazione responsabile della malattia è presente in uno dei genitori ed è già nota. La maggior parte dei casi di NF-2 sono il risultato di una mutazione. L'esame del DNA fetale, con ricerca del caratteristico polimorfismo conformazionale di una sequenza DNA alterata, costituisce un test prenatale attendibile. Nei casi familiari, la disponibilità di membri affetti e non dalla malattia consente l'analisi del linkage, che rende possibile una diagnosi prenatale abbastanza accurata.

596.2 • Sclerosi tuberosa

La sclerosi tuberosa (ST) è una malattia autosomica dominante a penetranza variabile, con una prevalenza di 1/6000. Mutazioni genetiche spontanee si verificano in circa il 75% dei casi. Studi di genetica molecolare hanno identificato due foci per il complesso ST. Il gene *TSC1* è localizzato sul cromosoma 9q34, e il gene *TSC2* sul cromosoma 16p13. Il trascritto 8.6-kb *TSC1* codifica per una proteina di 130kd chiamata *amartina*. Il gene *TSC2* codifica per la proteina *tuberina*. Amartina e tuberina agiscono in sincronia come un singolo complesso molecolare a livello dell'apparato del Golgi. La ST è una malattia eterogenea, caratterizzata da uno ampio spettro clinico, che va dal ritardo mentale grave associato a convulsioni disabilitanti a casi con intelligenza nella norma e assenza di crisi convulsive, spesso nell'ambito di una stessa famiglia. Di regola, la precocità dell'esordio dei sintomi di ST è collegata al rischio di ritardo mentale. La malattia colpisce diversi sistemi di organi oltre alla cute e al sistema nervoso tra cui il cuore, i reni, gli occhi, i polmoni e le ossa.

DIAGNOSI

La ST è diagnosticata in presenza di almeno due criteri maggiori oppure di uno maggiore e due minori. I criteri maggiori includono lesioni cutanee, lesioni oculari e cerebrali e tumori a carico di cuore, reni o polmoni. I criteri minori includono cisti ossee, polipi rettali, aree di rarefazione dello smalto dentale, anomalie della migrazione della sostanza bianca cerebrale, fibromi gengivali, amartomi nonrenali, chiazze retiniche acromiche, lesioni cutanee ipopigmentate dette "coriandoli" e cisti renali multiple.

MANIFESTAZIONI CLINICHE

LESIONI CUTANEE. Oltre il 90% dei casi mostra le tipiche macule ipomelanotiche a forma di foglia di frassino localizzate su tronco e arti. La visualizzazione delle macule ipomelanotiche è agevolata dall'uso di una lampada di Wood a luce ultravioletta, in particolare nel lattante (vedi Capitolo 553). La diagnosi richiede la presenza di almeno 3 macule ipomelanotiche. Gli adenomi sebacei si sviluppano tra i 4 e i 6 anni e inizialmente appaiono come minuscoli noduli rosa su naso e guance, talvolta confusi con acne (Fig. 596-3). In seguito, tendono a fondersi e ingrandirsi, assumendo un aspetto carnoso. Anche la cosiddetta *shagreen patch* (chiazza zigrinata) è caratteristica della ST e consiste in una lesione rilevata e ruvida, con una consistenza a buccia d'arancia, localizzata prevalentemente nella regione lombosacrale. I fibromi subungueali e periungueali originano dallo strato lucido delle dita e sono comuni nell'adolescenza.

LESIONI RETINICHE E CEREBRALI. Le lesioni retiniche si distinguono in due tipi: i tumori moriformi che originano intorno alla testa del nervo, lesioni grigie e piatte nella regione del disco (Fig. 596-4), e amartomi o aree di depigmentazione. Le più comuni manifestazioni neurologiche della ST includono convulsioni, deficit cognitivo e anomalie comportamentali (tra cui l'autismo). La lesione cerebrale caratteristica è costituita dai tuberi cerebrali. Essi sono localizzati sulle circonvoluzioni degli emisferi cerebrali e sono inoltre presenti nella regione subependimale, dove vanno incontro a calcificazione e proiezione nella cavità ventricolare, assumendo un aspetto a candela colante. I tuberi presenti nella regione del forame di Monro possono causare l'ostruzione del flusso del liquido cerebrospinale, con conseguente idrocefalo. Su piano microscopico, nei tuberi si osserva una riduzione del numero di neuroni, una proliferazione di astrociti e la presenza di neuroni giganti multinucleati dalla forma bizzarra. Le RM pesate in T_2 contribuiscono all'identificazione delle lesioni. In

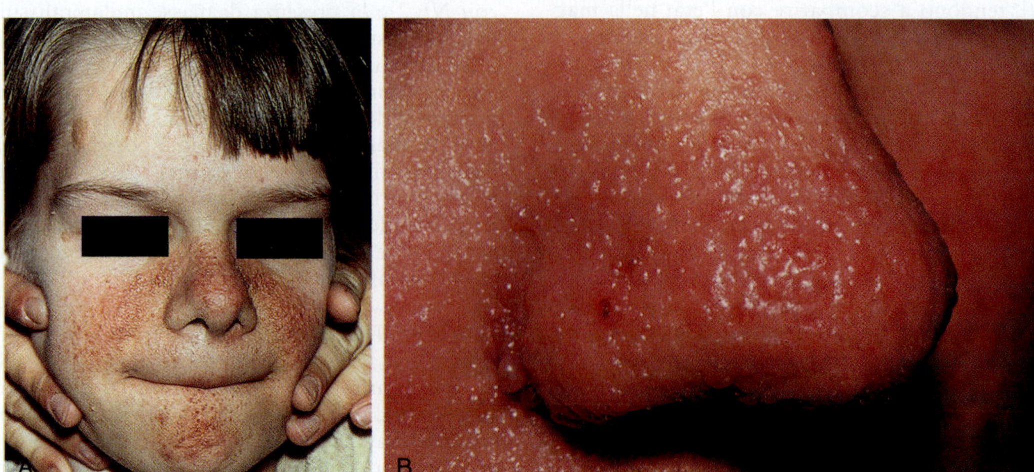

Figura 596-3. Sclerosi tuberosa. *A*, Adolescente con adenoma sebaceo dalla caratteristica distribuzione malare e lesioni al mento. *B*, Immagine ravvicinata delle lesioni nasali. (Tratta da Zitelli BJ, Davis HW: *Atlas of Pediatric Physical Diagnosis*, 4th ed. St. Louis, Mosby, 2002, p 509.)

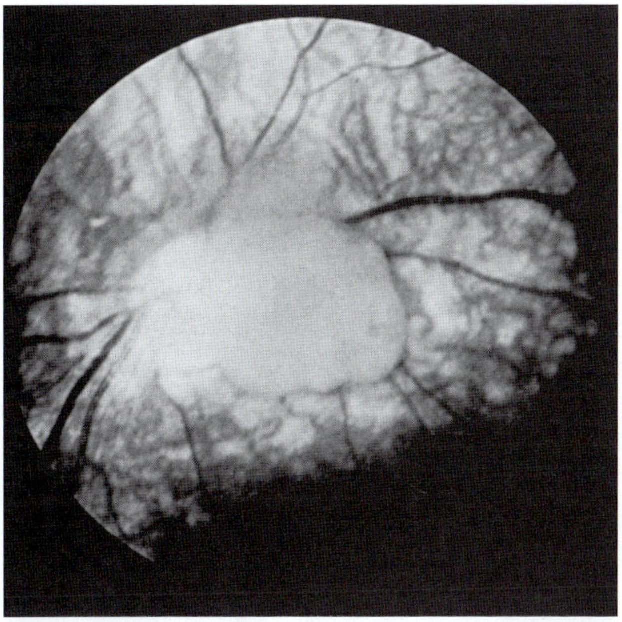

Figura 596-4. Lesione moriforme della retina in un paziente con sclerosi tuberosa.

generale, il numero di tuberi è direttamente collegato alla compromissione neurologica del paziente. I tumori cerebrali sono molto meno comuni rispetto alla NF, ma talvolta un tubero può trasformarsi in un astrocitoma subependimale maligno a cellule giganti. Dopo i 3-4 anni di età, la TC mostra tipicamente la presenza di tuberi calcificati nell'area periventricolare (Fig. 596-5). La ST può manifestarsi durante l'infanzia con spasmi infantili e EEG ipsaritmico. Le convulsioni sono talvolta difficili da controllare e, in uno stadio successivo, possono trasformarsi in epilessia mioclonica (vedi Capitolo 593). In Europa e Canada, gli spasmi infantili associati a ST sono trattati efficacemente con vigabatrin (e non con l'ormone adrenocorticotropo), ma negli Stati Uniti il farmaco non è disponibile. Nei bambini con ST e con spasmi infantili si riscontra un'elevata incidenza di deficit cognitivi, comportamento aggressivo e autismo. Molti altri pazienti con ST possiedono intelligenza nella norma e anomalie neurologiche minime.

LESIONI A CARICO DI ALTRI ORGANI. Circa il 50% dei bambini con ST presenta rabdomiomi cardiaci, individuabili nel feto a rischio mediante ecocardiogramma. I rabdomiomi possono essere numerosi o localizzarsi all'apice del ventricolo sinistro. Benché possano causare insufficienza cardiaca congestiva e aritmia, tendono a risolversi spontaneamente. Nei reni del 75-80% dei pazienti con età >10 anni si riscontrano angiomiolipomi, solitamente benigni. Cisti renali singole o multiple costituiscono un altro riscontro frequente. La lesione polmonare classica, più comune nelle femmine, è la linfangiomiomatosi.

DIAGNOSI

La diagnosi della ST si basa su di un elevato indice di sospetto durante la valutazione di un bambino con spasmi infantili. Una accurata ricerca delle lesioni cutanee e retiniche tipiche della malattia è indispensabile in tutti i pazienti con disturbo convulsivo. La TC o la RM della testa confermano la diagnosi nella maggior parte dei casi. La verifica genetica delle mutazioni *TSC1* e *TSC2* è attualmente disponibile ed è utile nei pazienti che non soddisfano tutti i criteri clinici. La possibilità di ricorrere alla diagnosi prenatale è offerta alla famiglie in cui è nota la presenza di una mutazione ST.

TRATTAMENTO

La gestione della malattia prevede il controllo delle convulsioni. Gli esami di base raccomandati includono l'ecografia renale, l'ecocardiogramma e la radiografia toracica, seguiti dai necessari follow-up. Sintomi e segni di aumento della pressione intracranica suggeriscono un'ostruzione del forame di Monro da parte di un tubero o di una trasformazione maligna di un tubero, tale complicanza richiede una verifica immediata e un tempestivo intervento chirurgico.

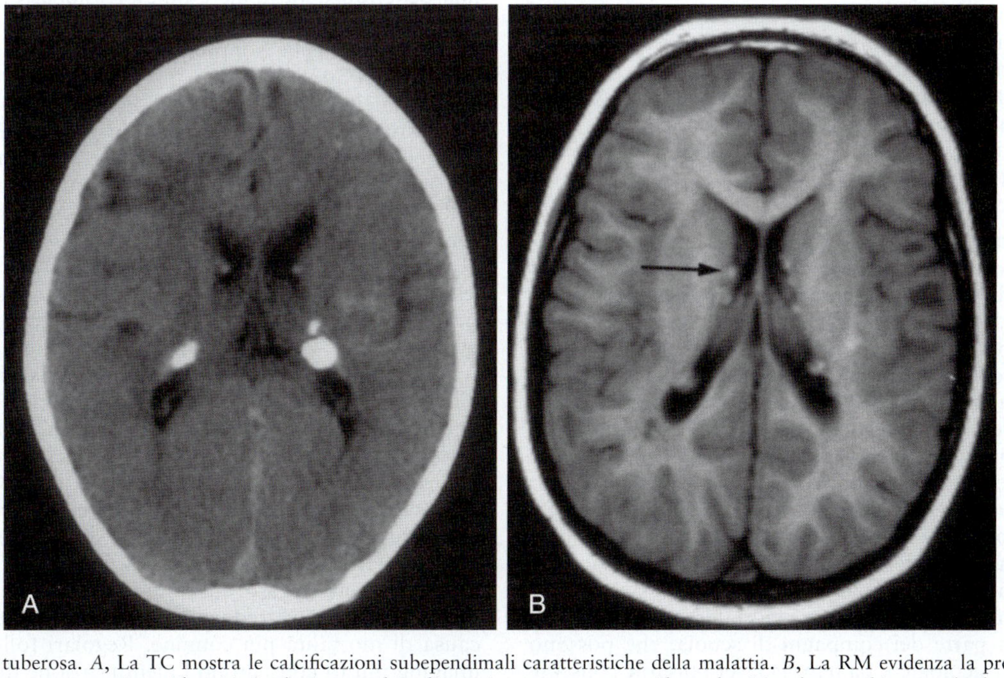

Figura 596-5. Sclerosi tuberosa. *A*, La TC mostra le calcificazioni subependimali caratteristiche della malattia. *B*, La RM evidenza la presenza di noduli subependimali multipli in uno stesso paziente (*freccia*). I tuberi parenchimali appaiono come aree a ridotta densità nel parenchima cerebrale sia nelle immagini TC sia in quelle RM.

596.3 • Sindrome di Sturge-Weber

Questa sindrome sporadica comprende una costellazione di sintomi e segni, che includono nevo facciale (macchia vino porto), convulsioni, emiparesi, episodi simil-ictus, calcificazioni intracraniche e, in molti casi, ritardo mentale. Si verifica in forma sporadica con una frequenza di circa 1/50 000 nati vivi.

EZIOLOGIA. Si ritiene che la malattia sia il risultato di uno sviluppo anomalo del letto vascolare primitivo negli stadi iniziali della vascolarizzazione, quando si verifica una riorganizzazione dell'apporto di sangue a cervello, meningi e volto, mentre l'ectoderma primitivo si differenzia in cute facciale e lobo occipitale del cervello. Nei pazienti portatori della sindrome, le sovrastanti leptomeningi risultano riccamente vascolarizzate, mentre il cervello sottostante diviene atrofico e calcificato, in particolare nello strato molecolare della corteccia.

MANIFESTAZIONI CLINICHE. Il nevo facciale è presente fin dalla nascita; solitamente unilaterale, è spesso localizzato nella parte superiore del volto o sulla palpebra, ma può riscontrarsi anche nella parte inferiore del volto, nel tronco, nella mucosa buccale o sulla faringe. Non tutti i bambini con nevi facciali sono affetti dalla sindrome di Sturge-Weber (vedi Capitolo 649). Buftalmo e glaucoma dell'occhio omolaterale costituiscono complicanze comuni. Il disturbo convulsivo si sviluppa nella maggior parte dei pazienti nel corso del primo anno di vita. Le convulsioni sono tipicamente focali tonico-cloniche, localizzate sul lato controlaterale rispetto al nevo facciale. Gli attacchi possono diventare refrattari agli anticonvulsivanti e, in molti casi, sono associati a un'emiparesi a lenta progressione. I frequenti episodi simil-ictus transitori o deficit visivi persistenti per diversi giorni (non collegati alle convulsioni) sono probabilmente il risultato di trombosi delle vene corticali nella regione colpita. Benché lo sviluppo neurologico appaia normale nel primo anno di vita, nella tarda infanzia si riscontrano ritardo mentale e gravi disturbi dell'apprendimento in almeno il 50% dei bambini, probabilmente a causa delle prolungate convulsioni generalizzate e della progressiva atrofia cerebrale, secondaria all'ipossia locale e all'assunzione di anticonvulsivanti.

DIAGNOSI. Nella maggior parte dei pazienti, la radiografia del cranio evidenzia un calcificazione intracranica nella regione occipitale, che assume un aspetto tortuoso. La TC mostra l'estensione della calcificazione, solitamente associata ad atrofia corticale unilaterale e dilatazione omolaterale del ventricolo laterale (Fig. 596-6). La RM è utile per delineare le dimensioni e la localizzazione della malformazione vascolare e diagnosticare la presenza di lesioni della sostanza bianca.

TRATTAMENTO. Il trattamento, che richiede un approccio multidisciplinare, mira a ottenere il controllo delle convulsioni e ad affrontare i disturbi comportamentali e di apprendimento. Le convulsioni a esordio infantile non risultano sempre associate a deficit dello sviluppo neurologico. Nei pazienti con disturbo convulsivo sotto controllo e sviluppo normale o pressoché normale, la gestione della malattia prevede l'assunzione di anticonvulsivanti e controlli periodici per diagnosticare eventuali complicanze, come glaucoma, buftalmo e anomalie comportamentali. Se le convulsioni sono refrattarie agli anticonvulsivanti, nella maggior parte dei centri specializzati si raccomanda la emisferectomia, in particolare nei primi 1-2 anni e se gli attacchi hanno origine prevalentemente da un emisfero. A causa del rischio di glaucoma, è opportuno effettuare misurazioni regolari della pressione endoculare mediante un tonometro. Il nevo facciale è spesso oggetto di prese in giro da parte dei compagni di scuola, che possono causare un trauma psicologico. La terapia laser pulsatile consente di ottenere ottimi risultati nello schiarire le macchie, in particolare se localizzate sulle fronte. A causa dell'elevata frequenza di disabilità evolutive, i pazienti richiedono spesso interventi educativi specifici.

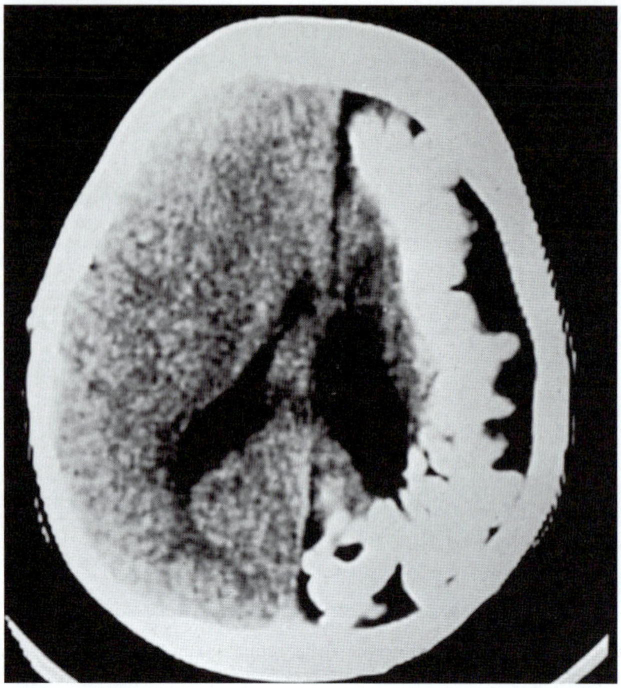

Figura 596-6. Immagine TC di un paziente con sindrome di Sturge-Weber, che mostra la presenza di calcificazione unilaterale e sottostante atrofia dell'emisfero cerebrale.

596.4 • Malattia di von Hippel-Lindau

Come la maggior parte delle sindromi neurocutanee, la malattia di von Hippel-Lindau colpisce diversi organi, inclusi il cervelletto, il midollo spinale, il bulbo, la retina, i reni, il pancreas e l'epididimo. Ereditata con modalità autosomica dominante, presenta una penetranza variabile e un'espressione ritardata. La malattia ha un'incidenza di 1/36 000 ed è causata da mutazioni della linea germinale del gene soppressore tumorale VHL, localizzato sul cromosoma 3p25-26.

Le principali caratteristiche della malattia includono emangioblastoma cerebellare e angiomi retinici. L'emangioblastoma cerebellare si manifesta nella prima età adulta (o in seguito) con sintomi e segni di un aumento della pressione intracranica. Un ridotto numero di pazienti presenta emangioblastoma del midollo spinale, causa di anomalie della propriocezione, disturbi della deambulazione e disfunzione vescicale. TC e RM mostrano una lesione cerebellare cistica con un nodulo vascolare murale. La rimozione chirurgica totale del tumore è risolutiva.

Circa il 25% dei pazienti con emangioblastoma cerebellare sviluppa angiomi retinici, caratterizzati da piccole masse di capillari dalle pareti sottili, irrorati da arteriole e venule tortuose. Poiché sono solitamente localizzati nella retina periferica, non compromettono la visione. L'essudato nella regione dell'angioma può causare distacco retinico e perdita visiva. Gli angiomi retinici sono trattati mediante fotocoagulazione e criocoagulazione, con buoni risultati.

La malattia è spesso associata a lesioni cistiche a carico di reni, pancreas, fegato ed epididimo. Anche l'associazione con feocromocitoma è frequente. Il carcinoma renale costituisce la causa di mortalità più comune. Regolari follow-up ed esami di imaging mirati consentono l'identificazione di queste lesioni allo stadio iniziale.

596.5 • Sindrome del nevo lineare

Questa malattia sporadica è caratterizzata dalla presenza di un nevo facciale e da anomalie neuroevolutive. Il nevo è localizzato sulla fronte o sul naso, solitamente lungo la linea mediana. Appena visibile durante l'infanzia, in seguito diviene ipercheratonico e assume un colore giallo-bruno. Più del 50% dei pazienti presenta un disturbo convulsivo e ritardo mentale. Le convulsioni possono essere di tipo generalizzato, mioclonico o motorio focale. I risultati della TC sono spesso normali, ma sono stati segnalati casi di riscontro di emimeganencefalia con alterazioni amartomatose. I segni neurologici focali più comuni includono emiparesi ed emianopsia omonima.

596.6 • Sindrome PHACE

L'acronimo PHACE indica la presenza contemporanea di malformazione della fossa *p*osteriore, emangioma (*hemangiomas*), anomalie *a*rteriose, *c*oartazione dell'aorta e altri difetti cardiaci e anomalie oculari (*eye abnormalities*). Emangiomi facciali di grandi dimensioni possono essere associati a malformazione di Dandy-Walker, anomalie vascolari (coartazione dell'aorta, aplasia o ipoplasia delle arterie carotidi, aneurismi carotidei, succlavia sinistra aberrante), glaucoma, cataratta, microftalmia, ipoplasia del nervo ottico e difetti della parete ventrale (fessure sternali). L'emangioma facciale è tipicamente omolaterale rispetto all'arco aortico. Si riscontra una predominanza femminile. Gli emangiomi delle vie aeree possono causare ostruzioni. L'interferone-α è utile nel trattamento degli emangiomi.

American Academy of Pediatrics Committee on Genetics: Health supervision for children with neurofibromatosis. *Pediatrics* 1995;96:368–372.
Cnossen MH, de Goede-Bolder A, van den Broek KM, et al: A prospective 10 year follow up study of patients with neurofibromatosis type 1. *Arch Dis Child* 1998;78:408–412.
Crino PB, Nathanson KL, Henske EP: The tuberous sclerosis complex. *N Engl J Med* 2006;355:1345–1356.
Gutmann DH, Aylsworth A, Carey JC, et al: The diagnostic evaluation and multidisciplinary management of neurofibromatosis 1 and neurofibromatosis 2. *JAMA* 1997;278:51–57.
Hofman KJ, Harris EL, Bryan RN, et al: Neurofibromatosis type 1: The cognitive phenotype. *J Pediatr* 1994;124:S1–S8.
Hurst RW, Newman SA, Cail WS: Multifocal intracranial MR abnormalities in neurofibromatosis. *AJNR Am J Neuroradiol* 1988;9:293–296.
Hymann MH, Whittemore VH: National Institutes of Health Consensus Conference: Tuberous sclerosis complex. *Arch Neurol* 2000;57:662–665.
Jozwiak S, Kawalec W, Dluzewska J, et al: Cardiac tumors in tuberous sclerosis: Their incidence and course. *Eur J Pediatr* 1994;153:155–157.
Kossoff EH, Buck C, Freeman JM: Outcomes of 32 hemispherectomies for Sturge-Weber syndrome worldwide. *Neurology* 2002;59:1735–1738.
Latif F, Tory K, Gmarra J, et al: Identification of the von Hippel-Lindau disease tumor suppressor gene. *Science* 1993;260:1317–1320.
Lazaro C, Gaona A, Ravella A, et al: Prenatal diagnosis of neurofibromatosis 1: From flanking RFLPS to intragene microsatellite markers. *Prenat Diagn* 1995;15:129–134.
Lovejoy FH, Boyle LE: Linear nevus sebaceous syndrome: Report of two cases and a review of the literature. *Pediatrics* 1973;52:382–387.
Maher ER, Kaelin WG Jr: von Hippel-Lindau disease. *Medicine* 1997;76:381–391.
Rizzo JF, Lessell S: Cerebrovascular abnormalities in neurofibromatosis type 1. *Neurology* 1994;44:1000–1002.
Roach ES, Williams MD, Laster MD: Magnetic resonance imaging in tuberous sclerosis. *Arch Neurol* 1987;44:301–303.
Seizinger BR, Martuza RL, Gusella JF: Loss of genes on chromosome 22 in tumorigenesis of human acoustic neuroma. *Nature* 1986;322:644–647.
Stumpf DA, Alksne JF, Annegers JF, et al: NIH Development Conference. Neurofibromatosis: Conference statement. *Arch Neurol* 1988;45:575–578.
Tan OT, Sherwood K, Gilchrest BA: Treatment of children with port-wine stains using the flashlamp-pulsed tunable dye laser. *N Engl J Med* 1989;320:416–421.

Capitolo 597 ■ Disturbi del movimento

Michael V. Johnston

I disturbi del movimento causano movimenti involontari e/o anomalie della postura, del tono, dell'equilibrio o del controllo della motricità fine. Il tipo di disturbo contribuisce alla localizzazione del processo patologico, mentre il suo esordio, l'età e il grado dell'anomalia dell'attività motoria aiutano a classificare il disturbo, orientando gli esami successivi.

597.1 • Atassie

L'atassia consiste nell'incapacità di eseguire movimenti coordinati e lineari, solitamente dovuta a un disturbo cerebellare e/o delle vie sensoriali delle colonne posteriori del midollo spinale. L'atassia, di tipo acuto a cronico (Tabb. 597-1 e 597-2), può essere generalizzata o coinvolgere prevalentemente la deambulazione, oppure mani e braccia. *Anomalie congenite* della fossa posteriore, come la sindrome di Dandy-Walker, la malformazione di Chiari e l'encefalocele, sono spesso associate ad atassia, a causa della distruzione o sostituzione del cervelletto (vedi Capitolo 592). L'**agenesia del verme cerebellare** si presenta nell'infanzia con ipotonia generalizzata e iporeflessia. Il ritardo nell'acquisizione delle tappe evolutive e l'atassia del tronco sono di comune riscontro. La **sindrome di Joubert** è un disturbo autosomico recessivo caratterizzato da agenesia del verme cerebellare, atassia, ipotonia, aprassia oculomotoria, disturbo della respirazione neonatale e ritardo mentale. Sono state identificate mutazioni del gene *AH11* (localizzato sul cromosoma 6), che codifica per la proteina Jouberina. Questo gene è espresso fortemente nel rombencefalo dell'embrione, in particolare nei neuroni che danno origine agli assoni del tratto corticospinale e i peduncoli cerebellari superiori (che nella sindrome di Joubert non si incrociano in maniera corretta). La RM è il metodo di elezione per l'esame di anomalie congenite di cervelletto, verme e strutture correlate. Nella sindrome di Joubert, la RM rivela un allargamento del quarto ventricolo a livello della giunzione tra mesencefalo e bulbo, che crea il "segno del dente molare".

TABELLA 597-1. Atassia acuta o ricorrente

Tumore cerebrale
Reazione di conversione
Ingestione di farmaci
Encefalite (troncoencefalica)
Disturbi genetici
Atassia ricorrente dominante
Atassia episodica di tipo 1
Atassia episodica di tipo 2
Malattia di Hartnup
Malattia delle urine a sciroppo d'acero
Deficit di piruvato deidrogenasi
Emicrania
Basilare
Vertigini parossistiche benigne
Disturbo postinfettivo/immune
Cerebellite postinfettiva acuta (varicella)
Sindrome di Miller Fisher
Sclerosi multipla
Encefalopatia mioclonica/neuroblastoma
Pseudoatassia (epilettica)
Trauma
Ematoma
Postconcussione
Occlusione vertebro-basilare
Disturbi vascolari
Emorragia cerebellare
Malattia di Kawasaki

TABELLA 597-2. Atassia cronica o progressiva

Tumori cerebrali
- Astrocitoma cerebellare
- Emangioblastoma cerebellare (malattia di von Hippel-Lindau)
- Ependimoma
- Medulloblastoma
- Tumori sopratentoriali

Malformazioni congenite
- Impronta basilare
- Aplasie cerebellari
- Aplasia dell'emisfero cerebellare
- Malformazione di Dandy-Walker
- Aplasia vermale
- Malformazione di Chiari

Atassie ereditarie
- A trasmissione autosomica dominante
- A trasmissione autosomica recessiva
  - Abetalipoproteinemia
  - Atassia-teleangiectasia
  - Atassia senza aprassia oculomotoria
  - Atassia con distonia episodica
  - Atassia di Friedreich
  - Malattia di Hartnup
  - Gangliosidosi GM_2 giovanile
  - Lipidosi sulfatidosi giovanile
  - Malattia delle urine a sciroppo d'acero
  - Sindrome di Marinesco-Sjögren
  - Deficit di piruvato deidrogenasi
  - Sindrome di Ramsay Hunt
  - Malattia di Refsum (HSMN IV)
  - Disturbi della catena respiratoria
- Trasmissione legata all'X
  - Adrenoleucodistrofia
  - Neuropatia ottica di Leber
  - Con demenza a esordio tardivo
  - Con sordità
  - Con sordità e perdita visiva

Tratta da Fenichel GM: *Clinical Pediatric Neurology*, 5th ed. Philadelphia, Elsevier, 2005, p 220.

Le *principali cause infettive* di atassia includono ascesso cerebrale, labirintite acuta e atassia cerebellare acuta. L'**atassia cerebellare acuta** si verifica prevalentemente nei bambini di 1-3 anni ed è diagnosticata per esclusione. Spesso l'insorgenza del disturbo segue di 2-3 settimane una malattia virale, come la varicella, l'infezione da coxsackievirus o echovirus, ed è considerata una risposta autoimmune all'agente virale che colpisce il cervelletto (vedi Capitoli 247, 250 e 602). L'esordio è improvviso e l'atassia del tronco può risultare talmente marcata da impedire al bambino di stare in piedi o di sedere. Il vomito può riscontrarsi nella fase iniziale, ma febbre e rigidità nucale sono assenti. Il nistagmo orizzontale è evidente in circa il 50% dei casi e la gravità della disartria nel caso il bambino sapesse già parlare può essere impressionante. L'esame del liquido cerebrospinale (LCS) è tipicamente normale all'esordio dell'atassia; una pleiocitosi linfocitica (10-30/mm^3) è comune. Durante il successivo decorso della malattia, la proteinorrachia subisce un moderato aumento. L'atassia comincia a migliorare dopo qualche settimana, ma può persistere fino a 2 mesi. La prognosi è eccellente; soltanto un ridotto numero di pazienti presenta sequele a lungo termine (disturbi comportamentali e del linguaggio, atassia e mancanza di coordinazione). Nel bambino piccolo, la **labirintite acuta** può essere difficile da distinguere dall'atassia cerebellare. Il disturbo è associato a infezioni dell'orecchio medio, intense vertigini, vomito e anomalie della funzione labirintica (evidenziate dal test calorico).

Le *cause tossiche di atassia* includono l'esposizione al tallio (usato come pesticida), l'assunzione di alcool e anticonvulsivanti, in particolare la fenitoina, quando il livello sierico supera i 30 μg/mL (120 μmol/L).

Nei casi di atassia si può riscontrare la presenza di *tumori cerebrali* (del cervelletto, del lobo frontale e neuroblastomi). I tumori del lobo frontale provocano atassia in seguito alla distruzione delle fibre che collegano il lobo frontale al cervelletto. I neuroblastomi possono essere associati a encefalopatia paraneoplastica, caratterizzata da atassia progressiva, spasmi mioclonici e opsoclono (oscillazioni orizzontali e verticali non ritmiche degli occhi).

Diversi *disturbi metabolici* sono caratterizzati da atassia, incluse l'abetalipoproteinemia, l'aciduria arginosuccinica e la malattia di Hartnup. L'**abetalipoproteinemia** (sindome di Bassen-Kornzweig) esordisce nell'infanzia, con steatorrea e deficit staturo-ponderale (vedi Capitolo 86.3). Lo striscio di sangue mostra acantocitosi e riduzione dei livelli sierici di colesterolo e trigliceridi; le β-lipoproteine sono assenti dal siero. I segni neurologici si evidenziano nella tarda infanzia e includono atassia, retinite pigmentosa, neurite periferica, anomalie della postura e del senso della vibrazione, debolezza muscolare e ritardo mentale. Nei pazienti con sintomi neurologici la vitamina E è indosabile.

Le *malattie degenerative* del sistema nervoso centrale (SNC) costituiscono un importante gruppo di disturbi atassici dell'infanzia, a causa delle conseguenze genetiche e della prognosi sfavorevole. La più comune è l'**atassia-teleangiectasia**, trasmessa con modalità autosomica recessiva, preannunciata dai sintomi di atassia, che esordiscono intorno ai 2 anni e progrediscono fino a causare la perdita della deambulazione nell'adolescenza (vedi Capitolo 125.2). L'atassia-teleangiectasia è causata da mutazioni del gene *ATM*, localizzato sul cromosoma 11q22-q23. ATM è una fosfatidilinositol-3 chinasi implicata nella fosforilazione delle proteine coinvolte nella riparazione del DNA e nel controllo del ciclo cellulare. L'aprassia oculomotoria dello sguardo, orizzontale, è definita come una difficoltà a fissare un oggetto, con conseguente tendenza a mancare il target a causa di movimenti laterali della testa, seguiti dal tentativo di rifissarlo. Sono di frequente riscontro anche strabismo, anomalie della saccade ipometrica e nistagmo. La teleangiectasia, che diviene evidente nella seconda infanzia, si riscontra sulla congiuntiva bulbare, sulla radice nasale, sulle orecchie e sulle superfici esposte degli arti. L'esame della cute mostra una perdita di elasticità. In più del 50% dei pazienti, le anomalie della funzione immunologica, spesso responsabili di infezioni sinopolmonari, includono una riduzione delle IgA sieriche e secretorie e dei livelli di IgG_2, IgG_4 e IgE. I bambini con atassia-teleangiectasia presentano un rischio da 50 a 100 volte superiore alla popolazione normale di sviluppare tumori linforeticolari (linfoma, leucemia e malattia di Hodgkin) e tumori cerebrali. Anomalie addizionali degli esami di laboratorio includono un aumento di incidenza di rotture cromosomiche, in particolare del cromosoma 14, e un aumento dei livelli di α-fetoproteina. Le infezioni e la disseminazione tumorale costituiscono le principali cause di mortalità.

L'**atassia di Friedreich**, ereditata con modalità autosomica recessiva, coinvolge i tratti spinocerebellari, le colonne dorsali del midollo spinale, i tratti piramidali, il cervelletto e il bulbo. La maggior parte dei pazienti è omozigote per un'espansione da ripetizione della tripletta GAA nella regione non codificante del gene che codifica per la proteina mitocondriale fratassina. Le mutazioni causano lesioni ossidative associate a un eccessivo accumulo di depositi di ferro mitocondriali. L'esordio dell'atassia è più tardivo rispetto all'atassia-teleangiectasia, ma solitamente avviene prima dei 10 anni. L'atassia progredisce lentamente, coinvolgendo maggiormente gli arti inferiori rispetto a quelli superiori. Il test di Romberg è positivo, mentre i riflessi tendinei profondi sono assenti (in particolare gli achillei); la riposta plantare è estensoria. I pazienti sviluppano un tipico eloquio esplosivo e disartrico; il nistagmo è presente nella maggioranza dei casi. Benché i pazienti possano apparire apatici, il livello intellettivo è risparmiato. Manifestano invece una significativa debolezza della muscolatura distale di mani e piedi. Si osserva tipicamente una marcata perdita dei sensi della vibrazione e della posizione, causata dalla degenerazione delle colonne posteriori e dalle alterazioni sensoriali indistinte a carico delle estremità distali degli arti. L'atassia di Friedreich è caratterizzata anche da anomalie scheletriche (come piede cavo) e alluce a martello, nonché da cifoscoliosi progressiva. I risultati degli esami elettrofisiologici, che includono i potenziali evocati visivi, uditivi e somatosensoriali, sono spesso anomali. La cardiomiopatia ipertrofica con progressione verso l'insufficienza cardiaca congestiva non trattabile costituisce la principale causa di mortalità. La terapia antiossidante con coenzima Q10 e vitamina E sembra rallentare la progressione in alcuni pazienti.

Esistono diverse varianti di *atassia spinocerebellare* simili all'atassia di Friedreich. La **malattia di Roussy-Levy** presenta, in aggiunta, atrofia dei muscoli degli arti inferiori, con una progressione della degenerazione analoga a quella osservata nella malattia di Charcot-Marie-Tooth. La **sindrome di Ramsay Hunt** presenta un'associata epilessia mioclonica. Si riscontrano inoltre più di 20 atassie spinocerebellari a trasmissione dominante, alcune delle quali esordiscono già nell'infanzia. Queste ultime includono le malattie associate alla tripletta CAG ripetuta (poliglutamina) e le espansioni non codificanti dei microsatelliti. Le atassie episodiche a trasmissione dominante causate dalla disfunzione dei canali di calcio e potassio si presentano con episodi di atassia e debolezza muscolare. Alcuni di questi disturbi rispondono all'acetazolamide. Le **atrofie olivopontocerebellari** (OPCA), a trasmissione dominante, includono atassia, paralisi dei nervi cranici e reperti sensoriali anomali nella seconda e terza decade, ma possono talvolta esordire nell'infanzia, con atassia a rapida progressione, nistagmo, disartria e convulsioni.

Altre forme di atassia degenerativa includono la **malattia di Pelizaeus-Merzbacher**, la **lipofuscinosi ceroide** e la **gangliosidosi** $\mathbf{GM_2}$ a esordio tardivo (vedi Capitolo 599). Rare forme di atassia cerebellare progressiva sono state descritte in associazione a **deficit di vitamina E**. Un certo numero di nuove forme di atassia progressiva ereditaria è stato definito a livello molecolare, incluse quelle causate da espansioni instabili da ripetizione di triplette nucleotidiche.

597.2 • Corea, atetosi, tremori

Il termine corea, "danza" in greco, si riferisce a movimenti irregolari, incontrollati e rapidi, spesso incorporati in gesti semi-intenzionali nel tentativo di mascherare l'anomalia, che provocano bizzarri movimenti di mani e braccia o in una camminata insolita. La classificazione della corea è riassunta nelle Tabelle 597-3 e 597-4. La **corea di Sydenham**, la più comune forma acquisita dell'infanzia, costituisce l'unica manifestazione neurologica della febbre reumatica (vedi Capitolo 182.1). La patogenesi è attribuita a una risposta autoimmune del SNC a streptococchi del gruppo A. La maggior parte dei bambini con corea di Sydenham presenta anticorpi antineuronali, che si sviluppano in risposta a infezioni da streptococchi β-emolitici. Gli anticorpi antineuronali, mediante un processo di reazione crociata, interagiscono con il citoplasma dei neuroni dei nuclei caudato e sottotalamico. La presenza di anticorpi antineuronali in alcuni pazienti in età pediatrica con tic e disturbi ossessivo-compulsivi (sintomi associati anche alla corea di Sydenham) suggerisce la possibilità che alcuni disturbi neuropsichiatrici infantili siano secondari a un processo autoimmune. Questi disturbi sono definiti con l'acronimo **PANDAS** (*Pediatric Autoimmune Neuropsychiatric Disorders Associated with Streptococcal Infections*, disturbi neuropsichiatrici infantili autoimmuni associati a infezioni da streptococchi). I principali reperti patologici, attribuiti alla risposta cellulare agli anticorpi antineuronali, consistono in vasculiti delle arteriole corticali con infiltrazione di cellule rotonde della sostanza bianca e grigia nell'area circostante. Sono prevalentemente colpiti la corteccia cerebrale, il nucleo caudato e i nuclei subtalamici. È probabile che la corea sia il risultato di un'iperattività funzionale del sistema dopaminergico.

Le tre principali manifestazioni cliniche della **corea di Sydenham** sono la corea, l'ipotonia e la labilità emotiva. La corea è solitamente simmetrica, ma i bambini possono presentare movimenti coreici limitati a un lato del corpo. I movimenti, rapidi e irregolari, coinvolgono prevalentemente il volto, il tronco e le estremità distali degli arti; tendono a trasmettersi da un gruppo muscolare all'altro; sono aggravati dallo stress, ma scompaiono durante il sonno. L'esordio può essere improvviso, ma tipicamente la corea manifesta un decorso a progressione lenta. L'ipotonia può costituire un segno prominente e, se combinata a grave corea, rende il bambino incapace di mangiare da solo, di vestirsi o di camminare. Anche il linguaggio è spesso coinvolto e risulta inintelligibile. Periodi di pianto incontrollabile e sbalzi di umore estremi sono tipici della malattia, forse in parte conseguenza dell'handicap motorio e del senso di disperazione. Diversi segni tipici sono associati a questa forma di corea: il "segno della mano da mungitrice" (stretta di mano prima debole, quindi serrata), la "mano coreica" (movimento a cucchiaio della mano estesa, con polso in flessione e dita in estensione), la protrusione involontaria della lingua che dura solo pochi secondi e il "segno di pronazione" (le braccia e i palmi si rivolgono verso l'esterno quando sono sollevati al di sopra del capo). La corea di Sydenham può persistere per diversi mesi, fino a 1-2 anni. Circa il 20% dei bambini sperimenta una recidiva entro due anni dall'episodio iniziale. I casi con segni minimi sono trattati in maniera conservativa, tentando di limitare al massimo lo stress. La corea invalidante è trattata con un trial di diazepam, seguito (in caso di fallimento) da acido valproico, fenotiazine o aloperidolo.

Benché le fenotiazine e l'aloperidolo risultino efficaci, l'utilizzo a lungo termine di questi farmaci può essere complicato dallo svilup-

TABELLA 597-3. Classificazione eziologica delle sindromi coreiche

COREA GENETICA
Malattia di Huntington
Malattia simil-Huntington 2 e altre sindromi simil-HD
Atrofia dentatorubropallidoluisiana
Neuroacantocitosi
Atassia-teleangiesctasia
Corea ereditaria benigna
Atassia spinocerebellare (di tipo 2, 3 o 17)
Coreoatetosi parossistica chinesigenica
LESIONI STRUTTURALI DEI GANGLI BASALI
Corea vascolare nell'ictus
Lesioni da massa (linfoma del SNC, tumori metastasici cerebrali)
Placche della sclerosi multipla
Mielinolisi extrapontina
DISTURBI PARAINFETTIVI E AUTOIMMUNI
Corea di Sydenham
Lupus eritematoso sistemico
Corea gravidica
Sindrome da anticorpi antifosfolipidi
Encefalite postinfettiva o postvaccinale
Corea paraneoplastica
COREA INFETTIVA
Encefalopatia HIV
Toxoplasmosi
Cisticercosi
Difterite
Endocardite batterica
Neurosifilide
Scarlattina
Encefalite virale (parotite, morbillo, varicella)
ENCEFALOPATIE METABOLICHE O TOSSICHE
Porfiria intermittente acuta
Ipo/ipernatremia
Ipocalcemia
Ipertiroidismo
Ipoparatiroidismo
Insufficienza epatica/renale
Avvelenamento da monossido di carbonio
Avvelenamento da manganese
Avvelenamento da mercurio
Avvelenamento da organofosfati
COREA INDOTTA DA FARMACI (VEDI TAB. 597-4)

Tratta da Cardoso F, Seppi K, Mair KJ, et al: Seminar on choreas. *Lancet* 2006; 5: 589-602.

TABELLA 597-4. Farmaci che possono indurre corea

AGENTI BLOCCANTI I RECETTORI DELLA DOPAMINA
Fenotiazine
Butirrofenoni
Benzamidi
FARMACI ANTIPARKINSONIANI
L-dopa
Agonisti della dopamina
Anticolinergici
FARMACI ANTIEPILETTICI
Fenitoina
Carbamazepina
Acido valproico
PSICOSTIMOLANTI
Amfetamine
Pemolina
Cocaina
CALCIOANTAGONISTI
Cinnarizina
Flunarizina
Verapamil
ALTRI
Litio
Baclofen
Digoxin
Antidepressivi triciclici
Ciclosporina
Steroidi/contraccettivi orali
Teofillina

Tratta da Cardoso F, Seppi K, Mair KJ, et al: Seminar on choreas. *Lancet* 2006; 5: 589-602.

po di un altro disturbo del movimento: la **discinesia tardiva**. Tale disturbo è caratterizzato da stereotipie facciali, come lo schioccare delle labbra e la protrusione e retrazione della lingua. I sintomi scompaiono gradualmente, ma in alcuni casi tendono a persistere dopo la sospensione della terapia. A causa del rischio di sviluppo di cardite reumatica (in particolare stenosi mitrale), nei pazienti con corea di Sydenham è opportuno il ricorso a una terapia quotidiana profilattica con penicillina, da proseguire fino all'età adulta. Una causa molto più rara di corea infantile, la *coreoatetosi parossistica chinesigenica*, è descritta nel Capitolo 594.

Il *lupus eritematoso sistemico* (LES) può presentarsi o essere associato a sintomi e segni neurologici, che includono convulsioni, sindromi organiche cerebrali (psicosi), meningite asettica e vari segni neurologici isolati, tra cui la corea. La corea può costituire il sintomo di presentazione di LES, in particolare in età pediatrica. Anticorpi antifosfolipidi sono presenti nel siero della maggior parte di questi pazienti. La presenza di anticorpi antifosfolipidi deve essere verificata in tutti i pazienti con corea, perché è associata a una elevata incidenza di occlusioni arteriose e venose.

La *malattia di Huntington* è un disturbo degenerativo del SNC, a trasmissione dominante, causato da una sequenza espansa della tripletta CAG in un gene localizzato sul cromosoma 4p16.3, risultato di mutazioni della proteina huntingtina. Tale proteina forma inclusioni anomale all'interno dei nuclei di neuroni e questa interazione può causare sequestro e riduzione dei livelli di proteine come la CBP (proteina legante le sequenze CREB), necessaria per attivare la trascrizione di altri geni. L'esordio dei sintomi della corea progressiva e della demenza presenile si verifica tipicamente tra i 35 e i 55 anni. Meno dell'1% dei casi esordisce nei bambini di età inferiore ai 10 anni, con rigidità, distonia e convulsioni. Il deterioramento mentale e i disturbi comportamentali sono rilevanti in età pediatrica. Le convulsioni tonico-cloniche sono comuni e resistenti agli anticonvulsivanti. I segni cerebellari sono presenti nel 50% dei pazienti, l'aprassia oculomotoria in circa il 20%. Il decorso della malattia è più rapido nei bambini, con una aspettativa di vita media di 8 anni (paragonata ai 14 dell'adulto). La TC, sebbene non diagnostica, mostra la riduzione del rapporto bifrontale/bicaudato, che indica l'atrofia di nucleo caudato e putamen. La RM mostra iperdensità del putamen negli adulti con la forma rigida acinetica. Non è disponibile alcuna terapia specifica per la malattia di Huntington ma, una volta confermata la diagnosi, il pediatra è chiamato a fornire un *counseling* genetico ai familiari, per chiarire i rischi futuri per nuove ricorrenze. Il test di biologia molecolare (ripetizione del trinucleotide CAG) è disponibile, ma negli Stati Uniti non è applicabile nei bambini al di sotto dell'età del consenso. I pazienti adulti presintomatici risultati positivi rispondono in maniera analoga ai pazienti con cancro quando la diagnosi è confermata.

Altre cause di corea includono convulsioni atipiche, intossicazione da farmaci (fenitoina, amitriptilina e flufenazina), convulsioni indotte da ormoni (contraccettivi orali, gravidanza/corea gravidica), malattia di Lyme, ipoparatiroidismo, ipertiroidismo e malattia di Wilson (vedi Capitolo 354.2).

L'**atetosi**, data da contorsioni distali degli arti, talvolta combinata a corea (coreoatetosi), rientra spesso nel quadro della paralisi cerebrale extrapiramidale causata da asfissia, ittero nucleare o disturbi metabolici genetici come l'aciduria glutarica. L'atetosi si evidenzia anche nei casi di paralisi cerebrale associata a prematurità. Corea e coreoatetosi possono insorgere dopo l'utilizzo dell'arresto della circolazione come tecnica di supporto per interventi cardiochirurgici complessi, o come complicanza di farmaci neurolettici dopamina-bloccanti come le fenotiazine. I pazienti con atetosi presentano spesso *rigidità* muscolare nei movimenti di flessione e estensione (in contrasto alla *spasticità*, in cui l'aumento del tono è dipendente dalla velocità). Come l'atetosi e la corea, la rigidità è il risultato della disfunzione dei gangli basali, mentre nella spasticità riflette la disfunzione dei motoneuroni superiori.

I **tremori** sono movimenti involontari caratterizzati da oscillazioni ritmiche di una parte del corpo, più evidenti a riposo o durante il movimento. Nel neonato a termine sano, i più comuni movimenti involontari sono definiti tremori fini (*jitteriness*), tremori ritmici di ampiezza identica intorno a un asse fisso. Tale comportamento, più evidente quando il neonato piange o mentre viene esaminato (riflesso di Moro), diviene anomalo se si verifica anche quando il neonato è sveglio e vigile o se persiste oltre la seconda settimana di vita. Le cause organiche di tremori fini includono sepsi, emorragia intracranica, encefalopatia ipossica, ipoglicemia, ipocalcemia, ipomagnesiemia, esposizione prenatale a marijuana (consumo da parte della madre) e sindrome da astinenza da narcotici.

Il *tremore essenziale* è una condizione familiare ereditata con modalità autosomica dominante. Può esordire durante l'infanzia e solitamente manifesta una progressione lenta. I tremori hanno una frequenza di 4-9Hz, coinvolgono prevalentemente le estremità distali degli arti superiori, sono tipicamente posturali e tendono a scomparire a riposo. Se il tremore impedisce al bambino di scrivere o complica le sue attività quotidiane, può essere alleviato da un trial di propanololo idrocloruro o primidone. Il tremore primitivo della scrittura è caratterizzato da movimenti a scatti che compaiono esclusivamente quando il paziente scrive, solitamente attenuabili da β-bloccanti anticolinergici.

I farmaci e le sostanze che possono causare tremore includono le amfetamine, l'acido valproico, i neurolettici, gli antidepressivi triciclici, la caffeina e la teofillina. I bambini in via di guarigione da una grave lesione cranica possono sviluppare un tremore prossimale aggravato dal movimento, che risponde al propanololo. Il tremore può costituire anche la manifestazione iniziale di un disturbo metabolico, come ipoglicemia, tirotossicosi, neuroblastoma e feocromocitoma. La malattia di Wilson si presenta spesso con tremore posturale associato a movimento cinetico. Questi pazienti possono sviluppare anche tremore a battito d'ali delle spalle con gli arti superiori in abduzione e i gomiti flessi. Nella sindrome distonia-parkinsonismo ereditaria si riscontra spesso tremore prossimale oltre ai movimenti distonici caratteristici. Il mioclono, definito come movimenti involontari improvvisi, brevi e a scatti, può sovrapporsi al tremore, causando tremore mioclonico, come osservato in seguito a lesione ipossica del cervelletto o in alcune malattie neurodegenerative.

597.3 • Distonia

La distonia è una sindrome caratterizzata dalla presenza di contrazioni muscolari sostenute, che causano torsioni, movimenti ripetitivi o posture anomale. Le principali cause includono asfissia perinatale (vedi Capitolo 99.5), ittero nucleare, distonia primaria generalizzata, effetti di farmaci, malattia di Wilson (degenerazione epatolenticolare), malattia di Hallervorden-Spatz e numerose altre mutazioni genetiche. La distonia può costituire una caratteristica prominente nei bambini con paralisi cerebrale extrapiramidale, conseguenza di una lesione dei gangli basali da asfissia, ittero nucleare o insulto derivato da un disturbo metabolico come l'aciduria glutarrica. Nei bambini più grandi o negli adolescenti, la distonia tende a svilupparsi gradualmente nel corso di molti anni in seguito a lesione dei gangli basali.

La **distonia generalizzata primaria**, nota anche come distonia da torsione o *distonia musculorum deformans* (DMD), è causata da un gruppo di disturbi genetici che cominciano a progredire durante l'infanzia. Una forma, frequente nella popolazione ebrea ashkenazita, è causata da una mutazione dominante del gene *DYT1*, che codifica per la proteina torsina A, legante l'adenosina trifosfato (ATP). La manifestazione iniziale della malattia durante l'infanzia è spesso una postura anomala unilaterale del piede, che assume una posizione estesa e ruotata, costringendo il bambino a camminare sulle punte. Poiché il movimento distonico è inizialmente intermittente ed è aggravato dallo stress, i pazienti sono spesso etichettati come isterici. Con il progredire della malattia, vengono coinvolti tutti e quattro gli arti e la muscolatura assiale, oltre ai muscoli facciali e linguali, che causano la compromissione di eloquio e deglutizione. Altre forme di distonia da torsione sono causate da mutazioni dei geni che codificano per la tirosina idrossilasi e l'ε-sarcoglicano, responsabili di una sindrome distonica mioclonica.

Sono stati identificati oltre una decina di loci per i geni della distonia da torsione. Uno di questi è responsabile della *distonia dopa-rispondente* (DRD), definita anche **distonia ereditaria progressiva con marcata variazione diurna**, o **malattia di Segawa**. Questa malattia a trasmissione dominante è più comune nelle femmine. Il gene per la distonia dopa-sensibile codifica per GTP-cicloidrolasi 1, enzima sintetico per il cofattore tetraidrobiopterina, richiesto per la sintesi dei neurotrasmettitori dopamina e serotonina. La distonia è solitamente diurna, migliora con il sonno ma può risultare invalidante durante il giorno. I casi a esordio precoce sono facilmente confusi con la paralisi cerebrale extrapiramidale. La DRD risponde a ridotte dosi quotidiane di levodopa (50-250 mg), somministrata assieme a un inibitore del catabolismo periferico. La DRD e la distonia causate da mutazioni di TH sono diagnosticali mediante ricerca dei metaboliti del neurotrasmettitore di serotonina e dopamina nell'LCS e misura dei livelli del cofattore biopterina.

La **distonia segmentale**, che include il crampo dello scrittore, il blefarospasmo e la distonia oromandibolare, è più comune negli adulti e tende a essere limitata a uno specifico gruppo muscolare. Si riscontra in pazienti affetti da forme genetiche di distonia da torsione o può avere un'origine idiopatica o acquisita, in seguito all'uso eccessivo di alcuni muscoli (come nei disturbi delle mani dei musicisti).

Alcuni **farmaci** possono causare una reazione distonica acuta nei bambini. In rari casi, dosi terapeutiche di fenitoina o carbamazepina provocano una distonia progressiva nei pazienti epilettici, in particolare se portatori di un'anomalia strutturale cerebrale. Alcuni bambini sperimentano una reazione idiosincratica alle fenotiazine, caratterizzata da una postura distonica acuta, talvolta confusa con l'encefalite. La somministrazione endovenosa di difenidramina (1-2 mg/kg/dose) consente una rapida remissione dei sintomi. Una grave rigidità, associata a febbre elevata e delirium, può rientrare nel quadro della **sindrome neurolettica maligna**, che si sviluppa qualche giorno dopo l'inizio della terapia con neurolettici.

La **malattia di Wilson** è un raro errore congenito del metabolismo del rame (incidenza: 1/40 000-1/100 000 nati vivi), trasmesso con modalità autosomica recessiva. È caratterizzato da cirrosi epatica e alterazioni degenerative del SNC, in particolare a livello dei gangli basali (vedi Capitolo 354.2). Il gene per la malattia di Wilson (*WND*) è stato mappato sul cromosoma 13q14-21. Mutazioni multiple di questo gene sono responsabili della variabilità di presentazione della malattia. La causa precisa non è nota, ma il meccanismo di base è collegato a una riduzione dell'escrezione biliare di rame, dovuta in parte a un difetto lisosomiale delle cellule epatiche. Nei bambini di età inferiore ai 10 anni, i sintomi e segni iniziali derivano da un'insufficienza epatica acuta o subacuta, spesso erroneamente diagnosticata come epatite infettiva. Le manifestazioni neurologiche della malattia di Wilson insorgono raramente prima dei 10 anni; il segno iniziale è solitamente la distonia progressiva. Compaiono poi i tremori agli arti, inizialmente unilaterali e in seguito generalizzati e invalidanti (tremore "a battito d'ali"). I segni di progressiva distruzione dei gangli basali includono scialorrea (incompetenza labiale responsabile di un sorriso fisso dato dalla retrazione del labbro superiore), disartria, disfonia, rigidità, contratture, distonia e coreoatetosi. L'anello di Kayser-Fleischer, visibile con la lampada a fessura, è patognomonico ed è il risultato della deposizione di rame nella membrana di Descemet. In assenza di trattamento, il paziente va incontro a demenza e coma, con conseguente decesso, entro qualche anno dall'esordio dei sintomi. Nei casi avanzati, la RM o la TC mostrano dilatazione ventricolare, con atrofia cerebrale e lesioni del talamo e dei gangli basali. Il trattamento della malattia di Wilson è discusso nel Capitolo 354.2.

La *malattia di Hallervorden-Spatz* è un raro disturbo degenerativo a trasmissione autosomica recessiva. Gli esami di linkage hanno localizzato il gene responsabile sul cromosoma 20p13. Molti pazienti presentano mutazioni della pantotenato chinasi 2 (PANK2), localizzate nei mitocondri neuronali; perciò il disturbo è chiamato anche neurodegenerazione associata a pantotenato chinasi. La malattia esordisce solitamente nell'infanzia, con distonia progressiva, rigidità e coreoatetosi. La spasticità, le risposte plantari in estensione, la disartria e il deterioramento intellettivo risultano evidenti durante l'adolescenza. La mortalità nella prima età adulta è elevata. La RM mostra lesioni del globo pallido, evidenziate dall'ipointensità del segnale nelle immagini pesate in T_2 (corrispondente a pigmenti ferrosi) e da un'area anteromediale di iperintensità (corrispondente a necrosi tissutale e edema), definita anche "segno dell'occhio di tigre". L'esame neuropatologico segnala l'eccessivo accumulo di pigmenti contenenti ferro nel globo pallido e nella substantia nigra.

La **terapia** della distonia ha subito notevoli progressi negli ultimi 10 anni. I bambini con distonia generalizzata, inclusi i casi con coinvolgimento dei muscoli della deglutizione, possono rispondere a dosi elevate di triesifenidile cloridrato. La dose iniziale di 2 mg/24 h è lentamente aumentata fino a 60-80 mg/24 h o fino alla comparsa di effetti collaterali indesiderati (ritenzione urinaria, confusione mentale o visione offuscata). Altri farmaci risultati efficaci includono carbamazepina, levodopa, bromocriptina e diazepam. La distonia segmentale, come il torcicollo, risponde spesso a iniezioni della tossina botulinica. Baclofen intratecale, somministrato per infusione continua da una pompa impiantata, è utile in alcuni casi. La chirurgia stereotassica (talamotomia, pallidotomia) consente di controllare molti effetti collaterali, mentre la stimolazione cerebrale bilaterale elettrica mediante elettrodi impiantati nel globo pallido contribuisce al trattamento dei bambini con grave distonia primaria generalizzata.

597.4 • Tic

I tic sono movimenti spasmodici, involontari, ripetitivi e stereotipati di tipo non ritmico, spesso esacerbati dallo stress, che coinvolgono qualsiasi gruppo muscolare. Sono classificabili in due sottogruppi: tic transitori dell'infanzia, tic cronici e sindrome di Gilles de la Tourette (TS). I **tic transitori** costituiscono la più comune anomalia del movimento nell'infanzia (vedi Capitolo

23). Sono più frequenti nei maschi e risultano spesso associati a un'anamnesi familiare positiva. Esempi comuni di tic sono gli ammiccamenti, i movimenti facciali o gli schiarimento della gola. Il disturbo persiste per settimane (ma meno di un anno) e non richiede terapia farmacologica. Il **disturbo da tic motori cronici** può persistere anche nella vita adulta. Tipicamente, i tic coinvolgono fino a tre gruppi muscolari simultaneamente. Il fatto che il gene per la TS possa essere espresso come tic transitori o tic motori cronici suggerisce una considerevole sovrapposizione tra le due condizioni patologiche.

La **sindrome di Gilles de la Tourette** è una condizione cronica, con una prevalenza di circa 1/2000 ed esordio tra i 2 e i 21 anni (vedi Capitolo 23). Nella maggior parte dei casi, è probabilmente ereditata con modalità autosomica dominante, ma il locus genetico non è stato ancora identificato con precisione. La TS è diagnostica nei bambini che presentano tic motori multipli in differenti parti del corpo, con almeno un tic vocale, che si protraggono, con intensità alterna, per almeno un anno, ed esordiscono prima dei 21 anni. Nei pazienti sono spesso presenti anche comportamento ossessivo-compulsivo e disturbo da deficit dell'attenzione/iperattività (ADHD). I tic motori sono associati a numerosi movimenti fluttuanti di faccia, palpebre, collo e spalle. Sono inoltre accompagnati da vocalizzazioni (tic verbali), che includono schiarimenti della gola, annusamento, coprolalia (parole oscene), tosse, ecolalia (ripetizione di parole rivolte al paziente), palilalia (ripetizione della proprie parole) ed ecocinesi (imitazione dei movimenti degli altri). Le vocalizzazioni sono incontrollabili e frequentemente compromettono le interazioni sociali del bambino con i suoi pari. Benché la TS sia una malattia cronica, la prognosi finale può essere determinata dalla gravità dei sintomi durante l'adolescenza.

Il ricorso alla **terapia farmacologica** deve essere preso in considerazione quando i tic e le vocalizzazioni interferiscono significativamente con la vita sociale e scolastica del bambino. I programmi di terapia comportamentale e di biofeedback si sono dimostrati utili in alcuni pazienti. Diversi studi hanno segnalato l'assunzione di farmaci stimolanti (metilfenidato) come causa della TS. In realtà, il metilfenidato può smascherare la TS ma non provocarla. Tutti i bambini con ADHD in terapia con farmaci stimolanti devono essere sottoposti ad attento monitoraggio per l'esordio di tic. La decisione di proseguire la terapia deve essere determinata dalla gravità dell'ADHD e dei tic. L'aloperidolo, un agente β-bloccante, è efficace nel trattamento di circa il 50% dei bambini con TS. La dose iniziale di 0,25 mg/24 h è aumentata progressivamente di 0,25 mg, fino a raggiungere una dose terapeutica compresa tra 2 e 6 mg/24 h (ma alcuni bambini possono tollerare dosi superiori). Gli effetti collaterali includono deficit cognitivo, letargia, affaticamento, depressione, irrequietezza, reazioni distoniche acute, parkinsonismo indotto dal farmaco, acatisia, discinesia tardiva e distonia tardiva. Altri farmaci utili sono penfluridolo, pimozide e clonidina. La clonidina, un α_2-agonista noradrenergico presinaptico, è somministrata alla dose iniziale di 0,05 mg/24 h, gradualmente aumentata fino a un massimo di 0,125-0,2 mg/24 h. Per cofntrollare i tic motori e verbali possono essere necessarie diverse settimane di terapia. I principali effetti collaterali includono letargia, affaticamento e sonnolenza. Circa il 50% dei pazienti con TS sperimenta sintomi ossessivo-compulsivi. L'antidepressivo triciclico clomipramina è efficace in circa il 60% dei pazienti. Altri utili antidepressivi includono sertralina, fluoxetina e fluvoxamina. Poiché la TS è un disturbo cronico associato a problemi sociali, comportamentali e dell'apprendimento, richiede la gestione da parte di un team multidisciplinare, coordinato dal pediatra.

Albin RL: Dominant ataxias and Friedreich ataxia: An update. *Curr Opin Neurol* 2003;16:507–514.

Burd L, Kerbeshian J, Berth A, et al: Long-term follow-up of an epidemiologically defined cohort of patients with Tourette syndrome. *J Child Neurol* 2001;16:431–437.

Cardoso F, Seppi K, Mair KJ, et al: Seminar on choleras. *Lancet Neurol* 2006;5:589–602.

Cervera R, Asherson RA, Font J, et al: Chorea in the antiphospholipid syndrome. Clinical, radiologic, and immunologic characteristics of 50 patients from our clinics and the recent literature. *Medicine (Baltimore)* 1997;76:203–212.

Dale RC, Heyman I, Surtees RAH, et al: Dyskinesias and associated psychiatric disorders following streptococcal infections. *Arch Dis Child* 2004;89:604–610.

Farr AK, Shalev B, Crawford TO, et al: Ocular manifestations of ataxia-telangiectasis. *Am J Ophthalmol* 2002;134:891–896.

Ferland RJ, Eyaid W, Collura RV, et al: Abnormal cerebellar development and axonal decussation due to mutations in AHI1 in Joubert syndrome. *Nat Genet* 2004;36:1126.

Hart PE, Lodi R, Rajagopalan B, et al: Antioxidant treatment of patients with Friedreich ataxia: Four-year followup. *Arch Neurol* 2005;62:621–626.

Hayflick SJ, Westaway SK, Levinson B, et al: Genetic, clinical, and radiographic delineation of Hallervorden-Spatz Syndrome. *N Engl J Med* 2003;348:33–40.

Holinski-Feder E, Jedele KB, Hörtnagel K, et al: Large intergenerational variation in age of onset in two young patients with Huntington's disease presenting as dyskinesia. *Pediatrics* 1997;100:896–898.

Hoon AH Jr, Freese PO, Reinhardt EM, et al: Age-dependent effects of trihexyphenidyl in extrapyramidal cerebral palsy. *Pediatr Neurol* 2001; 25:55–58.

Ichinose H, Ohye T, Takahashi E: Hereditary progressive dystonia with marked diurnal fluctuation caused by mutations in the GTP cyclohydrolase I gene. *Nat Genet* 1994;8:236–242.

Kids Move: *www.wemove.org/kidsmove/* [A good description of movement disorders in children and their treatment.]

Kupsch A, Beneccke R, Müller J, et al: Pallidal deep-brain stimulation in primary generalized or segmental dystonia. *N Engl J Med* 2006;355: 1978–1990.

Misbahuddin A, Warner TT: Dystonia: An update on genetics and treatment. *Curr Opin Neurol* 2001;14:471–475.

Pandolfo M: Friedreich ataxia. *Semin Pediatr Neurol* 2003;10:163–172.

Paulson H, Ammache Z: Ataxia and hereditary disorders. *Neurol Clin* 2001;19:759–782.

Schols L, Bauer P, Schmidt T, et al: Autosomal dominant cerebellar ataxias: Clinical features, genetics, and pathogenesis. *Lancet Neurol* 2004; 3:291–304.

Tarsy D, Simon DK: Dystonia. *N Engl J Med* 2006;355:818–829.

Vidailhet M, Vercueil L, Houeto JL, et al: Bilateral deep-brain stimulation of the globus pallidus in primary generalized dystonia. *N Engl J Med* 2005;352:459–467.

Zimprich A, Grabowski M, Asmus F, et al: Mutations in the gene encoding epsilon-sarcoglycan cause myoclonus-dystonia syndrome. *Nat Genet* 2001;29:66–69.

Zomorrodi A, Wald ER: Sydenham's cholera in Western Pennsylvania. *Pediatrics* 2006;117:e675–e679.

Capitolo 598 ■ Encefalopatie

Michael V. Johnston

L'encefalopatia è un disturbo generalizzato della funzione cerebrale, che può essere di tipo acuto o cronico, progressivo o statico. L'eziologia nei bambini include infezioni, esposizione a tossine (monossido di carbonio, farmaci, piombo), cause metaboliche e ischemiche. L'encefalopatia ipossica-ischemica è affrontata nel Capitolo 99.5.

598.1 • Paralisi cerebrale (vedi anche Capitoli 38 e 97.2)

L'espressione diagnostica paralisi cerebrale (PC) descrive un gruppo di sindromi motorie risultato di disturbi precoci dello sviluppo cerebrale, causate da un'ampia gamma di eziologie evolutive, genetiche, metaboliche, ischemiche, infettive e acquisite, che determinano fenotipi neurologici comuni. Storicamente, la PC è sempre stata considerata un'**encefalopatia statica**, ma questo termine non è del tutto corretto, perché alcune caratteristiche neurologiche si modificano o progrediscono nel corso del tempo. Benché la PC sia spesso associata a epilessia e ad anomalie dell'eloquio, della vista e dei deficit dell'intelletto, è la vulnerabilità selettiva del sistema cerebrale motorio a definire il disturbo. Molti adulti e bambini con PC hanno prestazioni scolastiche e professionali ad alto livello, senza mostrare i segni di disfunzione cognitiva solitamente impliciti nel termine *encefalopatia*.

EPIDEMIOLOGIA ED EZIOLOGIA. Con una prevalenza di 2/1000, la PC costituisce la più comune e costosa forma di disabilità motoria cronica a esordio infantile. Il Collaborative Perinatal Project ha monitorato circa 45 000 bambini, dalla vita fetale ai 7 anni, riscontrando che la maggior parte dei casi di PC era il risultato di parti a termine e senza complicanze, dopo una gravidanza e un travaglio normali. Nell'80% dei casi, i caratteri identificati suggerivano il ruolo patogenetico di fattori prenatali. Un numero significativo di bambini con PC presenta anomalie congenite esterne al sistema nervoso centrale (SNC). Meno del 10% mostra i segni di asfissia intrapartum. L'esposizione intrauterina a infezione materna (corioamnionite, infiammazione delle membrane placentari, infiammazione del cordone ombelicale, liquido amniotico maleodorante, sepsi materna, temperatura >38 °C durante il travaglio, infezione delle vie urinarie) è associata a un significativo aumento del rischio di PC in neonati con peso normale alla nascita. Elevati livelli di citochine infiammatorie si osservano nei campioni di sangue prelevati al momento del parto in neonati in seguito diagnosticati come affetti da PC. La prevalenza della PC aumenta nei neonati con basso peso alla nascita, in particolare se <1000 g, prevalentemente a causa di **emorragia intracerebrale** e **leucomalacia periventricolare** (*PeriVentricular Leukomalacia*, PVL). L'incidenza dell'emorragia intracerebrale è significativamente calata, mentre la PVL resta un problema rilevante. Nei neonati prematuri, quest'ultima patologia è il risultato dell'aumento di vulnerabilità dell'oligodendroglia immatura a stress ossidativi causati da ischemia o insulti infettivi/infiammatori. La presenza di anomalie della sostanza bianca (perdita di volume della sostanza bianca periventricolare, estese alterazioni cistiche, dilazione ventricolare, assottigliamento del corpo calloso) nella RM alla 40ª settimana gestazionale di neonati pretermine consente di prevedere lo sviluppo della PC entro i due anni. I tentativi di ridurre l'incidenza della PC nei neonati a termine dovrebbero essere diretti verso una migliore comprensione della biologia evolutiva fetale. È inoltre fondamentale sviluppare nuove strategie per garantire la protezione della vulnerabile sostanza bianca nei neonati prematuri.

MANIFESTAZIONI CLINICHE. I casi di PC sono generalmente classificati in diverse sindromi motorie principali, sulla base del coinvolgimento neurologico, della neuropatologia e dell'eziologia (Tab. 598-1). La classificazione fisiologica identifica l'anomalia motoria maggiore, mentre la tassonomia topografica segnala gli arti coinvolti. Inoltre, la PC è spesso associata a uno spettro di disabilità evolutive, che includono ritardo mentale, epilessia, anomalie visive, uditive, di linguaggio, cognitive e comportamentali. L'handicap motorio costituisce talvolta il problema minore del bambino.

L'**emiplegia spastica** causa una riduzione dei movimenti spontanei sul lato colpito e preferenza manuale controlaterale in uno stadio molto precoce. L'arto superiore è spesso più colpito rispetto all'arto inferiore e le difficoltà di manipolazione risultano evidenti entro il primo anno di vita. Solitamente il bambino non impara a camminare prima dei 18-24 mesi e manifesta un'andatura falciante. L'esame degli arti può rivelare arresto dello sviluppo, specialmente a livello di mano e unghie del pollice (in particolare in presenza di un'anomalia del lobo parietale controlaterale, area cerebrale che influenza la crescita degli arti). La spasticità negli arti colpiti è evidente e, a livello della caviglia, causa una deformità in equino-varismo del piede. Il bambino cammina spesso sulle punte a causa dell'aumento del tono, mentre l'arto superiore colpito assumere una postura distonica durante la corsa. Possono essere presenti clono della caviglia e segno di Babinski; l'iperreflessia e la debolezza di mano e piede in dorsiflessione sono evidenti. Circa un terzo dei pazienti con emiplegia spastica manifesta un disturbo convulsivo, che solitamente si sviluppa nei primo due anni di vita; circa il 25% presenta anomalie cognitive, incluso il ritardo mentale. TC e RM mostrano un emisfero cerebrale atrofico, con dilatazione del ventricolo laterale, controlaterale rispetto al lato degli arti colpiti. Per la maggior parte delle lesioni, la RM è molto più sensibile della TC, ma quest'ultima è utile per identificare calcificazioni associate a infezioni congenite. Un'importante causa di PC emiplegica è l'infarto cerebrale focale (ictus), secondario a tromboembolia intrauterina o perinatale, collegata a disturbi trombofilici, come la presenza di anticorpi anticardiolipina (vedi Capitolo 601). In questi casi, è possibile riscontrare un'anamnesi suggestiva di trombosi o disturbo della coagulazione e la valutazione della madre può fornire utili informazioni in vista di una futura gravidanza.

TABELLA 598-1. Classificazione della paralisi cerebrale e cause principali

Sindrome motoria	Neuropatologia	Cause principali
Diplegia spastica	Leucomalacia periventricolare (PVL)	Prematurità Ischemia Infezione Cause endocrine/metaboliche (per es. tiroide)
Quadriplegia spastica	PVL Encefalomalacia multicistica Malformazioni	Ischemia, infezione Cause endocrine/metaboliche, genetiche/evolutive
Emiplegia	Ictus: in utero o neonatale	Disturbi trombofilici Infezione Cause genetiche/evolutive Infarto emorragico periventricolare
Extrapiramidale (atetoide, discinetica)	Patologia: putamen, globo pallido, talamo, gangli basali	Asfissia Ittero nucleare Cause mitocondriali Cause genetiche/metaboliche

La **diplegia spastica** è una spasticità bilaterale che colpisce maggiormente gli arti inferiori rispetto ai superiori. Il disturbo è spesso notato per la prima volta quando il bambino comincia a gattonare, aiutandosi con le braccia in maniera corretta, ma trascinando passivamente le gambe. Una grave spasticità complica le operazioni di cambio del pannolino, a causa dell'eccessiva adduzione dell'anca. In caso di coinvolgimento della muscolatura paraspinale, il bambino non riesce a stare seduto. L'esame obiettivo rivela spasticità delle gambe associata a iperreflessia, clono della caviglia e segno di Babinski bilaterale. Quando il bambino è sospeso per le ascelle, mantiene la postura a forbice degli arti inferiori. Quando comincia a camminare, significativamente in ritardo rispetto alla media, tiene i piedi in posizione di equinovarismo e appoggia soltanto le punte. La diplegia spastica grave è caratterizzata anche da atrofia da disuso e compromissione della crescita degli arti inferiori e da crescita sproporzionata del torso superiore. La prognosi per lo sviluppo intellettuale è eccellente e la probabilità di sviluppare convulsioni minima. Il più comune riscontro neuropatologico è la leucomalacia periventricolare, in particolare nell'area dove le fibre che innervano le gambe decorrono attraverso la capsula interna. La RM è utile per valutare la gravità delle lesioni a carico della sostanza bianca e per escludere la presenza di altre lesioni cerebrali. Tecniche come l'imaging di diffusione tensiva (*Diffusion Tensor Imaging*, DTI) evidenziano specifiche anomalie delle fibre della sostanza bianca associate a diplegia spastica.

La **quadriplegia spastica** è la più grave forma di PC, a causa della marcata compromissione della funzionalità degli arti e dell'elevata associazione con ritardo mentale e convulsioni. Anche le difficoltà di deglutizione sono comuni, in seguito alla paralisi bulbare sopranucleare, responsabile spesso di polmonite da aspirazione. Le più frequenti lesioni evidenziate grazie all'esame anatomopatologico o alla RM sono una grave PVL e l'encefalomalacia multicistica corticale. L'esame neurologico mostra aumento del tono e spasticità in tutti e quattro gli arti, riduzione dei movimenti spontanei, iperreflessia e risposte plantari in estensione. Le contratture in flessione di ginocchia e gomiti sono spesso presenti nella tarda infanzia. Disabilità evolutive associate, come disturbi dell'eloquio e anomalie visive, sono particolarmente frequenti. I bambini con quadriparesi e atetosi sono spesso classificati come affetti da PC mista.

La **PC atetoide**, definita anche PC **coreoatetoide** o **extrapiramidale**, è meno comune della paralisi cerebrale spastica. I bambini colpiti appaiono ipotonici, non controllano i movimenti della testa e nel corso degli anni tendono a sviluppare un aumento del tono, con rigidità e distonia. L'allattamento è complicato dalla protrusione della lingua e dalla scialorrea. Il coinvolgimento dei muscoli orofaringei causa difficoltà di eloquio. Il linguaggio può essere del tutto assente, oppure il bambino tende a farfugliare e non controlla la modulazione della voce. I segni dei motoneuroni superiori sono generalmente assenti, le convulsioni sono rare e lo sviluppo intellettuale è solitamente normale. Questo tipo di PC, definito anche PC discinetica in Europa, è spesso collegato ad **asfissia neonatale**. La PC extrapiramidale secondaria ad asfissia intrapartum acuta è associata a lesioni bilaterali simmetriche del putamen posteriore e del talamo ventrolaterale. Tali lesioni sembrano correlate alla lesioni neuropatologica dei gangli basali chiamata *status marmoratus*. La PC atetoide può essere causata anche da **kernittero** secondario a un aumento del livello di bilirubina; in questi casi, la RM mostra lesioni bilaterali del globo pallido. La PC extrapiramidale può essere associata anche a lesioni del talamo e dei gangli basali causate da disturbi metabolici genetici, come disturbi mitocondriali e aciduria glutarrica. La RM e gli esami metabolici contribuiscono alla valutazione dei bambini con PC extrapiramidale, consentendo di formulare una corretta diagnosi eziologica.

DIAGNOSI. Un'anamnesi dettagliata e un accurato esame obiettivo devono escludere la presenza di un **disordine progressivo** del SNC, come una malattia degenerativa, un difetto metabolico, un tumore del midollo spinale o la distrofia muscolare. Nei pazienti con coinvolgimento lieve delle braccia o dei nervi cranici, deve essere presa in considerazione la possibile presenza di anomalie alla base del cranio o di altri disturbi a carico del midollo spinale cervicale. La RM cerebrale è indicata per determinare la localizzazione e l'estensione delle lesioni strutturali o l'associazione di malformazioni congenite; la RM spinale è utile in caso di sospetta patologia del midollo spinale. Gli esami di approfondimento includono l'esame dell'udito e della funzione visiva. La valutazione genetica deve essere effettuata nei pazienti con malformazioni congenite o difetti metabolici. Poiché la PC è solitamente associata a un'ampia varietà di disturbo evolutivi, il trattamento richiede un approccio multidisciplinare.

TRATTAMENTO. La gestione di questi pazienti è il risultato della collaborazione di un team multidisciplinare, composto da terapisti della riabilitazione e occupazionali, logopedisti, assistenti sociale, educatori e psicologi dell'età evolutiva. È importante insegnare ai genitori in che modo limitare gli effetti dell'anomalo tono muscolare durante le normali attività quotidiane del bambino, come mangiare, vestirsi, lavarsi e giocare. Devono inoltre essere istruiti a supervisionare l'esecuzione di specifici esercizi per prevenire l'insorgenza di contratture, in particolare a carico del tendine di Achille. Non è stato dimostrato che la fisioterapia o la terapia occupazionale *prevengano* lo sviluppo della PC nei bambini a rischio, né che *correggano* il deficit neurologico, ma queste terapie aiutano il bambino a sviluppare al massimo le sue potenzialità funzionali.

I pazienti con diplegia spastica sono inizialmente trattati utilizzando ausili e protesi, come tutori e apparecchi ortopedici. In caso di grave spasticità degli arti inferiori o lussazione dell'anca, è possibile ricorrere a procedure chirurgiche mirate a ridurre lo spasmo muscolare intorno al cingolo dell'anca, come la tenotomia degli adduttori o il trasferimento e rilascio dello psoas. In pazienti selezionati con grave diplegia spastica, la rizotomia, una procedura neurochirurgica che consiste nel sezionare una porzione di radici nervose sensitive, consente un notevole miglioramento (Fig. 598-1). Anche la tenotomia del tendine di Achille può risultare utile. La gestione della quadriplegia implica l'utilizzo di sedie a rotelle, speciali ausili per l'alimentazione, tastiere modificate e protesi per sedersi. Nei bambini con **PC emiplegica** si è dimostrata efficace l'applicazione di cinghie che bloccano il lato sano, che inducono un miglioramento del funzionamento del braccio e della mano sul lato colpito. Tale terapia indotta dal movimento è utile nei pazienti di ogni età.

La capacità di comunicazione può essere migliorata con l'uso dei simboli di Bliss, di tastiere parlanti e programmi computerizzati e ausili informatici appositamente realizzati per promuovere la funzione motoria e di linguaggio. Problemi comportamentali significativi possono interferire con lo sviluppo di un bambino con PC; l'assistenza di uno psicologo o di uno psichiatra può essere utile per la precoce identificazione e il trattamento di tali disturbi. Psicologi ed educatori contribuiscono anche alla diagnosi e alla gestione dei disturbi di apprendimento, dei deficit di attenzione e del ritardo mentale. Poiché strabismo, nistagmo e atrofia ottica sono comuni, la valutazione iniziale dovrebbe includere un esame oftalmologico. La disfunzione del tratto urinario inferiore richiede una precoce identificazione e terapia.

Per il trattamento della **spasticità** sono stati utilizzati diversi farmaci, tra cui il dantrolene sodio (orale), le benzodiazepine e il baclofen. Questi farmaci hanno modesti effetti benefici su alcuni pazienti, ma presentano una serie di effetti collaterali, come sedazione (le benzodiazepine) e riduzione della soglia convulsiva (baclofen). Il baclofen intratecale è stato usato con successo in pazienti selezionati con grave spasticità. questa terapia richiede un approccio multidisciplinare e regolari follow-up, per monitorare l'insorgenza di difetti del meccanismo di infusione e di complicanze (come infezioni).

L'iniezione della **tossina botulinica** in specifici gruppi muscolari per il trattamento della spasticità ha ottenuto una risposta positiva in molti pazienti. L'iniezione nelle ghiandole salivari consente di ridurre la scialorrea, riscontrata nel 10-30% dei pazienti e tradizionalmente trattata con agenti anticolinergici. I pazienti con rigidità, distonia e quadriparesi spastica talvolta rispondono alla somministrazione di levodopa. I bambini con distonia possono trarre beneficio da carbamazepina o trihexyphenidyl. L'ossigeno iperbarico non migliora le condizioni dei pazienti con PC.

598.2 • Encefalomiopatie mitocondriali*

Le malattie mitocondriali sono un gruppo eterogeneo di patologie causate da mutazioni del DNA nucleare (nDNA) o mitocondriale (mtDNA) (vedi Capitoli 80, 86 e 87). L'estrema variabilità dei fenotipi clinici e dell'età di insorgenza dipende dallo stadio evolutivo coinvolto e dai tessuti o sistemi colpiti. Sul piano biochimico, possono presentarsi con una monoenzimopatia tessuto-specifica o generalizzata, oppure con una multienzimopatia tessuto-specifica o generalizzata. Nella catena respiratoria, la fosforilazione ossidativa è mediata da 5 complessi enzimatici intramitocondriali (complessi I-V), responsabili della produzione dell'adenosina trifosfato (ATP) necessaria per la normale funzione cellulare. Il mantenimento e l'assemblaggio dei complessi della fosforilazione ossidativa richiedono la regolazione coordinata dei geni del DNA nucleare e mitocondriale. L'mtDNA umano è costituito da una piccola molecola a doppia elica, completamente sequenziata, che codifica per 13 proteine strutturali, subunità dei complessi della catena respiratoria, oltre ai due RNA ribosomiali (RNAs e 22tRNAs) necessari per la trasduzione. Il DNA nucleare è responsabile della sintesi di circa 70 subunità, del loro trasporto nei mitocondri (passando attraverso la membrana mitocondriale

*Scritto in collaborazione con Ingrid Tein.

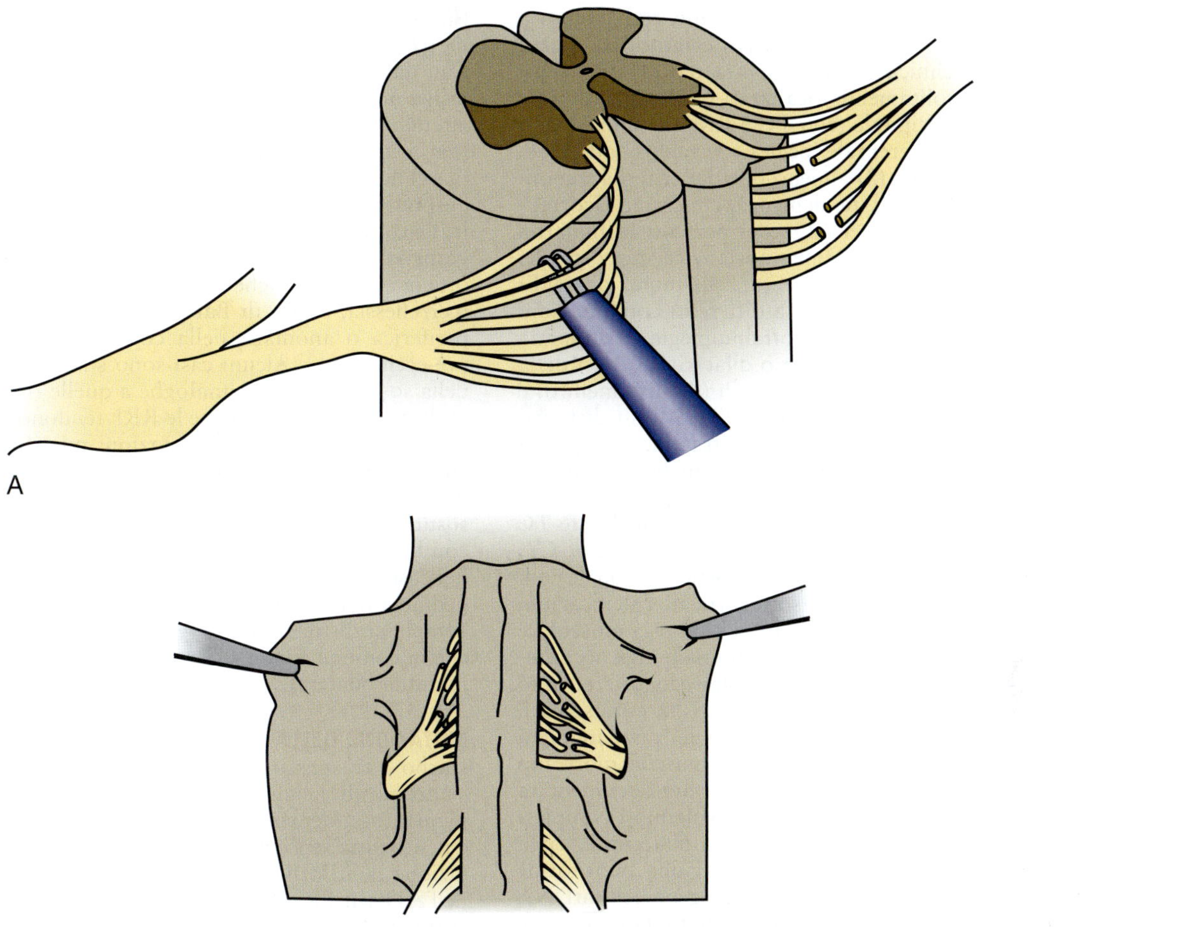

Figura 598-1. Rappresentazione schematica della tecnica di rizotomia dorsale selettiva. *A*, Dopo la laminectomia, la dura è aperta, per esporre le radici spinali dorsali. La stimolazione delle radici consente di identificare le anomalie di attività. *B*, Porzione di radici sezionata. (Tratta da Koman LA, Smith BP, Shilt JS: Cerebral palsy. *Lancet* 2004;363:1619-1631. Riprodotta per gentile concessione della Wake Forest University Orthopaedic Press.)

interna grazie alle proteine chaperone) e della coordinazione del loro corretto assemblaggio.

Il DNA mitocondriale differisce da quello nucleare per le seguenti ragioni: (1) il suo codice genetico è diverso da quello dell'nDNA; (2) poiché non contiene introni, immagazzina in maniera compatta le informazioni; (3) è maggiormente soggetto a mutazioni spontanee; (4) possiede meccanismi di riparazione meno efficienti; (5) è presente in centinaia o migliaia di copie per cellula ed è trasmesso per linea materna. Nel processo di formazione dello zigote, soltanto l'oocita contribuisce all'mtDNA. Se si verifica una mutazione dell'mtDNA nell'ovulo o nello zigote, può essere trasmessa in maniera casuale a successive generazioni di cellule. Alcuni ricevono solo pochi genomi mutanti o nessuno (omoplasmia normale o ceppo selvaggio), altri ricevono una popolazione mista di mtDNA **mutanti** e mtDNA **selvaggio** (**eteroplasmia**), altri ancora ricevono quasi esclusivamente genomi mutanti (omoplasmia mutante). L'eredità materna e l'eteroplasmia comportano le seguenti importanti implicazioni: (1) malgrado la trasmissione materna, entrambi i sessi sono colpiti; (2) l'espressione fenotipica di una mutazione dell'mtDNA dipende dalla proporzione relativa di genomi mutanti e di tipo selvaggio e richiede un numero critico minimo (effetto soglia); (3) al momento della divisione cellulare, la proporzione nelle cellule figlie può alterarsi (segregazione mitotica), determinando un corrispondente cambiamento fenotipico; (4) generazioni successive sono maggiormente colpite rispetto alle malattie autosomiche dominanti. Il numero critico di mtDNA mutanti necessario per l'effetto soglia varia sulla base della vulnerabilità tissutale ai disturbi del metabolismo ossidativo e dell'aumento di tale vulnerabilità determinato dalla crescita e dall'invecchiamento. I difetti della fosforilazione ossidativa possono essere classificati in tre categorie: (1) difetti dell'nDNA; (2) difetti dell'mtDNA; (3) difetti di comunicazione tra genoma nucleare e mitocondriale.

Utilizzando un sistema di classificazione più ampio, le malattie mitocondriali causate da difetti dell'nDNA includono: difetti del trasporto del substrato (deficit del trasportatore della carnitina nel plasmalemma, della carnitina palmitoil-trasferasi I e II, della carnitina acilcarnitina traslocasi); difetti dell'ossidazione del substrato (deficit del complesso piruvato deidrogenasi e della piruvato carbossilasi, difetti dell'ossidazione intramitocondriale degli acidi grassi); difetti del ciclo di Krebs (deficit di α-chetoglutarrato deidrogenasi, di fumarasi e di aconitasi); difetti della catena respiratoria (complessi I-V), che includono i difetti dell'accoppiamento ossidazione/fosforilazione (sindrome di Luft) e difetti del trasporto mitocondriale delle proteine. Queste patologie sono trasmesse con modalità mendeliana. Le malattie causate da difetti dell'mtDNA sono classificate in: disturbi dovuti a mutazioni puntiformi ereditate in linea materna (neuropatia ottica ereditaria di Leber, sindromi MELAS, MERRF e NARP); disturbi dovuti a delezioni o duplicazioni sporadiche (sindromi di Kearns-Sayre e di Pearson). Le malattie causate da difetti della comunicazione tra genoma nucleare e mitocondriale si trasmettono con modalità mendeliana e includono delezioni multiple dell'mtDNA (autosomiche dominanti) e sindromi da deplezione dell'mtDNA (solitamente autosomiche recessive).

ENCEFALOMIOPATIA MITOCONDRIALE, ENCEFALOMIOPATIA, ACIDOSI LATTICA ED EPISODI SIMIL-ICTUS (MELAS). I bambini con MELAS (*Mitochondrial encephalomphathy, encephalomyopathy, Lactic Acidosis, and Strokelike episodes*) possono apparire normali nei primi anni di vita, ma ben prestano cominciano a manifestare ritardo dello sviluppo cognitivo e motorio e bassa statura. La sindrome clinica è caratterizzata da: (1) ricorrenti episodi di simil-ictus, solitamente localizzati nei lobi temporale posteriore, parietale e occipitale (con TC e RM che dimostrano la presenza dell'anomalia cerebrale focale); (2) acidosi lattica e/o fibre rosse sfilacciate (RRF); (3) almeno due dei criteri seguenti: convulsioni focali o generalizzate; demenza; emicrania ricorrente; vomito. In una casistica, nel 62% dei pazienti la malattia esordiva prima dei 15 anni, con emianopsia o cecità corticale. La proteinorrachia risulta spesso aumentata. La mutazione MELAS 3243 può essere associata anche a differenti combinazioni di intolleranza allo sforzo, miopatia, oftalmoplegia, retinopatia pigmentosa, cardiomiopatia ipertrofica o dilatativa, difetti della conduzione cardiaca, sordità, endocrinopatia (diabete mellito) e disfunzione dei tubuli prossimali renali. MELAS è un disturbo progressivo, la cui presenza è segnalata nei fratelli. Gli episodi di simil-ictus conducono alla demenza (vedi anche il Capitolo 610.4).

L'ipoperfusione regionale può essere evidenziata mediante TC a emissione di un singolo fotone (*Single-Photon Emission CT*, SPECT). La neuropatologia rivela atrofia corticale, con lesioni simil-infarto nelle strutture corticali e sottocorticali, calcificazioni nei gangli basali e dilatazione ventricolare. La biopsia muscolare mostra solitamente la presenza di RRF. Le anomalie e gli accumuli mitocondriali, responsabili di angiopatia mitocondriale, sono dimostrati nelle cellule dei muscoli lisci dei vasi intramuscolari, nelle arteriole cerebrali, nelle cellule epiteliali e nei vasi sanguigni dei plessi coroidei. Gli esami biochimici dei muscoli mostrano in molti casi un deficit del complesso I, ma è stata documentata anche la presenza di difetti multipli, che coinvolgono i complessi I, III e IV. La trasmissione avviene in linea materna e, circa nell'80% dei pazienti, si riscontra una mutazione puntiforme altamente specifica, sebbene non esclusiva, del gene dell'mtDNA $tRNA^{Leu(UUR)}$ al nucleotide 3243. Il 7,5% presenta una mutazione puntiforme del gene $tRNA^{Leu(UUR)}$ al nucleotide 3271. È stata identificata una terza mutazione del gene $tRNA^{Leu(UUR)}$ al nucleotide 3252. Il tessuto di elezione per gli esami è quello muscolare, perché il numero dei genomi mutanti è superiore nel muscolo rispetto al sangue.

La prognosi dei pazienti è infausta. Sono stati tentati trial terapeutici con corticosteroidi e coenzima Q10. La riduzione della concentrazione sierica di lattato con dicloroacetato ha consentito un netto miglioramento in alcuni casi.

EPILESSIA MIOCLONICA E FIBRE ROSSE SFILACCIATE (MERRF). Questa sindrome *(Myoclonus Epilepsy and Ragged Red Fibres*, MERRF) è caratterizzata da progressiva epilessia mioclonica, miopatia mitocondriale e atassia cerebellare con disartria e nistagmo. L'esordio può avvenire nell'infanzia o nella vita adulta, mentre il decorso può risultare a lenta o rapida progressione. Le altre caratteristiche includono demenza, perdita uditiva neurosensoriale, atrofia ottica, neuropatia periferica e spasticità. Poiché alcuni pazienti manifestano anomalie della sensazione e piede cavo, la malattia può essere confusa con l'atassia di Friedreich. Un numero significativo di pazienti presenta una storia familiare positiva e bassa statura. La trasmissione avviene in linea materna.

I reperti patologici includono un aumento della concentrazione sierica di lattato, RRF evidenziate dalla biopsia muscolare e una marcata perdita neuronale e gliosi, in particolare a carico del nucleo dentato e del complesso olivare inferiore, con una fuoriuscita di cellule di Purkinje e neuroni del nucleo rosso. Possono riscontrarsi anche pallore dei cordoni posteriori del midollo spinale e degenerazione dei nuclei gracile e cuneato. La biochimica muscolare mostra difetti variabili dei complessi III, II e IV, I e IV, oppure soltanto del IV. Più dell'80% dei casi è causato da una mutazione eteroplasmica A con G al nucleotide 8344 del gene $tRNA^{Lys}$ dell'mtDNA. In altri pazienti è stata segnalata una mutazione C con T al nucleotide 8356 del gene $tRNA^{Lys}$.

Non è disponibile alcuna terapia. Il coenzima Q10 si è dimostrato utile in una madre e figlia con mutazione MERRF.

NEUROPATIA OTTICA EREDITARIA DI LEBER (LHON). Questa sindrome (*Leber Hereditary Optic Neuropathy*, LHON) è caratterizzata dalla comparsa, solitamente tra i 18 e i 30 anni, di perdita visiva acuta e subacuta, causata da una grave atrofia ottica bilaterale. Sono stati tuttavia segnalati casi di esordio più precoce (dai 5 anni). In almeno l'85% dei casi, i pazienti sono di sesso maschile. È ipotizzabile che un fattore correlato a X moduli l'espressione della mutazione puntiforme del DNA mitocondriale. Le caratteristiche oftalmologiche classiche includono microangiopatia teleangiectasia circumpapillare e pseudoedema del disco ottico. Caratteristiche variabili includono atassia cerebellare, iperreflessia, segno di Babinksi, sintomi psichiatrici, neuropatia periferica o anomalie della conduzione cardiaca (sindrome da pre-eccitazione). Alcuni casi sono stati associati a lesioni diffuse della sostanza bianca, analoghe a quelle riscontrate nella sclerosi multipla. L'acidosi lattica e le RRF tendono a essere assenti. Sono state descritte più di 11 mutazioni puntiformi dell'mtDNA, tra cui una transizione omoplastica di A a G al nucleotide 11,778 del gene ND4 del complesso I. Tale mutazione, che causa la sostituzione di un residuo di arginina a elevata conservazione con l'istidina nel 340° amminoacido, è responsabile del 50-70% dei casi in Europa e di circa il 90% dei casi in Giappone. Alcuni pedigree LHON con altre mutazioni puntiformi sono associati a complessi disturbi neurologici e possono presentare caratteristiche in comune con la sindrome MELAS e con la necrosi striatale infantile bilaterale.

MUTAZIONE DELLA SUBUNITÀ 6 DELL'ATPASI (NARP). Questo disturbo a trasmissione materna si presenta in due forme: con la sindrome di Leigh oppure con ritardo dello sviluppo, retinite pigmentosa, demenza, convulsioni, atassia, debolezza prossimale e neuropatia sensoriale (sindrome NARP). È causato da una mutazione puntiforme al nucleotide 8993 della subunità 6 del gene dell'ATPasi. La gravità della presentazione sembra strettamente correlata alla percentuale di mtDNA mutante nei leucociti. Non è disponibile alcun trattamento.

SINDROME DI KEARNS-SAYRE (KSS). I criteri per la KSS (*Kearns-Sayre Syndrome*) includono la seguente triade: (1) esordio prima dei 20 anni; (2) oftalmoplegia esterna progressiva (PEO) con ptosi; (3) retinopatia pigmentosa. È richiesta anche la presenza di almeno uno dei seguenti criteri: blocco cardiaco, sindrome cerebellare o proteinorrachia >100 mg/dL. Altre caratteristiche non specifiche ma comuni includono demenza, perdita uditiva neurosensoriale e anomalie endocrine multiple (bassa statura, diabete mellito e ipoparatiroidismo). Non è disponibile alcun trattamento per la KSS. La prognosi è infausta; l'applicazione di un pacemaker non riesce a impedire il decesso del paziente entro la terza o quarta decade. Presentazioni cliniche insolite includono l'acidosi renale tubulare e la sindrome di Lowe. Si riscontrano anche alcuni casi di sovrapposizione della KSS con episodi simil-ictus. La biopsia muscolare mostra RRF e fibre COX-negative. La maggior parte dei pazienti presenta delezioni dell'mtDNA, ma in alcuni casi si osservano duplicazioni. È possibile che si tratti di nuove mutazioni, responsabili della natura generalmente sporadica della KSS. Rari pedigree rivelano una trasmissione autosomica dominante.

La **PEO sporadica con RRF** è una condizione clinica benigna caratterizzata dall'esordio, nell'adolescenza o prima età adulta, di oftalmoplegia, ptosi e debolezza prossimale del cingolo pelvico. La progressione lenta di questa malattia è compatibile con una vita relativamente normale. La biopsia muscolare dimostra la presenza di RRF e fibre COX-negative. Circa il 50% dei pazienti con PEO ha delezioni dell'mtDNA; anamnesi familiare negativa.

MALATTIA DI LEIGH (ENCEFALOMIOPATIA NECROTIZZANTE SUBACUTA). Esistono almeno 4 cause note di malattia di Leigh geneticamente determinata: il deficit del complesso piruvato deidrogenasi; il deficit del complesso I; il deficit del complesso IV (COX) e il deficit del complesso V (ATPasi). Questi difetti possono verificarsi sporadicamente o essere ereditati con le seguenti modalità:

autosomica recessiva (deficit di COX); correlata alla X (deficit di PDH $E_1\alpha$); nella linea materna (mutazione 8993 dell'ATPasi 6 nel deficit del complesso V). Nella maggior parte dei casi, l'esordio avviene nell'infanzia, con disturbi dell'alimentazione e di deglutizione, vomito e deficit staturo-ponderale. È possibile riscontrare anche ritardo nell'acquisizione delle abilità linguistiche e motorie, convulsioni generalizzate, debolezza, ipotonia, atassia, tremori, segni piramidali e nistagmo. La caratteristica respirazione intermittente, associata a singhiozzi e sospiri, suggerisce una disfunzione troncoencefalica. Alcuni pazienti presentano oftalmoplegia esterna, ptosi, atrofia ottica e riduzione dell'acuità visiva. I risultati anomali di TC e RM consistono in aree simmetriche bilaterali di attenuazione nei gangli basali. Le alterazioni patologiche includono aree simmetriche di necrosi focale a carico di talamo, gangli basali, sostanza grigia tegmentale, regioni periventricolari e periacqueduttali del tronco e cordoni posteriori del midollo spinale. Sul piano microscopico, queste lesioni spongiformi mostrano cavitazione cistica con perdita neurale, demielinazione e proliferazione vascolare. L'aumento dei livelli sierici di lattato è caratteristico. La prognosi generale è infausta, ma un piccolo numero di pazienti sperimenta prolungati periodi di remissione. Non è disponibile alcun trattamento.

SINDROME DI REYE. Questa encefalopatia, sempre più rara, è caratterizzata da degenerazione grassa viscerale (steatosi microvescicolare) e anomalie mitocondriali e biochimiche compatibili con un disturbo del metabolismo mitocondriale (vedi Capitolo 358). La sindrome di Reye sporadica può verificarsi nel contesto della varicella, di un'infezione da virus B, dell'ingestione di salicilato, nella reazione idiosincratica di epatotossicità da acido valproico in individui con una predisposizione genetica e nella malattia da vomito giamaicana (causata dalla tossina ipoglicina).

La **sindrome ricorrente simil-Reye** si incontra in bambini con difetti genetici dell'ossidazione degli acidi grassi, come il deficit del trasportatore della carnitina nel plasmalemma, di carnitina palmitoil-trasferasi I e II, di carnitina acilcarnitina traslocasi, di acil-CoA deidrogenasi a catena media e lunga, di acil-CoA deidrogenasi e di L-3 idrossiacil-CoA deidrogenasi (o proteina trifunzionale). Questi disturbi, ereditati con modalità autosomica recessiva, si manifestano con ricorrente encefalopatia ipoglicemica e ipochetotica. Altri errori congeniti del metabolismo che si presentano con la sindrome di Reye includono i difetti del ciclo dell'urea (ornitina transcarbamilasi, carbamil fosfato sintetasi), alcune acidurie organiche (aciduria glutarrica di tipo I), difetti della catena respiratoria e difetti del metabolismo dei carboidrati (intolleranza al fruttosio).

598.3 • ALTRE ENCEFALOPATIE

ENCEFALOPATIA DA AIDS. L'encefalopatia costituisce una manifestazione comune e infausta dell'infezione da HIV in lattanti e bambini (vedi Capitolo 273). I segni neurologici nei pazienti con infezione congenita possono presentarsi nella prima infanzia o essere ritardati fino ai 5 anni. I principali segni e sintomi dell'encefalopatia da AIDS includono un arresto dello sviluppo cerebrale, ritardo evolutivo, debolezza muscolare con segni dei tratti piramidali, atassia, mioclono, paralisi pseudobulbare e convulsioni.

ENCEFALOPATIA DA PIOMBO. Vedi Capitolo 709.

ENCEFALOPATIA DA USTIONE. L'encefalopatia si sviluppa in circa il 5% dei bambini nella prime settimane di ricovero in ospedale in seguito a gravi ustioni (vedi anche Capitolo 74). Lo sviluppo del disturbo non è attribuito a una causa univoca, ma piuttosto a una combinazione di fattori, che includono anossia (inalazione di fumo, avvelenamento da monossido di carbonio, laringospasmo), anomalie elettrolitiche, batteriemia e sepsi, trombosi delle vene corticali con concomitante trauma alla testa, edema cerebrale, reazione da farmaci e stress emotivo. Le convulsioni costituiscono la principale manifestazione clinica dell'encefalopatia da ustione, ma possono riscontrarsi anche alterazione dello stato di coscienza, allucinazioni e coma. La gestione di questa forma di encefalopatia implica la ricerca della causa sottostante e il trattamento dell'ipossiemia, delle convulsioni, delle specifiche anomalie elettrolitiche o dell'edema cerebrale. La prognosi per il completo recupero neurologico è generalmente eccellente, in particolare se le convulsioni costituiscono l'anomalia principale.

ENCEFALOPATIA IPERTENSIVA. Nei bambini, l'encefalopatia ipertensiva è comunemente associata a malattia renale, come la glomerulonefrite acuta, la pielonefrite cronica e l'insufficienza renale allo stadio terminale (vedi Capitoli 445 e 535). In alcuni casi, l'encefalopatia ipertensiva costituisce la manifestazione iniziale di una sottostante malattia renale. Una marcata ipertensione sistemica causa vasocostrizione dei vasi cerebrali, con conseguente aumentata permeabilità vascolare, che determina aree di edema cerebrale focale e emorragia. L'esordio può essere acuto, con convulsioni e coma, o più indolente, con cefalea, sonnolenza e letargia, nausea e vomito, visione offuscata, cecità corticale transitoria ed emiparesi. L'esame del fondo oculare può non risultare diagnostico nei bambini, ma talvolta si riscontrano papilledema ed emorragia retinica. Le immagini pesate in T_2 della RM mostrano spesso un aumento dell'intensità del segnale nei lobi occipitali, corrispondente alla leucoencefalopatia posteriore reversibile, facilmente confondibile con un infarto cerebrale. Tali aree di iperintensità possono comparire anche in altre regioni cerebrali. Il trattamento è diretto al recupero di una stato normotensivo e al controllo delle convulsioni con i farmaci più opportuni.

ENCEFALOPATIA DA RADIAZIONI. Malgrado i considerevoli progressi nelle tecniche di irradiazione, che hanno consentito la drastica riduzione di seri effetti collaterali, l'encefalopatia da radiazioni resta una complicanza rilevante. Il rischio è maggiore nei pazienti molto piccoli che ricevono elevate dosi quotidiane. Radiazioni eccessive danneggiano l'endotelio dei vasi, causando un aumento della permeabilità vascolare, edema cerebrale ed emorragie. Il bambino può divenire improvvisamente irritabile e letargico, lamentare cefalea, o presentare convulsioni e segni neurologici focali. Occasionalmente, i pazienti sviluppano emiparesi dovuta a infarto secondario all'occlusione vascolare dei vasi cerebrali. Gli steroidi sono spesso utili nel ridurre l'edema cerebrale e trattare i segni neurologici. L'encefalopatia tardiva da radiazioni è caratterizzata da cefalea e segni neurologici focali a progressione lenta (che includono emiparesi e convulsioni). Alcuni bambini con leucemia linfatica acuta trattati con una combinazione di metotressato intratecale e irradiazione cranica sviluppano segni neurologici a mesi o anni di distanza; tali segni consistono in letargia crescente, perdita delle abilità cognitive, demenza, segni neurologici focali e convulsioni (vedi Capitolo 494). La TC mostra calcificazioni della sostanza bianca, e l'esame *post mortem* documenta una encefalopatia necrotizzante. Tale devastante complicanza del trattamento della leucemia ha condotto a una riconsiderazione dell'opportunità dell'irradiazione cranica nel trattamento di questi bambini.

SINDROME DI ZELLWEGER (SINDROME CEREBROEPATORENALE [CHRS]). Questo raro disturbo letale è ereditato con modalità autosomica recessiva. Costituisce il prototipo di un gruppo di disturbi perossisomali con sintomi, segni e anomalie biochimiche che tendono a sovrapporsi (vedi Capitolo 86.2). I bambini colpiti presentano una facies tipica, con fronte prominente e ampia fontanella anteriore. L'occipite è appiattito e i padiglioni auricolari sono dismorfici. Il quadro è solitamente completato da palato arcuato, cute del collo sovrabbondante, grave ipotonia e areflessia. L'esame oculare rivela movimenti nistagmoidi di rifissazione, cataratta bilaterale e atrofia ottica. Le convulsioni generalizzate esordiscono precocemente, associate a grave ritardo dello sviluppo globale e significativa perdita bilaterale dell'udito. La causa delle gravi anomalie neurologiche è collegata a un arresto della migrazione dei neuroblasti durante le fasi precoci dello sviluppo, con conseguente pachigiria cerebrale ed eterotopia neuronale (vedi Capitolo 592.7). L'epatomegalia è riscontrata subito dopo la nascita, spesso associata a ittero neonatale prolungato. I pazienti con sindrome di Zellweger sopravvivono raramente oltre il primo anno.

Alberman E, Peckham C: Cerebral palsy and perinatal exposure to neurotropic viruses. *BMJ* 2006;332:63–64.

Bax M, Tydeman C, Flodmark O: Clinical and MRI correlates of cerebral palsy. The European cerebral palsy study. *JAMA* 2006;269:1602–1608.

Bottos M, Feliciangeli A, Sciuto LS, et al: Functional status of adults with cerebral palsy and implications for treating children. *Dev Med Child Neurol* 2001;431:516–528.

Brunstrom JE: Clinical considerations on cerebral palsy and spasticity. *J Child Neurol* 2001;16:10–15.

Brunstrom JE, Bastion AJ, Wong M, et al: Motor benefit from levodopa in spastic quadriplegic cerebral palsy. *Ann Neurol* 2000;47:662–665.

Butler C, Darrah J: Effects of neurodevelopmental treatment (NDT) for cerebral palsy: An AACPDM evidence report. *Dev Med Child Neurol* 2001;43:778–790.

Chong SK: Gastrointestinal problems in the handicapped child. *Curr Opin Pediatr* 2001;13:441–446.

Croen LA, Grether JK, Curry CJ: Congenital abnormalities among children with cerebral palsy: More evidence for prenatal antecedents. *J Pediatr* 2001;138:804–810.

Edgar TS: Clinical utility of botulinum toxin in the treatment of cerebral palsy: Comprehensive review. *J Child Neurol* 2001;16:37–46.

Fitzgerald JJ, Tsegaye M, Vloeberghs MH: Treatment of childhood spasticity of cerebral origin with intrathecal baclofen: A series of 52 cases. *Br J Neurosurg* 2004;18:240–245.

Golomb MR, MacGregor DL, Domi T, et al: Presumed pre- or perinatal arterial ischemic stroke: Risk factors and outcomes. *Ann Neurol* 2001;50:163–168.

Gordon AM, Charles J, Wolf SL: Efficacy of constraint-induced movement therapy on involved upper-extremity use in children with hemiplegic cerebral palsy is not age-dependent. *Pediatrics* 2006;117:363–373.

Hagberg H, Mallard C: Effect of inflammation on central nervous system development and vulnerability. *Curr Opin Neurol* 2005;18:117–123.

Hansel DE, Hansel CR, Shindle MK, et al: Oral baclofen in cerebral palsy: Possible seizure potentiation? *Pediatr Neurol* 2003;29:203–206.

Harum KH, Hoon AH, Kato GJ, et al: Homozygous factor-V mutation as a genetic cause of perinatal thrombosis and cerebral palsy. *Dev Med Child Neurol* 1999;41:777–780.

Hoon AH, Freese PO, Reinhardt EM, et al: Age-dependent effects of trihexyphenidyl in extrapyramidal cerebral palsy. *Pediatr Neurol* 2001;25: 55–58.

Hoon AH, Lawrie WT, Melhem ER, et al: Diffusion tensor imaging of periventricular leukomalacia shows affected sensory cortex white matter pathways. *Neurology* 2002;59:752–756.

Hyland K: The lumbar puncture for diagnosis of pediatric neurotransmitter diseases. *Ann Neurol* 2003;54:S13–S17.

Inder TE, Wells SJ, Mogridge NB, et al: Defining the nature of the cerebral abnormalities in the premature infant: A qualitative magnetic resonance imaging study. *J Pediatr* 2003;143:171–179.

Jongerius PH, van den Hoogen JA, van Limbeek J, et al: Effect of botulism toxin in the treatment of drooling: A controlled clinical trial. *Pediatrics* 2004;114:620–627.

Kahana A, Rowley HA, Weinstein JM: Cortical blindness: Clinical and radiologic findings in reversible posterior leukoencephalopathy syndrome: Case report and review of the literature. *Ophthalmology* 2005;112:e7–e11.

Koman LA, Brashear A, Rosenfeld S, et al: Botulinum toxin type A neuromuscular blockade in the treatment of equinus foot deformity in cerebral palsy: A multicenter, open-label clinical trial. *Pediatrics* 2001;108: 1062–1070.

Koman LA, Smith BP, Shilt JS: Cerebral palsy. *Lancet* 2004;363:1619–1631.

Longo N: Mitochondrial encephalopathy. *Neurol Clin* 2003;21:817–831.

McLaughlin J, Bjornson KI, Temkin N, et al: Selective dorsal rhizotomy: Meta-analysis of three randomized controlled trials. *Dev Med Child Neurol* 2002;44:17–25.

Pavlakis SG, Phillips PC, Di Mauro S, et al: Mitochondrial myopathy, encephalopathy, lactic acidosis, and strokelike episodes: A distinctive clinical syndrome. *Ann Neurol* 1984;16:481–488.

Senner JE, Logemann J, Zecker S, et al: Drooling, saliva production, and swallowing in cerebral palsy. *Dev Med Child Neurol* 2004;46:801–806.

Shapiro SM: Definition of the clinical spectrum of kernicterus and bilirubin-induced neurologic dysfunction (BIND). *J Perinatology* 2005;25:54–59.

Sleigh G, Brocklehurst P: Gastrostomy feeding in cerebral palsy: A systematic review. *Arch Dis Child* 2004;89:534–539.

Ubhi T, Bhakta BB, Allgar V, et al: Randomised double blind placebo controlled trail of the effect of botulinum toxin on walking in cerebral palsy. *Arch Dis Child* 2000;83:481–487.

Woodward LJ, Anderson PJ, Austin NC, et al: Neonatal MRI to predict neurodevelopmental outcomes in preterm infants. *N Engl J Med* 2006;355: 685–694.

Capitolo 599 ■ Disturbi neurodegenerativi infantili Michael V. Johnston

I disturbi neurodegenerativi infantili comprendono un vasto numero di malattie eterogenee, risultato di specifici difetti genetici e biochimici o di infezioni virali croniche. Includono anche un gruppo di patologie dalla causa sconosciuta. I bambini con sospetto disturbo neurodegenerativo erano un tempo sottoposti a biopsia cerebrale e rettale (neurale), ma grazie all'avvento delle moderne tecniche di neuroimaging e di specifici esami biochimici o molecolari queste procedure invasive sono raramente necessarie. Le componenti principali della valutazione restano un'anamnesi dettagliata e un accurato esame obiettivo. La caratteristica distintiva delle malattie neurodegenerative è il **progressivo deterioramento** della funzione neurologica, con perdita del linguaggio, della visione, dell'udito o della locomozione, spesso in associazione a convulsioni, difficoltà di alimentazione e deficit cognitivo. L'età di esordio, la velocità della progressione e i principali reperti neurologici segnalano se la malattia coinvolge prevalentemente la sostanza bianca o grigia. Nel primo caso, i segni dei motoneuroni superiori sono prominenti, mentre nel secondo predominano le convulsioni e il coinvolgimento intellettivo e visivo. L'anamnesi conferma la regressione delle principali acquisizioni evolutive, mentre l'esame neurologico localizza il processo all'interno del sistema nervoso. Benché l'esito sia solitamente fatale e le terapie tentate finora si siano rivelate inefficaci, la formulazione di una corretta diagnosi è fondamentale per fornire ai genitori un *counseling* genetico ed elaborare una strategia preventiva. Il trapianto di midollo e le terapie genetiche e cellulari possono essere utili per prevenire la progressione della malattia in soggetti presintomatici. La prevenzione mediante diagnosi prenatale (amniocentesi o biopsia di villi coriali) è realizzabile in tutti i disturbi causati da un difetto enzimatico noto. La Tabella 599-1 riassume le modalità di trasmissione, i difetti biochimici e le specifiche anomalie diagnostiche dei disturbi neurodegenerativi ereditari. Una classificazione supplementare basata sull'età di esordio è presentata nella Tabella 599-2.

I disturbi neurodegenerativi ereditari includono le sfingolipidosi, la lipofuscinosi ceroide neuronale, la adrenoleucodistrofia e le sialidosi. Le sfingolipidosi sono caratterizzate dall'accumulo intracellulare di un normale componente lipidico della membrana cellulare, in seguito a un difetto del catabolismo di tale composto. Sono classificate in sei categorie: malattia di Niemann-Pick, malattia di Gaucher, gangliosidosi GM_1, gangliosidosi GM_2, malattia di Krabbe e leucodistrofia metacromatica. La malattia di Niemann-Pick e la malattia di Gaucher sono descritte nel Capitolo 86.4. Le malattie degenerative spinocerebellari (atassia di Friedreich, atassia-teleangiectasia, atrofia olivopontocerebellare e abetalipoproteinemia) e i disturbi degenerativi dei gangli basali (malattia di Huntington, distonia muscolare deformante, malattie di Wilson e di Hallervorden-Spatz) sono affrontate nel Capitolo 597. In questo capitolo, è approfondito un gruppo misto di malattie degenerative, che include la malattia di Pelizaeus-Merzbacher, la malattia di Alexander, la degenerazione spongiforme di Canavan, la malattia di Menkes, la sindrome di Rett e la panencefalite sclerosante subacuta.

TABELLA 599-1. Difetti ereditari e biochimici nei disturbi neurodegenerativi

DISTURBO NEURODEGENERATIVO	MODALITÀ DI TRASMISSIONE	DIFETTO BIOCHIMICO	CAMPIONE PER ANALISI
SFINGOLIPIDOSI	AR	β-galattosidasi	Siero, leucociti, fibroblasti cutanei
Gangliosidosi GM_1			
Gangliosidosi GM_2			
Malattia di Tay-Sachs	AR	Esosaminidasi A	Siero, leucociti, fibroblasti cutanei
Malattia di Sandhoff	AR	Esosaminidasi A e B	Siero, leucociti, fibroblasti cutanei
Malattia di Krabbe	AR	Galattocerebrosidasi	Leucociti e fibroblasti cutanei
Leucodistrofia metacromatica	AR	Arilsolfatasi A	Leucociti e fibroblasti cutanei
LIPOFUSCINOSI NEURONALE CEROIDE	AR	Palmitoil-proteina tioesterasi (PPT) Tripeptidil peptidasel 1 (TPP1)	EM di biopsia cutanea
ADRENOLEUCODISTROFIA	XLR	Ossidazione VLCFA	Plasma, fibroblasti cutanei
SIALIDOSI	AR	Neuraminidasi	Fibroblasti cutanei

AR, autosomica recessiva; EM, *Electron Microscopy* (microscopio elettronico); VLCFA, *Very Long Chain Fatty Acid* (acido grasso a catena molto lunga); XLR, *X-Linked Recessive* (recessiva correlata a X).

TABELLA 599-2. Alcune condizioni "intrinseche" associate a regressione dello sviluppo

ETÀ DI ESORDIO	MALATTIE	COMMENTI
<2 anni, con epatomegalia	Intolleranza al fruttosio	Vomito, ipoglicemia, disturbi dell'allattamento, deficit staturo-ponderale (in seguito all'assunzione di fruttosio)
	Galattosemia	Letargia, ipotonia, ittero, cataratta, ipoglicemia (in seguito all'assunzione di lattosio)
	Glicogenosi di tipo I-IV (malattie da accumulo del glicogeno)	Ipoglicemia, cardiomegalia (tipo II)
	Mucopolisaccaridosi tipo I e II	Lineamenti grossolani, rigidità articolare
	Malattia di Niemann-Pick, tipo infantile	Malattia della sostanza grigia, deficit staturo-ponderale
	Malattia di Tay-Sachs	Convulsioni, macchia rosso ciliegia, edema, lineamenti grossolani
	Sindrome di Zellweger (cerebroepatorenale)	Ipotonia, fronte alta, facies appiattita
	Malattia di Gaucher tipo II	Postura in estensione, irritabilità
	Sindromi da glicoproteine con deficit di carboidrati	Demielinizzazione, ipoplasia cerebellare
<2 anni, senza epatomegalia	Malattia di Krabbe	Irritabilità, postura in estensione, atrofia ottica e cecità
	Sindrome di Rett	Rallentamento della crescita della testa, perdita delle abilità manuali e della scrittura, compromissione del linguaggio, deambulazione aprassica; colpisce le femmine
	Malattia delle urine a sciroppo d'acero	Disturbi dell'allattamento, tremori, mioclono, epistotono
	Fenilchetonuria	Pigmentazione chiara, eczema, convulsioni
	Malattia di Menkes	Ipertonia, irritabilità, convulsioni, capelli fragili
	Encefalopatia necrotizzante subacuta di Leigh	Malattia della sostanza bianca
	Sindrome cerebro-oculofacioscheletrica (di Pena e Shokeir)	Riduzione della sostanza bianca, deficit staturo-ponderale
	Malattia di Canavan	Malattia della sostanza bianca
	Malattia di Pelizaeus-Merzbacher	Malattia della sostanza bianca
2-5 anni	Malattia di Niemann-Pick tipo III e IV	Epatosplenomegalia, difficoltà di deambulazione
	Malattia di Wilson	Malattia epatica, anello di Kayser-Fleischer; deterioramento cognitivo nello stadio avanzato
	Gangliosidosi di tipo II	Malattia della sostanza grigia
	Lipofuscinosi ceroide	Malattia della sostanza grigia
	Encefalopatie mitocondriali (epilessia mioclonica con fibre rosse sfilacciate [MERRF])	Malattia della sostanza grigia
	Atassia-teleangiectasia	Malattia dei gangli basali
	Malattia di Huntington (corea)	Malattia dei gangli basali
	Sindrome di Hallervorden-Spatz	Malattia dei gangli basali
	Leucodistrofia metacromatica	Malattia della sostanza bianca
	Adrenoleucodistrofia	Malattia della sostanza bianca, disturbi comportamentali, calo del rendimento scolastico, quadriparesi
5-15	Adrenoleucodistrofia	Stesso quadro della adrenoleucodistrofia nei bambini di 2-5 anni
	Sclerosi multipla	Malattia della sostanza bianca
	Lipofuscinosi ceroide neuronale, giovanile e adulta (malattie di Spielmeyer-Vogt e Kufs)	Malattia della sostanza grigia
	Malattia di Schilder	Malattia della sostanza bianca
	Malattia di Refsum	Neuropatia periferica, atassia, retinite pigmentosa
	Sialidosi II, forma giovanile	Macule rosso ciliegia, mioclono, atassia, lineamenti grossolani
	Panencefalite sclerosante subacuta	Encefalopatia diffusa, mioclono; può insorgere ad anni di distanza dal morbillo

Tratta da Kliegman RM, Greenbaum LA, Lye PS: *Practical Strategies in Pediatric Diagnosis and Therapy*, 2nd ed. Philadelphia, Elsevier/Saunders, 2004, p. 542.

599.1 • Sfingolipidosi

GANGLIOSIDOSI (VEDI ANCHE CAPITOLO 86.4)

I gangliosidi sono glicosfingolipidi, costituenti normali delle membrane sinaptiche e neuronali. La struttura di base del ganglioside GM_1 è composta da una catena oligosaccaride legata a un gruppo idrossile di ceramide e acido sialico legato al galattosio. I gangliosidi sono catabolizzati mediante clivaggio sequenziale delle molecole di zuccheri da parte di specifiche esoglicosidasi. Anomalie del catabolismo risultano in un accumulo di gangliosidi all'interno della cellula. I difetti di tale degradazione sono classificabili in due gruppi: gangliosidosi GM_1 e gangliosidosi GM_2.

GANGLIOSIDOSI GM_1. I tre sottotipi di gangliosidosi GM_1 sono classificati sulle base dell'età di presentazione: infantile (tipo 1), giovanile (tipo 2) e adulta (tipo 3). La malattia, ereditata con modalità autosomica recessiva, è il risultato di un marcato deficit di β-galattosidasi acida. Questo enzima può essere dosato su colture di fibroblasti o leucotici. Il gene che codifica per la β-galattosidasi acida è stato mappato sul cromosoma 3p14.2. La diagnosi prenatale è realizzabile mediante dosaggio della β-galattosidasi acida su colture di cellule amniotiche.

La ***gangliosidosi GM_1 infantile*** si presenta alla nascita o durante il periodo neonatale con anoressia, difficoltà di suzione e inadeguata crescita ponderale. Lo sviluppo globale è rallentato e le convulsioni prominenti. Il fenotipo presenta diversi caratteri in comune con la sindrome di Hurler: lineamenti grossolani, fronte prominente, radice nasale depressa, macroglossia e gengive ipertrofiche. La precoce epatosplenomegalia è il risultato dell'accumulo di istiociti schiumosi. La cifoscoliosi è evidenziata dalla malformazione a becco dei corpi vertebrali. L'esame neurologico rivela apatia, cecità progressiva, sordità, quadriplegia spastica e rigidità decerebrata. Nel 50% circa dei casi si osserva una **macchia rosso ciliegia** nella regione maculare, costituita da un anello opaco (composto da cellule ganglionari retiniche ripiene di sfingolipidi) che circonda la fovea, normalmente rossa (Fig. 599-1). Raramente i bambini sopravvivono oltre i 2-3 anni; la principale causa di mortalità è la polmonite da aspirazione.

La ***gangliosidosi GM_1 giovanile*** esordisce verso l'età di 1 anno. I sintomi iniziali includono mancanza di coordinazione, debolezza, atassia e regressione del linguaggio. In seguito, i reperti principali sono costituiti da convulsioni, spasticità, rigidità decerebrata e cecità. A differenza del tipo infantile, i pazienti solitamente non presentano né lineamenti grossolani né epatosplenomegalia. La radiografia delle vertebre lombari mostra una lieve malformazione a becco. Raramente i bambini sopravvivono oltre i 10 anni. La ***forma adulta della gangliosidosi GM_1*** è una malattia a progressione lenta, responsabile di spasticità, atassia, disartria e una graduale perdita della funzione cognitiva.

GANGLIOSIDOSI GM_2. Le gangliosidosi GM_2 costituiscono un gruppo eterogeneo di malattie a trasmissione autosomica recessiva, che include la malattia di Tay-Sachs (*Tay-Sachs Disease*, TSD), la malattia di Sandhoff, la gangliosidosi GM_2 giovanile e la gangliosidosi GM_2 adulta. La **malattia di Tay-Sachs** è prevalente nella popolazione ebrea ashkenazita, con una frequenza di portatori sani di circa 1/30. È causata da mutazioni del gene *HEXA*, localizzato sul cromosoma 15q23-q24. I bambini colpiti appaiono normali fino ai 6 mesi circa di età, fatta eccezione per una marcata reazione di trasalimento ai rumori, evidente fin dopo la nascita. Il ritardo nell'acquisizione delle tappe evolutive è seguito, entro il primo anno, dalla perdita della capacità di stare seduti, eretti e di vocalizzare. La precoce ipotonia evolve in progressiva spasticità. Il deterioramento inarrestabile conduce a convulsioni, cecità e sordità. Le macchie rosso ciliegia sono presenti in quasi tutti i pazienti (vedi Fig. 599-1). La macrocefalia si evidenzia entro il primo anno ed è provocata da un aumento del 200-300% del normale contenuto di gangliosidi GM_2 depositati nel cervello. Pochi bambini sopravvivono oltre i 3-4 anni; la mortalità è solitamente associata a broncopolmonite o a polmonite da aspirazione. Nei tessuti dei pazienti con TSD si riscontra un deficit dell'isoenzima esosaminidasi. Lo screening di massa per la diagnosi prenatale della TSD è un metodo preventivo efficace ed economico, perché il disturbo è ristretto a una popolazione specifica (ebrea ashkenazita). È disponibile inoltre un test affidabile ed economico per l'individuazione dei portatori sani (misura dell'esosaminidasi A in siero o leucociti). Nelle coppie a rischio (genitori eterozigoti) la malattia può essere diagnosticata nel primo trimestre di gravidanza mediante biopsia dei villi coriali.

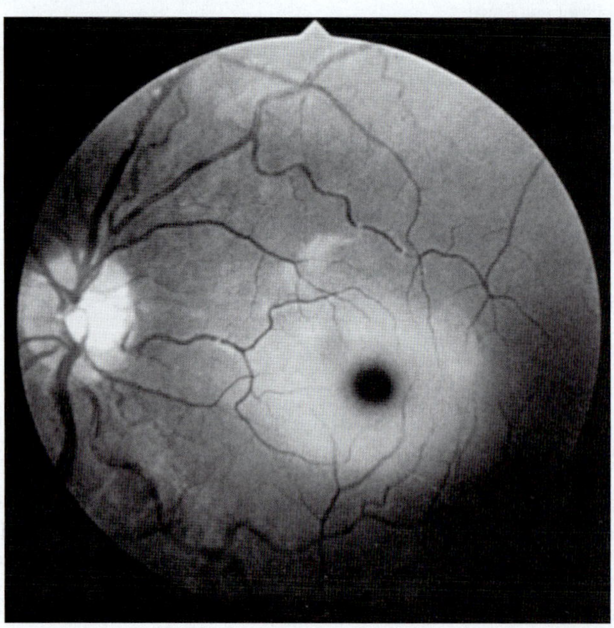

Figura 599-1. Macchia rosso ciliegia in un paziente con gangliosidosi GM_1. Notare l'anello biancastro di cellule ganglionari ripiene di sfingolipidi che circonda la fovea.

La **malattia di Sandhoff** ha una presentazione molto simile alla TDS, con progressiva perdita delle acquisizioni motorie e di linguaggio a iniziare dai 6 mesi di età. Nella maggior parte dei pazienti si riscontrano convulsioni, macchie rosso ciliegia, macrocefalia e faccia da bambola. Talvolta si osserva epatosplenomegalia. I potenziali evocati visivi sono normali nelle fasi precoci delle malattie di Sandhoff e TSD, ma in seguito divengono anomali o assenti. Le risposte evocate uditive troncoencefaliche mostrano latenze prolungate. La diagnosi di malattia di Sandhoff è stabilita sulla base del riscontro di un deficit di esosaminidasi A e B nel siero e nei leucociti. La mortalità entro i 3 anni è molto elevata. La malattia di Sandhoff è causata da mutazioni del gene HEXB, localizzato sul cromosoma 5q13.

La ***gangliosidosi GM_2 giovanile*** si sviluppa nella seconda infanzia, manifestandosi inizialmente come mancanza di coordinazione seguita da atassia. I segni di spasticità, l'atetosi, la perdita di linguaggio e le convulsioni insorgono gradualmente. La progressiva perdita visiva è associata ad atrofia ottica, ma le macchie rosso ciliegia sono presenti raramente. Si riscontra un deficit variabile di esosaminidasi (carenza da totale a pressoché assente). Il decesso sopraggiunge intorno ai 15 anni.

La ***gangliosidosi GM_2 adulta*** è caratterizzata da una miriade di segni neurologici, che includono atassia a lenta progressione, spasticità, distonia, atrofia dei muscoli prossimali e disartria. Solitamente, l'acuità visiva e la funzione intellettiva sono risparmiate. L'attività dell'esosaminidasi A, o A e B, è significativamente ridotta in siero e leucociti.

MALATTIA DI KRABBE (LEUCODISTROFIA A CELLULE GLOBOIDI). La malattia di Krabbe (*Krabbe Disease*, KD) è un raro disturbo neurodegenerativo a trasmissione autosomica recessiva, caratterizzato da grave perdita mielinica e dalla presenza di corpi globoidi nella sostanza bianca. Il gene per KD (*GALC*) è localizzato sul cromosoma 14q24.3-q32.1. La malattia è il risultato di un marcato deficit dell'enzima lisosomiale galattocerebroside β-galattosidasi, responsabile del clivaggio di galattosio dalla porzione ceramide del galattocerebroside. I disturbi sono provocati da una distruzione di mielina piuttosto che dalla sua anomala formazione. In circostanze normali, il processo di mielinizzazione inizia nel terzo trimestre, in coincidenza con un rapido aumento dell'attività cerebrale della galattocerebroside β-galattosidasi. Nei pazienti con KD, il galattocerebroside non può essere metabolizzato durante il normale turnover della mielina, a causa del deficit di galattocerebroside β-galattosidasi. L'iniezione di galattocerebroside nel cervello di animali sperimentali provoca la reazione a cellule globoidi. Un fenomeno simile è stato postulato anche negli esseri umani; il galattocerebroside non metabolizzato stimola la formazione di cellule globoidi, che riflette la distruzione delle cellule oligondendrogliali. Poiché tali cellule sono responsabili della produzione di mielina, la loro distruzione causa demielinizzazione, che determina un ulteriore aumento della produzione di galattocerebroside, innescando un circolo vizioso di distruzione della mielina.

I sintomi di KD, evidenti già nei primi mesi di vita, includono eccessiva irritabilità e pianto, episodi di iperpiressia inspiegabili, disturbi dell'allattamento, vomito e deficit staturo-ponderale. Negli stadi iniziali, ai bambini è spesso diagnosticata una colica o "allergia al latte", trattata cambiando marca di latte formulato. Le convulsioni generalizzate possono comparire precocemente. Nel corso della progressione della malattia, si evidenziano alterazioni del tono posturale, con rigidità e opistotono, e inattenzione visiva dovuta ad atrofia ottica. Negli stadi avanzati, si riscontrano cecità, sordità, assenza dei riflessi tendinei profondi e rigidità decerebrata. La TC cerebrale (senza mezzo di contrasto) può rivelare un aumento di densità simmetrico in talamo e nucleo caudato. La mortalità entro i primi 2 anni di vita è elevata. La RM e la risonanza magnetica spettroscopica sono utili per valutare l'estensione della demielinizzazione. Nei neonati asintomatici, il trapianto di cellule staminali da cordone ombelicale di donatori non imparentati può modificare favorevolmente il decorso della malattia.

La *KD a esordio tardivo* si manifesta nella fanciullezza o nell'adolescenza, con atrofia ottica e cecità corticale. Nelle fasi iniziali, la malattia è facilmente confusa con le adrenoleucodistrofie. I disturbi della deambulazione a lenta progressione, come spasticità e atassia, sono prominenti. Come nella KD classica, le cellule globoidi abbondano nella sostanza bianca e si riscontra un deficit di galattocerebroside β-galattosidasi nei leucociti. L'esame del liquido cerebrospinale (LCS) rivela un aumento del contenuto di proteine. A causa della demielinizzazione segmentale dei nervi periferici, la velocità di conduzione risulta marcatamente ridotta. I potenziali evocati visivi hanno un'ampiezza gradualmente decrescente, con assenza di risposta negli stadi terminali. I potenziali evocati uditivi sono caratterizzati dalla esclusiva presenza di onde I e II. TC e RM evidenziano la marcata riduzione di sostanza bianca, in particolare a livello di cervelletto e centro semi-ovale, mentre le fibre a U sottocorticali sono risparmiate. La diagnosi prenatale è realizzabile mediante verifica dell'attività della galattocerebroside β-galattosidasi sui villi coriali o su colture di cellule amniotiche.

LEUCODISTROFIA METACROMATICA (MLD). Questo disturbo del metabolismo della mielina (*Metachromatic LeukoDystrophy*, MLD), trasmesso con modalità autosomica recessiva, è caratterizzato da un deficit di attività dell'arilsolfatasi A. Sono state identificate diverse mutazioni del gene che codifica per arilsolfatasi A, localizzato sul cromosoma 22q13-13qter. È possibile la diagnosi mediante esame del DNA. L'assenza o la carenza di arilsolfatasi A determina l'accumulo di cerebroside solfato all'interno del rivestimento mielinico del sistema nervoso centrale (SNC) e periferico, dovuto all'impossibilità di scindere il solfato dal galattosil-3-solfato ceramide. Si ritiene che l'eccesso di cerebroside solfato causi la distruzione di mielina e oligodendroglia. La diagnosi prenatale della MLD è realizzabile mediante dosaggio dell'arilsolfatasi su villi coriali o coltura di cellule amniotiche. Il violetto di cresile colora in modo metacromatico i granuli di sulfatide; da questo prende il nome la malattia. Si distinguono sei sottotipi di MLD, classificati sulla base dell'età di esordio e del deficit enzimatico. Di seguito, sono approfondite tre forme: la classica o infantile, la giovanile e quella adulta.

La ***MLD infantile tardiva*** ha un esordio insidioso, con disturbi della deambulazione tra il primo e il secondo anno di vita. Inizialmente il bambino appare goffo e cade facilmente, ma in seguito alla progressione del disturbo ha bisogno di un supporto per camminare. Gli arti sono ipotonici e i riflessi tendinei profondi assenti o ridotti. Nei mesi seguenti, il bambino non riesce più a stare in piedi e il deterioramento della funzione intellettiva diviene evidente. L'eloquio è disarticolato e disartrico e il bambino appare apatico e passivo. La fissazione visiva è ridotta, si osserva nistagmo e l'esame della retina mostra atrofia ottica. Entro un anno dall'esordio della malattia, il bambino non riesce a stare seduto senza supporto e sviluppa una postura progressivamente decorticata. La pseudoparalisi bulbare compromette la deglutizione, rendendo necessaria una gastrostomia. Seguono l'insorgenza di *stupor* e il decesso entro i 5-6 anni in seguito a broncopolmonite o inalazione. La valutazione neurofisiologica mostra alterazioni progressive dei potenziali evocati visivi, uditivi e somatosensoriali, nonché una significativa riduzione della velocità di conduzione dei nervi periferici. TC e RM cerebrali mostrano una diffusa attenuazione simmetrica della sostanza bianca cerebellare e cerebrale. L'esame del LCS rivela un aumento del contenuto proteico. Il trapianto di midollo costituisce una promettente terapia sperimentale per la gestione della MLD infantile tardiva. Risultati positivi sono stati ottenuti solo in pazienti trattati nella fase precoce del decorso della malattia. L'esiguo numero di pazienti trattati e il follow-up troppo breve non consentono ancora di trarre conclusioni definitive sull'efficacia.

La ***MLD giovanile*** presenta molte caratteristiche in comune con la MLD infantile tardiva, ma l'esordio dei sintomi è ritardato fino ai 5-10 anni. L'insorgenza della malattia può essere preannunciata dal calo del rendimento scolastico e da alterazioni della personalità. Seguono incontinenza urinaria, disturbi della deambulazione e disartria. Il tono muscolare aumenta e possono evidenziarsi atassia, distonia o tremori. Negli stadi terminali, prevalgono le convulsioni generalizzate tonico-cloniche difficili da controllare. Raramente i pazienti sopravvivono oltre l'adolescenza.

La ***MLD adulta*** insorge tra la seconda e la sesta decade, con anomalie della memoria, disturbi psichiatrici e cambiamenti di personalità. Segni neurologici a lenta progressione, che includono spasticità, distonia, atrofia ottica e convulsioni generalizzate, obbligano infine il paziente a letto, in uno stato caratterizzato da postura decorticata e incoscienza.

599.2 • LIPOFUSCINOSI CEROIDI NEURONALI

Le lipofuscinosi ceroidi neuronali, trasmesse con modalità autosomica recessiva, costituiscono la più comune classe di malattie neurodegenerative infantili. Sono causate dall'accumulo di una sostanza autofluorescente nei lisosomi dei neuroni e di altri tessuti. Sono stati identificati singoli geni mutati in 6 forme.

Il ***tipo infantile (Haltia-Santavuori)*** esordisce verso la fine del primo anno di vita, con convulsioni miocloniche, deterioramento intellettivo e cecità. L'esame della retina evidenza l'atrofia ottica e la discolorazione bruna della macula. L'atassia cerebellare è marcata. L'elettroretinogramma (ERG) mostra tipicamente onde di ampiezza ridotta o assenti. Il decesso avviene entro i 10 anni. Il difetto genetico responsabile della forma infantile è stato localizzato sul cromosoma 1p32. Sono state inoltre identificate mutazioni del gene *CLN1*, che codifica per l'enzima lisosomiale palmitoil-proteina tioesterasi-1 (PPT).

Il ***tipo infantile tardivo (Jansky-Bielschowsky)*** è il più comune. La manifestazione iniziale, tra i 2 e i 4 anni, consiste in convulsioni miocloniche, in un bambino precedentemente sano. La demenza e l'atassia sono associate a una progressiva perdita di acuità visiva e a microcefalia. L'esame della retina mostra una marcata attenuazione dei vasi, anomalie granulose della pigmentazione periferica causate da spicule ossee nere, atrofia ottica e presenza di pigmento marrone nella regione maculare. L'ERG è anomalo già nelle fasi precoci della malattia, a causa dei depositi nell'area dei coni e bastoncelli della retina. I potenziali evocati visivi mostrano un caratteristico allargamento della risposta, seguito da assenza di onde con la progressione della malattia. Il materiale autofluorescente è depositato nei neuroni, nei fibroblasti e nelle cellule secretorie. L'esame al microscopio elettronico del materiale depositato nella biopsia cutanea o congiuntivale mostra tipicamente corpi curvilinei o un profilo a "impronte digitali". Sono state identificate mutazioni del gene *CLN2*, che codifica per tripeptidil peptidasi-1, essenziale per la degradazione di colecistochinina-8. Sono note anche mutazioni dei geni *CLN5*, *CLN6* e *CLN8*, che codificano per proteine costitutive di membrana ancora da caratterizzare con precisione.

Il ***tipo giovanile (Spielmeyer-Vogt)***, a esordio tra i 5 e i 10 anni, è caratterizzato da progressiva perdita visiva e coinvolgimento intellettivo. Le alterazioni del fundus oculare sono analoghe a quelle osservate nella forma infantile tardiva. L'ERG risulta anomalo precocemente e i potenziali evocati visivi mostrano inizialmente onde di ridotta ampiezza e più tardi un'assenza di onde con il progredire della malattia. Le convulsioni miocloniche sono meno importanti rispetto alla forma infantile tardiva, ma si osserva una postura gravemente distonica. L'aumento dei livelli di dolicolo nelle urine è un reperto non specifico. Nella maggior parte dei casi, la biopsia cutanea mostra le alterazioni ultrastrutturali. Sono state identificate mutazioni dei geni *CLN2* e *CLN3*.

599.3 • Adrenoleucodistrofia (vedi anche Capitolo 86.2)

Le adrenoleucodistrofie costituiscono un gruppo di disturbi degenerativi del SNC a trasmissione recessiva legata alla X, spesso associati a insufficienza corticosurrenale. L'*adrenoleucodistrofia classica* (ALD), considerata la forma più comune, diviene sintomatica tra i 5 e i 15 anni di età, con calo della prestazione scolastica, disturbi comportamentali e anomalie della deambulazione. La malattia è causata da un accumulo di acidi grassi a catena molto lunga nel tessuto neurale e surrenale, in seguito a mutazioni del gene *ABCD1*, che codifica per una proteina emi-trasportatrice ATP-legante localizzata sul cromosoma Xq28. La relazione tra ALD e il metabolismo degli acidi grassi a catena molto lunga non è stata ancora chiarita.

L'incidenza dell'ALD è di circa 1/20 000 maschi. Nel 40% degli emizigoti di sesso maschile, la malattia si presenta nella sua forma classica, come disturbo infiammatorio demielinizzante. Le convulsioni generalizzate sono comuni negli stadi precoci. I segni dei motoneuroni superiori includono quadriparesi spastica e contratture, atassia e gravi disturbi della deglutizione, secondari a paralisi pseudobulbare. Tali segni dominano gli stadi terminali della malattia. L'ipoadrenalismo è presente in circa il 50% dei casi; l'insufficienza surrenale, caratterizzata da un'anomala pigmentazione della cute (abbronzata senza esposizione al sole), può precedere l'esordio dei sintomi neurologici. TC e RM mostrano demielinizzazione periventricolare che inizia posteriormente e che avanza progressivamente nelle regioni anteriori della sostanza bianca cerebrale. Potenziali evocati visivi, uditivi e somatosensoriali sono inizialmente normali, ma in seguito mostrano latenze prolungate e onde anomale. Il decesso avviene entro 10 anni dall'esordio dei segni neurologici. Tuttavia, follow-up a lungo termine hanno dimostrato che il trapianto di midollo può prevenire la progressione della malattia, purché effettuato in uno stadio precoce, prima dell'insorgenza dei segni clinici. Anche la somministrazione dell'olio di Lorenzo, composto da gliceril trioleato e gliceril trierucato in proporzione di 4:1, nei bambini di età superiore ai 6 anni con RM cerebrale normale contribuisce a ridurre la probabilità di sviluppo di anomalie neurologiche.

L'***adrenomieloneuropatia*** si verifica nel 40% di pazienti maschi con adrenoleucodistrofia legata alla X. In questi casi, la malattia si presenta come un disturbo cronico del midollo spinale e dei nervi periferici, che esordisce con paraparesi spastica a progressione lenta, incontinenza urinaria e impotenza durante la terza e quarta decade, benché l'insufficienza surrenale possa essere presente fin dalla nascita. Casi di ALD tipica si sono verificati in famiglie in cui un individuo presentava adrenomieloneuropatia. Una delle principali difficoltà nella gestione dell'ALD legata alla X consiste nel fatto che individui di una stessa famiglia possono presentare decorsi clinici molto diversi. Per esempio, in una famiglia un bambino affetto da ALD classica era morto a 10 anni, un fratello presentava adrenomieloneuropatia a esordio tardivo e un terzo fratello era del tutto asintomatico. Gli esami di neuroimaging forniscono informazioni quantitative sulla progressione delle adrenoleucodistrofie, contribuendo a selezionare i pazienti idonei per il trapianto di midollo e migliorando il *counseling*.

L'***ALD neonatale***, a trasmissione autosomica recessiva, è caratterizzata da marcata ipotonia, grave ritardo psicomotorio ed esordio precoce delle convulsioni. La disattenzione visiva è secondaria all'atrofia ottica. I risultati degli esami della funzione surrenale sono normali, ma l'atrofia surrenale è evidente *post mortem*. La correzione dell'insufficienza surrenale non interrompe il deterioramento neurologico.

Oltre alle cosiddette leucodistrofie classiche, recentemente sono state identificate nuove malattie, grazie all'uso su larga scala della RM. La ***malattia della scomparsa della sostanza bianca*** o ***atassia infantile con ipomielinizzazione del SNC*** è un grave disturbo demielinizzante causato da mutazioni dei geni *eIF*, coinvolti nello scambio GDP/GTP. È interessante notare che in tali disturbi la demielinizzazione può essere scatenata dalla febbre o da uno spavento. Nel gruppo etnico indiano Ararwal è stata documenta la presenza di un disturbo genetico con megalencefalia, alterazioni diffuse della sostanza bianca con cisti temporali, declino cognitivo moderato e spasticità. Tale malattia è collegata a mutazioni del gene *MLC*.

599.4 • Sialidosi

La sialidosi, ereditata con modalità autosomica recessiva, è il risultato dell'accumulo di un complesso sialico acido-oligosaccaride, secondario a un deficit dell'enzima lisosomiale neuraminidasi. Il gene che codifica per la sialidasi lisosomiale è stato mappato sul cromosoma 6p21.3. Nei pazienti colpiti si riscontra un significativo aumento dell'escrezione di oligosaccaridi contenenti acido sialico nelle urine.

La ***sialidosi di tipo I***, detta anche **sindrome macchia rosso ciliegia-mioclono** (*Cherry Red Spot Myoclonus Syndrome*, CRSM), si presenta solitamente nella seconda decade con deterioramento visivo. L'esame della retina mostra la presenza di una macchia rosso ciliegia ma, a differenza dei pazienti con TSD, l'acuità visiva declina lentamente. Il mioclono agli arti è spesso progressivo e invalidante, fino a impedire la deambulazione. Le mioclonie, non controllabili con gli anticonvulsivanti, sono scatenate dal movimento volontario, dal tatto o da suoni. Convulsioni generalizzate che rispondono agli antiepilettici si riscontrano nella maggior parte dei pazienti.

La ***sialidosi di tipo II*** è classificata nelle forme infantile e giovanile, sulla base dell'età di presentazione. Oltre alle macchie rosso ciliegia e al mioclono, i pazienti presentano coinvolgimento somatico, con lineamenti facciali grossolani, offuscamento corneale (raro) e disostosi multiple (responsabili di una deformazione a becco delle vertebre lombari). L'esame dei linfociti mostra la presenza di vacuoli nel citoplasma; la biopsia epatica evidenzia vacuoli citoplasmatici nelle cellule di Kupffer e vacuoli legati alla membrana si riscontrano anche nel citoplasma delle cellule di Schwann. Tali reperti dimostrano la natura multiorgano della malattia. Non si osservano invece anomalie nei risultati degli esami di neuroimaging ed elettrofisiologici. Sono stati segnalati casi di pazienti sopravvissuti oltre la quinta decade.

Alcuni casi diagnosticati come sialidosi di tipo II sono il risultato di un deficit combinato di β-galattosidasi e α-neuraminidasi, secondario a una carenza di una "proteina protettiva" che previene la prematura degradazione intracellulare dei due tipi di enzimi menzionati. Sul piano clinico, i pazienti sono indistinguibili da quelli affetti da sialidosi II vera e propria (causata dal deficit isolato di α-neuraminidasi). Il disturbo può non essere riconosciuto se si effettua soltanto il test per β-galattosidasi, senza verificare l'attività di α-neuraminidasi nei fibroblasti.

599.5 • Disturbi vari

MALATTIA DI PELIZAEUS-MERZBACHER. La malattia include un gruppo di disturbi caratterizzati da nistagmo e anomalie della mielina. La forma classica, ereditata con modalità recessiva legata alla X, è causata da difetti del gene della proteina proteolipide (PLP), essenziale per la formazione di mielina e per la differenziazione degli oligodendrociti. Mutazioni dello stesso gene causano la paraparesi spastica familiare. La malattia è riconosciuta nell'infanzia per la presenza di nistagmo, movimenti erratici degli occhi e oscillazioni del capo. Il gene è localizzato sul cromosoma Xq22. La diagnosi molecolare è realizzabile mediante analisi della mutazione. Come nella maggior parte delle malattie legate alla X, la diagnosi molecolare della malattia di Pelizaeus-Merzbacher è complessa, perché soltanto nel 10-25% dei pazienti sono presenti mutazioni esoniche. Inizialmente il paziente manifesta ritardo nel raggiungimento delle principali tappe evolutive; in seguito compaiono atassia, coreoatetosi e spasticità. Atrofia ottica e disartria sono di comune riscontro. La mortalità nella seconda o terza decade è molto elevata. Il principale reperto patologico, la perdita di mielina con assoni integri, suggerisce un difetto nella funzione dell'oligodendroglia. Alcuni studi hanno segnalato un difetto genetico nella biosintesi del proteolipide apoproteina, coinvolta nella differenziazione e nel mantenimento degli oligodendrociti. La RM mostra un pattern simmetrico di mielinizzazione ritardata. I potenziali evocati multimodali segnalano già nelle fasi precoci della malattia in una perdita delle onde III-V in ABR. Questo dato è utile per diagnosticare il nistagmo nei maschi. I VEP mostrano latenze prolungate, mentre i SSEP rivelano l'assenza di risposte corticali o latenze ritardate. È stato dimostrato che un'ampia gamma di fenotipi, che includono la paraplegia spastica di tipo 2 e anomalie dei nervi periferici, può essere il risultato di mutazioni del gene PLP.

MALATTIA DI ALEXANDER. Questo raro disturbo sporadico causa macrocefalia progressiva nel primo anno di vita, secondaria a mutazioni del gene che codifica per la proteina gliale fibrillare acidica (*Glial Fibrillary Acidic Protein*, GFAP). L'esame istologico rivela la deposizione di corpi ialini eosinofili, distribuiti perivascolarmente nel cervello e al di sotto della pia madre. La degenerazione della sostanza bianca è particolarmente evidente a livello dei lobi frontali e la TC mostra una corrispondente attenuazione della sostanza bianca cerebrale. I bambini colpiti sviluppano una progressiva perdita della funzione intellettiva, spasticità e convulsioni non trattabili, responsabili del decesso entro i 5 anni.

DEGENERAZIONE SPONGIFORME DI CANAVAN. Vedi Capitolo 85.14.

MALATTIA DI MENKES. La malattia di Menkes (malattia dei capelli a cavaturacciolo) è un disturbo neurodegenerativo progressivo che si trasmette con modalità recessiva legata al sesso. Il gene responsabile codifica per una ATPasi di tipo P deputata al trasporto del rame; mutazioni della proteina sono associate a riduzione dei livelli sierici di rame e ceruplasmina, nonché a difetti dell'assorbimento e del trasporto del rame attraverso l'intestino. I sintomi esordiscono nei primi mesi di vita e includono ipotermia, ipotonia e convulsioni miocloniche generalizzate. I pazienti presentano una facies tipica, con guance rosee e piene e capelli fragili e scoloriti. L'esame microscopico dei capelli rivela diverse anomalie, tra cui la tricorressi nodosa (responsabili di fratture lungo lo stelo) e pili torti. Le rilevanti difficoltà di allattamento causano deficit staturo-ponderale. Le alterazioni neuropatologiche includono una degenerazione tortuosa della sostanza grigia, perdita dello strato granulare interno e necrosi delle cellule di Purkinje a livello cerebellare. In assenza di trattamento, il decesso avviene entro i 3 anni.

La terapia con rame-istidina può risultare efficace nel prevenire il deterioramento neurologico, in particolare se il trattamento è avviato nel periodo neonatale o, preferibilmente, in quello fetale. Il rame è essenziale negli stadi precoci dello sviluppo del SNC e la sua assenza è probabilmente responsabile delle alterazioni neuropatologiche. Il rame-istidina è somministrato per via sottocutanea alla dose di 50-150 μg di rame elementare/kg/24 h. La terapia deve proseguire per tutta la vita. I livelli sierici di rame e ceruloplasmina si normalizzano nel giro di 2-3 settimane.

La **sindrome del corno occipitale** è una displasia scheletrica causata da una diversa mutazione dello stesso gene coinvolto nella malattia di Menkes. Le due malattie sono spesso confuse, perché le anomalie biochimiche sono identiche, ma la sindrome del corno occipitale è relativamente più lieve. Un'accurata correlazione genotipo-fenotipo e trial clinici di terapia con rame consentono di chiarire eventuali dubbi.

SINDROME DI RETT (RS). A rigor di termini, questa sindrome (*Rett Syndome*, RS) non è una malattia degenerativa, ma un disturbo dello sviluppo cerebrale precoce, che colpisce prevalentemente le bambine. Nella prima infanzia, dopo un primo periodo neonatale relativamente normale, il paziente va incontro a regressione evolutiva e rallentamento della crescita cerebrale. La frequenza della malattia è di circa 1/15 000-1/22 000. La RS è causata da mutazioni di *MeCP2*, un fattore di trascrizione che si lega alle isole CpG metilate, silenziandone la trascrizione. Lo sviluppo può procedere normalmente fino al primo anno, quando si evidenziano il ritardo nelle tappe evolutive, la regressione del linguaggio e la microcefalia acquisita. I primi riscontri neurologici sono un'andatura atassica o tremori fini delle mani. La maggior parte dei bambini sviluppa una particolare respirazione sospirosa, con intermittenti periodi di apnea, talvolta associati a cianosi. Il tratti distintivi della sindrome di Rett, che appaiono tra i 2-3 anni, sono costituiti da ripetitivi movimenti delle mani, come se il paziente si lavasse le mani, e dalla perdita dell'uso intenzionale spontaneo delle mani. Il comportamento autistico è riscontrato in quasi tutti i pazienti. Convulsioni tonico-cloniche generalizzate si verificano nella maggior parte dei casi, ma solitamente sono ben controllate dai farmaci. I disturbi della suzione e la scarsa crescita ponderale sono comuni. Dopo un periodo iniziale di regressione neurologica, la malattia raggiunge un plateau, con persistenza del comportamento autistico. Il decesso avviene nell'adolescenza o nella terza decade. Aritmie cardiache possono provocare una morte improvvisa.

Gli esami *post mortem* hanno evidenziato una significativa riduzione del peso cerebrale (60-80% del normale), con un decremento del numero di sinapsi, associato a ridotta lunghezza e ramificazione dendritica. Il fenotipo può essere collegato alla mancata soppressione dell'espressione di geni normalmente silenti nella prime fasi dello sviluppo postnatale. Benché la sopravvivenza dei pazienti di sesso maschile con fenotipo RS classico sia rara, la genotipizzazione di ragazzi senza fenotipo classico ma con ritardo mentale e altre caratteristiche neurologiche atipiche ha consentito l'individuazione di un numero significativo di soggetti con mutazioni di *MeCP2*. La presenza di tali mutazioni è stata dimostrata anche in portatrici sane, femmine con sindrome di Angelman e maschi con encefalopatia fatale, sindrome di Klinefelter (47,XXY) e ritardo mentale familiare legato alla X.

PANENCEFALITE SCLEROSANTE SUBACUTA. Questa rara infezione progressiva da virus lento del SNC è causata da un virus simil-morbilloso (vedi Capitolo 243.1). Il numero di casi riportati è calato vertiginosamente a 0,06 casi/1 milione, parallelamente al declino dei casi di morbillo. Le manifestazioni cliniche iniziali includono cambiamenti della personalità, comportamento aggressivo e compromissione della funzione cognitiva. Le convulsioni miocloniche dominano il quadro clinico. Successivamente, si evidenziano convulsioni tonico-cloniche generalizzate, ipertonia e coreoatetosi, seguiti da paralisi bulbare progressiva, ipertermia e postura decerebrata. Già nelle fasi iniziali della malattia, l'esame del fundus oculare rivela papilledema in circa il 20% dei casi. Atrofia ottica, corioretinite e pigmentazione maculare si osservano nella maggior parte dei pazienti. La diagnosi è stabilita sulla base del decorso clinico tipico, associato alla presenza di uno dei seguenti criteri: (1) anticorpi contro il morbillo nel LCF; (2) un elettroencefalogramma caratteristico, con scariche di onde lente ad alto voltaggio e ritmo di fondo normale negli stadi iniziali; (3) reperti istologici tipici nella biopsia cerebrale o esame *post mortem*. Il trattamento con agenti antivirali è stato tentato senza successo. Il decesso sopraggiunge solitamente dopo 1-2 anni dall'esordio dei sintomi.

Aoki Y, Haginoya K, Munakata M, et al: A novel mutation in glial fibrillary acidic protein gene in a patient with Alexander disease. *Neurosci Lett* 2001;312:71–74.

Baram TZ, Goldman AM, Percy AK: Krabbe disease: Specific MRI and CT findings. *Neurology* 1986;36:111–115.

Berger J, Moser HW, Forss-Petter S: Leukodystrophies: Recent developments in genetics, molecular biology, pathogenesis and treatment. *Curr Opin Neurol* 2001;14:305–312.

Cooper JD: Progress towards understanding the neurobiology of Batten disease or neuronal ceroid lipofuscinosis. *Curr Opin Neurol* 2003;16: 121–128.

Couvert P, Bienvenu T, Aquaviva C: *MeCP2* is highly mutated in X-linked mental retardation. *Hum Mol Genet* 2001;10:941–946.

Dyken PR, Cunningham SC, Ward LC: Changing character of subacute sclerosing panencephalitis in the United States. *Pediatr Neurol* 1989;5:339–341.

Escolar ML, Poe MD, Provenzale JM, et al: Transplantation of umbilical-cord blood in babies with infantile Krabbe's disease. *N Engl J Med* 2005;352:2069–2080.

Gao H, Boustany RM, Espinola JA, et al: Mutations in a novel CLN6-encoded transmembrane protein cause variant neuronal ceroid lipofuscinosis in man and mouse. *Am J Hum Genet* 2002;70:324–335.

Gorospe JR, Singhal BS, Kainu T, et al: Indian Agarwal megalencephalic leukodystrophy with cysts is caused by a common *MLC1* mutation. *Neurology* 2004;62:878–882.

Hudson LD: Pelizaeus-Merzbacher disease and spastic paraplegia type 2: Two faces of myelin loss from mutations in the same gene. *J Child Neurol* 2003;18:616–624.

Julu PO, Kerr AM, Apartopoulos F, et al: Characterisation of breathing and associated central autonomic dysfunction in Rett disorder. *Arch Dis Child* 2001;85:29–37.

Kaye EM: Update on genetic disorders affecting white matter. *Pediatr Neurol* 2001;24:11–24.

Krivit W: Stem cell bone marrow transplantation in patients with metabolic storage disease. *Adv Pediat* 2002;49:359–378.

Moser HW, Dubey P, Fatemi A: Progress in X-linked adrenoleukodystrophy. *Curr Opin Neurol* 2004;17:263–269.

Percy AK, Lane JB: Rett syndrome: Clinical and molecular update. *Curr Opin Neurol* 2004;16:670–677.

Pshezhetsky AV, Richard C, Michaud L, et al: Cloning, expression and chromosomal mapping of human lysosomal sialidase and characterization of mutations in sialidoses. *Nat Genet* 1997;15:316–320.

Shapiro E, Krivit W, Lockman L, et al: Long-term effect of bone-marrow transplantation for childhood-onset cerebral X-linked adrenoleukodystrophy. *Lancet* 2000;356:713–718.

Schiffmann R, Brady RO: New prospects for the treatment of lysosomal storage diseases. *Drugs* 2002;62:733–742.

Schiffmann R, van der Knaap MS: The latest on leukodystrophies. *Curr Opin Neurol* 2004;17:187–192.

Staba SL, Escolar ML, Poe M, et al: Cord-blood transplants from unrelented donors in patients with Hurler's syndrome. *N Engl J Med* 2004;350: 1960–1968.

Suzuki K: Globoid cell leukodystrophy (Krabbe's disease): An update. *J Child Neurol* 2003;18:595–603.

Wisniewski KE, Kida E, Golabek AA, et al: Neuronal lipofuscinosis: Classification and diagnosis. *Adv Genet* 2001;45:1–34.

Vermeulen G, Seidl R, Mercimek-Mahmutoglu S, et al: Fright is a provoking factor in vanishing white matter disease. *Ann Neurol* 2005;57:560–563.

Capitolo 600 ■ Disturbi demielinizzanti del SNC Michael V. Johnston

I disturbi demielinizzanti del sistema nervoso centrale (SNC) causano encefalopatia acuta o remittente e altri segni multifocali di disfunzione cerebrale, troncoencefalica o midollare. Tali disturbi colpiscono la sostanza bianca, formata da fibre nervose ricoperte da mielina, un materiale isolante prodotto dagli oligondedrociti. A differenza delle leucodistrofie geneticamente determinate, i disturbi demielinizzanti provocano la degenerazione di sostanza bianca già formata, mediante meccanismi immunomediati. I principali disturbi demielinizzanti infantili sono la sclerosi multipla (SM) e l'encefalomielite acuta disseminata (ADEM). Le rare sindromi da attivazione dei macrofagi e la vasculite isolata del SNC possono essere talvolta confuse con la ADEM.

600.1 • Sclerosi multipla

La sclerosi multipla è un disturbo cronico e solitamente remittente caratterizzato da lesioni multiple a carico della sostanza bianca nel SNC, con tempi di insorgenza e localizzazioni differenti. La malattia è rara nella popolazione pediatrica; soltanto il 5% dei casi di SM si verifica prima dei 18 anni. La causa responsabile è ancora sconosciuta, ma si ipotizza un'interazione tra fattori genetici, immunologici e infettivi. In circa il 20% dei casi, si riscontra un'anamnesi di SM in un parente di primo grado. I più frequenti segni di presentazione sono debolezza unilaterale, con segni dei motoneuroni superiori, anomalie sensoriali, disturbi visivi o atassia. Parestesie che coinvolgono gli arti inferiori, le porzioni distali di mani e piedi e il volto sono di comune riscontro. I sintomi visivi includono diplopia, nistagmo o improvvisa perdita visiva dovuta a neurite ottica. Possono essere presenti anche cefalea, fatica, disartria, mielopatia e vescica neurogena, ma la compromissione della coscienza e l'encefalopatia sono rare. La **neuromielite ottica** (malattia di Devic) è una variante della SM classica caratterizzata dalla contemporanea presenza di *neurite ottica* e *mielite trasversa*. Benché la presenza della malattia sia sospettata già dall'episodio iniziale, la diagnosi può essere formulata soltanto dopo un secondo episodio clinico a distanza di almeno un mese o in seguito all'insorgenza di una nuova lesione della sostanza bianca dopo 3 mesi (dimostrata dalla RM).

La patologia della SM consiste nella demielinizzazione e nella formazione di placche. La biopsia e l'autopsia costituiscono gli unici test di laboratorio in grado di confermare con assoluta sicurezza la diagnosi di SM. La RM è l'esame di neuroimaging di elezione, poiché consente l'identificazione di piccole placche di 3-4 mm, in particolare se localizzate nel tronco encefalico e nel midollo spinale (Fig. 600-1). Le immagini pesate in T_2 mostrano la presenza di lesioni del corpo calloso e della sostanza bianca periventricolare in un'elevata percentuale di pazienti pediatrici. Il liquido cerebrospinale (LCS) contiene spesso bande oligoclonali.

Il **trattamento** di un attacco acuto di SM richiede spesso la somministrazione per via endovenosa di elevate dosi di metilprednisolone, che sono in grado di accelerare il recupero, ma non di alterare il decorso a lungo termine della malattia. Nei casi in cui la neurite ottica costituisce la prima manifestazione della SM, una terapia aggressiva con prednisone può ridurre il rischio di sviluppo a lungo termine della SM. La terapia riabilitativa è utile, in particolare per la gestione della vescica neurogena, in caso di coinvolgimento midollare. Come dimostrato dalla RM con mezzo di contrasto (gadolinio), le terapie con interferone possono limitare l'attività della malattia, riducendo il numero di nuove lesioni, la febbre e le recidive. Tali terapie, utili anche nei bambini, sono più efficaci se avviate tempestivamente. L'interferone β è l'agente più usato. Altri farmaci che interferiscono con la patologica infiammazione immunomediata e che sono stati efficaci nel trattare adulti con SM (immunomediata) includono: il glatiramer acetato, un polipeptide che mima la proteina mielinica basica; il fingolimod, modulatore orale del recettore della sfingosina-1-fosfato; il natalizumab, anticorpo monoclonale contro la molecola di adesione cellulare α4β1 integrina. La terapia con natalizumab è associata allo sviluppo di leucoencefalopatia multifocale progressiva.

La **prognosi** per i bambini con SM è simile a quella degli adulti; il recupero è spesso completo e la progressione della malattia tende a essere lenta, con lunghi periodi di remissione.

600.2 • Encefalomielite acuta disseminata

L'encefalomielite acuta disseminata (*Acute Disseminated EncephaloMyelitis,* ADEM) è un disturbo demielinizzante monofasico e

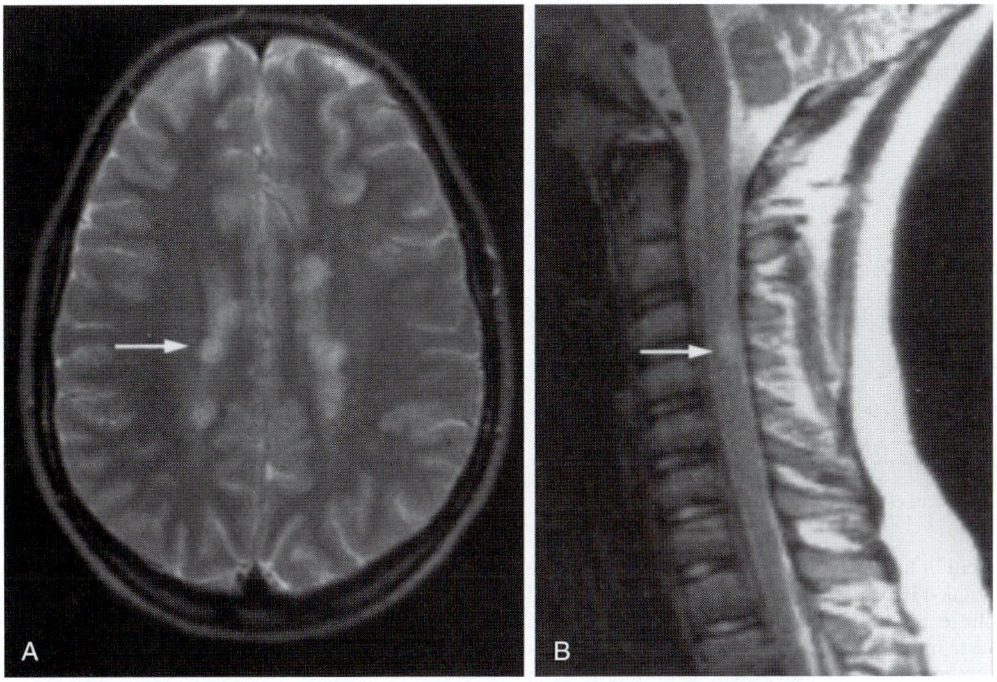

Figura 600-1. Sclerosi multipla. *A*, RM pesata in T_2 che mostra la presenza di caratteristiche lesioni multiple localizzate nella sostanza bianca (*freccia bianca*). *B*, Immagine pesata in T_1 della colonna vertebrale che evidenzia una placca demielinizzante nella regione mediocervicale (*freccia bianca*).

immunomediato, che può seguire a immunizzazioni o (più spesso) a infezioni come morbillo, rosolia, varicella, herpes zoster, parotite, *Mycoplasma pneumoniae* o, più comunemente, altre infezioni non specifiche del tratto respiratorio superiore. La documentazione di una precedente malattia non è necessaria per formulare la diagnosi. L'utilizzo su larga scala della RM ha consentito un più frequente riconoscimento della ADEM nei bambini con debolezza motoria, convulsioni acute o encefalopatia. Caratteristiche presenti o antecedenti includono febbre, letargia, debolezza, atassia, cefalea, convulsioni e altri segni sistemici. La malattia può progredire, con comparsa di delirio, coma, mielopatia e segni neurologici focali. La RM pesata in T_2 mostra tipicamente lesioni multifocali disseminate nella sostanza bianca, nei gangli basali, nel talamo e nel tronco, compatibili con edema, infiammazione e demielinizzazione. L'uso del gadolinio evidenzia ulteriormente tali lesioni (Fig. 600-2). Talvolta si riscontrano lesioni emorragiche della sostanza bianca. L'esame dell'LCS mostra pleocitosi monocitica e linfocitica.

Il **trattamento** con dosi elevate di corticosteroidi per via endovenosa può essere utile (metilprednisolone ev, 30 mg/kg/die per <30 kg, e 1 g/die per >30 kg, per 3-5 giorni, seguito da prednisolone orale, alla dose di 1 mg/kg/die, per 10 giorni). Sono state segnalate anche risposte positive al trattamento con immunoglobuline ev (IVIG). La prognosi dopo un episodio di ADEM è generalmente buona, con >70% di guarigioni complete senza esiti entro 6 mesi. Nella percentuale restante si riscontra disabilità residua. Sono stati segnalati casi di decesso nella fase acuta.

La **diagnosi differenziale** tra la SM e la ADEM monofasica in un bambino al primo episodio di demielinizzazione acuta del SNC è tutt'altro che semplice in assenza di ulteriori follow-up che verifichino l'insorgenza di episodi ricorrenti di SM. In un ridotto numero di bambini privi di lesioni addizionali, è stata formulata la diagnosi di ADEM recidivante, o DEM multifasica (*Multiphasic DEM*). La disponibilità di terapie che agiscono sulla progressione della SM rende particolarmente importante la formulazione di una diagnosi corretta e tempestiva. Gli elementi che contribuiscono a differenziare SM e ADEM sono riassunti nella Tabella 600-1. Nella SM, l'età di esordio è solitamente superiore ai 10 anni, mentre la ADEM tende a colpire bambini più piccoli. I pazienti con SM presentano spesso segni focali, in assenza di grave encefalopatia. Il riscontro di encefalopatia e livello di coscienza alterato suggerisce la ADEM. Anche la RM contribuisce alla diagnosi differenziale: lesioni localizzate a carico di corpo calloso e sostanza bianca periventricolare depongono a favore della SM, mentre lesioni di gangli basali, talamo o a livello della giunzione corticale tra sostanza bianca e grigia sono indicative di ADEM. Anche la comparsa di nuove lesioni dopo la risoluzione dell'episodio iniziale suggerisce la SM.

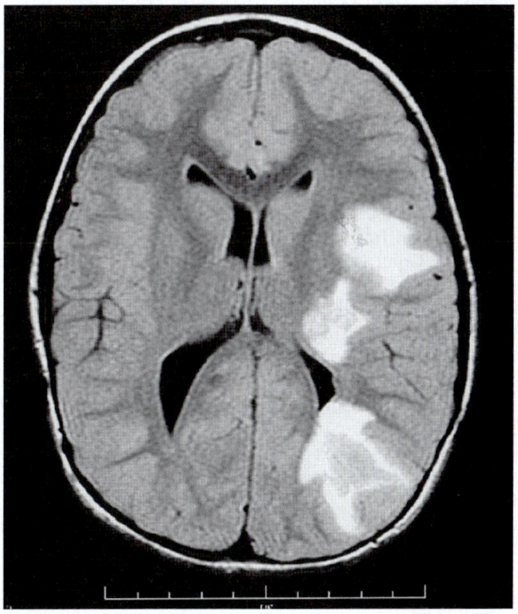

Figura 600-2. Sequenza FLAIR pesata in T_2 della RM cerebrale in un bambino con ADEM. Le aree iperintense (*in bianco*) indicano le zone di demielinizzazione e edema nella sostanza bianca sottocorticale e periventricolare, nonché nei gangli basali e nel talamo sul lato sinistro.

Le rare **sindromi da attivazione macrofagica genetiche** (*Macrophage Activation Syndromes*, **MAS**) possono essere confuse con la

TABELLA 600-1. Caratteristiche cliniche e risultati della RM per la diagnosi differenziale tra ADEM e primo attacco di SM

	ADEM	SM
Età	<10 anni	>10 anni
Stupor/coma	+	–
Febbre/vomito	+	–
Storia familiare	No	20%
Disturbi sensoriali	+	–
Neurite ottica	Bilaterale	Unilaterale
Manifestazioni	Polisintomatica	Monosintomatica
RM	Lesioni diffuse: gangli basali, talamo, giunzione sostanza bianca-grigia	Lesioni isolate: sostanza bianca periventricolare, corpo calloso
LCS	Pleocitosi (linfocitosi)	Bande oligoclonali
Risposta agli steroidi	+	+
Follow-up	Assenza di nuove lesioni	Nuove lesioni

La diagnosi finale della SM si basa sul follow-up e sulla RM. +, presenza probabile; –, presenza improbabile; ADEM, encefalomielite acuta disseminata; LCS, liquido cerebrospinale; SM, sclerosi multipla.

ADEM. Le MAS, tra cui la linfoistiocitosi emofagocitica familiare e la malattia di Chediak-Higashi, si presentano in bambini con manifestazioni cliniche e risultati della RM che suggeriscono la ADEM. Tuttavia, queste malattie continuano a progredire dopo la sospensione del trattamento con steroidi. Anche le anomalie della sostanza bianca e i deficit neurologici focali causati da vasculite isolata del SNC si possono confondere con la ADEM.

Alper G, Schor NF: Toward the definition of acute disseminated encephalitis of childhood. *Curr Opin Pediatr* 2004;16:637–640.

Brass SD, Caramanos Z, Santos C, et al: Multiple sclerosis vs acute disseminated encephalomyelitis in childhood. *Pediatr Neurol* 2003;29:227–231.

Dale RC, Branson JA: Acute disseminated encephalomyelitis or multiple sclerosis: Can the initial presentation help in establishing a correct diagnosis? *Arch Dis Child* 2005;90:636–639.

Dale RC, de Sousa C, Chong WK, et al: Acute disseminated encephalomyelitis, multiphasic disseminated encephalomyelitis and multiple sclerosis in children. *Brain* 2000;123:2407–2422.

Frohman EM, Racke MK, Raine CS: Multiple sclerosis—the plague and its pathogenesis. *N Engl J Med* 2006;354:942–955.

Kappos L, Antel J, Comi G, et al: Oral fingolimod (FYT720) for relapsing multiple sclerosis. *N Engl J Med* 2006;355:1124–1140.

Krupp LB: Multiple sclerosis in children. *J Pediatr* 2006;149:125–127.

Krupp LB, Macallister WS: Treatment of pediatric MS. *Curr Treat Options Neurol* 2005;7:191–199.

Langer-Gould A, Atlas SW, Green AJ, et al: Progressive multifocal leukoencephalopathy in a patient treated with natalizumab. *N Engl J Med* 2005;353:375–380.

Leake JAD, Albani S, Kao AS, et al: Acute disseminated encephalomyelitis in childhood: Epidemiologic, clinical and laboratory features. *Pediatr Infect Dis J* 2004;23:756–764.

McDonald WI, Compston A, Edan G, et al: Recommended diagnostic criteria for multiple sclerosis: Guidelines from the international panel on the diagnosis of multiple sclerosis. *Ann Neurol* 2001;50:121–127.

The Medical Letter: Natalizumab (Tysabri) for relapsing multiple sclerosis. *Med Lett Drugs Ther* 2005;47:13–15.

Miller DH: Brain atrophy, interferon beta, and treatment trials in multiple sclerosis. *Lancet* 2004;364:1463–1464.

Murray TJ: Diagnosis and treatment of multiple sclerosis. *BMJ* 2006;332: 525–527.

Polman CH, O'Connor PW, Havrdova E, et al: A randomized, placebo-controlled trial of natalizumab for relapsing multiple sclerosis. *N Engl J Med* 2006;899–910.

Shiraishi K, Higuchi Y, Ozawa K, et al: Clinical course and prognosis of 27 patients with childhood onset multiple sclerosis in Japan. *Brain Dev* 2005;27:224–227.

Stonehouse M, Gupte G, Wassmer E, et al: Acute disseminated encephalomyelitis: Recognition in the hands of general paediatricians. *Arch Dis Child* 2003;88:122–124.

Tardieu M, Mikaeloff Y: What is acute disseminated encephalomyelitis (ADEM)? *Eur J Paediatr Neurol* 2004;8:239–242.

Tenembaum, S, Chamoles N, Fejerman N: Acute disseminated encephalomyelitis, a long-term follow-up study of 84 pediatric patients. *Neurology* 2002;59:1224–1231.

Weng WC, Yang CC, Yu TW, et al: Multiple Sclerosis with childhood onset: Report of 21 cases in Taiwan. *Pediatr Neurol* 2006;35:327–334.

Whiting P, Harbord R, Main C, et al: Accuracy of magnetic resonance imaging for the diagnosis of multiple sclerosis: systematic review. *BMJ* 2006;332: 875–878.

Capitolo 601 ■ Sindrome da stroke acuto

Michael V. Johnston e Anne Comi

L'emiplegia secondaria a disturbo vascolare si verifica in età pediatrica con un'incidenza di 1-3/100 000 l'anno. Le cause sono differenti da quelle responsabili della malattia nell'adulto. I tipi di stroke prevalenti includono la trombosi arteriosa e venosa, l'emorragia intracranica, l'embolia arteriosa e altre condizioni patologiche varie. La causa dello stroke può essere stabilita in circa il 75% dei casi (Tab. 601-1). Data la mancanza di uniformità di presentazione delle sindromi da stroke, è opportuna una breve descrizione delle forme pediatriche prevalenti.

601.1 • Trombosi arteriosa/embolia

La trombosi arteriosa e l'embolia possono coinvolgere le arterie cerebrali principali (occlusione di carotide interna, media e arteria cerebrale posteriore) o quelle più piccole (Fig. 601-1). Alcuni processi trombotici colpiscono prevalentemente i grandi vasi, altri sono più comuni nelle piccole arterie. La **trombosi della carotide interna** può derivare da un'angolazione acuta dell'arteria (sulle montagne russe, dal barbiere, in un salone di bellezza, o in caso di abuso) oppure di un trauma della faringe posteriore (causato, per esempio, da una caduta su di una matita o dallo stecco di un ghiacciolo). La lesione produce una lacerazione della tonaca intima della parete del vaso, che può condurre alla formazione di un aneurisma dissecante. I sintomi cerebrali derivano dalla partenza di emboli dal trombo. I sintomi, il cui esordio può essere ritardato fino a 24 ore dopo l'incidente, includono una progressiva emiplegia flaccida, letargia e afasia (se è coinvolto l'emisfero dominante). Le convulsioni focali motorie costituiscono una complicanza comune. La dissezione di vasi del circolo vertebrale basilare può causare segni acuti di disfunzione troncoencefalica.

Un **ascesso retrofaringeo** può produrre un quadro clinico identico, ma in questo caso la trombosi arteriosa è il risultato di un'infiammazione della tonaca intima. L'angiografia cerebrale o la angiografia RM dimostrano la presenza dell'occlusione della carotide interna, mentre TC e RM evidenziano una lesione ipodensa lungo i contorni dell'area dell'infarto.

Anche l'**embolizzazione dei vasi cerebrali** può causare emiparesi acuta. Le anomalie cardiache costituiscono la più comune causa di stroke tromboembolico nei bambini. Le cause cardiache includono aritmie (in particolare fibrillazione atriale), mixoma, emboli paradossi attraverso un forame ovale pervio ed endocarditi batteriche responsabili di aneurisma micotico. Emboli costituiti da una bolla d'aria possono complicare un intervento chirurgico, mentre emboli grassi sono secondari a fratture delle ossa lunghe. Gli emboli settici possono evolvere in un'area focale di cerebrite, responsabile di ascesso cerebrale.

Nei bambini di età inferiore ai 2 anni, la **cardiopatia cianotica congenita** può causare trombosi, in particolare nell'arteria cerebrale media. Questi pazienti risultano particolarmente vulnerabili quando la saturazione di ossigeno cala significativamente in associazione a una malattia virale o alla disidratazione. Procedure cardiache, come il cateterismo o l'intervento di Fontan, possono provocare trombosi arteriosa in seguito a embolizzazione di un coagulo. Se si sospetta una causa cardiaca della trombosi arteriosa, si deve sottoporre il bambino a ecocardiografia.

TABELLA 601-1. Cause di ictus nei bambini

I. Cardiopatia
- A. Congenita
  - 1. Stenosi dell'aorta
  - 2. Stenosi mitralica
  - 3. Difetti settali ventricolari
  - 4. Dotto arterioso pervio
  - 5. Cardiopatia cianotica congenita con shunt destra-sinistra
- B. Acquisita
  - 1. Endocardite (batterica, lupus eritematoso sistemico)
  - 2. Malattia di Kawasaki
  - 3. Cardiomiopatia
  - 4. Mixoma atriale
  - 5. Aritmia
  - 6. Emboli paradossi attraverso il forame ovale pervio
  - 7. Febbre reumatica
  - 8. Protesi valvolare cardiaca

II. Anomalie ematologiche
- A. Emoglobinopatie
  - 1. Anemia falciforme
  - 2. Malattia falciforme
- B. Policitemia
- C. Leucemia/linfoma
- D. Trombocitopenia
- E. Trombocitosi
- F. Disturbi della coagulazione
  - 1. Deficit di proteina C
  - 2. Deficit di proteina S
  - 3. Fattore V di Leiden
  - 4. Deficit di antitrombina III
  - 5. Anticoagulante lupico
  - 6. Uso di contraccettivi orali
  - 7. Gravidanza e postpartum
  - 8. Coagulazione intravascolare disseminata
  - 9. Emoglobinuria parossistica notturna
  - 10. Protrombina G20210A (PT20210)
  - 11. Mutazioni trombofiliche del fattore V1691 GA
  - 12. Malattia infiammatoria intestinale (trombosi)

III. Disturbi infiammatori
- A. Meningite
  - 1. Virale
  - 2. Batterica
  - 3. Tubercolare
- B. Infezione sistemica
  - 1. Viremia
  - 2. Batteriemia
  - 3. Infezioni locali di testa e collo
- C. Infiammazione da sostanze stupefacenti
  - 1. Amfetamine
  - 2. Cocaina
- D. Malattia
  - 1. Lupus eritematoso sistemico
  - 2. Artrite reumatoide giovanile
  - 3. Arterite di Takayasu
  - 4. Connettivite mista
  - 5. Poliarterite nodosa
  - 6. Vasculite primaria del SNC
  - 7. Sarcoidosi
  - 8. Sindrome di Behçet
  - 9. Granulomatosi di Wegener

IV. Malattia metabolica associata a stroke
- A. Omocistinuria
- B. Pseudoxantoma elastico
- C. Malattia di Fabry
- D. Deficit di sulfito ossidasi
- E. Malattie mitocondriali
  - 1. MELAS
  - 2. Sindrome di Leigh
- F. Deficit di ornitina transcarbamilasi
- G. Metilenetetraidrofolato reduttasi termolabile (MTHFR C677T)

V. Processi vascolari intracerebrali
- A. Rottura di un aneurisma
- B. Malformazione arterovenosa
- C. Displasia fibromuscolare
- D. Malattia di Moyamoya
- E. Emicrania
- F. Vasospasmo da emorragia postsubaracnoidea
- G. Teleangiectasia emorragica ereditaria
- H. Sindrome di Sturge-Weber
- I. Dissezione dell'arteria carotide
- J. Post varicella
- K. Sindrome PHACE (vedi Capitolo 649)

VI. Trauma o altre cause esterne
- A. Maltrattamento
- B. Trauma cranico o al collo
- C. Trauma orale
- D. Embolia placentare
- E. Terapia ECMO

ECMO, *Extracorporeal Membrane Oxygenation* (ossigenazione della membrana extracorporea); MELAS, *Mitochondrial Encephalomyopathy, Lactic acidosis, and Stroke* (encefalomiopatia mitocondriale, acidosi lattica e ictus).
Tratta da Rivkin M: In Kliegman R (ed): *Practical Strategies in Pediatric Diagnosis and Therapy*. Philadelphia, WB Saunders, 1996.

I disturbi vascolari occlusivi costituiscono un'altra importante causa di emiplegia acuta nella popolazione pediatrica. L'**occlusione arteriosa con teleangiectasia** o **sindrome di Moyamoya** ("nuvola di fumo") presenta un angiogramma caratteristico (Fig. 601-2). La malattia è più comune nelle femmine e spesso esordisce con cefalea e segni bilaterali dei motoneuroni superiori. Può presentarsi anche con corea. Episodi intermittenti di attacchi ischemici transitori rischiano di causare segni neurologici progressivi e grave disabilità. Procedure chirurgiche per facilitare il flusso cerebrale (come impianto di shunt dall'arteria temporale superficiale all'arteria cerebrale media o posizionamento dell'arteria temporale superficiale sulla membrana aracnoidea) ottengono risultati variabili.

L'**anemia falciforme** è la più comune causa di stroke nei bambini afroamericani ed è associata a stenosi della porzione distale della carotide interna o della porzione prossimale dell'arteria cerebrale media. Oltre a evidenziare gli stroke, la RM rivela la presenza di infarti cerebrali silenti, potenzialmente responsabili di declino cognitivo, in un terzo dei bambini con anemia falciforme. Il trattamento trasfusionale cronico contribuisce a prevenire lo stroke in questo gruppo di pazienti.

I **disturbi della coagulazione** costituiscono un importante fattore di rischio. In oltre il 50% di bambini e neonati con tromboembolia cerebrale sono state identificate mutazioni del fattore V di Leiden e della protrombina, deficit della proteina C, S e dell'antitrombina III, nonché anticorpi antifosfolipidi (vedi Capitoli 478 e 479) (vedi Tab. 601-1).

L'**occlusione di piccole arterie** è associata anche a diabete mellito, neurofibromatosi, angiopatia post-varicella, irradiazione di testa e collo, assunzione di contraccettivi orali e abuso di sostanze stupefacenti (amfetamine, cocaina). I pazienti presentano segni neurologici unilaterali. Poiché l'area colpita dall'infarto è di piccole dimensioni, il recupero è spesso completo. I pazienti con *trombosi delle piccole arterie*, inclusi i vasi perforanti i muscoli striati, secondaria a poliarterite nodosa e omocistinuria manifestano un decorso progressivamente debilitante, caratterizzato da segni bilaterali ed elevata mortalità.

L'**arteriopatia cerebrale transitoria** è un processo non progressivo, solitamente autolimitante, responsabile di stenosi arteriosa intracranica unilaterale, spesso a carico dell'arteria media (Tab. 601-2, Fig. 601-3). L'associazione identificabile più comune è con la varicella. In circa il 75% dei casi si osserva un miglioramento o una stabilizzazione; la recidiva dell'infarto è un evento raro. L'arteriopatia cerebrale transitoria costituisce la più comune causa non progressiva di stroke nei bambini, con un esordio medio a 40 mesi di età (range 0,3-14,8).

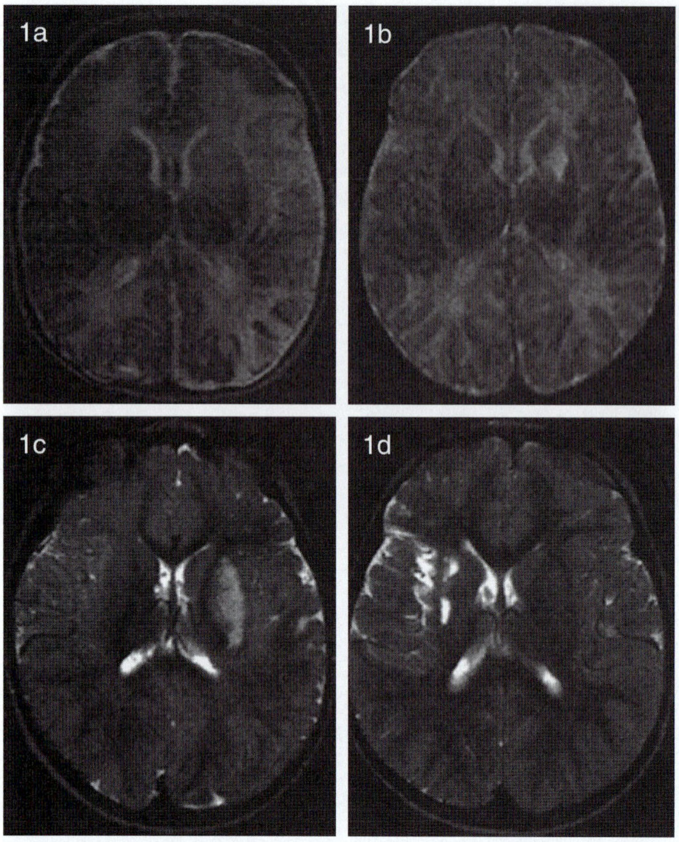

Figura 601-1. Immagini assiali pesate in T_2 dopo uno stroke ischemico a esordio neonatale (*a* e *b*) e infantile (*c* e *d*). Nella figura *a*, si osserva iperintensità anomala a livello dei nuclei caudato e lentiforme dei gangli basali (sul lato sinistro), del braccio posteriore della capsula interna e della corteccia cerebrale; si osserva anche perdita di differenziazione tra sostanza grigia e bianca. L'emiparesi presentata dal paziente si verifica tipicamente in caso di contemporaneo coinvolgimento di gangli basali, braccio posteriore della capsula interna e corteccia cerebrale. Nella figura *b*, si osserva iperintensità del nucleo lentiforme (gangli della base) e del braccio anteriore della capsula interna, in assenza di coinvolgimento del braccio posteriore della capsula interna e della corteccia cerebrale. Il bambino non presenta emiparesi; nessun neonato con coinvolgimento esclusivo dei gangli della base o della corteccia cerebrale, oppure con lesioni a carico dei gangli basali e del braccio posteriore della capsula interna o dei gangli basali e della corteccia cerebrale è destinato a sviluppare emiparesi. La figura *c* si riferisce invece a un paziente dopo uno stroke ischemico a esordio infantile. Mostra il coinvolgimento esclusivo dei gangli basali, mentre corteccia cerebrale e braccio posteriore della capsula interna sono risparmiati. Il paziente presenta emiparesi. La figura *d* mostra il coinvolgimento contemporaneo di braccio posteriore della capsula interna, gangli della base e corteccia cerebrale, in seguito a ictus ischemico a esordio infantile. Questa localizzazione è generalmente associata a emiparesi, ma alcuni bambini con tale distribuzione, incluso quello della figura, non sviluppano emiparesi. (Tratta da Boardman JP, Ganesan V, Rutherford MA, et al: Magnetic resonance image correlates of hemiparesis after neonatal and childhood middle cerebral artery stroke. *Pediatrics* 2005;115:321-326.)

601.2 • TROMBOSI VENOSA

Le trombosi dei seni venosi sono secondarie a cause settiche o non settiche (Tab. 601-3). I sintomi e segni possono evolversi nel giro di qualche giorno. Nei neonati sono caratteristici segni neurologici diffusi e convulsioni, mentre i segni neurologici focali sono prominenti nei bambini. È possibile riscontrare dilatazione delle vene craniche, fontanella anteriore sporgente, sintomi e segni di aumento della pressione intracranica.

Le **cause settiche** di trombosi dei seni venosi includono encefalite e meningite batteriche. L'emiplegia è una complicanza relativamente comune della **meningite batterica** causata da trombosi

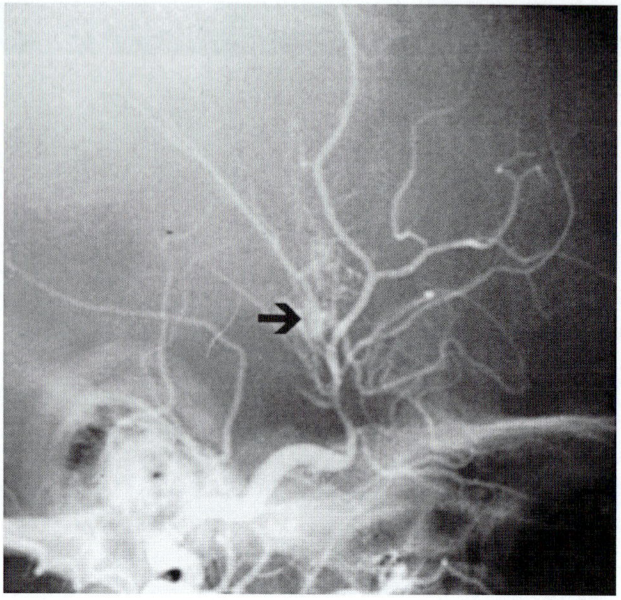

Figura 601-2. Angiogramma cerebrale che mostra un'arteriopatia idiopatica a carico della carotide interna sovraclinoidea, con classici vasi collaterali tipo Moyamoya (*freccia*).

TABELLA 601-2. Principali quadri clinici e radiologici nell'infarto cerebrale arteriopatico nell'infanzia

ARTERIOPATIA CEREBRALE TRANSITORIA

Definizioni

Imaging vascolare iniziale: stenosi focale unilaterale o segmentale; oppure occlusione che coinvolge la porzione distale della carotide interna e i segmenti iniziali e i rami dell'arteria cerebrale anteriore e/o media. In alcuni casi: stenosi assente o minima; la stenosi massima o l'occlusione sono osservate entro 3 mesi dall'imaging iniziale (Fig. 601-3 *A*, *B*). Imaging di follow-up a 6 mesi dall'ictus iniziale: assenza di progressione (o regressione) delle lesioni arteriose rispetto all'angiogramma a 3 mesi (Fig. 601-3 *B*, *C* e *D*)

Cause

Infiammatorie/infettive: virus varicella zoster, altri agenti (per es. borrelia, bartonella, enterovirus)?
Dissezione intracranica: traumatiche, infiammatorio-infettive?
Spasmo, tossine (cocaina?)
Fattori trombotici adiuvanti?
Alcune rare arteriopatie progressive si presentano allo stesso modo dell'arteriopatia cerebrale transitoria.

DISSEZIONE EXTRACRANICA

Definizioni

Imaging vascolare mostra: reperti angiografici di lume doppio, flap intimale, o pseudoaneurisma o infiltrazione lipidica (su RM assiali pesate in T_1), luminosità crescente nella parete arteriosa; sequela di trauma cervicale, cranico o dolore al collo, che precede di non più di 6 settimane i reperti angiografici di restringimento segmentale (o occlusione) delle arterie cervicali (Fig. 601-3 *E*, *freccia*); restringimento segmentale (o occlusione) delle arterie vertebrali a livello di C2, anche in assenza di causa traumatica nota.

Cause

Traumatica: accidentale-diretta, stiramento, trauma sottile (arteriopatia non progressiva); lesione non accidentale-sindrome del bambino scosso (arteriopatie progressive o non progressive)
Malattie del collagene +/− trauma (arteriopatia progressiva)

SINDROME DI MOYAMOYA

Definizioni

RM o angiografia con mezzo di contrasto mostrano restringimento o occlusione della porzione terminale di entrambe le carotidi interne (Fig. 601-3 *F*) e rete collaterale unilaterale o bilaterale di piccoli vasi, distale rispetto alle arterie occluse (Fig. 601-3 *F*, *frecce*)

Cause

Arteriopatie progressive e non progressive: genetiche-anemia falciforme, neurofibromatosi di tipo I; tossiche-radioterapia (in particolare nel contesto della neurofibromatosi di tipo I); infiammatorie/infettive-virus varicella zoster

*Definizioni elaborate di recente dall'International Pediatric Stroke Study Group. Cause distinte possono condurre a presentazioni clinico-radiologiche ed esiti analoghi. Al contrario, le stesse cause determinano talvolta quadri molto diversi. Di conseguenza, è molto difficile prevedere l'esito sulla base delle manifestazioni cliniche iniziali. Per evidenziare l'arteriopatia in caso di ictus, deve essere eseguita entro 24 ore angiografia RM.

Tratta da Sébire G: Transient cerebral arteriopathy in childhood. Lancet 2006; 368:8-10.

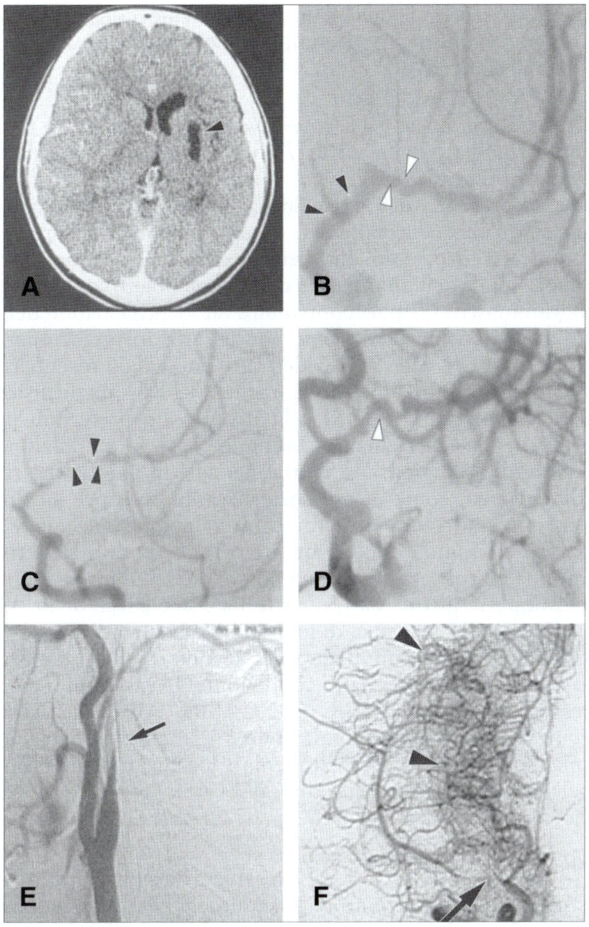

Figura 601-3. Quadro clinico e radiologico dell'infarto cerebrale infantile. Arteriopatia cerebrale transitoria in un bambino di 8 anni, che ha manifestato emiplegia destra 8 mesi dopo essere stato affetto da varicella. *A*, La TC mostra un piccolo infarto nell'area dei nuclei basali. *B*, L'angiogramma effettuato immediatamente dopo lo stroke mostra la stenosi segmentale irregolare della carotide sovraclinoidea (*frecce nere*) e dell'arteria silviana (*frecce bianche*). *C*, Tre mesi dopo lo stroke iniziale, si riscontra un peggioramento delle lesioni silviane. *D*, A 14 mesi di distanza, si nota un miglioramento rispetto all'angiogramma a 3 mesi (ma non rispetto a quello iniziale), con persistenza della stenosi dell'arteria silviana. Nei 5 anni seguenti non si verificheranno recidive dello stroke. *E*, Dissezione extracranica della carotide interna (*freccia*). *F*, Aspetto angiografico della sindrome di Moyamoya, con stenosi della carotide sovraclinoidea (*freccia*) e rete di sottili vasi collaterali distale rispetto all'arteria occlusa (*punte di freccia*). (Tratta da Sébire G: Transient cerebral arteriopathy in childhood. *Lancet* 2006;368:8-10.)

TABELLA 601-3. Cause e fattori di rischio associati alla trombosi dei seni venosi cerebrali

Condizioni protrombotiche genetiche	
	Deficit di antitrombina
	Deficit di proteina C e S
	Mutazione del fattore V di Leiden
	Mutazione della protrombina (sostituzione di A con G nella posizione 20210)
	Omocisteinemia causata da mutazioni genetiche della metilenetetraidrofolato reduttasi
Stati protrombotici acquisiti	
	Sindrome nefrotica
	Anticorpi antifosfolipidi
	Omocisteinemia
	Gravidanza
	Puerperio
Infezioni	
	Otite, mastoidite, sinusite
	Meningite
	Malattia infettiva sistemica
Malattia infiammatoria	
	Lupus eritematoso sistemico
	Granulomatosi di Wegener
	Sarcoidosi
	Malattia infiammatoria intestinale
	Sindrome di Behçet
Malattie ematologiche	
	Policitemia, primaria e secondaria
	Trombocitopenia
	Leucemia
	Anemia, inclusa l'emoglobinuria parossistica notturna
Farmaci	
	Contraccettivi orali
	Asparaginasi
Cause meccaniche, traumi	
	Trauma cranico
	Lesioni dei seni o alla vena giugulare, cateterismo giugulare
	Procedure neurochirurgiche
	Puntura lombare
Varie	
	Disidratazione, specialmente nei bambini
	Tumore

Tratta da Stam J: Thrombosis of the cerebral veins and sinuses. *New Engl J Med* 2005;352:1791-1798.

delle vene corticali superficiale e penetrante. Altre cause infettive sono l'**otite media,** la **mastoidite** con coinvolgimento dei vasi della dura madre e infezioni orbitali retrograde responsabili di **trombosi dei seni cavernosi.**

Le **cause non settiche** includono una **grave disidratazione**, in grado di provocare trombosi del seno sagittale superiore e delle vene corticali superficiali, secondarie a iperviscosità ematica. Altre possibili cause sono i disturbi responsabili di ipercoagulabilità, la cardiopatia cianotica congenita, l'anemia da deficit di ferro e la presenza di infiltrati leucemici nelle vene cerebrali. Nel 12-50% dei casi, si riscontrano **disturbi protrombotici**, inclusi i deficit degli inibitori della coagulazione (come la proteina C, la proteina S e l'antitrombina III) e gli stati procoagulanti come l'aumento dei livelli del fattore VIII, la resistenza alla proteina C attivata, mutazioni del fattore V di Leiden, anomalie della lipoproteina a, mutazioni del gene che codifica per la metilenetetraidrofolato reduttasi termolabile, aumento dei livelli di omocisteina a digiuno e la presenza di anticorpi anticardiolipina (vedi Capitoli 478 e 479). **Malformazioni vascolari** associate a compromissione del drenaggio venoso (come nella sindrome di Sturge-Weber) possono predisporre a infarti venosi ed episodi simil-stroke.

601.3 • Emorragia intracranica

L'emorragia intracranica può verificarsi nello spazio subaracnoideo o prevalentemente nel parenchima cerebrale. L'emorragia subaracnoidea è caratterizzata da grave cefalea, rigidità nucale e progressiva perdita di coscienza. L'emorragia intracerebrale, frequente nei neonati prematuri, causa segni neurologici focali e convulsioni (vedi Capitolo 99.2).

Le **malformazioni arterovenose**, risultato di anomalie dello sviluppo del letto capillare tra arterie e vene durante l'embriogenesi, causano disturbi del flusso sanguigno, responsabili di un'espansione dei vasi, con conseguente rottura venosa ed emorragia intracerebrale. Tali malformazioni sono solitamente localizzate negli emisferi cerebrali, ma anche nel cervelletto, nel tronco o nel midollo spinale. È possibile che restino asintomatiche per tutta la vita, ma eventuali rotture, con conseguente emorragia, rischiano di verificarsi a qualsiasi età. I bambini con malformazioni arterovenose presentano spesso un'anamnesi di convulsioni e disturbi simil-emicrania. L'emicrania classica si alterna da un lato all'altro, mentre la cefalea associata a malformazione arterovenosa colpisce sempre lo stesso lato. In circa il 50% dei casi, l'auscultazione del cranio rivela un rumore acuto. La rottura di una malformazione arterovenosa provoca grave cefalea, vomito, rigidità nucale causata dall'emorragia subaracnoidea, emiparesi progressiva e convulsioni focali o generalizzate. Gli angiomi cavernosi, spesso familiari, presentano un rischio minore di emorragia spontanea. La **malformazione della vena di Galeno** può causare insufficienza cardiaca congestizia secondaria allo shunting di grandi quantità di sangue o idrocefalo progressivo e aumento della pressione intracranica, secondari all'ostruzione delle vie di ricircolo del LCS. Tali malformazioni, difficili da correggere, sono associate a una prognosi infausta.

Nei bambini, gli **aneurismi cerebrali** sintomatici sono relativamente rari. A differenza dell'adulto, gli aneurismi infantili tendono a essere di grandi dimensioni e sono spesso localizzati alla biforcazione della carotide o nelle arterie cerebrali anteriore e posteriore (piuttosto che nel circolo di Willis). La dilatazione aneurismatica è il risultato di una debolezza congenita dei vasi e, in alcuni casi, di un deficit di collagene di tipo III. Nei bambini, si riscontra un'associazione tra aneurismi cerebrali, coartazione dell'aorta e malattia policistica renale bilaterale. La maggior parte degli aneurismi provoca un'emorragia nello spazio subaracnoideo (con conseguente cefalea, rigidità nucale e coma), ma è possibile riscontrare anche emorragia intracerebrale, con emiparesi progressiva. Anche i disturbi ematologici sono responsabili di ematoma intracerebrale, in particolare la porpora trombocitopenica e l'emofilia. Infine, un trauma può produrre emiparesi, dovuta all'emorragia intracerebrale o alla formazione di un ematoma subdurale o epidurale. La TC o la RM con mezzo di contrasto (gadolinio) e la angiografia RM sono utili per identificare malformazioni arterovenose di grandi dimensioni. L'angiografia cerebrale con visualizzazione dei quattro vasi è la tecnica di elezione per l'esame delle malformazioni arterovenose e degli aneurismi cerebrali.

601.4 • Diagnosi differenziale degli eventi simil-stroke

EZIOLOGIA E MANIFESTAZIONI CLINICHE. L'emiplegia alternante infantile è occasionalmente associata a emicrania, ma nella maggior parte dei casi la causa è sconosciuta. Si sviluppa nei bambini tra i 2 e i 18 mesi di età ed è caratterizzata da episodi intermittenti di emiplegia che si alternano sui due lati del corpo. In rari casi, entrambi i lati sono coinvolti durante un attacco. Coreoatetosi e movimenti distonici si osservano comunemente negli arti emiparetici. I segni regrediscono spontaneamente durante il sonno, ma ricompaiono al risveglio. L'emiplegia persiste da qualche minuto ad alcune settimane, per poi risolversi spontaneamente. La malattia ha tuttavia una prognosi infausta, con insorgenza di ritardo mentale progressivo e disabilità evolutive. I risultati degli esami di neuroimaging e metabolici sono negativi.

Diverse **malattie metaboliche** sono associate a episodi simil-stroke, inclusa l'encefalomielopatia mitocondriale (MELAS; vedi Capitolo 598.2), il deficit di ornitina transcarbamilasi, il deficit di piruvato deidrogenasi e l'omocistinuria.

La **paralisi di Todd** può essere inizialmente confusa con uno stroke. L'emiparesi segue una convulsione focale, me la debolezza e i segni neurologici scompaiono completamente entro 24 ore dalla convulsione. La causa di tale paralisi è sconosciuta, ma è ipotizzabile che sia il risultato di un fenomeno inibitorio, possibilmente collegato a una disfunzione dei neurotrasmettitori.

Altre cause di emiparesi includono **tumore cerebrale**, **encefalite** (in particolare da herpes), **encefalite postvirale focale** e **status epilettico**. In alcune casistiche pediatriche, è stata segnalata la presenza di **anomalie lipidiche** (come un aumento del livello di trigliceridi e una riduzione del livello di colesterolo ad alta densità) in circa il 20% dei casi di stroke inspiegabile. Le anamnesi familiari di questi bambini rivelano un aumento dell'incidenza di cardiopatie coronariche e malattie cerebrovascolari ischemiche precoci. Lo screening delle famiglie a rischio consente l'identificazione dei bambini per i quali è opportuna la prescrizione di una dieta specifica.

DIAGNOSI. L'anamnesi e l'esame obiettivo costituiscono le componenti principali della valutazione, mirata a identificare un sottostante processo patologico, eventuali segni di trauma o infezione, la presenza di una malattia ematologica o metabolica, di una sindrome neurocutanea, di un aumento della pressione intracranica o idrocefalo. La scelta degli esami di laboratorio si basa sui risultati dell'anamnesi e dell'esame obiettivo. L'elettroencefalogramma (EEG) può contribuire all'identificazione del processo patologico, ma raramente consente la formulazione della diagnosi. La TC è utile per evidenziare emorragie recenti o aree di infarto di grandi dimensioni, mentre la RM in diffusione o perfusione, l'angiografia RM e la RMV sono preferibili per la diagnosi precoce di ischemia cerebrale e per la valutazione dei vasi cerebrali. L'angiografia è utile nei casi in cui la RM risulta non diagnostica, come in presenza di vasculite o per localizzare la sede di un'emorragia intracranica. In tali circostanze, la tecnica di elezione è l'angiografia dei quattro vasi cerebrali. L'elettrocardiogramma e l'ecocardiogramma possono contribuire a escludere una cardiopatia intrinseca o un'aritmia come cause dello stroke. Per riassumere, in presenza di un bambino con sindrome da stroke inspiegabile, gli esami diagnostici devono essere organizzati in modo da escludere le seguenti condizioni: (1) vasculite o malattie del tessuto connettivo (ESR, C3, C4, RF, ANA); (2) disturbi lipidici; (3) disturbi di coagulazione; (4) malattie ematologiche (anemia falciforme, trombocitopenia); (5) malattie metaboliche (omocistinuria, malattia di Fabry, MELAS); (6) un'eziologia infettiva (meningite e encefalite).

TRATTAMENTO DELLO STROKE. Le terapie trombolitiche (con somministrazione di un attivatore tissutale del plasminogeno) sono utili entro 3 ore dall'attacco ischemico negli adulti, ma non sono state testate nei bambini. L'eparina a basso peso molecolare è talvolta utilizzata per trattare la trombosi dei seni venosi. Le controindicazioni all'uso di un agente antitrombotico includono significativa emorragia intracerebrale e ipertensione. Il trattamento di supporto prevede il controllo della pressione sanguigna e dei liquidi, il mantenimento della normoglicemia, il controllo della febbre e delle convulsioni. Il fattore VII ricombinante e attivato ha consentito di migliorare la prognosi negli adulti con emorragia intracerebrale. L'evacuazione chirurgica di coaguli di grandi dimensioni e di tessuto cerebrale edematoso è indicata in alcuni casi.

Nei neonati, il trattamento per la prevenzione di un secondo stroke non è solitamente necessario, perché il rischio di recidiva è molto basso. Nei bambini, il rischio è invece più elevato ed è spesso opportuno ricorrere a una terapia a lungo termine con dosi ridotte di acido acetilsalicilico. L'eparina a basso peso molecolare o il warfarin sono spesso utilizzati per diversi mesi a scopo preventivo in presenza di emboli cardiaci, dissezione di un aneurisma, stenosi di grado elevato di un'arteria cerebrale, gravi condizioni protrombotiche o inefficacia dell'acido acetilsalicilico. Regolari trasfusioni di sangue riducono l'incidenza di stroke nell'anemia falciforme. La terapia con immunosoppressori è spesso necessaria in presenza di vasculite. Il trattamento riabilitativo in seguito a stroke richiede un approccio multidisciplinare, che includa la logopedia, la fisioterapia, la terapia occupazionale, l'assistenza psicologica e il ricorso a tecniche educative specifiche.

Agner C, Weig SG: Arterial dissection and stroke following child abuse: Case report and review of the literature. *Childs Nerv Syst* 2005;21:416–420.

Baumer JH: Childhood arterial stroke. *Arch Dis Child* 2004;89:ep50–ep53.

Boardman JP, Ganesan V, Rutherford MA, et al: Magnetic resonance image correlates of hemiparesis after neonatal and childhood middle cerebral artery stroke. *Pediatrics* 2005;115:321–326.

Bourgeois M, Aicardi J, Goutières F: Alternating hemiplegia of childhood. *J Pediatr* 1993;122:673–679.

Danchaivijitr N, Cox TC, Saunders DE, Ganeson V: Evolution of cerebral arteopathics in childhood arterial ischemic stroke. *Ann Neurol* 2006;59: 620–626.
DeVeber G: Arterial ischemic strokes in infants and children: An overview of current approaches. *Semin Thromb Hemost* 2003;29:567–573.
DeVeber G, Andrew M, Adams C, et al: Cerebral sinovenous thrombosis in children. *N Engl J Med* 2001;345:417–423.
Duran R, Biner B, Demir M, et al: Factor V Leiden mutation and other thrombophilia markers in childhood ischemic stroke. *Clin Appl Thromb Hemost* 2005;11:83–88.
Fullerton HJ, Wu YW, Sidney S, Johnston SC: Risk of recurrent childhood arterial ischemic stroke in a population-based cohort: the importance of cerebrovascular imaging. *Pediatrics* 2007;119:495–501.
Haywood S, Liesner R, Pindora S, et al: Thrombophilia and first arterial ischaemic stroke: A systematic review. *Arch Dis Child* 2005;90:402–405.
Lanthier S, Armstrong D, Domi T, de Veber G: Post-varicella arteriopathy of childhood. *Neurology* 2005;64:660–663.
Lynch JK, Hirtz DG, DeVeber G, et al: Report on the National Institute of Neurological Diseases and Stroke Workshop on perinatal and childhood stroke. *Pediatrics* 2002;109:116–123.
Lynch JK, Nelson KB, Curry CJ, et al: Cerebrovascular disorders in children with the Leiden factor V mutation. *J Child Neurol* 2001;16:735–744.
Mayer SA, Brun NC, Begtrup K, et al: Recombinant activated factor VII for acute intracerebral hemorrhage. *N Engl J Med* 2005;352:777–785.
Mercuri E, Barnett A, Rutherford M, et al: Neonatal cerebral infarction and neuromotor outcome at school age. *Pediatrics* 2004;113:95–100.
Nowak-Göttl U, Günther G, Kurnik K, et al: Arterial ischemic stroke in neonates, infants and children: An overview of underlying conditions, imaging methods and treatment modalities. *Semin Thromb Hemost* 2003;29:405–414.
Rosenblum L: Management of stroke in childhood. *Br Med J* 2005;330: 1161–1162.
Scott RM, Smith JL, Robertson RL, et al: Long-term outcome in children with moyamoya syndrome after cranial revascularization by pial synangiosis. *J Neurosurg Pediatr* 2004;100:142–149.
Sebire G, Tabarki B, Saunders DE, et al: Cerebral venous sinus thrombosis in children: Risk factors, presentation, diagnosis and outcome. *Brain* 2005;128:477–489.
Stam J: Thrombosis of the cerebral veins and sinuses. *New Engl J Med* 2005;352:1791–1798.
Steen RG, Emudianughe T, Hankins GM, et al: Brain imaging findings in pediatric patients with sickle cell disease. *Radiology* 2003;228:216–225.
Wu YW, Miller SP, Chin K, et al: Multiple risk factors in neonatal sinovenous thrombosis. *Neurology* 2002;59:438–440.

Capitolo 602 ■ Infezioni del sistema nervoso centrale Charles G. Prober

Le infezioni costituiscono la più comune causa di febbre associata a segni e sintomi a carico del sistema nervoso centrale (SNC) in età pediatrica. Diversi microrganismi possono causare infezioni. Gli specifici patogeni sono identificabili e influenzati dall'età e dallo stato immunitario dell'ospite, nonché dagli aspetti epidemiologici. In linea generale, le infezioni virali del SNC sono molto più comuni delle infezioni batteriche; le infezioni fungine o parassitarie sono ancora più rare. Le infezioni causate da rickettsie (febbre maculosa delle Montagne Rocciose, *Ehrlichia*), benché poco comuni, assumono un ruolo importante in alcune circostanze epidemiologiche. Anche *Mycoplasma* spp. può causare infezioni del SNC, ma il suo contributo specifico è spesso difficile da determinare.

A prescindere dall'eziologia, la maggior parte dei pazienti con infezione del SNC presenta manifestazioni cliniche simili. I **sintomi comuni** (prevalentemente non specifici) includono cefalea, nausea, vomito, anoressia, irrequietezza, alterazione dello stato di coscienza e irritabilità. I **segni comuni** di infezione al SNC, oltre alla febbre, includono fotofobia, dolore e rigidità nucale, intorpidimento, *stupor*, coma, convulsioni e deficit neurologici focali. La gravità e la costellazione dei segni è determinata dallo specifico patogeno, dall'ospite e dell'area cerebrale colpita.

Le infezioni del SNC possono essere di tipo diffuso o focale. La meningite e l'encefalite costituiscono esempi di infezione diffusa. La meningite implica il coinvolgimento primario delle meningi, mentre l'encefalite segnala il coinvolgimento parenchimale. Poiché i confini anatomici sono spesso indistinti, i pazienti che manifestano un coinvolgimento contemporaneo di meningi e parenchima sono diagnosticati come affetti da meningoencefalite. L'ascesso cerebrale costituisce il migliore esempio di infezione focale del SNC. L'espressione neurologica di questa infezione è determinata dalla sede e dall'estensione dell'ascesso (vedi Capitolo 603).

La diagnosi di infezione diffusa del SNC si basa sull'esame del liquido cerebrospinale (LCS), prelevato mediante puntura lombare (PL). La Tabella 602-1 riassume le anomalie del LCS associate a vari disturbi del SNC.

602.1 • Meningite batterica acuta dopo il periodo neonatale

La meningite batterica è una delle infezioni potenzialmente più gravi che possono colpire lattanti e bambini, ed è associata ad alto rischio di complicanze e di morbilità a lungo termine. Nei lattanti febbrili, l'incidenza della meningite batterica è sufficientemente elevata da consigliarne l'inclusione nella diagnosi differenziale degli stati mentali alterati e degli altri segni di disfunzione neurologica.

EZIOLOGIA. Le cause di meningite batterica nel periodo neonatale (0-28 giorni) sono generalmente diverse da quelle che si riscontrano nei bambini più grandi (vedi Capitolo 109). I batteri responsabili della meningite nei neonati riflettono la flora gastrointestinale e genitourinaria materna, nonché l'ambiente al quale è esposto il bambino. I patogeni più comuni includono gli streptococchi dei gruppi B e D (enterococchi), i bacilli enterici Gram-negativi (*E. coli, Klebsiella*) e *Listeria monocytogenes*. Gli streptococchi del gruppo B, seguiti da *E. coli*, costituiscono le due più comuni cause di meningite neonatale. Gli streptococchi dei gruppi B e D e *Listeria* continuano a essere patogeni importanti per il SNC anche nel terzo mese di vita. In questo periodo, aumenta la prevalenza delle infezioni causate da *Streptococcus pneumoniae*, *Neisseria meningitidis* e *Haemophilus influenzae* tipo b.

Negli Stati Uniti, la più comune causa di meningite batterica nei bambini tra i 2 mesi e i 12 anni è *N. meningitidis*. Le meningiti batteriche provocate da *S. pneumoniae* e *H. influenzae* tipo b sono diventate molto più rare nei Paesi sviluppati dopo l'introduzione dell'immunizzazione universale contro questi patogeni a 2 mesi di età. La presenza di un'infezione da *S. pneumoniae* o *H. influenzae* tipo b deve essere presa in considerazione nei pazienti con vaccinazione incompleta o nei Paesi in via di sviluppo. Il rischio di infezioni provocate da questi due batteri aumenta anche nei pazienti con disturbi immunologici (infezione da HIV, deficit di sottoclassi delle IgG) o anatomici (disfunzione splenica, difetti o impianti cocleari).

Alterazioni delle difese dell'ospite dovute a difetti anatomici o deficit immunologici aumentano il rischio di meningite da patogeni meno comuni, come *Pseudomonas aeruginosa*, *Staphylococcus aureus*, stafilococchi coagulasi-negativi, *Salmonella* spp. e *Listeria monocytogenes*.

EPIDEMIOLOGIA. Uno dei maggiori rischi per l'insorgenza di meningite è costituito dall'assenza di immunità contro specifici patogeni associati al periodo infantile. Rischi addizionali includono una recente colonizzazione con batteri patogeni, il contatto stretto con individui con malattie invasive da *N. meningitidis* e *H. influenzae* tipo b (per es. negli asili nido, nei dormitori scolastici o in caserma), l'affollamento abitativo, la povertà, l'appartenenza alla razza afroamericana o nativa americana e il sesso maschile. La modalità di trasmissione è probabilmente per contagio diretto interpersonale, attraverso le secrezioni del tratto respiratorio. Nei lattanti e bambini con batteriemia occulta (vedi Capitoli 175 e

TABELLA 602-1. Reperti nel liquido cerebrospinale nelle malattie del sistema nervoso centrale

CONDIZIONE	PRESSIONE (MMH$_2$O)	LEUCOCITI (MM^3)	PROTEINE (MG/DL)	GLUCOSIO (MG/DL)	COMMENTI
Normale	**50-80**	**<5, ≥75% linfociti**	**20-45**	**>50 (o 75% glucosio sierico)**	
FORME COMUNI DI MENINGITE					
Meningite batterica acuta	Solitamente elevata (100-300)	100-10 000; solitamente 300-2000; PMN predominano	100-500	Ridotto <40 (<50% nel siero)	Organismi solitamente individuabili con colorazione Gram o coltura
Meningite batterica parzialmente trattata	Normale o elevata	5-10 000; PMN predominano, ma cellule mononucleate possono prevalere in caso di trattamento prolungato	100-500	Normale o ridotto	Organismi solitamente individuabili con colorazione Gram Il pretrattamento può rendere il LCS sterile. Il test di agglutinazione individua l'antigene
Meningite virale o meningoencefalite	Normale o leggermente elevata (80-150)	Raramente >1000. Conte di diverse migliaia nella encefalite equina e LCM	50-200	Solitamente normale; in alcuni casi virali ridotto <40, in particolare con parotite epidemica (15-20% dei casi)	L'encefalite da HSV è suggerita da convulsioni focali o reperti TC, EEG o RM focali. Enterovirus e HSV difficilmente identificabili nel LCS, ma individuabili con PCR del LCS
FORME DI MENINGITE MENO COMUNI					
Meningite tubercolare	Solitamente elevata	10-500; inizialmente predominano PMN, poi linfociti	100-300; più elevato in presenza di blocco liquorale	<50 nella maggior parte dei casi; cala ancora in assenza di trattamento	Su striscio non compaiono quasi mai microrganismi acido-resistenti, evidenziabili invece su colture di grandi volumi di LCS *Mycobacterium tuberculosis* individuato da PCR
Meningite fungina	Solitamente elevata	5-500; inizialmente predominano PMN, poi linfociti. Nella meningite criptococcica può riscontrarsi assenza di risposta infiammatoria	25-500	<50, cala ancora in assenza di trattamento	Lieviti ramificati possono essere visibili. Microrganismi individuabili su coltura. Antigene criptococcico può risultare positivo
Sifilide (acuta) e leptospirosi	Solitamente elevata	5-500 linfociti predominano	50-200	Solitamente normale	Sierologia LCS positiva. Spirochete non dimostrabili con tecniche tradizionali. Esame in campo denso talvolta positivo
Meningoencefalite amebica (*Naegleria*)	Elevata	1000-10 000 ed oltre; predominano PMN	50-500	Normale o leggermente ridotto	Ameba mobile evidenziabile nell'esame a goccia spessa del LCS a temperatura ambiente
ASCESSI CEREBRALI E PARAMENINGEI					
Ascesso cerebrale	Solitamente elevata (100-300)	5-200; LCS raramente acellulare, linfociti predominano; in caso di rottura dell'ascesso, PMN predomino e conta cellulare può raggiungere >100 000	75-500	Normale in assenza di rottura dell'ascesso nel sistema ventricolare	Microrganismi non rilevabili su striscio o coltura in assenza di rottura dell'ascesso nel sistema ventricolare
Empiema subdurale	Solitamente elevata (100-300)	100-5000; PMN predominano	100-500	Normale	Microrganismi non rilevabili su striscio o coltura, a meno che non sia presente anche meningite. Microrganismi rilevabili con puntura subdurale
Ascesso epidurale cerebrale	Normale o leggermente elevata	10-500; linfociti predominano	50-200	Normale	Microrganismi non rilevabili su striscio o coltura
Ascesso epidurale spinale	Solitamente bassa, con blocco spinale	10-100; linfociti predominano	50-400	Normale	Microrganismi non rilevabili su striscio o coltura
Da sostanze chimiche (farmaci, cisti dermoidi, mezzo di contrasto della mielografia)	Solitamente elevata	10-1000; PMN predominano	50-100	Normale o leggermente ridotto	Cellule epiteliali evidenziabili nel LCS con luce polarizzata in alcuni bambini con cisti dermoidi
CAUSE NON INFETTIVE					
Sarcoidosi	Normale o leggermente elevata	0-100; mononucleari	40-100	Normale	Assenza di reperti specifici
Lupus eritematoso sistemico con coinvolgimento SNC	Leggermente elevata	0-500; PMN predominano; linfociti talvolta presenti	100	Normale o leggermente ridotta	Microrganismi non rilevabili su striscio o coltura. Anticorpi per proteina P neuronale e ribosomiale nel LCS
Tumore, leucemia	Leggermente o molto elevata	0-100, mononucleari o cellule blastiche	50-1,000	Normale o ridotto (20-40)	Citologia talvolta positiva

LCS, liquido cerebrospinale; EEG, elettroencefalogramma; HSV, herpes simplex virus; PCR, *Polymerase Chain Reaction* (reazione a catena della polimerasi); PMN, *Polymorphonuclear Neutrophils* (neutrofili morfopolinucleati); LCM, coriomeningite linfocitaria..

176), il rischio di meningite aumenta di 85 volte per i meningococchi e di 12 volte per *H. influenzae* tipo b rispetto a quello per lo pneumococco.

L'aumento di rischio di meningite batterica nei nativi americani e negli eschimesi è attribuito a specifici difetti delle difese dell'ospite dovuti a un'alterazione della produzione di immunoglobulina in risposta a patogeni capsulati. Difetti del complemento (C5-C8) sono stati associati a infezioni meningococciche ricorrenti, mentre difetti del sistema properdinico sembrano collegati a un significativo rischio di malattia meningococcica letale. La disfunzione splenica (anemia falciforme) o l'asplenia (dovuta a trauma o difetto congenito) sono associate ad aumento del rischio di infezione da pneumococchi, *H. influenzae* tipo b e, più raramente, di sepsi meningococcica e meningite. Difetti dei linfociti T (congeniti o acquisiti in seguito a chemioterapia, AIDS o tumori maligni) determinano un aumento del rischio di contrarre infezioni del SNC da *L. monocytogenes*.

Perdite (congenite o acquisite) di LCS attraverso la barriera mucocutanea, come nei casi di difetto della linea mediana facciale (lamina cribriforme) e dell'orecchio medio (piatto stapediale) o di fistola dell'orecchio interno (finestra ovale, canale uditivo interno, acquedotto cocleare), o perdite di LCS attraverso una rottura delle meningi dovuta a frattura della base del cranio a livello della lamina cribriforme, sono associate a un aumento del rischio di meningite pneumococcica. Il rischio di meningite batterica da *S. pneumoniae* cresce (di 30 volte rispetto alla popolazione generale degli Stati Uniti) nei bambini con impianto cocleare, utilizzato nel trattamento della sordità. Seno dermico lombosacrale e meningocele sono associati a meningite da batteri enterici Gram-negativi e meningite stafilococcica. Infezioni di shunt del LCS aumentano il rischio di meningite da stafilococchi (in particolare delle specie coagulasi-negative) e da altri batteri a virulenza ridotta che tipicamente colonizzano la pelle.

***STREPTOCOCCUS PNEUMONIAE* (VEDI CAPITOLO 181).** L'epidemiologia delle infezioni causate da *S. pneumoniae* è stata drasticamente alterata dalla diffusione del vaccino pneumococcico coniugato 7-valente, introdotto negli Stati Uniti nel febbraio del 2000. Si raccomanda l'immunizzazione di routine per tutti i bambini di 23 mesi e per bambini più piccoli (a 2, 4, 6 e tra i 12 e i 15 mesi). L'immunizzazione ha come bersaglio questa fascia di età perché il picco dell'incidenza delle infezioni pneumococciche invasive si riscontra nei primi due anni di vita, con 228/100 000 casi tra i 6 e i 12 mesi. I bambini con infezione da HIV o con asplenia anatomica o funzionale secondaria ad anemia presentano un'incidenza di infezione da 20 a 100 volte superiore nei primi 5 anni di vita. Fattori di rischio addizionali per contrarre la meningite pneumococcica includono l'otite media, la sinusite, la polmonite, l'otorrea o rinorrea di LCS, la presenza di impianto cocleare e la malattia cronica GVHD post-trapianto di midollo osseo.

***NEISSERIA MENINGITIDIS* (VEDI CAPITOLO 190).** Cinque sottogruppi di meningococchi, A, B, C, Y e W-135, sono responsabili della malattia, che può essere di tipo sporadico o epidemico. Negli Stati Uniti, i sierogruppi B, C e Y sono responsabili del 30% dei casi circa, ma la distribuzione varia a seconda del luogo e dell'epoca. La malattia epidemica, in particolare nei Paesi in via di sviluppo, è solitamente causata dal sierogruppo A. I casi si verificano tutto l'anno, ma sono più frequenti in inverno e in primavera, successivamente alle infezioni da virus dell'influenza. Il trasporto nasofaringeo di *N. meningitidis* si verifica nell'1-15% degli adulti. La colonizzazione può durare settimane o mesi, mettendo a rischio in particolare i bambini piccoli non immuni. L'incidenza della malattia in associazione alla presenza di un caso indice nella famiglia è dell'1%, con un rischio 1000 volte superiore a quello della popolazione generale. Il rischio di insorgenza di casi secondari a contatto in asilo nido è di circa 1/1000. Nella maggior parte dei casi, i bambini contraggono l'infezione in seguito a contatto in asilo nido, contatto con un membro della famiglia colonizzato o con un altro paziente malato. Il tasso di infezione più elevato si riscontra nei bambini al di sotto dei 5 anni. Un secondo picco di incidenza si verifica tra i 15 e i 24 anni. Le matricole dei college che vivono nei dormitori hanno un'aumentata incidenza di infezioni in confronto ai coetanei che non vivono in college.

***HAEMOPHILUS INFLUENZAE* TIPO B (VEDI CAPITOLO 192).** Prima dell'introduzione obbligatoria della vaccinazione contro *H. influenzae* tipo b, negli Stati Uniti il 70% circa dei casi di meningite batterica nei primi 5 anni di vita era causato da questo patogeno. Le infezioni invasive colpivano prevalentemente i bambini tra i 2 mesi e i 2 anni, con un picco di incidenza tra i 6 e i 9 mesi. Il 50% dei casi si verificava nel primo anno di vita. Il rischio risultava notevolmente superiore in caso di contatto con pazienti affetti dalla malattia (in famiglia o asilo nido). Restano tuttora a rischio i soggetti con immunizzazione incompleta, che vivono nei Paesi in via di sviluppo o con risposta insufficiente al vaccino (come nei portatori di infezione da HIV).

ANATOMIA PATOLOGICA E FISIOPATOLOGIA. L'essudato purulento, di viscosità variabile, si distribuisce lungo le vene cerebrali, i seni venosi, la convessità cerebrale e cerebellare, i solchi, le scissure silviane, le cisterne basali e il midollo spinale. Può essere presente ventricolite (più frequente nei neonati), con batteri e cellule infiammatorie nel liquido ventricolare. Si possono riscontrare anche effusioni subdurali e, più raramente, empiema. Talvolta si osservano infiltrati perivascolari infiammatori o distruzione della membrana ependimale. Gli esami autoptici hanno consentito di evidenziare anche alterazioni vascolari e parenchimali cerebrali caratterizzate da infiltrati polimorfonucleari, che si estendono alla regione subintimale delle piccole arterie e vene, vasculite, trombosi delle vene corticali di piccolo calibro, occlusione dei principali seni venosi, arterite necrotizzante responsabile di emorragia subaracnoidea e, raramente, necrosi corticale cerebrale in assenza di trombosi identificabile. L'**infarto cerebrale**, risultato dell'occlusione vascolare dovuta all'infiammazione, al vasospasmo e alla trombosi, è una sequela frequente. L'infarto può essere microscopico o coinvolgere l'intero emisfero.

L'infiammazione dei nervi e delle radici spinali produce segni meningei, mentre l'infiammazione dei nervi cranici causa neuropatie dei nervi ottico, oculomotore, facciale e acustico. L'aumento della pressione intracranica (*IntraCranial Pressure*, ICP) provoca anche la paralisi del nervo oculomotore, secondaria alla presenza di compressione del nervo da parte del lobo temporale durante l'erniazione tentoriale. La paralisi del nervo abducente può costituire un segno non localizzato di ICP elevata.

L'**aumento dell'ICP** è dovuto a morte cellulare (edema cerebrale citotossico), aumento della permeabilità vascolare capillare indotto dalla citochine (edema cerebrale vasogenico) e, forse, ad aumento della pressione idrostatica (edema cerebrale intestiziale) secondario a ostruzione del riassorbimento del LCS nei villi aracnoidei o a ostruzione del flusso del liquor dai ventricoli. L'ICP può superare 300 mmH_2O. La perfusione cerebrale risulta ulteriormente compromessa se la pressione di perfusione (pressione arteriosa media meno l'ICP) scende al di sotto di 50 cmH_2O a causa della ipotensione sistemica secondaria alla riduzione del flusso sanguigno cerebrale. La sindrome da inappropriata secrezione dell'ormone antidiuretico (SIADH) può determinare una eccessiva ritenzione idrica, potenzialmente responsabile di aumento dell'ICP (vedi Capitolo 560). L'ipotonicità degli spazi extracellulari cerebrali causa edema citotossico secondario a rigonfiamento cellulare e lisi. L'erniazione del tentorio, della falce o del cervelletto solitamente non si verificano, perché l'aumento dell'ICP è trasmesso all'intero spazio subaracnoideo e si riscontra solo un lieve spostamento strutturale. Se le fontanelle sono ancora pervie, non sempre l'aumento dell'ICP è attenuato.

L'**idrocefalo** può costituire una complicanza acuta della meningite batterica. Nella maggior parte dei casi, si riscontra idrocefalo comunicante, dovuto all'ispessimento da aderenza dei villi aracnoidei intorno alle cisterne alla base del cervello, che interferisce con il normale riassorbimento di LCS. Meno frequentemente, l'idrocefalo ostruttivo si sviluppa in seguito a fibrosi e gliosi dell'acquedotto di Silvio o dei forami di Magendie e Luschka.

L'**aumento della proteinorrachia nel LCS** è in parte dovuto all'incremento della permeabilità vascolare della barriera ematoencefalica e alla perdita di liquido ricco di albumina dai capillari e dalle vene che attraversano lo spazio subdurale. La continua trasudazione può provocare effusioni subdurali, solitamente riscontrate nella fase più tardiva della meningite batterica acuta. L'**ipoglicorrachia** (calo dei livelli di glucosio nel LCS) è dovuta alla riduzione del trasporto di glucosio da parte del tessuto celebrale.

Il danno a carico della corteccia cerebrale è attribuibile a effetti focali o diffusi di un'occlusione vascolare (infarto, necrosi, acidosi lattica), ipossia, invasione batterica (cerebrite), encefalopatia tossica (tossine batteriche), aumento dell'ICP, ventricolite e trasudazione (effusioni subdurali). Questi fattori patologici provocano le seguenti manifestazioni cliniche: compromissione della coscienza, convulsioni, deficit dei nervi cranici, deficit motori e sensoriali, ritardo psicomotorio (a lungo termine).

PATOGENESI. Nella maggior parte dei casi, la meningite batterica è il risultato della disseminazione ematogena di microrganismi provenienti da una sede di infezione periferica; la **batteriemia** solitamente precede la meningite, o insorge contemporaneamente. La colonizzazione batterica del nasofaringe con microrganismi potenzialmente patogeni è solitamente all'origine della batteriemia. L'individuo portatore può risultare a lungo asintomatico, ma nella maggior parte dei pazienti la recente colonizzazione provoca una rapida invasione. Un'infezione virale del tratto respiratorio superiore precedente o contemporanea alla malattia rischia di potenziare la patogenicità dei batteri responsabili di meningite.

N. meningitidis e *H. influenzae* tipo b si legano ai recettori cellulari della mucosa epiteliale mediante pili e, dopo aver perforato la mucosa, entrano in circolo. *N. meningitidis* può essere trasportato attraverso la superficie mucosa all'interno di vacuolo fagocitico, successivamente a ingestione da parte della cellula epiteliale. La sopravvivenza batterica nel circolo sanguigno è favorita da capsule batteriche di grandi dimensioni, che interferiscono con la fagocitosi opsonica, aumentando la virulenza. Anche i difetti evolutivi della fagocitosi opsonica contribuiscono alla batteriemia. Nei bambini piccoli non immuni, il difetto può essere dovuto all'assenza di anticorpi anticapsulari IgM o IgG preformati, mentre nei pazienti immunodepressi vari deficit di fattori del complemento o del sistema properdinico interferiscono con l'efficacia della fagocitosi opsonica. Anche la disfunzione splenica può ridurre la fagocitosi opsonica a opera del sistema reticoloendoteliale.

I batteri accedono al LCS attraverso i plessi coroidei dei ventricoli laterali e le meningi, per poi circolare nel LCS extracerebrale e nello spazio subaracnoideo. Si moltiplicano rapidamente, perché le concentrazioni del complemento e di anticorpi del LCS non riescono a contenere la proliferazione batterica. Fattori chemiotattici evocano poi una risposta infiammatoria locale, caratterizzata da infiltrazione di polimorfonucleati. La presenza del lipopolisaccaride (endotossina) della parete cellulare di batteri Gram-negativi (*H. influenzae* tipo b, *N. meningitidis*) e di componenti della parete pneumococcica (acido teicoico, peptidoglicano) stimola una importante risposta infiammatoria, con produzione locale di fattore di necrosi tumorale, interleuchina 1, prostaglandina E e altri mediatori dell'infiammazione. La conseguente risposta infiammatoria è caratterizzata da infiltrazione neutrofila, aumento della permeabilità vascolare, alterazioni della barriera ematoencefalica e trombosi vascolare. Le lesioni cerebrali associate alla meningite non sono causate soltanto dal batterio, ma sono una conseguenza della reazione dell'ospite alla cascata infiammatoria avviata dalle componenti batteriche.

In rari casi, la meningite può seguire l'invasione batterica da un focolaio di infezione contiguo, come sinusite paranasale, otite media, mastoidite, cellulite orbitale, osteomielite vertebrale o craniale. Oppure la meningite può essere secondaria a introduzione del batterio mediante un trauma cranico penetrante, tratti del seno dermico o meningomielocele.

MANIFESTAZIONI CLINICHE. L'esordio della meningite acuta presenta due modalità predominanti. La presentazione più grave, e fortunatamente meno comune, è improvvisa e a rapida progressione, con shock, porpora, coagulazione intravascolare disseminata (*Disseminated Intravascular Coagulation*, DIC), riduzione del livello di coscienza, che progredisce verso il coma o il decesso entro 24 ore. Più spesso, la meningite è preceduta di alcuni giorni da febbre e sintomi gastrointestinali o del tratto respiratorio superiore, seguiti da segni non specifici di infezione del SNC, come crescente letargia e irritabilità.

I segni e sintomi di meningite sono collegati a reperti non specifici, associati a infezione sistemica e a manifestazioni di irritazione meningea, che includono: febbre, anoressia, cefalea, sintomi di infezione del tratto respiratorio superiore, mialgia, artralgia, tachicardia, ipotensione e vari segni cutanei, come petecchie, porpora o esantema eritematomaculare. L'irritazione meningea si manifesta con rigidità nucale, dolore alla schiena, **segno di Kernig** (flessione dell'anca di 90° e conseguente dolore con l'estensione dell'arto inferiore), **segno di Brudzinski** (involontaria flessione di ginocchia e anche, in seguito a flessione passiva del collo, con il soggetto in posizione supina). Nei bambini, in particolare se di età inferiore a 12-18 mesi, i segni di Kernig e Brudzinski non sono sempre presenti. La febbre, la cefalea e la rigidità nucale si riscontrano solo nel 40% degli adulti con meningite batterica. L'aumento dell'ICP è suggerito da: cefalea, emesi, diastasi (allargamento) delle suture o fontanella anteriore tesa o pulsante, paralisi del nervo oculomotore (anisocoria, ptosi) o abducente, ipertensione con bradicardia, apnea o iperventilazione, postura decorticata o decerebrata, *stupor*, coma o segni di erniazione. Il papilledema, raro nella meningite non complicata, suggerisce un processo cronico, come la presenza di un ascesso intracranico, di un empiema subdurale o dell'occlusione di un seno venoso durale. I segni neurologici focali sono solitamente dovuti a occlusione vascolare. L'infiammazione focale può provocare anche sofferenza dei nervi cranici ottico, oculomotore, abducente, facciale e acustico. Nel complesso, circa il 10-20% dei bambini con meningite batterica presenta segni neurologici focali.

Le **convulsioni** (focali o generalizzate) dovute a cerebrite, infarto o squilibri elettrolitici colpiscono il 20-30% dei pazienti. Le convulsioni che si verificano in coincidenza con la presentazione o entro i primi 4 giorni dall'esordio non hanno alcun significato prognostico. Le convulsioni che persistono oltre il quarto giorno di malattia e risultano difficili da controllare sono associate a prognosi sfavorevole.

Le **alterazioni dello stato mentale**, comuni tra i pazienti con meningite, sono attribuibili ad aumento dell'ICP, cerebrite o ipotensione. Le manifestazioni includono irritabilità, letargia, *stupor*, torpore e coma. I pazienti comatosi hanno una prognosi infausta. Manifestazioni addizionali includono fotofobia e *tache cérébrale* (dermografismo rosso, pronto e persistente), evidenziata strofinando la cute con un oggetto smusso e osservando la comparsa, entro 30-60 secondi di una stria rossa rilevata.

DIAGNOSI. La diagnosi di meningite piogenica acuta è confermata dall'analisi del LCS, che tipicamente rivela la presenza di microrganismi con colorazione Gram o coltura, di pleiocitosi neutrofila, elevazione della proteinorrachia e riduzione della concentrazione di glucosio (vedi Tab. 602-1). In caso di sospetta meningite batterica, è opportuno eseguire la PL, a meno che non sia presente una delle seguenti **controindicazioni:** (1) evidenza di aumento dell'ICP (oltre a fontanella sporgente), come paralisi del 3° o 6° nervo cranico, con depressione dello stato di coscienza, o ipertensione e bradicardia associate ad anomalie respiratorie (vedi Capitolo 591); (2) grave compromissione cardiopolmonare che richiede l'immediato ricorso a misure di rianimazione o in pazienti nei quali la posizione per la PL aggraverebbe ulteriormente la funzione cardiopolmonare; (3) infezioni cutanee nella sede della PL. La trombocitopenia costituisce una controindicazione relativa per la PL. Nei casi in cui è opportuno rimandare la PL, va avviata immediatamente una terapia antibiotica empirica. L'esordio della terapia non deve essere posposto alla realizzazione di una TC, per verificare la presenza di un ascesso cerebrale o di un aumento dell'ICP. La PL potrà essere effettuata successivamente al trattamento dell'ICP o alla esclusione della presenza di un ascesso.

Le emocolture devono essere eseguite in tutti i pazienti con sospetta meningite, perché consentono di rivelare il batterio responsabile nell'80-90% dei casi.

Puntura lombare (vedi anche Capitolo 591). In presenza di meningite, la conta leucocitaria nel LCS sale oltre $1000/mm^3$ e, tipicamente, si riscontra una predominanza neutrofila (75-95%). Il LCS appare torbido quando la conta leucocitaria eccede $200\text{-}400/mm^3$. I neonati sani possono presentare fino a 30 $leucociti/mm^3$ (solitamente <10), ma i bambini più grandi senza meningite batterica o virale hanno <5 $leucociti/mm^3$; in entrambi i gruppi di età si riscontra una predominanza di linfociti o monociti.

Una conta $<250/ mm^3$ può riscontrarsi fino al 20% dei pazienti con meningite batterica; la pleiocitosi può risultare assente nei pazienti con grave sepsi e meningite e costituisce un segno prognostico negativo. La pleiocitosi con predominanza linfocitica è talvolta presente durante lo stadio precoce della meningite batterica acuta; al contrario, la pleiocitosi neutrofila può essere osservata in pazienti negli stadi iniziali di una meningite virale. Il passaggio a una predominanza linfocitica-monocitica nella meningite virale si verifica invariabilmente entro 8-24 ore dalla PL iniziale. La colorazione Gram è positiva nel 70-90% dei pazienti con meningite batterica non trattata.

La valutazione di bambini con sospetta meningite batterica attraverso l'analisi del LCS ottenuto quando il paziente è già sotto terapia antibiotica (solitamente orale) costituisce una vera e propria sfida diagnostica. Si stima che il 20-25% dei bambini valutati per meningite batterica riceva già antibiotici. In questi casi, la colorazione Gram e la coltura possono risultare negative.

La pleiocitosi con predominanza neutrofila, l'aumento della proteinorrachia e la riduzione della concentrazione di glucosio nel LCS tendono a persistere per diversi giorni dopo l'esordio della terapia antibiotica. Di conseguenza, anche in caso di coltura negativa, può essere formulata la diagnosi presuntiva di meningite batterica. Alcuni medici testano la presenza di antigeni batterici nel LCS in caso di sospetta meningite batterica in un bambino pretrattato con antibiotici, ma tali test presentano limiti tecnici.

Una PL traumatica può complicare la diagnosi di meningite. La ripetizione della PL in uno spazio superiore tende a ottenere un liquor meno emorragico, ma solitamente tale liquor contiene anche globuli rossi. La colorazione Gram, i risultati della coltura e il livello di glucosio non sono alterati, ma una puntura traumatica altera l'interpretazione della conta leucocitaria e della concentrazione di proteine. Benché siano stati elaborati metodi per la presenza di globuli rossi, è più prudente affidarsi ai risultati batteriologici piuttosto che tentare l'interpretazione della conta leucocitaria e dei valori proteici di una PL traumatica.

Diagnosi differenziale. Oltre a *S. pneumoniae*, *N. meningitidis* e *H. influenzae* tipo b, molti altri microrganismi possono causare un'infezione generalizzata del SNC con manifestazioni cliniche analoghe. Tali microrganismi includono: batteri meno tipici, come *Mycobacterium tuberculosis*, *Nocardia* spp., *Treponema pallidum* (sifilide) e *Borrelia burgdorferi* (malattia di Lyme); miceti, come quelli endemici in aree geografiche specifiche (*Coccidioides, Histoplasma* e *Blastomyces*) e quelli responsabili di infezioni in ospiti debilitati (*Candida*, *Cryptococcus* e *Aspergillus*); parassiti, come *Toxoplasma gondii*, quelli responsabili di cisticercosi e virus (vedi Capitolo 602.2) (Tab. 602-2). Infezioni focali del SNC, inclusi ascessi cerebrali e ascessi parameningei (empiema subdurale, ascesso cranico e spinale epidurale), possono essere confusi con la meningite. In rari casi, malattie non infettive (come tumori maligni, connettiviti con vasculiti, esposizione a tossine) sono responsabili di infiammazioni generalizzate del SNC (vedi Tab. 602-2).

La determinazione della causa specifica dell'infezione è facilitata dall'esame del LCS mediante specifiche colorazioni (soluzione di Kinyoun per i micobatteri; inchiostro d'India per i funghi), dagli esami citologici, dalla ricerca degli antigeni (*Cryptococcus*), dalla sierologia (sifilide, West Nile virus, arbovirus, herpes simplex), dalle culture virali (Enterovirus) e dalla reazione polimerasica a catena (herpes simplex, Enterovirus e altri). Emocolture, TC e RM cerebrale, test sierologici e, in rari casi, biopsia cerebrale costituiscono altri utili test diagnostici.

La meningoencefalite virale acuta è l'infezione più facilmente confondibile con la meningite batterica (Tabb. 602-2 e 602-3). In linea generale, la prima appare meno grave della seconda, ma in entrambe le infezioni si riscontrano diversi gradi di serietà. Alcuni pazienti con meningite batterica manifestano segni e sintomi lievi, mentre alcuni pazienti con meningoencefalite virale possono risultare gravemente malati. I profili del LCS associati alle due malattie sono differenti, ma i risultati di alcuni test tendono a sovrapporsi (vedi Tab. 602-1).

TRATTAMENTO. L'approccio terapeutico in caso di presunta meningite batterica dipende dalla natura delle manifestazioni iniziali. In un bambino con malattia a rapida progressione nel corso di 24 ore, che non presenta aumento dell'ICP, è opportuno avviare il prima possibile la terapia antibiotica, dopo aver eseguito la PL. In presenza di segni di aumento dell'ICP o di reperti focali neurologici, gli antibiotici devono essere somministrati senza eseguire la PL e prima di ottenere i risultati della TC. L'aumento dell'ICP richiede un trattamento simultaneo (vedi Capitolo 67). È indicato anche il trattamento immediato dell'associata insufficienza multiorgano (vedi Capitolo 71), dello shock (vedi Capitolo 68) e della sindrome da distress respiratorio acuto (vedi Capitolo 69).

I pazienti con decorso subacuto, protratto per 4-7 giorni, devono essere anch'essi sottoposti a valutazione per aumento dell'ICP e per deficit neurologici focali. Cefalea unilaterale, papilledema e altri segni di elevazione dell'ICP suggeriscono una lesione focale, come un ascesso cerebrale o epidurale, oppure un empiema subdurale. In queste circostanze, la terapia antibiotica deve essere avviata prima della PL e della TC. In assenza di segni evidenti di un aumento dell'ICP, è invece opportuno procedere alla PL.

Terapia antibiotica iniziale. La scelta iniziale (empirica) della terapia in un bambino immunocompetente è influenzata dalla suscettibilità agli antibiotici di *S. pneumoniae* (Tab. 602-4). L'antibiotico selezionato deve raggiungere livelli batterici nel LCS. Malgrado alcune sostanziali differenze geografiche, la resistenza di *S. pneumoniae* agli antibiotici risulta globalmente in aumento. Negli Stati Uniti, il 25-50% dei ceppi di *S. pneumoniae* è resistente alla penicillina; una resistenza relativa (MIC = 0,1-1,0 μg/mL) è più comune di quella completa (MIC = 2,0 μg/mL). La resistenza al cefotaxima e al ceftriaxone si evidenzia fino al 25% degli isolati. Al contrario, la maggior parte dei ceppi di *N. meningitidis* è sensibile a penicillina e cefalosporine, sebbene siano stati segnalati rari isolati resistenti. Circa il 30-40% degli isolati di *H. influenzae* tipo b produce β-lattamasi e, di conseguenza, è resistente all'ampicillina. I ceppi che producono β-lattamasi sono sensibili alle cefalosporine ad ampio spettro.

In considerazione della frequente resistenza di *S. pneumoniae* ai farmaci β-lattamci, si raccomanda l'utilizzo della vancomicina (60 mg/kg/24 h, ogni 6 ore) come parte della terapia empirica iniziale. Anche le cefalosporine si sono dimostrate efficaci nel trattamento della meningite causata da *S. pneumoniae*, *N. meningitidis* e *H. influenzae* tipo b (cefotaxima: 200 mg/kg/24 h, ogni 6 ore; oppure ceftriaxone: 100 mg/kg/24 h una volta al giorno o 50 mg/kg/dose, ogni 12 ore). I pazienti allergici agli antibiotici β-lattamici (purché >1 mese di età) possono essere trattati con cloramfenicol (100 mg/kg/24 h ogni 6 ore). Alternativamente, è possibile tentare di desensibilizzare il paziente (vedi Capitolo 150).

In caso di sospetta infezione da *L. monocytogenes* in lattanti piccoli o con deficit dei linfociti T, è opportuna l'aggiunta di ampicillina (200 mg/kg/24 h, ogni 6 ore), perché le cefalosporine sono inattive contro *L. monocytogenes*. Trimetoprim-sulfametoxazolo per via endovenosa costituisce una valida alternativa pere il trattamento della *L. monocytogenes*.

Se il paziente è immunodepresso e si sospetta una meningite da Gram-negativi, la terapia iniziale dovrebbe includere ceftazidime e un aminoglicoside.

DURATA DELLA TERAPIA ANTIBIOTICA. La terapia di una meningite da *S. pneumoniae* penicillino-sensibile (priva di complicanze) con una cefalosporina di terza generazione o con penicillina endovenosa (400 000 U/kg/die, ogni 4-6 ore) si protrae per 10-14 giorni. Se l'isolato è resistente alla penicillina e alle cefalosporine di 3ª, generazione la terapia andrebbe completata con la vancomicina. La penicillina per via endovenosa (400 000 U/kg/die, per 5-7 giorni) costituisce il trattamento di elezione per la meningite da *N. meningitidis* non complicata. Il trattamento per la meningite da *H. influenzae* tipo b dovrebbe proseguire per 7-10 giorni. I pazienti che ricevono antibiotici orali o per via endovenosa prima della PL, e che non presentano un patogeno identificabile, ma mostrano segni di infezione batterica acuta sulla base del profilo del LCS, dovrebbero continuare a ricevere la terapia con ceftriaxone o cefotaxima per 7-10 giorni. In presenza di segni focali o di assenza di risposta al trattamento, si deve sospettare un focolaio parameningeo e si devono eseguire TC o RM.

La ripetizione di routine della PL non è indicata nei pazienti con meningite da *S. pneumoniae*, *N. meningitidis* o *H. influenzae* tipo b non complicata. L'esame del LCS deve essere ripetuto in alcuni neonati, nei pazienti con meningite batterica Gram-negativa o in caso di infezione causata da *S. pneumoniae* resistente ai β-lattamici. Il LCS dovrebbe risultare sterile entro 24-48 ore dall'inizio della terapia antibiotica.

La meningite dovuta a *Escherichia coli* o *P. aeruginosa* richiede la terapia con una cefalosporina di terza generazione attiva contro l'isolato *in vitro*. La maggior parte degli isolati di *E. coli* è sensibile a cefotaxima o ceftriaxone, e la maggior parte degli isolati di *P. aeruginosa* è sensibile a ceftazidime. Il trattamento della meningite batterica da Gram-negativi deve proseguire per 3 settimane, e per almeno 2 settimane dopo la sterilizzazione del LCS (che generalmente si verifica dopo 2-10 giorni di terapia).

TABELLA 602-2. Condizioni cliniche e agenti infettivi associati alla meningite asettica

VIRUS

Enterovirus (virus coxsackie, echovirus, poliovirus, enterovirus)
Arbovirus: equino orientale, occidentale, venezuelano; encefalite di St. Louis, encefalite Powassan e californiana, West Nile virus, febbre da zecche del Colorado
Herpes simplex (tipi 1, 2)
Herpes virus umano tipo 6
Virus varicella-zoster
Virus di Epstein-Barr
Parvovirus B19
Cytomegalovirus
Adenovirus
Vaiolo
Morbillo
Parotite epidemica
Rosolia
Influenza A e B
Parainfluenza
Rinovirus
Rabbia
Coriomeningite linfocitica
Rotavirus
Coronavirus
Virus dell'immudeficienza umana di tipo 1

BATTERI

Mycobacterium tuberculosis
Leptospira spp. (leptospirosi)
Treponema pallidum (sifilide)
Borrelia spp. (febbre recidivante)
Borrelia burgdorferi (malattia di Lyme)
Nocardia spp. (nocardiosi)
Brucella spp.
Bartonella spp. (malattia da graffio di gatto)
Rickettsia rickettsiae (febbre maculosa delle Montagne Rocciose)
Rickettsia prowazekii (tifo)
Ehrlichia canis
Coxiella burnetii
Mycoplasma pneumoniae
Mycoplasma hominis
Chlamydia trachomatis
Chlamydia psittaci
Chlamydia pneumoniae
Meningite parzialmente trattata

FOCOLAI PARAMENINGEI BATTERICI

Sinusite
Mastoidite
Ascesso cerebrale
Empiema subdurale-epidurale
Osteomielite cranica

FUNGHI

Coccidioides immitis (coccidioidomicosi)
Blastomyces dermatitidis (blastomicosi)
Cryptococcus neoformans (criptococcosi)
Histoplasma capsulatum (istoplasmosi)
Candida
Altri funghi (*Alternaria, Aspergillus, Cephalosporium, Cladosporium, Dreschlera hawaiiensis, Paracoccidioides brasiliensis, Petriellidium boydii, Sporotrichum schenckii, Ustilago* spp., *Zygomycetes*)

PARASSITI ASSOCIATI A EOSINOFILIA

Angiostrongylus cantonensis
Gnathostoma spinigerum
Baylisascaris procyonis
Strongyloides stercoralis
Trichinella spiralis
Toxocara canis
Taenia solium (cisticercosi)
Paragonimus westermani
Schistosoma spp.
Fasciola spp.

PARASSITI NON ASSOCIATI A EOSINOFILIA

Toxoplasma gondii (toxoplasmosi)
Acanthamoeba
Naegleria fowleri
Malaria

POSTINFETTIVE

Vaccini: rabbia, influenza, morbillo, poliovirus
Encefalite demielinizzante o allergica

SISTEMICHE O IMMUNOMEDIATE

Endocardite batterica
Malattia di Kawasaki
Lupus eritematoso sistemico
Vasculite, inclusa la poliarterite nodosa
Sindrome di Sjögren
Connettivite mista
Artrite reumatoide
Sindrome di Behçet
Granulomatosi di Wegener
Granulomatosi linfomatoide
Arterite granulomatosa
Sarcoidosi
Febbre mediterranea familiare
Sindrome di Vogt-Koyanagi-Harada

TUMORI MALIGNI

Leucemia
Linfoma
Carcinoma metastasico
Tumore del SNC (craniofaringioma, glioma, ependimoma, astrocitoma, medulloblastoma, teratoma)

FARMACI

Infezioni intratecali (da mezzo di contrasto, siero, antibiotici, agenti antineoplastici)
Agenti antinfiammatori non steroidei
Anticorpi monoclonali OKT3
Carbamazepina
Azatioprina
Immunoglobuline endovenose
Antibiotici (trimetoprim-sulfametoxazolo, sulfasalazina, ciprofloxacin, isoniazide)

VARIE

Avvelenamento da metalli pesanti (piombo, arsenico)
Corpi estranei (shunt, reservoir)
Emorragia subaracnoidea
Stato postictale
Stato post-emicrania
Sindrome di Mollaret (ricorrente)
Emorragia intraventricolare (neonatale)
Sindrome emofagocitica familiare
Post neurochirurgia
Cisti dermoide-epidermoide

Tratta da Cherry JD: Aseptic meningitis and viral meningitis. In Feigin RD, Cherry JD (editors): *Textbook of Pediatric Infectious Diseases*, 4th ed. Philadelphia, WB Saunders, 1998, p 450; and from Davis LE: Aseptic and viral meningitis. In Long SS, Pickering LK, Prober CG (editors): *Principles and Practice of Pediatric Infectious Disease*. New York, Churchill Livingstone, 1997, p 329; and from Kliegman RM, Greenbaum LA, Lye PS: *Practical Strategies in Pediatric Diagnosis Therapy*. 2nd ed. Philadelphia, Elsevier, 2004, p. 961.

Gli effetti collaterali della terapia antibiotica includono flebite, febbre da farmaci, eruzioni cutanee, emesi, candidosi orale e diarrea. Il ceftriaxone può causare pseudolitiasi della colecisti reversibile, individuabile mediante ecografia addominale. Tale complicanza, generalmente asintomatica, può essere associata a emesi e dolore al quadrante superiore destro.

Corticosteroidi. La rapida eliminazione dei batteri presenti nel LCS sterilizza efficacemente l'infezione meningea, ma causa il rilascio di prodotti tossici della lisi cellulare (endotossina della parete cellulare), responsabili dell'attivazione della cascata infiammatoria citochino-mediata. I risultanti edema e infiltrazione neutrofila rischiano di causare ulteriori lesioni neurologiche, aggravando i segni e sintomi a carico del SNC. Di conseguenza, nei pazienti con meningite batterica è utile la somministrazione di agenti in grado di limitare la produzione di mediatori infiammatori.

Nei bambini con più di 6 settimane affetti da meningite batterica acuta da *H. influenzae* tipo b, si raccomanda la somministrazione per via endovenosa di desametasone (0,15 mg/kg/

TABELLA 602-3. Classificazione delle encefaliti sulla base di cause e origine

I. INFEZIONI: VIRALI

A. Contagio: diretto da persona a persona
1. Parotite epidemica: frequente nelle popolazioni non immunizzate; spesso lieve
2. Morbillo: può avere gravi sequele
3. Enterovirus: frequente a tutte le età; più seria nei neonati
4. Rosolia: rara, sequele rare eccetto nella forma congenita
5. Gruppo degli herpes
a. Herpes simplex (tipo 1, 2, 6): relativamente comune; sequele frequenti; devastante nei neonati
b. Virus varicella-zoster: raro; sequele serie frequenti
c. Cytomegalovirus, congenito a acquisito: può avere sequele tardive nella forma congenita
d. Virus di Epstein-Barr (mononucleosi infettiva): raro
6. Poxvirus
a. Vaccinazione complicata e vaiolo: raro ma grave (lesione del SNC)
7. Parvovirus (eritema infettivo): raro
8. Influenza A e B
9. Adenovirus
10. Altri: reovirus, respiratorio sinciziale, parainfluenza, epatite B

B. Agenti da artropodi come vettori
Arbovirus: contagio all'uomo attraverso zanzare e zecche; epidemie stagionali. Le seguenti si verificano negli Stati Uniti: equina orientale, occidentale, venezuelana; St. Louis; West Nile; California; Powassan; Dengue; febbre da zecche del Colorado

C. Diffusione mediante animali a sangue caldo
1. Rabbia: saliva di animali domestici e non
2. Herpesvirus simiae (virus B): saliva delle scimmie
3. Coriomeningite linfocitaria: escrezioni dei roditori

II. INFEZIONI: NON VIRALI

A. Rickettsie: febbre maculosa delle Montagne Rocciose e tifo; componente encefalitica della vasculite cerebrale
B. *Mycoplasma pneumoniae*: intervallo di qualche giorno tra sintomi respiratori e cerebrali
C. Batteriche: meningite tubercolotica e altre meningiti batteriche spesso hanno una componente encefalitica
D. Da spirocheti: sifilide, congenita o acquisita; leptospirosi; malattia di Lyme
E. Malattia da graffio di gatto
F. Fungine: in pazienti immunocompromessi: criptococcosi; istoplasmosi; aspergillosi; mucormicosi; candidosi; coccidioidomicosi
G. Da protozoi: *Plasmodium*, *Trypanosoma*, *Naegleria* e *Acanthamoeba* spp.; *Toxoplasma gondii*
H. Da metazoi: trichinosi; echinococcosi; cisticercosi; schistosomiasi

III. PARAINFETTIVE: POSTINFETTIVE, ALLERGICHE

L'agente infettivo o uno dei suoi componenti contribuisce all'eziologia, ma l'agente intatto non è isolato in vitro dal SNC; in questo gruppo, sono particolarmente importanti nel produrre il danno tissutale osservato, la reazione cellulo-mediata e i complessi antigene-anticorpo-complemento

A. Associate a specifiche malattie (vedi I e II)

Morbillo	Rickettsie
Rosolia	Influenza A e B
Parotite epidemica	Varicella-zoster
Mycoplasma pneumoniae	

B. Associate a vaccini

Rabbia	Morbillo
Vaiolo	Febbre gialla

IV. MALATTIE UMANE DA VIRUS LENTI

Sembra dimostrato che virus acquisiti precocemente, non necessariamente individuabili durante la malattia acuta, contribuiscano allo sviluppo successivo di una malattia neurologica cronica (come si verifica nell'animale)
A. Panencefalite sclerosante subacuta; morbillo, rosolia?
B. Malattia di Creutzfeldt-Jakob (encefalopatia spongiforme)
C. Leucoencefalopatia multifocale progressiva
D. Kuru (solo nelle tribù della New Guinea)
E. Virus dell'immunodeficienza umana

V. SCONOSCIUTE

Questo gruppo include più dei due terzi dei casi di encefalite segnalati presso i Centers for Disease Control and Prevention, Atlanta, Georgia. La curva epidemica annuale di questi casi indica la responsabilità di Enterovirus e/o Arbovirus.

Il gruppo comprende malattie diagnosticate sulla base di criteri clinici (come la sindrome di Reye). Alcune classificazioni includono l'estinta encefalite di Von Economo (epidemica nel 1918-1928); l'encefalopatia mioclonica infantile; la retinomeningoencefalite con papilledema ed emorragia retinica; l'encefalomielite ricorrente (allergica o autoimmune); lo pseudotumor cerebri e la neuromiastenia epidemica.

Un quadro encefalitico può seguire l'ingestione o l'assorbimento di un certo numero di sostanze tossiche più o meno note (come l'ingestione di piombo e mercurio e l'assorbimento percutaneo di esaclorofene e γ-benzene esacloruro) come agente per la scabbia.

SNC, sistema nervoso centrale.
Modificata da Behrman RE (editor): *Nelson Textbook of Pediatrics*, 14th ed. Philadelphia, WB Saunders, 1992, p 667. From Kliegman RM, Greenbaum LA, Lye PS: *Practical Strategies in Pediatric Diagnosis and Therapy*, 2nd ed. Philadelphia, Elsevier, 2004, p. 967.

TABELLA 602-4. Antibiotici utilizzati nel trattamento della meningite batterica*

	NEONATI		
FARMACO	0-7 giorni	8-28 giorni	BAMBINI
Amikacina†‡	15-20 divisi ogni 12 ore	20-30 divisi ogni 8 ore	20-30 divisi ogni 8 ore
Ampicillina	200-300	300 divisi ogni 4-6 ore	300 divisi ogni 4-6 ore
Cefotaxima	100 divisi ogni 12 ore	150-200 divisi ogni 8-6 ore	200-300 divisi ogni 6-8 ore
Ceftriaxone§	–	–	100 divisi ogni 12 ore
Ceftazidime	150 divisi ogni 12 ore	150 divisi ogni 8 ore	150 divisi ogni 8 ore
Gentamicina†‡	5 divisi ogni 12 ore	7,5 divisi ogni 8 ore	7,5 divisi ogni 8 ore
Meropenem	–	–	120 divisi ogni 8 ore
Nafcillina	100-150 divisi ogni 8-12 ore	150-200 divisi ogni 8-6 ore	150-200 divisi ogni 4-6 ore
Penicillina G	250 000-450 000 divisi ogni 8 ore	450 000 divisi ogni 6 ore	450,000 divisi ogni 4-6 ore
Rifampicina	–	–	20 divisi ogni 12 ore
Tobramicina†‡	5 divisi ogni 12 ore	7,5 divisi ogni 8 ore	7,5 divisi ogni 8 ore
Vancomicina†‡	30 divisi ogni 12 ore	30-45 divisi ogni 8 ore	60 divisi ogni 6 ore

* Dosaggio in mg/kg/die.
† Dosi ridotte e intervalli più lunghi sono raccomandabili in neonati con basso peso.
‡ Si raccomanda il monitoraggio dei livelli sierici, per verificare che rientri nel range terapeutico.
§ L'uso nei neonati non è indicato.
Modificata da Klein JO: Antimicrobial treatment and prevention of meningitis. *Pediatr Ann* 1994;23:76; e da Kliegman RM, Greenbaum LA, Lye PS: *Practical Strategies in Pediatric Diagnosis and Therapy*, 2nd ed. Philadelphia, Elsevier, 2004, p 963.

dose ogni 6 ore, per 2 giorni). Nei bambini con meningite da *H. influenzae* tipo b che ricevono corticosteroidi si riscontrano una durata inferiore della febbre, livelli ridotti di lattato e di proteine nel LCS, e una riduzione della perdita uditiva sensorineurale. I dati relativi ai benefici dei corticosteroidi nel trattamento della meningite causata da altri batteri non sono conclusivi. Tuttavia, il trattamento precoce degli adulti con meningite batterica, in particolare pneumococcica, migliora la prognosi.

I corticosteroidi sembrano esercitare un effetto favorevole massimo se somministrati 1-2 ore prima dell'inizio della terapia antibiotica, ma risultano efficaci anche se somministrati contemporaneamente o a breve distanza dalla prima dose di antibiotici. Le complicanze dei corticosteroidi includono emorragia gastrointestinale, ipertensione, iperglicemia, leucocitosi e risalita della febbre dopo l'ultima dose.

Trattamento di supporto. Ripetute valutazioni neurologiche e mediche dei pazienti con meningite batterica sono essenziali per identificare segni precoci di complicanze cardiovascolari, cerebrali e metaboliche. È dunque opportuno monitorare la frequenza del polso, la pressione sanguigna e la frequenza respiratoria. Nelle prime 72 ore (quando il rischio di complicanze neurologiche è maggiore), si raccomanda di effettuare un approfondito esame neurologico, che includa la verifica dei riflessi pupillari, il livello di coscienza, la forza motoria, i segni dei nervi cranici e la presenza di convulsioni. Gli esami di laboratorio più importanti sono: misura dell'azotemia, della concentrazione sierica di sodio, cloruro, potassio e bicarbonato; diuresi e peso specifico urinario; esame emocromocitometrico con piastrine; in presenza di petecchie, porpora o sanguinamento anomalo, valutare la funzione di coagulazione (fibrinogeno, PT, PTT).

Inizialmente, non è opportuno somministrare nulla per via orale. Se il paziente è normovolemico, con pressione sanguigna normale, la somministrazione endovenosa di liquidi dovrebbe essere ridotta della metà o di due terzi rispetto alla dose di mantenimento (800-1000 $mL/m^2/24$ h), finché non viene esclusa la presenza di aumento dell'ICP o di SIADH. La normalizzazione del livello sierico di sodio consente la somministrazione di volumi normali di liquidi (1500-1700 $mL/m^2/24$ h). La restrizione di liquidi non è indicata in presenza di ipotensione sistemica, perché la riduzione della pressione sanguigna può determinare un calo della pressione di perfusione cerebrale, con conseguente ischemia. Lo shock deve essere trattato in maniera aggressiva, per prevenire la disfunzione cerebrale e di altri organi (necrosi tubulare acuta, sindrome da distress respiratorio acuta). I pazienti con shock, marcato aumento dell'ICP e convulsioni refrattarie devono essere ricoverati in un reparto di terapia intensiva, con accesso venoso centrale e arterioso per il monitoraggio dei segni vitali. I pazienti con shock settico richiedono la rianimazione con liquidi e la somministrazione di agenti vasoattivi (come dopamina e adrenalina; vedi Capitolo 176). In tali casi, l'obiettivo della terapia è di evitare l'ulteriore aumento dell'ICP, senza compromettere il flusso sanguigno o l'ossigenazione degli organi vitali.

Le complicanze neurologiche includono l'aumento dell'**ICP** con conseguente erniazione, convulsioni e aumento della circonferenza cranica, secondari a versamento subdurale e idrocefalo. I segni di aumento dell'ICP devono essere trattati tempestivamente con intubazione endotracheale e iperventilazione (per mantenere la pco_2 a 25 mmHg). In aggiunta 1 mg/kg di furosemide endovena e di mannitolo (0,5-1,0 g/kg) contribuiscono a ridurre l'ICP (vedi Capitolo 67). La furosemide riduce l'edema cerebrale mediante venodilatazione e diuresi, senza aumentare il volume ematico intracranico, mentre il mannitolo determina un gradiente osmotico tra cervello e plasma, trasferendo i liquidi dal SNC al plasma con conseguente escrezione durante la diuresi osmotica.

Le **convulsioni** costituiscono una complicanza comune durante il decorso della meningite batterica. La terapia immediata prevede la somministrazione endovenosa di diazepam (0,1-0,2 mg/kg/dose) o lorazepam (0,05-0,10 mg/kg/dose) e un attento monitoraggio del rischio di soppressione respiratoria. I livelli sierici di glucosio, calcio e sodio devono essere monitorati. La successiva somministrazione di fenitoina (dose di carico: 15-20 mg/kg; dose di mantenimento: 5 mg/kg/24 h) riduce il rischio di recidiva. La fenitoina è preferibile al fenobarbital, perché causa una minore depressione del SNC e permette la valutazione del livello di coscienza del paziente. I livelli sierici di fenitoina devono essere mantenuti nel range terapeutico (10-20 μg/mL).

COMPLICANZE. Durante il trattamento della meningite, le complicanze acute a carico del SNC includono: convulsioni, aumento dell'ICP, paralisi dei nervi cranici, stroke, erniazione cerebrale o cerebellare e trombosi dei seni venosi della dura madre.

La raccolta di liquido nello spazio subdurale si sviluppa nel 10-30% dei pazienti con meningite, ma risulta asintomatica nell'85-90% dei casi. Le **effusioni subdurali**, particolarmente comuni nei lattanti, causano un'estroflessione della fontanella anteriore, diastasi delle suture, aumento della circonferenza cranica, emesi, convulsioni, febbre e anomalie della transilluminazione cranica. La TC o la RM confermano la presenza di tali effusioni. In caso di aumento dell'ICP o di depressione del livello di coscienza, è opportuno trattare le effusioni subdurali sintomatiche mediante aspirazione attraverso la fontanella aperta (vedi Capitolo 591). La febbre isolata non costituisce un'indicazione sufficiente per l'aspirazione.

La SIADH insorge in alcuni pazienti con meningite, con conseguente iponatremia e riduzione dell'osmolarità sierica. Tale complicanza rischia di peggiorare l'edema cerebrale o di causare convulsioni iponatremiche (vedi Capitolo 55).

La febbre associata alla meningite batterica solitamente si risolve entro 5-7 giorni dall'esordio della terapia. In circa il 10% dei pazienti, si osserva **febbre prolungata** (oltre i 10 giorni), solitamente dovuta a un'infezione virale intercorrente, nosocomiale o secondaria all'infezione batterica, alla tromboflebite o alla reazione ai farmaci. Il termine febbre secondaria si riferisce alla recrudescenza dell'aumento della temperatura dopo un intervallo afebbrile. Nella valutazione di questi pazienti, è particolarmente importante verificare la presenza di un'infezione nosocomiale. Nei pazienti trattati per meningite da *N. meningitidis*, si riscontrano spesso pericardite e artrite. Il coinvolgimento di queste sedi può essere il risultato della disseminazione batterica o della deposizione di immunocomplessi. In generale, la pericardite o l'artrite infettive insorgono più precocemente durante il decorso della malattia rispetto alle malattie immunomediate.

Trombocitosi, eosinofilia e anemia possono svilupparsi durante la terapia per la meningite. L'anemia è talvolta dovuta a emolisi o soppressione midollare. La DIC tende a essere associata a un quadro di presentazione a rapida progressione ed è spesso riscontrata nei pazienti con shock e porpora. La combinazione di endotossiemia e grave ipotensione attiva la cascata coagulativa, mentre la contemporanea presenza di trombosi può causare cancrena periferica simmetrica.

PROGNOSI. Le terapie antibiotica e di supporto hanno consentito di ridurre a meno del 10% la mortalità in seguito a meningite batterica nel periodo neonatale. Il tasso di mortalità più elevato è associato a meningite pneumococcica. Gravi sequele neuroevolutive si riscontrano nel 10-20% dei pazienti, mentre il 50% presenta una sfumata morbilità neurocomportamentale. La prognosi risulta peggiore nei bambini con meno di 6 mesi o che presentano una elevata concentrazione di batteri o prodotti batterici nel LCS. Il rischio di sequele a lungo termine aumenta nei pazienti che continuano a presentare convulsioni dopo 4 giorni dall'esordio della terapia, oppure che manifestano coma o segni neurologici all'epoca della presentazione. Non risulta invece alcuna correlazione tra la durata dei sintomi prima della diagnosi e l'esito finale.

Le più comuni sequele neurologiche includono: perdita uditiva, ritardo mentale, convulsioni ricorrenti, ritardo nell'acquisizione del linguaggio, compromissione visiva e disturbi comportamentali. La **perdita uditiva sensorineurale**, causata dalla labirintite successiva all'infezione cocleare, è la più frequente sequela della meningite batterica e solitamente è già presente all'epoca della presentazione iniziale. Si riscontra nel 30% dei pazienti con meningite pneumococcica, nel 10% di quelli con meningite meningococcica e nel 5-20% di quelli con meningite da *H. influenzae* tipo b. La perdita uditiva può essere causata anche dall'infiammazione diretta del nervo acustico. Tutti i pazienti con meningite batterica devono essere sottoposti ad accurato esame audiologico prima della dimissione dall'ospedale (o subito dopo). Follow-up frequenti sono necessari nei pazienti con deficit uditivo.

PREVENZIONE. I due strumenti disponibili per ridurre il rischio di meningite batterica sono la prevenzione e la profilassi antibiotica dei contatti suscettibili. La disponibilità e l'applicabilità di tali approcci dipendono dal tipo di infezione.

Neisseria meningitidis. La chemioprofilassi è raccomandata per chiunque entri in contatto con pazienti affetti da meningite meningococcica, a prescindere dall'età e dallo stato di immunizzazione. La profilassi con rifampicina (10 mg/kg/dose ogni 12 ore, senza superare la dose massima di 600 mg, per 2 giorni dei contatti stretti) deve essere avviata immediatamente dopo l'identificazione di un caso di sospetta meningite o sepsi meningococcica. I contatti stretti sono i familiari del paziente, i contatti scolatici e il personale ospedaliero direttamente esposto alle secrezioni orali (rianimazione bocca-a-bocca, intubazione). Il sospetto di infezione nel paziente indice è sufficiente per avviare la profilassi, senza attendere la conferma batteriologica dell'infezione. Inoltre, chiunque sia entrato in contatto con il paziente deve essere istruito sull'identificazione dei precoci segni di malattia e avvisato sulla necessità di rivolgersi immediatamente al medico se questi sintomi compaiono.

Il vaccino quadrivalente (A,C,Y, W-135) coniugato (MCV-4; Menactra) è stato approvato dall'U.S. Food and Drug Administration. L'Advisory Committee on Immunization Practices (ACIP) ai Centers for Disease Control and Prevention (CDC) ne raccomanda la somministrazione di routine a tutti gli adolescenti di 11-12 anni. Questo vaccino è consigliato anche ai bambini ad alto rischio di età superiore ai 2 anni (con asplenia anatomica o funzionale, o deficit dei fattori terminali del complemento). L'uso del vaccino deve essere preso in considerazione anche nei bambini e adolescenti in college, in particolare se vivono in dormitori comuni, perché il rischio di contagio aumenta considerevolmente rispetto ai controlli della stessa età che invece vivono a casa. Infine, il vaccino può essere associato alla chemioprofilassi nei soggetti esposti all'infezione o durante epidemie.

***Haemophilus influenzae* tipo b.** Tutti gli individui entrati in contatto con un paziente affetto da malattia invasiva causata da *H. influenzae* tipo b devono essere sottoposti a profilassi con rifampicina, se un membro della famiglia con meno di 48 mesi non è completamente immunizzato o se un soggetto immunodepresso, di qualsiasi età, risiede nella casa. La definizione di contatto familiare si applica a chiunque risieda nella stessa casa del paziente o abbia trascorso un minimo di 4 ore con il caso indice almeno per 5 dei 7 giorni precedenti al ricovero. In caso di diagnosi sospetta, i membri familiari del paziente devono ricevere la rifampicina immediatamente, perché più del 50% dei casi familiari secondari si verifica nella prima settimana dopo il ricovero del caso indice.

La dose di rifampicina raccomandata è di 20 mg/kg/24 h (dose massima di 600 mg) in un'unica somministrazione, per 4 giorni. La rifampicina colora di rosso-arancio le urine e il sudore, macchia le lenti a contatto e riduce la concentrazione sierica di alcuni farmaci, come i contraccettivi orali. Il farmaco è controindicato in gravidanza.

L'introduzione dei vaccini coniugati contro *H. influenzae* tipo b ha consentito notevoli progressi nella prevenzione della meningite batterica infantile. Negli Stati Uniti sono attualmente disponibili 4 vaccini. Ciascun tipo è caratterizzato da profili differenti nella risposta anticorpale dei bambini immunizzati a 2-6 mesi di età, ma tutti e 4 garantiscono un livello di protezione contro le infezioni compreso tra il 70 e il 100%. L'efficacia risulta ridotta nella popolazione nativa americana, gruppo nel quale l'incidenza della malattia è particolarmente elevata. La vaccinazione contro *H. influenzae* tipo b è raccomandata in tutti i bambini con più di 2 mesi di età (vedi Capitolo 170).

Streptococcus pneumoniae. La somministrazione di routine del vaccino eptavalente coniugato contro *S. pneumoniae* è raccomandata nei bambini con meno di 2 anni. La dose iniziale è somministrata intorno ai 2 mesi. Dovrebbero ricevere il vaccino anche i bambini ad alto rischio, inclusi quelli con asplenia funzionale o anatomica, oppure con immunodeficienza (da HIV, da immunodeficienza primaria o da farmaci immunosoppressori).

602.2 • Meningoencefalite virale

La meningoencefalite virale è un processo infiammatorio acuto che coinvolge le meningi e, in grado variabile, il tessuto cerebrale. Si tratta di un'infezione relativamente comune, causata da un gran numero di agenti diversi (vedi Tab. 602-3). Nel LCS, si riscontra pleiocitosi e assenza di microrganismi alla colorazione Gram o coltura batterica di routine. Nella maggior parte dei casi, l'infezione è autolimitante, ma talvolta ha un'importante morbilità e un esito fatale.

EZIOLOGIA. Gli **Enterovirus** costituiscono la più comune causa di meningoencefalite. Fino a oggi, sono stati identificati più di 80 sierotipi di questi piccoli virus RNA. L'infezione ha una gravità variabile, dai casi più lievi con coinvolgimento quasi esclusivamente meningeo, alle gravi encefaliti responsabili di decesso o di sequele significative.

Gli **Arbovirus** sono agenti ospitati da artropodi, responsabili di alcuni casi di meningoencefalite durante i mesi estivi. Le zanzare e le zecche costituiscono i vettori più comuni, in grado di diffondere la malattia agli esseri umani e ad altri vertebrati, come i cavalli, dopo aver punto uccelli o altri piccoli animali infetti. L'encefalite può costituire la prima indicazione di un'epidemia incipiente. L'esposizione in ambiente rurale è la più frequente causa di contagio, ma focolai urbani e suburbani sono frequenti. Negli Stati Uniti, i più comuni arbovirus responsabili di infezione sono West Nile virus (WNV) e i virus dell'encefalite St. Louis e California (vedi Capitolo 264). West Nile virus è comparso per la prima volta negli Stati Uniti nel 1999 e, un'estate dopo l'altra, si è spostato dalla East coast alla West coast. Nel 2002, WNV ha causato la più grave epidemia di encefalite arbovirale mai descritta in Nord America, segnalata in 44 Stati e nel District of Columbia. Dal 1999 al 2005, WNV ha causato più di 19 000 casi in un totale di 46 Stati. L'infezione è trasmissibile anche mediante trasfusione di sangue, trapianto di organi o trasmissione verticale attraverso la placenta. La maggior parte dei bambini con WNV è asintomatica o presenta una malattia simil-virale non specifica. Soltanto circa l'1% sviluppa la malattia. Gli adulti sono colpiti più gravemente rispetto ai bambini.

Diversi membri della **famiglia degli herpes virus** possono causare meningoencefalite. L'herpes simplex di tipo 1 (HSV-1) è responsabile di encefalite grave e sporadica in adulti e bambini. Il coinvolgimento cerebrale è solitamente focale. In assenza di terapia antivirale, la progressione verso il coma e il decesso si verifica nel 70% dei casi. L'herpes simplex di tipo 2 (HSV-2) causa grave encefalite, con diffuso coinvolgimento cerebrale, nei neonati, che solitamente contraggono il virus dalla madre al momento del parto. Un forma lieve e transitoria di meningoencefalite può accompagnare l'infezione erpetica genitale negli adolescenti sessualmente attivi; nella maggior parte dei casi, queste infezioni sono causate da HSV-2. Il virus varicella-zoster (*Virus Varicella-Zoster*, VZV) può provocare l'infezione al SNC successivamente alla varicella. La più comune manifestazione del coinvolgimento cerebrale è l'atassia cerebellare, mentre la più grave è l'encefalite acuta. Dopo l'infezione primaria, VZV diviene latente nei gangli e nelle radici nervose spinali e craniali, manifestandosi successivamente come herpes zoster, talvolta associato a lieve meningoencefalite. L'infezione da Cytomegalovirus (CMV) del SNC può rientrare nel quadro di un'infezione congenita o di una malattia disseminata nei pazienti immunodepressi, ma non causa encefalite nei neonati e bambini sani. Il virus di Epstein-Barr (EBV) è stato associato a una miriade di sindromi a carico del SNC (vedi Capitolo 251). L'herpes virus 6 (HHV-6) può causare encefalite, in particolare negli ospiti immunocompromessi.

Il virus della parotite epidemica è un patogeno comune in regioni dove il vaccino non è diffuso. È responsabile di una meningoencefalite lieve, ma può causare sordità in seguito a danno dell'ottavo nervo cranico. Occasionalmente, la meningoencefalite è provocata da virus respiratori (adenovirus, virus dell'influenza e della parainfluenza), morbillo, rosolia o rabbia. Talvolta costituisce una complicanza delle vaccinazioni contro la polio, il morbillo, la parotite epidemica e la rosolia.

EPIDEMIOLOGIA. Il quadro epidemiologico della meningoencefalite virale è determinato dalla prevalenza degli Enterovirus, che costituiscono l'eziologia più comune. L'infezione da Enterovirus si diffonde per contagio diretto, con un periodo di incubazione di 4-6 giorni. Nei climi temperati, la maggior parte dei casi si verifica in estate e in autunno. Gli altri aspetti epidemiologici da considerare nei casi di meningite asettica causata da agenti diversi dagli Enterovirus includono la stagione, la geografia, le condizioni climatiche, l'esposizione ad animali e i fattori collegati ai patogeni specifici.

PATOGENESI E ANATOMIA PATOLOGICA. Il danno neurologico è causato dall'invasione diretta e dalla distruzione di tessuti neurali da parte di virus attivi o dalla reazione dell'ospite agli antigeni virali. Le sezioni tissutali cerebrali sono generalmente caratterizzate da congestione meningea e infiltrazione di cellule mononucleate, manicotti perivascolari di linfociti e plasmacellule, necrosi tissutale perivascolare con distruzione della mielina e lesioni neuronali, che includono neurofagia, proliferazione endoteliale e necrosi. Una marcata demielinizzazione associata a conservazione dei neuroni e degli assoni è considerata una encefalite "postinfettiva" o "allergica".

La corteccia cerebrale, in particolare del lobo temporale, è spesso gravemente colpita da HSV. Gli arbovirus tendono a colpire l'intero encefalo, mentre la rabbia manifesta una predilezione per le strutture basali. Il coinvolgimento di midollo spinale, radici nervose e nervi periferici è variabile.

MANIFESTAZIONI CLINICHE. La progressione e la gravità della malattia sono determinate dal grado di coinvolgimento meningeo e parenchimale, che dipende almeno in parte dall'eziologia specifica. Il decorso clinico di infezioni provocate dallo stesso patogeno varia considerevolmente a seconda dei pazienti. Alcuni bambini che sembrano presentare un'infezione lieve entrano in coma e muoiono improvvisamente. In altri casi, la malattia esordisce con febbre elevata, violente convulsioni con movimenti bizzarri, e allucinazioni alternate a brevi periodi di lucidità, ma è seguita da una guarigione completa.

L'esordio dell'infezione è spesso acuto, sebbene i segni e i sintomi cerebrali siano preceduti in molti casi da una malattia febbrile non specifica, che si protrae per qualche giorno. Nei bambini più grandi, le manifestazioni di presentazione includono cefalea e iperestesia, mentre nei lattanti includono irritabilità e letargia. La cefalea è solitamente frontale o generalizzata; gli adolescenti lamentano spesso dolore retrobulbare. Sono comuni anche febbre, nausea e vomito, fotofobia, dolore al collo, alla schiena e arti inferiori. A mano a mano che la temperatura corporea aumenta, può riscontrarsi torpore, che progredisce verso lo *stupor*, in combinazione a movimenti bizzarri e convulsioni. I segni neurologici possono essere stazionari, progressivi o fluttuanti. West Nile virus e gli Enterovirus nonpolio causano in alcuni casi lesioni delle cellule delle corna anteriori e paralisi flaccida. Si riscontrano talvolta perdita del controllo sfinterico e crisi emotive non provocate.

Gli esantemi spesso precedono o accompagnano i segni del SNC, in particolare in presenza di echovirus, virus coxsackie, VZV, morbillo, rosolia e, occasionalmente, West Nile virus. L'esame obiettivo rivela rigidità nucale, in assenza di significative alterazioni neurologiche localizzate, almeno all'esordio.

Specifiche forme o complicanze di infezioni virali che colpiscono il SNC includono la sindrome di Guillain-Barré, la mielite trasversa, l'emiplegia e l'atassia cerebellare.

DIAGNOSI. La diagnosi di encefalite virale è generalmente formulata sulla base della presentazione clinica di prodromi non specifici, seguiti da sintomi progressivi a carico del SNC. La diagnosi è supportata dall'esame del LCS, che solitamente mostra una lieve predominanza mononucleare (vedi Tab. 602-1). Altri test potenzialmente utili nella valutazione di un paziente con sospetta meningoencefalite includono l'elettroencefalogramma (EEG) e gli esami di neuroimaging. L'EEG mostra tipicamente attività diffusa a onde lente, senza alterazioni focali. TC e RM rivelano edema del parenchima cerebrale. Il riscontro di convulsioni focali o reperti focali su EEG, TC o RM (in particolare se coinvolgono i lobi frontali) suggerisce la presenza di encefalite da HSV.

Diagnosi differenziale. Un certo numero di condizioni patologiche responsabili di infiammazione del SNC simulano la meningite virale (vedi Tab. 602-2). Il principale gruppo di agenti infettivi alternativi da considerare è quello batterico. Nella maggior parte dei casi, i bambini affetti da meningite batterica acuta appaiono più gravi di quelli con infezione virale. Infezioni batteriche parameningee, come gli ascessi cerebrali o subdurali e l'empiema epidurale, possono presentare caratteristiche analoghe alle infezioni virali del SNC. Le infezioni causate da *M. tuberculosis*, *T. pallidum* (sifilide), *B. burgdorferi* (malattia di Lyme) e *Bartonella henselae* (associato alla malattia da graffio del gatto) tendono a presentare un decorso indolente. L'analisi del LCS e i test sierologici specifici sono necessari per distinguere tra questi patogeni.

Anche le infezioni dovute a funghi, rickettsie, micoplasmi, protozoi e altri parassiti devono essere incluse nella diagnosi differenziale. Solitamente, il sospetto della presenza di questi agenti è suggerito da sintomi associati, dalla località geografica dell'infezione o da fattori immuni dell'ospite.

Vari disturbi non infettivi possono associarsi a infiammazione del SNC e presentano manifestazioni che tendono a sovrapporsi a quelle della meningoencefalite virale. Tali disturbi includono i tumori maligni, le vasculiti delle connettiviti, l'emorragia intracranica e l'esposizione ad alcune tossine. Solitamente l'anamnesi e la verifica del coinvolgimento di altri organi consentono di escludere queste possibilità.

Reperti di laboratorio. Il LCS contiene da alcune a diverse migliaia di cellule per mm^3. Nelle fasi iniziali della malattia, le cellule sono spesso polimorfonucleati; in seguito, predominano le cellule mononucleate. Tale cambiamento del tipo cellulare prevalente è spesso dimostrato dall'esame di campioni di LCS prelevati a 8-12 ore di distanza. La concentrazione di proteine nel LCS tende a essere normale o leggermente elevata, ma può risultare molto alta in presenza di estesa distruzione cerebrale, come quella associata all'encefalite da HSV. La glicorrachia è solitamente normale, ma alcuni virus (come la parotite epidemica) causano una sostanziale depressione della concentrazione di glucosio.

Il LCS deve essere sottoposto a coltura per virus, batteri, funghi e micobatteri; in alcuni casi, sono indicati esami speciali per la ricerca di protozoi, micoplasmi e altri patogeni. La possibilità di isolare i virus nei bambini con meningoencefalite virale dipende dalla fase del decorso clinico in cui si ottiene il campione, dallo specifico agente eziologico, dal tipo di infezione (meningite o processo encefalitico localizzato) e dalla professionalità del laboratorio diagnostico. Isolare il virus è più facile nella fase iniziale della malattia. Gli Enterovirus tendono a essere più semplici da isolare, ma soltanto nel 70% dei casi circa si riscontrano nel LCS. Per aumentare la probabilità di identificare il patogeno virale responsabile, è opportuno prelevare campioni di secrezioni nasofaringee, feci e urine per l'esame colturale. L'isolamento del virus da una di queste sedi non consente la diagnosi eziologica, ma risulta altamente suggestivo. L'individuazione di DNA o RNA virale mediante reazione polimerasica a catena è utile nella diagnosi di infezioni del SNC causate da HSV ed Enterovirus. La sierologia del LCS è il test diagnostico di elezione per WNV.

Un campione di siero dovrebbe essere prelevato nella fase iniziale della malattia; se le colture virali non sono diagnostiche, il prelievo deve essere ripetuto dopo 2-3 settimane per gli esami sierologici. I metodi sierologici sono poco adatti alla diagnosi di infezioni causate da Enterovirus, a causa della presenza di un numero eccessivo di sierotipi. Tale approccio può essere utile per confermare la responsabilità di un sierotipo circolante già noto. I test sierologici consentono inoltre di determinare l'eziologia di infezioni non enterovirali, come quelle da arbovirus.

TRATTAMENTO. Fatta eccezione per l'utilizzo di aciclovir nell'encefalite da HSV (vedi Capitolo 249), il trattamento della meningoencefalite virale si limita a una terapia di supporto. I casi lievi richiedono soltanto un trattamento sintomatico. La cefalea e l'iperestesia sono alleviati con il riposo, la somministrazione di analgesici che non contengano acido acetilsalicilico, la riduzione della luce e del rumore nella stanza e dei visitatori. Il paracetamolo è raccomandato in presenza di febbre. Codeina, morfina e derivati delle fenotiazine sono talvolta necessari in presenza di dolore e vomito, ma il loro impiego nei bambini deve essere per quanto possibile limitato, perché possono indurre segni e sintomi ingannevoli. La somministrazione endovenosa di liquidi è talvolta necessaria a causa dell'inappetenza. I casi più gravi possono richiedere il ricovero ospedaliero in un reparto di terapia intensiva.

È importante anticipare ed essere preparati alla comparsa di convulsioni, edema cerebrale, difficoltà respiratorie, squilibri elettrolitici, aspirazione e asfissia, arresto cardiaco o respiratorio di origine centrale. Nei pazienti con grave encefalite è dunque necessario un attento monitoraggio. In presenza di aumento della pressione intracranica, può essere indicato inserire un trasduttore di pressione nello spazio epidurale. Il rischio di insufficienza cardiaca o respiratoria è molto elevato nei casi gravi. Inizialmente, tutti i farmaci, i liquidi e gli elettroliti sono somministrati per via parenterale. Negli stati di coma prolungato, è indicata anche l'alimentazione parenterale. La SIADH è comune nei disturbi del SNC acuti e la sua diagnosi precoce richiede il monitoraggio delle concentrazioni sieriche di sodio (vedi Capitolo 560). Per ridurre il rischio di convulsioni, è importante mantenere entro il range normale i livelli ematici di glucosio, magnesio e calcio. La comparsa di edema cerebrale e convulsioni richiede un trattamento aggressivo immediato.

PROGNOSI. La terapia riabilitativa è fondamentale nella fase di guarigione del paziente. Le infezioni virali del SNC possono essere seguite da mancanza di coordinazione motoria, disturbi convulsivi, sordità totale o parziale e disturbi comportamentali. Talvolta si riscontrano anche disturbi visivi dovuti alla corioretinopatia e all'ambliopia percettiva. L'impiego di ausili specifici e, talvolta, il ricovero in istituto possono rendersi necessari. Alcune sequele dell'infezione sono molto sfumate. Di conseguenza, la valutazione neuroevolutiva e quella audiologica devono essere incluse nei follow-up di routine dei bambini guariti da una meningoencefalite virale.

Nella maggior parte dei casi, la guarigione è completa, ma la prognosi dipende dalla gravità della malattia, dalla specifica causa e dall'età del bambino. In caso di malattia grave, con importante coinvolgimento parenchimale, la prognosi è sfavorevole, con potenziali deficit intellettivi, motori, psichiatrici, epilettici o uditivi. Le infezioni da HSV rischiano di causare sequele particolarmente gravi. Benché alcuni studi suggeriscano una prognosi a lungo termine peggiore nei lattanti che contraggono la meningoencefalite virale rispetto ai bambini più grandi, i dati clinici sembrano confutare tale tesi. Circa il 10% dei bambini con meno di 2 anni affetti da infezione enterovirale del SNC soffre di complicanze acute, come convulsioni, aumento della pressione intracranica o coma. Nella quasi totalità dei casi, l'esito neurologico a lungo termine è positivo.

PREVENZIONE. Negli Stati Uniti, la diffusione delle vaccinazione contro poliomielite, parotite epidemica, rosolia e varicella ha consentito la pressoché totale eliminazione delle complicanze di queste malattie. La disponibilità di programmi per la vaccinazione antirabbica degli animali domestici ha ridotto la frequenza dell'encefalite rabbica. Il controllo dell'encefalite da arbovirus ha avuto meno successo, perché non sono ancora disponibili i vaccini per le malattie arbovirali specifiche che si riscontrano in Nord America. L'eliminazione degli insetti vettori mediante programmi di disinfestazione consente tuttavia di ridurre l'incidenza di queste infezioni. Anche l'applicazione di repellenti antizanzare a base di DEET sulla cute esposta quando è all'aperto specialmente al tramonto o verso sera, o l'utilizzo di indumenti di protezione adeguati (magliette a manica lunga, calze) contribuisce a limitare i rischi.

602.3 • Meningiti eosinofile

La meningite eosinofila è definita dalla presenza di 10 o più eosinofili per mm^3 di LCS. La più comune causa mondiale di pleiocitosi eosinofila è l'infezione del SNC da elminti. In Paesi dove l'infestazione da elminti è rara, come gli Stati Uniti, la diagnosi differenziale delle pleiocitosi eosinofile del SNC è molto ampia.

EZIOLOGIA. Sebbene qualsiasi elminta che emigri nei tessuti possa causare la meningite eosinofila, il tipo di infezione più comune negli esseri umani è causato da *Angiostrongylus cantonensis* (verme del ratto) (vedi Capitolo 294). Altri parassiti responsabili includono *Gnathostoma spinigerum* (vedi Capitolo 294), *Baylisascaris procyonis*, *Ascaris lumbricoides*, *Trichinella spiralis*, *Toxocara canis*, *Toxoplasma gondii*, *Paragonimus westermani*, *Echinococcus granulosus*, *Schistosoma japonicum*, *Onchocerca volvulus* e *T. solium*. La meningite eosinofila può costituire anche una manifestazione insolita di una più comune infezione virale, batterica o fungina del SNC. Cause non infettive includono la sclerosi multipla, i tumori maligni, la sindrome ipereosinofila, la reazione a farmaci o uno shunt ventricolo-peritoneale.

EPIDEMIOLOGIA. *A. cantonensis* si riscontra nel Sud-est asiatico, nel Pacifico del Sud, in Giappone, a Taiwan, in Egitto, in Costa d'Avorio e a Cuba. L'infezione si acquisisce mangiando frutti di mare o molluschi (crudi o poco cotti) contenenti larve al terzo stadio. Le infezioni da *Gnathostoma* sono segnalate in Giappone, Cina, India, Bangladesh e Sud-est asiatico. Si acquisiscono mangiando pesce, rane, volatili o serpenti crudi.

MANIFESTAZIONI CLINICHE. Quando la meningite eosinofilica è il risultato di un'infestazione elmintica, il paziente si ammala 1-3 settimane dopo l'esposizione, perché i parassiti migrano dal tratto gastrointestinale al SNC. Reperti comuni includono febbre, eosinofilia periferica, vomito, dolore addominale, eruzioni cutanee lineari o pleurite. I sintomi neurologici includono cefalea, meningismo, atassia, paralisi dei nervi cranici e parestesie. La radicolite e la mielite possono provocare paraparesi o incontinenza.

DIAGNOSI. La diagnosi presuntiva di meningite eosinofila da elminti è formulata sulla base dell'anamnesi di viaggi e di possibile esposizione al parassita, e dei tipici reperti chimici di laboratorio.

TRATTAMENTO. Il trattamento è di supporto, perché l'infezione è autolimitante e il decorso della malattia non sembra influenzato dai farmaci antielmintici. In caso di cefalea e radicolite, è opportuno somministrare analgesici. Se presente, l'idrocefalo può essere attenuato mediante rimozione di LCS o impianto di uno shunt. Gli steroidi contribuiscono a ridurre la durata della cefalea nei pazienti adulti.

PROGNOSI. Nel 70% dei casi, il paziente può essere dimesso dall'ospedale entro 1-2 settimane. La mortalità associata alla meningite eosinofila è $<1\%$.

Meningite batterica acuta

Blazer S, Berant M, Alon U: Bacterial meningitis: Effect of antibiotic treatment on cerebrospinal fluid. *J Clin Pathol* 1983;80:386–387.

Bonsu BK, Harper MB: Fever interval before diagnosis, prior antibiotic treatment, clinical outcome for young children with bacterial meningitis. *Clin Infect Dis* 2001;32:566–572.

De Gans J, Van De Beek D, for the Europena Dexamethasone in adulthood bacterial meningitis study investigation: Dexamethasone in adults with bacterial meningitis. *N Engl J Med* 2002;347:1549–1556.

Enders A, Pannicke U, Berner R, et al: Two siblings with lethal pneumococcal meningitis in a family with a mutation in interleukin-1 receptor-associated kinase 4. *J Pediatr* 2004;145:698–700.

Gessner BD, Sutanto A, Linehan M, et al: Incidences of vaccine-preventable *Haemophilus influenzae* type b pneumonia and meningitis in Indonesian children: Hamlet-randomised vaccine-probe trial. *Lancet* 2005;365: 43–52.

Grimwood K, Anderson P, Anderson V, et al: Twelve year outcome following bacterial meningitis: Further evidence for persisting effects. *Arch Dis Child* 2000;83:111–116.

Healy CM, Baker CJ: The future of meningococcal vaccines. *Pediatr Infect Dis J* 2005;24:175–176.

Kilpi T, Anttila M, Kallio MJ, et al: Length of prediagnostic history related to the course and sequelae of childhood bacterial meningitis. *Pediatr Infect Dis J* 1993;12:184–188.

Kutz JW, Simon LM, Chennupati SK, et al: Clinical predictors for hearing loss in children with bacterial meningitis. *Arch Otolaryngol Head Neck Surg* 2006;132:941–945.

McIntyre PB, MacIntyre CR, Gilmour R, et al: A population based study of the impact of corticosteroid therapy and delayed diagnosis on the outcome of childhood pneumococcal meningitis. *Arch Dis Child* 2005;90:391–396.

Nigrovic LE, Kuppermann N, Macias CG, et al: Clinical prediction rule for identifying children with cerebrospinal fluid pleocytosis at very low risk of bacterial meningitis. *JAMA* 2007;297:52–60.

Ninis N, Phillips C, Bailey L, et al: The role of healthcare delivery in the outcome of meningococcal disease in children: Case-control study of fatal and non-fatal cases. *Br Med J* 2005;330:1475–1478.

Radetsky M: Duration of symptoms and outcome in bacterial meningitis: An analysis of causation and the implications of a delay in diagnosis. *Pediatr Infect Dis J* 1992;11:694–698.

Reefhuis J, Honein MA, Whitney CG, et al. Risk of bacterial meningitis in children with cochlear implants. *N Engl J Med* 2003;349:435–445.

Saha SK, Baqui AH, Darmstadt GL, et al: Invasive *Haemophilus influenzae* type B diseases in Bangladesh, with increased resistance to antibiotics. *J Pediatr* 2005;146:227–233.

Scheld WM, Koedel U, Nathan B, et al: Pathophysiology of bacterial meningitis: Mechanism(s) of neuronal injury. *J Infect Dis* 2002;186(Suppl 2):S225–S233.

Snape MD, Pollard AJ: Meningococcal polysaccharide-protein conjugate vaccines. *Lancet Infect Dis* 2005;5:21–30.

Swartz MN: Bacterial meningitis—A view of the past 90 years. *N Engl J Med* 2004;351:1826–1828.

Tunkel AR, Hartman BJ, Kaplan SL, et al: Practice guideline for the management of bacterial meningitis. *Clin Infect Dis* 2004;39:1267–1284.

Van de Beek D, de Gans J, Spanjaard L, et al: Clinical features and prognostic factors in adults with bacterial meningitis. *N Engl J Med* 2004;351:1849–1859.

Van de Beek D, de Gans J: Dexamethasone in adults with community-acquired bacterial meningitis. *Drugs* 2006;66:415–427.

Van de Beek D, de Gans J, Tunkel AR, Wijdicks EFM: Community-acquired bacterial meningitis in adults. *N Engl J Med* 2006;354:44–52.

Meningoencefalite virale

Bernit E, de Lamballerie X, Zandotti C, et al: Prospective investigation of a large outbreak of meningitis due to echovirus 30 during summer 2000 in Marseilles, France. *Medicine* 2004;83:245–253.

Glaser CA, Gilliam S, Schnurr D, et al: California Encephalitis Project, 1998–2000. In search of encephalitis etiologies: Diagnostic challenges in the California Encephalitis Project, 1998–2000. *Clin Infect Dis* 2003;36:731–742.

Glaser CA, Honarmand S, Anderson LJ, et al: Beyond viruses: clinical profiles and etiologies associated with encephalitis. *CID* 2006;43:1565–1577.

Hayes EB, O'Leary DR: West Nile infection: A pediatric perspective. *Pediatrics* 2004;113:1375–1381.

Rorabaugh ML, Berlin LE, Heldrich F, et al: Aseptic meningitis in infants younger than 2 years of age: Acute illness and neurologic complications. *Pediatrics* 1993;92:206–211.

Solomon T: Flavivirus encephalitis. *N Engl J Med* 2004;351:370–378.

Tyler KL: West Nile virus encephalitis in America. *N Engl J Med* 2001;344:1858–1859.

Yim R, Posfay-Barbe KM, Nolt D, et al: Spectrum of clinical manifestations of West Nile virus infection in children. *Pediatrics* 2004;114:1673–1675.

Meningiti eosinofile

Chotmongkol V, Sawanyawisuth K, Thavornpitak Y: Corticosteroids treatment of eosinophilic meningitis. *Clin Infect Dis* 2000;31:660–662.

Hsu W, Chen J, Chien C, et al: Eosinophilic meningitis caused by *Angiostrongylus cantonensis*. *Pediatr Infect Dis J* 1990;9:443–435.

Weller PF: Eosinophilic meningitis. *Am J Med* 1993;95:250–253.

Capitolo 603 ■ Ascesso cerebrale

Robert H.A. Haslam

Gli ascessi cerebrali possono insorgere nei bambini di qualsiasi età, ma sono più comuni nei neonati e nei bambini tra i 4 e gli 8 anni. Le cause includono embolizzazione dovuta a cardiopatia congenita con shunt destro-sinistro (in particolare tetralogia di Fallot), meningite, otite media cronica e mastoidite, sinusite, infezione dei tessuti molli di volto e cranio, cellulite orbitale, infezioni dentarie, ferite penetranti alla testa, stati di immunodeficienza e infezioni di shunt ventricolo-peritoneali.

ANATOMIA PATOLOGICA. Gli ascessi cerebrali sono distribuiti irregolarmente tra i due emisferi e più dell'80% dei casi sono equamente suddivisi tra lobi frontale, parietale e temporale. Gli ascessi cerebrali nel lobo occipitale, nel cervelletto e nel tronco encefalico sono responsabili del restante 20% dei casi. La maggior parte degli ascessi cerebrali è singolo, ma il 30% è multiplo e coinvolge più di un lobo. La patogenesi è indeterminata nel 10-15% dei casi. Un ascesso del lobo frontale è spesso causato dall'estensione di una sinusite o cellulite orbitaria, mentre gli ascessi localizzati nel lobo temporale o nel cervelletto sono frequentemente associati a otite media cronica e mastoidite. Gli ascessi provocati da ferite penetranti alla testa, solitamente singoli, sono causati dallo *Staphylococcus aureus*. Quelli secondari a embolia settica, cardiopatia congenita o meningite sono causati da diversi microrganismi patogeni.

EZIOLOGIA. I batteri responsabili includono gli streptococchi (*S. milleri*, *S. pyogenes* gruppo A o B, *S. pneumoniae*, *S. faecalis*), microrganismi anaerobi (cocchi Gram-positivi, *Bacteroides* spp., *Fusobacterium* spp., *Prevotella* spp., *Actinomyces* spp.) e i bacilli aerobi Gram-negativi (*Haemophilus aphrophilus*, *H. parainfluenzae*, *H. influenzae*, *enterobacter*, *E. coli*, *Proteus* spp.). Il *Citrobacter* è il più comune nei neonati. Nella maggior parte degli ascessi (70%) si riscontra un solo microrganismo; 2 nel 20% e 3 o più nel 10% dei casi. Negli ascessi associati a infezioni mucose (sinusite), è frequente la presenza di batteri anaerobi. Gli ascessi fungini (*Aspergillus*, *Candida*) sono più comuni nei pazienti immunocompromessi.

MANIFESTAZIONI CLINICHE. Gli stadi iniziali della cerebrite e della formazione dell'ascesso sono associati a sintomi non specifici, come febbre poco elevata, cefalea e letargia. Solitamente il significato di questi sintomi non è riconosciuto; la prescrizione di un antibiotico orale consente un miglioramento transitorio. Con il progredire del processo infiammatorio, possono comparire vomito, cefalea grave, convulsioni, papilledema, segni neurologici focali (emiparesi) e coma. L'ascesso cerebrale è caratterizzato da nistagmo, atassia ipsilaterale e dismetria, vomito e cefalea. In caso di rottura dell'ascesso nella cavità ventricolare, il paziente va solitamente incontro a shock e decesso.

DIAGNOSI. La conta dei globuli bianchi nel sangue periferico può risultare normale o elevata, mentre l'emocoltura è positiva in circa il 10% dei casi. L'esame del liquido cerebrospinale (LCS) ottiene risultati variabili; inizialmente, globuli bianchi e proteine possono risultare lievemente elevati o normali, mentre la concentrazione di glucosio appare talvolta ridotta. Le colture di LCS sono raramente positive, mentre l'aspirazione dell'ascesso è spesso diagnostica. Data la scarsa utilità dell'esame del LCS e il rischio di erniazione delle tonsille cerebellari, la puntura lombare non è indicata nei bambini con sospetto ascesso cerebrale. L'elettroencefalogramma (EEG) mostra rallentamento focale corrispondente, mentre gli studi con radionuclidi evidenziano nell'80% dei casi un'area di iperintensità dovuta alla distruzione della barriera ematoencefalica. La TC con mezzo di contrasto e la RM costituiscono i metodi più affidabili per dimostrare la presenza di una cerebrite e la formazione di una ascesso (Fig. 603-1). La RM è il test diagnostico di elezione. Le immagini TC con contrasto evidenziano una lesione parenchimale ipodensa, mentre le immagini RM pesate in T_2 segnalano un aumento dell'intensità del segnale. Nella TC con mezzo di contrasto, la cavità dell'ascesso appare come un lesione ad anello. La RM con gadolinio dimostra la presenza della capsula dell'ascesso.

TRATTAMENTO. La gestione iniziale dell'ascesso cerebrale, dopo una diagnosi tempestiva, prevede una terapia antibiotica basta sulla probabile patogenesi. Quando la causa è sconosciuta, solitamente si ricorre alla combinazione di vancomicina, una cefalosporina di terza generazione, e metronidazolo. Questa stessa terapia è iniziata se le cause più probabili sono otite media, sinusite o mastoidite. In caso di lesione o trauma alla testa o nel postoperatorio di un intervento neurochirurgico, è opportuna la somministrazione di vancomicina più una cefalosporina di terza generazione. Se la cardiopatia cianotica congenita costituisce un fattore predisponente, è raccomandata ampicillina-sulbactam da sola, o la combinazione di una cefalosporina di terza generazione più metronidazolo. Meropenem è efficace contro batteri Gram-negativi, anaerobi, stafilococchi e streptococchi, inclusi quelli resistenti agli antibiotici; può essere usato da solo in sostituzione della combinazione metronidazolo più un β-lattame. Tuttavia, meropenem non è efficace contro *S. aureus* meticillina-resistente ed esercita un'azione ridotta su *S. pneumoniae* penicillina-resistente; di conseguenza, se si sospetta la presenza di uno di questi microrganismi, la vancomicina deve essere inclusa nel trattamento iniziale. Gli ascessi secondari a infezione dello shunt ventricoloperitoneale possono essere inizialmente trattati con vancomicina e ceftazidime. Quando l'ascesso è causato da *Citrobacter meningitis* (come accade spesso nei neonati) si consiglia una cefalosporina di terza generazione, solitamente in combinazione con un aminoglicoside. Anche *Listeria monocytogenes* può provocare un ascesso cerebrale nel neonato; in caso di sospetto, l'ampicillina deve essere somministrata assieme alla cefalosporina. Nei pazienti immunocompromessi, si ricorre a una copertura antibiotica ad ampio spettro e, talvolta, a una terapia con amfotericina B.

L'ascesso cerebrale può essere trattato soltanto con antibiotici, senza ricorrere alla chirurgia, se non supera i 2 cm di diametro, la malattia è di breve durata (<2 settimane), non emergono né segni di aumento della pressione intracranica, né di compromissione neurologica. Se si opta per il solo trattamento antibiotico, esami di neuroimaging a cadenza settimanale consentono di verificare l'effettiva riduzione delle dimensioni dell'ascesso. Un ascesso incapsulato, in particolare se la lesione causa un effetto di massa o un aumento della pressione intracranica, deve essere trattato con una combinazione di terapia antibiotica e aspirazione. L'escissione chirurgica è raramente necessaria, perché la procedura è associata a morbilità superiore rispetto all'aspirazione. La chirurgia è indispensabile soltanto se l'ascesso supera i 2,5 cm di diametro o se contiene gas, se la lesione è multiloculata o localizzata nella fossa posteriore oppure se viene identificata la presenza di un fungo. Processi infettivi associati, come una mastoidite, una sinusite o un ascesso periorbitale, possono richiedere il drenaggio chirurgico. La durata della terapia antibiotica dipende dal microrganismo e dalla risposta al trattamento, ma solitamente non supera le 4-6 settimane.

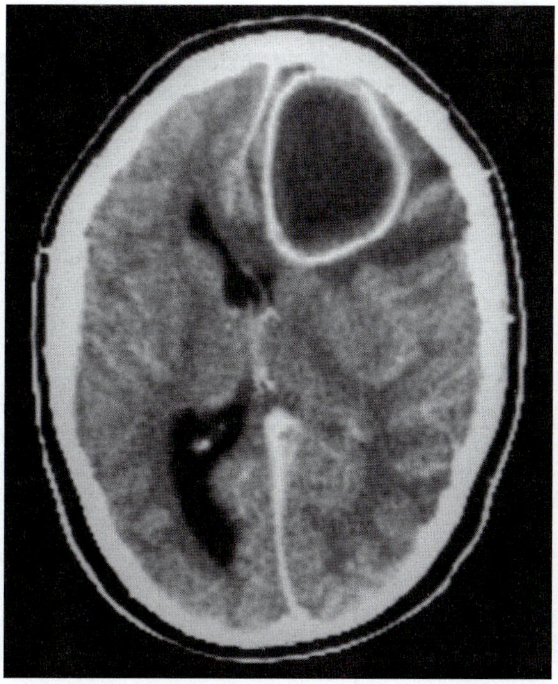

Figura 603-1. TC con mezzo di contrasto. Notare il voluminoso ascesso nel lobo frontale sinistro, responsabile di uno spostamento del cervello verso il lato destro. Poiché l'ascesso è localizzato nel lobo frontale, un'area "silente", il paziente non presentava segni neurologici.

PROGNOSI. La mortalità associata all'ascesso cerebrale è scesa significativamente al 15-20% grazie all'utilizzo delle tecniche di imaging (TC e RM) e al ricorso alle terapie antibiotiche e chirurgiche. I fattori associati ad una elevata mortalità includono l'età inferiore a un anno, la presenza di ascessi multipli; il coma, l'assenza di disponibilità della TC. Esiti a lungo termine si riscontrano in almeno il 50% dei sopravvissuti e includono emiparesi, convulsioni, idrocefalo, anomalie dei nervi cranici, disturbi comportamenti e di apprendimento.

Brook I: Aerobic and anaerobic bacteriology of intracranial abscesses. *Pediatr Neurol* 1992;8:210–214.

Goodkin HP, Harper MB, Pomeroy SL: Intracranial abscess in children: Historical trends at Children's Hospital Boston. *Pediatrics* 2004;113;1765–1770.

Saez-Lloreus XJ, Umana NA, Odio CN, et al: Brain abscesses in infants and children. *Pediatr Infect Dis J* 1989;8:449–458.

Sjolin J, Lilja A, Erikson N, et al: Treatment of brain abscess with cefotaxime and metronidazole: Prospective study on 15 consecutive patients. *Clin Infect Dis* 1993;17:857–863.

Smith RR: Neuroradiology of intracranial infection. *Pediatr Neurosurg* 1992;18:92–104.

Capitolo 604 ■ Pseudotumor cerebri

Robert H.A. Haslam

Lo pseudotumor cerebri è una sindrome clinica che mima il tumore cerebrale, caratterizzata da aumento della pressione intracranica (*IntraCranic Pressure*, ICP) oltre 200 mmH_2O nei lattanti e oltre 250 mmH_2O nei bambini più grandi. Il contenuto proteico e la conta cellulare nel liquido cerebrospinale (LCS) rientrano nella norma, così come le dimensioni ventricolari. La posizione dello pseudotumor è documentata dalla RM.

EZIOLOGIA. Le possibili spiegazioni dello sviluppo dello pseudotumor cerebri includono: alterazioni dell'assorbimento e della produzione di LCS, edema cerebrale, anomalie del controllo vasomotorio e del flusso sanguigno cerebrale, ostruzioni venose. Le cause sono numerose e includono: disturbi metabolici (galattosemia, ipoparatiroidismo, pseudoipoparatiroidismo, ipofosfatasia, prolungata terapia corticosteroidea o sua sospensione brusca, terapia con ormone della crescita, trattamento di un bambino gravemente denutrito, ipervitaminosi A, deficit di vitamina A, malattia di Addison, obesità, menarca, contraccettivi orali e gravidanza); infezioni (sesta malattia o *roseola infantum*, sinusite, otite media cronica e mastoidite, sindrome di Guillain-Barré), assunzione di farmaci (acido nalidixico, doxiciclina, minociclina, tetraciclina, nitrofurantoina); terapia con isotretinoina per la cura dell'acne, in particolare se combinata a tetracicline; disturbi ematologici (policitemia, anemia emolitica da causa marziale, sindrome di Wiskott-Aldrich); ostruzione del drenaggio intracranico secondaria a trombosi venosa (trombosi del seno laterale o del seno sagittale posteriore); ferite alla testa; ostruzione della vena cava superiore. Quando non è identificata una causa secondaria, la condizione viene classificata come "ipertensione endocranica idiopatica".

MANIFESTAZIONI CLINICHE. Il sintomo più frequente è la cefalea. Può riscontrarsi anche vomito, ma raramente in forma persistente e grave come nei casi di tumore della fossa posteriore. Sono segnalati spesso annebbiamento visivo transitorio e diplopia (secondaria alla paralisi del nervo abducente). Nella maggior parte dei casi, il paziente è vigile e non presenta sintomi generali. L'esame obiettivo rivela tipicamente una fontanella prominente e il segno di Macewen (la percussione del cranio produce un suono risonante, paragonato al "rumore di pentola fessa"), dovuto alla diastasi delle suture craniche. Il **papilledema** con allargamento della macchia cieca costituisce il segno più comune dopo la prima infanzia. L'ecografia evidenzia talvolta edema precoce del nervo ottico. Un difetto inferiore nasale può essere evidenziato al test dello schermo "formal tangent screen". La presenza di segni neurologici focali segnala un processo diverso dallo pseudotumor.

TRATTAMENTO. L'obiettivo principale del trattamento consiste nell'identificazione della causa sottostante. Non sono disponibili trial clinici in grado di guidare la terapia. Lo pseudotumor cerebri può costituire un disturbo autolimitante, ma le complicanze principali sono costituite da atrofia ottica e cecità. Nei pazienti obesi è opportuno iniziare una dieta e l'assunzione di farmaci sospetti deve essere immediatamente sospesa. In molti casi, il paziente richiede soltanto follow-up frequenti, per monitorare l'acuità visiva (verificabile anche mediante i potenziali evocati visivi in caso di necessità). La puntura lombare successiva alla TC o alla RM può avere una funzione diagnostica e terapeutica. L'ago spinale produce una piccola fessura nella dura madre, che consente la fuoriuscita del LCS dallo spazio subaracnoideo, riducendo l'ICP. Punture lombari addizionali e la rimozione di una quantità di liquido sufficiente a ridurre del 50% la pressione di apertura consentono talvolta la risoluzione del processo. In alcuni pazienti si è dimostrata efficace la somministrazione di acetazolamide (10-30 mg/kg/24 h) e corticosteroidi. La trombosi del seno può essere trattata con anticoagulanti. Nei rari casi di insorgenza di atrofia del nervo ottico, se gli approcci descritti si rivelano inefficaci, è necessario impiantare uno shunt lomboperitoneale o ricorrere alla decompressione subtemporale. In alcuni centri specialistici, viene realizzato l'intervento di fenestrazione della guaina del nervo ottico, per prevenire l'ulteriore perdita visiva. Se l'aumento della pressione intracranica è refrattario al trattamento, è opportuno ripetere gli esami neuroradiologici, per verificare la presenza di un **tumore a lenta crescita** o di un'**ostruzione di un seno venoso** non evidenziata in precedenza.

Baker R, Baumann R, Buncic J: Idiopathic intracranial hypertension (pseudotumor cerebri) in pediatric patients. *Pediatr Neurol* 1989;5:5–11.

Digre KB: Not so benign intracranial hypertension. *Br Med J* 2003;326: 613–614.

Shuper A, Snir M, Barash D: Ultrasonography of the optic nerves: Clinical application in children with pseudotumor cerebri. *J Pediatr* 1997;131:734–740.

Soler D, Cox T, Bullock P, et al: Diagnosis and management of benign intracranial hypertension. *Arch Dis Child* 1998;78:89–94.

Capitolo 605 ■ Patologie del midollo spinale

Robert H.A. Haslam

MARKER CUTANEI DI DISRAFISMO SPINALE OCCULTO (VEDI CAPITOLO 592.2)

Il disrafismo spinale occulto (*Occult Spinal Dysraphism*, OSD) comprende diverse anomalie, come risultato dell'incompleta fusione del tessuto molle, del tessuto osseo o delle componenti neurali della spina dorsale durante la neurulazione primaria o secondaria. Alcuni tipi di OSD, tra cui il *tethered cord*, la diastematomielia e la siringomielia, sono spesso associati a lesioni cutanee lombosacrali congenite della linea mediana. Tali lesioni includono lipomi, seni dermici, appendici, chiazze di capelli, deviazione della piega glutea, emangiomi e macchie a vino di porto. Tutti i bambini che presentano un neo congenito lungo la linea mediana lombosacrale devono essere sottoposti a esame neurologico completo. Le cosiddette macchie mongoliche e le fossette delle pieghe glutee non sono associate a OSD e non richiedono esami di approfondimento. I nei congeniti con elevata incidenza di OSD includono: appendici caudali (code), seni dermici al di sopra della piega glutea e lipomi. La presenza di due o più lesioni lungo la linea mediana è altamente suggestiva di OSD. La procedura diagnostica di elezione è la RM spinale.

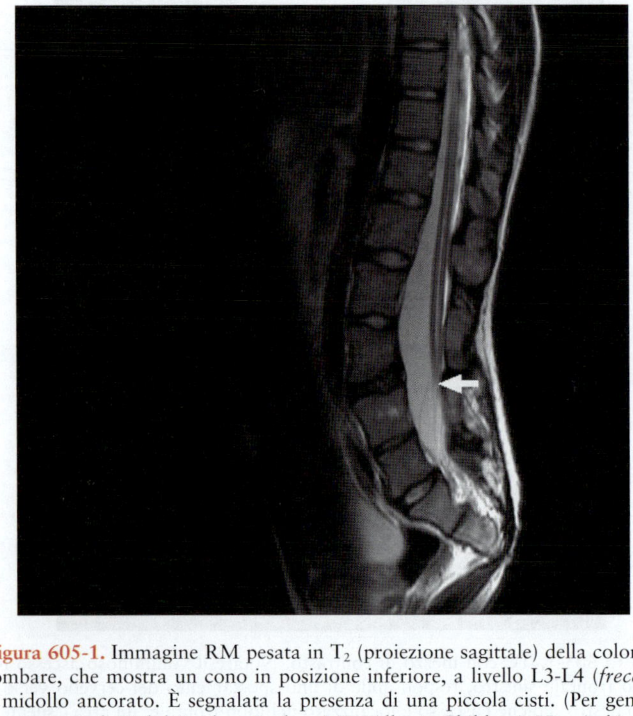

Figura 605-1. Immagine RM pesata in T_2 (proiezione sagittale) della colonna lombare, che mostra un cono in posizione inferiore, a livello L3-L4 (*freccia*) e midollo ancorato. È segnalata la presenza di una piccola cisti. (Per gentile concessione di Walid F. Abou Reslan, MD, Alberta Children's Hospital.)

605.1 • TETHERED CORD

Durante lo sviluppo fetale, il midollo spinale occupa l'intera estensione della colonna vertebrale, ma in seguito a una crescita differenziale il cono midollare assume infine la sua posizione a livello di L1. La normale regressione della porzione distale del midollo spinale embrionale produce un sottile filum terminale, attaccato al coccige. Come dimostrato dalla RM (Fig. 605-1), il midollo ancorato è il risultato della persistenza di un filum terminale inspessito, che ancora il cono a livello di L2, o inferiormente. In rari casi, il midollo ancorato sintomatico associato a lipoma o a un'altra anomalia congenita giace in posizione normale. I segni neurologici si sviluppano a causa dell'anomala tensione sul midollo spinale, che compromette l'apporto di sangue, in particolare durante i movimenti di flessione ed estensione. Il midollo ancorato può essere associato a filum terminale teso, diastematomielia, agenesia sacrale, lipoma intradurale, lipomielomeningocele e seno dermico.

MANIFESTAZIONI CLINICHE. In circa il 70% dei casi, l'ispezione del dorso rivela una lesione cutanea della linea mediana, come un lipoma, un ciuffo di peli, un'appendice caudale, un seno dermico o, più raramente, una macchia a vino di porto o un'area di iperpigmentazione della cute. La presentazione clinica è molto variabile; i segni possono risultare evidenti fin dalla nascita o essere ritardati fino all'età adulta. Talvolta i bambini manifestano una crescita asimmetrica di un piede o di una gamba, associata a piede equino talo-varo e a degenerazione muscolare dovuta alla prolungata denervazione. Alcuni pazienti presentano ritardo della deambulazione, altri tendono a camminare sulle punte, altri ancora manifestano una regressione della funzionamento degli arti inferiori. L'esame neurologico è caratterizzato da segni dei motoneuroni superiori alle gambe. Possono essere presenti anche anomalie della funzione vescicale con incontinenza e infezioni ricorrenti del tratto urinario, incontinenza fecale, stipsi e scoliosi progressiva. Il dolore agli arti inferiori è riscontrato comunemente nei bambini più grandi e negli adulti.

La radiografia diretta dei corpi vertebrali lombosacrali può mostrare un aumento della distanza interpeduncolare, emivertebre o malformazioni dei segmenti spinali anteriori. La RM delinea con precisione il livello del cono midollare e del filum terminale.

TRATTAMENTO. La transezione chirurgica del filum terminale ispessito interrompe la progressione dei segni neurologici e previene lo sviluppo di disfunzioni evolutive nei pazienti asintomatici. Il riancoraggio del midollo spinale è associato a deterioramento della funzione neurologica, inclusa la deambulazione; nella maggior parte dei casi, è secondario alla chiusura chirurgica di un mielomeningocele.

605.2 • DIASTEMATOMIELIA

La diastematomielia consiste nella duplicazione del midollo spinale, dovuta alla proiezione di un setto cartilagineo o osseo, originato da un corpo vertebrale posteriore. È il risultato di un disturbo della fusione neurale, con persistenza di tessuto mesodermico del primitivo canale neurenterico. Nel 50% dei casi, il difetto coinvolge le vertebre lombari (L1-L3) ed è associato ad anomalie dei corpi vertebrali, come i difetti di fusione, emivertebre, ipoplasia, cifoscoliosi, spina bifida e mielomeningocele.

MANIFESTAZIONI CLINICHE. Un'anomalia cutanea lungo la linea mediana della regione lombosacrale suggerisce la presenza di un difetto sottostante. Si ritiene che i segni neurologici siano il risultato della trazione esercitata durante i movimenti di flessione ed estensione della spina dorsale. La presentazione clinica della diastematomielia è molto variabile e, in alcuni casi, il paziente resta asintomatico. Più spesso, nei bambini in età prescolare si riscontrano anomalie unilaterali del piede equino talo-varo, alluce ad artiglio, atrofia del gastrocnemio, perdita della sensibilità al dolore e alla temperatura). In caso di decorso progressivo, insorgono ipostenia bilaterale e atrofia muscolare degli arti inferiori, mancanza dei riflessi achillei, incontinenza urinaria e dolore localizzato alla parte bassa della schiena. Le radiografie semplici delle vertebre possono non rivelare la presenza del setto, a causa dell'assenza di calcificazione. Di conseguenza, sono la TC o la RM a costituire gli strumenti diagnostici di elezione (Fig. 605-2).

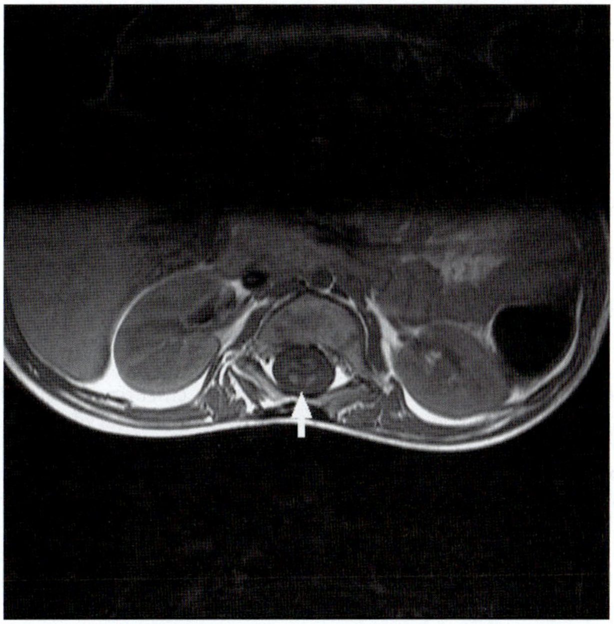

Figura 605-2. Immagine RM pesata in T_1 (proiezione assiale) del livello L1-L2, che mostra la divisione del midollo spinale (*freccia*) in un paziente con diastematomielia. (Per gentile concessione di Walid F. Abou Reslan, MD, Alberta Children's Hospital.)

TRATTAMENTO. Il trattamento dei pazienti sintomatici prevede l'escissione dello sperone o setto osseo e la lisi delle aderenze adiacenti.

605.3 • SIRINGOMIELIA

Il termine *siringomielia* indica la formazione patologica di una cavità cistica all'interno del midollo spinale, che può rimanere localizzata (forma non comunicante) o comunicare con i canali di circolazione del liquido cerebrospinale (LCS). Quando la cavità cistica si estende nel midollo, si parla di *siringobulbia*. La patogenesi della siringomielia comunicante non è nota, ma l'ipotesi prevalente suggerisce una costrizione del canale centrale a livello del forame magno durante l'embriogenesi. Il LCS fluisce caudalmente attraverso il canale ristretto, soprattutto durante i periodi di aumento della pressione intracranica (per es. in seguito a starnuti o tosse), provocando una dilatazione del canale centrale. La presenza di tale costrizione impedisce dunque al LCS di fluire in direzione cefalica. La siringomielia comunicante è frequentemente associata a malformazione di Chiari di tipo I, mentre la forma non comunicante è associata a tumori, eventi vascolari, traumi e aracnoidite.

MANIFESTAZIONI CLINICHE. Data la sua lenta evoluzione, la siringomielia è raramente sintomatica durante l'infanzia. L'interruzione della commessura anteriore a livello della colonna cervicale danneggia i tratti spinotalamici laterali, causando una perdita simmetrica della sensibilità al dolore e alla temperatura negli arti superiori, con conservazione della sensibilità superficiale (dissociazione della sensibilità). Il progressivo allargamento della cavità esercita una pressione sulle cellule delle corna anteriori e dei tratti corticospinali, con conseguente atrofia delle mani, assenza dei riflessi tendinei profondi degli arti superiori e segni dei motoneuroni superiori agli arti inferiori. Una scoliosi a rapida progressione può costituire la manifestazione iniziale della siringomielia. Ulcere trofiche associate ai disturbi vasomotori di mani e braccia segnalano la perdita della percezione del dolore.

DIAGNOSI. La TC con iniezione intratecale di metrizamide evidenzia l'allargamento del midollo spinale nella regione della cavità patologica. La tecnica diagnostica di elezione è la RM (Fig. 605-3).

TRATTAMENTO. La necessità dell'intervento chirurgico è stabilita sulla base della sede e della causa del difetto. L'intervento è raccomandato nei pazienti con siringomielia e scoliosi progressiva, o progressivo deterioramento sensitivo e motorio. La decompressione del forame magno e delle vertebre cervicali superiori è consigliata nei casi in cui la cavità è associata a una malformazione di Chiari di tipo I o II. Procedure alternative in grado di migliorare la funzione neurologica per periodi prolungati includono l'inserimento di un tappo tissutale nell'apertura del canale centrale, il drenaggio della cavità cistica nello spazio subaracnoideo e l'aspirazione percutanea della cisti. Nei pazienti asintomatici, si raccomandano esami neurologici e di imaging frequenti.

605.4 • TUMORI DEL MIDOLLO SPINALE

I tumori del midollo spinale, classificati sulla base della posizione anatomica (Fig. 605-4), costituiscono circa il 20% dei tumori neurassiali in età pediatrica. I **tumori intramidollari** originano nel midollo spinale e progrediscono lentamente, infiltrandosi nella regione cervicale. Il tipo più comune è l'astrocitoma a basso grado di malignità, seguito dal ganglioglioma e dall'ependimoma. I **tumori intradurali extramidollari** originano dal tessuto della cresta neurale e tendono a essere benigni. I tumori di quest'area includono neurofibromi, ganglioneuromi e meningiomi. I **tumori extradurali extramidollari** sono tipicamente lesioni metastasiche, in particolare neuroblastomi, sarcomi e linfomi.

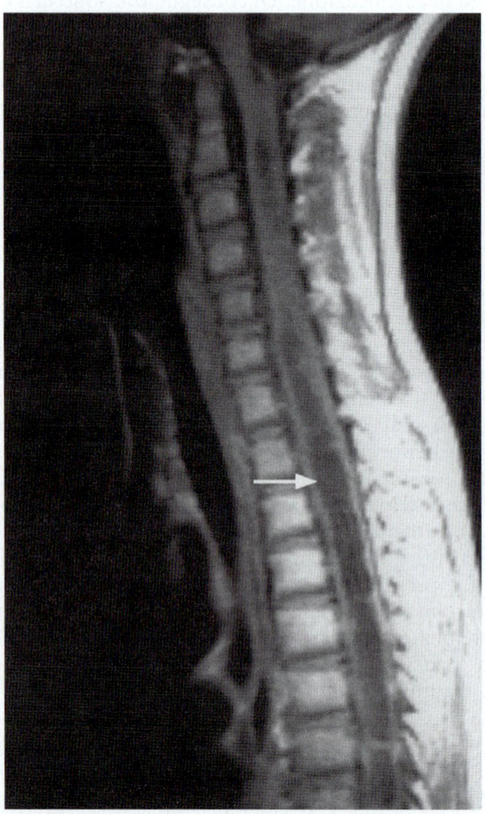

Figura 605-3. Immagine RM pesata in T_1 della colonna superiore, che mostra estesa siringomielia (*freccia bianca*).

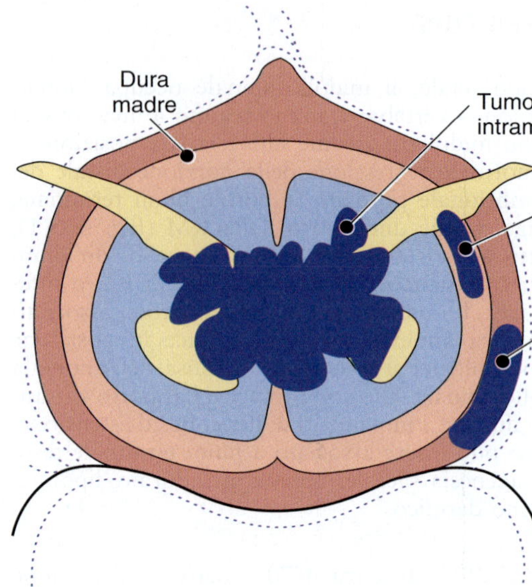

Figura 605-4. Diagramma della localizzazione dei tumori spinali nei bambini.

MANIFESTAZIONI CLINICHE. Nella maggior parte dei casi, a seconda della localizzazione, il tumore si presenta con una combinazione di disturbi della deambulazione, scoliosi, dolore alla schiena. I gliomi intramidollari crescono lentamente, causando progressive difficoltà di locomozione e disturbi sfinterici. I tumori gliali della colonna cervicale determinano segni dei motoneuroni inferiori alle braccia e segni dei motoneuroni superiori alle gambe. La denervazione dei muscoli intercostali causa una riduzione della mobilità della parete toracica, con conseguente tosse debole. La perdita della sensibilità al dolore e alla temperatura e della sensibilità superficiale è evidente negli arti inferiori e può essere dimostrata dai potenziali evocati somatosensoriali. Il sintomo di presentazione più frequente dei tumori extramidollari è il dolore alla schiena. Il bambino fa fatica ad addormentarsi e mantiene una postura a tripode. Se il tumore attacca una radice nervosa, si riscontrano dolore segmentale, parestesia e debolezza. I tumori extramidollari extradurali, poiché crescono rapidamente in uno spazio ristretto, tendono a causare un blocco acuto del flusso del LCS. In tali casi, il bambino presenta paraplegia flaccida, ritenzione urinaria e ano beante. Alcuni tumori extramidollari sono responsabili della sindrome di *Brown-Séquard*, che comprende debolezza omolaterale, spasticità e atassia, con perdita controlaterale della sensibilità al dolore e alla temperatura. Il papilledema è osservato in rari casi, solitamente in associazione a un marcato aumento dei livelli proteici nel LCS, che probabilmente interferisce con la sua normale circolazione.

DIAGNOSI. Una diagnosi tempestiva è fondamentale, perché l'intervento chirurgico consente di prevenire l'insorgenza di lesioni irreversibili. In circa il 40% dei casi, le radiografie di routine evidenziano anomalie come aumento della distanza interpeduncolare, distruzione o sclerosi dei corpi vertebrali adiacenti o dei peduncoli, allargamento del forame magno in caso di neurofibroma o ganglioneuroma (visualizzabile in proiezione obliqua). La **RM** costituisce l'esame diagnostico più importante. I tumori intramidollari causano un ispessimento fusiforme, talvolta con blocco completo del flusso di LCS (Fig. 605-5). I neurofibromi tendono a creare un'indentazione circolare della spina dorsale,

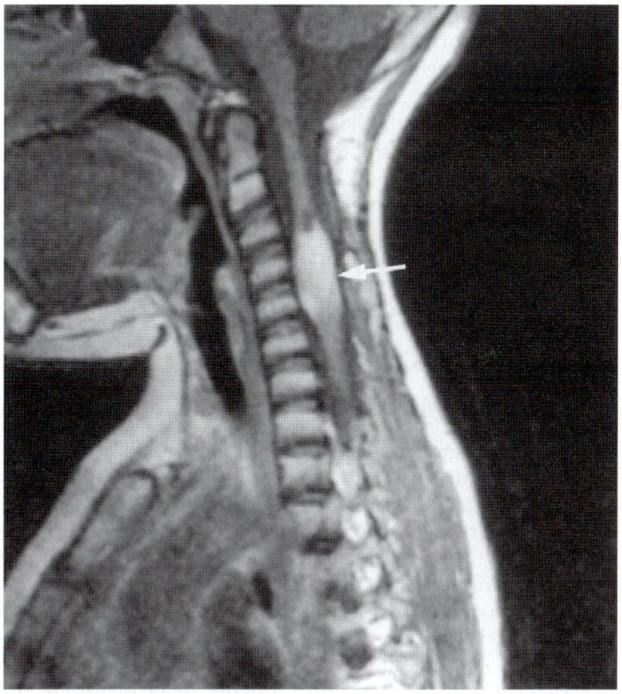

Figura 605-5. Immagine RM pesata in T_1 di un tumore del midollo spinale (*freccia bianca*). L'espansione fusiforme del midollo cervicale è evidenziata dall'iniezione ev di gadolinio.

mentre i tumori extramidollari provocano un blocco di gravità variabile.

TRATTAMENTO. Le moderne metodiche chirurgiche (microscopio chirurgico, tecniche di imaging, neurofisiologia intraoperatoria) consentono la rapida e sicura resezione della maggior parte dei tumori midollari. La rimozione chirurgica di tumori benigni è associata a una prognosi favorevole. La tipologia del tumore suggerisce l'opportunità o meno di ricorrere a una radioterapia e/o chemioterapia. Nei pazienti con neuroblastoma primario, che si presenta con paraplegia a esordio improvviso, secondaria alle metastasi nello spazio extradurale, un'immediata radioterapia può evitare il ricorso alla laminectomia.

605.5 • Traumi del midollo spinale (vedi anche Capitoli 62 e 99.3)

Le lesioni traumatiche del midollo spinale, rare in età pediatrica, presentano una gravità variabile (concussioni, lacerazioni, contusioni, transezioni). La prognosi dipende dall'estensione del trauma e dalla gestione immediata e a lungo termine. Le più comuni cause di lesione del midollo spinale nei bambini di età inferiore ai 10 anni includono: traumi da parto, maltrattamento (come nella sindrome del bambino scosso), incidenti automobilistici, ferite da arma da fuoco o di altro tipo, cadute da giostre o scivoli. Le lesioni spinali nei bambini più grandi avvengono solitamente in seguito a incidenti automobilistici o sportivi.

Circa il 20% delle lesioni non è associato ad anomalie radiologiche. Le lesioni **SCIWORA** (*Spinal Cord Injury WithOut Radiographic Injury*) sono quelle più comunemente riscontrate nei bambini e in molti casi sono il risultato di un grave trauma.

MANIFESTAZIONI CLINICHE. Una *grave lesione spinale* si manifesta con **shock spinale**, che comprende flaccidità, areflessia, perdita della sensibilità, bradicardia e ipotensione. Lo shock, risultato della disfunzione dell'attività sinaptica delle vie caudali rispetto alla lesione, può persistere fino a 4 settimane. Successivamente, si sviluppano movimenti flessori riflessi, seguiti da un'attività estensoria associata a iperreflessia, spasticità e vescica automatica. La *lesione spinale più lieve* è la tetraparesi transitoria secondaria a concussione, evidente per qualche secondo o minuto, con guarigione completa entro 24 ore. I bambini molto piccoli presentano un rischio più elevato di subire traumi alla colonna cervicale superiore, responsabili di circa l'80% delle lesioni nei bambini di età inferiore a 2 anni. Dopo gli 8-10 anni, la localizzazione delle lesioni è simile a quella riscontrata negli adulti.

Una lesione trasversa delle vertebre cervicali (a livello C1-C2) causa arresto respiratorio e decesso in assenza di supporto respiratorio. *Fratture o lussazioni a livello C5-C6* associate a lesioni del midollo spinale provocano tetraparesi flaccida, perdita della funzione sfinterica e livello di sensibilità corrispondente allo sterno superiore. Fratture o lussazioni nella regione toracica (T12-L1) possono causare la **sindrome del cono midollare**, che include perdita del controllo sfinterico rettale e vescicale, ipotonia flaccida e disturbi della sensibilità agli arti inferiori. Contusioni o emorragie possono provocare una **lesione centrale del midollo**, che tipicamente coinvolge gli arti superiori in modo più grave di quelli inferiori e determina segni del motoneurone superiore agli arti inferiori, e del motoneurone inferiore agli arti superiori, disfunzione vescicale e perdita della sensibilità a valle rispetto alla lesione. Il recupero delle funzioni è talvolta significativo, in particolare a livello degli arti inferiori.

TRATTAMENTO. Le lesioni del midollo spinale devono essere trattate mediante stabilizzazione e completa immobilizzazione della colonna vertebrale nel sito dell'incidente, utilizzando un collare cervicale di dimensioni adatte o stecche e cerotto. Il paziente va trasportato con una tavola spinale o barella rigida, adatta ai bambini, così da impedire la flessione del capo. È opportuno verificare la pervietà delle vie respiratorie e, se necessario, fornire assistenza respiratoria e trattare lo shock con plasma expander e con vasocompressori se necessario. L'uso degli steroidi è controverso, a causa dei seri effetti collaterali. Alcuni medici raccomandano di iniziare, entro 3 ore dalla lesione, una terapia con dosi elevate di steroidi, da proseguire per 24 ore (o per 48 ore se avviata 3-8 ore dopo la lesione). La dose iniziale di metilprednisolone (30 mg/kg in bolo) deve essere somministrata immediatamente, senza attendere il trasporto del paziente, seguita da 5,4 mg/kg h. Successivamente al trasporto, è opportuno effettuare radiografie della colonna in proiezione laterale e anteroposteriore. La RM è utilizzata in caso di sospetta lesione dei legamenti. TC e RM vengono usate se la diagnosi è incerta.

Dopo gli esami di imaging più opportuni, il trattamento chirurgico è diretto a stabilizzare le vertebre e prevenire ulteriori lesioni, ricorrendo se necessario a decompressione del midollo se interessato da una frattura o emorragia. Le fratture sono trattate con trazione, immobilizzazione e, in caso di lesione instabile, fusione dei corpi vertebrali. La laminectomia e l'ispezione midollare sono riservate ai casi di progressione dei segni neurologici o in presenza di una emorragia intramidollare o epidurale (suggerita da TC o RM).

Misure terapeutiche addizionali includono il trattamento dei disturbi vescicali o gastrointestinali, supporto nutrizionale, cure della cute e la definizione precisa di un programma riabilitativo multidisciplinare. La prognosi è direttamente collegata all'estensione della lesione. La guarigione può richiedere tempi prolungati (mesi o anni). Le lesioni centrali hanno una prognosi migliore di quelle responsabili di lesioni trasverse.

I pazienti con sindrome di Down tendono a presentare **instabilità atlantoassiale**, risultato della lassità dei legamenti trasversi, definita come una distanza superiore a 4,5 mm tra il processo odontoideo dell'epistrofeo e l'arco anteriore dell'atlante. La compressione del midollo spinale (mielopatia) può essere una conseguenza dell'instabilità atlanto-assiale. L'utilità di uno screening radiologico nei bambini con sindrome di Down, nel tentativo di predire l'insorgenza di lesioni spinali, è oggetto di controversie. Attualmente si raccomanda: (1) una radiografia laterale del collo in posizione neutrale, in flessione e in estensione a 3-5 anni, da ripetere successivamente per i soggetti con sindrome di Down (perché l'instabilità atlanto-assiale può insorgere durante i periodi di maggiore crescita); (2) non è opportuno che i bambini con instabilità atlanto-assiale pratichino sport rischiosi (come tuffi, calcio o atletica); (3) prima di effettuare operazioni chirurgiche o avviare programmi terapeutici che implicano la manipolazione attiva del collo, è necessario eseguire una radiografia; (4) i genitori e i terapisti devono saper riconoscere i segni e i sintomi di compressione midollare (dolore al collo, incontinenza urinaria e fecale, inclinazione del capo, disturbi della deambulazione, atassia, iperreflessia, debolezza, spasticità e quadriplegia); (5) nei pazienti con mielopatia, i risultati degli esami di laboratorio (radiografie del collo, TC, RM) suggeriscono la necessità di procedere all'intervento chirurgico.

PREVENZIONE. La prevenzione dei traumi midollari prevede l'utilizzo di cinture di sicurezza e attrezzature adeguate per limitare gli incidenti sportivi, seggiolini adatti per l'età e l'implementazione di regole strettamente correlate all'età negli sport di contrasto come rugby o calcio.

605.6 • MIELITE TRASVERSA

La mielite trasversa è caratterizzata dall'esordio improvviso di astenia progressiva e disturbi sensoriali agli arti inferiori. Nella maggior parte dei casi, l'anamnesi rivela una pregressa infezione virale, associata a febbre e malessere. Sono coinvolti diversi virus (Epstein-Barr, herpes, influenza, rosolia, parotite epidemica e varicella). Altri agenti infettivi includono la malattia di Lyme e *Mycoplasma pneumoniae*. Sono state proposte almeno tre teorie per spiegare la patogenesi della mielite trasversa: una risposta autoimmune cellulo-mediata; l'invasione virale diretta del midollo spinale; l'insorgenza di una vasculite autoimmune. L'esame patologico del midollo mostra marcato rammollimento e formazione di manicotti linfocitici, che sembrano confermare la base immunologica del disturbo.

MANIFESTAZIONI CLINICHE. I sintomi principali degli stadi precoci sono dolore addominale o nella parte bassa della schiena e parestesie degli arti inferiori. I muscoli degli arti inferiori appaiono deboli e flaccidi e si riscontra un livello di sensibilità, solitamente nella regione mediotoracica. Le sensibilità al dolore, alla temperatura e la sensibilità superficiale sono compromesse, mentre sono solitamente risparmiate la sensibilità della posizione articolare e vibratoria. I disturbi sfinterici sono comuni e richiedono spesso il cateterismo della vescica. Febbre e rigidità nucale si riscontrano fin dalle fasi iniziali della malattia. Il deficit neurologico evolve per 2-3 giorni, raggiungendo poi un plateau. La flaccidità si trasforma gradualmente in spasticità, con contemporaneo sviluppo di segni del motoneurone superiore alle gambe. La diagnosi differenziale include la meningite, la polineuropatia infettiva (sindrome di Guillain-Barré), la poliomielite, la neuromielite ottica (malattia di Devic), la neoplasia del midollo spinale, l'ascesso epidurale, il disturbo demielinizzante e la malformazione vascolare.

REPERTI DI LABORATORIO. L'esame del LCS mostra pleocitosi linfocitica moderata e un livello proteico normale o leggermente elevato. La RM è sempre indicata nei casi di sospetta mielite trasversa, per escludere la sclerosi multipla o una lesione midollare compressiva. Le anomalie RM della mielite trasversa includono ispessimento fusiforme, T_2 iperintenso e T_1 iso- o leggermente ipointenso esteso per almeno 3-4 vertebre, solitamente nella regione toracolombare.

TRATTAMENTO. La remissione spontanea, completa nel 40-50% dei casi, richiede un periodo di settimane o mesi. Deficit residui includono disfunzione sfinterica e debolezza degli arti inferiori. Il trattamento prevede la gestione dei disturbi sfinterici e la fisioterapia. Studi sperimentali hanno dimostrato che dosi elevate di metilprednisolone, somministrate precocemente, abbreviano la durata della malattia e ne migliorano la prognosi.

605.7 • MALFORMAZIONE ARTEROVENOSA

La malformazione arterovenosa del midollo spinale consiste in un insieme di vene tortuose e dilatate, solitamente localizzate sulla faccia dorsale del midollo toracico. La malformazione può causare sintomi neurologici per il suo effetto massa sul midollo o di un fenomeno di "furto" (il sangue è deviato nelle vene anomale, bypassando il midollo spinale, con perdita della funzione neurologica progressiva o transitoria). I pazienti presentano occasionalmente paraparesi acuta e deficit sensoriale dovuto all'emorragia subaracnoidea dovuta alla malformazione. Più comunemente, si osserva l'esordio graduale di anomalie della deambulazione, lombalgia e disfunzione sfinterica. I riflessi tendinei profondi sono assenti o ridotti agli arti inferiori, invece è presente il segno di Babinski. In circa un terzo dei casi, un angioma cutaneo della linea mediana si sovrappone alla malformazione arterovenosa e talvolta l'auscultazione rivela un rumore spinale. Le radiografie spinali mostrano erosione dei peduncoli. Per definire l'estensione della malformazione è necessario effettuare una mielografia con mezzo di contrasto e un'angiografia spinale selettiva. La malformazione è rimossa mediante asportazione utilizzando un microscopio chirurgico oppure è obliterata mediante embolizzazione.

Bracken MB, Shepard MJ, Holford TR, et al: Administration of methylprednisolone for 24 or 48 hours or tirilazad mesylate for 48 hours in the treatment of acute spinal cord injury. *JAMA* 1997;277:1597–1604.

Committee on Sports Medicine and Fitness 1994–1995, American Academy of Pediatrics: Atlantoaxial instability in Down syndrome: Subject review. *Pediatrics* 1995;96:151–154.

Defresne P, Meyer L, Tardieu M, et al: Efficacy of high dose steroid therapy in children with severe acute transverse myelitis. *J Neurol Neurosurg Psychiatry* 2001;71:272—274.

Guggisberg D, Hadj-Rabia S, Viney C, et al: Skin markers of occult spinal dysraphism in children: A review of 54 cases. *Arch Dermatol* 2004;140:1109–1115.

Jallo GI, Freed D, Epstein F: Intramedullary spinal cord tumors in children. *Childs Nerv Syst* 2003;19:641–649.

McDonald JW, Sadowsky C: Spinal-cord injury. *Lancet* 2002;359:417–425.

Michelson DJ, Ashwal S: Tethered cord syndrome in childhood: Diagnostic features and relationship to congenital anomalies. *Neurol Res* 2004;26:745–753.

Proctor MR: Spinal cord injury. *Crit Care Med* 2002;30(Suppl):S489–S499.

Riche MC, Modenesi-Freitas J, Djindjian M, et al: Arteriovenous malformations (AVM) of the spinal cord in children: Review of 38 cases. *Neuroradiology* 1982;22:171–180.

Sébire G, Hollenberg H, Meyer L, et al: High dose methylprednisolone in severe acute transverse myelopathy. *Arch Dis Child* 1997;76:167–168.

Parte XXVII ■ Disordini neuromuscolari

Harvey B. Sarnat

Capitolo 606 ■ Valutazione e diagnosi

La **patologia neuromuscolare** comprende le malattie dell'unità motoria con esclusione delle alterazioni della funzione muscolare date da lesioni centrali, come la spasticità. L'unità motoria è costituita da quattro elementi: il motoneurone, il cui corpo è localizzato nei nuclei del tronco cerebrale o nelle corna anteriori del midollo spinale; il suo assone, che insieme agli altri assoni forma il nervo periferico; la giunzione neuromuscolare; la fibra muscolare innervata da un singolo motoneurone. Le dimensioni dell'unità motoria variano nei differenti muscoli, in base alla precisione della funzione muscolare richiesta. Nei muscoli più grandi, come il gluteo e il quadricipite femorale, centinaia di fibre muscolari sono innervate da un unico motoneurone; nei piccoli muscoli deputati ai movimenti fini, come lo stapedio o i muscoli extraoculari, può predominare il rapporto 1:1. L'unità motoria è influenzata dal controllo sovrasegmentale o del primo motoneurone, che determina il tono muscolare, la precisione del movimento, l'inibizione reciproca dei muscoli antagonisti durante il movimento e la successione delle contrazioni muscolari necessarie per ottenere movimenti armoniosi e coordinati. Gli impulsi sovrasegmentali contribuiscono ad aumentare o inibire il riflesso monosinaptico dello stiramento; il fascio corticospinale esercita un'azione inibitoria su di esso.

Le patologie dell'unità motoria sono comuni nei bambini. Le malattie neuromuscolari possono essere geneticamente determinate, congenite o acquisite, acute o croniche, progressive o non ingravescenti. Dal momento che è disponibile una terapia specifica per molte di queste malattie, date le implicazioni genetiche e prognostiche, è importante una diagnosi precisa; è necessaria una conferma con indagini di laboratorio per la maggior parte di tali patologie, poiché possono presentare quadri clinici simili.

Molti loci cromosomici sono stati individuati per specifiche malattie neuromuscolari grazie a studi di linkage genetico e di isolamento e clonazione di alcuni geni specifici. In alcuni casi, come nella distrofia muscolare di Duchenne, il difetto genetico è stato identificato in una delezione di sequenze nucleotidiche con conseguente produzione di una proteina difettosa, la distrofina; in altri casi, come nella distrofia muscolare miotonica, il deficit genetico consiste nell'espansione o ripetizione, anziché nella delezione, di un codone (serie di tre nucleotidi consecutivi ripetuti, che codifica per un singolo aminoacido), con molte copie di un particolare codone, che in questo particolare caso si associa a un mRNA alterato. Alcune patologie presentano tratti autosomici dominanti e autosomici recessivi in famiglie differenti; questi distinti genotipi mendeliani possono essere il risultato di mutazioni differenti, che coinvolgono geni diversi (miopatia nemalinica), o di diverse mutazioni dello stesso gene nel medesimo locus cromosomico (miotonia congenita), nonostante caratteristiche fenotipiche comuni e quadri istopatologici alla biopsia muscolare simili. Tra le diverse miopatie mitocondriali clinicamente definite, sono state riconosciute specifiche delezioni del mtDNA e mutazioni puntiformi del tRNA. Le modalità di trasmissione e i loci cromosomici e mitocondriali delle malattie neuromuscolari che colpiscono più comunemente lattanti e bambini sono riassunti nella Tabella 607-1.

MANIFESTAZIONI CLINICHE

L'esame obiettivo del sistema neuromuscolare comprende la valutazione della massa muscolare, del tono e della forza. Tono e forza non vanno confusi: il **tono passivo** è l'estensione del movimento rispetto all'articolazione, mentre il **tono attivo** è la resistenza fisiologica al movimento. Nel lattante che viene sollevato in posizione seduta da quella sdraiata, il capo ciondolante è un segno di perdita di forza muscolare, non di una riduzione del tono. L'ipotonia può associarsi a una forza normale o ridotta. I muscoli ipertrofici possono essere deboli o aver conservato intatta la loro forza; muscoli sottili e ipotrofici possono essere deboli o presentare una forza inaspettatamente normale. La distribuzione di tali elementi è importante per la diagnosi. In linea generale, le miopatie sono caratterizzate da una distribuzione prossimale della perdita di forza e dell'ipotrofia muscolare (con l'unica eccezione della distrofia miotonica); le neuropatie hanno di solito una distribuzione distale (con l'unica eccezione dell'atrofia muscolare spinale) (Tab. 606-1). Il coinvolgimento dei muscoli faciali, della lingua, del palato e dei muscoli extraoculari fornisce un elemento prezioso per la diagnosi differenziale. I riflessi osteotendinei da stiramento sono generalmente assenti nelle neuropatie e nelle patologie del motoneurone e ridotti, ma conservati, nelle miopatie (vedi Tab. 606-1). Pochi elementi clinici specifici sono importanti per la diagnosi di alcune malattie neuromuscolari. Le fascicolazioni muscolari, spesso più evidenti a livello della lingua, sono segni di denervazione; le alterazioni della sensibilità sono indicative di neuropatia, mentre la facile affaticabilità è tipica delle malattie della giunzione neuromuscolare; la miotonia, infine, è specifica di poche miopatie.

Non sempre questi elementi permettono di distinguere una miopatia da una neuropatia. Il dolore muscolare, o mialgia, si associa a patologie acute di origine tanto muscolare quanto nervosa. Le mialgie sono tipiche sia della dermatomiosite acuta sia della polineuropatia acuta (sindrome di Guillain-Barré). Le distrofie muscolari e le atrofie muscolari spinali non si associano a dolore. Le mialgie possono manifestarsi anche in diverse patologie metaboliche del muscolo e nella miopatia ischemica. I crampi muscolari, sia all'esordio sia durante l'evoluzione di una patologia, possono verificarsi tanto nelle miopatie quanto nelle neuropatie.

I bambini che presentano debolezza durante l'ultima fase della vita fetale e nel periodo neonatale spesso hanno una mancata discesa dei testicoli. In condizioni normali i testicoli sono trazionati attivamente dalla parete addominale anteriore all'interno dello scroto da una coppia di cordoni costituiti da muscolo liscio e striato, detti gubernaculum. Il gubernaculum è indebolito in molte malattie neuromuscolari congenite, quali l'atrofia muscolare spinale, la distrofia miotonica e molte miopatie congenite.

Nei bambini con malattie neuromuscolari congenite il torace spesso ha una struttura a imbuto e le coste sono sottili e radiotrasparenti, a causa della debolezza dei muscoli intercostali durante lo sviluppo intrauterino. Questo fenomeno è tipico dell'atrofia muscolare spinale infantile, ma si osserva anche nella miopatia miotubulare, nella distrofia miotonica neonatale e in altre patologie (Fig. 606-1). Il peso alla nascita può essere basso per l'età gestazionale, a causa della ridotta massa muscolare.

L'ipotonia generalizzata e il ritardato sviluppo motorio sono le manifestazioni più comuni di presentazione delle malattie neuromuscolari nei lattanti e nei bambini piccoli (Tab. 606-2). Questi

TABELLA 606-1. Caratteristiche delle patologie del sistema motorio

	DEBOLEZZA*							
SEDE DELLA LESIONE	**VOLTO**	**ARTI SUPERIORI**	**ARTI INFERIORI**	**PROSSIMALE-DISTALE**	**RIFLESSI OSTEOTENDINEI**	**ELETTROMIOGRAFIA**	**BIOPSIA MUSCOLARE**	**ALTRO**
Centrale	0	+	+	> o =	Normale o ↑	Normale	Normale	Crisi comiziali, emiparesi e ritardo dello sviluppo
Corna anteriori	Tardivo	++++	++++	> o =	0	Fascicolazioni e fibrillazione	Pattern di denervazione	Fascicolazioni (lingua)
Nervo periferico	0	+++	+++	<	↓	Fibrillazioni	Pattern di denervazione	Deficit della sensibilità, aumento delle proteine nel liquor, ridotta velocità di conduzione nervosa, biopsia del nervo alterata
Giunzione neuromuscolare	+++	+++	+++	=	Normale	Risposta ridotta (miastenia); risposta aumentata e BSAP (botulismo)	Normale	Risposta alla neostigmina o edrofonio (miastenia); stipsi e pupille fisse (botulismo)
Muscolo	Variabile (da + a ++++)	++	+	>	↓	Potenziali di unità motoria di breve durata e di ampiezza ridotta e potenziali miopatici polifasici	Pattern miopatico†	Aumento dei livelli degli enzimi muscolari (variabile)

*Da + a ++++, secondo il grado di severità.
†Può anche avere un'unica caratteristica, come nella miopatia *central core*, nella miopatia nemalinica, nella miopatia miotubulare e nella sproporzione congenita del tipo di fibre.
BSAP (*Brief duration, Small Amplitude, overly abundant motor unit Potentials*), di breve durata, ridotta ampiezza, potenziali di unità motoria eccessivamente rappresentati.
Da Volpe J: *Neurology of the Newborn*, 4th ed. Philadelphia, WB Saunders, 2001, p 706.

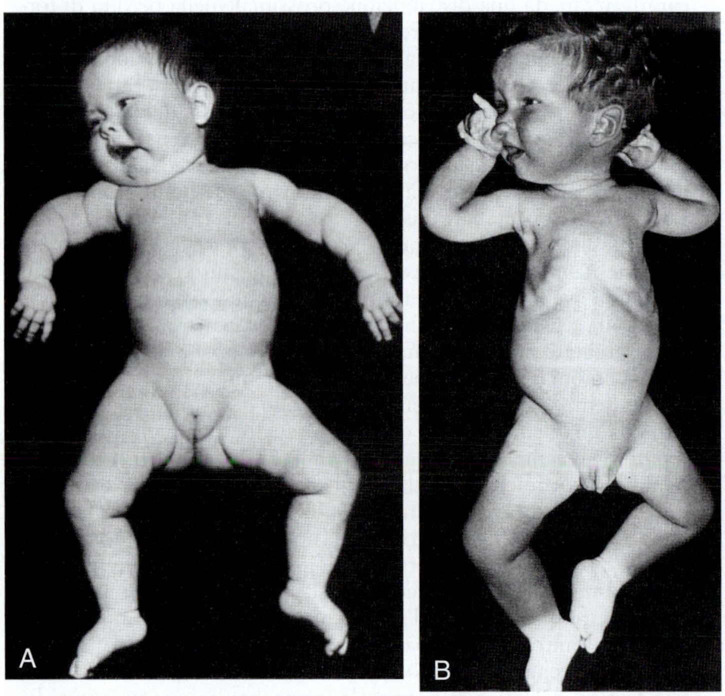

Figura 606-1. Atrofia spinale di tipo I (malattia di Werdnig-Hoffmann): tipiche posture in neonati di 6 settimane (*A*) e di 1 anno di vita (*B*), con debolezza e ipotonia congenite gravi. Si notino la postura a rana e l'intrarotazione degli arti inferiori ("a manico d'anfora") (*A*) o l'extrarotazione (*B*) delle spalle. Si osservino anche le retrazioni intercostali, più evidenti in *B*, e la normale espressione del volto. (Da Volpe J: *Neurology of the Newborn*, 4th ed. Philadelphia, WB Saunders, 2001, p 645.)

elementi possono anche essere l'espressione di patologie neurologiche, endocrinologiche e metaboliche, di sindrome di Down o essere manifestazioni neuromuscolari aspecifiche di malnutrizione o di malattie sistemiche croniche. Nei pazienti che sono sintomatici alla nascita, è frequente il riscontro di un'anamnesi prenatale positiva per riduzione dei movimenti fetali e ritardo dello sviluppo intrauterino. I disturbi dello sviluppo tendono a esordire lentamente e ad avere un andamento progressivo. La paralisi flaccida acuta nei lattanti più grandi e nei bambini presenta diverse diagnosi differenziali (Tab. 606-3).

ESAMI DI LABORATORIO

ENZIMI SIERICI. Molti enzimi lisosomiali, rilasciati dalle fibre muscolari danneggiate o degenerate, possono essere dosati nel siero. Il più utile è la **creatinchinasi (CK)**, che si trova in soli tre organi e che può essere separata nei corrispondenti isoenzimi: MM per il muscolo scheletrico, MB per il miocardio e BB per il cervello. La determinazione della CK sierica non è comunque il test di screening universale per le malattie neuromuscolari, poiché molte patologie dell'unità motoria possono non comportare un aumento enzimatico. Il livello di CK è tipicamente aumentato in alcune malattie, quali la distrofia muscolare di Duchenne, e l'entità dell'incremento è caratteristica di particolari quadri patologici.

MARCATORI GENETICI MOLECOLARI. Sono disponibili molti marcatori del DNA di miopatie e neuropatie ereditarie su campioni di sangue. Quando il quadro clinico è suggestivo per una particolare patologia, questi test possono permettere di formulare una dia-

TABELLA 602-2. Pattern di debolezza e relativa sede anatomica nel neonato flaccido

REGIONE ANATOMICA DELL'IPOTONIA	ALTERAZIONI CORRISPONDENTI	PATTERN DI DEBOLEZZA E ALTRI SEGNI
Sistema nervoso centrale	Alterazioni cromosomiche	Ipotonia centrale
	Errori congeniti del metabolismo	Prevalente ipotonia assiale
	Disgenesie cerebrali	Iperreflessia
	Traumi cerebrali, spinali	
Motoneurone	Atrofia muscolare spinale	Debolezza generalizzata; spesso risparmiati diaframma, muscolatura facciale, muscoli pelvici e sfinteri
Nervo	Neuropatie periferiche	Interessamento dei muscoli distali
		Debolezza con deperimento
Giunzione neuromuscolare	Sindromi miasteniche	Prevalente coinvolgimento dei muscoli bulbari e oculomotori
	Botulismo infantile	
Muscolo	Miopatie congenite	Predomina la debolezza
	Miopatie metaboliche	Muscolatura prossimale
	CMD	Iporeflessia
	Distrofia miotonica congenita	Blocchi articolari

CMD (*Congenital Muscular Dystrophy*), distrofia muscolare congenita.
Da Prasad AN, Prasad C: The floppy infant: Contribution of genetic and metabolic disorders. *Brain Dev* 2003; 27:457-476.

TABELLA 606-3. Diagnosi differenziale della paralisi flaccida acuta

ICTUS DEL TRONCO ENCEFALICO

ENCEFALITE DEL TRONCO

POLIOMIELITE ANTERIORE ACUTA
Da poliovirus
Da altri virus neurotropici

MIELOPATIA ACUTA
Processi occupanti spazio
Mielite trasversa acuta

NEUROPATIE PERIFERICHE
Sindrome di Guillain-Barré
Neuropatia post-vaccinica (rabbia)
Neuropatia difterica
Intossicazione da metalli pesanti, tossine biologiche o farmaci
Porfiria intermittente acuta
Neuropatia vasculitica
Neuropatia da gravi malattie
Neuropatia linfomatosa

ALTERAZIONI DELLA TRASMISSIONE NEUROMUSCOLARE
Miastenia grave
Tossine biologiche o industriali

MALATTIE MUSCOLARI
Ipokaliemia
Ipofosfatemia
Miopatia infiammatoria
Rabdomiolisi acuta
Trichinosi
Paralisi periodiche

Da Hughes RAC, Camblath DR: Guillain-Barré syndrome. *Lancet* 2005; 366:1653-1666.

gnosi definitiva, senza dover sottoporre il bambino a procedure più invasive, come la biopsia muscolare. Altri marcatori molecolari sono disponibili solo sul tessuto muscolare bioptico. Esami genetici sierologici, richiesti individualmente o in "gruppo", sono dispendiosi e possono non essere coperti dalle assicurazioni sanitarie negli Stati Uniti.

VELOCITÀ DI CONDUZIONE NERVOSA. La conduzione nervosa motoria e sensitiva può essere misurata elettrofisiologicamente utilizzando elettrodi di superficie. Neuropatie di vario genere si identificano per la ridotta velocità di conduzione. Con questo esame è possibile anche individuare la sede di un danno nervoso di origine traumatica. La conduzione nervosa alla nascita è circa la metà di quella dell'età adulta, valore che viene raggiunto intorno ai 2 anni di età. Sono disponibili tabelle che riportano i valori normali alle diverse età dell'infanzia, anche per i nati pretermine. Dal momento che tali studi misurano solo la conduzione delle fibre più veloci di un nervo, l'80% delle fibre del nervo deve essere compromessa affinché si possa evidenziare un rallentamento della velocità di conduzione.

ELETTROMIOGRAFIA (EMG). L'EMG, previo inserimento di un ago nel ventre muscolare, permette di registrare i potenziali elettrici del muscolo in diversi stati di contrazione. È meno utile in ambito pediatrico che nell'età adulta, in parte per le difficoltà tecniche connesse alla registrazione di tali potenziali nel bambino piccolo e in parte perché per avere risultati migliori è necessaria la collaborazione del paziente, per il completo rilassamento e per la contrazione massimale del muscolo, mentre i bambini nella maggior parte dei casi sono troppo spaventati per collaborare. Quadri elettromiografici caratteristici permettono di distinguere la denervazione da un problema di origine muscolare. Generalmente non si può formulare una diagnosi specifica di miopatia sulla base di questo solo esame, mentre è possibile rilevare alcune particolari condizioni, quali la miotonia. Un esame EMG può provocare un aumento transitorio del livello sierico di CK.

La combinazione dell'EMG con la stimolazione elettrica ripetitiva di un nervo motorio, inducendo il muscolo a produrre una risposta tetanica, è utile per dimostrare le risposte decrementali miasteniche. Per questi studi sono utilizzati i piccoli muscoli, come l'abduttore del quinto dito dell'eminenza ipotenar.

IMAGING MUSCOLARE. Lo studio del muscolo mediante l'ecografia, le scansioni TC e la RM è utile in molte malattie neuromuscolari. Sebbene queste metodiche non sempre siano in grado di fornire una diagnosi precisa, in mani esperte forniscono elementi aggiuntivi che consentono di seguire la progressione della malattia nel tempo. La RM, piuttosto utile nell'individuare miopatie infiammatorie di origine immune (dermatomiositi) o infettiva (virali, batteriche, parassitarie), rappresenta l'indagine di prima scelta per lo studio del midollo spinale, delle radici e dei plessi (per es. il plesso brachiale).

BIOPSIA MUSCOLARE. La biopsia muscolare è l'esame diagnostico più importante e specifico per la maggior parte delle malattie neuromuscolari, soprattutto se non si è giunti a una diagnosi definitiva con i test genetico-molecolari su sangue. La biopsia muscolare permette non solo di distinguere le neuropatie dalle miopatie, ma anche di precisare il tipo di miopatia e di identificare deficit enzimatici specifici. Il vasto laterale (quadricipite femorale) è il muscolo più spesso studiato. Il deltoide dovrebbe essere evitato nella maggior parte dei casi, poiché normalmente presenta un 60-80% di predominanza di fibre di tipo I, per cui la modalità di distribuzione dei diversi tipi di fibre è difficile da riconoscere. La biopsia muscolare è una semplice procedura ambulatoriale, che si può eseguire in anestesia locale con o senza il blocco del nervo femorale. In alcuni centri si preferisce ricorrere alle agobiopsie, che però, non essendo fatte per via transcutanea, richiedono un'incisione della cute simile a quella praticata per la biopsia a cielo aperto; si devono prelevare numerosi campioni per permettere un adeguato esame del tessuto e sono possibili solo piccoli prelievi. La quantità di tessuto prelevato con un'agobiopsia non è generalmente sufficiente per gli studi biochimici supplementari, come per evidenziare gli enzimi della catena respiratoria mitocondriale; è quindi preferibile una piccola, semplice, biopsia a cielo aperto.

Tutte le biopsie muscolari, in pediatria, richiedono studi istochimici su sezioni congelate di muscolo, poiché la maggior parte delle miopatie congenite e metaboliche non può essere diagnosticata sulla base di sezioni in paraffina, impiegando le tradizionali colorazioni istologiche. L'immunoistochimica è un utile supporto in alcuni casi, per esempio quando si tratta di dimostrare la distrofia in una sospetta malattia di Duchenne o la merosina nella distrofia muscolare congenita. Una parte dei campioni bioptici deve essere fissata in previsione di un'eventuale microscopia elettronica, ma l'ultrastruttura ha un valore diagnostico aggiuntivo solo in casi selezionati. L'interpretazione dei campioni di biopsia muscolare è complessa e deve essere eseguita da un patologo esperto. Una parte del tessuto muscolare congelato deve essere conservata di routine per eventuali analisi biochimiche (citopatie mitocondriali, carnitina palmitiltransferasi, maltasi acida).

BIOPSIA DEL NERVO. Il nervo più comunemente esaminato è quello surale, un nervo sensitivo puro, che innerva una piccola porzione di cute della superficie laterale del piede. Si può eseguire una biopsia completa o fascicolare. Quando si preleva il nervo surale dietro il malleolo laterale della caviglia, se ne ottiene la rigenerazione in più del 90% dei casi, per cui non si osserva un deficit sensitivo permanente. Il nervo surale è spesso coinvolto in molte neuropatie, le cui manifestazioni cliniche sono prevalentemente motorie.

La microscopia elettronica è utilizzata nella maggior parte delle biopsie di un nervo, poiché molte alterazioni morfologiche non sono apprezzabili con la risoluzione del microscopio ottico. Le preparazioni con colorazioni per le fibre nervose talora sono utili per dimostrare demielinizzazioni segmentali, rigonfiamenti assonali e altre anomalie specifiche, ma questa lunga procedura non viene effettuata di routine. Particolari colorazioni possono essere applicate a comuni sezioni di materiale da biopsia del nervo, congelate o in paraffina, per evidenziare la mielina, l'assoplasma o prodotti metabolici.

ELETTROCARDIOGRAMMA (ECG). La valutazione cardiaca è importante nel sospetto di una miopatia, poiché il miocardio può essere coinvolto nelle distrofie muscolari e nelle miopatie infiammatorie e metaboliche. L'ECG spesso individua precocemente una miocardiopatia o difetti di conduzione clinicamente asintomatici. Talora può essere indicato approfondire la valutazione cardiaca, eseguendo un ecocardiogramma e chiedendo la consulenza di un cardiologo pediatrico. Periodici controlli della funzionalità polmonare possono anche essere necessari nelle distrofie muscolari e in altre malattie croniche o progressive che interessano l'unità motoria.

Prasad AN, Prasad C: The floppy infant: Contribution of genetic and metabolic disorders. *Brain Dev* 2003;27:457–476.

Capitolo 607 ■ Disordini muscolari evolutivi

Miopatie congenite definisce un gruppo eterogeneo di **patologie neuromuscolari congenite**, per alcune delle quali tuttavia non è giustificata l'ipotesi di un coinvolgimento primitivo del muscolo. La maggior parte delle miopatie congenite è una condizione non progressiva, anche se alcuni pazienti possono andare incontro a un lento peggioramento clinico, che si accompagna a progressive alterazioni del reperto della biopsia muscolare. La maggior parte delle miopatie congenite è ereditaria, le altre sono sporadiche. Sebbene le caratteristiche cliniche, fenotipo compreso, possano far sospettare fortemente una miopatia congenita, la diagnosi definitiva si fonda sugli elementi istopatologici alla biopsia muscolare. Per i casi in cui il difetto genetico è stato identificato, la diagnosi può essere fatta sui linfociti del sangue periferico utilizzando specifici marcatori genetici. Le anomalie morfologiche e istochimiche permettono di differenziare le miopatie congenite dalle distrofie muscolari, dalle atrofie muscolari spinali e dalle neuropatie. Molte alterazioni ricordano fasi dello sviluppo embrionale del muscolo, suggerendo che alla base di queste vi siano anomalie della regolazione genetica dello sviluppo muscolare.

GENI MIOGENICI REGOLATORI E LOCI GENETICI DELLE PATOLOGIE MUSCOLARI EREDITARIE (TAB. 607-1)

I fattori di trascrizione delle proteine basiche con struttura "elica-giro-elica" (bHLH), comunemente associate a sequenze nucleotidiche di DNA, sono codificati da una famiglia di quattro geni regolatori miogenici. Questi geni regolano la differenziazione del muscolo striato a partire da qualsiasi cellula mesodermica indifferenziata. Il primo gene del sistema bHLH, che viene attivato per programmare la differenziazione del mioblasto, è il fattore miogenico 5 (*Myf5*). Il secondo gene, la *miogenina*, promuove la fusione dei mioblasti a formare i miotubi. L'*ercolina* (nota anche come *MYF6*) e il *MYOD1* sono gli altri due geni. *Myf5* non è in grado di determinare la differenziazione muscolare senza l'intervento della miogenina, di *MyoD* e di *MYF6*. Ciascuno di questi quattro geni può indurre l'espressione di almeno uno degli altri e, in particolari condizioni, è possibile anche l'autoinduzione. L'espressione di *MYF5* ed *ercolina* è transitoria durante le prime fasi dell'ontogenesi, ma si riattiva più avanti nella vita fetale e persiste nella vita adulta. Il locus umano del gene *MYOD1* si trova sul cromosoma 11, in prossimità del dominio associato con il rabdomiosarcoma embrionale. I geni che codificano per *Myf5* e per *ercolina* sono collocati sul cromosoma 12 e quello per la *miogenina* sul cromosoma 1. I geni miogenici vengono riattivati durante la rigenerazione muscolare, ripercorrendo il processo dello sviluppo; in particolare, *MyoD* è necessario per l'attivazione della cellula staminale miogenica (cellula satellite) nel muscolo adulto. Anche i geni *PAX3* e *PAX7* svolgono un ruolo importante nella biogenesi e interagiscono con ciascuno dei quattro geni basilari menzionati sopra. Un altro gene, la *miostatina*, è un inibitore dello sviluppo muscolare, che impedisce la differenziazione dei miociti. Il ruolo preciso dei geni miogenici nello sviluppo delle miopatie non è ancora stato definito con chiarezza. Le cellule satellite nel muscolo maturo, che mediano la rigenerazione, hanno la stessa origine metamerica delle cellule progenitrici muscolari embrionali.

607.1 • MIOPATIA MIOTUBULARE

L'espressione **miopatia miotubulare** indica un arresto della maturazione del muscolo fetale durante lo stadio miotubulare dello

TABELLA 607-1. Modalità di trasmissione e loci cromosomici o mitocondriali di malattie neuromuscolari di interesse pediatrico

PATOLOGIA	TRASMISSIONE	LOCUS
Distrofia muscolare di Duchenne/Becker	XR	Xp21.2
Distrofia muscolare di Emery-Dreifuss	XR	Xq28
Distrofia muscolare miotonica (Steinert)	AD	19q13
Distrofia muscolare facio-scapolo-omerale	AD	4q35
Distrofia muscolare dei cingoli	AD	5q
Distrofia muscolare dei cingoli	AR	15q
Distrofia muscolare congenita con deficit di merosina	AR	6q2
Distrofia muscolare congenita (Fukuyama)	AR	8q31-33
Miopatia miotubulare	XR	Xq28
Miopatia miotubulare	AR	Non noto
Miopatia nemalinica (NEM1)	AD	1q21-q23
Miopatia nemalinica (NEM2)	AR	2q21.2-q22
Miopatia nemalinica (NEM3)	AD, AR	1q42.1
Miopatia nemalinica (NEM4)	AD	9q13
Miopatia nemalinica (NEM5)	AR	19q13
Sproporzione congenita del tipo di fibre muscolari	AR, X-linked R	19p13.2, Xp23.12-p11.4, Xq13.1-q22.1; t(10; 17); sporadica
Miopatia *central core*	AD	19q13.1
Miotonia congenita (Thomsen)	AD	7q35
Miotonia congenita (Becker)	AR	7q35
Paramiotonia congenita	AD	17q13.1-13.3
Paralisi periodica iperkaliemica	AD	17q13.1-13.3
Paralisi periodica iperkaliemica	AD	1q31-q32
Glicogenosi II (Pompe; deficit della maltasi acida)	AR	17q23
Glicogenosi V (McArdle; deficit della miofosforilasi)	AR	11q13
Glicogenosi VII (Tarui; deficit della fosfofruttochinasi)	AR	1cenq32
Glicogenosi IX (deficit della fosfogliceratochinasi)	XR	Xq13
Glicogenosi X (deficit della fosfoglicerato mutasi)	AR	7p12-p13
Glicogenosi XI (deficit della lattato deidrogenasi)	AR	11p15.4
Deficit della carnitina muscolare	AR	Non noto
Deficit della carnitina-palmitil transferasi 2 muscolare	AR	1p32
Atrofia muscolare spinale (Werdnig-Hoffmann; Kugelberg-Welander)	AR	5q11-q13
Disautonomia familiare (Riley-Day)	AR	9q31-33
Neuropatia sensitivo-motoria ereditaria (Charcot-Marie-Tooth; Dejerine-Sottas)	AD	17p11.2
Neuropatia sensitivo-motoria ereditaria (di tipo assonale)	AD	1p35-p36
Neuropatia sensitivo-motoria ereditaria (Charcot-Marie-Tooth-X)	XR	Xq13.1
Miopatia mitocondriale (Kearns-Sayre)	Materna; sporadica	Singola, ampia delezione di mtDNA
Miopatia mitocondriale (MERRF)	Materna	Mutazione puntiforme del tRNA alla posizione 8344
Miopatia mitocondriale (MELAS)	Materna	Mutazione puntiforme del tRNA alle posizioni 3243 e 3271

AD, autosomica dominante; AR, autosomica recessiva; MELAS (*Mitochondrial Encephalomyopathy with Lactic Acidosis*), encefalomiopatia mitocondriale con acidosi lattica ed episodi simil-ictali; MERRF (*Mitochondrial Encephalomyopathy with Ragged-Red Fibers*), encefalopatia mitocondriale con fibre ragged red; mtDNA, acido desossiribonucleico mitocondriale; tRNA, acido ribonucleico transfer; XR, X-linked recessiva.

sviluppo, a 8-15 settimane di gestazione. Tale definizione è indicativa dell'aspetto morfologico delle miofibre: un groviglio di nuclei centrali collocati nel core del citoplasma, intorno al quale le miofibrille contrattili formano un cilindro (Fig. 607-1). Molti rifiutano tale interpretazione e preferiscono utilizzare la definizione più neutra di **miopatia centronucleare**, che però è troppo aspecifica, in quanto nuclei centrali si osservano anche in molte altre miopatie.

PATOGENESI. Nelle miofibre dei neonati con miopatia miotubulare sono presenti concentrazioni fetali costantemente elevate di vimentina e desmina, anche se non è stato possibile riprodurle in colture di miociti di pazienti. Queste proteine dei filamenti intermedi sono elementi del citoscheletro dei miotubi fetali che fanno aderire i nuclei e i mitocondri alle membrane del sarcolemma, in modo da garantire loro una posizione centrale. Durante le modificazioni dell'organizzazione intracellulare tipiche della maturazione, i nuclei si spostano verso la periferia e i mitocondri si ridistribuiscono tra le miofibrille. Contemporaneamente, vimentina e desmina diminuiscono: la prima scompare completamente, mentre la seconda rimane solo in piccole tracce. La persistenza di vimentina e desmina fetali nelle fibre muscolari può corrispondere a un meccanismo di "arresto della maturazione". Alcuni neonati con miopatia miotubulare presentano anche un difetto della trasmissione neuromuscolare simile a una miastenia secondaria. I miociti di pazienti, coltivati *in vitro* con fibre nervose, sviluppano una normale innervazione e maturano senza riprodurre le alterazioni patologiche che si osservano *in vivo*.

MANIFESTAZIONI CLINICHE. Al termine della gestazione si può verificare una riduzione dei movimenti fetali. Il polidramnios è una complicanza comune a causa della debolezza dei muscoli faringei fetali e dell'incapacità di deglutire il liquido amniotico. Alla nascita, i neonati affetti presentano masse muscolari ridotte a livello del tronco, dei cingoli e della muscolatura distale, grave ipotonia generalizzata e debolezza diffusa. Gli atti respiratori possono essere inefficaci, richiedendo un supporto ventilatorio. Può essere necessario un supporto nutrizionale per la debolezza muscolare che rende impossibili suzione e deglutizione. I testicoli sono spesso ritenuti. I muscoli faciali possono essere ipotonici, anche se questi soggetti non hanno la tipica facies della distrofia miotonica. La ptosi può essere un elemento predominante. L'oftamoplegia si osserva in pochi casi. Il palato può essere ogivale. La lingua è sottile, ma priva di fascicolazioni. I riflessi osteotendinei sono deboli o assenti. La miopatia miotubulare non si associa a miocardiopatia; le fibre muscolari mature del cuore hanno normalmente nuclei centrali. Non si associano anomalie congenite del sistema nervoso centrale o di altri apparati.

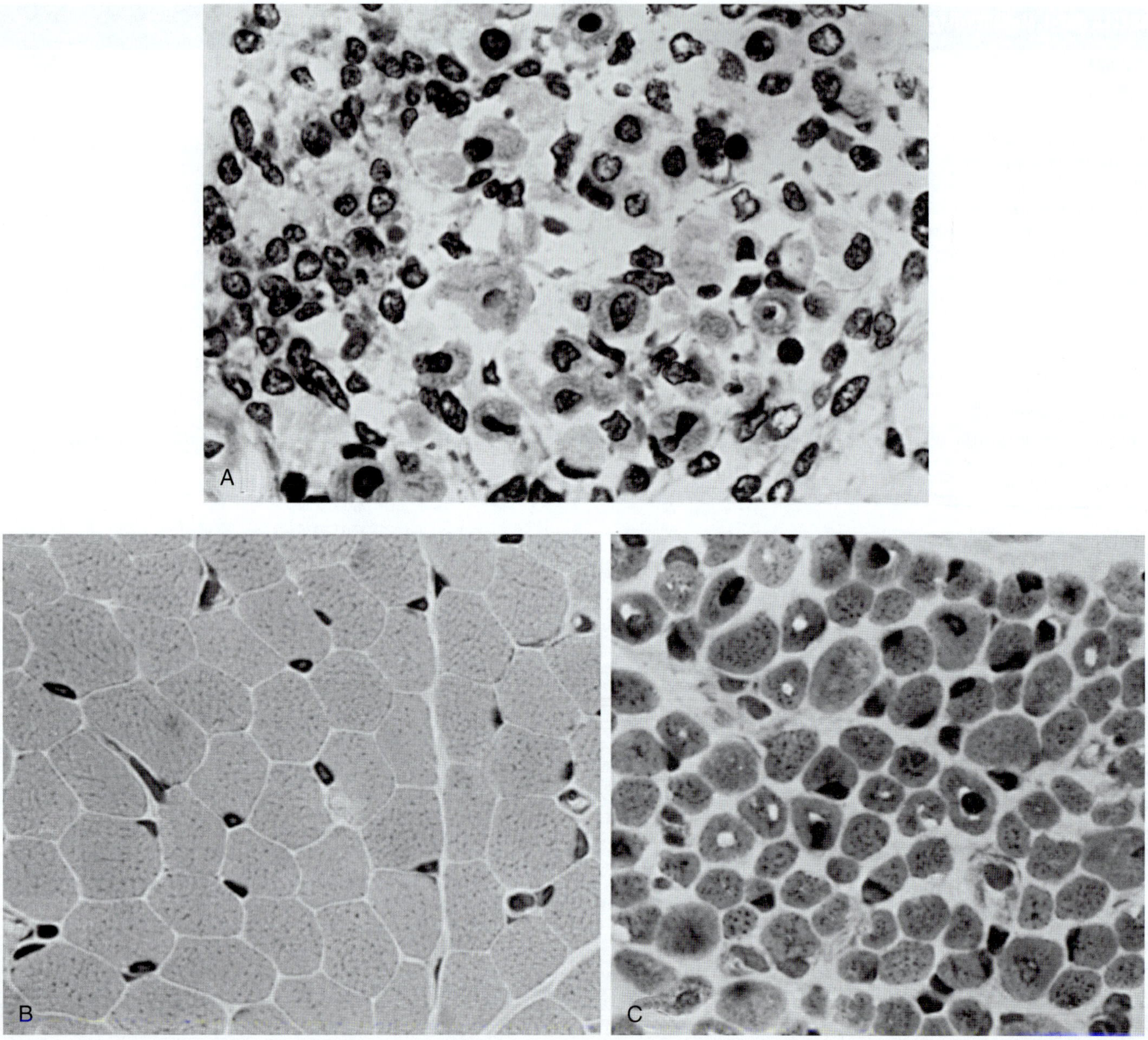

Figura 607-1. *A*, Sezione di muscolo di un feto umano di 14 settimane. *B*, Reperto normale di un neonato a termine. *C*, Neonato a termine con miopatia miotubulare X-linked recessiva. Le miofibre hanno grossi nuclei centrali nel feto e nella miopatia miotubulare; i nuclei sono localizzati alla periferia nella fibra muscolare del neonato a termine come nell'adulto (ematossilina-eosina, ×500).

I bambini più grandi e gli adulti possono sviluppare una miopatia centronucleare con debolezza muscolare variabile. Non è chiara la relazione fra questa malattia e la grave patologia neonatale.

ESAMI DI LABORATORIO. I livelli sierici della creatina chinasi (CK) sono normali. L'elettromiografia (EMG) non dimostra segni di denervazione; i risultati sono generalmente normali o denotano minime alterazioni miopatiche non caratteristiche nella prima infanzia. La velocità di conduzione nervosa può essere ridotta, ma in genere è normale. L'elettrocardiogramma (ECG) è normale. Le radiografie del torace non evidenziano cardiomegalia; le coste possono essere sottili.

DIAGNOSI. La biopsia muscolare è diagnostica alla nascita, anche nei prematuri. Più del 90% delle fibre muscolari è piccolo e presenta grossi nuclei vescicolari disposti in un unico groviglio, localizzati al centro del citoplasma. Gli spazi tra i nuclei sono colmati dal sarcoplasma contenente mitocondri. Le colorazioni immunoistochimiche per gli enzimi ossidativi e la glicogenesi dimostrano una distribuzione centrale delle attività enzimatiche, come nei miotubi fetali. I cilindri delle miofibrille rivelano una normale differenziazione immunoistochimica con colorazioni per l'adenosina trifosfato. Il tessuto connettivo del muscolo, i fusi, i vasi sanguigni, i nervi intramuscolari e le placche neuromuscolari sono maturi, come pure gli elementi ultrastrutturali, eccetto quelli che definiscono la malattia. Le fibre muscolari nella miopatia miotubulare presentano una spiccata positività per la vimentina e la desmina, non dimostrabili nel muscolo dei neonati normali. È disponibile il marcatore genetico molecolare su siero, utile non solo per confermare la diagnosi, ma anche per una diagnosi prenatale precoce.

GENETICA. La modalità di trasmissione più frequente di questa malattia, che colpisce i maschi, è X-linked recessiva. Le madri dei lattanti affetti sono clinicamente asintomatiche, nonostante la biopsia muscolare evidenzi modeste alterazioni. L'associazione genetica con il cromosoma X è localizzata sul sito Xq28, un locus differente da quello del gene Xp21 delle distrofie muscolari di Duchenne e Becker. È stata identificata una delezione nel gene responsabile *MTM1*, che codifica per una proteina detta miotubularina. *MTM1* appartiene a una famiglia di geni simili, i quali codificano per forme attive e non di fosfatidil inositolo-3-fosfatasi, che si associano in dimeri. La patogenesi risiede nella regolazione dell'attività enzimatica e nel legame con altre proteine, indotto dalle interazioni tra i dimeri. Sebbene sia coinvolto un unico gene, cinque distinte mutazioni puntiformi del gene *MTM1*, oltre alle 242 mutazioni note, sono responsabili solo del 27% dei casi. Molti alleli differenti possono determinare lo stesso quadro clinico. Sono note altre miopatie centronucleari, più rare, alcune autosomiche dominanti o recessive, che colpiscono entrambi i sessi, e altre sporadiche o con modalità di trasmissione non nota. Le forme recessive sono spesso distinte in forme a esordio precoce, con o senza oftalmoplegia, e in forme ad esordio tardivo senza oftalmoplegia. Le forme autosomiche dominanti, spesso lievi, possono non manifestarsi clinicamente fino all'età adulta e sono caratterizzate da debolezza muscolare diffusa lentamente progressiva e pseudoipertrofia muscolare generalizzata.

TRATTAMENTO. È possibile solo una terapia di supporto e palliativa.

PROGNOSI. Circa il 75% dei neonati con patologia severa muore nelle prime settimane o nei primi mesi di vita. Coloro che sopravvivono non hanno un decorso progressivo, ma presentano gravi handicap fisici, raramente camminano e rimangono gravemente ipotonici.

607.2 • Sproporzione congenita del tipo di fibre muscolari

La sproporzione congenita del tipo di fibre muscolari (CMFTD, *Congenital Muscle Fiber-Type Disproportion*) si manifesta sotto forma di miopatia isolata congenita, o in associazione con patologie diverse quali: miopatia nemalinica, fase precoce della malattia di Krabbe (leucodistrofia a cellule globoidi), prima della comparsa della neuropatia, ipoplasia cerebellare e diverse altre malformazioni cerebrali, sindrome alcolica fetale, alcune glicogenosi, molteplici deficit della solfatasi, sindrome di Lowe, miopatia con rigidità della colonna vertebrale e alcuni casi infantili di distrofia muscolare miotonica.

PATOGENESI. L'associazione della CMFTD con l'ipoplasia cerebellare suggerisce che la causa può essere un'anomala influenza sovrasegmentale sullo sviluppo dell'unità motoria durante la fase della differenziazione istochimica del muscolo tra la 20ª e la 28ª settimana di gestazione. Il tipo e le dimensioni delle fibre muscolari sono influenzati dall'innervazione e possono cambiare persino negli adulti. La CMFTD, pur non corrispondendo realmente a nessun stadio di sviluppo normale, sembra essere un'alterazione embriologica della differenziazione del tipo e delle dimensioni delle fibre.

MANIFESTAZIONI CLINICHE. Come condizione isolata, non associata ad altre patologie, la CMFTD è una malattia non progressiva presente alla nascita. I pazienti presentano ipotonia e debolezza muscolare generalizzate, ma la debolezza in genere non è severa. Insufficienza respiratoria e disfagia sono rare. Retrazioni muscolari sono presenti fin dalla nascita nel 25% dei pazienti. Lo scarso controllo del capo e un ritardo dello sviluppo con difficoltà ad acquisire le capacità motorie sono frequenti. Il bambino infine riesce a camminare, nonostante la deambulazione sia generalmente ritardata a 18-24 mesi. A causa dell'ipotonia, può verificarsi la sublussazione delle anche. Le masse muscolari sono ridotte. L'ipotrofia muscolare e l'ipotonia sono in proporzione maggiori della debolezza e durante l'esame obiettivo il bambino più risultare più forte del previsto. La miocardiopatia è una complicanza rara.

La facies dei bambini con CMFTD spesso desta sospetti, soprattutto quando il soggetto giunge all'osservazione del medico per un ritardo dello sviluppo e ipotonia muscolare. La testa è di forma allungata (dolicocefalia) ed è presente debolezza dei muscoli faciali. Il palato è generalmente ogivale. I muscoli ipotrofici del tronco e degli arti conferiscono un aspetto magro ed emaciato. Il fenotipo è molto simile a quello della miopatia nemalinica, che include anche la CMFTS tra i quadri patologici. I pazienti non lamentano mialgie. Il decorso clinico non è progressivo.

INDAGINI DI LABORATORIO. La CK sierica, l'ECG, l'EMG e le velocità di conduzione nervosa sono normali nella forma isolata. Se sono associate altre patologie, gli esami di laboratorio possono essere alterati in modo specifico.

DIAGNOSI. La CMFTD viene diagnosticata grazie alla biopsia muscolare, che dimostra una sproporzione sia delle dimensioni sia della relativa distribuzione immunoistochimica dei tipi di fibre: le fibre di tipo I, più numerose, sono generalmente piccole e quelle di tipo II ipertrofiche. Sono assenti la degenerazione delle miofibre e altri segni di miopatia primaria. La biopsia è diagnostica già alla nascita.

GENETICA. La maggior parte dei casi di CMFTD è sporadica, anche se in alcune famiglie è ben documentata una trasmissione autosomica recessiva e in altre è verosimile una trasmissione autosomica dominante. Le forme ereditarie sono geneticamente eterogenee. È stata riportata una mutazione nel gene del recettore dell'insulina in 19p13.2. La traslocazione t(10;17) è stata osservata in una famiglia. È stata descritta anche una trasmissione legata al cromosoma X con un linkage Xp23.12-p11.4 e Xq13.-q22.1. In tre famiglie con CMFTD, non correlate tra loro, è stata individuata una mutazione *missense* del gene dell'α-actina muscoloscheletrica (ACTA1), ma questa alterazione genetica è probabilmente presente in una minoranza dei casi. Nella forma di CMFTD associata all'ipoplasia cerebellare, il deficit genetico influisce sullo sviluppo cerebellare e l'alterazione muscolare è un effetto secondario.

TRATTAMENTO. Non è disponibile una terapia farmacologica. La fisioterapia può essere utile per rinforzare i muscoli nei pazienti che non eseguono sufficiente esercizio fisico durante le attività quotidiane. Le contratture muscolari congenite lievi spesso si correggono con esercizi che prevedono movimenti articolari di moderata entità e raramente si rendono necessarie protesi gessate o interventi chirurgici.

607.3 • Miopatia nemalinica

I bastoncelli nemalinici (dal greco *nema*, che significa "filo") sono strutture anomale, bastoncelliformi, simili a inclusioni all'interno delle fibre muscolari. Sono difficili da individuare istologicamente tramite la convenzionale colorazione con ematossilina-eosina, ma si osservano facilmente con tecniche specifiche. Non sono inclusioni di corpi estranei, ma consistono in un eccesso di materiale della banda Z, con ultrastruttura simile (Fig. 607-2). I bastoncelli, composti di actina, α-actinina, tropomiosina-3 e nebulina, possono essere la manifestazione di un'anomala reazione delle fibre muscolari a un insulto, poiché queste strutture sono di raro riscontro in altre patologie. Esse sono particolarmente numerose nella miopatia nota come miopatia nemalinica. Anche se la maggior parte di questi bastoncelli è localizzata nelle miofibrille (citoplasmatici), occasionalmente ne sono stati osservati a livello intranucleare con l'ausilio del microscopio elettronico.

MANIFESTAZIONI CLINICHE. Si riconoscono tre forme: neonatale, infantile e giovanile. La forma neonatale è severa e generalmente fatale alla nascita per insufficienza respiratoria. Gli elementi caratteristici della forma infantile sono: ipotonia e debolezza generalizzate, che possono interessare i muscoli respiratori e quelli

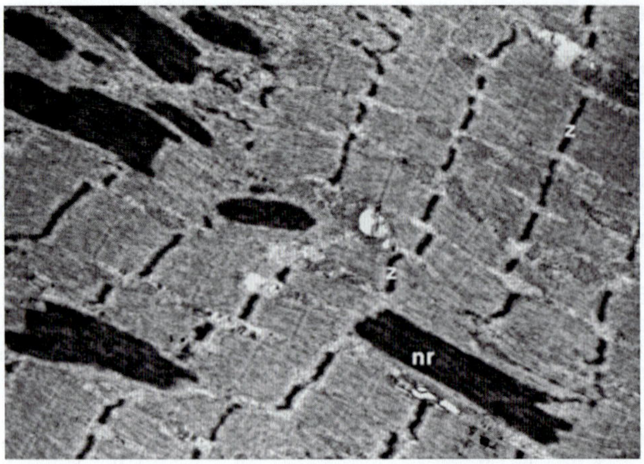

Figura 607-2. Immagine al microscopio elettronico del muscolo del paziente della Figura 607-4. In molte miofibrille si osservano bastoncelli nemalinici (nr) che hanno la stessa struttura delle normali bande Z (z) (×6000).

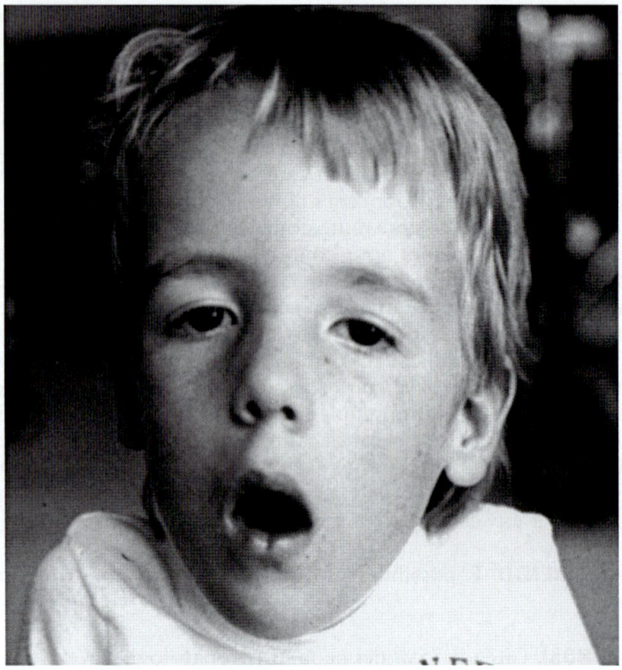

Figura 607-4. Forma infantile di malattia nemalinica in un bambino di 6 anni. La debolezza faciale e l'ipotrofia muscolare generalizzata sono importanti. È presente dolicocefalia. La bocca è generalmente aperta perché i masseteri sono troppo deboli per tenere sollevata la mandibola contro gravità più di qualche secondo.

d'innervazione bulbare, e masse muscolari gravemente ipotrofiche (Fig. 607-3). La testa è allungata (dolicocefalia) con palato ogivale o anche palatoschisi. Il soggetto può non riuscire a tenere la bocca chiusa per l'eccessiva debolezza dei muscoli della mandibola (Fig. 607-4). La madre spesso riferisce una riduzione dei movimenti fetali. I neonati soffrono di ipossia e disfagia. Può essere presente artrogriposi. I soggetti con miopatia nemalinica severa neonatale o infantile hanno una facies e un fenotipo difficilmente distinguibili da quelli della distrofia miotonica neonatale, ma le loro madri presentano una facies normale. La forma giovanile è la più lieve e non si associa a insufficienza respiratoria, mentre il fenotipo, incluso il coinvolgimento faciale, è simile a quello della forma infantile.

INDAGINI DI LABORATORIO. Il livello sierico di CK è normale o lievemente aumentato. La biopsia muscolare è diagnostica. Oltre ai caratteristici bastoncelli, si può osservare anche un quadro di CMFTD o almeno una predominanza di fibre di tipo I. In alcuni pazienti sono state osservate fibre di tipo I uniformi con poche o nessuna fibra di tipo II. Una degenerazione focale miofibrillare e un aumento degli enzimi lisosomiali sono stati riscontrati in pochi casi severi associati con sintomi progressivi. La presenza di bastoncelli intranucleari si correla con le manifestazioni cliniche più severe. I bastoncelli sono visibili al microscopio elettronico.

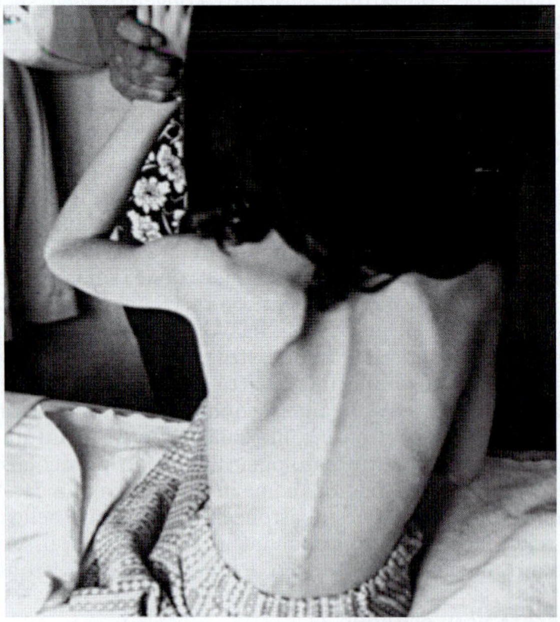

Figura 607-3. Schiena di una paziente di 13 anni affetta dalla forma giovanile della malattia nemalinica. I muscoli paravertebrali sono molto sottili e sono evidenti le scapole alate. Anche le masse muscolari degli arti sono ridotte in modo importante sia prossimalmente sia distalmente.

GENETICA. Vi sono forme di miopatia nemalinica autosomiche dominanti e recessive ed esiste anche una forma dominante X-linked che colpisce le bambine. Cinque geni sono associati a questa patologia. La miopatia nemalinica autosomica dominante di tipo 1 (NEM1) è stata mappata sul locus 1q21-23; il gene *TPM3* coinvolto produce una tropomiosina-a difettosa. Un'altra mutazione genetica (NEM2) al locus 2q21.2-q22 produce la *nebulina*, una grossa molecola necessaria anche per l'integrità della banda Z, ed è una forma autosomica recessiva. NEM3 è provocata da un difetto dell'actina-a e se ne conosce una variante sia autosomica dominante sia recessiva allo stesso locus 1q42.1. NEM4 è data da un difetto della β-tropomiosina al locus 9q13, trasmesso in modo autosomico dominante. Le alterazioni dell'α- e della β-tropomiosina sono rare e si verificano solo nel 3% dei pazienti con miopatia nemalinica. NEM5 è un difetto autosomico recessivo della troponina-T al locus 19q13, riscontrato solo nella popolazione Amish.

TRATTAMENTO E PROGNOSI. La terapia è di supporto. Coloro che sopravvivono sono costretti alla sedia a rotelle e sono generalmente incapaci di vincere la forza di gravità. Sono coinvolti sia i muscoli prossimali sia quelli distali. Può essere necessaria una gastrostomia per la disfagia cronica. Nella forma giovanile, i pazienti camminano e sono in grado di svolgere la maggior parte delle attività tipiche della vita quotidiana. La perdita di forza non è generalmente ingravescente, ma alcuni pazienti presentano maggiori difficoltà con il passare del tempo o entrano in una fase di indebolimento progressivo. La miocardiopatia è una complicanza infrequente, al contrario della polmonite.

607.4 • Miopatia central core e miopatia minicore

Questa malattia è trasmessa con modalità sia autosomica dominante sia recessiva, entrambe dovute alla stessa anomalia genetica al locus 19q13.1. Il gene trascrive per i recettori della rianodina (*RYR1*), un recettore tetramerico per un canale del calcio non voltaggio-dipendente del reticolo sarcoplasmatico. Mutazioni di questo gene sono responsabili anche dell'ipertermia maligna. Gli elementi caratteristici sia della forma dominante sia di quella recessiva sono l'ipotonia infantile, la debolezza muscolare prossimale, l'ipotrofia e il coinvolgimento dei muscoli faciali e flessori del collo. Sono frequenti le contratture a carico di ginocchia, anche e altre articolazioni, come pure lo sviluppo di cifoscoliosi e piede cavo, anche in assenza d'importante debolezza della muscolatura assiale o distale. L'incidenza delle anomalie cardiache è elevata. Il decorso non è progressivo, eccetto che per le retrazioni muscolari.

La malattia dal punto di vista anatomopatologico è caratterizzata da *central core* nelle fibre muscolari, in cui si distingue solo citoplasma granulare e amorfo con assenza di miofibrille e organuli. Le colorazioni immunoistochimiche dimostrano la mancanza di tutte le attività enzimatiche all'interno di questi core. Il valore sierico della CK è normale nella miopatia *central core*, tranne che durante le crisi d'ipertermia maligna (vedi Capitolo 610.2).

La miopatia *central core* è sostanzialmente correlata con l'ipertermia maligna, che può precedere la diagnosi della miopatia. Bisognerebbe prestare particolare attenzione a tutti i pazienti in cui si somministra un pretrattamento con dantrolene prima di un agente anestetico. L'utilizzo del salbutamolo in alcuni bambini con miopatia *central core* ha determinato un miglioramento della forza e della capacità vitale sotto sforzo per un periodo di 6 mesi, osservazione che richiede comunque ulteriori verifiche.

Varianti della forma *central core*, dette *minicore* e *multicore*, sono state descritte in alcune famiglie, ma la miopatia *minicore* è una malattia genetica diversa. Sono stati riportati casi con una mutazione simile nel gene RYR1, mentre altri presentano un difetto del gene della selenoproteina-N (*SEPN1*), che è implicato anche nella miopatia con rigidità della colonna vertebrale. I bambini con tale alterazione sono ipotonici nella prima infanzia e presentano un andamento benigno, ma spesso sviluppano cifoscoliosi progressiva o rigidità della colonna durante l'adolescenza. La variante uno è caratterizzata anche da oftalmoplegia esterna. Sono rari i casi di miopatia *minicore* che si associano a una miocardiopatia ipertrofica.

607.5 • Miopatie miofibrillari

La maggior parte delle miopatie miofibrillari non è sintomatica nell'infanzia, ma occasionalmente bambini più grandi e adolescenti possono presentare sintomi precoci come una debolezza muscolare prossimale e distale aspecifica. Vi è anche una forma infantile, che può essere responsabile di lieve ipotonia e debolezza muscolare neonatale con disfagia e insufficienza respiratoria severe e non proporzionate, che un tempo portavano a morte precoce. Si tratta tuttavia di una patologia non progressiva e alcuni pazienti vanno incontro a un miglioramento dopo i primi mesi di vita e nella prima infanzia, acquisendo la capacità di deglutire a 3 anni di età. La miocardiopatia può essere una complicanza in una minoranza dei casi. La diagnosi si basa sulla biopsia muscolare neonatale: alcuni sarcomeri delle fibre muscolari presentano una disorganizzazione e dissoluzione delle miofibrille, in vicinanza di altre aree di sarcomeri normali nella stessa fibra. Queste zone si associano ai filamenti delle bande Z e a incrementi focali di filamenti intermedi di desmina, miotilina e α-B-cristallina. È necessario sottoporre a indagine immunoistochimica e ultrastrutturale il materiale prelevato con la biopsia. La mutazione del gene della desmina è implicata nell'eziologia. In alcuni pazienti è stata riscontrata un'associazione con alterazioni mitocondriali.

607.6 • Malformazioni cerebrali e sviluppo muscolare

I lattanti con **ipoplasia cerebellare** sono ipotonici e presentano uno sviluppo ritardato, soprattutto nella capacità di eseguire movimenti non fini. Talvolta si ricorre alla biopsia muscolare per escludere una miopatia congenita. Un esame bioptico può evidenziare un ritardo della maturazione muscolare, una predominanza di un tipo di fibre o un CMFTD. Altre malformazioni cerebrali possono essere associate anche ad alterati pattern immunoistochimici, ma le lesioni sovratentoriali hanno minori probabilità di alterare lo sviluppo muscolare rispetto alle lesioni del tronco cerebrale o del cervelletto. Impulsi anomali discendenti lungo il tratto bulbospinale probabilmente alterano i pattern di trasmissione nervosa sul secondo motoneurone, che determinano la differenziazione istochimica del muscolo nella 20ª-28ª settimana di gestazione. Il tratto corticospinale non prende parte a tale evento non essendo ancora funzionante durante questa fase della vita fetale. In diverse distrofie muscolari congenite, tra cui la sindrome di Walker-Warburg, la malattia di Fukuyama e la sindrome muscolo-occhio-cervello o sindrome di Santavuori, sono presenti malformazioni cerebrali maggiori, quali la pachigiria e la lissencefalia.

607.7 • Amioplasia

L'assenza congenita di singoli muscoli è comune e spesso asimmetrica. Un'aplasia comune è quella del *muscolo palmare lungo* localizzato nella porzione ventrale dell'avambraccio, la cui assenza (riscontrabile nel 30% dei soggetti normali) è completamente compensata dagli altri flessori del polso. L'assenza unilaterale del *muscolo sternocleidomastoideo* è una delle cause di torcicollo congenito, mentre quella di uno dei *muscoli grandi pettorali* fa parte dell'anomalia di Poland.

Quando l'innervazione non si sviluppa, per esempio negli arti inferiori nei casi gravi di mielomeningocele, può accadere che neppure i muscoli si sviluppino. Nell'agenesia sacrale, i somiti anormali che non formano il corpo vertebrale possono anche non formare i muscoli dalla medesima lamina mesodermica, un disordine che porta a fenomeni di amioplasia segmentale. I muscoli scheletrici degli arti non vanno incontro a differenziazione a partire dai miomeri embrionali se non si sono formate le ossa lunghe. L'assenza di un osso lungo, come il radio, si accompagna a vari gradi di aplasia o ipoplasia dei muscoli associati, tra cui il *flessore radiale del carpo*. L'atrofia muscolare neurogenica della fase terminale è talora detta **amioplasia**, ma questo termine è semanticamente scorretto.

L'**amioplasia generalizzata** spesso causa la morte del feto, e i nati vivi raramente sopravvivono. Sulla base di studi genetici condotti su topi *knockout* si è ipotizzato che l'eziologia sia da ricercare nella mutazione di uno dei geni miogenici, che però non è ancora stata dimostrata negli esseri umani.

607.8 • Disgenesia muscolare (miopatia della sindrome di Proteus)

La **sindrome di Proteus** è dovuta a un'alterazione della crescita cellulare, a carico dei tessuti di origine ectodermica e mesodermica. La sua eziologia è sconosciuta, ma non ha una trasmissione di tipo mendeliano. Si manifesta con una crescita eccessiva e asimmetrica delle estremità, lesioni cutanee verrucose, vari tipi di angiomi, ispessimenti ossei, emimegaencefalia ed eccessiva crescita dei muscoli in assenza di debolezza. Dal punto di vista istologico, si riscontra una diffusa *disgenesia muscolare*. Accanto a zone muscolari normali ve ne sono altre patologiche che non rispettano i limiti anatomici. Il disturbo potrebbe dipendere dall'azione di fattori di crescita paracrini anomali.

607.9 • Ipotonia congenita benigna

L'ipotonia congenita benigna non è una patologia, ma un termine descrittivo con cui si indicano le ipotonie non progressive di origine non conosciuta dei neonati e dei bambini. L'ipotonia non è generalmente associata a debolezza o a ritardo dello sviluppo, sebbene alcuni bambini acquisiscano la destrezza dei movimenti più tardivamente. I riflessi tendinei da stiramento sono normali o ridotti. Non emergono alterazioni a carico dei nervi cranici e l'intelligenza è normale.

La **diagnosi** è fatta per esclusione, una volta che gli esami di laboratorio, tra cui la biopsia muscolare e l'indagine radiologica dell'encefalo (in particolare del cervelletto) hanno dato risultati normali (Tab. 606-2). Non è stata identificata alcuna base genetico-molecolare nota per questa sindrome.

La **prognosi** è generalmente buona; non è necessaria aluna terapia specifica. Non si sviluppano retrazioni. L'ipotonia persiste nell'età adulta. Il difetto non è sempre "benigno" come vorrebbe il suo nome, poiché una complicanza comune è la lussazione articolare recidivante, specialmente delle spalle. L'eccessiva mobilità della colonna può essere responsabile di danni da stiramento, compressione o di lesioni vascolari a carico delle radici nervose o del midollo; queste sono particolarmente pericolose per i pazienti che praticano attività ginniche o diventano acrobati, in quanto la lassità delle articolazioni non è associata a debolezza o dolore.

607.10 • Artrogriposi

L'**artrogriposi multipla congenita** non è una patologia, ma un termine descrittivo che indica la presenza di numerose retrazioni congenite (vedi Capitolo 681).

Clarke NF, North KN: Congenital fiber type disproportion—30 years on. *J Neuropathol Exp Neurol* 2003;62:977–989.

Goebel HH: Congenital myopathies in the new millennium. *J Child Neurol* 2005;20:94–101.

Gros J, Manceau M, Thomé V, et al: A common somitic origin for embryonic muscle progenitors and satellite cells. *Nature* 2005;435:954–958.

Jungbluth H, Sewry CA, Muntoni F: What's new in neuromuscular disorders? The congenital myopathies. *Eur J Paediatr Neurol* 2003;7:23–30.

Laing NC, Clarke NF, Dye DE, et al: Actin mutations are one cause of congenital fibre type disproportion. *Ann Neurol* 2001;56:689–691.

Pierson CR, Tomczak K, Agrawal P, et al: X-linked myotubular and centronuclear myopathies. *J Neuropathol Exp Neurol* 2005;64:555–564.

Quane KA, Healy JM, Keating KE, et al: Mutations in the ryanodine receptor gene in central core disease and malignant hyperthermia. *Nat Genet* 1993;5:51–55.

Quinlivan RM, Muller CR, Davis M, et al: Central core disease: clinical, pathological, and genetic features. *Arch Dis Child* 2003;88:1051–1055.

Relaix F, Rocancourt D, Mansouri A, et al: A Pax3/Pax7-dependent population of skeletal muscle progenitor cells. *Nature* 2005;435:948–953.

Sarnat HB: Cerebral dysgeneses and their influence on fetal muscle development. *Brain Dev* 1986;8:495–499.

Sarnat HB: Myopathy of the Proteus syndrome: Hypothesis of muscular dysgenesis. *Neuromuscul Disord* 1993;3:293–301.

Sarnat HB: Ontogenesis of striated muscle. In Polin RA, Fox WW (editors): *Neonatal and Fetal Medicine: Physiology and Pathophysiology,* vol. 2, 3rd ed. Philadelphia, WB Saunders, 2003, pp 1849–1870.

Schuelke M, Wagner KR, Stolz LE, et al: Myostatin mutation associated with gross muscle hypertrophy in a child. *N Engl J Med* 2004;350: 2682–2688.

Selcen D, Ohno K, Engel AG: Myofibrillar myopathy: Clinical, morphological and genetic studies in 63 patients. *Brain* 2004;127:439–451.

Wallgren-Pattersson C, Pelin K, Nowak KH, et al: Genotype-phenotype correlations in nemaline myopathy caused by mutations in the genes for nebulin and skeletal muscle α-actin. *Neuromuscul Disord* 2004;14: 461–470.

Wallgren-Pattersson C: Gene table: Congenital myopathies. *Eur J Paediatr Neurol* 2005;9:27–28.

Capitolo 608 ■ Distrofie muscolari

Il termine **distrofia** indica una crescita alterata e deriva dal greco *trophe*, che significa "nutrimento". La distrofia muscolare si distingue da qualunque altra patologia neuromuscolare fondamentalmente per quattro aspetti: è una miopatia primaria, ha una base genetica, il suo decorso è progressivo, la degenerazione e la morte delle fibre muscolari si verificano a un determinato stadio della malattia. Da questa definizione sono escluse le malattie neurogeniche quali l'atrofia muscolare spinale, le miopatie non ereditarie come la dermatomiosite, le miopatie congenite non progressive e non necrotizzanti come la sproporzione congenita dei tipi di fibre muscolari e le miopatie metaboliche ereditarie non progressive. Alcune miopatie metaboliche, pur potendo rientrare nella definizione di distrofia muscolare progressiva, ma non sono tradizionalmente classificate tra le distrofie (per es. deficit di carnitina muscolare). Tutte le distrofie muscolari potranno essere eventualmente classificate come miopatie metaboliche una volta che saranno stati meglio definiti i difetti biochimici.

Le distrofie muscolari sono un gruppo di malattie non correlate tra loro, ciascuna caratterizzata da una modalità di trasmissione differente, oltre che da un decorso clinico e da manifestazioni peculiari. Alcune sono gravi fin dalla nascita e portano a morte precoce; altre invece hanno un decorso lentamente progressivo nell'arco di diversi decenni, possono essere compatibili con una durata della vita normale o addirittura possono non diventare sintomatiche fino all'età adulta avanzata. Alcune categorie di distrofie, per esempio la distrofia muscolare dei cingoli, non sono malattie omogenee, ma piuttosto sindromi che comprendono diverse miopatie distinte. I rapporti tra le varie distrofie muscolari verranno chiariti dagli aspetti genetico-molecolari, più che da somiglianze o differenze relative agli aspetti clinici e istopatologici.

608.1 • Distrofie muscolari di Duchenne e di Becker

La **distrofia muscolare di Duchenne**, la più comune malattia neuromuscolare ereditaria, colpisce tutte le razze e tutti i gruppi etnici. I suoi elementi clinici caratteristici sono la perdita di forza muscolare progressiva, il deficit intellettivo, l'ipertrofia dei polpacci e la proliferazione di tessuto connettivo nel muscolo. La sua incidenza è di 1:3600 bambini nati vivi. Questa malattia si trasmette come carattere recessivo legato al cromosoma X; il gene alterato si trova sul locus Xp21 ed è uno dei geni più lunghi finora identificati. La **distrofia muscolare di Becker** è fondamentalmente simile a quella di Duchenne, essendo causata da un difetto genetico relativo allo stesso locus, ma clinicamente ha un decorso più lieve e prolungato.

MANIFESTAZIONI CLINICHE. I soggetti di sesso maschile di rado sono sintomatici alla nascita o nella prima infanzia, anche se alcuni presentano già ipotonia lieve. L'acquisizione delle prime capacità motorie grossolane, quali rotolarsi, sedersi e stare in piedi, è generalmente adeguata per l'età o può essere di poco ritardata. Lo scarso controllo del capo durante l'infanzia può essere il primo segno di debolezza muscolare. Di solito il bambino non ha una facies caratteristica, poiché la debolezza dei muscoli faciali è un evento tardivo. L'acquisizione della capacità di deambulare avviene spesso alla normale età di 12 mesi circa, ma la debolezza del cingolo pelvico può manifestarsi già intorno ai due anni d'età. I lattanti che muovono i primi passi possono assumere una postura lordotica quando stanno in posizione eretta, per compensare la debolezza dei glutei. Il segno di Gowers è precoce, spesso evidente a partire dai 3 anni e completamente espresso intorno ai 5-6 anni (vedi Fig. 591-2). A questa età compare anche un'andatura di Trendelenburg, o anserina.

Il periodo di tempo durante il quale il soggetto conserva la capacità di camminare è quanto mai variabile. Alcuni pazienti sono costretti alla sedia a rotelle all'età di 7 anni, mentre la maggior parte continua a deambulare, seppure con difficoltà crescente, fino ai 10 anni senza intervento ortopedico. Grazie agli apparecchi ortopedici, alla fisioterapia e talora a piccoli interventi chirurgici (allungamento del tendine d'Achille), la maggior parte di essi è in grado di camminare fino ai 12 anni. La deambulazione è importante non solo per posticipare la comparsa di depressione dell'umore, conseguente alla parziale perdita dell'autonomia, ma anche per la scoliosi che generalmente non diventa una complicanza maggiore, fintantoché il paziente conserva la capacità di camminare anche soltanto un'ora al giorno; spesso la scoliosi diventa rapidamente progressiva dopo che il paziente è costretto sulla sedia a rotelle.

L'inesorabile progressione della **perdita di forza** muscolare prosegue fino alla seconda decade di vita. La funzione dei muscoli distali è in genere relativamente ben conservata, permettendo al bambino di continuare a utilizzare le posate, la matita e la tastiera del computer. Il coinvolgimento dei muscoli respiratori si manifesta con tosse debole e inefficace, infezioni polmonari frequenti e riduzione del volume respiratorio. La debolezza dei muscoli faringei può portare a episodi di aspirazione, rigurgito nasale di liquidi e un timbro di voce aspirato o nasale. La funzione dei muscoli oculomotori rimane ben conservata. L'incontinenza, secondaria a debolezza degli sfinteri anale e uretrale, è un evento poco comune e tardivo.

Le **retrazioni muscolari** coinvolgono per lo più le caviglie, le ginocchia, le spalle e i polsi. La **scoliosi** è frequente. La deformità del torace compromette ulteriormente la capacità polmonare e determina compressione del cuore. La scoliosi, che generalmente progredisce più rapidamente quando il bambino non è più in grado di deambulare, può essere fastidiosa o dolorosa. L'aumento di volume dei polpacci (pseudoipertrofia) e la perdita di forza dei muscoli della coscia sono classici segni di malattia. L'aumento di volume dei polpacci è dovuto all'ipertrofia di alcune fibre muscolari, all'infiltrazione di grasso nel muscolo e alla proliferazione di collagene. Dopo i polpacci, la sede più frequentemente colpita dall'ipertrofia muscolare è la lingua, seguita dai muscoli dell'avambraccio. Non si osservano fascicolazioni della lingua. I muscoli sfinterici volontari sono raramente coinvolti.

A meno che le retrazioni della caviglia non siano severe, i riflessi achillei sono conservati fino agli stadi terminali. I riflessi rotulei possono essere presenti fino ai 6 anni circa, ma sono meno vivaci dei riflessi della caviglia e alla fine vengono persi. Agli arti superiori, il riflesso brachioradiale è generalmente più marcato di quelli dei bicipiti o tricipiti brachiali.

La **miocardiopatia**, con tachicardia persistente e insufficienza cardiaca, si osserva nel 50-80% dei pazienti affetti. La sua severità non correla necessariamente con il grado di debolezza dei muscoli scheletrici. Alcuni pazienti muoiono precocemente per miocardiopatia severa quando ancora hanno la capacità di camminare, mentre altri presentano un buon compenso cardiaco anche negli stadi più avanzati della malattia. Una disfunzione della muscolatura liscia, in particolare del tratto gastrointestinale, è un elemento di minore importanza, ma spesso trascurato.

Un **ritardo cognitivo** si osserva in tutti i pazienti, sebbene solo il 20-30% abbia un QI <70. La maggior parte di essi presenta difficoltà di apprendimento, che però in genere non impedisce di frequentare una classe regolare, talvolta con l'ausilio di insegnanti di sostegno. Una minoranza dei pazienti ha un ritardo mentale grave, che però non è correlato alla severità della miopatia. L'epilessia è lievemente più frequente che nella popolazione pediatrica generale. La distrofina è espressa nel cervello e nella retina, esattamente come nel muscolo striato e cardiaco, anche se il livello encefalico è più basso rispetto a quello muscolare. Questa distribuzione può spiegare alcune delle manifestazioni a carico del sistema nervoso centrale. Dal punto di vista neuropatologico si possono evidenziare anomalie dell'architettura corticale e delle diramazioni dendritiche; la RM rivela un'atrofia cerebrale nelle fasi avanzate della malattia. La degenerazione e la fibrosi muscolare sono indolori; non si osservano mialgie né spasmi muscolari e le calcificazioni del muscolo sono rare.

Il decesso avviene generalmente intorno ai 18-20 anni, per insufficienza respiratoria durante il sonno, insufficienza cardiaca incurabile, polmonite, raramente aspirazione o ostruzione delle vie aeree.

I soggetti con **distrofia muscolare di Becker** conservano la capacità di deambulare fino alla tarda adolescenza o all'inizio dell'età adulta. La pseudoipertrofia dei polpacci, la miocardiopatia e l'aumento della creatina chinasi (CK) sierica sono simili a quelli osservabili nei pazienti con la distrofia di Duchenne, mentre le difficoltà d'apprendimento sono meno frequenti. L'esordio della perdita di forza muscolare è più tardivo nella distrofia di Becker che in quella di Duchenne. Il decesso spesso si verifica dopo i 20 anni; meno della metà dei pazienti raggiunge i 40 anni e i sopravvissuti sono gravemente disabili.

ESAMI DI LABORATORIO. I livelli sierici di CK sono costantemente molto elevati nella distrofia muscolare di Duchenne, anche nelle fasi presintomatiche, come alla nascita; si riscontrano concentrazioni sieriche di 15 000-35 000 UI/L (valore normale <160 UI/L). Un livello di CK normale non è compatibile con la diagnosi di distrofia di Duchenne, anche se nelle fasi terminali della malattia, tale valore può essere considerevolmente più basso che negli anni precedenti, poiché vi è meno muscolo che va incontro a degenerazione. Si osserva inoltre un aumento di altri enzimi lisosomiali presenti a livello muscolare, quali l'aldolasi e l'aspartato aminotransferasi, che tuttavia sono meno specifici.

La valutazione cardiaca con ecocardiogramma, elettrocardiogramma (ECG) e radiografia del torace è essenziale e dovrebbe essere ripetuta periodicamente. Dopo la diagnosi, i pazienti dovrebbero essere regolarmente seguiti da un cardiologo pediatra.

L'elettromiografia (EMG) evidenzia la presenza di caratteristici elementi miopatici, ma non è specifica per la distrofia muscolare di Duchenne. Non è evidente denervazione. Le velocità di conduzione dei nervi motori e sensitivi sono normali.

DIAGNOSI. La PCR (*Polymerase Chain Reaction*, reazione a catena della polimerasi) su sangue per la mutazione del gene della distrofina è il primo esame da eseguire, se gli elementi clinici e la CK sierica sono suggestivi. Se la PCR è diagnostica, è possibile rimandare l'esecuzione della biopsia muscolare, ma se è normale e il sospetto clinico è elevato, l'esame immunoistochimico più specifico per la distrofina su campioni di muscolo prelevati tramite biopsia permette di riconoscere un terzo dei casi, che non avevano presentato anomalie alla PCR. La colorazione immunoistochimica di sezioni congelate di tessuto muscolare permette di apprezzare le differenze tra rod domain, estremità carbossilata (che si lega al sarcolemma) ed estremità aminica (che si lega ai miofilamenti di actina) della grossa molecola della distrofina, e può essere prognostico del decorso clinico, in grado di distinguere la distrofia di Duchenne da quella di Becker. Una debolezza muscolare più severa corrisponde all'interruzione della molecola di distrofina alla terminazione carbossilica anziché a quella aminica. È sempre necessaria la conferma della diagnosi con PCR su sangue o con biopsia muscolare. Si possono inoltre misurare i livelli di destroglicani e altre proteine regionali del sarcolemma, quali la merosina e i sarcoglicani, che talvolta risultano secondariamente ridotti.

La **biopsia muscolare** è diagnostica e dimostra alterazioni caratteristiche (Figg. 608-1 e 608-2). Le modificazioni miopatiche comprendono la proliferazione del connettivo endomisiale, degenerazione e rigenerazione diffuse delle miofibrille, infiltrati di cellule infiammatorie mononucleate che rappresentano una reazione alla necrosi delle fibre muscolari, lievi alterazioni strutturali delle fibre muscolari ancora funzionanti. La presenza di fibre ipercontratte probabilmente dipende da eventi necrotici segmentali avvenuti a un altro livello, che permettono l'ingresso di calcio dal sito di rottura della membrana del sarcolemma e provocano una contrazione della fibra per l'intera sua lunghezza. Le calcificazioni all'interno delle miofibre sono correlate con il deficit secondario di β-destroglicani.

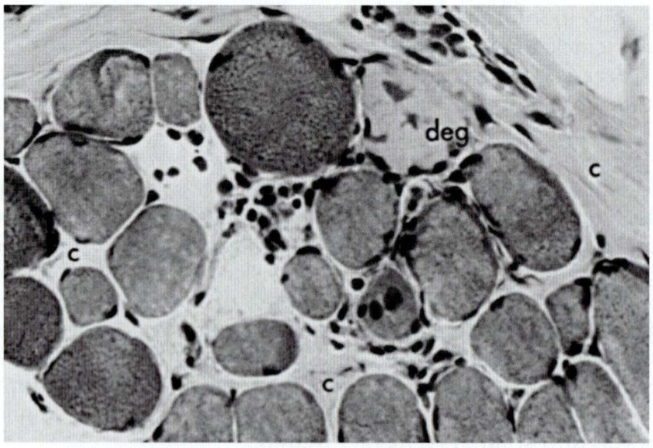

Figura 608-1. Biopsia muscolare di un bambino di 4 anni affetto da distrofia muscolare di Duchenne. Si osserva la presenza di fibre muscolari sia atrofiche sia ipertrofiche e di alcune fibre in degenerazione (deg). Il tessuto connettivo (c) tra le fibre è aumentato (ematossilina-eosina, ×400).

Talvolta, di fronte alla scelta se procedere o meno alla biopsia muscolare per stabilire una diagnosi, possono sorgere problemi. Se esiste una storia familiare di malattia, in particolare un fratello affetto la cui diagnosi è stata confermata, è probabile non sia necessario sottoporre a biopsia un paziente con aspetti clinici tipici della distrofia muscolare di Duchenne e un aumento della CK sierica. Anche il risultato della PCR può aiutare a decidere se eseguire o meno la biopsia muscolare. Un primo caso in una famiglia, anche se le caratteristiche cliniche sono tipiche, dovrebbe ricevere conferma diagnostica per escludere che non si tratti di un'altra miopatia con caratteristiche simili alla distrofia di Duchenne. I muscoli che vengono esaminati più comunemente sono il vasto laterale (quadricipite femorale) e il gastrocnemio.

EZIOLOGIA GENETICA E PATOGENESI. Anche se la modalità di trasmissione della distrofia muscolare di Duchenne è X-linked recessiva, nel 30% circa dei casi si osservano nuove mutazioni e la madre non è portatrice. La donna portatrice di solito non presenta debolezza muscolare né altre manifestazioni cliniche di malattia; occasionalmente si osservano femmine affette, che comunque, rispetto ai maschi, accusano una perdita di forza muscolare molto meno accentuata. Il riscontro di femmine sintomatiche si spiega con l'ipotesi di Lyon, secondo cui il cromosoma X normale può essere inattivato, mentre quello con la delezione genica è attivo (vedi Capitolo 80). Il quadro clinico completo della distrofia di Duchenne è stato osservato in alcune ragazze con sindrome di Turner, in cui l'unico cromosoma X presentava delezione del gene Xp21.

La condizione di portatrice asintomatica di distrofia di Duchenne si associa a un aumento dei livelli sierici di CK nell'80% dei casi. L'incremento del livello è generalmente dell'ordine di centinaia o alcune migliaia, ma non raggiunge mai i valori estremi riportati per i maschi affetti. Le ragazze portatrici della distrofia, in età prepubere, possono avere anch'esse un incremento dei valori di CK, che risultano più elevati a 8-12 anni. Circa il 20% delle portatrici ha livelli di CK normali. Se la madre di un bambino affetto presenta livelli di CK normali, è improbabile che la figlia possa essere riconosciuta come portatrice tramite la misurazione della CK. Nelle donne sospettate di essere portatrici la biopsia muscolare può diagnosticare un ulteriore 10% di portatrici in cui la CK non risultava aumentata; solo la diagnosi genetica specifica con PCR su sangue periferico è definitiva. Alcune portatrici possono soffrire di miocardiopatia senza manifestare alcun segno di perdita di forza della muscolatura striata.

La *distrofina*, proteina del citoscheletro di 427 kd, è codificata dal gene X sul locus Xp21.2. Questa proteina subsarcolemmale è legata alla membrana del sarcolemma che ricopre le bande A e M delle miofibrille ed è costituita da quattro distinte regioni o domini: la parte aminoterminale contiene 250 aminoacidi ed è correlata al sito di legame N-actina dell'α-actinina; il secondo

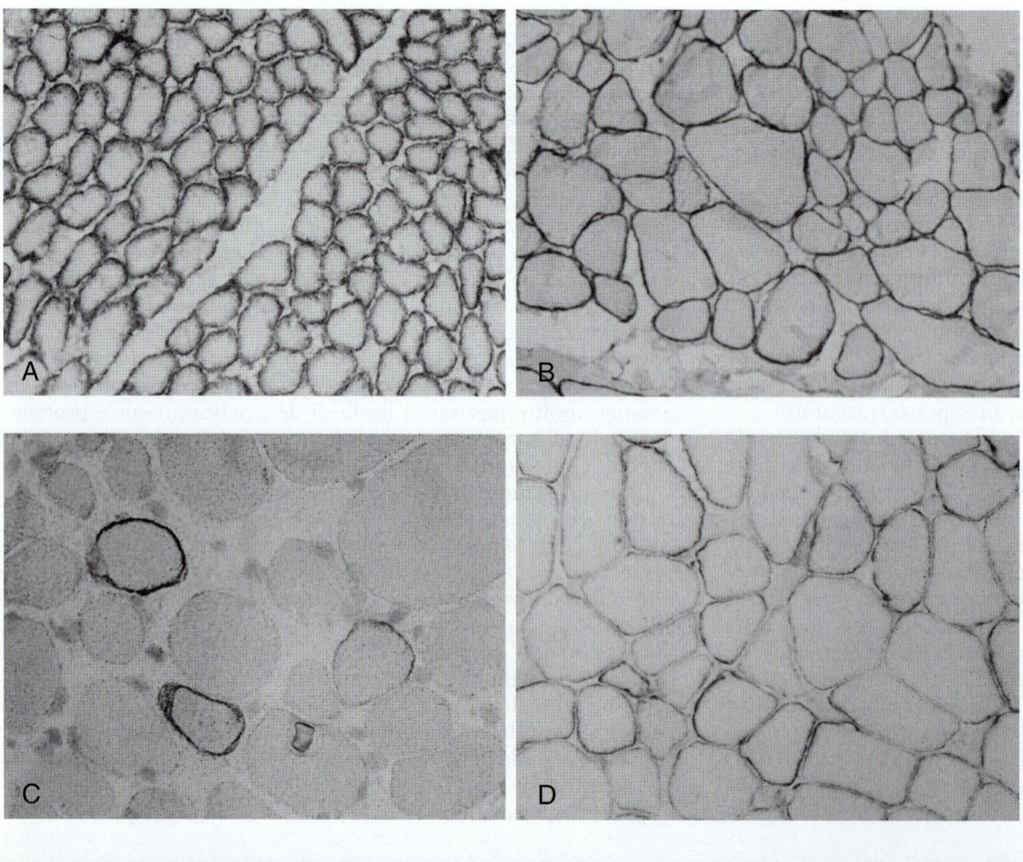

Figura 608-2. Immunoistochimica per la distrofina in biopsie muscolari di: un neonato normale a termine (*A*); un bambino di 10 anni con distrofia muscolare dei cingoli (*B*); un bambino di 6 anni con distrofia muscolare di Duchenne (*C*); un bambino di 10 anni con distrofia muscolare di Becker (*D*). Nel caso normale e nelle distrofie muscolari non X-linked, in cui la distrofina non è alterata, la membrane sarcolemmatiche di ciascuna fibra sono intensamente colorate, anche nelle fibre atrofiche e ipertrofiche. Nella distrofia di Duchenne, la maggior parte delle fibre non rivela la presenza di distrofina; alcune fibre sparse, dette "fibre revertant", presentano un'immunoreattività quasi normale. Nella distrofia di Becker, la distrofina alterata si distingue per una colorazione sottile e pallida del sarcolemma, in cui l'immunoreattività varia non solo tra le miofibrille ma anche lungo la circonferenza della singola fibra (×250).

dominio è il più grande, con 2800 aminoacidi, e contiene molte ripetizioni, che gli conferiscono una caratteristica forma a bastoncello; un terzo dominio, ricco di cisteina, è correlato alla porzione C-terminale dell'α-actinina; l'ultimo segmento C-terminale, di 400 aminoacidi, è tipico della distrofina e di una proteina correlata alla distrofina, codificata dal cromosoma 6.

Diverse sono le anomalie molecolari osservabili nelle distrofinopatie: delezioni intrageniche, duplicazioni o mutazioni puntiformi dei nucleotidi. Circa il 65% dei pazienti presenta una delezione, mentre solo il 7% ha una duplicazione. La sede o l'estensione delle anomalie intrageniche non sempre sono ben correlate con la gravità del fenotipo; in entrambe le forme (Duchenne e Becker) le mutazioni sono soprattutto in prossimità della parte centrale del gene e comprendono delezioni degli esoni 46-51. Le variazioni fenotipiche o cliniche si spiegano con l'alterazione della cornice di lettura del frammento di mRNA, che dà origine a molecole di distrofina instabili e tronche nella distrofia di Duchenne classica grave; le mutazioni che conservano la cornice di lettura del frammento, permettendo ancora la trascrizione delle sequenze a valle del gene, determinano la produzione di distrofina semifunzionante, che si manifesta clinicamente come distrofia di Becker. Una forma ancora più lieve con esordio in età adulta, detta in passato **miopatia dei quadricipiti**, è anch'essa provocata da una molecola di distrofina alterata. Lo spettro clinico delle distrofinopatie non comprende solo le forme classiche di Duchenne e Becker, ma spazia da una grave distrofia muscolare neonatale a bambini asintomatici con livelli sierici di CK costantemente elevati (>1 000 UI/L).

La proteina distrofina, la cui analisi richiede la biopsia muscolare, è evidenziabile con Western blot o studi immunoistochimici su sezioni di tessuto con anticorpi anti-distrofina, utilizzando il microscopio a fluorescenza o quello ottico (vedi Fig. 608-2). Nella distrofia di Duchenne classica si osservano livelli inferiori del 3% rispetto a quelli normali. Nella distrofia di Becker la distrofina ha un peso molecolare inferiore del 20-90% rispetto ai valori normali nell'80% dei pazienti; nel 15%, invece, è di dimensioni normali, ma presente in quantità ridotta e nel 5% è insolitamente grande per le eccessive duplicazioni o ripetizioni dei codoni. L'immunopositività selettiva di parti differenti della molecola di distrofina in sezioni di materiale bioptico permette di distinguere la forma di Duchenne da quella di Becker (Fig. 608-3). La dimostrazione di delezioni e duplicazioni può essere ottenuta anche su campioni di sangue con la più rapida tecnica della PCR, che identifica il 98% delle delezioni con l'amplificazione di 18 esoni, ma non è in grado di individuare le duplicazioni. La diagnosi può quindi essere confermata a livello genetico-molecolare sia con materiale bioptico sia con sangue periferico, nonostante circa un terzo dei ragazzi con distrofia di Duchenne o Becker abbia una PCR su sangue falsamente normale; tutti i casi di distrofinopatia sono diagnosticati con la biopsia muscolare.

Le stesse tecniche di analisi del DNA su sangue possono essere utilizzate per ricercare le portatrici tra i parenti a rischio, come sorelle e cugine, e per determinare se la madre è una portatrice o se si è verificata una nuova mutazione nell'embrione. È possibile eseguire una diagnosi prenatale alla 12ª settimana di gestazione tramite prelievo dei villi coriali per l'analisi del DNA con il Southern blot o la PCR; nei feti con distrofia di Duchenne abortiti la conferma si ottiene con colorazioni immunoistochimiche per la distrofina muscolare.

TRATTAMENTO. Anche se non esiste una terapia medica per questa malattia, né un modo per rallentarne la progressione, molto si può fare per trattarne le complicanze, migliorando così la qualità di vita dei bambini affetti. Lo **scompenso cardiaco** in fase iniziale spesso risponde bene alla digossina. Le **infezioni polmonari** dovrebbero essere trattate precocemente. I pazienti dovrebbero evitare di venire in contatto con bambini con infezioni respiratorie o altre malattie contagiose. Sono indicate l'immunizzazione contro i virus influenzali e le altre vaccinazioni di routine.

È importante mantenere un buono **stato nutrizionale**, ma dal momento che la distrofia muscolare di Duchenne non è dovuta a una carenza vitaminica, dosi eccessive di vitamine devono essere evitate. È importante un adeguato introito di calcio per combattere l'osteoporosi nei bambini costretti sulla sedia a rotelle; è inoltre possibile somministrare supplementi di fluoro, soprattutto se l'acqua della rete idrica locale non è arricchita con questo elemento. Questi bambini tendono a mangiare in modo eccessivo e ad aumentare di peso, in parte perché chi conduce una vita sedentaria consuma meno calorie di chi pratica attività fisica, in parte per effetto della depressione, che rappresenta un fattore aggiunto. L'obesità peggiora lo stato funzionale nei bambini con miopatia, poiché la già ridotta riserva di energia muscolare viene in parte persa per sollevare il peso del tessuto adiposo sottocutaneo in eccesso. Possono rendersi necessarie restrizioni dietetiche sotto stretto controllo medico.

La **fisioterapia** può ritardare, ma non prevenire la comparsa di retrazioni; queste ultime talvolta possono addirittura favorire la riabilitazione funzionale. Se le retrazioni impediscono l'estensione del polso oltre i 90 gradi e i muscoli degli arti superiori non sono abbastanza forti da vincere la forza di gravità, le retrazioni del polso si rivelano funzionalmente utili per fissare un arto altrimenti flaccido, permettendo al paziente di mangiare e scrivere. La correzione chirurgica della retrazione muscolare del polso, per quanto tecnicamente realizzabile, può risultare dannosa. La fisioterapia non è molto efficace per rinforzare la muscolatura, poiché i pazienti in genere hanno già speso la loro riserva di energia per le funzioni quotidiane e l'esercizio non è in grado di aumentare ulteriormente la forza muscolare; al contrario, un esercizio eccessivo può addirittura accelerare il processo di degenerazione delle fibre muscolari.

Un altro trattamento per i pazienti con distrofia di Duchenne consiste nell'utilizzo di prednisone, prednisolone, deflazacort e altri steroidi. I glucocorticoidi riducono l'apoptosi, o morte cellulare programmata, dei miotubuli durante l'ontogenesi e possono rallentare la necrosi delle miofibre nella distrofia muscolare. In genere la forza inizialmente migliora, ma le complicanze a lungo termine della terapia steroidea cronica, compresi il considerevole aumento di peso e l'osteoporosi, possono controbilanciare questi vantaggi o persino causare una debolezza muscolare maggiore di quella legata al decorso naturale della malattia. Per contro, in alcuni casi di distrofia di Duchenne il trattamento precoce con steroidi sembra comportare una prognosi migliore sia a breve sia a lungo termine e può consentire ai pazienti di conservare più a lungo la capacità di camminare. Per evitare complicanze tipiche dell'uso cronico, un protocollo prevede la somministrazione di prednisone (0,75 mg/kg/die) per i primi dieci giorni di ogni mese. Gli steroidi fluorurati, come il desametasone o il triamcinolone, andrebbero evitati poiché inducono miopatia alterando i depositi di ceramidi nei miotubuli.

608.2 • Distrofia muscolare di Emery-Dreifuss

La distrofia muscolare di Emery-Dreifuss, detta anche **distrofia muscolare scapoloperoneale o scapolo-omerale**, è una rara distrofia X-linked recessiva. Il locus genico è sul braccio lungo del cromosoma X, all'interno dell'ampia regione Xq28, comprendente altre mutazioni che causano la miopatia miotubulare, l'adrenoleucodistrofia neonatale e la sindrome di Bloch-Sulzberger o *incontinentia pigmenti*; è lontano dal gene della distrofia muscolare di Duchenne, che si trova sul braccio corto del cromosoma X. Un'altra forma di sindrome di Emery-Dreifuss, più rara, si trasmette invece come carattere autosomico dominante localizzato su 1q; pur essendo contraddistinta da segni e sintomi muscolari e cardiaci simili, essa può manifestarsi piuttosto tardi, nell'adolescenza o nella prima età adulta, e comportare il rischio di morte improvvisa per fibrillazione ventricolare.

L'esordio delle **manifestazioni cliniche** avviene tra i 5 e i 15 anni, ma la maggior parte dei pazienti sopravvive fino all'età adulta poiché la malattia ha un decorso lentamente progressivo. Non si instaura ipertrofia muscolare. Le retrazioni di polsi e caviglie si sviluppano precocemente e i muscoli diventano ipotrofici con distribuzione scapolo-omero-peroneale. Non è presente debolezza dei muscoli faciali; questa malattia è clinicamente distinta dalle

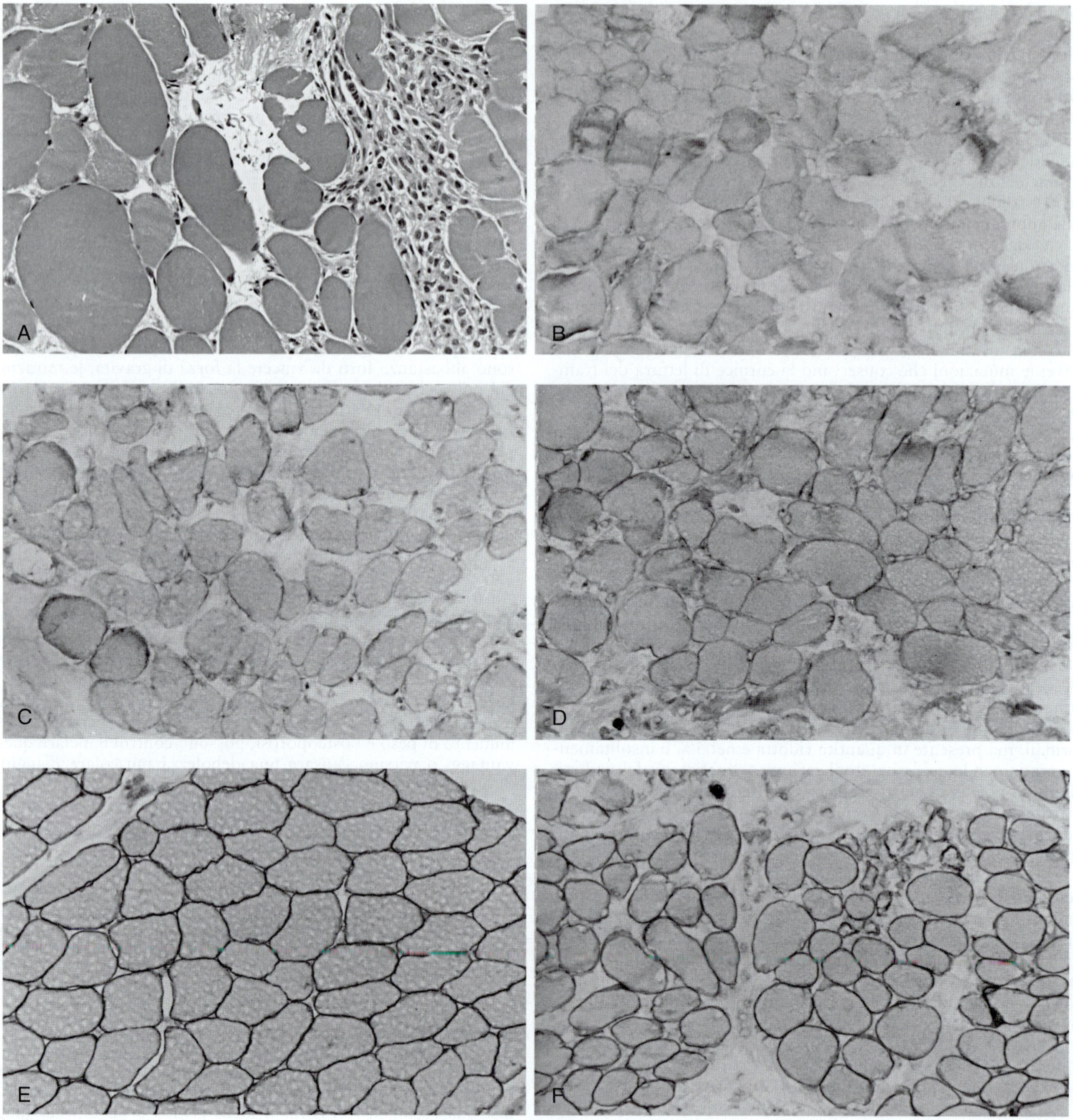

Figura 608-3. Biopsia del muscolo quadricipite femorale di un bambino di 4 anni affetto da distrofia di Becker. *A*, Le fibre presentano dimensioni molto diverse, sia nella forma atrofica sia in quella ipertrofica; sulla destra vi è una zona di degenerazione e necrosi con infiltrazione di macrofagi, simile alla distrofia muscolare di Duchenne (ematossilina-eosina, ×250). L'utilizzo di anticorpi diretti contro la distrofina nel rod domain (*B*), C-terminale (*C*) e amino-terminale (*D*) rivela una ridotta espressione della distrofina, ma non la sua completa mancanza; nella maggior parte delle fibre, di qualunque dimensione, contiene un po' di distrofina in alcune zone del sarcolemma, ma non per l'intera circonferenza, come si può osservare nelle sezioni traversali. La distrofina è comunque ridotta, rarefatta, a confronto con il quadro riscontrabile in un bambino normale di età paragonabile (*E*). *F*, Normale espressione della merosina in un paziente affetto da distrofia di Becker, sia nelle miofibre grandi sia in quelle piccole; la proteina è assente solo nelle fibre francamente necrotiche. Confrontare con la distrofia muscolare di Duchenne classica, illustrata nella Figura 608-2*C*, e con la Figura 608-5.

sindromi autosomiche dominanti scapolo-omerale e scapoloperoneale di origine neurogenica. La miotonia è assente e le facoltà cognitive sono normali. La miocardiopatia è severa e spesso porta al decesso, nella maggior parte dei casi per difetti di conduzione e fibrillazione ventricolare improvvisa, raramente per insufficienza cardiaca non trattabile. La CK è appena aumentata, elemento che aiuta a distinguere questa malattia dalle altre distrofie muscolari X-linked recessive.

Alla biopsia muscolare sono evidenti necrosi aspecifica delle miofibre e fibrosi dell'endomisio. La presenza di molte fibre centronucleari e l'atrofia selettiva delle fibre di tipo I possono creare confusione con la distrofia miotonica. Il gene difettoso della forma X-linked, chiamato emerina, è espresso sulla membrana nucleare interna, contrariamente a quanto avviene nelle altre distrofie, in cui il gene difettoso è espresso sulla membrana del sarcolemma; questa proteina protegge la membrana nucleare dagli stress meccanici che si verificano durante la contrazione muscolare. L'emerina può essere evidenziata con tecniche immunocitochimiche nella biopsia muscolare, per una diagnosi definitiva, oltre a poter essere riconosciuta come marcatore genetico nel sangue periferico. Le proteine difettose nella forma autosomica dominante sono la laminina-A e la laminina-C, che prendono parte alla costituzione della lamina nucleare, uno strato fibroso della membrana nucleare interna. Sono stati dimostrati diversi sottotipi e differenti mutazioni.

Il **trattamento** è di supporto, con particolare attenzione ai difetti di conduzione cardiaca, che possono richiedere la somministrazione di farmaci o il posizionamento di un pacemaker.

608.3 • DISTROFIA MUSCOLARE MIOTONICA

La distrofia muscolare miotonica (malattia di Steinert), ereditata come tratto autosomico dominante, è la seconda più comune distrofia muscolare nel Nord America, in Europa e in Australia, con un'incidenza nella popolazione generale di 1:30 000. La forma classica (DM1) è provocata da un'espansione del trinucleotide citosina-timina-guanina (CTG) sul cromosoma 19q13.3, nella regione 3′ non trascritta di DMPK, gene che codifica per la serina-treonina proteinchinasi. La seconda forma (DM2) si associa a un'instabile e ripetuta espansione di CTG sul cromosoma 3q21 di un introne del gene della proteina 9 del *zinc finger*. È inoltre stata identificata una terza e ultima forma (DM3), al locus 15q21-q24.

La distrofia miotonica è un esempio di difetto genetico che determina alterazioni a carico di più organi. Essa comporta non solo grave compromissione della muscolatura striata, ma anche il coinvolgimento della muscolatura liscia del tratto gastroenterico e dell'utero; la funzionalità cardiaca risulta alterata, e i pazienti presentano disfunzioni multiple, quali endocrinopatie, deficit immunologici, cataratta, facies dismorfica, problemi cognitivi e altre anomalie neurologiche.

MANIFESTAZIONI CLINICHE. Nel normale decorso della malattia, **tranne che nella grave forma neonatale**, i bambini alla nascita sembrano pressoché normali, anche se la debolezza dei muscoli faciali e l'ipotonia possono già essere segni precoci della distrofia. L'espressione faciale è tipica, con il labbro superiore a forma di V rovesciata, le guance incavate e i muscoli temporali festonati e concavi (Fig. 608-4). La testa può essere allungata; il palato è alto e ogivale, perché durante le ultime fasi della vita fetale i muscoli temporali e pterigoidei troppo deboli non esercitano forza laterale sufficiente per un normale sviluppo del cranio e del volto.

Durante i primi anni di vita l'ipotonia è lieve; con il passare del tempo, tuttavia, diventa sempre più evidente la progressiva ipotrofia dei muscoli distali, soprattutto a livello dei muscoli intrinseci della mano. Le eminenze tenar e ipotenar sono appiattite e si formano profonde scanalature tra le dita per l'atrofia dei muscoli interossei dorsali. I muscoli dorsali dell'avambraccio e quelli del compartimento anteriore della gamba diventano atrofici. La lingua è sottile e atrofica. La perdita di forza degli sternocleidomastoidei conferisce al collo un aspetto allungato, sottile e cilindrico. Infine, anche i muscoli prossimali possono diventare atrofici e le scapole diventano alate. La difficoltà nel salire le scale e il segno di Gowers compaiono progressivamente. I riflessi tendinei sono generalmente conservati.

La distribuzione distale della debolezza muscolare nella distrofia miotonica è un'eccezione al principio generale in base al quale le miopatie hanno una distribuzione prossimale, mentre le neuropatie una distribuzione distale. L'atrofia muscolare e la debolezza nella distrofia miotonica sono lentamente progressive nel corso dell'infanzia e dell'adolescenza e continuano nell'età adulta. È raro che i pazienti con distrofia miotonica perdano la capacità di camminare prima dell'età adulta, anche se possono essere necessari tutori o fasciature per stabilizzare le caviglie.

La **miotonia**, un elemento caratteristico che questa forma di distrofia ha in comune con poche altre miopatie, non si verifica durante l'infanzia e in genere non risulta clinicamente evidente neanche con l'elettromiografia fino a circa 5 anni di età. Solo in casi eccezionali i pazienti possono presentare la miotonia prima dei 3 anni. La miotonia consiste in un rilassamento molto lento del muscolo dopo una contrazione, che quest'ultima sia stata volontaria o indotta da un riflesso di stiramento o da una stimolazione elettrica. Durante l'esame obiettivo, la miotonia può essere dimostrata chiedendo al paziente di stringere forte i pugni e poi di aprire rapidamente le mani. Può essere indotta percuotendo l'eminenza tenar con un martelletto e si manifesta come contrazione involontaria del pollice sul palmo della mano. La miotonia può essere osservata anche a livello della lingua premendone il dorso con il bordo di un'abbassa lingua, manovra che determina la comparsa di profondi solchi che scompaiono rapidamente. La gravità della miotonia non va necessariamente di pari passo con il grado di perdita di forza e spesso i muscoli più deboli hanno solo lievi fenomeni miotonici. La miotonia è uno spasmo muscolare non doloroso. Nella distrofia miotonica le mialgie sono assenti.

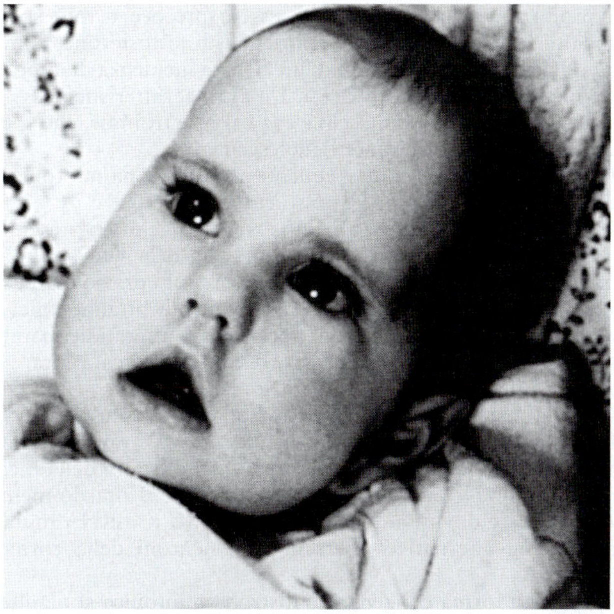

Figura 608-4. Debolezza faciale, labbro superiore a forma di V rovesciata e perdita della massa muscolare in corrispondenza delle fosse temporali sono tratti caratteristici della distrofia muscolare miotonica anche nella prima infanzia, come si può vedere in questa bambina di 8 mesi.

Il **linguaggio** nei pazienti con distrofia miotonica è spesso mal articolato e le parole sono mal pronunciate per il coinvolgimento dei muscoli faciali, della lingua e della faringe. Talora può insorgere disfagia. I bambini gravemente compromessi sono a rischio di sviluppare polmonite *ab ingestis*. La debolezza dei muscoli extraoculari può provocare oftalmoplegia esterna incompleta.

Il coinvolgimento della muscolatura liscia del **tratto gastrointestinale** provoca un rallentamento dello svuotamento gastrico, una peristalsi ridotta e stipsi. Alcuni pazienti presentano encopresi con debolezza dello sfintere anale. Le donne affette da distrofia miotonica possono avere contrazioni uterine inefficaci e anomale durante il travaglio e il parto.

Il **coinvolgimento cardiaco** si manifesta generalmente con blocco del sistema di conduzione del fascio del Purkinje e con turbe del ritmo, anziché con un quadro di miocardiopatia, al contrario di quanto avviene nella maggior parte delle altre distrofie muscolari.

Le **anomalie endocrinologiche** possono interessare diverse ghiandole e manifestarsi in qualunque momento durante il decorso della malattia, per cui è indicato effettuare una rivalutazione annuale dello stato endocrinologico. È comune l'ipotiroidismo, mentre l'ipertiroidismo è raro. L'insufficienza surrenalica può provocare crisi addisoniane fin dall'infanzia. Il diabete mellito è comune nei pazienti con distrofia miotonica; alcuni bambini hanno un alterato rilascio di insulina anziché un deficit della sua produzione. La pubertà può essere precoce o, più spesso, ritardata. L'atrofia testicolare e il deficit di testosterone, comuni negli adulti, sono responsabili di un'elevata incidenza di infertilità maschile. È rara l'atrofia ovarica. Un'altra caratteristica osservabile nei soggetti di sesso maschile è la calvizie frontale, che spesso inizia a manifestarsi durante l'adolescenza.

I **deficit immunitari** sono frequenti nella distrofia miotonica. Il livello di IgG plasmatiche è spesso ridotto.

Frequente è la **cataratta**, che può essere congenita o presentarsi in qualunque momento, durante l'infanzia o la vita adulta. Le forme precoci possono essere diagnosticate solo previo esame con lampada a fessura; si raccomandano controlli oftalmologici periodici. I potenziali evocati visivi sono spesso alterati nei bambini con distrofia miotonica e non si correlano con la cataratta. Non sono generalmente associate alterazioni della vista.

Circa la metà dei pazienti con distrofia miotonica presenta un **deficit cognitivo**, ma un ritardo mentale grave è raro; negli altri l'intelligenza è nella media o (raramente) al di sopra della media. L'epilessia non è comune. Il deficit cognitivo e il ritardo mentale possono essere dovuti a un accumulo di *DMPK* mRNA mutante e di splicing alternativo aberrante nei neuroni della corteccia cerebrale.

Una grave **forma congenita** di distrofia miotonica si manifesta in una minoranza di neonati figli di donne affette. Tutti i pazienti con questa grave malattia congenita fino a oggi hanno presentato la forma DM1. Il piede equino isolato o retrazioni congenite più estese a carico di diverse articolazioni possono coinvolgere qualunque arto e persino la colonna cervicale. Alla nascita sono evidenti ipotonia generalizzata e debolezza. È predominante la debolezza dei muscoli faciali. I neonati possono avere bisogno di un supporto nutrizionale o di ventilazione assistita per il deficit dei muscoli respiratori o per l'apnea (arresto respiratorio). Coloro che necessitano di ventilazione artificiale per meno di 30 giorni spesso sopravvivono, mentre quelli che richiedono un supporto ventilatorio prolungato hanno un rischio di mortalità neonatale del 25%. I bambini ventilati per meno di 30 giorni hanno migliori capacità motorie, di linguaggio e di attività in generale rispetto a quelli che hanno bisogno di ventilazione prolungata. Uno o entrambi gli emidiaframmi possono non essere funzionali. La presenza di gas nello stomaco e nell'intestino distende l'addome, in conseguenza della ridotta peristalsi da deficit della muscolatura liscia. La distensione addominale a sua volta può ulteriormente compromettere la respirazione e l'incapacità di svuotare il retto contribuisce ad aggravare la situazione.

ESAMI DI LABORATORIO. Il classico reperto elettromiografico della miotonia non si osserva nel lattante, mentre può comparire nei primi anni di vita o in età scolare. I livelli sierici di CK e degli altri enzimi muscolari possono essere normali o subire un lieve rialzo (nell'ordine delle centinaia di volte, non delle migliaia).

L'ECG dovrebbe essere eseguito a cadenza annuale nella prima infanzia. L'ecografia dell'addome può essere indicata nei bambini affetti per valutare la funzionalità diaframmatica. Possono inoltre essere necessari radiografie del torace e dell'addome ed esami con mezzo di contrasto per lo studio della motilità intestinale.

Si raccomanda di procedere a una valutazione endocrinologica per valutare la funzionalità tiroidea e surrenalica, oltre al metabolismo glucidico (test da carico con glucosio per verificare la tolleranza glucidica). Occorre inoltre determinare i livelli di immunoglobuline e, se necessario, effettuare esami immunologici più approfonditi.

DIAGNOSI. Il principale esame diagnostico è l'analisi del DNA per dimostrare l'anomala espansione della tripletta CTG. È anche possibile effettuare una diagnosi prenatale. La biopsia muscolare nei bambini più grandi dimostra la presenza di molte fibre muscolari con nuclei centrali e atrofia selettiva delle fibre di tipo I, ma le fibre in degenerazione generalmente sono poche e molto disperse e la fibrosi muscolare è di minima entità o assente. Le fibre intrafusali dei fusi muscolari sono anch'esse anomale. Nei bambini più piccoli con la forma comune della malattia, la biopsia può addirittura essere normale o tutt'al più non evidenziare necrosi delle fibre, aspetti che sono assolutamente in contrasto con quelli della distrofia di Duchenne. Nella forma di distrofia miotonica neonatale, la biopsia muscolare evidenzia un arresto della maturazione delle fibre a diversi stadi di sviluppo in alcuni soggetti e una sproporzione congenita dei tipi di fibre muscolari in altri. È probabile che la membrana sarcolemmatica delle fibre muscolari presenti anomale proprietà di polarizzazione elettrica, oltre a essere incapace di rispondere agli stimoli trofici dei motoneuroni. La biopsia muscolare in genere non è necessaria per la diagnosi, che nei casi tipici può essere posta sulla base delle sole manifestazioni cliniche.

GENETICA. L'alterazione genetica responsabile della distrofia muscolare miotonica è localizzata sul cromosoma 19, al locus 19q13; essa consiste nell'espansione del gene DM, che codifica per una serina-treonina chinasi (*DMPK*), con numerose ripetizioni del codone CTG. Le espansioni vanno da 50 a più di 2000, mentre gli alleli normali del gene hanno da 5 a 37 espansioni; più elevato è il numero di espansioni, più severa risulta l'espressione clinica (le espansioni maggiori si riscontrano nelle forme neonatali gravi). È raro che la malattia si manifesti in assenza di ripetizioni dimostrabili; forse si tratta di una correzione spontanea di una precedente espansione, anche se il fenomeno non stato ancora completamente chiarito. Un'altra distrofia miotonica (PROMM) è una entità clinica distinta della distrofia miotonia classica, ma con una patogenesi comune mediata da un mRNA mutato, che si associa ad almeno due differenti loci cromosomici. I difetti dello splicing dell'RNA sono responsabili della resistenza all'insulina e della miotonia nelle distrofie miotoniche.

Sia l'espressione clinica sia quella genetica possono variare tra fratelli o tra un genitore affetto e il figlio. Nella grave forma neonatale della malattia, la madre è il genitore che trasmette la malattia nel 94% dei casi, un fenomeno che non si spiega solo con l'aumentata infertilità maschile. Le analisi genetiche rivelano che questi bambini generalmente hanno molte più ripetizioni del codone CTG rispetto ai genitori con la forma più comune di malattia. La distrofia miotonica spesso presenta un pattern di **anticipazione** per cui la generazione successiva ha la tendenza ad avere una forma più grave di malattia rispetto alla precedente.

TRATTAMENTO. Anche se non esiste una terapia medica specifica, spesso è possibile trattare le complicanze cardiache, endocrinologiche, gastrointestinali e oculari. Nella forma neonatale della malattia la fisioterapia e il trattamento ortopedico delle contratture possono dare qualche beneficio.

È possibile combattere la miotonia e restituire la funzione somministrando farmaci che aumentano la soglia di depolarizzazione delle membrane muscolari, quali mexiletina, fenitoina, carbamazepina, procainamide e chinidina solfato. Poiché questi farmaci hanno anche un effetto cardiotropico, è importante procedere a una valutazione cardiologica prima di prescriverli. Fenitoina e carbamazepina sono somministrate a dosi simili a quelle previste per il loro utilizzo come antiepilettici (vedi Capitolo 593.4); bisognerebbe mantenere concentrazioni sieriche di 40-80 μmol/L per la fenitoina e 35-50 μmol/L per la carbamazepina. Se la disabilità del paziente è imputabile all'astenia più che alla miotonia, questi farmaci non hanno alcuna efficacia.

ALTRE SINDROMI MIOTONICHE. La maggior parte dei pazienti con miotonia ha una distrofia miotonica. La miotonia tuttavia non è specifica di questa malattia e si può osservare in altre condizioni più rare.

La **condrodistrofia miotonica** (**malattia di Schwartz-Jampel**) è una rara malattia congenita caratterizzata da ipertrofia muscolare generalizzata e perdita di forza. Il fenotipo dismorfico e l'aspetto radiolografico delle ossa lunghe richiamano alla mente la malattia di Morquio (vedi Capitolo 88), ma non si rilevano mucopolisaccaridi anomali. Sono presenti nanismo, anomalie articolari e blefarofimosi. Molti pazienti sono figli di consanguinei, osservazione suggestiva di ereditarietà autosomica recessiva. La proteina muscolare perlecan, codificata dal gene SJS1, un grosso proteoglicano eparansolfato delle membrane basali e delle cartilagini, è difettosa in alcuni casi di malattia di Schwartz-Jampel ed è responsabile sia dell'ipereccitabilità muscolare sia della condrodisplasia.

L'EMG evidenzia nelle fibre muscolari attività elettrica continua molto simile o identica alla miotonia. La biopsia muscolare evidenzia alterazioni miopatiche aspecifiche, che sono di minime entità in alcuni casi e notevoli in altri. Il sistema sarcotubulare è dilatato.

La **miotonia congenita** (**malattia di Thomsen**) è una canalopatia (Tab. 608-1) caratterizzata da perdita di forza e ipertrofia muscolare generalizzata, tanto che i bambini affetti sembrano dei culturisti. La miotonia è un aspetto predominante e può svilupparsi all'età di 2-3 anni, quindi prima che nella distrofia miotonica. La malattia è clinicamente stabile e sembra non progredire per molti anni. La biopsia muscolare mostra minime alterazioni patologiche e l'EMG evidenzia la miotonia. Sono state descritte diverse famiglie in cui l'ereditarietà è sia autosomica dominante (malattia di Thomsen) sia recessiva (malattia di Becker, da non confondere con la distrofia muscolare di Becker/Duchenne). Raramente la distrofia miotonica e la miotonia congenita coesistono nella stessa famiglia. La forma autosomica dominante e quella recessiva di miotonia congenita sono state mappate sullo stesso locus 7q35. Questo gene è importante per l'integrità dei canali del cloro del sarcolemma e delle membrane dei tubuli T.

La **paramiotonia** è una miotonia correlata alla temperatura, che si aggrava con il freddo e migliora con il caldo. I pazienti hanno difficoltà a nuotare nell'acqua fredda o in un clima rigido se non sono abbastanza protetti dai vestiti. La *paramiotonia congenita* (malattia di Eulenburg) è dovuta a un difetto genetico sul locus 17q13.1-13.3, lo stesso locus coinvolto nella paralisi periodica iperkaliemica. Diversamente dalla miotonia congenita, la paramiotonia è una malattia dei canali del sodio voltaggio-dipendenti, dovuta alla mutazione della subunità α. Anche la distrofia miotonica è una patologia del canale del sodio (vedi Tab. 608-1).

Nelle patologie del canale del sodio l'esercizio fisico intensifica la miotonia, mentre in quelle del canale del cloro, al contrario, l'attività fisica la allevia. Questo fenomeno può essere facilmente evocato durante l'esame obiettivo, chiedendo al paziente di chiudere gli occhi con forza per poi riaprirli, ripetutamente; questo esercizio diventa ogni volta più difficoltoso nelle malattie dei canali del sodio e più agevole nelle malattie dei canali del cloro.

608.4 • Distrofie muscolari dei cingoli

Questa denominazione viene attribuita a un gruppo di miopatie ereditarie progressive che colpiscono soprattutto i muscoli del cingolo pelvico e scapolare; talvolta anche i muscoli distali diventano atrofici e deboli. In alcune forme si sviluppano ipertrofia dei polpacci e retrazioni della caviglia, che possono creare confusione con la distrofia muscolare di Becker. Finora sono state descritte sedici forme genetiche di distrofia dei cingoli, ciascuna delle quali si manifesta in un differente locus genetico ed esprime diverse proteine alterate. Alcune comprendono malattie classificate tradizionalmente in altri gruppi, come i difetti della laminina A/C della membrana nucleare (vedi in precedenza la distrofia muscolare di Emery-Dreifuss) e alcune forme di distrofia muscolare congenita.

Le **manifestazioni cliniche** raramente cominciano a comparire prima dell'infanzia e possono manifestarsi anche più tardi, all'inizio dell'età adulta. Il dolore lombare può essere il sintomo di presentazione, perché la perdita di forza dei muscoli glutei costringe ad assumere una postura lordotica. Il paziente è generalmente costretto sulla sedia a rotelle intorno ai 30 anni. Il ritmo della progressione varia da una famiglia all'altra, ma è uniforme all'interno della stessa famiglia. Mentre la perdita di forza dei muscoli flessori ed estensori del collo è un dato costante, i muscoli faciali, della lingua e quelli con innervazione bulbare sono coinvolti raramente. Parallelamente al progredire della debolezza muscolare e dell'ipotrofia, si riducono i riflessi tendinei. È insolito osservare interessamento cardiaco. Le funzioni cognitive in genere sono conservate. La **diagnosi differenziale** clinica della distrofia muscolare dei cingoli comprende l'atrofia muscolare spinale giovanile (malattia di Kugelberg-Welander), la miastenia grave e le miopatie metaboliche.

La maggior parte delle distrofie muscolari dei cingoli è autosomica recessiva, ma alcune famiglie esprimono un tratto autosomico dominante; in quest'ultimo caso spesso il decorso è benigno, con deficit funzionali lievi.

L'EMG e la biopsia muscolare confermano il sospetto clinico di distrofia muscolare, ma nessuno di questi esami è specifico per porre una **diagnosi** definitiva senza l'ausilio di criteri clinici aggiuntivi. In alcuni casi, l'adalene, una glicoproteina del sarcolemma correlata alla distrofina, è deficitaria; questo specifico deficit può essere dimostrato alla biopsia muscolare con l'immunoistochimica. La CK sierica in genere è elevata, ma l'entità di questo incremento varia da una famiglia all'altra. L'ECG di solito è normale.

In una forma autosomica dominante di distrofia muscolare dei cingoli, il difetto genetico è stato localizzato sul braccio lungo

TABELLA 608-1. Canalopatie e malattie correlate

PATOLOGIA	MANIFESTAZIONI CLINICHE	MODALITÀ DI TRASMISSIONE	CROMOSOMA	GENE
Canalopatie del cloro				
Miotonia congenita				
Malattia di Thomsen	Miotonia	Autosomica dominante	7q35	*CLC1*
Malattia di Becker	Miotonia e debolezza	Autosomica recessiva	7q35	*CLC1*
Canalopatie del sodio				
Paramiotonia congenita	Paramiotonia	Autosomica dominante	17q13.1-13.3	*SCNA4A*
Paralisi periodica iperkaliemica	Paralisi periodica con miotonia e paramiotonia	Autosomica dominante	17q13.1-13.3	*CNA4A*
Paralisi periodica ipokaliemica	Paralisi periodica	Autosomica dominante	17q13.1-13.3	*SCNA4A*
Miotonie aggravate dal potassio				
Miotonia fluttuante	Miotonia	Autosomica dominante	17q13.1-13.3	*SCNA4A*
Miotonia permanente	Miotonia	Autosomica dominante	17q13.1-13.3	*SCNA4A*
Miotonia responsiva all'acetazolamide	Miotonia	Autosomica dominante	17q13.1-13.3	*SCNA4A*
Canalopatie del calcio				
Paralisi periodica ipokaliemica	Paralisi periodica	Autosomica dominante	1q31-32	Recettore della diidropiridina
Sindrome di Schwartz-Jampel (miotonia condrodistrofica)	Miotonia; dismorfismo	Autosomica recessiva	1q34.1-36.1	Perlecan
Rippling muscle disease	Muscolo costretto/rigido	Autosomica dominante	1q41	Caveolina-3
Sindrome di Anderson	Paralisi periodica, aritmia cardiaca, facies tipica	Autosomica dominante	17q23	KCNJ2-Kir2.1
Malattia di Brody	Ritardato rilassamento, senza evidenza di miotonia su EMG	Autosomica recessiva	16p12	Calcio ATPasi
Ipertermia maligna	Ritardato rilassamento indotto dagli anestetici	Autosomica dominante	19q13.1	Recettore della rianodina

ATPasi, adenosina trifosfatasi; EMG, elettromiografia.
Da Goldman L, Ausiello D: *Cecil Textbook of Medicine*, 22nd ed. Philadelphia, WB Saunders, 2004, p. 2392.

del cromosoma 5. La mutazione di una proteina associata alla distrofina nel complesso del sarcoglicano (sarcoglicanopatia) è responsabile di alcune forme autosomiche recessive di distrofia muscolare dei cingoli. L'adalene è un α-sarcoglicano, ma esistono anche altre forme di distrofia dei cingoli dovute a deficit di β-, γ- e δ-sarcoglicani. Nel muscolo liscio normale, l'α-sarcoglicano è sostituito da ε-sarcoglicano, mentre gli altri rimangono invariati.

Un altro gruppo di distrofie dei cingoli è dovuto a mutazioni alleliche del gene della disferlina (*DYSF*), gene che esprime una proteina essenziale per l'integrità del sarcolemma e che si pensa non sia associato con il complesso distrofina-glicoproteina. Siccome *DYSF* interagisce con la caveolina-3 o con calpaina-3, un suo deficit può essere secondario a deficit dei prodotti di questi altri geni. Sono stati dimostrati tratti autosomici recessivi (miopatia di Miyoshi) e autosomici dominanti; in entrambi i casi si tratta di miopatie lentamente progressive che esordiscono durante l'adolescenza o nella prima età adulta potendo interessare sia i muscoli distali sia quelli prossimali. La miocardiopatia è rara. Una CK sierica cronicamente elevata dell'ordine di migliaia di volte è un reperto tipico delle disferlinopatie. L'esame ultrastrutturale rivela una lamina basale ispessita in corrispondenza delle alterazioni del sarcolemma e la sostituzione del sarcolemma con molteplici strati di piccole vescicole. Le fibre rigenerate sono in numero superiore rispetto a quelle degenerate. Queste malattie in passato erano chiamate *iperCKemia* e *rippling muscle disease*, quest'ultima talora confusa con la miotonia.

608.5 • Distrofia muscolare facio-scapolo-omerale

La distrofia muscolare facio-scapolo-omerale, detta anche **malattia di Landouzy-Dejerine**, probabilmente non è un'unica entità nosologica, bensì un gruppo di patologie con manifestazioni cliniche simili. Normalmente è autosomica dominante; l'anticipazione genetica si osserva spesso nelle generazioni successive di una stessa famiglia, ogni volta con coinvolgimento progressivamente più grave e insorgenza sempre più precoce. La frequenza è di 1:20 000. Il meccanismo genetico della distrofia facio-scapolo-omerale autosomica dominante prevede la delezione completa di una sequenza tandem ripetuta (D4Z4) di 3,3 kb nella regione subtelomerica, sul locus 4q35. Un'area ripetuta strettamente omologa di 3,3 kb in prossimità del locus subtelomerico 10q26, con traslocazione cromosomica o conversione di sequenze tra queste due regioni, pare predisporre al riarrangiamento del DNA, che provoca la distrofia facio-scapolo-omerale.

MANIFESTAZIONI CLINICHE. Nella distrofia facio-scapolo-omerale sono i muscoli faciali e quelli del cingolo scapolo-omerale a essere colpiti dalla debolezza più precoce e più grave. La perdita di forza dei muscoli faciali differisce da quella della distrofia miotonica; anziché presentare un labbro superiore a forma di V rovesciata, nella distrofia facio-scapolo-omerale la bocca è arrotondata e come corrugata per la protrusione di entrambe le labbra. L'incapacità di chiudere completamente gli occhi durante il sonno è una comune manifestazione della perdita di forza dei muscoli faciali superiori; alcuni pazienti presentano inoltre debolezza dei muscoli extraoculari, anche se l'oftalmoplegia di rado è completa. La distrofia facio-scapolo-omerale è stata associata alla sindrome di Möbius in rare occasioni. La perdita di forza a carico dei muscoli della faringe e della lingua può essere assente, e in caso contrario non è mai così grave come quella riscontrabile a livello faciale. Possono associarsi una ipoacusia, spesso subclinica, e una vasculopatia retinica (indistinguibile dalla malattia di Coats), soprattutto nelle forme gravi con esordio nella prima infanzia.

Le scapole si presentano alate, caratteristica che spesso è già evidente nei bambini. Il profilo del deltoide è piatto o addirittura concavo, il bicipite e il tricipite brachiale sono ipotrofici e deboli. Anche i muscoli del cingolo pelvico e della coscia possono perdere forza e diventare atrofici, con comparsa del segno di Gowers e di un'andatura di Trendelenburg. La contratture articolari sono rare. Occasionalmente il primo sintomo può essere costituito dall'astenia delle dita e del polso. Un deficit del tibiale anteriore e del peroneo può provocare la caduta del piede, complicanza che peraltro di solito si verifica solo nelle forme avanzate caratterizzate da perdita di forza severa. La lordosi lombare e la cifoscoliosi sono complicanze comuni del coinvolgimento dei muscoli della colonna. La pseudoipertrofia del polpaccio non è patognomonica.

La distrofia muscolare facio-scapolo-omerale può talvolta essere una patologia non grave, che provoca un'invalidità lieve. Le manifestazioni cliniche possono non essere presenti nell'infanzia e comparire solo nella mezza età. Contrariamente alla maggior parte delle altre distrofie, è comune una distribuzione asimmetrica della debolezza muscolare.

ESAMI DI LABORATORIO. I livelli sierici di CK e altri enzimi sono molto variabili, andando da valori normali o quasi normali fino ad aumenti di diverse centinaia di volte. Si raccomanda di eseguire l'ECG, nonostante in genere non evidenzi anomalie. L'EMG rileva potenziali muscolari miopatici aspecifici. Ai fini della diagnosi sono indicati test molecolari sia nel singolo paziente, sia nei familiari.

DIAGNOSI E DIAGNOSI DIFFERENZIALE. La biopsia muscolare permette di distinguere più di una forma di distrofia facio-scapolo-omerale, in accordo con l'evidenza clinica dell'espressione *distrofie FSH*, che riunisce diverse malattie distinte. La biopsia muscolare e l'EMG permettono inoltre di distinguere una miopatia primitiva dalle malattie neurogeniche con analoga distribuzione del deficit muscolare. Gli elementi istopatologici caratteristici alla biopsia muscolare sono: un'estesa proliferazione del tessuto connettivo tra le fibre muscolari, un'importante variazione di dimensioni delle fibre, con presenza di molte miofibre ipertrofiche e atrofiche, e presenza di fibre sparse in degenerazione e rigenerazione. Si conosce inoltre una forma di distrofia muscolare facio-scapolo-omerale "infiammatoria", caratterizzata da estesi infiltrati linfocitari tra i fascicoli muscolari. Nonostante la somiglianza di questa forma con le miopatie infiammatorie come la polimiosite, non vi è evidenza di una malattia autoimmune e gli steroidi e gli immunosoppressori non modificano il decorso clinico. Una diagnosi istopatologica precisa ha importanti implicazioni terapeutiche. Il riscontro, durante la biopsia muscolare, di un quadro "infiammatorio" con cellule mononucleate in bambini di età inferiore ai 2 anni è generalmente indicativo di distrofia facio-scapolo-omerale.

TRATTAMENTO. La fisioterapia non è efficace per recuperare la forza o per rallentare la progressione della debolezza o dell'atrofia muscolare. Il piede cadente e la scoliosi possono trarre beneficio da un trattamento ortopedico. Per ottenere un miglioramento estetico dell'espressione del volto si può ricorrere alla chirurgia plastica, con impianto della fascia lata a livello del muscolo zigomatico e all'estremità zigomatica del muscolo quadrato del labbro superiore.

608.6 • Distrofia muscolare congenita

La dicitura "distrofia muscolare congenita", che di fatto è fuorviante poiché tutte le distrofie muscolari sono geneticamente determinate, viene utilizzata per indicare un gruppo di malattie distinte accomunate da un grave coinvolgimento alla nascita, ma anche, paradossalmente, da un decorso clinico in genere benigno. Di solito si trasmette come carattere autosomico recessivo.

MANIFESTAZIONI CLINICHE. I neonati spesso presentano contratture articolari o artrogriposi e ipotonia diffusa. Le masse muscolari hanno volume ridotto a livello del tronco e delle estremità. Il controllo del capo è scarso. Si può riscontrare un lieve interessamento dei muscoli faciali, ma oftalmoplegia, debolezza faringea e difficoltà di suzione sono rare. Solo una piccola percentuale di neonati presenta disfagia e necessita di supporto nutrizionale o gastrostomia. I riflessi tendinei possono essere ridotti o assenti. L'artrogriposi è comune in tutte le forme di distrofia muscolare congenita (vedi Capitolo 607.9). Le contratture congenite del gomito sono spesso associate alla distrofia muscolare congenita di Ullrich, dovuta a un difetto a carico di uno o più dei tre geni che codificano per il collagene VI, ciascuno in un locus differente.

La distrofia muscolare congenita detta di Fukuyama è la seconda distrofia muscolare più comune in Giappone (dopo quella di Duchenne) ed è stata osservata anche in bambini olandesi, tedeschi, scandinavi e turchi. Nella varietà Fukuyama, generalmente il coinvolgimento della muscolatura scheletrica si accompagna a grave miocardiopatia e a malformazioni cerebrali. I segni e sintomi correlati con l'interessamento di questi organi sono di notevole entità: cardiomegalia e insufficienza cardiaca, ritardo mentale, crisi comiziali, microcefalia e ritardo di accrescimento. Il difetto genetico della forma di Fukuyama è stato identificato in pazienti giapponesi al locus 8q31-33.

Il **coinvolgimento neurologico** può verificarsi anche in altre forme di distrofia muscolare congenita, oltre che in quella di Fukuyama. Lo stato mentale e neurologico sono gli elementi più variabili; un encefalo apparentemente esente da anomalie e un'intelligenza normale non escludono la diagnosi se vi sono altre manifestazioni indicative di questa miopatia. Le malformazioni cerebrali che possono verificarsi non sono di un solo tipo e vanno da una grave displasia (oloprosencefalia, lissencefalia) a quadri più lievi (agenesia del corpo calloso, eterotopia focale della corteccia cerebrale e della sostanza bianca sottocorticale, ipoplasia cerebellare). La distrofia muscolare congenita è strettamente correlata con la disgenesia cerebellare nella **sindrome di Walker-Warburg** e nella **malattia muscolo-occhio-cervello di Santavuori.** Dal punto di vista neuropatologico si osservano anomalie della migrazione dei neuroblasti nella corteccia cerebrale, nel cervelletto e nel tronco. Sono state dimostrate mutazioni genetiche della O-mannosilazione di un destroglicano, essenziale per la migrazione dei neuroblasti nel cervello fetale: *POMT1* e *POMTGnT1*. Un'altra forma distinta di distrofia muscolare congenita è caratterizzata da microcefalia e ritardo mentale.

ESAMI DI LABORATORIO. La CK presenta in genere un aumento moderato, che va da diverse centinaia ad alcune migliaia di UI/l, anche se talora si riscontra solo un rialzo di scarsa entità. L'EMG dimostra segni di miopatia aspecifici. Lo studio di tutte le forme di distrofia muscolare congenita dovrebbe includere una valutazione cardiologica e una radiografia dell'encefalo. La biopsia muscolare è essenziale per la diagnosi.

DIAGNOSI. La biopsia muscolare è diagnostica fin dal periodo neonatale. Un'estesa proliferazione del collagene endomisiale avvolge le singole fibre muscolari già alla nascita, fenomeno che anche sulle sezioni trasverse fa sembrare le fibre circondate da un involucro simile a un manicotto rigido, soprattutto durante la contrazione. Il tessuto connettivo e il grasso perimesiali risultano aumentati e l'organizzazione fascicolare del muscolo può essere sovvertita dalla fibrosi. Le colture tissutali di fibroblasti intramuscolari dimostrano un aumento della sintesi di collagene, ma una struttura normale. Le fibre muscolari hanno diametro variabile e molte presentano nuclei centrali, degenerazione miofibrillare e altre alterazioni della citoarchitettura. Si osservano fibre sparse in degenerazione e rigenerazione. Non si riscontrano infiltrati infiammatori né inclusioni anomale.

L'immunoreattività per la merosina (catena α_2 della laminina) nella regione del sarcolemma è assente in circa il 40% dei casi, mentre è normalmente espressa negli altri (Figg. 608-5 e 608-6).

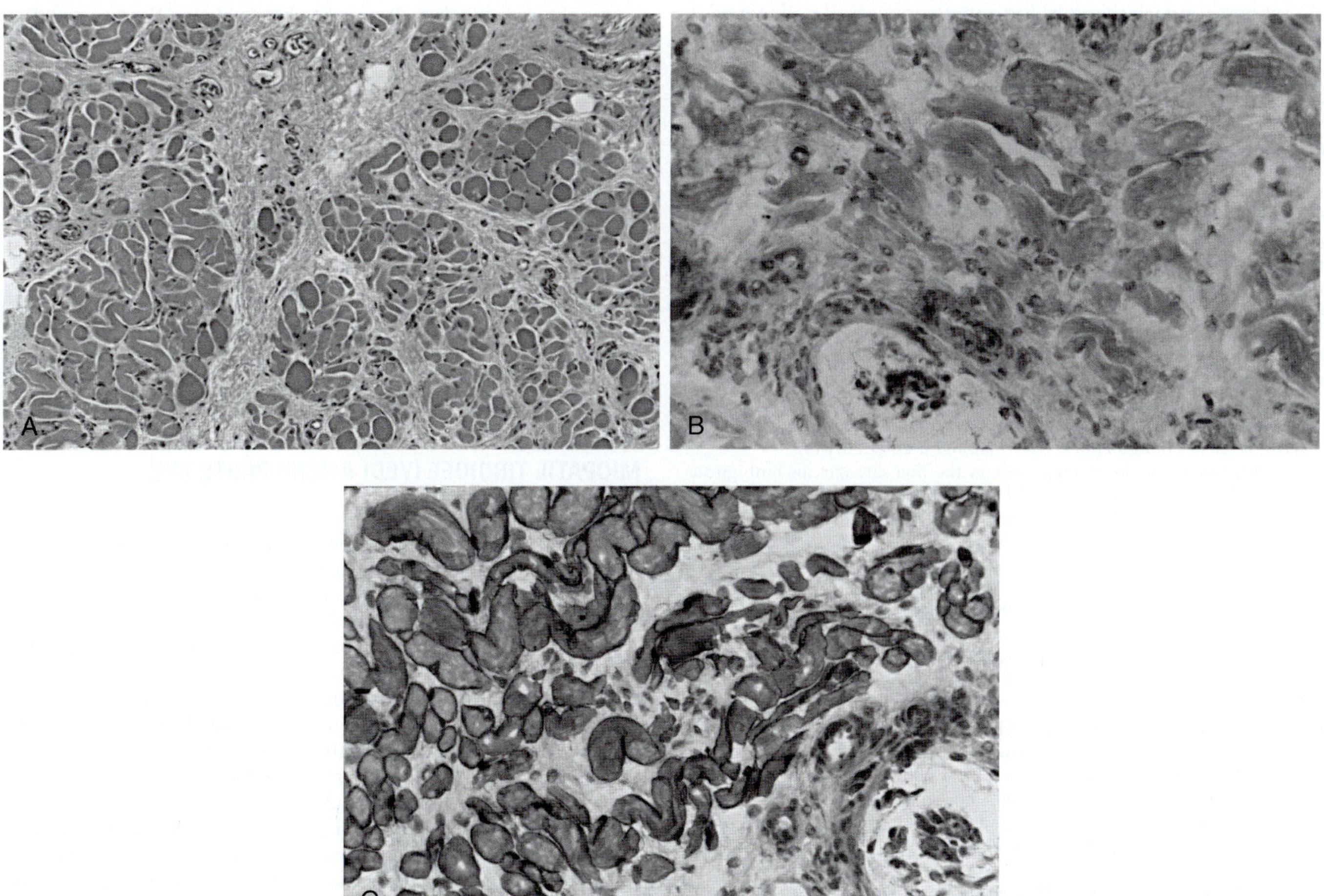

Figura 608-5. Biopsia di muscolo quadricipite femorale di una bambina di 6 mesi affetta da distrofia muscolare congenita associata a deficit di merosina (α_2-laminina). *A*, Dal punto di vista istologico, il muscolo è infiltrato da un'importante proliferazione di tessuto connettivo collagene; le miofibre hanno diametro variabile, ma quelle necrotiche sono rare. *B*, La merosina (α_2-laminina) non è espressa in nessuna fibra, neppure in quelle intrafusali del fuso neuromuscolare (in basso). *C*, Normale espressione della distrofina (rod domain). Confrontare con le Figure 608-2, 608-3 e 608-6.

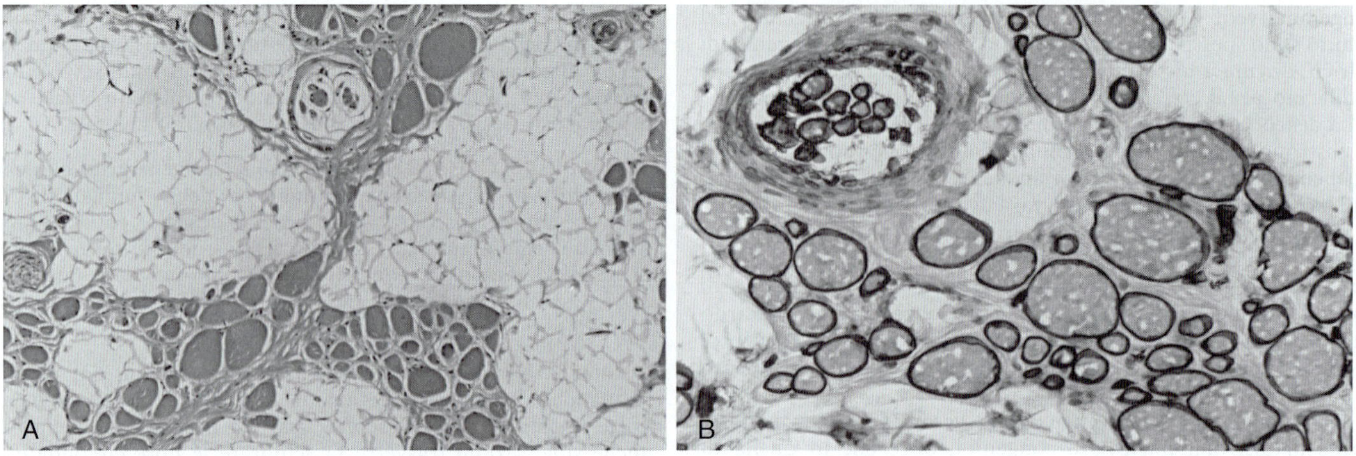

Figura 608-6. Biopsia di muscolo quadricipite femorale di una bambina di 2 anni affetta da distrofia muscolare congenita. *A*, L'architettura fascicolare del muscolo risulta gravemente alterata e il muscolo è sostituito da tessuto adiposo e fibroso; si osservano piccoli gruppi isolati di miofibre di varie dimensioni e un fuso muscolare (in alto). *B*, L'espressione della merosina è normale sia nelle fibre extrafusali, indipendentemente dalle loro dimensioni, sia in quelle intrafusali. La gravità della miopatia nella distrofia muscolare congenita non è correlata con la presenza o assenza di merosina. Confrontare con la Figura 608-5.

La merosina è una proteina che ancora la membrana del sarcolemma delle miofibre alla lamina basale o alla membrana basale; il suo deficit è dovuto a una mutazione del gene *LAMA2* sul locus 6q22-q23. La presenza o assenza di questa proteina, espressa anche nel cervello e nelle cellule di Schwann, non sempre correla con la gravità della miopatia o con la prognosi, ma i casi con deficit di merosina tendono a comportare un coinvolgimento cerebrale e una miopatia più gravi. L'adalene (α-destroglicano) può essere secondariamente ridotto in alcuni casi. Il collagene VI è selettivamente ridotto o assente nella malattia di Ullrich.

TRATTAMENTO. È possibile soltanto una terapia di supporto.

Anderson JH, Head SI, Rae C, et al: Brain function in Duchenne muscular dystrophy. *Brain* 2002;125:4–13.

Angelini C, Fanin N, Freda MP, et al: The clinical spectrum of sarcoglycanopathies. *Neurology* 1999;52:176–179.

Beenakker EAC, Fock JM, Van Tol MJ, et al: Intermittent prednisone therapy in Duchenne muscular dystrophy. *Arch Neurol* 2005;62:128–132.

Beltran Valero de Bernabe D, Currier S, Steinbrecher A, et al: Mutations in the O-mannosyltransferase gene *POMT1* give rise to the severe neuronal migration disorder Walter-Warburg syndrome. *Am J Hum Genet* 2002;71:1033–1043.

Bonne G, Muchin A, Helbling-Lecleerc A, et al: Clinical and genetical heterogeneity of laminopathies. *Acta Myologica* 2001;20:138.

Bushby KM, Beckmann JS: Pathogenesis in the non-sarcoglycan limb-girdle muscular dystrophies. *Neuromuscul Disord* 2003;13:80–90.

Campbell C, Sherlock R, Jacob P, Blayney M: Congenital myotonic dystrophy: Assisted ventilation duration and outcome. *Pediatrics* 2004;113: 811–816.

Colomer J, Iturriaga C, Bonne G, et al: Autosomal dominant Emery-Dreifuss muscular dystrophy; a new family with late diagnosis. *Neuromuscul Disord* 2002;12:19–25.

Compton AG, Cooper ST, Hill PM, et al: The syntrophin-dysbrevin subcomplex in human neuromuscular disorders. *J Neuropathol Exp Neurol* 2005;64:350–361.

Day JW, Richater K, Jacobsen JP, et al: Myotonic dystrophy type 2: Molecular, diagnostic and clinical spectrum. *Neurology* 2003;60:657–664.

Emery AEH: The muscular dystrophies. *Lancet* 2002;359:687–695.

Le Ber I, Martínez M, Campion D, et al: A non-DM1, non-DM2 multisystem myotonic disorder with frontotemporal dementia: Phenotype and suggestive mapping of the DM3 locus to chromosome 15q21-24. *Brain* 2004;127: 1979–1992.

Modoni A, Silvestri G, Pomponi MG, et al: Characterization of the pattern of cognitive impairment in myotonic dystrophy type 1. *Arch Neurol* 2004; 61:1943–1947.

Moxley RT, Meola G: Myotonic dystrophy. In Deymeer F (editor): Neuromuscular Disorders: From Basic Mechanisms to Clinical Management. *Monogr Clin Neurosci* 2000;18:61–78.

Muntoni F, Torelli S, Ferlini A: Dystrophin and mutations: One gene, several proteins, multiple phenotypes. *Lancet Neurol* 2003;2:731–740.

Nicole S, Vicart S, Davoine CS, et al: Mutations of perlecan, the major proteoglycan of basement membranes, cause Schwartz-Jampel syndrome: A new mechanism for myotonia? *Acta Myologica* 2001;20:130.

Rose MR: Neurological channelopathies. *BMJ* 1998;316:1104–1105.

Ruggieri V, Lubieniecki F, Meli F, et al: Merosin-positive congenital muscular dystrophy with mental retardation, microcephaly and central nervous system abnormalities unlinked to the Fukuyama muscular dystrophy and muscular-eye-brain loci: Report of three siblings. *Neuromuscul Disord* 2001;11:570–578.

van Deutekom JC, Baaker E, Lemmers RJ, et al: Evidence for subtelomeric exchange of 3.3 kb tandemly repeated units between chromosomes 4q35 and 10q26: Implications for genetic counselling and etiology of *FSHD1*. *Hum Mol Genet* 1996;5:1997–2003.

Zatz M, Starling A: Calpains and disease. *N Engl J Med* 2005;352:2413–2423.

Capitolo 608 ■ Miopatie endocrine e tossiche

MIOPATIE TIROIDEE (VEDI ANCHE PARTE XXV, SEZIONE 2)

La **tireotossicosi** determina debolezza della muscolatura prossimale e dimagramento, associati ad alterazioni elettromiografiche di tipo miopatico. La tiroxina si lega alle miofibrille e, se in eccesso, rende difficoltosa la contrazione muscolare. *L'ipertiroidismo* può provocare anche miastenia grave e paralisi periodica ipokaliemica.

L'**ipotiroidismo**, che sia congenito o acquisito, provoca importante ipotonia muscolare e perdita di forza a distribuzione prossimale. Anche se la manifestazione più tipica dell'ipotiroidismo è l'ipotrofia muscolare, una forma particolare, la sindrome di Kocher-Debré-Sémélaigne, è caratterizzata da pseudoipertrofia generalizzata dei muscoli colpiti. I bambini hanno un aspetto erculeo che ricorda la miotonia congenita. Nella miopatia ipotiroidea la creatina chinasi (CK) sierica è elevata, ma ritorna a valori normali dopo terapia sostitutiva a base di ormoni tiroidei.

La biopsia muscolare nell'ipotiroidismo dimostra alterazioni miopatiche acute, come la necrosi delle miofibre e talvolta nuclei centrali. Nell'ipertiroidismo, la biopsia muscolare rivela solo lievi alterazioni miopatiche aspecifiche, senza evidenza di necrosi delle miofibre.

Le alterazioni cliniche e patologiche della miopatia ipertiroidea e di quella ipotiroidea si risolvono dopo adeguato trattamento della malattia di base. Molti dei sintomi sistemici dell'ipertiroidismo, compresi la debolezza muscolare e l'oftalmoparesi, migliorano con la somministrazione di β-bloccanti.

Iperparatiroidismo (vedi Capitolo 574). La maggior parte dei pazienti con iperparatiroidismo primario sviluppa perdita di forza, facile affaticabilità, fascicolazioni e ipotrofia muscolare, che sono reversibili dopo l'asportazione dell'adenoma paratiroideo. La CK sierica e la biopsia muscolare sono normali, mentre l'elettromiografia può evidenziare alterazioni miopatiche aspecifiche. Una piccola percentuale di pazienti sviluppa una miotonia che può essere confusa con la distrofia miotonica.

MIOPATIA INDOTTA DA STEROIDI

Sia la malattia di Cushing sia la sindrome di Cushing iatrogena, dovuta alla somministrazione esogena di corticosteroidi, possono provocare una perdita di forza muscolare progressiva, non dolorosa e simmetrica, con aumento dei livelli di CK sierica, alterazioni miopatiche all'elettromiografia e alla biopsia muscolare (vedi Capitolo 578). Si può verificare una perdita selettiva dei filamenti di miosina. Gli steroidi 9α-fluorurati, come il desametasone, il betametasone e il triamcinolone, sono quelli che più facilmente provocano la *miopatia steroidea*. Il desametasone altera l'eccesso di ceramidi nei miotubi dei muscoli in via di sviluppo. Nei pazienti con dermatomiosite o altre miopatie trattate con steroidi talvolta è difficile capire se la perdita di forza muscolare sia indotta dalla malattia di base o dall'uso di steroidi, soprattutto se sono stati somministrati a lungo. Tutti i pazienti che hanno assunto steroidi per periodi di tempo prolungati sviluppano un'atrofia reversibile delle miofibre di tipo II; questo fenomeno è un *effetto degli steroidi*, ma si parla di miopatia steroidea soltanto in caso di progressione verso la miopatia necrotizzante. In età pediatrica sono a più elevato rischio i pazienti che necessitano di trattamento steroideo prolungato per asma, artrite reumatoide, dermatomiosite, lupus e altre patologie autoimmuni o infiammatorie, e quelli trattati per leucemia e altre malattie ematologiche. Miopatie acute o croniche possono essere provocate, oltre che dagli steroidi, anche dall'uso di altri farmaci (Tab. 609-1).

L'**iperaldosteronismo** (sindrome di Conn) provoca debolezza muscolare episodica e reversibile, simile a quella delle paralisi periodiche. La miopatia prossimale può diventare irreversibile nelle forme croniche. Durante gli attacchi acuti talvolta si possono osservare un aumento dei livelli di CK e persino mioglobinuria.

L'**aumento cronico dell'ormone della crescita** (talora assunto illecitamente da atleti adolescenti) o l'acromegalia determinano atrofia di alcune fibre e ipertrofia di altre, con degenerazione sparsa. Nonostante l'ormone della crescita stimoli la sintesi proteica, si osserva una riduzione dell'attività dell'ATPasi miofibrillare e dell'eccitabilità del sarcolemma, con conseguente diminuzione, anziché aumento, della forza delle corrispondenti masse muscolari aumentate di volume.

TABELLA 609-1. Miopatie tossiche

Infiammatorie
Cimetidina
D-Penicillamina
Procainamide
L-Triptofano
L-Dopa
Non infiammatorie necrotizzanti o vacuolari
Ipocolesterolemizzanti
Clorochina
Colchicina
Emetina
Acido ε-aminocaproico
Labetalolo
Ciclosporina e tacrolimus
Acido isoretinoico (analoghi della vitamina A)
Vincristina
Alcol
Rabdomiolisi e mioglobinuria
Ipocolesterolemizzanti
Alcol
Eroina
Amfetamine
Toluene
Cocaina
Acido ε-aminocaproico
Pentazocina
Fenciclidina
Ipertermia maligna
Alotano
Etilene
Dietiletere
Metossiflurano
Etilcloruro
Tricloroetilene
Gallamina
Succinilcolina
Mitocondriali
Zidovudina
Miotonia
Acido 2,4-*d*-clorofenossiacetico
Acido antracene-9-carbossiciclico
Ipocolesterolemizzanti
Clorochina
Ciclosporina
Perdita di miosina
Agenti bloccanti neuromuscolari non depolarizzanti
Glucocorticoidi somministrati ev

Da Goldman L, Ausiello D: *Cecil Textbook of Medicine*, 22nd ed, 2004, Saunders, Philadelphia, p 2399.

Hilton-Jones D, Squier M, Taylor D, et al: *Metabolic Myopathies*. Philadelphia, WB Saunders, 1995.

Mastaglia FL, Ojeda VJ, Sarnat HB, et al: Myopathies associated with hypothyroidism. *Aust N Z J Med* 1988;18:799–806.

Shee CD: Risk factors for hydrocortisone myopathy in acute, severe asthma. *Respir Med* 1990;84:229–233.

Capitolo 610 ■ Miopatie metaboliche

La diagnosi differenziale delle miopatie metaboliche è riportata nella Tabella 610-1.

610.1 • PARALISI PERIODICHE (POTASSIO-CORRELATE)

Episodi di ipostenia o paralisi reversibili, noti come **paralisi periodiche**, si associano a transitorie alterazioni dei livelli sierici di potassio (per lo più ipokaliemia, ma talora anche iperkaliemia). Tutte le forme familiari di paralisi periodica sono provocate da mutazioni di geni che codificano per i canali ionici sodio, calcio e potassio voltaggio-dipendenti nei muscoli (vedi Tab. 608-1). Durante gli attacchi, le miofibre non sono elettricamente eccitabili, anche se il sistema contrattile è normalmente sensibile agli ioni calcio. Si tratta di una malattia autosomica dominante. In alcuni pazienti la crisi è scatenata da pasti copiosi ricchi di carboidrati, insulina, adrenalina (anche indotta da stress emotivi), iperaldosteronismo o ipertiroidismo, somministrazione di amfotericina B o ingestione di liquirizia. Nella **paralisi periodica iperkaliemica**, i geni difettosi sono localizzati nel locus 17q13.1-13.3, lo stes-

TABELLA 610-1. Miopatie metaboliche e mitocondriali

DEFICIT DEL METABOLISMO DEL GLICOGENO
Tipo II: deficit di α-1,4 glucosidasi (maltasi acida)
Tipo III: deficit dell'enzima deramificante
Tipo IV: deficit dell'enzima ramificante
Tipo V: deficit di miofosforilasi (malattia di McArdle)*
Tipo VII: deficit di fosfofruttochinasi (malattia di Tarui)*
Tipo VIII: deficit di fosforilasi-b chinasi*
Tipo IX: deficit di fosfoglicerato chinasi*
Tipo X: deficit di fosfoglicerato mutasi*
Tipo XI: deficit di lattato deidrogenasi*
DEFICIT DEL METABOLISMO LIPIDICO
Deficit di carnitina palmitoiltransferasi*
Deficit primitivo sistemico/muscolare di carnitina
Deficit secondario di carnitina
Difetti della β-ossidazione
Farmaci (acido valproico)
DEFICIT DEL METABOLISMO PURINICO
Deficit di mioadenilato deaminasi*
MIOPATIE MITOCONDRIALI
Deficit del complesso piruvato-deidrogenasi (compresa la sindrome di Leigh)
Oftalmoplegia progressiva esterna
Forme autosomiche dominanti con multiple delezioni del DNA mitocondriale
Deficit del traslocatore 1 dell'adenina
TWINKLE
Deficit di gamma-polimerasi
Sindrome di Kearns-Sayre
Encefalopatia mitocondriale con episodi di acidosi lattica ed episodi simil-ictali
Epilessia mioclonica e fibre "rosse-irregolari"
Encefalomiopatia mitocondriale neurogastrointestinale
Sindrome con deplezione mitocondriale
Sindrome di Leigh e neuropatia, atassia, retinite pigmentosa
Deficit di succinato deidrogenasi*

*Questi deficit possono provocare scarsa tolleranza allo sforzo e mioglobinuria.
Da Goldman L, Ausiello D: *Cecil Textbook of Medicine*, 22nd ed. Philadelphia, WB Saunders, 2004, p 2392.

so della paramiotonia congenita, mentre nella **paralisi periodica ipokaliemica** si trovano nel locus 1q31-32.

Gli attacchi spesso esordiscono nell'infanzia e la malattia è quasi sempre sintomatica dopo i 10 anni, interessando ugualmente maschi e femmine. Durante l'infanzia, la paralisi periodica è un evento sporadico; i pazienti al risveglio sono incapaci di muoversi e recuperano la forza muscolare gradualmente nei minuti successivi o nell'arco di alcune ore. I muscoli che rimangono attivi anche durante il sonno, come il diaframma e il cuore, non sono interessati. Tra un attacco e l'altro, i pazienti sono normali, ma nel corso della vita adulta gli attacchi si fanno più frequenti e la malattia provoca una miopatia progressiva, con perdita di forza permanente anche nell'intervallo tra un attacco e l'altro. La frequenza degli attacchi durante l'infanzia solitamente è di uno alla settimana.

Alterazioni del potassio sierico si osservano solo durante la fase acuta, caratterizzata da paralisi, e si accompagnano a modificazioni dell'onda T all'elettrocardiogramma. L'ipokaliemia può essere secondaria ad alterazioni dei gradienti del calcio. Durante gli attacchi la creatina chinasi (CK) può andare incontro a un lieve aumento, mentre i livelli plasmatici di fosfato spesso diminuiscono. La biopsia muscolare è spesso normale negli intervalli tra un attacco e l'altro, ma durante gli attacchi si configura un quadro di miopatia vacuolare. Le modificazioni patologiche che caratterizzano le paralisi periodiche sono simili nei difetti tanto dei canali del sodio quanto di quelli del potassio, suggerendo che queste alterazioni derivino dagli episodi ripetuti di paralisi, anziché essere specifiche della singola canalopatia. I vacuoli sono formati da dilatazioni del reticolo sarcoplasmatico e invaginazioni dello spazio extracellulare nel citoplasma, e possono essere pieni di glicogeno. Non si verifica ipoglicemia.

TRATTAMENTO. Gli attacchi di paralisi da ipokaliemia rispondono bene alla somministrazione orale di potassio o anche di succhi di frutta contenenti potassio. Un basso introito di sodio e la somministrazione di acetazolamide, 125-250 mg due o tre volte al giorno nei bambini in età scolare, spesso sono in grado di impedire gli attacchi o almeno di ridurne la frequenza e la gravità. Anche la somministrazione di spironolattone, alla dose di 100-200 mg/die per os nei bambini in età scolare, può essere efficace.

610.2 • Ipertermia maligna

(Vedi anche i Capitoli 76 e 607.4.)

Questa sindrome, che generalmente si trasmette come carattere autosomico dominante, si manifesta in tutti i pazienti affetti da miopatia centrofibrillare, pur non essendo caratteristica esclusiva di tale patologia. Il gene coinvolto è localizzato nel locus 19q13.1 sia nella malattia centrofibrillare, sia nella forma senza evidenza di miopatia specifica. Sono almeno 15 le differenti mutazioni genetiche associate all'ipertermia maligna. Il gene interessato codifica per il recettore della rianodina, un canale a struttura tetramerica, che lascia passare gli ioni calcio nel reticolo sarcoplasmatico, in apposizione al canale del calcio voltaggio-dipendente del tubulo traverso. L'ipertermia maligna si osserva, per quanto raramente, nella malattia di Duchenne e nelle altre distrofie, nelle varie miopatie e in una sindrome isolata, non associata ad altre patologie muscolari. I bambini affetti possono presentare una facies caratteristica. Questa condizione può manifestarsi a qualunque età, anche nei neonati prematuri la cui madre è stata sottoposta ad anestesia generale per parto cesareo.

Gli episodi acuti sono scatenati dall'esposizione ad anestetici generali e occasionalmente ad anestetici locali. I pazienti sviluppano rapidamente febbre alta, rigidità muscolare e acidosi metabolica e respiratoria; la CK sierica aumenta fino a raggiungere le 35 000 UI/L. La mioglobinuria può provocare necrosi tubulare e insufficienza renale acuta.

La biopsia muscolare effettuata durante un episodio di ipertermia maligna o subito dopo permette di osservare necrosi delle fibre muscolari disperse, nota come rabdomiolisi. Nell'intervallo tra gli attacchi la biopsia muscolare dà risultati normali, in assenza di una miopatia cronica sottostante.

È importante riconoscere i pazienti a rischio di ipertermia maligna, poiché gli attacchi possono essere prevenuti con la somministrazione di dantrolene sodico prima dell'anestesia. Per identificare i pazienti a rischio, per esempio i fratelli, si ricorre alla prova della contrazione muscolare alla caffeina: un frammento di tessuto muscolare fresco immerso in un bagno salino viene attaccato a un misuratore di tensione e sottoposto all'effetto della caffeina e di altri farmaci; la comparsa di una contrazione anomala è diagnostica. L'alterazione del recettore è dimostrabile anche con l'analisi immunoistochimica su sezioni congelate ottenute mediante biopsia muscolare. Il gene alterato del recettore della rianodina è presente nel 50% dei pazienti; il test genetico è disponibile solo per questo gruppo. Tale recettore può inoltre essere evidenziato nella biopsia muscolare con l'immunoreattività. Un altro gene candidato è localizzato nel locus 1q31.

Oltre alla forma genetica di ipertermia maligna, alcuni farmaci possono provocare una rabdomiolisi acuta con mioglobinuria e possibile insufficienza renale, che però generalmente tendono a verificarsi in pazienti predisposti perché affetti da altre malattie metaboliche. L'acido valproico, per esempio, può provocare questa reazione in bambini con citopatie mitocondriali o con deficit di carnitina palmitoil-transferasi.

610.3 • Glicogenosi

(Vedi anche il Capitolo 87.1.)

La *glicogenosi I* (malattia di von Gierke) non è una vera miopatia, essendo provocata da un deficit della glucosio-6-fosfatasi epatica, enzima normalmente presente nel muscolo; ciononostante, i bambini affetti presentano ipotonia e una lieve debolezza muscolare le cui cause non sono state ancora chiarite.

La *glicogenosi II* (malattia di Pompe) è una malattia autosomica recessiva con deficit di maltasi acida, enzima lisosomiale della glicolisi. Delle 12 forme di glicogenosi note, il tipo II è l'unica caratterizzata dal deficit di un enzima lisosomiale. Il gene alterato si trova nel locus 17q23. Ne sono state descritte due forme: quella infantile è contraddistinta da una grave miopatia generalizzata e da miocardiopatia. I pazienti, che presentano cardiomegalia ed epatomegalia, sono diffusamente ipotonici e deboli. La CK sierica presenta un notevole aumento. La biopsia muscolare evidenzia una miopatia vacuolare con alterazione delle attività lisosomiali, quali le fosfatasi acida e alcalina. Il decesso si verifica generalmente nell'infanzia o nei primi anni di vita.

La forma dell'adolescente o dell'adulto è invece caratterizzata da una miopatia più moderata, senza cardiomegalia ed epatomegalia. Può non manifestarsi clinicamente fino all'adolescenza o l'inizio dell'età adulta, oppure essere sintomatica fin dalla prima infanzia, manifestandosi con debolezza muscolare e ipotonia. Anche nelle forme con esordio in età adulta avanzata, più della metà dei pazienti riferisce un deficit di forza muscolare sin dall'infanzia.

La CK sierica è molto elevata e la biopsia muscolare è diagnostica anche nelle fasi presintomatiche. La diagnosi di glicogenosi II viene confermata dalla valutazione quantitativa dell'attività della maltasi acida su biopsia del muscolo o del fegato. Una rara variante KM della forma più lieve del deficit di maltasi acida può presentare attività dell'enzima muscolare ai limiti inferiori, con riduzioni transitorie a valori al di sotto della soglia, ma le alterazioni evidenziabili alla biopsia muscolare sono simili, per quanto più moderate. La **malattia di Danon**, che si trasmette come carattere X-linked recessivo nel locus Xq24, è provocata da una carenza di proteina-2 della membrana lisosomiale (LAMP2), che provoca miocardiopatia ipertrofica, miopatia prossimale e ritardo mentale.

La ***glicogenosi III*** (malattia di Cori-Forbes), imputabile a un deficit dell'enzima deramificante (amilo-1,6-glucosidasi), è più comune di quanto si possa dedurre dalla frequenza con cui viene diagnosticata ed generalmente rappresenta la forma meno grave. In età pediatrica sono frequenti ipotonia, perdita di forza, epatomegalia e ipoglicemia a digiuno, che però spesso si risolvono spontaneamente, cosicché i pazienti diventano asintomatici nell'adolescenza e in età adulta. Altri pazienti presentano perdita di forza muscolare distale lentamente progressiva, cirrosi epatica, ipoglicemia ricorrente e insufficienza cardiaca, decorso cronico più severo osservabile soprattutto nella popolazione Inuit (eschimesi). Alla biopsia muscolare si possono riscontrare segni minori di miopatia, compresa la vacuolizzazione delle fibre muscolari.

La ***glicogenosi IV*** (malattia di Andersen) è un deficit dell'enzima ramificante, che determina la formazione di molecole di glicogeno anomale (amilopectina) nel fegato, nelle cellule reticoloendoteliali, nei muscoli scheletrici e nel miocardio. Ipotonia, perdita di forza generalizzata, ipotrofia muscolare e retrazioni muscolari sono i segni tipici del coinvolgimento muscolare. La maggior parte dei pazienti muore prima dei 4 anni di età per insufficienza epatica o cardiaca. Sono stati descritti anche alcuni casi di bambini che non presentavano manifestazioni neuromuscolari.

La ***glicogenosi V*** (malattia di McArdle), dovuta a un deficit della fosforilasi muscolare, si trasmette come carattere autosomico dominante nel locus 11q13. L'elemento clinico caratteristico è l'intolleranza allo sforzo, che provoca crampi, debolezza e mioglobinuria, mentre la forza è normale tra un attacco e l'altro. La CK sierica aumenta solo durante lo sforzo. Un dato clinico caratteristico è l'assenza del fisiologico aumento del lattato sierico durante il test ischemico, per l'incapacità di convertire il piruvato in lattato in condizioni di anaerobiosi *in vivo*. Il deficit di miofosforilasi può essere dimostrato sul tessuto muscolare bioptico sia istochimicamente sia biochimicamente. Alcuni pazienti hanno un difetto della fosforilasi-b chinasi muscolare (una fosforilasi attivante) monofosfato-dipendente. Il deficit di fosforilasi muscolare è stato il primo disturbo neuromuscolare diagnosticato con la RM spettroscopica, dalla quale si evince che il pH intramuscolare non diminuisce con lo sforzo e che non si verifica deplezione di ATPasi, ma la concentrazione di fosfocreatina va incontro a una riduzione eccessiva. Questa tecnica non invasiva può essere utile per alcuni pazienti, se il radiologo ha una certa esperienza con tale patologia.

Una **rara forma neonatale di deficit di miofosforilasi** rende l'alimentazione difficoltosa nella prima infanzia; può essere così grave da provocare il decesso in età neonatale oppure avere un decorso caratterizzato da debolezza lentamente progressiva, che simula una distrofia muscolare.

La prognosi a lungo termine è buona. I pazienti devono imparare a moderare l'attività fisica, ma non sviluppano gravi alterazioni miopatiche croniche né coinvolgimento cardiaco.

La ***glicogenosi VII*** (malattia di Tarui), provocata da un deficit della fosfofruttochinasi muscolare, si trasmette come malattia autosomica recessiva al locus 1cenq32; è più rara della glicogenosi V, con la quale ha in comune i sintomi di intolleranza allo sforzo, il decorso clinico e l'incapacità di convertire il piruvato in lattato. Per distinguere le due forme si ricorre allo studio biochimico sul tessuto muscolare prelevato mediante biopsia.

610.4 • MIOPATIE MITOCONDRIALI

(Vedi anche i Capitoli 87.4 e 598.2.)

Anomalie strutturali e funzionali dei mitocondri determinano alterazioni del metabolismo aerobico cellulare, della catena di trasporto degli elettroni e del ciclo di Krebs che possono provocare gravi patologie a carico dei muscoli, dell'encefalo e di altri organi. Le aberrazioni strutturali sono evidenziabili mediante esame al microscopio elettronico del campione di tessuto muscolare bioptico, che permette di osservare creste mitocondriali di forma anomala e fuse insieme a formare inclusioni paracristalline. Lo studio immunoistochimico della biopsia muscolare rivela la presenza di aggregati anomali di attività enzimatica ossidativa, miofibre sparse con perdita dell'attività della citocromo-C ossidasi, talora un aumento dei lipidi neutri imputabile a un blocco del metabolismo lipidico e fibre muscolari "ragged red", con accumuli di materiale membranoso al di sotto della membrana della fibra muscolare, evidenziabili con apposite colorazioni. Queste specifiche modificazioni istochimiche e ultrastrutturali sono più evidenti nei casi con mutazione puntiforme del tRNA mitocondriale. Ampie delezioni del DNA mitocondriale (mtDNA) pari a 5-7 kb (il singolo cromosoma mitocondriale ha 16,5 kb) si accompagnano a deficit del complesso enzimatico ossidativo della catena respiratoria, se è alterato meno del 2% dei mitocondri, anche se alla biopsia muscolare le alterazioni morfologiche o istochimiche risultano di minima entità o addirittura assenti, non rilevabili neppure con il microscopio elettronico; di conseguenza, per confermare la diagnosi si rendono necessari studi biochimici quantitativi del tessuto muscolare. Dal momento che la maggior parte delle subunità dei complessi della catena respiratoria è codificata dal DNA nucleare (nDNA) e non dal mtDNA, è possibile che si verifichi una trasmissione mendeliana autosomica anziché la trasmissione materna propria delle mutazioni puntiformi del mtDNA puro.

Sono state identificate diverse malattie mitocondriali distinte che colpiscono principalmente il muscolo striato oppure muscolo ed encefalo insieme; è possibile classificarle in malattie con fibre "ragged red" (Kearns-Sayre, MELAS [encefalopatia mitocondriale, acidosi lattica ed episodi simil-ictali], MERRF [*Myoclonic Epilepsy and Ragged Red Fibers*, epilessia mioclonica e fibre "ragged red"], oftalmoplegia esterna progressiva), associate con un difetto combinato dei complessi I e IV della catena respiratoria, e in malattie con fibre non irregolari (encefalopatia di Leigh, atrofia ottica ereditaria di Leber), associate a un coinvolgimento del complesso I o del IV singolarmente (nei bambini, è frequente un deficit combinato dei complessi III e V). La ***sindrome di Kearns-Sayre*** è caratterizzata dalla triade oftamoplegia esterna progressiva, degenerazione pigmentaria della retina ed esordio prima dei 20 anni; spesso si associano arresto cardiaco, deficit cerebellare e aumento delle proteine nel liquor. I potenziali evocati visivi sono alterati. I pazienti generalmente non lamentano debolezza ai muscoli del tronco o degli arti né disfagia. La maggior parte dei casi è sporadica.

L'*oftalmoplegia esterna cronica progressiva* può essere isolata o accompagnata da perdita di forza muscolare agli arti, disfagia e disartria. Alcuni pazienti presentano un quadro definito *oftalmoplegia plus*, caratterizzato da un coinvolgimento più esteso del sistema nervoso centrale. In alcune famiglie è stata osservata una trasmissione autosomica dominante, ma la maggior parte dei casi è sporadica.

Le ***sindromi MERRF*** e ***MELAS*** sono altre patologie mitocondriali che colpiscono i bambini. La seconda è caratterizzata da ridotto accrescimento, episodi di vomito, crisi ed eventi ischemici cerebrali ricorrenti, che provocano emiparesi, emianopsia o persino cecità corticale, e demenza. La malattia evolve come una patologia degenerativa e il decesso subentra nell'arco di pochi anni.

Altre patologie "degenerative" del sistema nervoso centrale che comprendono anche un quadro miopatico con anomalie mitocondriali sono l'**encefalopatia necrotizzante subacuta di Leigh** (vedi Capitolo 87.4) e la **malattia cerebroepatorenale (di Zellweger)** (vedi Capitolo 86.2). Un'altra miopatia mitocondriale conosciuta è provocata dal **deficit della citocromo-C ossidasi**. Anche la **distrofia muscolare oculofaringea** è essenzialmente una miopatia mitocondriale. La ***sindrome da deplezione mitocondriale della prima infanzia*** è caratterizzata da una grave riduzione delle attività enzimatiche ossidative in tutti e 5 i complessi; oltre alla diffusa debolezza muscolare, i neonati e i bambini presentano un coinvolgimento multisistemico, con insufficienza epatica, renale e cardiaca, encefalopatia e talvolta lesioni cutanee bollose o edema generalizzato. Vengono inoltre considerate di origine mitocondriale molte altre malattie rare di cui sono stati riportati solo pochi casi. Oggi è noto che alterazioni mitocondriali secondarie si osservano anche in un gran numero di malattie non mitocondriali, quali le miopatie autoimmuni infiammatorie e alcune malformazioni cerebrali, oltre a poter essere indotte da alcuni farmaci o tossine; pertanto, occorre essere cauti nel classificare le anomalie mitocondriali come difetti primitivi.

Il mtDNA è distinto dal DNA nucleare e viene ereditato esclusivamente per via materna; i mitocondri sono contenuti nel citoplasma dell'ovocita, ma non nella testa dello spermatozoo, l'unica porzione che prende parte alla fecondazione dell'ovocita. Le mutazioni del mtDNA sono 10 volte più numerose di quelle del DNA nucleare. Ciascun complesso degli enzimi respiratori del mitocondrio possiede subunità codificate dal mtDNA o dal nDNA. Il complesso II (succinato deidrogenasi, un enzima del ciclo di Krebs) possiede 4 subunità, tutte codificate nel DNA nucleare; il complesso III (ubiquinone o citocromo-b ossidasi) ne ha 9, di cui una sola è codificata dal mtDNA e 8 sono programmate dal DNA nucleare; il complesso IV (citocromo-c ossidasi) è caratterizzato da 13 subunità, delle quali solo 3 sono codificate da mtDNA. Per questo motivo, le malattie mitocondriali possono trasmettersi con modalità autosomica recessiva invece che con trasmissione strettamente materna, anche se tutti i mitocondri sono ereditati dalla madre.

Nella sindrome di Kearns-Sayre è stata identificata un'unica ampia deplezione del mtDNA, ma sono note altre varianti genetiche; nelle sindromi MERRF e MELAS sono state riconosciute mutazioni puntiformi a livello del tRNA (vedi Tab. 607-1).

Non esiste un trattamento specifico per le malattie mitocondriali, sebbene spesso, per cercare di sopperire ai deficit metabolici, si utilizzino empiricamente diversi "cocktail", comprendenti supplementi di carnitina, riboflavina, coenzima Q_{10}, acido ascorbico (vitamina C), vitamina E e altri antiossidanti. Anche se sono stati riportati alcuni dati aneddotici incoraggianti, finora non è stato pubblicato alcuno studio controllato che dimostri l'efficacia di questi trattamenti.

610.5 • MIOPATIE LIPIDICHE

(Vedi Capitolo 86.4.)

Considerati come organi del metabolismo energetico, i muscoli scheletrici sono le principali sedi del metabolismo degli acidi grassi a catena lunga, per via della loro massa voluminosa e della notevole densità dei mitocondri, nei quali gli acidi grassi vengono metabolizzati. Le malattie ereditarie del metabolismo lipidico, che provocano miopatie progressive, rappresentano un importante gruppo di malattie muscolari, relativamente comuni e spesso trattabili. L'aumento dei lipidi nelle miofibre si osserva alla biopsia muscolare di alcune, ma non di tutte, le miopatie mitocondriali ed è un segno di malattia specifico di costante riscontro, ma non è predittivo. Tra le malattie caratterizzate da fibre "ragged red", nella sindrome di Kearns-Sayre spesso si osserva un aumento dei lipidi neutri che, non essendo evidente nelle sindromi MERRF e MELAS, rappresenta un elemento diagnostico utile per il patologo.

Il ***deficit muscolare di carnitina*** è una malattia autosomica recessiva conseguente a un ridotto trasporto della carnitina assunta con la dieta attraverso la mucosa intestinale. La carnitina, introdotta con l'alimentazione ma anche sintetizzata nel fegato e nei reni a partire da lisina e metionina, è il fondamentale trasportatore di acidi grassi a catena lunga e media all'interno dei mitocondri del muscolo.

Il decorso clinico può essere caratterizzato da improvvise esacerbazioni di debolezza muscolare o può simulare una distrofia progressiva con sofferenza dei muscoli prossimali e talvolta coinvolgimento dei muscoli faciali, faringei e del miocardio. I sintomi generalmente esordiscono nella tarda infanzia o nell'adolescenza, ma possono anche non comparire prima dell'età adulta. Pur avendo una progressione lenta, la patologia può portare al decesso.

La CK sierica è lievemente aumentata. La biopsia muscolare rivela la presenza di vacuoli pieni di lipidi tra le fibre muscolari, oltre a cambiamenti aspecifici suggestivi di distrofia muscolare. I mitocondri possono apparire normali o meno. La carnitina dosata a livello del tessuto della biopsia è ridotta, mentre il livello sierico risulta normale.

Il **trattamento** arresta la progressione della malattia e può persino ripristinare la forza perduta, se la malattia non è troppo avanzata. La terapia consiste nella prescrizione di diete speciali a basso contenuto di acidi grassi a catena lunga. Gli steroidi possono aumentare il trasporto degli acidi grassi. Terapie specifiche con la somministrazione orale di L-carnitina a dosi elevate sono in grado di superare la barriera intestinale in alcuni pazienti. Alcuni soggetti migliorano anche con la somministrazione supplementare di riboflavina e altri sembrano trarre beneficio dall'assunzione di propranololo.

Il ***deficit sistemico di carnitina*** è una patologia dovuta a un'insufficiente produzione di carnitina a livello renale ed epatico e non a una miopatia primaria. Gli individui affetti da questa malattia autosomica recessiva presentano un quadro di miopatia prossimale progressiva e la biopsia muscolare rivela modificazioni simili a quelle osservabili nel deficit muscolare di carnitina; tuttavia la perdita di forza ha esordio più precoce e può essere già evidente alla nascita. Si può inoltre osservare fibroelastosi endocardica. Talvolta si verificano episodi di encefalopatia epatica acuta simili a quelli della sindrome di Reye. Gli episodi acuti sono complicati da ipoglicemia e acidosi metabolica.

La concentrazione di carnitina è ridotta a livello sierico, come nel muscolo e nel fegato. Una sindrome clinica analoga può rappresentare una complicanza della sindrome renale di Fanconi, dovuta a eccessiva perdita di carnitina attraverso le urine o per la dialisi cronica.

Il **trattamento** con la L-carnitina migliora il controllo della glicemia e i livelli sierici di carnitina, ma non corregge la chetosi o l'acidosi e non aumenta la resistenza allo sforzo.

Il ***deficit della carnitina palmitoiltransferasi (CPT) muscolare*** si manifesta con episodi di rabdomiolisi, coma e aumento della CK sierica, che possono configurare in quadro indistinguibile dalla sindrome di Reye. La CPT trasporta i residui di acil-coenzima A legati agli acidi grassi a lunga catena sulla carnitina, localizzata sulla membrana mitocondriale esterna, da cui verranno poi trasferiti all'interno dei mitocondri. La scarsa tolleranza allo sforzo e la mioglobinuria simulano le glicogenosi V e VII. L'entità dello sforzo in grado di scatenare un attacco varia da un soggetto all'altro, andando da una semplice passeggiata all'esercizio fisico intenso. La mioglobinuria è un segno incostante. Può manifestarsi ipoglicemia a digiuno. Alcuni pazienti presentano solo mialgie nella tarda adolescenza o nell'età adulta. Si tratta di una patologia a trasmissione autosomica recessiva, dovuta a un difetto sul cromosoma 1 al locus 1p32. Poiché l'acido valproico può scatenare rabdomiolisi acuta con mioglobinuria in pazienti con deficit di CPT, la sua somministrazione è da evitare nel trattamento delle crisi convulsive o dell'emicrania.

610.6 • MIOPATIA DA DEFICIT DI VITAMINA E

Il deficit di vitamina E (α-tocoferolo, un antiossidante importante per la produzione di superossido mitocondriale) provoca una miopatia molto simile alla distrofia muscolare negli animali da laboratorio. Nell'uomo sono state descritte una miopatia e una neuropatia da inadeguato introito di questo antiossidante. I pazienti con malassorbimento cronico, quelli sottoposti a dialisi per lungo tempo e i neonati prematuri che non ricevono supplementi di vitamina E sono soggetti particolarmente a rischio. Un trattamento con elevate dosi di vitamina E può correggere il deficit. È stata descritta anche una miopatia da ipervitaminosi E cronica.

Cannon SC: An expanding view for the molecular basis of familial periodic paralysis. *Neuromuscul Disord* 2000;12:533–543.
Chow CK: Vitamin E regulation of mitochondrial superoxide generation. *Biol Signals Recept* 2001;10:112–124.
Darin N, Oldfors A, Moslemi A-R, et al: Genotypes and clinical phenotypes in children with cytochrome-c-oxidase deficiency. *Neuropediatrics* 2003; 34:311–317.
Deschauer M, Wieser T, Zierz S: Muscle carnitine palmitoyltransferase II deficiency. Clinical and molecular genetic features and diagnostic aspects. *Arch Neurol* 2005;62:37–41.
Elpeleg O, Mandel H, Saada A: Depletion of the other genome-mitochondrial DNA depletion syndromes in humans. *J Mol Med* 2002;80:389–396.
Hagemans MLC, Winkel LPF, Van Doorn PA, et al: Clinical manifestations and natural course of late-onset Pompe disease in 54 Dutch patients. *Brain* 2005;128:671–677.
Kottlors M, Jaksch M, Ketelsen U-P, et al: Valproic acid triggers acute rhabdomyolysis in a patient with carnitine palmitoyltransferase type II deficiency. *Neuromuscul Disord* 2001;11:757–759.
Marín-García J, Goldenthal MJ, Sarnat HB: Probing striated muscle mitochondrial phenotype in neuromuscular disorders. *Pediatr Neurol* 2003; 29:26–33.
Nishino I, Yamamoto A, Sugie K, et al: Danon disease and related disorders. *Acta Myologica* 2001;20:120.
Sarnat HB, Marín-García J: Pathology of mitochondrial encephalomyopathies. *Can J Neurol Sci* 2005;32:152–166.
Schapira AHV: *Mitochondrial Function and Dysfunction*. New York, Academic Press, 2003.
Zimakas PJ, Rodd CJ: Glycogen storage disease type III in Inuit children. *CMAJ* 2005;172:355–358.

Capitolo 611 ■ Patologie della trasmissione neuromuscolare e del motoneurone

611.1 • MIASTENIA GRAVE

Questa malattia cronica è caratterizzata da una facile affaticabilità del muscolo striato. La causa più frequente è un blocco della giunzione neuromuscolare su base immunomediata. Il rilascio di acetilcolina (ACh) nella fessura sinaptica da parte del terminale assonico è normale, ma la membrana muscolare postsinaptica, o *placca motrice*, è meno responsiva del normale. Nella maggior parte dei casi di miastenia acquisita si ha un ridotto numero di recettori disponibili per l'ACh, per la presenza di anticorpi circolanti che si legano ai recettori. Generalmente la malattia è non ereditaria ed è di origine autoimmune. Una forma rara di miastenia grave familiare è probabilmente una malattia autosomica recessiva non associata alla presenza di anticorpi anti-recettore per l'ACh a livello plasmatico. Una forma familiare è dovuta a un deficit di ACh a livello della placca motrice terminale, detta AChE (*End plate ACh*). I neonati da madre miastenica possono presentare una sindrome miastenica neonatale transitoria, secondaria al passaggio attraverso la placenta di anticorpi diretti contro il recettore per l'ACh, da non confondere con la miastenia grave congenita (Tab. 611-1).

MANIFESTAZIONI CLINICHE. Nei bambini si distinguono tre varietà cliniche: la miastenia grave giovanile con esordio nell'infanzia, la miastenia congenita e la miastenia neonatale transitoria. Nella forma giovanile, la ptosi palpebrale e vari gradi di debolezza dei muscoli estrinseci dell'occhio sono i segni più precoci e costanti. I bambini più grandi possono lamentare diplopia e i più piccoli sono costretti a tenere aperti gli occhi con le dita o con i pollici se la ptosi è tanto severa da impedire la visione. Il riflesso fotomotore è conservato. Anche la disfagia e la debolezza della muscolatura facciale sono comuni e nella prima infanzia le difficoltà di alimentazione sono spesso il segno principale della miastenia. Altrettanto rilevante è la difficoltà del controllo del capo dovuta a un deficit dei muscoli flessori del collo. Anche se talvolta risultano colpiti solo i muscoli con innervazione bulbare, la malattia è sistemica e nella maggior parte dei casi l'ipostenia può interessare i muscoli dei cingoli e quelli distali delle mani. Non si osservano fascicolazioni, mialgie o deficit sensitivi. I riflessi osteotendinei possono essere ridotti, ma è raro che siano assenti.

La facile affaticabilità dei muscoli è il reperto caratteristico che permette di distinguere la miastenia dalla maggior parte delle altre malattie neuromuscolari. La ptosi aumenta progressivamente quando si chiede al paziente di tenere lo sguardo fisso verso l'alto per 30-90 s. Chi è affetto da questa patologia incontra grandi difficoltà nel tenere la testa sollevata dal piano del lettino mentre è disteso supino e riesce a vincere la forza di gravità soltanto per pochi secondi. Aprire e chiudere ripetitivamente le mani determina un rapido affaticamento dei muscoli della mano e i pazienti non possono tenere sollevate le braccia per più di 1-2 min, per l'affaticamento dei deltoidi. I sintomi si aggravano verso sera o per effetto della stanchezza. La disfagia può interferire con l'alimentazione e i muscoli della mascella si affaticano facilmente durante la masticazione.

Se non trattata, la miastenia grave è generalmente progressiva e può rappresentare una minaccia per la vita per il coinvolgimento dei muscoli respiratori e per il rischio di aspirazione, soprattutto se il bambino ha già altri problemi, per esempio un'infezione delle vie aeree superiori. La forma familiare della miastenia grave in genere non è progressiva.

I **figli di madri miasteniche** nel periodo neonatale possono presentare insufficienza respiratoria, incapacità a succhiare o deglutire, ipotonia generalizzata e debolezza; la loro attività motoria spontanea può essere limitata per diversi giorni o settimane, periodo durante il quale alcuni necessitano di un supporto ventilatorio e nutrizionale. Una volta che gli anticorpi anomali saranno scomparsi dal sangue e dal tessuto muscolare, i bambini recupereranno una forza normale e non presenteranno un rischio aumentato di sviluppare miastenia grave negli anni successivi. Questa sindrome della *miastenia grave neonatale transitoria* deve essere distinta dalla rara forma, spesso ereditaria, di **miastenia grave congenita**, non correlata con la miastenia materna, che è quasi sempre una malattia persistente senza possibilità di remissione spontanea (vedi Tab. 611-1).

Si distinguono tre **sindromi miasteniche congenite presinaptiche**, tutte autosomiche recessive; in alcune sono presenti gli anticorpi anti-MuSK. I bambini affetti presentano una debolezza dei muscoli estrinseci dell'occhio, di quelli faringei e respiratori e in seguito sviluppano anche un coinvolgimento dei muscoli del cingolo scapolare. L'**apnea** episodica è un problema nella

TABELLA 611-1. Caratteristiche cliniche, patologiche e neurofisiologiche di alcune sindromi miasteniche congenite

	LEMS	CMS-EA	DEFICIT DI ACHE DELLA PLACCA	MALATTIE DEL CANALE LENTO	MALATTIA DEL CANALE RAPIDO	DEFICIT DEL RECETTORE PER ACH
Modalità di trasmissione	AR-sporadica	AR	AR	AD	AR	AR
Sede del gene		17pter	3p24.2 (per il tipo 1c)	2q24-q32, 17p11-p12 & 17p13	17p13	17p13
Prodotto del gene		FIM	COLQ	CHRNA, CHRNB1 & CHRNE	CHRNE	CHRNE
Patogenesi/difetto	Autoimmune	Presinaptico	Sinaptico	Postsinaptico	Postsinaptico	Postsinaptico
Retrazioni	–	+	–	–	–	–
Riflessi osteotendinei	–	+	±	±	±	±
Manifestazioni precoci	+	+	+	Variabile	–	Variabile
Episodi di crisi	±	+	–	–	–	–
Risposta agli inibitori dell'ACh	–	+	–	–	+	+
Risposta al 3,4-DAP	Talvolta	–	–	–	Lieve risposta	+
Risposta alla chinidina	–	–	–	+	–	–
RS a bassa frequenza	Decremento	Decremento	Decremento	Decremento	Decremento	Decremento
RS ad alta frequenza	Incremento	Decremento	Decremento	Decremento	Decremento	Decremento
CMAP ripetitivi	–	–	+	+	–	–
Ampiezza del CMAP basale	+	–	–	–	–	–
MUP piccoli sull'elettromiografia	–	–	+	+	+	+
Biopsia muscolare	Normale	Normale	Alterata	Alterata	Normale	Alterata

AChE, acetilcolinesterasi; AD, autosomico dominante; AR, autosomico recessivo; CHRNA, subunità α del recettore dell'acetilcolina; CHRNB1, subunità β del recettore dell'acetilcolina; CHRNE, subunità ε del recettore dell'acetilcolina; CMAP, potenziale d'azione muscolare composto; CMS-EA (*Congenital Myasthenic Syndrome with Episodic Apnea*), sindrome miastenica congenita con episodi di apnea; COLQ, collagene Q; 3,4-DAP, 3,4-diaminopiridina; FIM (*Familial Infantile Myasthenia*), miastenia infantile familiare; LEMS (*Lambert-Eaton Myasthenic Syndrome*), sindrome miastenica di Lambert-Eaton; MUP (*Motor Unit Potential*), potenziale di unità motoria; RS (*Repetitive Stimulation*), stimolo ripetitivo; +, presente; –, assente; ±, dubbio.

Da Zafeiriou DI, Pitt M, de Sousa C: Clinical and neurophysiological characteristics of congenital myasthenic syndromes presenting in early infancy. *Brain Dev* 2004; 26: 47–52.

miastenia grave congenita. Un'altra forma sinaptica è provocata dall'assenza o da un grave deficit di AChE nella lamina basale della sinapsi e le forme postsinaptiche di miastenia sono causate da mutazioni dei geni per le subunità del recettore per l'ACh, che incidono sulla risposta sinaptica all'ACh. Un'anomalia dei recettori-canali per l'ACh, che si manifesta con un'elevata conduttanza e una chiusura troppo rapida, può essere il risultato di una mutazione puntiforme in una subunità del recettore, a carico di un unico residuo aminoacidico. I bambini con miastenia grave congenita non presentano crisi miasteniche e raramente hanno valori plasmatici elevati di anticorpi anti-ACh.

La miastenia grave talora può essere associata a ipotiroidismo, generalmente secondario a **tiroidite di Hashimoto**. È inoltre possibile l'associazione con altre malattie collagenopatie. Il timoma, che si riscontra in alcuni adulti, raramente accompagna la miastenia grave nei bambini; altrettanto raro è il carcinoma polmonare, che provoca la forma di miastenia propria soltanto dell'adulto, la **sindrome di Eaton-Lambert**. Nei bambini la miastenia grave postinfettiva è transitoria, generalmente fa seguito a un'infezione virale da varicella-zoster e si presenta entro 2-5 settimane come risposta autoimmune.

ESAMI DI LABORATORIO E DIAGNOSI. La miastenia grave è una delle poche malattie neuromuscolari in cui l'elettromiografia (EMG) è più specifica della biopsia muscolare ai fini della diagnosi. Si osserva un decremento della risposta dopo stimolazione ripetitiva del nervo; i potenziali muscolari diminuiscono rapidamente d'ampiezza finché il muscolo diventa refrattario a ulteriori stimoli. La velocità di conduzione motoria si mantiene normale. Questo tipico pattern EMG è il corrispettivo elettrofisiologico dell'esauribilità muscolare che si osserva clinicamente ed è reversibile con la somministrazione di un inibitore della colinesterasi. Il decremento può essere assente o difficile da dimostrare nei muscoli non coinvolti clinicamente. Questo fenomeno può indurre in errore negli stadi iniziali della malattia o nei pazienti che presentano solo un coinvolgimento dei muscoli estrinseci dell'occhio. Gli esami che prevedono l'applicazione di microelettrodi per lo studio dei potenziali di placca permettono di scoprire se il difetto di trasmissione è a livello pre- o post-sinaptico. Per la classificazione delle sindromi miasteniche congenite sono necessari studi elettrofisiologici particolari, quali la stima del numero di recettori per l'ACh e studi *in vitro* sulla funzione della placca. Questi studi specifici e le registrazioni patch-clamp delle proprietà cinetiche dei canali, disponibili solo presso centri specializzati, si eseguono su particolari prelievi bioptici di muscolo intercostale, comprendenti sia l'origine sia l'inserzione del muscolo. In caso di miastenia limitata ai muscoli estrinseci dell'occhio, all'elevatore della palpebra e ai muscoli faringei, l'EMG è generalmente normale se effettuato a livello dei muscoli delle estremità o del dorso, che sono invece diagnostici per la malattia generalizzata.

Gli **anticorpi anti-ACh**, che andrebbero dosati nel plasma, in realtà non sempre sono evidenziabili. Circa un terzo degli adolescenti affetti presenta un aumento degli anticorpi anti-recettore per l'ACh, che però in età prepubere è possibile dimostrare solo occasionalmente. Alcuni soggetti con miastenia giovanile, in cui non si riesce a rilevare la presenza di anticorpi anti-ACh nel siero, hanno anticorpi diretti contro il recettore per la tirosina chinasi (MuSK), anch'esso localizzato a livello della giunzione neuromuscolare, che sembra essere essenziale per lo sviluppo fetale della giunzione stessa. Alcuni casi di miastenia grave congenita sono dovuti non alla refrattarietà della membrana postsinaptica della giunzione neuromuscolare, come nella miastenia giovanile e dell'adulto, ma a insufficiente sintesi o rilascio di ACh a livello della membrana presinaptica. In alcuni casi si riscontra una mutazione del gene che codifica per l'enzima colina-acetiltransferasi ai fini della sintesi di ACh; in altri, vi è un insufficiente rilascio delle vescicole contenenti ACh. In questi pazienti il trattamento con gli inibitori della colinesterasi non è efficace.

Bisognerebbe sempre effettuare altri esami sierologici per le malattie autoimmuni, come la ricerca di anticorpi antinucleo e immunocomplessi. In caso di positività di queste indagini, dovrebbe essere in atto un più esteso coinvolgimento da malattia autoimmune, con vasculite o interessamento di altri tessuti oltre al muscolo. Si raccomanda di procedere sempre a una valutazione della funzionalità tiroidea. Il livello sierico della creatina chinasi (CK) è normale nella miastenia grave.

Il miocardio non è coinvolto e l'elettrocardiogramma è normale. La radiografia del torace spesso evidenzia un ingrandimento del timo dovuto a ipertrofia, e non alla presenza di un timoma. Tale alterazione dovrebbe essere comunque ulteriormente approfondita con l'esecuzione di una TC della parte anteriore del mediastino.

Il ruolo della biopsia muscolare convenzionale nella miastenia grave è controverso. Essa non è necessaria nella maggior parte dei casi, ma circa il 17% dei pazienti presenta alterazioni infiammatorie talora chiamate *linforragie*, che alcuni Autori interpretano come un disordine autoimmune misto, miastenico e polimiositico. La biopsia muscolare evidenzia un'atrofia aspecifica delle fibre di tipo II, simile a quella che si osserva nelle atrofie da non uso, nelle miopatie da assunzione prolungata di steroidi, nella polimialgia reumatica e in poche altre condizioni. L'esame ultrastrutturale della placca motrice evidenzia un assottigliamento delle pliche della membrana; i recettori dell'ACh sono localizzati a livello delle pliche postsinaptiche, come è stato dimostrato con la bungarotossina (veleno di serpente), che si lega in modo specifico ai recettori per l'ACh.

Il **test clinico diagnostico per la miastenia grave** prevede la somministrazione di un inibitore della colinesterasi a breve durata d'azione, generalmente il cloruro di edrofonio. La ptosi e l'oftalmoplegia migliorano entro pochi secondi e l'affaticabilità degli altri muscoli si riduce.

RACCOMANDAZIONI RELATIVE ALL'USO DEGLI INIBITORI DELLA COLINESTERASI COME TEST DIAGNOSTICO PER LA MIASTENIA GRAVE IN NEONATI E BAMBINI

PER BAMBINI DI 2 ANNI O PIÙ

1. Il bambino deve presentare una debolezza specifica che possa essere misurata, come ptosi palpebrale, disfagia o incapacità dei muscoli cervicali a sostenere il capo; la debolezza generalizzata aspecifica, senza alcun interessamento dei nervi cranici non è un criterio valido.
2. Occorre garantire un accesso venoso per rendere possibile la somministrazione di farmaci in caso di reazione avversa.
3. Si raccomanda il monitoraggio con elettrocardiogramma durante il test.
4. Si prepari una siringa con una dose di atropina solfato (0,01 mg/kg) e la si tenga pronta per una somministrazione ev al letto del paziente durante il test con l'edrofonio, qualora si rendesse necessario contrastare gli effetti muscarinici acuti dell'inibizione della colinesterasi (soprattutto crampi addominali e/o diarrea improvvisa da aumento della peristalsi, secrezioni tracheobronchiali profuse che possono ostruire le vie aeree, o (raramente) aritmie cardiache. Alcuni medici eseguono un pretrattamento con atropina in tutti i pazienti prima della somministrazione di edrofonio, ma questa pratica non è raccomandata a meno che non vi sia un'anamnesi positiva di sensibilità al farmaco. Occorre ricordare che una dose singola di atropina può provocare una midriasi pupillare prolungata (anche 14 giorni) dopo una singola dose e che gli effetti sulla pupilla della omotropina possono durare 4-7 giorni.
5. L'edrofonio cloridrato viene somministrato per via endovenosa. Si inizia con una dose di 0,04 mg/kg per accertarsi che il paziente non abbia una reazione allergica o che non sia particolarmente sensibile agli effetti collaterali muscarinici. Se questa dose è ben tollerata, la dose diagnostica da somministrare è di 0,1-0,2 mg/kg (dose massima singola pari a 10 mg, indipendentemente dal peso; in bambini di peso <30 kg, la dose massima è di 2 mg; la dose usuale per un bambino di 3-5 anni è di 5 mg). Nonostante le stesse dosi possano essere somministrate per via intramuscolare o sottocute, queste vie di somministrazione non sono raccomandate perché i risultati, molto più variabili per l'imprevedibilità dell'assorbimento, possono essere dubbi o falsamente negativi.
6. Gli effetti dovrebbero iniziare a manifestarsi entro 10 s e scomparire in 120 s; si raccomanda di quantificare la debolezza muscolare (valutando, per es. l'ampiezza dell'apertura palpebrale prima e dopo la somministrazione, il grado di oftalmoplegia esterna, la capacità di deglutire un sorso d'acqua).
7. Gli inibitori della colinesterasi con emivita prolungata, quali la piridostigmina, non sono generalmente efficaci per correggere in acuto la debolezza miastenica. È possibile ricorrere anche al test alla prostigmina (vedi oltre), che però potrebbe non essere definitivamente diagnostico come quello con l'edrofonio.

PER BAMBINI DI ETÀ INFERIORE AI 2 ANNI

1. I lattanti dovrebbero presentare uno specifico deficit astenico misurabile, come ptosi palpebrale, disfagia e incapacità dei muscoli cervicali a sostenere il capo; la debolezza generalizzata aspecifica, senza alcun interessamento dei nervi cranici, è meno semplice da valutare, anche se talora può essere considerata un criterio valido.
2. In caso di eventi avversi durante il test occorre iniziare un'infusione ev come via rapida di somministrazione dei farmaci.
3. Durante il test si raccomanda il monitoraggio elettrocardiografico.
4. Anche se il pretrattamento con atropina solfato per bloccare gli effetti muscarinici del test non è raccomandato, si dovrebbe comunque tenere a portata di mano una siringa già pronta. Se necessario, il farmaco va somministrato endovena alla dose di 0,1 mg/kg.
5. L'uso dell'edrofonio non è raccomandato in questa categoria di pazienti; infatti, non solo questo farmaco ha un effetto troppo breve per consentire una valutazione obiettiva, ma sembra aumentare l'incidenza di aritmie cardiache nei lattanti, soprattutto neonati.
6. La prostigmina metilsolfato viene somministrata per via intramuscolare alla dose di 0,04 mg/kg; se il risultato è negativo o dubbio, è possibile iniettare un'altra dose di 0,04 mg/kg 4 ore dopo la prima somministrazione (la dose usuale è di 0,5-1,5 mg). Il massimo effetto si osserva nel giro di 20-40 minuti. L'uso della prostigmina endovena è controindicato per il rischio di aritmie cardiache, compresa la fibrillazione ventricolare fatale, soprattutto nei bambini di pochi mesi.
7. Gli inibitori della colinesterasi a lunga durata d'azione somministrati per via orale, come la piridostigmina, non sono generalmente utili per valutare il beneficio immediato sulla debolezza miastenica, perché è difficile prevedere quando cominceranno ad agire e quanto durerà il loro effetto.

Dove dovrebbe essere effettuato il test? I luoghi più adatti sono un reparto di medicina d'urgenza, un reparto ospedaliero o, talvolta, lo studio medico; è di fondamentale importanza essere preparati a gestire eventuali complicanze, quali l'aritmia cardiaca o la crisi colinesterasica, come sottolineato in precedenza.

TRATTAMENTO. Alcuni pazienti con miastenia grave di lieve entità non necessitano di trattamento. Gli **inibitori della colinesterasi** sono i farmaci indicati nel trattamento di questa patologia. La neostigmina metilsolfato (0,04 mg/kg) può essere somministrata per via intramuscolare ogni 4-6 ore, ma la maggior parte dei pazienti assume neostigmina bromidrato per os, 0,4 mg/kg ogni 4-6 ore. Se il problema principale è la disfagia, il farmaco andrebbe somministrato circa 30 minuti prima dei pasti per migliorare la deglutizione. Una valida alternativa è la piridostigmina che, a fronte di dosaggi circa 4 volte maggiori di quelli della neostigmina, è dotata di una durata d'azione leggermente più lunga. Un sovradosaggio di anticolinesterasici provoca crisi colinergiche; l'atropina blocca gli effetti muscarinici, ma non quelli nicotinici, che provocano un ulteriore affaticamento della muscolatura scheletrica. Nella rara miastenia grave familiare provocata dall'assenza di AChE a livello della placca, gli anticolinesterasici non solo non sono efficaci, ma spesso aggravano la debolezza; questi pazienti possono essere trattati con efedrina o diaminopiridina, che aumentano il rilascio di ACh dagli assoni terminali.

Poiché la miastenia grave è una malattia autoimmune, il **trattamento a lungo termine** con steroidi, come il prednisone, può essere efficace. Occorre prendere in considerazione la timectomia, che può anche rappresentare un trattamento definitivo. L'intervento chirurgico è più efficace nei pazienti con un elevato titolo plasmatico di anticorpi anti-recettore dell'ACh e che sono sintomatici da meno di 2 anni, mentre non è indicato nelle forme congenite e familiari. Il trattamento dell'ipotiroidismo generalmente corregge la miastenia associata senza che vi sia bisogno di utilizzare anticolinesterasici o steroidi.

La **plasmaferesi**, pur essendo efficace in alcuni bambini (soprattutto in quelli che non rispondono agli steroidi), può dare una remissione dei sintomi solo temporanea. Le **immunoglobuline endovena** possono essere utili e andrebbero utilizzate prima della plasmaferesi, perché rappresentano un trattamento meno invasivo. Sia la plasmaferesi sia le immunoglobuline ev sembrano essere più efficaci in caso di elevati livelli di anticorpi anti-recettore per l'ACh. I pazienti refrattari possono rispondere al rituximab, un anticorpo monoclonale diretto contro l'antigene CD20 dei linfociti B.

I *neonati con miastenia grave transitoria trasmessa dalla madre* necessitano di anticolinesterasici solo per pochi giorni o, occasionalmente, poche settimane, soprattutto per permettere l'alimentazione. Di solito non sono necessari altri trattamenti.

COMPLICANZE. I bambini con miastenia grave non tollerano i farmaci che causano un blocco della trasmissione neuromuscolare, quali la succinilcolina e il pancuronio, e possono rimanere paralizzati per settimane dopo una sola somministrazione. L'anestesista deve valutare attentamente i pazienti miastenici che richiedono un anestetico chirurgico. Anche alcuni antibiotici, come gli aminoglicosidi (gentamicina e altri), possono aggravare la miastenia e andrebbero quindi evitati.

PROGNOSI. È difficile fare previsioni relativamente alla prognosi: alcuni pazienti vanno incontro a remissione spontanea dopo un periodo di mesi o anni, mentre altri presentano una malattia permanente, che si protrae nella vita adulta. Il decorso può essere migliorato con terapie immunosoppressive, timectomia e il trattamento dell'ipotiroidismo associato.

ALTRE CAUSE DI BLOCCO NEUROMUSCOLARE. Gli **organofosfati**, comunemente utilizzati come insetticidi, possono provocare una sindrome simil miastenica in bambini esposti a queste tossine (vedi Capitolo 58).

Il **botulismo** deriva dall'ingestione di cibo contenente la tossina del *Clostridium botulinum*, un bacillo anaerobio Gram-positivo, sporigeno (vedi Capitolo 207). Il miele rappresenta una comune fonte di contaminazione. Il periodo di incubazione è breve, della durata di poche ore, e i sintomi iniziali consistono in nausea, vomito e diarrea; ben presto si assiste al coinvolgimento dei nervi cranici, segnalato da diplopia, disfagia, difficoltà di suzione, debolezza della muscolatura facciale e assenza del riflesso mentoniero; infine si sviluppano ipotonia e debolezza generalizzate ed è possibile una progressione verso l'insufficienza respiratoria. Il blocco neuromuscolare è documentato con l'EMG eseguita sotto stimolazione ripetuta del nervo. Il supporto ventilatorio può essere necessario per alcuni giorni o per settimane, fino a completa eliminazione della tossina dall'organismo. Non sono disponibili antidoti specifici. La guanidina, 35 mg/kg/24 ore, può essere efficace per la debolezza dei muscoli estrinseci dell'occhio e degli arti, ma non per quella dei muscoli respiratori.

La **paralisi da puntura di zecca** deriva dall'alterazione del rilascio di ACh dagli assoni terminali, dovuto a una neurotossina che blocca la depolarizzazione; sono colpite anche le fibre nervose mieliniche di grosso calibro dei nervi motori e sensitivi. Questa tossina è prodotta dalla zecca dei boschi o dalla zecca del cane, un insetto comune nelle Montagne Rocciose e Appalachiane del Nord America. La zecca introduce la sua testa nella cute, generalmente a livello del cuoio capelluto, e la produzione di neurotossine è massima dopo circa 5-6 giorni. I sintomi motori comprendono debolezza, perdita di coordinazione e talvolta una paralisi ascendente simile a quella della sindrome di Guillain-Barré. I riflessi osteotendinei sono assenti. Sintomi sensitivi, come parestesie con sensazione di formicolio, possono verificarsi sul viso e agli arti. La diagnosi è confermata dall'EMG, dallo studio della conduzione nervosa e dall'isolamento della zecca. Occorre rimuovere il parassita completamente, avendo cura di non lasciarne la testa nella cute. Il paziente si ristabilisce in un periodo che va da alcune ore ad alcuni giorni.

611.2 • Atrofie muscolari spinali

Le atrofie spinali muscolari (SMA, *Spinal Muscolar Atrophy*) sono malattie degenerative dei motoneuroni, che esordiscono durante la vita fetale per poi aggravarsi nei primi anni di vita e nell'infanzia. Sebbene la progressiva denervazione del muscolo sia parzialmente compensata dalla reinnervazione da parte di unità motorie limitrofe, si vengono a formare unità motorie giganti, con conseguente atrofia delle fibre muscolari quando è coinvolta la reinnervazione di un motoneurone. Il motoneurone superiore non è colpito.

Le SMA vengono classificate in una grave forma neonatale (la cosiddetta **malattia di Werdnig-Hoffmann** o SMA di tipo 1), una forma intermedia con decorso progressivo più lento (SMA di tipo 2) e una forma giovanile più cronica, nota come **malattia di Kugelberg-Welander** o SMA di tipo 3. Una grave forma fetale, che generalmente conduce alla morte nel periodo perinatale, è stata descritta come SMA di tipo 0. Queste distinzioni sono cliniche, basate su età d'esordio, gravità della perdita di forza e decorso clinico; la biopsia muscolare non permette di distinguere il tipo 1 dal 2, mentre il tipo 3 presenta un pattern di denervazione/reinnervazione più simile a quello dell'età adulta. Il tipo 0 può presentare caratteristiche biologiche più simili alla miopatia miotubulare per un arresto della maturazione; nelle biopsie muscolari di pazienti con il tipo 1 e 2 si osservano anche miotubuli sparsi e altre fibre fetali immature, ma non in modo predominante. Circa il 25% dei pazienti ha la forma di tipo 1, il 50% quella di tipo 2 e il 25% quella di tipo 3; il tipo 0 è raro e si osserva in meno dell'1% dei pazienti. Alcuni soggetti presentano forme intermedie tra i tipi 1 e 2 o 2 e 3 in termini di andamento clinico. Una variante della SMA, la **malattia di Fazio-Londe**, è una forma di paralisi bulbare progressiva dovuta a una degenerazione dei motoneuroni a carico prevalentemente del tronco encefalico più che del midollo.

EZIOLOGIA. Alla base delle SMA vi è un patologico perpetuarsi del processo di morte cellulare programmata, che è normale nella vita embrionale. Il neuroectoderma primitivo produce in eccesso neuroblasti motori e altri neuroni, di cui però solo circa la metà sopravvive e matura trasformandosi in neuroni; le cellule in eccesso hanno invece un ciclo vitale breve e vanno incontro a degenerazione. Se i meccanismi preposti all'arresto fisiologico della morte cellulare programmata non intervengono entro un certo stadio, la morte neuronale può continuare nella vita fetale tardiva e nel periodo postnatale. Il gene del motoneurone superstite (SMN, *Survivor Motor Neuron*) arresta l'apoptosi (morte cellulare programmata) dei neuroblasti motori. Diversamente dalla maggior parte dei geni, che sono altamente conservati nell'evoluzione, l'*SMN* è presente solo nei mammiferi.

MANIFESTAZIONI CLINICHE. Gli elementi cardine della **SMA di tipo 1** sono grave ipotonia muscolare (Fig. 611-1), debolezza generalizzata, masse muscolari ipotrofiche, assenza dei riflessi osteotendinei, coinvolgimento della lingua, dei muscoli facciali e mascellari, con risparmio dei muscoli estrinseci dell'occhio e degli sfinteri. Il coinvolgimento del diaframma è tardivo. I lattanti sintomatici alla nascita possono soffrire di insufficienza respiratoria e sono incapaci di alimentarsi. Le retrazioni muscolari congenite, che vanno dal semplice piede equino all'artrogriposi generalizzata, si manifestano in circa il 10% dei neonati gravemente compromessi. Questi lattanti giacciono flaccidi, con scarsa capacità di movimento, e non riescono a opporsi alla forza di gravità (vedi Fig. 606-1); non sono in grado neppure di controllare il capo. Più dei due terzi muoiono nei primi due anni di vita, gli altri nella prima infanzia.

Nella **SMA di tipo 2**, i lattanti affetti sono generalmente in grado di succhiare il latte e deglutire, e la funzionalità respiratoria è adeguata nella prima infanzia. Questi bambini sviluppano una progressiva perdita di forza, ma alcuni sopravvivono fino all'età scolare o oltre, anche se costretti sulla sedia a rotelle elettrica e gravemente handicappati. La voce di timbro nasale e i problemi della deglutizione si sviluppano tardivamente. La scoliosi diventa la principale complicanza in molti pazienti con lunga sopravvivenza.

La **malattia di Kugelberg-Welander** è la forma più lieve di **SMA (tipo 3)** e i soggetti che ne sono colpiti possono apparire normali durante l'infanzia. La debolezza progressiva ha una distribuzione prossimale, con particolare coinvolgimento dei muscoli del cingolo scapolare. Il paziente è in grado di deambulare. È rara la comparsa di sintomi che denotano coinvolgimento dei muscoli con innervazione bulbare. Circa il 25% dei pazienti con questa forma di SMA presenta ipertrofia muscolare anziché ipotrofia, reperto che può facilmente creare confusione con la distrofia muscolare. La sopravvivenza è possibile senza grossi problemi fino all'età adulta. Le fascicolazioni sono un segno clinico specifico di denervazione muscolare; questo movimento vermicolare involontario e continuo, osservabile nei bambini magri a livello del deltoide, del bicipite brachiale e occasionalmente del quadricipite femorale, può essere mascherato dalla presenza di uno spesso pannicolo adiposo sottocutaneo. Le fascicolazioni sono meglio apprezzabili a livello della lingua, dove è praticamente assente il tessuto connettivo sottocutaneo, che separa i fasci muscolari dall'epitelio. Se i muscoli intrinseci della lingua sono contratti, come durante il pianto o la protrusione, le fascicolazioni sono più difficili da cogliere, rispetto a quando la lingua è rilassata.

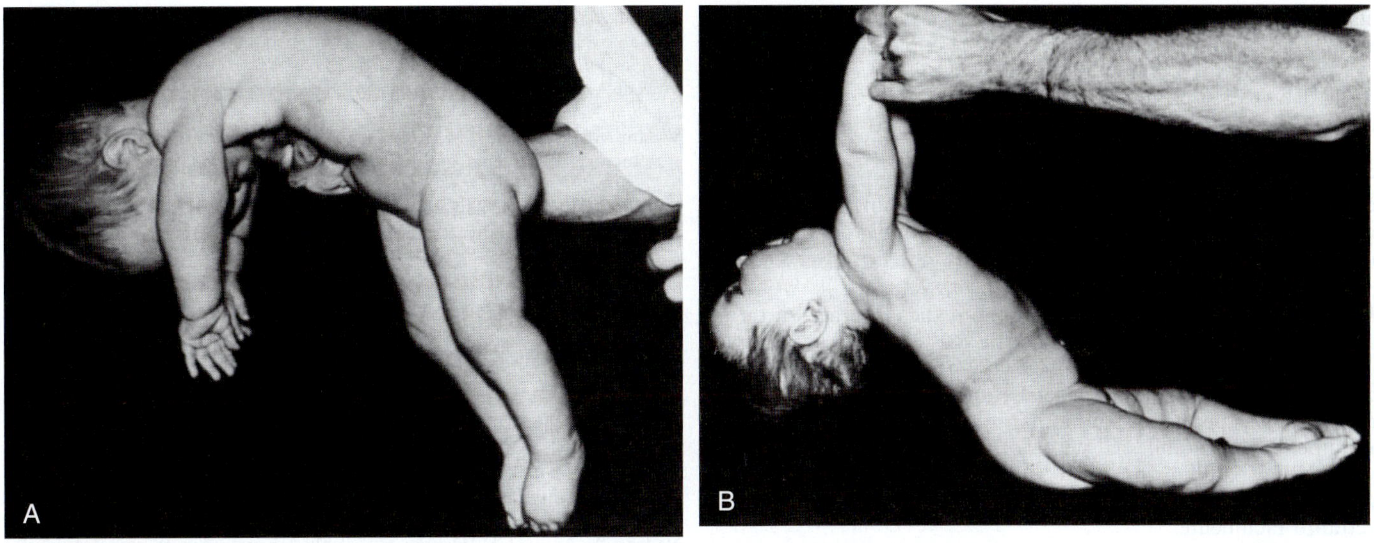

Figura 611-1. Atrofia muscolare spinale di tipo 1 (malattia di Werdnig-Hoffmann). Manifestazioni cliniche di debolezza degli arti e della muscolatura assiale in un lattante di 6 settimane, con grave debolezza e ipotonia dalla nascita. Si noti la marcata debolezza degli arti e del tronco quando il bambino viene sollevato dal ventre (*A*) e del collo quando viene sollevato in posizione seduta (*B*). (Da Volpe J: *Neurology of the Newborn*, 4th ed. Philadelphia, WB Saunders, 2001, p. 644.)

Nei bambini con SMA le dita in estensione spesso presentano un caratteristico tremore dovuto alle fascicolazioni e alla debolezza, che non va quindi confuso con il tremore di origine cerebellare. Le mialgie non sono caratteristiche delle SMA.

Il cuore non è coinvolto. L'intelligenza è normale e anzi i bambini affetti spesso sono più brillanti dei loro coetanei, poiché da una parte dedicano allo sviluppo delle capacità intellettive tutta l'energia che non possono sfogare nelle attività fisiche, e dall'altra sono più spesso a contatto con gli adulti, di cui assimilano il linguaggio, a causa delle ripercussioni sociali della malattia.

INDAGINI DI LABORATORIO. Il livello sierico di CK può essere normale, ma per lo più è moderatamente elevato, dell'ordine delle centinaia di UI; è raro il riscontro di un livello di CK dell'ordine di alcune migliaia di UI. Le velocità di conduzione dei nervi motori sono normali, eccetto che per un lieve rallentamento nelle fasi terminali della malattia; questa è una caratteristica importante, che permette di distinguere le SMA da una neuropatia periferica. L'EMG evidenzia potenziali di fibrillazione e altri segni di denervazione muscolare.

DIAGNOSI. Il test diagnostico più semplice e definitivo è la ricerca del marker molecolare per il gene *SMN* nel sangue periferico. La biopsia muscolare rivela un pattern caratteristico di denervazione perinatale, che è diverso da quello del muscolo maturo. Gruppi di fibre giganti di tipo I sono frammisti a fascicoli di fibre gravemente atrofiche appartenenti a entrambi i tipi istochimici (Fig. 611-2). Si osservano anche miofibre immature sparse che assomigliano a miotubuli. Nella SMA giovanile, il quadro può essere più simile a quello del muscolo adulto che è andato incontro a diversi cicli di denervazione e rigenerazione. Le modificazioni neurogeniche del muscolo possono essere dimostrate anche con l'EMG, ma i risultati nei bambini sono meno definitivi rispetto a quelli della biopsia. La biopsia del nervo surale occasionalmente evidenzia alterazioni neuropatiche sensitive lievi e la velocità di conduzione del nervo sensitivo può essere ridotta; è inoltre evidente un'ipertrofia degli assoni non mielinizzati. All'autopsia si osservano modeste alterazioni degenerative a carico dei neuroni sensitivi dei gangli delle radici dorsali e dei nuclei somatosensoriali del talamo, le quali tuttavia non si manifestano clinicamente con deficit sensitivi o parestesie. Le modificazioni neuropatologiche più evidenti sono l'estesa degenerazione neuronale e la gliosi nelle corna anteriori del midollo spinale e dei nuclei motori del tronco, soprattutto quello dell'ipoglosso.

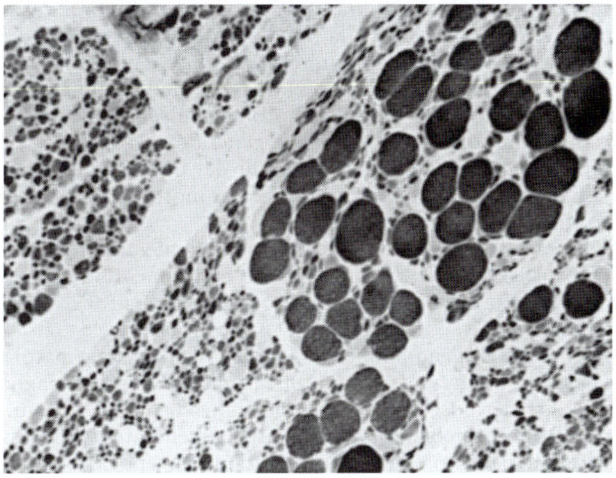

Figura 611-2. Biopsia muscolare di un neonato con atrofia muscolare spinale infantile. Si osservano gruppi di fibre giganti di tipo I (di colore scuro) tra fascicoli di miofibre gravemente atrofiche appartenenti a entrambi i tipi istochimici. Questo è il tipico quadro di denervazione perinatale del muscolo. ATPasi miofibrillare, preincubata a pH 4,6 (×400).

GENETICA. La diagnosi genetica molecolare con sonde di DNA su campioni di sangue periferico, biopsia muscolare o tessuto prelevato dai villi coriali è disponibile non solo per la diagnosi dei casi sospetti, ma anche per la diagnosi prenatale. Nella maggior parte dei casi è una malattia autosomica recessiva. La SMA, con un'incidenza di 10-15 casi su 100 000 nati vivi, colpisce tutti i gruppi etnici ed è la seconda patologia neuromuscolare in ordine di frequenza, dopo la distrofia muscolare di Duchenne. L'incidenza di eterozigoti per le SMA autosomiche recessive è di 1:50. Il locus genetico per tutte e tre le forme più comuni di SMA è sul cromosoma 5; una delezione al locus 5q11-q13 è indicativa di varianti della stessa malattia e non di malattie differenti. I geni *SMN* alterati contengono 8 esoni di 20 kb, esoni telomerici e centromerici che differiscono solo per 5 pb e producono un trascritto di 294 aminoacidi. Un altro gene, *NAIP* (*Neuronal Apoptosis Inhibitory gene*, gene che inibisce l'apoptosi neuronale), è localizzato a fianco di *SMN* e in alcuni casi si verifica una duplicazione invertita con due copie, telomerica e centromerica, di entrambi i geni; mutazioni isolate o delezioni di *NAIP* non provocano segni clinici di SMA e danno per lo più origine a un'isoforma non funzionante, priva degli aminoacidi C-terminali codificati dall'esone 7. Forme più lievi di SMA hanno più di due copie di *SMN2* e nei casi a esordio tardivo con delezione omozigote del gene *SMN1*, le copie di *SMN2* sono quattro. Un altro gene mappato sul locus 11q13-q21 può essere responsabile della precoce insufficienza respiratoria in alcuni pazienti.

Sono state descritte poche famiglie in cui la malattia si trasmette con modalità autosomica dominante; è stata inoltre segnalata una rara forma X-linked recessiva. È disponibile un test per riconoscere i portatori.

TRATTAMENTO. Non esiste alcuna terapia medica in grado di rallentare la progressione di queste malattie. La terapia di supporto comprende un'assistenza ortopedica con particolare attenzione alla scoliosi e alle retrazioni articolari, un supporto fisioterapico e meccanico per permettere ai bambini di mangiare e di essere il più indipendenti possibile dal punto di vista funzionale. La maggior parte dei bambini impara a usare la tastiera del computer con grande abilità, ma non è in grado di impugnare una matita altrettanto facilmente.

611.3 • Altre malattie dei motoneuroni

Le malattie del motoneurone sono rare nei bambini, con l'unica eccezione delle SMA. La *poliomielite* in passato era una delle principali cause di disabilità cronica, ma è diventata rara da quando è stata introdotta la vaccinazione obbligatoria (vedi Capitolo 246). Anche altri enterovirus, quali i virus *Coxsackie* ed *Echo*, o il virus attenuato del vaccino della polio possono causare un'infezione acuta dei motoneuroni con sintomi e segni simili alla poliomielite, sebbene generalmente più moderati. Specifici test con PCR e colture virali del liquor sono diagnostici. È inoltre possibile un'infezione dei motoneuroni da virus West Nile.

Nella rara **forma giovanile di sclerosi laterale amiotrofica**, dal decorso progressivo e sempre fatale, è clinicamente evidente un interessamento del primo e del secondo motoneurone, diversamente dalle SMA.

Le **malattie di Pena-Shokeir** e **Marden-Walker** sono patologie degenerative progressive dei motoneuroni, che si accompagnano a grave artrogriposi e anomalie congenite di diversi organi. Le **ipoplasie pontocerebellari** sono malattie degenerative progressive del sistema nervoso centrale che iniziano in epoca fetale; una forma coinvolge anche i motoneuroni con un quadro simile alle SMA, ma il gene *SMN* sul cromosoma 5 è normale.

I motoneuroni risultano coinvolti in molte malattie metaboliche del sistema nervoso, quali le gangliosidosi (malattia di Tay-Sachs), le ceroidolipofuscinosi (malattia di Batten) e la glicogenosi II (malattia di Pompe), nelle quali tuttavia i segni di denervazione possono essere minimi o mascherati dal più importante coinvolgimento di altre parti del sistema nervoso centrale o del muscolo.

Patologie della trasmissione neuromuscolare

Andrews PL: Autoimmune myasthenia gravis in childhood. *Semin Neurol* 2004;24:101–110.

Barisic N, Müller JS, Paucic-Kirincic E, et al: Clinical variability of CMS-EA (congenital myasthenic syndrome with episodic apnea) due to identical CHAT mutations in two infants. *Eur J Paediatr Neurol* 2005;9:7–12.

Dalakas MC: Intravenous immunoglobulin in autoimmune neuromuscular diseases. *JAMA* 2004;291:2367–2375.

Felice KJ, DiMario F, Conway SR: Postinfectious myasthenia gravis: Report of 2 cases. *J Child Neurol* 2005;20:441–444.

Harper CM: Congenital myasthenic syndromes. *Semin Neurol* 2004;24: 111–123.

Maselli RA, Kong DZ, Bowe CM, et al: Presynaptic congenital myasthenic syndrome due to quantal release deficiency. *Neurology* 2001;57:279–289.

Scherer K, Bedlack RS, Simel DL: Does this patient have myasthenia gravis? *JAMA* 2005;293:1906–1914.

Schmidt C, Abicht A, Krampfl K, et al: Congenital myasthenic syndrome due to a novel missense mutation in the gene encoding choline acetyltransferase. *Neuromuscul Disord* 2003;13:245–251.

Vincent A, McConville J, Farrugia ME, et al: Seronegative myasthenia gravis. *Semin Neurol* 2004;24:125–133.

Wylam ME, Anderson PM, Kuntz NL, Rodriguez V: Successful treatment of refractory myasthenia gravis using rituximab: A pediatric case report. *J Pediatr* 2003;143:674–677.

Zafeiriou DI, Pitt M, de Sousa C: Clinical and neurophysiological characteristics of congenital myasthenic syndromes presenting in early infancy. *Brain Dev* 2004;26:47–52.

Atrofie muscolari spinali

Chung BHY, Wong VCN, Ip P: Spinal muscular atrophy: survival pattern and functional status. *Pediatrics* 2004;114:e548–e553.

Grohmann K, Varon R, Stolz P, et al: Infantile spinal muscular atrophy with respiratory distress type 1 (SMARD1). *Ann Neurol* 2003;54:719–724.

Hardart MKM, Truog RD: Spinal muscular atrophy-type 1. *Arch Dis Child* 2003;88:848–850.

Kizilates SU, Talim B, Sel K, et al: Severe lethal spinal muscular atrophy variant with arthrogryposis. *Pediatr Neurol* 2005;32:201–204.

Nadeau A, Anjou GD, Debray FG, et al: A newborn with spinal muscular atrophy type 0 presenting with a clinicopathological picture of centronuclear myopathy. *Can J Neurol Sci* 2005;32(Suppl 1):S45.

Souchon F, Simard LR, Lebrun S, et al: Clinical and genetic study of chronic (types II and III) childhood onset spinal muscular atrophy. *Neuromuscul Disord* 1996;6:419–424.

Tachi N, Kikuchi S, Nozuka N, et al: A new mutation of *IGHMBP2* gene in spinal muscular atrophy with respiratory distress type 1. *Pediatr Neurol* 2005;32:288–290.

Capitolo 612 ■ Neuropatie sensitivo-motorie ereditarie

Le neuropatie sensitivo-motorie ereditarie (HMSN, *Hereditary Motor-Sensory Neuropathies*) sono un gruppo di malattie progressive dei nervi periferici. Il quadro clinico è in genere dominato dalla componente motoria, ma più tardivamente si può osservare anche un coinvolgimento sensitivo e autonomico.

612.1 • Atrofia muscolare peroneale (malattia di Charcot-Marie-Tooth; HMSN di tipo I)

Questa malattia è la neuropatia geneticamente determinata più comune, con una prevalenza globale di 3,8/100 000. Si trasmette come tratto autosomico dominante con una penetranza dell'83%; il gene alterato è localizzato sul locus 17p11.2. È stata descritta anche una trasmissione autosomica recessiva, che però è più rara. Il prodotto del gene interessato è la proteina mielinica periferica P22 (PMP22). Una forma ancora più rara di HMSN di tipo I associata al cromosoma X deriva da un difetto al locus Xq13.l, che provoca mutazioni nella connessina-32, la proteina delle *gap junction*.

MANIFESTAZIONI CLINICHE. La maggior parte dei pazienti è asintomatica fino alla tarda infanzia o prima adolescenza, anche se talvolta i bambini cominciano a presentare difficoltà di deambulazione già prima dei 2 anni di età. I nervi peroneale e tibiale sono i primi e i più gravemente coinvolti. I bambini affetti da questa malattia sono goffi, cadono facilmente o hanno tendenza a inciampare sui loro stessi piedi. L'esordio dei sintomi può essere tardivo e verificarsi oltre la quinta decade di vita.

I muscoli della loggia anteriore degli arti inferiori diventano atrofici conferendo alle gambe il caratteristico profilo a zampa di cicogna. L'atrofia muscolare si accompagna a una progressiva perdita di forza nella dorsiflessione della caviglia e talora a piede equino. Il processo è bilaterale, ma può essere leggermente asimmetrico. Malformazioni come il piede cavo si sviluppano invariabilmente per la denervazione dei muscoli intrinseci del piede, che contribuisce a destabilizzare ulteriormente la deambulazione. L'atrofia dei muscoli dell'avambraccio e della mano non è generalmente grave quanto quella che colpisce gli arti inferiori, ma nelle forme avanzate le contratture dei polsi e delle dita provocano la mano ad artiglio. La perdita di forza della muscolatura prossimale è un evento tardivo e generalmente lieve. I muscoli assiali non sono coinvolti.

La malattia è lentamente progressiva per tutta la vita, ma alcuni pazienti presentano un rapido deterioramento della funzionalità motoria nell'arco di pochi anni. La maggior parte dei pazienti conserva la capacità di camminare e ha una sopravvivenza normale, anche se si rendono necessari apparecchi ortopedici per stabilizzare le caviglie.

Il coinvolgimento sensitivo interessa soprattutto le grosse fibre nervose mieliniche, che veicolano la sensibilità propriocettiva e quella vibratoria, ma anche la soglia della percezione termodolorifica può aumentare. Alcuni bambini lamentano una sensazione di formicolio o bruciore ai piedi, mentre il dolore è raro. Poiché la massa muscolare è ridotta, i nervi risultano più vulnerabili ai traumi e alla compressione. L'interessamento delle fibre autonomiche può manifestarsi come uno scarso controllo vasomotorio, con comparsa di macchie o pallore sulla cute dei piedi e con la presenza di piedi freddi senza correlazione con la temperatura ambientale.

I nervi ingrossati spesso diventano palpabili. I riflessi osteotendinei sono assenti a livello distale. I nervi cranici non sono coinvolti. Il controllo degli sfinteri è conservato. La neuropatia autonomica risparmia il miocardio, il tratto gastrointestinale e la vescica. L'intelligenza è normale. Una mutazione puntiforme unica a livello di *PMP22* provoca anche una sordità progressiva per interessamento dei nervi acustici, ma questo è un evento generalmente più tardivo rispetto alla neuropatia periferica.

La **sindrome di Davidenkow** è una variante della HMSN di tipo I con distribuzione scapolo-omerale.

INDAGINI DI LABORATORIO E DIAGNOSI. Le velocità di conduzione motoria e sensitiva sono generalmente ridotte e talvolta risultano pari al 20% del normale tempo di conduzione. Nei casi di nuova diagnosi in cui non vi è una storia di familiarità, lo studio delle velocità di conduzione dovrebbe essere effettuato anche sui genitori.

L'elettromiografia (EMG) e la biopsia muscolare, pur senza essere generalmente necessarie per la diagnosi, dimostrano la presenza di molti cicli di denervazione e reinnervazione. Il livello sierico di creatina chinasi è normale. Nel liquido cerebrospinale si può riscontrare un aumento delle proteine, ma non sono presenti cellule.

La biopsia del nervo surale è diagnostica. Le fibre mielinizzate di grosso e medio calibro sono ridotte di numero, il collagene è aumentato ed è tipica la presenza di **formazioni a bulbo di cipolla** per la proliferazione del citoplasma delle cellule di Schwann intorno agli assoni. Questo quadro patologico è definito **neuropatia interstiziale ipertrofica.** Si osservano inoltre estese demielinizzazioni e remielinizzazioni segmentali.

La diagnosi molecolare genetica definitiva può essere fatta su sangue periferico.

TRATTAMENTO. La stabilizzazione delle caviglie è di primaria importanza; nelle prime fasi, spesso sono sufficienti degli stivaletti rigidi fino a metà polpaccio, soprattutto quando i pazienti camminano su superfici irregolari, come su ghiaccio, neve o pietre. Quando i flessori dorsali delle caviglie diventano più deboli, occorre adottare stecche di plastica leggera, che si estendono sotto la pianta del piede e dietro la caviglia; se indossati sotto le calze non risultano visibili, con grande vantaggio psicologico per il paziente. Quando la caduta del piede diventa completa possono essere necessari piccoli sostegni esterni per la gamba; in alcuni casi bisogna valutare la possibilità di effettuare un'artrodesi delle caviglie.

Si raccomanda di proteggere gli arti inferiori da eventi traumatici. Per prevenire le neuropatie da compressione, che si verificano durante il sonno nelle fasi più avanzate della malattia, si consiglia di sistemare dei cuscini sotto o tra le gambe. Le parestesie urenti dei piedi, peraltro poco frequenti, spesso rispondono alla somministrazione di fenitoina o carbamazepina. Non esiste un trattamento medico in grado di arrestare o rallentare la progressione della malattia.

612.2 • ATROFIA MUSCOLARE PERONEALE (DI TIPO ASSONALE)

Questa malattia è clinicamente simile alla HMSN di tipo I, ma caratterizzata da una progressione più lenta e da disabilità minore. L'EMG evidenzia una denervazione del muscolo. La biopsia del nervo surale rivela una degenerazione assonale, più che una demielinizzazione, e spirali dei processi delle cellule di Schwann tipici del tipo I. Il locus della malattia è sul cromosoma 1, a livello del locus 1p35-p36; si tratta di un'entità distinta dalla HMSN di tipo I, anche se entrambe le malattie si trasmettono come tratti autosomici dominanti.

612.3 • MALATTIA DI DÉJERINE-SOTTAS (HMSN DI TIPO III)

Questa neuropatia interstiziale ipertrofica a trasmissione autosomica dominante, pur essendo simile alla HMSN di tipo I, ha un decorso più grave. I sintomi compaiono nella prima infanzia e sono rapidamente progressivi. Le anomalie pupillari, come la scomparsa del riflesso fotomotore e la *pupilla di Argyll Robertson*, sono comuni. Alterazioni scheletriche, quali la cifoscoliosi e il piede cavo, complicano circa il 35% dei casi. I nervi risultano ipertrofici alla palpazione già nella prima infanzia.

Le formazioni a bulbo di cipolla che si osservano nella biopsia del nervo surale sono particolarmente pronunciate. Si può riscontrabile anche ipomielinizzazione.

Il locus genetico interessato, 17p11.2, è lo stesso della HMSN di tipo I o malattia di Charcot-Marie-Tooth. Le differenze cliniche e patologiche possono essere varianti fenotipiche della stessa malattia, analogamente alla situazione delle distrofie muscolari di Duchenne e Becker. È stata descritta anche una forma autosomica recessiva di malattia di Dejerine-Sottas, che però ancora non è stata ben documentata.

612.4 • SINDROME DI ROUSSY-LÉVY

Questa sindrome consiste nella combinazione di HMSN di tipo I e deficit cerebellare simile a quello dell'atassia di Friedreich, ma senza miocardiopatia.

612.5 • MALATTIA DI REFSUM

(Vedi Capitolo 86.2.)

Questa rara malattia è dovuta a un blocco enzimatico della β-ossidazione dell'acido fitanico ad acido pristanico. L'acido fitanico è un acido grasso ramificato che viene introdotto principalmente con la dieta: ne sono ricchi gli spinaci, le noci e il caffè. I livelli di acido fitanico sono enormemente aumentati nel plasma, nel liquido cerebrospinale e nel tessuto cerebrale. Il liquor mostra una dissociazione albuminocitologica con una concentrazione di proteine di 100-600 mg/dL.

L'esordio dei sintomi avviene generalmente tra i 4 e i 7 anni di età, con una neuropatia intermittente motoria e sensitiva. Si associano anche vari gradi di atassia, progressiva ipoacusia neurosensoriale, retinite pigmentosa e perdita della visione notturna, ittiosi e disfunzione epatica. Le velocità di conduzione motorie e sensitive sono ridotte. Il trattamento consiste in misure dietetiche e periodiche plasmaferesi.

612.6 • Malattia di Fabry

(Vedi Capitolo 86.4.)

Questa rara malattia correlata all'X provoca un accumulo di triesoso-ceramide per un deficit della ceramide triesosidasi, che stacca il galattosio terminale dalla triesoso-ceramide (ceramide-glucosio-galattosio-galattosio), con conseguente accumulo di questo lipide triesoso nei neuroni del sistema nervoso centrale (SNC), nelle cellule di Schwann e nelle cellule del perinervio, nei gangli del plesso mienterico, nella cute, nei reni, nelle cellule endoteliali e nella muscolatura liscia dei vasi sanguigni, nel cuore, nelle ghiandole sudoripare, nelle cornee e nel midollo osseo. È provocata da una mutazione *missense* che altera la struttura cristallografica dell'α-galattosidasi A.

MANIFESTAZIONI CLINICHE. La malattia si manifesta nella tarda infanzia o nell'adolescenza, con episodi ricorrenti di dolore urente e parestesie ai piedi e agli arti inferiori, così invalidanti da impedire al paziente di deambulare. Questi episodi sono spesso scatenati dalla febbre o dall'attività fisica. All'esame neurologico non sono evidenziabili deficit sensitivi o motori e i riflessi sono normali. Si osservano caratteristiche lesioni cutanee a livello della regione perineale, dello scroto, dei glutei e della zona periombelicale, simili a teleangectasie rosso-nere, piane o rilevate, che configurano il cosiddetto **angiocheratoma corporis diffusum**. Può essere presente ipoidrosi. Opacità corneale, cataratta e necrosi della testa del femore sono elementi che possono far parte del quadro clinico. La malattia è progressiva. Ipertensione e insufficienza renale compaiono generalmente in età adulta. Gli ictus ricorrenti sono dovuti alle alterazioni della parete vascolare. Il decesso spesso subentra nella quinta decade di vita per ischemia cerebrale o per insufficienza renale, ma una significativa morbilità può già verificarsi durante l'infanzia, anche senza gravi insufficienze d'organo.

ESAMI DI LABORATORIO. Le velocità di conduzione motorie e sensitive sono normali o di poco ridotte, a dimostrazione di un risparmio delle grosse fibre mieliniche. Le proteine nel liquido cerebrospinale sono normali. La proteinuria è un segno precoce di malattia.

In genere per ricercare le caratteristiche patologiche si ricorre dapprima alla biopsia della cute o del nervo surale. I glicosfingolipidi cristallizzati appaiono come *corpi zebrati* nei lisosomi delle cellule endoteliali, nei miociti della parete delle arteriole e nelle cellule di Schwann e sono visibili soprattutto con la microscopia elettronica. I nervi presentano una perdita selettiva delle piccole fibre mieliniche con relativo risparmio di quelle di ampie e medie dimensioni, diversamente da quanto avviene nella maggior parte delle neuropatie assonali, in cui le più coinvolte sono le grosse fibre mieliniche.

La valutazione del deficit enzimatico può essere fatta sui fibroblasti cutanei, sui leucociti o su altri tessuti. Questo test permette di individuare le donne portatrici asintomatiche e rappresenta quindi un semplice strumento per la diagnosi prenatale.

TRATTAMENTO. Per il trattamento specifico della malattia di Fabry, vedi Capitolo 86.4. La terapia medica delle neuropatie dolorose comprende la gestione delle fasi iniziali della malattia e la terapia diretta al controllo del dolore neuropatico a prescindere dall'eziologia. Il dolore può essere urente o associato a parestesie, iperalgesia (anomala risposta a stimoli dolorosi) o allodinia (sensazione dolorosa indotta da stimoli non dolorosi) (vedi Capitolo 77). Il dolore neuropatico è spesso controllato dall'uso di antidepressivi triciclici, mentre gli inibitori selettivi del reuptake della serotonina sono meno efficaci. Sono utili anche gli antiepilettici (carbamazepina, fenitoina, gabapentin, lamotrigina), come pure gli analgesici narcotici e non narcotici.

612.7 • Neuropatia assonale gigante

Questa rara malattia autosomica recessiva con esordio nella prima infanzia è una forma mista progressiva di neuropatia periferica e degenerazione della sostanza bianca centrale, simile alle leucodistrofie. Atassia e nistagmo si accompagnano a segni di neuropatia periferica progressiva. Molti bambini affetti hanno i capelli ricci, che microscopicamente presentano variazioni del diametro e attorcigliamento su se stesso del fusto, come nella malattia di Menkes, ma possono anche apparire normali. Rigonfiamenti focali degli assoni si osservano sia nel sistema nervoso periferico sia nel SNC, ma il rivestimento mielinico è intatto. La malattia è dovuta a una proliferazione generalizzata dei filamenti intermedi, compresi i neurofilamenti degli assoni, i filamenti gliali (per es. le fibre di Rosenthal) nell'encefalo, la citocheratina nei capelli e la vimentina nelle cellule di Schwann e nei fibroblasti. Si verificano mutazioni *nonsense* e *missense* o delezioni del gene *GAN*, con eterogeneità allelica, al locus 16q24. Queste mutazioni sono responsabili di un'alterata sintesi della proteina gigassonina, un componente della superfamiglia BTB/kelch del citoscheletro, fondamentale per il legame tra le proteine intermedie e la membrana cellulare. La risonanza magnetica dimostra la presenza di lesioni della sostanza bianca cerebrale simili a quelle che si osservano nelle leucodistrofie e la spettroscopia (MRS) rivela un aumento del rapporto colina/creatina e mioinositolo/creatina, a fronte di un rapporto N-acetil-aspartato/creatina normale, indicativi di demielinizzazione e proliferazione gliale senza perdita assonale. La gigassonina, espressa in diverse cellule neuronali, è localizzata nell'apparato di Golgi e nel reticolo endoplasmatico.

La diagnosi, posta con l'esame microscopico del capello e con la risonanza magnetica cerebrale e la spettroscopia, è confermata dalla biopsia del nervo e/o dallo studio genetico, se disponibile, del gene *GAN*.

612.8 • Neuropatia ipomielinica congenita

Questa malattia è imputabile a un'insufficiente mielinizzazione dei nervi motori e sensitivi periferici, ma non della sostanza bianca del SNC. Non è dovuta a una degenerazione o perdita di mielina precedentemente formata, e in questo si differenzia dalla leucodistrofia. Le cellule di Schwann sono preservate e gli assoni sono normali. Casi tra fratelli suggeriscono un'eredità di tipo autosomico recessivo. Sono state dimostrate mutazioni nei geni *MTMR2*, *PMP22*, *EGR2* e *MPZ* in diversi bambini affetti da questa neuropatia, che viene quindi considerata una sindrome anziché una singola malattia.

È una condizione presente sin dalla nascita; ipotonia e ritardo dello sviluppo sono gli elementi clinici distintivi. Alcuni pazienti presentano clinicamente un'insensibilità congenita al dolore. I nervi cranici sono poco coinvolti, l'insufficienza respiratoria e la disfagia sono complicanze rare. I riflessi osteotendinei sono assenti. In almeno la metà dei casi è presente artrogriposi alla nascita. Non è chiaro se si tratti di una malattia progressiva; la mielinizzazione dei nervi procede lentamente e rimane incompleta. Le velocità di conduzione dei nervi motori e sensitivi sono ridotte. La diagnosi è confermata dalla biopsia del nervo surale, che mette in luce un'insufficiente mielinizzazione delle grandi e piccole fibre e talvolta alterazioni ipertrofiche interstiziali reattive. La biopsia muscolare può evidenziare una lieve atrofia neurogenica, ma non le tipiche alterazioni dell'atrofia muscolare spinale. Non si osservano infiltrati infiammatori né nel muscolo né nel nervo. La terapia è solo di supporto.

612.9 • Neuropatia tomaculosa

Questa neuropatia ereditaria è caratterizzata da una produzione ridondante di mielina intorno a ogni assone in modo segmentale e irregolare, che determina la comparsa di rigonfiamenti tomaculosi (a forma di salsiccia) a livello delle singole fibre nervose mielinizzate. I nervi sono particolarmente inclini a sviluppare paralisi da compressione e i pazienti presentano mononeuropatie ricorrenti, secondarie a traumi minori. La malattia si trasmette come tratto autosomico dominante e il locus interessato è 17p11.2. Anche se la biopsia del nervo surale è diagnostica, si raccomanda di eseguire speciali preparazioni su sezioni di fibre per evidenziare più chiaramente le anomalie della mielina. Il difetto genetico consiste in una delezione di esoni in *PMP22*. La terapia è solo di supporto.

612.10 • Leucodistrofie

Diverse malattie ereditarie caratterizzate da degenerazione della sostanza bianca del SNC sono responsabili anche di neuropatie periferiche. Le più importanti sono la malattia di Krabbe (leucodistrofia a cellule globose), la leucodistrofia metacromatica e l'adenoleucodistrofia (vedi Capitolo 86).

Bruno C, Bertini E, Federico A, et al: Clinical and molecular findings in patients with giant axonal neuropathy (GAN). *Neurology* 2004;62:13–16.
Chance PF, Alderson MK, Leppig KA, et al: DNA deletion associated with hereditary neuropathy with liability to pressure palsies. *Cell* 1993;72:143–151.
Evgrafov OV, Mersiyanova I, Irobi J, et al: Mutant small heat-shock protein 27 causes axonal Charcot-Marie-Tooth disease and distal hereditary motor neuropathy. *Nat Genet* 2004;36:602–606.
Gordon N. Giant axonal neuropathy. *Dev Med Child Neurol* 2004;46:717–719.
Houlden H, Blake J, Reilly MM: Hereditary sensory neuropathies. *Curr Opin Neurol* 2004;17:569–577.
Kochanski A, Drac H, Kabzinska D, et al: A novel *MPZ* gene mutation in congenital neuropathy with hypomyelination. *Neurology* 2004;62:2122–2123.
Kovach MJ, Lin JP, Boyadjiev S, et al: A unique point mutation in the PMP22 gene is associated with Charcot-Marie-Tooth disease and deafness. *Am J Hum Genet* 1999;64:1580–1593.
Mendell JR, Sahenk Z: Painful sensory neuropathy. *N Engl J Med* 2003;348: 1243–1255.
Pleasure D: New treatments for denervating diseases. *J Child Neurol* 2005;20: 258–262.
Ries M, Gupta S, Moore DF, et al: Pediatric Fabry disease. *Pediatrics* 2005;115:344–255.
Shy ME: Charcot-Marie-Tooth disease: An update. *Curr Opin Neurol* 2004; 17:579–585.

TABELLA 613-1. Neuropatie tossiche e metaboliche

DA METALLI
Arsenico (insetticidi, erbicidi)
Piombo (vernici, batterie, stoviglie)
Mercurio (metallico, vapore)
Tallio (veleni per topi)
OCCUPAZIONALI/INDUSTRIALI
Acrilamide (cementazione, flocculazione)
Carbonio bisolfito (solventi)
Cianuro
Diclorofenossiacetato
Dimetilaminopropionitrito
Ossido di etilene (gas per sterilizzare)
Esacarboni (colla, solventi)
Esteri organofosforici (insetticidi, additivi del petrolio)
Policlorinato bifenile
Tetraclorbifenile
Tricloroetilene
DA FARMACI
Amiodarone
Cloramfenicolo
Clorochina
Cisplatino
Colchicina
Dapsone
Etambutolo
Etanolo
Oro
Idralazina
Isoniazide
Metronidazolo
Nitrofurantoina
Nucleosidi (agenti antiretrovirali ddC, ddI, d4T)
Penicillamina
Pentamidina
Fenitoina
Piridossina (eccesso)
Stilbamidina
Suramina
Talidomide
Vincristina
MALATTIE METABOLICHE
Malattia di Fabry
Malattia di Krabbe
Leucodistrofie
Porfiria
Malattia di Tangier
Tirosinemia
Uremia

Capitolo 613 ■ Neuropatie tossiche

Molte sostanze chimiche (organofosfati), tossine e farmaci sono in grado di provocare neuropatie periferiche (Tab. 613-1). L'effetto neurotossico dei metalli pesanti è ben noto. L'avvelenamento da piombo, soprattutto se cronico, provoca principalmente una neuropatia motoria selettiva a carico dei grossi nervi, come il peroneo comune, il radiale e il mediano, una condizione nota come **mononeurite multipla** (vedi Capitolo 709). L'arsenico provoca parestesie urenti dolorose e un quadro di polineuropatia motoria. L'esposizione a sostanze chimiche di origine industriale o utilizzate in ambito agricolo è una causa di neuropatia tossica meno comune nei bambini che negli adulti, ma gli insetticidi sono neurotossici sia per gli insetti sia per l'uomo e, se utilizzati sotto forma di spray in ambienti chiusi, possono venire inalati, provocando letargia, vomito, crisi epilettiche e neuropatia, soprattutto per esposizioni ripetute o prolungate nel tempo. I più esposti a questo rischio sono gli adolescenti e i bambini che lavorano nei Paesi in via di sviluppo. La tetradotossina, che viene generalmente ingerita mangiando piatti a base di pesce cotto contaminato, provoca la sindrome di Guillain-Barré.

Antimetaboliti e farmaci immunosoppressori, come la vincristina, il cisplatino e il paclitaxel, provocano polineuropatie come complicanza della chemioterapia. Questa causa "iatrogena" è la più frequente eziologia di neuropatia tossica nei bambini. In genere rappresenta una degenerazione assonale, più che una demielinizzazione primaria, contrariamente a quanto avviene nelle neuropatie autoimmuni.

L'uremia cronica è associata a neuropatia e miopatia tossiche. La neuropatia è imputabile agli eccessivi livelli circolanti di ormone paratiroideo. La riduzione dei livelli sierici di ormone paratiroideo si accompagna a un miglioramento clinico e a un ritorno ai valori normali delle velocità di conduzione nervosa.

Le neurotossine biologiche sono responsabili della paralisi da zecche, della difterite, del botulismo e delle forme di paralisi da avvelenamento da crostacei. Anche la malattia di Lyme, il virus West Nile, la lebbra, i virus herpetici (paralisi di Bell) e la rabbia provocano perdita di forza o paralisi dei nervi periferici o dei neuroni localizzati nelle corna anteriori del midollo. Diversi errori congeniti del metabolismo si associano a neuropatie periferiche per l'effetto tossico di alcuni metaboliti o per il deficit di altri (vedi Parte X e Tab. 613-1).

Capitolo 614 ■ Neuropatie autonomiche

Il coinvolgimento delle piccole fibre autonomiche, poco o per nulla mielinizzate, si può osservare in molte neuropatie periferiche; le manifestazioni autonomiche sono generalmente lievi o

TABELLA 614-1. Neuropatie autonomiche

SINDROME DI GUILLAIN-BARRÉ (GBS, *GUILLAIN-BARRÉ SYNDROME*) (VEDI CAPITOLO 615)
Forme autoimmuni non GBS
Paraneoplastiche (anticorpi nucleari antineuronali di tipo I)
Sindrome di Lambert-Eaton
Anticorpi diretti contro i recettori neuronali nicotinici per l'acetilcolina
Anticorpi diretti contro i canali del calcio P/Q
Altri autoanticorpi
Lupus eritematoso sistemico
Forme ereditarie
Autosomica dominante di tipo I
Autosomica recessiva di tipo II (malattia di Morvan)
Autosomica recessiva di tipo III (Riley-Day)
Autosomica recessiva di tipo IV (insensibilità congenita al dolore con anidrosi)
Tipo V (assenza di dolore)
Forme mataboliche
Malattia di Fabry
Diabete mellito
Malattia di Tangier
Porfiria
Forme infettive
HIV
Malattia di Chagas
Botulismo
Lebbra
Difterite
Altre forme
Sindrome della tripla A (Allgrove)
Neuropatia degli indiani Navajo
Neoplasie endocrine multiple di tipo 2b
Forme tossiche (vedi Tab. 613-1)

TABELLA 614-2. Test per la valutazione delle funzioni autonomiche

I test di valutazione della funzionalità del sistema autonomo permettono di studiare sia il sistema simpatico sia quello parasimpatico
FUNZIONALITÀ DEL SISTEMA PARASIMPATICO CARDIACO
Variabilità della frequenza cardiaca con la respirazione profonda (aritmia respiratoria sinusale); valutazione del tempo (*time-domain*) e della frequenza (*frequency-domain*)
Risposta della frequenza cardiaca alla manovra di Valsalva
Risposta della frequenza cardiaca durante la stazione eretta
FUNZIONALITÀ DEL SISTEMA SIMPATICO ADRENERGICO
Variazioni della pressione durante la stazione eretta (in piedi o con il tavolo oscillante)
Variazioni della pressione con la manovra di Valsalva
Microneurografia
FUNZIONALITÀ DEL SISTEMA SIMPATICO COLINERGICO
Test del sudore per valutare la termoregolazione
Test quantitativo del riflesso assale-sudomotore
Metodi di sweat imprint
Risposta delle simpatiche cutanee

Da Freeman R: Autonomic peripheral neuropathy. *Lancet* 2005;365:1259-1270.

TABELLA 614-3. Trattamento delle neuropatie autonomiche

PROBLEMA	PROVVEDIMENTO
Ipotensione ortostatica	Incremento della volemia e dell'apporto di sale
	Fluoridrocortisone (mineralcorticoidi)
	Midodrina (α-agonista)
Gastroparesi	Agenti procinetici (metoclopramide, domperidone, eritromicina)
Ipomotilità intestinale	Fibre, lassativi
Disfunzione urinaria	Svuotamenti programmati; cateterizzazione vescicale
Iperidrosi	Agenti anticolinergici (glicopirrolato, propantidina)
	Somministrazione sottocutanea di tossina botulinica

subcliniche. Alcune neuropatie autonomiche sono più sintomatiche e presentano vari gradi di coinvolgimento del sistema nervoso autonomo nella regolazione degli apparati cardiovascolare, gastrointestinale, genitourinario, termoregolatorio, sudoriparo e muscolare dell'iride.

Le diagnosi differenziali sono riportate nella Tabella 614-1, mentre i test per la valutazione della funzionalità del sistema nervoso autonomo sono elencati nella Tabella 614-2. La terapia generale delle disautonomie acquisite prevede il trattamento della malattia di base (lupus eritematoso sistemico, diabete) e la gestione a lungo termine delle manifestazioni specifiche per organo o apparato (Tab. 614-3). Fluttuazioni acute di sintomi autonomici si possono osservare nella sindrome di Guillain-Barré. Le rapide fluttuazioni di ipertensione o tachicardia in ipotensione o bradicardia dovrebbero essere valutate con attenzione e trattate rapidamente.

614.1 • Disautonomia familiare

La disautonomia familiare (sindrome di Riley-Day) è una malattia autosomica recessiva, comune negli ebrei dell'Europa orientale, in cui l'incidenza è di 1/10 000-20 000 e i portatori sono circa l'1%. È rara in altri gruppi etnici. Il difetto genetico è nel locus 9q31-q33. Il gene della disautonomia familiare è *IKBKAP*, con splicing aberrante e produzione di una proteina tronca. Questa a altre neuropatie autonomiche sono spesso indicate come **neurocristopatie**, poiché i tessuti compromessi sono principalmente quelli di derivazione della cresta neurale.

ANATOMIA PATOLOGICA. Questa malattia del sistema nervoso periferico è caratterizzata da una riduzione del numero di fibre amieliniche di piccolo calibro, che trasmettono la sensibilità termodolorifica e tattile e che mediano le funzioni autonomiche. Sono ridotte anche le fibre mieliniche afferenti di grosso calibro, che conducono gli impulsi dai fusi muscolari e dagli organi tendinei del Golgi. I nervi periferici e, soprattutto, quelli autonomici presentano un grado variabile di compromissione dimostrabile anatomicamente. Le papille linguali fungiformi (papille gustative) sono assenti o ridotte di numero. Il numero di cellule gangliari parasimpatiche a livello del plesso mienterico è ridotto. Si riscontra un'iperperfusione vascolare terminale nei tessuti, a fronte di un'ipoperfusione a livello degli organi e degli arti.

MANIFESTAZIONI CLINICHE. La malattia esordisce nei primi mesi di vita con difficoltà alla suzione e alla deglutizione. Si possono avere polmoniti *ab ingestis*. La difficoltà di alimentarsi rimane il sintomo principale anche durante l'infanzia. Possono verificarsi crisi di vomito. Nei neonati si può osservare sonnolenza episodica. Sono comuni l'eccessiva sudorazione e la presenza di chiazze cutanee eritematose, soprattutto durante i pasti o quando il paziente è agitato. I bambini sono a rischio per colpi di calore. L'iperidrosi episodica è dovuta a un'ipersensibilità chimica degli assoni sudomotori superstiti, più che all'iperattività delle ghiandole sudoripare. Nei primi 5 anni di vita sono comuni episodi di apnea, seguiti da una sincope. Via via che il bambino cresce, diventa evidente l'insensibilità al dolore e sono frequenti gli eventi traumatici. Sono comuni le ulcere corneali. Nuove eruzioni dei denti provocano ulcerazioni della lingua. La deambulazione è acquisita con ritardo o appare goffa o atassica per un deficit della sensibilità propriocettiva a partenza dai fusi muscolari. Probabilmente l'atassia è correlata più al deficit dei riflessi a partenza dai fusi muscolari e alla disfunzione del nervo vestibolare che non a una compromissione cerebellare. I riflessi osteotendinei sono assenti. La scoliosi è una grave complicanza nella maggior parte dei pazienti ed è generalmente progressiva. L'emissione di lacrime durante il pianto normalmente non si manifesta prima del secondo-terzo mese di vita, ma nei bambini con disautonomia familiare questa capacità può svilupparsi ancora più tardi o essere gravemente ridotta. Si osserva un'aumentata incidenza di incontinenza urinaria. Possono esservi bradicardia e altre aritmie e alcuni pazienti necessitano di impianto di pacemaker.

Circa il 40% dei pazienti ha crisi motorie generalizzate, alcune delle quali associate a ipossia acuta durante gli episodi di respiro trattenuto, altre associate a febbre alta, sebbene nella maggior parte dei casi sembrino verificarsi senza un evento scatenante. Poiché il controllo della temperatura corporea risulta carente, possono verificarsi sia ipotermia sia ipertermia. Le funzioni cognitive di solito sono compromesse, ma indipendentemente dall'epilessia. La pubertà è spesso ritardata, soprattutto nel sesso femminile. In caso di bassa statura, è possibile migliorare la velocità di crescita somministrando l'ormone della crescita. Il timbro di voce è spesso alterato o nasale.

Dopo i 3 anni iniziano le crisi autonomiche, generalmente caratterizzate da attacchi di vomito che durano 24-72 ore o talvolta anche diversi giorni. I conati di vomito, che si verificano ogni 15-20 minuti, si accompagnano a ipertensione, sudorazione profusa, comparsa di chiazze cutanee, agitazione e irritabilità. Può verificarsi una notevole distensione gastrica, che provoca dolore addominale e insufficienza respiratoria. L'ematemesi può complicare gli episodi più gravi di vomito.

La **sindrome di Allgrove** è una variante clinica, comprendente assenza di lacrime, acalasia, disautonomia con ipotensione ortostatica, vari disturbi del ritmo cardiaco e polineuropatia sensitivo-motoria, che generalmente si manifesta durante l'adolescenza. Può essere dovuta a una disfunzione colinergica.

ESAMI DI LABORATORIO. L'elettrocardiogramma rivela la presenza di intervalli QT allungati, che compensano la perdita del fisiologico accorciamento durante l'esercizio, per l'alterata regolazione autonomica della conduzione cardiaca. Le radiografie del torace evidenziano atelectasie e alterazioni polmonari simili alla fibrosi cistica. Il livello urinario dell'acido vanilmandelico è ridotto, mentre è aumentato quello dell'acido omovanillico. Il livello plasmatico della dopamina β-idrossilasi (l'enzima che converte la dopamina in adrenalina) è ridotto. La biopsia del nervo surale dimostra un numero ridotto di fibre non mieliniche. L'elettroencefalogramma è utile per studiare le crisi comiziali.

DIAGNOSI. L'infusione ev lenta di noradrenalina provoca una risposta pressoria esagerata. La risposta ipotensiva all'infusione di metacolina è aumentata. L'iniezione intradermica di istamina fosfato 1:1 000 non è in grado di provocare un normale riflesso assonale e localmente il dolore è assente o ridotto. Dal momento che la cute di un bambino normale reagisce più intensamente all'istamina, si dovrebbe utilizzare una diluizione di 1:10 000. L'instillazione di metacolina al 2,5% nel sacco congiuntivale provoca miosi nei soggetti con disautonomia familiare e nessun effetto evidente su una pupilla normale; questo è un segno aspecifico di denervazione parasimpatica dovuto a qualsiasi causa. In questo test la metacolina viene applicata in un solo occhio, mentre l'altro serve da controllo; le pupille vanno confrontate a intervalli di 5 min per 20 min. Il marcatore genetico su sangue per la diagnosi definitiva sarà disponibile in futuro.

TRATTAMENTO. Il trattamento sintomatico consiste in una particolare attenzione all'apparato respiratorio e a quello gastrointestinale, nell'uso topico di gocce di metilcellulosa o lubrificanti oculari come sostituti delle lacrime, per prevenire l'ulcerazione della cornea, nell'adozione di apparecchi ortopedici per la scoliosi e i problemi articolari e in un'adeguata terapia antiepilettica per le crisi. La clorpromazina, che, oltre a essere un efficace antiemetico, riduce l'agitazione e abbassa la pressione, può essere somministrata per via rettale, sotto forma di supposte, durante le crisi autonomiche. Si raccomanda di prevenire la disidratazione e i disturbi elettrolitici. Il betanecolo può essere un farmaco alternativo in caso di vomito protratto; è utile anche per l'enuresi, un'altra complicanza comune, e aumenta la produzione di lacrime. È importante prevenire i traumi, in quanto è assente il meccanismo protettivo rappresentato dal dolore. La scoliosi spesso richiede un trattamento chirurgico. Possono essere indicati i farmaci antiepilettici. Alcuni bambini necessitano di impianto di pacemaker. Il monitoraggio della pressione può essere importante in alcuni casi. Un approccio genetico al trattamento per ora non ancora disponibile, ma promettente, è l'utilizzo di un polifenolo per regolare l'espressione dei trascritti del gene *IKBKAP*.

PROGNOSI. La maggior parte dei pazienti muore durante l'infanzia, generalmente per insufficienza polmonare cronica o per aspirazione.

614.2 • Altre neuropatie autonomiche

NEUROPATIE DEL PLESSO MIENTERICO. Il *megacolon agangliare* (*malattia di Hirschsprung*) deriva da un mancato sviluppo embrionale dei neuroni parasimpatici sottomucosi e dei plessi mienterici di segmenti del colon e del retto. I nervi compresi tra gli strati circolari e longitudinali della muscolatura liscia della parete intestinale sono ipertrofici; sono assenti le cellule dei gangli (vedi Capitolo 329).

INSENSIBILITÀ CONGENITA AL DOLORE E ANIDROSI. Questa malattia ereditaria, con modalità di trasmissione non chiara, colpisce i maschi molto più frequentemente delle femmine e si manifesta nella prima infanzia. I pazienti hanno episodi di febbre alta in correlazione con temperature ambientali elevate, perché la sudorazione è assente. Sono frequenti le ustioni e i traumi per un'apparente perdita della capacità di percepire il dolore. L'intelligenza è normale. La biopsia nervosa rivela l'assenza quasi totale delle fibre amieliniche, che veicolano gli impulsi termodolorifici e mediano le funzioni autonomiche. Alcuni casi di neuropatia ipomielinizzante si presentano clinicamente con un'insensibilità congenita al dolore (vedi Capitolo 612.8). La risposta simpatica della cute e la valutazione elettrofisiologica sono i test diagnostici da eseguire nei casi associati a una mutazione del recettore TrKA per il fattore di crescita del nervo.

DISTROFIA SIMPATICA RIFLESSA. Questa malattia è una forma di causalgia locale, che generalmente coinvolge una mano o un piede, ma senza che vi sia corrispondenza anatomica con la distribuzione dell'innervazione periferica (vedi Capitolo 167.2). Un dolore urente continuo e l'iperestesia si associano a instabilità vasomotoria nelle zone colpite, con conseguente aumento della temperatura cutanea, arrossamento ed edema dovuti a vasodilatazione e iperidrosi. Nella forma cronica si osservano aree di cute atrofica, fredda e umida, oltre ad atrofia da non uso dei muscoli e dell'osso sottostanti. Occasionalmente può essere interessato più di un arto. Il dolore è invalidante ed esacerbato dal movimento di un'articolazione associata, anche se non sono evidenti segni di infiammazione articolare; l'immobilizzazione dà sollievo. Il più comune evento scatenante è un trauma locale, sotto forma di contusione, lacerazione, distorsione o frattura verificatasi giorni o settimane prima.

Per spiegare questo fenomeno sono state formulate diverse teorie patogenetiche. La più accreditata è quella di un'eccessiva attività riflessa del sistema autonomico in risposta agli insulti esterni; il blocco simpatico regionale spesso produce un sollievo temporaneo. Anche la fisioterapia è utile. Alcuni casi si risolvono spontaneamente dopo settimane o mesi, mentre quelli che continuano a essere sintomatici richiedono una simpatectomia. In alcuni pazienti si sospetta una componente psicogena, che è però difficile da dimostrare.

Anderson SL, Qiu J, Rubin BY: EGCG corrects aberrant splicing of IKAP mRNA in cells from patients with familial dysautonomia. *Biochem Biophy Res Commun* 2003;310:627–633.

Axelrod FB: Familial dysautonomia. *Muscle Nerve* 2004;29:352–363.

Freeman R: Autonomic peripheral neuropathy. *Lancet* 2005;365:1259–1270.

Gold-von Simson G, Rutkowski M, Berlin D, et al: Pacemakers in patients with familial dysautonomia—a review of experience with 20 patients. *Clin Autonom Res* 2005;15:15–20.

Hilz MJ, Axelrod FB, Bickel A, et al: Assessing function and pathology in familial dysautonomia: Assessment of temperature perception, sweating and cutaneous innervation. *Brain* 2004;127:2090–2098.
Kamboj MK, Axelrod FG, David R, et al: Growth hormone treatment in children with familial dysautonomia. *J Pediatr* 2004;144:63–67.

Capitolo 615 ■ Sindrome di Guillain-Barré

La sindrome di Guillain-Barré è una polineuropatia postinfettiva a carico soprattutto dei nervi motori, nonostante talvolta interessi anche quelli sensitivi e autonomici. Questa sindrome, che colpisce persone di tutte le età e non è ereditaria, è molto simile alle polineuropatie allergiche sperimentali indotte negli animali. La maggior parte dei pazienti presenta una neuropatia demielinizzante, ma in alcuni casi viene documentato un quadro di degenerazione assonale prevalente.

MANIFESTAZIONI CLINICHE. La paralisi in genere insorge a distanza di 10 giorni circa da un'infezione virale aspecifica. Tale infezione può essere caratterizzata anche soltanto da sintomi a carico dell'apparato gastroenterico (soprattutto da *Campylobacter jejuni*, ma pure da *Helicobacter pylori*) o delle vie aeree (soprattutto da *Mycoplasma pneumoniae*). Il virus West Nile, pur potendo essere a sua volta responsabile di una sindrome simile a quella di Guillain-Barré, per lo più interessa i motoneuroni determinando una patologia simile alla poliomielite. L'insorgenza della sindrome di Guillain-Barré è stata inoltre descritta dopo vaccinazione per la rabbia, l'influenza, la poliomielite (vaccino orale) ed è possibile dopo vaccinazione per l'infezione meningococcica.

La perdita di forza generalmente inizia a livello degli arti inferiori per poi estendersi al tronco, agli arti superiori e infine ai muscoli a innervazione bulbare, con un pattern noto come **paralisi ascendente di Landry**. I muscoli prossimali e distali sono coinvolti in modo relativamente simmetrico, ma un'asimmetria si riscontra in circa il 9% dei pazienti. L'esordio è graduale e progressivo nell'arco di giorni o settimane. Soprattutto nei casi a esordio improvviso, le fasi iniziali sono comunemente caratterizzate da disturbi della sensibilità tattile e dolore muscolare. I bambini affetti sono irritabili. La perdita di forza può progredire fino a incapacità o impossibilità a deambulare e, nelle fasi più avanzate, sfociare in una tetraplegia flaccida. Le parestesie sono rare. La diagnosi differenziale della perdita di forza acuta è riportata nella Tabella 606-3.

Il **coinvolgimento bulbare**, che si verifica in circa la metà dei casi, può presentarsi con un quadro di insufficienza respiratoria. Disfagia e perdita di forza a livello del viso sono spesso segni di compromissione respiratoria imminente; essi interferiscono con l'alimentazione e aumentano il rischio di aspirazione. Possono essere coinvolti i nervi facciali. Alcuni giovani pazienti possono presentare sintomi da meningite virale o da meningoencefalite. È raro che siano coinvolti i muscoli estrinseci dell'occhio, ma in una variante non comune l'interessamento dei nervi oculomotori e di altri nervi cranici è grave e compare precocemente. La **sindrome di Miller-Fisher** è caratterizzata da oftalmoplegia esterna acuta, atassia e areflessia. In alcuni casi si osserva papilledema, anche se non è clinicamente evidente una compromissione della vista. L'incontinenza o la ritenzione urinaria rappresentano una complicanza, per quanto transitoria, nel 20% circa dei casi. La sindrome di Miller-Fisher è sovrapponibile all'encefalite del tronco di Bickerstaff, che a sua volta presenta molte caratteristiche in comune con la sindrome di Guillain-Barré (per es. coinvolgimento del secondo motoneurone) e può quindi rappresentare un'evoluzione della stessa malattia di base.

I riflessi osteotendinei vanno perduti generalmente già nelle fasi precoci della malattia, ma talvolta sono conservati a lungo; questa variabilità può rendere il quadro confuso al momento della diagnosi. In alcuni casi anche il sistema nervoso autonomo può essere coinvolto. Possono verificarsi instabilità della pressione e della frequenza cardiaca, ipotensione posturale, episodi di grave bradicardia e talora di asistolia. È importante un monitoraggio cardiovascolare. In alcuni pazienti si rende necessario l'impianto di un pacemaker cardiaco temporaneo.

La **poliradicoloneuropatia cronica recidivante** (denominata anche poliradicoloneuropatia demielinizzante infiammatoria cronica) o la **poliradicoloneuropatia cronica progressiva** sono varianti croniche della sindrome di Guillain-Barré, che recidivano in modo intermittente o non migliorano per un periodo di mesi o anni. Circa il 7% dei bambini con sindrome di Guillain-Barré ha avuto una ricaduta acuta. I pazienti sono generalmente molto deboli e possono presentare una tetraplegia flaccida con o senza coinvolgimento dei muscoli bulbari e respiratori.

La ***sindrome di Guillain-Barré congenita***, di raro riscontro, si presenta con un quadro di ipotonia generalizzata, debolezza e areflessia neonatale, che soddisfa tutti i criteri elettrofisiologici e liquorali, in assenza di malattia neuromuscolare nella madre. Il trattamento può non essere necessario e si assiste a un graduale miglioramento nei primi mesi, senza evidenza di malattia residua dopo il primo anno di vita. In un caso, la madre aveva una colite ulcerosa trattata con prednisone e mesalamina dal settimo mese di gravidanza fino al termine.

ESAMI DI LABORATORIO E DIAGNOSI. Ai fini della diagnosi è fondamentale l'esame del liquido cerebrospinale, da cui emergono un aumento delle proteine, che risultano più del doppio rispetto al limite superiore della norma, un livello di glucosio normale e assenza di pleiocitosi. Si riscontrano meno di 10 globuli bianchi/mm^3. Gli esami colturali per la ricerca di batteri sono negativi ed è raro che si riescano a isolare virus specifici. La dissociazione tra un alto contenuto proteico del CSF e una riduzione delle cellule in un paziente con polineuropatia acuta o subacuta è diagnostico per sindrome di Guillain-Barré.

Le velocità di conduzione motoria sono molto ridotte e spesso anche il tempo di conduzione delle fibre sensitive è basso. L'elettromiografia dimostra la presenza di una denervazione acuta del muscolo. La creatina chinasi (CK) sierica può essere lievemente aumentata o normale. Gli anticorpi antigangliosidi, soprattutto anti-GM1 e GD1, subiscono un aumento in alcuni casi, soprattutto quando l'interessamento assonale è prevalente rispetto alla demielinizzazione, suggerendo che questi talora possano giocare un ruolo nella progressione e/o risoluzione della malattia (Tab. 615-1). In genere, la biopsia muscolare non è necessaria per la diagnosi; i reperti, normali allo stadio iniziale, dimostrano la presenza di atrofia da denervazione nelle fasi di cronicizzazione. La biopsia del nervo surale rivela demielinizzazione segmentale, infiammazione focale e degenerazione walleriana, ma in genere neppure questo esame è indispensabile ai fini della diagnosi.

Il test sierologico per le infezioni da *Campylobacter* e *Helicobacter* aiuta a chiarire la causa se ha un esito positivo, ma non

TABELLA 615-1. Classificazione della sindrome di Guillain-Barré e dei disordini correlati e dei tipici anticorpi antigangliosidi alla base della patologia

	ANTICORPI
Poliradicoloneuropatia demielinizzante infiammatoria acuta	Sconosciuti
Neuropatia assonale acuta motoria e sensitiva	GM1, GM1b, GD1a
Neuropatia assonale acuta motoria	GM1, GM1b, GD1a, GalNac-GD1a
Neuropatia acuta sensitiva	GD1b
Pandisautonomia acuta	
Varianti regionali	
Sindrome di Fisher	GQ1b, GT1a
Orofaringea	GT1a
Forme miste	
Forma mista Fisher/Guillain-Barré	GQ1b, GM1, GM1b, GD1a, GalNac-GD1a

Da Hughes RAC: Treatment of Guillain-Barré syndrome with corticosteroids: Lack of benefit? *Lancet* 2004;363:181-182.

modifica il piano terapeutico. La coprocoltura è generalmente negativa, poiché l'infezione è autolimitante e spesso dura solo 3 giorni circa, mentre la neuropatia si manifesta dopo la risoluzione della gastroenterite acuta.

TRATTAMENTO. I pazienti nella fase iniziale della malattia acuta dovrebbero essere ricoverati in ospedale per essere tenuti sotto controllo, poiché la paralisi ascendente può estendersi rapidamente ai muscoli respiratori già durante le prime 24 ore. I soggetti in cui la progressione è lenta, se stabili, possono essere semplicemente messi in osservazione e spesso vanno incontro a remissione spontanea dei disturbi senza bisogno di trattamento. Il trattamento della paralisi ascendente rapidamente progressiva si basa sulle immunoglobuline, somministrate ev per 2, 3 o 5 giorni; un protocollo comunemente raccomandato ne prevede la somministrazione alla dose di 0,4 mg/kg/die per 5 giorni consecutivi. La plasmaferesi e/o farmaci immunosoppressori sono valide alternative qualora le immunoglobuline ev si rivelassero inefficaci. Gli steroidi non sono di alcun beneficio. La somministrazione combinata di immunoglobuline e interferone è efficace in alcuni pazienti. Sono importanti le terapie di supporto, come la ventilazione assistita, la prevenzione delle piaghe da decubito nei bambini con tetraplegia flaccida e il trattamento delle sovrainfezioni batteriche.

Ci si avvale delle immunoglobuline ev anche per il trattamento della poliradicoloneuropatia cronica recidivante e della neuropatia progressiva cronica; una possibile alternativa è rappresentata dalla plasmaferesi (talvolta sono necessari 10 lavaggi al giorno). Sebbene la remissione di questi casi possa essere prolungata, talvolta nell'arco di pochi giorni, settimane o anche dopo alcuni mesi si osservano recidive, che però in genere rispondono a un altro ciclo di plasmaferesi. In alternativa si possono utilizzare steroidi o immunosoppressori, la cui efficacia è comunque meno prevedibile. Alte dosi di metilprednisolone somministrato per via endovenosa sono efficaci in alcuni casi. La prognosi è più incerta nelle forme croniche di Guillain-Barré che non nelle forme acute e in alcuni pazienti possono residuare deficit importanti.

Anche se viene rilevata la presenza del *Campylobacter jejuni* con la coprocoltura o con test sierologici, non è necessario trattare l'infezione, che si risolve spontaneamente, e l'utilizzo di antibiotici non modifica il decorso della polineuropatia.

Per il trattamento del dolore cronico neuropatico che fa seguito alla sindrome di Guillain-Barré, il farmaco più efficace è il gabapentin, seguito dalla carbamazepina, mentre non è necessario somministrare il fentanil.

PROGNOSI. Il decorso clinico è generalmente benigno, con un recupero spontaneo che inizia entro 2-3 settimane. La maggior parte dei pazienti recupera completamente la forza muscolare, anche se alcuni possono presentare un deficit di forza residuo. Di solito i riflessi osteotendinei sono l'ultima funzione a essere recuperata. Il miglioramento tende a seguire un ordine inverso a quello di presentazione: la funzione bulbare è la prima a migliorare, mentre da ultimo si verifica la risoluzione della perdita di forza agli arti inferiori. Il coinvolgimento bulbare e dei muscoli respiratori può portare al decesso del paziente, se la sindrome non viene riconosciuta e trattata. Anche se in genere la prognosi è buona poiché la maggior parte dei bambini recupera completamente, tre elementi clinici sono predittivi di prognosi severa con possibili sequele: l'interessamento dei nervi cranici, l'intubazione e una grave disabilità al momento della presentazione clinica. Un quadro elettrofisiologico che attesta un blocco di conduzione è predittivo di un buon andamento clinico. Studi di follow-up a lungo termine compiuti su pazienti in via di recupero, dopo un attacco di sindrome di Guillain-Barré, dimostrano che molti presentano una perdita assonale permanente, con o senza segni clinici residui di neuropatia cronica. La facile affaticabilità è uno dei più comuni sintomi cronici, da non confondere con la rapida esauribilità muscolare tipica della miastenia grave. Molti dei pazienti con la forma assonale della malattia che presentano un recupero lento nei primi sei mesi possono infine riprendere a camminare, anche se talvolta devono passare alcuni anni. L'EMG e lo studio della velocità di conduzione nervosa non sono necessariamente predittivi dell'andamento clinico.

Ammache Z, Afini AK, Brown CK, et al: Childhood Guillain-Barré syndrome: Clinical and electrophysiologic features predictive of outcome. *J Child Neurol* 2001;16:477–483.

Bradshaw DY, Jones HR: Pseudomeningoencephalitic presentation of pediatric Guillain-Barré syndrome. *J Child Neurol* 2001;16:505–508.

Centers for Disease Control and Prevention: Cluster of tick paralysis cases—Colorado, 2006. *MMWR* 2006;55:933–936.

Dornonville de la Coeur C, Jakobsen J: Residual neuropathy in long-term population-based follow-up of Guillain-Barré syndrome. *Neurology* 2005;64:246–253.

England JD, Asbury AK: Peripheral neuropathy. *Lancet* 2004;363:2151–2161.

Hiraga A, Mori M, Ogawara K, et al: Recovery patterns and long-term prognosis for axonal Guillain-Barré syndrome. *J Neurol Neurosurg Psychiatry* 2005;76:719–722; comment 622.

Hughes RAC: Treatment of Guillain-Barré syndrome with corticosteroids: Lack of benefit? *Lancet* 2004;363:181–182.

Jackson AH, Barquis GD, Shah BL: Congenital Guillain-Barré syndrome. *J Child Neurol* 1996;11:407–410.

Koller H, Kieseier BC, Jander S, Hartung HP: Chronic inflammatory demyelinating polyneuropathy. *N Engl J Med* 2005;352:1343–1356.

Korinthenberg R, Schessl J, Kirschner J, et al: Intravenously administered immunoglobulin in the treatment of childhood Guillain-Barré syndrome: A randomized trial. *Pediatrics* 2005;116:8–14.

Kountouras J, Deretzi G, Zavos C, et al: Association between *Helicobacter pylori* infection and acute inflammatory demyelinating polyradiculoneuropathy. *Eur J Neurol* 2005;12:139–143.

Pandey CK, Raza M, Tripathhi M, et al: The comparative evaluation of gabapentin and carbamazepine for pain management in Guillain-Barré syndrome patients in the intensive care unit. *Anesth Analg* 2005;101:220–225.

Press R, Mata S, Lolli F, et al: Temporal profile of anti-ganglioside antibodies and their relation to clinical parameters and treatment in Guillain-Barré syndrome. *J Neurol Sci* 2001;190:41–47.

Ramachandran R, Kuruvilla A: Guillain-Barré syndrome in children and adolescents: A retrospective analysis. *J Indian Med Assoc* 2004;102:480–482.

Schessl J, Koga M, Funakoshi K, et al: Prospective study on anti-ganglioside antibodies in childhood Guillain-Barré syndrome. *Arch Dis Child* 2007;92:48–52.

Van Koningsveld R, Schmitz PIM, van der Meche, et al: Effect of methylprednisone when added to standard treatment with intravenous immunoglobulin for Guillain-Barré syndrome: Randomized trial. *Lancet* 2004;363:192.

Winer JB: Bickerstaff's encephalitis and the Miller-Fisher syndrome. *J Neurol Neurosurg Psychiatry* 2001;71:433–435.

TABELLA 616-1. Cause di paralisi periferica acuta facciale

COMUNI
Virus herpes simplex di tipo 1*
Virus varicella-zoster*
INFEZIONI MENO COMUNI
Otite media ± colesteatoma
Malattia di Lyme
Virus di Epstein-Barr
Cytomegalovirus
Virus della parotite
Herpesvirus umano 6
Vaccino influenzale per via nasale
Mycoplasma
ALTRE CONDIZIONI MENO COMUNI
Traumi
Tumori
Ipertensione
Sindrome di Guillain-Barré
Sarcoidosi
Sindrome di Melkersson-Rosenthal†
Ribavirina
Interferone

*Implicati nella paralisi di Bell idiopatica.

†Granulomi non caseosi con edema facciale (labbra, palpebre), paralisi facciale ricorrente alternante, familiarità, emicrania o cefalea.

Capitolo 616 ■ Paralisi di Bell

La paralisi di Bell è una paralisi unilaterale acuta del nervo facciale, non associata ad altre neuropatie dei nervi cranici o a disfunzioni del tronco encefalico. È una malattia comune a tutte le età, dall'infanzia all'adolescenza, e di solito si sviluppa improvvisamente due settimane dopo un'infezione sistemica di origine virale. La precedente infezione in genere è dovuta a virus herpes simplex, virus varicella-zoster, virus di Epstein-Barr, malattia di Lyme, virus della parotite, *Mycoplasma* (Tab. 616-1). L'attivazione o la riattivazione del virus herpes simplex o varicella-zoster è la causa più comune di paralisi di Bell. Questa forma potrebbe essere determinata da una neurite demielinizzante postinfettiva del nervo faciale, su base allergica o immune. Può anche essere una neuropatia focale tossica o infiammatoria ed è stata associata con l'uso di ribavirina e interferone α nell'ambito del trattamento per l'epatite C.

MANIFESTAZIONI CLINICHE. La parte superiore e inferiore della faccia è paralizzata e l'angolo della bocca è piegato verso il basso. Il paziente non riesce a chiudere l'occhio dal lato colpito ed è a rischio di sviluppare una cheratite per esposizione della cornea durante la notte. In circa la metà dei casi viene persa la sensibilità dei due terzi anteriori della lingua dal lato coinvolto; questi reperti aiutano a stabilire i limiti anatomici della lesione, che può essere prossimale o distale rispetto alla corda del timpano, ramo del nervo faciale. In genere non si osservano intorpidimento né parestesie, ma in alcuni casi è stata riportata un'insensibilità della parte del volto omolaterale al deficit motorio, probabilmente dovuta a una compromissione autoimmune del trigemino e del faciale, di origine virale (soprattutto da herpesvirus) o postvirale. Sono stati messi a punto diversi sistemi di stadiazione della paralisi di Bell: Sunnybrook, House-Brackmann e Yanagihara.

TRATTAMENTO. La somministrazione orale di prednisone (1 mg/kg/die per una settimana e poi a scalare per un'altra settimana), iniziata entro i primi 3-5 giorni, determina un miglioramento. Dal momento che è stata riscontrata la presenza di virus herpes simplex nel fluido neurale del settimo nervo cranico, alcuni raccomandano anche la somministrazione di aciclovir o valaciclovir per via orale in aggiunta alla terapia steroidea. La decompressione chirurgica del canale faciale, che teoricamente dovrebbe creare più spazio per il nervo faciale edematoso, in realtà non è efficace. In alcuni casi cronici con scarso recupero si raccomanda la fisioterapia dei muscoli faciali, la cui efficacia tuttavia non è sicura. La somministrazione di metilcellulosa o di lubrificanti oculari è particolarmente importante di notte. Alcuni chirurghi plastici utilizzano la tossina botulinica per trattare la ptosi cronica unilaterale, ma questa tecnica ha scarse applicazioni nei pazienti pediatrici.

PROGNOSI. La prognosi è eccellente: più dell'85% dei casi guarisce spontaneamente, senza evidenza di ipostenia facciale residua, il 10% continua ad accusare una lieve debolezza e solo il 5% ha un deficit severo permanente. Nei pazienti che non recuperano nel giro di pochi giorni (deficit cronico), la valutazione elettrofisiologia del nervo faciale aiuta a determinare il grado di neuropatia e di rigenerazione. Nei casi cronici occorre prendere in esame altre possibili cause di neuropatia facciale, compresi i tumori del nervo faciale come lo schwannoma e il neurofibroma, l'infiltrazione del nervo da parte di cellule leucemiche o di un rabdomiosarcoma dell'orecchio medio, infarti o neoplasie del tronco encefalico ed eventi traumatici.

PARALISI FACCIALE ALLA NASCITA. In genere si tratta di una neuropatia dovuta alla compressione esercitata dal forcipe durante il parto e nella maggior parte dei casi guarisce spontaneamente in pochi giorni o settimane. L'***assenza congenita del muscolo depressore dell'angolo della bocca*** provoca un'asimmetria facciale, che diventa più evidente quando il bambino piange. Non è dovuta a una lesione del nervo, ma rappresenta solo un inconveniente estetico, che non compromette l'alimentazione. I neonati con la ***sindrome di Möbius*** possono avere una paralisi facciale bilaterale o, meno comunemente, unilaterale; questa sindrome in genere è provocata da infarti calcificati simmetrici verificatisi a livello del tegmento pontino e del midollo allungato durante la fase intermedia della gestazione o alla fine della vita fetale, anche se raramente può costituire un'anomalia di sviluppo del tronco encefalico.

Berg T, Jonsson L, Engstrom M: Agreement between the Sunnybrook, House-Brackmann and Yanagihara facial nerve grading systems in Bell's palsy. *Otol Neurotol* 2004;25:1020–1026.

Eidlitz-Markus T, Gilai A, Mimouri M, et al: Recurrent facial nerve palsy in pediatric patients. *Eur J Pediatr* 2001;160:659–663.

Furuta Y, Ohtani F, Aizawa, et al: Varicella-zoster virus reactivation is an important cause of acute peripheral facial paralysis in children. *Pediatr Infect Dis J* 2005;24:97–101.

Gilden DH: Bell's palsy. *N Engl J Med* 2004;351:1323–1331.

Holland NJ, Weiner GM: Recent developments in Bell's palsy. *BMJ* 2004;329:553–557.

Kisaki H, Hato N, Mizobuchi M, et al: Role of T-lymphocyte subsets in facial nerve paralysis owing to the reactivation of herpes simplex virus type 1. *Acta Laryngol* 2005;125:316–321.

Salinas RA, Alvarez G, Ferreira J: Corticosteroids for Bell's palsy (idiopathic facial paralysis). *Cochrane Database Syst Rev* 2004;4:CD001942.

Parte XXVIII ▪ Malattie dell'occhio

Capitolo 617 ▪ Crescita e sviluppo

Scott E. Olitsky, Denise Hug
e Laura P. Smith

Alla nascita le dimensioni dell'occhio di un neonato a pieno termine sono circa il 65% di quelle dell'adulto. La crescita postnatale è massima durante il primo anno, procede a una velocità rapida ma decrescente fino al terzo e successivamente continua più lentamente fino alla pubertà, dopo la quale l'occhio si modifica di poco. Le strutture anteriori sono relativamente grandi alla nascita, ma in seguito crescono di meno in proporzione a quelle posteriori. Ciò determina una progressiva modificazione della forma del globo oculare, che diventa più sferico.

Nel bambino piccolo la sclera è sottile e trasparente ed è di colore bluastro. La cornea è relativamente grande nei neonati (in media 10 mm) e raggiunge le dimensioni dell'adulto (circa 12 mm) entro l'età di 2 anni o prima. La sua curvatura tende ad appiattirsi con l'età, con la progressiva modificazione delle proprietà refrattive dell'occhio. Una cornea normale è perfettamente trasparente. Nei bambini nati prematuramente, la cornea può presentare un velo opaco transitorio. La camera anteriore nel neonato appare poco profonda e le strutture dell'angolo, importanti per il mantenimento della normale pressione intraoculare, devono andare incontro a un'ulteriore differenziazione dopo la nascita. L'iride, tipicamente di colore blu chiaro o grigio alla nascita nei soggetti bianchi, subisce un progressivo cambiamento di colore con l'aumentare della pigmentazione dello stroma nei primi 6 mesi di vita. Le pupille del neonato tendono a essere piccole e sono spesso difficili da dilatare. Spesso sono evidenti residui della **membrana pupillare** (capsula vascolare anteriore) all'esame oftalmoscopico, che appaiono come linee simili a una ragnatela che attraversano l'apertura pupillare, specialmente nei neonati pretermine.

Il cristallino del neonato è più sferico di quello di un adulto; il suo maggiore potere refrattivo consente di compensare la brevità relativa dell'occhio giovane. Il cristallino continua a crescere per tutta la vita; nuove fibre aggiunte alla periferia spingono continuamente le più vecchie verso il centro. Con l'invecchiamento, diventa progressivamente più denso e più resistente alle variazioni della forma durante l'accomodazione.

Il fondo oculare di un neonato è meno pigmentato di quello dell'adulto; la trama vascolare coroideale è ben visibile, mentre il disegno pigmentario retinico spesso presenta un aspetto punteggiato o chiazzato. In alcuni bambini piccoli di pigmentazione scura, il fondo oculare presenta una lucentezza grigia o opaca. Nel neonato i punti di riferimento maculari, in particolare il riflesso foveale alla luce, sono meno ben definiti e possono non essere facilmente evidenti. La retina periferica si presenta pallida o grigiastra, mentre la vascolarizzazione retinica periferica è immatura, specialmente nei prematuri. Il colore della testa del nervo ottico varia da rosso a leggermente pallido, talvolta grigiastro. Entro 4-6 mesi, l'aspetto del fondo oculare diventa molto simile a quello dell'occhio maturo.

In molti neonati si possono osservare emorragie retiniche superficiali, che di solito vengono assorbite prontamente e lasciano di rado effetti permanenti. La maggior parte delle **emorragie retiniche** correlate al parto si risolve entro 2 settimane, con completa risoluzione di tutte quante entro 4-6 settimane. Alla nascita si possono verificare anche emorragie congiuntivali, che sono riassorbite spontaneamente senza conseguenze.

Si possono inoltre osservare residui del sistema **vascolare ialoide primitivo** sotto forma di piccoli ciuffi o di strutture vermiformi che si proiettano dal disco (papilla di Bergmeister) o sotto forma di una stria sottile che attraversa il vitreo; in alcuni casi, rimane soltanto un piccolo punto (punto di Mittendorf) sulla parte posteriore della capsula del cristallino.

L'occhio del bambino piccolo è piuttosto iperopico. L'**ipermetropia** tende in genere ad aumentare dalla nascita fino ai 7 anni, per poi diminuire rapidamente fino all'età di 14 anni, nella quale si può osservare la sua eliminazione. Se il processo continua, si sviluppa la miopia. Una più lenta continuazione della diminuzione dell'ipermetropia, o dell'aumento della miopia, continua nella terza decade. Lo stato refrattivo, in qualunque epoca della vita, dipende dall'effetto netto di molti fattori: le dimensioni dell'occhio, lo stato del cristallino e la curvatura della cornea.

I neonati tendono a mantenere gli occhi chiusi per molto tempo, ma quelli normali possono comunque vedere, rispondere a variazioni dell'illuminazione e fissare punti di contrasto. L'acuità visiva stimata nei neonati è di circa 20/400. Una delle prime risposte a uno stimolo visivo formato è l'interesse per il volto della madre, evidente specialmente durante l'allattamento. Dalla seconda settimana di vita, il bambino dimostra un'attenzione più sostenuta nei confronti degli oggetti grandi, mentre dall'ottava-decima settimana può seguire un oggetto in un arco di 180 gradi. L'acuità migliora rapidamente e può raggiungere 20/30-20/20 entro i 2-3 anni.

Molti neonati normali possono presentare una coordinazione imperfetta dei movimenti oculari e dell'allineamento degli occhi durante i primi giorni e settimane di vita, ma un'appropriata coordinazione dovrebbe essere ottenuta entro 3-6 mesi, o di solito prima. La deviazione persistente di un occhio richiede una valutazione.

Spesso le lacrime non sono presenti con il pianto se non dopo 1-3 mesi. Nei pretermine il riflesso e la secrezione lacrimale basale sono ridotti e ciò favorisce la concentrazione dei farmaci applicati topicamente con il conseguente rapido seccarsi delle cornee.

Archer SM, Sondhi N, Helveston EM: Strabismus in infancy. *Ophthalmology* 1989;96:133–137.

Emerson MV, Pieramici DJ, Stoessel KM, et al: Incidence and rate of disappearance of retinal hemorrhage in newborns. *Ophthalmology* 2001;108: 33–39.

Isenberg SJ, Apt L, McCarty J: Development of tearing in preterm and term infants. *Arch Ophthalmol* 1998;116:773–776.

Khodadoust AA, Ziai M, Biggs SL: Optic disc in normal newborns. *Am J Ophthalmol* 1968;66:502–504.

Krishnamohan VK, Wheeler MB, Testa MA, et al: Correlation of postnatal regression of the anterior vascular capsule of the lens to gestational age. *J Pediatr Ophthalmol Strabismus* 1982;19:28–32.

Roarty JD, Keltner JL: Normal pupil size and anisocoria in newborn infants. *Arch Ophthalmol* 1990;108:94–95.

Spieres A, Isenberg SJ, Inkelis SH: Characteristics of the iris in 100 neonates. *J Pediatr Ophthalmol Strabismus* 1989;26:28–30.

Capitolo 618 ▪ Esame dell'occhio

Scott E. Olitsky, Denise Hug
e Laura P. Smith

L'esame dell'occhio fa abitualmente parte della valutazione pediatrica periodica a partire dal periodo neonatale. Il medico di assistenza primaria ha un ruolo molto importante nel riconoscere malattie oculari sia evidenti sia asintomatiche insidiose. Anche lo screening nelle scuole e i programmi comunitari possono risultare efficaci nell'identificazione precoce dei disturbi. L'American Academy of Ophtalmology raccomanda lo screening prescolare della vista come strategia per ridurne la perdita prevenibile (Tab. 618-1). L'esame dell'occhio dovrebbe essere effettuato dal pediatra durante le visite. Il bambino andrebbe esaminato dall'oculista ogniqualvolta si rilevi o si sospetti un'anomalia oculare significativa o un difetto della vista, così come occorrerebbe valutare i bambini che sono a elevato rischio di problemi oftalmologici, per esempio quelli con condizioni oculari geneticamente ereditate e varie malattie sistemiche.

L'esame di base, effettuato dal pediatra o dall'oculista, deve comprendere la misurazione dell'acuità visiva e dei campi visivi, la valutazione delle pupille, della motilità e dell'allineamento oculare, un esame esterno generale e l'esame oftalmoscopico dei mezzi di rifrazione e dei fondi. Quando indicati, la biomicroscopia (esame con lampada a fessura), la rifrazione citoplegica e la tonometria vengono effettuate dall'oculista. Per malattie particolari sono indicate anche procedure diagnostiche speciali, come l'ecografia, la fluorangiografia, l'elettroretinografia o i potenziali evocati visivi.

ACUITÀ VISIVA. Esistono molti test per l'acuità visiva. Quello utilizzato dipende dall'età e dalla capacità di collaborare del bambino, così come dalla preferenza e dall'esperienza del medico con lo stesso. Il test di acuità visiva più comune nei bambini piccoli consiste nella valutazione della loro capacità di fissare e seguire un oggetto di interesse. Se si usano oggetti target appropriati, questo riflesso può essere dimostrato a partire circa dalla sesta settimana di vita. Il test viene effettuato facendo sedere comodamente il bambino in grembo al genitore. L'oggetto, di solito un giocattolo dai colori vivaci, viene spostato lentamente da destra a sinistra. L'esaminatore osserva se gli occhi del bambino si girano verso l'oggetto e ne seguono il movimento; egli può quindi occludere con il pollice un occhio del bambino, in modo da valutarlo separatamente. Sebbene gli oggetti che producono suoni possano compromettere la purezza dello stimolo visivo, nella pratica i giocattoli che squittiscono o tintinnano accrescono l'attenzione e l'interesse del bambino nei confronti del test.

Il volto umano è un oggetto di interesse migliore rispetto ai giocattoli. L'esaminatore può sfruttare questo fatto muovendo il suo volto lentamente davanti a quello del bambino. Se non si riescono a generare appropriati movimenti di attenzione, il test andrebbe ripetuto con il volto del genitore come stimolo. Si dovrebbe tenere presente che anche i bambini con scarsa funzione visiva possono seguire un oggetto grande senza apparente difficoltà, specialmente se è affetto soltanto un occhio.

Una misurazione obiettiva dell'acuità visiva è solitamente possibile quando il bambino raggiunge i 2(1/2)-3 anni di vita. A questa età ci si serve di una figura schematica o di altre tavole oculari senza lettere. Si dovrebbe testare ciascun occhio separatamente, impedendo attentamente che l'occhio occluso sbirci. L'esaminatore dovrebbe tenere l'occlusore in posizione e osservare il bambino durante tutto il test il bambino, che andrebbe continuamente rassicurato e incoraggiato, perché potrebbe essere intimidito dalla procedura e temere di subire un "brutto voto" o una punizione in caso di errori.

Il **test della E**, in cui il bambino indica la direzione della lettera, è quello più diffusamente utilizzato nell'età prescolare. Le presentazioni destra-sinistra sono più confondenti rispetto a quelle alto-basso. Con l'esercizio preliminare, questo test può essere effettuato dalla maggior parte dei bambini di 3-4 anni di età.

Una **tavola dell'acuità visiva di Snellen** di tipo adulto può essere utilizzata a circa 5 o 6 anni, se il bambino conosce le lettere. In genere un'acuità visiva di 20/40 è accettata come normale per i bambini di 3 anni, quindi a 4 anni è tipica 20/30 ed entro i 5 o 6 anni la maggior parte dei bambini raggiunge 20/20.

Anche il **nistagmo optocinetico** (la risposta a una sequenza di oggetti in movimento, nistagmo "da treno") può essere impiegato per la valutazione dell'acuità visiva; esso può essere calibrato

TABELLA 618-1. Linee guida per lo screening della vista*

FUNZIONE	TEST RACCOMANDATI	CRITERI DI RIFERIMENTO	COMMENTI
DAI 3 AI 5 ANNI			
Acuità visiva a distanza	Lettere di Snellen Numeri di Snellen Test della E cadente HOTV test Test con figure Figure di Allen Esame LH	1. <4 su 6 corretti su linea di 6 m con valutazione di ciascun occhio a 3 m monocularmente (ossia <10/20 o 20/40) oppure 2. Differenza di due linee tra gli occhi, anche entro il range di passaggio (ossia 10/12,5 e 10/20 o 20/25 e 20/40)	1. I test sono elencati in ordine decrescente di difficoltà cognitiva; occorrerebbe scegliere il test più alto che il bambino è in grado di effettuare; in generale, a 3-5 anni andrebbero utilizzati il test della E cadente o l'HOTV test, mentre le lettere o i numeri di Snellen dai 6 anni in avanti. 2. Per tutti i test di acuità visiva si raccomanda una distanza di 3 m. 3. È preferibile una fila di figure anziché figure singole. 4. L'occhio non testato andrebbe occluso con un occlusore tenuto dall'esaminatore oppure con l'applicazione di un occlusore adesivo; occorre che l'esaminatore si assicuri che l'occhio non testato non possa sbirciare.
Allineamento oculare	Cover test unilaterale a 3 m oppure Random dot E stereo test a 40 cm (630 secondi di arco)	Qualunque movimento oculare <4 su 6 corretti	
DAI 6 ANNI IN AVANTI			
Acuità visiva a distanza	Lettere di Snellen Numeri di Snellen Test della E cadente HOTV test Test con figure Figure di Allen Esame LH	1. <4 su 6 corretti a 4,5 m con valutazione di ciascun occhio a 3 m monocularmente (ossia <10/15 o 20/30) oppure 2. Differenza di due linee tra gli occhi, anche entro il range di passaggio (ossia 10/10 e 10/15 o 20/20 e 20/30)	1. I test sono elencati in ordine decrescente di difficoltà cognitiva; occorrerebbe scegliere il test più alto che il bambino è in grado di effettuare; in generale, a 3-5 anni andrebbero utilizzati il test della E cadente o l'HOTV test, mentre le lettere o i numeri di Snellen dai 6 anni in avanti. 2. Per tutti i test di acuità visiva si raccomanda una distanza di 3 m. 3. È preferibile una fila di figure anziché singole figure. 4. L'occhio non testato andrebbe occluso con un occlusore tenuto dall'esaminatore oppure con l'applicazione di un occlusore adesivo; occorre che l'esaminatore si assicuri che l'occhio non testato non possa sbirciare.
Allineamento oculare	Cover test unilaterale a 3 m oppure Random dot E stereo test a 40 cm (630 secondi di arco)	Qualunque movimento oculare <4 su 6 corretti	

*Le linee guida di screening sono state sviluppate dalla AAP Section on Ophthalmology Executive Committee, 1991-1992; Robert D. Gross, MBA, MD, Chairman; Walter M. Fierson, MD, Jane D. Kivlin, MD, I. Matthew Rabinowicz, MD, David R. Stager, MD, Mark S. Ruttum, MD, AAPOS; e Earl R. Crouch, Jr., MD, American Academy of Ophthalmology.
Da Nelson LB: *Harley's Pediatric Ophthalmology*, 4th ed. Philadelphia, WB Saunders, 1998, p 84.

mediante target di varie dimensioni (righe o punti) o utilizzando un cilindro a distanze specifiche. Per studiare la funzione visiva in casi selezionati, possono essere inoltre utilizzati i potenziali evocati visivi, un metodo elettrofisiologico per la valutazione della risposta alla luce e a stimoli visivi speciali, come strisce calibrate o un'immagine a scacchiera. Si possono quindi menzionare i test della visione preferenziale, impiegati per misurare la vista nei bambini piccoli e grandi che non risultano in grado di rispondere ai test standard. Si tratta di una tecnica comportamentale basata sull'osservazione che, potendo scegliere, un bambino preferisce guardare disegni con pattern piuttosto che senza. I test della visione preferenziale non possono tuttavia essere direttamente correlati ai dati dell'acuità visiva standard. Dal momento che per tali test è necessaria la presenza di un esaminatore esperto, il loro impiego è spesso limitato a protocolli di ricerca che riguardano i bambini che ancora non sono in grado di parlare.

VALUTAZIONE DEL CAMPO VISIVO. Analogamente ai test di acuità visiva, la valutazione del campo visivo deve essere adattata all'età e alle capacità del bambino. L'esame formale (perimetria e scotometria) può spesso essere effettuato nei bambini di età scolare. L'esaminatore deve in genere basarsi su tecniche di confronto e sul conteggio delle dita nei quadranti del campo visivo. In molti bambini si può eseguire soltanto il test per attrazione, in cui l'esaminatore osserva la risposta nei confronti di oggetti familiari introdotti in ciascuno dei quattro quadranti del campo visivo di ciascuno occhio, a turno. Il biberon, un giocattolo preferito e un lecca-lecca sono oggetti di attenzione particolarmente efficaci. Questi metodi grossolani possono spesso identificare alterazioni diagnosticamente significative, come l'emianopsia bitemporale di una lesione del chiasma o l'emianopsia omonima di una lesione cerebrale.

TEST DELLA VISIONE DEI COLORI. Può essere realizzato quando il bambino è in grado di denominare o di rintracciare i simboli del test, che possono essere numeri oppure X, O, triangoli o altri. Questo test non è frequentemente necessario nei bambini piccoli, ma i genitori talvolta lo richiedono, in particolare se sembra che il bambino sia lento ad apprendere i colori. Spesso i genitori sono rassicurati dal fatto di sapere che i bambini con deficit della visione dei colori non sbagliano a denominare i colori stessi e che la "cecità per i colori" vera e propria è molto rara e non compatibile con la vista normale. Il deficit è comune nei maschi, ma raro nelle femmine. L'acromatopsia, un deficit totale con acuità visiva subnormale, nistagmo e fotofobia, è riscontrata occasionalmente. Una modificazione della discriminazione dei colori può essere un segno di una malattia del nervo ottico o della retina.

ESAME PUPILLARE. Comprende la valutazione delle reazioni diretta e consensuale alla luce, della reazione allo sguardo da vicino e della risposta all'illuminazione ridotta, notando le dimensioni e la simmetria delle pupille in tutte le condizioni. Particolare attenzione va prestata a differenziare la reazione alla luce da quella allo sguardo da vicino. Il bambino tende naturalmente a guardare in modo diretto la luce in avvicinamento, inducendo il riflesso per lo sguardo da vicino quando si cerca di testare soltanto la reazione alla luce; di conseguenza, si deve cercare in tutti i modi di controllare la fissazione. Il test con lampi di luce oscillante è particolarmente utile per identificare i deficit afferenti chiasmatici unilaterali o asimmetrici (vedi il paragrafo: "Pupilla di Marcus Gunn" nel Capitolo 621).

MOTILITÀ OCULARE. Viene testata facendo seguire al bambino un oggetto in varie posizioni di sguardo. Si valutano i movimenti di ciascun occhio individualmente (duzioni) e dei due occhi insieme (versioni, movimenti coniugati e convergenza). Per valutare l'allineamento ci si basa sulla simmetria dei riflessi della luce corneale e sulla risposta all'occlusione alternata degli occhi (vedi la discussione a proposito del cover test per lo strabismo nel Capitolo 622).

VISIONE BINOCULARE. La valutazione del grado di visione binoculare viene comunemente realizzata dall'oculista. Il Titmus test è probabilmente quello più frequentemente utilizzato; si mostra una serie di immagini tridimensionali al bambino mentre questo indossa un paio di occhiali Polaroid®. Il livello di difficoltà con cui le immagini possono essere identificate è correlato al grado di visione binoculare posseduto. Ci si può servire anche di altri test per riconoscere la presenza di adattamenti binoculari anormali secondari a deficit della vista o a strabismo.

ESAME ESTERNO. Inizia con l'ispezione generale in buona illuminazione, notando le dimensioni, la forma e la simmetria delle orbite; la posizione e il movimento delle palpebre; la posizione e la simmetria dei globi oculari. L'osservazione degli occhi e delle palpebre dall'alto consente di identificare un'asimmetria orbitale, masse palpebrali, una proptosi (**esoftalmo**) e pulsazioni anormali. Anche la palpazione è importante nell'individuazione di masse orbitali e palpebrali.

L'apparato lacrimale viene valutato ricercando segni di deficit lacrimali, iperafflusso di lacrime (**epifora**), eritema ed edema nella regione del sacco o della ghiandola lacrimale. Il sacco viene massaggiato per controllare l'eventuale esistenza di un reflusso quando si sospetta un'ostruzione. Si controllano anche la presenza e la posizione dei punti lacrimali.

Le palpebre e la congiuntiva vengono esaminate in modo specifico alla ricerca di lesioni, corpi estranei e segni di infiammazione; si dovrebbero anche notare la perdita e il malposizionamento delle ciglia. Quando necessario, le palpebre possono essere ribaltate nel modo seguente: (1) si invita il paziente a guardare in basso; (2) si afferrano le ciglia della palpebra superiore tra il pollice e l'indice di una mano; (3) si colloca uno specillo, un applicatore con punta di cotone o il pollice dell'altra mano in corrispondenza del margine superiore del piatto tarsale; (4) si tira la palpebra verso il basso e all'esterno, la si ribalta sopra lo specillo utilizzando lo strumento come fulcro. Corpi estranei sono comunemente localizzati nella concavità appena al di sotto del margine palpebrale e vengono esposti soltanto ribaltando completamente la palpebra.

Si valuta quindi il segmento anteriore dell'occhio con un'illuminazione focale obliqua, notando la lucentezza e la chiarezza della cornea, la profondità e la chiarezza della camera anteriore e le caratteristiche dell'iride. La transilluminazione del segmento anteriore aiuta nell'identificazione di opacità e nella dimostrazione dell'atrofia o dell'ipopigmentazione dell'iride; questi ultimi segni sono importanti quando si sospetta l'albinismo oculare. Quando necessario, si può utilizzare la colorazione con fluoresceina per diagnosticare abrasioni, ulcerazioni e corpi estranei.

BIOMICROSCOPIA (ESAME CON LAMPADA A FESSURA). Consente di osservare a elevato ingrandimento le varie strutture e una sezione ottica attraverso i mezzi di rifrazione dell'occhio: la cornea, l'umore acqueo, il cristallino e il vitreo. Le lesioni possono essere identificate e localizzate in base alla loro profondità all'interno dell'occhio; la risoluzione è sufficiente per riconoscere singole cellule infiammatorie nell'acqueo e nel vitreo. Con l'aggiunta di particolari lenti e prismi, anche l'angolo della camera anteriore e le regioni del fondo possono essere esaminati con la lampada a fessura. La biomicroscopia è spesso fondamentale nei traumi e nella valutazione di una irite e risulta utile anche nella diagnosi di malattie metaboliche dell'infanzia.

ESAME DEL FONDO OCULARE (OFTALMOSCOPIA). Viene realizzato al meglio con la pupilla dilatata, a meno che non vi siano controindicazioni neurologiche o di altro tipo. La tropicamide 0,5-1% e la fenilefrina 2,5% sono raccomandate come midriatici di breve durata: sono sicure nella maggior parte dei bambini, ma va riconosciuta la possibilità di effetti avversi sistemici. Per i bambini molto piccoli, possono essere consigliabili preparazioni più diluite. Iniziando con i punti di repere posteriori, il disco e la macula, i quattro quadranti vengono sistematicamente esaminati seguendo ciascuno dei gruppi vascolari principali alla periferia. Gran parte del fondo oculare può essere osservato se si ordina al bambino di guardare in alto e in basso e a destra e a sinistra. Anche con grande accuratezza, solo una parte limitata del fondo oculare può essere valutata con un oftalmoscopio diretto manuale, per cui è necessario un oftalmoscopio indiretto, con una fondamentale dilatazione completa della pupilla, per l'esame della parte più periferica.

RIFRAZIONE. Stabilisce lo stato refrattivo dell'occhio; il grado di miopia, ipermetropia o astigmatismo. La retinoscopia fornisce una determinazione obiettiva dell'entità di correzione necessaria e può essere effettuata a qualunque età. Nei bambini piccoli essa viene realizzata al meglio in cicloplegia. Per l'affinamento soggettivo della rifrazione si chiedono ai pazienti le preferenze nella potenza e nell'asse delle lenti correttive; ciò può essere realizzato in molti bambini in età scolare. La rifrazione e la determinazione dell'acuità visiva indossando lenti correttive appropriate sono fasi fondamentali nello stabilire se un paziente presenta un deficit visivo o un'ambliopia. Le videocamere di fotoscreening consentono al personale medico ausiliare di effettuare lo screening degli errori refrattivi anormali nei bambini ancora non in grado di parlare. L'accuratezza e l'utilità pratica di questi dispositivi sono ancora allo studio.

TONOMETRIA. Misura la pressione intraoculare; può essere effettuata con un apparecchio portatile indipendente o mediante il metodo di appianamento con la lampada a fessura. Metodi alternativi sono la tonometria pneumatica ed elettronica. Quando è necessaria una misurazione accurata della pressione in un bambino che non è in grado di collaborare, essa può essere effettuata con la sedazione o mediante l'anestesia generale. Una stima grossolana della pressione può essere fatta palpando il globo con gli indici posizionati l'uno accanto all'altro sulla palpebra superiore al di sopra del piatto tarsale.

American Academy of Ophthalmology Preferred Practice Patterns Committee, Pediatrics Ophthalmology Panel: Pediatric eye evaluations: Preferred practice pattern. Abstracts of Clinical Care Guidelines, April 7, 1998.

American Academy of Ophthalmology: *Preferred Practice Pattern: Comprehensive Pediatric Eye Evaluation.* San Francisco, American Academy of Ophthalmology, 1992.

American Academy of Pediatrics, Committee on Practice and Ambulatory Medicine, Section on Ophthalmology: Eye examination and vision screening in infants, children and young adults. *Pediatrics* 1996;98:153–157.

Donahue SP, Johnson TM, Ottar W, et al: Sensitivity of photoscreening to detect high-magnitude amblyogenic factors. *J AAPOS* 2002;6:86–91.

Fulton A: Screening preschool children to detect visual and ocular disorders. *Arch Ophthalmol* 1992;110:1553–1554.

Isenberg SJ: Clinical application of the pupil examination in neonates. *J Pediatr* 1991;118:650–652.

Reinecke RD: Screening 3-year olds for visual problems: Are we gaining or falling behind? *Arch Ophthalmol* 1986;104:245–248.

Salcido AA, Bradley J, Donahue SP: Predictive value of photoscreening and traditional screening of preschool children. *J AAPOS* 2005;9:114–120.

Simons K: Preschool vision screening: Rationale, methodology and outcome. *Surv Ophthalmol* 1996;41:3–30.

Teller DY, McDonald MA, Preston KI, et al: Assessment of visual acuity in infants and children: The acuity card procedure. *Dev Med Child Neurol* 1986;28:779–789.

Capitolo 619 ■ Anomalie della rifrazione e dell'accomodazione

Scott E. Olitsky, Denise Hug e Laura P. Smith

L'**emmetropia** è lo stato in cui i raggi paralleli della luce vengono messi a fuoco sulla retina con l'occhio a riposo (che non accomoda). Sebbene tale condizione ottica ideale sia comune, quella opposta, l'ametropia, si verifica spesso. Esistono tre tipi principali di **ametropia**: l'**ipermetropia**, la **miopia** e l'**astigmatismo**. La maggior parte dei bambini è fisiologicamente ipermetrope alla nascita, ma un numero significativo, specialmente i nati prematuramente, è miope e spesso presenta un certo grado di astigmatismo. Con la crescita lo stato refrattivo tende a modificarsi e dovrebbe essere valutato periodicamente.

La misurazione della rifrazione può essere effettuata in modo obiettivo o soggettivo. Nel metodo obiettivo si dirige un fascio di luce dal retinoscopio alla retina del paziente. A seconda del modo in cui la luce si comporta con il movimento del retinoscopio e della manipolazione con lenti di vario potere tenute davanti all'occhio, si può realizzare una rifrazione precisa. Questo esame può essere fatto a qualunque età, in quanto non richiede alcuna risposta da parte del paziente. Nei bambini piccoli e grandi in genere è più preciso effettuarlo dopo avere istillato gocce oculari che producono midriasi (dilatazione della pupilla) e cicloplegia (paralisi dell'accomodazione); quelle usate più comunemente sono la tropicamide, il ciclopentolato e l'atropina solfato. Nella rifrazione soggettiva, invece, si collocano le lenti davanti all'occhio e il paziente riferisce quali di esse forniscono l'immagine più nitida delle lettere sulla tavola. Questo metodo dipende dalla capacità del paziente di discriminare e comunicare, ma può essere utilizzato per alcuni bambini e può risultare utile per stabilire la migliore correzione refrattiva per quelli che sono già in grado di seguirlo.

IPERMETROPIA. Se i raggi paralleli di luce vengono messi a fuoco posteriormente alla retina con l'occhio a riposo, si ha l'ipermetropia, che può essere dovuta al fatto che il diametro anteroposteriore dell'occhio è troppo corto oppure il potere refrattivo della cornea o del cristallino è inferiore alla norma.

Nell'ipermetropia l'accomodazione viene utilizzata per mettere a fuoco gli oggetti nello sguardo da lontano e da vicino. Se lo sforzo accomodativo necessario non è troppo elevato, il bambino ha una visione nitida e non ha problemi con la visione da lontano e da vicino. Nell'ipermetropia di grado elevato, che richiede un maggiore sforzo accomodativo, la vista può essere offuscata e il bambino può lamentare una tensione oculare, cefalea o affaticamento. Lo strabismo, lo sfregamento degli occhi e la mancanza di interesse nella lettura sono frequenti manifestazioni. Se il fastidio indotto è sufficientemente elevato, il bambino può non sforzarsi di guardare bene e può sviluppare un'ambliopia bilaterale (ametropica). Può trovarsi associata anche l'esotropia (vedi la discussione sullo strabismo convergente e sull'esotropia accomodativa nel Capitolo 622). Se necessario, vengono prescritte lenti convesse (occhiali o lenti a contatto) di potere sufficiente da fornire una visione nitida e uno stato di benessere. Anche i bambini con elevati gradi di ipermetropia ma con una vista buona indosseranno volentieri gli occhiali, perché questi forniscono uno stato di benessere eliminando l'eccessiva accomodazione necessaria per vedere bene. Anche a quelli che non sono ancora in grado di parlare si dovrebbero prescrivere gli occhiali per elevati gradi di ipermetropia, per prevenire lo sviluppo di un'esotropia o un'ambliopia. Per i bambini con livelli normali d'ipermetropia nella maggior parte dei casi non è invece necessaria la correzione.

MIOPIA. Nella miopia i raggi paralleli di luce vengono messi a fuoco anteriormente alla retina. Ciò può essere dovuto al fatto che il diametro anteroposteriore dell'occhio è troppo lungo oppure il potere refrattivo della cornea o del cristallino è maggiore della norma. Il sintomo principale è la visione offuscata per gli oggetti lontani. Il punto remoto di visione nitida è variabile in modo inversamente proporzionale al grado di miopia, avvicinandosi all'occhio con l'aumentare della miopia. In caso di miopia di 1 diottria, per esempio, il punto remoto di visione nitida si trova a 1 mm dall'occhio, mentre con una miopia di 3 diottrie è soltanto a 1/3 di mm dall'occhio. Pertanto, i bambini miopi tendono a tenere vicini gli oggetti e il materiale di lettura, preferiscono stare vicini alla lavagna e possono non essere interessati alle attività lontane. Lo strabismo è comune, perché l'acuità visiva migliora quando l'apertura delle palpebre è ridotta.

La miopia è rara nei bambini piccoli e in età prescolare. È più comune in quelli con un'anamnesi di **retinopatia della prematurità**. È stata anche osservata una sua tendenza ereditaria e i bambini con genitori miopi dovrebbero essere esaminati precocemente. L'incidenza della miopia aumenta durante gli anni scolastici, specialmente nella preadolescenza e nell'adolescenza, e anche il suo grado cresce con l'età durante gli anni dello sviluppo.

Vengono prescritte lenti concave (occhiali o lenti a contatto) di potere appropriato in modo da fornire una visione nitida e comfort. Di solito vanno modificate periodicamente, talvolta ogni 1-2 anni, talvolta dopo pochi mesi. Secondo alcuni Autori, l'eccessiva accomodazione durante il lavoro da vicino favorirebbe la progressione della miopia. Seguendo questa teoria, alcuni medici raccomandano l'uso di agenti cicloplegici, lenti bifocali, ipocorrezione intenzionale degli errori refrattivi miopici o la rimozione obbligatoria degli occhiali da miopia per il lavoro da vicino, nel tentativo di ritardare la sua progressione. L'utilità di questo trattamento non è stata scientificamente dimostrata.

La correzione mediante il laser a eccimeri è stata approvata negli adulti dal 1995. La procedura LASIK (*Laser-Assisted In Situ Keratomileusis*) utilizza un microcheratomo o un laser a femtosecondi che forma un lembo epiteliale-stromale permettendo l'ablazione del tessuto corneale sottostante per correggere la vista; il lembo ricopre quindi l'area della cornea. La correzione risulta solitamente eccellente e stabile nel tempo. I rischi più grandi si hanno per elevati gradi di miopia (>10 diottrie) e comprendono starburst, aloni e immagini distorte o multiple (solitamente di notte). La più bassa incidenza di complicanze si ha con i chirurghi più esperti. Le attuali raccomandazioni per questa procedura e per le procedure più recenti sono disponibili alla pagina web www.aao.org/aao/education/library/recommendations/lasik.cfm.

Nella maggior parte dei casi la miopia non è dovuta a un'alterazione patologica dell'occhio ed è denominata miopia semplice o fisiologica. Alcuni bambini possono presentarne una patologica, una rara malattia causata da una lunghezza assiale patologicamente anormale dell'occhio, che è solitamente associata all'assottigliamento della sclera, della coroide e della retina e spesso a un certo grado di compromissione visiva incorreggibile. Si possono verificare lacerazioni o rotture della retina, perché questa si assottiglia sempre di più, portando allo sviluppo di distacchi retinici. La miopia può insorgere anche in seguito ad altre anomalie oculari, come il cheratocono, l'ectopia lentis, la cecità notturna congenita stazionaria e il glaucoma. La miopia è anche una delle principali caratteristiche della sindrome di Stickler.

ASTIGMATISMO. Nell'astigmatismo il potere refrattivo dei vari meridiani dell'occhio è diverso. La maggior parte dei casi è determinata da irregolarità della curvatura della cornea; alcuni sono dovuti ad alterazioni del cristallino. Gradi lievi di astigmatismo sono comuni e possono non produrre alcun sintomo, ma nei gradi più elevati può presentarsi una distorsione della vista. Per ricavare un'immagine più nitida, il soggetto con astigmatismo utilizza l'accomodazione o lo strabismo per ottenere l'effetto della capocchia di spillo. Tra i sintomi vi sono tensione oculare, cefalea e affaticamento. Per fornire la correzione ottica vengono utilizzate lenti cilindriche o sferiche, quando indicato. Gli occhiali possono risultare necessari in modo costante o solo part-time, a seconda del grado di astigmatismo e della gravità dei sintomi di accompagnamento. In alcuni casi si usano le lenti a contatto.

I bambini piccoli e grandi con irregolarità corneali secondarie a lesioni, emangiomi periorbitali e palpebrali e ptosi sono ad aumentato rischio di astigmatismo e di ambliopia associata.

ANISOMETROPIA. Quando lo stato refrattivo di un occhio è significativamente diverso da quello dell'altro occhio, si ha anisometropia. Se non viene corretta, è possibile che un occhio sia sempre fuori fuoco, portando allo sviluppo dell'ambliopia. L'identificazione e la correzione precoci sono fondamentali per ottenere lo sviluppo visivo normale in entrambi gli occhi.

ACCOMODAZIONE. Durante l'accomodazione, il muscolo ciliare si contrae, le fibre sospensorie del cristallino si rilassano e il cristallino assume una forma più arrotondata per fare convergere i raggi di luce nel fuoco della retina. L'ampiezza dell'accomodazione è massima durante l'infanzia e diminuisce gradualmente con l'età. La riduzione fisiologica della capacità accomodativa che si verifica con l'età è denominata presbiopia.

I disturbi dell'accomodazione nei bambini sono relativamente rari. Occasionalmente si osserva una presbiopia prematura nei più piccoli. La causa più comune di paralisi dell'accomodazione nei bambini è l'uso involontario o accidentale di sostanze cicloplegiche, per via topica o sistemica; tra queste vi sono i farmaci e i veleni anticolinergici, così come piante e sostanze vegetali dotate di tali effetti. Tra le cause neurogene compaiono invece lesioni che interessano il nervo oculomotore (terzo nervo cranico) in qualunque punto del suo decorso. La diagnosi differenziale comprende tumori, malattie degenerative, lesioni vascolari, traumi e malattie infettive. Tra le malattie sistemiche che possono determinare la compromissione dell'accomodazione rientrano il botulismo, la difterite, la malattia di Wilson, il diabete mellito e la sifilide. Anche la pupilla tonica di Adie può portare a un deficit dell'accomodazione dopo alcune patologie virali (vedi Capitolo 621). Un deficit apparente può essere di origine psicogena: è comune che un bambino finga di non essere in grado di leggere anche quando si può dimostrare che l'acuità visiva e la capacità di mettere a fuoco sono normali.

Brown NP, Koretz JF, Bron AJ: The development and maintenance of emmetropia. *Eye* 1999;13:83–92.

Klimek DL, Cruz OA, Scott WE, et al: Isoametropic amblyopia due to high hyperopia in children. *J AAPOS* 2004;8:310–313.

Kuo A, Sinatra RB, Donahue SP: Distribution of refractive error in healthy infants. *J AAPOS* 2003;7:174–177.

Larsson EK, Rydberg AC, Holmstrom GE: A population-based study of the refractive outcome in 10-year-old preterm and full-term children. *Arch Ophthalmol* 2003;121:1430–1436.

Mayer DL, Hansen RM, Moore BD, et al: Cycloplegic refractions in healthy children aged 1 through 48 months. *Arch Ophthalmol* 2001;119: 1625–1628.

Sakimoto T, Rosenblatt MI, Azar DT: Laser eye surgery for refractive errors. *Lancet* 2006;369:1432–1447.

Ton Y, Wysenbeek YS, Spierer A: Refractive error in premature infants. *J AAPOS* 2004;8:534–538.

Wilson SE: Use of lasers for vision correction of nearsightedness and farsightedness. *N Engl J Med* 2004;351:470–475.

Capitolo 620 ■ Disturbi della vista

Scott E. Olitsky, Denise Hug e Laura P. Smith

La grave compromissione della vista (visione corretta inferiore a 6/60) e la cecità nei bambini possono conoscere molte eziologie e possono essere dovute a deficit multipli che interessano qualsiasi struttura o funzione lungo le vie ottiche (Tab. 620-1). L'incidenza globale è di circa 2,5 ogni 100 000 bambini; la diffusione appare maggiore nei Paesi in via di sviluppo, nei neonati di basso peso alla nascita e nel primo anno di vita. Le cause più comuni sono prenatali e perinatali; le vie ottiche-cerebrali, il nervo ottico e i siti retinici risultano colpiti più spesso. Importanti origini perinatali comprendono malattie genetiche autosomiche recessive (più comuni), autosomiche dominanti e X-linked, così come l'ipossia e sindromi cromosomiche. Tra le determinanti perinatali/neonatali vi sono la retinopatia della prematurità, l'ipossia-ischemia e le infezioni. La grave compromissione che inizia nei bambini più

TABELLA 620-1. Cause di grave compromissione visiva o cecità nell'infanzia

CONGENITA
Ipoplasia o aplasia del nervo ottico
Displasia setto-ottica
Coloboma ottico
Idrocefalo congenito
Idroanencefalia
Porencefalia
Microencefalia
Encefalocele, in particolare occipitale
Anomalia di Morning glory
Aniridia
Macroftalmia/anoftalmia
Anomalia di Peters
Anomalia di Reiger
Membrana pupillare persistente
Glaucoma
Cataratta
Vitreo primario iperplastico persistente

FACOMATOSI
Sclerosi tuberosa
Neurofibromatosi (speciale associazione con il glioma ottico)
Sindrome di Sturge-Weber
Malattia di von Hippel-Lindau

TUMORI
Retinoblastoma
Glioma ottico
Meningioma periottico
Craniofaringioma
Glioma cerebrale
Astrocitoma
Tumori posteriori e intraventricolari complicati da idrocefalo
Pseudotumore cerebrale

MALATTIE NEURODEGENERATIVE
Malattia da accumulo cerebrale
Gangliosidosi, in particolare la malattia di Tay-Sachs, la variante di Sandhoff, gangliosidosi generalizzata
Altre lipidosi e lipofuscinosi ceroidi, in particolare le malattie a esordio tardivo come quella di Jansky-Bielschowsky e di Batten-Mayou-Spielmeyer-Vogt
Mucoplisaccaridosi, in particolare la sindrome di Hurler e la sindrome di Hunter
Leucodistrofie (malattie da dismielinizzazione), in particolare la leucodistrofia metacromatica e la malattia di Canavan
Sclerosi demielinizzante (malattie mielinoclastiche), specialmente la malattia di Schilder e la neuromielite ottica di Devic
Tipi speciali: malattia di Dawson, malattia di Leigh, sindrome di Bassen-Kornzweig, malattia di Refsum
Degenerazioni retiniche: retinite pigmentosa e sue varianti e tipo congenito di Leber
Atrofie ottiche: tipo congenito autosomico recessivo; tipi congeniti autosomici dominanti, malattia di Leber e atrofie associate ad atassia ereditaria: i tipi di Behr, di Marie e di Sanger-Brown

PROCESSI INFETTIVI/INFIAMMATORI
Encefalite, specialmente nelle sindromi infettive prenatali dovute a Toxoplasma gondii, Cytomegalovirus, virus della rosolia, *Treponema pallidum*, virus dell'herpes simplex
Meningite; aracnoidite
Corioretinite
Endoftalmite
Tracoma
Cheratite
Uveite

MALATTIE EMATOLOGICHE
Leucemia con interessamento del sistema nervoso centrale

MALATTIE VASCOLARI E CIRCOLATORIE
Collagenopatie vascolari
Malformazioni arterovenose: emorragia intracerebrale, emorragia subaracnoidea
Occlusione retinica centrale

TRAUMA
Contusione o avulsione dei nervi ottici, del chiasma, del globo oculare, della cornea
Contusione o lacerazione cerebrale
Emorragia intracerebrale, subaracnoidea o subdurale
Distacco di retina

FARMACI E TOSSINE
Chinino
Etambutolo
Metanolo
Molti altri

ALTRO
Retinopatia della prematurità
Sclerocornea
Reazione da conversione
Neurite ottica
Osteopetrosi

Modificata da Kliegman R: *Practical Strategies in Pediatric Diagnosis and Therapy*. Philadelphia, WB Saunders, 1996.

grandi può essere dovuta a tumori del sistema nervoso centrale o della retina, a infezioni, ipossia-ischemia, lesioni, malattie neurodegenerative o artrite reumatoide giovanile.

AMBLIOPIA. Consiste in una diminuzione dell'acuità visiva, unilaterale o bilaterale, che si verifica nei bambini con un'immaturità della vista dovuta al fatto che le immagini non cadono nella retina. L'immagine retinica non formata può avere luogo secondariamente a un occhio deviato (**ambliopia strabismica**), a un'ineguale necessità per la correzione della vista tra gli occhi (**ambliopia anisometropica**), a un elevato errore refrattivo in entrambi gli occhi (**ambliopia ametropica**) o a un'opacità dei mezzi di rifrazione all'interno dell'asse visivo (**ambliopia da deprivazione**).

In condizioni normali lo sviluppo dell'acuità visiva procede rapidamente nel periodo neonatale e nella prima infanzia. Qualunque fattore che interferisca con la formazione di un'immagine retinica nitida durante questo periodo evolutivo precoce può produrre un'ambliopia. L'ambliopia si può verificare soltanto durante il momento critico dello sviluppo, prima che la corteccia sia diventata visivamente matura, entro la prima decade di vita. Più giovane è il bambino, maggiore risulta la suscettibilità allo sviluppo dell'ambliopia.

La **diagnosi** viene confermata quando un esame oftalmoscopico completo evidenzia una ridotta acuità che non si spiega con un'anomalia organica. Se l'anamnesi e l'esame oftalmologico non risultano a favore della diagnosi di ambliopia in un bambino con vista scarsa, bisogna prendere in considerazione altre cause (neurologiche, psicologiche). Di solito l'ambliopia è asintomatica e viene identificata soltanto attraverso i programmi di screening, che risulta più semplice nei bambini più grandi. Tuttavia, è meno probabile che l'ambliopia si verifichi in un bambino più grande e inoltre essa appare anche maggiormente resistente al trattamento, a un'età maggiore, mentre risulta reversibile più rapidamente nei bambini più piccoli, in cui il sistema visivo è meno maturo. L'identificazione precoce e l'intervento tempestivo sono la chiave perché il trattamento dell'ambliopia abbia successo.

In genere il **trattamento** consiste innanzitutto nella rimozione di ogni opacità dei mezzi di rifrazione dell'occhio o nella prescrizione di occhiali appropriati, se necessari, in modo da potere produrre un'immagine retinica bene a fuoco in ciascun occhio. L'occhio sano viene quindi coperto (terapia occlusiva) o offuscato con occhiali o gocce (terapia di penalizzazione) per stimolare l'appropriato sviluppo visivo di quello colpito più gravemente. La terapia occlusiva può fornire un miglioramento più rapido della vista, ma alcuni bambini possono tollerare meglio la penalizzazione con l'atropina. Il trattamento migliore per qualsiasi paziente dovrebbe essere selezionato su base individuale. Gli obiettivi del trattamento dovrebbero essere conosciuti in modo completo e il trattamento andrebbe supervisionato attentamente. Lo stretto monitoraggio è essenziale, specialmente nei soggetti molto giovani, per evitare l'ambliopia nell'occhio sano. Molte famiglie hanno bisogno di rassicurazione e sostegno durante tutto il faticoso decorso del trattamento. In passato i bambini con un'ambliopia grave erano trattati con un bendaggio occlusivo a tempo pieno, ma i dati attuali suggeriscono che nei bambini di 3-7 anni si può praticare l'occlusione per 6 ore al giorno, associata a 1 ora di attività visive da vicino durante l'occlusione stessa. Ai bambini (3-7 anni) con un'ambliopia moderata possono invece essere prescritte 2 ore di occlusione se associate a 1 ora di attività visive da vicino.

DIPLOPIA. La diplopia, o visione doppia, è in genere secondaria all'errato allineamento degli assi visivi. L'occlusione di un occhio la migliora; comunemente i bambini interessati sono strabici, coprono un occhio con la mano oppure assumono un'anomala posizione del capo (lo inclinano o ruotano il volto da un lato) per alleviare la sensazione fastidiosa. Questi modi di comportarsi, specialmente nei bambini che ancora non sanno parlare, sono importanti segnali di diplopia. La sua comparsa giustifica una tempestiva valutazione; essa può segnalare l'esordio di un problema grave, come un aumento della pressione endocranica, un tumore cerebrale o una massa orbitale.

La diplopia monoculare è dovuta alla dislocazione del cristallino, a cataratta o a qualche difetto nei mezzi di rifrazione o nella macula.

SOPPRESSIONE. In presenza di strabismo, la diplopia insorge secondariamente al fatto che la medesima immagine cade su differenti regioni della retina in ciascun occhio. In un bambino visivamente immaturo si può verificare un processo nella corteccia che elimina l'incapacità di vedere doppio. Si tratta di un processo attivo denominato soppressione, che si sviluppa soltanto nei bambini. Sebbene la soppressione elimini il sintomo fastidioso della diplopia, è la potenziale consapevolezza della seconda immagine che tende a tenere gli occhi allineati in modo appropriato. Quando si sviluppa, la soppressione può permettere che uno strabismo intermittente diventi costante o che lo strabismo si sviluppi di nuovo in una fase successiva della vita, anche dopo un trattamento efficace durante l'infanzia.

AMAUROSI. L'amaurosi è la perdita parziale o totale della vista; di solito il termine è riservato alla compromissione profonda e alla cecità completa o quasi completa. Nel caso di un'amaurosi presente dalla nascita, nella diagnosi differenziale si deve dare primaria considerazione a malformazioni dello sviluppo, a lesioni conseguenti a un'infezione gestazionale o perinatale, all'anossia o all'ipossia, a un trauma perinatale e a malattie geneticamente determinate che possono interessare l'occhio stesso o le vie ottiche. Spesso la causa può essere rapidamente determinata mediante l'esame obiettivo oftalmico; esempi sono la macroftalmia grave, l'opacizzazione corneale, la cataratta densa, le cicatrici corioretiniche, i difetti maculari, la displasia della retina e la grave ipoplasia del nervo ottico. In altri casi, una malattia retinica intrinseca può non essere evidente all'esame oftalmoscopico iniziale oppure il difetto può interessare il cervello e non l'occhio. La valutazione neuroradiologica (TC o RM) ed elettrofisiologica (elettroretinografia) può risultare particolarmente utile in questi casi.

Un'amaurosi che si sviluppa in un bambino che in passato ha avuto una vista soddisfacente ha diverse implicazioni. In assenza di una malattia oculare evidente (cataratta, corioretinite, retinoblastoma, retinite pigmentosa), si devono considerare molte malattie neurologiche e sistemiche che possono interessare le vie ottiche. Un'amaurosi a esordio piuttosto rapido può indicare una encefalopatia (ipertensione), processi infettivi o parainfettivi, vasculite, emicrania, leucemia, tossine o trauma. Essa può essere determinata da una malattia demielinizzante acuta che interessa i nervi ottici, il chiasma o il cervello. In alcuni casi la perdita precipitosa della vista è secondaria a un aumento della pressione endocranica, a un idrocefalo rapidamente progressivo o alla disfunzione di uno shunt. La perdita del visus più lentamente progressiva suggerisce un tumore o una malattia neurodegenerativa. I gliomi del nervo ottico e del chiasma e i craniofaringiomi costituiscono considerazioni diagnostiche primarie nei bambini che mostrano una perdita progressiva del visus.

Le **manifestazioni cliniche** della compromissione del visus variano con l'età e con le capacità del bambino, con la modalità di esordio e con la lateralità e la gravità del deficit. Il primo segnale dell'amaurosi in un bambino può essere il **nistagmo** o lo **strabismo**, per cui il deficit visivo stesso rimane non diagnosticato per un certo tempo. Timidezza, goffaggine o modificazione del comportamento possono essere i segnali iniziali nei soggetti molto giovani. Il peggioramento nel rendimento scolastico e l'indifferenza verso le altre attività sono segni comuni nel bambino più grande. Spesso i bambini di età scolare cercano di nascondere la loro incapacità e, nel caso delle malattie a progressione molto lenta, possono non rendersi conto essi stessi della gravità del disturbo; alcuni percepiscono e riportano tempestivamente piccole alterazioni della vista.

Ogni segno di perdita della vista necessita di una valutazione oftalmica tempestiva ed esauriente. Per una completa definizione dell'amaurosi infantile e della sua causa possono essere necessarie indagini estese, che comportano una valutazione neurologica, test elettrofisiologici, procedure neuroradiologiche e talvolta esami metabolici e genetici. Inoltre si devono soddisfare gli speciali bisogni educativi, sociali ed emotivi connessi.

NICTALOPIA. La nictalopia, o cecità notturna, consiste in un deficit della vista in condizioni di illuminazione ridotta. In genere comporta la compromissione della funzione dei bastoncelli, in particolare nel tempo di adattamento al buio e nella soglia di percezione. Una cecità notturna congenita stazionaria può insorgere come malattia autosomica dominante, autosomica recessiva o recessiva X-linked. Può essere associata a miopia e a nistagmo. I bambini possono presentare particolare difficoltà ad andare a letto in stanze buie e ciò potrebbe essere scambiato per un disturbo comportamentale. Di solito la cecità notturna progressiva indica una degenerazione retinica, coroideale o vitreoretinica primaria o secondaria (vedi Capitolo 629); avviene anche nel deficit di vitamina A o in seguito all'assunzione di farmaci retinotossici come il chinino.

DISTURBI PSICOGENI. I disturbi della vista di origine psicogena sono comuni nei bambini in età scolare. Si riscontrano sia reazioni di conversione sia una simulazione volontaria. La manifestazione abituale consiste nel riferire la diminuzione dell'acuità visiva in uno o in entrambi gli occhi, oppure la riduzione del campo visivo. In alcuni casi il sintomo è costituito dalla diplopia o dalla poliopia (vedi Capitoli 21 e 24).

Importanti segnali per la diagnosi sono sentimenti inappropriati, smorfie eccessive, incostanza nel rendimento e suggestionabilità. Una visita oftalmologica completa è essenziale per differenziare tra i disturbi visivi organici e quelli funzionali.

Di solito i bambini affetti migliorano con rassicurazioni e incoraggiamenti. A volte è indicata l'assistenza psichiatrica e in tutti i casi l'approccio deve essere di sostegno e non punitivo.

DISLESSIA. Si tratta dell'incapacità di sviluppare la possibilità di leggere a un livello atteso nonostante un intelletto altrimenti normale. I termini disabilità nella lettura e dislessia sono spesso utilizzati in modo intercambiabile. La maggior parte dei soggetti dislessici presenta anche scarse abilità nella scrittura. La dislessia è un disturbo primario della lettura e dovrebbe essere distinto dalle difficoltà secondarie dovute al ritardo mentale, alla deprivazione ambientale o educativa e a malattie fisiche o organiche. Dal momento che non esiste alcun test standard, la diagnosi viene solitamente posta confrontando la capacità di lettura con l'intelligenza e con la lettura standard attesa. La dislessia è una malattia basata sul linguaggio e non è causata da alcun deficit oculare o dell'acuità visiva di per sé, né è attribuibile a un difetto nella motilità oculare o dell'allineamento binoculare. Sebbene la valutazione oftalmologica dei bambini con un problema di lettura sia raccomandata per diagnosticare e correggere ogni disturbo oculare concomitante, come un errore refrattivo, ambliopia o strabismo, non ci si può aspettare che il trattamento diretto agli occhi corregga la dislessia legata allo sviluppo (vedi Capitolo 32).

Dutton G, Cleary M: Should we be screening for and treating amblyopia? *Br Med J* 2003;327:1242–1243.
Holmes JM, Clarke MP: Amblyopia. *Lancet* 2006;367:1343–1351.
Olitsky SE, Nelson LB: Reading disorders in children. *Pediatr Clin North Am* 2003;50:213–224.
Pediatric Eye Disease Investigator Group: A randomized trial of atropine vs. patching for treatment of moderate amblyopia in children. *Arch Ophthalmol* 2002;120:268–278.
Pediatric Eye Disease Investigator Group: A randomized trial of prescribed patching regimens for treatment of severe amblyopia in children. *Ophthalmology* 2003;110:2075–2087.
Pediatric Eye Disease Investigator Group: A randomized trial of patching regimens for treatment of moderate amblyopia in children. *Arch Ophthalmol* 2003;121:603–611.
Pediatric Eye Disease Investigator Group: Randomized trial of treatment of amblyopia in children aged 7 to 17 years. *Arch Ophthalmol* 2005;123: 437–447.
Rahl JS, Cable N: Severe visual impairment and blindness in children in the UK. *Lancet* 2003;362:1359–1364.
Shaywitz SE, Shaywitz BA: The science of reading and dyslexia. *J AAPOS* 2003;7:158–166.
Simons K: Amblyopia characterization, treatment, and prophylaxis. *Surv Ophthalmol* 2005;50:123–166.

Capitolo 621 ■ Anomalie della pupilla e dell'iride

Scott E. Olitsky, Denise Hug e Laura P. Smith

ANIRIDIA. Il termine aniridia è improprio, perché il tessuto irideo di solito è presente, sebbene ipoplasico (Fig. 621-1). Due terzi dei casi sono trasmessi in modo dominante con un elevato grado di penetranza, mentre l'altro terzo è sporadico e si ritiene sia costituito da nuove mutazioni. La malattia è bilaterale nel 98% di tutti i pazienti, indipendentemente dalla modalità di trasmissione, e viene osservata in circa 1/50 000 persone.

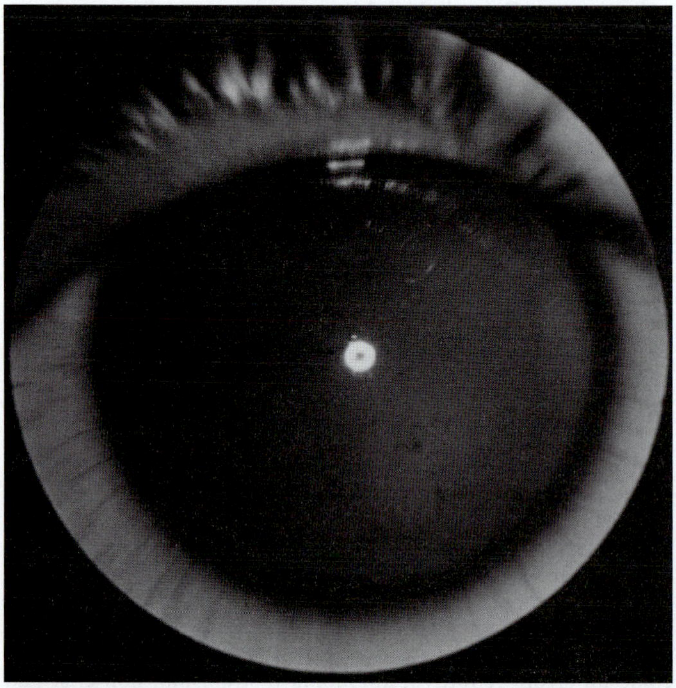

Figura 621-1. Aniridia. Tessuto irideo minimo. (Da Nelson LB, Spaeth GL, Nowinski TS, et al: Aniridia: A review. *Surv Ophthalmol* 1984;28:621-642.)

Si tratta di una malattia panoculare, che non dovrebbe essere considerata come un difetto isolato dell'iride. Ipoplasie della macula e del nervo ottico sono comunemente presenti e conducono a una diminuzione della vista e al nistagmo sensoriale. Nella maggior parte dei pazienti l'acuità visiva misurata è di 20/200, sebbene la vista possa occasionalmente essere migliore. Altre deformità oculari sono comuni e possono interessare il cristallino e la cornea, la quale può risultare piccola e sviluppare occasionalmente un infiltrato cellulare (panno) negli strati superficiali della parte periferica, che dal punto di vista clinico si presenta come un'opacizzazione grigia. Tra le anomalie del cristallino rientrano invece la formazione della cataratta e la lussazione parziale o totale. Un **glaucoma** si forma fino nel 75% dei casi.

Nel 20% dei pazienti con un'aniridia **sporadica** può comparire il **tumore di Wilms** (vedi Capitolo 499). Di particolare interesse è l'associazione tra l'aniridia, alcune anomalie genitourinarie, il ritardo mentale e una delezione parziale del braccio corto del cromosoma 11. Negli individui che presentano tali caratteristiche, l'insorgenza del tumore di Wilms è più comune. Si ritiene che soltanto i pazienti con aniridia sporadica siano a rischio di svilupparlo, sebbene esso si sia verificato in un paziente con aniridia familiare. Di solito si presenta prima dei 3 anni, per cui i bambini a rischio dovrebbero essere sottoposti a uno screening mediante ecografia renale ogni 3-6 mesi fino all'età di circa 5 anni.

Il gene per l'aniridia è stato localizzato alla regione 11p13. Questo gene può essere coinvolto nel dirigere in modo appropriato le interazioni tra il calice ottico, l'ectoderma di superficie e le cellule della cresta neurale durante l'iniziale formazione dell'iride e di altre strutture oculari.

COLOBOMA DELL'IRIDE. Questo difetto correlato allo sviluppo può presentarsi come un difetto in un settore dell'iride, un foro nella sua sostanza o un'incisura nel margine pupillare. I colobomi semplici sono frequentemente trasmessi come tratto autosomico dominante e possono verificarsi da soli o in associazione ad altre anomalie. Un coloboma si forma quando la fessura embrionale non si chiude in modo completo. A causa della localizzazione anatomica della fessura embrionale, il coloboma dell'iride è sempre localizzato inferiormente, conferendo all'iride un aspetto a "buco di serratura". Esso può essere l'unica parte visibile esternamente di una chiusura incompleta più ampia della fessura embrionale, che interessi anche il fondo oculare e il nervo ottico. Quando questo avviene, è probabile che la vista sia gravemente compromessa. Pertanto, tutti i bambini con il coloboma dell'iride dovrebbero essere sottoposti a un esame oftalmologico completo.

MICROCORIA. La microcoria (miosi congenita) consiste in una pupilla piccola che non reagisce alla luce o all'accomodazione e che si dilata poco o per nulla con i farmaci. La malattia può essere unilaterale o bilaterale. Nei casi bilaterali il grado di miosi può risultare differente in ciascun occhio, il quale può essere per il resto normale può mostrare altre anomalie del segmento anteriore. La microcoria congenita è solitamente trasmessa come tratto autosomico dominante, sebbene possa verificarsi in modo sporadico.

MIDRIASI CONGENITA. In questa malattia le pupille sembrano dilatate, non si stringono in modo significativo alla luce o allo sguardo da vicino e rispondono minimamente agli agenti miotici. L'iride è per il resto normale e i bambini affetti sono di solito in buona salute. Si dovrebbero escludere i traumi, una midriasi farmacologica e malattie neurologiche. Molti casi evidenti di midriasi congenita mostrano anomalie delle strutture centrali dell'iride e possono essere considerati come una forma di aniridia.

DISCORIA E CORECTOPIA. La discoria consiste in una pupilla di forma anormale, mentre nella corectopia l'anormalità sta nella posizione pupillare. Esse si possono verificare insieme o indipendentemente come anomalie congenite o acquisite.

La corectopia congenita è solitamente bilaterale e simmetrica e raramente si verifica come anomalia isolata; di solito si trova infatti accompagnata dalla lussazione del cristallino (ectopia lentis et pupillae), con il cristallino e la pupilla comunemente dislocati in direzioni opposte. L'ectopia lentis et pupillae è trasmessa come malattia autosomica recessiva; la consanguineità risulta comune.

Nella forma acquisita, la distorsione e lo spostamento della pupilla sono frequentemente dovute a un trauma o a un'infiammazione intraoculare. Il prolasso dell'iride dopo lesioni perforanti dell'occhio fa sì che la pupilla si sposti in direzione della perforazione. Sinechie posteriori (aderenze dell'iride al cristallino) sono comunemente osservate quando un'infiammazione da qualunque causa interessa il segmento anteriore.

ANISOCORIA. Consiste nella disuguaglianza tra le pupille. La differenza di dimensioni può essere dovuta a malattie locali o neurologiche. Di norma, se diviene più pronunciata con una illuminazione focale intensa o nello sguardo da vicino, vi è un difetto di costrizione pupillare e la pupilla più grande è anormale. Se l'anisocoria risulta invece peggiore in caso di una illuminazione ridotta, esiste un difetto di dilatazione e a essere anormale è la pupilla più piccola. Le origini neurologiche di anisocoria (lesioni parasimpatiche o simpatiche) devono essere differenziate da quelle locali come le sinechie (aderenze), i difetti congeniti dell'iride (colobomi, aniridia) e gli effetti farmacologici. Un'anisocoria centrale semplice può comparire in soggetti per il resto normali.

PUPILLA FISSA DILATATA. La diagnosi differenziale di una pupilla non reattiva dilatata comprende l'oftalmoplegia interna determinata da una lesione centrale o periferica, la pupilla di Hutchinson di erniazione transtentoriale, la pupilla tonica, il blocco farmacologico e l'iridoplegia secondaria a un trauma oculare.

La causa più comune di una pupilla non reattiva dilatata è l'istillazione accidentale o volontaria di un agente cicloplegico, in particolare l'atropina e le sostanze correlate. Le lesioni del sistema nervoso centrale, come il pinealoma, possono dare origine a un'oftalmoplegia interna nei bambini. Dal momento che la superficie esterna del nervo oculomotore trasporta le fibre responsabili della costrizione pupillare, la compressione del nervo lungo il suo decorso intracranico può essere associata a un'oftalmoplegia interna, anche prima dello sviluppo di ptosi o di un deficit della motilità oculare. Sebbene l'emicrania oftalmoplegica sia una causa comune di paralisi del terzo nervo cranico con interessamento pupillare nei bambini, nella diagnosi differenziale occorre anche prendere in considerazione un aneurisma intracranico. La **pupilla dilatata** di erniazione transtentoriale, che si verifica con una pressione endocranica crescente, è in genere unilaterale e di solito i pazienti appaiono evidentemente malati. Il test della pilocarpina può essere utile per differenziare l'iridoplegia neurologica dal blocco farmacologico. Nel caso dell'iridoplegia neurologica, la pupilla dilatata si costringe entro minuti dopo l'istillazione di una o due gocce di pilocarpina 0,5-1%; se la pupilla è stata dilatata con l'atropina, la pilocarpina non ha alcun effetto. Dato che la pilocarpina è un farmaco a lunga durata d'azione, questo test non deve essere utilizzato nelle situazioni acute, in cui i segni pupillari vanno attentamente monitorati. A causa della risposta pupillare consensuale alla luce, anche la cecità unioculare completa non determina una pupilla dilatata unilateralmente.

PUPILLA TONICA. Si tratta tipicamente di una pupilla ampia che reagisce scarsamente alla luce (la reazione può essere molto lenta o sostanzialmente nulla), poco e lentamente all'accomodazione e si ridilata in modo lento, tonico. Le caratteristiche della pupilla tonica sono spiegate dalla supersensibilità colinergica dello sfintere dopo una denervazione periferica (postgangliare) e una reinnervazione imperfetta. Un elemento distintivo è la sua sensibilità agli agenti colinergici diluiti. L'istillazione di pilocarpina 0,125% provoca una significativa costrizione della pupilla interessata e possiede un effetto scarso o nullo sul lato non coinvolto. La malattia è solitamente unilaterale.

La pupilla tonica può comparire dopo la fase acuta di una iridoplegia parziale o completa. Può venire osservata in seguito a un trauma dell'occhio o dell'orbita e può verificarsi in associazione a malattie tossiche o infettive. Nei soggetti della popolazione pediatrica la pupilla tonica è rara. Le cause principali sono i processi infettivi (principalmente le sindromi virali) e i traumi. Le sue caratteristiche possono anche essere osservate nei bambini piccoli e grandi con una disautonomia familiare (sindrome di Riley-Day), sebbene l'importanza di questi reperti sia stata messa in dubbio. La pupilla tonica è stata anche riportata nei bambini piccoli con la malattia di Charcot-Marie-Tooth. La sua comparsa in associazione alla diminuzione dei riflessi tendinei profondi nelle giovani donne è nota come **sindrome di Adie**.

PUPILLA DI MARCUS GUNN. Questo difetto pupillare afferente relativo indica un difetto di conduzione afferente asimmetrico, prechiasmatico. Viene dimostrato meglio mediante il test del lampo di luce oscillante, che consente il confronto delle risposte pupillari diretta e consensuale in entrambi gli occhi. Mentre il paziente fissa un bersaglio distante (per controllare l'accomodazione), una luce chiara focale viene diretta alternativamente su ciascun occhio a turno. In presenza di una lesione afferente, sia la risposta diretta alla luce nell'occhio affetto sia la risposta consensuale nell'altro occhio risultano subnormali. Spostando la luce all'occhio migliore o normale, entrambe le pupille reagiscono (si costringono) normalmente. Riportando la luce nuovamente all'occhio affetto, entrambe si ridilatano per un certo grado, riflettendo il deficit di conduzione. Si tratta di un test molto sensibile e utile per identificare e confermare la malattia del nervo ottico e della retina. Il test dà risultati anormali soltanto nel caso di una differenza "relativa" nelle proprietà di conduzione dei nervi ottici, per cui i pazienti con una malattia bilaterale e simmetrica del nervo ottico non mostreranno un difetto pupillare afferente. In alcuni bambini con ambliopia si può osservare un difetto afferente relativo subdolo.

SINDROME DI HORNER. I principali segni della paresi oculosimpatica (sindrome di Horner) sono una miosi omolaterale, una ptosi lieve e un enoftalmo apparente con una lieve elevazione della palpebra inferiore. I pazienti possono presentare anche una ridotta sudorazione facciale, un'aumentata ampiezza dell'accomodazione e una transitoria diminuzione della pressione intraoculare. Se la paralisi delle fibre simpatiche oculari si verifica prima dell'età di 2 anni, può comparire un'eterocromia dell'iride con ipopigmentazione sul lato affetto.

La paralisi oculosimpatica può essere causata da una lesione nel mesencefalo, nel tronco cerebrale, nel midollo spinale superiore, nel collo, nella fossa media o nell'orbita. La forma congenita, spesso nell'ambito della paralisi brachiale di Klumpke, è comune, sebbene i segni oculari, in particolare l'anisocoria, possano passare inosservati per anni. La sindrome di Horner è osservata anche in alcuni bambini dopo interventi chirurgici toracici, come quelli per cardiopatie congenite. La forma congenita della sindrome può verificarsi in associazione ad anomalie vertebrali e a cisti enterogene. In alcuni bambini piccoli e grandi, la sindrome di Horner è il segno di presentazione di un tumore nella regione mediastinica o toracica, in particolare del neuroblastoma. Cause rare della sindrome in età pediatrica sono rappresentate da lesioni vascolari. In alcuni casi non si riesce a identificare alcuna origine. Occasionalmente la malattia è familiare.

Quando l'origine è dubbia si dovrebbero effettuare ulteriori accertamenti, come la radiografia del torace, la TC, la RM della testa e del collo e il dosaggio delle catecolamine urinarie delle 24 ore. Talvolta l'esame di vecchie fotografie e vecchie cartelle cliniche può essere utile per stabilire l'età di esordio.

Il test con la cocaina è utile per la diagnosi della paralisi oculosimpatica; una pupilla normale si dilata entro 20-45 minuti dopo l'istillazione di una o due gocce di cocaina al 4%, mentre la pupilla miotica di una paresi oculosimpatica si dilata poco o per nulla. In alcuni casi si ha un'ipersensibilità da denervazione alla noradrenalina diluita; una o due gocce di una soluzione all'1% dilatano la pupilla affetta ma non quella normale. Inoltre, l'istillazione di idrossiamfetamina idrobromuro dilata la pupilla soltanto se il neurone simpatico postgangliare è integro.

REAZIONE PUPILLARE PARADOSSA. Alcuni bambini mostrano una costrizione paradossa delle pupille all'oscurità: quando la luce viene spenta si verifica una iniziale costrizione rapida, seguita dalla ridilatazione. Le risposte alla stimolazione diretta della luce e allo sguardo da vicino sono normali. Il meccanismo non è chiaro, ma la costrizione paradossa delle pupille in condizioni di luce ridotta può essere un segno di anomalie della retina o del nervo ottico. Il fenomeno è stato osservato nei bambini con cecità notturna stazionaria congenita, albinismo, retinite pigmentosa, amaurosi retinica congenita di Leber e malattia di Best. È stata riportata anche in soggetti con anomalie del nervo ottico, neurite ottica, atrofia ottica e forse ambliopia.

MEMBRANA PUPILLARE PERSISTENTE. L'involuzione della membrana pupillare e della capsula vascolare anteriore del cristallino si completa solitamente durante il quinto-sesto mese di sviluppo fetale. È comune osservare alcuni residui della membrana nei neonati, in particolare nei prematuri. Queste membrane sono strie non pigmentate di vasi obliterati che attraversano la pupilla e possono secondariamente attaccarsi al cristallino o alla cornea. I residui tendono ad atrofizzarsi nel tempo e solitamente non danno alcun disturbo. In alcuni casi, tuttavia, ne rimangono alcuni significativi, che oscurano la pupilla e interferiscono con la vista. Raramente si riscontra una pervietà degli elementi vascolari; la rottura dei vasi persistenti può portare a ifema.

Occorre prendere in considerazione l'intervento per ridurre al minimo l'ambliopia nei bambini con una membrana pupillare persistente e sufficientemente ampia da interferire con la vista nei primi mesi di vita. In alcuni casi i farmaci midriatici e la terapia occlusiva possono risultare efficaci, ma in altri può essere necessario l'intervento chirurgico per fornire un'apertura pupillare adeguata.

ETEROCROMIA. Nell'eterocromia le due iridi sono di colore differente (eterocromia delle iridi) oppure una porzione di una è di colore diverso dalla parte rimanente (eterocromia dell'iride). L'eterocromia semplice può verificarsi come caratteristica autosomica dominante. Quella congenita è una caratteristica anche della sindrome di Waardenburg, una malattia autosomica dominante caratterizzata principalmente dallo spostamento laterale del canto interno e dei punti lacrimali, da alterazioni pigmentarie (solitamente ciuffo bianco mediano e chiazze di ipopigmentazione della cute) e deficit dell'udito. Una variazione del colore dell'iride può essere secondaria a trauma, emorragia, infiammazione intraoculare (iridociclite, uveite), tumore intraoculare (specialmente retinoblastoma), corpo estraneo intraoculare, melanosi oculare, pregresso intervento chirurgico oculare e alcuni farmaci antiglaucoma.

ALTRE LESIONI DELL'IRIDE. Noduli ben distinti dell'iride, noti anche come **noduli di Lisch**, sono comunemente osservati nei pazienti con neurofibromatosi. I noduli di Lisch rappresentano amartomi melanocitici dell'iride e variano da aree pigmentate lievemente rilevate a escrescenze sferiche ben distinte. Dal momento che vengono riscontrati nel 92-100% dei soggetti di età superiore a 5 anni con neurofibromatosi, la loro identificazione con la lampada a fessura può aiutare a soddisfare i criteri necessari per confermare la diagnosi di questa malattia.

Nella leucemia si può riscontrare un'infiltrazione dell'iride, talvolta con **ipopion**, un accumulo di leucociti nella camera anteriore, che può preannunciare la recidiva o l'interessamento del sistema nervoso centrale.

La lesione dello **xantogranuloma giovanile** (nevoxantoendotelioma) si può realizzare nell'occhio sotto forma di una massa polposa giallastra o di una placca dell'iride. Possono esservi associati un ifema spontaneo (sangue nella camera anteriore), un glaucoma o un occhio rosso con segni di uveite. In tutti i bambini con ifema spontaneo si dovrebbero ricercare le lesioni cutanee dello xantogranuloma (vedi anche Capitolo 86.3). In molti casi la lesione oculare risponde alla terapia corticosteroidea topica.

LEUCOCORIA. Comprende qualunque riflesso pupillare bianco, o il cosiddetto riflesso dell'occhio di gatto. In ogni bambino con leucocoria le prime considerazioni diagnostiche sono cataratta, vitreo primario iperplasico persistente, retinopatia cicatriziale della prematurità, distacco della retina e retinoschisi, granulomatosi larvale e retinoblastoma (Fig. 621-2). Altre caratteristiche da considerare sono l'endoftalmite, l'emorragia organizzata del vitreo, l'oftalmopatia leucemica, la retinopatia essudativa (come nella malattia di Coats) e malattie meno comuni come il medulloepitelioma, la gliosi retinica massiva, lo pseudotumore retinico della malattia di Norrie, il cosiddetto pseudoglioma della sindrome di Bloch-Sulzberger, la displasia retinica e le lesioni retiniche delle facomatosi. Un riflesso bianco può anche essere osservato in caso di coloboma del fondo oculare, di ampie cicatrici corioretiniche atrofiche e di medullazione ectopica delle fibre del nervo retinico. La leucocoria costituisce un'indicazione per una valutazione tempestiva e completa.

Spesso la diagnosi può essere posta con l'esame diretto dell'occhio mediante oftalmoscopia e biomicroscopia. Le indagini ecografiche e radiologiche riescono spesso utili. In alcuni casi la diagnosi definitiva spetta all'anatomopatologo.

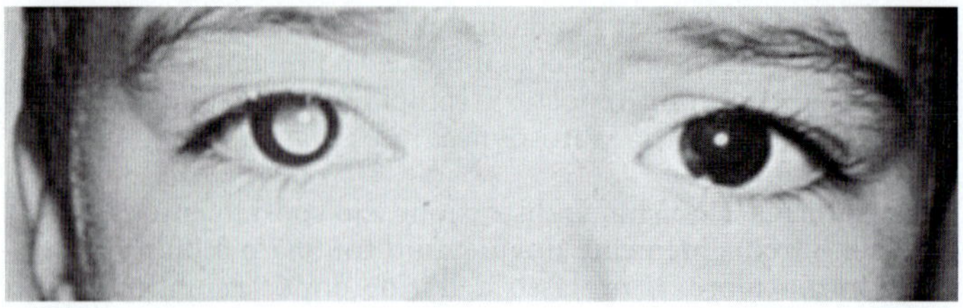

Figura 621-2. Leucocoria. Riflesso pupillare bianco in un bambino con retinoblastoma.

Cross HE: Ectopia lentis et pupillae. *Am J Ophthalmol* 1979;88:381–384.

Francois J: Differential diagnosis of leukokoria in children. *Ann Ophthalmol* 1978;10:1375–1378.

Frank JW, Kushner BJ, France TD: Paradoxic pupillary phenomenon: A review of patients with pupillary constriction to darkness. *Arch Ophthalmol* 1988;106:1564–1566.

Greenwald MJ, Folk ER: Afferent pupillary defects in amblyopia. *J Pediatr Ophthalmol Strabismus* 1983;20:63–67.

Ivanov I, Shuper A, Shohat M, et al: Aniridia: Recent achievements in paediatric practice. *Eur J Pediatr* 1995;154:795–800.

Jaffe N, Cassady JR, Filler RM, et al: Heterochromia and Horner syndrome associated with cervical and mediastinal neuroblastoma. *J Pediatr* 1975;87:75–77.

Jeffery AR, Ellis FJ, Repka MX, et al: Pediatric Horner syndrome. *J Am Assoc Pediatr Ophthalmol Strabismus* 1998;2:159–167.

Loewenfeld IE: "Simple, central" anisocoria: A common condition seldom recognized. *Trans Am Acad Ophthalmol Otolaryngol* 1977;83:832.

Maloney WF, Younge BR, Moyer NJ: Evaluation of the causes and accuracy of pharmacologic localization in Horner syndrome. *Am J Ophthalmol* 1980;90:394–402.

Thompson HS: Segmental palsy of the iris sphincter in Adie's syndrome. *Arch Ophthalmol* 1978;96:1615–1620.

Capitolo 622 ■ Disturbi del movimento e dell'allineamento degli occhi

Scott E. Olitsky, Denise Hug e Laura P. Smith

STRABISMO

Lo strabismo, o deviazione degli occhi, è uno dei disturbi oculari più comuni riscontrati nei bambini, dal momento che interessa circa il 4% di quelli con meno di 6 anni. Lo strabismo può portare alla perdita della vista (ambliopia) e può avere significative conseguenze psicologiche. La sua identificazione e trattamento precoci sono fondamentali per prevenire la compromissione permanente della vista. Il 30-50% dei bambini con strabismo sviluppa l'ambliopia. Il ripristino di un appropriato allineamento dell'asse visivo deve avvenire a una età precoce dello sviluppo visivo, per consentire a questi bambini di sviluppare una visione binoculare normale. Il termine strabismo significa "deviazione o sguardo obliquo". Nella sua discussione e caratterizzazione si utilizzano molti termini.

L'**ortoforia** è la condizione ideale di esatto equilibrio oculare. Implica che l'apparato oculomotore sia in perfetto equilibrio, così che gli occhi rimangano coordinati e allineati in tutte le posizioni di sguardo e a tutte le distanze. Anche quando la visione binoculare è impedita, come nel caso dell'occlusione di un occhio, individui realmente ortoforici mantengono un allineamento perfetto. L'ortoforia è riscontrata raramente, perché la maggior parte degli individui presenta una piccola deviazione latente (eteroforia).

L'**eteroforia** è appunto la tendenza latente degli occhi a deviare. Normalmente viene controllata da meccanismi fusionali che forniscono la visione binoculare o evitano la diplopia (visione doppia). L'occhio devia soltanto in certe condizioni, come affaticamento, malattia o stress oppure durante i test che interferiscono con il mantenimento di queste normali capacità fusionali (come coprire un occhio). Se il grado di eteroforia è ampio, può dare origine a sintomi fastidiosi, come una diplopia transitoria, cefalea o astenopia (tensione oculare). Un certo grado di eteroforia viene riscontrato anche negli individui normali; essa è solitamente asintomatica.

L'**eterotropia** è un errato allineamento degli occhi che risulta incostante. Si verifica a causa di un'incapacità del meccanismo fusionale di controllare la deviazione. Le tropie possono essere alternanti, possono interessare entrambi gli occhi o risultare unilaterali. In una tropia alternante ognuno dei due occhi può fissare ed entrambi deviano con uguale frequenza. Dal momento che ciascun occhio viene usato periodicamente, di solito la vista si sviluppa in maniera normale. La tropia unilaterale dà luogo a una situazione più seria, in quanto soltanto un occhio è costantemente disallineato. L'occhio non deviato diventa quello preferito, con la conseguente perdita della vista o l'ambliopia dell'altro.

Nei disallineamenti oculari è comune descrivere il tipo di deviazione, ciò che aiuta a prendere le decisioni riguardanti la causa e il trattamento dello strabismo. I prefissi eso-, exo-, iper- e ipo- vengono aggiunti ai termini foria e tropia per delineare ulteriormente il tipo di strabismo. Le esoforie e le esotropie sono deviazioni dirette verso l'interno o convergenti degli occhi, comunemente note come "occhi incrociati". Le exoforie e le exotropie sono invece deviazioni divergenti o rivolte verso l'esterno, popolarmente dette "occhi strabici". Le iperdeviazioni e le ipodeviazioni indicano rispettivamente la deviazione verso l'alto e verso il basso di un occhio. Nei casi di strabismo unilaterale, l'occhio che devia viene generalmente descritto del disallineamento (esotropia sinistra).

DIAGNOSI. Molte sono le tecniche utilizzate per valutare l'allineamento e il movimento degli occhi, al fine di aiutare nella diagnosi delle alterazioni dello strabismo. In un bambino con strabismo o con qualunque altra malattia oculare, la valutazione dell'acuità visiva è obbligatoria. In caso di diminuzione della vista in un occhio è necessario escludere lo strabismo o altre anomalie che possono essere difficili da distinguere in una breve valutazione di screening. Anche deviazioni di solo pochi gradi di ampiezza, troppo piccole per essere evidenti all'ispezione macroscopica, possono condurre all'ambliopia e a una grave perdita della vista.

I test del riflesso luminoso sulla cornea sono forse i test diagnostici più rapidi e di facile realizzazione per lo strabismo. Risultano particolarmente utili per i bambini che non collaborano e in quelli con scarsa fissazione oculare. Per effettuare il **test del riflesso corneale alla luce di Hirschberg**, l'esaminatore proietta una sorgente luminosa sulla cornea di entrambi gli occhi simultaneamente mentre il bambino guarda direttamente verso la luce. Andrebbe quindi confrontata la posizione del riflesso corneale alla luce in ciascun occhio. Negli occhi allineati, il riflesso appare simmetrico e, a causa della relazione tra la cornea e la macula, leggermente nasale al centro di ciascuna pupilla. In caso di strabismo, la luce riflessa è asimmetrica e appare spostata in un occhio. Nel test del riflesso corneale secondo il metodo di Krimsky si utilizzano prismi collocati al di sopra di uno o di entrambi gli occhi per allineare i riflessi luminosi. La quantità di prisma necessaria per l'allineamento serve a misurare il grado di deviazione. Sebbene questo sia un utile test di screening, può non identificare un angolo piccolo o uno strabismo intermittente.

Per i **cover test** per lo strabismo sono necessarie l'attenzione e la collaborazione del bambino, una buona capacità di movimento oculare e una vista sufficientemente buona in ciascun occhio. Se uno di questi requisiti è assente, i risultati possono non essere validi. Questi test comprendono il cover-uncover test e il cover test alternato. Nel cover-uncover test il bambino osserva un oggetto a distanza, preferibilmente 6 m. Per i bambini di età superiore a 3 anni comunemente si utilizza una tavola oculistica per la fissazione, mentre un giocattolo che fa rumore o un filmato aiuta a mantenere l'attenzione per il test nei più piccoli. Mentre il bambino osserva l'oggetto distante, l'esaminatore copre un occhio e studia il movimento dell'altro. Se non si verifica alcun movimento, non vi è apparente disallineamento di quell'occhio. Dopodiché la stessa procedura viene ripetuta sull'altro occhio. Quando invece si effettua il cover test alternato, l'esaminatore copre e scopre rapidamente ciascun occhio, muovendo l'occlusore da un occhio all'altro. Se il bambino presenta una deviazione oculare, l'occhio si muove rapidamente quando la copertura viene spostata all'altro. Entrambi i test andrebbero eseguiti con la fissazione da lontano e da vicino. Il cover-uncover test differenzia le tropie, o deviazioni manifeste, dalle deviazioni latenti, denominate forie.

MANIFESTAZIONI CLINICHE E TRATTAMENTO. La classificazione eziologica dello strabismo è complessa e si devono distinguere i tipi causativi; esistono forme comitanti e non comitanti.

Strabismo comitante. È il tipo più comune di strabismo. Di solito i singoli muscoli extraoculari non presentano alcun deficit. L'entità della deviazione è costante o relativamente costante nelle varie direzioni dello sguardo.

Lo **pseudostrabismo** (pseudoesotropia) è una delle ragioni più comuni per cui si richiede all'oculista pediatrico di valutare un bambino. Questa condizione è caratterizzata dalla falsa presenza di strabismo quando invece gli assi visivi sono allineati in modo accurato. Ciò può essere determinato da un setto nasale largo e piatto, da pieghe epicantiche prominenti o da una ridotta distanza interpupillare. L'osservatore può rilevare una minore quantità di sclera bianca medialmente rispetto a quella prevista, ricavandone l'impressione che l'occhio sia diretto verso il naso, specialmente quando il bambino guarda verso un lato o l'altro. Frequentemente i genitori commentano che quando il bambino guarda di lato l'occhio quasi scompare dalla vista. La pseudoesotropia si può differenziare da un disallineamento vero quando il riflesso corneale alla luce è centrato in entrambi gli occhi e quando il cover-uncover test non mostra alcun movimento di rifissazione. Dopo avere confermato la pseudoesotropia, i genitori possono essere rassicurati che l'esotropia scomparirà con la crescita, quando il setto nasale si fa più prominente e sposta le pieghe epicantiche, mentre la sclera mediale diventa proporzionale alla quantità visibile lateralmente. L'apparente deviazione scomparirà con lo sviluppo. Alcuni genitori ritengono erroneamente che il loro bambino abbia un'esotropia vera che si risolverà spontaneamente. Dato che questa può svilupparsi in un momento successivo nei bambini con pseudoesotropia, i genitori e i pediatri dovrebbero essere messi in guardia sulla necessità di una rivalutazione se l'apparente deviazione non migliora.

Le **esodeviazioni** sono il tipo più comune di disallineamento oculare nei bambini e rappresentano >50% di tutte le deviazioni oculari. Il termine *esotropia congenita* appare poco appropriato, dal momento che pochi tra i bambini cui è stata diagnosticata questa alterazione sono effettivamente nati con un'esotropia. La maggior parte dei casi riportati in letteratura ha pertanto considerato che questa malattia sia la stessa che si riscontra nei bambini con un esordio confermato prima dei 6 mesi e che alcuni osservatori hanno denominato *esotropia infantile*.

L'angolo caratteristico delle esodeviazioni congenite è ampio e incostante (Fig. 622-1). A causa dell'ampia deviazione, frequentemente si riscontra una fissazione crociata, uno stato in cui il bambino guarda a destra con l'occhio sinistro e a sinistra con l'occhio destro. Con la fissazione crociata non vi è la necessità che l'occhio devi dal naso (abduzione), perché l'occhio adducente viene utilizzato nello sguardo laterale; tale situazione simula una paralisi del sesto nervo cranico. L'abduzione può essere dimostrata dalla manovra degli occhi di bambola o occludendo un occhio per un breve periodo. I bambini con l'esotropia congenita tendono a presentare errori refrattivi simili a quelli dei bambini normali della stessa età, il che contrasta con il caratteristico livello elevato d'ipermetropia associata all'esotropia accomodativa. L'**ambliopia** è comune nei bambini con esotropia congenita.

L'obiettivo primario del trattamento nell'esotropia congenita è di eliminare o ridurre il più possibile la deviazione. Idealmente ciò porta a una vista normale in entrambi gli occhi, a occhi correttamente allineati e allo sviluppo della visione binoculare. Il trattamento precoce ha una maggiore probabilità di condurre allo sviluppo di tale visione, la quale aiuta a mantenere l'allineamento oculare a lungo termine. Dopo avere trattato l'eventuale ambliopia associata, si effettua l'intervento chirurgico per allineare gli occhi. Anche nel caso in cui l'allineamento tramite chirurgia abbia successo, comunemente compaiono deviazioni verticali nei bambini con un'anamnesi di esotropia congenita. Le due forme più comuni di deviazione verticale sono l'iperattività del muscolo obliquo inferiore e la deviazione verticale dissociata. Nella prima, il muscolo obliquo inferiore iperattivo produce uno spostamento verso l'alto dell'occhio più vicino al naso quando il paziente guarda di lato (Fig. 622-2). Nella deviazione verticale dissociata, invece, un occhio si sposta verso l'alto lentamente senza alcun movimento dell'altro. L'intervento chirurgico può essere necessario per trattare una o entrambe queste malattie.

È importante che i genitori si rendano conto che il successo dell'allineamento chirurgico iniziale è solo l'avvio del processo di trattamento. Dal momento che molti bambini possono sviluppare nuovamente lo strabismo o l'ambliopia, essi vanno strettamente monitorati durante il periodo della vita in cui la vista è ancora immatura.

L'*esotropia accomodativa* è definita come una "deviazione convergente degli occhi associata all'attivazione del riflesso accomodativo (focalizzante)". Essa si verifica solitamente in un bambino fra i 2 e i 3 anni di vita con un'anamnesi di incrociamento acquisito intermittente o costante. Un'ambliopia è presente nella maggior parte dei casi.

Nel meccanismo dell'esotropia accomodativa sono implicate un'ipermetropia non corretta, l'accomodazione e la convergenza accomodativa. L'immagine che arriva a un occhio ipermetrope è offuscata. Se l'entità dell'ipermetropia non è significativa, l'immagine offuscata può essere messa a fuoco mediante un'accomodazione (messa a fuoco del cristallino dell'occhio). L'accomodazione è strettamente collegata alla convergenza (gli occhi si dirigono verso l'interno). Se l'errore refrattivo ipermetropico di un bambino è ampio o se l'entità della convergenza che si verifica in risposta a ciascuna unità di sforzo accomodativo è elevata, si può sviluppare l'esotropia.

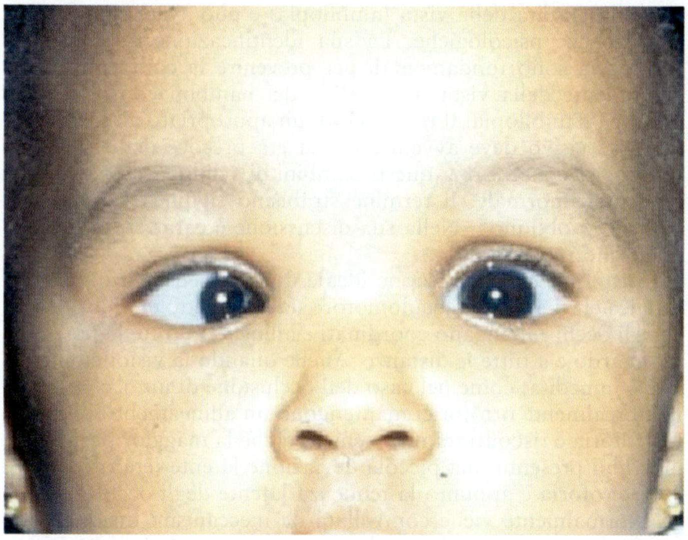

Figura 622-1. Esotropia congenita. Si noti l'ampio angolo di deviazione.

Per trattare l'esotropia accomodativa inizialmente si prescrive la correzione ipermetropica completa, con occhiali che eliminano la necessità del bambino di accomodare e quindi correggono l'esotropia (Fig. 622-3). Sebbene molti genitori siano inizialmente preoccupati che il loro bambino non vorrà indossarli, i vantaggi della visione binoculare e la diminuzione dello sforzo focalizzante necessario per vedere in modo nitido rappresenteranno un potente stimolo per renderli bene accetti. Talvolta la correzione ipermetropica completa raddrizza la posizione dell'occhio nella fissazione da lontano, ma lascia una deviazione residua nella fissazione da vicino; questa situazione può essere sottoposta a una semplice osservazione oppure può essere trattata mediante lenti bifocali, gocce antiaccomodative o intervento chirurgico.

È importante avvisare i genitori dei bambini con un'esotropia accomodativa che l'esodeviazione può apparentemente aumentare senza gli occhiali dopo la correzione iniziale. Frequentemente i genitori riferiscono che prima di indossare gli occhiali il bambino presentava un'esodeviazione piccola, mentre dopo averli tolti questa diventa piuttosto ampia e spesso imputano questo fenomeno agli occhiali. L'aumento apparente è tuttavia dovuto al fatto che il bambino utilizza l'appropriata quantità di sforzo accomodativo dopo avere indossato gli occhiali, quindi quando li toglie continua a praticare un tentativo di accomodazione per portare gli oggetti nel fuoco appropriato e questo aumenta l'esodeviazione.

La maggior parte dei bambini mantiene gli occhi diritti dopo il trattamento iniziale. Dal momento che in genere l'ipermetropia si riduce con l'età, molti pazienti non hanno più necessità di indossare gli occhiali per mantenere l'allineamento. In alcuni persiste un'esodeviazione residua anche con gli occhiali, la quale si verifica comunemente quando vi è un ritardo tra l'esordio dell'esotropia accomodativa e il trattamento. In altri pazienti l'esotropia può inizialmente essere eliminata con gli occhiali ma l'incrociamento si sviluppa nuovamente e non può essere corretto con essi. L'incrociamento non più correggibile con gli occhiali è

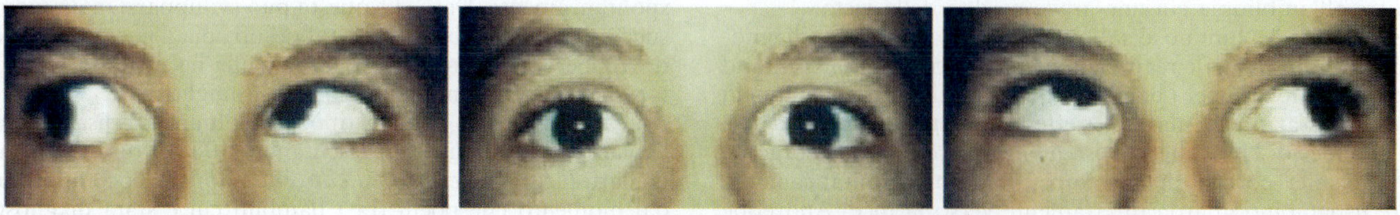

Figura 622-2. Iperattività del muscolo obliquo inferiore.

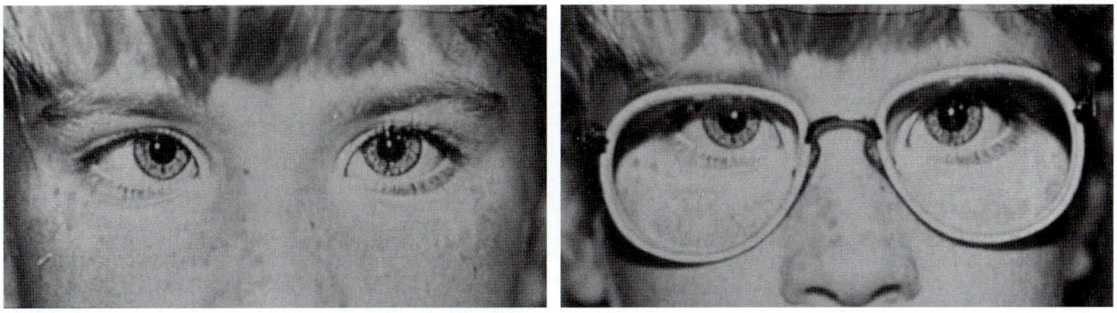

Figura 622-3. Esotropia accomodativa; controllo della deviazione con lenti correttive.

la porzione deteriorata o non accomodativa, per la quale può risultare indicato l'intervento chirurgico al fine di ripristinare la visione binoculare.

Le **exodeviazioni** sono il secondo tipo più frequente di disallineamento. La deviazione divergente può essere intermittente o costante. Quella intermittente è l'esodeviazione più comune nell'infanzia, caratterizzata dalla deviazione esterna di un occhio, che di solito si verifica quando il bambino fissa da lontano e che in genere risulta più frequente con l'affaticamento o con la malattia. L'esposizione alla luce chiara può provocare la chiusura riflessa dell'occhio isotropico. Dato che gli occhi inizialmente possono essere mantenuti diritti per la maggior parte del tempo, l'acuità visiva tende a essere buona in entrambi e la visione binoculare è normale.

L'età all'esordio dell'esotropia intermittente è variabile, ma è spesso compresa tra 6 mesi e 4 anni. La decisione di effettuare l'intervento chirurgico sul muscolo oculare si basa sull'entità e sulla frequenza della deviazione. Se risulta modesta e infrequente, è ragionevole sottoporre il bambino a osservazione, ma se l'esotropia è ampia o aumenta di frequenza, l'intervento chirurgico è indicato per mantenere la visione binoculare normale.

L'esotropia costante rare volte può essere congenita. L'esotropia congenita può associarsi a una malattia neurologica o ad anomalie dell'orbita ossea, come nella sindrome di Crouzon. L'esotropia che si verifica successivamente nella vita può rappresentare il peggioramento di un'esotropia intermittente che era presente nell'infanzia. L'intervento chirurgico può ripristinare la visione binoculare anche nei casi che durano da molto tempo.

Strabismo non comitante. Quando un muscolo oculare è paretico, paralizzato o ristretto, si verifica uno squilibrio muscolare in cui la deviazione dell'occhio varia a seconda della direzione dello sguardo. L'esordio recente di un muscolo paretico può essere suggerito dal sintomo della visione doppia che aumenta in una direzione, l'osservazione di una deviazione oculare che aumenta nel campo d'azione del muscolo paretico e un incremento della deviazione quando il bambino fissa con l'occhio paretico. È importante differenziare uno strabismo non comitante da una deviazione comitante, perché le forme non comitanti sono spesso associate a un trauma, a malattie sistemiche o ad anomalie neurologiche.

Paralisi del terzo nervo cranico. Nella popolazione pediatrica, le paralisi del terzo nervo cranico sono solitamente congenite. La forma congenita è spesso associata a un'anomalia dello sviluppo o a un trauma da parto. Queste paralisi nei bambini possono costituire un segno infausto e indicare un'anomalia neurologica come una neoplasia o un aneurisma endocranici. Tra le altre cause meno gravi rientrano lesioni infiammatorie o infettive, traumi cranici, sindromi postvirali ed emicranie.

Una paralisi del terzo nervo cranico, sia essa congenita o acquisita, di solito porta a exotropia e ipotropia o deviazione verso il basso dell'occhio affetto, così come a ptosi completa o parziale della palpebra superiore. Questo strabismo caratteristico è dovuto all'azione di muscoli non contrastati normali, il retto laterale e l'obliquo superiore. Se è interessato il ramo interno del terzo nervo cranico, si può osservare anche una dilatazione pupillare. I movimenti oculari sono solitamente limitati dal lato nasale, in elevazione e in depressione. Inoltre, i reperti clinici e il trattamento possono essere complicati nei casi congeniti e traumatici di paralisi del terzo nervo a causa dell'errata direzione delle fibre nervose che si rigenerano, nota come rigenerazione aberrante. Ciò determina movimenti paradossi della palpebra, dell'occhio e della pupilla, come l'elevazione della palpebra, la costrizione della pupilla o la depressione del globo oculare nel tentativo dello sguardo mediale.

Paralisi del quarto nervo cranico. Queste paralisi possono essere congenite o acquisite. Dato che il quarto nervo presenta un decorso intracranico, è suscettibile al danno secondario a un trauma cranico. Nei bambini, tuttavia, le paralisi sono più frequentemente congenite che traumatiche. Una paralisi del quarto nervo cranico determina la debolezza del muscolo obliquo superiore, che causa una deviazione verso l'alto dell'occhio, un'ipertropia. Dal momento che il muscolo antagonista, l'obliquo inferiore, è relativamente incontrastato, l'occhio affetto devia verso l'alto quando l'individuo guarda verso il naso. Tipicamente i bambini si presentano con il capo inclinato verso la spalla del lato opposto a quello dell'occhio colpito, il mento verso il basso e il volto rivolto verso la direzione opposta a quella affetta. La posizione della testa allontana l'occhio dall'area di massima azione del muscolo coinvolto e quindi riduce al minimo la deviazione e la visione doppia associata. Le inclinazioni del capo di lunga data possono portare a un'asimmetria facciale. L'ambliopia è rara, in quanto l'anomala postura del capo mantiene l'allineamento oculare. Non essendoci alcuna anomalia nei muscoli del collo, i tentativi di correzione dell'inclinazione del capo mediante esercizi e intervento chirurgico su questi muscoli risultano inefficaci. Il riconoscimento di una paresi obliqua superiore può comportare difficoltà, perché la deviazione del capo e dell'occhio può essere minima. L'intervento chirurgico sul muscolo oculare può essere effettuato per migliorare l'allineamento oculare ed eliminare la postura anomala.

Paralisi del sesto nervo cranico. Queste paralisi determinano un grave incrociamento degli occhi con una limitata capacità di spostare lateralmente l'occhio affetto. Frequentemente i bambini si presentano con il capo inclinato verso il muscolo paralizzato, una posizione che aiuta a conservare la visione binoculare. L'esotropia più ampia si osserva quando l'occhio viene spostato verso il muscolo colpito.

Le paralisi congenite del sesto nervo sono rare. La diminuzione dello sguardo laterale nei bambini è spesso associata ad altre malattie, come l'esotropia congenita o la sindrome da retrazione di Duane. Nei neonati si può verificare una paresi transitoria, che di solito si risolve spontaneamente entro 6 settimane. Si ritiene che un fattore contribuente sia l'aumento della pressione intracranica associata al travaglio e al parto.

Le paralisi acquisite nell'infanzia sono spesso un segno infausto, perché il sesto nervo è suscettibile all'aumentata pressione intracranica determinata da idrocefalo e da tumori intracranici. Tra le altre cause di deficit del sesto nervo nei bambini vi sono traumi, malformazioni vascolari, meningite e sindrome di Gradenigo. Una paralisi benigna, indolore e acquisita, può essere osservata nei bambini piccoli e in quelli più grandi, frequentemente preceduta da una malattia febbrile o da un'infezione del tratto respiratorio superiore e possibilmente ricorrente. Di solito si risolve in maniera completa. Sebbene non infrequenti, altre cause di paralisi acuta dovrebbero essere escluse prima di porre tale diagnosi.

SINDROMI DA STRABISMO. Alcuni speciali tipi di strabismo possiedono caratteristiche cliniche insolite. La maggior parte di queste malattie è determinata da anomalie strutturali dei muscoli extraoculari o dei tessuti adiacenti e produce disallineamenti non comitanti.

Doppia paralisi degli elevatori. Un deficit dell'elevazione monoculare nell'abduzione e nell'adduzione è denominato doppia paralisi degli elevatori. Può essere costituita da una paresi di entrambi gli elevatori, i muscoli retto superiore e obliquo inferiore, oppure da una possibile limitazione dell'elevazione dovuta a un muscolo retto inferiore fibrotico. Quando il bambino affetto fissa con l'occhio non paretico, l'altro è ipotropico e la palpebra superiore ipsilaterale può apparire ptosica. La fissazione con l'occhio paretico causa invece un'ipertrofia del non paretico e la scomparsa della ptosi (Fig. 622-4). Dal momento che la ptosi apparente è di fatto secondaria allo strabismo, la correzione dell'ipotropia la risolve.

Sindrome di Duane. Questa malattia congenita della motilità oculare è caratterizzata dalla retrazione del globo oculare in adduzione. Questo fatto viene attribuito all'assenza del nucleo del sesto nervo e a un'anomala innervazione del muscolo retto laterale, che porta a una contrazione dei muscoli retto mediale e laterale nel tentativo di adduzione dell'occhio affetto. Nello spettro della sindrome di Duane, i pazienti possono presentare la compromissione dell'abduzione, oppure lo spostamento dell'occhio interessato verso l'alto o verso il basso durante l'adduzione. Possono inoltre manifestare esotropia, exotropia o occhi relativamente diritti. Molti assumono una postura compensatoria del capo in modo da mantenere la visione singola. Alcuni sviluppano l'ambliopia. L'intervento chirurgico per migliorare l'allineamento o per ridurre un'evidente rotazione del volto può risultare utile in casi selezionati. La sindrome di Duane solitamente si verifica in modo sporadico; talvolta viene ereditata come tratto autosomico dominante. In genere compare come malattia isolata, ma può trovarsi in associazione ad altre varie anomalie oculari e sistemiche.

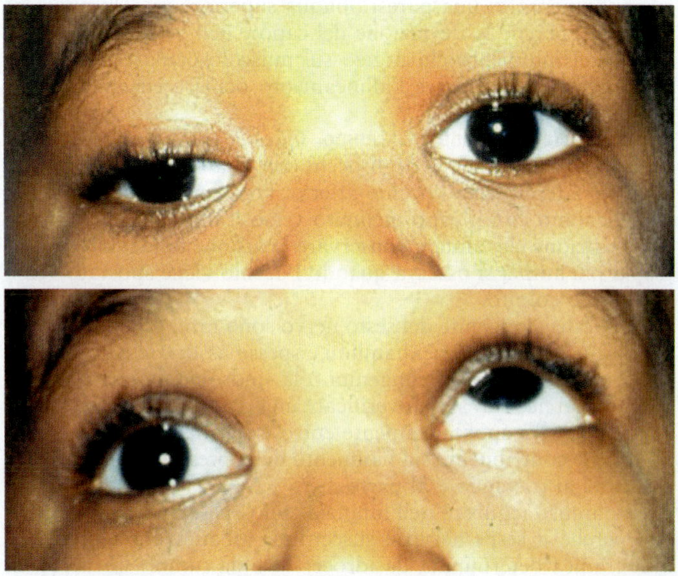

Figura 622-4. Doppia paralisi degli elevatori dell'occhio destro. Si noti la scomparsa della ptosi apparente durante la fissazione con l'occhio interessato.

Sindrome di Möbius. Le caratteristiche distintive della sindrome di Möbius sono la paresi facciale congenita e il deficit dell'abduzione. La paralisi è comunemente bilaterale, frequentemente asimmetrica e spesso incompleta, tendendo a risparmiare la parte inferiore del volto e il platisma. Possono svilupparsi ectropion, epifora e cheratopatia da esposizione. Il deficit dell'abduzione può invece risultare unilaterale o bilaterale. L'esotropia è comune. La causa rimane sconosciuta: non è chiaro se il difetto primario sia l'errato sviluppo dei nuclei del nervo cranico, l'ipoplasia dei muscoli o una combinazione di fattori centrali e periferici. Sono stati riportati alcuni casi familiari. Tra i deficit dello sviluppo associati si possono trovare la ptosi, la paralisi del palato e della lingua, la perdita dell'udito, i deficit dei muscoli pettorali e linguali, la micrognatia, la sindattilia, le dita soprannumerarie e l'assenza delle mani, dei piedi, delle dita delle mani o delle dita dei piedi. È indicata la correzione chirurgica dell'esotropia e si dovrebbe trattare l'eventuale ambliopia associata.

Sindrome di Brown. In questa sindrome l'elevazione dell'occhio in posizione addotta appare limitata (Fig. 622-5). L'occhio affetto può presentare anche un'associata deviazione verso il basso in adduzione. Può essere evidente una postura compensatoria del capo. Sono state descritte varie cause. Alcuni casi sono stati attribuiti ad anomalie strutturali, come un tendine obliquo superiore teso, l'accorciamento o l'ispessimento congenito della guaina del tendine obliquo superiore o trabecole di tessuto connettivo tra il tendine obliquo superiore e la troclea. La sindrome di Brown acquisita può fare seguito a un trauma dell'orbita che interessa la regione della troclea o a un intervento chirurgico sinusale. Può anche insorgere assieme a processi infiammatori, in particolare la sinusite e l'artrite reumatoide giovanile.

La sindrome di Brown infiammatoria acquisita può rispondere al trattamento con farmaci non steroidei o corticosteroidi. L'intervento chirurgico può essere utile per i bambini con sindrome di Brown congenita vera.

Sindrome di Parinaud. Con questo eponimo si indica una paralisi dello sguardo verticale, isolata o associata a paresi pupillare o nucleare dell'oculomotore (terzo nervo cranico). Comporta una lesione che interessa il tegumento mesencefalico. Tra i segni oftalmici di malattia del mesencefalo vi sono la paralisi dello sguardo verticale, la dissociazione delle risposte pupillari alla luce e alla messa a fuoco da vicino, la paralisi pupillomotoria generale, la corectopia, la discoria, i disturbi dell'accomodazione, la retrazione patologica della palpebra, la ptosi, la paresi del muscolo extraoculare e la paralisi della convergenza. Alcuni casi presentano spasmi associati della convergenza, nistagmo da retrazione convergente e nistagmo verticale, in particolare nel tentativo dello sguardo verticale. Le combinazioni di questi segni sono denominati sindrome dell'acquedotto di Silvio.

Una delle principali cause della paralisi dello sguardo verticale e dei segni mesencefalici associati nei bambini è il tumore dell'epifisi o del terzo ventricolo. La diagnosi differenziale comprende traumi e malattia demielinizzante. Nei bambini con idrocefalo, la compromissione dello sguardo verticale e la retrazione patologica palpebrale sono noti come il "segno del sole che tramonta".

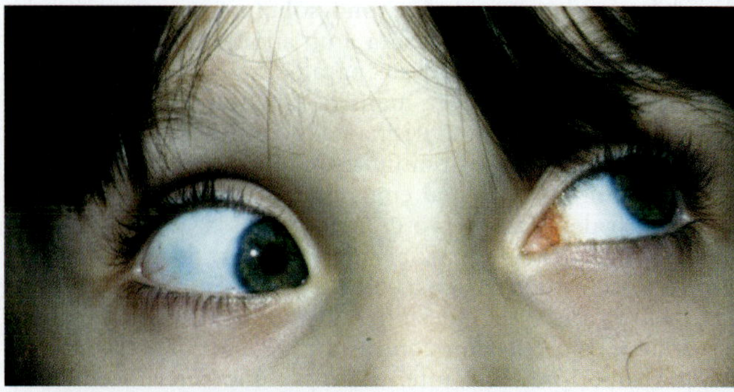

Figura 622-5. Sindrome di Brown dell'occhio destro.

Talvolta anche nei neonati sani si osserva un disturbo transitorio dello sguardo verticale.

APRASSIA OCULOMOTORIA CONGENITA

Questa malattia congenita dello sguardo coniugato è caratterizzata da un deficit nello sguardo orizzontale volontario, da un movimento compensatorio a scatti del capo e dalla conservazione di lenti movimenti di inseguimento e di riflessi oculari. Altre caratteristiche sono l'assenza della fase rapida (rifissazione) del nistagmo optocinetico e la deviazione opposta obbligata degli occhi alla rotazione del corpo. I bambini affetti in genere non sono in grado di guardare rapidamente verso un lato o l'altro in modo volontario in risposta a un comando o a un oggetto presentato in sede eccentrica, ma possono essere capaci di seguire un oggetto che si muove lentamente da un lato all'altro. Per compensare il difetto nei movimenti oculari laterali intenzionali, i bambini manifestano scosse del capo per mantenere gli occhi nella posizione desiderata e possono anche ammiccare ripetutamente nel tentativo di modificare la fissazione. I segni tendono a diventare meno vistosi con l'età.

La patogenesi dell'aprassia oculomotoria congenita è sconosciuta. Essa può fare seguito a una ritardata mielinizzazione delle vie motorie oculari. In pochi pazienti sono state riscontrate anomalie strutturali del sistema nervoso centrale, tra cui l'agenesia del corpo calloso e del verme cerebellare, la porencefalia, l'amartoma del forame di Monro e la macrocefalia. Molti bambini con questa malattia mostrano uno sviluppo motorio e cognitivo ritardato.

NISTAGMO

Il nistagmo (oscillazioni ritmiche di uno o di entrambi gli occhi) può essere causato da un'anomalia in uno dei tre meccanismi di base che regolano la posizione e il movimento degli occhi: la fissazione, lo sguardo coniugato, i meccanismi vestibolari. Inoltre, il nistagmo fisiologico può essere provocato mediante stimoli appropriati (Tab. 622-1).

Il **nistagmo sensoriale congenito** è generalmente associato ad anomalie oculari che conducono alla riduzione dell'acuità visiva; comuni malattie che portano al nistagmo a esordio precoce sono l'albinismo, l'aniridia, l'acromatopsia, la cataratta congenita, le lesioni maculari congenite e l'atrofia ottica congenita. In alcuni casi il nistagmo insorge come caratteristica dominante o X-linked senza evidenti anomalie oculari.

Il **nistagmo motorio idiopatico congenito** è caratterizzato da scosse oscillanti del capo con preponderanza della fissazione; il nistagmo risulta più grossolano in una direzione di sguardo che nell'altra, con la scossa verso quella direzione. Non sono presenti difetti anatomici che lo determinino e l'acuità visiva di solito è pressoché normale. Ci può essere un punto nullo in cui il nistagmo diminuisce e la vista migliora; si svilupperà allora una postura compensatoria del capo che colloca gli occhi nella posizione di nistagmo minore. La causa del nistagmo motorio idiopatico congenito è sconosciuta; in alcuni casi è familiare. L'intervento chirurgico sul muscolo oculare può essere effettuato per eliminare l'anomala postura del capo, portando il punto di visione migliore nello sguardo diritto.

Il **nistagmo acquisito** richiede una valutazione tempestiva e completa. Tipi patologici preoccupanti sono le oscillazioni sguardo-paretiche o sguardo-evocate delle malattie cerebellare, cerebrale o del tronco cerebrale.

Il **nistagmo retractorius** o **nistagmo convergente** consiste in scatti ripetuti degli occhi nell'orbita o di un occhio verso l'altro. Solitamente compare in caso di una paralisi verticale dello sguardo nell'ambito della sindrome di Parinaud (dell'acquedotto di Silvio). La malattia causale può essere neoplastica, vascolare o infiammatoria. Nei bambini il nistagmo retractorius suggerisce particolarmente la presenza di un pinealoma o di un idrocefalo.

Un approccio diagnostico al nistagmo è presentato nella Figura 622-6.

Lo **spasmus nutans** è un particolare tipo di nistagmo acquisito nell'infanzia (vedi anche Capitolo 597). Nella sua forma completa è caratterizzato dalla **triade** di nistagmo pendolare, testa ciondolante e torcicollo. Il nistagmo è caratteristicamente molto fine, molto rapido, orizzontale e pendolare; spesso è asimmetrico, talvolta unilaterale. Di solito i segni si sviluppano entro il primo o il secondo anno di vita. Le componenti della triade possono comparire in epoche diverse. In molti casi la malattia è benigna e autolimitata, di solito dura pochi mesi, talvolta anni. La causa della forma classica di spasmus nutans, che di solito si risolve spontaneamente, è sconosciuta. Alcuni bambini che presentano segni simili a quelli dello spasmus nutans hanno tumori cerebrali sottostanti, in particolare gliomi ipotalamici e del chiasma ottico. Di conseguenza si raccomandano un'appropriata valutazione neurologica e neuroradiologica e un attento monitoraggio dei bambini piccoli e grandi con nistagmo.

ALTRI MOVIMENTI OCULARI ANOMALI

Da tenere distinti rispetto al nistagmo vero vi sono alcuni speciali tipi di movimenti oculari anomali, in particolare l'opsoclono, la dismetria oculare e il flutter (Tab. 622-2).

OPSOCLONO. L'opsoclono e i movimenti coniugati atassici sono movimenti caotici, multidirezionali, non ritmici, spontanei. Gli occhi sembrano essere in agitazione, con raffiche di movimenti coniugati di ampiezza e direzione variabili. L'opsoclono è più spesso associato all'encefalite. Può essere il primo segno di un neuroblastoma.

DISMETRIA MOTORIA OCULARE. È analoga alla dismetria degli arti. Gli individui che ne sono affetti mostrano, nell'effettuare movimenti di rifissazione, una mancanza di precisione caratterizzata

TABELLA 622-1. Tipologie specifiche di nistagmo

TIPOLOGIA	DESCRIZIONE	MALATTIE ASSOCIATE
Nistagmo latente	Nistagmo saccadico coniugato verso l'occhio fissante	Deficit congeniti della vista, si verifica con l'occlusione dell'occhio
Nistagmo latente manifesto	Fase rapida verso l'occhio fissante	Strabismo, nistagmo idiopatico congenito
Alternante periodico	Cicli orizzontali o orizzontali-rotatori che cambiano direzione	Causato da malattie visive e neurologiche
Nistagmo tipo see-saw	Un occhio va in alto e ruota verso l'interno mentre l'altro scende e ruota verso l'esterno	Di solito associato a difetti del chiasma ottico
Nistagmo retractorius	Gli occhi si muovono a scosse posteriormente nell'orbita o l'uno verso l'altro	Causato dalla pressione sul tegumento mesencefalico (sindrome di Parinaud)
Nistagmo evocato dallo sguardo	Nistagmo a scatti in direzione dello sguardo	Causato da farmaci, lesione del tronco cerebrale o disfunzione labirintica
Nistagmo sguardo-paretico	Gli occhi si muovono a scatti posteriormente per mantenere lo sguardo eccentrico	Malattia cerebellare
Nistagmo che batte verso il basso	La fase rapida batte verso il basso	Malattia della fossa posteriore, farmaci
Nistagmo che batte verso l'alto	La fase rapida batte verso l'alto	Malattia cerebellare e del tronco cerebrale; alcune malattie visive
Nistagmo vestibolare	Scatti orizzontali-torsionali o orizzontali	Disfunzione del sistema vestibolare
Nistagmo asimmetrico o monoculare	Nistagmo verticale pendolare	Malattia della retina e delle vie ottiche
Spasmus nutans	Nistagmo fine, rapido, pendolare	Torcicollo, spasmo del capo; idiopatico o gliomi delle vie ottiche

Da Kliegman R: *Practical Strategies in Pediatric Diagnosis and Therapy*. Philadelphia, WB Saunders, 1996.

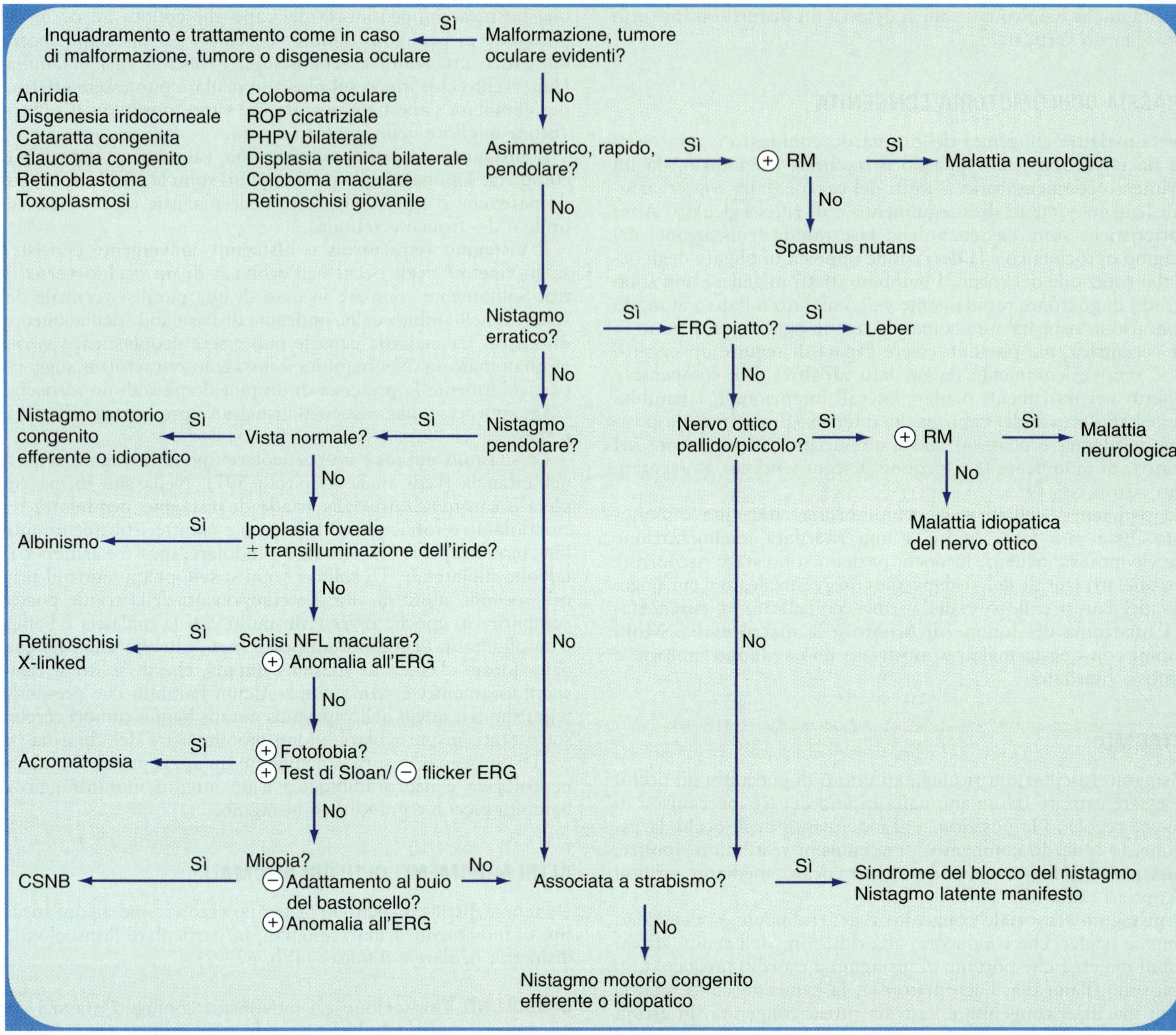

Figura 622-6. Algoritmo per l'inquadramento di un bambino con nistagmo. (+), positività; (−), negatività; CNNB, cecità notturna congenita stazionaria (*Congenital Stationary Night Blindness*); ERG, elettroretinogramma; NFL, strato della fibra nervosa (*Nerve Fiber Layer*); PHPV, vitreo primario iperplasico persistente (*Persistent Hyperplastic Primary Vitreous*); ROP, retinopatia della prematurità (*Retinopathy Of Prematurity*). (Da Nelson LB: *Harley's Pediatric Ophthalmology*, 4th ed. Philadelphia, WB Saunders, 1998, p 470.)

TABELLA 622-2. Forme specifiche di movimenti oculari diversi dal nistagmo

TIPO	DESCRIZIONE	MALATTIE ASSOCIATE
Opsoclono	Movimenti multidirezionali coniugati di frequenza e direzione variabili	Idrocefalo, malattie del tronco cerebrale e del cervelletto, neuroblastoma
Dismetria oculare	Spostamento in alto degli occhi alla fissazione rapida	Disfunzione cerebellare
Flutter oculare	Oscillazioni orizzontali con sguardo in avanti e talvolta con ammiccamento	Malattia cerebellare, idrocefalo o neoplasia del sistema nervoso centrale
Bobbing oculare	Scatto verso il basso dallo sguardo primario, che rimane per pochi secondi quindi ritorna in posizione	Malattia pontina
Mioclono oculare	Oscillazioni pendolari ritmiche in avanti e indietro degli occhi, con movimento muscolare non oculare sincrono	Danneggiamento del nucleo rosso, del nucleo olivare inferiore e del nucleo dentato ipsilaterale

Da Kliegman R: *Practical Strategies in Pediatric Diagnosis and Therapy*. Philadelphia, WB Saunders, 1996.

da uno spostamento verso l'alto (o verso il basso) degli occhi con diverse oscillazioni correttive in su e in giù guardando da un punto all'altro. La dismetria motoria oculare è un segno di malattia cerebellare o delle vie cerebellari.

OSCILLAZIONI A FLUTTER. Queste oscillazioni orizzontali intermittenti da e verso gli occhi possono verificarsi spontaneamente o per cambiamenti di fissazione. Sono caratteristiche della malattia cerebellare.

Abroms AD, Mohney BG, Rush DP, et al: Timely surgery in intermittent and constant exotropia for superior sensory outcome. *Am J Ophthalmol* 2001;131:111–116.

Holmes JM, Mutyala S, Maus TL, et al: Pediatric third, fourth, and sixth nerve palsies: A population-based study. *Am J Ophthalmol* 1999;127:388–392.
Hunter DG, Kelly JB, Buffenn AN, et al: Long-term outcome of uncomplicated infantile exotropia. *J AAPOS* 2001;5:352–356.
Ing M: Early surgical alignment for congenital esotropia. *Ophthalmology* 1983;90:132–135.
Lambert SR, Lynn M, Sramek J, et al: Clinical features predictive of successfully weaning from spectacles those children with accommodative esotropia. *J AAPOS* 2003;7:7–13.
Mohney BG, Huffaker RK: Common forms of childhood exotropia. *Ophthalmology* 2003;110:2093–2096.
Morris RJ, Scott WE, Dickey CF: Fusion after surgical alignment of longstanding strabismus in adults. *Ophthalmology* 1993;100:135–137.
Olitsky SE, Nelson LB: Strabismus disorders. In Nelson LB, Olitsky SE (editors): *Harley's Pediatric Ophthalmology,* 5th ed. Philadelphia, Lippincott Williams & Wilkins, 2005 pp 143–192.
Pediatric Eye Disease Investigator Group: Spontaneous resolution of early-onset esotropia: Experience of the Congenital Esotropia Observational Study. *Am J Ophthalmol* 2002;133:109–118.
Pranzatelli MR, Tate ED, Travelstead AL, et al: Immunologic and clinical responses to rituximab in a child with opsoclonus-myoclonus syndrome. *Pediatrics* 2005;115:e115–e119.
Strominger M: Nystagmus. In Nelson LB, Olitsky SE (editors): *Harley's Pediatric Ophthalmology,* 5th ed. Philadelphia, Lippincott Williams & Wilkins, 2005, pp 475–507.
Tarpey P, Thomas S, Sarvananthan N, et al: Mutations in FRMDT, a newly identified member of the FERM family, cause X: linked idiopathic congenital nystagmus. *Nature Genetics* 2006;38:1242–1244.

Capitolo 623 ■ Anomalie delle palpebre

Scott E. Olitsky, Denise Hug e Laura P. Smith

PTOSI. Nella blefaroptosi la palpebra superiore si abbassa al di sotto del suo livello normale. La ptosi congenita è di solito dovuta a una distrofia localizzata del muscolo elevatore, in cui le fibre muscolari striate sono sostituite da tessuto fibrotico. La malattia può risultare unilaterale o bilaterale e può essere familiare, trasmessa come tratto dominante.

Spesso i genitori commentano che l'occhio sembra più piccolo a causa della palpebra cadente. La piega palpebrale è ridotta o assente nel punto in cui il muscolo elevatore di norma si inserirebbe al di sotto della superficie cutanea. Dal momento che questo muscolo è sostituito da tessuto fibroso, la palpebra non si sposta completamente in basso quando lo sguardo vi viene rivolto (*lidlag*). Se la ptosi è grave, i bambini che ne sono affetti spesso tentano di sollevare la palpebra tirando su il sopracciglio o adattando una postura del capo con il mento verso l'alto per mantenere la visione binoculare. La **ptosi maxillo-palpebrale di Marcus Gunn** rappresenta il 5% delle ptosi nei bambini. In questa sindrome esiste un'anomala sincinesia tra il quinto e il terzo nervo cranico, che determina il sollevamento della palpebra con il movimento della mascella. L'ammiccamento è prodotto dalla masticazione o dalla suzione e può essere più evidente della ptosi stessa.

Sebbene la ptosi nei bambini sia spesso un reperto isolato, essa si può verificare in associazione ad altre malattie oculari o sistemiche. Tra le sistemiche vi sono la miastenia grave, la distrofia e il botulismo, mentre tra le oculari si trovano la ptosi meccanica secondaria a tumori palpebrali, la sindrome della blefarofimosi, la sindrome della fibrosi congenita, l'errato sviluppo combinato dell'elevatore e del retto superiore e la paralisi congenita o acquisita del terzo nervo cranico. Una ptosi di grado modesto è osservata nella sindrome di Horner (vedi Capitolo 621). Un esame oftalmico e sistemico completo sono pertanto importanti nella valutazione.

Nei bambini con ptosi può comparire l'**ambliopia**, che può essere secondaria al fatto che la palpebra copre l'asse visivo (deprivazione) o a un astigmatismo indotto (anisometropia). Quando è presente l'ambliopia, in genere dovrebbe essere trattata prima della ptosi stessa.

Il **trattamento** della ptosi nel bambino è indicato per eliminare un'anomala posizione del capo, migliorare il campo visivo, prevenire l'ambliopia e ripristinare un normale aspetto della palpebra. La scelta del momento per realizzare l'intervento dipende dal grado della ptosi, dalla sua gravità estetica e funzionale, dalla presenza o assenza di atteggiamenti posturali compensatori, dalle richieste dei genitori e dal giudizio del chirurgo. Il trattamento chirurgico viene stabilito in base all'entità della funzione dell'elevatore, la cui resezione può essere operata nei bambini con funzione da moderata a buona, mentre in quelli con funzione scarsa o assente può risultare necessaria una procedura di sospensione del frontale. Questa tecnica comporta il posizionamento di materiale di sospensione tra il muscolo frontale e il tarso della palpebra, consentendo con ciò ai pazienti di utilizzare più efficacemente il sopracciglio e il muscolo frontale per sollevare la palpebra. Dopo la correzione chirurgica rimane la preoccupazione per l'ambliopia, che andrebbe strettamente monitorata.

PIEGHE EPICANTICHE. Si tratta di pieghe cutanee verticali o oblique che si estendono su ciascun lato della radice nasale dall'area del sopracciglio o della palpebra e che ricoprono la regione del canto interno. Un certo grado di pieghe epicantiche è presente nella maggior parte dei bambini piccoli e diventa meno evidente con l'età. Le pieghe possono essere sufficientemente larghe da ricoprire la porzione mediale dell'occhio, portando in apparenza gli occhi a incrociarsi (pseudoesotropia). Le pieghe epicantiche sono una caratteristica comune di molte sindromi, tra cui aberrazioni cromosomiche (trisomie) e malattie monogeniche.

LAGOFTALMO. Si tratta di una malattia in cui la completa chiusura delle palpebre sul globo oculare risulta difficoltosa o impossibile. Può essere di origine paralitica, per una paralisi facciale con interessamento del muscolo orbicolare, oppure spastica, come nella tireotossicosi. Può essere strutturale quando la retrazione o l'accorciamento delle palpebre sono dovuti a una fibrosi cicatriziale o a un'atrofia secondaria a lesioni (ustioni) o a malattia. I bambini con membrana colloidale possono presentare un lagoftalmo temporaneo, determinato dall'effetto restrittivo della membrana sulle palpebre. Il lagoftalmo può accompagnare la proptosi o il buftalmo quando le palpebre, sebbene normali, non possono coprire efficacemente l'occhio ingrandito o protuberante. Un certo grado di lagoftalmo può verificarsi normalmente durante il sonno, ma il lagoftalmo funzionale può costituire un disturbo in un paziente in stato di incoscienza o debilitato.

Nei pazienti con lagoftalmo l'esposizione dell'occhio può portare a secchezza, infezione, ulcerazione o perforazione della cornea; ciò può determinare la perdita della vista e anche dell'occhio. Nel lagoftalmo la protezione dell'occhio con preparati a base di lacrime artificiali, unguento oftalmico o camere da applicare agli occhiali per mantenere inumidito e protetto l'occhio è fondamentale. I tamponi di garze devono essere evitati, perché la garza può provocare abrasioni della cornea. In alcuni casi la chiusura chirurgica delle palpebra (tarsorrafia) può essere necessaria per la protezione a lungo termine dell'occhio.

RETRAZIONI PALPEBRALI. La retrazione patologica della palpebra può essere miogena o neurogena. Quella miogena della palpebra superiore si verifica nella tireotossicosi, in cui è associata a tre segni classici: un aspetto di sguardo sbarrato (segno di Dalrymple), un ammiccamento scarso (segno di Stellwag) e un incompleto abbassamento della palpebra superiore durante lo sguardo verso il basso (segno di von Graefe).

La retrazione neurogena delle palpebre può comparire nelle malattie che colpiscono il mesencefalo anteriore. La retrazione palpebrale è una caratteristica della sindrome dell'acquedotto di Silvio. Nei bambini è un segno comune di idrocefalo. Si può verificare in caso di meningite. La retrazione paradossa è osservata nella sindrome maxillo-palpebrale di Marcus Gunn e possibilmente anche durante i tentativi di movimento oculare in seguito alla guarigione da una paralisi del terzo nervo cranico, in presenza di rigenerazione aberrante delle fibre del nervo oculomotore.

Lo sguardo sbarrato semplice e la retrazione palpebrale fisiologica o riflessa ("eye popping"), a differenza delle retrazioni palpebrali patologiche, si verificano nei bambini in risposta a un'improvvisa riduzione dell'illuminazione o come reazione a uno spavento.

ECTROPION, ENTROPION ED EPIBLEFARON. L'**ectropion** consiste nell'eversione del margine palpebrale; può portare a iperlacrimazione (epifora) e conseguente macerazione della cute palpebrale, infiammazione della congiuntiva esposta o cheratopatia superficiale da esposizione. Cause comuni sono la cicatrizzazione secondaria a un'infiammazione, ustioni o traumi oppure il deficit del muscolo orbicolare in seguito a una paralisi facciale; queste forme possono essere corrette chirurgicamente. La protezione della cornea è fondamentale. L'ectropion è presente anche in alcuni bambini con lo sviluppo difettoso del legamento cantale laterale, come può avvenire nella sindrome di Down.

L'**entropion** è l'inversione del margine palpebrale, che provoca fastidio e danno corneale dovuti al fatto che le ciglia sono dirette verso l'interno (trichiasi). Una causa primaria è la cicatrizzazione secondaria a una infiammazione, come quella che si verifica nel tracoma o come sequela della sindrome di Stevens-Johnson. Vi sono anche rare forme congenite. La correzione chirurgica è efficace in molti casi.

L'**epiblefaron** è comunemente osservato nell'infanzia e può essere confuso con l'entropion. Nell'epiblefaron, una piega di cute al di sotto delle ciglia della palpebra inferiore fa sì che esse siano dirette verticalmente e vengano a contatto con la cornea (Fig. 623-1). A differenza dell'entropion, il margine palpebrale non è di per sé ruotato verso la cornea. Di solito l'epiblefaron si risolve spontaneamente. Se inizia a comparire la cicatrizzazione corneale, può essere necessaria la correzione chirurgica.

BLEFAROSPASMO. Consiste nella chiusura spastica o ripetitiva delle palpebre che può essere determinata da una malattia irritativa della cornea, della congiuntiva o del nervo facciale, dall'affaticamento o da un errore refrattivo non corretto, oppure può costituire un tic comune. È indicato un esame completo alla ricerca delle cause patologiche, come trichiasi, cheratite, congiuntivite e corpi estranei. L'iniezione locale di tossina botulinica può produrre sollievo, ma frequentemente deve essere ripetuta.

BLEFARITE. Questa infiammazione dei margini palpebrali è caratterizzata da eritema e formazione di croste o squame; i sintomi abituali sono irritazione, bruciore e prurito. La malattia è solitamente bilaterale e cronica o ricorrente. Le due forme principali sono quella **stafilococcica** e quella **seborroica**. Nella prima l'ulcerazione del margine palpebrale è comune, le ciglia tendono a cadere e spesso si associano la congiuntivite e una cheratite superficiale. Nella blefarite seborroica le squame tendono a essere untuose, i margini palpebrali meno arrossati e di solito non compare l'ulcerazione. La blefarite si trova spesso di tipo misto.

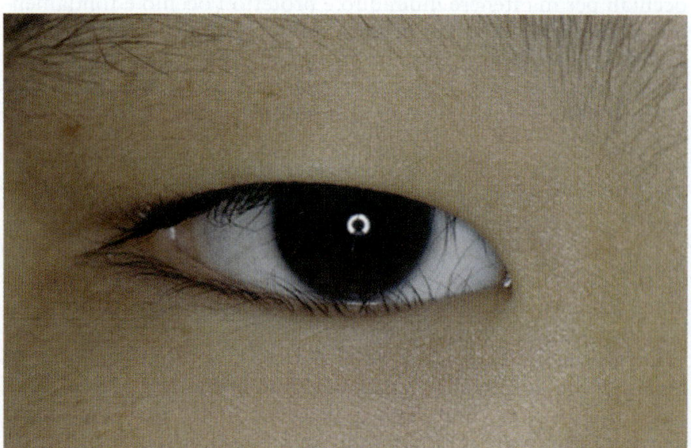

Figura 623-1. Epiblefaron.

Nel **trattamento** di entrambe le forme è importante una pulizia quotidiana completa dei margini palpebrali con un panno o un applicatore di cotone inumidito, per rimuovere le squame e le croste. La blefarite stafilococcica viene trattata con un antibiotico antistafilococcico applicato direttamente sui margini palpebrali. Quando il bambino presenta anche la seborrea, è importante il concomitante trattamento del cuoio capelluto.

La pediculosi delle ciglia può produrre un quadro clinico di blefarite. I pidocchi possono essere uccisi mediante l'applicazione di un unguento di petrolato di tipo oftalmico al margine palpebrale e alle ciglia. Le lendini dovrebbero essere asportate meccanicamente dalle ciglia. Occorre ricordare che la pediculosi è una malattia trasmessa sessualmente.

ORZAIOLO. L'infezione delle ghiandole palpebrali può essere acuta o subacuta; si osservano edema focale dolorabile e arrossamento. L'agente eziologico abituale è lo *Staphylococcus aureus*. Quando vengono coinvolte le ghiandole di Meibomio, la lesione viene denominata orzaiolo interno; l'ascesso tende a essere di grosse dimensioni e può crescere attraverso la cute o la superficie congiuntivale. Quando l'infezione interessa le ghiandole di Zeiss o di Moll, l'ascesso tende a essere più piccolo e più superficiale e cresce in corrispondenza del margine palpebrale, venendo quindi denominato orzaiolo esterno.

Il **trattamento** consiste in impacchi tiepidi con garze e, se necessario, nell'incisione e nel drenaggio chirurgici. Inoltre, spesso si utilizzano preparati antibiotici topici. In assenza di trattamento, l'infezione può trasformarsi in cellulite della palpebra o dell'orbita, sicché subentra la necessità di un'antibioticoterapia sistemica.

CALAZIO. Il calazio è un'infiammazione granulomatosa di una ghiandola di Meibomio caratterizzata da un nodulo non dolorabile solido nella palpebra superiore o inferiore. La lesione tende a essere cronica e si distingue dall'orzaiolo interno per l'assenza di segni di infiammazione acuta. Sebbene molti calazi si risolvano spontaneamente, l'asportazione può essere necessaria se diventano sufficientemente grandi da alterare la vista (inducendo astigmatismo attraverso la pressione sul globo oculare) oppure a scopo estetico. Nei pazienti con frequente formazione di calazi o in quelli con significative alterazioni corneali secondarie a una blefarite sottostante, può essere utile il trattamento con l'eritromicina sistemica.

COLOBOMA DELLA PALPEBRA. Questa deformità a fessura può variare da una piccola intaccatura o incisura del margine libero della palpebra a un ampio difetto che interessa la palpebra quasi interamente. Se la lacuna è estesa, l'esposizione può portare a una ulcerazione e a opacizzazioni corneali. È raccomandata la correzione chirurgica precoce del difetto palpebrale. Tra le altre deformità frequentemente associate ai colobomi palpebrali vi sono le cisti dermoidi o i dermolipomi sul globo oculare, che spesso compaiono in una posizione corrispondente al sito del difetto palpebrale. I colobomi possono anche essere associati a una malformazione facciale estesa, come nella disostosi mandibolofacciale (sindrome di Franceschetti o di Treacher Collins).

TUMORI DELLA PALPEBRA. Numerosi tumori della palpebra possono avere origine dalle strutture di superficie (epitelio e ghiandole sebacee). Nella prima infanzia possono comparire i nevi, la maggior parte dei quali è di tipo giunzionale. I nevi composti tendono a svilupparsi negli anni prepuberali e quelli dermici nella pubertà. I tumori epiteliali maligni (carcinoma basocellulare, carcinoma squamocellulare) sono rari nei bambini, ma la sindrome del nevo basocellulare e le lesioni maligne dello xeroderma pigmentoso e della sindrome di Rothmund-Thomson possono comparire nell'infanzia.

Altri tumori palpebrali originano dalle strutture più profonde (tessuto nervoso, vascolare e connettivo). Gli emangiomi capillari si trovano in modo particolarmente comune nei bambini (Fig. 623-2). Molti tendono a regredire spontaneamente, sebbene possano presentare una crescita rapida allarmante. Molte volte il trattamento migliore è l'osservazione del paziente, lasciando che avvenga la regressione spontanea (vedi Capitolo 649). Nel caso di una lesione in rapida espansione, che può causare l'ambliopia ostruendo l'asse visivo o inducendo l'astigmatismo, si dovrebbero prendere in considerazione i corticosteroidi, l'interferone o il trattamento chirurgico. Il nevo flammeo ("macchia di vino porto"), un emangioma non evolutivo, compare come lesione isolata o in associazione ad altri segni della sindrome di Sturge-Weber. I pazienti affetti andrebbero monitorati per lo sviluppo di un glaucoma. I linfangiomi dell'iride appaiono come masse solide alla nascita o poco dopo e tendono a ingrandirsi lentamente durante gli anni dello sviluppo. L'interessamento congiuntivale associato, che appare sotto forma di una massa congiuntivale serpiginosa, cistica, chiara, può fornire un indizio per la diagnosi. In alcuni casi non vi è alcun interessamento orbitale. Il **trattamento** consiste nell'asportazione chirurgica.

I neuromi plessiformi delle palpebre compaiono nei bambini con neurofibromatosi, avendo spesso la ptosi come primo segno. La palpebra può assumere un aspetto a forma di S. Le palpebre possono anche essere interessate da altri tumori, come il retinoblastoma, il neuroblastoma e il rabdomiosarcoma dell'orbita; queste malattie vengono discusse in altra sede.

Dray JP, Leibovitch I: Congenital ptosis and amblyopia: A retrospective study of 130 cases. *J Pediatr Ophthalmol Strabismus* 2002;39:222–225.
Drolet BA, Esterly NB, Frieden IJ: Hemangiomas in children. *N Engl J Med* 1999;341:173–181.
Gusek-Schneider GC, Martus P: Stimulus deprivation amblyopia in human congenital ptosis: A study of 100 patients. *Strabismus* 2000;8:261–270.

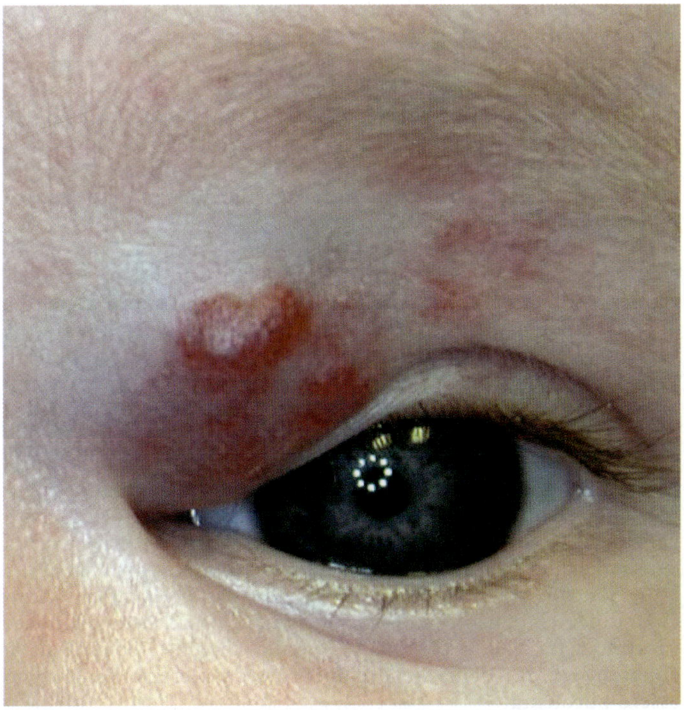

Figura 623-2. Emangioma capillare della palpebra. (Per gentile concessione di Amy Nopper, MD, e Brandon Newell, MD.)

Meisler DM, Raizman MB, Traboulsi EI: Oral erythromycin treatment for childhood blepharokeratitis. *J AAPOS* 2000;4:379–380.
Plager DA, Snyder SK: Resolution of astigmatism after surgical resection of capillary hemangiomas in infants. *Ophthalmology* 1997;104:1102–1106.
Sterker I, Grafe G: Periocular hemangiomas in childhood—functional and esthetic results. *Strabismus* 2004;12:103–110.
Wasserman BN, Sprunger DT, Helveston EM: Comparison of materials used in frontalis suspension. *Arch Ophthalmol* 2001;119:687–691.

Capitolo 624 ■ Malattie del sistema lacrimale

Scott E. Olitsky, Denise Hug e Laura P. Smith

IL FILM LACRIMALE. Questo film, che inumidisce l'occhio, è di fatto una struttura complessa costituita da tre strati. Lo strato più interno di mucina viene secreto dalle cellule caliciformi ed epiteliali della congiuntiva e dalla cellule acinari della ghiandola lacrimale. Conferisce stabilità e offre un punto di attacco per il film lacrimale alla congiuntiva e alla cornea. Lo strato acqueo intermedio costituisce il 98% del film lacrimale ed è prodotto dalla ghiandola lacrimale principale e da quelle accessorie; contiene vari elettroliti e proteine, nonché anticorpi. Lo strato lipidico più esterno è prodotto in gran parte dalle ghiandole sebacee di Meibomio della palpebra e ritarda l'evaporazione del film lacrimale. Le lacrime defluiscono medialmente nelle aperture dei punti lacrimali del margine palpebrale e scorrono attraverso i canalicoli nel sacco lacrimale e quindi attraverso il dotto nasolacrimale raggiungono il naso. I neonati pretermine presentano una ridotta secrezione lacrimale. Ciò può mascherare la diagnosi di un'ostruzione del dotto nasolacrimale e concentrare i farmaci applicati topicamente. La produzione di lacrime raggiunge i livelli dell'adulto in prossimità del termine.

DACRIOSTENOSI. L'ostruzione congenita del dotto nasolacrimale (CNLDO, *Congenital NasoLacrimal Duct Obstruction*), o dacriostenosi, è la malattia più comune del sistema lacrimale, verificandosi fino nel 6% dei neonati. È solitamente causata da un deficit della canalizzazione delle cellule epiteliali che formano il dotto nasolacrimale nel punto in cui questo entra nel naso (valvola di Hasner). I suoi segni possono essere presenti alla nascita, sebbene la malattia possa non diventare evidente prima dello sviluppo della normale produzione lacrimale. Tra essi vi sono un lago lacrimale eccessivo, l'iperafflusso di lacrime sulla palpebra e sulla guancia e il reflusso di materiale mucoide prodotto nel sacco lacrimale. Possono comparire un eritema o la macerazione della cute secondariamente all'irritazione o allo sfregamento prodotto dal grondare delle lacrime e dalle secrezioni. Se l'ostruzione è completa, questi segni possono essere gravi e continui, mentre se è solo parziale il dotto nasolacrimale può riuscire a fare defluire il film lacrimale basale. Tuttavia, nei periodi di incrementata produzione lacrimale (esposizione al freddo, al vento, alla luce del sole) o di aumentata chiusura dell'estremità distale del dotto (edema della mucosa nasale), l'iperafflusso di lacrime può diventare evidente o più alto.

I bambini con la CNLDO possono sviluppare un'infezione e un'infiammazione acute del sacco nasolacrimale (**dacriocistite**), l'infiammazione dei tessuti circostanti (**pericistite**) o raramente la cellulite periorbitale. In caso di dacriocistite, l'area del sacco appare edematosa, rossa e dolorabile e i pazienti possono presentare segni sistemici d'infezione come febbre e irritabilità.

Il **trattamento** primario dell'ostruzione nasolacrimale non complicata consiste in un ciclo di massaggio nasolacrimale, di solito 2-3 volte al giorno, accompagnato dalla detersione delle palpebre con acqua tiepida. In caso di drenaggio mucopurulento significativo si utilizzano antibiotici topici. La maggior parte dei casi di CNLDO si risolve spontaneamente; il 96% entro il primo anno di vita, mentre per gli altri si può effettuare il sondaggio del dotto nasolacrimale con uno specillo, il che comporta un tasso di guarigione del 90% circa.

La dacriocistite o la cellulite acuta richiede un trattamento precoce con antibiotici. In questi casi di solito è indicata una qualche forma d'intervento chirurgico definitivo.

Il **dacriocistocele** (mucocele) è una presentazione insolita di un sacco nasolacrimale non pervio, che è ostruito prossimalmente e distalmente. I dacriocistoceli si possono osservare alla nascita o poco dopo sotto forma di una massa sottocutanea bluastra appena al di sotto del tendine cantale mediale (Fig. 624-1). Il trattamento iniziale dovrebbe comprendere impacchi tiepidi e un massaggio delicato del sacco lacrimale. Se si sviluppa un'infezione, è necessaria la somministrazione sistemica di antibiotici. Il sondaggio del sistema nasolacrimale con uno specillo può in seguito essere necessario per prevenire un'ulteriore infezione o trattare la formazione di un ascesso.

Non tutti i casi di lacrimazione nei bambini piccoli e grandi sono dovuti all'ostruzione nasolacrimale. Essa può anche essere un segno di glaucoma, d'infiammazione intraoculare o d'irritazione esterna, come quella dovuta a un'abrasione corneale o a un corpo estraneo.

ALACRIMIA E "OCCHIO SECCO". Il deficit marcato di lacrime può verificarsi come difetto congenito isolato unilaterale o bilaterale oppure in associazione ad altre anomalie del sistema nervoso, come l'aplasia dei nuclei dei nervi cranici. Compare congenitamente nella disautonomia familiare (sindrome di Riley-Day) e nella forma anidrosica della displasia ectodermica. L'alacrimia si osserva nella **sindrome della tripla A** o **sindrome di Allgrove**, caratterizzata da un'insufficienza surrenale resistente all'ormone adrenocorticotropo, dall'acalasia del cardias esofageo e dall'alacrimia. I pazienti soffrono frequentemente di disturbi neurologici.

Un'anomalia acquisita di qualunque strato del film lacrimale può produrre un occhio secco. Tra le malattie comunemente acquisite che possono determinare un film lacrimale ridotto o instabile si trovano la sindrome di Sjögren, la sindrome di Stevens-Johnson, il deficit di vitamina A, il pemfigoide oculare, il tracoma, le ustioni chimiche, l'irradiazione e la disfunzione delle ghiandole di Meibomio. Ogni deficit lacrimale può portare all'ulcerazione, alla cicatrizzazione o all'infezione corneale. Il **trattamento** comprende la correzione della malattia sottostante, quando possibile, e la frequente istillazione di un preparato di lacrime artificiali. In alcuni casi è utile l'occlusione dei punti lacrimali, mentre nei casi gravi per proteggere la cornea può essere necessaria la tarsorrafia.

Honavar SG, Prakash VE, Rao GN: Outcome of probing for congenital nasolacrimal duct obstruction in older children. *Am J Ophthalmol* 2000;130:42–48.
Huebner A, Yoon SJ, Ozkinay F, et al: Triple A syndrome—clinical aspects and molecular genetics. *Endocr Res* 2000;26:751–759.
Kushner BJ: Congenital nasolacrimal system obstruction. *Arch Ophthalmol* 1982;100:597–600.
MacEwen CJ, Young JD: Epiphora during the first year of life. *Eye* 1991;5:596–600.
O'Driscoll TG: Alacrima. *Trans Ophthalmol Soc* 1975;95:13–14.
Schnall BM, Christian CJ: Conservative treatment of congenital dacryocele. *J Pediatr Ophthalmol Strabismus* 1996;33:219–222.
Young JD, MacEwen CJ: Managing congenital lacrimal obstruction in general practice. *Br Med J* 1997;315:293–296.

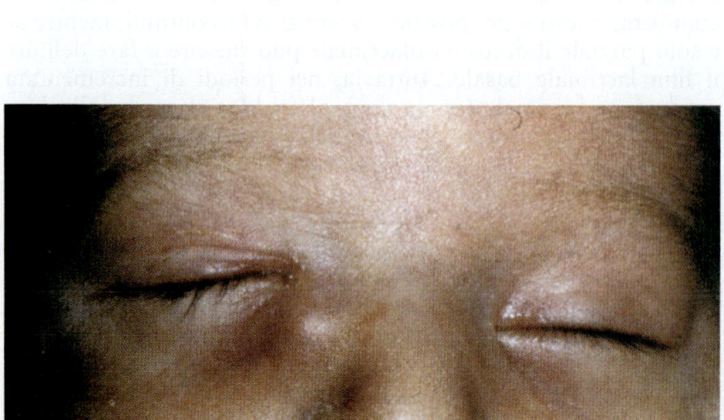

Figura 624-1. Dacriocistocele sotto il canto interno dell'occhio destro.

Capitolo 625 ■ Malattie della congiuntiva

Scott E. Olitsky, Denise Hug e Laura P. Smith

CONGIUNTIVITE

La congiuntiva reagisce a un'ampia serie di agenti batterici e virali, allergeni, irritanti, tossine e malattie sistemiche. La congiuntivite è comune nell'infanzia e può essere infettiva o non infettiva. La diagnosi differenziale di un occhio rosso comprende sedi congiuntivali e altre sedi oculari (Tab. 625-1).

OFTALMIA DEI NEONATI. Questa forma di congiuntivite, che si verifica in bambini con meno di 4 settimane di vita, è la malattia oculare più comune nei neonati. I suoi agenti eziologici sono molto differenti e presentano virulenza ed esiti molto variabili. L'istillazione di nitrato d'argento può portare a una lieve congiuntivite chimica autolimitata, mentre la *Neisseria gonorrhoeae* e la *Pseudomonas* sono in grado di provocare perforazione corneale, cecità e morte. Il rischio di congiuntivite nei neonati dipende dalle frequenze delle infezioni materne, dalle misure profilattiche, dalle circostanze durante il travaglio e il parto e dalle esposizioni ai microrganismi nel postpartum.

Epidemiologia. La congiuntivite nel periodo neonatale viene solitamente acquisita durante un parto vaginale e riflette le infezioni sessualmente trasmesse prevalenti nella comunità d'appartenenza. Nel 1880, il 10% dei bambini europei sviluppava una congiuntivite gonococcica alla nascita e a quell'epoca l'oftalmia neonatale era la principale causa di cecità. L'epidemiologia di questa malattia è cambiata radicalmente nel 1881, quando Crede riportò che l'istillazione di una soluzione di nitrato d'argento al 2% negli occhi dei neonati riduceva l'incidenza dell'oftalmia gonococcica dal 10 allo 0,3%.

Durante il ventesimo secolo, l'incidenza dell'oftalmia gonococcica dei neonati si è ridotta nei Paesi industrializzati secondariamente alla diffusione della profilassi con il nitrato d'argento e allo screening e al trattamento prenatali della gonorrea materna. Ora essa presenta un'incidenza dello 0,3/1000 nati vivi negli Stati Uniti, mentre la *Chlamydia trachomatis* è diventata il microrganismo più comunemente responsabile, con un'incidenza dell'8,2/1000 nati.

Manifestazioni cliniche. Le manifestazioni cliniche delle varie forme di oftalmia dei neonati non sono sufficientemente specifiche da consentire una diagnosi accurata. Sebbene l'epoca d'insorgenza e il carattere dei segni siano piuttosto tipici per ciascuna causa della malattia, esiste una significativa sovrapposizione e i medici non dovrebbero basarsi unicamente sui reperti clinici. Indipendentemente dalla sua origine, l'oftalmia neonatale è caratterizzata dall'arrossamento e dalla chemosi (edema) della congiuntiva, da edema delle palpebre e da secrezione, che può essere purulenta.

L'oftalmia dei neonati può portare alla cecità. L'infezione può essere associata a manifestazioni sistemiche che necessitano di

TABELLA 625-1. L'occhio rosso

MALATTIA	EZIOLOGIA	SEGNI E SINTOMI	TRATTAMENTO
Congiuntivite batterica	*Haemophilus influenzae*, *Haemophilus aegyptius*, *Streptococcus pneumoniae* *Neisseria gonorrhoeae*	Secrezione mucopurulenta unilaterale o bilaterale, vista normale, fotofobia Iniezione ed edema (chemosi) congiuntivale; sensazione di sabbia	Antibiotici topici, ceftriaxone parenterale per gonococco, *H. influenzae*
Congiuntivite virale	Adenovirus, echovirus, coxsackievirus	Come sopra, può essere emorragica, unilaterale	Autolimitata
Congiuntivite neonatale	*Chlamydia trachomatis*, gonococco, sostanze chimiche (nitrato d'argento), *Staphylococcus aureus*	Follicolo o papille congiuntivali palpebrali; come sopra	Ceftriaxone per il gonococco ed eritromicina per la *C. trachomatis*
Congiuntivite allergica	Esposizione a pollini stagionali o ad allergeni	Prurito, incidenza di chemosi (edema) bilaterale superiore a quella dell'eritema, papille tarsali	Antistaminici, steroidi, cromoglicato
Cheratite	Virus dell'herpes simplex, adenovirus, *S. pneumoniae*, *S. aureus*, *Pseudomonas*, *Acanthamoeba*, sostanze chimiche	Dolore grave, edema corneale, offuscamento, eritema del limbus, ipopion, cataratta; anamnesi di lenti a contatto con infezione amebica	Antibiotici specifici per le infezioni batteriche/fungine; cheratoplastica, aciclovir per l'herpes
Endoftalmite	*S. aureus*, *S. pneumoniae*, *Candida albicans*, intervento chirurgico o trauma associati	Esordio acuto, dolore, perdita del visus, edema, chemosi, arrossamento; ipopion e velo vitreo	Antibiotici
Uveite anteriore (iridociclite)	Artrite reumatoide giovanile, postinfettiva con artrite e rash, sarcoidosi, malattia di Behçet, malattia di Kawasaki, malattia infiammatoria intestinale	Unilaterale/bilaterale; eritema, arrossamento ciliare, pupilla irregolare, aderenze dell'iride; dolore, fotofobia, pupilla piccola, vista scarsa	Steroidi topici associati alla terapia della malattia primaria
Uveite posteriore (coroidite)	Toxoplasmosi, istoplasmosi, *Toxocara canis*	Assenza di segni di eritema, diminuzione della vista	Terapia specifica per il patogeno
Episclerite/sclerite	Malattia autoimmune idiopatica (per es. SLE, porpora di Schönlein-Henoch)	Dolore localizzato, eritema intenso, unilaterale; vasi sanguigni più grandi che nella congiuntivite; la sclerite può provocare perforazione del globo oculare	L'episclerite è autolimitante; steroidi topici per un rapido sollievo
Corpo estraneo	Esposizione professionale	Unilaterale, rosso, sensazione di sabbia; visibile o di dimensioni microscopiche	Irrigazione, rimozione; verificare se è presente ulcerazione
Blefarite	*S. aureus*, *Staphylococcus epidermidis*, seborroica, ostruzione del dotto lacrimale; raramente mollusco contagioso, *Phthirus pubis*, *Pediculus capitis*	Bilaterale, irritazione, prurito, iperemia, formazione di croste, interessa i margini palpebrali	Antibiotici topici, impacchi tiepidi
Dacriocistite	Ostruzione del sacco lacrimale: *S. aureus*, *H. influenzae*, pneumococco	Dolore, dolorabilità, eritema ed essudati nell'area del sacco lacrimale (inferomediale al canto interno); lacrimazione (epifora); possibile cellulite orbitale	Antibiotici sistemici, topici; drenaggio chirurgico
Dacrioadenite	*S. aureus*, *Streptococcus*, CMV, morbillo, EBV, enterovirus; trauma, sarcoidosi, leucemia	Dolore, dolorabilità, edema, eritema sopra l'area ghiandolare (palpebra superiore temporale); febbre, leucocitosi	Antibiotici sistemici; drenaggio degli ascessi orbitali
Cellulite orbitale (cellulite postsettale)	Sinusite paranasale: *H. influenzae*, *S. aureus*, *S. pneumoniae*, streptococchi Trauma: *S. aureus* Funghi: *Aspergillus*, *Mucor* spp. in caso di immunodeficienza	Rinorrea, chemosi, perdita della vista, movimento extraoculare doloroso, proptosi, oftalmoplegia, febbre, edema palpebrale, leucocitosi	Antibiotici sistemici; drenaggio degli ascessi orbitali
Cellulite periorbitale (cellulite presettale)	Trauma: *S. aureus*, streptococchi Batteriemia: pneumococco, streptococchi, *H. influenzae*	Eritema cutaneo, calore, vista normale, minimo interessamento dell'orbita; febbre, leucocitosi, aspetto tossico	Antibiotici sistemici

CMV, Cytomegalovirus; EBV, virus di Epstein-Barr (*Epstein-Barr Virus*); SLE, Lupus eritematoso sistemico (*Systemic Lupus Erythematosus*).
Da Behrman R, Kliegman R: *Nelson's Essentials of Pediatrics*, 3ª ed. Philadelphia, WB Saunders, 1998.

trattamento, per cui ogni neonato che sviluppa segni di congiuntivite necessita di valutazioni sistemica e oculare tempestive e globali per determinare l'agente causale dell'infezione e il trattamento appropriato.

L'esordio dell'infiammazione causata dalle gocce di nitrato d'argento di solito si verifica entro 6-12 ore dalla nascita, con risoluzione entro 24-48 ore. Il periodo di incubazione abituale per la congiuntivite da *N. gonorrhoeae* è di 2-5 giorni. L'infezione gonococcica può manifestarsi alla nascita o può essere ritardata oltre i 5 giorni di vita, a motivo della parziale soppressione dovuta alla profilassi oculare; può anche iniziare nell'infanzia dopo un contatto con dita contaminate degli adulti. L'epoca di esordio della malattia nel caso degli altri batteri è molto variabile.

La congiuntivite gonococcica inizia con una lieve infiammazione e una secrezione sieroematica. Entro 24 ore la secrezione diventa spessa e purulenta e compare un edema teso delle palpebre con una marcata chemosi. Se il trattamento appropriato viene ritardato, l'infezione può diffondersi e interessare gli strati più profondi delle congiuntive e della cornea. Tra le complicanze sono incluse l'ulcerazione e la perforazione corneale, l'iridociclite, le sinechie anteriori e raramente la panoftalmite. La congiuntivite causata dalla *C. trachomatis* (blenorrea da inclusione) può variare da una lieve infiammazione a un grave edema delle palpebre con abbondante secrezione purulenta. Il processo interessa principalmente le congiuntive tarsali; le cornee vengono raramente colpite. La congiuntivite dovuta allo *Staphylococcus aureus* o ad altri microrganismi è simile a quella prodotta dalla *C. trachomatis*. È raro che venga causata dalla *Pseudomonas aeruginosa*, quando viene acquisita nella nursery e risulta un processo potenzialmente grave. Questa congiuntivite è caratterizzata dalla comparsa, tra il 5° e il 18° giorno, di edema, eritema delle palpebre, secrezione purulenta, formazione di panno, endoftalmite, sepsi, shock e morte.

Diagnosi. La congiuntivite che compare dopo 48 ore andrebbe valutata per escludere una possibile causa infettiva. Si dovrebbe eseguire la colorazione di Gram della secrezione purulenta e il materiale andrebbe messo in coltura. Se si sospetta una causa virale, bisognerebbe praticare un tampone da sottoporre a terreni di coltura tissutale per l'isolamento del virus. Nella congiuntivite da clamidia, la diagnosi viene confermata esaminando le cellule epiteliali colorate con Giemsa prelevate mediante raschiamento dalla congiuntiva tarsale alla ricerca delle caratteristiche inclusioni intracitoplasmatiche; isolando i microrganismi da un tampone congiuntivale mediante speciali tecniche di coltura tissutale; tramite la colorazione con immunofluorescenza del materiale raschiato dalla congiuntiva alla ricerca delle inclusioni da clamidia; mediante un test per l'antigene o per il DNA della clamidia. La diagnosi differenziale comprende la dacriocistite da ostruzione congenita del dotto lacrimale con distensione del sacco lacrimale (dacriocistocele).

TRATTAMENTO. Nei bambini in cui si sospetta l'oftalmia gonococcica e in cui la colorazione Gram mostra i caratteristici diplococchi Gram-negativi intracellulari, il trattamento andrebbe iniziato immediatamente con ceftriaxone, 50 mg/kg/24 h in monosomministrazione senza superare i 125 mg. Inizialmente l'occhio dovrebbe anche essere irrigato con soluzione fisiologica ogni 10-30 minuti, aumentando gradualmente a intervalli di 2 ore finché la secrezione purulenta non si schiarisce. Un regime terapeutico alternativo comprende cefotaxima (100 mg/kg/24 h somministrati per via ev o im ogni 12 ore per 7 giorni oppure 100 mg/kg in monosomministrazione). Il trattamento viene protratto in caso di sepsi o interessamento di altre sedi extraoculari (meningite, artrite). La blenorrea da inclusione viene trattata con eritromicina per os (50 mg/kg/24 h suddivisa in quattro dosi) per 2 settimane. Questo cura la congiuntivite e può prevenire la conseguente polmonite da clamidia. La congiuntivite neonatale da *Pseudomonas* viene trattata con antibiotici sistemici, che comprendono un aminoglicoside, insieme all'irrigazione locale con soluzione fisiologica e unguento oftalmico a base di gentamicina. La congiuntivite stafilococcica richiede la meticillina parenterale e l'irrigazione locale con soluzione fisiologica.

PROGNOSI E PREVENZIONE. Se appropriatamente applicata, la profilassi oftalmica topica risulta altamente efficace, a meno che non vi sia un'infezione alla nascita. L'oftalmia gonococcica era una causa comune di cecità o di danno oculare permanente, prima della sua istituzione, che comprende l'instillazione alla nascita di gocce di eritromicina 0,5% o di nitrato d'argento 1% direttamente negli occhi aperti mediante contenitori monodose di cera o di plastica. L'irrigazione con soluzione fisiologica dopo l'applicazione di nitrato d'argento non è necessaria. Il nitrato d'argento non ha efficacia contro l'infezione attiva. Anche lo iodopovidone (soluzione al 2%) può essere un valido agente profilattico.

L'identificazione e il trattamento appropriato dell'infezione gonococcica materna sono diventati un elemento standard dell'assistenza prenatale di routine. Un bambino nato da una donna con un'infezione non trattata dovrebbe ricevere una singola dose di ceftriaxone, 50 mg/kg (massimo 125 mg) ev o im in aggiunta alla profilassi topica. La dose andrebbe ridotta per i neonati prematuri. Se il materiale gonococcico isolato dalla madre è penicillinosensibile, bisognerebbe usare la penicillina (50 000 U).

Né la profilassi topica né il trattamento topico prevengono la polmonite afebbrile che si verifica nel 10-20% dei neonati esposti alla *C. trachomatis*. Sebbene la congiuntivite da clamidia sia spesso una malattia autolimitata, la polmonite da clamidia può avere gravi conseguenze. È importante che i bambini con malattia da clamidia ricevano la terapia sistemica. Il trattamento con eritromicina delle donne gravide colonizzate può prevenire la malattia neonatale.

CONGIUNTIVITE PURULENTA ACUTA. È caratterizzata da un'iperemia congiuntivale più o meno generalizzata, edema, essudato mucopurulento, occhi incollati (palpebre appiccicate tra di loro al risveglio) e dolore e fastidio oculare di vario grado. Di solito è secondaria a un'infezione batterica. Le cause più frequenti sono un *Haemophilus influenzae* non tipizzabile (associato a un'otite media ipsilaterale), pneumococchi, stafilococchi e streptococchi. La congiuntivite purulenta batterica, specialmente dovuta a uno pneumococco o all'*H. influenzae*, può verificarsi in forma epidemica. Lo striscio e la coltura congiuntivale sono utili per differenziare i tipi specifici. Queste forme comuni di congiuntivite di solito rispondono bene agli impacchi tiepidi con garze sterili e all'istillazione topica frequente di gocce antibiotiche. La febbre purpurica brasiliana dovuta all'*Haemophilus aegyptius* si manifesta con congiuntivite e sepsi. La *N. gonorrhoeae* e la *Chlamydia* sono cause relativamente comuni di congiuntivite purulenta acuta nei bambini oltre il periodo neonatale, specialmente negli adolescenti. Queste infezioni richiedono indagini e trattamento specifici.

CONGIUNTIVITE VIRALE. È generalmente caratterizzata da una secrezione acquosa. Spesso si osservano alterazioni follicolari (piccoli aggregati di linfociti) nella congiuntivite palpebrale. La congiuntivite secondaria a un'infezione da adenovirus è relativamente comune, talvolta con interessamento corneale e faringite o polmonite. Si osservano anche epidemie di congiuntivite determinata da enterovirus, una variante che può essere emorragica. La congiuntivite emorragica acuta può essere epidemica, dovuta all'enterovirus CA24 o 70 e caratterizzata da occhi rossi edematosi e dolenti con secrezione acquosa emorragica. La congiuntivite virale è comunemente associata a infezioni virali sistemiche come esantemi infantili e in particolare il morbillo. Di solito la congiuntivite virale è autolimitata.

CHERATOCONGIUNTIVITE EPIDEMICA. È causata dall'adenovirus di tipo 8 ed è trasmessa per contatto diretto. Inizialmente si presenta con una sensazione di corpo estraneo sotto alle palpebre, con prurito e bruciore. Edema e fotofobia si sviluppano rapidamente e compaiono ampi follicoli ovali all'interno della congiuntiva. Frequentemente insorgono un'adenopatia preauricolare e una pseudomembrana sulla superficie congiuntivale. Possono inoltre svilupparsi infiltrati corneali subepiteliali, che possono provocare l'offuscamento della vista; questi di solito scompaiono, ma possono ridurre permanentemente l'acuità visiva. Le complicanze corneali sono meno frequenti nei bambini rispetto agli adulti. Nei bambini possono tuttavia trovarsi associate un'infezione delle alte vie respiratorie e una faringite. Non è disponibile alcuna terapia specifica per ridurre i sintomi o abbreviare il decorso della malattia, per cui occorre dare importanza alla prevenzione della sua diffusione. Il virus in fase di replicazione è presente nel 95% dei pazienti dopo 10 giorni dalla comparsa dei sintomi.

CONGIUNTIVITE MEMBRANOSA E PSEUDOMEMBRANOSA. Queste varianti possono essere riscontrate in numerose malattie. La congiuntivite membranosa classica è quella della difterite, accompagnata da un essudato ricco di fibrina che si forma sulla superficie congiuntivale e permea l'epitelio; la membrana viene rimossa con difficoltà e lascia aree escoriate sanguinanti. Nella congiuntivite pseudomembranosa, lo strato di essudato ricco di fibrina è superficiale e spesso può essere rimosso facilmente, lasciando una superficie liscia. Questa forma compare in molte infezioni batteriche e virali, tra cui le congiuntiviti stafilococcica, pneumococcica, streptococcica o da clamidia e nella cheratocongiuntivite epidemica. Viene riscontrata anche nella congiuntivite primaverile e nella malattia di Stevens-Johnson.

CONGIUNTIVITE ALLERGICA. Si trova solitamente accompagnata da un prurito intenso, lacrimazione acquosa trasparente ed edema congiuntivale. È comunemente stagionale. Gli impacchi freddi e le gocce decongestionanti forniscono un sollievo sintomatico. Anche gli stabilizzanti topici dei mastociti o gli inibitori delle prostaglandine possono risultare d'aiuto. In casi selezionati si utilizzano corticosteroidi topici sotto la supervisione oculistica.

CONGIUNTIVITE PRIMAVERILE. Di solito inizia nel periodo prepuberale e può essere ricorrente per molti anni; sembra che l'atopia possa essere implicata nella sua origine, ma la patogenesi è incerta. I sintomi abituali riguardano un estremo prurito e la lacrimazione. Ampie lesioni papillari, appiattite, ad acciottolato, sono caratteristiche (Fig. 625-1). Un essudato filamentoso e una pseudomembrana congiuntivale lattescente compaiono frequentemente. Possono essere riscontrate piccole lesioni rilevate della congiuntiva bulbare adiacente al limbus (forma limbale). Lo striscio dell'essudato congiuntivale evidenzia molti eosinofili. La terapia con corticosteroidi topici e impacchi freddi può fornire un certo sollievo. Gli stabilizzatori topici dei mastociti o gli inibitori delle prostaglandine risultano utili quando è necessario il controllo a lungo termine. L'uso prolungato di corticosteroidi andrebbe evitato.

SINDROME OCULOGHIANDOLARE DI PARINAUD. Rappresenta una variante della malattia da graffio di gatto ed è causata dalla *Bartonella henselae*, che viene trasmessa da gatto a gatto attraverso le pulci (vedi Capitolo 206). I gatti piccoli sono colpiti con maggiore probabilità rispetto a quelli adulti. L'uomo può essere infettato nel caso di un graffio, oppure i batteri possono passare dalla saliva del gatto al suo pelo durante la pulizia, per poi depositarsi sulla congiuntiva durante lo sfregamento degli occhi dopo avere toccato il gatto con le mani. La linfadenopatia e la congiuntivite sono segni caratteristici della malattia. Si possono sviluppare granulomi congiuntivali (Fig. 625-2). In genere

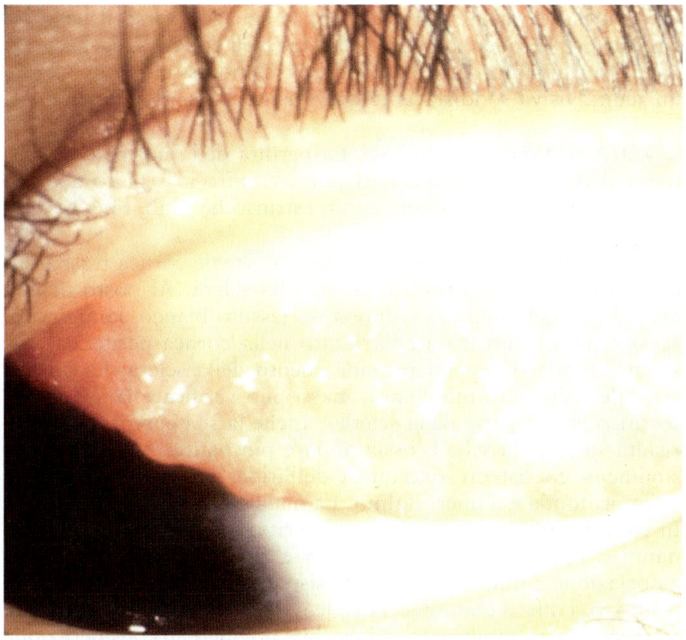

Figura 625-1. Congiuntivite primaverile.

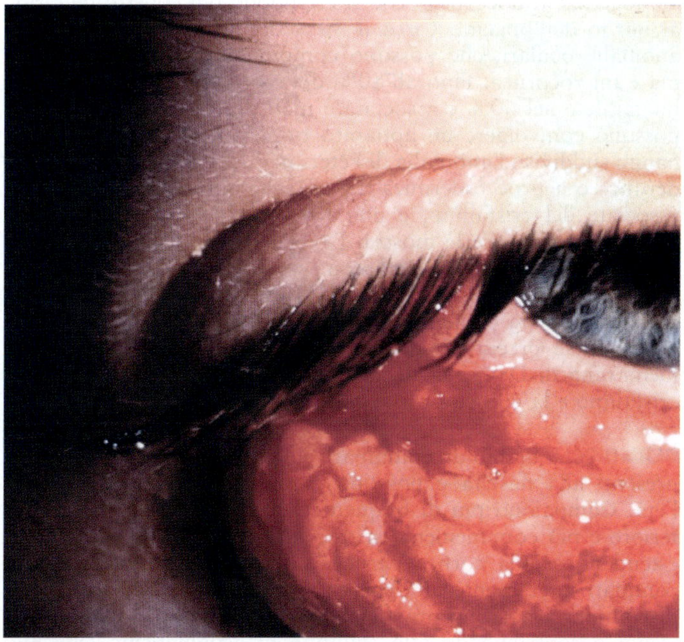

Figura 625-2. Granulomi congiuntivali nella sindrome oculoghiandolare di Parinaud.

il decorso è autolimitato, ma in alcuni casi si possono utilizzare gli antibiotici.

CONGIUNTIVITE CHIMICA. Può comparire quando una sostanza irritante entra nel sacco congiuntivale (come nella congiuntivite acuta ma benigna causata dal nitrato d'argento nei neonati). Altre comuni sostanze imputate sono i prodotti detergenti domestici, gli spray, il fumo, lo smog e gli inquinanti industriali. Gli alcali tendono a permanere nei tessuti congiuntivali e continuano a infliggere il danno per ore o giorni. Gli acidi precipitano le proteine nei tessuti e in questo modo producono immediatamente il loro effetto. In entrambi i casi, l'irrigazione rapida, completa e abbondante è fondamentale. Può verificarsi un esteso danno tissutale, persino la perdita dell'occhio, specialmente se l'agente lesivo è un alcale.

ALTRE MALATTIE CONGIUNTIVALI. L'emorragia sottocongiuntivale si manifesta con chiazze rosso chiaro o rosso scuro nella congiuntiva bulbare e può essere dovuta a una lesione o a una infiammazione. In genere si verifica in modo spontaneo. Occasionalmente può essere dovuta a tosse o a starnuti gravi. Rare volte può rappresentare la manifestazione di una discrasia ematica.

La pinguecola è una massa leggermente rilevata, di colore bianco-giallastro, sulla congiuntiva bulbare, di solito nella regione interpalpebrale. Rappresenta alterazioni degenerative elastiche e ialine della congiuntiva. Nessun trattamento è necessario se non per motivi estetici, nel qual caso la semplice asportazione risulta sufficiente.

Lo pterigio è una lesione congiuntivale triangolare carnosa che può sconfinare nella cornea. Tipicamente insorge nella regione interpalpebrale nasale. I reperti anatomopatologici sono simili a quelli della pinguecola. Lo sviluppo degli pterigi è riscontrato più comunemente negli individui che vivono vicino all'equatore. La rimozione è suggerita quando la lesione sconfina profondamente nella cornea, ma la recidiva è comune.

La cisti dermoide e il dermolipoma sono lesioni benigne, clinicamente simili nell'aspetto. Appaiono rotonde o ovali, rilevate, lisce, di dimensioni variabili. Il colore varia da bianco giallastro a rosa carne. La sede più frequente è il quadrante superiore esterno del globo oculare, ma insorgono comunemente anche vicino o a cavallo del limbus. Il dermolipoma è composto da tessuto adiposo e connettivo. Le cisti dermoidi possono contenere anche tessuto ghiandolare, follicoli piliferi e peli. L'asportazione per motivi estetici è possibile. I dermolipomi sono spesso collegati ai muscoli extraoculari, rendendo impossibile la loro completa rimozione senza sacrificare la motilità oculare.

Il nevo congiuntivale è una lesione piccola, leggermente rilevata, di pigmentazione variabile da rosa salmone chiaro a marrone scuro. È solitamente benigna, ma si consiglia un'attenta osservazione per la crescita progressiva o per alterazioni suggestive di malignità.

Il simblefaron è un'aderenza cicatriziale tra la congiuntiva della palpebra e il globo oculare; solitamente viene colpita la palpebra inferiore. Compare dopo interventi chirurgici o lesioni, specialmente ustioni da alcali, acidi o metalli liquidi. Costituisce una grave complicanza della sindrome di Stevens-Johnson. Può interferire con il movimento del bulbo oculare e può causare diplopia. Le aderenze dovrebbero essere separate e bisognerebbe impedire che le superfici escoriate si uniscano durante la guarigione. Possono essere necessari innesti di membrana mucosa orale.

Atik B, Thanh TTK, Luong VQ, et al: Impact of annual targeted treatment of infectious trachoma and susceptibility to reinfection. *JAMA* 2006;296: 1488–1497.

Centers for Disease Control and Prevention: Outbreak of bacterial conjunctivitis at a college—New Hampshire, January–March, 2002. *MMWR* 2002;51:205–208.

Centers for Disease Control and Prevention: Acute hemorrhagic conjunctivitis outbreak caused by coxsackievirus A24—Puerto Rico, 2003. *MMWR* 2004;53:632.

Chang DC, Grant GB, O'Donnell K, et al: Multistate outbreak of fusarium keratitis associated with use of a contact lens solution. *JAMA* 2006;296:953–963.

Everitt HA, Little PS, Smith PWF: A randomised controlled trial of management strategies for acute infective conjunctivitis in general practice. *BMJ* 2006;333:321–324.

Matoba A: Ocular viral infections. *Pediatr Infect Dis* 1984;3:358–368.

O'Hara MA: Ophthalmia neonatorum. *Pediatr Clin North Am* 1993;40: 715.

Rietveld RP, ter Riet G, Bindels PJE, et al: Predicting bacterial cause in infectious conjunctivitis: Cohort study on informativeness of combinations of signs and symptoms. *Br Med J* 2004;329:206–208.

Rose PW, Hamden A, Brueggemann AB, et al: Chloramphenicol treatment for acute infective conjunctivitis in children in primary care: A randomized double-blind placebo-controlled trial. *Lancet* 2005;366:37–42.
Shiuey Y, Ambati BK, Adamis AP, and the Viral Conjunctivitis Study Group: A randomized, double-masked trial of topical ketorolac versus artificial tears for treatment of viral conjunctivitis. *Ophthalmology* 2000;107: 1512–1517.
Weiss A, Brinser JH, Nazar-Stewart V: Acute conjunctivitis in childhood. *J Pediatr* 1993;122:10–14.

Capitolo 626 ■ Anomalie della cornea

Scott E. Olitsky, Denise Hug e Laura P. Smith

MEGALOCORNEA. Si tratta di un'anomalia simmetrica non progressiva caratterizzata da una cornea ingrandita (diametro >12 mm) e un segmento anteriore in cui non si trovano segni d'ipertensione oculare pregressa o concomitante. Spesso si ha una miopia elevata, che può portare alla diminuzione della vista. Una frequente complicanza è lo sviluppo di opacizzazioni del cristallino nella vita adulta. Tutte le modalità di ereditarietà sono state descritte, sebbene quella recessiva X-linked sia la più comune; pertanto questa malattia colpisce più frequentemente i maschi. Tra le anomalie sistemiche che possono trovarsi associate alla megalocornea vi sono la sindrome di Marfan, la craniosinostosi e la sindrome di Alport. La causa dell'ingrandimento della cornea e del segmento anteriore è sconosciuta, ma tra le possibili spiegazioni sono stati proposti un deficit della crescita del calice ottico e un arresto del glaucoma congenito. La regione sul cromosoma X responsabile di questa malattia è stata identificata.

L'ingrandimento patologico della cornea determinato dal glaucoma va differenziato dalla megalocornea. Qualunque aumento progressivo delle dimensioni corneali, specialmente quando viene accompagnato da fotofobia, lacrimazione o opacizzazione corneale, richiede una valutazione oftalmologica tempestiva.

MICROCORNEA. La microcornea, o microftalmia anteriore, consiste in una cornea abnormemente piccola nel contesto di un occhio per il resto relativamente normale. Può essere familiare, con una modalità di trasmissione più spesso dominante che recessiva. Più comunemente una cornea piccola è soltanto una caratteristica di un occhio che per il resto è anormale nello sviluppo oppure microftalmico; tra i difetti associati vi sono colobomi, microfachia, cataratta congenita, glaucoma e aniridia.

CHERATOCONO. Si tratta di una malattia a patogenesi sconosciuta caratterizzata dai progressivi assottigliamento e protrusione della cornea centrale, che assume una forma a cono. Sebbene siano note occorrenze familiari, la maggior parte dei casi è sporadica. Fattori patogenetici implicati sono stati lo sfregamento degli occhi e le lenti a contatto, ma le prove a supporto sono controverse. L'incidenza è più alta negli individui con atopia, sindrome di Down, sindrome di Marfan e retinite pigmentosa.

La maggior parte dei casi è bilaterale, ma l'interessamento può essere asimmetrico. Di solito la malattia si presenta e progredisce rapidamente durante l'adolescenza, per poi rallentare e stabilizzarsi quando i pazienti raggiungono uno sviluppo completa. Occasionalmente la membrana di Desçemet può essere tesa oltre il suo punto di rottura elastico, provocando appunto la rottura con un conseguente edema corneale improvviso e marcato (idrope acuta) e una diminuzione della vista. L'edema corneale si risolve man mano che le cellule endoteliali coprono l'area deficitaria. Si verifica un certo grado di cicatrizzazione corneale, ma l'acuità visiva è spesso migliore di quella precedente all'episodio iniziale. Tra i segni di cheratocono vi sono il segno di Munson (sporgenza della palpebra inferiore durante lo sguardo verso il basso) e l'anello di Fleischer (deposito di ferro nell'epitelio alla base del cono). Il trapianto corneale è indicato se non si può raggiungere un'acuità visiva soddisfacente con l'uso delle lenti a contatto.

OPACITÀ CORNEALI NEONATALI. La perdita della normale trasparenza della cornea nei neonati può avvenire in seguito a cause ereditarie intrinseche o ambientali estrinseche (Tab. 626-1).

SCLEROCORNEA. Nella sclerocornea la normale cornea trasparente è sostituita da un tessuto simile alla sclera. Al posto di una cornea ben delimitata si sviluppa un tessuto bianco, lanuginoso, spesso mal definito e vascolarizzato nella cornea periferica, che sembra fondersi con un prolungamento della sclera. La cornea centrale è di solito più chiara, ma si può verificare la sua totale sostituzione da parte della sclera e anche la sua curvatura spesso risulta simile alla sclera, ossia appare più piatta. Anomalie possibilmente coesistenti sono quelle dell'iride, una camera anteriore poco profonda e il microftalmo. La malattia di solito è bilaterale. In circa il 50% dei casi è stata descritta una ereditarietà dominante o recessiva. La sclerocornea è stata inoltre riportata in associazione a numerose malattie sistemiche, tra cui la deformità degli arti, i difetti craniofacciali e le malattie genitourinarie. Nella sclerocornea generalizzata si dovrebbe prendere in considerazione la cheratoplastica precoce nel tentativo di ripristinare il visus.

ANOMALIA DI PETERS. Si tratta di un'opacità centrale della cornea (leucoma) presente alla nascita (Fig. 626-1) e spesso associata ad aderenze iridocorneali che si estendono dal colletto dell'iride al bordo dell'opacità. Circa il 50% dei pazienti presenta altre anomalie oculari, che possono comprendere cataratta, glaucoma e microcornea. Fino all'80% dei casi la malattia può essere bilaterale e nel 60% è associata a malformazioni sistemiche che possono coinvolgere un apparato principale. Alcuni ricercatori hanno suddiviso l'anomalia di Peters in due tipi: una forma mesodermica o neuroectodermica (tipo I), che non mostra alterazioni associate del cristallino, e una forma ectodermica superficiale (tipo II), che invece le mostra. I reperti istologici comprendono un'assenza focale della membrana di Desçemet e dell'endotelio corneale nella regione dell'opacità. L'anomalia di Peters può essere determinata da un'incompleta migrazione e differenziazione delle cellule precursori dell'endotelio corneale centrale e della membrana di Desçemet o da un deficit della separazione tra il cristallino e la cornea primitivi durante l'embriogenesi.

DERMOIDI. I dermoidi epibulbari sono coristomi. Sono spesso presenti alla nascita e possono aumentare di dimensioni con l'età. Compaiono più di frequente nel quadrante temporale inferiore e più comunemente si dispongono a cavallo del limbus, estendendosi alla cornea periferica. Rare volte possono essere confinati interamente alla cornea o alla congiuntiva. I dermoidi epibulbari possono provocare disturbi visivi invadendo l'asse visivo o contribuendo allo sviluppo di astigmatismo, che può portare all'ambliopia.

Di solito un dermoide appare come una massa ben circoscritta rotondeggiante o ovale, grigia o giallo-rosata, con una superficie secca dalla quale possono protrudere peli corti. Può coinvolgere soltanto gli strati superficiali della cornea, sebbene l'interessamento a tutto spessore risulti comune. Tra le anomalie oculari associate vi sono i colobomi della palpebra e dell'iride, il microftalmo e i difetti retinici e coroidei. Il 30% dei dermoidi è inoltre associato ad anomalie sistemiche, molte delle quali comportano difetti dello sviluppo del primo arco branchiale (anomalie vertebrali, disostosi delle ossa facciali, anomalie dentali e sindrome di Goldenhar). I dermoidi epibulbari sono riscontrati nel 75% dei casi di sindrome di Goldenhar.

CHERATITE DENDRITICA. L'infezione della cornea da parte del virus dell'herpes simplex produce una lesione caratteristica dell'epitelio corneale denominata dendrite, che presenta un aspetto ramificato arboriforme dimostrabile mediante la co-

TABELLA 626-1. STUNMPED: diagnosi differenziale delle opacità corneali neonatali

DIAGNOSI	LATERALITÀ	OPACITÀ	PRESSIONE OCULARE	ALTRE ANOMALIE OCULARI	ANAMNESI NATURALE	EREDITARIETÀ
S: sclerocornea	Unilaterale o bilaterale	Vascolarizzata, si fonde con la sclera, più chiara al centro	Normale (o elevata)	Cornea plana	Non progressiva	Sporadica
T: lacerazioni (Tears) nell'endotelio e nella membrana di Desçemet						
Trauma da parto	Unilaterale	Edema diffuso	Normale	Possibile ifema, ecchimosi periorbitali	Spontaneo miglioramento in 1 mese	Sporadica
Glaucoma infantile	Bilaterale	Edema diffuso	Elevata	Megalocornea, fotofobia e lacrimazione, angolo anomalo	Progressiva se non trattata	Autosomica recessiva
U: ulcere						
Cheratite da herpes simplex	Unilaterale	Diffusa con difetto epiteliale a carta geografica	Normale	Nessuna	Progressiva	Sporadica
Rosolia congenita	Bilaterale	Disciforme o edema diffuso, assenza di una franca ulcerazione	Normale o elevata	Microftalmo, cataratta, chiazze di pigmento epiteliale	Stabile, può regredire	Sporadica
N: esposizione Neurotrofica	Unilaterale o bilaterale	Ulcera centrale	Normale	Anomalie palpebrali, neuropatia sensoriale congenita	Progressiva	Sporadica
M: metabolica (raramente presente alla nascita) (mucopolisaccaridosi IH, IS; mucolipidosi tipo IV)*	Bilaterale	Opacità diffusa, più densa alla periferia	Normale	Poche	Progressiva	Autosomica dominante
P: difetto corneale Posteriore	Unilaterale o bilaterale	Opacità diffusa, centrale o leucoma vascolarizzato	Normale o elevata	Sindrome del clivaggio della camera anteriore	Stabile, talvolta regressione precoce o vascolarizzazione	Sporadico, autosomico recessivo
E: distrofia Endoteliale						
Distrofia endoteliale ereditaria congenita	Bilaterale	Edema corneale diffuso, marcato ispessimento corneale	Normale	Nessuna	Stabile	Autosomica dominante o recessiva
Distrofia polimorfa posteriore	Bilaterale	Opacità diffusa, spessore corneale normale	Normale	Occasionali sinechie anteriori periferiche	Lentamente progressiva	Autosomica dominante
Distrofia stromale ereditaria congenita	Bilaterale	Opacità stromali lanuginose, lamellari; spessore corneale normale	Normale	Nessuna	Stabile	Autosomica dominante
D: dermoide	Unilaterale o bilaterale	Massa bianca vascolarizzata, pelo, arco lipidico	Normale	Nessuna	Stabile	Sporadico

*Mucopolisaccaridosi IH (sindrome di Hurler); mucopolisaccaridosi IS (sindrome di Scheie).
Da Nelson LB, Calhoun JH, Harley RD: *Pediatric Ophthalmology*, 3rd ed. Philadelphia, WB Saunders, 1991, p 210.

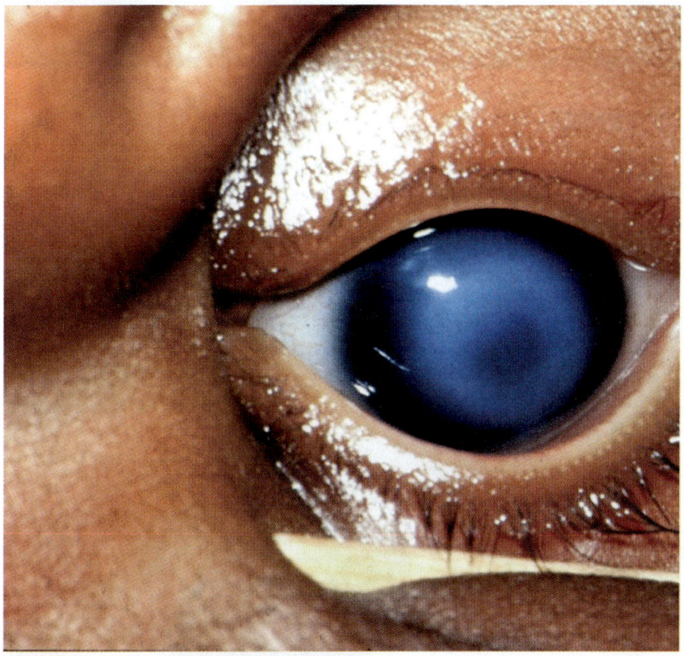

Figura 626-1. Anomalia di Peters. Opacità centrale in un paziente con anomalia di Peters.

lorazione con la fluoresceina. L'episodio acuto è associato a dolore, fotofobia, lacrimazione, blefarospasmo e iniezione congiuntivale. Il trattamento specifico può comprendere lo sbrigliamento meccanico dell'epitelio corneale interessato per rimuovere la sorgente d'infezione ed eliminare uno stimolo antigenico all'infiammazione nello stroma adiacente. Il trattamento medico comporta l'uso di trifluridina o di aciclovir sistemico. Inoltre, un agente cicloplegico è utile per alleviare il dolore dovuto allo spasmo del muscolo ciliare. Un trattamento antivirale topico eccessivamente aggressivo può essere di per sé tossico per la cornea e andrebbe evitato. L'infezione ricorrente e l'interessamento stromale profondo possono portare a una cicatrizzazione corneale e alla perdita della vista.

L'uso topico di corticosteroidi causa l'esacerbazione della malattia erpetica superficiale dell'occhio e può condurre a una perforazione della cornea; i colliri in cui si associano steroidi e antibiotici devono quindi essere evitati nel trattamento di un occhio rosso, a meno che non vi siano indicazioni ben definite per il loro utilizzo e una stretta supervisione durante la terapia.

I bambini nati da madri infettate dal virus dell'herpes simplex dovrebbero essere esaminati con attenzione, alla ricerca di segni di interessamento oculare. L'aciclovir endovenoso è necessario per il trattamento dell'herpes oculare nei neonati.

ULCERE CORNEALI. I segni e i sintomi abituali sono l'opacità corneale focale o diffusa, l'iperemia, l'edema della palpebra, il dolore, la fotofobia, la lacrimazione e il blefarospasmo. L'ipopion (pus nella camera anteriore) è comune. Le ulcere corneali richiedono un trattamento tempestivo. Sono dovute più di frequente a lesioni traumatiche che diventano infette secondariamente. Molti microrganismi sono in grado di contagiare la cornea. Uno dei più gravi è lo *Pseudomonas aeruginosa*, che può rapidamente distruggere il tessuto stromale e condurre alla perforazione corneale. Anche la *Neisseria gonorrhoeae* risulta particolarmente dannosa. Ulcere indolenti possono essere provocate da funghi, spesso in associazione all'uso delle lenti a contatto. In ciascun caso si devono studiare i raschiamenti corneali, nel tentativo di identificare l'agente infettivo e di determinare la terapia migliore. Sebbene il trattamento locale aggressivo sia in genere necessario per salvare gli occhi, in alcuni casi può occorrere anche il trattamento sistemico. La perforazione o la cicatrizzazione secondaria a un'ulcerazione corneale è una grave causa di cecità in tutto il mondo e si ritiene sia responsabile del 10% dei casi negli Stati Uniti.

Ulcere corneali inspiegate nei lattanti e nei bambini piccoli dovrebbero sollevare il dubbio di un deficit sensoriale, come nella sindrome di Riley-Day o in quella di Goldenhar-Gorlin, oppure di una malattia metabolica come la tirosinemia.

FLITTENE. Sono lesioni piccole, giallastre, leggermente rilevate, di solito localizzate nel limbo corneale; possono invadere la cornea ed estendersi centralmente. Una piccola ulcera corneale è spesso riscontrata in corrispondenza dell'apice della lesione in progressione, che ha posteriormente un fascicolo di vasi sanguigni. Sebbene in passato si ritenesse che rappresentasse un segno d'infezione tubercolinica sistemica, la cheratocongiuntivite flittenulare è attualmente considerata un'espressione morfologica d'ipersensibilità ritardata a diversi antigeni. Nei bambini, essa si verifica comunemente in seguito a una reazione d'ipersensibilità della congiuntiva o della cornea a prodotti batterici. Di solito il trattamento consiste nell'eliminazione della malattia sottostante, in genere la blefarite o la meibomianite stafilococcica e nella soppressione della risposta immunitaria con l'uso della terapia corticosteroidea topica. Talvolta dopo il trattamento rimangono un panno stromale superficiale e segni cicatriziali.

CHERATITE INTERSTIZIALE. Denota un'infiammazione dello stroma corneale, la cui causa più comune è costituita dalla sifilide. Questa malattia rappresenta per la precisione una delle manifestazioni tardive caratteristiche della sifilide congenita. Le alterazioni corneali in quest'ultima compaiono in due fasi. Quella acuta si presenta tra i 5 e i 10 anni di vita, con una cheratite intensa che può durare diversi mesi e determina una grave riduzione della vista. Gli effetti acuti della sifilide sono prevalentemente dovuti alla risposta immune dell'ospite, come infiltrati cellulari mononucleati, alterazioni vascolari proliferative e occasionalmente la formazione di granulomi. L'infiammazione profonda produce dolore, fotofobia, lacrimazione, iniezione pericorneale e opacità corneale. Questo episodio è seguito da una fase cronica con una significativa regressione dei reperti corneali, assieme a un parallelo miglioramento dell'acuità visiva. Sebbene i reperti corneali possano regredire nel tempo, persistono "vasi fantasma", che rappresentano alterazioni vascolari pregresse, nonché rimangono cicatrici corneali a chiazze, che segnano il passaggio della malattia.

La **sindrome di Cogan** è una cheratite interstiziale non luetica associata a perdita dell'udito e sintomi vestibolari. Sebbene la sua causa sia sconosciuta, si sospetta una vasculite sistemica. È necessario un trattamento precoce per evitare la perdita permanente dell'udito. Sia le alterazioni corneali sia l'interessamento uditivo possono rispondere all'uso di immunosoppressori.

Meno frequentemente la cheratite interstiziale viene determinata da altre malattie infettive, come la tubercolosi o la lebbra.

MANIFESTAZIONI CORNEALI DI MALATTIA SISTEMICA. Diverse malattie metaboliche producono alterazioni corneali distinte nell'infanzia. Nella cistinosi si depositano cristalli policromatici refrattivi in tutta la cornea. Depositi corneali che producono vari gradi di opacità compaiono anche in certi tipi di mucopolisaccaridosi (MPS), in particolare nella MPS IH (Hurler), nella MPS IS (Scheie), nella MPS I H/S (Hurler/Scheie composta), nella MPS IV (Morquio), nella MPS VI (Maroteaux-Lamy) e talvolta nella MPS VII (Sly). Gli stessi depositi possono inoltre svilupparsi nei pazienti con gangliosidosi GM_1 (generalizzata). Nella malattia di Fabry compaiono opacità fini che s'irradiano a spirale o a ventaglio e le alterazioni corneali possono risultare importanti nella identificazione dello stato di portatore. Un aspetto di opacità corneale a spruzzo può essere osservato anche nella sindrome di Bloch-Sulzbergere. Nella malattia di Wilson il segno corneale distintivo è l'anello di Kayser-Fleischer, un anello di colore marrone oro nella cornea periferica secondario alle alterazioni nella membrana di Desçemet. Anelli corneali pigmentati possono svilupparsi nei neonati con epatopatia colestatica. Alterazioni corneali possono formarsi nell'ipoparatiroidismo autoimmune e nella cheratopatia a bande nei pazienti con ipercalcemia. La cheratite transitoria può associarsi al morbillo e talvolta alla rosolia.

Beauchamp GR, Gillette TE, Friendly DS: Phlyctenular keratoconjunctivitis. *J Pediatr Ophthalmol Strabismus* 1981;18:22–28.

Comer RM, Daya SM, O'Keefe M: Penetrating keratoplasty in infants. *J AAPOS* 2001;5:285–290.

Dana MR, Moyes AL, Gomes JA, et al: The indications for and outcome in pediatric keratoplasty. A multicenter study. *Ophthalmology* 1995;102: 1129–1138.

Mackey DA, Buttery RG, Wise GM, et al: Description of X-linked megalocornea with identification of the gene locus. *Arch Ophthalmol* 1991;109: 829–833.

Mohandessan MM, Romano PE: Neuroparalytic keratitis in Goldenhar-Gorlin syndrome. *Am J Ophthalmol* 1978;85:111–113.

Reidy JJ: Congenital corneal opacities. *Ophthalmol Clin North Am* 1996;2: 199–213.

Traboulsi EI, Maumenee IH: Peters' anomaly and associated congenital malformations. *Arch Ophthalmol* 1992;110:1739–1742.

Yang LL, Lambert SR, Fernhoff PM, et al: Peters' anomaly: Associated congenital malformations and etiology. *Invest Ophthalmol Vis Sci* 1995;36:S41.

Yang LL, Lambert SR, Lynn MJ, et al: Long-term results of corneal graft survival in infants and children with Peters anomaly. *Ophthalmology* 1999;106:833–848.

Capitolo 627 ■ Anomalie del cristallino

Scott E. Olitsky, Denise Hug e Laura P. Smith

CATARATTA

La cataratta è una opacizzazione del cristallino (Fig. 627-1). Alcune forme sono clinicamente irrilevanti, mentre altre colpiscono significativamente la funzione visiva. L'incidenza della cataratta infantile è di circa 2/10000. Nel 50-60% dei casi si tratta di un difetto isolato; nel 20-25% fa parte di una sindrome; nella

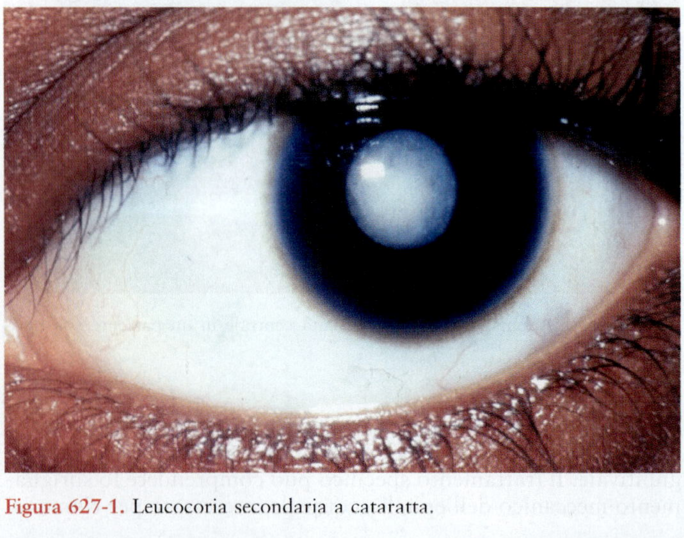

Figura 627-1. Leucocoria secondaria a cataratta.

percentuale rimanente è associata a difetti congeniti non oculari. È più comune nei neonati di basso peso alla nascita. Alcuni tipi sono associati a una malattia oculare o sistemica.

DIAGNOSI DIFFERENZIALE. La diagnosi differenziale della cataratta nei lattanti e nei bambini comprende un'ampia serie di malattie legate allo sviluppo, processi infettivi e infiammatori, malattie metaboliche e lesioni tossiche e traumatiche (Tab. 627-1). La cataratta si può anche sviluppare secondariamente a processi intraoculari, come una retinopatia della prematurità, un vitreo primario iperplastico persistente, il distacco della retina, una retinite pigmentosa e l'uveite. Infine, una certa percentuale nei bambini è di tipo ereditario (Fig. 627-2).

VARIANTI LEGATE ALLO SVILUPPO. Alcuni processi evolutivi iniziali possono portare a varie opacizzazioni congenite del cristallino. Puntini ben definiti o opacità bianche a placca interessano la regione sottocapsulare contigua. Piccole opacità della capsula posteriore possono essere associate a residui persistenti del sistema vascolare ialoide primitivo (il comune punto di Mittendorf), mentre quelle della capsula anteriore possono essere associate a strie persistenti della membrana pupillare o della tunica vascolare del cristallino. Le cataratte congenite di questo tipo sono solitamente stazionarie e raramente interferiscono con la vista; alcune sono progressive.

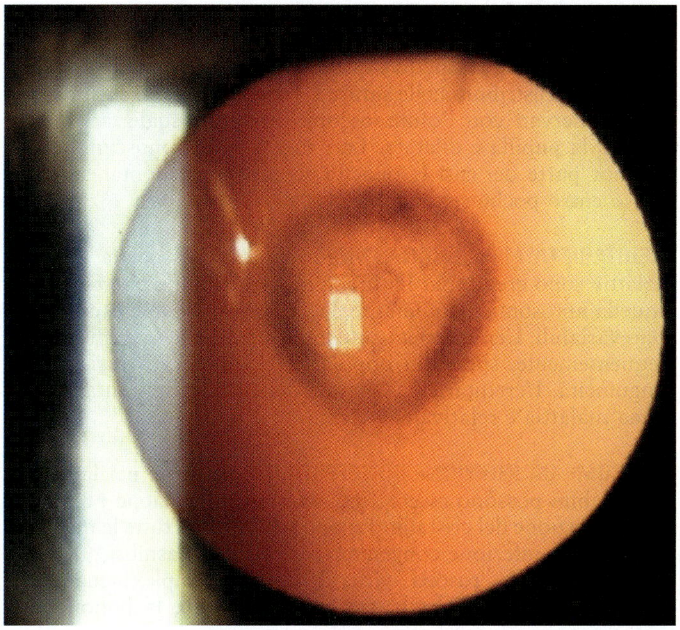

Figura 627-2. Cataratta lamellare centrale.

TABELLA 627-1. Diagnosi differenziale della cataratta

VARIANTI LEGATE ALLO SVILUPPO
Prematurità (vacuoli della sutura a Y) con o senza retinopatia della prematurità
MALATTIE GENETICHE
Ereditarietà mendeliana semplice
Autosomica dominante (più comune)
Autosomica recessiva
X-linked
Difetti cromosomici maggiori
Trisomie (13, 18, 21)
Sindrome di Turner (45X)
Sindrome da delezione (11p13, 18p, 18q)
Sindrome da duplicazione (31, 20p, 10q)
Malattie genetiche multisistemiche
Sindrome di Alport (perdita dell'udito, nefropatia)
Sindrome di Alström (sordità nervosa, diabete mellito)
Malattia di Apert (craniosinostosi, sindattilia)
Sindrome di Cockayne (senilità prematura, fotosensibilità cutanea)
Malattia di Conradi (condrodisplasia puntata)
Malattia di Crouzon (disostosi craniofacciale)
Sindrome di Hallermann-Streiff (microftalmia, naso piccolo appuntito, atrofia cutanea e ipotricosi)
Displasia ectodermica ipoidrosica (dentizione anomala, ipoidrosi, ipotricosi)
Ittiosi (malattia cheratinizzante con cute ispessita, squamosa)
Incontinentia pigmenti (anomalie dentali, ritardo mentale, lesioni cutanee)
Sindrome di Lowe (sindrome oculocerebrorenale: ipotonia, nefropatia)
Sindrome di Marfan
Sindrome di Meckel-Gruber (displasia renale, encefalocele)
Distrofia miotonica
Nail-patella syndrome (disfunzione renale, unghie displastiche, rotula ipoplasica)
Sindrome di Marinesco-Sjögren (atassia cerebellare, ipotonia)
Sindrome del carcinoma basocellulare nevoide (autosomica dominante, il carcinoma basocellulare insorge durante l'infanzia)
Anomalia di Peters (opacizzazioni corneali con disgenesia irido-corneale)
Sindrome di Reiger (displasia dell'iride, distrofia miotonica)
Sindrome di Rothmund-Thomson (poichiloderma: atrofia cutanea)
Sindrome di Rubinstein-Taybi (alluce largo, ritardo mentale)
Sindrome di Smith-Lemli-Opitz (sindattilia delle dita dei piedi, ipospadia, ritardo mentale)
Sindrome di Sotos (gigantismo cerebrale)
Displasia spondiloepifisaria (nanismo, tronco corto)
Sindrome di Werner (invecchiamento prematuro nella seconda decade di vita)
Errori congeniti del metabolismo
Abetalipoproteinemia (chilomicroni assenti, degenerazione retinica)
Malattia di Fabry (deficit di α-galattosidasi A)
Deficit di galattochinasi
Galattosemia (deficit di galattosio-1-fosfato uridiltrasferasi)
Omocistinemia (sublussazione del cristallino, ritardo mentale)
Mannosidosi (deficit di α-mannosidasi)
Malattia di Niemann-Pick (deficit di sfingomielinasi)
Malattia di Refsum (deficit di acido fitanico α-idrossilasi)
Malattia di Wilson (l'accumulo di rame porta a cirrosi e sintomi neurologici)
ENDOCRINOPATIE
Ipocalcemia (ipoparatiroidismo)
Ipoglicemia
Diabete mellito
INFEZIONI CONGENITE
Toxoplasmosi
Infezione da Cytomegalovirus
Sifilide
Rosolia
Infezione perinatale da virus dell'herpes simplex
Morbillo
Poliomielite
Influenza
Varicella-zoster
ANOMALIE OCULARI
Microftalmia
Coloboma
Aniridia
Disgenesia mesodermica
Membrana pupillare persistente
Lenticono posteriore
Vitreo primario iperplastico persistente
Sistema vascolare ialoide primitivo
MALATTIE VARIE
Dermatite atopica
Farmaci (corticosteroidi)
Radiazioni
Trauma
IDIOPATICA

PREMATURITÀ. Un particolare tipo di alterazione del cristallino osservata in alcuni neonati pretermine è la cosiddetta cataratta della prematurità. L'aspetto è quello di un raggruppamento di piccoli vacuoli distribuiti nelle suture a Y del cristallino, che possono essere osservati con l'oftalmoscopio e sono visualizzati meglio quando la pupilla è dilatata. La patogenesi è sconosciuta. Nella maggior parte dei casi le opacità scompaiono spontaneamente, spesso entro poche settimane.

EREDITARIETÀ MENDELIANA. Molte cataratte associate ad altre malattie sono ereditarie. La modalità più comune di ereditarietà è quella autosomica dominante, la cui penetranza ed espressività sono variabili. L'ereditarietà autosomica recessiva si verifica meno frequentemente, spesso in popolazioni con elevati tassi di consanguineità. L'ereditarietà X-linked delle cataratte non associate a una malattia è relativamente rara.

SINDROME DA INFEZIONE CONGENITA. Le cataratte nei lattanti e nei bambini possono essere secondarie a un'infezione prenatale. L'opacizzazione del cristallino si può verificare in tutte le maggiori sindromi da infezione congenita (per es. toxoplasmosi, Cytomegalovirus, sifilide, rosolia, virus dell'herpes simplex), ma anche in altre infezioni prenatali, tra cui il morbillo, la poliomielite, l'influenza, la varicella-zoster e il vaiolo.

MALATTIE METABOLICHE. La cataratta è una manifestazione principale di molte malattie metaboliche, in particolare di alcune alterazioni del metabolismo dei carboidrati, degli aminoacidi, del calcio e del rame. Una delle prime malattie da prendere in considerazione in ogni bambino con cataratta è una possibile **galattosemia** (vedi Capitolo 87.2). Nella galattosemia infantile classica, con deficit di galattosio-1-fosfato uridil trasferasi, la cataratta è tipicamente di tipo zonulare, con l'offuscamento o l'opacizzazione di uno o più strati perinucleari del cristallino e spesso anche del nucleo. Nelle sue fasi iniziali la cataratta in genere ha un aspetto distintivo a gocce d'olio ed è identificata meglio con la pupilla pienamente dilatata. Entro alcune settimane si può verificare la progressione fino all'opacizzazione completa. In caso di trattamento precoce (dieta priva di galattosio) le alterazioni del cristallino possono essere reversibili.

Nel **deficit di galattochinasi** la cataratta è l'unica manifestazione clinica, risulta solitamente zonulare e può comparire nei primi mesi o nei primi anni di vita o successivamente nell'infanzia.

Nei bambini con diabete mellito a esordio giovanile, le alterazioni del cristallino sono rare. Alcuni sviluppano opacità bianche "a fiocchi di neve", che possono progredire e maturare rapidamente, talvolta nel giro di giorni, specialmente durante l'adolescenza. Un evento antecedente può essere costituito dall'improvviso sviluppo di miopia causata da alterazioni della densità ottica del cristallino.

Opacità congenite del cristallino possono essere osservate nei bambini di madri diabetiche e prediabetiche. Anche l'ipoglicemia, nei neonati, può essere associata allo sviluppo precoce della cataratta, così come l'ipoglicemia chetosica.

L'associazione tra la cataratta e l'ipocalcemia è ben stabilita. Diverse opacità del cristallino possono essere osservate nei pazienti con ipoparatiroidismo.

La **sindrome oculocerebrale renale di Lowe** è associata alla cataratta nei bambini. I maschi affetti mostrano frequentemente una cataratta densa bilaterale alla nascita, spesso insieme a un glaucoma e a pupille miotiche. Opacità puntinate del cristallino si trovano spesso nelle femmine eterozigoti.

La caratteristica cataratta "a girasole" della **malattia di Wilson** non è osservata comunemente nei bambini. Varie opacità del cristallino possono essere notate nei bambini con alcuni tipi di sfingolipidosi, mucopolisaccaridosi e mucolipidosi, in particolare la malattia di Niemann-Pick, la mucosulfatidosi, la malattia di Fabry e l'aspartilglicosaminuria.

DIFETTI CROMOSOMICI. Opacizzazioni del cristallino di vario tipo si possono verificare in associazione a difetti cromosomici, tra cui le trisomie 13, 18 e 21, la sindrome di Turner e tutta una serie di sindromi da delezione (11p13, 18p, 18q) e duplicazione (3q, 20p, 10q).

FARMACI, AGENTI TOSSICI E TRAUMI. Dei vari farmaci e sostanze tossiche che possono produrre la cataratta, i corticosteroidi sono i più importanti nel gruppo di età pediatrico. Le cataratte steroide-correlate sono caratteristicamente opacità sottocapsulari posteriori del cristallino. L'incidenza e la gravità appaiono variabili. L'importanza relativa della dose, della modalità di somministrazione, della durata del trattamento e della sensibilità individuale è controversa e la patogenesi della cataratta steroide-indotta non è chiara. L'effetto sulla vista dipende dall'estensione e dalla densità dell'opacità. In molti casi l'acuità risulta compromessa solo in modo minimo o moderato. A volte le cataratte steroide-indotte possono essere reversibili. Tutti i bambini che ricevono un trattamento steroideo a lungo termine dovrebbero essere sottoposti a un esame oculistico periodico.

Il trauma oculare è una delle principali cause della cataratta nei bambini. L'opacizzazione del cristallino può essere secondaria a una contusione o a una lesione penetrante. Le cataratte costituiscono inoltre un'importante manifestazione dell'abuso di minore.

La formazione della cataratta dopo un'esposizione a radiazioni dipende dalla dose e dalla durata. Gli studi nell'adulto mostrano una occorrenza del 50% alla dose per cristallino di 15 Gy. L'esordio tardivo è la regola.

MALATTIE VARIE. La lista di sindromi e malattie multisistemiche associate all'opacità del cristallino e ad altre anomalie degli occhi è lunga (vedi Tab. 627-1).

Trattamento. Il trattamento di una cataratta che interferisce significativamente con la vista comprende: (1) la rimozione chirurgica del materiale del cristallino per fornire un asse visivo otticamente libero; (2) la correzione del conseguente errore refrattivo afachico con occhiali, lenti a contatto o un impianto di lente intraoculare; (3) la correzione dell'eventuale ambliopia da deprivazione sensoriale associata. Dal momento che l'uso degli occhiali può non essere possibile nei bambini dopo la rimozione della cataratta, il ricorso alle lenti a contatto per la riabilitazione visiva è una necessità medica. Il trattamento dell'ambliopia può costituire la fase più difficoltosa e impegnativa nella riabilitazione visiva dei lattanti o dei bambini con la cataratta.

Prognosi. La prognosi dipende da molti fattori, tra cui la natura della cataratta, la malattia sottostante, l'età all'esordio, l'età al momento dell'intervento e la presenza di anomalie oculari associate (per es. microftalmia, lesioni retiniche, atrofia ottica, glaucoma, nistagmo, strabismo). L'ambliopia persistente è la causa più comune dello scarso recupero della vista dopo un intervento chirurgico per cataratta nei bambini. In quelli che vi sono stati sottoposti possono svilupparsi malattie e complicanze secondarie, come sequele infiammatorie, membrane secondarie, glaucoma, distacco di retina e alterazioni nella lunghezza assiale dell'occhio. Tutte queste andrebbero prese in considerazione nella pianificazione del trattamento.

ECTOPIA LENTIS. Normalmente il cristallino è mantenuto sospeso dietro al diaframma dell'iride dalle fibre zonulari del corpo ciliare. Le anomalie del sistema sospensorio secondarie a un difetto dello sviluppo, a una malattia o a un trauma possono portare all'instabilità o alla dislocazione del cristallino. Quest'ultima viene classificata come lussazione (dislocazione-spostamento completo del cristallino) (Fig. 627-3) o sublussazione (spostamento parziale-spostamento o inclinazione del cristallino) (Fig. 627-4). I sintomi comprendono l'offuscamento del visus, spesso secondario ad alterazioni refrattive come la miopia, l'astigmatismo o l'ipermetropia afachica. Alcuni pazienti presentano diplopia. Un importante segno di spostamento è l'iridocinesi, un tremolio dell'iride determinato dalla perdita del suo abituale supporto. Inoltre, la camera anteriore può apparire più profonda della norma. Talvolta la regione equatoriale ("bordo") del cristallino

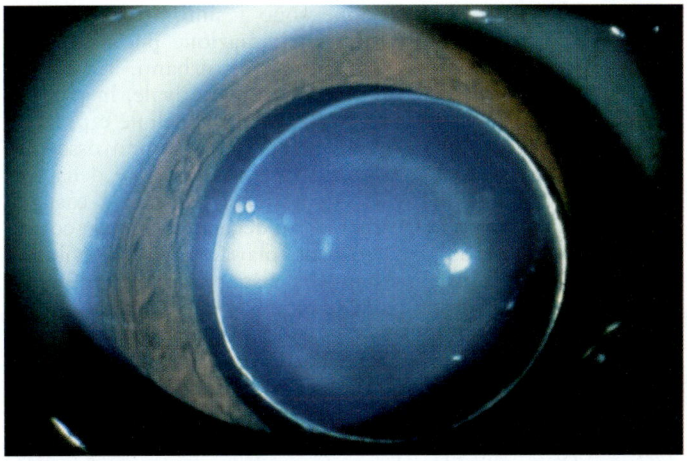

Figura 627-3. Lussazione completa del cristallino nella camera anteriore osservata nella sindrome di Weill-Marchesani.

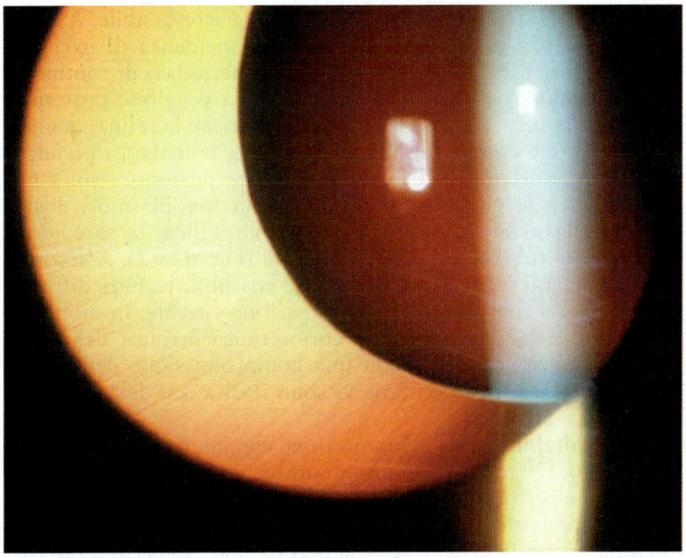

Figura 627-4. Sublussazione del cristallino nella sindrome di Marfan.

dislocato può essere visibile nell'apertura pupillare e all'oftalmoscopia può apparire come una mezzaluna nera. Inoltre, si può apprezzare la differenza tra le porzioni fachica e afachica quando ci si focalizza sul fondo oculare.

Diagnosi differenziale. Una delle principali cause di dislocazione è il trauma. Essa può verificarsi anche in seguito a una malattia oculare come l'uveite, un tumore intraoculare, un glaucoma congenito, la miopia elevata, la megalocornea, l'aniridia o in associazione a cataratta. Esistono anche forme ereditarie e forme associate a una malattia sistemica.

La dislocazione che si sviluppa come malattia oculare ereditabile non associata ad anomalie sistemiche è denominata ectopia lentis semplice e di solito viene trasmessa in maniera autosomica dominante. Il cristallino è in genere dislocato verso l'alto e temporalmente. L'ectopia può essere presente alla nascita o può apparire successivamente nella vita. Un'altra forma di dislocazione ereditabile è l'ectopia lentis et pupillae, in cui sia il cristallino sia la pupilla si trovano dislocati, di solito in direzioni opposte. Questa malattia è generalmente bilaterale e un occhio appare quasi l'immagine speculare dell'altro. Si tratta inoltre di una malattia recessiva, sebbene sia stata riportata un'espressione variabile con la mescolanza con l'ectopia lentis semplice.

Tra le **malattie sistemiche** associate alla dislocazione del cristallino vi sono la sindrome di Marfan, l'omocistinuria, la sindrome di Weill-Marchesani e il deficit di sulfito ossidasi. L'ectopia lentis si verifica in circa l'80% dei pazienti con una sindrome di Marfan e in circa il 50% di essi risulta evidente a partire dall'età di 5 anni. Nella maggior parte dei casi il cristallino risulta dislocato verso l'alto e temporalmente, è quasi sempre bilaterale e relativamente simmetrico. Nell'omocistinuria, invece, di solito è dislocato in basso e piuttosto nasalmente. Ciò si verifica precocemente nella vita e spesso appare evidente a partire dall'età di 5 anni. Nella sindrome di Weill-Marchesani la dislocazione è spesso verso il basso e in avanti e il cristallino tende a essere piccolo e rotondo.

L'ectopia lentis è anche associata occasionalmente ad altre malattie, tra cui le sindromi di Ehlers-Danlos, di Sturge-Weber, di Crouzon e di Klippel-Feil, l'ossicefalia e la disostosi mandibolofacciale. È stata descritta anche una sindrome di blefaroptosi ereditata con modalità dominante, miopia elevata ed ectopia lentis.

Trattamento e prognosi. La dislocazione del cristallino spesso comporta soltanto disturbi ottici. In alcuni casi, tuttavia, si possono sviluppare complicanze più gravi, come il glaucoma, l'uveite, il distacco della retina o la cataratta. Il trattamento deve essere personalizzato, a seconda del tipo di dislocazione, della sua causa e della presenza di eventuali malattie oculari o sistemiche complicanti. A molti pazienti si può fornire una correzione ottica con occhiali o lenti a contatto. La manipolazione del diaframma dell'iride con gocce di midriatici o miotici può talvolta aiutare a migliorare la vista. In casi selezionati, il trattamento migliore è la rimozione chirurgica del cristallino. In molti bambini il trattamento di un'eventuale ambliopia associata deve essere intrapreso precocemente. Inoltre, per quelli con ectopia lentis andrebbero prese precauzioni di sicurezza per prevenire lesioni dell'occhio.

MICROSFEROFACHIA. Con microsferofachia s'intende un cristallino piccolo, rotondo, che può comparire come un'anomalia isolata (probabilmente autosomica recessiva) o in associazione ad altre anomalie oculari, come l'ectopia lentis, la miopia o il distacco della retina (facilmente autosomica dominante). La microsferofachia può anche verificarsi in associazione a varie malattie sistemiche, tra cui la sindrome di Marfam, la sindrome di Weill-Marchesani, la sindrome di Alport, la disostosi mandibolofacciale e la sindrome di Klinefelter.

LENTICONO ANTERIORE. Si tratta di una rara malattia bilaterale in cui la superficie anteriore del cristallino sporge centralmente. Può essere accompagnato da opacità del cristallino o da altre anomalie oculari ed è una caratteristica importante della sindrome di Alport. L'aumentata curvatura dell'area centrale può causare una miopia grave.

LENTICONO POSTERIORE. Si verifica più comunemente del lenticono anteriore ed è caratterizzato dalla protuberanza circoscritta o ovale della capsula e della corteccia posteriori del cristallino limitata alla regione dei 2-7 mm centrali (assiali). Nelle fasi iniziali, mediante il test del riflesso rosso, può apparire come una goccia d'olio. Si verifica nei lattanti e nei bambini piccoli e tende ad aumentare con l'età. Di solito alla fine il materiale del cristallino all'interno e attorno alla sporgenza capsulare diventa opacizzato. Il lenticono posteriore solitamente compare come un'anomalia oculare isolata. In genere è unilaterale, ma può apparire anche bilaterale. Si ritiene che sia sporadico, sebbene in alcuni casi sia stata ipotizzata un'ereditarietà autosomica dominante. Nei bambini affetti possono essere necessari la correzione ottica, il trattamento dell'ambliopia e l'intervento chirurgico per la cataratta progressiva.

Anteby I, Isaac M, BenEzra D: Hereditary subluxated lenses: visual performances and long-term follow-up after surgery. *Ophthalmology* 2003; 110:1344–1348.

Bhatti TR, Dott M, Yoon PW, et al: Descriptive epidemiology of infantile cataracts in metropolitain Atlanta, GA, 1968–1998. *Arch Pediatr Adolesc Med* 2003;157:341–347.
Chugh KS, Sakhuja V, Agarwal A, et al: Hereditary nephritis (Alport's syndrome)—clinical profile and inheritance in 28 kindreds. *Nephrol Dial Transplant* 1993;8:690–695.
Fallaha N, Lambert SR. Pediatric cataracts. *Ophthalmol Clin North Am* 2001;14:479–492.
Khalil M, Saheb N: Posterior lenticonus. *Ophthalmology* 1984;91:1429–1430.
Levin AV, Edmonds SA, Nelson LB, et al: Extended-wear contact lenses for the treatment of pediatric aphakia. *Ophthalmology* 1988;95:1107–1113.
Peterseim MW, Wilson ME: Bilateral intraocular lens implantation in the pediatric population. *Ophthalmology* 2000;107:1261–1266.
Plager DA, Yang S, Neely D, et al: Complications in the first year following cataract surgery with and without IOL in infants and older children. *J AAPOS* 2002;6:9–14.
Tesser RA, Hess DB, Buckley EG: Pediatric cataracts and lens anomalies. In Nelson LB, Olitsky SE (editors): *Harley's Pediatric Ophthalmology*, 5th ed. Philadelphia, Lippincott Williams & Wilkins, 2005;255–284.

Capitolo 628 ■ Malattie del tratto uveale

Scott E. Olitsky, Denise Hug e Laura P. Smith

UVEITE (IRITE, CICLITE, CORIORETINITE). Il tratto uveale (la tonaca vascolare interna dell'occhio, costituita da iride, corpo ciliare e coroide) è soggetto a processi infiammatori in tutta una serie di malattie sistemiche, infettive e non infettive, e in risposta a fattori esogeni, tra cui traumi e agenti tossici (Tab. 628-1). L'infiammazione può colpire qualunque porzione del tratto uveale in modo preferenziale oppure tutte le parti insieme.

L'**irite** può comparire da sola o insieme all'infiammazione del corpo ciliare come iridociclite o in associazione a pars planite.

TABELLA 628-1. Uveite nell'infanzia

UVEITE ANTERIORE
Artrite reumatoide giovanile (pauciarticolare)
Sarcoidosi
Trauma
Tubercolosi
Malattia di Kawasaki
Colite ulcerosa
Postinfettiva (enterica o genitale) con artrite e rash
Da spirochete (sifilide, leptospirosi)
Iridociclite eterocromica (Fuchs)
Virale (herpes simplex, herpes zoster)
Spondilite anchilosante
Sindrome di Stevens-Johnson
Idiopatica
Farmaci
UVEITE POSTERIORE (COROIDITE, PUÒ INTERESSARE LA RETINA)
Toxoplasmosi
Parassiti (toxocariasi)
Sarcoidosi
Tubercolosi
Virale (rosolia, herpes simplex, HIV, Cytomegalovirus)
Panencefalite subacuta sclerosante
Idiopatica
UVEITE ANTERIORE E/O POSTERIORE
Oftalmia simpatica (trauma all'altro occhio)
Sindrome di Vogt-Koyanagi-Harada (sindrome uveo-otocutanea: poliosi, vitiligine, sordità, tinnito, uveite, meningite asettica, retinite)
Sindrome di Behçet
Malattia di Lyme

Dolore, fotofobia e lacrimazione sono i sintomi caratteristici dell'uveite anteriore acuta, ma l'infiammazione può realizzarsi anche in modo insidioso senza sintomi disturbanti. Tra i segni di uveite anteriore vi sono l'iperemia congiuntivale, in particolare nella regione perilimbare (flush ciliare), e cellule e proteine ("flare") nell'umore acqueo (Fig. 628-1). Si possono osservare anche depositi infiammatori sulla superficie anteriore della cornea (precipitati cheratici) e la congestione dell'iride. I casi più cronici possono comportare alterazioni degenerative della cornea (cheratopatia a banda), opacità lenticolari (cataratta), sviluppo di glaucoma e compromissione della vista. La causa dell'uveite anteriore è spesso oscura; nei bambini le prime patologie da considerare sono la malattia reumatoide, in particolare l'artrite reumatoide pauciarticolare, la malattia di Kawasaki, la sindrome di Reiter e la sarcoidosi. L'irite può essere secondaria a una malattia corneale, come la cheratite erpetica o l'ulcera corneale batterica o fungina, oppure a un'abrasione corneale o a un corpo estraneo. L'irite e l'iridociclite traumatiche sono particolarmente comuni nei bambini.

L'**iridociclite** che si verifica nei bambini con artrite merita un cenno particolare. A differenza della maggior parte delle forme di uveite anteriore, essa provoca raramente dolore, fotofobia o iperemia congiuntivale. La perdita della vista può non essere rilevata finché non si sia verificato un danno grave e irreversibile. A causa della mancanza di sintomi e dell'elevata incidenza di uveite in questi bambini, è necessario lo screening periodico di routine.

La **coroidite**, ossia l'infiammazione della porzione posteriore del tratto uveale, interessa costantemente anche la retina; quando entrambe sono colpite in maniera evidente, la malattia prende il nome di corioretinite. Le cause dell'uveite posteriore sono numerose e tra le più comuni si trovano la toxoplasmosi, l'istoplasmosi, la malattia da inclusione citomegalica, la sarcoidosi, la sifilide, la tubercolosi e la toxocariasi (Fig. 628-2). A seconda dell'eziologia, i segni d'infiammazione possono risultare diffusi o focali. Spesso compare anche una reazione vitreale. In molti tipi il risultato è la cicatrizzazione corioretinica atrofica delimitata da pigmentazione, spesso con una compromissione della vista. Tra le complicanze secondarie vi sono il distacco della retina, il glaucoma e la ftisi.

La **panoftalmite** è un'infiammazione che interessa tutte le parti dell'occhio. È frequentemente suppurativa, più spesso in seguito a una lesione perforante o a setticemia. Produce un dolore grave, la marcata congestione dell'occhio, l'infiammazione dei tessuti orbitali adiacenti e delle palpebre e la perdita della vista. In molti casi l'occhio viene perso nonostante il trattamento intensivo dell'infezione e dell'infiammazione. Possono infatti essere necessarie la sua enucleazione o l'eviscerazione dell'orbita.

L'**oftalmia simpatica** è un raro tipo di risposta infiammatoria che interessa l'occhio non danneggiato dopo una lesione penetrante. Può comparire a distanza di settimane, mesi o anche anni

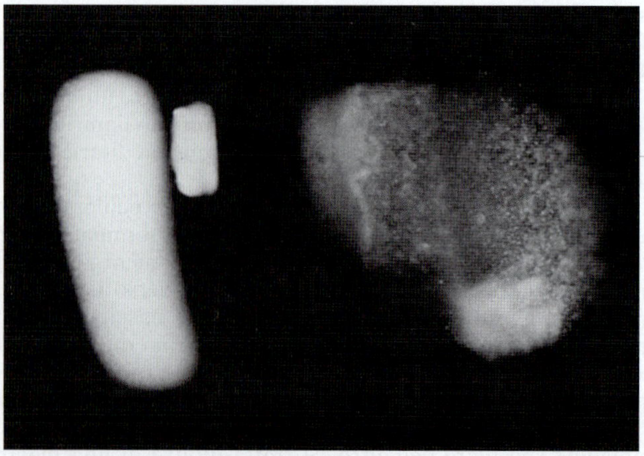

Figura 628-1. Cellula e flare nella camera anteriore. Il flare rappresenta il leakage di proteine. (Per gentile concessione di Peter Buch, CRA.)

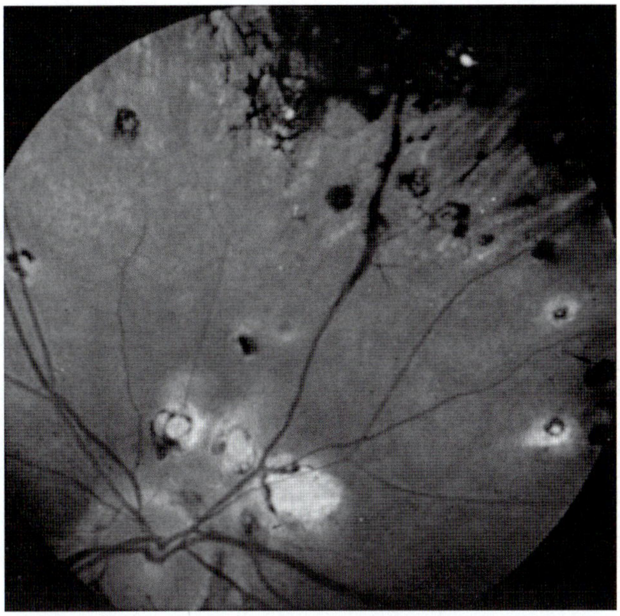

Figura 628-2. Cicatrici focali atrofiche e pigmentate della corioretinite.

dalla lesione. La causa più probabile è un fenomeno di ipersensibilità. Ne può conseguire la perdita della vista nell'occhio non danneggiato (simpatizzante). La rimozione dell'occhio lesionato previene lo sviluppo dell'oftalmia simpatica ma non arresta la progressione della malattia dopo che questa è insorta. Pertanto l'enucleazione andrebbe presa in considerazione se non vi è speranza di recupero visivo dopo una lesione grave.

Trattamento. Le varie forme d'infiammazione intraoculare sono trattate in funzione dei loro fattori causali. Quando l'infezione è dimostrata o sospetta, si utilizza l'appropriata terapia sistemica antimicrobica o antivirale. In alcuni casi è indicata l'iniezione intravitreale.

L'eliminazione dell'infiammazione è importante per ridurre il rischio di una grave perdita della vista, che spesso può diventare permanente. Se non viene trattato, il processo infiammatorio può portare allo sviluppo di cheratopatia a banda (deposito di calcio nella cornea), cataratta, glaucoma e danno retinico irreversibile. L'infiammazione anteriore può rispondere bene al trattamento con corticosteroidi topici, mentre i casi posteriori spesso richiedono una terapia sistemica. L'uso di corticosteroidi topici e sistemici può portare allo sviluppo di un glaucoma e della cataratta, cosicché per ridurre la loro necessità nei pazienti che abbisognano di un trattamento a lungo termine si utilizza frequentemente l'immunosoppressione sistemica. Tra gli agenti immunosoppressori comunemente utilizzati ci sono il metrotexato, la ciclosporina e gli inibitori del tumor necrosis factor. Si impiegano anche agenti cicloplegici, in particolare l'atropina, per ridurre l'infiammazione e prevenire l'aderenza dell'iride al cristallino (sinechie posteriori), specialmente nell'uveite anteriore. L'estesa formazione di sinechie posteriori può condurre a un glaucoma acuto ad angolo chiuso.

L'intervento chirurgico può risultare necessario per i pazienti che sviluppano un glaucoma a causa del processo patologico sottostante o per la necessità di un trattamento corticosteroideo. L'intervento per cataratta dovrebbe essere rimandato finché l'infiammazione non sia stata tenuta sotto controllo per un certo periodo di tempo, ma in ogni caso nei bambini con un'anamesi di uveite protratta esso può comportare un rischio significativo. Non vi è un accordo generale per quanto riguarda l'uso delle lenti oculari in questi pazienti.

Le **sindromi masquerade** possono talvolta simulare l'infiammazione intraoculare. Il retinoblastoma, la leucemia, la ritenzione di un corpo estraneo intraoculare, lo xantogranuloma giovanile e i distacchi della retina periferici possono produrre segni simili a quelli dell'uveite. Queste sindromi andrebbero tenute presenti nella valutazione di un paziente con sospetta uveite o se un soggetto non risponde come previsto al trattamento antinfiammatorio.

BenEzra D, Cohen E: Cataract surgery in children with chronic uveitis. *Ophthalmology* 2000;107:1255–1260.

Chu DS, Foster CS: Sympathetic ophthalmia. *Int Ophthalmol Clin* 2002; 42:179–185.

Holland GN, Stiehm ER: Special considerations in the evaluation and management of uveitis in children. *Am J Ophthalmol* 2003;135: 867–878.

Kadayifcilar S, Eldem B, Tumer B: Uveitis in childhood. *J Pediatr Ophthalmol Strabismus* 2003;40:335–340.

Kotaniemi K, Savolainen A, Karma A, et al: Recent advances in uveitis of juvenile idiopathic arthritis. *Surv Ophthalmol* 2003;48:489–502.

McCluskey P, Powell RJ: The eye in systemic inflammatory diseases. *Lancet* 2004;364:2125–2133.

Oren B, Sehgal A, Simon JW, et al: The prevalence of uveitis in juvenile rheumatoid arthritis. *J Am Assoc Pediatr Ophthalmol Strabismus* 2001;5:2–4.

Patel H, Goldstein D: Pediatric uveitis. *Pediatr Clin North Am* 2003; 50:125–136.

Rosenberg KD, Feuer WJ, Davis JL: Ocular complications of pediatric uveitis. *Ophthalmology* 2004;111:2299–2306.

Capitolo 629 ■ Malattie della retina e del vitreo

Scott E. Olitsky, Denise Hug e Laura P. Smith

RETINOPATIA DELLA PREMATURITÀ (ROP). La ROP (*Retinopathy Of Prematurity*) è una malattia complessa della vascolarizzazione retinica in fase evolutiva nei neonati prematuri. Può essere acuta (fasi iniziali) o cronica (fasi tardive). Le manifestazioni cliniche vanno da lievi alterazioni solitamente transitorie della retina periferica a una grave proliferazione progressiva, alla cicatrizzazione e al distacco della retina che può portare alla cecità. La ROP comprende tutti gli stadi della malattia e le sue sequele; il nome con cui era nota in passato, ossia fibroplasia retrolenticolare, descriveva soltanto gli stadi cicatriziali.

Patogenesi. A partire dalla 16ª settimana di gestazione, l'angiogenesi retinica normalmente procede dal disco ottico alla periferia, raggiungendo il bordo esterno della retina (in quel momento serrata) a livello nasale a circa 36 settimane ed estendendosi temporalmente a partire dalla 40ª settimana circa. La compromissione di tale processo comporta varie alterazioni patologiche e cliniche. La prima osservazione nella fase acuta è l'interruzione della vasculogenesi. Piuttosto che una graduale transizione dalla retina vascolarizzata a quella avascolare, avviene un'interruzione improvvisa dei vasi contrassegnata da una linea nella retina. La linea può quindi trasformarsi in una cresta composta da cellule mesenchimali ed endoteliali. La divisione e la differenziazione cellulare possono riprendere in un momento successivo e la vascolarizzazione della retina può proseguire. In alternativa, vi può essere la progressione a un'anomala proliferazione di vasi al di fuori del piano della retina, nel vitreo e al di sopra della superficie della retina. Successivamente possono comparire la cicatrizzazione e una trazione sulla retina che portano al suo distacco.

I fattori di rischio associati alla ROP non sono pienamente noti, ma la prematurità e l'immaturità retinica alla nascita rappresentano quelli principali. Alcuni ritengono che contribuiscano anche l'ossigenazione, il distress respiratorio, l'apnea, la bradicardia, la cardiopatia, un'infezione, l'ipercarbia, l'acidosi, l'anemia e la necessità di trasfusione. In genere, minore è l'età gestazionale, più basso è il peso corporeo e più malato è il bambino, maggiore risulta il rischio della ROP.

La patogenesi di base è ancora sconosciuta. L'esposizione all'ambiente extrauterino, che comprende concentrazioni necessariamente elevate di ossigeno inspirato, produce un danno cellulare, forse mediato dai radicali liberi. Successivamente, nel corso della malattia si sviluppa un'ipossia periferica e si producono fattori di crescita vascolo-endoteliali nella retina non vascolarizzata. Questi stimolano una vasculogenesi anormale e si può avere una neovascolarizzazione. A causa della funzione polmonare deficitaria, s'instaura uno stato di ipossia retinica relativa. Ciò provoca l'upregulation dei fattori di crescita vascolo-endoteliali, che nei bambini predisposti può determinare l'anomala crescita fibrovascolare. La neovascolarizzazione può quindi causare una cicatrizzazione e la perdita della vista.

Classificazione. La classificazione internazionale attualmente utilizzata della ROP descrive la localizzazione, l'estensione e la gravità della malattia. Per indicare la localizzazione, la retina viene suddivisa in tre zone concentriche, centrate sul disco ottico. La zona I, o posteriore o interna, si estende per una lunghezza pari a due volte la distanza disco-maculare, oppure per 30 gradi in tutte le direzioni dal disco ottico. La zona II, o intermedia, si estende dal margine esterno della zona I all'ora serrata nasalmente e all'equatore anatomico temporalmente. La zona III, la più esterna, è la mezzaluna residua che si spande dal bordo esterno della zona II all'ora serrata temporalmente. L'estensione della lesione viene descritta secondo il numero delle ore dell'orologio interessate.

Le fasi e la gravità del processo di malattia sono classificate in cinque stadi. Lo stadio 1 è caratterizzato da una linea di demarcazione che separa la retina vascolarizzata da quella avascolare. Questa linea si trova entro il piano della retina e appare relativamente piatta e bianca. Spesso si nota una ramificazione o un inarcamento anomalo dei vasi retinici che conducono alla linea. Lo stadio 2 è contraddistinto da una cresta; la linea di demarcazione è cresciuta, acquisendo altezza, profondità e volume ed estendendosi verso l'alto e l'esterno dal piano della retina. Lo stadio 3 vede la presenza di una cresta e lo sviluppo di tessuto fibrovascolare extraretinico (Fig. 629-1*A*). Lo stadio 4 comporta il distacco subtotale della retina causato dalla trazione dal tessuto proliferante nel vitreo o sulla retina. Questo stadio è suddiviso in due fasi: (a) distacco subtotale della retina che non coinvolge la macula e (b) coinvolgimento della macula. Lo stadio 5, infine, è il distacco totale della retina.

Quando alcuni segni di alterazioni vascolari retiniche posteriori accompagnano gli stadi attivi della ROP, si utilizza il termine

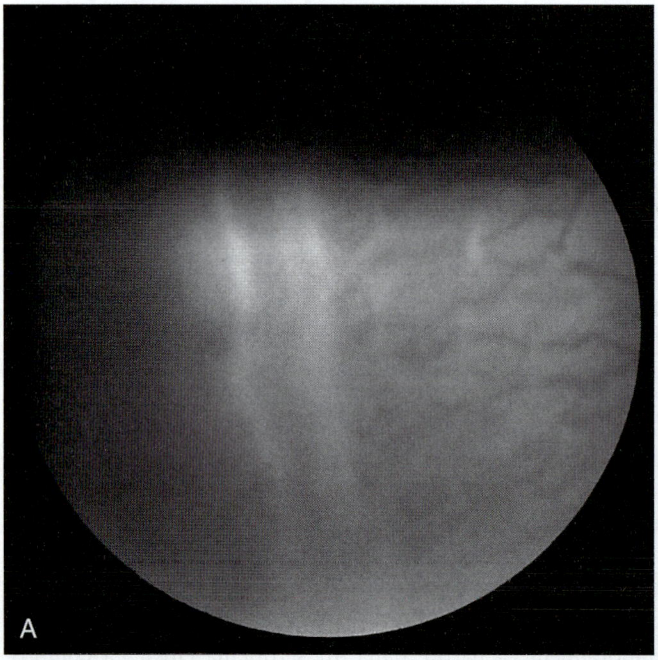

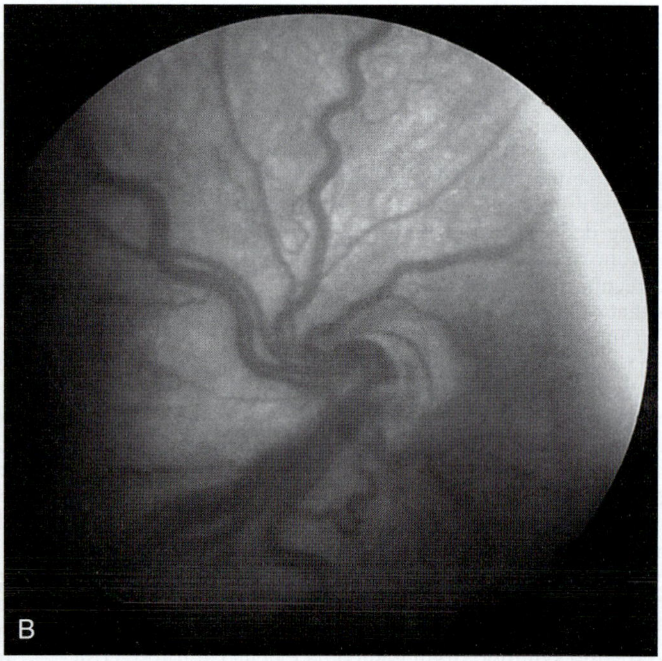

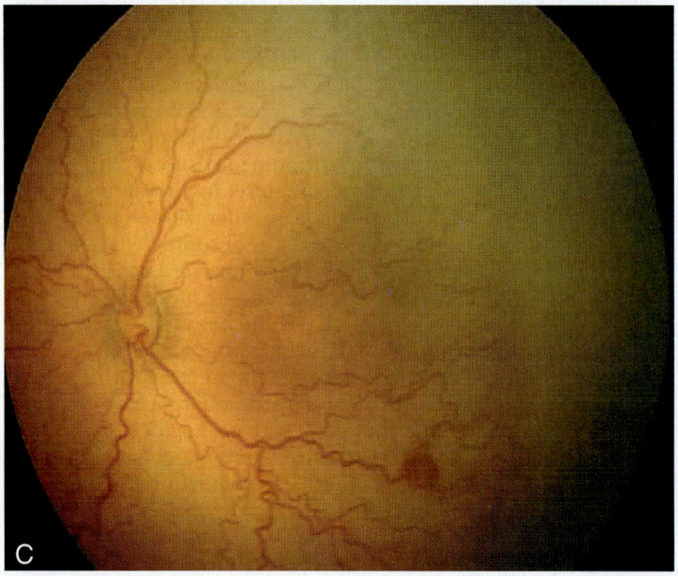

Figura 629-1. Retinopatia della prematurità (ROP). *A*, Nello stadio 3 sono presenti una cresta e tessuto vascolare extraretinico. *B*, I vasi retinici sono dilatati e tortuosi nella malattia plus della ROP attiva. *C*, Zona I, stadio ROP con malattia plus.

di "malattia plus" (Fig. 629-1*B*, *C*). I pazienti che raggiungono il punto della dilatazione e della tortuosità dei vasi retinici mostrano frequentemente anche reperti associati d'ingorgo dell'iride, rigidità pupillare e velo vitreo.

Manifestazioni cliniche e prognosi. In oltre il 90% dei neonati a rischio il decorso comporta l'interruzione e la regressione spontanei, con effetti residui scarsi o assenti o una disabilità visiva. Meno del 10% presenta la progressione a una malattia grave, con significativa vasoproliferazione extraretinica, cicatrizzazione, distacco della retina e compromissione della vista.

Alcuni bambini con una ROP interrotta o regredita manifestano linee di demarcazione residue, l'ipovascolarizzazione della retina periferica o una ramificazione anormale, tortuosità o raddrizzamento dei vasi retinici. In alcuni rimangono alterazioni pigmentarie retiniche, il dragging della retina (cosiddetto "dragged disc"), l'ectopia della macula, pieghe o rotture retiniche. Altri progrediscono al distacco totale della retina, che comunemente assume una configurazione a imbuto. Il quadro clinico è spesso quello di una membrana retrolentale, che produce la leucocoria (un riflesso bianco della pupilla). Alcuni pazienti sviluppano la cataratta, un glaucoma e segni di infiammazione. La fase terminale è spesso un occhio cieco dolente o ftisico degenerato. Lo spettro della ROP comprende anche la miopia, che è spesso progressiva e di grado significativo nell'infanzia. Anche l'incidenza di anisometropia, strabismo, ambliopia e nistagmo può essere aumentata.

Diagnosi. Sono consigliati esami oftalmologici seriali sistematici dei neonati a rischio. Le linee guida sono variabili, ma in genere comprendono i neonati di peso inferiore a 1500 g alla nascita e quelli nati prima della 31ª settimana di età gestazionale. Anche quelli con peso alla nascita superiore a 1500 g che però presentano un decorso clinico instabile e si ritiene siano a rischio elevato dovrebbero essere valutati per la ROP. L'esame iniziale andrebbe realizzato a 4-6 settimane di età cronologica o a 31-33 di età postconcezionale. La ROP viene più spesso diagnosticata 32-44 settimane dopo il concepimento. L'esame può essere stressante per i fragili neonati pretermine e le gocce dilatanti possono avere effetti collaterali indesiderati; pertanto la scelta del momento di attuazione dell'esame oculare deve essere effettuata con giudizio e i neonati vanno attentamente monitorati durante e dopo l'esame. Il follow-up si basa sui reperti iniziali e sui fattori di rischio, ma di solito dura 2 settimane o meno.

Trattamento. In casi selezionati, la crioterapia o la fotocoagulazione laser della retina avascolare riducono le più gravi complicanze della ROP progressiva. I perfezionamenti nelle tecniche chirurgiche vitreoretiniche hanno portato a un limitato successo nel riattacco della retina nei neonati con un distacco totale (ROP di stadio 5), ma i risultati sulla vista sono spesso deludenti. Lo studio Early Treatment for Retinopathy of Prematurity Cooperative ha riscontrato risultati strutturali e visivi migliorati con una soglia ridefinita per il trattamento. Questo studio ha dimostrato l'importanza della malattia plus e della presenza di un interessamento retinico posteriore per determinare quando trattare la ROP. Ha anche confermato che il laser è la **modalità di trattamento di scelta.** L'ablazione retinica periferica dovrebbe essere presa in considerazione per tutti gli occhi con una ROP di tipo 1. Esami seriali sono indicati per tutti quelli con una ROP di tipo 2; il trattamento viene preso in considerazione se quest'ultimo progredisce a tipo 1 o se la soglia della ROP si trasforma.

Prevenzione. La prevenzione della ROP dipende in definitiva da quella del parto prematuro e dei disturbi associati. Nonostante i progressi tecnologici e la meticolosa assistenza ai neonati ad alto rischio nelle nursery moderne, la ROP continua a verificarsi. L'ossigeno da solo non è sufficiente né necessario per produrre la ROP e il suo livello sicuro non è ancora stato determinato. Ogni neonato deve essere trattato con tutto ciò che occorre per supportare la vita e la funzione neurologica. Alcuni ricercatori hanno suggerito l'uso di vitamina E supplementare, per le sue proprietà antiossidanti, nei neonati a rischio di ROP, ma la sua efficacia non è stata dimostrata e a certe dosi può anche provocare effetti collaterali indesiderati (vedi Capitolo 97.2).

VITREO PRIMARIO IPERPLASTICO PERSISTENTE (PHPV). Il PHPV (*Persistent Hyperplastic Primary Vitreous*) comprende uno spettro di manifestazioni originate dalla persistenza di varie porzioni del sistema vascolare ialoide fetale e del tessuto fibrovascolare associato.

Patogenesi. Durante lo sviluppo dell'occhio, l'arteria ialoide si estende dal disco ottico alla parte posteriore del cristallino; invia rami nel vitreo e si ramifica per formare la porzione posteriore della capsula vascolare del cristallino. La porzione posteriore del sistema ialoide normalmente regredisce durante il settimo mese di vita fetale e la porzione anteriore a partire dall'ottavo mese. Piccoli residui del sistema, come un ciuffo di tessuto in corrispondenza del disco (papilla di Bergmeister) o una placca di tessuto sulla capsula posteriore del cristallino (punto di Mittendorf), sono reperti comuni in individui sani. Residui più estesi e complicanze associate costituiscono il PHPV. Sono descritte due forme principali, il PHPV anteriore e il PHPV posteriore. La variabilità è grande ed esistono forme miste o intermedie.

Manifestazioni cliniche. La caratteristica clinica abituale del PHPV anteriore è la presenza di una placca vascolarizzata di tessuto sulla superficie posteriore del cristallino in un occhio microftalmico o leggermente più piccolo della norma. La malattia è solitamente unilaterale e può verificarsi in neonati senza altre anomalie e senza un'anamnesi di prematurità. Il tessuto fibrovascolare tende a subire una graduale restrizione. I processi ciliari diventano allungati e la camera anteriore può divenire poco profonda. Di solito il cristallino appare più piccolo della norma e può essere chiaro, ma spesso si opacizza e si può rigonfiare o assorbire liquido. Possono essere presenti vasi ampi o anomali dell'iride. L'angolo della camera anteriore può manifestare anomalie. A volte la cornea può diventare opaca.

Il PHPV viene solitamente rilevato nella prima settimana o nel primo mese di vita. I segni più frequenti sono la leucocoria (riflesso pupillare bianco), lo strabismo e il nistagmo. Il decorso è solitamente progressivo e gli esiti sfavorevoli. Complicanze maggiori sono un'emorragia intraoculare spontanea, l'edema del cristallino causata dalla rottura della capsula posteriore e un glaucoma. Alla fine l'occhio può deteriorarsi.

Trattamento. L'intervento chirurgico viene realizzato nel tentativo di prevenire le complicanze, di conservare l'occhio e un aspetto estetico sufficientemente buono e, in alcuni casi, di recuperare la vista. Di solito comporta l'aspirazione del cristallino e l'asportazione del tessuto anomalo. Se si deve ottenere una vista soddisfacente, sono necessarie una correzione refrattiva e una terapia aggressiva dell'ambliopia. In alcuni casi l'occhio affetto viene enucleato, perché la distinzione tra questa massa bianca e il retinoblastoma può essere difficile. L'ecografia e la TC sono mezzi diagnostici utili.

Prognosi. Lo spettro del PHPV posteriore comprende veli fibrogliali attorno al disco e alla macula, membrane vitree e peduncoli contenenti residui dell'arteria ialoide che partono dal disco e pieghe retiniche meridionali. Si può verificare un distacco della retina per trazione. La vista può risultare compromessa, ma di solito l'occhio è conservato.

RETINOBLASTOMA (VEDI ANCHE CAPITOLO 502). Il retinoblastoma (Fig. 629-2) è il tumore maligno primitivo intraoculare più comune dell'infanzia. Si verifica in circa 1/15 000 nati vivi; negli Stati Uniti vengono diagnosticati 250-300 nuovi casi all'anno. La modalità di trasmissione può essere ereditaria o meno; non esiste una predilezione di sesso o di razza. La forma ereditaria è solitamente bilaterale e multifocale, mentre quella non ereditaria unilaterale e unifocale. Il 15% dei casi unilaterali è ereditario. I casi bilaterali in genere si presentano più precocemente rispetto agli altri. Spesso i tumori unilaterali appaiono di grosse dimensioni nel momento in cui vengono scoperti. L'età media alla diagnosi è di 15 mesi per i casi bilaterali, 25 mesi per quelli unilaterali. È raro che un bambino si presenti con un retinoblastoma dopo l'età di 3 anni. Raramente il tumore viene scoperto alla nascita, durante l'adolescenza o anche nell'età giovane adulta.

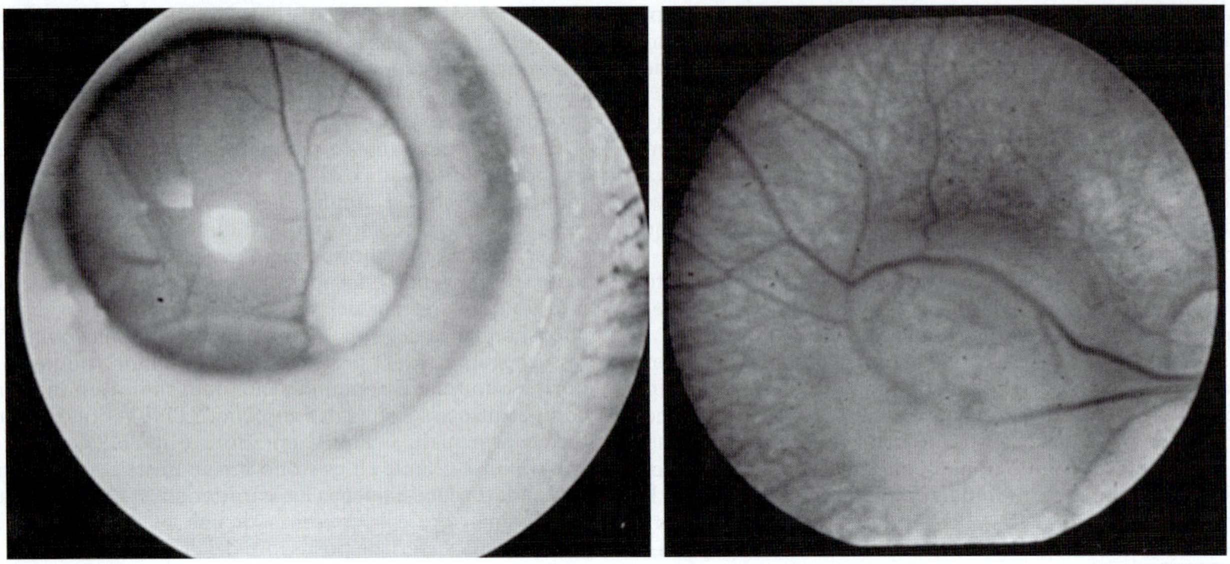

Figura 629-2. Retinoblastoma.

Manifestazioni cliniche. Le manifestazioni cliniche del retinoblastoma sono variabili, dipendendo dallo stadio in cui il tumore viene identificato; nella maggior parte dei pazienti il segno iniziale è un riflesso pupillare bianco (leucocoria), che compare a causa della riflessione della luce da parte del tumore bianco. Il secondo segno iniziale più frequente è lo strabismo. Tra i segni meno usuali vi sono lo pseudoipopion (cellule tumorali stratificate inferiormente davanti all'iride), determinato dalla disseminazione del tumore nella camera anteriore dell'occhio, l'ifema (sangue stratificato di fronte all'iride), conseguente alla neovascolarizzazione dell'iride, l'emorragia del vitreo e segni di cellulite orbitale. All'esame il tumore si mostra come una massa bianca, talvolta piccola e relativamente piatta, talvolta grande e protuberante. Può apparire nodulare. Possono essere evidenti un velo vitreo o una disseminazione tumorale.

Il gene del retinoblastoma è un gene soppressore recessivo localizzato sul cromosoma 13 in corrispondenza della regione 13q14. A causa della natura ereditaria del retinoblastoma, i membri della famiglia dei bambini affetti dovrebbero essere sottoposti a un esame oculistico completo e a counseling genetico. I neonati fratelli e figli dei pazienti affetti andrebbero inviati all'oculista poco dopo la nascita, quando la retina periferica può essere valutata senza la necessità di un esame in anestesia.

Diagnosi. Viene posta mediante l'osservazione diretta da parte di un oculista esperto. Test ausiliari come la TC o l'ecografia possono aiutare a confermarla e dimostrare la calcificazione all'interno della massa. Occasionalmente non si è in grado di porla in maniera definitiva e si deve prendere in considerazione la rimozione dell'occhio per evitare la possibilità di metastasi letali del tumore. Dal momento che la biopsia può favorire la diffusione del tumore, la conferma istologica prima dell'enucleazione non è possibile nella maggior parte dei casi. Pertanto la rimozione di un occhio cieco in cui la diagnosi di retinoblastoma sia probabile può essere appropriata.

Trattamento. La terapia è variabile a seconda delle dimensioni e della localizzazione del tumore e a seconda che questo sia unilaterale o bilaterale. I tumori avanzati possono venire trattati mediante l'enucleazione. Tra le altre modalità vi sono l'irradiazione a fasci esterni, la radioterapia con placche, la laser- o la crioterapia e la chemioterapia.

La prognosi dei bambini con un retinoblastoma dipende dalle dimensioni e dall'estensione del tumore. Se confinati all'occhio, la maggior parte dei tumori può essere trattata. La prognosi per la sopravvivenza a lungo termine è scarsa, se il tumore si è esteso nell'orbita o lungo il nervo ottico.

RETINITE PIGMENTOSA. Questa degenerazione retinica progressiva è caratterizzata da alterazioni pigmentarie, attenuazione arteriolare, di solito un certo grado di atrofia ottica e una progressiva compromissione della funzione visiva. La dispersione e l'aggregazione del pigmento retinico producono varie alterazioni visibili all'esame oftalmoscopico, che vanno da granulosità o chiazze del disegno del pigmento a caratteristici aggregati focali di pigmento con la configurazione delle spicole ossee (Fig. 629-3). Tra gli altri reperti vi sono la cataratta sottocapsulare, il glaucoma e il cheratocono.

La compromissione della visione notturna, o difficoltà all'adattamento al buio, è spesso la prima manifestazione clinica. La progressiva perdita della visione periferica, spesso sotto forma di uno scotoma ad anello in espansione o di una contrazione concentrica del campo, risulta abituale. Si può perdere la visione centrale. La funzione retinica, misurata dall'elettroretinografia (ERG), è caratteristicamente ridotta. Le manifestazioni esordiscono comunemente nell'infanzia. La malattia può essere autosomica recessiva, autosomica dominante o X-linked. È disponibile soltanto la terapia di supporto.

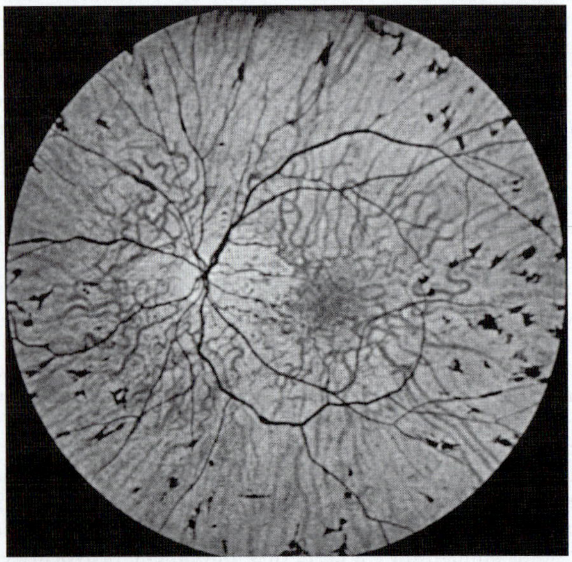

Figura 629-3. Retinite pigmentosa.

Una forma particolare di retinite pigmentosa è l'**amaurosi retinica congenita di Leber**, in cui le alterazioni retiniche tendono a divenire pleomorfe, con vari gradi di alterazione del pigmento, attenuazione arteriolare e atrofia ottica. La retina può apparire normale durante l'infanzia. La compromissione della vista di solito diventa evidente poco dopo la nascita; i reperti dell'ERG sono precocemente anormali e confermano la diagnosi.

Alcune degenerazioni retiniche pigmentarie secondarie risultano clinicamente simili alla retinite pigmentosa, ma devono essere differenziate da essa. Si sviluppano in un'ampia serie di malattie metaboliche, processi neurodegenerativi e sindromi multifattoriali. Tra gli esempi si trovano le alterazioni retiniche progressive delle mucopolisaccaridosi (in particolare le sindromi di Hurler, di Hunter, di Scheie e di Sanfilippo) e alcune gangliosidosi a esordio tardivo (malattie di Batten-Mayou, Spielmeyer-Vogt e Jansky-Bielschowsky), la degenerazione retinica progressiva associata all'oftalmoplegia esterna progressiva (sindrome di Kearns-Sayre) e le alterazioni simili alla retinite pigmentosa nelle sindromi di Laurence-Moon e di Bardet-Biedl. Anche le manifestazioni retiniche dell'abetalipoproteinemia (sindrome di Bassen-Kornzweig) e della malattia di Refsum assomigliano a quelle riscontrate nella retinite pigmentosa. La diagnosi di queste ultime due in un paziente con una presunta retinite pigmentosa è importante, perché il trattamento è possibile. Esiste anche un'associazione tra la retinite pigmentosa e la perdita dell'udito congenita, come nella sindrome di Usher.

MALATTIA DI STARGARDT (FUNDUS FLAVIMACULATUS). Questa malattia retinica autosomica recessiva è caratterizzata da una degenerazione maculare bilaterale lentamente progressiva e dalla compromissione della vista. Di solito compare all'età di 8-14 anni e nei bambini affetti spesso la diagnosi viene confusa con una perdita funzionale della vista. Il riflesso foveale è ridotto o appare grigiastro, si sviluppano macchie di pigmento nell'area maculare e alla fine compaiono depigmentazione maculare e atrofia corioretinica. Possono prodursi anche emorragie maculari. Alcuni pazienti presentano inoltre macchie bianche o gialle dietro la macula o alterazioni pigmentarie nella periferia. Il termine fundus flavimaculatus viene comunemente utilizzato per indicare la malattia di Stargardt, sebbene attualmente si riconosca che in realtà si tratta di due parti differenti nello spettro della stessa malattia. L'acuità visiva centrale è ridotta spesso a 20/200, ma non si osserva mai una perdita totale della vista. I reperti dell'ERG sono variabili. La malattia non è poi associata ad anomalie del sistema nervoso centrale e deve essere differenziata dalle alterazioni maculari di molte malattie metaboliche progressive. È stata identificata la mutazione genetica responsabile della distrofia maculare di Stargardt.

DEGENERAZIONE VITELLIFORME DI BEST. Questa distrofia maculare è caratterizzata da una lesione sottoretinica discoide di colore giallo o arancio nella macula che assomiglia al tuorlo intatto di un uovo fritto. La diagnosi viene solitamente posta all'età di 3-15 anni, con l'età media all'esordio di 6 anni. La vista è in genere normale a questo stadio. La malattia può progredire, con una possibile finale degenerazione ("strapazzamento") della lesione a tuorlo d'uovo e lo sviluppo di pigmentazione, atrofia corioretinica e compromissione della vista. La malattia di solito è bilaterale. Non esistono associazioni con anomalie sistemiche. L'ereditarietà è generalmente autosomica dominante. Nella degenerazione maculare vitelliforme la risposta dell'ERG è normale. I reperti elettro-oculografici appaiono anormali nei pazienti affetti e nei portatori e questo test è utile nella diagnosi e nel counseling genetico.

MACCHIA ROSSO CILIEGIA. A causa delle particolari caratteristiche istologiche della macula, alcuni processi patologici che colpiscono la retina producono un segno visibile all'oftalmoscopia noto come macchia rosso ciliegia, una macchia rossa chiara o opaca al centro della macula circondata e accentuata da un alone bianco-grigiastro o giallastro. L'alone è conseguente alla perdita della trasparenza dello strato delle cellule gangliari della retina secondario a un edema e/o all'accumulo dei lipidi. Dato che le cellule gangliari non sono presenti nella fovea, la retina attorno a quest'ultima è opacizzata ma trasmette il normale colore coroideale sottostante (rosso), giustificando la presenza della macchia. Una macchia rosso ciliegia tipicamente compare in alcune sfingolipidosi, principalmente nella malattia di Tay-Sachs (GM_2 tipo 1), nella variante di Sandhoff (GM_2 tipo 2) e nella gangliosidosi generalizzata (GM_1 tipo 1). Alterazioni maculari simili ma meno distintive si realizzano in alcuni casi di leucodistrofia metacromatica (lipidosi sulfatidica), in alcune forme di malattia di Niemann-Pick neuronopatica e in alcune mucolipidosi. La macchia rosso ciliegia che caratteristicamente compare in seguito a un'ischemia retinica secondaria a vasospasmo, contusione oculare o occlusione dell'arteria retinica centrale deve essere differenziata da quella della malattia neurodegenerativa.

FACOMI. Si tratta di lesioni che precorrono alterazioni amartomatose. Nella malattia di Bourneville (sclerosi tuberosa), la lesione oculare distintiva è cistica multinodulare, giallastra, refrattile che origina dal disco della retina; l'aspetto di questa lesione tipica è spesso paragonato a quello di una mora acerba (Fig. 629-4). Ugualmente caratteristiche e più comuni nella sclerosi tuberosa sono lesioni retiniche più piatte, da gialle a biancastre, di dimensioni variabili da piccoli punti a grandezze che possono quasi raggiungere quelle del disco ottico. Tali lesioni sono proliferazioni astrocitiche benigne. Raramente facomi retinici simili compaiono nella malattia (neurofibromatosi) di von Recklinghausen. Nella malattia di von Hippel-Lindau (angiomatosi della retina e del cervelletto), la lesione distintiva del fondo oculare è un emangioblastoma; questa lesione vascolare di solito compare sotto forma di una massa globulare rossastra con grosse arterie e vene appaiate che la attraversano da un lato e dall'altro. Nella sindrome di Sturge-Weber (angiomatosi encefalofacciale), l'anomalia del fondo oculare è un emangioma coroideale, che se anche può conferire un colore scuro all'area affetta del fondo, si può comunque osservare meglio alla fluorangiografia.

RETINOSCHISI. La retinoschisi ereditaria congenita, nota anche come retinoschisi giovanile X-linked, è una distrofia vitreoretinica bilaterale che compare precocemente nella vita, spesso nell'infanzia. È caratterizzata dalla divisione della retina in due strati, esterno e interno. Il reperto oftalmoscopico abituale nei maschi affetti è un sollevamento dello strato interno, più comunemente nel quadrante inferotemporale del fondo oculare, spesso con fori rotondi o ovali visibili nello strato interno. La schisi della fovea è virtualmente patognomonica ed è riscontrata in quasi il 100% dei pazienti. Dal punto di vista oftalmoscopico, appare negli stadi iniziali sotto forma di strie sottili e piccole nella membrana limitante interna. Queste strie si irradiano poi verso l'esterno come

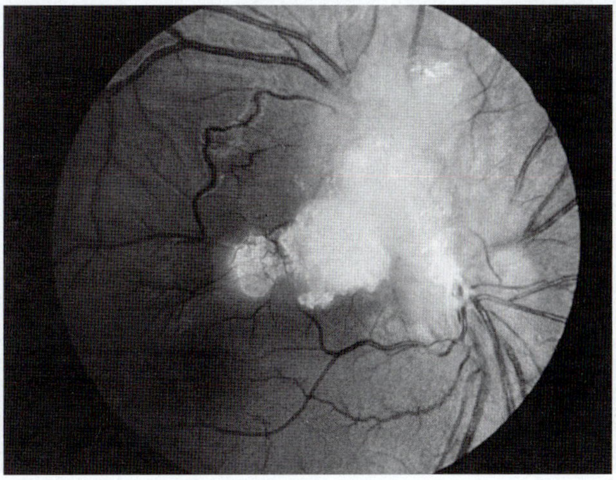

Figura 629-4. Facoma retinico della sclerosi tuberosa.

petali o a raggiera. In alcuni casi ha luogo un autentico distacco della retina o una emorragia vitreale.

La compromissione della vista può essere da lieve a grave; l'acuità visiva può peggiorare con l'età, ma spesso si conserva buona. Le femmine portatrici sono asintomatiche, ma gli studi di linkage possono risultare utili per identificarle.

DISTACCO DELLA RETINA. Consiste nella separazione degli strati esterni della retina dall'epitelio pigmentato retinico sottostante. Durante l'embriogenesi la retina e l'epitelio pigmentato retinico sono inizialmente separati, quindi nello sviluppo oculare si uniscono e sono mantenuti in apposizione tra loro da vari meccanismi fisiologici. Gli eventi patologici che determinano un distacco della retina riportano la retina-epitelio pigmentato retinico al loro stato originario separato. Il distacco può verificarsi come anomalia congenita, ma più spesso in seguito ad altre anomalie oculari o a un trauma. Ne sono descritti tre tipi e tutti si possono verificare nei bambini. I distacchi regmatogeni sono dovuti a una rottura nella retina che consente l'ingresso di liquido nello spazio sottoretinico. Nei bambini questi distacchi sono solitamente secondari a un trauma (come un abuso), ma possono anche insorgere in seguito alla miopia o a una ROP, oppure dopo un intervento chirurgico per cataratta congenita. I distacchi trazionali compaiono quando le membrane vitreoretiniche esercitano trazione sulla retina. Possono avere luogo nel diabete, nella malattia falciforme e nella ROP. I distacchi essudativi, infine, avvengono quando l'essudazione supera l'assorbimento, come si può osservare nella malattia di Coats, nel retinoblastoma e nell'infiammazione oculare.

Il segno di presentazione di un distacco di retina in un lattante o in un bambino può essere la perdita della vista, lo strabismo o il nistagmo secondari oppure una leucocoria (riflesso pupillare bianco). Oltre all'esame diretto dell'occhio, possono essere necessari speciali esami diagnostici come l'ecografia e tecniche di neuroimaging (TC, RM) per stabilire la causa e il trattamento appropriato. Il trattamento precoce risulta essenziale, per salvaguardare la vista.

MALATTIA DI COATS. Questa retinopatia essudativa di origine sconosciuta è caratterizzata dalla teleangectasia dei vasi retinici con fuoriuscita di plasma che forma essudati intraretinici e sottoretinici e da emorragie retiniche e distacco della retina (Fig. 629-5). La malattia di solito è unilaterale. Colpisce prevalentemente i maschi, in genere manifestandosi nella prima decade. Non è familiare e per la maggior parte si verifica in bambini altrimenti sani. I segni di presentazione più frequenti sono l'offuscamento della vista, la leucocoria e lo strabismo. Possono svilupparsi la rubeosi dell'iride, il glaucoma e la cataratta. Il **trattamento** con fotocoagulazione o crioterapia può risultare utile.

VITREORETINOPATIA ESSUDATIVA FAMILIARE (FEVR). La causa della FEVR (*Familial Exudative VitreoRetinopathy*), una malattia vascolare retinica progressiva, è sconosciuta, ma i reperti clinici e angiografici suggeriscono un'aberrazione dello sviluppo vascolare. L'avascolarizzazione della retina temporale periferica è un reperto significativo nella maggior parte dei casi, con l'improvvisa interruzione della rete capillare retinica nella regione dell'equatore. La zona avascolare spesso presenta un aspetto a cuneo o a V nel meridiano temporale e in essa si possono osservare una proliferazione gliale o un'atrofia retinocoroideale ben demarcata. Compaiono un'eccessiva ramificazione delle arterie e delle vene retiniche, la dilatazione dei capillari, la formazione di shunt arterovenosi, una neovascolarizzazione e un leakage dai vasi retinici della retina vascolarizzata più lontana. Di solito si trovano aderenze vitreoretiniche in corrispondenza del margine periferico della retina vascolarizzata. Trazione, dragging retinico e dislocazione temporale della macula, pieghe retiniche falciformi e distacco della retina sono comuni. Possono svilupparsi un essudato intraretinico o sottoretinico, un'emorragia retinica ed emorragie vitreali ricorrenti. I pazienti possono anche sviluppare cataratta e glaucoma. Si può presentare una compromissione della vista di gravità variabile. La malattia in genere è bilaterale e di solito costituisce una condizione autosomica dominante a penetranza incompleta. I familiari asintomatici spesso mostrano una zona di retina periferica avascolare.

I reperti possono assomigliare a quelli della ROP negli stadi cicatriziali, ma a differenza di questa la neovascolarizzazione della FEVR sembra svilupparsi a distanza di anni dalla nascita e la maggior parte dei pazienti non possiede un'anamnesi di prematurità, ossigenoterapia, lesione o infezione prenatale o postnatale, né anomalie legate allo sviluppo. La FEVR deve anche essere differenziata dalla malattia di Coats, dalla angiomatosi della retina, dall'uveite periferica e da altre malattie del segmento posteriore.

RETINOPATIA IPERTENSIVA. Negli stadi iniziali dell'ipertensione non sono osservabili alterazioni retiniche. Il restringimento generalizzato e l'irregolare riduzione delle arteriole costituiscono solitamente i primi segni nel fundus. Altre alterazioni comprendono l'edema retinico, emorragie a fiamma, macchie cotonose (infarti dello strato delle fibre nervose retiniche) e papilledema

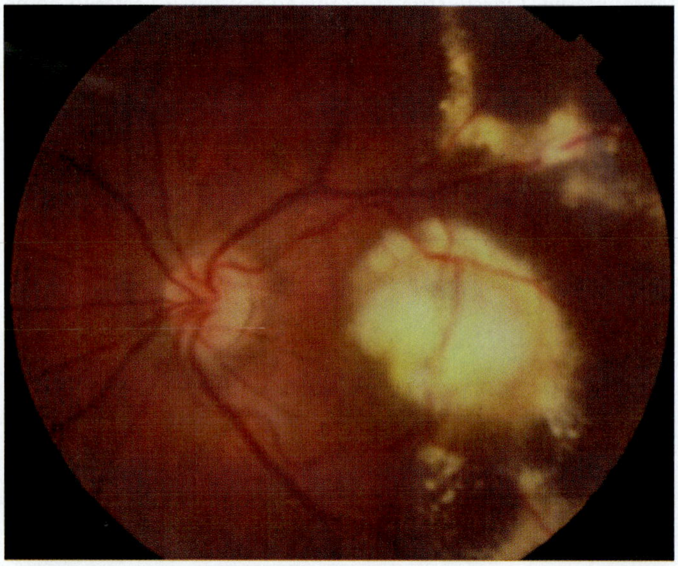

Figura 629-5. Malattia di Coats con essudato retinico massivo.

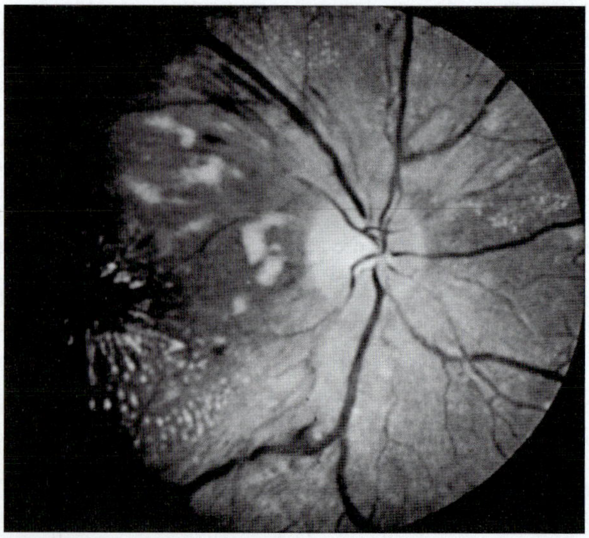

Figura 629-6. Retinopatia ipertensiva.

(Fig. 629-6). Queste alterazioni sono reversibili se l'ipertensione può venire controllata negli stadi iniziali, ma in quella presente da lungo tempo possono diventare irreversibili. L'ispessimento della parete vasale può produrre un aspetto a filo d'argento o di rame. Le alterazioni retiniche ipertensive nel bambino dovrebbero mettere in guardia il medico sulla presenza di nefropatia, feocromocitoma, collagenopatia e malattie cardiovascolari, in particolare la coartazione dell'aorta.

RETINOPATIA DIABETICA. Le alterazioni retiniche del diabete mellito sono classificate in non proliferative e proliferative. La retinopatia diabetica non proliferativa è caratterizzata da microaneurismi retinici, dilatazione venosa, emorragie retiniche ed essudati. I microaneurismi appaiono come piccoli punti rossi. Le emorragie possono essere puntiformi o a macchia, rappresentando sanguinamenti intraretinici profondi e a fiamma che interessano lo strato delle fibre nervose superficiali. Gli essudati tendono a essere profondi e ad assumere un aspetto cereo. Si possono trovare anche infarti delle fibre nervose superficiali denominati corpi citoidi o macchie cotonose, così come edemi retinici. Questi segni possono crescere e diminuire. Vengono osservati principalmente nel polo posteriore, attorno al disco e alla macula, all'interno del raggio d'azione dell'oftalmoscopia diretta. L'interessamento della macula può portare alla diminuzione della vista.

La retinopatia proliferativa, la forma più grave, è contraddistinta dalla neovascolarizzazione e dalla proliferazione di tessuto fibrovascolare sulla retina, che si estende nel vitreo. La neovascolarizzazione può comparire sul disco ottico, in qualche altro punto della retina o sull'iride e nell'angolo della camera anteriore (rubeosi dell'iride) (Fig. 629-7). La trazione su questi nuovi vasi porta a un'emorragia e infine alla cicatrizzazione. Le complicanze minacciose per la vista sono rappresentate da emorragie retiniche e vitreali, cicatrizzazione, trazione e distacco della retina. La neovascolarizzazione dell'iride può condurre a un glaucoma secondario se non viene trattata precocemente.

La retinopatia diabetica comporta l'alterazione e la mancata perfusione dei capillari retinici, un'ischemia retinica e una neovascolarizzazione, ma la sua patogenesi non è ancora stata completamente chiarita, in termini di localizzazione del meccanismo patogenetico primario (vasi retinici piuttosto che tessuto neuronale o gliale circostanti) o di fattori biochimici specifici coinvolti. Migliore appare il grado di controllo metabolico a lungo termine, minore di conseguenza risulta il rischio di retinopatia diabetica.

Dal punto di vista clinico, la prevalenza e il decorso della retinopatia sono correlati all'età del paziente e alla durata della malattia. Le alterazioni microvascolari identificabili sono rare nei bambini in età prepuberale, mentre la diffusione aumenta significativamente dopo la pubertà, specialmente dopo l'età di 15 anni. L'incidenza è bassa durante i primi 5 anni di malattia e cresce progressivamente in seguito; quella della retinopatia proliferativa diventa significativa dopo i 10 anni e il rischio della compromissione della vista si alza dopo i 15 anni o più. La valutazione oculistica periodica è raccomandata in tutti i pazienti con diabete mellito.

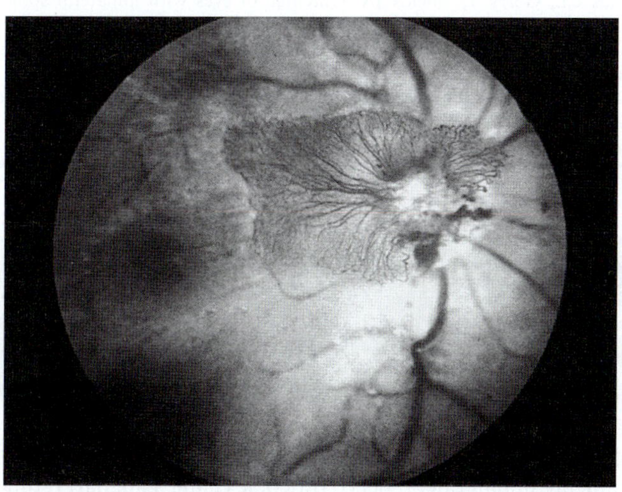
Figura 629-7. Retinopatia proliferativa diabetica con neovascolarizzazione del disco.

Oltre alla retinopatia, i pazienti con diabete a esordio giovanile possono sviluppare una neuropatia ottica, caratterizzata da edema del disco e offuscamento della vista, nonché la cataratta, anche in età precoce, talvolta con una progressione rapida.

Trattamento. L'edema maculare è la principale causa di perdita della vista nei soggetti diabetici; per ridurre il rischio di un calo continuato, può venire utilizzata la fotocoagulazione.

La retinopatia proliferativa provoca una diminuzione della vista più grave, fino a una perdita totale nonché alla perdita dell'occhio. I pazienti con la malattia proliferativa e che mostrano certe caratteristiche ad alto rischio dovrebbero essere sottoposti a una fotocoagulazione panretinica per conservare la visione centrale. Anche la neovascolarizzazione dell'iride viene trattata allo stesso modo, per arrestare lo sviluppo del glaucoma neovascolare.

La vitrectomia e altri interventi chirurgici oculari possono essere necessari nei pazienti con un'emorragia vitreale che non si risolve o con un distacco della retina per trazione. L'utilità di progressi tecnologici come le pompe d'infusione insulinica e i trapianti di pancreas nella prevenzione delle complicanze oculari è in corso di studio (vedi Capitolo 590).

ENDOCARDITE BATTERICA SUBACUTA. In un certo momento durante il decorso della malattia, la retinopatia è presente in circa il 40% dei casi di endocardite batterica subacuta. Le lesioni comprendono emorragie, emorragie con centro bianco (macchie di Roth), papilledema e raramente occlusione embolica dell'arteria retinica centrale.

MALATTIE EMATICHE. Nelle anemie primitive e secondarie la retinopatia può comparire sotto forma di emorragie e chiazze cotonose. Può essere coinvolta la vista, se l'emorragia si verifica nell'area maculare. Le emorragie possono essere lievi e soffici o dense e preretiniche. Nella policitemia vera le vene retiniche appaiono scure, dilatate e tortuose. Si possono osservare emorragie retiniche, edema retinico e papilledema. Nella leucemia le vene sono dilatate in maniera caratteristica, con restringimenti a salsicciotto; emorragie, in particolare con centri bianchi ed essudati, sono comuni durante lo stadio acuto. Nelle malattie falciformi le alterazioni del fundus comprendono tortuosità vascolare, occlusioni arteriose e venose, "chiazze salmone", depositi refrattili, lesioni pigmentate, anastomosi arteriolari-venose e neovascolarizzazione (con formazioni "a ventaglio di mare"), che talvolta portano a un'emorragia vitreale e al distacco della retina. I soggetti con emoglobinopatie Hb SC e Hb S-β-talassemia hanno un rischio maggiore di sviluppare la retinopatia rispetto a quelli con malattia da Hb SS. Si ritiene che lo stato più anemico dei pazienti con malattia SS offra una protezione nei confronti delle occlusioni vascolari nella retina.

RETINOPATIA TRAUMA-CORRELATA. Alterazioni retiniche possono comparire in pazienti che subiscono un trauma in altre parti del corpo. L'insorgenza di emorragie retiniche nei bambini che hanno subito un abuso fisico è ben documentata (Fig. 629-8; vedi Capitolo 36). Emorragie retiniche, sottoretiniche, sottoialoidi e vitreali sono state descritte nei bambini piccoli e giovani con un neurotrauma inflitto. Spesso non appaiono i segni di un trauma diretto all'occhio, alla regione perioculare o al capo. Questi casi possono essere dovuti a un violento scuotimento del bambino, cui può conseguire un danno retinico permanente.

Nei pazienti con un grave trauma compressivo cranico o toracico può comparire un'angiopatia retinica traumatica nota come **retinopatia di Purtscher**, caratterizzata da emorragia retinica, macchie cotonose, possibile edema del disco e riduzione della vista. La patogenesi è incerta, ma si trovano segni di occlusione arteriolare. Un quadro del fundus simile alla retinopatia di

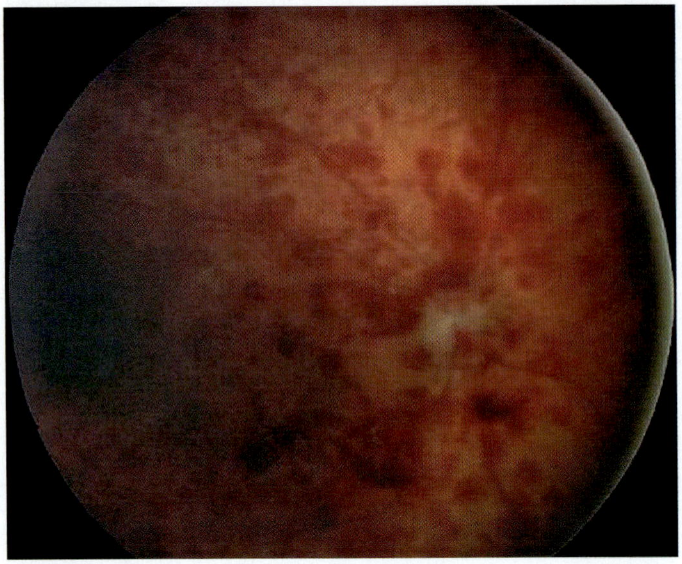

Figura 629-8. Sindrome da scuotimento del bambino (neurotrauma inflitto). Emorragie retiniche in più strati troppo numerose per potere essere contate nella lontana periferia.

Purtscher può essere riscontrato in diverse situazioni non traumatiche, come nella pancreatite acuta, nel lupus eritematoso e nel parto.

FIBRE NERVOSE MIELINIZZATE. La mielinizzazione delle fibre del nervo ottico normalmente termina a livello del disco, ma in alcuni individui si osserva più comunemente una mielinizzazione ectopica adiacente al disco, sebbene possano venire coinvolte le aree più periferiche della retina. Il quadro oftalmoscopico caratteristico è quello di una chiazza bianca focale con un margine a pennacchio o a colpo di pennello. Dato che in genere la macula non è coinvolta, la prognosi visiva è buona. Di solito l'unica anomalia oculare associata è un difetto relativo o assoluto del campo visivo corrispondente alle aree di mielinizzazione ectopica. Tuttavia, l'interessamento unilaterale esteso è stato associato a miopia ipsilaterale, ambliopia e strabismo. Nel caso di miopia elevata ipsilaterale e ambliopia, si dovrebbero istituire l'appropriata correzione ottica e la terapia occlusiva. Per ragioni sconosciute la malattia è più comunemente riscontrata nei pazienti con disostosi craniofacciale, ossicefalia, neurofibromatosi e sindrome di Down.

COLOBOMA DEL FONDO OCULARE. Il termine coloboma descrive un difetto come una lacuna, un'incisura, una fessura o un foro. Il tipico coloboma del fondo oculare è dovuto all'errata chiusura della fessura embrionale, che lascia una lacuna nella retina, nell'epitelio pigmentato retinico e nella coroide, esponendo la sclera sottostante. Il difetto può essere esteso, con interessamento del nervo ottico, del corpo ciliare, dell'iride e anche del cristallino, oppure può essere localizzato a una o più porzioni della fessura. L'aspetto abituale è quello di un'area bianca, cuneiforme, ben circoscritta, che si estende inferonasalmente al di sotto del disco, talvolta con suoi interessamento e sommersione. In alcuni casi si riscontra un'ectasia o una formazione di cisti nell'area del difetto. Difetti colobomatosi meno estesi possono comparire sotto forma di difetti corioretinici singoli o focali multipli a stampo, o come un'anomala pigmentazione del fondo oculare nella linea della fessura embrionale. I colobomi si possono sviluppare in uno o in entrambi gli occhi. Di solito un difetto del campo visivo corrisponde al difetto corioretinico. L'acuità visiva può venire compromessa, in particolare se il difetto interessa il disco o la macula.

I colobomi del fondo oculare si possono formare in modo isolato come difetti sporadici oppure come malattia ereditaria. Le anomalie colobomatose isolate sono comunemente ereditate in modo autosomico dominante con penetranza ed espressività molto variabili. I familiari dei pazienti affetti dovrebbero ricevere un appropriato counseling genetico. I colobomi possono anche essere associati ad anomalie come microftalmia, glioneuroma dell'occhio, ciclopia o encefalia. Compaiono in bambini con varie malattie cromosomiche, fra cui le trisomie 13 e 18, la triploidia, la sindrome degli occhi di gatto e la 4p-. I colobomi oculari si verificano anche in molte malattie multisistemiche, tra cui l'associazione CHARGE (C, coloboma; H, cardiopatia [*Heart disease*]; A, atresia coanale; R, ritardo di crescita e sviluppo e/o anomalie del sistema nervoso centrale; G, anomalie genetiche e/o ipogonadismo; E, anomalie dell'orecchio [*Ear*] e/o sordità); le sindromi di Joubert, Aicardi, Meckel, Warburg e Rubinstein-Taybi; il nevo sebaceo lineare; le sindromi della microftalmia di Goldenhar e Lenz; l'ipoplasia dermica focale di Goltz.

Abramson DH, Frank CM, Susman M, et al: Presenting signs of retinoblastoma. *J Pediatr* 1998;132:505–508.

Chang M, McLean IW, Merritt JC: Coats' disease: A study of 62 histologically confirmed cases. *J Pediatr Ophthalmol Strabismus* 1984;21:163–168.

Cryotherapy for Retinopathy of Prematurity Cooperative Group: 15-year outcomes following threshold retinopathy of prematurity. *Arch Ophthalmol* 2005;123:311–318.

Dass AB, Trese MT: Surgical results of persistent hyperplastic primary vitreous. *Ophthalmology* 1999;106:280–284.

Early Treatment Diabetic Retinopathy Research Study Group: Photocoagulation for diabetic macular edema. Early treatment diabetic retinopathy study report 1. *Arch Ophthalmol* 1985;103:1796–1806.

Early Treatment for Retinopathy of Prematurity Cooperative Group. Revised indications for the treatment of retinopathy of prematurity: Results of the early treatment for retinopathy of prematurity randomized trial. *Arch Ophthalmol* 2003;121:1684–1696.

Fierson W, Palmer E, Biglan A, et al: Screening examination of premature infants for retinopathy of prematurity. A joint statement of the American Academy of Pediatrics, the American Association for Pediatric Ophthalmology and Strabismus and the American Academy of Ophthalmology. *Pediatrics* 1997;100:273–274.

Hardwig P, Robertson DM: Von Hippel-Lindau disease: A familial, often lethal, multi-system phakomatosis. *Ophthalmology* 1984;91:263–270.

Hartong DT, Berson EL, Dryja TP: Retinitis pigmentosa. *Lancet* 2006;368:1795–1809.

Miyakulo H, Hashimoto K, Miyakulo S: Retinal vascular pattern in familial exudative vitreoretinopathy. *Ophthalmology* 1984;91:1524–1530.

Mohler CW, Fine SL: Long-term evaluation of patients with Best's vitelliform dystrophy. *Ophthalmology* 1981;88:688–692.

Noble KG, Carr RE: Leber's congenital amaurosis: A retrospective study of 33 cases and a histopathological study of one case. *Arch Ophthalmol* 1978;96:818–821.

Shalev B, Farr A, Repka MX: Randomized comparison of diode laser photocoagulation versus cryotherapy for threshold retinopathy of prematurity: Seven year outcome. *Am J Ophthalmol* 2001;132:76–80.

Shields CL, Gorry T, Shields JA: Outcome of eyes with unilateral sporadic retinoblastoma based on the initial external findings by the family and the pediatrician. *J Pediatr Ophthalmol Strabismus* 2004;41:143–149.

Weinberg DV, Lyon AT, Greenwald MJ, et al: Rhegmatogenous retinal detachments in children: Risk factors and surgical outcomes. *Ophthalmology* 2003;110:1708–1713.

Capitolo 630 ■ Anomalie del nervo ottico

Scott E. Olitsky, Denise Hug e Laura P. Smith

APLASIA DEL NERVO OTTICO. Questa rara anomalia congenita è tipicamente unilaterale. Il nervo ottico, le cellule gangliari retiniche e i vasi sanguigni retinici sono assenti. Di solito una tonaca durale vestigiale è collegata alla sclera in posizione normale, ma senza

contenere tessuto neurale. L'aplasia del nervo ottico compare tipicamente in modo sporadico e in soggetti per il resto normali. Si può verificare un'ampia varietà di anomalie oculari, ma i colobomi sono il reperto che si trova associato più frequentemente.

IPOPLASIA DEL NERVO OTTICO. L'ipoplasia del nervo ottico è una malattia non progressiva caratterizzata da un numero di assoni del nervo ottico inferiore alla norma, con elementi mesodermici e tessuto gliale di supporto normali. Nei casi tipici la testa del nervo è piccola e pallida, con un alone prepapillare pallido o pigmentato o un segno ad anello doppio.

Questa anomalia è associata a difetti della vista e dei campi visivi di gravità variabile, andando dalla cecità a una vista normale o quasi normale. Può trovarsi insieme ad anomalie sistemiche che più comunemente interessano il sistema nervoso centrale (SNC), per esempio difetti proteiformi quali l'idrocefalo o l'anencefalia oppure lesioni più focali compatibili con il continuo sviluppo del paziente; tuttavia l'ipoplasia unilaterale o bilaterale può essere riscontrata senza difetti concomitanti.

L'ipoplasia del nervo ottico è una caratteristica importante della **displasia setto-ottica di de Morsier**, una malattia dello sviluppo caratterizzata dall'associazione tra anomalie delle strutture della linea mediana del cervello e ipoplasie dei nervi ottici, del chiasma ottico e dei tratti ottici; tipicamente si osservano l'agenesia del setto pellucido, l'agenesia parziale o completa del corpo calloso e la malformazione del fornice, con un'ampia cisterna chiasmatica. I pazienti possono manifestare anomalie oftalmiche e difetti endocrini, che vanno dal panipopituitarismo a un deficit isolato dell'ormone della crescita, all'ipotiroidismo o al diabete insipido. L'ipoglicemia e le convulsioni neonatali sono importanti segni di presentazione nei bambini affetti.

La RM è la più indicata per la valutazione delle anomalie del SNC nei pazienti con una ipoplasia del nervo ottico. Durante questo esame, una particolare attenzione dovrebbe essere rivolta all'infundibolo pituitario, dove può venire riscontrata l'ectopia dell'ipofisi posteriore, che appare come un'assenza dell'infundibolo ipofisario con un anomalo spot luminoso in corrispondenza dell'area dell'infundibolo superiore. Questa anomalia è presente in circa il 15% dei pazienti e suggerisce un deficit di ormoni dell'ipofisi posteriore, che richiede un ulteriore inquadramento endocrinologico.

L'ipoplasia bilaterale subdola può essere difficile da diagnosticare solo in base all'aspetto del disco, perché non è possibile alcun confronto con l'occhio controlaterale non interessato. Tuttavia, è importante confermare la diagnosi, dato che ciò elimina la confusione con l'atrofia o il glaucoma e può spiegare la causa della diminuzione della vista in un paziente che non risponde alla terapia per l'ambliopia. La funzione endocrina andrebbe osservata attentamente nei pazienti con un'ipoplasia del nervo ottico.

L'origine di tale ipoplasia rimane incerta. Lesioni gestazionali precoci della struttura della linea mediana del SNC con un danno assonale secondario o la distruzione dei normali meccanismi di guida che influiscono sul nervo ottico e sui neuroni cerebrali possono risultare determinanti. L'ipoplasia del nervo ottico può comparire con una frequenza piuttosto aumentata nei bambini di madri diabetiche ed è stato associato all'uso materno di fenitoina, chinino, LSD (acido lisergico dietilammide) e alcol durante la gravidanza.

I bambini con **leucomalacia periventricolare** manifestano un'insolita forma di ipoplasia del nervo ottico. I nervi ottici mostrano un ampio calice all'interno di un disco ottico di dimensioni normali. Questa forma di ipoplasia compare secondariamente a una degenerazione transinaptica degli assoni nervosi causata dalla lesione bilaterale primaria nella radiazione ottica (leucomalacia periventricolare).

COLOBOMA DEL NERVO OTTICO. I colobomi del nervo ottico possono essere unilaterali o bilaterali. L'acuità visiva può andare dalla normalità alla cecità totale. Il coloboma si sviluppa secondariamente all'incompleta chiusura della fessura embrionale. Il difetto può produrre un'escavazione parziale o globale del disco ottico

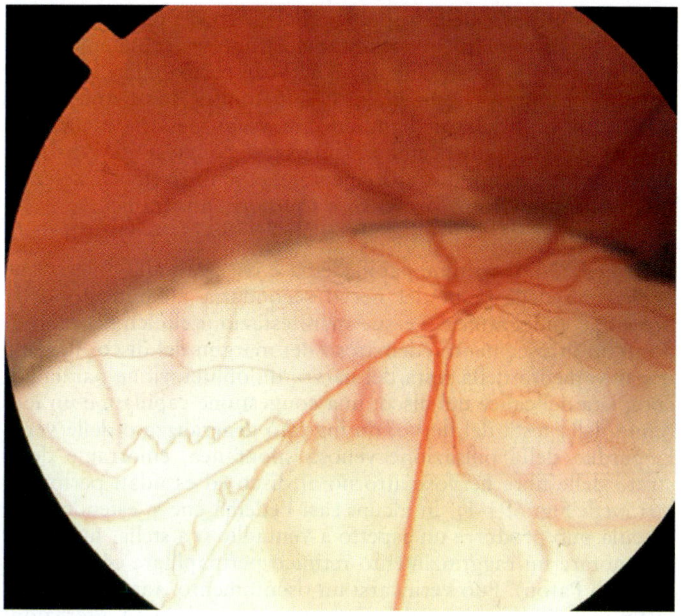

Figura 630-1. Coloboma del nervo ottico.

(Fig. 630-1). Possono anche verificarsi colobomi corioretinici e dell'iride. I colobomi del nervo ottico possono essere osservati in una moltitudine di anomalie oculari e sistemiche, tra cui l'associazione CHARGE (C, coloboma; H, cardiopatia [*Heart disease*]; A, atresia coanale; R, ritardo di crescita e sviluppo e/o anomalie del sistema nervoso centrale; G, anomalie genetiche e/o ipogonadismo; E, anomalie dell'orecchio [*Ear*] e/o sordità).

ANOMALIA DI MORNING GLORY. Con questo termine si indica una malformazione congenita del nervo ottico caratterizzata da un disco ingrandito, escavato a forma di imbuto con un margine rilevato, che assomiglia al convolvolo. Nella parte centrale del disco si trova tessuto gliale bianco. I vasi retinici sono anormali, appaiono alla periferia del disco e attraversano radialmente il margine rosa rilevato. Di solito si osservano chiazze pigmentarie della regione peripapillare. La maggior parte dei casi è unilaterale. Le femmine sono colpite in quantità doppia rispetto ai maschi. L'acuità visiva è di solito gravemente ridotta e in circa 1/3 degli occhi coinvolti avviene il distacco della retina. L'anomalia del disco a convolvolo è stata associata a un encefalocele basale nei pazienti con anomalie della parte centrale del volto. Si sono riscontrate anche anomalie della circolazione carotidea. La malattia di Moyamoya come reperto associato è stata descritto compiutamente.

DIVERSIONE PAPILLARE (TILTED DISC). In questa anomalia congenita l'asse verticale del disco ottico è diretto obliquamente, così che la porzione temporale superiore della testa del nervo risulta più prominente e anteriore rispetto a quella nasale inferiore del disco. I vasi retinici emergono dalla porzione temporale superiore del disco piuttosto che dal lato nasale. Spesso si nota una mezzaluna o un cono peripapillare. Si possono riscontrare difetti associati del campo visivo e un astigmatismo miopico. Il riconoscimento clinico della sindrome da diversione papillare è importante per evitare la confusione tra i suoi segni del disco e del campo visivo da quelli del papilledema e del tumore endocranico.

DRUSEN DEL NERVO OTTICO. Si ritiene che questi corpi acellulari e globulari originino da derivati assoplasmici di fibre nervose in via di disintegrazione. I drusen possono essere nascosti nel nervo ottico, producendo il sollevamento della sua testa (che può essere scambiata per un papilledema) oppure possono risultare parzialmente o completamente esposti, apparendo come corpi refrattili in corrispondenza della superficie del disco. In associazione ai drusen possono verificarsi difetti del campo visivo ed emorragie spontanee dello strato delle fibre nervose peripapillari. I drusen possono comparire come malattia autosomica dominante. Sono stati osservati anche in bambini con varie malattie neurologiche, tra cui la megalencefalia primaria, le convulsioni, i disturbi dell'apprendimento, il ritardo mentale, la schizofrenia, la sclerosi tuberosa, la sindrome di Down e i tumori endocranici.

PAPILLEDEMA. Il termine papilledema è riservato alla descrizione dell'edema della testa del nervo secondaria all'aumento della pressione endocranica. Le sue manifestazioni cliniche comprendono un offuscamento edematoso dei margini del disco, fullness o sollevamento della testa del nervo, un'obliterazione parziale o completa del calice del disco, una congestione capillare e un'iperemia della testa del nervo, un ingorgo generalizzato delle vene, la perdita della pulsazione venosa spontanea, emorragie dello strato delle fibre nervose attorno al disco ed essudati peripapillari (vedi Fig. 591-1). In alcuni casi l'edema che si estende nella macula può produrre un aspetto a ventaglio o a stella. Inoltre, si può notare un raggrinzimento retinico peripapillare concentrico (linee di Paton). Può verificarsi un oscuramento transitorio della vista, della durata di qualche secondo e associato ad alterazioni posturali. La vista, tuttavia, di solito è normale nel papilledema acuto. Normalmente, quando l'aumento della pressione endocranica si risolve, lo fa anche il papilledema e il disco ritorna a un aspetto normale o quasi entro 6-8 settimane. Il papilledema cronico sostenuto o l'ipertensione endocranica irrisolta che dura da lungo tempo possono, tuttavia, portare a un prematuro danno delle fibre nervose, ad alterazioni atrofiche del disco, alla cicatrizzazione maculare e alla compromissione della vista.

La *fisiopatologia* del papilledema è probabilmente la seguente: aumento del liquido cerebrospinale (LCS) subaracnoideo endocranico, crescita della pressione del LCS nella guaina del nervo ottico, incremento della pressione tissutale nel nervo ottico, stasi del flusso assoplasmico ed edema delle fibre nervose nella testa del nervo ottico, alterazioni vascolari secondarie e caratteristici segni oftalmoscopici della stasi venosa. Tra i segni neuro-oftalmici che si trovano insieme all'aumento della pressione endocranica nei lattanti e nei bambini vi sono la paralisi del sesto nervo cranico e l'esotropia associata, la retrazione palpebrale, la paresi dello sguardo verso l'alto, la deviazione tonica verso il basso degli occhi e il nistagmo convergente.

Le comuni **eziologie** del papilledema nell'infanzia sono i tumori endocranici e l'idrocefalo ostruttivo, l'emorragia endocranica, l'edema cerebrale del trauma, la meningoencefalite, l'encefalopatia tossica e alcune malattie metaboliche. Indipendentemente dalla causa, i segni di un'aumentata pressione endocranica a livello del disco ottico nella prima infanzia possono occasionalmente essere modificati dalla distensibilità del cranio giovane. In assenza di malattie associate a una precoce chiusura delle suture e a una precoce obliterazione della fontanella (craniosinostosi, malattia di Crouzon e sindrome di Apert), i bambini con un'aumentata pressione endocranica possono non sviluppare il papilledema.

Nella **diagnosi differenziale** del papilledema sono comprese alterazioni strutturali del disco (pseudopapilledema, pseudoneurite, drusen e fibre nervose mielinizzate), con cui esso può essere confuso, nonché l'edema del disco causato da una papillite associata a neurite ottica insieme ad altre sue alterazioni determinate dall'ipertensione e dal diabete mellito. A meno che l'emorragia retinica o l'edema non coinvolgano l'area maculare, la conservazione di una buona visione centrale e l'assenza di un difetto pupillare afferente (pupilla di Marcus Gunn) aiutano a differenziare il papilledema acuto dall'edema della testa del nervo ottico riscontrato nella neurite ottica acuta.

Il papilledema è un'emergenza neurologica. Esso può essere associato ad altri segni di ipertensione endocranica, come cefalea, nausea e vomito. Si dovrebbero realizzare indagini neuroradiologiche; se non vengono identificate masse endocraniche, bisognerebbe procedere alla rachicentesi lombare e alla determinazione della pressione del LCS.

NEURITE OTTICA. Si tratta di una qualunque infiammazione o demielinizzazione del nervo ottico con associazione di una compromissione funzionale. Il processo è solitamente acuto, con una perdita della vista rapidamente progressiva. Può essere unilaterale o bilaterale. Il dolore al movimento del globo oculare o alla palpazione del globo può precedere o accompagnare l'esordio dei sintomi visivi. Si presentano una ridotta acuità visiva, la diminuzione della visione dei colori e della sensibilità al contrasto, un difetto pupillare afferente relativo e una macula e una retina periferica normali.

Quando la porzione retrobulbare del nervo è interessata senza segni oftalmoscopici visibili in corrispondenza del disco, si parla di *neurite ottica retrobulbare*. Se vi sono segni oftalmoscopici di un'infiammazione della testa del nervo si usa il termine *papillite* o *neurite ottica intraoculare*. L'interessamento della retina e della papilla viene chiamato *neuroretinite* ottica.

Nell'infanzia la neurite ottica può comparire come malattia isolata o manifestazione di una malattia neurologica o sistemica. Può risultare secondaria a malattie infiammatorie (lupus eritematoso sistemico, sarcoidosi, malattia di Behçet, neurite ottica autoimmune), infettive (tubercolosi, sifilide, malattia di Lyme, meningite, encefalite virale o postinfettiva), tossiche o nutrizionali (metanolo, etambutolo, deficit di vitamina B_{12}). Può inoltre indicare una delle tante malattie demielinizzanti dell'infanzia (vedi Capitolo 600). Sebbene vi sia una significativa percentuale di adulti che dopo avere sperimentato un episodio di neurite ottica sviluppa in seguito altri sintomi associati a una sclerosi multipla, i bambini piccoli presentano un rischio apparentemente minore (il rischio di sclerosi multipla è del 19% entro i 20 anni). La neurite ottica bilaterale nei bambini può verificarsi insieme a una **neuromielite ottica** (**malattia di Devic**), caratterizzata da una perdita visiva bilaterale rapida e grave associata a una mielite trasversa e a paraplegia. La neurite ottica può anche essere secondaria a una tossina esogena o a un farmaco, così come a un'intossicazione da piombo o come complicanza del trattamento a lungo termine e ad alte dosi di cloramfenicolo o della terapia con vincristina. Di solito sono necessarie indagini neurologiche e oftalmologiche pediatriche estese, che comprendono la RM e la puntura lombare.

Nella maggior parte dei casi di neurite ottica acuta, un certo miglioramento della vista inizia entro 1-4 settimane dall'esordio, con una progressione fino alla norma o quasi entro settimane o mesi. Il decorso varia a seconda della causa. Sebbene la visione centrale possa ristabilirsi completamente, è frequente riscontrare difetti permanenti in altre aree (sensibilità al contrasto, colore, senso della luminosità e percezione del movimento). Le recidive possono realizzarsi soprattutto, ma non sempre, nei pazienti che continuano a sviluppare sclerosi multipla.

Un trial sul **trattamento** ha dimostrato che il metilprednisolone endovenoso ad alte dosi può aiutare a velocizzare il ripristino della vista nei giovani adulti e può prevenire lo sviluppo della sclerosi multipla in quelli a rischio. I corticosteroidi per via orale non dovrebbero essere somministrati, perché determinano un significativo aumento del tasso di recidiva. Non è noto fino a che punto i risultati del trial summenzionato possano valere anche per la neurite ottica infantile. Negli adulti in cui vengono riscontrate lesioni della sostanza bianca alla RM, il trattamento con interferone beta (1a o 1b) riduce l'incidenza della sclerosi multipla.

NEUROPATIA OTTICA DI LEBER. Questa malattia è caratterizzata da una perdita improvvisa della visione centrale che compare nella seconda e terza decade di vita, interessando primariamente i maschi giovani. Una microangiopatia telangectasica peripapillare caratteristica compare non solo nella fase presintomatica degli occhi interessati, ma anche in un elevato numero di figli asintomatici nella discendenza femminile. L'iperemia e un edema del disco contraddistinguono la fase acuta della perdita della vista. Di solito un occhio viene affetto prima dell'altro; si riscontrano una perdita del campo visivo e la compromissione della visione dei colori e con il tempo subentrano un'atrofia ottica progressiva e la perdita della vista. L'angiopatia tortuosa diventa meno evidente. Sebbene la funzione visiva dopo la perdita iniziale in genere rimanga stabile, si può verificare un recupero significativo e talvolta completo fino in 1/3 degli individui affetti. Questo recupero può richiedere diversi anni o decadi dall'episodio iniziale della perdita acuta della vista. L'angiopatia peripapillare, la mancanza di remissione a breve termine e il grado di simmetria servono per distinguere la maggior parte dei casi di malattia di Leber dalla neurite ottica della sclerosi multipla.

La neuropatia ottica di Leber è ereditata dalla madre ed è causata da un difetto del DNA mitocondriale citoplasmatico. Sono state riscontrate mutazioni puntiformi multiple nel DNA mitocondriale, che conducono allo sviluppo della malattia. Proprio a causa della sua natura mitocondriale, nei soggetti affetti si possono riscontrare altre malattie, che coinvolgono il muscolo scheletrico e cardiaco, incluse alcune alterazioni elettrocardiografiche.

ATROFIA OTTICA. Questo termine indica la degenerazione degli assoni del nervo ottico, con associazione di perdita funzionale. I segni oftalmoscopici sono il pallore del disco e la perdita di sostanza della testa del nervo, talvolta con un ingrandimento del calice del disco. Il difetto associato della vista varia a seconda della natura e della sede della malattia o della lesione primaria.

L'atrofia ottica è l'espressione comune di un'ampia varietà di processi patologici congeniti o acquisiti. L'origine può essere traumatica, infiammatoria, degenerativa, neoplastica o vascolare; i tumori endocranici e l'idrocefalo sono le principali cause nei bambini. In alcuni casi l'atrofia ottica progressiva è ereditaria. L'**atrofia ottica infantile ereditata con modalità dominante** è una forma eredodegenerativa relativamente lieve che tende a progredire nell'infanzia e nell'adolescenza. L'**atrofia ottica congenita ereditata con modalità autosomica recessiva** è una malattia rara che risulta evidente alla nascita o si sviluppa a una età molto precoce; il deficit visivo è solitamente grave. L'**atrofia ottica di Behr** è una forma ereditaria associata a un'ipertonia degli arti, un aumento dei riflessi tendinei profondi, un'atassia cerebellare lieve, un certo grado di deficit mentale e una possibile oftalmoplegia esterna. Questa malattia colpisce principalmente i maschi di 3-11 anni. Alcune forme di atrofia ottica eredodegenerativa sono associate a sordità neurosensoriale, come si può verificare in alcuni bambini con diabete mellito a esordio giovanile (insulinodipendente). In assenza di una causa evidente, l'atrofia ottica in un lattante o in un bambino giustifica indagini eziologiche estese.

GLIOMA DEL NERVO OTTICO. Il glioma del nervo ottico, più propriamente noto come **astrocitoma pilocitico giovanile**, è il tumore del nervo ottico più frequente nell'infanzia. Può svilupparsi nella porzione intraorbitale, intracanalicolare o endocranica del nervo e interessare spesso il chiasma.

Il tumore è un amartoma benigno citologico generalmente stazionario o solo lentamente progressivo. Le principali *manifestazioni cliniche* quando esso compare nella porzione intraorbitale del nervo sono la perdita unilaterale della vista, la proptosi e la deviazione dell'occhio; possono comparire un'atrofia ottica o una congestione del nervo ottico. L'interessamento del chiasma può essere accompagnato da difetti della vista e del campo visivo (spesso una emianopsia bitemporale), da un aumento della pressione endocranica, papilledema o atrofia ottica, disfunzione ipotalamica, disfunzione ipofisaria e talvolta nistagmo o strabismo. Gli astrocitomi pilocitici giovanili compaiono con maggiore frequenza nei pazienti con neurofibromatosi.

Il **trattamento** dei gliomi della via ottica è controverso. Di solito quello migliore consiste nell'osservazione periodica. La rimozione chirurgica può apparire appropriata quando il tumore è confinato alla porzione intraorbitale, intracanalicolare o prechiasmatica del nervo, oppure se un paziente presenta una proptosi esteticamente sgradevole e con una completa o quasi completa perdita della vista dell'occhio affetto. Quando è coinvolto il chiasma, la resezione di solito non è indicata, mentre può essere necessaria la radioterapia o la chemioterapia.

NEUROPATIE OTTICHE TRAUMATICHE. Un danno del nervo ottico può essere secondario a traumi diretti e indiretti. Il trauma diretto è dovuto a una lesione penetrante dell'orbita con recisione o contusione del nervo. Il trauma chiuso dell'orbita può portare anche a una grave perdita della vista, se la forza traumatica viene trasmessa al canale ottico e provoca la distruzione dell'apporto ematico alla porzione intracanalicolare del nervo. Il trattamento può comprendere corticosteroidi ad alte dosi o la decompressione del canale ottico.

Auw-Haedrich C, Staubach F, Witschel H: Optic disk drusen. *Surv Ophthalmol* 2002;47:515–532.

Balcer LJ: Optic neuritis. *N Engl J Med* 2006;354:1273–1280.

Birkebaek NH, Patel L, Wright NB, et al: Endocrine status in patients with optic nerve hypoplasia: Relationship to midline central nervous system abnormalities and appearance of the hypothalamic-pituitary axis on magnetic resonance imaging. *J Clin Endocrinol Metab* 2003;88:5281–5286.

Hickman SJ, Dalton CM, Miller DH, et al: Management of acute optic neuritis. *Lancet* 2002;360:1953–1962.

Hotchkiss ML, Green WR: Optic nerve aplasia and hypoplasia. *J Pediatr Ophthalmol Strabismus* 1979;16:225–240.

Kazarian EL, Gager WE: Optic neuritis complicating measles, mumps and rubella vaccination. *Am J Ophthalmol* 1978;86:544–547.

Massaro M, Thorarensen O, Liu GT, et al. Morning glory disc anomaly and moyamoya vessels. *Arch Ophthalmol* 1998;116:253–254.

Optic Neuritis Study Group: Visual function 5 years after optic neuritis. Experience of the optic neuritis treatment trial. *Arch Ophthalmol* 1997; 115:1545–1552.

Repka MX, Miller NR: Optic atrophy in children. *Am J Ophthalmol* 1988;106:191–193.

Skarf B, Hoyt CS: Optic nerve hypoplasia in children: Association with anomalies of the endocrine and CNS. *Arch Ophthalmol* 1984;102:62–67.

Weiss AH, Beck RW: Neuroretinitis in childhood. *J Pediatr Ophthalmol Strabismus* 1989;26:198–203.

Capitolo 631 ■ Glaucoma infantile

Scott E. Olitsky, Denise Hug e Laura P. Smith

Con il termine glaucoma si indica in generale il danno al nervo ottico con perdita del campo visivo causato o correlato a un aumento della pressione all'interno dell'occhio. Esso viene classificato in base all'età dell'individuo affetto all'esordio e all'associazione con altre malattie oculari o sistemiche. Il glaucoma che inizia entro i primi 3 anni di vita è denominato infantile (congenito); quello che inizia fra i 3 e i 30 anni è denominato giovanile.

Nel glaucoma primario la causa è un'anomalia isolata del sistema di drenaggio dell'occhio (rete trabecolare). In oltre il 50% dei casi il glaucoma infantile è primario. Al glaucoma secondario sono associate altre anomalie oculari o sistemiche, sebbene vi sia anche un difetto evolutivo simile a quello della rete trabecolare. Il glaucoma infantile primario si verifica con un'incidenza dello 0,03% (Tab. 631-1).

MANIFESTAZIONI CLINICHE. I sintomi del glaucoma infantile comprendono la classica triade costituita da epifora (lacrimazione), fotofobia (sensibilità alla luce) e blefarospasmo (strizzamento della palpebra) (Fig. 631-1). Ciascuno di questi può essere attribuito all'irritazione corneale. Solo circa il 30% dei bambini affetti manifesta il complesso sintomatologico classico. Tra i segni di glaucoma sono compresi l'edema corneale, gli ingrandimenti corneale e oculare e l'iniezione congiuntivale (Fig. 631-2).

La sclera e la cornea sono più elastiche nella prima infanzia che in seguito. Un aumento della pressione intraoculare, pertanto, porta a un'espansione del globo, inclusa la cornea, e allo sviluppo

TABELLA 631-1. Glaucomi infantili primitivi e secondari

I. GLAUCOMA PRIMARIO
- A. Glaucoma ad angolo aperto congenito
  - 1. Congenito
  - 2. Infantile
  - 3. A riconoscimento tardivo
- B. Glaucoma giovanile autosomico dominante
- C. Glaucoma primitivo ad angolo chiuso
- D. Associato ad anomalie sistemiche
  - 1. Sindrome di Sturge-Weber
  - 2. Neurofibromatosi di tipo 1 (NF-1)
  - 3. Sindrome di Stickler
  - 4. Sindrome oculocerebrorenale (di Lowe)
  - 5. Sindrome di Rieger
  - 6. Sindrome epatocerebrorenale
  - 7. Sindrome di Marfan
  - 8. Sindrome di Rubinstein-Taybi
  - 9. Glaucoma infantile associato a ritardo mentale e paralisi
  - 10. Displasia oculodentodigitale
  - 11. Glaucoma ad angolo aperto associato a microcornea e assenza dei seni frontali
  - 12. Mucopolisaccaridosi
  - 13. Trisomia 13
  - 14. Cutis marmorata teleangectasica congenita
  - 15. Sindrome di Warburg
  - 16. Sindrome di Kniest (displasia scheletrica)
  - 17. Sindrome di Michel
  - 18. Emiatrofia non progressiva
- E. Associata ad anomalie oculari
  - 1. Glaucoma congenito con anomalie dell'iride e pupillari
  - 2. Aniridia
    - a. Glaucoma congenito
    - b. Glaucoma acquisito
  - 3. Melanosi oculare congenita
  - 4. Sclerocornea
  - 5. Disgenesia iridotrabecolare
  - 6. Sindrome di Peters
  - 7. Disgenesia iridotrabecolare ed ectropion uveae
  - 8. Distrofia polimorfa posteriore
  - 9. Aumento idiopatico o familiare della pressione venosa episclerale
  - 10. Stafiloma corneale anteriore
  - 11. Microcornea congenita con miopia
  - 12. Distrofia endoteliale ereditaria congenita
  - 13. Ipoplasia stromale dell'iride ereditaria congenita

II. GLAUCOMA SECONDARIO
- A. Glaucoma traumatico
  - 1. Glaucoma acuto
    - a. Concussione dell'angolo
    - b. Ifema
    - c. Glaucoma a cellule fantasma
  - 2. Glaucoma a esordio tardivo con recessione dell'angolo
  - 3. Fistola arterovenosa
- B. Secondario a neoplasia intraoculare
  - 1. Retinoblastoma
  - 2. Xantogranuloma giovanile
  - 3. Leucemia
  - 4. Melanoma
  - 5. Melanocitoma
  - 6. Rabdomiosarcoma dell'iride
  - 7. Nevi aggressivi dell'iride
- C. Secondario a uveite
  - 1. Glaucoma ad angolo aperto
  - 2. Glaucoma ad angolo bloccato
    - a. Chiusura dell'angolo da sinechie
    - b. Iride bombata con blocco pupillare
- D. Glaucoma cristallino-indotto
  - 1. Sublussazione-dislocazione con blocco pupillare
    - a. Sindrome di Marfan
    - b. Omocistinuria
  - 2. Sferofachia a blocco pupillare
  - 3. Glaucoma facolitico
- E. Secondario a intervento chirurgico per cataratta congenita
  - 1. Blocco della rete trabecolare da parte di materiale del cristallino (acuto o subacuto)
  - 2. Blocco pupillare
  - 3. Glaucoma cronico ad angolo aperto associato a difetti dell'angolo
- F. Glaucoma steroide-indotto
- G. Secondario a rubeosi
  - 1. Retinoblastoma
  - 2. Malattia di Coats
  - 3. Medulloepitelioma
  - 4. Vitreoretinopatia essudativa familiare
- H. Glaucoma ad angolo chiuso secondario
  - 1. Retinopatia della prematurità
  - 2. Microftalmo
  - 3. Nanoftalmo
  - 4. Retinoblastoma
  - 5. Vitreo primario iperplastico persistente
  - 6. Membrana pupillare iride-cristallino congenita
- I. Glaucoma associato ad aumento della pressione venosa
  - 1. Fistola carotidea o durale-venosa
  - 2. Malattia orbitale
- J. Secondario a rosolia materna
- K. secondario a infezione intraoculare
  - 1. Toxoplasmosi ricorrente acuta
  - 2. Irite erpetica acuta

Da Nelson LB: *Harley's Pediatric Ophthalmology*, 4th ed., Philadelphia, WB Saunders, 1998, p 294.

di buftalmo ("occhio di bue"). Se la cornea continua a ingrandirsi, compaiono rotture nella membrana basale endoteliale (membrana di Desçemet) che possono condurre a una cicatrizzazione corneale permanente. Queste rotture della membrana di Desçemet (strie di Haab) sono visibili come linee edematose orizzontali che attraversano la cornea centrale o vi ruotano attorno. Raramente si verificano oltre i 3 anni di vita o in cornee di diametro inferiore ai 12 mm. La cornea diventa anche edematosa e opaca, con un aumento della pressione intraoculare. L'edema corneale porta a lacerazione e fotofobia. Il glaucoma dovrebbe essere preso in considerazione in un bambino con una sospetta ostruzione del dotto nasolacrimale che presenti uno di questi altri segni e sintomi.

I bambini con un glaucoma unilaterale in genere vengono individuati precocemente, perché si può notare la differenza delle dimensioni corneali tra i due occhi. Quando la malattia è bilaterale, i genitori possono non riconoscere le dimensioni aumentate. Molti di essi trovano anzi che gli occhi grandi siano attraenti e non cercano aiuto finché non si sviluppano altri sintomi.

La formazione di una piccola fossa nella testa del nervo ottico viene identificata mediante un esame oculare. Il nervo ottico di un bambino viene facilmente disteso dalla pressione eccessiva. Si verifica rapidamente un'escavazione centrale, profonda, che può regredire con la normalizzazione della pressione.

Alcuni lattanti e bambini con un glaucoma a esordio precoce presentano uno sviluppo errato più esteso del segmento anteriore dell'occhio. Le neurocristopatie comprendono uno spettro di malattie correlate a un anomalo sviluppo embrionale del segmento anteriore. Esse sono di solito bilaterali e possono comprendere anomalie dell'iride, della cornea e del cristallino. Altre anomalie oculari associabili a un glaucoma nei lattanti e nei bambini sono l'aniridia, la cataratta, la sferofachia e l'ectopia lentis. Il glaucoma si può anche sviluppare secondariamente a un vitreo primario iperplastico persistente o a una retinopatia della prematurità.

Anche i traumi, l'emorragia intraoculare, la malattia infiammatoria oculare e i tumori intraoculari sono importanti cause di glaucoma nella popolazione pediatrica. Le malattie sistemiche associate al glaucoma nei lattanti e nei bambini sono la sindrome di Sturge-Weber, la neurofibromatosi, la sindrome di Lowe, la sindrome di Marfan, la rosolia congenita e tutta una serie di sindromi cromosomiche.

Il glaucoma compare frequentemente nei bambini con un'anamnesi di cataratta congenita. Può inoltre svilupparsi fino nel 25%

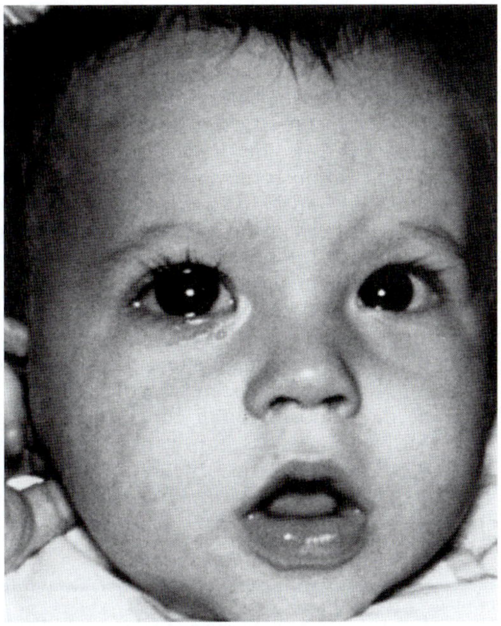

Figura 631-1. Lacrimazione dell'occhio destro causata da glaucoma. Si noti l'aumentato diametro corneale dell'occhio destro. (Da Nelson LB: *Harley's Pediatric Ophthalmology*, 4th ed. Philadelphia, WB Saunders, 1998, p 285.)

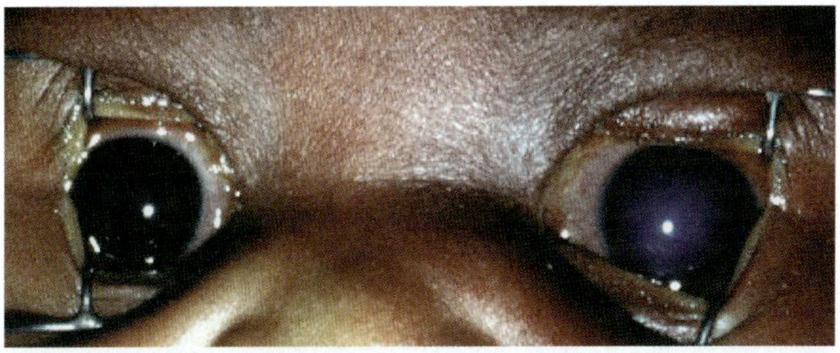

Figura 631-2. Glaucoma infantile. La cornea sinistra è ingrandita ed edematosa.

dei bambini che sono stati sottoposti in tenera età a un intervento chirurgico per cataratte. La causa del glaucoma afachico è sconosciuta, ma si ritiene che sia dovuto a una deformità coesistente della camera anteriore. I bambini trattati per cataratta vanno monitorati strettamente per questa temuta complicanza.

DIAGNOSI E TRATTAMENTO. La diagnosi di glaucoma infantile viene confermata in base al riconoscimento dei segni e dei sintomi. Sebbene la misurazione della pressione intraoculare possa risultare utile nel monitoraggio della risposta al trattamento, non si tratta di una parte essenziale del processo diagnostico. Dopo avere confermato la diagnosi, il trattamento viene iniziato tempestivamente. A differenza del glaucoma dell'adulto, in cui il farmaco è spesso la prima linea della terapia, per il glaucoma infantile il trattamento è principalmente chirurgico. Tra le procedure utilizzate vi sono l'intervento per ottenere un angolo della camera anteriore più normale (goniotomia e trabeculectomia), per creare un sito per la fuoriuscita dell'umore acqueo dall'occhio (trabeculectomia e posizionamento di seton) o per ridurre la sua produzione (ciclocrioterapia e ciclofotocoagulazione). In molti bambini sono frequentemente necessari diversi interventi per abbassare e mantenere adeguata la pressione intraoculare e la terapia medica a lungo termine può risultare necessaria. Anche i pazienti con anomalie oculari multiple e quelli con glaucoma afachico devono essere sottoposti a più interventi per ottenere e mantenere un adeguato controllo della pressione intraoculare. Sebbene la vista possa essere ridotta secondariamente al danno glaucomatoso del nervo ottico o alla cicatrizzazione corneale, l'ambliopia è la causa più comune di perdita della vista in questi bambini.

Beck AD, Freedman S, Kammer J, et al: Aqueous shunt devices compared with trabeculectomy with mitomycin-C for children in the first two years of life. *Am J Ophthalmol* 2003;136:994–1000.
Chen TC, Walton DS, Bhatia LS: Aphakic glaucoma after congenital cataract surgery. *Arch Ophthalmol* 2004;122:1819–1825.
Morad Y, Donaldson CE, Kim YM, et al: The Ahmed drainage implant in the treatment of pediatric glaucoma. *Am J Ophthalmol* 2003;135:821–829.
Neely DE, Plager DA: Endocyclophotocoagulation for management of difficult pediatric glaucomas. *J Am Assoc Pediatr Ophthalmol Strabismus* 2001;5:221–229.
Sidoti PA, Belmonte SJ, Liebmann JM, et al: Trabeculectomy with mitomycin-C in the treatment of pediatric glaucomas. *Ophthalmology* 2000;107:422–429.
Simon JW, Mehta N, Simmons ST, et al: Glaucoma after pediatric lensectomy/vitrectomy. *Ophthalmology* 1991;98:670–674.

Capitolo 632 ■ Anomalie dell'orbita

Scott E. Olitsky, Denise Hug e Laura P. Smith

IPERTELORISMO E IPOTELORISMO. L'ipertelorismo consiste in un'ampia separazione degli occhi o in un aumento della distanza interorbitale che può verificarsi come variante morfogenetica, deformità primitiva o fenomeno secondario in associazione ad anomalie correlate allo sviluppo, come un meningocele frontale o un encefalocele o la persistenza di una schisi facciale. Spesso è associato strabismo, generalmente esotropia e talvolta atrofia ottica.

Con il termine ipotelorismo si indica invece una diminuzione della distanza interorbitale, che si può sviluppare come variante morfogenetica isolata o insieme ad altre anomalie quali l'epicanto o l'oloprosencefalia, oppure secondariamente a una distrofia cranica, come la scafocefalia.

ESOFTALMO ED ENOFTALMO. La protrusione dell'occhio prende il nome di esoftalmo o proptosi ed è un comune indicatore di una malattia orbitale. Può essere causato da una scarsa profondità delle orbite, come in molte malformazioni craniofacciali, o da un aumento della massa tissutale all'interno dell'orbita, come nel caso di malattie neoplastiche, vascolari e infiammatorie. Tra le complicanze oculari si trovano la cheratopatia da esposizione, disturbi motori oculari e l'atrofia ottica con perdita della vista.

L'enoftalmo consiste nella dislocazione posteriore o nell'affossamento dell'occhio all'interno dell'orbita. Si può verificare in caso di frattura orbitale o di atrofia del tessuto orbitale.

INFIAMMAZIONE ORBITALE. La malattia infiammatoria che interessa l'orbita può essere primaria oppure secondaria a una malattia sistemica. L'infiammazione orbitale idiopatica (**pseudotumore orbitale**) rappresenta un ampio spettro di entità cliniche. I sintomi al momento della presentazione possono comprendere dolore, edema palpebrale, proptosi, occhio rosso e febbre. L'infiammazione può interessare un singolo muscolo extraoculare (miosite) o l'intera orbita. La sindrome dell'apice orbitale è una malattia grave che può coinvolgere anche il seno cavernoso e può comprimere o dislocare il nervo ottico. La confusione con la cellulite orbitale è comune, ma la differenziazione può essere posta in base all'assenza di una malattia sinusale associata, dal suo aspetto alla TC e dalla mancanza di miglioramento con gli antibiotici sistemici.

Lo pseudotumore orbitale è associato a lupus eritematoso sistemico, morbo di Crohn, miastenia grave e linfoma. Il **trattamento** comprende l'uso di corticosteroidi sistemici ad alte dosi. Spesso i sintomi migliorano considerevolmente poco dopo l'inizio del trattamento. Un interessamento bilaterale, un'uveite associata, un edema del disco e una recidiva dell'infiammazione non sono rari nella popolazione pediatrica. L'immunoterapia o la radioterapia possono essere necessarie per i casi resistenti o ricorrenti.

Si ritiene che l'**oftalmopatia tiroide-correlata** sia secondaria a un meccanismo immune, che porta a un'infiammazione e al deposito di mucopolisaccaridi e collagene nei muscoli extraoculari e nel grasso orbitale. L'interessamento di questi muscoli può condurre a uno strabismo restrittivo. La retrazione palpebrale può determinare l'esposizione e l'infezione della cornea oppure una sua perforazione. Il coinvolgimento dell'orbita posteriore può comprimere il nervo ottico. Il trattamento può comprendere l'uso di corticosteroidi sistemici, l'irradiazione dell'orbita, la chirurgia palpebrale, la chirurgia dello strabismo o la decompressione orbitale per eliminare i sintomi e proteggere la vista. Il grado di interessamento orbitale è spesso indipendente dallo stato della malattia sistemica (vedi anche Capitolo 569).

Altre malattie sistemiche che possono causare una malattia infiammatoria all'interno dell'orbita includono il linfoma, la sarcoidosi, l'amiloidosi, la poliartrite nodosa, il lupus eritematoso sistemico, la dermatomiosite, la granulomatosi di Wegener e lo xantogranuloma giovanile.

TUMORI DELL'ORBITA. Vari tumori compaiono all'interno e attorno all'orbita nell'infanzia. Tra quelli benigni i più frequenti sono le lesioni vascolari (principalmente emangiomi) (Fig. 632-1) e i dermoidi, mentre le più comuni neoplasie maligne comprendono il rabdomiosarcoma, il linfosarcoma e il neuroblastoma metastatico. I gliomi del nervo ottico sono più comunemente osservati nei pazienti con una neurofibromatosi e possono presentarsi con scarsa vista o proptosi. Il retinoblastoma può estendersi nell'orbita se scoperto tardivamente o se non sottoposto a trattamento. I teratomi sono tumori rari, che tipicamente crescono in modo rapido dopo la nascita e mostrano una proptosi esplosiva.

Gli effetti dei tumori orbitali variano a seconda della loro localizzazione e del pattern di crescita. I principali segni sono la proptosi, la resistenza al retroposizionamento dell'occhio e il peggioramento del movimento oculare. Può essere riscontrata una massa palpabile. Altri segni significativi sono la ptosi, la congestione della testa del nervo ottico, l'atrofia ottica e la perdita della vista. Un rumore anomalo e una pulsazione visibile del globo sono importanti segni di lesioni vascolari.

La valutazione dei tumori orbitali comprende l'ecografia, la RM e la TC. Nei bambini con segni di una lesione a massa va anche preso in considerazione uno pseudotumore. In casi selezionati può essere giustificata la biopsia incisionale o excisionale della lesione.

Gorospe L, Royo A, Berrocal T, et al: Imaging of orbital disorders in pediatric patients. *Eur Radiol* 2003;13:2012–2026.

Ohtsuka K, Hashimoto M, Suzuki Y: A review of 244 orbital tumors in Japanese patients during a 21-year period: Origins and locations. *Jpn J Ophthalmol* 2005;49:49–55.

Shields JA, Shields CL, Scartozzi R: Survey of 1264 patients with orbital tumors and simulating lesions: The 2002 Montgomery Lecture, part 1. *Ophthalmology* 2004;111:997–1008.

Yuen SJA, Rubin PAD: Idiopathic orbital inflammation. *Arch Ophthalmol* 2003;121:491–499.

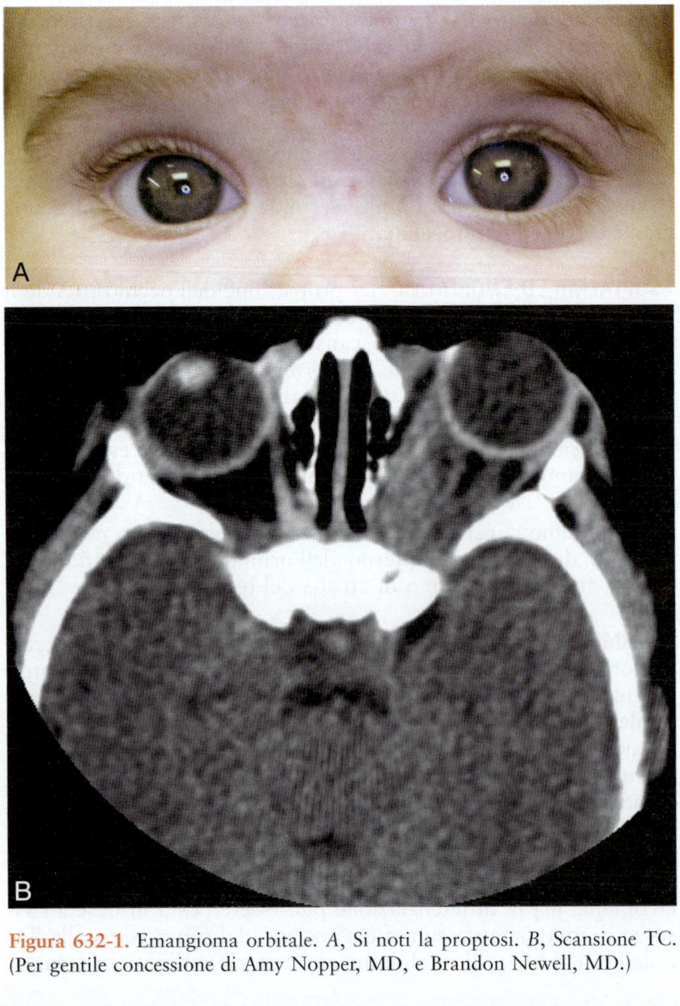

Figura 632-1. Emangioma orbitale. *A*, Si noti la proptosi. *B*, Scansione TC. (Per gentile concessione di Amy Nopper, MD, e Brandon Newell, MD.)

Capitolo 633 ■ Infezioni dell'orbita

Scott E. Olitsky, Denise Hug e Laura P. Smith

Le infezioni dell'orbita sono comuni nei bambini. È importante sapere distinguere le differenti forme d'infezione che si verificano nella regione orbitale, in modo da consentire una diagnosi e un trattamento tempestivi per prevenire la perdita della vista o la diffusione dell'infezione alle strutture intracraniche limitrofe (vedi Tab. 425-1).

DACRIOADENITE. La dacrioadenite, o infiammazione della ghiandola lacrimale, è rara nell'infanzia. Può comparire nel morbillo (nel quale caso di solito è acuta e bilaterale, con regressione in pochi giorni o settimane) o nella mononucleosi infettiva. Lo *Staphylococcus aureus* può produrre una dacrioadenite suppurativa. La dacrioadenite cronica è associata ad alcune malattie sistemiche, in particolare la sarcoidosi, la tubercolosi e la sifilide. Alcune malattie sistemiche possono produrre l'ingrandimento delle ghiandole lacrimali e salivari (sindrome di Mikulicz).

DACRIOCISTITE. Si tratta di un'infezione del sacco lacrimale. In genere è necessaria l'ostruzione del sistema nasolacrimale perché si sviluppi. La dacriocistite acuta si presenta con un arrossamento e un edema al di sopra della regione del sacco lacrimale. Viene trattata con impacchi tiepidi con garze e antibiotici sistemici. Ciò aiuta a controllare l'infezione, ma l'ostruzione di solito richiede un trattamento definitivo per ridurre il rischio di recidiva.

La dacriocistite può verificarsi nei neonati come complicanza di un dacriocistocele congenito. L'ostruzione del sistema nasolacrimale può risolversi dopo la guarigione dell'infezione.

CELLULITE PRESETTALE. L'infiammazione delle palpebre e dei tessuti periorbitali senza segni di un vero interessamento orbitale (come la proptosi o la limitazione del movimento oculare) è in genere nota come cellulite periorbitale o presettale ed è una forma di cellulite facciale. È comune nei bambini piccoli e può essere causata da batteriemia, trauma, ferita infetta o un ascesso della palpebra o della regione periorbitale (pioderma, orzaiolo, congiuntivite, dacriocistite, puntura d'insetto). I pazienti si presentano con un edema palpebrale, che può essere così intenso da rendere difficile la valutazione del globo. Prima dell'avvento della vaccinazione contro l'*Haemophilus influenzae* di tipo B, la causa più comune di cellulite presettale (facciale) pediatrica era la batteriemia determinata da questo microrganismo. Lo streptococco di gruppo A è una causa comune. L'esame clinico mostrerà un'assenza di proptosi, un normale movimento oculare e una funzione pupillare regolare. La TC dimostrerà un edema delle palpebre e dei tessuti sottocutanei anteriori al setto orbitale (Fig. 633-1). La terapia antibiotica e l'attento monitoraggio dei segni e dei sintomi e della progressione locale sono fondamentali.

CELLULITE ORBITALE. Si tratta di una malattia che comporta l'infiammazione dei tessuti dell'orbita, con proptosi, limitazione del movimento oculare, edema della congiuntiva (chemosi) e infiammazione ed edema delle palpebre con acuità visiva potenzialmente ridotta. L'età media è di circa 7 anni ma l'intervallo è di 10 mesi-18 anni. I pazienti spesso presentano un malessere con sintomi generali di tossicità, febbre e leucocitosi (vedi anche Capitolo 192).

La cellulite orbitale può fare seguito a un'infezione diretta dell'orbita da parte di una ferita, a un deposito metastatico di microrganismi in corso di batteriemia, o **più spesso** a un'estensione diretta o una diffusione venosa dell'infezione da siti contigui come palpebre, congiuntiva, globo, ghiandola lacrimale, sacco nasolacrimale o **più comunemente** dai seni paranasali (etmoidali). In alcuni casi un tumore primario o metastatico nell'orbita può produrre il quadro clinico della cellulite orbitale. La causa più comune di essa nei bambini è la sinusite paranasale. Tra i frequenti microrganismi patogeni sono compresi l'*H. influenzae*, lo *Staphylococcus aureus*, gli streptococchi β-emolitici di gruppo A, lo *Streptococcus pneumoniae* e batteri anaerobi.

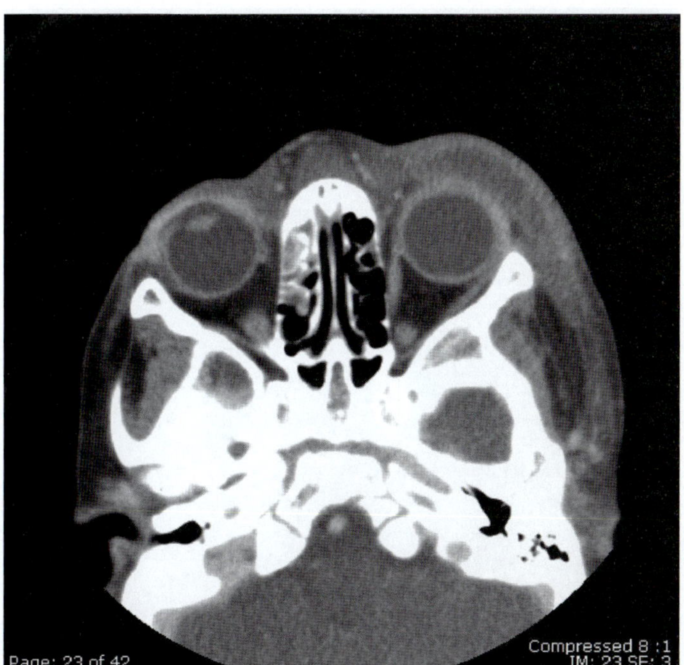

Figura 633-1. Scansione TC di un paziente con cellulite presettale.

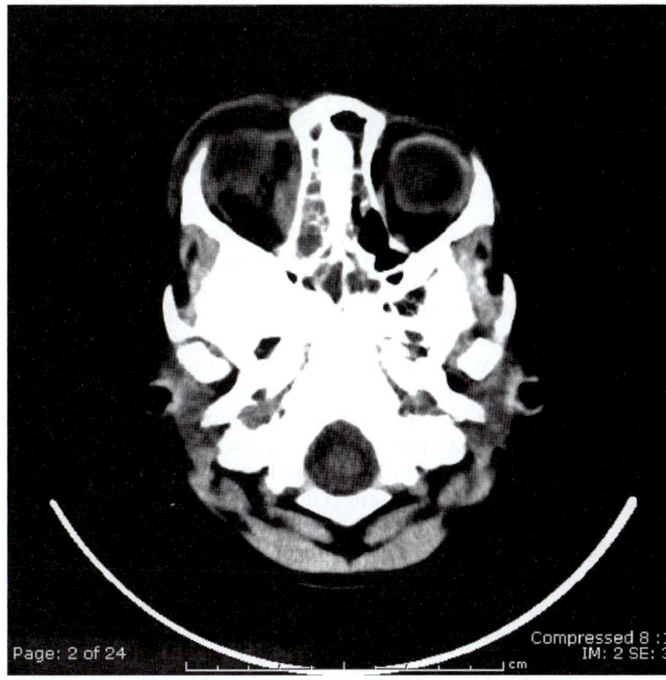

Figura 633-2. Scansione TC che dimostra un ascesso sottoperiostale lungo la parete mediale dell'orbita.

Il rischio di complicanze è elevato. L'interessamento del nervo ottico può portare alla perdita della vista. L'estensione dell'infezione dall'orbita alla cavità cranica può determinare la trombosi del seno cavernoso o la meningite, oppure un empiema epidurale o subdurale, o ancora ascessi cerebrali.

La cellulite orbitale deve essere riconosciuta tempestivamente e trattata in modo aggressivo (vedi Capitolo 192). Di solito sono indicate l'ospedalizzazione e la terapia antibiotica sistemica. In tutti i pazienti è necessaria la TC dell'orbita (incluso il SNC circostante), preferibilmente con un mezzo di contrasto endovenoso, per identificare un ascesso sottoperiostale o l'estensione endocranica. In assenza di segni di miglioramento o in presenza di segni di progressione può risultare necessario il drenaggio sinusale. In alcuni casi si può sviluppare un ascesso orbitale o sottoperiostale (Fig. 633-2), e quest'ultimo può richiedere il drenaggio urgente dell'orbita, che a volte può anche essere ritardato per consentire il miglioramento dopo l'inizio della terapia antibiotica (ampicillina/sulbactam) endovenosa ad alte dosi (200-400 mg/kg/24 h della componente di ampicillina ogni 4 o 6 h, con dose massima di 8 g ampicillina/24 h). La presentazione clinica e il decorso di ogni singolo paziente dovrebbero dettare la necessità e il momento più opportuni per drenare l'ascesso.

Ambati BK, Ambati J, Azar N, et al: Periorbital and orbital cellulitis before and after the advent of *Haemophilus influenzae* type B vaccination. *Ophthalmology* 2000;107:1450–1453.

Campolattaro BN, Lueder GT, Tychsen L: Spectrum of pediatric dacryocystitis: Medical and surgical management of 54 cases. *J Pediatr Ophthalmol Strabismus* 1997;34:143–153.

Garcia GH, Harris GJ: Criteria for nonsurgical management of subperiosteal abscess of the orbit: Analysis of outcomes 1988–1998. *Ophthalmology* 2000;107:1454–1456.

Greenberg MF, Pollard ZF: Medical treatment of pediatric subperiosteal orbital abscess secondary to sinusitis. *J AAPOS* 1998;2:351–355.

Nageswaran S, Woods CR, Benjamin Jr DK, et al: Orbital cellulitis in children. *Pediatr Infect Dis J* 2006;25:695–699.

Capitolo 634 ■ Traumi dell'occhio

Scott E. Olitsky, Denise Hug
e Laura P. Smith

Circa 1/3 dei casi di cecità nei bambini è secondario a un trauma. I bambini e gli adolescenti sono vittime di un numero sproporzionato di episodi di trauma oculare. I maschi di 11-15 anni di età sono i più esposti; in questo gruppo il numero di lesioni supera quello che occorre alle femmine con un rapporto di circa 4:1. La maggior parte è correlata a sport, piccoli dardi, altri oggetti lanciati, bastoncini, pietre, fuochi d'artificio, palline colorate e pistole a pallettoni ad aria compressa. Queste ultime causano lesioni oculari e orbitali particolarmente devastanti. Molti traumi sono evitabili (vedi Capitolo 61). Qualunque parte dell'orbita o del globo può essere interessata (Fig. 634-1).

ECCHIMOSI ED EDEMA DELLE PALPEBRE. Sono comuni dopo un trauma contusivo. L'emorragia nelle palpebre e nella regione periorbitale ("occhio nero" o "pesto") non ha solitamente conseguenze e si riassorbe spontaneamente, ma dovrebbe indurre a un attento esame dell'occhio alla ricerca di lesioni più serie, come la frattura a scoppio dell'orbita, un'emorragia intraoculare o la rottura del globo.

LACERAZIONI DELLE PALPEBRE. Necessitano di un trattamento scrupoloso. La lacerazione orizzontale della palpebra superiore può coinvolgere l'elevatore, il piatto tarsale o il setto orbitale. Una riparazione difettosa può portare a ptosi, distorsione della palpebra o erniazione del grasso orbitale. Le lacerazioni che coinvolgono i margini palpebrali richiedono una meticolosa apposizione chirurgica per prevenire intaccature, l'eversione o l'inversione del margine o alterazioni nell'orientamento delle ciglia che potrebbero portare a epifora (iperafflusso di lacrime), difetti di umidificazione della cornea e irritazione cronica. Le lacerazioni situate in prossimità del canto mediale possono coinvolgere il punto lacrimale, i canalicoli o il dotto nasolacrimale e richiedono la riparazione microchirurgica da parte di un chirurgo oftalmico esperto. In tutti i casi di lacerazione palpebrale l'esame del globo alla ricerca di lesioni perforanti è obbligatorio. Una riparazione primaria appropriata spesso ottiene risultati superiori della riparazione secondaria effettuata in un momento successivo.

ABRASIONI CORNEALI SUPERFICIALI. Quando l'epitelio corneale è graffiato, abraso o denudato, espone lo strato basale epiteliale sottostante e i nervi corneali superficiali. Ciò è accompagnato da dolore, lacrimazione, fotofobia e diminuzione della vista. Le abrasioni corneali sono individuate instillando la tintura di fluoresceina e ispezionando la cornea utilizzando una luce blu filtrata. Per questo esame è ideale la lampada a fessura, ma una lampada di Wood manuale risulta adeguata per i bambini piccoli.

Il **trattamento** di un'abrasione corneale è rivolto a promuovere la guarigione e ad alleviare il dolore. Le abrasioni sono trattate con frequenti applicazioni di un unguento antibiotico topico finché l'epitelio non sia completamente guarito. L'uso di una benda a semipressione non riduce il tempo di guarigione né il dolore, bensì una benda applicata in modo inappropriato può essa stessa abradere la cornea. Un agente cicloplegico topico (ciclopentolato idrocloruro 1%) può alleviare il dolore da spasmo ciliare nei pazienti con abrasioni ampie. Gli anestetici topici non dovrebbero essere somministrati a domicilio, perché ritardano la guarigione epiteliale e inibiscono il naturale riflesso di ammiccamento.

CORPO ESTRANEO AL DI SOPRA O ALL'INTERNO DELLA CORNEA O DELLA CONGIUNTIVA. Di solito produce un fastidio acuto, lacrimazione e infiammazione. La maggior parte dei corpi estranei può essere identificata all'esame in condizioni di buona illuminazione con l'aiuto dell'ingrandimento o con un set di oftalmoscopia diretta con lente positiva a elevato ingrandimento (+10 o +12). In molti casi risulta necessario l'esame con la lampada a fessura, specialmente se la particella è profonda e metallica. Alcuni corpi estranei congiuntivali tendono a posizionarsi sotto la palpebra superiore, causando una sensazione di corpo estraneo corneale quando vengono a contatto con il globo durante i movimenti delle palpebre; essi possono anche produrre abrasioni corneali lineari orientate verticalmente (Fig. 634-2). Il riscontro di queste abrasioni dovrebbe sollevare il dubbio di un siffatto corpo estraneo e può essere necessaria l'eversione della palpebra (vedi Capitolo 618). Se si sospetta un corpo estraneo, ma esso non

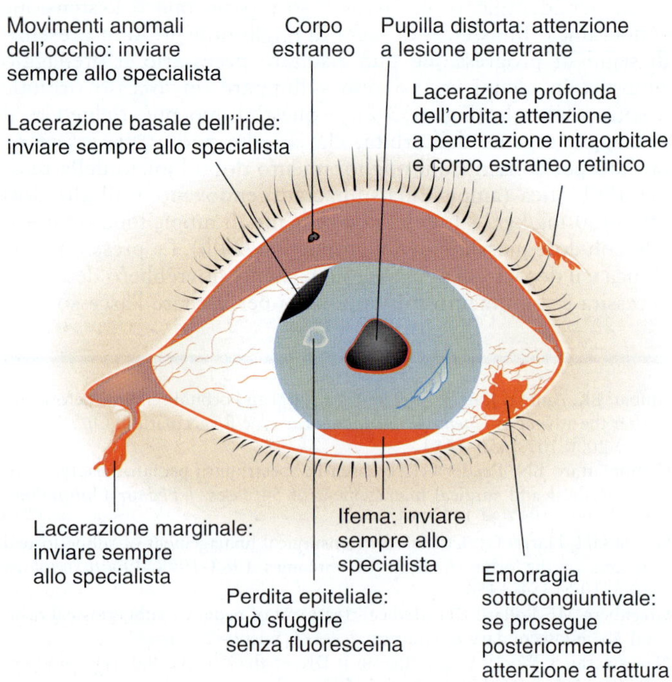

Figura 634-1. Occhio lesionato. (Da Khaw PT, Shah P, Elkington AR: Injury to the eye. *Br Med J* 2004;328:36-38.)

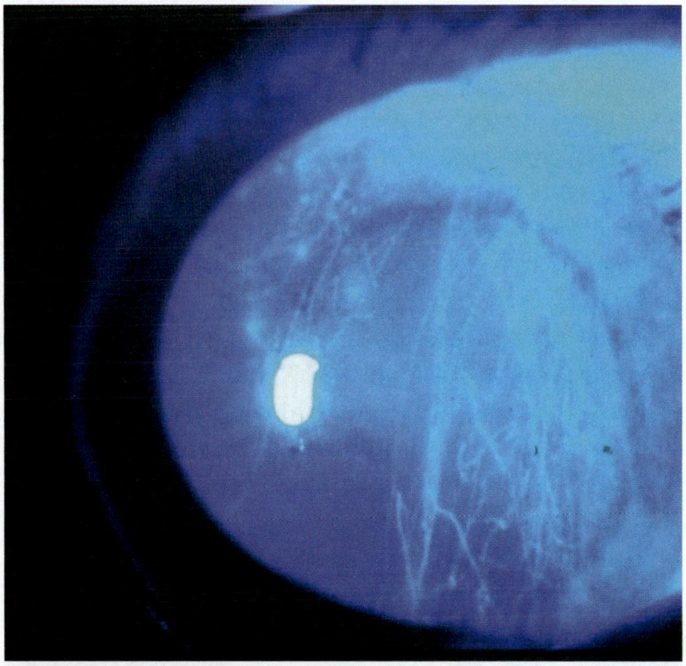

Figura 634-2. Abrasioni corneali lineari orientate verticalmente secondarie a un corpo estraneo sottostante alla palpebra superiore.

viene trovato, sono indicati ulteriori accertamenti. Se l'anamnesi suggerisce una lesione dovuta a una particella ad alta velocità, può essere necessario l'esame radiologico dell'occhio per esplorare la possibilità di un corpo estraneo intraoculare.

La rimozione di un corpo estraneo può essere facilitata dall'instillazione di una goccia di anestetico topico. Molti corpi estranei possono essere eliminati mediante l'irrigazione o un'asportazione con un applicatore con punta di cotone inumidito. Quelli che si sono conficcati dovrebbero essere trattati da un oculista. La rimozione di corpi estranei corneali può lasciare difetti epiteliali, che vengono trattati come abrasioni della cornea. I corpi metallici possono causare la formazione di ruggine nei tessuti corneali; l'esame da parte di un oculista 1 o 2 giorni dopo la rimozione è raccomandata, in quanto un anello di ruggine può richiedere un ulteriore trattamento (curettage).

IFEMA. Consiste nella presenza di sangue nella camera anteriore dell'occhio. Si può verificare in caso di lesione smussa o penetrante. Si manifesta come un livello di liquido rosso chiaro o scuro tra la cornea e l'iride o come una torbidità diffusa dell'umore acqueo. I bambini avvertono dolore e possono risultare sonnolenti. Il trattamento di solito comprende il riposo a letto, con la testa sollevata di 30-45 gradi per favorire la sedimentazione e il riassorbimento del sangue. L'ospedalizzazione e la sedazione possono essere necessarie per assicurare la compliance in alcuni bambini. Nella maggior parte dei casi, i midriatici topici, i corticosteroidi topici o orali o l'acido aminocaproico per os vengono adoperati per prevenire il risanguinamento. Il sanguinamento secondario in genere si verifica a distanza di 3-5 giorni dall'emorragia iniziale, aumentando il rischio di sequele. Il sangue nella camera anteriore può produrre un incremento della pressione intraoculare e macchie di sangue della cornea: complicanze che possono compromettere la vista. In tali casi possono essere necessarie l'evacuazione chirurgica del coagulo e l'irrigazione della camera anteriore. I pazienti con malattia o tratto falciforme sono a più elevato rischio di perdita acuta della vista secondaria all'aumentata pressione intraoculare o all'infarto del nervo ottico e possono richiedere un intervento più aggressivo. I soggetti con un'anamnesi di ifema traumatico hanno un'aumentata incidenza di glaucoma nel seguito della vita e andrebbero monitorati regolarmente.

LACERAZIONI E FERITE PERFORANTI DELLA CORNEA O DELLA SCLERA. Richiedono l'invio immediato all'oculista e la tempestiva riparazione chirurgica se l'occhio e la vista devono essere salvati. Importanti segni indicativi di una lesione perforante dell'occhio sono il collasso della camera anteriore, la distorsione e la dislocazione della pupilla e la protrusione di tessuto scuro (uvea) nella ferita. Il *trattamento di emergenza* consiste nel proteggere da ulteriori danni l'occhio lesionato mediante l'applicazione di un bendaggio sterile e di una copertura oculare rigida. Se questi presidi medici non sono disponibili, un'adeguata protezione oculare può essere creata con una tazzina di plastica o di Styrofoam o con un pezzo di cartone piegato in una scatola o in un cono. Bisognerebbe ridurre la manipolazione al minimo e non si dovrebbe istillare alcun farmaco se non sotto prescrizione oculistica.

ROTTURA DEL GLOBO. Se il globo è compresso lungo il suo diametro anteroposteriore con una forza sufficiente, si romperà in corrispondenza dei suoi punti deboli, che in genere comprendono l'area in cui la sclera e la cornea si incontrano (limbus), quelli in prossimità dei punti di inserzione dei muscoli retti e quelli in corrispondenza del sito di interventi chirurgici intraoculari pregressi. A differenza della maggior parte delle lesioni che comportano lacerazioni o perforazioni del globo, la forza necessaria per produrre una rottura della sclera ha molta più probabilità di causare un danno esteso e spesso permanente alla parte posteriore dell'occhio. Pertanto, la prognosi per il recupero della vista in queste lesioni è scarsa.

TRAUMA DEL NERVO OTTICO. La lesione del globo può produrre una neuropatia traumatica. Il danno indiretto al nervo ottico può avere luogo in seguito a un trauma smusso della fronte secondario a onde d'urto che attraversano il canale ottico. I pazienti possono presentarsi lamentando una diminuzione della vista. Più frequentemente, questi pazienti sono in stato d'incoscienza e l'unico segno indicativo della lesione può essere la presenza di un difetto papillare afferente. In questi casi il canale ottico dovrebbe essere studiato mediante le tecniche di imaging per ricercare l'esistenza di una frattura o di un ematoma. I corticosteroidi ad alte dosi a volte possono venire utilizzati, sebbene un recente trial nazionale non abbia dimostrato un miglioramento degli esiti visivi rispetto ai pazienti che non avevano ricevuto il trattamento.

LESIONI CHIMICHE. Le ustioni chimiche della cornea e dei tessuti annessi sono tra le emergenze oculari più urgenti. Le ustioni da alcali sono di solito più distruttive di quelle da acidi, perché gli alcali reagiscono con i grassi per formare saponi che danneggiano le membrane cellulari, consentendo l'ulteriore penetrazione degli alcali nell'occhio. In genere gli acidi causano un danno tissutale meno grave, più localizzato. L'epitelio corneale offre una moderata protezione nei confronti degli acidi deboli e il danno è lieve a meno che il pH non sia di 2,5 o inferiore. La maggior parte degli acidi più forti precipita le proteine tissutali, creando una barriera fisica che si oppone alla loro ulteriore penetrazione.

Le ustioni lievi da acidi o alcali sono caratterizzate da una iniezione congiuntivale e un edema e lievi erosioni corneali epiteliali. Lo stroma corneale può essere lievemente edematoso e la camera anteriore può presentare una reazione cellulare e flare da lievi a moderati. Con gli acidi forti, la cornea e la congiuntiva diventano rapidamente bianche e opache e l'epitelio corneale può sfaldarsi, lasciando uno stroma relativamente chiaro, con un aspetto che può inizialmente mascherare la gravità dell'ustione. Le ustioni gravi da alcali sono caratterizzate da un'opacizzazione corneale.

Il **trattamento di emergenza** di un'ustione chimica inizia con l'irrigazione immediata e abbondante con acqua o soluzione fisiologica. Lo sbrigliamento locale e la rimozione delle particelle estranee dovrebbero essere effettuati durante l'irrigazione. Quando la natura della lesione chimica è sconosciuta, l'uso della cartina per testare il pH è utile per determinare se l'agente era basico o acido. L'irrigazione dovrebbe proseguire per almeno 30 minuti o fino a che siano stati istillati 2 L per 2-4 ore di soluzione irrigante nei casi lievi o fino a 10 L nei casi gravi. Alla fine dell'irrigazione, il pH dovrebbe trovarsi nel range normale (7,3-7,7) e quindi andrebbe ricontrollato circa 30 minuti dopo per assicurarsi che non si sia modificato.

FRATTURE. Una frattura diretta del pavimento orbitale è una frattura del pavimento associata a una della rima orbitale, mentre una frattura indiretta del pavimento orbitale è isolata del pavimento ed è più comunemente nota come frattura a scoppio. Le fratture del pavimento sono comuni quando oggetti di dimensioni maggiori rispetto all'apertura orbitale, come palle, pugni o il cruscotto di un'automobile, colpiscono l'orbita, in particolare quella laterale inferiore.

Il segno clinico più evidente di una frattura del pavimento orbitale è la limitazione dello sguardo verso l'alto. Tra gli altri segni vi sono l'ecchimosi della palpebra inferiore, l'epistassi, l'enfisema orbitale e l'iperestesia della guancia ipsilaterale e del labbro superiore. Quest'ultimo segno è dovuto alla distruzione del nervo infraorbitale nel punto in cui esso attraversa il pavimento orbitale.

Le migliori tecniche di imaging per visualizzare le fratture orbitali sono la radiografia diretta e la TC. La proiezione di Waters mostra meglio il pavimento orbitale e il seno mascellare.

Il **trattamento** per i bambini con fratture orbitali acute comprende la profilassi antibiotica, decongestionanti nasali e pacchi di ghiaccio. In caso di intrappolamento dei muscoli extraoculari (con conseguente limitazione del movimento dell'occhio e diplopia) ed erniazione del grasso orbitale o dell'occhio stesso (con conseguente enoftalmo), può essere necessaria la riparazione chirurgica.

FERITE PENETRANTI DELL'ORBITA. Richiedono un'attenta valutazione per possibili danni all'occhio, al nervo ottico o al cervello. L'esame dovrebbe comprendere indagini per ricercare eventuali corpi estranei ritenuti. L'emorragia e l'infezione orbitale sono comuni e devono essere trattate come emergenze.

ABUSO DI MINORE (VEDI CAPITOLO 36). Si tratta di una delle principali cause di lesioni all'occhio e alla regione orbitale. La possibilità di un trauma non accidentale va presa in considerazione in ogni bambino con ecchimosi o lacerazione delle palpebre, emorragia all'intero occhio o del suo intorno, cataratta o dislocazione del cristallino, distacco della retina o frattura dell'orbita. Il neurotrauma infantile inflitto (sindrome da scuotimento del bambino) compare in seguito a violenti movimenti non accidentali ripetitivi, sfrenati, in accelerazione-decelerazione della testa e del collo, con o senza un trauma contusivo del capo in bambini di solito minori di 3 anni. Esso riguarda circa il 10% di tutti i casi di abuso di minore e comporta un tasso di mortalità che arriva al 25%. L'identificazione dell'abuso non è importante solo per trattare la patologia scoperta, ma anche per prevenire un abuso ulteriore e anche la morte. Le manifestazioni oculari sono numerose e possono avere un ruolo importante nel riconoscimento di questa condizione. L'emorragia retinica è il reperto oculistico più comune e si verifica a tutti i livelli della retina. Il suo aspetto aiuta a distinguere questa condizione da altre cause di emorragia retinica o dalle lesioni accidentali (Fig. 634-3). Le emorragie retiniche possono comparire senza una patologia endocranica associata.

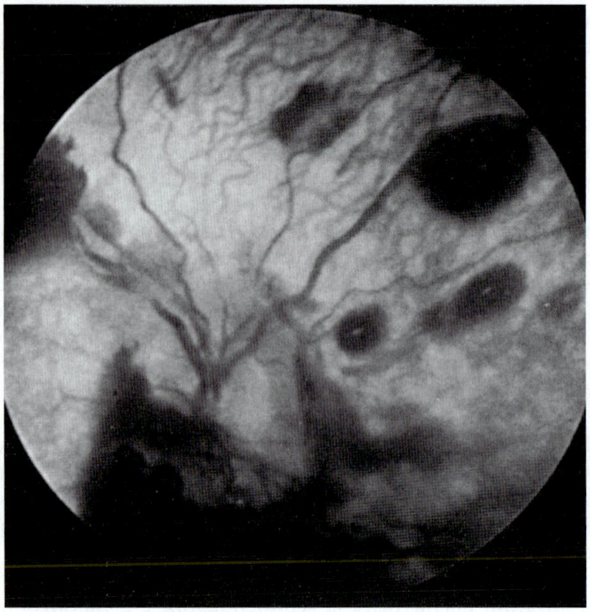

Figura 634-3. Emorragie retiniche con ematoma subdurale in un bambino che ha subito un abuso.

LESIONI CORRELATE A FUOCHI D'ARTIFICIO. Possono rappresentare i traumi oculari più devastanti nei bambini. Almeno 1/5 delle visite di pronto soccorso per lesioni correlate a fuochi d'artificio sono per un trauma oculare. Negli Stati Uniti, la massima parte di tali lesioni si verifica in concomitanza dell'Indipendence Day e la maggior parte ha luogo nonostante la supervisione degli adulti.

LESIONI OCULARI CORRELATE A SPORT E LORO PREVENZIONE. Sebbene le lesioni sportive si verifichino in tutti i gruppi di età, un numero molto più elevato di bambini e adolescenti partecipa a sport ad alto rischio rispetto agli adulti. Il maggiore numero di bambini partecipanti, la loro immaturità atletica e l'aumentata probabilità di un utilizzo inadeguato o inappropriato di protezioni oculari sono responsabili della spropositata quota di lesioni oculari (vedi Capitoli 687 e 691).

Negli Stati Uniti, gli sport con il più elevato rischio di lesioni oculari sono quelli in cui non si possono indossare protezioni, come la boxe, il wrestling e le arti marziali. Gli sport a elevato rischio comprendono quelli in cui si usano palle o dischi che si muovono velocemente, mazze, bastoni, racchette o frecce (baseball, hockey, lacrosse, sport con racchetta e tiro con l'arco) o comportano un contatto corporeo aggressivo (football e basket). In base al rischio e alla frequenza di partecipazione, la più elevata percentuale di lesioni oculari si osserva nel basket e nel baseball.

Alcune protezioni oculari concepite per un'attività specifica sono disponibili per la maggior parte degli sport. Per il basket, gli sport con racchetta e altre attività ludiche che non richiedono il casco o una maschera facciale, si suggerisce l'uso di occhiali in policarbonato modellati che vengono fissati alla testa mediante un nastro elastico. Anche per l'hockey, il football, il lacrosse e il baseball (specie per il battitore) sono disponibili maschere e protezioni in policarbonato. I bambini dovrebbero anche indossare occhiali sportivi sotto il casco. Per il baseball, gli occhiali e il casco andrebbero indossati per la battuta, la presa e la corsa alle basi; per le altre posizioni di solito sono sufficienti solo gli occhiali.

American Academy of Pediatrics Committee on Sports Medicine and Fitness, American Academy of Ophthalmology Committee on Eye Safety and Sports Ophthalmology: Protective eyewear for young athletes. *Pediatrics* 1996;98:311–313.

Buys YM, Levin AV, Enzenauer RW, et al: Retinal findings after head trauma in infants and young children. *Ophthalmology* 1992;99:1718–1723.

Egbert JE, May K, Kersten RC, et al: Pediatric orbital floor fracture: Direct extraocular muscle involvement. *Ophthalmology* 2000;107:1875–1879.

Forbes BJ, Christian CW, Judkins AR, et al: Inflicted childhood neurotrauma (shaken baby syndrome): Ophthalmic findings. *J Pediatr Ophthalmol Strabismus* 2004;41:80–88.

Khaw PT, Shah P, Elkington AR: Injury to the eye. *Br Med J* 2004;328:36–38.

Kivlin JD, Simons KB, Lazoritz S, et al: Shaken baby syndrome. *Ophthalmology* 2000;107:1246–1254.

Michael JG, Hug D, Dowd MD: Management of corneal abrasion in children: A randomized clinical trial. *Ann Emerg Med* 2002;40:67–72.

Morad Y, Avni I, Benton SA, et al: Normal computerized tomography of brain in children with shaken baby syndrome. *J AAPOS* 2004;8:445–450.

Serious eye injuries associated with fireworks—United States, 1990–1994. *MMWR* 1995;44:449–452.

Smith GA, Knapp JF, Barnett TM, et al: The rocket's red glare, the bombs bursting in air: Fireworks-related injuries to children. *Pediatrics* 1996;98:1–9.

Parte XXIX ▪ L'orecchio

Capitolo 635 ▪ Considerazioni generali e valutazione Joseph Haddad Jr.

MANIFESTAZIONI CLINICHE. Otto segni e sintomi sono principalmente associati a malattie dell'orecchio e dell'osso temporale.

L'**otalgia** di solito si associa a infiammazioni dell'orecchio esterno o medio, ma può rappresentare un dolore riferito in seguito al coinvolgimento dei denti, dell'articolazione temporomandibolare o faringe. Nei lattanti, il tirarsi o sfregarsi l'orecchio, associati a irritabilità generale o sonno insufficiente, specialmente in presenza di febbre, possono anche essere i soli segni di dolore all'orecchio. Il solo gesto di tirare l'orecchio non è diagnostico di patologia auricolare.

L'**otorrea purulenta** è un segno di otite esterna, otite media con perforazione della membrana timpanica MT, drenaggio dall'orecchio medio attraverso timpanostomia con posizionamento di un tubo o, raramente, drenaggio attraverso la fessura di un seno branchiale. Il drenaggio di materiale ematico può essere associato a infiammazione acuta o cronica (spesso con tessuto di granulazione), trauma, neoplasia, corpo estraneo o discrasia ematica. Un drenaggio chiaro suggerisce invece una perforazione della MT con effusione sierosa dall'orecchio medio o, raramente, una fuoriuscita di liquido cerebrospinale attraverso difetti (congeniti o traumatici) del condotto uditivo esterno o dell'orecchio medio.

La **perdita di udito** (ipoacusia) dipende da patologie a carico sia dell'orecchio esterno o medio (perdita di udito conduttiva) sia dell'orecchio interno, delle strutture retrococleari o delle vie uditive centrali (perdita dell'udito neurosensoriale). La sua causa più comune nei bambini è l'otite media (OM).

Un **rigonfiamento** intorno all'orecchio comunemente è conseguenza di un'infiammazione (per es. otite esterna, pericondrite, mastoidite), un trauma (per es. ematoma), masse cistiche benigne o neoplasie.

La **vertigine** è un tipo specifico di capogiro, che provoca un'illusoria sensazione di movimento. Il termine **capogiro** è meno specifico di "vertigine" e si riferisce a un alterato orientamento nello spazio. La vertigine è un disturbo raro nei pazienti pediatrici; il bambino o il genitore possono anche non accennare ai problemi di equilibrio se il medico non rivolge loro una domanda specifica. La causa più comune di capogiro nei bambini più piccoli è una patologia delle tube di Eustachio e dell'orecchio medio, ma la vera vertigine può essere provocata anche da labirintite, fistola perilinfatica attraverso l'orecchio medio e interno per trauma o difetto congenito dell'orecchio interno, colesteatoma della mastoide o dell'orecchio medio, neuronite vestibolare, vertigine parossistica benigna, malattia di Menier o patologia del sistema nervoso centrale. I bambini più grandi possono anche descrivere la sensazione che la stanza si muova o giri; i bambini più piccoli possono manifestare i problemi di equilibrio solo cadendo, inciampando o mostrando una certa goffaggine.

Il **nistagmo** può essere unidirezionale, orizzontale o a scosse. Di origine vestibolare, in genere è associato a vertigine.

È raro che i bambini descrivano spontaneamente gli **acufeni**, che tuttavia sono un disturbo comune, soprattutto in pazienti con patologia della tuba di Eustachio e dell'orecchio medio o con sordità neurosensoriale. I bambini possono descrivere gli acufeni se vengono specificamente interrogati in merito, senza trascurare la lateralità e la qualità del suono.

PARALISI FACCIALE. Il nervo facciale può essere deiscente nel suo decorso attraverso l'orecchio medio nel 50% dei pazienti. Un'infezione con infiammazione locale, più frequente nell'OM acuta, può portare a temporanea paralisi del nervo facciale. Altre possibili cause sono colesteatoma, paralisi di Bell, sindrome di Ramsay Hunt (herpes zoster ottico), malattia di Lyme, frattura, neoplasia, o infezione dell'osso temporale. La paralisi facciale congenita può essere dovuta a trauma da parto o ad anomalia congenita del settimo nervo cranico, come nella sindrome di Möbius o CHARGE (*Coloboma, Heart defects, Atresia choanae, Retarded growth, Genital hypoplasia, and Ear anomalies*, colobomi, difetti cardiaci, atresia coanale, ritardo della crescita, ipoplasia genitale e anomalie auricolari), oppure essere associata ad anomalie di altri nervi cranici e anomalie craniofacciali.

ESAME OBIETTIVO

L'esame completo, con particolare attenzione al capo e al collo, può rivelare una condizione predisponente o associata a patologia auricolare nei bambini. L'aspetto del volto e le caratteristiche del linguaggio possono costituire segni di un'anomalia dell'orecchio o dell'udito. Molte anomalie craniofacciali, come il palato leporino, la disostosi mandibolofacciale (sindrome di Treacher Collins) e la trisomia 21 (sindrome di Down), sono associate a patologie dell'orecchio e delle tube di Eustachio. La respirazione orale e l'iponasalità possono indicare un'ostruzione nasale o post nasale. L'**ipernasalità** è un segno di insufficienza velofaringea. Esaminando la cavità orofaringea si può scoprire una schisi palatale o una schisi sottomucosa (solitamente associata a uvula bifida), che predispongono entrambi a OM con effusione. Un tumore rinofaringeo che ostruisce il naso e la tuba di Eustachio può essere associato a OM.

La posizione del paziente per l'esame di orecchio, naso e gola dipende dall'età del paziente stesso e dalla sua capacità di cooperare, dal setting clinico e dalle preferenze dell'esaminatore. Il bambino può essere visitato su un lettino o in braccio a un genitore. La presenza di un genitore o di un assistente di solito è necessaria per ottenere risultati più attendibili, facendo sì che l'esaminato si muova il meno possibile (Fig. 635-1). Il lettino può essere utile per i bambini più grandi che non collaborano, o quando si esegue una qualche procedura, per esempio una valutazione microscopica o una timpanocentesi. Per diminuire

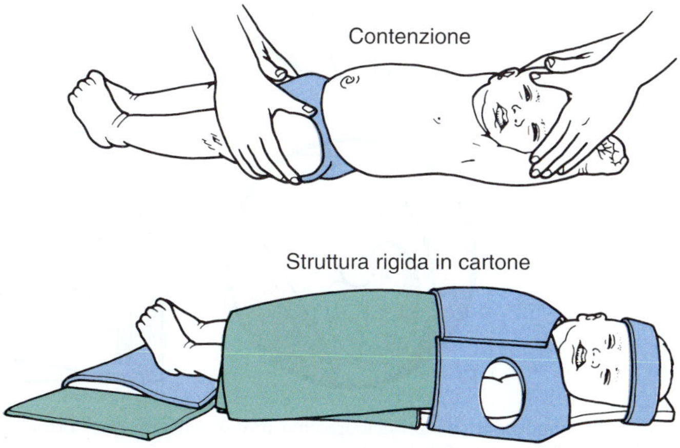

Figura 635-1. Metodi per tenere fermo un lattante durante l'esame obiettivo e procedure come la timpanocentesi o la miringotomia. (Da Bluestone CD, Klein JO: *Otitis media in Infants and Children*, 2nd ed. Philadelphia, WB Saunders, 1995, p. 91.)

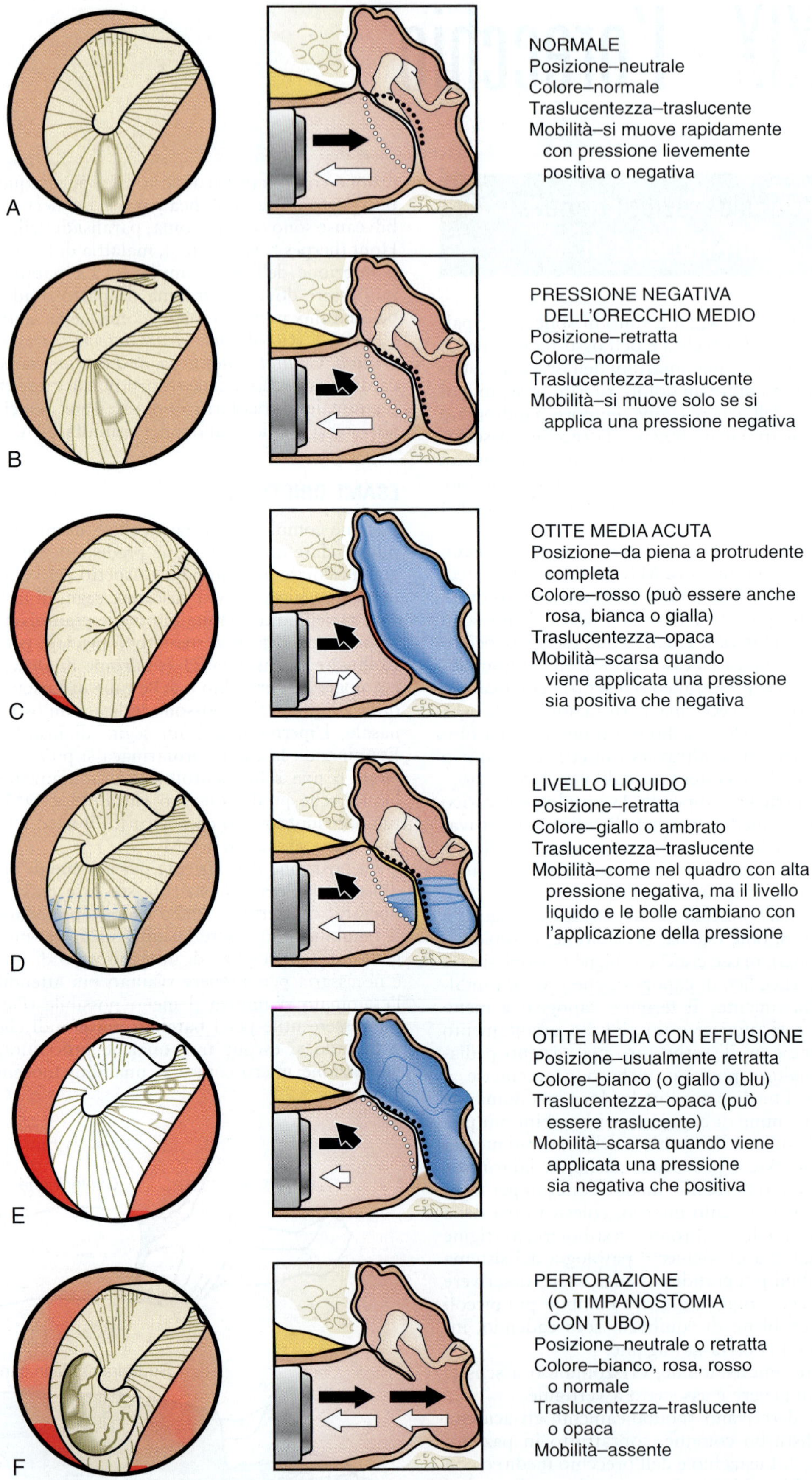

Figura 635-2. Condizioni comuni dell'orecchio medio, valutate con l'otoscopio. (Da Bluestone CD, Klein JO: *Otitis media in Infants and Children*, 3rd ed. Philadelphia, WB Saunders, 2001, p. 131.)

i movimenti, può essere d'aiuto avvolgere il bambino in un lenzuolo o usare una struttura contenitiva in cartone. Nella maggior parte dei casi è preferibile che lattanti e bambini piccoli vengano esaminati in braccio a un genitore; quest'ultimo può aiutare a ridurre i movimenti del bambino tenendogli la testa contro il proprio petto e, con l'altra mano, bloccandogli i polsi e le braccia incrociati sull'addome. Se necessario, potrà trattenere le gambe del paziente tra le ginocchia. Per evitare un trauma all'orecchio da movimento, l'esaminatore dovrebbe tenere l'otoscopio con la mano saldamente posizionata contro il viso o la testa del bambino, così che l'otoscopio si muova insieme al capo. Sollevando l'otoscopio ed esercitando una lieve trazione sul padiglione auricolare si raddrizza il canale auricolare, manovra che consente una migliore esposizione della MT.

Durante l'esame dell'orecchio, la ricerca di infezioni del padiglione auricolare e del meato uditivo esterno può aiutare nella valutazione delle complicanze dell'OM. L'otite esterna può essere dovuta alle secrezioni di un'OM acuta; l'infiammazione dell'area auricolare posteriore può indicare una periostite o un ascesso subperiostale che si estende dalle cellule aeree della mastoide. È necessario ricercare la presenza di depressioni preauricolari o di segni cutanei, perché i bambini colpiti hanno un'incidenza lievemente più alta di ipoacusia neurosensoriale.

Il **cerume** è uno strato di materiale idrorepellente e ceroso, che protegge il condotto uditivo ma può interferire con l'esame. In genere per rimuoverlo si utilizza la testa chirurgica dell'otoscopio, che permette il passaggio di un filo ad anello o di una curette smussata sotto visualizzazione diretta. Altri metodi, da adottare soltanto se la MT è integra, comprendono l'irrigazione delicata del canale auricolare con acqua calda o l'instillazione di una soluzione a base di perossido d'idrogeno diluito nel canale auricolare per pochi minuti, allo scopo di ammorbidire il materiale, che verrà poi aspirato o irrigato. Alcune preparazioni commerciali, come il polipeptide oleato-condensato trolamina, possono causare, per uso cronico, una dermatite del canale esterno, e devono essere utilizzate solo sotto controllo medico.

L'infiammazione dolorosa del condotto uditivo spesso è indicativa di otite esterna. Le anomalie del condotto uditivo esterno comprendono stenosi (comune nei bambini con trisomia 21), esosotosi ossea, otorrea e presenza di corpi estranei. Il colesteatoma dell'orecchio medio può manifestarsi nel condotto come un drenaggio intermittente di odore fetido, talvolta associato a detriti biancastri; il colesteatoma del condotto esterno può apparire come una massa bianca perlacea nella cute del canale stesso. Detriti bianchi o grigi nel condotto suggeriscono un'otite esterna micotica. I condotti uditivi dei neonati sono ripieni di vernice caseosa, molle e di colore giallo pallido, che dovrebbe scomparire rapidamente dopo la nascita.

La MT e la sua mobilità si valutano meglio con un otoscopio pneumatico. La MT normale è in posizione neutrale; una MT sporgente può essere causata da un aumento della pressione dell'aria nell'orecchio medio, con o senza pus o effusione nell'orecchio medio; un tamburo protrudente può impedire la visualizzazione del martello e dell'annulus. La retrazione della MT di solito indica una pressione negativa nell'orecchio medio, ma può dipendere anche da pregresse malattie dell'orecchio medio con fissazione degli ossicini, dei legamenti o della MT. In presenza di retrazione, il martello appare più evidente e l'incudine può essere più visibile posteriormente al martello.

La MT normale, di colore grigio argento, è simile alla carta cerata (Fig. 635-2). Una MT bianca o gialla può indicare effusione nell'orecchio medio. Una sola MT di colore rosso può non indicare alcuna patologia, perché i vasi sanguigni possono andare incontro a congestione in seguito a pianto, starnuti, o dopo essersi soffiati il naso. Una MT normale è traslucida e permette all'osservatore di visualizzare le strutture dell'orecchio medio: l'incudine, il promontorio, la finestra ovale e, spesso, il nervo timpanico. In presenza di effusione dell'orecchio medio, possono essere visibili un livello idroaereo o delle bolle (vedi Fig. 635-2). L'impossibilità di visualizzare le strutture dell'orecchio medio indica l'opacizzazione del tamburo, di norma provocata da ispessimento della MT, da effusione dell'orecchio medio o da entrambi. La valutazione della luce riflessa in genere non è d'aiuto, perché l'orecchio medio con effusione riflette la luce come l'orecchio normale.

La **mobilità della MT** è utile per valutare la pressione dell'orecchio medio e la presenza o assenza di liquido (vedi Fig. 635-2). Per eseguire un'otoscopia pneumatica si raccomanda di usare uno speculum di dimensioni tali da permettere un buona chiusura e il movimento dell'aria nel canale. Un anello di gomma intorno alla punta può aiutare a ottenere una migliore chiusura del canale. La pressione dell'orecchio medio è normale se la MT è in posizione neutrale e si muove vivacemente per effetto della pressione sia positiva che negativa.

La retrazione della MT è più frequente in presenza di pressione negativa dell'orecchio medio; se si applica una pressione positiva nel condotto uditivo, anche in presenza di pressione negativa moderata dell'orecchio medio, non c'è movimento visibile verso l'interno (vedi Fig. 635-1). Tuttavia, la pressione negativa intracanalare, prodotta da rilascio del bulbo di gomma dell'otoscopio pneumatico, può determinare il ritorno della MT in posizione neutrale. Una retrazione della MT si può verificare sia in presenza sia in assenza di liquido nell'orecchio medio, e se il liquido dell'orecchio medio è frammisto ad aria, la MT può conservare una certa mobilità. Il movimento della MT verso l'esterno è meno probabile in presenza di pressione negativa grave o di effusione dell'orecchio medio.

Se la pressione nell'orecchio medio è positiva ed è presente una certa quantità d'aria, la MT protrudente (*bulging*) si sposta quando si applica una pressione positiva, ma non quando si applica una pressione negativa. Nei bambini piccoli che piangono durante l'esame otoscopico, nei bambini più grandi con ostruzione nasale e negli stadi precoci della OM acuta si può riscontrare una MT completa e una pressione positiva dell'orecchio medio senza effusione. Quando il sistema delle cellule ciliate mastoidee dell'orecchio medio è pieno di liquido e l'aria è scarsa o addirittura assente, la mobilità della MT risulta notevolmente diminuita o assente in risposta all'applicazione di pressione positiva e negativa.

La **timpanocentesi**, o aspirazione dell'orecchio medio, è il metodo definitivo per verificare la presenza di effusione dell'orecchio medio e stabilirne il tipo: la procedura consiste nell'inserimento, attraverso la parte inferiore della MT, di un ago spinale del 18 collegato a una siringa o a un sifone di raccolta (Fig. 635-3). La coltura del condotto uditivo e la pulizia con alcol devono precedere la timpanocentesi e la coltura dell'aspirato dall'orecchio me-

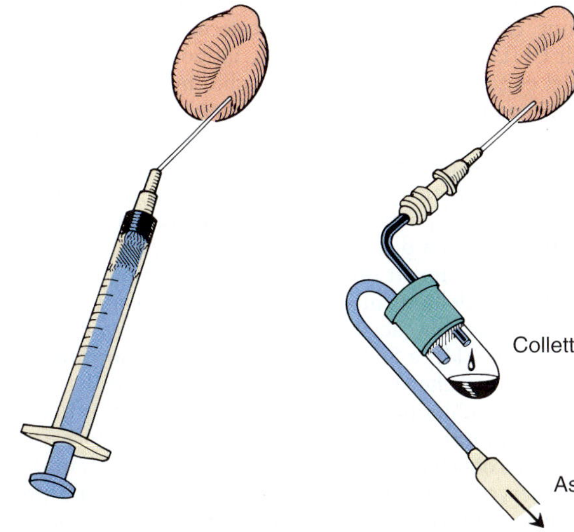

Figura 635-3. La timpanocentesi viene eseguita con ago sottile e una siringa da tubercolina (a sinistra) o un collettore Alden-Senturia. (Da Bluestone CD, Klein JO: *Otitis Media in Infants and Children*, 2nd ed. Philadelphia, WB Saunders, 1995, p. 127.)

dio; l'esecuzione di una coltura del condotto serve principalmente a stabilire se i microrganismi dell'orecchio medio provengono dal canale esterno o se si tratta di veri patogeni dell'orecchio medio.

Ulteriori indagini diagnostiche dell'orecchio e dell'udito comprendono la valutazione audiometrica, l'audiometria a impedenza (timpanometria), la riflettometria acustica e studi specializzati sulla funzionalità della tuba di Eustachio. Gli esami diagnostici per immagini, comprese la tomografia computerizzata e la risonanza magnetica, spesso forniscono ulteriori informazioni circa anomalie anatomiche e l'esistenza di processi infiammatori o neoplasie. Nell'esame di un bambino con un sospetto disturbo vestibolare, si deve considerare se eseguire una valutazione specialistica della funzione labirintica (vedi Capitolo 640).

Capitolo 636 ■ Ipoacusia

Joseph Haddad Jr.

INCIDENZA E FREQUENZA. Nonostante la varietà delle stime, basate su criteri diversi di definizione dei problemi uditivi, di età del gruppo indagato e di metodi di esame utilizzati, circa 1-2 neonati su 1000 nati presentano una ipoacusia neurale bilaterale moderata (30-50 dB), grave (50-70 dB) o profonda (>70 dB), incluso uno 0,5-1 su 1000 con ipoacusia bilaterale >75 dB. Inoltre, 1-2 bambini su 1000 possono manifestare un difetto più lieve o unilaterale; a 19 anni d'età l'incidenza raddoppia. Negli Stati Uniti, si riscontra una ipoacusia neurosensoriale (SNHL, *SensoryNeural Hearing Loss*) unilaterale >26 dB in 13/1000 bambini in età scolare e una SNHL >45 dB in 3/1000 bambini in età scolare. L'esordio della ipoacusia può verificarsi in qualsiasi momento dell'infanzia. Se si considera la meno grave o transitoria ipoacusia che comunemente accompagna la patologia dell'orecchio medio nei bambini piccoli, il numero dei pazienti pediatrici colpiti aumenta sostanzialmente.

TIPI DI IPOACUSIA. L'ipoacusia può avere un'origine periferica o centrale. L'**ipoacusia conduttiva** (**CHL**, *Conductive Hearing Loss*) è comunemente causata da alterazioni della trasmissione del suono attraverso l'orecchio esterno o medio, o da un'anomala trasduzione dell'energia sonora in attività nervosa nell'orecchio medio e nell'ottavo nervo. Può essere conduttiva, neurosensoriale o mista. La CHL, che nei bambini è il tipo più comune di ipoacusia, si verifica quando esiste un impedimento fisico alla trasmissione del suono nell'orecchio esterno e/o medio. Cause comuni di CHL sono atresia o stenosi, tappo di cerume o corpi estranei del condotto uditivo. Nell'orecchio medio, perforazione della membrana timpanica (MT), discontinuità o fissazione della catena degli ossicini, otite media (OM) con effusione, oteosclerosi e colesteatoma possono provocare CHL.

Un danno o un'alterazione dello sviluppo delle strutture dell'orecchio interno possono causare un'**ipoacusia neurosensoriale** (**SNHL**), dovuta a distruzione delle cellule ciliate per traumi acustici, malattia o agenti ototossici, malformazioni cocleari, fistola perilinfatica della membrana della finestra ovale o rotonda e lesioni della divisione acustica dell'ottavo nervo cranico. Una combinazione di CHL e SNHL è considerata una **sordità mista**.

Il deficit uditivo che origina lungo le vie uditive del sistema nervoso centrale, dalla porzione prossimale dell'ottavo nervo alla corteccia cerebrale, in genere viene considerato una **sordità centrale** (**o retrococleare**). Tumori o patologie demielinizzanti dell'ottavo nervo e dell'angolo cerebellopontino possono provocare un deficit d'udito, ma risparmiano l'orecchio esterno, medio e interno. Tali cause di perdita d'udito sono rare nei bambini. Altre forme di deficit uditivi centrali, conosciute come **disordini dell'elaborazione uditiva centrale**, comprendono quelli che rendono difficile, anche per i bambini con udito normale, ascoltare selettivamente in presenza di rumore, associare correttamente le informazioni provenienti dalle due orecchie, elaborare le parole quando sono lievemente distorte e decodificare le informazioni uditive quando vengono formulate più velocemente piuttosto che a una velocità inferiore. Questi deficit possono manifestarsi con scarsa attenzione, problemi di apprendimento o disturbi del comportamento in ambito scolastico. I bambini più grandi possono mettere in atto una serie di strategie per affrontare questi disturbi, e spesso sono importanti l'identificazione e la documentazione di patologie dell'elaborazione uditiva centrale, perché è possibile intervenire dal momento stesso in cui genitori e insegnanti si rendono conto che la scarsa attenzione del bambino dipende da un problema fisico.

EZIOLOGIA. L'eziologia di un difetto uditivo varia a seconda che l'ipoacusia sia conduttiva o neurosensoriale. La maggior parte delle CHL sono acquisite, e la causa più comune è la presenza di liquido nell'orecchio medio. Le cause congenite includono anomalie del padiglione auricolare, del condotto uditivo esterno, della MT e degli ossicini. È invece raro che responsabili di CHL siano un colesteatoma congenito o altre masse dell'orecchio medio. Anche perforazione della MT (per es. di origine traumatica o dovuta a OM), discontinuità degli ossicini (per es. infezioni, colesteatoma, trauma), timpanosclerosi, colesteatoma acquisito o masse nel condotto uditivo o nell'orecchio medio (per es. istiocitoma a cellule di Langerhans, tumori delle ghiandole salivari, rabdomiosarcoma) possono provocare una CHL. Malattie rare che colpiscono l'orecchio medio e l'osso temporale e che possono presentarsi con CHL sono: otosclerosi, osteopetrosi, displasia fibrosa e osteogenesi imperfetta.

La SHNL può essere congenita o acquisita. La forma acquisita può essere causata da fattori genetici, infettivi, autoimmuni, anatomici, traumatici, ototossici e idiopatici (Tabb. 636-1, 636-2, 636-3 e 636-4). I fattori di rischio riconosciuti sono all'origine del 50% circa dei casi di SNHL da moderata a profonda. La più comune causa infettiva di SNHL congenita è il **Cytomegalovirus** (**CMV**), che infetta 1/100 neonati negli Stati Uniti (vedi Capitolo 252); di questi, 6000-8000 neonati ogni anno presentano manifestazioni cliniche, che comprendono circa il 75% delle SNHL. Il CMV congenito richiede particolare attenzione, perché nelle sue forme sia sintomatiche sia asintomatiche è associato a ipoacusia, che può essere progressiva. Alcuni bambini con CMV congenito perdono improvvisamente l'udito residuo a 4-5 anni d'età. Le infezioni congenite, che rappresentano cause molto meno frequenti di SNHL, sono la toxoplasmosi e la sifilide. Il CMV congenito, la toxoplasmosi e la sifilide possono presentarsi anche con una SNHL a esordio tardivo, da qualche mesi ad alcuni anni dopo la nascita. La rosolia, che in passato costituiva la causa virale più frequente di SNHL, oggi è molto rara grazie a programmi di vaccinazione efficaci. Le infezioni intrauterine con virus dell'herpes simplex sono rare e la perdita di udito non è una manifestazione isolata.

Altre infezioni postnatali responsabili di SNHL sono la sepsi da streptococco di gruppo B e la meningite batterica, a qualsiasi età. *Streptococcus pneumoniae* rappresenta la causa più comune di meningite batterica con SNHL dopo il periodo neonatale, ma è diventato meno frequente da quando si somministra di routine il vaccino pneumococcico coniugato. *Haemophilus influenzae* di tipo b, che in passato era la causa più frequente di meningite con SNHL, ora, con il vaccino coniugato Hib, è raro. Rare infezioni responsabili di SNHL comprendono la malattia di Lyme, il parvovirus B19 e la varicella. Parotite, rosolia e morbillo, una volta tutte cause comuni di SNHL nei bambini, attualmente, grazie ai programmi di vaccinazione, sono rare.

I fattori genetici sono responsabili probabilmente di almeno il 50% dei casi di SNHL (vedi Tabb. 632-2 e 636-3). Queste patologie possono essere associate ad altre anomalie, far parte di una sindrome nota o presentarsi in forma isolata. La SNHL spesso si verifica in concomitanza con anomalie dell'orecchio e dell'occhio e malattie del sistema metabolico, muscoloscheletrico, tegumentario, renale e nervoso. Le perdite di udito **autosomiche dominanti**

TABELLA 636-1. Indicatori associati a ipoacusia neurosensoriale e/o conduttiva

PER NEONATI (NASCITA-28 GIORNI DI VITA) QUANDO NON SIA DISPONIBILE UNO SCREENING GENERALIZZATO

Anamnesi familiare di sordità infantile ereditaria neurosensoriale
Infezione intrauterina, dovuta a Cytomegalovirus, rosolia, sifilide, herpes simplex o toxoplasmosi
Anomalie craniofacciali, comprese quelle con alterazioni morfologiche del padiglione auricolare e del canale auricolare
Peso alla nascita <1500 g
Iperbilirubinemia sierica che richieda trasfusioni
Farmaci ototossici, tra cui gli aminoglicosidi, usati in numerosi cicli di terapia o in combinazione con diuretici dell'ansa
Meningite batterica
Punteggio di Apgar tra 0 e 4 a 1 minuto o tra 0 e 6 a 5 minuti
Ventilazione meccanica che duri ≥5 giorni
Segni tipici o altri reperti associati a una sindrome conosciuta che comprenda ipoacusia neurosensoriale e/o conduttiva

PER BAMBINI PICCOLI (ETÀ 29 GIORNI-2 ANNI) QUALORA SI RENDA NECESSARIO RIPETERE LO SCREENING

Sospetti dei genitori o del personale di assistenza riguardo a udito, linguaggio e/o ritardo dello sviluppo
Meningite batterica e altre infezioni associate a ipoacusia neurosensoriale
Trauma cranico con perdita di coscienza o frattura cranica
Segni tipici o altri reperti associati a sindrome nota che comprenda ipoacusia neurosensoriale e/o conduttiva
Farmaci ototossici, tra cui chemioterapici o aminoglicosidi, usati in numerosi cicli di terapia o in combinazione con diuretici dell'ansa
Otite media ricorrente o persistente con effusione, per almeno 3 mesi

PER BAMBINI (ETÀ 29 GIORNI-3 ANNI) CHE RICHIEDONO MONITORAGGIO PERIODICO DELL'UDITO

(Alcuni neonati e bambini, pur avendo superato un primo screening uditivo, possono richiedere un periodico monitoraggio dell'udito che valuti un'eventuale ipoacusia neurosensoriale a esordio ritardato e/o conduttiva. I pazienti con queste indicazioni richiedono una valutazione dell'udito almeno ogni 6 mesi fino all'età di 3 anni, e successivamente a intervalli appropriati.)

INDICATORI ASSOCIATI A IPOACUSIA NEUROSENSORIALE A ESORDIO RITARDATO

Anamnesi familiare di sordità infantile ereditaria
Infezione intrauterina, come Cytomegalovirus, rosolia, sifilide, herpes simplex, toxoplasmosi
Neurofibromatosi di tipo 2 e patologie neurodegenerative

INDICATORI ASSOCIATI A IPOACUSIA CONDUTTIVA

Otite media persistente o ricorrente con effusione
Deformità anatomiche e altre patologie con alterazione della funzione della tuba di Eustachio
Patologie neurodegenerative

Adattata da American Academy of Pediatrics, Joint Committee on Infant Hearing: Joint Committee on Infant Hearing 1994 Position Statement. *Pediatrics* 1995;95:152.

TABELLA 636-2. Tipi comuni di ipoacusia neurosensoriale ereditaria non sindromica

LOCUS	GENE	FENOTIPO UDITIVO
DFN3	*POU3F4*	Ipoacusia conduttiva dovuta a fissazione della staffa che mima l'otosclerosi. Si sovappone una SNHL progressiva
DFNA1	*DIAPH1*	Inizia con perdita delle basse frequenze nella prima decade di vita per poi coinvolgere tutte le frequenze, fino a produrre un audiogramma piatto con perdite profonde in tutto il range uditivo
DFNA2	*KCNQ4*	Perdita neurosensoriale simmetrica delle alte frequenze nella prima decade di vita e progressiva perdita di tutte le frequenze
	GJB3	Perdita neurosensoriale simmetrica delle alte frequenze che inizia nella terza decade di vita
DFNA6/14/38	*WFS1*	Perdita neurosensoriale delle basse frequenze a esordio precoce; circa il 75% dei familiari che segregano in modo dominante questo profilo uditivo è portatore di mutazioni missense nel dominio C-terminale della wolframina
DFNA10	*EYA4*	Progressiva perdita che inizia nella seconda decade di vita con un profilo uditivo da piatto a lievemente inclinato, che con l'età acquista una notevole pendenza
DFNA13	*COL11A2*	Perdita neurosensoriale congenita delle medie frequenze che mostra una progressione correlata all'età nel range uditivo
DFNA15	*POU4F3*	Perdita neurosensoriale progressiva bilaterale che comincia nella seconda decade di vita
DFNA20/26	*ACTG1*	Perdita neurosensoriale bilaterale progressiva che comincia nella seconda decade; con l'età la perdita aumenta con soglia che si sposta a tutte le frequenze, sebbene nella maggior parte dei casi si mantenga una configurazione pendente
DFNB1	*GJB2* *GJB6*	L'ipoacusia può essere da lieve a profonda. Il genotipo più comune, GJB6 35delG/35delG, è associato a SNHL da grave a profonda in circa il 90% dei bambini colpiti; una sordità da grave a profonda si osserva solo nel 60% dei bambini che sono portatori eterozigoti uno dell'allele 35delG e un altro della variante all'elica GJB2 che provoca SNHL; nei bambini portatori di mutazioni missense di due GJB2 che causano SNHL non si osserva sordità da grave a profonda
DFNB4	*SLC26A4*	DFNB4 e la sindrome di Pendred (vedi Tab. 636-3) sono allelici. La perdita di udito di DFNB4 è associata a dilatazione dell'acquedotto vestibolare e può essere uni- o bilaterale. Nelle alte frequenze, la perdita è da grave a profonda; nelle basse frequenze, il grado della perdita varia ampiamente. L'esordio può essere congenito (prelinguaggio), ma è comune anche una perdita progressiva dopo l'acquisizione del linguaggio
mtDNA 1555A>G	*12SrRNA*	La perdita d'udito può essere da lieve a profondo ma in genere è simmetrica; le più colpite sono le alte frequenze; una perdita a picco dell'udito si può verificare dopo una terapia con aminoglicosidi

Da Smith RJH, Bale JF Jr, Withe KR: Sensorineural hearing loss in children. *Lancet* 2005;365:879-890.

TABELLA 636-3. Tipi comuni di ipoacusia neurosensoriale sindromica

	GENE	FENOTIPO
DOMINANTE		
Waardenberg (WS1)	*PAX3*	I criteri diagnostici maggiori comprendono dystopia canthorum, ipoacusia congenita, eterocromia dell'iride, ciuffo bianco, e un parente affetto di primo grado. Circa il 60% dei bambini colpiti ha un'ipoacusia congenita; nel 90% dei casi è bilaterale.
Waardenberg (WS2)	*MITF*	I criteri diagnostici maggiori sono gli stessi della WS1 ma senza dystopia canthorum. Circa l'80% dei bambini colpiti ha un'ipoacusia congenita; nel 90% dei casi è bilaterale.
Branchio-otorenale	*EYA1*	I criteri diagnostici comprendono perdita di udito (98%), fossette preauricolari (85%) e anomalie branchiali (70%), renali (40%) e dell'orecchio esterno (30%). La perdita di udito può essere conduttiva, neurosensoriale, o mista, e di grado da lieve a profondo.
RECESSIVO		
Sindrome di Pendred	*SLC26A4*	I criteri diagnostici comprendono ipoacusia neurosensoriale che è congenita, non progressiva e da grave a profonda in molti casi, ma che può avere un esordio tardivo ed essere progressiva; dilatazione bilaterale dell'acquedotto vestibolare con o senza ipoplasia cocleare; anomalo test di dismissione di perclorato o gozzo.
Sindrome di Usher tipo 1 (USH1)	*USH1A, MYO7A, USH1C, CDH23*	I criteri diagnostici comprendono ipoacusia congenita, profonda e bilaterale, areflessia vestibolare e retinite pigmentosa (comunemente non diagnosticata fino a che la visione a tunnel e la nictalopia non diventano gravi tanto da essere evidenti
Sindrome di Usher tipo 2 (USH2)	*USH2A, USH2B, USH2C*	I criteri diagnostici comprendono ipoacusia bilaterale, congenita, da lieve a grave, e retinite pigmentosa; l'ipoacusia può essere percepita come progressiva nel tempo perché la percezione delle parole diminuisce in quanto diminuisce anche il visus, interferendo con la lettura subconscia delle labbra.
Sindrome di Usher tipo 3 (USH3)	*USH3*	I criteri diagnostici comprendono ipoacusia progressiva neurosensoriale successiva all'acquisizione del linguaggio, retinite pigmentosa a esordio tardivo, e alterazione variabile della funzione vestibolare.

Da Smith RJH, Bale JF Jr, White KR: Sensorineural hearing loss in children. *Lancet* 2005;365:879-890.

TABELLA 636-4. Patogeni infettivi implicati nell'ipoacusia neurosensoriale di interesse pediatrico

INFEZIONI CONGENITE
Cytomegalovirus
Virus della coriomeningite linfocitaria
Virus della rosolia
Toxoplasma gondii
Treponema pallidum
INFEZIONI ACQUISITE
Borrelia burgdorferi
Virus di Epstein-Barr
Haemophilus influenzae
Virus Lassa
Virus del morbillo
Virus della parotite
Neisseria meningitidis
Enterovirus non polio
Plasmodium falciparum
Streptococcus pneumoniae
Virus della varicella-zoster

Da Smith RJH, Bale JF Jr, Withe KR: Sensorineural hearing loss in children. *Lancet* 2005;365:879-890.

rendono conto di circa il 10% dei casi infantili di SNHL. La sindrome di Waardenburg (tipi I e II) e le sindromi branchio-oto-renali sono responsabili delle più comuni forme di SNHL imputabili a sindromi autosomiche dominanti. Per classificare i vari tipi di SNHL si utilizza un codice di quattro lettere e un numero, come segue: **DFN** = sordità, A = dominante, B = recessiva, numero = ordine di scoperta, per esempio DFNA 13. Altre condizioni autosomiche dominanti, oltre a quelle già indicate, sono: DFNA da 1 a 11, 13, 15, 17, 20, 22, 28, 36, 48, e mutazioni del gene cristallino (*CRYM*). Le SNHL genetiche **autosomiche recessive**, sia sindromiche sia non sindromiche, rappresentano circa l'80% di tutti i casi di SNHL nell'infanzia. La sindrome di Usher (tipi 1, 2, e 3), la sindrome di Pendred e la sindrome di Jervell e Lange-Nielsen (una forma della sindrome del Q-T lungo) sono tre dei tipi sindromici recessivi più comuni di SNHL. Altre condizioni autosomiche recessive comprendono: la sindrome di Alström, la sindrome di Bartter tipo 4, il deficit di biotinidasi e DFNB 1-4, 6-9, 12, 16, 18, 21-23, 28-31, 36, 37, 67. A differenza dei bambini con una sindrome ben riconoscibile o con anomalie dell'orecchio esterno, che vengono identificati come soggetti a rischio di perdere l'udito e di conseguenza sono tenuti sotto adeguato monitoraggio, i bambini non sindromici presentano una difficoltà maggiore. Mutazioni dei geni della connessina-26 e -30 sono state identificate nelle forme autosomiche tanto recessive (DNFB 1) quanto dominanti (DFNA 3), e anche, sporadicamente, in pazienti non sindromici con SNHL; fino al 50% delle SNHL non sindromiche può essere correlato a una mutazione della connessina-26. Mutazioni del gene *GJB2* co-localizzano con DFNA 3 e DFNB 1 i loci sul cromosoma 13, sono associate a una certa suscettibilità alla ipoacusia autosomica non sindromica e sono associate almeno al 30% dei casi di sordità congenita sporadica da grave a profonda e al 50% dei casi di sordità autosomica recessiva non sindromica. Malattie legate al sesso associate a SNHL, che si ritiene rappresentino ll'1-2% delle SNHL, comprendono la malattia di Norie, la sindrome digitale otopalatale, la sordità di Nance e la sindrome di Alport. Le anomalie cromosomiche come le trisomie 13-15, 18 e 21 possono essere accompagnate da alterazioni dell'udito. I pazienti con sindrome di Turner presentano una monosomia di tutto il cromosoma X o di una sua parte, e possono manifestare CHL, SNHL o ipoacusia mista. La perdita dell'udito può essere progressiva. Anche anomalie genetiche mitocondriali possono portare a SNHL (vedi Tab. 636-2).

Possono essere genetiche anche l'agenesia o malformazioni delle strutture cocleari, tra cui le anomalie di Scheibe, di Mondini (Fig. 636-1), di Alexander e di Michel, la dilatazione dell'acquedotto vestibolare e anomalie del canale semicircolare. Queste anomalie probabilmente compaiono prima dell'8ª settimana di gestazione dando luogo a un arresto del normale sviluppo, a sviluppo aberrante o a entrambi. Molte di queste anomalie sono state descritte anche in associazione con altre patologie congenite, come le infezioni intrauterine da CMV e rosolia. Queste anomalie sono molto comuni; nel 20% almeno dei bambini con SNHL si riscontrano, alla TC o alla RM, anomalie evidenti o lievi dell'osso temporale.

LA CHL PUÒ ESSERE ANCHE GENETICA. Condizioni, patologie o sindromi caratterizzate da anomalie craniofacciali possono essere associate a ipoacusia conduttiva e forse a SNHL. Le sindromi di Pierre Robin, di Treacher Collins, di Klippel-Feil, di Crouzon, la sindrome branchio-otorenale e l'osteogenesi imperfetta spesso sono associate a perdita dell'udito. Anomalie congenite che provocano CHL comprendono malformazioni degli ossicini e delle strutture dell'orecchio medio e atresia del condotto uditivo esterno.

Molte cause geneticamente determinate di deficit uditivo, sindromiche e non sindromiche, si esprimono soltanto a distanza

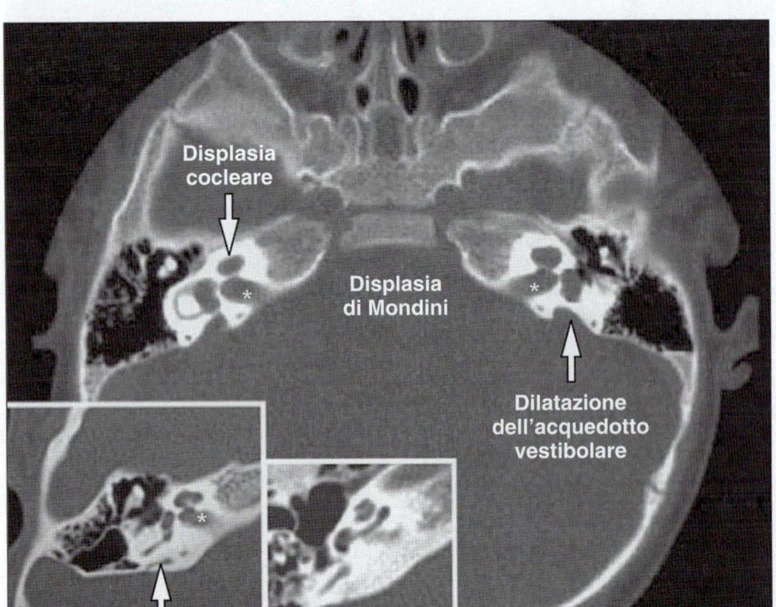

Figura 636-1. Displasia di Mondini alla TC dell'osso temporale in un bambino con sindrome di Pendred. La dilatazione dell'acquedotto vestibolare e la displasia cocleare sono entrambe presenti in questa sezione. Nel più ampio dei due riquadri, che raffigurano un osso temporale normale, l'acquedotto vestibolare è visibile ma molto più piccolo (*freccia*). La coclea appare normale, e nel riquadro più piccolo di una sezione assiale inferiore si può facilmente contare il numero previsto di giri cocleari (*nel condotto uditivo interno). (Da Smith RJH, Bale JF Jr, Withe KR: Sensorineural hearing loss in children. *Lancet* 2005;365:879-890.)

di un certo tempo dalla nascita. Le sindromi di Alport, Alström e Down, la malattia di Recklingausen e la sindrome di Hunter-Hurler sono malattie genetiche che possono presentare ipoacusia come manifestazione tardiva.

La SNHL si può verificare anche dopo l'esposizione a tossine, prodotti chimici e antibatterici. Nei primi mesi di gravidanza, l'embrione è particolarmente vulnerabile agli effetti delle sostanze tossiche. Anche i farmaci ototossici, tra cui gli aminoglicosidi, i diuretici dell'ansa e i chemioterapici (cisplatino), possono provocare SNHL. La forma congenita può comparire secondariamente a esposizione a farmaci come talidomide e retinoidi. Alcuni prodotti chimici, come chinina, piombo e arsenico, possono determinare perdita dell'udito prima e dopo la nascita.

Altre possibili cause sono i traumi, in particolare le fratture dell'osso temporale, la concussione dell'orecchio interno, il trauma cranico, quello iatrogeno (per es. chirurgia, ossigenazione con membrana extracorporea [ECMO]) e l'esposizione a radiazioni e rumore; nei bambini è invece raro che la causa della SNHL siano malattie immuni (sistemiche o limitate all'orecchio interno), anomalie metaboliche e neoplasie dell'osso temporale.

Un'ipoacusia improvvisa in un bambino precedentemente sano, peraltro rara, può essere dovuta a otite media o ad altre patologie dell'orecchio medio. Normalmente queste cause risultano chiare all'anamnesi e all'esame fisico. L'ipoacusia improvvisa in assenza di cause evidenti spesso è dovuta a eventi vascolari che colpiscono l'apparato cocleare o il nervo, come un'embolia o una trombosi (secondaria a condizioni protrombotiche). Ulteriori cause includono la fistola perilinfatica, i farmaci, un trauma e il primo episodio della sindrome di Menier.

EFFETTI DELL'IPOACUSIA. Gli effetti dell'ipoacusia dipendono tanto dalla natura e dal grado del deficit uditivo, quanto dalle caratteristiche del singolo paziente. L'ipoacusia può essere unilaterale o bilaterale; conduttiva, neurosensoriale o mista; lieve, moderata, grave o profonda; a esordio improvviso o graduale; stabile, progressiva o fluttuante; può inoltre interessare lo spettro acustico totalmente o parzialmente. Altri fattori, come il quoziente intellettivo, le condizioni mediche o fisiche (comprese le sindromi d'accompagnamento), il sostegno del nucleo familiare, l'età di esordio, l'età al momento dell'identificazione e la tempestività dell'intervento, incidono sull'impatto che l'handicap ha sul bambino.

La maggior parte dei bambini con problemi di udito ha una qualche capacità uditiva residua. Solo il 6% dei portatori di handicap uditivo presenta un'ipoacusia profonda bilaterale. Una perdita d'udito molto precoce può incidere sull'acquisizione del linguaggio, sullo sviluppo sociale ed emotivo, sul comportamento, sull'attenzione e sul rendimento scolastico. In alcuni casi i problemi di udito non vengono riconosciuti, perché i bambini colpiti hanno un udito sufficiente che permette loro di reagire ai suoni ambientali e apprendere il linguaggio, anche se, al momento del confronto con i compagni, in classe, non sono in grado di esprimere appieno tutte le loro potenzialità.

Anche un'ipoacusia lieve e monolaterale può avere ripercussioni negative sullo sviluppo di un bambino piccolo e sul rendimento scolastico. I bambini con tali problemi d'udito manifestano maggiori difficoltà quando le condizioni d'ascolto sono sfavorevoli (per es. rumori di sottofondo e acustica scarsa), come può succedere in un'aula scolastica. Coloro che sottovalutano l'impatto dei problemi d'udito sull'apprendimento dimenticano che la scuola è un contesto di tipo uditivo-verbale. In ogni bambino con difficoltà di parola e linguaggio, o con rendimento inferiore a quello dei coetanei, comportamento inadeguato o deficit di attenzione, bisognerebbe prendere in considerazione la possibilità di un'ipoacusia (Tab. 636-5).

I soggetti con ipoacusia moderata, grave o profonda, come peraltro quelli con altri deficit, spesso vengono destinati a classi o scuole per bambini con necessità particolari. Il trattamento uditivo e le scelte in merito alle modalità di comunicazione ed educazione devono essere individualizzate, perché questi bambini non rappresentano un gruppo omogeneo. È essenziale un approccio in team per la gestione del singolo caso, dato che ogni alunno e ogni nucleo familiare hanno esigenze e capacità diverse.

SCREENING DELL'UDITO. I deficit uditivi possono avere un impatto maggiore su un soggetto in via di sviluppo, e dato che l'identificazione precoce migliora la prognosi, si sono sostenuti ampiamente e fermamente programmi di screening. I dati provenienti dal programma di screening neonatale del Colorado suggeriscono che un lattante con deficit uditivi, se identificato e trattato entro

TABELLA 636-5. Handicap uditivo come funzione di livello di soglia uditiva media dell'orecchio migliore

LIVELLO MEDIO DI SOGLIA	DESCRIZIONE	CAUSE COMUNI	SUONI UDIBILI SENZA AMPLIFICAZIONE	GRADO DI HANDICAP (SE NON TRATTATO NEL PRIMO ANNO DI VITA)	PROBABILI ESIGENZE
0-15	Range normale	Ipoacusia conduttiva	Tutti i suoni delle parole	Nessuno	Nessuna
16-25	Perdita di udito lieve	Otite media, perforazione della MT, timpanosclerosi, disfunzione della tuba di Eustachio, SNHL	I suoni vocalici vengono percepiti chiaramente; il bambino può non cogliere le consonanti sorde	Lieve disfunzione uditiva nell'apprendimento del linguaggio. Difficoltà nella percezione di alcuni suoni del linguaggio articolato	Prendere in esame la necessità di un ausilio uditivo; lettura delle parole, training uditivo Logopedia Intervento chirurgico appropriato Posti preferenziali
25-30	Modesta	Otite media, perforazione della MT, timpanosclerosi, disfunzione grave della tromba di Eustachio, SNHL	Vengono uditi solo alcuni suoni del linguaggio articolato, vocali e consonanti sonore più forti	Disfunzione dell'apprendimento uditivo Lieve ritardo del linguaggio Lievi problemi della parola Disattenzione	Ausili uditivi Lettura delle labbra Training uditivo Logopedia Intervento chirurgico appropriato
30-50	Perdita di udito moderata	Otite cronica, anomalie del canale uditivo/orecchio medio, SNHL	Il bambino non coglie la maggior parte dei suoni del linguaggio articolato al normale livello di conversazione	Problemi della parola Ritardo nel linguaggio Disfunzione dell'apprendimento Disattenzione	Tutti i precedenti; in più, valutare la possibilità di inserimento in classi speciali
50-70	Perdita di udito grave	SNHL o perdita mista dovuta alla combinazione di patologia dell'orecchio medio e coinvolgimento neurosensoriale	Non sono uditi i suoni linguaggio articolato al normale livello di conversazione	Gravi problemi della parola Ritardo del linguaggio Disfunzione dell'apprendimento Disattenzione	Tutti i precedenti, probabile assegnazione a classi speciali
70+	Perdita di udito profonda	SNHL o mista	Non sono udite né le parole né altri suoni	Gravi problemi della parola Ritardo del linguaggio Disfunzione dell'apprendimento Disattenzione	Tutti i precedenti, probabile assegnazione a classi o scuole speciali

ANSI, American National Standards Institute; SNHL, perdita di udito neurosensoriale; MT, membrana timpanica.
Modificata Da Northern JL, Downs MP: *Hearing in Children*, 4th ed. Baltimore, Williams e Wilkins.

il sesto mese di vita, sarà in grado di sviluppare lo stesso livello di linguaggio dei coetanei che non presentano alcun problema (l'unica eccezione è rappresentata dai soggetti con ipoacusia bilaterale profonda). Si tratta di un dato significativo, che spinge a mettere a punto programmi di screening uditivo per tutti i neonati. L'American Academy of Pediatrics approva l'obiettivo dello screening uditivo universale in lattanti prima del terzo mese di vita, con intervento appropriato non oltre il sesto mese. Attualmente lo screening uditivo è attivo in 32 Stati degli Stati Uniti. Finché i programmi di screening non saranno instaurati ovunque, molti ospedali continueranno a usare criteri diversi per la ricerca dei casi di ipoacusia. Per decidere quali bambini sottoporre a indagine, alcuni usano il criterio del rischio elevato (vedi Tab. 636-1), altri esaminano tutti i pazienti che richiedono terapia intensiva e infine alcuni prendono in esame entrambe le categorie precedenti. Se si utilizza il criterio del rischio elevato sorge però un problema: in questo modo il 50% dei problemi d'udito passa inosservato, perché i lattanti non rientrano in alcuno dei criteri di alto rischio, pur avendo deficit uditivi, o sviluppano problemi uditivi solo dopo il periodo neonatale.

Le tecniche di screening consigliate sono l'analisi delle emissioni otoacustiche (OAE, *OtoAcoustic Emissions*) o i potenziali evocati uditivi del tronco dell'encefalo (ABR, *Auditory Brainstem evoked Responses*). Il test ABR, una risposta uditiva evocata elettrofisiologica che si correla strettamente con l'udito, è stato utilizzato con successo per studiare neonati e identificare successivamente il grado e il tipo di ipoacusia, dando prova di un buon rapporto costo-beneficio. I test OAE, impiegati con successo nella maggior parte dei programmi di screening mondiali, oltre a essere veloci, di facile gestione e poco costosi, forniscono indicazioni sensibili su un'eventuale ipoacusia. Non sono invece consigliati metodi di screening quali l'osservazione delle risposte comportamentali a rumori-tipo non calibrati, o sistemi automatizzati come il Crib-o-gram o la risposta uditiva in culla (in cui sensori di moto registrano il movimento del neonato in risposta al suono).

Molti bambini che sviluppano problemi uditivi dopo il periodo neonatale non vengono identificati dai programmi di screening neonatale. Spesso non vengono eseguiti ulteriori test di screening prima che il soggetto sia in età prescolare o abbia cominciato a frequentare la scuola materna. Medici di base e pediatri devono prestare grande attenzione ai segni e sintomi di ipoacusia infantile, affinché i bambini con problemi d'udito che sono sfuggiti alle indagini di screening possano essere identificati quanto prima.

Identificazione dei deficit uditivi. Dato che l'impatto del difetto acustico è maggiore su un neonato che non ha ancora sviluppato il linguaggio, l'identificazione, la diagnosi, la descrizione e il trattamento devono essere cominciati il prima possibile. In generale, i neonati con anamnesi pre- o perinatale a rischio (vedi Tab. 636-1), o quelli in cui il normale screening sia risultato negativo, devono essere strettamente monitorati da un audiologo esperto fino a ottenere una valutazione affidabile della funzione uditiva. I pediatri devono incoraggiare la famiglia a collaborare con i piani di follow-up. I soggetti nati a rischio, ma non sottoposti a test subito dopo la nascita (spesso per il trasferimento da un ospedale a un altro), devono essere sottoposti a un esame audiologico al terzo mese di vita.

I soggetti con problemi d'udito nati a rischio e sottoposti a test per l'ipoacusia, nell'ambito di uno screening uditivo neonatale, rappresentano solo una parte della popolazione pediatrica con problemi uditivi. I bambini con sordità congenita a trasmissione ereditaria autosomica recessiva o con infezioni congenite subcliniche spesso non sono identificati fino al primo-terzo anno di vita. Anche se, in genere, quelli con più grave ipoacusia vengono identificati a un'età più precoce, spesso il deficit viene alla luce troppo tardi, a un'età nella quale un intervento non può più portare a esiti ottimali. I bambini con udito normale sviluppano un linguaggio esteso al terzo-quarto anno di vita (Tab. 636-6) e mostrano comportamenti che rispecchiano una normale funzione uditiva (Tab. 636-7). Se questi criteri non vengono soddisfatti, occorre procedere a una valutazione audiologica. La preoccupazione dei genitori circa l'udito e qualunque ritardo nell'acquisizione del linguaggio articolato deve mettere in allarme il pediatra, perché i familiari sono i primi ad accorgersi di queste anomalie e la loro osservazione generalmente precede l'identificazione formale e la diagnosi di problemi d'udito dal sesto mese all'anno di vita.

TABELLA 636-6. Criteri per la richiesta di valutazione audiologica

ETÀ (MESI)	LINEE GUIDA DI RIFERIMENTO PER BAMBINI CON RITARDO DELLA PAROLA
12	Assenza di glossolalia differenziata o imitazione vocale
18	Assenza dell'uso di singole parole
24	Vocabolario di parole singole con ≤10 parole
30	<100 parole; nessuna combinazione di 2 parole; incomprensibile
36	<200 parole; assenza dell'uso di frasi telegrafiche; chiarezza <50%
48	<600 parole; assenza dell'uso di semplici frasi; chiarezza ≤80%

Da Matkin ND: Early recognition and referral of hearing-impaired children. *Pediatr Rev* 1984;6:151. Per gentile concessione di *Pediatrics*.

TABELLA 636-7. Linee guida per i bambini con sospetta ipoacusia

ETÀ (MESI)	SVILUPPO NORMALE
0-4	Si deve spaventare per suoni alti, quietarsi con la voce della mamma, sospendere momentaneamente la propria attività quando si produce un suono al livello di conversazione
5-6	Deve localizzare correttamente il suono presentato in un piano orizzontale e cominciare a imitare suoni almeno vocalizzare in risposta alle parole di un adulto
7-12	Deve localizzare correttamente il suono presentato in qualsiasi piano Deve reagire quando chiamato per nome, anche con un tono di voce basso
13-15	Deve voltarsi verso la fonte di un suono inaspettato o verso oggetti familiari o persone quando richiesto
16-18	Deve seguire semplici istruzioni senza suggerimenti gestuali o visivi; con l'esercizio, può raggiungere un gioco interessante posto sulla linea mediana quando gli si presenta un suono
19-24	Deve indicare parti del corpo quando richiesto; al 21°-24° mese può essere addestrato per eseguire un gioco audiometrico

Da Matkin ND: Early recognition and referral of hearing-impaired children. *Pediatr Rev* 1984;6:151. Per gentile concessione di *Pediatrics*.

VALUTAZIONE AUDIOLOGICA CLINICA. Anche nei bambini più piccoli è possibile procedere a una valutazione della funzionalità uditiva, ogni qualvolta sorga il sospetto di una ipoacusia. Le strategie di trattamento efficace per i bambini con deficit uditivo dipendono dall'identificazione precoce e dalla valutazione continua al fine di determinare l'entità della funzione uditiva residua. La cooperazione tra il pediatra e una figura specializzata in ambiti come l'audiologia, le patologie del linguaggio, l'educazione e lo sviluppo del bambino è necessaria per ottimizzare lo sviluppo uditivo-verbale. La terapia dei difetti uditivi infantili consiste nell'applicazione di un apparecchio acustico, nel monitoraggio dell'udito e delle capacità uditive, nella consulenza a genitori e familiari, nell'informazione alle insegnanti e nei rapporti con gli enti pubblici.

Audiometria. La tecnica di valutazione audiologica varia in funzione dell'età o del grado di sviluppo del bambino, del motivo della valutazione, della condizione o dell'anamnesi otologica del paziente stesso. Un audiogramma fornisce la descrizione fondamentale della sensibilità uditiva (Fig. 636-2). Le soglie uditive sono valutate in funzione della frequenza usando toni puri (senza onde) a ottavi d'intervallo da 250-8000 Hz. Di solito si utilizzano auricolari e si valuta l'udito per ogni orecchio separatamente. Gli auricolari (o altoparlanti) trasmettono **segnali per via aerea**: in questo modo è possibile ottenere informazioni circa la sensibilità dell'apparato uditivo. Gli stessi test sonori possono essere trasmessi all'orecchio attraverso un oscillatore collocato sul capo, in genere sulla mastoide. Tali segnali si propagano attraverso l'osso, perché le ossa craniche trasmettono le vibrazioni sotto forma di energia sonora direttamente all'orecchio interno, oltrepassando l'orecchio esterno e medio. In un orecchio normale, e anche nei bambini con SNHL, le soglie della conduzione dell'aria e dell'osso sono le stesse, a differenza di quanto avviene nei soggetti con

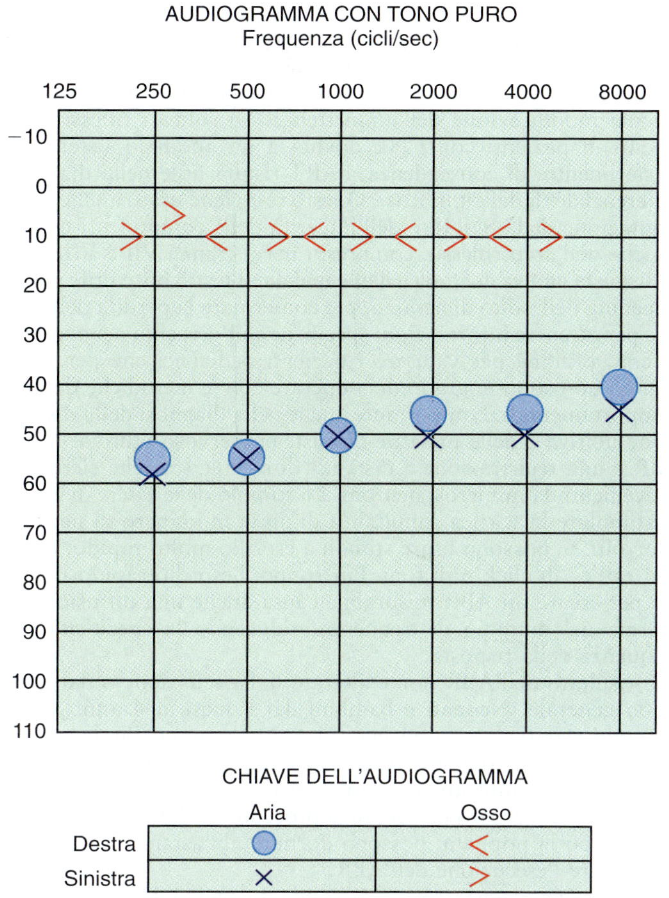

Figura 636-2. Audiogramma che rivela una ipoacusia conduttiva bilaterale. Audiogramma di tono puro

CHL. Questo fenomeno, definito **gap aria-osso**, fornisce una misura della perdita di udito, attribuibile a disfunzione dell'orecchio esterno o medio. Nell'ipoacusia mista, sono anomale le soglie di conduzione sia dell'aria sia dell'osso, con gap aria-osso.

Soglia di riconoscimento della parola. Un'altra misura utile per valutare la funzionalità uditiva è la soglia di riconoscimento della parola (SRT, *Speech Recognition Threshold*), ossia il livello più basso d'intensità a cui si ottiene un punteggio corretto per il 50%, in una prova di individuazione di vocaboli spondaici. I vocaboli spondaici sono parole bisillabe che hanno uguale accento su ogni sillaba, come baseball, hotdog e pancake. Affinché il risultato del test sia valido, gli ascoltatori devono avere familiarità con tutte le parole. La SRT deve corrispondere alla media delle soglie del tono puro a 500, 1000 e 2000 Hz, la media del tono puro (PTA, *Pure-Tone Average*). La SRT rappresenta un utile indicatore del potenziale del bambino di acquisire e usare il linguaggio articolato; serve anche per verificare la validità del risultato del test, perché nei bambini con ipoacusia di tipo non organico può essere presente una discrepanza tra PTA e SRT.

La batteria di base dei test si conclude con una valutazione della capacità del bambino di comprendere parole monosillabiche presentate a un livello di ascolto confortevole. I risultati di questo test di intelligibilità della parola aiuta nella diagnosi differenziale dei difetti uditivi e fornisce una misura della capacità uditiva del bambino, quando il linguaggio è presentato a livelli di intensità simili a quelli incontrati nell'ambiente.

Gioco audiometrico. Il test audiometrico è età-dipendente. Per bambini che corrispondono a un livello di sviluppo di 5-6 anni o più si possono utilizzare le metodiche dei test tradizionali, mentre per quelli dal trentesimo mese al quinto anno d'età si ricorre al gioco audiometrico. Le reazioni che si ottengono in genere consistono in attività motorie condizionate associate a un gioco, come far entrare dei blocchetti in una serie di buchi, infilare degli anelli su un piolo o completare un puzzle. La tecnica può essere utilizzata per ottenere un audiogramma attendibile in soggetti in età prescolare. Per quelli che non sono in grado di ripetere chiaramente le parole per la SRT e le prove di riconoscimento delle parole, si può utilizzare una serie di disegni con una risposta da indicare.

Audiometria con rinforzo visivo. Per bambini di età compresa tra il sesto e il trentesimo mese si usa comunemente l'audiometria con rinforzo visivo (VRA, *Visual reinforcement audiometry*). Questa tecnica consiste nell'osservare se l'esaminando gira la testa in risposta a uno stimolo di rinforzo rappresentato da un gioco animato (meccanico). Se i bambini sono correttamente condizionati, con opportuni suoni associati alla visione di giocattoli segnale, la VRA è in grado di stimare in modo attendibile la sensibilità uditiva per i toni e il suono delle parole. Nella maggior parte delle applicazioni della VRA, i suoni vengono trasmessi da altoparlanti in un campo sonoro, così che non si ottengono informazioni specifiche riguardo all'orecchio. Spesso si valuta un bambino piccolo per escludere un'ipoacusia che potrebbe interferire sullo sviluppo della parola e del linguaggio. I normali livelli di risposta di un bambino al campo sonoro indicano un udito sufficiente a questo scopo, nonostante sussista la possibilità che i livelli uditivi siano diversi da un orecchio all'altro.

Audiometria con osservazione del comportamento. Utilizzata come strumento di screening nei bambini di età <5 mesi, l'audiometria con osservazione del comportamento (BOA, *Behavioral Observation Audiometry*) è limitata a risposte riflesse, incondizionate, a suoni test complessi (non frequenza-specifici) come rumori, parole o musica, utilizzando segnali calibrati o un generatore di rumori non calibrati. I livelli di risposta possono variare notevolmente da un lattante all'altro e di solito non consentono di stimare in modo attendibile la sensibilità.

La valutazione di un bambino con sospetta ipoacusia non è completa finché non si eseguono una valutazione della soglia di udito del tono puro e la SRT (ossia un audiogramma attendibile) per ogni orecchio. BOA e VRA in ambiente sonoro valutano la responsività uditiva nell'orecchio che ha un udito migliore.

Valutazione dell'immittenza acustica. Questo esame standard, che rientra nella batteria di test audiologici clinici, comprende la timpanometria. Si tratta di una tecnica usata per una valutazione obiettiva che fornisca informazioni circa lo stato dell'orecchio medio. La timpanometria, che può essere eseguita in uno studio medico, semplifica la diagnosi e la gestione dell'OM con effusione, causa comune di ipoacusia da lieve a moderata nei bambini piccoli.

TIMPANOMETRIA. Con la timpanometria si ottiene un grafico che rappresenta la capacità dell'orecchio medio di trasmettere energia sonora (ammettenza, o compliance) o opporre resistenza alla trasmissione delle onde sonore (impedenza) in funzione della pressione dell'aria nel condotto uditivo esterno. Poiché la maggior parte degli strumenti della valutazione dell'immittenza acustica misurano l'ammettenza acustica, si usa il termine ammettenza. Gli stessi principi valgono a prescindere dall'unità di misura utilizzata.

Si inserisce una sonda nel condotto uditivo esterno in modo da ottenere una chiusura ermetica. La sonda provoca una variazione della pressione aerea, produce un tono e misura il livello pressorio del suono nel condotto uditivo attraverso i componenti della sonda. La pressione del suono misurata nel condotto uditivo, relativa all'intensità conosciuta del segnale della sonda, viene utilizzata per stimare l'ammettenza del condotto uditivo e del sistema dell'orecchio medio. L'ammettenza può essere espressa in un'unità chiamata millimho (mmho) o come volume d'aria (mL) con ammettenza acustica equivalente. Il test viene eseguito in modo che sia possibile stimare il volume d'aria racchiuso tra l'estremità della sonda e la MT. Per misurare l'ammettenza del solo orecchio medio, si deduce l'ammettenza acustica di questo volume di aria dalla misura totale dell'ammettenza. La stima del volume del condotto uditivo ha anche un'utilità diagnostica, perché un valore notevolmente elevato è in rapporto alla presenza di una soluzione di continuo della MT (perforazione o cannula).

Una volta sottratta l'ammettenza della massa d'aria nel condotto uditivo esterno, si suppone che la misura dell'ammettenza rimanente rispecchi accuratamente quella dell'intero sistema dell'orecchio medio. Il suo valore è ampiamente controllato dalla dinamica della MT. Anomalie della MT possono influire sulla forma del timpanogramma, ponendo in ombra anomalie mediali alla MT. Inoltre, la frequenza del tono della sonda, la velocità e la direzione del cambiamento di pressione dell'aria, e la pressione dell'aria con cui si è iniziato il timpanogramma, possono condizionare pesantemente i risultati.

Se la pressione dell'aria nel condotto uditivo è uguale a quella dell'orecchio medio, il sistema dell'orecchio medio funziona ottimamente. Quindi, la pressione del condotto uditivo che consente il maggior flusso di energia (ammettenza) deve fornire una valutazione ragionevole della pressione d'aria dell'orecchio medio. Questa pressione viene determinata trovando il punto massimo o il **picco di ammettenza** sul timpanogramma e riportandone il valore sull'asse x. Il valore sull'asse y che corrisponde al picco del timpanogramma è una stima del picco di ammettenza basato sulla timpanometria ad ammettenza (Tab. 636-8). Questa misura del picco talvolta è riferita a un'ammettenza acustica statica, anche se si pensa sia stimata in base a una misura dinamica (vedi Fig. 639-4*A*).

TIMPANOMETRIA NELL'OTITE MEDIA CON EFFUSIONE. I bambini che presentano un'OM con effusione hanno un ridotto picco di ammettenza o un picco pressorio timpanometrico negativo (vedi Fig. 639-4*C*). Tuttavia, nella diagnosi di effusione, la valutazione timpanometrica con la maggiore sensibilità e specificità riguarda la forma del timpanogramma più che il suo picco di pressione o ammettenza. Questa forma, talvolta indicata come gradiente o ampiezza timpanometrica, misura il grado di arrotondamento o l'**acutezza** del timpanogramma. Più arrotondato è il picco (o, in assenza di picco, un timpanogramma piatto), maggiore è la probabilità che sia presente un'effusione (vedi Fig. 639-4*B*). È importante conoscere lo strumento utilizzato, perché alcuni misurano automaticamente il gradiente, altri no.

TEST DEL RIFLESSO ACUSTICO. Anche il test del riflesso acustico (ART, *Acoustic Reflex Test*) fa parte della batteria dei test di immittenza. Con un orecchio medio correttamente funzionante, l'ammittenza in corrispondenza della MT cambia all'attivazione dello stapedio e dei muscoli tensori del timpano. In un orecchio sano il riflesso dello stapedio si verifica dopo l'esposizione a suoni forti. Gli strumenti di ammettenza sono progettati per presentare segnali attivanti il riflesso (toni puri di varie frequenze o rumori), sia per lo stesso orecchio sia per quello controlaterale, mentre monitorano l'ammettenza. Variazioni molto piccole dell'ammettenza, collegate da un punto di vista temporale con la presentazione del segnale, sono considerate il risultato di riflessi muscolari dell'orecchio medio. L'assenza dei cambiamenti dell'ammettenza può riscontrarsi quando l'ipoacusia è sufficiente a impedire al segnale di raggiungere l'altezza di livello necessaria per stimolare il riflesso, o quando una condizione dell'orecchio medio interferisce con la capacità dell'orecchio di monitorare una piccola modificazione dell'ammettenza. Di solito i riflessi sono assenti in pazienti con CHL dovuta a un anomalo sistema di trasferimento; di conseguenza, l'ART risulta utile nella diagnosi differenziale di deficit uditivo. Questo test viene usato anche nella valutazione della SNHL e dell'integrità delle componenti neurologiche dell'arco riflesso, compresi i nervi cranici VII e VIII.

TABELLA 636-8. Norme per il picco (statico) ammettenza (in mL) che usa una sonda di tono 226-Hz per bambini e adulti

		VELOCITA' DELLA CURVA DI PRESSIONE DELL'ARIA	
		≤50daPa/s*	200 daPa/s†
Bambini (3-5 anni)	Limite inferiore	0,30	0,36
	Medio	0,55	0,61
	Limite superiore	0,90	1,06
Adulti	Limite inferiore	0,56	0,27
	Medio	0,85	0,72
	Limite superiore	1,36	1,38

*Misurazione del volume del condotto uditivo basata sull'ammettenza al limite inferiore del timpanogramma.

†Misurazione del condotto uditivo basata sull'ammettenza al limite inferiore del timpanogramma per bambini e a +200 daPa per gli adulti.

daPa, decaPascal.

Adattata da Margolis RH, Shanks JE: Tympanometry: Basic principles of clinical application. In Rintelman WS (ed): *Hearing Assessment*, 2nd ed. Austin, TX, PRODED, 1991, pp. 179-245.

Risposta uditiva del tronco dell'encefalo. Il test ABR è utile per lo screening dell'udito di neonati, per confermare la perdita dell'udito e per ottenere informazioni specifiche sull'orecchio nei bambini piccoli, e infine per valutare i pazienti pediatrici che per varie ragioni non sono in grado di cooperare con le metodiche dei test comportamentali. È importante anche nella diagnosi della disfunzione uditiva e delle malattie del sistema nervoso uditivo. Il test ABR è una registrazione a distanza di piccole scariche elettriche provenienti da numerosi neuroni. Lo stimolo deve essere in grado di stimolare la scarica simultanea di un gran numero di neuroni coinvolti. Si possono usare stimoli a esordio molto rapido, come una raffica di click o di toni. Purtroppo, l'esordio rapido richiesto per creare un ABR misurabile causa anche una diffusione di energia nel dominio di frequenza, riducendo la specificità per frequenza della risposta.

Il risultato dell'ABR non è alterato dalla sedazione o dall'anestesia generale. Neonati e bambini dai 4 mesi ai 4 anni di età vengono sedati di routine per ridurre al minimo l'interferenza elettrica causata dall'attività muscolare durante il test. L'ABR può essere eseguito anche in sala operatoria su un paziente pediatrico anestetizzato per un'altra procedura. I lattanti di età <4 mesi, dopo la poppata, possono dormire abbastanza a lungo da permettere l'esecuzione dell'ABR.

L'ABR viene registrato con 5-7 onde. Le onde I, III e V possono essere ottenute in tutti i gruppi di età; le onde II e IV appaiono invece con minore frequenza. La latenza di ogni onda (tempo che precede il picco dell'onda dopo l'inizio dello stimolo) aumenta, e l'ampiezza diminuisce con la riduzione dell'intensità o altezza dello stimolo. La latenza diminuisce anche con l'aumentare dell'età; le onde più precoci, rispetto a quelle più tardive, raggiungono valori di latenza quando il paziente ha un'età molto inferiore.

Il test ABR ha due usi principali in pediatria: come test audiometrico, fornisce informazioni sulla capacità del sistema uditivo periferico di trasmettere informazioni al nervo acustico e oltre. Trova impiego anche nella diagnosi differenziale o nel monitoraggio della patologia del sistema nervoso centrale. Per l'audiometria, l'obiettivo è trovare la minima intensità di stimolo che provochi un ABR osservabile. Il rapporto tra l'intensità per varie onde serve anche per la diagnosi differenziale dei deficit uditivi. Un importante vantaggio della valutazione uditiva con il test ABR è che le stime della soglia specifica per l'orecchio possono essere ottenute su neonati o pazienti difficili da esaminare. Le soglie di ABR usando stimoli click si correlano meglio con il comportamento delle soglie uditive alle frequenze più alte (1000-4000 Hz); la responsività a basse frequenze richiede stimoli differenti (raffica di toni o click filtrati) o l'uso di mascheramenti, nessuno delle quali individua la regione di bassa frequenza della coclea in tutti i casi, e questo può influire sull'interpretazione.

Il test ABR non può valutare "l'udito". Esso riflette le risposte elettriche uditive dei neuroni che possono essere correlate al comportamento delle soglie uditive, ma un risultato normale di questo test suggerisce solo che il sistema uditivo, oltre il livello del tronco dell'encefalo, è responsivo allo stimolo utilizzato. Al contrario, un fallimento della risposta all'ABR indica un'alterazione della risposta sincrona del sistema, ma non comporta necessariamente una sordità. La risposta comportamentale al suono talvolta è normale quando non può essere evocato l'ABR, come nelle patologie neurologiche demielinizzanti. Il test ABR può essere usato per dedurre se e a quale livello esiste un difetto del sistema uditivo. Le perdite d'udito improvvise, progressive o unilaterali sono indicazioni per il test ABR. Sebbene si creda che le differenti onde dell'ABR riflettano l'attività in aumento dei livelli rostrali del sistema uditivo, i generatori neuronali della risposta non sono stati determinati in modo preciso. Ogni onda ABR oltre le onde più precoci probabilmente è il risultato di una serie di emissioni a molti livelli del sistema, e ogni livello del sistema probabilmente contribuisce a parecchie onde ABR. Stimoli con click ad alta intensità hanno un'applicazione neurologica. La morfologia della risposta dell'onda e delle latenze tra le onde vengono esaminate confrontandole con quadri conformi per l'età. La mancanza di onde ABR o un loro ritardo spesso hanno un significato diagnostico.

L'ABR e altre risposte elettriche sono estremamente complesse e difficili da interpretare. Sulla qualità della registrazione può influire una serie di fattori, tra cui il tipo di strumentazione, il setting, l'ambiente, il grado e la configurazione dell'ipoacusia e le caratteristiche del paziente. Quindi, il test e l'interpretazione dell'attività elettrofisiologia devono essere affidati a un audiologo qualificato, per evitare il rischio che conclusioni non attendibili o errate possano influire sulle decisioni terapeutiche.

Emissioni otoacustiche. In presenza di udito normale, le OAE originano dalle cellule ciliate della coclea e sono rilevabili tramite processi di amplificazione sensibile. Esse viaggiano dalla coclea attraverso l'orecchio medio fino al condotto uditivo esterno, dove possono essere rilevate usando microfoni miniaturizzati. Le OAE evocate transitorie (TEOAE, *Transient Evoked OAE*) possono essere utili per studiare l'integrità della coclea. Nel periodo neonatale è possibile rilevare OAE durante il sonno naturale, e le TEOAE possono essere utilizzate come screening per l'udito nei neonati e nei bambini, per ipoacusie intorno ai 30 dB. Esse richiedono meno tempo e sono meno complesse rispetto all'ABR e, nei bambini piccoli, sono più sensibili dei test comportamentali. Le TEOAE sono ridotte o assenti in presenza di varie disfunzioni dell'orecchio medio e interno. Sono assenti in pazienti con perdita di udito oltre i 30 dB e non sono utilizzate per determinare la soglia uditiva; inoltre, esse consentono di esaminare se è presente udito a più di 30-40 dB. Malattie come l'OM o anomalie congenite delle strutture dell'orecchio medio riducono la trasmissione delle TEOAE e possono erroneamente indicare una patologia cocleare. Se l'assenza di OAE induce a sospettare una perdita d'udito, prima si devono esaminare le orecchie alla ricerca di patologie evidenti, poi si deve eseguire il test ABR per confermare e identificare il tipo, il grado e la lateralità dell'ipoacusia.

Reflettometria acustica. La reflettometria acustica consiste nel collocare uno strumento a impugnatura manuale vicino all'apertura del condotto uditivo emettendo un suono di 80 dB a una frequenza variabile da 2000 a 4500 Hz, in un periodo di 100 ms. Lo strumento misura il livello totale di suono riflesso e trasmesso; alcuni medici lo trovano utile per misurare la presenza o l'assenza di liquido nell'orecchio medio; ne viene commercializzata anche una versione commerciale con la quale i genitori stessi possono tenere sotto controllo i liquidi nell'orecchio. Lo strumento non fornisce alcuna informazione circa l'udito; la presenza cronica di liquido deve spingere a eseguire una valutazione audiometrica.

TRATTAMENTO. In molte aree degli Stati Uniti lo screening uditivo ha reso comune la diagnosi precoce e il trattamento dei bambini con ipoacusia. La valutazione del grado di ipoacusia è possibile anche in bambini molto piccoli, e deve essere eseguita se un genitore sospetta questo problema. Tutti i bambini con un fattore noto di rischio per perdita di udito dovrebbero essere valutati tra il primo e il sesto mese di vita.

È necessario valutare il linguaggio dal momento in cui viene identificata un'ipoacusia per l'intero arco dello sviluppo. In tutti gli stadi della valutazione e del trattamento o della riabilitazione, sono richiesti la consulenza ai genitori e il loro coinvolgimento. Una sordità conduttiva spesso può essere corretta mediante il trattamento di un'effusione dell'orecchio medio (per es. posizionamento di un drenaggio timpanostomico nell'orecchio) o la correzione chirurgica dell'anomalo meccanismo di conduzione del suono. Nei bambini con SNHL un audiologo pediatrico deve valutare l'opportunità di ricorrere a un apparecchio acustico. Alcuni modelli possono essere adatti anche a lattanti al secondo mese. Lo screening dell'udito in Colorado ha dimostrato che l'identificazione e l'amplificazione prima del sesto mese di vita è molto importante ai fini dell'acquisizione del linguaggio articolato. In questi bambini, è necessario ripetere i test audiologici per identificare in modo attendibile il grado della perdita d'udito e per mettere a punto in modo ottimale l'uso di apparecchi acustici.

Neonati e bambini con ipoacusia congenita o a esordio precoce, prima dell'acquisizione del linguaggio, traggono beneficio dagli **impianti cocleari multicanale** (Fig. 636-3); tali strumenti oltrepassano la lesione dell'organo del Corti e consentono una stimolazione neuronale con un microfono esterno e un processore di segnali che trasforma lo stimolo uditivo in impulsi di radiofrequenza digitali. L'impianto cocleare prima dei 2 anni (e anche di 1 anno) migliora l'udito e il linguaggio, permettendo a più del 90% dei bambini di ricevere un'educazione tradizionale. La maggior parte sviluppa una percezione uditiva adeguata all'età e la capacità di articolare il linguaggio.

Una seria complicanza degli impianti cocleari è una frequenza eccessivamente alta di meningite meningococcica. Tutti i pazienti pediatrici che ricevono un impianto cocleare devono essere vaccinati con il vaccino PCV-7 (Tab. 636-9).

Quale sia l'approccio migliore per l'educazione dei bambini con ipoacusia significativa è ancora oggetto di dibattito. Dato che quello attuale è un mondo dominato dalla parola, alcuni hanno sostenuto un approccio puramente uditivo e orale alla terapia dell'udito. Tuttavia, dato che i bambini colpiti spesso sono lenti nello sviluppo delle capacità comunicative, molti sono i fautori di un approccio totale, basato sulla comunicazione; a seconda delle necessità individuali del bambino, questa tecnica

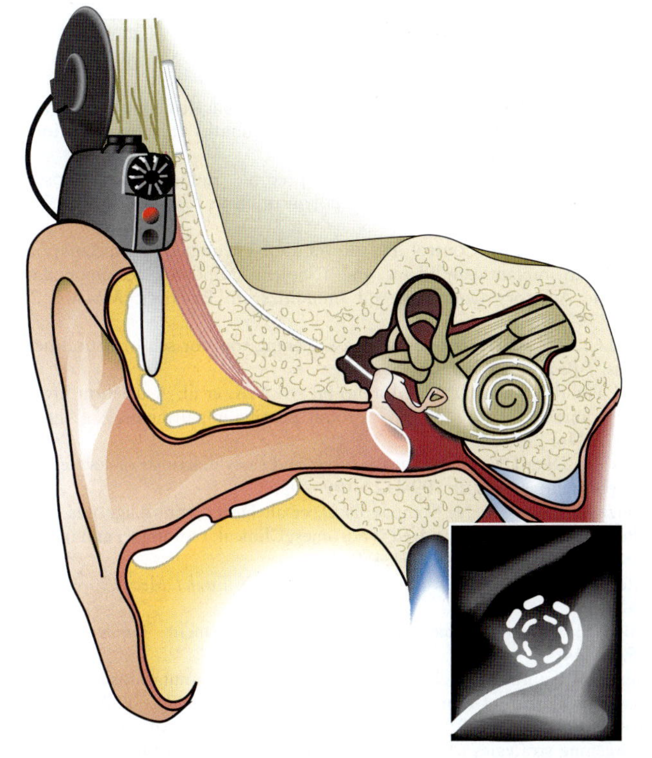

Figura 636-3. Tutti gli impianti cocleari hanno gli stessi componenti chiave: microfono, processore di parola e bobina di trasmissione, visibili in posizione retroauricolare in questo diagramma. Il microfono/processore di parola migliora i suoni ambientali e li digitalizza in segnali codificati. I segnali sono inviati alla bobina di trasmissione e inoltrati attraverso la cute all'apparecchio interno, impiantato nel cranio. Tale apparecchio a sua volta converte il codice in segnali elettronici, che vengono trasmessi attraverso il filo porta-elettrodi intorno alla coclea. Il riquadro mostra l'immagine radiografica del filo stimolatore porta-elettrodi. Riprodotta per gentile concessione di MED-EL Corporation, Innsbruck, Austria. (Da Smith RJH, Bale JF, Withe KR: Sensorineural hearing loss in children. *Lancet* 2005; 365:879-890.)

TABELLA 636-9. Programma di vaccinazione antipneumococcica per soggetti con impianti cocleari

ETÀ ALLA PRIMA DOSE DI PCV7 (MESI)*	SERIE PRIMARIE DI PCV7	DOSE ADDIZIONALE DI PCV7	DOSE DI PCV7
2-6	3 dosi, a partire dal 2° mese[†]	1 dose al 12°-15° mese di vita[‡]	Indicato a >24° mese di vita[§]
7-11	2 dosi, a partire dal 2° mese[†]	1 dose a partire dal 12°-15° mese di vita[‡]	Indicato a >24° mese di vita[§]
12-23	2 dosi, a partire dal 2° mese[**]	Non indicato	Indicato a >24° medi vita[§]
24-59	2 dosi, a partire dal 2° mese[**]	Non indicato	Indicato[§]
≥60	Non indicato[***]	Non indicato[***]	Indicato

*Un programma con un numero ridotto di dosi di vaccino coniugato pneumococcico totale eptavalente (PCV7) è indicato se il vaccino viene somministrato tardi o se la vaccinazione è incompleta. I bambini che hanno saltato una tappa della vaccinazione devono essere vaccinati in accordo alla ripresa del programma (CDC. Pneumococcal coniugate vaccine shortage resolved. *MMWR* 2003;52:446-447.)

[†]Per bambini vaccinati all'età di <1 anno, l'intervallo minimo fra le dosi è di 4 settimane.

[‡]La dose addizionale deve essere somministrata ≥8 settimane dopo che è stata completata la prima serie.

[§]Bambini di età <5 anni devono completare la prima serie di PCV7; si deve somministrare il vaccino pneumococcico polisaccaridico 23-valente (PPV23) a bambini >24 mesi a distanza di >8 settimane dall'ultima dose di PCV7 (CDC. Preventing pneumococcal desease among infants and young children: Reccomendations of the Advisory Committee on Immunization Practices. *MMWR* 2000;49 (No.RR-9).

[**]L'intervallo minimo fra le dosi è di 8 settimane.

[***]Generalmente il PCV7 non è raccomandato per bambini di età ≥5 anni.

Da Pneumoccocal Vaccination for cochlear implant candidates and recipients: Updated reccomendations of the Advisory Committee on Immunization Practices. *MMWR* 2003;52:739-740.

usa un approccio misto, che si avvale del linguaggio gestuale, dell'interpretazione dei movimenti labiali, dell'uso di apparecchi acustici e della parola. Il programma più adatto per ogni bambino dipende dal paziente, dalla famiglia di provenienza e dalle risorse a disposizione.

Counseling genetico. I familiari di bambini in cui è stata diagnosticata una SNHL, o una sindrome associata a SNHL e/o CHL, dovrebbero prendere in considerazione una consulenza genetica, durante la quale si affronta l'argomento della probabilità che tale problema si ripresenti nelle gravidanze successive. Il genetista può aiutare anche a stabilire la diagnosi.

Barsky-Firkser L, Sun S: Universal newborn hearing screenings: A three-year experience. *Pediatrics* 1997;99:1.

Ben-Yousef T, Ness SL, Madeo AC, et al: A mutation of *PCDH15* among Ashkenazi Jews with the type 1 Usher syndrome. *N Engl J Med* 2003; 348:1664–1670.

Biernath KR, Reefhuis J, Whitney CG, et al: Bacterial meningitis among children with cochlear implants beyond 24 months after implantation. *Pediatrics* 2006;117:284–289.

Capaccio P, Ottaviani F, Cuccarini V, et al: Sudden hearing loss and MTHFR 677C>T/1298A>C gene polymorphisms. *Genet Med* 2005;7:206–208.

Centers for Disease Control and Prevention: Pneumococcal vaccination for cochlear implant candidates and recipients: Updated recommendations of the Advisory Committee on Immunization Practices. *MMWR* 2003; 52:739–740.

Cox LC: Otoacoustic emissions as a screening tool for sensorineural hearing loss. *J Pediatr* 1997;130:685–686.

Del Castillo I, Villamar M, Moreno-Pelayo MA, et al: A deletion involving the connexin 30 gene in nonsyndromic hearing impairments. *N Engl J Med* 2002;346: 243–249.

Eilers RE, Oller DK: Infant vocalizations and early diagnosis of severe hearing impairment. *J Pediatr* 1994;124:199–203.

Fugazzola L, Cerutti N, Mannavola D, et al: Differential diagnoses between Pendred and pseudo-Pendred syndromes: Clinical, radiologic, and molecular studies. *Pediatr Res* 2002;51:479–484.

Gates GA, Miyamoto RT: Cochlear implants. *N Engl J Med* 2003;349:421–423.

Grote JJ: Neonatal screening for hearing impairment. *Lancet* 2000;355: 513–514.

Hinson JT, Fantin VR, Schönberger J, et al: Missense mutations in the BCS1L gene as a cause of Björnstad syndrome. *N Engl J Med* 2007;356:809–819.

Kemper AR, Downs SM: A cost-effectiveness analysis of newborn hearing screening strategies. *Arch Pediatr Adolesc Med* 2000;154:484.

Kennedy C, McCann D, Campbell MJ, et al: Universal newborn screening for permanent childhood hearing impairment: An 8 year follow up of a controlled trial. *Lancet* 2005;366:660–662.

Mason JA, Herrmann KR: Universal infant hearing screening by automated auditory brainstem response measurement. *Pediatrics* 1998;101:221–228.

Moeller MP: Early intervention and language development in children who are deaf and hard of hearing. *Pediatrics* 2000;106:E43.

Morell RJ, Kim HJ, Hood LJ, et al: Mutations in the connexin 26 gene (GJB2) among Ashkenazi Jews with nonsyndromic recessive deafness. *N Engl J Med* 1998;339:1500–1505.

Morton CC, Nance WE: Newborn hearing screening—a silent revolution. *N Engl J Med* 2006;354:2151–2164.

Nikolopoulos TP, Archbold SM, O'Donoghue GM: Does cause of deafness influence outcome after cochlear implantation in children? *Pediatrics* 2006;118:1350–1356.

Nikolopoulos TP, Dyar D, Archbold S, et al: Development of spoken language grammar following cochlear implantation in perlingually deaf children. *Arch Otolaryngol Head Neck Surg* 2004;130:629–633.

Niskar AS, Kieszak SM, Holmes A, et al: Prevalence of hearing loss among children 6 to 19 years of age. *JAMA* 1998;279:1071–1075.

Pirozzo S, Papinczak T, Glasziou P: Whispered voice test for screening for hearing impairment in adults and children: systematic review. *BMJ* 2003; 327:967–970.

Ramsden RT: Prognosis after cochlear implantation. *BMJ* 2004;328:419–420.

Reefhuis J, Honein MA, Whitney CG, et al: Risk of bacterial meningitis in children with cochlear implants. *N Engl J Med* 2003;349:435–445.

Schultz JM, Yang Y, Caride AJ, et al: Modification of human hearing loss by plasma-membrane calcium pump PMCA2. *N Engl J Med* 2005;352: 1557–1564.

Smith RJH: Deafness: from bedside to bench and back. *Lancet* 2002;360: 656–657.

Smith RJH, Bale JF Jr, White KR: Sensorineural hearing loss in children. *Lancet* 2005; 365:879–890.

Thomas MA, Der Kaloustian VM, Tewfik TL: Connexin mutation testing of children with nonsyndromic, autosomal recessive sensorineural hearing loss. *J Otolaryngol* 2004;33:189–192.

Thompson DC, McPhillips H, Davis RL, et al: Universal newborn hearing screening: Summary of evidence. *JAMA* 2001;286:2000–2010.

Waltzman SB, Roland T Jr: Cochlear implantation in children younger than 12 months. *Pediatrics* 2005;16:487–493.

Willems PJ: Genetic causes of hearing loss. *N Engl J Med* 2000;342:1101.

Wilson C, Roberts A, Stephens D: Aetiological investigation of sensorineural hearing loss in children. *Arch Dis Child* 205;90:307–309.

Wolf B, Spencer R, Gleason T: Hearing loss is a common feature of symptomatic children with profound biotinidase deficiency. *Pediatrics* 2002;140:242–246.

Yoshinaga-Itano C, Sedey AL, Coulter DK, et al: Language of early- and later-identified children with hearing loss. *Pediatrics* 1998;102:1161–1171.

Capitolo 637 ■ Malformazioni congenite

Joseph Haddad Jr.

L'orecchio esterno e medio, che derivano dal primo e dal secondo arco e solco branchiale, continuano a crescere durante la pubertà, mentre l'orecchio interno, che si sviluppa dall'otocisti, raggiunge le dimensioni e la forma tipiche dell'età adulta già nelle fasi intermedie dello sviluppo fetale. Gli ossicini derivano dal primo e dal secondo arco (martello e incudine), mentre la staffa proviene dal secondo arco e dalla capsula otica. Il martello e l'incudine raggiungono le dimensioni e la forma adulte alla 15ª settimana di gestazione, la staffa alla 18ª. Sebbene il padiglione auricolare, il condotto uditivo e la membrana timpanica (MT) continuino a crescere dopo la nascita, le anomalie congenite di queste strutture si sviluppano durante la prima metà della gestazione. Le malformazioni dell'orecchio esterno e medio possono essere associate a una serie di anomalie renali, a disostosi mandibolofacciale, microsomia emifacciale e altre malformazioni craniofacciali. Le anomalie del nervo facciale possono essere associate a ciascuna delle alterazioni congenite dell'orecchio e dell'osso temporale; le malformazioni dell'orecchio esterno e medio possono anche essere associate ad anomalie dell'orecchio interno e a ipoacusia sia conduttiva (CHL, *Conductive Hearing Loss*) sia neurosensoriale (SNHL, *SensoriNeural Hearing Loss*).

Le malattie congenite dell'orecchio possono essere lievi e di significato soprattutto estetico, oppure gravi, quando coinvolgono sia l'estetica sia la funzione. Tutti i bambini nati con una malformazione del padiglione auricolare, del condotto uditivo esterno o della MT devono essere sottoposti a una completa valutazione audiologica nel periodo neonatale. Per la valutazione e il trattamento sono necessari studi morfologici; nel paziente con altre anomalie craniofacciali un approccio multidisciplinare con altri specialisti può aiutare nella conduzione della terapia.

MALFORMAZIONI DEL PADIGLIONE AURICOLARE. Le gravi malformazioni dell'orecchio esterno sono rare, a differenza delle deformità minori, che sono invece frequenti. In circa l'1% dei bambini si verificano anomalie isolate dell'orecchio esterno. Una depressione simile a una fossa davanti all'elice e sopra il trago può rappresentare una cisti o un tratto fistoloso sottoepidermico. Queste patologie sono comuni, con una frequenza di circa 8/1000 bambini, e possono essere unilaterali, bilaterali e familiari. Le cisti richiedono la rimozione chirurgica solo se soggette a infezioni ricorrenti. I lembi cutanei accessori, che hanno un'incidenza di 1-2/1000, possono essere rimossi per ragioni estetiche con la semplice legatura, se attaccati con un peduncolo sottile; se però il peduncolo ha una base ampia o contiene cartilagine, il difetto deve essere asportato chirurgicamente. Un orecchio insolitamente prominente o "a pipistrello" dipende dalla mancanza della piega di cartilagine che forma l'anti elice; un miglioramento estetico è ottenibile nel periodo neonatale grazie all'applicazione di una struttura rigida (talvolta vengono usati fili metallici da saldatura) attaccata con suture cutanee adesive al padiglione e portata giorno e notte, per un periodo variabile da qualche settimana ad alcuni mesi. Una correzione estetica con otoplastica può essere presa in considerazione in bambini di età >5 anni, quando il padiglione ha raggiunto circa l'80% delle dimensioni adulte.

Il termine **microtia** può indicare lievi anomalie di dimensione, forma e localizzazione del padiglione auricolare e del condotto uditivo, o alterazioni più gravi, con solo piccole sporgenze della cute e della cartilagine e assenza dell'apertura del condotto uditivo; **anotia** indica invece l'assenza completa del padiglione auricolare e del condotto uditivo. In presenza di microtia le orecchie spesso hanno un'attaccatura più anteriore e più bassa rispetto alla norma, e la localizzazione e la funzione del nervo facciale può essere anomala. La chirurgia per la correzione della microtia viene presa in considerazione per ragioni sia estetiche sia funzionali; i bambini che possiedono parte del padiglione auricolare possono indossare occhiali normali, un apparecchio acustico e sentirsi di aspetto più normale. Se la microtia è grave, alcuni pazienti possono optare per la creazione e l'attacco di un orecchio protesico, che da un punto di vista estetico assomiglia molto a un orecchio vero. La correzione chirurgica di una microtia grave può richiedere una procedura in più fasi, fra cui il prelievo e il trapianto di cartilagine autogena di provenienza costale, e lembi locali di tessuto molle. La ricostruzione estetica dell'orecchio di solito si esegue tra i 5 e i 7 anni, nei soggetti ritenuti adatti a questo intervento, ed è preceduta dalla riparazione dell'atresia canalare.

STENOSI CONGENITA O ATRESIA DEL CONDOTTO UDITIVO ESTERNO. La stenosi o l'atresia del condotto uditivo spesso compaiono in associazione a malformazioni del padiglione auricolare e dell'orecchio medio; stenosi minori si possono verificare in forma isolata. In alcune sindromi genetiche, per esempio la trisomia 21, il condotto uditivo è stretto. Questi bambini devono essere sottoposti a una valutazione audiometrica il più precocemente possibile. La maggior parte dei bambini con CHL significativa secondaria ad atresia bilaterale porta apparecchi acustici a conduzione ossea per i primi anni di vita. La diagnosi, la valutazione e il piano chirurgico spesso richiedono l'ausilio della TC e talvolta della RM dell'osso temporale. Stenosi lievi del condotto uditivo non richiedono un intervento chirurgico, a meno che il paziente non sviluppi un'otite cronica esterna o un grave tappo di cerume, in grado di alterare l'udito.

Solitamente si prende in considerazione l'intervento di chirurgia ricostruttiva del condotto uditivo e dell'orecchio medio per atresia, in bambini con più di 5 anni che presentano deformità bilaterali con CHL significativa. L'obiettivo della chirurgia ricostruttiva è migliorare l'udito in modo da rendere inutile l'apparecchio acustico, oppure creare un condotto uditivo e un padiglione auricolare così che il bambino possa trarre un ulteriore beneficio da un apparecchio acustico a conduzione aerea. Per l'esecuzione dell'intervento chirurgico è richiesta la dimostrazione tomografica di una fessura adeguata dell'orecchio medio, degli ossicini e della mastoide; occorre inoltre considerare la posizione del nervo facciale, che spesso in questi soggetti si trova in sede anomala. In alcuni casi, durante la crescita, una possibile alternativa è l'uso di un apparecchio acustico ancorato all'osso (BAHA, *Bone-Anchored Hearing Aids*).

MALFORMAZIONI CONGENITE DELL'ORECCHIO MEDIO. I bambini possono avere malformazioni congenite dell'orecchio medio come difetto isolato o in associazione con altre alterazioni dell'osso temporale, specialmente del condotto uditivo e del padiglione auricolare, nell'ambito di una sindrome. I bambini interessati di solito presentano CHL, ma possono anche avere una forma mista con CHL e SNHL. La maggior parte delle malformazioni coinvolge gli ossicini, in particolare l'incudine. Altre anomalie meno comuni comprendono la persistenza dell'arteria stapedia, un bulbo giugulare "alto" e anomalie della forma e del volume della porzione aerata dell'orecchio medio e della mastoide; tutti presentano problemi di tipo chirurgico. A seconda del tipo di anomalia e della presenza di altre malformazioni, si può prendere in esame l'intervento chirurgico per migliorare l'udito.

MALFORMAZIONI CONGENITE DELL'ORECCHIO INTERNO. Le malformazioni congenite dell'orecchio interno sono state identificate e classificate grazie al miglioramento della diagnostica per immagini, specialmente TC e RM. Il 20% dei bambini con SNHL di vario grado ha anomalie anatomiche che vengono identificate con la TC e la RM. Le malformazioni congenite dell'orecchio interno solitamente sono associate a SNHL di vario grado, da lieve a profonda. Queste malformazioni possono presentarsi come anomalie isolate o in associazione con altre sindromi, anomalie genetiche o anomalie strutturali del capo e del collo. La diagnostica per immagine ha permesso di identificare, in associazione a SNHL, un allargamento degli acquedotti vestibolari; sebbene non esista una terapia per questa condizione, dal momento che in alcuni bambini essa può essere associata a SNHL progressiva, la diagnosi può avere un qualche valore prognostico.

La **fistola perilinfatica congenita** (**PLF**, *PeriLymphatic Fistula*) della membrana della finestra rotonda o ovale si può presentare come una SNHL a esordio rapido, fluttuante o progressiva, con o senza vertigini, e spesso si associa ad anomalie congenite dell'orecchio interno. Può essere richiesta l'esplorazione dell'orecchio medio per confermare questa diagnosi, perché non esiste un test diagnostico non invasivo che sia davvero affidabile. Può essere necessario riparare una PLF per prevenire la possibile diffusione di un'infezione dall'orecchio medio al labirinto, per stabilizzare l'ipoacusia e per attenuare il senso di vertigine, quando presente.

COLESTEATOMA CONGENITO. Un colesteatoma congenito appare solitamente come una struttura simil-cistica, biancastra, rotondeggiante, mediale rispetto a una MT intatta. Le cisti si osservano più frequentemente nella porzione anterosuperiore dell'orecchio medio, sebbene possano comparire anche in altre sedi, oltre che nella MT o nella cute del condotto uditivo. I bambini colpiti spesso non hanno un'anamnesi precedente di otite media (OM). Secondo una teoria patogenetica la cisti deriverebbe da un residuo congenito di tessuto epiteliale che persiste oltre la 33ª settimana di gestazione, quando normalmente scompare. Altre teorie la attribuiscono invece a metaplasia squamosa dell'orecchio medio, all'ingresso nell'orecchio medio di epitelio squamoso attraverso una lesione della membrana timpanica, a impianti ectodermici tra i residui del primo e del secondo arco branchiale, e a residui di detriti squamosi del liquido amniotico. Un colesteatoma, acquisito o congenito, va sospettato in presenza di sacche di retrazione profonda, detriti cheratinici, drenaggio cronico, tessuto di granulazione auricolare, oppure una massa posteriore o coinvolgente la MT. Oltre al fatto che si comporta come un tumore benigno, causando distruzione ossea locale, i detriti cheratinici del colesteatoma rappresentano un buon mezzo di coltura e possono diventare un focolaio infettivo di OM cronica. Le complicanze comprendono erosione della catena degli ossicini, caratterizzata da ipoacusia, erosione ossea dell'orecchio interno con vertigini o esposizione della dura madre, con conseguente meningite o ascesso cerebrale. Il colesteatoma deve essere rimosso chirurgicamente dopo l'esecuzione di una TC e una valutazione dell'udito, e l'appropriata terapia antibiotica. Poiché la forma congenita è una malattia aggressiva, la precoce rimozione chirurgica e uno stretto monitoraggio possono aiutare a prevenire un danno permanente a carico dell'orecchio medio e interno.

Capitolo 638 ■ Otite esterna

Joseph Haddad Jr.

In un lattante i due terzi esterni del condotto uditivo sono cartilaginei e il terzo interno è osseo, mentre in un bambino più grande e in un adulto solo il terzo esterno è cartilagineo. Nella porzione ossea, rispetto a quella cartilaginea, l'epitelio, oltre a essere più sottile, è saldamente ancorato al sottostante periostio e manca il tessuto sottocutaneo; follicoli piliferi, ghiandole sebacee e ghiandole apocrine sono scarsi o assenti. La cute dell'area cartilaginea, che presenta invece un derma e un tessuto sottocutaneo ben sviluppati, contiene follicoli piliferi, ghiandole sebacee e ghiandole apocrine. Le secrezioni altamente viscide delle ghiandole sebacee e le secrezioni acquose, pigmentate delle ghiandole apocrine presenti nella parte esterna del condotto si combinano con le cellule superficiali esfoliate della cute a formare il **cerume**, una sostanza protettiva, cerosa, idrorepellente.

La normale flora del condotto esterno è formata principalmente da batteri aerobi e include stafilococchi coagulasi-negativi, *Corynebacterium* (difteroidi), *Micrococcus*, talvolta anche *Staphylococcus aureus*, *Streptococcus viridans* e *Pseudomonas aeruginosa*. L'umidità eccessiva (piscina, bagni, aumento dell'umidità ambientale), la secchezza locale dovuta a un'insufficiente secrezione di cerume, la presenza di altre patologie cutanee (pregressa infezione, eczema o altre forme di dermatite) e i traumi (digitali, da corpo estraneo, da bastoncini di cotone) rendono la cute del condotto vulnerabile all'infezione da parte della normale flora o di batteri esogeni.

EZIOLOGIA. L'otite esterna (detta **orecchio del nuotatore**, sebbene si possa verificare anche in chi non nuota) è per lo più causata da *P. aeruginosa*, ma possono essere isolati anche *S. aureus*, *Enterobacter aerogenes*, *Proteus mirabilis*, *Klebsiella pneumoniae*, streptococco, stafilococco coagulasi-negativo, difteroide e miceti come la *Candida* e l'*Aspergillus*. L'otite esterna è causata da irritazione cronica e macerazione del condotto da umidità eccessiva. Può giocare un ruolo la perdita del cerume protettivo, ma anche un tappo di cerume che intrappola l'acqua all'interno del condotto uditivo può causare infezione. Infine, possono predisporre all'otite esterna anche l'infiammazione del condotto uditivo da herpesvirus o virus varicella-zoster, altri esantemi cutanei e l'eczema.

MANIFESTAZIONI CLINICHE. Il sintomo predominante è il dolore auricolare acuto, spesso grave, accentuato dalla manipolazione del padiglione auricolare o dalla pressione esercitata sul trago. Il dolore e la sensibilità possono essere sproporzionati al grado d'infiammazione, perché la cute del condotto uditivo esterno è strettamente aderente al sottostante pericondrio e periostio. Il prurito spesso precede il dolore e solitamente è caratteristico dell'infiammazione cronica del condotto o di otite esterna acuta in via di risoluzione. L'ipoacusia conduttiva può dipendere dall'edema della cute e della membrana timpanica (MT), da secrezioni sierose o purulente, oppure dall'ispessimento della cute del condotto associata a otite esterna cronica.

Edema del condotto uditivo, eritema e otorrea densa sono segni evidenti di malattia acuta. Il cerume solitamente è bianco e di consistenza morbida, mentre in condizioni normali è giallastro di consistenza più pastosa. Spesso il canale è così dolorante ed edematoso che non è possibile visualizzare adeguatamente l'intero condotto uditivo e la membrana timpanica e si deve attendere la scomparsa dell'edema acuto per l'esecuzione di un esame otoscopio completo. Se si può visualizzare la MT, essa appare normale o opaca. In risposta a una pressione negativa o positiva, la MT può avere una mobilità normale o, se ispessita, ridotta.

Altri reperti fisici possono comprendere linfonodi palpabili e doloranti nella regione periauricolare, oltre a eritema ed edema del padiglione auricolare e della cute periauricolare. È raro che si manifestino paralisi facciale o anomalie di altri nervi cranici, vertigini e/o ipoacusia neurosensoriale; se si verificano queste evenienze, è probabile un'**otite esterna necrotizzante (maligna)**. L'infezione invasiva dell'osso temporale e della base cranica richiede una coltura immediata, antibiotici per via endovenosa e indagini per immagini per valutare l'estensione della malattia. Può rendersi necessario l'intervento chirurgico per ottenere colture o eliminare il tessuto devitalizzato. *P. aeruginosa* è il microrganismo più frequentemente responsabile dell'otite esterna necrotizzante. Fortunatamente, si tratta di una malattia rara nell'infanzia, osservabile solo in associazione a immunosoppressione o malnutrizione grave. Negli adulti è associata a diabete mellito.

DIAGNOSI. L'otite esterna diffusa può essere confusa con la foruncolosi, l'**otite media (OM)** e la mastoidite. I **foruncoli** compaiono nella parte laterale, dotata di follicoli piliferi, del condotto uditivo. La foruncolosi di solito causa una tumefazione localizzata del condotto limitata a un quadrante, mentre l'otite esterna è associata a tumefazione concentrica e coinvolge l'intero condotto uditivo. Nell'OM, la MT può essere perforata, gravemente retratta o sporgente e immobile; di solito si riscontrano alterazioni dell'udito. Se l'orecchio medio drena attraverso una perforazione della MT o un tubo da timpanostomia, si può verificare un'otite esterna secondaria; se la MT non è visibile per drenaggio o tumefazione del condotto uditivo, è difficile distinguere l'OM acuta con drenaggio da un'otite esterna acuta. Il dolore alla manipolazione del padiglione e una linfoadenite significativa non sono caratteristiche comuni dell'OM, e questi reperti aiutano nella diagnosi differenziale. In alcuni pazienti con otite esterna, l'edema periauricolare è così esteso da spingere in avanti il padiglione, creando una condizione che può essere confusa con una **mastoidite** acuta e un ascesso sotto periosteo; nella mastoidite, la piega postauricolare va perduta, a differenza di quanto in genere avviene nell'otite esterna. Nella mastoidite acuta, è usuale un'anamnesi di OM e ipoacusia; è presente dolorabilità a livello mastoideo, non dovuta a movimento del padiglione auricolare; l'esame otoscopio può dimostrare un avvallamento della parete posteriore del condotto.

TRATTAMENTO. Preparazioni auricolari topiche contenenti neomicina (attiva contro i microrganismi Gram-positivi e alcuni Gram-negativi, soprattutto *Pseudomonas* spp.) e corticosteroidi sono molto efficaci nel trattamento della maggior parte delle forme di otite esterna acuta. Sono disponibili preparazioni più recenti di gocce auricolari (per es. ofloxacina e ciprofloxacina) che non contengono antibiotici potenzialmente ototossici. Se l'edema del condotto uditivo è marcato, il paziente può aver bisogno di una visita specialistica per una pulizia e l'eventuale posizionamento di un tampone. Alcuni consigliano di utilizzare corticosteroidi topici insieme agli antibiotici. Si può inserire un tampone nel condotto uditivo e applicare antibiotici topici 3 volte al giorno per 24-48 ore. Il tampone può essere rimosso dopo 2-3 giorni, momento in cui di solito l'edema del condotto è notevolmente ridotto e si riesce a vedere meglio il condotto uditivo e la MT. Si continuano quindi gli antibiotici topici per instillazione diretta. In presenza di dolore grave, per qualche giorno può essere necessario somministrare analgesici per via orale (per es. ibuprofene, codeina). In pazienti con otite esterna grave o ricorrente è necessaria una valutazione attenta delle condizioni sottostanti. Un approccio al trattamento è indicato nella Figura 638-1.

Non appena il processo infiammatorio diminuisce, una pulizia del condotto con aspirazione o cotton fioc, per rimuovere i detriti, migliora l'efficacia dei farmaci topici. Nelle infezioni subacute o croniche è essenziale effettuarla periodicamente. Nell'otite esterna acuta grave, associata a febbre e linfoadenite, possono essere indicati antibiotici per via orale o parenterale; occorre eseguire un esame colturale del materiale del condotto e, se necessario, modificare il trattamento antibiotico empirico sulla scorta di un antibiogramma. Un'infezione micotica del condotto uditivo esterno, o **otomicosi**, è caratterizzata da detriti morbidi e biancastri, talvolta con spore nere; il trattamento comprende la pulizia e

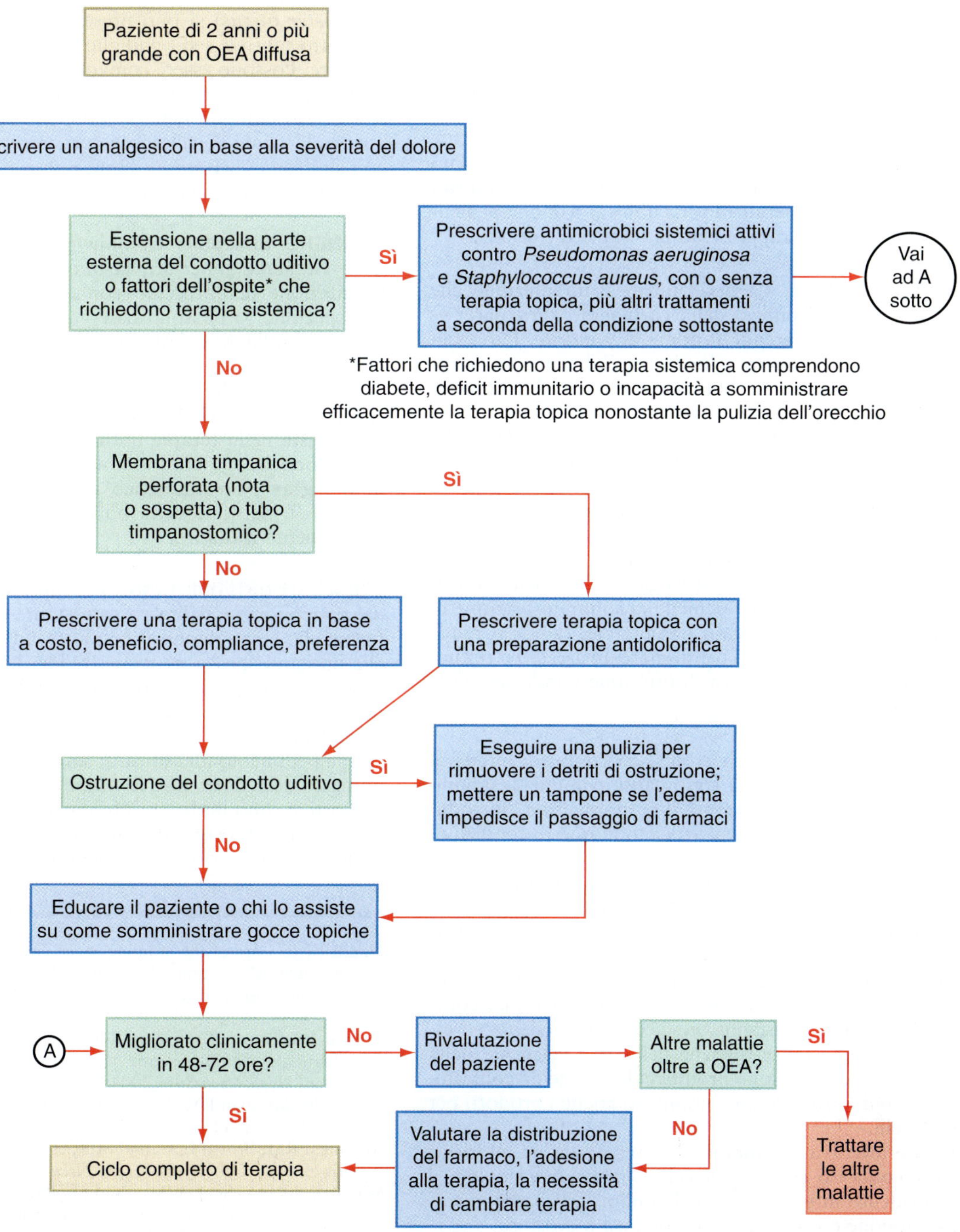

Figura 638-1. Diagramma per il trattamento dell'otite esterna acuta. (Da Rosenfeld RM, Brown L, Cannon CR et al: Clinical practice guideline: acute otitis externa. *Otolaryngol Head Neck Surg* 2006;134:S4-S23, © 2006 American Academy of Otolaryngology-Head and Neck Surgery Foundation, Inc.)

l'applicazione di soluzioni antimicotiche come il cotrimazolo o la nistatina; altri farmaci antimicotici sono m-cresil acetato al 25%, violetto di genziana al 2%, e timerosal 1:1000.

PREVENZIONE. La prevenzione dell'otite esterna può essere necessaria negli individui suscettibili alle recidive, in particolare nei bambini che nuotano. La profilassi più efficace consiste nell'instillazione di alcol diluito o acido acetico (2%) immediatamente dopo il bagno. Durante un episodio acuto di otite esterna, il paziente deve astenersi dal nuoto e le orecchie devono essere protette durante il bagno, perché non entri una quantità d'acqua eccessiva nel condotto uditivo.

ALTRE MALATTIE DELL'ORECCHIO ESTERNO

FORUNCOLOSI. La foruncolosi, causata da *S. aureus*, colpisce solo il terzo esterno del condotto uditivo, dove sono presenti follicoli piliferi. Per il trattamento delle forme lievi ci si avvale di antibiotici orali attivi contro lo *S. aureus*. Se si forma un ascesso, possono essere necessari incisione e drenaggio.

CELLULITE ACUTA. La cellulite acuta del padiglione auricolare e del condotto uditivo esterno di solito è provocata da uno streptococco di gruppo A e solo occasionalmente da *S. aureus*. La cute è rossa, calda e indurita, senza un bordo nettamente definito. Può essere presente febbre con essudato lieve o assente nel condotto. La somministrazione parenterale di penicillina G o di una penicillina penicillinasi-resistente rappresenta la terapia d'elezione.

PERICONDRITE E CONDRITE. La pericondrite è un'infezione che colpisce la cute e il pericondrio della cartilagine auricolare; se si estende alla cartilagine prende il nome di *condrite*. Può essere coinvolto anche il condotto uditivo, specialmente la parete laterale. Nelle fasi iniziali potrebbe essere difficile differenziare una pericondrite da una cellulite, perché entrambe sono caratterizzate dalla presenza di cute arrossata, edematosa e dolente. La causa principale di pericondrite/condrite e cellulite è un trauma (accidentale o iatrogeno, lacerazione o contusione), compreso il piercing dell'orecchio, soprattutto se eseguito attraverso la cartilagine. Il microrganismo isolato più spesso nella pericondrite e condrite è *Pseudomonas aeruginosa*, sebbene sia possibile ritrovare anche altri microrganismi Gram-negativi e, occasionalmente, Gram-positivi. Il trattamento richiede la somministrazione di antibiotici per via sistemica, spesso parenterale; talora si rende necessario l'intervento chirurgico per drenare un ascesso o rimuovere cute o cartilagine. In presenza di infezione è indispensabile togliere orecchini e piercing.

DERMATOSI. Varie dermatosi (seborroica, da contatto, infettiva, eczematoide o neurodermatoide) sono cause comuni di infiammazione del condotto uditivo esterno; il grattamento e l'introduzione di microrganismi infettanti provocano in queste condizioni un'otite esterna acuta.

La **dermatite seborroica** è caratterizzata da scaglie grasse che si sfaldano e si sbriciolano non appena si staccano dall'epidermide; sono frequenti modificazioni associate di cuoio capelluto, fronte, guance, sopracciglia, area retroauricolare e conca.

La **dermatite da contatto** del padiglione o del condotto uditivo può essere causata da orecchini o da farmaci topici come neomicina, che provocano eritema, vescicolazione, edema ed essudazione. Anche le sostanze tossiche dell'edera velenosa, della quercia e del sommacco possono produrre dermatite da contatto. In soggetti sensibili, possono essere implicati anche i prodotti per la cura dei capelli.

La **dermatite infettiva eczematoide** è causata da un'infezione purulenta del condotto esterno, orecchio medio o mastoide; il drenaggio purulento infetta la cute del condotto, il padiglione o entrambi. La lesione è essudativa, eritematosa o crostosa.

La **dermatite atopica** si verifica in bambini con un'anamnesi familiare o personale di allergia; il padiglione auricolare, in particolar modo la piega retroauricolare, si ispessisce, si squama e si escoria.

La **neurodermatite** si riconosce dall'intenso prurito e dall'epidermide eritematosa, ispessita, localizzata sulla conca e sull'orifizio del meato.

Il **trattamento** dipende dal tipo di dermatosi, ma deve comprendere un'appropriata medicazione topica, l'eliminazione della sorgente di infezione o del contatto, quando identificato, e il trattamento di qualsiasi problema dermatologico sottostante. In aggiunta agli antibiotici topici (o agli antimicotici), sono utili gli steroidi topici qualora si sospettasse dermatite da contatto, dermatite atopica o dermatite eczematoide.

VIRUS HERPES SIMPLEX. Il virus herpes simplex si può manifestare sotto forma di vescicole sul padiglione auricolare e sulle labbra. Quando le lesioni diventano crostose e secche, possono essere scambiate per impetigine. L'applicazione topica di soluzione al 10% di perossido di carbamide in glicerolo anidro è utile dal punto vista sintomatologico. La **sindrome di Ramsay Hunt** (***herpes zoster oticus***) si può presentare con vescicole erpetiche nel condotto uditivo e sul padiglione, oltre che con paralisi facciale e dolore. Possono essere coinvolti altri nervi cranici, specialmente l'ottavo. Il trattamento attualmente consigliato dell'herpes zoster oticus consiste nella somministrazione per via sistemica di antivirali, come l'aciclovir, e corticosteroidi. Il 50% dei pazienti con sindrome di Ramsay Hunt non riacquista completamente la funzione del nervo facciale.

MIRINGITE BOLLOSA. Comunemente associata a un'infezione delle vie aeree superiori, la miringite bollosa si presenta come un'infezione dell'orecchio con un dolore più grave del solito. All'ispezione, si possono osservare vescicole (bolle) emorragiche o sierose sulla MT. Talvolta è difficile differenziare la malattia dall'OM acuta, perché un'ampia bolla può essere confusa con la protusione della MT. I microrganismi coinvolti sono gli stessi che provocano l'OM acuta, sia batteri sia virus. Il trattamento consiste nella terapia antibiotica empirica e nella risoluzione del dolore. In aggiunta all'ibuprofene o alla codeina, in caso di dolore grave, un anestetico topico in gocce può dare qualche sollievo. L'incisione della bolla, seppure non necessaria, allevia rapidamente il dolore.

ESOSTOSI E OSTEOMI. L'esostosi rappresenta un'iperplasia benigna del pericondrio e dell'osso sottostante (vedi Capitolo 501.2). Le forme che coinvolgono il condotto uditivo colpiscono i soggetti che nuotano spesso in acque fredde. Le esostosi presentano una base ampia e spesso sono multiple e bilaterali. Gli osteomi sono neoplasie ossee benigne del condotto uditivo a eziologia incerta (vedi Capitolo 501.2). In genere solitari, si attaccano con un sottile peduncolo alla linea di sutura timpanosquamosa o timpanomastoidea. Entrambe le forme sono più frequenti nei maschi; le esostosi sono inoltre più frequenti degli osteomi. Si consiglia il trattamento chirurgico quando masse ampie provocano un accumulo di cerume, ostruzione del condotto uditivo o ipoacusia.

Haddad J Jr: Care of the draining ear in children. *Emerg Peds* 1995;8:75.

Nussinovitch M, Rimon A, Volovitz B, et al: Cotton-tip applicators as a leading cause of otitis externa. *Int J Pediatr Otolaryngol* 2004;68:433–435.

Roland PS, Eaton DA, Gross RD, et al: Randomized, placebo-controlled evaluation of Cerumenex and Murine earwax removal products. *Arch Otolaryngol Head Neck Surg* 2004;130:1175–1177.

Roland PS, Stroman DW: Microbiology of acute otitis externa. *Laryngoscope* 2002;112:1166–1177.

Rosenfeld RM, Brown L, Cannon CR, et al: Clinical practice guideline: acute otitis externa. *Otolaryngol Head Neck Surg* 2006;134:S4–S23.

Van Balen FAM, Smit WM, Zuithoff PA, et al: Clinical efficacy of three common treatments in acute otitis externa in primary care: randomized controlled trial. *BMJ* 2003;327:1201–1203.

Capitolo 639 ■ Otite media*

Joseph E. Kerschner

CONSIDERAZIONI GENERALI

Negli Stati Uniti, tra le malattie che portano un bambino in un ambulatorio medico, l'otite media (OM) è seconda solo al raffreddore comune. Il picco di incidenza e prevalenza si situa tra il 6° e il 20° mese di età. L'OM va tenuta in considerazione nella diagnosi differenziale della febbre, è il motivo più frequente per cui vengono prescritti antibiotici ai pazienti pediatrici e spesso rappresenta la ragione principale, se non l'unica, che induce a eseguire due tra gli interventi più frequenti nei lattanti e nei bambini piccoli: miringotomia con inserzione di tubi timpanostomici e adenoidectomia. Questa patologia ha la caratteristica di diventare cronica e recidivare. Più precoce è il primo episodio della malattia, maggiore sarà il disagio che il paziente dovrà in seguito affrontare, in termini di frequenza di recidiva, severità e persistenza di effusione dell'orecchio medio.

Spesso nei lattanti e nei bambini piccoli sono difficili una definizione e una diagnosi accurate (Tab. 639-1). I sintomi possono essere assenti o non immediatamente evidenti, soprattutto nella primissima infanzia e negli stadi cronici della malattia. La membrana timpanica può essere nascosta dal cerume, la cui rimozione talvolta è difficile e richiede tempo. Le anomalie della membrana timpanica possono essere lievi e difficili da apprezzare. Per tutti questi problemi, l'OM può sia sfuggire alla diagnosi sia essere sovradiagnosticata. Il suo significato, in termini di salute e benessere del bambino e di metodo ottimale di trattamento, rimane una questione aperta e discussa. Non esiste consenso tra gli specialisti circa il rapporto rischio/beneficio dei trattamenti disponibili, medici e chirurgici, e la possibilità di conseguenze a lungo termine. Sebbene l'OM possa essere responsabile di complicanze infettive serie, danni all'orecchio medio e interno, alterazioni dell'udito e problemi indiretti nello sviluppo linguistico, cognitivo e psicosociale, la maggior parte dei casi non è grave ed è autolimitantesi.

L'OM ha due componenti principali: un'infezione acuta, definita **otite media suppurativa o acuta (OMA)**, e un'infiammazione accompagnata da effusione, definita **otite media non suppurativa o secretiva**, o **otite media con effusione (OME)**. Questi due principali tipi di OM sono tra loro correlati: l'infezione acuta solitamente è seguita da un'infiammazione residuale e da effusione, che predispongono entrambe i bambini a infezioni ricorrenti. L'**effusione dell'orecchio medio** (MEE, *Middle-Ear Effusion*) è caratteristica sia dell'OMA sia dell'OME; in entrambe le condizioni, rappresenta l'espressione della sottostante infiammazione mucosa dell'orecchio medio. In bambini con OM l'infiammazione mucosa è presente anche nelle cellule aeree mastoidee, che si trovano in continuità con la cavità dell'orecchio medio: la MEE comporta ipoacusia conduttiva associata a OM. L'ipoacusia è variabile, dall'assenza di alterazioni a un livello di udito di 50 decibel (dB). Sono frequenti perdite di 21-30 dB. Sebbene la maggior parte dei singoli episodi di OM si risolva nel giro di alcune settimane, la MEE persiste per più di 3 mesi in circa il 10-25% dei casi.

TABELLA 639-1. Definizione di otite media acuta (OMA)

Una diagnosi di OMA richiede (1) un'anamnesi di esordio acuto di segni e sintomi, (2) la presenza di MEE e (3) segni e sintomi di infiammazione dell'orecchio medio.

La definizione di OMA include:
- Recente, solitamente brusco, esordio di segni e sintomi di infiammazione dell'orecchio medio e di MEE
- La presenza di MEE, indicata da ciascuno dei segni seguenti:
  - Bulging della MT
  - Limitata o assente mobilità della MT
  - Livello aria-liquido oltre la MT
  - Otorrea
- Segni o sintomi di infiammazione dell'orecchio medio, indicati da:
  - Distinto eritema della MT *o*
  - Distinta otalgia (disturbo chiaramente riferibile all'orecchio e che interferisce con le normali attività o il sonno)

OMA, otite media acuta; MEE (*Medium Ear Effusion*), effusione dell'orecchio medio; MT, membrana timpanica.

Da Subcommittee on Management of Acute Otitis Media: Diagnosis and management of acute otitis media. *Pediatrics* 2004;113:1451-1465.

EPIDEMIOLOGIA. I fattori ritenuti responsabili della comparsa di OM comprendono età, sesso, razza, fattori genetici, stato socioeconomico, tipo di latte usato nell'alimentazione neonatale, grado di esposizione al fumo di tabacco, frequenza con cui il soggetto entra in contatto con altri bambini, presenza o assenza di allergie respiratorie, stagione dell'anno e stato della vaccinazione antipneumococcica. I bambini con alcuni tipi di anomalie craniofacciali congenite sono particolarmente predisposti a OM.

Età. La probabilità di sviluppare almeno un episodio di OM è del 63-85% al 12° mese di età e del 66-99% al 24° mese. La percentuale di giorni con MEE è del 5-27% durante il primo anno di vita e del 6-18% durante il secondo anno. Le percentuali sono più alte dal 6° al 20° mese. Dopo i 2 anni, l'incidenza e la prevalenza di OM diminuiscono progressivamente, sebbene la malattia rimanga abbastanza frequente nei primi anni di scuola. La ragione più probabile della maggiore incidenza nei lattanti e nei bambini piccoli è da ricercare nelle minori difese immunitarie e nei fattori, meno favorevoli, relativi alla tuba di Eustachio, alla sua funzione e struttura. L'età d'esordio dell'OM è un importante fattore predittivo per lo sviluppo di un'OM recidivante e cronica: l'esordio in età più precoce comporta un aumento del rischio di contrarre questa malattia in fasi successive della vita.

Sesso. L'incidenza di OM è maggiore nei maschi rispetto alle femmine. In un ampio studio condotto a Pittsburgh sul rapporto tra OM e sviluppo infantile, che aveva comportato uno stretto monitoraggio in popolazioni diverse da un punto di vista sociodemografico, i bambini di sesso maschile avevano una media più alta di giorni con MEE rispetto alle bambine. Nella maggior parte degli studi sul trattamento dell'OM, i maschi risultano più colpiti e, confrontati con le femmine, presentano una percentuale notevolmente più alta di interventi rivolti ad attenuare gli effetti o a ridurre la recidiva di OM (per es. inserzione di un tubo timpanostomico, timpanoplastica, adenoidectomia): tutti questi dati supportano la tesi di una netta predilezione della malattia per i maschi, oltre a suggerire una maggiore severità nel sesso maschile.

Razza. L'otite media è particolarmente frequente e grave tra i nativi americani, gli Inuit e gli aborigeni australiani. Studi comparativi sulla frequenza di OM in bambini bianchi e neri hanno dato risultati contrastanti, ma dalla maggior parte di essi risulta una percentuale più alta nei bambini bianchi.

Fattori genetici. Si nota comunemente che le malattie dell'orecchio medio tendono a **ricorrere nella stessa famiglia**, e vari studi hanno suggerito che l'OM abbia una componente ereditaria. Esiste un maggior grado di concordanza per OM tra gemelli monozigoti rispetto ai dizigoti.

Status socioeconomico. La povertà è stata a lungo considerata un importante fattore favorente sia lo sviluppo sia la severità dell'OM. Si suppone che questo sia dovuto a fattori come affollamento, scarsa igiene, stato nutrizionale non ottimale, accesso limitato alle terapie e scarse risorse che non permettono di rispettare le prescrizioni mediche.

Latte materno vs latte formulato. La maggior parte degli studi sull'argomento ha scoperto che l'allattamento al seno esplica un effetto protettivo contro l'OM, probabilmente limitato, ma che può essere maggiore in bambini svantaggiati da un punto di vista socioeconomico. Tale effetto è attribuibile al latte stesso, più che al meccanismo di allattamento, come dimostra uno studio condotto su lattanti con palatoschisi in cui sia il latte materno sia quello formulato venivano somministrati con il biberon.

*Adattato dal capitolo di Jack L. Paradise, MD., presente nella 17ª edizione.

Esposizione al fumo di tabacco. È emersa una correlazione positiva tra la comparsa di OM e l'esposizione casalinga al fumo di tabacco in molti studi, ma non in tutti. Poiché il fumo casalingo si correla in modo inverso allo stato socioeconomico, è possibile una confusione con fattori socioeconomici, che complicano ulteriormente una corretta valutazione del rischio. Studi che hanno utilizzato misure oggettive per determinare l'esposizione indiretta al tabacco, come il livello di nicotina, hanno dimostrato un più significativo rapporto tra fumo di tabacco e OM. Questa evidenza suggerisce che l'esposizione al fumo di tabacco debba essere considerata un importante fattore di rischio nello sviluppo di OM.

Contatto con altri bambini. Molti studi hanno dimostrato uno stretto rapporto positivo tra la comparsa di OM e l'esistenza di un contatto ripetuto con altri bambini, sia a casa sia all'asilo. Lo stato socioeconomico familiare e il contatto con altri bambini costituiscono i due più importanti fattori di rischio identificabili per lo sviluppo di OM.

Stagionalità. Nei climi temperati, le più alte percentuali di comparsa dell'OM si osservano durante i mesi freddi e quelle più basse nei mesi caldi, in linea con l'andamento di comparsa delle infezioni delle vie aeree superiori. Nell'OM, è probabile che questi reperti dipendano dall'associazione significativa tra OM e malattie respiratorie virali.

Anomalie congenite. L'otite media, oltre a essere ubiquitaria tra i bambini con palatoschisi non corretta, presenta una notevole incidenza tra i bambini con palatoschisi sottomucosa, altre anomalie craniofacciali e sindrome di Down. La caratteristica comune a queste anomalie congenite è un deficit funzionale della tuba di Eustachio, che predispone alla patologia dell'orecchio medio.

Vaccinazione antipneumococcica. *Streptococcus pneumoniae*, o pneumococco, è il microrganismo patogeno più spesso identificato in pazienti con OM acuta. **Negli Stati Uniti** la vaccinazione neonatale con un vaccino antipneumococcico coniugato è una pratica standardizzata. Complessivamente, la riduzione dell'incidenza dell'OM con la vaccinazione sembra essere modesta, e il ricorso al medico e le prescrizioni antibiotiche per OM diminuiscono solo del 6-8%. Quindi, la vaccinazione non sembra avere la prerogativa di limitare episodi frequenti e la necessità d'intervento chirurgico con inserimento di tubi timpanostomici.

EZIOLOGIA

Otite media acuta. Con tecniche colturali standard si possono isolare i batteri patogeni dal liquido dell'orecchio medio in circa il 65-75% dei casi di OMA documentata; nei casi rimanenti, le colture batteriche mostrano l'assenza di crescita batterica o la presenza di microrganismi generalmente considerati non patogeni. Sono predominanti tre batteri patogeni: *S. pneumoniae* si trova in circa il 40% dei casi, *Haemophilus influenzae* in circa il 25-30% e *Moraxella catarrhalis* in circa il 10-15%. Altri patogeni che, insieme, sono responsabili di circa il 5% dei casi, sono lo streptococco di gruppo A, *Staphylococcus aureus* e batteri Gram-negativi. *S. aureus* e microrganismi Gram-negativi si trovano con maggiore frequenza in neonati e lattanti di pochi mesi ospedalizzati. A livello ambulatoriale, la distribuzione dei microrganismi patogeni in questi bambini piccoli è simile a quella dei bambini più grandi.

Nell'essudato dell'orecchio medio dei pazienti pediatrici con OMA si è riscontrata anche la presenza di **virus respiratori**, da soli o in associazione con batteri patogeni. Di questi virus, i più frequenti sono il rhinovirus e il virus respiratorio sinciziale (RSV, *Respiratory Syncytial Virus*). L'OMA è una complicanza nota della bronchiolite; gli aspirati dell'orecchio medio di bambini con bronchiolite contengono regolarmente batteri patogeni: se ne deduce che l'RSV è raramente, se mai, la sola causa dell'OMA. Utilizzando misure dei batteri vitali più precise rispetto alle tecniche colturali standard, per esempio i dosaggi basati sulla reazione a catena della polimerasi (PCR, *Polymerase Chain Reaction*), si può dimostrare una più alta percentuale di batteri patogeni. Non è chiaro se, in determinate circostanze, i virus da soli possano provocare OMA, o se il loro ruolo sia limitato alla fase di invasione batterica, e forse anche all'amplificazione del processo infiammatorio, che interferisce con la risoluzione dell'infezione batterica. I patogeni virali, oltre ad avere un impatto negativo sulla funzione della tromba di Eustachio, possono compromettere la funzione immunitaria locale, aumentare l'aderenza batterica e modificare la farmacocinetica, effetti questi che riducono l'efficacia dei farmaci antibiotici.

Otite media con effusione. I patogeni tipici dell'OMA possono essere evidenziati in circa il 30% dei bambini con OME usando tecniche colturali standard. Con i dosaggi basati sulla PCR, nel liquido dell'orecchio medio si è trovato DNA batterico vitale e/o RNA virale in maggior proporzione nei bambini con OME. Questi dati suggeriscono che i pazienti con OME non abbiano un'effusione sterile, come si pensava in precedenza. È quindi possibile che questi patogeni contribuiscano alla stimolazione dei processi infiammatori in corso nell'orecchio medio e possano anche giocare un ruolo nelle infezioni recidivanti attraverso la formazione di un biofilm.

PATOGENESI. L'otite media acuta solitamente è causata da patogeni batterici. Fondamentale per la comprensione della patogenesi dell'OM è prendere in esame altri fattori, come la tuba di Eustachio il sistema immunitario del bambino, il profilo dei fattori di rischio e le interazioni patogeni-ospite.

In circostanze normali, la tuba di Eustachio è passivamente chiusa e si apre per la contrazione del muscolo tensore del velo palatino. In relazione all'orecchio medio, essa ha tre funzioni principali: ventilazione, protezione e clearance. La più importante è la ventilazione. La mucosa dell'orecchio medio necessita di un continuo flusso d'aria dal rinofaringe attraverso la tuba di Eustachio. L'interruzione di questo processo di ventilazione a causa di un'ostruzione della tuba scatena una complessa risposta infiammatoria, che comprende metaplasia secretoria, compromissione del sistema di trasporto mucociliare ed effusione di liquido nella cavità timpanica. L'alterazione della ventilazione dell'orecchio medio è un fattore importante che contribuisce sia all'OME sia all'OMA. Ancora non si sa se l'infezione dell'orecchio medio possa svilupparsi in assenza di una preesistente ostruzione della tuba di Eustachio; se così fosse, senza dubbio l'infezione potrebbe rapidamente portare all'ostruzione della tuba per l'edema infiammatorio e l'accumulo di secrezioni dell'orecchio medio.

L'ostruzione della tuba di Eustachio può dipendere da fenomeni extraluminali, da edema infiammatorio della mucosa della tuba (attribuibile ad anomala funzione muscolare della tuba o a eccessiva compliance della parete tubarica) o da entrambi i fattori. La riduzione progressiva della compliance della parete tubarica con il progredire dell'età può aiutare a spiegare la minore frequenza dell'OM nei bambini più grandi. Nella patogenesi dell'OM può essere coinvolta anche la funzione di protezione e clearance della tuba di Eustachio. Pertanto, se le tube sono pervie o eccessivamente complianti, viene a mancare la funzione di protezione dell'orecchio medio dal reflusso di secrezioni infette rinofaringee, mentre un'alterazione della funzione di clearance mucociliare della tuba può contribuire all'infezione e alla sua persistenza. Il decorso orizzontale e la maggiore brevità della tuba, nei neonati e nei bambini più piccoli, posssono aumentare la possibilità di reflusso dal rinofaringe e ostacolare il drenaggio gravitazionale attraverso la tuba stessa. Un'altra possibile spiegazione del miglioramento della funzione della tuba di Eustachio e dell'incidenza di OM via via che il soggetto matura è l'aumento del diametro luminale, che riduce le possibilità di ostruzione e disfunzione tubarica.

Nei bambini con palatoschisi, in cui L'OM costituisce un reperto praticamente costante, il principale fattore che perpetua l'infiammazione dell'orecchio medio è la compromissione del meccanismo di apertura della tuba di Eustachio, dovuto forse a una compliance maggiore del normale della parete tubarica. Nei bambini con altre anomalie craniofacciali o con sindrome di Down la maggiore incidenza di OM è attribuita ad anomalie strutturali e/o funzionali della tuba di Eustachio; la valutazione istologica della tuba di Eustachio in queste popolazioni di pazienti dimostra tali anomalie.

Sebbene l'OM possa svilupparsi e persistere in assenza di infezioni manifeste delle vie aeree superiori, molti degli episodi cominciano in rapporto con un'infezione virale o batterica delle vie aeree superiori. In uno studio sui bambini di un asilo nido, si è osservata OMA in circa il 10-15% dei soggetti con malattie respiratorie causate da RSV, virus dell'influenza o adenovirus, e in circa il 10-15% di quelli con malattie respiratorie provocate da virus parainfluenzali, rinovirus o enterovirus. L'infezione virale delle vie aeree superiori comporta un rilascio di citochine e di mediatori dell'infiammazione, alcuni dei quali possono provocare una disfunzione della tuba di Eustachio. I virus respiratori possono anche aumentare la colonizzazione e l'aderenza dei batteri nel rinofaringe, compromettendo le difese immunitarie contro l'infezione batterica.

In alcuni bambini con OMA recidivante si è trovato un deficit di IgA, ma il significato di questo dato è discutibile, perché il deficit di IgA non è raro nei pazienti pediatrici senza OMA recidivante. Una carenza selettiva di sottoclassi di IgG (nonostante il normale livello di IgG totali) può essere trovato in bambini con OMA recidivante in associazione con infezione senopolmonare recidivante; queste carenze probabilmente sono alla base della suscettibilità all'infezione. Bambini con OM recidivante non associata a infezioni recidivanti in altre sedi raramente presentano un deficit immunologico identificabile. Ciononostante, la prova che lievi deficit immunitari giocano un ruolo nella patogenesi dell'OMA recidivante proviene da studi che riguardano le risposte anticorpali a vari tipi di infezione e immunizzazione; dall'osservazione che l'allattamento al seno, al contrario di quello artificiale, conferisce una protezione limitata contro la comparsa di OM in neonati con palatoschisi; e da studi in cui bambini piccoli con OMA recidivante ottengono una certa protezione dalla somministrazione intramuscolare di immunoglobuline antipolisaccaride batterico, o endovenosa di immunoglobuline policlonali. Questo dato, insieme al documentato decremento dell'incidenza di infezioni delle vie aeree superiori e OM a mano a mano che il sistema immunitario infantile matura, è indicativo dell'importanza, nella patogenesi dell'OM, del sistema immunitario innato.

Non esistono prove convincenti a supporto dell'ipotesi che l'allergia respiratoria sia un agente eziologico primario di OM; tuttavia, in bambini che manifestano sia allergia sia OM, è possibile che l'otite sia aggravata dall'allergia.

È sempre più evidente che il profilo dei rischi e le interazioni ospite-patogeno giocano un ruolo importante nella patogenesi dell'OM. Eventi come alterazioni della clearance mucociliare per ripetute esposizioni virali (per es. in un asilo) o per esposizione al fumo di tabacco, possono far sì che nella patogenesi dell'OM entrino in gioco patogeni meno virulenti. Esistono ampie prove che nei bambini che hanno frequenti contatti con i coetanei aumenta il rischio di colonizzazione batterica rinofaringea e di OM acuta da tipi batterici con resistenze multiple agli antibiotici, rendendo più difficile il trattamento e più probabile un prolungamento della malattia.

MANIFESTAZIONI CLINICHE. I segni e i sintomi di OMA sono quanto mai variabili, specialmente nei neonati e nei bambini piccoli. Può essere evidente il dolore all'orecchio, che spesso si manifesta con irritabilità, alterazioni del sonno o dell'alimentazione e talvolta con il gesto di stropicciarsi o tirarsi l'orecchio (vedi Tab. 639-1). La tendenza a tirarsi l'orecchio, tuttavia, ha una bassa sensibilità e specificità. Può anche essere presente febbre e, raramente, rottura della membrana timpanica con otorrea purulenta. Si possono manifestare inoltre sintomi sistemici o associati a infezioni delle vie aeree superiori, anche se talvolta la patologia è asintomatica; in quest'ultimo caso l'OMA è scoperta casualmente durante una visita routinaria. L'OME spesso non è accompagnata da pianto franco del bambino, ma da ipoacusia, la quale può manifestarsi come modificazione dei pattern linguistici, ma spesso, se lieve o unilaterale, rimane misconosciuta, in particolare nei bambini più piccoli. Le alterazioni dell'equilibrio possono essere associate a OME, e i bambini più grandi possono lamentarsi di lieve fastidio o della sensazione di avere l'orecchio tappato (vedi Capitolo 635).

ESAME DELLA MEMBRANA TIMPANICA

OTOSCOPIA. Per i medici, esclusi gli specialisti in otorinolaringoiatria che possono usare un microscopio operatorio, di solito la visualizzazione della membrana timpanica avviene per mezzo di un otoscopio. Sono disponibili due teste di otoscopio: **chirurgica** o **operatoria**, e **diagnostica** o **pneumatica**. La testa chirurgica include una lente che può ruotare su un ampio arco e una sorgente di luce aperta, che consente un facile accesso degli strumenti dell'esaminatore nel condotto uditivo esterno e alla membrana timpanica. L'uso della testa chirurgica, oltre a essere ottimale per rimuovere cerume o detriti sotto osservazione diretta, è necessaria per una timpanocentesi o una miringotomia. La testa diagnostica incorpora una lente più grande, una sorgente di luce chiusa e un foro a cui collegare un bulbo di gomma e un tubo. Quando si introduce lo speculum nel condotto uditivo esterno, occludendo quest'ultimo si crea una camera ermetica, formata dalla testa dell'otoscopio, dal bulbo o dal tubo, dallo speculum e dalla parte prossimale del condotto esterno. Sebbene l'esame dell'orecchio nei bambini piccoli sia una procedura relativamente invasiva, aggravata dalla mancanza di cooperazione da parte del paziente, bisogna fare in modo che provochi il minor dolore possibile. La parte esterna del condotto uditivo è rivestita da cute dotata di follicoli piliferi, tessuto adiposo sottocutaneo e cartilagine, che permettono di posizionare lo speculum senza causare troppo fastidio. La parte del condotto uditivo più vicina alla membrana timpanica è invece composta da osso e ricoperta solo dalla cute e non da strutture annesse o tessuto adiposo sottocutaneo; uno speculum spinto più in avanti e collocato in corrispondenza di questa zona spesso causa dolore e abrasioni cutanee. Usando uno speculum con punta di gomma o aggiungendo un piccolo manicotto di gomma alla sua punta di plastica è possibile ridurre al minimo il fastidio del paziente aumentando quindi la possibilità di ottenere un buon accesso e una chiusura ermetica.

Imparare a usare un otoscopio pneumatico è fondamentale per riuscire a valutare l'orecchio di un bambino e per fare una diagnosi accurata di OM (vedi Fig. 635-1). Comprimere e rilasciare il bulbo più volte permette di stimare il grado di mobilità della membrana timpanica in risposta a pressione positiva e negativa, valutando criticamente il liquido dell'orecchio medio, che è un segno distintivo sia di OMA sia di OME. Con entrambi i tipi di testa dell'otoscopio è fondamentale, per un'adeguata visualizzazione della membrana timpanica, una buona illuminazione.

PULIZIA DEL CONDOTTO UDITIVO. Se la membrana timpanica è nascosta dal cerume, quest'ultimo deve essere rimosso con la testa chirurgica dell'otoscopio sotto osservazione diretta, usando una curette di Buck (N-400-0). Eventuali residui possono poi essere eliminati con un applicatore di Farrell (N-2001-A), rivestendone la punta (triangolare in sezione traversa) con un pezzo di cotone asciutto o imbevuto d'alcol. In alternativa, si può esercitare un'aspirazione moderata, usando un tubo da aspirazione n. 5 o 7. Durante questa procedura può essere utile tenere il bambino in posizione prona, girandogli la testa a destra o a sinistra, in modo da pulire entrambe le orecchie. Un adulto, solitamente un genitore, può appoggiare una mano su ciascun gluteo del bambino e tenergli le anche contro il lettino, usando il proprio peso per impedirgli di muoversi, se necessario. Un altro adulto può bloccare la testa del bambino con una mano e le braccia con l'altra. Nei bambini più grandi, che di solito già a partire dai 5 anni sono in grado di collaborare, la pulizia del condotto uditivo esterno può essere eseguita più facilmente, in sicurezza, e in modo meno traumatico, con un lavaggio anziché con la rimozione meccanica, accertandosi prima che la membrana timpanica non sia perforata. Nella maggior parte dei casi le orecchie dei bambini tendono all'"autopulizia", per la migrazione squamosa della cute del condotto, e l'intervento di un genitore con bastoncini di cotone spesso aggrava la situazione, perché spinge il cerume più a fondo nel condotto rendendolo inoltre più compatto.

CARATTERISTICHE DELLA MEMBRANA TIMPANICA. Caratteristiche importanti della membrana timpanica sono il contorno, il colore, grado di lucentezza, le modificazioni strutturali e la mobilità. Le anomalie del contorno, che in condizioni normali è **leggermente concavo**, consistono in una sporgenza o protrusione (*bulging*) o, al contrario, in un'estrema retrazione. Il normale colore della membrana timpanica è **grigio-perla**. L'eritema può essere un segno di infiammazione o infezione, ma, a meno che non sia intenso, l'eritema da solo può anche dipendere dal pianto o da vasodilatazione. Un anormale aspetto biancastro della membrana può essere dovuto a cicatrizzazione o a presenza di liquido nella cavità dell'orecchio medio; il liquido può conferire anche un colore ambrato pallido o (raramente) bluastro. La membrana in genere è translucida, sebbene una certa opacità possa essere normale nei primi mesi di vita; più tardi, l'opacizzazione denota una cicatrizzazione, o, più comunemente, un'effusione sottostante. Le modificazioni strutturali comprendono cicatrici, perforazioni, tasche di retrazione e una complicanza dell'OM più grave, la formazione di colesteatoma. Di tutte le caratteristiche visibili della membrana timpanica, la mobilità è la più sensibile e specifica per determinare la presenza o l'assenza di MEE. La mobilità non è un fenomeno del tipo "tutto o niente"; sebbene l'assenza totale di mobilità, in assenza di perforazione della membrana timpanica, sia virtualmente sempre indicativa di MEE, il reperto più comune è una sostanziale alterazione della mobilità.

DIAGNOSI. La diagnosi corretta di OMA è importante per guidare le decisioni terapeutiche. Sebbene in molti casi una diagnosi accurata sia semplice, può rappresentare anche un compito impegnativo, specialmente in un paziente che non collabora. In base alle linee guida, gli elementi richiesti per la diagnosi di OM sono: (1) esordio recente e di solito acuto della malattia, (2) presenza di MEE, (3) segni e sintomi di infiammazione dell'orecchio medio, come eritema della membrana timpanica o otalgia (vedi Tab. 639-1). Secondo uno schema semplificato di diagnosi differenziale, si stabilisce diagnosi di OMA quando, oltre a MEE, un bambino evidenzia dolore all'orecchio, recente, clinicamente importante, o quando la membrana timpanica presenta un arrossamento marcato o una distinta protrusione o bulging (Fig. 639-1). La distinzione clinica tra OMA e OME nella maggior parte dei casi è semplice, ma poiché ciascuna delle due condizioni può evolvere nell'altra, senza reperti fisici chiaramente differenziativi, qualsiasi schema per distinguerle è, per certi versi, arbitrario. Ciononostante, considerato l'aumento delle resistenze batteriche, differenziare un'OMA da un'OME è importantissimo per la scelta del trattamento. Ovviamente, l'otorrea purulenta di esordio recente è indicativa di OMA; pertanto, la difficoltà di distinguere clinicamente l'OMA dall'OME è limitata ai casi in cui tale reperto non sia presente. Sia l'OMA senza otorrea sia l'OME sono accompagnate da segni fisici di MEE, per esempio la presenza di almeno due anomalie timpaniche su tre: colorazione bianca, gialla, ambrata o (raramente) bluastra; opacizzazione, a parte quella dovuta a cicatrizzazione; diminuzione o assenza di mobilità. In alternativa, nell'OME possono essere visibili sia un livello idroaereo sia delle bolle d'aria delineate da piccole quantità di liquido dietro alla membrana timpanica, condizione che spesso indica un'imminente guarigione.

A supportare una diagnosi di OMA piuttosto che di OME in un bambino con MEE può essere presente un'evidente protrusione o bulging della membrana timpanica, con o senza eritema d'accompagnamento. Come minimo, la MEE deve essere accompagnata da dolore all'orecchio di una certa rilevanza clinica. A meno che non sia intenso, il solo eritema è insufficiente potendo essere dovuto a pianto o vasodilatazione. Nell'OMA, il martello può essere nascosto e la membrana timpanica può assomigliare a una ciambella con una depressione centrale (Fig. 639-2). È raro che bolle superficiali nascondano la membrana timpanica o che questa possa avere un aspetto ad acciottolato. La **miringite bollosa** è una manifestazione fisica dell'OMA, non un'entità

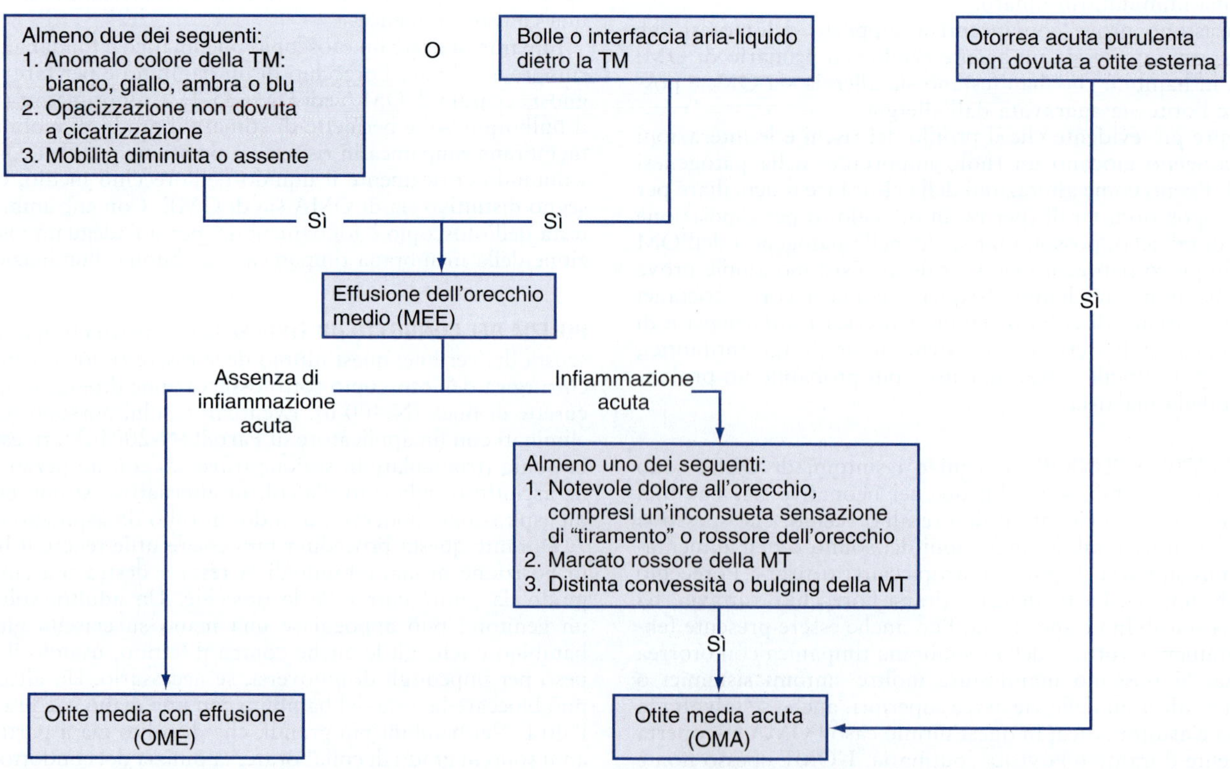

Figura 639-1. Algoritmo per la diagnosi differenziale da otite media acuta (OMA) e otite media con effusione (OME). MT, membrana timpanica.

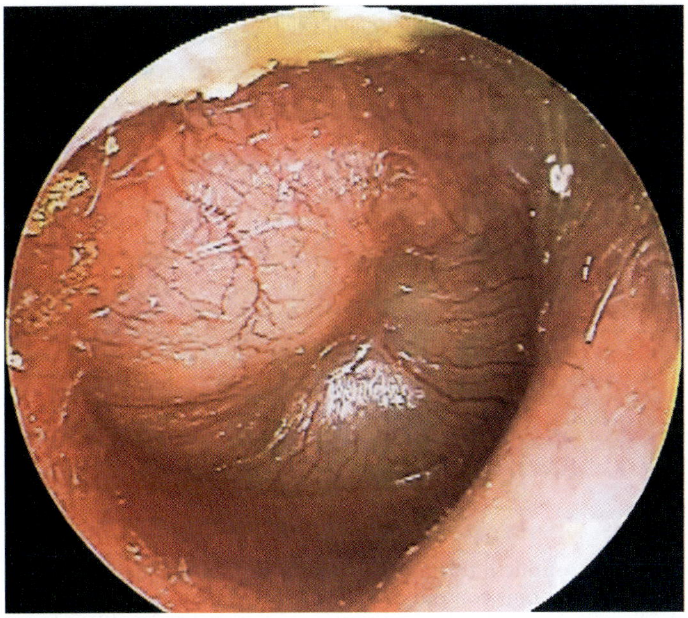

Figura 639-2. Membrana timpanica nell'otite media acuta (OMA).

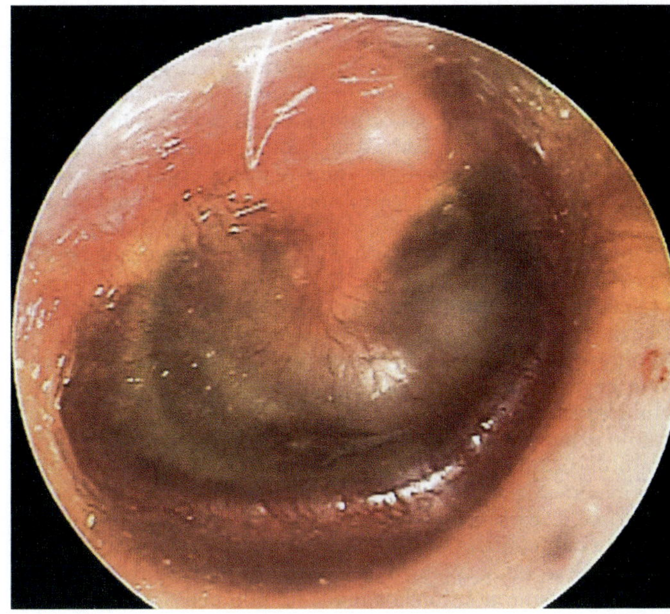

Figura 639-3. Membrana timpanica nell'otite media con effusione (OME).

eziologicamente distinta. La protrusione della membrana può diminuire alcuni giorni dopo l'esordio, anche se l'infezione può persistere.

Nell'OME la membrana timpanica non presenta protrusione oppure è retratta (Fig. 639-3); anche l'eritema è assente o lieve, ma può aumentare con il pianto o con un trauma superficiale del condotto uditivo esterno, che si può verificare durante la pulizia del condotto dal cerume. In bambini con MEE, ma senza sporgenza o protrusione della membrana timpanica, la presenza di un inequivocabile dolore all'orecchio è indicativo di OMA.

Comunemente, sia prima sia dopo gli episodi di OM, e anche in assenza di OM, la membrana timpanica può essere retratta come conseguenza di una pressione negativa dell'orecchio medio. Si presume che la causa del fenomeno sia da attribuire al fatto che la diffusione di aria dalla cavità dell'orecchio medio è più rapida rispetto alla sua sostituzione attraverso la tuba di Eustachio. Una retrazione lieve può non essere considerata patologica, nonostante in alcuni bambini sia accompagnata da lieve ipoacusia conduttiva. Un retrazione maggiore, invece, costituisce motivo di preoccupazione, come discusso nella sezione sulle sequele dell'OM.

TIMPANOMETRIA. La timpanometria, o **test di immettenza acustica**, è un test semplice, rapido, atraumatico che, se eseguito correttamente, offre un'evidenza oggettiva sulla presenza o assenza di MEE. Il timpanogramma fornisce informazioni, in termini elettroacustici, circa la **compliance** della membrana timpanica, che si ritiene possano essere approssimativamente equivalenti ai dati sulla mobilità della membrana timpanica, osservati direttamente durante l'indagine con l'otoscopio pneumatico. Il test si basa sul principio che l'assorbimento del suono da parte della membrana timpanica è inversamente proporzionale alla sua rigidità, e che la rigidità della membrana è minima, e di conseguenza la sua compliance è maggiore, quando le pressioni dell'aria che agiscono su ciascuna delle sue superfici (orecchio medio e condotto uditivo esterno) sono uguali. In termini semplici, qualsiasi fattore che provochi un irrigidimento della membrana timpanica, per esempio una cicatrice o del liquido nell'orecchio medio, riduce la compliance della membrana, che appare come un appiattimento della curva del timpanogramma. Un orecchio medio pieno di liquido di norma ha una membrana timpanica poco compliante: il tracciato del timpanogramma risulterà perciò appiattito.

I **timpanogrammi** possono essere suddivisi in tre categorie (Fig. 639-4). Un tracciato caratterizzato da un gradiente relativamente ripido, con un picco ad angolo acuto, e una pressione dell'aria dell'orecchio medio (localizzazione del picco in termini di pressione dell'aria) che si avvicina alla pressione atmosferica (Fig. 639-4*A*) (curva di tipo A), indica un orecchio medio normale. Un tracciato caratterizzato da un picco modesto o assente, o da una pressione dell'aria dell'orecchio medio negativa o indeterminata, e spesso definito come curva piatta o di tipo B (Fig. 639-4*B*), in genere indica un'anomalia dell'orecchio medio che provoca

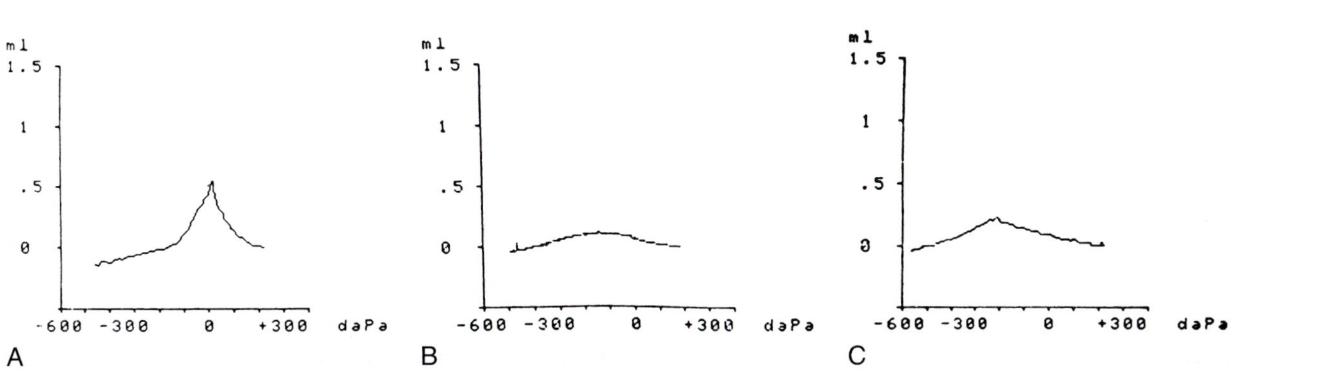

Figura 639-4. Timpanogramma ottenuto con Grason-Stadler GSI 33 Middle Ear Analyzer, che mostra (*A*) elevata ammettenza, gradiente ripido (cioè picco ad angolo acuto) e pressione dell'aria dell'orecchio medio vicina alla pressione atmosferica (0 decaPascal [daPa]); (*B*) bassa ammettenza e pressione dell'aria nell'orecchio medio indeterminata; e (*C*) ammettenza in una certa misura ridotta, gradiente graduale e pressione dell'aria nell'orecchio medio marcatamente negativa.

una riduzione della compliance della membrana timpanica. Di queste anomalie, la più comune nei lattanti e nei bambini è la MEE. Un tracciato caratterizzato da reperti intermedi – un picco talvolta modesto, spesso in associazione con un gradiente graduale (picco con angolo ottuso) o con una pressione negativa dell'aria dell'orecchio medio, o una combinazione di queste due caratteristiche (Fig. 639-4C) – può o meno essere associato a MEE, e deve essere considerato non diagnostico o equivoco. In generale, più il picco è basso, più graduale è la pendenza e più negativa è la pressione dell'aria dell'orecchio medio, maggiore è la probabilità di MEE.

Quando si legge un timpanogramma, è importante prestare attenzione alla misura. Un paziente con una perforazione della membrana timpanica o con un tubo timpanostomico pervio può avere un timpanogramma piatto di tipo B e un "alto volume". Il timpanometro misura e registra il volume del condotto uditivo esterno e, in presenza di una perforazione della membrana timpanica o di un tubo aperto da timpanostomia, il volume dell'orecchio medio e delle cellule aeree mastoidee. Un volume >1,0 mL suggerisce la presenza di una perforazione o di un tubo timpanostomico. Quindi, in un bambino con un tubo timpanostomico, un timpanogramma piatto con un volume <1,0 mL suggerisce un tubo chiuso o non funzionante e liquido nell'orecchio medio, mentre un timpanogramma piatto con un volume >1,0 mL fa pensare a un tubo timpanostomico pervio.

Sebbene la timpanometria sia assolutamente sensibile nella diagnosi di MEE, può presentare qualche limite, dovuto alla cooperazione del paziente, alla capacità del singolo operatore di gestire il test e all'età dell'esaminando, con risultati meno attendibili in bambini molto piccoli. L'uso della timpanometria può essere d'aiuto in screening ambulatoriali, per ovviare alla necessità di un esame otoscopico di routine in pazienti difficili in cui sia stata precedentemente visualizzata la membrana timpanica, asintomatici, e i cui timpanogrammi siano classificati come normali, e per identificare pazienti che richiedano ulteriore attenzione perché i loro timpanogrammi sono anomali. La timpanometria può essere utilizzata anche per confermare, migliorare o chiarire reperti otoscopici dubbi; per oggettivare la valutazione del follow-up di pazienti con patologia conosciuta dell'orecchio medio; infine, per convalidare la diagnosi otoscopica di MEE. Cosa molto importante, anche se si ritiene che la timpanometria sia predittiva di MEE, non è in grado di distinguere un'effusione da OME da una dovuta a OMA.

Sindrome otite media-congiuntivite. La presenza contemporanea di congiuntivite purulenta ed eritematosa e OM costituisce una sindrome nota, dovuta, nella maggior parte dei bambini, a *Haemophilus influenzae* non tipizzabile. La malattia spesso è presente in più membri della stessa famiglia, e colpisce bambini piccoli e lattanti. Gli antibiotici topici per via oculare sono inefficaci; il trattamento consiste nell'utilizzo di antibiotici per via orale (vedi oltre) efficaci contro *H. influenzae* non tipizzabile.

TRATTAMENTO

Trattamento dell'otite media acuta. I singoli episodi di OMA abitualmente vengono trattati con farmaci antibiotici. La preoccupazione circa l'incremento delle resistenze batteriche ha indotto alcuni Autori a consigliare di non prescrivere una terapia antibiotica, a meno che i sintomi non persistano per 2-3 giorni o si aggravino (Tab. 639-2).

Tre fattori depongono a favore del trattamento routinario con antibiotici dei bambini ritenuti affetti da OMA (vedi Tab. 639-1 e Fig. 639-2); innanzitutto i batteri sono responsabili della maggioranza dei casi; in secondo luogo, il miglioramento sintomatologico e la risoluzione dell'infezione si verificano più rapidamente e in modo più efficace con il trattamento antibiotico piuttosto che senza, anche se si ritiene che si possano risolvere pure i casi non trattati; infine, un pronto e adeguato trattamento antibiotico può prevenire lo sviluppo di complicanze suppurative. È verosimile che il netto declino delle complicanze negli ultimi cinquant'anni possa essere attribuito, almeno in parte, alla diffusione routinaria della terapia antibiotica per l'OMA. Nei Paesi Bassi, dove non si

TABELLA 639-2. Criteri per il trattamento iniziale con antibiotici o osservazione in bambini con OMA

ETÀ	DIAGNOSI CERTA	DIAGNOSI INCERTA
<6 mesi	Terapia antibiotica	Terapia ausiliaria
6 mesi-2 anni	Terapia antibiotica	Terapia ausiliaria se la malattia è grave *Opzione di osservazione se la malattia non è grave
≥2 anni	Terapia antibiotica *Opzione di osservazione se la malattia non è grave	*Opzione di osservazione

Questa tabella è stata modificata per gentile concessione del New York State Department of Health and the New York Region Otitis Project Committee.

*L'osservazione è un'opzione appropriata solo a patto che il follow-up sia garantito e si inizi la somministrazione degli antibiotici se i sintomi persistono o peggiorano. Si considera malattia non grave un'otalgia lieve o febbre <39 °C nelle ultime 24 ore. La malattia grave è caratterizzata da otalgia da moderata a grave o febbre ≥39 °C. Una diagnosi certa di OMA soddisfa tre criteri: (1) esordio rapido; (2) segni di MEE; (3) segni e sintomi di infiammazione dell'orecchio medio.

Da Subcommittee on Management of Acute Otitis Media: Diagnosis and managment of acute otitis media. *Pediatrics* 2004;113:1451-1465.

pratica di routine il trattamento antibiotico iniziale nella maggior parte dei bambini con più di 6 anni, e dove soltanto il 30% circa dei bambini con OMA viene trattato con antibiotici, l'incidenza della mastoidite acuta, sebbene bassa (in soggetti di età <14 anni, 3,8/100 000 persone all'anno), appare un po' più alta di quella riscontrabile in altri Paesi dove gli antibiotici vengono prescritti più spesso, che è di 1-2 episodi/100 000 persone all'anno. Il follow-up dei bambini dei Paesi Bassi può essere in generale più assiduo che in altri Paesi, compresi gli Stati Uniti, dove può accadere che una mancanza di miglioramento o un peggioramento dei sintomi vengano scoperti con minore tempestività.

Queste considerazioni sul trattamento dell'OMA con terapia antibiotica devono essere confrontate con i dati sul continuo aumento percentuale delle resistenze batteriche. Nei Paesi come i Paesi Bassi, dove, per il trattamento dell'OMA, l'utilizzo di antibiotici è meno frequente, la percentuale di resistenza batterica per i patogeni maggiori dell'OM è sostanzialmente inferiore a quella di Stati in cui per la cura dell'OMA si utilizzano di routine gli antibiotici. Dato che la maggior parte degli episodi di OM si risolve spontaneamente, le linee guida pubblicate dall'American Academy of Pediatrics consigliano di rispettare un periodo di "vigile attesa" o di osservazione, prima di trattare l'OMA con antibiotici (Tabb. 639-2 e 639 3; Fig. 639-5). L'aspetto più importante delle linee guida è che occorre garantire uno stretto follow-up dei pazienti per valutare la mancanza di risoluzione spontanea o il peggioramento dei sintomi, e trattare i pazienti con adeguati analgesici (paracetamolo o ibuprofene) durante il periodo d'osservazione. Possono essere efficaci per alleviare il dolore anche farmaci otologici per uso topico. Se si adotta la pratica della vigile attesa nei pazienti con OMA, vanno considerate la certezza della diagnosi, l'età del paziente e la severità della malattia. Di fronte ai pazienti più piccoli, di età <2 anni, si consiglia di trattare tutti i casi con diagnosi confermata di OMA. In pazienti molto piccoli, con meno di 6 mesi di vita, si deve trattare anche un presunto episodio di OMA, per il potenziale aumento della morbilità da complicanze infettive. È consigliata la terapia antibiotica anche in bambini di età compresa tra 6 e 24 mesi, che hanno una diagnosi dubbia di OM ma sono gravemente sofferenti, con una temperatura >39°C, otalgia significativa o segni tossici. I pazienti in questa fascia d'età, in cui la diagnosi sia dubbia e la malattia non sia grave, possono essere tenuti sotto osservazione con uno stretto follow-up per 2-3 giorni. Per i bambini di età >2 anni, si deve prendere in considerazione l'osservazione in tutti gli episodi di OM non grave o di diagnosi dubbia, riservando la terapia antibiotica ai casi di OMA grave, confermata.

RESISTENZE BATTERICHE. I batteri hanno una notevole capacità di sviluppare resistenza agli antibiotici; dal decennio scorso le resistenze batteriche sono un problema in aumento. I soggetti a maggiore rischio in tal senso sono i bambini con meno di 2

TABELLA 639-3. Antibiotici raccomandati per pazienti che sono stati inizialmente trattati con antibiotici o hanno fallito il periodo d'osservazione di 48-72 ore, o la terapia iniziale con antibiotici

TEMPERATURA ≥39 °C E/O GRAVE OTALGIA	ALLA DIAGNOSI PER PAZIENTI TRATTATI INIZIALMENTE CON ANTIBIOTICI		FALLIMENTO CLINICAMENTE DEFINITO DEL TRATTAMENTO A 48-72 ORE DALLA TERAPIA INIZIALE CON OPZIONE DI OSSERVAZIONE		FALLIMENTO CLINICAMENTE DEFINITO A 48-72 ORE DOPO INIZIALE TRATTAMENTO CON ANTIBIOTICI	
	RACCOMANDATO	ALTERNATIVA PER ALLERGIA ALLA PENICILLINA	RACCOMANDATO	ALTERNATIVA PER ALLERGIA ALLA PENICILLINA	RACCOMANDATO	ALTERNATIVA PER ALLERGIA ALLA PENICILLINA
No	Amoxicillina, 80-90 mg/kg/die	Non tipo 1: cefdinir, cefuroxima; tipo 1: azitromicina, claritromicina	Amoxicillina, 80-90 mg/kg/die	Non tipo 1: cefdinir, cefuroxima; tipo 1: azitromicina, claritromicina	Amoxicillina/acido clavulanico, 90 mg/kg/die di amoxicillina, con 6,4 mg/kg/die di acido clavulanico	Non tipo 1: ceftriaxone, 3 giorni; tipo 1: clindamicina
Sì	Amoxicillina/acido clavulanico, 90 mg/kg/die di amoxicillina, con 6,4 mg/kg/die di acido clavulanico	Ceftriaxone, 1 o 3 giorni	Amoxicillina/acido clavulanico, 90 mg/kg/die di amoxicillina, con 6,4 mg/kg/die di acido clavulanico	Ceftriaxone, 1 o 3 giorni	Ceftriaxone, 3 giorni	Timpanocentesi, clindamicina

Da Subcommittee on Managment of Acute Otitis Media: Diagnosis and management of acute otitis media. *Pediatrics* 2004;113:1451-1465.

anni d'età, quelli in contatto costante con ampi gruppi di coetanei, specialmente nell'ambito delle scuole materne, o quelli che hanno ricevuto una terapia antibiotica di recente. Le resistenze batteriche sono un problema particolare in relazione all'OM. Lo sviluppo di ceppi batterici resistenti e la loro rapida diffusione sono stati favoriti dalla pressione selettiva dovuta all'esteso utilizzo di antibiotici, somministrati nei bambini, il più delle volte, per OM. A questo si aggiunga che molti ceppi degli stessi batterii patogeni che comunemente provocano OMA sono resistenti ad alcuni degli antibiotici più utilizzati.

Sebbene i tassi di resistenza batterica varino da Paese a Paese, negli Stati Uniti circa il 40% dei ceppi non tipizzabili di *H. influenzae* e quasi tutti i ceppi di *M. catarrhalis* di solito sono resistenti alle aminopenicilline (ampicillina, amoxicillina). Nella maggior parte dei casi la resistenza è attribuibile alla produzione di β-lattamasi, e può essere superata associando l'amoxicillina a un inibitore della β-lattamasi, cioè l'acido clavulanico, o utilizzando un antibiotico β-lattamasi-stabile. Tuttavia, ceppi occasionali di *H. influenzae* non tipizzabili che non producono β-lattamasi sono resistenti alle aminopenicilline e ad altri antibiotici β-lattamici in virtù di alterazioni delle loro proteine di legame alla penicillina.

Non sono suscettibili alla penicillina circa il 50% circa dei ceppi di *S. pneumoniae*, divisi quasi equamente tra ceppi con resistenza intermedia alla penicillina e penicillino-resistenti (questi ultimi rendono il trattamento particolarmente problematico). Una più alta incidenza di resistenza si è osservata in bambini che frequentano scuole materne. La resistenza di *S. pneumoniae* alle penicilline e ad altri antibiotici β-lattamici è mediata non dalla produzione di β-lattamasi, ma da alterazioni delle proteine di legame della penicillina. Il grado di resistenza aumenta in risposta al numero di alterazioni di queste proteine, che sono almeno sei. Tuttavia, questo meccanismo di resistenza può essere superato se si raggiungono maggiori concentrazioni di antibiotici β-lattamici nella sede d'infezione per un tempo sufficiente. Molti ceppi penicillino-resistenti di *S. pneumoniae* sono resistenti anche ad altri antibiotici, compresi i sulfamidici, i macrolidi e le cefalosporine più recenti. La resistenza ai macrolidi, tra cui l'azitromicina e la claritromicina, da parte di *S. pneumoniae* è in rapido aumento (caratterizza circa il 30% dei ceppi). Ne sono stati identificati due meccanismi: il primo, mediato dal gene mef(A), implica una pompa di efflusso che diminuisce l'accumulo intracellulare di macrolidi, e conferisce un basso livello di resistenza; il secondo, mediato dal gene erm(B), implica la produzione di metilasi ribosomiali che modificano l'RNA ribosomiale, e comporta un elevato livello di resistenza. Il secondo meccanismo porta anche a resistenza alla clindamicina, che in genere è efficace contro i ceppi resistenti di *S. pneumoniae*. A differenza della resistenza agli antibiotici β-lattamici, la resistenza ai macrolidi può essere superata aumentando la dose. Nonostante la vancomicina in passato fosse considerata un antimicrobico infallibile nel trattamento di *S. pneumoniae*, sono stati identificati casi clinici di *S. pneumoniae* vancomicina-tolleranti e questo non fa che aumentare l'importanza e il pericolo della resistenza agli antibiotici.

TRATTAMENTO ANTIBIOTICO DI PRIMA SCELTA. Nella maggior parte dei casi, l'amoxicillina rimane il farmaco preferito per l'OMA non complicata, per le sue prestazioni eccellenti in termini di efficacia, palatabilità e basso costo (vedi Tab. 639-3). L'amoxicillina è il più efficace dei farmaci antibatterici orali disponibili contro ceppi di *S. pneumoniae* suscettibili o meno alla penicillina. Aumentare la dose dai tradizionali 40 mg/kg/die agli 80-100 mg/kg/die di solito si rivela utile contro ceppi con resistenza intermedia alla penicillina e alcuni penicillino-resistenti. Questa dose più elevata dovrebbe essere utilizzata soprattutto nei bambini di età >2 anni che abbiano da poco ricevuto un trattamento con β-lattamici o abbiano avuto contatto con molti altri bambini, perché in questi casi è più alta la prevalenza di ceppi di *S. pneumoniae* non suscettibili. Un limite dell'amoxicillina è che può essere inattivata dalla β-lattamasi prodotta da molti ceppi di *H. influenzae* non tipizzabile e dalla maggior parte dei ceppi di *M. catarrhalis*. Fortunatamente, episodi di OMA causati da questi patogeni, spesso, anche se non sempre, vanno incontro a risoluzione spontanea. Le allergie agli antibiotici penicillinici devono essere considerate come reazioni da ipersensibilità di tipo 1, che consistono in orticaria o anafilassi, e quelle che non rientrano in questa classificazione, come un rash. Per i bambini con reazione non di tipo 1 in cui la reazione crociata con le cefalosporine desta minori preoccupazioni, la terapia di prima istanza con cefdinir costituisce una scelta appropriata (vedi Tab. 639-3). In bambini con una reazione di tipo 1 o sensibilità nota alle cefalosporine, o in cui siano di notevole importanza la palatabilità o la comodità di somministrazione, l'azitromicina rappresenta una valida alternativa ai farmaci di prima linea. La resistenza al trimetoprim-sulfametoxazolo da parte di molti ceppi sia di *H. influenzae* sia di *S. pneumoniae*, e l'alta percentuale di insuccessi clinici riportata in bambini con OMA trattati inizialmente con questo antibiotico, costituiscono argomenti contro il suo utilizzo come terapia di prima scelta.

DURATA DEL TRATTAMENTO. La durata del trattamento dell'OMA è stata determinata in 10 giorni, apparentemente estrapolato sulla durata ottimale del trattamento penicillinico della faringite streptococcica. Tuttavia, 10 giorni possono essere decisamente troppi per alcuni bambini, e pochi per altri. Studi comparativi su trattamenti di maggiore e minore durata suggeriscono che spesso le terapie di breve durata sono inadeguate in bambini di età <6 anni, in particolarmente se hanno meno di 2 anni. Di conseguenza, per la maggior parte degli episodi infantili, è

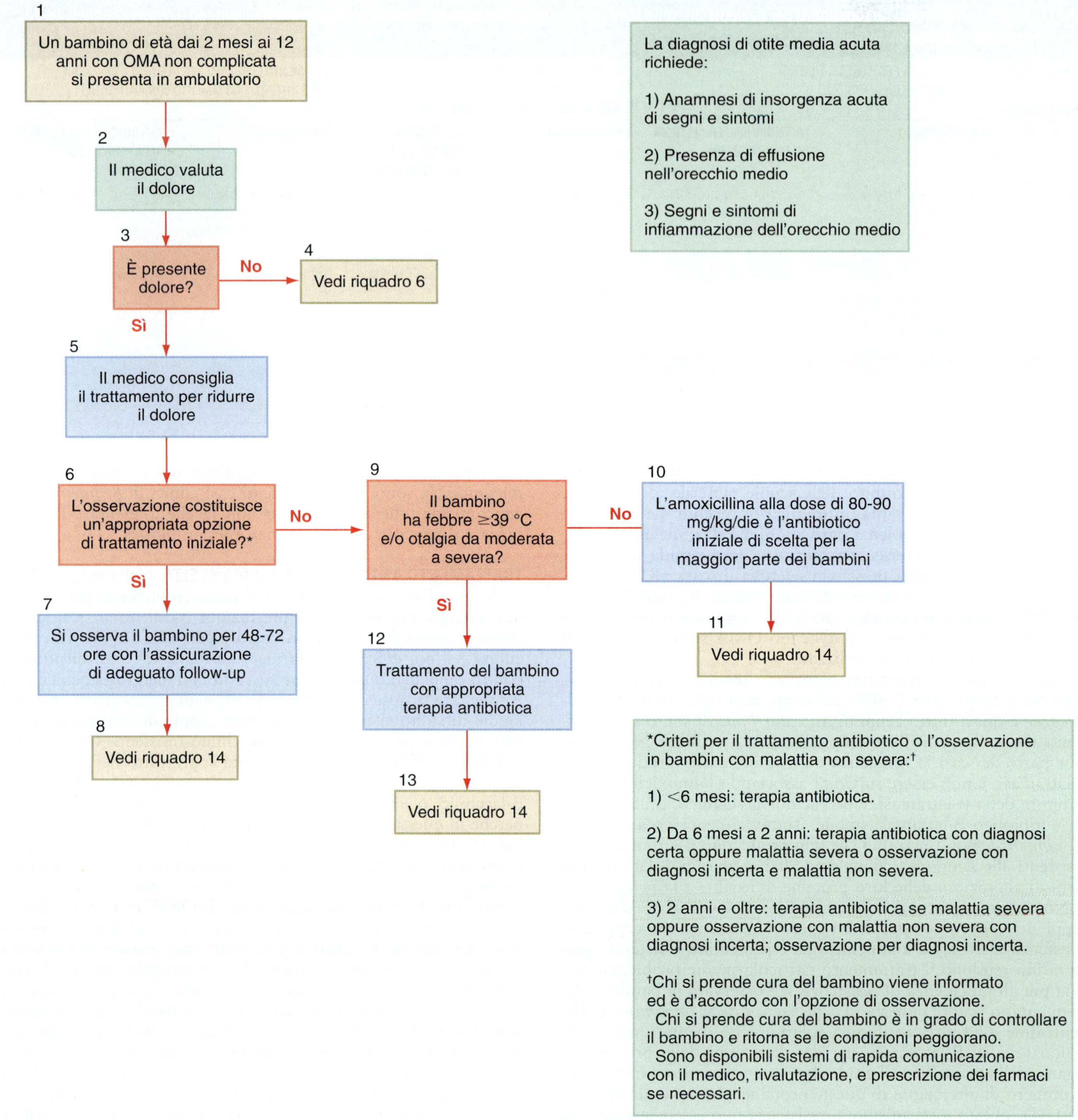

Figura 639-5. Trattamento dell'otite media acuta (OMA). (Da Subcommittee on Management of Acute Otitis Media: Diagnosis and managment of acute otitis media. *Pediatrics* 204;113:1451-1465.)

Continua

consigliabile una terapia che determini concentrazioni tissutali di antibiotico per almeno 10 giorni. Il trattamento per periodi più brevi, di 3-5 giorni, può essere indicato per bambini più grandi, con episodi lievi, che migliorano rapidamente; tuttavia, in questi casi, si potrebbe ragionevolmente argomentare che la semplice osservazione, senza terapia antibiotica, è preferibile. Trattamenti di durata >10 giorni potrebbero essere necessari per bambini molto piccoli, oltre che per pazienti pediatrici con episodi gravi o con una precedente esperienza di OM problematica.

FOLLOW-UP. Obiettivo principale del follow-up è valutare gli esiti del trattamento e differenziare le risposte inadeguate dalle recidive precoci. Di conseguenza, il giusto intervallo per il follow-up deve essere individualizzato. È consigliabile un controllo entro pochi giorni in bambini molto piccoli con episodio grave, o in bambini di qualsiasi età con dolore perseverante. Per lattanti o bambini piccoli che hanno avuto frequenti recidive, è adeguato un follow-up entro 2 settimane. A quest'epoca, la membrana timpanica probabilmente non è ancora tornata normale, ma dovrebbe comunque essere evidente un sostanziale miglioramento. In un bambino con un solo episodio sporadico di OMA e un rapido miglioramento sintomatico, è corretto effettuare un controllo un mese dopo il primo esame, e in bambini più grandi può non essere necessario alcun follow-up. Fatto molto importante,

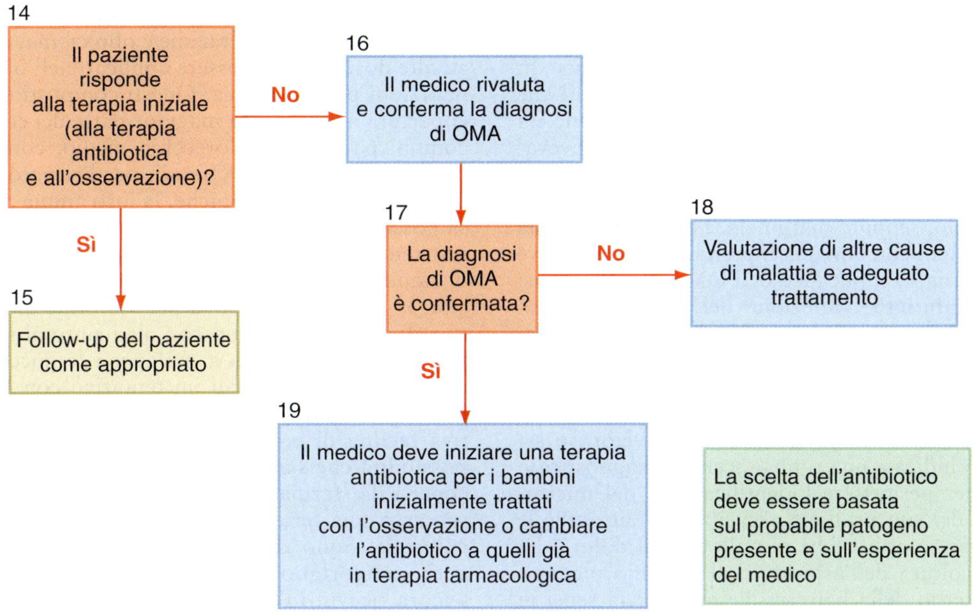

Figura 639-5. *Continua*

la persistenza della sola MEE dopo un episodio di OMA non costituisce un'indicazione a un trattamento ulteriore o di seconda scelta.

INSODDISFACENTE RISPOSTA ALLA TERAPIA DI PRIMA SCELTA. L'OMA è essenzialmente l'infezione di uno spazio chiuso, e la sua guarigione dipende dall'eradicazione del microrganismo patogeno e dal ripristino della ventilazione dell'orecchio medio. Fattori che contribuiscono a un'insoddisfacente risposta alla terapia di prima scelta, oltre all'inadeguata efficacia antibatterica, comprendono: scarsa compliance con il regime terapeutico, infezioni virali concomitanti o intercorrenti, persistente disfunzione della tuba di Eustachio e diminuita aerazione dell'orecchio medio, reinfezione da altre sedi per eradicamento incompleto dei patogeni dell'orecchio medio e difese dell'ospite immature o alterate. Nonostante i tanti fattori potenziali, è ragionevole il ricorso a un farmaco alternativo o di seconda scelta quando vi sia un inadeguato miglioramento dei sintomi o della condizione dell'orecchio medio, valutata dall'aspetto della membrana timpanica, o quando la persistenza di una rinorrea purulenta suggerisca che l'antibiotico utilizzato non aveva un'efficacia ottimale. Si possono utilizzare farmaci di seconda scelta quando l'OMA si sviluppa in bambini che abbiano già ricevuto antibiotici, presentino compromissione del sistema immunitario o abbiano sintomi gravi e precedente esperienza di OM problematica.

TRATTAMENTO DI SECONDA SCELTA. Se la terapia dell'OMA con antibiotici di prima scelta ha dato risultati inadeguati, sono utilizzabili vari farmaci di seconda scelta (vedi Tab. 639-3). I farmaci destinati al trattamento di seconda scelta devono essere efficaci contro i ceppi di *H. influenzae* produttori di β-lattamasi e di *M. catarrhalis*, e contro ceppi suscettibili e soprattutto non suscettibili di *S. pneumoniae*. Solo tre farmaci rispondono senz'altro ai requisiti: amoxicillina/acido clavulanico, cefuroxime/axetil e ceftriaxone per via intramuscolare. Dato che alte dosi di amoxicillina (80-100 mg/kg/die) sono efficaci contro la maggior parte dei ceppi di *S. pneumomiae*, e che l'aggiunta dell'acido clavulanico estende lo spettro della sua efficacia antibatterica anche a batteri produttori di β-lattamasi, alte dosi di amoxicillina/acido clavulanico sono particolarmente idonee alla terapia di seconda scelta per l'OMA. La formulazione amoxicillina/acido clavulanico 14:1 contiene una quantità di amoxicillina doppia rispetto alla precedente formulazione 7:1. La diarrea, soprattutto in lattanti e bambini piccoli, è un effetto collaterale frequente, ma in alcuni casi può essere attenuata utilizzando yogurt, e di solito non è così grave da richiedere la sospensione della terapia. Gli altri due farmaci presentano importanti limitazioni per l'utilizzo in bambini piccoli. Le sospensioni normalmente disponibili di cefuroxime/axetil non hanno un buon sapore e sono quindi poco accettate dai bambini. Il trattamento con ceftriaxone comporta dolore durante l'iniezione intramuscolare e un costo notevole; può essere necessario ripetere l'iniezione 1 o 2 volte a intervalli di 2-3 giorni per ottenere il grado di efficacia desiderato. Ciononostante, l'uso del ceftriaxone è adeguato nei casi gravi di OMA, quando non è realizzabile un trattamento orale, o, in casi altamente selezionati, dopo fallimento della terapia orale con farmaci di seconda istanza (per es. amoxicillina/acido clavulanico, cefuroxime/axetil), o quando, nell'aspirato da timpanocentesi diagnostica, si trova un ceppo di *S. pneumoniae* fortemente resistente. Il cefdinir non era ancora disponibile quando sono state formulate queste indicazioni. Tuttavia, la pratica clinica e l'efficacia del cefdinir suggeriscono che esso meriti considerazione come farmaco di seconda scelta, con uno spettro antibatterico simile a quello del cefuroxime/axetil, una buona percentuale di compliance e una certa palatabilità.

I macrolidi più recenti, claritromicina e azitromicina, hanno solo un'attività limitata contro ceppi non suscettibili di *S. pneumoniae* e contro ceppi di *H. influenzae* produttori di β-lattamasi. Tra le cefalosporine, oltre al cefuroxime/axetil e al cefdinir, sembra promettente la cefpodoxima. Tuttavia, la compliance può essere compromessa dalla scarsa palatabilità di questo farmaco. Il cefprozil possiede una minor stabilità alla β-lattamasi rispetto al cefuroxime o al cefpodoxime. Il ceflacor e il loracarbef hanno attività limitata contro batteri produttori di β-lattamasi e pneumococchi non suscettibili, e il ceflacor occasionalmente può provocare malattia da siero. Il cefixime ha un'attività eccellente contro i batteri produttori di β-lattamasi, ma limitata contro pneumococchi anche suscettibili alla penicillina. Il trimetoprim/sulfametoxazolo ha una così scarsa efficacia che non viene consigliato per il trattamento dell'OMA. Inoltre, questo farmaco può provocare (seppur raramente) reazioni gravi, come soppressione midollare o sindrome di Steven-Johnson. Anche l'eritromicina/sulfisoxazolo causa reazioni simili, oltre a non essere attiva contro pneumococchi non suscettibili alla penicillina. La clindamicina è attiva contro la maggior parte dei ceppi di *S. pneumoniae*, compresi quelli resistenti, ma non contro *H. influenzae* o *M. catarrhalis*; va perciò riservata a pazienti che abbiano un'infezione provocata da *S. pneumoniae* non suscettibile alla penicillina.

MIRINGOTOMIA E TIMPANOCENTESI. La miringotomia è un trattamento per l'OMA in uso da molto tempo, ma in genere non è necessaria nei pazienti pediatrici trattati con antibiotici. In un trial clinico limitato a bambini con OMA grave, quelli che ricevevano amoxicillina più miringotomia non presentavano un decorso complessivamente migliore rispetto a quelli che ricevevano solo amoxicillina, ma la popolazione dello studio non era così numerosa da escludere la possibilità che l'intervento chirurgico avesse qualche beneficio, seppure marginale. Le **indicazioni alla miringotomia** nei bambini con OMA comprendono dolore grave e refrattario, iperpiressia, complicanze dell'OMA quali paralisi facciale, mastoidite, labirintite, infezione del sistema nervoso centrale e compromissione immunologica. Questa procedura deve essere considerata una terapia di terza scelta in pazienti in cui, per un episodio di OMA, siano falliti due trattamenti antibiotici consecutivi. In bambini con OMA in cui la risposta clinica a una secondo trattamento antibiotico di seconda scelta vigoroso sia insoddisfacente, sono indicate una timpanocentesi diagnostica o una miringotomia, per permettere l'identificazione del microrganismo patogeno e del suo profilo di sensibilità. Entrambe le procedure possono essere utili anche per alleviare il dolore. La timpanocentesi con coltura dell'aspirato dall'orecchio medio è indicata anche all'interno della batteria d'esami per la sepsi in neonati con OMA con meno di 1 mese di vita, in cui siano presenti segni sistemici di malattia come febbre, vomito o letargia, e in cui di conseguenza la malattia non possa ritenersi limitata all'orecchio medio. Il CDC Working Group ha scritto: "In un'era di aumentate resistenze batteriche, i medici che trattano i bambini con OMA dovrebbero imparare a eseguire personalmente la timpanocentesi o almeno inviare subito i pazienti a un medico con questa capacità".

L'esecuzione della timpanocentesi può essere facilitata dall'uso di un aspiratore appositamente studiato per la timpanocentesi.

RECIDIVA PRECOCE DOPO IL TRATTAMENTO. La recidiva di OMA dopo un'apparente risoluzione può essere dovuta tanto a incompleta eradicazione dell'infezione dall'orecchio medio o dalle vie aeree superiori, quanto a reinfezione da parte dello stesso batterio o di uno diverso. La recidiva dopo parecchi giorni solitamente è dovuta allo stesso microrganismo, e di conseguenza si può fare riferimento alla risposta al trattamento dell'episodio precedente: se c'è stata risposta a un antibiotico di prima scelta, quel farmaco è ancora appropriato; se invece c'è stata risposta solo a un farmaco di seconda scelta, può essere opportuno, sin dall'inizio, l'uso di un farmaco di seconda scelta. Anche una recente terapia antibiotica predispone il paziente a una maggiore incidenza di microrganismi resistenti, che devono essere valutati nella scelta della terapia.

MIRINGOTOMIA E INSERIMENTO DI TUBI TIMPANOSTOMICI. Quando l'OMA è recidivante, nonostante un'appropriata terapia medica, è giustificato un suo trattamento chirurgico con l'inserimento di un tubo timpanostomico. Questa procedura è molto efficace nel ridurre la percentuale di OMA in pazienti con OM recidivante, nei quali può migliorare in modo significativo la qualità della vita. Fattori inerenti al singolo paziente, tra cui profilo del rischio, severità degli episodi di OMA, sviluppo ed età del bambino, anamnesi positiva per effetti collaterali da farmaci, concomitanti problemi medici e desideri dei genitori, hanno certamente un peso al momento di decidere se eseguire questa procedura. Tuttavia, quando un paziente richiede 3-4 cicli di antibiotici in un periodo di 6 mesi o va incontro a 5-6 episodi di OMA in 12 mesi, bisogna prospettare ai genitori un intervento chirurgico.

OTORREA DAL TUBO. Quando si sviluppa otorrea dal tubo timpanostomico, va preso in esame, come opzione di prima scelta, un trattamento per via topica. Con un tubo funzionante in sede, l'infezione può drenare e la possibilità che un episodio di OMA dia luogo a una complicanza seria è trascurabile. Le gocce topiche di quinolone, approvate dall'FDA per l'applicazione nell'orecchio medio in ambito pediatrico, sono formulate con ciprofloxacina/desametazone e ofloxacina, che, se somministrati ad alte dosi, possono essere applicati nell'orecchio medio in preparazioni per via topica. Questi composti offrono un'eccellente copertura anche per la maggior parte dei ceppi resistenti dei più comuni patogeni dell'orecchio medio, come *S. aureus* e *Pseudomonas aeruginosa*. Quindi, per l'elevato tasso di successo di queste preparazioni topiche, la loro ampia copertura, la più bassa possibilità che contribuiscano allo sviluppo di microrganismi resistenti, la relativa facilità di somministrazione, la mancanza di significativi effetti collaterali e la loro mancanza di ototossicità, la terapia antibiotica per via orale di solito va riservata ai casi di otorrea dal tubo con altri sintomi sistemici associati, in pazienti che tollerano a malapena le gocce otologiche o forse anche in pazienti in cui un tentativo con gocce otologiche per uso topico non abbia dato alcun risultato. Inoltre, per la relativa facilità di prelevare del liquido per l'esame colturale, e la possibilità che siano presenti altri patogeni (per es. miceti) non coperti dai farmaci per uso topico, sul paziente in cui non ha successo una terapia per uso topico si deve eseguire un esame colturale. Sono disponibili altre preparazioni otologiche, che però comportano un certo rischio di ototossicità o non hanno ancora ricevuto l'approvazione per l'utilizzo a livello dell'orecchio medio. Molte di queste preparazioni erano ampiamente utilizzate prima dello sviluppo delle attuali gocce di quinolone, ed erano generalmente considerate abbastanza sicure ed efficaci. In tutti i casi di otorrea dal tubo, è molto importante un'attenta igiene dell'orecchio, che consiste nell'eliminare le secrezioni del condotto uditivo esterno e nell'evitare il contatto dell'orecchio esterno con l'acqua. In alcuni casi le secrezioni molto dense e ostinate possono rappresentare un ostacolo alla terapia topica, perché i farmaci non sono in grado di distribuirsi alla sede d'infezione; l'aspirazione e la rimozione delle secrezioni, spesso eseguita da uno specialista otorinolaringoiatra, può essere essenziale. Quando i pazienti pediatrici con otorrea dal tubo non danno più segni di miglioramento con la tradizionale terapia ambulatoriale, può rendersi necessaria la rimozione del tubo e/o il ricovero in ospedale per un trattamento antibiotico per via parenterale.

TRATTAMENTO DELL'OTITE MEDIA CON EFFUSIONE

Per determinare il decorso di un episodio di OME, e per distinguere tra persistenza e recidiva, è necessaria una valutazione mensile fino alla guarigione; se l'effusione dura più di 3 mesi occorre valutare anche l'udito (vedi Fig. 639-1). Il razionale trattamento dell'OME dipende in misura notevole dalla comprensione della storia naturale e delle possibili complicanze e sequele. La maggior parte dei casi di OME si risolve senza trattamento in 3 mesi; pochi sono i dati disponibili in merito all'ulteriore decorso a lungo termine di bambini in cui l'OME non si risolve in questo periodo di tempo, e che non vengono sottoposti a intervento chirurgico. Al momento di prendere in esame il trattamento chirurgico dell'OME persistente con inserzione di tubo timpanostomico, è importante che il medico determini l'impatto dell'OME sul bambino. Sebbene l'ipoacusia sia la preoccupazione fondamentale, l'OME provoca nei bambini una serie di altre difficoltà, che vanno tenute in considerazione: predisposizione a OMA recidivante, dolore, disturbi dell'equilibrio e acufeni. Le sequele a lungo termine associate a OME includono: modificazioni patologiche dell'orecchio medio, atelettasia della membrana timpanica e formazione di tasche di retrazione, OM adesiva, discontinuità degli ossicini, colesteatoma e ipoacusia neurosensoriale. Sono noti anche gli effetti collaterali a lungo termine su linguaggio articolato e sviluppo cognitivo e psicosociale, anche se alcuni studi hanno dimostrato che l'impatto negativo a lungo termine dell'OME sullo sviluppo può essere scarso. A tale riguardo, è importante tenere conto della presentazione complessiva del bambino. Sebbene sia improbabile che l'OME che provoca ipoacusia unilaterale di grado lieve abbia effetti negativi a lungo termine su un bambino per altri versi sano e con uno sviluppo normale, anche un'ipoacusia lieve in un soggetto con altri ritardi dello sviluppo o della parola può costituire un fattore aggravante. Bambini con OME che persiste per più di 3 mesi meritano, come minimo, uno stretto monitoraggio dei livelli uditivi con una valutazione audiologica qualificata, una frequente valutazione delle tappe fondamentali dello sviluppo, compresa quella della parola e del linguaggio, e una particolare attenzione alla percentuale di recidiva di OMA.

VARIABILI CHE INFLUENZANO LE DECISIONI SUL TRATTAMENTO DELL'OTITE MEDIA CON EFFUSIONE. Le variabili legate al paziente che interferiscono con la decisione del trattamento da adottare per l'OME comprendono l'età del bambino, la frequenza e la severità di precedenti episodi di OMA e il tempo trascorso dall'ultimo episodio, lo sviluppo del linguaggio del bambino, la presenza o l'assenza di un'anamnesi di positività a effetti collaterali dei farmaci, problemi medici concomitanti, o fattori di rischio, come la frequenza di scuola materna o altro tipo di esposizione a malattie infettive, e i desideri dei genitori. Nel considerare il trattamento chirurgico dell'OME con inserimento di tubi timpanostomici, si sono notati particolari benefici in pazienti con OME persistente inframmezzata da episodi di OMA, perché i tubi generalmente guariscono entrambe le condizioni. Variabili legate alla malattia che occorre considerare nel trattamento dell'OME sono la mono- o bilateralità dell'effusione, la sua entità appurata, la durata, se nota, il grado di alterazione uditiva, la presenza o l'assenza di altri sintomi correlati (per es. acufeni, vertigini o disturbi dell'equilibrio) e la presenza o l'assenza di rinorrea mucopurulenta o purulenta che, se continua per più di 2 settimane, induce a pensare che la concomitante infezione del rinofaringe o del seno paranasale possa contribuire a perpetuare una condizione di scarsa ventilazione dell'orecchio medio.

TRATTAMENTO MEDICO. Gli antibiotici hanno un'efficacia definita ma limitata nella guarigione dell'OME, presumibilmente perché aiutano a eradicare l'infezione rinofaringea e/o l'infezione dell'orecchio medio asintomatica. Quindi, dal momento che apportano un beneficio a breve termine mentre d'altro canto contribuiscono allo sviluppo della resistenza batterica, il trattamento antibiotico di routine dell'OME, in precedenza consigliato da alcuni Autori, non sembra essere più una scelta condivisibile. Il trattamento deve essere, invece, limitato ai casi in cui sia evidente l'associazione con un'infezione delle vie aeree superiori o un'infezione dell'orecchio medio non trattata. A questo scopo, bisogna utilizzare il farmaco disponibile più efficace, come raccomandato per l'OMA.

L'efficacia dei corticosteroidi orali nell'OME probabilmente è massima a breve termine e le linee guida per la terapia dell'OME hanno stabilito che il rapporto rischio/beneficio sembra essere a loro sfavore. Le combinazioni di antistaminici e decongestionanti non sono efficaci nella terapia dei bambini con OME, ma la loro efficacia non è stata testata in pazienti con allergie ambientali. Gli antistaminici, i decongestionanti e i farmaci mucolitici hanno scarsa probabilità di essere efficaci. La terapia antiallergica può dimostrarsi d'aiuto nei bambini con OMR problematica, che presentano anche segni di allergia delle vie respiratorie superiori, ma mancano dati di supporto. Nei bambini senza evidenze di allergie non sono indicati i test per le allergie. La dilatazione delle tube di Eustachio con la manovra del Valsalva o con altri mezzi non si è rivelata efficace a lungo termine.

MIRINGOTOMIA E INSERIMENTO DI TUBI TIMPANOSTOMICI. Quando, nonostante un lungo periodo di vigile attesa, l'OME persiste per 3-6 mesi o più, in bambini con effusione monolaterale, si presenta l'opzione del trattamento chirurgico. La miringotomia senza inserimento di tubi permette di evacuare i fluidi presenti nell'orecchio medio e talvolta si rivela efficace; dato che l'incisione guarisce prima che la mucosa dell'orecchio medio ritorni normale, accade spesso che l'effusione ben presto si riformi. L'inserimento dei tubi offre la possibilità di ventilare l'orecchio medio per tutto il tempo in cui il drenaggio rimane funzionante e in sede, in media 12 mesi circa, e quasi sempre risolve l'ipoacusia conduttiva associata a OME. Episodi occasionali di ostruzione del lume e di estrusione prematura del tubo possono essere associati a otorrea. Il posizionamento di tubi, tuttavia, di norma consente la guarigione dell'OME infantile. Le sequele conseguenti all'estrusione del tubo consistono in perforazione residuale della membrana timpanica, timpanosclerosi, cicatrici atrofiche localizzate o diffuse della membrana timpanica, che possono predisporre allo sviluppo di atelettasia e/o a una tasca di retrazione o di entrambe le cose, di ipoacusia conduttiva residuale e colesteatoma. Fortunatamente, la più seria di queste sequele è raro che si verifichi. La recidiva con effusione dell'orecchio medio che fa seguito all'estrusione dei tubi è rara, soprattutto nei bambini più piccoli. Tuttavia, la maggior parte dei bambini senza sottostanti anomalie craniofacciali richiede solo un ciclo di inserimento di tubi timpanostomici, con modificazioni dello sviluppo che consentono un miglioramento delle condizioni dell'orecchio medio e la risoluzione dell'OME cronica al momento dell'estrusione del tubo. Dato che anche un'OME precedentemente persistente spesso va incontro a regressione spontanea nei mesi estivi, nella maggior parte dei bambini con OME per altri aspetti sani, è consigliabile l'attesa vigile durante l'estate. Infine, nel considerare il trattamento chirurgico dell'OME infantile, soprattutto nelle forme di malattia bilaterale e con ipoacusia, è stato dimostrato che il posizionamento di tubi timpanostomici consente di migliorare la qualità della vita.

COMPLICANZE DELL'OTITE MEDIA ACUTA. La maggior parte delle complicanze dell'OMA consiste nella diffusione dell'infezione alle strutture contigue o vicine e/o nello sviluppo di cronicità. Le complicanze suppurative sono relativamente rare nei bambini che vivono nei Paesi sviluppati, mentre sono tutt'altro che rare nei pazienti provenienti dagli strati sociali più bassi, in cui l'assistenza scarseggia o manca. Le complicanze dell'OMA possono essere classificate come intratemporali o intracraniche.

COMPLICANZE INTRATEMPORALI. Un'estensione diretta ma limitata dell'OM porta a complicanze all'interno dell'osso temporale: dermatite, perforazione della membrana timpanica, OM suppurativa cronica, mastoidite, ipoacusia, paralisi del nervo facciale, colesteatoma e labirintite.

DERMATITE INFETTIVA. La dermatite infettiva è un'infezione della cute del condotto uditivo esterno, dovuta alla contaminazione da parte delle secrezioni purulente provenienti dall'orecchio medio. La cute spesso è eritematosa, edematosa e dolente. Il trattamento consiste nell'igiene personale unita ad antibiotici per via sistemica o gocce otologiche, come per la terapia dell'OMA e dell'otorrea da tubo.

PERFORAZIONE DELLA MEMBRANA TIMPANICA. La rottura della membrana timpanica si può verificare con episodi di OMA e di OME. Sebbene il danno alla membrana timpanica di solito guarisca spontaneamente, in un piccolo numero di casi possono svilupparsi perforazioni croniche, che richiedono un ulteriore intervento chirurgico.

OTITE MEDIA CRONICA SUPPURATIVA. L'OM cronica suppurativa consiste in un'infezione persistente dell'orecchio medio con scarico attraverso una perforazione della membrana timpanica. La malattia inizia con un episodio di OMA con rottura della membrana. Le cellule aeree mastoidee sono sempre coinvolte. I più frequenti agenti eziologici sono *Pseudomonas aeruginosa* e *S. aureus*. Il trattamento dipende dai risultati dell'indagine microbiologica. Se non è presente un colesteatoma associato, è probabile che l'infezione si risolva con una terapia antibiotica parenterale combinata a un'assidua pulizia dell'orecchio; tuttavia, nei casi refrattari può essere richiesta la timpanomastoidectomia.

MASTOIDITE ACUTA. Tecnicamente, tutti i casi di OMA sono accompagnati da mastoidite, in virtù dell'infiammazione associata delle cellule aeree mastoidee. Tuttavia, nelle fasi precoci della malattia non sono presenti segni e sintomi di infezione mastoidea e in genere il processo infiammatorio è facilmente reversibile, con l'OMA, in risposta alla terapia antibiotica. La diffusione dell'infezione al periostio sovrastante, ma senza coinvolgimento dell'osso, costituisce una **mastoidite acuta con periosteite**. In questi casi, solitamente sono presenti segni di mastoidite, per esempio infiammazione dell'area retroauricolare, spesso con spostamento del lobo inferiormente e anteriormente (Tab. 639-4). La terapia con miringotomia e antibiotici per via parenterale, se istituita prontamente, di solito porta alla guarigione.

Nell'osteite acuta della mastoide, o mastoidite coalescente, l'infezione progredisce, provocando la distruzione delle trabecole ossee della mastoide (Fig. 639-6). Normalmente, ma non sempre, sono presenti segni e sintomi franchi di mastoidite. Nella petrosite acuta, l'infezione si estende ulteriormente fino a coinvolgere la porzione petrosa dell'osso temporale. Il sintomo principale è il dolore all'orecchio, dovuto all'irritazione della branca oftalmica del V nervo cranico; in seguito si instaura una paralisi del VI nervo cranico. La **sindrome di Gradenigo** è caratterizzata dalla triade di OM suppurativa, paralisi del muscolo retto esterno e dolore localizzato all'orbita ipsolaterale. È raro che l'infezione della mastoide si diffonda ai muscoli del collo, provocando un **ascesso di Bezold**.

Quando si sospetta una mastoidite, o la si diagnostica clinicamente, si deve eseguire una TC dell'osso temporale per chiarire ulteriormente la natura e l'estensione della malattia (vedi Fig. 639-6). La distruzione ossea della mastoide deve essere distinta dal semplice offuscamento delle cellule aeree mastoidee, che spesso è riscontrabile nei casi non complicati di OM. In tutte le varianti di mastoidite acuta, i più comuni agenti causali sono *S. pneumoniae*, *H. influenzae* non tipizzabile e *P. aeruginosa*. I bambini con osteite mastoidea acuta richiedono antibiotici per via endovenosa e mastoidectomia, la cui estensione dipende dal grado di diffusione del processo infiammatorio. Per quanto possibile, la scelta dell'antibiotico deve essere guidata dai reperti dell'indagine microbiologica.

Tutte le varianti della mastoidite si possono verificare anche nella forma subacuta o cronica. I sintomi sono analoghi ma un po' più lievi. La mastoidite cronica è sempre accompagnata da OM cronica suppurativa e talvolta risponde al trattamento conservativo consigliato per tale condizione. Nella maggior parte dei casi, tuttavia, è necessaria la mastoidectomia.

PARALISI FACCIALE. Il nervo facciale, nel suo passaggio attraverso l'orecchio medio e l'osso mastoideo, può essere colpito dall'infezione adiacente. La paralisi facciale come complicanza dell'OMA non è frequente, e spesso si risolve dopo miringotomia e trattamento antibiotico parenterale. La paralisi facciale in presenza di OMA richiede un'immediata attenzione, perché l'infezione prolungata può portare a paralisi facciale permanente, che può avere un effetto devastante sul bambino. Se si sviluppa paralisi facciale in un bambino con osteite mastoidea o con OM cronica suppurativa, occorre eseguire una mastoidectomia d'urgenza.

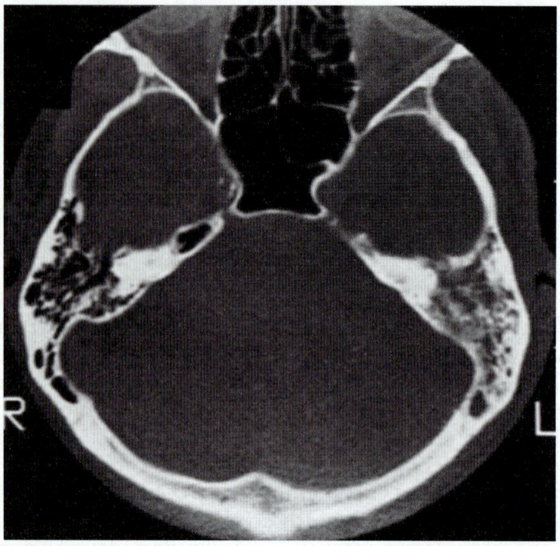

Figura 639-6. TC delle ossa temporali che dimostra un'osteite acuta alla mastoide sinistra con perdita dei setti tra le cellule aeree mastoidee, definita mastoidite acuta coalescente; la mastoide destra è normale. In questo caso è stato eseguito un intervento chirurgico mastoideo. (Da Bluestone CD, Klein JO [ed]: *Otitis Media in Infants and Children*, 3rd ed. Philadelphia, WB Saunders, 2001, p. 337.)

COLESTEATOMA ACQUISITO. Il colesteatoma consiste in una massa simil-cistica nell'orecchio medio o in altre porzioni pneumatizzate dell'osso temporale, delimitata da un epitelio squamoso stratificato cheratinizzato e contenente epitelio desquamato e/o cheratina (vedi Capitolo 637). Il colesteatoma acquisito, distinto dalla forma congenita, si sviluppa per lo più come complicanza di un'OM cronica di lunga durata. Tuttavia, questa patologia si può sviluppare anche da una tasca profonda di retrazione della membrana timpanica o come conseguenza di un impianto epiteliale nella cavità dell'orecchio medio, oppure dalla perforazione traumatica della membrana timpanica per l'inserimento di un tubo timpanostomico. I colesteatomi tendono a espandersi, causando riassorbimento osseo, e possono estendersi in direzione craniale, con conseguenze potenzialmente pericolose per la vita. Si deve sospettare un colesteatoma se l'otoscopia rivela una discreta opacità biancastra della membrana timpanica o un polipo che protrude attraverso un difetto della membrana, o detriti caseosi biancastri che ricoprono persistentemente la membrana timpanica, soprattutto nella parte superiore, oppure ancora se è dall'orecchio fuoriesce una secrezione maleodorante. Quando si sospetta un colesteatoma, si deve immediatamente consultare uno specialista otorinolaringoiatra. L'identificazione e il trattamento tardivi hanno conseguenze significative a lungo termine: necessità di un intervento chirurgico più esteso, ipoacusia permanente, lesione del nervo facciale, danno labirintico con perdita dell'equilibrio ed estensione intracranica. Per il trattamento del colesteatoma è necessario un intervento timpanomastoideo.

TABELLA 639-4. Diagnosi differenziale del coinvolgimento postauricolare della mastoidite acuta con periostite/ascesso

MALATTIA	SEGNI E SINTOMI POSTAURICOLARI				INFEZIONE DEL CONDOTTO ESTERNO	EFFUSIONE DELL'ORECCHIO MEDIO
	SOLCO*	ERITEMA	MASSA	DOLORABILITÀ		
Mastoidite acuta con periosteite	Può essere assente	Sì	No	Usuale	No	Usuale
Mastoidite acuta con ascesso sottoperiosteo	Assente	Sì	Possibile	Sì	No	Usuale
Periostite del padiglione auricolare con estensione postauricolare	Intatta	Sì	No	Usuale	No	No
Otite esterna con estensione postauricolare	Intatta	Sì	No	Usuale	Sì	No
Linfoadenite postauricolare	Intatta	No	Sì (circoscritta)	Possibile	No	No

*Solco postauricolare tra il padiglione auricolare e l'area postauricolare.
Da Bluestone CD, Klein JO (ed): *Otitis Media in Infants and Children*, 3rd ed. Philadelphia, WB Saunders, 2001, p. 333.

LABIRINTITE. È raro che una labirintite si verifichi come conseguenza della diffusione dell'infezione dall'orecchio medio e/o dalla mastoide nell'orecchio interno. Un colesteatoma o un'OM cronica suppurativa sono l'origine più frequente. I sintomi e i segni comprendono vertigini, acufeni, nausea, vomito, ipoacusia, nistagmo e impaccio dei movimenti. Il trattamento, rivolto alla patologia sottostante, deve essere intrapreso tempestivamente per preservare la funzione dell'orecchio interno e prevenire la diffusione dell'infezione.

COMPLICANZE INTRACRANICHE

Meningite, ascesso epidurale, ascesso subdurale, encefalite focale, ascesso cerebrale, trombosi del seno laterale (chiamata anche trombosi del seno sigmoideo) e idrocefalo otitico si possono sviluppare come complicanze di un'infezione acuta e cronica dell'orecchio medio e della mastoide, per estensione diretta, diffusione ematogena o tromboflebite. Spesso è implicata distruzione ossea adiacente alla dura madre e può essere presente colesteatoma. In un bambino con infezione dell'orecchio medio o della mastoide, la presenza di qualsiasi segno sistemico, come febbre, cefalea o letargia di grado estremo, oppure il reperto, all'esame fisico, di meningismo o di un segno del sistema nervoso centrale, devono indurre al sospetto di una complicanza intracranica.

Quando si sospetta una complicanza intracranica, si deve eseguire una puntura lombare solo dopo che le indagini morfologiche abbiano stabilito l'assenza di un effetto massa o di idrocefalo. Oltre all'esame del liquido cerebrospinale, anche la coltura dell'essudato dell'orecchio medio ottenuto con timpanocentesi può identificare il microrganismo in causa, rendendo inoltre più agevole la scelta del farmaco antibatterico; si deve eseguire la miringotomia per permettere il drenaggio dell'orecchio medio.

Occorre istituire con urgenza una terapia antibiotica, somministrata per via endovenosa in tutte le complicanze intracraniche, compreso il drenaggio di ogni ascesso. In presenza di mastoidite, deve essere eseguita quanto prima una mastoidectomia. In presenza di meningite come complicanza di OMA, gli esami devono essere volti a ricercare una possibile fistola perilinfatica.

La trombosi del seno laterale può essere complicata dalla disseminazione del trombo infetto, con successivi infarti settici in vari organi. La diagnosi è facilitata dalla RM. Può essere necessaria una mastoidectomia anche in assenza di osteite o di mastoidite coalescente, specialmente nel caso di propagazione ed embolizzazione del trombo infetto. Tuttavia, talvolta la mastoidite può essere trattata con posizionamento di un tubo timpanostomico e somministrazione di antibiotici per via endovenosa. Nel trattamento della trombosi del seno laterale si può inoltre prendere in considerazione la terapia anticoagulante; tuttavia, prima di iniziarla, è necessario consultare un otorinolaringoiatra, per stabilire se occorra effettuare un intervento chirurgico prima di somministrare anticoagulanti.

L'**idrocefalo otitico**, detto anche **ipertensione endocranica benigna** (pseudotumor cerebri), è una patologia non frequente, consistente nell'aumento della pressione endocranica senza dilatazione dei ventricoli cerebrali, che si verifica in associazione a OM acuta e cronica o a mastoidite (vedi Capitolo 604). La malattia, la cui patogenesi è incerta, è comunemente associata a trombosi del seno laterale; la fisiopatologia può comportare l'ostruzione a opera del trombo del drenaggio venoso intracranico nel collo, che si traduce in un aumento della pressione venosa cerebrale con conseguente aumento della pressione del liquido cerebrospinale. I sintomi sono quelli correlati all'aumento della pressione endocranica. I segni possono includere, oltre all'evidenza dell'OM, la paralisi di uno o entrambi i muscoli retti cutanei e papilledema. L'RM può confermare la diagnosi. Le misure terapeutiche comprendono l'utilizzo di antibiotici e farmaci come l'acetazolamide o la furosemide per ridurre la pressione intracranica, la mastoidectomia, punture lombari ripetute, lo shunt lomboperitoneale e lo shunt ventricoloperitoneale. Se non trattato, l'idrocefalo otitico può portare a perdita del visus secondaria ad atrofia ottica.

SEQUELE FISICHE

Le sequele fisiche di OM consistono in anomalie strutturali dell'orecchio medio riconducibili a una sua infiammazione di lunga durata. Nella maggior parte dei casi, queste sequele sono la conseguenza di un'infezione grave e/o cronica, ma talune possono dipendere anche da un'infiammazione presumibilmente non infettiva nel quadro di un'OME di lunga durata. Le varie sequele possono presentarsi isolatamente o interconnettersi in combinazioni diverse.

La **timpanosclerosi** consiste in placche biancastre della membrana timpanica e depositi nodulari nello strato sottomucoso dell'orecchio medio. Le alterazioni cui dà luogo sono ialinizzazione e deposizione di cristalli di calcio e fosforo. Si può associare a ipoacusia conduttiva, seppure raramente. Nei Paesi sviluppati, la causa più comune di timpanosclerosi è probabilmente il posizionamento di un tubo timpanostomico.

"**Atelettasia** della membrana timpanica" è una dicitura descrittiva con cui si indica una retrazione grave della membrana stessa, causata sia da un'alta pressione negativa che si esercita sull'orecchio medio, sia da perdita di rigidità e prolasso mediale della membrana, presumibilmente in conseguenza di una retrazione di lunga durata o di un'infiammazione cronica grave. Una tasca di retrazione consiste in un'area localizzata di atelettasia. L'atelettasia spesso è transitoria e in genere asintomatica, ma una tasca di retrazione profonda può portare a erosione degli ossicini e a otite adesiva, fungendo da focolaio per lo sviluppo di un colesteatoma. Nel caso di una tasca di retrazione profonda e di un'atelettasia insolita che si accompagna a sintomi come otalgia, acufeni o ipoacusia conduttiva, è necessario l'inserimento di un tubo timpanostomico.

L'**OM adesiva** consiste in una proliferazione di tessuto fibroso nella mucosa dell'orecchio medio, che può comportare un alterato movimento degli ossicini, rarefazione da osteite e discontinuità degli ossicini, perdita di udito conduttiva e colesteatoma. L'ipoacusia può essere suscettibile di correzione chirurgica.

Il **granuloma di colesterolo** è una condizione rara in cui la membrana timpanica appare di colorito blu scuro, per la presenza di un denso materiale granulomatoso nella cavità dell'orecchio medio. La condizione spesso è il risultato di un'OME di lunga durata, più che di un'infezione franca dell'orecchio medio. Poiché l'inserimento di un tubo timpanostomico non fornisce un sollievo soddisfacente, è necessario un intervento chirurgico sull'orecchio medio e sulla mastoide.

La **perforazione cronica** può svilupparsi dopo rottura spontanea della membrana timpanica durante un episodio di OMA, come sequela di OM cronica suppurativa, per trauma, o come conseguenza della mancata chiusura della membrana timpanica dopo estrusione di un tubo timpanostomico. Una perforazione cronica quasi sempre è suscettibile di riparazione chirurgica, solitamente dopo un certo periodo che il bambino è guarito dall'OM.

Un'**ipoacusia conduttiva** permanente può essere la conseguenza di ognuna delle condizioni appena descritte. Per quanto si tratti di un'evenienza rara, un'ipoacusia permanente neurosensoriale può manifestarsi in associazione con OM acuta o cronica, presumibilmente per diffusione dell'infezione o dei prodotti dell'infiammazione attraverso la finestra rotonda della membrana, o come conseguenza di una labirintite suppurativa.

POSSIBILI SEQUELE EVOLUTIVE

L'ipoacusia permanente nei bambini ha un impatto significativamente negativo sullo sviluppo, consistente soprattutto in un ritardo del linguaggio articolato. È difficile stabilire fino a che punto l'OM incida sullo sviluppo a lungo termine del bambino, e in merito a tale questione esistono studi contrastanti. Tuttavia, è verosimile che l'impatto sullo sviluppo sia maggiore in bambini con un'ipoacusia più grave, più prolungata e bilaterale, oltre che in pazienti che presentano altre difficoltà evolutive o fattori di rischio per ritardo evolutivo.

PREVENZIONE

Le misure generali per prevenire l'OM consistono nell'allattamento al seno, nell'evitare, per quanto possibile, la vicinanza a individui con infezioni delle vie respiratorie, nell'evitare il fumo di tabacco ambientale e nella vaccinazione antipneumococcica.

IMMUNOPROFILASSI

Il vaccino coniugato pneumococcico eptavalente riduce il numero complessivo degli episodi di OMA del 6-8% soltanto, ma diminuisce di un 57% gli episodi sierotipo-specifici. Sono state riscontrate riduzioni del 9-23% in bambini con anamnesi di episodi frequenti, e una riduzione del 20% in un certo numero di bambini sottoposti a inserimento di un tubo timpanostomico. Lo sviluppo di ulteriori vaccini contro i patogeni responsabili di OMA promette di migliorare la protezione complessiva. Anche il vaccino antinfluenzale può fornire una certa protezione dall'OM, ma sono necessari altri studi per chiarire fino a che punto sia efficace. L'immunizzazione passiva con la somministrazione di immunoglobuline esogene non è un'opzione praticabile, per il disagio, i rischi, i costi e gli inconvenienti che comporta.

PROFILASSI ANTIBATTERICA

In bambini con frequenti episodi di OMA, la profilassi antibatterica con dosi subterapeutiche di un'aminopenicillina o di un sulfamidico offre una protezione variabile contro le recidive di OMA (sebbene non contro l'OME). Tuttavia, dato che gli antibiotici concorrono alla resistenza batterica, attualmente i rischi di una prolungata profilassi antibiotica sembrano, in generale, superare i probabili benefici, soprattutto nei bambini che frequentano la scuola materna, i quali, in ogni caso, presentano un aumentato rischio di colonizzazione con multipli ceppi resistenti di *S. pneumoniae*. Ciononostante, la profilassi può costituire un'opzione appropriata per un paziente pediatrico con OMA recidivante che sia accudito in ambiente domiciliare e di solito lontano da altri bambini piccoli.

MIRINGOTOMIA E INSERIMENTO DI TUBI TIMPANOSTOMICI

In bambini con OME persistente, parecchi studi hanno dimostrato che la l'inserimento di tubi timpanostomici è efficace nel ridurre la successiva presenza di MEE, nel migliorare il livello dell'udito e anche nel ridurre la percentuale di recidiva di OMA. In bambini con OMA, vari studi hanno dimostrato che i tubi timpanostomici sono efficacissimi nel ridurre la percentuale di recidiva. Sia nell'OMA sia nell'OME, studi sulla qualità della vita nei pazienti pediatrici sottoposti a trattamento chirurgico hanno dimostrato un significativo miglioramento della stessa dopo il posizionamento di tubi timpanostomici.

Per un trattamento ottimale del singolo bambino gravemente colpito da OMA recidivante, è necessario adattare la terapia alle esigenze individuali, tenendo conto di una serie di fattori, tra cui severità degli episodi, profilo dei fattori di rischio, tolleranza alla terapia antibiotica, valutazione dell'udito, preferenze dei genitori e salute complessiva del bambino in via di sviluppo. Interventi ragionevoli sono: trattamento episodico con antibiotici, osservazione vigile negli episodi di OMA per cercare di ridurre l'uso complessivo di antibiotici, o invio a un ambito specialistico per l'inserimento di tubi timpanostomici.

ADENOIDECTOMIA

L'adenoidectomia è in una certa misura efficace nel ridurre il rischio di episodi ricorrenti sia di OMA sia di OME in bambini sottoposti all'inserimento di un tubo, in cui, dopo l'estrusione del tubo stesso, l'OM continui a rappresentare un problema. L'efficacia pare essere indipendente dalle dimensioni delle adenoidi, mentre è probabile sia correlata alla rimozione di un focolaio d'infezione. Nei bambini piccoli con OMA recidivante che non siano stati in precedenza sottoposti a inserimento di un tubo, solitamente non si consiglia l'adenoidectomia insieme all'inserimento del tubo, a meno che non si associno significativa ostruzione delle vie aeree nasali o rinosinusite recidivante, casi in cui si deve considerare la possibilità di eseguire un'adenoidectomia.

Acuin J: Chronic suppurative otitis media. *BMJ* 2002;325:1159–1160.

American Academy of Family Physicians; American Academy of Otolaryngology–Head and Neck Surgery; American Academy of Pediatrics Subcommittee on Otitis Media With Effusion: Otitis media with effusion. *Pediatrics* 2004;113:1412–1429.

American Academy of Pediatrics Subcommittee on Management of Acute Otitis Media: Diagnosis and management of acute otitis media. *Pediatrics* 2004;113:1451–1465.

Arguedas A, Dagan R, Pichichero M, et al: An open-label, double tympanocentesis study of levofloxacin therapy in children with, or at high risk for, recurrent or persistent acute otitis media. *Pediatr Infect Dis J* 2006;25: 1102–1108.

Bauchner H, Marchant CD, Bisbee A, et al: Effectiveness of Centers for Disease Control and Prevention recommendations for outcomes of acute otitis media. *Pediatrics* 2006;117:1009–1017.

Bluestone CD: Otitis media and congenital perilymphatic fistula as a cause of sensorineural hearing loss in children. *Pediatr Infect Dis J* 1988;7:S141.

Bodor FF: Systemic antibiotics for treatment of the conjunctivitis-otitis media syndrome. *Pediatr Infect Dis J* 1989;8:287–290.

Bodor FF, Marchant CD, Shurin PA, et al: Bacterial etiology of conjunctivitis–otitis media syndrome. *Pediatrics* 1985;76:26–28.

Fireman B, Black SB, Shinefield HR, et al: Impact of the pneumococcal conjugate vaccine on otitis media. *Pediatr Infect Dis J* 2003;22:10–16.

Garbutt J, Rosenbloom I, Wu J, et al: Empiric first-line antibiotic treatment of acute otitis in the era of the heptavalent pneumococcal conjugate vaccine. *Pediatrics* 2006;117:e1087–1094.

Hall-Stoodley L, Hu FZ, Gieske A, et al: Direct detection of bacterial biofilms on the middle-ear mucosa of children with chronic otitis media. *JAMA* 2006;296:202–211.

Hammaren-Malmi S, Saxen H, Tarkkanen J, et al: Adenoidectomy does not significantly reduce the incidence of otitis media in conjunction with the insertion of tympanostomy tubes in children who are younger than 4 years: A randomized trial. *Pediatrics* 2005;116:185–189.

Heikkinen T, Thint M, Chonmaitree T: Prevalence of various respiratory viruses in the middle ear during acute otitis media. *N Engl J Med* 1999;340:260–264.

Herbert RL, King GE, Bent JP: Tympanostomy tubes and water exposure. *Arch Otolaryngol Head Neck Surg* 1998;124:1118.

Isaacson G, Rosenfeld RM: Care of the child with tympanostomy tubes: A visual guide for the pediatrician. *Pediatrics* 1994;93:924.

Jose J, Coatesworth AP, Anthony R, et al: Life-threatening complications after partially treated mastoids. *BMJ* 2003;327:41–42.

Kerschner JE, Lindstrom DR, Pomeranz A, et al: Comparison of caregiver otitis media risk factor knowledge in suburban and urban primary care environments. *Int J Pediatr Otorhinolaryngol* 2005;69:49–56.

Koivunen P, Uhari M, Luotonen J, et al: Adenoidectomy versus chemoprophylaxis and placebo for recurrent acute otitis media in children aged under 2 years: Randomized controlled trial. *BMJ* 2004;328:487–490.

Marchetti F, Ronfani L, Nibali SC, et al: Delayed prescription may reduce the use of antibiotics for acute otitis media. *Arch Pediatr Adolesc Med* 2005;159:679–684.

McCormick DP, Chonmaitree T, Pittman C, et al: Nonsevere acute otitis media: A clinical trial comparing outcomes of watchful waiting versus immediate antibiotic treatment. *Pediatrics* 2005;115:1455–1465.

Palmu AAI, Herva E, Savolainen H, et al: Association of clinical signs and symptoms with bacterial findings in acute otitis media. *Clin Infect Dis* 2004;38:234–242.

Paradise JL, Elster BA, Tan L: Evidence in infants with cleft palate that breast milk protects against otitis media. *Pediatrics* 1994;94:853–860.

Paradise JL, Feldman HM, Campbell TF, et al: Tympanostomy tubes and developmental outcomes at 9 to 11 years of age. *N Engl J Med* 2007;356: 248–261.

Rovers MM, Glasziou P, Appelman CL, et al: Antibiotics for acute otitis media: a meta-analysis with individual patient data. *Lancet* 2006;368: 1429–1434.

Rovers MM, Schilder AGM, Zielhuis GA, et al: Otitis media. *Lancet* 2004;363:465–473.

Samuel J, Fernandes CMC, Steinberg JL: Intracranial otogenic complications: A persisting problem. *Laryngoscope* 1986;96:272.
Spiro DM, Tay KY, Arnold DH, et al: Wait-and-see prescription for the treatment of acute otitis media. *JAMA* 2006;296:1235–1241.
Stenstrom R, Pless IB, Bernard P: Hearing thresholds and tympanic membrane sequelae in children managed medically or surgically for otitis media with effusion. *Arch Pediatr Adolesc Med* 2005;159:1151–1156.
Subcommittee on Management of Acute Otitis Media: Diagnosis and management of acute otitis media. *Pediatrics* 2004;113:1451–1465.
Tonnaer ELGM, Graamans K, Sanders EAM, Curfs JHAJ: Advances in understanding the pathogenesis of pneumococcal otitis media. *Pediatr Infect Dis J* 2006;25:546–552.
Valtonen H, Tuomilehto H, Qvarnberg Y, et al: A 14-year prospective follow-up study of children treated early in life with tympanostomy tubes: Part 1: Clinical outcomes. *Arch Otolaryngol Head Neck Surg* 2005;131:293–298.
Valtonen H, Tuomilehto H, Qvarnberg Y, et al: A 14-year prospective follow-up study of children treated early in life with tympanostomy tubes: Part 2: Hearing outcomes. *Arch Otolaryngol Head Neck Surg* 2005;131:299–303.
Van Heerbeek N, Straetemans M, Wiertsema SP, et al: Effect of combined pneumococcal conjugate and polysaccharide vaccination on recurrent otitis media with effusion. *Pediatrics* 2006; 117:603–608.
Zapalac JS, Billings KR, Schwade ND, et al: Suppurative complications of acute otitis media in the era of antibiotic resistance. *Arch Otolaryngol Head Neck Surg* 2002;128:660–663.

Capitolo 640 ■ Orecchio interno e malattie del labirinto osseo

Joseph Haddad Jr.

I fattori genetici possono influire su anatomia e funzione dell'orecchio interno. Anche agenti infettivi, virus, batteri e protozoi, possono provocare un'alterazione della funzione, per lo più come sequela di un'infezione congenita o una meningite batterica. Altre malattie acquisite della capsula labirintica sono otosclerosi, osteopetrosi, istiocitosi a cellule di Langerhans, displasia fibrosa e altri tipi di displasia ossea. Tutte queste patologie possono provocare ipoacusia sia conduttiva sia neurosensoriale, oltre ad alterazione vestibolare. L'utilizzo dei vaccini attualmente disponibili riduce il rischio di meningite batterica e l'ipoacusia neurosensoriale associata.

VIRUS. La causa più comune di ipoacusia neurosensoriale nell'infanzia (SNHL, *SensoriNeural Hearing Loss*) è l'infezione congenita da Cytomegalovirus (CMV) (vedi Capitolo 252). L'utilizzo del ganciclovir in bambini molto piccoli con infezione congenita da CMV può stabilizzare l'ipoacusia o renderla reversibile. Altre cause virali di SHNL includono rosolia congenita e parotite acquisita, rosolia, morbillo e quinta malattia, provocata dal parvovirus B19. Anche molti altri virus sono occasionalmente associati a SNHL. In circa il 50% dei casi, l'ipoacusia, in genere bilaterale, sebbene asimmetrica, progredisce e peggiora nell'arco di settimane o addirittura anni.

Prima che fosse introdotto un vaccino efficace, la rosolia era responsabile di circa il 60% dei casi di SNHL infantili. Nei Paesi sviluppati la vaccinazione ne ha ridotto l'incidenza di circa il 97%. Analogamente, morbillo e parotite, negli Stati Uniti, sono ora cause rare di SNHL, grazie all'efficacia dei programmi di vaccinazione.

Anche l'encefalite da herpes simplex può essere associata a SNHL, soprattutto nei bambini con infezione congenita da herpesvirus. L'aciclovir e altri antivirali possono essere efficaci contro l'ipoacusia e le altre manifestazioni del sistema nervoso centrale (vedi Capitolo 242).

TOXOPLASMOSI. Il *Toxoplasma gondii* è un protozoo che può causare SNHL congenita. Negli Stati Uniti, ogni anno nascono circa 3000 bambini con toxoplasmosi congenita, e circa il 25% dei pazienti non trattati presenta SNHL. Se si documenta l'infezione materna durante il periodo fetale, la terapia medica può essere in grado di prevenire alcune manifestazioni cliniche, compresa l'SNHL del bambino (vedi Capitolo 287).

MENINGITE BATTERICA. Da quando è stato introdotto il vaccino contro *Haemophilus influenzae* tipo b, *Streptococcus pnueumoniae* e *Neisseria meningitidis* sono diventati le principali cause di meningite batterica nei bambini statunitensi. La perdita d'udito compare più frequentemente con *S. pneumoniae*, con un'incidenza del 15-20%. In circa il 60% dei casi l'ipoacusia è bilaterale, sebbene spesso asimmetrica. Se essa è già presente al momento della comparsa della meningite, e in particolare se è grave o profonda, la possibilità di un miglioramento significativo è bassa. Tuttavia, se l'ipoacusia si sviluppa dopo il ricovero per il trattamento e non è grave, sono possibili una stabilizzazione o un miglioramento. In alcuni bambini, anche alcuni anni dopo la meningite, si può verificare la progressione tardiva della SNHL. Negli Stati Uniti e in molti Paesi sviluppati, la meningite batterica è una delle principali cause di sordità profonda che induce a effettuare un impianto cocleare nei bambini. Si ritiene che l'introduzione del vaccino coniugato antipneumococcico ridurrà la SNHL da meningite pneumococcica.

Vari studi hanno dimostrato un trend favorevole del decorso e degli esiti dopo somministrazione di desametasone per la perdita d'udito e altri deficit neurologici associati a meningite batterica (vedi Capitolo 602.1), sebbene la sua efficacia, soprattutto per la meningite da *S. pneumoniae* e da *N. meningitidis*, in genere non sia statisticamente significativa, per il piccolo numero di casi del trial. Una metanalisi di 11 studi, condotta dal 1988 al 1996, ha dimostrato che il desametasone riduce la perdita d'udito grave associata a meningite da *H. influenzae* tipo b, in rapporto al tempo della somministrazione del farmaco (prima o insieme con gli antibiotici anziché dopo) o all'antibiotico usato. Per la meningite pneumococcica, dalla metanalisi è emerso che il desametasone risulta efficace solo se somministrato precocemente e solo per la perdita d'udito grave. Lo studio comprendeva anche qualche caso di meningite meningococcica, per verificare l'effetto del desametasone su questa patologia.

SIFILIDE. La sifilide congenita, causata da *Treponema pallidum*, può provocare SNHL nel 3-38% dei bambini colpiti (vedi Capitolo 215). L'incidenza esatta è difficile da accertare, perché la perdita d'udito può non svilupparsi fino all'adolescenza o anche fino all'età adulta. Una volta identificata la patologia, il trattamento con antibiotici e corticosteroidi può migliorare l'ipoacusia.

ALTRE MALATTIE DELL'ORECCHIO INTERNO. Per effetto della diffusione diretta dell'infezione, la **labirintite** può essere una complicanza di un'otite media acuta o cronica (OM) e di una mastoidite, oltre che di una meningite batterica, dovuta al passaggio nel labirinto del microrganismo attraverso il meato uditivo interno, il dotto endolinfatico, il dotto perilinfatico, i vasi, o per diffusione ematogena. Le manifestazioni cliniche della labirintite possono comprendere vertigini, alterazioni dell'equilibrio, dolore profondo all'orecchio, nausea, vomito, nistagmo e SNHL. La labirintite suppurativa acuta, caratterizzata da un esordio improvviso, grave, di questi sintomi, richiede una terapia antibiotica intensiva. Se è secondaria a OM, può essere necessario un intervento chirurgico per rimuovere il sottostante colesteatoma, oppure realizzare un drenaggio dell'orecchio medio o della mastoide, oltre alla terapia antibiotica. La labirintite sierosa acuta, con sintomi più lievi di vertigine o ipoacusia, può essere secondaria a infezioni dell'orecchio medio. Normalmente risponde bene alla terapia antibiotica e corticosteroidea, con miglioramento sia delle vertigini sia della perdita d'udito. La labirintite cronica, per lo più associata a colesteatoma, si manifesta con SNHL e alterazione vestibolare che si sviluppa con il tempo; è necessario un intervento chirurgico per rimuovere il colesteatoma. Seppure raramente, la labirintite cronica può complicare un'OM di lunga durata, con lo sviluppo lento di SNHL, di solito prima per le frequenze più alte e spesso con alterazione vestibolare. Inoltre, fenomeno di più frequente riscontro, i bambini con presenza cronica di liquido nell'orecchio medio spesso hanno un equilibrio instabile, che migliora immediatamente alla scomparsa del liquido stesso.

L'**otosclerosi**, una malattia autosomica dominante che colpisce solo le ossa temporali, provoca un'anomala crescita ossea che comporta fissazione della staffa alla finestra ovale, con ipoacusia progressiva. L'ipoacusia all'inizio è conduttiva, ma si può sviluppare una SNHL. Le più colpite sono le femmine di razza bianca, con esordio dell'otosclerosi durante l'adolescenza o in età giovane-adulta, spesso in rapporto con la gravidanza. Spesso è efficace un intervento chirurgico correttivo per sostituire la staffa con una protesi mobile.

L'**osteogenesi imperfetta** (OI) è una malattia sistemica che può coinvolgere sia l'orecchio medio sia l'orecchio interno (vedi Capitolo 699). L'ipoacusia insorge in circa il 20% dei bambini piccoli e nel 90% degli adulti con questa malattia. È per lo più di tipo conduttivo, per la presenza di anomalie degli ossicini, nonostante si possa verificare anche SNHL se sono colpite altre zone della capsula otica. Se la perdita d'udito è abbastanza grave, alla correzione chirurgica della fissità della staffa, può essere preferibile un apparecchio acustico, perché nei bambini con OI la stapedectomia può essere tecnicamente molto difficile, e la malattia e l'ipoacusia talvolta sono progressive.

L'**osteopetrosi**, una displasia scheletrica molto rara, può coinvolgere l'osso temporale, inclusi l'orecchio medio e gli ossicini, con ipoacusia da moderata a grave, solitamente di tipo conduttivo. Si può verificare anche paralisi facciale recidivante, in conseguenza di un'eccessiva deposizione ossea; a ogni recidiva si assiste a una progressiva riduzione del recupero della funzionalità facciale (vedi Capitolo 697).

Capitolo 641 ■ Lesioni traumatiche dell'orecchio e dell'osso temporale

Joseph Haddad Jr.

PADIGLIONE AURICOLARE E CONDOTTO UDITIVO ESTERNO. In alcuni sport i traumi del padiglione auricolare sono frequenti e la tempestività del drenaggio dell'ematoma può scongiurare un danno irreversibile. L'ematoma, caratterizzato da accumulo di sangue tra il pericondrio e la cartilagine, può essere la conseguenza di un trauma del lobo ed è comune soprattutto negli adolescenti che praticano il wrestling o il pugilato. È necessaria l'immediata aspirazione con ago o, quando l'ematoma è esteso o recidivante, l'incisione, il drenaggio e una fasciatura contenitiva per evitare una pericondrite, con conseguente perdita di cartilagine e deformità a cavolfiore dell'orecchio. Durante attività in cui sia possibile un traumatismo al capo, sarebbe opportuno indossare elmetti protettivi.

Il **congelamento** del padiglione auricolare deve essere trattato con un rapido riscaldamento della parte esposta, mediante irrigazioni calde o garze riscaldate.

Nei bambini è frequente la presenza di **corpi estranei** nel condotto uditivo esterno. Spesso è possibile rimuoverli in ambulatorio, senza anestesia generale, se il bambino è abbastanza grande da capire e cooperare ed è tenuto stretto adeguatamente: per visualizzare l'oggetto è necessario servirsi di una lampada al capo, un otoscopio con testa chirurgica o un otomicroscopio e per rimuoverlo, a seconda della sua forma, si utilizza un apposito strumentario ("pinza ad alligatore", ansa, curette smussa da cerume) oppure si ricorre all'aspirazione. Se il corpo estraneo è molto piccolo si può effettuare il lavaggio delicato del condotto uditivo con acqua alla temperatura corporea o con soluzione salina; questa procedura richiede però che la membrana timpanica sia intatta. I tentativi di asportare l'oggetto con la forza, senza una buona visuale e con strumenti inadeguati, oltre a spaventare il bambino, possono causare edema e sanguinamento del condotto uditivo, rendendo necessario un intervento in anestesia generale. Se l'estrazione di corpi estranei è difficoltosa, specialmente in caso di oggetti larghi, indovati profondamente e con edema associato del condotto uditivo, è preferibile praticare l'anestesia generale. Occorre estrarre con urgenza le pile a disco, da cui può fuoriuscire un liquido basico, gravemente lesivo per i tessuti. Nel caso di insetti penetrati nel condotto uditivo, prima si deve ucciderli con olio minerale o lidocaina, e solo successivamente procedere alla loro rimozione sotto visualizzazione otomicroscopica.

Dopo la rimozione di un corpo estraneo dal condotto uditivo, bisogna ispezionare attentamente la MT, per escludere una possibile perforazione traumatica o una preesistente effusione dell'orecchio medio. Se il corpo estraneo ha causato un'infiammazione acuta del condotto, si deve istituire la stessa terapia descritta per l'otite acuta esterna (vedi Capitolo 638).

MEMBRANA TIMPANICA E ORECCHIO MEDIO. La perforazione traumatica della MT di solito si verifica in conseguenza di una compressione esterna, come uno schiaffo, o della penetrazione di un corpo estraneo, per esempio un piccolo bastone o un bastoncino di cotone. La perforazione può essere lineare o stellata. Quando è dovuta a compressione, si localizza per lo più nella porzione anteriore della pars tensa, mentre se è imputabile a corpo estraneo può trovarsi in qualsiasi quadrante della MT. In assenza di otorrea suppurativa non sono necessari antibiotici per via sistemica e farmaci per via topica. È importante valutare e monitorare l'udito del paziente, per assicurarsi che si verifichi una guarigione spontanea, peraltro piuttosto frequente. Se nel giro di qualche mese la MT non guarisce, si deve prendere in considerazione la riparazione chirurgica con innesto. Per tutto il tempo in cui è presente la perforazione, si può manifestare otorrea, quando l'acqua penetra dall'orecchio medio nel condotto uditivo, durante il nuoto o il bagno, ed è pertanto necessario prendere alcune precauzioni. Le perforazioni dovute alla penetrazione di corpi estranei guariscono meno facilmente di quelle dovute a compressione. L'esame audiometrico rivela un'ipoacusia conduttiva (CHL, *Conductive Hear Loss*), con un gap aria-acqua maggiore rispetto a perforazioni più ampie. È indicata l'immediata esplorazione chirurgica se la lesione si accompagna a uno o più dei seguenti segni: vertigine, nistagmo, acufeni gravi, ipoacusia da moderata a grave, otorrea di liquido cerebrospinale (LCS). Al momento dell'esplorazione, è necessario ispezionare gli ossicini, specialmente la staffa, perché possono essere dislocati o fratturati, e cercare eventuali oggetti taglienti eventualmente penetrati attraverso la finestra ovale o rotonda. Se invece la staffa è sublussata, è dislocata nella finestra ovale o è penetrata attraverso la finestra rotonda o ovale, si manifesta un'ipoacusia neurosensoriale (SNHL, *SensoriNeural Hear Loss*). I bambini non devono usare da soli i bastoncini di cotone, perché il rischio che si provochino un trauma all'orecchio è elevato, e anzi potranno maneggiare piccoli oggetti solo sotto la supervisione dei genitori.

La **fistola perilinfatica** (**PLF**, *PeriLymphatic Fistula*) può verificarsi dopo improvviso trauma pressorio o aumento della pressione del LCS. Deve essere sospettata in un bambino che sviluppi un'improvvisa SNHL o vertigini dopo aver praticato attività fisica o un'immersione in acque profonde, aver fatto un viaggio in aereo, aver suonato uno strumento a fiato o aver subito un trauma significativo al capo. La perdita caratteristicamente si verifica a livello della finestra ovale o rotonda, e può essere associata ad anomalie congenite di queste strutture o ad anomalie anatomiche della coclea o dei canali semicircolari. Sebbene accada talvolta che una PLF si chiuda spontaneamente, si consiglia comunque l'immediata riparazione chirurgica della fistola per controllare le vertigini e fermare una qualsiasi progressione della SNHL; anche un intervento tempestivo può non essere in grado di trattare la SNHL. Poiché non si conosce un test affidabile per la PLF, si rende necessaria l'esplorazione dell'orecchio medio per la diagnosi e il trattamento.

FRATTURE DELL'OSSO TEMPORALE. I bambini vanno particolarmente soggetti a fratture della base cranica, che di solito coinvolgono l'osso temporale. Nelle lesioni del capo, va preso in considerazione anche un trauma dell'osso temporale e si deve valutare la condizione dell'orecchio e dell'udito. Le fratture dell'osso temporale sono per il 70-80% longitudinali e si manifestano comunemente con emorragia dovuta a lacerazione del condotto uditivo esterno o della membrana timpanica; ecchimosi postauricolare (**segno di Battle**), emotimpano (sangue dietro alla membrana timpanica intatta), CHL da perforazione della MT, emotimpano o lesione degli ossicini, esordio ritardato di paralisi facciale (che di solito migliora spontaneamente) e temporanea fuoriuscita di LCS dal naso o dalle orecchie (attraverso le tube di Eustachio). Le fratture trasversali dell'osso temporale hanno una prognosi più grave rispetto a quelle longitudinali, e spesso sono associate a immediata paralisi facciale. Quest'ultima può migliorare se è causata dall'edema, ma se non c'è evidenza di guarigione clinica e la valutazione del nervo facciale è sfavorevole, si consiglia spesso la decompressione chirurgica del nervo. Se il nervo facciale è stato sezionato, la decompressione chirurgica e l'anastomosi offrono la possibilità di un certo recupero funzionale. Le fratture trasversali danno luogo anche a grave SNHL, vertigini, nistagmo, acufeni, nausea e vomito associato a perdita della funzionalità cocleare e vestibolare, emotimpano, emorragia dal condotto uditivo esterno (evenienza peraltro rara) e otorrea di LCS sia nel condotto uditivo esterno sia dietro alla MT, che può uscire dal naso attraverso la tuba di Eustachio.

In caso di frattura dell'osso temporale, sospettata o confermata dalle radiografie, è indicato un cauto esame del padiglione auricolare e del condotto uditivo; con le fratture dell'osso temporale sono comuni lacerazioni o avulsioni del tessuto molle. L'energica rimozione di coaguli ematici dal condotto uditivo esterno o la timpanocentesi non sono indicate, perché può spostare ulteriormente gli ossicini o esacerbare una perdita di LCS. In pazienti con frattura della base cranica e otorrea e rinorrea di LCS, non è possibile determinare l'efficacia di una terapia antibiotica profilattica per la prevenzione della meningite, perché a oggi gli studi compiuti al riguardo sono inficiati da BIAS. Se il paziente non ha febbre e il drenaggio non è torbido, si consiglia un'osservazione attenta senza antibiotici. L'intervento chirurgico è riservato ai bambini in cui bisogna procedere alla riparazione di una perforazione della MT che non guarisce, a quelli con dislocazione della catena degli ossicini o laddove si renda necessaria la decompressione del nervo facciale. Una SNHL può anche essere la conseguenza di un trauma alla testa senza frattura visibile dell'osso temporale (concussione labirintica).

TRAUMA ACUSTICO. Dipende dall'esposizione a suoni di alta intensità (fuochi d'artificio, spari, musica rock, macchinari pesanti) e si manifesta inizialmente con un decremento temporaneo della soglia dell'udito, per lo più a 4000 Hz all'esame audiometrico, e acufeni. Se il suono è compreso tra 85-140 dB, l'ipoacusia è temporanea (dopo un concerto rock), ma l'ipoacusia e gli acufeni possono diventare permanenti con l'esposizione cronica al rumore; le più coinvolte sono le frequenze tra 3000 e 6000 Hz. Rumori improvvisi, estremamente forti (>140 dB), di breve durata, con componenti di picco alte (spari, bombe), possono causare un'ipoacusia permanente anche dopo un'unica esposizione. Le misure preventive consistono nel proteggere l'orecchio evitando l'esposizione cronica a rumori forti. I genitori dovrebbero essere informati dei danni del trauma acustico dovuto ai rumori ambientali o all'abitudine di ascoltare musica ad alto volume con gli auricolari, e dovrebbero prendere delle misure per ridurre al minimo l'esposizione.

Hough JVD, Stuart WD: Middle ear injuries in skull trauma. *Laryngoscope* 1968; 78:899–937.

Capitolo 642 ■ Tumori dell'orecchio e dell'osso temporale

Joseph Haddad Jr.

Il sospetto di tumori dell'orecchio e dell'osso temporale può sorgere dal riscontro di una massa nell'orecchio medio o in sede mastoidea, e di segni di emorragia o distruzione locale. La TC o la RM fungono da guida alla biopsia, effettuata allo scopo di confermare la diagnosi e stabilire il regime di trattamento.

I tumori benigni del condotto uditivo esterno consistono negli osteomi e nella displasia fibrosa monostotica e poliostotica. Gli osteomi si presentano come masse nel condotto uditivo e richiedono la rimozione solo in presenza di alterazioni dell'udito o otite esterna; gli osteomi possono essere clinicamente confusi con esostosi (vedi Capitolo 501.2).

Il **granuloma eosinofilo**, che può comparire isolatamente o fare parte della istiocitosi a cellule di Langerhans (vedi Capitolo 507), deve essere sospettato in pazienti con otalgia, otorrea (talvolta ematica), ipoacusia, tessuto anomalo nell'orecchio medio o nel condotto uditivo e reperti radiografici di una lesione distruttiva dell'osso temporale nettamente delimitata. La diagnosi definitiva è fatta con la biopsia. A seconda della sede, può essere trattato con escissione chirurgica, curettage o irradiazione locale. Se la lesione fa parte della presentazione sistemica dell'istiocitosi a cellule di Langerhans, oltre alla terapia locale (intervento chirurgico con o senza irradiazione) è indicata la chemioterapia. Se la lesione dell'osso temporale è singola, isolata o fa parte di una malattia multisistemica, è necessario un follow-up a lungo termine.

I sintomi e i segni del rabdomiosarcoma, che origina nell'orecchio medio o nel condotto uditivo, comprendono una massa o un polipo nell'orecchio medio o nel condotto, emorragia dall'orecchio, otorrea, otalgia, paralisi facciale e ipoacusia. Possono essere coinvolti altri nervi cranici. La diagnosi viene formulata sulla base della biopsia, ma per determinare l'estensione della malattia si ricorre alla TC e alla RM dell'osso temporale della base cranica e del cervello. Il trattamento comprende di solito una combinazione di chemioterapia, radioterapia e chirurgia (vedi Capitolo 501).

Anche il linfoma non Hodgkin e la leucemia possono, seppure raramente, presentarsi nell'osso temporale. Sebbene una neoplasia primitiva dell'orecchio medio sia molto rara nei bambini, è possibile riscontrare un carcinoma adenoide cistico, un adenocarcinoma o un carcinoma a cellule squamose. I tumori benigni dell'osso temporale comprendono i tumori glomici. I segni e i sintomi iniziali dei più frequenti tumori rinofaringei (angiofibroma, rabdomiosarcoma, carcinoma epidermoide) possono essere associati a esordio insidioso di otite media cronica con effusione (spesso unilaterale). Per la diagnosi precoce di questi tumori è necessario un alto indice di sospetto.

Parte XXX ▪ La cute

Capitolo 643 ▪ Morfologia della cute

Joseph G. Morelli

EPIDERMIDE. L'epidermide matura è un tessuto epiteliale stratificato costituito prevalentemente da cheratinociti. La funzione dell'epidermide è proteggere l'organismo dall'ambiente esterno e prevenire la perdita di acqua. Il processo di differenziazione epiteliale causa la formazione di una barriera funzionale con il mondo esterno. I cheratinociti sono composti in larga misura da filamenti di cheratina, proteine che appartengono alla famiglia dei filamenti intermedi. Le cheratine predominanti espresse all'interno dei cheratinociti mutano con la differenziazione cellulare. L'epidermide è costituita da quattro strati istologicamente riconoscibili. Lo strato basale è formato da cellule colonnari che giacciono sulla giunzione dermo-epidermica. I cheratinociti basali sono connessi alla giunzione dermo-epidermica mediante emidesmosomi e sono adesi a se stessi e alle cellule dello strato spinoso tramite giunzioni desmosomiche, gap e aderenti. Il ruolo del cheratinocita basale è quello di fornire continuamente cheratinociti all'epidermide tramite differenziazione normale e di fungere da serbatoio di cellule atte a riparare il danno epidermico. Il secondo strato è costituito da 3 o 4 file di cellule spinose che hanno il compito di avviare la formazione della barriera epidermica e la sintesi della vitamina D. Lo strato successivo è costituito da 2 o 3 file di cellule dall'aspetto granulare la cui funzione è continuare il processo di creazione della barriera epidermica e preparare la formazione dello strato corneo, che è costituito da più strati di cellule morte e altamente compatte. Le cellule morte sono costituite prevalentemente da cheratine con legame disolfuro. Gli spazi intercellulari sono composti da lipidi idrofobi, prevalentemente ceramidi. Mano a mano che lo strato corneo viene ricostituito, il vecchio strato corneo viene perso in un processo rigidamente regolato. Il normale processo di differenziazione epidermica dalla cellula basale alla perdita dello strato corneo impiega 28 giorni.

In aggiunta ai cheratinociti l'epidermide contiene altri 3 tipi di cellule. I melanociti sono cellule formanti il pigmento, responsabili del colore della cute e della protezione dai raggi ultravioletti. I melanociti epidermici derivano dalla **cresta neurale** e migrano nella cute durante la vita embrionale; risiedono nell'epidermide interfollicolare e nei follicoli piliferi e aumentano di numero mediante mitosi o migrazione di cellule aggiuntive nell'epidermide. Queste cellule producono organelli intracellulari (melanosomi) contenenti melanina. Nell'unità di melanina epidermica ci sono approssimativamente 1 melanocita per 36 cheratinociti. I melanosomi vengono quindi trasferiti attraverso i dendriti dei melanociti ai cheratinociti. Le cellule di Merkel sono recettori meccanosensoriali del tatto ad adattamento lento di tipo 1. Le cellule di Langerhans sono cellule dendritiche del sitema fagocitario mononucleato che risultano riconoscibili al microscopio elettronico grazie a un organulo specifico, il granulo di Birbeck. Queste cellule derivano dal midollo osseo e partecipano alle reazioni immunitarie della cute, esercitando un ruolo attivo nella presentazione e nell'elaborazione dell'antigene.

La giunzione dell'epidermide e del derma è la zona della membrana basale. Questa struttura complessa è il risultato del contributo delle cellule epidermiche e di quelle mesenchimali. La giunzione dermo-epidermica si estende dalla membrana plasmatica delle cellule basali alla regione superiore del derma. Dal punto di vista ultrastrutturale, la membrana basale appare come una struttura trilaminare, costituita da una lamina lucida immediatamente adiacente alla membrana plasmatica delle cellule basali, una lamina densa centrale e la lamina sub-basale sul lato dermico della lamina densa. Numerose strutture interne a questa zona fungono da ancoraggio dell'epidermide al derma. La membrana plasmatica delle cellule basali contiene placche elettron-dense note come emidesmosomi; i tonofilamenti scorrono all'interno delle cellule basali per inserirsi in questi siti. Gli emidesmosomi sono costituiti da 180 e 230 kd antigeni del pemfigoide bolloso, integrine $\alpha6\beta4$ e $\alpha3\beta1$ e plectina. I filamenti di ancoraggio originano nella membrana plasmatica, principalmente vicino agli emidesmosomi, e si inseriscono nella lamina densa. Le fibrille di ancoraggio, costituite prevalentemente da collagene di tipo VII, si estendono dalla lamina densa nel derma più superficiale dove si inseriscono in placche di ancoraggio.

DERMA. Il derma conferisce alla cute la maggior parte delle sue proprietà meccaniche. Forma una struttura di supporto forte, flessibile, fibrosa tra l'epidermide e il grasso sottocutaneo. È costituito da fibre di collagene, elastina e reticolina inserite in una sostanza di base amorfa; contiene i vasi sanguigni, i vasi linfatici, i mastociti, le strutture neurali, le ghiandole sudoripare eccrine e apocrine, i follicoli piliferi, le ghiandole sebacee e il muscolo liscio. Morfologicamente, il derma può essere diviso in 2 strati: lo strato papillare superficiale che si interpone alle creste epidermiche e lo strato reticolare più profondo che giace sotto il derma papillare. Lo strato papillare è meno denso e più cellulare, mentre quello reticolare sembra più compatto a causa della ruvida rete di fibre di collagene ed elastina interallacciate.

La cellula dermica predominante è un fibroblasto fusiforme responsabile della sintesi del collagene, delle fibre di elastina e dei mucopolisaccaridi. Sono presenti anche istiociti fagocitici, mastociti e leucociti mobili. La sostanza di base gelatinosa funge da mezzo di supporto per i componenti fibrillari e cellulari nonché quale sede di conservazione di una porzione sostanziale dell'acqua corporea. Sia l'epidermide sia il derma ricevono nutrienti dai vasi sanguigni dermici.

TESSUTO SOTTOCUTANEO. Il pannicolo, o tessuto sottocutaneo, è costituito da cellule adipose e setti fibrosi che lo dividono in lobuli e lo ancorano alla fascia sottostante e al periostio. In questo stato, che funge da sede di deposito dei lipidi, da isolante per conservare il calore corporeo e da cuscinetto protettivo contro i traumi, sono presenti anche vasi sanguigni e nervi.

ANNESSI. Queste strutture derivano da aggregati delle cellule epidermiche che si specializzano durante il primo sviluppo embrionale. Piccoli abbozzi (germi epiteliali primitivi) compaiono nel terzo mese fetale e danno vita ai follicoli piliferi, alle ghiandole sebacee e apocrine e alle sporgenze di attacco dei muscoli erettori dei peli. Le ghiandole sudoripare eccrine derivano da una crescita epidermica verso il basso separata che si verifica nel secondo mese fetale e sono completamente formate entro il quinto mese. La formazione delle unghie inizia nel terzo mese di vita intrauterina.

FOLLICOLI PILIFERI. Il follicolo è la struttura più importante del complesso pilare, che include la ghiandola sebacea, il muscolo erettore del pelo e, nelle aree come le ascelle, una ghiandola apocrina. I follicoli piliferi sono distribuiti su tutta la cute, eccetto i palmi delle mani, le piante dei piedi, le labbra e il glande del pene; se vengono distrutti, non possono rigenerarsi. I singoli follicoli si estendono dalla superficie dell'epidermide al derma profondo. Il follicolo pilifero è diviso in quattro segmenti: l'infundibolo, che si estende dalla superficie cutanea all'apertura del dotto sebaceo; l'istmo, che va dall'apertura del dotto sebaceo alla sporgenza; il follicolo inferiore tra la sporgenza e il bulbo pilifero e infine il bulbo pilifero. La sporgenza si trova sul punto di inserimento del muscolo erettore del pelo e rappresenta il sito delle cellule staminali cutanee. Il destino di differenziazione di queste cellule staminali è in parte controllato da *c-myc*. Il bulbo è il luogo in cui le cellule della matrice e la papilla dermica partecipano alla formazione e al mantenimento del pelo. Le parti in via di accrescimento comprendono il fusto del pelo e le guaine di supporto.

Nell'uomo, la crescita del pelo è ciclica con periodi alterni di crescita (**anagen**) e di riposo (**telogen**). La durata della fase anagen varia da mesi ad anni. Alla nascita, tutti i peli si trovano nella fase anagen. In seguito l'attività generativa perde la sincronia per cui prevale un modello generale casuale di crescita e caduta. In ogni momento, ≈85% dei peli si trova nella fase anagen. I capelli in genere crescono circa 1 cm/mese.

I peli si distinguono in lanugine fetale, peli terminali e vello. La lanugine è sottile e corta; questi peli vengono persi prima della fine della gestazione e verso la 36ª-40ª settimana sono sostituiti dal vello. I peli terminali sono lunghi e grossi e sono presenti sul cuoio capelluto, nella barba, sulle ciglia e sopracciglia nonché nell'area ascellare e pubica. Il vello è costituito da peli corti, morbidi e spesso non pigmentati ed è distribuito sul resto del corpo. Durante la pubertà, la stimolazione degli ormoni androgeni causa la mutazione dei peli pubici, ascellari e della barba da vello a peli terminali.

GHIANDOLE SEBACEE. Queste ghiandole sono presenti in tutte le zone tranne il palmo della mano, la pianta e il dorso del piede, e sono numerose soprattutto sul volto, nella regione superiore del torace e sulla schiena. I loro dotti si aprono nei follicoli piliferi tranne che sulle labbra, sul prepuzio e sulle piccole labbra, dove emergono direttamente sulla superficie muscolare. Queste ghiandole olocrine sono strutture sacculari spesso ramificate e lobulate e consistono di uno strato basale proliferativo di piccole cellule piatte periferiche alla massa centrale delle cellule lipidizzate. Queste ultime si disintegrano mano a mano che si spostano verso il dotto e formano la secrezione lipidica nota come sebo, che consiste di detriti cellulari, trigliceridi, fosfolipidi ed esteri di colesterolo. Le ghiandole sebacee dipendono dalla stimolazione ormonale e sono attivate dagli androgeni durante la pubertà. Le ghiandole sebacee fetali vengono stimolate dagli androgeni materni e la loro secrezione lipidica, insieme alle cellule desquamate dello strato corneo, forma la vernice caseosa.

GHIANDOLE APOCRINE. Le ghiandole apocrine si trovano in ascelle, areole, aree perianali e genitali nonché nella regione periombelicale. Queste strutture grandi, spiralizzate e tubulari secernono continuamente un liquido lattiginoso inodore che viene secreto in risposta agli stimoli adrenergici, di solito in seguito a stress emozionale. La decomposizione batterica del sudore apocrino è responsabile dell'odore sgradevole associato alla perspirazione. Le ghiandole apocrine restano quiescenti fino alla pubertà, quando aumentano di dimensioni e ha inizio la secrezione in risposta all'attività androgena. La parte secretoria della ghiandola è costituita da un singolo strato di cellule racchiuse da uno strato di cellule mioepiteliali contrattili. Il dotto è rivestito da un doppio strato di cellule cuboidali e si apre nel complesso pilosebaceo. Benché le ghiandole apocrine non siano deputate alla termoregolazione, sono coinvolte in determinati processi patologici.

GHIANDOLE SUDORIPARE ECCRINE. Queste ghiandole sono distribuite sull'intera superficie corporea, compresi i palmi delle mani e le piante dei piedi, dove sono più abbondanti. Quelle che si trovano sulla cute rivestita da peli rispondono agli stimoli termici e servono per regolare la temperatura corporea apportando acqua alla superficie cutanea per l'evaporazione; al contrario, le ghiandole sudoripare sui palmi delle mani e sulle piante dei piedi rispondono prevalentemente a stimoli fisiopsicologici.

Ogni ghiandola eccrina consiste di una spirale secretoria situata nel derma reticolare o nell'adipe sottocutaneo e di un dotto secretorio che si apre sulla superficie cutanea. Utilizzando una lente di ingrandimento è possibile individuare pori sudoripari sulle creste epidermiche dei palmi e delle dita delle mani, ma questi non sono prontamente individuabili altrove. Due tipi di cellule compongono la spirale secretoria a strato singolo: piccole cellule scure e grandi cellule chiare. Queste poggiano su uno strato di cellule mioepiteliali contrattili e su una membrana basale. Le ghiandole sono provviste di fibre nervose simpatiche, ma il mediatore farmacologico della sudorazione è l'acetilcolina invece dell'adrenalina. Il sudore è composto da acqua, sodio, potassio, calcio, cloro, fosforo, lattato e piccole quantità di ferro, glucosio e proteine. La composizione varia in base alla velocità di sudorazione ma è sempre ipotonica nei bambini normali.

UNGHIE. Le unghie sono strutture epidermiche protettive specializzate che formano placche convesse, traslucide e aderenti sulle superfici dorsali distali delle dita di mani e piedi. La lamina ungueale, che deriva da una matrice metabolicamente attiva di cellule in moltiplicazione situate sotto la plica ungueale posteriore, cresce a una velocità di ≈1 cm ogni 3 mesi. La lamina ungueale è vincolata dalle pliche ungueali laterali e posteriore; un piccolo eponichio (la cuticola) protrude dalla plica posteriore su un'area bianca a mezzaluna chiamata lunula. Il colore rosa riflette il letto vascolare sottostante.

Eckes B, Krieg T: Regulation of connective tissue homeostasis in the skin by mechanical forces. *Clin Exp Rheumatol* 2004;22:S73–S76.

Groscurth P: Anatomy of sweat glands. *Curr Prob Dermatol* 2002;30:1–9.

Honeycutt KA, Koster MI, Roop DR: Genes involved in stem cell fate decisions and commitment to differentiation play a role in skin disease. *J Investig Dermatol Symp Proc* 2004;9:261–268.

Marks R: The stratum corneum barrier: The final frontier. *J Nutr* 2004;134: 2017S–2021S.

McCarthy DJ: Anatomic consideration of the human nail. *Clin Podiatr Med Surg* 2004;4:477–491.

McMillan Jr, Akiyama M, Shimizu H: Epidermal basement membrane zone components: Ultrastructure, distribution and molecular interactions. *J Dermatol Sci* 2003;31:169–177.

Thiboutot D: Regulation of human sebaceous glands. *J Invest Dermatol* 2004; 123:1–12.

Capitolo 644 ■ Valutazione del paziente

Joseph G. Morelli

ANAMNESI ED ESAME OBIETTIVO. Benché molte malattie della cute siano prontamente riconosciute mediante semplice ispezione, per una valutazione accurata spesso occorrono l'anamnesi e un esame obiettivo. È necessario esaminare con attenzione in condizioni di illuminazione adeguata l'intera superficie corporea, le membrane mucose, la congiuntiva, i peli e le unghie. Bisogna notare il colore, il turgore, la consistenza, la temperatura e l'umidità della cute così come la crescita, la consistenza, il calibro e la lucidità dei peli e delle unghie. Le lesioni cutanee devono essere palpate, ispezionate e classificate sulla base di morfologia, dimensioni, colore, consistenza, compattezza, configurazione, ubicazione e distribuzione. È necessario inoltre stabilire se le alterazioni sono da ricondursi a una lesione primitiva o se il modello clinico è stato alterato da un fattore secondario come un'infezione, un trauma o una terapia.

Le lesioni primitive vengono classificate come macule, papule, chiazze, placche, noduli, tumori, vescicole, bolle, pustole, pomfi e cisti. Una **macula** rappresenta un'alterazione del colore della cute ma non può essere palpata. Quando la lesione è >1 cm, viene usato il termine **chiazza**. Le **papule** sono lesioni solide palpabili <0,5-1 cm, mentre i **noduli** hanno un diametro superiore. I **tumori** sono solitamente più grandi dei noduli e variano considerevolmente in termini di mobilità e di consistenza. Le **vescicole** sono lesioni rilevate, piene di liquido, con diametro <0,5 cm; quando sono più grandi vengono definite **bolle**. Le **pustole** contengono materiale purulento. I **pomfi** sono lesioni palpabili con la parte superiore piatta, di dimensioni, durata e configurazione variabili, che rappresentano raccolte dermiche di liquido edematoso. Le **cisti** sono lesioni circoscritte con la parete spessa, situate in profondità nella cute; sono ricoperte da epidermide normale e contengono materiale liquido o semisolido. In genere, le aggregazioni di papule vengono definite **placche**.

Le lesioni primitive possono trasformarsi in lesioni secondarie oppure, con il passare del tempo, è possibile che si sviluppino lesioni secondarie laddove prima non esisteva una lesione primitiva. Generalmente, le lesioni primitive sono più utili ai fini diagnostici rispetto a quelle secondarie. Queste ultime includono scaglie, ulcere, erosioni, escoriazioni, ragadi, croste e cicatrici. Le **scaglie** sono costituite da strati compressi di cellule dello strato corneo che vengono ritenute sulla superficie cutanea. Le **erosioni** comprendono la perdita focale di epidermide e guariscono senza lasciare cicatrici. Le **ulcere** si estendono nel derma e tendono a guarire lasciando cicatrici. Le lesioni ulcerate inflitte dai graffi hanno spesso una configurazione lineare e angolata e vengono definite **escoriazioni**. Le **ragadi** sono causate da spaccatura o fenditura della cute; di solito si verificano sulla cute malata. Le **croste** sono costituite da accumuli addensati e trattenuti di sangue, siero, pus e detriti epiteliali sulla superficie di una lesione trasudante. Le **cicatrici** sono lesioni terminali che possono essere sottili, depresse e atrofiche, in rilievo e ipertrofiche oppure piane e flessibili; sono costituite da tessuto connettivo fibroso. La **lichenificazione** è un ispessimento della cute con accentuazione delle normali linee cutanee, causata da un'irritazione cronica (sfregamento, grattamento) o da infiammazione.

Se dopo un attento esame la diagnosi non è chiara, possono essere indicate una o più procedure diagnostiche.

BIOPSIA CUTANEA. In alcuni casi per fare una diagnosi è necessaria una biopsia cutanea. La biopsia con punch è una procedura semplice, relativamente indolore e di solito fornisce una quantità di tessuto adeguata per l'esame se viene prelevato un campione appropriato. La selezione di una lesione primitiva recente e ben sviluppata è estremamente importante per ottenere una diagnosi accurata. La biopsia deve presentare un rischio relativamente ridotto di danneggiare le strutture dermiche sottostanti. Dopo aver pulito il sito, la cute viene anestetizzata applicando una pomata contenente lidocaina e prilocaina e/o tramite iniezione intradermica di lidocaina all'1-2% con o senza epinefrina, con un ago 27 o 30 G. Un punch da 3 o 4 mm viene premuto saldamente contro la cute e ruotato fino a raggiungere la profondità corretta. Tutti e tre gli strati (epidermide, derma e fascia superficiale sottocutanea) devono essere contenuti nel plug. Il plug deve essere sollevato delicatamente con il forcipe o estratto con un ago e separato dal tessuto sottostante con forbici tipo Iris. L'emorragia viene arrestata applicando una pressione salda e suturando. Il campione bioptico deve essere collocato in una soluzione di formaldeide al 10% in vista del trattamento appropriato.

LAMPADA DI WOOD. La lampada di Wood trasmette luce ultravioletta prevalentemente con una lunghezza d'onda di 365 nm. L'esame, che viene eseguito in una camera buia, è utile per rilevare macule ipopigmentate e determinate infezioni micotiche superficiali del cuoio capelluto. Una fluorescenza blu-verde è individuabile alla base di ogni fusto pilifero in caso di ectothrix e in alcune infezioni da endothrix. Le scaglie e le croste possono apparire di colore giallo pallido, ma non vi è segno di infezione micotica. Le lesioni dermatofitiche della cute (tinea corporis) non mostrano fluorescenza; le macule della tinea versicolor, invece, alla lampada di Wood, sono caratterizzate da una fluorescenza dorata. L'eritrasma, un'infezione intertriginosa causata da *Corynebacterium minutissimum*, può presentare una fluorescenza rosa-arancione, mentre la *Pseudomonas aeruginosa* alla lampada di Wood appare giallo-verde. Aree discrete di pigmento alterato possono spesso essere visualizzate più chiaramente utilizzando una lampada di Wood, in particolare se l'alterazione pigmentaria è epidermica. Le lesioni iperpigmentate appaiono più scure, mentre quelle ipopigmentate (sclerosi tuberosa) sono più chiare della cute circostante.

PREPARAZIONE DI IDROSSIDO DI POTASSIO (KOH). Questa preparazione offre un sistema rapido e affidabile per individuare elementi micotici di lieviti e dermatofiti. Per un recupero ottimale dei miceli e delle spore, le lesioni squamose devono essere grattate sul bordo attivo. Le vescicole vanno scoperchiate e la parte superiore della vescica deve essere pinzata e posta su un vetrino per l'esame. Nella tinea capitis, occorre prelevare i capelli infetti dal follicolo; le scaglie prelevate dal cuoio capelluto in genere non contengono miceli. Si aggiungono al campione poche gocce di KOH al 20%, che viene quindi delicatamente scaldato su una lampada ad alcol finché comincia a sobbollire; in alternativa, può essere concesso un tempo più lungo (≈10-20 min) per la dissoluzione della cheratina. Alla soluzione KOH è possibile aggiungere anche dimetil sulfossido (DMSO). La preparazione viene esaminata sotto una luce a intensità ridotta per rilevare la presenza di elementi micotici.

STRISCIO DI TZANCK. È utile nella diagnosi di alcune infezioni virali (herpes simplex, varicella, herpes zoster, eczema erpetico) e per l'individuazione di cellule acantolitiche nel pemfigo. È necessario rompere una vescicola recente, intatta e far drenare il liquido. La base della vescicola viene quindi grattata con uno strumento dai bordi smussati, facendo attenzione a non far sanguinare la lesione in maniera troppo abbondante; il materiale viene strisciato su un vetrino trasparente e lasciato asciugare all'aria. È preferibile la colorazione di Giemsa, ma anche la colorazione di Wright è accettabile. Le cellule a pallone (*balloon*) e le cellule giganti multinucleate consentono di formulare la diagnosi di infezione da herpes virus; le cellule epidermiche acantolitiche sono caratteristiche del pemfigo.

Il test di fluorescenza diretta è più sensibile e specifico. I cheratinociti vengono grattati dalla base della vescicola come precedentemente descritto. Il laboratorio colora il vetrino con anticorpi marcati specifici per il virus della varicella zoster o il virus dell'herpes simplex. L'osservazione del vetrino con un microscopio a fluorescenza documenta la presenza del virus specifico all'interno delle cellule. La PCR per gli herpes virus è rapida, sicura, specifica e sensibile.

STUDI DI IMMUNOFLUORESCENZA. Gli studi di immunofluorescenza cutanea possono essere usati per rilevare anticorpi fissati su tessuto a componenti della cute e al complemento; i modelli di colorazione caratteristici sono specifici di determinate malattie cutanee. Il siero può essere usato per identificare gli anticorpi circolanti. I campioni cutanei per le preparazioni destinate all'immunofluorescenza diretta devono essere prelevati dai siti interessati tranne che nelle malattie in cui è necessaria cute perilesionale o cute non danneggiata (Tab. 644-1). Si ottiene un campione per biopsia punch e il tessuto viene posto in uno speciale mezzo di trasporto o immediatamente congelato in azoto liquido per il trasporto e la conservazione. Le sezioni criostatiche sottili del campione vengono incubate con anticorpi coniugati con fluorescina agli antigeni specifici.

Il siero dei pazienti può essere esaminato mediante tecniche di immunofluorescenza indiretta utilizzando come substrato sezioni di cute umana normale, labbra di cavia o esofago di scimmia. Il substrato viene incubato con siero fresco o congelato sottoposto a scongelamento e quindi con globulina antiumana coniugata con fluorescina. Se il siero contiene anticorpi verso i componenti epiteliali, è possibile vederne il modello di colorazione specifico all'analisi con microscopio a fluorescenza. Mediante diluizione seriale si può stimare il titolo di anticorpi circolanti.

TABELLA 644-1. Reperti al microscopio a immunofluorescenza nelle malattie cutanee immunomediate

MALATTIA	CUTE INTERESSATA	CUTE NON INTERESSATA	IF DIRETTA	IF INDIRETTA	ANTICORPI CIRCOLANTI
Dermatite erpetiforme	Negativa	Positiva	IgA granulari +/− C nel derma papillare	Assenti	IgA anti-reticolina nel 20-70%. Anticorpi antiendomisio (IgA, IgG) e antitransglutaminasi se coesiste malattia celiaca
Pemfigoide bolloso	Positiva	Positiva	IgG lineari e C a banda in BMZ, occasionalmente IgM, IgA, IgE	IgG in BMZ nel 70%	Assenti
Pemfigo (tutte le varianti)	Positiva	Positiva	IgG negli spazi intercellulari dell'epidermide tra cheratinociti	IgG nello spazio intercellulare	Assenti
Pemfigo foliaceo	Positiva	Positiva	IgG a glicoproteina desmosomiale, desmogleina 1	Come nell'IF diretta	Assenti
Herpes gestationis	Positiva	Positiva	C3 in BMZ, occasionalmente IgG	IgG anti-BMZ	Assenti
Dermatosi lineare bollosa da IgA (dermatosi bollosa cronica dell'infanzia)	Positiva	Positiva	IgA lineari in BMZ, occasionalmente C	IgA rari, basso titolo, anti-BMZ	Assenti
Lupus eritematoso discoide	Positiva	Negativa	IgG, IgM, IgA lineari e C3 in BMZ (banda del lupus)	Assenti	ANA negativo
Lupus eritematoso sistemico	Positiva	Variabile; esposta al sole, 30-50%; non esposta, 10-30%	IgG, IgM lineari, C3 in BMZ (banda del lupus)	Assenti	ANA Anti-Ro (SSA) Anti-RNP Anti-DNA Anti-Sm
Porpora di Henoch-Schönlein	Positiva	Positiva	IgA attorno alle pareti dei vasi	Assenti	Fattore reumatoide IgA, occasionalmente

ANA, anticorpo antinucleare; BMZ, zona della membrana basale sulla giunzione dermoepidermica; C, complemento; IF, risultati all'immunofluorescenza; Ig, immunoglobuline.

Mtuasim DF, Adams BB: Immunofluorescence in dermatology. *J Am Acad Dermatol* 2001;45:822–824.

Weston WL, Lane AT, Morelli JG: Evaluation of children with skin disease. In *Color Textbook of Pediatric Dermatology.* St. Louis, Mosby, 2002.

644.1 • MANIFESTAZIONI CUTANEE DI MALATTIE SISTEMICHE

Determinate malattie presentano caratteristiche cutanee peculiari, spesso quale segno di esordio, che possono facilitare la valutazione di pazienti complessi (Tab. 644-2).

MALATTIE DEL TESSUTO CONNETTIVO

LUPUS ERITEMATOSO. Il lupus eritematoso (LE; vedi Capitolo 157) è una malattia infiammatoria autoimmune idiopatica che può essere multisistemica o confinata alla cute.

Lupus eritematoso sistemico. L'LE sistemico (LES) è una malattia multisistemica infiammatoria cronica. Viene diagnosticato quando sono presenti 4 su 11 criteri ben definiti (vedi Capitolo 157). Tre dei criteri riguardano manifestazioni cutanee. Il primo criterio è il classico rash malare o "a farfalla" (Fig. 644-1); deve essere distinto da altre cause di "viso arrossato", in particolare da dermatite seborroica, dermatite atopica e rosacea. Il secondo criterio è un rash discoide. Il terzo criterio è un'eruzione maculare e papulare eritematosa fotosensibile (Fig. 644-2). Altre manifestazioni cutanee associate ma non diagnostiche includono lesioni purpuree, livedo reticularis, ulcerazioni mucose, fenomeno di Raynaud e alopecia senza formazione di tessuto cicatriziale.

L'LE cutaneo mostra vari gradi di atrofia epidermica, occlusione dei follicoli piliferi e alterazione vacuolare sulla giunzione dermoepidermica infiammata. Il deposito di immunoglobuline (IgM, IgG) e complemento nella cute lesa può confermare la diagnosi (vedi Tab. 644-1). Nella maggior parte dei pazienti con LES viene rilevata presenza di immunodepositi nella cute esposta al sole e non lesa (lupus band test). Il trattamento delle lesioni cutanee include la protezione dal sole e l'uso topico di corticosteroidi di intensità da lieve a media.

Lupus eritematoso neonatale. L'LE neonatale (LEN; vedi Capitolo 157.1) si presenta durante le prime settimane o nei primi mesi di vita sotto forma di placche anulari, eritematose, squamose, tipicamente su testa, collo e parte superiore del tronco (Fig. 644-3). La luce ultravioletta può esacerbare o scatenare le lesioni cutanee. Il LEN viene spesso diagnosticato erroneamente come eczema infantile, dermatite seborroica o tinea corporis. Il trasferimento passivo di anticorpi anti-IgG materni (anti-Ro/La, SS-A/SS-B) causa lesioni cutanee transitorie; i livelli di anticorpi scemano entro il sesto mese e in genere ciò determina la scomparsa del rash. Un blocco cardiaco congenito si verifica nel 30% dei neonati affetti, ma solo il 10% dei bambini colpiti presenta anomalie sia cutanee sia cardiache. Le manifestazioni extracutanee non cardiache come anemia, trombocitopenia e malattia epatica con colestasi sono rare. È indicata un'analisi degli anticorpi materni (anticorpi antinucleari [ANA]).

Lupus eritematoso discoide. L'LE discoide (LED) è raro nella prima infanzia e si presenta nella tarda adolescenza. Le manifestazioni cutanee caratteristiche del LED sono placche croniche, eritematose, squamose, atrofiche, teleangiectasiche (Fig. 644-4) sulla cute esposta al sole che spesso guarisce con formazione di cicatrici e depigmentazione. I tratti extracutanei possono comprendere il coinvolgimento della mucosa nasale e orale, degli occhi e delle unghie. La **diagnosi differenziale** include altre fotodermatosi come l'eruzione polimorfa alla luce, l'eruzione primaverile giovanile e la dermatomiosite giovanile. Esiste una sovrapposizione distinta tra LES e LED con caratteristiche istopatologiche comuni e fotoesacerbazione; la maggior parte dei pazienti con LED presenta esami di laboratorio normali e non progredisce a malattia sistemica. Può essere utile l'uso topico di creme solari e steroidi. La somministrazione intralesionale di steroidi e di antimalarici per bocca (idrossiclorochina) viene adottata nei casi di malattia severa.

DERMATOMIOSITE GIOVANILE. Le manifestazioni cutanee caratteristiche sono spesso il primo segno di dermatomiosite giovanile (JDMS; vedi Capitolo 158). Un'eruzione non ben definita, da eritematosa a violacea, squamosa e minimamente pruriginosa si presenta in aree maggiormente esposte alla luce come il viso, la parte superiore del tronco e gli estensori degli arti. Un interessamento perioculare circoscritto da parte di questo rash **eliotropo** può conferire l'aspetto da "procione", soprattutto nei bambini piccoli. Le papule caratteristiche sulle nocche (**papule di Gottron**) suggeriscono la diagnosi in assenza di debolezza muscolare associata (Fig. 644-5). Altre manifestazioni cutanee includono teleangiectasia del margine gengivale e delle pliche ungueali, ipercheratosi palmare ("mani da meccanico") e un'eru-

TABELLA 644-2. Caratteristiche dei segni cutanei di malattie sistemiche

MALATTIA	ETÀ DI ESORDIO	LESIONI CUTANEE	DISTRIBUZIONE	VALUTAZIONI DIAGNOSTICHE	SEGNI/SINTOMI ASSOCIATI	DIAGNOSI DIFFERENZIALE
Lupus eritematoso sistemico	Qualsiasi	Placche eritematose; porpora palpabile; livedo reticularis; fenomeno di Raynaud; porpora trombocitopenica e non trombocitopenica	Fotodistribuzione; viso "malare"	Panel ANA Anti-DNA a doppio filamento Leucopenia/linfopenia Trombocitopenia Livelli di complemento Analisi delle urine	Artrite Nefrite Cerebrite Sierosite	Dermatite seborroica Rosacea Dermatite atopica Dermatomiosite giovanile Vasculite
Lupus discoide	Adolescenti	Placche anulari squamose; atrofia; depigmentazione	Fotodistribuzione	ANA	Formazione di cicatrici	Lupus cutaneo subacuto Eruzione polimorfa alla luce Dermatomiosite giovanile
Lupus neonatale	Dalla nascita a 6 mesi	Placche anulari, eritematose, squamose	Fotodistribuzione; testa/collo	ANA Anti-Ro	Blocco cardiaco Trombocitopenia	Tinea capitis Dermatite atopica Dermatite seborroica
Dermatomiosite giovanile	Qualsiasi	Macule squamose, da eritematose a violacee; papule discrete sulle nocche	Viso periocularе; cingolo scapolare; estensori degli arti; nocche; palmi	ANA Jo-1 Ab Aldolasi CK LDH	Debolezza muscoli prossimali Calcificazioni Vasculopatia	Dermatite atopica Dermatite allergica da contatto Lupus eritematoso Esantema virale Eruzione da farmaci
Porpora di Henoch-Schönlein	Bambini e adolescenti	Papule e placche purpuriche	Natiche; arti inferiori	Analisi delle urine Bun/Cr Biopsia cutanea	Dolore addominale Artrite	Vasculite Eruzione da farmaci Edema emorragico infantile Esantema virale
Malattia di Kawasaki	Neonati e bambini	Placche eritematose da maculopapulari a orticariose; eritema, edema, desquamazione acrale e inguinale	Diffusa	Leucocitosi ESR PCR Trombocitosi	Lingua a fragola Congiuntivite Linfadenopatia Complicazioni cardiovascolari	Sindrome virale Eruzione da farmaci Malattia stafilococcica/streptococcica
Malattia intestinale infiammatoria	Bambini e adolescenti	Afte; eritema nodoso; pioderma gagrenoso; tromboflebite	Ulcere orali; ragadi perianali	VES Trombocitosi Anomalie radiografiche	Dolore addominale Diarrea Crampi Artrite Congiuntivite	Sindrome di Behçet Vasculite *Yersinia colitis*
Sindrome di Sweet	Qualsiasi	Placche eritematose, edematose, infiltrate	Diffusa	Biopsia cutanea Leucocitosi VES	Febbre Malattie similinfluenzali Congiuntivite	Infezione Orticaria Eritema multiforme Vasculite orticariosa
Graft vs host disease	Qualsiasi	Acuta: eritema, papule, vescicole, bolle	Testa e collo; palmi/piante; diffusa	Biopsia cutanea Funzione epatica	Febbre Mucosite Epatite	Eruzione da farmaci Esantema infettivo
Reazione di ipersensibilità	Qualsiasi	Eritema; macule orticariose e placche	Diffusa	Funzione epatica Eosinofilia Linfocitosi atipica	Edema periorale Linfadenopatia Febbre Epatite	Sindrome di Stevens-Johnson Esantema infettivo
Reazione tipo malattia da siero	Qualsiasi	Placche edematose, purpuriche	Acrale; diffusa	VES	Febbre Linfadenopatia Artrite, nefrite	Malattia di Kawasaki Malattia del tessuto connettivo

ANA, anticorpi antinucleari; CK, creatinchinasi; PCR, proteina C reattiva; VES, velocità di eritrosedimentazione; LDH, lattato deidrogenasi.

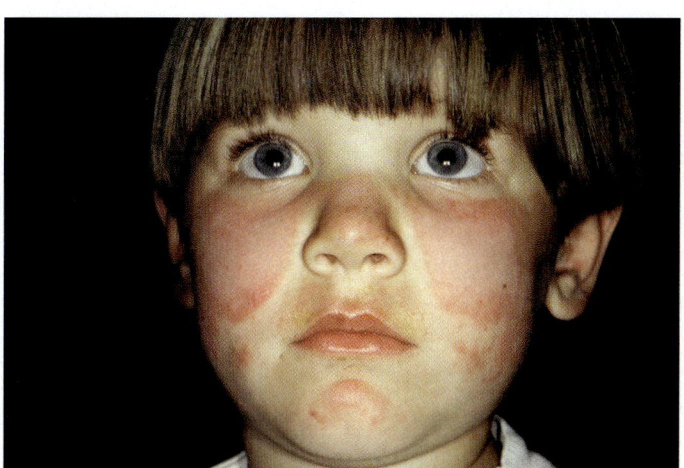

Figura 644-1. Rash malare del lupus eritematoso sistemico (LES).

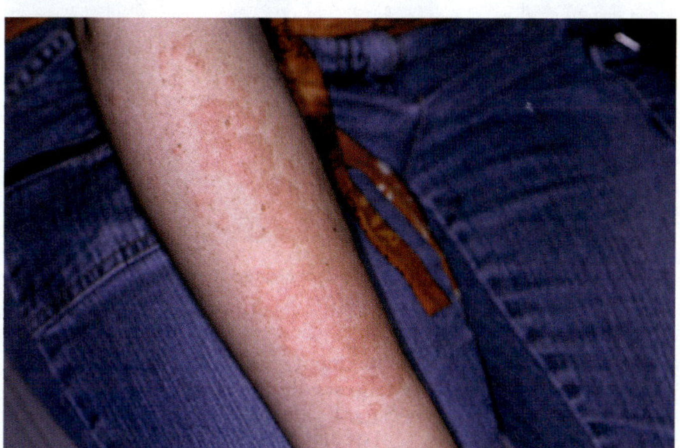

Figura 644-2. Rash fotosensibile del lupus eritematoso sistemico (LES).

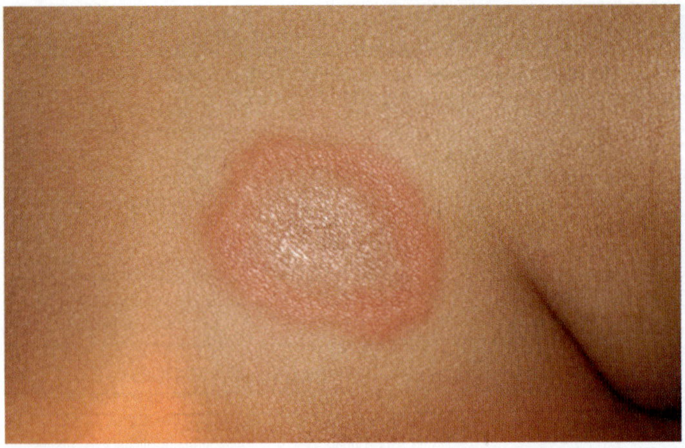

Figura 644-3. Placca anulare nel lupus eritematoso neonatale (LEN).

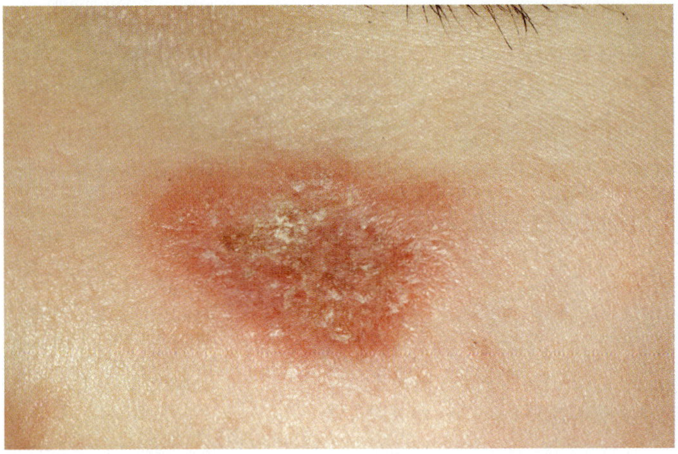

Figura 644-4. Placca squamosa eritematosa del lupus eritematoso discoide (LED).

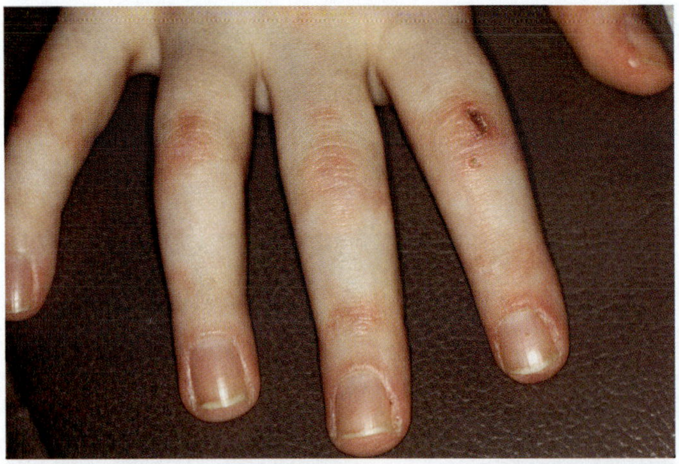

Figura 644-5. Papule di Gottron nella dermatomiosite giovanile.

zione poichilodermatosa (depigmentazione e teleangiectasia) sul cingolo scapolare ("segno dello scialle"). I tratti cutanei possono precedere la malattia sistemica. La **diagnosi differenziale** include dermatite atopica, altre malattie del tessuto connettivo, lichen planus, reazioni a farmaci ed esantemi infettivi. La scarsità del prurito nella JDMS può contribuire a eliminare alcune ipotesi. La cute lesa mostra atrofia epidermica e degenerazione vacuolare in corrispondenza della giunzione dermoepidermica. La JDMS si distingue dalla dermatomiosite dell'adulto sia nella presentazione sia nella prognosi. I pazienti pediatrici presentano maggiori problemi con vasculopatia gastrointestinale e calcificazioni cutanee, ma non mostrano un rischio aumentato di sviluppare neoplasie maligne.

La terapia include la somministrazione per via sistemica di immunosoppressivi steroidei e non steroidei; la fotoprotezione topica è fondamentale per prevenire le esacerbazioni cutanee.

SCLERODERMIA. Il termine *sclerodermia* descrive due entità separate. Una è una malattia sistemica (sclerosi sistemica progressiva [SSP]; vedi Capitolo 159), mentre l'altra è strettamente cutanea (**morfea**). La presentazione più frequente della morfea è costituita da chiazze circoscritte solitarie o multiple di eritema che evolvono in placche indurite, sclerotiche e atrofiche (Fig. 644-6), guariscono tardivamente o "si estinguono" con alterazione del pigmento. La morfea può interessare qualsiasi area della cute ma, quando è confinata alla regione frontale del cuoio capelluto, alla fronte e alla regione centrale del viso formando una fascia lineare, viene definita **sclerodermia lineare** o "en coup de sabre". Questa forma della patologia ha una prognosi sfavorevole per l'associata atrofia muscoloscheletrica sottostante che può essere causa di deturpazione estetica. La morfea lineare su un'articolazione può causare una limitazione della mobilità (Fig. 644-7). La **diagnosi differenziale** include granuloma anulare, necrobiosi lipoidea, sclerosi lichenoide e malattia di Lyme tardiva (acrodermatite cronica

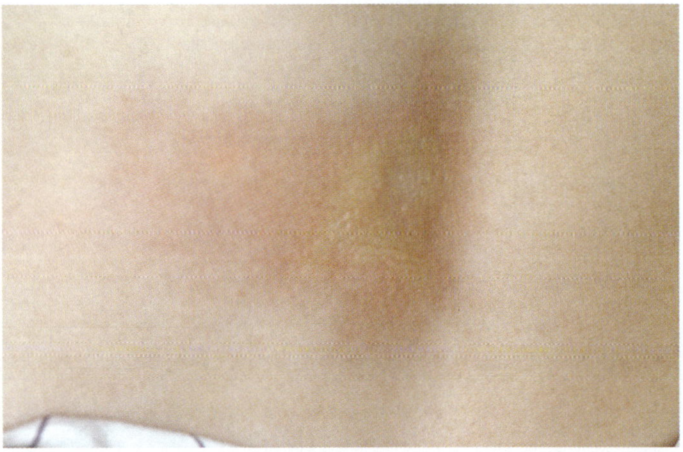

Figura 644-6. Placca eritematosa, iperpigmentata della morfea precoce.

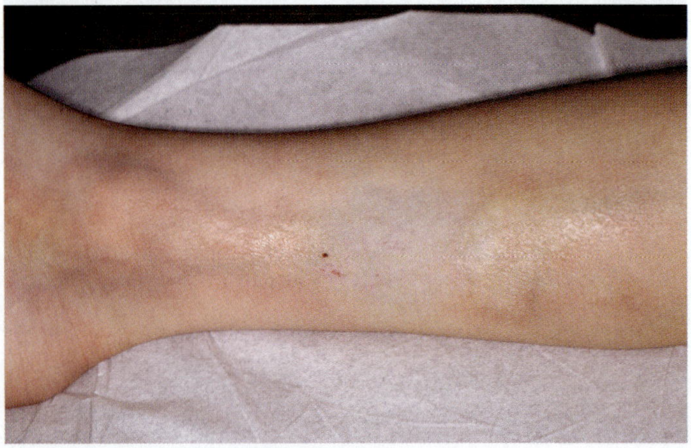

Figura 644-7. Morfea lineare con coinvolgimento sopra la caviglia.

atrofizzante). Si rileva ispessimento o sclerosi del derma con degenerazione del collagene. La morfea tende a persistere con un'espansione graduale verso l'esterno sulla cute fino a cessazione spontanea o indotta della fase infiammatoria a distanza di mesi o anni. La terapia topica con calcipotriene e UVA-1 può arrestare la progressione e contribuire ad abbreviare il decorso della malattia. Per mantenere la mobilità articolare è necessaria la fisioterapia. Un'alterazione significativa postinfiammatoria del pigmento può persistere per anni. La morfea pansclerotica è una variante disabilitante grave.

La sclerosi sistemica progressiva si presenta spesso con alterazioni acrali (sclerodattilia, ulcerazione, teleangiectasia delle pliche ungueali o fenomeni di Raynaud) e altre alterazioni di tipo cutaneo (naso affilato, cute periorale corrugata o "facies da sclerodermia") (vedi Capitolo 159). Le sindromi sovrapposte come la CREST (calcinosi, fenomeno di Raynaud, dismotilità esofagea, sclerodattilia e teleangiectasie) e la malattia del tessuto connettivo misto possono includere alcuni tratti fisici e di laboratorio della sclerodermia.

VASCULITI

Le vasculiti (vedi Capitolo 166) comprendono un ampio gruppo di malattie caratterizzate da una sovrapposizione considerevole con le patologie del tessuto connettivo. L'infiammazione immunomediata di vasi sanguigni di dimensioni variabili può essere causata da uno stato infiammatorio sottostante, da un'infezione, da un trattamento farmacologico o da una neoplasia maligna. I tratti clinici comuni includono lesioni cutanee **purpuriche non trombocitopeniche palpabili**, artrite, febbre, mialgia, spossatezza e calo ponderale nonché una elevata velocità di eritrosedimentazione. Il coinvolgimento degli organi extracutanei include le articolazioni, i polmoni, i reni e il sistema nervoso centrale.

PORPORA DI HENOCH-SCHÖNLEIN (VASCULITE DA IGA). La porpora di Henoch-Schönlein (HSP) è una vasculite che si presenta con lesioni purpuriche soprattutto sulle natiche e sulle estremità inferiori dei bambini in età scolare (Fig. 644-8). L'**edema emorragico infantile** (IHE; definito anche edema emorragico acuto dell'infanzia) condivide alcune caratteristiche cliniche con l'HSP, ma si presenta nei neonati e nei bambini piccoli. L'IHE è caratterizzato da papule e placche purpuriche circoscritte al tronco e agli arti ma, contrariamente all'HSP, interessa comunemente il volto e non comporta un altro coinvolgimento organico. L'IHE può fare seguito a un'infezione recente e si manifesta con edema periferico e febbre; i pazienti con HSP sono generalmente apiretici. L'HSP deve inoltre essere distinto dalle cause infettive di lesioni cutanee purpuriche come la meningococcemia, la febbre maculosa delle Montagne Rocciose e gli esantemi virali purpurici come quelli causati da enterovirus, nonché dall'artrite reumatoide giovanile e da altre vasculiti. La diagnosi è confermata dall'osservazione all'analisi di immunofluorescenza di IgA nelle pareti dei vasi sanguigni.

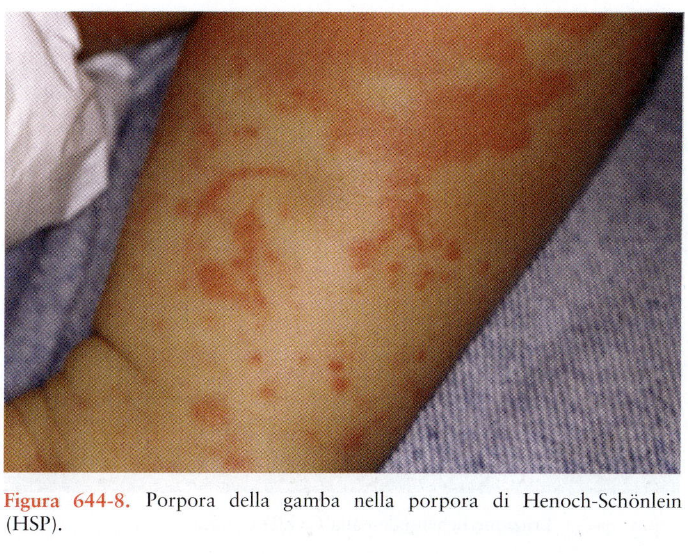

Figura 644-8. Porpora della gamba nella porpora di Henoch-Schönlein (HSP).

MALATTIA DI KAWASAKI. La malattia di Kawasaki (KD; vedi Capitolo 165) è una diagnosi clinica fondata su manifestazioni cutanee ed extracutanee. L'eruzione cutanea della KD può essere polimorfa e presentarsi in vario modo con chiazze orticarioidi, maculopapulari o morbilliformi e placche localizzate al tronco e gli arti, ma un coinvolgimento precoce con eritema e desquamazione nella regione perineale/inguinale può costituire una prima indicazione per la diagnosi. L'edema acrale e la desquamazione sono tratti prominenti ma tipicamente si manifestano in una fase più tardiva. La congiuntivite (non purulenta) spesso senza coinvolgimento del limbo e le placche linguali ("lingua a fragola bianca") che cadono per lasciare spazio a chiazze eritematose denudate con una papilla prominente ("lingua a fragola") sono tratti mucocutanei classici. I riscontri istopatologici sulla cute sono aspecifici e in generale non aiutano a escludere altre diagnosi differenziali come un esantema virale o batterico o una reazione a farmaci.

MALATTIA DI BEHÇET. La malattia di Behçet (vedi Capitolo 160) è una patologia polisistemica che include ulcerazioni orali e genitali e malattia oculare (uveite, iridociclite recidivante). Una stomatite aftosa ricorrente è presente in circa il 98% dei pazienti e in genere rappresenta il sintomo iniziale. Le ulcerazioni genitali possono assomigliare ad afte e presentarsi sul pene e sullo scroto; nelle bambine possono essere particolarmente dolorose. Altre potenziali manifestazioni cutanee includono follicolite, lesioni purpuriche, eritema nodoso e formazione di pustole in seguito a venipuntura o trauma cutaneo (**patergia**). La **diagnosi differenziale** delle lesioni orali comprende stomatite aftosa recidivante, herpes simplex e sindromi oculocutanee meno comuni (sindrome MAGIC [ulcere orali e genitali con flogosi della cartilagine]). La biopsia cutanea rivela vasculite leucocistoclastica o linfocitica. Le lesioni orali possono rispondere ai collutori che includono corticosteroidi, antistaminici, antibiotici e analgesici.

MALATTIE GASTROINTESTINALI

MALATTIA INFIAMMATORIA INTESTINALE. La **colite ulcerosa** (vedi Capitolo 333) si presenta con manifestazioni cutanee fino nel 30% dei pazienti. Le ulcere aftose sono comuni e possono peggiorare con esacerbazioni gastrointestinali. L'eritema nodoso, che viene rilevato fino nel 10% dei pazienti, si manifesta con noduli eritematosi caldi, spesso localizzati alle estremità distali inferiori. Il pioderma gangrenoso è un processo focale, ulcerativo, che presenta bordi distintivi, infiammati ed erosi e un centro purulento, paludoso. Nei pazienti con colite ulcerosa si rileva anche tromboflebite con una frequenza aumentata. Nella maggior parte dei casi, il trattamento dello stato patologico di base migliora le conseguenze cutanee.

Il **morbo di Crohn**, o enterite regionale (vedi Capitolo 333), classicamente si presenta con ragadi perianali e lembi cutanei, ascessi, seni e fistole; che possono essere i segni d'esordio della patologia. Analogamente alla colite ulcerosa, si rileva una maggiore frequenza di afte, eritema nodoso e pioderma gangrenoso ed è possibile ottenere un miglioramento trattando la malattia di base. All'analisi istopatologica di routine viene rilevata infiammazione granulomatosa non caseosa; quando l'osservazione viene effettuata su cute non contigua al tratto intestinale si parla di **morbo di Crohn metastatico**. Le lesioni metastatiche possono presentarsi sotto forma di placche o noduli localizzati, solitari o multipli, che possono trovarsi sulle superfici perianali, periorali e su altre superfici cutanee, comprese le cicatrici e i siti di ileostomia. La terapia standard include farmaci immunosoppressivi, supporto nutrizionale e intervento chirurgico per le complicazioni.

MANIFESTAZIONI CUTANEE DI NEOPLASIA MALIGNA

Le metastasi cutanee possono presentarsi come noduli solidi in qualsiasi sito della cute. A volte, i modelli distintivi di reazione paraneoplastica possono causare rash evidenti. Alcune sindromi genetiche presentano un rischio aumentato di malignità che può essere inizialmente suggerito da segni cutanei.

SINDROME DI SWEET. Nota anche come dermatosi neutrofila febbrile acuta, la sindrome di Sweet (vedi Capitolo 166.5) si presenta all'improvviso con placche o noduli dolenti, eritematosi ed edematosi su qualsiasi area della cute, spesso accompagnati da febbre, anemia e leucocitosi. La diagnosi è confermata dalla presenza di un denso infiltrato neutrofilo senza evidenza di vasculite. La **diagnosi differenziale** include pioderma gangrenoso, cellulite, eritema multiforme, sindrome di Behçet ed eritema nodoso. L'eziologia della malattia di Sweet è sconosciuta ma può essere dovuta a una reazione di ipersensibilità ad antigeni batterici, virali o tumorali e presentarsi in associazione alla malattia di Behçet. Benché la sindrome di Sweet possa presentarsi senza un'eziologia identificabile, è necessario investigare la presenza di infezione o di neoplasia maligna. Nei bambini, la sindrome di Sweet è stata associata a otite media, osteomielite, meningite asettica, HIV e leucemia. Negli adulti, il 15% dei pazienti presenta una malattia maligna associata, in generale ematologica. La sindrome di Sweet è sensibile ai corticosteroidi orali.

ERITEMA NECROLITICO MIGRANTE. L'eritema necrolitico migrante (ENM), o **sindrome da glucagonoma**, è un eritema migrante caratteristico che può essere il sintomo di una neoplasia sottostante, come un tumore pancreatico delle cellule α. Le chiazze e le placche eritematose policistiche su tronco, arti e inguine si presentano in associazione a glossite e cheilite. Livelli elevati di glucagone, intolleranza al glucosio e ipoaminoacidemia confermano la diagnosi e la resezione del tumore conduce a risoluzione del rash.

Altre manifestazioni cutanee che possono segnalare una neoplasia maligna sottostante includono prurito, ittiosi, acanthosis nigricans, orticaria, pemfigo ed eritroderma.

REAZIONI CUTANEE NELL'AMBITO DELL'IMMUNOSOPPRESSIONE

La diagnosi differenziale nei pazienti immunosoppressi deve includere reazioni a farmaci, eziologie infettive e malattia del trapianto contro l'ospite (GVHD); le somiglianze cutanee e istologiche possono essere motivo di confusione. La maggior parte delle reazioni a farmaci sono leggere eruzioni morbilliformi o esantematose con conseguenze cliniche scarse. L'identificazione del farmaco sospetto può essere difficile per i molti farmaci usati in questa popolazione. I tratti che contribuiscono a identificare i farmaci sospetti includono insorgenza del rash in seguito all'esposizione, tipo di distribuzione e diffusione, sintomi associati e dati di laboratorio. Le eruzioni da farmaci esordiscono sul tronco 7-10 giorni dopo l'esposizione, si diffondono perifericamente, sono associate a prurito e, meno frequentemente, a febbre, artralgia e linfoadenopatia. L'eosinofilia può sostenere una diagnosi di eruzione da farmaci ma può essere assente in caso di soppressione del midollo osseo. Le penicilline, i sulfamidici, le cefalosporine, gli antinfiammatori non steroidei, gli anticonvulsivanti e, talvolta, gli animoglicosidi sono responsabili comuni. Le eruzioni da farmaci possono risolversi nonostante l'uso continuato dell'agente responsabile oppure progredire e causare un coinvolgimento più grave. Sono indicati un'anamnesi farmacologica accurata, l'eliminazione di tutti i farmaci sospetti non essenziali o la sostituzione con medicinali di una classe diversa e il trattamento del prurito con emollienti, steroidi topici, antistaminici e preparati antiprurito. Le biopsie cutanee sono raramente utili per distinguere le eruzioni cutanee da farmaco dagli esantemi infettivi, benché la GVHD, se sufficientemente avanzata, possa avere manifestazioni istopatologiche distintive.

GRAFT VS HOST DISEASE, MALATTIA DEL TRAPIANTO CONTRO L'OSPITE. La GVHD (vedi Capitolo 136) può avere un'espressione cutanea importante oltre alle manifestazioni extracutanee caratteristiche come febbre, mucosite, diarrea ed epatite. La GVHD può essere confusa con una reazione a farmaci o con un esantema infettivo a causa dell'eruzione maculopapulare eritematosa aspecifica che spesso esordisce a livello focale per poi divenire generalizzata. I tratti che possono suggerire GVHD includono momento dell'eruzione (tipicamente 1-3 settimane dopo il trapianto al momento della ricostituzione ematopoietica), esordio su testa e collo incluse le orecchie e successiva diffusione al tronco, agli arti, ai palmi delle mani e alle piante dei piedi. La GVHD cronica, che si manifesta in ≈20% dei sopravvissuti a lungo termine a un trapianto, si riscontra con maggiore frequenza nei pazienti che hanno precedentemente sofferto di GVHD acuta. Le manifestazioni cutanee della GVHD cronica sono distintive con predominanza di placche squamose sclerotiche, depigmentate e papule lichenoidi (Fig. 644-9). La terapia include immunosoppressione sistemica integrata da applicazione topica di steroidi, antistaminici, antiprurito ed emollienti. La malattia cronica può anche rispondere a fotochemioterapia (PUVA), UVA-1, plasmaferesi e talidomide. Gli immunomodulatori topici come il tacrolimus possono rivelarsi efficaci. La GVHD può svilupparsi anche in contesti sensibili diversi dal trapianto, come nel neonato gravemente immunocompromesso o nel bambino molto piccolo in risposta a trasfusione terapeutica di prodotti ematici non irradiati, nel feto con immunodeficienza congenita e con passaggio transplacentare di linfociti materni nonché nel bambino più grande con neoplasia maligna che abbia ricevuto prodotti ematici non irradiati.

REAZIONI MULTISISTEMICHE A FARMACI (VEDI CAPITOLO 150)

La maggior parte delle reazioni cutanee che derivano dall'uso di farmaci per via sistemica è confinata alla cute e si risolve senza conseguenze dopo la sospensione dell'angente responsabile. Le eruzioni farmacologiche più gravi possono essere pericolose per la sopravvivenza e il riconoscimento rapido è fondamentale (vedi Capitolo 653).

RASH DA FARMACI CON EOSINOFILIA E SINTOMI SISTEMICI (SINDROME DRESS). Questa sindrome è stata in passato definita sindrome da ipersensibilità agli anticonvulsivi e sindrome da pseudolinfoma. Classicamente è riscontrata 1-4 settimane dopo l'esposizione iniziale a un anticonvulsivo aromatico e spesso si presenta con la triade **febbre**, **rash** ed **epatite**. Il rash cutaneo è caratterizzato da un'eruzione di placche coalescenti pruriginose e diffuse, da eritematose a orticarioidi. Questa eruzione cutanea

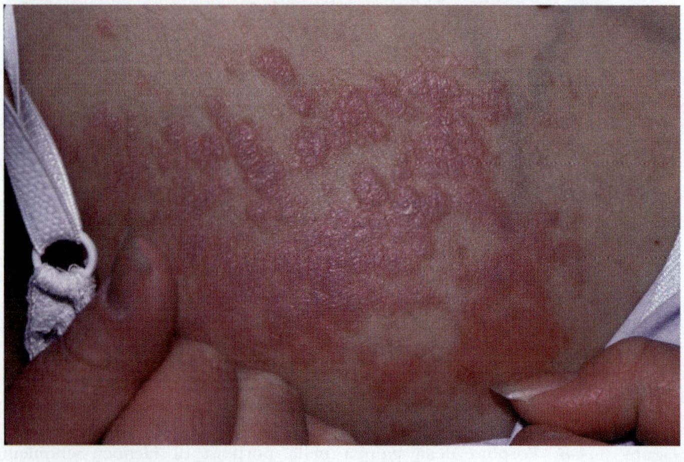

Figura 644-9. Eruzione lichenoide nalla GVHD cronica.

accentuata può essere accompagnata da edema perioculare prominente, linfoadenopatia cervicale, faringite e malessere. In circa il 30% dei pazienti si verifica eosinofilia. La presenza di linfocitosi atipica è comune. L'epatite che varia da un leggero aumento delle transaminasi epatiche a un'insufficienza epatica franca può essere accompagnata da nefrite interstiziale, polmonite ed encefalite. Tiroidite a insorgenza tardiva (parecchi mesi) e ipotiroidismo possono verificarsi in conseguenza di anticorpi antimicrosomiali diretti contro le perossidasi tiroidee coinvolte nel metabolismo dei farmaci. Un difetto ereditario della via dell'idrolasi epossidica, nel caso degli anticonvulsivi, conduce ad accumulo di metaboliti tossici, che reagiscono ai linfociti. Gli anticonvulsivi con una struttura aromatica distintiva (carbamazepina, fenobarbital, fenitoina) comportano un elevato rischio di scatenare la sindrome da ipersensibilità negli individui sensibili e nei loro parenti di primo grado. La **diagnosi differenziale** include la sindrome di Stevens-Johnson, un esantema virale o una GVHD nel contesto clinico appropriato. Oltre agli anticonvulsivi, alla prima esposizione i sulfamidici possono provocare sintomi simili a causa di anomalie delle vie della glutatione transferasi. Molti altri antibiotici sono stati indicati come responsabili di questa sindrome.

La sospensione del farmaco costituisce l'intervento terapeutico primario e il trattamento sintomatico del prurito e/o del dolore è universale. La terapia con corticosteroidi orali può essere molto utile, in particolare nel contesto di un coinvolgimento epatico o renale nella sindrome da ipersensibilità. Il ruolo delle immunoglobuline endovenose nella sindrome da ipersensibilità non è chiaro. È importante una consulenza sul maggior rischio comportato da questo tipo di farmaci e sul rischio per i fratelli. Le reazioni da ipersensibilità possono ripresentarsi, sia a carico della cute sia in altri apparati, parecchio tempo dopo che il farmaco è stato sospeso e dopo un miglioramento iniziale; ciò impone un attento follow-up per parecchi mesi.

REAZIONE SIMILE ALLA MALATTIA DA SIERO. La reazione tipo malattia da siero (SSLR) si presenta con placche coalescenti da orticarioidi a purpuriche, con bordi netti ed edema/eritema acrale, spesso in associazione ad artrite, linfoadenopatia e febbre. Contrariamente alla malattia da siero (vedi Capitolo 149), sono tipicamente assenti le evidenze di laboratorio di immunocomplessi circolanti e il coinvolgimento multisistemico della vasculite. La **diagnosi differenziale** include la malattia di Kawasaki, le patologie del tessuto connettivo e la sindrome da ipersensibilità. La SSLR si osserva soprattutto dopo l'esposizione a cefaclor. La causa è sconosciuta, ma si sospetta un metabolita tossico. Contrariamente alla reazione da ipersensibilità, la SSLR tipicamente si verifica in seguito a esposizioni ripetute al farmaco. Si raccomandano il trattamento sintomatico e la sospensione del farmaco.

Boh EE: Neonatal lupus erythematosus. *Clin Dermatol* 2004;22:125–128.

Klein-Gitelman M, Reiff A, Silverman ED: Systemic lupus erythematosus in childhood. *Rheum Dis Clin North Am* 2002;28:561–577.

Lee SJ: New approaches for preventing and treating chronic graft-versus-host disease. *Blood* 2005;105:4200–4206.

Poyrazoglu HM, Per H, Gunduz Z, et al: Acute hemorrhagic edema of infancy. *Pediatr Int* 2003;45:697–700.

Seghal VN, Srivastava G, Aggarwal AK, et al: Localized scleroderma/morphea. *J Dermatol* 2002;41:467–475.

Tas S, Simonart T: Management of drug rash with eosinophilia and systemic symptoms (DRESS syndrome): An update. *Dermatology* 2003;206: 353–356.

Ting TV, Hashkes PJ: Update on childhood vasculitis. *Curr Opin Rheumatol* 2004;16:560–565.

Van Gysel D, de Waard-van der Spek FB, Oranje AP: Childhood discoid lupus erythematosus: Report of five new cases and review of the literature. *J Eur Acad Dermatol Venereol* 2002;16:143–147.

Zipitis CS, Baildam EM, Ramanan AV: Treatment approaches to juvenile dermatomyositis. *Expert Opin Pharmacother* 2004;5:1509–1515.

Capitolo 645 ■ Principi di terapia

Joseph G. Morelli

Una cura competente della cute richiede una diagnosi specifica, conoscenza del corso naturale della malattia e capacità di distinguere le lesioni primarie da quelle secondarie. Se la diagnosi è incerta, è preferibile optare per un trattamento leggero piuttosto che per uno troppo aggressivo. Anche quando la diagnosi è chiara, una dermatite acuta può inizialmente richiedere una terapia delicata e blanda.

Quando si utilizzano farmaci topici, il veicolo è importante quanto l'agente terapeutico specifico. Le **lesioni trasudanti acute** rispondono meglio alle compresse di garze umide, seguite da lozioni o creme. Se la cute è **secca e ispessita** oppure quando occorre trattare reazioni allergiche da contatto probabilmente dovute a un componente di un farmaco topico, è preferibile un unguento. I gel e le soluzioni sono utili soprattutto per il cuoio capelluto e le altre aree rivestite da peli. Il sito interessato è molto importante poiché il veicolo migliore può non essere cosmeticamente o funzionalmente appropriato, come per esempio un unguento sul viso o sulle mani. Nella scelta del veicolo occorre inoltre tenere conto della preferenza del paziente poiché la compliance è scarsa se il farmaco risulta inaccettabile per il soggetto interessato. Sono stati sviluppati sistemi di somministrazione in schiuma accettabili dal punto di vista cosmetico, ma al momento i prodotti disponibili in questa forma sono pochi.

La maggior parte delle **lozioni** sono miscele liquide di acqua e olio. Dopo che l'acqua è evaporata, la piccola quantità residua di olio ricopre la cute. Alcune lozioni in sospensione sono costituite da acqua e polvere insolubile; l'evaporazione dell'acqua raffredda la cute, che resta rivestita da un sottile film di polvere. Le **creme** sono emulsioni di olio e acqua, vischiose, non liquide (contengono più olio delle lozioni). Gli **unguenti** contengono oli e una quantità di acqua minima o addirittura nulla; sono untuosi al tatto, lubrificano la cute secca, trattengono l'acqua e possono essere occlusivi. Gli unguenti senza acqua di solito non richiedono conservanti perché i microrganismi necessitano dell'acqua per sopravvivere.

La terapia dovrebbe essere la più semplice possibile e andrebbero fornite precise istruzioni scritte sulla frequenza e sulla durata dell'applicazione. I medici dovrebbero acquisire familiarità con uno o due preparati per ciascuna categoria e imparare a servirsene nella maniera più appropriata. Va evitata la prescrizione di farmaci brevettati non specifici che possono contenere agenti sensibilizzanti. Alcuni preparati, come gli antistaminici topici e gli anestetici sensibilizzanti, non sono mai indicati.

BENDAGGI UMIDI. I bendaggi umidi rinfrescano e asciugano la cute per evaporazione e la ripuliscono rimuovendo croste ed essudati, che causano ulteriore irritazione se non vengono eliminati. Riducono le sensazioni di prurito, bruciore e i dolori pungenti e sono indicati per le dermatiti umide o trasudanti con infiammazione acuta. Benché alla soluzione sia possibile aggiungere varie sostanze astringenti e antisettiche, le compresse inumidite con acqua di rubinetto fresca o tiepida sono altrettanto efficaci. I bendaggi realizzati con più strati di Kerlix®, garza o cotone soffice possono essere saturati di acqua e riumidificati ogniqualvolta necessario. Le compresse andrebbero applicate per 10-20 minuti almeno ogni 4 ore e il trattamento dovrebbe essere proseguito per 24-48 ore.

In alternativa, è possibile imbibire d'acqua mutandoni lunghi da uomo in cotone e strizzarli il più possibile. Queste devono quindi essere sistemate sul bambino e coperte con un pigiama asciutto, se possibile un pigiama con i piedi. Il bambino deve essere lasciato dormire così. Questo metodo può essere utilizzato tutte le notti per una settimana.

OLI DA BAGNO, COLLOIDI, SAPONI. Gli oli da bagno apportano scarsi benefici nel trattamento dei bambini. Offrono un leggero effetto idratante ma incrementano il rischio di provocarsi una ferita durante il bagno. Possono infatti rendere scivolosa la superficie della vasca, causando la caduta di un adulto o di un bambino durante l'ingresso nella stessa. È possibile prescrivere soluzioni da bagno a base di catrame, che possono essere utili per la psoriasi e per la dermatite atopica. I colloidi come l'amido in polvere o la farina d'avena colloidale producono un effetto lenitivo e in alcuni pazienti riducono il prurito quando vengono aggiunti all'acqua del bagno. La farina d'avena colloidale oleata contiene olio minerale e derivati della lanolina che lubrificano la cute secca. Anche questi prodotti, però, possono rendere scivolosa la superficie della vasca. I comuni saponi possono essere irritanti ed essiccare la cute se i pazienti hanno la cute disidratata o una dermatite. I saponi sintetici sono molto meno irritanti. Si raccomanda di evitare il sapone quando la cute è molto infiammata. Alcuni pazienti trovano lenitivi i detergenti privi di lipidi contenenti alcol cetilico.

LUBRIFICANTI. I lubrificanti, come le lozioni, le creme e gli unguenti, possono essere usati come emollienti per la cute secca e come veicoli per gli agenti topici come i corticosteroidi e i cheratolitici. In generale, gli unguenti sono gli emollienti più efficaci. Sono disponibili numerose preparazioni commerciali in aggiunta ai prodotti standard come petrolato, crema contenente stearina e lanolina nonché unguenti idrofili. Alcuni pazienti non tollerano gli unguenti mentre altri possono essere sensibilizzati a un componente del lubrificante; alcuni conservanti delle creme (soprattutto i paraben) sono sensibilizzanti. Queste preparazioni possono essere applicate più volte al giorno, se necessario. L'effetto migliore si raggiunge quando si utilizzano sulla cute umida immediatamente dopo il bagno o la doccia. Le lozioni contenenti mentolo e canfora in un veicolo emolliente possono essere impiegate per controllare il prurito e la secchezza.

SHAMPOO. Speciali shampoo contenenti zolfo, acido salicilico, zinco e selenio solfuro sono utili nel caso di desquamazione del cuoio capelluto. La maggior parte degli shampoo contiene surfattanti e detergenti. Gli shampoo contenenti catrame sono utili per la psoriasi e per la dermatite seborroica grave e andrebbero usati con la frequenza necessaria a controllare la desquamazione. Occorre spiegare ai pazienti di lasciare la schiuma a contatto con il cuoio capelluto per 5-10 minuti.

LOZIONI IN SOSPENSIONE. Queste lozioni sono utili agenti antiprurito; consistono in una sospensione di polvere in un veicolo liquido. Per la lubrificazione è possibile aggiungere olio idrosolubile. Questi preparati possono essere utilizzati efficacemente in combinazione con compresse umide nelle dermatiti essudative. L'evaporazione della lozione produce raffreddamento e la polvere depositata sulla cute assorbe l'umidità.

POLVERI. Le polveri sono igroscopiche e fungono da agenti assorbenti nelle aree di eccessiva sudorazione. Allo stato asciutto, le polveri riducono la frizione tra due superfici. Sono particolarmente utili nelle aree intertriginose e tra le dita dei piedi, dove la frizione e il movimento possono causare macerazione e abrasione. Le polveri grossolane possono formare incrostazioni, pertanto è necessario che le particelle siano fini e inerti, a meno che nella formulazione non sia stato incorporato un farmaco.

PASTE. Contengono una polvere fine in un mezzo rappresentato da un unguento e non vengono prescritte spesso nell'odierna terapia dermatologica; in alcune situazioni, tuttavia, possono essere usate efficacemente per proteggere la cute vulnerabile o danneggiata. Le paste dense all'ossido di zinco sono blande e inerti e possono essere applicate nell'area del pannolino per prevenire un'ulteriore irritazione dovuta a dermatite da pannolino. La pasta all'ossido di zinco deve essere applicata in un strato sottile in modo da rivestire completamente la cute ed è più facilmente eliminabile con olio minerale che con acqua e sapone.

AGENTI CHERATOLITICI. Gli agenti contenenti urea sono idrofili; idratano lo strato corneo e rendono la cute più elastica. Inoltre, dato che l'urea dissolve i legami idrogeno e la cheratina epidermica, è efficace nel trattamento delle malattie che causano desquamazione. Concentrazioni comprese tra il 10 e il 40% sono disponibili in molte lozioni e creme commerciali, applicabili una o due volte al giorno in base alla tolleranza. L'acido salicilico è un efficace agente cheratolitico e può essere incorporato in vari veicoli con concentrazioni fino al 6% da applicarsi da 2 a 3 volte al giorno. I preparati a base di acido salicilico non andrebbero utilizzati nei neonati, su aree superficiali estese o su cute disepitelizzata; l'assorbimento percutaneo può causare salicilismo. Gli α-idrossiacidi, in particolare l'acido lattico e l'acido glicolico, sono disponibili nei preparati commerciali oppure possono essere incorporati in un unguento in concentrazioni fino al 12%. Alcune creme contengono sia urea sia acido lattico. I preparati a base di α-idrossiacidi sono utili per il trattamento delle malattie cheratinizzanti e possono essere applicati una o due volte al giorno. Alcuni pazienti lamentano sensazione di bruciore; in questo caso, la frequenza dell'applicazione deve essere ridotta.

COMPOSTI CATRAMATI. I catrami si ottengono da carbone bituminoso, scisti, petrolato (catrame di carbone) e legno. Esercitano un'azione antiprurito e astringente e sembrano promuovere la normale cheratinizzazione. Possono essere utili nell'eczema cronico e nella psoriasi e si può incrementarne l'efficacia esponendo l'area interessata a luce ultravioletta (UV) dopo aver rimosso il catrame. I catrami non devono essere usati per le lesioni infiammatorie acute. Spesso risultano inaccettabili in quanto possono macchiare ed emanano un odore sgradevole. Possono essere incorporati in shampoo, oli da bagno, lozioni e unguenti. Una preparazione adatta ai pazienti in età pediatrica è il liquor carbonis detergens al 2-5% in crema o unguento. I gel di catrame e gli oli leggeri per il corpo contenenti catrame sono preparati cosmetici relativamente gradevoli che causano una colorazione minima della cute e dei tessuti. I catrami possono inoltre essere incorporati in un veicolo con corticosteroidi topici. La frequenza dell'applicazione varia da 1 a 3 volte al giorno, in base alla tolleranza. Molti bambini rifiutano di usare preparazioni a base di catrame perché macchiano e hanno un cattivo odore.

AGENTI ANTIMICOTICI. Questi agenti sono disponibili sotto forma di polveri, lozioni, creme e unguenti per il trattamento delle infezioni dermatofitiche e da lieviti. La nistatina, la naftifina e l'amfotericina B sono specifici per *Candida albicans* e sono inefficaci in altre infezioni micotiche. Il tolnaftato è efficace contro i dermatofiti ma non contro i lieviti. Lo spettro d'azione della ciclopiroxolamina include i dermatofiti, *Malassezia furfur* e *Candida albicans*. Gli azoli – clotrimazolo, econazolo, ketoconazolo, miconazolo, oxiconazolo e sulconazolo – hanno uno spettro altrettanto ampio. Rispetto agli azoli, la terbinafina ha un'attività superiore contro i dermatofiti ma inferiore contro i lieviti. Per la maggior parte delle infezioni fungine, gli agenti antimicotici topici devono essere applicati 1 o 2 volte al giorno. Sono tutti caratterizzati da un basso potenziale di sensibilizzazione; tuttavia, gli additivi come conservanti e stabilizzanti presenti nei veicoli possono causare dermatiti allergiche da contatto. Gli unguenti contenenti acido benzoico al 6% e acido salicilico al 3% sono potenti agenti cheratolitici e sono stati impiegati anche nel trattamento delle infezioni dermatofitiche. La comparsa di reazioni irritanti è comune.

ANTIBIOTICI TOPICI. Gli antibiotici topici sono stati usati per molti anni nel trattamento delle infezioni cutanee locali, sebbene la loro efficacia sia stata messa in dubbio, salvo che per la mupirocina. Gli unguenti sono i veicoli di elezione e, in generale, combinazioni con altri agenti topici come i corticosteroidi non sono consigliabili. Ogniqualvolta possibile, si raccomanda di identificare l'agente eziologico e trattarlo in maniera specifica. Gli antibiotici di largo impiego come preparati sistemici devono essere evitati per il rischio di sensibilizzazione. È necessario ricordare il potenziale di sensibilizzazione di determinati altri antibiotici, come la neomicina e il nitrofurazone. La mupirocina è l'agente topico più efficace al momento disponibile ed è tanto efficace quanto l'eritromicina orale nel trattamento dell'impetigine da lieve a moderata. La polisporina e la bacitracina non sono altrettanto efficaci quanto la mupirocina e gli antibiotici orali.

CORTICOSTEROIDI TOPICI. I corticosteroidi topici sono potenti agenti antinfiammatori ed efficaci antiprurito. Risultati terapeutici soddisfacenti sono stati ottenuti in una vasta gamma di malattie cutanee. I corticosteroidi possono essere suddivisi in 7 diverse categorie in base alla potenza, ma praticamente è possibile usare 4 categorie: ridotta, moderata, alta e massima (Tab. 645-1). I preparati con potenza ridotta includono l'idrocortisone, il desonide e l'idrocortisone butirrato. I composti con potenza media comprendono amcinonide, betametasone, flurandrenolide, fluocinolone, mometasone furoato e triamcinolone. Gli steroidi topici ad alta potenza includono fluocinonide e alcinonide. Il betametasone dipropionato e il clobetasol propionato sono preparati superpotenti e devono essere prescritti con cautela. Alcuni di questi composti sono formulati in diversi gradi di potenza in base all'efficacia clinica e al grado di vasocostrizione. I medici che utilizzano steroidi topici dovrebbero acquisire familiarità con i preparati di ciascuna classe.

Tutti i corticosteroidi possono essere ottenuti in veicoli diversi, tra cui creme, unguenti, soluzioni, gel e aerosol. Alcuni sono disponibili in schiuma. L'assorbimento è maggiore nel caso di unguento o gel, ma il veicolo va scelto sulla base del tipo di malattia e del sito interessato. La frequenza di applicazione deve essere determinata in base alla potenza del preparato e alla gravità del rash. In genere, l'applicazione di uno strato sottile due volte al giorno è sufficiente. Gli effetti locali avversi includono atrofia cutanea, strie, teleangiectasie, eruzioni acneiformi, porpora, ipopigmentazione e incremento della crescita dei peli. Gli effetti collaterali sistemici degli steroidi topici si manifestano con l'uso cronico e includono deficit di accrescimento, cataratta e soppressione della funzionalità surrenale.

In circostanze selezionate, i corticosteroidi possono essere somministrati mediante iniezione intralesionale (cisti dell'acne, cheloidi, placche psoriasiche, alopecia areata, reazioni persistenti a punture d'insetto). Questo metodo di somministrazione è riservato ai medici esperti.

AGENTI ANTINFIAMMATORI NON STEROIDEI TOPICI. Per il trattamento della dermatite atopica e di altri stati infiammatori si possono utilizzare agenti antinfiammatori inibenti la calcineurina che inibiscono l'attivazione delle cellule T, vale a dire il pimecrolimus e il tacrolimus. Non presentano gli effetti locali avversi evidenziati con altri steroidi a uso topico. L'effetto locale più frequentemente riscontrato in seguito all'applicazione è una sensazione pungente. La loro forza equivale solo a quella degli steroidi topici di intensità media. Vanno usati con cautela in quanto esperimenti su animali e studi clinici hanno evidenziato un rischio aumentato di malignità (linfoma).

SCHERMI SOLARI. I filtri solari in genere sono di due tipi: (1) quelli come l'ossido di zinco e il biossido di titanio che assorbono tutte le lunghezza d'onda dello spettro UV e dello spettro visibile e (2) un gruppo di sostanze chimiche eterogenee che assorbono in maniera selettiva l'energia di varie lunghezze d'onda all'interno dello spettro UV. Alcune protezioni solari permettono l'abbronzatura senza ustione; altre prevengono entrambe. Oltre allo spettro della luce che viene bloccato, altri fattori da considerare includono l'accettabilità cosmetica, il potenziale di sensibilizzazione, la permanenza sulla cute durante il nuoto o con il sudore, la frequenza di applicazione necessaria e il costo. Gli ingredienti delle protezioni solari includono acido para-aminobenzoico (PABA) con etanolo, esteri PABA, cinnamati e benzofenone. Questi bloccano la trasmissione della maggior parte delle lunghezze d'onda solari UVB e alcune UVA. Il parsol 1789/avobenzone è più efficace nel bloccare gli UVA. Sono disponibili protettori per le labbra che assorbono la gamma dei raggi UVB. Gli schermi solari si distinguono in base al fattore di protezione solare (FPS). I fattori di protezione si calcolano confrontando la quantità di tempo necessaria a sviluppare una lieve ustione utilizzando una protezione solare con la quantità di tempo che occorre, invece, senza la protezione solare. Per evitare una bruciatura, la maggior parte dei soggetti con cute chiara necessita almeno di un FPS pari a 15. Più alto è l'FPS, migliore è la protezione contro i raggi UVB. Gli schermi solari non proteggono contro i raggi UVA. L'efficacia di questi agenti dipende dal rispetto delle istruzioni per l'uso. Per poter superare la barriera dell'epidermide, gli schermi solari chimici vanno applicati almeno 30 minuti prima dell'esposizione al sole. La maggior parte dei pazienti con eruzioni da fotosensibilità richiede una protezione da parte di agenti che assorbono i raggi UVB; i soggetti con porfiria, eruzioni fototossiche e alcuni tipi di orticaria solare richiedono agenti con uno spettro di prevenzione più ampio (vedi Capitoli 147 e 655).

Benché gli schermi solari conferiscano una fotoprotezione e possano ridurre lo sviluppo di nevi, non proteggono da tutti i tipi di radiazioni UV dannose. È importante evitare l'esposizione nelle ore più calde della giornata, quando il sole è più intenso. Gli indumenti e i cappelli offrono una protezione aggiuntiva.

LASERTERAPIA. La laserterapia pulsata viene impiegata con risultati variabili nel trattamento di chiazze vinose, acne volgare ed emangiomi. I laser a luce pulsata producono una luce che viene prontamente assorbita dall'ossiemoglobina, producendo fototermolisi. L'irradiazione ad alta energia consente l'ablazione di piccoli vasi sanguigni, mentre quella a bassa energia può stimolare la produzione cutanea di procollagene. I laser a luce pulsata sono molto efficaci contro le chiazze vinose del viso.

TABELLA 645-1. Intensità dei glucocorticoidi topici

POTENZA RIDOTTA
Idrocortisone 1%
Desonide 0,05%
INTENSITÀ MODERATA
Aclometasone dipropionato 0,05%
Betametasone valerato 0,1%
Flucinolone acetonide 0,01%
Idrocortisone valerato 0,2%
Mometasone furoato 0,1%
Triamcinolone acetonide 0,25%, 0,1%
INTENSITÀ ELEVATA
Amcinonide 0,1% crema
Betametasone dipropionato 0,05%
Desossimetasone 0,25% crema
Fluocinonide 0,05% crema, unguento
Alcinonide 0,1% crema
INTENSITÀ MASSIMA
Betametasone dipropionato (nel veicolo ottimizzato)
Clobetasol propionato 0,05%
Diflorasone diacetato 0,05%
Alobetasolo propionato 0,05%

Da Weston WL, Lane AT, Morelli JG: *Color Textbook of Pediatric Dermatology*, 2nd ed. St. Louis, Mosby, 1996, p 360.

Bergstrom KG, Arambula K, Kimball AB: Medication formulation affects quality of life: A randomized single-blind study of clobetasol propionate foam 0.05% compared with a combined program of clobetasol cream 0.05% and solution 0.05% for the treatment of psoriasis. *Cutis* 2003;72:407–411.

Huang DB, Ostrosky-Zeichner L, Wu JJ, et al: Therapy of common superficial fungal infections. *Dermatol Ther* 2004;17:517–522.

Moloney FJ, Collins S, Murphy GM: Sunscreens: Safety, efficacy and appropriate use. *Am J Clin Dermatol* 2002;3:185–191.

Nghiem P, Pearson G, Langley RG: Tacrolimus and pimecrolimus: From clever prokaryocytes to inhibiting calcineurin and treating atopic dermatitis. *J Am Acad Dermatol* 2002;46:228–241.

Schnopp C, Holtmann C, Stock S, et al: Topical steroids under wet-wrap dressings in atopic dermatitis—a vehicle controlled trial. *Dermatology* 2002;204:56–59.

Capitolo 646 ■ Malattie del neonato

Joseph G. Morelli

Le lesioni evanescenti minori del neonato, in particolare quando sono floride, possono causare preoccupazioni ingiustificate. La maggior parte delle entità è relativamente comune, benigna e transitoria e non richiede terapia.

IPERPLASIA SEBACEA. Papule bianco-giallastre minute e abbondanti si osservano frequentemente su fronte, naso, labbro superiore e guance del neonato a termine e rappresentano ghiandole sebacee iperplasiche (Fig. 646-1). Queste piccole papule rimpiccioliscono gradualmente e scompaiono del tutto entro le prime settimane di vita.

MILIO. Il milio è costituito da cisti epidermiche superficiali incluse contenenti materiale cheratinizzato laminato. La lesione è una papula compatta, con diametro di 1-2 mm, di colore bianco perlaceo opalescente. Il milio può presentarsi a qualsiasi età ma nei neonati in genere è disseminato sul volto e sulle gengive nonché sulla linea mediana del palato, dove le lesioni vengono definite perle di Epstein. Il milio si esfolia spontaneamente nella maggior parte dei neonati e può essere ignorato; le lesioni che si manifestano sulle cicatrici o sui siti di traumi nei bambini più grandi possono essere aperte con delicatezza e il contenuto asportato con un ago sottile.

VESCICHE DA SUZIONE. La presenza di bolle superficiali isolate o disseminate sugli arti superiori del neonato alla nascita è probabilmente indotta da una vigorosa suzione della parte interessata in utero. I siti più frequenti sono il lato radiale dell'avambraccio, il pollice e l'indice. Queste bolle si risolvono rapidamente senza conseguenze e devono essere distinte dai calli da suzione che si osservano sulle labbra nei primi mesi e sono causati da una combinazione di edema intracellulare e ipercheratosi. La diagnosi può essere confermata osservando il neonato succhiare l'area interessata.

CUTIS MARMORATA. Quando un neonato viene esposto a temperature ambientali basse, sulla maggior parte della sua superficie corporea può comparire un disegno vascolare cutaneo evanescente, reticolato, simile a pizzo, di colore blu e/o rosso. Questa alterazione vascolare rappresenta una risposta vasomotoria fisiologica accentuata che scompare con l'aumentare dell'età, benché a volte sia visibile anche nei bambini più grandi. Una cutis marmorata persistente e pronunciata si presenta nella malattia di Menkes, nella disautonomia familiare e nelle sindromi di Cornelia Le Lange, Down e trisomia 18. La cutis marmorata teleangiectasica congenita è clinicamente simile, ma le lesioni appaiono più intense, possono essere segmentarie, sono persistenti e si possono associare a perdita di tessuto dermico, atrofia epidermica e ulcerazione.

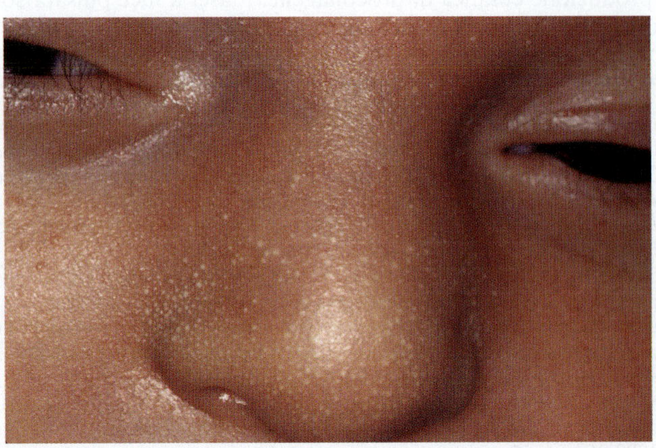

Figura 646-1. Iperplasia sebacea. Piccole papule bianco-giallastre sul naso di un neonato.

VARIAZIONE DI COLORE AD "ARLECCHINO". Questo evento vascolare raro ma marcato si verifica nell'immediato periodo neonatale ed è massimamente frequente nei neonati con peso alla nascita ridotto. Probabilmente riflette uno squilibrio nel meccanismo autonomo di regolazione vascolare. Quando il neonato viene posizionato su un fianco, il corpo si divide longitudinalmente in una metà superiore pallida e una metà inferiore rossa. Il cambiamento di colore dura solo qualche minuto e talvolta interessa solo una parte del tronco o del viso. Un cambiamento di posizione del neonato può invertire il modello. L'attività muscolare causa arrossamento generalizzato e annulla il differenziale di colore. Possono verificarsi episodi ripetuti, ma non indicano uno squilibrio autonomo permanente.

MACCHIA COLOR SALMONE (NEVUS SIMPLEX). Le macchie salmone sono piccole macule vascolari di colore rosa pallido, che si presentano più frequentemente sulla glabella, sulle palpebre, sul labbro superiore e nell'area nucale nel 30-40% dei neonati normali. Queste lesioni, che rappresentano un'**ectasia vascolare** localizzata, persistono per parecchi mesi e possono diventare più visibili durante il pianto o le variazioni della temperatura ambientale. La maggior parte delle lesioni sul viso alla fine scolorisce e scompare completamente benché spesso ciò non accada per quelle che occupano l'intera fronte centrale. In generale, le lesioni sulla regione posteriore del collo e sulle aree occipitali sono persistenti. Le lesioni facciali non devono essere confuse con una chiazza vinosa, che è una lesione permanente. La macchia salmone è generalmente simmetrica, con lesioni su entrambe le palpebre e sui due lati della linea mediana. Le chiazze vinose sono spesso più grandi e unilaterali e in genere terminano lungo la linea mediana (vedi Capitolo 649).

MACCHIE MONGOLICHE. Queste lesioni maculari blu o grigio ardesia hanno margini definiti in maniera variabile; si presentano prevalentemente nell'area presacrale ma possono comparire anche sul lato posteriore delle cosce, sulle gambe, sulla schiena e sulle spalle (Fig. 646-2). Possono essere solitarie o numerose e spesso interessano aree estese. Oltre l'80% dei neonati neri, asiatici e dell'India orientale presenta queste lesioni, mentre l'incidenza nei neonati di razza bianca è <10%. Il colore caratteristico di queste macule è dovuto alla collocazione dermica dei melanociti contenenti melanina (melanocitosi mediodermica) che si presume abbiano subito un arresto durante la loro migrazione dalla cresta neurale all'epidermide. In genere le macchie mongoliche spariscono durante i primi anni di vita perché la cute sovrastante si scurisce. Non si verifica degenerazione maligna. Le lesioni numerose e diffuse, in particolare quelle nei siti anomali, difficilmente spariscono. L'aspetto caratteristico e l'esordio congenito permettono di distinguere queste macchie dai lividi derivanti da abuso sui bambini.

ERITEMA TOSSICO. Questa eruzione evanescente, benigna e autolimitata si verifica in ≈50% dei neonati a termine; i neonati prematuri vengono colpiti con frequenza minore. Le lesioni sono papule o pustole compatte, bianco/giallastre, di 1-2 mm, con un contorno eritematoso (Fig. 646-3). A volte, l'eritema a chiazze è l'unica manifestazione. Le lesioni possono essere sparse o numerose e raggruppate in più siti o ampiamente disperse su gran parte della superficie corporea. In genere, i palmi delle mani e le piante dei piedi vengono risparmiati. La massima incidenza si verifica nel secondo giorno di vita, ma nuove eruzioni possono comparire durante i primi giorni quando il rash si acutizza e impallidisce. A volte, nei prematuri, l'insorgenza può essere ritardata di alcuni giorni o settimane. Le pustole si formano sotto lo strato corneo

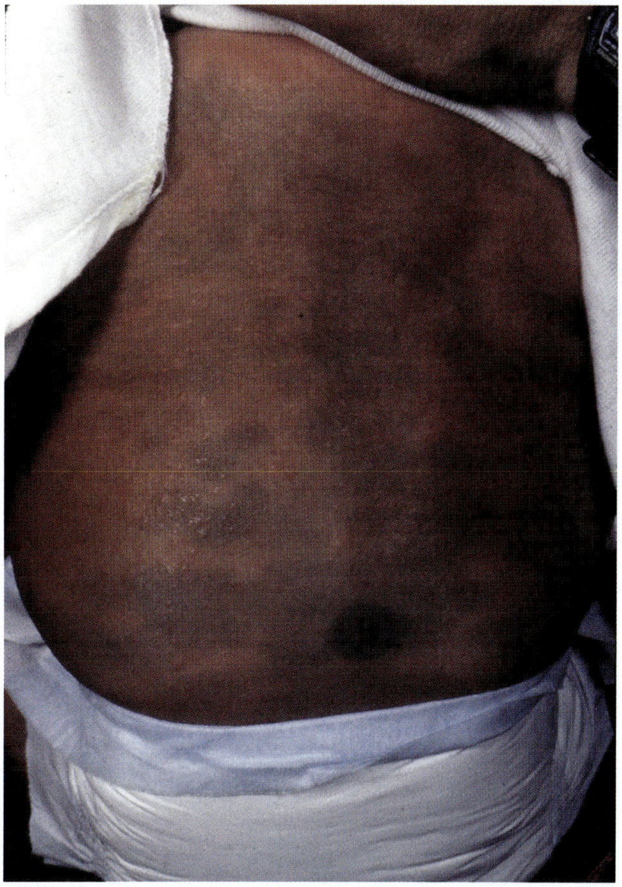

Figura 646-2. Ampia macchia mongolica sulla schiena di un neonato. (Per gentile concessione dell'archivio didattico del Fitzsimons Army Medical Center.)

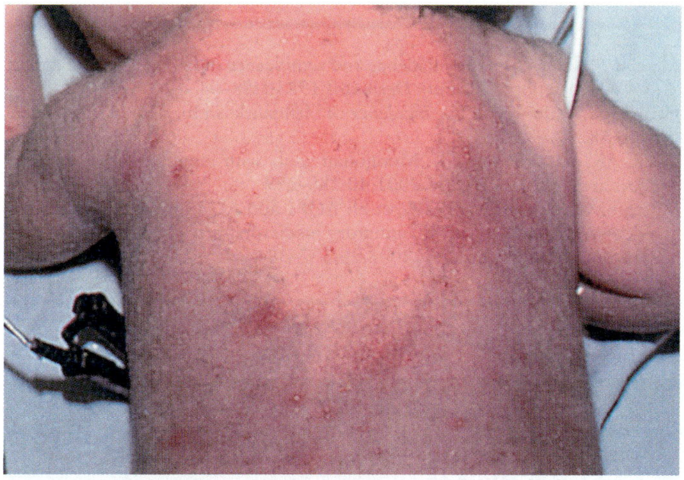

Figura 646-3. Eritema tossico sul tronco di un neonato.

o più in profondità nell'epidermide e rappresentano raccolte di eosinofili che si accumulano attorno alla porzione superiore del follicolo pilosebaceo. La presenza di **eosinofili** può essere dimostrata negli strisci del contenuto intralesionale sottoposti a colorazione di Wright. Le colture sono sterili.

La causa dell'eritema tossico è sconosciuta. Le lesioni possono mimare il pioderma, la candidosi, l'herpes simplex, la melanosi pustolosa neonatale transitoria e la miliaria, ma è possibile distinguerle grazie al caratteristico infiltrato di eosinofili e per l'assenza di organismi sullo striscio colorato. Il decorso è breve e non occorre terapia. Anche l'incontinentia pigmenti e la follicolite pustolosa eosinofila sono caratterizzate da infiltrazione eosinofila, ma possono essere distinte in base a distribuzione, tipo istologico e cronicità.

MELANOSI PUSTOLOSA TRANSITORIA NEONATALE. La melanosi pustolosa, più comune tra i bambini neri che tra i bianchi, è una dermatosi transitoria, benigna, autolimitata, di eziologia sconosciuta, caratterizzata da 3 tipi di lesioni: (1) pustole superficiali evanescenti; (2) pustole lacerate con un collaretto di squame fini, a volte con una macula centrale iperpigmentata; e (3) macule iperpigmentate (Fig. 646-4). Le lesioni sono presenti alla nascita e uno o tutti i tipi possono essere riscontrati con una distribuzione profusa o rada. Le pustole rappresentano la fase iniziale della malattia e le macule quella tardiva. Raramente la fase pustolosa dura più di 2-3 giorni, mentre le macule iperpigmentate possono persistere fino a 3 mesi. I siti prediletti sono la regione anteriore del collo, la fronte e la regione lombare, ma possono essere colpiti anche il cuoio capelluto, il tronco, gli arti, i palmi delle mani e le piante dei piedi.

La fase attiva mostra una pustola intracorneale o sottocorneale piena di **leucociti polimorfonuclati**, detriti e qualche eosinofilo. Le macule sono caratterizzate solo da un'accentuata melanizzazione delle cellule epidermiche. Per distinguere queste pustole da quelle dell'eritema tossico e del pioderma è possibile usare colture e strisci in quanto esse non contengono batteri o aggregati densi di eosinofili. Non occorre terapia.

ACROPUSTOLOSI INFANTILE. L'acropustolosi infantile generalmente si presenta a 2-10 mesi di età; a volte le lesioni vengono notate alla nascita. I soggetti di sesso maschile e razza nera hanno una predisposizione ma possono essere colpiti i neonati di entrambi i sessi e di tutte le razze. La causa è sconosciuta.

Inizialmente le lesioni sono papule eritematose discrete che diventano vescicolopustolose entro 24 ore e successivamente formano una crosta prima di guarire. Causano un intenso prurito e in genere l'eruzione recente è accompagnata da agitazione e irritabilità. Le sedi predilette sono i palmi delle mani e le piante e i lati dei piedi, dove le lesioni possono svilupparsi in abbondanza. Un'eruzione meno densa può essere osservata sul dorso di mani e piedi, caviglie e polsi. Talvolta le pustole si presentano anche in altre parti del corpo. Ogni episodio dura da 7 a 14 giorni, durante i quali le pustole continuano ad apparire a gruppi. Dopo una remissione di 2-4 settimane, segue una nuova eruzione. Questo modello ciclico continua per circa 2 anni; la risoluzione permanente è spesso preceduta da intervalli di remissione più lunghi tra i periodi di attività. Per il resto, i neonati con acropustolosi stanno bene.

Gli strisci del contenuto intralesionale sottoposti a colorazione di Wright mostrano abbondanza di neutrofili oppure, occasionalmente, una predominanza di eosinofili. All'analisi istologica si notano pustole neutrofile, sottocorneali, ben circoscritte, con o senza eosinofili.

Nei neonati, la **diagnosi differenziale** include melanosi pustolosa neonatale transitoria, eritema tossico, milio, candidosi cutanea e pustolosi stafilococcica. Nei lattanti e nei bambini fino ai 4-5 anni di età tra le considerazioni diagnostiche occorre includere la scabbia (e una storia di precedente infezione da scabbia è comune), eczema disidrosico, psoriasi pustolosa, dermatosi pustolosa subcornea e malattia mano-piede-bocca. Nei casi equivoci si raccomanda di eseguire un trial terapeutico con uno scabicida.

La **terapia** è volta a ridurre al minimo il disagio per i bambini. I preparati corticosteroidei a uso topico e gli antistaminici orali riducono il prurito e l'irritabilità del bambino. Il dapsone 2 mg/kg/24 h assunto per bocca due volte al giorno si è dimostrato efficace ma presenta effetti collaterali potenzialmente gravi – in particolare anemia emolitica e metemoglobinemia – e dovrebbe essere usato con cautela.

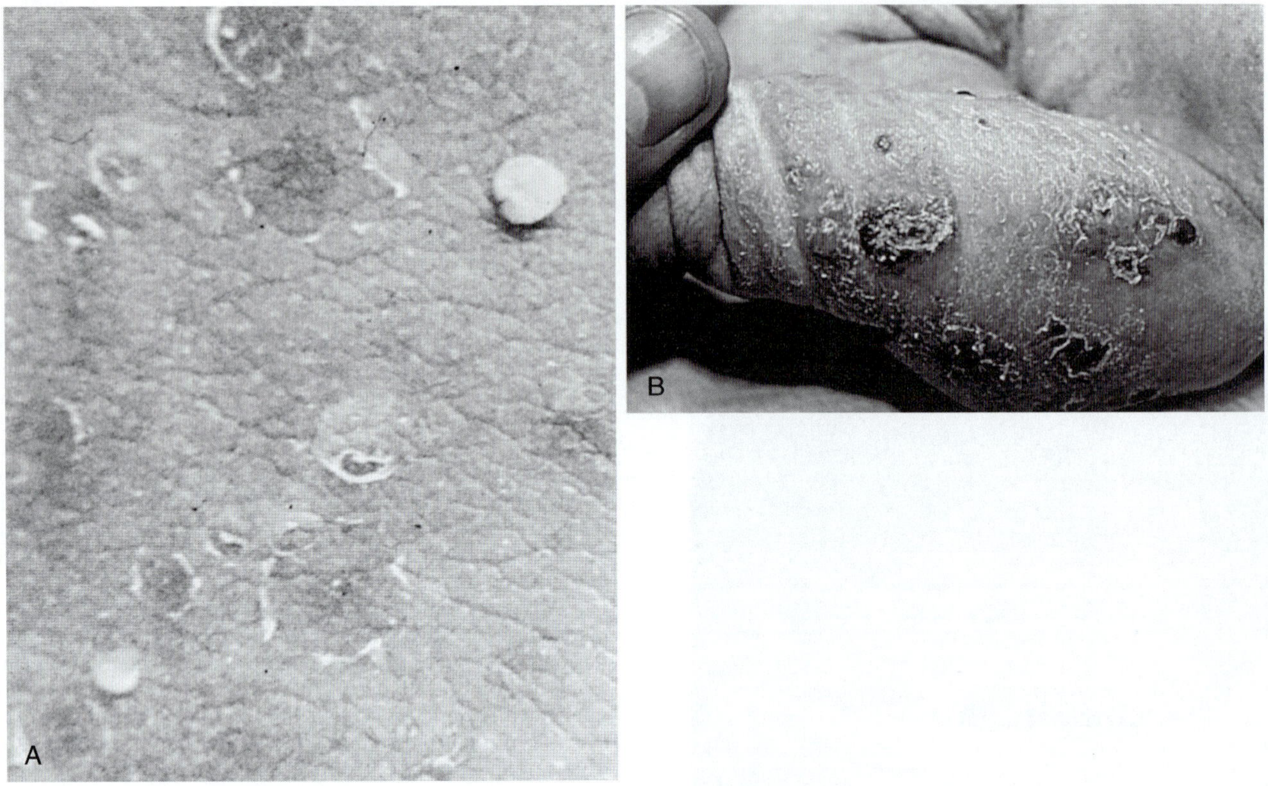

Figura 646-4. *A* e *B*, Melanosi pustolosa neonatale transitoria con pustole, anelli squamosi e macule iperpigmentate.

FOLLICOLITE PUSTOLOSA EOSINOFILA. Viene descritta come un gruppo ricorrente di papulopustole follicolari, pruriginose, coalescenti su viso, tronco e arti. Il cinquanta per cento dei pazienti presenta eosinofilia periferica superiore al 5% e circa 1/3 (32%) mostra leucocitosi (>10 000/mm^3).

Tra tutti i casi, quelli riguardanti i neonati sono <10%. L'aspetto clinico e istologico di questa malattia nei neonati assomiglia fortemente a quello degli adulti immunocompententi, a parte eccezioni minori. Nei neonati, le lesioni sono più evidenti sul cuoio capelluto, benché si presentino anche sul tronco e sugli arti e talvolta sui palmi delle mani e sulle piante dei piedi. L'aspetto anulare e policiclico classico con ingrossamento centrifugo non si osserva nei neonati. Gli adulti presentano un infiltrato eosinofilo che invade le ghiandole sebacee e la guaina della radice esterna dei follicoli piliferi, spesso con conseguente spongiosi nella guaina della radice esterna. Nella maggior parte dei neonati, tuttavia, l'infiltrato eosinofilo è perifollicolare, senza spongiosi nella guaina della radice esterna. Date le osservazioni cliniche e il decorso leggermente differenti negli adulti immunocompetenti rispetto ai neonati o ai pazienti con AIDS, è stato proposto di **sottoclassificare** la follicolite pustolosa eosinofila (FPE) in una forma classica, una correlata a virus dell'immunodeficienza umana e una infantile. La **diagnosi differenziale** include eritema tossico del neonato, acropustolosi infantile, psoriasi pustolosa localizzata, follicolite pustolosa e melanosi pustolosa neonatale transitoria.

La patogenesi della FPE è epidemiologicamente collegata all'attività delle ghiandole sebacee, in quanto le lesioni si manifestano con la massima frequenza in associazione ai follicoli piliferi nelle aree con un'elevata densità di ghiandole sebacee. La maggior parte delle teorie sostiene la partecipazione di meccanismi immunologici nell'eziologia delle lesioni. I fattori eziologici proposti per l'FPE includono un metabolita generato dalla ciclo-ossigenasi con proprietà chemiotattiche, una risposta esagerata ai saprofiti e ai dermatofiti della cute che conduce a infiltrazione eosinofila e distruzione del follicolo; oppure autoanticorpi diretti contro la sostanza intercellulare dell'epidermide inferiore o il citoplasma delle cellule basali dell'epidermide e la guaina esterna dei follicoli piliferi.

La risposta della FPE alla terapia è variabile; non esiste un trattamento specifico che rappresenti la terapia di elezione. Gli antimicrobici e gli shampoo medicati si sono rivelati inefficaci; i corticosteroidi topici a potenza media sono moderatamente efficaci nel trattamento delle lesioni sul cuoio capelluto dei neonati (vedi Tab. 645-1).

Alper JC, Holmes LB: The incidence and significance of birthmarks in a cohort of 4,641 newborns. *Pediatr Dermatol* 1983;1:58–68.
Jacobs AH, Walton RG: The incidence of birthmarks in the neonate. *Pediatrics* 1976;58:218–222.
Leung AK, Kao CP, Lee TK: Mongolian spots with involvement of the temporal area. *Int J Dermatol* 2001;40:288–289.
Marchini G, Stabi B, Kankes K, et al: AQP1 and AQP3, psoriasin and nitric oxide synthases 1–3 are inflammatory mediators in erythema toxicum neonatorum. *Pediatr Dermatol* 2003;20:377–384.

Capitolo 647 ■ Difetti cutanei

Joseph G. Morelli

FOSSETTE. Depressioni cutanee sulle prominenze ossee e nell'area sacrale, a volte associate a fossette e solchi, possono presentarsi nei bambini normali o in quelli con sindromi dismorfologiche. Le fossette possono svilupparsi in utero in seguito all'interposizione di tessuto tra una prominenza ossea marcata e la parete uterina, con conseguente minore formazione di tessuto sottocutaneo. Un'anomalia autosomica dominante benigna rara si presenta con fossette bilaterali in prossimità dell'acromion, in associazione a delezione del braccio lungo del cromosoma 18. Le fossette tendono a presentarsi sulla rotula nella rosolia congenita, sugli aspetti laterali delle ginocchia e dei gomiti nella sindrome da deficit della muscolatura addominale (*prune-belly syndrome*), sulla superficie pretibiale nei soggetti affetti da nanismo camptomelico e a forma di H sul mento in caso della sindrome di Freeman-Sheldon (*whistling-face syndrome*).

Le fossette sacrali sono comuni e possono presentarsi come manifestazione isolata o nel contesto di sindromi multiple, tra cui la sindrome di Bloom, la sindrome di Smith-Lemli-Opitz, la sindrome da delezione 4p, la spina bifida occulta e la diastematomielia. Le dimensioni elevate (>5 mm), una distanza aumentata dall'ano (>2,5 cm) o l'associazione a una massa o ad altre stigmate cutanee (peli, aplasia cutis, emangioma) devono far aumentare il sospetto di un sottostante **disrafismo spinale**. Le lesioni piccole si possono associare a seno dermico sottostante, ma non ad aumento di disrafismo spinale occulto. L'ecografia durante i primi tre mesi di vita, prima che avvenga l'ossificazione degli elementi posteriori della regione inferiore della colonna vertebrale, può costituire un metodo economicamente conveniente e non invasivo per valutare eventuali anomalie spinali lombosacrali associate.

CUTE SOVRABBONDANTE. Le pliche flaccide della cute devono essere distinte dai difetti congeniti del tessuto elastico o del collagene come la cutix laxa, la sindrome di Ehlers-Danlos o lo pseudoxanthoma elasticum. La cute sovrabbondante sulla regione posteriore del collo è comune nelle sindromi di Turner, Noonan, Down e Klippel-Feil nonché nella monosomia 1p36; pliche più generalizzate della cute si presentano nei neonati con trisomia 18 e nel nanismo disarmonico.

BRIGLIE AMNIOTICHE COSTRITTIVE. Le briglie costrittive parziali o complete causano difetti agli arti e alle dita e si riscontrano in 1/10 000-1/45 000 neonati altrimenti sani. Queste briglie tissutali sono causate prevalentemente dalla rottura del sacco amniotico, con conseguente imbrigliamento di parti fetali, in particolare gli arti, in bande amniotiche fibrotiche indurite. Questo evento è probabilmente sporadico e presenta un rischio di recidiva trascurabile. La formazione di briglie costrittive è associata a trauma addominale, amniocentesi e difetti ereditari del collagene come la sindrome di Ehlers-Danlos o l'osteogenesi imperfetta.

Le briglie adesive interessano l'area craniofacciale e sono associate a difetti gravi quali encefalocele e schisi facciale; derivano da un'estesa fusione tra parti fetali turbate e una membrana amniotica intatta. I difetti craniofacciali non sembrano essere causati da briglie amniotiche ma sono il risultato di una sequenza di scissione vascolare con o senza adesione cefaloamniotica (vedi Capitolo 108).

Il **limb-body wall complex** (LBWC) richiede una scissione vascolare in una fase precoce dello sviluppo che coinvolga numerose strutture embrionali; include almeno due delle seguenti tre caratteristiche: esencefalia o encefalocele con schisi facciale, toracoschisi e/o addominoschisi e difetti a carico degli arti. La rottura amniotica può essere la causa di scissione vascolare embrionale, con conseguente LBWC; tuttavia, è stata riferita LBWC anche in assenza di rottura amniotica.

SENI E DEPRESSIONI PREAURICOLARI. La presenza di depressioni e seni nella regione anteriore al padiglione auricolare può essere il risultato della fusione imperfetta dei tubercoli del primo e del secondo arco branchiale. Queste anomalie possono essere unilaterali o bilaterali e possono essere familiari, sono più comuni nelle bambine e nella razza nera e talvolta si associano ad altre anomalie delle orecchie e del viso. Depressioni preauricolari si osservano nella displasia **branchio-otorenale** (gene EYA-1), una malattia autosomica dominante che consiste in malformazioni dell'orecchio esterno, fistole branchiali, perdita dell'udito e anomalie renali. Quando i tratti fistolosi divengono cronicamente infetti, si possono formare cisti da ritenzione che possono drenare in maniera intermittente; queste lesioni possono richiedere l'escissione.

TRAGHI ACCESSORI. Un trago accessorio si presenta tipicamente come una singola papula peduncolata color carne nella regione preauricolare anteriore al trago. Meno comunemente, i traghi accessori sono multipli o bilaterali e possono essere situati nell'area preauricolare, sulla guancia lungo la linea della mandibola (Fig. 647-1) o sulla parte laterale del collo anteriormente al muscolo sternocleidomastoideo. Contrariamente al resto del padiglione auricolare, che si sviluppa dal secondo arco branchiale, il trago e i traghi accessori derivano dal primo arco branchiale. I traghi accessori possono presentarsi come difetti isolati oppure far parte delle sindromi cromosomiche del primo arco branchiale che includono anomalie delle orecchie e del volto come cheiloschisi, palatoschisi e ipoplasia mandibolare. Un trago accessorio è sempre presente nella **sindrome oculoauricolovertebrale** (sindrome di Goldenhar). È appropriata l'escissione chirurgica.

SCHISI BRANCHIALE, CISTI E SENI DEL DOTTO TIREOGLOSSO. Cisti e seni sul collo possono formarsi lungo 1ª, 2ª, 3ª o 4ª schisi branchiale in seguito a una chiusura inadeguata durante la vita embrionale. Le cisti della 2ª fessura branchiale sono le più comuni. Le lesioni possono essere unilaterali o bilaterali (2-3%) e possono aprirsi sulla superficie cutanea o drenare nella faringe. La presenza di infezione secondaria è un'indicazione alla terapia antibiotica sistemica. Queste anomalie possono essere ereditate come tratti autosomici dominanti.

Le fistole e le cisti tireoglosse sono difetti simili situati vicino o sulla linea mediana del collo; possono estendersi alla base della lingua. Un segno patognomonico è il movimento verticale della massa durante la deglutizione e la protrusione della lingua. In circa la metà dei bambini interessati, si presenta sotto forma di massa infetta nella regione superiore del collo, a livello della linea mediana. Le cisti alla base della lingua possono essere distinte da una tiroide linguale non discesa mediante scintigrafia. Contrariamente alle cisti branchiali, una cisti del dotto tireoglosso si presenta spesso in seguito a un'infezione del tratto respiratorio superiore (vedi Capitolo 564).

CAPEZZOLI SOVRANNUMERARI. I capezzoli accessori solitari o multipli possono avere una distribuzione unilaterale o bilaterale lungo una linea che corre dalla plica ascellare anteriore all'area inguinale. Sono più frequenti nei bambini neri (3,5%) che nei bianchi (0,6%). I capezzoli accessori possono essere dotati o meno di areola e si possono confondere con nevi congeniti. Vengono asportati per ragioni estetiche. Raramente subiscono degenerazione maligna. Nei bambini con capezzoli sovrannumerari possono verificarsi anche anomalie renali o del tratto urinario e anomalie ematologiche (vedi Capitolo 551).

APLASIA CUTIS CONGENITA (ASSENZA CONGENITA DELLA CUTE). L'assenza congenita della cute si riscontra solitamente sul cuoio capelluto sotto forma di ulcere multiple o solitarie (70%), non infiammatorie, ben demarcate, ovali o circolari, con dimensioni di 1-2 cm. L'aspetto delle lesioni varia in base al momento

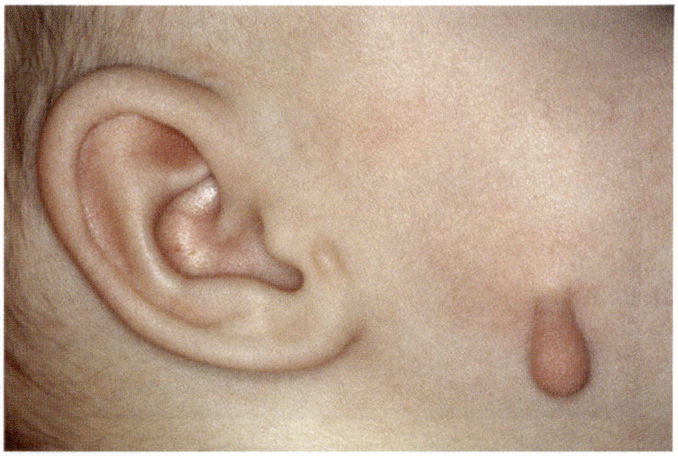

Figura 647-1. Trago accessorio sulla guancia lungo la linea mascellare.

di insorgenza durante lo sviluppo intrauterino. Quelle che si formano all'inizio della gestazione possono guarire prima del parto e assumere l'aspetto di una cicatrice atrofica, fibrotica, con alopecia associata, mentre i difetti più recenti possono presentarsi come ulcere. Il più delle volte, le lesioni si presentano sul vertice in posizione immediatamente laterale alla linea mediana, ma difetti simili possono manifestarsi anche sul viso, sul tronco e sugli arti, dove spesso sono simmetrici. La profondità delle ulcere varia. Possono essere coinvolti l'epidermide e il derma superiore con formazione di una cicatrice minima e perdita dei peli oppure il difetto può estendersi al derma profondo, al tessuto cutaneo e, raramente, al periostio, al cranio e alla dura madre. Le lesioni possono essere circondate da un colletto di peli (Fig. 647-2).

Non esiste una teoria unica che spieghi tutte le lesioni dell'aplasia cutis congenita. La diagnosi viene formulata sulla base delle osservazioni fisiche indicative di alterazione, in utero, dello sviluppo cutaneo. Le lesioni, che sono talvolta attribuite per errore agli elettrodi applicati sul cuoio capelluto o a trauma ostetrico, sembrano invece essere dovute a vari fattori, tra cui fattori genetici, teratogeni, compromissione della vascolarizzazione della cute e trauma.

Sebbene la maggior parte degli individui con aplasia cutis congenita non presenti altre anomalie, queste lesioni possono essere associate ad anomalie fisiche isolate o a sindromi malformative, tra cui le sindromi di Opitz, Adams-Oliver e oculocerebrocutanee, di Johanson-Blizzard, da microdelezione 4p e X-p22, trisomia 13-15 e difetti dei cromosomi 16-18. L'aplasia cutis congenita può essere riscontrata in associazione a una malformazione embrionale manifesta o sottostante, come il meningomielocele, la gastroschisi, l'omfalocele o il disrafismo spinale. L'aplasia cutis congenita associata a *fetus papyraceus* (mummificazione del feto) sembra essere dovuta a eventi ischemici o trombotici a carico della placenta e del feto. La formazione di vescicole, la fragilità cutanea e/o l'assenza o la deformità delle unghie associate ad aplasia cutis congenita costituiscono segni evidenti di **epidermolisi bollosa**. L'aplasia cutis può essere confusa con una lesione traumatica della cute causata da dispositivi di monitoraggio e con le chiazze atrofiche spontanee (anetoderma) della prematurità.

Le complicazioni principali sono emorragia, infezione locale secondaria e meningite. Se il difetto è piccolo, la guarigione si verifica senza conseguenze rilevanti, con una riepitelializzazione graduale e formazione di una cicatrice atrofica glabra nell'arco di diverse settimane. I difetti ossei di piccole dimensioni in genere si chiudono spontaneamente nel primo anno di vita. Difetti del cuoio capelluto ampi o numerosi possono richiedere l'escissione. I difetti localizzati sul tronco e sugli arti, anche quando di grandi dimensioni, in genere riepitelizzano e formano cicatrici atrofiche, che possono essere ritoccate in seguito.

DISPLASIA ECTODERMICA FACCIALE FOCALE (APLASIA CUTIS CONGENITA BITEMPORALE, DISPLASIA ECTODERMICA DEL VOLTO). Questa malattia rara è caratterizzata da lesioni atrofiche congenite simili a cicatrici, localizzate sulle tempie. La sudorazione è assente sui difetti, il terzo laterale delle sopracciglia è rado e sulla fronte sono presenti rughe verticali lineari. Sono state documentate un'ereditarietà autosomica dominante e una autosomica recessiva; entrambi i sottogruppi di pazienti non presentano anomalie facciali associate. I pazienti con **sindrome di Setleis** presentano cicatrici bitemporali associate a facies leonina, anomalie del ponte nasale e attaccatura dei capelli frontale bassa. Lo sviluppo e la crescita sono normali.

IPOPLASIA DERMICA FOCALE (SINDROME DI GOLTZ). Questa rara malattia congenita mesoectodermica ed ectodermica è caratterizzata da displasia del tessuto connettivo della cute e dello scheletro. Si presenta con numerosi papillomi molli iperpigmentati. Altre manifestazioni cutanee includono lesioni atrofiche lineari; ipopigmentazione e iperpigmentazione reticolate; teleangiectasie; assenza congenita di cute; angiofibromi che si presentano come escrescenze verrucose; papillomi di labbra, lingua, regione periorale, vulva, ano e aree inguinale, ascellare e periombelicale. L'alopecia parziale, i disturbi della sudorazione e le unghie distrofiche sono ulteriori anomalie ectodermiche meno comuni. I difetti scheletrici più frequenti includono sindattilia, clinodattilia, polidattilia e scoliosi. L'**osteopatia striata** è caratterizzata da sottili strie verticali parallele osservate ai raggi X nelle metafisi delle ossa lunghe; queste strie sono fortemente caratteristiche di ipoplasia dermica focale ma non sono patognomoniche. Caratteristiche sono anche molte anomalie oculari, le più comuni delle quali sono i colobomi, lo strabismo, il nistagmo, la microftalmia. Una statura ridotta, difetti dentali, anomalie dei tessuti molli e modelli dermatoglifici peculiari sono altri tratti comuni. Occasionalmente si presenta deficit mentale.

Il 90% dei casi si riscontra nelle bambine e ciò suggerisce un gene dominante legato al cromosoma X, letale nei bambini emizigoti. Il difetto primario può essere dovuto a deficit del collagene causato da un difetto fibroblastico.

DISCHERATOSI CONGENITA (SINDROME DI ZINSSER-ENGMAN-COLE). Questa rara sindrome familiare è classicamente costituita dalla triade comprendente iperpigmentazione reticolata della cute (Fig. 647-3), unghie distrofiche e leucoplachia delle membrane mucose in associazione ad anomalie immunologiche ed ematologiche. I pazienti con discheratosi congenita mostrano inoltre segni di invecchiamento prematuro e un rischio aumentato di sviluppare una neoplasia, in particolare a cellule squamose. La discheratosi congenita può essere recessiva legata al cromosoma X (gene DKC-1), autosomica dominante (gene hTERC) o autosomica recessiva causata da geni non ancora definiti. L'esordio

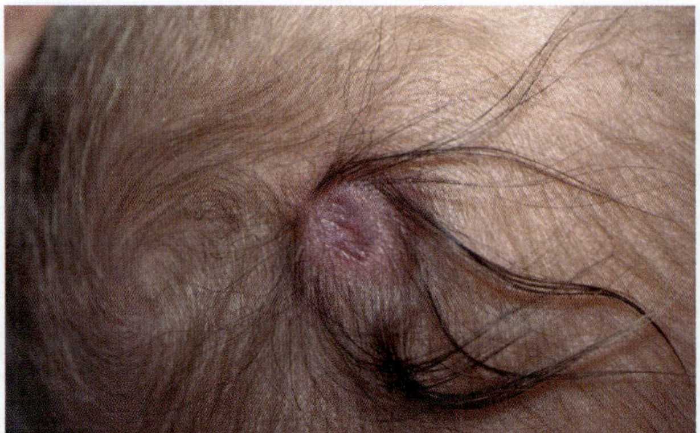

Figura 647-2. Lesione solitaria del vertice del cuoio capelluto causata da aplasia cutis congenita con colletto di capelli.

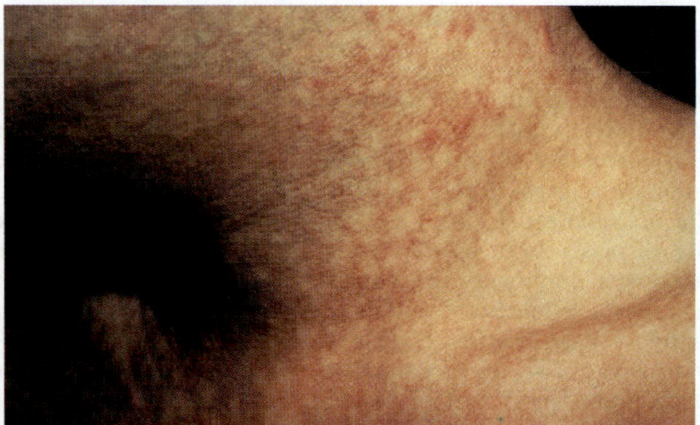

Figura 647-3. Depigmentazione reticolata sul collo del paziente con discheratosi congenita.

avviene nell'infanzia, in genere sotto forma di **distrofia ungueale**. Le unghie diventano atrofiche e corrugate longitudinalmente con progressione a pterigio e perdita completa dell'unghia. In genere, le alterazioni cutanee si manifestano dopo la comparsa di quelle ungueali e sono costituite da pigmentazione reticolata grigio-bruna, atrofia e teleangiectasia, in particolare su collo, faccia e torace. Ulteriori caratteristiche sono iperidrosi e ipercheratosi dei palmi delle mani e delle piante dei piedi, capelli radi e facile formazione di vescicole su mani e piedi. La blefarite, l'ectropion e l'eccessiva lacrimazione derivante da atresia dei dotti lacrimali sono manifestazioni occasionali. La leucocheratosi orale può dare origine a un carcinoma a cellule squamose. Possono essere interessate altre membrane mucose tra cui quelle congiuntivale, uretrale e genitale. Infezione, comparsa di neoplasie maligne e insufficienza midollare sono comuni e il decesso prima dei 40 anni è tipico.

CUTIS VERTICIS GYRATA (CIRCONVOLUZIONI LINEARI DELLA NUCA). Questa insolita alterazione del cuoio capelluto, più comune nei soggetti di sesso maschile, può essere presente sin dalla nascita oppure svilupparsi durante l'adolescenza. Il cuoio capelluto è caratterizzato da pliche elevate circonvolute, con uno spessore di 1-2 cm, di solito sull'asse fronto-occipitale. Contrariamente alla cute lassa delle altre malattie, le circonvoluzioni in genere non vengono appiattite con la trazione. La cutis gyrata primitiva può essere associata a ritardo mentale e si riscontra nella pachidermoperiostosi. La cutis gyrata secondaria può essere dovuta a malattie infiammatorie croniche, tumori, nevi e acromegalia.

Brousseau VJ, Solares CA, Xu M, et al: Thyroglossal duct cysts: Presentation and management in children versus adults. *Int J Pediatr Otorhinolaryngol* 2003;67:1285–1290.

Brown J, Schwartz RA: Supernumerary nipples: An overview. *Cutis* 2003;71:344–346.

Henriques JG, Pianetti G, Henriques KS, et al: Minor skin lesions as markers of occult spinal dysraphisms—prospective study. *Surg Neurol* 2005;63:S8–S12.

Marrone A, Dokai I: Dyskeratosis congenital: Molecular insights into telomerase function, aging and cancer. *Expert Rev Mol Med* 2004;20:1–23.

Miller TD, Metry D: Multiple accessory tragi as a clue to the diagnosis of the oculo-auriculo-vertebral (Goldenhar) syndrome. *J Am Acad Dermatol* 2004;50:S11–S13.

Scheinfeld NS, Silverberg NB, Weinberg JM, et al: The preauricular sinus: A review of its clinical presentation, treatment, and associations. *Pediatr Dermatol* 2004;21:191–196.

Werler MM, Louik C, Mitchell AA: Epidemiologic analysis of maternal factors and amniotic band defects. *Birth Defects Res A Clin Mol Teratol* 2003;67:68–72.

Capitolo 648 ■ Displasie ectodermiche

Joseph G. Morelli

Le displasie ectodermiche (ED, *Ectodermic Dysplasia*) rappresentano un gruppo eterogeneo di malattie caratterizzate da una costellazione di difetti, che colpiscono due o più delle seguenti strutture: denti, cute e annessi compresi peli, unghie, ghiandole eccrine e sebacee. Sono state descritte 170 displasie ectodermiche, ma la maggior parte di esse è rara e solo 30 sono state definite geneticamente.

DISPLASIA ECTODERMICA ANIDROTICA (IPOIDROTICA) Questa sindrome si manifesta con una triade di difetti: assenza parziale o completa delle ghiandole sudoripare, dentizione anomala e ipotricosi. Attualmente esistono 4 tipi riconosciuti di displasia ectodermica anidrotica (Tab. 648-1).

TABELLA 648-1. I quattro tipi di displasia ectodermica anidrotica noti

DISPLASIA ECTODERMICA ANIDROTICA	EREDITARIETÀ	DIFETTO GENETICO
ED-1	Recessiva legata al cromosoma X	Ectodisplasina A (EDA)
ED-anidrotica (DEAR)	Autosomica recessiva	Recettore anidrotico dell'ectodisplasina A
(DEARADD)		Gene death EDAR-associato
ED-3 (DEAR)	Autosomica dominante	Recettore anidrotico dell'ectodisplasina A
ED-anidrotica con immunodeficienza	Recessiva legata al cromosoma X	IKK-gamma (NEMO)

Nella ED-1, i soggetti maschi colpiti non sudano e possono sperimentare episodi di febbre alta negli ambienti caldi, che talvolta vengono erroneamente interpretati come febbre di origine sconosciuta. Questo si verifica soprattutto nell'infanzia, quando le alterazioni facciali sono difficili da apprezzare. A volte la diagnosi può essere formulata utilizzando il test amido-iodio, palmare, o una biopsia del cuoio capelluto. La biopsia del cuoio capelluto è la più sensibile e ha una specificità del 100%. La facies tipica è caratterizzata da prominenza della regione frontale, ipoplasia malare, ponte nasale appianato, columella rientrata, labbra spesse ed estroflesse, cute periorbitale iperpigmentata e orecchie prominenti con l'attaccatura bassa (vedi Fig. 648-1). La cute sull'intera

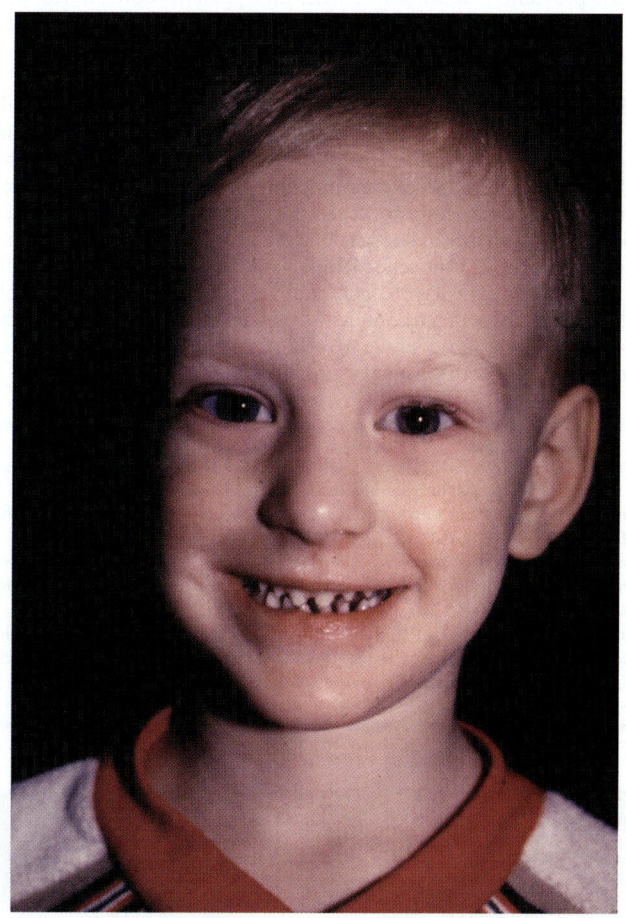

Figura 648-1. La displasia ectodermica ipoidrotica è caratterizzata da orecchie appuntite, peli sottili, iperpigmentazione periorbitale, ipoplasia mediofacciale e denti conici. (Per gentile concessione dell'archivio didattico Fitzsimons Army Medical Center.)

superficie del corpo appare secca, percorsa da rughe sottili e ipopigmentata, spesso con un pattern venoso prominente. Una desquamazione cutanea estesa costituisce un'indicazione clinica per la diagnosi nel periodo neonatale. La scarsità di ghiandole sebacee può spiegare la secchezza della cute. I capelli sono radi, sottili e scarsamente pigmentati; le sopracciglia e le ciglia rade o assenti. Anche gli altri peli del corpo sono radi o assenti. La crescita dei peli sessuali è normale. L'anodonzia o ipodonzia con denti molto spaziati e conici è un tratto costante (vedi Fig. 648-1). Si osservano anomalie otorinolaringoiatriche e oftalmologiche secondarie alla ridotta produzione di saliva e lacrime. L'incidenza delle malattie atopiche in questi bambini è elevata. Il reflusso gastroesofageo è comune e può esercitare un ruolo nella mancata crescita, che si osserva nel 20% dei casi. In genere, lo sviluppo sessuale è normale. Storicamente, si è registrato un tasso di mortalità infantile del 30%. Le bambine colpite da questa patologia presentano manifestazioni cliniche assenti o minime.

Le osservazioni cliniche nella displasia ectodermica anidrotica autosomica recessiva sono identiche alla forma recessiva legata al cromosoma X, tranne per il fatto che le bambine sono interessate tanto quanto i soggetti di sesso maschile. Nella forma autosomica dominante, gli aspetti clinici si rilevano in entrambi i sessi e sono simili alla forma recessiva legata al cromosoma X, ma molto più lievi. La displasia ectodermica ipoidrotica con deficit immunitario mostra riscontri simili sia per quanto concerne la sudorazione sia in merito allo sviluppo di peli e unghie, in associazione a **disgammaglobulinemia**. Si registra una mortalità significativa causata da infezioni ricorrenti.

La **terapia** per questi bambini include la protezione dall'esposizione a temperature ambientali elevate. È necessaria una valutazione precoce dei denti in modo da approntare protesi cosmetiche e per consentire una nutrizione adeguata. L'uso di lacrime artificiali previene i danni alla cornea nei pazienti con difetto della lacrimazione. L'alopecia può imporre l'uso di una parrucca per migliorare l'aspetto.

DISPLASIA ECTODERMICA IDROTICA (SINDROME DI CLOUSTON). I tratti salienti di questa malattia autosomica dominante sono unghie distrofiche, ipoplasiche o assenti, capelli radi e ipercheratosi palmare e plantare. Sono comuni congiuntivite e blefarite. La dentizione e la sudorazione sono sempre normali. In alcuni soggetti è stata notata assenza di sopracciglia e ciglia e iperpigmentazione su ginocchia, gomiti e nocche. Responsabili di questa malattia sono mutazioni del gene GJB6, che codifica per la proteina coinvolta nella formazione della connessina 30 delle gap junction. È stata descritta una malattia simile associata a sordità con mutazioni del gene GJB2 che codifica per la proteina connessina 26.

Carrol ED, Gennery AR, Flood TJ, et al: Anhidrotic ectodermal dysplasia and immunodeficiency: The role of NEMO. *Arch Dis Child* 2003;88:340–341.

Lamartine J: Toward a new classification of ectodermal dysplasias. *Clin Exp Dermatol* 2003;28:351–355.

Rousse C, Siegfried E, Breer W, et al: Hair and sweat glands in families with hypohidrotic ectodermal dysplasia: Further characterization. *Arch Dermatol* 2004;140:850–855.

Van Steensel MA, Steijlen PM, Bladergroen RS, et al: A phenotype resembling the Clouston syndrome with deafness is associated with a novel missense GJB2 mutation. *J Invest Dermatol* 2004;123:291–293.

Capitolo 649 ■ Lesioni vascolari

Joseph G. Morelli

Le lesioni vascolari infantili possono essere suddivise in difetti vascolari congeniti (malformazioni e tumori), alterazioni benigne acquisite e malattie genetiche. Le alterazioni a carattere familiare possono consistere in malformazioni arteriose, capillari, linfatiche e venose (Tab. 649-1).

DIFETTI VASCOLARI CONGENITI. I difetti vascolari congeniti si dividono in malformazioni presenti alla nascita e tumori, che, solitamente, si manifestano durante il primo o secondo mese di vita.

MALFORMAZIONI VASCOLARI. Le malformazioni vascolari sono causate da errori nella formazione del vaso sanguigno nel corso dello sviluppo intrauterino. Tali malformazioni non regrediscono, ma, anzi, si estendono lentamente. Esse prendono il nome dal vaso sanguigno ove si manifesta principalmente la lesione (Tab. 649-2). La Tabella 649-3 aiuta a distinguere le malformazioni vascolari dagli emangiomi puri.

MALFORMAZIONI CAPILLARI (ANGIOMA PIANO). L'angioma piano (detto anche *nevus flammeus* o "macchia di vino di porto") è congenito. Si tratta di una malformazione vascolare costituita da capillari cutanei maturi dilatati. Le lesioni sono maculari, a margini irregolari, di colore rosa-violaceo e di varie dimensioni (Fig. 649-1). Di solito esse si manifestano nella regione del capo e del collo, nella maggior parte dei casi, monolateralmente. A tali lesioni può associarsi anche l'interessamento delle membrane mucose. A mano a mano che il bambino cresce, avvicinandosi all'età adulta, l'angioma piano può assumere un colore più intenso e scuro e un aspetto a ciottolato. Si può avere, talvolta, la formazione di aree rilevate, che tendono a sanguinare spontaneamente.

È necessario distinguere gli angiomi piani puri dalle più comuni malformazioni vascolari, rappresentate dalle macchie color salmone dei neonati, le quali, al contrario, sono lesioni transitorie (vedi Capitolo 646). Nei casi in cui l'angioma piano sia localizzato nell'area trigeminale del volto (in particolare, attorno alle palpebre), va sempre considerata, ai fini di una diagnosi differenziale, la sindrome di Sturge-Weber (glaucoma, angioma venoso leptomeningeo, epilessia, emiparesi controlaterale rispetto alla lesione facciale, calcificazioni endocraniche) (vedi Capitolo 596.3). Per prevenire ulteriori danni oculari è fondamentale effettuare uno screening precoce del glaucoma. Gli angiomi piani possono anche costituire la prima manifestazione neonatale della sindrome di Klippel-Trenaunay e, più raramente, di altre sindromi, quali la sindrome di Cobb (malformazioni arterovenose spinali, angioma piano), nonché le sindromi di Proteus, di Beckwith-Wiedemann e di Bonnet-Dechaume-Blanc. In assenza di anomalie associate, la morbosità causata da tali lesioni può includere problemi estetici che si accompagnano a un'immagine di sé scadente, a ipertrofia delle strutture sottostanti e a emorragie traumatiche.

Il **trattamento** più efficace per gli angiomi piani è il laser pulsato a colori (*Pulsed Dye Laser*, PDL). Tale terapia interagisce esclusivamente con l'emoglobina, all'interno della lesione, evitando, in tal modo, che il tessuto sano circostante sia sottoposto a un danno termico. Dopo tale trattamento, la consistenza e la pigmentazione della cute restano generalmente inalterate, senza esiti cicatriziali. La terapia può essere intrapresa durante l'infanzia, quando la superficie da trattare ha una minore estensione. I risultati migliori si ottengono durante il primo anno di età. È possibile, inoltre, usare prodotti cosmetici per mascherare le lesioni.

MALFORMAZIONI VENOSE. Tra le malformazioni venose vi sono quelle con esclusivo interessamento venoso, gli angiocheratomi (venula ipercheratosica) e la cutis mormorata teleangiectasica congenita (cute marmorea teleangiectasica congenita).

Le malformazioni esclusivamente venose vanno da noduli contenenti una massa di venule (Fig. 649-2) ad anomalie venose estese e diffuse, che possono essere caratterizzate sia da una componente superficiale, che ricorda le varici, sia da malformazioni venose più profonde. Le malformazioni venose nodulari sono frequentemente confuse con gli emangiomi. Le malformazioni venose possono essere distinte in base alla loro presenza alla nascita e all'assenza sia di rapida proliferazione, sia di tendenza alla regressione. L'asportazione chirurgica è il trattamento più

TABELLA 649-1. Anomalie vascolari familiari associate a mutazioni genetiche identificate

CONDIZIONE PATOLOGICA	CROMOSOMA	GENE	FUNZIONE
Teleangiectasia emorragica ereditaria	9q3 12q	Endoglina, ALK-1	Proteine leganti il TGF-β
Malformazioni cavernose cerebrali	7q (variante ispanica) 7p 3q	KRIT 1	Via di trasduzione del segnale della RAPIA GTPasi
Tumori glomici familiari			
Paragangliomi	11q23		
Glomangioma disseminato cutaneo	1p21-22		
Linfedema familiare	5q34-q35	VEGFR3 (FLT4)	Sviluppo linfatico
Malformazione venosa familiare	9p	Tie-2	Interazione tra cellule endoteliali e cellule della muscolatura liscia
Emangioma familiare	5q33-34	VEGFR	

Da Blei F: Vascular anomalies: From bedside to bench and back again. *Curr Prob Pediatr Adolesc Health* 2002;32:67-102.

TABELLA 649-2. Malformazioni vascolari

TIPO	ESEMPI
Capillare	Macchia di vino di porto (angioma piano)
Venoso	Malformazione venosa Angiocheratoma circoscritto (venula ipercheratosica) Cutis marmorata telangiectasica congenita (flebectasia congenita)
Arterioso	Malformazione arterovenosa
Linfatico	Malformazione dei piccoli vasi linfatici (*lymphangioma circumscriptum*) Malformazione dei grandi vasi linfatici (igroma cistico)

adatto per le malformazioni vascolari nodulari superficiali. Nei casi di malformazioni venose più grandi i trattamenti risultano, nella migliore delle ipotesi, difficili o addirittura impossibili. La scleroterapia percutanea con iniezione diretta di polidocanolo in forma di microschiuma, effettuata con controllo eco-color-Doppler, è utile in molti pazienti, compresi quelli affetti da sindrome di Klippel-Trenaunay.

Angiocheratoma circoscritto. Sono state descritte diverse forme di angiocheratomi. Gli angiocheratomi, caratterizzati da ectasia dei vasi dermici superficiali e da ipercheratosi dell'epidermide soprastante, assomigliano a emangiomi piatti con una superficie verrucosa irregolare. L'angiocheratoma circoscritto è una rara lesione, solitaria o multipla, caratterizzata da una placca o da placche di papule di colore violaceo o noduli con superficie verrucosa. Tali lesioni prediligono gli arti. Qualora si voglia intervenire, la terapia di scelta è l'escissione chirurgica.

Cute marmorea teleangiectasica congenita (flebectasia congenita). Questa anomalia vascolare benigna, che si evidenzia già alla nascita, è caratterizzata da una dilatazione dei capillari superficiali e delle vene. Le aree cutanee coinvolte sono caratterizzate da un reticolo vascolare, di colore rosso o violaceo, che assomiglia alla cute marmorea fisiologica, ma che si presenta con aspetto più pronunciato e relativamente uniforme (Fig. 649-3). Le lesioni possono essere circoscritte a un singolo arto e a una porzione del

TABELLA 649-3. Principali differenze fra gli emangiomi e le malformazioni vascolari.

	EMANGIOMI	MALFORMAZIONI VASCOLARI (CAPILLARI, VENOSE, LINFATICHE, ARTERIOSE E ARTEROVENOSE PURE O COMPLESSE-COMBINATE)
Quadro clinico	Variabilità nella visibilità alla nascita Successiva rapida crescita Lenta involuzione spontanea	Di solito visibile alla nascita (le MAV possono essere quiescenti) Crescita proporzionale alla crescita cutanea (o lenta progressione); persistenza per tutta la vita
Rapporto tra i sessi F:M	Da 3:1 a 5:1 e 7:1 per i casi gravi	1:1
Reperti istopatologici	Stadio proliferativo: iperplasia delle cellule endoteliali e delle cellule positive per l'actina delle CML (*SMC-actin+cells*) Membrana basale multilaminare Maggior contenuto di mastociti in involuzione	Endotelio piatto Membrana basale sottile Spesso pareti irregolarmente attenuate (MV, ML)
Reperti radiologici	Lesione ad alta velocità di flusso dimostrabile mediante eco-doppler Massa tumorale con lacune di flusso dimostrabili con la RM Tumore lobulato dimostrabile con arteriografia	Flusso lento (MC, ML, MV) o flusso rapido (MAV) dimostrabile con Eco-doppler RM: maggior segnale in T2 quando il flusso è lento (ML, MV); lacune di flusso evidenziabili in T1 e T2 quando il flusso è rapido (MAV) L'esame arteriografico delle MAV dimostra fistole arterovenose
Alterazioni ossee	Raramente si rileva l'effetto della massa, con distorsione ma senza invasione	MV a basso flusso: distorsioni ossee, assottigliamento, iposviluppo MC a basso flusso: ipertrofia ML a basso flusso: distorsione, ipertrofia e invasione dell'osso MAV a flusso rapido: distruzione, raramente lesioni litiche estese, Malformazioni combinate (per es. a basso flusso [MCVL, sindrome di Klippel-Trenaunay] o ad flusso rapido [MCAV, sindrome di Parkes-Weber]): eccessiva crescita delle ossa degli arti, gigantismo
Esame immunoistochimico di campioni bioptici	*Emangioma proliferativo*: elevata espressione di PCNA, collagenasi di tipo IV, VEGF, urochinasi, e bFGF *Emangioma involutivo*: elevato TIMP-1, elevato bFGF	Assenza di espressione di PCNA, collagenasi tipo IV, urochinasi, VEGF, e bFGF Una forma familiare (rara) di MV legata a una mutazione genica su 9p (VMCM1)
Ematologia	Assenza di coagulopatie (la sindrome di Kasabach-Merritt è una complicanza di altri tumori vascolari dell'infanzia; per esempio, dell'emangioendotelioma kaposiforme e dell'angioma a ciuffi, con una componente di ML)	Nei casi di MV a flusso lento o ML o MLV può esservi una CIL con rischio di emorragie (CID)

MAV, malformazione arterovenosa; bFGF, fattore di crescita basale dei fibroblasti (*basic fibroblast growth factor*); MCAV, malformazione arterovenosa capillare; MCVL, malformazione venosa linfatica capillare; MC malformazione capillare/macchia di vino di porto; CID, coagulazione intravascolare disseminata; CIL, coagulopatia intravascolare localizzata; ML, malformazione linfatica; RM, risonanza magnetica; PCNA, antigene nucleare delle cellule proliferanti (*proliferating cell nuclear antigen*); CML, cellula muscolare liscia; TIMP, inibitore tessutale della metalloproteinasi (*tissue inhibitor of metalloproteinase*); VEGF, fattore di crescita dell'endotelio vascolare (*vascular endothelial growth factor*); MV, malformazione venosa.
Da Eichenfield LF, Frieden IJ, Esterly NB: *Textbook of Neonatal Dermatology*. Philadelphia, WB Saunders, 2001, p 337.

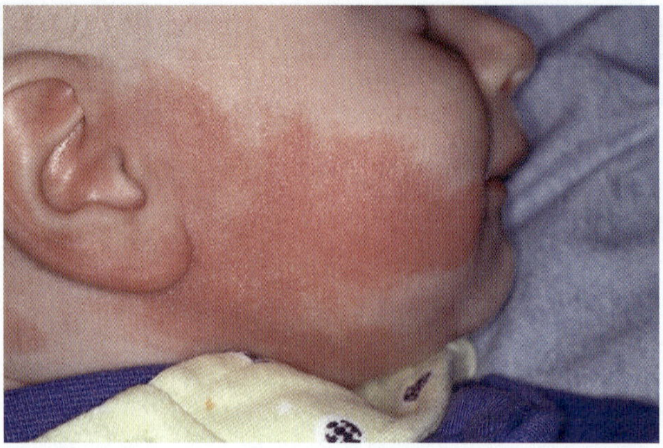

Figura 649-1. Malformazione capillare. Macula di colore rosato sulla guancia di un neonato.

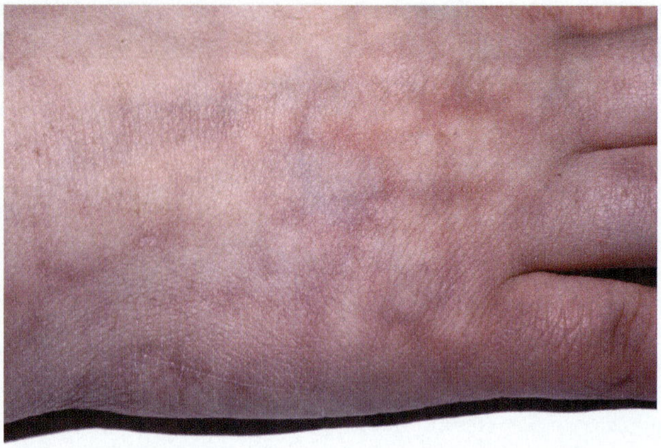

Figura 649-3. Aspetto chiazzato della cutis marmorata telangiectasica congenita, sulla mano destra.

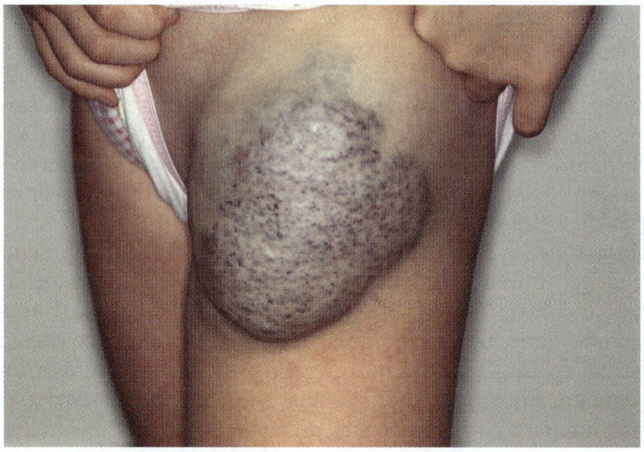

Figura 649-2. Malformazione venosa nodulare sulla gamba di un adolescente.

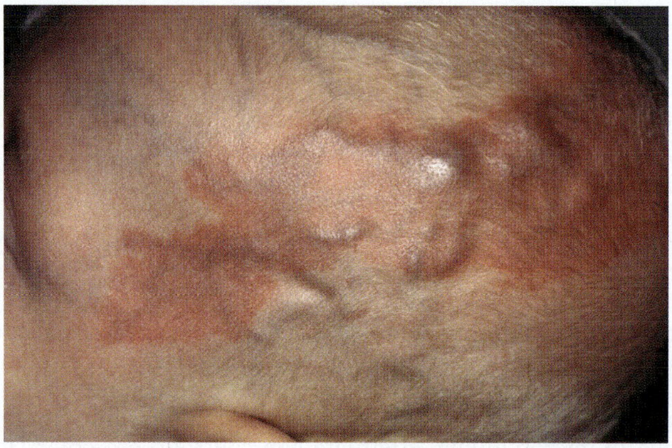

Figura 649-4. Malformazione arterovenosa (MAV) in associazione a "macchie di vino di porto" sul cuoio capelluto di un neonato.

tronco, ma possono essere anche più estese. Tale condizione morbosa può essere associata a un angioma piano. Le lesioni aumentano durante le variazioni della temperatura ambientale, l'attività fisica o il pianto. In alcuni casi, il tessuto cutaneo sottostante è iposviluppato e possono manifestarsi delle ulcere nell'ambito delle bande reticolate. Raramente può essere osservato un ritardo di sviluppo osseo, accanto ad altre anomalie congenite. Non è indicata nessuna terapia specifica. Soltanto i casi vascolari lievi possono andare incontro a un graduale miglioramento.

MALFORMAZIONI ARTEROVENOSE (MAV). Tali malformazioni sono costituite da collegamenti diretti tra arterie e vene, senza la normale interposizione di un letto capillare (Fig. 649-4). Le MAV cutanee sono rarissime. Esse sono diagnosticabili in base al rilievo dell'evidente pulsazione arteriosa. Molti medici considerano erroneamente tutte le malformazioni vascolari come MAV.

MALFORMAZIONI LINFATICHE (VEDI CAPITOLO 489).

SINDROMI DI KLIPPEL-TRENAUNAY (KT) E DI KLIPPEL-TRENAUNAY-WEBER (KTW). La sindrome di Klippel-Trenaunay consiste in una malformazione vascolare che interessa la cute e che, insieme all'ipertrofia dell'osso e dei tessuti molli e alle alterazioni venose, costituisce la triade di alterazioni di questo disturbo non ereditario (Fig. 649-5). L'anomalia, presente alla nascita, interessa, generalmente, l'arto inferiore, ma può colpire più di un arto, insieme a parti del tronco o del volto. L'ingrandimento dei tessuti molli può essere graduale e può interessare tutto l'arto, una sua porzione oppure solo alcune dita. La lesione vascolare, nella mag-

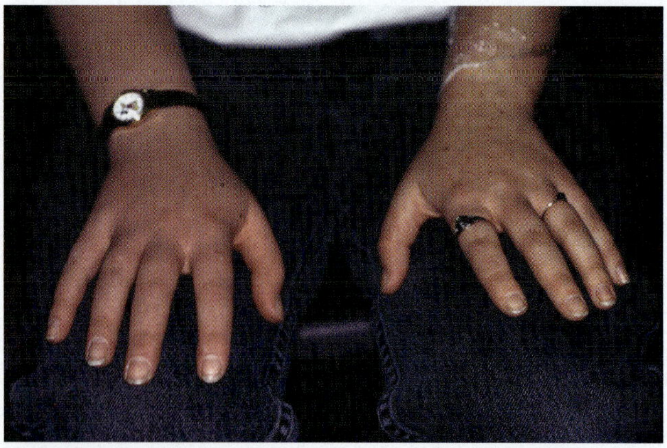

Figura 649-5. Eccessiva crescita del braccio e della mano destri in un adolescente con sindrome di Klippel-Trenaunay.

gior parte dei casi, consiste in una malformazione capillare, in genere localizzata nell'area di ipertrofia. Il sistema venoso profondo può essere assente o ipoplasico. In superficie possono essere presenti ectasie venose e/o lesioni linfatiche vescicolari. Varicosità venose, con parete spessa, divengono tipicamente evidenti, omolateralmente alla malformazione vascolare, dopo che il bambino ha incominciato a camminare. In presenza di una concomitante MAV, si parla di una KTW. Queste condizioni patologiche possono essere confuse con la sindrome di Maffucci oppure, se la lesione vascolare superficiale è minima, con la malattia di Milroy. Possono manifestarsi dolore, tumefazione dell'arto e cellulite. Rare complicanze possono essere le tromboflebiti, le lussazioni articolari, la gangrena dell'arto affetto, l'insufficienza cardiaca, l'ematuria derivante dalla presenza di angiomi nelle vie urinarie, le rettorragie da lesioni gastrointestinali, le lesioni polmonari e le malformazioni dei vasi linfatici. I reperti arteriografici, venografici, nonché quelli di TC e RM, possono delineare l'estensione dell'anomalia; nondimeno, una terapia chirurgica radicale o palliativa è spesso difficile. La scleroterapia percutanea, guidata dall'eco-color-Doppler, è utile, quando il quadro è dominato dalla componente malformativa venosa. Le indicazioni all'effettuazione di indagini radiologiche dei visceri dipendono dalla valutazione clinica. Interventi di supporto consistono in bendaggi compressivi sulle varicosità. Il trattamento chirurgico può essere d'aiuto in pazienti attentamente selezionati. Le discrepanze di lunghezza degli arti inferiori devono essere trattate con ortosi, allo scopo di prevenire lo sviluppo di deformità del rachide. Quando tali discrepanze sono rilevanti può, alla fine, essere necessario il ricorso a interventi chirurgici ossei correttivi

FACOMATOSI PIGMENTO-VASCOLARE. La facomatosi pigmento-vascolare è una rara alterazione caratterizzata dall'associazione di una malformazione capillare e da lesioni melanocitiche. Tipicamente, la malformazione capillare è estesa e le lesioni pigmentarie associate possono consistere in melanocitosi dermica (macchie mongoliche) e macchie color caffellatte, oppure manifestarsi come *nevus spilus* (nevo punteggiato lentigginoso). Le lesioni cutanee non pigmentate che possono verificarsi in questi casi sono il *nevus anemicus* e i nevi epidermici. In rari casi possono essere presenti anomalie sistemiche

NEVUS ANEMICUS. Sebbene sia presente alla nascita, il nevus anemicus può non essere rilevabile fino alla prima infanzia. La lesione consiste in macchie pallide, solitarie o numerose e nettamente delimitate, che, nella maggior parte dei casi, si presentano sul tronco, ma che possono anche essere riscontrate sul collo o sugli arti. Questi nevi, pur potendo simulare le placche di vitiligine, il leucoderma o difetti pigmentari nevoidi, possono essere facilmente distinti in base alla loro reazione all'energico strofinamento, che evoca la comparsa di una linea eritematosa e un aspetto rosso lucente nella cute normale che circonda la lesione, mentre la cute del nevus anemicus non si arrossa. La diagnosi può essere fatta anche mediante diascopia. La pressione sulla cute, effettuata mediante un vetrino, porterà a un oscuramento dei bordi della lesione. I vasi cutanei appaiano istologicamente normali, ma i vasi sanguigni all'interno del nevo non reagiscono all'iniezione di vasodilatatori. Si è ipotizzato che il pallore persistente possa dipendere da una prolungata vasocostrizione adrenergica localizzata.

TUMORI VASCOLARI. Tra i tumori vascolari figurano gli emangiomi (i più frequenti tumori in età infantile), gli angiomi a ciuffi, gli emangioendoteliomi kaposiformi, gli emangiomi congeniti a rapida involuzione (*Rapidly Involuting Congenital Hemangiomas*, RICH) e gli emangiomi congeniti non involutivi (*Non-Involuting Congenital Hemangiomas*, NICH).

Emangiomi. Gli emangiomi sono amartomi proliferativi dell'endotelio vascolare, che possono essere presenti alla nascita o che, più comunemente, si manifestano nel primo mese di vita, si ingrandiscono in modo prevedibile e, quindi, vanno incontro a involuzione spontanea. Gli emangiomi sono i più frequenti tumori dell'età infantile, in quanto si verificano nell'1-2% dei neonati e, in particolare, nel 10% dei neonati bianchi, nel corso del primo anno di vita. Gli emangiomi devono essere classificati come superficiali, profondi o misti. Non devono essere impiegati termini come "a fragola" o "cavernosi". Il marcatore immunoistochimico GLUT-1 permette di distinguere gli emangiomi dagli altri tumori vascolari dell'infanzia. Gli angiomi superficiali presentano un colorito rosso vivo, sono lesioni rilevate, comprimibili e nettamente demarcate, che possono presentarsi in qualsiasi parte del corpo (Figg. 649-6 e 649-7). Sebbene siano talora presenti alla nascita, più spesso appaiono nel primo bimestre di vita, annunciati da un'area eritematosa o bluastra, oppure pallida, che, in seguito, va incontro a una trasformazione, assumendo le caratteristiche tipiche della teleangiectasia, prima di andare incontro alla fase di espansione. La manifestazione di esordio può essere, talvolta, rappresentata da un'ulcerazione del perineo o delle labbra. Il sesso femminile è maggiormente colpito di quello maschile. Le sedi di più frequente comparsa sono il viso, il cuoio capelluto, il dorso e la parte anteriore del torace; le lesioni possono essere solitarie o multiple. Il volto può essere interessato nelle sedi frontotemporale, mascellare, mandibolare e frontonasale. Gli emangiomi situati più profondamente sono più diffusi e meno definiti rispetto agli angiomi superficiali. Le lesioni, in questi casi, sono cistiche, non mobili o comprimibili. La cute soprastante può apparire di colorito normale o bluastro (Fig. 649-8). Nella maggior parte dei casi gli emangiomi sono di tipo misto, con componente sia superficiale sia profonda. Gli emangiomi, dopo una fase di rapida espansione, seguita da un periodo stazionario, vanno infine incontro a involuzione spontanea. La regressione può essere prevista quando la lesione incomincia a presentare aree biancastre o di colorito grigio pallido, indicative di fibrosi. Il decorso di una particolare lesione è imprevedibile, ma circa il 60% di queste lesioni raggiunge la massima involuzione entro l'età di 5 anni e il 90-95% entro l'età di 9 anni. L'involuzione spontanea non è correlabile con le dimensioni o con la sede, ma sembra che le lesioni labiali

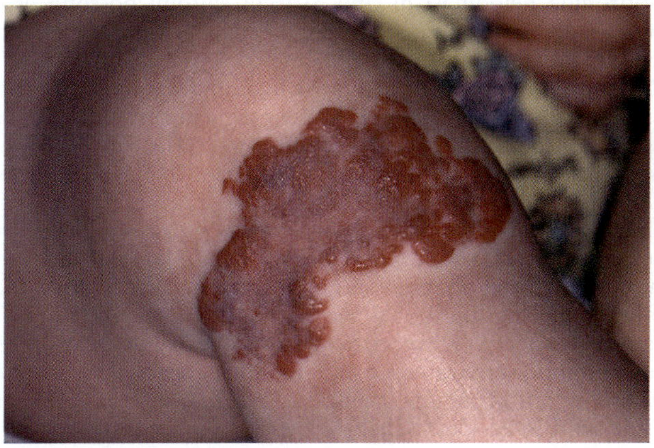

Figura 649-6. Emangioma superficiale sul ginocchio destro.

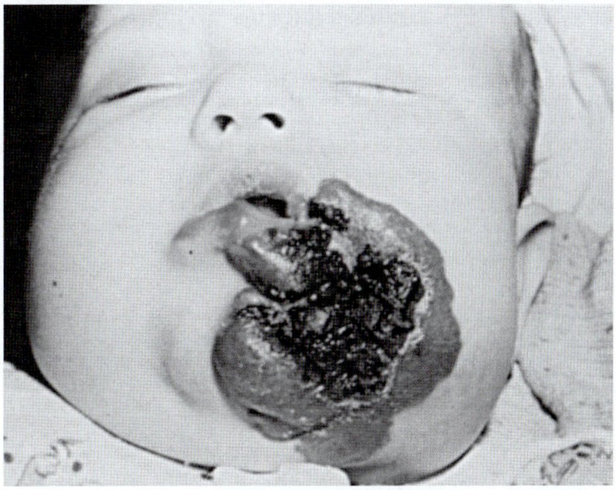

Figura 649-7. Ampio emangioma con ulcera centrale, in cui si è formata una crosta.

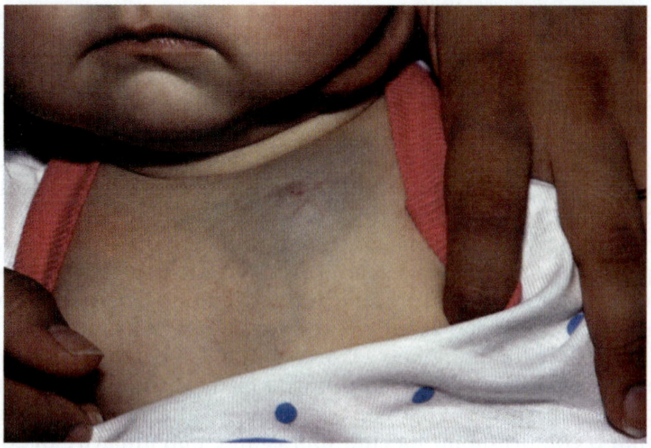

Figura 649-8. Emangioma profondo del torace.

persistano in una maggiore percentuale di casi. Tra le possibili complicanze figurano le ulcere, le infezioni secondarie e, raramente, le emorragie (Tab. 649-4). La localizzazione di una lesione può interferire con una funzione vitale (per es. con la vista, se è coinvolta la palpebra; con la minzione, se è coinvolta l'uretra). Gli emangiomi con distribuzione "a barba" possono associarsi a interessamento delle prime vie respiratorie o a interessamento subglottico. I sintomi respiratori devono far pensare a una lesione tracheobronchiale. Gli emangiomi di grandi dimensioni possono essere complicati da un coesistente ipotiroidismo, causato dalla iodotironina deiodinasi di tipo 3, i cui sintomi possono essere difficili da rilevare in questo gruppo di età. Altre caratteristiche preoccupanti sono indicate nella Tabella 649-5.

Nel paziente consueto, che non va incontro a gravi complicanze o a crescita estesa delle lesioni, con conseguente grave distruzione tessutale e aspetto sfigurato, il trattamento consiste nella semplice osservazione: poiché, infatti, quasi tutte le lesioni regrediscono spontaneamente, la terapia è raramente indicata e, anzi, può causare ulteriori danni. I pazienti hanno bisogno di interventi ripetuti di rassicurazione e di sostegno. Dopo l'involuzione spontanea, molti pazienti presentano piccoli difetti cosmetici residuali, quali teleangiectasie, ipopigmentazione, depositi fibroadiposi e cicatrici in zone in precedenza ulcerate. Le teleangiectasie residue possono essere trattate con PDL. Altri difetti possono essere risolti o ridotti al minimo mediante adeguati interventi plastici, se i pazienti lo desiderano.

TABELLA 649-4. Complicanze degli emangiomi e loro trattamento

REPERTI CLINICI	TRATTAMENTO CONSIGLIATO
Grave ulcerazione/macerazione	Consigliare un regime di lavaggi per due volte al giorno Impacchi di bicarbonato di sodio diluito Possibile impiego del laser a colori con pompaggio a lampada flash (*flashlamp-pumped-pulsed dye laser*) Possibile impiego di corticosteroidi per via orale Possibile impiego di creme al metronidazolo
Emorragia (al di fuori del KMP)	Applicazione di creme emostatiche Terapia compressiva eventualmente associata embolizzazione
Emangioma con sequele oculari	Bendaggio oculare (sotto supervisione specialistica) Somministrazione di corticosteroidi per via topica/intralesionale/orale
Emangioma subglottico	Corticosteroidi per via orale eventualmente associati a laser KTP (potassio titanil fosfato) È necessaria la tracheotomia
KMP	Corticosteroidi, acido aminocaproico, vincristina, interferone-α ed eventuale embolizzazione
Emangioma epatico ad alto flusso	Corticosteroidi o interferone eventualmente in associazione a embolizzazione

KMP, fenomeno di Kasabach-Merritt.
Da Blei F: Vascular anomalies: From bedside to bench and back again. *Curr Prob Pediatr Adolesc Health* 2002;32:67-102.

TABELLA 649-5. Elementi clinici di attenzione associati agli emangiomi

REPERTI CLINICI	VALUTAZIONE CONSIGLIATA
Emangioma facciale che interessa una parte rilevante del volto	Valutazione volta alla ricerca di una sindrome PHACES: RM per svelare un eventuale emangioma orbitario eventualmente accompagnato da malformazione della fossa posteriore Valutazione cardiologica e oculistica Valutazione volta a evidenziare anomalie della linea mediana: rafe sopraombelicale, atresia sternale, palatoschisi, anomalie tiroidee
Emangiomi cutanei con distribuzione a barba	Valutazione volta a evidenziare eventuali angiomi a livello delle vie respiratorie, specialmente in caso di stridore
Emangioma perioculare	RM dell'orbita Valutazione oculistica
Lesione vascolare paraspinale della linea mediana	Esame ecografico o RM per evidenziare un eventuale disrafismo spinale occulto
Emangiomatosi (piccoli emangiomi cutanei multipli)	Valutazione volta a evidenziare eventuali emangiomi parenchimali, soprattutto epatici e del SNC Ricerca del sangue occulto nelle feci
Emangioma di grandi dimensioni, in particolare epatico	Eco-doppler RM Prove di funzione tiroidea
Fremito e/o soffio associati a un emangioma	Considerare una valutazione cardiologica e un'ecografia per escludere un'eventuale insufficienza aortica RM per valutare l'estensione e le caratteristiche del flusso
Inclinazione della testa	Valutare adeguatamente in rapporto alla sede specifica della lesione e, inoltre, considerare il ruolo della terapia fisica
Ritardo di sviluppo	Considerare i possibili effetti collaterali della terapia corticosteroidea (miopatia, variazioni ponderali) Considerare i possibili effetti collaterali della terapia con interferone (in particolare, la diplegia spastica)

PHACES, P-*posterior fossa abnormalities* (anomalie della fossa posteriore), H-*hemangioma* (emangioma), A-*arterial abnormalities* (anomalie arteriose), C-*cardiac abnormalities* (anomalie cardiache), E-*eye abnormalities* (anomalie oculari), S-*sternal abnormalities* (anomalie sternali); RM, risonanza magnetica.
From Blei F: Vascular anomalies: From bedside to bench and back again. *Curr Prob Pediatr Adolesc Health* 2002;32:67-102.

Nei rari casi in cui sia necessario un intervento chirurgico, se la lesione è molto superficiale, può essere utile una terapia precoce con PDL per ridurre la crescita dell'emangioma. Il PDL, inoltre, è utile anche per il trattamento degli emangiomi ulcerati di piccole dimensioni (meno di 4-5 cm). L'applicazione di fasce elastiche può ridurre l'entità della distorsione tessutale derivante dalla rapida crescita; tale terapia, però, è appropriata solo in casi selezionati, quando siano presenti ampi emangiomi. Raramente, le lesioni emangiomatose possono esercitare un'azione meccanica nei riguardi di strutture vitali, interferendo con funzioni come la vista, la respirazione, la defecazione, la minzione o la nutrizione. In altri casi, talora le lesioni possono provocare gravi alterazioni sfiguranti, a causa della loro rapida crescita.

Se diventa necessario un ulteriore trattamento, è efficace un ciclo di prednisolone (2-3 mg/kg/24 ore) nella maggior parte dei neonati. La cessazione della crescita e talvolta la regressione della lesione possono essere evidenti dopo circa 2-4 settimane di terapia. Quando si sia ottenuta una risposta, la dose dovrà essere ridotta gradualmente L'iniezione intralesionale di corticosteroidi, nelle mani di un medico esperto in questo intervento, può essere anch'essa in grado di indurre una rapida involuzione di un emangioma localizzato. Può essere efficace anche la terapia con α-interferone (IFN-α), la quale, tuttavia, avendo mostrato di dare origine, nel 10% dei casi, a diplegia spastica, deve essere utilizzata soltanto nella cura degli emangiomi pericolosi per la sopravvivenza e refrattari alla terapia corticosteroidea.

Tra le sindromi associate con gli emangiomi figurano la sindrome **PHACES** (P-posterior fossa abnormalities [anomalie della fossa posteriore], H-hemangioma [emangioma], A-arterial abnormalities [anomalie arteriose], C-cardiac abnormalities [anomalie cardiache], E-eye abnormalities [anomalie oculari],

S-sternal abnormalities [anomalie sternali]) (consistente in difetti della fossa posteriore quali la malformazione di Dandy-Walker o ipoplasia cerebellare, la presenza di un grande emangioma a placca sul viso, anomalie arteriose quali aneurismi e conseguenti ictus, coartazione aortica, anomalie oculari e difetti del rafe mediano a livello sternale, come depressioni o cicatrici), la **sindrome di Gorham** (emangiomi cutanei associati a osteolisi massiva) e la **sindrome di Bannayan-Riley-Ruvalcaba** (macrocefalia, lipomi, emangiomi, con trasmissione ereditaria autosomica dominante).

Emangiomatosi diffusa. Si tratta di una condizione morbosa in cui si ha la distribuzione diffusa di numerosi emangiomi. La cute, di solito, si presenta con molti piccoli emangiomi rossi a carattere papuloso (Fig. 649-9). La maggior parte dei neonati affetti presenta angiomatosi neonatale benigna, con emangiomi cutanei diffusi e assenza di evidente interessamento viscerale. L'emangiomatosi neonatale diffusa consiste nell'associazione di molti emangiomi cutanei con lesioni simili negli organi interni. Gli emangiomi interni possono interessare qualsiasi viscere: le sedi maggiormente interessate sono il fegato, il tratto gastrointestinale, il sistema nervoso centrale e i polmoni. Nei casi di emangiomatosi neonatale benigna, è probabile la regressione spontanea delle lesioni. I neonati con emangiomatosi neonatale diffusa si presentano compromessi alla nascita, di solito. In questi casi, è indicato procedere a esami TC ed ecografici per stabilire l'estensione dell'interessamento viscerale o neurologico. Si tratta di una condizione morbosa spesso fatale, a causa del manifestarsi di insufficienza cardiaca ad alta gittata, di emorragie viscerali, di patologia respiratoria ostruttiva o di compressione dei tessuti del sistema nervoso centrale. Il trattamento consiste nella somministrazione sistemica di corticosteroidi, eventualmente in associazione con vincristina, IFN-α, intervento chirurgico o terapia radiante, nonché terapia di supporto con prodotti del sangue per contrastare il consumo di eritrociti, di piastrine e di fattori della coagulazione.

Angioma a ciuffi. Gli angiomi a ciuffi sono definiti, istologicamente, da ciuffi distinti "a palla di cannone" costituiti da vasi sanguigni del derma. Si osservano due varianti cliniche. La classica, più frequente, è costituita da una placca scura rosso-bluastra a lenta espansione, circondata da lesioni satelliti. In oltre il 50% dei casi, le lesioni, che non tendono a regredire, interessano la testa e il collo. Una variante meno comune si presenta come un nodulo vascolare solitario (Fig. 649-10). La distinzione clinica, rispetto a una malformazione venosa nodulare, è difficile. Secondo i dati disponibili, queste lesioni possono andare incontro a regressione spontanea.

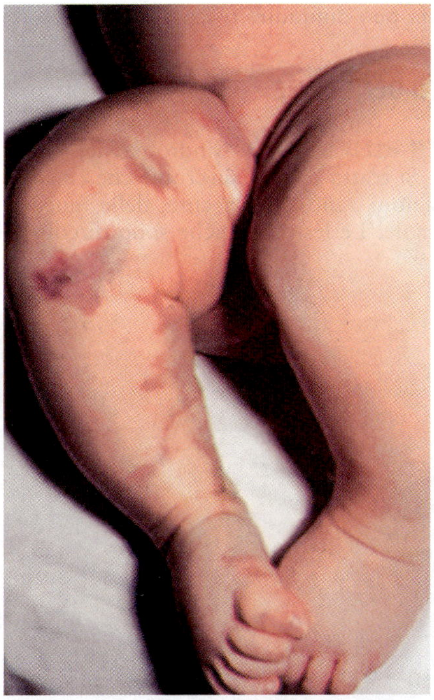

Figura 649-9. Emangiomatosi neonatale disseminata della cute (e del fegato). (Da Eichenfield LF, Frieden IJ, Esterly NB: *Textbook of Neonatal Dermatology*. Philadelphia, WB Saunders, 2001, p 340.)

Emangioendotelioma kaposiforme. L'emangioendotelioma kaposiforme è una lesione assai aggressiva che, sebbene non sia di natura maligna, può risultare letale. Le lesioni, in genere solitarie, fisse e di colore porpora scuro, non vanno incontro a regressione spontanea.

Sia gli angiomi a ciuffi, sia gli emangioendoteliomi Kaposiformi, sono lesioni difficili da trattare. Sono stati provati, con risultati estremamente variabili, tutti i trattamenti utilizzati per gli emangiomi. La sindrome di Kasabach-Merritt si osserva quasi esclusivamente nei casi di angiomi a ciuffi e in associazione agli emangioendoteliomi kaposiformi.

Sindrome di Kasabach-Merritt. Si tratta di una sindrome che mette in pericolo la vita dei pazienti e che consiste nell'associazione di un angioma a ciuffo a rapido accrescimento, o di un emangioendotelioma kaposiforme, con trombocitopenia, anemia emolitica microangiopatica e coagulopatia da consumo cronica. Le manifestazioni cliniche sono evidenti, in genere, nel primo periodo infantile. La lesione vascolare è, di solito, cutanea; solo raramente essa è localizzata nei visceri. Il difetto piastrinico associato può condurre a una improvvisa emorragia, accompagnata da ecchimosi, petecchie e rapido aumento delle dimensioni della lesione. Da ciò può derivare una grave anemia emorragica o da emolisi microangiopatica. Vi è trombocitopenia, ma il midollo osseo contiene un numero aumentato di megacariociti maturi o immaturi. La trombocitopenia è stata attribuita al sequestro o all'aumento di distruzione di piastrine all'interno della lesione. È relativamente frequente il reperto di ipofibrinogenemia e di diminuzione dei fattori coagulativi soggetti a consumo (vedi Capitolo 484.6).

Il **trattamento** comprende la terapia della trombocitopenia, dell'anemia e della coagulopatia da consumo, mediante la somministrazione di piastrine e la trasfusione di emazie e di plasma fresco congelato. La terapia eparinica è controversa, ma alcuni pazienti ne hanno tratto beneficio, in associazione alle trasfusioni. Il trattamento della sindrome di Kasabach-Merritt prevede anche l'escissione chirurgica delle piccole lesioni, la somministrazione di corticosteroidi per via sistemica, l'embolizzazione, la terapia radiante, nonché la somministrazione di vincristina, di acido aminocaproico, di ciclofosfamide, di pentossifillina o di IFN-α ricombinante. Il tasso di mortalità è rilevante.

Emangioma congenito a rapida involuzione (*Rapidly Involuting Congenital Hemangioma*, RICH). Gli emangiomi congeniti a rapida involuzione, per definizione, sono presenti già alla nascita. Essi si presentano come noduli violacei rilevati con vene ectasiche, oppure noduli grigiastri con teleangiectasie soprastanti, circon-

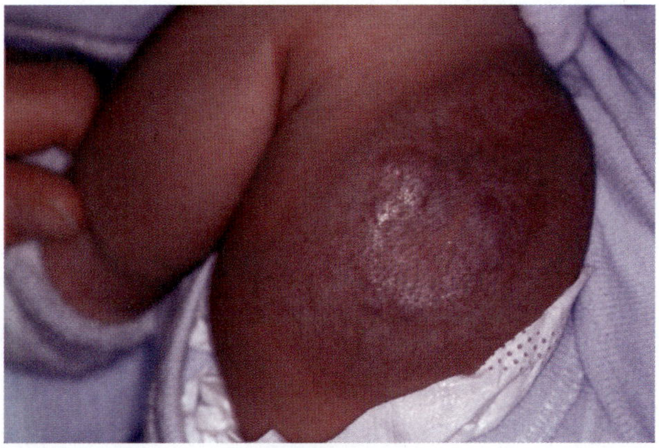

Figura 649-10. Angioma nodulare a ciuffi presente sulla coscia sinistra.

date da un margine pallido prodotto dalla vasocostrizione; in alternativa, le lesioni possono presentarsi come lesioni cutanee infiltrative con colorito violaceo. Esse non vanno incontro a una rapida fase di crescita e manifestano involuzione spontanea entro l'età di 1 anno.

Angioma congenito non involutivo (Non-Involuting Congenital Hemangioma, NICH). Come nel caso del RICH, queste lesioni vascolari solitarie sono presenti alla nascita. Esse sono placche di forma rotonda od ovalare con aree pallide in sede centrale o periferica e grossolane teleangiectasie sovrapposte. Anche queste lesioni non vanno incontro a una rapida fase di crescita, ma neppure a un'involuzione spontanea. Da un punto di vista nosografico sono, forse, meglio classificabili come malformazioni, anziché come neoplasie.

DISORDINI VASCOLARI BENIGNI ACQUISITI

GRANULOMA PIOGENO (EMANGIOMA CAPILLARE LOBULARE). Un granuloma piogeno è una piccola formazione papulosa, sessile o peduncolata, di colorito rosso brillante, che, spesso, presenta un visibile colletto epiteliale (Fig. 649-11). La superficie può essere crostosa e coperta di essudato, oppure completamente epitelizzata. I granulomi piogeni possono crescere rapidamente, ulcerarsi e sanguinare facilmente a seguito di traumi, in quanto consistono di tessuto di granulazione esuberante. Si tratta di lesioni relativamente frequenti nei bambini, in particolare sul viso, sulle braccia e sulle mani. Le lesioni localizzate sulle sole dita o sulla mano possono apparire come noduli sottocutanei. I granulomi piogeni possono insorgere in sedi traumatizzate, ma, spesso, manca il precedente anamnestico di un trauma. Clinicamente, essi somigliano a piccoli emangiomi e, spesso, sono da essi indistinguibili. Microscopicamente, una lesione precoce somiglia a un emangioma capillare in fase precoce. La formazione a colletto alla base del tumore e l'edema in sede stromale possono consentire la distinzione rispetto a un emangioma capillare.

I granulomi piogeni sono benigni, ma molto fastidiosi, poiché sanguinano con facilità in occasione di traumi e possono recidivare se asportati in modo incompleto. Dopo l'escissione chirurgica possono svilupparsi numerose papule satelliti, soprattutto nella regione interscapolare. Le lesioni di piccole dimensioni possono regredire a seguito di cauterizzazione con nitrato d'argento; le lesioni maggiori richiedono l'escissione e l'elettrocoagulazione della base del granuloma. Le lesioni piccole, inferiori a 5 mm, possono essere trattate con laser a colori con pompaggio a lampada flash (*flashlamp-pumped-pulsed dye laser*).

ANGIOCHERATOMA DI MIBELLI. L'angiocheratoma di Mibelli è caratterizzato da papule e noduli squamosi del diametro di 1-8 mm e di colorito rosso, purpureo o nero, con aspetto verrucoso, che compaiono sul dorso delle dita delle mani e dei piedi, sui gomiti e sulle ginocchia. Meno spesso, le lesioni interessano i palmi delle mani, le piante dei piedi e le orecchie. In molti pazienti, l'insorgenza è preceduta da congelamento o geloni. Questi noduli tendono a sanguinare copiosamente dopo una ferita e possono andare incontro a involuzione in risposta a traumi. Un'eradicazione efficace è possibile mediante crioterapia, elettrocoagulazione, escissione o ablazione mediante laser.

ANGIOMI A RAGNO. Un nevo a ragno vascolare (*nevus aracneus*) consiste di un'arteria nutritiva centrale con molti vasi dilatati che si irradiano da essa, con un'area circostante di eritema, di diametro variabile da pochi millimetri fino a diversi centimetri (Fig. 649-12). La pressione sul vaso centrale provoca lo sbiancamento della lesione; le pulsazioni visibili nei nevi maggiori rappresentano una prova dell'origine arteriosa della lesione. Gli angiomi a ragno sono associati a condizioni in cui vi sono in circolo maggiori concentrazioni di estrogeni, come avviene nella cirrosi epatica nella gravidanza; nondimeno, queste lesioni si verificano fino nel 15% dei bambini normali in età prescolare e fino nel 45% dei bambini in età scolare. Le sedi predilette nei bambini sono il dorso della mano, l'avambraccio, il volto e le orecchie. Le lesioni spesso regrediscono spontaneamente dopo la pubertà. Se si desidera l'asportazione, il metodo di scelta è il PDL (laser pulsato a colori), che consente di ottenere una risoluzione del 90% nell'ambito di un singolo trattamento.

TELEANGIECTASIA GENERALIZZATA ESSENZIALE. La teleangiectasia generalizzata essenziale è un'anomalia rara, presumibilmente nevoide, la cui causa è sconosciuta. Essa può insorgere sia nella fanciullezza sia nell'età adulta, manifestandosi, particolarmente sugli arti, con teleangiectasie retiformi a chiazze, che, talora, progrediscono fino a interessare grandi aree di superficie corporea. La condizione morbosa deve essere distinta dalle teleangiectasie secondarie derivanti da malattie del connettivo, dallo xeroderma pigmentosum, dal poichiloderma e dall'atassia-telangectasia. Il trattamento con il PDL è efficace.

TELEANGIECTASIA UNILATERALE NEVOIDE. Questa rara entità nosologica è caratterizzata da manifestazioni di teleangiectasia con distribuzione monolaterale, soprattutto sul volto, sul collo, sul torace e sulle braccia. La forma acquisita si manifesta, soprattutto, nel sesso femminile, con l'inizio del ciclo mestruale o durante la gravidanza. Quando ha inizio a seguito della gravidanza, la teleangiectasia può diminuire o scomparire dopo il parto.

ALTERAZIONI GENETICHE

BLUE RUBBER BLEB NEVUS. "Sindrome del nevo bolloso angiomatoso". Si tratta di una sindrome che consiste in numerose malformazioni venose della cute, delle mucose e del tratto gastrointestinale. Le lesioni tipiche sono di colore blu-porpora

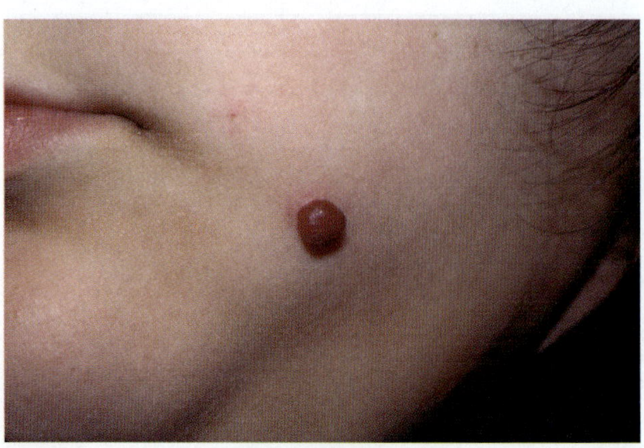

Figura 649-11. Granuloma piogeno nella guancia sinistra.

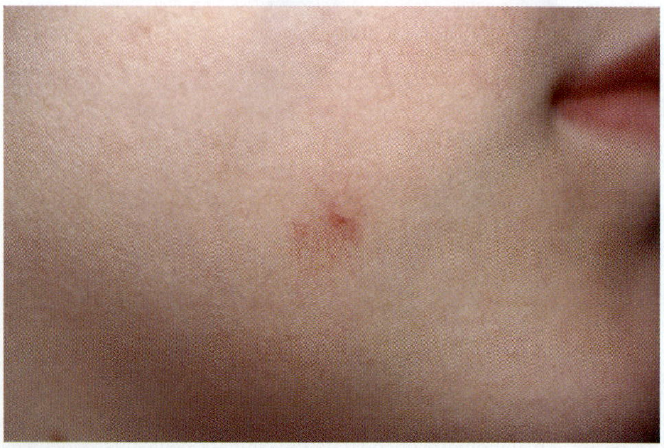

Figura 649-12. Teleangiectasia a ragno, con una componente arteriolare visibile al centro.

e di consistenza gommosa; le dimensioni possono variare da pochi millimetri ad alcuni centimetri di diametro. Talora le lesioni sono dolenti o dolorabili. I noduli, a volte presenti alla nascita, compaiono di solito nella fanciullezza. Le nuove lesioni possono continuare a svilupparsi per tutta la durata della vita. Possono, inoltre, comparire lesioni grandi e irregolari, con effetti sfiguranti. Le lesioni, che possono raramente essere localizzate nel fegato, nella milza e nel sistema nervoso centrale, oltre che nella cute e nel tratto gastrointestinale, di solito non vanno spontaneamente incontro a involuzione. Eventuali emorragie gastrointestinali ricorrenti possono condurre a grave anemia. Un effetto palliativo può essere raggiunto mediante l'escissione dell'intestino interessato.

SINDROME DI MAFFUCCI. L'associazione di numerose malformazioni vascolari e, talora, anche linfatiche con *encondromi nodulari* nella porzione metafisaria o diafisaria delle ossa lunghe è denominata sindrome di Maffucci. Nelle encondromatosi sono state identificate delle mutazioni che coinvolgono il recettore del PTH/PTHrP di tipo 1. Le lesioni vascolari consistono, tipicamente, in masse sottocutanee di consistenza molle, comprimibili, asintomatiche e di colorito da bluastro a purpureo. Queste masse crescono proporzionalmente all'accrescimento corporeo del bambino e si stabilizzano con il raggiungimento dell'età adulta. Può aversi anche l'interessamento delle membrane mucose o dei visceri. L'esordio avviene durante la fanciullezza. Le lesioni ossee possono produrre deformità degli arti e fratture patologiche. Una complicanza può essere costituita dalla trasformazione maligna degli encondromi (condrosarcoma, angiosarcoma) o dall'insorgenza di neoplasie maligne primitive (neoplasie ovariche e pancreatiche, fibrosarcomi e gliomi) (vedi Capitolo 501).

TELEANGIECTASIA EREDITARIA EMORRAGICA (MALATTIA DI OSLER-WEBER-RENDU). Si tratta di un'alterazione ereditaria trasmessa come carattere autosomico dominante. Un gene coinvolto nella malattia codifica per l'endoglina, una glicoproteina di membrana presente sulle cellule endoteliali, la quale lega il fattore di crescita trasformante β (*transforming growth factor*-β). I bambini colpiti dalla malattia possono andare incontro a episodi ricorrenti di epistassi, prima della scoperta delle caratteristiche lesioni della cute e delle membrane mucose. Le lesioni mucocutanee, che, di solito, compaiono al momento della pubertà, consistono in macule, papule o lesioni "a ragno", di colorito da rosso a porpora e della grandezza di 1-4 mm, demarcate da margini netti e composte, ciascuna, da un intreccio compatto di vasi tortuosi teleangiectasici. Sono interessati, di solito, la mucosa nasale, le labbra, la lingua; meno spesso, le lesioni si manifestano sul viso, sulle orecchie, sulle palme delle mani e sul letto ungueale. Le ectasie vascolari possono insorgere anche in sede congiuntivale, laringea, faringea, nel tratto gastrointestinale, nella vescica, nella vagina, nei bronchi, nel cervello e nel fegato.

L'emorragia massiva, che è la complicanza più grave, può dar luogo a grave anemia. Il sanguinamento può avvenire dal naso, dalla bocca, dal tratto genitourinario e dai polmoni; spesso, però, l'epistassi è l'unica manifestazione, che si verifica nell'80% dei pazienti. Circa il 15-20% dei pazienti con malformazioni arterovenose polmonari va incontro a ictus causato da ascessi embolici. Le persone con teleangiectasia ereditaria emorragica presentano normali concentrazioni dei fattori della coagulazione e un meccanismo coagulativo inalterato. In assenza di complicanze gravi, la durata della vita è normale. Le lesioni locali possono essere asportate temporaneamente con cauterizzazione chimica o con elettrocoagulazione. Interventi chirurgici più rilevanti possono rendersi necessari in caso di lesioni in sedi critiche, quali il polmone o il tratto gastrointestinale. L'anemia deve essere trattata con terapia marziale.

TELEANGIECTASIA EREDITARIA BENIGNA. Si tratta di una rara alterazione, ereditata come carattere autosomico dominante, che si sviluppa nel corso dell'infanzia. Le aree maggiormente interessate sono il volto, la parte superiore del tronco e le braccia. Questa condizione morbosa presenta un andamento progressivo, ma resta limitata alla cute.

ATASSIA-TELEANGIECTASIA (VEDI CAPITOLO 125.2). Questo disturbo (sindrome di Louis-Bar) è trasmesso come tratto autosomico recessivo, a seguito di una mutazione nel gene ATM. La caratteristica teleangiectasia si manifesta a circa 3 anni di età, in primo luogo nella congiuntiva bulbare e, successivamente, sul ponte del naso, sulle regioni zigomatiche, sull'orecchio esterno, sul palato duro, sulla parte anterosuperiore del torace, nonché sulle fosse antecubitale e poplitea. Altri segni cutanei sono rappresentati da macchie color caffellatte, incanutimento prematuro e alterazioni sclerodermiche. Come parte del quadro clinico, sono stati descritti anche atassia cerebellare progressiva, deterioramento neurologico, infezioni senopolmonari e neoplasie maligne.

ANGIOCHERATOMA CORPORIS DIFFUSUM (MALATTIA DI FABRY) (VEDI CAPITOLO 86.4). Questo errore congenito del metabolismo (concernente l'α-galattosidasi) è un disturbo recessivo legato al cromosoma X, con penetranza completa nel sesso maschile e penetranza variabile nelle femmine portatrici. Gli angiocheratomi insorgono prima della pubertà e si manifestano, in gran numero, in corrispondenza dei genitali, dell'anca, della natica, della coscia, nonché nella regione ombelicale e inguinale. Le lesioni consistono in papule di colorito da rosso a nero-bluastro e del diametro di 0,1-3 mm, le quali possono presentare una superficie ipercheratosica. Si osservano teleangiectasie nella mucosa e nella congiuntiva. Al microscopio ottico tali angiocheratomi appaiono come spazi vascolari riempiti di sangue, dilatati e ricoperti da endotelio. Nei macrofagi, nei fibrociti e nelle cellule endoteliali sono dimostrabili depositi lipidici granulari.

Ulteriori manifestazioni cliniche consistono in episodi ricorrenti di febbre e di dolore lancinante, con cianosi e arrossamento delle estremità degli arti, parestesie della mano e del piede, opacità della cornea rilevabili mediante l'esame con lampada a fessura (biomicroscopio), nonché ipoidrosi.

Generalmente le cause immediate del decesso consistono in lesioni renali e cardiache. L'alterazione biochimica consiste in un deficit dell'enzima lisosomiale α-galattosidasi, con conseguente accumulo di ceramide triesossido nei tessuti, in particolare nell'endotelio vascolare, e con escrezione urinaria della molecola. Lesioni cutanee simili sono state descritte anche in un altro disturbo legato a enzimi lisosomiali, il deficit di α-L-fucosidasi, come pure nella sialidosi, una malattia da accumulo associata a deficit di neuraminidasi (la terapia è trattata nel Capitolo 86.4).

Bayrak-Toydemir P, Mao R, Lewin S, et al: Hereditary hemorrhagic telangiectasia: An overview of diagnosis and management in the molecular era for clinicians. *Genet Med* 2004;6:175–191.

Cabrera J, Cabrera J Jr, Garcia-Olmedo A, et al: Treatment of venous malformations with sclerosant in Microfoam form. *Arch Dermatol* 2003;139:1409–1416.

Chang MW: Updated classification of hemangiomas and other vascular anomalies. *Lymphat Res Biol* 2003;1:259–265.

Haggstrom A, Lammer E, Schneider R, et al: Patterns of infantile hemangiomas: new clues to hemangioma pathogens and embryonic facial development. *Pediatr* 2005;117:698–703.

Hopyan S, Gokgoz N, Poon R, et al: A mutant PTH/PTHrP type I receptor in enchondromatosis. *Nat Genet* 2002;30:306–310.

Leung AK, Rafaat M: Benign neonatal hemangiomatosis. *Pediatr Dermatol* 2003;20:161–163.

Lyons LL, North PE, Mac-MouneLai F, et al: Kaposiform hemangioendothelioma: A study of 33 cases emphasizing its pathologic, immunophenotype, and biologic uniqueness from juvenile hemangiomas. *Am J Surg Pathol* 2004;28:559–568.

Mohrenschlager M, Henkel V, Ring J: Fabry disease: More than angiokeratomas. *Arch Dermatol* 2004;140:1526–1528.

Nahm WK, Moise S, Eichenfield LF, et al: Venous malformations in blue rubber bleb nevus syndrome: Variable onset of presentation. *J Am Acad Dermatol* 2004;50:S101–S106.

Perlman S, Becker-Catania S, Gatti RA: Ataxia-telangiectasia: Diagnosis and treatment. *Semin Pediatr Neurol* 2003;10:173–182.

Wananukul S, Nuchprayoon I, Seksarn P: Treatment of Kasabach-Merritt syndrome: A stepwise regimen of prednisolone, dipyramidole, and interferon. *Int J Dermatol* 2003;42:741–748.

Waner M, North PE, Scherer KA, et al: The nonrandom distribution of facial hemangiomas. *Arch Dermatol* 2003;139:869–875.

Capitolo 650 ■ Nevi cutanei

Joseph G. Morelli

I nevi sono lesioni cutanee caratterizzate istopatologicamente da raccolte di tipi cellulari ben differenziati normalmente presenti nella cute. I nevi vascolari sono descritti nel Capitolo 649. I nevi melanocitici sono suddivisi in due grandi gruppi: quelli che compaiono dopo la nascita (nevi acquisiti) e quelli che sono presenti alla nascita (nevi congeniti).

NEVI MELANOCITICI ACQUISITI. I nevi melanocitici sono costituti da grappoli benigni di nevociti che originano in seguito a un'alterazione e a proliferazione dei melanociti in corrispondenza della giunzione dermoepidermica.

Epidemiologia. Il numero di nevi melanocitici acquisiti aumenta gradualmente durante l'infanzia, bruscamente durante l'adolescenza e più lentamente nella prima età adulta; si stabilizza tra i 30 e i 40 anni e poi si riduce lentamente. Il numero medio di nevi melanocitici nell'adulto varia in base alla genetica, al colore della cute e all'esposizione al sole. Maggiore è il numero di nevi presenti, più elevato è il rischio di sviluppare un **melanoma**. L'esposizione al sole durante l'infanzia, soprattutto se intensa e poco regolare in individui con cute chiara, e la propensione a ustionarsi e a ricoprirsi di efelidi invece di abbronzarsi sono determinanti importanti del numero di nevi melanocitici che si svilupperanno. Nonostante la cute chiara e la propensione a coprirsi di lentiggini e a riportare ustioni solari, i bambini con i capelli rossi sviluppano meno nevi degli altri. L'aumento del numero di nevi è inoltre associato a immunosoppressione e a chemioterapia.

Manifestazioni cliniche. I nevi nevocellulari hanno un'anamnesi ben definita e vengono classificati come **giunzionali**, **composti** o **dermici** in base alla posizione dei nevociti presenti nella cute. Nell'infanzia, >90% dei nevi è di tipo giunzionale: si verifica una proliferazione di melanociti in corrispondenza della giunzione tra epidermide e derma con formazione di nidi di cellule. I nevi giunzionali compaiono in qualsiasi parte del corpo con diverse tonalità di marrone; sono relativamente piccoli, discreti, piani e di forma variabile. I nevociti melanizzati hanno configurazione cuboidale o epitelioide e si presentano a grappoli sul lato epidermico della membrana basale. Benché alcuni nevi, in particolare quelli localizzati sui palmi delle mani, le piante dei piedi e i genitali, restino giunzionali per tutta la vita, la maggior parte di essi diventa composta mano a mano che i melanociti migrano nel derma papillare per formare nidi sulla giunzione dermoepidermica e all'interno del derma. Se i melanociti giunzionali cessano di proliferare, i nidi di melanociti restano esclusivamente all'interno del derma, formando un nevo intradermico. Con la maturazione, i nevi composti e intradermici possono diventare rilevati, a cupola, verrucosi o peduncolati. Le lesioni leggermente rilevate di solito sono composte; quelle chiaramente rilevate, invece, generalmente sono intradermiche. Con l'età, i nidi melanocitici dermici regrediscono e i nevi gradualmente scompaiono.

Prognosi e terapia. I nevi pigmentati acquisiti sono benigni, ma una percentuale molto ridotta subisce trasformazione maligna. Le modificazioni sospette come rapido aumento di dimensioni, sviluppo di lesioni satellite, screziature di colore, in particolare con tonalità rosse, brune, grigie, nere e blu, *incontinentia pigmenti*, dentellatura o irregolarità dei bordi, alterazioni nella consistenza come desquamazione, erosione, ulcerazione e indurimento e linfoadenopatia regionale sono indicazioni per l'escissione e per una valutazione istopatologica. La maggior parte di queste alterazioni è dovuta a irritazione, infezione o maturazione; lo scurimento, il graduale aumento di dimensioni e l'elevazione di solito si verificano durante l'adolescenza e non costituiscono motivo di preoccupazione. Due alterazioni benigne comuni sono i nevi clonali (nevi a "uovo fritto") e i nevi anulari. I nevi clonali sono di colore marrone chiaro con centro scuro in rilievo e rappresentano l'alterazione clonale di un sottoinsieme di nevociti all'interno della lesione. I nevi anulari sono piani e chiari, con un anello marrone scuro, e si osservano prevalentemente sul cuoio capelluto (Fig. 650-1). Deve essere valutata la presenza di fattori di rischio per lo sviluppo di melanoma e la volontà dei genitori riguardo all'asportazione del nevo. Se vi sono dubbi sulla natura benigna di un nevo, l'escissione è una procedura ambulatoriale sicura e semplice e può essere giustificata per alleviare l'ansia.

NEVI MELANOCITICI ATIPICI. I nevi melanocitici atipici si presentano sia in un contesto di predisposizione familiare autosomica dominante al melanoma (sindrome del melanoma familiare, sindrome del nevo displastico, sindrome del nevo di Clark (BK mole) sia come eventi sporadici. Solo il 2% di tutti i melanomi pediatrici insorge in soggetti con questa sindrome familiare; il 10% dei pazienti che presenta questa sindrome sviluppa un melanoma prima dei 20 anni. Melanomi maligni sono stati osservati in bambini con sindrome del nevo displasico già a 10 anni di età. Il rischio di sviluppare un melanoma è essenzialmente del 100% nei soggetti con sindrome del nevo displasico che presentino due famigliari che abbiano sofferto di melanomi. Il termine sindrome del nevo atipico descrive le lesioni che interessano gli individui senza storia familiare autosomica dominante di melanoma ma con >50 nevi, alcuni dei quali atipici. Il rischio di melanoma nel corso della vita associato ai nevi displastici in questo contesto è compreso tra il 5 e il 10%.

I nevi atipici tendono a essere grandi (5-15 mm) e ad avere una forma da rotonda a ovale. Presentano margini irregolari, colore variegato e una parte della lesione è in rilievo. Questi nevi sono più frequenti sul tronco posteriore, ciò suggerisce che un'esposizione al sole discontinua e intensa influisce sulla loro genesi. Possono presentarsi anche in aree protette dal sole come le mammelle, le natiche e il cuoio capelluto. In genere, non si sviluppano fino alla pubertà, benché le lesioni sul cuoio capelluto possano essere presenti anche prima. I nevi atipici mostrano una proliferazione disordinata di melanociti intraepidermici atipici, infiltrazione linfocitica, fibroplasia e angiogenesi. Per identificare i soggetti colpiti può essere utile ottenere una documentazione istopatologica dell'alterazione displasica tramite biopsia. È prudente asportare i nevi atipici borderline nei bambini immunocompromessi o nei soggetti sottoposti a radioterapia o ad agenti chemioterapici. Benché la chemioterapia sia stata associata allo sviluppo di un numero maggiore di nevi melanocitici, non è sta-

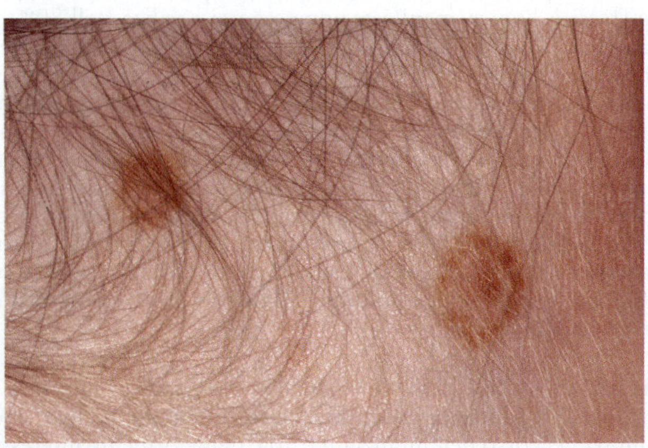

Figura 650-1. Nevi anulari sul cuoio capelluto.

ta direttamente collegata a un maggior rischio di sviluppare un melanoma. La soglia per la rimozione di nevi clinicamente atipici è anche più bassa nei siti difficili da osservare, come il cuoio capelluto. Tutti i bambini affetti dovrebbero essere sottoposti a un esame completo della cute ogni 6-12 mesi. Una mappatura fotografica dei nevi costituisce un utile ausilio per seguirne le modificazioni. I genitori andrebbero adeguatamente informati sull'importanza della protezione e sulla necessità di evitare il sole, oltre che istruiti a riconoscere i primi segni di melanomi attraverso una verifica attenta da effettuare, con regolarità, ogni 3-4 mesi circa.

NEVO MELANOCITICO CONGENITO. Nevi melanocitici congeniti sono presenti in circa l'1% dei neonati. Questi nevi sono stati classificati in base alle loro dimensioni: i nevi congeniti giganti hanno un diametro >20 cm (dimensioni nell'adulto) o occupano >5% della superficie corporea, i nevi congeniti piccoli hanno un diametro <2 cm e i nevi intermedi si collocano tra questi due estremi. I nevi congeniti sono caratterizzati dalla presenza di nevociti nel derma reticolare inferiore, tra le fibre di collagene, attorno agli annessi cutanei, ai nervi e ai vasi nel derma inferiore e occasionalmente si estendono nell'adipe sottocuticolare. La loro identificazione è spesso dubbia poiché possono presentare i tratti istologici di comuni nevi giunzionali, composti o intradermici. Alcuni nevi non presenti alla nascita mostrano i tratti istopatologici dei nevi congeniti; questi non vanno considerati come congeniti. Può inoltre essere difficile distinguere clinicamente i nevi congeniti da altri tipi di lesioni pigmentate, data la difficoltà dei genitori di individuare i nevi presenti dalla nascita. La diagnosi differenziale comprende le macchie mongoliche, le macchie a caffellatte, gli amartomi del muscolo liscio e la melanocitosi dermica (nevi di Ota e Ito).

I siti di predilezione dei nevi congeniti piccoli sono la parte inferiore del tronco, la regione superiore della schiena, le spalle, il torace e gli arti prossimali. Le lesioni possono essere piane, rilevate, verrucose o nodulari e assumere varie tonalità di marrone, blu o nero. Data la difficoltà nell'identificare con certezza i nevi congeniti piccoli, i dati riguardanti il loro potenziale maligno sono controversi e tendono a essere sopravvalutati. La reale incidenza del melanoma nei nevi congeniti, soprattutto quelli con dimensioni ridotte e medie, è sconosciuta. L'asportazione di tutti i nevi congeniti piccoli non è giustificata in quanto la possibilità di sviluppare un melanoma da questo tipo di nevo prima della pubertà è minima. Prima di decidere se rimuovere o meno un nevo occorre valutare con attenzione diversi fattori: la sua posizione e la possibilità di monitorarlo clinicamente, il potenziale di formazione di una cicatrice, la presenza di altri fattori di rischio per il melanoma e la presenza di tratti clinici atipici.

I nevi pigmentati congeniti giganti (<1/20 000 nati) si presentano soprattutto sul tronco posteriore (Fig. 650-2) ma possono comparire anche sul capo o sulle estremità. Questi nevi rivestono un significato particolare per la loro associazione con la melanocitosi leptomeningea (melanocitosi neurocutanea) e per la tendenza a sviluppare melanomi maligni. Il coinvolgimento leptomeningeo si verifica soprattutto quando il nevo si trova sulla testa o sulla linea mediana del tronco, in particolare quando è associato a numerosi nevi melanocitici "satellite" (>20 lesioni). I nevociti all'interno delle leptomeningi e del parenchima cerebrale possono causare un aumento della pressione intracranica, idrocefalo, convulsioni, ritardo e deficit motori ed evolvere in melanoma. La natura maligna può essere identificata mediante un attento esame citologico del liquido cerebrospinale per la ricerca di cellule contenenti melanina. La RMN mostra melanosi leptomeningea asintomatica in circa il 30% dei soggetti che presentano un nevo congenito gigante. Si stima che l'incidenza complessiva di melanoma maligno sviluppatosi da un nevo congenito gigante è compresa tra il 5 e il 10%. La metà dei melanomi che originano all'interno di un nevo congenito gigante si sviluppa entro i 5 anni di età. Il tasso di mortalità è del 45%. Il trattamento dei nevi congeniti giganti resta controverso e deve coinvolgere genitori, pediatra, dermatologo e chirurgo plastico. Se il nevo si trova sulla testa o sulla colonna vertebrale, una RMN può consentire di rilevare melanosi neurale; in questo caso è inutile rimuovere il nevo. In assenza di melanosi neurale, un'escissione precoce e una riparazione supportata da espansori tissutali o innesto di tessuto possono ridurre il carico di nevociti e pertanto il potenziale di sviluppare un melanoma, ma a costo di numerosi interventi chirurgici potenzialmente sfiguranti. I nevociti in profondità nei tessuti sottocutanei possono sottrarsi all'escissione. L'esecuzione di biopsie casuali del nevo non sono utili, mentre è indicata una biopsia per i noduli in espansione. Si raccomanda un follow-up ogni 6 mesi per cinque anni e quindi ogni 12 mesi. Le fotografie in serie del nevo possono essere utili per rilevarne le alterazioni.

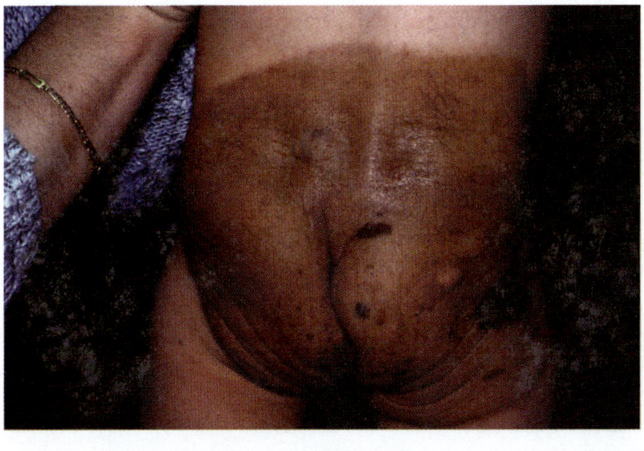

Figura 650-2. Nevo melanocitico congenito grande a "costume da bagno".

MELANOMA. I melanomi maligni rappresentano l'1-3% di tutte le neoplasie maligne pediatriche e costituiscono la forma di tumore più frequente nei giovani adulti di età compresa tra 25 e 29 anni. Dal 1973 l'incidenza è aumentata del 150%. Il melanoma si sviluppa prevalentemente nei soggetti di razza bianca, sulla testa e sul tronco nei maschi e sugli arti nelle femmine. I fattori di rischio per lo sviluppo del melanoma includono la presenza di sindrome del melanoma atipico familiare o xeroderma pigmentoso, un numero aumentato di nevi melanocitici acquisiti o nevi atipici, carnagione chiara, eccessiva esposizione al sole, specialmente se alla luce solare intensa in maniera discontinua, anamnesi personale o familiare (parente di primo grado) di melanoma, presenza di nevo congenito gigante e immunosoppressione. Nei bambini che in precedenza non accusavano disturbi, la radiazione UV è responsabile della maggior parte dei melanomi. Meno del 5% dei melanomi infantili si presenta all'interno di nevi congeniti giganti o nei soggetti con sindrome del melanoma atipico familiare. Nel 40-50% dei casi, la lesione si sviluppa su un sito in cui non vi era alcun nevo apparente (lesione amelanotica). Il tasso di mortalità è correlato prevalentemente allo spessore del tumore e al grado di invasività nella cute. Il tasso complessivo di mortalità raggiunge circa il 40% sia che si sviluppi nel bambino sia che insorga nell'adulto. Data la mancanza di una terapia efficace, le misure migliori sono la prevenzione e l'individuazione precoce. È fondamentale evitare l'esposizione al sole durante le ore più calde, ossia tra le 10 e le 15, utilizzare indumenti protettivi come cappelli, abiti a maniche lunghe e pantaloni, fare uso di protezioni solari. Il riconoscimento precoce prevede esami fotografici e clinici frequenti per i pazienti a rischio (sindrome del nevo displasico) e una risposta sollecita alle alterazioni rapide nei nevi (dimensioni, forma, colore, infiammazione, sanguinamento o formazione di croste e sensibilizzazione). La regola dell'ABCD (asimmetria, bordi irregolari, colore variabile e diametro >6 mm), che costituisce un utile strumento di screening per gli adulti, può non essere altrettanto efficace nei bambini.

NEVO ALONATO. I nevi alonati si manifestano soprattutto nei bambini e nei giovani adulti, in particolare sulla schiena (Fig.

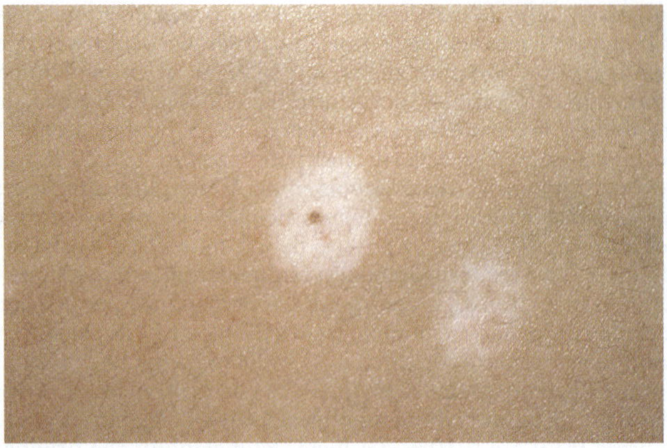

Figura 650-3. Nevo alonato ben sviluppato.

650-3). L'esordio dell'alone può coincidere con la pubertà o con la gravidanza. Numerosi nevi pigmentati sviluppano spesso contemporaneamente un alone. La successiva scomparsa del nevo centrale nell'arco di più mesi costituisce il decorso naturale e l'area depigmentata può venire o meno ripigmentata. L'escissione o l'esame istopatologico sono indicati solo quando la natura della lesione centrale è dubbia. Occasionalmente, un nevo melanocitico acquisito si sviluppa su una zona periferica di depigmentazione lungo un periodo variabile da giorni a settimane. Oltre ai nevociti, si osserva un denso infiltrato infiammatorio di linfociti e istiociti. L'alone pallido riflette la scomparsa dei melanociti. Questo fenomeno è associato a nevi congeniti, nevi blu, nevi di Spitz, nevi displasici, neurofibromi, melanomi maligni primitivi e secondari, e occasionalmente a poliosi, sindrome di Vogt-Koyanagi-Harada e anemia perniciosa. I pazienti con vitiligine presentano un'incidenza aumentata di nevi alonati. I soggetti con nevi alonati hanno anticorpi circolanti contro il citoplasma dei melanociti e dei nevociti.

NEVO DI SPITZ (NEVO A CELLULE FUSIFORMI ED EPITELIOIDI). Il nevo di Spitz si presenta con la massima frequenza nei primi vent'anni di vita sotto forma di papula rosa-rossa, liscia, a cupola, compatta e glabra su viso, spalle e arti superiori (Fig. 650-4). nella maggior parte dei casi le lesioni hanno un diametro <1 cm, ma possono raggiungere anche i 3 cm. Raramente si presentano sotto forma di lesioni multiple raggruppate. Alterazioni simili all'osservazione sono il granuloma piogeno, l'emangioma, il nevo nevocellulare, lo xantogranuloma giovanile e il carcinoma basocellulare; queste entità sono istologicamente differenziabili. Può essere difficile distinguere istopatologicamente il nevo di Spitz dal melanoma maligno perché l'atipia nucleare è un tratto comune, soprattutto dopo una recidiva locale del nevo. La difficoltà deriva dal fatto che molti altri tipi clinici di nevi melanocitici presentano un aspetto istologico simile. Una recidiva locale dopo l'escissione può verificarsi fino nel 5% dei casi. Se un nevo alimenta il sospetto clinico che potrebbe trattarsi di un melanoma, si raccomanda una biopsia escissionale dell'intera lesione. Se i margini dell'escissione di un nevo di Spitz risultano positivi, è prudente procedere a una nuova escissione del sito per evitare difficoltà nell'interpretazione istopatologica della lesione in futuro.

NEVO LENTIGGINOSO ZOSTERIFORME (LENTIGGINE AGGREGATA). Questo nevo è una raccolta unilaterale, lineare, a banda, di numerose macule brune o nere di 2-10 mm, su viso, tronco o arti. Il nevo può essere presente alla nascita oppure svilupparsi durante l'infanzia. Si rileva una quantità aumentata di melanociti nelle creste allungate dell'epidermide.

NEVUS SPILUS (NEVO LENTIGGINOSO MACULATO). Questo nevo è una macchia bruna e piana all'interno della quale si rilevano elementi melanocitici piani più scuri o rilevati di colore marrone (Fig. 650-5). I nevi spilus variano notevolmente per dimensioni e possono presentarsi in qualsiasi parte del corpo. Il colore della componente maculare può variare da marrone chiaro a marrone scuro e il numero di lesioni più scure può essere ridotto o significativo. Il nevus spilus è raro alla nascita e viene comunemente acquisito intorno al primo anno di vita o nella primissima infanzia. Gli elementi scuri all'interno di questa lesione sono solitamente presenti nella fase iniziale e tendono ad aumentare di numero gradualmente con il passare del tempo. Le macule più scure rappresentano nevociti in posizione giunzionale o dermica; la macchia presenta un numero aumentato di melanociti secondo un modello epidermico lentigginoso. Il potenziale maligno di questi nevi è incerto; il nevo spilus si riscontra più comunemente nei pazienti con melanoma che nei soggetti di controllo corrispondenti. Questi nevi non vanno escissi, a meno che non si notino tratti atipici o alterazioni cliniche recenti.

NEVO DI OTA. Il nevo di Ota è più comune tra i soggetti di sesso femminile, gli asiatici e i pazienti neri. È costituito da una macchia permanente composta da macule blu, nere e brune parzialmente confluenti. L'intensità della pigmentazione può variare di giorno in giorno e con il tempo la lesione può ingrandirsi e diventare più scura. Talvolta alcune aree del nevo sono rilevate. I nevi maculari sono simili alle chiazze mongoliche per colore e si manifestano unilateralmente in aree di competenza della prima e della seconda divisione del nervo trigemino. Il nevo di Ota differisce dalla chiazza mongolica non solo per la sua distribuzione ma anche per l'aspetto, che è punteggiato piuttosto che uniforme. Entrambe sono forme di melanocitosi mediodermiche. Il nevo di Ota presenta una maggiore concentrazione di melanociti

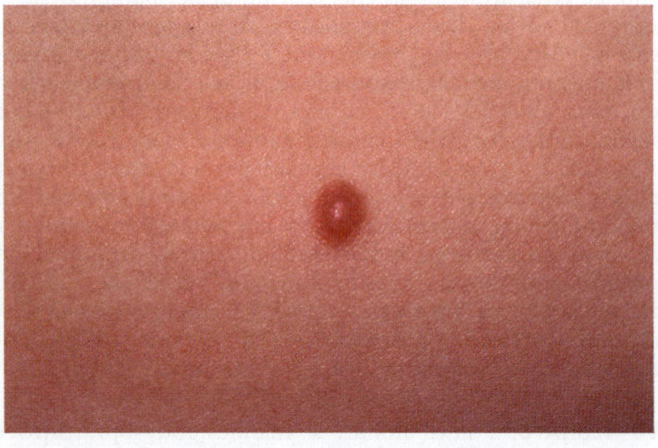

Figura 650-4. Nevo di Spitz rosso a cupola.

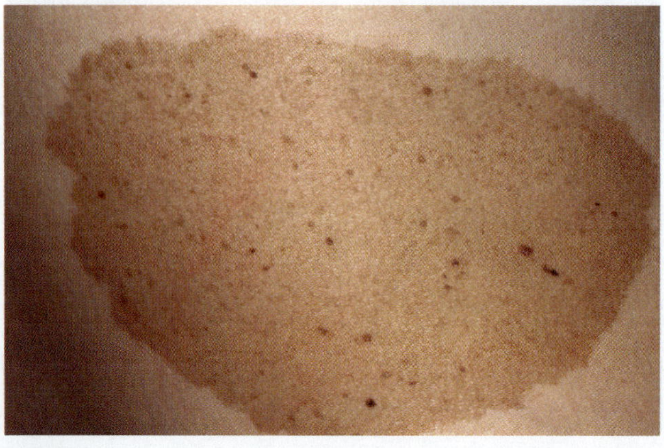

Figura 650-5. Nevus spilus.

dermici allungati e dendritici localizzati nella parte superiore del derma invece che in quella inferiore. A volte queste lesioni sono presenti alla nascita; in altri casi possono svilupparsi nel primo o nel secondo decennio di vita. In alcuni pazienti si osserva un coinvolgimento non uniforme di congiuntiva, palato duro, faringe, mucosa nasale, mucosa buccale o membrana timpanica. La degenerazione maligna è rarissima. La laserterapia può ridurre efficacemente la pigmentazione.

Il **nevo di Ito** è localizzato nelle regioni sopraclavicolare, scapolare e del deltoide. Tende ad avere una distribuzione più diffusa e a essere meno macchiettato del nevo di Ota. Rappresenta anch'esso una forma di melanocitosi mediodermica. L'unico trattamento disponibile consiste nel mascherare il nevo con cosmetici o laserterapia.

NEVI BLU. Il nevo blu comune è una papula solitaria, asintomatica, liscia, a cupola, di colore da blu a blu grigio e diametro <10 mm, che si presenta sul dorso di mani e piedi. Raramente tali nevi formano grandi placche. Il nevo blu è quasi sempre acquisito, spesso durante l'infanzia, ed è più comune nei soggetti di sesso femminile. Dal punto di vista microscopico, è caratterizzato da gruppi di melanociti fusiformi intensamente pigmentati nel derma. È un nevo benigno.

Il nevo blu cellulare ha tipicamente un diametro di 1-3 cm e si presenta più frequentemente sulle natiche e nell'area sacrococcigea. Oltre ai gruppi di melanociti dendritici dermici profondamente pigmentati, nel derma si osservano isole cellulari composte da grandi cellule fusiformi che possono estendersi al grasso sottocutaneo. Si può osservare un continuum istologico dai nevi blu ai nevi blu cellulari. Un nevo combinato è l'associazione di un nevo blu con un nevo melanocitico sovrastante.

Il colore blu-grigio caratteristico di questi nevi è un effetto ottico causato dalla melanina dermica. Le lunghezze d'onda maggiori della luce visibile penetrano fino al derma profondo, dove vengono assorbite dalla melanina; la luce blu con lunghezza d'onda più corta non riesce a penetrare in profondità e viene riflessa all'osservatore.

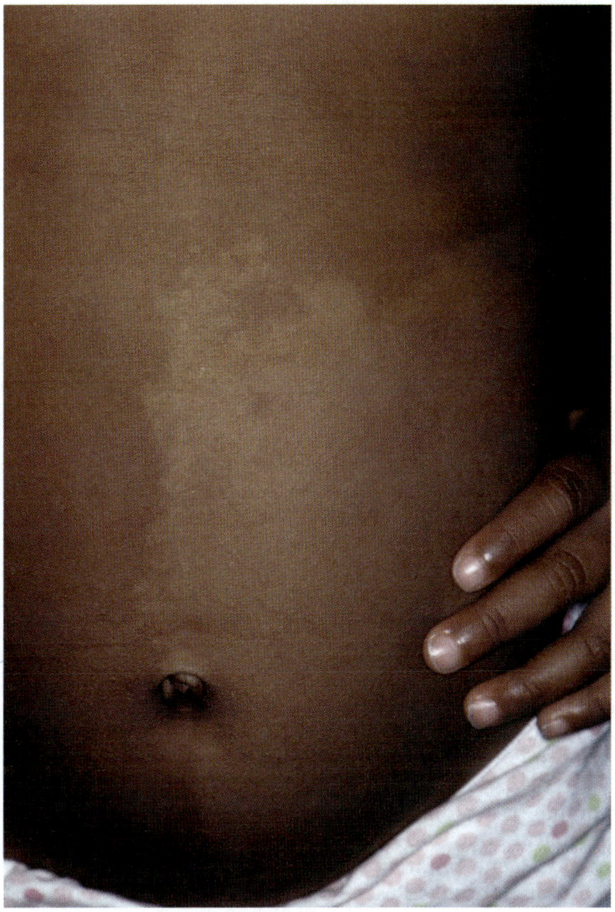

Figura 650-6. Grande nevo depigmentato dell'addome.

NEVUS DEPIGMENTOSUS (NEVO ACROMICO). In genere questi nevi sono presenti alla nascita; sono chiazze e striature ipopigmentate maculari localizzate, spesso con bordi bizzarri e irregolari (Fig. 650-6). Clinicamente possono somigliare all'ipomelanosi di Ito, tranne per il fatto che sono più localizzati e spesso unilaterali. Le lesioni piccole possono assomigliare, inoltre, alle macchie a "foglia di frassino" della sclerosi tuberosa. Sembra che rappresentino un difetto focale nel trasferimento di melanosomi ai cheratinociti.

NEVI EPIDERMICI. Possono essere visibili alla nascita oppure svilupparsi nei primi mesi o anni di vita. Interessano entrambi i sessi in uguale misura e di solito si presentano sporadicamente. Sono lesioni amartomatose caratterizzate da iperplasia dell'epidermide e/o degli annessi in un'area focale della cute.

Vengono classificati in diverse varianti, in base alla morfologia e all'estensione del nevo nonché alla struttura epidermica predominante. Il nevo epidermico inizialmente può apparire come una chiazza decolorata, leggermente squamosa che, con la maturazione, diviene più lineare, ispessita, verrucosa e iperpigmentata. Una distribuzione estesa e diffusa delle lesioni è detta *sistematizzata*, mentre una distribuzione estesa e bilaterale è detta *ittiosi istrice* (Fig. 650-7). I tipi morfologici comprendono papillomi pigmentati, spesso a distribuzione lineare; strie ipercheratosiche unilaterali che interessano un arto ed eventualmente una porzione del tronco; placche iperpigmentate vellutate e lesioni ipercheratosiche a spirale o marmorate in placche, localizzate o su aree estese del corpo lungo le linee di Blaschko. Una variante verrucosa lineare infiammatoria è marcatamente pruriginosa e tende a diventare eritematosa, desquamante e incrostata.

Il modello istologico evolve con la maturazione della lesione, ma un'iperplasia epidermica di vario grado è evidente in tutte

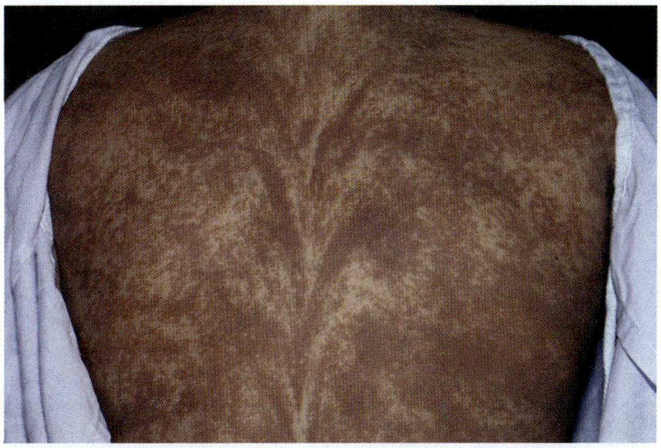

Figura 650-7. Nevo epidermico (ittiosi tipo istrice).

le fasi dello sviluppo. In una particolare lesione può prevalere l'uno o l'altro degli annessi dermici. Questi nevi vanno distinti dal lichen striatus, dal linfangioma circoscritto, dalle macchie zigrinate della sclerosi tuberosa, dai nevi pelosi congeniti, dalla porocheratosi lineare, dal lichen planus lineare, dalla psoriasi lineare, dallo stadio verrucoso dell'*incontinentia pigmenti* e dal nevo sebaceo (Jadassohn). Gli agenti cheratolitici come l'acido retinoico o l'acido salicilico possono essere moderatamente efficaci nel ridurre la desquamazione e nel controllare il prurito, ma il trattamento definitivo richiede un'escissione a tutto spessore; la recidiva è comune quando si tenta una rimozione più superficiale. In alternativa, il nevo può essere lasciato intatto. I nevi epidermici sono talvolta associati ad altre anomalie della cute e dei tessuti molli, degli occhi e degli apparati nervoso, cardiovascolare, muscoloscheletrico e urogenitale. In questi casi, definiti come sindrome del nevo epidermico, viene espresso un fenotipo a mosaico. Questa sindrome, tuttavia, non costituisce un'entità clinica distinta. Le sindromi ben definite che comprendono un tipo di nevo epidermico e anomalie definite alla nascita comprendono la sindrome di **Proteus** e la sindrome CHILD (emidisplasia congenita con eritroderma ittiosiforme e difetti agli arti).

Nevo sebaceo (Jadassohn). Si tratta di una placca relativamente piccola, nettamente demarcata, ovale o lineare, rilevata, di colore giallo-arancione, che generalmente appare glabra e si osserva sulla testa e sul collo dei neonati (Fig. 650-8). Occasionalmente può presentarsi sul tronco. Benché dal punto di vista istopatologico sia caratterizzata da un'abbondanza di ghiandole sebacee, presenta, di fatto, tutti gli elementi della cute. Nella prima infanzia il nevo sebaceo è frequentemente piatto e non evidente. Con la maturità, in genere durante l'adolescenza, le lesioni divengono verrucose e costellate da grossi noduli gommosi. Le variazioni dell'aspetto clinico riflettono il modello istologico, che è caratterizzato da un grado variabile di ipercheratosi, iperplasia dell'epidermide, follicoli piliferi malformati e spesso una profusione di ghiandole sebacee e presenza di ghiandole apocrine ectopiche. Si ritiene che questi nevi si formino da cellule staminali epiteliali primitive pluripotenziali, che possono differenziarsi in vari **tumori epiteliali**. Di conseguenza, durante l'età adulta, questi nevi sono spesso complicati da neoplasie maligne secondarie e tumori benigni degli annessi, soprattutto carcinomi basocellulari e siringocistoadenomi papilliferi. Nei nevi sebacei sono state osservate delezioni nel gene PTCH, il difetto del gene putativo nel carcinoma basocellulare. Il **trattamento di elezione** è l'escissione totale prima dell'adolescenza. I nevi sebacei associati a difetti del sistema nervoso centrale, scheletrici e oculari rappresentano una variante della sindrome del nevo epidermico.

Nevo di Becker (melanosi di Becker). Questa forma di nevo si riscontra soprattutto nei maschi, durante l'infanzia o l'adolescenza, inizialmente come macchia iperpigmentata. La lesione comunemente sviluppa ipertricosi, limitata all'area di iperpigmentazione, ed evolve in una placca unilaterale, leggermente ispessita, irregolare e iperpigmentata. Le sedi più comuni sono la parte superiore del dorso e del braccio (Fig. 650-9). Il nevo mostra un numero aumentato di melanociti basali e iperplasia epidermica variabile. La melanosi di Becker è comunemente associata ad amartoma del muscolo liscio, e può apparire come una leggera elevazione o un lieve indurimento delle papule perifollicolari. Sfregando le lesioni è possibile che si verifichi una contrazione del muscolo liscio con erezione dei peli. Il nevo è benigno, non vi è rischio di degenerazione maligna e raramente si associa ad altre anomalie.

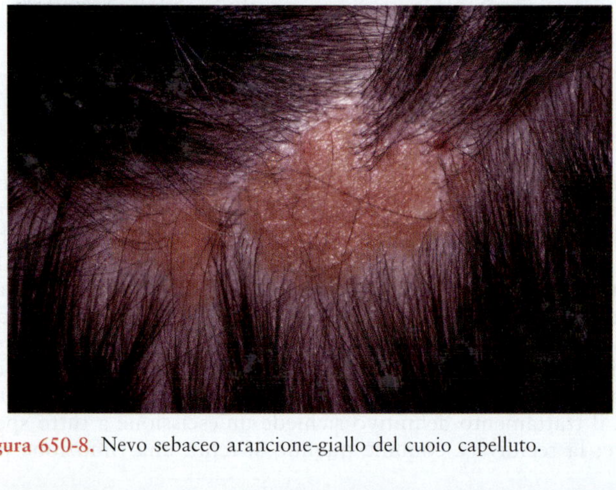

Figura 650-8. Nevo sebaceo arancione-giallo del cuoio capelluto.

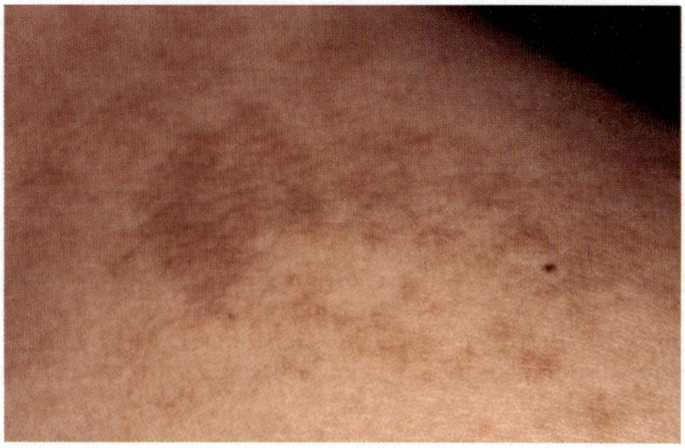

Figura 650-9. Nevo di Becker sulla spalla di un soggetto maschio adolescente.

NEVO COMEDONICO. Si tratta di un nevo organoide raro di origine epiteliale costituito da placche lineari di follicoli occlusi che simulano comedoni; i nevi comedonici possono essere presenti alla nascita o comparire durante l'infanzia. L'occlusione cornea rappresenta detriti cheratinosi all'interno dei follicoli pilosebacei dilatati e malformati. Le lesioni sono generalmente unilaterali e possono svilupparsi in qualsiasi sede. Raramente sono associate ad altre malformazioni congenite, tra cui difetti scheletrici, anomalie cerebrali e cataratta. Benché queste lesioni siano spesso asintomatiche, alcuni individui sperimentano infiammazione recidivante, che causa formazione di cisti, fistole e cicatrici. Non esiste una terapia efficace ad eccezione dell'asportazione a tutto spessore; una terapia palliativa di lesioni più estese può consistere nell'applicazione regolare di preparazioni a base di acido retinoico.

NEVI DEL TESSUTO CONNETTIVO. Si tratta di un amartoma di collagene, elastina e/o glicosaminoglicani della matrice extracellulare dermica. Può presentarsi come difetto solitario oppure come manifestazione di una malattia associata. Questi nevi possono manifestarsi in qualsiasi sede ma sono più comuni su schiena, natiche, braccia e cosce. Sono formati da placche color cute, avorio o giallo, di 2-15 cm di diametro, costituite da molte piccole papule o noduli raggruppati, spesso difficili da apprezzare visivamente a causa delle leggere variazioni di colore. Alla palpazione, le placche hanno una consistenza gommosa o ad acciottolato. I reperti bioptici sono variabili e includono aumento e/o degenerazione o frammentazione del collagene dermico, del tessuto elastico o della sostanza basale. Lesioni simili che compaiono nella sclerosi tuberosa sono definite macchie zigrinate; queste ultime tuttavia sono costituite solo da una quantità eccessiva di collagene. L'associazione di molti piccoli nevi papulari del tessuto connettivo con osteopoichilosi è definita dermatofibrosi lenticolare disseminata (**sindrome di Buschke Ollendorf**).

AMARTOMI DEL MUSCOLO LISCIO. Questo amartoma è un'anomalia dello sviluppo che deriva da iperplasia della muscolatura liscia (muscolo erettore del pelo) associata ai follicoli piliferi. Di solito risulta evidente alla nascita o subito dopo e si presenta come una placca color carne o leggermente pigmentata associata a ipertricosi sul tronco o sugli arti (Fig. 650-10). Talvolta, sfregando la superficie è possibile provocare un'elevazione transitoria o un'increspatura della lesione causate dalla contrazione dei fasci muscolari. L'amartoma del muscolo liscio può essere confuso con il nevo pigmentato congenito, ma la distinzione è importante poiché non comporta rischio di melanoma maligno e non deve essere rimosso.

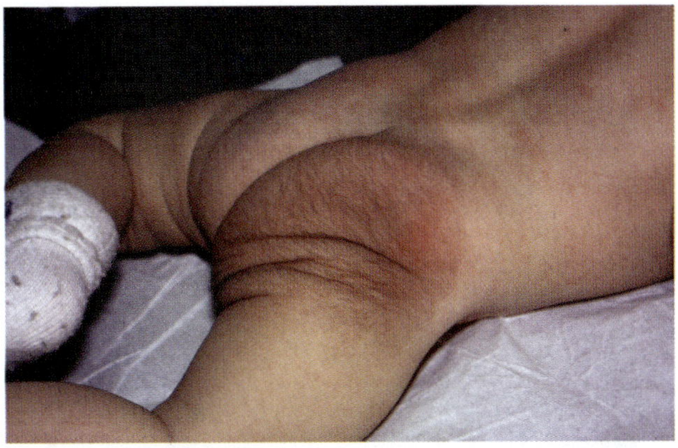

Figura 650-10. Grande amartoma del muscolo liscio sulla natica.

Bauer J, Garbe C: Acquired melanocytic nevi as risk factor for melanoma development. A comprehensive review of epidemiological data. *Pigment Cell Res* 2003;16:297–306.
Chan HH, Kono T: Nevus of Ota: Clinical aspects and management. *Skinmed* 2003;2:89–96.
Dahlstrom JE, Scolyer RA, Thompson JF, Jain S: Spitz naevus: Diagnostic problems and their management implications. *Pathology* 2004;36:452–457.
De Snoo FA, Bergman W, Gruis NA: Familial melanoma: A complex disorder leading to controversy of DNA testing. *Fam Cancer* 2003;2:109–116.
Ferrari A, Bono A, Baldi M, et al: Does melanoma behave differently in younger children than in adults? A retrospective study of 33 cases of childhood melanoma from a single institution. *Pediatrics* 2005;115:649–654.
Herron MD, Vanderhooft SL, Smock K, et al: Proliferative nodules in congenital melanocytic nevi: A clinicopathologic and immunohistochemical analysis. *Am J Surg Pathol* 2004;28:1017–1025.
Huynh PM, Glusac EJ, Bolognia JL: The clinical appearance of clonal nevi (inverted type A nevi). *Int J Dermatol* 2004;43:882–885.
Marghoob AA, Dusza S, Oliveria S, et al: Number of satellite nevi as a correlate for neurocutaneous melanocytosis in patients with large congenital melanocytic nevi. *Arch Dermatol* 2004;140:171–173.
Miller AJ, Mihm Jr. MC: Melanoma. *N Engl J Med* 2006;355:51–65.
Pappo AS: Melanoma in children and adolescents. *Eur J Cancer* 2003;39: 2651–2661.
Vidaurri-dela Cruz H, Tamayo-Sanchez L, Duran-McKinster C, et al. Epidermal nevus syndrome: Clinical findings in 35 patients. *Pediatr Dermatol* 2004;21:432–439.
Whiteman DC, Brown RM, Purdie DM, et al: Prevalence and anatomical distribution of naevi in young Queensland children. *Int J Cancer* 2003;106: 930–933.
Zaal LH, Mooi WJ, Klip H, Vander Horst CM: Risk of malignant transformation of congenital melanocytic nevi: a retrospective nationwide study from the Netherlands. *Plast Reconstr Surg* 2005;116:1902–1909.

Capitolo 651 ■ Lesioni iperpigmentate

Joseph G. Morelli

ALTERAZIONI DELLA PIGMENTAZIONE. La pigmentazione normale richiede la migrazione di melanoblasti dalla cresta neurale alla giunzione dermoepidermica, processi enzimatici per formare il pigmento, componenti strutturali per contenere il pigmento (melanosomi) e trasferimento del pigmento ai cheratinociti circostanti. L'iperpigmentazione cutanea può essere generalizzata o localizzata e può derivare da una varietà di difetti in ognuno dei processi elencati. Alcune di queste aberrazioni sono la manifestazione di una malattia sistemica, altre rappresentano difetti di sviluppo generalizzati o focali e altri ancora possono essere aspecifici oppure derivare da un'infiammazione cutanea.

EFELIDI. Si tratta di macule marrone chiaro o scuro, generalmente con diametro <3 mm e margine scarsamente definito, che si presentano nelle aree esposte al sole come il volto, la parte superiore del dorso, le braccia e le mani. Sono indotte dall'esposizione al sole, in particolare durante l'estate, e possono sbiadire o scomparire durante l'inverno. Sono più comuni nei soggetti con capelli rossi e biondi e fanno la prima apparizione in età prescolare. Dal punto di vista istologico, sono caratterizzate da un aumento del pigmento melanina nelle cellule epidermiche basali, che presentano processi dendritici più numerosi e più grandi rispetto ai melanociti della cute circostante che risulta più chiara. La mancanza di proliferazione melanocitica o il prolungamento delle creste interpapillari epidermiche le distingue dalle lentiggini. Le efelidi sono state identificate come fattore di rischio per il melanoma indipendentemente dai nevi melanocitici.

LENTIGGINI. Le **lentiggini**, spesso confuse con le efelidi o i nevi giunzionali, sono piccole (<3 cm) macule rotonde di colore marrone scuro, che possono comparire su qualsiasi parte del corpo. Non sono correlate all'esposizione al sole e sono permanenti. Dal punto di vista istologico, presentano un allungamento delle creste interpapillari epidermiche, a bastoncello, con un numero aumentato di melanociti e depositi epidermici densi di melanina. Non si osservano nidi di melanociti. Le lesioni sono benigne e, se limitate, possono essere considerate una manifestazione normale.

La **lentigginosi profusa** è costituita da innumerevoli piccole macchie pigmentate che sono presenti alla nascita o compaiono durante l'infanzia. Non si associa ad alcuna anomalia e le membrane mucose vengono risparmiate. La **sindrome di LAMB** (complesso di Carney), una patologia neoplastica endocrina multipla, è caratterizzata dalla presenza di lentiggini su viso e vulva, mixoma atriale, mixomi mucocutanei e nevi blu (gene PRKAR1). La **sindrome delle lentiggini multiple (LEOPARD)** è una malattia autosomica dominante che consiste nella distribuzione generalizzata e simmetrica di lentiggini (Fig. 651-1) associata ad anomalie all'elettrocardiogramma, ipertelorismo oculare, stenosi polmonare, anomalie dei genitali (criptorchidismo, ipogonadismo, ipospadia), ritardo di crescita e sordità neurosensoriale (gene PTPN11). Altri tratti includono miocardiopatia ipertrofica ostruttiva e pectus excavatum o carenato.

La **sindrome di Peutz-Jeghers** è caratterizzata da macule melanotiche sulle labbra e sulle membrane mucose e da poliposi gastrointestinale (GI). Viene ereditata come tratto autosomico dominante (gene STK11). L'insorgenza si osserva nel periodo neonatale e nella prima infanzia, quando sulle labbra e sulla mucosa buccale compaiono macule pigmentate. In genere il diametro delle macule è di pochi millimetri, ma può arrivare fino a 1-2 cm. Qualche volta le chiazze compaiono anche su palato, gengive, lingua e mucosa vaginale. Lesioni cutanee possono svilupparsi su naso, mani e piedi, attorno a bocca, occhi e ombelico, e possono apparire sotto forma di bande longitudinali o ipopigmentazione

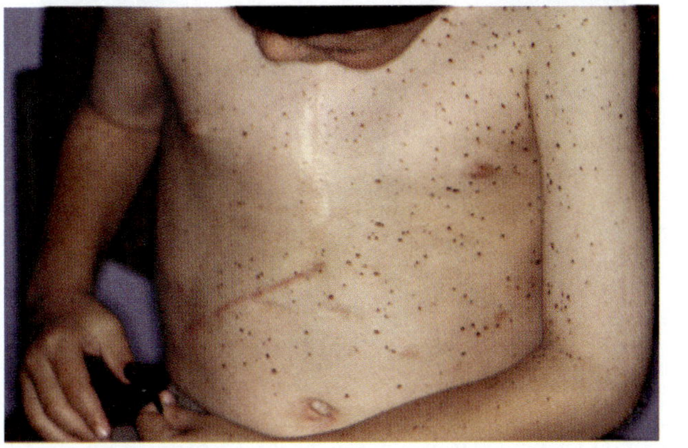

Figura 651-1. Lentiggini multiple nella sindrome LEOPARD.

diffusa delle unghie. Le macule pigmentate spesso scompaiono dalle labbra e dalle cute, durante la pubertà e in età adulta, mentre generalmente permangono sulle superfici mucose. Le macule mucose buccali sono il tratto più costante della malattia; in alcune famiglie, tuttavia, si hanno membri affetti esclusivamente da alterazioni del pigmento. Minime variazioni di pigmentazione, che compaiono in età adulta, senza coinvolgimento intestinale, si verificano sporadicamente.

Solitamente, la poliposi interessa il digiuno e l'ileo ma può presentarsi anche nello stomaco, nel duodeno, nel colon e nel retto (vedi Capitolo 342). Dolore addominale episodico, diarrea, melena e intussuscezione sono complicazioni frequenti. I pazienti presentano un rischio significativamente aumentato di sviluppare, in giovane età, sia tumori del tratto gastrointestinale sia altre neoplasie. Il cancro gastrointestinale è stato riscontrato in circa il 2-3% dei pazienti; il rischio relativo di neoplasia maligna del tratto gastrointestinale è pari a 13, mentre il rischio relativo di altre neoplasie maligne, tra cui tumori ovarici, cervicali e testicolari, è pari a 9. La sindrome di Peutz-Jeghers deve essere distinta da altre sindromi associate a lentiggini multiple (sindrome di Laugier-Hunziker), dalle comuni efelidi, dalla sindrome di Gardner e dalla sindrome di Cronkhite-Canada, una malattia caratterizzata da poliposi gastrointestinale, alopecia, onicodistrofia e pigmentazione diffusa dei palmi, degli aspetti volari delle dita e del dorso delle mani. In alcuni casi, il **trattamento** delle macule melanotiche di Peutz-Jeghers ha dato esiti positivi con più laser differenti.

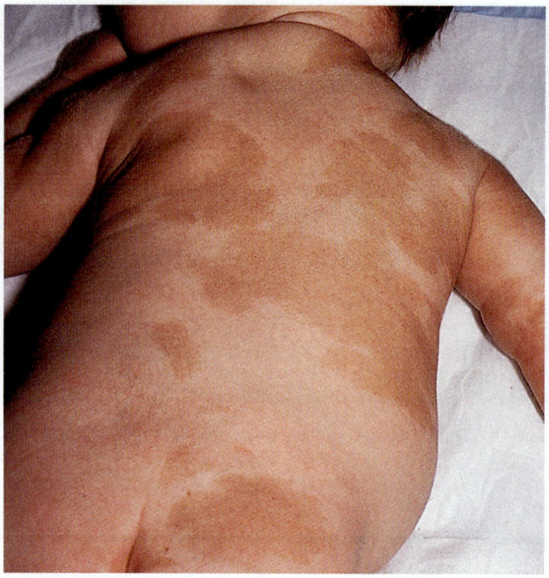

Figura 651-3. Macchie caffelatte multiple in un bambino con sindrome di McCune-Albright. (Da Eichenfield LF, Frieden IJ, Esterly NB: *Textbook of Neonatal Dermatology*. Philadelphia, WB Saunders, 2001, p 373.)

MACCHIE CAFFELATTE. Sono lesioni maculari uniformemente iperpigmentate e nettamente demarcate, con tonalità che variano in base al grado di pigmentazione del soggetto interessato: sono color bronzo o marrone chiaro nei bambini di razza bianca e possono essere scure in quelli di razza nera (Figg. 651-2 e 651-3). Le macchie caffelatte variano moltissimo per dimensioni; possono essere grandi e coprire una parte significativamente ampia del tronco o degli arti. I bordi sono generalmente uniformi, ma talvolta si presentano molto irregolari. Le lesioni sono caratterizzate da un numero aumentato di melanociti e melanina nell'epidermide ma mancano le creste reticolate a bastoncello tipiche delle lentiggini. Da una a tre macchie caffelatte sono comuni nei bambini normali; circa il 10% dei bambini sani, infatti, ha questo tipo di macchie. Esse possono essere presenti alla nascita oppure svilupparsi durante l'infanzia.

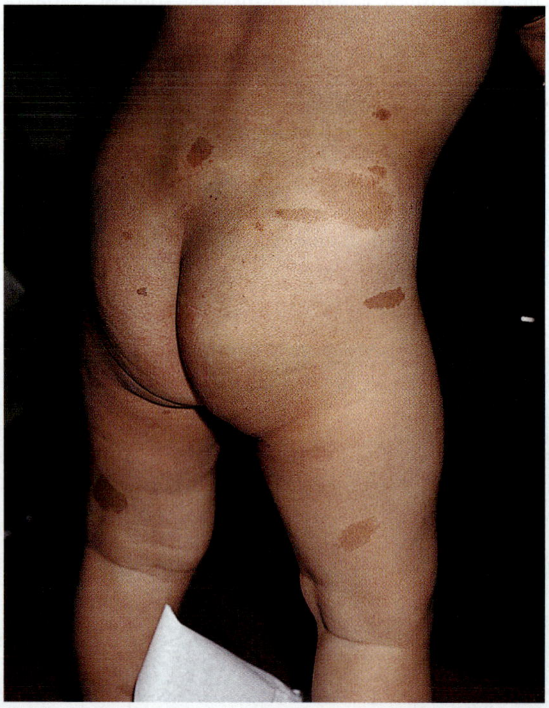

Figura 651-2. Macchie caffelatte multiple su un bambino con NF-1. (Da Eichenfield LF, Frieden IJ, Esterly NB: *Textbook of Neonatal Dermatology*. Philadelphia, WB Saunders, 2001, p 372.)

Le macchie caffelatte grandi e spesso asimmetriche, con bordi irregolari, sono caratteristiche dei pazienti con la sindrome di McCune-Albright (gene GNAS1) (vedi Capitolo 563.6) una patologia che comprende displasia fibrosa poliostotica, che conduce a fratture patologiche, pubertà precoce e numerose endocrinopatie iperfunzionali. L'iperpigmentazione maculare può essere presente alla nascita o svilupparsi nella tarda infanzia(vedi Fig. 651-3). La pigmentazione cutanea è tipicamente più estesa sul lato con l'interessamento osseo più grave.

Neurofibromatosi di tipo 1 (malattia di von Recklinghausen). La macchia caffelatte è il segno cutaneo distintivo più comune di questa sindrome neurocutanea autosomica dominante (gene della neurofibromina) (vedi Fig. 651-2; Capitolo 596.1). Lesioni simili si manifestano anche in altre malattie, tra cui ulteriori tipi di neurofibromatosi, ma in queste altre patologie le macchie caffelatte non sono il tratto saliente del disturbo e pertanto non sono diagnostiche (Tab. 651-1). La presenza di 5 o più macchie caffelatte di diametro >5 mm in bambini in età prepuberale oppure di 6 o più macchie caffelatte di diametro >15 mm in pazienti di età postpuberale costituisce criterio di diagnosi. Le macchie caffelatte multiple producono comunemente un aspetto lentigginoso delle aree non esposte al sole come le ascelle (segno di Crowe), le regioni inguinale e inframammaria e l'area sotto il mento.

INCONTINENTIA PIGMENTI (MALATTIA DI BLOCH-SULZBERGER). Questa rara malattia, multisistemica, ectodermica ed ereditaria comprende anomalie dermatologiche, dentali e oculari. Il fenotipo è prodotto da mosaicismo funzionale provocato da inattivazione X casuale di un gene dominante legato al cromosoma X che è letale nei maschi (gene IKK-gamma/NEMO). Questa supposizione è sostenuta dalla rarità di soggetti maschi affetti, dalla trasmissione da femmina a femmina e dall'elevata frequenza di aborti spontanei nelle femmine portatrici.

Manifestazioni cliniche. La malattia comprende quattro fasi, ma non è detto che compaiano tutte in uno stesso paziente. La **prima fase** è evidente alla nascita o nelle prime settimane di vita e consiste nella presenza di strie lineari eritematose e di placche vescicolose (Fig. 651-4), che sono più pronunciate sugli arti e sulla circonferenza del tronco. Le lesioni possono essere confuse con quelle

TABELLA 651-1. Malattie con macchie caffelatte

Neurofibromatosi 1 e 2
Sindrome di McCune-Albright
Sindrome di Silver-Russel
Atassia teleangiectasica
Anemia di Fanconi
Sclerosi tuberosa
Sindrome di Bloom
Sindrome nel nevo basocellulare
Malattia di Gaucher
Sindrome di Chédiak-Higashi
Sindrome di Hunter
Sindrome di Maffucci
Sindrome del neuroma mucosale multiplo
Sindrome di Watson
Sindrome di Proteus
Sindrome di Turner
Sindrome con cromosoma ad anello
Sindrome di Jaffe-Campanacci

dell'*herpes simplex*, dell'impetigine bollosa o della mastocitosi, ma la configurazione lineare è altamente specifica. Dal punto di vista istopatologico sono presenti edema epidermico e vescicole intraepidermiche piene di **eosinofili**. Gli eosinofili infiltrano anche l'epidermide adiacente e il derma. È comune un'eosinofilia ematica fino al 65% della conta leucocitaria. In generale, la prima fase si risolve entro il quarto mese di età, sebbene si possano verificare ricadute con la comparsa di recidive di breve durata nel corso di malattie febbrili. Nella **seconda fase**, mano a mano che le vescicole sugli arti distali si risolvono, diventano secche e ipercheratotiche e formano placche verrucose. Tali placche raramente interessano il tronco o il viso e in genere regrediscono entro 6 mesi. Sono caratteristiche l'iperplasia epidermica, l'ipercheratosi e la papillomatosi. La **terza fase o fase pigmentaria** rappresenta l'elemento distintivo dell'*incontinentia pigmenti*. Generalmente si sviluppa nell'arco di settimane o mesi e può sovrapporsi alle fasi precedenti, essere evidente alla nascita o, più comunemente, manifestarsi nelle prime settimane di vita. L'iperpigmentazione è più spesso evidente sul tronco che sugli arti ed è distribuita in spirali maculari, chiazze reticolate, macchie e strie lineari che seguono le linee di Baschko. Le ascelle e l'inguine sono sempre interessati. Le sedi coinvolte non sono necessariamente quelle precedentemente interessate dalle lesioni vescicolari e verrucose. Le lesioni pigmentate, una volta presenti, persistono per tutta l'infanzia. Generalmente cominciano a sbiadire nella prima adolescenza e spesso si risolvono entro i 16 anni. Talvolta la pigmentazione resta permanentemente, soprattutto nella regione inguinale. Dal punto di vista istopatologico, la lesione presenta degenerazione vacuolare delle cellule basali dell'epidermide e melanina nei melanofagi del derma superiore, quale conseguenza dell'incontinenza del pigmento. Nella **quarta fase**, quale manifestazione tardiva dell'*incontinentia pigmenti*, si hanno macchie o strie glabre, anidrotiche e ipopigmentate che possono svilupparsi anche prima che si sia risolta l'iperpigmentazione della terza fase. Le lesioni compaiono principalmente sul lato flessore delle gambe e meno frequentemente sulle braccia e sul tronco.

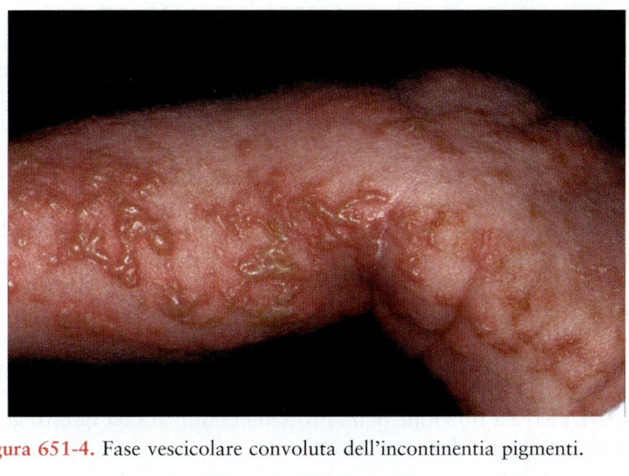

Figura 651-4. Fase vescicolare convoluta dell'incontinentia pigmenti.

Circa l'80% dei bambini colpiti presenta anche altre anomalie. L'alopecia, che può causare cicatrici, essere a chiazze o diffusa, è più frequente sul vertice e si manifesta fino nel 40% dei pazienti. I capelli possono essere privi di lucentezza, ispidi e ruvidi. Le anomalie dentali, che sono presenti fino nell'80% dei pazienti, persistono per tutta la vita e sono costituite da dentizione tardiva, ipodonzia, denti conici e inclusione. Manifestazioni a carico del sistema nervoso centrale, tra cui ritardo dello sviluppo cognitivo e motorio, convulsioni, microcefalia, spasticità e paralisi, si osservano fino in un terzo dei bambini interessati. Anomalie oculari, come neovascolarizzazione, microftalmo, strabismo, atrofia del nervo ottico, cataratta e masse retrolenticolari, si presentano in più del 30% dei bambini. Ciononostante, più del 90% dei pazienti ha un'acuità visiva normale. Tra le alterazioni meno comuni figurano la distrofia ungueale (presenza di croste, fossette) e difetti scheletrici.

La diagnosi di *incontinentia pigmenti* viene formulata su basi cliniche, benché siano stati definiti criteri maggiori e minori a sostegno della diagnosi. L'esame alla lampada di Wood può essere utile nei bambini più grandi e negli adolescenti per evidenziare le anomalie del pigmento.

Trattamento. Poiché le lesioni cutanee sono benigne, la scelta delle indagini strumentali e la pianificazione della terapia dipendono dalla presenza di particolari anomalie non cutanee. L'elevata incidenza di anomalie maggiori associate richiede una consulenza genetica.

ALTERAZIONI DEL PIGMENTO POSTINFIAMMATORIE. L'infiammazione cutanea può essere causa di iperpigmentazione o ipopigmentazione. In genere, l'alterazione del pigmento fa seguito a una reazione infiammatoria grave, ma può derivare anche da una dermatite lieve. I bambini con carnagione scura hanno una maggiore probabilità di andare incontro a queste alterazioni rispetto a quelli con carnagione chiara. Benché la pigmentazione alterata possa persistere per settimane o mesi, è possibile rassicurare i pazienti sul fatto che queste lesioni siano in genere temporanee.

Amos CL, Keitheri-Cheteri MB, Sabripour M, et al: Genotype-phenotype correlations in Peutz-Jeughers syndrome. *J Med Genet* 2004;41:327–333.

Bruckner AL: Incontinentia pigmenti: A window to the role of NF-kappaB function. *Semin Cutan Med Surg* 2004;23:116–124.

De Schepper S, Boucneau J, Lambert J, et al: Pigment cell-related manifestations in neurofibromatosis type 1: An overview. *Pigment Cell Res* 2005; 18:13–24.

Listernick R, Charrow J: Neurofibromatosis-1 in childhood. *Adv Dermatol* 2004;20:75–115.

Lumbroso S, Paris F, Sultan C: McCune-Albright syndrome: Molecular genetics. *J Pediatr Endocrinol Metab* 2002;15(Suppl 3):875–882.

Sandrini F, Stratakis C: Clinical and molecular genetics of Carney complex. *Mol Genet Metab* 2003;78:83–92.

Sarkozy A, Conti E, Diglio MC, et al: Clinical and molecular analysis of 30 patients with multiple lentigines LEOPARD syndrome. *J Med Genet* 2004;41:e68.

Capitolo 652 ■ Lesioni ipopigmentate

Joseph G. Morelli

ALBINISMO. I diversi tipi di albinismo oculocutaneo congenito (OCA, *OculoCutaneous Albinism*) sono caratterizzati da assenza parziale o completa di produzione di melanina in cute, peli e occhi, nonostante la presenza di melanociti normali per numero, struttura e distribuzione. Si possono dividere in due classi principali: quelli con anomalia funzionale delle proteine coinvolte nella formazione e nel trasferimento della melanina, e quelli con difetti dei melanosomi (Tab. 652-1). La tirosinasi è un enzima contenente rame, che catalizza varie fasi della biosintesi di melanina (vedi Capitolo 85.2). Le varianti tirosinasi-positive sono caratterizzate da scurimento del bulbo pilifero all'incubazione con tirosina.

OCA1. L'OCA1 è caratterizzato da un'attività tirosinasica molto ridotta o assente. **L'OCA1A** , la forma più severa, è caratterizzato dall'assenza di pigmento visibile nei capelli, nella cute e negli occhi (Fig. 652-1); si manifesta con fotofobia, nistagmo, acuità visiva ridotta, capelli bianchi e cute bianca. Le iridi sono blu-grigie alla luce obliqua e rosa intenso alla luce riflessa. **L'OCA1B**, o albinismo mutante giallo, si presenta alla nascita con capelli bianchi, cute rosa e occhi grigi. Questo tipo ha una prevalenza particolarmente elevata nella comunità Amish. Progressivamente, tuttavia, i capelli divengono giallo-rossi, la cute si scurisce leggermente con l'esposizione al sole e le iridi possono accumulare un po' di pigmento marrone, con un risultante miglioramento nell'acuità visiva. Sono presenti fotofobia e nistagmo moderati. **L'OCATS** è un tipo di albinismo sensibile alla temperatura. La tirosinasi anomala ha un'attività ridotta a 35-37 °C. Pertanto, le regioni più fredde del corpo, come gli arti e la testa, si pigmentano in una certa misura, mentre altre aree restano depigmentate.

L'**OCA2** varia da un fenotipo quasi normale a un albinismo molto simile al tipo 1. Si tratta della forma più comune di albinismo osservata in tutto il mondo. La melanina presente alla nascita è minima o assente, ma il pigmento, in particolare quello rosso-giallo, può accumularsi durante l'infanzia, e conferire alla cure una colorazione giallo paglia o leggermente scura, nei soggetti di razza bianca. Possono svilupparsi nevi pigmentati. Con l'età, si verifica un progressivo miglioramento dell'acuità visiva e del nistagmo. I pazienti di razza nera possono presentare una colorazione giallo-bruna della cute, efelidi marrone scuro nelle aree esposte al sole e una colorazione bruna delle iridi. **L'OCA bruno** è una variante allelica dell'OCA2. Le sindromi di Prader-Willi e di Angelma, che comprendono anche ipopigmentazione, hanno delezioni che coinvolgono il gene dell'OCA2.

OCA3 (ROSSASTRO). L'OCA3 si osserva prevalentemente nei pazienti di origine asiatica. È caratterizzato da capelli rossi, cute bruno-rossastra, nevi pigmentati, efelidi, occhi da rosso-brunastri a bruni, nistagmo, fotofobia e ridotta acuità visiva.

TABELLA 652-1. Geni associati a ipopigmentazione

DISORDINE	DIFETTO GENETICO
Albinismo oculocutaneo	
OCA1	Tirosinasi
OCA2	Proteina P
OCA3	TRP-1
OCA4	MATP
Sindrome di Hermansky-Pudlak	
Tipo 1	HPS-1 Topo (orecchio pallido)
Tipo 2	Subunità HPS-2 b3A della AP3
Tipo 3	HPS-3 Topo (color cacao)
Tipo 4	HPS-4 Topo (orecchio chiaro)
Tipo 5	HPS-5 Topo (occhio rosso 2)
Tipo 6	HPS-6 Topo (occhio rosso)
Sindrome di Chédiak-Higashi	CHS1/LYST
Piebaldismo	Recettore C-KIT
	Eterozigosi per SLUG
Sindrome di Waardenburg	
Tipo 1	Eterozigosi per PAX-3
Tipo 2	MITF
Tipo 3	Omozigosi per PAX-3
Tipo 4	SOX-10
	Endotelina 3
	Recettore dell'endotelina B

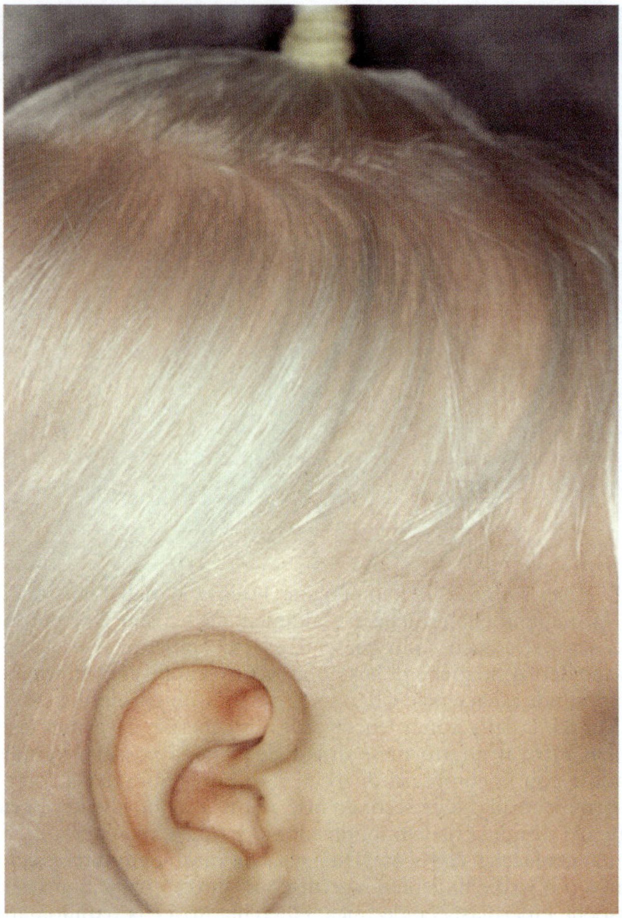

Figura 652-1. Cute e capelli bianchi nell'albinismo oculocutaneo di tipo 1 (OCA1).

OCA4. È una rara forma di OCA con reperti clinici simili alla OCA2.

La **sindrome di Cross-McKusick-Breen** è una forma di albinismo tirosinasi-positivo, con anomalie oculari, ritardo, spasticità e atetosi. Il difetto genetico non è stato identificato.

A causa dell'assenza della normale protezione da parte di quantità adeguate di melanina epidermica, i soggetti con albinismo sono predisposti a sviluppare cheratosi attinica e carcinomi cutanei, secondari al danno cutaneo causato dai raggi ultravioletti. I pazienti con questa patologia dovrebbero indossare indumenti protettivi e applicare creme ad alta protezione (vedi Capitolo 655), durante l'esposizione alla luce solare.

OCA CON ANOMALIE MELANOSOMIALI (VEDI TAB. 652-1). La **sindrome di Hermansky-Pudlak** è un insieme di disordini genetici, autosomici recessivi, caratterizzati da albinismo oculocutaneo, accumulo di ceroide nei lisosomi e sanguinamento prolungato. Nei topi sono attualmente riconosciuti 16 loci genetici distinti, che producono fenotipi mutanti per il colore della pelliccia, associati a difetti piastrinici. Nell'uomo, sono stati identificati sei di questi deficit.

La **sindrome di Chédiak-Higashi** (CHS; vedi Capitolo 129) è un altra anomalia genetica associata a disfunzione degli organelli correlati ai lisosomi. I pazienti con la CHS presentano ipopigmentazione della cute, degli occhi e dei capelli; tempo di emorragia prolungato e predisposizione agli ematomi; infezioni ricorrenti; alterazione della funzione dei linfociti natural killer; neuropatia periferica. La CHS è causata da mutazione del gene CHS1/LYST. La funzione della proteina codificata da questo gene non è attualmente ben conosciuta.

ANOMALIE DELLA MIGRAZIONE DEI MELANOBLASTI (VEDI TAB. 652-1)

PIEBALDISMO. Questo disturbo congenito autosomico dominante è caratterizzato da chiazze amelanotiche nettamente demarcate, che colpiscono più frequentemente la fronte, la parte anteriore del cuoio capelluto (dando luogo a una ciocca bianca sulla fronte), il tronco ventrale, i gomiti e le ginocchia. Possono essere presenti isole di pigmentazione normale o più scura della norma all'interno delle aree amelanotiche (Fig. 652-2). Le placche sono il risultato dell'assenza localizzata e permanente dei melanociti. Il quadro di depigmentazione deriva da un difetto di migrazione dei melanoblasti dalla cresta neurale, durante lo sviluppo. La ragione per cui il piebaldismo è un processo localizzato e non generalizzato resta sconosciuta. Il piebaldismo deve essere differenziato dalla vitiligine, che può essere progressiva e non è abitualmente congenita, dal nevo acromico, e dalla sindrome di Waardenburg.

SINDROME DI WAARDENBURG. Anche la sindrome di Waardenburg si presenta, alla nascita, con aree localizzate di cute e capelli depigmentati. Ne esistono quattro tipi. La caratteristica del tipo 1 è la presenza di un ciuffo bianco sulla fronte, che si osserva nel 20-60% dei pazienti. Solo il 15% dei soggetti colpiti ha aree di cute depigmentata. La sordità si verifica nel 9-37%, l'eterocromia dell'iride nel 20% e il monosopracciglio (*synophrys*) nel 17-69%. In tutti i pazienti con sindrome di Waardenburg di tipo 1 si osserva *dystopia cantorum*. La Waardenburg di tipo 2 è simile a quella di tipo 1, salvo il fatto che nel tipo 2 non si evidenzia *dystopia cantorum* e si verifica una maggiore incidenza di sordità. La sindrome di Waardenburg di tipo 3, detta anche sindrome di Klein-Waardenburg, è simile alla Waardenburg di tipo 1, salvo il fatto che i pazienti presentano anche anomalie degli arti. La Waardenburg di tipo 4 è chiamata anche sindrome di Shah-Waardenburg. I soggetti colpiti hanno tutti il morbo di Hirschsprung. La *dystopia cantorum* è osservata di rado in questi pazienti.

COMPLESSO DELLA SCLEROSI TUBEROSA (GENI TSC1, TSC2, TUBEROS SCLEROSIS COMPLEX) (VEDI CAPITOLO 596.2). Si tratta di una malattia multisistemica, che colpisce prevalentemente i tessuti derivati dall'ectoderma, ma che coinvolge anche gli organi di origine mesodermica ed endodermica, in particolare gli occhi, i reni e il cuore. La **classica triade clinica** è data da lesioni cutanee in associazione a epilessia e ritardo mentale.

Eziologia ed epidemiologia. È una patologia autosomica dominante, osservata in circa 1/300 000 persone, con una penetranza di circa il 100%. Il prodotto del TSC2 è la tuberina, che ha un'omologia di sequenza con una proteina attivante la GTPasi e che può avere un ruolo nella regolazione della crescita cellulare, agendo come gene soppressore della crescita. IL TSC1 (amartina) è ritenuto agire come soppressore della crescita. Circa il 60% dei casi è dovuto a nuove mutazioni.

Manifestazioni cliniche. I quattro principali **segni diagnostici** della TSC sono manifestazioni cutanee. Le lesioni a **foglia di frassino**, singole o multiple, si osservano più spesso sul tronco (Fig. 652-3), ma insorgono anche sul volto e sugli arti. Possono inoltre essere presenti piccole macule ipopigmentate, simili a confetti, che rappresentano aree localizzate di melanizzazione inadeguata. Le lesioni ipopigmentate possono essere presenti alla nascita o insorgere nei primi mesi di vita e possono essere difficilmente apprezzabili nei bambini dalla cute più chiara. Gli **angiogiofibromi** sono i marcatori cutanei della sclerosi tuberosa più comunemente osservati; le lesioni compaiono sul volto a partire dalla prima infanzia. Queste papule rosso-brune o color carne, lisce, brillanti, teleangiectasiche, di 1-10 mm, possono estendersi dal solco nasolabiale, alle guance e al collo (Fig. 652-4). La presenza di teleangiectasie e la mancanza di comedoni e di pustole aiuta a distinguere questa eruzione dall'acne volgare. Simili noduli fibromatosi possono essere sparsi sulla fronte, sul tronco e sugli arti. Nella zona lombosacrale, si possono osservare grosse placche del colore della cute, irregolarmente ispessite, con una pellicola arancione o una trama ad acciottolato (nevi del tessuto connettivo/ **macchie a pelle di zigrino**). Queste sono presenti alla nascita, ma la maggior parte dei pazienti con nevi del tessuto connettivo non ha una TSC. Con la pubertà, emergono fibromi periugueali duri, color carne, nelle pliche ungueali di alcuni bambini (Fig. 652-5); possono anche insorgere fibromi gengivali, non associati alla somministrazione di farmaci anticonvulsivanti. Le macchie caffe-

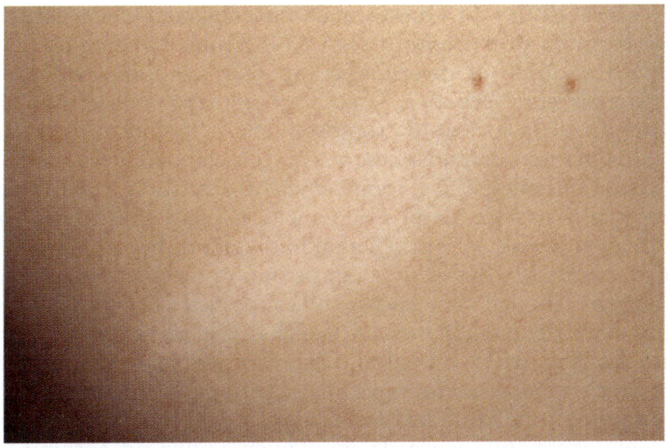

Figura 652-3. Macule a foglia di frassino nel complesso della sclerosi tuberosa (TSC).

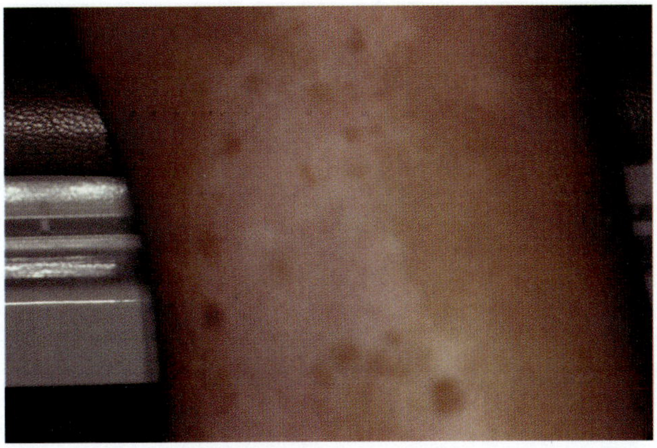

Figura 652-2. Macule depigmentate con isole di iperpigmentazione nel piebaldismo.

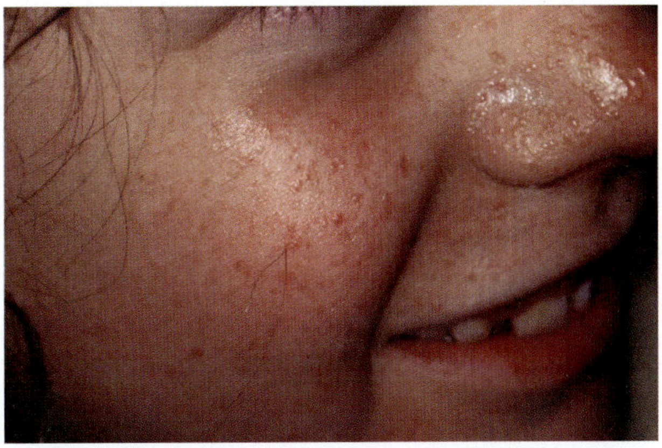

Figura 652-4. Angiofibromi faciali nel complesso della sclerosi tuberosa (TSC).

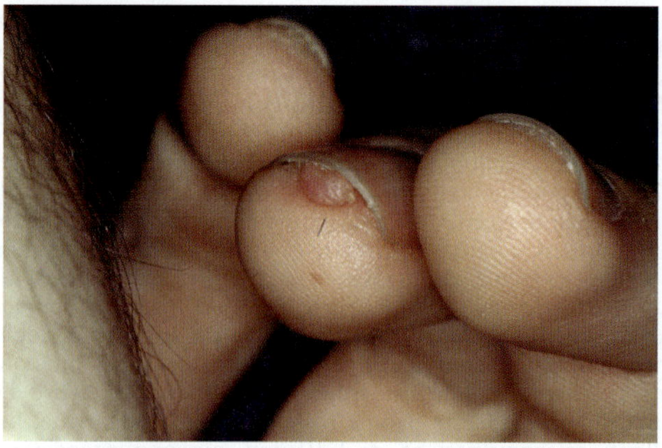

Figura 652-5. Fibromi periungueali nel complesso della sclerosi tuberosa (TSC).

latte insorgono con maggiore frequenza, ma non sono numerose come nella neurofibromatosi. Il deficit mentale colpisce il 60-70% dei pazienti; quasi tutti sono epilettici. L'epilessia si osserva anche in circa il 70% dei pazienti senza ritardo mentale; esordisce nella prima infanzia, o poco dopo, e spesso si aggrava progressivamente. Nel 50% dei lattanti affetti, sono presenti **rabdomiomi** cardiaci, che regrediscono di solito spontaneamente; l'ostruzione meccanica è una complicanza inusuale. Raramente, il sintomo di presentazione della sclerosi tuberosa è l'ematuria, causata da un **angiolipoma renale**, che è caratteristico di questa patologia.

IPOMELANOSI DI ITO. Questa malattia congenita della cute colpisce bambini di entrambi i sessi ed è frequentemente associata a difetti a carico di diversi apparati. Non vi sono evidenze di una trasmissione genetica; sono stati riportati mosaicismo cromosomico e traslocazioni cromosomiche. L'ipomelanosi di Ito è attualmente una diagnosi descrittiva, più che definitiva.

Le lesioni cutanee, nell'ipomelanosi di Ito, sono generalmente presenti alla nascita ma possono anche essere acquisite nei primi 2 anni di vita; esse sono simili a un'immagine al negativo di quelle dell'*incontinentia pigmenti*, e consistono in macule ipopigmentate, bizzarre, modellate, disposte sulla superficie corporea in volute nettamente demarcate, strie o macchie che seguono le linee di Blaschko (Fig. 652-6). I palmi delle mani, le piante dei piedi e le membrane mucose sono risparmiati. L'ipopigmentazione rimane invariata durante l'infanzia, ma scompare nell'età adulta. Il grado di depigmentazione varia da ipopigmentazione ad acromia. Lo sviluppo di alterazioni pigmentarie non è preceduto da lesioni infiammatorie, né vescicolari, come avviene nell'*incontinentia pigmenti*. Le aree ipopigmentate mostrano melanociti più piccoli e in numero inferiore, oltre che un numero ridotto di granuli di melanina nello strato basale della cellula, rispetto alla norma. Sono assenti cellule infiammatorie e *incontinentia pigmenti*.

Le anomalie associate più comuni coinvolgono il sistema nervoso e comprendono ritardo mentale (70%), convulsioni (40%), microcefalia (25%) e ipotonia muscolare (15%). Il sistema muscoloscheletrico è il secondo coinvolto in ordine di frequenza, con comparsa di scoliosi e deformità toraciche e degli arti. Nel 25% dei pazienti sono presenti anomalie oftalmologiche minori (strabismo, nistagmo), e nel 10% disturbi cardiaci. La diagnosi differenziale comprende il nevo depigmentoso sistematizzato, che è una leucodermia stabile non associata a manifestazioni sistemiche. La differenziazione dall'*incontinentia pigmenti*, in particolare nel quarto stadio ipopigmentato, è critica per il counseling genetico, poiché questa, a differenza della melanosi di Ito, è ereditaria.

VITILIGINE

Epidemiologia ed eziologia. La patogenesi della vitiligine non è nota. È stato suggerito che i melanociti vengano distrutti a causa dell'accumulo di intermedi tossici della sintesi della melanina. Vi sono prove in vitro che alcuni di questi metaboliti possano essere letali per i melanociti.

Una seconda ipotesi suggerisce che fattori neurochimici danneggino i melanociti e causino depigmentazione; il che spiegherebbe il pattern di coinvolgimento della vitiligine segmentaria, che segue approssimativamente il decorso di un dermatomero.

Una terza ipotesi, forse la più importante, suggerisce che anomalie immunologiche siano responsabili delle alterazioni della vitiligine. L'80% dei pazienti con malattia attiva ha anticorpi contro un antigene di superficie delle cellule pigmentate di melanoma. Questi autoanticorpi sembrano essere citotossici per i melanociti. Vi è anche una correlazione tra l'attività della malattia e il titolo di anticorpi sierici antimelanociti. Le forme genetiche di vitiligine sono probabilmente correlate alla forma immunologica. Sono stati identificati diversi loci di suscettibilità alla vitiligine (AIS1, AIS2, AIS3, SLEV1).

Manifestazioni cliniche. Vi sono due sottotipi di vitiligine: generalizzata (tipo A) e localizzata (tipo B), che sono probabilmente due malattie distinte. In circa il 50% di tutti i pazienti con vitiligine, la patologia esordisce prima dei 18 anni di età e nel 25% si ha depigmentazione prima degli 8 anni. La maggior parte dei bambini colpiti presenta la forma generalizzata, ma il tipo localizzato è più comune tra i bambini che tra gli adulti. I pazienti con la forma generalizzata si presentano usualmente con un quadro nettamente simmetrico di macchie e zone bianche (Fig. 652-7), i cui margini possono essere abbastanza pigmentati. Le chiazze tendono a essere acrali e/o periorifiziali. Qualche volta quasi tutta la superficie cutanea diviene depigmentata: in questo caso si parla di vitiligine totale.

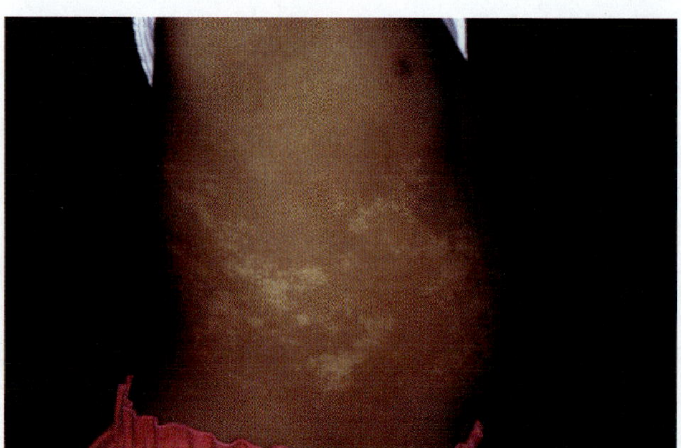

Figura 652-6. Strie ipopigmentate marmoriformi sull'addome, nell'ipomelanosi di Ito.

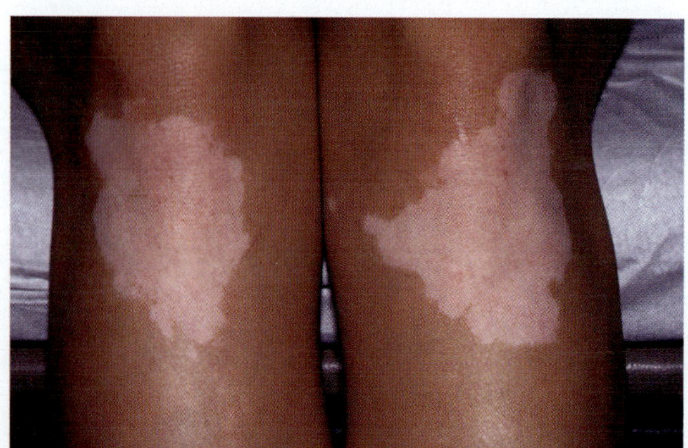

Figura 652-7. Aree di vitiligine nettamente demarcate, simmetriche, depigmentate.

Esistono diverse varietà di vitiligine localizzata. Nella vitiligine segmentaria, le aree depigmentate sono limitate a una distribuzione dermatomerica. Un'altra forma di vitiligine localizzata è il fenomeno del nevo alonato (*halo nevus*), in cui un neo benigno sviluppa anelli depigmentati alla periferia. Anche l'incanutimento prematuro dei capelli (canizie) è stato considerato una forma di vitiligine focale.

Nei pazienti con vitiligine si verificano numerose **malattie autoimmuni**, tra cui il morbo di Addison, la tiroidite di Hashimoto, l'anemia perniciosa, il diabete mellito, l'ipoparatiroidismo e la sindrome autoimmune polighiandolare con deficit selettivo di IgA. Sono state osservate, inoltre, altre malattie con possibili difetti immunitari, come l'alopecia areata e la morfea.

La **sindrome di Vogt-Koyanogi-Harada** è una forma di vitiligine associata a uveite, disacusia, meningoencefalite e depigmentazione di cute, capelli, sopracciglia e ciglia. Nella **sindrome di Alezzandrini**, la vitiligine è associata a degenerazione tapetoretinica e a sordità.

L'esame al microscopio ottico delle lesioni precoci mostra lievi alterazioni infiammatorie. Nel corso del tempo, nei melanociti si verificano alterazioni degenerative che portano alla loro completa scomparsa.

La diagnosi differenziale della vitiligine comprende le altre cause di leucodermia acquisita diffusa. Le diagnosi problematiche più comuni sono la tinea versicolor e l'ipopigmentazione postinfiammatoria.

Trattamento. Le aree localizzate di vitiligine possono rispondere agli steroidi topici ad elevata potenza, al tacrolimus topico o al piperolimus topico. Nei pazienti con coinvolgimento più esteso, il trattamento d'elezione è la luce ultravioletta B a banda stretta (UVB) (UVB311). In tutte le forme di vitiligine, la risposta alla terapia è lenta, e impiega da molti mesi ad alcuni anni. Coloro che non sono interessati al trattamento possono utilizzare cosmetici coprenti. Tutte le aree di vitiligine sono suscettibili di danno solare e si deve stare molto attenti a ridurre il più possibile l'esposizione solare delle aree affette. La remissione spontanea può essere osservata in una piccola percentuale di casi.

Au KS, Williams AT, Gambello MJ, et al: Molecular genetics of tuberous sclerosis complex: From bench to bedside. *J Child Neurol* 2004;19:699–709.

Herane MI: Vitiligo and leukoderma in children. *Clin Dermatol* 2003; 21:283–295.

Kihiczak TI, Fox MD, Janniger CK, et al: Piebaldism: An update. *Int J Dermatol* 2004;43:716–719.

Newton VE: Clinical features of Waardenburg syndrome. *Adv Otorhinolaryngol* 2002;61:201–208.

Okulicz JF, Shah RS, Schwartz RA, et al: Oculocutaneous albinism. *J Eur Acad Dermatol Venereol* 2003;17:251–256.

Scheinfeld NS: Syndromic albinism: A review of genetics and phenotype. *Dermatol Online J* 2003;9:5.

Silverberg NB, Lin P, Travis L, et al: Tacrolimus ointment promotes repigmentation of vitiligo in children: A review of 57 cases. *J Am Acad Dermatol* 2004;51:760–766.

Taibjee SM, Bennett DC, Moss C: Abnormal pigmentation in hypomelanosis of Ito and pigmentary mosaicism: The role of pigmentary genes. *Br J Dermatol* 2004;151:269–282.

Capitolo 653 ■ Malattie vescicolobollose

Joseph G. Morelli

Molte malattie sono caratterizzate da lesioni vescicolobollose e variano considerevolmente come eziologia, età d'esordio e caratteristiche. La morfologia della vescicola spesso fornisce un indizio sulla localizzazione della lesione nella cute. Le vescicole localizzate negli **strati epidermici** sono a parete sottile, relativamente flaccide e si rompono facilmente. Le **vescicole subepidermiche** sono tese, a parete spessa e più durature. La biopsia delle vescicole può essere diagnostica, poiché il livello di clivaggio endocutaneo e i fenomeni associati, come la natura dell'infiltrato infiammatorio, sono caratteristici per i diversi disordini. Altre procedure diagnostiche, come l'immunofluorescenza e la microscopia elettronica, possono spesso aiutare a distinguere disordini vescicolobollosi con reperti istopatologici quasi identici (Tab. 653-1).

ERITEMA MULTIFORME. L'eritema multiforme (EM) presenta numerose manifestazioni morfologiche cutanee, che variano da macule eritematose, papule, vescicole, bolle o placche orticarioidi fino a macchie di eritema confluente. L'eruzione compare più comunemente nei pazienti tra i 10 e i 30 anni ed è usualmente asintomatica, sebbene possano essere presenti bruciore o prurito. La diagnosi di EM viene posta in base al riconoscimento della lesione tipica: papule a forma di ciambella, a bersaglio (iride o occhio di bue) con margine esterno eritematoso, un anello interno pallido e un centro porpora scuro o necrotico (Figg. 653-1 e 653-2).

L'EM è caratterizzato da un'eruzione cutanea improvvisa, simmetrica, localizzata più comunemente sulla superficie estensoria delle estremità superiori; le lesioni sono relativamente sparse sul volto, sul tronco e sulle gambe. L'eruzione spesso esordisce con macule rosse o placche orticarioidi, che si espandono in senso centrifugo fino a formare lesioni con diametro fino a 2 cm, con centro scuro o necrotico. Le lesioni di un particolare episodio si manifestano tipicamente entro 72 ore e per quanto riguarda la loro posizione rimangono fisse. Possono comparire lesioni orali, con una predilezione per il margine vermiglio delle labbra e la mucosa buccale, ma le altre superfici mucose sono risparmiate.

TABELLA 653-1. Sedi di formazione delle vesciche e indagini diagnostiche per i disturbi vescicolobollosi

DISTURBO	SEDE DI CLIVAGGIO DELLA VESCICA	INDAGINI DIAGNOSTICHE
Acrodermatite enteropatica	IE	Livelli di Zn
Impetigine bollosa	GL	Striscio, coltura
Pemfigoide bolloso	SE (giunzionale)	Immunofluorescenza diretta e indiretta
Candidosi	SC	Preparazione di KOH, coltura
Dermatite erpetiforme	SE	Immunofluorescenza diretta
Dermatofitosi	IE	Preparazione di KOH, coltura
Eczema disidrosico	IE	Istopatologia di routine
EB semplice	IE	Microscopia elettronica, mappatura in immunofluorescenza
Mani e piedi	IE	Microscopia elettronica, mappatura in immunofluorescenza
EB giunzionale (letale)	SE (giunzionale)	Microscopia elettronica, mappatura in immunofluorescenza
EB distrofica recessiva	SE	Microscopia elettronica, mappatura in immunofluorescenza
EB distrofica dominante	SE	Microscopia elettronica, mappatura in immunofluorescenza
Ipercheratosi epidermolitica	IE	Istopatologia di routine
Eritema multiforme	SE	Istopatologia di routine
Eritema tossico	SC, IE	Striscio per ricerca eosinofili
Incontinentia pigmenti	IE	Striscio per ricerca eosinofili
Punture di insetto	IE	Istopatologia di routine
Dermatosi lineare a IgA	SE	Immunofluorescenza diretta
Mastocitosi	SE	Striscio per ricerca mastociti
Miliaria cristallina	IC	Istopatologia di routine
Melanosi pustolare neonatale	SC, IE	Striscio per ricerca di cellule
Pemfigo foliaceo	GL	Immunofluorescenza diretta e indiretta Striscio di Tzanck
Pemfigo volgare	SB	Immunofluorescenza diretta e indiretta Striscio di Tzanck
Scabbia	IE	Spazzolato
SSS stafilococcica	GL	Istopatologia di routine
Necrolisi epidermica tossica	SE	Istopatologia di routine
Vesciche virali	IE	Striscio di Tzanck per le infezioni da virus erpetici

EB, epidermolisi bollosa; GL, strato granulare; IC, intracorneo; IE, intraepidermico; KOH, idrossido di potassio; SB, soprabasale; SC, sottocorneo; SE, sottoepidermico; SSS, *Scalded Skin Syndrome*, sindrome della cute ustionata.

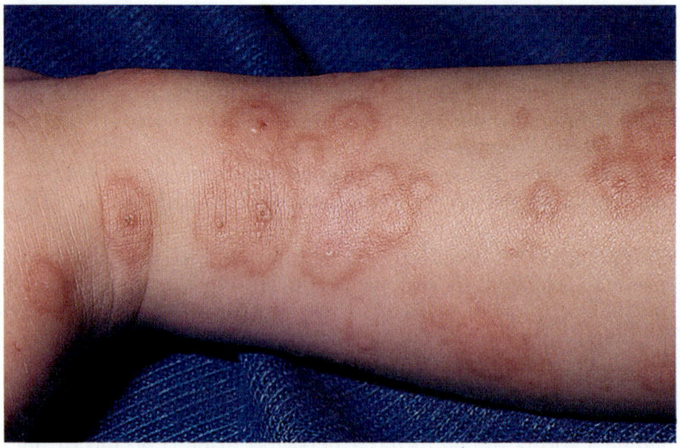

Figura 653-1. Papule fisse precoci con una zona scura centrale sul dorso della mano di un bambino con eritema multiforme da virus dell'herpes simplex. (Da Weston WL, Lane AT, Morelli J: *Color Textbook of Pediatric Dermatology*, 3rd ed, St. Louis, Mosby, 2002, p 156.)

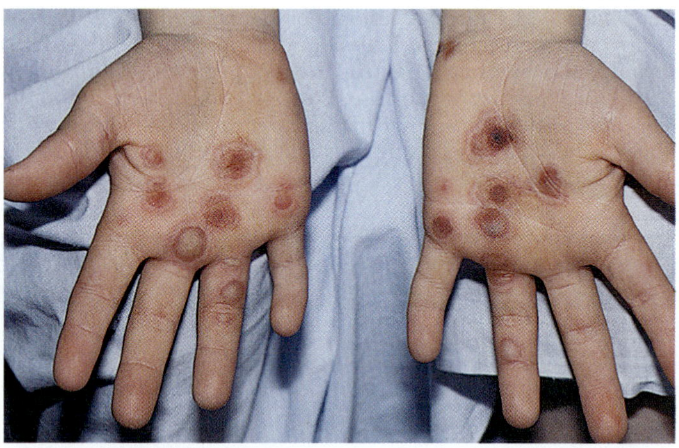

Figura 653-2. Lesioni "a bersaglio" o "a iride" con la caratteristica zona centrale scura, sui palmi delle mani di un bambino con eritema multiforme da virus dell'herpes simplex. (Da Weston WL, Lane AT, Morelli J: *Color Textbook of Pediatric Dermatology*, 3rd ed, St. Louis, Mosby, 2002, p 156.)

Sono generalmente assenti sintomi prodromici. Le lesioni si risolvono tipicamente senza sequele in circa 2 settimane e non compare progressione verso la sindrome di Stevens-Johnson.

Sebbene l'EM possa presentarsi inizialmente con lesioni orticariodi, a differenza dell'orticaria, le singole lesioni di EM non scompaiono entro 24 ore. È stata descritta anche una reazione simil-malattia da siero (SSLR, *Serum Sickness-Like Reaction*) al cefacloro, che si presenta con lesioni simili all'EM. Sebbene le lesioni possano sviluppare un centro da scuro a porpora, nella maggior parte dei casi l'eruzione della SSLR indotta da cefaclor è pruriginosa, transitoria e migrante, ed è probabilmente orticaria e non un vero EM.

La **diagnosi differenziale** di EM comprende anche il pemfigoide bolloso, il pemfigo, la dermatosi lineare IgA, la malattia del trapianto contro l'ospite, l'eruzione bollosa da farmaci, l'orticaria, le infezioni virali come l'herpes simplex, la malattia di Reiter, la malattia di Kawasaki, la malattia di Behçet, la vasculite allergica, l'eritema anulare centrifugo e la poliarterite nodosa. Un EM che coinvolga principalmente la mucosa orale può essere confuso con il pemfigoide bolloso, il pemfigo volgare, il lichen planus vescicolobolloso o erosivo, la sindrome di Behçet, la stomatite aftosa ricorrente e la gengivostomatite erpetica primaria.

Tra i numerosi fattori implicati nell'eziologia dell'EM, l'infezione da parte del virus dell'herpes simplex (HSV) è la più comune. L'HSV labiale e, meno comunemente, l'HSV genitale, sono stati osservati nel 60% degli episodi di EM e sono ritenuti i responsabili di quasi tutti gli episodi di EM ricorrente, spesso in associazione all'esposizione solare (Fig. 653-3). Gli antigeni e il DNA dell'HSV sono presenti nelle lesioni cutanee dell'EM, ma sono assenti nella cute non lesionale. La presenza degli antigeni leucocitari umani (HLA, *Human Leukocyte Antigens*) B62, B35 e DR53 si associa a un aumentato rischio di EM indotto da HSV, in particolare della forma ricorrente. La maggior parte dei pazienti ha un singolo episodio autolimitante di EM. Le lesioni dell'EM ricorrente indotto dall'HSV si sviluppano tipicamente 10-14 giorni dopo l'esordio di eruzioni ricorrenti di HSV, presentano un aspetto simile nei vari episodi, ma possono variare quanto a frequenza e durata in un dato paziente. Nei soggetti suscettibili, non tutti gli episodi di HSV ricorrente evolvono in EM.

La patogenesi dell'EM non è chiara, ma può essere una risposta immunitaria cellulomediata, specifica dell'ospite, a uno stimolo antigenico, che risulta in un danno dei cheratinociti. Le citochine rilasciate dalle cellule mononucleari attivate e dai cheratinociti possono contribuire alla morte delle cellule epidermiche e ai sintomi costituzionali.

I reperti microscopici dell'EM, così come l'aspetto macroscopico dell'eruzione cutanea, sono variabili, ma possono essere di aiuto nella diagnosi. Le lesioni precoci mostrano tipicamente un lieve edema intercellulare, rari cheratinociti discheratosici, vacuolizzazione basale dell'epidermide, e un infiltrato linfoistiocitico perivascolare con edema, nel derma superiore. Le lesioni più mature mostrano un'accentuazione di queste caratteristiche, con sviluppo di esocitosi linfocitaria e di un intenso infiltrato mononucleare perivascolare e interstiziale, nel terzo superiore del derma. Nei casi gravi, l'intera epidermide diviene necrotica.

Il trattamento dell'EM è di supporto. Gli emollienti topici, gli antistaminici sistemici e i farmaci antinfiammatori non steroidei non variano il decorso della malattia, ma possono fornire un sollievo sintomatologico. Non esistono studi prospettici non controllati che giustifichino l'uso di corticosteroidi nel trattamento dell'EM; anzi, la terapia steroidea può facilitare la replicazione dell'HSV e rendere gli episodi di EM può frequenti o continui. La profilassi con aciclovir orale, somministrato per 6 mesi, può essere efficace nel controllo degli episodi ricorrenti di EM associato a HSV. Alla sospensione dell'aciclovir, sia l'HSV sia l'EM possono recidivare, anche se gli episodi possono essere meno frequenti e più lievi.

SINDROME DI STEVENS-JOHNSON. Nella sindrome di Stevens-Johnson le lesioni cutanee in genere esordiscono come macule

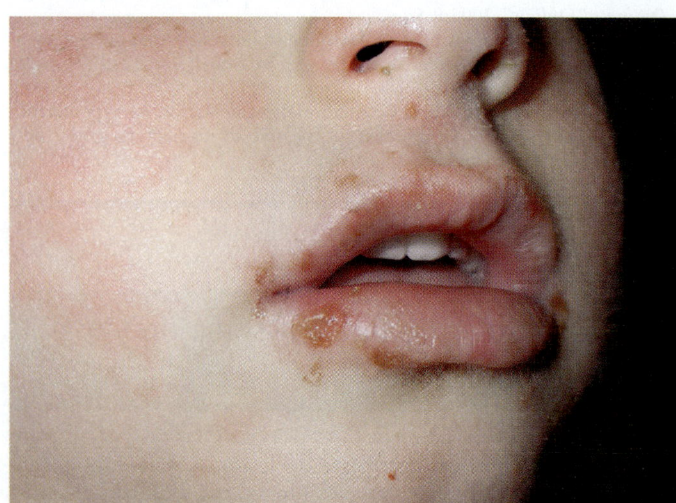

Figura 653-3. Infezione labiale ricorrente da virus dell'herpes simplex (HSV).

eritematose che rapidamente, e in modo variabile, sviluppano una necrosi centrale sino a formare vescicole, bolle e aree di esfoliazione sul volto, sul tronco e sugli arti. Le lesioni cutanee sono tipicamente più diffuse rispetto a quanto accade nell'EM e sono accompagnate dal coinvolgimento di **due o più superfici mucose**, in particolare gli occhi, la cavità orale, le vie aeree superiori o l'esofago, il tratto gastrointestinale o la mucosa anogenitale. I segni di presentazione sono spesso rappresentati da bruciore, edema ed eritema della labbra e della mucosa buccale, seguiti dallo sviluppo di bolle, ulcerazioni e croste emorragiche. Le lesioni possono essere precedute da una malattia similinfluenzale delle alte vie respiratorie. Il dolore delle ulcerazioni mucose è spesso intenso, ma la sensibilità cutanea è minima o assente, in contrasto con l'epidermolisi tossica. Possono verificarsi ulcerazione corneale, uveite anteriore, panoftalmite, bronchite, polmonite, miocardite, epatite, enterocolite, poliartrite, ematuria e necrosi tubulare acuta, che porta a insufficienza renale. Le bolle e le erosioni cutanee disseminate possono esitare in un'aumentata perdita di liquidi e in un elevato rischio di superinfezione batterica e di sepsi. Le nuove lesioni compaiono in gruppi e la guarigione completa può richiedere 4-6 settimane; possono residuare cicatrici oculari, compromissione della vista e stenosi di esofago, bronchi, vagina, uretra e ano. Nella sindrome di Stevens-Johnson le anomalie non specifiche agli esami di laboratorio comprendono leucocitosi, aumento della velocità di eritrosedimentazione e, occasionalmente, incremento delle transaminasi e riduzione dei valori di albumina. La **necrolisi epidermica tossica** è il disturbo più grave, nello spettro clinico della malattia, poiché comporta una notevole tossicità sistemica e necrolisi estesa delle membrane mucose e di >30% della superficie corporea.

Il *Mycoplasma pneumoniae* è l'agente causale infettivo che con maggiore certezza è stato dimostrato essere responsabile della sindrome di Stevens-Johnson. I farmaci, in particolare gli antinfiammatori non steroidei e gli anticonvulsivanti, sono gli agenti che più comunemente precipitano la sindrome di Stevens-Johnson e la necrolisi epidermica tossica.

Trattamento. Il trattamento della sindrome di Stevens-Johnson è di supporto e sintomatico. I farmaci potenzialmente dannosi devono essere sospesi appena possibile. È indispensabile una consulenza oculistica, poiché le sequele oculari, come la cicatrizzazione corneale, possono portare a perdita della vista. Gli steroidi topici possono ridurre la morbilità oculare. Le lesioni orali andrebbero trattate con collutori e garze con glicerina. Le lesioni vaginali dovrebbero essere tenute sotto osservazione e trattate per prevenire la stenosi o l'occlusione vaginale. Gli anestetici topici (difenidramina, diclonina e lidocaina viscosa) possono lenire il dolore, in particolare quando applicati prima dei pasti. Le lesioni cutanee esfoliate possono essere pulite con soluzione salina o impacchi di soluzione di Burow. La terapia antibiotica è indicata per le infezioni batteriche secondarie documentate. Il trattamento può richiedere il ricovero in un'unità di terapia intensiva, la somministrazione endovenosa di liquidi, un supporto nutrizionale; utilizzo di biancheria da letto particolare (pelli di pecora) o materassi ad acqua-aria; applicazione quotidiana di soluzione salina o di impacchi di soluzione di Burow, garze di paraffina o di idrogel per ricoprire le aree esfoliate, impacchi di salina su palpebre, labbra o naso, analgesici e cateterizzazione vescicale (quando necessaria). È essenziale un esame quotidiano per escludere infezioni e lesioni oculari, che costituiscono la principale causa di morbilità a lungo termine. Gli antibiotici sistemici sono indicati per le infezioni urinarie o cutanee e nel sospetto di batteriemia, poiché le infezioni sono la principale causa di morte. Gli antibiotici sistemici in via profilattica, tuttavia, non sono necessari. Sebbene i corticosteroidi siano talvolta utilizzati nei casi precoci e severi di sindrome di Stevens-Johnson, non si è a conoscenza di alcuno studio prospettico in doppio cieco che ne valuti l'efficacia. La maggior parte degli Autori ne scoraggia l'uso, a causa delle segnalazioni di aumentata morbilità e mortalità (sepsi) dovute alla loro somministrazione. Sono state utilizzate anche immunoglobuline endovena (1,5-2,0 g/kg/die per 3 giorni) e molti le ritengono efficaci.

NECROLISI EPIDERMICA TOSSICA

EPIDEMIOLOGIA ED EZIOLOGIA. La necrolisi epidermica tossica non ha patogenesi nota, ma sembra si tratti di un fenomeno di ipersensibilità che porta a un danno a carico principalmente dello strato basale dell'epidermide. Il danno epidermico sembra risultare dall'apoptosi dei cheratinociti Fas-mediata. Questa patologia è scatenata da molti degli stessi fattori responsabili della sindrome di Stevens-Johnson, in particolar modo farmaci come i sulfonamidi, l'amoxicillina, il fenobarbital, l'idantoina, il butazone e l'allopurinolo. La necrolisi epidermica tossica è definita da (1) formazione di vescicole diffuse e di eritema morbilliforme o confluente, associato a sensibilizzazione cutanea; (2) assenza di lesioni a bersaglio; (3) esordio improvviso e generalizzazione nell'arco di 24-48 ore; (4) reperti istologici di necrosi epidermica a tutto spessore e di infiltrato dermico minimo o assente. Questi criteri caratterizzano la necrolisi epidermica tossica come entità diversa dall'EM; tuttavia, alcuni autori sostengono che la necrolisi epidermica tossica rappresenti la forma più severa di EM.

MANIFESTAZIONI CLINICHE. I prodromi consistono in febbre, malessere, sensibilizzazione cutanea localizzata ed eritema diffuso. L'infiammazione delle palpebre, della congiuntiva, della bocca e dei genitali può precedere le lesioni cutanee. Possono svilupparsi bolle flaccide, sebbene questa non sia una caratteristica predominante. Tipicamente, l'epidermide si stacca a tutto spessore in ampi lembi. È presente il **segno di Nikolsky** (disepitelizzazione della cute con una lieve pressione), ma solo nelle aree di eritema. La guarigione avviene nell'arco di 14 o più giorni. La cicatrizzazione, soprattutto se interessa gli occhi, può causare opacità della cornea. Il decorso può essere inesorabilmente progressivo, complicato da grave disidratazione, squilibri elettrolitici, shock e infezioni secondarie localizzate o setticemia. Si può anche verificare la perdita delle unghie e dei capelli. La morbilità a lungo termine comprende alterazioni della pigmentazione cutanea, problemi oculari (assenza di lacrimazione, cicatrici congiuntivali, perdita delle ciglia) e stenosi delle superfici mucose. La **diagnosi differenziale** include la necrolisi combustiforme stafilococcica (SSSS, *Staphylococcal Scalded Skin Syndrome*) in cui il piano di clivaggio delle vesciche è intraepidermico, la reazione di rigetto del trapianto verso l'ospite, le ustioni chimiche, le eruzioni da farmaci, la sindrome da shock tossico e il pemfigo.

La **sindrome da ipersensibilità agli anticonvulsivanti** (sindrome DRESS, *Drug Rash, Eosinophilia, Systemic Symptoms* [eruzione da farmaci, eosinofilia, sintomi sistemici]) è una reazione multisistemica che compare da 4 settimane circa a 3 mesi dopo l'inizio dell'assunzione di fenitoina, carbamazepina, fenobarbital o primidone. Sebbene inizialmente sia stata descritta in associazione a terapia anticonvulsivante, sono stati implicati anche altri farmaci, in particolare gli antibiotici. L'eruzione mucocutanea può essere identica a quella dell'EM, della sindrome di Stevens-Johnson o della necrolisi epidermica tossica, ma la reazione comprende tipicamente anche linfadenopatia, febbre, danno epatico, renale e polmonare, eosinofilia e leucocitosi.

TRATTAMENTO. È fondamentale individuare lo specifico fattore eziologico. Quando il disturbo è indotto da farmaci, occorre interrompere il prima possibile la somministrazione del farmaco responsabile. Il trattamento è simile a quello delle ustioni severe e può essere effettuato al meglio in un reparto per grandi ustionati (vedi Capitolo 74). Può comprendere stretto isolamento per protezione, accurato ripristino di liquidi ed elettroliti, utilizzo di un materasso ad acqua-aria e colture quotidiane. Una terapia antibiotica sistemica è indicata quando c'è un'infezione secondaria sospetta o manifesta. Il trattamento della cute consiste nel lavaggio con soluzione salina isotonica o soluzione di Burow. I bendaggi di origine biologica o con idrogel alleviano il dolore e riducono la perdita di liquidi. Sono spesso necessari narcotici per ridurre il dolore. Possono essere necessarie cure dentarie e orali, come per l'EM maggiore. A causa del meccanismo immunitario, sono stati utilizzati glucocorticoidi sistemici e immunoglobuline endovena con apparente successo. Ciononostante, questo trattamento rimane controverso.

DISTURBI MECCANOBULLOSI

EPIDERMOLISI BOLLOSA. Le malattie classificate sotto questo termine generico comprendono un gruppo eterogeneo di alterazioni vescicolose congenite ed ereditarie. Differiscono per gravità e prognosi, caratteristiche cliniche e istologiche e tipo di ereditarietà, ma sono tutte caratterizzate da induzione di vescicole conseguenti a traumi e dall'esacerbazione di queste durante le stagioni calde. I disturbi possono essere classificati in tre gruppi maggiori, ognuno dei quali comprende diversi sottogruppi: (1) epidermolisi bollosa semplice (EBS), (2) epidermolisi bollosa giunzionale (JEB, *Junctional Epidermolysis Bullosa*) ed (3) epidermolisi bollosa distrofica (DEB, *Dystrophic Epidermolysis Bullosa*) (Tab. 653-2).

Epidermolisi bollosa semplice (EBS). Si tratta di un disturbo autosomico dominante, non cicatriziale. Il difetto, nella maggior parte dei tipi di epidermolisi bollosa semplice, è nella cheratina 5 o 14, che costituisce i filamenti intermedi dei cheratinociti basali. Le bolle intraepidermiche risultano dalla citolisi delle cellule basali.

Nelle variante di **Koebner**, in genere le bolle sono presenti alla nascita o compaiono durante il periodo neonatale. Le sedi di predilezione sono mani, piedi, gomiti, ginocchia, gambe e cuoio capelluto. Le lesioni intraorali sono minime; le unghie, raramente distrofiche, possono cadere ma solitamente ricrescono; la dentizione è normale. Le bolle guariscono con formazione di cicatrici o di milio, minima o assente. La propensione alle vescicole si riduce con l'età e la prognosi a lungo termine è buona. Le bolle dovrebbero essere drenate con un ago, lasciandone intatto il tetto per proteggere la cute sottostante. Le erosioni possono essere coperte con rivestimenti semipermeabili.

L'EBS localizzata di mani e piedi (tipo di Weber-Cockayne) si presenta spesso quando il bambino comincia a camminare; l'esordio può tuttavia essere ritardato fino alla pubertà o all'inizio dell'età adulta, quando si indossano calzature più pesanti o il piede è soggetto a traumi maggiori. Le bolle sono in genere limitate alle mani e ai piedi (Fig. 653-4); raramente insorgono altrove, come sulla superficie dorsale delle braccia e della cresta

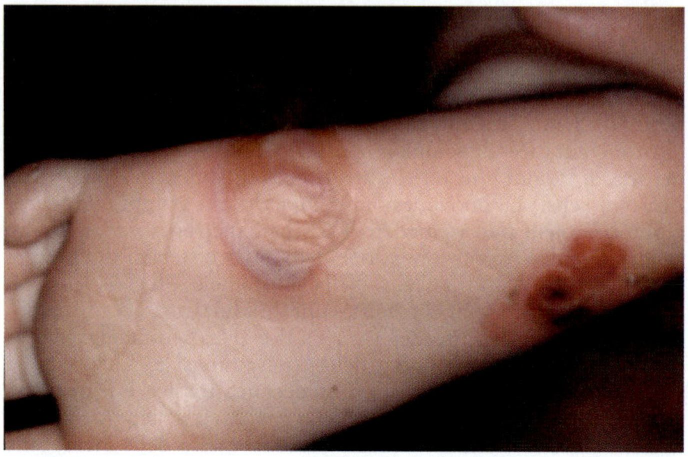

Figura 653-4. Grandi bolle sul piede in un caso di epidermolisi bollosa semplice.

TABELLA 653-2. Aspetto clinico e diagnosi di alcuni sottotipi di EB nel periodo neonatale

SOTTOTIPO DI EB (EREDITARIETÀ ABITUALE)	CARATTERISTICHE CLINICHE		DIAGNOSI: MICROSCOPIA ELETTRONICA (ME), IMMUNOISTOCHIMICA E MAPPATURA ANTIGENICA IN IMMUNOFLUORESCENZA (IF)
	Cutanea	**Extracutanea**	
EB semplice, di Koebner (AD)	Vescicazione da lieve a moderata, spesso generalizzata Cicatrici rare, milio CLAS	Occasionalmente vesciche su mucose	ME: Clivaggio intradermico; alterazione dei filamenti di cheratina IF: BPAG1 (BP230), BP-180 (BPAG2, collagene XVII), integrina α6β4, laminina 10, laminina 5, collagene di tipo IV (antigene EBA) alla base della bolla
EB semplice di Weber-Cockayne (AD)	Vesciche lievi, spesso localizzate, talvolta nei primi 24 mesi, ma spesso durante la prepubertà	Coinvolgimento mucoso raro	ME: Clivaggio nello strato basale IF: Come nella EB semplice di Koebner
EB semplice di Dowling-Meara (AD)	Vescicazione da moderata a severa, inizia generalizzata quindi raggruppata (erpetiforme) Milio Distrofia e perdita delle unghie CLAS	Lievi vesciche a livello delle mucose	ME: Clivaggio nello strato basale; filamenti di cheratina agglutinati IF: Come nella EB semplice di Koebner
EB giunzionale, tipo non-Herlitz (AR)	Vescicazione moderata Cicatrici atrofiche Distrofia ungueale	Lieve vescicazione delle mucose Ipoplasia dello smalto	ME: Clivaggio nella lamina lucida; riduzione variabile degli emidesmosomi IF: Colorazione assente con 19-DEJ-1 (unceina); colorazione variabile con GB3 e altri anticorpi laminina 5, inclusi 46 e K140; BPAg1 (BP230) BP180 (BPAG2, collagene XVII), integrina α6β4 sul tetto delle vesciche Laminina 10, collagene di tipo IV, collagene di tipo VII (antigene EBA) alla base della bolla
Giunzionale, tipo Herlitz (AR)	Vesciche generalizzate severe Scarsa tendenza alla guarigione, tessuto di granulazione Cicatrizzazione, distrofia ungueale, CLAS	Grave vescicazione delle mucose Coinvolgimento GI comune Coinvolgimento laringeo con ostruzione delle vie aeree Coinvolgimento urologico	ME: Clivaggio nella lamina lucida; emidesmosomi ridotti o assenti; placche dense sottobasali assenti IF: Assenza di colorazione con 19-DEJ-1 (unceina) e GB3 (laminina 5) e assenza di colorazione con altri anticorpi laminina 5, inclusi 46 e K140.BPAG1 (BP230) e BP180 (BPAG2, collagene di tipo XVII) sul tetto delle vesciche Laminina 10, collagene di tipo IV e di tipo VII alla base della bolla
EB giunzionale con atresia pilorica (AR)	Vescicazione severa CLAS	Polidramnios Atresia pilorica, coinvolgimento urologico: ostruzione ureterovescicale, idronefrosi	ME: Clivaggio nella lamina lucida e nella membrana basale; emodesmosomi piccoli IF: BPAG1 (BP230) e BP180 (BPAG2, collagene di tipo XVII) sulla sul tetto delle vesciche Laminina 10, collagene di tipo IV e di tipo VII alla base della bolla 19-DEJ-1 assente (unceina), integrina α6β4 assente o ridotta
EB distrofica dominante (AD)	Vescicazione da moderata a severa (ma può essere più severa nel periodo neonatale) Milio, cicatrici CLAS Distrofia ungueale	Lieve vescicazione delle mucose	ME: Clivaggio sotto la lamina densa; riduzione variabile delle fibrille di ancoraggio IF: BPAG1 (BP230)BP-180 (BPAG2, collagene di tipo XVII), integrina α6β4, laminina 10, collagene di tipo IV alla base della bolla Colorazione normale, variabile o assente per il collagene di tipo VII (antigene EBA)
EB distrofica recessiva di Hallopeau-Siemens (AR)	Vescicazione severa Milio, cicatrici CLAS	Grave vescicazione delle mucose Coinvolgimento GI comune Coinvolgimento urologico	ME: Clivaggio sotto la lamina densa; fibrille di ancoraggio assenti IF: BPAG1 (BP230)BP-180 (BPAG2, collagene di tipo XVII), α6β4 integrina, laminina 10, collagene di tipo IV alla base della vescica Colorazione variabile o assente per il collagene di tipo VII (antigene EBA)

AD, autosomico dominante; AR, autosomico recessivo; CLAS, *Congenital Localized Absence of Skin* (assenza localizzata congenita di cute); EB, epidermolisi bollosa; GI, gastrointestinale.
Da Eichenfield LF, Frieden IJ, Esterly NB: *Textbook of Neonatal Dermatology*. Philadelphia, WB, Saunders, 2001, p 159.

tibiale. Il disturbo varia da lievemente disabilitante a gravemente invalidante durante le esacerbazioni severe.

La **variante di Dowling-Meara** (erpetiforme) è caratterizzata da vesciche raggruppate simili a quelle dell'herpes simplex (Fig. 653-5). Durante l'infanzia, la formazione di bolle può essere severa ed estesa, coinvolgere le membrane mucose ed esitare nella perdita delle unghie, in formazione di milio, e in lievi alterazioni pigmentate, senza cicatrizzazione. Dopo il primo mese di vita, le temperature elevate non sembrano esacerbare più la formazione di bolle. Può svilupparsi ipercheratosi delle superfici palmari e plantari, ma generalmente la condizione migliora con l'età.

L'**EBS-distrofia muscolare** è una rara variante di EBS associata a distrofia muscolare. È causata da mutazioni del gene che codifica la plectina, una proteina emidesmosomiale.

EPIDERMOLISI BOLLOSA GIUNZIONALE (JEB). Il tipo Herlitz è una patologia autosomica recessiva potenzialmente fatale. Il neonato che ne è affetto solitamente presenta vesciche alla nascita o le sviluppa durante il periodo neonatale; le lesioni interessano soprattutto la zona periorale, il cuoio capelluto, l'area del pannolino e il torace. Al contrario delle altre varianti di epidermolisi bollosa, le mani e i piedi tendono a essere relativamente risparmiati, con l'eccezione delle falangi distali e delle lamine ungueali, che sono distrofiche o cadono per non ricrescere più. Il coinvolgimento delle membrane mucose può essere severo e, in molti bambini affetti, sono state documentate ulcerazioni dell'epitelio respiratorio, gastrointestinale e genitourinario, anche se meno frequentemente che nei casi gravi di epidermolisi bollosa distrofica autosomica recessiva. La guarigione è lenta, e possono persistere a lungo granulomi vegetanti. Le ampie placche macerate ed erose (Fig. 653-6) possono divenire la porta di ingresso di batteri e la setticemia è una causa frequente di morte. Nelle zone di vescicazione ricorrente si può osservare una lieve atrofia. È caratteristico un difetto di dentizione, con perdita precoce dei denti come risultato di carie incontrollate. Sono quasi sempre presenti anche ritardo della crescita e anemia resistente. Oltre alle infezioni, sono cause comuni di decesso la cachessia e l'insufficienza circolatoria. La maggior parte dei pazienti muore entro i primi tre anni di vita.

La variante **non-Herlitz** è un gruppo eterogeneo di disordini. La vescicazione può essere severa nel periodo neonatale, rendendo ardua la differenziazione dal tipo Herlitz. Possono essere osservate tutte le condizioni associate al tipo Herlitz, ma sono in genere più lievi. L'epidermolisi bollosa atrofica generalizzata benigna è inclusa tra le varianti del tipo non Herlitz. Un'altra variante di JEB non-Herlitz si associa ad **atresia del piloro**.

In tutti i tipi di epidermolisi bollosa giunzionale si osserva una bolla sottoepidermica all'esame al microscopio ottico, mentre la microscopia elettronica mostra un piano di clivaggio nella lamina lucida, tra la membrana plasmatica delle cellule basali e

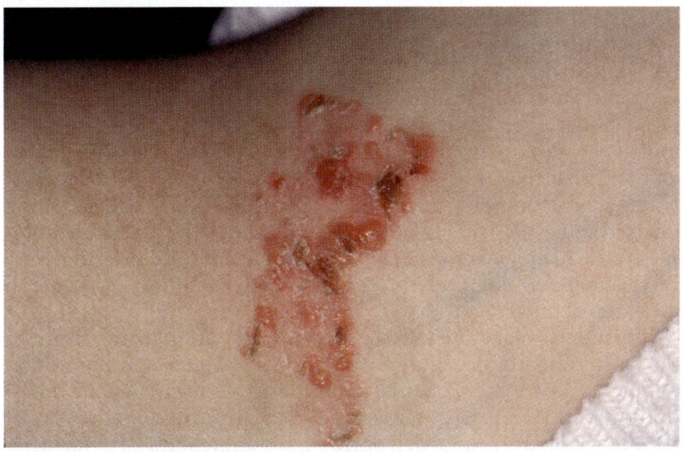

Figura 653-5. Vescicole raggruppate su cute eritematosa, in un caso di epidermolisi bollosa semplice di Dowling-Meara.

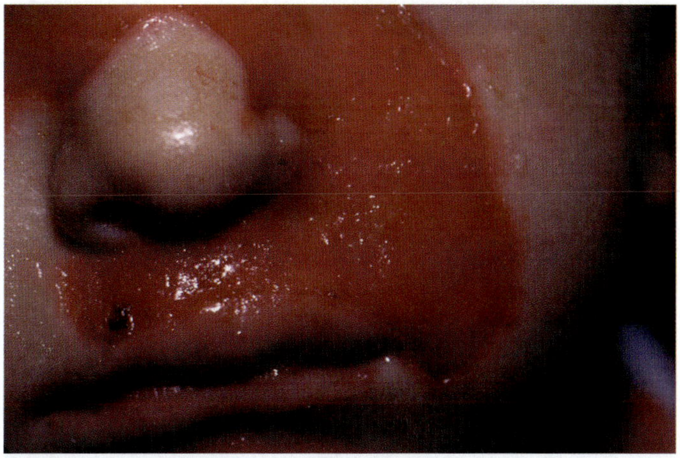

Figura 653-6. Tessuto di granulazione senza guarigione, in un caso di epidermolisi bollosa giunzionale.

la lamina basale. In micrografia elettronica si osservano filamenti di ancoraggio assenti o nettamente ridotti. Nel tipo Herlitz e in alcuni casi della variante non-Herlitz, il difetto è nella laminina 5, una glicoproteina associata ai filamenti di ancoraggio al di sotto degli emidesmosomi. Nella JEB non-Herlitz, sono state descritte anomalie anche in altri componenti degli emidesmosomi, come l'antigene del pemfigoide bolloso 2, e Col17A1. Nella JEB con atresia del piloro, il difetto è nell'integrina $\alpha 6\beta 4$.

Il **trattamento** dell'epidermolisi bollosa giunzionale è di supporto. La dieta deve fornire adeguato apporto calorico e un'appropriata supplementazione di ferro. Le infezioni devono essere trattate tempestivamente. Possono essere necessarie trasfusioni di emazie concentrate, se il paziente non risponde alla terapia con ferro ed eritropoietina. I trapianti di cute con tecniche di ingegneria tissutale (cute artificiale derivata da cheratinociti e fibroblasti umani) possono essere utili.

EPIDERMOLISI BOLLOSA DISTROFICA (DEB). Tutte le forme di epidermolisi bollosa distrofica sono causate da mutazioni del collagene VII, uno dei componenti principali delle fibrille di ancoraggio, che legano la membrana basale e l'epidermide sovrastante alle loro basi dermiche. La bolla è sottoepidermica in tutti i tipi di DEB. Il tipo e la localizzazione della mutazione determinano la gravità del fenotipo.

L'**epidermolisi bollosa distrofica dominante** (**DDEB**) è la forma più comune di DEB. Lo spettro della DDEB è variabile. Le vesciche possono essere presenti alla nascita, sono spesso limitate e si formano caratteristicamente sulle prominenze ossee acrali. Le lesioni guariscono rapidamente, con comparsa di cicatrici soffici e grinzose, di milio e alterazioni della pigmentazione (Fig. 653-7). Sono comuni anomalie ungueali e perdita delle unghie. In molti casi, il processo bolloso è lieve e causa una minima limitazione dell'attività, senza compromettere la crescita e lo sviluppo. Il coinvolgimento delle membrane mucose tende a essere minimo.

La **dermolisi bollosa transitoria** del neonato colpisce un raro sottogruppo di pazienti con malattia distrofica autolimitante; nella maggior parte dei casi l'ereditarietà è autosomica dominante. La formazione di bolle alla nascita tende a essere generalizzata, ma cessa entro i primi 1-2 anni. La risoluzione clinica delle bolle e l'alterata distribuzione del collagene di tipo VII, definita da un punto di vista immunoistochimico, si verificano contemporaneamente.

La variante **distrofica recessiva** (**RDEB-Hallopeau-Siemens**) è la forma più invalidante di epidermolisi bollosa, anche se lo spettro clinico è ampio. Alcuni pazienti presentano bolle, cicatrici e formazione di milio principalmente su mani, piedi, gomiti e ginocchia (Fig. 653-8). Altri alla nascita hanno erosioni estese con formazione di bolle che ostacolano seriamente le cure e l'alimentazione del neonato. Le lesioni delle mucose sono comuni e

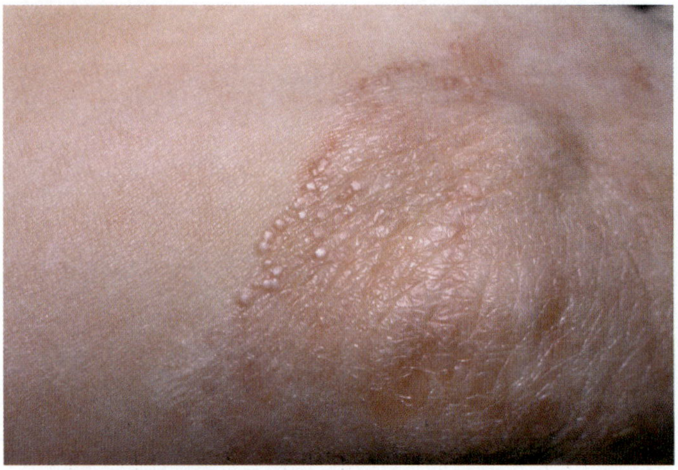

Figura 653-7. Cicatrizzazione con formazione di milio sul ginocchio, nell'epidermolisi bollosa distrofica.

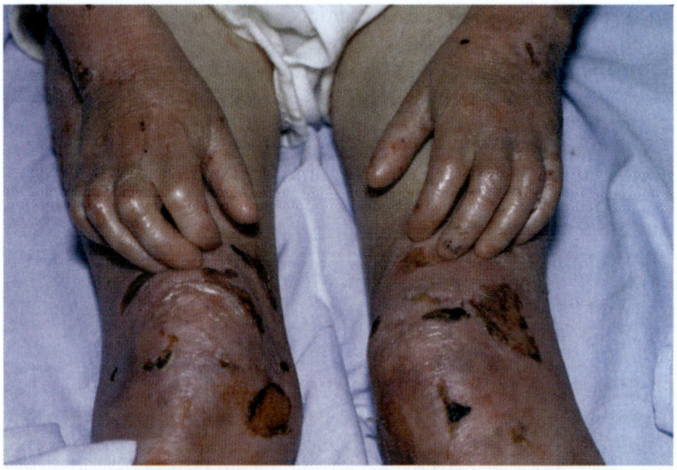

Figura 653-8. Grave cicatrizzazione delle mani e delle ginocchia nell'epidermolisi bollosa distrofica recessiva.

possono provocare grave deprivazione nutrizionale, anche nei bambini più grandi, ritardandone la crescita. Durante l'infanzia, la qualità di vita può essere seriamente compromessa a causa delle erosioni e delle stenosi esofagee, della cicatrizzazione della mucosa orale, delle contratture in flessione delle articolazioni, secondarie alla cicatrizzazione tegumentaria, dello sviluppo di carcinomi cutanei e della fusione digitale (Fig. 653-9).

Sebbene la cute divenga meno sensibile ai traumi con l'età, le deformità progressive e permanenti complicano il trattamento, e la prognosi, complessivamente, non è buona. Vanno evitati i cibi che possono traumatizzare la mucosa orale ed esofagea. Se si sviluppa cicatrizzazione esofagea, possono essere necessarie una dieta semiliquida e dilatazioni esofagee. L'escissione delle stenosi o l'interposizione di un tratto di colon possono essere necessarie per ridurre l'ostruzione esofagea. Nei lattanti, un grave coinvolgimento orofaringeo può richiedere l'utilizzo di speciali dispositivi per l'alimentazione, come il tubo gastrostomico. La terapia continuativa con ferro per l'anemia, la terapia antibiotica intermittente per le infezioni secondarie, che sono una causa comune di morte, e gli interventi chirurgici periodici per la separazione delle falangi possono ridurre la morbilità. Negli Stati Uniti, i trapianti di cute da ingegneria tissutale, contenenti cheratinociti e fibroblasti, hanno apportato un certo beneficio.

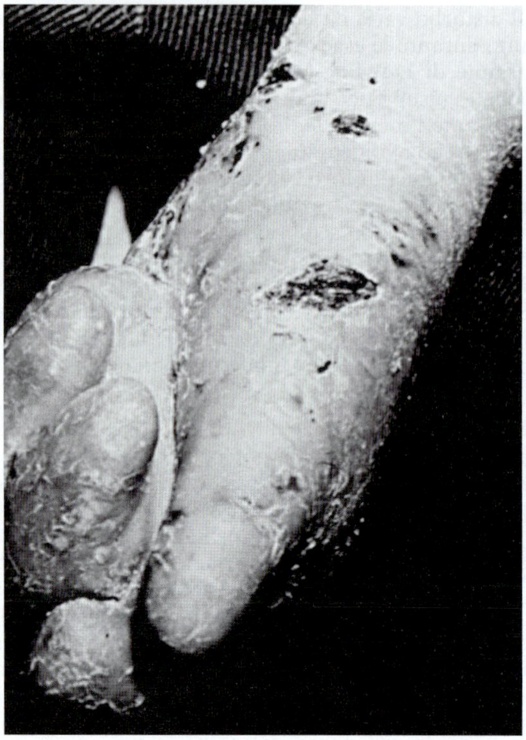

Figura 653-9. Deformità a guanto da pugile della mano, nell'epidermolisi bollosa distrofica.

DISTURBI IMMUNOBOLLOSI

PEMFIGO VOLGARE. Solitamente esordisce con ulcere orali dolorose, che possono essere l'unica manifestazione della malattia per settimane o mesi. Successivamente, emergono grandi bolle flaccide su cute non eritematosa, più comunemente su volto, tronco, punti di pressione, inguine e ascelle. È presente il **segno di Nikolsky**. Le lesioni si rompono e si allargano perifericamente, provocando aree dolorose denudate ed escoriate, con scarsa tendenza alla guarigione. Quando avviene, la guarigione è senza cicatrici, mentre è comune l'iperpigmentazione. Possono svilupparsi lesioni maleodoranti, verrucose e granulomatose, in sede di rottura delle bolle, in particolare nelle pieghe cutanee; quando questa condizione si fa più pronunciata, si parla più propriamente di pemfigo vegetante.

La biopsia viene effettuata di preferenza su una bolla piccola e recente, che si rivela sovrabasale (intraepidermica) e che contiene cellule epidemiche acantoliche, disperse, senza ponti intercellulari e pertanto senza possibilità di contatto reciproco. Gli anticorpi IgG diretti contro la sostanza epidermica intercellulare producono un quadro caratteristico all'immunofluorescenza diretta, sia della cute colpita sia di quella non coinvolta, in praticamente tutti i soggetti studiati. I titoli di anticorpi IgG sierici verso la sostanza intercellulare dell'epidermide correlano con il decorso clinico, in molti pazienti; pertanto, determinazioni seriate possono avere valore predittivo. Gli anticorpi del pemfigo sono patogenetici. L'antigene riconosciuto dagli anticorpi del pemfigo volgare è una glicoproteina da 130-kd nota come desmogleina III, che è complessata dalla placoglobina, una placca proteinica dei desmosomi. Le desmogleine sono un sottogruppo delle caderine, molecole di adesione cellulare.

Il **pemfigo volgare neonatale** si sviluppa in utero, come risultato del trasferimento placentare degli anticorpi materni in donne con pemfigo volgare attivo, sebbene ciò possa verificarsi anche quando la madre è in fase di remissione. Elevati titoli di anticorpi del pemfigo volgare prima del parto, e un'aumentata attività della malattia nella madre, correlano con una prognosi fetale infausta e con la morte del feto.

La **diagnosi differenziale** comprende l'eritema multiforme, il pemfigoide bolloso, la sindrome di Stevens-Johnson e la necrolisi epidermica tossica. Dato che il decorso può portare rapidamente a disabilità, malnutrizione e morte, è essenziale una diagnosi precoce. La malattia viene meglio controllata inizialmente con terapia corticosteroidea sistemica ad alte dosi. Le terapie con azatioprina, ciclofosfamide, metotrexate e sali d'oro sono tutte risultate efficaci negli schemi di mantenimento. Le immunoglobuline endovena, somministrate ciclicamente, possono essere di beneficio nei pazienti che non rispondono agli steroidi.

PEMFIGO FOLIACEO. Questo rarissimo disturbo è caratterizzato da vescicazione intraepidermica; la sede del clivaggio è situata più in alto, nell'epidermide, piuttosto che a livello sovrabasale, come nel pemfigo volgare. Le vescicole superficiali si rompono rapidamente, lasciando erosioni circondate da eritema, che guarisce con croste e desquamazione (Fig. 653-10). È presente il **segno di Nikolsky**. Le lesioni focali sono in genere localizzate al cuoio capelluto, al volto, al collo e alla parte superiore del tronco. Le lesioni delle membrane mucose sono scarse o assenti. I pazienti lamentano frequentemente prurito, dolore e bruciore. Quando è generalizzata, l'eruzione può somigliare alla dermatite esfoliativa o a qualsiasi disturbo bolloso cronico; le placche eritematose localizzate simulano dermatite seborroica, psoriasi, impetigine, eczema o lupus eritematoso. Il decorso clinico è variabile, ma è generalmente più benigno di quello del pemfigo volgare. Il **fogo selvagem**, che è endemico in alcune zone del Brasile, è identico clinicamente, istopatologicamente e immunologicamente, al pemfigo foliaceo.

È diagnostico il ritrovamento di una bolla acantolitica intraepidermica negli strati alti dell'epidermide. È imperativo selezionare per la biopsia una lesione precoce. Gli anticorpi epidermici intercellulari legati al tessuto e circolanti si legano a una porzione da 50-kD della glicoproteina desmosomiale da 160-kD, la desmogleina I. Alla soppressione della malattia mediante terapia corticosteroidea sistemica segue solitamente la remissione a lungo termine. In alcuni casi, è sufficiente una preparazione topica a base di dapsone o di steroidi.

PEMFIGOIDE BOLLOSO. Il pemfigoide bolloso insorge raramente nei bambini, ma deve essere considerato nella diagnosi differenziale di qualsiasi disordine bolloso cronico.

Manifestazioni cliniche. Tipicamente, le bolle si presentano a gruppi, su cute normale, eritematosa, eczematosa oppure orticarioide; esse compaiono prevalentemente sulle superfici flessorie delle estremità, sulle ascelle e a livello dell'inguine e della parte centrale dell'addome. I neonati presentano coinvolgimento delle superfici palmari, plantari e del volto, più frequentemente rispetto ai bambini più grandi. Le lesioni singole variano molto per dimensioni, sono tese e piene di liquido sieroso, che può diventare emorragico o torbido. Le lesioni orali insorgono meno frequentemente e sono meno gravi rispetto al pemfigo volgare, ma si osservano più comunemente nei bambini che negli adulti con pemfigoide bolloso. L'eruzione può essere accompagnata da prurito, bruciore ed edema sottocutaneo, sebbene i sintomi sistemici non siano predominanti.

Diagnosi e diagnosi differenziale. Il materiale bioptico deve essere raccolto da una bolla recente, insorta su base eritematosa. Istopatologicamente, si possono osservare una bolla sottoepidermica e un infiltrato infiammatorio dermico, prevalentemente eosinofilo. Nelle sezioni di una bolla o della cute periorale, nella zona della membrana basale, si può dimostrare una banda di immunoglobuline (solitamente IgG) e di C3 con metodi di immunofluorescenza diretta. Gli studi in immunofluorescenza indiretta del siero danno un risultato positivo in circa il 70% dei casi, per anticorpi IgG diretti verso la zona della membrana basale; il loro titolo, tuttavia, non correla bene con il decorso clinico. La **diagnosi differenziale** comprende l'eritema bolloso multiforme, il pemfigo, la dermatosi lineare a IgA, l'eruzione bollosa da farmaci, la dermatite erpetiforme, l'infezione da *herpes simplex* e l'impetigine bollosa, che possono essere differenziate mediante esame istologico, studi di immunofluorescenza e colture. Le bolle tese e ampie del pemfigoide bolloso possono generalmente essere distinte da quelle più piccole e flaccide del pemfigo volgare. I target principali per gli anticorpi del pemfigoide bolloso sono proteine del peso molecolare di 230 180-kD. La proteina da 230-kD è parte dell'emidesmosoma, mentre l'antigene da 180-kD si localizza sia sull'emidesmosoma sia sulla lamina lucida superiore ed è una proteina della transmembrana di collagene.

Trattamento. Il pemfigoide bolloso può essere controllato con successo mediante terapia topica o sistemica con corticosteroidi orali, da sola o in associazione ad azatioprina e dapsone. Il clobetasolo topico migliora i sintomi con minimi effetti collaterali. La patologia di solito si risolve in maniera definitiva.

DERMATITE ERPETIFORME. La dermatite erpetiforme è caratterizzata da piccole papule e vescicole simmetriche, raggruppate, eritematose, urenti e intensamente pruriginose. L'eruzione è pleomorfa e comprende lesioni eritematose, orticariodi, papulari, vescicolose e bollose. Le sedi di elezione sono le ginocchia, i gomiti, le spalle, le natiche e il cuoio capelluto; sono generalmente risparmiate le mucose. Possono svilupparsi lesioni emorragiche sulle superfici palmari e plantari. Quando il prurito è intenso, le escoriazioni possono essere il solo segno visibile (Fig. 653-11).

Eziologia. Nella dermatite erpetiforme, gli anticorpi IgA sono diretti contro la transglutaminasi epidermica. Nell'85-95% dei pazienti è presente un'enteropatia glutine-sensibile (vedi Capitolo 335.2). Nelle papille dermiche si osservano vescicole sottoepider-

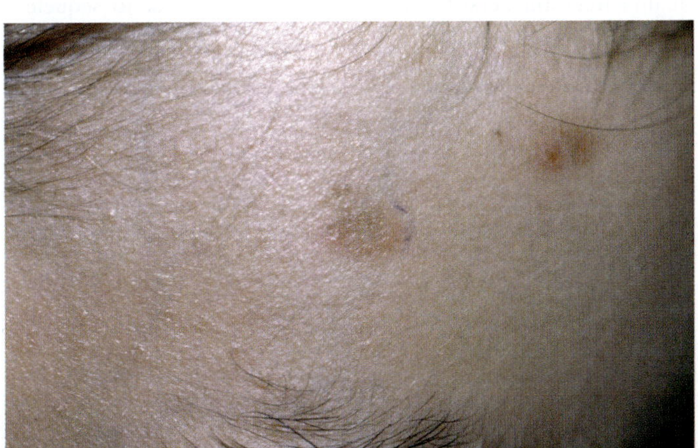

Figura 653-10. Erosioni superficiali nel pemfigo foliaceo.

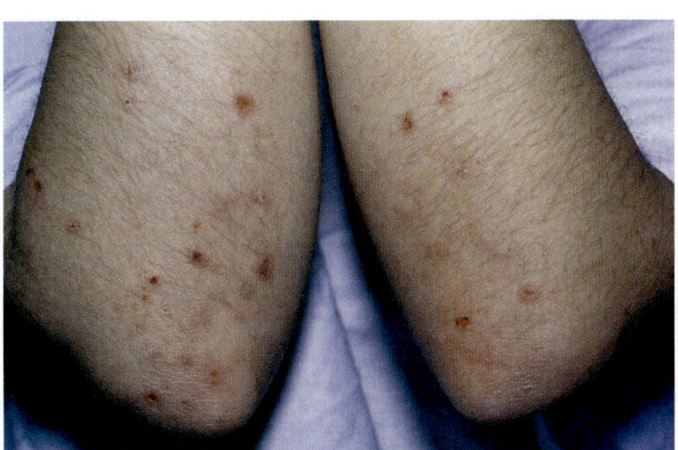

Figura 653-11. Escoriazioni multiple intorno ai gomiti, nella dermatite erpetiforme.

miche, composte prevalentemente da neutrofili. Tramite esame in immunofluorescenza, si possono riscontrare IgA e C3 nelle estremità delle papille dermiche della cute normale e perilesionale e nella regione della sublamina densa della giunzione dermoepidermica. Il frequente ritrovamento di immunocomplessi e di autoanticorpi nel siero, e l'associazione con l'antigene di istocompatibilità HLA-B8 in circa l'85% dei pazienti suggeriscono un meccanismo immunologico. Nel 70% dei pazienti con dermatite erpetiforme associata a enteropatia da glutine si trovano anticorpi anti-endomisio del muscolo liscio. I titoli anticorpali correlano con la severità della malattia intestinale e decrescono rapidamente quando si istituisce una dieta priva di glutine.

Trattamento. La dermatite erpetiforme può mimare altre malattie bollose croniche e può assomigliare anche alla scabbia, all'orticaria papulosa, a punture di insetto, alla dermatite da contatto e all'eczema papuloso. Il trattamento più efficace consiste nella somministrazione orale di dapsone (0,5-2,0 mg/kg/die in una o due somministrazioni). Questo farmaco dà sollievo immediato al prurito intenso, ma deve essere utilizzato con cautela a causa dei possibili gravi effetti collaterali (metaemoglobinemia, emolisi e sindrome da ipersensibilità [sindrome da sulfone]). Possono essere utili anche misure locali contro il prurito. La biopsia digiunale è indicata per diagnosticare l'enteropatia sensibile al glutine, poiché le manifestazioni cutanee possono precedere il malassorbimento. L'enteropatia risponde alla dieta priva di glutine più rapidamente di quanto facciano le lesioni cutanee.

DERMATOSI LINEARE A IGA (DERMATOSI BOLLOSA CRONICA DELL'INFANZIA). Questa rara dermatosi è più comune nella prima decade di vita, con un picco di incidenza durante l'età prescolare. L'eruzione consiste in molteplici bolle grandi e tese, piene di liquido limpido o emorragico, che si sviluppano su cute normale, eritematosa o orticarioide. Le sedi di elezione sono i genitali e le natiche (Fig. 653-12), la regione periorale e il cuoio capelluto. Le bolle "a salsiccia" possono essere disposte ad anello o a rosetta, intorno a una crosta centrale (Fig. 653-13). Placche eritematose con margini a spirale, circondate da bolle intatte, possono svilupparsi su ampie aree. Il prurito può essere assente o molto intenso e non compaiono segni e sintomi sistemici. Non è presente enteropatia da glutine.

Eziologia. Le bolle sottoepidermiche sono infiltrate da una varietà di cellule infiammatorie. Si possono osservare ascessi neutrofilici nelle estremità delle papille dermiche, indistinguibili da quelli della dermatite erpetiforme. Gli infiltrati possono anche essere in gran parte eosinofili, analogamente al pemfigoide. Pertanto, per una diagnosi definitiva, sono necessari esami in immunofluorescenza diretta; la cute lesionale o perilesionale dimostra una deposizione lineare di IgA, e talvolta di C3, a livello della

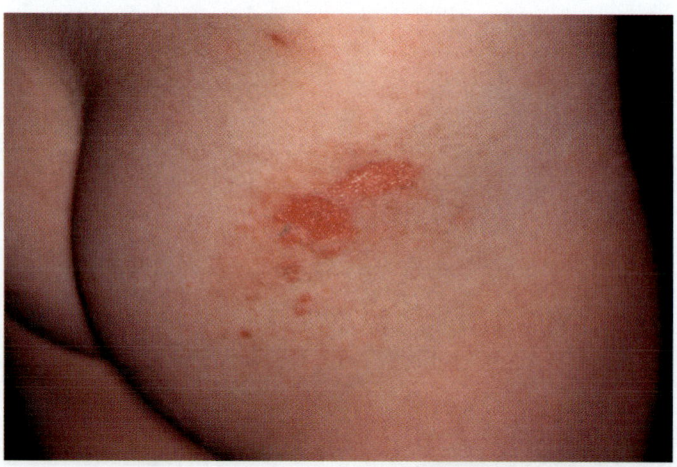

Figura 653-12. Erosioni su cute eritematosa conseguente a perdita del tetto della bolla, nella dermatosi lineare a IgA.

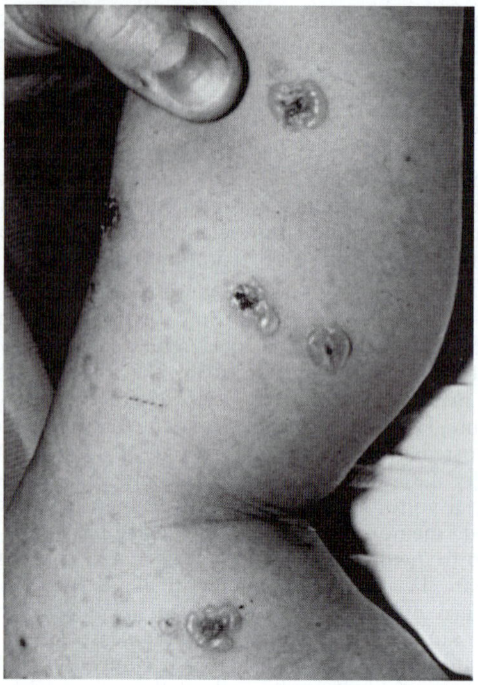

Figura 653-13. Vesciche a rosetta intorno a una crosta centrale, tipiche della dermatosi lineare a IgA (dermatosi cronica bollosa dell'infanzia).

giunzione dermoepidermica. I risultati dell'immunofluorescenza sono a volte positivi per anticorpi circolanti. La microscopia immunoelettronica ha localizzato gli immunoreagenti a livello della sublamina densa, sebbene sia anche stato osservato un pattern combinato di sublamina densa e lamina lucida. La dermatosi lineare a IgA è una malattia eterogenea con anticorpi diretti contro molteplici antigeni. I tre antigeni più comunemente riconosciuti sono LAD285, BP230 e BP180. Le IgA lineari possono essere osservate anche nelle eruzioni da farmaci. La maggior parte dei casi di IgA lineari indotte da farmaci è correlata alla vancomicina. L'eruzione può essere distinta istopatologicamente e in immunofluorescenza dal pemfigo, dal pemfigoide bolloso, dalla dermatite erpetiforme e dall'eritema multiforme. La colorazione di Gram e le colture escludono la diagnosi di impetigine bollosa. La mancata formazione di bolle in risposta ai traumi la differenzia dall'epidermolisi bollosa.

Trattamento. Molti pazienti rispondono favorevolmente al dapsone orale (vedi dermatite erpetiforme). I bambini che non rispondono al dapsone possono trarre beneficio dalla terapia orale con corticosteroidi o con una combinazione di questi farmaci. Il decorso abituale è di 2-4 anni, sebbene alcuni bambini soffrano di una malattia persistente o ricorrente; non vi sono sequele a lungo termine.

Ahmed AR, Dahl MV: Consensus statement on the use of intravenous immunoglobulin therapy in the treatment of autoimmune mucocutaneous blistering diseases. *Arch Dermatol* 2003;139:1051–1059.

Allen J, Wojnarosia F: Linear IgA disease: The IgA and IgG response to dermal antigens demonstrates a chiefly IgA response to LAD285 and a dermal 180-kDa protein. *Br J Dermatol* 2003;149:1055–1058.

Bello YM, Falabella AF, Schachner LA: Management of epidermolysis bullosa in infants and children. *Clin Dermatol* 2003;21:278–282.

Gannon BA: Epidermolysis bullosa: Pathophysiology and nursing care. *Neonatal Netw* 2004;23:25–32.

Lee WC, Leung JL, Fung CW, et al: Spectrum of anticonvulsant hypersensitivity syndrome: Controversy of treatment. *J Child Neurol* 2004; 19:619–623.

Metry DW, Jung P, Levy ML: Use of intravenous immunoglobulin in children with Stevens-Johnson syndrome and toxic epidermal necrolysis: Seven cases and review of the literature. *Pediatrics* 2003;112:1430–1436.

Ng PP, Sun YJ, Tan HH, et al: Detection of herpes simplex virus genomic DNA in various subsets of Erythema multiforme by polymerase chain reaction. *Dermatology* 2003;207:349–353.

Pfendner EG, Nakano A, Pulkkinen L, et al: Prenatal diagnosis for epidermolysis bullosa: A study of 144 consecutive pregnancies at risk. *Prenatal Diagn* 2003;23:447–456.

Williams PM, Conklin RJ: Erythema multiforme: A review and contrast from Stevens-Johnson syndrome/toxic epidermal necrolysis. *Dent Clin North Am* 2005;49:67–76.

Capitolo 654 ■ Disordini eczematosi

Joseph G. Morelli

I disordini cutanei eczematosi sono caratterizzati da essudazione, lichenificazione e prurito. Le lesioni eczematose acute presentano eritema, gemizio, essudato e formazione di microvescicole all'interno dell'epidermide. Le lesioni croniche sono generalmente ispessite, asciutte e squamose con segni cutanei grossolani (lichenificazione) e pigmentazione alterata. Nei bambini insorgono diversi tipi di eczema; il più comune è la **dermatite atopica** (vedi Capitolo 144), sebbene anche la dermatite seborroica, la dermatite allergica e da contatto, l'eczema nummulare e la dermatite vescicolosa di mani e piedi (disidrosi) siano relativamente comuni in età pediatrica. Diverse dermatiti pruriginose possono divenire eczematose in sede di grattamento. La cute atopica è sensibile a molti fattori che peggiorano il prurito, come i saponi, la lana, l'eccessivo riscaldamento e gli allergeni alimentari.

Dopo aver effettuato la diagnosi di eczema, è importante classificare l'eruzione in modo più specifico per poterla trattare nella maniera più appropriata. La chiave interpretativa è spesso fornita da dati anamnestici pertinenti. In alcuni casi, il decorso e il carattere dell'eruzione ne permettono la classificazione. Le alterazioni istologiche sono relativamente aspecifiche, ma tutti i tipi di dermatite eczematosa sono caratterizzati da edema intraepidermico, noto come spongiosi.

DERMATITE DA CONTATTO. Questa forma di eczema può essere suddivisa in dermatite irritativa, che è dovuta a un danno aspecifico alla cute, e dermatite allergica da contatto, in cui il meccanismo è una reazione da ipersensibilità ritardata. Delle due, la dermatite irritativa è più frequente nei bambini, in particolare durante i primi anni di vita.

La **dermatite irritativa da contatto** può essere causata da un contatto prolungato o ripetuto con varie sostanze, tra cui saliva, succo di limone, bagnoschiuma, detergenti, materiali abrasivi, saponi forti e prodotti farmaceutici. La saliva è probabilmente uno dei fattori scatenanti più comuni; può causare una dermatite del volto o delle pieghe cutanee nei lattanti che ne producono molta o nei bambini ritardati. I bambini più grandi che si leccano abitualmente, e spesso inconsapevolmente, le labbra a causa della secchezza, possono sviluppare un rash periorale acceso e demarcato (Fig. 654-1). Tra gli irritanti esogeni, il succo di limone, i prodotti farmaceutici e i bagnoschiuma sono relativamente comuni. Anche l'eccessivo accumulo di sudore e umidità, dovuto all'uso di scarpe occludenti, può causare una dermatite irritativa.

La dermatite irritativa da contatto può essere confusa con la dermatite atopica o con la dermatite allergica da contatto. Un'anamnesi dettagliata e la considerazione delle sedi coinvolte, dell'età del bambino e degli agenti con cui è venuto a contatto forniscono di solito indizi sugli agenti eziologici. La propensione a sviluppare una dermatite irritativa varia considerevolmente tra i bambini; alcuni possono rispondere a insulti minimi, rendendo difficile identificare l'agente causale dall'anamnesi. In genere, la dermatite irritativa da contatto si risolve dopo la rimozione dello stimolo e un trattamento temporaneo con preparazione cortico-

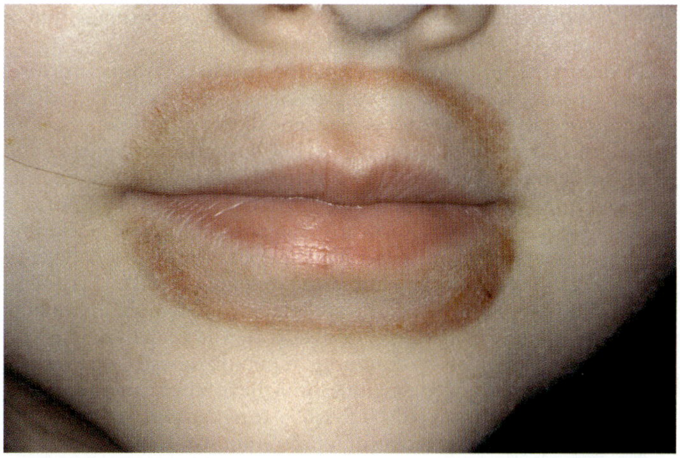

Figura 654-1. Dermatite irritativa da contatto periorale dovuta a inumidimento delle labbra con la lingua.

steroidee per uso topico (vedi Capitolo 645). L'educazione del paziente e dei genitori sulle cause della dermatite da contatto è essenziale per il successo della terapia.

La **dermatite da pannolino** può essere considerata il prototipo delle dermatite irritativa da contatto. Come reazione all'iperidratazione della cute, alla frizione, alla macerazione e al contatto prolungato con urine e feci, con saponi non asportati bene e con preparazioni topiche, la cute nell'area del pannolino può divenire eritematosa e squamosa, spesso con lesioni papulovescicolari o bollose, fissurazioni ed erosioni (Fig. 654-2). L'eruzione può essere focale o confluente, ma le pieghe genitocrurali sono spesso risparmiate. Possono insorgere papule croniche ipertrofiche, a sommità piana, e noduli infiltrativi. L'infezione batterica o micotica secondaria è comune. Il fastidio può essere marcato a causa di un'intensa infiammazione. Quando l'eruzione è persistente o resistente a semplici misure terapeutiche, andrebbero prese in considerazione condizioni quali la dermatite allergica da contatto, la dermatite seborroica, la psoriasi, la candidosi, la dermatite

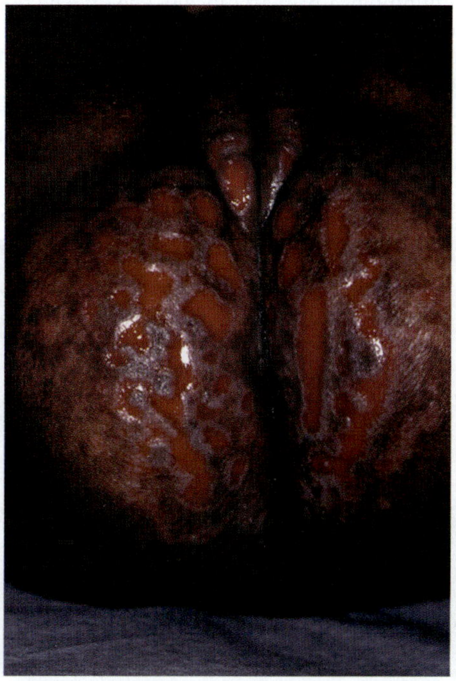

Figura 654-2. Grave dermatite erosiva da pannolino.

atopica e malattie rare come l'istiocitosi X (istiocitosi a cellule di Langerhans) e l'acrodermatite enteropatica.

La dermatite da pannolino risponde spesso a semplici misure; alcuni neonati hanno una predisposizione per la dermatite da pannolino e il trattamento può essere difficile. L'effetto dannoso dell'iperidratazione della cute e del contatto prolungato con feci e urine può essere ovviato con un cambio più frequente del pannolino. Si deve evitare il lavaggio eccessivo, poiché porta a screpolature e al peggioramento della dermatite. Il pannolini monouso contenenti un materiale superassorbente possono aiutare a mantenere un ambiente relativamente asciutto. Frequenti applicazioni topiche di agenti ad effetto barriera blandamente protettivi (petrolato o pasta all'ossido di zinco) possono essere sufficienti a prevenire la dermatite. Quando queste misure non bastano a ottenere la guarigione, una lieve applicazione di unguento all'idrocortisone allo 0,5-1,0% topico, dopo ogni cambio di pannolino, per un periodo di tempo limitato, è spesso efficace. Complicanze secondarie possono derivare dall'uso prolungato di cortisonici, specialmente da composti fluorinati. Prima di iniziare tale terapia, si dovrebbe escludere la possibilità di una dermatite da candida. L'**infezione da Candida** può essere diagnosticata per la cute rosso-rosa con numerose pustole e papule di 1-2 mm alla periferia della dermatite. Il trattamento con un agente anticandida topico può essere utile.

La **dermatosi plantare giovanile** è una forma comune di dermatite da contatto irritativa, che insorge prevalentemente nei bambini in età prepuberale. La dermatite coinvolge caratteristicamente le superfici di appoggio, può essere pruriginosa o dolorosa e causa un aspetto lucido della cute plantare (Fig. 654-3). La fissurazione più divenire estesa e causare un fastidio notevole. Tale dermatite è causata dall'alternanza di idratazione eccessiva e rapida perdita di umidità, che provocano desquamazione della cute e fissurazione dello strato corneo. I bambini affetti hanno spesso iperidrosi, indossano calzature sintetiche occlusive e sottopongono i loro piedi a un asciugamento rapido senza idratazione. L'applicazione immediata di uno strato spesso di un preparato emolliente, quando si tolgono calze e scarpe o dopo il nuoto, generalmente previene questa condizione.

La **dermatite allergica da contatto** è una reazione di ipersensibilità mediata da linfociti T, provocata dall'applicazione di un antigene sulla superficie cutanea. L'antigene penetra nella cute, dove viene coniugato con una proteina cutanea, e il complesso aptene-proteina è trasportato ai linfonodi regionali da cellule di Langerhans che presentano l'antigene. Nei linfonodi avviene una risposta immunologica primaria locale, che diviene poi generalizzata, presumibilmente a causa della disseminazione di linfociti T sensibilizzati. La sensibilizzazione richiede diversi giorni e, quando è seguita da un nuovo stimolo antigenico, si manifesta come dermatite allergica da contatto. Può verificarsi una distribuzione generalizzata anche se una quantità sufficiente di antigene raggiunge la circolazione. Una volta avvenuta la sensibilizzazione, ogni nuovo stimolo antigenico può provocare una reazione infiammatoria entro 8-12 ore; la sensibilizzazione a un particolare antigene persiste in genere per molti anni.

La dermatite allergica da contatto acuta è una dermatite eritematosa, eczematosa, intensamente pruriginosa che, se severa, può essere edematosa e vescicolobollosa. La condizione cronica ha le caratteristiche di un eczema di lunga durata: lichenificazione, desquamazione, fissurazione e alterazioni pigmentarie. La distribuzione dell'eruzione spesso fornisce un indizio per la diagnosi. I sensibilizzanti volatili colpiscono generalmente le aree esposte, come il volto e le braccia. La bigiotteria, gli agenti topici, gli indumenti e le piante causano dermatite nei punti di contatto.

La **dermatite da *Rhus toxicodendrum*** (edera velenosa, sommacco velenoso, quercia velenosa) è spesso vescicolobollosa e può essere distinta dalle strie lineari di vescicole che si formano nei punti in cui la cute è venuta a contatto con le piante (Fig. 654-4). Il liquido dalle vescicole cutanee rotte non diffonde l'eruzione; tuttavia, gli antigeni conservati sulla cute, sotto le unghie e sugli abiti possono scatenare nuove placche di dermatite se non vengono rimossi tramite lavaggio con acqua e sapone. Gli antigeni possono essere trasportati anche dagli animali sul loro pelo. L'allergene della linfa (oleoresina) è presente sulle foglie vive e morte e la sensibilizzazione a una pianta provoca reazioni crociate con le altre).

La **dermatite da nickel** si sviluppa solitamente in seguito al contatto con gioielli o fibbie metalliche di indumenti e si osserva più frequentemente sui lobi auricolari, nei casi in cui, per mantenere aperto il foro, sono stati utilizzati supporti per orecchini contenenti nickel invece che materiali non metallici o di acciaio inossidabile. Le fibbie metalliche sui pantaloni causano spesso una malattia a localizzazione periombelicale (Fig. 654-5). Alcuni bambini sono particolarmente sensibili al nickel, e manifestano eruzioni anche quando vengono a contatto con tracce minime all'interno di gioielli in oro.

La **dermatite da calzature** colpisce caratteristicamente il dorso e le dita dei piedi, risparmiando gli spazi interdigitali; solitamente è simmetrica. Altre forme di dermatite allergica da contatto, al contrario della dermatite irritativa, coinvolgono raramente le superfici palmoplantari. Gli allergeni comuni sono gli antiossidanti,

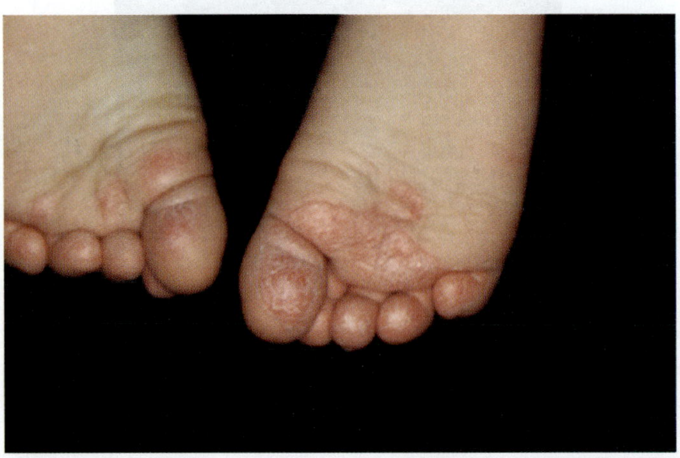

Figura 654-3. Dermatosi plantare giovanile arrossata e desquamante.

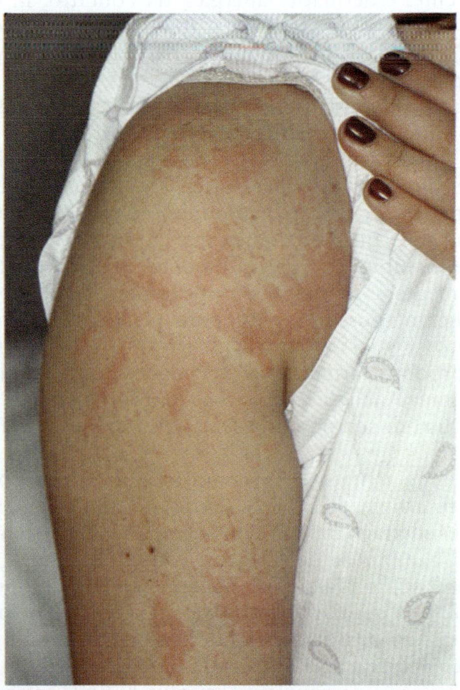

Figura 654-4. Lesioni lineari nella dermatite da edera velenosa.

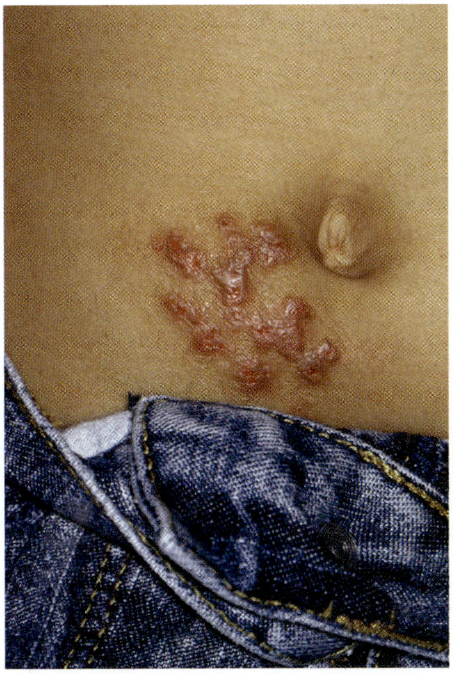

Figura 654-5. Dermatite cronica periombelicale da nickel.

gli acceleratori nella gomma delle scarpe e i sali di cromo presenti nella cute colorata o nelle tinture per scarpe. Queste sostanze vengono spesso liberate dall'eccessiva sudorazione.

I capi d'abbigliamento contengono numerosi sensibilizzanti, tra cui tinture, mordenti, finiture di fabbricazione, fibre, resine e soluzioni di lavaggio. La tinta può essere mal fissata all'abito e liberata dalla sudorazione, come lo sono le resine di formaldeide parzialmente fissate. Anche gli elastici degli indumenti sono una causa frequente di dermatite da contatto.

I farmaci topici e i cosmetici possono essere allergeni non sospetti, in particolare se il farmaco è utilizzato per una dermatite preesistente. Gli agenti causali più comuni sono la neomicina, il timerosal, gli antistaminici e gli anestetici topici, i conservanti e l'etilendiamina, uno stabilizzatore presente in molti farmaci. Tutti i tipi di cosmetici possono causare dermatite del volto; il coinvolgimento delle palpebre è caratteristico della sensibilizzazione al solvente dello smalto per unghie.

La dermatite da contatto può essere confusa con altri tipi di eczema, dermatofitosi e malattie vescicolobollose. Il patch test può chiarire l'eziologia. Il principio essenziale, nel **trattamento**, è l'eliminazione del contatto con l'allergene. La dermatite acuta risponde all'applicazione di compresse fredde e di un unguento steroideo topico. Può essere utile un antistaminico per os. Le reazioni bollose acute massive o le reazioni che causano edema perioculare o genitale, come quelle da edera velenosa, possono richiedere un trattamento di due settimane con corticosteroidi orali a scalare. Se si è instaurata un'infezione secondaria, dovrebbe essere somministrata un'appropriata terapia antibiotica per via sistemica. La terapia desensibilizzante è raramente indicata.

ECZEMA NUMMULARE. Questo disturbo non è correlato agli altri tipi di eczema ed è caratterizzato da placche eczematose dalla forma simile a una moneta. Le sedi più comuni sono le superfici estensorie delle estremità (Fig. 654-6), le natiche e le spalle. Le placche sono relativamente separate, umide, vescicolose, intensamente pruriginose ed essudative; quando croniche, divengono frequentemente ispessite e lichenificate. La causa è sconosciuta. Molto spesso, queste lesioni vengono confuse con quelle della *tinea corporis*, ma le placche dell'eczema nummulare sono distinguibili per la mancanza di un bordo rilevato e nettamente circoscritto, per l'assenza di organismi fungini alla esame con

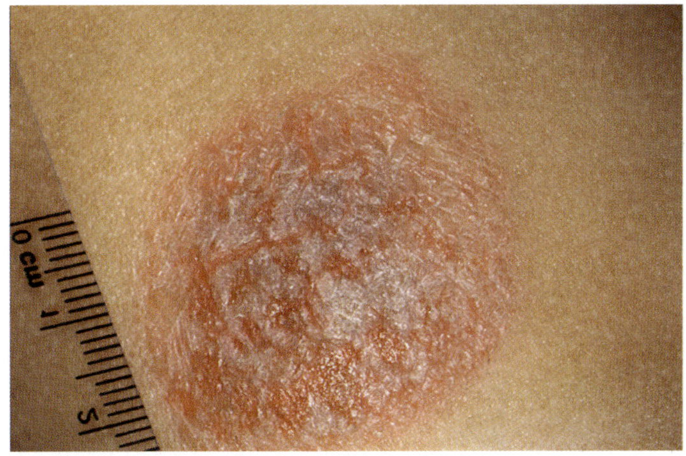

Figura 654-6. Placche separate, essudanti di dermatite nummulare.

idrossido di potassio (KOH) e per il frequente sanguinamento o gemizio con il grattamento. L'infezione secondaria è comune. Il controllo del prurito si ottiene generalmente con preparazioni a base di corticosteroidi fluorinati. Le garze impregnate di steroidi possono trattare e allo stesso tempo fungere da barriera protettiva per queste placche eczematose circoscritte. Un antistaminico può essere utile, specialmente di notte. Gli antibiotici sono indicati per le infezioni secondarie.

PITIRIASI ALBA. Insorge prevalentemente nei bambini; le lesioni sono ipopigmentate, rotonde o ovali, con zone maculari o leggermente rilevate e squame finemente aderenti (Fig. 654-7). Possono essere leggermente eritematose e relativamente ben definite, ma mancano di un margine nettamente demarcato. Le lesioni insorgono sul volto, sul collo, sulla parte superiore del tronco e sulla porzione prossimale delle braccia. Il prurito è minimo o assente. La causa è sconosciuta, ma l'eruzione sembra essere esacerbata dalla secchezza ed è spesso considerata una forma lieve di eczema. La pitiriasi alba viene spesso diagnosticata erroneamente come vitiligine, *tinea versicolor* o *tinea corporis*. Le lesioni compaiono e scompaiono, ma alla fine si risolvono. L'applicazione di un emolliente può migliorare la situazione; se il prurito è fastidioso, si può usare uno steroide topico a bassa potenza. Spesso occorrono mesi prima che la pigmentazione torni nella norma.

LICHEN SIMPLEX CRONICO. Questa lesione è caratterizzata da una placca unica e circoscritta cronica, pruriginosa ed eczematosa, solitamente lichenificata e iperpigmentata (Fig. 654-8). Le sedi più comuni sono la superficie posteriore del collo, il dorso del piede, i polsi e le caviglie. Sebbene l'evento scatenante possa essere una

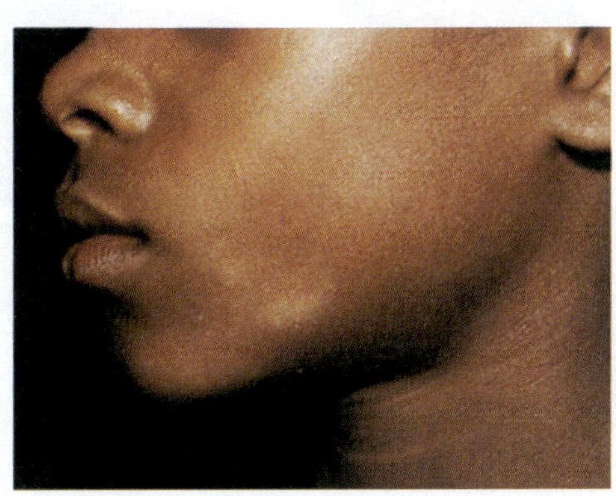

Figura 654-7. Lesioni ipopigmentate, a chiazze, con margini diffusi, caratteristiche della pitiriasi alba.

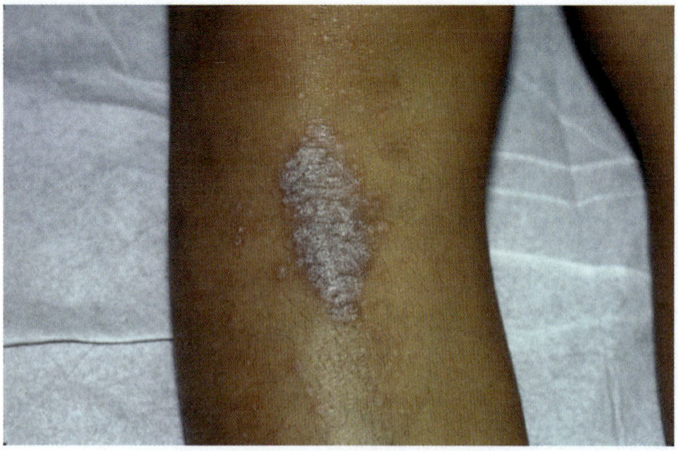

Figura 654-8. Placca ispessita di lichen simplex cronico.

lesione transitoria, come una puntura di insetto, il trauma da sfregamento e grattamento è responsabile della persistenza della placca. Per consentire la guarigione è necessario controllare il prurito. Una preparazione topica a base di corticosteroidi fluorinati è spesso utile; occorre evitare l'irritazione costante della cute. Può essere necessaria una copertura per evitare il grattamento.

DERMATITE VESCICOLOSA DI MANI E PIEDI (ECZEMA DISIDROSICO, DISIDROSI, POMFOLICE). Si tratta di un disturbo caratterizzato dalla presenza di vescicole ricorrenti, talvolta stagionale, delle mani e dei piedi; insorge a tutte le età ma è poco comune nell'infanzia. La patogenesi è sconosciuta; non sono stati identificati fattori genetici, sebbene sia stata osservata un'aumentata incidenza di atopia nei pazienti e nei loro famigliari. La malattia è caratterizzata da gruppi ricorrenti di piccole vescicole intensamente pruriginose sulle mani e sui piedi. Le sedi di predilezione sono le superfici palmari e plantari, e la parte laterale delle dita. Le lesioni primarie non sono infiammatorie e contengono un liquido limpido che, a differenza del sudore, ha una pH fisiologico e contiene proteine. Possono insorgere vescicole e bolle più grandi (Fig. 654-9), e, a causa del grattamento, sono frequenti macerazione e infezioni secondarie. La fase cronica è caratterizzata da placche ispessite e fissurate che possono causare un notevole fastidio. L'iperidrosi è comune in molti pazienti, ma l'associazione può essere casuale. La diagnosi è clinica. Il disturbo può essere confuso con la dermatite allergica da contatto, che solitamente, però, colpisce le superfici dorsali e non quelle volari, e con la dermatofitosi, che può essere distinta tramite una reazione al KOH del tetto della vescicola e con colture appropriate.

Quando localizzata a mani e piedi, nella fase acuta, la patologia risponde all'applicazione di medicazioni umide seguite da una preparazione topica corticosteroidea. Il controllo della fase cronica è difficile; possono essere indicati lubrificanti contenenti agenti cheratolitici lievi, in associazione con preparazioni a base di corticosteroidi fluorinati potenti. L'infezione batterica secondaria deve essere trattata con un antibiotico appropriato per via sistemica. I pazienti andrebbero informati sulla possibilità di recidive e istruiti a proteggersi mani e piedi dagli effetti dannosi dell'eccessiva sudorazione, di agenti chimici, di saponi aggressivi e clima sfavorevole. Purtroppo non è possibile prevenire le recidive o predirne la frequenza.

DERMATITE SEBORROICA. Questa patologia infiammatoria cronica è più comune nella prima infanzia e nell'adolescenza e rispecchia la distribuzione, l'ampiezza e l'attività delle ghiandole sebacee. La causa è sconosciuta, così come il ruolo delle ghiandole sebacee nella malattia. Non è noto nemmeno se la dermatite seborroica infantile e dell'adolescenza siano la stessa entità o due entità distinte. Non vi sono evidenze che i bambini con dermatite seborroica infantile sviluppino una dermatite seborroica da adolescenti. Un'eruzione generalizzata con le caratteristiche della dermatite seborroica è comune nei bambini e negli adolescenti con infezione da HIV.

Manifestazioni cliniche. Il disturbo può insorgere nel primo mese di vita ed essere molto fastidioso soprattutto nel primo anno. La prima manifestazione, talvolta l'unica, può essere una desquamazione con formazione di croste del cuoio capelluto, diffusa o focale, talvolta chiamata crosta lattea (Fig. 654-10). Una dermatite grassa, squamosa, eritematosa e papulosa, generalmente non pruriginosa, può coinvolgere il volto, il collo, le zone retroauricolari, le ascelle e l'area del pannolino. La dermatite può essere a macchie o focale o può diffondersi coinvolgendo quasi tutto il corpo (Fig. 654-11). Sono comuni alterazioni pigmentarie postinfiammatorie, in particolari nei bambini neri. Quando la desquamazione diviene pronunciata, la patologia può assomigliare alla psoriasi e, talvolta, ne viene distinta con difficoltà. Deve essere considerata la possibilità di una coesistente dermatite atopica qualora vi sia una dermatite acuta essudativa con prurito; nel primissimo periodo di vita è spesso impossibile separare queste due patologie. Una dermatite simil-seborroica non trattabile, con diarrea cronica e arresto dell'accrescimento, può riflettere una disfunzione del sistema immunitario. Un quadro cronico simil-seborroico, che risponda scarsamente al trattamento, può essere causato anche da infiltrati istiocitari cutanei in neonati con **istiocitosi X a cellule di Langerhans**. La dermatite seborroica è una manifestazione cutanea comune dell'**AIDS** nei giovani adulti,

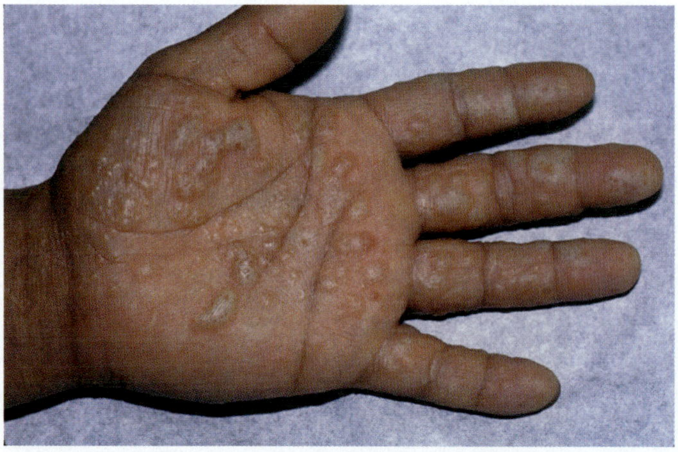

Figura 654-9. Lesioni vescicolari palmari dell'eczema disidrosico con grandi bolle.

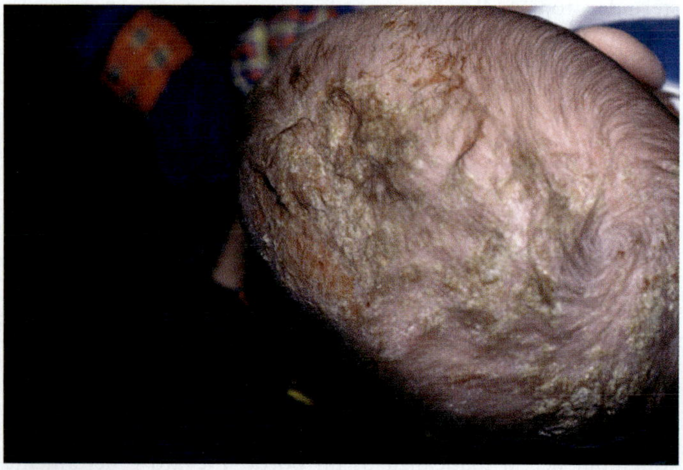

Figura 654-10. Crosta lattea in un lattante.

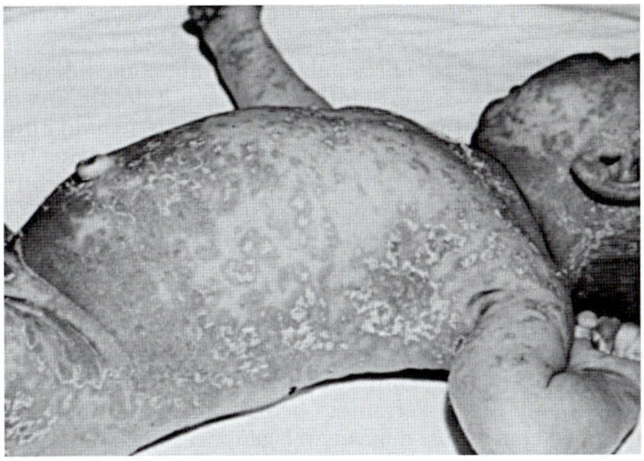

Figura 654-11. Dermatite seborroica diffusa.

ed è caratterizzata da squame spesse e grasse sul cuoio capelluto e da grandi placche eritematose e ipercheratosiche sul volto, sul torace e sui genitali.

Durante l'adolescenza, la dermatite seborroica è più localizzata e può essere limitata al cuoio capelluto e alle aree intertriginose. Si possono osservare anche blefarite marginale e interessamento del canale uditivo esterno. Le alterazioni del cuoio capelluto possono variare da una desquamazione diffusa, brunastra, ad aree focali di croste ispessite, untuose e giallastre con eritema sottostante. La perdita di capelli è comune e il prurito può essere assente o marcato. Quando la dermatite è severa, possono insorgere eritema e desquamazione a livello dell'attaccatura frontale dei capelli, delle superfici mediali delle sopracciglia e dei solchi nasolabiali e retroauricolari. Possono comparire placche rosse e squamose a livello delle ascelle, della regione inguinale, della fenditura glutea e dell'ombelico. Sulle estremità, le placche seborroiche possono essere più eczematose e meno eritematose e demarcate.

Eziologia. La *Malassezia furfur* è stata considerata un agente causale, sebbene il suo ruolo nell'eziologia della dermatite seborroica infantile sia poco chiaro. La diagnosi differenziale comprende la psoriasi, la dermatite atopica, la dermatofitosi e la candidosi. Sono comuni infezioni batteriche secondarie e candidosi sovrapposta.

Trattamento. Le lesioni del cuoio capelluto andrebbero controllate con uno shampoo antiseborroico (solfuro di selenio, zolfo, acido salicilico, zinco piritione, catrame), utilizzato quotidianamente, se necessario. Le lesioni infiammatorie rispondono di solito alla terapia corticosteroidea topica. Gli agenti immunomodulanti topici (tacrolimus, pimecrolimus), approvati per il trattamento della dermatite atopica nei bambini di età superiore a 2 anni (vedi Capitolo 144), possono essere utili nel trattamento di altri disturbi eczematosi, come la dermatite seborroica. I dubbi sull'assorbimento sistemico e sulla potenziale immunosoppressione sono maggiori nella popolazione più giovane, tipicamente colpita da dermatite seborroica. Sono stati impiegati in terapia anche gli agenti antimicotici topici, attivi contro la *Malassezia*. Garze umide dovrebbero essere applicate sulle lesioni essudanti o fissurate, prima dell'utilizzo di un unguento steroideo. Molti pazienti necessitano dell'uso continuativo di uno shampoo antiseborroico. La risposta alla terapia è solitamente rapida, a meno che non vi siano fattori complicanti o la diagnosi sia errata.

Brydensholt Halkjaer L, Loland L, Buchvald FF, et al: Development of atopic dermatitis during the first 3 years of life. *Arch Dermatol* 2006;142:561–566.
Faergemann J: Treatment of seborrheic dermatitis with oral terbinafine? *Lancet* 2001;358:170.
Fergusson DM, Horwood J, Shannon FT: Early solid feeding and recurrent childhood eczema: A 10-year longitudinal study. *Pediatrics* 1990; 86:541–546.
Krafchik BR: Eczematous disorders. In Eichenfield LF, Frieden IJ, Esterly NB (editors): *Textbook of Neonatal Dermatology.* Philadelphia, WB Saunders, 2001, p 241.
Paller AS: Use of non-steroidal topical immunomodulators for the treatment of atopic dermatitis in the pediatric population. *J Pediatr* 2001; 138:163–168.
Rothe M, Grant-Kels J: Diagnostic criteria for atopic dermatitis. *Lancet* 1996;348:769–770.
Tollesson A, Frithz A, Stenlund K: *Malassezia furfur* in infantile seborrheic dermatitis. *Pediatr Dermatol* 1997;14:423–425.

Capitolo 655 ■ Fotosensibilità

Joseph G. Morelli

La fotosensibilità denota una reazione cutanea qualitativamente o quantitativamente abnorme alla luce solare o artificiale.

ERITEMA SOLARE ACUTO. La più comune reazione da fotosensibilità osservata nei bambini è l'eritema solare acuto. L'ustione è causata principalmente dalle radiazioni UVB (lunghezza d'onda 290-320 nm). La luce solare contiene molte più radiazioni UVA (320-400 nm) che UVB, ma gli UVA devono essere assorbiti in quantità molto maggiori, rispetto agli UVB, per provocare eritema solare.

Fisiopatologia e manifestazioni cliniche. Le radiazioni con lunghezza inferiore a 300 nm sono in gran parte assorbite dall'epidermide, mentre quelle con lunghezza d'onda superiore ai 300 nm vengono trasmesse per la maggior parte al derma dopo un assorbimento variabile da parte della melanina cutanea. La suscettibilità alle radiazioni UV varia nei bambini in base al tipo di cute (quantità di pigmentazione) (Tab. 655-1). L'immediato inscurimento del pigmento è dovuto al processo foto-ossidativo indotto dalle radiazioni UVA della melanina esistente, e al suo trasferimento dai melanociti ai cheratinociti. Questo effetto dura generalmente per alcune ore e, come per le lampade abbronzanti a UVA, non è fotoprotettivo. Gli effetti indotti dagli UVB compaiono 6-12 ore dopo la prima esposizione e raggiungono un picco dopo 24 ore; comprendono eritema, sensibilizzazione, edema e vescicolazione (Fig. 655-1). Le specie ossidative reattive generate dagli UVB inducono un danno della membrana dei cheratinociti e sono coinvolte nella patogenesi dell'ustione solare. Una parte della vasodilatazione osservata nell'eritema indotto da UVB è mediata dalle prostaglandine E2 e F2. La melanogenesi ritardata, causata dalle radiazioni UVB, inizia entro 2-3 giorni e dura diversi giorni o qualche settimana. La produzione di nuova melanina nei melanociti, il trasferimento di melanina dai melanociti ai cheratinociti, l'aumento delle dimensioni e dell'arborizzazione dei melanociti e l'attivazione dei melanociti quiescenti danno luogo alla melanogenesi tardiva. Questo effetto riduce la sensibilità cutanea allo sviluppo di eritema, da due a tre volte circa. Gli ulteriori effetti e le possibili complicanze dell'esposizione solare comprendono aumento di spessore dello strato corneo oltre che recidiva o esacerbazione dell'*herpes simplex* labiale, del lupus eritematoso e di molti altri disordini (Tab. 655-2).

TABELLA 655-1. Tipi di cute in base alla reazione all'esposizione solare

CEPPO DEMOGRAFICO	ANAMNESI DI USTIONI E ABBRONZATURA
I Capelli rossi, efelidi, origine celtica	Si ustiona sempre con facilità, non si abbronza
II Cute e capelli chiari, occhi azzurri, caucasico	Solitamente si ustiona, si abbronza poco
III Caucasico con la cute più scura	Talvolta si ustiona, abbronzatura graduale marrone chiaro
IV Origine mediterranea	Ustioni minime o assenti, si abbronza sempre
V Medio Oriente-caucasico, messicano	Raramente si ustiona, si abbronza uniformemente raggiungendo un colorito marrone scuro
VI Neri	Non si ustiona mai, pigmentazione nera

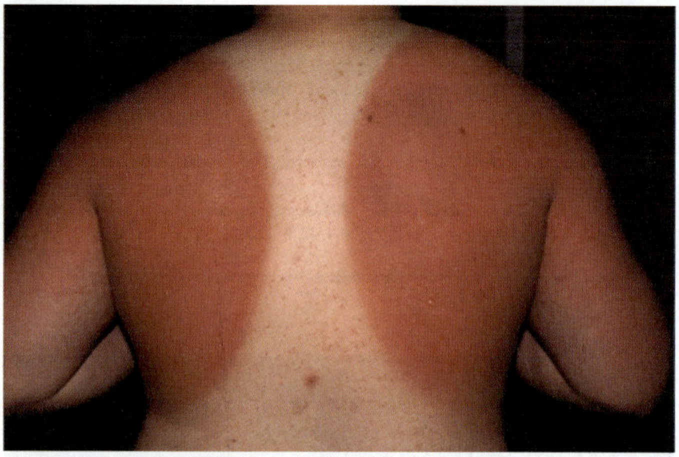

Figura 655-1. Ustione solare. Eritema severo, ben demarcato.

TABELLA 655-2. Reazioni cutanee alla luce solare
USTIONI SOLARI
ERUZIONI DA FARMACI FOTOINDOTTE
I farmaci sistemici comprendono tetracicline, psoraleni, clorotiazidl, sulfonamidi, barbiturici, griseofulvina, tiazidici, chinidina, fenotiazine
Gli agenti topici comprendono derivati del catrame, psoraleni, salicilanilidi alogenati (saponi), oli profumati (per es. olio di bergamotto), creme solari (per es. PABA, cinnamati, benzofenoni)
ERUZIONI FOTOTOSSICHE DA FARMACI
Dosi elevate degli agenti che causano eruzioni fotoallergiche; acido nalidixico, 5-fluorouracile, psoraleni, furosemide, farmaci antinfiammatori non steroidei (naproxene, piroxicam), sulfonamidi, tetracicline, fenotiazine, furocumarinici (per es. lime, limone, carota, sedano, aneto, pastinaca, prezzemolo)
MALATTIE GENETICHE CON FOTOSENSIBILITÀ
Xeroderma pigmentoso
Sindrome di Bloom
Sindrome di Cockayne
Sindrome di Rothmund-Thomson
ERRORI CONGENITI DEL METABOLISMO
Porfirie
Morbo di Hartnup
MALATTIE INFETTIVE ASSOCIATE A IPERSENSIBILITÀ
Infezione ricorrente da herpes simplex
Esantemi virali (fotodistribuzione accentuata, per es. varicella)
MALATTIE CUTANEE ESACERBATE O PRECIPITATE DALLA LUCE
Lichen planus
Malattia di Darier
Lupus eritematoso
Dermatomiosite
Sclerodermia
Granuloma anulare
Psoriasi
Eritema multiforme
Sarcoidosi
Dermatite atopica
Malattia di Hailey-Hailey
Pemfigo
Acne rosacea
Pemfigoide bolloso
DEFICIT DI PROTEZIONE DA MANCANZA DI PIGMENTO
Vitiligine
Albinismo oculocutaneo
Fenilchetonuria
Sindrome di Chédiak-Higashi
Sindrome di Hermansky-Pudlak
Sindrome di Waardenburg
Piebaldismo

Trattamento. Le ustioni solari acute e gravi devono essere trattate con compresse imbevute di acqua fredda. I corticosteroidi topici e gli inibitori delle prostaglandine orali, come l'ibuprofene e l'indometacina, possono ridurre l'eritema e il dolore, ma devono essere somministrati prima dell'esposizione o quando l'ustione è in fase iniziale. Una volta raggiunto il picco di eritema, questi farmaci offrono uno scarso beneficio. I farmaci contenenti anestetici topici sono piuttosto inefficaci e potenzialmente pericolosi, per la loro tendenza a causare dermatite da contatto. In fase desquamativa è efficace un blando emolliente.

Prognosi e prevenzione delle sequele. Le sequele a lungo termine dell'esposizione cronica e intensa alla luce solare non si osservano di frequente nei bambini, ma la maggior parte degli individui riceve più del 50% della quantità totale di UV della sua vita entro i primi vent'anni di età. Pertanto, i pediatri hanno un ruolo fondamentale nell'educazione di pazienti e genitori sugli effetti dannosi, sul rischio potenziale di malignità e sui danni cutanei irreversibili causati dall'esposizione eccessivamente prolungata al sole e alle lampade abbronzanti. Nella cute danneggiata dal sole si verificano con maggior frequenza invecchiamento precoce, elastosi senile, cheratosi attinica, carcinomi squamocellulari e basocellulari, oltre che melanomi. In particolare, le ustioni vescicolose in età pediatrica e nell'adolescenza incrementano significativamente il rischio di sviluppare un melanoma maligno. La migliore protezione solare consiste nell'evitare il sole; vale a dire che bisogna ridurre al minimo il tempo di esposizione nello ore centrali della giornata (dalle 10 alle 15), stare all'ombra e indossare indumenti protettivi, compresi cappelli a larghe tese. La protezione può essere aumentata da un'ampia varietà di agenti schermanti. Gli schermi solari fisici opachi (ossido di zinco, diossido di titanio) bloccano la luce UV, mentre le sostanze chimiche (acido paraminobenzoico [PABA], esteri del PABA, salicilati, benzofenoni, dibenzoilmetani, cinnamato) assorbono le radiazioni dannose. I benzofenoni e i dibenzoilmetani forniscono una protezione sia per lo spettro UVA sia per l'UVB. Anche le vitamine C ed E, aggiunte alla crema protettiva, possono essere utili a ridurre la formazione di specie reattive dell'ossigeno. I bambini con fototipo cutaneo da I a III (vedi Tab. 655-1) necessitano di creme solari con fattore di protezione (SPF, *Sun Protection Factor*) di almeno 15. Per SPF si intende la quantità minima di luce solare necessaria a provocare eritema cutaneo dopo l'applicazione della crema, divisa per la quantità necessaria senza uso di crema.

REAZIONI DA FOTOSENSIBILITÀ. Gli agenti fotosensibilizzanti, in associazione con una particolare lunghezza d'onda della luce, causano una dermatite che può essere classificata come reazione fototossica o fotoallergica. Il contatto della cute con l'agente sensibilizzante può avvenire esternamente, internamente tramite somministrazione enterale o parenterale, o per sintesi di fotosensibilizzanti da parte dell'ospite in risposta alla somministrazione di un farmaco.

Le reazioni fotoallergiche avvengono solo in una piccola percentuale di persone esposte ad agenti fotosensibilizzanti e alla luce, e richiedono un intervallo di tempo perché abbia luogo la sensibilizzazione. Successivamente, la dermatite compare entro 24 ore circa dalla riesposizione all'agente fotosensibilizzante e alla luce. La dermatite fotoallergica è una reazione da ipersensibilità ritardata mediata da linfociti T, in cui il farmaco, agendo come aptene, può combinarsi con una proteina cutanea formando la sostanza antigenica. Le reazioni fotoallergiche variano quanto a morfologia e possono insorgere su cute parzialmente coperta o esposta alla luce. Alcune importanti categorie di farmaci e sostanze chimiche responsabili di reazioni da fotosensibilità sono elencate nella Tabella 655-2.

Le reazioni fototossiche insorgono in tutti coloro che accumulano quantità sufficienti di un farmaco fotosensibilizzante o di una sostanza chimica nella cute. Non è necessaria una precedente sensibilizzazione. La dermatite si sviluppa dopo l'esposizione alle radiazioni dello spettro di 285-450 nm. L'eruzione è limitata alle aree esposte alla luce e spesso è simile a un eritema solare di notevoli dimensioni, ma può essere anche orticariode o bollosa ed esita in iperpigmentazione postinfiammatoria. Tutti i farmaci che causano reazioni fotoallergiche possono provocare anche una dermatite fototossica se somministrati in dosi sufficientemente elevate. Numerosi altri farmaci e agenti di contatto possono causare reazioni fototossiche, in particolare i furocumarinici fitoderivati (vedi Tab. 655-2). La differenziazione dalla dermatite da contatto causata dal veleno dell'edera o della quercia può essere difficile, sebbene nella dermatite da contatto il prurito sia un sintomo importante. Nella fitofotodermatite predomina il bruciore, che è confinato alle zone esposte al sole, e risparmia le palpebre superiori, le aree al di sotto del naso e del mento e le aree retroauricolari. L'iperpigmentazione postinfiammatoria si sviluppa rapidamente ed è abitualmente il segno con cui si presenta la patologia.

La fotodermatite causata da farmaci o sostanze chimiche può essere diagnosticata tramite il *photopatch test*, ma gli strumenti per questa procedura diagnostica non sono diffusamente disponibili. Per fare una diagnosi sono sufficienti un elevato indice di sospetto combinato con la valutazione del quadro di distribuzione dell'eruzione e un'anamnesi positiva per l'applicazione o l'ingestione di un agente fotosensibilizzante noto. La terapia consiste nella sospensione dei farmaci responsabili o nell'evitare l'esposizione al sole. Le reazioni severe possono necessitare di una terapia steroidea sistemica per un breve periodo.

PORFIRIE (VEDI CAPITOLO 91). Sono disordini congeniti o acquisiti, dovuti a specifiche mutazioni a carico di enzimi implicati nella via biosintetica dell'eme. Sono diversi quanto a manifestazione clinica; le varianti più frequenti nei bambini sono due ed entrambe hanno come caratteristica dominante la fotosensibilità. I segni e i sintomi possono essere trascurabili durante l'inverno, quando l'esposizione solare è minima.

La **porfiria eritropoietica congenita** (**morbo di Günther**) è un raro disturbo autosomico recessivo causato da un deficit di uroporfirinogeno III cosintetasi. Si presenta nei primi mesi di vita con un'intensa sensibilità alla luce, che può causare ripetute eruzioni bollose severe che esitano in cicatrici mutilanti (Fig. 655-2). Nelle zone esposte alla luce si sviluppano **iperpigmentazione**, ipercheratosi, vescicolazione e fragilità cutanea. Ulteriori manifestazioni caratteristiche sono l'**irsutismo** nelle aree lievemente coinvolte, l'**alopecia** cicatriziale in quelle colpite più gravemente, urine da rosa a rosse, denti marroni, anemia emolitica, splenomegalia e aumento di uroporfirina I nelle urine, nel plasma e negli eritrociti, e di coproporfirina I nelle feci. L'urina dei pazienti affetti appare di colore rosa-rossastro alla lampada di Wood.

La **protoporfiria eritropoietica** viene ereditata come carattere autosomico dominante ed è dovuta a una ridotta attività della ferrochelatasi, che converte la protoporfirina in eme. La fotosensibilità diviene evidente nella prima infanzia e si manifesta con dolore,

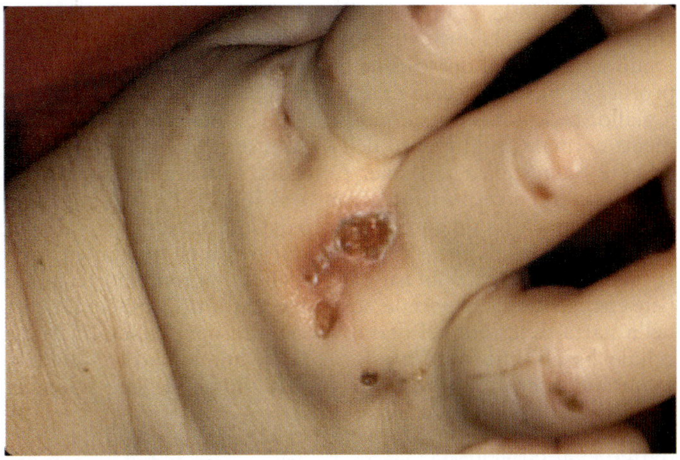

Figura 655-2. Ulcerazioni con croste in un lattante con porfiria congenita eritropoietica.

parestesie e sensazione urente entro 30 minuti dall'esposizione al sole, seguiti da eritema, edema, orticaria e, raramente, vescicole, sulle zone esposte alla luce. Le alterazioni ungueali consistono in opacizzazione della lamina, onicolisi, dolore e ipersensibilità. La reazione cutanea acuta può essere accompagnata da lievi sintomi sistemici consistenti in malessere, brividi e febbre. L'esposizione ricorrente al sole provoca una dermatite eczematosa cronica con cute ispessita e lichenificata, specialmente sulle articolazioni interfalangee (Fig. 655-3*A*, oltre che eritema violaceo persistente, ulcere e cicatrici atrofiche crostose punteggiate o lineari sul volto (Fig. 655-3*B*) e sui margini auricolari. La pigmentazione, l'ipertricosi, la fragilità cutanea e la mutilazione sono rare. L'epatopatia è generalmente lieve. I sintomi spesso migliorano spontaneamente dopo i 10-11 anni di età.

Le lunghezze d'onda della luce principalmente responsabili dello scatenamento delle reazioni cutanee, nella porfiria, si trovano nella regione dei 400 nm. I vetri delle finestre che trasmettono lunghezze d'onda >320 nm non sono protettivi, e le luci artificiali di una certa lunghezza d'onda possono essere patogene. I pazienti devono evitare la luce solare diretta, indossare indumenti protettivi e utilizzare agenti schermanti che blocchino efficacemente le lunghezze d'onda lesive. La **somministrazione** di β-carotene riduce la fluorescenza della molecola di porfirina dando un colorito giallo alla cute; la sua efficacia nel ridurre la fotosensibilità nei pazienti con protoporfiria ha inizio dopo 1-3 mesi ed è variabile.

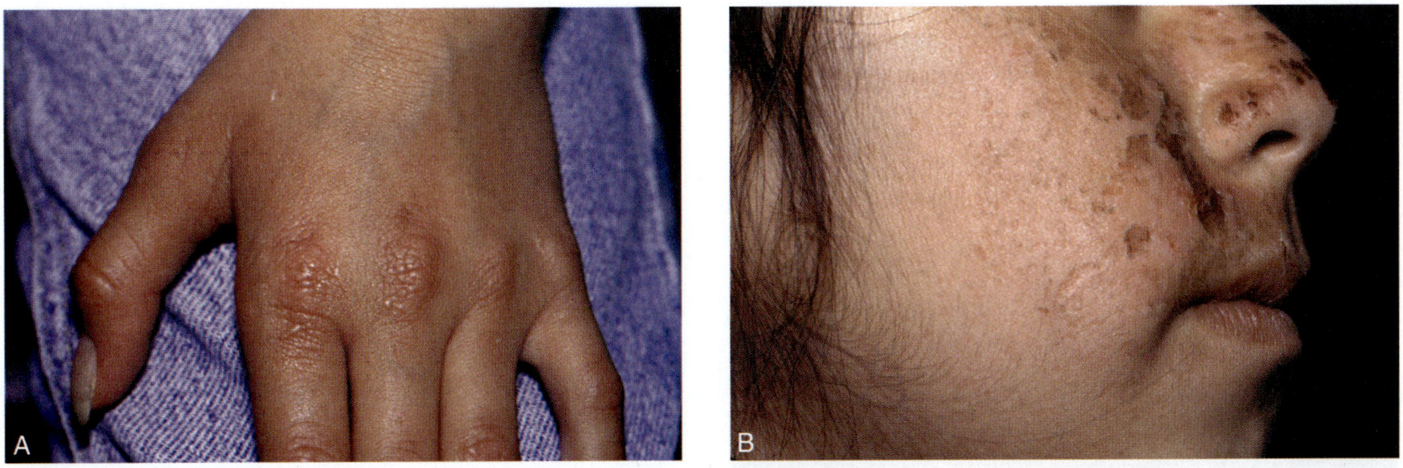

Figura 655-3. *A*, Ispessimento eritematoso a livello dell'articolazione metacarpo-falangea, nella porfiria eritropoietica. *B*, Croste lineari e cicatrici nella porfiria eritropoietica.

MILIUM COLLOIDE. È un raro disturbo asintomatico che insorge sul volto (naso, labbro superiore, parte superiore delle guance) e può estendersi al dorso delle mani e al collo come un'eruzione profusa di piccole papule dure, raggruppate, di colore da avorio a giallo. Le lesioni compaiono prima della pubertà su cute altrimenti normale, a differenza della variante adulta che si sviluppa su cute danneggiata dal sole. L'esordio può seguire un'ustione solare acuta o un'esposizione cronica al sole. Nella maggior parte dei casi la malattia raggiunge il picco entro 3 anni, rimanendo poi invariata, sebbene ci possa essere una regressione spontanea dopo la pubertà. Le alterazioni istopatologiche comprendono accumuli ben circoscritti di materiale eosinofilo fissurato, principalmente nella parte superiore del derma a contatto con l'epidermide. Le cellule basali, che sono trasformate in questi corpi colloidali, sembrano essere abnormemente suscettibili alla degenerazione in seguito all'esposizione attinica.

HYDROA VACCINIFORME. Questo disturbo vescicolobolloso è molto più comune nei bambini che nelle bambine, esordisce nella prima infanzia e può risolversi con la pubertà. Il picco di incidenza si ha in primavera e in estate. Entro alcune ore dall'esposizione solare compaiono macule eritematose e pruriginose localizzate a orecchie, naso, labbra, guance e superfici dorsali di mani e avambracci. Le lesioni si trasformano progressivamente in papule molli e pungenti e in vescicole o bolle emorragiche. Le lesioni severe dell'hydroa vacciniforme sono simili alle vescicole della varicella. Divengono ombelicate, ulcerate e crostose e guariscono con cicatrici puntinate e teleangiectasie. Durante la fase acuta si notano occasionalmente febbre e malessere. Istopatologicamente, le lesioni mostrano vescicole multiloculari intradermiche, che portano a necrosi focale epidermica e dermica. Inizialmente si osserva un infiltrato perivascolare di cellule mononucleate, che successivamente circonda le aree di necrosi. Questa eruzione deve essere distinta dalla protoporfiria eritropoietica, che raramente presenta vescicole. La patogenesi dell'hydroa vacciniforme è sconosciuta, ma lesioni tipiche sono state riprodotte con dosi ripetute di radiazioni UVA o UVB. Durante la fase infiammatoria dell'eruzione può essere utile l'impiego di un **corticosteroide topico**. Possono inoltre rivelarsi efficaci anche schermi solari profilattici ad ampio spettro, trattamenti di UBV a basso dosaggio e terapia con psoralene e UVA (PUVA). Il β-carotene e gli antimalarici talvolta sono di beneficio.

PRURIGO ATTINICA. È una fotodermatite cronica famigliare, ereditata come tratto autosomico dominante, che compare con una certa frequenza tra i Nativi Americani del Nord e Sud America. Il primo episodio insorge generalmente nella prima infanzia, da alcune ore a due giorni dopo un'intensa esposizione solare. La maggior parte dei pazienti è di sesso femminile ed è sensibile alle radiazioni UVA. Le lesioni sono papule eritematose intensamente pruriginose, sul volto (Fig. 655-4), sul labbro inferiore, sulle estremità distali e, nei casi severi, sulle natiche. Quelle localizzate al volto possono guarire lasciando minuscole cicatrici punteggiate o lineari. Le lesioni divengono spesso croniche, senza periodi di guarigione completa, e si uniscono a formare placche eczematose che lichenificano e possono sviluppare infezioni secondarie. Le caratteristiche associate che distinguono questo disturbo da altre fotoeruzioni e da dermatiti atopiche comprendono cheilite, congiuntivite e alopecia traumatica della metà esterna del sopracciglio. La prurigo attinica è una patologia cronica che persiste generalmente in età adulta, ma talvolta può migliorare spontaneamente nella tarda adolescenza. Le protezioni solari ad ampio spettro possono essere utili per prevenire l'eruzione, ma gli antimalarici e il β-carotene conferiscono una protezione scarsa o nulla. I **corticosteroidi topici** alleviano il prurito e l'infiammazione.

ORTICARIA SOLARE. È un disturbo raro, indotto dalle radiazioni UV o visibili. L'orticaria solare primaria è probabilmente mediata da un'ipersensibilità allergica di tipo 1 a un allergene cutaneo o circolante indotto dall'irradiazione, che porta a degranulazione mastocitaria e rilascio di istamina. Questa reazione insorge entro 5-10 minuti dall'esposizione, svanisce entro 1-2 ore ed è caratterizzata da diffusa e grave comparsa di pomfi (Fig. 655-5), che può portare ad astenia, cefalea, nausea, sincope o broncospasmo. Gli antistaminici anti-H_1 possono essere utili per prevenire o risolvere l'eruzione. L'orticaria solare secondaria è dovuta a fotosensibilizzazione da parte di sostanze chimiche o farmaci sistemici esogeni e qualche volta può essere un segno di presentazione della protoporfiria eritropoietica. Il **trattamento** consiste nell'evitare la lunghezza d'onda della luce e/o nel sospendere il farmaco fotosensibilizzanti.

ERUZIONE ATTINICA POLIMORFA. Questa patologia compare più comunemente nei soggetti di sesso femminile di età inferiore ai 30 anni. La prima eruzione si manifesta tipicamente dopo un'esposizione solare prolungata durante la primavera o l'estate. L'esordio dell'eruzione è ritardato di ore o giorni dopo l'esposizione e dura diversi giorni o alcune settimane. Le aree coinvolte tendono a essere simmetriche e sono caratteristiche di un dato paziente; comprendono alcune, ma non tutte, le zone esposte o poco coperte della cute, su viso, collo, parte superiore del torace ed estremità distali. Le lesioni hanno varie morfologie ma più comunemente si presentano come papule eritematose o populovescicole pruriginose, di 2-5 mm, raggruppate, oppure come placche eritematose di diametro >5 cm. Nella maggior parte dei casi si ha una sensibilizzazione alle radiazioni UVA, sebbene alcune manifestazioni siano indotte da UVB. Gli approcci **terapeutici** comprendono l'evitamento del sole, le creme protettive ad

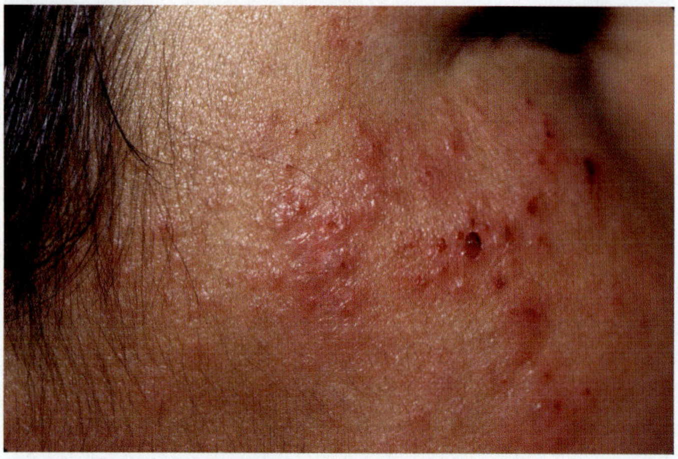

Figura 655-4. Papule eritematose ed escoriate nella prurigo attinica.

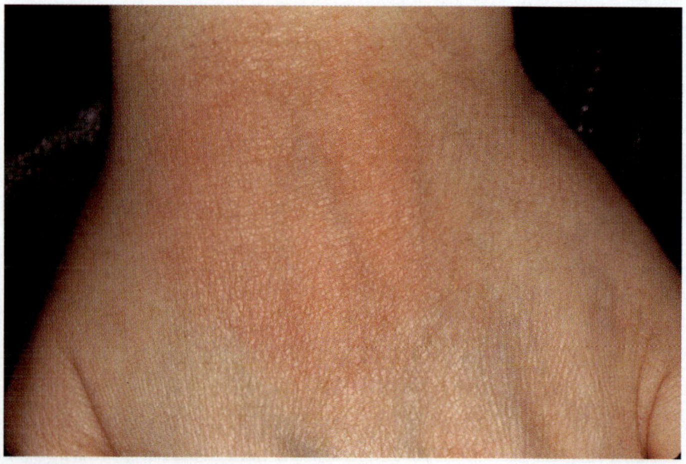

Figura 655-5. Orticaria dopo 5 minuti dall'esposizione a una radiazione artificiale ultravioletta A.

ampio spettro, i corticosteroidi topici o sistemici, il β-carotene, la nicotinamide, gli antimalarici o la fototerapia UVB o PUVA profilattica.

SINDROME DI COCKAYNE. L'esordio di questa malattia autosomica recessiva è caratterizzato dalla comparsa, approssimativamente all'età di 1 anno, di un eritema facciale con distribuzione a farfalla, dopo l'esposizione al sole, seguito dalla perdita di tessuto adiposo e dallo sviluppo di cute sottile, atrofica e iperpigmentata, in particolare al volto. Le caratteristiche associate comprendono nanismo, ritardo mentale, orecchie grandi e sporgenti, arti lunghi, mani e piedi sproporzionatamente grandi, che sono talvolta freddi e cianotici, naso sottile, carie dentarie, marcia instabile con tremori, limitazione della mobilità articolare, sordità progressiva, cataratta, degenerazione retinica, atrofia ottica, sudorazione e lacrimazione ridotte, incanutimento precoce. Segue una demielinizzazione diffusa ed estesa del sistema nervoso centrale e periferico, e i pazienti generalmente muoiono di vasculopatia ateromasica prima della terza decade. Vi sono tre tipi di sindrome di Cockayne. Il tipo I (gene CSA) è meno severo del tipo II (gene CSB). Nel tipo III (XP-CS) si ha complementazione con lo xeroderma pigmentoso dei gruppi B, D o G. La fotosensibilità è dovuta a una ridotta velocità di riparazione del danno indotto dagli UV, specialmente nelle regioni di trascrizione attiva del DNA. La sindrome si distingue dalla progeria (vedi Capitolo 90) per la fotosensibilità e le anomalie oculari.

XERODERMA PIGMENTOSO. È una rara malattia autosomica recessiva dovuta a un difetto nella riparazione dell'escissione nucleotidica. Sono stati riconosciuti sette gruppi di complementazione, in base all'incapacità di ogni singolo gruppo di riparare la parte di DNA danneggiata. La lunghezza d'onda della luce che induce il danno del DNA varia da 280 a 340 nm. Le alterazioni cutanee si osservano per la prima volta durante l'età neonatale o nella prima infanzia, nelle aree esposte al sole, come il volto, il collo, le mani e le braccia; le lesioni possono insorgere, tuttavia, anche in altre sedi, tra cui il cuoio capelluto. Le manifestazioni cutanee sono rappresentate da eritema, desquamazione, bolle, croste, efelidi, teleangiectasie, cheratosi (Fig. 655-6), carcinomi basocellulari e squamocellulari, e melanomi maligni. Le manifestazioni oculari comprendono fotofobia, lacrimazione, blefarite, simblefaron, cheratite, opacità corneali, tumori delle palpebre e possibile esito in cecità. Nel 20% circa dei pazienti, possono svilupparsi anomalie neurologiche come deterioramento mentale e sordità neurosensoriale.

Lo xeroderma pigmentoso è una patologia grave e mutilante; l'aspettativa di vita è spesso ridotta. Le famiglie affette dovrebbero ricevere un counseling genetico. Il difetto può essere ricercato nella coltura di cellule provenienti dal liquido amniotico. I bambini colpiti dovrebbero essere protetti totalmente dall'esposizione solare; anche nei bambini con malattia lieve occorre utilizzare indumenti protettivi, occhiali da sole, e una protezione solare opaca ad ampio spettro. Sono dannose, inoltre, la luce proveniente da fonti fluorescenti non schermate e la luce solare che attraversa i vetri delle finestre. Sono fondamentali l'identificazione e la rimozione precoci delle lesioni maligne.

SINDROME DI ROTHMUND-THOMSON. Questa sindrome è nota anche come poichiloderma congenito, a causa delle gravissime alterazioni cutanee (Fig. 655-7). È ereditata come tratto autosomico recessivo. In due terzi circa dei pazienti si trovano mutazioni nel gene RECQL4. Le altre mutazioni che causano la sindrome di Rothmund-Thomson (RTS) sono sconosciute. Le alterazioni cutanee si possono osservare già all'età di 3 mesi. Compaiono placche di eritema ed edema sulle guance, sulla fronte, sulle orecchie, sul collo, sulla porzione dorsale delle mani, sulle superfici estensorie delle braccia e sulle natiche, che vengono poi gradualmente sostituite da placche reticolari, atrofiche, iperpigmentate e teleangiectasiche. La sensibilità alla luce è presente in molti casi, e l'esposizione al sole può provocare la formazione di bolle. Le aree coinvolte, tuttavia, non sono strettamente fotodistribuite. Sono comuni bassa statura; mani e piedi piccoli; sopracciglia, ciglia e pelo pubico e ascellare rado; capelli radi, fini, con incanutimento precoce o alopecia; anomalie delle ossa; ipogenitalismo. Può anche insorgere cataratta in età precoce. La maggior parte dei pazienti presenta uno sviluppo mentale nella norma. Sulla cute esposta possono manifestarsi cheratosi e carcinomi squamocellulari. L'associazione più pericolosa è con l'osteosarcoma. Insorge nei pazienti con RTS con mutazione del gene RECQL4.

MORBO DI HARTNUP (VEDI CAPITOLO 85.5). È un raro errore congenito del metabolismo, a ereditarietà autosomica recessiva. Gli amminoacidi neutri, incluso il triptofano, non vengono trasportati attraverso l'epitelio dell'orletto a spazzola dell'intestino e dei reni, portando a un difetto di sintesi della nicotinamide e alla comparsa di una **sindrome** fotoindotta **simil-pellagrosa.** Le urine mostrano un aumento delle quantità di amminoacidi monoamino carbossilici. I segni cutanei, che precedono le manifestazioni neurologiche, esordiscono durante i primi mesi di vita, quando si osserva un'eruzione eczematosa, occasionalmente vescicolobollosa, sul volto e sulle estremità, con una fotodistribuzione a guanto e a calza. Possono sopravvenire iperpigmentazione e ipercheratosi, che sono intensificate dall'ulteriore esposizione alla luce solare. Riacutizzazioni episodiche possono essere precipitate da malattie febbrili, esposizione al sole, stress emotivo e scarsa nutrizione. Nella maggior parte dei casi, lo sviluppo mentale è normale, ma

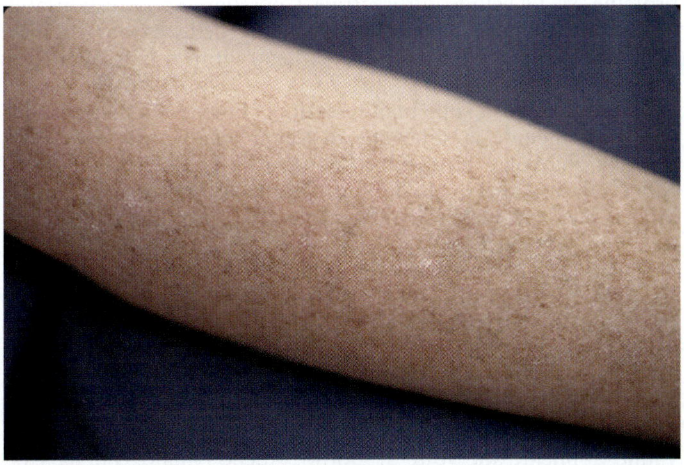

Figura 655-6. Depigmentazione e cheratosi attinica in un bambino con xeroderma pigmentoso.

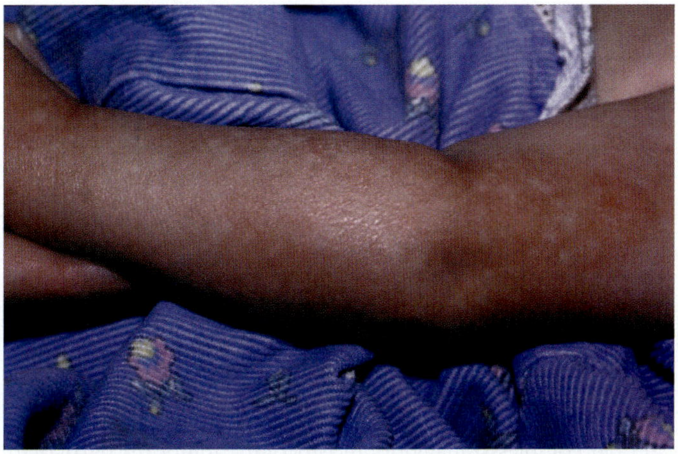

Figura 655-7. Poichilodermia sul braccio di un bambino con sindrome di Rothmund-Thomson.

alcuni pazienti presentano instabilità emotiva e atassia cerebellare episodica. I sintomi neurologici sono pienamente reversibili. La somministrazione di nicotinamide e la protezione dalla luce solare conducono a un miglioramento sia delle lesioni cutanee sia delle manifestazioni neurologiche.

SINDROME DI BLOOM. Il difetto, nella sindrome di Bloom (gene BLM), è ereditato in maniera autosomica recessiva. Il gene BML è un'elicasi del tipo RECQ. I pazienti sono sensibili alle radiazioni UV e hanno un tasso di rotture cromosomiche e scambi tra cromatidi fratelli marcatamente elevato. Durante l'infanzia si sviluppano eritema e teleangiectasie con distribuzione a farfalla sul volto, in seguito all'esposizione a luce solare. Possono svilupparsi un'eruzione bollosa sulle labbra e un eritema teleangiectasico su mani e avambracci. Possono essere presenti macchie a caffelatte e macule ipopigmentate. Si osservano generalmente bassa statura pre e postnatale e una facies tipica, con naso e orecchie prominenti e viso piccolo e stretto. L'intelligenza può essere nella media o leggermente inferiore alla media. In tutti i pazienti si osserva immunodeficienza, che si manifesta con infezioni auricolari e polmonari ricorrenti. È comune malassorbimento intestinale. I bambini affetti da questa patologia hanno una tendenza insolita a sviluppare tumori solidi e neoplasie linforeticolari.

Beattie PE, Dawe RS, Ibbotson SH, et al: Characteristics and prognosis of idiopathic solar urticaria: A cohort of 87 cases. *Arch Dermatol* 2003;139:1149–1154.

Demko CA, Boraeski EA, Debanne SM, et al: Use of indoor tanning facilities by white adolescents in the United States. *Arch Pediatr Adolesc Med* 2003;157:854–860.

Dummer R, Ivanova K, Scheidegger EP, et al: Clinical and therapeutic aspects of polymorphous light eruption. *Dermatology* 2003;207:93–95.

Han A, Maibach H: Management of acute sunburn. *Am J Clin Dermatol* 2004;5:39–47.

Hojyo-Tomoka MT, Vega-Memije ME, Cortes-Franco R, et al: Diagnosis and treatment of actinic prurigo. *Dermatol Ther* 2003;16:40–44.

Kaneko H, Kondo N: Clinical features of Bloom syndrome and function of the causative gene, BLM helicase. *Expert Rev Mol Diagn* 2004;4:393–401.

Kauppinen R: Porphyrias. *Lancet* 2005;365:241–252.

Lin JY, Selim MA, Shea CR, et al: UV photoprotection by combination topical antioxidants vitamin C and vitamin E. *J Am Acad Dermatol* 2003;48: 866–874.

Magnoldo T, Sarasin A: Xeroderma pigmentosum: From symptoms and genetics to gene-based therapy. *Cells Tissue Organs* 2004;177:189–198.

Murphy GM: Diagnosis and management of the porphyrias. *Dermatol Ther* 2003;16:57–64.

Oskay T, Erder C, Anadolu R, et al: Juvenile colloid milium associated with conjunctival and gingival involvement. *J Am Acad Dermatol* 2003;49: 1185–1188.

Spivak G: The many faces of Cockayne syndrome. *Proc Natl Acad Sci U S A* 2004;101:15273–15274.

Wang LL, Gannavarapu A, Kozinetz CA, et al: Association between osteosarcoma and deleterious mutations in the RECQL4 gene in Rothmund-Thomson syndrome. *J Natl Cancer Inst* 2003;95:669–674.

Capitolo 656 ■ Malattie dell'epidermide

Joseph G. Morelli

PSORIASI. Questa patologia cronica dell'epidermide, piuttosto comune, si manifesta entro le prime due decadi di vita in circa il 30% dei soggetti colpiti. Poiché il disturbo è più comune nelle famiglie con anamnesi positiva, è stata ipotizzata un'ereditarietà di tipo multifattoriale. Si riscontra inoltre un'associazione con i geni del complesso maggiore di istocompatibilità (in particolare CW6). Il principale gene di suscettibilità della psoriasi, chiamato PSORS1, si estende per un intervallo di 70 Kb sul cromosoma 6, intorno al gene per la desmina. Altri geni di suscettibilità sono stati identificati sui cromosomi 17q, 4q, 1q e 3q e definiti rispettivamente PSORS2, 3, 4 e 5. La psoriasi è caratterizzata dalla proliferazione e anomala differenziazione dei cheratinociti, nonché dall'infiltrazione infiammatoria di derma ed epidermide. L'anomalia primaria consiste spesso in un difetto del sistema immunitario, responsabile di un aumento del turnover epidermico secondario.

Manifestazioni cliniche. Le lesioni consistono in papule eritematose e coalescenti, che formano placche dai bordi ben marcati e irregolari. In assenza di trattamento, tali chiazze vengono ricoperte da scaglie desquamanti color argento o biancastre, con una consistenza caratteristica che ricorda la mica (Fig. 656-1*A*). La rimozione delle scaglie può causare un sanguinamento puntiforme (**segno di Auspitz**). La risposta di **Koebner** (o isomorfica), che consiste nella comparsa di nuove lesioni nella sede del trauma, ha un'importante funzione diagnostica. Le lesioni possono interessare qualsiasi parte del corpo, ma le sedi d'elezione sono il cuoio capelluto, le ginocchia, i gomiti, l'ombelico, la piega interglutea superiore e i genitali. Le lesioni del cuoio capelluto possono essere facilmente confuse con la dermatite seborroica, la dermatite atopica o la tinea capitis. Piccole lesioni a goccia sul volto si riscontrano comunemente. Un altro segno diagnostico utile è dato dal coinvolgimento delle unghie, che presentano depressioni puntiformi, si sfaldano e si distaccano dal letto ungueale (onicolisi), assumendo una colorazione da giallo a marrone, causata dall'accumulo di squame subungueali (Fig. 656-1*B*).

La psoriasi è rara nei neonati, ma può risultare grave, essere difficile da diagnosticare e non rispondere alla terapia. Le lesioni iniziali tendono a coinvolgere l'area del pannolino, mimando una dermatite seborroica, una dermatite eczematosa da pannolino, una dermatite streptococcica perianale o una candidosi. La diagnosi definitiva può richiedere una biopsia o una prolungata osservazione. Altre forme rare comprendono la psoriasi eritrodermica, la psoriasi localizzata o generalizzata e quella lineare.

La **psoriasi guttata** è una variante che colpisce prevalentemente in età pediatrica, caratterizzata da un'eruzione profusa di piccole lesioni ovali o rotonde, morfologicamente identiche alle placche più grandi della psoriasi (Fig. 656-1*C*). Le sedi di elezione sono il tronco, il volto e le porzioni prossimali degli arti. L'esordio segue spesso un'infezione **streptococcica**. In questi casi, è utile eseguire una coltura orofaringea e ottenere i titoli sierologici. La psoriasi guttata è stata osservata anche in seguito a infezione streptococcica perianale, infezioni virali, ustioni solari e sospensione di una terapia sistemica con corticosteroidi. In un ospite geneticamente suscettibile, le lesioni possono essere indotte da cellule T $CD4^+$, inizialmente attivate da esotossine streptococciche pirogeniche, che agiscono come superantigeni. Tali antigeni provengono dalla gola o dalla cute. Alcune delle cellule T attivate riconoscono la proteina streptococcica M della cute e sembrano presentare una reattività incrociata con una cheratina anomala, omologa alla proteina M. Le cellule autoreattive T possono essere responsabili della formazione e della cronicizzazione delle lesioni cutanee, facilmente confondibili con gli esantemi virali o con la pitiriasi lichenoide cronica (PCL).

Diagnosi. Si basa sulle manifestazioni cliniche. La diagnosi differenziale include la sindrome di Reiter (che a differenza della psoriasi coinvolge le membrane mucose), la PLC e la pitiriasi rubra pilare. In caso di dubbio, l'esame istopatologico di una lesione non sottoposta a trattamento rivela le caratteristiche alterazioni psoriasiche.

Trattamento. L'approccio terapeutico varia a seconda dell'età del bambino, del tipo di psoriasi, della sede interessata e dell'estensione della malattia. Traumi fisici e chimici della cute andrebbero evitati per quanto possibile (vedi risposta di Koebner).

Si distinguono tre fasi del trattamento. La **prima fase** è **topica** e prevede la somministrazione di corticosteroidi di media o alta potenza (vedi Capitolo 645). I preparati meno potenti ma efficaci vanno applicati due volte al giorno. Anche l'analogo della vitamina D calcipotriene, per via topica, è efficace, ma sembra agire sul metabolismo del calcio 100 volte meno rispetto al calcitriolo.

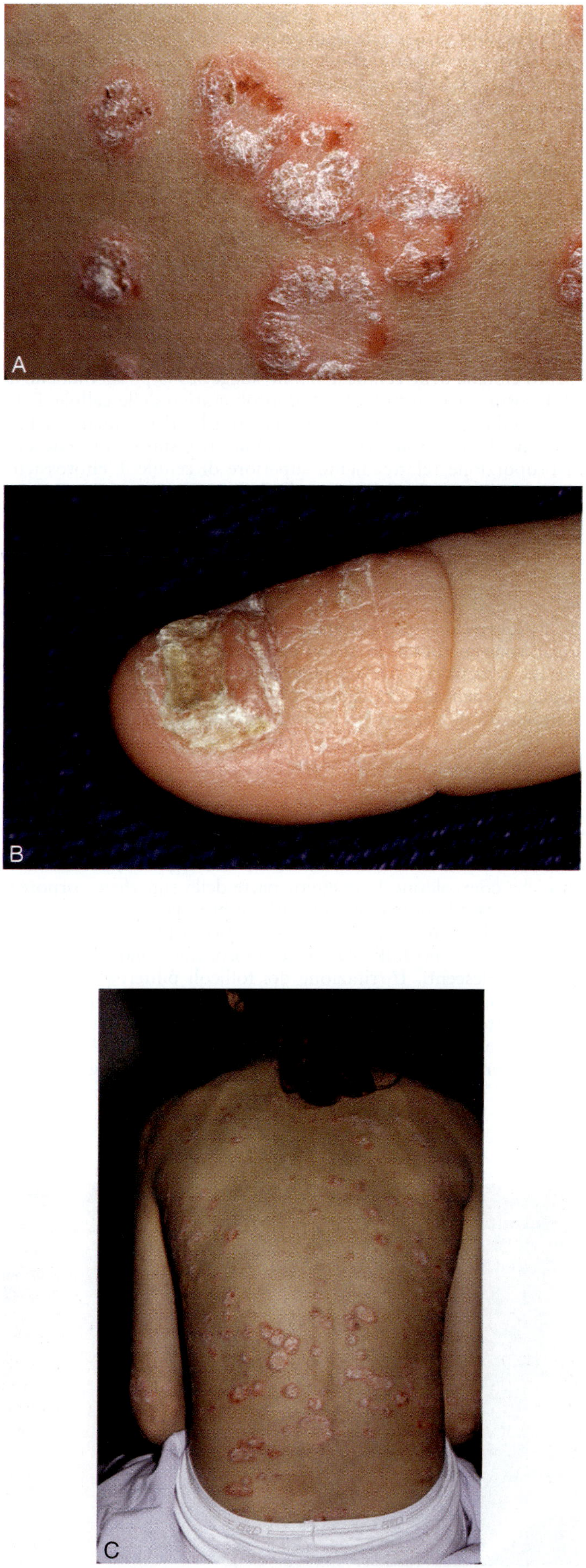

Figura 656-1. *A*, Placche della psoriasi cronica. *B*, Distrofia ungueale. *C*, Psoriasi guttata a distribuzione diffusa sul tronco.

Il calcipotriene può causare bruciore e dolore, perciò il suo utilizzo in età pediatrica è piuttosto limitato. Una strategia comune consiste nell'utilizzare il calcipotriene due volte al giorno durante i primi cinque giorni della settimana, ricorrendo invece a uno steroide topico due volte al giorno durante il weekend. Anche il tazarotene, un retinoide topico, può essere utile, usato da solo o in combinazione con altri preparati. Si possono impiegare anche i preparati a base di catrame e l'antralina. Per il trattamento delle lesioni del cuoio capelluto, l'applicazione di una soluzione salina fenolata, seguita da uno shampoo al catrame, è efficace nella rimozione delle scaglie. Una volta ottenuta la riduzione delle scaglie, è consigliabile applicare un corticosteroide in forma di schiuma, lozione, soluzione o gel.

La **seconda fase** del trattamento prevede la **fototerapia**. Le radiazioni UVB maggiormente utilizzate a scopo terapeutico nei bambini sono i raggi ultravioletti di tipo B a banda stretta (UVB 311 nm). Questi ultimi hanno un'efficacia paragonabile alle radiazioni UVA con associazione di psoraleni (PUVA), ma non presentano gli effetti collaterali caratteristici degli psoraleni. Il ricorso alla fototerapia è opportuno nei casi più gravi, successivamente al fallimento della terapia topica. Si tratta tuttavia di un trattamento molto lungo, disponibile solo in alcuni centri specialistici.

La **terza fase** consiste nella **terapia sistemica**, necessaria soltanto in un ristretto numero di casi. Il metotrexato, i retinoidi orali e la ciclosporina sono utilizzabili nelle rare forme gravi e generalizzate. La somministrazione orale di retinoidi può essere combinata alla fototerapia. Le lesioni ungueali sono difficili da curare, ma talvolta rispondono al tazarotene topico. Le terapie potenzialmente benefiche includono il trattamento localizzato di placche resistenti (mediante radiazioni UVB a lunghezza d'onda di 308 nm), l'inibizione del fattore di necrosi tumorale con etanercept e l'inibizione dei linfociti T della memoria (CD45RO+). Efalizumab, un anticorpo monoclonale diretto contro le interazioni con le cellule T, migliora l'esito delle forme da moderate a gravi negli adulti (il suo utilizzo non è raccomandato in età pediatrica, *N.d.C.*).

Prognosi. È migliore nei bambini che presentano una forma circoscritta. La psoriasi è una malattia cronica, caratterizzata da remissioni ed esacerbazioni. L'artrite costituisce la principale complicanza extracutanea.

PITIRIASI LICHENOIDE. Storicamente, questa definizione includeva le forme di pitiriasi lichenoide acuta (PLA, pitiriasi lichenoide e varioliforme acuta [PLEVA], malattia di Mucha-Habermann) e la pitiriasi lichenoide cronica (PLC). La distinzione tra il decorso acuto e cronico dovrebbe basarsi più sull'aspetto morfologico delle lesioni (spesso emorragiche o necrotiche nella PLA) che sulla durata della malattia. Non si evidenzia alcuna correlazione tra il tipo di lesione al momento dell'esordio dell'eruzione e la durata della malattia. Diversi pazienti presentano contemporaneamente lesioni acute e croniche, mentre in alcuni casi si osserva una transizione da una forma all'altra. La pitiriasi lichenoide si manifesta comunemente nella seconda e terza decade d'età; in circa il 30% dei casi, la malattia esordisce prima dei 20 anni.

Manifestazioni cliniche. La PLC si presenta con un'eruzione generalizzata di papule multiple, rossastre o porpora, rapidamente ricoperte da sottile squame argentee, che raggiungono il diametro di 3-5 mm (Fig. 656-2). Le lesioni sono asintomatiche o causano un leggero prurito. Solo occasionalmente appaiono infiltrate, vescicolari, emorragiche e crostose. Nel giro di 2-6 settimane, le papule si scuriscono e appiattiscono, trasformandosi infine in una macula iperpigmentata o ipopigmentata. Le lesioni, che tendono a risolversi senza cicatrici, colpiscono in prevalenza il tronco e gli arti, mentre solitamente risparmiano il volto, le superfici palmoplantari, il cuoio capelluto e le membrane mucose. L'eruzione persiste per alcuni mesi o anni ed è caratterizzata da lesioni polimorfe nei diversi stadi di evoluzione. Sul piano istologico, la PLC presenta uno strato corneale ispessito e paracheratosico; spongiosi epidermica; un infiltrato superficiale perivascolare di macrofagi e linfociti $CD8^+$, che può espandersi

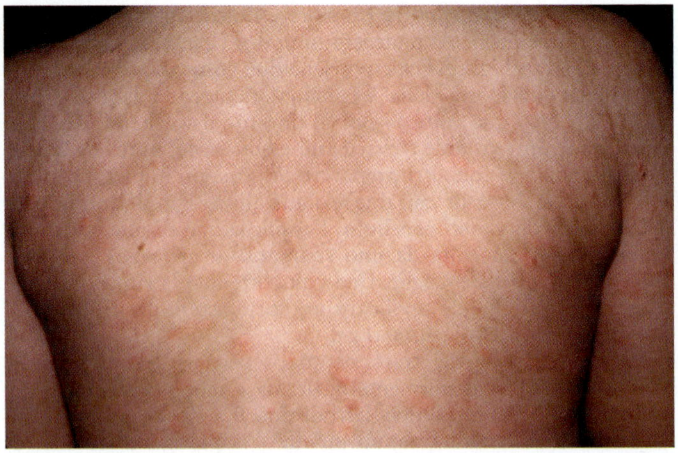

Figura 656-2. Placche diffuse ricoperte da fine desquamazione nella pitiriasi lichenoide cronica.

nell'epidermide; un piccolo numero di eritrociti stravasati nel derma papillare.

La PLA si presenta con un'improvvisa eruzione di vescicole pustolose, che in seguito sviluppano un centro purpurico, ricoperte da una crosta scura e circondate da un anello eritematoso (Fig. 656-3). I sintomi sistemici, presenti per 2-3 giorni dopo l'eruzione iniziale, includono febbre, malessere, cefalea e artralgia. Come nella PLC, le lesioni si distribuiscono in maniera diffusa sul tronco e sulle estremità. Le singole lesioni si risolvono in qualche settimana, lasciando talvolta cicatrici vaioliformi; eruzioni successive determinano il caratteristico aspetto polimorfo. La malattia, solitamente autolimitante, si protrae per alcune settimane o mesi. Le alterazioni istopatologiche della PLA riflettono il suo decorso più grave rispetto alla PLC. L'edema intercellulare o intracellulare dell'epidermide può condurre alla degenerazione dei cheratinociti. Un denso infiltrato di cellule mononucleari perivascolari può estendersi verso l'alto nell'epidermide, oppure verso il basso nel derma reticolare. Ulteriori caratteristiche comprendono edema delle cellule endoteliali e stravaso degli eritrociti nell'epidermide e nel derma. Lo sviluppo di vascolite è una complicanza rara. La **diagnosi differenziale** è con la psoriasi guttata, la pitiriasi rosea, l'eruzione da farmaci, la sifilide secondaria, gli esantemi virali e il lichen planus. La biopsia cutanea contribuisce ad escludere altre diagnosi.

È stata descritta una rara forma di PLA, che si presenta con febbre e placche ulceronecrotiche fino a 1 cm di diametro, più comuni sulla parte anteriore del tronco e sulle superfici flessorie della porzione prossimale degli arti superiori. Possono svilupparsi anche artrite e superinfezione delle lesioni cutanee da *Staphylococcus aureus*. Le lesioni ulceronecrotiche, miste alle papule, si risolvono in qualche settimana, lasciando una cicatrice ipopigmentata. Sul piano istopatologico, si osserva talvolta la comparsa di vascolite leucocitoclastica. L'eruzione può somigliare all'eritema multiforme, ma generalmente risparmia le membrane mucose.

Eziologia. La causa della pitiriasi lichenoide è sconosciuta. Eruzioni sporadiche hanno condotto alla ricerca di un agente infettivo, mai identificato. Anche la possibile trasmissione interumana non è stata dimostrata. La malattia potrebbe costituire una reazione di ipersensibilità a un organismo infettivo. Meccanismi cellulomediati sembrano importanti nella patogenesi, perché la maggior parte degli infiltrati cellulari è costituita da cellule citotossiche/soppressori. Studi immunoistologici e sul riarrangiamento clonale delle cellule T hanno suggerito la possibilità che la PLA costituisca un processo linfoproliferativo delle cellule T. In due bambini, l'evoluzione della malattia ha determinato la formazione di un linfoma cutaneo a cellule T. È stato ipotizzato che la proporzione relativamente superiore di cellule T citotossiche rispetto alle cellule T helper nelle lesioni PLA, se paragonate a quelle delle papulosi linfomatoidi o dei linfomi a cellule T, rifletta la maggior efficacia della risposta dell'ospite nella PLA.

Trattamento. In generale, la pitiriasi lichenoide deve essere considerata una condizione benigna, che non altera la salute del bambino. Se il paziente è asintomatico, il trattamento si limita all'utilizzo di un lubrificante per eliminare l'eccesso di scaglie. Gli steroidi topici sono inefficaci. In alcuni casi, l'eritromicina (30-50 mg/kg/die per 2 mesi) si è rivelata utile. Anche l'esposizione al sole può risultare benefica. Le radiazioni UVB a banda stretta costituisco il **trattamento di elezione** nei casi di **eruzione diffusa** e pruriginosa. La rara forma ulceronecrotica febbrile può richiedere la somministrazione di corticosteroidi sistemici.

CHERATOSI PILARE. Questa eruzione papulare piuttosto comune presenta un'estensione variabile, da poche lesioni sparse localizzate prevalentemente alla faccia estensoria degli arti, a lesioni diffuse che coinvolgono la maggior parte della superficie corporea, in particolare la porzione estensoria di braccia e cosce, le guance e i glutei. La cute assume un caratteristico aspetto a pelle d'oca. Le papule, di tipo follicolare e scaglioso, non sono infiammatorie né coalescenti. L'irritazione dei follicoli piliferi può causare un eritema che circonda le papule cheratosiche (Fig. 656-4). In un sottogruppo di pazienti, la cheratosi pilare è associata a telangiectasia facciale e a uleritema ofriogene. Poiché le lesioni sono accentuate da secchezza cutanea, tendono a peggiorare nel corso dell'inverno. Sono più frequenti nei pazienti con dermatite

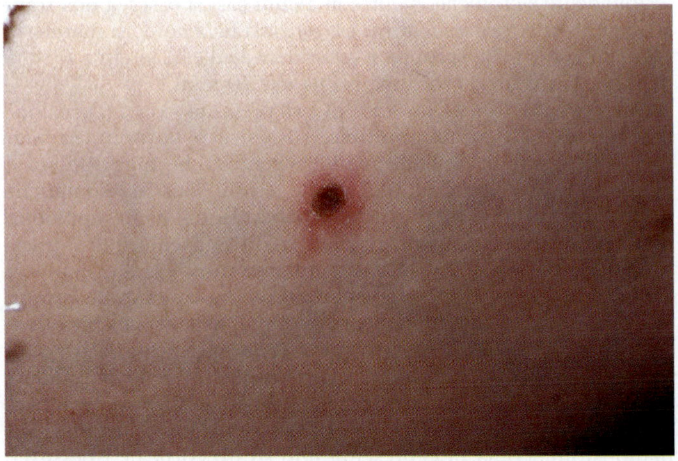

Figura 656-3. Lesione necrotica con orletto eritematoso nella pitiriasi lichenoide acuta.

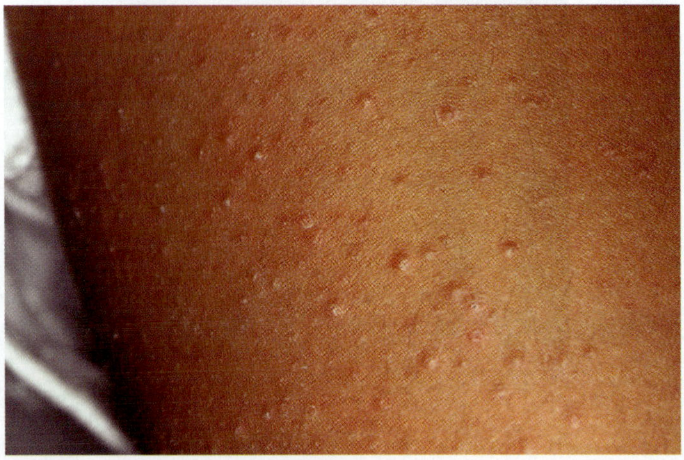

Figura 656-4. Tappi cheratosici follicolari circondati da eritema nella cheratosi pilare.

atopica e durante l'infanzia e la prima età adulta, mentre tendono a recedere nella terza decade. Eruzioni lievi o localizzate sono **trattate** mediante lubrificazione con un blando emolliente. Lesioni più pronunciate o diffuse richiedono la regolare applicazione di una crema al 10-40% di urea o di un preparato a base di acido α-idrossico, come una lozione o crema all'acido lattico. La terapia può migliorare i sintomi ma non è curativa.

LICHEN SPINULOSUS. Questo raro disturbo dalla causa sconosciuta colpisce prevalentemente i bambini, in particolare di sesso maschile. Le lesioni consistono in placche irregolari e ben definite con proiezioni spinose e cheratinose, che protrudono dagli orifizi dei follicoli pilosebacei. Le placche possono comparire in qualsiasi parte del corpo e risultano spesso distribuite simmetricamente su tronco, gomiti, ginocchia e sulle facce estensorie degli arti. Benché talvolta eritematose, le lesioni sono solitamente del colore della cute. I follicoli cheratosici sono nettamente palpabili. La patologia si distingue facilmente dalla cheratosi pilare perché in quest'ultima le lesioni non sono mai raggruppate in placche; può essere invece più spesso confusa con l'eczema papulare.

Solitamente il **trattamento** non è necessario. Per motivi estetici, si utilizzano lubrificanti a base di urea (10-40%), che in genere sono efficaci nell'appiattire le lesioni. Nella maggior parte dei casi, le placche scompaiono spontaneamente nel giro di qualche mese o anno.

PITIRIASI ROSEA. Questa comune eruzione benigna colpisce prevalentemente i bambini e i giovani adulti. Prodromi come febbre, malessere, artralgia e faringite possono precedere l'eruzione, ma raramente i bambini lamentano questi sintomi. La causa della malattia è sconosciuta, ma si sospetta un agente virale e si discute sulla possibile implicazione dell'herpesvirus umano 7.

Manifestazioni cliniche. L'eruzione generalizzata è spesso preceduta dalla comparsa, in qualunque parte del corpo, della **chiazza madre**, una lesione rotonda o ovale, spesso, ma non sempre, identificabile per le sue grandi dimensioni. Tali chiazze hanno un diametro che varia da 1 a 10 cm, sono anulari e presentano un bordo rilevato ricoperto da scaglie fini e aderenti. Circa 5-10 giorni dopo la comparsa della chiazza madre, si evidenzia un'eruzione simmetrica e diffusa, che coinvolge prevalentemente il tronco e la porzione prossimale degli arti (Fig. 656-5). Quando la malattia è estesa, possono essere coinvolti il viso, il cuoio capelluto e la porzione distale degli arti, oppure, nella forma cosiddetta inversa di pitiriasi rosea, i sintomi possono colpire soltanto queste sedi. Le lesioni possono comparire in gruppi e persistere diversi giorni; quelle tipiche hanno forma ovale o rotonda con diametro inferiore a 1 cm, risultano lievemente rilevate e presentano una colorazione rosa-bruno. Le scaglie sottili che le rivestono conferiscono alla cute un aspetto caratteristico. Alcune lesioni si risolvono nella zona centrale, formando un collaretto di scaglie aderenti solo alla periferia. Varianti più rare sono rappresentate da lesioni anulari di grandi dimensioni, papulari, vescicolari, emorragiche e urticanti. L'asse lungo di ciascuna lesione è solitamente allineato con le linee di clivaggio della cute, creando sul dorso un tipico pattern detto ad **albero di Natale**. Tale tendenza a seguire le linee cutanee è particolarmente evidente nelle pieghe ascellari anteriore e posteriore e nell'area sopraclavicolare. La durata dell'eruzione varia da 2 a 12 settimane. Le lesioni possono essere asintomatiche o risultare da lievemente a intensamente pruriginose.

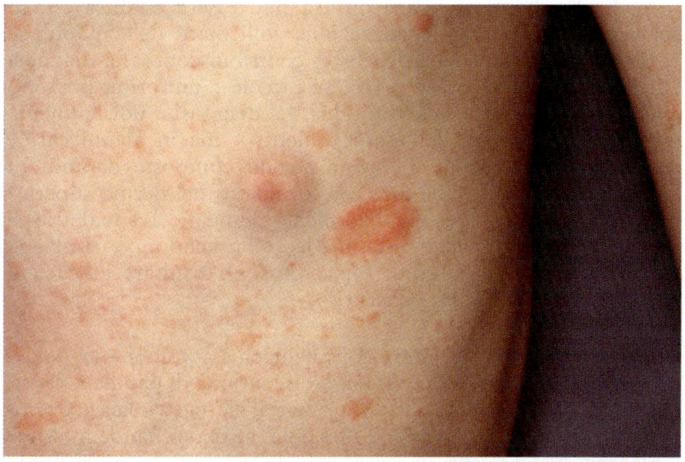

Figura 656-5. Chiazza madre circondata da pitiriasi rosea.

Diagnosi. È di tipo clinico. La chiazza madre può essere confusa con una tinea corporis, ma è possibile distinguere le due patologie con un test che utilizzi un preparato a base di idrossido di potassio. L'eruzione generalizzata assomiglia a diverse altre malattie, tra cui la sifilide secondaria, l'eruzione da farmaci, gli esantemi virali, la psoriasi guttata, la PCL e l'eczema.

Trattamento. Nei pazienti asintomatici non è richiesta alcuna terapia. Se la desquamazione è importante, può essere sufficiente ricorrere a un blando emolliente. È possibile alleviare il prurito con una lozione lubrificante a base di canfora e mentolo, oppure mediante somministrazione di un antistaminico orale per garantire una maggiore sedazione soprattutto nel corso della notte, quando il prurito risulta più fastidioso. Qualche volta, per alleviare il prurito, può essere necessaria l'applicazione topica di un corticosteroide non fluorinato. Dopo che l'eruzione si è risolta, l'ipopigmentazione o l'iperpigmentazione postinfiammatorie possono essere pronunciate, in particolare nei soggetti di razza nera; queste alterazioni scompaiono nelle settimane o nei mesi successivi.

PITIRIASI RUBRA PILARE. Questa rara dermatosi cronica ha spesso un esordio insidioso, con desquamazione diffusa ed eritema del cuoio capelluto, ed è difficilmente distinguibile dalla dermatite seborroica e dall'ipercheratosi spessa dei palmi delle mani e delle piante dei piedi (Fig. 656-6*A*). Altre localizzazioni comuni sono i gomiti e le ginocchia. La lesione primaria caratteristica è una piccola papula acuminata cupoliforme, di colorazione rosata o rossa, con un tappo centrale di cheratina che chiude il follicolo pilifero. Masse di papule coalescenti formano ampie placche eritematose ben demarcate, di colorazione arancio, all'interno delle quali si distinguono isole di cute normale, che creano un effetto bizzarro. Le tipiche papule localizzate sul dorso delle falangi prossimali sono facilmente palpabili. Nella cavità orale possono riscontrarsi placche o papule grigiastre che somigliano al lichen planus. Le alterazioni ungueali mimano quelle della psoriasi. La **diagnosi differenziale** comprende l'ittiosi, la dermatite seborroica, il cheratoderma di palmi delle mani e piante dei piedi e la psoriasi.

Eziologia. La causa è sconosciuta. Alcuni casi dell'infanzia sono probabilmente provocati da una forma genetica a trasmissione autosomica dominante, ma la maggior parte dei casi è sporadica. La biopsia cutanea aiuta a distinguere la malattia dalla psoriasi e dalla dermatite seborroica.

Trattamento. I numerosi protocolli terapeutici consigliati sono difficili da valutare perché la patologia ha un decorso imprevedibile, con alterne esacerbazioni e remissioni. Nei casi più lievi è sufficiente la lubrificazione. Retinoidi orali e topici sono prescritti di frequente. Nell'infanzia, la prognosi per una guarigione definitiva è relativamente buona.

MALATTIA DI DARIER (CHERATOSI FOLLICOLARE). Questo raro disordine genetico, ereditato con modalità autosomica dominante (gene ATP2A2), esordisce generalmente nella tarda infanzia. Le lesioni tipiche sono costituite da piccole papule color carne, non sempre follicolari. Le lesioni acquisiscono una crosta gialla maleodorante e confluiscono per formare ampie placche vegetative grigio-brune (Fig. 656-7). Le sedi più frequentemente coinvolte sono il viso, il collo, le spalle, il torace, la schiena e le superfici flessorie degli arti con distribuzione simmetrica. Papule, fissure, croste e ulcere possono comparire anche sulle membrane mucose di labbra, lingua, mucosa buccale, faringe, laringe e vulva.

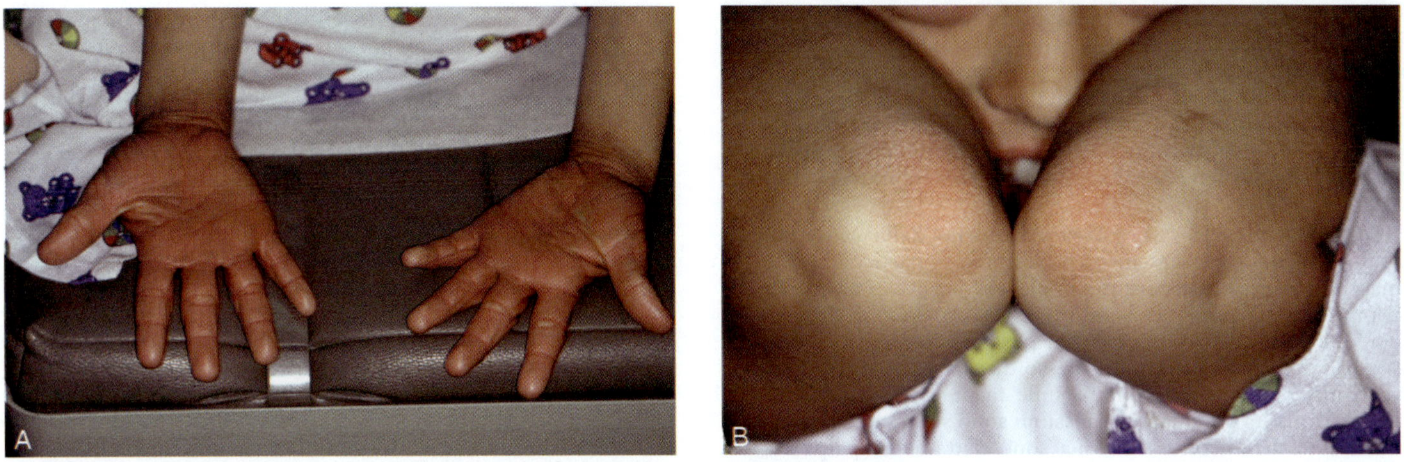

Figura 656-6. *A*, Ipercheratosi palmare di colore arancio nella pitiriasi rubra pilare (PRP). *B*, Lesioni al gomito nella PRP.

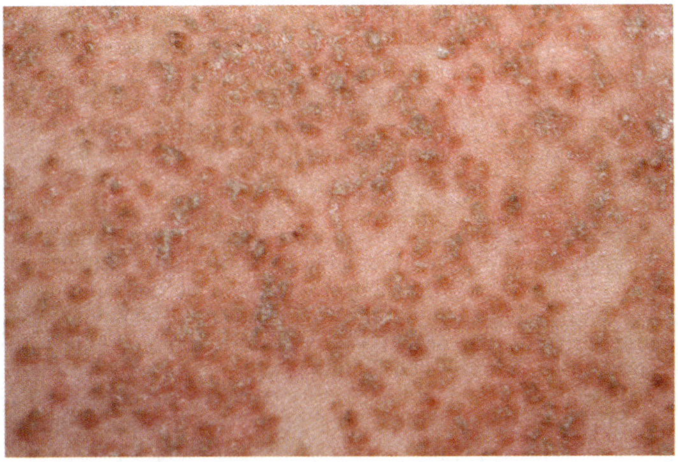

Figura 656-7. Papule coalescenti in ampie placche sulla schiena di un paziente con malattia di Darier.

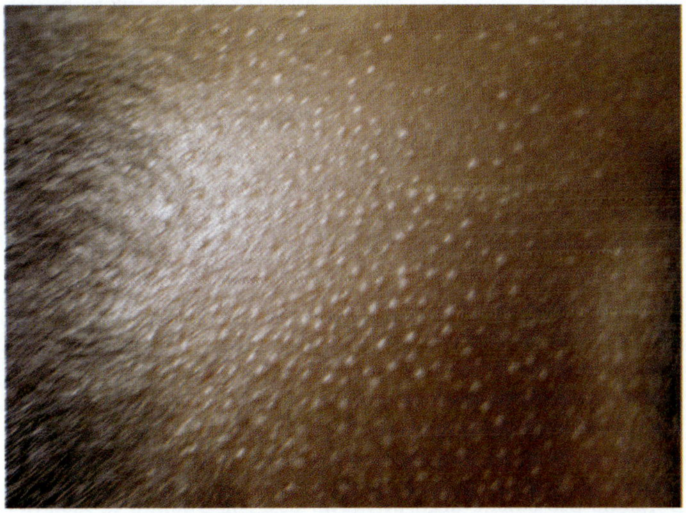

Figura 656-8. Papule uniformi e leggermente ipopigmentate nel lichen nitidus.

variabili sono l'ipercheratosi palmare e plantare e la distrofia ungueale con ipercheratosi subungueale. Talvolta si riscontrano prurito severo, infezione secondaria, cattivo odore e aggravamento della dermatosi in seguito all'esposizione al sole. La malattia di Darier è facilmente confondibile con la dermatite seborroica o le verruche piane giovanili. Le seguenti alterazioni istologiche assumono un valore diagnostico: ipercheratosi, separazione intraepidermica con formazione di fessure sovrabasali e cellule epidermiche discheratosiche.

Il **trattamento** è non specifico. Alcuni pazienti rispondono all'acido retinoico, con o senza bendaggio occlusivo. Le forme severe della malattia possono essere controllate con la somministrazione orale di retinoidi sintetici. L'insorgenza di un'infezione secondaria richiede la detersione locale e la somministrazione di antibiotici per via sistemica. I sintomi tendono a peggiorare durante i mesi estivi.

LICHEN NITIDUS. Questa eruzione cronica e benigna è caratterizzata da piccole papule appiattite, non mobili e lucenti, di dimensioni uniformi (1-2 mm), che solitamente hanno lo stesso colore della cute, ma talvolta assumono una colorazione rossastra o rosea. Negli individui di razza nera appaiono spesso ipopigmentate (Fig. 656-8). Le sedi d'elezione sono i genitali, l'addome, il torace, l'avambraccio, il polso e la faccia interna delle cosce. Le lesioni possono essere rade o numerose, raggruppate in placche di grandi dimensioni. Un attento esame obiettivo rivela spesso la presenza di papule lineari disposte in strie (fenomeno di Koebner), che assumono un importante valore diagnostico perché si riscontrano solo in un numero molto limitato di patologie. Il lichen nitidus può manifestarsi a qualsiasi età e la causa è sconosciuta. Fatta eccezione per il prurito, talvolta severo, i pazienti sono solitamente asintomatici e costituzionalmente sani. Le lesioni sono spesso confondibili con quelle del lichen planus e in rari casi le due forme coesistono.

Anche la cheratosi pilare diffusa può essere confusa con il lichen nitidus, ma la localizzazione follicolare delle papule e l'assenza del fenomeno di Koebster contribuiscono alla diagnosi differenziale. Le verruche piane, se piccole e uniformi, possono talvolta somigliare al lichen nitidus. La diagnosi è normalmente formulata sulla base dell'esame obiettivo, ma in alcuni casi è necessaria una biopsia. Le papule sono composte da nidi di linfociti e istiociti ben circoscritti, localizzati nel derma superiore e circondati da creste epidermiche allungate. La malattia si protrae per alcuni mesi o anni, ma le lesioni tendono a risolversi completamente. Gli steroidi topici possono risultare efficaci in particolare nell'attenuare il prurito.

LICHEN STRIATUS. Questa eruzione benigna e autolimitante consiste in una banda lineare continua o discontinua di papule a distribuzione zosteriforme. La lesione primaria, piatta e violacea, è ricoperta da fini scaglie. Aggregati di papule formano bande multiple o placche. Nei pazienti di razza nera, le lesioni possono risultare ipopigmentate. L'eziologia e la motivazione della distribuzione lineare sono sconosciute. L'eruzione evolve per alcuni giorni o settimane, in bambini per il resto in buona salute, e rimane stazionaria per settimane o mesi, per poi risolversi senza sequele. La malattia è solitamente asintomatica, ma alcuni bambini lamentano prurito. La distrofia ungueale può comparire quando l'eruzione coinvolge la piega ungueale posteriore e la matrice (Fig. 656-9).

Il lichen striatus viene talvolta confuso con altre patologie. La placca iniziale può somigliare all'eczema papulare o al lichen nitidus, finché la configurazione lineare non diviene evidente. Il lichen planus lineare e la psoriasi lineare spesso si associano a lesioni isolate caratteristiche, sparse in altre parti del corpo. I nevi epidermici lineari sono lesioni permanenti, solitamente più ipercheratosiche e iperpigmentate rispetto a quelle del lichen striatus. Se il prurito è intenso, può essere alleviato con una lozione lubrificante contenente mentolo e canfora o con un blando corticosteroide.

LICHEN PLANUS. Questo disturbo è raro nei bambini più piccoli e poco comune in quelli più grandi. La lesione primaria è una papula poligonale violacea, dai contorni ben demarcati, con linee sottili o scaglie biancastre sulla superficie. Le papule tendono a confluire, formando ampie placche (Fig. 656-10). Il prurito è talvolta molto intenso e il paziente, grattandosi, causa la formazione di nuove papule (fenomeno di Koebner), tanto che se ne possono spesso individuare delle linee. Le localizzazioni più comuni sono le superfici flessorie del polso, l'avambraccio e la faccia interna della coscia. Le lesioni delle membrane mucose consistono tipicamente in papule biancastre a capocchia di spillo, che confluiscono per formare un fine reticolato sulla mucosa orale e talvolta su labbra e lingua.

Il **lichen planus eruttivo acuto** è probabilmente la forma più comune nei bambini. Le lesioni compaiono in modo esplosivo, come negli esantemi virali, e si diffondono rapidamente, coinvolgendo la maggior parte della superficie corporea. La malattia può essere anche ipertrofica, lineare, bollosa, atrofica, anulare, follicolare, erosiva e ulcerativa. Nelle forme croniche si riscontra talvolta un coinvolgimento ungueale, raro in età pediatrica. Il disturbo può persistere per mesi o anni, ma la forma eruttiva acuta è più probabile che regredisca definitivamente. L'intensa iperpigmentazione tende a persistere a lungo dopo la risoluzione delle lesioni. I reperti istopatologici di lichen planus sono specifici e la biopsia è indicata quando la diagnosi è dubbia.

Il **trattamento** è diretto ad alleviare l'intenso prurito e a migliorare le lesioni cutanee. Spesso si rivela utile la somministrazione orale di antistaminici. Le lesioni cutanee rispondono bene alla regolare applicazione topica di un corticosteroide. In rari casi, quando le lesioni sono particolarmente diffuse e resistenti alla terapia, è necessario ricorrere a corticosteroidi sistemici. Anche la fototerapia si è rivelata utile nel caso di lesioni estese.

POROCHERATOSI. Questa rara malattia, cronica e progressiva, può presentarsi in forme diverse: placche isolate, porocheratosi lineare, lesioni ipercheratosiche palmari e plantari, lesioni eruttive diffuse e porocheratosi attinica superficiale. Quest'ultima forma, probabilmente indotta da un'eccessiva esposizione al sole, si verifica più comunemente nelle donne. Altre forme di porocheratosi sono più frequenti nei soggetti di sesso maschile e tendono a esordire nell'infanzia. Le sedi maggiormente coinvolte sono gli arti, il viso, il collo e i genitali. La lesione primaria è una piccola papula cheratosica che si allarga alla periferia, creando una depressione centrale, con i margini che formano un orletto rilevato (Fig. 656-11). La configurazione delle placche può essere rotonda, ovale o a spirale. I bordi rilevati sono divisi da una sottile scanalatura, da cui protrudono piccole proiezioni di cheratina. L'area centrale, liscia e secca, è sclerotica e assume una colorazione giallastra, grigia o pigmentata, mentre i bordi sono di colore grigio scuro, marrone o nero.

La **diagnosi differenziale** include le verruche, i nevi epidermici, il lichen planus, il granuloma anulare e l'elastosi perforante serpiginosa. La biopsia cutanea rivela la presenza della lamella cornoide (composta da cellule dello strato corneo con nuclei), responsabile del caratteristico aspetto lineare della lesione. Il decorso della malattia è lentamente progressivo, ma relativamente asintomatico. In alcuni casi è stata segnalata una degenerazione maligna in carcinoma squamocellulare. Nessun trattamento si è dimostrato universalmente efficace. Le lesioni possono rispondere

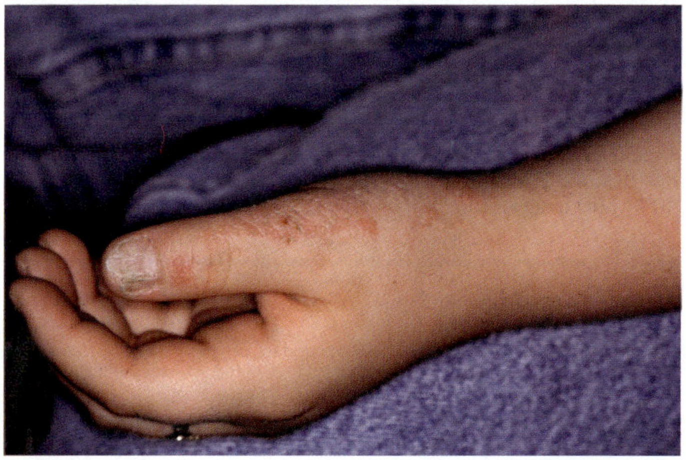

Figura 656-9. Lichen striatus con distrofia ungueale.

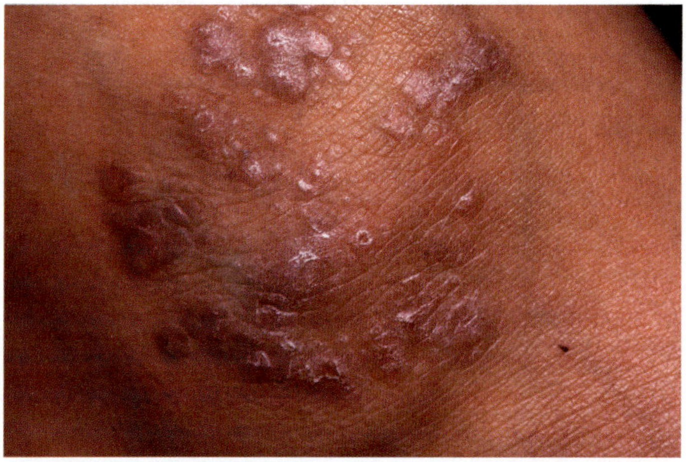

Figura 656-10. Papule poligonali appiattite, color porpora, nel lichen planus.

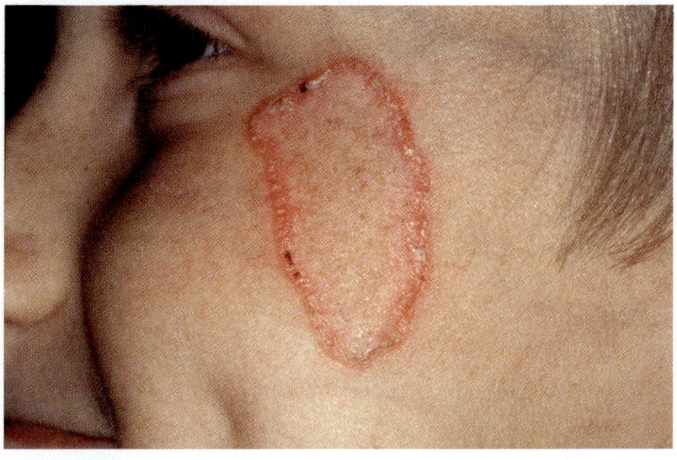

Figura 656-11. Ampie placche di porocheratosi di Mibelli, con bordi rilevati e centro depresso.

a un **trattamento** con azoto liquido, retinoidi topici, fluorouracile (5-FU) e imiquimod.

ACRODERMATITE PAPULOSA INFANTILE (SINDROME DI GIANOTTI-CROSTI). Questa eruzione caratteristica si associa occasionalmente a malessere, febbre e ad altri lievi sintomi sistemici. Il picco di incidenza è nella prima infanzia. Si verifica solitamente in forma sporadica, ma sono state segnalate epidemie della malattia. La lesione cutanea consiste in una papula monomorfa, generalmente non pruriginosa, appiattita, rosso scuro o ramato, di dimensioni variabili da 1 a 10 mm (Fig. 656-12). Le papule compaiono in gruppi, ma, benché profuse, restano discrete, formando un'eruzione simmetrica su volto, glutei e arti, compresa la regione palmoplantare. Le papule assumo spesso l'aspetto di vesciche, ma non contengono liquido; talvolta divengono emorragiche. Sugli arti si possono osservare linee di papule (**fenomeno di Koebner**). Il tronco è relativamente risparmiato, così come il cuoio capelluto e le membrane mucose. Linfoadenopatia generalizzata ed epatomegalia (nei soggetti con viremia da epatite B) costituiscono gli unici altri reperti anomali. L'eruzione si risolve spontaneamente in circa 15-60 giorni. Se presenti, l'epatomegalia e la linfoadenopatia possono persistere per diversi mesi. In Italia, quest'eruzione è stata inizialmente associata all'infezione primaria da epatite B. L'aumento dei valori delle transaminasi sieriche e della fosfatasi alcalina, in assenza di concomitante iperbilirubinemia, è insolito. La biopsia cutanea è aspecifica ed è caratterizzata da un infiltrato mononucleare perivascolare e da edema dell'endotelio capillare.

La malattia è solitamente benigna e, negli Stati Uniti, non è associata all'epatite. L'eruzione è stata riscontrata in bambini affetti dal virus di Epstein-Barr, dal coxsackievirus A16, da virus parainfluenzale, da altre infezioni virali o in seguito a vaccinazione. L'acrodermatite papulosa può essere confusa con il lichen planus, l'eritema multiforme, l'istiocitosi X e la porpora di Henoch-Schönlein.

ACANTHOSIS NIGRICANS. È caratterizzata da placche iperpigmentate, vellutate e ipercheratosiche, solitamente localizzate su collo, ascelle (Fig. 656-13), regione inframammaria, inguine, parte interna delle cosce e regione anogenitale. Le alterazioni istologiche sono più simili a quelle della papillomatosi e dell'ipercheratosi piuttosto che a quelle dell'acantosi e dovute all'eccessiva produzione di pigmento. Classicamente, la malattia è stata associata all'obesità, a farmaci come l'acido nicotinico, a endocrinopatie (in particolare diabete mellito e sindromi iperandrogeniche o ipogonadiche), a disturbi genetici causati dalla mutazione dei fattori di crescita dei fibroblasti. In alcuni casi la patologia è di origine familiare, con trasmissione autosomica dominante. L'acanthosis nigricans si riscontra nel 7% dei bambini ed è generalmente associata a obesità. Negli adulti è spesso associata a tumori maligni, ma questa complicanza è rara in età pediatrica.

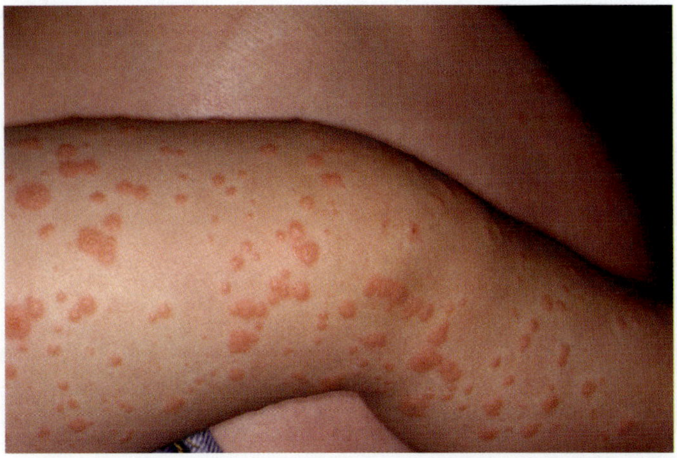

Figura 656-12. Numerose papule rosse e appiattite nella sindrome di Gianotti-Crosti.

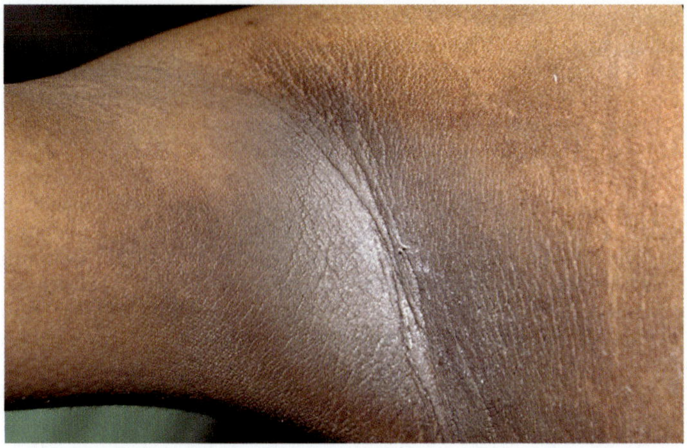

Figura 656-13. Iperpigmentazione vellutata dell'ascella nell'acanthosis nigricans.

Le lesioni cutanee appaiono come una manifestazione della resistenza all'insulina o di mutazioni dei fattori di crescita dei fibroblasti. La gravità clinica e le caratteristiche istopatologiche della malattia correlano positivamente con il grado di iperinsulinemia. La resistenza all'insulina e l'iperinsulinemia compensatoria possono causare l'attivazione dei recettori dei fattori di crescita insulino-simili, che promuovono la crescita epidermica. Nella forma maligna degli adulti, l'iperinsulinemia e la secrezione dei fattori di crescita possono risultare patogenetici.

I sintomi cutanei sono particolarmente difficili da trattare, ma possono essere migliorati con una terapia palliativa del disturbo soggiacente. In presenza di obesità, si raccomanda una riduzione del peso. Anche l'applicazione di una crema a base di urea al 40% può essere utile.

Amer A, Fischer H: Azithromycin does not cure pityriasis rosea. *Pediatrics* 2006;117:1702–1705.

Capon F, Trembath RC, Barker JN: An update on the genetics of psoriasis. *Dermatol Clin* 2004;22:339–347.

Chuh AA, Chan HH, Zawar V: Is human herpes virus 7 the causative agent of pityriasis rosea?—a critical review. *Int J Dermatol* 2004;43:870–875.

Eberting CL, Javor E, Gorden P, et al: Insulin resistance, acanthosis nigricans and hypertriglycidemia. *J Am Acad Dermatol* 2005;52:341–344.

Gerbig AW: Treating keratosis pilaris. *J Am Acad Dermatol* 2002;47:457–458.

Gibson LE: Acanthosis nigricans. *Mayo Clin Proc* 2004;79:1571.

Gordon KB, Papp KA, Hamilton TK, et al: Efalizumab for patients with moderate to severe plaque psoriasis. *JAMA* 2003;290:3073–3080.

Ito N, Ohshima A, Hashizume H, et al: Febrile ulceronecrotic Mucha-Habermann's disease managed with methylprednisolone semipule and subsequent methotrexate therapy. *J Am Acad Dermatol* 2003;49:1142–1148.

Lane JE, Guill MA: Juvenile pityriasis rubra pilaris. *Pediatr Dermatol* 2004;21:512–513.

Lewkowicz D, Gottlieb AB: Pediatrics psoriasis and arthritis. *Dermatol Ther* 2004;17:364–375.

Orru S, Giuressi E, Carcassi C, et al: Mapping of the major psoriasis-susceptibility locus (PSORS1) in a 70-Kb interval around the corneodesmin gene (CDSN). *Am J Hum Genet* 2005;76:164–171.

Schön MP, Boehncke WH: Psoriasis. *N Engl J Med* 2005;352:1899–1912.

Stulberg DL, Wolfrey J: Pityriasis rosea. *Am Fam Physician* 2004;69:87–91.

Tilly JJ, Drolet BA, Esterly NB: Lichenoid eruptions in children. *J Am Acad Dermatol* 2004;51:606–624.

Tyring S, Gottlieb A, Papp K, et al: Etanercept and clinical outcomes, fatigue, and depression in psoriasis: double-blind placebo-controlled randomised phase III trial. *Lancet* 2006;367:29–35.

Capitolo 657 ■ Disordini della cheratinizzazione

Joseph G. Morelli

MALATTIE DELLA CORNEIFICAZIONE. Le malattie della corneificazione, conosciute anche come **ittiosi**, costituiscono un gruppo primario di patologie ereditarie, caratterizzate sul piano clinico da desquamazione e su quello istopatologico da ipercheratosi. Sono solitamente diagnosticate in base al pattern di ereditarietà, agli aspetti clinici, alle anomalie associate e alle alterazioni istopatologiche (Tab. 657-1). Poiché alcune di queste patologie causano deturpazione, con conseguente notevole disagio psicosociale, la diagnosi precoce è indispensabile per prevederne il possibile decorso e la prognosi e per garantire il counseling ai pazienti e alle famiglie.

FETO ARLECCHINO. Questo raro disturbo della cheratinizzazione raggruppa probabilmente diversi genotipi con manifestazioni cliniche analoghe.

Alla nascita, la cute appare ispessita, corrugata e fissurata, con placche dure distribuite sull'intera superficie corporea, che sfigurano i lineamenti del viso e bloccano le dita.

Le orbite sono oscurate da grave ectropion e chemosi, orecchie e naso sono appiattiti, le labbra appaiono everse e socchiuse. Unghie e capelli possono essere assenti. La mobilità articolare è ridotta; le mani e i piedi appaiono fissi e ischemici. I neonati colpiti sono soggetti a gravi infezioni cutanee e presentano difficoltà respiratorie e della suzione. Nella maggior parte dei casi, il decesso avviene nei primi giorni o nelle prime settimane di vita, ma alcuni neonati sopravvivono oltre il periodo infantile, pur presentando grave ittiosi e una compromissione neurologica di entità variabile.

L'ectropion e l'eclabium tendono a risolversi, e le placche indurite e screpolate sono sostituite da sottili scaglie, circondate da eritema.

TABELLA 657-1. Disordini della corneificazione che solitamente si presentano nelle prime settimane di vita

DISTURBO	EREDITARIETÀ	CARATTERISTICHE CLINICHE	MUTAZIONE	DIAGNOSI
Ittiosi arlecchino	AR	Scaglie spesse con fessurazioni	Sconosciuta	Clinica
Collodion baby	Solitamente AR	Membrana di collodio lucida	Varie	Clinica
Ittiosi recessiva legata all'X	Recessiva legata al cromosoma X	Membrana di collodio Possono essere presenti anomalie dei genitali	Solfatasi steroidea	Colesterol solfato nel plasma
Ittiosi lamellare	Solitamente AR	Membrana di collodio	Transglutaminasi I Altro	Clinica
Eritrodermia ittiosiforme congenita	AR	Membrana di collodio	Sconosciuta	Clinica
Ipercheratosi epidermolitica	AD	Scaglie e vesciche	Cheratine 1,10, 2e	Clinica e istologica
Ittiosi istrice	AD	Placche e ipercheratosi	Sconosciuta	Clinica
Ruvidità cutanea familiare	AR	Ruvidità superficiale	Sconosciuta	Clinica e istologica
Sjögren-Larsson	AR	Ispessimento cutaneo variabile Ritardo mentale e dello sviluppo Diplegia spastica Convulsioni Macchie "brillanti"	Deidrogenasi aldeide grassa (FAD)	Clinica e colture di fibroblasti per FAD
Difetto di deposito di lipidi neutri	AR	Membrana di collodio o eritrodermia ittiosiforme	Riciclo del triacilglicerolo in diacilglicerolo	Striscio cutaneo per PMN vacuolati
Netherton	AR	Eritrodermia ittiosiforme Capelli radi, spesso deficit staturo-ponderale	SPINKS Sconosciuta	Clinica; esame del capello nell'infanzia Clinica e microscopia del capello; contenuto di zolfo
Tricotiodistrofia	AR	Membrana di collodio Capelli che si spezzano	Trascrizione del DNA, riparazione genetica	
Sindrome KID	AD o AR	Cute eritrodermatosa o ispessita, con papule	Sconosciuta	Clinica; potenziali evocati uditivi
Sindrome CHILD	Dominante legata al cromosoma X	Alopecia Scaglie unilaterali giallastre Emidisplasia Difetti degli arti	3β-idrossisteroide deidrogenasi Proteina legante l'emopamil	Clinica
Conradi-Hünermann	Dominante legata al cromosoma X	Scaglie spesse e psoriasiformi con eritrodermia, lungo le linee di Blaschko Accorciamento della porzione prossimale degli arti	Proteina legante l'emopamil	Clinica
Ittiosi follicolare	Solitamente recessiva legata al cromosoma X	Ipercheratosi follicolare prominente Alopecia Fotofobia	Sconosciuta	Clinica
Sindrome CHIME	AR	Placche eritematose ittiosiche Difetti cardiaci; facies tipica Colobomi retinici	Sconosciuta	Clinica
Gaucher	AR	Membrana di collodio Epatosplenomegalia	β-glucocerebrosidasi	Clinica; colture di fibroblasti

AD, autosomica dominante; AR, autosomica recessiva; CHILD, emidisplasia congenita con eritrodermia ittiosiforme e difetti degli arti; CHIME, colobomi oculari, difetti cardiaci, dermatosi ittiosiforme, ritardo mentale e anomalie delle orecchie; KID, cheratite con ittiosi e sordità; PMN, neutrofili polimorfonucleati.

Da Eichenfield LF, Frieden IJ, Esterly NB: *Textbook of Neonatal Dermatology*. Philadelphia, WB Saunders, 2001, p. 277.

Quasi tutti i casi sono ereditati come caratteri autosomici recessivi, ma è possibile riscontrare nuove mutazioni autosomiche dominanti. Le anomalie morfologiche più comuni sono l'ipercheratosi, l'accumulo di gocce lipidiche nei corneociti e l'assenza dei normali granuli lamellari. Si ritiene che il difetto alla base di tutte le forme sia un'anomalia dei granuli lamellari, responsabile della desquamazione.

Il **trattamento** iniziale prevede l'assunzione di liquidi per evitare la disidratazione causata dalla perdita d'acqua transepidermica, l'utilizzo di un'incubatrice con aria umidificata e riscaldata, l'applicazione di pomate ed emulsioni e l'assunzione orale di retinoidi. È inoltre opportuno prestare una particolare cura all'igiene.

I sopravvissuti alla terapia retinoide sviluppano grave eritrodermia ittiosiforme congenita. La diagnosi prenatale è realizzabile mediante fetoscopia, biopsia cutanea fetale o esame microscopico di cellule prelevate dal liquido amniotico tra la 17ª e la 21ª settimana di gestazione.

COLLODION BABY. Alla nascita, i neonati affetti da questa malattia sono ricoperti da una membrana spessa e tesa, simile a collodio o carta oleosa (Fig. 657-1), che in seguito cade. Il disturbo è solitamente una manifestazione dell'eritrodermia ittiosiforme o di ittiosi lamellare. Come nel caso del feto arlecchino, il *collodion baby* sembra costituire il fenotipo unico di diversi genotipi. In rari casi, si riscontra un'evoluzione verso altre forme di ittiosi o di malattia di Gaucher.

Un piccolo sottogruppo di pazienti non presenta altri sintomi, né sviluppa la malattia cutanea cronica. I neonati colpiti manifestano ectropion, appiattimento di naso e orecchie, labbra fisse con configurazione a O. I capelli possono essere assenti o perforare il rivestimento corneo.

I primi atti respiratori del bambino provocano lo sfaldamento della membrana, che, poco dopo la nascita, comincia a desquamarsi a grossi lembi. La completa eliminazione della membrana richiede diverse settimane, ma in alcuni casi se ne forma una nuova in aree localizzate.

La morbilità e la mortalità neonatale possono essere causate da infezioni cutanee, polmonite da aspirazione (di materiale squamoso), ipotermia o disidratazione ipernatremica dovuta all'eccessiva perdita di liquidi transcutanea causata dall'aumento della permeabilità cutanea.

L'esito è incerto e non è possibile formulare alcuna prognosi circa il successivo sviluppo dell'ittiosi. Il **trattamento** prevede il mantenimento di un elevato livello di umidità nell'ambiente e l'applicazione di lubrificanti non occlusivi atti ad agevolare lo sfaldamento della membrana.

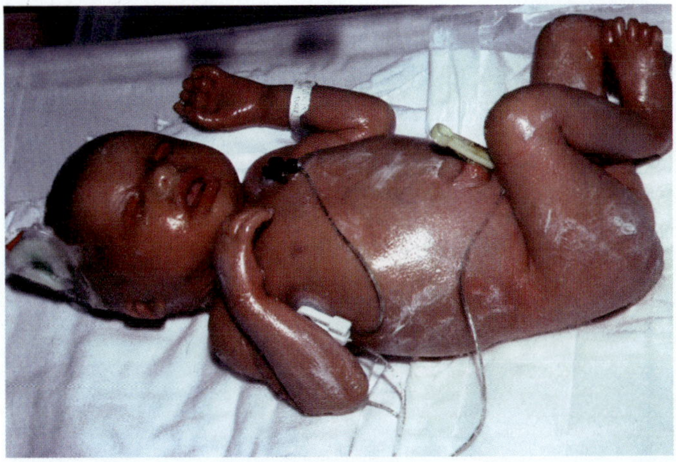

Figura 657-1. Aspetto tipico del collodion baby.

ITTIOSI LAMELLARE ED ERITRODERMIA ITTIOSIFORME CONGENITA (NON BOLLOSA). Si riscontrano due forme principali di ittiosi ereditaria autosomica recessiva; entrambe si presentano già alla nascita (o poco dopo) e si manifestano con eritrodermia, desquamazione o membrana di collodio.

Successivamente allo sfaldamento della membrana di collodio (se presente), l'ittiosi lamellare evolve in ampie squame scure, di forma quadrilaterale, libere ai margini e adese al centro. La desquamazione è spesso pronunciata e coinvolge l'intera superficie somatica, incluse le aree flessorie (Fig. 657-2). Il volto è in genere colpito gravemente, con ectropion e orecchie piccole e deformi. I palmi delle mani e le piante dei piedi sono spesso ipercheratosici. I capelli possono essere radi e fini, mentre denti e superfici mucose appaiono normali. A differenza dell'eritrodermia ittiosiforme congenita, l'eritema è minimo. Nessuna delle due forme prevede la formazione di vesciche. L'**ittiosi lamellare autosomica recessiva (ARLI)** costituisce un disturbo eterogeneo sul piano clinico e genetico. In circa il 50% dei casi, sono state riscontrate mutazioni del gene TGM1, che codifica per la transglutaminasi. Mutazioni di TGM1 si osservano anche nell'eritrodermia ittiosiforme congenita.

L'**eritrodermia ittiosiforme congenita** tende a essere persistente; le squame, sebbene generalizzate, sono più sottili e biancastre rispetto a quelle dell'ittiosi lamellare (Fig. 657-3). L'ipercheratosi si nota in particolare intorno alle ginocchia, ai gomiti e alle caviglie. I palmi delle mani e le piante dei piedi sono uniformemente

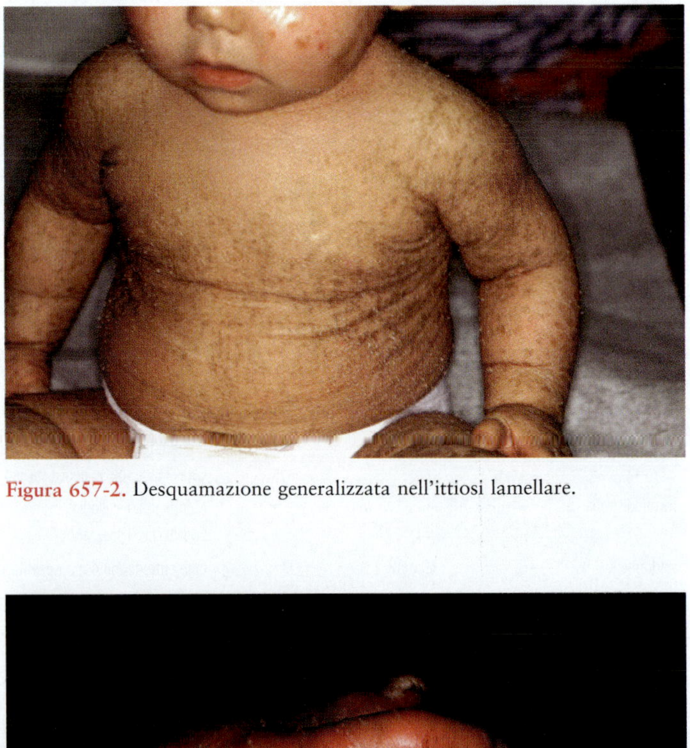

Figura 657-2. Desquamazione generalizzata nell'ittiosi lamellare.

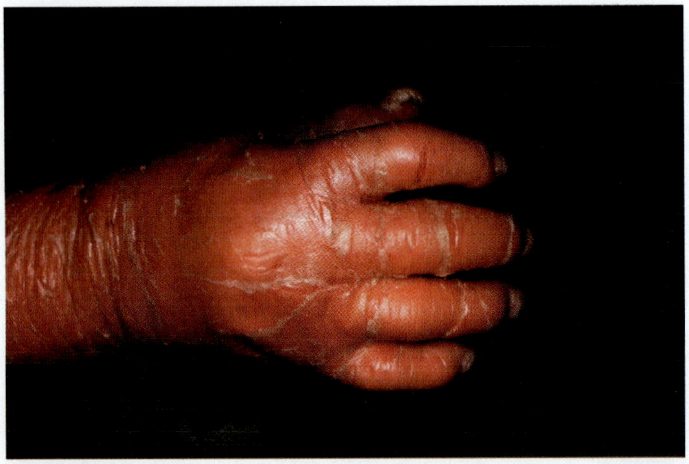

Figura 657-3. Grave eritema e desquamazione nell'eritrodermia ittiosiforme congenita.

ipercheratosici. I pazienti hanno capelli radi, alopecia cicatriziale e distrofia ungueale.

L'ittiosi lamellare è caratterizzata da uno strato corneo marcatamente ispessito e da lieve e irregolare ispessimento epidermico. L'eritrodermia ittiosiforme congenita presenta un ispessimento epidermico maggiore, con paracheratosi, ma l'ipercheratosi e l'ipergranulosi sono meno pronunciate rispetto all'ittiosi lamellare. Nell'eritrodermia ittiosiforme congenita si nota un evidente aumento del tasso di produzione di cellule epidermiche, ben superiore al lieve incremento riscontrabile nei pazienti con ittiosi lamellare.

Il prurito può essere grave e scarsamente controllabile con i farmaci. L'aspetto poco attraente del bambino e il cattivo odore provocato dalla colonizzazione batterica delle scaglie macerate rischiano di creare seri problemi psicologici. Il disagio può essere alleviato mantenendo l'ambiente umido in inverno e ricorrendo all'aria condizionata in estate. La generosa e frequente applicazione di agenti emollienti e cheratolitici come l'acido lattico o glicolico (al 5%), l'urea (al 10-40%) e l'acido retinoico (in crema allo 0,1%) consente di attenuare la desquamazione, ma questi agenti tendono a bruciare se la cute è fissurata. L'assunzione orale di **retinoidi** ha un effetto benefico, ma non altera il difetto alla base della malattia, dunque deve essere proseguita a tempo indeterminato. I rischi a lungo termine di questi composti (effetti teratogeni e tossicità ossea) ne limitano perciò l'utilità. L'ectropion richiede un trattamento oftalmologico e, in alcuni casi, un intervento plastico.

ITTIOSI VOLGARE. Questo disturbo può avere un'origine autosomica dominante o poligenetica. Mutazioni semidominanti del gene della filaggrina sono state segnalate in alcune famiglie. I pazienti eterozigoti presentano una forma lieve, a penetranza incompleta. Con un'incidenza di circa 1/300 nati vivi, l'ittiosi volgare è il **più comune** disturbo della cheratinizzazione. L'esordio avviene generalmente nel primo anno di vita. Nella maggior parte dei casi, l'unico sintomo è una lieve ruvidità cutanea. Qualche volta la malattia può presentarsi con l'aspetto del *collodion baby*. La desquamazione è più marcata sulle superfici estensorie degli arti, in particolare quelli inferiori (Fig. 657-4). Le superfici flessorie sono risparmiate, e anche addome, collo e volto risultano relativamente poco colpiti. Altri sintomi piuttosto comuni sono la cheratosi pilare, in particolare agli arti superiori e alle cosce, l'accentuazione delle linee palmari, l'ipercheratosi di palmi delle mani e piante dei piedi e l'atopia. La desquamazione è più pronunciata durante i mesi invernali e può risolversi completamente nelle stagioni calde. I disturbi tendono ad attenuarsi e anche a sparire con l'età. Non si osserva l'associazione con anomalie di capelli, denti, superfici mucose o di altri apparati.

Le alterazioni istopatologiche differiscono da quelle degli altri tipi di ittiosi, perché l'ipercheratosi è associata a una riduzione o all'assenza dello strato granulare. Al microscopio elettronico, si osserva la presenza di granuli di cheratoialina insolitamente piccoli e friabili nelle cellule dell'epidermide. Il tasso di proliferazione epidermica è nella norma. L'ipercheratosi è dovuta alla difettosa desquamazione. La profilaggrina è clinicamente anomala, ma non sono state identificate mutazioni nel gene della profilaggrina.

La desquamazione può essere attenuata con l'applicazione quotidiana di un emolliente o di lubrificante contenente urea (10-40%), acido salicilico o un acido α-idrossi come l'acido lattico (al 5-12%).

ITTIOSI LEGATA AL CROMOSOMA X. L'ittiosi legata al cromosoma X colpisce quasi esclusivamente i soggetti di sesso maschile, ma le pazienti portatrici sane possono manifestare fini scaglie argentee sulla porzione inferiore delle gambe. La cute appare screpolata alla nascita, ma tale sintomo solitamente scompare entro il terzo-sesto mese di vita. La desquamazione è maggiormente pronunciata ai lati del collo, nella parte inferiore del volto, nelle aree preauricolari, nel tronco anteriore e agli arti, in particolare le gambe. Le aree flessorie di gomiti (Fig. 657-5) e ginocchia sono solitamente risparmiate, ma talvolta risultano lievemente coinvolte. In rari casi, palmi delle mani e piante dei piedi possono apparire leggermente ispessiti. Il disturbo peggiora gradualmente, con aggravamento dei sintomi e diffusione progressiva. La cheratosi pilare non è presente, né si osserva un aumento dell'incidenza di atopia. **Opacità corneali profonde**, che non interferiscono con la visione, tendono a svilupparsi nella tarda infanzia o nell'adolescenza e costituiscono un utile marker della malattia perché possono essere presenti anche nelle portatrici sane di sesso femminile. Il **criptorchidismo** si riscontra in circa il 25% dei maschi colpiti. Alcuni pazienti presentano caratteristiche addizionali, come la **sindrome di Kallmann** (gene KAL1) e la **condroplasia puntata** (geni per l'arisolfatasi e EPB), dovute a mutazioni di geni contigui. Il rischio di cancro testicolare può risultare aumentato.

Si osservano ipercheratosi dello strato corneo, uno strato granulare ben sviluppato ed epidermide iperplastica. Il tasso di proliferazione epidermica è nella norma. L'ipercheratosi è dovuta alla ritenzione di corneociti e al ritardo nella dissoluzione dei dischi dei desmosomi. L'ittiosi legata all'X implica un deficit di solfatasi steroidea, che idrolizza in colesterolo il colesterol solfato e gli altri steroidi solfati. Il colesterol solfato si accumula nello strato corneo e nel plasma, causando ipercheratosi in seguito all'inibizione della proteolisi desmosomiale. L'aumento dei livelli di colesterol solfato può essere dimostrato nel siero, nelle membrane eritrocitarie, nelle cellule epidermiche e nelle scaglie dei maschi colpiti. La riduzione dell'attività dell'enzima solfatasi steroidea è diagnosticabile nei fibroblasti, nei cheratinociti, nei leucociti e, nella fase prenatale, negli amniociti o nelle cellule dei villi coriali. Nelle famiglie colpite, il soggetto di sesso maschile

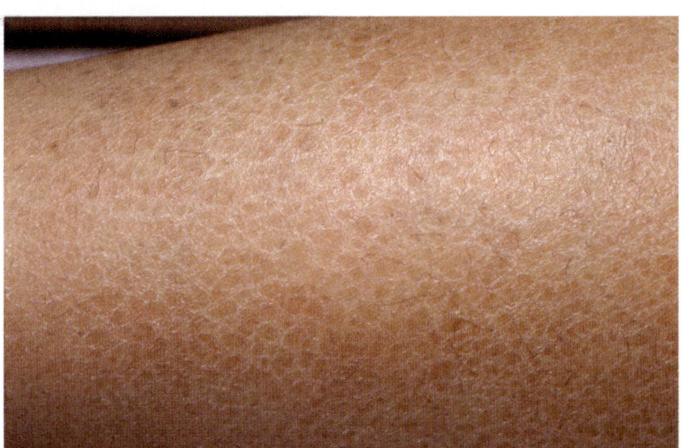

Figura 657-4. Presenza di scaglie a livello pretibiale nell'ittiosi volgare.

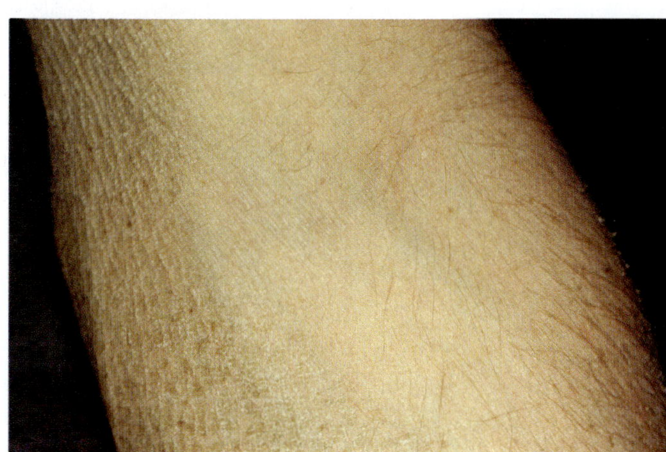

Figura 657-5. Fossa antecubitale risparmiata nell'ittiosi legata al cromosoma X.

affetto è individuabile mediante analisi degli enzimi di restrizione su coltura di villi coriali o amniociti, oppure mediante ibridazione in situ, che identifica, nella fase prenatale, le delezioni del gene che codifica per la solfatasi steroidea nelle cellule dei villi coriali. Il deficit placentare della solfatasi steroidea nelle madri portatrici può determinare una riduzione dei valori di estriolo in urine e siero, un travaglio prolungato e l'insensibilità dell'utero a ossitocina e prostaglandine.

L'applicazione quotidiana di emollienti e di un lubrificante a base di urea (10-40%) costituisce di solito il **trattamento** più efficace. Forme alternative di terapia includono l'applicazione notturna, con bendaggio occlusivo, di acido lattico (al 5%) in una base emolliente e di propilene glicol (al 40-60%) in acqua.

IPERCHERATOSI EPIDERMOLITICA (ERITRODERMIA ITTIOSIFORME CONGENITA BOLLOSA). L'ipercheratosi epidermolitica è ereditata con modalità autosomica dominante, ma in molti casi risulta sporadica. L'esordio avviene alla nascita, con **eritrodermia generalizzata** e grave ipercheratosi (Fig. 657-6). Le scaglie sono piccole, dure e verrucose. Tipiche linee ipercheratosiche parallele compaiono sulle superfici flessorie articolari, tra cui le ascelle, le fosse poplitea e antecubitale, collo e anche. L'eritema si attenua dopo l'infanzia, ma l'ipercheratosi persiste nella vita adulta. La formazione ricorrente di vesciche può essere disseminata nel neonato e complicare la diagnosi differenziale con gli atri disturbi bollosi. Tali vesciche si accentuano in aree sedi di traumi (come ginocchia, gomiti e arti inferiori), ma non costituiscono più un problema dopo i 7-8 anni di età. Palmi delle mani e piante dei piedi possono risultare ispessiti, mentre i capelli, le unghie, le mucose e le ghiandole sudoripare sono normali. L'infezione batterica secondaria è una complicanza comune, che richiede un'appropriata terapia antibiotica. I pazienti più gravi possono presentare ectropion e deformità delle orecchie.

L'istopatologia, che assume un valore diagnostico, consiste in ipercheratosi, un marcato ispessimento dello strato granulare con aumento del numero di granuli cheratoiali, spazi liberi intorno ai nuclei e confini cellulari indistinti nell'epidermide superiore. L'esame al microscopio elettronico rivela la presenza di agglomerati di filamenti intermedi di cheratina; molti desmosomi risultano attaccati soltanto a un cheratinocita invece di connettere i cheratinociti circostanti. È stato dimostrato che l'ipercheratosi epidermolitica è causata da difetti nella cheratina 1 o 10 codificata nel cromosoma 12p, dove si raggruppano i geni della cheratina di tipo II. Questi tipi di cheratina sono necessari per formare i filamenti intermedi nelle cellule degli strati soprabasali dell'epidermide. Le forme localizzate della malattia possono somigliare al nevo epidermico (**ittiosi istrice**) o a cheratodermia palmare e plantare, ma condividono le tipiche alterazioni istopatologiche dell'ipercheratosi epidermolitica. La diagnosi prenatale per le famiglie affette è possibile mediante esame delle cellule del DNA estratto dai villi coriali o da amniociti, purché sia nota la specifica mutazione del genitore affetto dalla malattia.

Il trattamento è difficile. Nel periodo prenatale, la morbilità aumenta in seguito a prematurità, sepsi e squilibri idroelettrolitici. La colonizzazione batterica secondaria alla macerazione delle scaglie produce un cattivo odore caratteristico, controllabile in parte con l'uso di detergenti antibatterici. Cicli di antibiotici orali sono generalmente necessari. Gli agenti cheratolitici sono spesso mal tollerati. I retinoidi orali possono consentire un significativo miglioramento, anche a dosi relativamente ridotte.

ITTIOSI LINEARE CIRCONFLESSA. Questa rara patologia a ereditarietà autosomica recessiva è presenta già alla nascita o esordisce nei primi mesi di vita, con eritema generalizzato e desquamazione. Tronco e arti presentano eritema diffuso e lesioni sovrapposte ipercheratosiche policicliche e serpiginose (Fig. 657-7), alcune delle quali dotate di un caratteristico doppio margine scaglioso. La lichenificazione o l'ipercheratosi tendono a persistere nelle fosse antecubitale e poplitea. Volto e cuoio capelluto possono rimanere eritematosi e desquamanti. In più del 50% dei pazienti, sono state descritte deformità del fusto del capello, più comunemente tricorressi invaginata. Questo tipo di ittiosi è caratteristico dei pazienti con **sindrome di Netherton**. L'esame istopatologico rivela alterazioni psoriasiformi non specifiche.

ERITROCHERATODERMIA VARIABILE. Questo raro ed eterogeneo disturbo autosomico dominante si presenta solitamente nei primi mesi di vita, progredisce nell'infanzia e tende a stabilizzarsi nell'adolescenza. In alcuni pazienti sono state identificate mutazioni del gene della connessina 31 e 30.3. La malattia è caratterizzata da placche ipercheratosiche ben delimitate, con bordi geografici, che si sviluppano in aree di cute normale (Fig. 657-8*A*) o all'interno di chiazze eritematose. La forma e le dimensioni di tali chiazze variano nel giro di qualche giorno, ora o minuto. Tendono inoltre a migrare (Fig. 657-8*B*) e possono gradualmente divenire ipercheratosiche e fisse. Sebbene distribuite in maniera generalizzata, le chiazze sono rade. Le principali localizzazioni sono il volto, i glutei, l'ascella e le superfici estensorie degli arti. Palmi delle mani e piante dei piedi possono risultare ispessiti, mentre capelli, unghie e denti sono normali. L'istopatologia rivela ipercheratosi, papillomatosi e iperplasia irregolare dell'epidermide.

L'eritrocheratodermia simmetrica progressiva è una malattia autosomica dominante che si presenta nell'infanzia con ampie placche eritematose simmetriche, ipercheratosiche e ricoperte di fini scaglie. Compare prevalentemente su arti, glutei, volto, cavi-

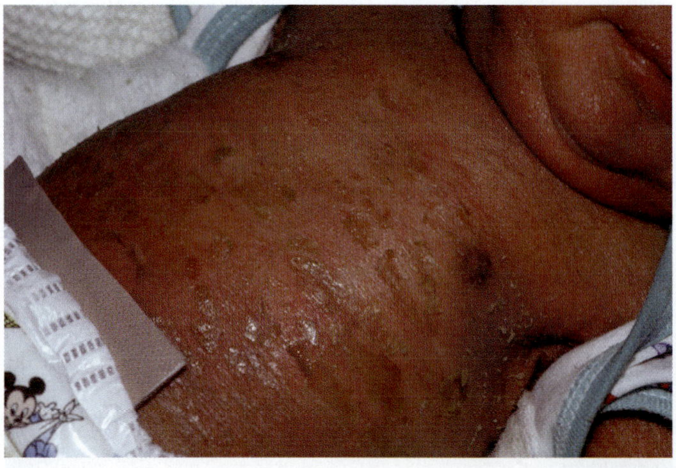

Figura 657-6. Erosioni superficiali e ipercheratosi nell'ipercheratosi epidermolitica.

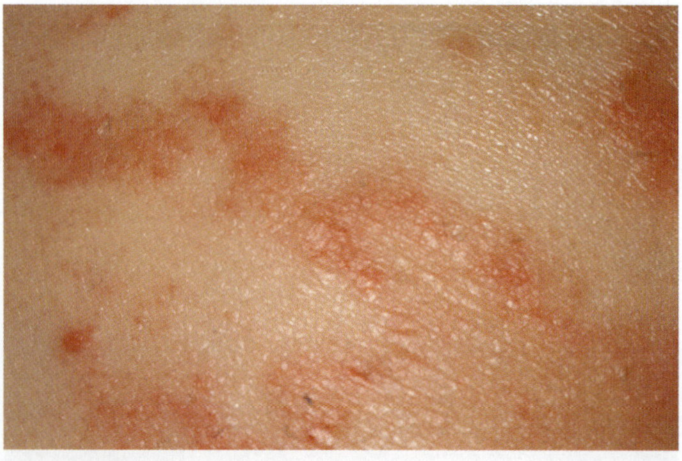

Figura 657-7. Lesioni eritematose, serpiginose e ipercheratosiche, nell'ittiosi lineare circonflessa.

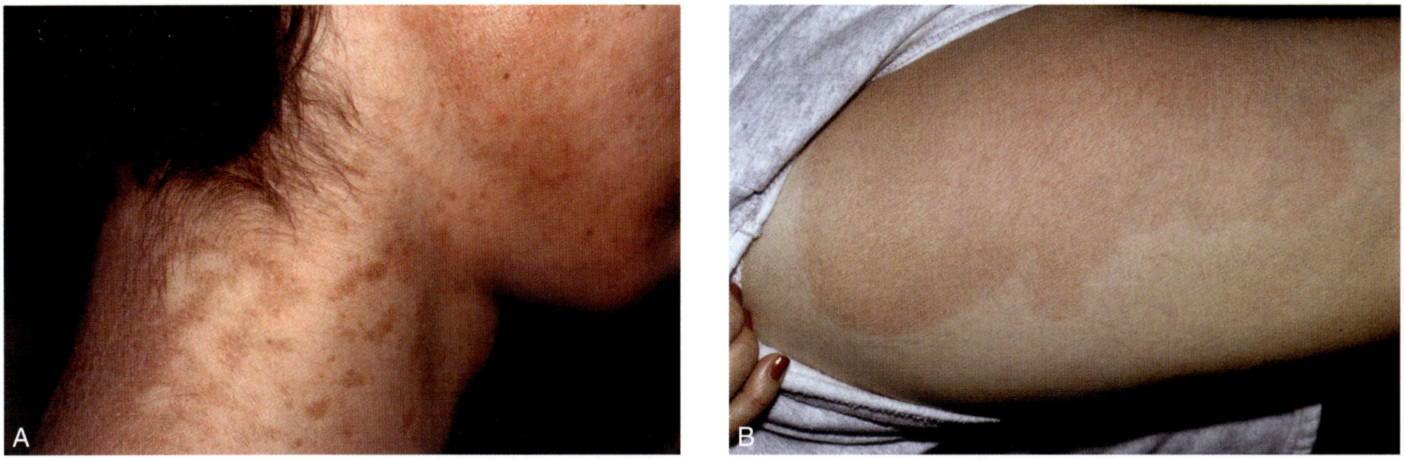

Figura 657-8. *A*, Placche ipercheratosiche fisse nell'eritrocheratodermia variabile. *B*, Lesione eritematosa migrante nell'eritrocheratodermia variabile.

glie e polsi. È presente anche cheratodermia palmoplantare. La principale caratteristica distintiva rispetto alla patologia precedente è la mancanza di eritema variabile. Le due malattie possono essere manifestazioni dello stesso disturbo, ma in alcuni pazienti con eritrocheratodermia simmetrica progressiva sono state individuate mutazioni del gene LOR (normale nella EKV).

DERMATOSI ITTIOSIFORME. Diverse sindromi che includono l'ittiosi sono state classificate come entità diagnostiche rare ma distinte.

Sindrome di Sjögren-Larsson. Questo errore congenito del metabolismo, a trasmissione autosomica recessiva, causa ittiosi, ritardo mentale e spasticità. L'ittiosi è generalizzata, ma appare più accentuata sulle superfici flessorie e sulla parte inferiore dell'addome. Consiste in eritrodermia, scaglie sottili, scaglie di dimensioni maggiori raggruppate in placche e ipercheratosi scura. È possibile riscontrare anche una lieve ipercheratosi palmoplantare. Le alterazioni cutanee sono talvolta identiche alle altre forme di ittiosi, perciò la diagnosi è spesso ritardata fino all'esordio dei sintomi neurologici. La presenza di macchie brillanti nell'area della fovea costituisce un importante segno oftalmologico utile sul piano diagnostico. Il ritardo nello sviluppo motorio e del linguaggio è solitamente osservato nel primo anno di vita, mentre nei primi tre anni si evidenziano diplegia o tetraplegia spastica, epilessia e ritardo mentale. Alcuni pazienti riescono a camminare con l'aiuto di tutori, ma nella maggior parte dei casi sono confinati sulla sedia a rotelle. Il difetto primario è un'anomalia nell'ossidazione degli alcol grassi, risultato di un deficit di aldeide deidrogenasi, un componente del complesso enzimatico alcol-nicotinamide adenin dinucleotide ossidoreduttasi. Questo deficit può essere dimostrato con colture di fibroblasti cutanei di pazienti affetti e portatori sani. La diagnosi prenatale è realizzabile mediante prelievo di cellule dei villi coriali o amniociti dei feti affetti. L'aumento della concentrazione urinaria di leucotriene B4 (LTB4) costituisce un criterio diagnostico più semplice; gli inibitori di 5-lipossigenasi sono stati utilizzati per ridurre il prurito.

Sindrome di Netherton. Questo disturbo autosomico recessivo è caratterizzato da ittiosi (solitamente lineare circonflessa, ma occasionalmente anche eritrodermia ittiosiforme di tipo congenito o lamellare), tricorressi invaginata o altre anomalie del fusto del capello e diatesi atopica. Nei pazienti sono state identificate mutazioni del gene SPINK 5, che codifica per un inibitore della serina proteasi. L'ittiosi è presente già nei primi 10 giorni di vita e può apparire estremamente marcata intorno a occhi, bocca e area perineale. L'eritrodermia risulta spesso intensificata successivamente a infezioni. I bambini possono presentare deficit staturo-ponderale, ricorrenti infezioni batteriche e candidosi, aumento dei livelli sierici di IgE e marcata disidratazione ipernatremica. Le più frequenti manifestazioni allergiche sono l'orticaria, l'angioedema, la dermatite atopica e l'asma. I capelli sono radi, corti e fragili (Fig. 657-9); anche sopracciglia, ciglia e peli corporei appaiono anomali. Tali caratteristiche alterazioni pilari sono evidenziabili al microscopio luminoso. Nel neonato, le anomalie delle ciglia sono le più facili da identificare.

Sindrome di Refsum (vedi Capitolo 86.2). Questo disturbo multisistemico, ereditato con modalità autosomica recessiva, diviene sintomatico nella seconda o nella terza decade di vita. L'ittiosi, relativamente lieve, può essere generalizzata e somiglia all'ittiosi volgare; in alcuni casi coinvolge anche i palmi delle mani e le piante dei piedi. I reperti più caratteristici della patologia sono polineurite cronica con progressiva paralisi e atassia, retinite pigmentosa atipica, anosmia, sordità, anomalie ossee e alterazioni dell'elettrocardiogramma. La diagnosi è formulata mediante analisi lipidica ematica o cutanea, che rivela l'aumento dei livelli di acido fitanico. Il difetto è stato localizzato sul gene PAHK. L'acido fitanico deriva esclusivamente dalla clorofilla assunta attraverso l'alimentazione, perciò l'eliminazione dalla dieta di verdure ricche di questo acido consente di ottenere un miglioramento clinico.

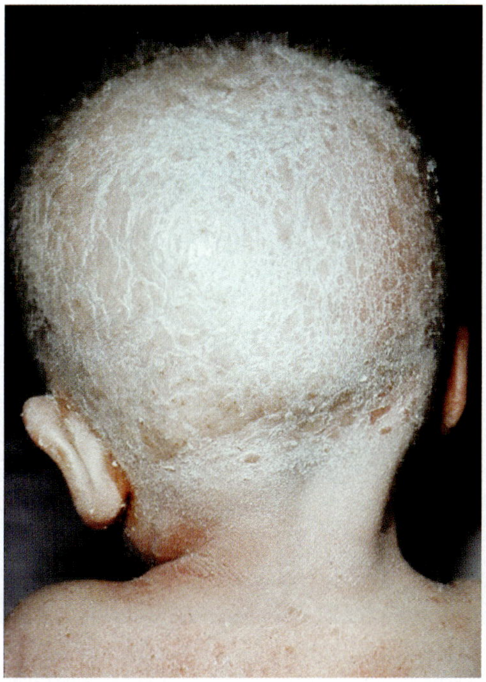

Figura 657-9. Capelli molto corti e scaglie spesse nella sindrome di Netherton.

Condrodisplasia puntata (vedi Capitolo 86.2). Questa definizione include diversi disturbi geneticamente eterogenei, caratterizzati da ittiosi e alterazioni ossee, in particolare la sindrome di Conradi-Hünermann-Happle (proteina che si lega all'isomerasi sterol-delta[8]-delta[7] [EBP]), una forma dominante legata al cromosoma X che colpisce esclusivamente i soggetti di sesso femminile, la condrodisplasia puntata recessiva legata al cromosoma X (che coinvolge il gene per l'arisolfatasi) e il nanismo rizomelico (trasmesso con modalità autosomica recessiva). La quasi totalità dei pazienti affetti dalla forma dominante legata al cromosoma X e il 25% circa di quelli con la forma recessiva presentano lesioni cutanee di gravità variabile (dall'eritema diffuso con desquamazione alla lieve ipercheratosi). La condrodisplasia rizomelica puntata è associata a cataratta, ipertelorismo, atrofia del nervo ottico, sproporzionata brevità della porzione prossimale degli arti, ritardo psicomotorio, deficit staturo-ponderale e spasticità. La mortalità nell'infanzia è molto elevata. Nei pazienti con condrodisplasia rizomelica si riscontrano diverse disfunzioni degli enzimi perossisomali. I soggetti affetti dalla forma dominante legata al cromosoma X presentano già alla nascita un accorciamento asimmetrico e variabile degli arti e una caratteristica eruzione ittiosiforme. Placche cheratinizzate spesse e adese, di colore giallastro, sono distribuite su tutto il corpo, con una disposizione a spirale. Le alterazioni istologiche includono un'ipercheratosi che penetra in profondità nei follicoli capillari. Tipicamente, l'eruzione si risolve nell'infanzia, ma può essere sostituita da atrofodermia follicolare o alopecia a chiazze.

Ulteriori caratteristiche, comuni a tutte le varianti, comprendono cataratta e anomalie della facies, con sella nasale e bozze frontali prominenti. Il difetto patognomonico, da cui deriva la definizione condrodisplasia puntata, consiste nella presenza di epifisi punteggiate nello scheletro cartilagineo. Questa alterazione, osservata in diversi disturbi ereditari, è spesso associata a deficit perossisomale e a disturbi della biosintesi del colesterolo, ma tende a sparire entro i 3-4 anni di età.

L'elenco delle sindromi rare responsabili di ittiosi include anche i disturbi seguenti: cheratite con ittiosi e sordità (sindrome KID, che coinvolge il gene per la connessina 26); ittiosi con alterazioni capillari (pattern a bande alla luce polarizzata) e ridotto contenuto di zolfo (tricotiodistrofia); deficit multiplo di solfatasi; malattia da deposito di lipidi neutri con ittiosi (sindrome di Chanarin-Dorfman, che coinvolge il gene CG158); e sindrome CHILD (Fig. 657-10) (emidisplasia congenita con eritrodermia ittiosiforme e deformità degli arti, gene NSDHL).

CHERATODERMIA PALMOPLANTARE. L'eccessiva ipercheratosi di palmi delle mani e piante dei piedi può costituire la manifestazione di un disturbo cutaneo congenito, di tipo focale o generalizzato, oppure è il risultato di una malattia cutanea cronica, come la psoriasi, l'eczema, la pitiriasi rubra pilare, il lupus eritematoso o la malattia di Reiter. I nomi di ciascuna sindrome derivano dalla modalità di trasmissione, dai reperti istopatologici, dai difetti biochimici o da elementi descrittivi.

Ipercheratosi palmoplantare diffusa (tipo di Unna-Thost, di Vorner). Fino a poco tempo fa, l'ipercheratosi del tipo di Unna-Thost e quella del tipo di Vorner erano considerate due entità distinte, sebbene clinicamente non differenziabili. Sul piano istologico, la diagnosi era formulata sulla base del riscontro di ipercheratosi epidermolitica, assente nel tipo di Unna-Thost e presente in quello di Vorner. Oggi si ritiene che questi due disturbi siano varianti di una stessa patologia causata da mutazioni della cheratina (geni KRT1 e 9). Questo disturbo autosomico dominante si presenta nei primi mesi di vita, con eritema a rapida progressione, che conduce alla comparsa di placche scagliose ipercheratosiche e ben delimitate su palmi delle mani (Fig. 657-11) e piante dei piedi. Le placche, i cui margini sono spesso arrossati, tendono a estendersi lungo le facce laterali di mani e piedi, nonché sulla faccia volare di polsi e talloni. È solitamente presente l'iperidrosi, mentre capelli, denti e unghie sono normali. Le forme striata (geni DSG1, DSP e KRT1) e puntata di ipercheratosi palmare e plantare costituiscono entità distinte.

Mal di Meleda (gene slurp-1). Questa rara malattia progressiva, a trasmissione autosomica recessiva, è caratterizzata da eritema e presenza di spesse scaglie su palmi, dita, piante dei piedi e superfici flessorie di polsi, ginocchia e gomiti. Possono riscontrarsi anche iperidrosi, ispessimento ungueale o coilonichia ed eczema.

Cheratodermia mutilante (Sindrome di Vohwinkel). Questa malattia progressiva, a trasmissione autosomica dominante, include ipercheratosi palmoplantare ad alveare, che risparmia gli archi; cheratosi lineare e a forma di stella di mare su dorso delle mani, delle dita, dei piedi e sulle ginocchia; costrizione anulare delle dita, che talvolta conduce all'autoamputazione. Può riscontrarsi alopecia in grado variabile. Sono state identificate due forme: la Vohwinkel con ittiosi è causata da mutazioni del gene LOR, mentre la Vohwinkel con sordità è attribuita a mutazioni della connessina 26.

Sindrome di Papillon-Lefèvre (gene della catepsina C). Questa ipercheratosi eritematosa autosomica recessiva colpisce i palmi delle mani e le piante dei piedi, ma talvolta si estende, nella tarda infanzia, alle superfici dorsali di mani e piedi, ai gomiti e alle ginocchia. La cheratodermia palmoplantare può essere diffusa, striata o puntata. La sindrome è caratterizzata da un'infiammazione periodontale che, se non trattata, conduce alla perdita dei denti entro i 4-5 anni di età.

Questa forma di cheratodermia rientra anche nel quadro di alcuni tipi di ittiosi e di displasia ectodermica. La sindrome di

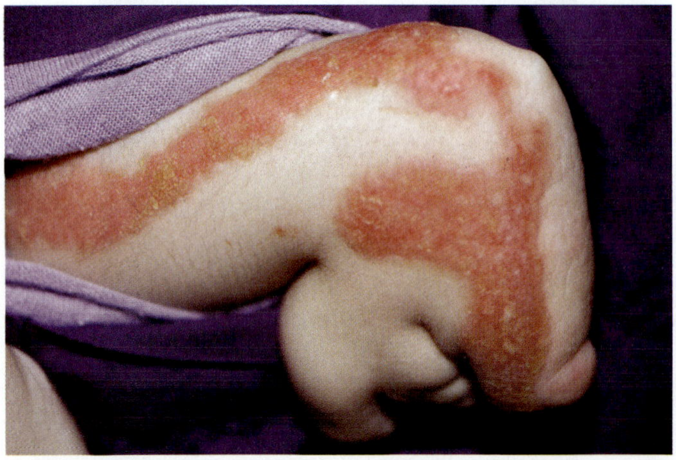

Figura 657-10. Displasia dell'arto ed eruzione ittiosiforme nella sindrome CHILD (emidisplasia congenita con eritrodermia ittiosiforme e deformità degli arti).

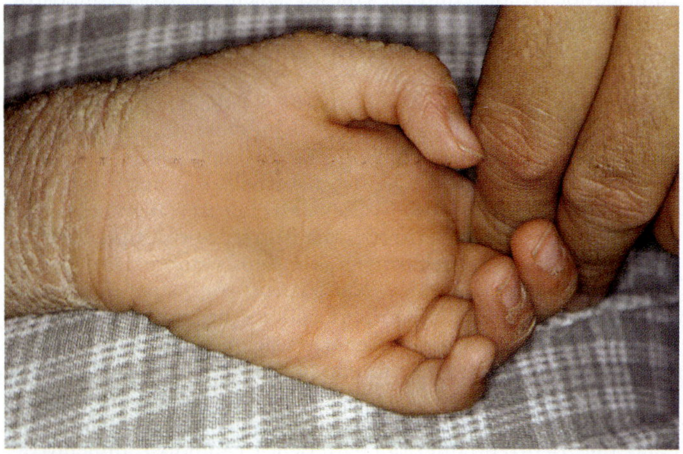

Figura 657-11. Cheratoderma palmare con alterazioni epidermolitiche visibili alla biopsia.

Richner-Hanhart è una cheratodermia autosomica recessiva responsabile di ulcere corneali, ritardo mentale progressivo e deficit della tirosina aminotrasferasi, che causa tirosinemia. La pachionichia congenita, trasmessa con modalità autosomica dominante, presenta un'espressione variabile. La forma classica di tipo 1 (sindrome di Jadassohn-Lewandowski) è dovuta a mutazioni del gene per la cheratina 16. La malattia provoca onicogrifosi, cheratoderma palmoplantare, ipercheratosi follicolare (in particolare di gomiti e ginocchia) e leucocheratosi orale. La distrofia ungueale, che costituisce la caratteristica più evidente, può essere presente già alla nascita o svilupparsi molto precocemente. Le unghie, ispessite e tubolari, presentano un sollevamento del margine libero che forma una copertura conica sopra un ammasso di detriti cheratosici subungueali. Infezioni ricorrenti del perionichio possono provocare il distacco dell'unghia. Il disturbo più costantemente presente nei pazienti con questa sindrome è la cheratordemia palmare e plantare. Caratteristiche associate includono iperidrosi di palmi delle mani e piante dei piedi, erosioni e bolle localizzate nelle stesse aree. Alcuni pazienti presentano un difetto cellulomediato selettivo nel riconoscere e processare la *Candida*. La rimozione chirurgica delle unghie e l'escissione della matrice si sono dimostrate utili in un certo numero di pazienti.

Il **trattamento** è identico in tutte le forme e prescinde dalla causa della patologia. Nei casi lievi, può essere sufficiente una terapia con emollienti. Agenti cheratolitici come l'acido salicilico, l'acido lattico e creme a base di urea sono talvolta necessari. L'assunzione orale di retinoidi costituisce il trattamento di elezione nei casi gravi, che non rispondono alla terapia topica.

DiGiovanna JJ: Ichthyosiform dermatoses: So many disorders, so little progress. *J Am Acad Dermatol* 2004;51:S31–S34.
Lane EB, McLean WH: Keratins and skin disorders. *J Pathol* 2004;204: 355–366.
McClean WH: Epithelial Genetics Group. Genetic disorders of palm skin and nail. *J Anat* 2003;202:133–141.
Richard G: Molecular genetics of the ichthyoses. *Am J Med Genet* 2004;15: 32–44.
Shwayder T: Disorders of keratinization: Diagnosis and management. *Am J Clin Dermatol* 2004;5:17–29.
Smith FJD, Irvine AD, Terron-Kwiatkowski A, et al: Loss of function mutations in the gene encoding filaggrin cause ichthyosis vulgaris. *Nat Genet* 2006;38:337–342.
Van Steensel MA: Gap junction diseases of the skin. *Am J Med Genet* 2004;15: 12–19.

Capitolo 658 ■ Malattie del derma

Joseph G. Morelli

CHELOIDE. Il cheloide è un aggregato benigno di tessuto connettivo, denso e ben delimitato, che si forma nel derma successivamente a traumi. Le lesioni, aderenti e rilevate, hanno una consistenza compatta e gommosa e assumono una colorazione rosea. Risultano sensibili o pruriginose. Le localizzazioni più frequenti sono il volto, i lobi delle orecchie (Fig. 658-1), il collo, le spalle, il tronco superiore, lo sterno e la parte inferiore delle gambe. I cheloidi sono generalmente indotti da traumi, come scottature, piercing delle orecchie, ustioni e procedure chirurgiche. Alcuni individui sembrano essere maggiormente predisposti alla formazione di cheloidi. In alcuni casi, una predisposizione familiare (a trasmissione recessiva o dominante) o la presenza di corpi estranei nelle ferite sembrano svolgere un ruolo patogenetico. I cheloidi costituiscono inoltre una rara caratteristica delle sindromi di Ehlers-Danlos, Rubinstein-Taybi e della pachidermoperiostosi. In presenza di cheloidi o cicatrici ipertrofiche, la formazione di nuovo collagene richiede tempi molto più lunghi rispetto alle lesioni che cicatrizzano normalmente. Il cheloide è composto da fibre di collagene ialinizzate, disposte a spirale e intrecciate.

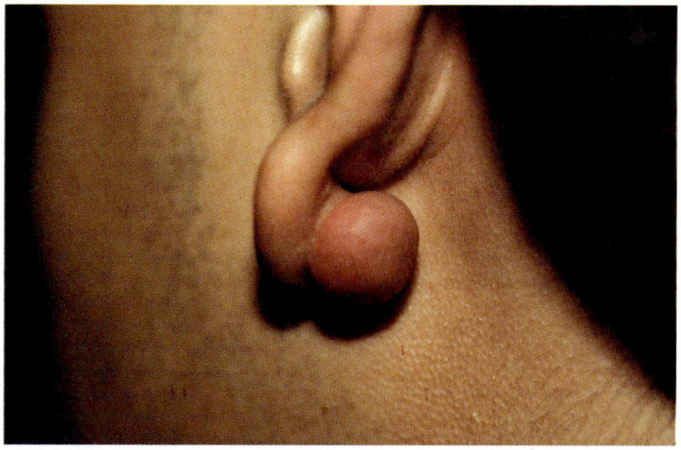

Figura 658-1. Cheloide sul lobo dell'orecchio conseguente a piercing.

È opportuno distinguere i cheloidi dalle cicatrici ipertrofiche, che restano confinate alla sede della lesione e regrediscono gradualmente con il trascorrere del tempo. Le dimensioni dei cheloidi recenti possono ridursi in seguito all'iniezione, a intervalli di 4 settimane, di una sospensione di triamcinolone (10-40 mg/mL). In alcuni casi, è necessario ricorrere a una sospensione più concentrata. I cheloidi più grandi o di vecchia data possono richiedere l'escissione chirurgica, seguita dall'iniezione intralesionale di un corticosteroide. L'escissione da sola è controindicata a causa del rischio di **recidive** nella stessa sede, tuttavia i cheloidi ai lobi delle orecchie rispondono meglio all'asportazione chirurgica. In alcuni pazienti, è utile l'applicazione topica quotidiana di un gel a base di silicone, per diverse ore al giorno e per varie settimane.

STRIAE CUTIS DISTENSAE (SMAGLIATURE). Sono costituite da sottili bande eritematose e depresse di cute atrofica, che assume infine una consistenza liscia e una colorazione argentea e opalescente. Compaiono comunemente in aree soggette a distensione, come la parte bassa della schiena (Fig. 658-2), i glutei, le cosce, il seno, l'addome e le spalle. Le cause più frequenti sono una rapida crescita, la gravidanza, l'obesità, la malattia di Cushing o prolungate terapie con corticosteroidi. La formazione di strie è comune nell'adolescenza, ma tali smagliature tendono ad attenuarsi nel tempo. Le strie presentano una notevole somiglianza con le cicatrici atrofiche.

ATROFIA INDOTTA DA CORTICOSTEROIDI. Il trattamento topico o sistemico con corticosteroidi può causare atrofia cutanea, in par-

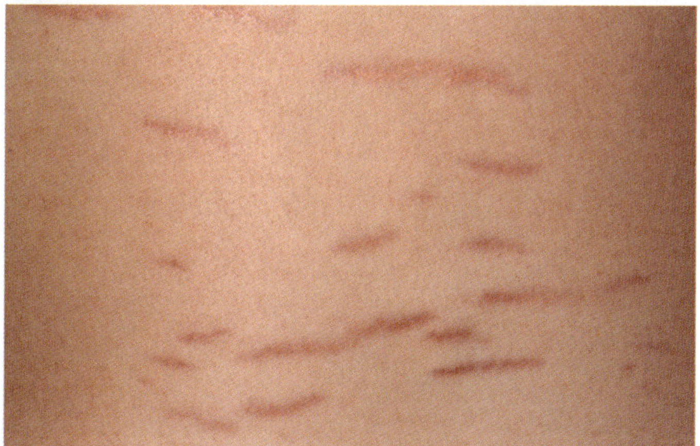

Figura 658-2. Strie sulla schiena di un adolescente.

ticolare se si applica un corticosteroide potente con bendaggio occlusivo o nelle aree intertriginose per un periodo prolungato. La cute colpita appare fragile, liscia, sottile e semitrasparente, con teleangiectasie e perdita dei solchi cutanei normali. Sul piano istopatologico, si osserva un assottigliamento dell'epidermide. Gli spazi tra il collagene e le fibre elastiche sono ridotti, determinando un derma più compatto ma sottile. Il meccanismo responsabile implica l'inibizione della sintesi di collagene di tipo I, di proteine non collagenose e del contenuto proteico totale della cute; la progressiva riduzione dei proteoglicani del tessuto dermico e di glicosaminoglicani; un'ischemia indotta dalla prolungata vasocostrizione. L'applicazione topica di retinoidi consente di rimediare alle alterazioni biochimiche indotte dagli steroidi, nel tessuto connettivale del derma dei topi privi di pelo, preservando il benefico effetto antiinfiammatorio.

GRANULOMA ANULARE. Questa comune dermatosi si verifica prevalentemente nei bambini e nella prima età adulta. Le lesioni tipiche sono papule eritematose benigne, di consistenza compatta e liscia, che si allargano gradualmente, per formare placche anulari di diversi centimetri, dotate di un bordo papulare e di un'area centrale leggermente atrofica o depigmentata. Le lesioni possono comparire in qualsiasi parte del corpo, ma le membrane mucose sono risparmiate. Le localizzazioni più frequenti includono il dorso delle mani (Fig. 658-3) e dei piedi. Le lesioni anulari sono spesso confuse con quelle della tinea corporis, a causa dei bordi rilevati, ma differiscono da queste per l'assenza di squame. Le lesioni papulari, un'altra variante, possono simulare i noduli reumatoidi, in particolare se le papule sono raggruppate su dita e gomiti. La forma papulare disseminata, provocata talvolta dalla luce, è rara nei bambini. Il granuloma anulare sottocutaneo, particolarmente comune in età pediatrica, tende a comparire su cuoio capelluto e arti, soprattutto nell'area pretibiale. Le lesioni consistono in noduli compatti, generalmente non dolenti, dello stesso colore della cute. Il granuloma anulare perforante è caratterizzato dallo sviluppo di un centro giallastro in alcune delle lesioni papulari, conseguenza dell'eliminazione transepidermica del collagene alterato.

Talvolta la diagnosi richiede una biopsia. Le lesioni consistono in granulomi con un'area centrale di collagene necrotico, depositi di mucina, un infiltrato periferico a palizzata di linfociti, istiociti e corpi estranei cellulari giganti. Il quadro ricorda quello della necrobiosi lipoidea e dei noduli reumatici, ma sottili differenze istologiche consentono solitamente la formulazione della diagnosi corretta. La causa del granuloma anulare è sconosciuta. I bambini colpiti appaiono solitamente sani. Alcuni casi di granuloma anulare, in particolare la forma generalizzata, sono stati associati al **diabete mellito**. L'eruzione persiste per mesi o anni, ma la risoluzione spontanea e priva di sequele è comune e, nel 75% dei pazienti, avviene entro due anni. L'applicazione topica di un potente preparato corticosteroide o l'iniezione intralesionale di un corticosteroide può favorire la regressione, ma è possibile optare per il non intervento.

NECROBIOSI LIPOIDEA. Questo raro disturbo si presenta con papule eritematose, che evolvono in placche sclerotiche irregolari e ben delimitate, di colorazione giallastra, con teleangiectasie centrali e margine violaceo. Desquamazione, formazione di croste e ulcerazione sono frequenti. Le lesioni compaiono più comunemente in area pretibiale (Fig, 658-4) e tendono a espandersi nel corso degli anni, ma possono riscontrarsi lunghi periodi di quiescenza o la completa guarigione con cicatrizzazione.

Aree scarsamente definite di collagene necrotico si osservano in tutto il derma, principalmente nella parte bassa, associate a depositi di mucina. Un infiltrato granulomatoso linfoistiocitico a palizzata circonda le aree di collagene disordinato e necrobiotico. Alcune lesioni appaiono maggiormente granulomatose, con limitata necrobiosi del collagene. La diagnosi differenziale clinica è con gli xantomi, la morfea, il granuloma anulare, l'eritema nodoso e il mixedema pretibiale. Una percentuale compresa tra il 50 e il 75% dei pazienti presenta **diabete mellito.** La necrobiosi lipoidea si verifica nello 0,3% della totalità dei pazienti diabetici. Le lesioni persistono malgrado l'adeguato controllo del diabete, ma migliorano leggermente con l'applicazione topica di steroidi potenti o con l'iniezione locale di un corticosteroide.

LICHEN SCLEROSO. Si presenta inizialmente con papule indurite e brillanti, color avorio, spesso circondate da un anello violaceo. La superficie mostra una dilazione degli orifizi dei dotti pilosebacei o sudoripari, ostruiti da tappi di cheratina giallastri o marroni. La coalescenza delle papule conduce alla formazione di placche irregolari di dimensioni variabili, che possono sviluppare bolle emorragiche ai margini. Negli stadi più avanzati, l'atrofia causa la formazione di placche depresse, dalla superficie raggrinzita. Questo disturbo, più frequente nelle ragazze, si localizza preferibilmente in sede vulvare (Fig. 658-5), perianale e perineale. Un coinvolgimento esteso può provocare una placca atrofica e sclerotica, con forma a clessidra, con conseguente contrazione delle labbra e stenosi dell'introito. In circa il 20% delle pazienti, perdite vaginali precedono le lesioni vulvari. Nei ragazzi, prepuzio e glande risultano spesso coinvolti, solitamente in associazione a fimosi; la maggior parte dei maschi affetti non è stata circoncisa alla nascita. Altre sedi comunemente coinvolte sono la parte superiore del tronco, il collo, le ascelle, le superfici flessorie dei polsi e le aree intorno all'ombelico e agli occhi. Il prurito può essere intenso.

Nei bambini, il disordine è frequentemente confuso con la morfea focale (vedi Capitolo 159), con la quale può coesistere. Se presente nell'area genitale, rischia di essere erroneamente attribuito ad

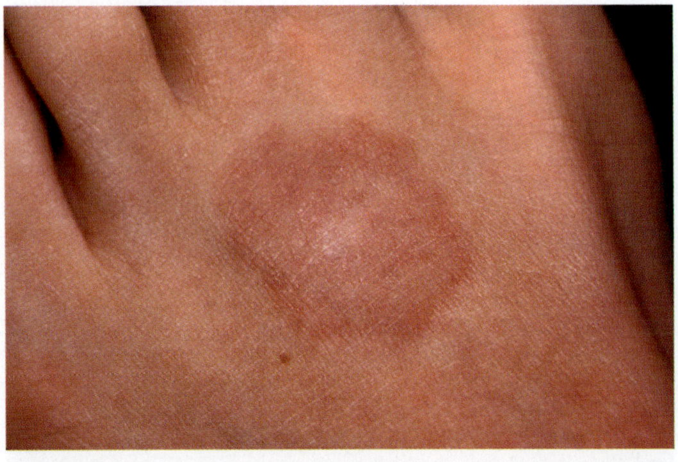

Figura 658-3. Lesione anulare con bordi papulari rilevati e depressione centrale, caratteristica del granuloma anulare.

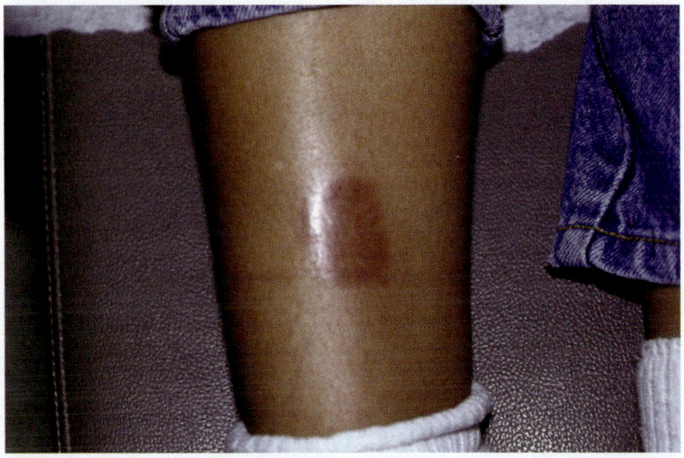

Figura 658-4. Placca sclerotica giallastra di necrobiosi lipoidea sullo stinco.

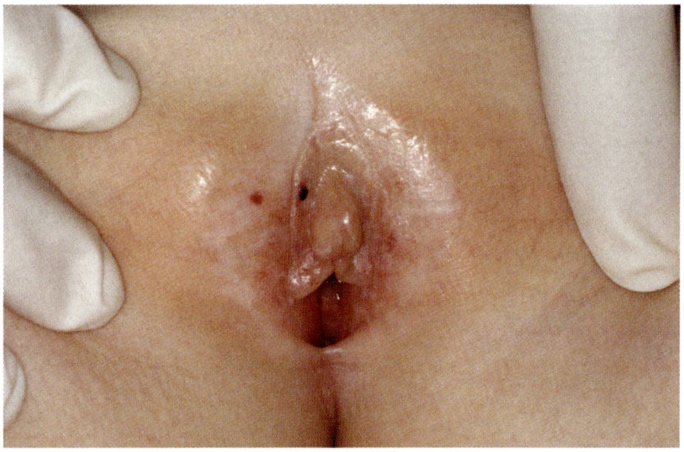

Figura 658-5. Placca perivaginale emorragica color avorio.

abuso sessuale. La biopsia assume un valore diagnostico, rivelando l'ipercheratosi con occlusione follicolare, la degenerazione idropica delle cellule basali, un infiltrato linfocitico dermico a banda, collagene omogeneizzato e assottigliamento delle fibre elastiche nel derma superiore. Possono svilupparsi leucoplachia e carcinoma squamocellulare. L'applicazione locale di **corticosteroidi topici potenti** allevia il prurito e consente la risoluzione delle lesioni, incluse quelle dell'area genitale. Terapie alternative prevedono l'utilizzo di tacrolimus e pimecrolimus topici.

SCLEREDEMA (SCLEREDEMA ADULTORUM, SCLEREDEMA DI BUSCHKE). Circa il 30% dei casi di scleredema compare prima dei 10 anni di età. L'esordio è improvviso, con grave edema localizzato al volto e al collo, che si diffonde rapidamente, coinvolgendo il torace e le braccia con una distribuzione "a maglia"; addome e gambe sono solitamente risparmiate. Il volto assume un aspetto simile a quello di una statua di cera o di una maschera. Le aree interessate risultano dure e legnose al tatto, non mostrano il segno della fovea dopo compressione e non sono nettamente demarcate da cute sana. La cute sovrastante mantiene un colorito normale e non appare atrofica. Il coinvolgimento sistemico, che è raro, prevede ispessimento della lingua, disartria, disfagia, limitazione dei movimenti oculari e articolari, oltre che effusioni pleuriche, pericardiche e peritoneali. Si possono osservare anche anomalie elettrocardiografiche.

Nel 65-90% dei casi, la malattia segue di qualche giorno o settimana un'infezione, come tonsillite, faringite, influenza, scarlattina, morbillo, parotite epidemica, impetigine o cellulite. La maggior parte dei casi fa seguito a un'infezione streptococcica. L'esordio può essere anticipato dai seguenti prodromi: febbre, artralgia, mialgia e malessere. L'esordio nei pazienti diabetici può risultare insidioso. I reperti di laboratorio non sono di alcun aiuto. Tuttavia, alcuni casi sono associati a paraproteinemia dell'immunoglobulina (Ig)G o IgA. La biopsia cutanea mostra un aumento dello spessore del derma, secondario all'edema e all'omogeneizzazione dei fasci di collagene, separati da ampi spazi interfibrosi. Colorazioni particolari contribuiscono all'identificazione di aumenti dei mucopolisaccaridi nel derma.

La fase attiva della malattia persiste per 2-8 settimane; la risoluzione completa e spontanea si verifica solitamente entro 6 mesi-2 anni. La ricorrenza degli attacchi è insolita. Questa patologia deve essere differenziata da sclerodermia, morfea, mixedema, trichinosi, dermatomiosite, sclerema neonatorum e necrosi adipose sottocutanee. Non è disponibile alcuna terapia specifica.

PROTEINOSI LIPOIDE (MALATTIA DI URBACH-WIETHE, IALINOSI CUTANEA E MUCOSA) [GENE ECM-1]. Questo disordine a trasmissione autosomica recessiva consiste nell'infiltrazione di materiale ialino nella cute, nella cavità orale, nella laringe e negli organi interni. Nella prima infanzia, il sintomo notato più precocemente è spesso la raucedine. Le lesioni cutanee esordiscono in età infantile e consistono in papule giallastre e noduli, che tendono a confluire in placche localizzate su volto, avambraccio, collo, genitali, dorso delle dita e cuoio capelluto, dove causano alopecia a chiazze. Depositi simili si riscontrano anche su labbra, superficie inferiore della lingua, fauci, ugola, epiglottide e corde vocali. La lingua è ingrandita e risulta compatta alla palpazione. Il paziente può essere incapace di protrudere la lingua. La manifestazione clinica più caratteristica è la presenza di noduli traslucidi lungo i margini della palpebra, che ne causano l'ispessimento. Cicatrici simili vaiolose possono comparire sul volto. Nei punti di frizione, come gomiti e ginocchia, si riscontrano noduli ipercheratosici e ipertrofici. I palmi delle mani possono apparire diffusamente ispessiti. La malattia progredisce fino alla prima età adulta, ma la prognosi è buona. Il coinvolgimento della laringe, in particolare nell'infanzia, può causare una compromissione respiratoria, che richiede la tracheotomia. Disturbi associati includono anomalie dentarie, epilessia e parotite ricorrente, conseguenza delle infiltrazioni del dotto di Stensen. Virtualmente ogni organo può essere coinvolto. Non è disponibile alcun trattamento specifico.

Sul piano istologico, si osservano tipicamente dilatazione dei vasi sanguigni del derma e infiltrazione di materiale ialino eosinofilo lungo le pareti capillari e intorno alle ghiandole sudoripare. La diffusa presenza di materiale ialino in fasci omogenei nel derma superiore causa l'ispessimento del derma. Gli infiltrati contengono sia lipidi sia mucopolisaccaridi. Un'ossificazione simmetrica nella regione temporale mediale, laterale alla sella turcica, è patognomonica se osservata alla radiografia, ma non è sempre presente. Il difetto biochimico è localizzato nella proteina-1 della matrice extracellulare.

ATROFIA MACULARE (ANETODERMIA). L'anetodermia è caratterizzata da aree circoscritte di cute lassa, con perdita di sostanza dermica. Questo disturbo può non essere associato ad alcuna malattia sottostante (atrofia maculare primaria), oppure si sviluppa in seguito a un processo infiammatorio cutaneo (atrofia maculare secondaria), come sifilide, lupus eritematoso, acne, varicella, lebbra, orticaria pigmentosa o follicolite da *Staphylococcus epidermidis*. Le dimensioni delle lesioni variano da 0,5 a 1 cm di diametro e, se infiammatorie, possono risultane inizialmente eritematose. Successivamente divengono più sottili, raggrinzite, ipopigmentate oppure bianco-bluastre. Le lesioni tendono a protrudere ma, alla palpazione, rientrano facilmente nel tessuto sottocutaneo, a causa dell'atrofia dermica. Le localizzazioni più frequenti includono il tronco, le cosce, la parte superiore delle braccia e, meno comunemente, il collo e il volto. Le lesioni restano invariate tutta la vita e nuove lesioni spesso continuano a svilupparsi per anni. Non è disponibile alcun trattamento efficace.

All'esame istopatologico, tutte le forme di atrofia maculare mostrano una perdita focale di tessuto elastico, ma quest'alterazione è identificabile soltanto utilizzando colorazioni particolari. L'elastolisi può essere dovuta al rilascio di elastasi dalle cellule infiammatorie (come i macrofagi), in contatto con le fibre elastiche. La diagnosi differenziale è con morfea, lichen scleroso, ipoplasia dermica focale, cicatrici atrofiche o lesioni nello stadio finale della dermatosi bollosa cronica.

CUTE LASSA (DERMATOMEGALIA, ELASTOLISI GENERALIZZATA). La cute lassa costituisce un gruppo eterogeneo di disordini, di tipo autosomico recessivo (gene per la fibulina 5), autosomico dominante (geni per l'elastina e la fibulina 5) o acquisito. La cute lassa acquisita può svilupparsi in seguito a una malattia febbrile o a patologie infiammatorie cutanee, come il lupus eritematoso o l'eritema multiforme, l'amiloidosi, l'orticaria, l'angioedema e le reazioni di ipersensibilità alla penicillina, o in neonati le cui madri assumevano penicillina.

Manifestazioni cliniche. Possono riscontrarsi ampie pieghe di tessuto lasso, oppure le alterazioni, analoghe all'anetoderma, risultano lievi e di estensione limitata. I pazienti con cute lassa severa presentano una facies tipica: cute rugosa e prematuramente invecchiata; guance cadenti, che conferiscono un aspetto

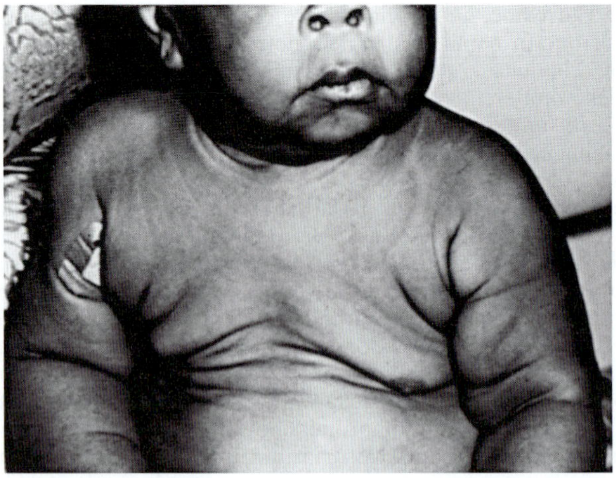

Figura 658-6. Pieghe cutanee pendule in un bambino con cute lassa. Si osservino il labbro superiore allungato e il naso rivolto verso l'alto.

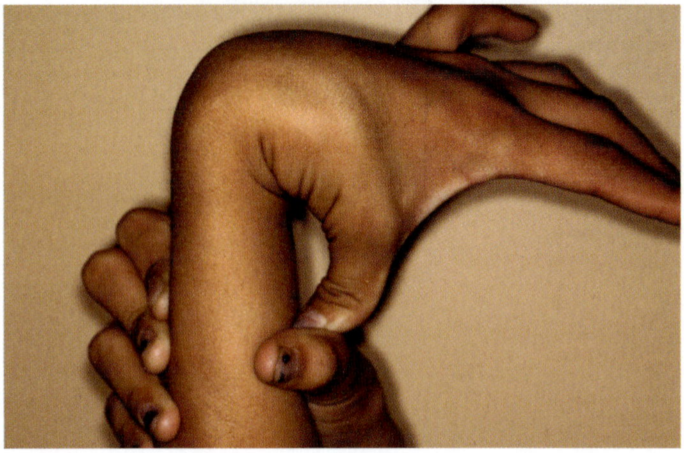

Figura 658-7. Iperestensibilità articolare nella sindrome di Ehlers-Danlos classica.

"da mastino" (Fig. 658-6); naso a uncino con narici invertite; columella breve; labbro superiore allungato; palpebre inferiori rovesciate. La cute è lassa su tutta la superficie corporea e può sembrare un vestito fuori misura. A differenza della sindrome di Ehlers-Danlos, **non sono presenti** l'iperelasticità e ipermobilità delle articolazioni. Il pianto dei neonati affetti può essere rauco, probabilmente a causa della lassità delle corde vocali. L'elasticità della cute è normale. Sul piano istologico, il tessuto elastico del derma risulta ridotto, con frammentazione, distensione e raggruppamento delle fibre elastiche.

La forma dominante della cute lassa può svilupparsi a qualsiasi età; generalmente è benigna e influisce soprattutto sul piano estetico. Se presente fin dall'infanzia, può essere associata a ritardo della crescita intrauterina, lassità legamentosa e ritardo nella chiusura delle fontanelle. Talvolta si riscontrano anche enfisema polmonare e lievi manifestazioni cardiovascolari. Al contrario, i pazienti con la più comune forma recessiva della malattia sono soggetti a gravi complicanze, come ernie multiple, prolasso rettale, atonia diaframmatica, diverticoli dei tratti gastrointestinale e genitourinario, cor polmonare, enfisema, pneumotorace, stenosi periferica dell'arteria polmonare e dilatazione aortica. Le caratteristiche facciali tipiche includono fessure palpebrali rivolte verso il basso, naso ampio e schiacciato, orecchie grandi. Sono comuni anche le anomalie scheletriche, le carie dentali, il ritardo di crescita e sviluppo. L'aspettativa di vita di questi pazienti risulta ridotta.

Le alterazioni cutanee tipiche della cute lassa si osservano anche in associazione a molte altre patologie, come la sindrome di Debarsy, la sindrome di Lenz-Majewski, il nanismo iperostosico, la sindrome SCARF (anomalie scheletriche, craniostenosi, cute lassa, ambiguità genitale, ritardo psicomotorio e dimorfismi facciali), la sindrome della pelle rugosa e la sindrome di Costello.

SINDROME DI EHLERS-DANLOS (EDS). Questo gruppo geneticamente eterogeneo di disordini del tessuto connettivo colpisce bambini che alla nascita appaiono normali, ma che in seguito sviluppano iperelasticità cutanea, fragilità della cute e dei vasi sanguigni, ritardo di cicatrizzazione delle ferite e ipermobilità articolare (Fig. 658-7). Il difetto di base è un deficit quantitativo del collagene fibrillare. Si distinguono 6 forme cliniche della sindrome.

Forma classica (geni COL5a1, COL5a2, COL1a1) [In precedenza: EDS di tipo I-grave, EDS di tipo II-mite]. Questo disordine autosomico dominante è caratterizzato da nascita prematura, dovuta a rottura delle membrane, iperelasticità e fragilità cutanea, facilità alle ecchimosi, ipermobilità articolare grave e generalizzata, scoliosi e prolasso della valvola mitralica. Lacerazioni minime rischiano di causare ferite aperte, che lasciano cicatrici ampie, atrofiche e papiracee. Ulteriori manifestazioni cutanee sono pseudotumori molluscoidi nei punti di pressione, secondari all'accumulo di tessuto connettivo. L'aspettativa di vita non risulta ridotta.

Forma ipermobile (COL3A1) [In precedenza: EDS di tipo III]. Questo disordine a trasmissione autosomica dominante si presenta con grave ipermobilità articolare e manifestazioni cutanee minime. Il dolore muscoloscheletrico è comune e l'osteoartrite può svilupparsi precocemente.

Forma vascolare (COL3A1) [In precedenza: EDS di tipo IV-arteriosa o ecchimotica]. Questo disordine autosomico dominante causa un pronunciato assottigliamento del derma, con conseguente prominenza della rete venosa sottostante. La cute presenta un'iperestensibilità minima, mentre le articolazioni non risultano ipermobili (con qualche eccezione durante l'infanzia). La morbilità e la riduzione dell'aspettativa di vita sono una conseguenza dei seguenti fattori: prematurità, ecchimosi estese provocate da traumi, elevata incidenza di cheloidi, rotture della parete intestinale e in particolare del colon, rotture uterine durante la gravidanza, rotture dei grandi vasi, aneurisma aortico dissecante e ictus. Si raccomanda ai pazienti di evitare la gravidanza, i traumi cutanei e le attività che determinano un aumento della pressione intracranica in seguito alla manovra di Valsalva (come suonare la tromba).

Cifoscoliosi (deficit di lisil idrossilasi [gene PLOD]) [In precedenza: EDS di tipo VI]. I pazienti con questa forma autosomica recessiva presentano iperestensibilità articolare, ipotonia, cifoscoliosi, fragilità corneale, cheratocono, iperelasticità cutanea e fragilità ossea. Il dosaggio dell'attività della lisil idrossilasi negli amniociti consente di formulare la diagnosi prenatale. L'individuazione di una riduzione dell'attività della lisil idrossilasi in colture di fibroblasti cutanei conferma la diagnosi.

Forma tipo artrocalasia (COLA1A-tipo A, COL1A2-tipo B) [In precedenza: EDS tipo VII A e B-artrocalasia multipla congenita]. Il tipo A è un disturbo autosomico dominante, caratterizzato da bassa statura, marcata iperestensibilità articolare e tendenza alla lussazione, moderata iperelasticità e tendenza alle contusioni. Il tipo B è un disturbo autosomico dominante che prevede iperelasticità cutanea e marcata ipermobilità articolare.

Forma tipo dermatosparassi (tipo 1 collageno N-peptidasi) [In precedenza: EDS tipo VII C]. Questa malattia autosomica recessiva include rottura prematura delle membrane, ritardo nella chiusura delle fontanelle, fragilità e lassità cutanea, tendenza alle contusioni, ritardo di crescita, arti corti, ernia ombelicale e una facies caratteristica con micrognatia, mascelle prominenti e palpebre gonfie.

Diagnosi differenziale. La sindrome di Ehlers-Danlos può essere confusa con la cute lassa, sebbene le due malattie presentino caratteristiche molto diverse. I pazienti con cute lassa hanno pieghe cutanee di tessuto ridondante, mentre nella sindrome di Ehlers-Danlos la cute risulta iperestensibile e ritorna in sede quando viene stirata. A causa della marcata fragilità capillare, nella sindrome di Ehlers-Danlos traumi di lieve entità portano a ecchimosi, emorragie, lenta cicatrizzazione e formazione di cicatrici atrofiche e papiracee, in particolare su fronte, parte inferiore delle gambe e punti di pressione. In questi pazienti, le procedure chirurgiche sono rischiose e la deiscenza delle ferite è comune.

PSEUDOXANTOMA ELASTICO. Questo disturbo primario del tessuto elastico presenta 4 forme, con considerevole sovrapposizione tra i diversi tipi.

Manifestazioni cliniche. Il **tipo I autosomico dominante** (gene ADCC6) presenta un'estesa compromissione delle aree flessorie, grave malattia retinica che conduce alla cecità e disfunzione dell'arteria coronaria. Il **tipo I autosomico recessivo** (gene ADCC6) comprende la patologia delle aree flessorie cutanee e una lieve malattia retinica. Possono essere presenti anche ipertensione e sanguinamento gastrointestinale. Il **tipo II autosomico dominante** è generalmente benigno e caratterizzato primariamente dalle alterazioni cutanee. I disturbi oculari sono lievi e la malattia vascolare è rara. Talvolta si riscontra iperestensibilità articolare, sclera blu e palato ad arco. Il **tipo II autosomico recessivo** presenta grave lassità cutanea, in assenza di segni di coinvolgimento sistemico.

L'esordio delle manifestazioni cutanee avviene solitamente nell'infanzia, ma le alterazioni causate dalle lesioni precoci sono spesso lievi e difficili da riconoscere. Papule giallastre asintomatiche, a disposizione lineare o reticolata, conferiscono alla cute un aspetto a "**pelle di pollo**". Tali lesioni caratteristiche, del diametro di 1-2 mm, possono confluire in placche. Le localizzazioni più comuni sono l'area flessoria del collo (Fig. 658-8), le pieghe ascellari e inguinali, l'ombelico, le cosce, le fosse antecubitale e poplitea. Il volto è solitamente risparmiato. Con l'aggravarsi delle lesioni, la cute acquisisce una consistenza vellutata e perde progressivamente elasticità. Le lesioni delle membrane mucose coinvolgono le labbra, la cavità buccale, il retto e la vagina. Si riscontrano inoltre alterazioni del tessuto connettivo della tonaca media e intima dei vasi sanguigni, della membrana di Bruch della retina, di endocardio e pericardio. Tali anomalie possono provocare disturbi visivi, strie angioidi della retina, claudicazione intermittente, occlusione cerebrale e coronarica, ipertensione ed emorragie del tratto gastrointestinale, dell'utero o delle superfici mucose. Nelle donne affette aumenta il rischio di aborto nel primo trimestre. Il coinvolgimento arterioso solitamente subentra in età adulta, ma la claudicazione e l'angina possono riscontrarsi già nella prima infanzia. Non è disponibile alcun trattamento efficace. La terapia laser può contribuire alla prevenzione dell'emorragia retinica.

Patologia e patogenesi. L'esame istopatologico rivela la presenza di fibre elastiche raggruppate, frammentate e gonfie nel terzo inferiore e intermedio del derma, che si colorano positivamente per il calcio. In prossimità delle fibre elastiche alterate, il collagene è presente in quantità ridotta e le sue fibre appaiono scisse. L'anomala calcificazione delle fibre elastiche della lamina interna delle arterie è responsabile di un restringimento del lume dei vasi sanguigni.

ELASTOSI PERFORANTE SERPIGINOSA. Questo insolito disordine cutaneo è caratterizzato da papule cheratosiche di 1-3 mm, di consistenza compatta e dello stesso colore della cute, che tendono a raggrupparsi in anelli o archi nell'area posterolaterale del collo e sugli arti (Fig. 658-9). Più raramente, compaiono anche su volto e tronco. L'esordio avviene solitamente nell'infanzia o nell'adolescenza. La papula consiste in un'area circoscritta di iperplasia epidermica, che comunica con il derma sottostante mediante uno stretto canale. Materiale elastosico estrude dal canale. Nel derma superiore, e in particolare nelle papille, si nota un rilevante aumento della quantità e delle dimensioni delle fibre elastiche. L'anomalia primaria è probabilmente un difetto dell'elastina, che provoca una risposta cellulare responsabile dell'eliminazione del tessuto elastico anomalo. In circa il 30% dei casi, la malattia è associata a osteogenesi imperfetta, sindrome di Marfan, pseudoxantoma elastico, sindrome di Ehlers-Danlos, sindrome di Rothmund-Thomson e sindrome di Down. Anche la terapia con penicillamina può causare questa patologia. La diagnosi differenziale è con tinea corporis, granuloma anulare perforante, collagenosi reattiva perforante, lichen planus, dermatite serpiginosa e porocheratosi di Mibelli. Non è disponibile alcun trattamento efficace, ma le lesioni sono asintomatiche e scompaiono spontaneamente.

COLLAGENOSI PERFORANTE REATTIVA. Questa malattia si presenta solitamente nella prima infanzia, con piccole papule sulle aree dorsali di mani a avambracci, gomiti, ginocchia e, talvolta, viso e tronco. Il disturbo è spesso familiare ed ereditabile con modalità autosomica recessiva. Durante un periodo di diverse settimane, le papule aumentano di dimensioni, fino a 5-10 mm, divengono ombelicate e sviluppano un tappo centrale di cheratina (Fig. 658-10). Le lesioni isolate si risolvono spontaneamente nell'arco di 2-4 mesi, lasciando una macula o cicatrice ipopigmentata. Tuttavia, le lesioni possono recidivare in gruppi, andare incontro al fenomeno di Koebner o riformarsi in risposta a basse temperature e traumi superficiali, come abrasioni, punture di insetti e acne. Il collagene del derma papillare è contenuto all'interno di una perforazione a forma di tazza dell'epidermide. Il cratere centrale contiene cellule infiammatorie picnotiche e detriti di cheratina. Il processo sembra il risultato dell'eliminazione transepidermica del collagene alterato. L'applicazione topica di acido retinoico può ridurre il numero delle lesioni.

XANTOMI (VEDI CAPITOLO 86).

MALATTIA DI FABRY (VEDI CAPITOLO 86).

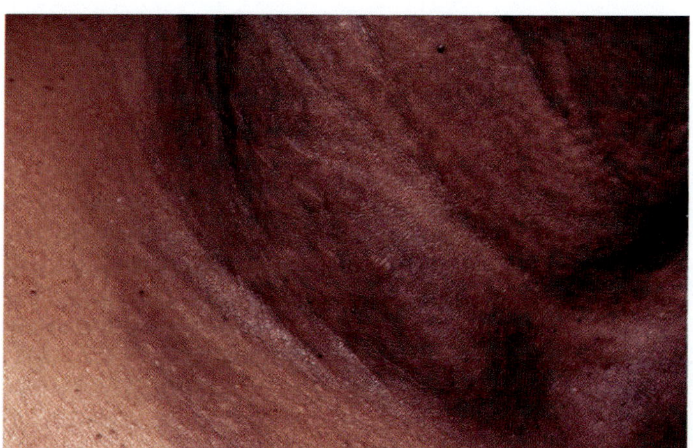

Figura 658-8. Placca confluente di cute zigrinata nello pseudoxantoma elastico.

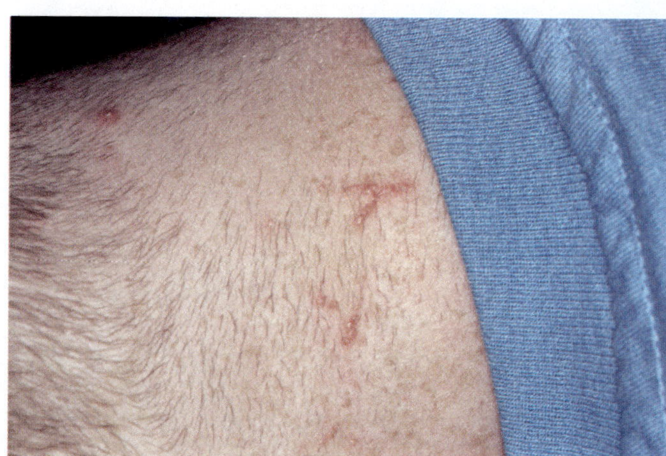

Figura 658-9. Papula cheratosica arcuata nell'elastosi perforante serpiginosa.

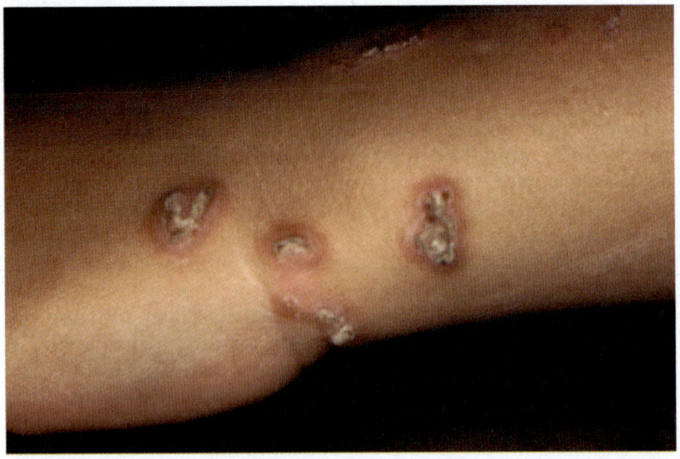

Figura. 658-10. Papule ipercheratosiche nella collagenosi reattiva perforante.

MUCOPOLISACCARIDOSI (VEDI ANCHE CAPITOLO 88). In molti di questi disturbi, gli aspetti caratteristici, ma non specifici, sono dati da cute spessa, ruvida e poco elastica, in particolare agli arti, e da irsutismo generalizzato. Nelle sindromi di Scheie e Morquio si osservano teleangiectasie su volto, avambracci, tronco e gambe. In alcuni pazienti con sindrome di Hunter si riscontrano papule o noduli color avorio, di consistenza compatta e rugosi in superficie, raggruppati in placche simmetriche sulla parte superiore del tronco (Fig. 658-11), di braccia e cosce. Solitamente queste insolite lesioni esordiscono nella prima decade di vita e in alcuni casi scompaiono spontaneamente.

MASTOCITOSI. Il termine mastocitosi include un'ampia gamma di disturbi di gravità variabile, da noduli cutanei isolati a diffusa infiltrazione della cute con coinvolgimento sistemico (Tab. 658-1). Tutti i disturbi sono caratterizzati da aggregati di mastociti nel derma. Il fattore di crescita dei mastociti, secreto dai cheratinociti, stimola la proliferazione di tali cellule e incrementa la produzione di melanina da parte dei melanociti. La mastocitosi può essere dovuta all'alterazione del metabolismo cutaneo del fattore di crescita dei mastociti, dunque è probabile che il disturbo abbia una natura iperplastica piuttosto che neoplastica.

Manifestazioni cliniche. I bambini colpiti dalla malattia lamentano un intenso prurito. I segni sistemici del rilascio di istamina, come ipotensione, sincope, mal di testa, arrossamenti episodici, tachicardia, asma, coliche e diarrea si presentano con maggiore frequenza nelle forme più gravi di mastocitosi. L'arrossamento è di gran lunga il sintomo più comune. Le manifestazioni locali e sistemiche della malattia sono causate, almeno in parte, dal rilascio di istamina ed eparina da parte dei granuli dei mastociti. Benché l'eparina sia presente in quantità significativa nei mastociti, i disturbi della coagulazione sono rari. La prostaglandina D_2 o i suoi metaboliti sembrano esacerbare l'arrossamento. I livelli sierici di triptasi sono spesso elevati.

I mastocitomi sono lesioni solitarie di 1-5 cm di diametro; possono essere presenti dalla nascita o comparire nella prima infanzia, in qualunque parte del corpo. Inizialmente le lesioni si possono presentare come bolle o pomfi ricorrenti ed evanescenti che talvolta confluiscono in placche infiltrate gommose, di colore giallastro, rosato o marrone (Fig. 658-12). La superficie acquisisce una consistenza a pelle d'arancia e appare iperpigmentata. Lo sfregamento o il trauma dei noduli possono causare un rigonfiamento della lesione od orticazione (segno di Darier), conseguenza del rilascio locale di istamina; in rari casi, si evidenziano segni sistemici del rilascio di istamina. Agenti farmacologici possono esacerbare i sintomi (Tab. 658-2). La **diagnosi differenziale** include impetigine bollosa ricorrente, nevi e xantogranuloma giovanile. I mastocitomi regrediscono spontaneamente nella prima infanzia. Per attenuare i sintomi, le lesioni più gravi possono essere trattate con steroidi topici superpotenti. In rari casi, si sviluppano lesioni multiple.

TABELLA 658-1. Classificazione delle mastocitosi*

MASTOCITOSI CUTANEE
1. Orticaria pigmentosa
Forma infantile classica
Forma cronica, con mutazioni SCF
2. Mastocitosi cutanea diffusa
3. Mastocitoma cutaneo
MASTOCITOSI SISTEMICHE (IN ASSENZA DI MALATTIA DI AHNMD O LEUCEMIA A MASTOCITI)
1. Mastocitosi sistemica indolente
2. Mastocitosi sistemica subacuta
MASTOCITOSI SISTEMICHE CON AHNMD
1. Sindrome mieloproliferativa
2. Sindrome mielodisplasica
3. Leucemia mieloide acuta
4. Linfoma non Hodgkin
MASTOCITOSI SISTEMICHE AGGRESSIVE
LEUCEMIA A MASTOCITI
SARCOMA A MASTOCITI
MASTOCITOMA EXTRACUTANEO

*Classificazione adottata dall'Organizzazione Mondiale della Sanità.
AHNMD, disturbo ematologico non da mastociti
Adattata da Carter MC, Metcalfe DD: Paediatric mastocytosis. *Arch Dis Child* 2002;86:315-319.

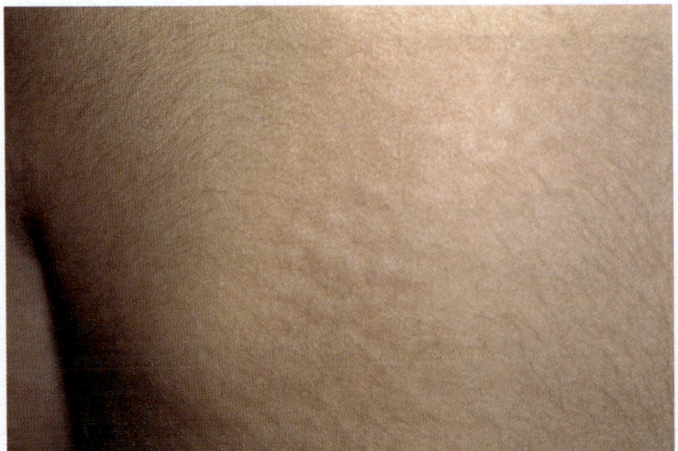

Figura 658-11. Papule color avorio localizzate sulla parte alta della schiena nella sindrome di Hunter.

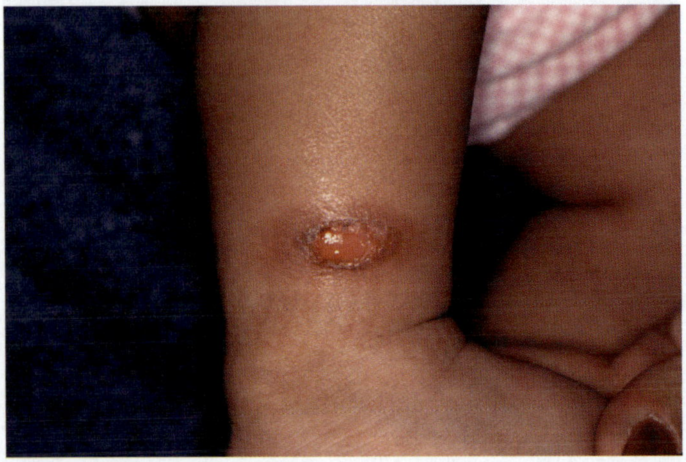

Figura 658-12. Mastocitoma isolato parzialmente bolloso.

TABELLA 658-2. Agenti farmacologici e stimoli fisici che possono esacerbare il rilascio del mediatore dei mastociti nei pazienti con mastocitosi

STIMOLI IMMUNOLOGICI
Veleno di insetti (IgE mediato)
Anafilatossine derivate dal complemento
Peptidi biologici (sostanza P, somatostatina)
Polimeri (dextran)
STIMOLI NON IMMUNOLOGICI
Stimoli fisici (temperature estreme, frizione, luce solare)
Farmaci
Acido acetilsalicilico e analgesici non steroidei*
Tiamina
Ketorolac trometamina
Alcol
Narcotici (codeina, morfina)*
Metodi di contrasto radiografici (contenenti iodina)

*Problematica in meno del 10% dei pazienti.
Da Carter MC, Metcalfe DD: Paediatric mastocytosis. *Arch Dis Child* 2002;86:315-319.

L'**orticaria pigmentosa** è la forma più comune di mastocitosi; ne esistono due tipi. Nell'orticaria pigmentosa infantile, le lesioni sono presenti dalla nascita, ma più frequentemente compaiono a gruppi nei primi mesi, o entro i due anni. Dopo i 3-4 anni, è raro che insorgano nuove lesioni. In alcuni casi, le lesioni precoci bollose o orticanti recedono, per poi recidivare nella stessa sede, trasformandosi infine in lesioni fisse e iperpigmentate. In altri casi, le lesioni iniziali risultano iperpigmentate. Solitamente la vescicazione si interrompe entro i 2 anni di età. Le singole lesioni sono di tipo maculare, papulare o nodulare e hanno dimensioni variabili da qualche millimetro a diversi centimetri; presentano bordi scarsamente definiti (Fig. 658-13) e assumono una colorazione giallastra o marrone. Le lesioni nodulari più ampie hanno una caratteristica consistenza a buccia d'arancia. Spesso a distribuzione simmetrica, le lesioni dell'orticaria pigmentosa possono essere rade o numerose. Le regioni palmare e plantare, il viso e le membrane mucose sono talvolta risparmiate. Grattandosi, il paziente provoca la rapida comparsa di eritema e vescicazione; anche il dermografismo della cute normale è comune. Il secondo tipo di orticaria pigmentosa può esordire in qualsiasi momento dall'infanzia all'età adulta. Questa forma, associata a mutazioni del fattore delle cellule staminali, non si risolve e nuove lesioni continuano a svilupparsi per tutto l'arco di vita. I pazienti rischiano di sviluppare un coinvolgimento sistemico.

La diagnosi differenziale è con eruzioni da farmaci, degenerazioni pigmentose post infiammatorie, xantogranuloma giovanile, nevi pigmentati, efelidi, xantomi, orticaria cronica, punture di insetti e impetigine bollosa.

Prognosi. In tutti i pazienti affetti dalla forma infantile classica di orticaria pigmentosa si assiste alla remissione spontanea e l'incidenza di coinvolgimento sistemico è molto ridotta. Se le lesioni continuano a svilupparsi oltre i 4 anni di età, il paziente è affetto dalla forma cronica della malattia, con mutazione del fattore delle cellule staminali e maggior rischio di coinvolgimento sistemico.

MASTOCITOSI CUTANEA DIFFUSA. Questa variante è caratterizzata dall'assenza di lesioni discrete iperpigmentate e dal diffuso coinvolgimento della cute. I pazienti appaiono solitamente normali alla nascita e cominciano a sviluppare il disturbo dopo i primi mesi di vita. In rari casi, la malattia si presenta con intenso prurito generalizzato, in assenza di alterazioni cutanee visibili. La cute solitamente appare ispessita, di colore giallastro o roseo, con aspetto a buccia d'arancia e consistenza flaccida. Le alterazioni superficiali sono accentuate nelle aree flessurali. Bolle ricorrenti (Fig. 658-14), prurito intrattabile e vampate (flushing) sono comuni, così come il coinvolgimento sistemico. La malattia può essere causata da una mutazione del fattore delle cellule staminali differente da quella responsabile dell'orticaria pigmentosa cronica. Per controllare i sintomi può essere necessario ricorrere al trattamento con raggi ultravioletti (UV)A-1 o UVA associati a psoraleni (PUVA).

La teleangiectasia eruttiva maculare persistente è un'altra variante caratterizzata da macule teleangiectasiche iperpigmentate, solitamente localizzate al tronco; le lesioni non provocano orticaria se strofinate. Questa forma della malattia si riscontra prevalentemente in adolescenti e adulti.

MASTOCITOSI SISTEMICA. Questo disturbo è contrassegnato da un anomalo incremento del numero dei mastociti nei tessuti diversi da quello cutaneo. Si sviluppa in circa il 5-10% dei pazienti affetti da mastocitosi associata a mutazione del fattore delle cellule staminali, ed è più comune negli adulti che nei bambini. Le lesioni ossee, talvolta silenti, sono rilevabili radiologicamente come aree osteoporotiche o osteosclerotiche, localizzate prevalentemente nello scheletro assiale. Il coinvolgimento del tratto gastrointestinale può causare diarrea e steatorrea. Infiltrati nelle mucose sono evidenziabili mediante esame con bario o biopsia intestinale. Si osserva anche ulcera peptica. L'infiltrazione di mastociti e la fibrosi possono causare epatosplenomegalia. È stata descritta anche la proliferazione di mastociti in linfonodi, reni, adipe perisurrenalico e midollo osseo. In circa un terzo dei pazienti si osservano anomalie del sangue periferico, come anemia, leucocitosi ed eosinofilia. Infine, può insorgere leucemia a mastociti.

Trattamento. Il rossore può essere esacerbato da bagni troppo caldi, dallo sfregamento vigoroso della cute, dall'assunzione di alcol e da alcuni farmaci, come codeina, acido acetilsalicilico, morfina, atropina, ketorolac, tubocurarina, colorazioni radio-

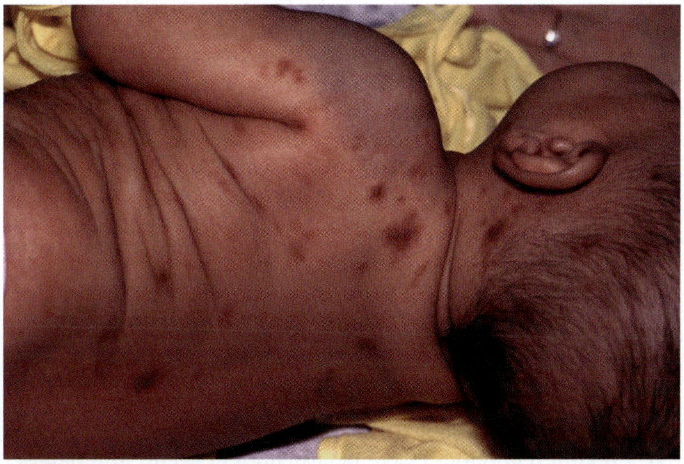

Figura 658-13. Lesioni papulari iperpigmentate nell'orticaria pigmentosa.

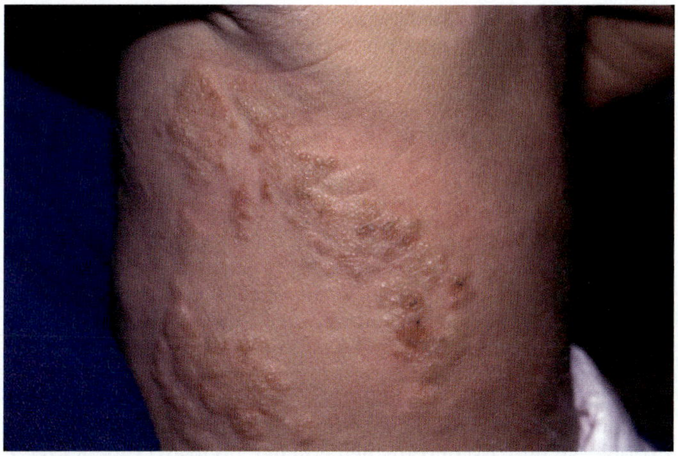

Figura 658-14. Grave vescicazione nella mastocitosi cutanea diffusa.

grafiche contenenti iodina e polimixina B (vedi Tab. 658-2). È quindi consigliabile evitare questi fattori scatenanti. Nei pazienti sintomatici è possibile ricorrere al trattamento palliativo con antistaminici orali. I farmaci di elezione per il trattamento iniziale dei segni sistemici del rilascio di istamina sono gli antagonisti dei recettori H1 (idrossizina). In caso di inefficacia di questa terapia, la somministrazione di antagonisti dei recettori H2 può contribuire ad alleviare il prurito o l'ipersecrezione gastrica. Steroidi topici superpotenti attenuano l'orticaria e la formazione di vesciche. L'assunzione orale di agenti stabilizzanti dei mastociti, come cromolyn sodico o chetotifene, può risultare efficace contro la diarrea, i crampi addominali e alcuni sintomi sistemici come la cefalea o il dolore muscolare.

Bercovitch L, Terry P: Pseudoxanthoma elasticum 2004. *J Am Acad Dermatol* 2004;51:S13–S14.

Carter MC, Metcalfe DD: Paediatric mastocytosis. *Arch Dis Child* 2002;86: 315–319.

Chan I: The role of extracellular matrix protein 1 in human skin. *Clin Exp Dermatol* 2004;29:52–56.

Kelly AP: Medical and surgical therapies for keloids. *Dermatol Ther* 2004;17:212–218.

Renaud-Vilmer C, Cavelier-Balloy B, Porcher R, et al: Vulvar lichen sclerosis: Effect of long-term topical application of a potent steroid on the course of the disease. *Arch Dermatol* 2004; 140:709–712.

Valent P, Sperr WR, Schwartz LB, et al: Diagnosis and classification of mast cell proliferative disorders: Delineation from immunologic diseases and non-mast cell hematopoetic neoplasms. *J Allergy Clin Immunol* 2004;114:3–11.

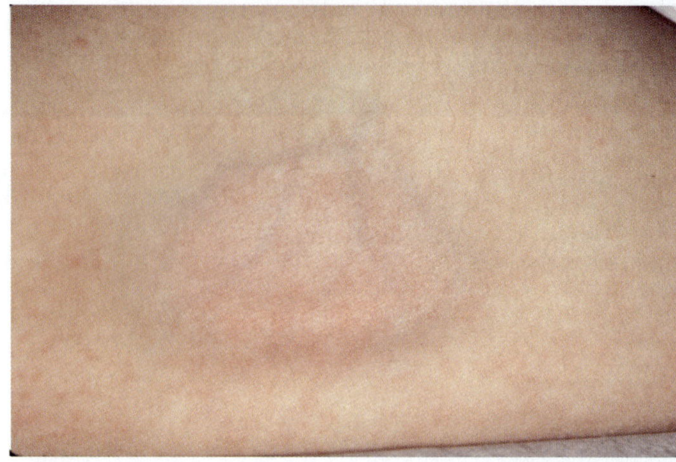

Figura 659-1. Atrofia adiposa localizzata con eritema secondario all'iniezione di uno steroide.

TABELLA 659-1. Eziologia dell'eritema nodoso

VIRUS	
	Epstein-Barr, epatite B, parotite epidemica
MICOSI	
	Coccidioidomicosi, istoplasmosi
BATTERI E ALTRI AGENTI INFETTIVI	
	Streptococco del gruppo A, *tubercolosi, **Yersinia*, malattia da graffio di gatto, lebbra, leptospirosi, tularemia, micoplasma, malattia di Whipple, linfogranuloma venereo, psittacosi
ALTRO	
	Sarcoidosi, malattia infiammatoria dell'intestino, *contraccettivi orali contenenti estrogeni, *lupus eritematoso sistemico, sindrome di Behçet, acne grave, malattia di Hodgkin, linfoma, sulfonamidi, bromidi, malattia di Sweet, gravidanza

*Comune.

Capitolo 659 ■ Malattie del tessuto sottocutaneo

Joseph G. Morelli

Le malattie che colpiscono il tessuto sottocutaneo sono solitamente caratterizzate da necrosi e/o infiammazione. Possono costituire un evento primario, o la risposta secondaria a vari stimoli o processi patologici. Questi disturbi non sono diagnosticabili sulla base delle alterazioni istopatologiche, che possono rispecchiare semplicemente lo stadio della lesione al momento della biopsia. I principali criteri diagnostici sono l'aspetto e la distribuzione delle lesioni, i sintomi associati, i risultati degli esami di laboratorio, la storia naturale e i fattori esogeni scatenanti i disturbi.

ATROFIA INDOTTA DA CORTICOSTEROIDI. L'iniezione intradermica di un corticosteroide può causare una profonda atrofia, associata ad alterazioni pigmentarie superficiali e a teleangiectasie (Fig. 659-1). Tali disturbi compaiono circa 2 settimane dopo l'iniezione e possono protrarsi per mesi. L'area del deltoide è la più suscettibile a questa complicanza.

PANNICULITE. L'infiammazione del tessuto grasso sottocutaneo può coinvolgere in primo luogo il lobulo adiposo o, alternativamente, il setto fibroso che suddivide i lobuli in compartimenti. La panniculite lobulare che risparmia la vascolarizzazione sottocutanea include la panniculite post-steroidea, il lupus eritematoso profondo, la panniculite pancreatica, il deficit di α_1-antitripsina, la necrosi del tessuto adiposo sottocutaneo del neonato, lo sclerema neonatorum, la panniculite da freddo, la sarcoidosi sottocutanea e la panniculite factizia. La panniculite lobare con vasculite è presente nell'eritema indurato e, occasionalmente, nel morbo di Crohn (vedi Capitolo 333.2). Una panniculite a predominanza infiammatoria, localizzata al setto, che risparmia la vascolarizzazione, si può riscontrare nell'eritema nodoso (Tab. 659-1 e Fig. 659-2), nella necrobiosi lipoidea, nella sclerosi sistemica progressiva (vedi Capitolo 159) e nel granuloma anulare subcutaneo (vedi Capitolo 656). La panniculite settale con vasculite si osserva prevalentemente nella vasculite leucocitoclastica e nella poliarterite nodosa (vedi Capitolo 166).

La **panniculite post steroidea** si osserva nei bambini che avevano assunto in precedenza, per periodi relativamente brevi, dosi elevate di corticosteroidi per via orale. Una o due settimane dopo la sospensione della terapia, noduli sottocutanei multipli compaiono su guance, tronco e braccia. Eritematosi e dello stesso colore della cute, i noduli hanno dimensioni variabili da 0,5 a 4 cm e possono risultare pruriginosi. Il meccanismo alla base della reazione infiammatoria nel tessuto adiposo è sconosciuto. Non è necessario alcun **trattamento** perché le lesioni si risolvono spontaneamente senza cicatrizzazione, entro qualche mese.

Il **lupus eritematoso profondo** (panniculite lupica) si presenta con un numero variabile di placche o noduli color porpora, con diametro compreso tra 1 e 3 cm. Le lesioni, ben definite e compatte, sono localizzate prevalentemente su volto, glutei o sulle porzioni prossimali degli arti. Il disturbo può manifestarsi in pazienti affetti da lupus eritematoso sistemico o discoide, e può precedere o seguire lo sviluppo delle altre lesioni cutanee. La cute soprastante è solitamente normale, ma in alcuni casi appare atrofica, poichilodermica o ipercheratosica (Fig. 659-3). Le lesioni possono essere dolorose e ulcerate. Dopo la guarigione, resta spesso una lieve depressione o, più raramente, un'area di anetoderma sensibile e rosata. Le alterazioni istopatologiche sono specifiche e contribuiscono alla diagnosi in assenza di altre lesioni cutanee tipiche del lupus eritematoso. I test per la ricerca degli anticorpi antinucleari e della banda lupica sono solitamente positivi. I noduli tendono a essere persistenti. Gli agenti antimalarici (idrossiclorochina) costituiscono il **trattamento di elezione**. La

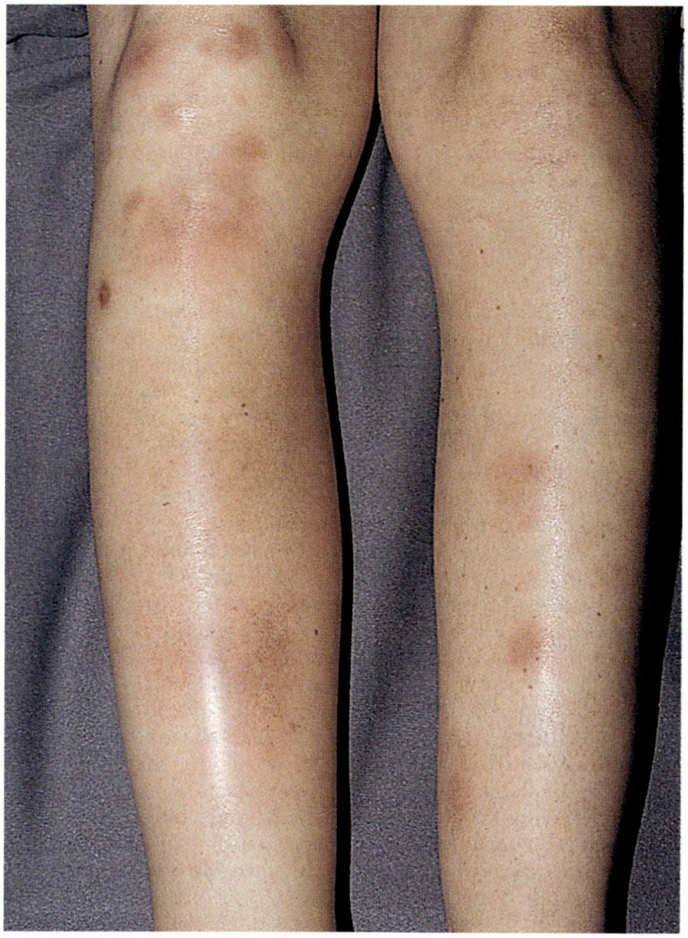

Figura 659-2. Noduli rossi sensibili al tatto, con bordi indistinti, in un'adolescente con eritema nodoso. (Da Weston AL, Lane AT, Morelli JG: *Color Textbook of Pediatric Dermatology,* 3rd ed. St. Louis, Mosby, 2002, p 212.)

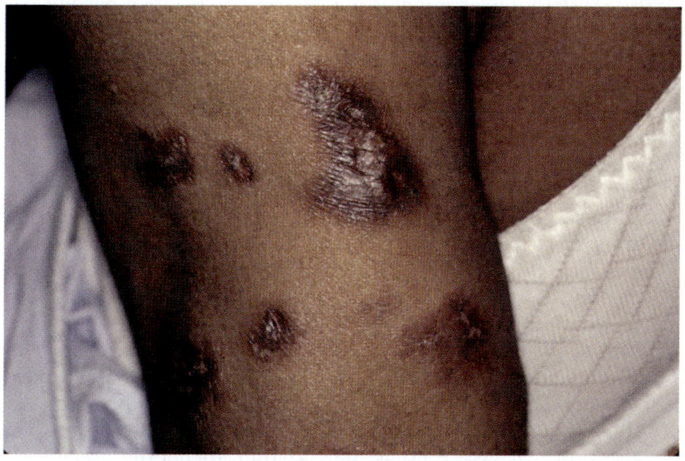

Figura 659-3. Nodulo profondo in un paziente con lupus profundus, associato alla lesione ipercheratosica del lupus eritematoso disseminato.

somministrazione intralesionale di corticosteroidi può aggravare la lipoatrofia residua. Gli agenti immunosoppressivi sono indicati solo per il trattamento delle altre gravi manifestazioni del lupus eritematoso sistemico (LES). È opportuno inoltre evitare l'esposizione al sole e i traumi.

Il **deficit di α_1-antitripsina** può presentarsi con aree cellulitiche o sensibili, noduli arrossati sul tronco o sulle porzioni prossimali degli arti (vedi Capitolo 390), che tendono a ulcerarsi spontaneamente, rilasciando un liquido giallastro e oleoso. In alcuni pazienti, i traumi costituiscono un fattore scatenante. Gli individui colpiti presentano un grave deficit omozigote o, più raramente, un deficit parziale dell'inibitore della proteasi α_1-antitripsina, che inibisce l'attività di tripsina, elastasi, serina proteasi, collagenasi, fattore VIII e callicreina. La panniculite può essere associata ad altre manifestazioni della malattia, come enfisema panacinare, epatite non infettiva, cirrosi, vasculite cutanea persistente, orticaria da freddo o angioedema acquisito. La diagnosi può essere confermata dal riscontro di una riduzione del livello dell'attività dell'α_1-antitripsina nel siero. Alcuni pazienti rispondono al dapsone o all'infusione di un concentrato dell'inibitore di α_1-antitripsina ottenuto da donatori.

La **panniculite pancreatica** compare più comunemente nelle regioni pretibiali, su cosce o glutei e si manifesta con noduli sensibili, talvolta fluttuanti, che possono rilasciare una sostanza oleosa giallastra. La malattia colpisce prevalentemente i soggetti di sesso maschile ed è associata all'alcolismo, ma si riscontra anche in pazienti con pancreatite conseguente a colelitiasi o traumi addominali, con rottura di una pseudocisti pancreatica, con adenocarcinoma duttale o carcinoma delle cellule acinari del pancreas. Le caratteristiche associate includono artropatia e sinovite (in particolare delle caviglie), eosinofilia, polisierosite e lesioni ossee dolorose, con necrosi midollare. Le alterazioni microscopiche consistono in focolai multipli di necrosi lipoidea, che contengono cellule fantasma prive di nucleo e dotate di pareti spesse e scure. Un infiltrato infiammatorio polimorfo circonda le aree di necrosi lipoidea. La patogenesi della panniculite, di tipo multifattoriale, implica la liberazione nella circolazione degli enzimi lipolitici lipasi, tripsina e amilasi, responsabili del danneggiamento della membrana degli adipociti e della lipolisi intracellulare. Non si riscontra però alcuna correlazione tra l'insorgenza della panniculite e la concentrazione sierica degli enzimi pancreatici.

La **necrosi del tessuto adiposo sottocutaneo** è un disturbo infiammatorio che si verifica prevalentemente nelle prime 4 settimane di vita, in neonati nati a termine o post-termine. La patologia è stata attribuita ad asfissia perinatale o a difficoltà durante il travaglio o il parto. Le lesioni tipiche consistono in placche o noduli eritematosi violacei, di consistenza gommosa o compatta, che compaiono solitamente su guance, glutei, schiena, cosce o parte superiore delle braccia (Fig. 659-4). Le lesioni, focali o diffuse, sono generalmente asintomatiche, ma talvolta risultano sensibili al tatto durante la fase acuta. Le seguenti alterazioni istopatologiche assumono un valore diagnostico: necrosi adiposa; infiltrato cellulare granulomatoso composto da linfociti, istiociti, cellule giganti multinucleate e fibroblasti; fessure a disposizione radiale di trigliceridi cristallini nelle cellule adipose e nelle cellule giganti multinucleate. Depositi di calcio si riscontrano comunemente nelle aree di necrosi adiposa. In età pediatrica, la malattia può essere dovuta a una lesione ischemica secondaria a preeclampsia materna, trauma da parto, asfissia o ipotermia prolungata. Tuttavia, in molti casi non si evidenzia alcun fattore scatenante. La predisposizione a tale patologia è stata attribuita a differenze di composizione tra il tessuto sottocutaneo dei neonati e quello dei bambini più grandi e degli adulti. L'adipe neonatale solidifica a temperature relativamente elevate a causa della maggior concentrazione di acidi grassi saturi a elevato punto di fusione come gli acidi palmitico e stearico.

In assenza di complicanze, le lesioni regrediscono spontaneamente entro qualche settimana o mese, solitamente senza lasciare cicatrici né atrofia. I depositi di calcio che si formano occasionalmente nelle aree di necrosi adiposa rischiano di determinare rotture e drenaggio di materiale liquido. Una complicanza rara ma potenzialmente fatale è l'**ipercalcemia**, che si presenta a 1-6 mesi con letargia, inappetenza, vomito, deficit staturo-ponderale, irritabilità, convulsioni, accorciamento dell'intervallo QT o insufficienza renale. L'origine dell'ipercalcemia è sconosciuta. La necrosi del tessuto adiposo sottocutaneo può essere confusa con

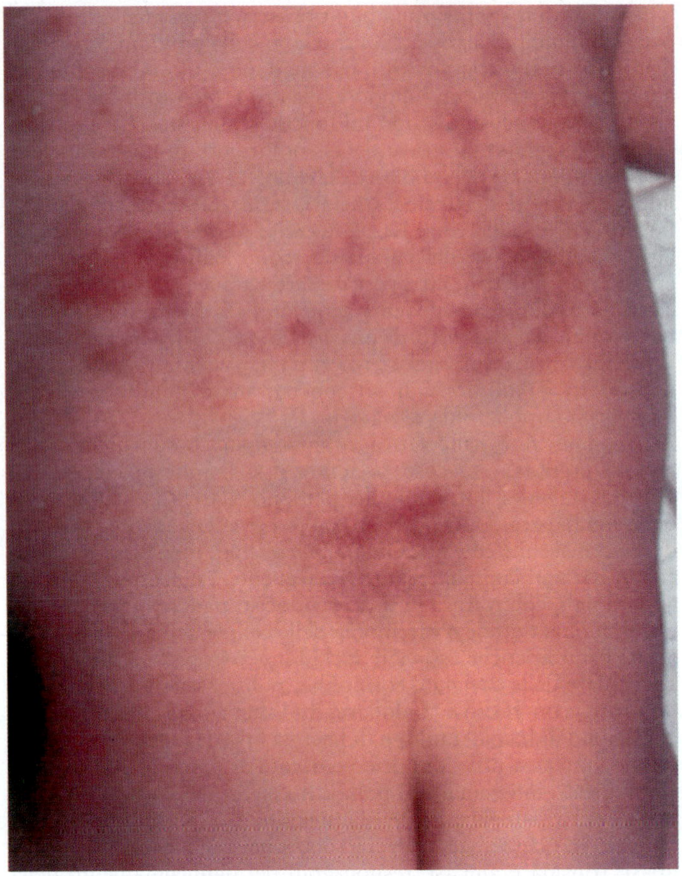

Figura 659-4. Infiltrato nodulare rosso porpora sulla schiena, causato da necrosi del tessuto adiposo sottocutaneo.

sclerema neonatorum, panniculite, cellulite o ematoma. Poiché le lesioni sono autolimitanti, in assenza di complicanze non è necessaria alcuna terapia. L'aspirazione con ago di lesioni fluttuanti può prevenire eventuali rotture e la conseguente formazione di cicatrici. Il trattamento dell'ipercalcemia mira a favorire l'escrezione renale di calcio, mediante idratazione e somministrazione di furosemide. È opportuno inoltre limitare l'apporto dietetico di calcio e vitamina D. La riduzione dell'assorbimento intestinale e dell'alterazione del metabolismo della vitamina D si possono ottenere mediante somministrazione di corticosteroidi.

Lo **sclerema neonatorum** è un insolito disturbo del tessuto adiposo, che si presenta all'improvviso in neonati pretermine e gravemente compromessi, con un indurimento della cute, che assume una consistenza legnosa e una colorazione bianco-giallastra. Al tatto, la cute risulta fredda e non depressibile. Il volto assume un'espressione che ricorda una maschera e la mobilità articolare può venire compromessa dalla mancanza di elasticità cutanea. Le alterazioni istopatologiche dello sclerema neonatorum consistono in un aumento delle dimensioni delle cellule adipose e dello spessore dei setti del tessuto connettivo fibroso. A differenza della necrosi del tessuto adiposo sottocutaneo, con cui questa patologia va in diagnosi differenziale, nello sclerema neonatorum generalmente non si riscontrano necrosi adiposa, infiammazione, cellule giganti, né cristalli di calcio. Nella quasi totalità dei casi, il disturbo è associato a una grave malattia, come sepsi, cardiopatia congenita, anomalie congenite multiple o ipotermia. La comparsa dello sclerema nel paziente è considerata un segno prognostico infausto. L'esito dipende dalla risposta alla terapia della malattia soggiacente.

La **panniculite da freddo** causa la comparsa di lesioni, localizzate prevalentemente alle guance, in seguito alla prolungata esposizione a basse temperature, o alla prolungata applicazione su di un'area cutanea di un oggetto freddo, come un cubetto di ghiaccio, una borsa d'acqua fredda o un ghiacciolo. Entro qualche ora, o al massimo dopo un paio di giorni, si sviluppano placche indurite o noduli eritematosi e bluastri, che persistono per 2-3 settimane, per poi scomparire senza lasciare segni. La recidiva della lesione è comune, perciò è fondamentale informare i genitori sul trattamento più opportuno. L'esame istopatologico rivela un infiltrato di cellule linfoidi o istiocitiche intorno ai vasi sanguigni nella giunzione tra derma e epidermide; entro 3 giorni, alcune delle cellule adipose si rompono e confluiscono in strutture cistiche. La panniculite da freddo può essere confusa con la cellulite facciale causata da *Haemophilus influenzae* di tipo b. A differenza della cellulite buccale, l'area può risultare fredda al tatto, il paziente non ha febbre e appare in buone condizioni di salute. Il **gelone** è una lesione da freddo acuta o cronica, caratterizzata da placche edematose simmetriche, eritematose o color porpora, nelle aree esposte al freddo, tipicamente le zone acrali (porzioni distali di mani e piedi, orecchie, volto) (vedi Capitolo 75). Le lesioni si sviluppano 12-24 ore dopo l'esposizione alle basse temperature e possono essere associate a prurito, bruciore o dolore. La formazione di vesciche e l'ulcerazione sono rare. Il meccanismo responsabile della malattia sembra essere il vasospasmo delle arteriole, dovuto all'esposizione al freddo, con conseguente ipossiemia e infiammazione perivascolare mononucleare localizzata. Il congelamento è estremamente doloroso e, sul piano istopatologico, coinvolge l'epidermide, il derma e l'adipe sottocutaneo. Il meccanismo patogenetico della panniculite da freddo, simile a quello della necrosi del tessuto adiposo sottocutaneo, è collegato alla maggiore facilità di solidificazione dell'adipe neonatale, secondaria alla presenza di una percentuale più elevata di acidi grassi saturi.

La **panniculite factizia** è il risultato dell'iniezione sottocutanea, da parte del paziente stesso o per procura, di una sostanza estranea di vario tipo, come materiali organici (latte o feci), farmaci come oppioidi o pentazocina, sostanze oleose (paraffina, olio minerale) o il polimero sintetico povidone. Sul piano clinico, si osserva la comparsa di placche indurite, ulcere o noduli che tendono a liquefarsi e drenano. I reperti istopatologici dipendono dal tipo di sostanza iniettata, ma includono la presenza di cristalli birifrangenti, cisti oleose circondate da fibrosi e infiammazione, e una reazione infiammatoria acuta, con necrosi adiposa. Tipicamente, i vasi sanguigni sono risparmiati.

LIPODISTROFIA. Diverse malattie rare sono associate a perdita del tessuto adiposo, con una distribuzione parziale o generalizzata.

Lipodistrofia parziale. Può essere familiare o acquisita. La perdita di tessuto adiposo non è preceduta da una fase infiammatoria e l'esame istopatologico rivela soltanto l'assenza dell'adipe sottocutaneo.

Si distinguono 3 forme di lipodistrofia familiare parziale.

Il **tipo 1 (di Kobberling)** è caratterizzato da perdita di tessuto adiposo confinata alle estremità e ai glutei. La distribuzione adiposa su volto, collo e tronco può risultare normale o aumentata. Si osservano talvolta iperlipidemia, diabete mellito insulino-resistente e xantomi eruttivi. Il gene responsabile è sconosciuto, ma la malattia colpisce soltanto le donne.

Il **tipo 2 (di Dunnigan)** è causato da mutazioni del gene per la laminina A/C. La distribuzione adiposa è normale nell'infanzia, ma l'atrofia esordisce nell'adolescenza. La lipodistrofia si osserva su tronco, glutei ed estremità. Il tessuto adiposo si accumula su viso e collo, ma talvolta anche alle ascelle, su schiena, grandi labbra e regione infra-addominale. Si sviluppano diabete mellito insulino-resistente e ipertrigliceridemia, ma i livelli di colesterolo e di lipoproteine ad alta densità sono bassi. La malattia colpisce indifferentemente uomini e donne, ma la formulazione della diagnosi è più complessa negli uomini, a causa del loro habitus corporeo.

Il **tipo 3** è causato da mutazioni del gene per il recettore gamma attivatore della proliferazione perossisomale. La lipodistrofia colpisce gli arti e i glutei. Sono presenti anche diabete mellito insulino-resistente, amenorrea primaria, acanthosis nigrans, ipertensione e infiltrazione adiposa del fegato.

La **lipodistrofia parziale acquisita** (sindrome di Barraquer-Simons) è una malattia rara, che colpisce prevalentemente le donne. La perdita adiposa comincia nell'infanzia o nell'adolescenza e interessa volto, collo, braccia, torace e addome superiore. Su fianchi e gambe si osserva un eccesso di grasso, in particolare nelle donne. La riduzione dei livelli di C3 si riscontra nella quasi totalità dei casi. È inoltre presente il fattore nefritico C3, che stabilizza la C3 convertasi, consentendo l'attivazione della via alternativa del complemento e la riduzione del livello di C3. Possono svilupparsi glomerulonefrite e altre malattie autoimmuni. Il diabete mellito insulino-resistente è raro.

LIPODISTROFIA GENERALIZZATA. Può essere congenita o acquisita. Il tipo congenito è presente in 2 forme.

Il **tipo 1 (lipodistrofia congenita di Berardinelli-Seip di tipo 1 [BSCL1])** è un disturbo a trasmissione autosomica recessiva causato da mutazioni del gene per 1-acilglicerol-3-fosfato-0-aciltrasferasi (AGPAT2).

Il **tipo 2 (lipodistrofia congenita di Berardinelli-Seip di tipo 2 [BSCL2])**, anch'esso autosomico recessivo, è causato da mutazioni del gene per la seipina.

La lipodistrofia marcata esordisce dopo la nascita o nella prima infanzia. Si osservano diabete mellito, ipertrigliceridemia, steatosi epatica, acanthosis nigricans e ipertrofia muscolare. La BSCL2 ha un fenotipo più grave, responsabile del decesso del paziente in circa il 15% dei casi.

Anche la **lipodistrofia acquisita generalizzata** è più comune nelle donne. Nel 25% dei pazienti, la malattia si presenta con una panniculite infiammatoria; in un altro 25% con una malattia autoimmune associata (solitamente la dermatomiosite giovanile); nel restante 50% non si riscontra alcuna malattia associata. La perdita adiposa comincia nella prima infanzia o nell'adolescenza e coinvolge la maggior parte del corpo. I bambini colpiti manifestano un appetito vorace. Nella maggior parte dei pazienti, si sviluppano acanthosis nigricans e steatosi epatica, con un 20% di progressione verso la cirrosi.

La **lipoatrofia localizzata** è una malattia idiopatica che esordisce con un'atrofia anulare alle caviglie, una depressione a banda semicircolare del diametro di 2-4 cm sulle cosce o, più raramente, con una placca bluastra e depressa, con margine eritematoso, a diffusione centrifuga, su addome e inguine superiore. La malattia colpisce prevalentemente i bambini giapponesi.

La **lipoatrofia da insulina** si verifica dopo 6 mesi-2 anni dall'inizio dell'assunzione di dosi relativamente elevate di insulina. Solitamente si nota la comparsa di una depressione o di una fossetta nella sede dell'iniezione, ma la perdita adiposa può estendersi oltre quest'area, causando la formazione di un'ampia placca depressa. La biopsia rivela una marcata riduzione o l'assenza di tessuto sottocutaneo, senza infiammazione né fibrosi. In alcuni pazienti si osserva ipertrofia. In questi casi, le sezioni istopatologiche mostrano che il collagene del derma intermedio è sostituito da cellule adipose ipertrofiche. È ipotizzabile che il meccanismo responsabile di questa forma di lipoatrofia consista in una reazione incrociata degli anticorpi dell'insulina con le cellule adipose. L'incidenza della malattia si è drasticamente ridotta in seguito alla diffusione dell'utilizzo di insulina purificata. Le lesioni possono essere prevenute anche modificando di frequente la sede dell'iniezione.

Garg A: Acquired and inherited lipodystrophies. *N Engl J Med* 2004;350:1220–1234.

McBean J, Sable A, Maude J, et al: Alpha1-antitrypsin deficiency panniculitis. *Cutis* 2003;71:205–209.

Ng PP, Tan SH, Tan T: Lupus erythematosus panniculitis: A clinicopathologic study. *Int J Dermatol* 2002;41:88–90.

Tran JT, Sheth AP: Complications of subcutaneous fat necrosis of the newborn: A case report and review of the literature. *Pediatr Dermatol* 2003;20:257–261.

Van der Zee JA, van Hillegersberg R, Toonstra J, et al: Subcutaneous nodules pointing towards pancreatic disease: Pancreatic panniculitis. *Dig Surg* 2004;21:275–276.

Wimmershoff MB, Hohenleutner U, Landthaler M: Discoid lupus erythematosus and lupus profundus in childhood: Report of two cases. *Pediatr Dermatol* 2003;20:140–145.

Capitolo 660 ■ Disordini delle ghiandole sudoripare Joseph G. Morelli

Le ghiandole eccrine, disseminate sulla quasi totalità della superficie cutanea, costituiscono il principale strumento di raffreddamento del corpo, attraverso l'evaporazione dell'acqua in sudore. Tali ghiandole, prive di qualsiasi legame anatomico con i follicoli piliferi, secernono un'elevata quantità di sudore acquoso inodore. Al contrario, la distribuzione delle ghiandole apocrine è limitata ad ascelle, cute anogenitale, ghiandole mammarie, ghiandole ceruminose dell'orecchio, ghiandole di Moll della palpebra e specifiche aree del volto e del cuoio capelluto. Il dotto della ghiandola apocrina penetra nel follicolo pilosebaceo a livello dell'infundibolo e secerne una piccola quantità di un complesso liquido vischioso che, se alterato da microorganismi, produce un caratteristico odore acre. Alcuni dei disordini che colpiscono i due tipi di ghiandole sudoripare sono patogeneticamente simili, mentre altri risultano specifici.

ANIDROSI. L'anidrosi neuropatica è il risultato di un difetto della via neurale di attivazione del sudore dal centro di controllo cerebrale alle fibre nervose periferiche efferenti. I disturbi caratterizzati da anidrosi generalizzata includono tumori dell'ipotalamo e lesioni del pavimento del terzo ventricolo. Le lesioni pontine o midollari possono causare anidrosi del lato ipsilaterale di volto o collo e anidrosi ipsilaterale o controlaterale del resto del corpo. L'anidrosi della cute innervata può essere associata a neuropatie segmentali o periferiche causate da lebbra, amiloidosi, diabete mellito, neurite alcolica o siringomielia. Anche diversi disturbi autonomici sono associati all'alterazione della funzione delle ghiandole sudoripare eccrine.

I farmaci anticolinergici (come atropina e scopolamina) possono paralizzare le ghiandole sudoripare. L'intossicazione acuta con barbiturici o diazepam può produrre necrosi delle ghiandole sudoripare, con conseguente anidrosi, associata o meno a eritema e bolle. Nei pazienti con **displasia ectodermica anidrosica**, le ghiandole eccrine sono pressoché assenti, mentre nell'**assenza localizzata congenita** sono presenti solo in aree cutanee circoscritte. I disturbi infiltranti o distruttivi in grado di causare atrofia delle ghiandole sudoripare mediante pressione o cicatrizzazione includono scleroderma, acrodermatite cronica atrofizzante, radiodermatite, ustioni, sindrome di Sjögren, mieloma multiplo e linfoma. L'ostruzione delle ghiandole sudoripare può riscontrarsi nella miliaria e in alcuni disturbi infiammatori e iperacheratosici, come ittiosi, psoriasi, *lichen planus*, pemfigo, porocheratosi, dermatite atopica e dermatite seborroica. L'occlusione dei pori può insorgere anche in seguito all'applicazione topica di alluminio, sali di zirconio, formaldeide o glutaraldeide.

I disordini associati ad anidrosi provocata da meccanismi d'azione sconosciuti includono disidratazione; overdose tossica da piombo, arsenico, tallio, fluorina o morfina; uremia; cirrosi; disturbi endocrini come malattia di Addison, diabete mellito, diabete insipido o ipertiroidismo; patologie ereditarie come la malattia di Fabry, la sindrome di Franceschetti-Jadassohn (che combina caratteristiche dell'*incontinentia pigmenti* e della displasia ectodermica anidrosica) e l'anidrosi familiare con neurolabirintite.

L'anidrosi può essere completa, ma in molti casi il disturbo che, sul piano clinico, appare come anidrosi consiste in realtà in un'**ipoidrosi** causata dall'anidrosi di molte ma non tutte le ghiandole eccrine. Le ghiandole rimanenti presentano talvolta iperidrosi compensatoria localizzata, in particolare in presenza di diabete mellito e miliaria. La complicanza principale dell'anidrosi è l'**ipertermia**, riscontrata prevalentemente nella displasia ectodermica anidrosica, in neonati pretermine sani o in neonati a termine che presentano immaturità delle cellule eccrine.

IPERIDROSI. I diversi disturbi associati ad aumento della produzione di sudore eccrino possono essere classificati in due sottogruppi: nel primo, meccanismi neurali causano un'anomalia della via dai centri regolatori alle ghiandole sudoripare; nel secondo, i disturbi sono il risultato di effetti diretti sulle ghiandole sudoripare, in assenza di mediazione neurale (Tab. 660-1). L'eccessiva sudorazione di palmi della mani e piante dei piedi in risposta a stimoli emotivi (iperidrosi volare) e la sudorazione ascellare possono rispondere alle seguenti terapie: applicazione, con bendaggio occlusivo per varie ore, di una soluzione di cloruro di alluminio al 20% esaidrato in alcol etilico; ionoforesi; iniezione con tossina botulinica; assunzione per via orale di anticolinergici; simpatectomia lombare o cervicotoracica nei casi più gravi e refrattari.

MILIARIA. È il risultato della ritenzione di sudore secondaria all'occlusione dei dotti sudoripari, causata da un tappo di cheratina. La pressione retrograda può determinare una rottura del dotto e la fuoriuscita di sudore, che si diffonde nell'epidermide e/o nel derma. Nella maggior parte dei casi, l'eruzione è indotta da temperature molto elevate associate a umidità, ma può essere provocata anche da febbre alta. I bambini troppo coperti possono sviluppare il disturbo anche nei mesi invernali.

Nella **miliaria cristallina**, una profusione di vesciche chiare a punta di spillo, asintomatiche e non infiammatorie, compare improvvisamente su ampie aree della superficie corporea, residuando, dopo la guarigione, una desquamazione tendente al marrone (Fig. 660-1). La diagnosi differenziale con le altre forme di disordini con formazione di vesciche si basa sulla limpidezza del liquido, la superficialità delle vescicole e l'assenza di infiammazione. Questo tipo di miliaria si verifica con maggior frequenza nei neonati, a causa di una relativa immaturità e scarsa pervietà dei dotti sudoripari, e in seguito all'abitudine di mantenere caldo-umido l'ambiente in cui vive il neonato. La miliaria cristallina si riscontra anche in pazienti più grandi con iperpiressia. Sul piano istopatologico, si rileva la presenza di una vescica intra o subcorneale, in comunicazione con il dotto sudoriparo.

La **miliaria rubra** è un'eruzione più superficiale, caratterizzata da minute papulovescicole eritematose, che possono causare una sensazione di pizzicore. Le lesioni sono solitamente localizzate nelle sedi di occlusione o nelle aree flessorie, come il collo, l'inguine e l'ascella, in cui la frizione ha probabilmente un ruolo nella patogenesi. La macerazione e la lacerazione della cute coinvolta sono frequenti. Questo tipo di lesione può essere confusa o sovrapporsi alle altre eruzioni da pannolino, come candidosi e follicoliti. Le lesioni della miliaria rubra sono però extrafollicolari. Sul piano istopatologico si osservano aree focali di spongiosi e la formazione, in prossimità dei dotti sudoripari, di vescicole spongiotiche, che generalmente contengono un tappo di cheratina. Tale tappo si forma soltanto negli stadi avanzati della malattia e, di conseguenza, non costituisce la causa primaria dell'ostruzione dei dotti. È ipotizzabile invece che l'ostruzione iniziale sia provocata dalla dilazione delle cellule dei dotti piliferi, forse secondaria all'assorbimento di acqua. Attacchi ripetuti di miliaria rubra possono condurre alla **miliaria profonda**, dovuta alla rottura dei dotti piliferi a livello della giunzione dermoepidermica. Gravi ed estese forme di miliaria rubra o profonda possono provocare un'alterazione nella regolazione del calore. Le lesioni della miliaria rubra rischiano inoltre di infettarsi, in particolare in neonati malnutriti o debilitati, con conseguente sviluppo di **periporite stafilogene**, causata dal coinvolgimento delle ghiandole sudoripare.

Tutte le forme di miliaria rispondono bene al raffreddamento del paziente mediante regolazione della temperatura ambientale e rimozione degli indumenti eccessivamente pesanti. Nei pazienti con febbre, è utile anche la somministrazione di antipiretici. Gli agenti topici sono solitamente inefficaci e rischiano di esacerbare l'eruzione.

BROMIDROSI. L'odore corporeo particolarmente intenso e sgradevole che caratterizza la bromidrosi è il risultato di un'alterazione del sudore apocrino o eccrino. La bromidrosi apocrina si sviluppa dopo la pubertà, per la formazione di acidi grassi a catena corta e ammoniaca, in seguito all'azione di difteroidi anaerobici sul sudore ascellare apocrino. La bromidrosi eccrina

TABELLA 660-1. Cause dell'iperidrosi

CORTICALI	**Vasomotorie**
Fattori emotivi	Lesioni da freddo
Disautonomia familiare	Fenomeno di Raynaud
Eritroderma ittiosiforme congenito	Artrite reumatoide
Epidermolisi bollosa	**Neurologiche**
Nail-patella syndrome	Ascessi
Sindrome di Jadassohn-Lewandowsky	Disautonomia familiare
Pachionichia congenita	Postencefalitiche
Cheratoderma palmoplantare	Tumori
IPOTALAMICHE	**Varie**
Farmaci	Sindrome di Chédiak-Higashi
Antipiretici	Compensatorie
Emetici	Fenilchetonuria
Insulina	Feocromocitoma
Meperidina	Vitiligine
Esercizio fisico	**MIDOLLARI**
Infezioni	Sudorazione gustativa fisiologica
Defervescenza	Encefaliti
Malattie croniche	Granulosi rubra del naso
Metaboliche	Siringomielia
Astenia	Toracentesi
Diabete mellito	**SPINALI**
Iperpituitarismo	Transectomia spinale
Ipertiroidismo	Siringomielia
Ipoglicemia	**ALTERAZIONI DEL FLUSSO SANGUIGNO**
Obesità	Sindrome di Maffucci
Porfiria	Fistola arteriovenosa
Gravidanza	Sindrome di Klippel-Trenaunay
Rachitismo	Tumore glomico
Scorbuto infantile	Nevo blu gommoso
Cardiovascolari	
Insufficienza cardiaca	
Shock	

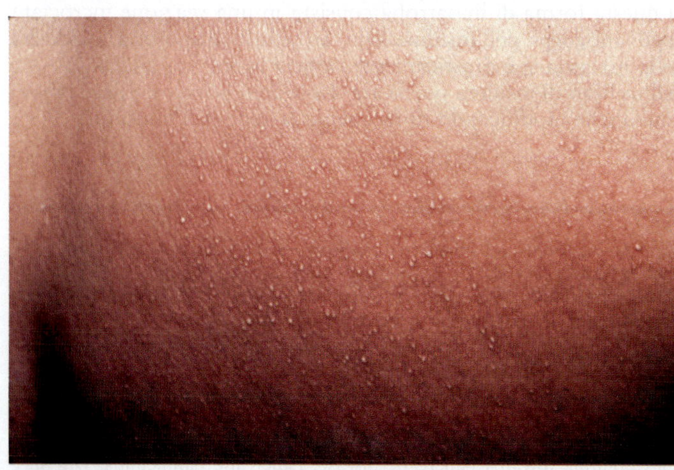

Figura 660-1. Vesciche superficiali chiare nella miliaria cristallina.

è causata dalla degradazione microbiologica dello strato corneo, ammorbidito dall'eccessiva sudorazione. Le aree più colpite sono le piante dei piedi e le zone intertriginose. Il **trattamento** prevede la detersione con saponi germicidi, e l'applicazione topica di clindamicina, eritromicina, alluminio, zirconio o sali di zinco. I preparati per uso topico a base di cloruro di alluminio sono particolarmente utili per contrastare la bromidrosi eccrina. I fattori predisponenti includono iperidrosi, temperature elevate, obesità, intertrigine e diabete mellito.

IDROSOADENITE SUPPURATIVA. Questo disturbo cronico, infiammatorio e suppurativo, delle ghiandole apocrine colpisce le ascelle, l'area anogenitale e, occasionalmente, il cuoio capelluto, la faccia posteriore dell'orecchio, il seno nelle donne e l'area periombelicale. L'esordio delle manifestazioni cliniche, talvolta preceduto da prurito o fastidio, avviene solitamente nella pubertà o nella prima età adulta. I noduli eritematosi, singoli o multipli, gli ascessi profondi e le cicatrici contratte sono confinati alla aree cutanee contenenti ghiandole apocrine. Nei casi di malattia grave o cronica, si sviluppano tragitti fistolosi, ulcere e spesse bande fibrotiche lineari. L'idrosoadenite suppurativa tende a persistere per molti anni, con l'alternarsi di remissioni parziali e recidive. Le complicanze includono cellulite, ulcerazione e ascessi in grado di perforare le strutture adiacenti, con formazione di fistole nell'uretra, nella vescica, nel retto o nel peritoneo. In alcuni pazienti, si sviluppa artrite infiammatoria episodica. In una minoranza di casi, si osserva la cosiddetta triade di occlusione follicolare, che include acne e perifollicolite del capo. Le lesioni precoci sono spesso confuse con cisti epidermiche infette, foruncoli, scrofuloderma, actinomicosi, malattia da graffio del gatto, granuloma inguinale o linfogranuloma venereo. La localizzazione in aree del corpo che presentano ghiandole apocrine suggerisce idrosoadenite. Quando il coinvolgimento è limitato alla regione anogenitale, il disturbo può essere difficile da distinguere dal morbo di Crohn.

Le lesioni precoci sono caratterizzate dalla presenza di un tappo di cheratina nei dotti apocrini o nell'orifizio del follicolo pilifero, e da una distensione cistica del follicolo. Generalmente (ma non necessariamente), il processo patologico si estende alle ghiandole apocrine. Le alterazioni successive includono un'infiammazione all'interno e intorno alle ghiandole apocrine e la presenza di gruppi di cocchi all'interno delle ghiandole e nel derma adiacente. Le cicatrici rischiano di obliterare gli annessi cutanei. L'esordio della malattia è probabilmente attribuibile all'ostruzione dei dotti delle ghiandole apocrine da parte di detriti di cheratina. Lo sviluppo di un'infezione batterica, in particolare da *Staphylococcus aureus*, *Streptococcus milleri*, *Escherichia coli* o streptococchi anaerobici, contribuisce alla progressiva dilatazione al di sotto dell'ostruzione, responsabile della rottura del dotto, dell'infiammazione, dei tragitti fistolosi e delle cicatrici deturpanti. La patogenesi dell'idrosoadenite suppurativa è controversa.

È opportuno che il paziente eviti gli indumenti aderenti, che rischiano di esacerbare il disturbo. Il **trattamento** con retinoidi topici o con antibiotici topici, come clorexidina, eritromicina o clindamicina, può risultare efficace nella fase precoce e non dolente della malattia. Gli antibiotici sistemici, scelti sulla base della coltura batterica (solitamente stafilococchi e streptococchi) e dei test di sensibilità, andrebbero somministrati nella fase acuta. Se il paziente ha più di 8 anni, la terapia empirica prevede la somministrazione di tetraciclina, doxiciclina o minociclina; anche la clindamicina e le cefalosporine sono efficaci. Alcuni pazienti richiedono un trattamento a lungo termine con tetraciclina o eritromicina. Nella fase precoce della malattia, l'iniezione intralesionale di triamcinolone acetonide (5-10 mg/mL) è spesso utile. Per ridurre la fibrosi e le cicatrici nei pazienti refrattari agli antibiotici, si consiglia l'associazione di prednisone, alla dose di 40-60 mg/die per 7-10 giorni, da ridurre gradualmente non appena l'infiammazione inizia a regredire. In alcuni pazienti, è possibile somministrare contraccettivi orali a elevato rapporto estrogeno-progesterone e un ridotto grado di androgenicità del progesterone, oppure retinoidi orali. L'applicazione di impacchi caldi favor
prossimi a
controllo
a procedu

MALATTI
donne, s
vita, cor
regione
da stre
apocrir
della c
prurigi
di tap
dotti
apocr
parac
dura
pazi
l'applicazione top...

Boer A: Patterns histopathologic of Fox-Fordyce disease. *Am J Dermatopathol* 2004;26:482-492.

Cheshire WP, Freeman R: Disorders of sweating. *Semin Neurol* 2003;23:399-406.

Kamada A, Saga K, Jimbow K: Apoeccrine sweat obstruction as a cause of Fox-Fordyce disease. *J Am Acad Dermatol* 2003;48:453-455.

Capitolo 661 ■ Anomalie dei capelli

Joseph G. Morelli

Le anomalie dei capelli e dei peli in neonati e bambini possono essere causate da disturbi intrinseci della crescita dei capelli/peli, difetti metabolici o biochimici, dermatosi infiammatorie o anomalie strutturali del fusto. La crescita eccessiva e anomala dei peli è detta ipetricosi o irsutismo. L'**ipertricosi** è la crescita eccessiva di peli in sedi non appropriate, mentre l'**irsutismo** consiste in una modalità maschile androgeno-dipendente di crescita dei peli in una donna. Il termine **ipotricosi**, invece, designa una crescita pilifera deficitaria. La perdita dei capelli, parziale o completa, è definita alopecia, classificabile come non cicatriziale o cicatriziale; quest'ultima forma è rara in età pediatrica e, se presente, è spesso dovuta a malattie infiammatorie protratte o non trattate, come il pioderma o la *tinea capitis*.

IPERTRICOSI

L'ipertricosi, rara nei bambini, può essere localizzata o generalizzata, permanente o transitoria. Può avere diverse cause, alcune delle quali sono elencate nella Tabella 661-1.

IPOTRICOSI E ALOPECIA

Alcuni dei disturbi associati all'ipertricosi e all'alopecia sono elencati nella Tabella 661-2. L'alopecia vera è raramente congenita; nella maggior parte dei casi è collegata a dermatosi infiammatoria, fattori meccanici, assunzione di farmaci, infezioni, endocrinopatie, disturbi nutrizionali o del ciclo capillare. Qualsiasi condizione infiammatoria del cuoio capelluto, come la dermatite atopica o seborroica, se sufficientemente grave rischia di causare alopecia parziale, che recede in seguito al trattamento della malattia responsabile, a meno che i follicoli piliferi non siano stati danneggiati permanentemente.

...ll'ipertricosi

...pelosi, falangi pelose o irsutismo generalizzato

...nte

...rticosteroidi, neomicina o polimixina B con idrocortisone, ciclosporina, androgeni, ...clorobenzene, minoxidil, psoraleni, penicillamina, streptomicina

...EVI

...o pigmentato congenito, nevo peloso, nevo di Becker, amartoma muscolare liscio congenito, ...coda di fauno associato a diastematomielia

...URBI ENDOCRINI

...rilizzazione o tumori ovarici, sindrome di Cushing, acromegalia, ipertiroidismo, ipotiroidismo, iperplasia surrenale congenita, tumori surrenalici, disgenesia gonadica, pseudoermafroditismo maschile, tumori non secernenti l'ormone endocrino, sindrome dell'ovaio policistico

DISTURBI CONGENITI E GENETICI

Ipertricosi lanuginosa, mucopolisaccaridosi, leprecaunismo o sindrome dello gnomo, lipodistrofia congenita generalizzata, sindrome di de Lange, trisomia 18, sindrome di Rubinstein-Taybi, sindrome di Bloom, emiipertrofia congenita, fibromatosi gengivale con ipertricosi, sindrome di Winchester, diabete lipoatrofico (sindrome di Lawrence-Seip), sindrome fetale da idantoina, sindrome alcolica fetale, porfiria eritropoietica congenita o variegata (nella aree esposte al sole), porfiria cutanea tardiva (nelle aree esposte al sole), sindrome di Cowden, sindrome di Seckel, sindrome di Gorlin, trisomia 3q parziale, sindrome di Ambra

TABELLA 661-2. Disordini associati ad alopecia e ipotricosi

Alopecia congenita totale: anomalia autosomica recessiva isolata, progerie, displasia ectodermica idrotica, sindrome di Moynahan, atrichia con cisti di cheratina, sindrome di Baraitser

Alopecia congenita localizzata: aplasia cutanea, alopecia triangolare, nevo epidermico, amartoma del follicolo capillare, emiatrofia facciale (sindrome di Romberg), calvizie di tipo maschile

Ipotricosi ereditaria: ipotricosi con cheratosi pilare, sindrome di Marie-Unna, fenilchetonuria, aciduria argino succinica, iperlisinemia, omocistinuria, oroticoaciduria, sindrome di Cockayne, sindrome di Rothmund-Thomson, discheratosi congenita, sindrome di Seckel, ipoplasia cartilagine-capelli, sindrome di Conradi, pachionichia congenita, sindrome di Hallermann-Streiff, sindrome di Treacher Collins, ipotricosi displasia oculodentodigitale, sindrome orofaciodigitale, *incontinentia pigmenti*, ipoplasia dermica focale, cheratosi follicolare, epidermolisi bollosa, displasia ectodermica, ittiosi, perdita di capelli anagen

Alopecia diffusa di origine endocrina: ipopituitarismo, ipotiroidismo, ipoparatiroidismo, ipertiroidismo, diabete mellito

Alopecia di origine nutrizionale: marasma, kwashiorkor, carenza di ferro, carenza di zinco (acrodermatite enteropatica), enteropatia sensibile al glutine, deficit di acidi grassi essenziali, deficit di biotinidasi

Disturbi del ciclo dei capelli: effluvio telogen

Alopecia tossica: effluvio anagen

Alopecia autoimmune: alopecia areata

Alopecia traumatica: alopecia da trazione, tricotillomania

Alopecia cicatriziale: lupus eritematoso, *lichen planus pilaris*, pseudopelade, sclerodermia, dermatomiosite, infezioni (da cherion, favo, tubercolosi, sifilide, follicolite, leishmaniasi, herpes zoster, varicella), acne cheloide, mucinosi follicolare, pemfigoide cicatriziale, lichen scleroso e atrofico, sarcoidosi

Anomalie del fusto del capello: monilethrix, pili annulati, pili torti, tricorressi invaginata, tricorressi nodosa, sindrome dei capelli lanosi, malattia di Menkes, tricotiodistrofia, sindrome tricodento-ossea, sindrome tricorinofalangea, sindrome dei capelli non pettinabili (capelli a fibra di vetro, pili trianguli e canalicoli)

La perdita dei capelli in età infantile viene suddivisa in quattro categorie: diffusa congenita, congenita localizzata, acquisita diffusa e acquisita localizzata.

La forma più comune in età pediatrica è quella acquisita localizzata. Si riscontrano prevalentemente tre disturbi: l'alopecia traumatica, l'alopecia areata e la *tinea capitis*.

ALOPECIA TRAUMATICA (ALOPECIA DA TRAZIONE, COMPULSIONE A STRAPPARSI I CAPELLI, TRICOTILLOMANIA)

ALOPECIA DA TRAZIONE. L'alopecia da trazione è dovuta a traumi dei follicoli capillari, causati da particolari acconciature come coda di cavallo o trecce troppo strette, e dall'uso di fasce, elastici, arricciacapelli o bigodini (Fig. 661-1). In aree circoscritte ai margini del cuoio capelluto, si osservano papule follicolari infiammate e capelli spezzati; tali alterazioni possono accompagnarsi a linfoadenopatia regionale. Bambini e genitori devono essere incoraggiati a evitare gli oggetti che possono causare traumi al capello e, se necessario, a cambiare pettinatura; in caso contrario si può arrivare alla cicatrizzazione dei follicoli piliferi.

COMPULSIONE A STRAPPARSI I CAPELLI. In età pediatrica, questa compulsione costituisce una reazione acuta a stress emotivi. Si osserva anche in associazione a tricotillomania, in presenza di disturbi psichiatrici più gravi.

TRICOTILLOMANIA. La compulsione a tirarsi, attorcigliarsi e strapparsi i capelli causa la formazione di aree di perdita capillare incompleta, localizzate nella parte posteriore della testa o nelle aree occipitali e parietali. Qualche volta, il paziente si strappa anche ciglia, sopracciglia e peli del corpo. Alcune placche di alopecia hanno contorni lineari. I capelli rimasti nelle aree di alopecia hanno una lunghezza variabile (Fig. 661-2) e presentano una tipica punta smussa data dalla rottura. Il cuoio capelluto appare solitamente normale, ma talvolta si riscontrano emorragie, croste (Fig. 661-3) e follicolite cronica. La tricofagia, con conseguente formazione di **tricobezoari**, costituisce una complicanza comune. L'incidenza del disturbo è del 3% nelle ragazze e dell'1% nei maschi.

I criteri elencati nel *Diagnostic and Statistical Manual of Mental Disorders* includono una visibile perdita di capelli attribuibile

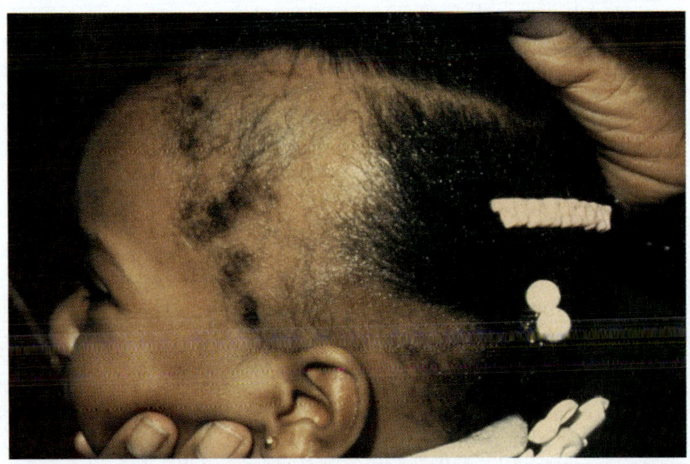

Figura 661-1. Alopecia da trazione.

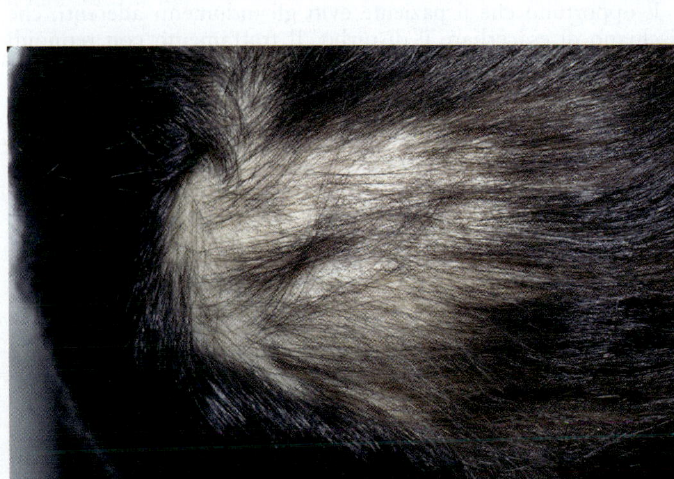

Figura 661-2. Capelli strappati a lunghezze variabili.

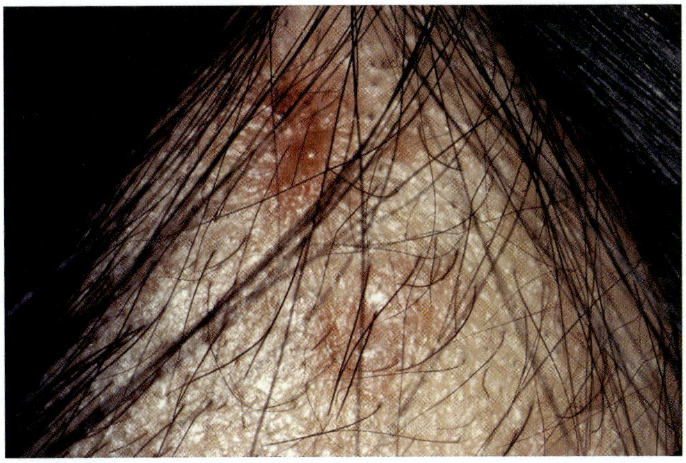

Figura 661- 3. Emorragia e formazione di crosta secondaria alla compulsione a strapparsi i capelli.

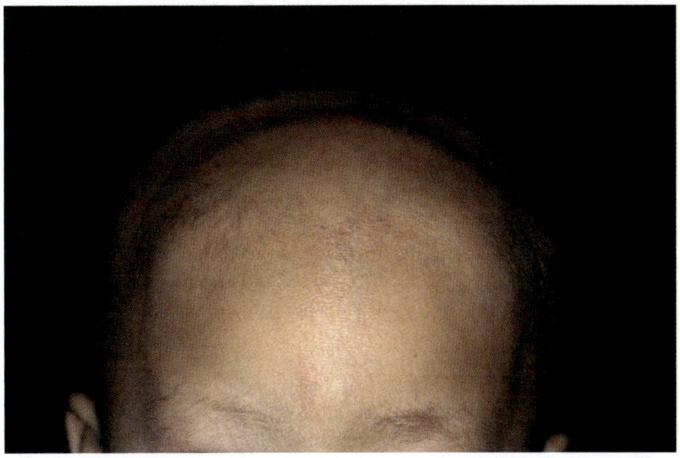

Figura 661-5. Alopecia totale (perdita di capelli completa).

alla trazione; un senso crescente di tensione immediatamente prima di strapparsi i capelli; gratificazione o sollievo durante l'atto; assenza di allucinazioni, deliri o disturbi infiammatori cutanei. Le alterazioni istologiche includono coesistenza di follicoli normali e danneggiati, emorragia perifollicolare, atrofia di alcuni follicoli e trasformazione in catagen dei capelli. Negli stadi più avanzati può insorgere fibrosi perifollicolare. A lungo termine, traumi ripetuti rischiano di determinare un danno irreversibile e alopecia permanente. La diagnosi differenziale è con la compulsione a strapparsi i capelli, la *tinea capitis* e l'alopecia areata.

In alcuni pazienti, la **tricotillomania** è un'espressione di un **disturbo ossessivo-compulsivo**. In tali casi, la somministrazione di clomipramina, fluoxetina o trazodone si è dimostrata efficace, in particolare se combinata a terapia comportamentale.

ALOPECIA AREATA. L'alopecia areata è caratterizzata dalla rapida e completa perdita di capelli in chiazze ovali o circolari (Fig. 661-4) o dalla perdita dei peli in altre aree del corpo. Nell'alopecia totale, il cuoio capelluto risulta completamente privo di capelli (Fig. 661-5); l'alopecia universale colpisce sia il cuoio capelluto sia i peli del corpo. L'incidenza dell'alopecia areata nella popolazione è dell'1%. Più del 50% dei pazienti ha meno di 20 anni.

Manifestazioni cliniche. La perdita dei capelli avviene solitamente in cerchi ben definiti. La cute nelle aree colpite appare normale. La biopsia su campioni prelevati dalle aree attive rivela un infiltrato perifollicolare di cellule infiammatorie rotonde. L'alopecia areata è associata ad atopia; alterazioni ungueali come fessurazioni (Fig. 661-6), increspature, opacizzazioni, chiusura del margine ungueale, distrofia e lunula rossa; cataratta o opacizzazione del cristallino; **malattie autoimmuni** come tiroidite di Hashimoto, malattia di Addison, anemia perniciosa, colite ulcerante, miastenia grave, malattia vascolare del collagene e vitiligine. Un aumento dell'incidenza dell'alopecia aerata è stato segnalato in pazienti con sindrome di Down (fino al 5-10%).

Eziologia. La causa dell'alopecia areata è sconosciuta. Sono stati suggeriti fattori precipitanti come stress e fattori emotivi, ma quest'ipotesi resta da confermare. Il 10-20% dei pazienti presenta una storia familiare di alopecia areata. La rara ma evidente associazione con le malattie autoimmuni suggerisce una patogenesi autoimmune. Nel siero di alcuni pazienti si riscontrano anticorpi contro la tiroglobulina, le cellule parietali e le ghiandole surrenali; è stata dimostrata anche la presenza di autoanticorpi contro gli antigeni dei follicoli dei capelli.

Diagnosi differenziale e prognosi. La diagnosi differenziale è con *tinea capitis*, dermatite seborroica, tricotillomania, alopecia traumatica e lupus eritematoso. Il decorso della malattia è imprevedibile, ma la risoluzione spontanea entro 6-12 mesi è frequente, in particolare se le chiazze di alopecia sono di dimensioni relativamente ridotte. Le recidive sono tuttavia comuni. I segni prognostici più sfavorevoli sono l'esordio precoce, una perdita di

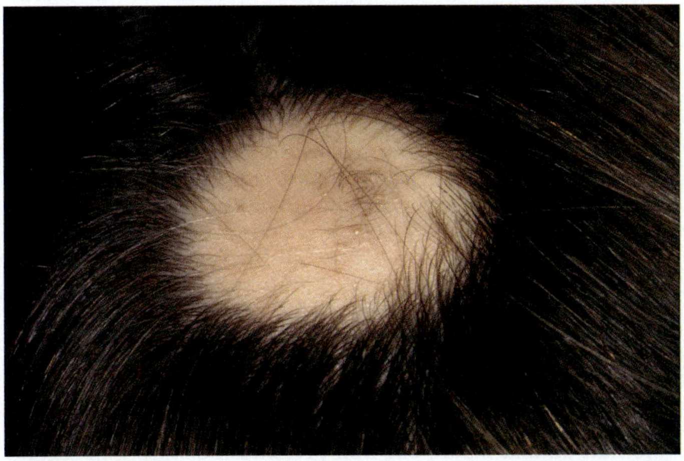

Figura 661-4. Chiazze circolari di alopecia areata; il cuoio capelluto appare normale.

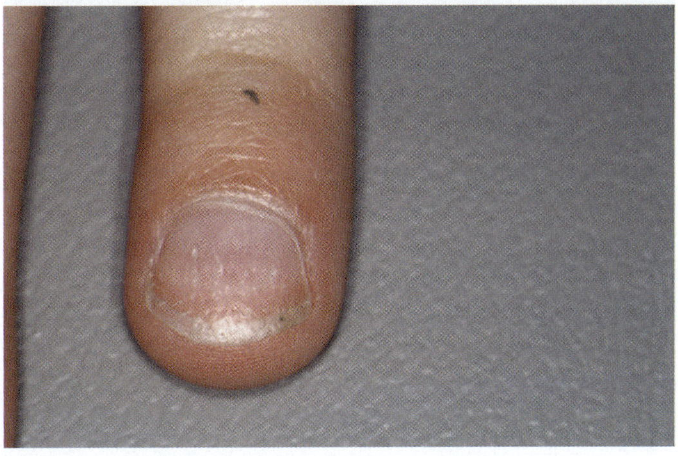

Figura 661- 6. Fessurazioni ungueali multiple nell'alopecia areata.

capelli estesa e prolungata, numerosi episodi ricorrenti e atrofia associata. La risoluzione è meno probabile nelle forme universale, totale e ofiasica (una forma di alopecia che colpisce le zone occipitale e temporale; Fig. 661-7).

Trattamento. È difficilmente valutabile a causa del decorso imprevedibile della malattia. L'utilizzo topico, con occlusione notturna, di corticosteroidi fluorinati ad alta potenza è efficace in alcuni pazienti. Iniezioni intradermiche di steroidi possono riuscire a stimolare la ricrescita locale, ma questa modalità di trattamento è difficilmente praticabile nei bambini molto piccoli o in presenza di perdita di capelli estesa. La terapia sistemica con corticosteroidi è stata talvolta associata a risultati positivi, ma si discute sull'opportunità di prolungare questo tipo di cura, i cui effetti collaterali costituiscono un serio deterrente. Altre terapie risultate talvolta efficaci includono l'antralina con contatto breve, l'applicazione topica di minoxidil e la sensibilizzazione da contatto con acido squarico dibutilestere o difenciprone. In linea generale, genitori e pazienti possono essere rassicurati sulla remissione spontanea della malattia. A volte, i capelli ricresciuti appaiono inizialmente più chiari e sottili, ma le loro caratteristiche tendono a normalizzarsi.

PERDITA DI CAPELLI DIFFUSA ACQUISITA

EFFLUVIO TELOGEN. Si presenta con la perdita improvvisa di consistenti quantità di capelli, spesso mentre il paziente si pettina o si lava la testa. Tale caduta è il risultato della prematura conversione in capelli telogen dei capelli anagen (in crescita), che normalmente costituiscono l'80-90% del totale. La perdita si nota da 6 settimane a 3 mesi dopo una causa precipitante, come il parto, un episodio febbrile, un intervento chirurgico, una perdita ematica acuta (inclusa una donazione), un'improvvisa e grave perdita di peso, la sospensione di una terapia corticosteroidea a dosi elevate o dell'assunzione di contraccettivi orali, uno stress emotivo. L'effluvio telogen è inoltre responsabile della perdita di capelli del lattante nei primi mesi di vita. La frizione delle lenzuola può esacerbare il problema, in particolare in presenza di cute atopica e pruriginosa. Non si riscontra alcuna reazione infiammatoria; i follicoli sono integri e la presenza di bulbi telogen può essere dimostrata al microscopio. L'alopecia è raramente grave, poiché solitamente non coinvolge più del 50% del cuoio capelluto. I genitori possono dunque essere rassicurati sulla probabile ricrescita di capelli normali entro circa 6 mesi.

ALOPECIA TOSSICA (EFFLUVIO ANAGEN). L'effluvio anagen è una grave, acuta e diffusa inibizione della crescita dei follicoli anagen, con conseguente perdita dell'80-90% dei capelli, che appaiono distrofici e si spezzano facilmente. La perdita è diffusa e rapida (1-3 settimane dopo la terapia), ma temporanea, perché i capelli cominciano a ricrescere non appena l'assunzione dell'agente tossico viene interrotta. Le cause dell'effluvio anagen includono radiazioni, agenti chemioterapici come gli antimetaboliti, agenti alchilanti e inibitori mitotici, tallio, tiouracile, eparina, cumarinici, acido borico, e ipervitaminosi A.

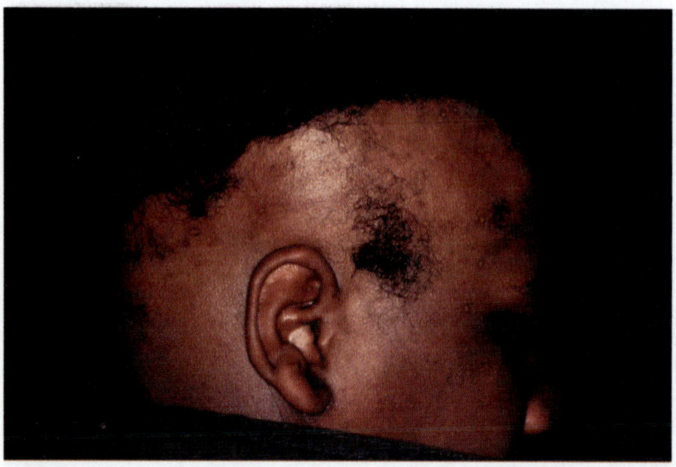

Figura 661-7. Alopecia ofiasica.

PERDITA DI CAPELLI CONGENITA DIFFUSA. L'estrema sottigliezza congenita dei capelli è collegata all'ipoplasia del follicolo o a difetti strutturali del fusto.

DIFETTI STRUTTURALI DEL CAPELLO. I difetti strutturali a carico del fusto del capello possono essere congeniti, riflettere aberrazioni biochimiche note o essere collegati a pratiche di igiene personale dannose. I difetti sono dimostrabili mediante un esame al microscopio dei capelli colpiti, in particolare con microscopio elettronico a scansione.

TRICORESSI NODOSA. La tricorressi nodosa cronica è una malattia a trasmissione autosomica dominante. I capelli appaiono secchi, fragili, opachi, con noduli grigio-bianchi disposti irregolarmente lungo il fusto (Fig. 661-8*A*). Il difetto è dovuto a fratture del fusto nei punti dei nodi, causate da lesioni cellulari della corteccia del capello. La tricorressi nodosa si osserva anche nei bambini con sindrome di Menkes, tricotiodistrofia e aciduria argininosuccinica.

Tricorressi nodosa acquisita. Questo disturbo, causato nella maggior parte dei casi da rotture dei capelli, si presenta in due forme. I difetti prossimali sono più comuni nei bambini neri, in cui il disturbo non è l'alopecia ma l'assenza di crescita dei capelli. I capelli sono corti e presentano scanalature longitudinali, nodi e noduli visibili al microscopio. La facilità di rottura è dimostrabile con una leggera trazione del fusto. Si riscontra spesso un'anamnesi familiare positiva per la patologia. È ipotizzabile che il problema sia causato da una combinazione tra predisposizione genetica e traumi meccanici dovuti ad acconciature, permanenti, utilizzo di phon e piastre. I pazienti devono evitare tali procedure dannose, limitandosi a utilizzare una spazzola con setole naturali e un pettine a denti larghi. Il disturbo è autolimitante, con risoluzione entro 2-4 anni se il paziente si attiene alle raccomandazioni del medico. La tricorressi nodosa distale si osserva con maggior frequenza nei bambini asiatici o di razza bianca. La porzione distale del capello appare assottigliata, lacerata e scolorita; macchie bianche, spesso confuse con uova di pidocchi, si notano lungo il fusto. L'osservazione su vetrino mostra punti di eccessiva fragilità e rottura e difetti che conferiscono al pelo la caratteristica forma a "pennello". La malattia può colpire anche aree localizzate di barba e baffi. I disturbi possono migliorare evitando pratiche dannose, spuntando con regolarità i capelli e utilizzando balsami e creme specifici.

PILI TORTI. I pazienti presentano capelli radi, fragili e di lunghezza variabile sull'intero cuoio capelluto. A causa di un difetto strutturale, il fusto capillare appare appiattito e scanalato a intervalli irregolari, nonché attorcigliato intorno al proprio asse in grado variabile. Gli arricciamenti minori che si osservano nel capello normale non devono essere confusi con il disturbo. La curvatura del follicolo è responsabile dell'appiattimento e della rotazione del fusto. La malattia si trasmette con modalità autosomica dominante o recessiva, ma il difetto genetico responsabile è tuttora sconosciuto. Le **sindromi** in cui le anomalie del fusto descritte sono associate ad altre anomalie cutanee e sistemiche includono la malattia di Menkes, la sindrome di Bazex, la sindrome di Bjornstad (pili torti in associazione a sordità), la displasia ectodermica di Crandall e Rapp-Hodgkin e la tricotiodistrofia.

SINDROME DI MENKES (TRICOPOLIDISTROFIA). I pazienti di sesso maschile, portatori del tratto recessivo legato al cromosoma X, sono nati da una madre che non presenta il disturbo, in seguito a una gravidanza nella norma. I disturbi neonatali includono ipotermia, ipotonia, disturbi della suzione, convulsioni e deficit

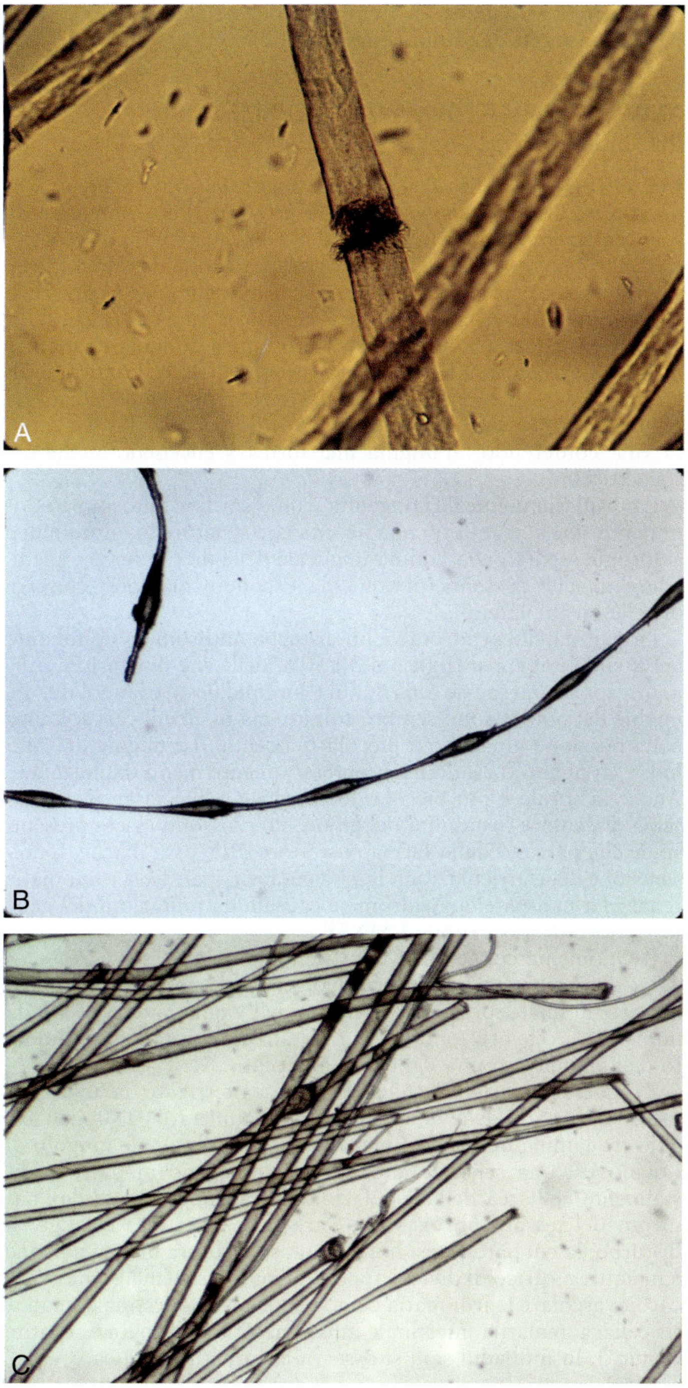

Figura 661-8. *A*, Frattura microscopica del capello nella tricorressi nodosa. *B*, Fusto a corona nel monilethrix. *C*, Anomalia a coppa del capello nella sindrome di Netherton.

staturo-ponderale. I capelli, normali o radi alla nascita, sono sostituiti da capelli sottili, corti, fragili e chiari, che possono presentare caratteristiche di tricorressi nodosa, pili torti o monilethrix. Il paziente presenta guance piene, cute ipopigmentata e radice nasale appiattita. Nella prima infanzia si comincia a notare un progressivo ritardo psicomotorio. La sindrome è causata da mutazioni del gene ATP7A, che codifica per una proteina ATPasi di trasporto del rame, responsabile di una maldistribuzione del rame nel corpo. L'assorbimento di rame attraverso l'orletto a spazzola dell'intestino tenue aumenta, mentre il trasporto da queste cellule al plasma è deficitario, con conseguente riduzione della quantità totale di rame immagazzinato nel corpo. La somministrazione parenterale di rame è efficace, purché avviata nei primi due mesi di vita.

MONILETHRIX. Questo difetto del fusto capillare, ereditato con modalità autosomica dominante, è caratterizzato da un'età di esordio, una gravità e un decorso variabili. Sono state identificate mutazioni delle cheratine HBI e HB6. Il capello appare secco, opaco e fragile; tende a spezzarsi spontaneamente o in seguito a lievi traumi. Oltre al cuoio capelluto, possono essere coinvolti anche peli corporei e pubici, ciglia e sopracciglia. Il monilethrix può essere presente fin dalla nascita, ma nella maggior parte dei casi i capelli appaiono inizialmente normali, per poi essere sostituiti da capelli anomali nei primi mesi di vita. Talvolta, il disturbo esordisce nell'infanzia. Papule follicolari possono comparire sulla nuca, nell'area occipitale e, occasionalmente, sull'intero cuoio capelluto. Capelli corti e fragili, che emergono dai tappi di cheratina follicolari, assumono un caratteristico aspetto a rosario. Possono essere presenti anche cheratosi pilare e coilonichia ungueale di mani e piedi. Al microscopio è evidente l'aspetto a rosario del fusto capillare, caratterizzato da nodi ellittici separati da internodi più stretti (Fig. 661-8*B*). Tali nodi non sono presenti su tutti i capelli, ma anche i capelli dall'aspetto normale tendono a spezzarsi. Per limitare le rotture, si consiglia al paziente di manipolare i capelli con delicatezza. Il trattamento è generalmente inefficace.

TRICOTIODISTROFIA. I capelli sono radi, corti, fragili e distribuiti in maniera non uniforme; possono essere colpite anche le ciglia e le sopracciglia. Al microscopio, il capello appare appiattito, ripiegato e di diametro variabile; presenta inoltre scanalature longitudinali e nodi simili a quelli della tricorressi nodosa. Al microscopio polarizzato, si nota una caratteristica alternanza di bande scure e chiare. Nei capelli anormali, il contenuto di cistina è superiore alla norma di oltre il 50%, a causa di una maggiore riduzione e dell'alterazione nella composizione delle proteine a elevato contenuto di zolfo della matrice. La tricotiodistrofia può riscontrasi isolata o in associazione a varie sindromi complesse, che includono ritardo mentale, bassa statura, ittiosi, distrofia ungueale, carie dentali, cataratta, calo della fertilità, anomalie neurologiche e ossee, immunodeficienza. Alcuni pazienti manifestano fotosensibilità e una compromissione dei meccanismi di riparazione del DNA (analoga a quella riscontrata nei pazienti con xeroderma pigmentoso di gruppo D); tuttavia, l'incidenza di tumori cutanei non risulta aumentata. I pazienti con tricotiodistrofia hanno una facies caratteristica, con mento poco pronunciato, orecchie protrudenti, voce stridula; sono inoltre accomunati da una personalità socievole ed estroversa. La tricoschisi, una frattura perpendicolare del fusto, è tipica di molte sindromi associate alla tricotiodistrofia. La rottura perpendicolare del fusto è stata descritta anche in associazione ad altre anomalie, in particolare il monilethrix.

TRICORESSI INVAGINATA (CAPELLI A CANNA DI BAMBÙ). Questo disturbo, che si riscontra prevalentemente in associazione alla sindrome di Netherton (vedi Capitolo 656), è caratterizzata da capelli radi, corti e fragili, che crescono poco. È segnalato anche in altre dermatosi ittiosiformi. La porzione distale del capello è invaginata nella porzione prossimale a coppa, formando un rigonfiamento nodoso e fragile (Fig. 661-8*C*).

PILI ANNULATI. Il fusto si presenta a bande alternate chiare e scure. Al microscopio ottico, la regione del fusto che appare luminosa in luce riflessa risulta invece scura in luce trasmessa, per la presenza di aggregati focali di cavità anomale piene di aria all'interno del fusto. Il capello non è fragile. Il difetto può essere sporadico o trasmesso con modalità autosomica dominante. Gli pseudopili annulati costituiscono una variante normale del capello biondo; la presenza di bande è un effetto ottico determinato dalla refrazione e dalla riflessione della luce dal fusto parzialmente appiattito e torto.

CAPELLI LANOSI. Questo disordine, trasmesso con modalità autosomica recessiva o dominante, si presenta alla nascita, con capelli crespi, in un neonato non di razza nera. Il nevo lanoso è una forma sporadica che coinvolge una porzione circoscritta del

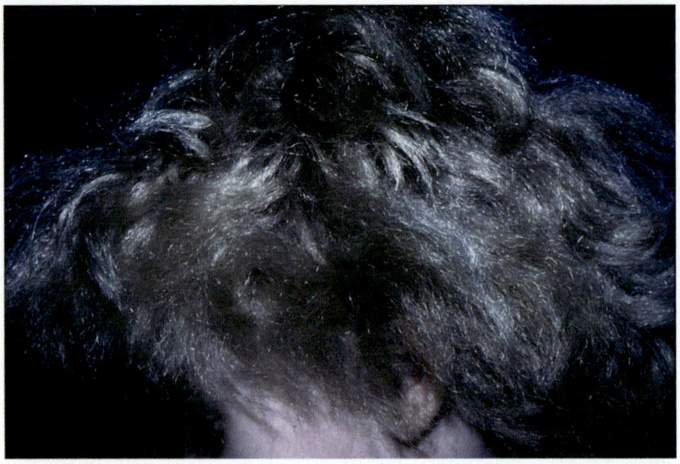

Figura 661-9. Capelli disordinati color biondo argenteo nella sindrome dei capelli non pettinabili.

cuoio capelluto. I capelli colpiti sono sottili, crespi e chiari; la loro crescita è rallentata. Al microscopio il capello appare ovale e attorcigliato intorno al proprio asse a 180°.

SINDROME DEI CAPELLI NON PETTINABILI (CAPELLI A "FIBRE DI VETRO"). I capelli, spesso color biondo argenteo (Fig. 661-9), appaiono disordinati e si spezzano facilmente in seguito agli inutili tentativi del paziente di domarli. Si tratta probabilmente di un disordine a trasmissione autosomica dominante. Ciglia e sopracciglia sono normali. Si riscontra costantemente una depressione longitudinale lungo il fusto, e la maggior parte dei follicoli e dei fusti risultano triangolari (*pili trianguli et canaliculi*). La forma del capello varia a seconda della lunghezza, e ciò lo rende ingovernabile.

Alexis AF, Dudda-Subramanya R, Sinha AA: Alopecia areata: Autoimmune basis of hair loss. *Eur J Dermatol* 2004;14:364–370.

Hantash BM, Schwartz RA: Traction alopecia in children. *Cutis* 2003;71: 18–20.

Harrison S, Sinclair R: Optimal management of hair loss (alopecia) in children. *Am J Clin Dermatol* 2003;4:757–770.

Harrison S, Sinclair R: Telogen effluvium. *Clin Exp Dermatol* 2002;27: 389–395.

Liang C, Kraemer KH, Morris A: Characterization of tiger tail banding and hair shaft abnormalioties in trichothiodystrophy. *J Am Acad Dermatol* 2005;52:224–232.

Norris D: Alopecia areata: Current state of knowledge. *J Am Acad Dermatol* 2004;51:S16–S17.

Nuss MA, Carlisle D, Hall M, et al: Trichotillomania: A review and case report. *Cutis* 2003;72:191–196.

Tay YK, Levy ML, Metry DW: Trichotillomania in childhood: Case series and review. *Pediatrics* 2004;113:e494–e498.

Wiedemeyeer K, Schill WB, Loser C: Diseases on hair follicles leading to hair loss part I: Nonscarring alopecias. *Skinmed* 2004;3:209–214.

Capitolo 662 ■ Malattie delle unghie

Joseph G. Morelli

Le anomalie ungueali in età pediatrica possono costituire le manifestazioni di una malattia cutanea generalizzata o localizzata all'area periungueale, di una malattia sistemica, di traumi o di infezioni batteriche o micotiche localizzate. Rientrano inoltre tra gli effetti collaterali di alcune terapie farmacologiche e sono comuni in molti disordini congeniti (Tab. 662-1).

ANOMALIE NELLA FORMA O NELLE DIMENSIONI DELLE UNGHIE

L'**anonichia** è l'assenza della lamina ungueale, solitamente secondaria a un disturbo congenito o a un trauma. Può comparire da sola o associata a malformazioni delle dita. La **coilonichia**, letteralmente "unghia a cucchiaio", è un'alterazione dell'unghia che consiste nella perdita del suo contorno normale, per la presenza di una lamina ungueale appiattita e concava. In alcuni casi, il disordine è trasmesso con modalità autosomica dominante, mentre in altri è associato ad anemia da carenza di ferro, sindrome di Plummer-Vinson o emocromatosi. Nei bambini sani, la lamina ungueale può essere relativamente sottile per i primi 1-2 anni di vita, conferendo all'unghia una forma a cucchiaio anche nei soggetti sani.

La **displasia ungueale congenita** è un disordine autosomico dominante, che si manifesta alla nascita con striature longitudinali e assottigliamento della lamina ungueale delle dita di mani e piedi. L'unghia, che presenta platonichia e coilonichia, può crescere oltre le pieghe laterali.

La **nail-patella syndrome** è un disturbo autosomico dominante nel quale l'unghia si riduce al 30-50% delle sue dimensioni normali e presenta spesso una lunula piramidale o triangolare. Le unghie del pollice sono sempre colpite, ma in alcuni casi soltanto nella porzione ulnare (più piccola o assente). Le unghie dal dito indice al mignolo risultano progressivamente meno danneggiate. Anche la rotula è più piccola del normale e questa anomalia rischia di causare instabilità del ginocchio. Possono essere presenti spine che partono dalla faccia posteriore delle ossa iliache, iperestensione delle articolazioni, lassità cutanea, iperidrosi e anomalie renali. La nail-patella syndrome è causata da mutazioni del gene del fattore di trascrizione LMX1B.

Pachionichia congenita (vedi Capitolo 657).

La **deformità da tic**, che coinvolge uno o entrambi i pollici, consiste in una depressione al centro dell'unghia, attraversata da numerose creste orizzontali. È il risultato del continuo sfregamento dell'unghia con una delle dita adiacenti.

L'ippocratismo digitale (**clubbing**) è caratterizzato da: ingrossamento dei tessuti delle falangi distali; un aumento >180° dell'angolo tra lamina ungueale e piega ungueale prossimale (angolo di Lovibond); una sensazione spugnosa spingendo in basso e distalmente nell'area dell'articolazione interfalangea, data dall'aumento del tessuto fibrovascolare tra la matrice e la falange. Il disturbo, la cui patogenesi non è nota, si riscontra in associazione a malattie a carico di diversi apparati, come il sistema polmonare, cardiovascolare (cardiopatia cianogena), gastrointestinale (malattia celiaca, malattia intestinale infiammatoria), ed epatico (epatite cronica). In individui sani si osserva la forma idiopatica.

ALTERAZIONI DEL COLORE DELLE UNGHIE

La **leuconichia** è un'opacità della lamina ungueale, che assume una colorazione bianca uniforme, striata o punteggiata. Tale anomalia del colore costituisce l'unica alterazione rilevabile. Il disturbo può essere di origine traumatica, oppure associato a

TABELLA 662-1. Malattie congenite con difetti ungueali

Unghie grandi: pachionichia congenita, sindrome di Rubinstein-Taybi, emiipertrofia
Unghie piccole o assenti: displasie ectodermiche, nail-patella syndrome, discheratosi congenita, ipoplasia dermica focale, ipoplasia cartilagine-capelli, sindrome di Ellis-van Creveld, sindrome di Larsen, epidermolisi bollosa, *incontinentia pigmenti*, sindrome di Rothmund-Thomson, sindrome di Turner, briglia poplitea, trisomia 13, trisomia 18, sindrome di Gorlin-Pindborg, delezione del braccio lungo del cromosoma 21, sindrome otopalatodigitale, sindrome fetale da alcool, sindrome fetale da idantoina, facies elfica, anonichia, acrodermatite enteropatica
Altro: difetto congenito di allineamento dell'alluce, distrofia familiare delle unghie

infezioni come la lebbra e la tubercolosi, a dermatosi come il lichen planus e la malattia di Darier, a patologie maligne come il morbo di Hodgkin, l'anemia e l'avvelenamento da arsenico (linee di Mees). In rari casi, la leuconichia è trasmessa con modalità autosomica dominante e può essere associata a cisti epidermiche congenite, calcoli renali e sordità. Le linee di Muehrcke, associate all'ipoalbuminemia, sono bande bianche, parallele e accoppiate, che non cambiano posizione in seguito alla crescita dell'unghia. Nelle unghie di Lindsay (**half-and-half nails**), la porzione prossimale dell'unghia è bianca, mentre il 20-50% distale è rosso, rosa o marrone; tale particolare colorazione è comune nei pazienti con nefropatia, ma può costituire anche una variante normale. Nelle unghie bianche di Terry, tipiche della **cirrosi**, l'intera lamina o il suo estremo prossimale assumono un aspetto a vetro smerigliato e una colorazione biancastra, mentre la porzione distale dell'unghia (per 1-2 mm) mantiene un colore rosato normale. Tale anomalia è associata a ipoalbuminemia.

La **pigmentazione nera** dell'intera lamina ungueale o la presenza di bande lineari (malanonichia striata) è comune nei soggetti afroamericani (90%) e asiatici (10-20%), mentre è insolita nei bianchi (<1%). Nella maggior parte dei casi, la presenza del pigmento (melanina prodotta dai melanociti di un nevo giunzionale nella matrice e nel letto ungueale) non ha alcuna conseguenza. In caso di estensione o alterazione della pigmentazione, è opportuno effettuare una biopsia, per valutare la possibilità di una trasformazione maligna.

Unghie bluastre o verdastre possono essere il risultato di un'infezione da Pseudomonas (Fig. 662-1), in particolare in associazione a onicolisi o paronichia cronica. La colorazione è dovuta alla presenza di detriti subungueali e al pigmento piocianina prodotto dagli organismi batterici.

La **sindrome delle unghie gialle** si manifesta con ispessimento e curvatura eccessiva, assenza di lunula e crescita rallentata. Nella maggior parte dei casi, la malattia colpisce la totalità delle unghie. Malattie sistemiche associate includono bronchiectasia, chilotorace ed edema focale di arti e volto. Le manifestazioni di questa sindrome sono attribuite a un deficit del drenaggio linfatico, secondario a ipoplasia dei vasi linfatici.

Le **emorragie subungueali** sono spesso il risultato di traumi minori, ma possono essere associate anche a endocardite batterica subacuta, vasculite, artrite reumatoide grave, ulcera peptica, ipertensione, glomerulonefrite cronica, cirrosi, scorbuto, trichinosi, neoplasie maligne e psoriasi.

SEPARAZIONE DELL'UNGHIA

L'**onicolisi** consiste nello scollamento della lamina dal letto ungueale distale. Le cause più comuni sono: traumi, esposizione cronica all'umidità, iperidrosi, uso di cosmetici, psoriasi, infezioni micotiche (onicosi distale), dermatite atopica o da contatto, porfiria, assunzione di farmaci (bleomicina, vincristina, retinoidi, indometacina, clorpromazina) e fototossicità idiopatica indotta da tetracicline (Fig. 662-2) o cloramfenicolo.

Le **linee di Beau** sono solchi trasversali della lamina ungueale (Fig. 662-3), causati da una temporanea interruzione della formazione della lamina. Le linee compaiono a qualche settimana di distanza dall'evento responsabile del disturbo. Nella maggior parte dei neonati, tra la 4ª e la 6ª settimana si osserva l'apparizione di una linea unica, che si sposta in direzione distale in seguito alla crescita dell'unghia; è ipotizzabile che tale linea rifletta i cambiamenti metabolici successivi al parto. Nel bambino più grande, le linee di Beau indicano solitamente traumi ripetuti o una transitoria interruzione di attività della matrice, secondaria ad una malattia sistemica, come morbillo, parotide epidemica, polmonite o deficit di zinco. Nell'**onicomadesi**, le linee di Beau sono responsabili di una separazione del letto ungueale (Fig. 662-4).

ALTERAZIONI UNGUEALI ASSOCIATE A MALATTIE CUTANEE

In molti casi, le alterazioni ungueali sono associate ad altre malattie. Le anomalie tipiche della **psoriasi** includono: solchi, onicolisi, colorazione giallo-marrone e ispessimento. Le alterazioni del lichen planus includono: papule violacee nella piega ungueale prossimale

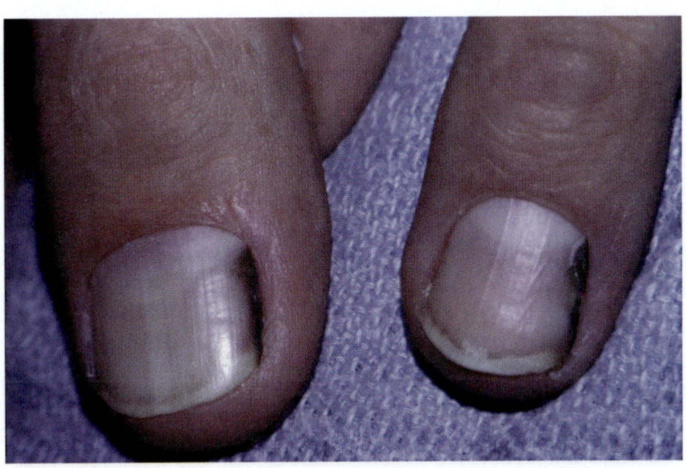

Fig. 662-1. Colorazione verde/nera del margine delle unghie secondaria a infezione da pseudomonas.

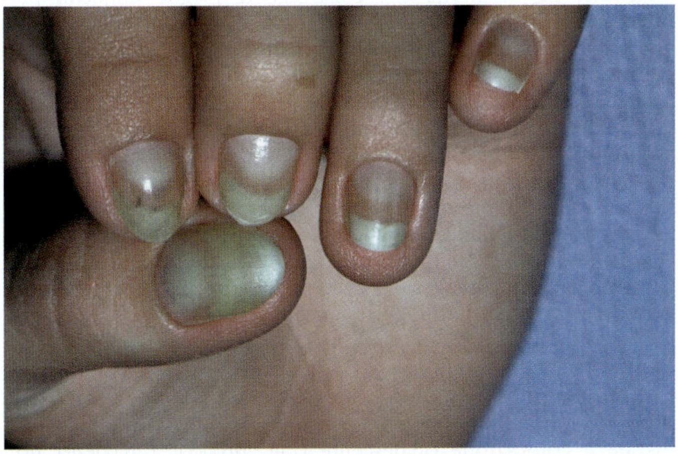

Fig. 662-2. Onicolisi distale secondaria all'uso di tetracicline orali e all'esposizione a luce ultravioletta.

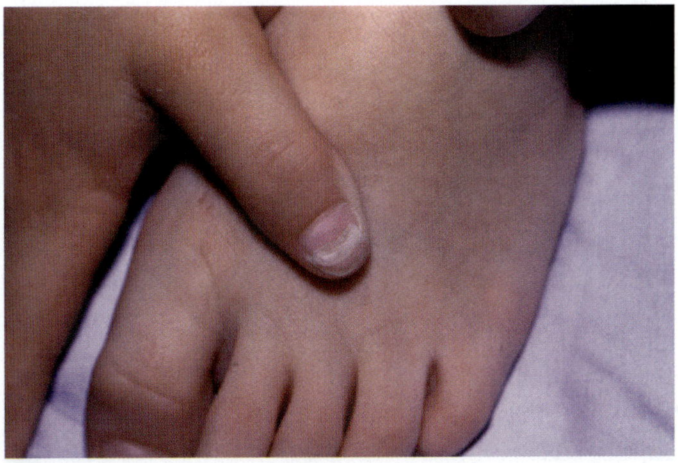

Figura 662-3. Linee di Beau. Lesione longitudinale dell'unghia.

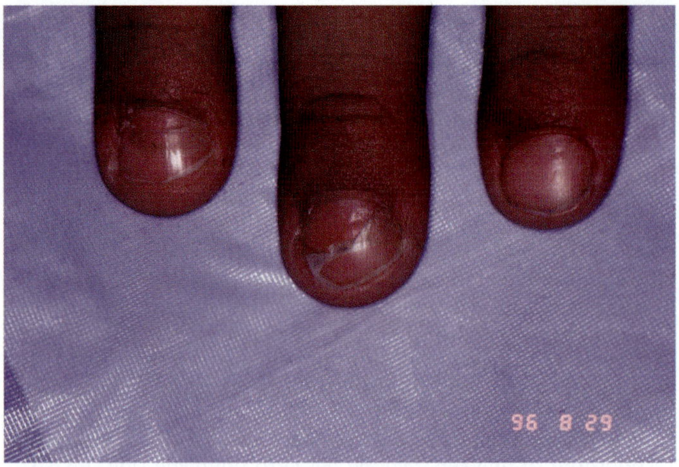

Figura 662-4. Onicomadesi. Separazione prossimale dal letto ungueale.

e nel letto, leuconichia, fessure longitudinali, assottigliamento dell'intera lamina ungueale e formazione di pterigio (anomala adesione della cuticola alla lamina ungueale o, in caso di distruzione focale della lamina, al letto ungueale). La malattia di Reiter può causare: un indurimento eritematoso doloroso della base della piega ungueale; una desquamazione paracheratosica subungueale; ispessimento, opacizzazione o formazione di creste sulla lamina ungueale. La dermatite che coinvolge le pieghe ungueali può provocare distrofia, irruvidimento o formazione di solchi. Le alterazioni ungueali sono più comuni nella dermatite atopica rispetto alle altre forme di dermatite che colpiscono le mani. La malattia di Darier è caratterizzata da strie rosse o bianche, che si estendono longitudinalmente e attraversano la lunula. Nel punto in cui le strie incontrano l'estremo distale dell'unghia, è talvolta presente un'incisura a forma di V. Può riscontrarsi anche leuconichia totale. File trasversali di piccole fossette sono caratteristiche dell'alopecia aerata. Nei casi più gravi, l'intera superficie dell'unghia risulta ruvida al tatto. I pazienti con acrodermatite enteropatica possono presentare solchi trasversali (linee di Beau) e distrofia ungueale, provocati dalla dermatite periungueale.

TRACHIONICHIA (DISTROFIA DELLE 20 UNGHIE). La trachionichia è caratterizzata da formazione di creste longitudinali e formazione di fossette, fragilità, assottigliamento, comparsa di un'intaccatura distale e colorazione opalescente (Fig. 662-5). I pazienti non presentano malattie cutanee o sistemiche associate, né manifestano altri difetti ectodermici. La sua occasionale associazione con l'alopecia aerata ha suggerito la possibilità che la trachionichia rifletta un'anomala risposta immunologica alla matrice ungueale. Studi istopatologici suggersicono invece che la malattia sia una manifestazione di lichen planus, psoriasi o infiammazione spongiotica (eczematosa) della matrice ungueale. La diagnosi differenziale è con infezioni micotiche, psoriasi, alterazioni ungueali dell'alopecia aerata e distrofia ungueale secondaria a eczema. L'eczema e le infezioni micotiche causano raramente alterazioni simultanee sulla totalità delle unghie. Il disordine è autolimitante, con remissione entro l'età adulta.

INFEZIONI DELLE UNGHIE

Le **infezioni micotiche** delle unghie sono classificate in 4 tipi. L'onicomicosi bianca superficiale si presenta con una decolorazione uniforme o punteggiata della superficie delle unghie dei piedi. È causata prevalentemente dall'invasione della lamina ungueale da parte di *Trichophyton mentagrophytes*. Tale organismo può essere raschiato via con una lama, ma il trattamento preferibile consiste nell'applicazione topica di un agente antimicotico a base di azoli. L'onicomicosi subungueale distale si presenta con focolai di onicolisi al di sotto della lamina distale o lungo il solco ungueale laterale, seguiti dallo sviluppo di ipercheratosi e discolorazione giallo-marrone. Il processo si estende in direzione prossimale, con conseguente ispessimento della lamina, sgretolamento (Fig. 662-6) e separazione dal letto. *Trichophyton rubrum*, e occasionalmente *T. mentagrophytes*, invadono le dita dei piedi; l'infezione alle dita delle mani è quasi esclusivamente causata da *T. rubrum*, talvolta associato a desquamazione della superficie plantare del piede e spesso di una mano. Tali dermatofiti si individuano più facilmente nell'area prossimale del letto ungueale o nella adiacente porzione ventrale della lamina. Le **terapie topiche** (come una lacca a base di ciclopirox all'8%) sono efficaci in caso di infezioni di una sola unghia. Grazie alla loro emivita lunga, terbinafina o itraconazolo sono efficaci ricorrendo a terapia pulsata (1 settimana al mese, per 3-4 mesi). Entrambi gli agenti menzionati sono preferibili a griseofulvina, fluconazolo o chetoconazolo. I rischi, in particolare l'epatotossicità, e i costi della terapia orale devono essere soppesati con i benefici di un disordine che causa soltanto problemi estetici.

L'onicomicosi bianca prossimale subungueale si verifica quando l'organismo, generalmente *T. rubrum*, penetra nell'unghia attraverso la piega ungueale, causando la colorazione giallo-bianca di porzioni della superficie inferiore della lamina ungueale. La superficie dell'unghia non è coinvolta. Il disturbo si verifica quasi esclusivamente in pazienti immunocompromessi ed è una delle manifestazioni più facilmente riconoscibili dell'AIDS.

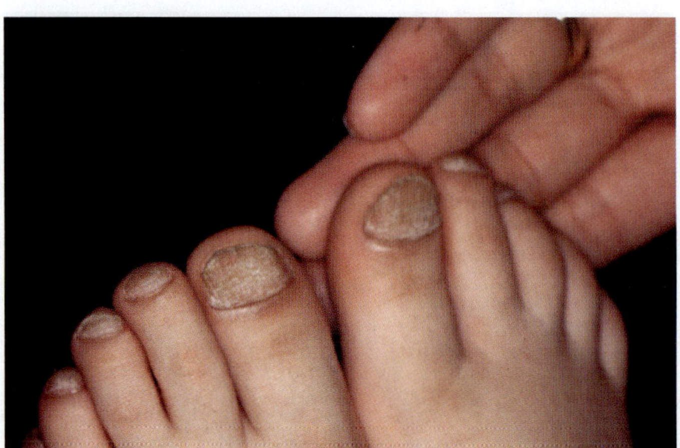

Figura 662-5. Distrofia di tutte le unghie nella trachionichia.

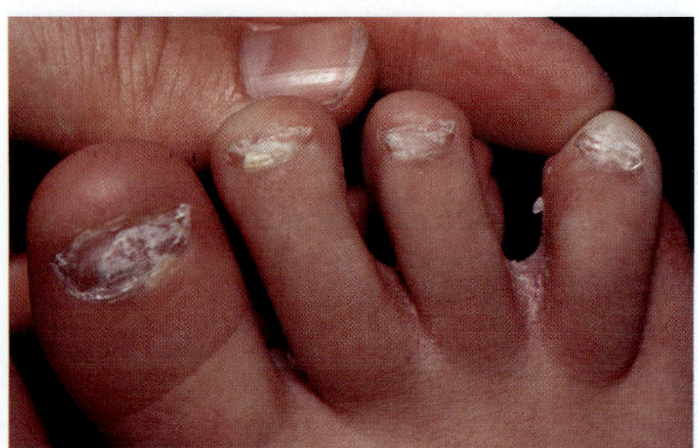

Figura 662-6. Discolorazione, ipercheratosi e sgretolamento dell'unghia secondari a infezione da dermatofiti.

L'onicomicosi da *Candida* coinvolge l'intera lamina ungueale in pazienti con candidiasi mucocutanea. È comune anche nei pazienti con AIDS. L'organismo, generalmente *Candida albicans*, entra distalmente o lungo le pieghe laterali, coinvolgendo rapidamente l'intero spessore della lamina ungueale e causando ispessimento, sgretolamento e deformità della lamina. Gli agenti antimicotici topici a base di azoli sono sufficienti per il trattamento dell'onicomicosi da *Candida* in un ospite immunocompetente, mentre in presenza di deficit immunitari è necessario ricorrere ad agenti orali.

PARONICHIA

La paronichia è un'infiammazione acuta o cronica, che generalmente coinvolge 1 o 2 pieghe ungueali delle dita. La paronichia acuta si presenta con eritema, sensazione di calore, edema e sensibilità della piega prossimale, solitamente in seguito all'invasione di stafilococchi o streptococchi (Fig. 662-7). Impacchi caldi e antibiotici orali (clindamicina o amoxicillina più acido clavulanico) sono generalmente efficaci; l'incisione o il drenaggio sono occasionalmente necessari. Lo sviluppo della paronichia cronica è una conseguenza della prolungata immersione in acqua (come nel bambino che si succhia il pollice; Fig. 662-8), dell'esposizione a soluzioni irritanti, di traumi o di malattie (come il fenomeno di Raynaud, le malattie vascolari del collagene o il diabete). La tumefazione della piega ungueale prossimale è seguito dalla separazione dell'unghia dalla lamina e dalla suppurazione. Corpi estranei penetrati nel derma si trasformano in un focolaio di infiammazione e infezione da *Candida* e da flora batterica mista. Il successo del trattamento della paronichia cronica richiede una combinazione dei seguenti elementi: attenzione ai fattori predisponenti; abitudine ad asciugarsi accuratamente le mani; applicazione di una soluzione di timolo al 4%; ricorso ad agenti antiinfiammatori, antibatterici e antimicotici topici.

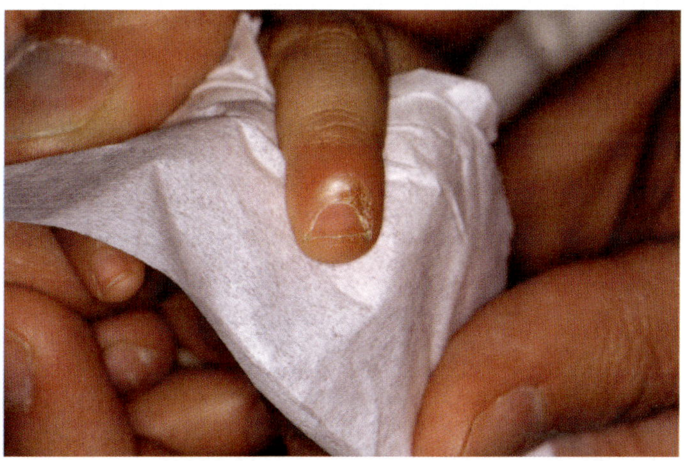

Figura 662-7. Paronichia acuta secondaria a *Staphylococcus aureus*.

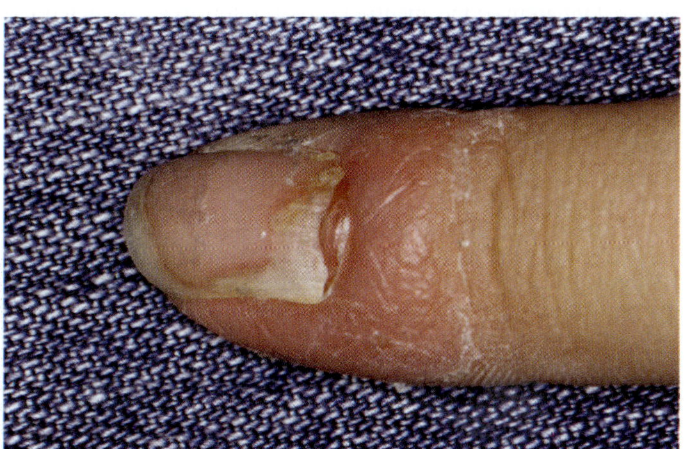

Figura 662-8. Paronichia cronica con eritema e separazione laterale della piega ungueale.

L'unghia incarnita è il risultato della penetrazione nei tessuti molli del margine laterale dell'unghia o di spicole che si separano dalla lamina ungueale. Nei casi acuti, si riscontrano eritema, edema e dolore localizzato solitamente all'alluce. Episodi ricorrenti possono condurre alla formazione di tessuto di granulazione. I fattori predisponenti includono: (1) difetti congeniti di allineamento (specialmente a carico dell'alluce); (2) compressione del lato dell'alluce da parte della scarpa, in particolare se l'alluce è insolitamente lungo e le pieghe ungueali laterali prominenti; (3) scorretta modalità curvilinea di taglio delle unghie. La **gestione** del disordine include l'abitudine a indossare scarpe comode e a tagliare le unghie solo quando crescono oltre il margine superiore del dito. Possono essere utili anche impacchi caldi e antibiotici orali (in presenza di cellulite della piega laterale). Nei casi gravi e ricorrenti, è talvolta richiesta l'applicazione di nitrato d'argento sul tessuto granulomatoso, l'avulsione dell'unghia o l'escissione della faccia laterale, seguita da matricectomia.

TUMORI DELL'AREA PARONICHIALE

I tumori dell'area paronichiale includono granulomi piogenici, cisti mucose, esostosi subungueali e nevi giunzionali. I fibromi periungueali che compaiono nella tarda infanzia suggeriscono la diagnosi di sclerosi tuberosa.

Fawcett RS, Linford S, Stullberg DL: Nail abnormalities: Clues to systemic disease. *Am Fam Physician* 2004;69:1417–1424.

Fistarol SK, Itin PH: Nail changes in genodermatoses. *Eur J Dermatol* 2002;12:119–128.

Grover C, Khandpur S, Reddy BS, et al: Longitudinal nail biopsy: Utility in 20-nail dystrophy. *Dermatol Surg* 2003;29:1125–1129.

Gupta AK, Ryder JE, Skinner AR: Treatment of onychomychosis: Pros and cons of antifungal agents. *J Cutan Med Surg* 2004;8:25–30.

Herzberg AJ: Nail manifestations of systemic diseases. *Clin Podiatr Med Surg North Am* 2004;21:631–640.

Lembach L: Pediatric nail disorders. *Clin Podiatr Med Surg North Am* 2004;21:641–650.

Rockwell PG: Acute and chronic paronychia. *Am Fam Physcian* 2001;63:1113–1116.

Scheinfeld NS: Trachyonychia: A case report and review of manifestations, associations and treatments. *Cutis* 2003;71:299–302.

Capitolo 663 ■ Disordini delle membrane mucose Joseph G. Morelli

Le membrane mucose possono essere colpite da disturbi dello sviluppo, infezioni, malattie cutanee croniche e acute, genodermatosi, tumori maligni e benigni. In questo capitolo sono approfondite alcune delle più comuni malattie specifiche delle membrane mucose.

CHEILITE. Nella maggior parte dei casi, l'infiammazione delle labbra (cheilite) e degli angoli della bocca (cheilite angolare o perlèche) (Fig. 663-1) è causata da secchezza, dalla formazione di screpolature e dall'abitudine di leccarsi le labbra. Anche l'eccessiva salivazione e la scialorrea, in particolare in bambini con deficit neurologici, possono determinare un'irritazione cronica.

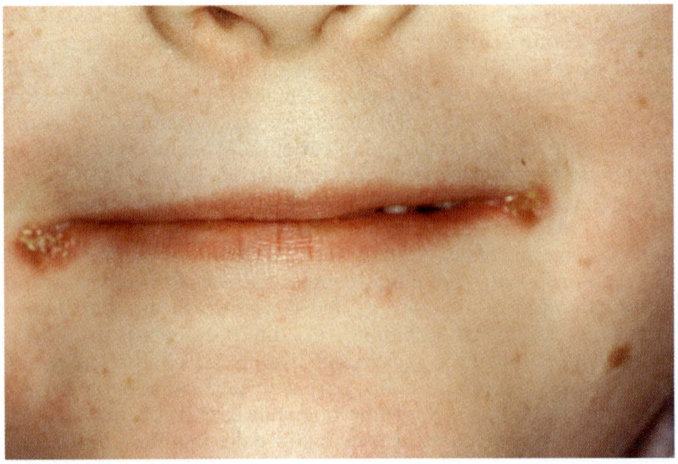

Figura 663-1. Cheilite angolare.

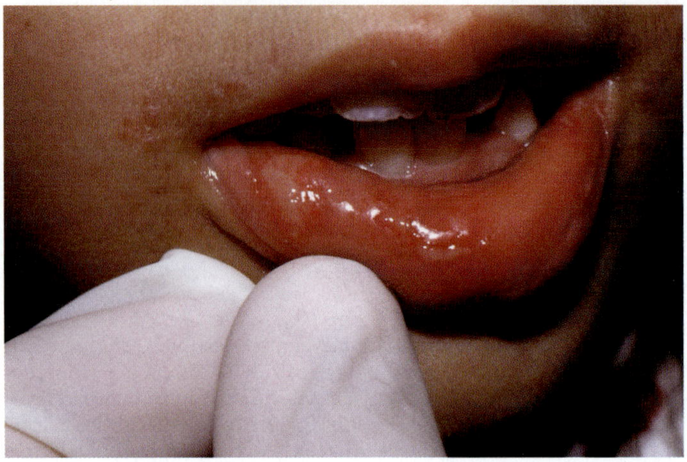

Figura 663-3. Ulcera aftosa sul labbro inferiore.

Le lesioni della candidosi orale (mughetto) possono estendersi occasionalmente agli angoli della bocca. La frequente applicazione di una blanda pomata a base di petrolato garantisce una protezione. La candidosi deve essere trattata con un adeguato agente antimicotico, mentre la dermatite da contatto della cute periorale richiede l'applicazione topica di un corticosteroide leggero e il frequente utilizzo di vaselina o di un emolliente analogo.

GRANULI DI FORDYCE. Si tratta di piccole papule giallo-bianche, del tutto asintomatiche, che compaiono sul bordo vermiglio delle labbra e della mucosa buccale. Tali ghiandole sebacee ectopiche si riscontrano in individui sani e non richiedono alcuna terapia.

MUCOCELE. Le cisti da ritenzione di muco sono papule bluastre non dolenti, tese e fluttuanti, del diametro di 2-10 mm, localizzate su labbra (Fig. 663-2), lingua, palato o mucosa buccale. La ritenzione della secrezione mucosa è il risultato della rottura traumatica del dotto di una ghiandola salivare minore. Le cisti localizzate sul pavimento buccale sono dette ranule quando implicano il coinvolgimento dei dotti sublinguali o salivari. Oscillazioni delle dimensioni sono comuni e le lesioni possono scomparire temporaneamente in seguito a rottura traumatica. La recidiva è prevenuta mediante escissione del mucocele.

STOMATITE AFTOSA (ULCERA AFTOSA DELLA BOCCA). È costituita da ulcere dolorose, singole o multiple, sulla mucosa labiale (Fig. 663-3), buccale, linguale, sublinguale, palatale o gengivale. Le lesioni possono esordire come papule dure ed eritematose, che si erodono rapidamente, formando ulcere necrotiche ben circoscritte, con un essudato fibroso e circondate da un anello eritematoso. Le ulcere aftose minori, non superiori a 2-10 mm di diametro, guariscono spontaneamente in 7-10 giorni. Le ulcere più grandi, con diametro superiore a 10 mm, si risolvono in 10-30 giorni. Un terzo tipo di ulcerazione aftosa, di aspetto erpetiforme, si presenta con lesioni raggruppate di 1-2 mm, che tendono a confluire in placche, e guariscono in 7-10 giorni. In circa un terzo dei pazienti con lesioni ricorrenti si riscontra un'anamnesi familiare positiva per il disordine. (Vedi Capitolo 312 per la diagnosi differenziale.)

L'eziologia della stomatite aftosa è probabilmente multifattoriale; il disturbo costituisce probabilmente la manifestazione orale di diverse malattie. Un'alterazione della regolazione locale del sistema immunologico cellulomediato, successiva all'attivazione e all'accumulo di cellule T citotossiche, può contribuire alla lesione mucosa localizzata. L'idea che la stomatite aftosa sia una manifestazione dell'infezione da *herpes simplex* è un luogo comune errato. Infezioni erpetiche ricorrenti restano localizzate alle labbra e raramente attraversano la giunzione mucocutanea; il coinvolgimento della mucosa orale si riscontra solo nelle infezioni primarie.

Il **trattamento** della stomatite aftosa è palliativo. La maggior parte dei casi lievi non richiede alcuna terapia. Il dolore, in particolare durante i pasti, può essere alleviato con l'uso di un anestetico topico, come la lidocaina, o mediante sciacqui con una soluzione composta da difenidramina elisir, lidocaina viscosa e un antacido orale. Subito dopo l'assunzione di un anestetico locale è importante evitare cibi o bevande troppo caldi. I corticosteroidi topici in una formulazione aderente alla mucosa possono contribuire a ridurre l'infiammazione, mentre l'uso di collutori a base di tetraciclina accelera la guarigione. Nei casi più gravi e debilitanti, è utile ricorrere a una terapia sistemica con corticosteroidi, colchicina, cimetidina o dapsone.

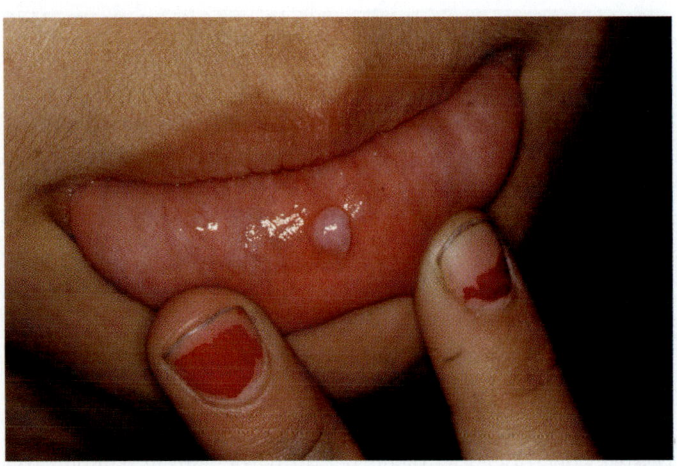

Figura 663-2. Mucocele sul labbro inferiore.

SINDROME DI COWDEN (SINDROME DEGLI AMARTOMI MULTIPLI). Questo disordine, a trasmissione autosomica dominante, si presenta solitamente nella seconda o terza decade, con papule lisce biancastre o rosa sulle mucose labiale, palatale, buccale e gengivale. La sindrome è causata da mutazioni del gene soppressore tumorale PTEN. La coalescenza dei fibromi benigni è responsabile del particolare aspetto a ciottolato. Numerose papule color carne si sviluppano sul volto, in particolare attorno a bocca, naso e orecchie. Nella maggior parte dei casi, si tratta di trichilemmomi, neoplasie benigne del follicolo pilifero. Reperti associati includono papule cheratosiche acrali, gozzo, polipi gastrointestinali, noduli fibrocistici della mammella e carcinoma mammario o tiroideo.

PERLE DI EPSTEIN (CISTI GENGIVALI DEL NEONATO). Consistono in cisti bianche contenenti cheratina, localizzate sulla mucosa palatale o alveolare di circa l'80% dei neonati. Non causano alcun sintomo e generalmente scompaiono nel giro di qualche settimana.

LINGUA A CARTA GEOGRAFICA (GLOSSITE MIGRANTE BENIGNA). Questa particolare forma di glossite consiste nella presenza sul dorso della lingua di placche rosse, lisce e irregolari, dai contorni ben demarcati, causate da atrofia transitoria delle papille filiformi della superficie epiteliale, spesso con margini grigi e rilevati, composti da papille filiformi di spessore superiore al normale (Fig. 663-4). Sintomi come un leggero bruciore o irritazione risultano talvolta fastidiosi. L'esordio è rapido e la distribuzione delle placche può modificarsi velocemente, anche nel corso di qualche ora o giorno. Alcuni pazienti hanno l'impressione che il disturbo sia esacerbato dallo stress e dall'assunzione di cibi caldi o piccanti. L'istologia della lingua a carta geografica è simile a quella della psoriasi pustolosa. Non è necessaria alcuna terapia e l'unico intervento richiesto è la rassicurazione del paziente.

LINGUA SCROTALE (FESSURATA). Circa l'1% dei lattanti e il 2,5% dei bambini presentano molte pieghe con solchi profondi sulla superficie dorsale della lingua, che le conferiscono un aspetto grinzoso o a ciottolato. Alcuni casi sono congeniti, causati da un'incompleta fusione delle due metà della lingua; altri, invece, si sviluppano in associazione a infezioni, traumi, malnutrizione o deficit di vitamina A. Molti pazienti con lingua fessurata presentano anche una lingua a carta geografica. Particelle di cibo possono restare intrappolate nelle fessure, determinando irritazione, infiammazione e alitosi. Si raccomanda perciò al paziente di pulire accuratamente la lingua con uno spazzolino a setole morbide o utilizzando un collutorio.

LINGUA NERA VILLOSA. Il dorso della lingua è ricoperto da una patina scura, causata da iperplasia e allungamento delle papille filiformi. La crescita eccessiva di batteri cromogeni e di funghi e residui pigmentati intrappolati che adsorbono placche microbiche e cheratina desquamante possono contribuire alla colorazione scura. Le alterazioni esordiscono solitamente nella parte posteriore della lingua, per poi estendersi anteriormente sul dorso. Il disordine è più comune negli adulti, ma può manifestarsi anche durante l'adolescenza. I fattori predisponenti includono una scarsa igiene orale e un'eccessiva crescita batterica, trattamenti con antibiotici sistemici come la tetraciclina (che favorisce la crescita di *Candida* spp.) e l'abitudine al fumo. La terapia prevede unicamente il miglioramento delle pratiche igieniche e l'utilizzo di uno spazzolino a setole morbide.

LEUCOPLACHIA ORALE VILLOSA. Questo disturbo, prevalentemente asintomatico, insorge nel 25% circa dei pazienti con AIDS, mentre è raro nella popolazione pediatrica. Si presenta con un ispessimento e un'accentuazione delle normali pieghe verticali dei margini laterali della lingua. La mucosa appare bianca e irregolarmente ispessita, ma rimane morbida. Talvolta i sintomi possono diffondersi alla superficie ventrale, al pavimento buccale, ai pilastri tonsillari e alla faringe. La malattia è causata dal virus di Epstein-Barr, presente nello strato superiore dell'epitelio colpito. Le placche sono prive di potenziale maligno. Il disordine si riscontra prevalentemente nei pazienti con HIV, ma può svilupparsi anche in individui immunodepressi per altre ragioni (come un trapianto d'organo, la leucemia o la chemioterapia). Tale patologia è generalmente asintomatica e non richiede alcun trattamento.

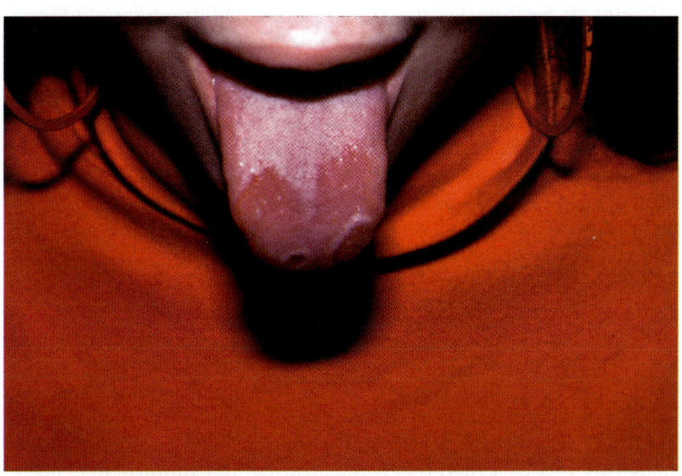

Figura 663-4. Lingua a carta geografica.

GENGIVITE ULCEROSA NECROTIZZANTE ACUTA (STOMATITE DI VINCENT, GENGIVITE FUSOSPIRILLARE, "TRENCH MOUTH"). Questo disordine si presenta con ulcere perforate, necrosi e sanguinamento delle papille interdentali. Una pseudomembrana biancogrigiastra può ricoprire le ulcerazioni. Le lesioni possono diffondersi, coinvolgendo la mucosa buccale, le labbra, la lingua, le tonsille e la faringe; sono talvolta associate a dolore dentale, bocca amara, febbricola e linfoadenopatia. Nella maggior parte dei casi, il disturbo si presenta nella seconda o terza decade, in seguito a scarsa igiene orale, scorbuto o pellagra. È stato ipotizzato che un'associazione sinergica tra i microrganismi fusospirillari (*Fusobacterium nucleatum*) e *Borrelia vincentii* contribuisca alla patogenesi.

La **noma** è una grave forma di stomatite gangrenosa fusospirillare, che si presenta prevalentemente in bambini malnutriti di età tra i 2 e i 5 anni, precedentemente colpiti da una delle seguenti malattie: morbillo, scarlattina, tubercolosi, tumori maligni o immunodeficienza. Papule rosse, dure e dolenti, si sviluppano sul margine alveolare, seguite da ulcerazione e distruzione gangrenosa mutilante del tessuto della regione oronasale. La patologia può coinvolgere anche il cuoio capelluto, il collo, le spalle, il perineo e la vulva. La ***noma neonatorum*** si presenta nel primo mese di vita, con lesioni gangrenose su labbra, naso, bocca e regione anale. I neonati colpiti sono spesso piccoli per l'età gestazionale, malnutriti, prematuri e si ammalano facilmente, in particolare in seguito a sepsi da *Pseudomonas aeruginosa*. La gestione della malattia implica il supporto nutrizionale, lo sbrigliamento conservativo di tessuti molli necrotici, la somministrazione empirica di antibiotici ad ampio spettro, come penicillina e metronidazolo, e di antibiotici attivi contro Pseudomonas in caso di *noma neonatorum*.

Akintoye SO, Greenberg MS: Recurrent aphthous stomatitis. *Dent Clin North Am* 2005;49:31–47.

Baurmash HD: Mucocoeles and ranulas. *J Oral Maxillofac Surg* 2003; 61:369–378.

Folayan MO: The epidemiology, etiology, and pathology of acute necrotizing gingivitis associated with malnutrition. *J Contemp Dent Pract* 2004; 5:28–41.

Laskin DM, Giglio JA, Rippert ET: Differential diagnosis of tongue lesions. *Quintessence Int* 2003;34:331–342.

Capitolo 664 ■ Infezioni cutanee batteriche Joseph G. Morelli

L'infezione cutanea batterica è la diagnosi singola più comune tra i bambini con problemi cutanei ed è responsabile del 17% di tutte le visite cliniche. L'infezione cutanea batterica più comune nel bambino è l'impetigine, che riguarda il 10% circa di tutte le patologie cutanee.

IMPETIGINE

Vedi Capitoli 182 e 180.

MANIFESTAZIONI CLINICHE

Impetigine non bollosa. Esistono due forme classiche di impetigine: non bollosa e bollosa. L'**impetigine non bollosa** riguarda più del 70% dei casi. Le lesioni esordiscono tipicamente sulla cute del viso o delle estremità, in presenza di un trauma. Le lesioni più comuni che precedono l'impetigine non bollosa comprendono punture di insetto, abrasioni, lacerazioni, varicella, scabbia e ustioni. Inizialmente si forma una minuscola vescicola o pustola, che rapidamente evolve a crosta color miele, generalmente di diametro inferiore a 2 cm (Fig. 664-1). L'infezione si può diffondere ad altre parti del corpo attraverso le dita, i vestiti e gli asciugamani. Le lesioni sono asintomatiche o poco dolorose e possono essere circondate da eritema; di solito sono assenti segni sistemici. Il prurito è presente solo occasionalmente; l'adenopatia regionale si riscontra nel 90% dei casi e la leucocitosi in circa il 50%. In genere la patologia si risolve spontaneamente senza residuare cicatrice, in circa 2 settimane; non è quindi necessario alcun trattamento. La **diagnosi differenziale** dell'impetigine non bollosa comprende infezioni virali (*herpes simplex*, varicella-zoster), fungine (*tinea corporis*, kerion) e parassitarie (scabbia, *pediculosis capitis*), che possono tutte impetiginizzare.

Staphylococcus aureus è il microrganismo più frequente nell'impetigine non bollosa negli Stati Uniti; *Streptococcus* β-Emolitico di gruppo A (SBEA) è implicato nello sviluppo di alcune lesioni. *Staphylococcus* generalmente diffonde dal naso alla cute normale, e poi la infetta. Al contrario, lo SBEA colonizza la cute in media 10 giorni prima dello sviluppo dell'impetigine. Lo SBEA colonizza poi il nasofaringe, in media 2-3 settimane dopo la comparsa della lesione impetiginosa. La cute funge da sorgente di SBEA e da probabile sorgente primaria per la diffusione dell'impetigine. Le lesioni dell'impetigine non bollosa che provocano la crescita colturale di stafilococchi non sono distinguibili clinicamente da quelle dovute invece a SBEA. Mentre *S. aureus* può essere coltivato in vitro da lesioni impetiginose di bambini di tutte le età, lo SBEA è coltivato molto più frequentemente da bambini in età prescolare, ma è raro prima dei 2 anni, eccetto che nelle aree ad alta endemia. Sono diversi i tipi di *Staphylococcus* che provocano l'impetigine non bollosa, ma generalmente non appartengono al gruppo 2, che è associato invece alla Staphylococcal Scalded Skin Syndrome (SSSS) e alla sindrome da shock tossico. Nelle lesioni non bollose si trovano più frequentemente diversi sierotipi di SBEA, denominati "ceppi dell'impetigine", diversi da quelli che causano faringite.

Impetigine bollosa. Si tratta di un'infezione che riguarda principalmente neonati e bambini molto piccoli. L'impetigine bollosa è sempre provocata da *S. aureus*; circa l'80% appartiene al gruppo 2, e di questo il 60% è rappresentato dal tipo 71, mentre la maggior parte dei rimanenti è dei tipi 3A, 3B, 3C e 55. La malattia è caratterizzata da bolle flaccide, trasparenti, più frequenti sulla cute del viso, dei glutei, del tronco, del perineo e delle estremità. L'**impetigine bollosa del neonato** può esordire nella zona del pannolino. Le bolle si rompono facilmente, lasciando un'erosione superficiale, umida e a bordo esiguo. Eritema circostante e adenopatia regionale sono generalmente assenti. Contrariamente a quelle dell'impetigine non bollosa, le lesioni dell'impetigine bollosa rappresentano una manifestazione della SSSS localizzata, e si sviluppano su cute integra.

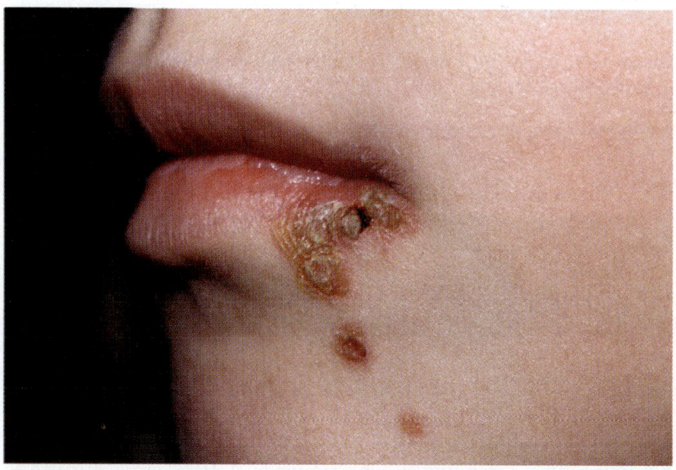

Figura 664-1. Lesioni impetiginose multiple crostose ed essudanti.

DIAGNOSI. Colture di liquidi provenienti da una bolla intatta o da croste umide forniscono informazioni sull'agente eziologico; se il paziente ha un aspetto sofferente, è necessario approntare anche emocolture. Le lesioni delle bolle impetiginose mostrano formazione di vescicole nella regione subcorneale o granulare, neutrofili e occasionalmente cellule acantolitiche nella bolla, spongiosi, edema del derma papillare, e un infiltrato misto di linfociti e neutrofili intorno ai vasi sanguigni del plesso superficiale. Se si escludono i casi in cui si può coltivare lo stafilococco dalle bolle o, meno frequentemente, lo si può osservare con la colorazione Gram, è impossibile differenziare le bolle impetiginose dal pemfigo fogliaceo o dalla dermatosi pustolosa subcorneale. L'impetigine non bollosa presenta reperti istopatologici simili a quelli della variante bollosa, eccetto che la formazione delle bolle è minima.

La **diagnosi differenziale** dell'impetigine bollosa nel neonato include l'epidermolisi bollosa, la mastocitosi bollosa, l'infezione erpetica e la SSSS. Nei bambini più grandi devono essere considerati anche dermatite allergica da contatto, ustioni, eritema multiforme, dermatosi cronica bollosa dell'infanzia, pemfigo e pemfigoide bolloso, soprattutto se le lesioni non rispondono alla terapia.

COMPLICANZE. Complicanze potenziali, anche se molto rare, dell'impetigine bollosa e non bollosa sono rappresentate da osteomielite, artrite settica, polmonite e setticemia. In bambini con lesioni cutanee localizzate, per altro sani, è molto raro trovare un'emocoltura positiva. In circa il 10% dei pazienti con impetigine non bollosa, e raramente dopo un'impetigine bollosa, è stata riportata cellulite. La malattia streptococcica occasionalmente è seguita da linfangite, linfoadenite suppurativa, psoriasi guttata e scarlattina. Non esiste correlazione tra il numero delle lesioni e il coinvolgimento clinico dei linfatici o lo sviluppo di cellulite in associazione all'impetigine streptococcica.

L'infezione con ceppi nefritogeni di SBEA può portare a **glomerulonefrite acuta post-streptococcica** (vedi Capitolo 511.1). Il carattere clinico delle lesioni dell'impetigine non è predittivo di sviluppo di glomerulonefrite post-streptococcica. Il gruppo di età colpito con maggiore frequenza è quello compreso tra i 3 e i 7 anni. Il periodo latente tra l'esordio dell'impetigine e lo sviluppo della glomerulonefrite è in media 18-21 giorni, che è più lungo del periodo di latenza di 10 giorni dopo una faringite. La glomerulonefrite post-streptococcica si verifica epidemicamente dopo un'infezione faringea o cutanea. Le epidemie associate a impetigine sono causate dai gruppi M2, 49, 53, 55, 56, 57 e 60. Ceppi di SBEA associati a impetigine endemica negli Stati Uniti hanno un potenziale patogeno renale scarso o assente. La febbre reumatica acuta non si verifica in seguito a impetigine.

TRATTAMENTO. Il trattamento antibiotico per via topica o sistemica è superiore al placebo. La pomata a base di mupirocina possiede attività battericida per l'inibizione reversibile della isoleuciltransfer RNA sintetasi batterica. Applicata topicamente 3 volte al giorno per 7-10 giorni, ha un'efficacia uguale o maggiore, con meno effetti collaterali, rispetto all'eritromicina etilsuccinato per via orale, alla dose di 30-50 mg/kg/die per 7-10 giorni. Sono stati registrati rari casi di resistenza batterica alla mupirocina, ma la maggior parte dei pazienti era stata trattata irregolarmente o a scopo profilattico per più di 2 settimane. Anche l'acido fusidico per uso topico può essere efficace.

Si preferisce la terapia sistemica con un antibiotico orale β-lattamasi-resistente nei pazienti con interessamento diffuso, quando le lesioni sono vicine alla bocca, dove il farmaco può avere contatto con la mucosa orale, o nei casi con evidente interessamento degli strati più profondi, comprese cellulite, foruncolosi, formazione di ascesso o linfoadenite suppurativa. Nelle zone in cui *S. aureus* non manifesta resistenza all'eritromicina, l'eritromicina etilsuccinato (40 mg/kg/die divisi in 3-4 dosi giornaliere, per 7 giorni) o l'eritromicina estolato (30 mg/kg/die in 3-4 dosi giornaliere) rappresentano la **terapia orale elettiva**. Se nella comunità è diffusa la resistenza all'eritromicina, antibiotici alternativi efficaci nei bambini per il trattamento dell'impetigine sono dicloxacillina, amoxicillina più acido clavulanico, clindamicina, e cefalosporine come cefalexina, ceflacor, cefadroxil, cefprozil o cefpodoxime. La scelta tra questi farmaci può essere fatta in base a fattori di costo, disponibilità locale e compliance. I macrolidi claritromicina e azitromicina possono essere vantaggiosi soprattutto nei casi di intolleranza all'eritromicina, ma non offrono una percentuale di guarigione superiore all'eritromicina stessa. Non ci sono dati che suggeriscano che una terapia protratta per 10 giorni sia migliore di una della durata di 7 giorni. Se non si ottiene una risposta soddisfacente entro 7 giorni è necessario eseguire una coltura da tampone, sollevando il bordo della crosta. Se si trova un microrganismo resistente, è necessario somministrare un antibiotico adeguato per altri 7 giorni.

INFEZIONI DEL TESSUTO SOTTOCUTANEO

Fra le infezioni del tessuto molle si distinguono principalmente forme non necrotizzanti e forme necrotizzanti. Le prime rispondono alla sola terapia antibiotica, mentre le seconde richiedono, oltre alla terapia antibiotica, la rapida rimozione chirurgica di tutto il tessuto necrotico. Le infezioni necrotizzanti del tessuto molle sono patologie potenzialmente pericolose per la vita, caratterizzate da rapida distruzione del tessuto locale e da tossicità sistemica. La necrosi tissutale si differenzia poi dalla cellulite. In quest'ultima, il processo infiammatorio infettivo coinvolge il tessuto sottocutaneo, ma non lo distrugge. Le infezioni necrotizzanti del tessuto molle caratteristicamente si presentano con scarsi segni cutanei precoci, in rapporto alla rapidità e al grado di distruzione del tessuto sottocutaneo.

CELLULITE. La cellulite è caratterizzata da infezione e infiammazione del tessuto connettivo lasso, con coinvolgimento limitato del derma e relativo risparmio dell'epidermide. Una lesione cutanea dovuta a trauma pregresso, chirurgia, o a una preesistente lesione cutanea, predispongono a cellulite. La cellulite è anche più frequente in individui immunosoppressi, con stasi linfatica o diabete mellito.

Eziologia. Gli agenti eziologici più comuni sono *Streptococcus pyogenes* e *S. aureus*. Occasionalmente sono microrganismi causali anche *Streptococcus pneumoniae*, streptococchi di gruppo G e C, streptococchi di gruppo B nei neonati, o, raramente, *Escherichia coli*. In pazienti immunocompromessi o diabetici, possono essere coinvolti molti altri agenti batterici o micotici, soprattutto *Pseudomonas aeruginosa*, *Aeromonas hidrophila* e, occasionalmente, altri enterobatteri, *Legionella* spp., *Mucorales*, particolarmente *Rhizopus* spp., *Mucor* spp., *Absidia* spp. e *Criptococcus neoformans*. Bambini con sindrome nefrotica recidivante possono sviluppare cellulite da *Eschirichia coli*. In bambini dal terzo mese fino a 3-5 anni, *Haemophilus influenzae* di tipo b è stato una causa importante di cellulite facciale, ma la sua incidenza è significativamente diminuita dopo l'istituzione di un'efficace vaccinazione contro questo microrganismo.

Manifestazioni cliniche. La cellulite si presenta clinicamente come un'area edematosa, calda, eritematosa e dolente. I margini laterali tendono a essere indistinti, perché il processo è situato profondamente nella cute, coinvolgendo principalmente il tessuto sottocutaneo e poi il derma. Premendo si può produrre una fossetta (fovea). Sebbene non sia possibile una distinzione certa in ogni singolo paziente, la cellulite da *S. aureus* tende a essere più localizzata e può suppurare, mentre le infezioni da *S. pyogenes* (streptococco di gruppo A) tendono a diffondersi più rapidamente e possono associarsi a linfangite. Sono frequenti adenopatia regionale, segni sistemici e sintomi di febbre, di raffreddamento e malessere. Le complicanze della cellulite comprendono ascesso sottocutaneo, batteriemia, osteomielite, artrite settica, tromboflebite, endocardite e fascite necrotizzante. Un'infezione da *S. pyogenes* può essere seguita anche da linfangite o glomerulonefrite.

Diagnosi. Nel 25% dei casi di cellulite, aspirati dalle sede dell'infiammazione, biopsia cutanea ed emocolture permettono di identificare l'organismo in causa. L'ottenimento di un campione contenente il microrganismo causale si ha in circa il 30% dei casi in cui la sede d'origine della cellulite è apparente, come per esempio un'abrasione o un'ulcera. Un aspirato eseguito nel punto di massima infiammazione è in grado di isolare il microrganismo responsabile più spesso rispetto a uno eseguito sui margini della lesione. Il mancato isolamento del microrganismo è dovuto principalmente a un basso numero di microrganismi nella lesione.

Trattamento. La terapia empirica della cellulite dovrebbe basarsi sulla storia della malattia, su localizzazione e caratteristiche della cellulite, sull'età e sullo stato immunitario del paziente. In un neonato, la cellulite richiede una valutazione completa della sepsi e una successiva terapia empirica per via endovenosa con un antibiotico antistafilococcico β-lattamasi-stabile, come la meticillina (la vancomicina è un'altra possibilità), e un aminoglicosidico, come la gentamicina, o una cefalosporina come il cefotaxime. Il trattamento della cellulite in un lattante o in un bambino con meno di 5 anni necessita di una copertura per *S. pyogenes* e *S. aureus*, così come per *H. influenzae* di tipo b e *S. pneumoniae*. La valutazione dovrebbe includere un'emocultura e, se il bambino ha meno di 1 anno, se sono presenti segni di tossicità sistemica o se non sia possibile un adeguato esame, anche una puntura lombare. Nella maggior parte dei casi di cellulite a un'estremità, indipendentemente dall'età, la causa è rappresentata da *S. aureus* e da *S. pyogenes*, ed è altamente improbabile la presenza batteriemia in bambini altrimenti sani. In caso si sospetti una sepsi sono necessarie emocolture. In assenza di febbre, adenopatia e di altri segni sistemici (conta dei leucociti <15 000), è possibile iniziare il trattamento della cellulite di un'estremità per via orale, ambulatorialmente, con una penicillina penicillinasi-resistente come la dicloxacillina o la cloxacillina, o una cefalosporina di prima generazione come la cefalexina, oppure, se si sospetta uno stafilococco resistente alla meticillina, con la clindamicina. Se non si nota miglioramento, o se la malattia progredisce significativamente nelle prime 24-48 ore di trattamento, è necessario passare alla terapia per via parenterale. In presenza di febbre, linfoadenopatia o segni sistemici, la terapia va somministrata per via parenterale sin dall'inizio. Nella maggior parte dei casi, l'oxacillina e la nafcillina sono efficaci, ma in presenza di tossicità sistemica significativa si deve prendere in considerazione la possibilità di aggiungere clindamicina o vancomicina. Dal momento in cui si registra una significativa diminuzione di eritema, di calore, di edema e di febbre, il trattamento del paziente va protratto per altri 10 giorni su base ambulatoriale. Immobilizzando e tenendo sollevato l'arto colpito, particolarmente se nella fase precoce di terapia, si può aiutare a ridurre tumefazione e dolore.

FASCITE NECROTIZZANTE. La fascite necrotizzante è un'infezione del tessuto sottocutaneo che coinvolge lo strato profondo della fascia superficiale ma risparmia in gran parte l'epidermide, la fascia profonda e il muscolo adiacenti.

Eziologia. Relativamente pochi microrganismi possiedono una virulenza tale da provocare fascite necrotizzante quando agiscono da soli. La maggior parte delle infezioni fulminanti, associata a sindrome da shock tossico e a un'alta percentuale di casi fatali, è causata da *S. pyogenes* (vedi Capitolo 182). La fascite necrotizzante streptococcica si può verificare in assenza di sindrome tossica shock-simile, ed è raramente fatale, ma può essere associata a considerevole morbilità. La fascite necrotizzante può occasionalmente essere provocata da *S. aureus*, *Clostridium perfrigens*, *Clostridium septicus*, *Pseudomonas aeruginosa*, *Vibrio* spp., soprattutto *Vibrio vulnificus*, e da miceti dell'ordine dei *Mucorales*, in particolare *Rhizopus* spp., *Mucor* spp. e *Absidia* spp. In rare occasioni sono stati riportati casi di fascite necrotizzante da streptococchi di gruppo non-A, o di gruppo B, C, F, o G, *S. pneumoniae*, o *H. influenzae* di tipo b. La fascite necrotizzante può anche essere polimicrobica. Nella maggior parte dei casi, la necrosi tissutale è causata da un insieme di batteri anaerobi, aerobi o facoltativi. I batteri aerobi o facoltativi più comuni sono rappresentati da alcune specie di streptococchi emolitici o non emolitici di gruppo non-A, *S. aureus*, *E. coli*, *Enterobacter* spp., e varie altre *Enterobacteriaceae* e *Pseudomonas* spp. Gli anaerobi presenti sono simili a quelli trovati negli ascessi sottocutanei: *Bacteroides* spp., *Poststreptococcus* spp., *Peptococcus* spp., *Prevotella* spp., *Porphyromonas* spp., *Clostridium* spp. e *Fusobacteriium* spp. Le infezioni dovute a un solo microrganismo o alla combinazione di alcuni di essi devono essere distinte clinicamente l'una dall'altra, sebbene lo sviluppo di **crepitio** segnali la presenza di *Clostridium* spp., o di bacilli Gram-negativi come *E. coli*, *Klesbiella*, *Proteus* e *Aeromonas*.

Epidemiologia. La fascite necrotizzante si può verificare in ogni parte del corpo. Le sedi più frequenti, tuttavia, sono le estremità, l'addome e la regione perineale. Frequenti condizioni predisponenti nei neonati sono l'onfalite e la balanite dopo circoncisione. L'incidenza della fascite necrotizzante è più alta nei soggetti con immunocompromissione sistemica o tissutale locale, nei pazienti diabetici, neoplastici o portatori di patologie vascolari periferiche, in quelli che sono stati sottoposti a interventi chirurgici, nei soggetti che abusano di sostanze per via endovenosa, o in coloro che sono in trattamento con farmaci immunosoppressori, particolarmente con corticosteroidi. L'infezione può comparire anche in individui sani dopo una piccola lesione da puntura, abrasioni o lacerazioni, o in seguito a trauma contusivo, interventi chirurgici, in particolare all'addome, al perineo e al tratto gastrointestinale o genitourinario, oppure a causa di un'iniezione con ago ipodermico. A partire dalla metà degli anni '80, si è verificata una ripresa di infezioni fulminanti necrotizzanti del tessuto molle da *S. pyogenes*, che possono manifestarsi in individui precedentemente sani, con minima o non apparente compromissione dell'integrità immunologica cutanea. La fascite necrotizzante da *S. pyogenes* può comparire dopo superinfezione di lesioni varicellose. Questi bambini tendono a presentare un esordio, una recrudescenza o una persistenza di febbre elevata e di segni di tossicità, dopo il terzo o quarto giorno di varicella.

Manifestazioni cliniche. La fascite necrotizzante esordisce in maniera acuta con edema locale, eritema, dolorabilità e calore. La febbre è quasi sempre presente; dolore, dolorabilità e segni sistemici sono sproporzionati rispetto ai segni cutanei, specialmente con il coinvolgimento della fascia e del muscolo. Linfangite e linfadenite sono solitamente assenti. L'infezione si diffonde lungo il piano della fascia superficiale e inizialmente vi sono pochi segni cutanei che possano suggerire la gravità e l'estensione della necrosi tissutale sottocutanea che si sta verificando. Le alterazioni cutanee possono comparire dopo 24-48 ore, per trombosi vascolare e ischemia cutanea. Reperti clinici precoci comprendono eritema ed edema cutanei mal definiti, che si estendono oltre l'area eritematosa. Sono segni ulteriori la formazione di bolle ripiene inizialmente di liquido paglierino, e più tardi di liquido da bluastro a emorragico, e iscurimento del tessuto colpito dal rosso, al porpora, al blu. In seguito all'ischemia e alla necrosi, si sviluppano anestesia cutanea e, infine, franca gangrena tissutale e perdita di sostanza. La formazione di vescicole o bolle, ecchimosi, crepitio, anestesia e necrosi sono segni infausti e indicano uno stadio avanzato della malattia. I bambini con lesioni varicellose possono all'inizio non mostrare segni cutanei di superinfezione da *S. pyogens* invasivo, quali eritema o edema. La fascite necrotizzante può essere associata a tossicità sistemica significativa, compresi shock, insufficienza d'organo e decesso. L'evoluzione della patologia, in questo quadro, può essere rapida, portando a morte nel giro di qualche ora. I pazienti con coinvolgimento della fascia muscolare superficiale e profonda tendono a manifestare forme più acute, con coinvolgimento sistemico, e vanno incontro a una progressione più rapida della malattia, rispetto a quelli in cui l'infezione si limita esclusivamente al tessuto sottocutaneo soprafasciale. Una **sindrome compartimentale** può svilupparsi a un'estremità; si manifesta con edema duro, dolore al movimento e perdita della sensibilità e del polso distali. Si tratta di un'emergenza chirurgica.

Diagnosi. La diagnosi definitiva viene fatta con l'esplorazione chirurgica, che deve essere eseguita precocemente, non appena si ponga il sospetto. La fascia necrotica e il tessuto sottocutaneo sono grigiastri e offrono una scarsa resistenza al sondaggio con sonda smussa. Sebbene la RM aiuti a delineare l'estensione e i piani tissutali coinvolti, questa procedura non deve ritardare l'intervento chirurgico. Sezioni congelate di campioni bioptici ottenuti nelle fasi precoci dell'infezione possono aiutare la gestione della malattia riducendo il tempo necessario per la diagnosi e stabilendo i margini di coinvolgimento. La colorazione di Gram del tessuto può essere particolarmente utile per evidenziare file di cocchi Gram-positivi, indicativi di infezione da *S. pyogenes*.

Trattamento. Sono indispensabili una precoce terapia di supporto, la rimozione chirurgica del tessuto necrotico e la somministrazione di antibiotici per via parenterale. Tutto il tessuto necrotico deve essere rimosso fino al sanguinamento dei bordi, e solitamente è indicato ripetere l'operazione entro 24-36 ore, per confermare che non sia rimasto tessuto necrotico. In molti casi, può essere necessario ripetere questa procedura più volte finché non cessa la formazione di tessuto necrotico. È fondamentale anche la pulizia quotidiana della ferita.

Non appena possibile va iniziata la terapia antibiotica per via parenterale, con farmaci ad ampio spettro, contro tutti i potenziali agenti patogeni. La maggior parte degli specialisti consiglia l'utilizzo iniziale di penicillina, ampicillina o nafcillina, insieme a clindamicina e a un aminoglicoside, per la copertura contro *S. pyogenes* e l'ampia varietà di potenziali patogeni anaerobi e Gram-negativi. Si aggiunge spesso la clindamicina, per inibire la sintesi proteica di nuove tossine batteriche necrotizzanti.

Prognosi. Il tasso di mortalità combinato tra i bambini e gli adulti con fascite necrotizzante e sindrome tossica shock-simile dovuta a *S. pyogenes* è del 60%. Tuttavia, nei bambini e nei casi con sindrome tossica shock-simile non complicata la morte è meno frequente.

STAPHYLOCOCCAL SCALDED SKIN SYNDROME, SSSS (MALATTIA DI RITTER)

MANIFESTAZIONI CLINICHE. La Staphylococcal Scalded Skin Syndrome (SSSS) si verifica soprattutto in neonati e bambini con meno di 5 anni, e comprende una serie di patologie che vanno dall'impetigine bollosa localizzata a forme cutanee generalizzate con coinvolgimento sistemico. L'esordio del rash può essere preceduto da malessere, febbre, irritabilità e intensa dolorabilità cutanea. Si sviluppa poi un **eritema scarlattiniforme** diffuso, accentuato nelle zone di flessione e intorno agli orifizi. Le congiuntive sono infiammate e talvolta diventano purulente. La cute, intensamente eritematosa, può rapidamente acquisire un aspetto rugoso e, nei casi severi, compaiono erosioni e bolle sterili, flaccide e diffuse. Sono caratteristiche la formazione di prominente eritema circumorale e di croste e fessurazioni intorno a occhi, bocca e naso. Durante questo stadio si possono avere aree di distacco epidermico in seguito a lieve sfregamento (segno di Nikolsky) (Fig. 664-2). Quando si ha il distacco di ampi lembi di epidermide si evidenziano aree scoperte brillanti e umide, dapprima alle pieghe e successivamente sulla maggior parte della superficie corporea; ciò può portare a infezione secondaria della cute, sepsi e alterazioni dei liquidi e degli elettroliti. La fase desquamativa inizia dopo 2-5 giorni dalla comparsa dell'eritema;

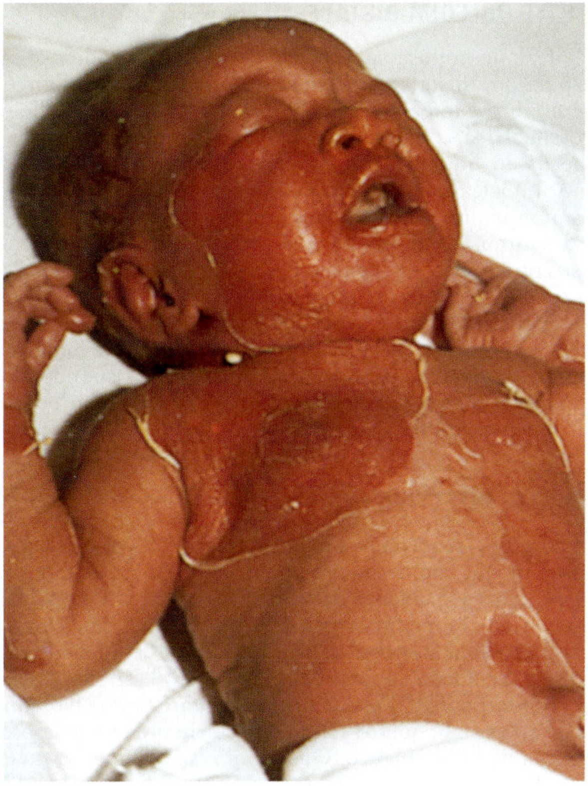

Figura 664-2. Neonato con Staphylococcal Scalded Skin Syndrome (SSSS).

la guarigione si verifica senza cicatrici in 10-14 giorni. I pazienti possono presentare faringite, congiuntivite ed erosioni superficiali delle labbra, ma la mucosa orale è risparmiata. Alcuni pazienti hanno un aspetto sofferente, mentre altri stanno abbastanza bene, se si esclude la marcata dolorabilità cutanea.

Una presunta forma **abortiva** della malattia si presenta con un eritroderma diffuso, molle, scarlattiniforme, accentuato nelle aree flessurali, ma che non progredisce fino alla formazione di bolle. In questi pazienti il segno di Nikolsky può essere assente. Sebbene l'esantema sia simile a quello streptococcico della scarlattina, sono assenti lingua a fragola e petecchie palatali. La SSSS può essere confusa con varie altre malattie bollose ed esfolianti, come l'impetigine bollosa, l'epidermolisi bollosa, l'ipercheratosi epidermolitica, il pemfigo, le eruzioni da farmaci, l'eritema multiforme e la necrolisi epidermica da farmaci. Quest'ultima può essere distinta in base all'anamnesi positiva per ingestione di farmaci, la presenza del segno di Nikolsky solo nelle sedi di eritema, l'assenza di croste periorali, la necrosi epidermica a tutto spessore, e un piano di clivaggio situato a maggiore profondità nell'epidermide.

EZIOLOGIA E PATOGENESI. La SSSS è causata principalmente da stafilococchi di gruppo 2, particolarmente i ceppi 71 e 55, che sono presenti in sedi localizzate dell'infezione. I foci d'infezione comprendono il nasofaringe e, meno frequentemente, l'ombelico, il tratto urinario, un'abrasione superficiale, congiuntiva e sangue. Le manifestazioni cliniche della SSSS sono mediate dalla diffusione per via ematogena, in assenza di specifici anticorpi antitossina, delle tossine stafilococciche epidermolitiche o esfolianti A o B. Le tossine hanno riprodotto la malattia sia in modelli animali sia in volontari umani. Una ridotta clearance renale delle tossine può giustificare il fatto che la malattia è molto frequente nei neonati e nei bambini molto piccoli. La tossina epidermolitica A è termostabile ed è codificata da geni cromosomici batterici. La tossina epidermolitica B è termolabile ed è codificata su un plasmide di 37,5 kb. La sede di clivaggio delle vescicole è subcorneale, attraverso lo strato granulare. Le tossine epidermolitiche paiono produrre una rottura dello strato granulare attraverso il legame con la desmogleina I dei desmosomi. I dati suggeriscono che le tossine fanno parte della famiglia delle serinoproteasi tripsina-simili, e che esercitano la loro azione tramite proteolisi.

DIAGNOSI. Le bolle intatte sono regolarmente sterili, diversamente da quelle dell'impetigine bollosa, ma è necessario ottenere colture da tutte le sedi sospette di infezione localizzata, oltre all'emocoltura, per identificare la sede dell'elaborazione delle tossine epidermolitiche. Lo scollamento subcorneale dello strato granulare può essere identificato con la biopsia cutanea. È caratteristica l'assenza di un infiltrato infiammatorio. Nei casi che richiedono una diagnosi rapida, lo strato corneale esfoliato può essere osservato su un campione bioptico coagulato di epidermide desquamata. Con la preparazione di Tzanck si possono osservare anche cellule acantolitiche sparse, evidenti nelle bolle fissurate.

TRATTAMENTO. Nei casi di coinvolgimento localizzato, è necessaria una terapia sistemica per via orale, o parenterale, con una penicillina semisintetica penicillinasi-resistente, perché di solito gli stafilococchi sono resistenti alla penicillina. Si può aggiungere la clindamicina per inibire la sintesi della proteina batterica (tossina). La cute deve essere delicatamente inumidita e detersa. L'applicazione di un emolliente permette la lubrificazione e diminuisce il fastidio. Non è necessaria terapia antibiotica topica. La guarigione solitamente è rapida, ma eventuali complicanze, come eccessiva perdita di liquidi, squilibrio elettrolitico, alterazione della termoregolazione, polmonite, setticemia e cellulite, possono provocare un aumento della morbilità.

ECTIMA (VEDI CAPITOLI 182 E 202)

L'ectima assomiglia all'impetigine non bollosa per quanto riguarda l'esordio e le manifestazioni, ma gradualmente evolve verso un'infezione più profonda e più cronica. La lesione iniziale è una vescicola o una vescicolopustola, con una base eritematosa, che si approfonda attraverso l'epidermide nel derma, formando un'ulcera con margini rilevati. L'ulcera viene ricoperta da una crosta secca, strettamente aderente (Fig. 664-3), che contribuisce alla persistenza dell'infezione e alla formazione di cicatrici. Le lesioni, che si localizzano principalmente alle gambe, possono diffondersi per autoinoculazione e avere un'ampiezza fino a 4 cm. I fattori predisponenti sono scarsa igiene, malnutrizione e lesioni pruriginose, come punture di insetti, scabbia o pediculosi, soggette a frequente grattamento. Le complicanze includono linfangite, cellulite e, raramente, glomerulonefrite poststreptococcica. L'agente eziologico è in genere lo streptococco β-emolitico di gruppo A; anche *S. aureus* viene coltivato dalla maggior parte delle lesioni, ma si tratta probabilmente di un agente patogeno secondario. Le croste devono essere ammorbidite con garze calde

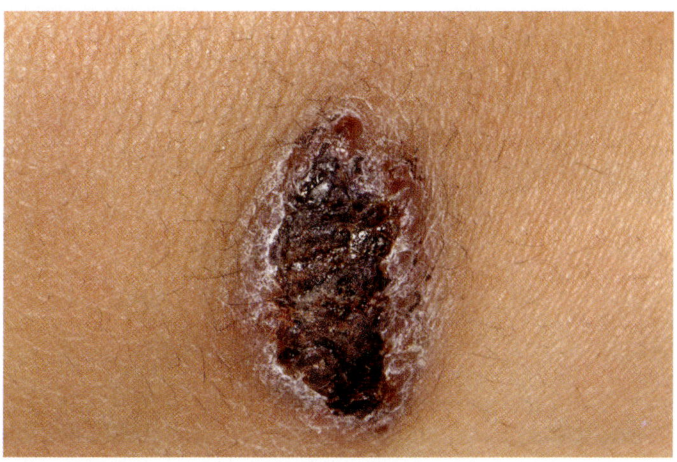

Figura 664-3. Crosta secca, strettamente aderente nell'ectima.

e poi rimosse. È indicata una terapia antibiotica sistemica, come per l'impetigine; quasi tutte le lesioni rispondono al trattamento con penicillina.

L'**ectima gangrenosa** è un'ulcera necrotica ricoperta da un'escara grigio-nera. È frequentemente un segno della sepsi da *P. aeruginosa* e di solito si verifica in pazienti immunodepressi. L'ectima gangrenosa compare nel 6% dei pazienti con infezione sistemica da *P. aeruginosa*, ma può verificarsi anche come infezione cutanea primaria da inoculazione. La lesione esordisce come una macula rossa o purpurea che si trasforma in vescicola e poi si ulcera. La cute circostante ha un colorito variabile da rosa a violaceo. Le ulcere perforanti sviluppano bordi rilevati con una zona centrale depressa, ricoperta da una crosta densa e nera. Le lesioni possono essere singole o multiple. I pazienti con batteriemia comunemente presentano lesioni in aree apocrine. Lesioni clinicamente simili si possono sviluppare anche dopo un'infezione con altri agenti, quali *S. aureus*, *A. hydrophila*, *Enterobacter* spp., *Proteus* spp., *Burkholderia cepacia*, *Serratia marcescens*, *Aspergillus* spp., *Mucorales*, *E. coli* e *Candida* spp. Si verifica un'invasione delle tonache media e avventizia delle vene del derma, ma non delle arterie. L'intima e il lume sono risparmiati. Occorre eseguire emocolture e colture da biopsie cutanee, ed è necessario avviare, il prima possibile, una terapia empirica ad ampio spettro, per via sistemica, che sia attiva anche contro *Pseudomonas*.

PIODERMA BLASTOMICOSI-SIMILE (PYODERMA VEGETANS)

Si tratta di un'esuberante reazione cutanea a un'infezione batterica, principalmente nei bambini malnutriti e immunodepressi. Gli organismi più frequentemente isolati dalle lesioni sono *S. aureus* e lo streptococco di gruppo A, ma parecchi altri microrganismi sono stati associati a queste lesioni, compresi *P. aeruginosa*, *Proteus mirabilis*, difteroidi, *Bacillus* spp. e *C. perfringens*. È caratteristica la presenza di placche iperplastiche localizzate alle estremità e ricoperte da croste, che talvolta si formano dalla coalescenza di molti ascessi puntiformi, purulenti e crostosi (Fig. 664-4). Possono manifestarsi ulcerazioni e fistole e possono comparire ulteriori lesioni in zone distanti dalla sede di inoculazione. È frequente una linfoadenopatia regionale, ma non febbre. L'indagine istopatologica rivela un'iperplasia pseudoepiteliomatosa e ascessi composti da neutrofili e/o eosinofili. Mancano di solito cellule giganti. La **diagnosi differenziale** comprende infezioni micotiche profonde, particolarmente la blastomicosi e la tubercolosi, e infezioni micobatteriche atipiche. Si dovrebbe escludere un'immunodeficienza sottostante e la scelta dell'antibiotico andrebbe guidata dall'antibiogramma, perché la risposta a questi farmaci è spesso scarsa.

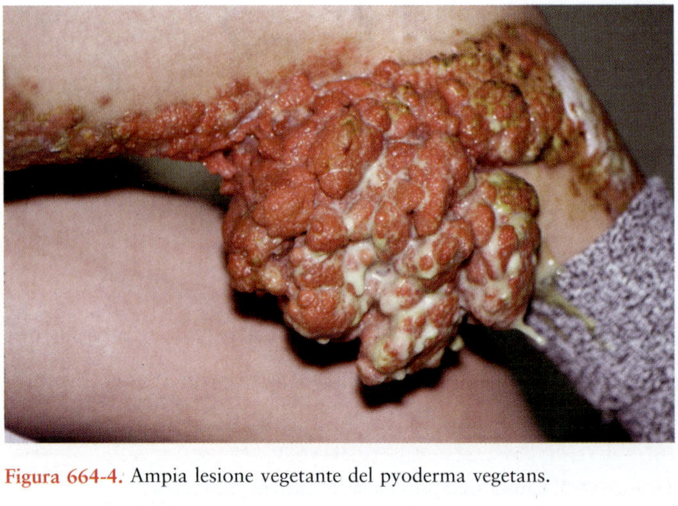

Figura 664-4. Ampia lesione vegetante del pyoderma vegetans.

DATTILITE BOLLOSA DISTALE

È un'infezione bollosa superficiale del cuscinetto adiposo volare della porzione distale delle dita. La patologia può coinvolgere più di un dito e interessare anche la superficie volare delle falangi prossimali, la zona palmare e le dita dei piedi. Le bolle sono ripiene di un liquido acquoso purulento che contiene leucociti polimorfonucleati e catene di cocchi Gram-positivi. I pazienti in genere non hanno anamnesi positiva per traumi, e di solito sono assenti sintomi sistemici. Non si è riscontrata glomerulonefrite post-streptococcica in seguito a dattilite bollosa distale. L'infezione è causata più frequentemente dallo streptococco di gruppo A, ma anche dallo streptococco β-emolitico di gruppo B e da *S. aureus*. Se non trattate, le bolle possono continuare a ingrandirsi ed estendersi all'area paronichiale. L'infezione risponde all'incisione e al drenaggio, e a una terapia di 10 giorni con penicillina o eritromicina per via sistemica.

DERMATITE INFETTIVA PERIANALE

Si presenta più frequentemente nei maschi (70% dei casi) tra i 6 e i 10 anni di età, con dermatite perianale (90% dei casi) e prurito (80% dei casi). L'incidenza della dermatite infettiva perianale non è nota con precisione, ma varia da 1 su 2000 a 1 su 218 pazienti visitati. L'eruzione è superficiale, eritematosa, ben delimitata, non indurita, e confluente a partire dall'ano verso l'esterno. Nella fase acuta (<6 settimane), il rash tende a diventare rosso vivo, umido e sensibile al tatto. In questo stadio può essere presente una pseudomembrana di colore bianco. Quando il rash comincia a diventare cronico, l'eruzione perianale può consistere di fissurazioni dolorose, secrezioni mucose secche o placche simili a quelle della psoriasi, con crosta periferica gialla. Nelle femmine l'eruzione perianale può essere associata a vulvovaginite. Nei maschi, può essere coinvolto anche il pene. Circa il 50% dei pazienti manifesta dolore rettale, descritto più comunemente come un bruciore interno in sede anale durante la defecazione, e il 33% presenta feci striate di sangue. Frequentemente, come risposta all'infezione, il paziente tende a ritenere le feci. I soggetti colpiti possono manifestare anche psoriasi guttata. Nonostante la possibilità di indurimento locale ed edema, sono assenti sintomi sistemici come febbre, cefalea e malessere; ciò suggerisce l'assenza, come nella cellulite, di coinvolgimento sottocutaneo. La diffusione della dermatite infettiva perianale ad altri membri della famiglia è frequente, particolarmente quando fanno il bagno insieme o usano la stessa acqua.

La **diagnosi differenziale** della dermatite infettiva perianale comprende la psoriasi, la dermatite seborroica, la candidosi, l'ossiuriasi, un abuso sessuale e la malattia intestinale infiammatoria. La differenziazione può essere effettuata con l'indagine colturale, che evidenzierà una crescita, da moderata a consistente, di streptococco di gruppo A (SBEA). La dermatite infettiva perianale può essere causata anche da *S. aureus*. I bambini con colonizzazione perianale asintomatica mostrano una bassa crescita di SBEA su agar sangue. Anche gli studi sugli antigeni diretti per lo SBEA sono molto sensibili (89%), ma possono risultare falsamente negativi nelle fasi precoci della malattia. La ricerca dell'antistreptolisina O o dell'anti-DNasi B su siero di pazienti in fase acuta o convalescenti non è utile per fare diagnosi. Vanno eseguite colture con prelievi dal caso di riferimento e dai membri della famiglia; sono raccomandate inoltre colture di follow-up, per documentare la guarigione dopo un certo periodo di terapia.

Il **trattamento** per 10 giorni con penicillina per via orale provoca la risoluzione della dermatite e dei sintomi nella maggior parte dei pazienti; sono state ripetute recidive nel 40-50% dei casi, il che sottolinea la necessità di uno stretto follow-up che comprenda la ripetizione delle colture. L'eritromicina estolato e l'etilsuccinato rappresentano un'eccellente alternativa per i soggetti allergici alla penicillina, o per quelli infettati da *S. aureus*. Anche la clindamicina è stata utilizzata con successo nel trattamento della dermatite perianale recidivante. La mupirocina è stata utilizzata in associazione ad antibiotici orali per trattare le recidive, ma non è stata valutata come farmaco unico per la terapia.

ERISIPELA (VEDI CAPITOLO 182)

FOLLICOLITE

L'agente eziologico più frequente di questa infezione superficiale del follicolo pilifero è *S. aureus* (impetigine di Bockhart). Occasionalmente sono chiamati in causa gli stafilococchi coagulasi-negativi. Le lesioni sono tipicamente piccole pustole, separate, a forma di cupola, con una base eritematosa, localizzate all'imbocco del canale pilosebaceo (Fig. 664-5). La crescita dei peli non viene compromessa e le lesioni guariscono senza residuare cicatrici. Le sedi più colpite sono il cuoio capelluto, i glutei e le estremità. Fattori favorenti possono essere rappresentati da scarsa igiene, macerazione e drenaggio da ferite e ascessi. La follicolite si può verificare anche in conseguenza di una terapia con catrame o dell'uso di bendaggi occlusivi. L'ambiente umido favorisce la proliferazione batterica. In pazienti con virus HIV, *S. aureus* può produrre chiazze eritematose confluenti con pustole satelliti nelle zone intertriginose, e placche violacee composte da pustole follicolari superficiali nel cuoio capelluto, nelle ascelle o all'inguine. *Candida* può provocare papule follicolari satellite e pustole che circondano chiazze eritematose di intertrigine, e *Malassenzia furfur* produce papule perifollicolari eritematose, pruriginose, di 2-3 mm, e pustole sul dorso, sul petto e alle estremità, soprattutto in pazienti con diabete mellito o in terapia con corticosteroidi o antibiotici. La diagnosi viene fatta con l'esame del materiale raschiato dalle lesioni e trattato con idrossido di potassio. Per la diagnosi di *Malassezia* può essere necessaria una biopsia cutanea, che dimostra aggregati di lieviti e ife corte e ramificate ("maccheroni e polpette") in corrispondenza dell'imbocco follicolare allargato, misti a detriti cheratinici.

L'agente eziologico della follicolite può essere identificato dalla colorazione di Gram e dalla coltura del materiale purulento proveniente dall'orifizio follicolare. Il **trattamento** della follicolite comprende detergenti antibiotici topici come la clorexidina o l'esaclorofene. La terapia antibiotica topica è usualmente sufficiente per i casi lievi, ma quelli più severi possono richiedere l'uso di antibiotici penicillinasi-resistenti per via sistemica, come la dicloxacillina o la cefalexina. Nella follicolite cronica recidivante, l'applicazione giornaliera di una lozione o di un gel a base di benzoil perossido può facilitare la guarigione.

La follicolite da microrganismi Gram-negativi si verifica soprattutto in pazienti con acne volgare trattata per lungo tempo con antibiotici ad ampio spettro per via sistemica. Una forma pustolosa superficiale, causata da *Klesbiella*, *Enterobacter*, *E. coli* o *P. aeruginosa*, compare intorno al naso e si diffonde alle guance e al mento. Una forma profonda e nodulare di follicolite localizzata su viso e tronco è causata da *Proteus* spp. Per stabilire la diagnosi è necessaria la coltura dei follicoli infetti. Il **trattamento** consiste nell'incisione e nel drenaggio della lesione profonda e nella scelta di un antibiotico orale basata sull'antibiogramma del microrganismo patogeno. Per i casi severi e recidivanti è utile l'acido retinoico 13-cis, alla dose di 1 mg/kg/die, ma deve essere somministrato solo da medici esperti, per i suoi effetti collaterali.

La **sicosi della barba** è una forma ricorrente, più profonda e più severa, di follicolite infiammatoria causata da *S. aureus*, che coinvolge anche le strutture più profonde del follicolo. Papule follicolari eritematose e pustole si sviluppano sul mento, sul labbro superiore e sull'angolo della mandibola, soprattutto in giovani maschi neri. Le papule possono confluire in placche e la guarigione può comportare la formazione di cicatrici. I soggetti colpiti sono spesso portatori di *S. aureus*. Il **trattamento** con garze imbevute di soluzione salina e antibiotici per via topica, come per esempio la mupirocina, generalmente sterilizza la lesione. Nei casi più estesi e resistenti è necessaria una terapia con antibiotici β-lattamasi-resistenti per via sistemica, e l'eliminazione di *S. aureus* dalle sedi di diffusione.

La **follicolite da "hot tub"** (vasca calda per trattamenti rilassanti) è attribuibile a *P. aeruginosa*, soprattutto al sierotipo O-11. Le lesioni sono costituite da papule pruriginose e pustole o noduli di colore variabile dal rosso al violaceo, che si sviluppano 8-48 ore dopo l'esposizione, e che sono più dense nelle zone coperte dal costume da bagno (Fig. 664-6). I pazienti occasionalmente sviluppano febbre, malessere e linfoadenopatia. Il microrganismo è facilmente isolabile dal pus. L'eruzione solitamente si risolve in modo spontaneo in 1-2 settimane, spesso lasciando un'iperpigmentazione postinfiammatoria. In pazienti adolescenti con sintomi sistemici andrebbe valutato l'utilizzo di antibiotici per via sistemica (ciprofloxacina). I bambini immunodepressi sono suscettibili alle complicanze della follicolite da *Pseudomonas* (cellulite) e devono evitare le "hot tub".

FORUNCOLI E CARBONCHIO

Queste lesioni follicolari possono originare da una precedente follicolite o insorgere sin dall'inizio come noduli perifollicolari eritematosi, dolenti, a base profonda. Sebbene le lesioni siano inizialmente dure, sono seguite da necrosi e suppurazione centrale, che porta alla rottura e alla fuoriuscita del tessuto necrotico centrale e alla distruzione del follicolo (Fig. 664-7). La guarigione comporta la formazione di cicatrici. Le sedi di elezione sono le aree pelose del volto, del collo, delle ascelle, dei glutei e dell'inguine. Il dolore può essere intenso se la lesione è situata in una zona in cui la cute sia relativamente fissa, come nel canale uditivo esterno o sulle cartilagini nasali. I pazienti con foruncoli solitamente non presentano sintomi sistemici; si può verificare occasionalmente batteriemia. Raramente le lesioni sul labbro superiore o sulle guance possono portare a trombosi del

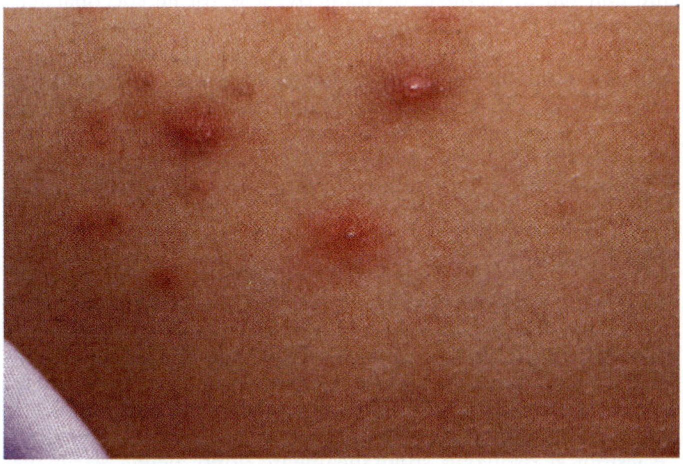

Figura 664-5. Follicolite. Pustole follicolari multiple.

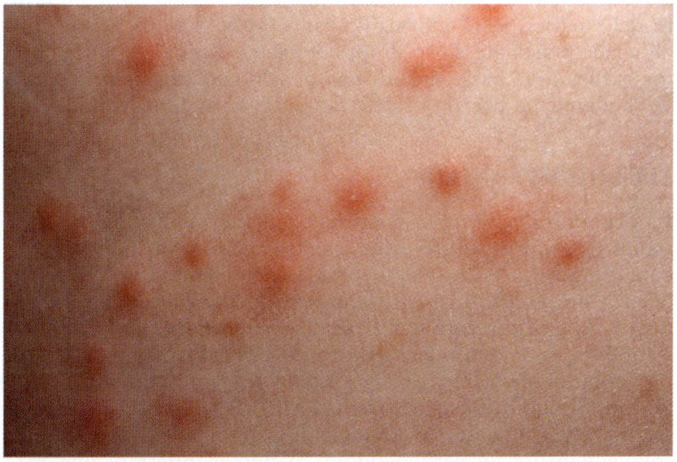

Figura 664-6. Papule e pustole nella follicolite da "hot tub".

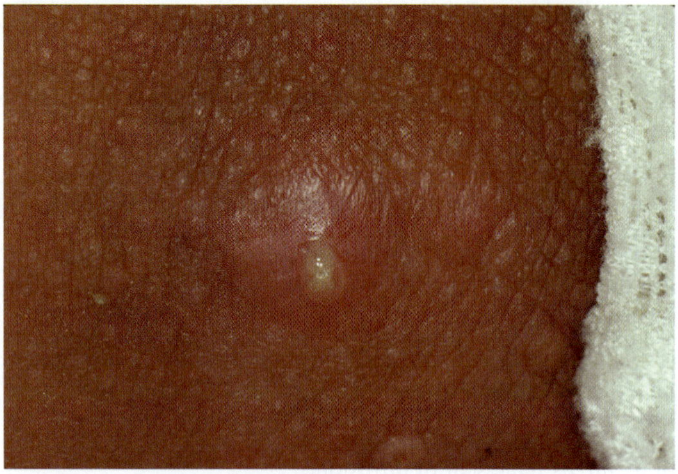

Figura 664-7. Rottura e fuoriuscita di pus in un foruncolo.

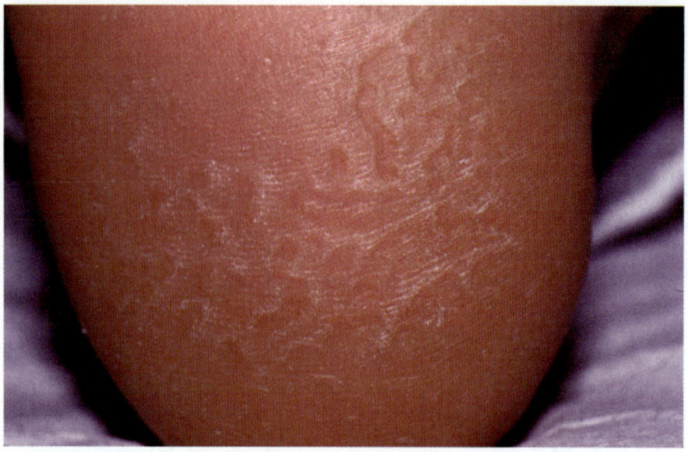

Figura 664-8. Erosioni superficiali dello strato corneo nella cheratolisi puntata.

seno cavernoso. L'infezione di un gruppo contiguo di follicoli, con multipli punti di drenaggio, accompagnata da alterazioni infiammatorie del sottostante tessuto connettivo, viene definita carbonchio. Il carbonchio si può accompagnare a febbre, leucocitosi e batteriemia.

EZIOLOGIA. L'agente eziologico è di solito *S. aureus*, che penetra attraverso la cute abrasa perifollicolare. Le condizioni che favoriscono la comparsa di foruncoli sono obesità, iperidrosi, macerazione, frizione e dermatite preesistente. La foruncolosi è più frequente anche in individui con iposideremia, diabete, malnutrizione, infezione da HIV, o altre condizioni di immunodeficienza. La foruncolosi ricorrente si associa spesso alla presenza di *S. aureus* a livello di narici, ascelle, perineo, o allo stretto contatto con un membro della famiglia portatore. Occasionalmente possono essere responsabili di foruncoli o carbonchio altri batteri o miceti; sono indicati colorazione di Gram e coltura del pus.

TRATTAMENTO. Comprende l'utilizzo regolare di detergenti antimicrobici e l'uso di vestiti comodi, per ridurre al minino i fattori che predispongono alla formazione dei foruncoli. L'applicazione frequente di garze caldo-umide può facilitare il drenaggio delle lesioni. Le lesioni ampie possono essere drenate con una piccola incisione. Il carbonchio e i foruncoli voluminosi o multipli richiedono un trattamento per via sistemica con antibiotici penicillinasi-resistenti, come la cloxacillina per via orale o l'oxacillina per via parenterale. I pazienti allergici alla penicillina possono essere trattati con cefalosporine, clindamicina o eritromicina. Lo stato di portatore può temporaneamente essere eliminato con l'applicazione di una pomata a base di mupirocina sulla parte anteriore delle narici per 5 giorni. Possono essere d'aiuto l'attenzione all'igiene personale, l'uso di un detergente antibatterico, la somministrazione a basse dosi di una penicillina antistafilococcica o di clindamicina per via orale e frequenti lavaggi delle mani.

CHERATOLISI PUNTATA

La cheratolisi puntata si manifesta più frequentemente in climi umidi tropicali e subtropicali, particolarmente in individui con cute dei piedi cronicamente umida, per esempio come conseguenza di iperidrosi, uso prolungato di stivali o immersioni in acqua. Le lesioni consistono di erosioni superficiali, di forma irregolare, di 1-7 mm, dello strato corneo della pianta del piede, particolarmente nelle zone che sostengono il peso del corpo (Fig. 664-8). Si può evidenziare una colorazione brunastra delle zone coinvolte. La malattia è solitamente asintomatica, ma provoca frequentemente un cattivo odore. Si può manifestare una rara variante dolorosa, sotto forma di placche ispessite, con colore variabile dal rossastro al violaceo, che si aggiungono alle lesioni puntate caratteristiche. L'agente eziologico più frequente è una specie di *Corynebacterium*. Dalle lesioni sono stati isolati anche *Actinomycetes*, *Dermatiphilus* e micrococchi. Evitando l'umidità e la macerazione si ottiene una lenta e spontanea risoluzione dell'infezione. I regimi terapeutici efficaci comprendono l'applicazione topica di glutaraldeide tamponata al 2%, una soluzione di formaldeide al 20% in un emolliente a base di petrolato, eritromicina, clindamicina e imidazolici.

ERITRASMA

Si tratta di un'infezione superficiale benigna e cronica, causata da *Corynebacterium minutissimum*. I fattori predisponenti sono calore, umidità, obesità, macerazione cutanea e scarsa igiene. Circa il 20% dei pazienti presenta un coinvolgimento degli spazi interdigitali dei piedi. Altre sedi colpite frequentemente sono le zone umide e intertriginose come il pube e le ascelle. Qualche volta sono coinvolte le regioni inframammaria e perineale. Caratteristiche della malattia sono chiazze nettamente demarcate, a bordi irregolari, lievemente squamose, di colorito rosso-marrone. L'unico sintomo costante è rappresentato da un moderato prurito. Il *C. minutissimum* è un complesso di microrganismi correlati che producono porfirine, che alla luce ultravioletta appaiono fluorescenti e di colore rosso corallo brillante. La diagnosi si effettua con facilità; l'eritrasma si differenzia da un'infezione dermatofitica e dalla *tinea versicolor* mediante l'esame con lampada di Wood. Sedute di 20 ore alla lampada di Wood, inoltre, possono rimuovere le porfirine idrosolubuli. La colorazione della cute con blu di metilene o Gram rivela le forme coccobacillari pleiomorfe e filamentose.

La maggior parte dei casi presenta colonizzazione, è asintomatica e non richiede terapia. Un **trattamento** efficace si può ottenere con eritromicina, clindamicina o miconazolo per via topica, con unguento solfosalicilico, o con eritromicina per via orale per 10-14 giorni. Si possono evitare recidive utilizzando frequentemente un antibatterico.

ERISIPELOIDE

Questa rara infezione cutanea è causata dall'inoculazione di *Erysipelothrix rhusiophatiae* da animali, uccelli e pesci contaminati o dai loro prodotti. La forma più frequente è quella cutanea localizzata, caratterizzata da macchie ben demarcate, romboidi, da eritematose a violacee, nella sede di inoculazione. I sintomi locali generalmente non sono severi, mentre quelli sistemici sono rari. Le lesioni si risolvono spontaneamente dopo alcune settimane, ma possono recidivare nella stessa sede o comparire in altre zone, settimane o mesi più tardi. La forma cutanea diffusa si manifesta con lesioni in numerose aree del corpo, oltre che nella sede di inoculazione; anch'essa è autolimitante. La forma sistemica, causata da diffusione per via ematica, si accompagna a sintomi generali e può comprendere endocardite, artrite settica, infarto cerebrale e ascesso, meningite e versamento pleurico. La diagnosi è confermata dalla biopsia cutanea, che rivela microrganismigram-positivi, e dalla coltura. Il **trattamento** d'elezione è rappresentato dall'eritromicina o dalla penicillina per via parenterale.

TUBERCOLOSI CUTANEA (VEDI ANCHE CAPITOLI 212 E 214)

L'infezione tubercolare cutanea è presente in tutto il mondo, particolarmente in associazione con infezione da HIV, malnutrizione e scarse condizioni sanitarie. La tubercolosi cutanea primaria è rara negli Stati Uniti, ma si verifica con frequenza maggiore nei neonati e nei bambini. L'incidenza complessiva della tubercolosi cutanea tra tutte le forme di tubercolosi negli Stati Uniti è dell'1-2%. Tutte le forme di patologie cutanee sono causate da *Mycobacterium tuberculosis*, da *Mycobacterium bovis* e, occasionalmente, dal bacillo di Calmette-Guérin (BCG), una forma attenuata di *M. bovis*. Le manifestazioni dovute a un determinato microrganismo sono indistinguibili dalle altre. In seguito all'invasione della cute, entrambi i micobatteri si moltiplicano intracellularmente all'interno dei macrofagi, portando progressivamente alla malattia, o sono controllati dalla reazione immunitaria dell'ospite.

La lesione primaria, l'ulcera tubercolare, appare quando *M. tuberculosis* o *M. bovis* riescono a penetrare nella cute o nelle membrane mucose in seguito a un trauma. Le sedi elettive sono viso, arti inferiori e genitali. La lesione iniziale si sviluppa 2-4 settimane dopo l'introduzione del microrganismo all'interno del tessuto danneggiato. Gradualmente, una papula rosso-marrone si ingrandisce, sino a formare un'ulcera poco profonda, dura e nettamente demarcata. Può essere presente un ascesso satellite. Alcune lesioni si ricoprono di una crosta simile a quella dell'impetigine, mentre altre si ammassano e diventano verrucose ai margini. La lesione primaria compare nel 30% dei casi come un'ulcera indolore su congiuntiva, gengiva o palato e, occasionalmente, come paronichia acuta asintomatica. Circa 3-8 settimane dopo l'inoculazione, compare un'adenopatia satellite indolore che può essere accompagnata da linfangite, linfadenite o perforazione della superficie cutanea, con formazione di uno **scrofuloderma**. Nel 10% dei casi si sviluppa un **eritema nodoso**. Le lesioni non trattate guariscono con cicatrice in circa 12 mesi, ma possono riattivarsi, formare un *lupus vulgaris* o, raramente, progredire verso la forma miliare acuta.

Sono possibili colture di *M. tuberculosis* o *M. bovis* dalla lesione cutanea e dai linfonodi locali, ma la colorazione acido resistente delle sezioni istologiche, particolarmente nel caso di un'infezione ben controllata, spesso non rivela la presenza del microrganismo. La **diagnosi differenziale** è ampia e comprende ulcera sifilitica, infezioni profonde micotiche o micobatteriche atipiche, lebbra, tularemia, malattia da graffio di gatto, sporotricosi, nocardiosi, leismaniasi, reazioni da sostanze estranee come lo zirconio, il berillio, le suture di seta o di nylon, talco o amido, acne rosacea papulosa, e lupus miliare disseminato facciale. La guarigione spontanea con cicatrici coincide con l'immunizzazione, a questo punto le lesioni cutanee e i linfonodi infetti possono diventare calcificati. È indicata la terapia antitubercolare (vedi Capitolo 212).

L'inoculazione cutanea diretta del bacillo tubercolare in individui precedentemente infetti, con un grado di immunità da moderato a elevato, produce inizialmente una piccola papula con infiammazione circostante. La **cute verrucosa tubercolare** (tubercolosi verrucosa) compare quando la papula diventa ipercheratosica e verrucosa, e numerose papule adiacenti confluiscono o una singola papula si espande perifericamente a formare una placca verrucosa con crosta, essudativa, e di colore da rosso-bruno a violaceo. L'estensione irregolare dei margini della placca produce un bordo serpiginoso. I bambini manifestano molto più frequentemente la lesione alle estremità inferiori dopo un trauma e il contatto con materiale infetto come escreato o terreno. I linfonodi regionali sono coinvolti solo raramente. La guarigione spontanea con cicatrizzazione atrofica si verifica lentamente, in mesi o anni; le lesioni guariscono gradualmente anche con la terapia antitubercolare.

Il ***lupus vulgaris*** è una rara forma cronica e progressiva di tubercolosi cutanea, che si sviluppa in individui con una reattività tubercolinica da moderata ad alta, indotta da una precedente infezione. L'incidenza è maggiore in climi freddi e umidi, particolarmente nelle femmine. Il *lupus vulgaris* si sviluppa in conseguenza di un'estensione diretta da articolazioni o linfonodi sottostanti, per via linfatica o ematica, o, raramente, per inoculazione cutanea del vaccino BCG. Più frequentemente segue un'adenite cervicale o una tubercolosi polmonare. Circa il 33% dei casi è preceduto da scrofuloderma, e il 90% dei casi si manifesta sulla testa e sul collo e in particolare sul naso o sulle guance. È raro il coinvolgimento del tronco. Una tipica lesione solitaria consiste di una papula molle, rosso-bruna, che alla diascopia presenta un colore a "gelatina di mela". L'espansione periferica della papula o, occasionalmente, la coalescenza di numerose papule, dà origine a una lesione di forma irregolare e di dimensioni variabili. Si possono sviluppare una o più lesioni tra cui noduli o placche piani e serpiginosi, ipertrofici e verrucosi, o di aspetto edematoso. La guarigione spontanea inizia centralmente e, caratteristicamente, le lesioni ricompaiono nella zona atrofica. È tipica la cronicità e sono comuni persistenza e progressione delle placche per parecchi anni. Nel 40% dei casi di *lupus vulgaris* si riscontra linfoadenite, e nel 10-20% è presente infezione di polmoni, ossa o articolazioni. Masse vegetanti e ulcerazioni che coinvolgono la mucosa nasale, orale o congiuntivale, il palato, le gengive o l'orofaringe possono causare deformità estese. Si può sviluppare, generalmente dopo parecchi anni di malattia, un carcinoma squamocellulare con un potenziale metastatico relativamente elevato. Dopo un temporaneo deficit immunitario, soprattutto in seguito a morbillo (*lupus exanthematicus*), si possono formare lesioni multiple in sedi distali, in conseguenza della diffusione per via ematogena da un focolaio latente dell'infezione. L'esame istopatologico mostra un granuloma tubercolare senza caseificazione; è estremamente difficile individuare i microrganismi. La **diagnosi differenziale** comprende sarcoidosi, infezioni micobatteriche atipiche, blastomicosi, cromoblastomicosi, actinomicosi, leismaniasi, sifilide terziaria, lebbra, *lichen planus* ipertrofico, psoriasi, lupus eritematoso, linfocitoma e malattia di Bowen. Le lesioni di piccole dimensioni possono essere asportate. Solitamente la terapia con farmaci antitubercolari interrompe la diffusione e favorisce l'involuzione della patologia.

Lo **scrofuloderma** è causato da ingrossamento, formazione di un ascesso freddo e rottura di un linfonodo, più frequentemente della catena cervicale, con estensione alla cute sovrastante. Si possono sviluppare ulcere lineari o serpiginose, fistole dissecanti e tragitti sottocutanei costellati di noduli molli. La guarigione spontanea può richiedere anni; possono residuare cheloidi cordoniformi. Può anche svilupparsi un *lupus vulgaris*. Lo scrofuloderma di un linfonodo cervicale spesso origina nella laringe e, in passato, era associato all'assunzione di latte contenente *M. bovis*. Le lesioni possono originare anche da una sottostante infezione a livello articolare, tendineo, osseo o epididimale. La **diagnosi differenziale** comprende gomma sifilitica, infezioni micotiche profonde, actinomicosi e idrosoadenite suppurativa. Il decorso è indolente e tipicamente mancano segni sistemici. La terapia antitubercolare è solitamente efficace.

La **tubercolosi orifiziale** si presenta sulle membrane mucose e sulla cute periorifiziale dopo autoinoculazione del micobattere dalle sedi di infezione progressiva. Rappresenta un segno di malattia interna avanzata e comporta una prognosi infausta. Le lesioni si manifestano come noduli dolorosi, giallastri o rossi, che formano ulcere perforanti con infiammazione ed edema della mucosa circostante. Il **trattamento** consiste nell'identificazione della sorgente d'infezione e nella terapia antitubercolare.

La **tubercolosi miliare** (tubercolosi primaria ematogena) raramente si presenta in sede cutanea e si verifica molto più frequentemente nei neonati e in individui immunodepressi in seguito a chemioterapia o a infezioni con virus del morbillo o HIV. L'eruzione consiste in gruppi di minute macule, papule o vescicole, simmetricamente distribuite, da eritematose a purpuree. Le lesioni possono ulcerare, drenare, ricoprirsi di croste e formare tragitti fistolosi o gomme sottocutanee, specialmente in bambini malnutriti con alterazioni immunitarie. Sono comuni segni e sintomi sistemici e possono comparire reazioni leucemoidi o anemia aplastica. In una lesione attiva si identifica facilmente il bacillo tubercolare. È necessario prevenire un decorso fulminante ed è indicata una terapia antitubercolare aggressiva.

Ascessi tubercolari metastatici, singoli o multipli (**gomme tubercolari**) possono svilupparsi sulle estremità e sul tronco, in seguito a diffusione ematogena da un focolaio primario di infezione, durante un periodo di immunodepressione, particolarmente in bambini malnutriti e immunodepressi. I noduli sottocutanei fluttuanti, non dolenti, eritematosi, possono ulcerare e formare fistole.

La **vaccinazione con BCG** produce caratteristicamente una papula circa 2 settimane dopo la vaccinazione. La papula si ingrandisce, tipicamente si ulcera in 2-4 mesi, e guarisce lentamente con la formazione di una cicatrice. In circa 1-2 vaccinazioni per milione si verificano complicanze causate specificamente da BCG, tra cui linfoadenite regionale, *lupus vulgaris*, scrofuloderma e formazione di ascesso sottocutaneo.

I **tubercolidi** sono reazioni cutanee che mostrano caratteristiche istologiche di tipo tubercolare ma che non contengono micobatteri individuabili. Le lesioni appaiono in un ospite che solitamente presenta reattività tubercolinica da moderata a importante, anamnesi di precedente tubercolosi di altri organi, e solitamente risponde alla terapia antitubercolare. La causa dei tubercolidi è scarsamente conosciuta. La maggior parte dei pazienti è in buone condizioni di salute, senza chiari segni della malattia al momento dell'eruzione. Il tubercolide più frequentemente osservato è quello papulonecrotico. Gruppi recidivanti di papule rosso scuro, sterili, dure, simmetricamente distribuite e asintomatiche appaiono sul lato estensore degli arti, sul dorso delle mani e dei piedi e sui glutei. Le papule possono presentare un'ulcerazione centrale e andare incontro a guarigione, residuando cicatrici depresse, circolari, nettamente delimitate. La durata dell'eruzione è variabile, ma di solito la patologia scompare prontamente dopo il trattamento dell'infezione primaria. Il lichen scrofoloso, un'altra forma di tubercolide, è caratterizzato da papule asintomatiche, raggruppate, dalle dimensioni di una capocchia di spillo, spesso follicolari, di colore rosa o rosso, che formano placche discoidali, soprattutto sul tronco. La guarigione avviene senza cicatrici.

L'infezione micobatterica atipica può causare lesioni cutanee nei bambini. *Mycobacterium marinum* si trova nei pesci d'acqua salata, d'acqua dolce e nei pesci affetti da malattia. Negli Stati Uniti si acquisisce soprattutto dalle vasche di pesci tropicali e in piscina. Un'abrasione traumatica della cute rappresenta la porta d'ingresso del microrganismo. Circa 3 settimane dopo l'inoculazione, si sviluppa una singola papula rossastra che si ingrandisce lentamente fino a formare un nodulo violaceo o, occasionalmente, una placca verrucosa (Fig. 664-9). La lesione talvolta si rompe e si forma un'ulcera ricoperta da crosta o un ascesso suppurante. Noduli sporotricoidi eritematosi lungo i linfatici possono anch'essi suppurare e drenare. Le lesioni sono più comuni su gomiti, ginocchia e piedi dei nuotatori e su mani e dita nelle infezioni da acquario. Sono assenti segni e sintomi sistemici. Talvolta i linfonodi regionali si ingrandiscono leggermente, ma non si rompono. Raramente l'infezione diventa disseminata, e ciò accade soprattutto nei soggetti immunodepressi. Il campione bioptico di una lesione completamente sviluppata mostrerà un infiltrato granulomatoso con architettura tubercoloide, e, con appropriate colorazioni, in genere si possono identificare microrganismi intracellulari negli istiociti. Il trattamento più efficace comprende tetraciclina, minociclina, e rifampicina in associazione a etambutolo. L'applicazione di calore nelle sedi colpite può essere un'ulteriore presidio terapeutico. La guarigione spontanea con cicatrici è prevedibile entro un periodo di tempo che va da diversi mesi a due anni (vedi Capitolo 214).

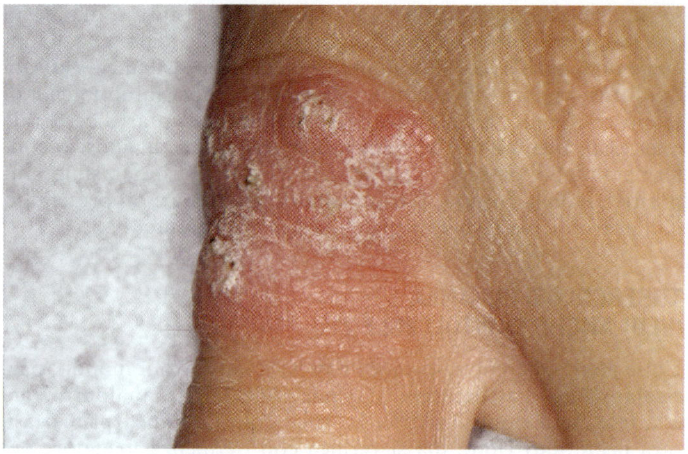

Figura 664-9. Placca violacea e verrucosa da infezione da *Mycobacterium marinum*.

Mycobacterium kansasii causa principalmente malattie polmonari, mentre il coinvolgimento cutaneo è raro e si verifica più spesso nei soggetti immunodepressi. Più comunemente si sviluppano noduli sporotricoidi dopo l'inoculazione in corrispondenza di cute traumatizzata. Le lesioni si possono sviluppare come placche ulcerate, crostose o verrucose. Il microrganismo è relativamente sensibile alla terapia antitubercolare, che deve essere scelta sulla base dell'antibiogramma.

M. scrofulaceum causa linfoadenite cervicale (scrofuloderma) nei bambini piccoli, tipicamente nella regione sottomandibolare. I noduli si ingrandiscono nel corso di parecchie settimane, si ulcerano e drenano. La reazione locale non è circoscritta, non dolente, sono assenti segni sistemici, e non c'è evidenza di coinvolgimento polmonare o di altri organi. Altri micobatteri atipici, tra cui *M. avium*, *M. kansasii* e *M. fortuitum*, possono provocare un quadro simile. Il **trattamento** prevede l'asportazione e la somministrazione di farmaci antitubercolari (vedi Capitolo 214).

Mycobacterium ulcerans provoca un nodulo sottocutaneo non doloroso dopo l'inoculazione su cute abrasa. La maggior parte delle infezioni si verifica in bambini che vivono nelle foreste pluviali tropicali. Il nodulo solitamente si ulcera, sviluppa bordi non ben definiti, e può diffondere su ampie aeree, soprattutto alle estremità. La necrosi locale del tessuto adiposo sottocutaneo produce una panniculite settica localizzata, che è caratteristica. L'ulcera persiste per mesi o anni prima di guarire spontaneamente con cicatrice e talvolta con linfedema. Sono assenti sintomi sistemici e linfoadenopatia. La diagnosi viene fatta sulla scorta di colture del microrganismo a 32-33 °C. Il **trattamento d'elezione** è la precoce escissione della lesione. Impacchi caldi e chemioterapia orale possono essere utili in alcuni pazienti.

Il complesso di *M. avium*, composto da più di 20 sottotipi, causa più frequentemente infezioni polmonari croniche. Talvolta si verificano linfadenite cervicale e osteomielite; raramente dopo l'inoculazione primaria compaiono papule o ulcere purulente alle gambe. Le lesioni cutanee possono rappresentare un segno precoce di infezione disseminata e si presentano sotto varie forme: papule eritematose, pustole, noduli, ascessi, ulcere, panniculite e diffusione sporotricoide lungo i linfatici. Per il trattamento, vedi Capitolo 214.

Il gruppo di *M. fortuitum* è composto da due microrganismi: *M. fortuitum* e *M. chelonei*. Questi microrganismi causano malattie in ospiti immunocompetenti principalmente per inoculazione primaria cutanea in seguito a una lesione traumatica, un'iniezione o un intervento chirurgico. Dopo 4-6 settimane dall'inoculazione si sviluppa un nodulo, un ascesso o cellulite. In un ospite immunocompromesso si possono formare numerosi noduli sottocutanei, che si rompono e drenano. Il **trattamento** si basa sull'identificazione del microrganismo con antibiogramma.

Barbagallo J, Tager P, Ingleton R, et al: Cutaneous tuberculosis: Diagnosis and treatment. *Am J Clin Dermatol* 2002;3:319–328.

Herbst R: Perineal streptococcal dermatitis/disease: Recognition and management. *Am J Clin Dermatol* 2003;4:555–560.

Johnston GA: Treatment of bullous impetigo and staphylococcal scalded skin syndrome in infants. *Expert Rev Anti Infect Ther* 2004;3:439–446.

Konig S, Verhagen AP, van Suijlekom-Smit, et al: Interventions in impetigo. *Cochrane Database Syst Rev* 2004;2:CD003261.

Lewis FM, Marsh BJ, von Reyn CF: Fish tank exposure and cutaneous infections due to Mycobacterium marinum: Tuberculin skin testing, treatment and prevention. *Clin Infect Dis* 2003;37:390–397.

Luelmo-Aguilar J, Santandreu MS: Folliculitis: Recognition and management. *Am J Clin Dermatol* 2004;5:301–310.

Lyon M, Doehring MC: Blistering distal dactylitis: A case series in children under nine months of age. *J Emerg Med* 2004;26:421–423.

Morris A: Cellulitis and erysipelas. *Clin Evid* 2003;10:1878–1883.

Patel GK: Treatment of staphylococcal scalded skin syndrome. *Expert Rev Anti Infect Ther* 2004;2:575–587.

Recih HL, Williams-Fadeyi D, Naik NS, et al: Nonpseudomonal ecthyma gangrenosum. *J Am Acad Dermatol* 2004;50:S114–S117.

Sladden MJ, Johnston GA: Common skin infections in children. *Br Med J* 2204;329:95–99.

Wong CH, Wang US: The diagnosis of necrotizing fasciitis. *Curr Opin Infect Dis* 2005;18:101–106.

Capitolo 665 ■ Infezioni cutanee da miceti

Joseph G. Morelli

TINEA VERSICOLOR

Questa comune, innocua, cronica infezione micotica dello strato corneo è causata dal lievito dimorfico *Malassenzia furfur*. I sinonimi *Pityrosporum ovale* e *P. orbicolare* erano usati in passato per identificare il microrganismo in causa.

EZIOLOGIA. *M. furfur* fa parte della flora indigena, soprattutto nella forma di lievito, e si trova particolarmente in aree cutanee ricche di sebo. Quando compare la malattia, si assiste alla proliferazione di forme filamentose. I fattori predisponenti comprendono un ambiente caldo-umido, un'eccessiva sudorazione, l'occlusione, l'ipercortisolemia, l'immunosoppressione, la malnutrizione e una suscettibilità geneticamente determinata. La malattia è più frequente negli adolescenti e nei giovani adulti.

MANIFESTAZIONI CLINICHE. Le lesioni hanno un colore molto variabile. Nei soggetti caucasici sono tipicamente rossicce-marroni, mentre nei neri possono presentarsi ipo- o iperpigmentate. Le caratteristiche macule sono ricoperte da fini squame. Spesso iniziano in sede perifollicolare, si allargano e si fondono per formare chiazze confluenti, più comunemente sul collo, sulla parte superiore del torace, sul dorso e sugli arti superiori (Fig. 665-1). Le lesioni al volto sono frequenti negli adolescenti; occasionalmente compaiono sull'avambraccio, sul dorso, sulle mani e sul pube. Può essere presente o meno un modesto prurito. Sul dorso, sul petto e talvolta sugli arti può verificarsi una variante papulopustolosa perifollicolare della malattia.

DIAGNOSI. L'indagine con la lampada di Wood dimostra una fluorescenza giallo-oro. Risulta diagnostico il trattamento con l'idrossido di potassio (KOH) di materiale proveniente dalla lesione, dove si evidenziano gruppi di spore a parete spessa e

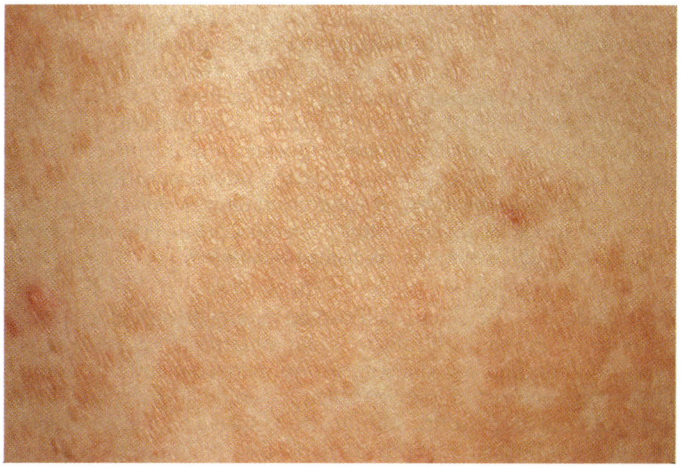

Figura 665-1. Macule nettamente delimitate, iperpigmentate, di varie dimensioni, sulla porzione superiore del tronco, caratteristiche della tinea versicolor.

una miriade di piccole, spesse ife spigolose, che configurano una quadro a "maccheroni e polpette". Frequentemente è necessaria la biopsia cutanea, con un'indagine colturale e l'uso di una colorazione speciale per i miceti (acido periodico-Schiff), per porre la diagnosi nei casi di un coinvolgimento follicolare primario. I microrganismi e i detriti cheratinici possono essere osservati al microscopio negli osti dilatati dei follicoli.

La tinea versicolor deve essere distinta dalle infezioni da dermatofiti, dalla dermatite seborroica, dalla pitiriasi alba e dalla sifilide secondaria. Se il paziente ha rimosso con uno scrub il materiale desquamante, possono essere mimate malattie pigmentarie non desquamanti, come le alterazioni pigmentarie postinfiammatorie. La follicolite da *M. furfur* deve essere distinta da altre forme di follicolite.

TRATTAMENTO. In questa malattia possono venire utilizzati con successo molti agenti terapeutici. Il microrganismo patogeno, tuttavia, un normale saprofita umano, non viene eradicato dalla cute e la malattia recidiva in soggetti predisposti. Un'adeguata terapia topica comprende una sospensione di solfuro di selenio applicata durante la notte per 1 settimana e poi per 1 notte a settimana per 4 settimane. Si può altrimenti applicare una crema contenente imidazolo o terbinafina 2 volte al giorno per 2-4 settimane. Oppure può risultare più conveniente una terapia per via orale e si può impiegare con successo il ketoconazolo o il fluconazolo, 400 mg ripetuti in una settimana, o l'itraconazolo, 200 mg/die per 5-7 giorni. Anche gli episodi recidivanti continuano a rispondere rapidamente alla terapia. Ci si può servire di una terapia di mantenimento con il solfuro di selenio applicato di notte, 1 volta alla settimana.

DERMATOFITOSI

Le dermatofitosi sono provocate da un gruppo strettamente correlato di miceti filamentosi, con una particolare propensione a invadere lo strato corneo, i capelli e le unghie. I 3 generi principali responsabili delle infezioni sono *Trichophyton*, *Microsporum* ed *Epidermophyton*.

EZIOLOGIA. *Trichophyton* spp. provoca lesioni di tutti i tessuti cheratinizzati, compresi la cute, le unghie e i capelli. *T. rubrum* è il più frequente dermatofita patogeno; *Microsporum* spp. invade principalmente i capelli ed *Epidermophyton* spp. la cute intertriginosa. Le infezioni da dermatofiti sono note con il termine **tinea**, seguito dal nome latino della sede anatomica coinvolta. I dermatofiti sono classificati anche in base alla fonte e al loro habitat naturale. I funghi acquisiti dal terreno vengono chiamati geofili; infettano sporadicamente l'uomo, provocando una reazione infiammatoria. I dermatofiti di origine animale sono invece detti zoofili e la loro trasmissione può avvenire per contatto diretto o indirettamente attraverso peli animali o vestiario. Gli animali infetti sono spesso asintomatici. I dermatofiti trasmessi dall'uomo sono detti antropofili. Queste infestazioni vanno da forme croniche di lieve entità a malattie infiammatorie acute. Le infezioni da *Epidermophyton* vengono trasmesse solo dall'uomo, ma varie specie di *Tricophyton* e *Microsporum* possono essere acquisite sia dall'uomo sia da fonti non umane.

EPIDEMIOLOGIA. Le difese dell'ospite hanno una grande importanza per la gravità dell'infezione. La malattia tende a essere più severa in individui con diabete mellito, neoplasie linfoidi, immunosoppressione e stati ipercortisolemici, come la sindrome di Cushing. Alcuni dermatofiti, soprattutto le specie zoofile, tendono a provocare nell'uomo una più grave risposta infiammatoria di tipo suppurativo. La maggior parte delle persone infettate acquisisce un certo grado di resistenza alla reinfezione e può presentare una risposta da ipersensibilità ritardata. Non è stato dimostrato un rapporto, tuttavia, tra il livello di anticorpi e la resistenza all'infezione. La frequenza e la gravità delle lesioni dipendono anche dal luogo geografico, dalla sensibilità genetica dell'ospite e dalla virulenza del ceppo di dermatofiti. Ulteriori fattori locali predisponenti sono un trauma cutaneo, l'idratazione della cute con la macerazione, l'occlusione e la temperatura elevata.

Occasionalmente, in individui sensibilizzati, compare un'eruzione cutanea secondaria nota come dermatofitide o a reazione "ID", che è stata attribuita ad antigeni micotici circolanti derivati dall'infezione primaria. L'eruzione è caratterizzata da papule raggruppate (Fig. 665-2) e vescicole, nonché, a volte, pustole sterili. Possono comparire anche lesioni orticariodi simmetriche e un'eruzione più generalizzata di tipo maculopapulare, che è più spesso associata a tinea pedis, ma si può verificare anche in caso di tinea capitis.

DIAGNOSI. Le procedure diagnostiche valide per le varie malattie da dermatofiti comprendono l'esame dei capelli infetti con la lampada di Wood, l'indagine microscopica di preparazioni di materiale infetto trattato con KOH e l'identificazione colturale dell'agente eziologico. I capelli infetti da *Microsporum* spp. evidenziano una fluorescenza brillante blu-verde. La maggior parte dei capelli infettatti da *Tricophyton* non manifesta invece fluorescenza.

MANIFESTAZIONI CLINICHE. La **tinea capitis** è un'infezione dermatofitica del cuoio capelluto, assai spesso provocata da *Tricophyton tonsurans*, occasionalmente da *Microsporum canis* e, molto meno di frequente, da altri *Microsporum* e specie di *Tricophyton*. È particolarmente comune nei bambini neri dai 4 ai 14 anni. Nelle infezioni da *Microsporum* e in alcune da *Tricophyton* le spore sono distribuite come una guaina intorno allo stelo del capello (infezione **ecotrix**), mentre *T. tonsurans* produce un'infezione all'interno dello stelo (**endotrix**). Le infezioni endotrix possono continuare oltre la fase anagen della crescita del capello, fino alla fase telogen e più cronicamente rispetto alle infezioni ecotrix, che persistono solo durante la fase anagen. *T. tonsurans* è una specie antropofila trasmessa all'uomo assai spesso dal contatto con capelli infetti e cellule epiteliali che si trovano sulla superficie delle sedie in teatri e cinema, di cappelli e pettini. Le spore dermatofitiche possono anche venire trasportate dall'aria nell'ambiente intorno e tra compagni di classe e familiari si è riscontrata un'alta percentuale di trasporto. *M. canis* è una specie zoofila che viene trasmessa da cani e gatti.

La presentazione clinica della tinea capitis varia a seconda dell'agente infettante. Il quadro prodotto da *Microsporum audouinii*, la causa più comune di tinea capitis negli anni '40 e '50, è caratterizzato inizialmente da una piccola papula alla base di un follicolo pilifero. L'infezione si diffonde quindi in periferia, formando una placca circolare eritematosa e squamosa (**ringworm**), in cui i capelli infetti diventano fragili e si spezzano. Si sviluppano numerose placche confluenti di alopecia e i pazienti possono soffrire di un notevole prurito. Questa infezione non è tuttavia più frequente negli Stati Uniti. Infezioni endotrix come quelle provocate da *T. tonsurans* creano un quadro simile a una "tigna con punti neri", contraddistinto inizialmente da molte piccole macchie circolari di alopecia in cui appaiono capelli spezzati in corrispondenza del follicolo pilifero (Fig. 665-3). Un'altra variante clinica si presenta con una desquamazione diffusa, accompagnata da una perdita minima di capelli. Sussiste una certa somiglianza con altre patologie, quali la dermatite seborroica, la psoriasi o la dermatite atopica (Fig. 665-4). *T. tonsurans* può provocare un'alopecia cronica più diffusa. La linfoadenopatia è comune (Fig. 665-5). Una risposta infiammatoria severa produce notevoli masse granulomatose (**kerion**), spesso costellate da pustole (Fig. 665-6*A*). Sono frequenti febbre, dolore e adenopatia regionale e possono residuare una cicatrice permanente e alopecia (Fig. 665-6*B*). Anche il microrganismo zoofilo *M. canis* o il geofilo *Microsporum gypseum* possono essere responsabili della formazione di kerion. Il **favo** è una forma cronica di tinea capitis, rara negli Stati Uniti, provocata dal fungo *Trichophyton schoenleinii*. Il favo inizia con papule giallo-rosse all'imbocco dei follicoli, che poi si espandono e si fondono per formare delle chiazze crostose, giallastre, che mostrano una fluorescenza verde opaco alla lampada di Wood.

La tinea capitis si può confondere con la dermatite seborroica, la psoriasi, l'alopecia aerata, la tricotillomania e con certe

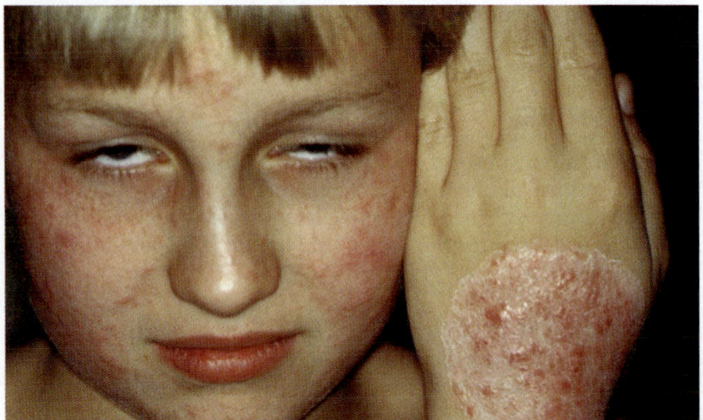

Figura 665-2. Autoreazione o reazione "ID". Eruzione papulare del volto associata a severa tinea della mano.

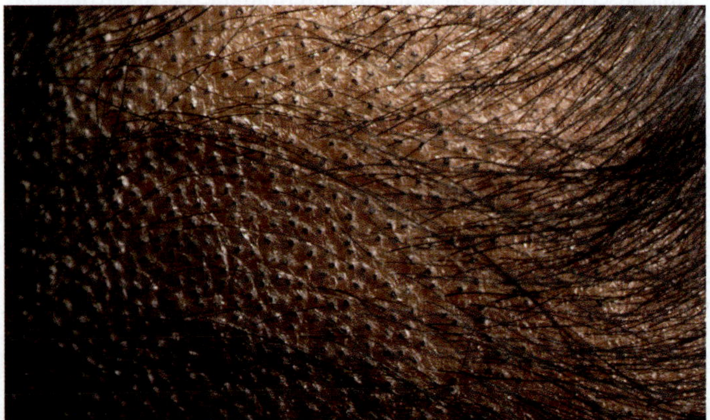

Figura 665-3. Aspetto della tinea "a punti neri" con zone di alopecia del cuoio capelluto.

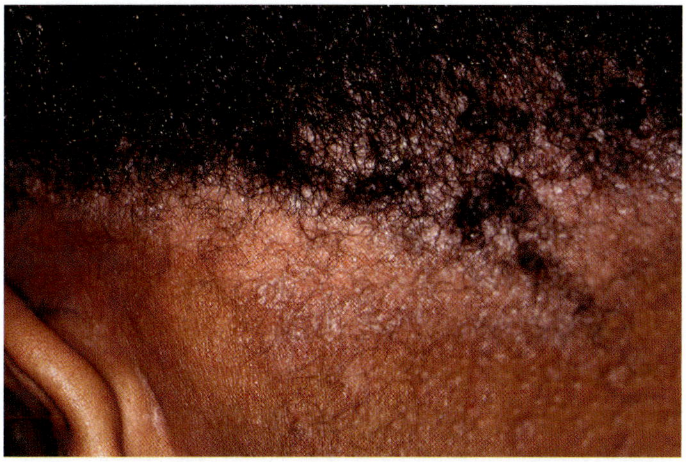

Figura 665-4. Tinea capitis che mima la dermatite seborroica.

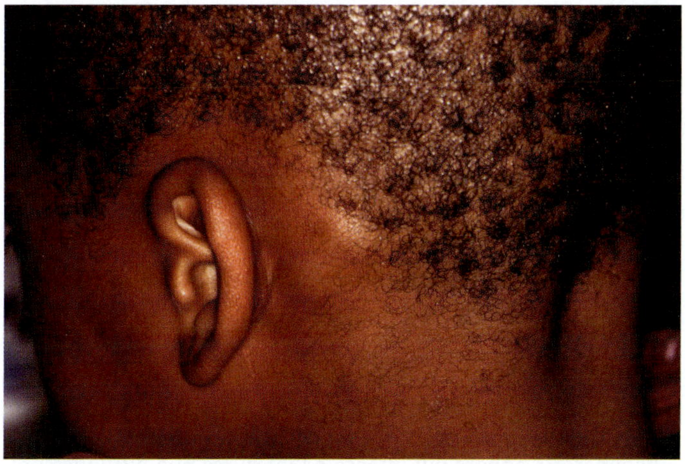

Figura 665-5. Linfoadenopatia associata a tinea capitis.

patologie distrofiche dei capelli. Quando l'infiammazione è pronunciata, come nel kerion, si deve valutare attentamente anche la presenza di un'eventuale infiammazione batterica primaria o secondaria. Negli adolescenti, il tipo di alopecia focale e con aspetto "tarmato", associata a una sifilide secondaria, può assomigliare alla tinea capitis. Se compare una cicatrice, nella diagnosi differenziale vanno considerati anche il lupus eritematoso discoide e il lichen plano pilare.

L'esame microscopico di una preparazione di capello infetto ottenuto dal bordo attivo di una lesione, trattato con KOH, rivela minuscole spore che circondano lo stelo nelle infezioni da *Microsporum* e catene di spore dentro lo stelo nelle infezioni da *T. tonsurans*. Nelle squame non sono in genere visibili elementi micotici. Una diagnosi eziologica specifica di tinea capitis è possibile con l'allestimento di colture di capelli infetti spezzati in un terreno di Sabouraud, addizionato a reagenti che inibiscono la crescita degli altri microrganismi. In questo modo l'identificazione può richiedere 2 o più settimane.

La somministrazione orale di griseofulvina microcristallina (20 mg/kg/die) è il **trattamento** raccomandato per tutte le forme di tinea capitis. Può essere necessario per 8-12 settimane e va sospeso solo dopo che l'esame colturale del fungo risulta negativo. Il proseguimento per un altro mese dopo la negativizzazione colturale minimizza il rischio di recidiva. Le reazioni collaterali alla griseofulvina sono rare, ma comprendono nausea, vomito, cefalea, discrasia ematica, fototossicità ed epatotossicità. L'itraconazolo orale viene adoperato nei casi resistenti, intolleranti o allergici alla griseofulvina. Si somministra per 4-6 settimane al dosaggio di 3-5 mg/kg/die ai pasti. Le capsule sono preferibili allo sciroppo, che può provocare diarrea. Anche la terbinafina appare efficace al dosaggio 3-6 mg/kg/die per 4-6 settimane o meglio con una somministrazione pulsata, sebbene abbia un'attività limitata nei confronti di *M. canis*. Né l'itraconazolo né la terbinafina sono approvati dalla Food and Drug Administration (FDA) per il trattamento delle dermatofitosi nei bambini. La terapia topica da sola è inutile, ma può essere importante come coadiuvante, in quanto diminuisce la diffusione delle spore. Avviene di frequente il trasporto di dermatofiti da parte di familiari asintomatici. Pertanto, il trattamento sia del paziente sia dei potenziali portatori con uno shampoo sporicida può accelerare la risoluzione clinica. Può risultare utile un lavaggio vigoroso con uno shampoo contenente solfuro di selenio al 2,5%, zinco piritione o ketonazolo. Non è necessario tagliare i capelli.

La **tinea corporis**, un'infezione della cute glabra, esclusi il palmo della mano, la pianta del piede e l'inguine, può essere provocata dalla maggior parte delle specie dermatofitiche, sebbene i più frequenti agenti eziologici siano costituiti da *T. rubrum* e da *T. mentagrophytes*. Nei bambini sono abituali anche le infezioni da *M. canis*. La tinea corporis può comparire per contatto diretto con persone infette o con squame o capelli infetti presenti sulle superfici ambientali. Le infezioni da *M. canis* vengono trasmesse solitamente da animali domestici contagiati.

La più tipica lesione clinica comincia come una papula o una placca secca, mediamente eritematosa, elevata, squamosa, che si diffonde in maniera centrifuga e si distrugge centralmente fino a formare una caratteristica lesione anulare, responsabile del

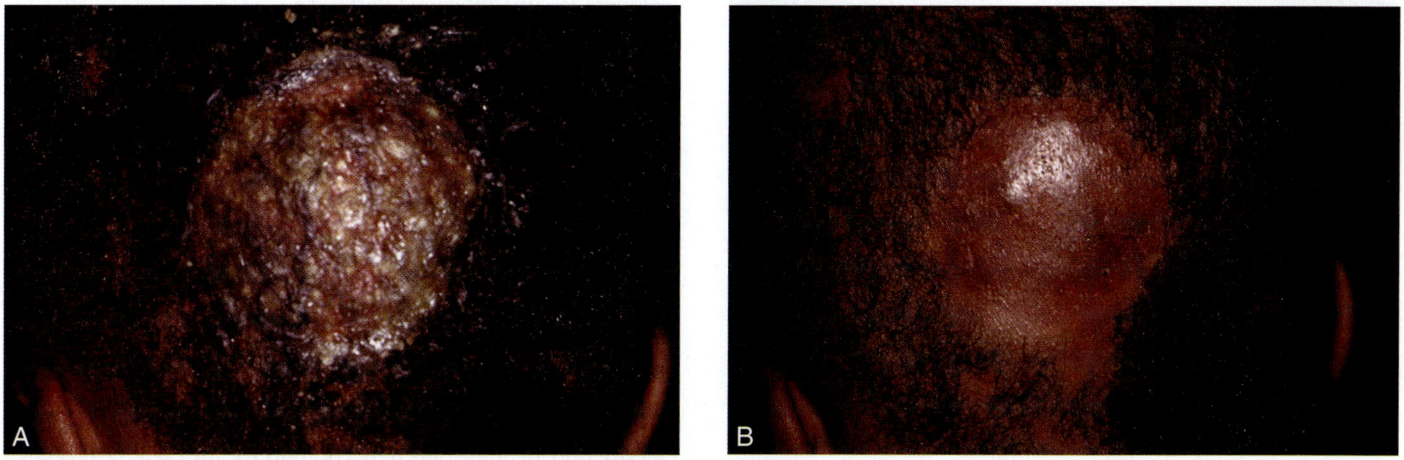

Figura 665-6. *A*, Kerion. Massa granulomatosa del cuoio capelluto. *B*, Cicatrizzazione post kerion.

termine inglese "ringworm" [letteralmente: "verme ad anello", *N.d.C.*] (Fig. 665-7). Le placche con bordi sopraelevati possono spandersi su vaste aree. Un'altra variante è rappresentata da gruppi di pustole. La maggior parte delle lesioni guarisce spontaneamente in diversi mesi, ma alcune possono cronicizzarsi. Non sempre si verifica la risoluzione centrale (Fig. 665-8) e gradi diversi della risposta immune dell'ospite possono comportare una notevole varietà di manifestazioni cliniche. Possono comparire, per esempio, lesioni granulomatose definite **granuloma di Majocchi**, dovute alla penetrazione del microrganismo lungo il follicolo pilifero fino al livello del derma, con la produzione di follicolite e perifollicolite micotiche (Fig. 665-9), nonché lesioni kerion-simili riferite a una tinea profonda. Il granuloma di Majocchi è più frequente dopo un inappropriato trattamento con corticosteroidi topici, specialmente quelli appartenenti alla classe superpotente.

Molte lesioni cutanee, sia infettive sia non infettive, vanno differenziate da quelle tipiche della tinea corporis. Quelle che vengono confuse più di frequente sono il granuloma anulare, l'eczema nummulare, la pitiriasi rosea, la psoriasi, la dermatite seborroica, l'eritema cronico migrante e la tinea versicolor. È sempre necessario, qualora si sospetti un'infezione micotica, l'esame microscopico di preparati trattati con KOH e l'indagine colturale. La tinea corporis di solito non rivela fluorescenza, se viene osservata con la lampada Wood.

La tinea corporis risponde abitualmente al **trattamento** con un farmaco antimicotico topico (per es. imidazoli, terbinafina, naftifina), somministrato 2 volte al giorno per 2-4 settimane. In casi di malattia particolarmente severa o estesa, può essere richiesto un ciclo di trattamento orale con la griseofulvina microcristallina per 4 settimane. L'itraconazolo, somministrato per via orale per 1-2 settimane, ha fornito ottimi risultati in molti casi.

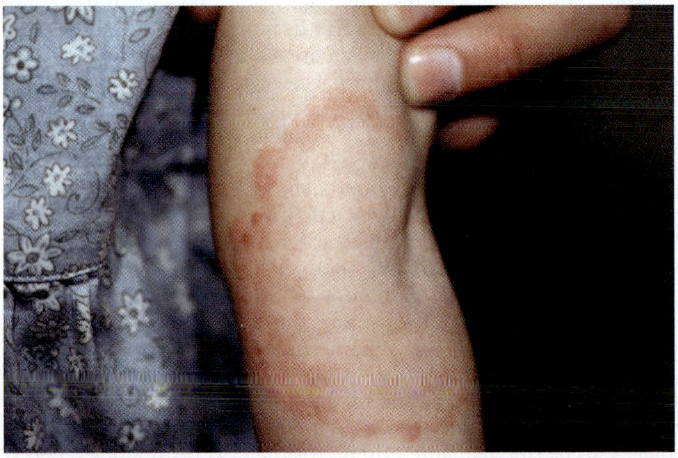

Figura 665-7. Placca anulare di tinea corporis con attenuazione centrale.

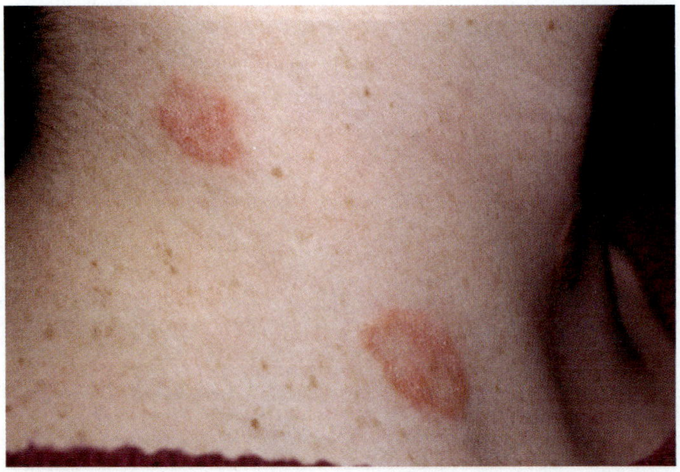

Figura 665-8. Minima attenuazione centrale in una tinea corporis.

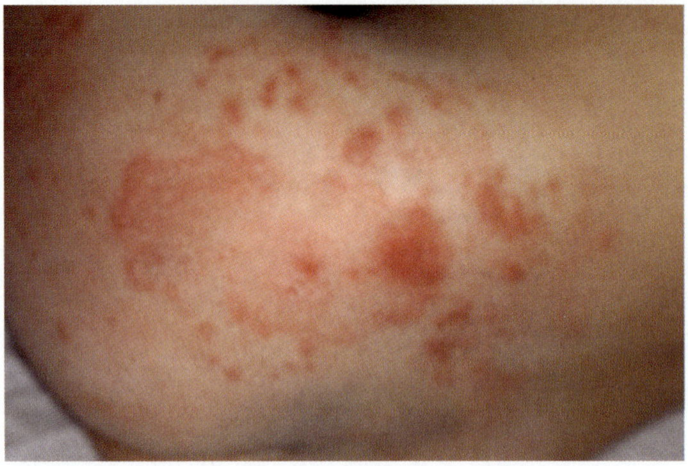

Figura 665-9. Papula follicolare e pustola in un granuloma di Majocchi dopo l'utilizzo di uno steroide topico superpotente.

La **tinea cruris**, un'infezione del pube, si verifica assai spesso negli adolescenti maschi ed è solitamente causata dalle specie antropofile *Epidermophyton floccosum* o *Tricophyton rubrum*, ma occasionalmente anche dalle specie zoofile di *T. mentagrophytes*.

La lesione clinica iniziale è una piccola macchia eritematosa, sopraelevata, squamosa, situata sulla superficie interna della coscia. Essa si espande perifericamente, spesso con lo sviluppo di numerose minuscole vescicole a livello del margine esterno. Alla fine si formano macchie bilaterali, irregolari, nettamente delimitate, con una zona centrale squamosa iperpigmentata. In alcuni casi, particolarmente nelle infezioni con *T. mentagrophytes*, la reazione infiammatoria appare più intensa e l'infezione può diffondersi oltre la regione crurale. Il pene di solito non viene coinvolto e questo dato differenzia la tinea dalla candidiasi. Il prurito inizialmente può essere severo, ma si attenua quando diminuisce la reazione infiammatoria. Una sovrainfezione batterica può modificare l'aspetto clinico e possono coesistere l'eritrasma o la candidiasi. La tinea cruris è più frequente nelle persone obese e in quelle con una sudorazione eccessiva e che indossano abiti stretti.

La diagnosi è confermata dall'esame colturale e dalla dimostrazione di ife settate su preparati di cute lesa trattati con KOH. La tinea cruris deve essere differenziata dall'intertrigine, dalla dermatite allergica da contatto, dalla candidiasi e dall'eritrasma. In presenza di una reazione infiammatoria severa, è necessario escludere la superinfezione batterica.

Ai pazienti va consigliato d'indossare biancheria intima comoda e di cotone. È raccomandato il **trattamento topico** con un imidazolo per le infezioni severe, soprattutto perché questo gruppo di composti risulta valido nelle forme miste, da dermatofiti e Candida. L'infezione dermatofitica pura può essere trattata anche con tolnaftato.

La **tinea pedis** (piede d'atleta), un'infezione degli spazi interdigitali e della pianta del piede, è rara nei bambini piccoli, ma si verifica con una certa frequenza nei maschi preadolescenti e adolescenti. Gli agenti eziologici usuali sono *T. rubrum*, *T. mentagrophytes* e *E. floccosum*.

Più di frequente, gli spazi interdigitali laterali (dal terzo al quarto e dal quarto al quinto dito) e la fessura subdigitale sono fissurati, con macerazione ed esfoliazione della cute circostante (Fig. 665-10). Sono caratteristici dolorabilità, prurito e un cattivo odore persistente. Queste lesioni possono diventare croniche. Questo tipo di infezione può comportare un crescita eccessiva della flora batterica, compresi *Micrococcus sedantarius*, *Brevi-*

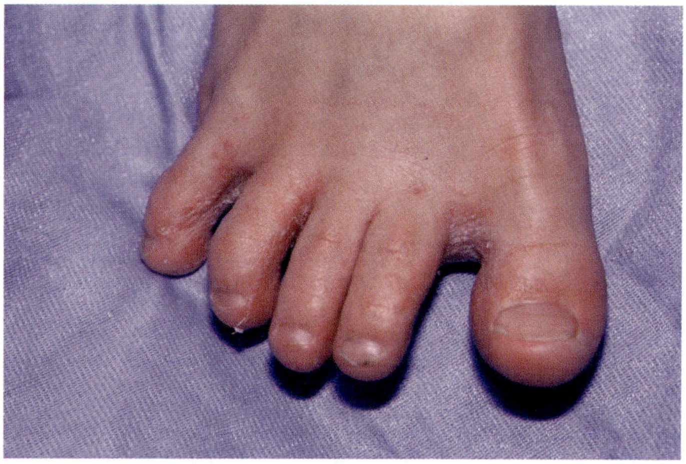

Figura 665-10. Tinea pedis interdigitale.

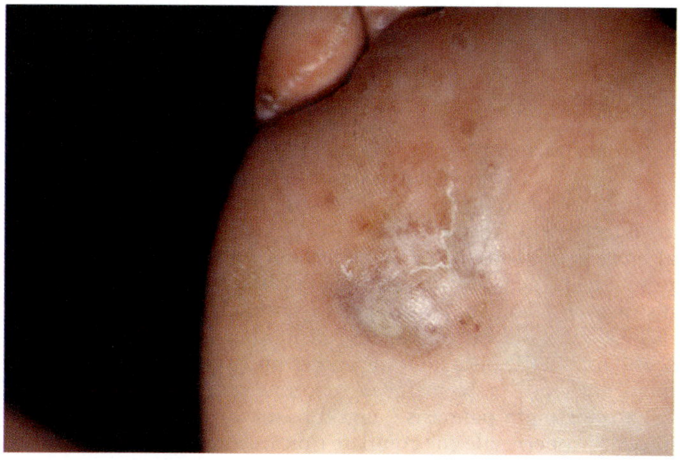

Figura 665-12. Tinea pedis vescicolobollosa.

bacterium epidermidis e microrganismi Gram-negativi. Meno spesso compare un'ipercheratosi cronica diffusa della pianta del piede, con solo un modesto eritema (Fig. 665-11). In molti casi vengono coinvolti entrambi i piedi e una mano. Questo tipo d'infezione è più refrattario al trattamento e tende a recidivare. Nel caso di infezione da *T. mentgrophytes* può comparire un tipo di reazione infiammatoria vescicolare, più frequente nei bambini piccoli. Queste lesioni coinvolgono ogni parte del piede, compresa la superficie dorsale e in genere sono circoscritte. Le papule iniziali evolvono a vescicole e bolle che possono anche pustolizzarsi (Fig. 665-12). Una serie di fattori, come calzature occlusive e clima caldo-umido, favorisce l'infezione. La tinea pedis può venire trasmessa nelle docce e nelle piscine.

La tinea pedis va differenziata dalla semplice macerazione e dall'esfoliazione degli spazi interdigitali, frequente nei bambini. Le infezioni da *Candida albicans* e da batteri vari (eritrasma) possono creare confusione, o possono coesistere con la tinea pedis. All'indagine microscopica di preparazioni colturali trattate con KOH possono essere visualizzati i miceli fungini.

Il **trattamento** delle infezioni lievi comprende semplici misure, come per esempio evitare calzature occlusive, asciugare con attenzione la cute dei bambini tra le dita dopo il bagnetto e usare una polvere adsorbente antimicotica come lo zinco undecilenato. La terapia topica con imidazoli è adeguata nella maggior parte dei casi. Ciascuno di questi farmaci è efficace anche contro le infezioni da Candida. Nelle forme dermatofitiche non complicate può essere utilizzato anche il tolnaftato. Possono essere necessarie parecchie settimane di terapia e infezioni modeste e croniche, particolarmente quelle provocate da *T. rubrum*, possono recidivare. In alcuni pazienti la terapia orale con la griseofulvina può risultare opportuna, ma sono comuni le recidive.

La **tinea unguium** è un'infezione dermatofitica della superficie ungueale. Colpisce più spesso i pazienti con la tinea pedis, ma può comparire anche come infezione primaria. Può essere provocata da un certo numero di dermatofiti, tra i quali *T. rubrum* e *T. mentagrophytes* sono i più frequenti.

La forma più superficiale di tinea unguium (per es. una onicomicosi superficiale bianca) è dovuta a *T. mentagrophytes*. Si manifesta con una macchia singola o multipla, di colorito bianco e irregolare, sulla superficie delle unghie, non associata all'infiammazione del paronichio o a un'infezione profonda. *T. rubrum* generalmente provoca un'infezione più invasiva, subungueale, che inizia in corrispondenza dei margini laterali distali delle unghie ed è spesso preceduta da una paronichia lieve. Gli strati intermedio e ventrale dell'unghia e le zone intorno al letto ungueale rappresentano le sedi di infezione. L'unghia inizialmente diventa giallastra e lentamente spessa e fragile e quindi si stacca dal letto ungueale (Fig. 665-13). Nelle fasi avanzate dell'infezione, le unghie possono mutare il colorito in marrone scuro fino a nero e possono incrinarsi o rompersi.

La tinea unguium deve essere differenziata da varie malattie distrofiche delle unghie. Le modificazioni dovute a trauma, psoriasi, lichen planus, eczema e trachionichia possono tutte venire confuse con la tinea unguium. L'infezione delle unghie da *C.*

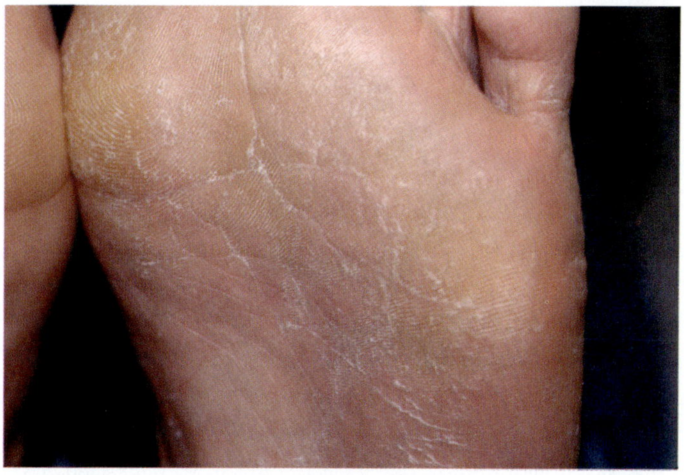

Figura 665-11. Tinea pedis diffusa, con eritema minimo.

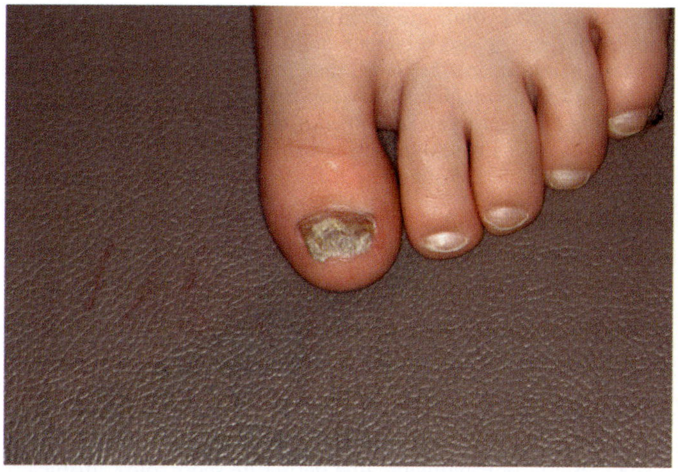

Figura 665-13. Unghia ipercheratosica nell'onicomicosi.

albicans presenta diverse caratteristiche distintive e una tumefazione ungueale decisamente più pronunciata. È necessario l'esame colturale e microscopico di un sottile strato di materiale dell'unghia infetta, preferibilmente dalle zone più profonde, dopo un trattamento con KOH. Può essere richiesto un ulteriore esame per dimostrare la presenza del fungo.

La lunga emivita dell'itraconazolo nell'unghia ha portato a trial promettenti, basati sull'utilizzo del farmaco per periodi brevi, intermittenti (il doppio della dose normale per 1 settimana al mese per 3-4 mesi). Anche la terbinafina orale si è dimostrata promettente per il trattamento dell'onicomicosi. La sua somministrazione 1 volta al giorno per 12 settimane risulta più efficace dell'itraconazolo fatto assumere in modo intermittente. La griseofulvina e l'applicazione di agenti micostatici topici sul letto ungueale sono spesso inefficaci e non vengono consigliati.

La **tinea nigra palmaris** è una rara ma caratteristica infezione micotica superficiale che compare tipicamente nei bambini e negli adolescenti. È causata dal fungo dimorfico *Exophiala werneckii*, che conferisce una colorazione grigio-nera al palmo colpito. La lesione caratteristica è una macula iperpigmentata ben definita. Desquamazione ed eritema sono rari e le lesioni appaiono asintomatiche. La tinea nigra viene spesso confusa con un nevo giunzionale, un melanoma o una macchia delle forme da contatto. La terapia prevede l'uso di un antimicotico imidazolico.

INFEZIONI DA CANDIDA (CANDIDOSI, CANDIDIASI E MONILIASI) (VEDI CAPITOLO 231)

I lieviti dimorfici del genere *Candida* sono ubiquitari nell'ambiente, ma *C. albicans* provoca usualmente candidosi nei bambini. Questo lievito non fa parte della flora cutanea indigena, bensì occupa di frequente la cute in modo transitorio e può colonizzare come microrganismo saprofita il tubo digerente e la vagina. Certe condizioni ambientali, soprattutto temperatura e umidità elevate, si associano a un aumento della frequenza dell'isolamento di *C. albicans* dalla cute. Molte specie batteriche inibiscono il suo sviluppo, mentre l'alterazione della normale flora in corso di terapia antibiotica può essere responsabile di una crescita eccessiva del lievito.

CANDIDOSI ORALE (MUGHETTO). Vedi Capitolo 231.

CANDIDOSI VAGINALE. Vedi Capitoli 231 e 119. *C. albicans* è un'abitante della vagina nel 5-10% delle donne e la candidosi vaginale non è rara nelle adolescenti. Vari fattori possono predisporre a questa infezione, compresi una terapia antibiotica, una terapia corticosteroidea, il diabete mellito, la gravidanza e l'uso di contraccettivi orali. L'infezione si manifesta con la comparsa di macchie bianche tipo formaggio sulla mucosa vaginale eritematosa e con abbondanti perdite vaginali bianco-giallastre. Può presentarsi in forma relativamente lieve o comportare notevoli infiammazione ed esfoliazione dei genitali esterni e della cute circostante, con evoluzione verso la formazione di vescicole e ulcere. Le pazienti spesso si lamentano di marcati prurito e bruciore vaginali. Prima di iniziare il trattamento, la diagnosi deve essere confermata dall'indagine microscopica e/o colturale. L'infezione può essere eradicata dall'inserimento di ovuli vaginali, supposte, creme o schiuma a base di nistatina o imidazolo. Se questi prodotti risultano inefficaci, si aggiunge il fluconazolo in una dose unica da 150 mg.

CANDIDOSI CUTANEA CONGENITA. Vedi Capitolo 231.

DERMATITE DA CANDIDA DELL'AREA DEL PANNOLINO. Si tratta di un disturbo ubiquitario nei neonati e, sebbene relativamente benigno, è spesso frustrante per la sua tendenza a recidivare. I neonati predisposti sono in genere portatori di *C. albicans* a livello del tratto digerente e la presenza di cute calda, umida, occlusa in corrispondenza del pannolino costituisce un ambiente ottimale per la sua crescita. Normalmente una dermatite seborroica, atopica o irritativa da contatto costituisce la porta d'ingresso del lievito.

La manifestazione clinica primaria consiste in una placca intensamente eritematosa, confluente, con un bordo indentato e un contorno nettamente demarcato. Si forma dalla confluenza di numerose papule e vescicolopustole. Pustole satelliti situate sulla cute contigua sono un segno distintivo delle infezioni localizzate da Candida. In genere è interessata la cute perianale, inguinale, perineale e dell'addome inferiore (Fig. 665-14). Nei maschi possono essere coinvolti anche tutto lo scroto e il pene, con una balanite erosiva della cute perimeatale. Nelle femmine le lesioni si possono localizzare sulla mucosa vaginale e sulle grandi labbra. In alcuni neonati il processo generalizzato può rappresentare una reazione al fungo (ipersensibilità).

La **diagnosi differenziale** comprende altre eruzioni della zona del pannolino, che possono coesistere con l'infezione da Candida. Per questa ragione è importante confermare la diagnosi sulla scorta di un esame colturale o microscopico di una preparazione trattata con KOH.

Il **trattamento** consiste nell'applicazione, 2 volte al giorno, di una crema contenente un preparato imidazolico. La combinazione di un corticosteroide e di un antimicotico può essere giustificata se l'infiammazione è severa, ma può confondere la situazione in assenza di una diagnosi certa. Il farmaco corticosteroide non deve esser continuato per più di qualche giorno. Può essere di aiuto la protezione della zona del pannolino con l'applicazione di una pasta all'ossido di zinco sopra alla preparazione antimicotica. La pasta si rimuove più facilmente con olio minerale piuttosto che con acqua e sapone. Man mano che la dermatite da pannolino guarisce, le reazioni micotiche gradualmente diminuiscono o possono venire trattate con una preparazione a modesto contenuto corticosteroideo. In presenza di frequenti recidive, può risultare efficace la prescrizione di un ciclo di terapia antimicotica per via orale, per diminuire la popolazione dei lieviti nel tratto gastrointestinale. Alcuni neonati sembrano essere ospiti recettivi di *C. albicans* e possono riacquisire il microrganismo da un adulto colonizzato.

CANDIDOSI INTERTRIGINOSA. Si verifica più frequentemente nelle ascelle e nel pube, sul collo (Fig. 665-15), sotto le mammelle, nelle zone cutanee sotto pliche addominali pendule, nell'ombelico e nelle pieghe glutee. Le lesioni tipiche sono rappresentate da ampie aree confluenti di cute eritematosa, umida, esfoliata, con un bordo irregolare, macerato, squamoso. Sono caratteristiche lesioni satelliti, consistenti in piccole vescicole o pustole su una base eritematosa. Con il tempo, le lesioni intertriginose da Candida possono lichenificare, seccarsi e formare placche squamose. Le lesioni si sviluppano sulla cute soggetta a irritazione e macerazione. La superinfezione risulta più frequente nelle situazioni caratterizzate da un'eccessiva sudorazione, specialmente nei bambini obesi e in quelli con malattie sottostanti come il diabete mellito.

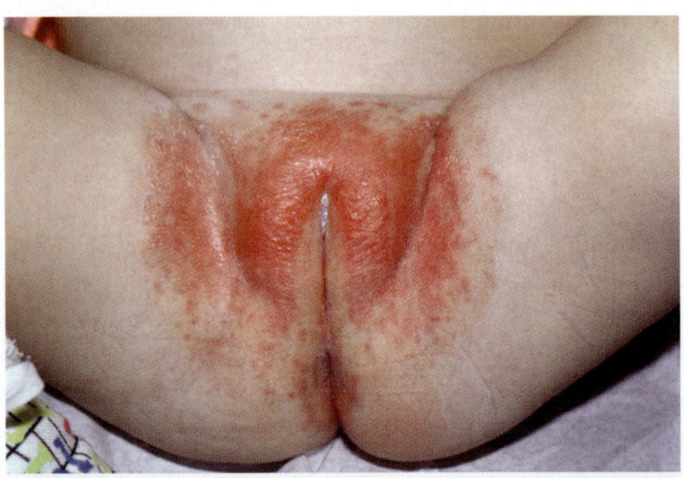

Figura 665-14. Placca eritematosa confluente causata da infezione da Candida.

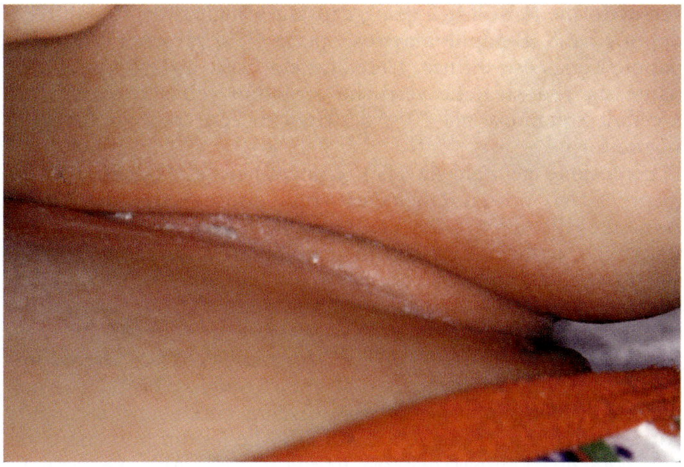

Figura 665-15. Candidosi intertriginosa del collo.

Una patologia simile, la candidosi interdigitale, compare comunemente in individui in cui le mani sono costantemente immerse nell'acqua. Tra le dita compaiono fissurazioni che mostrano un centro rosso, delimitate da un margine epiteliale di colore bianco. Lesioni simili tra le dita dei piedi possono essere secondarie all'uso di calzature occlusive. Il trattamento è lo stesso delle altre infezioni da Candida.

CANDIDOSI PERIANALE. La dermatite perianale si sviluppa nelle zone cutanee irritate da occlusione, costante umidità, scarsa igiene, fissurazioni anali e prurito da ossiuriasi. Si può verificare una superinfezione da *Candida albicans* specialmente in bambini trattati con antibiotici o corticosteroidi orali. La cute interessata diventa eritematosa, macerata ed escoriata e le lesioni sono identiche a quelle dell'intertrigine da Candida o della dermatite da pannolino. L'applicazione di un antimicotico topico, oltre a un miglioramento dell'igiene, risultano solitamente efficaci. Anche le malattie sottostanti, come l'ossiuriasi, devono essere trattate (vedi Capitolo 290).

PARONICHIA E ONICHIA DA CANDIDA. Vedi Capitolo 662.

GRANULOMA DA CANDIDA. Si tratta di una rara risposta a un'infezione cutanea invasiva da Candida. Le lesioni appaiono come placche crostose, verrucose e proiezioni simili a piccole corna sul cuoio capelluto, viso e zone distali degli arti. I pazienti colpiti possono presentare difetti singoli o multipli del meccanismo immunitario e sono spesso refrattari alla terapia topica. Un farmaco attivo contro la Candida per via sistemica può essere necessario per eradicare l'infezione o istituire una terapia palliativa.

Chan YC, Friedlander SF: New treatment for tinea capitis. *Curr Opin Infect Dis* 2004;17:97–103.

Fleece D, Gaughan JP, Aronoff SC: Griseofulvin versus terbinafine in the treatment of tinea capitis: A meta-analysis of randomized, clinical trials. *Pediatrics* 2004;114:1312–1315.

Foster KW, Ghannoum MA, Elewski BE: Epidemiologic surveillance of cutaneous fungal infection in the United States from 1999 to 2002. *J Am Acad Dermatol* 2004;50:748–752.

Gupta AK, Cooper EA, Ryder JE, et al: Optimal management of fungal infection of the skin, hair, and nails. *Am J Clin Dermatol* 2004;5:225–237.

Gupta AK, Ryder JE, Johnson AM: Cumulative meta-analysis of systemic antifungal agents for the treatment of onychomycosis. *Br J Dermatol* 2004;150:537–544.

Gupta AK, Ryder JE, Skinner AR: Treatment of onychomycosis: Pros and cons of antifungal agents. *J Cutan Med Surg* 2004;8:25–30.

Schwartz RA: Superficial fungal infections. *Lancet* 2004;364:1173–1182.

Capitolo 666 ■ Infezioni cutanee virali

Joseph G. Morelli

VERRUCA

Il papillomavirus umano (HPV, *Human PapillomaVirus*) provoca uno spettro di malattie che vanno dalle verruche al carcinoma a cellule squamose della cute e delle membrane mucose, compresa la laringe (vedi Capitolo 387.2). Gli HPV sono classificati in base al genere, alla specie e al tipo. Attualmente se ne conoscono oltre 200 tipi ed è noto l'intero genoma di 100 di questi. L'incidenza di tutti i tipi di verruche è maggiore nei bambini e negli adolescenti. L'HPV si trasmette per contatto diretto e autoinoculazione; ha luogo anche la trasmissione tramite fomiti. Le manifestazioni cliniche dell'infezione compaiono un mese dopo l'inoculazione e dipendono dal tipo di HPV, dalla sede d'inoculazione, dallo stato immunitario dell'ospite e dalla parte anatomica colpita.

MANIFESTAZIONI CLINICHE. Le verruche cutanee si sviluppano nel 5-10% dei bambini. Le **verruche comuni** (*verruca vulgaris*), causate più frequentemente dall'HPV dei tipi 2 e 4, compaiono più spesso sulle dita e sul dorso delle mani (Fig. 666-1), sulle aree paronichiali, sul viso, sulle ginocchia e sui gomiti. Si tratta di papule ben circoscritte, con una superficie irregolare, ruvida, cheratosica, che se sollevata spesso rende visibili molti punti neri che rappresentano capillari dermici trombizzati. Le **verruche periungueali** risultano molte volte dolorose e possono diffondersi al di sotto della lamina ungueale, separandola dal letto ungueale (Fig. 666-2). Le **verruche plantari**, sebbene simili a quelle comuni, sono causate dal tipo 1 di HPV e si trovano di solito allo stesso livello della superficie della pianta del piede, per la costante pressione dovuta al peso del corpo. Quando diventano ipercheratosiche (Fig. 666-3) possono essere dolorose. Lesioni simili (palmari) si possono verificare anche nel palmo delle mani. Si tratta di lesioni nettamente demarcate, spesso con un grosso anello calloso. Talvolta, prima di poterne apprezzare il contorno, deve essere rimossa la superficie del materiale cheratosico. Numerose verruche contigue (HPV di tipo 4) possono fondersi per formare una larga placca, il cosiddetto mosaico verrucoso. La verruca piana (*verruca plana*), provocata dall'HPV dei tipi 3 e 10, è costituita da papule solo lievemente elevate, minimamente ipercheratosiche, che in genere hanno un diametro <3 mm e possono variare nel colore dal rosa al marrone. Si possono trovare in abbondanza in corrispondenza del volto, delle braccia, del dorso delle mani e delle ginocchia. La distribuzione di numerose lesioni lungo una linea di trauma cutaneo è una caratteristica utile per la diagnosi

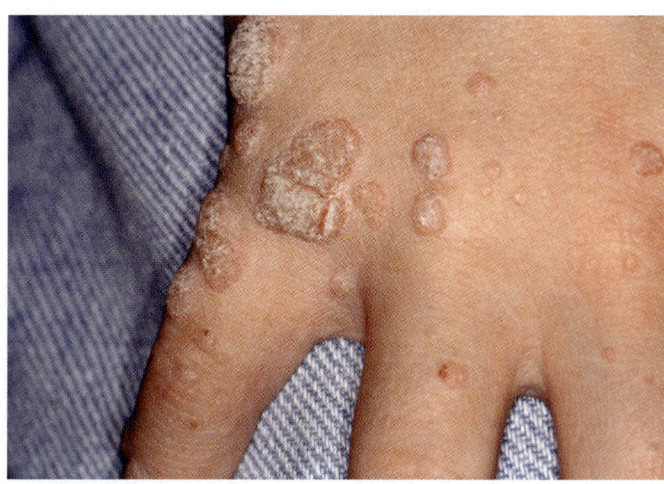

Figura 666-1. Papule verrucose sul dorso della mano.

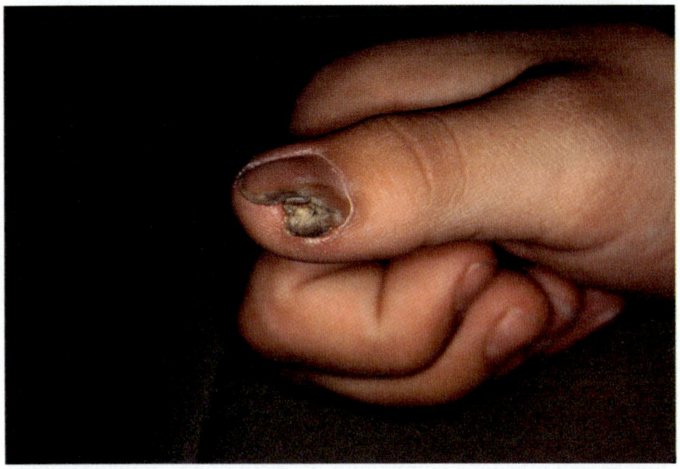

Figura 666-2. Verruca periungueale con alterazione della crescita dell'unghia.

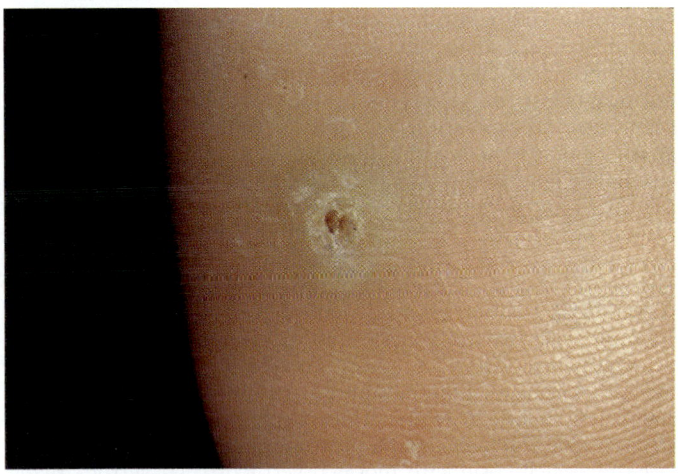

Figura 666-3. Verruca plantare ipercheratosica.

(Fig. 666-4). Le lesioni possono essere disseminate nell'area della barba e sulle gambe con la rasatura e dall'attaccatura dei capelli sul cuoio capelluto, per l'uso del pettine. L'**epidermodisplasia verruciforme** (EVER1, 2 geni), causata principalmente dall'HPV dei tipi 5 e 8 (β-papillomavirus, specie 1), si presenta con molte papule verrucose diffuse. L'ereditarietà è sia autosomica dominante sia recessiva. Le verruche evolvono verso un **carcinoma a cellule squamose** nel 10% dei pazienti con epidermodisplasia verruciforme.

L'**infezione genitale da HPV** compare in adolescenti sessualmente attivi, più comunemente come conseguenza di un'infezione da HPV dei tipi 6 e 11. Il **condiloma acuminato** (verruche mucose) è costituito da lesioni papillomatose umide e carnose, che compaiono sulla mucosa perianale (Fig. 666-5), sulle grandi labbra, sull'orifizio vaginale e sul rafe perineale, sul corpo, sulla corona e sul glande del pene. Occasionalmente provoca un'ostruzione del meato uretrale o dell'orifizio vaginale. Dato che si localizza in aree intertriginose, può diventare umido e friabile. Se non trattato, il condiloma prolifera e diventa confluente, formando con il tempo ampie masse a cavolfiore. Le lesioni possono comparire anche su labbra, gengive, lingua e congiuntiva. Le verruche genitali nei bambini possono manifestarsi dopo un'inoculazione durante la nascita attraverso un canale del parto infetto, come conseguenza di un abuso sessuale, o per diffusione accidentale da verruche cutanee. Una percentuale significativa di verruche genitali nei bambini contiene tipi di HPV che sono usualmente isolati dalle verruche cutanee. L'infezione da HPV della cervice possiede il maggiore rischio di sviluppare un carcinoma, particolarmente se è dovuta ai tipi di HPV 16, 18, 31, 33, 35, 39, 45, 52, 59, 67, 68 o 70. Il papilloma laringeo (respiratorio) contiene gli stessi tipi di HPV di quello anogenitale. Si ritiene che la trasmissione avvenga da un'infezione genitale da HPV materna ai neonati, che aspirano il virus durante la nascita.

ANATOMIA PATOLOGICA. I vari tipi di verruche hanno in comune alcune alterazioni di base, quali l'iperplasia delle cellule epidermiche e la vacuolizzazione dei cheratinociti spinosi, che possono contenere inclusioni nucleari basofile (particelle virali). Le verruche sono confinate nell'epidermide e non hanno "radici". Varie altre modificazioni istologiche sono rappresentate da paracheratosi, papillomatosi e inclusioni citoplasmatiche eosinofile, che si ritengono formate da cheratoialina alterata. Gli individui con alterazioni dell'immunità cellulo-mediata sono particolarmente suscettibili all'infezione da HPV. In risposta all'infezione compaiono anticorpi, che hanno però uno scarso effetto protettivo.

DIAGNOSI DIFFERENZIALE. Le verruche comuni sono assai spesso confuse con il mollusco contagioso. Può essere difficile distinguere le verruche plantari e palmari dalla cheratosi puntata, dai duroni e dai calli. A differenza di questi ultimi le verruche cancellano le normali caratteristiche cutanee. Le verruche piane

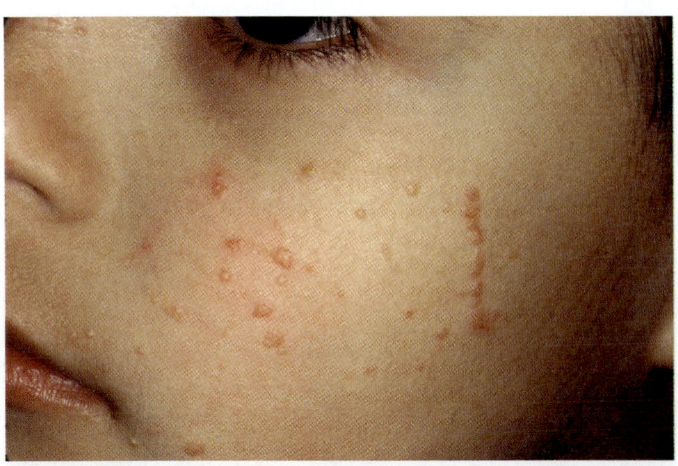

Figura 666-4. Verruche piane multiple sul volto, con le lesioni distribuite sulla linea del trauma.

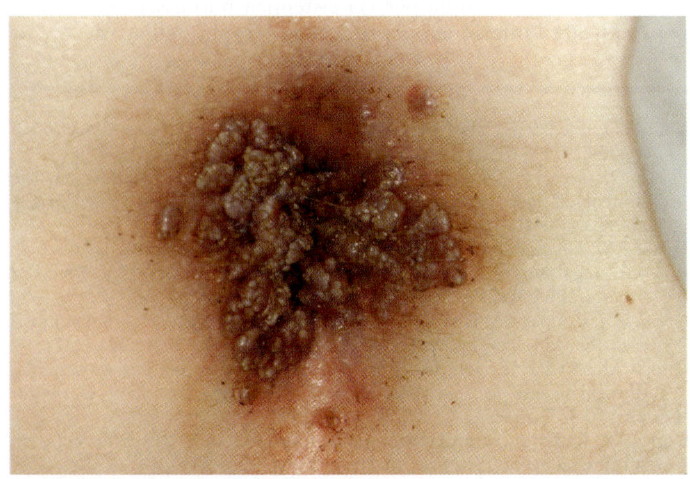

Figura 666-5. Condiloma acuminato in un bambino in corrispondenza dell'area perineale.

giovanili mimano il lichen planus, il lichen nitidus, l'angiofibroma, il siringoma, il milium e l'acne. Il condiloma acuminato può assomigliare al condiloma piano della sifilide secondaria.

TRATTAMENTO. Varie misure terapeutiche risultano efficaci nel trattamento delle verruche. Oltre il 50% di queste scompare spontaneamente in 2 anni. Le verruche sono lesioni epidermiche e non producono cicatrice, a meno che non vengano trattate chirurgicamente o in modo eccessivamente aggressivo. Le lesioni ipercheratosiche (verruca comune, plantare, palmare) rispondono meglio alla terapia se si stacca delicatamente la porzione cheratosica fino a rendere evidenti i capillari trombizzati; se si prosegue compare sanguinamento. Il trattamento è più efficace se viene eseguito regolarmente e frequentemente (ogni 2-4 settimane).

Le verruche comuni possono essere eliminate con l'applicazione di azoto liquido o con un trattamento con laser a colori pulsato. L'applicazione giornaliera di acido salicilico in collodio elastico è un metodo lento ma indolore, efficace in parecchi pazienti. Le verruche plantari e palmari possono essere trattate con cerotti di acido salicilico al 40%, che vanno applicati per periodi di 5 giorni intervallati da 2 giorni di riposo. Dopo la rimozione del cerotto e il lavaggio prolungato con acqua tiepida può essere rimossa la parte cheratosica con uno strumento smerigliato o pietra pomice. Risulta molto valido anche un cerotto occlusivo senza farmaci per diverse settimane. Il condiloma risponde meglio ad applicazioni settimanali di podofillina al 25% in tintura di benzoino, da lasciare sulle verruche per 4-6 ore e poi rimuovere con un lavaggio. Le verruche cheratinizzate vicine ai genitali (glutei) non rispondono alla podofillina. Appare utile anche l'imiquimod (crema al 5%), applicato 3 volte alla settimana, che risulta indicato per le verruche genitali ma è stato adoperato con successo anche per trattare verruche in altre sedi. Per quelle non genitali, l'imiquimod deve essere applicato giornalmente. Per i bambini con verruche multiple, che non rispondono ad altri trattamenti, è stata usata anche la cimetidina alla dose di 30-40 mg/kg/die. Ci si può avvalere pure dell'immunoterapia con acido squarico o antigeni di Candida intralesionali. Un nastro occlusivo applicato direttamente sulla verruca e lasciato in loco per 6 giorni consecutivi, con successivi lavaggio e abrasione con pietra pomice, ha avuto successo nel trattamento se ripetuto a cicli settimanali per 2 mesi. Inoltre, l'α-lattoalbumina-acido oleico umano per via topica applicato giornalmente per 3 settimane è una terapia promettente per il papilloma. Con ciascun tipo di terapia, è necessario proteggere la cute sana circostante dalla forte irritazione.

MOLLUSCO CONTAGIOSO

Il poxvirus che provoca il mollusco contagioso è un grosso virus con DNA a doppio filamento che si replica nel citoplasma della cellula epiteliale dell'ospite. I tre tipi possono essere differenziati sulla base dell'aspetto clinico, della localizzazione delle lesioni, dell'età e del sesso del paziente. Il virus di tipo 1 provoca la maggior parte delle infezioni. La malattia si acquisisce per contatto diretto con una persona infetta oppure da fomiti e si diffonde per autoinoculazione. I bambini in età scolare altrimenti sani e gli individui immunosoppressi sono le categorie colpite più di frequente. Il periodo di incubazione è stimato a ≥2 settimane.

MANIFESTAZIONI CLINICHE. Papule separate, perlacee, lisce e colore della cute, a forma di cupola, variano per dimensione da 1 a 5 mm. Presentano al centro una tipica ombelicatura, da cui può fuoriuscire un tappo di materiale caseoso. Le papule possono comparire in qualunque zona del corpo, ma le sedi di predilezione sono il viso, le palpebre, il collo, le ascelle e le cosce (Fig. 666-6). Si possono presentare negli adolescenti in grappoli, a livello genitale o inguinale e, in soggetti sessualmente attivi, si possono associare ad altre malattie veneree. Le lesioni nei bambini coinvolgono comunemente l'area genitale, ma nella maggior parte dei casi non sono acquisite per trasmissione sessuale. Le papule possono essere accompagnate da un modesto eritema circostante o da una dermatite eczematosa (Fig. 666-7). Le lesioni in pazienti con AIDS tendono a essere ampie e numerose, particolarmente sul viso. Lesioni esuberanti possono essere trovate anche nei bambini con leucemia e altre immunodeficienze. I bambini con dermatite atopica sono suscettibili di un coinvolgimento diffuso nelle aree della dermatite. Si osserva un'eruzione pustolosa nella sede delle lesioni individuali da mollusco (Fig. 666-8). Non si tratta di un'infezione batterica secondaria, ma di una reazione immunologica al virus del mollusco e non va trattata con antibiotici. Come esito di questo tipo di reazione, spesso sono visibili cicatrici atrofiche.

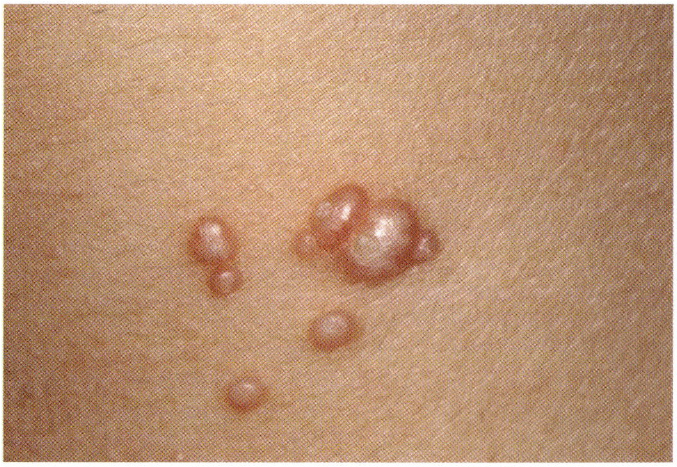

Figura 666-6. Mollusco raggruppato.

DIAGNOSI DIFFERENZIALE. Include tricoepitelioma, carcinoma a cellule basali, ghiandole sebacee ectopiche, siringoma, idrocistoma, cheratoacantoma e discheratoma verrucoso. Negli individui con AIDS la criptococcosi può essere indistinguibile clinicamente dal mollusco contagioso. Raramente, coccidioidomicosi, istoplasmosi o infezioni da *Penicillium marneffei* si confondono con lesioni mollusco-simili in un ospite immunocompromesso.

ANATOMIA PATOLOGICA E DIAGNOSI. L'epidermide è iperplasica e ipertrofica, si estende nel sottostante derma e si proietta sulla superficie cutanea. La papula da mollusco consiste in una massa aderente e lobulata di cellule epidermiche infettate dal virus. Inclusioni eosinofile di origine virale (corpi del mollusco o di Henderson-Patterson) diventano più vistosi man mano che le cellule migrano dallo strato basale verso quello corneo. La parte centrale del materiale, che è composta da cellule contenenti il virus, può essere prelevata da una lesione ed esaminata al microscopio dopo un trattamento con idrossido di potassio al 10% o con colorazione di Wright o di Giemsa. Una massa capsulata, rotondeggiante,

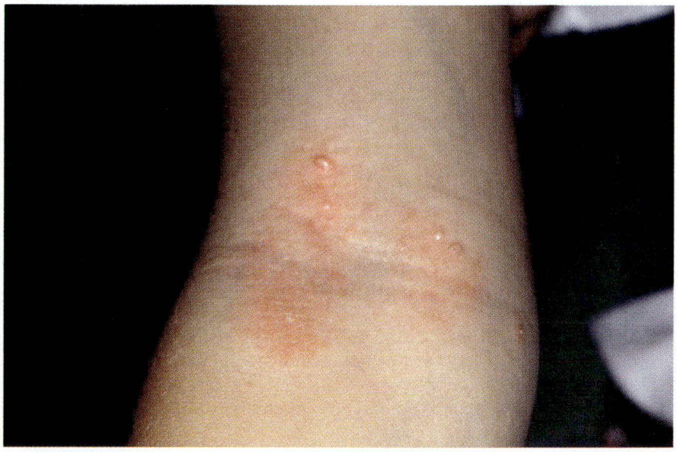

Figura 666-7. Mollusco con dermatite circostante.

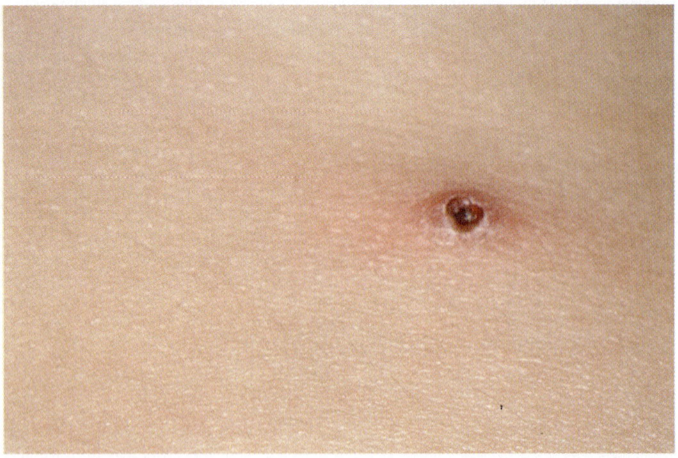

Figura 666-8. Mollusco infiammato. Papula crostosa nella sede di un mollusco precedente.

di cellule omogenee, spesso con lobuli identificabili, risulta diagnostica. Nella maggior parte degli individui infetti si ritrovano anticorpi specifici contro il virus del mollusco contagioso, ma il loro significato immunologico è incerto. Si ritiene che l'immunità cellulo-mediata sia importante nella difesa dell'ospite.

TRATTAMENTO. Il mollusco contagioso è una malattia autolimitante. Un attacco ha la durata media di 6-9 mesi, tuttavia le lesioni possono persistere per anni, possono diffondersi in sedi lontane ed essere trasmesse ad altre persone. I pazienti colpiti devono essere consapevoli di non dovere condividere l'acqua del bagno e gli asciugamani fino alla guarigione. L'infezione può espandersi rapidamente e produrre centinaia di lesioni in bambini con dermatite atopica o immunodeficienti. Nei bambini abbastanza grandi da sopportare un dolore modesto, il **trattamento di elezione** è rappresentato dal curettage. Nei bambini più piccoli si può applicare sulla lesione la cantaridina, coperta con un cerotto per prevenire la diffusione dell'agente responsabile delle vesciche. Nella sede di applicazione si forma una vescica e il mollusco viene rimosso con essa. Occorre evitare l'uso della cantaridina sul volto. Per il bambino e i famigliari, il mollusco al volto è più fastidioso esteticamente; l'applicazione topica di imiquimod è efficace e non eccessivamente irritante. Il mollusco è una malattia epidermica e non deve essere trattata in modo aggressivo, tanto da portare alla formazione di cicatrici.

Bellew SG, Quartarolo N, Janniger CK: Childhood warts: An update. *Cutis* 2004;73:379–384.

De Villiers EM, Fauquet C, Broker TR, et al: Classification of papillomaviruses. *Virology* 2004;324:17–27.

Dupin N: Genital warts. *Clin Dermatol* 2004;22:481–486.

Focht DR III, Spicer C, Fairchok MP: The efficacy of duct tape vs cryotherapy in the treatment of verruca vulgaris (the common wart). *Arch Pediatr Adolesc Med* 2003;156:971–974.

Grussendorf-Conen EI, Jacobs S: Efficacy of imiquimod 5% cream in the treatment of recalcitrant warts in children. *Pediatr Dermatol* 2002;19:263–266.

Gustafsson L, Leijonhufvud I, Aronsson A, et al: Treatment of skin papillomas with topical a-lactalbumin-oleic acid. *N Engl J Med* 2004;350: 2663–2672.

Majewski S, Jablonska S: Why epidermodysplasia verruciformis—a rare genetic disease—has raised such great interest. *Int J Dermatol* 2004;43: 309–311.

Molina AC, Fleischer AB, Feldman SR: Patient demographics and utilization of health care services for molluscum contagiosum. *Pediatr Dermatol* 2004;21:628–632.

Silverberg NB: Warts and molluscum in children. *Adv Dermatol* 2004; 20:23–73.

Capitolo 667 ■ Punture e infestazioni da artropodi

Joseph G. Morelli

PUNTURE DA ARTROPODI

Le punture da artropodi sono un'evenienza comune nei bambini e talvolta pongono problemi diagnostici. Un paziente può non essere consapevole della fonte delle lesioni o negare di essere stato punto, rendendo difficoltosa l'interpretazione dell'eruzione. In questi casi, la conoscenza delle abitudini, del ciclo vitale e dei segni clinici degli artropodi più comuni che colpiscono l'uomo possono aiutare a porre una diagnosi corretta. Le classi principali di artropodi che provocano una lesione cutanea nell'uomo sono elencate nella Tabella 667-1.

MANIFESTAZIONI CLINICHE. Il tipo di reazione che si verifica dopo il morso di un artropode dipende dalla sua specie e dall'età e reattività dell'ospite umano. Gli artropodi possono causare una lesione con vari meccanismi, tra i quali: il trauma meccanico, come il morso lacerante di una mosca tse-tse; l'invasione dei tessuti dell'ospite, come nella miasi; la dermatite da contatto, come per l'esposizione ripetuta ad antigeni di scarafaggio; la reazione granulomatosa da ritenzione di parti dell'apparato buccale; la trasmissione di malattie sistemiche; l'iniezione di sostanze citotossiche irritanti o farmacologicamente attive, quali ialuronidasi, proteasi, peptidasi e fosfolipasi nel veleno del pungiglione; l'induzione di anafilassi. La maggior parte delle reazioni alle punture dipende dalla formazione di anticorpi contro sostanze antigeniche della saliva o del veleno. Il tipo di reazione è determinato principalmente dal grado della precedente esposizione alla stessa specie o a una specie correlata di artropodi. Se una persona viene punta per la prima volta non si sviluppa alcuna reazione. Talvolta, però, compare un'immediata reazione petecchiale, come nei neonati dopo punture di zanzare. Dopo punture ripetute, invece, si sviluppa sensibilità, con la comparsa di una papula pruriginosa (Fig. 667-1) 24 ore dopo la puntura stessa. Questa è la reazione più comune nei bambini più piccoli. Con esposizioni ripetute e prolungate si può sviluppare, pochi minuti dopo la puntura, un pomfo, seguito 24 ore dopo dalla formazione di una papula; questa successione di reazioni si osserva comunemente nei bambini più grandi. Negli adolescenti e negli adulti, si può formare solo il pomfo, senza la reazione papulare ritardata. Infine, quando una persona diventa insensibile alla puntura, non compare alcuna reazione. Questo stadio di non reattività si mantiene solo fino a che il soggetto continua regolarmente a venire punto. Gli individui in cui si sviluppa un'orticaria papulare sono nella fase di transizione tra lo sviluppo di una reazione papulare ritardata primaria e quello di una reazione orticarioide immediata.

Le punture di artropodi si possono verificare come lesione solitaria, multipla o diffusa, in rapporto alle abitudini alimentari dell'agente in causa. Le pulci tendono a mordere il proprio ospite parecchie volte in una zona piccola, limitata, mentre le zanzare sono portate ad attaccarlo casualmente, in sedi sparse. Le reazio-

TABELLA 667-1. Artopodi che causano patologia cutanea nell'uomo

Classe Aracnidi (quattro paia di zampe): pidocchi, ragni, zecche
Classe Chilopodi: centipedi
Classe Diplopodi: millepiedi
Classe Insetti (tre paia di zampe):
Ordine Ditteri: zanzare, mosche
Ordine Sifonatteri: pulci
Ordine Imenotteri: formiche, api, vespe
Ordine Anopluri: pidocchio
Ordine Emitteri: cimice dei letti, kissing bug
Ordine Coleotteri: coleotteri
Ordine Lepidotteri: farfalle, tarme

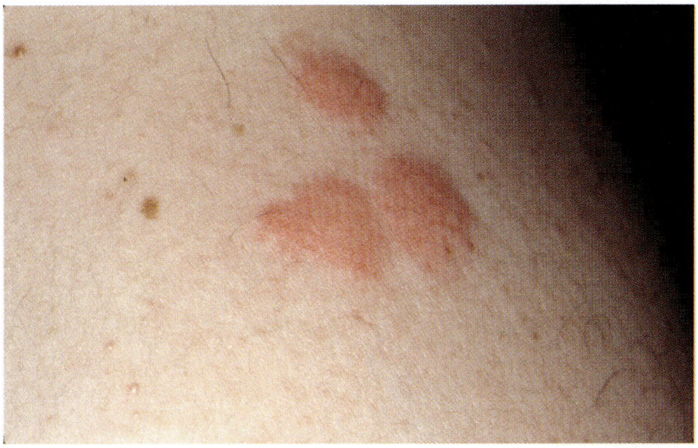

Figura 667-1. Papule pruriginose dopo puntura di cimice dei letti.

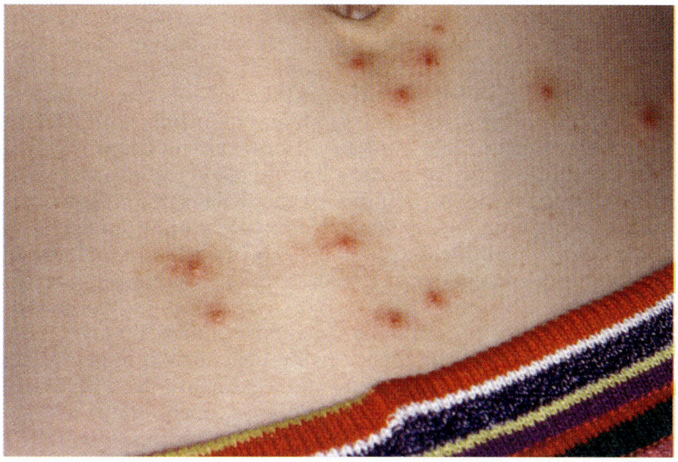

Figura 667-2. Papule rosso-marroni, nell'orticaria papulare.

ni di ipersensibilità ritardata alle punture d'insetto, prevalenti nei giovani e in coloro che non hanno mai avuto un contatto, sono caratterizzate da papule dure, persistenti, che possono diventare iperpigmentate e spesso si escoriano e si coprono di una crosta. Il prurito può essere lieve o severo, transitorio o persistente. In genere è visibile un punto centrale, che però scompare non appena la lesione invecchia o viene grattata. L'ipersensibilità immediata è caratterizzata da un pomfo eritematoso, evanescente, che può essere ricoperto da una piccola vescicola se l'edema è marcato. Certi coleotteri producono una lesione bollosa attraverso l'azione della cantaridina e vari insetti, come anche alcuni coleotteri e ragni, possono provocare noduli emorragici e ulcere. Le punture agli arti inferiori, rispetto a quelle localizzate in altre sedi, possono più facilmente essere severe o persistenti, o diventare bollose. Le complicanze delle punture di artropodi comprendono lo sviluppo di impetigine, follicolite, cellulite, linfangite e gravi reazioni anafilattiche, particolarmente dopo il morso di certi imenotteri. Le modificazioni istopatologiche risultano variabili e dipendono dall'artropode, dall'età della lesione e dalla reattività dell'ospite. Le lesioni orticarioidi acute tendono a mostrare una vescicolazione centrale con numerosi eosinofili. Le papule più frequentemente evidenziano un edema del derma e un infiltrato infiammatorio misto, perivascolare superficiale e profondo, spesso con numerosi eosinofili. Talvolta l'infiltrato cellulare dermico diventa così denso da fare sospettare un linfoma. La ritenzione di parti dell'apparato buccale può stimolare una reazione da corpo estraneo di tipo granulomatoso.

L'**orticaria papulare** si realizza principalmente nella prima decade di vita, durante i mesi più caldi dell'anno. Gli agenti più frequenti sono mosche, acari, cimici dei letti, moscerini, zanzare, pulci e pidocchi degli animali. Gli individui affetti hanno soprattutto lesioni transitorie in vari stadi di evoluzione, da papule a esordio ritardato a pomfi a esordio immediato. La lesione più caratteristica è una papula edematosa, rosso-marrone (Fig. 667-2). Una lesione individuale di solito inizia come un pomfo che, a sua volta, è sostituito da una papula. Una puntura può scatenare la stessa reazione in zone distanti, in sedi di punture quiescenti, sotto forma di macule eritematose, papule o placche orticarioidi. Dopo una stagione o due, la reazione evolve da un'ipersensibilità transitoria a una reazione orticarioide di ipersensibilità primariamente immediata.

Una delle più comuni punture d'insetto è quella dovuta alla pulce dell'uomo, del gatto e del cane (famiglia delle *Pulicidae*). Le uova, solitamente deposte in zone polverose e fissurate del parquet, danno origine a larve, che poi si trasformano in bozzoli. Lo stadio di bozzolo può persistere per più di 1 anno e la pulce emerge in risposta alle vibrazioni dei passi, ciò che motiva l'assalto che frequentemente subisce un nuovo proprietario di un'abitazione che era rimasta disabitata. Le pulci del cane adulto possono vivere senza cibarsi di sangue per circa 60 giorni. Gli attacchi sono più probabili quando le pulci non hanno accesso al loro ospite usuale; si trovano pulci del gatto o del cane più voraci e problematiche visitando l'area frequentata dall'animale domestico, piuttosto che per il contatto diretto con lui. I morsi delle pulci tendono a essere raggruppati in linee o in gruppi casuali. Spesso le pulci non sono visibili sul corpo dell'animale. La diagnosi dei morsi di pulci è aiutata dall'esame del materiale proveniente dalla cuccia degli animali; i detriti si trovano scuotendolo in un sacchetto di plastica ed esaminandone il contenuto, per cercare le pulci o le loro uova, larve o feci.

TRATTAMENTO. Il trattamento è volto ad alleviare il prurito con antistaminici orali e impacchi freddi. Possono venire usati anche corticosteroidi per via topica, mentre gli antistaminici per via topica sono potenti sensibilizzanti e non vanno adoperati. Un breve periodo di terapia corticosteroidea per via sistemica può risultare d'aiuto se compaiono alcune reazioni severe, particolarmente intorno agli occhi. I repellenti per gli insetti con dietiltoluamide (DEET) possono fornire una protezione moderata contro zanzare, pulci, mosche, acari e zecche, ma sono relativamente inefficaci contro vespe, api e calabroni. Il DEET, per essere efficiente, va applicato sulla cute esposta e sugli abiti. La protezione più valida contro le zanzare, il pidocchio del corpo umano e altri artropodi ematofagi, è l'uso del DEET e di vestiario impregnato di permetrina. Tuttavia queste misure non valgono contro la mosca della sabbia flebotoma, che trasmette la leismaniasi.

È necessario uno sforzo per identificare ed eradicare l'agente eziologico. Gli animali domestici vanno attentamente ispezionati. Occorre decontaminare i vespai, le grondaie e altri luoghi della casa o degli annessi frequentati da animali e uccelli e anche le fessure dei battiscopa, i materassi, i tappeti, i mobili e le cucce dove dormono gli animali. Agenti efficaci nella disinfestazione della casa dalle pulci comprendono il lindano, i piretroidi e i tiocianati organici. Gli animali infestati dalle pulci possono essere trattati con polveri contenenti rotenone, piretroidi, malatione o metossicloro.

INFESTAZIONI

SCABBIA. La scabbia è causata dalla penetrazione della femmina dell'acaro *Sarcoptes scabiei* var. *hominis* e dal suo rilascio di sostanze tossiche o antigeniche. Il fattore più importante che determina la diffusione della malattia è il contatto fisico e la sua durata con un individuo affetto. I bambini e i partner sessuali di una persona affetta sono i più a rischio. La scabbia è trasmessa solo raramente da altri mezzi di diffusione, in quanto il parassita isolato muore in 2-3 giorni.

Manifestazioni cliniche. In un ospite immunocompetente, la scabbia è frequentemente annunciata da un intenso prurito, in particolare notturno. Il primo segno dell'infestazione spesso consiste in papule di colorito rosso, di 1-2 mm, alcune delle quali escoriate, con crosta o desquamazione. Le classiche lesioni sono rappresentate dai cunicoli filiformi (Fig. 667-3), che però possono non risultare visibili nei bambini. Nei neonati sono relativamente frequenti bolle e pustole. L'eruzione può comprendere anche pomfi, papule, vescicole e una dermatite eczematosa (Fig. 667-4). Spesso vengono colpiti il palmo delle mani, la pianta dei piedi, il viso, il cuoio capelluto. Nei bambini più grandi e negli adolescenti il quadro clinico è simile a quello dell'adulto, in cui le sedi preferite sono gli spazi interdigitali, le superfici flessorie dei polsi, le pieghe ascellari anteriori, le caviglie, i glutei, l'ombelico e la zona della cintura, il pube, i genitali nel maschio e le areole nelle donne. La testa, il collo, i palmi delle mani e le piante dei piedi vengono invece generalmente risparmiati. Noduli rosso-marrone, più spesso localizzati nelle aree coperte come ascelle, pube e genitali, predominano nella variante meno comune, la scabbia nodulare. Se non trattata, la scabbia può portare a dermatite eczematosa, impetigine, ectima, follicolite, foruncolosi, cellulite, linfangite e reazioni "ID". I bambini, per l'impetiginizzazione streptococcica della scabbia, possono sviluppare una glomerulonefrite. In alcune aree tropicali la scabbia è la causa sottostante del pioderma. All'iniziale infestazione segue un periodo di latenza di circa un mese, per cui può mancare il prurito e le lesioni possono essere relativamente poco apparenti, in soggetti a rischio che sono portatori asintomatici. In caso di reinfestazione, inoltre, si notano reazioni agli antigeni del parassita nel giro di ore.

Eziologia e patogenesi. Una femmina adulta del parassita misura circa 0,4 mm in lunghezza, possiede 4 paia di zampe e ha un corpo emisferico caratterizzato da rughe trasversali, aculei marroni e setole sulla superficie dorsale. Un maschio è circa la metà, con una configurazione simile. Dopo la fecondazione sulla superficie cutanea, una femmina gravida produce una sostanza cheratolitica e un cunicolo nello strato corneo, spesso formando una fossetta poco profonda in 30 min. Gradualmente estende questo tratto di 0,5-5 mm/die lungo il confine con lo strato granuloso. Deposita da 1 a 3 uova e numerose palline formate da feci (scibale) al giorno. Quando la deposizione delle uova è completata, in 4-5 settimane, essa muore all'interno del cunicolo. Le uova si schiudono in 3-5 giorni, rilasciando delle larve che si muovono verso la superficie per diventare ninfe. Raggiungono la maturità in 2-3 settimane, poi si accoppiano e le femmine gravide invadono la cute per completare il loro ciclo vitale.

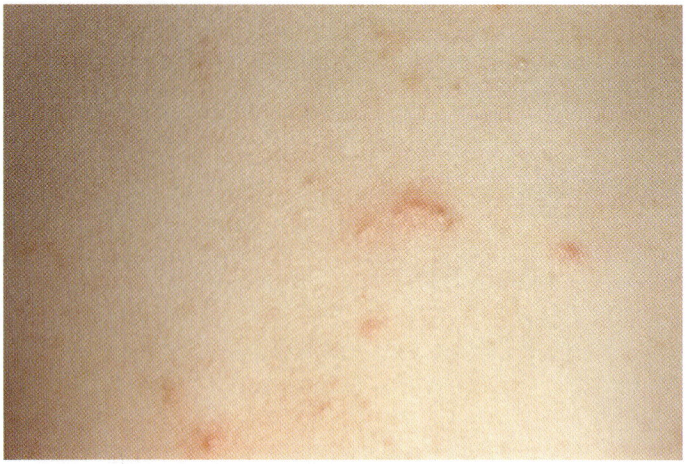

Figura 667-3. Classico cunicolo della scabbia.

Diagnosi. Spesso è clinica, ma viene confermata dall'identificazione microscopica di parassiti (Fig. 667-5*A*), uova e scibale (Fig. 667-5*B*) nei detriti epiteliali. Il materiale è assai spesso positivo, se ottenuto dai cunicoli o da papule fresche. Un metodo affidabile è l'applicazione di una goccia di olio minerale in una lesione, raschiandola poi con una lama n. 15 e trasferendo l'olio e il materiale raschiato su di un vetrino.

La **diagnosi differenziale** dipende dal tipo di lesioni presenti. I cunicoli sono virtualmente patognomonici di scabbia umana. Le lesioni papulovescicolari possono venire confuse con orticaria papulare, scabbia canina, varicella, esantemi virali, eruzioni da farmaci, dermatite erpetiforme e seborroica e, nei neonati con lesioni prevalentemente bollose, possono essere sospettate le meno comuni patologie bollose dell'infanzia. Spesso la scabbia nodulare è scambiata per orticaria pigmentosa e istiocitosi a cellule di Langerhans. Il quadro istopatologico della scabbia nodulare, che consiste in un infiltrato perivascolare profondo, denso, formato da linfociti, istiociti, plasmacellule e cellule mononucleate atipiche, può mimare neoplasie linfoidi maligne.

Trattamento. L'applicazione di crema alla permetrina al 5% o di una crema o lozione al lindano all'1% sull'intero corpo, dal collo in giù, con particolare attenzione per le zone intensamente

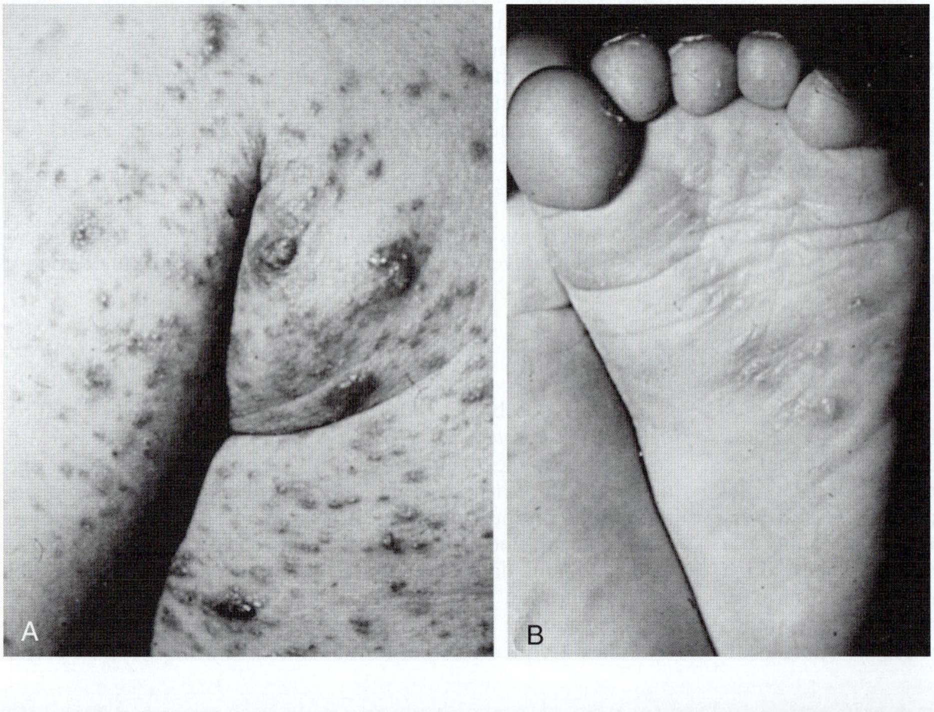

Figura 667-4. *A*, Dermatite eczematosa, papule e noduli della scabbia umana. *B*, Lesioni vescicolo-pustolose della scabbia sulla pianta dei piedi di un neonato.

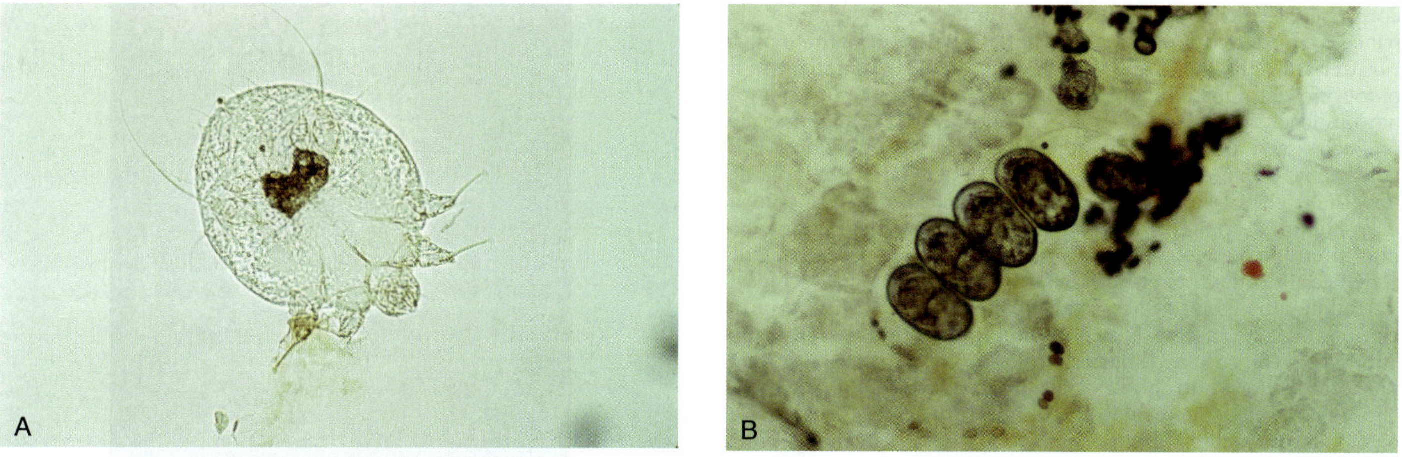

Figura 667-5. *A*, Acaro della scabbia dell'uomo, ottenuto per grattamento. *B*, Uova e scibale di acaro della scabbia.

coinvolte, rappresenta la terapia standard. Spesso nei neonati la scabbia coinvolge zone al di sopra del collo, richiedendo quindi anche un trattamento del cuoio capelluto. Si lascia la medicazione sulla cute per 8-12 ore. Se necessario, si può ripetere l'applicazione entro una settimana per un altro periodo di 8-12 ore. Dato che il lindano è potenzialmente neurotossico, la vulnerabilità dei neonati per quanto riguarda l'assorbimento percutaneo obbliga alla cautela nel prescrivere questo farmaco. I segni di tossicità da lindano comprendono nausea, vomito, stanchezza, tremori, irritabilità, disorientamento, crisi epilettiche e compromissione respiratoria. L'assorbimento sistemico e la tossicità possono essere minimizzati evitando l'applicazione su cute calda e sudata e la ripetizione del trattamento nei 7 giorni successivi, nonché non utilizzando il farmaco in bambini sottopeso o malnutriti o che presentino estese aree infiammate, escoriate o con un'infiammazione cutanea secondaria. La crema di permetrina al 5% è un farmaco lievemente più efficace rispetto al lindano contro la scabbia, ma è più caro. Presenta uno scarso assorbimento, viene rapidamente metabolizzato dalle esterasi tissutali e ha inoltre una tossicità molto bassa. Per neonati con meno di 2 mesi, la terapia alternativa include lo zolfo al 6% in petrolato applicato per tre periodi consecutivi di 24 ore. La pomata allo zolfo sporca e ha un cattivo odore, macchia gli abiti e comunemente provoca una dermatite irritativa. In anni recenti sono stati pubblicati studi non controllati sulla sua efficacia e sicurezza. Per i neonati un'alternativa migliore è rappresentata dalla crema alla permetrina al 5%. La crema o la lozione al crotamitone non è consigliata, perché meno efficace e tossica.

La trasmissione dei parassiti è improbabile oltre le 24 ore dal trattamento. Il prurito, dovuto a ipersensibilità agli antigeni parassitari, può persistere per alcuni giorni e può essere alleviato dall'uso di preparazioni corticosteroidee per via topica. Se invece persiste oltre due settimane dopo il trattamento e compaiono inoltre nuove lesioni, il paziente va riesaminato alla ricerca di parassiti. I noduli sono estremamente resistenti al trattamento e possono richiedere alcuni mesi per la risoluzione. Occorre trattare l'intera famiglia e chi si prende cura del bambino infestato. Devono essere accuratamente lavati i vestiti, la biancheria da letto e gli asciugamani.

Scabbia norvegese. Questa variante della scabbia umana è molto contagiosa e si verifica principalmente in individui mentalmente e fisicamente debilitati, particolarmente quelli ricoverati in istituti o con sindrome di Down, in pazienti con scarsa sensibilità cutanea (lebbra, spina bifida), in soggetti con malattie sistemiche severe (leucemia, diabete) e in quelli immunosoppressi (infezione da HIV). Chi ne viene colpito è infestato da una miriade di parassiti che vivono sulle croste e sulle squame esfoliate della cute e del cuoio capelluto. Le unghie possono diventare sottili e distrofiche. I detriti subungueali sono densamente popolati da parassiti. L'infestazione è spesso accompagnata da una linfoadenopatia generalizzata e da eosinofilia. Sono presenti una massiva ortocheratosi e una paracheratosi con numerosi parassiti sparsi, iperplasia epidermica psoriasiforme, foci di spongiosi e ascessi neutrofili. Si ritiene che la scabbia norvegese costituisca una scarsa risposta immune dell'organismo all'ospite. Il trattamento è difficile e richiede scrupolose misure di isolamento, rimozione delle spesse squame e applicazioni ripetute ma attente di prodotti antiparassitari. Nei casi refrattari, particolarmente in pazienti con infezione da HIV, è stata utilizzata con successo una terapia con dose unica di ivermectina, ma la Food and Drug Administration (FDA) non ha approvato questo farmaco per il trattamento della scabbia o per qualsiasi applicazione in bambini con meno di 5 anni.

Scabbia canina. Viene provocata da *S. scabiei* var. *canis*, il parassita del cane associato alla rogna. Nell'uomo l'eruzione, che si acquisisce il più delle volte accudendo un cucciolo infestato, consiste di minuscole papule, vescicole, pomfi e placche escoriate eczematose. Non sono presenti cunicoli, perché il parassita di rado vive nello strato corneo dell'uomo. Il rash cutaneo è pruriginoso e predilige le braccia, il petto e l'addome, che sono le zone abituali di contatto con i cani. L'esordio è improvviso, usualmente segue l'esposizione di 1-10 giorni e risulta dallo sviluppo di una reazione di ipersensibilità agli antigeni parassitari. È raro trovare parassiti o uova nel materiale che proviene dal grattamento della cute dell'uomo. La malattia è autolimitante, in quanto l'uomo non costituisce un ospite preferito. Generalmente risultano sufficienti il cambio e il lavaggio degli abiti. Diviene necessario l'allontanamento o il trattamento dell'animale infestato. Può essere utile una terapia sintomatica per il prurito. In rari casi in cui il parassita si ritrovi nel materiale grattato da un bambino colpito, può essere eradicato dalle stesse misure applicate per la scabbia umana.

Altri parassiti che occasionalmente pungono l'uomo comprendono la pulce penetrante, o acaro del genere *Trombicula* (*Eutrombicula alfreddugesi*), che preferisce vivere sull'erba, sugli arbusti, sulle viti e sugli steli dei cereali. Le larve hanno un apparato buccale uncinato, che permette alle pulci di attaccarsi alla cute, ma non di scavare cunicoli per succhiare il sangue, la maggior parte delle volte sulle parti inferiori delle gambe. Parassiti degli uccelli possono colpire persone in stretto contatto con polli o gerbilli domestici. L'uomo può occasionalmente essere infestato da parassiti aviari presenti in un nido vicino a una finestra, in un attico, in una ventola del riscaldamento o un condizionatore d'aria. La dermatite è variabile e comprende gruppi di papule, pomfi e lesioni vescicolari su polsi, collo, mammelle, ombelico e pieghe ascellari anteriori. Una ricerca prolungata è spesso necessaria prima di trovare la causa e la fonte della dermatite.

PEDICULOSI. Tre tipi di pidocchi sono parassiti obbligati dell'uomo: il pidocchio del corpo o degli abiti (*Pediculum humanus corporis*), il pidocchio del capo (*Pediculus humanus capitis*) e il pidocchio del pube (*Phthirus pubis*). Solo il pidocchio del corpo serve come vettore di malattia umana (tifo, febbre delle trincee, febbre ricorrente). I pidocchi del corpo e del capo hanno caratteristiche fisiche simili: sono lunghi circa 2-4 mm, mentre il pidocchio del pube è lungo solo 1-2 mm ed è invece più sviluppato in larghezza, assomigliando a un granchio. La femmina del pidocchio vive per circa 1 mese e deposita 3-10 uova al giorno nell'uomo. Il pidocchio del corpo, inoltre, generalmente lascia le uova nelle cuciture degli abiti o in prossimità di queste. Le uova o le lendini si appiccicano ai capelli o alle fibre degli abiti, ma non direttamente al corpo; si schiudono quindi in 1-2 settimane e richiedono un'altra settimana per maturare. Dopo la schiusa, le lendini rimangono attaccate ai capelli come sacchetti vuoti di chitina. Le larve dischiuse da poco muoiono se non trovano cibo entro 24 ore e, successivamente, in pochi giorni. Sia le larve sia i pidocchi adulti si nutrono di sangue umano, iniettando i loro succhi salivari nell'ospite e depositando il loro materiale fecale sulla cute. I sintomi dell'infestazione non compaiono immediatamente, ma si sviluppano man mano che un individuo si sensibilizza. Il segno distintivo di tutti i tipi di pediculosi è il prurito.

La **pediculosi del corpo** è rara nei bambini, eccetto che in condizioni di igiene scarsa, specialmente nei climi più freddi, quando gli abiti vengono cambiati meno regolarmente. Il parassita si trasmette principalmente da un letto o un abito contaminati. La lesione primaria è una piccola macula o papula rossa intensamente pruriginosa, con un punto centrale emorragico, localizzata su tronco, spalle o glutei. Lesioni ulteriori comprendono escoriazioni, pomfi e placche eczematose secondariamente infettate. Un'infestazione massiva può essere associata a sintomi sistemici come febbre, malessere e cefalea. L'infestazione cronica può portare a un quadro noto come "cute del vagabondo", che si manifesta con placche iperpigmentate, desquamate, lichenificate, più di frequente sul tronco. Solo transitoriamente si ritrovano pidocchi sulla cute, mentre si stanno alimentando. In tutti gli altri momenti essi vivono nelle cuciture degli abiti. Le lendini aderiscono strettamente alle fibre del tessuto e possono rimanere vitali per oltre un mese; si schiudono poi a contatto del calore del corpo dell'ospite quando i vestiti vengono nuovamente indossati. La terapia consiste nel miglioramento dell'igiene e nel lavaggio con acqua bollente di tutti i vestiti infestati e della biancheria del letto. Una temperatura uniforme di 65 °C, secca o umida, per 15-30 minuti, uccide tutte le uova o i pidocchi. In alternativa, se il vestiario è riposto per 2 settimane a 25-30 °C, le uova si schiudono e le larve muoiono. Per le persone che non sono in grado di cambiare abbigliamento, si possono rovesciare i vestiti e trattarli con polvere a base di lindano al 10%. L'effetto dura per 1 mese. Possono essere usate una crema a base di permetrina o una lozione a base di lindano, applicate per 8-12 ore, per eradicare ogni uovo e pidocchio presenti sui capelli.

La **pediculosi del capo** è un'infestazione da pidocchi intensamente pruriginosa a livello del cuoio capelluto. Le modalità più frequenti di trasmissione sono il contatto diretto testa-testa e tramite altri mezzi. Nei mesi estivi in molte aree degli Stati Uniti e per tutto il tempo dell'anno ai tropici, per la trasmissione della pediculosi rivestono un ruolo assai importante lo scambio di pettine, spazzola o asciugamani. Le uova traslucide, di 0,5 mm, lasciate in corrispondenza della porzione prossimale del fusto del capello, aderiscono al fusto stesso (Fig. 667-6). Una lendine può essere spostata lungo il capello o staccata dal fusto con le dita. Come conseguenza di un trauma da grattamento, possono comparire pioderma secondario con compattamento di capelli tra loro e linfoadenopatia cervicale e occipitale. La perdita dei capelli non è dovuta alla pediculosi, ma al pioderma secondario. La pediculosi del capo è la causa più frequente di numerosi casi di pioderma del cuoio capelluto, particolarmente in ambienti tropicali. I pidocchi risultano quasi invisibili, ma si possono trovare le lendini sui capelli, più frequentemente nella regione occipitale e dietro le orecchie, raramente sulla barba o nei peli pubici. Talora si può riscontrare una dermatite sul collo o sul padiglione auricolare. Anche sul tronco si può sviluppare una reazione analoga, che consiste in chiazze e placche eritematose. Per ragioni sconosciute, il pidocchio del capo raramente infesta gli afroamericani.

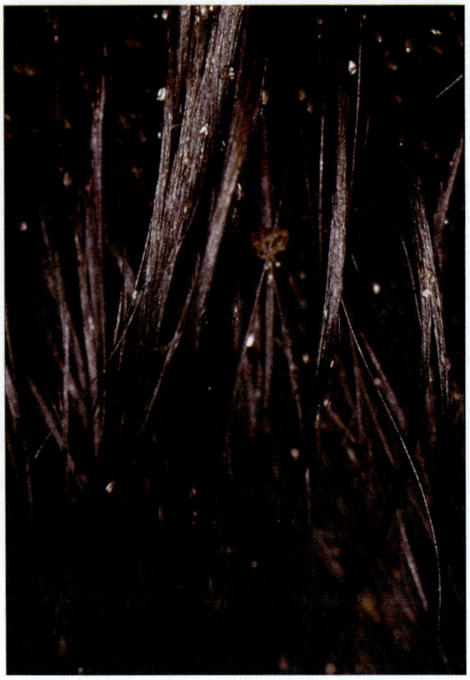

Figura 667-6. Lendini intatte su un capello umano.

Spazzolare e pettinare regolarmente i capelli aiuta a ridurre il numero dei pidocchi e delle uova e a minimizzare la severità dell'infestazione. I **trattamenti** comprendono una crema alla permetrina all'1% applicata per 10 minuti, ripetendo l'operazione dopo 7-10 giorni; uno shampoo alla permetrina naturale; uno shampoo al lindano all'1% da applicare per 10 minuti e da ripetere dopo 7-10 giorni. Il malatione allo 0,5% in isopropanolo è approvato dalla FDA per il trattamento della pediculosi del capo e deve essere applicato sui capelli asciutti fino a bagnarli tutti insieme al cuoio capelluto e quindi va lasciato in sede per 12 ore. Questo prodotto è infiammabile ed è necessaria un'estrema cautela per evitare fiamme libere. Il malatione può essere usato nei casi di resistenza alla piretrina e alla permetrina. Il malatione, simile allo shampoo al lindano, non è indicato nei neonati e nei lattanti. Tutti i membri della famiglia devono essere trattati allo stesso momento. Le lendini possono essere rimosse con un pettine a denti molto stretti dopo l'applicazione di un asciugamano umido sulla testa per 30 minuti. Gli abiti e la biancheria del letto vanno lavati in acqua molto calda o a secco; le spazzole e i pettini devono essere buttati o lavati con un prodotto antiparassitario per 15 minuti e poi sciacquati in acqua bollente.

La **pediculosi del pube** viene trasmessa per contatto cute-cute o per contatto sessuale con un individuo infestato; la probabilità di acquisire il pidocchio durante un rapporto sessuale è di circa il 95%. L'infestazione si riscontra abitualmente negli adolescenti, sebbene anche bambini piccoli possano occasionalmente acquisire il pidocchio del pube sulle ciglia. Il paziente riferisce un prurito da moderato a severo e può sviluppare un pioderma secondario da grattamento. Le escoriazioni tendono a essere molto superficiali e l'incidenza dell'infezione secondaria è inferiore rispetto a quella della pediculosis corporis. Le macule cerulee sono macchie grigio-acciaio, di solito del diametro di 1 cm, che possono comparire nell'area pubica e sul petto, sull'addome e sulle cosce. Lendini ovali translucide, fermamente attaccate al fusto del pelo, possono essere visibili a occhio nudo o possono essere identificate facilmente con una lente di ingrandimento o con un esame microscopico (vedi Fig. 667-6). Se si passano le dita attraverso i peli infestati, talvolta si può percepire una sorta di granulosità, come conseguenza della presenza di lendini aderenti. Riesce difficile individuare il pidocchio adulto, a causa del suo basso livello di attività e per il suo corpo più piccolo e translucido rispetto a quello del pidocchio del corpo o del capo. Dato che il pidocchio del pube può occasionalmente spostarsi, o essere trasportato in sedi diverse da altri mezzi di diffusione, occorre esaminare tutti i peli terminali del tronco, delle cosce, della regione ascellare, della barba e delle ciglia, per cercare eventuali lendini. Va considerata anche la possibilità della coesistenza di altre malattie veneree.

Il **trattamento** con un'applicazione di 10 minuti di una preparazione di piretrina di solito è efficace. Dopo 7-10 giorni può essere necessario un secondo trattamento. Lo shampoo a base di lindano, che richiede un tempo di posa di 10 minuti, costituisce una scelta alternativa, ma la crema o la lozione al lindano non sono più consigliate per il trattamento della pediculosi pubica. L'infestazione delle ciglia è risolta con petrolato applicato 3-5 volte per 24 ore per 8-10 giorni. Anche i vestiti, gli asciugamani e la biancheria del letto possono essere contaminati con peli infestati e vanno lavati con acqua o a secco.

DERMATITE DEL NUOTATORE. La dermatite del nuotatore è una dermatosi notevolmente pruriginosa caratterizzata da papule infiammatorie che si sviluppano in 12 ore dopo un bagno in acqua salata, soprattutto sulle parti del corpo coperte dal costume da bagno. L'eruzione è stata descritta principalmente in rapporto ai bagni nelle acque della Florida e dei Caraibi. Le lesioni, che possono comprendere pustole, vesciche e placche orticarioidi, sono più numerose nei soggetti che tengono addosso i costumi da bagno per un periodo prolungato dopo che sono usciti dall'acqua. L'eruzione può essere accompagnata da sintomi sistemici di fatica, malessere, febbre, freddo, nausea e cefalea; in un'ampia serie, circa il 40% dei bambini con meno di 16 anni ha presentato febbre. La durata del prurito e dell'eruzione cutanea è di 1-2 settimane. Le lesioni consistono in un infiltrato superficiale e profondo perivascolare e interstiziale di linfociti, eosinofili e neutrofili. L'eruzione sembra legata a una reazione di ipersensibilità allergica al veleno delle larve di un tipo di meduse (*Linuche unguiculata*). Il trattamento è ampiamente sintomatico. I corticosteroidi topici a elevata potenza possono essere utili in alcuni pazienti.

Chosidow O: Scabies. *N Engl J Med* 2006;354:1718–1727.
Demain JG: Papular urticaria and things that bite in the night. *Curr Allergy Asthma Rep* 2003;4:291–303.
Frankowski BL: American Academy of Pediatrics guidelines for the prevention and treatment of head lice infestation. *Am J Manag Care* 2004;10:S-69–S272.
Heukelbach J, Feldmeier H: Scabies. *Lancet* 2006;367:1767–1774.
Huynh TH, Norman RA: Scabies and pediculosis. *Dermatol Clin* 2004;22:7–11.
Roberts RJ: Head lice. *N Engl J Med* 2002;346:1645–1650.
Roberts RJ, Burgess IF: New head-lice treatments: Hope or hype? *Lancet* 2005;365:8–10.
Steen CJ, Carbonaro PA, Schwartz RA: Arthropods in dermatology. *J Am Acad Dermatol* 2004;50:819–842.
Walton SF, Holt DC, Currie RJ, et al: Scabies: New future for a neglected disease. *Adv Parasitol* 2004;57:309–376.

Capitolo 668 ■ Acne

Joseph G. Morelli

ACNE VOLGARE

L'acne, particolarmente la forma comedonica, colpisce l'80% degli adolescenti.

PATOGENESI. Le lesioni dell'acne volgare si sviluppano al livello dei follicoli sebacei, formati da una grande ghiandola sebacea multilobulare che secerne il suo prodotto nel canale follicolare. La lesione iniziale è rappresentata da un microcomedone, che si evolve poi a comedone. Questo è formato da un sacco follicolare dilatato, delimitato da un epitelio, ripieno di materiale cheratinico lamellare, di lipidi e di batteri. Un comedone aperto, chiamato anche **punto nero**, è un orifizio pilosebaceo dilatato che permette la visualizzazione del tappo. Un comedone aperto si infiamma più raramente rispetto a uno chiuso o con l'estremità bianca, che presenta solo un'apertura a capocchia di spillo. La papula infiammatoria o il nodulo si sviluppano dalla rottura del comedone, che riversa il contenuto follicolare nel derma adiacente, inducendo una risposta infiammatoria neutrofila. Se la reazione infiammatoria è vicina alla superficie, si sviluppa una papula o una pustola, mentre se l'infiltrato infiammatorio si localizza più profondamente nel derma, si forma un nodulo. Le lesioni nodulocistiche dipendono dalla suppurazione e da un'occasionale reazione a cellule giganti alla cheratina e al pelo. Non si tratta di vere cisti, ma di masse liquefatte di detriti infiammatori.

Le alterazioni patogenetiche primarie dell'acne sono: 1) un'anomala cheratinizzazione dell'epitelio follicolare, con la conseguente occlusione del lume follicolare da parte delle cellule cheratinizzate; 2) un aumento della produzione di sebo da parte delle ghiandole sebacee; 3) la proliferazione follicolare di *Propionibacterium acnes*; 4) l'infiammazione. L'acne comedonica (Fig. 668-1), particolarmente della zona centrale del volto, è spesso il primo segno di maturazione puberale. Alla pubertà, la ghiandola sebacea s'ingrandisce e aumenta la produzione di sebo in risposta all'incremento dell'attività degli androgeni di origine principalmente surrenalica. La maggior parte dei pazienti con acne non presenta significative alterazioni endocrine. Probabilmente un'iperresponsività del sebocita agli androgeni determina la severità dell'acne in un determinato individuo. I sebociti e i cheratinociti follicolari contengono 5α-reduttasi, e 3β- e 17β-idrossisteroido deidrogenasi, che sono in grado di metabolizzare gli androgeni. Un significativo numero di donne con acne (25-50%), particolarmente quelle con un'acne papulo pustolosa relativamente lieve, notano che questa si accentua circa una settimana prima delle mestruazioni. La patogenesi di questo fenomeno è sconosciuta.

Il sebo appena formato consiste di una miscela di trigliceridi, cere, esteri, squalene ed esteri dello sterolo. I normali batteri follicolari producono lipasi che idrolizzano i trigliceridi del sebo in acidi grassi liberi. Quelli con catene di media lunghezza (C8-C14) possono fungere da fattori scatenanti della reazione infiammatoria. Il sebo costituisce anche un substrato favorevole per la proliferazione batterica. *Propionibacterium acnes* è ampiamente responsabile della formazione di acidi grassi liberi. Esiste una correlazione tra la sua riduzione e il miglioramento dell'acne volgare. È probabile che proteasi, ialuronidasi ed enzimi idrolitici batterici producano materiali extracellulari biologicamente attivi, che aumentano la permeabilità dell'epitelio follicolare. I fattori chemiotattici rilasciati dai batteri intrafollicolari attraggono neutrofili e monociti. Gli enzimi lisosomiali dei neutrofili, rilasciati

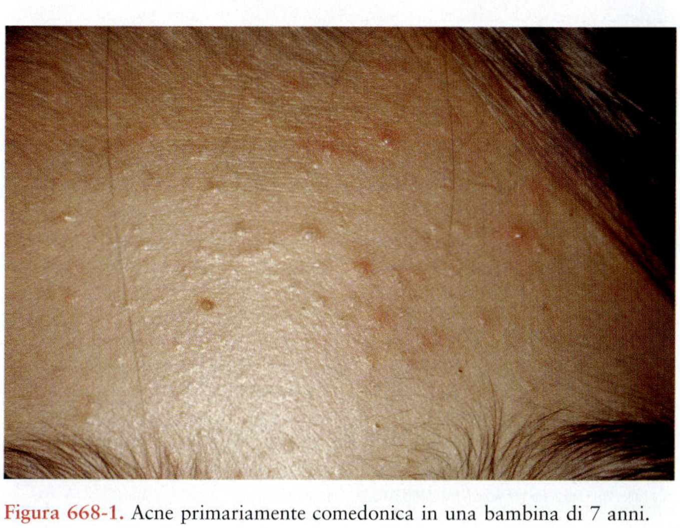

Figura 668-1. Acne primariamente comedonica in una bambina di 7 anni.

durante il processo di fagocitosi batterica, alterano successivamente l'integrità della parete follicolare e aumentano la reazione infiammatoria.

MANIFESTAZIONI CLINICHE. L'acne volgare è caratterizzata da 4 tipi di lesioni di base: comedoni aperti e chiusi, papule, pustole (Fig. 668-2) e lesioni nodulo-cistiche (Fig. 668-3 e Tab. 668-1). Possono essere predominanti uno o più tipi. Nelle forme più lievi, che spesso si vedono nelle prime fasi dell'adolescenza, le lesioni sono limitate a comedoni nella porzione centrale del volto, ma possono coinvolgere anche il torace, la parte superiore del dorso e la zona deltoidea. Una predominanza di lesioni sulla fronte, particolarmente di comedoni chiusi, è attribuibile spesso all'uso prolungato di preparazioni grasse per i capelli (acne da brillantina) (Fig. 668-4). Un marcato coinvolgimento del tronco è più frequente nei maschi. Le lesioni spesso guariscono con un temporaneo eritema postinfiammatorio e un'iperpigmentazione. In rapporto alla severità, alla profondità e alla cronicità del processo, possono essere presenti cicatrici infossate, atrofiche o ipetrofiche. La diagnosi di acne raramente pone difficoltà, sebbene verruche piane, follicolite e altri tipi di acne possano essere confusi con quella volgare.

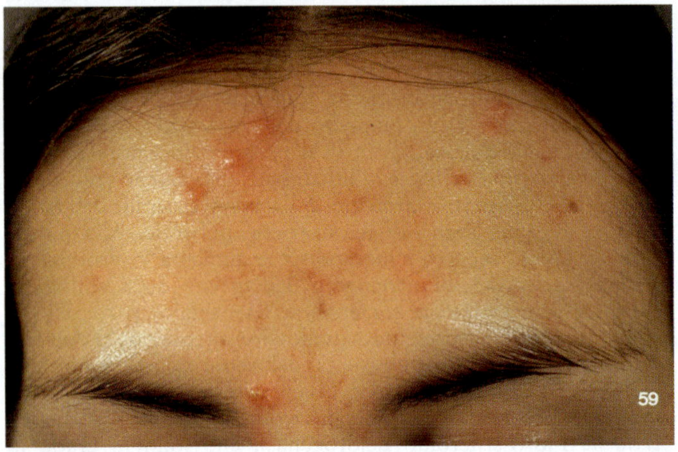

Figura 668-2. Papule e pustole infiammatorie.

TRATTAMENTO. Non ci sono dati che dimostrino che il trattamento precoce, a eccezione dell'isotretinoina, modifichi il decorso dell'acne. Tuttavia, con un'adeguata terapia di mantenimento da continuare fino alla scomparsa spontanea del processo patologico, l'acne può essere controllata e si possono prevenire gravi cicatrici. La terapia deve essere individualizzata e aiuta a prevenire la formazione del microcomedone attraverso la riduzione dell'ipercheratosi follicolare, della produzione di sebo, della popolazione del *P. acnes* negli orifizi follicolari e della produzione di acidi grassi liberi. L'iniziale controllo dura almeno 6-8 settimane, a seconda della severità (Tab. 668-2). È importante anche tenere conto dell'impatto emotivo potenzialmente grave dell'acne sull'adolescente.

Il pediatra dovrebbe essere consapevole della correlazione, spesso scarsa, tra la severità dell'acne e l'impatto psicosociale, particolarmente negli adolescenti. Dato che gli adolescenti sono molto preoccupati del loro aspetto, offrire un trattamento anche ai più giovani, in cui l'acne è lieve, può aumentare l'autostima.

Dieta. Pochi dati dimostrano che l'ingestione di particolari alimenti possa scatenare l'acne. Quando un paziente è convinto che

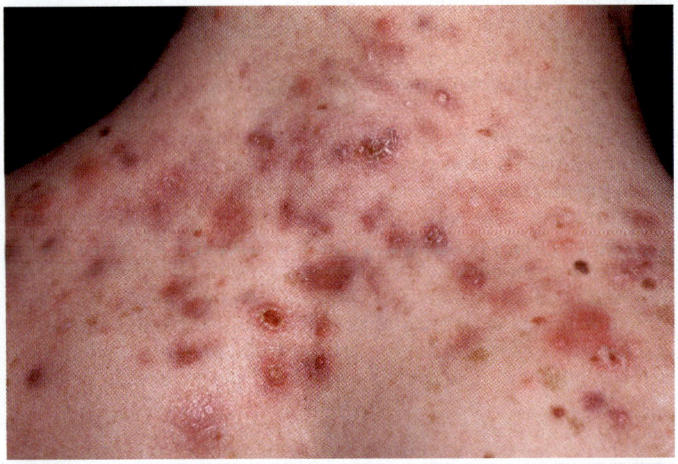

Figura 668-3. Severa acne nodulocistica.

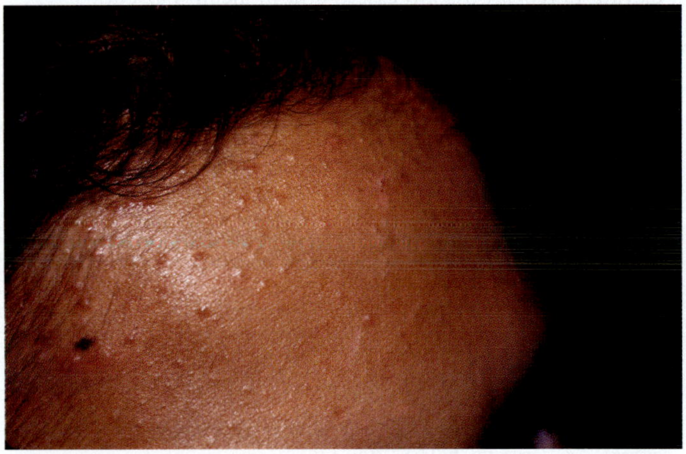

Figura 668-4. Acne da brillantina lungo l'attaccatura dei capelli.

TABELLA 668-1. Classificazione dell'acne

SEVERITÀ	DESCRIZIONE
Lieve	I comedoni (lesioni non infiammatorie) sono le lesioni principali. Possono essere presenti papule e pustole, ma piccole e in scarso numero (generalmente 10).
Moderata	Moderato numero di papule e pustole (10-40) e comedoni (10-40). Può essere presente anche un lieve interessamento del tronco.
Moderatamente severa	Sono presenti numerose papule e pustole (40-100), usualmente con molti comedoni e occasionalmente lesioni nodulari infiammate più ampie, più profonde (oltre 5). Le aree diffuse interessate coinvolgono il viso, il torace e il dorso.
Severa	Acne nodulo-cistica e acne conglobata con molte spesse lesioni dolorose nodulari o pustolose, insieme a molte papule, pustole e comedoni più piccoli.

Da James WD: Clinical practice. Acne. *N Engl J Med* 2005;352:1463-1472.

TABELLA 668-2. Regime di trattamento tipico per l'acne

ACNE COMEDONICA
Retinoide topico o
Acido azelaico

ACNE PAPULOPUSTOLOSA LIEVE
Retinoide topico più
Benzoil perossido o
Antibiotico topico o
Antibiotico orale

ACNE PAPULOPUSTOLOSA SEVERA O NODULARE
Retinoide topico più
Benzoil perossido e antibiotici orali o
Isotretinoina 1 mg/kg/die

certi cibi la esacerbino, è meglio sospendere tali alimenti. Non è necessario, tuttavia, imporre ingiustificate restrizioni dietetiche.

Clima. Il clima influenza l'acne, nel senso che frequentemente essa migliora durante la stagione estiva e peggiora in inverno. In estate la remissione può essere correlata, in parte, alla relativa assenza di stress. In molte persone la tensione emotiva e la fatica esacerbano infatti l'acne; il meccanismo non è chiaro, ma si pensa sia legato a un aumento della risposta corticosurrenalica.

Igiene. La pulizia con acqua e sapone rimuove i lipidi della superficie e rende la cute di aspetto meno oleoso, ma non è stato dimostrato che i lipidi superficiali abbiano un ruolo nella genesi delle lesioni acneiche. Con il lavaggio si ottiene solo di seccare la cute e di eseguire un peeling superficiale e si può utilizzare qualsiasi sapone lieve o astringente. Lavaggi ripetuti possono essere dannosi, perché irritano e screpolano la cute. I detergenti che contengono abrasivi e cheratolitici, come lo zolfo, il resorcinolo e l'acido salicilico, possono rimuovere temporaneamente il sebo dalla superficie cutanea. Essi consentono un lavaggio delicato e un effetto di peeling, nonché limitano le lesioni a livelli moderati. Non sono in grado, tuttavia, di prevenire la formazione dei microcomedoni. Non esistono dati che dimostrino che le preparazioni contenenti alcol o esaclorofene abbiano un effetto riducente sull'acne, in quanto i batteri di superficie non sono coinvolti nella patogenesi. I cosmetici grassi e le preparazioni per i capelli vanno sospesi, in quanto possono peggiorare un'acne preesistente e provocare un'ulteriore ostruzione dell'orifizio follicolare. La manipolazione e lo schiacciamento delle lesioni al volto provocano la rottura di quelle intatte e una reazione infiammatoria localizzata.

Terapia topica. Tutte le preparazioni topiche devono essere usate per 6-8 settimane prima di verificarne l'efficacia. I retinoidi possono venire adoperati da soli per le forme lievi, ma spesso una terapia combinata è più efficace. Una combinazione diffusa ma efficace è rappresentata dall'uso di un gel a base di benzoil perossido al mattino e di un retinoide alla sera.

RETINOIDI. Nell'acne volgare il **primo trattamento** dovrebbe essere un retinoide topico. Questi farmaci hanno molteplici azioni, comprese l'inibizione della formazione di numerosi microcomedoni, la riduzione dei comedoni maturi, la diminuzione delle lesioni infiammatorie e la produzione di una normale desquamazione dell'epitelio follicolare. I retinoidi devono essere applicati giornalmente in tutte le zone affette. I principali effetti collaterali sono costituiti dall'irritazione e dalla secchezza. Inizialmente non tutti i pazienti ne tollerano l'uso giornaliero, per cui risulta prudente cominciare la terapia a giorni alterni o ogni tre giorni, per poi aumentare lentamente la frequenza delle applicazioni, se vengono ben tollerate. La tretinoina, l'adapalene e il tazarotene (Tab. 668-3) sono i retinoidi disponibili. Hanno più o meno tutti la stessa efficienza, sebbene l'adapalene sia meno irritante e il tazarotene sia lievemente più efficace nell'acne comedonica.

BENZOIL PEROSSIDO. Il benzoil perossido è primariamente un agente antibatterico. Il suo vantaggio rispetto agli antibiotici topici è di non aumentare la resistenza batterica. Risulta disponibile in molteplici formulazioni e concentrazioni. Quelle in gel sono preferibili per la loro migliore stabilità e per il più consistente rilascio di principio attivo. Lozioni e saponi vengono utilizzati per coprire ampie superfici, quali il torace e il dorso. I principali effetti collaterali sono l'irritazione e la secchezza, come quelli dei retinoidi. Il benzoil perossido può anche decolorare gli abiti.

ANTIBIOTICI TOPICI. Gli antibiotici topici sono indicati per il trattamento dell'acne infiammatoria. La clindamicina e l'eritromicina sono quelli utilizzati più comunemente, ma non sono efficaci come il benzoil perossido o gli antibiotici per via orale. Non vanno usati in monoterapia, perché non inibiscono la formazione del microcomedone e possono indurre una resistenza antimicrobica. Irritazione e secchezza generalmente sono inferiori a quelle che si verificano con i retinoidi o il benzoil perossido.

ACIDO AZELAICO. L'acido azelaico (crema al 20%) ha modeste proprietà amtimicrobiche e cheratolitiche.

Terapia sistemica. Gli antibiotici, specialmente le tetracicline e i loro derivati (vedi Tab. 668-3), sono indicati per il trattamento dei pazienti che non tollerano o non hanno risposto ai farmaci per via topica, che presentano un'acne infiammatoria papulo pustolosa da moderata a severa e nodulocistica e che hanno propensione per le cicatrici. Le tetracicline e i loro derivati agiscono riducendo la crescita e il metabolismo del *P. acnes*. Possiedono inoltre proprietà antinfiammatorie. Per la maggior parte dei pazienti adolescenti, la terapia va iniziata con due somministrazioni al giorno per almeno 6-8 settimane, seguite da un graduale decremento della dose minima efficace. I farmaci vanno sempre fatti assumere in combinazione con i retinoidi per uso topico, ma non con gli antibiotici topici. L'assorbimento della tetraciclina è inibito dagli alimenti, dal latte, dalla supplementazione di ferro, dal gel di idrossido di alluminio e dai sali di calcio-magnesio. Vanno assunti a stomaco vuoto 1 ora prima o 2 ore dopo i pasti. La minociclina e la doxiciclina possono invece essere assunte durante i pasti. Gli effetti collaterali di questi farmaci sono rari e comprendono candidiasi vaginale, particolarmente in chi assume tetracicline insieme ai contraccettivi orali, irritazione gastrointestinale, reazioni fototossiche, comprese l'onicolisi e una colorazione marrone delle unghie, ulcerazioni esofagee, inibizione della crescita scheletrica fetale e della colorazione dei denti in crescita, ciò che quindi preclude il loro utilizzo durante la gravidanza e nei bambini con meno di 8 anni. La doxiciclina è il più fotosensibilizzante tra i derivati tetraciclinici. Raramente, la minociclina provoca vertigini, ipertensione endocranica, colorazione bluastra di cute e mucose, epatite e una sindrome lupus-simile. Una possibile complicanza del prolungato uso sistemico degli antibiotici è rappresentata dalla proliferazione di microrganismi Gram-negativi, particolarmente *Enterobacter*, *Klesbiella*, *Eschirichia coli* o *Pseudomonas aeruginosa*, che producono una grave follicolite refrattaria.

Le donne che presentano acne e anomalie ormonali, non responsive alla terapia antibiotica, o che non sono candidate alla terapia con l'isotretinoina, possono essere trattate con una terapia ormonale, di cui i contraccettivi orali costituiscono la forma primaria. Si è dimostrato efficace anche lo spironolattone.

La isotretinoina (acido 13-cis-retinoico) è indicata per l'acne nodulocistica severa e per quella da moderata a grave che non ha risposto alla terapia convenzionale. Il dosaggio raccomandato è di circa 0,5-1,0 mg/kg/die. Un trattamento standard, negli Stati Uniti, prevede 16-20 settimane, al termine delle quali circa il 40% dei pazienti è guarito, il 45% necessita di farmaci convenzionali topici o orali per mantenere un adeguato controllo e il 20% presenta recidive e necessita di un ulteriore ciclo. Dosaggi di 0,5 mg/kg/die o una dose cumulativa di 120 mg/kg sono associati a una percentuale significativamente maggiore d'insuccesso terapeutico e di recidiva. Se il processo patologico non è in remissione due mesi dopo il primo ciclo, è necessario considerarne un secondo. L'isotretinoina riduce le dimensioni e la secrezione delle ghiandole sebacee, normalizza la cheratinizzazione follicolare, previene la formazione di nuovi microcomedoni, diminuisce la popolazione del *P. acnes* ed esercita un effetto antinfiammatorio.

Il suo utilizzo ha molti effetti collaterali. L'isotretinoina è altamente **teratogena** e **assolutamente controindicata** durante la gravidanza. È inoltre necessario evitare una gravidanza per i 6 mesi successivi all'interruzione della terapia. Sono richieste 2 o 3 forme di controllo delle nascite e un test di gravidanza mensile. Le preoccupazioni per i casi di gravidanza nonostante gli avvertimenti hanno suggerito un programma di registrazione da parte del produttore, iPLEDGE (www.ipledgeprogram.com), che richiede, per la prescrizione di isotretinoina, l'iscrizione del medico e un accurato screening di gravidanza delle pazienti. Molte presentano cheilite, xerosi, epistassi periodica e blefarocongiuntivite e risulta comune anche un incremento dei valori del colesterolo e dei trigliceridi. Prima di cominciare la terapia è importante escludere l'iperlipidemia e preesistenti patologie epatiche ed è necessario richiedere un controllo delle indagini di laboratorio 4 settimane dopo l'inizio. Effetti collaterali meno comuni ma significativi comprendono artralgie, mialgie, un temporaneo diradamento dei capelli, paronichia, un'aumentata suscettibilità agli eritemi solari, la formazione di granulomi piogenici e la colonizzazione della cute da *Staphylococcus aureus*, che porta a impetigine, secondariamente a dermatite infetta e a

TABELLA 668-3. Farmaci per il trattamento dell'acne

FARMACI	DOSE	EFFETTI COLLATERALI	ALTRE CONSIDERAZIONI
AGENTI TOPICI			
Retinoidi			
Tretinoina	Applicata una volta al giorno alla notte; concentrazione di 0,025-0,1% disponibile**	Irritazione	Disponibile generico
Adapalene	Applicato una volta al giorno, di notte o al mattino, 0,01%§§	Minima irritazione	
Tazarotene*	Applicato una volta al giorno la notte, 0,05, 0,1%	Irritazione	Dati limitati suggeriscono che il tarazotene sia più efficace rispetto alle alternative
Antimicrobici			
Benzoil perossido, solo o con lo zinco, 2,5-10%	Applicato una o due volte al giorno	Il benzoil perossido può decolorare gli abiti e le lenzuola	Farmaco da banco; la concentrazione al 2,5-5% è efficace come quella al 10% e secca meno la cute
Clindamicina, eritromicina†	Applicate una o due volte al giorno	Possibile resistenza	Più efficaci per lesioni infiammatorie (più che per i comedoni); possibilità di resistenza se usate da sole
Combinazione di benzoil perossido e clindamicina o eritromicina	Applicati una o due volte al giorno		Combinazione più efficace degli antibiotici topici da soli; limitato lo sviluppo di resistenza; l'uso di un singolo prodotto in combinazione è meno costoso e appare ugualmente efficace
ALTRI AGENTI TOPICI			
Acido azelaico, sodio sulfacetamide-solfuro, acido salicilico†	Applicati una o due volte al giorno	Ben tollerati	Buon trattamento adiuvante o alternativo
ANTIBIOTICI ORALI‡			
Tetraciclina§	250-500 mg una o due volte al giorno	Disturbi gastrointestinali, pseudotumor cerebri	Non costoso; dosaggio limitato da prendere a stomaco vuoto: una dose di 20 mg solo antinfiammatoria; dati limitati sull'efficacia
Doxiciclina§	50-100 mg una o due volte al giorno	Fototossicità, pseudotumor cerebri	
Minociclina§	50-100 mg una o due volte al giorno	Iperpigmentazione dei denti, della mucosa orale e della cute; reazioni lupus-simili con trattamenti di lunga durata, pseudotumor cerebri	
Trimetropim-sulfametoxazolo	Una dose (160 mg di trimetropim e 800 mg di sulfametoxazolo) due volte al giorno	Necrolisi epidermica tossica ed eruzioni allergiche	Il trimetropin può essere usato da solo alla dose di 300 mg due volte al giorno; disponibili dati limitati
Eritromicina†	250-500 mg da due a quattro volte al giorno	Disturbi gastrointestinali	Resistenza problematica, efficacia limitata
AGENTI ORMONALI¶			
Spironolattone§	50-200 mg divisi in due dosi	Irregolarità mestruali, dolorabilità mammaria	Dosi maggiori più efficaci, ma provocano più effetti collaterali; meglio se usato in combinazione con contraccettivi orali
Contraccettivi orali contenenti estrogeni	Giornalieri	Potenziali effetti collaterali, compresa tromboembolia	
RETINOIDI ORALI			
Isotretinoina‖	0,5-1,0 mg/kg/die divisi in dosi	Difetti alla nascita; è essenziale l'aderenza a un programma di prevenzione della gravidanza descritto dalla produzione di farmaci, compresi due test iniziali di gravidanza negativi. Sono possibili di frequente o costituiscono importanti effetti collaterali: ipertrigliceridemia, elevati livelli dei test di funzionalità epatica, anomalie della visione notturna, ipertensione endocranica benigna, secchezza della mucosa di labbra, naso, occhi e bocca, e della cute, infezioni stafilococciche secondarie; eseguire indagini di laboratorio sul profilo lipidico e la funzionalità epatica mensilmente fino alla stabilizzazione del dosaggio	Percentuale di recidiva più alta se il paziente all'inizio del trattamento ha meno di 16 anni, se l'acne è molto severa e coinvolge il tronco o se il farmaco è usato da donne adulte

*Il tazarotene è in categoria gravidanza X: controindicato in gravidanza.
†Clindamicina, eritromicina e acido azelaico sono nella categoria gravidanza B: non ci sono evidenze di rischio per l'essere umano.
‡Antibiotici orali sono indicati per malattia da moderata a severa; per il trattamento dell'acne di torace, dorso, spalle; in pazienti con malattia infiammatoria in cui combinazioni topiche abbiano fallito o non siano tollerate.
§Questo farmaco è nella categoria gravidanza D: evidenze positive di rischio nell'essere umano.
¶Gli agenti ormonali sono per uso esclusivo delle donne.
‖L'isotretinoina è in categoria gravidanza X: controindicata. Deve essere usata solo in pazienti con acne severa che non rispondono alla combinazione di antibiotici orali e terapia topica.
**Come crema, gel o lozione.
§§Come crema o gel.
Modificata da James WD: Clinical practice: Acne. *N Engl J Med* 2005;352:1463-1472.

follicolite del cuoio capelluto. Raramente, dopo più di un ciclo di terapia con l'isotretinoina, si sviluppano lesioni iperostotiche della colonna vertebrale. L'uso concomitante della tetraciclina e della isotretinoina è controindicato, perché entrambi i farmaci, ma particolarmente l'associazione dei due, possono provocare un'ipertensione endocranica benigna. Nonostante non sia stato stabilito un rapporto causa-effetto, le modificazioni dell'umore e la depressione e/o il suicidio indotti dal farmaco hanno imposto uno stretto controllo medico prima e durante la prescrizione.

Terapia chirurgica. Iniezioni intralesionali di basse dosi (3 mg/mL) di glicocorticoidi di potenza medio-alta (per es. triamcinolone) con un ago di calibro 30 o una siringa da tubercolina possono accelerare la comparsa di lesioni dolorose, individuali, nodulocistiche. Per minimizzare le cicatrici vanno presi in considerazione la dermoabrasione o il laser, ma solo dopo che il processo attivo è diventato quiescente.

Il ruolo del laser a colori pulsato nel trattamento dell'acne infiammatoria è controverso e non convincente.

ACNE DA FARMACI

I pazienti in età puberale e postpuberale che vengono sottoposti a una terapia sistemica con glicocorticoidi sono predisposti all'acne da steroidi. Questa follicolite monomorfa si verifica primariamente su volto, collo, torace (Fig. 668-5), spalle, parte superiore del dorso, braccia e raramente sul cuoio capelluto. L'esordio avviene dopo circa 2 settimane dall'inizio della terapia. Le lesioni sono

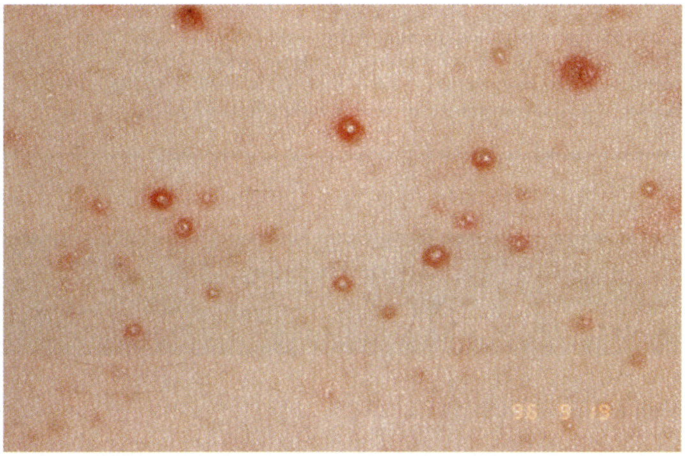

Figura 668-5. Eruzione papulare monomorfa di acne da steroidi.

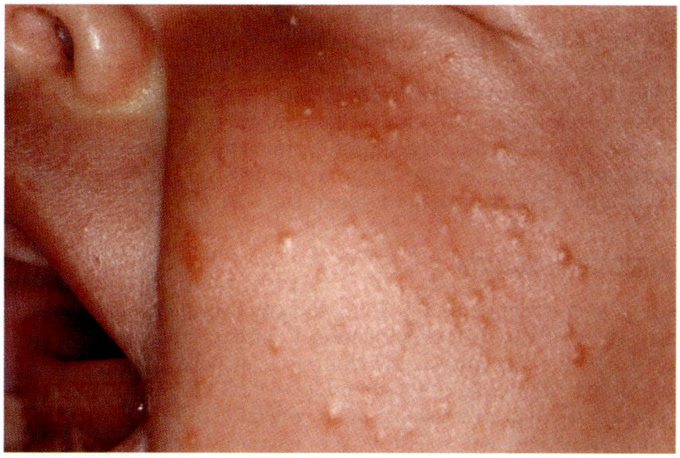

Figura 668-6. Acne comedonica in un neonato.

piccole, formate da papule eritematose o pustole che possono manifestarsi numerose e sono tutte nello stesso stadio di sviluppo. Successivamente possono comparire comedoni, ma le lesioni nodulocistiche e le cicatrici sono rare. Il prurito è occasionale. Nonostante l'acne da steroidi sia relativamente refrattaria se si continua la terapia, l'eruzione può rispondere all'uso della tretinoina e di un gel al benzoil perossido.

Altri **farmaci** che possono indurre **lesioni acneiformi** in individui sensibili sono l'isoniazide, la fenitoina, il fenobarbital, il trimetadione, il carbonato di litio, gli androgeni (steroidi anabolizzanti) e la vitamina B_{12}.

ACNE DA ALOGENI

La somministrazione di farmaci contenenti ioduri o bromuri o, raramente, l'ingestione di quantità massive di preparazioni a base di vitamine e minerali o di "cibi dietetici" contenenti iodio, come il fuco, possono indurre un'acne da alogeni. Le lesioni spesso presentano una notevole infiammazione. La sospensione dell'agente responsabile e appropriate terapie topiche usualmente ottengono ragionevoli risultati terapeutici.

CLORACNE

La cloracne è dovuta al contatto esterno, all'inalazione o all'ingestione di idrocarburi aromatici alogenati, compresi i bifenili polialogenati e le diossine. Le lesioni sono primariamente comedoniche, mentre quelle infiammatorie appaiono infrequenti, sebbene possano comunque comprendere papule, pustole, noduli e cisti. La guarigione si realizza lasciando cicatrici atrofiche o ipetrofiche. Vengono coinvolti più comunemente il volto, le regioni retroauricolari, il collo, le ascelle, i genitali e il torace. Il naso spesso viene risparmiato. Nei casi di esposizione severa si possono associare epatite, produzione di porfirine, formazioni di bolle sulla cute esposta al sole, iperpigmentazione, ipertricosi e iperidrosi palmare e plantare. Retinoidi topici o orali possono risultare opportuni, mentre il benzoil perossido e gli antibiotici di solito sono inefficaci.

ACNE NEONATALE

Circa il 20% dei neonati normali sviluppa almeno qualche comedone nel primo mese di vita. Comedoni chiusi predominano sulle guance e sulla fronte (Fig. 668-6); occasionalmente si riscontrano comedoni aperti e papulopustole. La causa dell'acne neonatale è sconosciuta, ma è stata attribuita a un passaggio transplacentare di androgeni materni, all'iperattività dei surreni neonatali e a un'ipersensibilità neonatale agli ormoni androgeni. Nel giro di qualche mese le ghiandole sebacee ipertrofiche vanno incontro a involuzione spontanea e così anche l'acne. Di solito non è necessario alcun **trattamento**. Le lesioni possono comunque venire trattate efficacemente con la tretinoina e/o il benzoil perossido per uso topico.

ACNE INFANTILE

L'acne infantile si presenta abitualmente dopo il primo anno di vita, sia nei maschi sia nelle femmine. Le lesioni acneiche sono più numerose, pleiomorfe, severe e persistenti di quelle dell'acne neonatale (Fig. 668-7). Comedoni aperti e chiusi predominano sul volto. Papule e pustole compaiono di frequente, ma solo occasionalmente si sviluppano lesioni nodulocistiche. Nel 10-15% dei casi si notano cicatrici butterate. Il decorso può essere relativamente breve, oppure le lesioni possono persistere per molti mesi, sebbene l'eruzione generalmente si risolva intorno ai 3 anni. L'uso di un gel topico a base di benzoil perossido e di tretinoina di solito porta alla risoluzione in poche settimane. Solo talvolta è necessaria l'eritromicina per via orale. Un bambino con un'acne refrattaria giustifica la ricerca di una fonte anomala di androgeni, come un tumore virilizzante o un'iperplasia surrenalica congenita.

ACNE TROPICALE

Nei climi tropicali si manifesta una forma severa di acne, che si ritiene sia dovuta al caldo intenso e all'umidità. L'idratazione del

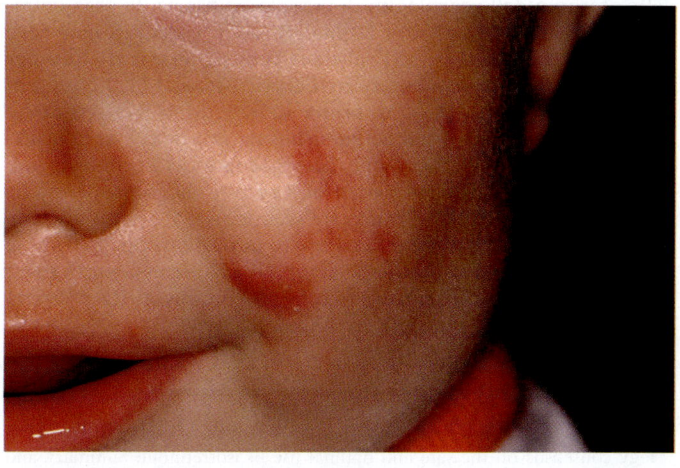

Figura 668-7. Acne infantile infiammatoria.

poro del dotto pilosebaceo può accentuare l'occlusione del dotto. Gli individui colpiti tendono ad avere un'anamnesi precedente di acne giovanile, che è quiescente al momento dell'eruzione. Le lesioni si verificano soprattutto su tutto il dorso, sul torace, sui glutei e sulle cosce, con una predominanza di papule suppurate e di noduli. Come complicanza può comparire un'infezione secondaria da *S. aureus*. Se non vengono eliminati i fattori ambientali, l'eruzione è refrattaria alla terapia dell'acne.

ACNE CONGLOBATA

L'acne conglobata è una malattia infiammatoria cronica progressiva che compare principalmente nel maschio adulto, più comunemente di razza bianca che non nera, ma che può cominciare durante l'adolescenza. I pazienti di solito hanno un'anamnesi positiva per una preesistente acne volgare. La lesione principale è il nodulo, sebbene spesso vi sia una miscela di comedoni con multipli pori, papule, pustole, noduli, cisti, ascessi e dissezione sottocutanea con formazione di molteplici canalicoli. Una grave cicatrizzazione è caratteristica. Il viso è relativamente risparmiato, ma oltre al dorso e al torace possono essere coinvolti i glutei, l'addome, le braccia e le cosce. Sintomi sistemici e anemia possono accompagnare il processo infiammatorio. Di frequente nel materiale che proviene dalle lesioni si ritrovano lo stafilococco coagulasi-positivo e lo streptococco emolitico, ma questi non sembrano essere primariamente coinvolti nella patogenesi. Occasionalmente si realizza un'acne conglobata in associazione con un'idrosoadenite suppurativa e una cellulite dissecante del cuoio capelluto (come la triade d'occlusione follicolare) e può essere complicata da un'artrite erosiva e una spondiloartrite anchilosante. Le indagini endocrine non appaiono significative. La terapia di routine dell'acne è generalmente inefficace. Per sopprimere l'intensa attività infiammatoria può invece essere necessaria una terapia sistemica con corticosteroidi. L'isotreitinoina è la soluzione più efficace per molti pazienti, ma dopo il suo inizio può comportare una riacutizzazione in alcuni pazienti.

ACNE FULMINANTE (ACNE ULCERATIVA FEBBRILE ACUTA)

L'acne fulminante è caratterizzata dall'esordio brusco di estese lesioni infiammatorie acneiche con tendenza ulcerativa, sul dorso e sul torace di maschi adolescenti. La caratteristica distintiva è la tendenza a formare ampi noduli, fino a placche essudative, necrotiche, ulcerate, crostose. Le lesioni spesso risparmiano il viso e guariscono con una cicatrice. Nella maggior parte dei pazienti si ha una precedente anamnesi di acne papulopustolosa lieve o di acne nodulare. I sintomi e i segni sistemici sono comuni e comprendono febbre, debilitazione, artralgie, mialgie, perdita di peso e leucocitosi. L'emocultura è sterile. Lesioni di un **eritema nodoso** talvolta si sviluppano in area pretibiale. Lesioni **ossee di tipo osteolitico** possono formarsi in corrispondenza della clavicola, dello sterno e delle cartilagini di crescita epifisarie; le ossa colpite appaiono normali o, con la guarigione, presentano una lieve sclerosi o un ispessimento. I salicilati possono essere d'aiuto per le mialgie, le artralgie e la febbre. I corticosteroidi (1,0 mg/kg di prednisone) sono i farmaci di prima scelta e dopo una settimana si aggiunge l'isotretinoina. Se quest'ultima non può essere utilizzata, risulta efficace il dapsone. Si sospendono i corticosteroidi dopo 6 settimane. Gli antibiotici non sono indicati, a meno che non vi siano i segni di un'infezione secondaria. Rispetto all'acne conglobata, quella fulminante compare in pazienti più giovani, è più esplosiva all'esordio, è associata più di frequente a segni sistemici e a lesioni crostose ulcerate e meno comunemente presenta comedoni con teste multiple o coinvolge il viso.

Goldsmith LA, Bolognia JL, Callen JP, et al: Amercian Academy of Dermatology consensus on the safe and optimal use of isotretinoin: Summary and recommendations. *J Am Acad Dermatol* 2004;50:900–906.
Gollnick H, Cunliffe W: Management of acne: A report from the global alliance to improve outcomes in acne. *J Am Acad Dermatol* 2003;49:S1–S37.
Haider A, Shaw JC: Treatment of acne vulgaris. *JAMA* 2004;292:726–735.
James WD: Clinical practice. Acne. *N Engl J Med* 2005;352:1463–1472.
Webster GF: Laser treatment of acne. *Lancet* 2003;362:1342.

Capitolo 669 ■ Tumori della cute

Joseph G. Morelli

Vedi anche Capitoli 505 e 650.

CISTI DA INCLUSIONE EPIDERMICA (CISTI EPIDERMOIDE). Le cisti epidermoidi sono le formazioni nodulari più frequenti nei bambini. Si tratta di noduli nettamente circoscritti, di forma rotondeggiante, duri, mobili, sovrastati da cute di colorito normale (Fig. 669-1), spesso con una fossetta centrale o un punto che è il poro ostruito, dilatato, di un follicolo pilosebaceo. Le cisti epidermoidi si formano più di frequente sul volto, sul collo, sul torace o sulla parte superiore del dorso e possono infiammarsi periodicamente e secondariamente infettarsi, soprattutto in associazione con l'acne volgare. La parete della cisti può anche rompersi e indurre una reazione infiammatoria del derma. Questa parete è derivata dall'infundibolo follicolare. La cavità è riempita da una massa di materiale cheratinizzato stratificato, che può avere una consistenza caseosa. Le cisti epidermoidi possono derivare dall'occlusione di follicoli pilosebacei, dall'impianto di cellule epidermiche nel derma come risultato di una lesione che penetra l'epidermide e dai resti di cellule epidermiche. Cisti epidermoidi multiple possono essere presenti nella sindrome di Gardner e nella sindrome del carcinoma nevoide a cellule basali. È indicata l'escissione delle cisti, particolarmente se si infettano spesso, con la rimozione dell'intero sacco e del suo contenuto. Una cisti fluttuante, infetta, deve essere trattata con un antibiotico efficace contro *Staphylococcus aureus*. Dopo che l'infiammazione si è risolta, la cisti può essere rimossa.

MILIUM. Si tratta di una cisti cheratinica subepidermica di 1-2 mm, dura, bianco perlacea o giallastra. I *milia neonatorum* sono stati discussi nel Capitolo 646. I grani di milium secondari si verificano in associazione a malattie bollose subepidermiche, dopo una dermoabrasione o altre lesioni della cute. Si tratta di cisti da ritenzione causate dall'iperproliferazione di un epitelio lesionato e sono istologicamente indistinguibili dalle forme pri-

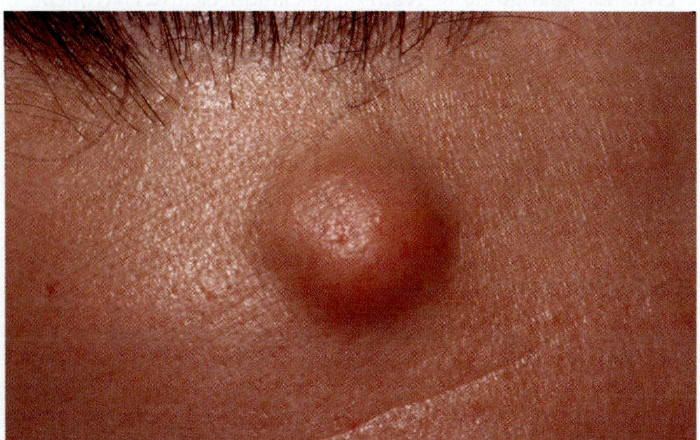

Figura 669-1. Cisti color carne sulla fronte.

marie. I grani che si sviluppano dopo le lesioni bollose derivano usualmente dal dotto delle ghiandole sudoripare merocrine, ma possono svilupparsi anche dal follicolo pilifero, dal dotto sebaceo o dall'epidermide. I grani di milium differiscono dalla cisti epidermoide solo per le piccole dimensioni e la localizzazione superficiale.

CISTI PILARE (CISTI TRICHILEMMALE). Può essere clinicamente indistinguibile da una cisti epidermoide. Si presenta come un nodulo liscio, duro, mobile, soprattutto del cuoio capelluto (Fig. 669-2). Queste cisti occasionalmente si sviluppano su volto, collo o tronco; si possono infiammare e occasionalmente suppurare e ulcerare. La parete della cisti è composta da cellule epiteliali con indistinti collegamenti intercellulari. Lo strato di cellule periferiche della parete mostra una struttura a palizzata, che manca nelle cisti epidermoidi. Non è presente uno strato granulare. La cavità cistica contiene materiale cheratinico omogeneo eosinofilo e nel 25% dei casi si trovano foci di calcificazione. La propensione a sviluppare una cisti pilare e una cisti epidermoide, tumori dermoidi, fibromi, lipomi o osteomi, può essere associata alla poliposi del colon o all'adenocarcinoma nella sindrome di Gardner. Le cisti pilari si staccano facilmente dal derma.

PILOMATRICOMA. È il secondo più comune nodulo nei bambini, un tumore benigno di 3-30 mm duro, solitario, dermico profondo o sottocutaneo, localizzato su capo, collo o arti superiori. L'epidermide sottostante di solito è normale. La neoplasia può occasionalmente essere localizzata più superficialmente, tingendo la cute sovrastante di blu-rosso (Fig. 669-3). I pazienti con pilomatricoma e distrofia miotonica hanno una maggiore probabilità di andare soggetti a tumori multipli e di manifestare un andamento familiare. In generale, tuttavia, i pilomatricomi non sono ereditari. Da un punto di vista istopatologico, isole irregolari di cellule epiteliali si tovano radicate in uno stroma cellulare. Nel 75% dei tumori ci sono depositi di calcio. I pilomatricomi sono dovuti a mutazioni della β-catenina.

TRICOEPITELIOMA. Si tratta di una papula di 2-8 mm liscia, rotondeggiante, dura, ricoperta da cute di colorito normale, che deriva da follicoli piliferi immaturi. I tricoepiteliomi in genere compaiono singolarmente sul volto del bambino o del giovane adulto. I tricoepiteliomi multipli si trasmettono con eredità autosomica dominante, compaiono nell'infanzia o nell'adolescenza e gradualmente aumentano di numero in ambito naso-facciale, nasale, frontale e sul labbro superiore, nonché occasionalmente sul cuoio capelluto, sul collo e sulla parte superiore del tronco. Da un punto di vista microscopico, questi tumori benigni sono caratterizzati da cisti cornee composte di una zona centrale completamente cheratinizzata circondata da cellule basofile in un contesto ghiandolare. Può risultare utile una terapia con imiquimod per via topica. L'escissione chirurgica è la sola altra terapia.

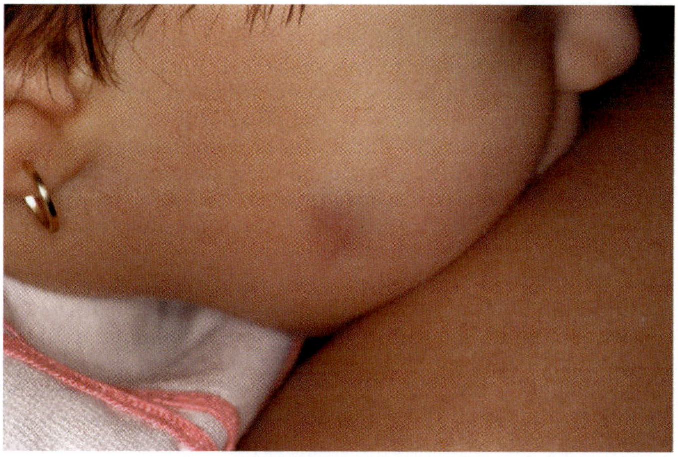

Figura 669-3. Pilomatricoma. Tumore duro con sovrastante colorazione bluastra della cute.

CISTI ERUTTIVE DEL VELLO. Si tratta di papule follicolari ricoperte da una cute di colorito normale, di 1-3 mm, asintomatiche, molli, situate sul torace (Fig. 669-4). Possono ricoprirsi di una crosta o ombelicare. L'occlusione di follicoli piliferi anomali a livello infundibulare porta alla ritenzione di peli in una dilatazione cistica rivestita da epitelio, in corrispondenza della porzione prossimale del follicolo. La maggior parte dei casi è cronica, ma si sono riscontrate regressioni spontanee.

STEATOCISTOMA MULTIPLO. Questa condizione si presenta usualmente durante l'adolescenza o la giovane età adulta, con numerosi noduli cistici di consistenza da molle a dura, aderenti alla cute sottostante e con un diametro variabile da 3 mm a 3 cm. Se punte, le cisti possono drenare materiale oleoso o caseoso. Le sedi di predilezione comprendono la regione sternale, ascellare, le braccia e la cute scrotale. La parete della cisti ripiegata più volte è tappezzata sulla superficie interna da uno strato corneo, omogeneo, eosinofilo, mentre manca uno strato granulare. Lobuli appiattiti della ghiandola sebacea sono spesso visibili nella parete della cisti e nella cavità cistica possono essere presenti peli lanuginosi.

SIRINGOMA. I tumori benigni conosciuti come siringomi sono piccole papule di consistenza molle e con la cute di colorito normale

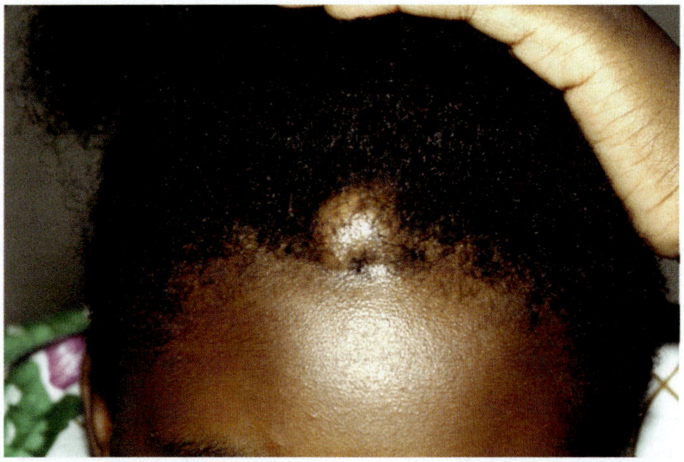

Figura 669-2. Cisti pilare della zona anteriore del cuoio capelluto.

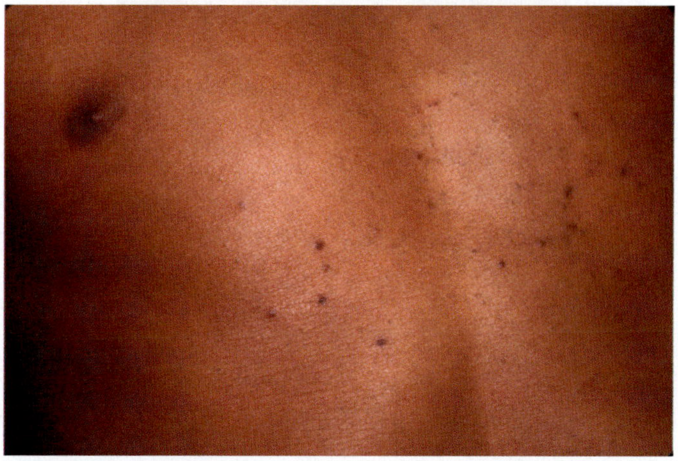

Figura 669-4. Cisti eruttiva del vello. Papule multiple sul torace.

o giallo-marrone che si sviluppano sul volto, particolarmente sulle regioni periorbitali (Fig. 669-5). Altre sedi di predilezione comprendono le ascelle e le aree ombelicale e pubica. Spesso si formano durante la pubertà e sono più frequenti nelle femmine. Siringomi eruttivi compaiono in gruppo sulla zona anteriore del tronco durante l'infanzia o l'adolescenza. Il siringoma deriva dal dotto intraepidermico di una ghiandola sudoripara. I siringomi spesso hanno solo una rilevanza estetica. Le lesioni sparse possono essere escisse, ma spesso sono troppo numerose per essere rimosse.

FIBROMA DIGITALE INFANTILE. Si tratta di un nodulo liscio, di consistenza dura, eritematoso o ricoperto da una cute di colorito normale, sulla superficie laterale delle falangi distali delle dita delle mani e dei piedi. Oltre l'80% dei tumori si manifesta nell'infanzia ed essi possono essere presenti alla nascita. Le lesioni possono apparire solitarie o multiple e presentarsi come tumori "kissing" sul dito opposto. Solitamente risultano asintomatici, ma si può verificare la deformità del dito in flessione. Da un punto di vista clinico, le lesioni assomigliano a fibroma, leiomioma, angiofibroma, fibrocheratoma digitale acquisito, dito accessorio o cisti mucosa. La diagnosi viene confermata dal ritrovamento di numerosi fibroblasti fusati che contengono piccole inclusioni citoplasmatiche rotondeggianti, dense, eosinofile, composte da una serie di filamenti di astina. La recidiva locale dopo un'escissione semplice si verifica nel 75% dei pazienti. Dato che il tumore non metastatizza e può regredire spontaneamente in 2-3 anni, si consiglia un atteggiamento di vigile attesa. Se compare un impedimento funzionale o la deformità in flessione del dito diventa evidente, è indicata un'immediata escissione.

DERMATOFIBROMA (ISTIOCITOMA). Questo tumore dermico benigno può essere peduncolato, nodulare (Fig. 669-6) o piatto, è di solito ben circoscritto e di consistenza dura, ma occasionalmente può apparire molle alla palpazione. La cute sovrastante è in genere iperpigmentata, ma può essere lucida o cheratosica e s'increspa quando si pizzica il tumore. I dermatofibromi variano da 0,5 a 10 mm, si presentano più frequentemente sugli arti e di solito appaiono asintomatici, anche se talvolta danno prurito. Sono composti da fibroblasti, collagene giovane e maturo, capillari

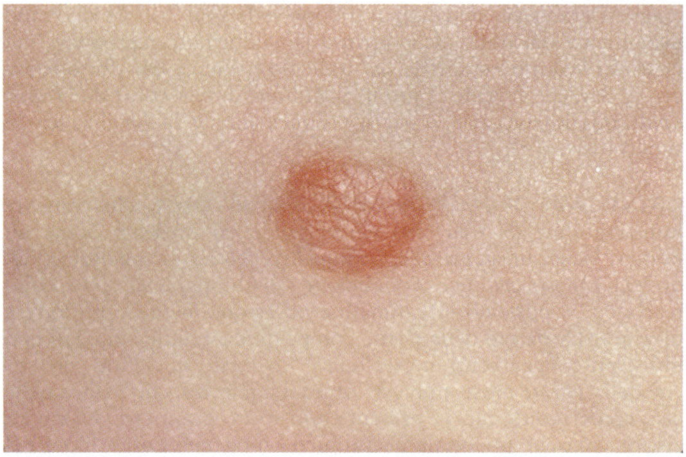

Figura 669-6. Dermatofibroma. Variante nodulare rosso-marrone.

e istiociti in varie proporzioni, formando un nodulo nel derma con contorni scarsamente definiti. La loro causa è sconosciuta, ma pare che un trauma, una puntura d'insetto o una follicolite possano indurre una fibroplasia reattiva. La diagnosi differenziale comprende cisti epidermiche da inclusione, xantogranuloma giovanile, cicatrice ipertrofica e neurofibromi. I dermatofibromi possono essere escissi o lasciati intatti, a seconda del desiderio del paziente. In genere persistono indefinitamente.

XANTOGRANULOMA GIOVANILE. Si tratta di una papula tondeggiante, gialla, rosa o arancione, oppure di un nodulo (Fig. 669-7) con un diametro di dimensioni variabili da 5 mm a 4 cm. Questi noduli sono dieci volte più comuni nelle persone di razza bianca che in quelle di razza nera. Le sedi di predilezione sono il cuoio capelluto, il volto e la parte superiore del tronco; possono erompere in profusione o rimanere lesioni isolate. Le lesioni nodulari sono caratterizzate istologicamente da un infiltrato dermico di istiociti pieni di lipidi, frammisti a cellule infiammatorie e cellule giganti di Touton. Le lesioni possono assomigliare clinicamente a un'orticaria papulonodulare pigmentosa, dermatofibromi o agli xantomi dell'iperlipoproteinemia, ma possono distinguersi istologicamente da queste entità.

I neonati interessati sono quasi sempre altrimenti normali, con livelli lipidici plasmatici non elevati. Nel 20% dei pazienti con xantogranuloma giovanile si trovano anche macchie a caffelatte. Gli infiltrati xantogranulomatosi si verificano occasionalmente nei tessuti oculari. Possono comportare glaucoma, ifema, uveite, eterocromia dell'iride, irite o una proptosi improvvisa. Un'età

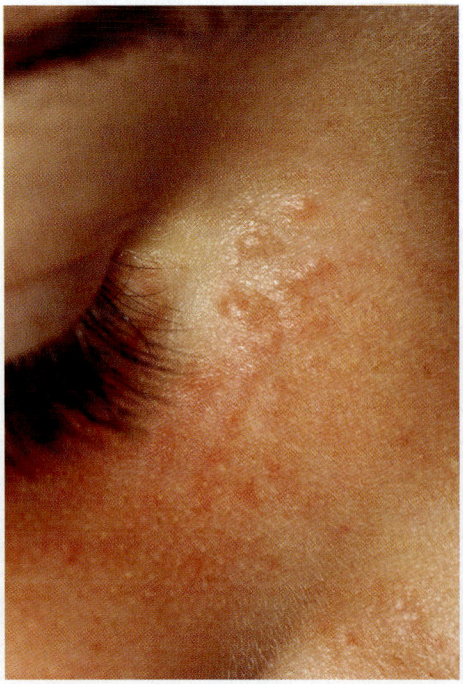

Figura 669-5. Siringomi. Multiple papule giallastre in prossimità degli occhi.

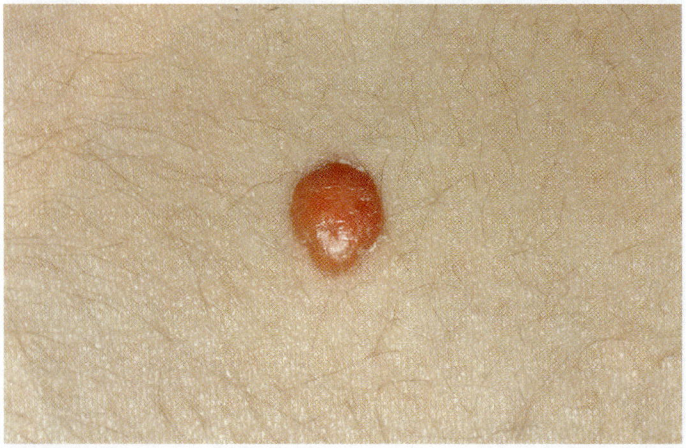

Figura 669-7. Xantogranuloma giovanile. Papula arancione solitaria.

inferiore a 2 anni, lesioni multiple e una localizzazione perioculare possono aumentare le preoccupazioni per il coinvolgimento intraoculare. Pare ci sia un'associazione tra il xantogranuloma giovanile, la neurofibromatosi e la leucemia infantile o più frequentemente la leucemia mieloide cronica giovanile. Non è necessario rimuovere queste lesioni benigne, perché la maggior parte regredisce spontaneamente nei primi anni di vita. Possono residuare pigmentazione e atrofia.

LIPOMA. Questo accumulo benigno di tessuto adiposo compare sul tronco, sul collo o sulle porzioni prossimali degli arti. I lipomi sono masse sottocutanee molli, comprimibili, lobulate. Occasionalmente possono verificarsi lesioni multiple, come nella sindrome di Gardner. Atrofia, calcificazione, liquefazione o modificazioni xantomatose possono talvolta complicare il decorso. Un lipoma è formato da normali cellule adipose circondate da una sottile capsula di tessuto connettivo. I lipomi rappresentano un difetto estetico e possono essere asportati chirurgicamente. Quelli multipli, identici ai singoli, costituiscono una patologia ereditaria, a trasmissione autosomica dominante, e spesso appaiono nella terza decade di vita in pazienti con lipomatosi multipla familiare. I lipomi possono presentarsi in sede intra-addominale, intramuscolare e sottocutanea. La lipomatosi congenita si manifesta nei primi mesi di vita con ampie masse sottocutanee di tessuto adiposo sul torace, con estensione nel muscolo scheletrico. La lipomatosi congenita può essere anche una manifestazione della sindrome di Proteus. Gli angiolipomi in genere appaiono come numerosi noduli sottocutanei, indolori, sulle braccia o sul tronco.

EPITELIOMA A CELLULE BASALI (CARCINOMA A CELLULE BASALI). Il carcinoma a cellule basali è raro nei bambini in assenza di una condizione predisponente, come la sindrome del carcinoma nevoide a cellule basali, lo xeroderma pigmentoso, il nevo sebaceo di Jadassohn, l'assunzione di arsenico o l'esposizione a radiazioni. Le lesioni sono rappresentate da papule teleangiectasiche lisce, perlacee, rosa, che si allargano lentamente e possono sanguinare o ulcerarsi. Le sedi preferite sono il volto, il cuoio capelluto e la parte superiore del tronco. La diagnosi differenziale comprende il granuloma piogenico, il nevo nevocellulare, la cisti epidermica da inclusione, il comedone chiuso, il dermatofibroma e un tumore degli annessi. A seconda della sede di comparsa e delle patologie associate, sono in genere risolutivi l'elettrodissecazione e il curettage o la semplice escissione. Se il tumore recidiva, se ha un diametro di 2 cm, è localizzato in aree anatomiche problematiche come la parte mediale del volto o le orecchie, oppure, se si tratta di un tipo istologicamente aggressivo, il trattamento più appropriato è l'intervento chirurgico di Mohs sotto controllo microscopico.

SINDROME DEL CARCINOMA NEVOIDE A CELLULE BASALI (SINDROME DEL NEVO A CELLULE BASALI, SINDROME DI GORLIN). Questa sindrome autosomica dominante dipende da un gene sul cromosoma 9q22.3, con un'incidenza di 1 su 60 000. Questo gene soppressore tumorale è una parte della via di segnalazione hedgehog ed è importante nel determinare il pattern embrionale e il destino cellulare in una serie di strutture dell'embrione in via di sviluppo. Le mutazioni nel gene patched umano producono una disregolazione di numerosi geni coinvolti nell'organogenesi e nella carcinogenesi. Di conseguenza, la sindrome comprende un ampio spettro di difetti, che coinvolgono la cute, gli occhi, il sistema nervoso centrale ed endocrino e le ossa. Le caratteristiche principali sono carcinomi a cellule basali a esordio precoce e cisti mandibolari. Circa il 20% dei soggetti in cui si sviluppa un carcinoma a cellule basali prima dei 19 anni presenta questa sindrome. I carcinomi a cellule basali appaiono tra la pubertà e i 35 anni, appartenendo a un gruppo di tumori che variano per dimensioni, colore e numero, ma possono essere difficili da distinguere da altri tipi di lesioni cutanee. Le sedi predilette sono la cute periorbitale, il naso, gli zigomi e il labbro superiore, ma le lesioni possono svilupparsi sul tronco e sugli arti e non essere limitate alle aree esposte al sole. Possono ulcerarsi, sanguinare, coprirsi di una crosta e manifestare segni di invasione locale. Ulteriori reperti cutanei sono rappresentati da piccoli grani di milium, cisti epidermiche, lesioni pigmentate, irsutismo, fossette palmari e plantari.

La facies dei pazienti con questa sindrome è caratterizzata da una protuberanza temporoparietale, da creste sopraorbitali prominenti, da una radice nasale larga, da ipertelorismo oculare o *dystopia canthorum* e da prognatismo. Sono presenti cisti cheratinizzate (cheratocisti odontogeniche) nel mascellare e nella mandibola della maggior parte dei pazienti. Le loro dimensioni variano da pochi mm a parecchi cm, comportano un'alterazione dello sviluppo dei denti e causano dolore, ingrossamento della mandibola, deformità facciali, erosione ossea, fratture patologiche e tragitti fistolosi suppuranti. I difetti ossei, come un anomalo sviluppo delle costole, la spina bifida, la cifoscoliosi e il brachimetacarpalismo si verificano nei 2/3 dei pazienti, mentre anomalie oculari come cataratta, glaucoma, colobomi, strabismo e cecità compaiono in circa 1/4 di essi. Alcuni maschi presentano ipogonadismo, con testicoli assenti o non distesi. Sono state riportate anche malformazioni renali. Le manifestazioni neurologiche comprendono calcificazioni della falx cerebri, crisi epilettiche, ritardo mentale, parziale agenesia del corpo calloso, idrocefalo e ipoacusia neurosensoriale. È inoltre aumentata l'incidenza di medulloblastoma, ameloblastoma della cavità orale, fibrosarcoma della mandibola, teratoma, cistoadenoma, fibroma cardiaco, fibroma ovarico e rabdomiosarcoma a esordio fetale.

Il **trattamento** richiede la partecipazione di vari specialisti, in rapporto ai singoli problemi clinici. I carcinomi a cellule basali non devono essere trattati con radioterapia. La maggior parte dei carcinomi a cellule basali ha un decorso clinico benigno e spesso è impossibile rimuoverli in toto. Quelli con crescita aggressiva e quelli delle zone centrali del volto, tuttavia, vanno rimossi prontamente. I retinoidi orali possono essere utili, in alcuni pazienti, a prevenire lo sviluppo di nuovi tumori. È indicata anche una consulenza genetica.

SINDROME DEL NEUROMA MUCOSO (NEOPLASIA ENDOCRINA MULTIPLA TIPO IIB). La sindrome del neuroma mucoso, autosomica dominante, è caratterizzata da un habitus astenico o marfanoide con scoliosi, *pectus excavatum*, piede cavo e ipotonia muscolare. La sindrome è dovuta a mutazioni del dominio della tirosina chinasi del gene RET. I pazienti hanno labbra spesse, aperte e il prognatismo dei tessuti molli simula un'acromegalia. Sono presenti neuromi o neurofibromi mucosi multipli sotto forma di noduli rosa, peduncolati o sessili, sul terzo anteriore della lingua, a livello delle commessure labiali, sulla mucosa orale e sulla congiuntiva palpebrale. Reperti comuni sono rappresentati anche da difetti oftalmologici e da una ganglioneuromatosi intestinale con diarrea ricorrente. Vi è un'alta incidenza di carcinoma tiroideo midollare associato a elevati livelli di calcitonina, a feocromocitoma e a iperparatiroidismo. Sono necessari periodici test di screening per i tumori maligni associati.

Dehner LP: Juvenile xanthogranuloma in the first two decades of life: A clinicopathologic study of 174 cases with cutaneous and extracutaneous manifestations. *Am J Surg Pathol* 2003;27:579–583.

Gorlin RJ: Nevoid basal cell carcinoma (Gorlin) syndrome. *Genet Med* 2004;6:530–539.

High A, Zedan W: Basal cell nevus syndrome. *Curr Opin Oncol* 2005; 17:160–166.

Marin-Gutzke M, Sanchez-Olaso A, Berenguer B, et al: Basal cell carcinoma in childhood after radiation therapy: A case report and review. *Ann Plast Surg* 2004;53:593–595.

Pirousmanesh A, Reinisch JF, Gonzalez-Gomez I, et al: Pilomatrixoma: A review of 346 cases. *Plast Reconstr Surg* 2003;112:1784–1789.

Zelger B, Zelger BG, Burgdorf WH: Dermatofibroma—a critical review. *Int J Surg Pathol* 2004;12:333–344.

Capitolo 670 ■ Dermatosi nutrizionali

Joseph G. Morelli

ACRODERMATITE ENTEROPATICA. Si tratta di una rara malattia autosomica recessiva causata dall'incapacità di assorbire una sufficiente quantità di zinco dagli alimenti. Il difetto genetico è a livello del gene SLC39A4, specifico per il trasportatore intestinale dello zinco. I segni e i sintomi iniziali di solito compaiono nei primi mesi di vita, spesso dopo il passaggio dall'allattamento al seno a quello con latte di mucca. L'eruzione consiste in lesioni cutanee vescicolo-bollose, eczematose, secche, squamose o psoriasiformi, distribuite simmetricamente nelle aree periorale, acrale e perineale (Fig. 670-1*A* e *B*) e su guance, ginocchia e gomiti (Fig. 670-2*A* e *B*). I capelli spesso mostrano una peculiare tonalità rossastra ed è caratteristica un'alopecia di grado variabile. Le manifestazioni oculari comprendono fotofobia, congiuntivite, blefarite e distrofia corneale, rilevabile con un esame a lampada a fessura. Manifestazioni associate comprendono diarrea cronica, stomatite, glossite, paronichia, distrofia ungueale, ritardo della crescita, irritabilità, ritardata guarigione delle ferite, infezioni batteriche intercorrenti e superinfezioni da *Candida albicans*. La funzione dei linfociti e l'eliminazione dei radicali liberi sono alterati. Senza trattamento il decorso è cronico e intermittente, ma spesso inesorabilmente progressivo. Nei casi di malattia meno severa possono essere manifesti solo il ritardo della crescita e dello sviluppo.

La **diagnosi** è confermata sulla scorta dei vari reperti clinici e del ritrovamento di bassi livelli plasmatici di zinco. Le modificazioni istopatologiche della cute sono aspecifiche e comprendono paracheratosi e pallore della porzione superiore dell'epidermide. La varietà delle manifestazioni di questa sindrome può essere dovuta al fatto che lo zinco ha un ruolo in numerose vie metaboliche, comprese quelle di rame, proteine, acidi grassi essenziali e prostaglandine, e inoltre rientra nella composizione di molti metalloenzimi.

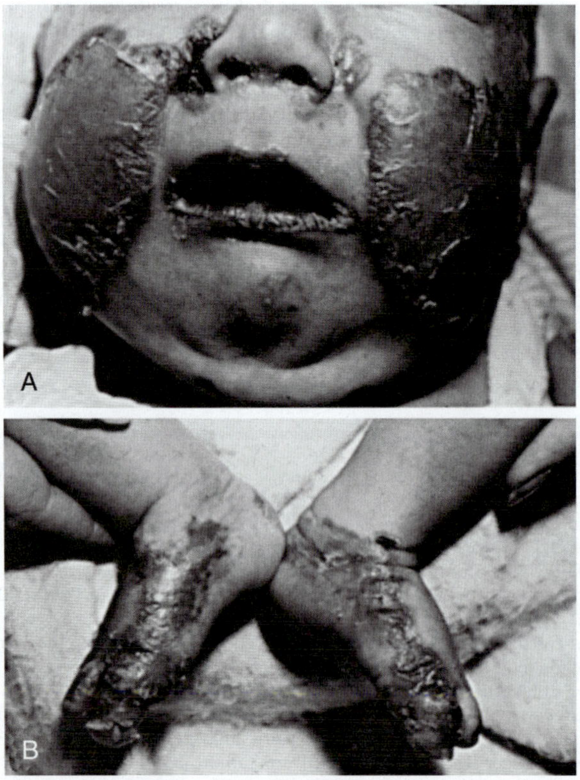

Figura 670-1. *A*, Lesioni facciali psoriasiformi della dermatite da deficit di zinco. *B*, Lesioni similari sul piede con distrofia ungueale secondaria.

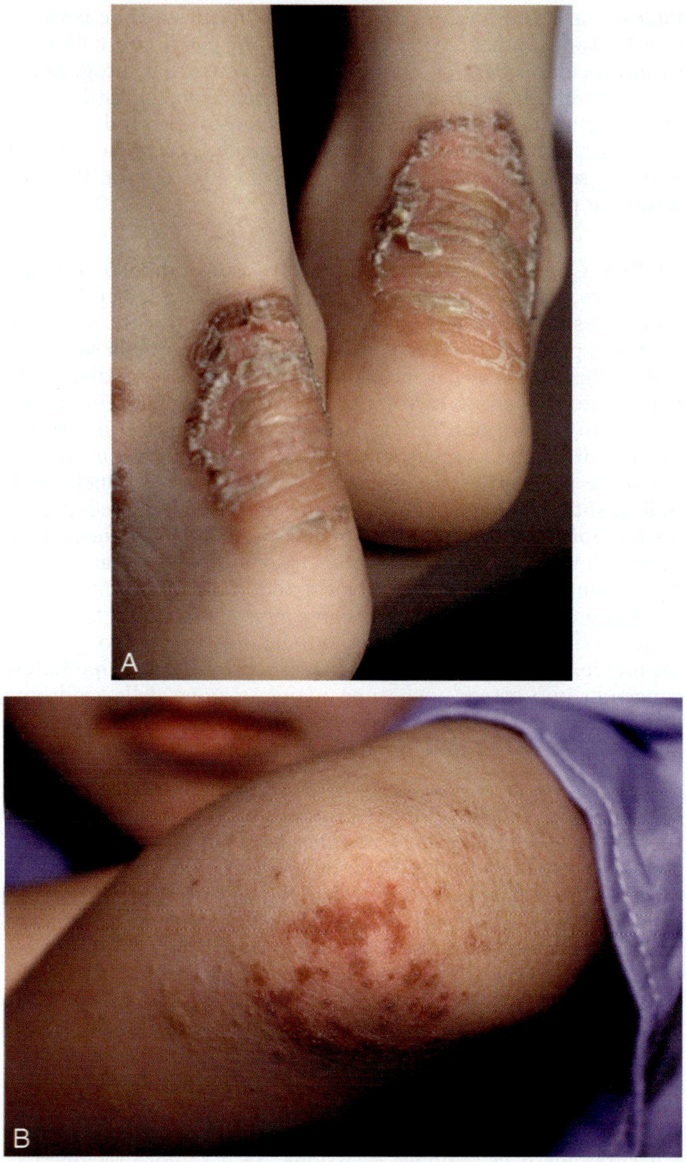

Figura 670-2. *A*, Lesione psoriasiforme della dermatite da deficit di zinco sulle anche. *B*, Lesioni simili sui gomiti.

Il **trattamento** elettivo è rappresentato dalla terapia orale con composti contenenti zinco. Il dosaggio ottimale varia dai 50 mg giornalieri di zinco solfato, acetato o gluconato per i neonati, agli oltre 150 mg/die per i bambini. I livelli plasmatici dello zinco devono essere monitorati per individualizzare la dose. La terapia con lo zinco abolisce rapidamente le manifestazioni della malattia. Una sindrome che assomiglia all'acrodermatite enteropatica è stata osservata in pazienti con un deficit secondario di zinco causato da una nutrizione parenterale di lunga durata senza una supplementazione di zinco o da sindromi malassorbitive croniche. Un rash simile è stato riportato anche in neonati alimentati con latte materno, che contiene scarse quantità di zinco e in quelli con la malattia delle urine a sciroppo d'acero, aciduria organica, deficit essenziale di acidi grassi, severa malnutrizione proteica (kwashiorkor) e fibrosi cistica.

DEFICIT ESSENZIALE DI ACIDI GRASSI. Il deficit causa una dermatite generalizzata, squamosa, composta da placche ispessite, eritematose, desquamanti. Negli animali l'eruzione è stata indotta sperimentalmente con una dieta priva di acidi grassi; inoltre, è stata osservata in pazienti con severo un malassorbimento cronico, come nella sindrome dell'intestino corto e nei casi di una dieta o di un'alimentazione parenterale priva di acidi grassi. Sono carenti l'acido linoleico (18:2 n-6) e arachidonico (20:4 n-6) e nel plasma si trova un metabolita anomalo, l'acido 5,8,11-eicosatrienoico (20:3 n-9). Ulteriori manifestazioni comprendono l'alopecia, la trombocitopenica e un deficit di accrescimento. Lo strato corneo della cute è microscopicamente fissurato, la funzione di barriera della cute è alterata ed è aumentata la perdita transepidermica di acqua. L'applicazione topica di acido linoleico, presente nei semi di girasole e nell'olio di cartamo, può migliorare le manifestazioni cliniche e biochimiche della cute. È necessaria un'alimentazione adeguata.

KWASHIORKOR. Una grave deprivazione di proteine e aminoacidi essenziali, in associazione a un adeguato introito calorico può portare al kwashiorkor, soprattutto al momento dello svezzamento, per una dieta a base principalmente di grano, riso o fagioli (vedi Capitolo 43). Nei casi lievi in bambini bianchi, dapprima si sviluppa un eritema cutaneo, che si evolve verso una fine desquamazione lungo le linee cutanee naturali e nell'area pretibiale, sulla superficie esterna delle cosce e sul dorso. Nei bambini neri i reperti precoci caratteristici comprendono pallore circumorale, depigmentazione cutanea e sviluppo di chiazze purpuree. Con l'avanzare della malattia appaiono placche ceree, violacee, leggermente sopraelevate, ben delineate, particolarmente nell'area del pannolino e nelle sedi sottoposte a pressione, come ginocchia, gomiti, anche e tronco. Nei casi severi si sviluppano erosioni e fessure lineari (Fig. 670-3). La cute esposta al sole, i piedi e la superficie dorsale delle mani sono relativamente risparmiate. Le unghie sono sottile e molli, i capelli radi, sottili e depigmentati, con la presenza, talvolta, di un'alternanza di bande chiare e scure che riflettono periodi alterni di nutrizione adeguata e inadeguata. Le manifestazioni cutanee possono assomigliare molto a quelle della dermatite enteropatica. I livelli plasmatici dello zinco spesso sono bassi e, in alcuni casi, le lesioni cutanee dello kwashiorkor guariscono più rapidamente con l'applicazione topica dello zinco.

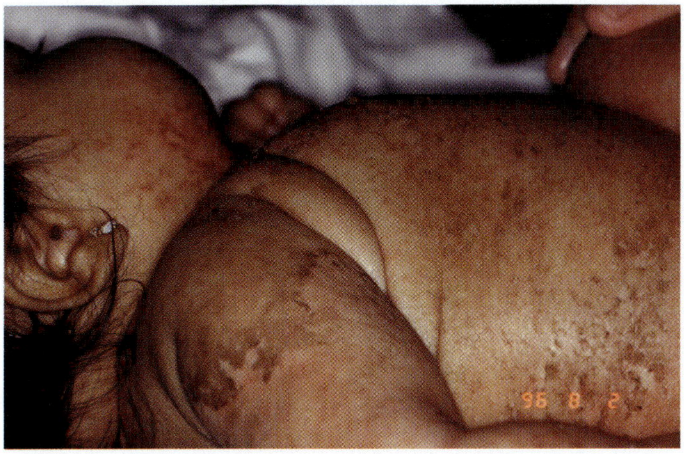

Figura 670-3. Erosioni e desquamazione nel kwashiorkor.

FIBROSI CISTICA (VEDI CAPITOLO 400). Dal 5 al 10% dei pazienti con fibrosi cistica sviluppa una malnutrizione proteica cronica. Nei neonati con fibrosi cistica e malnutrizione il rash cutaneo è raro, ma può comparire al sesto mese. L'eruzione iniziale consiste di papule eritematose, desquamanti, che progrediscono in 1-3 mesi verso placche desquamanti estese. Il rash è accentuato intorno alla bocca e nel perineo e agli arti (inferiori > superiori). Può essere riscontrata alopecia, ma non sono coinvolte le membrane mucose e le unghie.

PELLAGRA (VEDI CAPITOLO 46). Si presenta con edema, eritema e bruciature della cute esposta al sole su viso, collo e superficie dorsale delle mani, degli avambracci e dei piedi. Le lesioni della pellagra possono essere provocate anche da ustioni, pressione, frizione e infiammazione. L'eruzione sul volto frequentemente segue una distribuzione a farfalla e la dermatite intorno al collo è stata denominata "collare di Casal". Si sviluppano vesciche e squame e la cute diventa sempre più secca, ruvida, ispessita, fissurata e iperpigmentata. Le infezioni cutanee possono risultare particolarmente severe. La pellagra compare in soggetti con un insufficiente introito dietetico o un malassorbimento di niacina e/o triptofano. Anche la somministrazione di isoniazide, 6-mercaptopurina o 5 fluorouracile può provocare la pellagra. Il cardine della terapia consiste nella supplementazione con la nicotinamide e nell'evitare il sole.

SCORBUTO (DEFICIT DI VITAMINA C O ACIDO ASCORBICO) (VEDI CAPITOLO 47). Si presenta inizialmente con ipercheratosi follicolare e spiralizzazione dei peli della parte superiore di braccia, dorso, glutei e arti inferiori. Possono comparire anche un eritema perifollicolare e un'emorragia, particolarmente sulle gambe, fino alla formazione di ampie zone emorragiche, edema ed eritema gengivale, stomatite ed ematomi subperiostei. Il metodo migliore per confermare la diagnosi clinica di scorbuto è un ciclo di supplementazione con vitamina C.

DEFICIT DI VITAMINA A (VEDI CAPITOLO 45.1). Questo deficit si presenta inizialmente con un'alterazione dell'adattamento visivo al buio. Le alterazioni cutanee comprendono xerosi, ipercheratosi e iperplasia dell'epidermide, particolarmente l'allineamento dei follicoli piliferi e delle ghiandole sebacee. Nei casi severi la desquamazione può essere notevole.

Darmstadt GL: The skin and nutritional disorders in the newborn. *Eur J Pediatr Dermatol* 1998;8:221.

Heygi J, Schwartz RA, Heygi V: Pellagra: Dermatitis, dementia, and diarrhea. *Int J Dermatol* 2004;43:1–5.

Oumeish OY, Oumeish I: Nutritional skin problems in children. *Clin Dermatol* 2003;21:260–263.

Perafan-Riveros C, Franca LF, Alves AC, et al: Acrodermatitis enteropathica: A case report and review of the literature. *Pediatr Dermatol* 2002;19:426–431.

KWASHIORKOR. Una grave deprivazione di proteine [illegible] [illegible], in [illegible]

Figura [illegible] Kwashiorkor.

Parte XXXI ■ Malattie delle ossa e delle articolazioni

Sezione 1 — Problemi ortopedici

Capitolo 671 ■ Crescita e sviluppo

Harish S. Hosalkar e Lawrence Wells

Nel bambino, i pattern di crescita e di sviluppo sono spesso specifici del singolo individuo e pertanto la definizione di ciò che è normale presenta potenziali ramificazioni. Statisticamente, si definisce normale il 95% di una popolazione che ricade entro due deviazioni standard della media rispetto a ogni determinata misura. La sfida per il chirurgo ortopedico che si occupa di pazienti pediatrici è comprendere quali deviazioni dalla norma avranno maggiore probabilità di sfociare in un deficit funzionale, una deformità progressiva o un'artrosi degenerativa prematura dolorosa. I termini utilizzati per descrivere alcune comuni deviazioni dalla norma sono elencati nella Tabella 671-1.

Le anomalie congenite possono essere classificate come:

a. **problemi di produzione**, comprendenti anomalie causate da malformazioni, displasie o soluzioni di continuo che non si risolvono spontaneamente;
b. **problemi di packaging** (contenimento in utero), consistenti in deformità imputabili a cause meccaniche compresi il posizionamento e il modellamento in utero, che di solito si risolvono con il tempo.

POSIZIONAMENTO IN UTERO. Nel neonato, può essere evidente l'impronta della posizione in utero, talvolta scambiata per un'anomalia. Il posizionamento in utero produce contratture temporanee di muscoli e articolazioni e altera l'allineamento torsionale delle ossa lunghe, specialmente di quelle delle estremità inferiori. I neonati normali a termine possono avere contratture in flessione di anca e ginocchio fino a 20-30°, che tendono a risolversi entro i 4-6 mesi di età. L'anca neonatale ruota esternamente in estensione fino a 80-90° e ha una limitata rotazione interna, pari a circa 0-10°. La gamba spesso presenta una rotazione interna (torsione tibiale interna) e i piedi sono supinati in seguito all'avvolgimento dei loro margini mediali contro l'aspetto posterolaterale della coscia opposta. La gamba posta superiormente in utero può presentare maggiori alterazioni rispetto a quella posta inferiormente. Anche il viso può essere deformato, mentre la colonna e gli arti superiori sono meno interessati dalla posizione in utero. Gli effetti del posizionamento in utero, pertanto, sono di origine fisiologica, anche se possono causare preoccupazione nei genitori. Possono trascorrere 3-4 anni prima che gli effetti del posizionamento in utero si risolvano del tutto.

TABELLA 671-1. Terminologia delle anomalie

TERMINE	DESCRIZIONE
Congenito	Anomalia evidente alla nascita
Deformazione	Una struttura normalmente formata che viene deformata da forze meccaniche
Deformità	Una parte del corpo di forma alterata rispetto al normale, al di fuori del range normale
Evolutiva (developmental)	Un'anomalia che si verifica nel corso del tempo e che può non essere presente o evidente alla nascita
Interruzione (disruption)	Una struttura fino a quel momento sviluppatasi normalmente, che cessa di svilupparsi o viene distrutta o rimossa
Displasia	Un tessuto anormale o strutturalmente anomalo
Malformazione	Una struttura il cui sviluppo è anormale; assenza di sviluppo o differenziazione embriologici che risulta in una struttura anormale o assente

ACCRESCIMENTO E SVILUPPO

Considerare accrescimento e sviluppo facilita la formulazione di strategie di trattamento volte a conservare o ripristinare un normale potenziale di crescita. L'accrescimento non è una caratteristica costante, ma è soggetto a molte variabili, tra le quali genetica, alimentazione, salute generale, stato endocrino, forze meccaniche ed età fisiologica. L'applicazione di forze allo scheletro in accrescimento può migliorare o peggiorare le deformità nei bambini. L'accrescimento varia anche tra due regioni anatomiche e persino tra due ossa della stessa regione.

La formazione di osso o ossificazione si verifica in due modi differenti:

ossificazione encondrale, in cui le cellule mesenchimali si raggruppano e vanno incontro a un processo di condrogenesi per formare cartilagine che matura e ipertrofizza, si calcifica e quindi viene sostituita da tessuto osseo. La maggior parte delle ossa dello scheletro assiale e appendicolare si forma in questo modo;
ossificazione intramembranosa, in cui si formano osteoblasti per differenziazione diretta di cellule mesenchimali senza precursore o modello cartilagineo. In questo modo si formano le ossa piatte del cranio e la clavicola.

Centri di ossificazione:

centri di ossificazione **primari**: all'inizio del periodo fetale i condrociti della diafisi delle ossa lunghe formano i centri primari, e la crescita a partire da questi centri allunga l'osso a lungo termine;
centri di ossificazione **secondari**: questi compaiono nella condroepifisi e per la maggior parte compaiono dopo la nascita. Dirigono la formazione dell'osso nel corso della crescita.

I centri di ossificazione presenti tipicamente nel nato a termine sono il femorale distale, il tibiale prossimale, il calcaneare e il talare.

Le **ossa lunghe tipiche** si dividono nelle seguenti parti:

cartilagine di accrescimento, che è la cartilagine di crescita situata all'estremità dell'osso;
epifisi, che è tipicamente il centro di ossificazione secondario;
metafisi, che rappresenta la parte di osso adiacente alla cartilagine di accrescimento dal lato opposto all'articolazione;
diafisi, che è la parte centrale delle ossa lunghe.

Le ossa lunghe delle estremità (omero, radio-ulna, femore, tibia-perone) hanno cartilagini di accrescimento a ciascuna estremità. Le estremità di ciascun osso lungo sono composte dalle epifisi, rivestite dalla cartilagine articolare, che formano le relative articolazioni. Le epifisi sono all'inizio quasi del tutto cartilaginee e nel corso della crescita vanno progressivamente incontro a ossificazione. Anche la cartilagine articolare contribuisce alla crescita delle epifisi. L'anello pericondrale, che circonda le cartilagini di accrescimento, come anche il pericondrio intorno alle epifisi e il periostio, che circonda le regioni metafisarie e diafisarie dell'osso, contribuiscono alla crescita apposizionale o circonferenziale. Le ossa senza cartilagini di accrescimento (bacino, scapola, ossa del carpo, ossa del tarso) crescono per crescita ossea apposizionale dai relativi pericondrio e periostio circostanti. Altre ossa (metacarpi, metatarsi, falangi, colonna) crescono secondo una combinazione di ossificazione apposizionale ed encondrale.

TAPPE IMPORTANTI DELL'ACCRESCIMENTO E DELLO SVILUPPO

Alcune importanti considerazioni sulla crescita muscoloscheletrica sono riassunte nella Tabella 671-2.

PATTERN DI CRESCITA DELLE ESTREMITÀ SUPERIORI E INFERIORI

L'estremità superiore cresce longitudinalmente in primo luogo a partire dalle cartilagini di accrescimento in direzione opposta al gomito; il contributo della cartilagine di accrescimento omerale prossimale e delle cartilagini di accrescimento radiali e ulnari distali è maggiore rispetto a quello delle cartilagini di accrescimento in prossimità del gomito. Ciò è l'esatto contrario rispetto al pattern di crescita dell'estremità inferiore in cui gran parte della crescita longitudinale avviene intorno al ginocchio, a livello delle cartilagini di accrescimento femorale distale e tibiale prossimale (Fig. 671-1).

Nell'articolazione dell'anca, l'acetabolo si forma con la convergenza di tre centri di ossificazione primari (ischio, ilio e pube), mentre nel femore prossimale si verifica una confluenza della cartilagine di accrescimento femorale prossimale e della cartilagine di accrescimento del grande trocantere nei primi anni di vita.

TABELLA 671-2. Considerazioni sullo sviluppo scheletrico

- Una statura anormale può essere considerata "proporzionata" o "sproporzionata" rispetto al rapporto tra statura da seduto e altezza sottoischiatica (*arti inferiori*).
- Normalmente la lunghezza delle due braccia tese (*arm span*) è quasi uguale alla statura in posizione eretta.
- La testa è sproporzionatamente grande alla nascita e il rapporto tra lunghezza della testa e lunghezza totale è di circa 1:4 alla nascita, passando a 1:7,5 alla maturità scheletrica.
- Le estremità inferiori rappresentano il 15% circa della lunghezza alla nascita e il 30% alla maturità scheletrica.
- Il tasso di aumento dell'altezza e della crescita non è costante e varia con gli scatti di crescita.
- A partire dai 5 anni, l'altezza alla nascita di solito raddoppia e il bambino ha un'altezza pari al 60% circa di quella dell'adulto. Il bambino ha un'altezza pari all'80% di quella finale a 9 anni. Nel corso della pubertà, l'altezza in posizione eretta aumenta di circa 1 cm al mese.
- L'età ossea è più importante dell'età cronologica per determinare il futuro potenziale di crescita.

MATURAZIONE DELL'ANDATURA

La maturazione del sistema nervoso centrale contribuisce significativamente allo sviluppo dell'andatura. All'inizio della deambulazione, il bambino mantiene un'andatura a base allargata con iperflessione dell'anca e del ginocchio, senza oscillazione reciproca della braccia e con un contatto iniziale del tallone. A partire dai 2 anni di età, si riduce la base dell'andatura, inizia

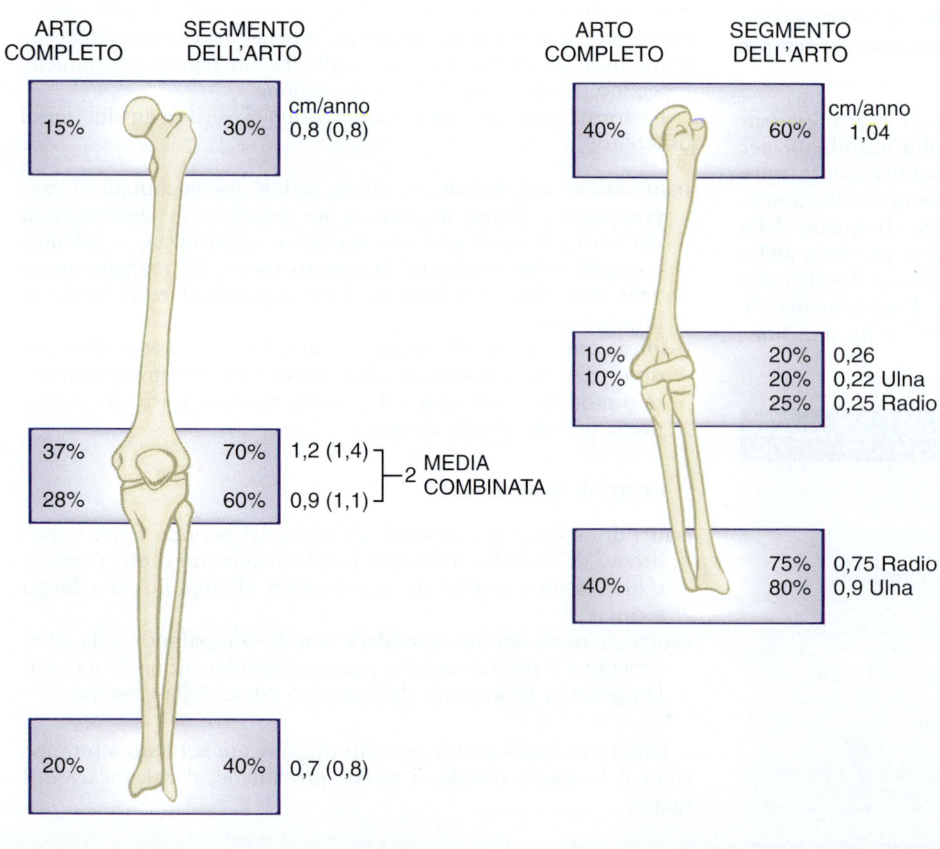

Figura 671-1. Contributo (%) di ciascuna cartilagine di accrescimento alla crescita globale delle estremità. (Da Morrissy R, Weinstein S [ed]: *Lovell and Winter's Pediatric Orthopedics*, 5th ed. Philadelphia, Lippincott Williams & Wilkins, 2001.)

l'oscillazione reciproca delle braccia e il contatto iniziale avviene con il tallone: ne deriva un aumento della lunghezza del passo e della velocità. Di solito i pattern cinetici di tipo adulto iniziano a svilupparsi a partire dai 3 anni e i parametri di tempo-distanza raggiungono i valori dell'adulto a partire da 7 anni circa, con lo sviluppo di un pattern di andatura pienamente maturo.

Ballock RT, O'Keefe RJ: The biology of the growth plate. *J Bone Joint Surg Am* 2003;85:715–726.
Davids JR: Normal gait and assessment of gait disorders. In Morrissy R, Weinstein S (editors): *Lovell and Winter's Pediatric Orthopedics,* 5th ed. Philadelphia, Lippincott Williams & Wilkins, 2001, pp 131–156
Dimeglio A: Growth in pediatric orthopedics. In Morrissy R, Weinstein S (editors): *Lovell and Winter's Pediatric Orthopedics,* 5th ed. Philadelphia, Lippincott Williams & Wilkins, 2001, pp 33–62.
Frick SL: Normal growth and development in pediatric orthopedics. In Dormans JP (editor): *Pediatric Orthopedics: Core Knowledge in Orthopedics.* Philadelphia, Mosby, 2005, pp 1–14.
Ogden J: Anatomy and physiology of skeletal development. In Catterall A (editor): *Skeletal Injury in the Children,* 3rd ed. New York, Springer-Verlag, 2000, pp 1–37.
Song KM, Little DG: Peak height velocity as a maturity indicator for males with idiopathic scoliosis. *J Pediatr Orthop* 2000;20:286–288.
Westh RN, Menelaus MB: A simple calculation for the timing of the epiphyseal arrest. *J Bone Joint Surg Br* 1981;63:117–119.

Capitolo 672 ■ Valutazione del bambino

Harish S. Hosalkar e Lawrence Wells

Un'anamnesi dettagliata e un esame obiettivo completo sono di inestimabile valore nella valutazione di un bambino con un problema ortopedico. A fornire informazioni sul bambino possono essere diverse figure, tra cui genitori, nonni, tutori, fratelli o sorelle e allenatori; le informazioni ottenute si rivelano molto importanti, specialmente per i bambini più piccoli e per i lattanti. A seconda della natura e della severità del problema possono essere necessari un imaging radiografico e talvolta anche esami di laboratorio appropriati.

ANAMNESI. Un'anamnesi completa deve tener conto in dettaglio dell'anamnesi prenatale, perinatale e postnatale. L'anamnesi prenatale deve comprendere i problemi sanitari materni tra cui fumo, assunzione prenatale di vitamine, abuso di farmaci o droghe, consumo di alcol, diabete, rosolia e infezioni sessualmente trasmesse. L'anamnesi prenatale e perinatale deve comprendere informazioni su durata della gravidanza, parto prematuro, durata del travaglio, tipo di travaglio (indotto o spontaneo), presentazione fetale, evidenza di qualsiasi segno di sofferenza fetale al momento del parto, necessità di somministrazione di ossigeno dopo il parto, lunghezza e peso alla nascita, punteggio di Apgar, tono muscolare alla nascita, anamnesi alimentare e durata dell'ospedalizzazione. Per quanto riguarda i lattanti e i bambini più piccoli, è importante valutare la presenza delle tappe dello sviluppo o un loro eventuale ritardo per ciò che riguarda postura, locomozione, desterità, attività sociali e linguaggio. L'anamnesi medica e chirurgica deve comprendere qualsiasi pregressa procedura e i problemi medici significativi, soprattutto nei pazienti con sintomi cronici. Le domande specificamente ortopediche devono essere focalizzate sui disturbi articolari e muscolari, oltre che sui problemi relativi allo scheletro appendicolare e assiale. Devono essere ricercate opportunamente informazioni su dolore o altri sintomi relativi a tutte queste aree (Tab. 672-1). L'anamnesi familiare può fornire indizi su possibili disordini genetici come sindromi congenite, distrofia muscolare, displasie scheletriche e altre anomalie dell'apparato muscoloscheletrico. L'anamnesi familiare può anche avere un ruolo rispetto allo sviluppo atteso del bambino.

TABELLA 672-1. Caratterizzazione del dolore e del sintomo di presentazione

1. ***Sede:*** se il dolore è localizzato a un particolare segmento o coinvolge un'area più grande.
2. ***Intensità:*** di solito rispetto a una scala del dolore da 1 a 10.
3. ***Qualità:***
   i. Il dolore tumorale è spesso di intensità costante, progressivo e notturno;
   ii. Il dolore notturno è particolarmente suggestivo di osteoma osteoide;
   iii. Il dolore da infiammazione e infezione è di solito continuo.
4. ***Esordio:*** (è stato acuto e correlato a un trauma specifico oppure insidioso?): un dolore acuto e una storia di trauma sono più comunemente associati alle fratture.
5. ***Durata:*** se transitorio, della durata di pochi minuti, o se prolungato per ore o per giorni. Un dolore che duri per più di 3-4 giorni è più suggestivo di un problema sottostante severo.
6. ***Progressione:*** stabile, che aumenta o diminuisce.
7. ***Irradiazione:*** un dolore che si irradia alle estremità superiori o inferiori oppure la presenza di insensibilità, formicolio o perdita di forza richiedono indagini diagnostiche appropriate.
8. ***Fattori aggravanti:*** qualsiasi attività come nuoto o immersioni o con qualsiasi posizione particolare.
9. ***Fattori allevianti:*** il dolore è alleviato da riposo, calore e/o farmaci? Condizioni come spondilolisi, malattia di Scheuermann, spondiloartropatia infiammatoria, strappi muscolari o le sindromi da sforzo (overuse) migliorano con il riposo a letto.
10. ***Andatura e postura:*** disturbi associati a dolore.

ESAME OBIETTIVO. L'esame obiettivo ortopedico deve comprendere un accurato esame dell'apparato muscoloscheletrico, come anche una valutazione neurologica completa. Tale esame consiste nell'ispezione, palpazione e valutazione del movimento, della stabilità e dell'andatura. Occorre inoltre eseguire un'indagine neurologica di base comprendente l'esame sensitivo, la funzione motoria e la valutazione dei riflessi, in base all'età e allo sviluppo del bambino. L'esame obiettivo ortopedico richiede conoscenze di base dell'anatomia, in quanto sono coinvolti archi di movimento, allineamento e stabilità, come anche un glossario di termini base in modo da standardizzare la comunicazione rispetto ai segni e sintomi del paziente. L'esame obiettivo comprende un'accurata valutazione dei sistemi muscoloscheletrico e neurologico, oltre a un appropriato esame obiettivo generale. Molti disordini muscoloscheletrici comuni possono essere diagnosticati in base alla sola anamnesi e al solo esame obiettivo. L'esame dell'apparato muscoloscheletrico si articola in quattro fasi: ispezione, palpazione, valutazione dell'arco di movimento articolare e valutazione dell'andatura nei bambini che deambulano.

ISPEZIONE. Il primo esame del bambino inizia con l'ispezione, nel corso della quale il medico deve usare le linee guida elencate nella Tabella 672-2.

TABELLA 672-2. Linee guida per l'ispezione di un bambino con un problema muscoloscheletrico

- Il paziente deve essere *a suo agio con un'adeguata esposizione e in un'area bene illuminata* (per evitare di lasciarsi sfuggire alcuni importanti segni fisici). I lattanti o i bambini piccoli possono essere esaminati in grembo ai genitori, in modo che si sentano più sicuri e disposti a collaborare.
- È importante osservare come il paziente si muove nella stanza prima e durante l'esame, oltre che durante le diverse manovre. Occorre controllare anche *equilibrio, postura e andatura.*
- L'*esame obiettivo generale* deve comprendere la ricerca di rash cutanei, macchie caffelatte, chiazze pelose, fossette, cisti, ciuffi di peli o segni di difetti della linea mediana che possono indicare un problema sottostante severo e che necessitano di una revisione diagnostica.
- Occorre notare l'*habitus corporeo generale,* compresi segni di cachessia, pallore e deficit nutrizionali.
- È importante prestare attenzione a qualsiasi evidente asimmetria della colonna, alle deformità assiali o appendicolari, allo scompenso del tronco e alle evidenze di spasmo o contratture muscolari. Il *test del bending in avanti* è utile per valutare asimmetrie e movimento della colonna.
- È essenziale eseguire e documentare un *esame neurologico completo.* Occorre eseguire e registrare la valutazione della sensibilità, della funzione motoria e dei riflessi.
- Si raccomanda di annotare qualsiasi *discrepanza della lunghezza degli arti,* come anche la presenza di *atrofia muscolare.*
- In tutti i casi occorre osservare l'arco di movimento di tutte le articolazioni, la loro stabilità e qualsiasi evidenza di iperlassità, i polsi periferici e la presenza di linfoadenopatia.

PALPAZIONE. La palpazione della regione interessata deve comprendere la valutazione a livello locale di temperatura e calore, dolore, presenza di masse o tumefazioni, evidenza di rigidità, spasticità o contrattura, deformità ossee o articolari e la valutazione dell'asse anatomico dell'arto, e infine la valutazione della lunghezza degli arti.

Le **contratture** consistono nella perdita di mobilità di un'articolazione da cause congenite o acquisite e sono imputabili a fibrosi dei tessuti molli periarticolari o all'interessamento dei muscoli che attraversano l'articolazione. Le contratture congenite sono comuni nell'**artrogriposi** (vedi Capitolo 681). La spasticità, che rappresenta un aumento anormale del tono muscolare associato a iperreflessia, è comune nella paralisi cerebrale.

La **deformità** di un osso o di un'articolazione è una forma o posizione anormale e fissa, da cause congenite o acquisite. È importante valutarne il tipo, la sede e il grado nel corso dell'esame obiettivo, come pure stabilire se la deformità sia fissa o se possa essere corretta attivamente o passivamente e se siano presenti spasmo muscolare associato, dolore locale o dolore nel corso del movimento. A seconda del piano della deformità, questa può essere definita in **varo** (apice discosto dalla linea mediana) o in **valgo** (apice verso la linea mediana) (sul piano coronale o frontale) o deformità in **flessione** (**recurvatum**) (sul piano sagittale). Nello scheletro assiale, con particolare riguardo alla colonna, la deformità può essere definita come scoliosi, cifosi, iperlordosi e cifoscoliosi.

ARCO DI MOVIMENTO. Quando si esamina un'articolazione è importante valutare e registrare l'arco di movimento attivo e passivo. L'arco di movimento deve sempre essere confrontato con quello del lato opposto tendente verso l'arco di movimento normale. Una valutazione oggettiva andrebbe idealmente eseguita con un goniometro e quindi registrata.

Di seguito si indicano i differenti termini per i movimenti articolari:

Abduzione: allontanamento dalla linea mediana.
Adduzione: avvicinamento alla linea mediana.
Flessione: movimento di piegamento dalla posizione iniziale.
Estensione: movimento di piegamento verso la posizione iniziale.
Supinazione: rotazione dell'avambraccio in modo da avere il palmo della mano rivolto verso l'alto.
Pronazione: rotazione dell'avambraccio in modo da avere il palmo della mano rivolto verso il basso.
Inversione: rotazione del retropiede verso l'interno.
Eversione: rotazione del retropiede verso l'esterno.
Rotazione interna: rotazione all'interno verso l'asse del corpo.
Rotazione esterna: rotazione all'esterno lontano dall'asse del corpo.

VALUTAZIONE DEL CAMMINO. I bambini tipicamente iniziano a camminare tra i 12 e i 16 mesi. La deambulazione precoce è caratterizzata da una falcata corta, una cadenza rapida e una bassa velocità con una base d'appoggio allargata. Il ciclo del passo è una singola sequenza di funzioni di un arto, che comprende il tempo tra l'appoggio a terra del tallone destro seguito dal distacco da terra delle dita del piede sinistro, l'appoggio a terra del tallone sinistro e il distacco da terra delle dita del piede destro, e termina con l'appoggio a terra del tallone destro. I cinque eventi descrivono un ciclo del passo e comprendono due fasi: appoggio e oscillazione. La fase di appoggio è il periodo durante il quale il piede è a contatto con il terreno; quella di oscillazione è la parte del ciclo del passo durante la quale un arto si trova in posizione avanzata, senza contatto con il terreno (vedi Capitolo 671).

Alcuni termini importanti utilizzati nella descrizione del ciclo del cammino sono i seguenti:

Cadenza: numero di passi al minuto.
Lunghezza del passo: distanza ricoperta durante un passo.
Periodo del passo: il tempo misurato da un evento in un piede allo stesso evento nell'altro piede.
Periodo di falcata: il tempo intercorso tra appoggio a terra del tallone di un piede e successivo appoggio a terra del tallone dello stesso piede.
Lunghezza della falcata: distanza totale ricoperta da un appoggio a terra di un tallone all'appoggio a terra dello stesso tallone.

È necessaria la maturazione neurologica per lo sviluppo del cammino e il normale avvicendamento delle tappe dello sviluppo. Nel soggetto in età pediatrica, il cammino varia con la maturazione neurologica. I bambini più piccoli di solito camminano con una maggiore flessione dell'anca e del ginocchio, con braccia flesse e una base d'appoggio più ampia rispetto a quelli più grandi. Con la progressione in senso cefalocaudale della maturazione neurologica, aumentano l'efficienza e la scioltezza della deambulazione. Le caratteristiche del cammino di un bambino di 7 anni sono simili a quelle di un adulto. Quando sono presenti anomalie neurologiche (come nella paralisi cerebrale), il delicato sistema di controllo del cammino è alterato portando allo sviluppo di riflessi patologici e a movimenti anomali.

Deviazioni rispetto a un cammino normale si verificano in diverse condizioni ortopediche. I disordini che causano perdita di forza muscolare (per es. spina bifida, distrofia muscolare), spasticità (per es. paralisi cerebrale) o contratture (per es. artrogriposi) portano ad anomalie del cammino. Altre cause di disturbi del cammino comprendono zoppia, dolore, variazioni torsionali (cammino a punte intraruotate ed extraruotate), cammino sulle punte, anomalie articolari e disparità di lunghezza degli arti inferiori.

ZOPPIA

L'esecuzione accurata di anamnesi ed esame obiettivo è il primo passo per l'identificazione precoce del problema di base che provoca una zoppia. Quest'ultima può essere **dolorosa** (**antalgica**) o non dolorosa, e la diagnosi differenziale deve tenere conto di diverse cause, benigne e severe (anca settica, neoplasia). In caso di cammino doloroso, la fase di appoggio è abbreviata in quanto il bambino riduce il tempo in cui carica il peso sull'arto dolente. In caso di cammino non doloroso, indicativo di una perdita di forza muscolare prossimale o di instabilità dell'anca, la fase di appoggio è uguale nel lato interessato e in quello non interessato, ma il bambino tenderà ad appoggiarsi o a spostare il centro di gravità sull'estremità interessata per mantenere l'equilibrio. Se il disordine è bilaterale, causa un'andatura anserina.

I disordini più comunemente responsabili di un cammino anormale sono diversi, a seconda dell'età del paziente. La diagnosi differenziale della zoppia varia in base all'età (Tab. 672-3) o al meccanismo (Tab. 672-4). Anche i disordini neurologici, specialmente quelli del midollo spinale o dei nervi periferici, possono causare zoppia e difficoltà del cammino. L'andatura antalgica è prevalentemente il risultato di un trauma, di un'infezione o di una frattura patologica. L'andatura di Trendelenburg è generalmente dovuta a disordini congeniti, dello sviluppo o muscolari. In alcuni casi una zoppia può essere dovuta anche a cause non scheletriche come torsione testicolare, ernia inguinale e appendicite.

DORSALGIA

Rispetto agli adulti, le indagini diagnostiche per la dorsalgia del bambino sono estese e aggressive già in una fase molto più precoce dell'evoluzione della sintomatologia. I bambini hanno spesso una patologia scheletrica specifica come causa della dorsalgia. Nella popolazione pediatrica, una storia di dorsalgia persistente deve essere considerata seriamente e spesso richiede ulteriori indagini. Le cause più frequenti di dorsalgia nel bambino sono traumi, spondilolisi e spondilolistesi e infezioni. La Tabella 678-1 elenca le cause più comuni di dorsalgia nell'infanzia. È importante notare che la probabilità di trascurare le neoplasie e le lesioni similtumorali che causano dorsalgia nel bambino è tutt'altro che remota, a meno che non venga eseguita una valutazione clinica

TABELLA 672-3. Cause comuni di zoppia in base all'età

ETÀ	ANTALGICA	TRENDELENBURG	DISCREPANZA TRA ARTI INFERIORI
1-3 anni	Infezione Artrite settica Anca Ginocchio Osteomielite Discite Trauma occulto Frattura (bambino ai primi passi) Neoplasia	Lussazione dell'anca (DDH) Malattia neuromuscolare Paralisi cerebrale Poliomielite	–
4-10 anni	Infezione Artrite settica Anca Ginocchio Osteomielite Discite Sinovite transitoria, anca LCPD Coalizione tarsale Disordini reumatologici JRA Trauma Neoplasia	Lussazione dell'anca (DDH) Malattia neuromuscolare Paralisi cerebrale Poliomielite	+
Adolescenza (≥11 anni)	SCFE Disordini reumatologici JRA Trauma: frattura, sforzo Coalizione tarsale Neoplasia		+

DDH (*Developmental Dysplasia of the Hip*), displasia evolutiva dell'anca; JRA (*Juvenile Rheumatoid Arthritis*), artrite reumatoide giovanile; LCPD (*Legg-Calvé-Perthes Disease*), malattia di Legg-Calvé-Perthes; SCFE (*Slipped Capital Femoral Epiphysis*), epifisiolisi femorale; –, assente; +, presente.
Da Thompson GH: Gait disturbances. In Kliegman RM (ed): *Practical Strategies of Pediatric Diagnosis and Therapy*. Philadelphia, WB Saunders, 1996, pp 757-778.

TABELLA 672-4. Diagnosi differenziale della zoppia

ANTALGICA	TRENDELENBURG
CONGENITA Coalizione tarsale	**EVOLUTIVA** DDH Discrepanza di lunghezza degli arti inferiori
ACQUISITA LCPD SCFE	**NEUROMUSCOLARE** Paralisi cerebrale Poliomielite
TRAUMA Distorsioni, stiramenti, contusioni Fratture Occulta Frattura del bambino ai primi passi Abuso	
NEOPLASTICA Benigna Cisti ossea unicamerata Osteoma osteoide Maligna Sarcoma osteogenico Sarcoma di Ewing Leucemia Neuroblastoma Neoplasie del midollo spinale	
INFETTIVA Artrite settica Artrite reattiva Osteomielite Acuta Subacuta Discite	
REUMATOLOGICA Artrite reumatoide giovanile Sinovite monoarticolare dell'anca (sinovite tossica transitoria)	

DDH (*Developmental Dysplasia of the Hip*), displasia evolutiva dell'anca; LCPD (*Legg-Calvé-Perthes Disease*), malattia di Legg-Calvé-Perthes; SCFE (*Slipped Capital Femoral Epiphysis*), epifisiolisi femorale.
Da Thompson GH: Gait disturbances. In Kliegman RM (ed): *Practical Strategies of Pediatric Diagnosis and Therapy*. Philadelphia, WB Saunders, 1996, pp 757-778.

completa con indagini adeguate, quando necessario. Le cause non ortopediche di dorsalgia comprendono IVU, nefrolitiasi e polmonite.

VALUTAZIONE NEUROLOGICA. Dell'esame muscoloscheletrico pediatrico fa parte un'accurata valutazione neurologica (vedi Capitolo 591), che esamini le tappe motorie, la forza muscolare, la sensibilità, il tono muscolare e i riflessi osteotendinei profondi. La valutazione neurologica deve anche comprendere la colonna e identificare la presenza di deformità come scoliosi e cifosi, esaminando inoltre la mobilità della colonna. Può essere necessario l'esame di specifici nervi periferici.

Con la maturazione del sistema nervoso, la corteccia cerebrale in via di sviluppo normalmente inibisce i riflessi primitivi che sono spesso presenti alla nascita (vedi Capitolo 591). Pertanto, la persistenza di questi riflessi oltre una certa età indica la presenza di anomalie neurologiche. I riflessi osteotendinei profondi che vengono esaminati più frequentemente sono i riflessi bicipitale, tricipitale, rotuleo e achilleo. Occorre identificare e documentare una perdita di forza muscolare localizzata o diffusa. In tutti i casi di disordini neuromuscolari sono obbligatori un'attenta valutazione e un accurato *grading* della forza muscolare.

Un sistema di grading della forza muscolare di uso comune si basa su una scala da 0 a 5:

Grado 0: non è identificabile alcuna contrazione muscolare.
Grado 1: presenza di tracce di contrazione, a malapena identificabili clinicamente.
Grado 2: movimento attivo con eliminazione della gravità.
Grado 3: movimento attivo contro gravità.
Grado 4: movimento attivo contro gravità e una certa resistenza.
Grado 5: movimento attivo contro una resistenza piena.

INDAGINI RADIOLOGICHE. Le radiografie di routine sono il primo passo per la valutazione della maggior parte dei disordini muscoloscheletrici. Le tecniche di imaging avanzate comprendono procedure particolari come la scintigrafia muscolare, l'ecografia, la TC, la RM e la PET (*Positron Emission Tomography*, tomografia a emissione di positroni).

RADIOGRAFIE SENZA CONTRASTO. Il primo passo è costituito dalle radiografie di routine, che consistono in una proiezione anteroposteriore e in una laterale dell'area interessata, compresa un'articolazione in alto e in basso. Immagini di confronto del lato opposto, se non interessato, possono essere utili nelle situazioni difficoltose, ma non sempre sono necessarie. È importante che il medico sia a conoscenza delle normali varianti radiologiche dello scheletro. Diverse sincondrosi possono essere considerate erroneamente delle fratture. Possono rendersi necessari ulteriori studi di imaging in un paziente con un aspetto radiografico "normale" ma con dolore o sintomi persistenti, se si sospetta una neoplasia.

IMAGING CON RADIOISOTOPI. Una scintigrafia ossea evidenzia informazioni fisiologiche più che anatomiche e si basa sull'emissione di energia da parte di radioisotopi iniettati nel paziente. Le indicazioni comprendono un'artrite settica o un'osteomielite in fase precoce, una necrosi avascolare, i tumori (osteoma osteoide), le lesioni metastatiche, le fratture occulte e da stress, e i casi di abuso.

La scintigrafia *total body* (Tecnezio-99) è utile sia per identificare le lesioni ossee (infiammatorie, tumorali, fratture da stress) sia per valutare l'attività biologica delle lesioni ossee primitive. La vascolarizzazione tumorale può essere dedotta in base alle immagini della fase di flusso e del pool ematico. La scintigrafia con gallio o indio ha un'elevata sensibilità per le infezioni locali. La scintigrafia con Tallio-201 cloruro possiede una sensibilità >90% e un'accuratezza dell'80-90% nell'identificare lesioni tumorali maligne di ossa o tessuti molli.

ECOGRAFIA. L'ecografia è priva di radiazioni ionizzanti, non necessita della somministrazione di mezzo di contrasto, non ha effetti biologici dannosi e può essere ripetuta ogniqualvolta sia necessario. L'attrezzatura è portatile e le immagini possono essere eseguite su qualsiasi piano. Gli svantaggi di questa metodica sono i seguenti: l'osso non viene penetrato dagli ultrasuoni, le immagini statiche sono di difficile interpretazione e i risultati sono operatore-dipendenti. Le principali indicazioni per l'ecografia sono lo studio fetale delle estremità e della colonna, compresa la diagnosi di anomalie congenite come la disostosi spondilocostale, l'osteogenesi imperfetta, la displasia evolutiva dell'anca, i versamenti articolari, il disrafismo spinale *neonatale* occulto, i corpi estranei nei tessuti molli e le cisti poplitee del ginocchio.

RISONANZA MAGNETICA (RM). La RM è la modalità di imaging di scelta per definire ulteriormente l'esatta estensione anatomica della maggior parte delle lesioni muscoloscheletriche. Oltre a non fare uso di radiazioni ionizzanti, si ritiene che non produca effetti biologici negativi. Permette di ottenere eccellenti immagini anatomiche dell'apparato muscoloscheletrico, compresi i tessuti molli, le cavità midollari, il midollo spinale e il cervello. Particolarmente utile per le lesioni dei tessuti molli, permette di definire la lesione e la sua estensione (indicando l'entità dell'interessamento delle strutture neurovascolari e delle cartilagini di accrescimento). I piani tissutali sono ben delineati e permettono una valutazione più accurata della lesione o dell'invasione tumorale delle strutture adiacenti. È possibile visualizzare le strutture cartilaginee e distinguerne le differenti forme (la cartilagine articolare del ginocchio può essere distinta dalla fibrocartilagine del menisco). La RM è utile per visualizzare le articolazioni non ossificate nella popolazione pediatrica, compresi spalla, gomito e anca del lattante. Distingue inoltre le alterazioni fisiologiche che si verificano a livello del midollo osseo rispetto all'età e a malattie come la necrosi avascolare.

La RM può essere preziosa per valutare la necrosi ossea avascolare, infezioni e infarti ossei, del midollo spinale e delle radici nervose, lesioni dei nervi periferici e neoplasie ossee e dei tessuti molli. Essendo in grado di definire la regione di interesse su piani multipli (assiale, sagittale e frontale), è vantaggiosa per la definizione dell'estensione di diversi tumori. È la migliore modalità per la dimostrazione dell'estensione dei tumori intraossei, per la valutazione dell'interessamento di strutture neurovascolari critiche e per la valutazione dell'estensione neoplastica nei tessuti molli. È inoltre possibile utilizzare la RM dinamica con mezzo di contrasto per monitorare la risposta alla chemioterapia e identificare *skip lesion* e lesioni satelliti.

ANGIOGRAFIA RM (MRA. MAGNETIC RESONANCE ANGIOGRAPHY). Questa metodica diagnostica ha ampiamente sostituito l'angiografia di routine nella valutazione preoperatoria delle lesioni vascolari e dei tumori ossei. Permette una buona visualizzazione dei rami vascolari periferici e della neovascolarizzazione tumorale nei pazienti con neoplasie ossee primitive. È inoltre utile per dimostrare la compressione e l'inglobamento dei vasi principali da parte della massa tumorale. Mentre la RM può essere in molti casi sufficiente per la diagnosi di grossi trombi tumorali, è stato raccomandato di aggiungere MRA ed ecografia alla RM nella pianificazione preoperatoria di un intervento conservativo in casi come gli osteosarcomi del bacino, specialmente se è presente una risposta insoddisfacente alla chemioterapia.

TOMOGRAFIA COMPUTERIZZATA (TC). La TC ha migliorato la valutazione di diversi disordini muscoloscheletrici. Con questa tecnica sono possibili immagini frontali, sagittali e assiali, compresa una ricostruzione tridimensionale che può essere utile per valutare le lesioni complesse dello scheletro assiale e appendicolare; essa permette di visualizzare l'anatomia ossea in dettaglio e le relazioni tra ossa e strutture contigue. Alcuni dei disordini muscoloscheletrici pediatrici valutabili con la TC sono coalizione tarsale, osso navicolare accessorio, infezioni, arresto della cartilagine di coniugazione, osteoma osteoide, pseudoartrosi, tumori ossei e dei tessuti molli, spondilolisi e spondilolistesi.

La TC è superiore alla RM nella valutazione dell'interessamento osseo e della distruzione corticale (anche alterazioni sfumate), comprese calcificazione o ossificazione e frattura. La valutazione della cavità acetabolare e dell'anatomia ossea del bacino è critica nei tumori periacetabolari; la TC può essere un'utile aggiunta alla RM. I migliori studi di imaging per la diagnosi e la valutazione delle metastasi polmonari e della risposta di queste lesioni alla chemioterapia rimangono sia la TC spirale (HCT) sia la TC ad alta risoluzione (HRCT, *Hight Resolution Computed Tomography*) (l'HCT è più sensibile della HRCT per la diagnosi delle metastasi polmonari).

TOMOGRAFIA A EMISSIONE DI POSITRONI (PET). L'imaging funzionale per mezzo della PET è stato riconosciuto come un'importante modalità di imaging e come esame complementare a TC/RM che fornisce informazioni metaboliche preziose in molte applicazioni oncologiche. La PET con ^{18}F-fluorodesossiglucosio (FDG) valuta l'aumento del metabolismo del glucosio nei sarcomi. L'esame con FDG-PET dei sarcomi ossei in età pediatrica dimostra un'alterazione significativa della risposta alla chemioterapia neoadiuvante. Indicazioni cliniche potenzialmente utili della FDG-PET sono il monitoraggio della terapia e la diagnosi delle recidive metastatiche.

INDAGINI DI LABORATORIO. Talvolta si rendono necessari anche gli esami di laboratorio nella valutazione di un bambino con un disordine muscoloscheletrico. Questi possono comprendere un emocromo completo, la VES, la proteina C-reattiva, la sierologia della malattia di Lyme, un'emocoltura e la coltura di materiale prelevato da ferite, articolazioni, periostio e tessuto osseo per la diagnosi di malattie infettiva come un'artrite settica o un'osteomielite. Può essere necessario il dosaggio di fattore reumatoide, anticorpi antinucleo e HLA B27 nei bambini con un sospetto disordine reumatologico. L'esame di creatina chinasi, aldolasi, aspartato aminotransferasi e distrofina è indicato nei bambini con un sospetto disordine del muscolo striato come la distrofia muscolare di Duchenne o Becker.

Beebe AC, Kerpsack JM: Pediatric musculoskeletal examination. In Dormans JP (editor): *Pediatric Orthopedics: Core Knowledge in Orthopedics.* Philadelphia, Mosby, 2005, pp 15–35.

Herring JA: The orthopedic examination: A comprehensive overview. In Herring JA (editor): *Tachdjian's Pediatric Orthopedics,* 3rd ed. Philadelphia, WB Saunders, 2002, pp 25–61.

Herring JA: The limping child. In Herring JA (editor): *Tachdjian's Pediatric Orthopedics,* 3rd ed. Philadelphia, WB Saunders, 2002, pp 83–94.

Herring JA: Imaging. In Herring JA (editor): *Tachdjian's Pediatric Orthopedics,* 3rd ed. Philadelphia, WB Saunders, 2002, pp 127–168.

Hosalkar HS, Garg S, Pollack A, Dormans JP: The diagnostic accuracy of MRI vs. CT imaging for osteoid osteoma in children. *Clin Orthop* 2005;433:171–177.

Hosalkar HS, Moroz L, Drummond DS, Finkel RS: Neuromuscular disorders of infancy and childhood and arthrogryposis. In Dormans JP (editor): *Pediatric Orthopedics: Core Knowledge in Orthopedics,*. Philadelphia, Mosby, 2005, pp 454–482.

Jones DHA, Hosalkar HS, Jones S: The orthopaedic management of osteogenesis imperfecta. *Curr Orthop* 2002;16:374–388.

Staheli LT: Normative data in pediatric orthopaedics. *J Pediatr Orthop* 1996;16:561–562.

Sutherland DH, Olsten R, Cooper L, et al: The development of gait. *J Bone Joint Surg Am* 1980;62:336–353.

Capitolo 673 ■ Piede e dita del piede

Harish S. Hosalkar, David A. Spiegel e Richard S. Davidson

Le anomalie delle strutture ossee e articolari del piede possono essere congenite, dello sviluppo, neuromuscolari o infiammatorie. I problemi relativi al piede e/o alle dita del piede possono associarsi a numerose malattie e sindromi del tessuto connettivo; le sindromi da sforzo sono di frequente riscontro nei giovani atleti. I sintomi possono comprendere dolore e difficoltà a portare le calzature; sono comuni le preoccupazioni estetiche. Il piede può essere suddiviso in **avampiede** (dita e ossa del metatarso), **piede intermedio** (cuneiformi, scafoide e cuboide) e **retropiede** (talo o astragalo e calcagno). Mentre l'articolazione tibiotarsica (caviglia) permette la flessione plantare e la dorsiflessione del piede, l'articolazione sottoastragalica (tra astragalo e calcagno), orientata obliquamente, permette inversione ed eversione. L'inversione rappresenta una combinazione di flessione plantare e varo, mentre l'eversione comprende la dorsiflessione e il valgo del piede. L'articolazione sottoastragalica è particolarmente importante per il cammino su superfici irregolari. Le articolazioni astragaloscafoidea e calcaneocuboidea connettono il piede intermedio con il retropiede.

673.1 • Metatarso addotto

Il metatarso addotto, comune nei neonati, consiste nell'adduzione dell'avampiede relativamente al retropiede; quando invece l'avampiede è supinato e addotto, prende il nome di metatarso varo (Fig. 673-1). La causa più comune è il modellamento intrauterino; la deformità è bilaterale nel 50% dei casi. Come per le altre deformità posizionali intrauterine del piede, l'anca deve sempre essere esaminata con attenzione.

MANIFESTAZIONI CLINICHE. L'avampiede è addotto (occasionalmente supinato), mentre il piede intermedio e il retropiede sono normali. Il margine laterale del piede è convesso e la base del 5° osso metatarsale appare sporgente. L'arco di movimento a livello della caviglia e delle articolazioni sottotalari è normale. Occorre documentare sia l'entità sia il grado di flessibilità. Quando si osserva il piede dalla superficie plantare, una linea tracciata attraverso il punto medio del tallone (e parallela a esso) dovrebbe normalmente estendersi attraverso il 2° dito. La flessibilità viene valutata stabilizzando il retropiede e il piede intermedio in posizione neutra con una mano e applicando una pressione sulla 1ª testa metatarsale con l'altra. Nel bambino che cammina con un metatarso addotto non corretto si possono verificare un'andatura a punte intraruotate e difficoltà a portare le calzature. Un sottogruppo di pazienti presenterà anche una deformità dinamica in adduzione dell'alluce (alluce varo), spesso più evidente durante la deambulazione. Questa di solito migliora spontaneamente e non richiede trattamento.

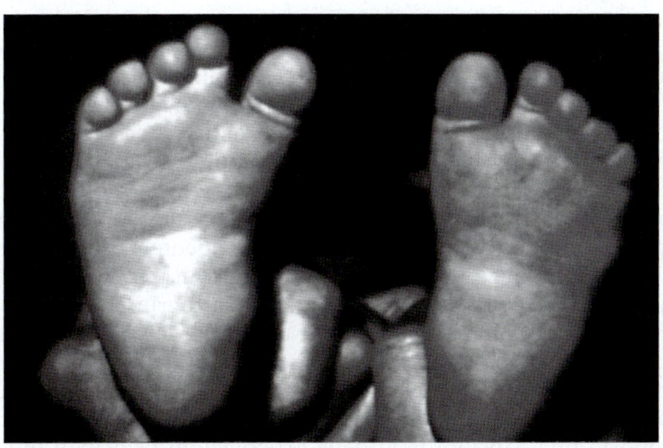

Figura 673-1. Aspetto clinico del metatarso addotto con piede normale dal lato opposto.

INDAGINI RADIOLOGICHE. Le indagini radiologiche non sono necessarie di routine. Radiografie in proiezione anteroposteriore e laterale, in carico o in carico simulato, sono indicate in pazienti di 1-3 anni o in bambini più grandi con deformità residue. Le radiografie in proiezione anteroposteriore dimostrano un'adduzione dei metatarsi a livello dell'articolazione tarsometatarsale e un aumento dell'angolo intermetatarsale tra il 1° e il 2° metatarso.

TRATTAMENTO. Il trattamento del metatarso addotto si basa sulla rigidità della deformità; la maggior parte dei bambini risponde al trattamento conservativo. Si possono osservare deformità flessibili e ipercorrette in abduzione con manipolazioni passive. I piedi che si correggono fino alla posizione neutra possono trarre beneficio da esercizi di stretching e dal mantenimento in una posizione leggermente ipercorretta con un'ortesi o con scarpe "a biscotto". Questi ausili devono essere portati sempre (22 ore al giorno) e la condizione va rivalutata dopo 4-6 settimane. Se si nota un miglioramento, si può continuare il trattamento; in caso contrario, occorre prendere in considerazione l'utilizzo di gessi seriati. Quando si esegue un esercizio di stretching su un piede con metatarso addotto, occorre fare attenzione a mantenere il retropiede in allineamento da neutro a leggermente in varo, onde evitare di creare un retropiede valgo. I piedi che non possono essere corretti fino a raggiungere una posizione neutra possono trarre beneficio da gessi seriati; i migliori risultati si ottengono quando il trattamento viene iniziato prima degli 8 mesi di vita. Oltre allo stretching dei tessuti molli, l'obiettivo è quello di modificare la crescita a livello delle cartilagini di accrescimento e stimolare il rimodellamento con una correzione permanente. Una volta ripristinati flessibilità e allineamento, si raccomandano generalmente ortesi o scarpe correttive per un ulteriore periodo di tempo. Un alluce varo dinamico di solito migliora spontaneamente e non è necessario alcun trattamento attivo.

Il trattamento chirurgico può essere preso in considerazione in quel piccolo sottogruppo di pazienti con deformità residue sintomatiche che non hanno risposto ai trattamenti precedenti. Per eseguire l'intervento chirurgico in genere si attende che il bambino abbia 4-6 anni di età. L'aspetto estetico rappresenta spesso un problema e il dolore o l'incapacità di indossare certi tipi di calzature possono talvolta portare i pazienti a desiderare l'intervento. Le opzioni per il trattamento chirurgico consistono nel rilascio dei tessuti molli o in un'osteotomia. L'intervento di osteotomia (piede intermedio o più metatarsi) ha la maggiore probabilità di consentire un allineamento permanente.

673.2 • Piede calcaneovalgo

Il piede calcaneovalgo è un'anomalia comune nel neonato, secondaria al posizionamento in utero. A livello del retropiede si possono osservare una dorsiflessione e un'eversione eccessive, mentre l'avampiede può essere abdotto. Può essere associata una torsione tibiale esterna.

MANIFESTAZIONI CLINICHE. Il bambino tipicamente si presenta con il piede dorsiflesso ed evertito e occasionalmente il dorso del piede è in contatto con la superficie anterolaterale dell'arto inferiore. La flessione plantare e l'inversione sono spesso limitate. Come in altre deformità posizionali intrauterine, bisogna esaminare accuratamente l'anca; se vi è qualche sospetto, occorre valutare se eseguire un'ecografia delle anche. Il piede calcaneovalgo può essere confuso con un astragalo verticale congenito ed essere associato a un'incurvatura posteromediale della tibia, per quanto si tratti di un'eventualità rara. Una deformità in calcaneovalgo è osservabile anche in bambini più grandi, caratteristicamente in quelli con squilibrio neuromuscolare da perdita di forza o paralisi dei muscoli gastrocnemio e soleo (poliomielite, mielomeningocele).

INDAGINI RADIOLOGICHE. Le indagini radiologiche di solito non sono necessarie, ma devono essere prese in considerazione se la deformità non si corregge spontaneamente o con un trattamento precoce. Radiografie in proiezione anteroposteriore e laterale con una radiografia laterale del piede in massima flessione plantare talvolta permettono di distinguere tra piede calaneovalgo e astragalo verticale. Se si sospetta un'incurvatura posteromediale della tibia, sono necessarie radiografie in proiezione anteroposteriore e laterale della tibia e del perone.

TRATTAMENTO. I casi lievi di piede calcaneovalgo, in cui è presente alla nascita un arco di movimento passivo completo, non richiedono trattamento attivo e di solito si risolvono entro la prima settimana di vita. Un programma di stretching leggero, focalizzato sulla flessione plantare e l'inversione, è raccomandato nei casi caratterizzati da una certa limitazione del movimento. Se tale limitazione della mobilità è spiccata, si possono prendere in considerazione gessi seriati per ripristinare la mobilità e l'allineamento. Nel trattamento del piede calcaneovalgo è raro che si renda necessario il gesso. Il trattamento di quei casi associati a incurvatura posteromediale della tibia è simile.

673.3 • PIEDE EQUINOVARO (PIEDE TORTO)

Con l'espressione "piede equinovaro" o "piede torto" si indica una deformità consistente nel disallineamento del complesso calcaneo-astragalo-scafoideo. Per ricordare le componenti di questa deformità si può fare ricorso alla sigla **CAVE** (cavo, addotto, varo, equino). Anche se questa è soprattutto una deformità del retropiede, sono presenti flessione plantare (cavo) del 1° raggio e adduzione dell'avampiede/piede intermedio rispetto al retropiede. Il retropiede è in varo ed equino. Il piede equinovaro può essere posizionale, congenito o associato a diverse altre entità patologiche (neuromuscolari o sindromiche).

Il **piede equinovaro posizionale** è un piede normale che è rimasto in una posizione abnorme in utero e che appare flessibile all'esame neonatologico. La **forma congenita** ha severità variabile, mentre il piede equinovaro associato a malattie neuromuscolari o a sindromi è tipicamente rigido e di trattamento più difficoltoso. Il piede equinovaro è estremamente comune nei pazienti con mielodisplasia e artrogriposi.

Il piede torto congenito si osserva in circa 1/1000 nati. Anche se sono state proposte numerose teorie, l'eziologia è multifattoriale e probabilmente include gli effetti di fattori ambientali in un ospite geneticamente suscettibile. Il rischio è di circa 1:4 quando un genitore e un fratello (o una sorella) hanno un piede torto. Più comune nei maschi (2:1), è bilaterale nel 50% dei casi. L'anatomia patologica comprende sia una morfologia tarsale anomala (deviazione plantare e mediale della testa e del collo dell'astragalo) sia la presenza di relazioni anomale tra le ossa tarsali su tutti e 3 i piani, oltre a contratture associate dei tessuti molli degli aspetti plantare e mediale del piede.

MANIFESTAZIONI CLINICHE. È necessario eseguire un esame obiettivo completo per escludere problemi muscoloscheletrici e neuromuscolari concomitanti. Occorre esaminare la colonna per ricercare segni di disrafismo occulto. L'esame del piede torto del lattante evidenzia un avampiede cavo e addotto e un retropiede varo ed equino (Fig. 673-2). Il grado di flessibilità è variabile e tutti i pazienti presentano atrofia del polpaccio. In un sottogruppo di casi si osservano torsione tibiale interna e una discrepanza di lunghezza degli arti inferiori (accorciamento dell'estremità ipsilaterale).

VALUTAZIONE RADIOGRAFICA. Si raccomanda l'esecuzione di radiografie anteroposteriore e laterale, spesso con il piede mantenuto nella posizione di massima correzione. È possibile effettuare misurazioni radiografiche multiple per descrivere il disallineamento tra le ossa tarsali. Lo scafoide non ossifica fino ai 3-6 anni di vita, per cui il punto focale dell'interpretazione radiografica è il rapporto tra i segmenti del piede. Un comune aspetto radiografico è il "parallelismo" tra le linee tracciate lungo l'asse dell'astragalo e del calcagno sulla radiografia laterale, che indicano il varismo del retropiede. Molti clinici ritengono che non siano necessarie radiografie per la valutazione e il trattamento del piede torto nei lattanti e riservano queste indagini ai bambini più grandi con deformità persistente o recidivante.

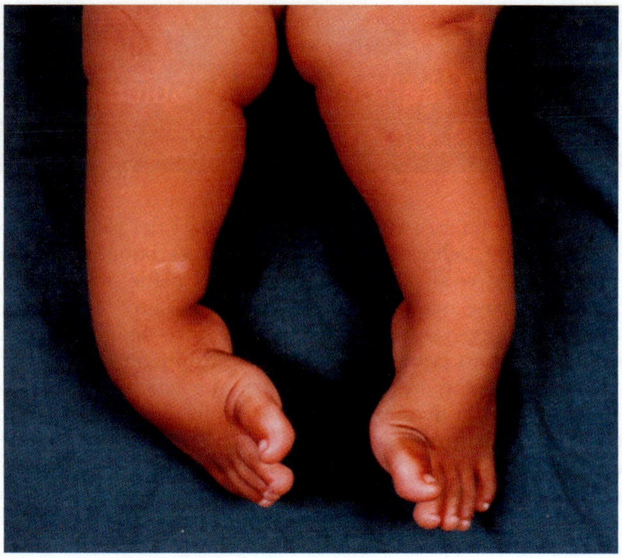

Figura 673-2. Immagine clinica che evidenzia una deformità del piede torto.

TRATTAMENTO. In tutti i bambini si inizia con un trattamento non operatorio, che deve essere instaurato non appena possibile, dopo la nascita. Le tecniche comprendono bendaggi e strapping, manipolazioni e gessi seriati e trattamenti funzionali. In passato una significativa percentuale di pazienti trattati con manipolazioni e gessi richiedeva in seguito un rilascio chirurgico, che veniva di solito eseguito fra i 3 e i 12 mesi di età. Anche se molti piedi rimangono bene allineati dopo il rilascio chirurgico, una significativa percentuale di pazienti necessita di ulteriori interventi per la presenza di deformità residue o per una recidiva. La rigidità rimane un problema al follow-up a lungo termine. Il dolore non è comune nell'infanzia e nell'adolescenza, ma può manifestarsi in età adulta. Questi problemi hanno fatto sì che si sviluppasse un notevole interesse per metodi meno invasivi di trattamento della deformità. Il metodo Ponseti per il trattamento del piede torto, comprendente una tecnica specifica con manipolazioni e gessi seriati, può essere definito "minimamente invasivo" più che "non operatorio". L'ordine di correzione segue l'acronimo mnemonico **CAVE**. Si eseguono gessi settimanali e di solito ne sono necessari da 5 a 10. La deformità più difficile da correggere è l'equinismo del retropiede e nel 90% circa dei pazienti è necessaria una tenotomia percutanea ambulatoriale del tendine d'Achille. Dopo la tenotomia il paziente porta per 3 settimane un gesso lungo con il piede in massima abduzione (70°) e in massima dorsiflessione, dopodiché inizia un programma comprendente l'uso di ortesi. Un'ortesi in abduzione viene indossata tutto il tempo per 3 mesi e quindi solo la notte per 3-5 anni. Un sottogruppo di pazienti richiede il trasferimento del tendine del tibiale anteriore sull'osso cuneiforme medio in seguito a una recidiva. Anche se la maggior parte dei pazienti richiede qualche tipo di intervento, le procedure sono di minima entità in confronto al rilascio chirurgico, che comporta una capsulotomia delle articolazioni principali (e l'allungamento de muscoli) per riposizionare in sede le articolazioni. Il risultato del metodo di Ponseti è eccellente fino a 40 anni di follow-up. È essenziale la compliance rispetto al programma di trattamento con le ortesi; le recidive sono comuni se l'ortesi non viene portata secondo le raccomandazioni. Il trattamento funzionale, o "metodo francese", consiste in manipolazioni giornaliere (sotto la supervisione di un fisioterapista) e nell'applicazione di un bendaggio elastico, oltre che in una mobilizzazione passiva continua (è necessaria una macchina) durante il sonno. Anche se i primi risultati sono promettenti, questo metodo richiede molto impegno professionale e non è chiaro se in futuro avrà maggiore diffusione negli Stati Uniti. Questi metodi minimamente invasivi hanno un maggiore successo quando il trattamento viene iniziato alla nascita o nei primi mesi di vita.

Il riallineamento chirurgico ha un ruolo ben preciso nel trattamento del piede torto, specialmente in quella minoranza di piedi torti congeniti in cui il trattamento non operatorio o quello minimamente invasivo non hanno dato alcun beneficio, e nei piedi torti neuromuscolari e sindromici che hanno la caratteristica di essere rigidi. In tali casi, i metodi non operatori come la tecnica di Ponseti potrebbe essere utile per ridurre l'entità dell'intervento necessario. Gli approcci chirurgici più comuni comprendono un rilascio delle articolazioni interessate (riallineamento delle ossa tarsali), un allungamento delle unità muscolotendinee posteromediali accorciate e, di solito, il posizionamento del piede nella postura corretta mediante l'applicazione di chiodi. La procedura specifica deve essere adattata alle caratteristiche peculiari di ciascuna deformità. Nei bambini più grandi con piedi torti non trattati o in quelli in cui si osserva una recidiva o una deformità residua, possono essere necessarie procedure ossee (osteotomie), oltre alla chirurgia dei tessuti molli. La tripla artrodesi è riservata agli interventi di salvataggio, nei casi con deformità e dolore del piede di adulti e adolescenti.

673.4 • ASTRAGALO VERTICALE CONGENITO

L'astragalo verticale congenito è una deformità del piede non frequente in cui il piede intermedio è lussato dorsalmente sul retropiede. Il 60% circa dei casi è idiopatico e il rimanente 40% è associato a una patologia neuromuscolare o a una sindrome. Le cause neurologiche comprendono mielodisplasia, *tethered cord* (midollo ancorato) e agenesia sacrale. Altre condizioni associate comprendono artrogriposi, sindrome di Larsen e anomalie cromosomiche (trisomia 13-15, 19). A seconda dell'età alla diagnosi, la diagnosi differenziale può comprendere il piede calcaneovalgo, l'astragalo obliquo (l'articolazione astragaloscafoidea si riduce passivamente), il piede piatto flessibile con tensione del tendine d'Achille e la coalizione tarsale.

MANIFESTAZIONI CLINICHE. L'astragalo verticale congenito prende anche il nome di **piede a sedia a dondolo** (Fig. 673-3) o a pantofola persiana. La superficie plantare è convessa e la testa dell'astragalo sporge lungo il margine mediale del piede intermedio. L'avampiede è dorsiflesso (lussato dorsalmente rispetto al retropiede) e abdotto relativamente al retropiede, mentre il retropiede è in equino e in valgo. È presente una contrattura associata dei tessuti molli anterolaterali (tibiale anteriore, estensori delle dite del piede) e posteriori (tendine d'Achille, peronei). La deformità è tipicamente rigida. È necessario un accurato esame obiettivo per identificare tutte le anomalie neurologiche e/o muscoloscheletriche coesistenti.

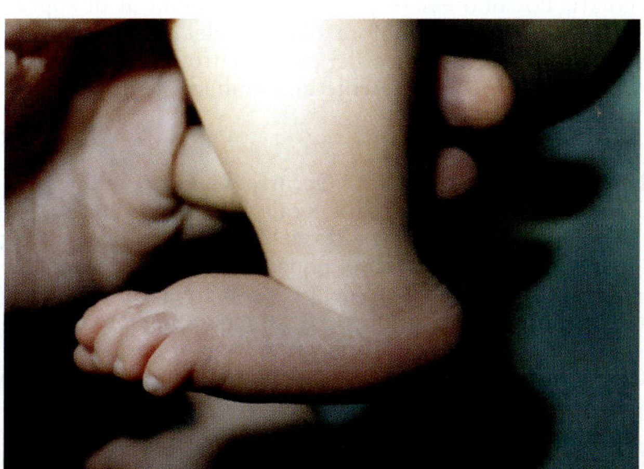

Figura 673-3. Piede a pantofola persiana o a sedia a dondolo in un caso di astragalo verticale congenito.

VALUTAZIONE RADIOGRAFICA. In caso di sospetto diagnostico occorre eseguire radiografie in proiezione anteroposteriore, laterale e in massima flessione plantare. La proiezione in flessione plantare ha lo scopo di determinare se la sublussazione o la lussazione dorsale del piede intermedio sul retropiede sono riducibili passivamente. Anche se lo scafoide non ossifica fino ai 3-6 anni di età, è possibile valutare il rapporto tra astragalo e 1° osso metatarsale.

TRATTAMENTO. Il trattamento, consistente in manipolazioni e gessi seriati, viene iniziato subito dopo la nascita. Innanzitutto si esegue un tentativo di ridurre la lussazione dorsale dell'avampiede/piede intermedio sul retropiede. Una volta raggiunto questo obiettivo, è possibile concentrarsi sullo stretching delle contratture dell'avampiede. Queste deformità sono tipicamente rigide e nella maggior parte dei casi richiedono un intervento chirurgico. In tali casi, il gesso favorisce lo stretching dei tessuto molli contratti. L'intervento, di solito eseguito tra i 6 e i 12 mesi di vita, comporta l'esecuzione di un rilascio dei tessuti molli con una procedura in una o due fasi. Una componente coinvolge il rilascio/allungamento dei tessuti molli anteriori contratti insieme a una riduzione aperta dell'articolazione astragaloscafoidea, mentre l'altra consiste nel rilascio posteriore con allungamento delle unità muscolotendinee contratte. Di solito si esegue una fissazione con fili di Kirschner per mantenere l'allineamento. Nel postoperatorio si usa il gesso per un periodo di tempo variabile; spesso i pazienti necessitano di un'ortesi per periodi prolungati, a seconda della diagnosi di base. Per le deformità residue o ricorrenti nei bambini più grandi, le opzioni comprendono un'artrodesi sottoastragalica o una tripla artrodesi.

673.5 • PES PLANUS IPERMOBILE (PIEDE PIATTO FLESSIBILE)

Il piede piatto è una diagnosi comune; è stato stimato che possa esserne affetto fino al 23% della popolazione, a seconda dei criteri diagnostici adottati. Ne esistono tre tipi: flessibile, con contrattura del tendine d'Achille e rigido. L'espressione "piede piatto" descrive un'alterazione della forma del piede, con diverse anomalie dell'allineamento tra le ossa tarsali. È presente un'eversione del complesso sottoastragalico. Il retropiede è allineato in valgo ed è presente un'infossatura del piede intermedio a livello dell'articolazione scafocuneiforme e/o dell'articolazione astragaloscafoidea. L'avampiede è abdotto relativamente al retropiede; la testa dell'astragalo è scoperta e sporge lungo il margine plantare e mediale del piede intermedio/retropiede. Mentre il pes planus ipermobile o flessibile rappresenta una comune causa di preoccupazione per i genitori, è raro che questi bambini siano sintomatici. Il piede piatto, comune nei neonati e nei bambini ai primi passi, è associato a una lassità legamentosa fisiologica. Si può osservare un miglioramento tra i 5 e i 10 anni di età, con lo sviluppo dell'arco longitudinale. Il piede piatto è meno comune nelle società in cui non si indossano scarpe nel corso della prima e seconda infanzia. È raccomandata una scarpa dalla suola flessibile. Il piede piatto flessibile che persiste nell'adolescenza e nell'età adulta è di solito associato a lassità legamentosa familiare ed è presente in altri membri della famiglia.

MANIFESTAZIONI CLINICHE. I pazienti presentano tipicamente un arco longitudinale normale se vengono esaminati in posizione di scarico del peso, ma l'arco scompare sotto carico. Il retropiede collassa in valgo e l'infossatura del piede intermedio diviene evidente. Si osserva comunemente una lassità legamentosa generalizzata. L'arco di movimento deve essere valutato a livello sia dell'articolazione sottoastragalica sia della tibiotarsica ed è normale nei pazienti con piede piatto flessibile. Quando si esamina l'arco di movimento a livello della caviglia, il piede deve sempre essere invertito mentre si valuta la dorsiflessione. Se il piede è in posizione neutra o in eversione, si può verificare una dorsiflessione spuria attraverso il piede intermedio, che maschera una contrattura del tendine d'Achille. Se vi è una limitazione del movimento sottoastragalico, il piede piatto non è ipermobile/flessibile e occorre considerare altre diagnosi come la coalizione tarsale e l'artrite reumatoide giovanile. Talvolta vi può essere dolore e/o formazione di callo al di sotto della testa dell'astragalo medialmente. Occorre inoltre valutare le calzature, in quanto possono presentare un'eccessiva usura lungo il bordo mediale.

VALUTAZIONE RADIOGRAFICA. Di solito non sono indicate radiografie di routine del piede piatto flessibile asintomatico. Per la valutazione della deformità sono necessarie radiografie sotto carico (anteroposteriore e laterale). Alla radiografia in anteroposteriore, è presente un allargamento dell'angolo tra l'asse longitudinale dell'astragalo e del calcagno, indicativo di un eccessivo valgo del tallone. La proiezione laterale evidenzia una distorsione della normale relazione (una linea diritta) tra l'asse lungo dell'astragalo e il 1° metatarso con un'infossatura dell'articolazione astragaloscafoidea o dell'articolazione scafocuneiforme, risultando in un appiattimento dell'arco longitudinale mediale normale (Fig. 673-4).

TRATTAMENTO. Nonostante la storia naturale del piede piatto flessibile rimanga sconosciuta, non vi sono prove certe che questa condizione dia luogo a problemi o disabilità a lungo termine. Pertanto, il trattamento è riservato a quel piccolo sottogruppo di pazienti che sviluppano sintomi. I pazienti con dolore del retropiede o quelli con problemi a indossare le calzature possono trarre beneficio da un'ortesi come un supporto mediale per l'arco plantare. I casi severi, spesso associati a un disordine del connettivo come la sindrome di Ehlers-Danlos o la sindrome di Down, possono trarre beneficio da un'ortesi personalizzata come l'UCBL (University of California Biomechanics Laboratory) per migliorare il controllo del retropiede e prevenire il collasso dell'arco plantare. Anche se un'ortesi può alleviare i sintomi, non vi sono evidenze che suggeriscano alcun cambiamento permanente della forma del piede o un allineamento delle ossa tarsali. I pazienti con piede piatto flessibile e tensione del tendine d'Achille devono essere trattati con esercizi di stretching ed eventualmente può rendersi necessario un allungamento chirurgico del muscolo. Per i pochi pazienti con dolore persistente è possibile prendere in esame il trattamento chirurgico. L'allungamento della colonna laterale, che affronta tutte le componenti della deformità, ha suscitato notevole interesse. La procedura consiste in un'osteotomia del calcagno e nell'inserimento di un innesto di osso trapezoide. Si rende necessario l'allungamento del tendine di Achille, spesso seguito da un'osteotomia in flessione plantare del cuneiforme mediale. Questa procedura conserva la mobilità delle articolazioni del retropiede, al contrario dell'artrodesi sottoastragalica o tripla. Anche se un'artrodesi del retropiede è in grado di correggere adeguatamente la deformità, il trasferimento dello stress sulle articolazioni adiacenti può causare alterazioni degenerative dolorose tardive. Un'altra possibilità è quella di inserire uno spaziatore nel seno del tarso per bloccare l'eversione a livello dell'articolazione sottoastragalica. Possibili complicanze di queste procedure sono la sinovite e l'allentamento dell'impianto.

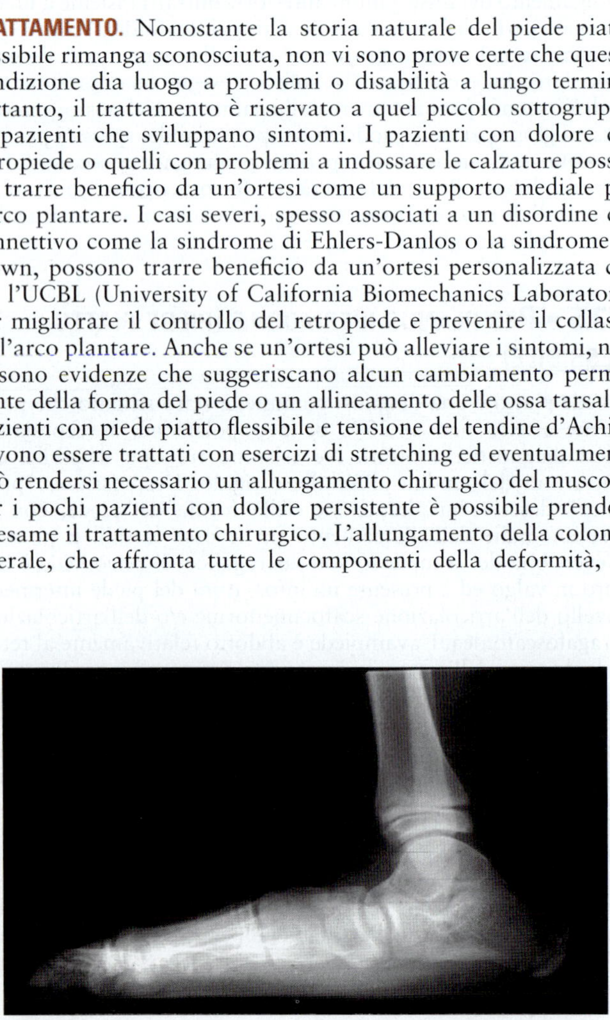

Figura 673-4. Radiografia in carico laterale che evidenzia aspetti di piede piatto.

673.6 • COALIZIONE TARSALE

La coalizione tarsale, nota anche come **piede piatto spastico peroneale**, è caratterizzata da un piattismo rigido e doloroso e da spasmo dei muscoli peroneale ma senza una vera spasticità. Essa rappresenta una fusione congenita o una mancata segmentazione tra due o più ossa tarsali. Qualsiasi condizione che alteri il normale scorrimento e il normale movimento rotatorio dell'articolazione sottoastragalica può causare il quadro clinico di una coalizione tarsale; quest'ultima pertanto può essere attribuibile a malformazioni congenite, artrite o patologie infiammatorie, infezioni, neoplasie e traumi.

Le coalizioni tarsali più comuni si verificano a livello della faccetta astragalocalcaneare mediale (sottoastragalica) e tra il calcagno e lo scafoide (calcaneoscafoidea). Le coalizioni possono essere fibrose, cartilaginee o ossee. La coalizione tarsale, che si verifica nell'1% circa della popolazione generale, sembra trasmettersi come un tratto autosomico dominante con penetranza quasi completa. Il 60% circa delle coalizioni calcaneoscafoidee e il 50% delle coalizioni della faccetta astragalocalcaneare mediale è bilaterale.

MANIFESTAZIONI CLINICHE. Il 25% circa dei pazienti diviene sintomatico, caratteristicamente nella seconda decade di vita. Anche se il piede piatto e una diminuzione della mobilità sottoastragalica potrebbero essere stati presenti fin dalla prima infanzia, l'esordio dei sintomi può essere correlato all'ulteriore limitazione del movimento che si verifica in seguito all'ossificazione di una barra cartilaginea. I tempi di ossificazione sono diversi per le coalizioni astragaloscafoidea (3-5 anni di età), calcaneoscafoidea (8-12 anni) e astragalocalcaneare (12-16 anni). Si osserva comunemente dolore del retropiede, in particolare nella regione del sinus tarsi, ma anche sotto la testa dell'astragalo. I sintomi, correlati all'attività, sono spesso aumentati dalla corsa o dalla deambulazione prolungata, specialmente su superfici irregolari. Possono essere presenti dolorabilità al di sopra del sito della coalizione e/o dolore all'esame del movimento sottoastragalico. L'aspetto clinico del piede piatto si osserva sia sotto carico sia in scarico. È presente una limitazione del movimento sottoastragalico.

VALUTAZIONE RADIOGRAFICA. Occorre eseguire radiografie in proiezione anteroposteriore e laterale in carico e una radiografia obliqua del piede. La coalizione calcaneoscafoidea è meglio valutabile con la radiografia obliqua. La radiografia laterale può evidenziare un allungamento del processo anteriore del calcagno, noto come "segno del formichiere". Il modo migliore per valutare la coalizione astragalocalcaneare è tramite una proiezione di Harris (assiale) del tallone. Alla radiografia laterale vi possono essere un restringimento della faccetta posteriore dell'articolazione sottoastragalica o una linea a C lungo il profilo mediale della volta astragalica e lungo il profilo inferiore del sustentaculum tali ("segno della C"). Si osserva con una certa frequenza una sporgenza dell'aspetto anteriore dell'astragalo alla proiezione laterale, derivante da un'alterazione della distribuzione dello stress.

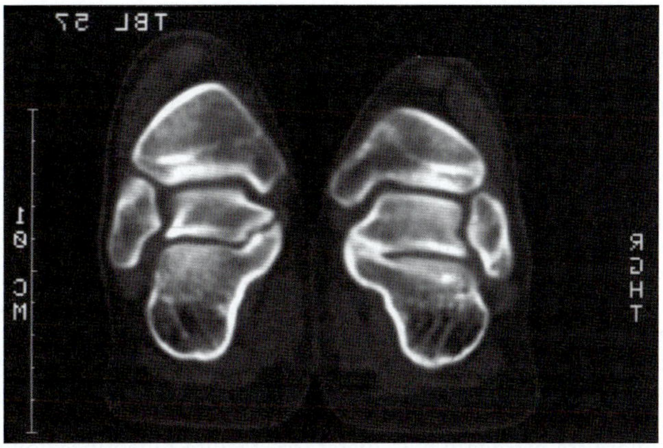

Figura 673-5. TC del complesso astragalocalcaneare che dimostra una coalizione tarsale.

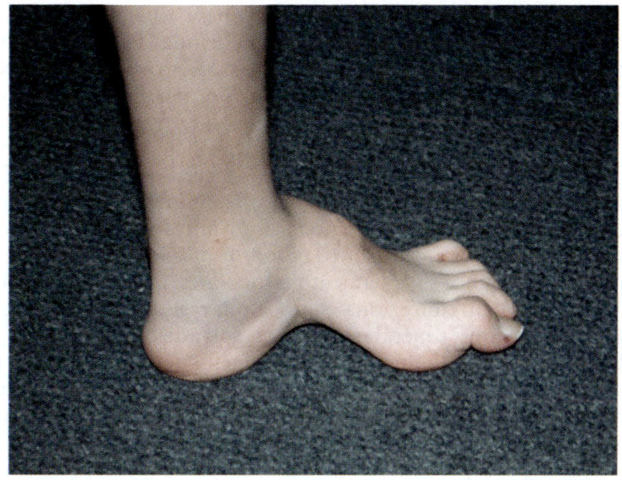

Figura 673-6. Immagine clinica di pes cavus.

Questo aspetto non implica la presenza di un'artrite degenerativa. Un'irregolarità a livello delle superfici ossee subcondrali è osservabile in pazienti con una coalizione cartilaginea, mentre in quelli con coalizione ossea si riscontra un ponte osseo ben formato. Una coalizione fibrosa può richiedere ulteriori studi di imaging per la diagnosi. Anche se le radiografie senza contrasto possono essere diagnostiche, la TC è la modalità di imaging di scelta quando si sospetta una coalizione (Fig. 673-5); oltre a permettere la diagnosi, questa metodica contribuisce a definire il grado di interessamento articolare nei pazienti con coalizione astragalocalcaneare. Per quanto si tratti di un'evenienza infrequente, è possibile osservare più di una coalizione tarsale nello stesso paziente.

TRATTAMENTO. Il trattamento delle coalizioni tarsali sintomatiche varia a secondo del tipo e dell'estensione della coalizione, dell'età del paziente e della presenza e dell'entità dei sintomi. Necessario soltanto per le coalizioni sintomatiche, esso inizialmente consiste nella limitazione dell'attività e nell'uso di farmaci antinfiammatori non steroidei (FANS), con o senza un plantare. Nei pazienti con sintomi più pronunciati può rendersi necessaria l'immobilizzazione in un gesso a stivaletto per 4-6 settimane. Per coloro che presentano dolore cronico nonostante un ciclo adeguato di terapia conservativa, si deve prendere in considerazione un intervento chirurgico (resezione della coalizione, osteotomia o artrodesi). Per la coalizione calcaneoscafoidea, si sono dimostrate efficaci la resezione e l'interposizione del muscolo estensore breve delle dita. Il trattamento chirurgico delle coalizioni astragalocalcaneari si basa sul grado di interessamento articolare, definito in base alla TC. Nei pazienti in cui l'interessamento articolare è <50%, si può prendere in considerazione la resezione della coalizione con interposizione di tessuto adiposo o di una porzione del tendine del flessore dell'alluce. In caso di interessamento esteso dell'articolazione e/o di alterazioni degenerative, la scelta migliore potrebbe essere una tripla artrodesi. Il ruolo dell'osteotomia nel trattamento della coalizione tarsale è attualmente in fase di studio.

673.7 • PIEDE CAVO

Il cavismo è una deformità che consiste nella flessione plantare dell'avampiede o del piede intermedio rispetto al retropiede e può interessare l'intera parte anteriore del piede oppure soltanto la colonna mediale. Il risultato è un'elevazione dell'arco longitudinale (Fig. 673-6); spesso si sviluppa una deformità del retropiede per compensare l'anomalia primaria dell'avampiede. Anche se si può verificare un piede cavo familiare, la maggior parte dei pazienti con questa deformità avrà una causa neuromuscolare di base. L'obiettivo iniziale è di escludere (e trattare) qualsiasi causa sottostante. Queste diagnosi possono essere correlate ad anomalie del midollo spinale (disrafismo occulto, *tethered cord*, poliomielite, mielodisplasia) e dei nervi periferici (neuropatie motorie e sensoriali ereditarie come la malattia di Charcot-Marie-Tooth, la malattia di Dejerine-Sottas, la malattia di Refsum). Se un piede cavo unilaterale è più probabile sia associato a un'anomalia intraspinale occulta, l'anomalia bilaterale di solito suggerisce una malattia nervosa o muscolare sottostante. Il piede cavo si osserva comunemente in associazione a una deformità del retropiede. Nel piede cavovaro, la deformità più comune nei pazienti con una neuropatia motoria o sensoriale ereditaria, la perdita di forza e lo squilibrio muscolare progressivi si traducono nella flessione plantare del primo raggio/colonna mediale. Perché il piede appoggi a terra con tutta la pianta, il retropiede deve ruotare in varismo. Nel piede equinocavo il retropiede è in equino, mentre in quello calcaneocavo (di solito presente nella poliomielite o nella mielodisplasia) il retropiede è in calcaneus (eccessiva dorsiflessione).

TRATTAMENTO. Innanzitutto occorre identificare qualsiasi eziologia sottostante: solo così sarà possibile mettere a punto un trattamento specifico. In caso di deformità lievi, lo stretching della fascia plantare ed esercizi di rinforzo muscolare possono essere utili per rallentare la progressione. Talvolta per stabilizzare il piede e migliorare la deambulazione occorre applicare un'ortesi caviglia-piede. Il trattamento chirurgico è indicato per le deformità progressive o sintomatiche che non hanno risposto agli interventi conservativi. Nel caso di una condizione neuromuscolare progressiva, si osserva comunemente una recidiva della deformità e possono rendersi necessarie altre procedure per mantenere un piede plantigrado. Bisogna informare in modo dettagliato i genitori sul processo patologico e sui benefici attesi dall'intervento. Lo scopo della chirurgia è ripristinare il movimento e l'allineamento e migliorare l'equilibrio muscolare. Nelle deformità più lievi, può essere sufficiente il rilascio dei tessuti molli della fascia plantare, spesso associato a trasferimento tendineo. Nei pazienti con deformità ossea fissa dell'avampiede/piede intermedio e/o del retropiede, possono essere richieste una o più osteotomie per il riallineamento. Talvolta è necessaria una tripla artrodesi (calcaneo-cuboidea, astragalo-scafoidea e sottoastragalica) per le forme più severe (o per la recidiva delle deformità) nei pazienti più grandi.

673.8 • OSTEOCONDROSI/APOFISITE

Per quanto si tratti di un'evenienza rara, una necrosi avascolare idiopatica può essere osservata a livello dello scafoide tarsale (**malattia di Köhler**) oppure della 2ª o 3ª testa metatarsale (**infrazione di Freiberg**). Queste condizioni, generalmente autolimitate, danno luogo a dolore correlato all'attività che talvolta può essere disabilitante. Il trattamento, stabilito in base alla gravità dei sintomi, consiste comunemente nella limitazione dell'attività. Nei pazienti con malattia di Köhler, un gesso corto di gamba (6-8 settimane) è in grado di fornire un miglioramento significativo. I pazienti con infrazione di Freiberg possono trarre beneficio da un periodo in gesso e/o da calzature ortopediche come quelle con suola *rocker-bottom*, suola rigida o una barra metatarsale. Occasionalmente possono verificarsi alterazioni degenerative dopo il graduale processo di guarigione e un intervento chirurgico è necessario soltanto in un sottogruppo di pazienti. Le procedure comprendono uno sbrigliamento articolare, un innesto osseo, un'osteotomia di ridirezionamento o un'escissione subtotale o completa della testa metatarsale e una sostituzione articolare.

L'**apofisite**, ossia l'infiammazione a livello dell'inserzione di un gruppo muscolare da carico tensivo ripetitivo, è più comune nei periodi di rapida crescita. Questi stress risultano in microfratture a livello del sito di inserzione fibrocartilagineo, associate a infiammazione. L'apofisite calcaneare (**malattia di Sever**) è la causa più comune di tallonite nei bambini; il trattamento consiste in modifiche dell'attività, FANS, esercizi di stretching del tendine d'Achille e anche nell'adozione di solette per il tallone e di supporti per l'arco plantare. La **malattia di Iselin**, meno frequente, rappresenta un'apofisite della base del 5° metatarso (peroneo breve). Se i sintomi sono unilaterali o non si osserva alcuna risposta al trattamento, occorre eseguire uno studio radiografico.

673.9 • Ferite penetranti del piede

La maggior parte delle ferite penetranti del piede può essere trattata adeguatamente in Pronto Soccorso. Il **trattamento** consiste in un'accurata irrigazione e un richiamo di vaccino antitetanico, se necessario; molti medici raccomandano una terapia antibiotica. Per mezzo di tale approccio, la maggior parte dei casi guarirà senza complicanze. Un sottogruppo di casi può sviluppare una cellulite, per lo più causata da *Staphylococcus aureus*, che rende necessaria la somministrazione di antibiotici per via endovenosa, con o senza drenaggio chirurgico. Le infezioni profonde, peraltro infrequenti, possono essere associate ad artrite settica o osteomielite. I microrganismi più comuni sono *S. aureus* e *Pseudomonas*; il trattamento comprende un completo sbrigliamento chirurgico seguito da un breve (10-14 giorni) ciclo di antibiotici per via generale. Anche se le radiografie senza contrasto permettono di visualizzare qualsiasi frammento metallico, può essere necessaria l'ecografia per identificare gli oggetti in vetro o in legno. L'esplorazione e la rimozione dei corpi estranei non sono richieste di routine, ma possono essere necessarie se sono presenti sintomi, in caso di recidiva o se si sospetta un'infezione. Dolore e/o disturbi della deambulazione sono più probabili nel caso di oggetti situati in superficie, sotto la pianta del piede. Una situazione particolare è costituita da una ferita penetrante provocata da un chiodo attraverso una vecchia calzatura da ginnastica. In questo caso, poiché sussiste un rischio elevato di infezione da *Pseudomonas*, occorre procedere a un'irrigazione accurata e uno sbrigliamento in anestesia generale, seguiti da antibiotici sistemici per 10-14 giorni.

673.10 • Deformità delle dita del piede

ALLUCE VALGO GIOVANILE

L'alluce valgo giovanile, più comune nelle femmine, è tipicamente associato a lassità legamentosa familiare. È comune un'anamnesi familiare positiva. Nell'eziologia entrano in gioco vari fattori, i più importanti dei quali sono i fattori genetici, la lassità legamentosa, il piede piatto, l'uso di scarpe a punta con uno spazio ristretto per le dita e occasionamente la spasticità (paralisi cerebrale).

MANIFESTAZIONI CLINICHE. Sono presenti una sporgenza della 1ª articolazione metatarsofalangea e, spesso, un eritema da irritazione cronica. L'alluce è in valgo e in genere pronato; si nota un allargamento dell'avampiede. Si osserva comunemente anche un piede piatto, con o senza una contrattura associata del tendine d'Achille. Anche se l'aspetto estetico è forse la principale preoccupazione, i pazienti possono presentare dolore nell'area della 1ª articolazione metatarsofalangea e/o difficoltà a indossare le calzature.

VALUTAZIONE RADIOGRAFICA. Occorre eseguire radiografie anteroposteriori e laterali in carico del piede. Alla proiezione anteroposteriore, le misurazioni comunemente eseguite consistono nelle relazioni angolari tra il 1° e il 2° metatarso (angolo metatarsale, normale <10°) e tra il 1° metatarso e la falange prossimale (angolo dell'alluce valgo, normale <25°). Bisogna inoltre documentare l'orientamento della 1ª articolazione metatarsocuneiforme mediale. Alla radiografia laterale, il rapporto angolare tra astragalo e 1° metatarso facilita l'identificazione di un'interruzione a livello del piede intermedio, associata a piede piatto. Le radiografie sono più utili nella pianificazione chirurgica che per stabilire la diagnosi.

TRATTAMENTO. Il trattamento conservativo dell'alluce valgo dell'adolescente consiste principalmente nella modifica delle calzature, in modo che si adattino alla larghezza dell'avampiede. I pazienti devono evitare di indossare calzature con un scarso spazio per le dita (scarpe a punta) e/o con il tacco alto. Da evitare sono anche quelle a punta (con uno spazio per le dita ristretto) e/o con tacco alto. Talvolta si consigliano anche altri accorgimenti, come una tomaia morbida, una soletta per l'alluce varo o una soletta per il tallone. In presenza di un piede piatto, può essere utile un'ortesi per ripristinare l'arco longitudinale mediale. Si raccomandano esercizi di stretching per il trattamento delle contratture del tendine d'Achille. Rimane invece ancora da stabilire l'utilità dei tutori notturni. Il trattamento chirurgico è riservato ai pazienti con dolore persistente e debilitante nei quali un ciclo di terapia conservativa non si è dimostrato efficace. La chirurgia, oltre a non essere raccomandabile a scopi puramente estetici, viene di solito rimandata fino al raggiungimento della maturità scheletrica, per ridurre il rischio di recidive. Le radiografie sono essenziali durante la pianificazione preoperatoria per valutare sia l'entità della deformità (angolo dell'alluce valgo, angolo intermetatarsale, angolo articolare metatarsale distale) sia le caratteristiche associate come l'obliquità della 1ª articolazione metatarsocuneiforme mediale. Il trattamento chirurgico spesso consiste nel rilascio dei tessuti molli e/o in una procedura di riequilibrio a livello della 1ª articolazione metatarsofalangea, e in un'osteotomia singola o doppia del 1° metatarso per ridurre la larghezza del piede e riallineare le articolazioni lungo la colonna mediale dell'avampiede. Un'artrodesi della 1ª articolazione metatarsofalangea può essere indicata nei pazienti con spasticità, allo scopo di prevenire le recidive.

DITA CURVE

Un dito curvo è causato dalla contrattura del muscolo flessore lungo della dita, con flessione a livello dell'articolazione metatarsofalangea e delle articolazioni interfalangee associata a deviazione mediale del dito. Il dito si trova di solito sotto il suo vicino, e i più coinvolti sono il 4° e 5° dito. La deformità è raramente sintomatica e non richiede un trattamento attivo (stretching, tutore o bendaggi). La maggior parte dei casi migliora con il tempo e un sottogruppo si risolverà completamente. Nei rari casi con dolore cronico o irritazione cutanea, si può prendere in considerazione il rilascio del muscolo flessore lungo delle dita a livello dell'articolazione interfalangea distale.

ACCAVALLAMENTO DEL 5° DITO

Il dito mignolo varo congenito o 5° dito varo consiste in una dorsiflessione e adduzione del 5° dito, che si sovrappone caratteristicamente al 4°. È inoltre presente una deformità rotatoria del dito e l'unghia tende a essere rivolta verso l'esterno. Questa deformità è di solito bilaterale e può avere una base genetica. I sintomi sono frequenti e comprendono dolore del dorso del dito in seguito all'uso di calzature. Il trattamento conservativo non si è dimostrato efficace. Nei pazienti sintomatici sono state descritte diverse opzioni ricostruttive, che comportano tutte il rilascio della contrattura del tendine estensore a livello della capsula dell'articolazione metatarsofalangea (dorsale, dorsomediale o completa). Sono state eseguite una rimozione parziale della falange prossimale e la creazione di una sindattilia tra 4° e 5° dito in associazione al rilascio.

POLIDATTILIA

La polidattilia, la più comune deformità congenita, si osserva in circa 2/1000 nati vivi ed è bilaterale nel 50% dei casi. Può essere preassiale (alluce) o postassiale (5° dito) e occasionalmente è presente la duplicazione di una delle dita centrali. Anomalie associate si osservano nel 10% circa dei casi di polidattilia preassiale e nel 20% dei casi di polidattilia postassiale. Un terzo dei pazienti presenta anche polidattilia della mano. Le condizioni che possono essere associate comprendono la sindrome di Ellis-Van Creveld (displasia condroectodermica), il deficit longitudinale della tibia e la sindrome di Down. Il dito soprannumerario può essere rudimentale o ben formato; le radiografie senza contrasto del piede consentono la definizione dell'anatomia e la valutazione di tutte le anomalie ossee coesistenti. Il trattamento, indicato per motivi estetici e per permettere l'uso di calzature standard, consiste nella rimozione chirurgica del dita soprannumerario, procedura che viene eseguita di solito quando il paziente ha dai 9 ai 12 mesi di età. Le dita rudimentali possono essere asportate anche prima, ma non dovrebbero essere "strappate via".

SINDATTILIA

La sindattilia comprende l'unione delle dita tramite una plica, che può essere incompleta o completa (estesa alla punta delle dita), con la possibile confluenza delle unghie. Spesso l'anamnesi familiare è positiva; quelli più frequentemente interessati sono il 3° e il 4° dito. I sintomi sono estremamente rari e sono infrequenti le preoccupazioni estetiche. Il trattamento è necessario soltanto per un sottogruppo di pazienti che presentano una polidattilia associata (Fig. 673-7); in tali casi, si asporta il dito esterno e la cute in eccesso facilita il rivestimento della ferita chirurgica. Se la sindattilia non interessa il dito soprannumerario, questo può essere mantenuto sotto osservazione senza asportarlo. Nei pazienti con sindrome di Apert può essere osservata una sindattilia complessa.

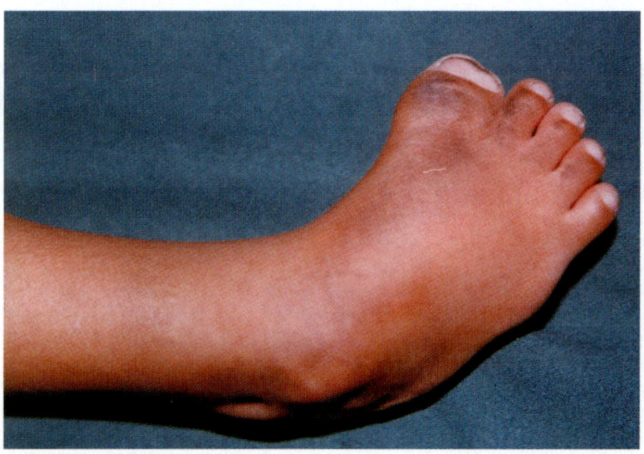

Figura 673-7. Quadro clinico di polisindattilia che interessa l'alluce.

DITO A MARTELLO

Un dito a martello consiste in una flessione dell'articolazione interfalangea prossimale, con o senza flessione dell'articolazione interfalangea distale; l'articolazione metatarsofalangea può essere iperestesa. Questa deformità si differenzia da un dito curvo per l'assenza di rotazione. È interessato più frequentemente il 2° dito, sul cui dorso può svilupparsi una callosità dolorosa, nel punto in cui sfrega contro la scarpa. La terapia conservativa è raramente efficace e per i casi sintomatici si raccomanda la chirurgia. Nella maggior parte dei casi sarà sufficiente il rilascio dei tendini flessori. Alcuni Autori hanno raccomandato un trasferimento del tendine flessore sull'estensore. Nei casi severi con rigidità significativa, specialmente nei pazienti più grandi, possono essere necessarie una resezione parziale o completa della falange prossimale e una fusione dell'articolazione interfalangea prossimale.

DITO A MAGLIO

Il dito a maglio consiste in una contrattura in flessione dell'articolazione interfalangea distale e deriva dall'accorciamento congenito del tendine del flessore lungo delle dita. I pazienti possono sviluppare una callosità dolorosa sulla superficie plantare dell'ultima falange. Dal momento che la terapia conservativa di solito non è efficace, è necessario l'intervento chirurgico per i pazienti con sintomi cronici. Per le deformità flessibili nei bambini piccoli, è raccomandato il rilascio del tendine del flessore lungo delle dita. Per le deformità rigide nei soggetti più grandi, si possono prendere in considerazione la resezione della testa della falange media o l'artrodesi dell'articolazione interfalangea distale.

DITO AD ARTIGLIO

La deformità del dito ad artiglio consiste nell'iperestensione a livello dell'articolazione metatarsofalangea e nella flessione delle articolazioni interfalangea prossimale e distale, spesso associata a sublussazione dorsale dell'articolazione metatarsofalangea. La maggior parte dei casi è associata a un disordine neurologico sottostante, come la malattia di Charcot-Marie-Tooth. L'eziologia deriva di solito dallo squilibrio muscolare dovuto al reclutamento dei tendini estensori per compensare la perdita di forza del muscolo tibiale anteriore. In caso di trattamento elettivo è necessaria la chirurgia. La procedura eseguita con maggiore frequenza è il trasferimento del tendine dell'estensore delle dita (o dell'alluce) sulla testa metatarsale, insieme alla capsulotomia dorsale dell'articolazione metatarsofalangea e alla fusione dell'articolazione interfalangea prossimale (articolazione interfalangea dell'alluce).

BANDE ANULARI

Bande di tessuto amniotico associate ad *amniotic disruption syndrome* (sequenza di rottura amniotica precoce, sindrome della banda di costrizione congenita, sindrome della banda anulare) possono intrecciarsi con le estremità causando uno spettro di problemi che vanno dall'amputazione in utero (Fig. 673-8) a un anello di costrizione lungo un dito (Fig. 673-9) (vedi Capitolo 108). Questi anelli, se abbastanza profondi, possono causare un'ostruzione del flusso arterioso o venoso. Anche se i problemi riguardanti la vitalità dei tessuti sono meno comuni, l'edema derivante da un ostruzione del ritorno venoso rappresenta spesso un disturbo di una certa entità. Il trattamento delle bande anulari di solito prevede l'osservazione; tuttavia, può essere necessario eseguire d'urgenza il rilascio circonferenziale della banda se il flusso arterioso è ostruito oppure può essere effettuato un trattamento elettivo per eliminare la congestione venosa.

MACRODATTILIA

La macrodattilia rappresenta un aumento delle dimensioni delle dita e può manifestarsi come problema isolato o in associazio-

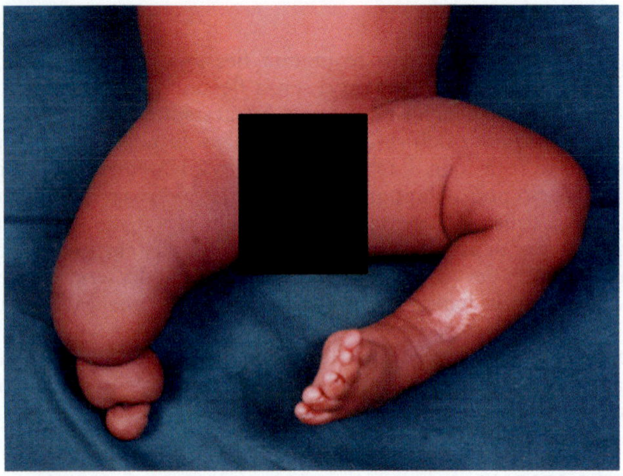

Figura 673-8. Sindrome della banda di costrizione e amputazione congenita.

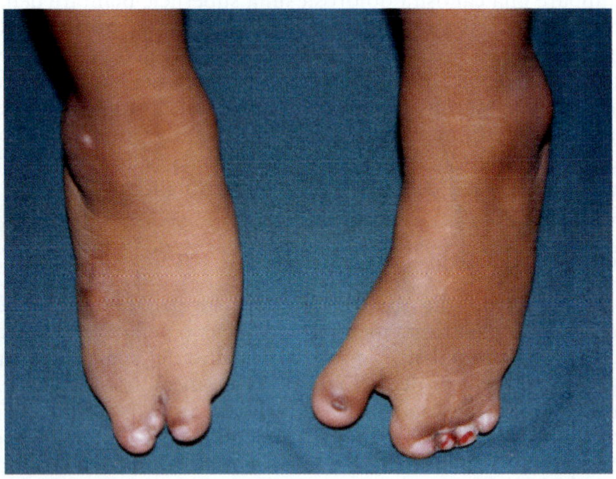

Figura 673-9. Sindrome della banda di costrizione con coinvolgimento dei piedi.

ne a diverse altre condizioni come la sindrome di Proteus (Fig. 673-10), la neurofibromatosi, la sclerosi tuberosa e la sindrome di Klippel-Trenaunay-Weber. Questa condizione deriva da una deregolazione dell'accrescimento ed è presente iperplasia di uno o più dei tessuti sottostanti (osseo, nervoso, linfatico, vascolare, fibroadiposo). La macrodattilia della dita del piede è osservabile in forma isolata (gigantismo localizzato) o associata a ingrandimento di tutto il piede. Oltre ai problemi estetici, i pazienti possono avere difficoltà a indossare calzature standard. Il trattamento consiste nell'osservazione, qualora possibile. Si tratta di un'anomalia difficile da trattare chirurgicamente, che spesso dà luogo a complicanze. Nell'interessamento di un singolo dito, l'opzione preferibile può essere una resezione del raggio (metatarso compreso). Se l'interessamento è di grado più esteso, è necessaria la riduzione di volume dei vari tessuti. Spesso si esegue un arresto della crescita delle strutture ossee sottostanti. Sono comuni rigidità e problemi della ferita chirurgica. Il tasso di recidive è elevato e può rendersi necessaria più di una riduzione di volume. I pazienti talvolta preferiscono un'amputazione, se il processo non è controllabile con procedure meno estese.

ESOSTOSI SUBUNGUEALE

Un'esostosi subungueale è una massa di tessuto osseo normale che si proietta dalla superficie dorsale e mediale di un dito, al di sotto dell'unghia. L'eziologia è sconosciuta, ma può essere

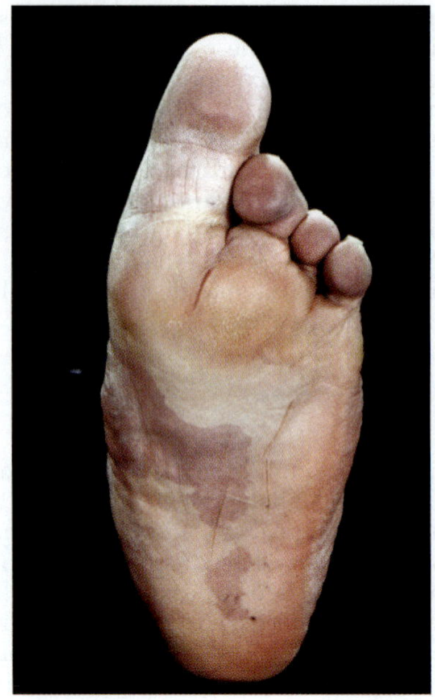

Figura 673-10. Macrodattilia dell'alluce in un caso di sindrome di Proteus.

correlata a traumi minori ripetuti. L'alluce è il dito più spesso interessato. I pazienti si presentano con dolore e l'unghia può essere sollevata. La lesione, dimostrabile con le radiografie senza contrasto e istologicamente, consiste in un tessuto osseo normale con un cappuccio fibrocartilagineo. Il trattamento delle lesioni sintomatiche è l'escissione e il tasso di recidiva è dell'ordine del 10%.

UNGHIA INCARNITA

L'unghia incarnita, relativamente comune nei lattanti e nei bambini piccoli, di solito interessa il margine mediale o laterale dell'alluce. I sintomi comprendono irritazione e dolore cronici e in alcuni casi si osservano infezioni ricorrenti. Se le misure conservative, tra cui modifiche delle calzature, impacchi caldi e un taglio appropriato dell'unghia, non controllano i sintomi, si deve valutare l'opportunità di rimuovere chirurgicamente una parte dell'unghia.

673.11 • PIEDE DOLOROSO

La diagnosi differenziale del piede doloroso in varie fasce d'età è mostrata nella Tabella 673-1. Oltre all'anamnesi e all'esame obiettivo, particolarmente utili a scopo diagnostico sono le ra-

TABELLA 673-1. Diagnosi differenziale del dolore del piede in base all'età

0-6 anni	6-12 anni	12-20 anni
Scarpe inadatte	Scarpe inadatte	Scarpe inadatte
Corpo estraneo	Malattia di Sever	Frattura da stress
Frattura	Enteropatia (artrite reumatoide giovanile)	Corpo estraneo
Osteomielite	Corpo estraneo	Unghia incarnita
Leucemia	Scafoide accessorio	Metatarsalgia
Ferita penetrante	Coalizione tarsale	Fascite plantare
Prelievo di sangue	Sarcoma di Ewing	Osteocondrosi (necrosi avascolare)
Dattilite	Piede piatto ipermobile	Freiberg
Artrite reumatoide giovanile	Trauma (distorsioni, fratture)	Köhler
	Ferita penetrante	Tendinite del tendine d'Achille
		Trauma (distorsioni)
		Verruche plantari
		Coalizione tarsale

diografie senza contrasto. Talvolta possono essere necessarie metodiche di imaging più sofisticate.

673.12 • Scarpe

Nei bambini di 1-2 anni e in quelli più grandi, è consigliabile una scarpa con suola flessibile. Questa raccomandazione è almeno in parte basata su studi da cui emerge che lo sviluppo dell'arco longitudinale sembra essere migliore nelle società dove non si fa uso di scarpe. Scarpe ben imbottite e in grado di assorbire le sollecitazioni sono utili nel bambino e nell'atleta adolescente allo scopo di ridurre le probabilità di sviluppare una sindrome da stress. Altrimenti, di solito si fa ricorso a calzature apposite solo dinanzi ad anomalie di allineamento dei segmenti del piede o se vi sono sintomi da una condizione sottostante. Sono disponibili numerosi tipi di calzature modificate.

Akcali O, Tiner M, Ozaksoy D: Effects of lower extremity rotation on prognoses of flexible flatfoot in children. *Foot Ankle Int* 2000;21:72–74.

Bhone WH: Tarsal coalition. *Curr Opin Pediatr* 2001;13:29–35.

Chang CH, Kumar SJ, Riddle EC, Glutting J: Macrodactyly of the foot. *J Bone Joint Surg Am* 2002;84:1189–1194.

Coughlin MJ: Lesser toe abnormalities. *Instr Course Lect* 2003;52:421–444.

Furdon SA, Donlon CR: Examination of the newborn foot: Positional and structural abnormalities. *Adv Neonatal Care* 2002:2:248–258.

Giannini BS, Ceccarelli F, Benedetti MG, et al: Surgical treatment of flexible flatfeet in children: A four-year follow-up study. *J Bone Joint Surg Am* 2001; 83:78–79.

Herzenberg JE, Radler C, Bor N: Ponseti versus traditional methods of casting for idiopathic clubfoot. *J Pediatr Orthop* 2002;22:517–521.

Ippolito E, Fraracci L, Farsetti P, et al: The influence of treatment on the pathology of clubfoot. CT study at maturity. *J Bone Joint Surg Br* 2004;86:574–580.

Lin CJ, Lai KA, Kuan TS, et al: Correlating factors and clinical significance of flexible flatfeet in preschool children. *J Pediatr Orthop* 2001;21:378–382.

Lincoln TL, Suen PW: Common rotational variations in children. *J Am Acad Orthop Surg* 2003;11:312–320.

Lokiec F, Ezra E, Krasin D, et al: A simple and efficient surgical technique for subungual exostosis. *J Pediatr Orthop* 2001;21:76–79.

Mazzocca AD, Thomson JD, Deluca PA, Romness MJ: Comparison of the posterior approach versus the dorsal approach in the treatment of congenital vertical talus. *J Pediatr Orthop* 2001;21:212–217.

Morcuende JA, Dolan LR, Dietz FR, Ponseti IV: Radical reduction in the rate of extensive corrective surgery for clubfeet using the Ponseti method. *Pediatrics* 2004;113:376–380.

Morley SE, Smith PJ: Polydactyly of the feet in children: Suggestions for surgical management. *Br J Plast Surg* 2001;54:34–38.

Noonan KJ, Richards BS: Nonsurgical management of idiopathic clubfoot. *J Am Acad Orthop Surg* 2003;11:392–402.

Roye DP Jr, Roye BD. Idiopathic congenital talipes equinovarus. *J Am Acad Orthop Surg* 2002;10:239–248.

Thometz J: Tarsal coalition. *Foot Ankle Clin* 2000;5:103–118.

Capitolo 674 ■ Deformità torsionali e angolari

Harish S. Hosalkar, Purushottam A. Gholve e Lawrence Wells

674.1 • Normale sviluppo degli arti

I pediatri valutano di routine i problemi di allineamento dell'arto inferiore e la morfologia del piede. La conoscenza del normale sviluppo degli arti è essenziale per riconoscere le condizioni patologiche. Durante la 7ª settimana di vita intrauterina, l'arto inferiore ruota medialmente per portare l'alluce verso la linea mediana. L'articolazione dell'anca si forma a partire dall'11ª settimana; il femore prossimale e l'acetabolo continuano a svilupparsi fino alla chiusura delle cartilagini di accrescimento, che avviene nell'adolescenza. Alla nascita il collo femorale è ruotato in avanti di 40°: questa rotazione prende il nome di antiversione (l'angolo tra l'asse del collo femorale e l'asse transcondiloideo). Insieme all'antiversione aumenta anche la rotazione interna dell'anca. L'antiversione femorale si riduce a 15-20° dagli 8-10 anni di età. La seconda causa di rotazione dell'arto inferiore si trova a livello tibiale. I lattanti possono avere 30° di rotazione mediale della tibia, e a partire dalla maturità la rotazione avviene tra 5° di rotazione mediale e 15° di rotazione laterale (Fig. 674-1). Un'eccessiva rotazione mediale della tibia viene definita torsione tibiale mediale. La torsione mediale è la differenza angolare tra l'asse del ginocchio e l'asse transmalleolare. Una rotazione mediale o laterale oltre ±2 deviazioni standard (DS) dalla media è considerata anormale e quindi rappresenta una deformità.

Una rotazione dell'arto è osservabile anche a livello del piede. Le anomalie possono consistere in un'adduzione o un'abduzione eccessive. Nel corso della crescita scheletrica è presente una rotazione laterale sia nel segmento femorale sia nel segmento tibiale; pertanto, la torsione tibiale mediale e l'antiversione femorale nei bambini migliorano con il tempo. La torsione tibiale laterale di solito peggiora con la crescita. La deformità torsionale può essere semplice, se interessa un unico segmento, oppure complessa, se ne coinvolge diversi. Le deformità complesse possono essere aggiuntive (per es. torsione tibiale interna e torsione femorale interna) o compensatorie (per es. torsione tibiale esterna e torsione femorale interna).

Il normale angolo tibiofemorale alla nascita presenta 10-15° di varismo fisiologico. L'allineamento raggiunge gli 0° verso i 18 mesi e tra i 3 e i 4 anni di età si raggiunge un valgismo fisiologico fino a 12° (Fig. 674-2). La persistenza del varismo oltre i 2 anni di età può essere patologica. In generale, il 95% dei casi di varismo e valgismo fisiologici del ginocchio tipici dell'età evolutiva si risolvono con la crescita; ciò è vero anche per i bambini con varismo o valgismo fisiologici più pronunciati, nonostante alcuni casi possano non correggersi completamente fino all'adolescenza.

674.2 • Valutazione

L'anamnesi deve essere focalizzata su esordio, progressione, limitazioni funzionali, precedenti trattamenti, evidenza di disordini neuromuscolari e qualsiasi dettaglio anamnestico familiare significativo. Un'anamnesi dettagliata è importante per giungere a una diagnosi.

L'esame obiettivo consiste nella determinazione dell'esatto profilo torsionale ed è utile nella diagnosi del livello e della severità di qualsiasi problema torsionale. Questo profilo comprende: (1) angolo di progressione del piede, (2) antiversione femorale, (3) versione tibiale con angolo coscia-piede e (4) valutazione dell'adduzione e dell'abduzione del piede.

ANGOLO DI PROGRESSIONE DEL PIEDE

La posizione dell'arto nel corso della deambulazione è espressa come angolo di progressione del piede (FPA, *Foot Progression Angle*), ossia come differenza angolare tra l'asse del piede e la direzione in cui il bambino sta camminando. L'FPA rappresenta la somma delle rotazioni di femore, tibia e piede; per misurarlo di solito si chiede al bambino di camminare nel corridoio dell'ambulatorio (Fig. 674-3). Alla rotazione verso l'interno del piede viene assegnato un valore negativo, a quella verso l'esterno un valore positivo. L'FPA normale nei bambini e negli adolescenti è di 10° (range 13-20°). L'FPA serve soltanto a stabilire se il soggetto presenta una deambulazione a punte intraruotate o extraruotate.

ANTIVERSIONE FEMORALE

La misurazione della rotazione dell'anca con il bambino in posizione prona, l'anca in flessione o estensione neutrale, le cosce

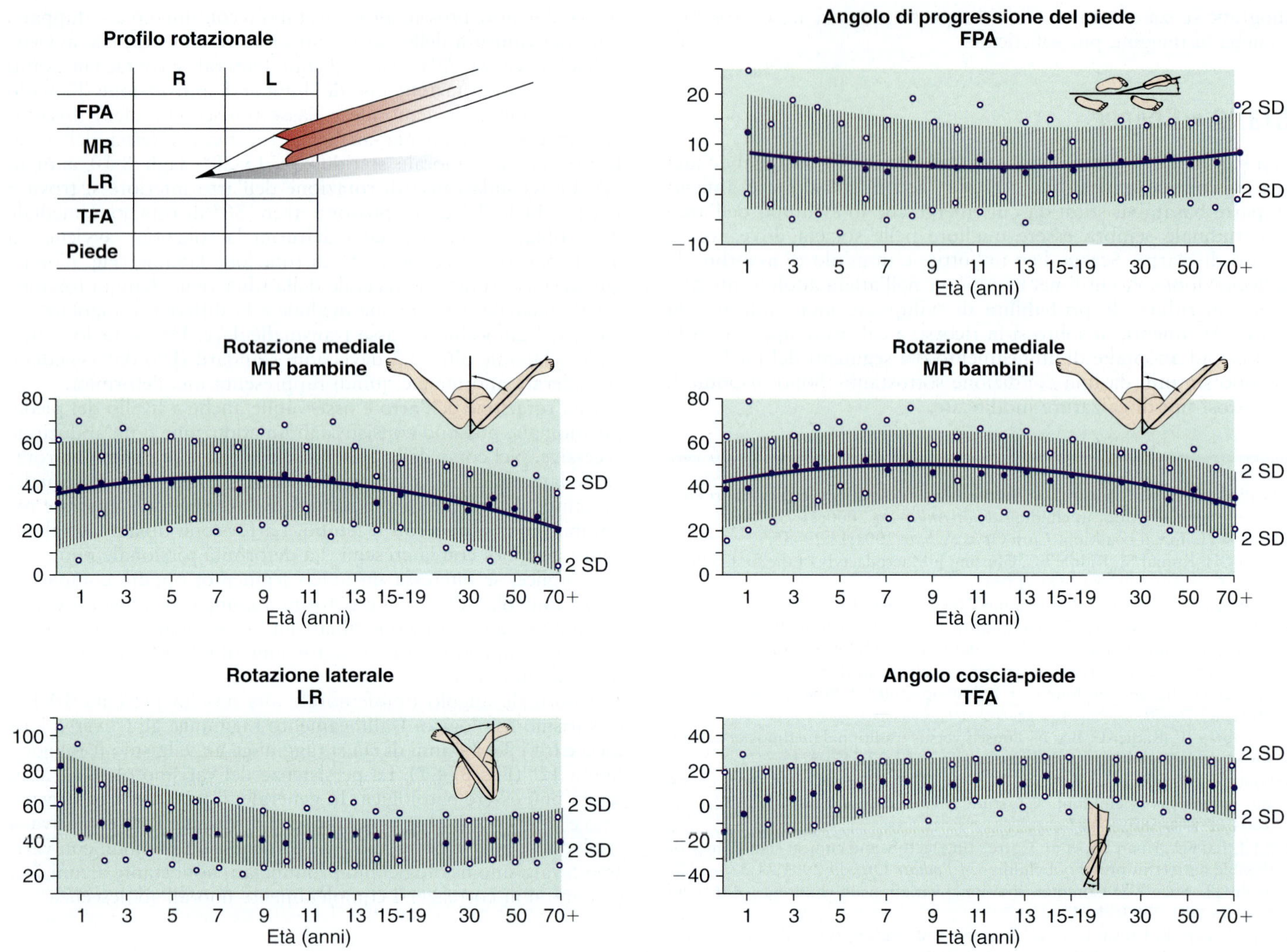

Figura 674-1. Grafico del profilo rotazionale dalla nascita alla maturità. Tutti i grafici comprendono 2 deviazioni standard dalla media per l'angolo di progressione del piede (FPA, *Foot Progression Angle*), per la rotazione femorale mediale e laterale (maschi e femmine) e per l'angolo coscia-piede (TFA, *Thigh-Foot Angle*). MR (*Medial Rotation*), rotazione mediale; R (*Right*), destra; L (*Left*), sinistra. (Da Morrissey RT, Weinstein SL [ed]: *Lovell and Winter's Pediatric Orthopaedics*, 3rd ed. Philadelphia, Lippincott Williams & Wilkins, 1990.)

unite e le ginocchia flesse a 90° permette la valutazione indiretta dell'antiversione (Fig. 674-4). Vengono esaminate entrambe le anche allo stesso tempo. Con la rotazione ipsilaterale della gamba si produce una rotazione interna dell'anca, mentre la rotazione controlaterale dà luogo a una rotazione esterna. Un'eccessiva antiversione aumenta la rotazione interna e, viceversa, la retroversione aumenta la rotazione esterna.

ROTAZIONE TIBIALE

La rotazione tibiale si misura mediante l'angolo transmalleolare (TMA, *TransMalleolar Angle*). Il TMA è l'angolo tra l'asse longitudinale della coscia e una linea perpendicolare all'asse del malleolo mediale e laterale (Fig. 674-5). In assenza di deformità del piede, si preferisce l'angolo coscia-piede (TFA, *Thigh Foot Angle*) (Fig. 674-6), che si misura con il bambino in posizione prona ed è compreso tra l'asse longitudinale della coscia e l'asse longitudinale del piede. Esso serve per determinare lo stato rotazionale della tibia e del retropiede. Alla rotazione interna si assegna un valore negativo, a quella esterna un valore positivo. La rotazione interna indica una torsione tibiale interna, mentre la rotazione esterna rappresenta una torsione tibiale esterna. I lattanti hanno un angolo medio di −15° (range da −35 a 40°) in conseguenza della normale posizione in utero. Dalla seconda infanzia fino alla vita adulta, il TFA medio è di 10° (range da −15 a 30°). La differenza tra TMA e TFA è una misura della rotazione del retropiede.

FORMA E POSIZIONE DEL PIEDE

Il piede deve essere osservato in posizione prona ed eretta, qualunque sia la deformità ricercata. Si utilizza la linea bisettrice del tallone (HBL, *Heel Bisector Line*) per valutare le deformità in adduzione e in abduzione del piede. L'HBL è una linea che divide il tallone in due metà uguali lungo l'asse longitudinale (Fig. 674-7). Normalmente si estende fino al 2° dito. Quando l'HBL è mediale rispetto al 2° dito l'avampiede è abdotto, mentre quando è laterale al 2° dito l'avampiede è addotto.

È inoltre importante valutare ogni bambino affetto per l'associazione con displasia dell'anca e con problemi neuromuscolari (paralisi cerebrale).

674.3 • DEFORMITÀ TORSIONALI

TORSIONE FEMORALE INTERNA

Un'eccessiva antiversione femorale è la deformità che più comunemente si presenta come **deambulazione con intrarotazione**

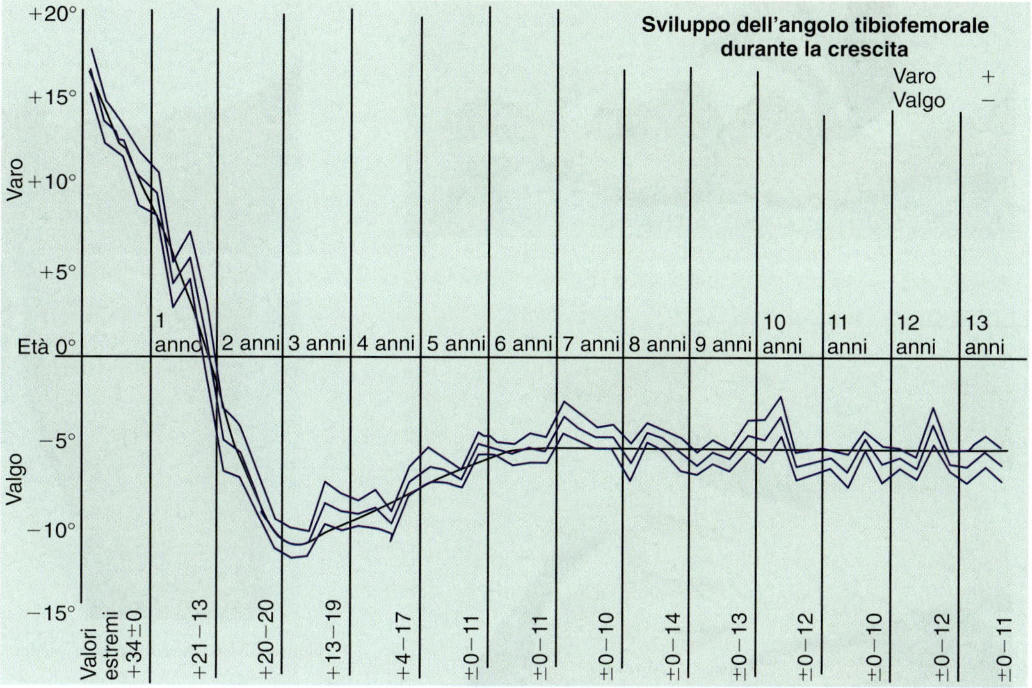

Figura 674-2. Normale allineamento coronale in base all'età. (Da Salenius P, Vanka E: The development of the tibiofemoral angle in children. *J Bone Joint Surg Am* 1975;57:259-261.)

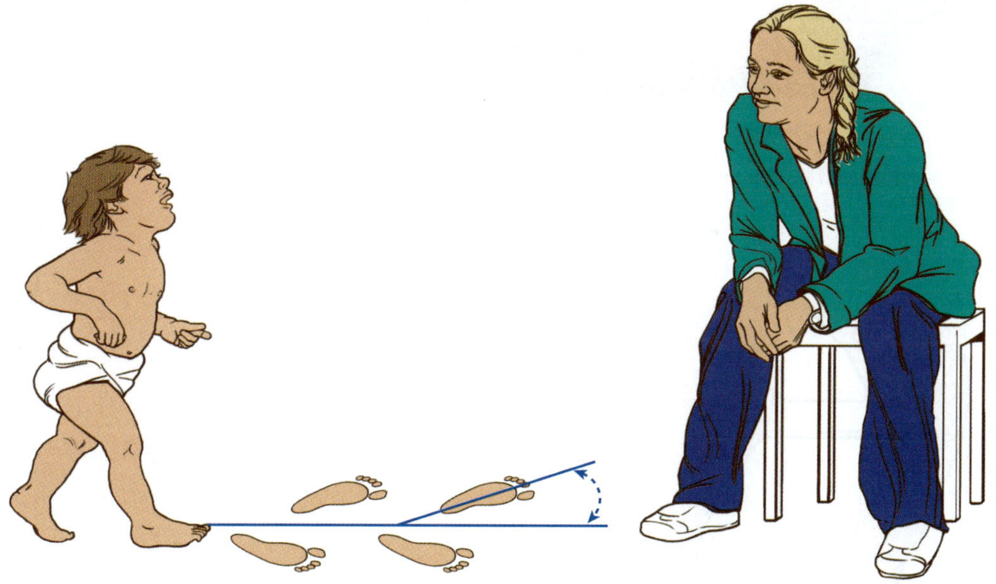

Figura 674-3. Angolo di progressione del piede. L'asse lungo del piede viene confrontato con la direzione in cui il bambino sta camminando: se l'asse lungo del piede è diretto all'esterno, l'angolo è positivo; se il piede è diretto all'interno, l'angolo è negativo ed è indicativo di cammino a punte intraruotate. (Da Thompson GH: Gait disturbances. In Kliegman RM [ed]: *Practical Strategies in Pediatric Diagnosis and Therapy*. Philadelphia, Elsevier/Saunders, 2004.)

delle punte. Si verifica più spesso nelle femmine che nei maschi (2:1), nella fascia di età da 3 a 6 anni. L'eziologia della torsione femorale è una questione controversa. Alcuni la considerano congenita e ritengono derivi da un'antiversione femorale infantile persistente, mentre altri sono del parere che venga acquisita secondariamente a una posizione seduta viziata. Alcuni bambini hanno l'abitudine di sedere in posizione a W o di dormire proni. All'esame obiettivo, la maggior parte dei bambini con questa condizione presenta una lassità legamentosa generalizzata. L'esame del cammino rivela una rotazione interna di tutto l'arto inferiore. La rotazione interna dell'anca supera i 70° e di conseguenza la rotazione esterna è limitata a 10-20°. Le rotule sono rivolte all'interno quando il piede è diritto ed è presente una rotazione esterna compensatoria della tibia.

La diagnosi è clinica e viene posta in base all'esame obiettivo; la TC permette di effettuare misurazioni obiettive, che però sono indicate raramente. Il trattamento consiste per lo più nell'osservazione e nella correzione della posizione seduta anormale: tale correzione può essere difficile da ottenere nei bambini in età prescolare e di solito non si verifica prima dell'età scolare. La torsione di solito si corregge con la crescita entro gli 8-10 anni di età. Alcune indicazioni all'intervento operatorio sono una deformità persistente, un aspetto estetico inaccettabile, un deficit funzionale, un'antiversione >45° e l'assenza di rotazione esterna oltre la posizione neutra. L'intervento chirurgico consiste in un'osteotomia di derotazione del femore.

TORSIONE TIBIALE INTERNA

La torsione tibiale mediale si presenta con **deambulazione con intrarotazione delle punte** ed è comunemente associata a metatarso varo congenito, ginocchio valgo o antiversione femorale. Questa condizione si osserva di solito nel corso del 2° anno di vita. Alla nascita, il malleolo mediale si trova normalmente dietro il malleolo laterale, ma a partire dall'età adulta si inverte con la tibia a 15° di rotazione esterna. Clinicamente, questi pazienti

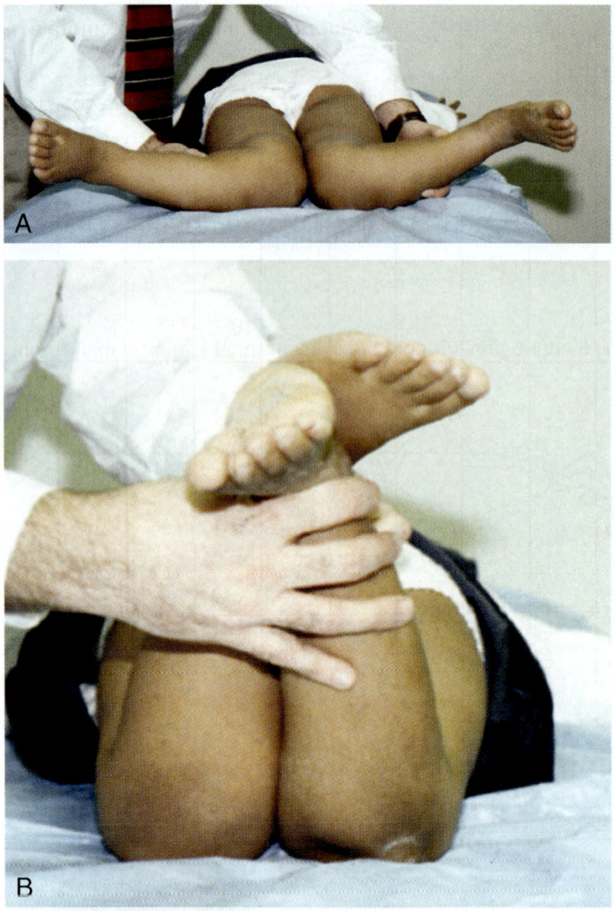

Figura 674-4. Antiversione misurata mediante rotazione mediale (*A*) e laterale dell'anca (*B*).

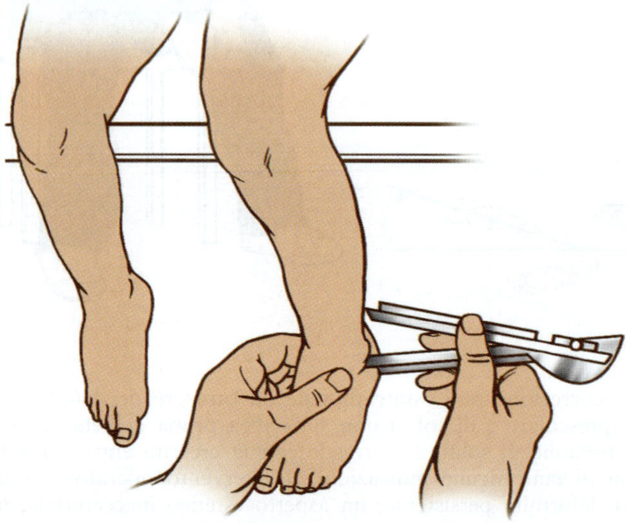

Figura 674-5. L'angolo transmalleolare viene misurato con il paziente seduto sul bordo del tavolo, i condili femorali allineati con il lato del tavolo. L'angolo tra una linea tracciata tra i malleoli mediale e laterale e il margine del tavolo deve essere esterno di 30° circa. (Da Bleck EE: *Orthopaedic Management in Cerebral Palsy*. London, MacKeith Press, 1987, p. 55.)

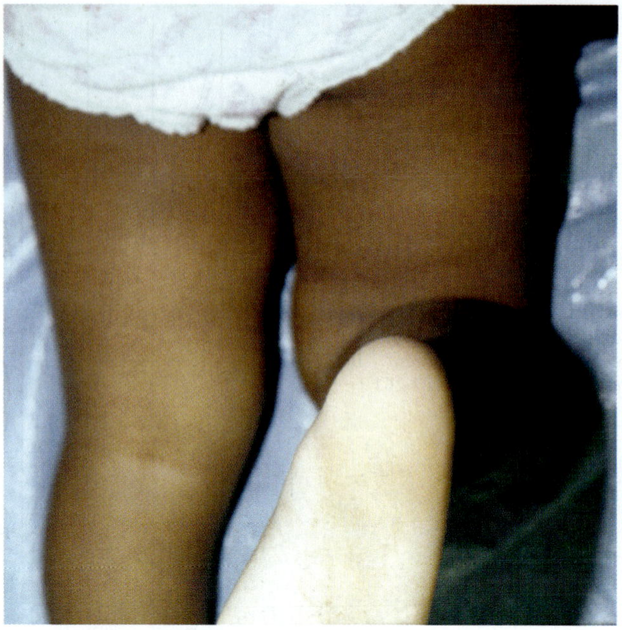

Figura 674-6. Angolo coscia-piede.

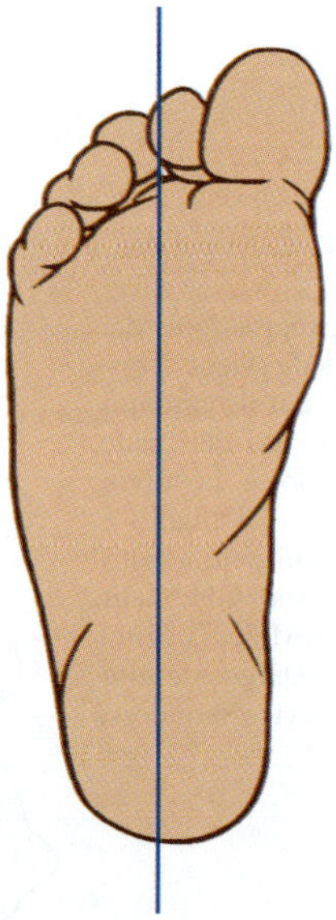

Figura 674-7. Dimostrazione schematica della linea bisettrice del tallone.

presentano una riduzione di TFA e TMA. Il trattamento consiste essenzialmente nell'osservazione e nella rassicurazione, perché si prevede una risoluzione spontanea nel corso di una crescita e uno sviluppo normali. Un miglioramento significativo di solito non si verifica prima che il bambino inizi a stare in piedi da solo e a camminare senza aiuto. In seguito si può osservare una correzione anche a 4 anni di età e in alcuni bambini entro gli 8-10 anni di età. Oltre all'osservazione, è stato tentato l'uso di ortesi per torsioni >40°. La deformità persistente con deficit funzionale viene trattata con un'osteotomia sovramalleolare.

TORSIONE FEMORALE ESTERNA

La torsione femorale esterna può far seguito a un'epifisiolisi della testa femorale (SCFE, *Slipped Capital Femoral Epiphysis*); la soglia per l'esecuzione di radiografie delle anche in bambini con più di 10 anni è bassa. La retrotorsione femorale, se di origine idiopatica, è di solito bilaterale. Il disordine è associato a una **deambulazione con extrarotazione delle punte** e a un aumento dell'incidenza di artrosi degenerativa. L'esame obiettivo evidenzia un'eccessiva rotazione esterna dell'anca e una limitazione della rotazione interna. L'anca ruota esternamente fino a 70-90°, mentre la rotazione interna è soltanto di 0-20°. Se viene identificata una SCFE, il trattamento è chirurgico e qualsiasi retroversione femorale prossimale migliora con il rimodellamento nel corso della crescita successiva. Occasionalmente, una retroversione femorale persistente successiva a una SCFE può produrre un deficit funzionale come una deambulazione con extrarotazione severa delle punte e una difficoltà all'opposizione delle ginocchia in posizione seduta. Quest'ultimo problema può essere disabilitante nelle ragazze durante la pubertà; in tal caso, potrebbe essere necessaria un'osteotomia di derotazione.

TORSIONE TIBIALE ESTERNA

La torsione tibiale laterale, meno comune della rotazione mediale, è spesso associata a un piede calcaneovalgo. Può essere compensatoria rispetto a un'antiversione femorale persistente, idiopatica o secondaria a una tensione della banda iliotibiale. Poiché durante la crescita naturale si verifica una rotazione della tibia verso l'esterno, questa deformità può peggiorare con il tempo. Clinicamente, la rotula è rivolta esternamente quando il piede è diritto. TFA e TMA sono aumentati. Vi può essere un'instabilità femororotulea associata con dolore del ginocchio. Anche se si può verificare un certo grado di correzione con la crescita, i bambini estremamente sintomatici necessitano di un'osteotomia sovramalleolare, che di solito viene eseguita entro i 10-12 anni di età.

ADDUZIONE DEL METATARSO

Questa deformità si presenta con adduzione dell'avampiede e inversione di tutti i metatarsi. Dal 10 al 15% dei casi è associato a displasia dell'anca. La prognosi è buona e la maggior parte dei pazienti migliora con l'intervento conservativo. Per valutare il grado della deformità si utilizza l'HBL. I piedi, che sono flessibili e correggibili fino alla posizione neutra, vengono trattati con esercizi di stretching. Per i casi non completamente correggibili si fa ricorso a gessi seriati. Le deformità rigide, non essendo correggibili con lo stretching, sono trattate con una capsulotomia mediale della 1ª articolazione metatarsocuneiforme e con il rilascio dei tessuti molli entro i 2 anni di età. Le osteotomie della base del metatarso vengono di solito eseguite dopo i 6 anni di età (vedi Capitolo 673.1).

674.4 • DEFORMITÀ SUL PIANO CORONALE

Varismo e valgismo sono comuni deformità pediatriche del ginocchio. I valori normali per l'età dell'angolo del ginocchio sono presentati nella Figura 674-2. La curvatura della tibia è comune nel corso del 1° anno, il varismo del ginocchio è frequente nel 2° anno e il valgismo del ginocchio è più evidente tra i 3 e i 4 anni di età.

GINOCCHIO VARO

Il ginocchio varo fisiologico è una comune associazione torsionale secondaria alla posizione in utero. Con una crescita e uno sviluppo normali ci si attende una risoluzione spontanea. La persistenza del varismo oltre i 2 anni di età può essere patologica. Le diverse cause sono una malattia del metabolismo osseo (deficit di vitamina D, rachitismo, ipofosfatasia), arresto asimmetrico della crescita (trauma, infezione, tumore, malattia di Blount), displasia ossea (nanismo, displasia metafisaria) e disordini congeniti e neuromuscolari (Tab. 674-1). Per prudenza, occorre differenziare il varismo fisiologico dalla malattia di Blount (Tab. 674-2), oltre che dal rachitismo e dalla displasia scheletrica. Nel rachitismo sono presenti le classiche alterazioni ossee con allargamento e aspetto "liso" della metafisi e allargamento della cartilagine di accrescimento (vedi Capitolo 48).

TABELLA 674-1. Classificazione del ginocchio valgo

FISIOLOGICO
CRESCITA ASIMMETRICA
Tibia vara (malattia di Blount)
Infantile
Giovanile
Dell'adolescente
Displasia fibrocartilaginea focale
Lesione della cartilagine di accrescimento
Trauma
Infezione
Tumore
DISORDINI METABOLICI
Deficit di vitamina D (rachitismo nutrizionale)
Rachitismo vitamina D-resistente
Ipofosfatasia
DISPLASIA SCHELETRICA
Displasia metafisaria
Acondroplasia
Encondromatosi

Modificata da Thompson GH: Angular deformities of the lower extremities. In Chapman MW (ed): *Operative Orthopedics*, 2nd ed. Philadelphia, JB Lippincott, 1993, pp. 3131-3164.

TABELLA 674-2. Diagnosi differenziale del ginocchio varo

Varismo fisiologico	Malattia di Blount
Deformità ampia e simmetrica	Angolazione asimmetrica, discontinua e "acuta"
Angolo tra metafisi e diafisi <11°	Angolo tra metafisi e diafisi >11°
Aspetto normale della cartilagine di accrescimento tibiale prossimale	Inclinazione mediale dell'epifisi
	Allargamento della cartilagine di accrescimento
	Frammentazione della metafisi
Assenza di spostamento laterale significativo	Spostamento laterale significativo

TIBIA VARA

La tibia vara idiopatica o **malattia di Blount** è un'anomalia della crescita dell'aspetto mediale dell'epifisi tibiale prossimale, che porta ad angolazione in varo e a rotazione mediale della tibia (Fig. 674-8). L'incidenza è maggiore nelle bambine obese di razza nera che hanno un membro della famiglia affetto, che hanno iniziato a camminare presto o che risiedono in certe aree geografiche come la parte sudorientale degli Stati Uniti. È stata classificata in tre tipi a seconda dell'età di esordio: infantile (1-3 anni), giovanile (4-10 anni) e dell'adolescente (11 anni o più). Le forme giovanile e dell'adolescente sono comunemente associate a tibia vara a esordio tardivo. Anche se la sua causa esatta rimane sconosciuta, la tibia vara può essere secondaria alla soppressione della crescita dovuta a un eccesso di forze compressive attraverso l'aspetto mediale del ginocchio.

La forma infantile è la più comune; le sue caratteristiche comprendono la predominanza nelle donne nere, l'interessamento bilaterale nell'80% circa dei casi, la presenza di una sporgenza metafisaria mediale, la torsione tibiale interna e una differenza di lunghezza tra gli arti inferiori (LLD, *Leg-Lenght Discrepancy*). Le caratteristiche delle forme giovanili e dell'adolescente (esordio tardivo) comprendono la predominanza nei maschi neri, di altezza normale o superiore al normale, l'interessamento bilaterale nel 50% circa dei casi, una deformità in varismo del ginocchio lentamente progressiva, il dolore come disturbo primario iniziale più che la deformità in sé, l'assenza di una sporgenza metafisaria mediale prossimale palpabile, una torsione tibiale interna minima, una lieve lassità del legamento collaterale mediale e una LLD lieve. Il gruppo infantile ha la maggiore probabilità di andare incontro a una progressione.

Occorre eseguire una radiografia anteroposteriore in posizione eretta di entrambe le estremità inferiori con le rotule in avanti e una radiografia laterale dell'estremità interessata (Fig. 674-9).

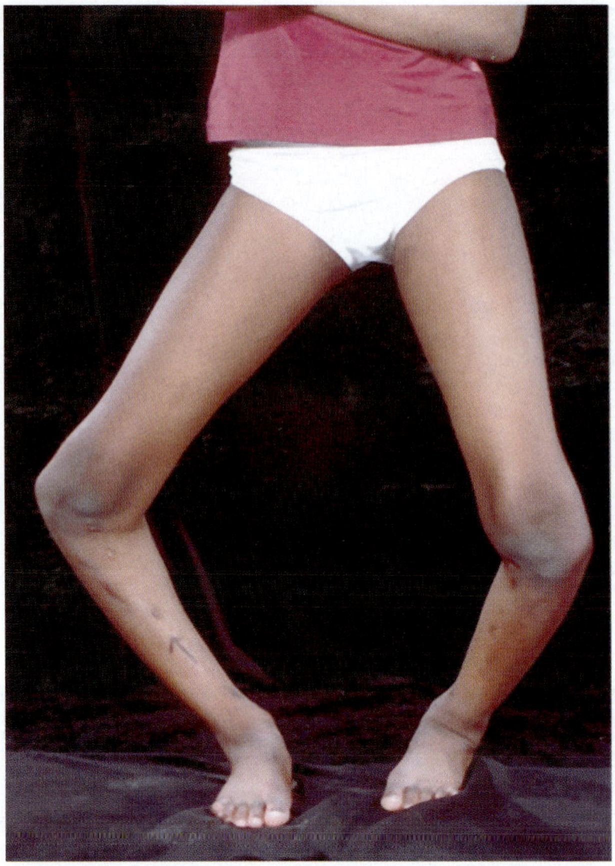

Figura 674-8. Varismo di entrambe le ginocchia nella malattia di Blount infantile.

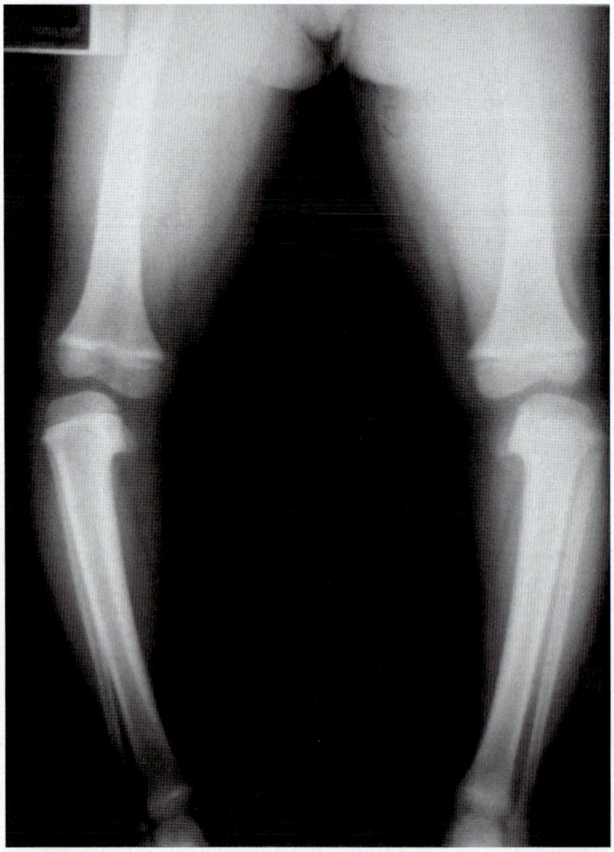

Figura 674-9. Radiografia anteroposteriore di entrambe le ginocchia nella malattia di Blount.

Sono preferibili le radiografie sotto carico in quanto permettono una presentazione prossimale della deformità clinica. Si può misurare l'angolo tra metafisi e diafisi, utile per distinguere il varismo del ginocchio fisiologico dal varismo tibiale precoce (Fig. 674-10). Langenskiöld ha sviluppato una classificazione in 6 stadi in base all'aspetto radiografico (Fig. 674-11): i fattori da considerare sono la presenza di frammentazione epifisaria, la sporgenza (*beaking*) dell'epifisi tibiale mediale, la depressione del piatto tibiale mediale e la formazione di una barra ossea. Talvolta possono essere necessarie un'artrografia, una TC con ricostruzione tridimensionale o una RM per valutare il menisco, la superficie articolare della tibia prossimale, compresa l'inclinazione posteromediale, o l'integrità della cartilagine di accrescimento tibiale prossimale.

Il **trattamento** varia in base allo stadio della malattia, all'età del bambino e al tipo di presentazione (deformità primitiva o ricorrente). Nei bambini di età <3 anni con stadio di Langenskiöld <3, l'uso di un'ortesi è efficace e può prevenire la progressione nel 50% dei casi. È raccomandato un trial massimale di 1 anno di trattamento ortotico. Se non si ottiene la correzione completa dopo 1 anno o se si verifica una progressione in questo periodo di tempo, può essere indicata un'osteotomia correttiva. Le altre indicazioni al trattamento chirurgico sono i bambini con più di 4 anni di età, uno stadio di Langenskiöld >3 e la presenza di deformità severe. La procedura di scelta di solito è l'osteotomia in valgo tibiale prossimale con un'osteotomia diafisaria peroneale associata. Nella tibia vara a esordio tardivo, la correzione è necessaria anche per ripristinare l'asse meccanico del ginocchio. Anche l'elevazione dell'emipiatto tibiale con la correzione dell'inclinazione posteromediale rappresenta una modalità di trattamento, in caso di recidiva.

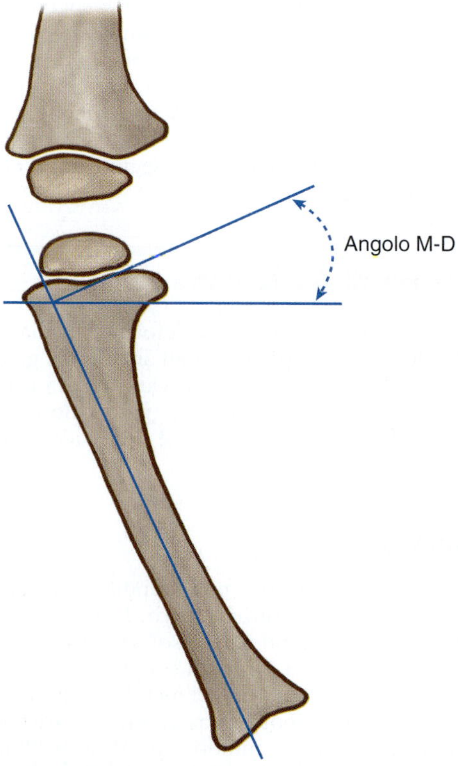

Figura 674-10. Angolo tra metafisi e diafisi (M-D). Tracciare una linea sulla radiografia attraverso la cartilagine di accrescimento tibiale prossimale; tracciarne quindi un'altra lungo la corticale tibiale laterale. Infine, tracciare una linea perpendicolare alla linea che decorre lungo la diafisi, come indicato dal diagramma. (Da Morrissey RT, Weinstein SL [ed]: *Lovell and Winter's Pediatric Orthopedics*, 3rd ed. Philadelphia, Lippincott Williams & Wilkins, 1990.)

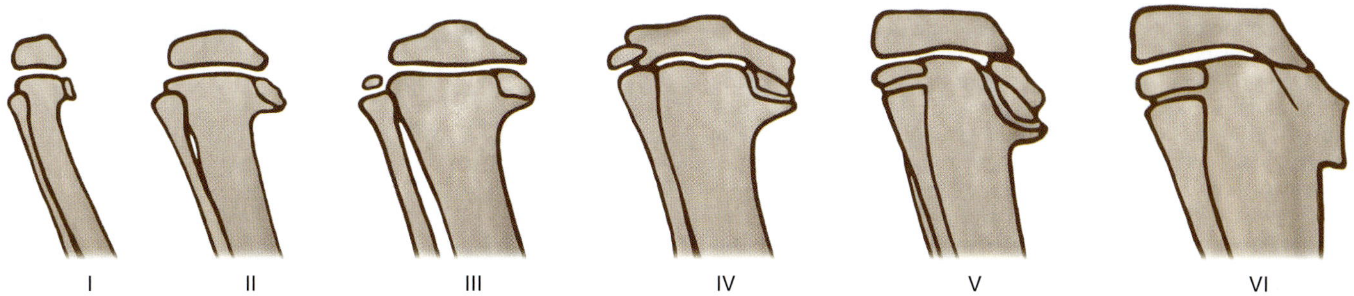

Figura 674-11. Stadi della malattia di Blount infantile. (Da Langeskiöld A: Tibia vara (osteochondrosis deformans tibiae): A survey of 23 cases. *Acta Chir Scand* 1952;103:1.)

GINOCCHIO VALGO

Un valgismo normale viene raggiunto entro i 4 anni di età. Poiché sono possibili variazioni fino a 15° entro i 6 anni, fino a quest'età il valgismo fisiologico ha una buona probabilità di correzione. La distanza intermalleolare con il ginocchio approssimato è normalmente di 2 cm, mentre nella deformità in valgo severa può raggiungere i 10 cm. Le condizioni patologiche che portano al valgismo sono le malattie del metabolismo osseo (rachitismo, osteodistrofia renale), la displasia scheletrica, l'arresto post-traumatico della cartilagine di coniugazione, i tumori e le infezioni. L'aumento del valgismo a livello del ginocchio provoca una deviazione laterale dell'asse meccanico con stretching dell'aspetto mediale del ginocchio che causa dolore. Le deformità >15° verificatesi dopo i 6 anni di età è improbabile si correggano con la crescita e richiedono quindi un trattamento chirurgico. Nel soggetto con immaturità scheletrica, si tenta la correzione tramite emiepifisiodesi epifisaria tibiale mediale. Nel soggetto scheletricamente maturo è necessaria un'osteotomia al centro della rotazione o dell'angolazione, situato di solito a livello del femore distale. Per la pianificazione preoperatoria in genere sono necessarie radiografie in anteroposteriore sotto carico di tutto l'arto inferiore.

674.5 • DEFORMITÀ CONGENITE ANGOLARI DELLA TIBIA E DEL PERONE

CURVATURA TIBIALE POSTEROMEDIALE

La causa della curvatura tibiale posteromediale congenita è sconosciuta. Di solito si associa a piede calcaneovalgo, raramente a valgismo secondario della tibia. Questa curvatura ha un buon potenziale di correzione con la crescita e quindi non richiede alcun intervento precoce. Tuttavia, nonostante la correzione dell'angolazione, permane un accorciamento residuo della tibia e del perone. L'inibizione media della crescita è del 12-13% (range 5-27%). La differenza di lunghezza degli arti inferiori alla maturità è in media di 4 cm (range 3-7 cm). La diagnosi di curvatura è confermata dalle radiografie, che mostrano l'angolatura posteromediale senza altre anomalie ossee. La deformità in calcaneovalgo del piede migliora con lo stretching o con una calzatura ortopedica e occasionalmente con un'ortesi caviglia-piede. Una differenza degli arti inferiori predetta <4 cm viene trattata con un'epifisiodesi della gamba normale appropriata per l'età; se invece tale discrepanza è >4 cm si utilizza un'associazione di epifisiodesi controlaterale e allungamento ipsilaterale. Per il valgismo distale può rendersi necessaria un'osteotomia correttiva, da eseguirsi nello stesso tempo della correzione della LLD.

CURVATURA TIBIALE ANTEROMEDIALE (EMIMELIA POSTASSIALE)

L'**emimelia peroneale** è la causa più comune di curvatura anteromediale della tibia. Il deficit peroneale può presentarsi con un'assenza completa del perone o con uno sviluppo parziale a livello sia prossimale sia distale. È associata a deformità di femore, ginocchio, tibia, caviglia e piede. Il femore è corto e presenta un'ipoplasia condilare laterale che causa un'instabilità rotulea e una deformità in valgismo del ginocchio. La tibia presenta una curvatura anteromediale con riduzione del potenziale di crescita. Gli obiettivi principali del trattamento sono la stabilizzazione della caviglia e la correzione delle deformità del piede. La caviglia assomiglia a un'articolazione a tipo enartrosi con instabilità laterale. Le deformità del piede sono caratterizzate dall'assenza delle dita laterali, piede equino-cavo-varo e coalizione tarsale.

Sono state descritte diverse opzioni chirurgiche; il trattamento viene scelto in base alle esigenze dell'individuo e alle preferenze dei genitori. Il modo migliore per trattare un piede con deformità severa potrebbe essere un'amputazione di Syme o di Boyd, con protesi applicata già a un anno di vita. Nel piede che può essere conservato, la LLD viene trattata con un'epifisiodesi dell'arto controlaterale o con un allungamento dell'arto ipsilaterale.

CURVATURA TIBIALE ANTEROLATERALE

La curvatura tibiale anterolaterale è associata a pseudoartrosi congenita della tibia. Il 50% dei pazienti ha una neurofibromatosi, mentre solo il 10% dei pazienti con neurofibromatosi presenta questa lesione. La pseudoartrosi caratteristicamente interessa il terzo medio e il terzo distale della tibia. Boyd ha classificato questa patologia in gradi di severità progressiva a seconda della presenza di alterazioni cistiche e displasiche. Il trattamento per questa condizione è stato molto frustrante, con risultati scadenti. Per la prevenzione delle fratture è stato raccomandato l'uso precoce di ortesi, che però non ha avuto successo. Per ottenere l'unione sono stati tentati molti tipi di intervento chirurgico, come l'innesto *onlay* singolo e doppio con fissazione rigida interna, l'inserimento di un chiodo intramidollare con o senza innesto osseo e persino l'uso di un fissatore di Ilizarov. Con l'avvento della microchirurgia, sono stati utilizzati innesti vitali di perone con risultati variabili. A causa della scarse probabilità di unione efficace e della considerevole LLD, può essere preferibile un'amputazione sotto il ginocchio con riabilitazione precoce. È importante non effettuare alcun tentativo di osteotomia per la correzione della curvatura tibiale.

DEFICIT TIBIALE LONGITUDINALE

Questa patologia, dal pattern ereditario autosomico dominante, è stata classificata in quattro tipi, a seconda della parte mancante della tibia. Le altre anomalie associate sono deformità del piede, displasia dell'anca e sinfalangismo delle dita. Il trattamento verte intorno alla presenza di *anlage* tibiale prossimale e a un meccanismo funzionale del quadricipite. Nella deformità di tipo Ia, l'*anlage* tibiale prossimale è assente e si raccomanda una disarticolazione del ginocchio con protesizzazione. Nei tipi

Ib e II, l'*anlage* tibiale è presente e il trattamento consiste in un'amputazione precoce secondo Syme, seguita da una sinostosi del perone con la tibia e da una protesizzazione sotto il ginocchio. Il tipo III, peraltro raro, viene trattato principalmente con l'amputazione secondo Syme e la protesizzazione. La deformità di tipo IV è associata a diastasi della caviglia, che richiede la stabilizzazione della caviglia e la correzione della LLD in un tempo successivo.

Arazi M, Ogun TC, Memik R: Normal development of the tibiofemoral angle in children: A clinical study of 590 normal subjects from 3 to 17 years of age. *J Pediatr Orthop* 2001;21:264–267.

Cahuzac JP, Vardon D, Sales de Gauzy J: Development of the clinical tibiofemoral angle in normal adolescents: A study of 427 normal subjects from 10 to 16 years of age. *J Bone Joint Surg Br* 1995;77:729–732.

Davids JR, Blackhurst DW, Allen BL Jr: Radiographic evaluation of bowed legs in children. *J Pediatr Orthop* 2001;21:257–263.

Do TT: Clinical and radiographic evaluation of bowlegs. *Curr Opin Pediatr* 2001;13:42–46.

Doyle BS, Volk G, Smith CI: Infantile Blount's disease: Long-term follow-up of surgically treated patients at skeletal maturity. *J Pediatr Orthop* 1996;16:469–476.

Feldman MD, Schoenecker PL: Use of metaphyseal-diaphyseal angle in the evaluation of bowed legs. *J Bone Joint Surg Am* 1993;75:1602–1609.

Heath CH, Staheli LT: Normal limits of knee angle in white children—genu varum and genu valgum. *J Pediatr Orthop* 1993;13:259–262.

Henderson RC, Kemp GJ, Greene WB: Adolescent tibia vara: Alternatives for operative treatment. *J Bone Joint Surg Am* 1992;74:342–350.

Henderson RC, Kemp GJ, Hayes PRL: Prevalence of late-onset tibia vara. *J Pediatr Orthop* 1993;13:255–258.

Johnston CE II: Infantile tibia vara. *Clin Orthop* 1990;255:13–23.

Ruwe PA, Gage JR, Ozonoff MB, et al: Clinical determination of femoral anteversion: A comparison of established techniques. *J Bone Joint Surg Am* 1992;74:820–830.

Salenius P, Vankka E: The development of the tibiofemoral angle in children. *J Bone Joint Surg Am* 1975;57:259–261.

Staheli LT: Rotational problems in children. *Am Acad Orthop Surg Instr Course Lect* 1994;43:199–209.

Stevens PM, Maguire M, Dales MD, et al: Physeal stapling for idiopathic genu valgum. *J Pediatr Orthop* 1999;19:645–649.

Thompson GH: Angular deformities of the lower extremities in children. In Chapman MW (editor): *Operative Orthopedics*, 3rd ed. Philadelphia, JB Lippincott, 2001, pp 4287–4335.

Thompson GH: Gait disturbances. In Kliegman RM (editor): *Practical Strategies in Pediatric Diagnosis and Therapy*, 2nd ed. Philadelphia, WB Saunders, 2003, pp 823–843.

Wallach DM, Davidson RS: Pediatric lower limb disorders. In Dormans JP (editor): *Core Knowledge in Orthopaedics: Pediatric Orthopaedics*. Philadelphia, Mosby, 2005, pp 197–223.

Wallach DM, Davidson RS: Pediatric lower limb disorders. In Dormans JP (editor): *Pediatric Orthopaedics and Sports Medicine: The Requisites in Pediatrics*. Philadelphia, Mosby, 2005, pp 246–272.

Capitolo 675 ■ Differenza di lunghezza degli arti inferiori

Harish S. Hosalkar, Purushottam A. Gholve e David A. Spiegel

Una differenza di lunghezza degli arti inferiori può derivare da diverse condizioni congenite o acquisite (Tab. 675-1) e anche se fino al 25% della popolazione americana può avere una differenza >1 cm, soltanto una piccola percentuale ne ha una di 2 cm. La principale conseguenza è l'asimmetria dell'andatura. Si osserva un aumento del movimento verticale del bacino e la deambulazione comporta un maggiore dispendio energetico. Anche se si può sviluppare una piccola curva lombare compensatoria, vi sono poche evidenze a sostegno della teoria che la differenza della lunghezza degli arti inferiori causi dorsalgia, scoliosi strutturale o artrosi degenerativa. L'obiettivo del trattamento è avere una differenza <2-2,5 cm alla maturità scheletrica, e per ottenerlo sono disponibili diversi metodi di trattamento. La conoscenza dell'eziologia sottostante, insieme a un follow-up regolare per valutare la crescita degli arti e la maturità scheletrica, permette al medico di proiettare la discrepanza alla maturità scheletrica e di pianificare il trattamento. Un sottogruppo di pazienti presenta anomalie concomitanti degli organi interni o del sistema muscoloscheletrico, che vanno identificate e trattate.

TABELLA 675-1. Cause della differenza di lunghezza degli arti inferiori

CAUSE CONGENITE
Difetti di crescita
Deficit focale del femore prossimale
Pseudoartrosi congenita della tibia
Emimelia peroneale (vedi Fig. 675-8)
Tumori/malattie ossee
Displasia scheletrica
Esostosi ereditarie multiple
Neurofibromatosi
Encondromatosi (malattia di Ollier)
Osteogenesi imperfetta
Vascolari
Sindrome di Klippel-Trenaunay-Weber
Sindrome di Silver-Russell
Varie
Coxa vara congenita
Sindrome di Proteus
CAUSE ACQUISITE
Traumatiche
Fratture sovrapposte
Fratture epifisarie con danno della cartilagine di accrescimento
Evolutive
Displasia evolutiva dell'anca
Neoplastiche
Tumori maligni
Tumori che attraversano l'epifisi
Neurologiche
Mielodisplasia
Paralisi cerebrale
Infezioni/cause infiammatorie
Artrite settica dell'anca
Osteomielite
Artrite reumatoide
Varie
Coxa vara acquisita
Obliquità fissa del bacino nella scoliosi

DIAGNOSI E ASPETTI CLINICI. L'asimmetria dell'andatura è il disturbo più frequente. La diagnosi è posta con l'esame obiettivo e le radiografie specializzate consentono di quantificare la differenza e di seguirla nel tempo. La discrepanza tra i due arti può essere correlata all'accorciamento osseo e/o alla deformità angolare (accorciamento reale), alla contrattura dei tessuti molli a livello di anca, ginocchio o caviglia (accorciamento apparente) o a una combinazione di questi. Altri fattori contribuenti comprendono la sublussazione o la lussazione articolare (anca) e una riduzione dell'altezza del piede (congenita o neuromuscolare). È necessario un accurato esame radiologico per identificare tutti i fattori contribuenti. Esistono diversi metodi clinici per misurare la lunghezza degli arti. Gli Autori di questo capitolo preferiscono eseguire un esame in posizione eretta, in cui blocchi di varie dimensioni vengono posizionati sotto la gamba più corta fino a rimettere il bacino in posizione orizzontale (Fig. 675-1). Un me-

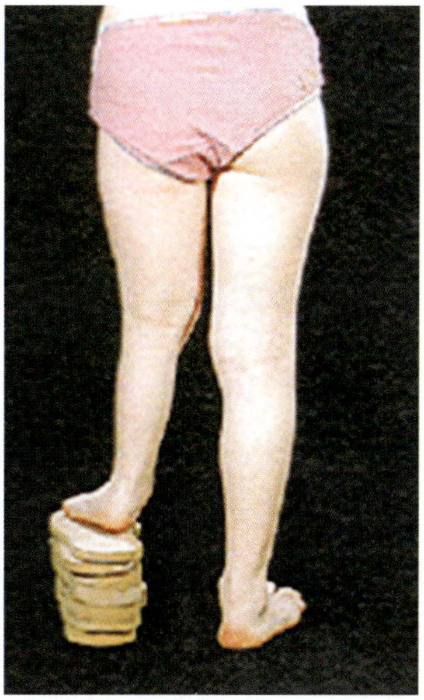

Figura 675-1. Esame con blocchi sotto l'arto inferiore corto fino a livellamento del bacino.

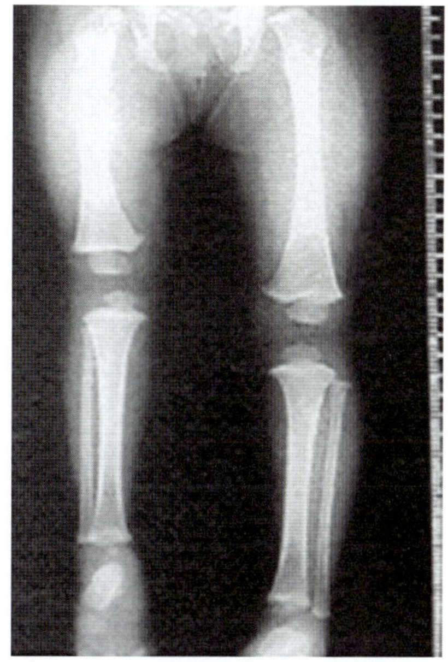

Figura 675-2. Scanografia che dimostra l'esatta differenza di lunghezza degli arti inferiori.

todo alternativo consiste nel misurare la lunghezza di ciascuna gamba con il paziente supino. Utilizzando un metro a nastro si misura la distanza tra la spina iliaca anterosuperiore e il malleolo mediale. Questi metodi dovrebbero essere ragionevolmente accurati in assenza di cause "apparenti" di discrepanza. Oltre a usare uno o entrambi questi metodi, occorre valutare l'arco di movimento di anca, ginocchio e caviglia per identificare qualsiasi causa di un'apparente differenza di lunghezza. Una contrattura in abduzione (o adduzione) fissa di 10° dell'anca crea un'apparente differenza di lunghezza di 2-3 cm. Allo stesso modo, una contrattura in flessione dell'anca e/o del ginocchio creerà un accorciamento apparente dell'estremità, mentre una contrattura in equino della caviglia darà luogo a un allungamento apparente. Una scoliosi lombare rigida (contrattura sovrapelvica) creerà un'obliquità del bacino e di conseguenza gli arti inferiori non avranno la stessa lunghezza. Una volta quantificata la differenza, occorre seguirla a intervalli regolari; in genere si eseguono valutazioni a intervalli di 6-12 mesi.

VALUTAZIONE RADIOGRAFICA. La valutazione radiografica completa l'esame clinico; entrambi sono tipicamente utilizzati quando si devono prendere decisioni riguardo al trattamento. La stessa tecnica deve essere utilizzata longitudinalmente per massimizzarne l'accuratezza. Sono disponibili quattro differenti metodiche. La rönt-teleradiografia è una singola esposizione di entrambe le estremità inferiori (in posizione eretta) e richiede una cassetta lunga. Si posiziona un regolo sulla lastra e si eseguono misurazioni dirette, calcolando un errore da ingrandimento del 6%. Comporta il vantaggio di permettere la valutazione delle deformità angolari. La sua indicazione primaria è nei bambini più piccoli. L'ortoradiografia consiste in tre esposizioni separate di anche, ginocchi e caviglie su una cassetta lunga. Con il paziente supino, si posiziona sulla cassetta un regolo per la misurazione della lunghezza delle ossa. Non vi è errore da ingrandimento. Tuttavia, il paziente deve giacere immobile per tre esposizioni, cosa spesso difficile da ottenere in un bambino piccolo. Anche la scanografia consiste in tre esposizioni separate di anche, ginocchia e caviglie su una cassetta con un regolo radiografico; la differenza consiste nel fatto che si utilizza una cassetta piccola (Fig. 675-2). Non vi è errore da ingrandimento; per contro, i pazienti devono rimanere immobili per tre esposizioni e non è possibile valutare le deformità angolari. Anche se la TC è la tecnica più accurata, la valutazione richiede tempo e la tecnica non è disponibile nella maggior parte dei centri. Oltre a quantificare la discrepanza, è essenziale determinare l'età scheletrica (età ossea). Una radiografia anteroposteriore della mano e del polso viene di solito eseguita a ogni visita e confrontata con gli standard dell'atlante di Greulich e Pyle allo scopo di stabilire l'età scheletrica. Anche se sono disponibili tecniche più accurate, la maggior parte di esse richiede tempo ed è poco pratica per un uso routinario. Il range di variabilità con l'uso dell'atlante è di circa 9 mesi, quindi il metodo è più accurato quando sono stati raccolti diversi dati in tempi successivi.

TRATTAMENTO. Le opzioni di trattamento comprendono l'osservazione, una calzatura con rialzo o un'ortesi personalizzata, una procedura di accorciamento dell'arto (accorciamento acuto vs accorciamento graduale per arresto della crescita), una procedura di allungamento dell'arto o una combinazione di queste. Nei deficit congeniti (femore, tibia, perone), un'amputazione precoce del piede è spesso la scelta migliore per il trattamento di una discrepanza severa prevedibile e permette di ottenere l'esito funzionale più soddisfacente. Oltre all'entità della differenza predetta alla maturità scheletrica, sono considerazioni importanti l'altezza che si prevede il paziente raggiungerà in età adulta (stimata in base ai membri della famiglia) e i desideri del paziente e dei suoi genitori. Le linee guida generali per il trattamento sono le seguenti.

Le differenze di lunghezza fino a 2,5 cm possono essere trattate con l'osservazione o con un rialzo. È possibile inserire all'interno della calzatura fino a 1 cm, e aggiungere all'esterno della scarpa fino a 5 cm. Non è necessaria una correzione completa della discrepanza e l'altezza del rialzo dovrebbe essere corretta in base all'andatura e al comfort del paziente. Come misura temporanea, prima del trattamento definitivo, si può utilizzare un'ortesi.

Se il divario tra i due arti è di 2-5 cm, si raccomanda un'epifisiodesi nei pazienti scheletricamente immaturi, mentre in un paziente scheletricamente maturo si può eseguire un accorciamento in un solo tempo operatorio. L'epifisiodesi consiste in un arresto temporaneo o permanente della crescita a livello di una o più cartilagini di coniugazione. È più comune optare per un arresto permanente della crescita qualora siano disponibili dati sufficienti per predire accuratamente quando eseguire la procedura. Il 65% circa della crescita dell'estremità inferiore deriva dal femore distale (37%, 9 mm/anno) e dalla tibia prossimale (28%, 6 mm/anno). Tipicamente i maschi crescono fino ai 16

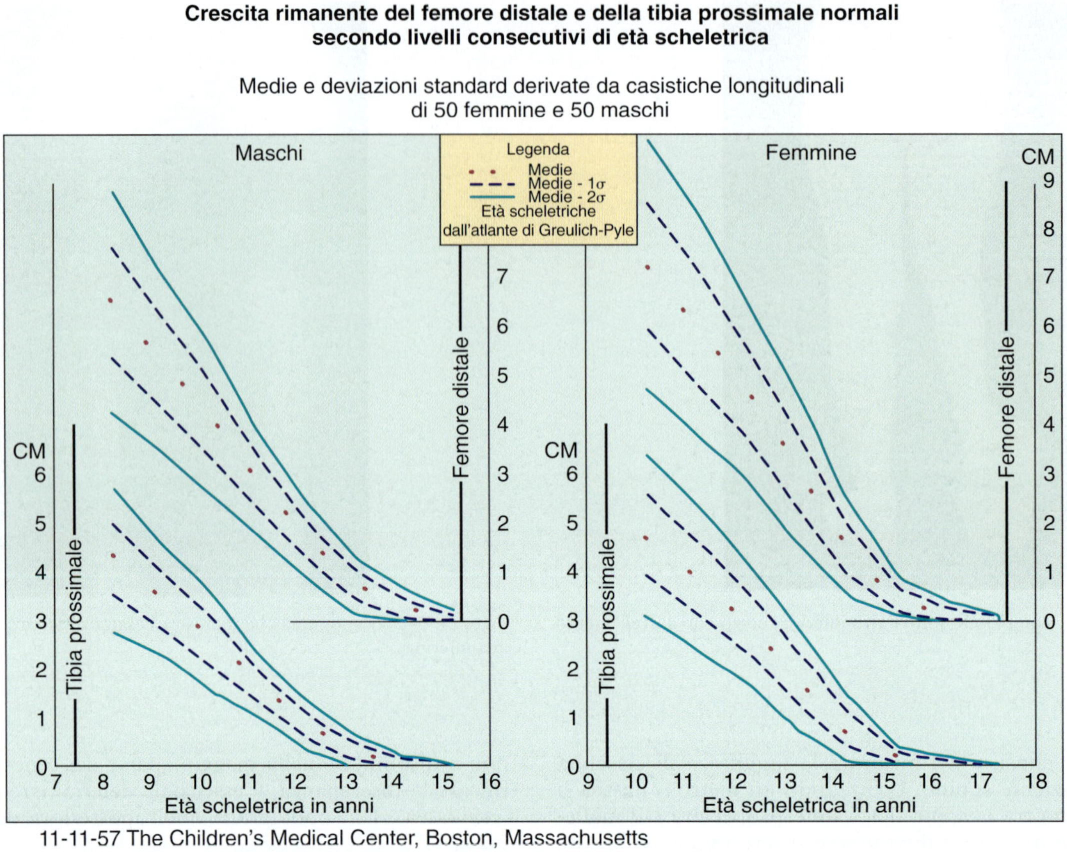

Figura 675-3. Grafici della crescita rimanente per maschi e femmine. I grafici della crescita rimanente per maschi e femmine sono diversi. La correzione reale si basa sulla crescita dell'arto più corto. Per utilizzare correttamente il grafico, occorre calcolare la differenza di lunghezza alla maturità e la percentuale di ritardo di crescita dell'arto più corto. (Modificata da Anderson M, Green WT, Messner MB: Growth and predictions of growth in lower extremities. *J Bone Joint Surg Am* 1963;45:1-4.)

anni di età, le femmine fino ai 14 anni. Pertanto, l'esecuzione di un'epifisiodesi sia del femore distale sia della tibia prossimale in un paziente con 3 anni di crescita restanti deve permettere una correzione di almeno 4,5 cm. Le tecniche utilizzate per determinare il timing dell'epifisiodesi sono il metodo di Menelaus ("regola pratica"), il metodo di Green e Anderson, il grafico a linea diritta di Moseley e il metodo moltiplicatore (Figg. 675-3, 675-4 e 675-5). La tecnica chirurgica più comune è l'epifisiodesi percutanea, in cui la cartilagine di coniugazione viene eliminata con un trapano e una curette sotto intensificazione d'immagine. Si tratta di una procedura ambulatoriale con poche complicanze. Un'alternativa è rappresentata dall'inserimento di viti attraverso la cartilagine di coniugazione. Se i dati a disposizione non sono sufficienti o se la diagnosi di base è associata a un pattern di crescita non prevedibile si può prendere in esame una tecnica reversibile. L'inserzione di graffe nella cartilagine di coniugazione consiste nell'applicazione di una o più graffe attraverso entrambi i lati della cartilagine di coniugazione; una volta ottenuto il riequilibrio degli arti, la loro rimozione permetterà la ripresa della crescita. Quando il paziente è scheletricamente maturo o se si ritiene opportuno attendere la maturità prima di intraprendere il trattamento, l'accorciamento in un solo tempo può essere l'opzione preferibile. Questo intervento viene tipicamente eseguito a livello del femore (ne sono state descritte diverse tecniche), dato l'elevato rischio di complicanze (sindrome compartimentale, problemi neurovascolari) associati all'accorciamento di tibia e perone.

Per differenze di lunghezza >5 cm, l'allungamento dell'arto più corto è la procedura di scelta. Un'eccezione potrebbe essere rappresentata da una discrepanza secondaria alla crescita eccessiva di un arto, che quindi viene accorciato allo scopo di conservare le proporzioni corporee. I pazienti con discrepanza predetta >8-10 cm richiedono spesso una o più procedure di allungamento degli arti (a diversi anni di distanza), con o senza epifisiodesi. La tecnica più comunemente utilizzata per l'allungamento di un arto consiste nell'inserimento di un fissatore esterno, sia un fissatore ad anello come quello di Ilizarov sia un sistema monolaterale (Fig. 675-6). Una volta resecato l'osso a livello della giunzione tra metafisi e diafisi, si procede a un graduale allungamento mediante distrazione a livello della corticotomia. Il tasso di allungamento è in genere pari a 1 mm/die e occorre circa 1 mese in fissatore per ogni centimetro di lunghezza ottenuto. In ogni seduta è possibile ottenere un allungamento massimo pari al 15-25% della lunghezza originale dell'osso. Un vantaggio del fissatore circolare è la possibilità di correggere allo stesso tempo le deformità angolari esistenti. Le complicanze comprendono infezione del tratto di inserimento del chiodo (la più frequente), infezione della ferita, ipertensione, sublussazione articolare, contratture muscolari, consolidamento prematuro, ritardo dell'unione, problemi correlati all'impianto e fratture in seguito alla sua rimozione. Infine, l'amputazione precoce e l'uso di un'ortesi possono garantire la migliore funzionalità a lungo termine nei pazienti in cui si prevedono discrepanze in eccesso di 18-20 cm, in particolare se sono presenti contemporaneamente

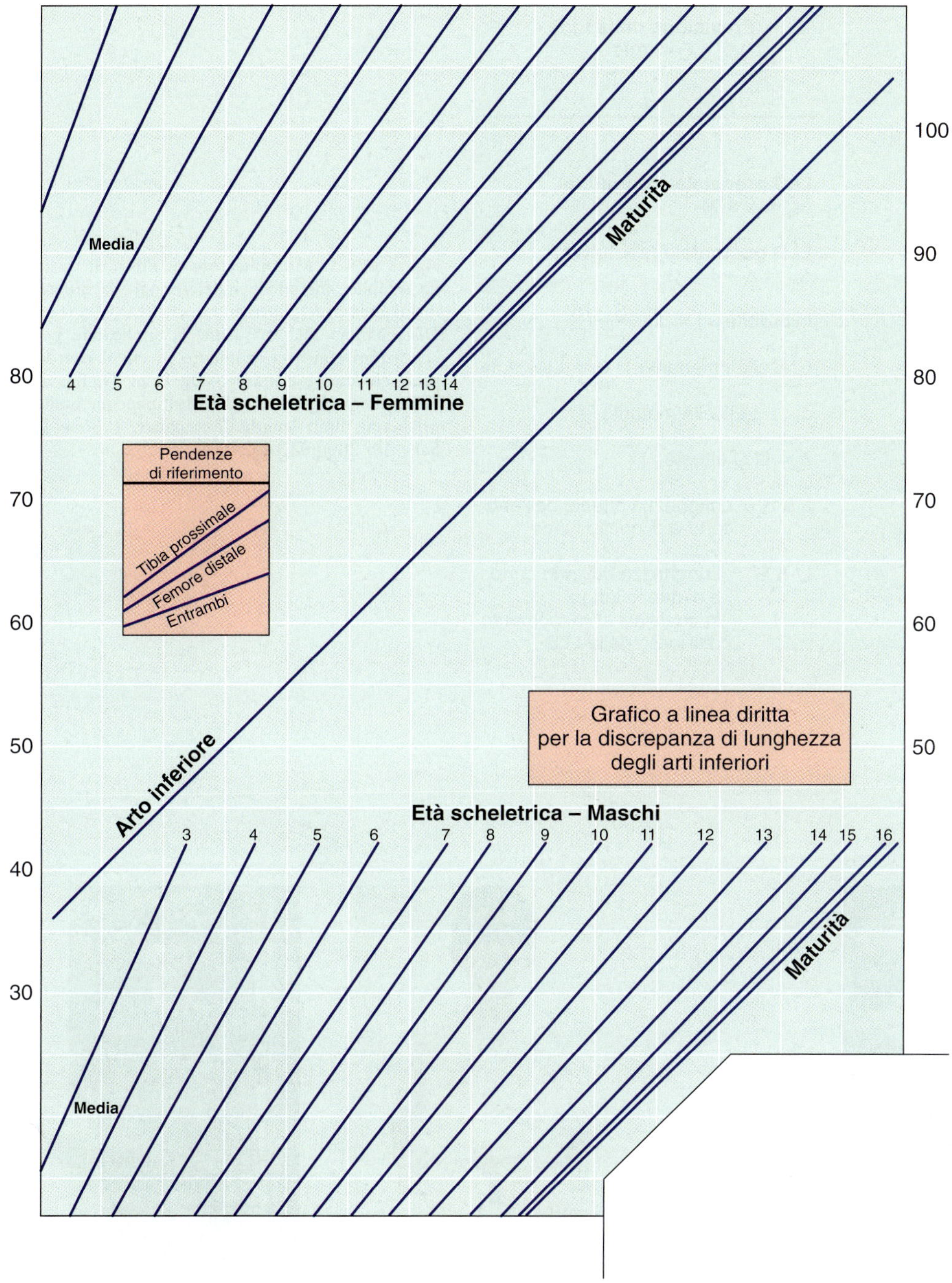

Figura 675-4. Grafico a linea diritta di Moseley per la valutazione della differenza di lunghezza degli arti inferiori. Questo grafico permette la correlazione simultanea tra arto normale, arto più corto ed età ossea del bambino. Predice accuratamente la lunghezza di ciascuna estremità alla maturità scheletrica. Le pendenze di riferimento sono utilizzate come guida per determinare quando deve essere eseguito un trattamento appropriato. (Da Moseley CF: A straight-line graph for leg-length discrepancies. *J Bone Joint Surg Am* 1977;59:174-179.)

deformità o deficit del piede ipsilaterale (Figg. 675-7 e 675-8). L'alternativa sarebbe una serie di procedure ricostruttive multiple, da effettuarsi nell'arco di tutta l'infanzia e l'adolescenza. Occorre tuttavia tenere presente l'impatto di procedure multiple sullo sviluppo psicosociale del bambino quando si formula il piano di trattamento per questi casi complessi.

Anderson M, Messner M, Green W: Distribution of lengths of the normal femur and tibia in children from one to eighteen years of age. *J Bone Joint Surg* 1964;46:1197–1202.

Beumer A, Lampe HI, Swierstra BA, et al: The straight line graph in limb length inequality: A new design based on 182 Dutch children. *Acta Orthop Scand* 1997;68:355–360.

Coppola C, Maffulli N: Limb shortening for the management of leg length discrepancy. *J R Coll Surg Edinb* 1999;44:46–54.

Gabriel KR, Crawford AH, Roy DR, True MS: Percutaneous epiphysiodesis. *J Pediatr Orthop* 1994;14:358–362.

Gruelich WW, Pyle SI: *Radiographic Atlas of Skeletal Development of the Hand and Wrist,* 2nd ed. Stanford, CA, Stanford University Press, 1959.

Horton GA, Olney BW: Epiphysiodesis of the lower extremity: Results of the percutaneous technique. *J Pediatr Orthop* 1996;16:180–182.

Little DG, Nigo L, Aiona MD: Deficiencies of current methods for the timing of epiphysiodesis. *J Pediatr Orthop* 1996;16:173–179.

Menelaus MB: Correction of leg length discrepancy by epiphyseal arrest. *J Bone Joint Surg Br* 1996;48:336–339.

Moseley CF: Leg length discrepancy. In Morrissey RT, Weinstein SL (editors): *Lovell and Winter's Pediatric Orthopaedics.* Philadelphia, Lippincott Williams & Wilkins, 2000, pp 1105 1150.

Moltiplicatore per maschi e femmine (Paley et al. 1999)

Maschi		Femmine	
Età	**Moltiplicatore**	**Età**	**Moltiplicatore**
0	5,08	0	4,63
0,4	4,01	0,3	4,01
1	3,24	1	2,97
1,3	2,99	2	2,39
2	2,59	3	2,05
3	2,23	3,3	2,00
4	2,00	4	1,83
5	1,83	5	1,66
6	1,68	6	1,53
7	1,57	7	1,43
8	1,47	8	1,33
9	1,38	9	1,26
10	1,31	10	1,19
11	1,24	11	1,13
12	1,18	12	1,07
13	1,12	13	1,03
14	1,07	14	1,00
15	1,03	15	1,00
16	1,01	16	1,00
17	1,00		
18	1,00		

Previsione della LLD Formule

LLD prenatale (congenita)

$\Delta_m = \Delta \times M$

LLD postnatale (evolutiva)

$\Delta_m = \Delta + I \times G$

Inibizione $\approx I = 1 - \dfrac{S - S^\bullet}{L - L^\bullet}$

Crescita rimanente $= G = L(M - 1)$

Δ_m = LLD alla maturità

Δ = LLD attuale

L & S = Lunghezza attuale dell'arto corto e di quello lungo

$L^\bullet$ & $S^\bullet$ = Lunghezza dell'arto corto e di quello lungo in qualsiasi altro momento dall'inizio della LLD

Figura 675-5. Moltiplicatore di Plyer. Si tratta di un semplice metodo per determinare la differenza di lunghezza degli arti inferiori (LLD, *Leg-Length Discrepancy*) alla maturità. È applicabile per le condizioni con accorciamento in cui il ritardo di accrescimento è costante. (Da Paley D, Bhave A, Herzenberg JE, Bowen JR: Multiplier methods for predicting limb length discrepancy. *J Bone Joint Surg Am* 2000;82;1432-1446.)

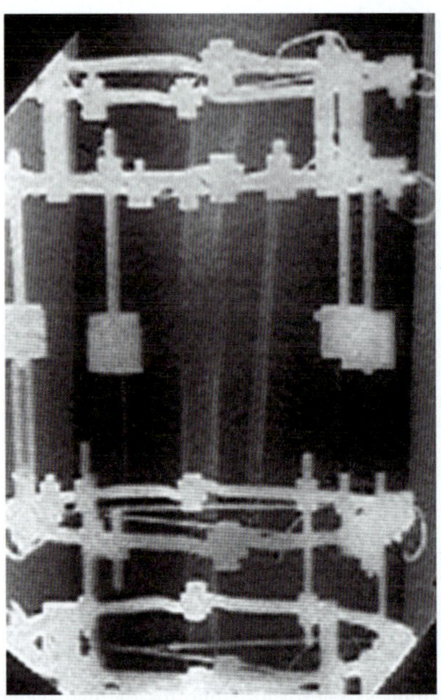

Figura 675-6. Dispositivo di Ilizarov che dimostra l'allungamento dell'osso per osteogenesi da distrazione.

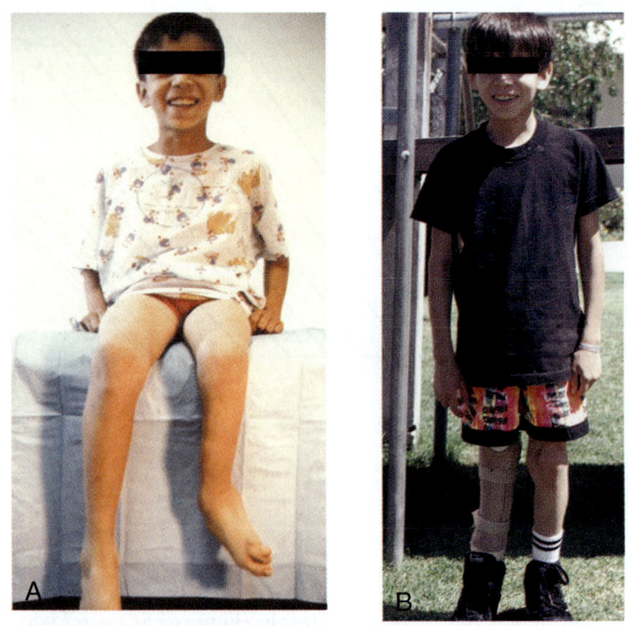

Figura 675-7. Differenza di lunghezza degli arti inferiori (*A*), compensata con protesi di estensione (*B*).

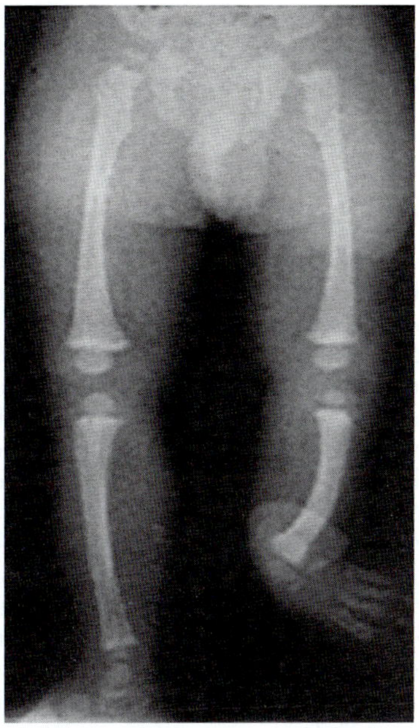

Figura 675-8. Radiografia anteroposteriore di emimelia peroneale con differenza di lunghezza degli arti inferiori.

Paley D, Bhave A, Herzenberg JE, Bowen JR: Multiplier method for predicting limb-length discrepancy. *J Bone Joint Surg Am* 2000;82:1432–1446.
Pritchett JW: Comparison of methods for prediction of lower-extremity growth. *J Bone Joint Surg Am* 2001;83:1108–1110.
Stanitski DF: Limb-length inequality: Assessment and treatment options. *J Am Acad Orthop Surg* 1999;7:143–153.
Stanitski DF, Bullard M, Armstrong P, Stanitski CL: Results of femoral lengthening using the Ilizarov technique. *J Pediatr Orthop* 1995;15:224–231.
Westh RN, Menelaus MB: A simple calculation for the timing of epiphyseal arrest: A further report. *J Bone Joint Surg Br* 1981;63:117–119.

Capitolo 676 ■ Il ginocchio

Harish S. Hosalkar e Lawrence Wells

SVILUPPO NORMALE DEL GINOCCHIO

Il ginocchio è un'articolazione sinoviale principale che si sviluppa tra il 3° e il 4° mese di vita fetale. I centri di ossificazione secondari si formano tra il 6° e il 9° mese di vita fetale per il femore distale e tra l'8° mese di vita fetale e il 1° mese di vita postnatale per la tibia superiore. Il centro di ossificazione rotuleo compare tra il 2° e il 4° anno di vita nelle femmine e tra il 3° e il 5° nei maschi.

ARCO DI MOVIMENTO NORMALE

Il ginocchio completamente esteso di norma si trova in posizione neutra. L'arco di movimento normale si estende dalla posizione neutra a circa 140° e la maggior parte dell'attività si svolge nell'arco di flessione di 0-70°. In un bambino è considerata normale un'iperestensione fino a 10-15°.

Il ginocchio, la più grande articolazione del corpo, è un tipo modificato di articolazione sinoviale (diartrosi) a cerniera, che può effettuare anche una rotazione di qualche grado. Esso è costituito da tre articolazioni riunite in una sola: una intermedia tra rotula e femore e due (una laterale, l'altra mediale) tra i condili femorale e tibiale. Il femore distale ha una forma a camme che gli consente di effettuare movimenti di scivolamento e a cerniera. I principali elementi di contenimento sono i legamenti collaterali mediale e laterale, i legamenti crociati anteriore e posteriore e i menischi mediale e laterale. Il ginocchio è circondato da diverse borse in quanto i tendini circostanti decorrono in gran parte paralleli alle ossa ed esercitano una trazione sull'articolazione del ginocchio nel senso della lunghezza.

Il dolore al ginocchio è uno dei più comuni disturbi di presentazione nei bambini più grandi e negli adolescenti. È comunemente correlato a un trauma, ma può anche avere un esordio insidioso. Al dolore è spesso associato un versamento articolare. A seconda dell'eziologia del processo intrarticolare, il liquido raccolto nella cavità articolare può essere sangue (emartro da trauma o da emofilia), infiammatorio (artrite reumatoide giovanile) o purulento (artrite settica). La presenza di globuli di grasso nel sangue aspirato da un emartro suggerisce una frattura occulta. Versamenti ricorrenti possono indicare un'alterazione interna cronica come una lacerazione meniscale. L'aspirazione del liquido articolare è spesso necessaria non solo per stabilire la diagnosi, ma anche per eliminare i sintomi (vedi Capitolo 684).

PROBLEMI DEL GINOCCHIO IN ETÀ PEDIATRICA

676.1 • Menisco laterale discoide

Il menisco laterale discoide (DLM, *Discoid Lateral Meniscus*) è una variante anatomica del menisco laterale che può essere asintomatica oppure causare uno scatto durante i movimenti del ginocchio. Ne esistono tre tipi. Il 1° è il **tipo con legamento di Wrisberg**, in cui il menisco laterale non è connesso con il piatto tibiale posteriormente, ma possiede un legamento meniscofemorale, o legamento di Wrisberg, che collega il corno posteriore del menisco laterale alla superficie laterale del condilo femorale mediale. Tale legamento impedisce lo scivolamento del menisco durante l'estensione del ginocchio, producendo una scatto a ogni escursione del menisco e causandone ipertrofia e irregolarità. Il 2° è il **tipo completo**, caratterizzato da un ispessimento del menisco laterale, che non si sposta internamente ed esternamente rispetto al centro dell'articolazione e possiede connessioni periferiche normali. Il 3° infine è il **tipo incompleto**, che è più piccolo rispetto al tipo completo e non riempie il compartimento laterale.

La causa del DLM non è chiara, ma potrebbe consistere nell'assenza della sequenza embriologica di degenerazione del centro del menisco. Il menisco normale possiede connessioni lungo i propri margini e slitta anteriormente e posteriormente con i movimenti del ginocchio, mentre un menisco discoide è meno mobile e può lacerarsi. Talvolta sono assenti le connessioni periferiche intorno all'aspetto posterolaterale del menisco, consentendone lo spostamento anomalo in avanti con la flessione del ginocchio, che produce un suono simile a uno schiocco.

Il sintomo di presentazione usuale è quello di uno scatto del ginocchio che viene sia udito sia percepito dal bambino o dai genitori. Questo sintomo, di più frequente riscontro nei bambini di età >6 anni, di solito non è doloroso e non impedisce al soggetto di svolgere una vita attiva. Un secondo tipo di presentazione è quella di un bambino che non ha sintomi a carico del ginocchio, ma si presenta (spontaneamente o dopo un trauma) con dolore, sensazione di scatto, schiocco o blocco localizzati lungo la linea articolare laterale. L'esame obiettivo può evidenziare un versamento e una dolenzia di lieve entità, con senso di ripienezza a livello della linea articolare laterale e crepitio con il movimento. I sintomi comprendono uno scatto palpabile con la flessione e l'estensione del ginocchio. L'esaminatore avverte una sporgenza lungo la linea articolare laterale, come se il menisco tendesse a protrudere oltre il margine tibiale. Con il movimento del ginocchio, il menisco scatta nell'incisura intercondiloidea e la sporgenza scompare.

La radiografia anteroposteriore del ginocchio può evidenziare un allargamento dell'aspetto laterale dell'articolazione del ginocchio. Altri aspetti radiografici comprendono l'appiattimento del condilo femorale laterale (con aspetto squadrato) e una depressione a coppa dell'aspetto laterale del piatto tibiale. Per una diagnosi definitiva sono necessarie la RM o l'artroscopia.

TRATTAMENTO. Molti bambini con menisco discoide non richiedono alcun trattamento. Questi soggetti devono essere seguiti e trattati soltanto se accusano dolore o perdita del movimento. L'intervento chirurgico può essere preso in considerazione quando il DLM causa blocco, tumefazione, perdita del movimento, impossibilità di correre o di praticare attività sportive. Il trattamento consiste nell'escissione delle lacerazioni e nella risagomatura del menisco per via artroscopica (Fig. 676-1). Talvolta è possibile riparare o ricostruire l'instabilità meniscale. Se le altre procedure non hanno successo può rendersi necessaria un'escissione completa.

676.2 • Cisti poplitea

Le cisti poplitee (**cisti di Baker**) sono di comune osservazione nei bambini, in cui hanno caratteristiche diverse che negli adulti. Si tratta di masse cistiche ripiene di materiale gelatinoso che si sviluppano nella fossa poplitea, sono di solito asintomatiche e non sono correlate a patologia intrarticolare. Di solito si verifica una risoluzione spontanea, anche se il processo può richiedere diversi anni.

La presentazione usuale è quella di una massa dietro il ginocchio che può essere abbastanza grande quando viene notata per la prima volta. In genere non vi sono sintomi di alterazioni interne del ginocchio. L'esame obiettivo rivela una massa di consistenza dura nella fossa poplitea, spesso localizzata medialmente e di solito distale rispetto alla cresta poplitea. La massa appare più evidente con il ginocchio in estensione e quando il paziente è in posizione prona.

Il più comune sito di origine è la borsa del gastrocnemio e del semimembranoso; anche un'ernia attraverso la parte posteriore della capsula articolare del ginocchio è un'origine frequente. Istologicamente, le cisti vengono classificate come fibrose, sinoviali, infiammatorie o transizionali. La transilluminazione della cisti all'esame obiettivo è un semplice test diagnostico. Le radiografie del ginocchio sono normali e devono essere effettuate per diagnosticare altre lesioni come osteocondromi, osteocondrite dissecante e neoplasie maligne. La diagnosi deve essere confermata con l'ecografia (per distinguere una massa solida da una lesione cistica) o con l'aspirazione. Nella maggior parte dei casi, non è necessario alcun intervento in quanto spesso queste cisti si risolvono spontaneamente. L'escissione chirurgica è indicata soltanto quando i sintomi sono severi e limitanti e non si sono risolti dopo diversi mesi. La presenza di una massa solida individuata all'esame obiettivo o alla RM rende necessaria l'esplorazione.

676.3 • Osteocondrite dissecante

L'osteocondrite dissecante si verifica quando un'area ossea adiacente alla cartilagine articolare diviene avascolare e infine si separa dall'osso sottostante. L'esatta eziologia non è nota; tuttavia, le cause di fratture osteocondrali del condilo femorale comprendono la compressione da parte di una spina tibiale alta, traumi diretti che causano compattamento, forze rotatorie e forze di compressione articolare. La forma giovanile può rappresentare un disturbo dello sviluppo epifisario, con piccole isole ossee accessorie separate dall'epifisi. È stata suggerita una predisposizione familiare. Le lesioni sono per la maggior parte localizzate sulla porzione laterale del condilo femorale mediale, sebbene possano interessare anche il condilo femorale laterale o la rotula. L'aspetto anatomopatologico caratteristico della lesione consiste in un'area di necrosi avascolare contraddistinta da una fissurazione da entrambi i lati, con ischemia e fibrosi della cartilagine ialina sovrastante di grado variabile.

MANIFESTAZIONI CLINICHE E DIAGNOSI. Il più comune disturbo di presentazione è un vago dolore al ginocchio. In caso di distacco del frammento, si possono osservare crepitio, schiocco, cedimento e occasionalmente blocco del ginocchio, con o senza un lieve versamento articolare. I segni fisici, peraltro minimi, possono comprendere dolorabilità perirotulea, atrofia del quadricipite e dolore lieve nell'ambito dell'arco di movimento. Il test di Wilson è considerato un esame diagnostico specifico: si esegue flettendo il ginocchio a 90°, ruotando completamente la tibia medialmente e quindi estendendo gradualmente il ginocchio. Quando il test è positivo, è presente dolore a 30° di flessione, localizzato al di sopra del condilo femorale mediale, anteriormente.

Di solito la lesione si rende evidente alle radiografie anteroposteriore, laterale e in proiezione a tunnel (*notch view*) del ginocchio. Le lesioni precoci si presentano con una piccola area di radiotrasparenza a livello della superficie articolare, mentre quelle più avanzate formano un segmento ben delimitato di osso subcondrale separato dal condilo da una linea radiotrasparente. Nei bambini più piccoli possono comparire piccoli focolai di ossificazione oltre il margine del nucleo di ossificazione principale. Con la rivascolarizzazione l'osso guarisce spontaneamente. Con l'aumentare dell'età, aumenta il rischio di frattura della cartila-

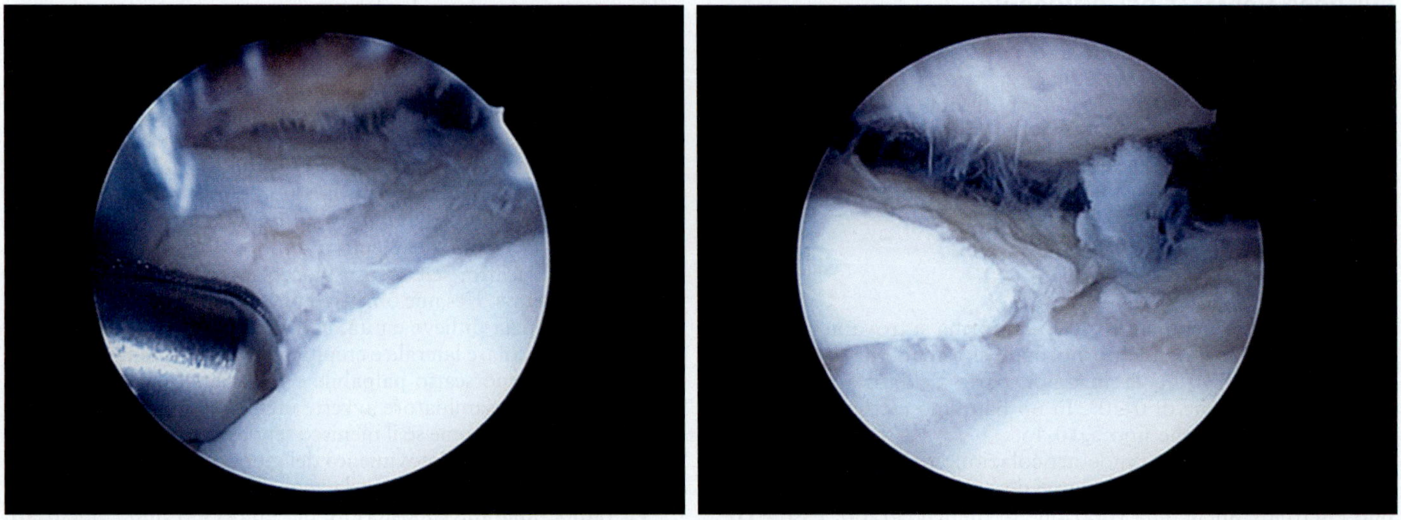

Figura 676-1. Immagine artroscopica di un menisco discoide e *shaving* artroscopico con meniscectomia.

gine articolare e di separazione del frammento osseo, che danno origine a un corpo libero intrarticolare.

La TC delinea l'estensione e la sede della lesione, oltre a fornire indicazioni sul grado di distacco. La RM è utile per determinare l'integrità della cartilagine articolare e la stabilità della lesione. L'artroscopia è il metodo più affidabile per la valutazione dello stato della lesione (Fig. 676-2). I fattori comunemente associati a una prognosi favorevole sono un gruppo d'età più giovane, una lesione di piccole dimensioni, una sede non sottoposta a carico e l'assenza di spostamento. La progressione dell'osteocondrite dissecante si articola in quattro stadi. Nello stadio I si osserva una piccola area di compressione subcondrale, nello stadio II un frammento parzialmente distaccato, nello stadio III un frammento completamente distaccato, che però rimane nella sede di origine, e nello stadio IV un frammento libero nella cavità articolare.

TRATTAMENTO. Il trattamento iniziale dell'osteocondrite dissecante, nei bambini con cartilagini di accrescimento aperte, consiste nell'osservazione con una restrizione dell'attività sufficiente per la risoluzione dei sintomi. Le lesioni più stabili guariscono spontaneamente nel giro di diversi mesi. Le lesioni di stadio I e II sono trattate con la modificazione dell'attività, esercizi isometrici e un immobilizzatore del ginocchio. Una volta confermata la guarigione con radiografie di follow-up, il paziente può fare ritorno ai normali livelli di attività. L'artroscopia è indicata nei pazienti in cui il trattamento conservativo è inefficace e in quelli con segni, sintomi e altre indagini diagnostiche suggestivi di una lesione instabile. Per trattare le lesioni di stadio III si effettua la trapanazione e la stabilizzazione con fili di Kirschner o chiodi. Le lesioni di stadio IV, se di piccole dimensioni, sono trattate con l'escissione, mentre le lesioni più grandi o quelle che interessano aree sottoposte a carico vengono sostituite o sottoposte a fissazione interna. Nei casi molto severi con distacco di ampi frammenti, può essere necessario l'innesto di osso e cartilagine. Dopo l'intervento i pazienti seguono un programma di fisioterapia e possono o meno fare ritorno ai livelli di attività preoperatori. Un trattamento precoce ed efficace dell'osteocondrite dissecante spesso previene la recidiva dei sintomi in età adulta, anche se alcune lesioni molto severe possono divenire sintomatiche nelle fasi successive della vita.

676.4 • MALATTIA DI OSGOOD-SCHLATTER

Questa patologia è caratterizzata da dolore in corrispondenza della tuberosità tibiale, in un bambino in fase di crescita. Il tendine rotuleo si inserisce sulla tuberosità tibiale, che è un'estensione dell'epifisi tibiale prossimale. Si suppone che la malattia di Osgood-Schlatter sia un'apofisite da trazione della cartilagine di accrescimento della tuberosità tibiale e del tendine rotuleo adiacente. Insorge nella tarda infanzia o nell'adolescenza, soprattutto negli atleti, ed è probabilmente dovuta a ripetuti microtraumi tensivi. Si verifica in soggetti di età compresa tra i 10 e i 15 anni; l'esordio nelle femmine avviene circa 2 anni prima che nei maschi. È più comune nei maschi.

Si tratta di un disturbo autolimitato nella maggior parte dei pazienti, che si risolve con la maturità scheletrica. Il sintomo più frequente è il dolore in corrispondenza della tuberosità tibiale e spesso appare preoccupante l'edema a livello della tuberosità. Il dolore è esacerbato dal movimento, ma spesso persiste anche a riposo. L'esame obiettivo rivela un dolore a punto a livello della tuberosità tibiale e della porzione distale del tendine rotuleo. Spesso si osserva un aumento della sporgenza della tuberosità tibiale, che appare di consistenza dura. Di solito le radiografie sono l'unica indagine diagnostica necessaria (Fig. 676-3). Talvolta si può notare un'ossificazione frammentaria della tuberosità tibiale, che spesso rappresenta una variante normale. Alcuni casi possono essere associati a rotula alta.

Possono essere necessari riposo, restrizione dell'attività e occasionalmente un immobilizzatore del ginocchio, in associazione a un programma di esercizi isometrici e di flessibilità. È importante rassicurare sia i diretti interessati sia i loro genitori, se temono che la tumefazione della tuberosità sia un segno di neoplasia maligna. La completa risoluzione dei sintomi attraverso la guarigione fisiologica (chiusura delle cartilagini di coniugazione) della tuberosità tibiale può richiedere dai 12 ai 24 mesi. È raro che si renda necessaria la rimozione di ossicini dalla tuberosità in pazienti con sintomi disabilitanti persistenti. Le complicanze sono rare e comprendono la chiusura precoce della tuberosità tibiale con deformità in recurvatum e, eventualità ancora più remota, la rottura del tendine rotuleo o avulsione della tuberosità tibiale.

PROBLEMI ROTULEOFEMORALI

La stabilità dell'articolazione rotuleofemorale dipende dall'equilibrio tra legamenti contenitivi, forze muscolari e anatomia ar-

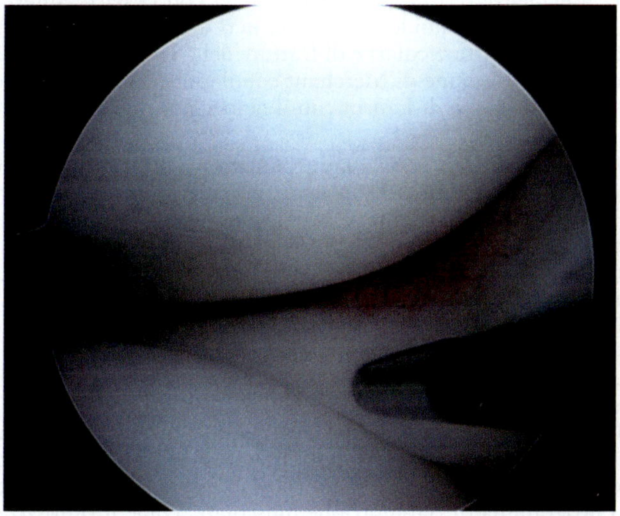

Figura 676-2. Classica immagine artroscopica di osteocondrite dissecante.

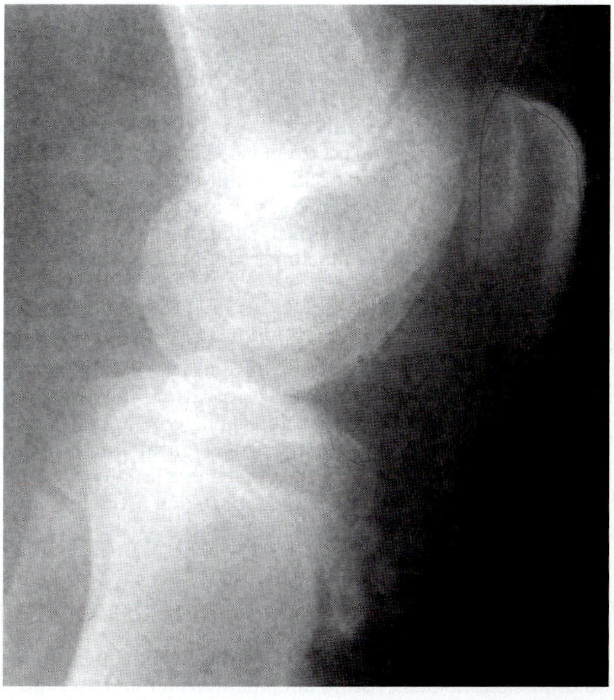

Figura 676-3. Radiografia laterale del ginocchio che evidenzia un'apofisite della tuberosità tibiale nella malattia di Osgood-Schlatter.

ticolare del solco rotuleofemorale. I fattori che contribuiscono all'instabilità rotuleofemorale comprendono insufficienza del quadricipite, torsione femorale interna, assottigliamento capsulare mediale, ipoplasia condiloidea e genu valgum.

La rotula possiede un polo inferiore a V che la guida lungo il solco nel femore distale. La forza dei muscoli che esercitano una trazione attraverso il meccanismo quadricipitale e il tendine rotuleo non agisce in linea retta in quanto il tendine rotuleo ha una direzione leggermente inclinata rispetto alla linea del quadricipite: si tratta del cosiddetto angolo Q. Questo movimento laterale, insieme al movimento dei legamenti contenitivi, tende a spostare la rotula in una direzione laterale. È necessario il muscolo vasto mediale per contrastare le forze che si esercitano lateralmente. Un'anomalia di uno qualsiasi o di alcuni di questi fattori può alterare la funzione dell'articolazione rotuleofemorale. Un'eccessiva instabilità di tale articolazione può manifestarsi come lussazione acuta della rotula, sublussazione o lussazione ricorrente della rotula, lussazione abituale e lussazione cronica.

676.5 • Sindrome idiopatica del dolore anteriore del ginocchio dell'adolescente

Nota in precedenza come condromalacia rotulea, la sindrome idiopatica del dolore anteriore del ginocchio dell'adolescente è una patologia comune che si presenta con dolore al ginocchio. Questa dicitura è stata inizialmente utilizzata per descrivere un'alterazione della superficie articolare della rotula. Comune nelle ragazze durante l'adolescenza, è spesso correlata all'attività e scarsamente localizzata e può causare disabilità. In base a ogni evidenza la superficie articolare risulta in realtà normale. La causa di dolore al ginocchio, che comunemente si presenta all'inizio della pubertà, è sconosciuta. Un paziente con dolore non spiegabile del ginocchio anteriore rappresenta una sfida diagnostica e terapeutica per il chirurgo ortopedico.

MANIFESTAZIONI CLINICHE E DIAGNOSI. I sintomi sono di solito scatenati da attività fisiche vigorose come la corsa. Di solito non esiste una storia di trauma precedente. Non vi sono sintomi meccanici associati come blocco articolare, cedimento articolare o versamento articolare ricorrente.

Occorre valutare l'arco di movimento attivo e passivo del ginocchio, l'allineamento dell'estremità inferiore, la stabilità del ginocchio, lo scorrimento della rotula, le aree di dolorabilità locale e l'andatura, allo scopo di identificare qualsiasi causa evidente di dolore o instabilità del ginocchio. Le radiografie di routine, comprese le proiezioni anteroposteriore, laterale e a tunnel, non sono particolarmente utili per stabilire le cause di dolore anteriore del ginocchio nell'adolescente, eccetto per il fatto che possono eliminare altre eziologie. Nel gruppo degli adolescenti, nei casi sospetti, si raccomanda di prendere in esame l'esecuzione di radiografie dell'anca per escludere un'epifisiolisi della testa femorale, che può presentarsi come un dolore indefinito al ginocchio.

TRATTAMENTO. La storia naturale del dolore anteriore del ginocchio è quella di una spontanea risoluzione nel giro di alcuni anni. Il trattamento, prevalentemente conservativo, può consistere in esercizi di flessibilità, esercizi di rafforzamento (esercizi isometrici per il quadricipite), fisioterapia con applicazione di caldo e freddo, l'uso di ortesi e farmaci antinfiammatori non steroidei (FANS). Si può prevedere una percentuale di successo del 70-90%. La valutazione artroscopica dell'articolazione del ginocchio e rotuleofemorale è raramente necessaria.

676.6 • Sublussazione e lussazione della rotula

La lussazione ricorrente della rotula è definita come più di un episodio di lussazione della rotula documentato da un osservatore o descritto chiaramente dal paziente. L'espressione "sublussazione rotulea ricorrente" non è adeguatamente definita, ma allude a più di un episodio di sublussazione rotulea senza una lussazione franca. La lussazione abituale della rotula si definisce come una lussazione che si verifica ogniqualvolta il ginocchio è flesso, mentre una lussazione cronica della rotula è una lussazione che non si riduce mai per tutto l'arco di movimento del ginocchio.

La sublussazione e la lussazione traumatiche della rotula possono verificarsi in seguito a un trauma diretto. La sublussazione o lussazione abituale è di solito dovuta a un ginocchio displasico con contrattura della porzione laterale del meccanismo quadricipitale. In questo caso, la rotula si lussa lateralmente a ogni flessione del ginocchio. Il più comune fattore eziologico della lussazione ricorrente della rotula è il disallineamento laterale del meccanismo quadricipitale. Diverse sono le sindromi associate a instabilità rotulea, tra cui sindrome di Down, sindrome di Turner, sindrome del trucco Kabuki e sindrome di Rubinstein-Taybi.

MANIFESTAZIONI CLINICHE E DIAGNOSI. La diagnosi è di solito suggerita dai riscontri all'esame obiettivo. Dopo una lussazione acuta, vi può essere un emartro da lacerazione capsulare o da frattura osteocondrale. Se il bambino giunge all'osservazione del medico poco dopo aver subito una lussazione, si possono riscontrare dolenzia pararotulea e un versamento di grado lieve.

L'esame di un bambino con una rotula che non scorre correttamente, e quindi predisposta alla lussazione, spesso può mettere in evidenza una sublussazione terminale della rotula quando il ginocchio viene portato in estensione completa. Vi può essere dolenzia alla palpazione sulla superficie inferiore della faccetta laterale della rotula. Occorre osservare il tragitto della rotula nel corso della flessione del ginocchio a partire da una posizione di estensione completa. Nel paziente con instabilità, la rotula devia lateralmente non appena il ginocchio inizia a flettersi, per poi deviare medialmente con un'ulteriore flessione. Questo spostamento laterale della rotula seguito da un movimento mediale è denominato *J tracking*. Un altro segno classico è il *segno dell'apprensione di Fairbanks*: con il ginocchio flesso a 30°, l'esaminatore sposta manualmente la rotula ottenendo una sensazione soggettiva di sublussazione, con il risultato che il paziente afferra la mano dell'esaminatore per prevenire una lussazione da manipolazione.

È importante valutare il profilo torsionale del paziente per escludere possibili anomali rotatorie del femore, della tibia o di entrambi.

Gli studi radiografici possono aiutare a identificare i fattori che contribuiscono alla lussazione ricorrente della rotula o dopo una lussazione acuta. Occorre eseguire le proiezioni anteroposteriore, laterale e tangenziale di profilo (ottenuta in flessione completa) della rotula per la ricerca di una frattura osteocondrale dal condilo femorale mediale o dalla rotula stessa. Sono utili anche la proiezione di MacNab (con il ginocchio in flessione a 40°), che, oltre a evidenziare i rapporti della rotula con la parte anteriore del solco intercondiloideo femorale, può dimostrare la presenza di corpi liberi intrarticolari e di fratture della rotula o del condilo laterale, la proiezione di Merchant con il ginocchio in flessione a 45° e la proiezione di Laurin con il ginocchio in flessione a 20°.

TRATTAMENTO. Una lussazione traumatica della rotula deve essere trattata inizialmente con un immobilizzatore del ginocchio per il comfort del paziente. Dopo alcuni giorni, il paziente deve iniziare esercizi di rinforzo isometrici per il quadricipite e con la risoluzione del dolore potrà eseguire esercizi di rinforzo ancora più energici. Una volta terminata l'immobilizzazione (che dura circa 6 settimane), il programma di esercizi isometrici deve essere proseguito fino alla completa riabilitazione del ginocchio. Grazie a questo metodo, il 75% circa dei pazienti non presenta lussazioni ricorrenti.

Il trattamento iniziale della lussazione ricorrente della rotula deve essere conservativo. Se la lussazione della rotula è dovuta a uno squilibrio muscolare dinamico, può essere efficace un specifico programma di riabilitazione muscolare, come il rinforzo del muscolo vasto mediale. Può essere utile un'ortesi che stabilizzi la rotula, anche se il meccanismo di azione e l'efficacia rimangono ancora da chiarire.

La stabilizzazione operatoria può rendersi necessaria se gli episodi di lussazione si ripetono continuamente o se il trattamento conservativo della sublussazione rotulea non dà alcun risultato. L'approccio chirurgico nei bambini in fase di crescita prevede il riallineamento del meccanismo quadricipitale, di solito in associazione con un rilascio laterale e con la creazione di un contenimento rotuleo mediale. Il riallineamento del meccanismo estensorio è ottenibile intervenendo sul muscolo stesso, cambiandone l'inserzione sulla rotula o modificando la connessione della rotula con la tibia. A seconda dell'estensione dell'interessamento, si può eseguire un rilascio laterale in artroscopia, con o senza una ricostruzione dei tessuti molli, con una procedura di riallineamento. Se necessario, per ovviare alle anomalie torsionali del femore o della tibia si ricorre a un'osteotomia rotatoria del femore distale o della tibia prossimale, più raramente di entrambi.

Ahn JH, Shim JS, Hwang CH, et al: Discoid lateral meniscus in children: Clinical manifestations and morphology. *J Pediatr Orthop* 2001;21:812–816.
Bensahel H, Souchet P, Pennecot GF, et al: The unstable patella in children. *J Pediatr Orthop* 2000;9:265–270.
Davids JR: Pediatric knee: Clinical assessment and common disorders. *Pediatr Clin North Am* 1996;43:1067–1090.
Ganley TJ, Kolze EA, Gregg JR: Pediatric sports medicine. In Dormans JP (editor): *Pediatric Orthopedics: Core Knowledge in Orthopedics*. Philadelphia, Mosby, 2005, pp 138–158.
Ganley TJ, Lou JE, Pryor K, Gregg JR: Sports medicine. In Dormans JP (editor): *Pediatric Orthopedics and Sports Medicine: The Requisites in Pediatrics*. Philadelphia, Mosby, 2004, pp 273–298.
Hamer AJ: Pain in the hip and knee. *Br Med J* 2004;328:1067–1069.
Herring JA: Disorders of the knee. In Herring JA (editor): *Tachdjian's Pediatric Orthopedics*, 3rd ed. Philadelphia, WB Saunders, 2002, pp 789–837.
Kocher MS, DiCanzio J, Zurakowski D, et al: Diagnostic performance of clinical examination and selective magnetic resonance imaging in the evaluation of intraarticular knee disorders in children and adolescents. *Am J Sports Med* 2001;29:292–296.
Stanitski CL: Instructional course lecture: Anterior knee pain syndromes in the adolescent. *J Bone Joint Surg Am* 1993;75:1407–1416.
Vahasarja V, Kinnunen P, Lanning P, et al: Operative realignment of patellar malalignment in children. *J Pediatr Orthop* 1995;15:281–285.
Van Rhijn LW, Jansen EJ, Pruijs HE: Long-term follow-up of conservatively treated popliteal cysts in children. *J Pediatr Orthop* 2000;9:62–64.

Capitolo 677 ■ L'anca

Harish S. Hosalkar, David Horn, Jared E. Friedman e John P. Dormans

Quella dell'anca è un'articolazione chiave dell'arto inferiore e le sue esigenze funzionali richiedono una grande stabilità associata a un'ampia escursione, che permetta un movimento poliassiale, comprendente flessione, estensione, abduzione, adduzione, rotazione interna ed esterna e circumduzione. Da un punto di vista anatomico, l'articolazione dell'anca è un'enartrosi tra testa femorale e acetabolo. Testa femorale e acetabolo sono in stretta relazione e pertanto altamente dipendenti l'uno dall'altro per lo sviluppo e la crescita.

CRESCITA E SVILUPPO

L'articolazione dell'anca inizia a svilupparsi intorno alla 7ª settimana di gestazione, quando compare una fessura nel mesenchima della gemma dell'arto primitivo. Queste cellule precartilaginee si differenziano in una testa femorale e in un acetabolo, che risultano completamente formati a partire dall'11ª settimana di gestazione. Alla nascita, l'acetabolo neonatale è completamente composto di cartilagine, con un sottile margine fibrocartilagineo denominato *labrum*.

La cartilagine ialina ipercellulare dell'acetabolo è in continuità con le cartilagini triradiate, che dividono e interconnettono le tre componenti ossee del bacino (ilio, ischio e pube). La forma concava dell'articolazione dell'anca dipende dalla presenza di una testa femorale sferica.

Diversi sono i fattori che determinano la profondità dell'acetabolo, tra cui la crescita interstiziale all'interno della cartilagine acetabolare, la crescita apposizionale sotto il pericondrio e la crescita delle ossa adiacenti (ilio, ischio, pube). Nel neonato, l'intero femore prossimale è una struttura cartilaginea a forma di testa femorale, con grande e piccolo trocantere. Le tre principali aree di crescita sono la cartilagine di accrescimento, la cartilagine di accrescimento del grande trocantere e l'istmo del collo femorale. Tra il 4° e il 7° mese di vita compare il centro di ossificazione femorale prossimale (al centro della testa femorale), che continua a ingrandirsi, insieme al suo *anlage* cartilagineo, fino alla vita adulta, quando rimane soltanto un sottile strato di cartilagine articolare. Durante il periodo della crescita, lo spessore della cartilagine che circonda questo nucleo osseo si riduce gradualmente, insieme allo spessore della cartilagine acetabolare. Sulla crescita del femore prossimale influiscono la trazione muscolare, le forze trasmesse attraverso l'articolazione dell'anca, la normale nutrizione dell'articolazione, la circolazione e il tono muscolare. Alterazioni di questi fattori possono causare profondi cambiamenti nello sviluppo del femore prossimale.

VASCOLARIZZAZIONE

La vascolarizzazione dell'epifisi della testa femorale (CFE, *Capital Femoral Epiphysis*) è complessa, il cui pattern cambia con l'allungamento del collo femorale, la cartilagine di accrescimento, la graduale ossificazione del femore prossimale e dell'acetabolo. Il femore prossimale è vascolarizzato da vasi intraossei (*in primis* l'arteria circonflessa femorale mediale) ed extraossei (Fig. 677-1). I vasi del retinaculum (extraossei) decorrono sulla superficie del collo femorale, ma sono intracapsulari in quanto penetrano nell'epifisi dalla periferia; ciò rende l'apporto vascolare vulnerabile al danno derivante da un'artrite settica, traumi, trombosi e altri insulti vascolari.

677.1 • DISPLASIA EVOLUTIVA DELL'ANCA

La displasia evolutiva dell'anca (DDH, *Development Dysplasia of the Hip*) è uno spettro di anomalie a carico dell'anca in accrescimento. Con l'espressione "displasia acetabolare", d'altra parte, si indica una morfologia e uno sviluppo anormali dell'acetabolo. La **sublussazione** dell'anca è definita come un contatto parziale tra la testa femorale e l'acetabolo, mentre la **lussazione** si riferisce a un'anca senza contatto tra le superfici articolari dell'anca. La gamma delle presentazioni della DDH varia da una displasia acetabolare semplice (la testa femorale può essere ritenuta all'interno di un acetabolo inadeguato) a una displasia acetabolare con sublussazione (la testa femorale si allontana leggermente dalla parete acetabolare mediale), fino a una lussazione dell'articolazione dell'anca (una completa perdita di contatto tra la testa femorale e l'acetabolo).

La DDH si classifica in due gruppi principali: tipica e teratologica. La forma tipica si presenta in soggetti altrimenti normali o in quelli senza sindromi o condizioni genetiche definite. Le lussazioni dell'anca teratologiche di solito hanno cause identificabili e si verificano prima della nascita.

EZIOLOGIA, INCIDENZA E FATTORI DI RISCHIO

Anche se molti studi di screening sui neonati suggeriscono che un certo grado di instabilità dell'anca possa permanere in 1 caso su 100-250, le anche davvero lussate o lussabili sono molto meno

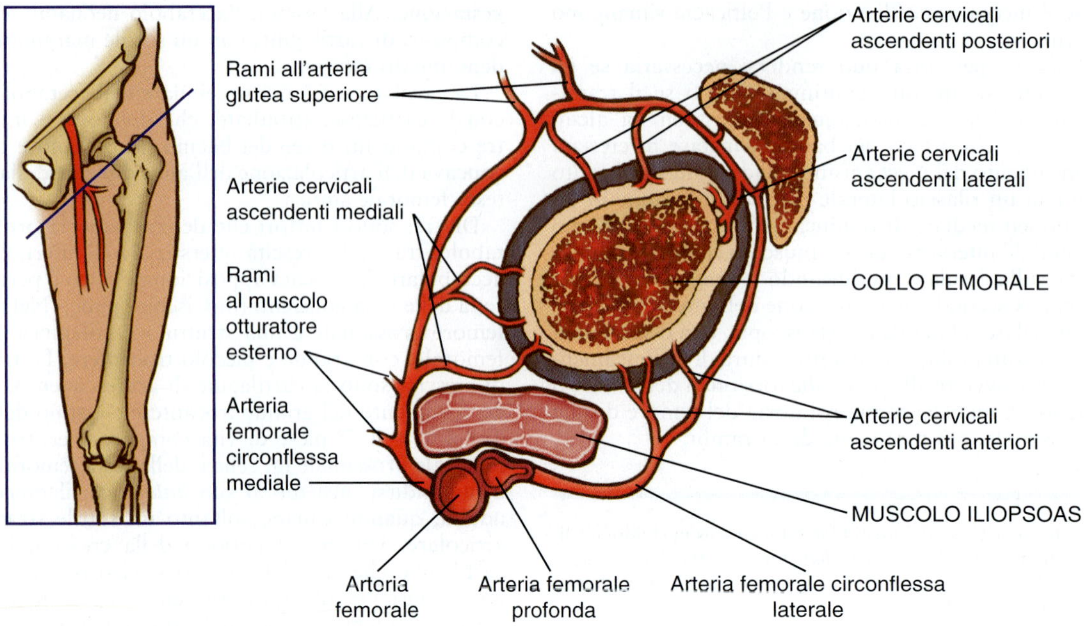

Figura 677-1. Diagramma dell'anatomia vascolare del femore prossimale.

frequenti, essendo presenti in 1-1,5/1000 nati vivi. L'eziologia della DDH è multifattoriale e comprende sia fattori genetici sia fattori ambientali intrauterini. Si osserva una marcata variabilità geografica ed etnica. L'incidenza riportata in base all'area geografica va da 1,7/1000 neonati in Svezia a 75/1000 in Iugoslavia fino a 188,5/1000 in un distretto del Manitoba, Canada. L'incidenza della DDH nei neonati cinesi e africani è quasi dello 0%, mentre è dell'1% per la displasia dell'anca e dello 0,1% per la lussazione dell'anca nei neonati bianchi. Queste differenze potrebbero essere dovute a fattori ambientali, come le pratiche di puericultura, più che a una predisposizione genetica. Tradizionalmente i genitori africani e asiatici trasportano i neonati tenendoli contro il proprio corpo, sostenuti da uno scialle, per cui le anche del bambino sono flesse, abdotte e libere di muoversi. Questa usanza mantiene le anche nella posizione ottimale per la stabilità e il modellamento dinamico dell'acetabolo in via di sviluppo da parte della testa femorale cartilaginea. Al contrario, i bambini che crescono in tutt'altro contesto culturale, tra i Nativi Americani e nell'Europa orientale, dove l'incidenza di DDH è relativamente elevata, sono sempre stati avvolti in indumenti costrittivi che mantengono le anche in estensione; questa posizione aumenta la tensione dell'unità tendine-muscolo psoas, potendo predisporre le anche a spostarsi e infine a lussarsi lateralmente e superiormente.

FATTORI DI RISCHIO DELLA DDH

Un'anamnesi familiare positiva per DDH si osserva nel 12-33% dei pazienti interessati. La DDH è più comune nelle femmine (80%), forse per la loro maggiore sensibilità agli ormoni materni come la relaxina, che aumentano la lassità legamentosa. Anche se soltanto il 2-3% di tutti i neonati nasce con una presentazione podalica, il tasso di podalismo è del 16-25% per i pazienti con DDH. Qualsiasi condizione che porti a uno spazio intrauterino più ristretto, che limita i normali movimenti fetali, può essere associata a DDH. Queste condizioni comprendono oligoidramnios, un elevato peso alla nascita e la primiparità. L'elevato tasso di associazione della DDH con altre anomalie da modellamento intrauterino, come il torcicollo e l'adduzione del metatarso, avvalora la teoria che il "fenomeno dell'affollamento" abbia un ruolo patogenetico. L'anca sinistra è la più colpita; nella posizione fetale più comune, è proprio l'anca sinistra quella solitamente forzata in adduzione contro il sacro della madre. Altri bambini con una più elevata incidenza di DDH sono quelli nati da parto cesareo e quelli ricoverati in reparti speciali dopo la nascita.

ANATOMIA PATOLOGICA

Se l'anca non è lussata alla nascita, tutte le componenti specifiche dell'articolazione dell'anca, tranne il legamento rotondo e la capsula articolare, di solito appaiono relativamente normali. Le lussazioni teratologiche sono spesso accompagnate da un acetabolo piccolo e poco profondo e da rigidità dell'articolazione dell'anca alla nascita. Nella tipica DDH non trattata, si può verificare una deformità secondaria all'alterata crescita dell'anca. Queste alterazioni possono comprendere ipertrofia della cartilagine laterale dell'acetabolo (formazione di un neolimbo), ipertrofia del legamento rotondo, lassità capsulare, costrizione a clessidra della capsula articolare dell'anca e ipertrofia del legamento acetabolare trasverso, oltre a un'eccessiva antiversione femorale. È essenziale che il medico curante sia consapevole di queste alterazioni per un trattamento efficace della DDH.

PRESENTAZIONE CLINICA

NEONATO. La diagnosi di DDH nel neonato si pone evocando il segno di Ortolani o di Barlow, oppure individuando alterazioni significative della morfologia dell'anca all'esame ecografico. L'esame obiettivo deve essere eseguito con il lattante svestito e supino, disteso su un lettino piano, in un ambiente caldo e confortevole.

La manovra di provocazione di **Barlow** valuta la possibilità di lussazione di un'anca non lussata. L'esaminatore adduce l'anca flessa e spinge delicatamente la coscia posteriormente, tentando di lussare la testa femorale (Fig. 677-2). Se il test è positivo, si percepirà lo scivolamento della testa femorale fuori dall'acetabolo. Quando l'esaminatore smette di esercitare la spinta prossimale, si può percepire il rientro dell'anca nell'acetabolo.

Il test di **Ortolani** è la manovra contraria rispetto al test di Barlow e consiste nel tentativo di ridurre un'anca lussata (Fig. 677-3). L'esaminatore afferra la coscia del bambino tra pollice e indice e con il 4° e 5° dito solleva il grande trocantere abducendo contemporaneamente l'anca. Quando il test è positivo, la testa femorale scivola nella cavità articolare con un "clunk" delicato che è palpabile ma di solito non udibile. Deve essere una manovra delicata e non forzata.

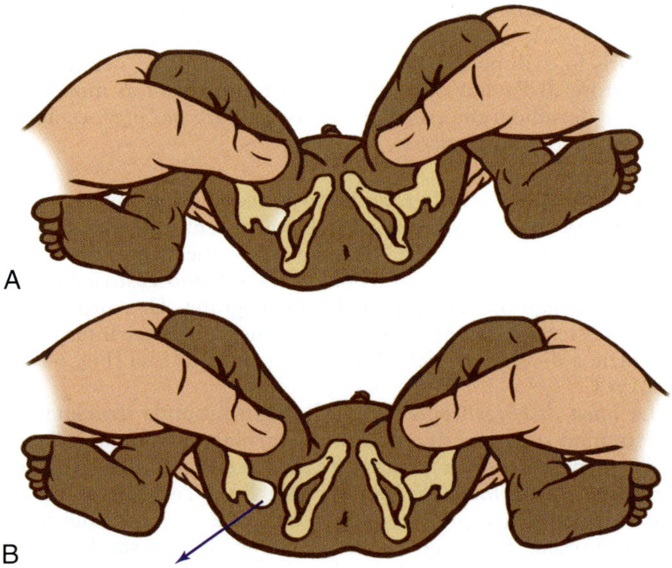

Figura 677-2. Il test di provocazione di Barlow si esegue con le ginocchia e le anche del paziente in flessione. *A*, Afferrare delicatamente gli arti del paziente; con la coscia in adduzione, l'esaminatore esercita una forza diretta posteriormente. *B*, Questo test è positivo in un'anca lussabile.

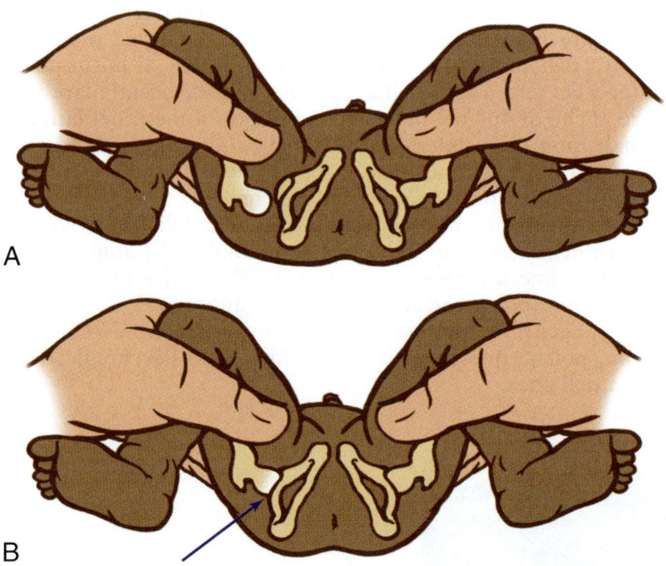

Figura 677-3. La manovra di Ortolani è il segno che la testa femorale si sposta fuori e dentro l'acetabolo. *A*, L'esaminatore afferra la coscia del paziente e abduce delicatamente l'anca sollevando il grande trocantere con due dita. *B*, Quando il test è positivo, la testa femorale lussata ricade nell'acetabolo con un clunk percepibile successivamente all'abduzione dell'anca.

Il **click dell'anca** è la sensazione (o suono) di elevata intensità che si percepisce al termine dell'abduzione nel corso del test per la DDH con le manovre di Barlow e Ortolani. Classicamente è diverso dal clunk dell'anca, che viene percepito con l'entrata e l'uscita della testa femorale dall'articolazione. I click dell'anca di solito hanno origine dal legamento rotondo, talvolta dalla fascia lata o dal tendine dello psoas, e non sono indicativi di una significativa anormalità dell'anca.

LATTANTE. Quando il neonato entra nella 2-3ª settimana di vita, compaiono altri segni di DDH.

Quando l'anca non è più riducibile, compaiono specifici segni fisici, compresi una limitazione dell'abduzione dell'anca, un apparente accorciamento della coscia, una localizzazione prossimale del grande trocantere, un'asimmetria delle pliche glutee o della coscia (Fig. 677-4) e un movimento a pistone dell'anca. Una limitazione dell'abduzione è il segno più affidabile di lussazione dell'anca.

L'accorciamento della coscia, il *segno di Galeazzi*, si apprezza nel modo migliore ponendo entrambe le anche in flessione a 90° e confrontando l'altezza dei ginocchi alla ricerca di un'asimmetria (Fig. 677-5). Un'asimmetria delle pliche glutee e della coscia è suggestiva di DDH, pur potendo essere presente nel 10% dei lattanti normali. Un'altra indagine utile è il *test di Klisic*, in cui l'esaminatore pone il 3° dito sopra il grande trocantere e il dito indice della stessa mano sulla spina iliaca anterosuperiore. Nell'anca normale una linea immaginaria tracciata tra le due dita punta verso l'ombelico. Nell'anca lussata il trocantere si trova più in alto e la linea si proietta a metà strada tra l'ombelico e il pube (Fig. 677-6).

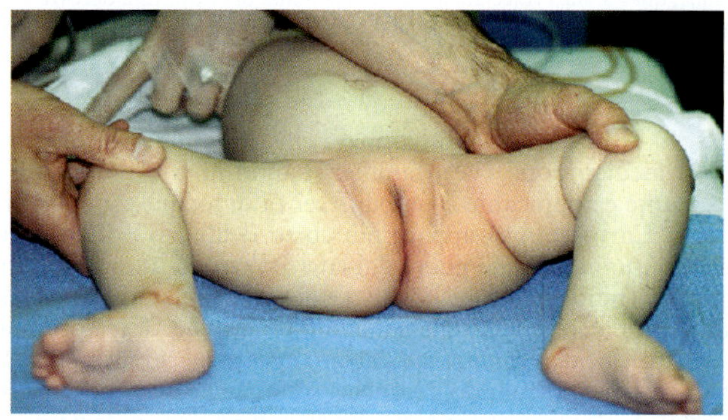

Figura 677-4. Asimmetria delle pliche della coscia in un bambino con displasia evolutiva dell'anca.

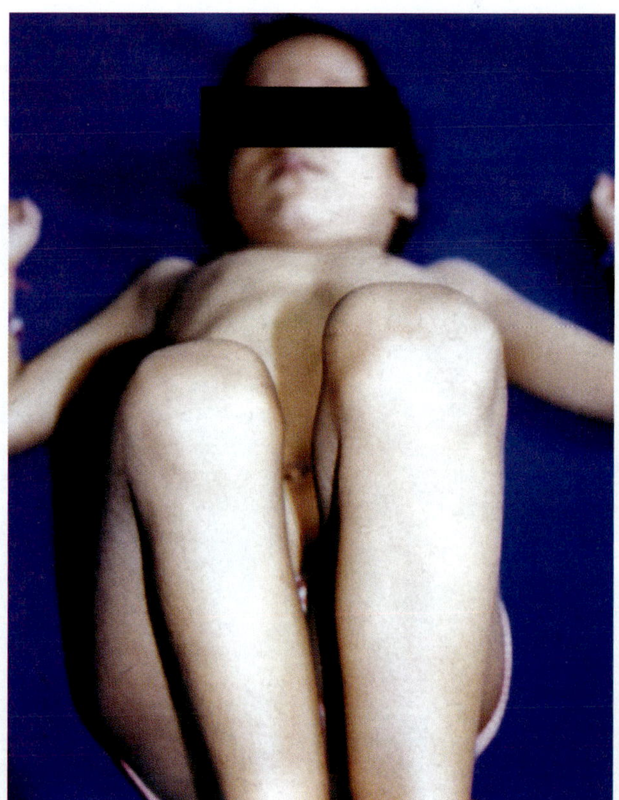

Figura 677-5. Segno di Galeazzi positivo in un caso di displasia evolutiva dell'anca non trattata.

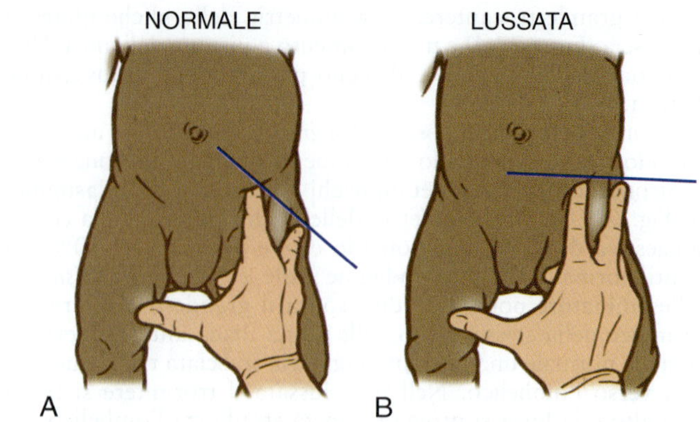

Figura 677-6. Test di Klisic. *A*, In un'anca normale, una linea immaginaria tracciata verso il basso attraverso la punta del dito indice posizionato sulla cresta iliaca del paziente e la punta del dito medio posizionato sul grande trocantere del paziente deve puntare verso l'ombelico. *B*, In caso di lussazione dell'anca, questa linea tracciata attraverso la punta delle due dita decorre sotto l'ombelico in quanto il grande trocantere è più alto del normale.

BAMBINO CHE CAMMINA. Il bambino che cammina spesso si presenta al medico dopo che i familiari hanno notato un'andatura ondeggiante e zoppicante o una differenza di lunghezza degli arti inferiori. L'arto colpito appare più corto dell'altro e il soggetto tende a camminare sulle punte dal lato affetto. In questi bambini il segno di Trendelenburg è positivo e di solito si osserva un'andatura di Trendelenburg. Come nel bambino più piccolo, è presente una limitazione dell'abduzione dal lato affetto e le ginocchia sono a livelli differenti quando le anche sono in flessione (segno di Galeazzi). Un'eccessiva lordosi, che si sviluppa secondariamente all'alterazione della meccanica dell'anca, è comune e spesso costituisce il sintomo di presentazione.

ALTERAZIONI RADIOGRAFICHE

ECOGRAFIA. Nei lattanti con meno di 6 mesi di vita l'acetabolo e il femore prossimale sono prevalentemente cartilaginei, non sono visibili radiograficamente e sono meglio visualizzabili all'ecografia. Oltre alla valutazione morfologica, l'ecografia consente una valutazione dinamica della stabilità dell'articolazione dell'anca (Figg. 677-7*A*, *B*). Questa indagine può essere usata per monitorare lo sviluppo dell'acetabolo, in particolare nei neonati con tutore di Pavlik, oltre a consentire di ridurre al minimo il numero di radiografie eseguite e di identificare più precocemente un fallimento terapeutico.

RADIOGRAFIA. Le radiografie sono raccomandate nel lattante allorché avviene l'ossificazione dell'epifisi femorale prossimale, di solito entro i 4-6 mesi. Nei soggetti di questa età, gli esami radiografici si sono dimostrati più efficaci, meno costosi e meno dipendenti dall'operatore rispetto all'ecografia. Una proiezione anteroposteriore dell'immagine del bacino può essere interpretata grazie a diverse classiche linee tracciate su di essa (Fig. 677-8 da *A* a *C*).

La *linea di Hilgenreiner* è una linea orizzontale tracciata tra le estremità superiori di entrambe le cartilagini triradiate (l'area radiotrasparente nella profondità dell'acetabolo). Perpendicolare a essa è la *linea di Perkins*, una linea verticale tracciata attraverso la parte più laterale del margine ossificato del tetto dell'acetabolo. Il nucleo di ossificazione della testa femorale deve essere localizzato nel quadrante inferiore mediale dell'intersezione di queste due linee. La *linea di Shenton* è una linea ricurva tracciata dall'aspetto mediale del collo femorale fino al margine inferiore del ramo pubico superiore; in un bambino con anche normali ha un profilo continuo, mentre in un bambino con DDH è formata da due archi separati e viene quindi definita "interrotta". L'*indice acetabolare* è l'angolo formato dalla linea di Hilgenreiner e una linea tracciata dalla profondità della cavità acetabolare fino alla parte più laterale del margine ossificato del tetto dell'acetabolo. Quest'angolo consente di misurare lo sviluppo del tetto osseo dell'acetabolo. L'indice acetabolare può essere anche di 40° nel neonato, ma dopo i 4 mesi, nel lattante normale, non deve superare i 30°. Nel bambino più grande, un parametro utile per misurare la posizione dell'anca è l'*angolo centro-margine*, formato dall'intersezione della linea di Perkins e da una linea che unisce il margine laterale dell'acetabolo con il centro della testa femorale. Nei bambini di 6-13 anni, è stato riportato come normale un angolo >19°, mentre nei bambini di 14 o più anni è considerato tale un angolo >25°. Occorre eseguire anche radiografie dell'anca in abduzione e rotazione interna, poiché queste proiezioni evidenziano l'eventuale riducibilità dell'anca.

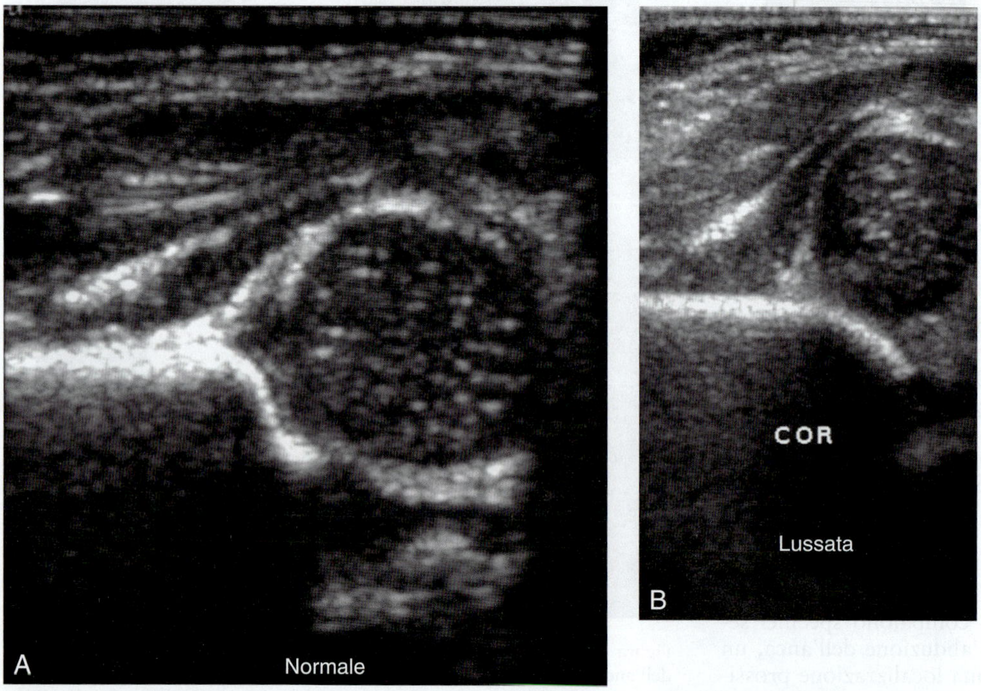

Figura 677-7. Immagini ecografiche normali di un lattante (*A*) a confronto con un caso di displasia evolutiva dell'anca (*B*).

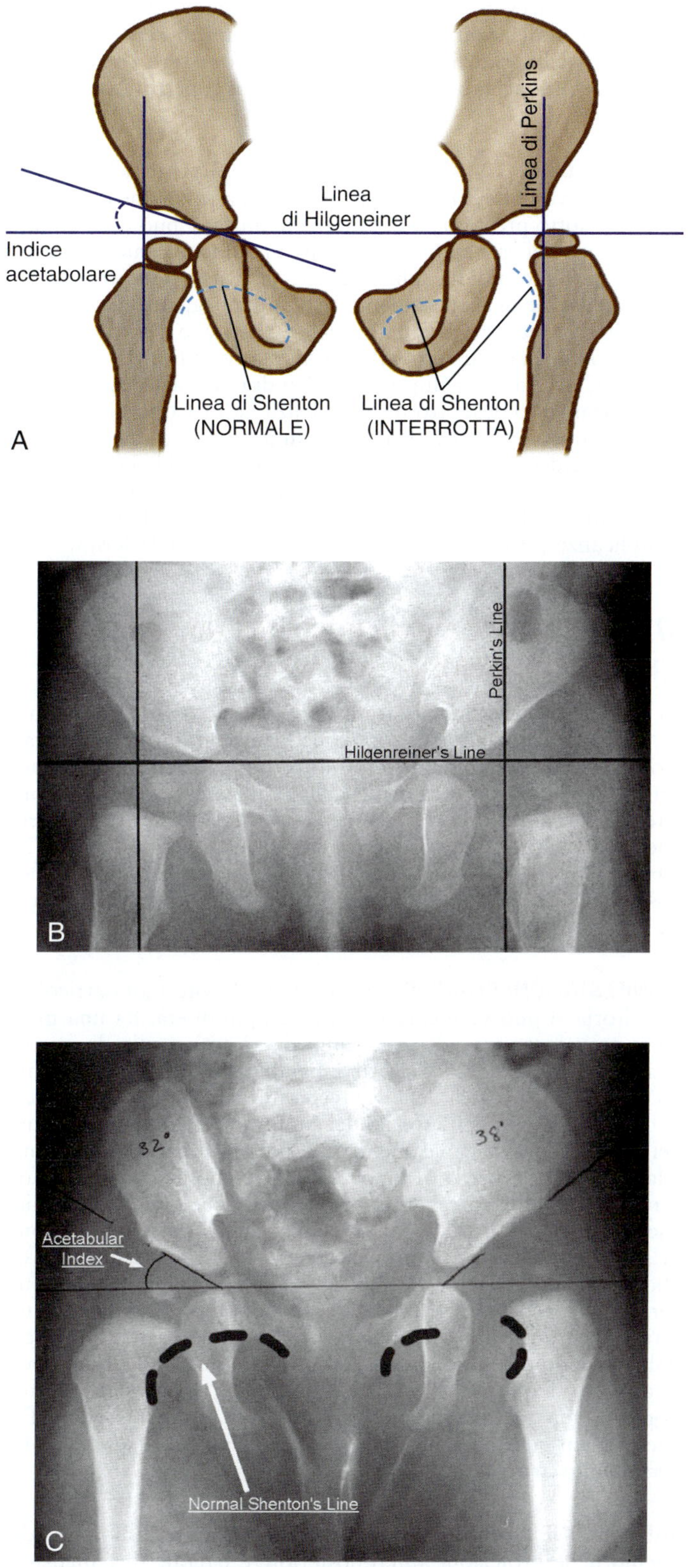

Figura 677-8. Le misure radiografiche sono utili per la valutazione della DDH. La linea di Hilgenreiner (*Hilgenreiner Line*) passa attraverso le cartilagini triradiate. La linea di Perkins (*Perkins Line*) è tracciata perpendicolarmente alla linea di Hilgenreiner al margine laterale dell'acetabolo. Il nucleo di ossificazione della testa femorale dovrebbe essere situato nel quadrante mediale inferiore all'intersezione di queste due linee. La linea di Shenton ha un andamento curvo lungo la metafisi femorale e si unisce con il margine interno del pube formando un angolo smusso. Nel bambino con DDH, questa linea è formata da due archi separati e viene quindi definita "interrotta". L'indice acetabolare (*Acetabular Index*) è l'angolo tra una linea tracciata lungo il margine dell'acetabolo e la linea di Hilgenreiner; è in media di 27,5° nei neonati normali e diminuisce con l'età. *Normal Shenton's Line*, linea di Shelton normale.

TRATTAMENTO

Scopo del trattamento della DDH è ottenere e mantenere una riduzione concentrica della testa femorale all'interno dell'acetabolo onde fornire l'ambiente ottimale per il normale sviluppo sia della testa femorale sia dell'acetabolo. Più la diagnosi di DDH è tardiva, più difficile risulta raggiungere questo obiettivo, minore è il potenziale di rimodellamento dell'acetabolo e del femore prossimale e più si rendono necessari trattamenti complessi.

NEONATI E LATTANTI DI ETÀ INFERIORE AI 6 MESI DI VITA. L'ideale sarebbe che la diagnosi di DDH avvenisse nella nursery neonatale. Nel neonato non è utile l'uso di tripli pannolini o di pannolini che provocano abduzione; essi di solito sono inefficaci e danno alla famiglia un falso senso di sicurezza. Per tutti i gradi di displasia dell'anca in neonati altrimenti normali si ricorre al divaricatore di Pavlik, che rimane lo strumento più usato in tutto il mondo (Fig. 677-9), nonostante oggi siano disponibili anche altre ortesi (splint di Van Rosen, cuscino di Frejka). Esso va prontamente applicato ai lattanti di 1-6 mesi di vita con displasia dell'anca, sublussazione o lussazione. Mantenendo l'anca positiva al test di Ortolani in un divaricatore di Pavlik per un periodo di 6 settimane, giorno e notte, l'instabilità dell'anca si risolve nel 95% dei casi. Dopo i 6 mesi di età, il tasso di fallimento di questo apparecchio è >50% in quanto il bambino diventa sempre più attivo e mobile; sono necessarie visite e rivalutazioni frequenti per accertarsi che il divaricatore sia indossato correttamente.

BAMBINI DA 6 MESI A 2 ANNI DI ETÀ. Se la diagnosi è stata tardiva, obiettivo principale del trattamento sarà ottenere e mantenere la riduzione dell'anca senza danneggiare la testa femorale.

Le *riduzioni chiuse* vengono eseguite in sala operatoria, in anestesia generale. L'anca viene mobilizzata per determinare l'arco di movimento nel quale rimane ridotta, che viene poi confrontato con l'arco di movimento massimo per stabilire una "zona di sicurezza" (Fig. 677-10). Un'artrografia eseguita al momento della riduzione è molto utile per valutare la profondità e la stabilità della riduzione (Fig. 677-11). La riduzione è mantenuta

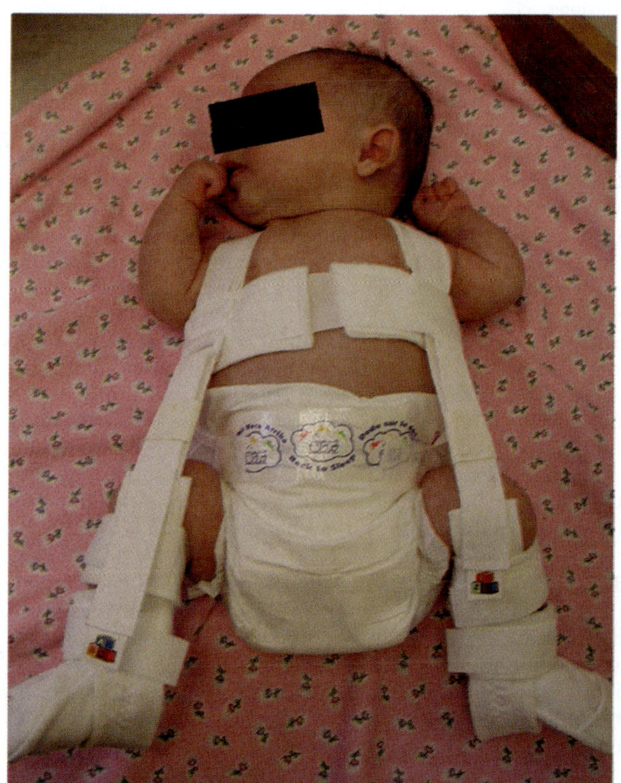

Figura 677-9. Divaricatore di Pavlik.

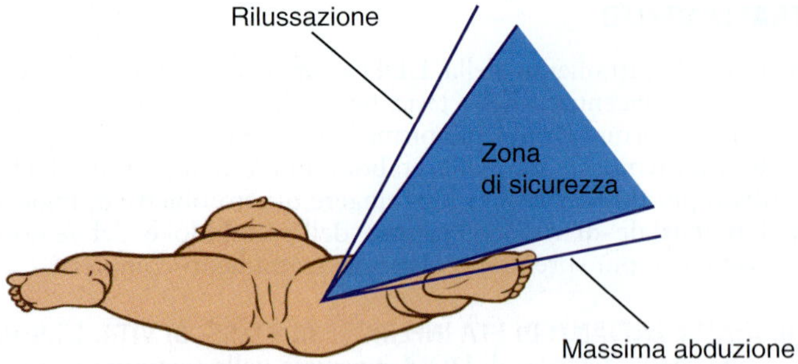

Figura 677-10. Illustrazione schematica della zona di sicurezza di Ramsey.

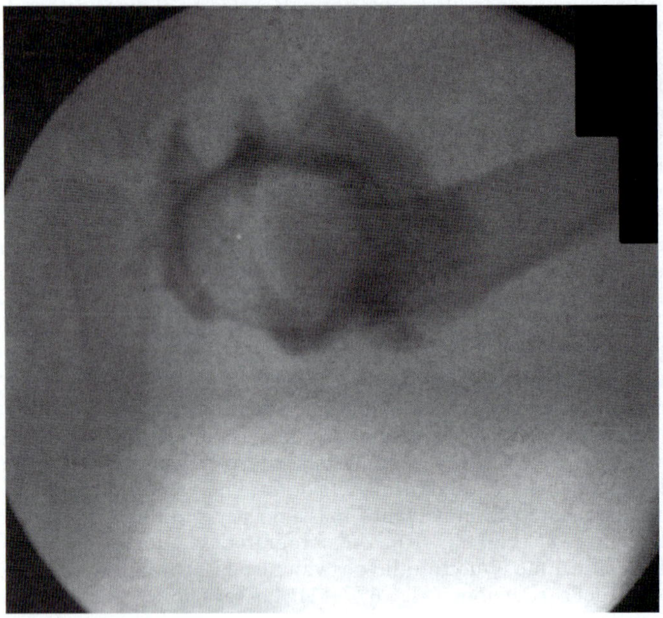

Figura 677-11. Artrografia di un'anca ridotta che serve a valutare la stabilità della riduzione.

con un gesso accuratamente modellato, e la "posizione umana" in flessione e abduzione moderate è quella preferita. Dopo la procedura, si possono eseguire una TC con scansione singola, una RM o un'ecografia per la conferma della riduzione. Dodici settimane dopo la riduzione chiusa, il gesso viene rimosso e sostituito da un'ortesi in abduzione da utilizzare giorno e notte per 2 mesi, finché lo sviluppo acetabolare non sarà normale. Se non si ottiene un'anca stabile con una riduzione chiusa, occorre eseguire una *riduzione aperta*. Nei pazienti di età <2 anni, raramente è necessaria una procedura acetabolare o femorale secondaria. Il potenziale di sviluppo acetabolare dopo una riduzione chiusa o aperta è eccellente e continua a distanza di 4-8 anni dalla procedura.

C'è infine chi raccomanda una *trazione*, seguita da una riduzione chiusa o aperta, per il trattamento dei lattanti più grandi con lussazione dell'anca nei quali il tentativo di riduzione con divaricatore di Pavlik è fallito o nei bambini di età >9 mesi.

BAMBINI DI ETÀ SUPERIORE AI 2 ANNI. Il trattamento dei bambini di età compresa tra i 2 e i 6 anni con lussazione dell'anca è più difficile. In questo gruppo di pazienti si rende spesso necessaria la riduzione aperta.

Nei bambini con più di 3 anni di età, l'accorciamento femorale per evitare un'eccessiva pressione sul femore prossimale consente tassi molto più bassi di disturbi della crescita del femore prossimale rispetto alla trazione preliminare seguita da una riduzione aperta. Nei bambini tra i 2 e i 3 anni, dal momento che il potenziale si sviluppo acetabolare è marcatamente diminuito, può essere necessaria una contemporanea procedura acetabolare in associazione alla riduzione aperta. I bambini di età >3 anni al momento della riduzione di solito devono essere sottoposti a una procedura acetabolare per un'adeguata copertura della testa femorale.

SEQUELE E COMPLICANZE. La principale complicanza della DDH è la necrosi avascolare della testa femorale. La riduzione della testa femorale sotto pressione o in estrema abduzione può determinare l'occlusione dei vasi epifisari e causare un infarto totale o parziale della testa femorale. Fa subito seguito la rivascolarizzazione, ma se la cartilagine di accrescimento è stata danneggiata gravemente, possono conseguirne anomalie della crescita e dello sviluppo. Pertanto, l'anca è più vulnerabile a questa complicanza prima dei 4-6 mesi, quando si sviluppa il nucleo di ossificazione.

Il trattamento descritto in precedenza ha lo scopo di minimizzare questa complicanza. Per mezzo di diversi trattamenti appropriati, l'incidenza di necrosi avascolare nella DDH si è ridotta al 5-15%. Altre complicanze della DDH comprendono la rilussazione, una sublussazione residua, una displasia dell'acetabolo e complicanze postoperatorie, tra cui l'infezione della ferita.

677.2 • Sinovite monoarticolare transitoria (sinovite tossica)

La sinovite monoarticolare transitoria, o sinovite tossica dell'anca, è una causa comune di zoppia nel bambino normale. È caratterizzata dall'esordio acuto di dolore, zoppia e lieve limitazione del movimento, specificamente dell'abduzione e della rotazione interna. Tuttavia, occorre escludere un'artrite settica e un'osteomielite dell'anca prima di confermare questa diagnosi (vedi Capitoli 683 e 684). L'origine della sinovite tossica è incerta; alcune possibili cause sono una sindrome virale sistemica attiva o recente, un trauma e un'ipersensibilità allergica.

MANIFESTAZIONI CLINICHE. Anche se la sinovite monoarticolare transitoria si può verificare in tutti i gruppi di età, ha una maggiore prevalenza tra i 3 e gli 8 anni di età (età media di esordio 6 anni). Il 70% circa di tutti i bambini affetti ha presentato un'infezione aspecifica delle vie respiratorie di durata superiore a 7-14 giorni prima dell'esordio dei sintomi. Questo esordio acuto dei sintomi consiste tipicamente in dolore localizzato all'inguine, alla coscia anteriore o al ginocchio, oltre che in un dolore non traumatico della parte anteriore della coscia o del ginocchio, che può essere riferito a partire dall'anca. Questi bambini sono di solito deambulanti; l'anca in genere non è mantenuta flessa, abdotta o ruotata lateralmente, a meno che non sia presente un versamento articolare significativo. I bambini con sinovite monoarticolare transitoria deambulano con un'andatura zoppicante e dolorosa. Inoltre, sono spesso afebbrili o hanno una febbre lieve, al di sotto dei 38 °C. I valori di laboratorio sono relativamente normali, ma talvolta si osserva un lieve aumento della VES. Mentre l'artrocentesi produce risultati normali, è comune un versamento articolare di 1-3 mL.

VALUTAZIONE RADIOGRAFICA. Si possono eseguire radiografie del bacino nelle proiezioni anteroposteriore e laterale di Lauenstein (a rana), che di solito sono normali. L'ecografia dell'anca evidenzia un versamento nell'articolazione dell'anca. L'aspirazione del fluido articolare sotto guida ecografica può essere necessaria per rivelare la presenza di un'anca settica in alcuni casi clinici. Anche la scintigrafia ossea con Tecnezio o la RM sono estremamente utili per escludere la presenza di determinate lesioni, tra cui artrite settica, tumori, fratture, epifisiolisi della testa femorale (SCFE, *Slipped Capital Femoral Epiphysis*) o una malattia di Legg-Calvé-Perthes (LCPD, *Legg-Calvé-Perthes Disease*) in fase iniziale. La presenza di febbre elevata, rifiuto del cammino e un aumento della VES, della proteina C-reattiva e della conta leucocitaria sono tutti criteri di rischio elevato per un'artrite settica.

TRATTAMENTO. Il trattamento della sinovite monoarticolare transitoria dell'anca è sintomatico. Le terapie raccomandate comprendono la limitazione dell'attività e lo scarico del peso fino alla scomparsa del dolore. I farmaci antinfiammatori e analgesici possono abbreviare la durata del dolore. La maggior parte dei bambini guarisce completamente nel giro di 3 settimane.

677.3 • Malattia di Legg-Calvé-Perthes

La LCPD è una patologia a carico della testa femorale, di eziologia sconosciuta, consistente nell'interruzione temporanea della vascolarizzazione del nucleo osseo dell'epifisi femorale prossimale, che determina un'alterazione della crescita epifisaria e una deformità della testa femorale.

EZIOLOGIA

L'eziologia della LCPD rimane sconosciuta. Sono state proposte come cause infezioni, traumi e sinovite transitoria, ma il loro ruolo non è stato provato. Sono stati identificati fattori che determinano trombofilia, un'aumentata tendenza allo sviluppo di trombosi e ipofibrinolisi e una ridotta tendenza alla lisi dei trombi. La mutazione del fattore V di Leiden, il deficit delle proteine C e S, l'anticoagulante lupico, gli anticorpi anticardiolipina, l'antitripsina e l'attivatore del plasminogeno possono avere un ruolo nell'anomalia del meccanismo della coagulazione.

I bambini con LCPD presentano un ritardo della maturazione scheletrica e sono più bassi del normale. Sono state segnalate anomalie degli ormoni tiroidei e dei fattori di crescita insulino-simili. Altri fattori associati comprendono il disordine da iperattività o deficit di attenzione, influenze ereditarie e influenze ambientali (tra cui la nutrizione). Gli aspetti istologici della CFE rivelano diversi stadi di necrosi e riparazione ossea. Sono stati proposti due possibili meccanismi per la necrosi tissutale; le alterazioni vascolari possono essere l'evento o gli eventi primari, oppure vi può essere un disordine primitivo della cartilagine epifisaria con conseguente collasso e necrosi.

La necrosi avascolare della testa femorale, non correlata alla LCPD, può essere sporadica, ma occasionalmente si verifica come disordine autosomico dominante. La maggior parte dei casi si presenta in età adulta, ma il 10-20% dei casi può esordire a un'età <20 anni. I casi familiari possono essere dovuti a una mutazione del gene del collagene di tipo II.

PATOGENESI DELLA DEFORMITÀ

Nella LCPD la deformità può verificarsi in seguito a quattro meccanismi.

Il 1° consiste in un disturbo di crescita della CFE e della cartilagine di accrescimento; un arresto centrale della cartilagine di accrescimento porta alla formazione di un collo corto (coxa brevis) e a un'eccessiva crescita trocanterica, mentre un suo arresto laterale inclina la testa esternamente e in valgo, con eccessiva crescita trocanterica.

Il 2° meccanismo coinvolge il processo di riparazione stesso; la deformità può comparire in seguito al processo di riparazione asimmetrica e alle sollecitazioni applicate alla testa femorale.

Il 3° meccanismo è correlato al processo patologico. Gli strati superficiali della cartilagine articolare continuano a "crescere eccessivamente" in quanto sono nutriti dal liquido sinoviale. Tuttavia, gli strati profondi sono devitalizzati dal processo patologico, con collasso trabecolare epifisario e deformità.

Il 4° meccanismo è iatrogeno, causato dal tentativo di contenere, sia chirurgicamente sia non chirurgicamente, una testa femorale non contenibile.

EPIDEMIOLOGIA

L'incidenza globale di LCPD negli Stati Uniti è di circa 1/1200 bambini. Questa patologia è più comune nei maschi rispetto alle femmine, con un rapporto di 4-5:1. Il suo picco di incidenza si situa tra i 4 e gli 8 anni; è stata riportata in pazienti di 2-12 anni di età. Nel 10% circa dei pazienti si può osservare un interessamento bilaterale, ma i CFE presentano solitamente gradi diversi di collasso.

PRESENTAZIONE CLINICA

Il più comune sintomo di presentazione è una **zoppia** di durata variabile. Il dolore, se presente, è di solito correlato all'attività e può essere localizzato a livello dell'inguine oppure riferito alla parte anteromediale della coscia o alla regione del ginocchio. Se il medico non si rende conto che il dolore alla coscia o al ginocchio nel bambino può essere secondario alla patologia dell'anca, la diagnosi può essere ulteriormente ritardata. È meno comune che l'esordio della malattia sia molto più acuto e associato all'impossibilità di camminare. I genitori spesso riferiscono che i sintomi sono stati scatenati da un evento traumatico.

ESAME OBIETTIVO

Un'andatura antalgica può essere particolarmente evidente alla fine della giornata, dopo un'attività intensa. I movimenti dell'anca, in particolare la rotazione interna e l'abduzione, sono limitati. Nelle prime fasi della malattia, la limitazione dell'abduzione è secondaria alla sinovite e allo spasmo muscolare del gruppo degli adduttori; tuttavia, con il tempo e le conseguenti deformità che possono svilupparsi, essa può divenire permanente. Può essere presente una lieve contrattura in flessione dell'anca (10-20°). È possibile riscontrare un'atrofia dei muscoli della coscia, del polpaccio o delle natiche, da disuso secondario al dolore. Può essere presente un'apparente differenza di lunghezza tra gli arti inferiori, dovuta a una contrattura in adduzione, o un reale accorciamento dell'arto interessato, a causa del collasso della testa femorale o dell'inibizione della crescita. Il classico bambino con LCPD è piccolo, magro, estremamente attivo (corre e salta in continuazione).

ASPETTI RADIOGRAFICI

Le radiografie di routine sono il primo strumento diagnostico nella LCPD. Le proiezioni in anteroposteriore e quelle laterali di Lauenstein (a rana) sono utilizzate per la diagnosi, la stadiazione, la prognosi e il follow-up della malattia, e per valutare i risultati del trattamento (Fig. 677-12*A*, *B*). Per seguire il decorso della malattia è particolarmente importante che tutte le radiografie siano esaminate in sequenza e confrontate con le radiografie precedenti, così da valutare lo stadio del processo riparativo e determinare la costanza dell'estensione dell'interessamento epifisario. In assenza di alterazioni radiografiche, in particolare nelle prime fasi della malattia, una scintigrafia ossea con Tecnezio-99m può rivelare la condizione avascolare della CFE. La RM è sensibile per la diagnosi degli infarti ossei, ma non è in grado di delineare con precisione gli stadi della guarigione. Il suo ruolo nel trattamento della LCPD non è stato definito. L'artrografia può dimostrare qualsiasi appiattimento della testa femorale e il fenomeno della *hinge abduction* con l'abduzione della gamba.

STADI RADIOGRAFICI. La LCPD è stata suddivisa in quattro stadi radiografici: iniziale, di frammentazione, di riossificazione (o riparazione) e residuale (o di guarigione). Nello stadio iniziale, le alterazioni radiografiche comprendono una diminuzione delle dimensioni del centro di ossificazione, una lateralizzazione della testa femorale con allargamento dello spazio articolare mediale, una frattura subcondrale e irregolarità della cartilagine di accrescimento. Nello stadio della frammentazione, l'epifisi appare frammentata, con aree di aumentata radiotrasparenza e radiodensità. Nel corso dello stadio di riossificazione, la densità ossea ritorna normale mediante neoformazione ossea. Lo stadio residuale è contraddistinto dalla riossificazione della testa femorale,

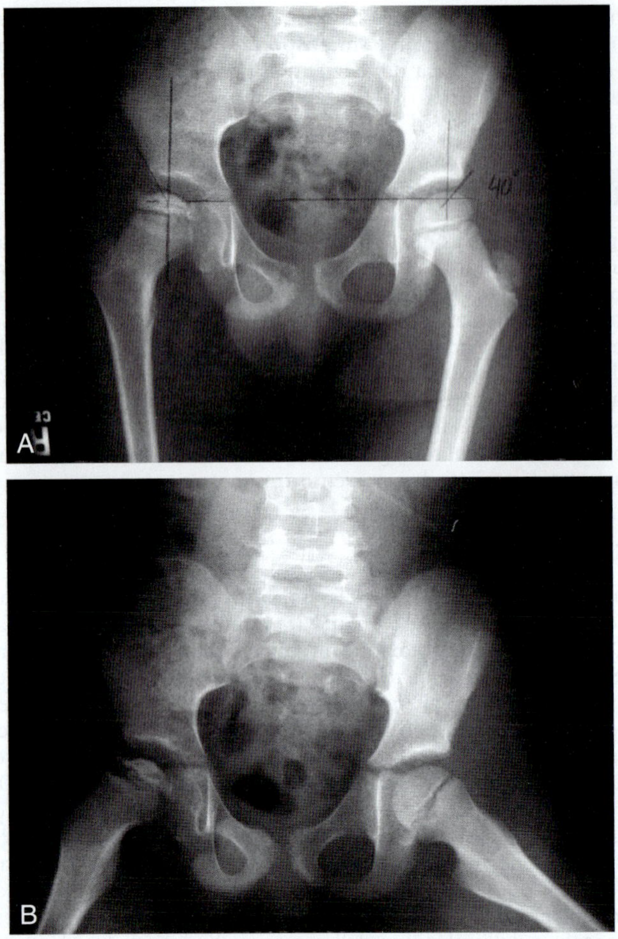

Figura 677-12. *A*, Radiografia anteroposteriore del bacini che evidenzia una frammentazione epifisaria dell'anca destra, caratteristicamente della fase di frammentazione della LCPD. *B*, La proiezione laterale a rana dimostra una frattura subcondrale, un aumento della densità della testa femorale e un certo grado di collasso.

dal graduale rimodellamento della forma della testa femorale fino alla maturità scheletrica e dal rimodellamento dell'acetabolo.

SISTEMI DI CLASSIFICAZIONE. *Catterall* ha proposto una classificazione in quattro gruppi, basata sul grado di CFE e una serie di segni radiografici di "testa a rischio", con un elevato grado di variabilità interosservatore. Le anche del gruppo I presentano un interessamento anteriore del 25%, assenza di sequestro e assenza di anomalie metafisarie. Le anche del gruppo II sono interessate fino al 50%, con una chiara demarcazione tra i segmenti colpiti e quelli indenni. Possono essere presenti cisti metafisarie. Le anche del gruppo III presentano un interessamento fino al 75% con un ampio sequestro. Nel gruppo IV, è coinvolta l'intera testa femorale.

Una classificazione in due gruppi si basa sull'estensione della frattura sottocondrale che corrisponde all'entità del successivo riassorbimento. Nel gruppo A di *Salter-Thompson*, è interessata meno della metà della testa femorale (gruppi I e II di Catterall), mentre nel gruppo B è coinvolta più di metà della testa femorale (gruppi III e III di Catterall). Il principale fattore che determina la distinzione tra i gruppi A e B è la presenza o assenza di una colonna laterale dell'epifisi vitale. Questa colonna laterale intatta (gruppo II di Catterall, gruppo A) può difendere l'epifisi dal collasso e dalla conseguente deformità.

Uno svantaggio di tale classificazione è che non tutti i pazienti ricevono una diagnosi precoce durante la fase della frattura subcondrale.

Il sistema del pilastro laterale di *Herring*, la classificazione radiografica più utilizzata per determinare trattamento e prognosi durante la fase attiva della malattia (Fig. 677-13), si basa su

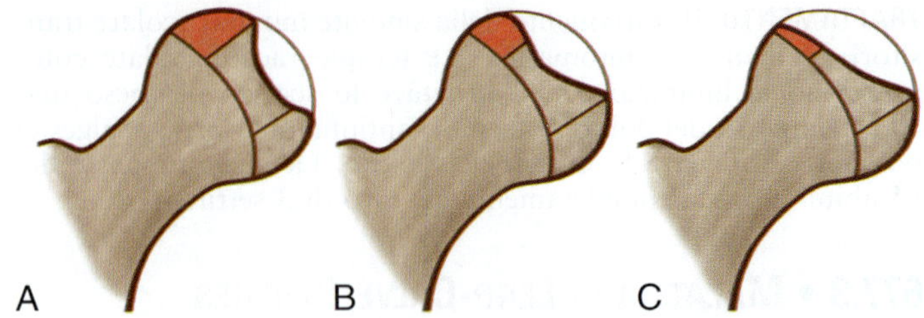

Figura 677-13. Classificazione del pilastro laterale per la LCPD. *A*, Il pilastro laterale non è interessato. *B*, Permane più del 50% dell'altezza del pilastro laterale. C, Permane meno del 50% dell'altezza del pilastro laterale.

diverse radiografie eseguite nella fase precoce della frammentazione. Il sistema di classificazione del pilastro laterale per la LCPD valuta la forma dell'epifisi della testa femorale alla radiografia anteroposteriore dell'anca. La testa è suddivisa in tre sezioni o pilastri: il pilastro laterale occupa il 15-30% della larghezza della testa, il pilastro centrale il 50% circa e il pilastro mediale il 20-35%. A seconda del grado di interessamento del pilastro laterale si distinguono tre gruppi: nel gruppo A il pilastro laterale è radiograficamente normale; nel gruppo B esso presenta un certo grado di radiotrasparenza ma conserva >50% della sua altezza; nel gruppo C il pilastro laterale è più radiotrasparente che nel gruppo B e conserva <50% della sua altezza.

FATTORI PROGNOSTICI. Determinati segni radiografici, noti come "segni a rischio", sono associati a risultati sfavorevoli. Questi comprendono il segno di Gage, una radiotrasparenza della metafisi e dell'epifisi laterale, una calcificazione laterale all'epifisi, una sublussazione laterale della CFE e una cartilagine di accrescimento orizzontale.

STORIA NATURALE E PROGNOSI

Da un punto di vista prognostico, gli studi di follow-up a lungo termine dei pazienti con LCPD evidenziano come la maggior parte delle anche non presenti problemi fino alla 5ª decade di vita. La maggior parte dei pazienti è attiva, non presenta dolore e ha un buon arco di movimento. La deformità e la congruenza alla maturità e l'età all'esordio sono i principali fattori prognostici per la LCPD. I bambini che sviluppano segni e sintomi prima dell'età di 5 anni tendono a guarire senza problemi residui. I pazienti con più di 9 anni di età alla presentazione hanno di solito una prognosi sfavorevole. Il potenziale di rimodellamento è più elevato nei bambini più piccoli; la forma della testa femorale può significativamente migliorare fino alla maturità. L'estensione dell'interessamento della CFE e la durata del processo patologico sono ulteriori fattori associati a una prognosi sfavorevole. Le anche classificate come gruppi di Catterall III e IV, gruppo B di Salter-Thompson e gruppo C del pilastro laterale sono a rischio di una prognosi sfavorevole.

TRATTAMENTO

Obiettivo del trattamento nella LCPD è creare una testa femorale sferica e ben coperta, con un arco di movimento dell'anca vicino a quello normale. I due principi terapeutici fondamentali sono il mantenimento dell'arco di movimento e il contenimento acetabolare della testa femorale durante il periodo attivo della malattia. I metodi terapeutici comprendono la semplice osservazione, il trattamento sintomatico intermittente, il contenimento, la chirurgia definitiva della deformità e la chirurgia tardiva per l'osteomielite.

TRATTAMENTO NON OPERATORIO. La pietra angolare del trattamento è un atteggiamento conservativo, in particolare con limitazione dell'attività e fisioterapia per mantenere l'arco di movimento dell'anca. I pazienti con dolore severo possono trarre beneficio da un breve periodo di riposo a letto con trazione. Sono stati utilizzati ortesi in abduzione per mantenere la testa femorale all'interno dell'acetabolo. L'ortesi in abduzione più utilizzata è l'ortesi Atlanta Scottish Rite. Questi apparecchi, concepiti per il contenimento mediante la sola abduzione, senza rotazione interna fissa, sono considerati inefficaci e non vengono usati comunemente.

TRATTAMENTO OPERATORIO. Il contenimento chirurgico può prevedere un approccio dal lato femorale, dal lato acetabolare o da entrambi i lati dell'articolazione dell'anca. La procedura più comune è l'*osteotomia in varo* del femore prossimale. L'*osteotomia pelvica* nella LCPD si suddivide in tre categorie: osteotomie rotazionali acetabolari, procedure *shelf*, spostamento mediale o osteotomie di Chiari. Tutte queste procedure possono essere associate a un'osteotomia femorale prossimale in varo quando non è possibile ottenere il contenimento di una deformità severa della testa femorale mediante la sola osteotomia femorale pelvica o prossimale in varo.

677.4 • Epifisiolisi della testa femorale

La SCFE è una patologia dell'anca che interessa gli adolescenti, per lo più tra i 12 e i 15 anni di età, e consiste nello spostamento della CFE rispetto alla metafisi, attraverso la zona dello strato ipertrofico della cartilagine di accrescimento.

CLASSIFICAZIONE

La SCFE può essere classificata applicando tre diversi criteri: temporale, in base all'esordio dei sintomi (acuto, cronico, acuto su cronico); funzionale, in base alla capacità del paziente di caricare il peso (stabile o instabile); morfologico, in base all'entità dello spostamento dell'epifisi femorale relativamente al collo (lieve, moderato o severo), valutato con misurazioni su immagini radiografiche o TC.

Viene considerata **SCFE acuta** quella che si verifica in un paziente con sintomi prodromici per ≤3 settimane e deve essere distinta da una separazione puramente traumatica dell'epifisi in un'anca precedentemente normale (una vera frattura di Salter-Harris di tipo I). Il paziente con spostamento acuto presenta di solito un certo dolore prodromico a livello inguinale, della coscia o del ginocchio e riferisce un trauma relativamente minore (una torsione o una caduta), che di norma non è tanto violento da produrre una frattura acuta di questa severità. L'osteonecrosi è una significativa e frequente complicanza della SCFE acuta, con un'incidenza riportata del 17-47%.

La **SCFE cronica** è la forma più frequente di presentazione. Caratteristicamente, un adolescente si presenta con una storia di pochi mesi di un dolore vago a livello di inguine, parte superiore o inferiore della coscia, e zoppia. Le radiografie evidenziano in misura variabile una migrazione posteriore dell'epifisi femorale e un rimodellamento del collo femorale nella stessa direzione; l'estremità superiore del femore sviluppa un'"inclinazione (*bending*) del collo".

I bambini con **SCFE acuta su cronica** possono avere caratteristiche proprie di entrambe le estremità dello spettro. I sintomi prodromici sono stati presenti per più di 3 settimane con un'improvvisa esacerbazione del dolore. Le radiografie dimostrano un rimodellamento del collo femorale e un ulteriore spostamento dell'epifisi della testa femorale oltre il punto di rimodellamento del collo femorale.

La classificazione imperniata sulla stabilità, che separa i pazienti in base alla capacità di camminare, è più utile per prevedere la prognosi e stabilire un piano di trattamento. La SCFE è considerata "stabile" quando il bambino è in grado di camminare con o senza grucce. Un bambino con SCFE "instabile" non riesce a camminare né con le grucce né senza. I pazienti con SCFE instabile hanno una prevalenza molto più elevata di osteonecrosi (fino al 50%) rispetto a quelli con SCFE stabile (quasi lo 0%): è probabile che ciò sia dovuto al danno vascolare venutosi a determinare al momento dello spostamento iniziale. La SCFE può inoltre essere classificata in base al grado di spostamento della CFE sul collo femorale.

La differenza angolare tra testa e diafisi è <30° negli spostamenti lievi, tra i 30 e i 60° negli spostamenti moderati e >60° negli spostamenti severi, rispetto al lato controlaterale normale.

EZIOLOGIA

È stato ipotizzato che i fattori meccanici creati dalla retroversione relativa o vera del collo femorale, l'orientamento dell'epifisi della testa femorale e della cartilagine di coniugazione rispetto al collo femorale e l'alterazione della forza meccanica della cartilagine di accrescimento, del periostio e dell'anello pericondrale nel corso dell'adolescenza abbiano tutti un ruolo nell'eziologia dell'epifisiolisi della testa femorale. È stato dimostrato che una riduzione della normale antiversione femorale, una reale retroversione della testa femorale e un orientamento più obliquo della cartilagine di accrescimento durante l'adolescenza sono tutti fattori che concorrono a un aumento della forza di scivolamento a livello della cartilagine di accrescimento femorale prossimale, oltre a poter essere associati a usura della cartilagine di accrescimento.

I bambini obesi hanno spesso una retroversione del collo femorale, che appare diretto più posteriormente di quello di altri bambini. Le forze fisiologiche che si esercitano a livello del femore prossimale, nel corso di normali attività fisiche, nei pazienti obesi possono essere di entità tale da causare usura della cartilagine di accrescimento. È stata sospettata un'eziologia endocrinologica per l'epifisiolisi femorale, in base alla comune associazione di questa condizione all'obesità e, almeno nei maschi, a caratteristiche di ipogonadismo e al fatto che questa condizione si manifesta più frequentemente durante lo scatto di crescita adolescenziale. Altre evidenze di un'associazione con una disfunzione endocrina sono suggerite dalla frequente associazione della SCFE con ipotiroidismo primitivo e secondario, panipopituitarismo, condizioni di ipogonadismo, osteodistrofia renale e terapia con ormone della crescita. Nel corso della pubertà, l'ormone della crescita aumenta l'attività fisiologica della cartilagine di accrescimento e ne determina un rapido accrescimento longitudinale, che a sua volta comporta l'allargamento e l'indebolimento della cartilagine di accrescimento femorale prossimale.

EPIDEMIOLOGIA

L'incidenza annuale della SCFE è di 2/100 000 casi nella popolazione generale. L'incidenza va da 0,2/100 000 nel Giappone orientale a 10,08/100 000 negli Stati Uniti nordorientali. Nelle popolazioni afroamericane e polinesiane è stato riportato un aumento dell'incidenza di SCFE. L'obesità è il fattore più strettamente associato allo sviluppo di SCFE; il 65% circa dei pazienti sono al di sopra del 90° percentile nelle curve peso per altezza. Esiste una ben precisa predilezione per il sesso maschile e per l'anca sinistra. In almeno il 60% dei casi è stata riportata una bilateralità, che quasi nella metà dei pazienti può essere presente al momento della presentazione iniziale.

PRESENTAZIONE CLINICA

I pazienti con SCFE di solito si presentano all'attenzione del medico lamentando dolore a livello dell'anca interessata o dell'inguine, un'alterazione dell'arco di movimento dell'anca e anomalie della deambulazione. È invece infrequente che il paziente accusi soltanto un dolore del ginocchio mediale che può essere riferito al ginocchio attraverso i nervi otturatore e femorale.

I segni e i sintomi variano a seconda che i sintomi siano cronici, acuti sul cronico o acuti; che l'epifisiolisi sia stabile o instabile; che la deformità risultante sia più o meno severa; che siano o meno presenti complicanze come l'osteonecrosi o la condrolisi.

Nella *SCFE cronica stabile* il paziente descrive un dolore intermittente localizzato all'inguine, nella parte mediale della coscia o nella regione sovrarotulea anteriore del ginocchio. Il dolore, tipicamente descritto come sordo e vago, è esacerbato dall'attività fisica come la corsa o gli sport. L'esordio del dolore può avere durata variabile da diverse settimane a diversi mesi. Il paziente continua a camminare, ma presenta un'andatura antalgica con zoppia associata. L'esame obiettivo dell'anca affetta rivela una limitazione della rotazione interna, dell'abduzione e della flessione. L'esaminatore nota comunemente che l'anca affetta è flessa, che la coscia tende a ruotare sempre più esternamente (segno del ginocchio-ascella; Fig. 677-14) e che la flessione è limitata.

I pazienti che si presentano con epifisiolisi *acuta instabile* o *acuta sul cronico* caratteristicamente riferiscono l'esordio improvviso di un dolore severo simile a quello di una frattura nell'area dell'anca affetta, di solito in seguito a un trauma minore da caduta o da torsione. La *forma acuta* si manifesta con l'esordio acuto di un dolore severo e con disfunzione dell'anca in un paziente in precedenza asintomatico. L'esame obiettivo dimostra una rotazione esterna e un accorciamento dell'arto interessato, con rifiuto del carico da parte del paziente.

Dal momento che il 25% circa dei pazienti ha alcune evidenze di epifisiolisi controlaterale alla presentazione iniziale, l'anca controlaterale deve sempre essere valutata con grande attenzione dal medico curante, sia clinicamente sia radiograficamente.

ASPETTI RADIOGRAFICI

RADIOGRAFIE. Le radiografie in proiezione anteroposteriore e laterale sono il primo e spesso unico studio di imaging necessario per la valutazione di un'epifisiolisi. Gli aspetti radiografici più comuni comprendono un allargamento e un'irregolarità della cartilagine di accrescimento, una riduzione dell'altezza epifisaria nel centro dell'acetabolo, un'area a forma di mezzaluna con densità aumentata nella porzione prossimale del collo femorale e il "segno *blanch* di Steel", corrispondente alla doppia densità creata dal collo femorale spostato in avanti al di sopra della testa femorale.

Nel soggetto sano la linea di Klein, una retta tracciata lungo la corticale superiore del collo femorale sulla radiografia in anteroposteriore, interseca la parte laterale dell'epifisi della testa femorale. Con lo spostamento progressivo dell'epifisi che si verifica nella SCFE, l'entità della linea di Klein che interseca l'epifisi diminuisce, rispetto all'anca non interessata, e alla fine la linea manca del tutto l'intersezione con l'epifisi femorale prossimale (Fig. 677-15). Una vera proiezione radiografica laterale dell'anca (*cross-table* laterale) definisce meglio l'estensione dello spostamento posteriore dell'epifisi femorale.

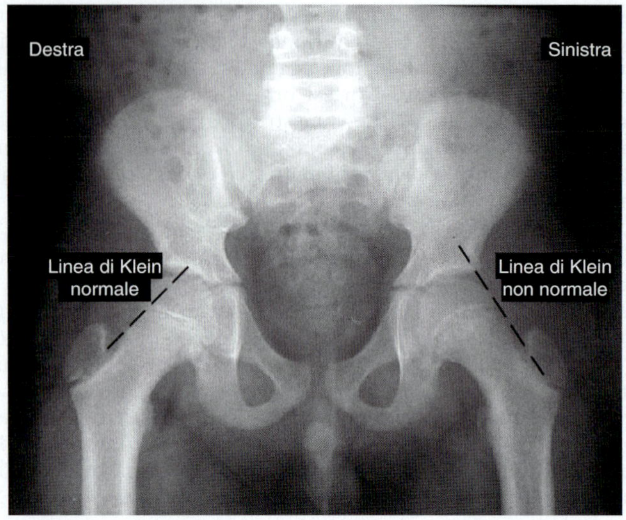

Figura 677-15. Illustrazione della linea di Klein.

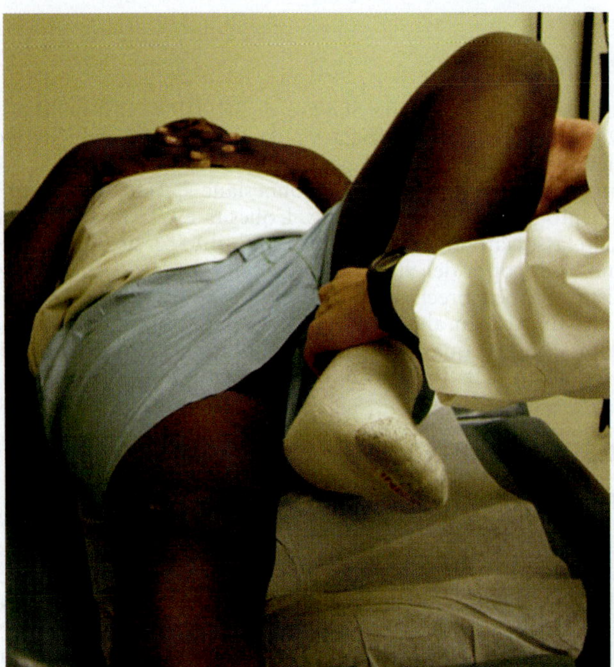
Figura 677-14. Progressiva rotazione esterna osservata con la flessione: segno del ginocchio-ascella.

TOMOGRAFIA COMPUTERIZZATA. La TC può essere utilizzata per la conferma dello spostamento epifisario e per misurare con precisione l'entità dello spostamento nei pazienti con sintomi suggestivi di SCFE, ma senza la relativa documentazione alla radiografia.

SCINTIGRAFIA OSSEA CON TECNEZIO 99M. La scintigrafia ossea evidenzia un aumento della captazione nella cartilagine di accrescimento femorale prossimale dell'anca interessata, una riduzione della captazione in presenza di osteonecrosi e un aumento della captazione nello spazio articolare in presenza di condrolisi.

TRATTAMENTO

Esistono tre tipi di trattamento: uno che mira alla prevenzione di un ulteriore spostamento, uno che ha lo scopo di ridurre il grado di spostamento e infine un trattamento di salvataggio.

TRATTAMENTO PER LA PREVENZIONE DI UN ULTERIORE SPOSTAMENTO. Per prevenire un ulteriore spostamento si ricorre all'immobilizzazione in gesso a spica, associata a fissazione *in situ* con chiodo o vite e a un'epifisiodesi con innesto osseo. Il termine *in situ* significa che non si fa alcun tentativo di ridurre lo spostamento tra epifisi e collo femorale. L'inserimento di un chiodo *in situ* ha lo scopo di stabilizzare l'epifisi prossimale rispetto al collo femorale, impedendo così un ulteriore spostamento (Fig. 677-16).

Dopo la fissazione, è fondamentale la conferma radiografica che il mezzo usato per la fissazione non sia penetrato nello spazio articolare. Se ci si attiene alle linee guida e ai principi di trattamento, è possibile stabilizzare quasi tutte le SCFE mediante l'inserimento percutaneo di una singola vite cannulata di 6,5-7,5 mm. La fissazione *in situ* con chiodo e vite accelera la chiusura della cartilagine di crescita interessata.

TRATTAMENTO PER RIDURRE IL GRADO DI SPOSTAMENTO. La tecnica per ridurre il grado di spostamento consiste nella manipolazione chiusa prima della stabilizzazione della cartilagine di crescita e delle osteotomie del femore prossimale, eseguita o contemporaneamente alla stabilizzazione della cartilagine di accrescimento o dopo la chiusura della cartilagine di accrescimento. Le osteoto-

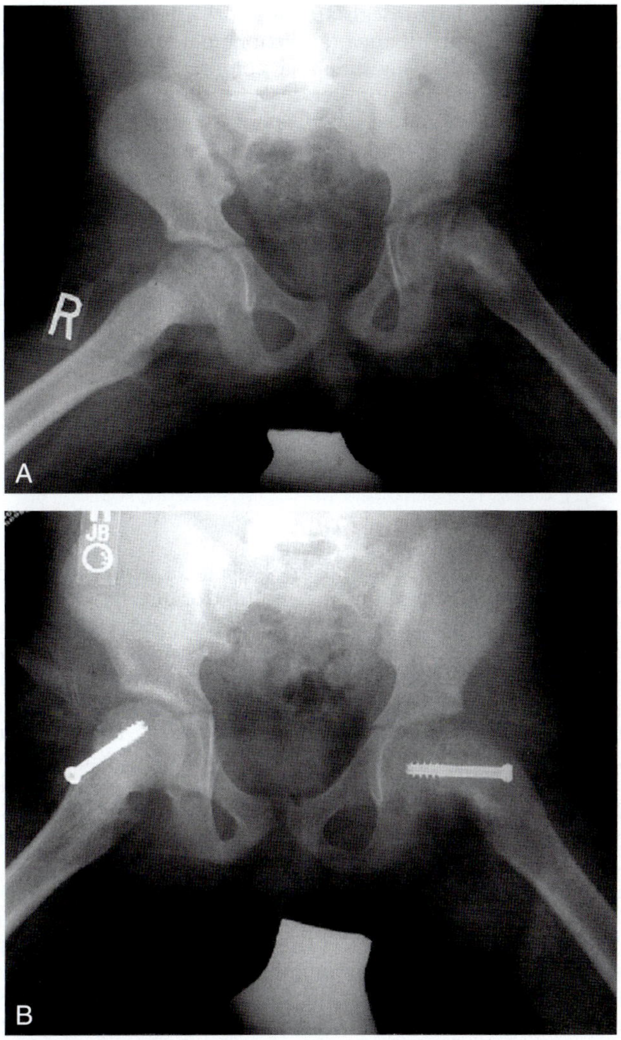

Figura 677-16. Radiografie preoperatoria (*A*) e postoperatoria (*B*) che illustrano l'inserimento *in situ* di un chiodo in un caso di epifisiolisi della testa femorale.

mie del femore prossimale nella SCFE sono state studiate come procedure di riallineamento attraverso le quali si può ottenere il ripristino di un più normale rapporto tra testa femorale, collo femorale, diafisi e acetabolo.

PROCEDURE DI SALVATAGGIO. Se la testa femorale va incontro a deformazione severa e l'articolazione diviene rigida e dolorosa in seguito a osteonecrosi o condrolisi, sono indicate procedure di salvataggio per eliminare il dolore e migliorare la funzione.

L'artrodesi dell'anca è raccomandata negli adolescenti e nei giovani adulti.

INSERIMENTO PROFILATTICO DI UN CHIODO NELL'ANCA CONTROLATERALE

La prevalenza di spostamento controlaterale, anche in un paziente asintomatico, fa sì che molti raccomandino l'inserimento profilattico di un chiodo. Nei pazienti con SCFE associata a disordini endocrini e metabolici noti, in cui il rischio di uno spostamento controlaterale è estremamente elevato, può essere appropriato l'inserimento profilattico di un chiodo nell'anca controlaterale.

COMPLICANZE

Osteonecrosi e condrolisi sono le due complicanze più severe della SCFE. L'osteonecrosi, o necrosi avascolare, si verifica di solito in seguito a un danno dei vasi del retinacolo. Quest'ultimo può essere causato da una forza traumatica iniziale, soprattutto nelle anche instabili, dalla manipolazione forzata di una SCFE acuta o instabile, dalla compressione esercitata da un ematoma intracapsulare, oppure manifestarsi come un danno diretto nel corso di un intervento chirurgico. Forme iniziali di osteonecrosi possono comparire anche dopo fissazione interna, per effetto di un'interruzione dei vasi sanguigni intraepifisari. La condrolisi, d'altra parte, è una dissoluzione acuta della cartilagine articolare dell'anca. Anche se questa complicanza non ha cause chiare, si ritiene sia associata alle epifisiolisi più severe, si verifichi con maggiore frequenza negli afroamericani e nelle femmine e sia associata alla protrusione di chiodi o viti al di fuori della testa femorale.

Catterall A: The natural history of Perthes disease. *J Bone Joint Surg Br* 1971;53:37–53.

Dobbs MT, Weinstein SL: Natural history and long-term outcomes of slipped capital femoral epiphysis. *Am Acad Orthop Surg Instr Course Lect* 2001;50:571–575.

Erol B, Dormans JP: Hip disorders. In Dormans JP (editor): *Pediatric Orthopedics: Core Knowledge in Orthopedics,* Philadelphia, Mosby, 2005, pp 224–264.

Guille JT, Pizzutillo PD, MacEwen GD: Developmental dysplasia of the hip from birth to six months. *J Am Acad Orthop Surg* 2000;8:232–242.

Hamer AJ: Pain in the hip and knee. *Br Med J* 2004;328:1067–1069.

Haynes DJ: Developmental dysplasia of the hip: Etiology, pathogenesis and examination and physical findings in the newborn. *Am Acad Orthop Surg Instr Course Lect* 2001;50:535–540.

Hennrikus WL: Developmental dysplasia of the hip: Diagnosis and treatment in children younger than 6 months. *Pediatr Ann* 1999;28:740–746.

Herring JA, Neustadt JB, Williams JJ, et al: The lateral pillar classification of Legg-Calvé-Perthes disease. *J Pediatr Orthop* 1992;12:143–150.

Kocher MS, Zurakowski D, Kasser JR: Differentiating between septic arthritis and transient synovitis of the hip in children: An evidence-based clinical prediction algorithm. *J Bone Joint Surg Am* 1999;81:1662–1670.

Liu YF, Chen WM, Lin YF, et al: Type II collagen gene variants and inherited osteonecrosis of the femoral head. *N Engl J Med* 2005;352:2294–2301.

Loder RT, Aronsson DD, Dobbs MT, et al: Slipped capital femoral epiphysis. *Am Acad Orthop Surg Instr Course Lect* 2001;50:555–570.

Lowry CA, Donoghue VB, Murphy JF: Auditing hip ultrasound screening of infants at increased risk of developmental dysplasia of the hip. *Arch Dis Child* 2005;90:579–581.

Lubicky JP: Chondrolysis and avascular necrosis: Complications of slipped capital femoral epiphysis. *J Pediatr Orthop* 1996;5:162–167.

Martinez AG, Weinstein SL, Dietz FR: The weight-bearing abduction brace for the treatment of Legg-Calvé-Perthes disease. *J Bone Joint Surg Am* 1992;74:12–21.

Moseley CF: Developmental hip dysplasia and dislocation: Management of the older child. *Am Acad Orthop Surg Instr Course Lect* 2001;50: 547–553.

Noonan KJ, Price CT, Kupiszewski SJ, et al: Results of femoral varus osteotomy in children older than 9 years of age with Perthes disease. *J Pediatr Orthop* 2001;21:198–204.

Reynolds RA: Diagnosis and treatment of slipped capital femoral epiphysis. *Curr Opin Pediatr* 1999;11:80–83.

Roovers EA, Boere-Boonekamp MM, Castelein RM, et al: Effectiveness of ultrasound screening for developmental dysplasia of the hip. *Arch Dis Child Fetal Neonatal Ed* 2005;90:F25–F30.

Roy DR: Current concepts in Legg-Calvé-Perthes disease. *Pediatr Ann* 1999;28:748–752.

Tamai J, Erol B, Dormans, JP: Hip disorders. In Dormans JP, Bell, LM (editors): *Pediatric Orthopedics and Sports Medicine: The Requisites in Pediatrics*. St. Louis, MO, Mosby, 2004, pp 175–212.

Thompson GH, Price CT, Roy D, et al: Legg-Calvé-Perthes disease: Current concepts. *Am Acad Orthop Surg Instr Course Lect* 2002;51:367–384.

US Preventive Services Task Force: Screening for developmental dysplasia of the hip: recommendation statement. *Pediatrics* 2006;117:898–902.

Warner WC Jr, Beaty JH, Canale ST: Chondrolysis after slipped capital femoral epiphysis. *J Pediatr Orthop* 1996;5:168–172.

Willis RB: Developmental dysplasia of the hip: Assessment and treatment before walking age. *Am Acad Orthop Surg Instr Course Lect* 2001;50:541–545.

Woolacott NF, Puhan MA, Steurer J, Kleijnen J: Ultrasonography in screening for developmental dysplasia of the hip in newborns: Systemic review. *Br Med J* 2005;330:1413–1415.

Capitolo 678 ■ La colonna vertebrale

David A. Spiegel, Harish S. Hosalkar e John P. Dormans

Le anomalie della colonna vertebrale possono essere presenti alla nascita (congenite) oppure svilupparsi nel corso dell'infanzia o dell'adolescenza (evolutive). Mentre le alterazioni dell'allineamento della colonna rappresentano un problema estetico per il paziente e la sua famiglia, alcune curve progressive possono essere associate a disfunzione cardiopolmonare, dolore e perdita dell'equilibrio da seduti (non deambulanti). La diagnosi precoce non solo facilita il trattamento, ma permette anche di identificare e trattare i problemi viscerali e/o neurologici coesistenti che possono essere associati alla deformità vertebrale. Una classificazione delle comuni anomalie della colonna vertebrale è presentata nella Tabella 678-1.

La **scoliosi** è una deformità tridimensionale descritta per lo più come una curvatura laterale della colonna sul piano frontale. Anche se nella maggior parte dei casi non ha un'eziologia dimostrabile (ed è quindi idiopatica), può essere congenita oppure associarsi a diverse malattie o sindromi neuromuscolari. Può inoltre essere secondaria a una deformità infrapelvica come una differenza di lunghezza degli arti inferiori o una contrattura dei tessuti molli intorno all'anca (abduzione o adduzione).

TABELLA 678-1. Classificazione delle deformità vertebrali

SCOLIOSI
Idiopatica
Infantile
Giovanile
Dell'adolescente
Congenita
Mancata formazione
Vertebre cuneiformi
Emivertebre
Mancata segmentazione
Barra unilaterale
Vertebra a blocco
Mista
Neuromuscolare
Malattie neuropatiche
Motoneurone superiore
Paralisi cerebrale
Degenerazione spinocerebellare (atassia di Friedreich, malattia di Charcot-Marie-Tooth)
Siringomielia
Tumore del midollo spinale
Trauma del midollo spinale
Motoneurone inferiore
Poliomielite
Atrofia muscolare spinale
Miopatie
Distrofia muscolare di Duchenne
Artrogriposi
Altre distrofie muscolari
Sindromi
Neurofibromatosi
Sindrome di Marfan
Compensatoria
Differenza di lunghezza degli arti inferiori
CIFOSI
Cifosi posturale (flessibile)
Malattia di Scheuermann
Cifosi congenita
Mancata formazione
Mancata segmentazione
Mista

Adattata dal Terminology Committee, Scoliosis Research Society: A glossary of scoliosis terms. *Spine* 1976;1:57.

Sul piano laterale (sagittale), la colonna presenta curvature normali a livello delle regioni cervicale (lordotica o convessa anteriormente), toracica (cifosi o confessa posteriormente) e lombare (lordosi) per mantenere le relazioni dei segmenti corporei relative alle forze di gravità. Mantenere il centro di gravità è importante per l'equilibrio e per ridurre al minimo l'attività muscolare (conservazione dell'energia) necessaria per conservare la postura eretta. Una linea verticale (gravità) a piombo dalla 7ª vertebra cervicale in condizioni normali deve passare attraverso l'angolo posterosuperiore del sacro. I disordini dell'allineamento sagittale comprendono l'ipercifosi toracica e l'iperlordosi lombare. L'**ipercifosi toracica** si osserva più frequentemente nei pazienti con **cifosi posturale** o **malattia di Scheuermann**. L'iperlordosi lombare può essere associata a spondilolistesi o essere secondaria a contratture in flessione dell'anca.

678.1 • Scoliosi idiopatica

EZIOLOGIA ED EPIDEMIOLOGIA. L'eziologia della scoliosi idiopatica è sconosciuta ma probabilmente multifattoriale. La genetica ha un ruolo ed è stata suggerita un'ereditarietà dominante legata al sesso, autosomica dominante e multifattoriale. Un'anamnesi familiare positiva non aiuta a prevedere il comportamento di una singola curva. Le anomalie individuate nel tessuto connettivo, nel muscolo e nell'osso sembrano essere secondarie. La melatonina e la calmodulina possono avere effetti indiretti; anche i fattori neurologici sono importanti. Sono state documentate lievi alterazioni della funzione vestibolare, oculare e propriocettiva, da cui si deduce che le anomalie dell'equilibrio potrebbero avere un ruolo.

La scoliosi idiopatica viene classificata, a seconda dell'età all'esordio, in infantile (rara, dalla nascita a 3 anni), giovanile (3-10 anni) e dell'adolescente (11 anni e oltre). La scoliosi idiopatica dell'adolescente è la più comune (circa 70%). La prevalenza della scoliosi (curva >10°) è del 2-3% circa; tuttavia, lo 0,3% circa avrà una curva >20°. Mentre l'incidenza è più o meno simile nei maschi e nelle femmine per le piccole curve (<10°), le ragazze hanno un rischio 10 volte superiore di sviluppare una curva >30°.

MANIFESTAZIONI CLINICHE. I pazienti di solito si presentano con un'alterazione dell'aspetto estetico, che viene notata dai familiari e/o dagli amici o viene alla luce nel corso di un esame di screening, in ambito scolastico o medico. Anche se non è tipica, una dorsalgia può essere occasionalmente associata alla scoliosi. Sono necessari un'anamnesi e un esame obiettivo accurati in quanto quella di scoliosi idiopatica è una diagnosi di esclusione. Il paziente viene valutato in posizione eretta, sia di fronte sia di lato, per identificare qualsiasi asimmetria della parete del torace, del tronco e/o delle spalle. Un'asimmetria della parete posteriore del torace al *bending* anteriore (test di Adams) è l'anomalia più precoce (Fig. 678-1). La rotazione dei corpi vertebrali verso la convessità si traduce in una rotazione esterna e in una sporgenza delle relative coste posteriormente. La parete toracica anteriore può essere appiattita sulla concavità a causa della rotazione interna della parete toracica e delle coste. Le caratteristiche associate possono comprendere elevazione della spalla, uno spostamento laterale del tronco, un'apparente discrepanza di lunghezza degli arti inferiori. Il paziente deve essere valutato anche di lato. La scoliosi idiopatica determina caratteristicamente una perdita della normale cifosi toracica nella regione della curva (lordosi toracica relativa). Occorre sempre eseguire un accurato esame neurologico. Un sottogruppo di curve deve essere associato a una diagnosi neurologica sottostante, specialmente nei pazienti che si presentano nella prima infanzia e negli anni giovanili (il 20% hanno un'anomalia intraspinale associata). L'indice di sospetto è aumentato in presenza di dorsalgia o di sintomi neurologici, macche caffelatte, una fossetta sacrale, anomalie cutanee della linea

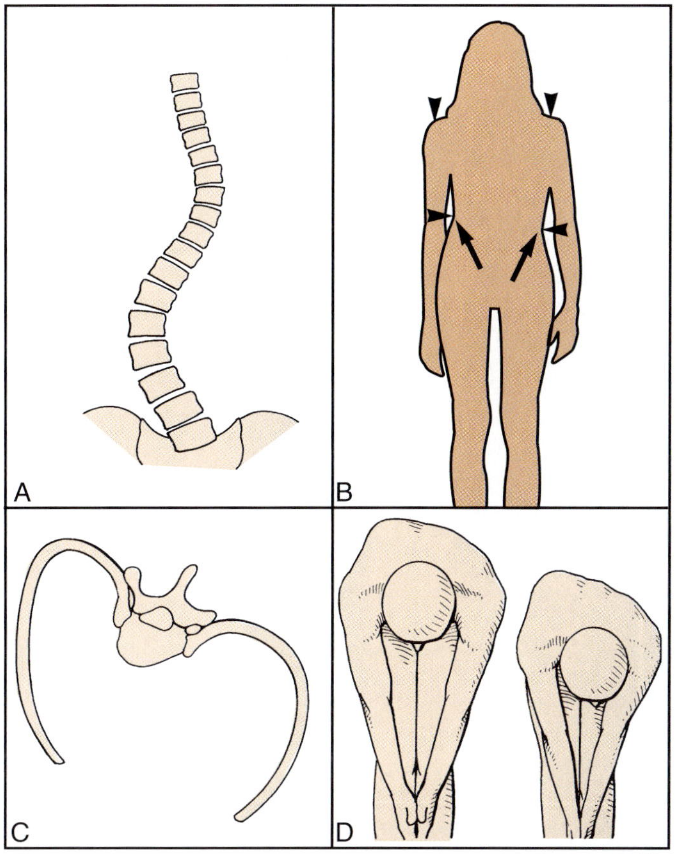

Figura 678-1. Alterazioni strutturali osservabili nella scoliosi idiopatica. *A*, Via via che la curvatura aumenta, si sviluppano alterazioni della configurazione del corpo vertebrale sia nella regione della curva primitiva sia nella regione della curva compensatoria. *B*, Sono comuni asimmetrie dell'altezza delle spalle, della linea della vita e della distanza tra gomito e fianco. C, La rotazione vertebrale e l'associato spostamento posteriore delle coste dal lato convesso della curva sono responsabili della caratteristica deformità della parete toracica nei pazienti con scoliosi. *D*, Nell'esame di screening scolastico per la scoliosi, il paziente si piega in avanti a livello della vita. È evidente un'asimmetria delle coste, anche di grado minore. (Da Scoles PV: Spinal deformity in childhood and adolescence. In Behrman RE, Vaughn VC III [ed]: *Nelson Textbook of Pediatrics, Update 5*. Philadelphia, WB Saunders, 1989.)

mediana come un ciuffo di peli o una lesione (*tag*) cutanea, una deformità unilaterale del piede o un pattern di curva atipico.

Osservando il tronco di lato, è possibile valutare il grado di cifosi e lordosi. La regione superiore della colonna toracica normalmente presenta una curva arrotondata e poco accentuata che si estende in basso alla regione mediotoracica. Negli adolescenti è comune una schiena curva flessibile che si corregge facilmente quando il soggetto si alza in piedi. Un'angolazione in avanti acuta, improvvisa o accentuata nella regione toracica o toracolombare è indicativa di una deformità cifotica patologica. In posizione eretta, la colonna lombare inferiore è di norma concava (lordotica). L'entità della lordosi varia con l'età e da un individuo all'altro. I bambini hanno normalmente una minore lordosi cervicale e una maggiore lordosi lombare degli adulti o degli adolescenti.

Oltre allo screening nel corso di visite regolari presso un ambulatorio di medicina generale, sono diffusi in Nord America programmi di screening che fanno uso del test del bending in avanti di Adams per identificare qualsiasi asimmetria della regione toracica e/o lombare. In alcuni programmi si impiega anche uno scoliometro (Orthopaedic Systems Inc.) per misurare il grado di asimmetria, e il numero di gradi utilizzati per l'invio al centro di riferimento varia caratteristicamente da 5 a 7. Il tasso di invio al centro di riferimento di questi programmi va dal 3 al 30%. Il follow-up di pazienti adulti con scoliosi non trattata a esordio tardivo rivela un rischio aumentato di dorsalgia da lieve a moderata e di dispnea (maggiore con un apice toracico e un angolo di Cobb >80°).

VALUTAZIONE RADIOGRAFICA. Si raccomandano radiografie in posizione eretta, di elevata qualità, in proiezione anteroposteriore (AP) e laterale della colonna *in toto* come valutazione iniziale dei pazienti con segni clinici suggestivi di deformità spinale. Alla radiografia AP, il grado di curvatura è determinato dal metodo di Cobb, consistente nel misurare l'angolo tra vertebra terminale superiore e inferiore (all'interno della curva) (Fig. 678-2). Dopo aver tracciato una linea passante per il piatto vertebrale superiore di ciascuna vertebra terminale, si misura l'angolo tra le linee perpendicolari a ognuna di queste linee. Anche se le indicazioni all'esecuzione di una RM sono variabili, questa modalità è utile quando si sospetta una causa sottostante per la scoliosi in base all'età (curve giovanili, infantili), a caratteristiche anomale dell'anamnesi e dell'esame obiettivo e ad aspetti radiografici atipici (pattern della curva e/o aspetti specifici). Le caratteristiche **radiografiche atipiche** comprendono pattern della curva insoliti come una curva toracica sinistra, curve toraciche doppie, curve toraciche alte, allargamento del canale spinale e alterazioni erosive o displasiche dei corpi vertebrali o delle coste. Alla radiografia laterale, un aumento della cifosi toracica o un'assenza di lordosi segmentaria possono essere suggestivi di un'anomalia neurologica sottostante.

TRATTAMENTO. La decisione di trattare o meno il paziente si basa sulla storia naturale; le opzioni comprendono l'osservazione, l'uso del busto e la stabilizzazione chirurgica. In generale, le curve toraciche idiopatiche possono non dar luogo ad alterazioni significative della funzione cardiopolmonare fino a quando non hanno raggiunto gli 80-90°; pertanto, le curve di minore entità rappresentano principalmente un problema estetico. Studi a lungo termine hanno suggerito che la dorsalgia possa essere un problema più significativo per i pazienti con curve non trattate di maggiore entità. Il rischio di progressione della curva dipende dall'entità della crescita restante (età, situazione rispetto al menarca, stadio di Tanner, segno di Risser), dall'entità della curva e dal sesso. Le curve hanno una maggiore probabilità di progredire se sussiste una significativa possibilità che la crescita continui (premenarca, stadio I o II di Tanner, Risser 0 o 1). Le ragazze prima del menarca con curve di 20-30° hanno un rischio significativamente più elevato di progressione delle ragazze che presentano curve simili 2 anni dopo il menarca; la progressione della curva è probabile nel primo gruppo e infrequente nel secondo. I ragazzi con curve della stessa entità sembrano avere un rischio analogo di progressione quando sono giudicati in base ad altri standard di maturazione; tuttavia, la valutazione della maturazione scheletrica nei ragazzi è più difficile. Le curve toraciche <30° raramente progrediscono dopo la maturità scheletrica, mentre quelle >45-50° possono continuare ad aggravarsi di circa 1° all'anno nel corso della vita. Le curve lombari hanno una maggiore probabilità di progredire e possono causare dolore nel corso della vita adulta.

Il trattamento chirurgico è di solito indicato per pazienti scheletricamente immaturi con curve toraciche progressive >45° e per pazienti scheletricamente maturi con curve toraciche >50-55°. Le curve lombari hanno una maggiore probabilità di progressione e la stabilizzazione chirurgica può essere offerta per curve anche di soli 35-40° se è presente un inestetismo significativo, per lo più una deviazione del tronco. Gli obiettivi della chirurgia sono arrestare la progressione della deformità, migliorare l'aspetto estetico e ottenere una colonna equilibrata, riducendo al minimo nello stesso tempo il numero di segmenti vertebrali da stabilizzare. Si usano impianti che applicano forze meccaniche agli elementi ossei per correggere una deformità sia sul piano frontale sia sul piano laterale, per assicurare un normale equilibrio spinale frontale e sagittale e per mantenere la correzione in modo che non siano necessari un gesso o un'ortesi postoperatoria. La maggior parte delle procedure viene eseguita posteriormente e la tipica strumentazione spinale comprende due barre ancorate alla colonna mediante ganci, fili e/o viti

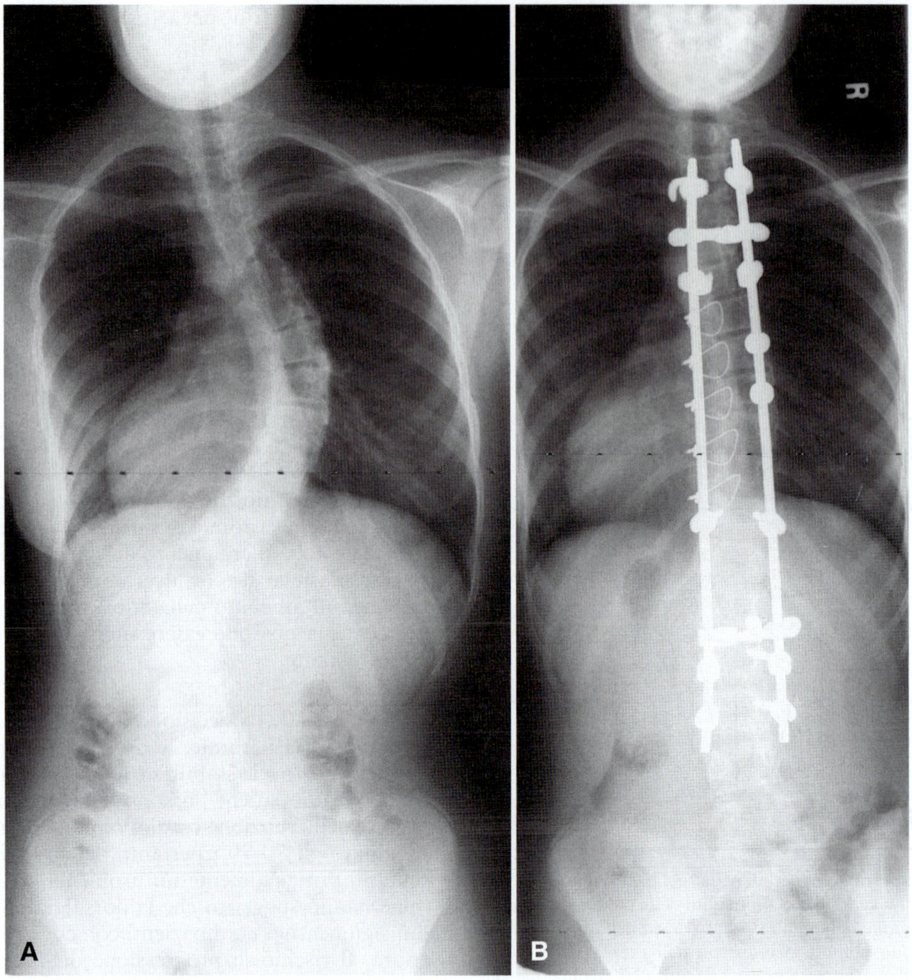

Figura 678-2. Radiografia preoperatoria in posizione eretta e in proiezione anteroposteriore di una ragazza di 14 anni con immaturità scheletrica che ha sviluppato una scoliosi toracica destra di 68° e una scoliosi lombare sinistra di 53°. *A*, Il tronco era deviato a destra e la spalla sinistra era leggermente abbassata. Dato il rischio di progressione futura, la paziente è stata trattata con una fusione vertebrale posteriore strumentata da T3 a L3, con correzione della curva toracica destra a 20° e della curva lombare sinistra a 10°. *B*, L'equilibrio coronale della colonna è stato ripristinato e l'altezza delle spalle è stata mantenuta.

(vedi Fig. 678-2). Una procedura di rilascio e fusione anteriore, eseguita per via toracotomica o con esposizione toracolombare, è indicata per le curve isolate toracolombari e lombari, per le curve più rigide (migliorano la correzione), per i pazienti scheletricamente immaturi (per prevenire il *crankshaft* dovuto alla continua crescita anteriore) e per i pazienti in cui è più elevata la probabilità di non ottenere un'artrodesi con il solo approccio posteriore (neurofibromatosi, mielomeningocele). Per le curve toracolombari e lombari idiopatiche, è possibile eseguire in alternativa una fusione anteriore con strumentazione (di solito con viti inserite nel corpo vertebrale connesse a 1-2 barre) al fine di salvare i segmenti coinvolti nel movimento lombare.

Diverse tecniche sono in corso di valutazione per il trattamento della scoliosi idiopatica. La chirurgia toracoscopica è stata utilizzata per eseguire un rilascio e una fusione anteriore; con questa tecnica si possono inserire anche impianti spinali anteriori. Le indicazioni alla chirurgia vertebrale toracoscopica sono in continua evoluzione. Inoltre, ha suscitato un certo interesse lo sviluppo di tecniche per guidare e controllare la crescita della colonna, con l'obiettivo di arrestare la progressione della curva (e ottenere un certo grado di correzione), onde evitare una successiva fusione vertebrale in pazienti con elevato rischio di progressione. La tecnica comprende l'inserimento in aperto o toracoscopico di graffe metalliche nei corpi vertebrali (attraverso ogni spazio discale intervertebrale o zona di crescita) per mantenere la colonna in posizione corretta guidando e controllando la crescita sulla convessità della curva.

678.2 • Scoliosi congenita

La scoliosi congenita deriva da una crescita e da uno sviluppo anormali della colonna vertebrale, presumibilmente dovuti a eventi intrauterini verificatisi intorno alla 6ª settimana di gestazione. Vi può essere una mancata formazione (vertebre cuneiformi o emivertebre), parziale o completa, una mancata segmentazione (barre non segmentate unilaterali), parziale o completa, o una combinazione delle due anomalie (Fig. 678-3). Si possono verificare una o più anomalie dei corpi vertebrali, da sole o in combinazione.

Con lo sviluppo della colonna (compresi gli elementi nervosi) e dei visceri intorno alla 6ª settimana in utero, i pazienti con scoliosi congenita presentano spesso anche anomalie viscerali e intraspinali. Una volta diagnosticata un'anomalia congenita della colonna, è prioritario escludere malformazioni di altri sistemi d'organo. Le anomalie genitourinarie, presenti nel 20-40% dei bambini con scoliosi congenita, comprendono agenesia renale unilaterale, duplicazione ureterale, rene a ferro di cavallo e anomalie genitali. Il 2% circa dei questi pazienti ha un'uropatia ostruttiva silente che può essere potenzialmente fatale. Occorre eseguire un'ecografia renale il prima possibile in tutti i bambini con scoliosi congenita e possono rendersi necessari anche altri studi di imaging (TC, RM). Le anomalie cardiache sono presenti nel 10-25% dei pazienti. Si raccomanda un'accurata valutazione cardiologica; alcuni medici consigliano un'ecocardiografia di routine. Il 20-40% circa dei pazienti può presentare un'anomalia intraspinale. Nei neonati con anomalie cutanee in corrispondenza

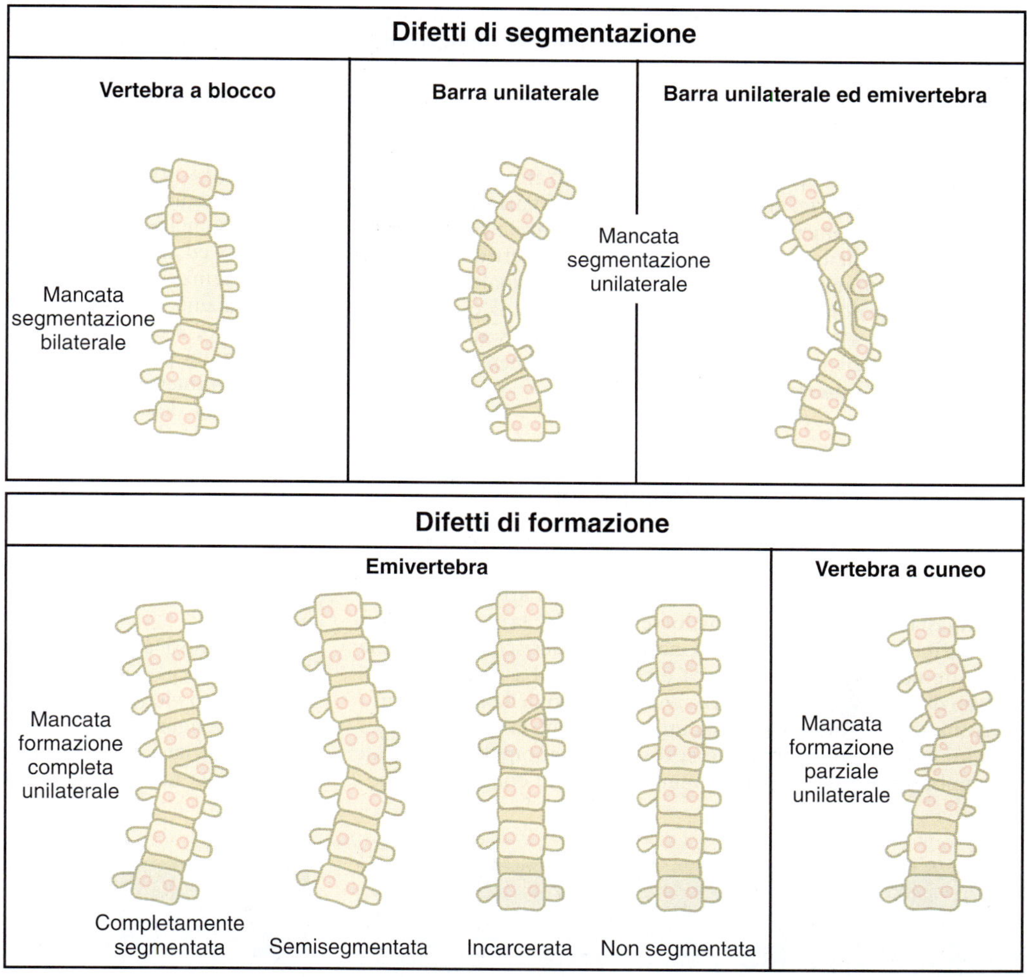

Figura 678-3. Difetti di segmentazione e formazione possono verificarsi durante lo sviluppo della colonna. (Da McMaster MJ: Congenital scoliosis. In Weinstein SL [ed]: *The Pediatric Spine: Principles and Practice*, 2nd ed. Philadelphia, Lippincott Williams & Wilkins, 2001, p. 163.)

della colonna vertebrale può essere utile un'ecografia per escludere un disrafismo spinale occulto. La RM è di solito raccomandata nel corso del trattamento. Disrafismo spinale è un termine generale applicato a queste lesioni (vedi Capitoli 592 e 605), tra cui diastematomelia, malformazioni con schisi midollare spinale, lipomi intraspinali (intradurale o extradurali), cisti aracnoidee, teratomi, fistole dermoidi, bande fibrose e tensione del filum terminale. Le anomalie cutanee osservabili nei pazienti con disrafismo spinale chiuso comprendono ciuffi di peli, tag o fossette cutanee, fistole ed emangiomi. La maggior parte di queste lesioni diviene clinicamente evidente in seguito alla tensione (*tethering*) del midollo spinale, i cui sintomi comprendono dorsalgia e/o cruralgia, atrofia del polpaccio, deformità unilaterale progressiva del piede (specialmente in cavovaro) e disfunzione intestinale o vescicale.

Il rischio di progressione dipende dal potenziale di crescita di ogni anomalia, che può variare considerevolmente, per cui è necessario un costante follow-up radiografico. La progressione di queste curve è più pronunciata durante i periodi di rapida crescita, cioè nei primi 2-3 anni di vita e durante lo scatto di crescita puberale. La forma più severa di scoliosi congenita è una barra non segmentata unilaterale con un'emivertebra controlaterale. In questa anomalia, la colonna è fusa da un lato (barra non segmentata) e ha un centro di crescita (emivertebra) dall'altro lato, allo stesso livello. Si osserva una curva rapidamente progressiva e tutti i pazienti di solito necessitano di stabilizzazione chirurgica. Una barra unilaterale non segmentata è inoltre associata a progressione significativa e nella maggior parte dei casi richiede l'intervento chirurgico. Mentre una barra non segmentata può non essere radiograficamente evidente, le coste adiacenti sulla concavità possono essere fuse, fornendo un indizio diagnostico. Un'emivertebra isolata deve essere seguita con attenzione e molte di queste forme, se non tutte, sono associate a una deformità progressiva che richiede l'intervento chirurgico. Al contrario, una vertebra a blocco isolata ha uno scarso potenziale di crescita e raramente richiede un trattamento.

La diagnosi precoce e l'immediato trattamento delle curve progressive sono essenziali. L'uso di un busto non è indicato nella maggior parte delle curve congenite a causa della loro natura strutturale, eccetto che in rari casi in cui l'obiettivo è il controllo di una curva di compenso flessibile in un'altra area della colonna. Il trattamento delle curve progressive è un'artrodesi spinale preventiva, e spesso è necessaria una fusione spinale sia anteriore sia posteriore. Altre procedure che sono utilizzate in pazienti selezionati comprendono una fusione posteriore isolata (talvolta una fusione *in situ*), un'emiepifisiodesi convessa (soltanto un lato della colonna viene fuso per consentire un certo grado di correzione della deformità con la crescita) e un'escissione parziale o completa dell'emivertebra (di solito nella colonna lombare). L'artrodesi spinale deve essere idealmente eseguita prima che si sviluppi una deformità significativa, in quanto la correzione intraoperatoria è difficile da ottenere e il rischio di complicanze neurologiche è elevato.

Quando sono interessati diversi livelli della colonna toracica, specialmente in presenza di coste fuse tra loro, una deformità toracica tridimensionale progressiva può limitare lo sviluppo e la funzione polmonare, determinando una sindrome da insufficienza toracica. La migliore descrizione di questa sindrome è l'incapacità della parete toracica di sostenere una respirazione normale. Una sindrome da insufficienza toracica può essere osservata in pazienti con diverse condizioni note come la sindrome di Jarcho-Levin (displasia spondilocostale o spondilotoracica) e la sindrome di Jeune (distrofia toracica con asfissia). Attualmente, vi è interesse per una tecnica di trattamento di questi casi chiamata **toracoplastica di espansione**, in cui la gabbia toracica viene gradualmente espansa nel tempo mediante un allungamento progressivo della parete toracica sulla concavità della deformità spinale (o in alcuni casi su entrambi i lati della colonna). La procedura consiste nell'accesso mediante toracotomia a cuneo, seguito dall'inserimento di una costa protesica espandibile verticale in titanio. L'impianto viene quindi distratto (allungato) a intervalli regolari (Fig. 678-4). L'obiettivo primario è quello di correggere gradualmente la deformità della parete toracica per migliorare la funzione polmonare, mentre l'obiettivo secondario è la correzione di un'eventuale deformità spinale associata. Questa tecnica non è attualmente approvata per il trattamento della scoliosi in assenza di insufficienza toracica e sono necessari ulteriori studi per meglio precisare (ed eventualmente allargare) le indicazioni di questa nuova tecnica.

678.3 • Scoliosi neuromuscolare, sindromi genetiche e scoliosi compensatoria

SCOLIOSI NEUROMUSCOLARE. La scoliosi è di riscontro frequente nei bambini con malattie neuromuscolari come la paralisi cerebrale, le distrofie muscolari e altre miopatie, l'atrofia muscolare, l'atassia di Friedreich, il mielomeningocele, la poliomielite e l'artrogriposi. Eziologia e storia naturale differiscono da quelle osservate nella scoliosi idiopatica e congenita. La maggior parte dei casi deriva da perdita di forza e/o squilibrio della muscolatura del tronco, e in molti pazienti ha un ruolo anche la spasticità. Nei pazienti con mielomeningocele si osservano anomalie vertebrali concomitanti. La scoliosi neuromuscolare è più comune nei soggetti non deambulanti; può essere diagnosticata anche nel 68% dei pazienti non deambulanti con paralisi cerebrale e in più del 90% di quelli con distrofia muscolare di Duchenne. Il pattern più comune è una lunga curva a "C", spesso associata a obliquità pelvica. In generale, il decorso clinico dipende dalla severità dell'interessamento neuromuscolare e dalla natura del processo patologico sottostante (specialmente se progressivo).

Le conseguenze di una scoliosi progressiva nei pazienti neuromuscolari incidono tanto sulla funzionalità (equilibrio in posizione seduta ed eretta) quanto sulla facilità dell'assistenza; in alcuni casi, la funzione viscerale può essere compromessa. I pazienti in carrozzina possono aver bisogno di sostenere il tronco con un braccio, il che riduce la funzionalità dell'estremità superiore. Un'obliquità pelvica associata fa sì che la pressione si eserciti in modo asimmetrico nella posizione seduta, il che può limitare la tollerabilità della posizione seduta ed eventualmente provocare decubiti a livello ischiatico. Le curve severe talvolta sono associate a riduzione della riserva polmonare, specialmente quando l'apice è a livello della colonna toracica, complicando i problemi respiratori preesistenti. La pressione esercitata dalla gabbia toracica sulla cresta iliaca può provocare dolore nelle curve toracolombari di maggiore entità. I pazienti che conservano una capacità marginale di camminare possono perderla in seguito alla scoliosi.

La diagnosi è sospettata in base all'esame obiettivo. La diagnosi precoce è utile in quanto i risultati sono ottimali se il trattamento viene completato prima che l'entità e la rigidità della curva divengano severe. Se il paziente è in grado di camminare l'esame avviene con le modalità descritte nel paragrafo dedicato alla scoliosi idiopatica; in caso contrario, con il paziente seduto

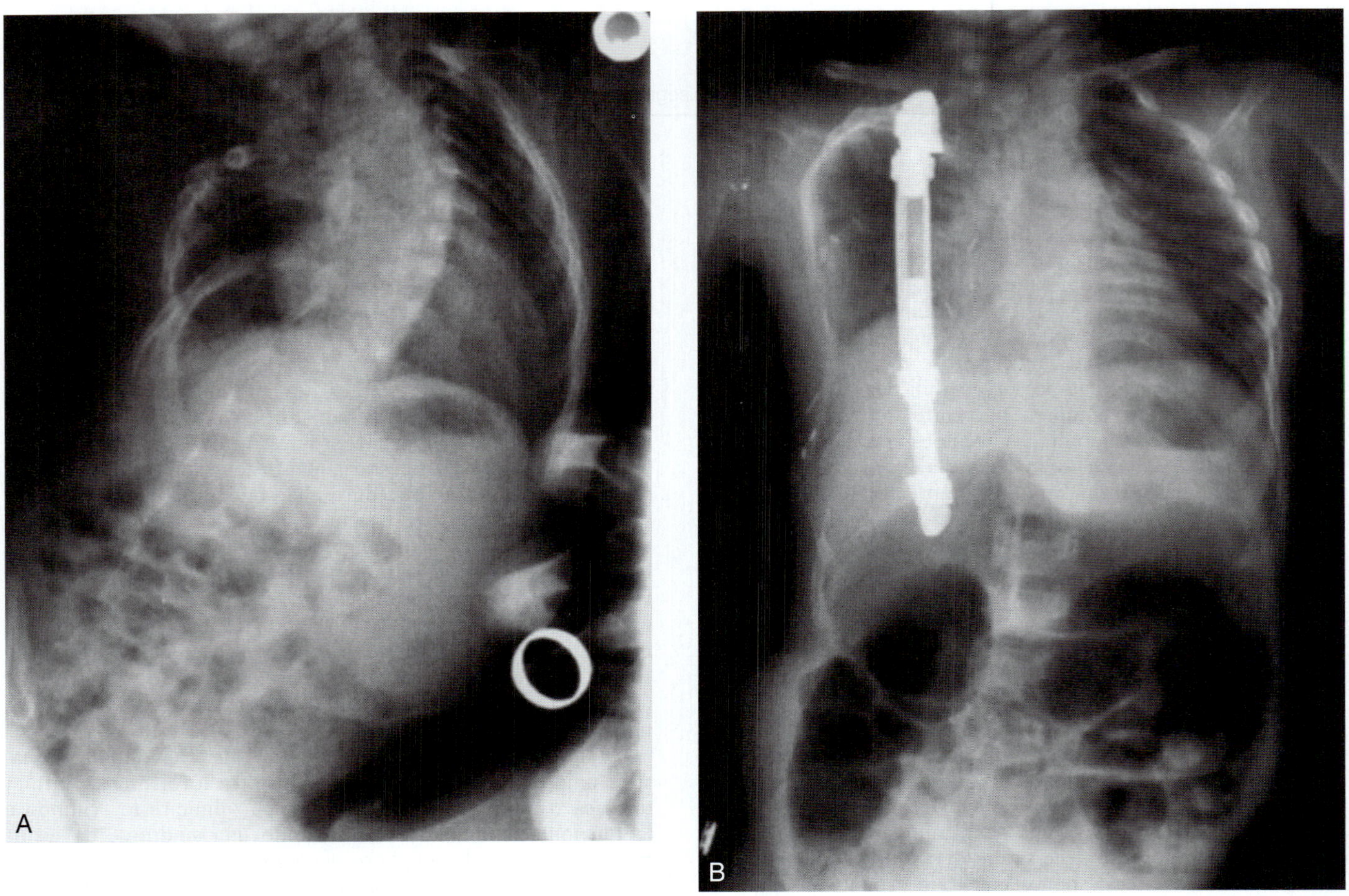

Figura 678-4. *A*, Radiografia preoperatoria in proiezione anteroposteriore di un bambino di 7 mesi con scoliosi congenita e coste fuse insieme. Una ricostruzione tridimensionale alla TC del torace di questo bambino ha stimato un volume polmonare di 173,2 mL^3. *B*, Radiografia anteroposteriore dopo impianto di una costa protesica in titanio espandibile verticalmente e dopo diverse espansioni nell'arco di 33 mesi. Il volume polmonare misura attualmente 330,3 mL^3, pari a un aumento del 90,7%. (Da Gollogly S, Smith JT, Campbell RM: Determining lung volume with three-dimensional reconstructions of CT scan data: A pilot study to evaluate the effects of expansion thoracoplasty on children with severe spinal deformities. *J Pediatr Orthop* 2004;23:323-328.)

con il tronco eretto (con o senza sostegno), si esamina la schiena prestando attenzione a qualsiasi asimmetria. Questi soggetti spesso necessitano di un sostegno manuale per mantenere la posizione seduta con il tronco eretto. Se si osserva una qualunque asimmetria, occorre eseguire radiografie nelle proiezioni anteroposteriore e laterale, in posizione seduta (con il tronco eretto).

Il **trattamento** della scoliosi neuromuscolare dipende dall'età del paziente, dalla diagnosi di base e dal grado di progressione. L'obiettivo è ottenere o mantenere una curva dritta al di sopra di un bacino in asse, specialmente nei pazienti in carrozzina, e intervenire tempestivamente, prima che l'entità della curva e la sua rigidità aumentino. Al contrario della scoliosi idiopatica e congenita, le curve neuromuscolari continuano a progredire dopo la maturità scheletrica. In generale, curve >40-50° continuano a peggiorare nel tempo. Anche se il trattamento con il busto non arresta la progressione a lungo termine, questa strategia può servire a rallentare il ritmo di progressione, in attesa che sia possibile mettere in atto un trattamento più definitivo. Dal momento che i busti standard utilizzati per la scoliosi idiopatica sono poco tollerati nei pazienti neuromuscolari, si raccomandano spesso ortesi spinali morbide o sedute modificate. Oltre a rallentare la progressione, queste ortesi migliorano sia l'equilibrio da seduti (funzione dell'estremità superiore) sia la tolleranza alla posizione seduta, e facilitano l'assistenza. In generale, si propone un'artrodesi spinale ai pazienti con curve progressive >40-50°. Le indicazioni differiscono in qualche misura a seconda della diagnosi di base. In presenza di distrofia muscolare di Duchenne si propone l'intervento quando la curva supera i 20-30°, prima che un significativo declino della funzione polmonare o cardiaca precluda l'intervento. Le indicazioni alla fusione spinale nei pazienti con quadriplegia spastica, specialmente per quelli con ritardo mentale severo, sono piuttosto controverse. In questo gruppo di pazienti le indicazioni, che comunque devono essere individualizzate, caratteristicamente comprendono una perdita funzionale documentata, difficoltà nell'assistenza o disagio cronico. I pazienti con curve simili a quelle osservate nella scoliosi idiopatica, che sono di solito in grado di camminare, sono trattati con principi e tecniche chirurgiche simili. Invece, quelli non in grado di camminare, che spesso presentano obliquità pelvica, di solito vengono sottoposti a una fusione spinale estesa dalla colonna toracica superiore al bacino. Si utilizza la fissazione segmentaria per aumentare il più possibile la rigidità (ogni livello della curva serve da punto di fissazione) e il costrutto tipico consiste nell'inserimento a ogni livello di fili sublaminari, connessi a una o due barre spinali. Tali barre si estendono verso il basso nella parte posteriore dell'ilio, permettendo una fissazione attraverso l'articolazione lombosacrale. Dopo questa procedura di solito non è necessario l'uso del busto. Anche se le complicanze sono relativamente frequenti rispetto ai pazienti con scoliosi non neuromuscolare, la letteratura esistente suggerisce che la maggior parte dei casi tragga beneficio in termini di funzione e facilità di assistenza. L'ideale sarebbe che questo intervento venisse eseguito presso centri con esperienza significativa (per es. da chirurghi vertebrali esperti, con anestesia, in un reparto di terapia intensiva).

SINDROMI/DISORDINI GENETICI. Esempi rappresentativi di questo gruppo eterogeneo di diagnosi sono la neurofibromatosi, l'osteogenesi imperfetta, le malattie del tessuto connettivo (sindrome di Marfan, sindrome di Ehlers-Danlos), la sindrome di Prader-Willi e molte altre. Nei pazienti con queste diagnosi, il medico curante deve esaminare la colonna di routine. Come con altri tipi di scoliosi, follow-up e trattamento si basano su età del paziente, grado di deformità, eventuale riscontro di una progressione e diagnosi di base.

SCOLIOSI COMPENSATORIA. La differenza di lunghezza degli arti inferiori è comune e di solito associata a una piccola curva lombare compensatoria (vedi Capitolo 675). Questa è una causa di falsi positivi nelle valutazioni di screening. Un'inclinazione del bacino verso il lato più corto si associa a una curva lombare (convessità dalla parte opposta alla gamba più corta). Vi sono poche evidenze che una piccola curva lombare compensatoria metta il paziente a rischio di progressione o sia causa di lombalgia. Dal momento che i bambini con arti inferiori di lunghezza differente possono avere anche una scoliosi idiopatica o congenita, occorre eseguire una radiografia in posizione eretta, con uno spessore sotto il piede dal lato più corto, per correggere la discrepanza e livellare il bacino. Se la curva scompare con la correzione della discrepanza degli arti inferiori, si può porre diagnosi di curva compensatoria. Un'alternativa è una radiografia AP con il paziente in posizione seduta. Nelle patologie neuromuscolari come poliomielite o paralisi cerebrale, una contrattura in adduzione o abduzione dell'anca (contrattura infrapelvica fissa) può essere compensata da una scoliosi lombare per mantenere l'equilibrio in posizione eretta o seduta. Nei pazienti che camminano, una contrattura fissa di 10° determina una differenza apparente degli arti inferiori di 3 cm.

678.4 • Cifosi (dorso curvo)

La colonna toracica normale ha una cifosi di 20-50° secondo la tecnica di Cobb (T3-12); gli individui con cifosi di grado più elevato possono presentarsi per problemi estetici, dorsalgia o entrambe le cose. Una cifosi toracica che superi la gamma di valori normali prende il nome di ipercifosi. La deformità può essere flessibile (cifosi posturale) o rigida (malattia di Scheuermann, cifosi congenita, altre cause). Molte condizioni possono essere associate a ipercifosi e le categorie comprendono le cifosi post-traumatiche (da frattura spinale), postinfettive (batterica, tubercolare, micotica), metaboliche (osteogenesi imperfetta, osteoporosi), iatrogene (post-laminectomia, post-radioterapia), neuromuscolari, neoplastiche e congenite/evolutive. Alcuni esempi di condizioni congenite o evolutive sono le collagenopatie (sindrome di Marfan) e diversi tipi di displasia (neurofibromatosi, acondroplasia, mucopolisaccaridosi). La valutazione e il trattamento dipendono dalla diagnosi di base e dal grado di deformità; occorre inoltre considerare se la deformità è progressiva e se sono presenti sintomi.

CIFOSI FLESSIBILE (CIFOSI POSTURALE)

La cifosi posturale è un problema estetico comune, che spesso viene notato da familiari e amici. Gli adolescenti con questa anomalia possono correggere la curva volontariamente. Una radiografia laterale in posizione eretta rivelerà un aumento della cifosi, senza alcuna alterazione patologica delle vertebre coinvolte. Una radiografia laterale in iperestensione in posizione supina mostrerà una correzione completa. Non vi sono evidenze che la cifosi posturale progredisca a deformità strutturale o che successivamente si associ a dorsalgia o ad altri sintomi. Occorre rassicurare il paziente. Un programma di esercizi di iperestensione toracica può essere utile per rafforzare i muscoli estensori della colonna, mentre l'uso del busto o la chirurgia non rientrano nel trattamento di questa condizione.

CIFOSI STRUTTURALE

MALATTIA DI SCHEUERMANN. La malattia di Scheuermann, la forma più comune di ipercifosi strutturale, può verificarsi a livello della colonna toracica o toracolombare. Oltre all'ipercifosi, questa condizione è per definizione caratterizzata dalla cuneizzazione (>5°) di 3 o più corpi vertebrali consecutivi all'apice della deformità in una radiografia laterale. Gli aspetti radiografici associati sono irregolarità dei piatti vertebrali e nodi di Schmorl. I campioni istologici hanno dimostrato un pattern alterato di ossificazione encondrale, ma rimane da chiarire se questi aspetti siano primitivi (genetici o metabolici) o secondari (da sovraccarico meccanico). Anche se l'eziologia resta sconosciuta, è probabile che siano coinvolte forze meccaniche in un individuo geneticamente suscettibile. L'incidenza riportata va dallo 0,4 al 10% e i maschi sono colpiti più delle femmine.

MANIFESTAZIONI CLINICHE. È presente un'ipercifosi della colonna toracica, tipicamente associata a un profilo acuto, mentre l'apice della deformità si trova spesso nella colonna toracica inferiore. I pazienti non sono in grado di correggere volontariamente la deformità. Il dolore è un disturbo abbastanza comune ed è tipicamente lieve nell'area dell'apice della cifosi. I sintomi sono intermittenti, raramente severi, e talvolta limitano certe attività. I sintomi neurologici sono infrequenti.

VALUTAZIONE RADIOGRAFICA. Si eseguono radiografie standard nelle proiezioni anteroposteriore e laterale (Fig. 678-5). Per la proiezione laterale si raccomanda una tecnica specifica standardizzata, in cui il paziente tiene le braccia piegate sul torace. Oltre agli aspetti diagnostici già menzionati, si osserva comunemente una lieve scoliosi, mentre è meno frequente identificare una spondilolistesi sulla proiezione laterale.

TRATTAMENTO. Il trattamento dipende dall'età del paziente, dal grado di deformità e dalla presenza di sintomi. La storia naturale della malattia di Scheuermann sembra essere relativamente benigna. Le prime segnalazioni facevano pensare che alterazioni degenerative e dolore significativi fossero comuni con le curve in eccesso di 75°, mentre altri studi riferiscono un esito più benigno. Anche se gli adulti con malattia di Scheuermann non trattata possono presentare una dorsalgia più intensa, la prevalenza di dorsalgia sembra non essere differente rispetto a quella della popolazione generale. I pazienti possono scegliere occupazioni più sedentarie, ma non sembrano differire dalla popolazione generale in quanto ad autostima, partecipazione ad attività quotidiane e ricreative e livello di istruzione. Le deformità cifotiche >90° hanno una maggiore probabilità di essere esteticamente inaccettabili, sintomatiche e progressive; quelle >100° possono essere associate a disfunzione polmonare.

Esistono poche linee guida assolute per il trattamento e le decisioni devono essere individualizzate. I pazienti immaturi da un punto di vista scheletrico che presentano una deformità lieve possono trarre beneficio da un programma di esercizi in iperestensione, ma gli effetti di questa strategia sulla storia naturale devono ancora essere documentati. Se resta più di un anno di crescita e la cifosi è >55-60° può essere utile un'ortesi. Si raccomanda un corsetto di Milwaukee (esteso fino al collo) per le curve con un apice al di sopra di T7, mentre le curve con un apice posto più in basso lungo la colonna possono spesso essere trattate con un'ortesi toracolombare. Si raccomanda che il paziente indossi l'apparecchio fino a 23 ore al giorno. Talvolta si possono utilizzare gessi seriati (o un programma di esercizi di stretching) per ottenere flessibilità prima di adottare l'ortesi. Quest'ultima ha lo scopo di prevenire la progressione, mentre è meno frequente un miglioramento permanente dell'allineamento. Quando l'ortesi è efficace, le radiografie evidenziano spesso una ricostituzione dell'altezza vertebrale anteriore (inversione della cuneizzazione), che determina un miglioramento permanente dell'allineamento. Non si trattano i pazienti maturi da un punti di vista scheletrico con dolore scarso o assente e un aspetto estetico accettabile. Nei pazienti con deformità progressiva >70-80° non soddisfatti del proprio aspetto estetico e in quelli con dorsalgia persistente nonostante il trattamento conservativo si può prendere in considerazione una fusione vertebrale finale. Di solito è necessaria una fusione dalla colonna toracica superiore alla colonna lombare superiore. Alcuni chirurghi eseguono una semplice fusione vertebrale posteriore strumentata, mentre altri raccomandano il rilascio vertebrale anteriore e la fusione, seguiti da una fusione vertebrale posteriore strumentata.

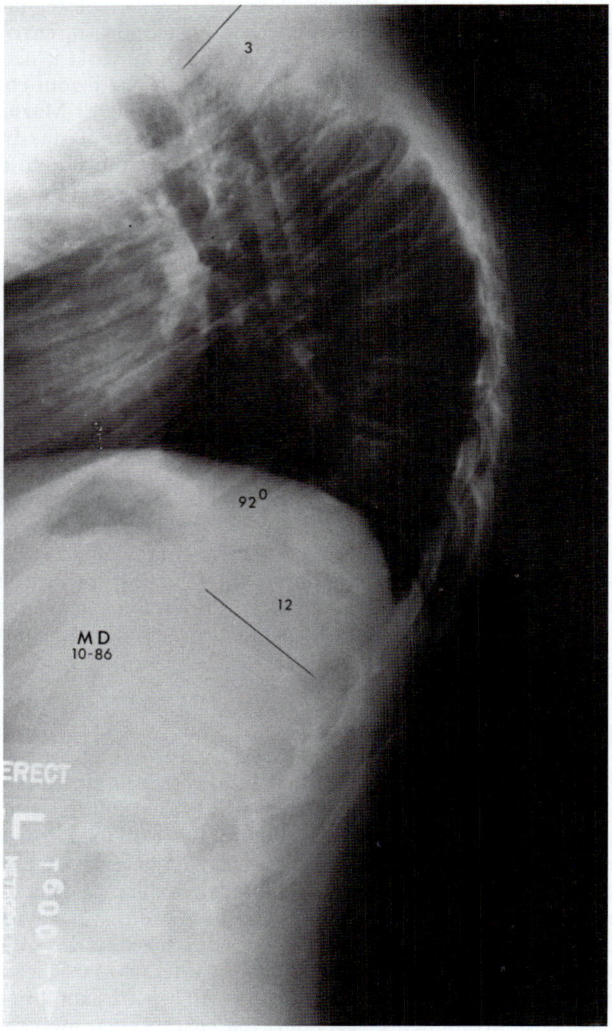

Figura 678-5. Radiografia laterale in posizione eretta di un ragazzo di 14 anni con cifosi di Scheuermann severa. Questa misura 92° tra T3 e T12. Si noti la cuneizzazione delle vertebre a T6, T7, T8 e T9. La cifosi toracica normale è ≤40°.

CIFOSI CONGENITA

La cifosi congenita deriva da malformazioni vertebrali congenite. In caso di mancato sviluppo anteriore (tipo I), non si forma una parte del corpo vertebrale. La cifosi che ne deriva, presente alla nascita, progredisce rapidamente e determina comunemente una disfunzione neurologica, se non trattata. La disfunzione del midollo spinale di solito è causata dalla compressione del midollo spinale all'apice della deformità. Il tipo II consiste in una mancata segmentazione anteriore, in cui due vertebre sono fuse anteriormente. Con la continua crescita degli elementi posteriori della colonna si sviluppa spesso una cifosi progressiva. Il tipo II è meno associato a un deficit neurologico; tuttavia, i pazienti devono essere seguiti attentamente e il trattamento si rende necessario in un numero significativo di casi. Come nella scoliosi congenita, bisogna escludere anomalie di altri apparati.

Il trattamento dipende dal tipo di malformazione, dal grado di deformità e dall'eventuale presenza di sintomi neurologici. Le ortesi sono per lo più inutili e l'intervento chirurgico (artrodesi vertebrale) di solito è l'unica opzione di trattamento efficace. Dal momento che la storia naturale è così sfavorevole per le cifosi di tipo I, in genere si procede alla fusione vertebrale subito dopo la diagnosi. Si eseguono per lo più una fusione anteriore e una fusione vertebrale posteriore, con o senza strumentazione. L'ideale sarebbe stabilizzare la colonna prima che si stabilisca una deformità severa. La costotrasversectomia è un altro approccio possibile (Fig. 678-6). Anche le deformità di tipo II richiedono una stabilizzazione vertebrale nella maggior parte dei casi, ma con una mancata segmentazione vi è meno urgenza. Spesso è possibile seguire i pazienti per un certo periodo di tempo prima che si renda necessario l'intervento e in alcuni casi non è richiesto alcun trattamento.

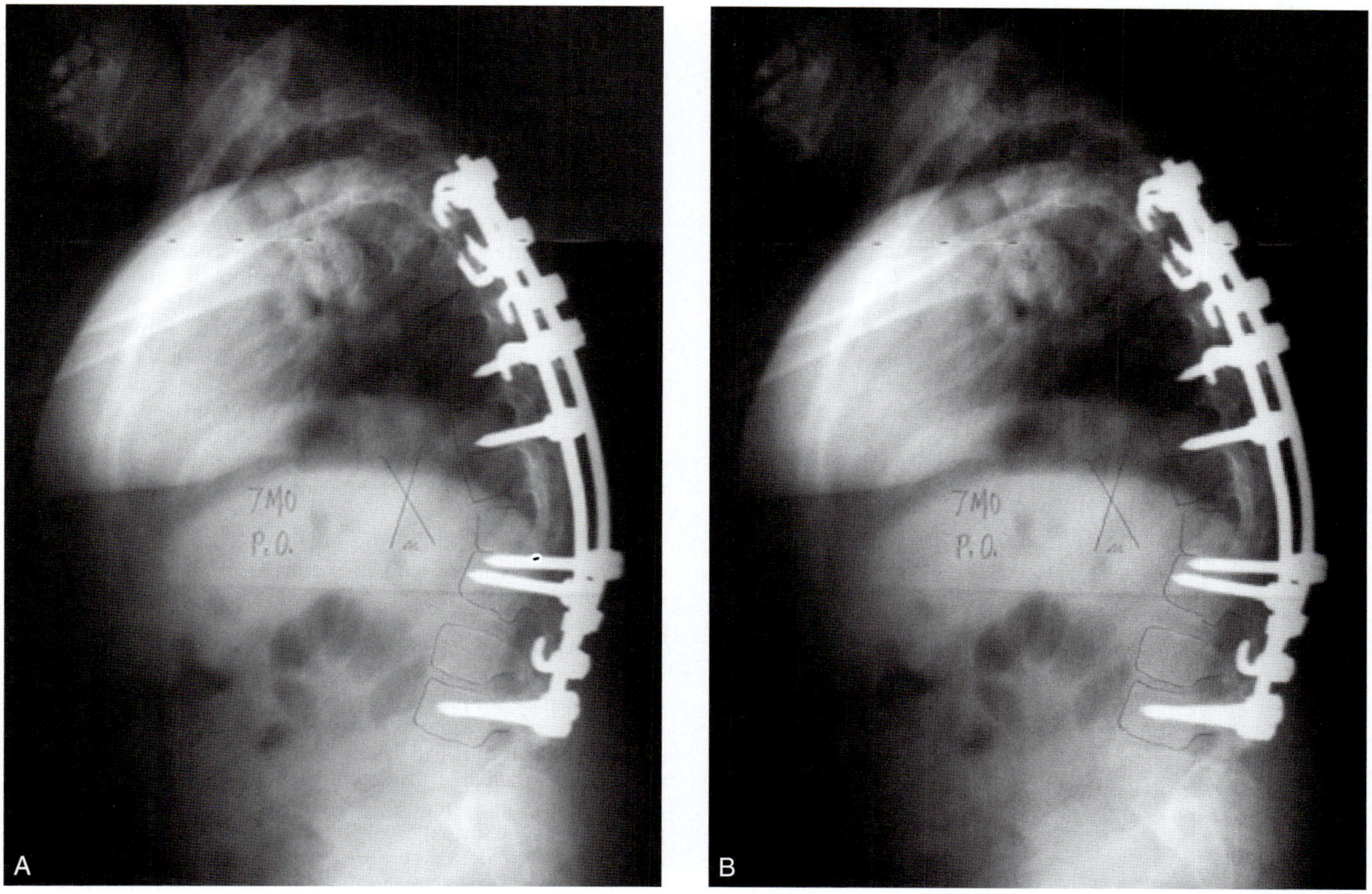

Figura 678-6. Radiografie della colonna di un ragazzo di 11 anni con cifosi progressiva secondaria a cifosi congenita di tipo I. *A*, Radiografia preoperatoria che evidenzia una deformità cifotica di 61° con emivertebra posteriore intrappolata in T11. *B*, Radiografia laterale 7 mesi dopo l'escissione dell'emivertebra con approccio solo posteriore mediante costotrasversectomia, con fissazione vertebrale segmentaria da T5 a L3. La cifosi postoperatoria misurava 41°. (Da Smith JT, Gollogly S, Dunn HK: Simultaneous anterior-posterior approach through a costotransversectomy for the treatment of congenital kyphosis and acquired kyphoscoliotic deformities. *J Bone Joint Surg Am* 2005;87:2281-2289.)

678.5 • Dorsalgia nei bambini

La dorsalgia è un disturbo relativamente frequente nei bambini e negli adolescenti e la diagnosi differenziale è molto ampia (Tab. 678-2). Sono necessari un'anamnesi e un esame obiettivo accurati, spesso associati a imaging, per escludere qualsiasi processo patologico di base nei pazienti con dolore persistente.

VALUTAZIONE CLINICA. Al momento di raccogliere l'anamnesi bisogna innanzitutto annotare la sede, il carattere e la durata dei sintomi. Occorre ricercare qualsiasi storia di trauma acuto o attività fisiche ripetitive. Un dolore costante, non alleviato dal riposo e che sveglia il paziente dal sonno ha maggiori probabilità di essere secondario a un'infezione o a una neoplasia. È preoccupante anche la presenza di segni sistemici (febbre, brividi) o sintomi costituzionali (calo ponderale, malessere). Bisogna inoltre individuare i sintomi di una disfunzione neurologica, interrogando i pazienti sulla presenza di qualsiasi sintomo radicolare, alterazioni del cammino, perdita di forza, alterazioni della sensibilità e anomalie della funzionalità intestinale e/o vescicale. L'esame obiettivo comprende una completa valutazione muscoloscheletrica e neurologica, e il paziente deve essere adeguatamente esposto per l'esame obiettivo. Si raccomanda di prestare attenzione a qualsiasi alterazione dell'allineamento sul piano frontale o sagittale e di valutare l'arco di movimento in flessione, estensione e bending laterale. Si deve chiedere ai bambini più piccoli di raccogliere un oggetto da terra per valutare la flessione della colonna. I pazienti con dolore alla flessione (compressione sulla colonna spinale anteriore) possono presentare un'anomalia del corpo vertebrale o del disco come una discite. I pazienti con dolore da estensione (compressione sugli elementi posteriori) possono avere una spondilolistesi o altri problemi degli elementi posteriori. La palpazione rivelerà qualsiasi area di dolorabilità e/o spasmo muscolare. La palpazione dell'estremità superiore delle ali iliache mentre il paziente è in piedi permette di valutare la lunghezza delle gambe. Occorre eseguire anche un esame dell'addome e, nelle femmine, può essere necessaria una valutazione ginecologica, dal momento che problemi a questo livello possono dar luogo a dolore riferito alla colonna. Una patologia a livello dell'articolazione sacroiliaca può occasionalmente simulare una lombalgia e questa articolazione deve essere messa sotto stress mediante compressione delle ali iliache o con rotazione esterna a livello dell'anca. Si deve procedere a un'accurata valutazione neurologica. Oltre all'esame muscolare manuale e alla valutazione di sensibilità e propriocezione, occorre esaminare il riflesso addominale superficiale strofinando delicatamente la cute di ciascuno dei quattro quadranti che circondano l'ombelico. In condizioni normali l'ombelico si sposterà verso l'area stimolata. Il risultato del test è normale se si ottiene una risposta simmetrica a entrambi i lati della linea mediana, anche se il riflesso non è elicitabile da un lato. Un test anomalo suggerisce la presenza di una lieve anomalia della funzione del midollo spinale, per lo più una siringomielia. Il test di sollevamento della gamba diritta valuta la tensione esercitata sulle radici spinali inferiori, ricercando un'ernia discale o uno scivolamento dell'apofisi vertebrale.

VALUTAZIONE RADIOGRAFICA E DI LABORATORIO. Innanzitutto si raccomandano radiografie della regione della colonna vertebrale interessata, nelle proiezioni anteroposteriore e laterale. In caso di lombalgia si devono eseguire anche proiezioni oblique destra e sinistra. Nei pazienti con esame neurologico normale, una TC

TABELLA 678-2. Diagnosi differenziale della dorsalgia

INFIAMMATORIA/INFETTIVA
Discite
Osteomielite vertebrale (piogenica, tubercolare)
Ascesso epidurale spinale
Pielonefrite
Pancreatite
REUMATOLOGICA
Artrite reumatoide giovanile pauciarticolare
Sindrome di Reiter
Spondilite anchilosante
Artrite psoriasica
EVOLUTIVA
Spondilolisi
Spondilolistesi
Malattia di Scheuermann
Scoliosi
TRAUMATICA (ACUTA O RIPETITIVA)
Anomalie di anca/bacino
Ernia del disco
Sindromi da uso eccessivo
Fratture vertebrali da stress
Instabilità della colonna cervicale superiore
NEOPLASTICA
Tumori vertebrali
Benigni
Granuloma eosinofilo
Cisti ossea aneurismatica
Osteoma osteoide
Osteoblastoma
Maligni
Sarcoma osteogeno
Leucemia
Linfoma
Tumore metastatico
Midollo spinale, gangli e radici nervose
Tumore intramidollare del midollo spinale
Catena del simpatico
Ganglioneuroma
Ganglioneuroblastoma
Neuroblastoma
ALTRE CAUSE
Patologia intraddominale o pelvica
Puntura lombare
Reazione da conversione
Osteoporosi giovanile

ossea a emissione di fotone singolo (SPECT, *Single-Photon Emission Computed Tomography*) può servire a diagnosticare una reazione da stress o una spondilolisi. La RM è particolarmente utile quando sono presenti segni e sintomi neurologici. La TC è l'esame di scelta per la definizione delle lesioni ossee. Quando sono presenti segni sistemici o sintomi costituzionali, occorre eseguire un emocromo completo e determinare VES e proteina C-reattiva. In certi casi, sono indicate le indagini di laboratorio per le forme giovanili di artrite reumatoide (artrite reumatoide giovanile e spondilite anchilosante).

678.6 • Spondilolisi e spondilolistesi

La **spondilolisi** rappresenta un difetto unilaterale o bilaterale della pars interarticularis, il segmento osseo che connette le faccette articolari superiore e inferiore. Si tratta di una condizione acquisita, che si presenta nel 4-6% circa della popolazione adulta e che si ritiene derivare da stress ripetitivi in iperestensione, per cui la faccetta articolare inferiore impatta con la pars interarticularis. La condizione si sviluppa come una frattura da stress, che quindi progredisce in molti casi a pseudoartrosi. I pazienti con un'eccessiva lordosi lombare possono essere predisposti e la spondilolisi è più comune negli atleti che eseguono gesti tecnici comprendenti l'iperestensione ripetitiva della colonna, in particolare ginnasti, giocatori di football americano (specialmente il lineman interno), sollevatori di pesi e lottatori. È stata avanzata l'ipotesi di una componente genetica. La lesione è particolarmente comune a livello di L5, ma può essere identificata anche nei livelli lombari superiori. Circa il 5% dei casi di spondilolisi svilupperà un ulteriore scivolamento della vertebra interessata sulla vertebra sottostante (spondilolistesi). La storia naturale è variabile. Anche se un sottogruppo di casi rimane asintomatico, la spondilolisi è una causa comune di dorsalgia negli adolescenti.

La **spondilolistesi**, ossia lo scivolamento di una vertebra su un'altra, è anch'essa più comune a livello di L5. Nei bambini e negli adolescenti, i tipi più comuni sono le forme displasica (congenita) e istmica (derivante da una frattura da stress). Può presentare quattro gradi di gravità, stabiliti in base all'entità dello spostamento vertebrale: grado 1 (<25%), grado 2 (25-50%), grado 3 (50-75%), grado 4 (75-100%) e grado 5 (spostamento completo o spondiloptosi). I segni fisici dipendono anche dal grado di rotazione sagittale della vertebra superiore su quella inferiore.

MANIFESTAZIONI CLINICHE. I pazienti sintomatici con spondilolisi di solito si presentano con lombalgia meccanica che può irradiarsi alle natiche, con o senza spasmo dei muscoli flessori della gamba. I sintomi radicolari non sono frequenti. Il dolore è esacerbato dall'iperestensione della colonna. L'esame obiettivo può rivelare una limitazione della flessibilità lombare, oltre a dolore alla palpazione sui processi spinosi della vertebra interessata. Un importante segno clinico è lo spasmo dei muscoli flessori della gamba, che determina una lieve contrattura e spesso dolore durante l'esame dell'arco di movimento.

I pazienti con spondilolistesi, oltre alla lombalgia, possono presentare anche sintomi neurologici (radiculopatia o disfunzione intestinale/vescicale) da compressione della cauda equina o delle radici nervose. Si riscontrano di solito una perdita della mobilità spinale e spesso alterazioni del cammino. Le natiche appaiono appiattite (sacro inclinato più verticalmente, cifosi lombosacrale) e l'addome può essere sporgente. Spesso è presente un dislivello palpabile tra i processi spinosi dei livelli interessati, soprattutto se lo slittamento è di grado elevato. Oltre a un completo esame della colonna (è comunemente associata una scoliosi), è essenziale un accurato esame neurologico.

VALUTAZIONE RADIOGRAFICA. La valutazione iniziale della regione lombare deve comprendere l'esecuzione di radiografie di elevata qualità in proiezione anteroposteriore, laterale e obliqua. Si eseguono radiografie in posizione eretta in proiezione anteroposteriore e laterale se sono presenti anche aspetti suggestivi di scoliosi o ipercifosi (Figg. 678-7 e 678-8). Nei pazienti con radiografie normali, una SPECT ossea può servire a diagnosticare una spondilolistesi allo stadio iniziale, prima che si instauri una pseudoartrosi. Una TC a sezioni sottili può fornire ulteriori informazioni per stabilire la presenza di un difetto della pars interarticularis. La RM è indicata in presenza di segni o sintomi di interessamento della cauda equina o delle radici nervose.

TRATTAMENTO. Mentre i pazienti asintomatici con spondilolisi non richiedono un trattamento attivo, quelli con dolore sono trattati modificando l'attività, con la fisioterapia (tesa soprattutto al rinforzo della muscolatura addominale e paraspinale) e con analgesici non narcotici. L'uso di un'ortesi lombosacrale modificata, che riduce la lordosi lombare e immobilizza la colonna, può portare a una più rapida risoluzione dei sintomi. L'apparecchio viene indossato per 3-4 mesi. Il paziente deve inoltre astenersi dall'attività sportiva fino alla risoluzione dei sintomi. Anche se nella maggior parte dei casi si assiste a una risoluzione dei sintomi, la spondilolisi guarisce soltanto in un piccolo numero di pazienti che hanno ricevuto una diagnosi prima di sviluppare un difetto della pars interarticularis. Si propone l'intervento quando le misure precedenti non sono state sufficienti a controllare i sintomi. Se la spondilolisi è a livello di L5, è indicata una fusione vertebrale posteriore da L5 a S1. Nei casi, peraltro non frequenti,

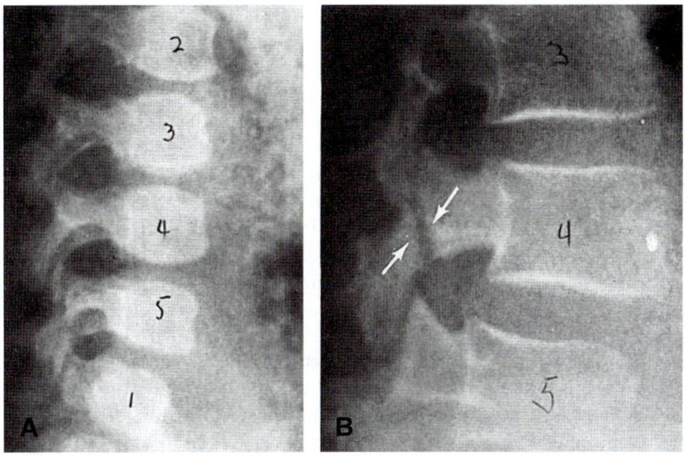

Figura 678-7. *A*, Colonna normale a 9 mesi di età. *B*, Spondilolisi di L4 a 10 anni di età. (Da Silverman FN, Kuhn JP: *Essentials of Caffrey's Pediatric X-Ray Diagnosis*. Chicago, Year Book Medical Publishers, 1990, p. 94.)

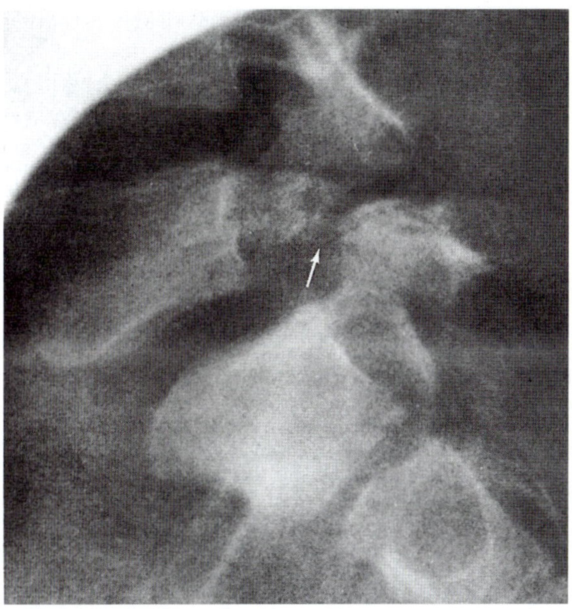

Figura 678-8. Difetto della pars interarticularis (*freccia*) dell'arco neurale di L5 (spondilolisi) che ha permesso al corpo di L5 di scivolare anteriormente (spondilolistesi) sul corpo di S1. (Da Silverman FN, Kuhn JP: *Essentials of Caffrey's Pediatric X-Ray Diagnosis*. Chicago, Year Book Medical Publishers, 1990, p. 95.)

in cui il difetto è situato a un livello più elevato della colonna lombare, si possono prendere in esame metodiche per la riparazione del difetto. In caso di successo, queste procedure permetteranno di evitare la fusione chirurgica delle due vertebre. Le raccomandazioni per il trattamento della spondilolistesi dipendono dall'età del paziente, dalla presenza di sintomi (dolore e/o neurologici), dal grado di deformità e, in misura minore, dai problemi estetici. Per le lesioni di basso grado (slittamento <50%), il trattamento è simile a quello della spondilolisi. Dal momento che può verificarsi uno scivolamento progressivo in un sottogruppo di pazienti con immaturità scheletrica, si raccomanda generalmente un follow-up ogni 6-12 mesi e occorre eseguire periodicamente una radiografia standard in proiezione laterale della colonna lombare. Per gli scivolamenti di basso grado con sintomi persistenti nonostante le misure conservative, può avere successo una fusione vertebrale senza altri interventi. Ai pazienti con immaturità scheletrica e scivolamento >50% si deve proporre l'intervento chirurgico, considerata l'elevata tendenza di questi casi alla progressione. L'approccio chirurgico a questi scivolamenti di grado elevato, con e senza disfunzione neurologica, è diverso da un chirurgo all'altro, da un centro all'altro. Il concetto principale è quello di stabilizzare il segmento instabile della colonna. Le procedure di comune esecuzione sono la fusione vertebrale posteriore e la fusione vertebrale anteriore e posteriore, con o senza strumentazione vertebrale, con o senza un tentativo di riduzione della deformità. I sintomi neurologici possono risolversi con la stabilizzazione e talvolta si esegue la decompressione degli elementi nervosi nell'ambito della procedura di stabilizzazione.

678.7 • Infezione dello spazio discale

Sia la discite sia l'osteomielite vertebrale possono essere considerate come varianti dipendenti dall'età della spondilite infettiva. La discite si osserva generalmente in soggetti di età <5 anni, mentre l'osteomielite vertebrale si verifica nei bambini più grandi e negli adolescenti. I pazienti nel range di età più basso hanno canali vascolari comunicanti tra il piatto vertebrale e lo spazio vascolare discale, il che spiega la prevalenza di discite. Con la chiusura di tali canali l'infezione rimane confinata alla vertebra.

Lo *Staphylococcus aureus* è il microrganismo di più comune riscontro nel sangue (raramente) o nel liquido aspirato dallo spazio discale (occasionalmente). Altri microrganismi sono la *Kingella kingae*, lo streptococco di gruppo A e l'*Escherichia coli*. Un microrganismo viene isolato da qualsiasi sito soltanto nel 50-60% dei pazienti.

MANIFESTAZIONI CLINICHE. È necessario un elevato indice di sospetto per porre la diagnosi di discite. Oltre alla dorsalgia e/o alla febbre, i pazienti possono presentare malessere, mentre i bambini da 1 a 3 anni possono sviluppare una zoppia o rifiutarsi di camminare o mettersi seduti. Nel tentativo di ridurre il dolore associato ai movimenti della colonna, questa viene mantenuta in una posizione rigida e vi può essere anche un sostegno rappresentato dallo spasmo dei muscoli paraspinali. Vi può essere dolore locale a carico dei processi spinosi. In particolare, la flessione della colonna comprime gli elementi anteriori della colonna ed è associata a un aumento del dolore. Per condurre accertamenti in tal senso si chiede al bambino di raccogliere un oggetto da terra. Si riscontra una perdita della normale lordosi lombare. Tra le manifestazioni neurologiche, peraltro rare, si può osservare la perdita di forza. I pazienti possono essere afebbrili e anche se l'emocromo può essere normale, la VES e la proteina C-reattiva sono di solito elevate. I bambini più grandi possono presentare febbre e dolore addominale simile a quello di un ascesso dello psoas.

VALUTAZIONE RADIOGRAFICA. Gli aspetti radiografici caratteristici, tra cui restringimento dello spazio discale e irregolarità dei piatti vertebrali adiacenti, si sviluppano 2-3 settimane dopo l'esordio dei sintomi. La diagnosi può essere stabilita precocemente mediante una scintigrafia ossea con tecnezio o con la RM; quest'ultima è particolarmente utile per diagnosticare gli ascessi ed escludere un'osteomielite vertebrale.

TRATTAMENTO. Una volta posta la diagnosi, il trattamento sintomatico comprende la limitazione dell'attività, analgesici e l'immobilizzazione in un'ortesi spinale. Dal momento che l'emocoltura e le colture del materiale dello spazio discale sono spesso negative, l'eziologia della discite è stata oggetto di controversie. La maggior parte delle evidenze depone a favore di un'eziologia batterica; si raccomanda quindi che il trattamento comprenda un ciclo di 4-6 settimane di antibiotici efficaci contro lo *S. aureus*, somministrati dapprima per via endovenosa (inizialmente per 1-2 settimane), poi per os. La biopsia con guida TC dello spazio discale non è necessaria di routine, ma viene di solito riservata ai bambini che non rispondono al trattamento antibiotico iniziale. Il trattamento chirurgico è di solito necessario a fini diagnostici, nei pazienti che non rispondono alla terapia iniziale, o per il drenaggio di un ascesso.

678.8 • Ernia del disco intervertebrale/ scivolamento dell'apofisi vertebrale

L'ernia del disco intervertebrale e lo scivolamento dell'apofisi vertebrale sono estremamente rari nei bambini e infrequenti negli adolescenti. Segni e sintomi sono abbastanza simili a quelli degli adulti. Anche se l'eziologia resta sconosciuta, i fattori predisponenti per entrambe queste patologie possono comprendere degenerazione discale, malformazione congenita, fattori genetici e ambientali. Entrambe sono lesioni occupanti spazio che possono comprimere gli elementi nervosi. Mentre l'ernia del disco comporta caratteristicamente una protrusione (raramente un frammento libero) di materiale nucleare nel canale midollare, lo scivolamento dell'apofisi vertebrale consiste nella protrusione di una parte dell'anello apofisario, con o senza un frammento osseo attaccato.

MANIFESTAZIONI CLINICHE. I sintomi dell'ernia del disco intervertebrale negli adolescenti sono simili a quelli degli adulti, e spesso è presente una storia di trauma. Un sottogruppo di pazienti presenta anomalie congenite della colonna lombosacrale. Il principale disturbo è la dorsalgia e gli eventuali sintomi radicolari generalmente compaiono in una fase più avanzata. La dorsalgia è spesso peggiorata dalla tosse o dall'evacuazione. All'esame obiettivo, sono comuni uno spasmo dei muscoli paraspinali e una riduzione dell'arco di movimento. Anche se nella maggior parte dei pazienti sono assenti segni conclamati di interessamento neurologico, di solito il test di sollevamento della gamba diritta risulta positivo. Quando presenti, i sintomi neurologici spesso non sono correlati al livello dell'ernia del disco. Al momento di formulare la diagnosi differenziale, si deve sempre sospettare un tumore intraspinale.

VALUTAZIONE RADIOGRAFICA. Le radiografie spesso evidenziano una perdita della lordosi lombare e una curva lombare (non una vera scoliosi) dovute allo spasmo muscolare. Occasionalmente si notano alla radiografia alterazioni degenerative e/o perdita dell'altezza del disco intervertebrale. La RM è l'indagine più indicata a scopi diagnostici, mentre la TC è utile soprattutto per visualizzare un frammento parzialmente ossificato associato a uno scivolamento ipofisario.

TRATTAMENTO. Il trattamento iniziale è conservativo nella maggior parte dei pazienti e incentrato su riposo, modificazione dell'attività, analgesici e fisioterapia. Un'ortesi può fornire un ulteriore sollievo sintomatico. Non è indicato il riposo completo a letto. Il ruolo degli steroidi per via epidurale deve ancora essere determinato. Il trattamento chirurgico deve essere considerato quando le misure conservative sono fallite o quando è presente una grave sindrome con deficit neurologico o della cauda equina, sia inizialmente sia durante l'evoluzione del decorso clinico. Purtroppo bambini e adolescenti rispondono meno favorevolmente alla terapia conservativa rispetto agli adulti e una significativa percentuale richiederà l'intervento chirurgico. La tecnica chirurgica consiste in una laminectomia e un'escissione subtotale del disco per decomprimere gli elementi nervosi. In caso di scivolamento dell'apofisi vertebrale, si utilizza un approccio similare, ma si rende necessario rimuovere anche i frammenti di osso e cartilagine, il che spesso richiede una laminectomia bilaterale per risolvere in modo completo la patologia. Anche se i risultati iniziali sono eccellenti nella maggior parte dei pazienti, dalla letteratura si deduce che fino a un terzo dei pazienti può avere sintomi ricorrenti di dorsalgia o di dolore delle gambe, al follow-up a lungo termine. Può essere necessaria una fusione vertebrale quando è presente un'instabilità clinica.

678.9 • Tumori

Una dorsalgia può essere il più comune sintomo di presentazione nei bambini con tumore della colonna vertebrale o del midollo spinale. Altri sintomi associati comprendono perdita di forza delle estremità inferiori, scoliosi e perdita del controllo degli sfinteri. La maggior parte dei tumori è benigna (vedi Capitolo 501): osteoma osteoide, osteoblastoma, cisti ossea aneurismatica e granuloma eosinofilo. I tumori maligni della colonna vertebrale possono essere ossei (osteosarcoma o sarcoma di Ewing), interessare il midollo spinale e i nervi simpatici o parasimpatici (ganglioneuroma, ganglioneuroblastoma, neuroblastoma) o infine essere metastatici (eventualità peraltro remota). Oltre a eseguire radiografie di elevata qualità, nella maggior parte dei casi, prima di elaborare un piano di trattamento, si utilizzano altre tecniche di imaging, come la scintigrafia ossea (localizzazione, ricerca di altre lesioni), la RM (estensione nei tessuti molli, compressione neurologica) e la TC (eccellenti dettagli ossei). Per la diagnosi è di solito necessaria una biopsia; il trattamento dei tumori della colonna vertebrale può richiedere un approccio multidisciplinare e dovrebbe essere effettuato in centri con esperienza nella terapia di queste lesioni.

Scoliosi idiopatica

Cassar-Pullicino VN, Eisenstein SM: Imaging in scoliosis: What, why and how? *Clin Radiol* 2002;57:543–562.

Do T, Fras C, Burke S, et al: Clinical value of routine preoperative magnetic resonance imaging in adolescent idiopathic scoliosis: A prospective study of three hundred and twenty-seven patients. *Bone Joint Surg Am* 2001;83:577–579.

Dobbs M, Lenke LG, Szymanski DA, et al: Prevalence of neural axis abnormalities in patients with infantile idiopathic scoliosis. *J Bone Joint Surg Am* 2002;84:2230–2234.

Edgar M: A new classification of adolescent idiopathic scoliosis. *Lancet* 2002;360:270–271.

Goldberg CJ, Moore DP, Fogarty EE, et al: Adolescent idiopathic scoliosis: The effect of brace treatment on the incidence of surgery. *Spine* 2001;26:42–47.

Karol LA: Effectiveness of bracing in male patients with idiopathic scoliosis. *Spine* 2001;26:2001–2005.

Lenke LJ, Betz RR, Harms J, et al: Adolescent idiopathic scoliosis. A new classification to determine the extent of spinal arthrodesis. *J Bone Joint Surg Am* 2001;83:1169–1181.

Little DG, Song KM, Katz D, et al: Relationship of peak height velocity to other maturity indicators in idiopathic scoliosis in girls. *J Bone Joint Surg Am* 2000;82:685–693.

Merola AA, Haher TR, Brkaric M, et al: A multi-center study of the outcomes of the surgical treatment of adolescent idiopathic scoliosis using the Scoliosis Research Society (SRS) outcome instrument. *Spine* 2002;27:2046–2051.

Song KM, Little DG: Peak height velocity as a maturity factor for males with idiopathic scoliosis. *J Pediatr Orthop* 2000;20:286–288.

Sponseller PD: Sizing up scoliosis. *JAMA* 2203;289:608–609.

Weinstein SL, Dolan LA, Spratt KF, et al: Health and function of patients with untreated idiopathic scoliosis. *JAMA* 2003;289:559–567.

Scoliosi congenita/Cifosi

Basu PS, Elsebaie H, Noordeen MH: Congenital spinal deformity: A comprehensive assessment at presentation. *Spine* 2002;27:2255–2259.

Campbell RM, Hell-Vocke AK: Growth of the thoracic spine in congenital scoliosis after expansion thoracoplasty. *J Bone Joint Surg Am* 2003;85:409–420.

Campbell RM, Smith MD, Mayes TC, et al: The characteristics of thoracic insufficiency syndrome associated with fused ribs and congenital scoliosis. *J Bone Joint Surg Am* 2003;85:399–408.

Deviren V, Bervin S, Smith JA, et al: Excision of hemivertebrae in the management of congenital scoliosis involving the thoracic and thoracolumbar spine. *J Bone Joint Surg Br* 2001;83:496–500.

Gollogly S, Smith JT, Campbell RM: Determining lung volume with three-dimensional reconstructions of CT scan data. *J Pediatr Orthop* 2004;24:323–328.

Kim YJ, Otsuka NY, Flynn JM, et al: Surgical treatment of congenital kyphosis. *Spine* 2001;26:2251–2257.

McMaster MJ, Singh H: The surgical management of congenital kyphosis and kyphoscoliosis. *Spine* 2001;26:2146–2154.

Smith JT, Gollogly S, Dunn HK: Simultaneous anterior-posterior approach through a costotransversectomy for the treatment of congenital kyphosis and acquired kyphoscoliotic deformities. *J Bone Joint Surg Am* 2005;87:2281–2289.

Suh SW, Sarwark JF, Vora A, et al: Evaluating congenital spine deformities for intraspinal anomalies with magnetic resonance imaging. *J Pediatr Orthop* 2001;21:525–531.

Scoliosi neuromuscolare

Jones KB, Sponseller PD, Shindle MK, et al: Longitudinal parental perceptions of spinal fusion for neuromuscular spine deformity in patients with totally involved cerebral palsy. *J Pediatr Orthop* 2003;23:143–149.
Spiegel DA, Flynn JM, Stasikelis PJ, et al: Curve patterns in Chiari I malformation and/or syringomyelia. *Spine* 2003;28:2139–2146.
Westerlund LE, Gill SS, Jjarosz TS, et al: Posterior-only unit rod instrumentation and fusion for neuromuscular scoliosis. *Spine* 2001;26:1984–1989.

Cifosi

Boseker EH, Moe JH, Winter RB, Koop SE: Determination of "normal" thoracic kyphosis: A roentgenographic study of 121 "normal" children. *J Pediatr Orthop* 2000;20:796–798.
Papegelopoulos PJ, Klassen RA, Peterson HA, et al: Surgical treatment of Scheuermann's disease with segmental compression instrumentation. *Clin Orthop* 2001;386:139–149.
Poolman RW, Been HD, Ubags LH: Clinical outcome and radiographic results after operative treatment of Scheuermann's disease. *Eur Spine J* 2002;11:561–569.

Dorsalgia

Balague F, Dudler J, Nordin M: Low-back pain in children. *Lancet* 2003;361: 1403–1404.
Feldman DS, Hedden DM, Wright JG: The use of bone scan to investigate back pain in children and adolescents. *J Pediatr Orthop* 2000;20:790–795.
Jones GT, Macfarlane GJ: Epidemiology of low back pain in children and adolescents. *Arch Dis Child* 2005;90:312–316.
Parisini P, DiSilvestre M, Greggi T, et al: Lumbar disc excision in children and adolescents. *Spine* 2001;26:1997–2000.
Speed C: Low back pain. *Br Med J* 2004;328:1119–1121.
Watson KD, Papageorgiou AC, Jones GT, et al: Low back pain in schoolchildren: the role of the mechanical and psychosocial factors. *Arch Dis Child* 2003;88:12–17.

Spondilolisi e spondilolistesi

Grzegorzewski A, Kumar SJ: In situ posterolateral spine arthrodesis for grades III, IV, and V spondylolisthesis in children and adolescents. *J Pediatr Orthop* 2000;20:506–511.
Lenke LG, Bridwell KW: Evaluation and surgical treatment of high-grade isthmic dysplastic spondylolisthesis. *Instr Course Lect* 2003;52:525–532.

Infezione dello spazio discale

Brown R, Hussain M, McHugh K, et al: Discitis in young children. *J Bone Joint Surg Br* 2001;83:106–211.
Early S, Kay R, Tolo V: Childhood diskitis. *J Am Acad Orthop Surg* 2003;11:413–420.
Fernandez M, Carroll CL, Baker CJ: Discitis and vertebral osteomyelitis in children: An 18-year review. *Pediatrics* 2000;105:1299–1304.
Garron E, Veihweger E, Launay F, et al: Nontuberculous spondylodiscitis in children. *J Pediatr Orthop* 2002;22:321–328.
Nussinovitch M, Sokolover N, Volovitz B, Amir J: Neurologic abnormalities in children presenting with diskitis. *Arch Pediatr Adolesc Med* 2002; 156:1052–1054.

Capitolo 679 ■ Il collo

David A. Spiegel, Harish S. Hosalkar, John P. Dormans e Denis S. Drummond

679.1 • Torcicollo

Torcicollo è il termine usato per descrivere i segni fisici consistenti nell'inclinazione laterale del collo e della testa sul lato sinistro o destro, in associazione alla rotazione della testa e del collo dal lato opposto. Il torcicollo non è una diagnosi, ma piuttosto una manifestazione di una varietà di condizioni di base (Tab. 679-1).

TABELLA 679-1. Diagnosi differenziale del torcicollo

CONGENITO
Torcicollo muscolare
Deformità posizionale
Emivertebra (colonna cervicale)
Fusione atlanto-occipitale unilaterale
Sindrome di Klippel-Feil
Assenza unilaterale del muscolo sternocleidomastoideo
Pterygium colli
TRAUMATICO
Lesioni muscolari (muscoli cervicali)
Sublussazione atlanto-occipitale
Sublussazione atlantoassiale
Sublussazione C2-C3
Sublussazione rotatoria
Fratture
INFIAMMATORIO
Linfoadenite cervicale
Ascesso retrofaringeo
Osteomielite vertebrale cervicale
Artrite reumatoide
Sublussazione spontanea (iperemia, edema) con infezione adiacente della testa e del collo (sindrome della sublussazione rotatoria): sindrome di Grisel
Polmonite del lobo superiore
NEUROLOGICO
Disturbi visivi (nistagmo, paresi del muscolo obliquo superiore)
Reazioni distoniche da farmaci (fenotiazine, aloperidolo, metoclopramide)
Tumore del midollo spinale cervicale
Tumore della fossa cranica posteriore
Siringomielia
Malattia di Wilson
Dystonia muscolorum deformans
Spasmus nutans
ALTRI
Calcificazione acuta dei dischi cervicali
Sindrome di Sandifer (reflusso gastroesofageo, ernia iatale)
Torcicollo parossistico benigno
Tumori ossei (granuloma eosinofilo)
Tumore dei tessuti molli
Isteria

La maggior parte dei casi diagnosticati alla nascita o subito dopo rappresenta un **torcicollo muscolare congenito** (CMT, *Congenital Muscular Torticollis*). Anche se l'eziologia è sconosciuta, questa deformità può derivare da un anormale posizionamento in utero e comporta la retrazione del muscolo sternocleidomastoideo. La biopsia muscolare e la RM suggeriscono che il torcicollo congenito possa essere causato da una sindrome compartimentale intramuscolare. Un trauma muscolare intrauterino da compressione e/o stiramento può creare un'ischemia localizzata, che a sua volta determina fibrosi e retrazione. È stata riportata una base familiare del torcicollo come anche dell'aplasia muscolare ereditaria. Una retrazione del muscolo sternocleidomastoideo sinistro determina un'inclinazione della testa a sinistra e una rotazione verso destra e viceversa. Il CMT è definito in base alla presenza di una massa palpabile (tessuto fibroso) all'interno del muscolo sternocleidomastoideo, aspetto che tuttavia è presente in circa la metà dei pazienti. La massa scompare nel corso della prima infanzia, sostituita da una banda fibrosa. Segni associati comprendono plagiocefalia e asimmetria facciale, che si risolvono entrambe con il ripristino della mobilità cervicale. I pazienti possono presentare deformità muscoloscheletriche posizionali come metatarso addotto e piedi calcaneovalghi (vedi Capitoli 673.1 e 673.2). Il 5-8% circa dei pazienti presenta inoltre una displasia dell'anca. Nonostante non siano stati stabiliti gli standard per lo screening dei pazienti con esame dell'anca normale, occorre prendere in considerazione un'ecografia (all'età di 1 mese) o una radiografia dell'anca (all'età di 4-5 mesi).

Il torcicollo nei neonati può inoltre derivare da anomalie vertebrali congenite; le radiografie anteroposteriore e laterale della colonna cervicale sono indicate quando i tipici aspetti clinici associati al torcicollo muscolare congenito sono assenti o la deformità non risponde al trattamento. Un programma di stretching dovrebbe essere efficace in più del 90% dei pazienti con torcicollo muscolare congenito, specialmente se il trattamento viene iniziato nei primi 3 mesi di vita. Per i pazienti in cui la diagnosi è stata tardiva o per quelli in cui il programma di stretching non ha corretto la deformità, si deve prendere in considerazione il rilascio chirurgico del muscolo sternocleidomastoideo. Prima di eseguire l'intervento si può attendere che il bambino abbia raggiunto 1-1,5 anni di età, per ottenere la massima correzione spontanea della plagiocefalia. Dopo il rilascio chirurgico, il movimento può migliorare fino ai primi anni dell'adolescenza. Il trattamento chirurgico determina una funzione adeguata e un aspetto estetico accettabile in più del 90% dei pazienti. Se la diagnosi e il trattamento sono precoci, la chirurgia dovrebbe essere necessaria in una minoranza di casi.

La valutazione del torcicollo diviene più complessa quando sono assenti i segni tipici associati al CMT (massa e/o retrazione del muscolo sternocleidomastoideo), non si osserva la tipica risposta clinica o la deformità insorge in un'età più tardiva. In tali casi, saranno utili un'anamnesi e un esame obiettivo accurati e, spesso, il parere di un oftalmologo e/o un neurologo. Occorre eseguire un'indagine radiologica e in un sottogruppo di casi può essere necessaria anche una RM del cervello e della colonna cervicale. La diagnosi differenziale è ampia (vedi Tab. 679-1). Lo **spostamento rotatorio atlantoassiale** rappresenta uno spettro di disordini da disallineamento rotazionale (da sublussazione a lussazione) tra atlante C1 ed epistrofeo (C2): la definizione migliore è "rigidità patologica dell'arco di movimento articolare". La fissazione rotatoria atlantoassiale è la completa perdita di movimento che si manifesta come torcicollo, con perdita della rotazione cervicale passiva. Il disallineamento può dapprima essere riducibile, ma dopo un periodo di settimane o mesi la deformità diviene fissa e irriducibile. Pertanto, diagnosi e trattamento precoci sono essenziali. La condizione è per lo più secondaria a infezione/infiammazione dei tessuti delle vie respiratorie superiori, del collo e/o della faringe (**sindrome di Grisel**). Anche i traumi, di solito minori, possono portare allo sviluppo di uno spostamento rotatorio. Questa condizione complica talvolta le procedure chirurgiche a carico di orofaringe, orecchio o naso. Per valutare nel modo migliore il disallineamento rotazionale di questa articolazione si fa ricorso alla TC, in cui le immagini assiali sono ottenute attraverso la colonna cervicale superiore in posizioni differenti (rotazione destra e sinistra). Questa indagine non solo permette di stabilire la diagnosi, ma determina se lo spostamento può essere ridotto passivamente. Uno spostamento "fisso" persiste con la testa in posizioni differenti. Se il paziente viene osservato entro pochi giorni dall'esordio dei sintomi, si può tentare con un ciclo di analgesici e un collare morbido. I pazienti con sintomi che durano da più di una settimana vengono spesso ricoverati in ospedale per la somministrazione di analgesici, rilassanti muscolari e un periodo di trazione cervicale. Se queste misure non riducono lo spostamento, si può tentare con la trazione mediante halo. Se l'articolazione è riducibile, i pazienti vengono caratteristicamente immobilizzati per almeno 6 settimane in un corsetto con halo. I pazienti con deformità fissa possono necessitare di una fissazione atlantoassiale posteriore per stabilizzare l'articolazione.

Il **torcicollo neurogeno**, peraltro infrequente, è imputabile a tumori della fossa posteriore o del tronco encefalico, siringomielia e malformazione di Arnold-Chiari. Oltre all'esame neurologico, è necessaria la RM del cervello e della colonna cervicale per stabilire la diagnosi. Anche il **torcicollo parossistico dell'infanzia** è infrequente e può essere dovuto a disfunzione vestibolare. Gli episodi possono durare da minuti a giorni e il lato della deformità può alternarsi. La condizione è autolimitata e non è necessario alcun trattamento specifico, a parte l'esclusione di altre diagnosi curabili. Il torcicollo può essere osservato anche in associazione a discite o osteomielite vertebrale, artrite reumatoide giovanile, calcificazione dei dischi cervicali, problemi visivi (strabismo da paralisi dei muscoli extraoculari), condizioni simil-tumorali e nei pazienti con paralisi cerebrale e reflusso gastroesofageo cronico (sindrome di Sandifer).

679.2 • Sindrome di Klippel-Feil

La sindrome di Klippel-Feil consiste nella fusione congenita (mancata segmentazione) di uno o più segmenti mobili cervicali e la maggior parte dei pazienti presenta anomalie congenite della colonna cervicale (Fig. 679-1) a livello della giunzione craniocer-

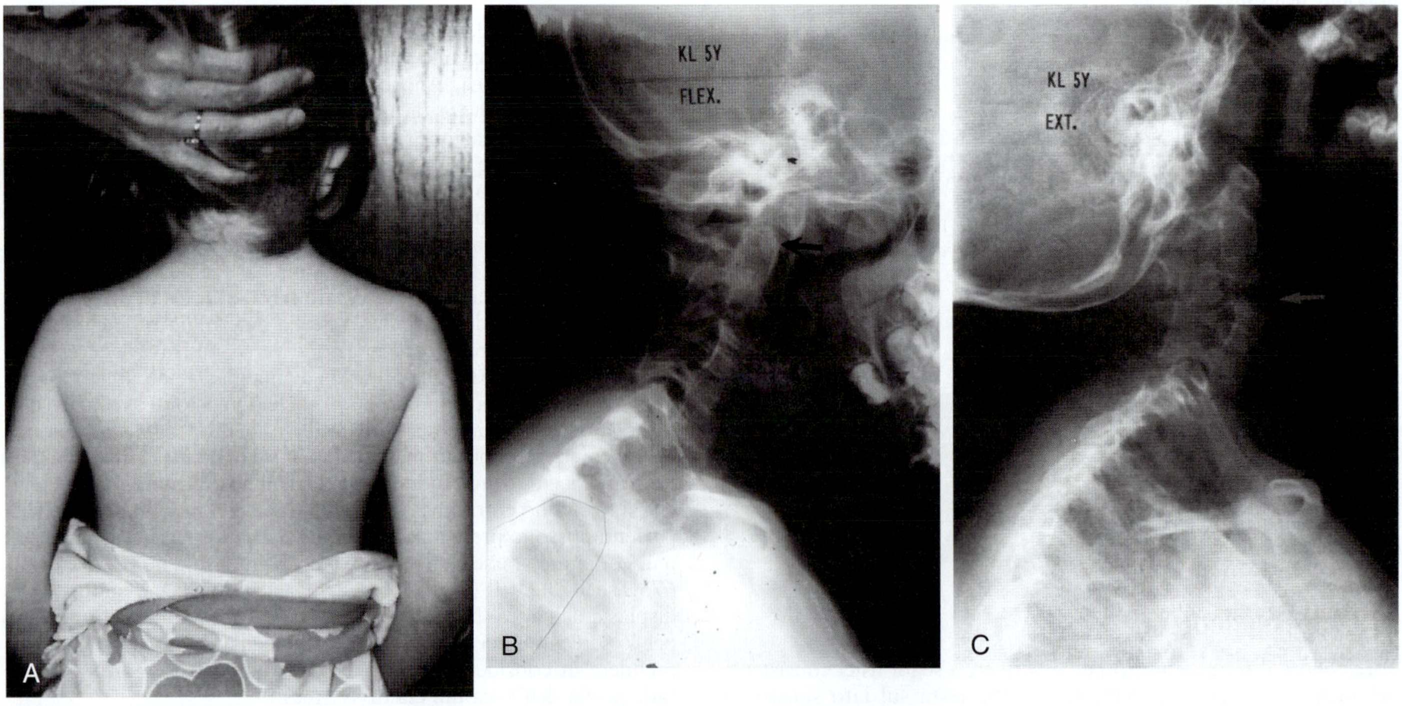

Figura 679-1. Quadro clinico di un bambino di 5 anni con sindrome di Klippel-Feil. *A*, Si notino il collo corto e l'attaccatura del capelli bassa. Le radiografie della colonna cervicale (*B*, flessione; *C*, estensione) dimostrano la presenza di fusione congenita e instabilità spinale (*freccia*). (Da Drummond DS: Pediatric cervical instability. In Weisel SE, Boden SD, Wisnecki RI [ed]: *Seminars in Spine Surgery*. Philadelphia, WB Saunders, 1996, pp. 292-309.)

vicale (occipite-C2), della colonna subassiale (al di sotto di C2) o di entrambe. La triade clinica di collo corto, attaccatura dei capelli bassa e limitazione dei movimenti del collo si osserva soltanto nella metà circa dei pazienti. Esiste una forte associazione con anomalie congenite del tratto genitourinario (30-40%), tra cui un sistema collettore doppio, aplasia renale e rene a ferro di cavallo. Anomalie associate possono essere presenti nel sistema uditivo, nell'asse nervoso, nell'apparato cardiovascolare e in quello muscoloscheletrico. La deformità di Sprengel (elevazione congenita della scapola) è un aspetto comunemente associato e più del 50% dei pazienti sviluppa una scoliosi. Dal momento che possono essere presenti anomalie congenite in più di una regione della colonna, si eseguono di routine radiografie della colonna toracica e lombosacrale. Queste alterazioni cervicali sono osservabili anche in pazienti con sindrome di Goldenhar, sindrome di Mohr, sindrome VACTERL e sindrome alcolica fetale.

I segni fisici caratteristici comprendono un'attaccatura dei capelli bassa e un collo corto con pterigio. Di solito è presente una riduzione della mobilità cervicale, anche se il grado della limitazione dipende dalla sede e dal numero di livelli fusi e può esserne difficile l'identificazione in pazienti affetti solo in misura minima. Il torcicollo può essere tenuto sotto osservazione. La valutazione iniziale deve comprendere le proiezioni anteroposteriore, laterale e obliqua della colonna cervicale. L'aspetto caratteristico è una fusione congenita di 2 o più vertebre (mancata segmentazione); possono essere interessate diverse vertebre. I sintomi, più comuni negli adulti che nei bambini o negli adolescenti, comprendono dolore e/o disfunzione neurologica. Anomalie degenerative dolorose dei dischi e/o delle faccette articolari possono derivare da un'alterazione degli stress meccanici e può svilupparsi un'ipermobilità o un'instabilità a livello dei segmenti mobili adiacenti a quelli fusi. Un'eccessiva mobilità segmentaria (instabilità) può divenire clinicamente evidente sotto forma di radiculopatia o mielopatia, e può verificarsi anche una compressione del tronco encefalico. Anche una stenosi spinale, evolutiva o acquisita, può determinare dolore e/o compressione neurologica. Le proiezioni laterali in flessoestensione possono servire a identificare i segmenti con eccessiva mobilità e se sono presenti sintomi neurologici è utile la RM. Può essere necessario un intervento chirurgico per decomprimere gli elementi nervosi e/o stabilizzare i segmenti della colonna cervicale.

679.3 • Anomalie e instabilità cervicali

Una o più anomalie della giunzione craniovertebrale e/o della colonna cervicale inferiore (sindrome di Klippel-Feil) sono osservabili in forma isolata o in associazione con altre patologie (sindromi genetiche, displasie scheletriche, connettivopatie, malattie metaboliche). Queste possono essere congenite, derivando da una mutazione dei geni homeobox, o evolutive. Anche se la maggior parte dei casi decorre asintomatica e sfugge alla diagnosi, un sottogruppo può mettere il paziente a rischio di danni neurologici basati sull'instabilità o sulla stenosi. Le cause più frequenti di instabilità cervicale nei bambini sono classificabili in base all'eziologia (Tab. 679-2).

Nei pazienti con associazioni note occorre valutare la colonna cervicale. Altri possono presentarsi con dolore e/o sintomi neurologici. Tra i segni fisici si osserva una limitazione della mobilità cervicale, con o senza anomalie neurologiche. Nella colonna cervicale superiore, flessione ed estensione si verificano a livello dell'articolazione tra occipite e C1, mentre la rotazione si verifica a livello dell'articolazione atlantoassiale (C1-C2). Entrambe le articolazioni sono prive di una stabilità ossea intrinseca e dipendono invece dall'integrità dei legamenti e delle capsule articolari per contenere la mobilità. L'instabilità può determinare una compressione del tronco dell'encefalo e/o del midollo spinale. Le anomalie della giunzione craniovertebrale comprendono fusione occipitoatlantoidea (occipitalizzazione dell'atlante), impressione e invaginazione basilare e vertebre accessorie. Un'aplasia o ipoplasia dell'atlante o dell'epistrofeo possono determinare un'instabilità atlantoassiale. La presenza di un **os odontoideum** rappresenta una discontinuità della parte media del dente dell'epistrofeo e la parte superiore del dente si muove insieme all'anello di C1, restringendo lo spazio disponibile per il midollo spinale e spesso mettendo a rischio di lesioni lo stesso midollo. Anche se l'eziologia dell'os odontoideum è ancora controversa, si sospetta un'origine traumatica.

TABELLA 679-2. Cause di instabilità cervicale pediatrica

CAUSE	SOTTOTIPI
Congenite	***Vertebrali*** (anomalie ossee)
	Difetti cranio-occipitali (vertebre occipitali, impressione basilare, displasie occipitali, ipoplasia condiloidea, atlante occipitalizzato)
	Difetti atlantoassiali (aplasia dell'arco dell'atlante, aplasia del processo odontoideo)
	Anomalie subassiali (mancata segmentazione e/o fusione, spina bifida, spondilolistesi)
	Legamentose oppure
	Anomalie combinate presenti alla nascita come elementi di aberrazioni somatogeniche
	Disordini ***sindromici*** (per es. sindrome di Down, sindrome di Klippel-Feil, sindrome della delezione di 22q11.1, sindrome di Larsen, sindrome di Marfan, sindrome di Ehlers-Danlos)
Acquisite	***Traumi***
	Infezioni (piogeniche/granulomatose)
	Tumori (compresa la neurofibromatosi)
	Malattie ***infiammatorie*** (per es. artrite reumatoide giovanile)
	Osteocondrodisplasie (acondroplasia, displasia diastrofica, displasia metatropica, displasia spondiloepifisaria)
	Malattie da ***accumulo*** (mucopolisaccaridosi)
	Disordini ***metabolici*** (rachitismo)
	Varie (tra cui osteogenesi imperfetta, post-chirurgia)

I segni e i sintomi fisici variano a seconda della sede di compressione. I pazienti possono lamentare cefalea e/o cervicalgia e avere sintomi di compressione neurologica. La valutazione radiografica inizia con le proiezioni anteroposteriore, laterale e a bocca aperta (odontoidea), cui si possono aggiungere proiezioni laterali in flessione ed estensione. La TC fornisce i migliori dettagli ossei ed è utile per definire qualunque anomalia. La RM, comprese le immagini dinamiche in flessione ed estensione, è la scelta migliore per valutare la compressione neurologica. Il trattamento sintomatico può essere utile; tuttavia, i pazienti con instabilità cervicale e/o compressione neurologica richiedono la decompressione e/o la stabilizzazione chirurgica.

SINDROME DI DOWN. L'iperlassità legamentosa caratteristica della sindrome di Down può determinare un'instabilità o un'ipermobilità a livello delle articolazioni occipitoatlantoidea o atlantoassiale nel 10-30% dei pazienti (vedi Capitolo 81). Questi soggetti possono inoltre presentare concomitanti anomalie congenite o evolutive della colonna cervicale, come occipitalizzazione dell'atlante, ipoplasia dell'arco dell'atlante, invaginazione basilare e os odontoideum. Un'instabilità del livello C1-2 si osserva nel 40% dei bambini con sindrome di Down. L'instabilità atlanto-occipitale può essere altrettanto comune in questa popolazione, al punto che è stata riportata anche nel 61% dei casi. Nonostante la storia naturale di questo spettro patologico rimanga sconosciuta, un sottogruppo di pazienti sviluppa una disfunzione neurologica (o ne è a rischio significativo). Tutti i pazienti devono essere esaminati con anamnesi ed esame obiettivo (a intervalli regolari) e con almeno una serie di radiografie della colonna cervicale, comprendenti una proiezione laterale in flessione ed estensione. Anche se le raccomandazioni specifiche possono variare nei diversi stati, prima della partecipazione alle Olimpiadi per i diversamente abili è necessario uno screening clinico e radiografico. La diagnosi clinica di disfunzione neurologica può rappresentare una sfida; lievi segni e sintomi clinici, come una ridotta tolleranza allo sforzo e anomalie del cammino tra cui tendenza a inciampare o cadere, possono essere i primi segni di una mielopatia. Clono e iperreflessia sono identificabili all'esame obiettivo. La valutazione della funzionalità sensitiva e motoria può essere abbastanza difficile in questa popolazione e nella maggior parte dei pazienti è necessaria la presenza di anomalie cliniche e radiografiche (radiografie, RM) perché si possa valutare un sospetto interessamento neurologico.

Anche se un'ipermobilità dell'articolazione occipitoatlantoidea è presente in più del 50% dei bambini con sindrome di Down, la maggior parte di essi non sviluppa un'instabilità né sintomi neurologici. I rapporti a livello di questa articolazione sono difficili da misurare in modo affidabile sulle radiografie e la RM può essere utile per chiarire il significato di qualsiasi aspetto radiografico dubbio. A suscitare una maggiore preoccupazione clinica è l'articolazione atlantoassiale. L'intervallo atlanto-odontoideo (ADI, *Atlanto-Dens Interval*) viene utilizzato per diagnosticare l'ipermobilità o l'instabilità. La spazio tra il dente e l'anello anteriore di C1 (ADI) viene misurato sulle radiografie laterali in posizione neutra, in flessione e in estensione (Fig. 679-2).

Un ADI normale nei bambini con sindrome di Down misura <4,5 mm. Si fa diagnosi di ipermobilità con un ADI tra 4,5 e 10 mm; un ADI >10 mm rappresenta un'instabilità che comporta un serio rischio di lesioni neurologiche. La RM è indicata per la ricerca di una compromissione neurologica nei pazienti con instabilità radiografica. L'interessamento della colonna subassiale, meno comune, è caratteristico degli adulti con sindrome di Down. Le alterazioni degenerative e/o l'instabilità possono determinare dolore, radiculopatia e mielopatia.

Le raccomandazioni per la sorveglianza della potenziale instabilità cervicale nei bambini con sindrome di Down sono di vario tipo. Gli Autori di questo capitolo raccomandano una serie di radiografie della colonna cervicale (proiezioni in flessoestensione comprese) per i bambini con sindrome di Down. Occorre procedere a un esame neurologico su base annuale. Nei pazienti con esame clinico normale bisogna eseguire radiografie in flessione ed estensione ad anni alterni. I soggetti con segni o sintomi anormali devono essere sottoposti a RM. In questo modo è possibile dare consigli sul livello di attività fisica più appropriato e identificare il piccolo sottogruppo con lassità/instabilità progressiva o interessamento neurologico franco. I pazienti con radiografie normali e che risultano normali anche sotto il profilo

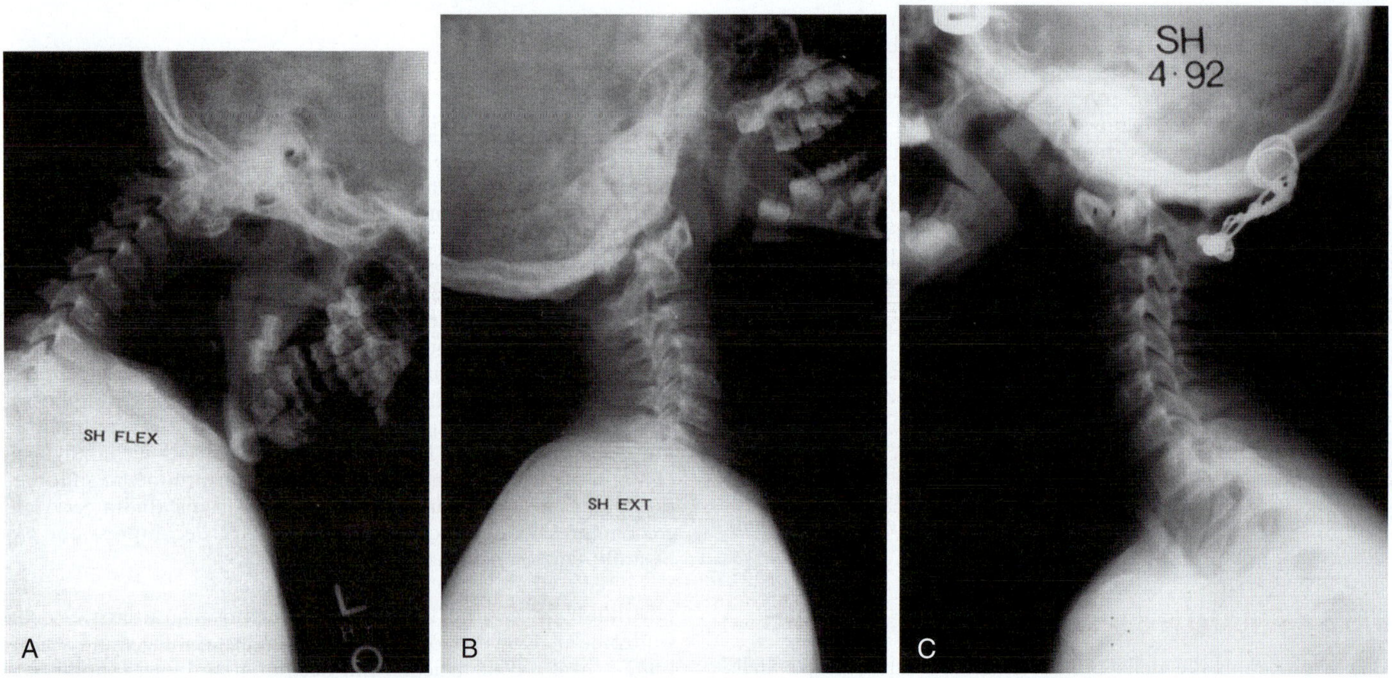

Figura 679-2. Radiografie in flessione (*A*) ed estensione (*B*), che evidenziano ipermobilità e sublussazione atlantoassiale in un caso di sindrome di Down. *C*, L'instabilità e i sintomi sono stati alleviati da un'artrodesi occipitoassiale.

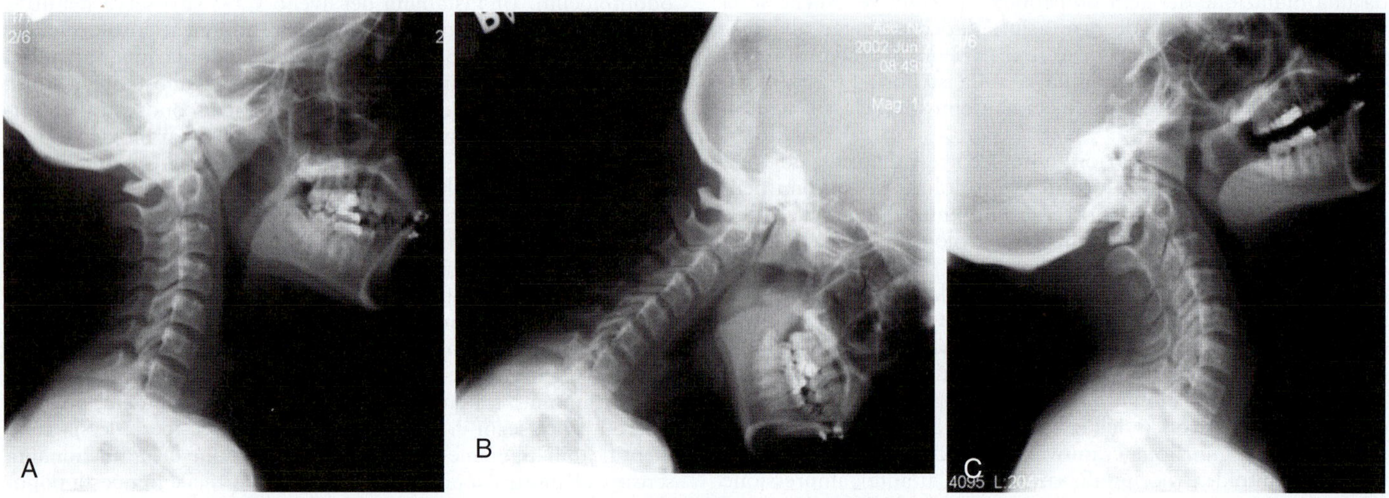

Figura 679-3. Radiografie della colonna cervicale che evidenziano platibasia e instabilità occipitocervicale e atlantoassiale in un bambino con sindrome della delezione di 22q11.2. *A*, Radiografia in posizione neutra. *B*, Flessione. *C*, Estensione. (Da Drummond DS: Pediatric cervical instability. In Weisel SE, Boden SD, Wisnecki RI [ed]: *Seminars in Spine Surgery*. Philadelphia, WB Saunders, 1996, pp. 292-309.)

neurologico non sono soggetti ad alcuna limitazione di attività. Quelli che ricevono una diagnosi di ipermobilità devono evitare gli sport di contatto e altre attività ad alto rischio che potrebbero aumentare il rischio di traumi alla colonna cervicale. Il piccolo sottogruppo con interessamento neurologico o instabilità e trauma neurologico imminente è invece candidato alla fusione. In questa popolazione la fusione cervicale posteriore è gravata da un rischio estremamente elevato di complicanze maggiori, tra cui morte, deterioramento neurologico e pseudoartrosi con o senza riassorbimento dell'innesto.

SINDROME DELLA DELEZIONE 22Q11.2. La delezione cromosomica anomala 22q11.2 è una comune sindrome genetica che comprende un ampio spettro di anomalie tra cui anomalie cardiache, palatali e immunologiche. Sono comuni le anomalie radiografiche della colonna cervicale superiore.

In tutti i pazienti si nota almeno una variante evolutiva dell'occipite o della colonna cervicale. Le varianti occipitali osservate comprendono platibasia e impressione basilare. Le varianti dell'atlante sono un aspetto dismorfico, un arco posteriore aperto e l'occipitalizzazione, mentre le varianti dell'epistrofeo consistono in un dente dell'epistrofeo dismorfico e "*C2 swoosh*". In questi pazienti si nota una gamma di fusioni tra vertebre cervicali, la più comune delle quali è C2-3. Un aumento della mobilità segmentaria della colonna cervicale si nota in più della metà dei pazienti e più di un terzo presenta un aumento della mobilità segmentaria a vari livelli.

Considerata la frequente presenza di varianti della colonna cervicale superiore nella sindrome da delezione 22q11.1 (Fig. 679-3), si raccomanda l'uso di tecniche di imaging avanzate della colonna cervicale superiore e un follow-up regolare dei pazienti per chiarirne il decorso clinico.

Adams SB Jr, Flynn JM, Hosalkar HS: Torticollis in an infant caused by hereditary muscle aplasia. *Am J Orthop* 2003;32:556–558.
Cheng JC, Tang SP, Chen TM, et al: The clinical presentation and outcome of treatment of congenital muscular torticollis in infants—a study of 1086 cases. *J Pediatr Surg* 2000;35:1091–1096.
Cheng JC, Wong MW, Tang SP, et al: Clinical determinants of the outcome of manual stretching in the treatment of congenital muscular torticollis in infants: A prospective study of eight hundred and twenty-one cases. *J Bone Joint Surg Am* 2001;83:679–687.
Clarke RA, Catalan G, Diwan AD, et al. Heterogeneity in Klippel-Feil syndrome: A new classification. *Pediatr Radiol* 1998;28:967–974.
Collins A, Jankovic J: Botulinum toxin injection for congenital muscular torticollis presenting in children and adults. *Neurology* 2006;67:1083–1085.
Copley LA, Dormans JP: Cervical spine disorders in infants and children. *J Am Acad Orthop Surg* 1998;6:204–214.
Dai L, Yuan W, Ni B, et al: Os odontoideum: Etiology, diagnosis and management. *Surg Neurol* 2000;53:106–109.
Drummond DS, Hosalkar HS. Treatment of cervical instability. In Clark CR (editor): *The Cervical Spine,* 4th ed. The Cervical Spine Research Society, 2005, pp 427–447.
Guille JT, Sherk HH: Congenital osseous anomalies of the upper and lower cervical spine in children. *J Bone Joint Surg Am* 2002;84:277–288.
Gupta AK, Roy DR, Conlon ES: Torticollis secondary to posterior fossa tumors. *J Pediatr Orthop* 1996;16:505–507.
Hensinger RN, Lang JE, MacEwen GD: Klippel-Feil syndrome: A constellation of associated anomalies. *J Bone Joint Surg Am* 1974;56:1246–1253.
Hosalkar HS, Gill IS, Gujar P, Shaw BA: Familial torticollis with polydactyly: Manifestation in three generations. *Am J Orthop* 2001;30:656–658.
Martinez-Lage JF, Morales T, Fernandez Cornejo V: Inflammatory C2-3 subluxation: A Grisel's syndrome variant. *Arch Dis Child* 2003;88:628–629.
Mezue WC, Taha ZM, Bashir EM: Fever and acquired torticollis in hospitalized children. *J Laryngol Otol* 2002;116:280–284.
Pang D, Li V: Atlantoaxial rotatory fixation: Part III of a prospective study of the clinical manifestation, diagnosis, management, and outcome of children with atlantoaxial rotatory fixation. *Neurosurgery* 2005;57:952–972.
Pizzutillo PD, Woods M, Nicholson L, et al: Risk factors in Klippel-Feil syndrome. *Spine* 1994;19:2110–2116.
Ricchetti ET, States L, Hosalkar HS, et al: Radiographic study of the upper cervical spine in the 22q11.2 deletion syndrome. *J Bone Joint Surg Am* 2004;86:1751–1760.
Segal LS, Drummond DS, Zarotti RM, et al: Complications of posterior arthrodesis of the cervical spine in patients who have Down syndrome. *J Bore Joint Surg [Am]* 1991;73(10):1547–1554.
Snyder EM, Coley BD: Limited value of plain radiographs in infant torticollis. *Pediatrics* 2006;118:e1779–e1784.

Capitolo 680 ■ Arto superiore

Roger Cornwall

SPALLA

L'articolazione della spalla è un'enartrosi che differisce dall'anca in quanto la glenoide (la cavità articolare della spalla) è molto più piccola e meno profonda dell'acetabolo, mentre la testa omerale è molto più grande rispetto alla glenoide di quanto lo sia la testa femorale rispetto all'acetabolo. Tale differenza permette alla spalla un arco di movimento molto più ampio rispetto a quello dell'anca, ma predispone anche all'instabilità, in quanto la stabilità della spalla dipende dalle inserzioni muscolari e legamentose più che dalla congruità articolare. L'ampio arco di movimento dell'articolazione gleno-omerale è aumentato da una sostanziale mobilità scapolotoracica, che consente all'arto superiore una notevole libertà d'azione nello spazio tridimensionale.

PARALISI DEL PLESSO BRACHIALE ALLA NASCITA. I traumi del plesso brachiale possono verificarsi prima o durante il parto, di solito in seguito a un meccanismo di stretching, e sono spesso associati a un feto di grosse dimensioni e a distocia di spalla (vedi Capitolo 99). La loro incidenza, pari a 1-3/1000 nati vivi, è la stessa in tutto il mondo nonostante le pratiche del parto e la qualità delle cure siano ampiamente variabili. Le più colpite sono le radici superiori (C5, C6 e, in misura variabile, C7), con paralisi o perdita di forza di spalla, gomito e polso. Il braccio rimane in una posizione caratterizzata da adduzione e rotazione interna della spalla, estensione del gomito e flessione del polso (posizione della mancia del cameriere). Può essere interessato l'intero plesso, con paralisi totale dell'arto superiore. L'interessamento isolato della parte inferiore del plesso (C8-T1) è molto rara. La lesione può essere di diversa gravità, da una neuroaprassia o un semplice stiramento del nervo fino alla completa rottura o avulsione della radice nervosa dal midollo spinale. Il 30-40% circa dei bambini non trattati può avere deficit residui.

Trattamento. Le fratture a carico della clavicola e dell'omero possono simulare una paralisi del plesso brachiale e devono essere valutate. Una terapia fisica o occupazionale per le lesioni del plesso brachiale deve essere istituita a 3 settimane di età per mantenere l'arco di movimento passivo e promuovere l'uso del braccio. Se il bicipite non mostra alcun segno di recupero entro i 3 mesi di età o, al contrario, presenta una perdita sostanziale di forza che persiste a 5 mesi di età, è altamente probabile una rottura o avulsione delle radici nervose e sono indicati l'esplorazione chirurgica e l'innesto nervoso del plesso brachiale. La RM e le indagini elettrodiagnostiche non sempre sono affidabili in questa situazione.

Una displasia e una lussazione di spalla (analoga alla displasia evolutiva dell'anca) possono verificarsi in lattanti e bambini in seguito allo squilibrio muscolare e necessitare di riduzione artroscopica o aperta e di riequilibrio muscolare. I bambini più grandi con perdita di forza residua nell'abduzione e nella rotazione esterna della spalla possono trarre beneficio da un trasferimento tendineo. L'osteotomia è riservata ai bambini con articolazione gleno-omerale severamente deformata e deficit funzionale da persistente retrazione della spalla in rotazione interna.

DEFORMITÀ DI SPRENGEL. La deformità di Sprengel, o elevazione congenita della scapola, è un'anomalia dello sviluppo che consiste in una scapola elevata e una limitazione dei movimenti scapolotoracici. La scapola si forma nelle fasi precoci dell'embriogenesi posteriormente alla 4ª vertebra cervicale, per poi discendere, durante lo sviluppo, al di sotto della 7ª vertebra cervicale. Una mancata discesa, uni- o bilaterale, costituisce appunto la deformità di Sprengel. La severità della deformità dipende dalla sede della scapola e dalle anomalie associate. Nei **casi lievi** la scapola è semplicemente ruotata, con una sporgenza palpabile o visibile corrispondente all'angolo scapolare superomediale nella regione del muscolo trapezio. La funzione è generalmente buona. Nei **casi moderati**, essa è più alta sul collo e unita alla colonna da un legamento omovertebrale anormale o anche da osso. I movimenti della spalla, in particolare l'abduzione, sono limitati. Nei **casi severi**, la scapola è piccola e posizionata sul collo posteriormente e il collo può presentare uno pterigio. La maggior parte dei pazienti presenta anomalie associate dell'apparato muscoloscheletrico, specialmente della colonna (tra cui l'**anomalia di Klippel-Feil** con fusione congenita delle vertebre cervicali [vedi Capitolo 679]), motivo per cui è importante procedere alla valutazione della colonna.

Trattamento. Nei casi lievi il trattamento non è generalmente necessario, anche se l'angolo scapolare superomediale sporgente e antiestetico può essere asportato. Nei casi più severi, il riposizionamento chirurgico della scapola con riequilibrio dei muscoli parascapolari può migliorare significativamente la funzione e l'aspetto estetico.

LUSSAZIONE DELLA SPALLA. La lussazione gleno-omerale traumatica è un trauma comune negli adolescenti, ma insolito nei bambini più piccoli (vedi Capitolo 686.2), nei quali è più frequente una frattura della cartilagine di accrescimento prossimale dell'omero. La lussazione, in genere anteriore, dà luogo a una rotazione forzata e una rotazione esterna. I legamenti, le capsule e i muscoli di supporto ne risultano danneggiati, predisponendo a una lussazione ricorrente. Minore è l'età del paziente al momento della lussazione iniziale, più è probabile la recidiva della lussazione.

Trattamento. Dopo una riduzione chiusa della lussazione, la spalla viene immobilizzata in adduzione e rotazione interna per 4-6 settimane. In seguito, si inizia la riabilitazione per recuperare l'arco di movimento rinforzando al contempo i muscoli che stabilizzano la spalla. L'elevata probabilità di lussazioni ricorrenti negli adolescenti rappresenta un argomento a favore della riparazione chirurgica precoce del danno capsulare e dei legamenti, allo scopo di ripristinare la stabilità anatomica dell'articolazione gleno-omerale.

GOMITO

L'articolazione del gomito è posta tra l'omero prossimalmente e l'ulna e il radio distalmente. La flessione e l'estensione del gomito si verificano grazie alle articolazioni ulno-omerale e radio-omerale, mentre pronazione e supinazione sono consentite dall'articolazione radioulnare. A differenza della spalla, il movimento del gomito è limitato dalla complessa anatomia ossea, anche se i robusti legamenti sui versanti mediale e laterale assicurano la stabilità di questa articolazione. Il gomito tende alla rigidità, con scarsa tolleranza alla formazione di tessuto cicatriziale in seguito a un trauma o a un intervento.

GOMITO DELLA BAMBINAIA (PRONAZIONE DOLOROSA). La pronazione dolorosa è una sublussazione di un legamento più che una sublussazione o lussazione della testa del radio. L'estremità prossimale del radio, o capitello del radio, è ancorata all'ulna prossimale dal legamento anulare, che si avvolge come un laccio a partire dall'ulna intorno al capitello del radio per poi inserirsi di nuovo sull'ulna. Se il radio viene trazionato distalmente, il legamento anulare può scivolare prossimalmente dal capitello del radio inserendosi nell'articolazione tra il capitello del radio e l'omero (Fig. 680-1). Il trauma si produce caratteristicamente

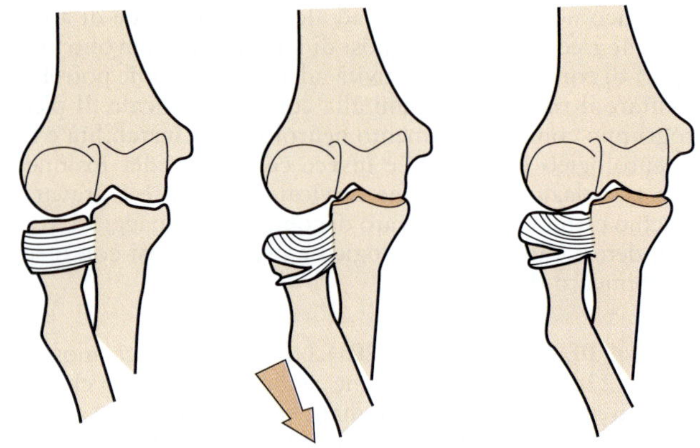

Figura 680-1. Pronazione dolorosa (gomito della bambinaia). Il legamento anulare si lacera parzialmente quando il braccio viene trazionato. La testa del radio si sposta distalmente e quando si smette di esercitare la trazione il legamento entra nell'articolazione. (Da Rang M: *Children's Fractures*, 2nd ed. Philadelphia, JB Lippincott, 1983, p. 193.)

quando il braccio subisce una forza di trazione longitudinale, come quando un bambino che cade viene afferrato per il braccio o tirato per la mano. La lesione di solito si verifica nei bambini di 1-3 anni, mentre è rara dopo i 5 anni. La sublussazione del legamento anulare produce immediatamente dolore e limitazione della supinazione. La flessione e l'estensione del gomito non sono limitate e l'edema è generalmente assente. La diagnosi si pone in base all'anamnesi e all'esame obiettivo in quanto le radiografie sono caratteristicamente normali.

Trattamento. Per ridurre il legamento anulare si ruota l'avambraccio in supinazione esercitando pressione sul capitello radiale. Si può percepire un "click" o un "clunk" palpabile. Il bambino recupera immediatamente la supinazione attiva e di solito prova un sollievo immediato dal dolore. Non è necessaria l'immobilizzazione, ma possono verificarsi sublussazioni ricorrenti del legamento anulare e i genitori devono evitare attività che implichino una trazione sul gomito. I genitori possono imparare le manovre di riduzione per gli episodi ricorrenti onde evitare di rivolgersi ogni volta al pronto soccorso o all'ambulatorio del pediatra. La sublussazione ricorrente oltre i 5 anni di età è rara. La sublussazione irriducibile tende a guarire spontaneamente con risoluzione graduale dei sintomi in un periodo che va da qualche giorno a qualche settimana; la chirurgia è raramente indicata.

MALATTIA DI PANNER. La malattia di Panner colpisce l'osso e la cartilagine del capitello dell'aspetto laterale dell'omero distale. Un'alterazione idiopatica del flusso sanguigno a livello osseo può far sì che il capitello collassi, configurando un quadro simile a quello della malattia di Legg-Calvé-Perthes dell'anca; in alternativa, un trauma ripetuto può dar luogo alla frammentazione e separazione di osso e cartilagine, come nell'osteocondrite dissecante. Il processo tende a verificarsi in adolescenti impegnati in sport di lancio come il baseball o che comportano un carico sulle braccia come la ginnastica (vedi Capitolo 86.7). In questi casi, il capitello subisce elevate forze di compressione sia da stress in valgo sul gomito nel corso del lancio, sia da carico assiale diretto imposto da un peso sull'estremità superiore. I sintomi sono inizialmente dolore e limitazione del movimento, in particolare l'impossibilità di estendere completamente il braccio. Il gomito può essere tumefatto e si può udire un crepitio. Alle radiografie si osserva un'area di radiotrasparenza o una franca frammentazione del capitello. La RM è utile per determinare l'estensione dell'interessamento osseo e l'integrità della cartilagine articolare. Osso e cartilagine possono distaccarsi dal capitello e formare corpi liberi all'interno dell'articolazione.

Trattamento. Riposo e astensione dalle attività di carico o di lancio possono consentire la risoluzione dei casi allo stadio iniziale. Nei casi più avanzati la guarigione può talvolta essere favorita dalla trapanazione o dall'innesto chirurgico, effettuato per favorire la crescita vascolare. Quando si sviluppano corpi liberi intrarticolari che provocano sintomi meccanici, è necessaria la rimozione artroscopica o aperta.

POLSO

Il polso è la complessa articolazione compresa tra radio e ulna da una parte e le ossa del carpo dall'altra. Il radio e le ossa carpali hanno forma irregolare e sono interconnesse con precisione per permettere sia la mobilità sia la stabilità. L'articolazione radioulnare distale consente la rotazione dell'avambraccio intorno al suo asse. L'articolazione tra ulna e ossa carpali è rivestita e sostenuta dal complesso fibrocartilagineo triangolare, che è analogo al menisco del ginocchio e può andare incontro a traumi. Un'alterazione dell'anatomia o delle relazioni tra queste ossa può causare disfunzione meccanica con dolore, rigidità e perdita funzionale.

CISTI SINOVIALE. Essendo un'articolazione sinoviale, l'articolazione del polso è lubrificata dal liquido sinoviale, prodotto dal rivestimento sinoviale dell'articolazione e mantenuto all'interno dell'articolazione dalla capsula articolare. Un difetto della capsula può permetterne lo stravaso dall'articolazione nei tessuti molli, con formazione di una cisti. In realtà, il termine "cisti" è errato in quanto questa raccolta extrarticolare di liquido non ha un vero e proprio rivestimento. Il difetto capsulare può verificarsi come evento traumatico, anche se è raro che un trauma faccia parte della storia di presentazione. Il liquido normalmente fuoriesce dall'articolazione nello spazio tra scafoide e semilunare, formando una cisti localizzata sull'aspetto dorsoradiale del polso. Le cisti possono verificarsi anche in altre sedi, per esempio nell'aspetto volare del polso o nel palmo della mano in seguito allo stravaso di liquido dalle guaine del tendine del flessore. Nei bambini di solito esse non sono dolorose; nei casi in cui il dolore è presente non è chiaro se sia la cisti a causarlo. La diagnosi è di solito evidente all'esame obiettivo, specialmente se la lesione è transilluminabile. Una tenosinovite dell'estensore e la presenza di muscoli anomali può simulare una cisti, ma la radiografia o la RM non sono necessarie di routine. L'ecografia è uno strumento efficace e non invasivo per confermare la diagnosi e rassicurare il paziente e i familiari.

Trattamento. Fino all'80% delle cisti nei bambini di età <10 anni si risolve spontaneamente entro un anno dalla comparsa. Se la cisti è dolorosa o fastidiosa e se il bambino ha più di 10 anni, può essere necessario il trattamento. La semplice aspirazione del liquido ha un elevato tasso di recidive e risulta dolorosa per i pazienti pediatrici, considerato l'ago piuttosto grosso necessario per prelevare il liquido gelatinoso. L'escissione chirurgica, compresa l'escissione del peduncolo che connette la cisti alla sua articolazione di origine, ha un tasso di successo elevato, anche se la cisti può recidivare.

DEFICIT LONGITUDINALE RADIALE. L'ipoplasia congenita o assenza dell'aspetto radiale dell'avambraccio, del polso e della mano è denominata collettivamente deficit longitudinale radiale; l'espressione "mano torta radiale", peraltro ormai caduta in disuso, si riferisce alla rassomiglianza visiva della condizione con il piede torto (che in realtà ha una patologia di base differente). Il deficit può presentare vari gradi di severità, da un radio un po' più corto del normale, con una leggera deviazione radiale del polso, fino alla completa assenza de radio e del pollice con lussazione del polso, un'ulna corta e ricurva e dita e gomito disfunzionali. La condizione è sporadica nella maggior parte dei casi, anche se il deficit radiale è classicamente associato a sindromi sistemiche, in particolare anemia di Fanconi, sindrome dell'assenza del radio e trombocitopenia, associazione VACTERL e sindrome di Holt-Oram (Tab. 680-1). Pertanto, in ogni bambino con deficit radiale si rendono necessarie indagini genetiche complete e una valutazione multispecialistica.

TABELLA 680-1. Sindromi comunemente associate a deficit radiale

SINDROME	CARATTERISTICHE
Holt-Oram	Difetti cardiaci, soprattutto difetti del setto interatriale
TAR	Sindrome della trombocitopenia e dell'assenza del radio; la trombocitopenia è presente alla nascita, ma migliora con il tempo
VACTERL	(*Vertebral abnormalities, Anal atresia, Cardiac abnormalities, Tracheoesophageal fistula, Esophageal atresia, Renal defects, radial dysplasia, Lower limb abnormalities*), anomalie vertebrali, atresia anale, anomalie cardiache, fistola tracheoesofagea, atresia esofagea, difetti renali, displasia radiale, anomalie degli arti inferiori
Anemia di Fanconi	Anemia aplastica non presente alla nascita, che compare dopo i 6 anni di età; fatale senza trapianto di midollo osseo; per la diagnosi precoce è disponibile un test di challenge di rottura cromosomica

Da Trumble T, Budoff J, Cornwall R (ed): *Core Knowledge in Orthopedics: Hand, Elbow, Shoulder*. Philadelphia, Elsevier, 2005, p. 425.

Trattamento. Subito dopo la nascita si prescrivono lo stretching passivo e l'uso di un tutore per la deviazione radiale del polso. Nei casi lievi in cui il radio è un po' più corto e il pollice è presente e funzionale, può essere sufficiente il trattamento conservativo. Se invece il radio parzialmente o totalmente assente, è necessaria la chirurgia per centralizzare il carpo sull'estremità dell'ulna. Se il pollice è meno sviluppato ma possiede un'articolazione caropometacarpale stabile, la ricostruzione chirurgica del pollice può aumentare la funzionalità del pollice. Se però il pollice non ha un'articolazione carpometacarpale stabile o addirittura è assente, la pollicizzazione dell'indice (riposizionamento dell'indice nella posizione del pollice) fornisce risultati eccellenti. Una mano con tre dita e un pollice è funzionalmente ed esteticamente preferibile a una mano con quattro dita ma senza pollice. Gli interventi vengono programmati in modo che la ricostruzione sia completa entro i 18 mesi di età, per permettere al bambino di imparare a usare le mani e i polsi ricostruiti fin dalla più tenera età.

MANO E DITA

Mano, dita e pollice funzionano come un complesso apparecchio elettrobiomeccanico con enormi potenzialità funzionali ma scarsa tolleranza a eventuali alterazioni. Le mani consentono al bambino di esplorare il mondo circostante e di conseguenza rappresentano strumenti importanti per il suo sviluppo funzionale e sociale. I traumi delle mani sono comuni nei pazienti pediatrici; tra le anomalie congenite, le malformazioni della mano e dell'arto superiore sono le più frequenti dopo i difetti cardiaci.

LESIONI DELLA PUNTA DELLE DITA. I bambini piccoli sono affascinati dai cardini delle porte, dalle portiere delle automobili e da altri spazi ristretti, il che rende molto comuni i traumi da schiacciamento della punta delle dita. La lesione può variare da un semplice ematoma subungueale all'amputazione completa della punta del dito. Le radiografie sono importanti per escludere la presenza di fratture. Quelle della cartilagine di coniugazione associate a lesioni del letto ungueale sono **fratture aperte** e comportano un rischio elevato di osteomielite, arresto della crescita e deformità se non vengono trattate prontamente con sbrigliamento chirurgico e riduzione formale. Le fratture della parte più distale della falange distale sono comuni e richiedono un trattamento specifico, non molto diverso da quello previsto per le lesioni dei tessuti molli. Il trattamento della lesione dei tessuti molli dipende dal tipo di trauma. Per la sutura bisogna utilizzare solo punti riassorbibili, in quanto la rimozione di una sutura dalla punta del dito di un bambino piccolo può richiedere la sedazione o l'anestesia generale. Se si forma un ematoma subungueale ma l'unghia è normale e non è presente una frattura da spostamento, l'unghia non deve essere rimossa per una riparazione del letto ungueale. Un'unghia lacerata o avulsa deve invece essere rimossa; in tal caso, il letto ungueale e la cute devono essere riparati con punti assorbibili e l'unghia (o, se questa manca, un pezzo di foglio metallico) deve essere riposizionata sotto l'eponichio per prevenire la formazione di aderenze cicatriziali dell'eponichio al letto ungueale che impedirebbero la ricrescita dell'unghia. Se la punta del dito è completamente amputata, il trattamento dipende dal livello di amputazione e dall'età del bambino. Le amputazioni distali di cute e tessuto adiposo nei bambini di età <2 anni possono essere riparate con un innesto composito, che ha una ragionevole possibilità di sopravvivenza. Amputazioni simili in bambini più grandi possono guarire anche senza sostituzione della cute fintantoché l'osso non è esposto e l'area implicata è piccola. Esistono diverse procedure di ricopertura per le amputazioni lungo la porzione media dell'unghia. Le amputazioni a livello del margine prossimale dell'unghia o prossimali rispetto a esso devono essere inviate con urgenza a un centro di reimpianto, dove verrà valutata la possibilità di un intervento di reimpianto microvascolare. In tal caso, occorre conservare tutte le parti amputate, avvolgerle in una garza imbevuta di soluzione fisiologica posta in un contenitore impermeabile, immerso in acqua ghiacciata. Il ghiaccio non deve mai essere a diretto contatto con la parte, in quanto può causare un danno osmotico e termico severo.

POLIDATTILIA. La polidattilia consiste nella presenza di una o più dita o parti di dita soprannumerarie; può essere postassiale, cioè sul bordo ulnare della mano, preassiale, cioè sul bordo radiale della mano, oppure centrale, cioè tra dita adiacenti. La polidattilia postassiale presenta spesso una trasmissione autosomica dominante e può interessare sia le mani sia i piedi. Nei casi lievi, il dito soprannumerario è un escrescenza cutanea o un elemento mobile con osso e un'unghia, ma connesso alla mano solo da un sottile peduncolo. Tali dita possono essere legate con un punto di sutura già nel reparto di neonatologia, anche se talvolta permane un residuo che richiede un'escissione chirurgica formale. La polidattilia postassiale può consistere in un piccolo dito interamente duplicato, che richiede un'amputazione e una ricostruzione formale, di solito a un anno di età. La polidattilia preassiale, o duplicazione del pollice, varia da una duplicazione dell'unghia del pollice a un pollice completamente duplicato con falangi extra. L'anomalia muscoloscheletrica di base è complessa e richiede una ricostruzione chirurgica formale, ottenuta combinando parti di ciascun pollice.

La polidattilia centrale è un'anomalia complessa associata a deformità delle dita "normali" e richiede una ricostruzione chirurgica formale. La polidattilia può essere associata a un'ampia varietà di sindromi (Tab. 680-2).

SINDATTILIA. All'inizio dello sviluppo la mano è una struttura a forma di spatola; solo in seguito si verifica l'apoptosi che permette la formazione delle singole dita. La sindattilia, ossia la mancata separazione di dita adiacenti, può essere classificata come semplice (unione della dita soltanto attraverso la cute) o complessa (unione di cute, tendini e ossa), parziale (dita palmate, in cui soltanto l'aspetto prossimale è congiunto) o completa (fusione delle dita in tutta la loro lunghezza, comprese le unghie). Può essere un reperto isolato o associato a un'ampia varietà di sindromi (Tab. 680-3). La sindattilia tra dita di lunghezza ineguale (pollice e indice, indice e medio, anulare e mignolo) causa tensione e deformità del dito più lungo e deve essere riparata chirurgicamente nei primi mesi di vita. La separazione del dito medio dall'anulare può invece avvenire più tardi, di solito dopo che il paziente ha compiuto l'anno di età.

TABELLA 680-2. Sindromi associate a polidattilia

Sindrome di Carpenter	Sindrome della trisomia 13
Sindrome di Ellis-Van Creveld	Sindrome Orofaciodigitale
Sindrome di Meckel-Gruber	Sindrome di Rubinstein-Taybi
Polisindattilia	

TABELLA 680-3. Sindromi associate a sindattilia

Sindrome di Apert	Trisomia 21
Sindrome di Carpenter	Sindrome idantoinica fetale
Sindrome di De Lange	Sindrome di Laurence-Moon-Biedl
Sindrome di Holt-Oram	Pancitopenia di Fanconi
Sindrome orofaciodigitale	Trisomia 13
Polisindattilia	Trisomia 18

POLLICE E DITA A SCATTO. I tendini flessori del pollice e della dita attraversano tunnel fibrosi composti da una serie di pulegge sulla superficie volare della dita. Questi tunnel, per motivi che non sono ben chiari, possono divenire rigidi a livello della puleggia più prossimale o della 1[a] anulare. Il tendine sottostante diventa edematoso e non scivola più sotto la puleggia. Nei bambini, il dito più comunemente interessato è il pollice. In passato si riteneva che questo fosse un problema congenito, ma gli studi prospettici di screening condotti su un gran numero di neonati non hanno rilevato neppure un caso in questa fascia di età. È raro riscontrare traumi all'anamnesi e la condizione spesso non è dolorosa. La funzione globale raramente è limitata. Un pollice a scatto si presenta caratteristicamente con l'impossibilità di estendere completamente l'articolazione interfalangea del pollice. Nel tendine del muscolo flessore lungo del pollice, alla base del pollice, si può percepire un nodulo palpabile. Altre condizioni possono simulare un pollice a scatto, tra cui la deformità "pollice nel palmo" della paralisi cerebrale. Un sintomo analogo nelle altre dita è molto meno comune e può essere associato a condizioni infiammatorie come l'artrite reumatoide giovanile.

Trattamento. La risoluzione spontanea del pollice a scatto può verificarsi anche nel 30% dei casi diagnosticati prima che il paziente compisse un anno di vita. La risoluzione spontanea oltre questa età non è comune. Le iniezioni di corticosteroidi sono efficaci negli adulti, ma non nei bambini, e comportano il rischio di un danno dei nervi digitali adiacenti. Il rilascio chirurgico della 1[a] puleggia anulare è curativo e in genere viene eseguito a 1-3 anni di età. Il trattamento di dita a scatto diverse dal pollice nei bambini comprende la valutazione e il trattamento di qualsiasi processo infiammatorio sottostante e, in alcuni casi, la decompressione chirurgica della guaina dei flessori.

Chan O, Hughes T: Hand. *Br Med J* 2005;330:1073–1075.
Dao KD, Shin AY, Billings A, et al: Surgical treatment of congenital syndactyly of the hand. *J Am Acad Orthop Surg* 2004;12:39–48.
Farsetti P, Weinstein SL, Caterini R, et al: Sprengel's deformity: Long-term follow-up study of 22 cases. *J Pediatr Orthop B* 2003;12:202–210.
Good CR, MacGillivray JD: Traumatic shoulder dislocation in the adolescent athlete: Advances in surgical treatment. *Curr Opin Pediatr* 2005;17: 25–29.
Kobayashi K, Burton KJ, Rodner C, et al: Lateral compression injuries in the pediatric elbow: Panner's disease and osteochondritis dissecans of the capitellum. *J Am Acad Orthop Surg* 2004;12:246–254.
Kozin SH: Upper-extremity congenital anomalies. *J Bone Joint Surg Am* 2003; 85:1564–1576.
McAdams TR, Moneim MS, Omer GE Jr: Long-term follow-up of surgical release of the A(1) pulley in childhood trigger thumb. *J Pediatr Orthop* 2002;22:41–43.
Pondaag W, Malessy MJ, van Dijk JG, Thomeer RT: Natural history of obstetric brachial plexus palsy: A systematic review. *Dev Med Child Neurol* 2004;46:138–144.
Rayan GM, Frey B: Ulnar polydactyly. *Plast Reconstr Surg* 2001;107: 1449–1457.
Wang AA, Hutchinson DT: Longitudinal observation of pediatric hand and wrist ganglia. *J Hand Surg [Am]* 2001;26:599–602.
Waters PM: Update on management of pediatric brachial plexus palsy. *J Pediatr Orthop* 2005;25:116–126.

Capitolo 681 ■ Artrogriposi

Harish S. Hosalkar e Denis S. Drummond

DEFINIZIONE

L'artrogriposi multipla congenita (AMC) è un'anomalia del neonato che comporta la presenza fin dalla nascita di molte articolazioni ricurve (Fig. 681-1). "Artrogriposi" è un termine descrittivo e non una diagnosi esatta, in quanto le possibili cause sottostanti sono almeno 150. L'incidenza della forma classica è di circa 1/10 000 nati vivi. I tre tipi principali sono:

AMC classica, a carico principalmente degli arti, in cui i muscoli sono deficitari o assenti (amioplasia) (Fig. 681-2);

artrogriposi in associazione con una disfunzione neurologica maggiore (encefalo, midollo spinale, cellule del corno anteriore o nervi periferici) o una miopatia (distrofia muscolare congenita, miopatia tossica);

artrogriposi in associazione con altre anomalie maggiori e sindromi specifiche come la displasia diastrofica e la distrofia craniocarpotarsale (Tab. 681-1).

ASPETTI CLINICI

Sono presenti deformità articolari multiple con deficit muscolare ma sensibilità normale. Si riscontra rigidità di diverse articolazioni che in ciascun caso deriva sia dalla presenza di muscoli corti e tesi sia da retrazioni capsulari. Può essere presente uno pterigio sul lato flessorio delle articolazioni retratte (Fig. 681-3). Spesso la patologia è caratterizzata dall'assenza o dalla fibrosi di alcuni muscoli o gruppi muscolari. Nella maggior parte dei casi lo sviluppo intellettuale è normale. La forma classica (AMC) comporta il coinvolgimento di tutti e quattro gli arti, nonostante possa colpire anche solo gli arti superiori o quelli inferiori. Una variante autosomica dominante denominata artrogriposi distale colpisce mani e piedi, con deformità severe ma con retrazioni di scarsa entità, più prossimali; la scoliosi è una possibile evoluzione. Oltre alle retrazioni articolari multiple, sono quanto mai caratteristiche la mancanza di solchi cutanei (arti cilindrici o tubulari) e la presenza di profonde fossette sulle articolazioni (Fig. 681-4). Si osserva una lussazione delle articolazioni, per lo più delle anche, ma talvolta anche del ginocchio, mentre è raro un coinvolgimento del tronco. Possono essere presenti altre anomalie congenite come criptorchidismo, ernie e gastroschisi.

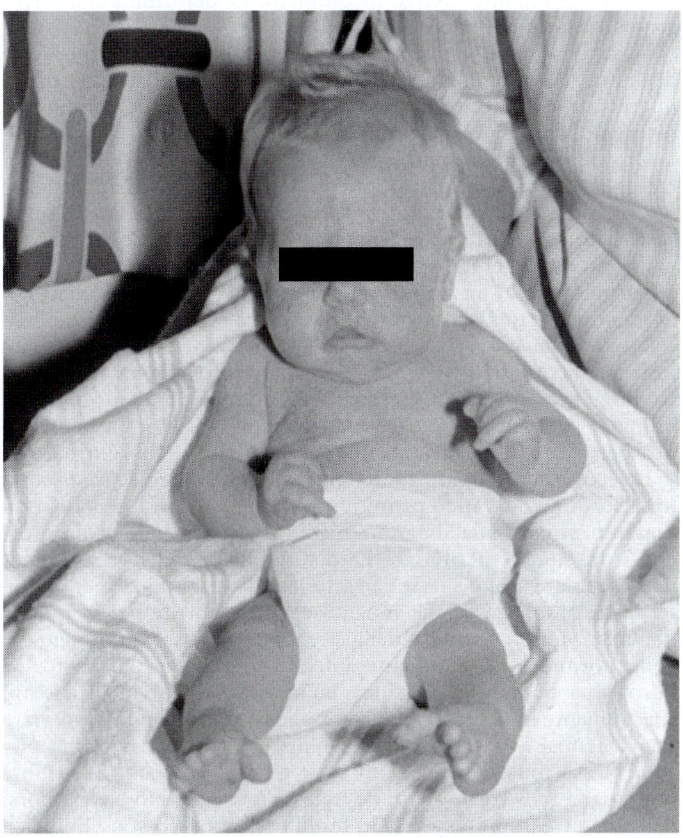

Figura 681-1. Artrogriposi multipla congenita. Neonato prematuro di 32 settimane con gravi retrazioni multiple congenite e neuropatia congenita severa. (Da HS, Moroz L, Drummond DS, Finkel R: Neuromuscular disorders of infancy and childhood and arthrogryposis. In Dormans JP [ed]: *Pediatric Orthopaedics: Core Knowledge in Orthopedics*. Philadelphia, Mosby, 2005.)

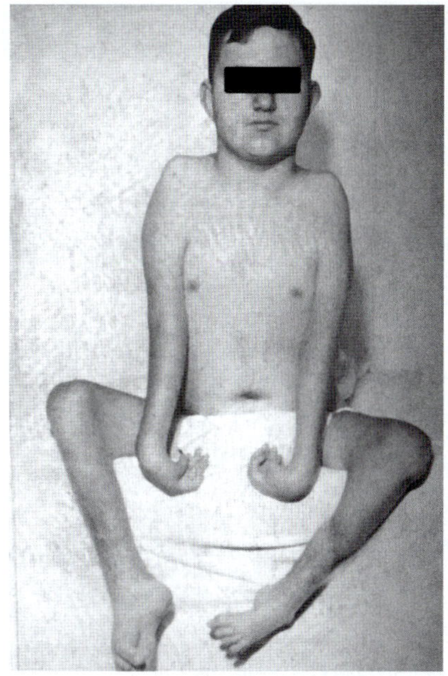

Figura 681-2. Caratteristiche dell'artrogriposi sono le retrazioni articolari e l'assenza di solchi cutanei e infossature profonde a livello delle articolazioni. (Da Hosalkar HS, Moroz L, Drummond DS, Finkel R: Neuromuscular disorders of infancy and childhood and arthrogryposis. In Dormans JP [ed]: *Pediatric Orthopedics: Core Knowledge in Orthopedics*. Philadelphia, Mosby, 2005.)

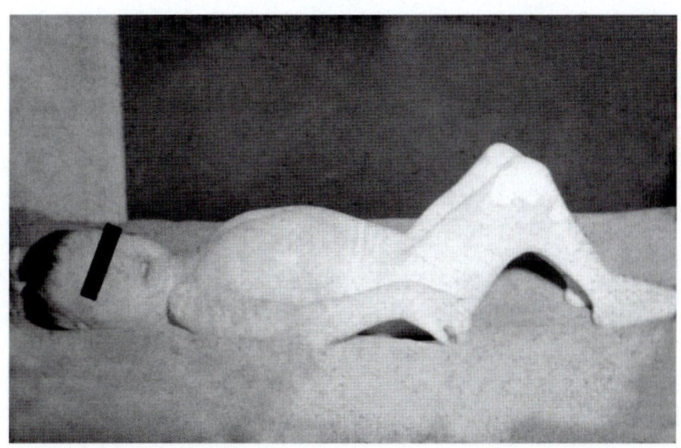

Figura 681-3. Flessione fissa delle ginocchia in un ragazzo con artrogriposi multipla congenita. (Da Hosalkar HS, Moroz L, Drummond DS, Finkel R: Neuromuscular disorders of infancy and childhood and arthrogryposis. In Dormans JP [ed]: *Pediatric Orthopedics: Core Knowledge in Orthopedics*. Philadelphia, Mosby, 2005.)

TABELLA 681-1. Associazioni eziologiche dell'artrogriposi

ARTROGRIPOSI DA PATOLOGIE DEL SISTEMA NERVOSO
- Deficit delle cellule delle corna anteriori del midollo
- Deficit generalizzati delle corna anteriori del midollo
- Disordine/danno strutturale cerebrale
- Sede incerta

(Le condizioni di spasticità sono escluse)

SINDROMI DI ARTROGRIPOSI DISTALE
- Tipo I dominante distale
- Tipo IIa dominante distale (sindrome di Gordon)
- Tipo IIe distale
- Dismorfismo digitotalare
- Distribuzione distale, tipo non specificato

SINDROMI CON PTERIGIO
- Sindrome degli pterigi multipli
- Sindrome degli pterigi multipli letale
- Sindrome dello pterigio popliteo
- Ptosi, scoliosi, pterigi
- Sindrome dello pterigio antecubitale (Liebenberg)

MIOPATIE
- Distrofia muscolare di Emery-Dreifuss
- Ipotonia, miopatia, retrazioni lievi

ANOMALIE DELLE ARTICOLAZIONI E DEI TESSUTI CONTIGUI
- Aracnodattilia contratturale congenita
- Sindrome di Freeman-Sheldon
- Lassità o ipertonicità con lussazione intrauterina e retrazioni
- Sindrome di Larsen
- Displasia spondiloepimetafisaria con lassità articolare
- Trisomia 18, parto podalico in estensione con lussazione bilaterale dell'anca
- Fratelli o sorelle con omero bifido, ipertelorismo e lussazione delle articolazioni di anche e ginocchia

DISORDINI SCHELETRICI
- Displasia distrofica
- Displasia parastremmatica
- Displasia di Kniest
- Displasia metatropica
- Displasia camptomelica
- Sindrome di Schwartz
- Sindrome alcolica fetale con sinostosi
- Osteogenesi imperfetta con ossa ricurve/retrazioni

FATTORI MATERNI/INTRAUTERINI
- Sindrome alcolica fetale con retrazioni
- Infezioni
- Lupus eritematoso sistemico materno non trattato
- Costrizione fetale intrauterina
- Deformità (pressione)
- Stravaso di liquido amniotico
- Gravidanze multiple
- Tumori intrauterini
- Disruption (bande)

VARIE
- Pseudotrisomia 18 con retrazioni
- Sindrome della pseudotalidomide di Roberts
- Sordità con retrazioni distali
- Associazione VACTERL
- Anomalie multiple e retrazioni non altrimenti specificate
- ARC*

SINGOLA ARTICOLAZIONE
- Campomelica
- Sinfangilismo
- Dito "a scatto"

*Artrogriposi, acidosi tubulare renale, colestasi.
Modificata da Mennen U, Van Heest A, Ezaki MB et al: Arthrogryposis multiplex congenita. *J Hand Surg [Br]* 2005;30:5:468-474.
© 2005 The British Society for Surgery of the Hand.

EZIOLOGIA

L'AMC ha un'eziologia multifattoriale. I fattori che tendenzialmente producono immobilità del feto possono contribuire alle retrazioni congenite: tra questi, anomalie strutturali dell'utero (utero bifido, grossi fibromi), oligoidramnios, aumento della pressione intrauterina, compressione meccanica del feto, deboli movimenti fetali, presentazione podalica e prematurità. È stata ipotizzata anche un'eziologia infiammatoria o infettiva (infiammazione articolare, muscolare, midollare o cerebrale, rosolia nei primi mesi di gravidanza e infezione da virus sconosciuti). L'opinione prevalente è che la condizione primaria sia rappresentata dalla degenerazione focale delle cellule del corno anteriore, nei primi mesi di gestazione. Una donna gravida trattata con curaro per tetano severo ha partorito un bambino con artrogriposi.

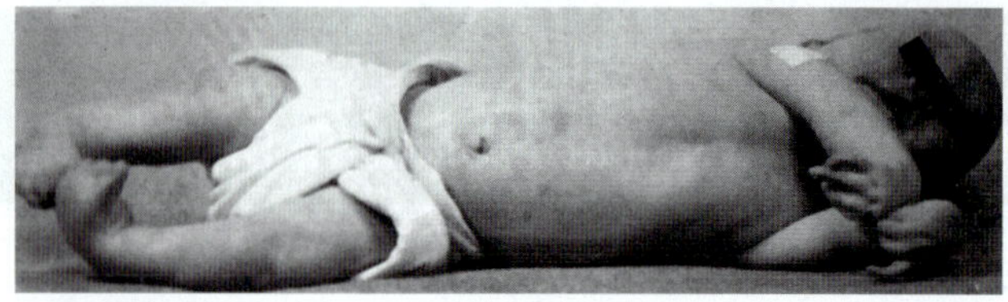

Figura 681-4. Caratteristica assenza di solchi cutanei e arti tubulari. (Da Hosalkar HS, Moroz L, Drummond DS, Finkel R: Neuromuscular disorders of infancy and childhood and arthrogryposis. In Dormans JP [ed]: *Pediatric Orthopedics: Core Knowledge in Orthopedics*. Philadelphia, Mosby, 2005.)

DIAGNOSI

L'esame obiettivo rimane il sistema migliore per stabilire la diagnosi di artrogriposi. Gli Autori di questo capitolo hanno individuato alcuni fattori che spesso si rivelano utili per la diagnosi; anche se non si tratta di criteri assoluti, sono comunque un valido ausilio se considerati insieme.

A differenza delle patologie che causano paralisi, le deformità articolari dell'AMC sono di solito rigide fin dall'inizio, con un arco di movimento passivo incompleto. Le deformità dell'artrogriposi tendono a essere simmetriche.

La severità delle retrazioni in genere aumenta verso la periferia degli arti. Le articolazioni più prossimali tendono a essere meno interessate e il tronco è spesso risparmiato. Le deformità più severe di solito si verificano nelle mani e nei piedi.

Ortopedico, neurologo, genetista e pediatra devono collaborare alla diagnosi e al trattamento di questa condizione. Sono raccomandate le radiografie delle estremità interessate con il coinvolgimento articolare, in quanto possono dimostrare anomalie ossee congenite e perdita del tessuto adiposo sottocutaneo e dei muscoli. Le radiografie della colonna *in toto* permettono di identificare qualsiasi anomalia vertebrale. La TC/RM dell'encefalo e della colonna sono utili per accertare o escludere un interessamento strutturale del sistema nervoso centrale. L'elettromiografia e studi di conduzione nervosa, peraltro di utilità limitata, sono stati impiegati per distinguere la forma neuropatica periferica dalle varianti miopatiche.

È necessaria una biopsia del muscolo scheletrico se si sospetta un disordine miopatico primitivo, a meno che i test genetici non rendano possibile la diagnosi mediante l'esame molecolare del DNA dal sangue periferico. La determinazione della creatinchinasi plasmatica può servire a escludere disturbi miopatici; è preferibile che questo esame venga eseguito a partire dal 3° giorno di vita, quando i valori della creatinchinasi saranno rientrati nella norma dopo l'aumento iniziale conseguente al parto. Se l'ecografia prenatale identifica un'assenza di movimenti fetali, specialmente in associazione con polidramnios, si può sospettare una diagnosi di artrogriposi. L'analisi istologica rivela una piccola massa muscolare con fibrosi e tessuto adiposo tra le fibre muscolari. Aspetti miopatici e neuropatici possono sovrapporsi nello stesso campione. I tessuti molli periarticolari sono fibrotici. Il counseling genetico, con analisi dei cromosomi e studio del collagene, deve essere preso in considerazione laddove non sia immediatamente evidente una patologia neuromuscolare periferica ben precisa.

La diagnosi differenziale è riportata nella Tabella 681-2.

TABELLA 681-2. Diagnosi differenziale delle retrazioni congenite

PATOLOGIE	DIAGNOSI DIFFERENZIALE
Neurogeni	Spina bifida e patologie vertebrali
	Mielodisplasia
	Agenesia sacrale e lombare
	Atrofia muscolare spinale
	Neuropatia fetale (tossica, infettiva)
Miopatici	Distrofia miotonica congenita
	Distrofia muscolare congenita
	Miopatia congenita/fetale
	Miastenia fetale (trasferimento passivo di anticorpi da madre con miastenia grave)
Tessuto connettivo	Sindrome di Marfan
	Sindrome di Ehlers-Danlos
Varie	Sindrome di Freeman-Sheldon
	Sindrome di Turner
	Sindrome di Edward
	Sindrome dello pterigio
	Nanismo diastrofico

PROGNOSI

Il medico deve essere in grado di formulare una prognosi generale e un piano di trattamento, una volta stabilita la diagnosi di AMC. Vi possono essere pochi movimenti motori funzionali verso la periferia dell'arto. Una vigorosa terapia occupazionale e l'applicazione di splint per la mano e gessi seriati possono migliorare l'arco di movimento e la funzionalità della mano in molti casi di AMC in cui l'eziologia non sia quella di una patologia progressiva (amioplasia). La chirurgia, in casi selezionati, è necessaria per ottenere una posizione più neutra del polso e delle dita, così da sfruttare la limitata forza muscolare per ottenere un vantaggio biomeccanico ottimale.

La recidiva di una deformità corretta è alquanto comune e si verifica con la crescita in un arto le cui strutture periarticolari sono incapaci di stretching. I bambini con artrogriposi presentano alcuni fattori positivi su cui è possibile far leva per un trattamento efficace.

L'instabilità articolare non è un problema nell'AMC, a differenza di quanto avviene in altre condizioni paralitiche.

Grazie a un approccio coordinato e d'équipe al trattamento spesso si assisterà solo a un lieve deterioramento rispetto alle condizioni alla nascita. Spesso vi è risparmio centrale e un tronco relativamente normale.

Si prevede che il bambino senza anomalie del SNC abbia un'intelligenza nella norma e, se sufficientemente motivato, possa dare il suo contributo all'efficacia del trattamento.

PRINCIPI DI TRATTAMENTO ORTOPEDICO DEI PAZIENTI CON ARTROGRIPOSI E RETRAZIONI CONGENITE MULTIPLE

È necessario visitare i pazienti quanto prima e iniziare tempestivamente il trattamento delle deformità in quanto alcuni risponderanno molto bene a fisioterapia, stretching e uso dei tutori.

L'**equilibrio muscolare**, che rispetto ad altre patologie neuromuscolari paralitiche di solito rappresenta un problema minore ed è più facile da raggiungere, dovrebbe essere stabilito se sono disponibili muscoli per il trasferimento. La **recidiva della deformità** è la regola, in quanto i tessuti molli densi e non elastici intorno alle articolazioni non si allungano adeguatamente con la crescita. Queste strutture sono considerate la chiave per un trattamento efficace dell'artrogriposi nel bambino in accrescimento. La massima correzione ottenibile in sicurezza deve essere raggiunta al momento dell'intervento. L'uso di cunei o gessi correttivi aggiunge ben poco al trattamento. **Arco di movimento:** i risultati dello stretching per l'arco passivo di movimento sono variabili. Un trattamento aggressivo può determinare un apprezzabile aumento del limitato arco di movimento articolare oppure avere un impatto trascurabile. Tuttavia, l'arco di movimento può spesso essere trasformato in una posizione funzionalmente migliore. **Interessamento centrifugo:** la severità della deformità aumenta verso la periferia dell'arto e le articolazioni meno prossimali tendono a essere meno interessate. Nella maggior parte dei casi si può osservare un risparmio centrale del tronco. **Scopo del trattamento:** l'obiettivo principale è ottenere il massimo guadagno funzionale per ciascun paziente. I requisiti minimi sono la deambulazione indipendente, l'autonomia della cura di sé e, idealmente, in futuro, la capacità di ottenere un impiego soddisfacente. **Stadiazione e timing delle procedure chirurgiche:** il massimo beneficio dalla ricostruzione chirurgica di un arto con artrogriposi si ottiene con un'accurata stadiazione delle procedure. Le deformità disabilitanti e le retrazioni vanno corrette nel primo stadio. Le articolazioni principali devono quindi essere poste in un arco di movimento funzionale più adatto alle esigenze del paziente.

Nello stadio finale, talvolta si rendono necessari trasferimenti tendinei per portare la forza motrice a un'articolazione che è stata posta in posizione ottimale. L'articolazione del gomito è quanto mai adatta ai trasferimenti tendinei ed è opinione diffusa che consenta risultati soddisfacenti.

ARTI INFERIORI

Interessamento del piede. È noto che nell'artrogriposi le deformità più severe si verificano nel piede. La deformità con rigidità del piede consiste di solito in un piede torto o deformità in equinovarismo e, meno frequentemente, in una deformità da astragalo verticale congenito. Lo scopo del trattamento è la conversione del piede rigido e deformato in un piede rigido plantigrado.

La correzione del *retropiede ha la precedenza* su quella dell'avampiede. *Esercizi (gessi) seriati* possono talvolta produrre un certo grado di correzione. Se durante il trattamento appare chiaro che l'approccio conservativo è destinato al fallimento, occorre considerare la chirurgia, preferibilmente quando il bambino è pronto a camminare.

Si raccomanda un *rilascio posteromediale e posterolaterale esteso*. Se il piede non si corregge neppure con il rilascio tissutale più esteso o se il problema recidiva nel giro di 2 anni, si può prendere in esame una talectomia. La tecnica e l'apparecchio di Ilizarov offrono l'opportunità di correggere queste deformità mediante una distrazione graduale e la successiva neoistiogenesi (Fig. 681-5). L'applicazione di questo fissatore nel piede pediatrico è stato abbastanza efficace e soddisfacente. Nei bambini più grandi con deformità in equinovarismo negletta o recidivata, la correzione preferibile consiste in una **tripla artrodesi.** In rari casi di recidiva della deformità dopo tripla artrodesi (a livello della caviglia), può essere proposta un'**artrodesi pantalare** mediante una facile conversione della tripla artrodesi.

Articolazione del ginocchio. La flessione e l'estensione fisse, entrambe presentazioni comuni della deformità del ginocchio, devono essere trattate inizialmente con ripetuti stretching e l'applicazione di tutori. L'obiettivo è quello di ottenere un ginocchio diritto e di mantenerlo tale mediante un tutore. L'estensione del ginocchio è considerata la chiave per ottenere successivamente la deambulazione. Se un ginocchio flesso viene trascurato, è probabile che ne conseguano retrazioni posturali in flessione dell'anca. L'associazione di retrazioni dell'anca e del ginocchio non è compatibile con una deambulazione adeguata.

Trattamento non chirurgico: manipolazioni e gessi hanno avuto successo in un'ampia popolazione di bambini piccoli trattati dagli Autori. È importante sottolineare che, anche se l'arco di movimento passa a una posizione più estesa, il range non aumenta. Sebbene non sia possibile ottenere un'estensione completa, le articolazioni del ginocchio sono di solito stabili e lievi deformità in flessione sono per lo più compatibili con un buon pattern di deambulazione.

Trattamento chirurgico: le deformità che non rispondono allo stretching dei tessuti molli possono richiedere un intervento chirurgico. È consigliabile pianificare il timing della chirurgia del ginocchio in associazione al piano di trattamento del piede. Per

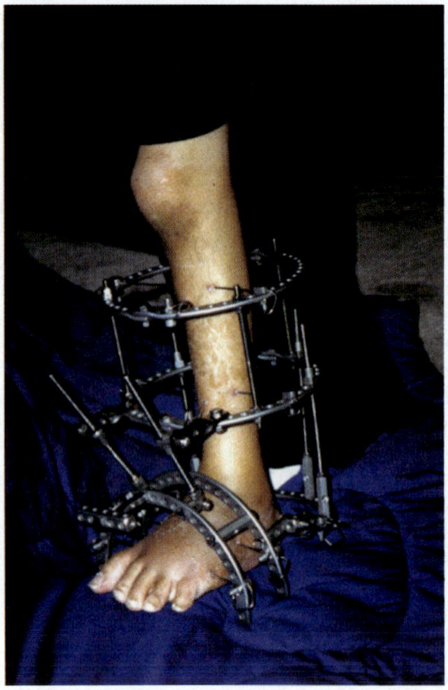

Figura 681-5. Sistema di fissazione di Ilizarov per la correzione della retrazione della caviglia. Per gentile concessione di Richard Davidson, Children's Hospital of Philadelphia.

esempio, se il piede richiede un'immobilizzazione con il ginocchio flesso, la correzione del ginocchio deve essere programmata dopo la flessione del piede; per contro, se il ginocchio è in estensione fissa, è preferibile correggere l'estensione del ginocchio prima di intervenire sul piede, in modo che sia possibile immobilizzare il piede con il ginocchio flesso.

L'iperestensione fissa del ginocchio può rispondere abbastanza bene a ripetuti interventi di stretching e a gessi seriati. Nei casi severi che non rispondono allo stretching, può essere necessario un rilascio muscolare esteso con plastica del quadricipite per correggere la posizione del ginocchio. È probabile che a lungo termine occorra applicare tutori e supporti per il ginocchio. Il fissatore di Ilizarov rappresenta un'utile alternativa al rilascio chirurgico in caso di fallimento della chirurgia, specialmente nel bambino più grande.

Articolazione dell'anca. Un sintomo consueto nei pazienti con artrogriposi congenita è la rigidità dell'anca in flessione, abduzione e rotazione esterna. I due aspetti più comuni dell'anca sono le retrazioni fisse e la lussazione dell'anca.

È importante correggere la deformità del ginocchio prima di tentare qualsiasi intervento e correzione chirurgici dell'anca. Se la correzione del ginocchio viene eseguita in una fase precoce, i risultati della correzione della deformità dell'anca sono incoraggianti.

Trattamento chirurgico:

Bambino in fase di accrescimento: la correzione completa non è facilmente ottenibile con le procedure di rilascio dei tessuti molli. Con la crescita scheletrica di solito le recidive sono inevitabili.

Bambino con maturità scheletrica: se il paziente può camminare con una lordosi compensatoria, è preferibile attendere fino alla maturità scheletrica per poter sperare in una correzione duratura con un'osteotomia subtrocanterica.

L'artrogriposi può causare una **lussazione unilaterale o bilaterale** delle anche. La lussazione è di solito stabile e, se il bacino è ben bilanciato, compatibile con un cammino adeguato. Il trattamento della lussazione dell'anca spesso non è facile perché la riduzione chiusa invariabilmente fallisce e alla riduzione aperta fanno seguito di solito una rigidità e una persistente deformità in flessione. La diagnosi talvolta è clinicamente difficile in quanto la marcata rigidità può costituire un fattore limitante per la dimostrazione clinica dell'instabilità dell'anca. Se le anche sono lussate, nella maggior parte dei casi non sono riducibili in abduzione e in tal caso non si devono applicare tutori, che potrebbero causare necrosi avascolare. Le **lussazioni bilaterali** tendono a essere alte e stabili, sono di solito simmetriche e mantengono il bacino abbastanza in equilibrio, caratteristiche spesso compatibili con un cammino adeguato; può essere preferibile astenersi da qualunque trattamento in quanto spesso non è possibile ottenere un risultato soddisfacente da entrambi i lati, mentre si rischia di aumentare la rigidità e quindi anche le probabilità di una nuova lussazione. In caso di **lussazione unilaterale**, sussiste il rischio di obliquità pelvica progressiva e di scoliosi secondaria. Gli Autori di questo capitolo, pertanto, ritengono spesso utile ridurre l'anca lussata, specialmente nel lattante e nel bambino piccolo. La riduzione aperta deve essere eseguita non appena il paziente è in buone condizioni di salute e le retrazioni in flessione del ginocchio sono sotto controllo. Un ritardo eccessivo rende la procedura più complessa tecnicamente e la riduzione più difficile da ottenere.

ARTI SUPERIORI. A differenza del trattamento degli arti inferiori, in cui il raggiungimento di una deambulazione indipendente è l'obiettivo principale, il trattamento delle estremità superiori nell'artrogriposi richiede notevole cautela in quanto la prognosi dipende di più dall'estensione della deformità e dall'intelligenza del bambino. Le esigenze minime del paziente sono la capacità di alimentarsi e la cura personale.

Inoltre, al contrario di quanto avviene con gli arti inferiori, dove non è possibile rimandare l'intervento per il rischio di ritardo della deambulazione, le operazioni chirurgiche sugli arti superiori possono essere posposte per diversi anni. È interessante notare come i bambini con artrogriposi sviluppino una notevole capacità di utilizzare gli arti superiori nonostante la complessità di queste deformità, dando prova di una destrezza sorprendente; pertanto, i pro e i contro dell'intervento chirurgico, se necessario, devono essere soppesati con molta attenzione in questi casi.

Pianificazione. *I due arti devono essere considerati come unità.* Come principio generale, occorre ricordare che l'arco di movimento può essere cambiato ma non aumentato. Al termine del trattamento è ragionevole aspettarsi che il paziente sia in grado di portare una mano alla bocca e l'altra all'ano, ma anche di opporre entrambe le mani. Questa è una considerazione importante in quanto i bambini con deformità e perdita di forza severe delle mani dipendono dall'uso concomitante di entrambe le mani (opposizione bimanuale) per eseguire qualsiasi compito che le persone normali eseguono con una mano sola. Inoltre, il paziente deve essere in grado di alzarsi da una sedia.

Le articolazioni della spalla e del gomito devono essere considerate come unità. La rotazione della spalla è un fattore importante dal quale dipende in larga misura l'asse di movimento dell'articolazione del gomito. Pertanto, se si prevede di effettuare un intervento sul gomito per consentire alla mano di raggiungere la bocca, bisogna al contempo correggere anche una spalla fissa e ruotata internamente in modo severo.

La fisioterapia, insieme all'uso di stretching e tutori, è molto importante per ottenere la mobilità di articolazioni rigide. Si rende necessaria una valutazione dettagliata da parte di un fisioterapista e un terapista occupazionale prima di intraprendere qualsiasi intervento chirurgico, e quest'ultimo, se possibile, non andrebbe eseguito in pazienti di età <4 anni.

Spalla. La deformità tipica consiste in adduzione e rotazione interna. Anche se la perdita di forza a livello della spalla è comune, questi bambini possono sviluppare in misura notevole movimenti "trucco" e quindi l'intervento chirurgico raramente è indicato. La stessa adduzione non è problematica in quanto di solito è presente un'abduzione passiva sufficiente per la cura di sé e la chirurgia di rado è necessaria. La rotazione interna fissa della spalla in alcuni casi può compromettere l'asse del movimento del gomito. Nei casi severi, si può eseguire una semplice osteotomia di rotazione esterna a livello dell'omero superiore per portare avambraccio e mano in una posizione più funzionale.

Gomito. Di solito le due deformità più comuni del gomito sono la retrazione in estensione fissa e la retrazione in flessione fissa. Entrambe rispondono bene allo stretching e alla fisioterapia e possono essere adeguatamente controllate nell'infanzia. Una volta che il bambino ha imparato a camminare, attività come la deambulazione con le grucce, la pulizia personale e l'alzarsi da una sedia richiedono essenzialmente un'estensione attiva del gomito. Pertanto, è importante non danneggiare inavvertitamente il meccanismo di estensione attiva nel tentativo di migliorare la flessione attiva. La flessione passiva può essere ottenuta chirurgicamente con un rilascio dei tessuti molli posteriori del gomito, con l'allungamento del tricipite e un rilascio capsulare posteriore e del legamento collaterale. In questo modo è possibile ripristinare un arco di movimento molto utile e nella maggior parte dei casi non sono necessarie altre procedure. Nei soggetti in cui è possibile stabilire un valore di aumentata flessione attiva, una forza attiva può essere apportata in vari modi, tra cui una plastica flessoria di Steindler e un trasferimento del tricipite o del grande pettorale.

In molti casi, le retrazioni dei tessuti molli del gomito e dell'avambraccio possono essere corrette con il fissatore di Ilizarov.

Polso e mano. Il polso è spesso interessato da una retrazione in flessione e anche le dita possono essere ricurve e rigide. Altrettanto comune è la deformità in adduzione del pollice (pollice nel palmo). Manipolazioni, stretching e tutori (specialmente se applicati quanto prima) possono essere molto importanti per stabilire mobilità e range di movimento. È interessante notare come la posizione flessa del polso sia molto funzionale e possa non richiedere l'intervento. Sono state descritte correzioni chirurgiche (tra cui una carpectomia parziale o completa) che spesso però sono associate a un'elevata incidenza di recidive della deformità con la crescita. La rigidità delle dita è difficilissima da correggere in questi casi e la chirurgia è indicata raramente. La maggior parte dei pazienti si adatta assai bene alla rigidità delle dita e ha capacità funzionali davvero impressionanti. Il rilascio degli adduttori del pollice e l'allargamento dello spazio tra le dita sono molto utili per correggere la deformità del pollice. Al momento della maturità scheletrica si può prendere in considerazione l'artrodesi del polso per un miglioramento funzionale o estetico.

COLONNA VERTEBRALE. Compatibilmente con il principio secondo cui la severità della rigidità e della deformità aumenta verso la periferia degli arti e che le aree più centrali o prossimali sono le meno coinvolte, un tronco diritto, flessibile e ben bilanciato è una risorsa importante. Nell'artrogriposi si osserva frequentemente una scoliosi, a causa di un'elevata incidenza di curve congenite (vedi Capitolo 678).

Scoliosi idiopatica. La scoliosi genetica o idiopatica sembra manifestarsi con la stessa frequenza nei pazienti con artrogriposi e nella popolazione generale. La progressione e il comportamento di una curva idiopatica nell'artrogriposi sembrano essere uguali a quelli degli altri bambini, anche se può essere più disabilitante a causa delle deformità periferiche coesistenti.

Scoliosi paralitica. Lunghe curve scoliotiche paralitiche si osservano talvolta in bambini con il classico tipo neuropatico di artrogriposi. Alcune forme di distrofia muscolare congenita comprendono una componente di "colonna rigida". La curva viene tipicamente osservata prima del 2° anno di vita e progredisce diventando lunga, severa e infine rigida. Un busto adeguatamente controllato è il trattamento di scelta nei bambini piccoli, anche se l'intervento chirurgico può rendersi necessario nei casi progressivi.

Scoliosi congenita. Queste curve sono comuni nell'artrogriposi, forse a causa di altre anomalie congenite di frequente riscontro nell'artrogriposi. Sono state osservate mancata formazione vertebrale e mancata segmentazione, oltre a una deformità di Klippel-Feil. Queste curve devono essere tenute sotto stretta osservazione; in presenza di curve progressive asimmetriche può essere indicato un trattamento aggressivo come una fusione chirurgica precoce.

Scoliosi associata a obliquità pelvica. È frequentemente associata a una deformità trascurata delle anche che si traduce in un'obliquità femoropelvica e che sarebbe potenzialmente evitabile. In particolare, occorre sorvegliare e correggere una deformità unilaterale dell'anca. Il tronco può quindi essere mantenuto flessibile e diritto.

Abu-Sa'da O, Barbar M, Al-Harbi N, Taha D: Arthrogryposis renal tubular acidosis and cholestasis (ARC) syndrome: Two new cases and review. *Clin Dermatol* 2005;14:191–196.

Brunner R, Hefti F, Tgetgel JD: Arthrogrypotic joint contracture at the knee and the foot: Correction with a circular frame. *J Pediatr Orthop* 1997;6:192–197.

Burglen L, Amiel J, Violet L, et al: Survival motor neuron gene deletion in the arthrogryposis multiplex congenita–spinal muscular atrophy association. *J Clin Invest* 1996;98:1130–1132.

Fixsen J: Arthrogryposis multiplex congenita. In Benson MK, MF Macnicol MF, Parsch K (editors): *Children's Orthopaedics and Fractures.* Philadelphia, Churchill Livingstone, 2002, pp 293–298.

Hall JG: Genetic aspects of arthrogryposis. *Clin Orthop* 1985;194:44–53.

Hall JG: Arthrogryposis multiplex congenita: Etiology, genetics, classification, diagnostic approach, and general aspects. *J Pediatr Orthop* 1997;6: 159–166.

Hosalkar HS, Moroz L, Drummond DS, Finkel R: Neuromuscular disorders of infancy and childhood and arthrogryposis. In Dormans J (editor): *Pediatric Orthopedics: Core Knowledge in Orthopedics.* Philadelphia, Mosby, 2005, pp 454–482.

Mennen U, Van Heest A, Ezaki MB: Arthrogryposis multiplex congenita. *J Hand Surg [Br]* 2005;30:468–474.

Murray C, Fixsen JA: Management of knee deformity in classical arthrogryposis multiplex congenita (amyoplasia congenita). *J Pediatr Orthop* 1997;6:186–191.

Capitolo 682 ■ Fratture comuni

Purushottam A. Gholve, Harish S. Hosalkar e Lawrence Wells

I traumi sono cause importanti di morte e disabilità nei bambini di età superiore a un anno. Diversi fattori rendono le fratture dello scheletro immaturo diverse da quelle che interessano lo scheletro maturo. Anatomia, biomeccanica e fisiologia dall'apparato scheletrico pediatrico sono differenti da quelle tipiche degli adulti: ne derivano notevoli differenze relativamente a pattern di frattura (Fig. 682-1), problemi diagnostici e tecniche di trattamento (che nel paziente pediatrico mirano a preservare la funzione senza interferire con la crescita).

Alle radiografie possono essere visibili linee epifisarie, rarefazione, linee di crescita dense, fratture congenite e pseudofratture, tutti aspetti che creano confusione e talvolta rendono difficoltosa l'interpretazione di una frattura. La maggior parte delle fratture nei bambini guarisce bene anche senza un trattamento attento; ciò ha portato operatori inconsapevoli a trascurare il fatto che altre fratture possono avere un esito disastroso se affidate a mani inesperte. Le peculiarità dell'apparato scheletrico infantile predispongono i bambini a traumi diversi da quelli degli adulti. Le differenze importanti sono la presenza della cartilagine periossea, della cartilagine di accrescimento e di un periostio più spesso, robusto e osteogenico, che produce nuovo tessuto osseo (callo) a un ritmo più rapido e in maggiore quantità. Altre caratteristiche dei pazienti pediatrici sono una testa sproporzionatamente grande rispetto al corpo, una gabbia toracica flessibile, la mancanza di protezione per intestino tenue e colon e l'apertura delle cartilagini di accrescimento. L'osso in età pediatrica presenta una bassa densità, dovuta a un minore contenuto in minerali, e una maggiore porosità, riconducibile a un maggior numero di canali

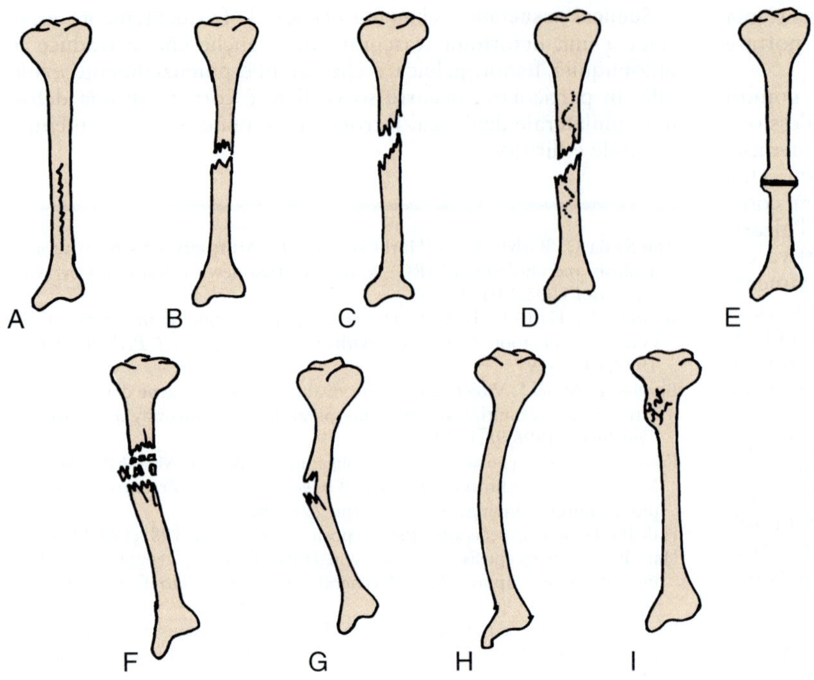

Figura 682-1. Schema dei pattern di frattura. *A*, Linea di frattura longitudinale parallela all'asse osseo. *B*, Linea di frattura trasversale perpendicolare all'asse osseo. *C*, Linea di frattura obliqua ad angolo con l'asse osseo. *D*, Linea di frattura spirale che decorre in modo curvilineo rispetto all'asse osseo. *E*, Estremità ossee fratturate e compattate, compresse l'una contro l'altra. *F*, Frammentazione comminuta dell'osso in tre o più parti. *G*, Curvatura a legno verde dell'osso con frattura del lato convesso. *H*, Deformazione plastica con curvatura dell'osso. *I*, Frattura toroidale (a fibbia). (Da White N, Sty R: Radiological evaluation and classification of pediatric fractures. *Clin Pediatr Emerg Med* 2002;3:94-105.)

di Havers e canali vascolari. Queste differenze determinano un modulo di elasticità più basso e una forza di piegamento minore che negli adulti. L'osso del bambino può cedere se sottoposto sia a tensione sia a compressione; le linee di frattura non si propagano come negli adulti, per cui vi è una minore probabilità di fratture comminute.

Traumi articolari, lussazioni e rotture dei legamenti sono infrequenti nei bambini. È più probabile un danno a carico di una cartilagine di accrescimento contigua. I corpi mammillari interdigitati e l'anello pericondrale aumentano la resistenza della cartilagine di accrescimento. Da un punto di vista biomeccanico, quest'ultima non è resistente come i legamenti o l'osso metafisario. Essa è più resistente alla trazione e meno alle forze di torsione. Il periostio aderisce poco alla diafisi mentre è strettamente aderente alla parte periferica della cartilagine di accrescimento. Il periostio di solito risulta sempre traumatizzato in caso di fratture, ma ha minori probabilità di andare incontro a una rottura completa per tutta la sua circonferenza in quanto poco aderente alla diafisi. Questo manicotto periosteo (cerniera periostea) rende meno esteso lo spostamento delle fratture e facilita la riduzione. Lo spesso periostio può inoltre fungere da ostacolo alle riduzioni chiuse, in particolare se la frattura è penetrata nel periostio, o alla riduzione di una cartilagine di accrescimento spostata.

682.1 • Caratteristiche peculiari delle fratture pediatriche

RIMODELLAMENTO DELLA FRATTURA

Il rimodellamento è la terza e ultima fase del processo biologico che porta alla guarigione delle fratture, preceduta dalla fase infiammatoria e riparativa. Consiste nella combinazione di deposizione ossea apposizionale sulla concavità della deformità, riassorbimento sulla convessità e crescita asimmetrica della cartilagine di accrescimento. Pertanto, l'accuratezza della riduzione è un po' meno importante che negli adulti (Fig. 682-2). I tre principali fattori che influiscono sul potenziale della correzione angolare sono l'età scheletrica, la distanza rispetto all'articolazione e l'orientamento rispetto all'asse articolare. Le deformità rotatoria e angolare non in asse con il movimento articolare hanno una minore probabilità di andare incontro a rimodellamento. L'entità della crescita restante fornisce le basi del rimodellamento; i bambini piccoli hanno un maggiore potenziale di rimodellamento. Le fratture adiacenti a una cartilagine di accrescimento vanno incontro al rimodellamento maggiore, sempre che la deformità si trovi sul piano dell'asse di movimento di quella articolazione. Le fratture distanti dal gomito e quelle vicine al ginocchio hanno il maggiore potenziale di rimodellamento, in quanto queste cartilagini di accrescimento forniscono la massima crescita ossea. Ci si può aspettare che il rimodellamento avvenga nell'arco di molti mesi dopo il trauma fino alla maturità scheletrica. Questa viene raggiunta nelle femmine tra i 13 e i 15 anni e nei maschi tra i 14 e i 16 anni di età.

ECCESSO DI CRESCITA

La stimolazione della cartilagine di accrescimento da parte dell'iperemia associata alla guarigione della frattura causa un eccesso di crescita, di solito evidente nelle ossa lunghe come il femore. L'accelerazione della crescita di solito si osserva per 6 mesi-1 anno dopo il trauma e non si associa a un eccesso continuo e progressivo di crescita, a meno che non sia complicata da una rara malformazione arterovenosa. Le fratture femorali nei bambini di età <10 anni frequentemente si associano a un eccesso di crescita di 1-3 cm. Per compensare l'eccesso di crescita previsto si preferisce un'apposizione ossea a baionetta. Tale fenomeno porta comunque a una lunghezza uguale o pressoché uguale degli arti, al termine del rimodellamento della frattura. Dopo i 10 anni di età, l'eccesso di crescita è un problema minore e si raccomanda l'allineamento anatomico. Nelle fratture della cartilagine di coniugazione, la stimolazione della crescita è associata all'uso di impianti o di strumenti di fissazione che possono causare uno stimolo cronico alla crescita longitudinale.

DEFORMITÀ PROGRESSIVA

I traumi delle cartilagini di accrescimento possono essere complicati da deformità progressive con la crescita. La causa più comune è la chiusura parziale o completa della cartilagine di accrescimento, che si traduce in una deformità angolare, un accorciamento o entrambi. L'arresto parziale può essere periferico, centrale o combinato. La gravità della deformità dipende dalla cartilagine di accrescimento coinvolta e dall'entità della crescita rimanente. TC e RM sono importanti sia per valutare gli arresti parziali sia per formulare il trattamento (Fig. 682-3).

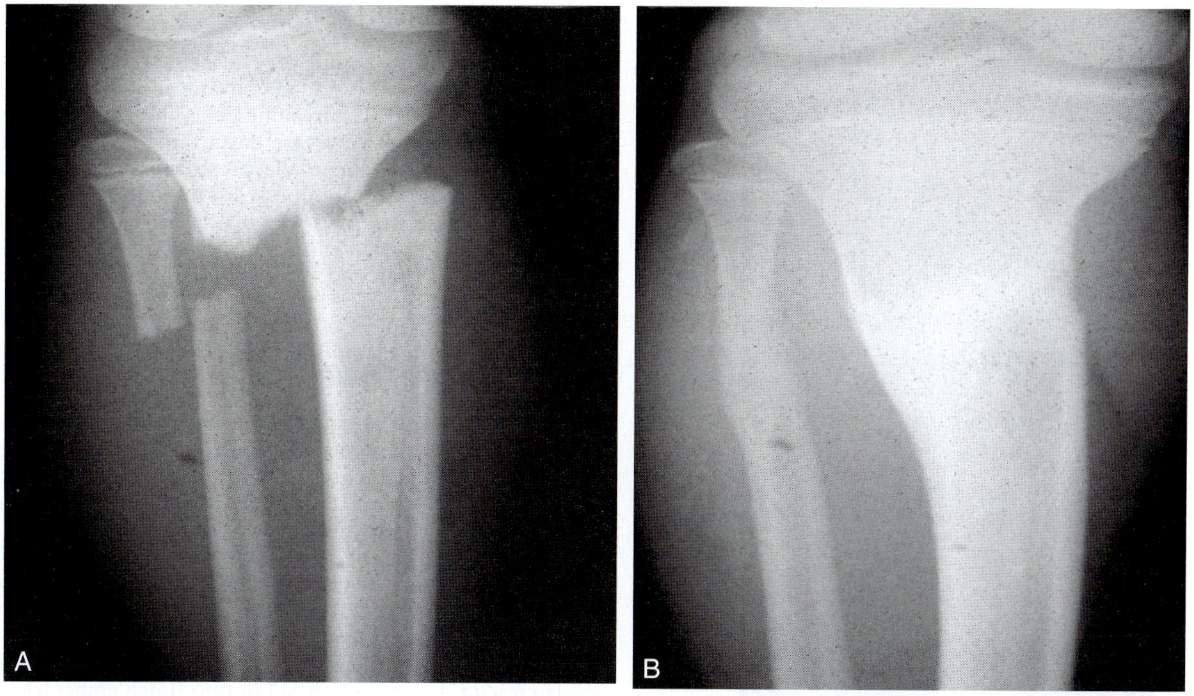

Figura 682-2. Il rimodellamento nei bambini è spesso esteso, come in questa frattura tibiale prossimale, al momento del trauma (*A*) e un anno dopo (*B*). (Da Dormans JP: *Pediatric Orthopedics: Introduction to Trauma*. Philadelphia, Mosby, 2005, p. 38.)

GUARIGIONE RAPIDA

Le fratture pediatriche guariscono più rapidamente di quelle degli adulti, per effetto del potenziale di crescita dei bambini e del periostio più spesso e attivo. Con l'avvicinarsi dell'adolescenza e della maturità, la velocità della guarigione diminuisce e diviene simile a quella di un adulto. La guarigione rapida comporta tuttavia un risvolto negativo, in quanto provoca rifratture.

682.2 • PATTERN DI FRATTURA PEDIATRICA

I diversi pattern di frattura pediatrica rispecchiano le caratteristiche dell'apparato scheletrico infantile. La maggior parte delle fratture pediatriche può essere trattata con metodi chiusi e guarisce perfettamente.

DEFORMITÀ PLASTICA

La deformità plastica è tipica dei bambini e limitata a questa categoria di pazienti. Più comune nell'ulna, occasionalmente si riscontra anche nel perone. La frattura si verifica per effetto di una forza che produce un cedimento microscopico dal lato tensile dell'osso e non si propaga al lato concavo. Quest'ultimo presenta anche un cedimento microscopico in compressione. L'osso si angola oltre il suo limite elastico, ma l'energia non è tale da produrre una frattura. Pertanto, alle radiografie non risulta visibile alcuna linea di frattura (Fig. 682-4). La deformità plastica è permanente e un'angolatura ulnare <20° si correggerà con la crescita.

FRATTURA TOROIDALE O A FIBBIA

Un cedimento in compressione dell'osso di verifica di solito alla giunzione tra metafisi e diafisi, specialmente nel radio distale (Fig. 682-5). Il trauma viene denominato "frattura toroidale" a causa della sua somiglianza con la modanatura in rilievo (toro) che circonda la base di una colonna greca classica. Queste fratture

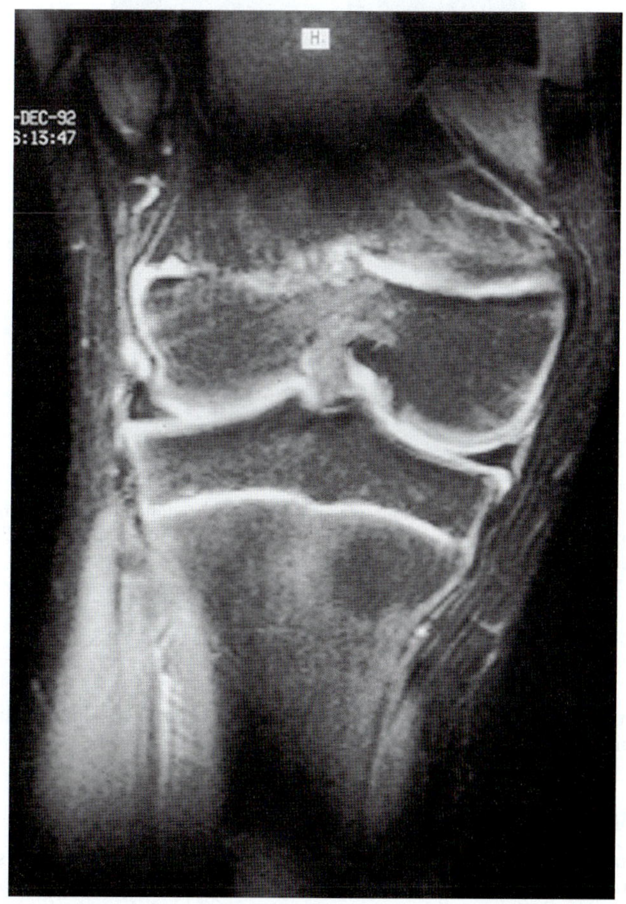

Figura 682-3. RM con sequenza a gradiente di eco, che rivela una barra a livello della cartilagine di accrescimento femorale distale. (Da Dormans JP: *Pediatric Orthopedics: Introduction to Trauma*. Philadelphia, Mosby, 2005, p. 43.)

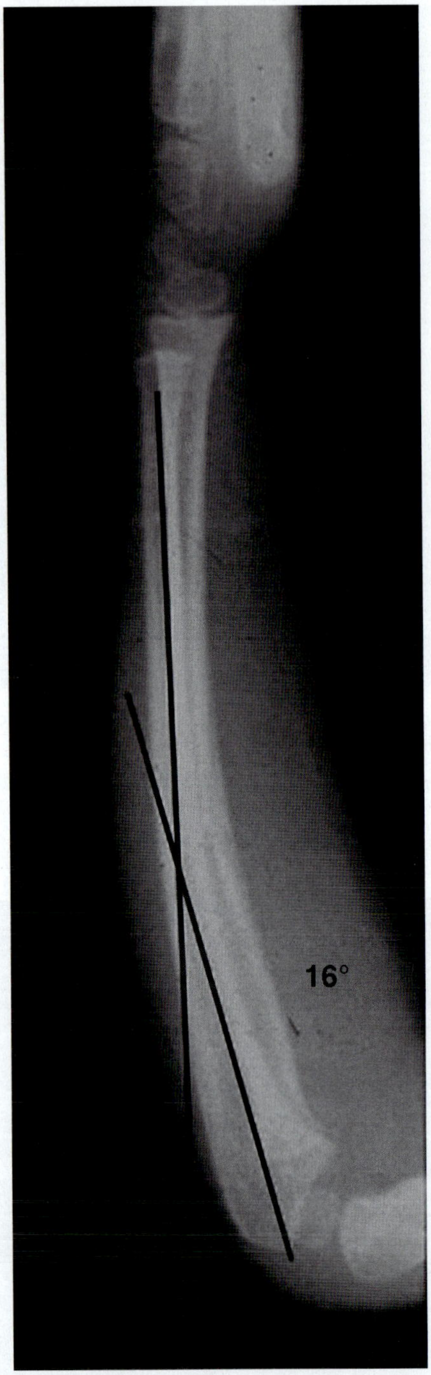

Figura 682-4. La deformazione plastica è un microcedimento della tensione senza linea di frattura visibile. (Per gentile concessione di John Flynn, Children's Hospital, Philadelphia, PA.)

sono di per sé stabili e guariscono in 3-4 settimane con la semplice immobilizzazione.

FRATTURA A LEGNO VERDE

Queste fratture si verificano quando l'osso si piega e cede sul lato tensile (convesso). La linea di frattura non si estende al lato concavo dell'osso. Il lato concavo presenta segni di un cedimento microscopico con deformazione plastica. È necessario rompere l'osso dal lato concavo in quanto la deformazione plastica lo fa ritornare alla posizione deformata.

FRATTURE COMPLETE

Le fratture dette complete, che attraversano tutto lo spessore dell'osso, possono essere classificate in spirali, trasverse o oblique, a seconda della direzione delle linee di frattura. Le fratture spirali di solito sono create da una forza di rotazione e la loro riduzione è facile grazie alla presenza di una cerniera periostea intatta. Le fratture oblique si localizzano nella diafisi a 30° rispetto all'asse dell'osso e sono di per sé instabili. Le fratture trasverse si verificano in seguito a una forza di piegamento su tre punti e si riducono facilmente utilizzando il periostio intatto del lato concavo.

FRATTURE EPIFISARIE

I traumi dell'epifisi coinvolgono la cartilagine di accrescimento. Esiste sempre un potenziale di deformazione e quindi è necessaria l'osservazione a lungo termine. La cartilagine di accrescimento radiale distale è quella più frequentemente interessata. Salter e Harris (SH) hanno suddiviso i traumi epifisari in cinque gruppi (Tab. 682-1 e Fig. 682-6), elaborando un sistema di classificazione che facilita la previsione della prognosi e offre linee guida per il trattamento. Le fratture di SH di tipo I e II di solito possono essere trattate con tecniche di riduzione chiusa e non richiedono un allineamento perfetto in quanto tendono a rimodellarsi con la crescita. Le fratture di SH di tipo II dell'epifisi femorale distale richiedono una riduzione anatomica. Le fratture epifisarie di tipo III e IV sono a carico della superficie articolare e necessitano di un allineamento anatomico per prevenire qualsiasi dislivello e riallineare le cellule di crescita della cartilagine di accrescimento. In genere le fratture di tipo V non vengono inizialmente diagnosticate, ma si presentano in epoche successive con disturbi della crescita. Altri traumi dell'epifisi sono quelli con avulsione della tuberosità tibiale e delle inserzioni muscolari del bacino. Le fratture osteocondrali vengono considerate anche traumi della cartilagine di accrescimento che non coinvolgono direttamente la cartilagine di accrescimento stessa.

VIOLENZA SUI BAMBINI

Il chirurgo ortopedico vede il 30-50% dei bambini sottoposti ad abuso fisico. Si deve sospettare una violenza nei bambini non deambulanti con fratture delle ossa lunghe degli arti inferiori (vedi Capitolo 36). Non esiste un pattern o un tipo di frattura che sia patognomonico di abuso; qualsiasi tipo di frattura può derivare da un trauma non accidentale. Sono suggestive di trauma intenzionale le fratture di femore in bambini non deambulanti, le fratture angolari della metafisi femorale distale, le fratture costali posteriori, quelle a carico del processo spinoso della scapola e le fratture prossimali d'omero. È essenziale esaminare tutto lo scheletro in ogni caso sospetto, in quanto da tale indagine possono emergere altre fratture in differenti stadi di guarigione. Da un punto di vista radiografico, possono simulare segni di abuso alcune malattie sistemiche come l'osteogenesi imperfetta, l'osteomielite, la malattia di Caffey e le fratture da stress. Molti ospedali si avvalgono di un team multidisciplinare preposto alla valutazione e al trattamento dei pazienti vittime di violenze. Negli Stati Uniti è obbligatorio segnalare questi casi alle agenzie di welfare sociale.

682.3 • FRATTURE DELLE ESTREMITÀ SUPERIORI

FRATTURE DELLE FALANGI

I diversi pattern di frattura delle falangi nei bambini comprendono fratture diafisarie, della cartilagine di accrescimento e della parte finale della falange distale. Il meccanismo traumatico è un colpo diretto sul dito o caratteristicamente un dito intrappolato in una porta (vedi Capitolo 680). I traumi da schiacciamento

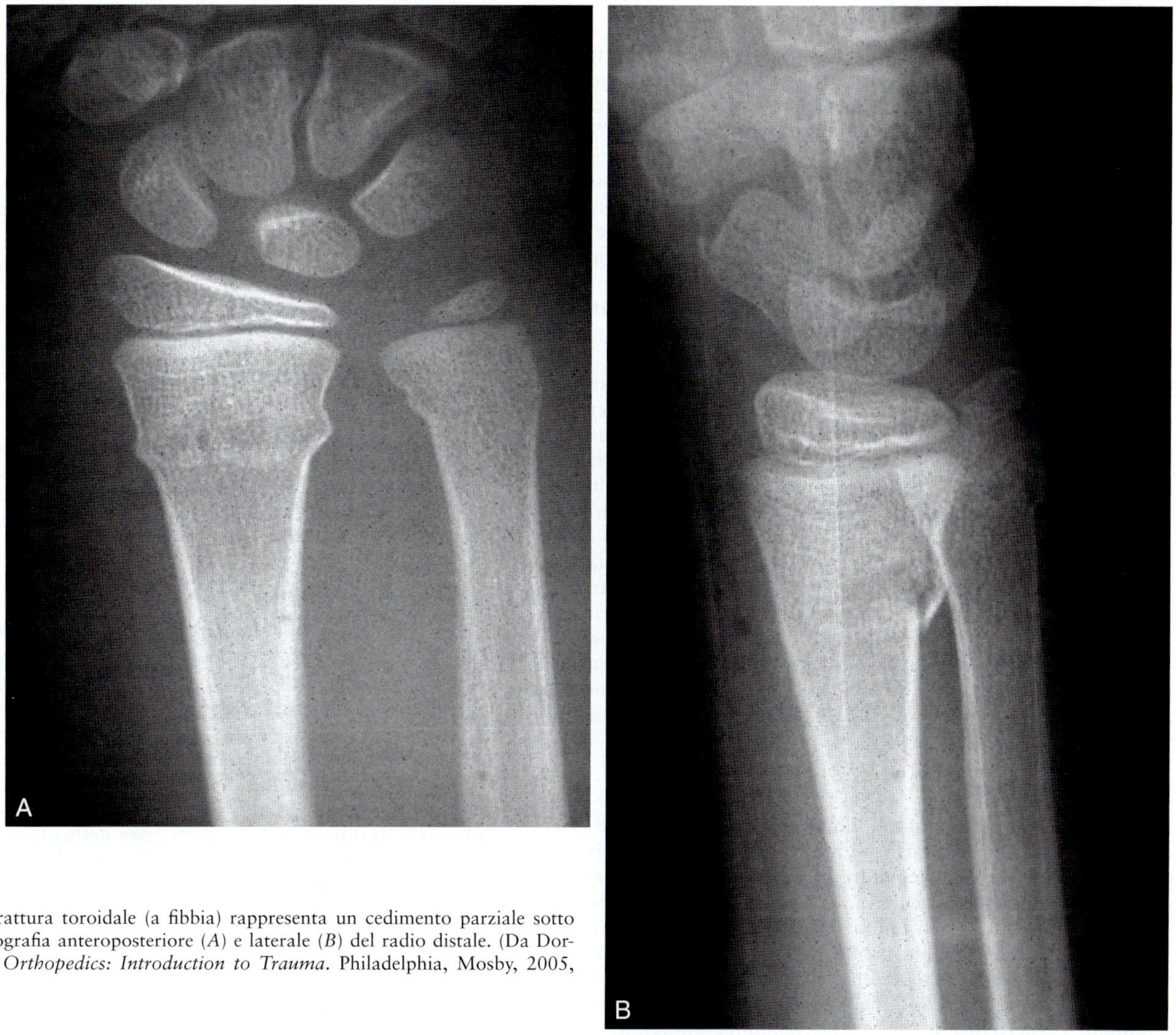

Figura 682-5. La frattura toroidale (a fibbia) rappresenta un cedimento parziale sotto compressione: radiografia anteroposteriore (*A*) e laterale (*B*) del radio distale. (Da Dormans JP: *Pediatric Orthopedics: Introduction to Trauma*. Philadelphia, Mosby, 2005, p. 37.)

TABELLA 682-1. Classificazione di Salter-Harris

TIPO DI SALTER-HARRIS	CARATTERISTICHE
I	Separazione attraverso la cartilagine di accrescimento, di solito attraverso le zone delle colonne cellulari ipertrofiche e in degenerazione
II	Frattura attraverso una porzione della cartilagine di accrescimento che però si estende nelle metafisi
III	Frattura attraverso una porzione della cartilagine di accrescimento che si estende nell'epifisi e all'interno dell'articolazione
IV	Frattura che attraversa metafisi, cartilagine di accrescimento ed epifisi
V	Trauma da schiacciamento della cartilagine di accrescimento

della falange distale si presentano con una grave comminuzione dell'osso sottostante (frattura della parte finale della falange distale o *tuft fracture*), rottura del letto ungueale e trauma significativo dei tessuti molli. Il migliore trattamento di questi traumi consiste in antibiotici, profilassi del tetano e irrigazione con soluzione fisiologica. Un dito a martello consiste nell'impossibilità di estendere la parte distale del dito, in conseguenza di un trauma in iperestensione. Rappresenta una frattura in avulsione della cartilagine di coniugazione della falange distale. Il trattamento consiste nell'immobilizzare in estensione il dito con un tutore per 3-4 settimane. I traumi della cartilagine di accrescimento delle falangi medie e prossimali sono trattati allo stesso modo con immobilizzazione in tutore. Le fratture diafisarie, che siano oblique, spirali o trasverse, devono essere valutate per una deformità angolare e rotatoria con il dito in flessione. Qualsiasi malrotazione o deformità angolare richiede una correzione per una funzionalità ottimale della mano. Queste deformità vengono corrette con una riduzione chiusa e, se instabili, richiedono la stabilizzazione.

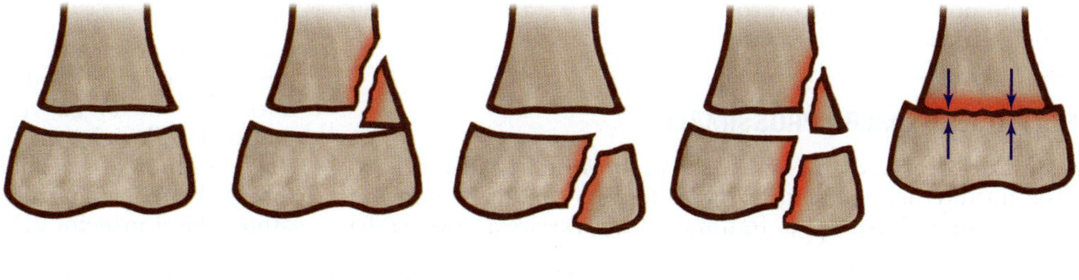

Figura 682-6. Classificazione di Salter-Harris delle fratture della cartilagine di accrescimento, tipi I-V.

FRATTURE DELL'AVAMBRACCIO

Le fratture di polso e avambraccio, molto comuni nei bambini, rappresentano quasi la metà di tutte le fratture che si osservano nel soggetto con immaturità scheletrica. Il meccanismo traumatico più frequente è la caduta su una mano protesa. L'80% delle fratture di avambraccio coinvolgono radio distale e ulna, il 15% il terzo medio e le restanti sono rare fratture del terzo prossimale della diafisi radiale o ulnare. Nella maggior parte dei casi si tratta di fratture toroidali o a legno verde. La frattura toroidale è una frattura impattata con edema ed emorragia minimi. Il modo migliore per trattarle è con un gesso corto per l'avambraccio (sotto il gomito) e di solito guariscono in 3-4 settimane. Le fratture a fibbia del polso sono state trattate in modo efficace con un tutore rimovibile.

Le fratture diafisarie possono essere più difficili da trattare perché i limiti di una riduzione accettabile sono più stretti che per le fratture distali del radio. Una malunione significativa di una frattura diafisaria dell'avambraccio può portare a una perdita permanente di pronazione e supinazione, con difficoltà funzionali. L'esame obiettivo deve essere incentrato sul trauma dei tessuti molli, previa esclusione di qualsiasi interessamento neurovascolare. Le radiografie in proiezione anteroposteriore e laterale dell'avambraccio e del polso confermano la diagnosi. Le fratture con spostamento e angolate, che vengono sottoposte a riduzione chiusa con manipolazioni in anestesia generale, richiedono l'immobilizzazione in gesso al di sopra del gomito per almeno 6 settimane. La perdita di riduzione e le fratture instabili rendono necessaria una riduzione aperta con fissazione interna.

FRATTURE DI OMERO DISTALI

Alle fratture in prossimità dell'omero si dedica maggiore attenzione in quanto è necessario un trattamento più aggressivo per ottenere un buon risultato. Molti traumi sono intrarticolari, interessano la cartilagine di accrescimento e possono raramente dare luogo a malunione o non unione. L'omero distale si sviluppa da una serie di centri di ossificazione, che possono venire scambiati per fratture da un occhio inesperto. Un'attenta valutazione radiografica è parte integrante della diagnosi e del trattamento dei traumi dell'omero distale. Le fratture comuni comprendono la separazione dell'epifisi omerale distale (frattura transcondiloidea), fratture sopracondiloidee dell'omero distale e fratture epifisarie del condilo mediale o laterale. Il meccanismo del trauma è la caduta sul braccio esteso. L'esame obiettivo comprende la valutazione della sede e dell'estensione della tumefazione dei tessuti molli, l'esclusione di qualsiasi lesione neurovascolare, in particolare l'interessamento del nervo interosseo anteriore o un'evidenza di sindrome compartimentale. La frattura transcondiloidea nei neonati deve far sorgere il sospetto di violenza. Per la diagnosi sono necessarie radiografie in proiezione anteroposteriore e laterale dell'estremità coinvolta. Se la frattura non è visibile, ma è presente un'alterazione dei rapporti tra omero, radio e ulna o si osserva un segno del cuscinetto adiposo posteriore, occorre sospettare una frattura transcondiloidea o una frattura occulta. Per un'ulteriore conferma possono essere necessari studi di imaging come TC, RM ed ecografia.

In generale, le fratture distali d'omero richiedono che venga ripristinato l'allineamento anatomico, necessario ai fini della prevenzione delle deformità e di una crescita e uno sviluppo normali. Il metodo preferito è la riduzione chiusa, da sola o in associazione con la fissazione percutanea. La riduzione aperta è necessaria per le fratture non riducibili con metodi chiusi. Riduzioni inadeguate possono portare a cubito varo, cubito valgo e, raramente, a non unione o instabilità del gomito.

FRATTURE DI OMERO PROSSIMALE

Le fratture di omero prossimale, che rappresentano meno del 5% delle fratture nei bambini, di solito derivano da una caduta sul braccio esteso. Il pattern di frattura tende a variare a seconda del gruppo di età. I bambini di età <5 anni hanno una frattura di SH di tipo I, quelli di 5-10 anni vanno soggetti a fratture metafisarie e i i ragazzi di età >11 anni hanno una frattura di SH di tipo II. L'esame comprende un'accurata valutazione neurologica, specialmente del nervo ascellare. La diagnosi si pone in base alle radiografie in anteroposteriore della spalla. Per escludere la presenza di una lussazione, si esegue una proiezione ascellare. Le fratture di SH di tipo I non richiedono riduzione in quanto hanno un'ottima capacità rimodellante, ed è sufficiente una semplice immobilizzazione per 2-3 settimane in un bendaggio a sospensione. L'omero prossimale contribuisce per l'80% alla crescita dell'omero. Le fratture metafisarie di solito non necessitano di riduzione, a meno che l'angolazione non sia >50°. Una riduzione chiusa con immobilizzazione in bendaggio sospeso è un trattamento adeguato per la frattura. Per le fratture di SH di tipo II con angolazione <30° e uno spostamento <50% si ricorre al bendaggio a sospensione. Le fratture con spostamento sono trattate con riduzione chiusa e ulteriore stabilizzazione in caso di instabilità. Talvolta occorre effettuare una riduzione chiusa a causa della penetrazione del frammento di frattura attraverso il deltoide o dell'interposizione del tendine bicipitale.

FRATTURE DELLA CLAVICOLA

Le fratture neonatali si verificano in seguito a un trauma diretto nel corso del parto, per lo più attribuibile alla presenza di un bacino ristretto o di una distocia di spalla. Esse possono essere inizialmente trascurate e manifestarsi con una pseudoparalisi. Le fratture dell'infanzia sono di solito conseguenza di una caduta sulla spalla interessata o di un trauma diretto della clavicola. La loro sede più comune è la giunzione tra terzo medio e terzo laterale della clavicola. La diagnosi viene formulata in base alla presenza di dolore in corrispondenza della clavicola. È importante un esame neurovascolare completo per la diagnosi di qualsiasi **trauma del plesso brachiale** associato. Una radiografia anteroposteriore della clavicola dimostra la frattura e può evidenziare una sovrapposizione dei frammenti. I traumi della cartilagine di accrescimento possono verificarsi attraverso la parte mediale o laterale della cartilagine di accrescimento e talvolta non è facile distinguerli dalla lussazione dell'articolazione acromioclavicolare o sternoclavicolare. Per definire meglio il trauma possono essere necessari ulteriori studi di imaging, per esempio una TC. Il trattamento della maggior parte delle fratture della clavicola consiste nell'applicazione di un bendaggio a 8, che permette l'estensione delle spalle e riduce al minimo la sovrapposizione dei frammenti di frattura. Le fratture delle cartilagini di accrescimento sono trattate con una semplice immobilizzazione in bendaggio a sospensione, senza alcun tentativo di riduzione. Spesso non si ottiene l'allineamento anatomico, che peraltro non è necessario. Le fratture guariscono rapidamente, in 3-6 settimane. Di solito in questi bambini è visibile una massa palpabile, costituita dal callo osseo; questo si rimodella in modo soddisfacente in 6-12 mesi. Si ottiene sempre un ripristino completo della mobilità della spalla e della funzionalità della spalla.

682.4 • FRATTURE DELLE ESTREMITÀ INFERIORI

FRATTURA DELL'ANCA

Le fratture dell'anca nei bambini, che rappresentano meno dell'1% di tutte le fratture di interesse pediatrico, derivano da traumi ad alta energia e sono spesso associate a traumi cranici, toracici o addominali. Il loro trattamento dà luogo a un tasso di complicanze che può raggiungere il 60%, a una necrosi avascolare globale nel 50% dei casi e a una percentuale di malunioni intorno al 30%. La vascolarizzazione esclusiva delle testa femorale è all'origine dell'elevato tasso di necrosi avascolare. Le fratture sono classificabili come separazioni transepifisarie, fratture transcervicali, fratture cervicotrocanteriche e fratture intertocanteriche. I principi del trattamento comprendono la riduzione anatomica in urgenza (aperta o chiusa), una fissazione interna stabile (evitando se possibile la cartilagine di coniugazione) e un gesso a spica.

FRATTURE DEL BAMBINO DI 1-4 ANNI

Le fratture del bambino ai primi passi (*toddler fracture*) si verificano in tenera età, in pazienti deambulanti. Il range di età per questa frattura è tipicamente intorno a 1-4 anni. Il trauma tende a verificarsi dopo cadute o movimenti in torsione apparentemente non pericolosi, spesso senza testimoni. I bambini in questo gruppo di età sono di solito incapaci di descrivere in modo chiaro il meccanismo traumatico o di indicare con precisione l'area anatomica del trauma. Le radiografie possono non evidenziare una frattura; la diagnosi si basa sull'esame obiettivo. Il sintomo classico è il rifiuto del carico, che può manifestarsi con il rifiuto di poggiare a terra l'estremità affetta o con vivaci proteste. Le proiezioni anteroposteriore e laterale di tibia e perone possono evidenziare una frattura spirale senza spostamento della metafisi tibiale distale. Spesso è utile una proiezione obliqua, in quanto la linea di frattura può essere visibile soltanto in una delle tre proiezioni. Una scintigrafia ossea trifasica con tecnezio può essere utile per escludere infezioni come un'artrite settica e un'osteomielite. La frattura è trattata con un gesso al di sopra del ginocchio per circa 3 settimane.

FRATTURE DELLA DIAFISI TIBIALE E PERONEALE

La tibia è l'osso dell'arto inferiore che più comunemente va incontro a frattura nei bambini. Questa frattura in genere deriva da un trauma diretto. La maggior parte delle fratture tibiali è associata a una frattura di perone e l'età media alla presentazione è di 8 anni. Il bambino presenta dolore, edema e deformità dell'arto interessato e non riesce a caricare. L'esame neurovascolare distale è importante nell'ambito della valutazione generale. Le radiografie nelle proiezioni anteroposteriore e laterale devono comprendere ginocchio e caviglia. La riduzione chiusa e l'immobilizzazione sono metodi di trattamento standard. La maggior parte delle fratture va incontro a guarigione completa e i bambini di solito presentano ottimi risultati. Le fratture aperte devono essere più volte sottoposte a irrigazione e a sbrigliamento. Il modo migliore di trattare le fratture con trauma dei tessuti molli particolarmente severo è la fissazione esterna. La guarigione richiede più tempo nelle fratture aperte che in quelle chiuse.

FRATTURE DELLA DIAFISI FEMORALE

Le fratture del femore sono comuni nei bambini. Tutti i gruppi di età, dalla prima infanzia all'adolescenza, possono essere interessati. Il meccanismo traumatico varia da traumi di tipo rotatorio a bassa energia a traumi ad alta velocità in incidenti con veicoli a motore. Le fratture di femore nei bambini di età <2 anni devono suscitare il sospetto di violenza. È necessario un esame obiettivo completo per escludere altri traumi e valutare le condizioni neurovascolari. In caso di trauma a elevata energia, la presenza di qualsiasi segno di instabilità emodinamica deve indurre l'esaminatore a ricercare altre fonti di emorragia. Le radiografie del femore nelle proiezioni anteroposteriore e laterale dimostrano la frattura. Si esegue una radiografia anteroposteriore del bacino per escludere qualsiasi frattura associata a questo livello. Il trattamento delle fratture diafisarie varia in base al gruppo d'età, come descritto nella Tabella 682-2.

TABELLA 682-2. Opzioni di trattamento nelle varie età (frattura di diafisi femorale)

OPZIONI DI TRATTAMENTO	0-2 anni	3-5 anni	6-10 anni	>11 anni
Gesso a spica	X	X		
Trazione e gesso a spica		X	X	X
Chiodo intramidollare		X	X	X
Fissatore esterno		X*	X*	X*
Vite o placca		X	X	X

*Frattura aperta.

Modificata da Wells L: Trauma related to the lower extremity. In Dormans JP (ed): *Pediatric Orthopaedics: Core Knowledge in Orthopaedics*. Philadelphia, Mosby, 2005, p. 93.

FRATTURE TRIPLANARI E DI TILLAUX

Questi pattern di frattura, che si presentano alla fine del periodo di crescita, sono imputabili alla forza relativa della giunzione tra osso e cartilagine di accrescimento e alla chiusura asimmetrica della cartilagine di accrescimento tibiale. Le fratture vengono dette triplanari in quanto hanno componenti coronali, sagittali e trasversali (Fig. 682-7). La frattura di Tillaux è una frattura da avulsione dell'aspetto anterolaterale dell'epifisi tibiale distale. Radiografie e imaging con TC e ricostruzioni tridimensionali sono necessarie per analizzare la geometria della frattura. La frattura triplanare interessa la superficie articolare e quindi richiede la riduzione anatomica, ulteriormente stabilizzata con la fissazione interna. Il trattamento della frattura di Tillaux consiste nella riduzione chiusa. La riduzione aperta è raccomandata se residua un dislivello intrarticolare.

FRATTURE METATARSALI

Le fratture metatarsali, comuni nei bambini, di solito derivano da un trauma diretto al dorso del piede. I traumi ad alta energia o le fratture multiple della base del metatarso sono associate a edema significativo. Occorre mantenere un elevato indice di sospetto per la sindrome compartimentale del piede e, se indicato, misurare le pressioni compartimentali. La diagnosi si pone in base alle radiografie del piede nelle proiezioni anteroposteriore, laterale e obliqua. La maggior parte delle fratture metatarsali può essere trattata in modo chiuso con gesso sotto al ginocchio. Il carico è consentito secondo tolleranza. Le fratture con spostamento possono richiedere una riduzione chiusa o aperta con fissazione interna. I fili di Kirschner lisci per via percutanea di solito assicurano una fissazione interna sufficiente per queste fratture. In caso di aumento della pressione compartimentale, è necessario il rilascio chirurgico di tutti i compartimenti del piede.

FRATTURE DELLE FALANGI DELLE DITA DEL PIEDE

Le fratture che interessano dal 2° al 5° dito del piede sono comuni e di solito secondarie a traumi diretti. Si verificano comunemente quando il bambino è a piedi nudi. Le dita appaiono edematose, ecchimotiche e dolenti; si può notare una lieve deformità. La diagnosi è radiografica. L'emorragia suggerisce la possibilità di una frattura aperta. Le dita del piede dal 2° al 5° di solito non richiedono una riduzione chiusa, a meno che non vi sia uno spostamento significativo. Al bisogno, la riduzione può di solito essere ottenuta con trazione longitudinale del dito. Di solito non è necessario il gesso. La fasciatura del dito fratturato con un dito adiacente stabile (*"buddy" taping*) di solito permette un allineamento soddisfacente ed elimina i sintomi. Può essere utile che il paziente usi grucce e cammini sul tallone per diversi giorni, fino alla scomparsa dell'edema dei tessuti molli e del dolore.

682.5 • TRATTAMENTO OPERATORIO

Il 4-5% delle fratture pediatriche richiede l'intervento chirurgico. Le comuni indicazioni al trattamento operatorio nei bambini e negli adolescenti comprendono: (1) fratture della cartilagine di coniugazione con spostamento, (2) fratture intra-articolari con spostamento, (3) fratture instabili, (4) bambino con traumi multipli, (5) fratture aperte, (6) impossibilità di ottenere una riduzione adeguata in bambini più grandi, (7) impossibilità di mantenere una riduzione adeguata e (8) alcune fratture patologiche.

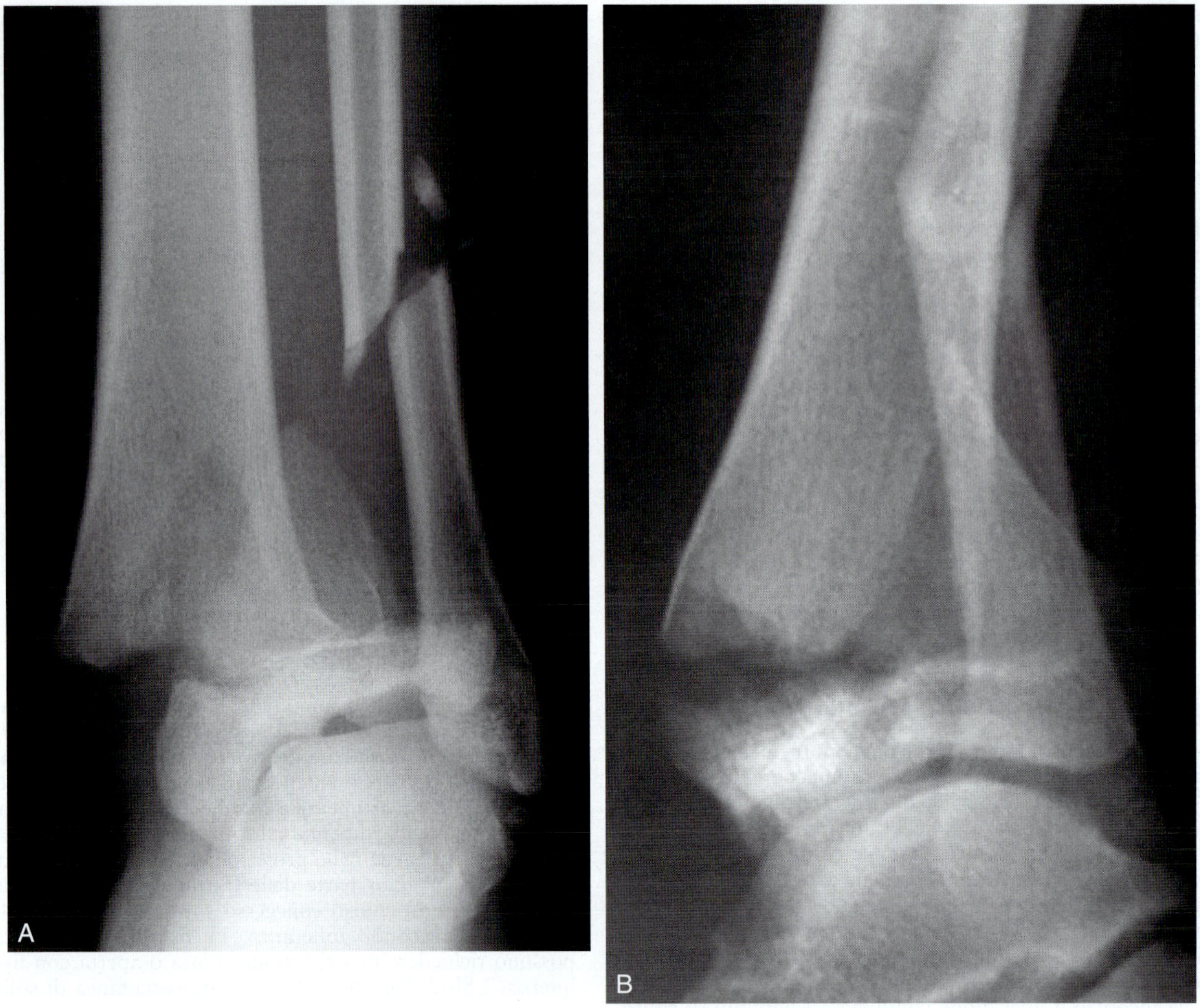

Figura 682-7. La frattura triplanare è una frattura transizionale: radiografie in proiezione anteroposteriore (*A*) e laterale (*B*). (Da Dormans JP: *Pediatric Orthopedics: Introduction to Trauma*. Philadelphia, Mosby, 2005, p. 38.)

Lo scopo dell'intervento è di ottenere un allineamento anatomico e una stabilità relativa. La fissazione rigida non è necessaria quanto una mobilizzazione precoce negli adulti. Inoltre, il costrutto relativamente stabile può essere supplementato con un'immobilizzazione esterna. Le fratture di SH di tipo III e IV richiedono un allineamento anatomico e, se instabili, la fissazione interna (con fili di Kirschner lisci, preferibilmente evitando di attraversare la cartilagine di coniugazione). Le riduzioni chiuse multiple di una frattura epifisaria sono controindicate in quanto possono causare un danno permanente alle cellule germinali della cartilagine di coniugazione.

TABELLA 682-3. Indicazioni comuni alla fissazione esterna nelle fratture pediatriche

1. Fratture aperte di grado II e III
2. Fratture associate a ustioni severe
3. Fratture con perdita di tessuti molli che richiede innesti cutanei o lembi liberi
4. Fratture con necessità di distrazione come quelle con significativa perdita di tessuto osseo
5. Fratture instabili del bacino
6. Fratture pediatriche in associazione con traumi cranici e spasticità
7. Fratture associate a riparazione o ricostruzione vascolare o nervosa

TECNICHE CHIRURGICHE

È importante prestare molta attenzione ai tessuti molli e alla cute. Le altre indicazioni alla riduzione aperta e alla fissazione interna sono le fratture instabili della colonna, le fratture ipsilaterali del femore, i traumi neurovascolari che richiedono una riparazione e, talvolta, le fratture aperte di femore e tibia. La riduzione chiusa e la fissazione minimamente invasiva sono usate specificamente per le fratture sovracondiloidee dell'omero distale, per le fratture delle falangi e per le fratture del collo femorale. Il mancato allineamento anatomico con metodi chiusi rappresenta un'indicazione alla riduzione aperta.

Le principali indicazioni alla fissazione esterna sono elencate nella Tabella 682-3. I vantaggi di questa tecnica comprendono l'immobilizzazione rigida delle fratture, l'accesso alle ferite aperte per un trattamento continuo e una più facile mobilizzazione del paziente per il trattamento di altri traumi e per il trasporto, in vista di procedure diagnostiche e terapeutiche. La maggior parte delle complicanze conseguenti alla fissazione esterna è costituita da infezioni del tratto di inserimento dei chiodi, da un'osteomielite cronica e dalla recidiva della frattura dopo rimozione dei chiodi.

682.6 • COMPLICANZE DELLE FRATTURE NEI BAMBINI

Le complicanze specifiche dei bambini sono l'allineamento scorretto e la correzione con la crescita naturale, l'arresto della crescita della cartilagine di accrescimento, la crescita eccessiva e la recidiva della frattura causata dalla rapida guarigione della frattura. Un allineamento scorretto e l'angolazione tardiva sono problemi comuni nelle fratture della metafisi tibiale prossimale. L'arresto della crescita della cartilagine di accrescimento può causare deformità angolare o accorciamento. Le deformità angolari vengono corrette mediante emiepifisiodesi o osteotomia. Per trattare l'accorciamento si ricorre all'epifisiodesi della gamba controlaterale, se la maturità scheletrica è vicina, oppure all'allungamento dell'arto più corto. Le recidive della frattura causano una maggiore deformità e possono richiedere una riduzione aperta. Altre complicanze sono distrofia simpatica riflessa, instabilità legamentosa, malunione, mancata unione, embolia adiposa e lesioni neurovascolari.

682.7 • VALUTAZIONE DELL'ESITO

Una valutazione empirica e soggettiva porta a conclusioni erronee e rende difficoltoso raffrontare gli esiti ottenuti con quelli di altri studi. Le tre scale usate per valutare differenti modalità di trattamento dei traumi muscoloscheletrici sono l'Activities Scale for Kids, la Pediatric Functional Health Outcomes Instrument e la Pediatric Outcome Data Collection Instruments.

L'American Academy of Orthopaedic Surgeons ha sviluppato il Pediatric Functional Health Outcomes Instrument come esempio della misurazione dello stato di salute.

Bandyopandhyay S, Yen K: Non-accidental fractures in child maltreatment syndrome. *Clin Pediatr Emerg Med* 2002;3:145–152.

Beaty JH, Kasser JR (editors): *Rockwood and Wilkins' Fractures in Children*, 5th ed. Philadelphia, JB Lippincott, 2001.

Bohm ER, Bubbar V, Hing KY, et al: Above- and below-the-elbow plaster casts for distal forearm fractures in children. *J Bone Joint Surg* 2006;88-A:1–8.

Cummings RJ: Paediatric femoral fracture. *Lancet* 2005;365:1116–1117.

Davidson JS, Brown DJ, Barnes SN, et al: Simple treatment for torus fractures of the distal radius. *J Bone Joint Surg Br* 2001;83:1173–1175.

Della-Giustina K, Della-Giustina DA: Emergency department evaluation and treatment of pediatric orthopedic injuries. *Emerg Med Clin North Am* 1999;17:895–922.

Flynn JM, Kolze EA: Upper extremity injuries. In Dormans JP (editor): *Pediatric Orthopaedics: Core Knowledge in Orthopaedics*. Philadelphia, Mosby, 2005, pp 47–84.

Flynn JM, Nagda S: Upper extremity injuries. In Dormans JP (editor): *The Requisites in Pediatrics: Pediatric Orthopaedics and Sports Medicine*. Philadelphia, Mosby, 2005, pp 21–48.

Green NE, Swiontkowski MF (editors): *Skeletal Trauma in Children*, 3rd ed., vol. 3. Philadelphia, WB Saunders, 2001.

Horn DB, Wells L, Tamai J: Lower extremity fractures. In Dormans JP (editor): *The Requisites in Pediatrics: Pediatric Orthopaedics and Sports Medicine*. Philadelphia, Mosby, 2005, pp 49–92.

Kocher MS, Waters PM, Micheli LJ: Upper extremity injuries in the pediatric athlete. *Sports Med* 2000;30:117–135.

Overly F, Steele DW: Common pediatric fractures and dislocations. *Clin Pediatr Emerg Med* 2002;3:106–117.

Plint AC, Perry JJ, Correll R, et al: A randomized, controlled trial of removable splinting versus casting for wrist buckle fractures in children. *Pediatrics* 2006;117:691–697.

Salter RB, Harris WR: Injuries involving the epiphyseal plate. *J Bone Joint Surg Am* 1963;45:587–622.

Skaggs DL, Mirzayan R: The posterior fat pad sign in association with occult fracture of the elbow in children. *J Bone Joint Surg Am* 1999;81:1429–1433.

Thompson GH, Haber LL: Upper extremity fractures in the pediatric patients. In Fitzgerald RH Jr, Kaufer H, Malkani A (editors): *Orthopaedics*. St. Louis, Mosby, 2002, pp 484–494.

Wells L, Millman JE: Trauma related to the lower extremity. In Dormans JP (editor): *Pediatric Orthopaedics: Core Knowledge in Orthopaedics*. Philadelphia, Mosby, 2005, pp 85–115.

Wright JG, Wang EEL, Owen JL, et al: Treatments for paediatric femoral fractures: A randomized trial. *Lancet* 2005;365:1153–1162.

Capitolo 683 ■ Osteomielite

Richard Lampe

Le infezioni ossee nei bambini sono importanti in quanto possono causare disabilità permanente. La frequenza delle infezioni scheletriche è maggiore nei lattanti e nei bambini di 1-4 anni rispetto ai pazienti pediatrici più grandi. Nei più giovani, la diagnosi di osteomielite, fatta prima che si sviluppi un'infezione estesa, e l'immediata istituzione di un appropriato trattamento medico e chirurgico riducono al minimo i danni permanenti. Il rischio è maggiore se la cartilagine di accrescimento è danneggiata.

EZIOLOGIA. I batteri sono i patogeni più comuni nell'ambito delle infezioni scheletriche acute. Nell'osteomielite, lo *Staphylococcus aureus* è il più comune microrganismo infettante per tutti i gruppi di età, compresi i neonati. Anche lo streptococco di gruppo B e i bacilli enterici Gram-negativi (*Escherichia coli*) sono patogeni importanti nei neonati; lo streptococco di gruppo A è responsabile di meno del 10% di tutti i casi. Dopo i 6 anni di età, la maggior parte dei casi di osteomielite è causata da *S. aureus*, *Streptococcus* o *Pseudomonas aeruginosa*. I casi di infezione da *Pseudomonas* sono correlati quasi esclusivamente a ferite penetranti del piede, con inoculo diretto di *P. aeruginosa* dall'imbottitura schiumosa della scarpa nell'osso o nella cartilagine, che evolve in un'osteocondrite. *Salmonella* spp. e *S. aureus* sono i due più comuni patogeni responsabili di osteomielite nei bambini. La *Kingella kingae* può essere sporadica o manifestarsi in cluster causando osteomielite o artrite settica.

L'infezione da micobatteri atipici, *S. aureus* o *Pseudomonas*, può verificarsi in seguito a traumi penetranti. Le infezioni da miceti si verificano di solito nell'ambito di una malattia disseminata multisistemica; l'osteomielite da *Candida* talvolta complica una fungemia nei neonati con o senza cateteri vascolari a permanenza. Un'infezione virale primitiva delle ossa è estremamente rara.

L'eziologia microbica risulta confermata nel 75% circa dei casi di osteomielite. Una pregressa terapia antibiotica e l'effetto inibitorio del pus sulla crescita batterica possono spiegare la frequente negatività delle colture.

EPIDEMIOLOGIA. L'osteomielite è comune nei bambini più piccoli; il 30% circa dei casi si verifica prima dei 2 anni di età e il 50% prima dei 5 anni. Le infezioni ossee sono più comuni nei maschi che nelle femmine, di solito con un rapporto di 2:1. Il comportamento dei ragazzi può predisporre a eventi traumatici. Tranne che per l'aumentata incidenza dell'infezione scheletrica nei pazienti con malattia a cellule falciformi, non esiste una predisposizione all'osteomielite basata sulla razza.

La maggior parte delle infezioni in bambini precedentemente sani è di origine ematogena. Un trauma minore chiuso, un comune evento che precede l'osteomielite, si verifica in circa il 30% dei pazienti. L'infezione ossea può far seguito a traumi penetranti o a fratture aperte. L'infezione ossea successiva a chirurgia ortopedica è infrequente. Anche una riduzione delle difese dell'ospite aumenta il rischio di infezione scheletrica. Altri fattori di rischio sono elencati nella Tabella 683-1.

PATOGENESI. La peculiare anatomia e circolazione sanguigna delle estremità delle ossa lunghe spiegano la predilezione per la localizzazione dei batteri che si diffondono per via ematogena. Nella metafisi le arterie nutritive si ramificano in capillari non anastomizzati al di sotto della cartilagine di accrescimento formando un ansa molto stretta prima di entrare nei sinusoidi venosi che drenano nel midollo osseo. Il flusso sanguigno in quest'area è lento e crea l'ambiente ideale per la disseminazione batterica. Una volta stabilitosi un focolaio batterico, i fagociti migrano nel sito e producono un essudato infiammatorio (ascesso metafisario). La produzione di enzimi proteolitici, radicali tossici dell'ossigeno e

TABELLA 683-1. Microrganismi isolati nei pazienti con osteomielite e relative associazioni cliniche

ASSOCIAZIONE CLINICA PIÙ COMUNE	MICRORGANISMO
Microrganismo più comune in qualsiasi tipo di osteomielite	*Staphylococcus aureus* (suscettibile o resistente alla meticillina)
Infezione associata a corpo estraneo	Stafilococchi coagulasi-negativi o *Propionibacterium* spp.
Comune nelle infezioni nosocomiali	*Enterobacteriaceae*, *Pseudomonas aeruginosa*, *Candida* spp.
Associata a morsi, lesioni diabetiche del piede e piaghe da decubito	Streptococchi e/o batteri anaerobi
Malattia a cellule falciformi	*Salmonella* spp., *S. aureus* o *Streptococcus pneumoniae*
Infezione da HIV	*Bartonella henselae* o *Bartonella quintana*
Morsi umani o animali	*Pasteurella multocida* o *Eikenella corrodens*
Pazienti immunocompetenti	*Aspergillus* spp., *Candida albicans* o *Mycobacteria* spp.
Popolazioni in cui è prevalente la tubercolosi	*Mycobacterium tuberculosis*
Popolazioni in cui sono endemici questi patogeni	*Brucella* spp., *Coxiella burnetii*, miceti che si trovano in specifiche aree geografiche (coccidioidomicosi, blastomicosi, istoplasmosi)

Da Lew DP, Waldvogel FA: Osteomyelitis. *Lancet* 2004; 364:369-379.

TABELLA 683-2. Distribuzione delle ossa interessate nell'osteomielite ematogena acuta

OSSO	N.	%
Tibia	107	24,3
Femore	105	23,8
Omero	58	13,2
Perone	26	5,9
Radio	17	3,9
Ulna	10	2,3
Vertebre	9	2,0
Ossa del piede	33	7,5
Ossa pelviche	30	6,8
Ossa della mano	27	6,1
Ossa del torace	13	2,9
Ossa craniche	6	1,4

Basata su una casistica non pubblicata di 372 pazienti con 441 infezioni ossee.

citochine causa una riduzione della tensione di ossigeno e del pH, osteolisi e distruzione dei tessuti. Con la progressione dell'essudato infiammatorio, la pressione aumenta la diffusione nello spazio sottoperiosteo attraverso lo spazio metafisario poroso, mediante i canali di Havers e di Volkmann. L'essudato purulento presente sotto il periostio può sollevare la membrana periostea della superficie ossea, riducendo ulteriormente l'apporto ematico alla corticale e alla metafisi.

Nei neonati e nei lattanti, i vasi sanguigni transepifisari connettono la metafisi e l'epifisi, per cui è comune che il materiale purulento entri nello spazio articolare dalla metafisi. Questa estensione attraverso la cartilagine di accrescimento può determinare una crescita anormale e una deformità ossea o articolare. Al termine del primo anno di vita si forma la cartilagine di accrescimento, che oblitera i vasi transepifisari. Una volta formatasi la cartilagine di accrescimento, si può avere un interessamento articolare nelle articolazioni in cui la metafisi è intrarticolare (anca, caviglia, spalla e gomito) e il pus penetra nello spazio articolare.

Nella tarda infanzia il periostio diviene più aderente: questo fenomeno favorisce il deflusso del pus lungo il periostio. Con la chiusura della cartilagine di accrescimento, che avviene nella tarda adolescenza, l'osteomielite ematogena inizia per lo più nella diafisi, da cui può diffondersi all'intero canale intramidollare.

MANIFESTAZIONI CLINICHE. I segni e sintomi di osteomielite sono altamente dipendenti dall'età del paziente e all'inizio sono spesso subdoli.

I neonati possono presentare pseudoparalisi o dolore con il movimento dell'estremità affetta. Metà dei neonati non presenta febbre e non dare segno di sofferenza. I lattanti e i bambini più grandi hanno una maggiore probabilità di sviluppare febbre, dolore e segni localizzati come edema, eritema e calore locale. Con l'interessamento delle estremità inferiori, si osserva zoppia o rifiuto del cammino in circa metà dei pazienti.

Il dolore locale a livello di un osso lungo può essere un segno importante. Edema ed eritema locale con un'osteomielite possono significare una diffusione al di fuori della metafisi nello spazio sottoperiosteo, con una risposta infiammatoria secondaria dei tessuti molli.

Nell'osteomielite sono interessate principalmente le ossa lunghe (Tab. 683-2); femore e tibia, ugualmente affetti, insieme costituiscono quasi la metà dei casi. Le ossa delle estremità superiori comprendono un quarto di tutti i casi. Le ossa piatte sono interessate con minore frequenza.

Di solito vi è un solo sito di interessamento osseo o articolare. L'infezione colpisce diverse ossa in meno del 10% dei casi; l'eccezione è rappresentata dall'osteomielite dei neonati, in cui due o più ossa sono interessate in quasi la metà dei casi. I bambini con sintomi subacuti e segni focali nell'area metafisaria (di solito la tibia) possono avere un **ascesso di Brodie**, che alla radiografia risulta radiotrasparente e circondato da osso reattivo.

I pazienti con osteomielite e coltura negativa possono avere un quadro clinico più benigno ma rispondono bene alla terapia empirica antistafilococcica.

DIAGNOSI. In tutti i casi di sospetta osteomielite occorre eseguire un'emocoltura. L'aspirazione per la colorazione di Gram e per la coltura quando l'anamnesi e i segni e sintomi clinici sono fortemente indicativi di osteomielite restano le tecniche diagnostiche definitive e forniscono campioni ottimali per la coltura di conferma della diagnosi. Nella sospetta osteomielite, è necessario utilizzare un ago in acciaio che penetri la corticale fino alla metafisi. Se nello spazio sottoperiosteo si incontra del pus, non occorre proseguire oltre. L'inoculo diretto di campioni clinici in contenitori per emocoltura aerobica può migliorare l'isolamento della *Kingella kingae*, soprattutto se mantenuto per una settimana. Con l'aspirazione di pus dall'osso si ottiene il migliore campione per la coltura batteriologica dell'infezione. Per identificare la *K. kingae* può essere necessario ricorrere alla reazione a catena della polimerasi (PCR, *Polymerase Chain Reaction*).

Non esistono esami di laboratorio specifici per l'osteomielite. Test come la conta leucocitaria e la formula leucocitaria, la VES e la proteina C-reattiva sono molto sensibili per le infezioni ossee, ma sono aspecifici e quindi non hanno alcuna utilità per distinguere un'infezione scheletrica da altri processi infiammatori. La conta leucocitaria e la VES possono essere nella norma nei primi giorni dell'infezione e quindi risultati normali non escludono la diagnosi di infezione scheletrica. Valori elevati della VES e della proteina C-reattiva possono essere utili per valutare la risposta alla terapia o identificare le complicanze.

Valutazione radiografica. Gli studi radiografici hanno un ruolo cruciale nella valutazione dell'osteomielite. Radiografie convenzionali, ecografia, TC, RM e scintigrafia possono tutte contribuire alla diagnosi. Le radiografie sono spesso utilizzate per la valutazione iniziale per escludere altre cause come un trauma e corpi estranei. La RM, rivelatasi un esame molto sensibile e specifico, è ampiamente utilizzata per la diagnosi. La sequenza degli studi scintigrafici o RM è determinata da età, sede e presentazione clinica.

STUDI RADIOGRAFICI. Entro 72 ore dall'esordio dei sintomi di osteomielite, le radiografie della sede interessata (utilizzando la tecnica per i tessuti molli), confrontate, se necessario, con quelle dell'estremità opposta, possono evidenziare uno spostamento dei piani muscolari profondi dalla metafisi adiacente, causato dall'edema dei tessuti profondi. Alterazioni ossee di tipo litico non sono visibili radiograficamente finché non è andato distrutto il 30-50% della matrice ossea. Le ossa tubulari lunghe non evidenziano alterazioni di tipo litico per 7-14 giorni dopo l'esordio dell'infezione. Le ossa piatte e irregolari possono richiedere ancora più tempo.

TC e RM. La TC, oltre a dimostrare anomalie delle ossa e dei tessuti molli, è ideale per visualizzare gas presenti nei tessuti molli. La

RM è la migliore tecnica radiografica di imaging per l'identificazione di ascessi e per la distinzione tra infezioni delle ossa e quelle dei tessuti molli. La RM è molto precisa nel visualizzare i dettagli anatomici della raccolta purulenta sottoperiostea e dell'accumulo di materiale purulento nel midollo osseo e nelle metafisi, in vista di un possibile intervento chirurgico. Nell'osteomielite acuta, il materiale purulento e l'edema appaiono scuri con ridotta intensità del segnale nelle immagini pesate in T1, mentre il tessuto adiposo appare brillante (Fig. 683-1); l'opposto si osserva con le immagini pesate in T2. Il segnale del tessuto adiposo può essere diminuito con tecniche di soppressione per il tessuto adiposo per migliorare la visualizzazione. Anche la somministrazione di gadolinio può potenziare la RM. Cellulite e tragitti fistolosi appaiono come aree di elevata intensità del segnale nelle immagini pesate in T2.

La RM sembra avere un valore predittivo positivo simile a quello della scintigrafia nell'osteomielite acuta. È particolarmente utile nella valutazione dell'osteomielite vertebrale e nella discite in quanto permette una netta demarcazione tra corpo vertebrale e disco cartilagineo.

Studi scintigrafici. La scintigrafia può essere utile nelle sospette infezioni ossee, specialmente se si ipotizzano focolai multipli. Il mezzo di contrasto utilizzato (scintigrafia ossea trifasica) è il Tecnezio-99 metilene difosfonato (^{99m}Tc). L'osteomielite causa aumento della vascolarizzazione, infiammazione e aumento dell'attività osteoblastica, facendo aumentare la concentrazione di ^{99m}Tc. Qualsiasi area caratterizzata dall'aumento del flusso sanguigno o dell'infiammazione può intensificare la captazione di ^{99m}Tc nella 1ª e nella 2ª fase, ma nell'osteomielite questo fenomeno avviene nella 3ª fase (4-6 ore). La scintigrafia trifasica con ^{99m}Tc ha un'eccellente sensibilità (84-100%) e specificità (70-96%) nell'osteomielite ematogena e può identificare un'osteomielite entro 24-48 ore dall'esordio dei sintomi. La sensibilità nei neonati è molto più bassa a causa della scarsa mineralizzazione ossea. I vantaggi comprendono l'infrequente necessità di sedazione, costi inferiori, la possibilità di studiare tutto lo scheletro per la ricerca di focolai multipli e di eseguire numerose scansioni dopo una sola iniezione.

Diagnosi differenziale. La diagnosi differenziale dell'osteomielite comprende i traumi, sia accidentali sia non accidentali. I bambini con leucemia presentano comunemente dolore osseo o articolare come sintomo iniziale. Il neuroblastoma con interessamento osseo può essere scambiato per un'osteomielite. Occorre considerare i tumori ossei primitivi, in cui tuttavia febbre e altri segni di malattia sono generalmente assenti, eccetto che nel sarcoma di Ewing. Osteomielite cronica ricorrente (CRMO, *Chronic Recurrent Multifocal Osteomyelitis*) e sinovite, acne, pustolosi, iperostosi e osteite sono condizioni non infettive rare nei bambini, caratterizzate da infiammazione osteoarticolare ricorrente e differenti condizioni cutanee, pustolosi palmoplantare, psoriasi, acne severa, dermatosi neutrofila (sindrome di Sweet) e pyoderma gangrenosum. La CRMO, che colpisce le bambine (4:1) con un picco a 10 anni di età, può essere associata ad artrite, sacroiliite, malattia infiammatoria intestinale e granulomatosi di Wegener. Alcune lesioni sono asintomatiche, ma la maggior parte è dolorosa. I fattori che permettono di porre diagnosi sono la presenza di più di 2 lesioni con osteolisi e circondate da sclerosi, una durata >6 mesi e un'istologia caratteristica (peraltro non sempre necessaria).

TRATTAMENTO. Il trattamento ottimale delle infezioni scheletriche richiede lo sforzo collaborativo di pediatri, chirurghi ortopedici e radiologi.

Terapia antibiotica. La terapia antibiotica empirica iniziale si basa sulla conoscenza dei probabili patogeni batterici nelle varie

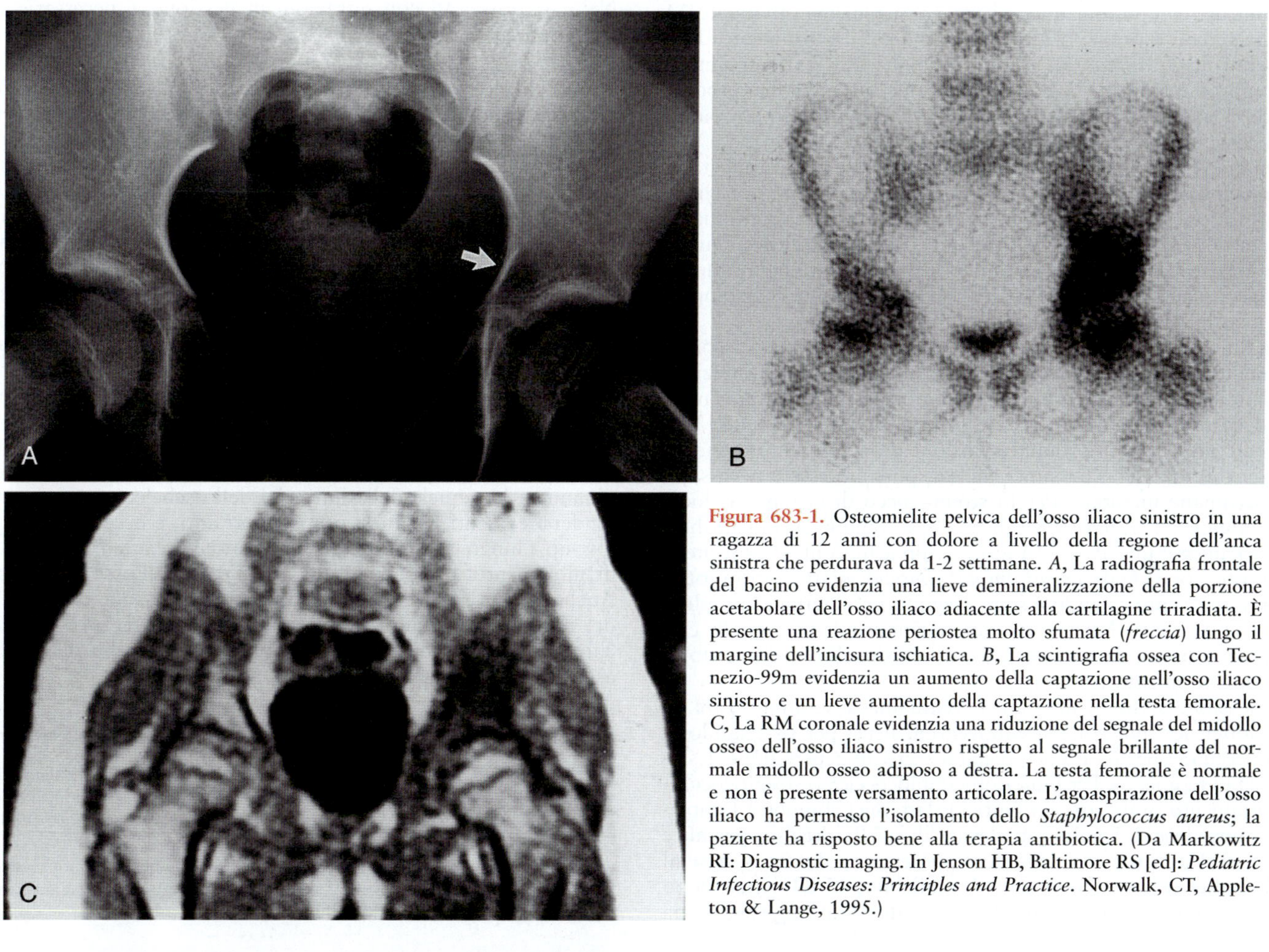

Figura 683-1. Osteomielite pelvica dell'osso iliaco sinistro in una ragazza di 12 anni con dolore a livello della regione dell'anca sinistra che perdurava da 1-2 settimane. *A*, La radiografia frontale del bacino evidenzia una lieve demineralizzazione della porzione acetabolare dell'osso iliaco adiacente alla cartilagine triradiata. È presente una reazione periostea molto sfumata (*freccia*) lungo il margine dell'incisura ischiatica. *B*, La scintigrafia ossea con Tecnezio-99m evidenzia un aumento della captazione nell'osso iliaco sinistro e un lieve aumento della captazione nella testa femorale. *C*, La RM coronale evidenzia una riduzione del segnale del midollo osseo dell'osso iliaco sinistro rispetto al segnale brillante del normale midollo osseo adiposo a destra. La testa femorale è normale e non è presente versamento articolare. L'agoaspirazione dell'osso iliaco ha permesso l'isolamento dello *Staphylococcus aureus*; la paziente ha risposto bene alla terapia antibiotica. (Da Markowitz RI: Diagnostic imaging. In Jenson HB, Baltimore RS [ed]: *Pediatric Infectious Diseases: Principles and Practice*. Norwalk, CT, Appleton & Lange, 1995.)

età, sui risultati della colorazione di Gram del materiale aspirato e su altre considerazioni. Nei neonati, una penicillina attiva contro lo stafilococco, come la nafcillina o l'oxacillina (150-200 mg/kg/24 ore suddivisi ogni 6 ore, ev) e una cefalosporina ad ampio spettro, come la cefotaxima (150-200 mg/kg/24 ore suddivisi ogni 8 ore, ev), forniscono una copertura per *S. aureus*, streptococco di gruppo B e bacilli Gram-negativi. Se si sospetta lo *Staphylococcus* meticillinoresistente, si sostituisce la nafcillina con la vancomicina. Al posto della cefalosporina si può utilizzare un aminoglicoside, ma gli antibiotici aminoglicosidici hanno una ridotta attività antibatterica nei siti con ridotta tensione d'ossigeno e basso pH, condizioni presenti nelle infezioni tissutali. Se il neonato è un piccolo prematuro o ha un catetere venoso centrale, deve essere presa in considerazione la possibilità di infezione batterica nosocomiale (*Pseudomonas* o stafilococchi coagulasi-negativi) o di infezione micotica nosocomiale (*Candida*). Nei lattanti e nei bambini più grandi i principali patogeni sono lo *S. aureus* e lo streptococco. La cefazolina (100-150 mg/kg/24 ore suddivisi ogni 8 ore, ev) o la nafcillina (150-200 mg/kg/24 ore suddivisi ogni 6 ore) forniscono una copertura contro questi patogeni. Se si sospetta lo *Staphylococcus* meticillinoresistente, si sostituisce la nafcillina con la vancomicina. È inoltre possibile somministrare cefotaxima (200 mg/kg/24 ore suddivisi ogni 8 ore, ev) e ceftriaxone ai pazienti non vaccinati contro l'*Haemophilus influenzae* di tipo b.

Situazioni particolari rendono necessario discostarsi dalle consuete scelte di antibiotici empirici. Nei pazienti affetti da malattia a cellule falciformi con osteomielite sono comuni patogeni i batteri enterici Gram-negativi (*Salmonella*) come pure *S. aureus*; si utilizza quindi una cefalosporina ad ampio spettro come la cefotaxima (200 mg/kg/24 ore suddivisi ogni 8 ore), oltre a un antibiotico attivo contro lo stafilococco. La clindamicina (40 mg/kg/24 ore suddivisi ogni 6 ore, ev) è un'utile alternativa nei pazienti allergici ai β-lattamici. Oltre a una buona attività antistafilococcica, la clindamicina ha un'ampia attività contro gli anaerobi ed è utile per il trattamento delle infezioni secondarie a traumi penetranti o a fratture composte. Clindamicina e vancomicina (40 mg/kg/24 suddivisi ogni 6 ore, ev) sono alternative per il trattamento delle infezioni da *S. aureus* meticillinoresistente. Nei pazienti immunocompromessi si inizia di solito una terapia combinata, come vancomicina e ceftazidima, o piperacillina/clavulanato e un aminoglicoside. *K. kingae* di solito risponde alla cefotaxima.

Quando si identifica il patogeno, se necessario si apportano le appropriate correzioni della terapia. Se il patogeno non viene identificato e condizioni del paziente migliorano, si continua la terapia con l'antibiotico scelto in precedenza. Se viene identificato un patogeno e le condizioni del paziente non migliorano, si devono prendere in considerazione la riaspirazione o la biopsia e la possibilità di una patologia non infettiva.

La durata della terapia antibiotica è individualizzata a seconda del microrganismo isolato e del decorso clinico. Per le infezioni causate da *S. aureus* o da bacilli Gram-negativi, la durata minima della terapia antibiotica è 28 giorni, a condizione che (1) il paziente presenti una pronta risoluzione di segni e sintomi (entro 5-7 giorni) e (2) la VES si normalizzi; possono essere necessarie 4-6 settimane in totale. Per lo streptococco di gruppo A, lo *S. pneumoniae* o l'*H. influenzae* di tipo b, si somministrano antibiotici per un minimo di 10-14 giorni, applicando gli stessi criteri. Per l'osteocondrite da *Pseudomonas* sono adeguati 7 giorni totali dopo l'intervento quando è stato eseguito un curettage completo dei tessuti infetti. I pazienti immunocompromessi e quelli con infezione causata da micobatteri o miceti di solito necessitano di cicli di trattamento prolungati.

È possibile prendere in esame l'eventualità di somministrare gli antibiotici non più per via endovenosa, bensì per os quando le condizioni del paziente si sono stabilizzate, in genere dopo 1 settimana di terapia ev. Per l'infezione stafilococcica o streptococcica il trattamento orale con antibiotici β-lattamici comporta l'impiego di una dose 2-3 volte più elevata di quella prevista per altre infezioni. L'adeguatezza della dose può essere valutata in base al **titolo battericida sierico** o **titolo di Schlichter**, 45-60 minuti dopo una dose di sospensione o 60-80 minuti dopo una capsula o una compressa. Si considera auspicabile un titolo battericida sierico di 1:8 o più. Il trattamento per os riduce il rischio di infezioni nosocomiali correlate a una terapia endovenosa prolungata, è più comodo per i pazienti e permette il trattamento al di fuori dell'ospedale, se è possibile assicurarsi la compliance dei pazienti. In alternativa, per completare la terapia a domicilio, si può fare ricorso alla terapia endovenosa extraospedaliera con un catetere venoso centrale.

La CRMO richiede il trattamento di qualsiasi disordine primitivo. Nel trattamento della CRMO rientra anche l'utilizzo del prednisone; se i corticosteroidi non sono efficaci, in alcuni pazienti si è dimostrato efficace l'infliximab.

Terapia chirurgica. Il trattamento chirurgico delle infezioni dello scheletro non è stato oggetto di studi prospettici randomizzati di confronto tra le procedure chirurgiche. Quando si ottiene una secrezione francamente purulenta dall'aspirazione sottoperiostea o metafisaria, di solito è indicato il drenaggio chirurgico. L'intervento chirurgico è spesso indicato anche dopo un trauma penetrante e quando si sospetta la presenza di un corpo estraneo ritenuto. Il drenaggio chirurgico è obbligatorio per l'osteomielite della testa femorale con interessamento dell'articolazione dell'anca.

Il trattamento dell'osteomielite cronica consiste nella rimozione chirurgica dei tragitti fistolosi e dei sequestri, se presenti. Si prosegue con la terapia antibiotica per diversi mesi o più a lungo, finché i segni e sintomi clinici e il quadro radiografico non indicano l'avvenuta guarigione.

Fisioterapia. Il ruolo principale della fisioterapia è preventivo. Se si permette a un bambino di giacere sdraiato con un'estremità in flessione, entro pochi giorni può svilupparsi una limitazione dell'estensione. L'estremità affetta deve essere mantenuta in estensione con sacchetti di sabbia, tutori o, se necessario, con un gesso; quest'ultimo è indicato anche in caso di potenziale frattura patologica. Dopo 2-3 giorni, quando il dolore si riduce, si possono iniziare esercizi di mobilizzazione passiva nell'arco di movimento, da proseguire fino alla ripresa della normale attività. Nei casi trascurati con retrazioni in flessione, è necessaria una fisioterapia prolungata.

PROGNOSI. Se si esegue un drenaggio del materiale purulento e si instaura un'appropriata terapia antibiotica, il miglioramento di segni e sintomi è rapido. Un mancato miglioramento o il peggioramento entro 72 ore rende necessario riconsiderare la correttezza della terapia antibiotica, valutare la necessità dell'intervento chirurgico o rivedere la diagnosi. I reattanti della fase acuta possono essere utili per monitorare il processo. La proteina C-reattiva sierica tipicamente si normalizza entro 7 giorni dall'inizio del trattamento, mentre la VES aumenta tipicamente per 5-7 giorni, quindi si riduce lentamente, con una brusca diminuzione dopo 10-14 giorni. Il fatto che uno di questi due reattanti della fase acuta non seguano il decorso usuale deve suscitare il dubbio che la terapia possa non essere adeguata. La recidiva della malattia e lo sviluppo di un'infezione cronica dopo il trattamento di verificano in meno del 10% dei pazienti.

Dal momento che i bambini sono in uno stato di crescita dinamico, le sequele delle infezioni dello scheletro possono non rendersi evidenti per mesi o anni; pertanto, è necessario un follow-up a lungo termine, dedicando particolare attenzione all'arco di movimento articolare e alla lunghezza dell'osso interessato. Anche se non sono disponibili dati attendibili sulle conseguenze del ritardo del trattamento, sembra che una terapia medica e chirurgica iniziata entro una settimana dall'esordio dei sintomi assicuri una prognosi migliore.

Bocchini C, Hulten KG, Mason Jr. EO, et al: Panten-valentine leukodicin genes are associated with enhanced inflammatory response and local disease in acute hematogenous *Staphylococcus aureus* osteomyelitis in children. *Pediatrics* 2006;117:433–440.

Connolly LP, Connolly SA, Druback LA, et al: Acute hematogenous osteomyelitis of children: Assessment of skeletal scintigraphy-based diagnosis in the era of MRI. *J Nucl Med* 2002;43:1310–1316.

Deutschmann A, Mache CJ, Bodo K, et al: Successful treatment of chronic recurrent multifocal osteomyelitis with tumor necrosis factor-α blockage. *Pediatrics* 2005;116:1231–1233.
Fernandez M, Carrol CL, Baker CJ: Discitis and vertebral osteomyelitis in children: An 18-year review. *Pediatrics* 2000;105:1299–1304.
Floyed RL, Steele RW: Culture-negative osteomyelitis. *Pediatr Infect Dis J* 2003;22:731–735.
Gomez M, Maraqa N, Alvarez A, et al: Complications of outpatient parenteral antibiotic therapy in childhood. *Pediatr Infect Dis J* 2001;20:541–543.
Gonzales BE, Teruya J, Mahoney Jr. DH, et al: Venous thrombosis associated with staphylococcal osteomyelitis in children. *Pediatrics* 2006;117: 1675–1679.
Huber AM, Lam PY, Duffy CM, et al: Chronic recurrent multifocal osteomyelitis: Clinical outcomes after more than five years of follow-up. *J Pediatr* 2002;141:198–203.
Ibia EO, Imoisili M, Pikis A: Group A ß-hemolytic streptococcal osteomyelitis in children. *Pediatrics* 2003;112:e22–e26.
Jurik AG: Chronic recurrent multifocal osteomyelitis. *Semin Musculoskelet Radiol* 2004;8:243–253.
Kiang KM, Ogunmodede F, Juni BA, et al: Outbreak of osteomyelitis/septic arthritis caused by *Kingella kingae* among child care center attendees. *Pediatrics* 2005;116:e206–e213.
Lew DP, Waldvogel FA: Osteomyelitis. *Lancet* 2004;364:369–379.
Maraqa NF, Gomez MM, Rathore MH: Outpatient parenteral antimicrobial therapy in osteoarticular infections in children. *J Pediatr Orthop* 2002;22:506–510.
Martinez-Aguilar G, Hammerman WA, Mason EO Jr, Kaplan SL: Clindamycin treatment of invasive infections caused by community-acquired, methicillin-resistant and methicillin-susceptible *S. aureus* in children. *Pediatr Infect Dis J* 2003;22:593–598.
Nelson JD: Bugs, drugs and bones: A pediatric infectious disease specialist reflects on management of musculoskeletal infections. *J Pediatr Orthop* 1999;19:141–142.
Saigal G, Azouz EM, Abdenour G: Imaging of osteomyelitis with special reference to children. *Semin Musculoskelet Radiol* 2004;8:255–265.
Shih HN, Shih LY, Wong YC: Diagnosis and treatment of subacute osteomyelitis. *J Trauma* 2005;58:83–87.
Verdier I, Gayet-Ageron A, Ploton C, et al: Contribution of a broad range polymerase chain reaction to the diagnosis of osteoarticular infections caused by *Kingella kingae*. *Pediatr Infect Dis J* 2005;24:692–696.
Yagupsky P: *K. kingae* infections of the skeletal system in children: Diagnosis and therapy. *Expert Rev Anti Infect Ther* 2004;2:787–794.
Yagupsky P, Erlich Y, Ariela S, et al: Outbreak of *Kingella kingae* skeletal system infections in children in daycare. *Pediatr Infect Dis J* 2006;25:526–532.

Capitolo 684 ■ Artrite suppurativa (artrite settica) Richard Lampe

Le infezioni suppurative delle articolazioni nei lattanti e nei bambini possono causare disabilità permanente. La frequenza dell'artrite suppurativa (denominata anche artrite settica) è maggiore nei lattanti e nei bambini di 1-4 anni di età che nei soggetti più grandi. Nei bambini più piccoli una diagnosi tempestiva, prima che si sviluppi un'infezione diffusa, e l'immediata istituzione di un'appropriata terapia medica e chirurgica riducono al minimo ulteriori danni alla sinovia, alla cartilagine adiacente e all'osso.

EZIOLOGIA. Nell'artrite suppurativa lo spettro microbico è vario, anche se l'infezione da *Staphylococcus aureus* è la più comune. L'*Haemophilus influenzae* di tipo b era implicato in più della metà dei casi di artrite batterica nei lattanti prima dell'introduzione del vaccino coniugato, ma ora è infrequente. Lo streptococco di gruppo A e lo *Streptococcus pneumoniae* (pneumococco) storicamente causano il 10-20% de casi. Oggi, con il miglioramento dei metodi diagnostici (coltura e PCR), la *Kingella kingae* è stata riconosciuta come un agente eziologico relativamente comune. Negli adolescenti sessualmente attivi il gonococco è una causa comune di artrite settica e tenosinovite, che colpisce di solito le piccole articolazioni o può manifestarsi come infezione monoarticolare di una grande articolazione (ginocchio).

Le infezioni micotiche di solito fanno parte di una malattia disseminata multisistemica. Un'artrite da *Candida* può complicare un'infezione sistemica in neonati con o senza cateteri vascolari a permanenza. Le infezioni articolari primitive sono rare, ma un'artrite accompagna molte sindromi virali (parvovirus, parotite epidemica, vaccini vivi per la rosolia), suggerendo una patogenesi immunomediata.

Un'eziologia microbica è confermata nel 65% circa dei casi di artrite suppurativa. Una pregressa terapia antibiotica e l'effetto inibitorio del pus sulla crescita batterica possono spiegare questa bassa percentuale di isolamento batterico. Inoltre, alcuni casi trattati come artrite batterica sono in realtà artriti reattive postinfettive gastrointestinali o genitourinarie (vedi Capitolo 156) e non infezioni primitive. La malattia di Lyme causa un'artrite più simile a un disordine reumatologico, tipicamente non suppurativa.

EPIDEMIOLOGIA. L'artrite suppurativa è più comune nei bambini piccoli: metà dei casi si verifica entro i 2 anni di vita e tre quarti di tutti i casi si verificano entro i 5 anni di età. Adolescenti e neonati sono a rischio di artrite settica gonococcica.

La maggior parte delle infezioni in bambini altrimenti sani è di origine ematogena. L'infezione articolare può fare seguito a lesioni o procedure penetranti, come traumi, artroscopia, interventi di protesizzazione articolare, iniezione intrarticolare di corticosteroidi e interventi di chirurgia ortopedica, anche se si tratta di un'evenienza poco frequente. Anche i pazienti immunocompromessi e quelli con artropatie reumatologiche hanno un rischio aumentato di infezione articolare.

PATOGENESI. Un'artrite suppurativa si verifica principalmente in seguito alla disseminazione ematogena nello spazio sinoviale. È invece meno frequente che i microrganismi penetrino nello spazio articolare per inoculazione diretta o estensione da un focolaio contiguo. La membrana sinoviale, possedendo una ricca vascolarizzazione ed essendo priva di membrana basale, rappresenta un ambiente ideale per la disseminazione ematogena. La presenza di endotossina batterica nello spazio articolare stimola la produzione di citochine (fattore di necrosi tumorale α, interleuchina 1) all'interno dell'articolazione, scatenando una cascata infiammatoria. Le citochine stimolano la chemiotassi dei neutrofili nello spazio articolare, dove vengono rilasciati da parte dei neutrofili enzimi proteolitici ed elastasi che danneggiano la cartilagine. Anche gli enzimi proteolitici rilasciati dalle cellule sinoviali e dai condrociti contribuiscono alla distruzione di cartilagine e tessuto sinoviale. La ialuronidasi batterica degrada l'acido ialuronico nel liquido sinoviale, rendendo il liquido meno viscoso e riducendone il potere di lubrificazione e protezione della cartilagine articolare. Il danno della cartilagine può avvenire in seguito all'aumentata frizione: questo vale soprattutto per le articolazioni che sopportano il carico. L'aumento della pressione all'interno dello spazio articolare, dovuto all'accumulo di materiale purulento, può compromettere la vascolarizzazione e indurre una necrosi da pressione della cartilagine. La distruzione di sinovia e cartilagine è imputabile a una combinazione di enzimi proteolitici e fattori meccanici.

MANIFESTAZIONI CLINICHE. I segni e i sintomi dell'artrite suppurativa dipendono dall'età del paziente. Quelli precoci possono essere subdoli, soprattutto nei neonati. L'artrite suppurativa nei neonati e nei lattanti è spesso associata a osteomielite adiacente, dovuta alla diffusione transepifisaria dell'infezione (vedi Capitolo 683).

I lattanti e i bambini più grandi possono avere febbre e dolore, con segni di localizzazione come edema, eritema e calore a livello dell'articolazione interessata. Con l'interessamento delle articolazioni del bacino e delle estremità inferiori, si osservano spesso zoppia o rifiuto di camminare.

Eritema ed edema della cute e dei tessuti molli al di sopra della sede dell'infezione si osservano più precocemente nell'artrite suppurativa che nell'osteomielite, dal momento che la sinovia infetta ed edematosa è più superficiale, a differenza della metafisi che è localizzata più in profondità. L'artrite suppurativa dell'anca rappresenta un'eccezione a causa della sede profonda dell'articolazione dell'anca.

Le articolazioni dell'arto inferiore sono colpite nel 75% di tutti i casi di artrite suppurativa (Tab. 684-1). Gomito, polso e spalla sono interessati nel 25% dei casi, mentre è raro che l'infezione coinvolga le piccole articolazioni. Le infezioni suppurative di anca, spalla, gomito e caviglia nei lattanti e nei bambini più grandi possono essere associate a un'osteomielite adiacente del femore prossimale, dell'omero prossimale, del radio prossimale e della tibia distale poiché la metafisi si estende all'interno dell'articolazione.

DIAGNOSI. Occorre eseguire un'emocoltura in tutti i casi di sospetta artrite settica. L'aspirazione del liquido articolare per la colorazione di Gram e la coltura se la storia clinica indica un'artrite suppurativa rimangono le tecniche diagnostiche definitive, che forniscono i campioni più adatti per la coltura di conferma della diagnosi. L'aspirazione è agevole per la maggior parte dei grandi spazi articolari, ma l'anca può porre problemi tecnici; la guida ecografica è senz'altro d'aiuto. Se non si ottiene del fluido, si inietta un mezzo di contrasto e si esegue una radiografia per essere certi che la punta dell'ago si trovi nella cavità articolare. L'aspirazione del materiale purulento presente nell'articolazione fornisce il campione più adatto per la coltura batteriologica dell'infezione. Se si sospetta un gonococco, occorre eseguire anche le colture anale, cervicale e faringea. Oltre all'immediato inoculo su un terreno di coltura solido, l'inoculo del campione in provette da emocoltura può aumentare l'isolamento di *K. kingae*.

L'analisi del liquido sinoviale per la determinazione della conta cellulare, del tipo cellulare, del contenuto proteico e del contenuto di glucosio ha un'utilità limitata in quanto anche le malattie infiammatorie non infettive, come la febbre reumatica e l'artrite reumatoide, possono causare una reazione esuberante con aumento delle cellule e delle proteine e riduzione del glucosio. Le caratteristiche del liquido sinoviale nell'artrite suppurativa possono suggerire un'infezione ma non sono abbastanza specifiche perché si possa escludere un'infezione.

Non esistono test di laboratorio specifici per l'artrite suppurativa. Esami come la conta dei globuli bianchi e la formula leucocitaria, VES e proteina C-reattiva sono molto sensibili per le infezioni articolari, ma non sono specifici e possono non permettere di distinguere un'infezione da altri processi infiammatori. La conta leucocitaria e la VES possono essere normali durante i primi giorni dell'infezione e risultati normali degli esami non escludono di per sé la diagnosi di artrite suppurativa. Il monitoraggio dell'aumento della VES e della proteina C-reattiva possono essere utili per valutare la risposta alla terapia o identificare le complicanze.

Valutazione radiografica. Gli studi radiografici hanno un ruolo cruciale nella valutazione dell'artrite suppurativa. Le radiografie convenzionali, l'ecografia, la RM, la TC e la scintigrafia possono tutte contribuire alla diagnosi.

TABELLA 684-1. Distribuzione delle articolazioni interessate da artrite suppurativa acuta

ARTICOLAZIONE	N.	%
Ginocchio	309	39,6
Anca	173	22,2
Gomito	109	14,0
Caviglia	104	13,3
Spalla	37	4,7
Polso	34	4,4
Sacroiliaca	5	0,6
Interfalangea	4	0,5
Metatarsale	3	0,4
Acromioclavicolare	1	0,1
Sternoclavicolare	1	0,1
Metacarpale	1	0,1

Basata su una casistica non pubblicata di 725 pazienti con 781 infezioni articolari.

STUDI RADIOGRAFICI. Nell'artrite suppurativa le radiografie possono evidenziare un allargamento della capsula articolare, edema dei tessuti molli e obliterazione delle normali linee adipose. Le radiografie dell'anca possono evidenziare uno spostamento mediale del muscolo otturatore della pelvi (segno dell'otturatore), spostamento laterale o obliterazione delle linee adipose glutee ed elevazione della linea di Shenton con un allargamento dell'arco.

ECOGRAFIA. L'ecografia è particolarmente utile per l'identificare un versamento articolare e le raccolte di fluidi nei tessuti molli e nelle regioni sottoperiostee. Oltre a essere altamente sensibile nell'identificare i versamenti articolari, soprattutto nell'articolazione dell'anca, dove le radiografie possono essere normali in più del 50% dei casi di artrite suppurativa dell'anca, può servire come ausilio nell'esecuzione di un'agoaspirazione dell'anca.

TOMOGRAFIA COMPUTERIZZATA E RISONANZA MAGNETICA. Sia la TC sia la RM possono essere utili per confermare la presenza di liquido articolare in pazienti con sospetta osteoartrite. La RM può inoltre servire per escludere un'osteomielite adiacente.

Nell'artrite suppurativa la scintigrafia trifasica con Tecnezio-99 metilene difosfonato evidenzia una captazione simmetrica su entrambi i lati dell'articolazione, limitata alle strutture ossee adiacenti all'articolazione. La scintigrafia è utile anche per la valutazione dell'articolazione sacroiliaca.

Diagnosi differenziale. La diagnosi differenziale dell'artrite suppurativa dipende dall'articolazione o dalle articolazioni interessate e dall'età del paziente. Per l'anca occorre prendere in considerazione la sinovite tossica, la malattia di Legg-Perthes-Calvé, l'epifisiolisi della testa femorale, l'ascesso dello psoas, un'osteomielite del femore prossimale, del bacino o delle vertebre. Per il ginocchio, invece, bisogna valutare la possibilità di un'osteomielite femorale distale o tibiale prossimale, un'artrite reumatoide pauciarticolare e dolore riferito dall'anca. Altre condizioni come traumi, cellulite, piomiosite, anemia a cellule falciformi, emofilia e porpora di Schonlein-Henoch possono simulare un'artrite purulenta. Quando sono interessate diverse articolazioni, occorre considerare la malattia da siero, una malattia vascolare del collagene, la febbre reumatica e la porpora di Schönlein-Henoch. Un'artrite reattiva, che fa seguito a varie infezioni batteriche (gastrointestinali o genitali) e parassitarie, a faringite streptococcica o a epatite virale, può assomigliare a un'artrite suppurativa acuta (vedi Capitolo 156).

TRATTAMENTO. Il trattamento ottimale dell'artrite suppurativa richiede lo sforzo congiunto di pediatri, chirurghi ortopedici e radiologi.

Terapia antibiotica. La terapia antibiotica empirica iniziale si basa sulla conoscenza dei probabili patogeni batterici alle varie età, sui risultati della colorazione di Gram del materiale aspirato e su altre considerazioni ancora. Nei neonati, una penicillina antistafilococcica, come la nafcillina o l'oxacillina (150-200 mg/kg/24 ore suddivisi ogni 6 ore, ev) e una cefalosporina ad ampio spettro, come la cefotaxima (200 mg/kg/24 ore suddivisi ogni 8 ore, ev) forniscono una copertura per *S. aureus*, streptococco di gruppo B e bacilli Gram-negativi. Se il neonato è un piccolo prematuro o ha un catetere venoso centrale, bisogna considerare la possibilità di un'infezione nosocomiale da batteri (*Pseudomonas aeruginosa* o stafilococchi coagulasi-negativi) o da miceti (*Candida*).

Nei bambini con artrite suppurativa, una terapia empirica contro *S. aureus*, streptococchi e *K. kingae* deve comprendere la somministrazione di cefazolina (100-150 mg/kg/24 ore suddivisi ogni 8 ore) o nafcillina (150-200 mg/kg/24 ore suddivisi ogni 6 ore).

La clindamicina (40 mg/kg suddivisi ogni 6 ore) e la vancomicina (40 mg/kg/24 ore suddivisi ogni 6 ore, ev) sono alternative nel caso di infezioni da *S. aureus* meticillinoresistenti. Nei pazienti immunocompromessi si inizia di solito una terapia in associazione, per esempio con vancomicina e ceftazidima o con penicilline ad ampio spettro e inibitori della β-lattamasi associati a un aminoglicoside. L'aggiunta alla terapia antibiotica di desametasone per 4 giorni sembra essere utile nei bambini con artrite settica.

Una volta identificato il patogeno, se necessario si apportano gli opportuni cambiamenti della terapia antibiotica. Se non viene identificato un patogeno e le condizioni del paziente migliorano, si prosegue la terapia con l'antibiotico prescelto inizialmente. Se non viene identificato un patogeno e le condizioni del paziente non migliorano, occorre prendere in considerazione una nuova aspirazione oppure la possibilità di una patologia non infettiva.

La durata della terapia antibiotica va individualizzata a seconda del microrganismo isolato e del decorso clinico. Da 10 a 14 giorni sono di solito sufficienti per streptococchi, pneumococco e *K. kingae*; una terapia più prolungata può essere necessaria per *S. aureus* e altre infezioni da Gram-negativi. La normalizzazione della VES e della proteina C-reattiva e un esame obiettivo normale consentono di sospendere la terapia antibiotica.

Terapia chirurgica. L'infezione dell'anca è considerata un'emergenza chirurgica a causa della vulnerabilità della vascolarizzazione della testa femorale. Per le altre articolazioni può essere necessaria l'aspirazione quotidiana del liquido sinoviale. In generale, sono sufficienti 1-2 aspirazioni. Se il liquido continua ad accumularsi dopo 4-5 giorni, è necessaria un'artrotomia. Al momento dell'intervento, l'articolazione viene irrigata con soluzione fisiologica sterile. Non si instillano antibiotici perché sono irritanti per il tessuto sinoviale e con la somministrazione sistemica se ne ottengono comunque concentrazioni adeguate nel liquido sinoviale.

PROGNOSI. Quando si drena il materiale purulento e si somministra un'adeguata terapia antibiotica, il miglioramento dei segni e dei sintomi è rapido. Un mancato miglioramento o un peggioramento entro 72 ore richiedono che il medico metta in discussione la correttezza della terapia antibiotica prescelta e della diagnosi, valutando se sia necessario procedere a un intervento chirurgico. I reattanti della fase acuta possono essere utili per monitorare la terapia; se uno qualsiasi di esse non segue il decorso consueto, questo dovrebbe suscitare dubbi sull'adeguatezza della terapia. La recidiva della malattia e lo sviluppo di un'infezione cronica dopo il trattamento si verificano in meno del 10% dei pazienti.

Dal momento che i bambini sono in uno stato dinamico di crescita, le sequele delle infezioni scheletriche possono non essere evidenti per mesi o anni; è pertanto necessario un follow-up a lungo termine che valuti con particolare attenzione l'arco di movimento articolare e la lunghezza ossea. Anche se mancano dati attendibili sull'impatto del ritardo terapeutico sugli esiti, sembra che l'inizio della terapia medica e chirurgica entro una settimana dall'esordio dei sintomi si associ a una prognosi migliore.

Bonheffer J, Haeberle B, Schaad UB, Heininger U: Diagnosis of hematogenous osteomyelitis and septic arthritis: 20 years experience at the University Children's Hospital Basel. *Swiss Med Wkly* 2001;131:575–581.

Centers for Disease Control and Prevention: Osteomyelitis/septic arthritis caused by *Kingella kingae* among day care attendees—Minnesota. *MMWR* 2003;53:241–243.

Nelson JD: Bugs, drugs and bones: A pediatric infectious disease specialist reflects on management of musculoskeletal infections. *J Pediatr Orthop* 1999;19:141–142.

Odio CM, Ramirez T, Arias G, et al: Double blind, randomized, placebo-controlled study of dexamethasone therapy for hematogenous septic arthritis in children. *Pediatr Infect Dis J* 2003;22:883–888.

Ross JJ, Hu LT: Septic arthritis of the pubic symphysis. *Medicine* 2003;82: 340–345.

Schirtliff ME, Mader JT: Acute septic arthritis. *Clin Microbiol Rev* 2002; 15:527–544.

Wang CL, Wang SM, Yang YJ, et al: Septic arthritis in children: Relationship of causative pathogens, complications, and outcome. *J Microbiol Immunol Infect* 2003;36:41–46.

Sezione 2 — Medicina dello sport

Capitolo 685 ■ Epidemiologia e prevenzione dei traumi

Gregory L. Landry e Kelsey Logan

Il Surgeon General's Healthy People 2010 Objectives sottolinea l'importanza di un'attività fisica da moderata a vigorosa su base regolare per tutti gli adolescenti. L'attività fisica ha effetti favorevoli su ipertensione, obesità e livelli lipidici sierici nei giovani. Negli adulti, l'attività fisica è associata a tassi più bassi di malattia cardiovascolare, diabete di tipo 2, osteoporosi e cancro del colon e della mammella.

I medici dovrebbero spronare i propri pazienti all'attività fisica, adattandola a seconda del loro stato di salute. Uno sforzo particolare va fatto per cercare di inserire l'attività fisica nello stile di vita di quelli con minori tassi di attività fisica e partecipazione allo sport, compresi i bambini con necessità sanitarie speciali e quelli appartenenti a gruppi socioeconomici svantaggiati. I medici hanno la responsabilità non solo di promuovere l'attività fisica, ma anche di fornire certificati per la partecipazione agli sport e per la diagnosi e riabilitazione dei traumi.

Negli Stati Uniti circa 30 milioni di bambini e adolescenti partecipano a sport organizzati. Circa 3 milioni di traumi si verificano ogni anno se si definisce trauma il tempo perso a causa dell'attività sportiva. I decessi nello sport sono rari, e la maggior parte delle morti non dovute a traumi è imputabile a cardiopatie (vedi Capitolo 436). In generale, la percentuale di traumi sportivi e la loro severità aumentano con l'età e con lo sviluppo puberale, in relazione alla maggiore velocità, forza e intensità della competizione.

Il riconoscimento dei meccanismi traumatici e l'applicazione di regole che riducono la probabilità di un meccanismo traumatico, compresa la penalizzazione del gioco pericoloso, hanno ridotto la percentuale di traumi con conseguenze catastrofiche. Negli Stati Uniti tassi dei traumi sono stati inoltre ridotti dalla rimozione dei rischi ambientali, come i trampolini nella ginnastica e le basi stazionarie (rispetto al breakaway) nel softball, e modificano i tassi di traumi cranici nei tornei di calcio aggiungendo water break e riducendo i tempi di gioco. Inoltre, una riabilitazione appropriata in caso di traumi riduce il rischio che questi tornino a verificarsi in futuro. L'allenamento prestagionale degli atleti delle scuole superiori, in particolare per ciò che riguarda velocità, agilità, salto e flessibilità, si associa alla riduzione del tasso dei traumi nel calcio e dei traumi gravi del ginocchio nelle atlete. Le tradizionali manovre di stretching o di massaggio non riducono il rischio di lesioni o di affaticamento muscolare, ma il bendaggio dell'anca è particolarmente utile per prevenire nuovi traumi della caviglia. Un ambito per applicare alcune di queste strategie preventive e per identificare traumi e problemi medici non sottoposti a riabilitazione che potrebbero ostacolare la partecipazione agli sport è l'esame preliminare per la partecipazione all'attività sportiva (PSE, *Prepartecipation Sport Examination*).

ESAME PRELIMINARE PER LA PARTECIPAZIONE ALL'ATTIVITÀ SPORTIVA

Il PSE, che viene eseguito mediante un'anamnesi e un esame obiettivo specifici, deve comprendere uno screening muscoloscheletrico. Esso identifica possibili problemi nell'1-8% degli atleti e preclude l'attività sportiva a meno dell'1% di essi. Il PSE non sostituisce la valutazione annuale completa, volta a individuare i comportamenti potenzialmente pericolosi per gli adolescenti, come la promiscuità sessuale, l'uso di droghe, il suicidio e la violenza. Gli scopi del PSE sono i seguenti: identificare le condizioni mediche che inducono a rimandare l'attività sportiva o addirittura rappresentano una controindicazione in tal senso, a causa di un rischio di trauma o di morte; identificare eventuali patologie non ancora diagnosticate; diagnosticare condizioni mediche che necessitano di ulteriore valutazione o riabilitazione prima che il paziente possa praticare sport; fornire una guida alla partecipazione agli sport per i pazienti con condizioni mediche e infine soddisfare gli obblighi legali e assicurativi. Se possibile, il PSE dovrebbe essere associato alla visita annuale completa, con particolare riferimento all'assistenza preventiva (vedi Capitoli 5 e 12).

Le indicazioni sulla frequenza con la quale un giovane debba essere sottoposto a PSE differiscono nei vari Stati (si parla degli Stati Uniti), variando da una frequenza annuale a una visita in occasione del passaggio a un nuovo livello scolastico (junior high, senior high, college). Come minimo, ogni giovane atleta altrimenti sano dovrebbe essere sottoposto ogni anno a una visita ad interim focalizzata. Il momento ottimale per il PSE è 3-6 settimane prima dell'inizio dell'attività.

ANAMNESI ED ESAME OBIETTIVO. Le componenti essenziali del PSE sono l'anamnesi e un esame obiettivo medico e muscoloscheletrico focalizzati di screening. I problemi eventualmente individuati richiedono ulteriori indagini (Tabb. 685-1 e 685-2). In assenza di sintomi, non è necessario alcun test di laboratorio.

Il 75% dei segni e sintomi significativi è identificabile con l'anamnesi; è importante proporre un questionario standard non solo al giovane atleta, ma anche ai genitori, in quanto il diretto interessato può non conoscere o dimenticare aspetti importanti della propria storia medica. Il questionario deve comprendere

TABELLA 685-1. Esame preliminare per la partecipazione all'attività sportiva

COMPONENTE DELL'ESAME OBIETTIVO	CONDIZIONE DA IDENTIFICARE
Segni vitali	Ipertensione, cardiopatie, bradi/tachicardia
Altezza e peso	Obesità, disordini del comportamento alimentare
Visus e dimensioni pupillari	Cecità legale, occhio assente, anisocoria, ambliopia
Linfonodi	Malattie infettive, neoplasie maligne
Esame obiettivo cardiaco (in piedi e in posizione supina)	Soffi cardiaci, interventi chirurgici pregressi, aritmie
Esame obiettivo polmonare	Broncospasmo ricorrente e indotto dall'esercizio, pneumopatia cronica
Addome	Organomegalia, masse addominali
Cute	Malattie contagiose (impetigine, herpes, infezioni stafilococciche e streptococciche)
Esame obiettivo genitourinario	Varicocele, testicoli non discesi, tumori, ernia
Esame obiettivo muscoloscheletrico	Traumi acuti e cronici, anomalie fisiche (scoliosi)

TABELLA 685-2. Condizioni mediche e possibilità di praticare sport*

CONDIZIONE	PUÒ PARTECIPARE
Instabilità atlantoassiale (instabilità dell'articolazione tra le vertebre cervicali 1 e 2)	Sì, qualificato
Spiegazione l'atleta deve essere sottoposto a valutazione del rischio di trauma midollare spinale durante l'attività sportiva.	
Disordine emorragico	Sì, qualificato
Spiegazione l'atleta deve essere sottoposto a valutazione.	
Patologia cardiovascolare	
Cardite (infiammazione del cuore)	No
Spiegazione la cardite può causare morte improvvisa in seguito allo sforzo.	
Ipertensione	Sì, qualificato
Spiegazione i pazienti con ipertensione essenziale significativa devono evitare il sollevamento pesi, body building e l'allenamento per il potenziamento muscolare. Quelli con ipertensione secondaria o ipertensione essenziale severa devono essere sottoposti a valutazione.	
Cardiopatie congenite	Sì, qualificato
Spiegazione i pazienti con forme lievi possono fare sport senza limitazioni; quelli con forme severe o moderate o che sono stati sottoposti a intervento devono essere sottoposti a valutazione. La 26ª Conferenza di Bethesda ha definito le forme lievi, moderate e severe per le comuni lesioni cardiache.	
Aritmie	Sì, qualificato
Spiegazione i pazienti con sintomi (dolore toracico, sincope, vertigini, dispnea o altri sintomi di possibile aritmia) o evidenze di insufficienza mitralica all'esame obiettivo devono essere sottoposti a valutazione. Tutti gli altri possono partecipare senza limitazioni.	
Soffio sistolico	Sì, qualificato
Spiegazione se il soffio è innocente (non indica una cardiopatia), si permette una piena partecipazione all'attività. Altrimenti, l'atleta richiede una valutazione (vedi Cardiopatia congenita e Prolasso mitralico).	
Paralisi cerebrale	Sì, qualificato
Spiegazione l'atleta richiede una valutazione.	Sì
Diabete mellito	
Spiegazione possono essere praticati tutti gli sport con un'adeguata attenzione alla dieta, alla glicemia, all'idratazione e alla terapia insulinica. La glicemia deve essere monitorata ogni 30 minuti durante un'attività continua e 15 minuti dopo il termine dell'attività.	
Diarrea	Non qualificato
Spiegazione a meno che la malattia sia lieve, non è permessa alcuna partecipazione, in quanto la diarrea può aumentare il rischi di disidratazione e di malattia da calore. Vedi Febbre.	
Disordini del comportamento alimentare	Sì, qualificato
Anoressia nervosa	
Bulimia nervosa	
Spiegazione prima di partecipare a un'attività sportiva, i pazienti con questi disordini devono essere sottoposti a valutazione medica e psichiatrica.	
Occhi	Sì, qualificato
Atleta con un solo occhio funzionale	
Perdita di un occhio	
Distacco di retina	
Pregressa chirurgia oculare o trauma oculare severo	
Spiegazione un atleta con un solo occhio funzionale ha un'acuità visiva con la migliore correzione <20/40 nell'occhio con l'acuità peggiore. Questi atleti, come peraltro quelli privi di un occhio, avrebbero una disabilità significativa se l'occhio migliore subisse un trauma severo. Alcuni atleti che in precedenza hanno subito un intervento chirurgico all'occhio o che hanno avuto un trauma oculare severo possono correre maggiori rischi di trauma a causa dell'indebolimento dei tessuti oculari. L'uso di apposite protezioni per gli occhi può permettere la partecipazione alla maggior parte degli sport, ma è importante effettuare una valutazione caso per caso.	

TABELLA 685-2. Condizioni mediche e possibilità di praticare sport – *continua*

CONDIZIONE	PUÒ PARTECIPARE
Febbre	No
Spiegazione la febbre può aumentare lo sforzo cardiopolmonare, ridurre la capacità massimale d'esercizio, rendere la malattia da calore più probabile e aumentare la tensione ortostatica durante l'attività fisica. Anche se raramente, la febbre può inoltre accompagnare una miocardite o altre infezioni che rendono potenzialmente pericolosa l'attività fisica.	
Malattia da calore, storia di	Sì, qualificato
Spiegazione a causa dell'aumentata probabilità di recidiva, l'atleta necessita di una valutazione individuale, utile per determinare la presenza di condizioni predisponenti e stabilire una strategia preventiva.	
Epatite	Sì
Spiegazione dal momento che questa patologia comporta rischi minimi per gli altri, l'atleta può praticare tutti gli sport se il suo stato di salute lo permette. Occorre sempre bendare con cura le lesioni cutanee e l'équipe medica sportiva deve usare precauzioni universali quando manipola sangue o fluidi corporei con sangue visibile.	
Virus dell'immunodeficienza umana	Sì
Spiegazione dal momento che questa patologia comporta rischi minimi per gli altri, l'atleta può praticare tutti gli sport se il suo stato di salute lo permette. Occorre sempre bendare con cura le lesioni cutanee e l'équipe medica sportiva deve usare precauzioni universali quando manipola sangue o fluidi corporei con sangue visibile.	
Rene, assenza di un	Sì, qualificato
Spiegazione l'atleta necessita di una valutazione individuale per gli sport che comportano contatto, anche limitato, e collisione.	
Epatomegalia	Sì, qualificato
Spiegazione se l'epatomegalia è acuta, occorre evitare le attività sportive a causa del rischio di rottura. Se l'epatomegalia è cronica, è necessaria una valutazione individuale prima di praticare sport che comportino contatto, anche limitato, e collisione.	
Neoplasia maligna	Sì, qualificato
Spiegazione l'atleta deve essere sottoposto a una valutazione individuale.	Sì, qualificato
Disordini muscoloscheletrici	
Spiegazione l'atleta deve essere sottoposto a una valutazione individuale.	
Disordini neurologici	Sì, qualificato
Anamnesi di trauma cranico o spinale severo, concussione severa o ripetuta o craniotomia	
Spiegazione l'atleta deve essere sottoposto a una valutazione individuale per gli sport che comportano collisione e contatto, e anche per gli sport senza contatto se sono presenti deficit cognitivi o mentali. La ricerca supporta un approccio conservativo al trattamento della concussione.	
Disordine convulsivo ben controllato	Sì
Spiegazione il rischio di convulsioni durante l'attività è minimo.	
Disordine convulsivo non ben controllato	Sì, qualificato
Spiegazione l'atleta deve essere sottoposto a una valutazione individuale per gli sport che comportano collisione e contatto, anche limitato. Devono inoltre essere evitati i seguenti sport senza contatto: tiro con l'arco, tiro al bersaglio con armi da fuoco, nuoto, sollevamento pesi, allenamento di rinforzo muscolare o sport che comportano di trovarsi a una certa altezza da terra, poiché in questi casi una crisi convulsiva costituirebbe un pericolo per sé o per gli altri.	
Obesità	Sì, qualificato
Spiegazione a causa del rischio di malattia da calore, gli obesi richiedono un'accurata acclimatazione e idratazione.	
Ricevente di trapianto d'organo	Sì, qualificato
Spiegazione l'atleta deve essere sottoposto a una valutazione individuale.	
Ovaio, assenza di un	Sì
Spiegazione il rischio di danni severi all'ovaio restante è minimo	
Malattie respiratorie	
Compromissione polmonare, compresa la fibrosi cistica	Sì, qualificato
Spiegazione l'atleta deve essere sottoposto a una valutazione individuale, ma in generale tutti gli sport possono praticati se l'ossigenazione rimane soddisfacente durante un test fisico graduato. I pazienti con fibrosi cistica necessitano di acclimatazione e di una buona idratazione per ridurre il rischio di malattia da calore.	
Asma	Sì
Spiegazione con una terapia e un'educazione appropriate, soltanto gli atleti con l'asma più severa necessitano di limitare la partecipazione agli sport.	
Infezione acuta delle vie respiratorie superiori	Sì, qualificato
Spiegazione un'ostruzione delle vie respiratorie superiori può influire sulla funzionalità polmonare. L'atleta deve essere sottoposto a una valutazione individuale per tutte le forme tranne quelle lievi. Vedi Febbre.	
Malattia a cellule falciformi	Sì, qualificato
Spiegazione l'atleta necessita di valutazione individuale. In generale, se lo stato della malattia lo permette, possono essere praticati tutti gli sport tranne quelli che richiedono uno sforzo strenuo, collisione e contatto. Devono essere evitati un eccessivo riscaldamento, la disidratazione e il raffreddamento.	
Trait falciformi	Sì
Spiegazione è improbabile che persone con trait falciformi possano avere un rischio aumentato di morte improvvisa o altri problemi medici nel corso della partecipazione ad attività atletiche, eccetto che nelle condizioni estreme di calore, umidità e forse l'altitudine elevata. Queste persone, come tutti gli atleti, devono essere accuratamente condizionate, acclimatate e idratate per ridurre tutti i possibili rischi.	
Patologie cutanee (impetigine, foruncoli, herpes simplex, scabbia, mollusco contagioso)	Sì, qualificato
Spiegazione se il paziente è contagioso non deve essere permessa la partecipazione a ginnastica su tappeto, arti marziali, lotta o altri sport con collisione, contatto o limitato contatto.	
Splenomegalia	Sì, qualificato
Spiegazione un paziente con splenomegalia acuta deve evitare tutti gli sport a causa del rischio di rottura della milza. Un paziente con splenomegalia cronica necessita di una valutazione individuale prima di praticare sport di collisione, contatto o di contatto limitato.	
Testicolo non disceso, oppure assenza di un testicolo	Sì
Spiegazione alcuni sport possono richiedere l'uso di una conchiglia protettiva.	

*Questa tabella è intesa per l'uso da parte di personale medico e non medico. "Necessità di valutazione" significa che un medico con conoscenze ed esperienza in materia deve valutare la sicurezza di un determinato sport per un atleta con una delle condizioni elencate. A meno che non venga diversamente dichiarato, ciò è dovuto al vario grado di severità della malattia, al rischio di trauma per gli sport specifici elencati nelle Tabelle 685-3 e 685-4 o a entrambe le cose. Da American Academy of Pediatrics, Committee on Sports Medicine and Fitness: Medical conditions affecting sports participation. *Pediatrics* 2001;107:1206-1207.

domande su pregressi problemi medici, chirurgici, cardiaci, polmonari, neurologici, dermatologici, visivi, psicologici, muscoloscheletrici e mestruali, come anche su altre malattie, farmaci, allergie, vaccinazioni e dieta. I problemi più comunemente identificati sono i **traumi non riabilitati**. È indicato uno studio dei traumi precedenti, comprendente i test diagnostici, il trattamento e lo stato funzionale presente.

La **morte improvvisa** durante l'attività sportiva può derivare da una cardiopatia non identificata come una miocardiopatia ipertrofica o altre miocardiopatia, anomalie dei vasi coronarici o la rottura aortica nella sindrome di Marfan (vedi Capitolo 700). In molti casi nessuno era a conoscenza della cardiopatia sottostante e la morte rappresenta il suo primo segno (vedi Capitolo 436). Radiografia toracica, elettrocardiogramma (ECG) ed ecocardiogramma (ECO) non sono raccomandati come test di screening di routine. Se sorge un **sospetto** di cardiopatia, giustificato da una storia di sincope, presincope, palpitazioni, dispnea eccessiva allo sforzo o una storia familiare di una condizione come una miocardiopatia ipertrofica o un QT prolungato o una sindrome di Marfan, la valutazione deve essere completa e comprendere un ECG con 12 derivazioni, un ECO, un Holter o un monitoraggio per la cattura degli eventi e un test da stress con monitoraggio elettrocardiografico. Per i pazienti con cardiopatia accertata che intendono fare sport il medico deve formulare le sue raccomandazioni in collaborazione con un cardiologo.

L'American Academy of Pediatrics ha indicato le **controindicazioni** e le **limitazioni** all'attività sportiva per diverse condizioni mediche (vedi Tab. 685-2). Gli sport possono inoltre essere classificati in base all'intensità (Tab. 685-3) e al contatto (Tab. 685-4). Talvolta gli atleti decidono di proseguire l'attività sportiva professionistica anche contro il parere del medico. La sezione 504(a) del Rehabilitation Act del 1973 proibisce la discriminazione nei confronti degli atleti disabili se hanno le capacità o le abilità richieste per praticare uno sport competitivo. Tale principio è stato ribadito dall'Americans with Disabilities Act del 1990. Un atleta dilettante non ha il diritto assoluto di decidere se praticare sport competitivi. La partecipazione a sport competitivi è considerata un privilegio, non un diritto. La sentenza Knapp vs Northwestern University ha stabilito che "difficili decisioni mediche su complessi problemi medici possono essere prese da medici responsabili che esercitano un giudizio prudente (che sarà necessariamente conservativo quando le evidenze scientifiche mancano o sono conflittuali) e basato sulle raccomandazioni di specialisti o sulle linee guida stabilite da un'équipe di esperti".

American Academy of Pediatrics: Medical conditions affecting sports participation. *Pediatrics* 2001;107:1205–1209.

American Academy of Pediatrics, American Academy of Family Physicians, American Medical Society for Sports Medicine, American Orthopedic Society for Sports Medicine, American Osteopathic Association for Sports Medicine: *Preparticipation Physical Evaluation Monograph*, 3rd ed. Minneapolis, MN: McGraw-Hill Medical Publishing, 2004.

TABELLA 685-3. Classificazione degli sport in base all'intensità

INTENSITÀ DA ELEVATA A MODERATA		
RICHIESTE STATICHE E DINAMICHE DA ELEVATE A MODERATE	**RICHIESTE DINAMICHE DA ELEVATE A MODERATE E RICHIESTE STATICHE RIDOTTE**	**RICHIESTE STATICHE DA ELEVATE A MODERATE E RICHIESTE DINAMICHE RIDOTTE**
Pugilato*	Badminton	Tiro con l'arco
Canottaggio	Baseball	Corse automobilistiche
Sci di fondo	Basket	Immersione
Ciclismo	Hockey su prato	Equitazione (salto)
Sci di discesa	Lacrosse	Atletica (lancio)
Scherma	Orieentering	Ginnastica
Football	Maratona	Karate o judo
Hockey su ghiaccio	Racquetball	Corse in motocicletta
Rugby	Calcio	Rodeo
Corsa (sprint)	Squash	Vela
Pattinaggio in velocità	Nuoto	Salto con gli sci
Polo acquatico	Tennis da tavolo	Sci d'acqua
Lotta	Tennis	Sollevamento pesi
	Pallavolo	
BASSA INTENSITÀ (RIDOTTE RICHIESTE STATICHE E DINAMICHE)		
Bowling		
Cricket		
Curling		
Tiro al bersaglio		

*La partecipazione non è raccomandata dall'American Academy of Pediatrics.

Da American Academy of Pediatrics, Committee on Sports Medicine and Fitness:Medical conditions affecting sports participation. *Pediatrics* 2001;107:1208.

TABELLA 685-4. Classificazione degli sport per contatto

CONTATTO O COLLISIONE	CONTATTO LIMITATO	SENZA CONTATTO
Basket	Baseball	Tiro con l'arco
Pugilato*	Ciclismo	Badminton
Immersione	Cheerleading	Culturismo
Hockey su prato	Canoa o kayak	Canoa o kayak
Football	(fiumi)	(laghi)
Tackle	Scherma	Canottaggio
Hockey su ghiaccio†	Atletica	Curling
Lacrosse	Salto in alto	Ballo
Arti marziali	Salto con l'asta	Danza classica
Rodeo	Hockey su campo sintetico	Danza moderna
Rugby	Football	Jazz
Salto con gli sci	Flag	Atletica
Calcio	Ginnastica	Lancio del disco
Pallamano a squadre	Pallamano	Lancio del giavellotto
Polo acquatico	Equitazione	Lancio del peso
Lotta	Racquetball	Golf
	Pattinaggio	Orienteering‡
	Su ghiaccio	Sollevamento pesi
	In linea	Maratona
	A rotelle	Tiro al bersaglio
	Sci	Salto con la corda
	Fondo	Corsa
	Discesa	Vela
	Sci d'acqua	Immersione con respiratore
	Skateboard	Nuoto
	Snowboard	Tennis da tavolo
	Softball	Tennis
	Squash	Atletica leggera
	Frisbee	Sollevamento pesi
	Pallavolo	
	Windsurf o surf	

*La partecipazione non è raccomandata dall'American Academy of Pediatrics.

†L'American Academy of Pediatrics raccomanda di limitare l'entità del contatto corporeo per i giocatori di hockey di età ≤15 anni o meno per ridurre i traumi.

‡Una gara in cui i concorrenti usano mappa e bussola per orientarsi in un territorio non familiare.

Da American Academy of Pediatrics, Committee on Sports Medicine and Fitness: Medical conditions affecting sports participation. *Pediatrics* 2001;107:1205.

Anderson SJ: Sports injuries. *Curr Prob Pediatr Adolesc Health Care* 2005;35:105–176.

Jonhagen S, Ackermann P, Erikssin T, et al: Sports massage after eccentric exercise. *Am J Sports Med* 2004;32:1499–1503.

MacAuley D, Best TM: Reducing risk of injury due to exercise. *Br Med J* 2002;325:451–452.

Olsen OE, Myklebust G, Engebretsen L, et al: Exercises to prevent lower limb injuries in youth sports: Cluster randomized controlled trial. *Br Med J* 2005;330:449–452.

Capitolo 686 ■ Trattamento dei traumi muscoloscheletrici Gregory L. Landry

MECCANISMI TRAUMATICI

TRAUMI ACUTI. La maggior parte dei traumi muscoloscheletrici sono distorsioni, stiramenti e contusioni. La storia del trauma può essere poco chiara, ma è particolarmente utile nella valutazione dei traumi del ginocchio e della spalla. I traumi più severi, indicativi di alterazioni strutturali, possono presentarsi con segni e sintomi acuti e immediati come tumefazione, deformità, perdita di forza o della sensibilità, incapacità di continuare il gioco, incapacità di camminare senza zoppia, uno schiocco doloroso udibile, blocco meccanico dell'articolazione o sensazione di instabilità. Si dice **distorsione** il trauma di un legamento o di una capsula articolare, mentre uno **stiramento** è un trauma di un muscolo o di un tendine e una **contusione** è una lesione da schiacciamento di schiacciamento di qualsiasi tessuto molle. Le distorsioni sono suddivise in gradi da 1 a 3, dove *grado 1* significa che alcune fibre sono state lacerate ma senza evidenze di lassità del legamento all'esame obiettivo, *grado 2* indica che si sono lacerate varie fibre (ma non tutte) con una certa lassità del legamento ma con un buon arresto finale e infine *grado 3* implica una lacerazione di tutte le fibre, nella quale l'esame obiettivo dei legamenti determina un arresto finale piuttosto cedevole. Anche gli stiramenti sono suddivisi in gradi da 1 a 3, dove il *grado 1* provoca un dolore lieve all'esame del muscolo e una scarsissima perdita di forza, il *grado 2* causa maggiore dolore e una moderata perdita di forza all'esame del muscolo e il *grado 3* rappresenta una completa rottura del muscolo o del tendine, che determinano una marcata perdita di forza e talvolta un difetto palpabile nel muscolo o nel tendine stessi.

TRAUMI DA STRESS (OVERUSE). Le sindromi da stress, che interessano muscoli, tendini, ossa, borse, cartilagini e nervi, sono causate da microtraumi ripetitivi che superano la capacità di riparazione dell'organismo. I traumi da stress si verificano in tutti gli sport, ma con particolare frequenza in quelli che comportano movimenti ripetitivi (nuoto, corsa, tennis, ginnastica). I fattori possono essere classificati in estrinseci (errori di allenamento, superficie di gioco o equipaggiamento inadeguati) e intrinseci (anatomia o condizioni mediche dell'atleta). L'errore di allenamento è il fattore identificato più spesso. All'inizio del programma di esercizi, gli atleti possono violare la "regola del 10%", cioè aumentare la durata o l'intensità degli esercizi di più del 10% alla settimana. I fattori intrinseci comprendono fattori biomeccanici anormali (differenza di lunghezza degli arti inferiori, pes planus, pes cavus, coalizione tarsale, tallone valgo, torsione tibiale esterna, antiversione femorale), squilibri muscolari, assenza di flessibilità e condizioni mediche (decondizionamento, deficit nutrizionali, amenorrea, obesità). Occorre indagare sulle caratteristiche dell'allenamento e, in particolare, interrogare i corridori su calzature, ortosi, superficie del campo di corsa, su quante miglia percorrono alla settimana o sul tempo che dedicano alla corsa durante la settimana, sugli allenamenti in velocità o in salita, oltre che sui traumi e sulla riabilitazione precedenti. Una volta identificati, i fattori causali possono essere eliminati o modificati in modo che, dopo la riabilitazione, l'atleta non faccia ritorno allo stesso regime di attività subendo così un nuovo trauma.

Per gli atleti impegnati in allenamenti eccessivi che causano lesioni da stress, di solito non è necessario sospendere tutti gli esercizi. È indicato un programma di riabilitazione inteso a velocizzare il ritorno all'attività sportiva riducendo al minimo l'esposizione a una nuova lesione. L'identificazione precoce di un trauma da stress rende necessario introdurre un minor numero di modifiche nel regime di allenamento.

Gli obiettivi del trattamento sono il controllo del dolore e dello spasmo per riabilitare flessibilità, forza, endurance e deficit propriocettivi (Tab. 686-1). In molti traumi da stress, il ruolo dell'infiammazione nel processo è minimo. Nella maggior parte dei traumi tendinei il termine "tendinite" è obsoleto, dal momento che l'infiammazione o non esiste o è di minima entità a livello tendineo, da un punto di vista istopatologico, mentre sono presenti cicatrici e tessuti anomali. Oggi per la maggior parte di queste entità il termine corretto usato è "tendinopatie" e probabilmente i farmaci antinfiammatori hanno un ruolo di secondo piano (ammesso che siano utili) nel trattamento, eccetto che come analgesici.

VALUTAZIONE INIZIALE DELL'ESTREMITÀ TRAUMATIZZATA

Inizialmente, l'esaminatore deve determinare l'entità dei polsi periferici e del tasso di riempimento capillare come anche la funzione motoria e sensitiva macroscopiche per valutare l'entità del danno neurovascolare. La priorità iniziale è il mantenimento della stabilità vascolare e scheletrica.

TABELLA 686-1. Stadiazione dei traumi da stress

GRADO	SINTOMI PER DETERMINARE IL GRADO	TRATTAMENTO
I	Dolore soltanto dopo l'attività Non interferisce con la performance o l'intensità dell'allenamento Dolenzia generalizzata Scompare prima della sessione di allenamento successiva	Modifica dell'attività, considerare cross-training, programma di riabilitazione a domicilio
II	Dolore minimo con l'attività Non interferisce con la performance Dolenzia più localizzata	Modifica dell'attività, cross-training, programma di riabilitazione a domicilio
III	Dolore che interferisce con attività e performance Area di dolorabilità definita Di solito scompare tra una sessione di allenamento e l'altra	Modificazione significativa dell'attività, incoraggiare fortemente il cross-training, programma di riabilitazione a domicilio e fisioterapia ambulatoriale
IV	Dolore con le attività della vita quotidiana Il dolore non scompare tra una sessione di allenamento e l'altra Marcata interferenza con la performance e con l'intensità dell'allenamento	Interrompere temporaneamente l'attività, solo cross-training, analgesici per os, programma di riabilitazione a domicilio e fisioterapia ambulatoriale intensiva
V	Il dolore interferisce con le attività della vita quotidiana Segni di lesioni dei tessuti (per es. edema) Sintomi cronici o ricorrenti	Interruzione prolungata dell'attività, solo cross-training, analgesici orali, programma di riabilitazione domiciliare e fisioterapia ambulatoriale intensiva

I *criteri per un'attenzione immediata e un rapido consulto ortopedico* comprendono la compromissione vascolare, la compromissione nervosa e la frattura aperta. La ferita esposta deve essere ricoperta con garza sterile imbevuta di soluzione fisiologica e l'arto traumatizzato va protetto con un'imbottitura e sostenuto con un tutore. Occorre comprimere qualsiasi sito emorragico. Altri criteri comprendono una lacerazione profonda in corrispondenza di un'articolazione, una lussazione non riducibile, una lacerazione di grado III (completa) di un'unità muscolotendinea e fratture con spostamento e angolazione significativa (dipende dall'osso interessato, dal grado di spostamento e di angolazione e dallo stato neurovascolare dell'estremità).

TRANSIZIONE DAL TRATTAMENTO IMMEDIATO AL RITORNO IN CAMPO

La riabilitazione di un trauma muscoloscheletrico deve iniziare il giorno stesso del trauma.

Fase 1: *Limitare altri danni, controllare edema e dolore e minimizzare le perdite di forza e flessibilità. Per ottenere questi obiettivi si fa ricorso a un apparecchio* appropriato come grucce o a un bendaggio a fionda, ghiaccio, compressione, elevazione e analgesia. Le grucce, staffe (air stirrup) per la distorsione della caviglia, i bendaggi sospensivi per i traumi del braccio e i bendaggi elastici compressivi (12-24 cm circa) sono interventi ragionevoli a livello ambulatoriale. Si pone una borsa del ghiaccio direttamente sulla cute per 20 minuti, 3-4 volte al giorno, fino a risoluzione dell'edema. La compressione limita ulteriormente l'emorragia e l'edema ma non deve essere tanto stretta da ostacolare la perfusione. Il sollevamento dell'estremità favorisce il ritorno venoso e riduce l'edema. Per l'analgesia sono indicati i corticosteroidi o il paracetamolo. Il rinforzo isometrico e gli esercizi per l'arco di movimento non dolorosi devono essere iniziati quanto prima. Il dolore inibisce la completa contrazione muscolare; si ha un decondizionamento se il dolore e l'inattività che ne derivano persistono per un periodo che va da alcuni giorni ad alcune settimane, ritardando la guarigione. È utile fornire al diretto interessato spiegazioni sulla natura del trauma e sulle caratteristiche specifiche degli esercizi di riabilitazione, comprendenti istruzioni scritte e illustrazioni degli esercizi.

Fase 2: *Migliorare la forza e l'arco di movimento (flessibilità) permettendo nel frattempo la guarigione delle strutture traumatizzate.* Si rimuovono gli apparecchi protettivi quando la forza e la flessibilità del paziente migliorano e le attività della vita quotidiana non causano dolore. La flessibilità può quindi essere migliorata da un programma di stretching specifico, mantenuto per 15-20 s per 3-5 ripetizioni, 1-2 volte al giorno. In questo trattamento è utilissimo un fisioterapista o un preparatore atletico. Quando il soggetto scende in campo può aver bisogno di apparecchi protettivi per diversi mesi. Nuoto, water jogging e cyclette sono buoni esercizi anaerobici grazie ai quali è possibile mantenere la fitness cardiovascolare e al tempo stesso consentire all'estremità traumatizzata di riposare o essere utilizzata senza dolore.

Fase 3: *Raggiungere una forza e una flessibilità quasi normali delle strutture lesionate e migliorare ulteriormente o mantenere la fitness cardiovascolare.* Forza ed endurance migliorano dapprima in condizioni controllate con bande elastiche, poi con l'uso di pesi e attrezzi senza limitazioni. L'allenamento propriocettivo permette all'atleta di sviluppare nuovamente un senso cinestesico, di importanza fondamentale per la funzione e la stabilità articolare.

Fase 4: *Ritorno all'attività sportiva, anche agonistica, senza restrizioni.* Quando l'atleta ha raggiunto flessibilità, forza, propriocezione ed endurance quasi normali, può iniziare esercizi sportivi specifici. Il paziente passerà dal programma di riabilitazione alla riabilitazione funzionale appropriata per lo sport. Non è corretto sostituire alla riabilitazione la partecipazione allo sport; piuttosto, vi dovrebbe essere un ritorno funzionale progressivo per gradi a un programma di piena attività/gioco. Per esempio, un giocatore di basket in fase di recupero dopo un trauma alla caviglia potrebbe iniziare un programma di cammino-corsa-sprint prima di fare ritorno alle competizioni. In qualsiasi momento di questa progressione, se compare dolore, l'atleta deve fermarsi, applicare ghiaccio, evitare di correre per 1-2 giorni, continuare gli esercizi per la caviglia e quindi riprendere la corsa a minore intensità, aumentando lo sforzo gradualmente.

LINEE GUIDA PER IL RIPOSO RELATIVO E IL RITORNO ALL'ATTIVITÀ SPORTIVA. "Riposo relativo" significa che l'atleta può fare tutto quello che vuole finché le strutture traumatizzate non causano dolore durante l'attività o nelle 24 ore successive. Allenarsi oltre la soglia del dolore ritarda la guarigione.

DIAGNOSI DIFFERENZIALE DEL DOLORE MUSCOLOSCHELETRICO

Processi traumatici, reumatologici, infettivi, ematologici, psicologici e oncologici possono dare luogo a dolore muscoloscheletrico come disturbo di presentazione. Sintomi come astenia, calo ponderale, rash, disturbi articolari multipli, febbre, malattie croniche o recenti e persistenza del dolore suggeriscono una diagnosi diversa da quella di un trauma correlato allo sport. Un'incongruenza tra storia del paziente ed esame obiettivo deve portare a un'ulteriore valutazione. Una revisione negativa dei sistemi d'organo con una storia di trauma compatibile con i segni e i sintomi fisici suggerisce una causa correlata all'attività sportiva.

Khan KM, Cook JL, Kannua P, et al: Time to abandon the "tendonitis" myth. *Br Med J* 2002;324:626–627.

Sharma P, Maffulli N: Tendon injury and tendinopathy: Healing and repair. *J Bone Joint Surg Am* 2005;87:187–202.

686.1 • TRAUMI DELLA CARTILAGINE DI ACCRESCIMENTO

Il 20% dei traumi sportivi pediatrici osservati al pronto soccorso sono fratture; di queste, il 25% coinvolge una cartilagine di accrescimento (vedi Capitolo 682). La crescita nelle ossa lunghe si verifica in tre aree ed è suscettibile ai traumi. L'osso immaturo può andare incontro a trauma acuto a livello delle cartilagini di accrescimento (fratture di Salter-Harris), superficie articolare (osteocondrite dissecante) o apofisi (fratture da avulsione). I maschi vanno incontro a fratture della cartilagine di accrescimento due volte più spesso delle femmine: la massima incidenza delle fratture è durante il picco della velocità di crescita (femmine 12 ±2,5 anni, maschi 14 ±2 anni). La cartilagine di accrescimento è un'area di crescita da pressione, responsabile della crescita ossea longitudinale. L'apofisi, una sporgenza ossea in corrispondenza di un'inserzione tendinea, è invece un'area di crescita da trazione. L'epifisi è l'estremità di un osso lungo, distale o prossimale rispetto all'osso lungo, e contiene cartilagine articolare a livello dell'articolazione.

I traumi più comuni che interessano le **cartilagini di accrescimento** sono quelli a livello del radio distale, seguiti dalle fratture falangee e tibiali distali. Il 94% delle fratture dell'avambraccio da skateboard, pattini in linea e ciclomotore coinvolge il radio distale. I traumi della cartilagine di accrescimento a livello del ginocchio (femore distale, tibia prossimale) sono rari. Un'alterazione della crescita in seguito a un trauma della cartilagine di accrescimento è in funzione della sede e della parte della cartilagine di accrescimento coinvolta. Questi fattori incidono sulla probabilità che si formi una barra a livello della cartilagine di accrescimento, portando all'arresto della crescita a questo livello. Le aree che contribuiscono maggiormente alla crescita longitudinale delle estremità superiori sono l'omero prossimale e il radio/ulna distale; nelle estremità inferiori, sono il femore distale e la tibia/perone prossimale. I traumi di queste aree hanno una maggiore probabilità di causare disturbi della crescita rispetto ai traumi delle cartilagini di accrescimento all'estremità opposta di queste ossa lunghe. Il tipo di frattura della cartilagine di accrescimento relativo al rischio di disturbo della crescita è descritto dal sistema di classificazione di Salter-Harris (vedi Tab. 686-1). Un trauma di grado I ha una minore probabilità di portare a un disturbo della crescita e il grado V è il tipo di frattura che ha maggiore probabilità di causare un disturbo della crescita.

L'**osteocondrite dissecante** (OCD) interessa l'osso subcondrale e la superficie articolare sovrastante. Con la necrosi avascolare dell'osso subcondrale, la superficie articolare può appiattirsi, rammollirsi o frammentarsi. L'eziologia è sconosciuta, ma può essere correlata a un trauma da stress ripetitivo in alcuni pazienti. nei bambini e negli adolescenti; il 51% delle lesioni si verifica sull'aspetto laterale del condilo femorale mediale, il 17% sul condilo laterale e il 7% sulla rotula. Un interessamento bilaterale è riportato nel 13-30% dei casi. Altre articolazioni in cui si osserva spesso un'OCD sono la caviglia (astragalo), il gomito (di solito con interessamento del capitello) e la testa del radio. L'OCD classicamente colpisce gli atleti nel 2° decennio di vita. La presentazione più comune è un dolore del ginocchio poco localizzato. Raramente è presente una storia di trauma acuto recente. Alcune lesioni da OCD sono asintomatiche (diagnosticate alle radiografie di routine), mentre altre si manifestano con dolore da versamento articolare, riduzione del range di movimento e sintomi meccanici (blocco, crepitio, schiocco). L'attività di solito esacerba il dolore.

L'esame obiettivo può non evidenziare alcun segno specifico. Talvolta è possibile suscitare dolore a livello del condilo interessato mediante palpazione profonda con il ginocchio flesso. La diagnosi si pone generalmente con le radiografie (Fig. 686-1). Si deve eseguire una radiografia con proiezione a tunnel per una migliore visualizzazione dei due terzi posteriori del condilo femorale. I pazienti con OCD vanno inviati al chirurgo ortopedico per un'ulteriore valutazione.

Le **fratture da avulsione** si verificano quando una contrazione muscolare forzata distacca l'apofisi dall'osso e sono più

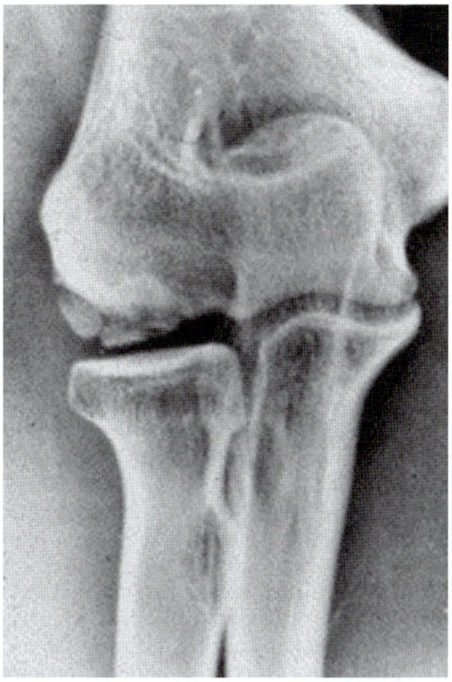

Figura 681-1. Osteocondrite dissecante, gomito. (Da SJ: Sports injuries. *Curr Prob Pediatr Adolesc Health* 2005;35:105-176.)

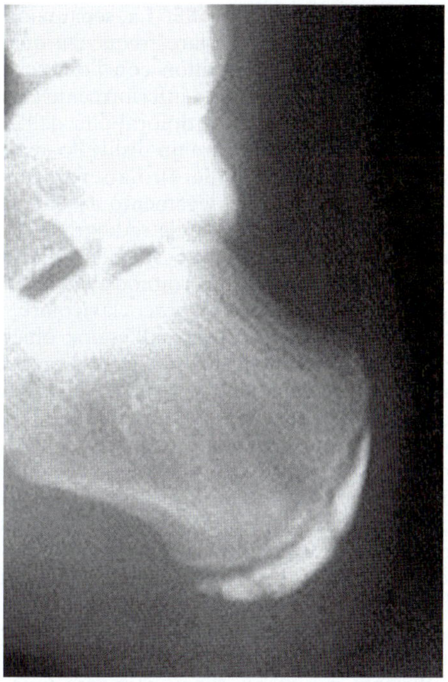

Figura 686-3. Apofisite calcaneare (malattia di Sever). (Da Anderson SJ: Sports injuries. *Curr Prob Pediatr Adolesc Health* 2005;35:105-176.)

frequenti intorno all'anca (Fig. 686-2). Un aumento cronico della trazione a livello dell'inserzione tra muscolo e apofisi può causare un microtrauma ripetitivo e dolore a livello dell'apofisi. Le aree più comunemente interessate sono il ginocchio (malattia di Osgood-Schlatter e malattia di Sindig-Larsen), la caviglia (malattia di Sever) (Fig. 686-3) e l'epicondilo mediale (gomito della Little League). L'apofisite da trazione del ginocchio e della caviglia sono potenzialmente trattabili nell'ambito delle cure primarie. L'obiettivo principale del trattamento è ridurre al minimo tanto l'intensità quanto la frequenza del dolore e

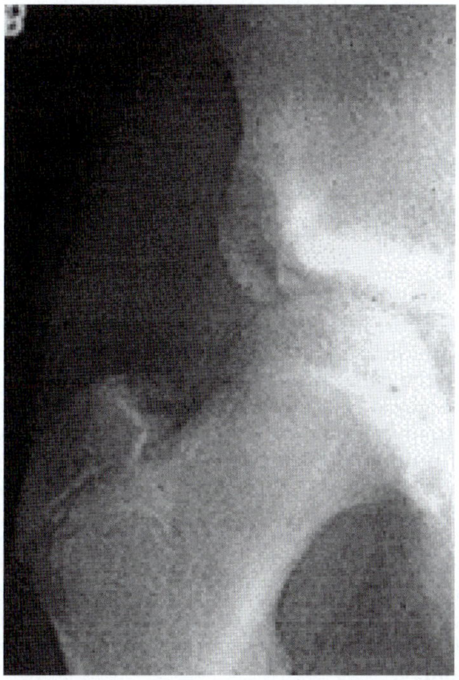

Figura 686-2. Avulsione della spina iliaca anteroinferiore. (Da Anderson SJ: Lower extremity injuries in youth sports. *Pediatr Clin North Am* 2003;49:627-641).

della disabilità. Sono appropriati gli esercizi che aumentano la forza, la flessibilità e la resistenza dei muscoli inseriti sull'apofisi utilizzando il principio del riposo relativo. I sintomi possono durare per 12-24 mesi se non trattati e scompaiono con il rallentamento della crescita.

Wall E, Von Stein D: Juvenile osteochondritis dissecans. *Orthop Clin North Am* 2003;34:341–353.

Zalavras C, Nikolopoulou G, Essin D, et al: Pediatric fractures during skateboarding, roller skating, and scooter riding. *Am J Sports Med* 2005;33:568–573.

686.2 • Traumi della spalla

Il dolore della spalla associato a sintomi irradiati lungo il braccio deve suggerire la possibilità di un concomitante trauma del collo. Il dolore cervicale e il dolore o la limitazione dell'arco di movimento a livello cervicale rendono necessari l'immobilizzazione della colonna cervicale e il trasferimento dell'atleta per un'ulteriore valutazione. Se non sono presenti dolore cervicale, dolorabilità o limitazione del movimento della colonna cervicale, la spalla è la sede del trauma primitivo.

FRATTURE DI CLAVICOLA

Uno dei più comuni traumi della spalla è una frattura di clavicola, che di solito si verifica per caduta sulla parte laterale della spalla, su una mano sporta in fuori o per trauma diretto. L'80% delle fratture interessa il terzo medio della clavicola; in tal caso il trattamento consiste nell'uso di una fionda per il braccio. Le fratture del terzo mediale e laterale senza spostamento sono di solito trattate conservativamente. Se vi è spostamento, le fratture del terzo mediale e laterale richiedono un consulto ortopedico in quanto comportano una più elevata incidenza di osteoartrosi acromioclavicolare (laterale) e di interessamento della cartilagine di accrescimento (mediale).

SEPARAZIONE ACROMIOCLAVICOLARE. La separazione acromioclavicolare si verifica con particolare frequenza quando l'atleta subisce un colpo diretto all'acromion con l'omero in posizione addotta, colpo che forza l'acromion inferiormente e medialmente. I pazienti presentano una discreta dolorabilità dell'articolazione acromioclavicolare e possono avere un dislivello evidente tra clavicola distale e acromion (Fig. 686-4). La separazione acromioclavicolare di **tipo I** coinvolge il legamento acromioclavicolare e non è associata a deformità visibile; le radiografie sono normali. La manovra di incrociare il braccio sul petto causa un dolore acuto a livello dell'articolazione acromioclavicolare. Nei traumi di **tipo II**, a carico del legamento coracoclavicolare, la clavicola distale appare un po' più sporgente all'esame obiettivo, ma le radiografie sono di solito normali (può essere presente un lieve allargamento dell'articolazione acromioclavicolare). I traumi di tipo I e tipo II sono trattati in modo conservativo. Per il controllo del dolore sono utili un bendaggio in sospensione e analgesici. Non appena il dolore è sotto controllo, si iniziano esercizi per l'arco di movimento. Con il miglioramento dell'arco di movimento senza dolore si possono iniziare gli esercizi di rinforzo dei muscoli di cuffia dei rotatori, deltoide e trapezio. Il tempo di norma richiesto per il ritorno all'attività sportiva è di 1-2 settimane per il tipo I e di 2-4 settimane per il tipo II. Il ritorno in campo è possibile quando l'articolazione acromioclavicolare non è dolente, la spalla ha un range di movimento del tutto normale e il paziente ha forza sufficiente per essere funzionalmente protetto da una collisione o da una caduta ed eseguire le manovre necessarie per lo sport. Nei traumi di **tipo III** la lacerazione legamentosa è più severa, con distacco della fascia trapezio-deltoidea dalla clavicola distale. Tali traumi vanno trattati chirurgicamente soltanto in rari casi e per lo più per motivi estetici. La maggior parte può essere gestita come i traumi acromioclavicolari di tipo I e II. Nei **tipi IV, V** e **VI** vi è un peggioramento progressivo della lacerazione legamentosa e fasciale, con spostamento clavicolare sempre più accentuato. Fortunatamente, questi traumi sono rari, anche se richiedono la riparazione chirurgica. Se è presente una frattura d'omero, in corrispondenza della frattura si riscontra dolorabilità a punto. Se si percepisce un crepitio, è necessario immobilizzare il braccio in un bendaggio a sospensione e trasferire il paziente in un reparto d'emergenza.

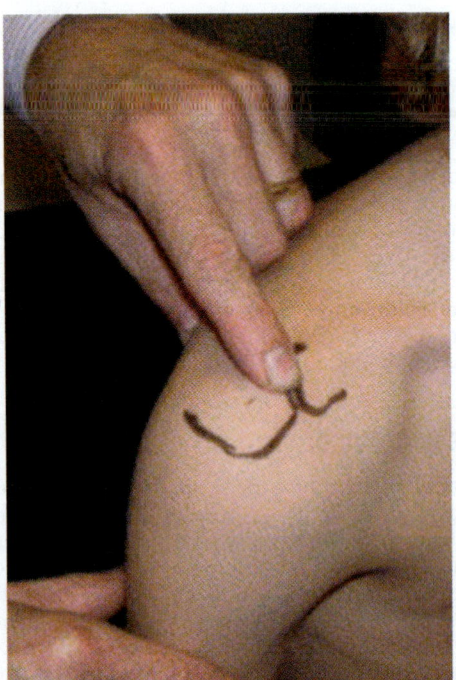

Figura 686-4. Palpazione dell'articolazione acromioclavicolare. (Da Anderson SJ: Sports injuries. *Curr Prob Pediatr Adolesc Health* 2005;35:105-176.)

LUSSAZIONE ANTERIORE

I comuni meccanismi traumatici sono la caduta su una mano stesa con il braccio diritto o il contatto con un altro giocatore con la spalla abdotta a 90° e ruotata forzatamente all'esterno. Un esempio dell'ultimo meccanismo è un giocatore di football americano che placca l'avversario soltanto con il braccio. I pazienti lamentano un dolore severo e riferiscono che la spalla è "uscita dalla sua sede" o si è "spostata". I pazienti con lussazione anteriore non ridotta presentano un'area infossata al di sotto dell'acromion e una sporgenza nella porzione anteriore della spalla, causata dallo spostamento anteriore della testa dell'omero. Occorre valutare la presenza di una sensibilità anormale della regione deltoidea laterale (nervo ascellare) e della superficie estensoria dell'avambraccio prossimale (nervo muscolocutaneo), e la capacità di contrarre la parte media del deltoide (abduzione contro resistenza) e il bicipite isometricamente. È indicato un tentativo di ridurre la lussazione anteriore, se non è presente crepitio. Una volta ridotta la lussazione, se le radiografie evidenziano una posizione normale, si suggerisce l'immobilizzazione per una settimana circa. Il periodo di immobilizzazione è controverso, ma la maggior parte dei medici dello sport ritiene importanti gli esercizi per l'arco di movimento e di rinforzo. Con il rafforzamento dei muscoli della cuffia dei rotatori, un rinforzo progressivo si verifica con gradi maggiori di abduzione e rotazione esterna. I pazienti possono fare ritorno all'attività sportiva quando forza, flessibilità e propriocezione sono uguali a quelle del lato non interessato, risultato che permette loro di proteggere la spalla ed eseguire le attività sportive specifiche senza dolore. Nella maggior parte dei casi la chirurgia non è raccomandata, a meno che la spalla non si sia lussata almeno tre volte. Una riparazione precoce può essere presa in considerazione per gli atleti che praticano sport di collisione ad alto rischio che comportano un tasso di recidive molto elevato.

TRAUMA DELLA CUFFIA DEI ROTATORI

La cuffia dei rotatori è formata dai muscoli sopraspinato, sottospinato, piccolo rotondo e sottoscapolare. Il muscolo sopraspinato è quello più frequentemente traumatizzato. La *tendinopatia della cuffia dei rotatori* si manifesta come dolore della spalla all'acme dell'arco di movimento. Tale dolore è di solito poco localizzato e può essere riferito all'area del deltoide. Dopo un esordio talvolta, insidioso, peggiora con l'attività ma spesso è presente a riposo, anche di notte. L'esame della forza dei muscoli della cuffia produce dolore e può dimostrare una certa perdita di forza rispetto alla spalla non traumatizzata. La tendinopatia del sopraspinato produce dolore all'abduzione attiva nella posizione del "barattolo vuoto" in cui il paziente abduce il braccio a 90°, lo flette in avanti a 30 gradi anteriormente al piano sagittale e ruota internamente l'omero. Il **trattamento** comprende ghiaccio, una modifica della tecnica, riposo, stretching, rinforzo della cuffia dei rotatori e dei muscoli superiori del dorso, fisioterapia e analgesici. La prevenzione comprende l'astensione da sforzi eccessivi, una tecnica appropriata e rinforzo ed esercizi di stretching. Talvolta, questa patologia è denominata *sindrome da compressione della cuffia dei rotatori* negli adulti, a causa della compressione della cuffia da parte delle strutture ossee poste superiormente rispetto a essa. Il dolore della cuffia dei rotatori nei giovani atleti è quasi sempre secondario a instabilità gleno-omerale. Il solo stretching può peggiorare il dolore e l'aspetto più importante della riabilitazione è il rinforzo dei muscoli della cuffia.

Le lacerazione del labrum glenoideo può presentare analogie con una tendinopatia della cuffia dei rotatori. Una delle lesioni più comuni, chiamata lesione **SLAP** (*Superior Labrum Anterior and Posterior*), è difficile da diagnosticare clinicamente. Un dolore della spalla che si accompagna a click o *catching* è sospetto per una lacerazione del labrum. Le radiografie sono di solito normali. L'artrografia RM è l'esame preferibile per la visualizzazione di queste lesioni.

La *frattura da stress dell'omero prossimale* (epifisiolisi), una rara causa di dolore della spalla prossimale, si sospetta quando il dolore della spalla non risponde alle misure di routine. Un esordio graduale di dolore profondo della spalla si verifica nel giovane (cartilagini di accrescimento epifisarie aperte) atleta che esegue movimenti ripetitivi al di sopra della testa, come nel baseball o nel tennis, ma senza storia di un trauma. A livello dell'omero prossimale si nota la presenza di dolore; la diagnosi è confermata dal riscontro di una cartilagine di accrescimento epifisaria allargata a livello radiografico, di un aumento della captazione alla scintigrafia o di un edema della cartilagine di accrescimento alla RM. Il trattamento consiste nel riposo a partire dal momento del trauma per 6-8 settimane.

Bradley JP, Elkousy H: Decision-making: Operative versus nonoperative treatment of acromioclavicular joint injuries. *Clin Sports Med* 2003;2:277–290.
Luime JJ, Verhagen AP, Miedema HS, et al: Does this patient have an instability of the shoulder or a labrum lesion? *JAMA* 2004;292:1989–1998.
Wasserlauf BL, Paletta GA Jr: Shoulder disorders in the skeletally immature throwing athlete. Orthop Clin North Am 2003;34:427–437.

686.3 • Traumi del gomito

TRAUMI ACUTI

La più comune lussazione di gomito è quella posteriore. Il meccanismo traumatico è la caduta all'indietro sul braccio sporto in fuori con il gomito esteso. La lussazione ha la prerogativa potenziale di compromettere l'arteria brachiale. La presenza di un polso radiale e ulnare normale è il migliore indicatore di integrità vascolare dell'estremità superiore distale. Si nota un'evidente deformità, con l'olecrano marcatamente spostato dietro l'omero distale. La riduzione si esegue esercitando una lieve trazione longitudinale all'avambraccio, accompagnata da una delicata pressione verso l'alto sull'omero distale. Se la riduzione non è possibile, il braccio deve essere protetto con una fasciatura e posto in un bendaggio in sospensione e il paziente deve essere trasportato in un reparto d'emergenza. I traumi del gomito possono compromettere i nervi radiale, mediano e ulnare.

Le *fratture omerali sovracondiloidee* possono derivare dallo stesso meccanismo traumatico delle lussazioni di gomito ed essere complicate da un trauma concomitante dell'arteria brachiale e, in misura minore, dei nervi mediano, radiale e ulnare. Dopo queste fratture può svilupparsi una sindrome compartimentale acuta (Fig. 686-5).

Un trauma del gomito può causare emorragia della borsa olecranica risultando in una *borsite olecranica*, la quale raramente richiede l'aspirazione e può essere trattata con ghiaccio, analgesia e bendaggi compressivi. Un'imbottitura adeguata, oltre a essere confortevole, è utile per la prevenzione di nuovi traumi.

FRATTURE CRONICHE

Le fratture da stress si verificano principalmente negli sport di lancio e in quelli che richiedono una flessione o un'estensione ripetitiva del polso oppure un carico del peso sulle mani (ginnastica). "Gomito della Little League" è l'espressione generica con cui si indicano problemi differenti del gomito.

Il lancio di un oggetto a un'altezza superiore a quella della spalla crea uno stress in vago del gomito con apertura mediale dell'articolazione e forze compressive laterali.

Il dolore mediale del gomito è un disturbo comune dei giovani lanciatori a causa del sovraccarico ripetitivo in valgo dei gruppi muscolari flessori/pronatori del polso e delle loro inserzioni sull'apofisi mediale. Nei preadolescenti, i cui centri di ossificazione secondaria sono in via di maturazione, è probabile un'*apofisite da trazione dell'epicondilo mediale*. I pazienti presentano dolore lungo l'epicondilo mediale, esacerbato dallo stress in valgo o dalla flessione e pronazione del polso contro resistenza. Il trattamento comprende l'astensione dai lanci per 4-6 settimane, esercizi di rinforzo non dolorosi e stretching del gruppo dei flessori/pronatori, seguiti da 1-2 settimane di un programma funzionale progressivo di lanci con riabilitazione accelerata. Questo problema deve essere trattato con il riposo a causa del rischio di mancato consolidamento dell'apofisi e di dolore cronico. Se si verifica un dolore acuto, bisogna prendere in esame la possibilità di una *frattura da avulsione dell'epicondilo mediale*. Occorre eseguire radiografie in qualsiasi lanciatore con dolore acuto del gomito (Fig. 686-6). Se l'epicondilo mediale è avulso, è indicata una consulenza ortopedica. Negli adolescenti più grandi e nei giovani adulti con l'apofisi fusa, la struttura vulnerabile è il *legamento collaterale ulnare* (UCL, *Ulnar Collateral Ligament*); le lacerazioni dell'UCL si osservano di solito nei lanciatori di baseball (*pitcher*), ma sono riscontrabili in qualsiasi sport di lancio. Si può apprezzare una lassità allo stress in valgo del gomito flesso a 30°. Spesso sono necessarie una RM o un'ecografia per valutare l'integrità dell'UCL. In presenza di una lacerazione completa, è indicata la riparazione chirurgica se l'atleta vuole continuare la sua carriera di pitcher. La disfunzione del nervo ulnare può essere una complicanza del sovraccarico in valgo, che si verifica in seguito a tutte le patologie precedentemente discusse.

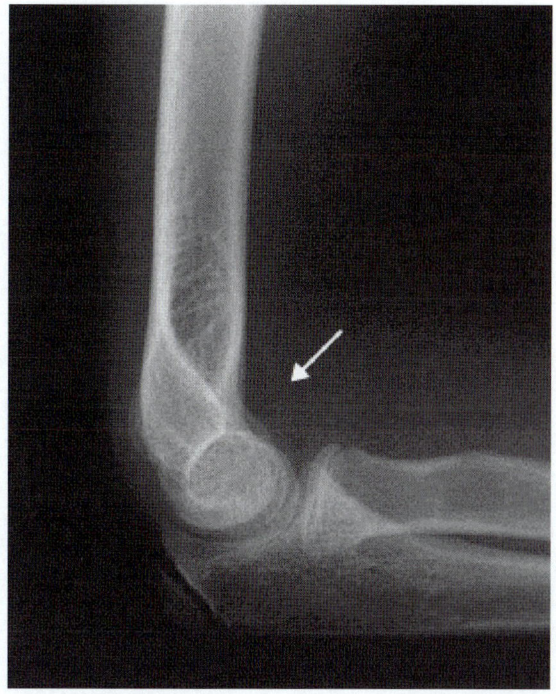

Figura 686-5. Deflessione del cuscinetto adiposo coronoideo con versamento articolare (segno del cuscinetto adiposo) che evidenzia una frattura. (Da Gomez JE: Upper extremity injuries in youth sports. *Pediatr Clin N Am* 2002;49:593-626.)

Il dolore della parte laterale del gomito può essere causato dalla compressione durante il movimento di lancio a livello dell'articolazione tra radio e capitello. La *malattia di Panner* è un'osteocondrosi del capitello che si presenta tra i 7 e i 12 anni (Fig. 686-7), mentre l'*OCD* del capitello esordisce all'età di 13-16 anni (vedi Fig. 686-1). Queste due entità possono rappresentare un continuum della stessa malattia. Anche se i pazienti con entrambe le condizioni si presentano con un esordio insidioso di dolore laterale del gomito esacerbato dai movimenti di lancio, i pazienti con OCD presentano sintomi meccanici (blocco, scatto) e, più frequentemente, una riduzione dell'arco di movimento. Per contro, i pazienti con malattia di Panner non presentano sintomi meccanici e spesso hanno un arco di movimento normale. La prognosi della malattia di Panner è ottima e il trattamento con-

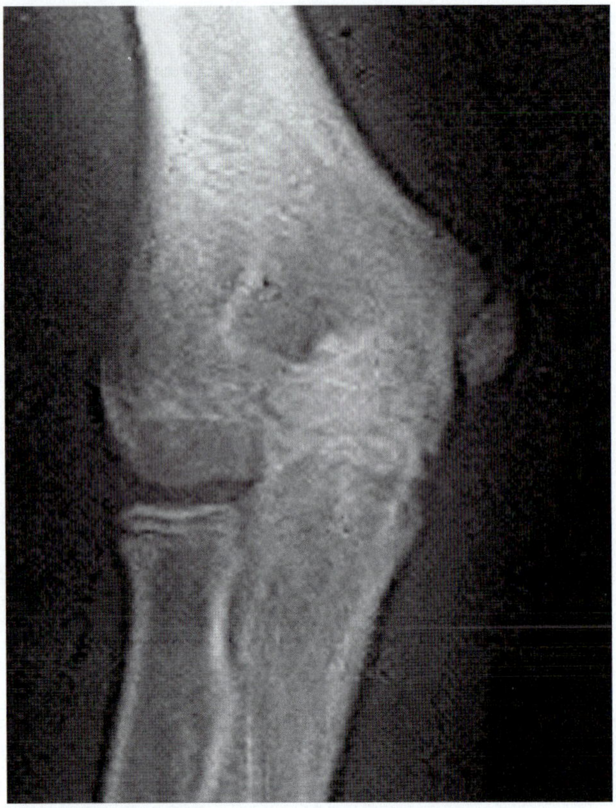

Figura 686-6. Epicondilite mediale. (Da Anderson SJ: Sports injuries. *Curr Prob Pediatr Adolesc Health* 2005;35:105-176.)

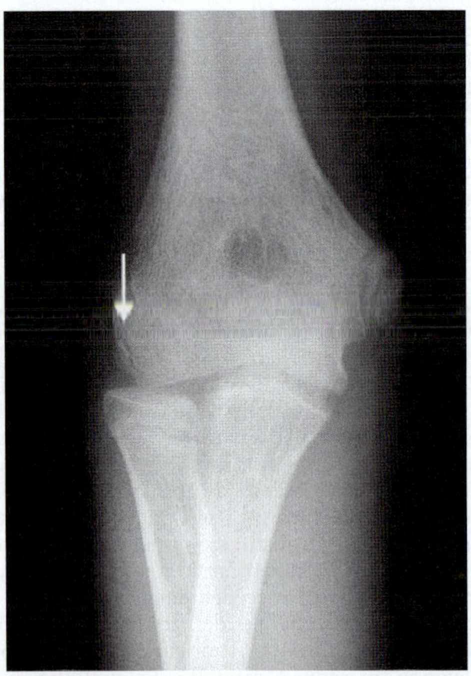

Figura 686-7. Malattia di Panner. Si notino la frammentazione del capitello omerale e l'appiattimento della superficie articolare (*freccia*). (Per gentile concessione di Ralph J. Curtis, MD. Da Gomez JE: Upper extremity injuries in youth sports. *Pediatr Clin N Am* 2002;49:593-626.)

siste i riposo relativo (senza lanci), una breve immobilizzazione e ripetute radiografie, eseguite nell'arco di 6-12 settimane, per valutare il rimodellamento osseo. L'OCD richiede una consulenza ortopedica.

L'*epicondilite laterale*, o "gomito del tennista", è la più comune lesione da stress del gomito nell'adulto, mentre è rara nei bambini e negli adolescenti. Si tratta di una tendinopatia dell'inserzione dei muscoli estensori sull'epicondilo laterale. Il dolore è elicitabile sull'epicondilo laterale e si percepisce alla flessione passiva del polso e all'estensione del polso contro resistenza. Il trattamento comprende riposo relativo, analgesia ed esercizi specifici di stretching e rinforzo. La riabilitazione funzionale, come il ritorno al tennis, deve essere graduale e progressiva.

I traumi del gomito non possono essere prevenuti da esercizi di rinforzo e di stretching prestagionali. Per la prevenzione dei traumi del gomito nei lanciatori le due misure più importanti sono limitare il numero di lanci e raccomandare ad atleti, allenatori e giocatori di fermarsi immediatamente non appena provano dolore al gomito. Se il dolore persiste, è necessaria una valutazione medica. È stato raccomandato che un giovante pitcher ogni settimana non esegua più di 200 lanci e non partecipi a più di due gare; il numero massimo di lanci per gara deve essere pari all'età del pitcher espressa in anni moltiplicata per 6.

Altri problemi meno comuni che causano dolore del gomito sono la neuropatia ulnare, la tendinite tricipitale e l'apofisite dell'olecrano, oltre ai corpi liberi intrarticolari.

Assendelft W, Green S, Buchbinder R, et al: Tennis elbow. *Br Med J* 2003; 327:329–330.

Petty DH, Andrews JR, Fleisig GS, Cain EL: Ulnar collateral ligament reconstruction in high school baseball players: Clinical results and injury risk factors. *Am J Sports Med* 2004;32:1158–1164.

686.4 • Traumi della regione lombare

La **spondilolisi**, una causa comune di lombalgia negli atleti, è una frattura da stress della pars interarticularis (vedi Capitolo 678.6). Si può verificare a qualsiasi livello vertebrale ma è più frequente a L4 o L5. L'incidenza negli atleti adolescenti valutati per lombalgia è del 13-47%. Oltre all'iperestensione acuta, che provoca una frattura acuta, il meccanismo traumatico è un difetto congenito o un'ipoplasia della pars, che viene esacerbata dal carico in estensione lombare o da una frattura da stress imputabile a un carico ripetitivo in estensione. La danza classica, il sollevamento pesi, la ginnastica e il football americano sono esempi di attività fisiche che comportano un carico ripetitivo in estensione della colonna lombare; si può verificare in qualsiasi attività in cui vi è un carico ripetitivo in estensione, compreso il nuoto. I pazienti spesso si presentano con dolore a esordio insidioso; tuttavia, vi può essere un trauma precipitante come una caduta o un singolo episodio di iperestensione. Il dolore peggiora con l'estensione, può irradiarsi alle natiche e finire per influire negativamente sulle attività della vita quotidiana. Il riposo o la posizione supina di solito alleviano il dolore. All'esame obiettivo, il dolore è riprodotto con l'estensione lombare in posizione eretta, specialmente se si sta in piedi su una gamba sola (test in iperestensione su una gamba sola). Si possono osservare una limitazione della flessione in avanti della colonna e una tensione dei muscoli posteriore della coscia. L'esame neurologico deve essere normale. È presente dolore ben localizzato alla palpazione profonda appena lateralmente al processo spinoso dal lato affetto, di solito a livello di L4 o L5. La diagnosi è confermata dal riscontro di un difetto della pars alla radiografia obliqua della colonna lombare, difetto che si osserva raramente nelle proiezioni anteroposteriore e laterale. La SPECT ossea è necessaria per la conferma diagnostica se le radiografie sono normali. Una TC senza contrasto può essere utile per identificare il grado di interessamento osseo e talvolta viene utilizzata per valutare la guarigione. Il **trattamento** comprende antidolorifici e restrizione dell'attività; inoltre, nella maggior parte dei casi è importante la riabilitazione, che consiste in esercizi di rinforzo per il tronco, stretching dei flessori dell'anca e stretching dei muscoli posteriori della coscia. L'uso di un'ortosi antilordotica è controverso e probabilmente più efficace per la spondilolisi associata a frattura da stress. Si instaura una *spondilolistesi* quando sono presenti difetti bilaterali della pars e si verifica uno spostamento o scivolamento in avanti di una vertebra rispetto alla vertebra sottostante (vedi Capitolo 678.6).

La *sindrome delle faccette* presenta la stessa anamnesi e lo stesso esame obiettivo della spondilolisi, essendo causata da instabilità o trauma delle faccette articolari, posteriormente alla pars interarticularis e all'interfaccia tra processi articolari superiori e inferiori. La diagnosi può essere stabilita identificando le anomalie delle faccette alla TC o per esclusione, eseguendo una radiografia e una scintigrafia non diagnostiche per escludere una spondilolisi.

Spondilolisi, spondilolistesi e sindrome delle faccette sono lesioni posteriori rispetto ai corpi vertebrali. Il **trattamento** delle lesioni degli elementi posteriori è conservativo, volto alla riduzione dell'attività di carico in estensione, spesso per 2-3 mesi. Camminare, nuotare e andare in bicicletta sono esercizi consigliati durante la riabilitazione.

L'**ernia del disco lombare** si presenta come lombalgia che peggiora alla flessione in avanti, alla flessione laterale e con una prolungata posizione seduta, specialmente in automobile. Rispetto agli adulti, nei bambini e negli adolescenti ha minori probabilità di produrre una sciatalgia (vedi Capitolo 678.8). L'esame obiettivo talvolta mette in luce segni minimi, ma che possono comprendere un test di sollevamento della gamba tesa positivo, dolore alla flessione in avanti ed eventualmente una riduzione della forza, della sensibilità o dei riflessi osteotendinei profondi a livello della gamba. Vi può essere dolorabilità dei processi spinosi vertebrali a livello del disco. La RM di solito conferma la diagnosi clinica. Se l'ernia non è massiva e il dolore non è intrattabile, il trattamento di scelta è l'analgesia e la fisioterapia. Raramente sono necessari riposo a letto o un intervento chirurgico.

Uno **stiramento** o una **contusione lombare acuta** si presentano dopo un evento precipitante. L'esame obiettivo rivela una dolenzia diffusa laterale rispetto alla colonna. Il **trattamento** comprende analgesici, massaggi e fisioterapia, secondo tolleranza. Dalla storia naturale dello stiramento lombare acuto negli adulti si desume che il 50% dei pazienti migliora in una settimana, l'80% in un mese e il 90% in due mesi, indipendentemente dalla terapia. È probabile che il decorso della lombalgia nei giovani atleti sia simile.

La **sacroileite** si presenta con un dolore lombare di solito cronico, ma occasionalmente associato a una storia di trauma. Il **test di Patrick**, che consiste nel porre il piede dal lato affetto sul ginocchio del lato opposto (anca flessa a 90°), stabilizzare la cresta iliaca del lato opposto e ruotare esternamente l'anca sul lato affetto (spingendo il ginocchio in basso e lateralmente), di solito è positivo. È indicata una radiografia delle articolazioni sacroiliache e, se i risultati sono positivi, occorre ricercare una patologia reumatologica (spondilite anchilosante, artrite reumatoide giovanile, colite ulcerosa). Il **trattamento** consiste nel riposo relativo, nella somministrazione di FANS e nella fisioterapia. La spondilite anchilosante è più probabile se l'esordio della lombalgia è avvenuto prima dei 40 anni, se vi è rigidità mattutina che migliora con l'attività e se il dolore ha un esordio graduale e dura da meno di 3 mesi.

Altre cause di lombalgia, ossia infezioni (osteomielite, discite) e neoplasie, devono essere prese in considerazione nei pazienti con febbre, calo ponderale, altri segni costituzionali o una mancata risposta alla terapia iniziale. L'osteomielite dell'area lombare o del bacino è spesso, ma non sempre, associata a febbre.

Jones GT, Macfarlane GJ: Epidemiology of low back pain in children and adolescents. *Arch Dis Child* 2005;90:312–316.

686.5 • Traumi di anca e bacino

I traumi di anca e bacino rappresentano una piccola percentuale dei traumi sportivi, ma possono essere severi e richiedono una diagnosi immediata. La patologia dell'anca può manifestarsi con dolore al ginocchio nonostante un esame obiettivo normale.

Nei bambini, la causa più comune è la *sinovite transitoria*, la quale di solito si presenta con l'esordio acuto di zoppia, con il bambino che rifiuta di usare la gamba colpita e con dolore all'arco di movimento all'esame obiettivo. Vi può essere una storia di trauma minore. Si tratta di una condizione autolimitante che di solito si risolve in 48-72 ore.

Anche la *malattia di Legg-Calvé-Perthes* (necrosi avascolare della testa del femore) si presenta durante l'infanzia con un esordio insidioso di zoppia e dolore dell'anca (vedi Capitolo 677.3).

Fino alla maturazione dello scheletro, gli atleti più giovani vanno soggetti ai traumi ipofisari (per es. la spina iliaca anterosuperiore). Un'*apofisite* deriva da uso eccessivo o da trauma diretto. Le *fratture da avulsione* si verificano in adolescenti che praticano sport che richiedono improvvisi ed esplosivi scatti di velocità (Fig. 686-8); i grandi muscoli si contraggono e producono una forza maggiore rispetto a quella dell'inserzione muscolare sull'apofisi. Le sedi più comuni di fratture da avulsione (e i relativi muscoli inseriti) sono la spina iliaca anterosuperiore (sartorio), la spina iliaca anteroinferiore (retto femorale), il piccolo trocantere (ileopsoas) e la tuberosità ischiatica (muscoli posteriori della coscia). I sintomi comprendono tumefazione e dolore localizzati, con una riduzione della forza e dell'arco di movimento. È necessario uno studio radiografico. Il **trattamento** iniziale comprende ghiaccio, analgesici, riposo ed esercizi per l'arco di movimento non dolorosi. Per la deambulazione sono di solito necessarie le grucce. Di solito non è indicato un intervento chirurgico, considerato che queste fratture, anche se ampie o con spostamento, guariscono bene nella maggior parte dei casi. Il contatto con l'osso intorno ad anca e bacino provoca ematomi sottoperiostei dolorosi, chiamati *hip pointer*. Il trattamento sintomatico consiste in riposo, applicazione di ghiaccio, analgesici e protezione da nuovi traumi.

L'*epifisiolisi della testa del femore* si presenta di solito nella fascia di età dagli 11 ai 15 anni, durante il periodo di rapida crescita lineare ossea (vedi Capitolo 677.4).

Una *frattura da stress del collo del femore* può presentarsi con un vago dolore progressivo dell'anca in un atleta che pratica uno sport di resistenza. Le ragazze con la triade dell'atleta femmina sono particolarmente a rischio. La diagnosi deve sempre essere tenuta presente nell'atleta che corre e che presenta un vago dolore

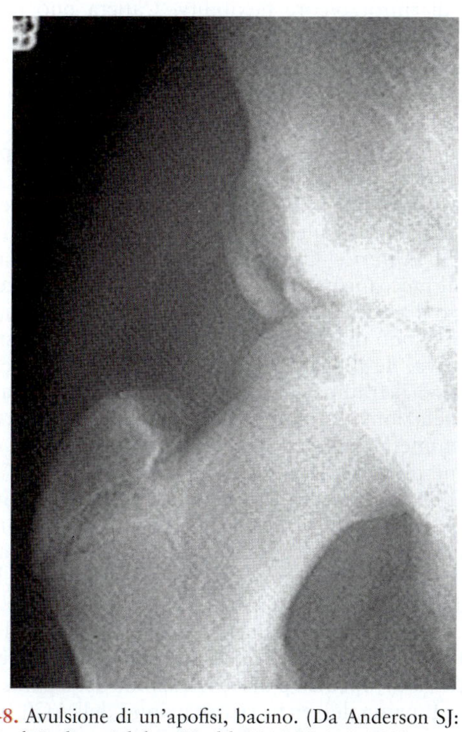

Figura 686-8. Avulsione di un'apofisi, bacino. (Da Anderson SJ: Sports injuries. *Curr Prob Pediatr Adolesc Health* 2005;35:105-176.)

della parte anteriore della coscia. All'esame obiettivo il dolore può essere suscitato dalla distensione passiva dei flessori dell'anca e dalla rotazione dell'anca. Se le radiografie non dimostrano una reazione periostea compatibile con una frattura da stress, possono essere necessarie una scintigrafia ossea o una RM. Occorre richiedere una consulenza ortopedica nelle fratture da stress del collo del femore, a causa della loro predisposizione alla mancato consolidamento e allo spostamento in seguito a un trauma minore o alla prosecuzione del carico. Queste fratture comportano un rischio aumentato di necrosi avascolare della testa del femore.

L'*osteitis pubis* è un'infiammazione della sinfisi pubica che può essere causata da un eccessivo movimento di va e vieni laterale del bacino. Anche se si può osservare in chi pratica qualunque sport che comporti la corsa, è più comune negli sport che richiedono un maggiore uso dei muscoli adduttori, come hockey, calcio e rollerblade. Gli atleti si presentano caratteristicamente con un vago dolore inguinale che può essere uni- o bilaterale. All'esame obiettivo è presente dolorabilità in corrispondenza della sinfisi e talvolta sugli adduttori prossimali. Il test di valutazione della forza dell'adduzione provoca fastidio. Prima che si riscontrino evidenze radiografiche (irregolarità, sclerosi, allargamento della sinfisi pubica con osteolisi) possono passare anche 6-8 settimane dalla comparsa dei sintomi; scintigrafia ossea e RM sono più sensibili per le alterazioni precoci. Può essere necessario il riposo relativo per 6-12 settimane. Alcuni pazienti richiedono l'iniezione di corticosteroidi come terapia aggiuntiva.

Possono verificarsi *lacerazioni del labrum acetabolare* a livello dell'anca, analoghe alle lacerazioni del labrum glenoideo nella spalla. Gli atleti possono avere una storia di trauma e lamentare un dolore intenso a livello della parte anteriore dell'anca, associato a una sensazione di click o catching. La diagnosi clinica è difficile; l'artrografia RM è utile per la diagnosi.

La *sindrome dell'anca a scatto* è causata dal tendine del muscolo ileopsoas, che passa al di sopra della parte anteriore della capsula articolare dell'anca, o dall'ITB, che passa sopra il grande trocantere. Comune nei ballerini e nei corridori, si può verificare sotto forma di trauma acuto o trauma da stress (caso più frequente). Gli atleti si presentano con un click o uno scatto dell'anca, più o meno dolorosi, di solito localizzati nella parte anteriore o laterale e in profondità nell'anca. L'esame obiettivo spesso è in grado di riprodurre i sintomi. Di solito le radiografie non sono necessarie per l'accertamento diagnostico. Il **trattamento** comprende analgesia, riposo relativo, una valutazione biomeccanica ed esercizi di rinforzo/core flexibility. L'atleta può fare ritorno all'attività non appena riesce a tollerarla.

686.6 • Traumi del ginocchio

Il ginocchio è il sito muscoloscheletrico che causa più comunemente disturbi nell'adolescenza. Traumi acuti del ginocchio che causano disabilità immediata sono probabilmente dovuti a frattura, lussazione rotulea, lesione del legamento crociato anteriore (ACL, *Anterior Cruciate Ligament*) o a una lacerazione meniscale. Il meccanismo traumatico è di solito un evento sotto carico. Dopo il trauma, se il giocatore non riesce a caricare entro pochi minuti, sono più probabili una frattura o una lesione interna significativa. Se il soggetto è in grado di caricare e ritornare alla gara dopo il trauma, una lesione grave è improbabile. Se si verifica tumefazione del ginocchio a distanza di diverse ore dal trauma, la tumefazione è probabilmente dovuta a un emartro e a una lesione più severa.

Il trauma che ha maggiori probabilità di verificarsi in associazione con un emartro è una lesione dell'**ACL**. Le lesioni dell'ACL di solito si verificano in seguito a un trauma diretto, atterrando e perdendo l'equilibrio dopo un salto, cambiando velocemente direzione durante la corsa, o in seguito a un trauma in iperestensione. Sono spesso presenti una tumefazione e instabilità significative. La maggior parte degli atleti con tale lesione necessitano di una consulenza ortopedica e di ricostruzione del legamento. L'uso di un'ortesi funzionale senza ricostruzione dell'ACL aumenta il rischio di lesione meniscale e di instabilità ricorrente.

Le **lesioni del legamento crociato posteriore** derivano da un trauma diretto sulle regione della tibia prossimale, come quella che si produce nell'impatto contro un cruscotto di automobile o in una caduta sulle ginocchia, durante una partita di pallavolo. Si tratta comunque di lesioni rare, che di solito non vengono trattate chirurgicamente.

Le **lesioni del legamento collaterale mediale** sono imputabili a un trauma in valgo sulla parte esterna del ginocchio. Le lesioni isolate del *legamento collaterale* laterale, peraltro infrequenti, derivano da uno stress in varo significativo. Le lesioni isolate del collaterale, essendo extrarticolari, non devono produrre un versamento articolare importante o una disabilità significativa. A prescindere dalla loro severità, le lesioni isolate dei collaterali mediale e laterale sono sottoposte a un trattamento non chirurgico con riabilitazione aggressiva.

Le **lacerazioni meniscali** si verificano in seguito agli stessi meccanismi che determinano le lesioni dell'ACL. Si associano a enartrosi, dolore sulla linea articolare e spesso dolore alla flessione completa. La consulenza ortopedica è indicata quando si sospetta una lacerazione meniscale.

Le **lussazioni rotulee** si verificano per lo più come lesioni non da contatto quando i muscoli del quadricipite si contraggono forzatamente per estendere il ginocchio mentre la gamba è ruotata verso l'esterno. La lussazione rotulea è la seconda causa più comune di enartrosi. La rotula è quasi sempre lussata lateralmente e questo movimento lacera il retinacolo rotuleo mediale, causando emorragia intrarticolare. Episodi ricorrenti di instabilità rotulea sono associati a minore tumefazione. L'instabilità rotulea viene trattata non chirurgicamente, con una ginocchiera che stabilizza la rotula e con un programma di riabilitazione aggressiva.

Il medico deve ricercare i versamenti e le deformità evidenti e, di fronte a qualsiasi deformità, trasferire il paziente per un trattamento d'emergenza, dopo averne valutato lo stato neurovascolare. Se non sono presenti deformità grossolane e lo stato neurovascolare è integro, le manovre iniziali sono un'estensione passiva completa e un delicato stress in valgo sul ginocchio in estensione. Una lassità del ginocchio allo stress in valgo in estensione completa indica che sia l'ACL sia il legamento collaterale mediale sono lesionati. Bisogna controllare la capacità del paziente di contrarre il quadricipite. Se questa manovra causa dolore o risulta impossibile, se ne deduce una lesione del meccanismo estensorio. Una dolorabilità sulla parte mediale della rotula, sul retinacolo mediale e/o sul tubercolo degli adduttori si associa a lussazione rotulea. Una dolorabilità a punto è compatibile con una frattura o una lesione della struttura sottostante; una lacerazione meniscale mediale può manifestarsi come dolorabilità lungo la linea articolare mediale, la quale tuttavia non è specifica di una lacerazione del menisco mediale. Un dolore o una limitazione della flessione o dell'estensione passiva mentre si ruota la tibia (test di McMurray o di McMurray modificato) implicano una lesione meniscale, come anche altre manovre (Fig. 686-9). Una lesione del legamento si manifesta come dolore o lassità con la manovra appropriata.

TRATTAMENTO INIZIALE DEI TRAUMI ACUTI DEL GINOCCHIO

Se un paziente non tollera il carico o presenta segni clinici di instabilità, occorre immobilizzare il ginocchio, prescrivere l'uso di stampelle ed eseguire uno studio radiografico. Se la rotula è lussata, si può ottenerne la riduzione con l'estensione del ginocchio. Si rendono necessarie le radiografie previste dalle cosiddette **regole del ginocchio di Ottawa** per i pazienti pediatrici con lesioni del ginocchio che presentano uno qualsiasi di questi segni o sintomi: dolorabilità isolata della rotula, dolore della testa del perone, incapacità di flettere il ginocchio a 90° e incapacità di caricare immediatamente e in pronto soccorso per quattro gradini (a prescindere dalla zoppia). Gli immobilizzatori della gamba in estensione non offrono sostegno strutturale e sono usati solo per dare maggiore comfort al paziente. Nel caso si utilizzi un'ortesi, è consigliabile che sia articolata per la stabilizzazione di una le-

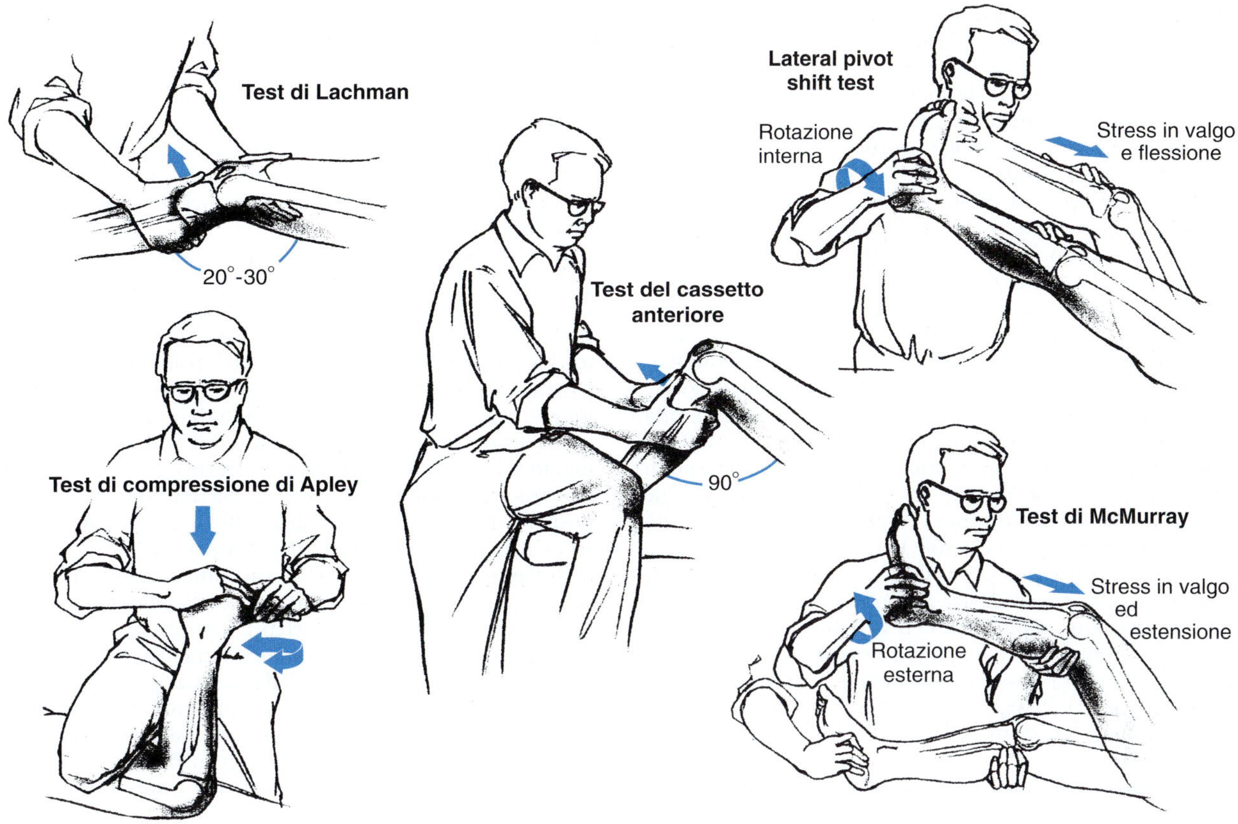

Figura 686-9. Manovre per l'esame obiettivo. Quello qui raffigurato è il ginocchio destro. Le manovre comprendono: test di Lachman, manovra del cassetto anteriore, *lateral pivot shift test*, manovra in compressione di Apley e test di McMurray. Il test di Lachman, il cui scopo è individuare le lesioni del legamento crociato anteriore (ACL, *Anterior Cruciate Ligament*), si esegue con il paziente supino e il ginocchio flesso a 20-30°. Il test del cassetto anteriore, che individua le lesioni dell'ACL, si esegue con il paziente supino e il ginocchio a 90° di flessione. Il *lateral pivot shift test* si esegue con il paziente supino, l'anca flessa a 45° e il ginocchio in estensione completa; si applica una rotazione interna mentre il ginocchio è flesso a 40° con stress in valgo (spingendo medialmente l'esterno del ginocchio). Il test di compressione di Apley, utilizzato per valutare l'integrità del menisco, si esegue con il paziente prono e il ginocchio dell'esaminatore posto sulla parte posteriore della coscia del paziente; si ruota esternamente la tibia esercitando su di essa una forza compressiva diretta verso il basso. Il test di McMurray, utilizzato per valutare l'integrità meniscale, si esegue con il paziente supino e l'esaminatore in piedi dal lato del ginocchio affetto. (Da Solomon DH, Simel DL, Bates DW et al: Does this patient have a torn meniscus or ligament of the knee? *JAMA* 2001;286:1610.)

sione in cui sono interessati sia l'ACL sia il legamento collaterale mediale. L'arto inferiore deve essere mantenuto in elevazione e per la compressione occorre una benda elastica.

TRAUMI CRONICI

La **sindrome da stress femororotuleo** (PFSS, *PatelloFemoral Stress Syndrome*) è la causa più comune di dolore anteriore del ginocchio. La PFSS è nota anche come sindrome del dolore rotuleofemorale o disfunzione rotuleofemorale (vedi Capitolo 676). Si tratta di una diagnosi di esclusione utilizzata per descrivere un dolore anteriore del ginocchio che non ha altre origini patologiche identificabili. Il dolore è di solito difficile da localizzare. I pazienti indicano un'area diffusa a livello del ginocchio anteriore come origine del dolore, oppure possono percepirlo come proveniente da dietro la rotula. Il dolore, comunemente bilaterale, spesso peggiora nel salire le scale, dopo essere stati seduti per periodi prolungati, dopo essersi accovacciati o dopo la corsa. Non vi deve essere una storia di tumefazione significativa, in quanto questa indicherebbe una lesione più seria. È comune una storia di cambiamento dell'attività: per esempio, può avvenire che l'atleta si alleni su terreni diversi da quello consueto, introduca modifiche nello schema di allenamento o si dedichi a nuove attività. L'esame obiettivo deve comprendere la valutazione della posizione in piedi da fermo e del cammino per valutare l'allineamento degli arti, la muscolatura e iperpronazione del piede medio. Occorre valutare la flessibilità dei muscoli posteriori della coscia, della banda ileotibiale e del gastrocnemio, in quanto quando queste strutture sono in tensione aumenta lo stress attraverso l'articolazione femororotuleo. Si deve inoltre esaminare l'arco di movimento dell'anca per escludere una patologia a questo livello. Una dolorabilità rotulea mediale o un dolore alla compressione dell'articolazione femororotulea confermano la diagnosi in assenza di versamento e di altri segni positivi all'esame obiettivo. La PFSS è una diagnosi clinica di solito trattata senza imaging. Il **trattamento** è focalizzato sulla valutazione e sul miglioramento della flessibilità, della forza e delle anomalie della deambulazione. In presenza di iperpronazione del piede medio (valgo della caviglia), nuove calzature o l'uso di supporti per l'arco plantare migliorano la meccanica femororotulea e attenuano il dolore. Per il controllo del dolore si può ricorrere ad applicazioni di ghiaccio e a un analgesico. All'inizio della riabilitazione è importante una riduzione dell'attività globale o degli allenamenti. Al ritorno all'attività, si raccomanda di partire con il 50% della durata e intensità consueta del lavoro, aumentandole gradualmente del 10% alla settimana fino a raggiungere la piena attività. È essenziale una riabilitazione di mantenimento attraverso esercizi da svolgere a domicilio per prevenire le recidive. La chirurgia è raramente indicata.

La **malattia di Osgood-Schlatter** è un'apofisite da trazione che si verifica a livello dell'inserzione del tendine rotuleo sulla tuberosità tibiale (vedi Capitolo 676). Dal momento che è correlata anche all'uso eccessivo del meccanismo estensorio, il **trattamento** è lo stesso della PFSS. Si può ricorrere a una protezione imbottita per proteggere la tuberosità tibiale dai traumi diretti. La complicanza più comune è di tipo estetico: la tuberosità tibiale può essere leggermente sporgente dal lato affetto (o da entrambi se la malattia è bilaterale). I pazienti devono astenersi dallo sport soltanto in caso di zoppia.

La **malattia di Sinding-Larsen-Johansson** è un'apofisite da trazione che si verifica al polo inferiore della rotula e colpisce con maggiore frequenza chi pratica la pallavolo e il basket. Il **trattamento** è simile a quello della malattia di Osgood-Schlatter. La tendinopatia rotulea (ginocchio del saltatore) è dovuto a microtraumi ripetitivi subiti dal tendine rotuleo di solito a livello del polo inferiore della rotula. Nel 10% dei casi è interessato il tendine del quadricipite al di sopra della rotula. È associata agli sport di salto, pur essendo osservabile anche nei corridoi. Il **trattamento** è simile a quello della PFSS. Il riposo relativo è più importante nella tendinopatia rotulea in quanto il dolore cronico è associato ad alterazioni irreversibili del tendine. La **sindrome da frizione della banda iliotibiale** (ITB, *IleoTibial Band*) è la causa più comune di dolore cronico laterale del ginocchio. Generalmente non associata a tumefazione o instabilità, è dovuta alla frizione dell'ITB lungo la parte laterale del ginocchio, che dà luogo a una borsite. Il dolore viene evocato lungo l'ITB, nel suo decorso sul condilo femorale laterale o all'inserzione a livello del tubercolo di Gerdy, lungo il piatto tibiale laterale. Inoltre, si nota una tensione dell'ITB con il test di Ober. Durante l'esecuzione di quest'ultimo test, l'atleta giace sul fianco ed estende l'anca (del lato opposto a quello su cui giace) con il ginocchio flesso, mentre l'esaminatore gli sostiene la caviglia a mezz'aria; l'eventuale spostamento del ginocchio inferiormente implica un'ITB flessibile e la negatività del test; se invece il ginocchio e la gamba rimangono a mezz'aria, l'ITB è tesa e il test risulta positivo. I principi di **trattamento** sono gli stessi indicati per la PFSS, con la differenza che viene dato maggior peso al miglioramento della flessibilità dell'ITB.

Agel J, Arendt EA, Bershadsky B: Anterior cruciate ligament injury in national collegiate athletic association basketball and soccer: A 13-year review. *Am J Sports Med* 2005;33:524–530.

LaBotz M: Patellofemoral syndrome: Diagnostic pointers and individualized treatment. *Phys Sportsmed* 2004;32:7.

Vaquero J, Vidal C, Cubillo A: Intra-articular traumatic disorders of the knee in children and adolescents. *Clin Orthop* 2005;432:97–106.

686.7 • DOLORE DELLA GAMBA: SHIN SPLINT, FRATTURE DA STRESS E SINDROME COMPARTIMENTALE CRONICA

Le lesioni da stress a carico delle ossa degli arti inferiori si verificano in un continuum da una lesione lieve (*shin splint*) a una frattura da stress. Tutte sono conseguenza di un uso eccessivo. Lo **shin splint**, noto anche come sindrome da stress tibiale mediale, si presenta con dolore lungo la tibia mediale o entrambe le tibie ed è il più comune trauma da uso eccessivo della gamba. All'inizio il dolore compare verso la fine dell'esercizio, ma è destinato a peggiorare e a presentarsi sempre più precocemente se l'attività fisica continua senza riabilitazione. Si riscontra una dolorabilità diffusa dal terzo medio alla metà della tibia mediale distale. Qualsiasi dolorabilità focale o della tibia prossimale deve far sorgere il sospetto di una frattura da stress. Lo shin splint di solito può essere distinto da una **frattura tibiale da stress** in cui la dolorabilità è più focalizzata (2-5 cm) e severa. Lo shin splint e la frattura da stress rappresentano un continuum nell'ambito dei traumi da stress della tibia e sono considerati correlati alla trazione del muscolo soleo sulla tibia.

La diagnosi può essere posta in base all'anamnesi e all'esame obiettivo. Gli aspetti radiografici della tibia sono normali in caso di shin splint e fratture tibiali da stress nelle prime settimane dopo il trauma. In seguito, le radiografie possono dimostrare una reazione periostea se è presente una frattura da stress. La sensibilità delle radiografie può essere aumentata eseguendo quattro proiezioni della tibia: anteroposteriore, laterale ed entrambe le proiezioni oblique. La scintigrafia ossea, che è l'esame più sensibile per la diagnosi delle fratture da stress, denota una captazione del tracciante discreta a livello della sede o delle sedi della frattura da stress. Un'aumentata captazione è osservabile in presenza di shin splint, ma con un pattern fusiforme lungo la superficie periostea. Se i risultati della scintigrafia ossea sono normali, la diagnosi è probabilmente quella di shin splint o di sindrome compartimentale cronica (CCS, *Chronic Compartment Syndrome*). In molti centri medici la RM ha sostituito la scintigrafia ossea in quanto strumento diagnostico più sensibile per le fratture da stress delle ossa lunghe.

Il **trattamento** dello shin splint è analogo, con riposo relativo, correzione degli errori di allenamento e delle disfunzioni della catena cinetica e, spesso, uso di calzature da corsa più adeguate. La fitness può essere mantenuta con attività in scarico come nuoto, bicicletta e jogging acquatico. Con lo shin splint, dopo 7-10 giorni, i pazienti possono di solito iniziare il programma di walk-jogging. Se il dolore si esacerba, devono passare 2-3 giorni liberi da dolore prima che si possa riprendere il programma di walk-jogging. Si devono usare ghiaccio tutti i giorni e analgesici per il controllo del dolore. Nei pazienti che tendono all'iperpronazione possono possono essere utili ortesi o nuove calzature. Talvolta sono benefici lo stretching dei flessori plantari e il rinforzo dei dorsiflessori della caviglia. Si raccomandano 7-10 giorni senza dolore prima di iniziare le marce di allenamento.

La **CCS** si verifica negli atleti che praticano la corsa, di solito durante un periodo di strenuo allenamento. È dovuta all'ipertrofia muscolare e all'aumento della pressione intracompartimentale connessa all'esercizio. Di solito è presente un periodo libero dal dolore di circa 10 minuti, all'inizio dell'esercizio, prima dell'esordio di un dolore pulsante costante difficile da localizzare, che persiste da qualche minuto ad alcune dopo l'attività fisica ed è alleviato dal ghiaccio e dall'elevazione. Nei casi classici, è presente una perdita di sensibilità del piede associata a pressione elevata nel compartimento muscolare corrispondente. Il compartimento muscolare più colpito è quello anterolaterale, con compressione del nervo peroneale. L'esame obiettivo in ambulatorio è spesso normale, ma possono essere presenti anche perdita di forza dell'estensore lungo dell'alluce e una riduzione della sensibilità nello spazio interdigitale tra il 1° e il 2° dito del piede.

Se si sospetta una CCS, è indicato l'invio dal chirurgo appropriato (ortopedico o vascolare) che misuri la pressione intracompartimentale. Il trattamento è chirurgico e richiede la fasciotomia o la fasciectomia per ridurre la pressione.

Pell RF 4th, Khanuja HS, Cooley GR: Leg pain in the running athlete. *J Am Acad Orthop Surg* 2004;12:396–404.

686.8 • TRAUMI DELLA CAVIGLIA

Quelli della caviglia sono i traumi atletici più comuni. L'85% è rappresentato da distorsioni e l'85% di queste sono traumi in inversione (piede appoggiato con il perone laterale che si sposta verso il suolo), il 5% sono traumi in eversione (piede appoggiato con il malleolo mediale che si sposta verso il terreno), mentre il 10% sono traumi associati.

ESAME OBIETTIVO E SCALA DI VALUTAZIONE DEL TRAUMA

Nei casi evidenti di frattura o lussazione, è prioritario valutare lo stato neurovascolare muovendo la parte il meno possibile. Se non vi sono evidenti deformità, il passo successivo è la ricerca di edemi, ecchimosi e varianti anatomiche. Le sedi chiave da palpare per la ricerca della dolorabilità sono il perone per tutta la sua lunghezza, i malleoli mediali e laterali, la base del 5° metatarso, le linee articolari anteriore, mediale e laterale, lo scafoide e il complesso del tendine d'Achille. È indicata la valutazione dell'arco attivo di movimento (il paziente da solo) in dorsiflessione, flessione plantare, inversione ed eversione, e dell'arco di movimento contro resistenza.

I test di provocazione hanno lo scopo di valutare l'integrità dei legamenti, ma in un paziente con una caviglia marcatamente edematosa e dolente sono difficili da eseguire a causa dello spasmo muscolare e della difesa involontaria. Sono quindi molto utili sul campo prima che si siano verificati un edema e un'emorragia significativi. Il test del cassetto anteriore valuta la traslazione dell'astragalo e la competenza del legamento astragaloperoneale anteriore. Il test di stress in inversione esamina la competenza dei legamenti astragaloperoneale anteriore e calcaneoperoneale (Fig. 686-10). In una situazione acuta, si esamina l'integrità dei legamenti tibioperoneali e della sindesmosi tibioperoneale con il test di compressione della sindesmosi (*squeezing test*). Un dolore alla compressione (*squeezing*) della parte inferiore della gamba implica una lesione della membrana interossea e della sindesmosi tra tibia e perone, rendendo più sospetta una lesione severa. Gli atleti con questo tipo di lesioni non tollerano alcun carico, oltre a presentare un dolore severo alla rotazione esterna del piede. Talvolta si verifica una lussazione del tendine peroneale contemporaneamente a una distorsione della caviglia. Per valutare l'instabilità del tendine peroneale, l'esaminatore esercita una pressione da dietro il tendine peroneale con eversione contro resistenza e flessione plantare: questa manovra farà scattare il tendine anteriormente. Se si sospetta una lesione della sindesmosi o una lussazione peroneale acuta, occorre una consulenza ortopedica.

RADIOGRAFIE

Si eseguono proiezioni della caviglia in anteroposteriore e in laterale, oltre che del mortaio tibiale, quando i pazienti hanno dolore nell'area dei malleoli, sono incapaci di caricare o presentano dolorabilità ossea posteriormente a livello della tibia distale o del perone distale. Le regole per la caviglia di Ottawa sono utili per individuare i pazienti che necessitano di uno studio radiografico (Fig. 686-11). Quando i pazienti presentano dolore nell'area del piede medio o dolorabilità ossea in corrispondenza dello scafoide o del 5° metatarso, occorre eseguire uno studio completo del piede (proiezioni anteroposteriore, laterale e obliqua). È importante differenziare una frattura da avulsione del 5° metatarso prossimale dalla frattura di Jones del 5° metatarso prossimale (un'area di radiotrasparenza a circa 2 cm dall'estremità prossimale). La prima viene trattata come una distorsione della caviglia; la seconda si associa a un aumentato rischio di mancato consolidamento e richiede una consulenza ortopedica. La *frattura della volta dell'astragalo* si manifesta come una distorsione della caviglia

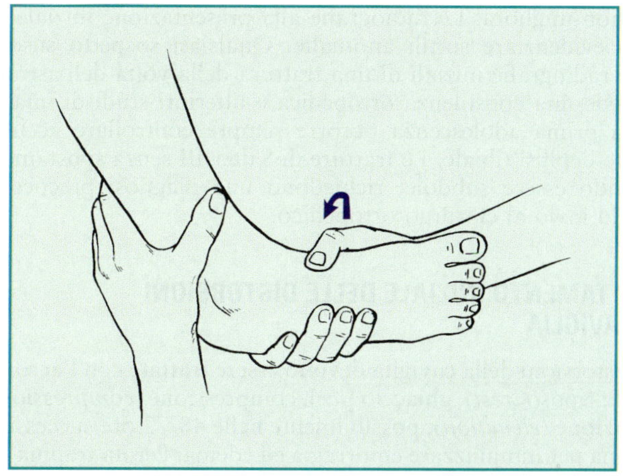

Figura 686-10. Test da stress in inversione per l'instabilità della caviglia. (Da Hergenroeder AC: Diagnosis and treatment of ankle sprains. A review. *Am J Dis Child* 1990;144:809.)

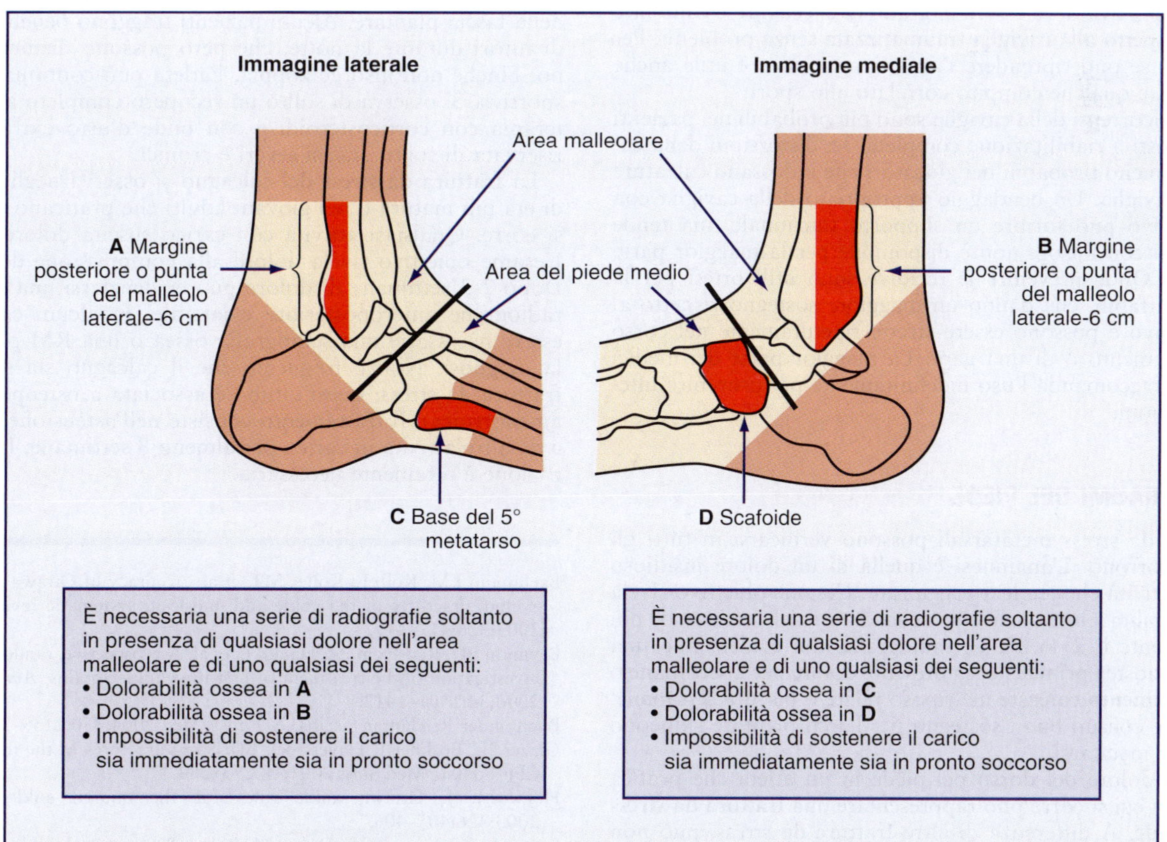

Figura 686-11. Regole per la caviglia di Ottawa. (Da Bachmann LM, Kolb E, Koller MT et al: Accuracy of Ottawa ankle rules to exclude fractures of the ankle and midfoot; systematic review. *Br Med J* 2003;326:417-419.)

che non migliora. Le radiografie alla presentazione iniziale possono evidenziare sottili anomalie. Qualsiasi sospetto suscitato dalle radiografie iniziali di una frattura della volta dell'astragalo richiede una consulenza ortopedica e ulteriori studi di imaging. Nella prima adolescenza occorre sempre controllare accuratamente l'epifisi tibiale. Le fratture di Salter III senza spostamento, potendo essere subdole, richiedono una diagnosi precoce e il rapido invio al chirurgo ortopedico.

TRATTAMENTO INIZIALE DELLE DISTORSIONI DI CAVIGLIA

Le distorsioni della caviglia devono essere **trattate** con l'acronimo RICE: riposo (*rest*), ghiaccio (*ice*), compressione (*compression*) ed elevazione (*elevation*), possibilmente nelle 48-72 ore successive al trauma per minimizzare emorragia ed edema. Per un trauma della caviglia si utilizzano grucce e un bendaggio elastico, anche se altri sistemi di compressione come una staffa funzionano molto bene; questi permettono un carico precoce con protezione e possono essere rimossi per la riabilitazione. È importante iniziare un programma di riabilitazione quanto prima.

RIABILITAZIONE. La riabilitazione dovrebbe iniziare il giorno del trauma; nei pazienti con dolore al movimento, si può iniziare il rinforzo isometrico. I deficit importanti da correggere sono la perdita della dorsiflessione, la perdita di forza dei muscoli peroneali e la diminuzione della propriocezione: finché non saranno stati eliminati, l'anca sarà vulnerabile a un nuovo trauma. Perché si possa concludere che un atleta è pronto per la corsa si deve avere un arco di movimento completo e una forza quasi completa rispetto al lato non traumatizzato. Caricando sul lato non traumatizzato, l'atleta deve saltare 8-10 volte, se è in grado di farlo. Se gli è possibile farlo senza dolore, può iniziare a correre. Iniziando con il jogging e passando da metà a tre quarti della velocità e finalmente alle accelerazioni, l'atleta deve fermarsi in caso di dolore o zoppia significativa. Infine, prima di ritornare all'attività sportiva deve essere in grado di accelerare e cambiare direzione rispetto alla caviglia traumatizzata senza problemi. Per determinare se può riprendere l'attività agonistica è utile anche fargli eseguire qualche compito correlato allo sport.

I traumi ricorrenti della caviglia sono più probabili nei pazienti non sottoposti a riabilitazione completa. Le distorsioni della caviglia sono meno probabili nei giocatori che indossano calzature alte sulla caviglia. Un bendaggio appropriato della caviglia con nastro adesivo può fornire un supporto funzionale, ma tende ad allentarsi con l'uso e non è disponibile per la maggior parte degli atleti. Onde prevenire le recidive sono utili ortesi per la caviglia adattabili, che danno un maggiore sostegno rispetto al nastro adesivo e possono essere strette ripetutamente nel corso di un allenamento o di una gara. La maggior parte dei medici sportivi ne raccomanda l'uso indefinitamente per prevenire ulteriori distorsioni.

686.9 • TRAUMI DEL PIEDE

Le **fratture da stress metatarsali** possono verificarsi in tutti gli atleti che corrono. L'anamnesi è quella di un dolore insidioso durante l'attività che tende a peggiorare. L'esame obiettivo rivela una dolorabilità punto a livello della diafisi del metatarso, più frequentemente il 2° o 3°. Le radiografie non evidenziano una reazione periostea prima che sia presente dolore per 2 settimane o più. Il **trattamento** consiste nel riposo relativo per 6-8 settimane. Le calzature con un buon sostegno per l'arco plantare riducono lo stress sui metatarsi.

Un vago dolore del dorso del piede in un atleta che pratica uno sport in cui si corre può rappresentare una **frattura da stress dello scafoide.** A differenza di altre fratture da stress, può non essere ben localizzato all'esame obiettivo. Se è presente qualsiasi dolorabilità intorno allo scafoide, si deve sospettare una frattura da stress. Poiché possono passare molte settimane prima che sia visibile alle radiografie, occorre eseguire una scintigrafia ossea o una RM a fini diagnostici. Dal momento che questa frattura è ad alto rischio di mancato consolidamento, il **trattamento** usuale consiste nell'immobilizzazione e nello scarico dell'arto. Si deve eseguire una TC per documentare una completa guarigione dopo il periodo di immobilizzazione.

La **malattia di Sever** (apofisite calcaneare), che colpisce l'inserzione del tendine di Achille sul calcagno, si presenta sotto forma di dolore correlato all'attività (vedi Fig. 686-3). Più comune nei maschi (2:1), spesso è bilaterale e di solito si presenta tra gli 8 e i 13 anni. È possibile elicitare la dolorabilità a livello dell'inserzione del tendine di Achille sul calcagno, in particolare comprimendo il tallone ("squeeze test" positivo). La malattia di Sever è associata a tensione del tendine di Achille e a iperpronazione del piede medio con maggiore stress sui flessori plantari del piede. Il **trattamento** comprende riposo relativo, ghiaccio, massaggi, stretching e rinforzo del tendine di Achille. La correzione dell'iperpronazione del piede medio con ortesi, supporto per l'arco plantare o calzature migliori è importante nella maggior parte degli atleti con malattia di Sever. Se il piede è in posizione neutra o se l'iperpronazione è lieve, un plantare da 0,6 cm è utile per scaricare il tendine di Achille e la sua inserzione. Con un trattamento ottimale, i sintomi migliorano in 4-8 settimane. In generale, se non vi è zoppia durante l'attività sportiva, i giovani atleti devono poter gareggiare anche con la malattia di Sever.

La **fascite plantare** è un trauma da uso eccessivo che determina degenerazione dell'aponeurosi plantare. Questa diagnosi, rara nei bambini prepuberi, è più probabile nell'adolescente o nel giovane adulto. Gli atleti riferiscono dolore del tallone con l'attività che peggiora con i primi passi della giornata o dopo diverse ore di scarico dell'arto. È possibile elicitare una dolorabilità sulla tuberosità calcaneare mediale. È utile il riposo relativo dalle attività in carico. Gli atleti sviluppano la fascite plantare quando indossano calzature con inadeguato supporto per l'arco plantare. Il dolore è spesso alleviato da nuove calzature o dall'uso di supporti semirigidi per l'arco plantare. È utile lo stretching dei polpacci e della fascia plantare. Alcuni pazienti traggono beneficio dall'uso di tutori durante la notte, che però possono disturbare il sonno. Finché non insorge zoppia, l'atleta può continuare l'attività sportiva. Si osserva di solito un recupero completo a 6 mesi. La terapia con corticosteroidi e con onde d'urto extracorporee è riservata di solito ai casi severi e cronici.

La **frattura da stress del calcagno** si osserva negli adolescenti di età più matura o nei giovani adulti che praticano sport in cui si corre. Qualsiasi attività con carico suscita dolore al tallone. L'esame obiettivo rivela dolore alla compressione del calcagno. Dopo 2-3 settimane di dolore può evidenziarsi una sclerosi alle radiografie anteroposteriore e laterale. In alcuni casi possono essere necessarie una scintigrafia ossea o una RM per precisare la diagnosi. Non è frequente che il calcagno sia sede di una frattura da stress; quest'ultima è associata a osteopenia (donna amenorroica). Il **trattamento** consiste nell'astensione dalla corsa e da altre attività in carico per almeno 8 settimane. L'immobilizzazione è raramente necessaria.

Bachmann LM, Kolb E, Koller MT, et al: Accuracy of Ottawa ankle rules to exclude fractures of the ankle and mid-foot; systematic review. *Br Med J* 2003;326:417–419.

Beynnon BD, Renström PA, Haugh L, et al: A prospective, randomized clinical investigation of the treatment of first-time ankle sprains. *Am J Sports Med* 2006;34:1401–1412.

Buchbinder R: Plantar fascitis. *N Engl J Med* 2004;350:2159–2166.

Glazer JL, Brukner P, Haverstock BD: Stress fractures of the foot and ankle. Clin Podiatr Med Surg 2001;18:273–284.

Heyworth J: Ottawa ankle rules for the injured ankle. *Br Med J* 2003;326:405–406.

Kennedy JG, Knowles B, Dolan M, Bohne W: Foot and ankle injuries in the adolescent runner. *Curr Opin Pediatr* 2005;17:34–42.

Capitolo 687 ■ Traumi della testa e del collo Gregory L. Landry

TRAUMI CRANICI

In ambito scolastico, le concussioni si verificano in più di 62 000 atleti ogni anno, e il football è responsabile del 63% dei casi. Lievi traumi cerebrali possono verificarsi con o senza perdita di coscienza. La maggior parte delle concussioni che si verificano in ambito sportivo non è associata a perdita di coscienza e attualmente si considera concussione *qualsiasi* decremento della funzione neurologica o cognitiva dopo un evento traumatico (Tab. 681-1) (vedi Capitolo 67).

La concussione da sport è un complesso processo fisiopatologico che interessa il cervello, indotto da forze biomeccaniche traumatiche. Definizione, valutazione e trattamento si sono evoluti significativamente negli ultimi 35 anni. Sono state pubblicate scale graduate per la valutazione della severità della concussione, anche se persistono controversie a causa delle diverse linee guida. Nel marzo del 2005, il 2nd International Symposium on Concussion in Sport ha concluso che tali scale non andrebbero più utilizzate, in quanto la valutazione e le decisioni su quando ritornare all'attività sportiva dovrebbero essere guidate dalla risposta individuale. Se si sospetta una concussione, il soggetto deve sospendere l'attività sportiva ed essere valutato da un punto di vista medico. Un monitoraggio regolare nelle prime ore successive al trauma è importante. Il Symposium ha suggerito ai medici di avvalersi di uno strumento di valutazione denominato SCAT (*Sport Concussion Assessment Tool*) durante la valutazione dell'atleta.

Come guida del trattamento, le concussioni possono essere classificate come semplici o complesse. La forma più comune è quella semplice, responsabile di un trauma che si risolve entro 7-10 giorni e non comporta complicanze. Le concussioni semplici non richiedono test neuropsicologici e raramente rendono necessari studi di neuroimaging. L'atleta deve astenersi dallo sport finché non diventa asintomatico, dopodiché il ritorno all'attività sarà graduale. È inoltre importante per la guarigione il "riposo cognitivo", durante il quale i giovani atleti limitano lo sforzo nel corso delle attività quotidiane di routine come anche nei compiti a casa.

Il ritorno alle gare deve avvenire attraverso una serie di compiti successivi, che può essere affrontato solo da un soggetto asintomatico:

- **Riposo fino alla scomparsa dei sintomi**
- **Attività anaerobica leggera; bisogna astenersi dall'allenamento contro resistenza**
- **Allenamento sport-specifico**
- **Allenamento senza contatto**
- **Allenamento a contatto completo**
- **Gara**

In presenza di sintomi di concussione (vedi Tab. 687-1), si raccomanda di ritornare al compito precedente per almeno 24 ore. Il paziente non deve far uso di farmaci per il trattamento dei sintomi.

Le concussioni complesse causano sintomi o alterazioni cognitive persistenti. Rientrano in questo gruppo gli atleti con sintomi da concussioni multiple. Possono essere presenti sintomi neurologici focali. I sintomi da alterazioni cognitive comprendono scarsa attenzione o concentrazione, alterazioni della memoria, irritabilità, ansia, depressione dell'umore, disturbi del sonno, cefalea lieve persistente, capogiri e/o intolleranza per le luci intense o i rumori forti. Lo sforzo tipicamente esacerba i sintomi da concussione. In questo gruppo gli accertamenti diagnostici sono più estesi e consistono in una valutazione neuropsicologica formale. Questi pazienti devono essere inviati a medici specializzati nel trattamento di questo tipo di lesione.

TABELLA 687-1. Segni e sintomi di concussione

MEMORIA O ORIENTAMENTO
Disorientamento spazio-temporale
Il soggetto non ricorda più la fase di gioco, gli avversari o il punteggio di gara
Confusione generale
SINTOMI
Cefalea
Vertigini
Sensazione di ottundimento
Sensazione di confusione
Sensazione di essere "lenti"
Visione di "stelle" o luci lampeggianti
Tinnito
Sonnolenza
Visione offuscata
Perdita di campo visivo
Diplopia
Nausea
SEGNI FISICI
Scarsa coordinazione
Scarso equilibrio
Sguardo "invetriato"/vuoto
Vomito
Rallentamento della parola
Lentezza nel rispondere alle domande
Lentezza nel seguire le istruzioni
Facile distraibilità/scarsa concentrazione
Emozioni insolite/inappropriate (per es. riso, pianto)
Alterazioni della personalità
Comportamento inappropriato sul campo di gioco (per es. correre nella direzione sbagliata)
Significativa riduzione delle capacità di gioco rispetto a prima dell'incidente

Modificata da Canadian Academy of Sport Medicine Concussion Committee: Guidelines for assessment and management of sport-related concussion. *Clin J Sport Med* 2000;10:210, per gentile concessione.
Da Landry GL: Central nervous system trauma management of concussions in athletes. *Pediatr Clin N Am* 2002;49:723-741.

Nella concussione, TC e RM sono di solito normali. Gli studi di neuroimaging, che di solito non sono necessari nelle concussioni semplici, devono invece essere utilizzati in caso di sospetta patologia strutturale intracranica dovuta a un problema focale rilevato all'esame neurologico o a sintomi che tendono a peggiorare. Il rischio di una patologia intracranica aumenta in presenza di vomito continuato, cefalea prolungata, amnesia anterograda persistente (scarsa memoria a breve termine), convulsioni, punteggio della Glasgow Coma Scale <15 e segni di frattura della base cranica o frattura cranica infossata.

TRAUMI CERVICALI

I traumi cervicali più comuni sono quelli dei tessuti molli (contusioni, stiramenti muscolari e distorsioni tendinee). Tuttavia, quando un atleta lamenta un dolore cervicale della linea mediana o nell'arco di movimento, presenta deficit neurologici focali o ha perso coscienza, bisogna ipotizzare una frattura cervicale. Si raccomanda di immobilizzare la colonna cervicale ed eseguire radiografie in proiezione anteroposteriore, laterale, obliqua e a bocca aperta, prima di rimuovere l'immobilizzatore. Se non sono possibili flessione ed estensione attiva, occorre eseguire una TC (vedi Capitolo 67).

Esiste spesso una sovrapposizione tra distorsione, stiramento e contusione cervicale. Diversi sono i segni radiografici indicativi di instabilità (allargamento interspinoso, sublussazione vertebrale, frattura vertebrale da compressione, perdita della lordosi cervicale). La RM, in quanto molto sensibile, deve essere utilizzata per diagnosticare e definire i traumi legamentosi e midollari spinali. Dopo un esame radiografico negativo per una frattura (comprendente le proiezioni dinamiche in flessione ed estensione), il collo può essere immobilizzato in un collaretto morbido per il comfort. Riposo e farmaci antinfiammatori sono utili nei traumi minori. Il collaretto viene eliminato gradualmente e si iniziano esercizi utili per l'arco di movimento. L'atleta può fare ritorno alle gare una volta recuperato l'arco di movimento con forza completa e una funzione cervicale sport-specifica. È importante seguire un programma di condizionamento cervicale per prevenire le recidive.

Le lesioni dei dischi cervicali in ambito sportivo di solito derivano da una flessione laterale non controllata. I traumi cervicali sono meno comuni delle lesioni discali lombari e sono infrequenti nei pazienti pediatrici. La maggior parte dei problemi a livello dei dischi cervicali si risolve nel giro di diversi mesi con riposo iniziale, immobilizzazione, farmaci antinfiammatori, modifiche dell'attività e trazione cervicale. Dopo il miglioramento dei sintomi si iniziano esercizi per l'arco di movimento e successivamente di rinforzo.

TRAUMI DEL PLESSO BRACHIALE

Il plesso brachiale comprende i nervi che originano da C5-T1 ed emergono dalla colonna vertebrale nella triangolo profondo del collo. La parte superiore del collo (C5-6) può subire una contusione o uno stiramento quando si gioca a football con il tackling di spalla o in seguito a flessione forzata della testa di lato. Le manifestazioni comprendono bruciore e parestesie unilaterali e perdita di forza del braccio, di solito con distribuzione C5-6 che si manifesta con l'incapacità di flettere anteriormente o abdurre la spalla. Questi sintomi spesso si risolvono spontaneamente nel giro di qualche minuto. La presenza di sintomi bilaterali, come una quadriplegia transitoria, è un'indicazione alla sospensione dell'attività sportiva fino all'esecuzione di una RM. Se il paziente presenta una sensazioni di "bruciore" ricorrente, è indicata una RM della colonna cervicale.

Guskiewicz KM, McCrea M, Marshall SW, et al: Cumulative effects associated with recurrent concussion in collegiate football players. *JAMA* 2003;290:2549–2554.

Kirkwood MW, Yeates KO, Wilson PE: Pediatric sport-related concussion: a review of the clinical management of an oft-neglected population. *Pediatrics* 2006;117:1359–1371.

Landry GL: Central nervous system trauma management of concussions in athletes. *Pediatr Clin N Am* 2002;49:723–741.

McCrea M, Guskiewicz KM, Marshall SW, et al: Acute effects and recovery time following concussion in collegiate football players. *JAMA* 2003;290:2556–2562.

McCrory P, Johnson K, Meeuwise W, et al: Summary and agreement statement of the 2nd International Conference on Concussion in Sport, Prague 2004. *Clin J Sports Med* 2005;15:48–55.

Smits M, Dippel DWJ, de Haan GG, et al: External validation of the Canadian CT head rule and the New Orleans criteria for CT scanning in patients with minor head injury. *JAMA* 2005;294:1519–1525.

Stiell IG, Clement CM, Rowe BH, et al: Comparison of the Canadian CT head rule and the New Orleans criteria in patients with minor head injury. *JAMA* 2005;294:1511–1518.

Zmurko MG, Tannoury TY, Tannoury CA, Anderson DG: Cervical sprains, disc herniations, minor fractures, and other cervical injuries in the athlete. *Clin Sports Med* 2003;22:513–521.

Capitolo 688 ■ Traumi da calore

Gregory L. Landry

La malattia da calore è la terza causa principale di morte negli atleti di scuola superiore negli Stati Uniti. Si tratta di un continuum di segni e sintomi clinici che possono essere da lievi (stress da calore) a fatali (colpo di calore) (vedi Capitolo 68). I bambini sono più vulnerabili degli adulti, rispetto ai quali hanno un rapporto tra superficie corporea e massa corporea maggiore e producono più calore per chilogrammo di peso corporeo durante l'attività fisica, oltre a presentare un tasso di sudorazione più basso, in quanto la temperatura alla quale inizia l'emissione di sudore è più elevata. Possono richiedere più tempo per acclimatarsi ad ambienti molto caldi e umidi (tipicamente quasi 8-12 giorni consecutivi di esposizione per 30-45 minuti). Hanno anche una minore risposta della sete rispetto agli adulti e possono non consumare abbastanza liquidi durante l'attività fisica per prevenire la disidratazione.

Generalmente si classifica la malattia da calore in tre categorie (crampi da calore, esaurimento da calore, colpo di calore). Tuttavia, tutte e tre queste forme sono accomunate dal fatto che i sintomi si sovrappongono e progrediscono con l'aumento della temperatura del nucleo corporeo. I **crampi da calore**, il disturbo da calore più comune, di solito si verificano nella disidratazione lieve e/o nella deplezione di sali, interessando di solito i muscoli posteriori della gamba e quelli del polpaccio. Essi tendono a verificarsi tardivamente nel corso dell'attività, per effetto dell'affaticamento muscolare e delle maggiori perdite d'acqua e sodio. Rispondono alla reidratazione orale con la somministrazione di una soluzione elettrolitica e a uno stretching leggero. L'atleta può fare ritorno in campo quando non è alterata la capacità di performance. La **sincope da calore** consiste in uno svenimento dopo un esercizio prolungato, attribuibile a una scarso tono vasomotorio e a una deplezione di volume intravascolare, e risponde alla somministrazione di fluidi, al raffreddamento e alla posizione supina. L'**edema da calore** è un edema lieve delle mani e dei piedi che si verifica all'inizio dell'esposizione al calore; si risolve con l'acclimatazione. La **tetania da calore** consiste in parestesie o spasmi carpopedali causati dall'iperventilazione correlata al calore; risponde al trasferimento del soggetto in un ambiente più fresco e alla diminuzione della frequenza respiratoria (o al *rebreathing*, che consiste nel respirare in un sacchetto). L'**esaurimento da calore** è una malattia moderata con temperatura del nucleo corporeo di 37,7-39,4 °C. Naturalmente la performance è alterata ma, se presente, la disfunzione del sistema nervoso centrale (SNC) è di grado lieve. Essa si manifesta sotto forma di cefalea, nausea, vomito, vertigini, ortostasi, perdita di forza, orripilazione e talvolta sincope. Il **trattamento** consiste nel trasferimento in un ambiente più fresco, nel raffreddamento del corpo con ventilatori, nella rimozione dei vestiti in eccesso e nell'applicazione di ghiaccio su inguine e ascelle. Se il soggetto non è in grado di tollerare la reidratazione orale, sono indicati liquidi per via endovenosa. I pazienti devono essere monitorati (compresa la misurazione della temperatura rettale) per la ricerca dei segni di un colpo di calore. Se non si ottiene un rapido miglioramento, si raccomanda il trasporto in pronto soccorso.

Il **colpo di calore** è una patologia severa che si manifesta con disturbi del SNC e potenziali danni ai tessuti. Si tratta di un'emergenza medica, il cui tasso di mortalità è del 50%. Il colpo di calore, caratterizzato da sudorazione profusa, è correlato allo sport e a sforzi intensi, mentre il colpo di calore "classico", con cute calda e secca, ha un esordio più lento (giorni) nei soggetti anziani o con malattia cronica. La temperatura rettale è di solito >40 °C. Si verificano danni significativi a cuore, cervello, fegato, reni e muscoli, con possibili conseguenze fatali in assenza di trattamento.

Il **trattamento** consiste nel raffreddamento immediato di tutto il corpo tramite immersione in acqua fredda. Occorre tenere costantemente sotto controllo vie aeree, respirazione, circolazione, temperatura del nucleo corporeo e situazione del SNC. Il raffreddamento rapido va interrotto quando la temperatura del nucleo corporeo raggiunge i 38,3-38,9 °C. La somministrazione di fluidi per via endovenosa alla velocità di 800 mL/m^2 nella prima ora con soluzione fisiologica o lattato di Ringer migliora il volume intravascolare e la capacità dell'organismo di eliminare il calore. È necessario il trasporto immediato in pronto soccorso.

TABELLA 688-1. Restrizione dell'attività per differenti livelli di stress da calore

WBGT		
°C	°F	RESTRIZIONE DELL'ATTIVITÀ
<24	<75	Sono consentite tutte le attività, ma bisogna essere pronti a cogliere i prodromi di patologie correlate al calore in caso di sforzi fisici prolungati
24,0-25,9	75,0-78,6	Periodi di riposo all'ombra prolungati; favorire l'assunzione di liquidi ogni 15 minuti
26-29	79-84	I soggetti non acclimatati e quelli ad alto rischio devono interrompere l'attività; tutti gli altri devono limitarsi (non partecipare a gare su lunga distanza, ridurre la durata delle altre attività)
>29	>85	Sospendere tutte le attività atletiche

La WBGT (*Wet Bulb Globe Temperature*) non è la temperatura ambiente. Essa indica la temperatura a bulbo umido, un indice di stress da calore ambientale misurabile sul campo con uno psicrometro. Questo strumento, disponibile in commercio, si compone di tre termometri. Il primo (bulbo umido [WB]) monitora l'umidità, il secondo [G] si trova all'interno di una sfera cava nera (globo) e serve per monitorare l'irraggiamento, mentre il terzo è un semplice termometro (temperatura [T]) per misurare la temperatura ambiente. L'indice di stress da calore si calcola come WBGT = 0,7 temperatura WB ≶ 0,2 temperatura G + 0,1 temperatura T. Si noti che il 70% dello stress è dovuto all'umidità, il 20% all'irraggiamento e soltanto il 10% alla temperatura ambiente.

Da American Academy of Pediatrics, Committee on Sports Medicine and Fitness: Climatic heat stress and the exercising child and adolescent. *Pediatrics* 2000;106:159.

Prima del ritorno all'attività fisica occorre l'autorizzazione del medico.

In tutte le patologie da calore è comune la disidratazione; pertanto, le misure volte alla prevenzione della disidratazione possono prevenire anche la malattia da calore. La sete non è un buon indicatore delle condizioni di idratazione in quanto comincia a farsi sentire a una disidratazione del 2-3%. Bisogna raccomandare agli atleti di idratarsi bene prima dell'esercizio e di bere ogni 20 minuti durante l'attività sportiva (140 mL per 40 kg di peso corporeo, 260 mL per 90 kg e 300-460 per un peso >60 kg). Occorre raccomandare agli allenatori di mettere a disposizione degli atleti acqua fredda a volontà. Durante un allenamento di football, pause programmate ogni 20-30 minuti togliendo i caschi per eliminare il calore possono ridurre la quantità cumulativa di esposizione al calore. Gare e allenamenti devono essere programmati per il mattino presto o nel tardo pomeriggio per evitare la parte più calda del giorno. Sono state pubblicate linee guida sulle modifiche dell'attività relativamente alla temperatura a bulbo umido (Tab. 688-1). Indossare un vestiario appropriato, come pantaloni corti e magliette, senza casco può migliorare l'eliminazione del calore. Pesarsi prima e dopo l'allenamento può essere utile per determinare la quantità di liquido che occorre assumere per sostituire le perdite (circa 220 g per ogni 450 g di perdita di peso).

L'acqua è un liquido adeguato per la maggior parte degli individui che si allenano per meno di un'ora, anche se vi sono evidenze che i bambini ne bevono di più quando è dolcificata e aromatizzata. I liquidi con elettroliti e carboidrati sono più importanti per gli individui che si allenano per più di un'ora. La maggior parte degli atleti non deve assumere compresse contenenti sali minerali, per l'elevato rischio di ipernatremia e di ritardo dello svuotamento gastrico. Queste compresse però possono essere utili in un individuo con un elevato tasso di sudorazione o crampi da calore ricorrenti. L'attività prolungata (maratona) con la sola assunzione di acqua comporta per l'atleta un rischio di iponatremia.

Almond CSD, Shin AY, Fortescue EB: Hyponatremia among runners in the Boston marathon. *N Engl J Med* 2005;15:1150–1156.

American Academy of Pediatrics, Committee on Sports Medicine and Fitness: Climatic heat stress and the exercising child and adolescent. *Pediatrics* 2000;106:158–159.

Bytomski JR, Squire DL: Heat illness in children. *Curr Sports Med Rep* 2003;2:320–324.

Capitolo 689 ■ Problemi mestruali e rischio di osteopenia nelle atlete

Gregory L. Landry

Particolare preoccupazione destano l'eccessiva attività atletica nelle giovani donne e i suoi effetti sulla funzione riproduttiva e sullo stato minerale osseo, in particolare quando l'attività eccessiva è associata a restrizione calorica (vedi Capitoli 27 e 115).

La maggior parte della massa ossea viene acquisita entro la fine della seconda decade di vita (vedi Capitolo 705). Il 60-70% della massa ossea adulta è geneticamente determinata, mentre il resto dipende da tre fattori controllabili: attività fisica, assunzione di calcio e steroidi sessuali, in primo luogo estrogeni. L'attività fisica promuove la mineralizzazione ossea nella maggior parte delle giovani donne e deve essere incoraggiata. Nelle femmine con disordini del comportamento alimentare e in quelle che svolgono un'attività fisica tale da causare un'eccessiva perdita di peso con amenorrea o oligomenorrea, l'attività fisica può nuocere all'acquisizione di minerale osseo determinando una riduzione della contenuto minerale osseo o **osteopenia**.

Nello specifico, a incidere negativamente sulla mineralizzazione ossea è l'amenorrea (assenza di mestruazioni per 3 o più mesi consecutivi), che può dipendere da schemi alimentari anormali o disordini del comportamento alimentare. Quando disordini del comportamento alimentare, amenorrea e osteoporosi si verificano insieme, formano la **"triade della donna atleta"**. Nel corso delle visite mediche generali e di quelle che precedono la partecipazione ad attività sportive occorre ricercare con particolare attenzione qualsiasi segno di tale triade.

L'**amenorrea** nelle atlete è di solito causata dallo stress dell'allenamento o da una combinazione di allenamento e disordini del comportamento alimentare. L'amenorrea da attività fisica deve sempre essere una diagnosi di esclusione. Altre cause da escludere sono gravidanza, tumori ipofisari, anomalie della tiroide, sindrome dell'ovaio policistico, uso di steroidi anabolizzanti ed effetti collaterali di altri farmaci.

Il basso livello di estrogeni che caratterizza l'amenorrea non solo predispone la donna atleta a osteopenia, ma mette a rischio di fratture da stress, specialmente della colonna e delle estremità inferiori. Se non controllata, la perdita ossea è parzialmente irreversibile nonostante la ripresa delle mestruazioni, la terapia sostitutiva con estrogeni o i supplementi di calcio. Lo screening di routine della densità minerale ossea non è indicato, ma nei casi severi può fungere da guida per il trattamento e il ritorno all'attività.

Le atlete con amenorrea possono riavere un'ovulazione normale e le mestruazioni. Per ottenere questo risultato di solito sono necessari la riduzione dell'attività fisica e/o l'aumento dell'introito calorico. Tuttavia, molte rifiutano di ridurre l'attività, e in tal caso si rende necessario proporre altri metodi, come la supplementazione ormonale. Il counseling nutrizionale è importante per aiutare l'atleta a sviluppare un piano per aumentare l'introito calorico. Occorre correggere l'assunzione di calcio proponendosi l'obiettivo di raggiungere almeno i 1500 mg/die. Se l'amenorrea è presente da >6 mesi, si raccomanda la supplementazione ormonale. Tre sono i disordini del comportamento alimentare che possono presentarsi nel contesto di un'amenorrea: anoressia nervosa, che si manifesta come un peso <85% del peso ideale stimato con evidenze di denutrizione sotto forma di bradicardia, ipotermia e ipotensione ortostatica o tachicardia ortostatica; bulimia nervosa, che si manifesta con peso ridotto o normale e fluttuazioni del peso più ampie di quanto ci si aspetterebbe in base all'introito calorico e all'attività fisica riportati; disturbi del comportamento alimentare non altrimenti specificati, con alcuni aspetti dell'anoressia nervosa o della bulimia nervosa, anche se per la diagnosi di una delle due condizioni non sono soddisfatti tutti i criteri del manuale *Diagnostic and Statistical Manual of Mental Disorders*, 4ª edizione (vedi Capitolo 27). La maggior parte delle atlete che sviluppano il terzo tipo di disturbo del comportamento alimentare rientra in quello viene talvolta denominato "disturbo del comportamento alimentare atipico". Possono essere presenti contemporaneamente diversi sintomi e comportamenti anomali, da un'eccessiva restrizione delle calorie o dei grassi alle abbuffate e al vomito. Gli indizi di questo problema sono calo ponderale, restrizione alimentare, depressione, astenia, peggioramento della performance atletica, preoccupazione per le calorie e il peso. L'atleta può evitare le occasioni che implicano l'assunzione di alimenti oppure può fingere di mangiare, nascondendo il cibo per poi gettarlo via. Segni e sintomi comprendono deplezione dei tessuti adiposi, ipotrofia muscolare, bradicardia rispetto alla frequenza cardiaca consueta, ipotensione ortostatica, stipsi, intolleranza al freddo, ipotermia, disturbi della motilità gastrica e, in alcuni casi, presenza di lanugine. Le anomalie elettrolitiche possono causare aritmie cardiache. I problemi psichiatrici (depressione, ansia, rischio di suicidio) hanno un'aumentata incidenza in questa popolazione.

Per il **trattamento** dei disordini del comportamento alimentare, è fondamentale il controllo dei sintomi. Il primo passo è indurre l'atleta a prendere atto dei propri comportamenti anormali e del peso inadeguato. In generale, non si raccomanda l'attività fisica se il peso corporeo è <85% rispetto ai valori ideali stimati, anche se vi possono essere alcune eccezioni, specialmente se l'atleta è eumenorroica. Se l'atleta non riesce a riprendere peso soltanto con l'alimentazione e con la consulenza medica, è necessario un supporto psicologico.

Nella maggior parte dei casi le atlete inizialmente non ammettono il problema e possono essere inconsapevoli delle gravi conseguenze fisiche cui vanno incontro. Una strategia utile è quella di parlare con loro sottolineando con tatto i problemi legati alla performance. Spiegare loro che questo comportamento alimentare comporta diminuzione della forza, della resistenza e della concentrazione può fornire incentivi al trattamento. Spesso è necessario coinvolgere la famiglia dell'atleta e incoraggiare la diretta interessata a rivelare ai propri cari le informazioni necessarie. Nell'approccio multidisciplinare al trattamento dei disturbi del comportamento alimentare è importante una consulenza psicologica o psichiatrica: mentre il medico tiene sotto controllo la salute fisica dell'atleta, lo specialista psicologo/psichiatra si occupa degli aspetti mentali del disturbo del comportamento alimentare.

American Academy of Pediatrics Committee on Sports Medicine and Fitness: Medical concerns in the female athlete. *Pediatrics* 2000;106:610–612.
Birch K: Female athlete triad. *Br Med J* 2005;330:244–246.
Greydanus DE, Patel DR: The female athlete before and beyond puberty. *Pediatr Clin N Am* 2002;49:553–580.
Warren MP, Shantha S: The female athlete. *Best Pract Res Clin Endocrinol Metab* 2000;14:37–53.

Capitolo 690 ■ Ausili ergogenici

Gregory L. Landry

Gli ausili ergogenici sono sostanze utilizzate migliorare la performance, la maggior parte delle quali sono supplementi non soggetti a regolamentazione. Negli Stati Uniti il 1994 Dietary Supplement and Health Education Act ha limitato la possibilità della Food and Drug Administration (FDA) di regolamentare qualsiasi prodotto etichettato come supplemento. Molti agenti hanno effetti collaterali significativi senza proprietà ergogeniche accertate. Nell'aprile del 2005, l'American Academy of Pediatrics ha pubblicato una dichiarazione di ferma condanna del loro uso nei bambini e negli adolescenti.

Gli **steroidi anabolizzanti** (**AAS**, *Anabolic-Androgenic Steroids*) sono stati utilizzati a dosaggi superiori a quelli fisiologici per la loro capacità di aumentare la massa e la forza muscolare. Essi possiedono significativi effetti collaterali endocrinologici, come riduzione della conta degli spermatozoi e atrofia testicolare negli uomini e irregolarità mestruali e virilizzazione nelle donne. I problemi epatici comprendono aumento delle aminotransaminasi e della γ-glutamil transferasi, ittero colestatico, epatite peliosica e diverse neoplasie, tra cui il carcinoma epatocellulare. Vi sono evidenze che gli AAS possono anche causare problemi cardiovascolari, tra cui un aumento della pressione arteriosa, una riduzione delle lipoproteine a elevata densità, un aumento delle lipoproteine ad alta densità, un aumento dell'omocisteina e una riduzione della tolleranza al glucosio. Gli effetti psicologici comprendono aggressività, vari disordini della personalità e diversi altri problemi psicologici (ansia, paranoia, depressione, stati maniacali, psicosi). I segni e sintomi fisici comprendono ginecomastia, atrofia testicolare, ittero, acne e striae rubrae. Le donne possono presentare irsutismo, voce più profonda e alopecia di tipo maschile.

I **precursori del testosterone** (noti anche come pro-ormoni) comprendono androstenedione e diidroepiandrosterone (DHEA). Il loro uso nella popolazione adolescente è notevolmente aumentato in associazione alle segnalazioni dell'uso da parte di atleti di alto profilo. Si tratta di androgenizzanti, ma non è stato provato che siano anabolizzanti. Se hanno qualche effetto anabolizzante, questo deriva dall'aumento della produzione di testosterone. Essi aumentano anche la produzione di metaboliti degli estrogeni. Gli effetti collaterali sono simili a quelli degli AAS e superano di gran lunga qualsiasi effetto di tipo ergogenico. A partire dal gennaio 2005, negli Stati Uniti, queste sostanze non possono essere vendute senza prescrizione.

La **creatina** è un aminoacido immagazzinato principalmente nei muscoli scheletrici. La sua caratteristica principale è la capacità di rifosforilare l'adenosina difosfato ad adenosina trifosfato, aumentando in questo modo la performance muscolare. Il suo uso è aumentato, specialmente da quando altri supplementi sono stati ritirati dal mercato. Negli Stati Uniti il 30% dei giocatori di football delle scuole superiori ne ha fatto uso. Vi sono evidenze che la creatina aumenti la forza e la performance nello sforzo massimale quando utilizzata in allenamento. Non vi sono invece prove che influisca sull'idratazione o sulla regolazione della temperatura. I dubbi sul fatto che possa causare nefrite non sono stati confermati da studi controllati. Tuttavia, esistono pochi studi a lungo termine che valutano l'uso della creatina.

American Academy of Pediatrics: American Academy of Pediatrics policy statement: Use of performance enhancing substances. *Pediatrics* 2005;115:1103–1106.
The Medical Letter: Performance-enhancing drugs. Med Lett 2004;46:57–60.
Miah A: Doping and the child: An ethical policy for the vulnerable. *Lancet* 2005;366:874–876.
Tokish JM, Kocher MS, Hawkins RJ: Ergogenic aids: A review of basic science, performance, side effects, and status in sports. *Am J Sports Med* 2004;32:1543–1553.

Capitolo 691 ■ Sport esaminati singolarmente e traumi associati

Gregory L. Landry

GINNASTICA. I ginnasti iniziano a 5-6 anni di età e raggiungono i massimi livelli agonistici intorno ai 15 anni, spesso ritirandosi entro i 20 anni. I maschi tendono ad avere più traumi degli arti superiori, mentre le femmine vanno più soggette a traumi a livello degli arti inferiori. Oltre alle lesioni meccaniche o traumatiche, le ginnaste tendono ad avere un ritardo del menarca e possono presentare un'amenorrea o un'oligomenorrea ipotalamiche, associate a basso peso corporeo. La tipica conformazione corporea, che si manifesta con una riduzione del peso per altezza, associata ad amenorrea o oligomenorrea, suggerisce che la riduzione della densità ossea sia un problema per le ginnaste di alto livello. Nella maggior parte di esse, la densità ossea tende a essere elevata, fenomeno che si ritiene secondario alle attività ripetitive ad alto impatto; ciononostante, le fratture da stress sono un problema significativo. La bassa statura che caratterizza i ginnasti di entrambi i sessi è probabilmente dovuta alla selezione effettuata a monte e non è il risultato degli allenamenti.

Problemi comuni sono le lesioni traumatiche acute, come la distorsione della caviglia, e le lesioni croniche da uso eccessivo, come fratture da stress del polso e della colonna. La loro incidenza aumenta con il livello di abilità ed è maggiore negli esercizi a terra. Il dolore del polso da carico cronico sull'estremità superiore può essere causato da una frattura di Salter I da stress del radio distale, che si presenta tipicamente sull'aspetto dorsale radiale del polso ed è peggiorata dall'estensione passiva e dalla palpazione. Altre lesioni del polso comprendono lacerazioni del complesso fibrocartilagineo triangolare, fratture dello scafoide, cisti sinoviali dorsali e lesioni del legamento carpale. Il **trattamento** comprende in quasi tutti i casi l'immobilizzazione per un certo periodo, l'applicazione di ghiaccio e la somministrazione di analgesici. Se il dolore persiste, la diagnosi corretta può essere posta mediante RM o artroscopia per escludere lacerazioni intrarticolari, corpi liberi o instabilità legamentosa. Il pediatra deve inviare il paziente da uno specialista della mano in caso di trauma del polso che non migliora con il riposo. La lassità legamentosa può predisporre a lussazione di gomito o spalla e a distorsione della caviglia. I problemi della colonna comprendono spondilolisi (frattura da stress della pars interarticularis) e spondilolistesi (vedi Capitolo 678.6) a causa del carico ripetitivo in estensione.

NUOTO. Nei nuotatori di livello agonistico il trauma della spalla è la più comune lesione da uso eccessivo. La spalla del nuotatore, che consiste in una combinazione di borsite sottoacromiale e tendinite della cuffia dei rotatori, di solito del tendine del sopraspinato, si manifesta con un dolore insidioso alla spalla. Tale dolore, causato dalla borsite sottoacromiale, può essere suscitato dal test di compressione di Hawkin, mediante flessione passiva in avanti dell'omero a 90°, seguita dalla rotazione interna dell'omero. La tendinite del sopraspinato suscita dolore durante l'abduzione attiva tra 60 e 100° e la manovra cosiddetta di "svuotamento del barattolo", in cui il paziente ruota internamente l'omero a riposo e quindi solleva il braccio su un piano a metà tra flessione e abduzione. Il **trattamento** comprende applicazione del ghiaccio, modifica della tecnica di bracciata, riposo relativo e rinforzo muscolare della cuffia dei rotatori e dei muscoli dorsali superiori. Ai fini della prevenzione occorre evitare un rapido aumento del carico di allenamento, adottare una tecnica appropriata ed eseguire esercizi di rinforzo.

BASEBALL. I traumi da lancio di gomito e spalla (specialmente nei *pitcher*) sono i più comuni nel baseball (vedi Capitoli 686.2 e 686.3). È importante non solo limitare il numero di lanci, ma raccomandare a giocatori, allenatori e atleti di fermarsi immediatamente quando avvertono dolore del gomito e, qualora quest'ultimo persistesse, di rivolgersi al medico. È stato stabilito che un giovane lanciatore non dovrebbe eseguire più di 200 lanci alla settimana e che il numero massimo di lanci per gara sia pari all'età del lanciatore in anni moltiplicata per 6. I decessi nel baseball, peraltro rari, sono riconducibili a trauma toracico causato dalla palla (**commotio cordis**) (vedi Capitolo 436) o a trauma cranico causato dalla palla o dalla mazza. I caschi da battitore devono essere indossati correttamente, nel tentativo di prevenire i traumi del viso e della testa.

DANZA. Questa attività molto impegnativa può essere associata a ritardo del menarca e a disturbi del comportamento alimentare nelle ballerine (vedi Capitolo 689). Si verificano traumi acuti, per lo più a carico delle estremità inferiori. Come con qualsiasi attività ripetitiva, sono probabili lesioni da uso eccessivo; la chiave consiste in una diagnosi corretta e anche nel considerare la disfunzione della catena cinetica che può aver contribuito a tale lesione. Un ballerino può avere una distorsione della caviglia non riabilitata e quindi risparmiare la gamba sede della lesione, procurandosi in questo modo una frattura da stress della tibia controlaterale. I problemi del piede comprendono fratture metatarsali da stress, ematomi subungueali, formazione di callosità e di cisti sinoviali, sesamoiditi e fascite plantare. Una domanda che i giovani ballerini e i loro genitori possono rivolgere al medico è quella relativa alla possibilità di danzare **sulle punte**; a tal fine, l'età media è 12 anni. Questa decisione andrebbe presa dopo l'esecuzione di un test funzionale: il soggetto viene considerato pronto quando può salire sulle punte e mantenere la posizione, senza apparire instabile e privo di forza, e senza provare dolore. I problemi della caviglia consistono nelle sindromi da compressione anteriore e posteriore, causate degli estremi dell'arco di movimento raggiunti rispettivamente nel *grand plié* e nella danza sulle punte. I problemi dell'anca comprendono sia la sindrome dello scatto mediale, causata dal tendine dell'ileopsoas che scorre sopra la parte anteriore della capsula articolare dell'anca, sia una tendinite (piriforme, ileopsoas, retto femorale). La **sindrome del piriforme**, che si verifica spesso a causa della rotazione esterna ripetitiva dell'anca necessaria nella danza, si può manifestare sotto forma di dolore della natica e dell'anca e con una sciatalgia.

LOTTA. I lottatori presentano ampie fluttuazioni ponderali per soddisfare gli standard agonistici basati sul peso. Tali fluttuazioni sono associate a digiuno con disidratazione, seguito da abbuffate.

Le prese della lotta possono causare traumi in seguito a varie forze o torsioni applicate alle estremità e alla colonna; i lanci che avvengono durante la lotta e le conseguenti cadute possono produrre concussioni, distorsione cervicale o traumi spinali. Le due sedi più comuni di trauma sono anca e ginocchio. Sensazioni di bruciore e formicolio possono essere dovute a plessopatia brachiale (vedi "Football").

La sublussazione della spalla è comune. I pazienti sono spesso consapevoli della lussazione e del riposizionamento in sede della spalla (vedi Capitolo 686.2). I traumi della mano, di solito non severi, consistono nelle distorsioni ricorrenti delle articolazioni metacarpofalangee e interfalangee prossimali. Il trattamento dei traumi della mano consiste nell'uso di tutori e nel bendaggio.

I traumi del ginocchio, comuni e potenzialmente severi, comprendono borsite prerotulea, distorsioni mediali e laterali e lacerazioni del menisco mediale e laterale (vedi Capitolo 686.6). La borsite prerotulea è causata da un impatto traumatico acuto o ricorrente contro il tappeto. Si sviluppa un edema sulla rotula e i pazienti non presentano limitazioni del movimento, tranne che per la flessione completa. Se la cute si è lacerata, occorre prendere in considerazione una borsite settica. Il medico deve cercare di distinguere la borsite traumatica dalla borsite infetta, che può richiedere l'aspirazione della borsa. Il **trattamento** della borsite traumatica comprende imbottiture protettive, ghiaccio, FANS e talvolta, se la flessione è limitata, aspirazione. La borsectomia si rende necessaria di rado, se si verificano diverse recidive.

I problemi **dermatologici** comprendono herpes simplex (herpes gladiatorum), impetigine, foruncolosi o follicolite stafilococcica, micosi superficiali e dermatite da contatto; le prime due sono controindicazioni alla lotta fino a quando l'infezione non è più contagiosa. In caso di infezioni erpetiche ricorrenti, si devono somministrare farmaci antivirali per os.

FOOTBALL. Tra gli sport più praticati, il football è uno di quelli con i più elevati tassi di traumi. Tuttavia, in termini di severità dei traumi, quantificata in base ai giorni persi, le lesioni che si verificano nel football in media sono meno gravi di quelle associate a molti altri sport. In gran parte dei casi si tratta di distorsioni, stiramenti e contusioni che, se trattati appropriatamente, determinano un'astensione relativamente breve dalla pratica sportiva.

Anche se la maggior parte dei traumi sportivi catastrofici negli Stati Uniti si è verificata proprio nel football, i traumi severi sono rari. Si definisce catastrofico un trauma fatale o grave con o senza disabilità funzionale severa permanente. Sono disabilitanti i traumi della colonna cervicale e quelli cerebrali.

I traumi cranici e cervicali nel football comprendono concussione, distorsione cervicale e plessopatia brachiale, quest'ultima riferita come sensazione di bruciore o formicolio a livello degli arti superiori. I traumi della colonna lombare che si manifestano sotto forma di lombalgia possono rappresentare una spondilolisi. I traumi della spalla possono causare lussazione gleno-omerale (nella maggior parte dei casi lussazioni anteriori), separazioni acromioclavicolari e fratture clavicolari e omerali.

Le **contusioni** dei muscoli del braccio e della coscia sono comuni e possono causare grandi ematomi se non vengono trattate in modo aggressivo. In assenza di fratture, nei primi giorni il **trattamento** consiste nell'applicazione del ghiaccio e nella compressione durante la maggior parte delle ore del giorno, al fine di impedire all'ematoma di espandersi; in seguito l'infortunato dovrà eseguire esercizi non dolorosi di rinforzo e stretching fino al ripristino della funzionalità iniziale, dopodiché il medico potrà autorizzare il ritorno al contatto. Quando l'ematoma persiste, in particolare se al suo interno si forma un secondo ematoma, si può sviluppare una miosite ossificante.

I problemi muscoloscheletrici più comuni al momento della valutazione prestagionale sono i traumi del ginocchio, affrontati nel Capitolo 686.6.

Sono possibili distorsioni della caviglia; il rischio che il trauma si ripeta può essere ridotto dalla riabilitazione e dall'uso di un sostegno rimovibile per la caviglia. La distorsione della prima articolazione metatarsofalangea (*turf toe*) è causata dalla dorsiflessione forzata nel gioco su terreni artificiali con calzature leggere e flessibili. Il **trattamento** comprende ghiaccio, FANS, un'ortesi per limitare l'estensione dell'alluce e riposo. Il turf toe può essere una lesione in grado di compromettere non solo la stagione agonistica, ma persino la carriera di un calciatore.

HOCKEY SU GHIACCIO. L'hockey è uno sport di collisione associato a traumi causati dall'impatto del disco o della mazza sul giocatore o dal contatto corporeo con gli avversari, con il ghiaccio o con le delimitazioni del campo, che producono contusioni, lacerazioni, fratture, distorsioni o concussioni. Per ridurre il rischio di trauma il giocatore deve adottare un'attrezzatura adeguata (casco con maschera per il viso) e applicare una serie di regole sul contatto corporeo pericoloso (contatto da dietro, colpire alto, colpire di taglio e colluttazione).

I traumi specifici dello hockey comprendono distorsioni della caviglia (dorsiflessione, eversione e rotazione esterna, diversamente dalla consueta distorsione in inversione in altri sport), stiramento degli adduttori dell'anca, osteite pubica e diversi traumi della spalla da contatto corporeo. Questi ultimi comprendono distorsione acromioclavicolare, lussazione di spalla e fratture di clavicola. I traumi più severi sono quelli cranici e cervicali.

BASKET E PALLAVOLO. I comuni gesti tecnici di questi due sport comprendono presa di una palla con le mani, salto, movimenti di rotazione, corsa inframmezzata da arresti improvvisi, tutti movimenti che aumentano il rischio di traumi della caviglia, del ginocchio e delle dita.

I traumi da uso eccessivo del ginocchio comprendono la **tendinite rotulea** ("ginocchio del saltatore") e l'**apofisite da trazione** (malattia di Osgood-Schlatter). Come in altri sport che prevedono l'atto di saltare, si possono verificare distorsioni acute dei legamenti (collaterale mediale, con o senza interessamento del legamento crociato anteriore).

La distorsione della caviglia è il trauma più comune, di solito causato da inversione con flessione plantare, che sottopone a notevole tensione i legamenti laterali. Una frattura da avulsione della base del 5° metatarso a livello dell'inserzione del tendine del peroneo breve è un'altra conseguenza dei traumi in inversione della caviglia. La tendinite del tendine di Achille è un'altra comune lesione da uso eccessivo. Il dolore del piede può essere dovuto a borsite retrocalcaneare, tendinite del tibiale posteriore, scafoide tarsale accessorio, periostite calcaneare, fascite plantare, frattura da stress dello scafoide tarsale, frattura da stress di Jones del 5° metatarso, sesamoidite, formazione di vesciche, ematoma subungueale e paronichia.

CORSA. I problemi della corsa sono di solito riconducibili a traumi da uso eccessivo correlati a squilibrio muscolare, deformità scheletriche minori o inadeguata flessibilità, forza, endurance o propriocezione. Nella corsa l'impatto del piede varia a ogni passo, potendo essere da 3 a 8 volte il peso corporeo dell'atleta. La maggior parte dei problemi è dovuta a errori compiuti durante l'allenamento quando il corridore aumenta la distanza o l'intensità dello sforzo fisico troppo rapidamente. Variazioni anatomiche minori (disallineamento), che non causano problemi a riposo, possono predisporre a traumi in sedi specifiche (stress rotuleofemorale, iperpronazione). Anche la fatica muscolare, la temperatura ambientale e la superficie del campo (erba o cemento rigido) contribuiscono ai traumi. La prevenzione dei traumi è possibile con esercizi di rinforzo muscolare in caso di traumi pregressi. L'uso di calzature da corsa di buona qualità che si adattino al piede è un passo preliminare essenziale. Sono importanti le calzature specifiche per il sesso in quanto le ragazze generalmente hanno un retropiede più stretto. I soggetti con iperpronazione severa necessitano di una calzatura di controllo del movimento per un supporto massimale del retropiede e dell'arco plantare a livello della parte mediana della suola. I soggetti con iperpronazione lieve necessitano di una calzatura in grado di assicurare stabilità, con supporto extra e un'imbottitura a livello della parte centrale della suola. I soggetti con supinazione hanno invece bisogno di una calzatura dotata di imbottitura in grado di assorbire di più lo shock a livello della parte centrale della suola, una forma più ricurva e un supporto minimo per l'arco plantare.

Possono verificarsi **fratture da stress** di collo femorale, rami pubici inferiori, area subtrocanterica, diafisi femorale prossimale, tibia prossimale, perone, scafoide, metatarsi, sesamoidi e apofisi calcaneare. Nei corridori possono manifestarsi fratture da stress delle ossa dell'arto inferiore. La più comune è a livello dei metatarsi, della tibia e del perone. Quelle più preoccupanti in termini di mancato consolidamento sono le fratture della tibia prossimale anteriore, del collo femorale e dello scafoide tarsale. Gli stiramenti muscolari sono frequenti nei muscoli posteriori della coscia, seguiti da quadricipite, adduttori dell'anca, soleo e muscoli gastrocnemi. Una tendinite che interessa il tendine e della sua guaina è comune nel tendine d'Achille, seguito da tendini del tibiale posteriore, peronei, ileopsoas e muscoli posteriori della coscia prossimali. L'infiammazione del tendine d'Achille, che tende a divenire cronica, inizialmente può migliorare durante una corsa; caratterizzata da dolorabilità e crepitio se è acuta e modularità se è cronica, deve essere differenziata da un borsite retrocalcaneare. Il **trattamento** comprende l'identificazione della causa di base e l'astinenza temporanea dalla corsa (iniziare il cross-training), una soletta per il tallone, stretching del tendine d'Achille e FANS.

Il dolore anteriore del ginocchio è di solito dovuto a una sindrome da stress femororotuleo (**ginocchio del corridore**), che deriva da un eccesso di movimento dinamico, di solito laterale, del tendine rotuleo in relazione al solco intracondiloideo femorale. Il **trattamento** consiste nello stretching del quadricipite e dei muscoli posteriori della coscia ed eventualmente della banda ileotibiale, in esercizi di rinforzo del quadricipite, nell'applicazione del ghiaccio e nel riposo relativo. Le ortesi per il piede possono essere indicate se il trattamento appena esposto non produce alcun miglioramento. Il dolore posteriore del ginocchio può essere causato da stiramento del gastrocnemio, quello posteromediale da fratture da stress tibiali prossimali o da una tendinite del semimembranoso o del semitendinoso, mentre il dolore laterale del ginocchio può essere dovuto a sindrome della banda ileotibiale e a tendinite del popliteo. La **sindrome della banda ileotibiale** può essere una combinazione di borsite e tendinite dovuta alla frizione meccanica della banda (un'estensione del muscolo tensore della fascia lata) sull'epicondilo femorale laterale.

Con la dicitura **shin splint**, o sindrome da stress tibiale mediale, si indica il dolore a livello della tibia mediale, condizione che deve essere distinta dalle fratture tibiali da stress e dalle sindromi compartimentali croniche (vedi Capitolo 686.7). La sindrome da stress tibiale mediale si verifica di solito nei corridori con iperpronazione che hanno iniziato da poco l'attività. Il **trattamento** comprende la corsa su superfici morbide, la scelta di calzature appropriate ed eventualmente l'uso di ortesi, FANS e riposo relativo (o cross-training). Le sindromi compartimentali croniche interessano i compartimenti posteriori o anteriori profondi, causando dolore pulsante locale limitato al gruppo muscolare (senza coinvolgimento dell'osso). Classicamente, il dolore inizia non appena l'atleta comincia a correre ed è alleviato dal riposo; rende impossibile proseguire l'allenamento, limitando così il rischio di un danno nervoso permanente. La diagnosi si pone misurando l'aumento delle pressioni intracompartimentali nel corso dell'attività fisica.

La **fascite plantare** è un'infiammazione della struttura di supporto dell'arco longitudinale riconducibile al carico ciclico ripetitivo causato dall'appoggio del piede a terra. Il dolore, che si manifesta con il primo passo fuori da letto al mattino e aumenta con la corsa, è localizzato sull'aspetto mediale del tallone. La fascite è associata all'uso di calzature vecchie e consumate con uno scarso supporto plantare. Il **trattamento** comprende stretching del polpaccio, calzature appropriate, tutori notturni, iniezione di corticosteroidi, riposo relativo e massaggio con ghiaccio del tallone. La frattura da stress calcaneare deve essere presa in considerazione, soprattutto nella maratoneta amenorroica.

CALCIO. Nel calcio, i traumi comprendono tutte le lesioni correlate alla corsa, come abrasioni, contusioni, stiramenti muscolari e distorsioni dei legamenti (caviglia, ginocchio), in parte a causa del contatto corpo a corpo, alle cadute, alla corsa e ai calci. I problemi dell'anca sono contusioni della cresta iliaca (*hip pointer*), apofisite della cresta iliaca e dolore inguinale cronico (stiramento muscolare, ernia, osteite del pube). Le fratture da stress del collo femorale, l'epifisiolisi del collo femorale e le fratture da avulsione del bacino o del femore devono essere considerate nella diagnosi differenziale, come pure le cause insolite di dolore dell'anca. Nel calcio possono verificarsi tutte le altre lesioni delle estremità superiori e inferiori.

Nel calcio sono frequenti le **concussioni**, che possono portare a disfunzione neurocognitiva; esse sono dovute al contatto con l'avversario, con il palo della porta o con il terreno di gioco. L'American Academy of Pediatrics raccomanda che i ragazzi che giocano a calcio riducano al minimo i colpi di testa, fintantoché non si avranno maggiori informazioni sui rischi di questa pratica in età pediatrica. Occorre inoltre insegnare una corretta tecnica dei colpi di testa; sui lanci lunghi, il giocatore che riceve la palla la blocca con il petto o con le gambe, non con la testa; i difensori calciano la palla davanti ai centrocampisti o attaccanti in modo che questi la raggiungano e la blocchino con i piedi; i giocatori devono evitare di colpire la palla di testa all'indietro verso la porta (con estensione cervicale); gli arbitri, come in tutti gli sport, devono mantenere il gioco sotto controllo e penalizzare le azioni pericolose. Dopo una concussione, il calciatore deve seguire le linee guida per poter far ritorno in campo.

TENNIS. I traumi degli arti inferiori si verificano con una frequenza due volte superiore rispetto ai traumi degli arti superiori e, in generale, il tasso di traumi è simile nei maschi e nelle femmine. Le aree più soggette a traumi nel tennis comprendono muscoli e tendini del gomito, spalla, dorso, polso e addome. Il rischio aumenta con l'allenamento intenso, con traumi pregressi non riabilitati e relativi deficit di flessibilità, forza e resistenza, e con una tecnica inadeguata. I traumi acuti delle estremità inferiori comprendono distorsioni a livello di caviglia, ginocchio, gamba e inguine. Possono verificarsi lesioni da uso eccessivo della schiena e delle estremità inferiori e superiori. I pattern traumatici degli arti inferiori sono correlati al fatto che nei giocatori molto abili vi è una media di 8 cambiamenti di direzione per punto, che impongono carichi eccentrici e concentrici alle estremità inferiori. Per quanto riguarda la schiena, i traumi sono correlati ai marcati e rapidi cambiamenti di carico e direzione associati al servizio, con la spalla, il gomito e il polso che si spostano a velocità che possono arrivare rispettivamente 1700, 900 e 350°/s, in modo ripetitivo. I traumi possono essere correlati a un'attrezzatura inadeguata, come una racchetta troppo grande, oppure all'apprendimento delle tecniche, come colpire con effetto o con forza prima di avere acquisito un corretto coordinamento e una tecnica appropriata per i colpi di base. I traumi da uso eccessivo comprendono le fratture da stress di omero, ulna e metacarpi, e l'apofisite da trazione del calcagno, della tuberosità tibiale (malattia di Osgood-Schlatter) e dell'epicondilo omerale mediale.

La tendinite della cuffia dei rotatori, causata da un uso eccessivo ripetitivo, può essere correlata a instabilità gleno-omerale anteroposteriore. Può essere presente anche una sublussazione dell'articolazione gleno-omerale. La tendinite del bicipite può presentarsi come dolore anteriore della spalla.

Il **gomito del tennista**, o epicondilite laterale, è dovuto a sovraccarico ripetitivo del meccanismo di estensione/supinazione del polso, soprattutto dell'estensore radiale breve del carpo (vedi Capitolo 686-3). L'epicondilite mediale è causata dal sovraccarico ripetitivo dei gruppi muscolari flessori/pronatori. Il fenomeno può interessare secondariamente il legamento collaterale mediale, che però è raramente la sede del trauma primario. L'apofisite epicondilare mediale può essere associata a disfunzione del nervo ulnare se è presente una frattura da avulsione. L'apofisite dell'olecrano, simile alla malattia di Osgood-Schlatter, è caratterizzata da dolore dell'olecrano all'estensione del gomito.

I problemi del polso sono cisti sinoviali dorsali, sinovite della capsula articolare radiocarpale (limitazione), attrito degenerativo (lacerazioni) del complesso fibrocartilagineo triangolare e fratture dell'uncino dell'uncinato.

Il **trattamento** di base comprende riposo relativo, analgesici, applicazione di ghiaccio, riabilitazione, apprendimento della meccanica corretta, uso di racchette di dimensioni appropriate, uso di ortesi protettive che controbilanciano la forza (gomito, polso), esercizi di rinforzo e ritorno graduale al gioco. Le iniezioni di corticosteroidi nei gruppi muscolari estensori/supinatori per il "gomito del tennista" non sono raccomandate in quanto l'esito a un anno è meno buono che nei pazienti trattati con la riabilitazione.

SCI. I traumi sono correlati alle cadute (concussioni, contusioni, lacerazioni) e ai meccanismi specifici dello sci. In generale, i traumi sono diminuiti, in parte grazie al miglioramento dell'attrezzatura (scarponi, attacchi, racchette da sci) e delle condizioni delle piste. È stato raccomandato che bambini e adolescenti indossino caschi per lo sci o lo snowboard.

I traumi del pollice derivanti da cadute con questo dito in abduzione e iperestensione causano una distorsione del legamento collaterale ulnare (pollice dello sciatore). Le lacerazioni complete con apertura a 45° dell'articolazione richiedono l'intervento chirurgico, mentre aperture di grado minore possono essere trattate con un gesso a spica per il pollice per 4 settimane. Può essere presente anche una frattura di Salter-Harris di tipo III; se vi è spostamento della frattura epifisaria, richiede la riduzione aperta e la fissazione interna.

I traumi dell'estremità inferiore comprendono fratture (spesso spirali) della tibia (*boot top*) e distorsioni della caviglia e del legamento crociato anteriore, con o senza frattura dell'eminenza tibiale. Un emartro è presente nelle fratture e nelle lesioni del menisco e del legamento crociato anteriore. Il **trattamento** è discusso nel Capitolo 676.

American Academy of Pediatrics Committee on Sports Medicine and Fitness: Injuries in youth soccer: A subject review. *Pediatrics* 2000;105:659–661.

American Academy of Pediatrics Committee on Sports Medicine and Fitness: The management of minor closed head injury in children. *Pediatrics* 1999;104:1407–1415.

Bisset L, Beller E, Jull G, et al: Mobilisation with movement and excercise, corticosteroid injection, or wait and see for tennis elbow: randomised trial. *BMJ* 2006;333:939–941.

Boutis K, Komar L, Jaramillo D, et al: Sensitivity of a clinical examination to predict need for radiography in children with ankle injuries: A prospective study. *Lancet* 2001;358:2118–2121.

Christopher NC, Congeni J: Overuse injuries in the pediatric athlete: Evaluation, initial management, and strategies for prevention. *Clin Pediatr Emerg Med* 2002;3:118–128.

Committee on Sports Medicine and Fitness: Climatic heat stress and the exercising child and adolescent. *Pediatrics* 2000;106:158–159.

Committee on Sports Medicine and Fitness: Medical concerns in the female athlete. *Pediatrics* 2000;106:610–613.

Committee on Sports Medicine and Fitness: Medical conditions affecting sports participation. *Pediatrics* 2001;107:1205–1209.

Heidt RS, Sweeterman LM, Carlonas Richelle L, et al: Avoidance of soccer injuries with preseason conditioning. *Am J Sport Med* 2000;28:659–662.

Hoffman JR, Mower WR, Wolfson AB, et al: Validity of a set of clinical criteria to rule out injury to the cervical spine in patients with blunt trauma. *N Engl J Med* 2000;343:94–99.

Maron BJ, Shirani J, Poliac LC, et al: Sudden death in young competitive athletes. Clinical, demographic, and pathological profiles. *JAMA* 1996;276:199–204.

McClain LG, Reynolds S: Sports injuries in a high school. *Pediatrics* 1989;84:446–450.

McCrory PR: Brain injury and heading in soccer. *Br Med J* 2003;327:351–352.

Nysted M, Drogset JO: Trampoline injuries. *Br J Sports Med* 2006;40:984–987.

Smidt N, van der Windt DAWM: Tennis elbow in primary care. *BMJ* 2006;333:927–928.

Smidt N, van der Windt DAWM, Assendelft JJ, et al: Corticosteroid injections, physiotherapy, or a wait-and-see policy for lateral epicondylitis: A randomized controlled trial. *Lancet* 2002;359:657–662.

Solomon DH, Simel DL, Bates DW, et al: Does this patient have a torn meniscus or ligament of the knee? *JAMA* 2001;286:1610–1620.

Speed CA: Corticosteroid injections in tendon lesions. *Br Med J* 2001;323:382–386.

University Interscholastic League-Preparticipation Physical Evaluation, 2002. Search www.uil.utexas.edu/index.html. Go to Athletics, then to Athletic forms, then Preparticipation Physical Evaluation.

Warren WL, Bailes JE: On the field evaluation of athletic head injuries. *Clin Sports Med* 1998;17:13–26.

Sezione 3 — Displasie scheletriche

Capitolo 692 ■ Considerazioni generali

William A. Horton e Jacqueline T. Hecht

Quando si parla di displasie scheletriche, displasie ossee e osteocondrodisplasie ci si riferisce a un gruppo geneticamente e clinicamente eterogeneo di disordini dello sviluppo e della crescita dello scheletro. La loro prevalenza è stimata in circa 1/4000 nati. Esse si possono suddividere in osteodisplasie, come l'osteogenesi imperfetta (vedi Capitolo 699), e condrodisplasie; queste ultime derivano da mutazioni di geni che sono essenziali per lo sviluppo e la crescita dello scheletro. Il quadro clinico è dominato dalle anomalie scheletriche. Le manifestazioni possono essere limitate alle ossa, ma nella maggior parte dei casi sono interessati anche altri tessuti. I disordini possono essere letali già in utero o lievi, con segni che passano inosservati.

Le condrodisplasie si distinguono da altre forme di ipostaturalità per una sproporzione delle manifestazioni scheletriche. L'importanza della cartilagine nella formazione dell'osso è sottolineata nella Figura 692-1. Esse si dividono in forme in cui i pazienti hanno prevalentemente arti corti e forme in cui i pazienti hanno prevalentemente il tronco più corto. Nel tentativo di definire l'estensione dell'eterogeneità clinica sono state individuate più di 100 entità distinte. Molti di questi disordini derivano da mutazioni di un gruppo di geni relativamente piccolo, i "geni della condrodisplasia".

Un International Working Group on Bone Dysplasias li ha classificati in gruppi basati su cause genetiche, se note, o sulle analogie riscontrabili negli aspetti clinici e radiografici, che spesso implicano una patogenesi comune e una base genetica comune, se la causa è sconosciuta (Tab. 692-1). I gruppi di condrodisplasie meglio definite, come quelli dell'acondroplasia e della collagenopatia di tipo II, contengono una serie graduale di disordini la cui severità varia da molto elevata a minima. Ciò può essere vero per altri gruppi via via che sempre più mutazioni vengono identificate e si comincia a delineare lo spettro completo dei fenotipi clinici associati alle mutazioni di un determinato gene. Questi disordini sono fenotipi clinici distribuiti lungo spettri di anomalie fenotipiche associate a mutazioni di particolari geni. Per le mutazioni di alcuni geni, come COL2A1, la distribuzione è abbastanza continua, con fenotipi clinici che trapassano l'uno nell'altro attraverso un ampio range. Esiste invece una sovrapposizione clinica molto

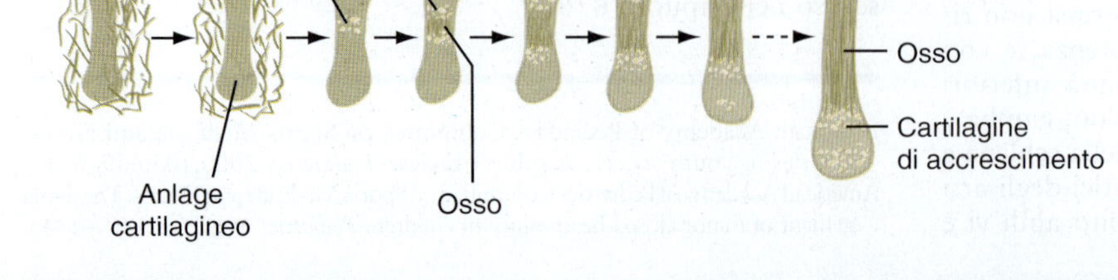

Figura 692-1. Importanza della cartilagine nella formazione dell'osso. (Da Horton WA: Skeletal development: Insights from targeting the mouse genome. *Lancet* 2005;362:560.)

TABELLA 692-1. Genetica delle displasie scheletriche

LOCUS GENICO	LOCALIZZAZIONE CROMOSOMICA	PROTEINA	FUNZIONE DELLA PROTEINA	FENOTIPO CLINICO	OMIM	MECCANISMO DELLA MALATTIA	EREDITARIETÀ
COL2A1	12q13.1-q13.3	Catena α_1 del collagene di tipo II	Proteina della matrice cartilaginea	Acondrogenesia di tipo II	200610	Dominante negativo	AD*
				Ipocondrogenesia	200610	Dominante negativo	AD*
				SED congenita	183900	Dominante negativo	AD
				Displasia di Kniest	156550	Dominante negativo	AD
				SED a esordio tardivo		Dominante negativo	AD
				Displasia di Stickler	108300	Aploinsufficienza	AD
SEDL	Xp22.2-p22.1	Sedlina	Trasportatore intracellulare	SED tardiva X-linked	313400	Perdita funzionale	XLR
COL11A1	1p21	Catena α_1 del collagene di tipo XI	Proteina della matrice cartilaginea	Displasia Stickler-simile	184840	Dominante negativo	AD
COL11A2	6p21.3	Catena α_2 del collagene di tipo XI	Proteina della matrice cartilaginea	Displasia Stickler-simile	215150	Perdita funzionale	AR
COMP	19p12-p13.1	Proteina oligomerica della matrice cartilaginea	Proteina della matrice cartilaginea	Pseudoacondroplasia	177170	Dominante negativo	AD
				MED	600969	Dominante negativo	AD
COL9A2	1p32.2-p33	Catena α_2 del collagene di tipo IX	Proteina della matrice cartilaginea	MED	600969	Dominante negativo	AD
COL9A3	20q13.3	Catena α_3 del collagene di tipo IX	Proteina della matrice cartilaginea	MED	600969	Dominante negativo	AD
MATN3	2p24-p23	Matrilina 3	Proteina della matrice cartilaginea	MED	600969	Dominante negativo	AD
COL10A1	6q21-q22.3	Catena α_1 del collagene di tipo X	Proteina della matrice cartilaginea ipertrofica	Condrodisplasia metafisaria di Schmid	156500	Aploinsufficienza	AD
FGFR3	4p16.3	Recettore FGF 3	Recettore della tirosina chinasi per i FGF	Displasia tanatofora I	187600	Guadagno funzionale	AD*
				Displasia tanatofora II	187610	Guadagno funzionale	AD*
				Acondroplasia	100800	Guadagno funzionale	AD
				Ipocondroplasia	146000	Guadagno funzionale	AD
PTHR1	3p21-p22	Recettore del PTHrP	Recettore del PTH e del PTHrP accoppiato alla proteina G	Condrodisplasia metafisaria di Jansen	156400	Guadagno funzionale	AD
DTDST	5q32-q33	Trasportatore del DTD solfato	Trasportatore transmembrana del solfato	Acondrogenesia 1B	600972	Perdita funzionale	AR*
				Atelosteogenesia II	256050	Perdita funzionale	AR*
				Displasia diastrofica	222600	Perdita funzionale	AR
SOX9	17q24.3-q25.1	SRY box 9	Fattore di trascrizione	Displasia camptomelica	114290	Aploinsufficienza	AD
CBFA1[†]	6p21	Subunità α del core binding factor	Fattore di trascrizione	Displasia cleidocranica	119600	Aploinsufficienza	AD
LMX1B	9q34.1	Fattore di trascrizione		Nail-patella syndrome	161200	Aploinsufficienza	AD
CTSK	1q21	Catepsina K	Enzima	Picnodisostosi	265800	Perdita funzionale	AR
RMPR	9p21-p12	Mitocondriale Endoribonucleasi che processa l'RNA	Enzima che processa l'RNA	CHH	250250	Perdita funzionale	AR

*Di solito letale.
[†]Denominato anche RUNX2.
AD, autosomico dominante; AR, autosomico recessivo; CHH (*Cartilage-Hair Hypoplasia*), ipoplasia cartilagine-capelli; DTD (*Diastrophic Dysplasia*), displasia diastrofica; FGF (*Fibroblast Growth Factor*), fattore di crescita dei fibroblasti; MED (*Multiple Epiphyseal Dysplasia*), displasia epifisaria multipla; PTH (*ParaThyroid Hormone*), paratormone; PTHrP (*PTH-related Protein*), proteina correlata al paratormone; SED (*SpondyloEpiphyseal Dysplasia*), displasia spondiloepifisaria; SRY (*Sex-determining Region of the Y chromosome*), regione determinante il sesso del cromosoma Y.

minore per le mutazioni di alcuni altri geni, come *FGFR3*, in cui la distribuzione è discontinua. Dal momento che la maggior parte degli Autori e la maggior parte degli studi di riferimento si riferiscono a questi disordini come a entità distinte, si continua a usare queste definizioni,

Anche se alcune condrodisplasie possono essere facilmente diagnosticate, la maggior parte di esse richiede l'analisi di informazioni fornite da anamnesi, esame obiettivo, radiografie dello scheletro, anamnesi familiare e test di laboratorio. Il processo comprende il riconoscimento di pattern complessi caratteristici dei differenti disordini (Tabb. 692-2, 692-3, 692-4 e 692-5). Le descrizioni complete dei disordini e le relative referenze si possono trovare sul sito internet On-Line Mendelian Inheritance (vedi Biliografia).

MANIFESTAZIONI CLINICHE

MANIFESTAZIONI CORRELATE ALL'ACCRESCIMENTO. Il segno distintivo di tutte le condrodisplasie è la statura sproporzionatamente bassa. Anche se con questa espressione si intende indicare una sproporzione tra arti e tronco, la maggior parte dei disordini presenta un certo accorciamento di entrambi e una leggera spro-

TABELLA 692-2. Principali problemi associati alle displasie scheletriche

PROBLEMA	ESEMPIO
Letalità*	Displasia tanatofora
Anomalie associate[†]	Sindrome di Ellis-Van Creveld
Bassa statura	Comune a quasi tutte
Lussazioni della colonna cervicale	Sindrome di Larsen
Severa curvatura degli arti	Displasia metafisaria, tipo Schmid
Curvature della colonna	Displasia metatropica
Piede torto	Displasia diastrofica
Fratture	Osteogenesi imperfetta
Polmoniti, aspirazioni	Displasia camptomelica
Compressione del midollo spinale	Acondroplasia
Problemi articolari (anche, ginocchia)	La maggior parte delle displasie scheletriche
Ipoacusia	Comuni (massima nella palatoschisi)
Miopia/cataratte	Sindrome di Stickler
Immunodeficienza[‡]	Cartilage-hair hypoplasia, displasia immuno-ossea di Schimke
Immagine corporea negativa	Variabile, ma comune a tutte
Sex reversal	Displasia camptomelica

*Causata soprattutto alla riduzione severa delle dimensioni toraciche.
[†]Vedi Tabella 692-3.
[‡]Almeno 4 ulteriori disordini, che interessano tutti le metafisi, possono comportare un'immunodeficienza.

TABELLA 692-3. Anomalie associate nelle displasie scheletriche

ANOMALIA	ESEMPIO
Difetti cardiaci	Sindrome di Ellis-Van Creveld, sindrome di Jeune
Polidattilia	Polidattilia con coste corte, tipo di Maiewski
Palatoschisi	Displasia diastrofica
Cisti auricolari	Displasia distrofica
Compressione del midollo spinale	Acondroplasia
Encefalocele	Displasia dissegmentaria
Emivertebre	Displasia dissegmentaria
Micrognazia	Displasia camptomelica
Displasia ungueale	Sindrome di Ellis-Van Creveld
Denti conici, oligodontia	Sindrome di Ellis-Van Creveld
Frenuli orali multipli	Sindrome di Ellis-Van Creveld
Dentinogenesi imperfetta	Osteogenesi imperfetta
Fossette cutanee pretibiali	Displasia camptomelica
Cataratta, distacco di retina	Sindrome di Stickler
Atresia intestinale	Saldino-Noonan
Cisti renali	Saldino-Noonan
Camptodattilia	Displasia diastrofica
Craniosinostosi	Displasia tanatofora
Ittiosi	Condrodistrofia puntata
Pollice dell'autostoppista	Displasia diastrofica
Capelli radi	Ipoplasia cartilagine-capelli
Ipertelorismo	Sindrome di Robinow
Ipoplasia del ponte nasale	Acrodisostosi
Agenesia clavicolare	Displasia cleidocranica
Ipoplasia genitale	Sindrome di Robinow
Appendice caudale	Displasia metatropica
Onfalocele	Sindrome di Beemer-Langer
Sclera blu	Osteogenesi imperfetta

TABELLA 692-4. Nanismo neonatale fatale

SOLITAMENTE FATALE*
Acondrogenesia (tipi diversi)
Displasia tanatofora
Polidattilia con coste corte (tipi diversi)
Acondroplasia omozigote
Displasia camptomelica
Displasia dissegmentaria, tipo di Silverman-Handmaker
Osteogenesi imperfetta, tipo II
Ipofosfatasia (forma congenita)
Condrodisplasia puntata (forma rizomelica)

SPESSO FATALE
Distrofia toracica con asfissia (sindrome di Jeune)

OCCASIONALMENTE FATALE
Sindrome di Ellis-Van Creveld
Displasia diastrofica
Nanismo metatropico
Displasia di Kniest

*Nella maggior parte di questi disordini sono stati riportati alcuni pazienti con sopravvivenza prolungata.

porzione può essere difficile da apprezzare nei bambini prematuri, obesi o edematosi. Si dovrebbe sospettare un accorciamento sproporzionato degli arti se gli arti superiori non raggiungono l'emipelvi in età infantile o la parte superiore della coscia nelle età successive. Collo corto, torace stretto e addome sporgente segnalano invece un accorciamento sproporzionato del tronco. La sproporzione scheletrica è in genere accompagnata da bassa statura (statura e peso al di sotto del terzo percentile); queste misure possono talvolta rientrare in un range da normale a basso nelle prime fasi di determinate condizioni.

L'accorciamento sproporzionato può riguardare differenti segmenti del corpo; il pattern specifico rappresenta talvolta un indizio utile per una diagnosi specifica. L'accorciamento è maggiore nei segmenti prossimali (parte superiore di braccia e gambe) nell'acondroplasia, nel qual caso si parla di **accorciamento rizomelico**. Un accorciamento sproporzionato dei segmenti intermedi (avambraccio e gamba) è denominato **accorciamento mesomelico**; l'**accorciamento acromelico** interessa mani e piedi.

TABELLA 692-5. Condizioni con nanismo solitamente non letali diagnosticabili alla nascita o entro i primi mesi di vita

PIÙ COMUNI
Acondroplasia
Osteogenesi imperfetta (tipi I, III, IV)
Displasia congenita spondiloepifisaria
Displasia diastrofica
Sindrome di Ellis-Van Creveld

MENO COMUNI
Condrodisplasia puntata (alcune forme)
Displasia di Kniest
Displasia metatropica
Displasia mesomelica di Langer

Con alcune eccezioni, esiste una forte correlazione tra l'età all'esordio e la severità clinica. Molte delle condrodisplasie neonatali letali sono già evidenti all'ecografia prenatale di routine eseguita al termine del primo trimestre di gravidanza (vedi Tab. 692-4). Esistono tabelle standard che indicano la giusta lunghezza delle ossa lunghe nel corso della gestazione; si osservano spesso discrepanze tra diametro biparietale del cranio e lunghezza delle ossa lunghe. Molti disordini si rendono evidenti alla nascita, mentre altri si manifestano nel primo anno di vita, nella prima infanzia o, più raramente, nella seconda infanzia o nelle età successive.

MANIFESTAZIONI NON CORRELATE ALL'ACCRESCIMENTO. La maggior parte dei pazienti presenta anche problemi non correlati all'accrescimento. Le deformità scheletriche, come un'anormale mobilità articolare, protuberanze a livello e intorno alle articolazioni e deformità angolari, sono comuni e di solito simmetriche. Le anomalie scheletriche possono influire negativamente sui tessuti non scheletrici. Una riduzione dell'accrescimento alla base del cranio e dei peduncoli vertebrali riduce le dimensioni del canale spinale nell'acondroplasia e può contribuire alla compressione del midollo spinale. Le coste corte incidono sul volume toracico, compromettendo la respirazione dei pazienti con condrodisplasie caratterizzate da tronco corto. La palatoschisi è comune in molti disordini, fatto che presumibilmente rispecchia un deficit di crescita palatale.

Le manifestazioni possono non essere correlate allo scheletro, dovute all'espressione di geni mutanti nei tessuti non scheletrici. Ne sono esempi il distacco di retina nella displasia spondiloepifisaria congenita, il *sex reversal* nella displasia camptomelica, le malformazioni cardiache congenite nella sindrome di Ellis-Van Creveld, l'immunodeficienza nell'ipoplasia cartilagine-capelli e la disfunzione renale nella distrofia toracica con asfissia. Questi problemi non scheletrici forniscono utili indizi per una diagnosi specifica e devono essere trattati clinicamente (vedi Tab. 692-3).

ANAMNESI FAMILIARE E RIPRODUTTIVA. L'anamnesi familiare permette di identificare i parenti affetti; si può osservare un pattern di ereditarietà mendeliana. Dal momento che la presentazione può variare in alcuni disordini, occorre identificare gli aspetti clinici che potrebbero essere correlati al disordine. Bisogna dedicare particolare attenzione a gradi lievi di bassa statura, aspetto sproporzionato, deformità e altre manifestazioni come un'osteoartrosi precoce in quanto potrebbero essere trascurati. L'esame obiettivo dei parenti può essere utile, come pure la revisione delle loro fotografie, radiografie e cartelle mediche.

Un'anamnesi riproduttiva può rivelare una pregressa natimortalità, morti fetali e altri esiti anormali della gravidanza derivanti da una displasia scheletrica. Complicanze della gravidanza, come polidramnios o riduzione dei movimenti fetali, sono comuni nelle displasie ossee, specialmente nelle varianti neonatali letali.

Anche se la maggior parte delle displasie scheletriche è genetica, in genere non si osserva un'anamnesi familiare del disordine. Nuove mutazioni sono comuni per le patologie autosomiche dominanti, soprattutto per quelle letali nel periodo neonatale (displasia tanatofora, osteogenesi imperfetta). La maggior parte dei casi di acondroplasia deriva da nuove mutazioni. Il mosaicismo delle cellule germinali, in cui un genitore ha cloni di cellule germinali mutanti, è stato osservato nell'osteogenesi imperfetta e in altri disordini dominanti. Un'anamnesi familiare negativa si osserva di solito nelle malattie recessive. È disponibile la diagnosi prenatale per le patologie per le quali è stato identificato un locus genetico. L'appropriatezza del test dipende da molti fattori e per queste famiglie è necessario un counseling genetico.

ASPETTI RADIOGRAFICI. La valutazione radiografica di una condrodisplasia deve comprendere la radiografia di tutto lo scheletro. Occorre tentare in tutti i modi di identificare le ossa e le parti (epifisi, metafisi, diafisi) specificamente interessate. Se possibile, si raccomanda di esaminare radiografie eseguite a età diverse in quanto le alterazioni radiografiche evolvono nel tempo. Le radiografie eseguite prima della pubertà sono generalmente più informative in quanto la chiusura puberale delle epifisi oblitera molti dei segni necessari per una diagnosi radiografica.

DIAGNOSI

Se un lattante o un bambino ha bassa statura con caratteristiche sproporzionate, la diagnosi si pone confrontando il quadro clinico osservato (definito principalmente in base alla storia clinica, familiare e gestazionale, all'esame obiettivo e alla valutazione radiologica) con fenotipi clinici di disordini ben documentati. I pediatri devono essere in grado di raccogliere gran parte di queste informazioni e, con la consulenza di un radiologo, fare diagnosi delle condrodisplasie più comuni. Numerosi sono i testi di riferimento e i database online che forniscono informazioni sulle patologie e liste complete delle referenze attuali. Per le malattie meno comuni e per i lattanti e i bambini il cui fenotipo non corrisponde esattamente con i fenotipi clinici ben stabiliti, è necessaria la consulenza di esperti in questo campo.

Gli esami di laboratorio non si sono dimostrati utili nella diagnosi delle condrodisplasie, a eccezione dell'osteogenesi imperfetta, in cui l'analisi della sintesi del collagene da parte dei fibroblasti cutanei facilita la diagnosi. L'osteogenesi imperfetta, pur non essendo una condrodisplasia, rientra spesso nella diagnosi differenziale, specialmente per i neonati con deformità scheletriche severe (vedi Capitolo 699). Nei pazienti con pseudoacondroplasia e displasie epifisarie multiple in cui sono state osservate mutazioni della COMP (*Cartilage Oligomeric Matrix Protein*, proteina oligomerica della matrice cartilaginea) sono stati individuati ridotti livelli plasmatici di questa proteina.

I test di genetica molecolare per le condrodisplasie possono essere utili, specialmente per quei disordini in cui si verificano mutazioni ricorrenti (l'acondroplasia tipica ha la stessa mutazione *FGFR3*). È disponibile il test per le mutazioni dell'acondroplasia; la diagnosi di solito è clinica. La maggiore utilità del test può essere nella diagnosi prenatale per le coppie in cui entrambi i genitori hanno un'acondroplasia tipica (eterozigote). Essi hanno un rischio del 25% per la molto più severa acondroplasia eterozigote, identificabile con l'analisi delle mutazioni. Un altro esempio è costituito dai disordini dovuti alle mutazioni di *DTDST*, che sono ereditati secondo una modalità autosomica recessiva; in tali casi è stato trovato un numero limitato di alleli mutanti. Le mutazioni eventualmente identificate nel paziente devono caratterizzare anche i genitori e vanno utilizzate per la diagnosi prenatale. Tuttavia, le mutazioni della condrodisplasia nella maggior parte dei casi tendono a disperdersi tra i geni dell'ospite e possono essere specifiche per quella famiglia. Questo fenomeno ne rende più difficile l'identificazione e attualmente riduce l'utilità di tale esame a scopi diagnostici.

Molte condrodisplasie sono caratterizzate da alterazioni istologiche distintive della cartilagine di accrescimento. Talvolta i tessuti ottenuti dalla biopsia o eliminati da una procedura chirurgica sono utili da un punto di vista diagnostico. È infrequente porre una diagnosi istologicamente se non è già sospettata sul piano clinico. Un'eccezione è costituita dalle condrodisplasie neonatali letali, in cui il feto abortito va incontro a macerazione, per cui la valutazione clinica e radiografica rende difficile la diagnosi.

GENETICA MOLECOLARE. Sono stati identificati diversi geni per la condrodisplasia (vedi Tab. 694-1), che codificano diverse categorie di proteine, compresi le proteine della matrice cartilaginea, i recettori transmembrana, i trasportatori di ioni e i fattori di trascrizione. Il numero di loci genici identificati è più piccolo di quanto si potrebbe supporre in base al numero dei fenotipi clinici riconosciuti. La maggior parte dei pazienti ha disordini che mappano in meno di dieci loci; mutazioni di due loci (*COL2AI* e *FGFR3*) comprendono più del 50% dei casi. Vi può essere un numero limitato di geni la cui funzione è fondamentale per lo sviluppo scheletrico, in particolare per la crescita lineare dell'osso; mutazioni a questo livello danno origine a un'ampia gamma di fenotipi clinici di condrodisplasia.

Le mutazioni dei loci *COL2AI* e *FGFR3* presentano caratteristiche genetiche differenti. Le mutazioni *COL2AI* sono distribuite in tutto il gene con pochi casi di recidive in persone non correlate. Al contrario, quelle di *FGFR3* sono limitate a pochi siti all'interno del gene, e la comparsa di nuove mutazioni in tali siti, in persone non correlate, è la regola. Esiste una forte correlazione tra fenotipo clinico e sito di mutazione per le mutazioni di *FGFR3*, ma non di *COL2AI*.

FISIOPATOLOGIA. Le mutazioni della condrodisplasia agiscono attraverso diversi meccanismi. La maggior parte di quelle che interessano le proteine della matrice cartilaginea causano malattia quando soltanto uno dei due alleli del gene rilevante è mutato (aploinsufficienza). Queste mutazioni di solito agiscono attraverso un meccanismo dominante negativo in virtù del quale i prodotti proteici dell'allele mutante interferiscono con l'assemblaggio e la funzione delle molecole multimeriche contenenti i prodotti proteici dell'allele normale e dell'allele mutante. La molecola del collagene di tipo II è una tripla elica composta di tre catene di collagene, che sono i prodotti del gene *COL2AI* del collagene di tipo II. Quando le catene sia dell'allele mutante sia dell'allele normale si combinano a formare triple eliche, la maggior parte delle molecole contiene almeno una catena mutante. Non è noto quante catene mutanti siano necessarie per produrre una molecola disfunzionale ma, a seconda della mutazione, una sola potrebbe essere sufficiente.

Le mutazioni che interessano il collagene di tipo X differiscono dal modello appena descritto. Esse mappano sulla regione della catena responsabile del riconoscimento della catena; le catene devono riconoscersi a vicenda prima di assemblarsi nelle molecole di collagene. Si ritiene che le mutazioni interrompano questo processo. Ne consegue che nessuna delle catene mutanti viene incorporata nelle molecole. Questo meccanismo è quello dell'aploinsufficienza in quanto i prodotti dell'allele mutane sono funzionalmente assenti e l'allele normale è insufficiente per una normale funzione. Le mutazioni dei geni di trasporto ionico agiscono attraverso una perdita di funzione dei trasportatori. In alternativa, le mutazioni dei recettori transmembrana studiate fino a ora sembrano agire attraverso un guadagno funzionale; i recettori mutanti iniziano i segnali in una maniera costitutiva indipendente dai loro ligandi normali.

Indipendentemente dal meccanismo genetico, le mutazioni da ultimo alterano l'ossificazione encondrale, il processo biologico responsabile dello sviluppo e della crescita lineare dello scheletro (vedi Fig. 692-1). Nelle condrodisplasie è stata infatti descritta un'ampia gamma di anomalie morfologiche della cartilagine di accrescimento scheletrica, la struttura anatomica in cui si verifica l'ossificazione encondrale.

TRATTAMENTO

Il primo passo è quello di porre una diagnosi corretta: in questo modo è possibile fare previsioni prognostiche e anticipare i problemi medici e chirurgici associati a una particolare patologia. La diagnosi permette la distinzione tra disordini letali e non letali in un neonato a termine o prematuro (vedi Tabb. 692-4 e 692-5). Una prognosi sfavorevole per la sopravvivenza a lungo termine può essere un argomento contro l'adozione di misure salvavita estreme per la displasia tanatofora o l'acondrogenesia di tipo Ib o II, mentre tali misure possono essere indicate per i soggetti con displasia congenita spondiloepifisaria o displasia distrofica, che hanno una buona prognosi se sopravvivono al periodo neonatale.

Dal momento che non esiste una terapia definitiva per normalizzare la crescita ossea in nessuno di questi disordini, il medico deve mirare alla prevenzione e alla correzione delle deformità scheletriche, al trattamento delle complicanze non scheletriche, al counseling genetico e ad aiutare i pazienti e le famiglie ad affrontare la malattia. Poiché ogni malattia comporta una serie di problemi specifici, il trattamento deve essere adattato caso per caso. Le informazioni mediche per alcuni disordini sono reperibili sul sito web Medical Information on Dwarfism (vedi Bibliografia).

Esistono diversi problemi comuni a molte condrodisplasie per cui si possono fare raccomandazioni generali. Nella maggior parte delle condrodisplasie, i pazienti devono evitare gli sport di contatto e altre attività che possono causare traumi o stress delle articolazioni. Questi soggetti fin dall'infanzia devono adottare corrette abitudini alimentari, al fine di prevenire l'obesità o tenere sotto controllo il sovrappeso nell'età adulta. Occorre iniziare con l'igiene dentale molto presto per ridurre al minimo i problemi di affollamento e allineamento dei denti. I bambini e i loro parenti devono avere l'opportunità di partecipare a gruppi di supporto come la Little People of America e la Human Growth Foundation.

Per aumentare la lunghezza delle ossa sono stati utilizzati due approcci controversi. L'allungamento chirurgico degli arti, impiegato per alcune patologie, ha ottenuto i maggiori successi nell'acondroplasia, in cui i tessuti non scheletrici tendono a essere ridondanti e facilmente distensibili. Di solito la procedura viene eseguita nel corso dell'adolescenza. In diversi disordini sono state somministrate anche dosi farmacologiche di ormone della crescita umana simili a quelle usate per il trattamento della sindrome di Turner, ma i risultati di questo tentativo sono stati poco chiari.

Bibliografia

Apajasalo M, Sintonen H, Rautonen J, et al: Health-related quality of life patients with genetic skeletal dysplasias. *Eur J Pediatr* 1998;157:114–121.

Hall JG, Froster-Iskenius UG, Allanson JE: *Handbook of Normal Physical Measurements*. Oxford, Oxford University Press, 1989.

Horton WA: Skeletal development: insights from targeting the mouse genome. *Lancet* 2005;362:560–569.

Horton WA, Hecht JT: Chondrodysplasias: general concepts and diagnostic and management considerations. In Royce PM, Steinmann B (editors): *Connective Tissue and Its Disorders, Molecular, Genetic and Medical Aspects*, 2nd ed. New York, Wiley-Liss, 2002, p 901.

Krakow D, Williams J, Poehl M, et al: Use of three-dimensional ultrasound imaging in the diagnosis of prenatal-onset skeletal dysplasias. *Ultrasound Obstet Gynecol* 2003;21:465–472.

Lachman RS: Neurologic abnormalities in the skeletal dysplasias: A clinical and radiological perspective. *Am J Med Genet* 1997;69:33–43.

Rimoin DL, Lachman RS Unger S: Chondrodysplasias. In Rimoin DL, Connor JM, Pyeritz RE, Korf BR (editors): *Emery and Rimoin's Principles and Practice of Medical Genetics,* 4th ed. New York, Churchill Livingstone, 2002, p 4071.

Spranger J, Maroteaux P: The lethal osteochondrodysplasias. *Adv Hum Genet* 1995;19:1–103.

Spranger JW, Brill PW, Poznansk A: *Bone Dysplasias. An Atlas of Genetic Disorders of Skeletal Development,* 2nd ed. New York, Oxford University Press, 2002.

Taybi H, Lachman RS: *Radiology of Syndromes, Metabolic Disorders, and Skeletal Dysplasias,* 4th ed. New York, Mosby, 1996.

Risorse online

Medical Information on Dwarfism: Available at *medical.lpaonline.org* (accessed 9/14/06).

On-Line Mendelian Inheritance in Man (OMIM): Available at *www.ncbi.nlm.nih.gov/entrez/query.fcgi?db=OMIM* (accessed).

Capitolo 693 ■ Disordini delle proteine della matrice cartilaginea

William A. Horton e Jacqueline T. Hecht

Alcuni disordini delle ossa e delle articolazioni derivano da disturbi funzionali delle proteine della matrice cartilaginea. Essi ricadono in quattro gruppi, corrispondenti principalmente alle proteine difettose: tre proteine del collagene e non-collagene COMP (*Cartilage Oligomeric Matrix Protein*, proteina oligomerica della matrice cartilaginea) e la matrilina 3. I fenotipi clinici differiscono non solo da un gruppo e l'altro, ma anche all'interno di un singolo gruppo, specialmente in quello della displasia spondiloepifisaria (SED, *SpondyloEpiphyseal Dysplasia*). In alcuni gruppi esiste una sostanziale variabilità della severità clinica.

DISPLASIE SPONDILOEPIFISARIE

Con la dicitura "displasia spondiloepifisaria" si indica un gruppo eterogeneo di disordini caratterizzato da accorciamento del tronco e, in misura minore, degli arti. La severità varia dall'acondrogenesia di tipo II alla leggermente meno severa ipocondrogenesia (entrambi i tipi sono però letali nel periodo perinatale) alla SED congenita e alle sue varianti, compresa la displasia di Kniest (che sono evidenti alla nascita e di solito non letali), fino alla SED a esordio tardivo (che può non venire identificata fino all'adolescenza o anche oltre). I segni radiografici caratteristici sono l'anormale sviluppo dei corpi vertebrali e delle epifisi, l'estensione del quale corrisponde alla gravità clinica. Tutte le SED derivano da mutazioni eterozigoti di *COL2AI* e sono disordini autosomici dominanti. Le mutazioni sono sparse in tutto il gene; esiste una scarsa correlazione tra sede della mutazione e fenotipo clinico risultante. Per i casi familiari, la diagnosi prenatale è possibile se si identifica la mutazione. La displasia immuno-ossea di Schimke può rappresentare un'eccezione in quanto è un disordine autosomico recessivo caratterizzato da bassa statura, macule iperpigmentate, facies insolita, proteinuria e insufficienza renale progressiva, ischemia cerebrale e un difetto dei linfociti T con linfopenia e infezioni ricorrenti.

DISPLASIE SPONDILOEPIFISARIE LETALI. L'acondrogenesia di tipo II (OMIM 200610) è caratterizzata da severo accorciamento del collo, del tronco e (in particolare) degli arti inferiori e da una testa grande e molle. Idrope fetale e prematurità sono comuni; i pazienti nascono morti o muoiono subito dopo la nascita. L'ipocondrogenesi (OMIM 200610), tipicamente letale nel periodo neonatale, è un fenotipo clinico intermedio tra l'acondrogenesia di tipo II e la SED congenita.

La severità delle alterazioni radiografiche è correlata alla severità clinica (Fig. 693-1). Entrambe le condizioni danno luogo a ossa tubulari corte e larghe con metafisi a coppa. Le ossa pelviche sono ipoplasiche e quelle craniche non sono ben mineralizzate. I corpi vertebrali sono scarsamente ossificati nell'intera colonna vertebrale nell'acondrogenesia di tipo II e nella colonna cervicale e sacrale nell'ipocondrogenesi. I peduncoli vertebrali sono ossificati in entrambe le forme.

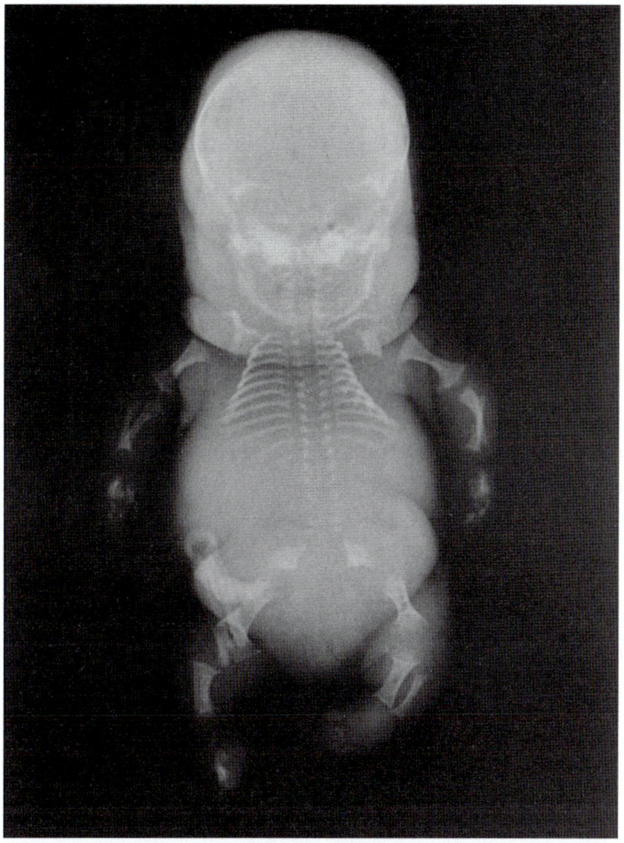

Figura 693-1. Neonato nato morto con acondrogenesia di tipo II. Si noti la scarsa ossificazione della volta cranica, dei corpi vertebrali e del sacro, l'ipoplasia delle ossa pelviche e le ossa tubulari brevi con metafisi a coppa.

DISPLASIA SPONDILOEPIFISARIA CONGENITA. Il fenotipo del gruppo, la SED congenita (OMIM 183900), è evidente alla nascita. Testa e viso sono di solito normali, ma è comune una palatoschisi. Il collo è corto e il torace è a barile (Fig. 693-2). Sono comuni una cifosi e un'accentuazione della normale lordosi lombare. I segmenti prossimali degli arti sono più corti delle mani e dei piedi, che spesso appaiono normali. Alcuni neonati hanno un piede torto o sono ipotonici.

Le radiografie dello scheletro del neonato rivelano ossa tubulari corte, ritardo dell'ossificazione dei corpi vertebrali e delle epifisi prossimali degli arti (Fig. 693-3). Sono evidenti un'ipoplasia del processo odontoideo, un bacino corto e quadrato con una sinfisi pubica scarsamente ossificata e lievi irregolarità delle metafisi.

I bambini di solito hanno tappe dello sviluppo normali; nella prima infanzia è tipica la comparsa di un'andatura anserina. Le complicanze che si manifestano in età infantile consistono in una compromissione respiratoria per le deformità vertebrali e una compressione del midollo spinale da instabilità cervicomidollare. La sproporzione e la brevità degli arti peggiorano progressivamente con l'età e l'altezza in età adulta va da 95 a 128 cm. La miopia è tipica; gli adulti sono predisposti al distacco di retina. Nell'età adulta si verifica un'osteoartrosi precoce che richiede una protesizzazione articolare chirurgica.

DISPLASIA DI KNIEST. La variante di displasia di Kniest (OMIN 156550) si presenta alla nascita con tronco e arti corti associati a viso piatto, occhi prominenti, ingrandimento delle articolazioni, palatoschisi e piede torto. Le radiografie evidenziano difetti vertebrali e ossa tubulari corte, con irregolarità epifisarie e ingrossamento metafisario che dà origine a un aspetto a manubrio.

Lo sviluppo motorio è spesso ritardato a causa delle deformità articolari, anche se l'intelligenza è normale. Si sviluppano comunemente ipoacusia e miopia nel corso dell'infanzia e come complicanza tardiva si può avere un distacco di retina. L'ingrossamento articolare progredisce nel corso dell'infanzia divenendo doloroso; è accompagnato da retrazioni in flessione e atrofia muscolare, che può diventare disabilitante prima dell'adolescenza.

DISPLASIA SPONDILOEPIFISARIA A ESORDIO TARDIVO. Questo termine si riferisce a un fenotipo clinico lieve o molto lieve caratterizzato da statura leggermente bassa associata a lievi anomalie epifisarie e vertebrali alle indagini radiografiche. Si osserva tipicamente nel corso dell'infanzia o dell'adolescenza ma può passare

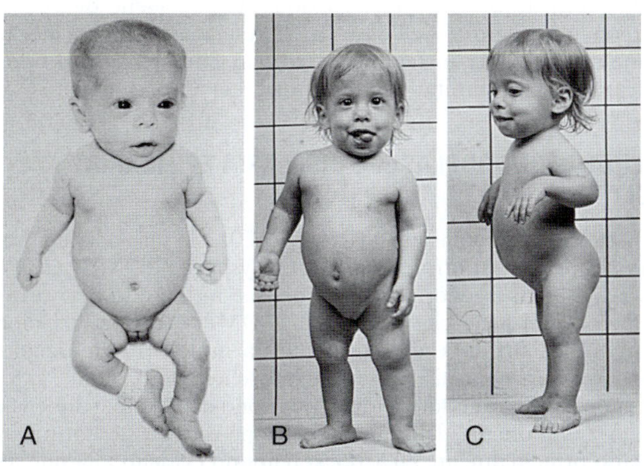

Figura 693-2. Displasia spondiloepifisaria congenita come appare nei lattanti (*A*) e nella prima infanzia (*B*, *C*). Si notino le estremità corte, le mani relativamente normali, il viso piatto e la lordosi accentuata.

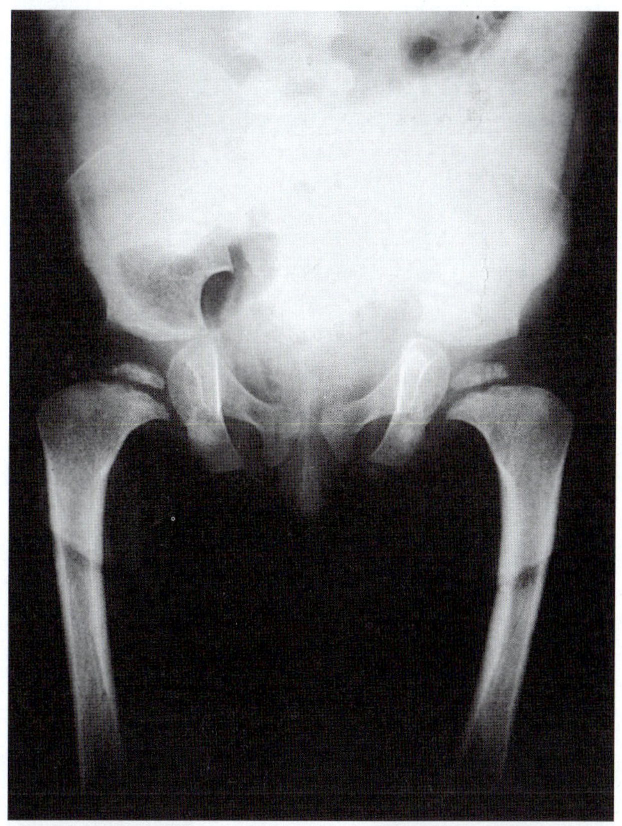

Figura 693-3. Radiografia del bacino in una displasia spondiloepifisaria congenita che evidenzia un bacino quadrato, epifisi della testa femorale ipoplasiche e collo femorale largo e corto.

inosservata fino all'età adulta, quando compare un'osteoartrosi precoce. Si tratta di entità nosologica distinta dalla SED tardiva, clinicamente simile ma che deriva da una mutazione del gene SEDL X-linked.

DISPLASIA DI STICKLER (OSTEOARTRO-OFTALMOPATIA EREDITARIA)

La bassa statura non è una caratteristica della displasia di Stickler (OMIM 184840). Questa patologia assomiglia alla SED per via delle sue manifestazioni articolari e oculari. Mutazioni dei geni che codificano il collagene di tipo XI, che interagisce funzionalmente con il collagene di tipo II, sono state identificate in disordini Stickler-simili (OMIM 184840, OMIM 215150). La displasia di Stickler è spesso identificata nel neonato a causa della palatoschisi e della micrognatia (anomalia di Pierre-Robin). Tipiche dei neonati sono una miopia severa e complicanze oftalmologiche ulteriori, tra cui una degenerazione coroidoretinica e del vitreo; il distacco di retina è comune nel corso dell'infanzia (Fig. 693-4). Un'ipoacusia neurosensoriale può insorgere nel corso dell'adolescenza, quando iniziano anche i sintomi dell'osteoartrosi. Occorre riservare particolare attenzione alle complicanze oculari, anche nell'infanzia.

DISPLASIA METAFISARIA DI SCHMID

La displasia metafisaria di Schmid (OMIM 156500) rientra in un gruppo numeroso di condrodisplasie in cui le anomalie metafisarie predominano negli aspetti radiografici. Si presenta tipicamente nella prima infanzia con bassa statura di grado lieve, incurvamento delle gambe e un'andatura anserina (Fig. 693-5); si

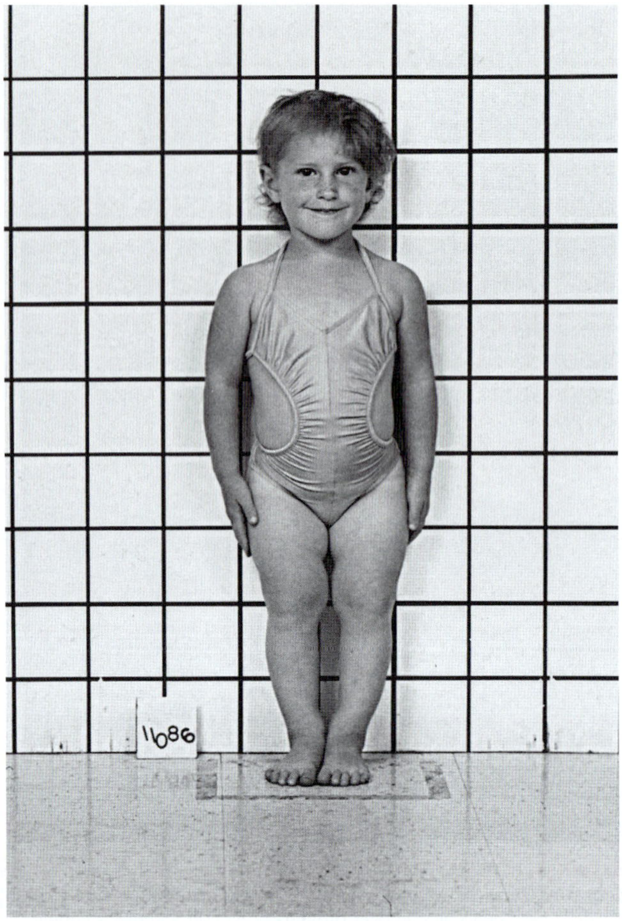

Figura 693-5. Paziente di sesso femminile con displasia metafisaria, tipo Schmid. La facies è normale e la statura è leggermente ridotta. È presente una tibia vara di grado lieve.

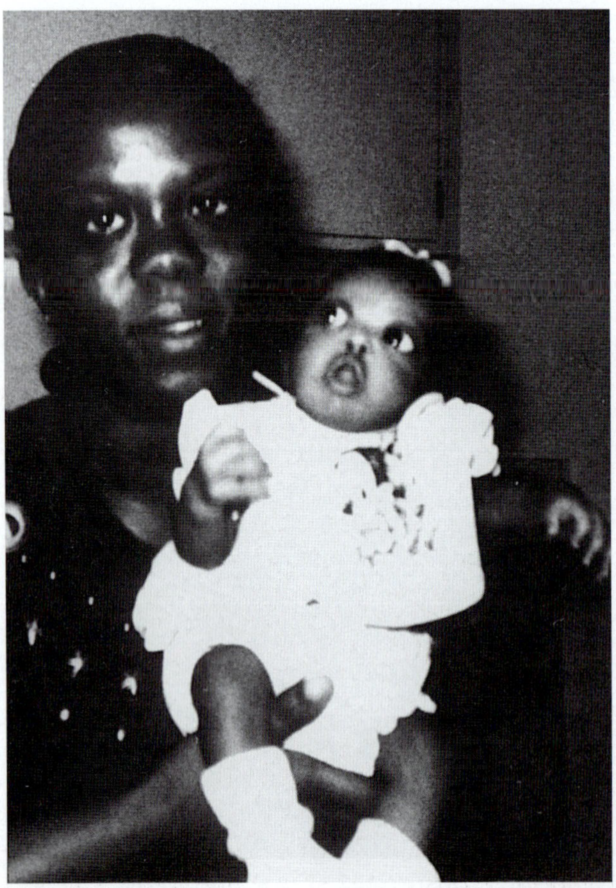

Figura 693-4. Sindrome di Stickler in madre e figlio. La facies è piatta e gli occhi sono prominenti.

può inoltre osservare un ingrossamento delle articolazioni, come il polso. Le radiografie evidenziano svasatura e mineralizzazione irregolare delle metafisi delle ossa tubulari degli arti prossimali (Fig. 693-6). Di solito è presente coxa vara, che può richiedere la correzione chirurgica. La bassa statura diviene più evidente con l'età e interessa gli arti inferiori più di quelli superiori; le manifestazioni sono limitate allo scheletro.

La condrodisplasia metafisaria di Schmid, autosomica dominante, è dovuta a mutazioni eterozigoti del gene che codifica il collagene di tipo X. La distribuzione del collagene di tipo X è ristretta alla regione dell'osso in accrescimento in cui la cartilagine si trasforma in tessuto osseo; ciò può spiegare perché le alterazioni siano limitate alle metafisi.

PSEUDOACONDROPLASIA E DISPLASIA EPIFISARIA MULTIPLA

La pseudoacondroplasia (OMIN 177170) e la displasia epifisaria multipla (MED, *Multiple Epiphyseal Dysplasia*) (OMIN 600969) sono due distinti fenotipi riuniti insieme in quando derivano da mutazioni del gene che codifica la COMP. Autosomiche dominanti, sono entrambe caratterizzate da mutazioni eterozigoti. I fenotipi clinici sono limitati ai tessuti scheletrici.

I neonati con pseudoacondroplasia sono di aspetto e dimensioni medie. Le anomalie della deambulazione e la bassa statura interessano principalmente gli arti e si rendono evidenti alla fine della prima infanzia. La bassa statura, che diviene sempre più marcata via via che il bambino cresce, è associata a lassità articolare generalizzata (Fig. 693-7). Le mani sono corte, larghe e deviate in

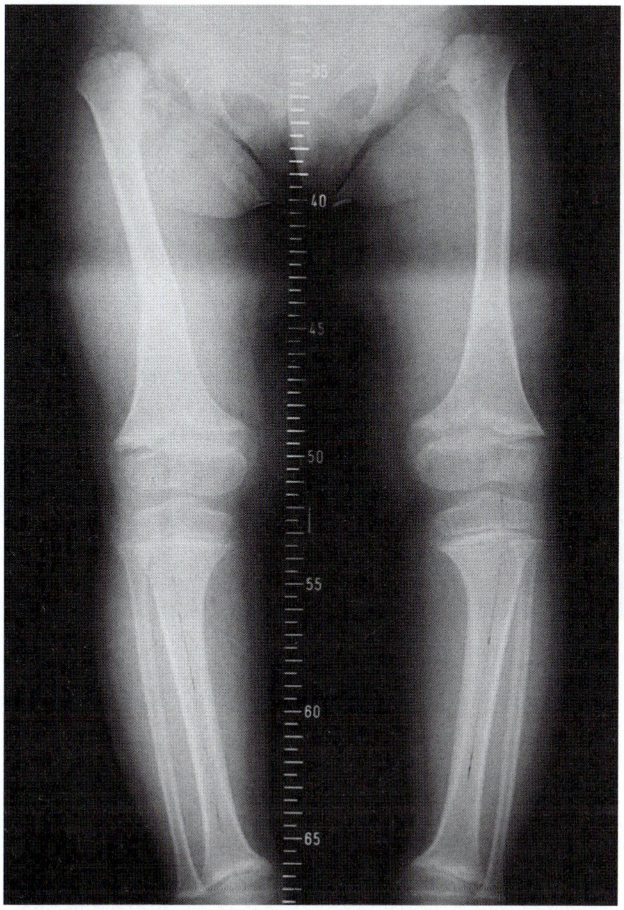

Figura 693-6. Radiografia delle estremità inferiori nella displasia metafisaria di Schmid che evidenza corte ossa tubulari e svasatura e irregolarità delle metafisi, epifisi della testa femorale e collo femorale anormali. Le epifisi sono normali. È presente coxa vara.

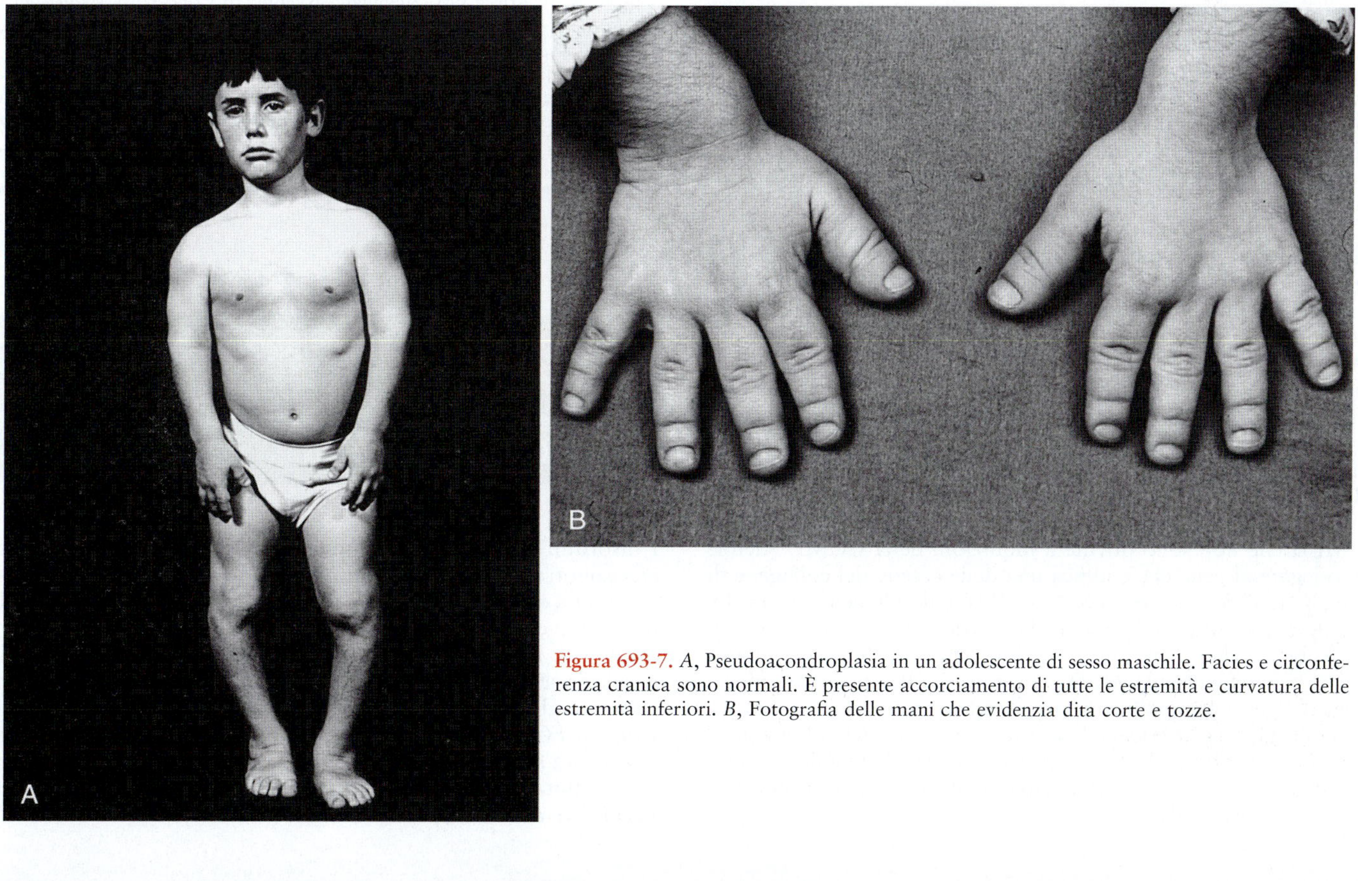

Figura 693-7. *A*, Pseudoacondroplasia in un adolescente di sesso maschile. Facies e circonferenza cranica sono normali. È presente accorciamento di tutte le estremità e curvatura delle estremità inferiori. *B*, Fotografia delle mani che evidenzia dita corte e tozze.

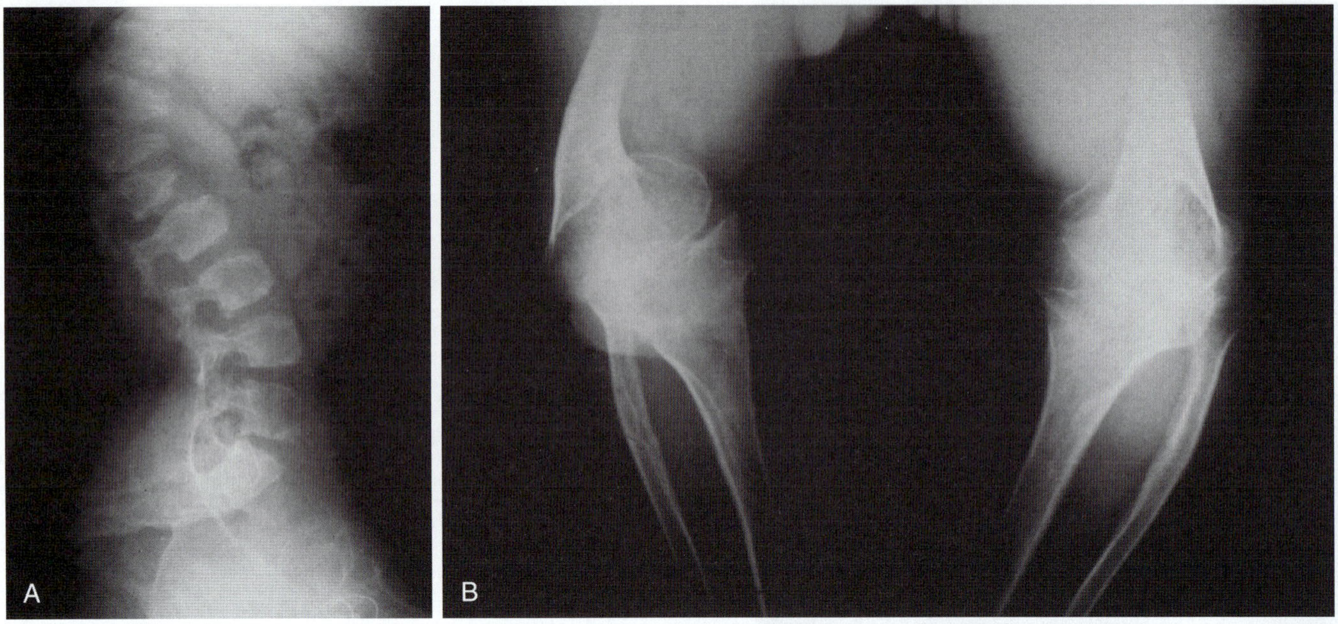

Figura 693-8. *A*, Radiografia laterale della colonna toracolombare con pseudoacondroplasia che evidenzia la protrusione centrale dell'aspetto anteriore delle vertebre toraciche lombari superiori e toraciche inferiori. Si notino la riduzione dell'altezza dei corpi vertebrali (platispondilia) e la lordosi secondaria. *B*, Radiografia dell'estremità inferiore di un paziente con pseudoacondroplasia che evidenzia metafisi di grandi dimensioni, epifisi poco formate e marcata curvatura delle ossa lunghe.

direzione ulnare; gli avambracci sono ricurvi. Le tappe evolutive e l'intelligenza sono di solito normali. Durante l'infanzia si sviluppano un'iperlordosi lombare e una deformità del ginocchio, che richiedono spesso la correzione chirurgica. Il dolore è comune nelle articolazioni che sopportano il carico nell'infanzia e nell'adolescenza: ne deriva un'osteoartrosi alla fine del 2° decennio di vita. Gli adulti hanno un'altezza variabile da 105 a 128 cm.

Le radiografie scheletriche evidenziano anomalie caratteristiche dei corpi vertebrali e di epifisi e metafisi delle ossa tubulari (Fig. 693-8).

Il fenotipo ME presenta anomalie scheletriche che interessano in modo predominante le epifisi, come si deduce dalle radiografie. Due classiche forme sono il tipo di Fairbank, severo, e il tipo di Ribbing, lieve. Dal momento che in entrambi i tipi si osserva una sovrapposizione delle caratteristiche cliniche e si riscontrano le mutazioni della COMP, essi possono essere considerati varianti cliniche.

Il fenotipo clinico più severo ha il suo esordio nell'infanzia con bassa statura di grado lieve e arti corti, dolore delle articolazioni che sopportano il carico e un'andatura anserina. Le radiografie evidenziano un'ossificazione epifisaria ritardata e irregolare. Gli individui con malattia più lieve possono non venire riconosciuti fino all'adolescenza o all'età adulta. Le alterazioni radiografiche talvolta sono limitate alle epifisi della testa femorale e in quest'ultimo caso la MED lieve deve essere distinta dalla malattia di Legg-Calvé-Perthes bilaterale. Un'osteoartrosi precoce delle anche e dei ginocchi è la principale complicanza negli adulti con MED. L'altezza degli adulti va da 136 a 151 cm.

Vi sono famiglie con manifestazioni cliniche e radiografiche di MED che non sono dovute a mutazioni della COMP. Alcune sono legate al gene che codifica una delle catene del collagene di tipo IX. È stato suggerito che la COMP e il collagene di tipo IX interagiscano funzionalmente nella matrice cartilaginea: ciò spiegherebbe perché mutazioni di geni differenti producano quadri simili. Nei pazienti con MED sono state inoltre osservate mutazioni dei geni che codificano per un'altra proteina della matrice del collagene, la matricina 3, e il trasportatore del solfato della distrofia distrofica. Nei casi familiari di pseudoacondroplasia e di MED derivate da una mutazione della COMP, è disponibile la diagnosi prenatale.

Boerkoel CF, O'Neill S, Andre JL, et al: Manifestations and treatment of Schimke immuno-osseous dysplasia: 14 new cases and a review of the literature. *Eur J Pediatr* 2000;159:1–7.

Briggs MD, Mortier GR, Cole WG, et al: Diverse mutations in the gene for cartilage oligomeric matrix protein in a pseudoachondroplasia-multiple epiphyseal dysplasia disease spectrum. *Am J Hum Genet* 1998;62:311–319.

Horton WA, Hecht JT: Chondrodysplasias: Disorders of cartilage matrix proteins. In Royce PM, Steinmann B (editors): *Connective Tissue and Its Disorders, Molecular, Genetic and Medical Aspects,* 2nd ed. New York, Wiley-Liss, 2002, p 909.

Kennedy J, Jackson G, Ramsden S, et al: COMP mutation screening as an aid for the clinical diagnosis and counseling of patients with a suspected diagnosis of pseudoachondroplasia or multiple epiphyseal dysplasia. *Eur J Hum Genet* 2005;13:547–555.

Capitolo 694 ■ Disordini dei recettori transmembrana

William A. Horton e Jacqueline T. Hecht

I disordini dei recettori transmembrana derivano da mutazioni eterozigoti dei geni che codificano *FGFR3* (recettore 3 del fattore di crescita dei fibroblasti) e *PTHR* (recettore del paratormone). Le mutazioni causano l'attivazione dei recettori in assenza di ligandi fisiologici, il che accentua la normale funzione recettoriale della regolazione negativa della crescita ossea. Le mutazioni agiscono aumentando questa funzione negativa. Nel gruppo della mutazione di *FGFR3*, in cui i fenotipi clinici vanno da severo a lieve, la severità sembra correlata al grado di attivazione del recettore. Sia la mutazione di *PTHR* sia (in particolare) la mutazione di *FGFR3* tendono a ripetersi in individui non correlati.

GRUPPO DELL'ACONDROPLASIA

Il gruppo dell'acondroplasia, che rappresenta una notevole percentuale di pazienti con condrodisplasie, comprende: la displasia tanatofora (TD, *Thanatophoric Dysplasia*), la più comune condrodisplasia letale con un'incidenza di 1/35 000 nascite, l'acondroplasia, la più comune condrodisplasia non letale con un'incidenza di 1/15 000-1/40 000 nascite, e l'ipocondroplasia. Tutte e tre queste forme comportano mutazioni in un piccolo numero di siti del gene *FGFR3*. Esiste una forte correlazione tra sito di mutazione e fenotipo clinico.

DISPLASIA TANATOFORA. La TD (OMIM 187600, OMIN 187610) si presenta in utero o al momento della nascita. Nel primo caso, l'ecografia a metà gravidanza o nel periodo successivo evidenzia una grossa testa e arti molto corti; la gestazione è spesso caratterizzata da polidramnios e parto prematuro. Il fenotipo alla nascita è contraddistinto da arti molto corti, collo corto, torace lungo e stretto e testa grossa con ipoplasia della parte centrale della faccia (Fig. 694-1). Si osserva talvolta la deformità cranica a quadrifoglio nota come **Kleeblattschädel**. A causa del torace piccolo, i neonati hanno difficoltà respiratorie severe: nonostante un'assistenza respiratoria intensiva, la prognosi a lungo termine è sfavorevole.

Le radiografie dello scheletro permettono di distinguere due forme leggermente differenti denominate TD I e TD II. Nella più comune TD I, le radiografie evidenziano un'ampia volta cranica con una base piccola, marcato assottigliamento e appiattimento dei corpi vertebrali meglio visualizzabile alla proiezione laterale, coste molto corte, ipoplasia severa delle ossa pelviche e ossa tubulari molto corte e ricurve con metafisi svasate (Fig. 694-2). I femori appaiono ricurvi e a forma di cornetta del telefono. La TD II si distingue in quanto il femore è più lungo e dritto.

Il fenotipo clinico della TD II si associa a mutazioni che mappano sul codone 650 di *FGFR3* causando la sostituzione di una molecola di lisina con un acido glutammico; ciò attiva la tirosina chinasi di un recettore che trasmette segnali a vie intracellulari. La sostituzione di una molecola di lisina del codone 650 con una molecola di metionina si associa a un fenotipo clinico intermedio tra TD e acondroplasia, noto come acondroplasia severa con ritardo evolutivo e acanthosis nigricans o SADDAN (*Severe Achondroplasia with Developmental Delay and Acanthosis Nigricans*). Le mutazioni del fenotipo TD I mappano soprattutto in due regioni nel dominio extracellulare del recettore, dove sostituiscono altri aminoacidi con residui cisteinici. Si ritiene che

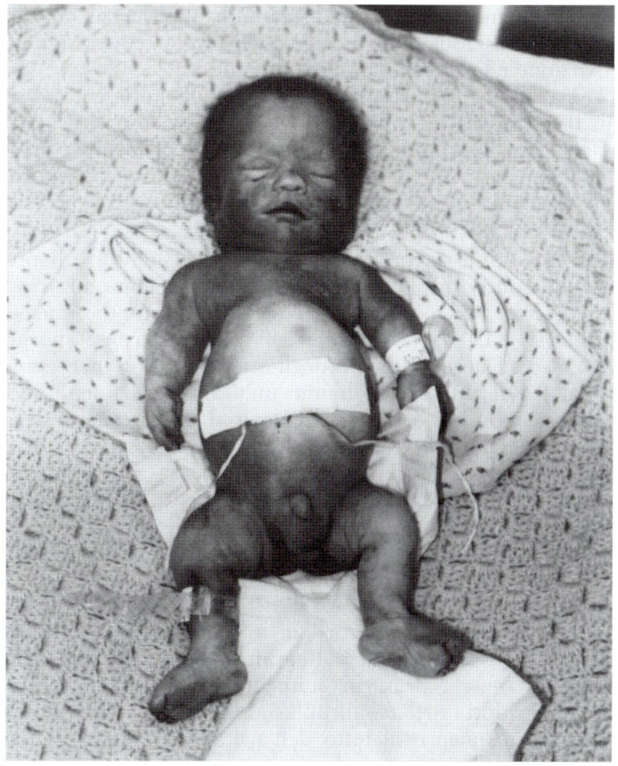

Figura 694-1. Neonato nato morto con displasia tanatofora. Gli arti sono molto corti; quelli superiori si estendono soltanto per due terzi dell'addome. Il torace stretto accentua la sporgenza dell'addome. La testa è relativamente grande.

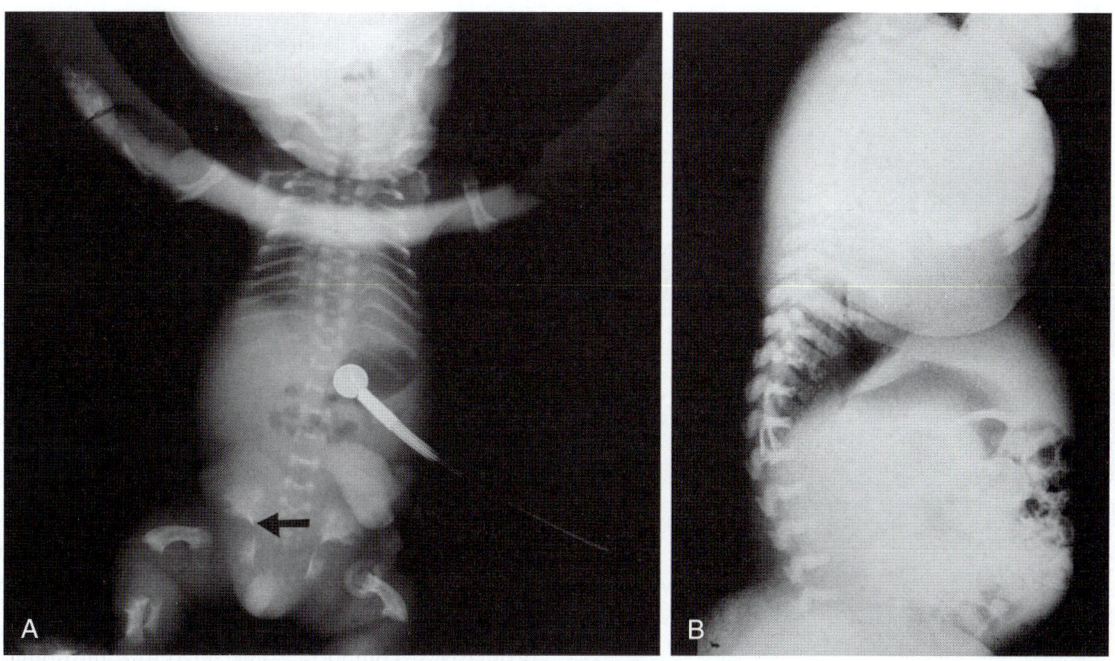

Figura 694-2. *A*, Radiografia di un neonato con displasia tanatofora. Si notino gli speroni acetabolari mediali (*freccia nera*), l'ipoplasia delle ossa iliache, i femori ricurvi con protrusione arrotondata dei femori prossimali, l'ipoplasia del torace e i corpi vertebrali sottili. *B*, Radiografia laterale della colonna toracolombare nella displasia tanatofora, che evidenzia un marcato appiattimento vertebrale e coste corte. È presente un difetto di ossificazione della porzione centrale dei corpi vertebrali.

i residui cisteinici liberi formino legami disulfidrici che favoriscono la dimerizzazione delle molecole del recettore, determinando l'attivazione e la trasmissione del segnale.

TD I e TD II rappresentano nuove mutazioni da genitori normali. Il rischio di recidiva è basso. Dal momento che i codoni mutati nella TD sono mutevoli per ragioni sconosciute e a causa del rischio teorico di mosaicismo delle cellule germinali, si propone ai genitori la diagnosi prenatale per le gravidanze successive.

ACONDROPLASIA. L'acondroplasia (OMIM 100800) è il prototipo delle condrodisplasie. Si presenta tipicamente alla nascita con arti corti, tronco lungo e stretto, testa di grandi dimensioni e ipoplasia della parte centrale del viso con fronte sporgente (Fig. 694-3). L'accorciamento degli arti è maggiore nei segmenti prossimali e le dita spesso hanno una configurazione a tridente. La maggior parte delle articolazioni è iperestensibile, ma l'estensione è limitata a livello del gomito. Si osserva spesso un gibbo toracolombare. Di solito, la lunghezza alla nascita è di poco inferiore al normale, ma occasionalmente rientra nel *range* normale.

Diagnosi. Le radiografie dello scheletro confermano la diagnosi (Fig. 694-4). Le ossa della volta cranica sono di grandi dimensioni, mentre la base cranica e le ossa del viso sono piccole. I peduncoli vertebrali sono corti in tutta la colonna vertebrale, come si può osservare alla radiografia laterale. La distanza interpeduncolare, che di norma aumenta dalla 1ª alla 5ª vertebra lombare, è ridotta nell'acondroplasia. Le ossa iliache sono corte e arrotondate, mentre il tetto dell'acetabolo è piatto. Le ossa tubulari sono corte con metafisi leggermente irregolari e svasate. Il perone è sproporzionatamente lungo rispetto alla tibia.

Manifestazioni cliniche. I bambini di solito hanno un ritardo delle tappe motorie ed è frequente che non camminino fino ai 18-24 mesi: ciò è dovuto all'ipotonia e alla difficoltà meccanica di mantenere in equilibrio una testa così grossa su un tronco di dimensioni normali e su estremità corte. L'intelligenza è normale, a meno che non si sviluppino complicanze a carico del sistema nervoso centrale. Quando il bambino inizia a camminare, il gibbo di solito viene sostituito da un'esagerata lordosi lombare.

Lattanti e bambini con acondroplasia di solito si trovano al di sotto degli standard di peso e altezza normali per l'età e possono essere valutati utilizzando le apposite tabelle per l'acondroplasia. L'altezza da adulti tipicamente va dai 118 ai 145 cm per i maschi e dai 112 ai 136 cm per le femmine. Per aumentare l'altezza sono stati utilizzati l'allungamento chirurgico degli arti e il trattamento con ormone della crescita umano; entrambi i trattamenti sono controversi.

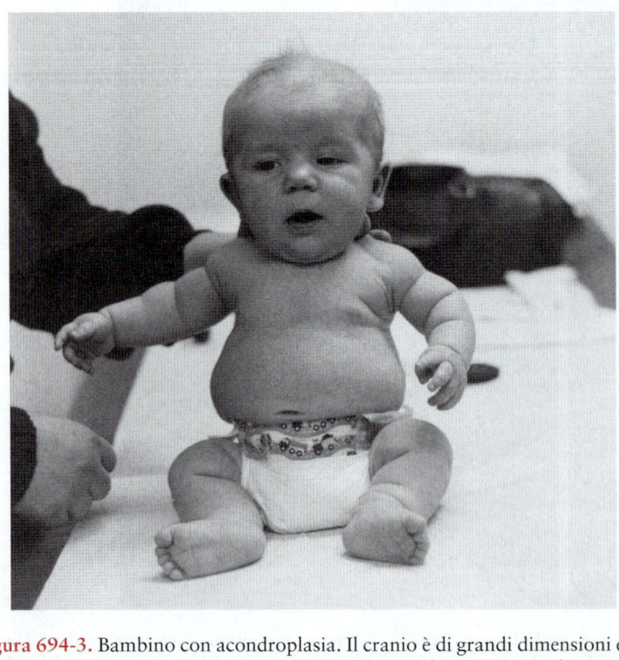

Figura 694-3. Bambino con acondroplasia. Il cranio è di grandi dimensioni e la fronte sporgente. Il ponte nasale è piuttosto piatto e il torace è piccolo rispetto all'addome. Si notino i solchi della parte mediale di braccio e avambraccio, che riflettono l'incurvamento nei punti di massima concavità degli arti.

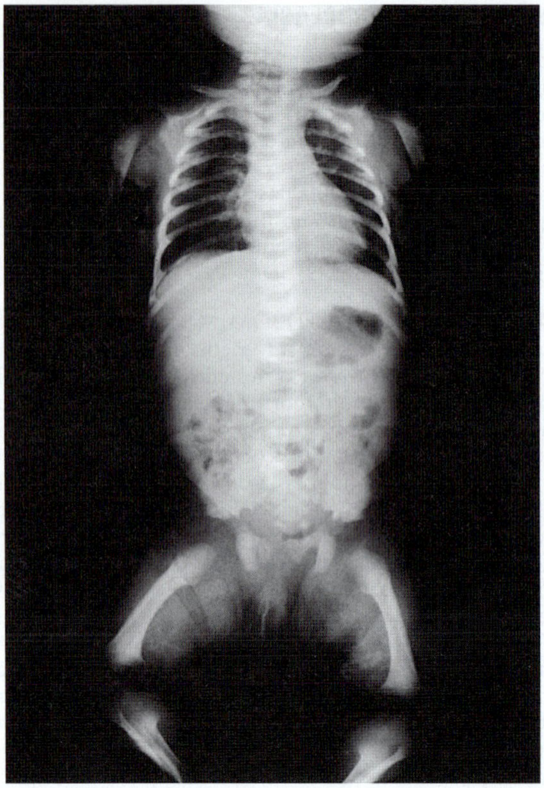

Figura 694-4. Radiografia di un neonato con acondroplasia che evidenzia un restringimento interpeduncolare dalla 1ª alla 5ª vertebra lombare, ossa iliache corte e arrotondate e tetto acetabolare piatto. Le ossa tubulari sono corte, con lievi irregolarità delle metafisi.

Virtualmente tutti i lattanti e i bambini con acondroplasia hanno una testa di grandi dimensioni, anche se solo una parte di essi presenta un vero idrocefalo. È necessario monitorare accuratamente sia la circonferenza cranica, utilizzando standard sviluppati per l'acondroplasia, sia la funzione neurologica in generale. Il canale spinale è stenotico e si può avere una compressione del midollo spinale a livello del forame magno e della colonna lombare. Il primo caso si osserva di solito nei lattanti e nei bambini più piccoli; può essere associato a ipotonia, scarso accrescimento, quadripartesi, apnee centrali e ostruttive e morte improvvisa. In caso di stenosi severa può rendersi necessaria la correzione chirurgica. La stenosi della colonna lombare di solito non si presenta fino alla prima età adulta. I sintomi comprendono parestesie, perdita della sensibilità e claudicatio. La perdita del controllo degli sfinteri vescicale e anale può essere una complicanza tardiva.

È comune l'incurvamento delle gambe, che può richiedere una correzione chirurgica. Altri problemi comuni comprendono affollamento dentale, difficoltà di articolazione del linguaggio, obesità e frequenti episodi di otite media che possono contribuire all'ipoacusia.

Genetica. Tutti i pazienti con acondroplasia tipica hanno mutazioni del codone 380 del gene *FGFR3*. La mutazione mappa sul dominio transmembrana del recettore e si ritiene determini dimeri del recettore che aumentano i segnali del recettore, con la conseguenza di un'inibizione della crescita lineare. L'acondroplasia si comporta come un tratto autosomico dominante; la maggior parte dei casi deriva da una nuova mutazione da genitori normali.

A causa dell'elevata frequenza di acondroplasia tra le condizioni che determinano nanismo, è un fatto relativamente comune che adulti con acondroplasia si sposino tra loro. Tali coppie hanno un rischio del 50% di trasmettere la propria condizione a ciascun figlio o figlia, come anche un rischio del 25% di **acondroplasia omozigote**. Quest'ultima condizione presenta una severità intermedia tra la displasia tanatofora e l'acondroplasia eterozigote ed è di solito letale nel periodo neonatale. È disponibile la diagnosi prenatale, che è stata utilizzata per la diagnosi di acondroplasia omozigote.

IPOCONDROPLASIA. L'ipocondroplasia (OMIM 146000) è simile all'acondroplasia ma più lieve. Di solito, non viene scoperta prima dei 3-4 anni di vita, quando si rende evidente una bassa statura dovuta agli arti corti. I bambini affetti hanno una costituzione fisica tozza e una lieve protrusione delle bozze frontali. Le alterazioni radiografiche sono lievi e compatibili con il fenotipo lieve dell'acondroplasia. Le complicanze sono rare; alcuni pazienti non ricevono mai una diagnosi. Negli adulti l'altezza da adulti va da 116 a 146 cm. In molti pazienti con ipocondroplasia è stata identificata una mutazione del codone 540 del gene *FGFR3*. Nell'ipocondroplasia esiste un'eterogeneità genetica e si attende l'identificazione di altri loci genetici.

DISPLASIA METAFISARIA DI JANSEN

La condrodisplasia metafisaria di Jansen (OMIM 156400) è una condrodisplasia rara con ereditarietà dominante, caratterizzata da accorciamento severo degli arti associato a facies insolita. Talvolta si accompagna a piede torto e ipercalcemia. Alla nascita, è possibile effettuare una diagnosi in base a questi segni cinici e alle radiografie, che evidenziano ossa tubulari corte con caratteristiche anomalie metafisarie consistenti in aspetto svasato, mineralizzazione irregolare, frammentazione e allargamento dello spazio delle cartilagini di accrescimento. Le epifisi sono normali.

Con l'età le articolazioni si ingrandiscono e perdono mobilità. A livello di anche e ginocchia si sviluppano retrazioni in flessione, che si traducono in una postura flessa in avanti. L'intelligenza è normale, anche se vi può essere ipoacusia.

La condrodisplasia metafisaria di Jansen è causata da mutazioni attivanti del PTHR1. Questo recettore transmembrana, accoppiato alla proteina G, funge da recettore sia per il PTH sia per il PTHrP. La segnalazione attraverso questo recettore pone un freno alla differenziazione terminale dei condrociti in una fase critica della crescita ossea. Dal momento che le mutazioni attivano il recettore, esse aumentano l'effetto di freno rallentando quindi la crescita ossea. Nella condrodisplasia di Blomstrand si osservano mutazioni del PTHR1 che determinano una perdita di funzione; gli aspetti clinici della condrodisplasia di Blomstrand sono identici a quelli della condrodisplasia metafisaria di Jansen.

American Academy of Pediatrics Committee on Genetics: Health supervision for children with achondroplasia. *Pediatrics* 1995;95:443–451.

Ho NC, Guarnieri M, Brant LJ, et al: Living with achondroplasia: Quality of life evaluation following cervico-medullary decompression. *Am J Med Genet* 2004;131:163–167.

Horton WA, Lunstrum GP: Fibroblast growth factor receptor 3 mutations in achondroplasia and related forms of dwarfism. *Rev Endocr Metab Disord* 2002;3:381–385.

Hunter AG, Bankier A, Rogers JG, et al: Medical complications of achondroplasia: A multicentre patient review. *J Med Genet* 1998;35:705–712.

Pauli RM, Horton VK, Glinski LP, et al: Prospective assessment of risks for cervicomedullary-junction compression in infants with achondroplasia. *Am J Hum Genet* 1995;56:732–744.

Schipani E, Langman CB, Parfitt AM, et al: Constitutively activated receptors for parathyroid hormone and parathyroid hormone-related peptide in Jansen's metaphyseal chondrodysplasia. *N Engl J Med* 1996;335:708–714.

Capitolo 695 ■ Disordini dei trasportatori di ioni

William A. Horton e Jacqueline T. Hecht

In ordine di gravità decrescente, i disordini dei trasportatori di ioni comprendono l'acondrogenesia di tipo 1B, l'atelosteogenesia di tipo II e la displasia diastrofica. Essi derivano dalla perdita funzionale del trasportatore di ione solfato denominato trasportatore di ione solfato della displasia diastrofica (DTDST, *Diastrophic Dysplasia Sulfate Transporter*), noto anche come SLC26A2 (membro 2 della famiglia 26 dei trasportatori di soluti). Questa proteina trasporta ioni solfato nelle cellule ed è importante per i condrociti che aggiungono gruppi solfato ai proteoglicani di nuova sintesi destinati alla matrice extracellulare della cartilagine. I proteoglicani della matrice sono responsabili di molte delle proprietà che consentono alla cartilagine di fungere da stampo per lo sviluppo dello scheletro. Le manifestazioni cliniche derivano da una difettosa solfatazione dei proteoglicani della cartilagine.

Sono stati identificati diversi alleli mutanti per il gene *DTDST*, che alterano in modo variabile la funzione del trasportatore. I disordini sono recessivi e richiedono la presenza di due alleli mutanti. Il fenotipo è determinato dalla combinazione degli alleli mutanti; alcuni alleli sono presenti in più di un disordine.

DISPLASIA DIASTROFICA (OMIM 22600). Questo disturbo ben caratterizzato viene riconosciuto alla nascita in base alla presenza di estremità molto corte, piede torto e mani corte con spostamento prossimale del pollice con aspetto "ad autostoppista" (Fig. 695-1). Le mani sono di solito deviate in direzione ulnare. La fusione ossea delle articolazioni metacarpofalangee (sinfalangismo) è comune, come anche la limitazione dei movimenti di molte articolazioni, tra cui anca, ginocchio e caviglia. L'orecchio esterno spesso si infiamma subito dopo la nascita; l'infiammazione si risolve spontaneamente ma residuano una fibrosi e una retrazione dell'orecchio (deformità auricolare "a cavolfiore"). Molti neonati hanno una palatoschisi.

Le radiografie rivelano ossa tubulari corte e larghe con metafisi svasate ed epifisi piatte e irregolari (Fig. 695-2).

L'epifisi della testa femorale è ipoplasica, mentre la testa femorale è larga. Ulna e perone sono sproporzionatamente corti. I centri carpali possono essere evolutivamente avanzati; il 1° metacarpo è tipicamente ovoidale e i metatarsi hanno una torsione mediale. Vi possono essere anomalie vertebrali, tra cui fessure della lamina vertebrale cervicale e diminuzione delle distanze interpeduncolari nella colonna lombare.

Le complicanze, principalmente ortopediche, tendono a essere severe e progressive. La deformità del piede torto nel neonato resiste ai trattamenti usuali e sono frequenti diversi interventi correttivi. Nella prima infanzia si sviluppa tipicamente una scoliosi che richiede spesso diversi interventi chirurgici per il controllo e che spesso compromette la funzione respiratoria nei bambini più grandi. Nonostante i problemi ortopedici, i pazienti hanno tipicamente un'aspettativa di vita normale e raggiungono un'altezza da adulti nell'ambito dei 105-130 cm, a seconda della severità della scoliosi. Sono disponibili curve di crescita per la displasia diastrofica. Alcuni pazienti, affetti in modo lieve, presentano bassa statura e retrazioni articolari, non hanno piede torto o palatoschisi e pertanto nessuna alterazione radiografica. Il fenotipo lieve tende a recidivare nelle famiglie; il rischio di recidiva di questa condizione autosomica recessiva è del 25%. Per la diagnosi prenatale si può ricorrere all'ecografia, ma se nel paziente o nei genitori sono identificabili le mutazioni di DTDST, è possibile anche utilizzare tecniche di genetica molecolare.

ACONDROGENESIA DI TIPO 1B (OMIN 600972) E ATELOSTEOGENESI DI TIPO II (OMIM 256050). Entrambe le condizioni sono rare condrodisplasie letali recessive. La più severa è l'acondrogenesia di

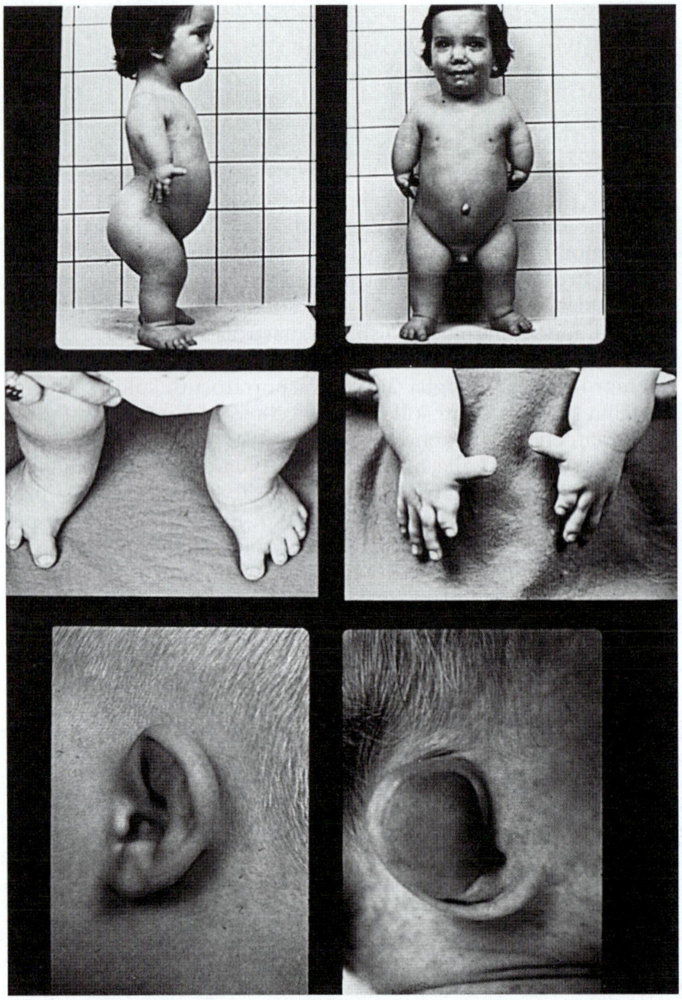

Figura 695-1. Bambino con displasia diastrofica. Le estremità sono drasticamente accorciate (*in alto*). Si osserva comunemente piede torto (*al centro a sinistra*). Le dita sono corte, specialmente l'indice; il pollice è caratteristicamente prossimale e ha un aspetto "ad autostoppista" (*al centro a destra*). La parte superiore dell'elice dell'orecchio diviene edematoso 3-4 settimane dopo la nascita (*in basso a sinistra*); questa infiammazione si risolve spontaneamente, lasciando una deformità "a cavolfiore" del padiglione (*in basso a destra*).

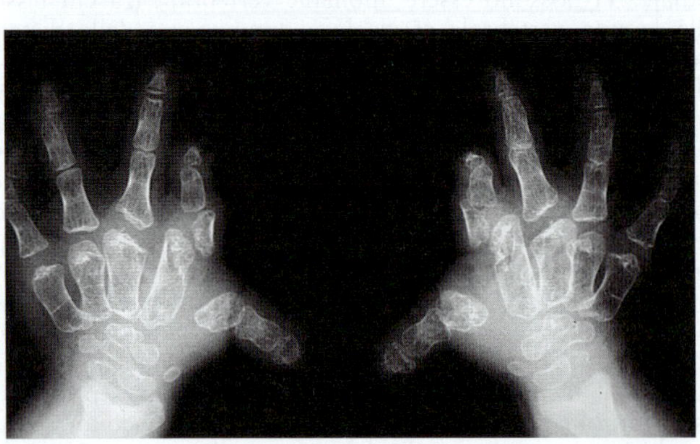

Figura 695-2. Radiografia delle mani nella displasia diastrofica. I metacarpi e le falangi sono irregolari e corti. Il primo osso metacarpale è ovoidale.

tipo 1B, contraddistinta da un severo deficit di sviluppo dello scheletro, di solito identificato in utero o dopo un aborto. Gli arti sono estremamente corti e la testa è molle. Le radiografie scheletriche evidenziano un'ossificazione scarsa o assente di ossa craniche, corpi vertebrali, perone e ossa della caviglia. Il bacino è ipoplasico e le coste sono corte. Il femore è corto e presenta un aspetto trapezoidale con metafisi irregolari.

I bambini con atelosteogenesia di tipo II nascono morti o muoiono subito dopo la nascita; la prematurità è frequente. Presentano arti molto corti, specialmente i segmenti prossimali. Si possono osservare piede torto e lussazione del gomito e del ginocchio. Alle radiografie si osserva un'ipoplasia dei corpi vertebrali, soprattutto a livello della colonna cervicale e lombare. Femore e omero sono ipoplasici e presentano un aspetto a bastone. Le ossa distali degli arti, compresi ulna e perone, sono scarsamente ossificate.

Entrambi i disordini hanno un rischio di recidiva del 25% e sono potenzialmente diagnosticabili in utero con l'analisi delle mutazioni se nei genitori sono identificati gli alleli mutanti. La diagnosi prenatale dovrebbe essere possibile grazie all'ecografia fetale.

Hall BD: Diastrophic dysplasia: Extreme variability within a sibship. *Am J Med Genet* 1996;63:28–33.

Makitie O, Kaitila I: Growth in diastrophic dysplasia. *J Pediatr* 1997;130: 641–646.

Newbury-Ecob R: Atelosteogenesis type 2. *J Med Genet* 1998;35:49–53.

Rossi A, Superti-Furga A: Mutations in the diastrophic dysplasia sulfate transporter (DTDST) gene (SLC26A2): 22 novel mutations, mutation review, associated skeletal phenotypes, and diagnostic relevance. *Hum Mutat* 2001;17:159–171.

Capitolo 696 ■ Disordini dei fattori di trascrizione William A. Horton e Jacqueline T. Hecht

Tre sono i disordini dei fattori di trascrizione che sono causa di displasia ossea. Uno, la displasia camptomelica, è classificato storicamente tra le condrodisplasie. Gli altri due, la displasia cleidocranica e la *nail-patella syndrome*, sono considerati disostosi o anomalie di singole ossa. I geni mutanti che codificano questi fattori di trascrizione, rispettivamente *SOX9*, *CBFA1* (*RUNX2*) e *LMX1B*, rientrano in famiglie di geni molto più ampie. Per esempio *SOX9* è un membro della famiglia *SOX* di geni correlati al gene *SRY* (regione determinante il sesso del cromosoma Y); CBFA1 (*RUNX2*) appartiene alla famiglia *runt* dei geni di fattori di trascrizione, mentre *LMX1B* è uno dei geni della famiglia genica dell'omeodominio LIM.

Tutti e tre i disordini sono dominanti e causati da un'aploinsufficienza dei rispettivi prodotti genici. Per i casi familiari di displasia cleidocranica e *nail-patella syndrome*, la diagnosi prenatale è possibile se si identificano le mutazioni. La displasia camptomelica deriva da nuove mutazioni e ha un basso rischio di recidiva nelle gravidanze successive.

DISPLASIA CAMPTOMELICA. Evidente già nel neonato, la displasia camptomelica (OMIM 114290) è caratterizzata da incurvamento delle ossa lunghe (specialmente di tibia e perone), ossa corte, difficoltà respiratoria e altre anomalie tra cui difetti della colonna cervicale, del sistema nervoso centrale, cuore e reni. Sono stati riportati diversi casi di *sex reversal* in maschi XY. Le radiografie confermano l'incurvamento e spesso evidenziano ipoplasia delle scapole e delle ossa del bacino (Fig. 696-1). I soggetti affetti di solito muoiono per distress respiratorio nel periodo neonatale. Le complicanze nei bambini e negli adolescenti che sopravvivono comprendono bassa statura con cifoscoliosi progressiva, apnee ricorrenti, infezioni respiratorie e difficoltà dell'apprendimento.

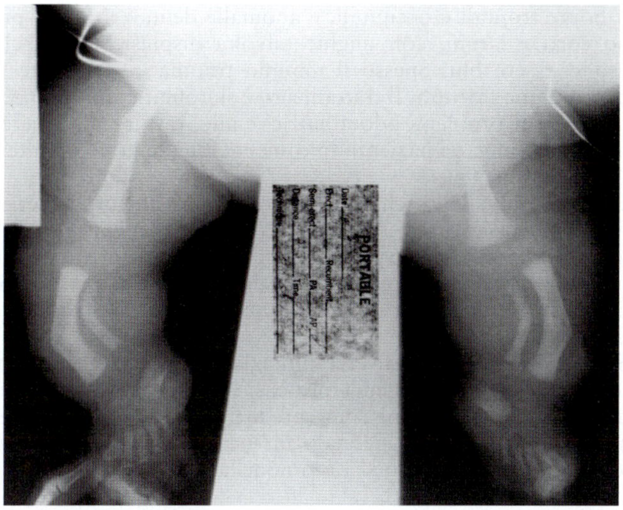

Figura 696-1. Radiografia delle estremità inferiori di un bambino con displasia camptomelica. Si noti l'incurvamento del femore, non particolarmente spesso rispetto alla tibia e al perone, incurvati e spessi.

DISPLASIA CLEIDOCRANICA. La diagnosi della displasia cleidocranica (OMIM 114290) nel neonato è possibile grazie ai seguenti segni: spalle cadenti, delle fontanelle aperte, fronte sporgente, lieve ipostaturalismo e anomalie dentali (Fig. 696-2). Le radiografie rivelano ipoplasia o assenza delle clavicole, ritardo dell'ossificazione delle ossa craniche con centri di ossificazione multipli (ossa wormiane) e ritardo dell'ossificazione delle ossa pelviche. Il decorso è di solito non complicato, eccetto che per le lussazioni, specialmente delle spalle, e le anomalie dentali (denti soprannumerari) che richiedono il trattamento.

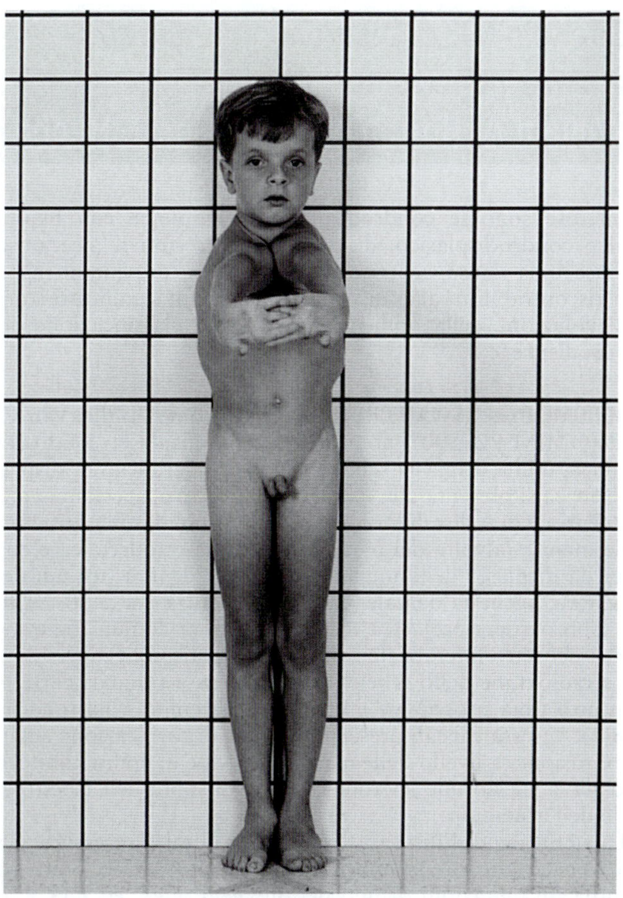

Figura 696-2. Displasia cleidocranica che evidenzia un'approssimazione del cingolo scapolare sulla linea mediana. Si notino la fronte alta e sporgente e l'ipertelorismo.

NAIL-PATELLA SYNDROME. Displasia delle unghie, assenza o ipoplasia della rotula, anomalie del gomito e speroni delle ossa iliache caratterizzano la *nail-patella syndrome* (OMIM 119600), denominata anche osteo-onicodisostosi. Alcuni pazienti hanno una nefrite simile alla glomerulonefrite cronica. Esiste un ampio spettro di severità; in alcuni pazienti si presenta nella prima infanzia, mentre altri sono asintomatici o si rivolgono al medico in età adulta.

Dryer SD, Zhou G, Baldini A, et al: Mutations in *LMX1B* cause abnormal skeletal patterning and renal dysplasia in nail patella syndrome. *Nat Genet* 1998;19:47–50.

Mansour S, Offiah AC, McDowall S, et al: The phenotype of survivors of camptomelic dysplasia. *J Med Genet* 2002;39:597–602.

Meyer J, Sudbeck P, Held M, et al: Mutational analysis of the *SOX9* gene in camptomelic dysplasia and autosomal sex reversal: Lack of genotype/phenotype correlations. *Hum Mol Genet* 1997;6:91–98.

Mundlos S, Otto F, Mundlos C, et al: Mutations involving the transcription factor CBFA1 cause cleidocranial dysplasia. *Cell* 1997;89:773–779.

Capitolo 697 ■ Disordini da alterato riassorbimento osseo William A. Horton e Jacqueline T. Hecht

Le displasie ossee, la maggior parte delle quali sono rare, possono essere accompagnate da aumento della densità ossea. L'osteopetrosi, che ha molti sottotipi, la picnodisostosi e probabilmente altre displasie ossee derivano da un difetto del riassorbimento osseo.

OSTEOPETROSI

Sono state descritte due forme principali di osteopetrosi: una forma severa autosomica recessiva (OMIM 259700) e una lieve autosomica dominante (OMIM 166600). Nella maggior parte dei pazienti con la malattia recessiva si riscontrano anomalie della funzione degli osteoclasti, dovute a mutazioni di un gene che codifica una subunità specifica degli osteoclasti della pompa protonica vacuolare (TCIRG1). Nella forma dominante invece le mutazioni riguardano il gene che codifica la proteina del canale del cloro, CLCN7. Entrambi i tipi di mutazioni alterano l'acidificazione, necessaria per la normale funzione degli osteoclasti.

La forma severa viene di solito diagnosticata nella prima infanzia o anche più precocemente sulla base della presenza di macrocefalia, epatosplenomegalia, sordità, cecità e anemia severa. Le radiografie evidenziano dapprima una sclerosi ossea diffusa, poi il caratteristico aspetto di "osso all'interno di altro osso". Con il tempo, i bambini tipicamente vanno incontro a scarso accrescimento, ritardo psicomotorio, peggioramento delle neuropatie craniche e anemia. Sono comuni problemi dentali, osteomielite della mandibola e fratture patologiche. I pazienti con le forme più severe muoiono nel corso della prima infanzia; gli altri raramente superano il 2° decennio di vita. I pazienti che sopravvivono oltre la prima infanzia di solito presentano disturbi dell'apprendimento, ma possono anche avere un'intelligenza normale nonostante l'ipoacusia e i problemi visivi.

MANIFESTAZIONI CLINICHE. La maggior parte delle manifestazioni è dovuta al mancato rimodellamento delle ossa in crescita, che causa il restringimento dei forami dei nervi cranici e la compressione degli spazi midollari, con la comparsa di complicanze secondarie, come una disfunzione del nervo ottico e del nervo facciale, e anemia accompagnata da ematopoiesi extramidollare compensatoria a livello epatico e splenico.

La forma autosomica dominante di osteopetrosi (malattia di Albers-Schönberg, osteopetrosi tarda o malattia delle ossa di marmo) si presenta di solito nel corso dell'infanzia o dell'adolescenza con fratture e anemia lieve e, meno frequentemente, con disfunzione dei nervi cranici, anomalie dentali o osteomielite della mandibola. Le radiografie dello scheletro rivelano un aumento generalizzato della densità ossea e *clubbing* delle metafisi (Fig. 697-1). L'alternanza di bande dense e radiotrasparenti produce un aspetto a sandwich dei corpi vertebrali. Le alterazioni radiografiche sono talvolta di riscontro accidentale in adulti e adolescenti altrimenti asintomatici.

TRATTAMENTO. Alcuni pazienti con osteopetrosi severa hanno risposto al trapianto di midollo osseo. Sono stati utilizzati con qualche beneficio anche il calcitriolo e l'interferone γ. Nei pazienti che sopravvivono oltre la prima infanzia è importante il trattamento sintomatico, come le cure odontoiatriche, le trasfusioni per l'anemia e la terapia antibiotica per le infezioni.

PICNODISOSTOSI

Una displasia ossea autosomica recessiva, la picnodisostosi (OMIM 265800), si presenta nella prima infanzia con arti corti, facies caratteristica, fontanella anteriore aperta, cranio grosso con bozze frontali e occipitali, e anomalie dentali. Mani e piedi sono corti e larghi, con unghie talvolta displasiche. Le sclere possono essere blu. Spesso il minimo trauma è sufficiente per provocare una frattura. Il trattamento è sintomatico, rivolto principalmente ai problemi odontoiatrici e alle fratture. In genere la prognosi è buona e i pazienti tipicamente raggiungono un'altezza di 130-150 cm.

Le radiografie dello scheletro mostrano un aumento generalizzato della densità ossea. Al contrario di quanto avviene in molti disordini di questo gruppo, le metafisi sono normali. Altre alterazioni comprendono la presenza di suture ampie e ossa wormiane a livello del cranio, una mandibola piccola e un'ipoplasia delle falangi distali.

Sono state osservate diverse mutazioni del gene che codifica la catepsina K, una cisteina proteasi altamente espressa negli osteoclasti. Le mutazioni sono predittive di una perdita della funzione enzimatica, suggerendo un'incapacità degli osteoclasti di degradare la matrice ossea e rimodellare l'osso.

Charles JM, Key LL: Developmental spectrum of children with congenital osteopetrosis. *J Pediatr* 1998;132:371–374.

Gelb BD, Shi GP, Chapman HA, et al: Pycnodysostosis, a lysosomal disease caused by cathepsin K deficiency. *Science* 1996;273:1236–1238.

Gerritsen EJ, Vossen JM, Fasth A, et al: Bone marrow transplantation for autosomal recessive osteopetrosis: A report from the Working Party on Inborn Errors of the European Bone Marrow Transplantation Group. *J Pediatr* 1994;125:896–902.

Tolar J, Teitelbaum SL, Orchard PJ: Osteopetrosis, mechanisms of disease review. *N Engl J Med* 2004;351:2839–2849.

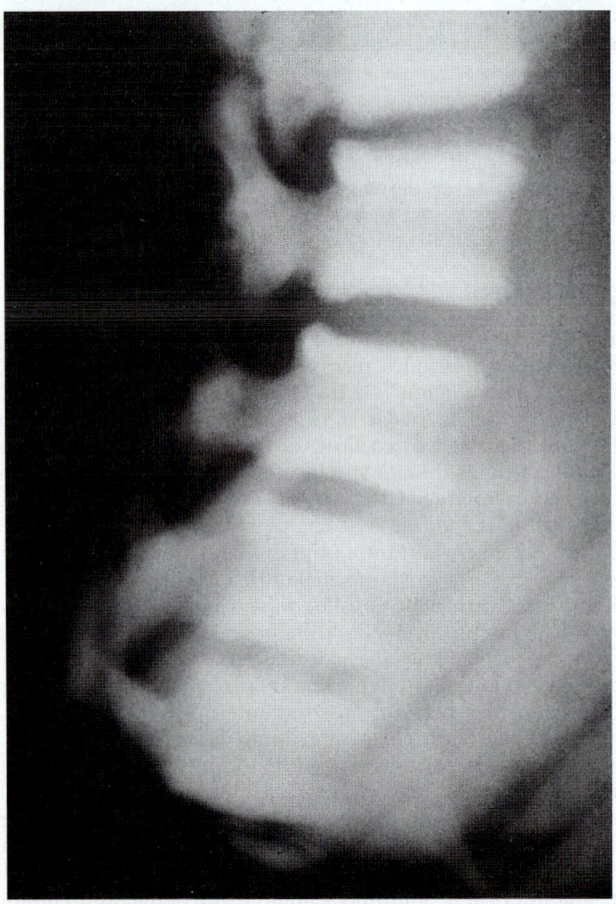

Figura 697-1. Radiografia laterale che evidenzia l'aspetto di "osso all'interno di altro osso" caratteristico dell'osteopetrosi.

Capitolo 698 ■ Disordini con difetto di base poco noto o sconosciuto

William A. Horton e Jacqueline T. Hecht

Numerose sono le condrodisplasie, o patologie con fenotipo clinico condrodisplasico, di cui sono poco noti il meccanismo di base o la causa genetica. Molte di esse presentano aspetti non riscontrabili in altri disordini e hanno un significato storico nell'evoluzione della nomenclatura e della classificazione delle condrodisplasie.

SINDROME DI ELLIS-VAN CREVELD. La sindrome di Ellis-Van Creveld (OMIM 225500), nota anche come displasia condroectodermica, è una displasia scheletrica ed ectodermica. La displasia scheletrica si presenta alla nascita con arti corti, specialmente nei segmenti medi e distali, accompagnati da polidattilia postassiale delle mani e talvolta dei piedi. La displasia ectodermica è costituita da displasia delle unghie e anomalie dentali (tra cui denti neonatali, agenesia dentale, caduta prematura dei denti e difetti del labbro superiore). Tra le manifestazioni comuni figurano i difetti del setto interatriale e altre cardiopatie congenite.

Le radiografie dello scheletro rivelano ossa tubulari corte (soprattutto tibia prossimale e ulna) con estremità a bastone (Fig. 698-1). Le ossa carpali presentano centri di ossificazione aggiuntivi e fusione; a livello delle mani sono evidenti epifisi coniformi. Si osserva spesso uno sperone osseo al di sopra dell'aspetto mediale dell'acetabolo.

La sindrome di Ellis-Van Creveld, autosomica recessiva, si verifica per lo più tra i membri della comunità Amish. Sono state identificate mutazioni di uno dei due geni, *EVC* ed *EVC2*, che mappano molto vicino l'uno all'altro sul cromosoma 4p. Le funzioni dei prodotti genici sono sconosciute. Il 30% circa dei pazienti muore per problemi cardiaci o respiratori durante la pri-

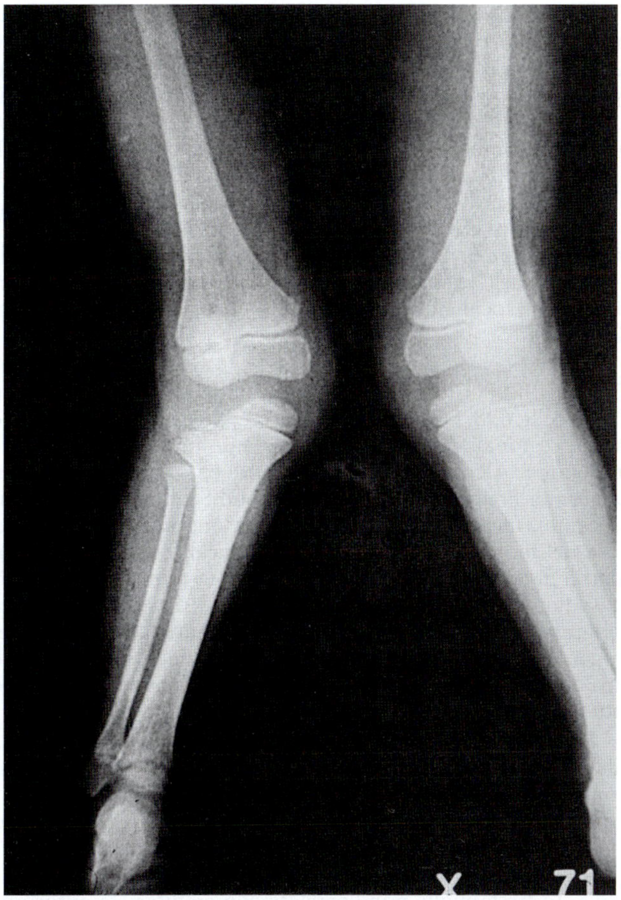

Figura 698-1. Radiografia delle estremità inferiori nella sindrome di Ellis-Van Creveld. Le ossa tubulari sono corte e il perone prossimale è corto. L'ossificazione è ritardata nelle epifisi tibiali laterali, con deformità in valgo del ginocchio.

ma infanzia. L'aspettativa di vita è altrimenti normale e l'altezza da adulti va da 109 a 152 cm.

DISTROFIA TORACICA CON ASFISSIA. La distrofia toracica con asfissia (OMIM 208500), o sindrome di Jeune, è una condrodisplasia autosomica recessiva simile alla sindrome di Ellis-Van Creveld. I neonati affetti, caratterizzati da un torace lungo e stretto e da insufficienza respiratoria associata a ipoplasia polmonare, spesso vanno incontro a decesso. Altre manifestazioni neonatali comprendono arti leggermente corti e polidattilia postassiale. La condizione è stata mappata sul cromosoma 15q13, ma l'identità del locus non è nota.

Le radiografie scheletriche evidenziano coste molto corte con espansione anteriore. Le ossa tubulari degli arti sono corte con estremità bulbose; nelle ossa delle mani si osservano epifisi coniformi. Le ossa iliache sono corte e squadrate, con uno sperone sopra l'aspetto mediale dell'acetabolo.

Se i bambini affetti sopravvivono al periodo neonatale, la funzione respiratoria di solito migliora con la crescita della gabbia toracica. Un intervento di espansione laterale del torace migliora la crescita delle coste e permette alla parete toracica di raggiungere dimensioni maggiori. Spesso si sviluppa una disfunzione renale progressiva nel corso della seconda infanzia. Sono stati riportati anche malassorbimento intestinale e disfunzione epatica.

SINDROME POLIDATTILIA/COSTE CORTE. Ne sono state descritte quattro forme (tipi I-IV) (OMIM 263530, 263520, 263510, 269860), tutte letali nel periodo neonatale. I neonati si presentano con distress respiratorio, un torace estremamente piccolo, arti molto corti, polidattilia e vari difetti non scheletrici. Le radiografie dimostrano coste molto corte e ossa tubulari con alterazioni caratteristiche per ciascun tipo. Tutti e quattro le forme sono autosomiche recessive.

IPOPLASIA CARTILAGINE-CAPELLI. L'ipoplasia cartilagine-capelli (CHH, *Cartilage-Hair Hypoplasia*) (OMIN 250250), detta anche condrodisplasia metafisaria-tipo di McKusick, viene diagnosticata nel 2° anno di vita a causa del deficit di accrescimento degli arti, accompagnato da svasatura della parte inferiore della gabbia toracica, sterno sporgente e incurvamento delle gambe. Mani e piedi sono corti e le dita sono molto corte con estrema lassità legamentosa. I capelli sono sottili, radi e chiari, le unghie ipoplasiche. La cute è ipopigmentata.

Le radiografie evidenziano ossa tubulari corte con metafisi a coppa e svasate, irregolarmente mineralizzate (Fig. 698-2). Il ginocchio è più interessato dell'anca e il perone è sproporzionatamente più lungo della tibia. Metacarpi e falangi sono corti e larghi. Le radiografie spinali rivelano una lieve platispondilia.

Le manifestazioni non scheletriche associate a CHH comprendono deficit immunitari (anomalie dei linfociti T, neutropenia, leucopenia e suscettibilità alla varicella; i bambini possono anche andare incontro a complicanze in seguito alla vaccinazione antivaiolosa e antipolio), malassorbimento, celiachia e morbo di Hirschprung. Gli adulti, che raggiungono un'altezza di 107-157 cm, sono a rischio di neoplasie maligne, in particolare tumori cutanei e linfoma.

La CHH ha un'ereditarietà autosomica recessiva. Anche se rara, la sua massima prevalenza si osserva nelle popolazioni Amish e finlandese. Essa deriva da mutazioni di un gene che codifica una componente RNA di grandi dimensioni e non tradotta di un complesso enzimatico coinvolto nell'elaborazione dell'RNA mitocondriale (RMRP). La perdita di questo prodotto genico può alterare l'elaborazione dell'RNA ribosomiale 5.8S, interferendo con la traduzione proteica e il controllo della mitosi. Le mutazioni di RMRP, di solito associate a CHH tipica, sono state occasionalmente osservate in pazienti con fenotipi clinici più lievi che non presentano le caratteristiche extrascheletriche tipiche

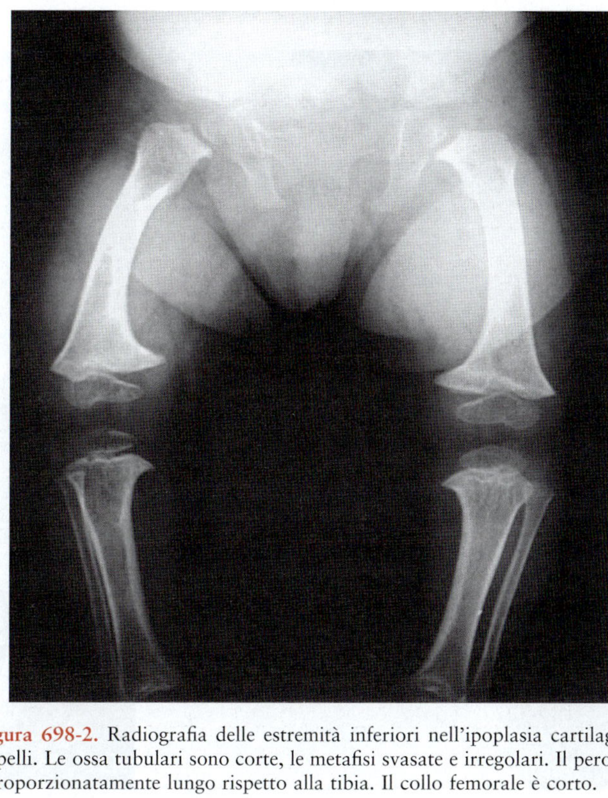

Figura 698-2. Radiografia delle estremità inferiori nell'ipoplasia cartilagine-capelli. Le ossa tubulari sono corte, le metafisi svasate e irregolari. Il perone è sproporzionatamente lungo rispetto alla tibia. Il collo femorale è corto.

della CHH. Se la mutazione è identificabile nel paziente o nei genitori, è possibile la diagnosi prenatale.

DISPLASIA METATROPICA. Esistono almeno due tipi di displasia metatropica (OMIM 156530, 250600): una forma autosomica dominante e una autosomica recessiva. Indipendentemente dal tipo, i neonati si presentano con un tronco lungo e stretto ed estremità corte. Dalla base della colonna si diparte talvolta un'appendice simile a una coda. È comune un'ipoplasia dell'odontoide, che può essere associata a instabilità cervicale. Alla fine della prima infanzia compare una cifoscoliosi, che progredisce nel corso della seconda infanzia, diventando spesso così severa da compromettere la funzione cardiopolmonare. Le articolazioni sono di grandi dimensioni e presentano una perdita progressiva della mobilità, con l'eccezione delle mani. Si sviluppano spesso retrazioni a livello di anche e ginocchi nel corso della seconda infanzia. I bambini con forme severe talvolta muoiono in giovane età per insufficienza respiratoria; ciononostante i pazienti di solito sopravvivono, anche se da adulti possono divenire disabili a causa delle deformità muscoloscheletriche progressive. L'altezza degli adulti va da 110 a 120 cm.

Le radiografie scheletriche evidenziano alterazioni caratteristiche, dominate da una platispondilia severa e da ossa tubulari corte con metafisi espanse e deformate con aspetto a manubrio (Fig. 698-3). Le ossa pelviche sono ipoplasiche e presentano un aspetto ad alabarda a causa di una piccola incisura ischiatica e di un'incisura sopra il margine laterale dell'acetabolo.

DISPLASIA SPONDILOMETAFISARIA-TIPO DI KOZLOWSKI. Il tipo di Kozlowski della displasia spondilometafisaria (OMIM 184252) si presenta nella prima infanzia con bassa statura di grado lieve che interessa principalmente il tronco e con andatura anserina. Mani e piedi possono essere corti e tozzi. Le radiografie mostrano un appiattimento dei corpi vertebrali. Le metafisi delle ossa tubulari sono allargate e irregolarmente mineralizzate, soprattutto a livello del femore prossimale. Le ossa pelviche presentano una lieve ipoplasia.

Durante l'adolescenza si può sviluppare una scoliosi. Il disordine è altrimenti non complicato e le manifestazioni sono limitate allo scheletro. Gli adulti raggiungono un'altezza di 130-150 cm.

Il tipo di Kozlowski di displasia spondilometafisaria è un disordine autosomico dominante. In diversi disordini dello sviluppo scheletrico sono state osservate mutazioni dei geni che codificano le proteine filamina A e filamina B: mutazioni della filamina A nelle sindromi otopalatodigitali di tipo 1 e 2, nella displasia frontometafisaria e nella sindrome di Melnick-Needles (OMIM 311300, 304120, 305620, 309350); mutazioni della filamina B nella sindrome di Larsen e nell'atelosteogenesi letale perinatale di tipo I e III (OMIM 150250, 108720, 108721). Le filamine connettono funzionalmente le proteine strutturali extracellulari e intracellulari, legando in questo modo le cellule al loro microambiente locale, che è essenziale per lo sviluppo e la crescita dello scheletro.

OSTEOCONDROSI GIOVANILI. Le osteocondrosi giovanili, riassunte nella Tabella 698-1, sono un gruppo eterogeneo di disordini in cui disturbi regionali della crescita ossea causano artropatie non infiammatorie. Alcune comportano dolore e dolorabilità localizzati (malattia di Freiberg, malattia di Osgood-Schlatter, osteocondrite dissecante), mentre altre danno luogo a una limitazione non dolorosa del movimento articolare (malattia di Legg-Calvé-Perthes, malattia di Scheuermann). La crescita ossea può essere interrotta, con sviluppo di deformità. La diagnosi è di solito confermata radiograficamente e il trattamento è sintomatico. Si ritiene che la patogenesi di questi disordini coinvolga la necrosi ischemica dei centri di ossificazione primari e secondari. Anche se sono state descritte forme familiari, questi disordini di solito sono sporadici.

MALATTIA DI CAFFEY (IPEROSTOSI CORTICALE INFANTILE). Si tratta di un raro disordine di eziologia sconosciuta caratterizzato da iperostosi corticale con infiammazione della fascia e del muscolo contigui. È spesso sporadico, ma sono state riportate sia un'ereditarietà autosomica dominante sia un'ereditarietà autosomica recessiva. In tre famiglie non correlate con ereditarietà autosomica dominante è stato osservato un linkage con mutazioni del gene *COLIA1* (che codifica la catena α1 del collagene di tipo I.

È stato descritto un esordio prenatale e più spesso postnatale. L'esordio prenatale può essere lieve (autosomico dominante) o severo (autosomico recessivo). La malattia prenatale severa è caratterizzata da tipiche lesioni ossee, polidramnios, idrope

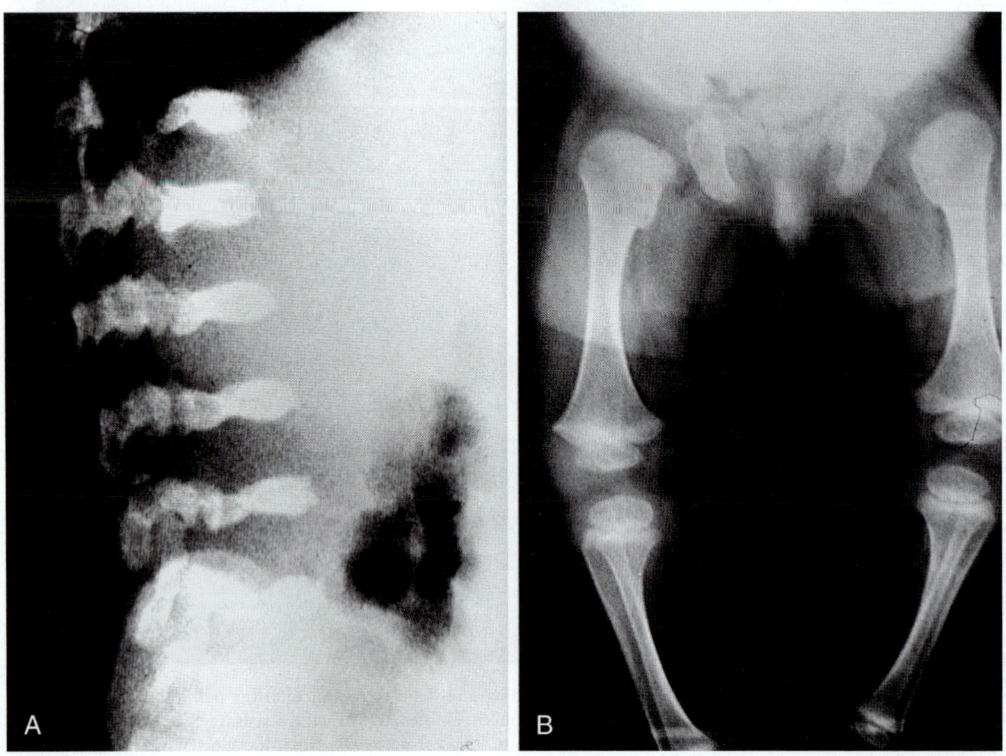

Figura 698-3. *A*, Radiografia della colonna toracolombare laterale nella displasia metatropica che evidenzia una severa platispondilia. *B*, Radiografia delle estremità inferiori nella displasia metatropica che evidenziano ossa tubulari corte con allargamento delle metafisi. Il femore ha un aspetto a manubrio.

TABELLA 698-1. Osteocondrosi giovanili

EPONIMO	REGIONE INTERESSATA	ETÀ ALLA PRESENTAZIONE
Malattia di Legg-Calvé-Perthes	Epifisi della testa femorale	3-12 anni
Malattia di Osgood-Schlatter	Tuberosità tibiale	10-16 anni
Malattia di Sever	Calcagno	6-10 anni
Malattia di Freiberg	Testa del 2° metatarso	10-14 anni
Malattia di Scheuermann	Corpi vertebrali	Adolescenza
Malattia di Blount	Aspetto mediale dell'epifisi tibiale prossimale	Infanzia o adolescenza
Osteocondrite dissecante	Regioni subcondrali di ginocchio, anca, gomito e caviglia	Adolescenza

fetale, distress respiratorio severo, prematurità ed elevata mortalità. L'esordio nella primissima infanzia (<6 mesi, in media 10 settimane) è quello più comune; le manifestazioni comprendono l'esordio improvviso di irritabilità, edema dei tessuti molli contigui che precede l'ispessimento corticale delle ossa sottostanti, febbre e anoressia. L'edema è doloroso con un indurimento di consistenza lignea ma con eritema o calore minimi; la suppurazione è assente. Vi sono remissioni e recidive non prevedibili; un episodio può durare da 2 settimane a 3 mesi. Le ossa più comunemente interessate sono mandibola (75%) (Fig. 698-4), clavicola e ulna. Se la tumefazione non è visibile o non è accentuata, la diagnosi può non essere evidente.

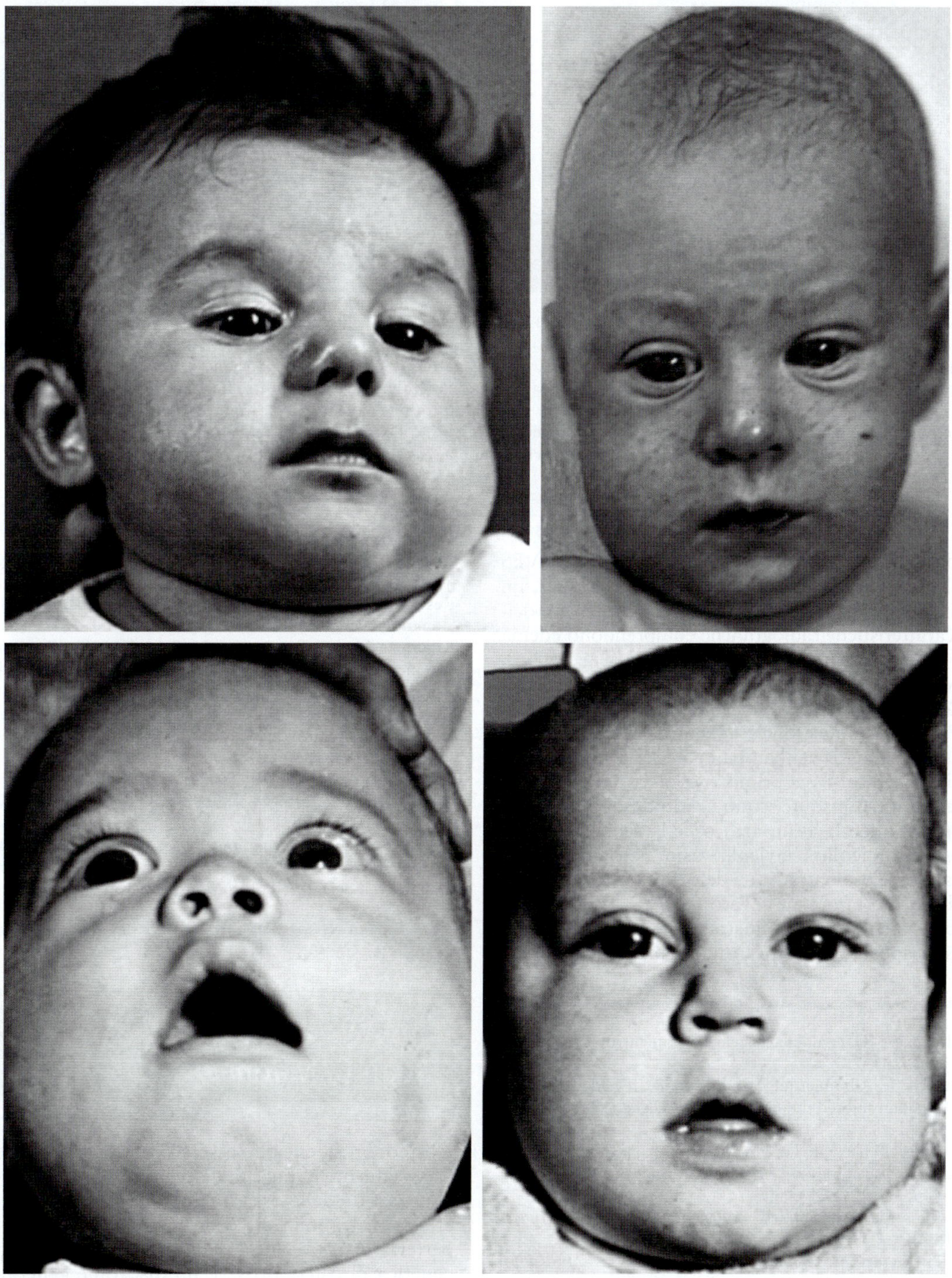

Figura 698-4. Facies dei pazienti con iperostosi corticale infantile. In quasi tutti i casi, le alterazioni sono comparse prima del 5° mese di vita. Tumefazione unilaterale della guancia sinistra e del lato sinistro della mandibola in un lattante di 12 settimane di vita. (Da Kuhn JP, Slovis TL, Haller JO: *Caffey's Pediatric Diagnostic Imaging*, 10th ed., vol. 2, Philadelphia, Mosby, 2004, p. 2363.)

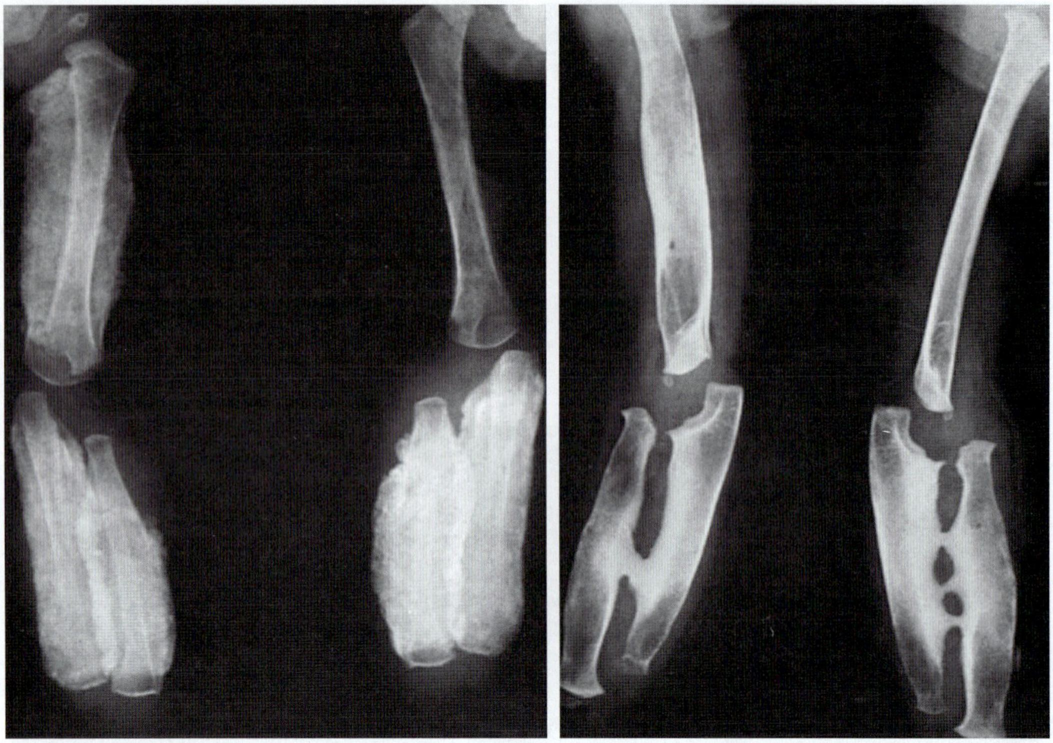

Figura 698-5. Ponti ossei residui tra radio e ulna nell'iperostosi corticale infantile. *A*, Ispessimento corticale massivo bilaterale di radio e ulna a 4 mesi e mezzo di età. La pressione esercitata dall'ispessimento osseo esterno ha forzato la testa del radio lateralmente e in fuori rispetto al gomito. *B*, A 12 mesi e mezzo, 9 mesi dopo l'esordio, tutte le ossa affette sono ancora molto ingrandite, in gran parte per effetto dell'espansione della cavità midollare, anche se permangono residui del precedente ispessimento corticale. La testa del radio è ancora lussata bilateralmente e la diafisi radiale è ora fissata in questa posizione ectopica da ponti ossei solidi tra la diafisi radiale e la diafisi ulnare, un unico ponte osseo a destra e tre a sinistra. A 32 mesi, questi ponti sono ancora intatti, anche se il loro diametro è leggermente diminuito. È possibile che questi ponti ossei rappresentino l'ossificazione di parti della membrana interossea. (Da Kuhn JP, Slovis TL, Haller JO: *Caffey's Pediatric Diagnostic Imaging*, 10th ed., vol. 2, Philadelphia, Mosby, 2004, p. 2365.)

Le **anomalie di laboratorio** comprendono un aumento della VES e della fosfatasi alcalina sierica, come pure, in alcuni pazienti, un aumento dei livelli di prostaglandina E. Vi possono essere trombocitosi e anemia. Le **caratteristiche radiografiche** comprendono edema dei tessuti molli e calcificazioni e iperostosi corticale (Fig. 698-5). Tutte le ossa possono essere colpite, a eccezione delle falangi o dei corpi vertebrali. La **diagnosi differenziale** comprende altre cause di iperostosi, come l'intossicazione cronica da vitamina A, l'infusione prolungata di prostaglandina E nei bambini con pervietà del dotto di Botallo congenita, i tumori ossei primitivi e lo scorbuto.

Le **complicanze**, peraltro insolite, sono costituite da una pseudoparalisi con interessamento di un arto o della scapola, versamenti pleurici (costa), torcicollo (clavicola), asimmetria mandibolare, fusione ossea (coste o ulna/radio) e deformità angolari delle ossa (comuni nell'esordio prenatale severo).

Il **trattamento** consiste nella somministrazione di indometacina e, in caso di scarsa risposta a questo farmaco, prednisone.

Beck M, Roubicek M, Rogers JG, et al: Heterogeneity of metatropic dysplasia. *Eur J Pediatr* 1983;140:231–237.

da Silva EO, Janovitz D, de Albuquerque SC: Ellis-van Creveld syndrome: Report of 15 cases in an inbred kindred. *J Med Genet* 1980;17:349–356.

Davis JT, Long FR, Adler BH, et al: Lateral thoracic expansion for Jeune syndrome: Evidence of rib healing and new bone formation. *Ann Thorac Surg* 2004;77:445–448.

Glorieux FH: Caffey disease: An unlikely collagenopathy. *J Clin Invest* 2005;115:1142–1144.

Hall CM, Elcioglu NH: Metatropic dysplasia lethal variants. *Pediatr Radiol* 2004:34:66–74.

Krakow D, Robertson SP, King LM, et al: Mutations in the gene encoding filamin B disrupt vertebral segmentation, joint formation and skeletogenesis. *Nat Genet* 2004;36:405–410.

Makitie O, Sulisalo T, de la Chapelle A, et al: Cartilage-hair hypoplasia. *J Med Genet* 1995;32:39–43.

Restrepo S, Sanchez AM, Palacios E: Infantile cortical hyperostosis of the mandible. *Ear Nose Throat J* 2004;83:454–455.

Ridanpaa M, van Eenennaam H, Pelin K, et al: Mutations in the RNA component of RNase MRP cause a pleiotropic human disease, cartilage-hair hypoplasia. *Cell* 2001;104:195–203.

Ruiz-Perez VL, Ide SE, Strom TM, et al: Mutations in a new gene in Ellis-van Creveld syndrome and Weyers acrodental dysostosis. *Nat Genet* 2000;24:283–286.

Schweiger S, Chaoui R, Tennstedt C, et al: Antenatal onset of cortical hyperostosis (Caffey disease): Case report and review. *Am J Med Genet* 2003;120A:547–552.

Sharrard WJW: Abnormalities of the epiphyses and limb inequality. In Sharrard WJW (editor): *Paediatric Orthopaedics and Fracture*, 3rd ed. Oxford, Blackwell Scientific Publications, 1993, p 719.

Capitolo 699 ■ Osteogenesi imperfetta

Joan C. Marini

L'osteoporosi, che può essere sia acquisita sia ereditaria, si associa classicamente a fragilità dell'apparato scheletrico e a suscettibilità alle fratture delle ossa lunghe o alla compressione vertebrale per effetto di traumi lievi o di scarsa importanza. L'osteogenesi imperfetta (OI) (malattia delle ossa di vetro), la più comune causa genetica di osteoporosi, è un disordine generalizzato del tessuto connettivo, il cui spettro è estremamente ampio, andando da una forma letale nel periodo perinatale a una forma lieve la cui diagnosi può essere equivoca in età adulta.

EZIOLOGIA. Difetti strutturali o quantitativi del collagene di tipo I causano lo spettro clinico completo dell'OI. Il collagene di tipo I è la componente primaria della matrice extracellulare ossea e cutanea. Nel 10% dei casi clinicamente indistinguibili dall'OI non è possibile dimostrare un difetto molecolare del collagene di tipo I. Alcuni di essi si associano a un collagene biochimicamente normale e probabilmente rappresentano un'eterogeneità genetica. Altri casi si associano a un collagene estremamente modificato e a displasia ossea severa/letale simile all'OI: essi sono causati da mutazioni *null* recessive di un enzima modificante il collagene, la prolil 3-idrossilasi 1 (codificata dal gene *LEPRE1* sul cromosoma 134.1) o della sua proteina associata, la CRTAP.

EPIDEMIOLOGIA. L'OI è una patologia autosomica dominante che si verifica in tutti i gruppi razziali ed etnici. La sua incidenza nella prima infanzia è di circa 1/20 000, simile all'incidenza della forma lieve di tipo I.

ANATOMIA PATOLOGICA. Le mutazioni strutturali del collagene causano un'anomalia globale del tessuto osseo nell'OI. La matrice ossea contiene fibrille di collagene di tipo I anormali e livelli relativamente aumentati di collagene di tipo III e V. Inoltre, sono presenti in quantità ridotta molte altre proteine della matrice ossea. I cristalli di idrossiapatite depositati su questa matrice sono scarsamente allineati all'asse lungo delle fibrille.

PATOGENESI. Il collagene di tipo I è un eterotrimero, composto da due catene α1(I) e una catena α2(I). Le catene sono sintetizzate sotto forma di molecole di procollagene con brevi estensioni globulari a entrambe le estremità del dominio dell'elica centrale. Il dominio dell'elica è composto da ripetizioni ininterrotte della sequenza Gly-X-Y, dove Gly è la glicina, X è spesso la prolina e Y è spesso l'idrossiprolina. La presenza di glicina ogni terzo residuo è cruciale per la formazione dell'elica, in quanto la sua piccola catena laterale può adattarsi al poco spazio disponibile nel trimero elicoidale. Le catene sono assemblate in eliche utilizzando siti cruciali di allineamento nell'estensione carbossil-terminale. La formazione dell'elica quindi procede in modo lineare in direzione carbossiaminica. Contemporaneamente all'assemblaggio e alla formazione dell'elica, le catene sono glicosilate a livello dei residui di lisina.

I difetti strutturali del collagene sono prevalentemente di due tipi: l'80% è rappresentato da mutazioni puntiformi che causano sostituzioni dei residui di glicina dell'elica o dei residui cruciali del propeptide C da parte di altri aminoacidi, mentre il 20% è dato da difetti di unione di un singolo esone (*splicing*). L'OI di tipo I, clinicamente lieve, comporta un difetto quantitativo con mutazioni *null* in un allele α1(I). Questi pazienti producono collagene normale in quantità ridotta.

Le sostituzioni della glicina nelle due catene α hanno relazioni genotipo-fenotipo distinte. Un terzo delle mutazioni della catena α1 è letale, in particolare le sostituzioni con catene laterali cariche o ramificate che incidono sulla stabilità dell'elica. Due regioni uniformemente letali nel terzo carbossilico di α1(I) si allineano con le principali regioni di legame del ligando dell'elica del collagene. Le sostituzioni della glicina in α2(I) sono prevalentemente non letali. Le mutazioni letali si verificano in 8 regioni regolarmente spaziate lungo la catena che si allineano con le regioni di legame per i proteoglicani della matrice a livello della struttura della matrice del collagene di ordine superiore, la fibrilla.

L'OI classica è una patologia autosomica dominante. Alcune ricorrenze familiari sono causate da mosaicismo dei genitori per mutazioni dominanti del collagene. Una piccola percentuale di casi simili all'OI è rappresentata da difetti recessivi del complesso di proteine responsabili della prolil 3-idrossilazione del collagene di tipo I.

MANIFESTAZIONI CLINICHE. L'OI è caratterizzata dalla triade fragilità ossea, sclere blu e sordità precoce. Un tempo era classificata in due categorie, "congenita" (forme identificabili alla nascita) e "tarda" (forme identificabili nelle età successive), suddivisione che però non spiegava la variabilità riscontrabile in questa patologia. La classificazione di Sillence suddivide l'OI in quattro tipi in base a criteri clinici e radiografici. Sono stati proposti altri tipi sulla base di distinzioni istologiche.

Osteogenesi imperfetta di tipo I (lieve). Questa forma piuttosto lieve si osserva con una certa frequenza in grandi famiglie. Molti membri di famiglie con OI di tipo I hanno sclere blu, fratture ricorrenti nell'infanzia e sordità presenile (30-60%). Tanto il tipo I quanto il tipo IV si suddividono in sottotipi A e B, a seconda dell'assenza (A) o della presenza (B) di **dentinogenesi imperfetta**. Altre possibili anomalie del tessuto connettivo comprendono facilità al sanguinamento, lassità articolare e bassa statura di grado lieve rispetto ad altri membri della famiglia. Le fratture, che derivano da traumi lievi o moderati, si riducono dopo la pubertà.

Osteogenesi imperfetta di tipo II (letale nel periodo perinatale). Questi bambini possono nascere morti o morire nel primo anno di vita. Il peso alla nascita e la lunghezza sono scarsi per l'età gestazionale. Lo scheletro e altri tessuti connettivi sono estremamente fragili. Si verificano numerose fratture intrauterine delle ossa lunghe, che alle radiografie hanno un aspetto "accartocciato". Sono presenti una micromelia e un incurvamento delle estremità molto marcati; le gambe sono mantenute in abduzione ad angolo retto rispetto al corpo, nella posizione "a zampe di rana". Le numerose fratture conferiscono alle coste un aspetto nodulare, mentre il torace di piccole dimensioni contribuisce all'insufficienza respiratoria. Il cranio è grande rispetto al corpo, con un aumento del diametro delle fontanelle anteriore e posteriore. Le sclere hanno un colore grigio-blu.

Osteogenesi imperfetta di tipo III (progressivamente deformante). Questa è la più severa forma non letale di OI, che causa una significativa disabilità fisica. Peso alla nascita e lunghezza sono spesso inferiori alla norma. Di solito si verificano fratture in utero. Si riscontrano una macrocefalia relativa e facies triangolare (Fig. 699-1). Dopo la nascita, le fratture sono causate da traumi di

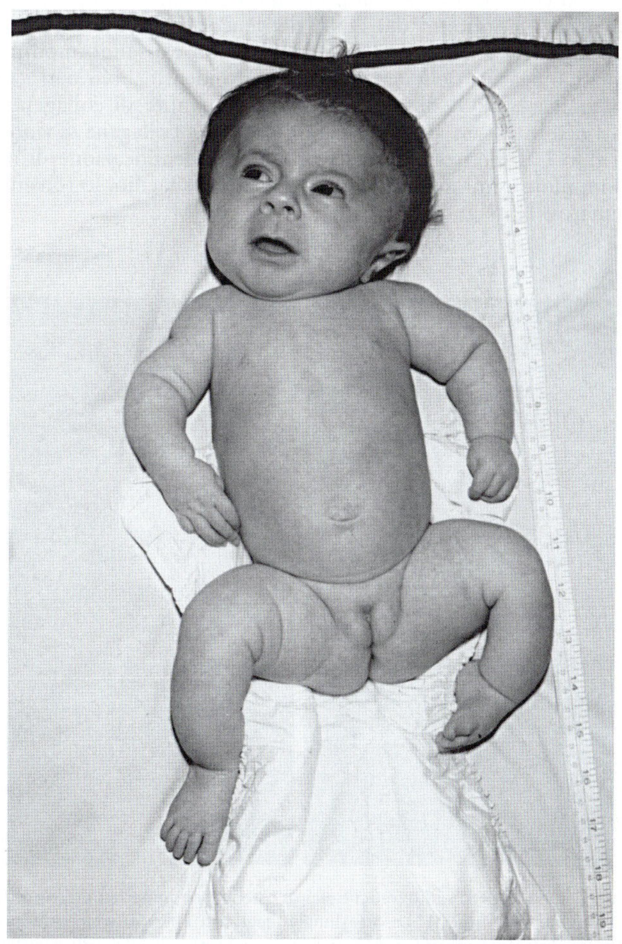

Figura 699-1. Bambino con osteogenesi imperfetta di tipo III che presenta estremità curve e corte, deformità toracica e macrocefalia relativa.

poco conto e dopo la guarigione residuano deformità. La disorganizzazione della matrice ossea produce un aspetto "a popcorn" a livello delle metafisi (Fig. 699-2). La gabbia toracica è svasata alla base e sono frequenti le deformità del petto. Praticamente tutti i pazienti di tipo III hanno scoliosi e compressione vertebrale. L'accrescimento scende al di sotto della curva normale entro il primo anno; tutti i pazienti di tipo III hanno una statura estremamente bassa. I colore delle sclere varia dal bianco al blu.

Osteogenesi imperfetta di tipo IV (moderatamente severa). I pazienti con OI di tipo IV possono presentarsi alla nascita con fratture in utero o incurvamento delle ossa lunghe degli arti inferiori, oltre che con fratture ricorrenti dopo l'inizio della deambulazione. La maggior parte dei bambini ha un incurvamento moderato anche in caso di fratture infrequenti. I bambini con OI di tipo IV richiedono interventi ortopedici e riabilitativi, ma di solito sono in grado di camminare. L'incidenza delle fratture diminuisce dopo la pubertà. Da un punto di vista radiografico, sono presenti osteoporosi, svasatura delle metafisi e compressioni vertebrali. I pazienti di tipo IV hanno una bassa statura di grado moderato. Il colore delle sclere può essere blu o bianco.

Osteogenesi imperfetta di tipo V (callo iperplasico), di tipo VI (difetto di mineralizzazione) e di tipo VII (autosomica recessiva). È stata avanzata la proposta di classificare in tipi distinti piccoli gruppi di pazienti con OI clinica di tipo IV, ma con caratteristiche peculiari alla biopsia ossea. In questi soggetti, che costituiscono il 5% circa della popolazione con OI, lo screening per le mutazioni del collagene è negativo. I pazienti di tipo V hanno anche un callo iperplasico, calcificazioni della membrana interossea dell'avambraccio e una banda radiopaca metafisaria. Il tipo VII mappa sul cromosoma 3p22-24 ed è un difetto ipomorfico del CRTAP.

INDAGINI DI LABORATORIO. La diagnosi è confermata dagli studi biochimici del collagene, dalla sequenziazione del cDNA con fibroblasti coltivati da una biopsia cutanea a stampo oppure dalla sequenziazione diretta del DNA dei leucociti. Le mutazioni nel terzo aminico delle catene di collagene, non causando modificazioni significative delle catene, non sono identificabili con i test biochimici. Nell'OI di tipo I, la ridotta quantità di collagene di tipo I determina un aumento del rapporto tra collagene di tipo III e di tipo I all'elettroforesi delle proteine. L'identificazione di mutazioni puntiformi in base alla sequenziazione facilita lo screening familiare e la diagnosi prenatale.

L'OI severa è identificabile prima della nascita mediante un'ecografia di livello II, già alla 16ª settimana di gestazione. È possibile confondere l'OI con la displasia tanatofora. L'ecografia fetale può non identificare l'OI di tipo IV e raramente identifica l'OI di tipo I. Per i casi ricorrenti, si può effettuare la biopsia dei villi coriali per studi biochimici o molecolari. Gli amniociti producono risultati falsi positivi nelle analisi biochimiche, ma in determinati casi possono essere utilizzati per studi molecolari.

Nel periodo neonatale, i livelli normali o aumentati di fosfatasi alcalina presenti nell'OI permettono di distinguere questa patologia dall'ipofosfatasia.

COMPLICANZE. Morbilità e mortalità dell'OI dipendono dalle complicanze cardiopolmonari. Nei pazienti pediatrici si verificano polmoniti ricorrenti e un declino della funzione respiratoria, mentre negli adulti si osserva un cuore polmonare.

Le complicanze neurologiche comprendono invaginazione basilare, compressione del tronco encefalico, idrocefalo e siringoidromelia. La maggior parte dei bambini con OI di tipo III e IV ha un'invaginazione basilare, ma la compressione del tronco encefalico è infrequente. L'invaginazione basilare è più evidente alla TC spirale della giunzione craniocervicale (Fig. 699-3).

TRATTAMENTO. Non esiste un trattamento per l'OI. Per la forma severa non letale, la riabilitazione fisica attiva nei primi anni permette ai bambini di raggiungere un livello funzionale più elevato che con il solo trattamento ortopedico. I pazienti pediatrici con OI di tipo I e alcuni con OI di tipo IV deambulano spontaneamente. I bambini con OI di tipo III e IV severa traggono beneficio dall'uso di tutori lunghi per gli arti inferiori in materiale plastico, ausili per la deambulazione e un programma di nuoto e riabilitazione. I soggetti con malattia severa dipendono dalla sedia a rotelle per la mobilità, pur potendo acquisire un certo grado di autonomia negli spostamenti e nella cura della propria persona. Gli adolescenti possono richiedere un sostegno psicologico per problemi di immagine corporea.

Il trattamento ortopedico dell'OI ha l'obiettivo di trattare le fratture e correggere le deformità che incidono negativamente sulla funzionalità. Le fratture devono essere trattate immediatamente con tutori o gesso; esse guariscono bene e si consiglia di rimuovere il gesso quanto prima allo scopo di minimizzare l'oste-

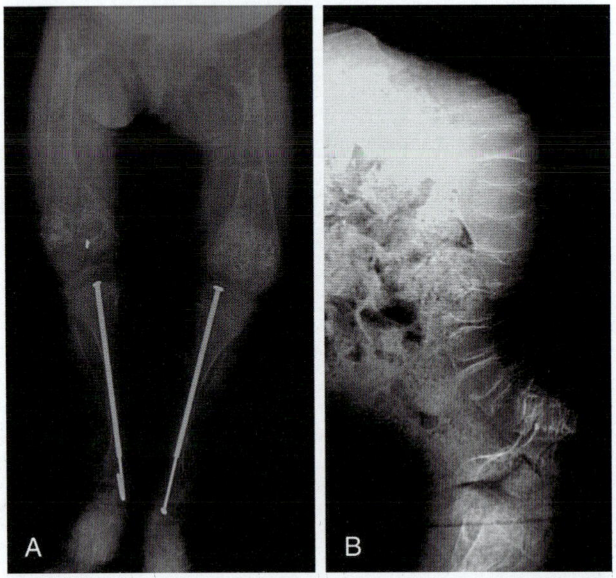

Figura 699-2. Aspetti radiografici tipici di osteogenesi imperfetta di tipo III in un bambino di 6 anni. *A*, Le ossa lunghe degli arti inferiori sono osteoporotiche con svasatura metafisaria, aspetto "a popcorn" a livello delle cartilagini di accrescimento e presenza di chiodi intramidollari. *B*, I corpi vertebrali sono compressi e osteoporotici.

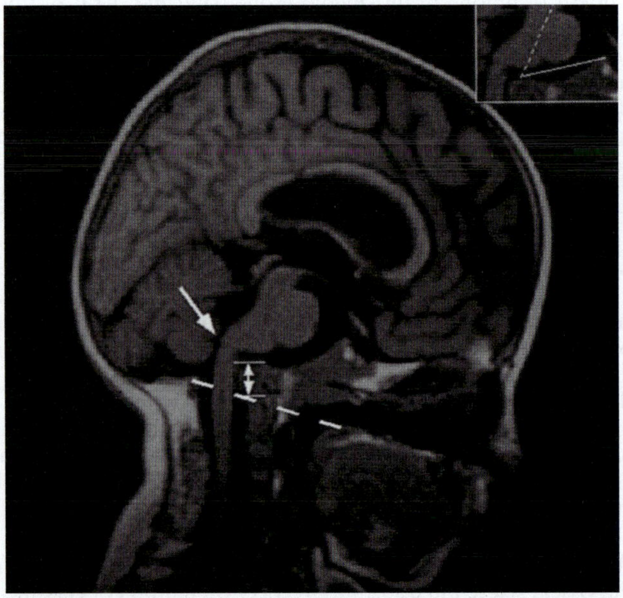

Figura 699-3. Aspetto tipico dell'invaginazione basilare alla RM sagittale di un bambino sintomatico con osteogenesi imperfetta di tipo III. È presente un'invaginazione dell'odontoide sopra la linea di Chamberlain che causa compressione e deviazione a livello della giunzione pontomidollare (*freccia*).

oporosi da immobilizzazione. La correzione delle deformità delle ossa lunghe richiede una procedura osteotomica e l'inserimento di un chiodo intramidollare.

Il trattamento con supplementi di calcio o fluoro o con calcitonina non migliora l'OI. L'ormone della crescita migliora l'istologia ossea nei bambini che rispondono al farmaco (di solito i tipi I e IV). Un breve ciclo di trattamento dei bambini con OI con bifosfonati (pamidronato ev o olpadronato per os) è di qualche beneficio. I bifosfonati riducono il riassorbimento osseo da parte degli osteoclasti; i pazienti con OI avranno un volume maggiore di tessuto osseo, che però continuerà a contenere il collagene difettoso. I bifosfonati sono più utili per le vertebre (osso trabecolare) che per le ossa lunghe (osso corticale). Il trattamento per 1-2 anni determina un aumento dei parametri DEXA L1-4 e, cosa più importante, migliora le compressioni vertebrali e l'area vertebrale in genere, con il risultato di prevenire o ritardare la scoliosi. Il rischio relativo di fratture delle ossa lunghe subisce una modesta riduzione. Tuttavia, il trattamento prolungato non solo indebolisce le proprietà fisiche delle ossa lunghe, ma aumenta i mancati consolidamenti dopo interventi di osteotomia. I bifosfonati non hanno alcun effetto sui punteggi di mobilità, sulla forza muscolare o sul dolore osseo. Limitando la durata del trattamento a 2-3 anni tra la prima e la seconda infanzia è possibile ottenere i massimi benefici riducendo al minimo gli effetti negativi sulle proprietà dell'osso corticale. I benefici sembrano persistere a distanza di diversi anni dal trattamento. Gli effetti collaterali comprendono un anormale rimodellamento delle ossa lunghe, osteonecrosi della mandibola e una fragilità ossea simile a quella dell'osteopetrosi.

PROGNOSI. L'OI è una condizione cronica che limita sia l'aspettativa di vita sia i livelli funzionali. I bambini con OI di tipo II di solito muoiono entro un periodo variabile tra alcuni mesi e l'anno di vita. Occasionalmente, un soggetto con gli aspetti radiografici del tipo II e un deficit estremo di accrescimento può sopravvivere fino all'adolescenza. I pazienti con OI di tipo III hanno un'aspettativa di vita ridotta; alcuni muoiono per cause polmonari nella prima infanzia; altri picchi si registrano nell'adolescenza e nella quarta decade di vita. I tipi I e IV sono compatibili con un'aspettativa di vita normale.

I soggetti con OI di tipo III di solito dipendono dalla carrozzina. Con una riabilitazione aggressiva, possono raggiungere una certa autonomia e la capacità di deambulare tra le mura domestiche. I bambini con OI di tipo IV di solito riescono a deambulare fuori casa, in completa autonomia o con ausili appositi.

COUNSELING GENETICO. L'OI è una patologia autosomica dominante; il rischio che un individuo affetto trasmetta il gene alla progenie è del 50%. Un bambino affetto ha in genere una malattia di severità uguale a quella del genitore; tuttavia, esiste una variabilità di espressione e la condizione del bambino può essere più o meno grave di quella del genitore.

Per una coopia apparentemente non affetta, il rischio di avere un secondo figlio con OI è empiricamente del 5-7%, corrispondente alla probabilità statistica che un genitore abbia un mosaicismo della linea germinale. La mutazione del collagene nel genitore non affetto è presente in alcune cellule germinali e può manifestarsi anche nei tessuti somatici. Se i test genetici rivelano che uno dei due genitori è portatore di un mosaicismo, il rischio di recidiva può giungere al 50%.

Antoniazzi F, Bertoldo F, Mottes M, et al: Growth hormone treatment in osteogenesis imperfecta with quantitative defect of type I collagen synthesis. *J Pediatr* 1996;129:432–439.

Barnes AM, Chang W, Morello R, et al: Deficiency of cartilage-associated protein in recessive lethal osteogenesis imperfecta. *N Engl J Med* 2006; 355:2757–2764.

Cabral WA, Chang W, Barnes AM, et al: Prolyl 3-hydroxylase 1 deficiency causes a recessive metabolic bone disorder resembling lethal/severe osteogenesis imperfecta. *Nat Genet* 2007;39:359–365.

Glorieux FH, Rauch F, Plotkin H, et al: Type V osteogenesis imperfecta: A new form of brittle bone disease. *J Bone Miner Res* 2000;15:1650–1658.

Glorieux FH, Rauch F, Ward LM, et al: Alendronate in the treatment of pediatric osteogenesis imperfecta. *J Bone Miner Res* 2004;19(Suppl 1):S12.

Glorieux FH, Ward LM, Rauch F, et al: Osteogenesis imperfecta type VI: A form of brittle bone disease with a mineralization defect. *J Bone Miner Res* 2002;17:30–38.

Letocha A, Cintas HL, Troendle JF, et al: Controlled trial of pamidronate in children with types III and IV osteogenesis imperfecta confirms vertebral gains but not short-term functional improvement. *J Bone Miner Res* 2005;20:977–986.

Marini JC: Should children with osteogenesis imperfecta be treated with bisphosphonates? *Nat Clin Prac Endo & Metab* 2006;2:14–15.

Marini JC, Hopkins E, Glorieux FH, et al: Positive linear growth and bone responses to growth hormone treatment in children with types III and IV osteogenesis imperfecta. *J Bone Miner Res* 2003;18:237–243.

Plotkin H, Rauch F, Bishop NJ: Pamidronate treatment of severe osteogenesis imperfecta in children under 3 years of age. *J Clin Endocrinol Metab* 2000;85:1846–1850.

Sakkers R, Kok D, Engelbert R, et al: Skeletal effects and functional outcome with olpadronate in children with osteogenesis imperfecta: A 2-year randomized placebo-controlled study. *Lancet* 2004;363:1427–1431.

Capitolo 700 ■ Sindrome di Marfan

Luther K. Robinson ed Emily Fitzpatrick

La sindrome di Marfan è una patologia a ereditarietà autosomica dominante con penetranza quasi completa ma espressività variabile. La sua incidenza è di circa 1 su 5000-10 000 nati; quasi il 30% dei neonati affetti è il risultato di nuove mutazioni sporadiche. La diagnosi di sindrome di Marfan si basa sulle caratteristiche cliniche, alcune delle quali dipendono dall'età e dal grado di maturazione.

PATOGENESI. La patogenesi è correlata a una biosintesi anormale della fibrillina 1, una proteina extracellulare di 350 kD, il maggiore costituente delle microfibrille che formano l'impalcatura dell'elastina e hanno una funzione di ancoraggio in tessuti non elastici come l'avventizia aortica e il legamento sospensore dell'occhio. Il locus genico per la fibrillina 1 (*FBNI*) si trova nel braccio lungo del cromosoma 15 (15q21). Il gene si compone di 65 esoni e finora ne sono state descritte più di 600 mutazioni, distribuite per tutta la sua lunghezza, ognuna delle quali è unica per una determinata famiglia. La distribuzione relativamente uniforme delle mutazioni lungo *FBNI* probabilmente contribuisce alla variabilità fenotipica del disordine. Tuttavia, le correlazioni fenotipo-genotipo non sempre sono evidenti ed esiste una significativa variabilità intrafamiliare da cui si deduce che fattori epigenetici, modificanti il gene o ambientali influiscono sull'espressione della malattia. Le mutazioni associate alla più severa variante neonatale della sindrome di Marfan si raggruppano negli esoni 26-27 e 31-32. Le mutazioni negli esoni 59-65 possono essere associate a una malattia più lieve nel 40% dei pazienti, che inoltre non presentano una patologia aortica.

Anche la regolazione del fattore di crescita trasformante β da parte della fibrillina può contribuire alle varie manifestazioni della sindrome di Marfan. In effetti, i pazienti con mutazioni eterozigoti del recettore del fattore di crescita trasformante β presentano manifestazioni Marfan-simili con un gene della fibrillina normale. La sindrome risultante (**sindrome aneurismatica di Loeys-Dietz**) ha in comune con la sindrome di Marfan molte caratteristiche, cui si aggiungono ipertelorismo, ugola bifida e vasculopatia più aggressiva, compresa la presenza di tortuosità arteriose e di rottura aortica, con dimensioni aortiche inferiori a quelle osservate nella sindrome di Marfan.

MANIFESTAZIONI CLINICHE. La diagnosi di sindrome di Marfan si basa sul pattern globale delle malformazioni (tipicamente scheletriche, cardiovascolari, oculari); molte manifestazioni sono dipendenti dall'età o dal grado di maturazione. L'alta statura può essere presente alla nascita e persistere fino all'età adulta. Una riduzione del tessuto adiposo sottocutaneo può suggerire uno scarso accrescimento nella prima infanzia. Ipotonia e lassità legamentosa possono indicare ritardi evolutivi, ma la performance cognitiva in genere è normale per la famiglia.

La **sindrome di Marfan neonatale (infantile, congenita)** è più severa dei casi osservati nei bambini più grandi e può essere clinicamente simile all'aracnodattilia contrattuale congenita, presentandosi con ipotonia, aracnodattilia, lassità legamentosa, lussazioni e retrazioni in flessione. Il viso è allungato e la cute lassa, con diminuzione del ritorno elastico. Le orecchie talora sono grandi e pieghevoli. L'esame oculare può evidenziare megalocornea, iridodonesi o una franca lussazione del cristallino. L'esame cardiologico spesso rivela soffi da prolasso mitralico con o da insufficienza aortica, mentre una dilatazione della radice aortica può essere documentata tramite l'ecocardiografia.

I bambini più grandi presentano, oltre a statura elevata, un viso sottile e allungato, con mandibola stretta e affollamento dentale (Fig. 700-1). Le anomalie oculari, che rispecchiano il difetto del tessuto connettivo, comprendono sclere blu, miopia (nel 60% degli individui affetti) e lassità del legamento sospensore con iridodonesi. L'esame alla lampada a fessura già nella primissima infanzia consente la diagnosi di lussazione del cristallino, che può essere congenita. L'iridodonesi è un segno clinico utile, ma nei casi di sospetta sindrome di Marfan occorre richiedere una consulenza oftalmologica con esame alla lampada a fessura anche in assenza di anomalie oculari grossolane, in quanto possono essere presenti miopia, aumento della pressione intraoculare o distacco di retina.

L'esame dell'apparato muscoloscheletrico evidenzia una dolicostenomelia (arti lunghi e sottili) e un *arm span* (rapporto tronco e arto superiore) esagerato rispetto all'altezza (>1,05 volte). Il segmento inferiore (distanza dal pube al tallone) è maggiore rispetto a quello superiore (altezza meno il segmento inferiore) e contribuisce alla diminuzione del rapporto segmento superiore:segmento inferiore (Us/Ls). Le caratteristiche della mano, che sono aspecifiche, comprendono dita lunghe, sottili (aracnodattilia) e iperestensibili. Il pollice può essere addotto attraverso il palmo ristretto (segno di Steinberg) e sovrapporsi in modo apprezzabile al 5° dito quando si circonda il polso con queste due dita (segno del polso) (Figg. 700-2 e 700-3).

Le coste, lunghe e sottili, possono contribuire a varie anomalie sternali tra cui il pectus excavatum ("torace a imbuto") o il pectus carinatum ("petto di piccione"). Il rischio di scoliosi negli adolescenti è aumentato.

Il difetto del tessuto connettivo contribuisce all'aumento della distensibilità del parenchima polmonare e della dura e aumenta i rischi rispettivamente di pneumotorace spontaneo ed estasia durale.

I **difetti cardiovascolari progressivi** contribuiscono alla sostanziale morbilità della sindrome di Marfan; l'ecocardiografia ha migliorato la diagnosi precoce dei pazienti a rischio di complicanze cardiache. Una dilatazione aortica progressiva, accompagnata o meno dall'evidenza auscultatoria di malattia aortica, si verifica nell'80-100% degli individui affetti e può essere congenita.

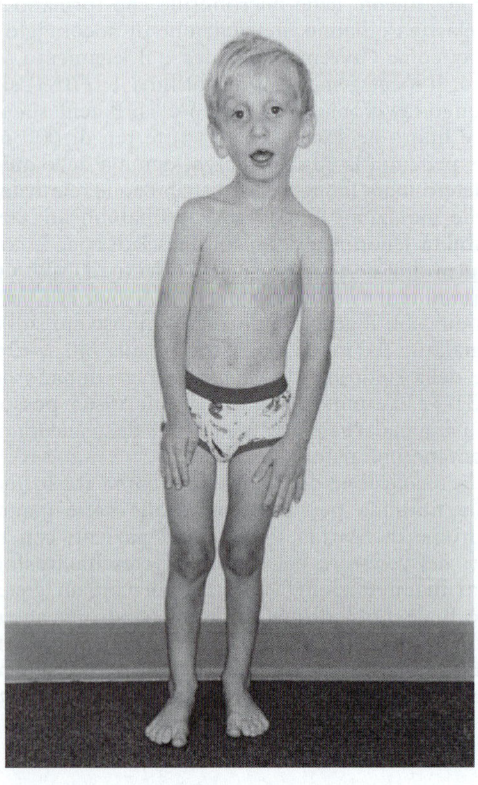

Figura 700-1. Sindrome di Marfan. Si notino il viso allungato, le palpebre cadenti, l'evidente dolicostenomelia e la lieve scoliosi.

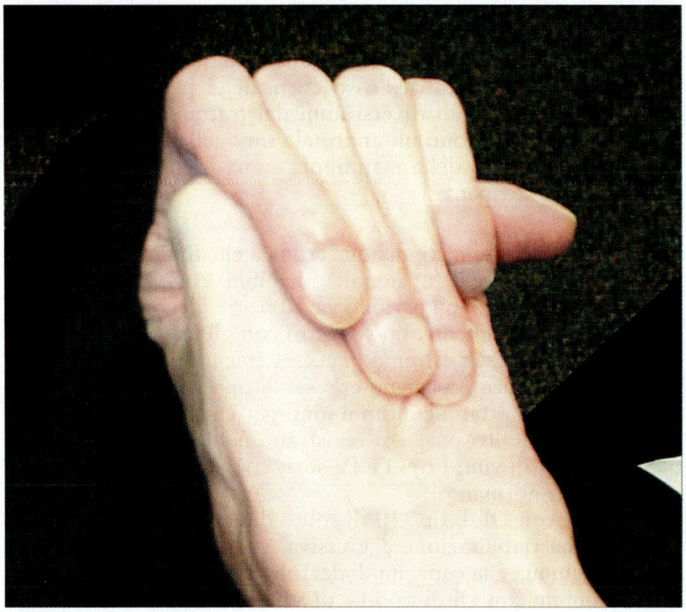

Figura 700-2. "Segno del pollice": quando la mano viene stretta a pugno senza assistenza, tutta l'unghia del pollice si proietta al di fuori del margine della mano. (Da Zitelli BJ: Picture of the month. *Arch Pediatr Adolesc Med* 2005;159:721-723.)

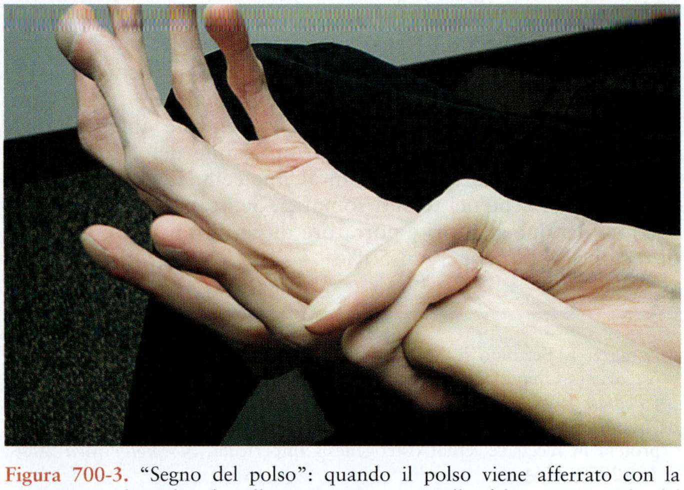

Figura 700-3. "Segno del polso": quando il polso viene afferrato con la mano controlaterale, il pollice si sovrappone alla falange terminale del 5° dito. (Da Zitelli BJ: Picture of the month. *Arch Pediatr Adolesc Med* 2005;159:721-723.)

Un'insufficienza aortica conclamata è meno comune nei bambini che negli adulti, forse perché la distensione raggiunge un'entità e una durata tali da causare una disfunzione aortica soltanto in età successiva. Il prolasso della valvola mitrale, frequente quanto la dilatazione aortica, tende a essere progressivo, a differenza delle lesioni più statiche del prolasso della mitrale idiopatico. Il prolasso della mitrale, la causa più comune di morbilità nei bambini con sindrome di Marfan, può manifestarsi con aritmie, insufficienza cardiaca, tromboembolia o endocardite. Un'insufficienza mitralica si manifesta nel 50% circa dei pazienti affetti di età <20 anni.

DIAGNOSI. La diagnosi di sindrome di Marfan si basa su criteri clinici (Tab. 700-1). In generale, la diagnosi di una mutazione nuova o sporadica richiede che siano presenti le principali manifestazioni del disordine. Nei casi con un parente di primo grado inequivocabilmente affetto, le manifestazioni più lievi con almeno una malformazione maggiore confermano la diagnosi. L'alta statura con un rapporto Us/Ls elevato o un aumento del rapporto *arm span*:altezza (>1,05) è la caratteristica di presentazione più costante. L'ecocardiografia o la RM dovrebbero dimostrare almeno una dilatazione della radice aortica insolita rispetto all'età. Altre anomalie, come prolasso della valvola mitrale, insufficienza mitralica o insufficienza aortica, possono fornire una conferma. Un esame alla lampada a fessura è indicato in tutti i casi sospetti. È importante notare che soltanto il 60-70% dei pazienti che soddisfano i criteri clinici per la sindrome di Marfan ha mutazioni note del gene della fibrillina, mentre il 12% dei pazienti che non soddisfano tali criteri ha una mutazione per la fibrillina.

La **diagnosi differenziale** comprende omocistinuria, sindrome di Loeys-Dietz, dissezione aortica familiare, ectopia del cristallino familiare e sindrome MASS (miopia, prolasso della valvola mitrale, lieve dilatazione aortica, strie cutanee, aspetti scheletrici tipo Marfan). La MASS è causata da una diversa mutazione del gene della fibrillina. Altre condizioni che occorre escludere sono sindrome di Stickler, sindrome del prolasso mitralico idiopatico, sindrome dell'aracnodattilia contrattuale congenita, necrosi mediale cistica isolata dell'aorta (sindrome di Erdheim) e sindrome di Shprintzen-Goldberg (craniosinostosi-aracnodattilia).

Per poter escludere il deficit di cistationina sintetasi (omocistinuria) sono necessari studi specifici sugli aminoacidi e le indagini di laboratorio devono documentare un test al cianuro nitroprussiato negativo. Le tecniche di genetica molecolare come l'analisi diretta delle mutazioni o del linkage genetico contribuiscono alla diagnosi nelle famiglie in cui è nota una mutazione o in un individuo che soddisfa in modo stretto i criteri diagnostici. Dal 30 al 40% dei pazienti che soddisfano i criteri diagnostici per la sindrome di Marfan ha test di genetica molecolare negativi, mentre il 10-12% degli individui con fenotipi simili ma distinti come il fenotipo MASS o la sindrome dell'ectopia del cristallino può avere mutazioni del gene della fibrillina.

TRATTAMENTO. La terapia è focalizzata sulla prevenzione delle complicanze e sul counseling genetico. Considerata la potenziale complessità del trattamento richiesto da alcuni individui affetti, sono preferibili visite periodiche presso un centro multidisciplinare con esperienza nel campo della sindrome di Marfan.

TABELLA 700-1. Criteri diagnostici per la sindrome di Marfan

Caso indice
- Se l'anamnesi genetica/familiare non è significativa, criteri maggiori in 2 o più sistemi d'organo differenti e interessamento di un terzo sistema d'organo
- Se viene identificata una mutazione nota come causa della sindrome di Marfan in altri pazienti, un criterio maggiore in un sistema d'organo e interessamento di un secondo sistema d'organo

Parente di un caso indice che soddisfa in modo indipendente questi rigidi criteri diagnostici
- Presenza di un criterio maggiore nell'anamnesi familiare, un criterio maggiore in un sistema d'organo e interessamento di un secondo sistema d'organo

Sistemi d'organo

Apparato scheletrico

Almeno 4 dei seguenti costituiscono un criterio maggiore nell'apparato scheletrico:
- Pectus carinatum
- Pectus excavatum con necessità di intervento chirurgico
- Riduzione del rapporto segmento superiore:segmento inferiore o *arm span*:altezza >1,05
- Segni del polso e del pollice
- Scoliosi >20° o spondilolistesi
- Riduzione dell'estensione dei gomiti (<170°)
- Spostamento del malleolo mediale che causa pes planus
- Protrusio acetabulae di qualsiasi grado (accertata radiograficamente)

Criteri minori
- Pectus excavatum di severità moderata
- Ipermobilità articolare
- Palato ogivale con affollamento dentale
- Facies caratteristica (dolicocefalia, ipoplasia malare, enoftalmo, retrognazia, rime palpebrali rivolte verso il basso)

Per l'interessamento dell'apparato scheletrico, devono essere presenti almeno 2 aspetti che contribuiscono ai criteri maggiori o 1 aspetto dell'elenco che contribuisce al criterio maggiore e 2 criteri minori

Sistema oculare

Criterio maggiore
- Ectopia del cristallino

Criteri minori
- Cornea anormalmente piatta
- Aumento della lunghezza assiale del bulbo oculare
- Iride ipoplasica o muscolo ciliare ipoplasico, che causano una riduzione della miosi

Per l'interessamento del sistema oculare devono essere presenti almeno 2 criteri minori

Sistema cardiovascolare

Criteri maggiori (uno qualsiasi dei seguenti)
- Dilatazione dell'aorta ascendente, con o senza insufficienza aortica, che interessa almeno i seni di Valsalva
- Dissecazione dell'aorta ascendente

Criteri minori
- Prolasso della valvola mitrale con o senza insufficienza mitralica
- Dilatazione dell'arteria polmonare principale, in assenza di stenosi valvolare o stenosi polmonare periferica o qualsiasi altra causa ovvia, in un paziente di età <40 anni
- Calcificazione dell'annulus mitralico in paziente di età <40 anni
- Dilatazione o dissecazione dell'aorta toracica discendente o dell'aorta addominale in paziente <50 anni

Per l'interessamento dell'apparato cardiovascolare, deve essere presente soltanto 1 dei criteri minori

Sistema polmonare

Criteri maggiori
- Nessuno

Criteri minori
- Pneumotorace spontaneo
- Bolle apicali

Per l'interessamento del sistema polmonare, deve essere presente soltanto 1 criterio minore

Cute e tegumenti

Criteri maggiori
- Nessuno

Criteri minori
- Strie atrofiche senza marcato aumento di peso, gravidanza o stress ripetitivo
- Ernie ricorrenti o da incisione

Per l'interessamento della cute e dei tegumenti, deve essere presente soltanto 1 criterio minore

Dura madre

Criterio maggiore
- Ectasia durale lombosacrale

Criteri minori
- Nessuno

Anamnesi familiare/genetica

Criteri maggiori (uno qualsiasi dei seguenti)
- Avere un genitore o figlio/a che soddisfa questi criteri diagnostici in modo indipendente
- Presenza di una mutazione di *FBN1*, nota per causare la sindrome di Marfan
- Presenza di un aplotipo intorno a *FBN1* ereditato da un membro della famiglia, noto per essere associato a sindrome di Marfan diagnosticata in modo inequivocabile nella famiglia

Criteri minori
- Nessuno

Da Judge DP, Dietz HC: Marfan's syndrome. *Lancet* 2005; 366: 1965-1976.

Il pediatra deve collaborare con sottospecialisti pediatri per coordinare un approccio razionale all'expectant monitoraggio e trattamento di potenziali complicanze. Sono necessarie valutazioni annuali per complicanze potenziali come valvulopatie cardiache, scoliosi o problemi oftalmologici. La fisioterapia può migliorare il tono neuromuscolare nella prima infanzia. Occorre raccomandare una moderata attività fisica aerobica non traumatica come il nuoto o la bicicletta, secondo tolleranza, scoraggiando invece gli sforzi di notevole entità a causa dello stress che l'aumento della gittata cardiaca impone all'aorta. Prima dei trattamenti odontoiatrici o di altre procedure invasive si rende necessaria la profilassi dell'endocardite. Il blocco β-adrenergico con farmaci come propranololo o atenololo può rallentare la progressione della dilatazione aortica e ridurre i rischi di eventi cardiaci catastrofici. Attualmente, si sta introducendo il losartan, un bloccante del recettore di tipo 1 dell'angiotensina II e un agonista del TGF-β, come agente aggiuntivo che potrebbe rivelarsi efficace nel trattamento della malattia aortica. La dissezione aortica acuta può essere trattata con un innesto composito.

Il trattamento ottimale dell'adolescente gravida con sindrome di Marfan non è stato ancora stabilito. Il rischio che la gestazione peggiori le anomalie cardiovascolari rappresenta un problema. Anche se mancano dati rappresentativi, donne giovani con manifestazioni cardiache minori o una lieve dilatazione della radice aortica possono tollerare la gravidanza con prognosi buona tanto per la madre quanto per il bambino. Le pazienti con dilatazione aortica conclamata devono essere sottoposte a monitoraggio ecocardiografico a intervalli regolari. Anche se la teratogenicità del blocco β-adrenergico non è stata dimostrata, i bambini esposti nel periodo prenatale, figli di donne con sindrome di Marfan trattate con β-antagonisti, devono essere monitorati nel periodo neonatale per problemi indotti dai farmaci quali ipotensione, bradicardia e ipoglicemia.

PROGNOSI. La longevità nella sindrome di Marfan risulta minore rispetto agli standard della popolazione, principalmente a causa dell'aumentato rischio di complicanze cardiovascolari. La dilatazione della radice aortica e dell'aorta ascendente, che è progressiva, può portare a formazione di aneurismi e aumentare il rischio di dissezione aortica. Questo e altri aspetti, oltre a sollevare problemi medici, causano stress psicologici nel bambino affetto e nei suoi genitori, soprattutto durante l'adolescenza. La consapevolezza di tali conseguenze e l'invio ai servizi di sostegno possono favorire un approccio positivo a questa condizione.

COUNSELING GENETICO. La sindrome di Marfan, essendo una patologia ereditaria, rende obbligatorio il counseling genetico per il rischio di recidive. Il 15-30% circa dei casi è costituito dai primi individui affetti della loro famiglia. I padri di questi casi sporadici sono, in media, più anziani di 7-10 anni rispetto ai padri della popolazione generale. L'età paterna induce a pensare che questi casi rappresentino nuove mutazioni dominanti con rischi minimi di recidiva per la futura prole dei genitori normali. Pochi casi di mosaicismo gonadico in un genitore fenotipicamente normale richiedono un counseling di un genetista esperto in merito al rischio di recidiva. Tuttavia, ogni figlio di un individuo affetto ha un rischio del 50% di ereditare il cromosoma 15 con la mutazione della sindrome di Marfan e quindi di avere la malattia. Il counseling per il rischio genetico deve essere effettuato da personale che vanti una certa esperienza nei problemi che questa malattia cronica e disabilitante comporta.

American Academy of Pediatrics Committee on Genetics: Health supervision of children with Marfan syndrome. *Pediatrics* 1996;98:978–982.

Boileau C, Jondeau G, Babron M-C, et al: Autosomal dominant Marfan-like connective-tissue disorder with aortic dilation and skeletal anomalies not linked to the fibrillin genes. *Am J Hum Genet* 1993;53:46–54.

Collod G, Babron M-C, Jondeau G, et al: A second locus for Marfan syndrome maps to chromosome 3p24.2-p25. *Nat Genet* 1994;8:264–268.

DePaepe A, Devereux RB, Dietz HC, et al: Revised criteria for Marfan syndrome. *Am J Med Genet* 1996;62;417–426.

Franke U, Furthmayr H: Marfan's syndrome and other disorders of fibrillin. *N Engl J Med* 1994;330:1384–1385.

Gelb BD: Marfan's syndrome and related disorder—more tightly connected than we thought. *N Engl J Med* 2006;355:841–844.

Glesby MJ, Pyeritz RE: Association of mitral valve prolapse and systemic abnormalities of connective tissue: A phenotypic continuum. *JAMA* 1989;262:523–528.

Gross DM, Robinson LK, Smith LT, et al: Severe perinatal Marfan syndrome. *Pediatrics* 1989;84:83–89.

Habashi JP, Judge D, Holm TM, et al: Losartan, an ATI antagonist prevents aortic aneurysm in a mouse model of Marfan syndrome. *Science* 2006; 312:117–121.

Judge DP, Dietz HC: Marfan's syndrome. *Lancet* 2005;366:1965–1976.

Loeys BL, Chen J, Neptune ER, et al: A syndrome of altered cardiovascular, craniofacial, neurocognitive and skeletal development caused by mutations in TGFBR1 or TGFBR2. *Nat Genet* 2005;37:275–281.

Palz M, Tiecke F, Booms P, et al: Clustering of mutation associated with mild Marfan-like phenotypes in the 3′ region of FBN1 suggests a potential genotype phenotype correlation. *Am J Med Genet* 2000;91:212–221.

Pereira L, Levran O, Ramirez F, et al: A molecular approach to stratification of cardiovascular risk in families with Marfan syndrome. *N Engl J Med* 1994;331:148–153.

Rossiter JP, Morales AJ, Repke JT, et al: A prospective longitudinal evaluation of pregnancy in the Marfan syndrome. *Am J Obstet Gynecol* 1995;173:1599–1606.

Shores J, Berger KR, Murphy EA, Pyeritz RE: Progression of aortic dilatation and the benefit of long-term β-adrenergic blockade in Marfan's syndrome. *N Engl J Med* 1994;330:1335–1341.

Tierney ESS, Feingold B, Printz BF, et al: Beta-blocker therapy does not alter the rate of aortic root dilation in pediatric patients with Marfan syndrome. *J Pediatr* 2007;150:77–82.

Sezione 4 — Malattie del metabolismo osseo — Russell W. Chesney

Capitolo 701 ■ Struttura, crescita e regolazione ormonale dell'osso

Vedi anche Capitoli 48 e 571.

L'osso è un organo dinamico soggetto a un rapido turnover, in grado di sopportare il carico e gli stress di varie attività fisiche. Esso si deposita (modellamento) e si riforma (rimodellamento) continuamente. È la principale riserva di calcio, fosforo e magnesio nell'organismo umano. I disordini che alterano quest'organo e il processo di mineralizzazione sono denominati malattie del metabolismo osseo.

Dal momento che la crescita ossea e i tassi di turnover sono elevati nel corso dell'infanzia, molti aspetti clinici di queste patologie sono più marcati nei bambini che negli adulti.

Lo scheletro umano è formato da una matrice proteica, in gran parte composta di una proteina contenente collagene, l'osteoide, sulla quale si deposita una fase minerale cristallina. Anche se l'osteoide contenente collagene costituisce il 90% delle proteine dell'osso, sono presenti altre proteine, tra cui l'osteocalcina, che contiene acido γ-carbossiglutamico. La sintesi dell'osteocalcina dipende dalle vitamine K e D; negli stati caratterizzati da elevato turnover osseo, i valori di osteocalcina sierica sono spesso elevati.

La matrice microfibrillare dell'osteoide permette la deposizione di cristalli di fosfato di calcio altamente organizzati, tra cui idrossiapatite [$Ca_{10}(PO_4)_6 \cdot 6H_2O$] e fosfato ottacalcico [$Ca_8(H_2PO_4)_6 \cdot 5H_2O$], oltre ai meno organizzati fosfato di calcio amorfo, carbonato di calcio, sodio, magnesio e citrato. L'idrossiapatite si trova in profondità nella matrice ossea, mentre il fosfato di calcio amorfo riveste la superficie del tessuto osseo neoformato o rimodellato.

Nel bambino la crescita ossea avviene attraverso il processo di calcificazione delle cellule cartilaginee presenti alle estremità dell'osso. Secondo le concentrazioni di calcio e fosfato prevalenti nel liquido extracellulare, il minerale si deposita nei condrociti destinati alla mineralizzazione. La funzione principale dell'asse endocrino vitamina D-paratormone (PTH) è quella di mantenere le concentrazioni di calcio e fosfato nel liquido extracellulare a livelli tali da permettere la mineralizzazione.

Anche altri ormoni sembrano regolare la crescita e la mineralizzazione della cartilagine, tra cui l'ormone della crescita, che agisce attraverso i fattori di crescita insulino-simili, gli ormoni tiroidei, l'insulina, la leptina, gli androgeni e gli estrogeni durante lo scatto di crescita puberale. Concentrazioni sovrafisiologiche di glucocorticoidi alterano la funzione della cartilagine e la crescita ossea e aumentano il riassorbimento osseo.

L'omeostasi del fosfato è regolata dal rene in quanto il suo assorbimento intestinale è quasi totale ed è l'eliminazione renale a determinarne il livello sierico. Un eccessivo assorbimento intestinale di fosfato causa una riduzione dei livelli sierici di calcio ionizzato e un aumento della secrezione di PTH (che provocano fosfaturia), riducendo pertanto i livelli sierici di fosfato e permettendo l'aumento dei livelli di calcio. L'ipofosfatemia blocca la secrezione di PTH e favorisce la sintesi renale di 1,25-diidrossivitamina D (1,25[OH]$_2$D); quest'ultima promuove anche un maggiore assorbimento intestinale di fosfato.

I tassi di formazione di tessuto osseo sono coordinati con le variazioni del metabolismo minerale sia nell'intestino sia nel rene. Un'inadeguata assunzione con la dieta o un insufficiente assorbimento intestinale di calcio causa una riduzione dei livelli sierici di questo minerale e della sua frazione ionizzata; ciò funge da segnale per la sintesi e la secrezione del PTH, determinando un maggiore riassorbimento osseo per aumentare i livelli sierici di calcio, il riassorbimento di calcio a livello del tubulo distale e la sintesi renale di 1,25-diidrossivitamina D (1,25[OH]$_2$D) o calcitriolo, il metabolita più attivo della vitamina D (Fig. 701-1). In questo modo, l'omeostasi del calcio è controllata a livello intestinale in quanto è la disponibilità di 1,25[OH]$_2$D che da ultimo determina la frazione di calcio ingerita che verrà assorbita.

Il pattern di crescita ossea consiste in un'accelerazione della crescita (lunghezza) degli arti durante la preadolescenza, un aumento della crescita (lunghezza) del tronco (colonna vertebrale) durante la prima fase dell'adolescenza e un aumento della deposizione di minerale osseo nella tarda adolescenza. L'uso dell'assorbimetria a raggi X a energia duale (DEXA, *Dual-Energy X-ray Absorptiometry*) o, meno spesso, della TC quantitativa permette di determinare sia del contenuto minerale sia la densità ossea nei soggetti sani e nei bambini con malattie del metabolismo osseo. La DEXA espone il paziente a una dose di radiazioni inferiore rispetto a una radiografia toracica.

Per valutare le malattie del metabolismo osseo e il rachitismo è necessario conoscere il metabolismo della vitamina D (vedi Fig. 701-1). La cute contiene 7-deidrocolesterolo, convertito a vitamina D_3 dai raggi ultravioletti; durante questo processo vengono prodotti anche altri steroli della vitamina D inattivi (vedi Capitolo 48). La vitamina D_3 viene quindi trasportata in circolo fino al fegato da una proteina legante la vitamina D (DBP, *vitamin D-Binding Protein*); la DBP lega tutte le forme di vitamina D. La concentrazione plasmatica di vitamina D libera o non legata è molto più bassa del livello dei metaboliti della vitamina D legati alla DBP.

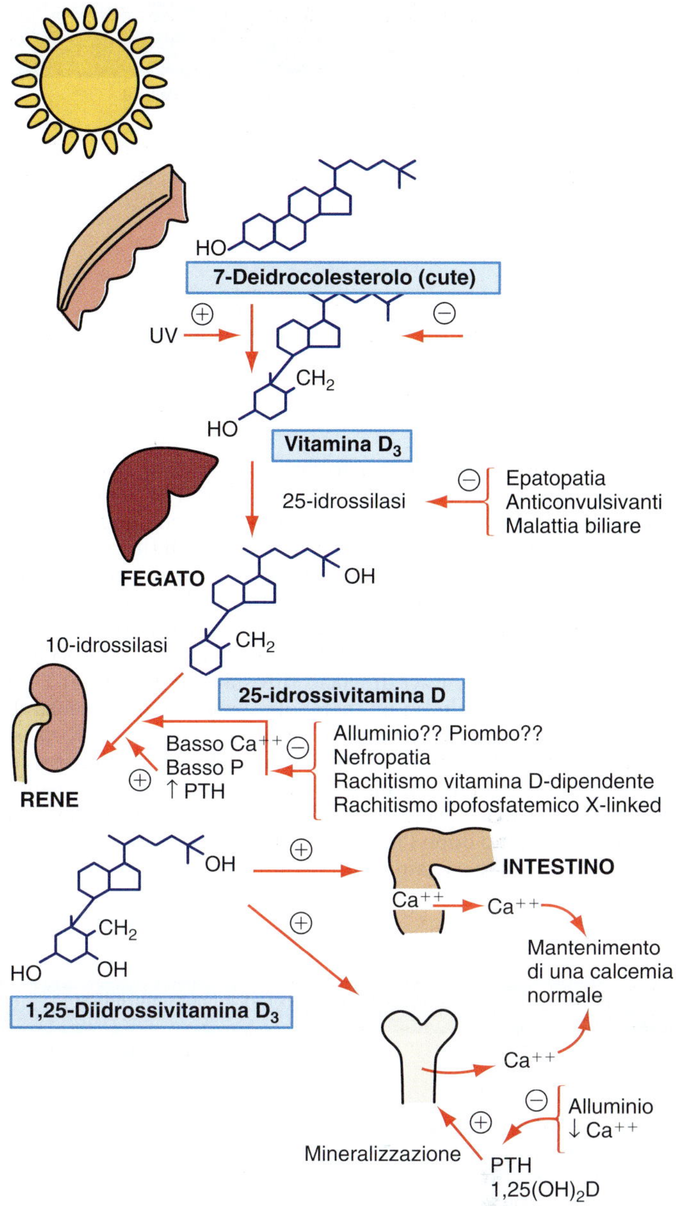

Figura 701-1. Via metabolica della vitamina D, che mostra la sua conversione a 1,25(OH)$_2D_3$ e a 24,25(OH)$_2D_3$. La vitamina D_2 (ergosterolo), di origine vegetale, sembra andare incontro a passaggi metabolici analoghi.

La vitamina D può entrare nella via metabolica anche in seguito all'ingestione di vitamina D_2 (ergocalciferolo) o D_3 (colecalciferolo), che vengono entrambe assorbite a livello intestinale grazie all'azione dei sali biliari. Dopo l'assorbimento, la vitamina D ingerita viene trasportata dai chilomicroni al fegato, dove, insieme alla vitamina D_3 di origine cutanea, è convertita a 25-diidrossivitamina D (25[OH]$_2$D) dall'azione di un enzima microsomiale epatico che richiede ossigeno, NADPH e magnesio per idrossilare la vitamina D in corrispondenza del 25° atomo di carbonio. La 25(OH)D viene quindi trasportata dalla DBP ai reni, dove va incontro a ulteriori tappe metaboliche. La 25(OH)D è il principale metabolita circolante della vitamina D negli esseri umani (Tab. 701-1). Dal momento che la sua sintesi viene scarsamente regolata dal feedback, i suoi livelli plasmatici aumentano in estate e scendono in inverno. Un elevato introito di vitamina D aumenta i livelli plasmatici di 25(OH)D di molte volte rispetto ai valori normali, nonostante lo stesso composto progenitore di vitamina D venga assorbito dal tessuto adiposo.

Nel rene, la 25(OH)D subisce un'ulteriore idrossilazione, a seconda della concentrazione sierica prevalente di calcio, fosfato

TABELLA 701-1. Valori metabolici plasmatici della vitamina D in soggetti sani

METABOLITA	VALORE PLASMATICO
Vitamina D_2	1-2 ng/mL
Vitamina D_3	1-2 ng/mL
$25(OH)D_2$	4-10 ng/mL
$25(OH)D_3$	12-40 ng/mL
25(OH)D totale	15-50 ng/mL
$24,25(OH)_2D$	1-4 ng/mL
$1,25(OH)_2D$	
Prima infanzia	70-100 pg/mL
Seconda infanzia	30-50 pg/mL
Adolescenza	40-80 pg/mL
Età adulta	20-35 pg/mL

e PTH. Se i livelli di calcio o fosfato sono ridotti o se i livelli di PTH sono elevati, si attiva l'enzima 25(OH)D-1-idrossilasi e si forma $1,25(OH)_2D$. Questo metabolita circolante, che corrisponde soltanto allo 0,1% dei livelli di 25(OH)D (vedi Tab. 701-1), agisce sull'intestino aumentando il trasporto attivo di calcio e stimola l'assorbimento di fosfato. Dal momento che la 1α-idrossilasi è un enzima mitocondriale regolato con un feedback rigido, la sintesi di $1,25(OH)_2D$ declina con il ritorno alla normalità dei livelli sierici di calcio o fosfato. Il $1,25(OH)_2D$ in eccesso viene convertito in un metabolita inattivo. In presenza di concentrazioni sieriche normali o elevate di calcio o fosforo, si attiva la 25(OH)D-24-idrossilasi, producendo 24,25-diidrossivitamina D ($24,25[OH]_2D$), una via che permette lo smaltimento della vitamina D in eccesso; i livelli sierici di $24,25(OH)_2D$ (1-5 ng/mL) aumentano dopo l'ingestione di grandi quantità di vitamina D. Anche se l'ipervitaminosi D e la produzione di metaboliti inattivi possono verificarsi dopo la somministrazione per os (vedi Capitolo 48), un'estesa esposizione cutanea alla luce solare non produce solitamente livelli tossici di $25(OH)D_3$, fenomeno che fa pensare a una regolazione naturale della produzione di questo metabolita nel tessuto cutaneo.

I livelli sierici di $1,25(OH)_2D$ sono più elevati nei bambini che negli adulti, non vanno soggetti a variabilità stagionale e raggiungono un picco nel 1° anno di vita e ancora durante lo scatto di crescita puberale. Questi valori devono essere interpretati alla luce dei valori sierici prevalenti di calcio, fosfato e PTH, e rispetto all'intero profilo dei metaboliti della vitamina D.

Il deficit di minerali impedisce il normale processo di deposizione di minerali nel tessuto osseo. Se si verifica un carenza di minerali nella cartilagine di accrescimento, la crescita rallenta e l'età ossea è ritardata, una condizione nota come rachitismo. Una scarsa mineralizzazione dell'osso trabecolare che determina una maggiore percentuale di osteoide non mineralizzato corrisponde all'osteomalacia. Il rachitismo si osserva soltanto nei bambini in crescita prima della fusione delle epifisi, mentre l'osteomalacia è presente a tutte le età. Tutti i pazienti con rachitismo hanno un'osteomalacia, ma non tutti i pazienti con osteomalacia soffrono di rachitismo. Queste condizioni non devono essere confuse con l'osteoporosi, che comporta un'uguale perdita di volume osseo e contenuto minerale (vedi Capitolo 705).

Il rachitismo può essere dovuto a deficit di calcio o di fosfato. Dal momento che sia gli ioni calcio sia gli ioni fosfato costituiscono il minerale osseo, l'insufficienza di uno dei due ioni nel liquido extracellulare che bagna la superficie di mineralizzazione del tessuto osseo determina rachitismo e osteomalacia. I due tipi di rachitismo sono indistinguibili in base alle manifestazioni cliniche (Tab. 701-2). Il rachitismo può verificarsi anche in presenza di un deficit minerale nonostante adeguati depositi di vitamina D. Un vero deficit di calcio della dieta si osserva in alcune aree

TABELLA 701-2. Varianti cliniche del rachitismo e delle condizioni correlate

TIPO	LIVELLI SIERICI DI CALCIO	LIVELLI SIERICI DI FOSFORO	ATTIVITÀ DELLA FOSFATASI ALCALINA	CONCENTRAZIONE URINARIA DI AMINOACIDI	GENETICA	DIFETTO GENICO NOTO
I. Deficit di calcio con iperparatiroidismo secondario (carenza di vitamina D, bassi livelli di 25(OH)D e assenza di stimolazione per livelli più elevati di $1,25(OH)_2D$)						
1. Assenza di vitamina D						
a. Assenza di esposizione alla luce solare	N o B	B	A	A		
b. Carenza dietetica di vitamina D	N o B	B	A	A		
c. Congenita	N o B	B	A	A		
2. Malassorbimento della vitamina D	N o B	B	A	A		
3. Epatopatie	N o B	B	A	A		
4. Farmaci anticonvulsivanti	N o B	B	A	A		
5. Osteodistrofia renale	N o B	B	A	V		
6. Tipo I vitamina D-dipendente	B	N o B	A	A	AR	Sì
II. Deficit primario di fosfato (nessun iperaparatiroidismo secondario)						
1. Ipofosfatemia primitiva genetica	N	B	A	N	XD, AD	Sì
2. Sindrome di Fanconi						
a. Cistinosi	N	B	A	A	AR	Sì
b. Tirosinosi	N	B	A	A	AR	Sì
c. Sindrome di Lowe	N	B	A	A	XR	Sì
d. Acquisita	N	B	A	A		
3. Acidosi tubulare renale prossimale di tipo II	N	B	A	N		Sì
4. Ipofosfatemia oncogena	N	B	A	N		Sì
5. Deficit o malassorbimento di fosfato						
a. Iperalimentazione parenterale	N	B	A	N		
b. Ridotta assunzione di fosfato	N	B	A	N		
III. Resistenza terminale d'organo alla $1,25(OH)_2D_3$						
1. Tipo II vitamina D-dipendente (diverse varianti)	B	B o N	A	A	AR	Sì
IV. Condizioni correlate simili al rachitismo						
1. Ipofosfatasia	N	N	B	Aumento della fosfoetanolamina	AR	Sì
2. Disostosi metafisaria						
a. Tipo di Jansen	A	N	A	N	AD	Sì
b. Tipo di Schmid	N	N	N	N	AD	Sì

A, autosomica; D, dominante; A, aumentato; B, basso; N, normale; R, recessiva; V, variabile; X, X-linked.

dell'Africa mentre è raro in Europa e nell'America settentrionale. Una forma di rachitismo da deficit di fosfato può verificarsi in lattanti che hanno assunto per periodi prolungati sali di alluminio che sequestrano il fosfato come trattamento delle coliche o del reflusso gastroesofageo: ne deriva la sindrome da deplezione di fosfato.

Capitolo 702 ■ Condrodistrofia primaria (displasia metafisaria)

Questa condizione autosomica dominante è caratterizzata da incurvamento delle gambe, bassa statura e un'andatura anserina che compaiono in assenza di anomalie di calcemia, fosfatemia, attività della fosfatasi alcalina o dei metaboliti della vitamina D. Nella condrodisplasia metafisaria (*tipo di Jansen*) si osservano metafisi a coppa e di aspetto "consumato", che nel tempo sviluppano calcificazioni di tipo marmorizzato alle estremità distali dell'osso. Può essere presente ipercalcemia, con valori sierici di 13-15 mg/mL. Anche la colonna può presentare deformazioni, dovute alla crescita irregolare delle vertebre. Per quanto riguarda la causa molecolare di questa sindrome, sono state identificate tre diverse mutazioni del recettore del paratormone di tipo I, oltre ad alcuni geni a valle che possono contribuire alla patogenesi. Il *tipo di Schmid* è meno severo, anche se l'aspetto radiografico delle ginocchia e l'estremo incurvamento degli arti inferiori ricordano i segni clinici osservati nei pazienti con ipofosfatemia familiare. In questa forma si riscontrano difetti del collagene di tipo X e le anomalie delle anche sono più debilitanti che nella condrodisplasia metafisaria di Jansen. I pazienti con entrambi i tipi di condrodisplasia metafisaria hanno bassa statura per tutta la vita.

La disostosi metafisaria, o *malattia di Pyle*, deriva da difetti dell'ossificazione encondrale e del rimodellamento metafisario. Le estremità delle ossa lunghe sono allargate, nella tipica configurazione "a fiasco di Erlenmeyer". La bassa statura non è necessariamente caratteristica e i livelli sierici di minerali sono normali. Spesso si sviluppa una facies leonina se sono interessate le ossa facciali. La disostosi metafisaria può essere un aspetto clinico della sindrome di Shwachman-Diamond, un raro disordine autosomico recessivo caratterizzato da neutropenia, insufficienza esocrina pancreatica, disfunzione del midollo osseo e talvolta complicanze ematologiche severe (vedi Capitolo 448). Come approccio terapeutico è stato utilizzato il trapianto allogenico di midollo, che però ha dato risultati variabili.

Allo stato attuale non sono disponibili altre forme di trattamento realmente efficaci per le condrodistrofie o la disostosi.

Capitolo 703 ■ Ipofosfatasia

L'ipofosfatasia è un disordine autosomico recessivo che dà luogo a reperti radiografici simili a quelli del rachitismo ed è causato da una ridotta attività sierica della fosfatasi alcalina. È un errore congenito del metabolismo consistente in un deficit dell'attività dell'isoenzima della fosfatasi alcalina aspecifica (fegato/osso/rene) (TNSALP, *Tissue Non-Specific ALkaline Phosphatase*), a fronte di un'attività normale degli isoenzimi intestinale e placentare. Singole mutazioni puntiformi del gene impediscono l'espressione dell'attività di questo enzima *in vitro* e ne indicano la necessità per una normale mineralizzazione dello scheletro. Delle 100 mutazioni del gene finora identificate una notevole percentuale è rappresentata da mutazioni nonsenso, nonostante siano state osservate anche mutazioni *splice-site*, piccole delezioni e mutazioni *frame-shift*. L'unico fenotipo associato è l'ipofosfatasia. Alcuni pazienti possono avere un deficit di regolazione di questo enzima anziché una mutazione.

Per quanto riguarda la gravità della malattia, si riscontra una certa eterogeneità. Alcuni casi si manifestano alla nascita e la diagnosi può essere posta già in utero grazie all'esame radiografico del feto. La patologia può manifestarsi in forma neonatale o perinatale letale (ipofosfatasia letale congenita), in una forma infantile severa o in una forma più lieve tipica dell'infanzia o della tarda adolescenza (ipofosfatasia tarda). La forma letale è caratterizzata da un aspetto "tarlato" delle estremità delle ossa lunghe, da un deficit severo dell'ossificazione in tutto lo scheletro e da marcato accorciamento delle ossa lunghe. I pazienti con malattia lieve possono presentare incurvamento delle gambe e bassa statura di grado variabile. L'ipercalcemia è comune nelle forme neonatali e infantili, e dal momento che non si verifica accumulo di calcio da parte dei condrociti maturi, i pazienti possono sembrare affetti da rachitismo.

Manifestazioni cliniche insolite comprendono ossa wormiane nella volta cranica, scarsa calcificazione delle ossa frontali, parietali e occipitali e perdita prematura dei denti decidui o permanenti, a causa dell'ipoplasia del cemento dentale. Nella forma infantile si osserva anche nefrocalcinosi, dovuta all'ipercalcemia; altre sue caratteristiche sono dolore osseo, frequenti fratture, lievi deformità scheletriche e la perdita prematura dei denti. Il difetto metafisario consiste in ossificazione irregolare, aree con deficit a stampo e *cupping* metafisario.

Nell'ipofosfatasia, si ritrovano grandi quantità di fosfoetanolamina nelle urine in quanto questa sostanza non può essere degradata in assenza di attività TNSALP. Per lo stesso motivo risultano aumentati anche i livelli plasmatici di pirofosfato inorganico e di piridossal-5-fosfato (PLP). I livelli di PLP sono utili nella diagnosi differenziale dell'ipofosfatasia, in quanto tendono a essere più bassi del normale nella maggior parte delle altre malattie ossee. Le convulsioni nei pazienti con le forme letale e infantile possono essere correlate a un deficit del metabolismo della piridossina. Sebbene non sia stata ancora messa a punto una terapia risolutiva, l'infusione di plasma ricco di fosfatasi alcalina si è rivelata utile a promuovere la guarigione dell'osso in studi a breve termine. Il trapianto di midollo osseo si è dimostrato efficace utilizzando donatori con valori normali di TNSALP. Il decorso clinico di questa patologia spesso migliora spontaneamente con la crescita del bambino, anche se nella forma infantile si può verificare una morte precoce da insufficienza renale o disordini del movimento toracico (*flail chest*) con evoluzione in polmonite. Quei pochi pazienti che si presentano con pattern clinici e radiografici identici hanno un'attività della fosfatasi alcalina sierica normale. La loro malattia, denominata *pseudoipofosfatasia*, può dipendere dalla presenza di un isoenzima mutante della fosfatasi alcalina che reagisce con substrati artificiali in ambiente alcalino (in provetta) ma non con substrati naturali *in vivo*.

Capitolo 704 ■ Iperfosfatasia

L'iperfosfatasia è caratterizzata da un aumento eccessivo dell'isoenzima osseo della fosfatasi alcalina nel siero e un significativo ritardo di crescita. La proliferazione osteoide nella parte sottoperiostea dell'osso determina la separazione del periostio dalla corticale. Sono comuni incurvamento e ispessimento delle diafisi, insieme a osteopenia. La malattia di solito esordisce entro i 2-3 anni di vita, quando una deformità dolorosa delle estremità causa deambulazione anomala e talvolta fratture. Altri aspetti comuni comprendono pectus carinatum, cifoscoliosi e logoramento delle coste. Il cranio è grande e le ossa che lo compongono sono ispessite (allargamento della diploe) e talvolta deformate. L'interessamento cranico può portare a ipoacusia progressiva e profonda. Radiograficamente, la texture ossea è variabile: aree radiopache contraddistinte da un aspetto a batuffolo di lana pettinata-cotone sono frammiste ad aree radiotrasparenti e di demineralizzazione generalizzata. Le ossa lunghe appaiono cilindriche, perdono il modellamento delle metafisi e contengono pseudocisti con un alone osseo denso.

In questo disordine autosomico recessivo i livelli sierici di calcio e fosfato sono normali, mentre l'attività urinaria della peptidasi dell'aminoacido leucina e i livelli sierici di fosfatasi acida sono aumentati. Si tratta di una patologia spesso chiamata *malattia di Paget giovanile*, in quanto, come nella malattia di Paget a esordio in età adulta, la calcitonina può ridurre il rapido turnover osseo osservato in questo disordine; nel bambino, il disordine è più generalizzato e simmetrico. La forma cosiddetta giovanile si distingue dalla malattia di Paget classica in quanto l'istologia ossea denota la perdita del normale rimodellamento dell'osso corticale e l'assenza del classico pattern a mosaico di osso lamellare riscontrabile nella patologia dell'adulto. Pertanto, l'espressione "malattia di Paget giovanile" non è corretta. È stato riportato un caso in cui una terapia intensiva con bifosfonato (ibandronato) per via endovenosa, somministrato in un periodo di 3 anni, ha arrestato la progressione dell'iperfosfatasia idiopatica, prevenendo la deformità e la disabilità e migliorando la situazione uditiva.

L'*iperfosfatasia transitoria* si verifica tra i 2 mesi e i 2 anni di età, non ha manifestazioni associate, a parte alcuni lievi sintomi gastrointestinali, e si riscontra di solito nel corso di indagini di laboratorio di routine (screening) per altri disturbi non correlati. Sono aumentate sia la frazione isoenzimatica epatica sia quella epatica; non vi sono altre manifestazioni di disfunzione epatica o ossea. La causa è sconosciuta. La risoluzione avviene di solito nel giro di 4-6 mesi.

L'*iperfosfatemia familiare*, un disordine autosomico dominante, è un'altra condizione benigna che si distingue dalla forma transitoria infantile per l'aumento persistente e asintomatico dei livelli sierici di fosfatasi alcalina.

Una variante autosomica dominante più severa, l'*iperplasia scheletrica espansile* è caratterizzata da sordità a esordio precoce, perdita prematura dei denti, progressivo allargamento iperostosico delle ossa lunghe con dolore a carico delle falangi delle mani, ipercalcemia episodica e aumento del rimodellamento osseo. È rilevante un difetto del gene che codifica l'attivazione del recettore per il fattore nucleare γB (NF-γB). Questo gene sembra essere necessario per l'osteogenesi e il difetto causa un aumento dell'attività di NF-γB nello scheletro.

Capitolo 705 ■ Osteoporosi

L'osteoporosi è il più comune disordine osseo dell'adulto, ma è relativamente infrequente nel bambino. In questa condizione alla diminuzione del volume osseo fa riscontro un'incidenza di fratture molto aumentata. Al contrario dell'osteomalacia, che consiste in una scarsa mineralizzazione a fronte di un volume osseo normale, le sezioni istologiche in tutte le forme di osteoporosi rivelano un grado normale di mineralizzazione ma una riduzione del volume osseo, specialmente di osso trabecolare (osso vertebrale). Per definizione, l'osteoporosi è caratterizzata anche da una ridotta quantità di tessuto osseo (denominata osteopenia), che si associa a fratture non traumatiche (patologiche). L'osteoporosi infantile può essere primitiva o secondaria (Tab. 705-1). Le forme primitive possono essere ulteriormente suddivise in disordini ereditari del tessuto connettivo, tra cui osteogenesi imperfetta, sindrome di Bruck, sindrome osteoporosi-pseudoglioma, sindrome di Ehlers-Danlos, sindrome di Marfan, omocistinuria e osteoporosi idiopatica giovanile. Le forme secondarie di osteoporosi comprendono vari disordini neuromuscolari, malattie croniche, squilibri endocrini ed errori del metabolismo congeniti oppure indotti da farmaci, comprese l'intolleranza proteica lisinurica e la malattia di Gaucher.

TABELLA 705-1. Rischi di osteoporosi

DISORDINI ENDOCRINI
Ipogonadismo femminile
Sindrome di Turner
Amenorrea ipotalamica (triade della donna atleta)
Anoressia nervosa
Insufficienza ovarica prematura e primitiva
Terapia con medrossiprogesterone acetato depot
Recettore α degli estrogeni; mutazioni
Iperprolattinemia
Ipogonadismo maschile
Insufficienza gonadica primitiva (sindrome di Klinefelter)
Insufficienza gonadica secondaria (ipogonadismo ipogonadotropo idiopatico)
Pubertà ritardata
Ipertiroidismo
Iperparatiroidismo
Ipercortisolismo (terapeutico o morbo di Cushing)
Deficit di ormone della crescita
DISORDINI GASTROINTESTINALI
Sindromi da malassorbimento (fibrosi cistica, celiachia)
Malattia infiammatoria intestinale
Ittero ostruttivo cronico
Cirrosi biliare primitiva e altre cirrosi
Alattasia
Gastrectomia subtotale
DISORDINI DEL MIDOLLO OSSEO
Trapianto di midollo osseo
Linfoma
Leucemia
Anemie emolitiche (anemia a cellule falciformi, talassemia)
Mastocitosi sistemica
DISORDINI DEL TESSUTO CONNETTIVO/OSSEO
Osteoporosi giovanile
Osteogenesi imperfetta
Sindrome di Ehlers-Danlos
Sindrome di Marfan
Omocistinuria
Displasia fibrosa
Pregresse o ricorrenti fratture a basso impatto
FARMACI
Alcol
Eparina
Glucocorticoidi
Tiroxina
Anticonvulsivanti
Agonisti dell'ormone di rilascio della gonadotropina
Ciclosporina
Chemioterapia
Fumo di sigaretta
DISORDINI VARI
Immobilizzazione (paralisi cerebrale, atrofia muscolare spinale)
Artrite reumatoide
Nefropatie
Triade della donna atleta
Scarsa assunzione di calcio con la dieta
Malattia di Gaucher

Quando non è possibile identificare alcuna causa evidente, né primitiva né secondaria, occorre prendere in considerazione l'*osteoporosi idiopatica giovanile*, specialmente in presenza delle seguenti caratteristiche cliniche: esordio prima della pubertà, dolore a carico delle ossa lunghe e della regione lombare, fratture vertebrali, fratture delle ossa lunghe e dei metatarsi, un aspetto slavato della colonna e dello scheletro degli arti e un miglioramento dopo la pubertà. Le ossa trabecolari come quelle della colonna e i metatarsi vanno particolarmente soggetti a fratture atraumatiche.

In generale, i valori ematici di minerali, metaboliti della vitamina D, fosfatasi alcalina e paratormone sono normali. La valutazione del contenuto minerale osseo e della densità ossea mediante assorbimetria a raggi X a energia duale (DEXA, *Dual-*

Energy X-ray Absorptiometry) o, meno spesso, con TC quantitativa produce valori marcatamente ridotti. Sono state utilizzate con un certo successo diverse modalità terapeutiche (tra cui supplementi di calcio per os, calcitriolo, bifosfonati e calcitonina) in condizioni individuali, ma è difficile giudicare l'effetto di questi trattamenti in quanto si può avere guarigione spontanea dopo l'esordio della pubertà in >75% dei casi.

L'*osteoporosi-pseudoglioma* è un disordine autosomico-recessivo che si manifesta con età variabile all'esordio, riduzione della massa ossea, fratture durante l'infanzia e anormale sviluppo oculare; il gene difettoso è stato mappato sul cromosoma 11q12-13. La mutazione rappresenta una perdita funzionale del gene per la proteina 5 correlata al recettore delle lipoproteine a bassa densità. È interessante notare come mutazioni con guadagno funzionale risultino in un prodotto genico che aumenta la densità ossea.

Occorre sottolineare le implicazioni che una demineralizzazione significativa o l'osteoporosi infantile hanno sul ciclo vitale. Gli eventi durante l'infanzia influenzano il picco di massa ossea e la tarda adolescenza è un periodo in cui si assiste a un rapido accumulo di minerale osseo. Inoltre, anche se il picco di massa ossea viene raggiunto entro i 20-35 anni di età (a seconda dell'osso in cui viene misurato), il contributo durante l'infanzia è considerevole. È stato dimostrato che diversi valori incidono sulla massa ossea: vitamina D (400-800 UI al giorno), assunzione di calcio (>1200 mg/die negli adolescenti) e attività fisica che comporti un carico nel corso dell'infanzia. L'attività fisica comportante aumenta la formazione di tessuto osseo e ne riduce il riassorbimento. Un altro fattore che può impedire alla massa ossea di raggiungere il picco è il consumo di alcol e tabacco. Eccellenti fonti di calcio alimentare sono soprattutto il latte e i derivati del latte, ma anche il pesce con le spine, i vegetali a foglia verde e le bevande con supplemento di calcio (succo d'arancia). Agli individui con deficit di lattasi si possono somministrare yogurt e formaggio. Dal momento che l'osteoporosi a esordio in età adulta sembra derivare da diversi fattori genetici, che formano in tal modo una complessa interazione su basi genetiche, non sono disponibili interventi specifici durante l'infanzia in grado di influire sulla massa ossea.

Il trattamento dell'osteoporosi secondaria consiste soprattutto nel trattamento del disordine sottostante, quando possibile. L'ipogonadismo deve essere trattato con terapia ormonale sostitutiva, specialmente nelle donne magre e atletiche. L'assunzione di calcio deve essere aumentata a 1500-2000 mg/die. Nell'osteoporosi indotta da glucocorticoidi, è fondamentale sottolineare l'importanza di usare la più bassa dose possibile per prevenire l'attività della malattia (malattia intestinale infiammatoria) con una terapia a giorni alterni o con un'applicazione topica, e con l'uso di glucocorticoidi per via inalatoria nell'asma. Sono appropriate anche diete speciali per gli errori congeniti del metabolismo. La celiachia, che può essere molto diffusa negli adulti con osteoporosi, deve essere ricercata e trattata in modo corretto (vedi Capitolo 335.8). Si è dimostrato efficace il trattamento con bifosfonati, che inibiscono il riassorbimento osseo di certi casi di osteoporosi secondaria (indotta da glucocorticoidi) e con esordio nell'età adulta. La terapia con bifosfonati è utile anche nell'osteogenesi imperfetta e nella paralisi cerebrale.

Beier F, LuValle P: The cyclin D1 and cyclin A genes are targets of activated PTH/PTHrP receptor in Jansen's metaphyseal chondrodysplasia. *Mol Endocrinol* 2002;16:2163–2173.

Birch K: Female athlete triad. *Br Med J* 2005;330:244–246.

Boyden LM, Mao J, Belsky J, et al: High bone density due to a mutation in LDL-receptor related protein 5. *N Engl J Med* 2002;346:1513–1521.

Cundy T, Wheadon L, King A: Treatment of idiopathic hyperphosphatasia with intensive bisphosphonate therapy. *J Bone Miner Res* 2004;19:703–711.

Fewtrell MS: Bone densitometry in children assessed by dual x ray absorptiometry: Uses and pitfalls. *Arch Dis Child* 2003;88:795–798.

Gordon CM, Bachrach LK, Carpenter TO: Bone health in children and adolescents. *Curr Prob Pediatr Adolesc Health Care* 2004;34:221–248.

Hsu JW, Vogelsang G, Jones RJ, Brodsky RA: Bone marrow transplantation in Shwachman-Diamond syndrome. *Bone Marrow Transplant* 2002;30: 255–258.

Ioannidis JPA, Ralston SH, Bennett ST, et al: Differential genetic effects of *ESR1* gene polymorphisms on osteoporosis outcomes. *JAMA* 2004;292: 2105–2114.

Jonsson KB, Zahradnik R, Larsson T, et al: Fibroblast growth factor 23 in oncogenic osteomalacia and X-linked hypophosphatemia. *N Engl J Med* 2003;348:1656–1663.

Kholsa S: Parathyroid hormone plus alendronate—a combination that does not add up. *N Engl J Med* 2003;349:1277–1279.

Loud KJ, Gordon CM: Adolescent bone health. *Arch Pediatr Adolesc Med* 2006;160:1026–1032.

Mumm S, Jones J, Finnegan P, Whyte MP: Hypophosphatasia: Molecular diagnosis of Rathbun's original case. *J Bone Miner Res* 2001;16:1724–1727.

Scholes D, LaCroix AZ, Ichikawa LE, et al: Change in bone mineral density among adolescent women using and discontinuing depot medroxyprogesterone acetate contraception. *Arch Pediatr Adolesc Med* 2005;159: 139–144.

Solomon CG: Bisphosphonates and osteoporosis. *N Engl J Med* 2002; 346:642.

Stenson WF, Newberry R, Lorenz R, et al: Increased prevalence of celiac disease and need for routine screening among patients with osteoporosis. *Arch Intern Med* 2005;165:393–399.

Van der Sluis IM, de Ridder MAJ, Boot AM, et al: Reference data for bone density and body composition measured with dual energy x-ray absorptiometry in white children and young adults. *Arch Dis Child* 2002;87: 341–347.

Whyte MP, Hughes AE: Expansile skeletal hyperphosphatasia is caused by a 15-base pair tandem duplication in TNFRSF11A encoding RANK and is allelic to familial expansile osteolysis. *J Bone Miner Res* 2002;17:26–29.

Whyte MP, Wenkert D, Clements KL, et al: Bisphosphonate-induced osteopetrosis. *N Engl J Med* 2003;349:457–463.

Parte XXXII ▪ Rischi ambientali per la salute

Capitolo 706 ▪ Effetti biologici delle radiazioni nei bambini Thomas L. Slovis

PRINCIPI DI BASE

L'esposizione a radiazioni può essere naturale o ambientale (prodotta dall'uomo). Negli Stati Uniti la maggior parte delle radiazioni ambientali proviene dal gas radon (55%); i raggi cosmici e altri radionuclidi terrestri primordiali contribuiscono per un ulteriore 16%. Per il 28% delle radiazioni prodotte dall'uomo, le procedure mediche costituiscono la componente principale (15%). Alcune procedure di imaging tuttavia non causano radiazioni (Tab. 706-1) e non tutte le modalità che fanno uso di radiazioni ne espongono il bambino alla stessa quantità (Tab. 706-2).

Le indagini di medicina nucleare e la tomografia a emissione di positroni sono descritte in base alla quantità di radioattività iniettata. Le unità di dose assorbita, secondo la definizione della International Commission of Radiation Units, sono il **rad**, introdotto negli anni '60, e il **gray** (Gy), introdotto nel 1985. In radioprotezione si utilizzano le quantità *dose equivalente* e *dose efficace*, la cui vecchia unità è il **rem**, mentre la nuova è il **sievert** (Sv) (Tab. 706-3). Non tutte le radiazioni possiedono gli stessi effetti sul tessuto biologico a parità di dose: le particelle alfa e i protoni determinano un danno significativamente maggiore rispetto alle radiazioni γ (raggi X). Nell'imaging diagnostico si utilizzano raggi X. Ogni dose presenta un modificatore, per es. dose cutanea, dose corporea, dose d'organo o dose efficace. La **dose efficace** tiene conto dei tessuti specifici e della loro radiosensibilità.

EFFETTI BIOLOGICI DELLE RADIAZIONI

Gli effetti biologici delle radiazioni sono suddivisi in due tipi. Gli **effetti deterministici** sono caratterizzati da una dose soglia; per esempio, la cataratta non compare dopo un'esposizione acuta inferiore a 200 rad o nell'esposizione cronica inferiore a 500 rad (Tab. 706-4). Non sono stati riportati effetti deterministici dovuti alle dosi generalmente utilizzate in radiodiagnostica, sebbene le procedure invasive più recenti abbiano portato a maggiori effetti cutanei. Gli **effetti stocastici** (casuali) sono invece più preoccupanti, perché si possono verificare a qualunque dose; in altre parole, non esiste una dose soglia e la probabilità di un effetto cresce

TABELLA 706-1. Modalità di imaging

MODALITÀ	SORGENTE
Radiografia diretta	Radiazioni (raggi X)
Ecografia	Fasci di ultrasuoni
Tomografia computerizzata	Radiazioni (raggi X)
Risonanza magnetica	Campo magnetico
Medicina nucleare	Radiazioni (isotopo iniettato)
Tomografia a emissione di positroni	Radiazioni (isotopo iniettato)

TABELLA 706-2. Dose di radiazioni per varie tecniche di imaging

ESAME	mrad o mrem	SITO DI MISURAZIONE
Torace: 2 proiezioni	10-20	Entrata (cute)
Addome: 2 proiezioni	50-100	Entrata (cute)
Fluoroscopia		
Non pulsata	300-500/min	Entrata (cute)
Pulsata	100-150/min	Entrata (cute)
Tomografia computerizzata†		
Cranio	6000 (2000-3000)	Diametro medio del phantom di 16 cm
Addome	3000 (1000)	Diametro medio del phantom di 32 cm
Medicina nucleare‡ (^{99m}TcMAG3-renale)	120	Dose efficace
Tomografia a emissione di positroni‡ (BDG cerebrale)	185	Dose efficace, corpo intero

*La radiazione di fondo è di circa 1 mrad/die (300 mrad/anno).
†Scansione spiegata come TC dose index (TCDI). La prima dose è in caso di fattori per adulto; la seconda tra parentesi è l'esame aggiustato per i bambini.
‡Espressa come dose efficace. Si tratta di linee guida approssimative per la dose somministrata a un soggetto di 5 anni con normale funzione renale.
FDG, (F-18) fluoro-2-desossiglucosio; ^{99m}TcMAG3, ^{99m}tecnezio mercaptoacetiltriglicina.
Da Valentin J: Radiation dose to patients from radiopharmaceuticals: (Addendum 2 to ICRP Publication 53) ICRP Publication 80 Approved by the Commission in September 1997. *Ann ICRP* 1998; 28:1.

TABELLA 706-3. Unità di misura delle radiazioni

UNITÀ	RADIOATTIVITÀ	DOSE ASSORBITA	DOSE EQUIVALENTE	ESPOSIZIONE
Unità comuni	curie (Ci)	rad	rem	roentgen (R)
Unità recenti	becquerel (Bq)	gray (Gy)	sievert (Sv)	coulomb/kg

EQUIVALENTI DI CONVERSIONE

1 millicurie (mCi)	= 37 megabecquerel (MBq)*
100 rad	= 1 Gy
1 rad	= 1 cGy
100 rem	= 1 Sv
1 rem	= 10 mSv

La dose di fondo è di circa 1 millirad/die

*Per convertire mBq a mSv, usare la tabella di conversione:
1 mrad = millirad = 1/1000 di rad.
*rem = rad × fattore di radiazione; pesando per raggi γ e raggi X questo fattore è 1.
rem = rad × 1.

TABELLA 706-4. Tassi di dose deterministica

DANNO	SOGLIA APPROSSIMATIVA
Cute	
Eritema transitorio	200 rad (2 Gy)
Desquamazione secca	1000 rad (10 Gy)
Desquamazione umida	1500 rad (15 Gy)
Epilazione temporanea	200 rad (2 Gy)
Epilazione permanente	700 rad (7 Gy)
Occhi	
Cataratta	>200 rad (2 Gy)

Modificata da Hall EJ: *Radiobiology for the Radiologist*, 5th ed. Philadelphia, Lippincott Williams & Wilkins, 2000.

con l'aumentare della dose. Questi effetti possono essere originati da una qualunque radiazione che colpisca tessuti vulnerabili (soprattutto il DNA, ma anche il citoplasma può essere a rischio) e provochi un danno irreversibile. Essi portano al modello della **linear no dose threshold** (LNT), secondo il quale il danno da radiazioni si amplifica in modo lineare con l'aumento della dose. Tale modello sottolinea anche che nessun livello di esposizione a radiazioni può essere considerato sicuro in modo assoluto.

Le radiazioni possono dare origine a mutazioni genetiche, carcinogenesi e morte cellulare. Gli effetti biologici sono dovuti principalmente al danno immediato al DNA attraverso l'interazione degli elettroni fast recoil dovuta all'assorbimento di raggi X (1/3 del danno) oppure secondario alla formazione di radicali liberi. Dato che circa l'80% della cellula è costituito di acqua, la maggior parte dell'energia ivi depositata determina la produzione di radicali liberi dell'acqua. Le reazioni sono rapide (da 10^{-18} a 10^{-3} secondi). Una dose di 1 rad determina circa 10^{3} ionizzazioni per tipo cellulare. Le alterazioni biochimiche e fisiologiche che seguono richiedono ore o giorni, mentre l'induzione del tumore necessita di molti anni.

Le manifestazioni del danno del DNA sono variabili. La cellula che contiene il DNA danneggiato può morire; la morte cellulare (apoptosi) è del resto un meccanismo per eliminare le cellule gravemente danneggiate e potenzialmente mutabili. Il danno a un paio di basi è l'effetto più prevalente e meno significativo. Sebbene le rotture di un singolo filamento di DNA di solito abbiano scarsa importanza biologica, in quanto i filamenti vengono riparati tramite il filamento opposto come stampo, se la riparazione avviene in modo errato può comparire una mutazione.

La rottura di entrambi i filamenti (l'evento meno comune) è più problematica. Il risultato finale sembra dipendere dalla vicinanza della rottura in ciascun filamento. Se le rotture sono molto distanti, le riparazioni avvengono come nel caso di quelle di un filamento singolo, ma se invece sono opposte l'una all'altra (oppure sono separate soltanto da poche paia di basi), la riparazione è più difficile senza uno stampo. Questo tipo di rottura è il meccanismo dell'uccisione cellulare, del danno cromosomico, delle mutazioni e della carcinogenesi indotti da radiazioni.

In caso di danno del DNA, si producono aberrazioni cromosomiche, con una conseguente *aberrazione instabile* (di solito letale per le cellule in fase di divisione) o *aberrazione stabile*. Quest'ultima può portare a una mancata riunione dei cromosomi (che genera delezioni) oppure essi si possono riarrangiare in modo anomalo, come una traslocazione reciproca o un'aneuploidia. Sebbene sia logico pensare che tali anomalie determinino poi mutazioni che possono attivare oncogeni o proto-oncogeni o originare mutazioni in geni soppressori tumorali (vedi Capitolo 492), pochi tumori radioindotti mostrano in realtà traslocazioni specifiche che sarebbero associate all'attivazione di specifici oncogeni o geni soppressori tumorali noti. Un'eccezione è il carcinoma papillare della tiroide indotto da radiazioni, che probabilmente è dovuto all'attivazione dell'oncogene RET (vedi Capitolo 506).

La **carcinogenesi da radiazioni** sembra essere un processo multifasico progressivo costituito da tre stadi indipendenti: alterazioni morfologiche, immortalità cellulare e tumorigenicità. L'esposizione a radiazioni induce un'instabilità genomica cellulare, che viene trasmessa alla progenie della cellula con un conseguente continuo aumento del tasso di sviluppo di alterazioni genetiche nelle generazioni successive della cellula irradiata (Fig. 706-1).

Uno studio longitudinale sul rischio in vita di sviluppare un cancro in eccesso da irradiazione ha preso in considerazione alcuni sopravvissuti alla bomba atomica, seguendo oltre 86 000 di essi per oltre 50 anni dall'esposizione. Le dosi delle radiazioni individuali furono stimate considerando la localizzazione della persona in relazione alla distanza dall'epicentro e le condizioni di protezione. La maggior parte dell'esposizione proveniva da radiazioni γ dirette, con una certa percentuale derivata da neutroni. L'età al momento dell'esposizione influenza la sensibilità ai tumori indotti da radiazioni (Fig. 706-2). Rispetto agli adulti di età media, i bambini hanno una sensibilità a carcinogenesi radioindotta di 10 volte superiore e i neonati più giovani risultano maggiormente sensibili rispetto ai bambini più grandi. A causa dei maggiori rischi associati al carcinoma mammario e tiroideo, le femmine appaiono più sensibili rispetto ai maschi.

Le dosi utilizzate in radiodiagnostica per le scansioni TC multislice coincidono in parte con le basse dosi assorbite dai sopravvissuti alla bomba atomica che hanno poi sviluppato un carcinoma (Fig. 706-3). È stato stimato che il rischio nel corso della vita di un tumore in seguito a TC del cranio e dell'addome nei bambini è di 1:1000. L'avvento dei sistemi di comunicazione per l'archiviazione delle immagini digitali (*Picture Archiving Communication Systems*, PACS) può rendere impossibile determinare se il paziente abbia ricevuto la dose di radiazioni "più bassa possibile" (*As Low As Reasonably Achievable*, ALARA).

Un'**aumentata vulnerabilità biologica** è osservata nel feto esposto in utero a radiazioni dirette alla madre. I risultati di uno studio caso controllo condotto a metà degli anni '90 che confrontava la frequenza dell'esposizione intrauterina alle radiazioni nei bambini deceduti per tumore maligno infantile con quella di bambini morti per altre cause misero in evidenza che l'irradiazione in utero era associata a un rischio di morte da leucemia più alto del 92% prima dell'età di 10 anni e da altre malattie maligne incrementato del 180%. Anche un follow-up condotto a distanza di 20 anni riscontrò un aumento del rischio relativo (1,38) di tumore nell'infanzia associato all'irradiazione in utero.

Il feto e i bambini piccoli sono più vulnerabili al tumore da radiazioni perché: (1) stanno crescendo rapidamente, con molte cellule in attività mitotica; (2) questi tumori, a eccezione della leucemia, necessitano di molto tempo per svilupparsi e i bambini hanno davanti a sé una vita più lunga; (3) l'effetto cumulativo delle radiazioni dura per tutta la vita.

La maggior parte dei tumori infantili insorge in modo sporadico, ma il 10-15% dei casi presenta una forte componente familiare. Le malattie che sono associate alla sensibilità alle radiazioni sono elencate nella Tabella 706-5.

RIDUZIONE DELLE RADIAZIONI DIAGNOSTICHE NON NECESSARIE NEI BAMBINI OTTENENDO ANCORA IMMAGINI DIAGNOSTICHE: UNA DOPPIA RESPONSABILITÀ

La scelta dell'esame appropriato è una responsabilità del medico prescrivente e può comportare la consultazione con il radiologo pediatra. Organizzazioni come l'American College of Radiology possiedono linee guida radiologiche basate sull'evidenza. La medicina basata sull'evidenza ha mostrato una scarsa resa dell'inquadramento radiologico (inclusa la TC) di un bambino con un singolo episodio convulsivo senza altre anomalie neurologiche. Ciò si verifica in maniera particolare in assenza di un'anamnesi precedente di comportamento o personalità anormali o di alterazioni dello sviluppo. La TC non identifica tante anomalie come la RM e in più comporta l'uso di radiazioni. La RM individua inoltre molto più facilmente subdole alterazioni di anomalie congenite o acquisite. Pertanto, **a eccezione** di una situazione di urgenza, è appropriato realizzare la RM entro un periodo di tempo ragionevole, anziché effettuare due esami (TC seguita da RM).

TABELLA 706-5. Sindromi ereditarie nell'uomo associate a sensibilità ai raggi X

Atassia-teleangiectasia
Sindrome da nevoide basocellulare
Sindrome di Cockayne
Sindrome di Down
Anemia di Fanconi
Sindrome di Gardner
Sindrome da rottura di Nijmegan
Sindrome di Usher

Modificata da Slovis TL, Berdon WE, Hall EJ: The effects of radiation on children. In Kuhn JP, Slovis TL, Haller JO (editors): Caffey's *Pediatric Diagnostic Imaging*, 10th ed. Philadelphia, Mosby, 2003, pp 1-13; e Hall EJ: *Radiobiology for the Radiologist*, 5th ed. Philadelphia, Lippincott Williams & Wilkins, 2000, p 45.

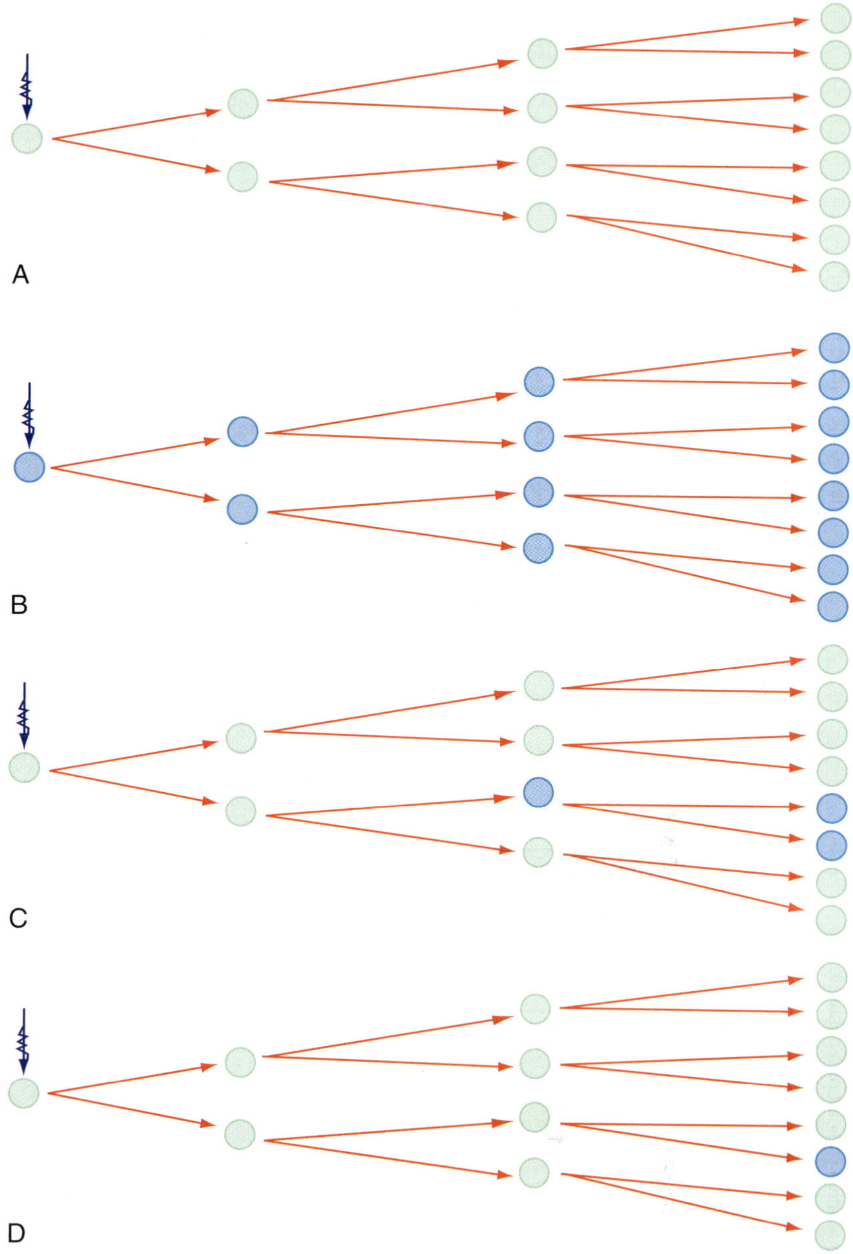

Figura 706-1. Schema della mutagenesi indotta da radiazioni. I *cerchi vuoti* rappresentano le cellule native normali, mentre i *cerchi pieni* le cellule mutate. *A*, La maggior parte delle cellule in una popolazione irradiata conserverà il fenotipo nativo. *B*, Esempio di una cellula direttamente mutata dopo l'esposizione a radiazioni; la mutazione è trasmessa a tutta la sua progenie. *C* e *D* sono esempi di mutazioni che originano come conseguenza d'instabilità genomica indotta dalle radiazioni. La cellula irradiata e la sua progenie immediata sono di tipo nativo, ma la frequenza con cui le mutazioni si verificano nelle cellule discendenti più lontane della cellula irradiata è elevata. (Da Little JB: Ionizing radiation. In Kufe DW, Pollock RE, Weichselbaum RR, et al [editors]: *Holland-Frei Cancer Medicine*, 6th ed. Ontario, BC Decker, 2003, capitolo 19, figura 19.3, per gentile concessione.)

È stato stimato che il 30% delle indagini con la TC non è necessario, è ridondante o può essere sostituito da un'altra modalità che non produce radiazioni. Il dialogo tra il medico prescrivente e il radiologo pediatra è fondamentale. Entrambi hanno simili preoccupazioni, non vogliono che sfugga alcuna anomalia. Il medico prescrivente non desidera non scoprire una lesione acuta e vuole essere sicuro che il paziente effettui l'esame, mentre il radiologo necessita di scoprire tutto anche riducendo la dose di radiazioni (ottenendo cioè una immagine non diagnostica).

RIDUZIONE DELLE RADIAZIONI NELLA TC

La fonte più comune di radiazioni mediche è la TC. Si è passati da uno scanner single slice a scanner che possono ottenere fino a 64 slice in tempi inferiori al secondo. Le immagini hanno un dettaglio eccellente, includendo la ricostruzione multiplanare e 3D dei dati acquisiti, sebbene la dose di radiazioni per esame sia in aumento. Se un tempo si avevano 10-12 immagini in 30 minuti, attualmente se ne ottengono centinaia in meno di un minuto. Fare di più non è necessariamente utile nei bambini, perché essi sono più sensibili alle radiazioni rispetto agli adulti. Simili settaggi della TC ed esposizioni nei bambini portano a una dose relativamente più alta di radiazioni rispetto a quella somministrata agli adulti (la dose efficace per gli organi è infatti più elevata), perché i raggi X a minore energia che sarebbero assorbiti nel campo vicino in un adulto attraversano il bambino per intero, irradiando tutti gli organi. Si stima che agli stessi parametri la dose necessaria in una TC del cranio di un neonato sia 4 volte maggiore della dose di un adulto. Con l'imaging addominale la dose è aumentata soltanto di 2/3.

Il compito del radiologo è di adattare l'esame al paziente pediatrico. Si può dire se ciò viene realizzato osservando i parametri della corrente del tubo (milliamperaggio/secondo-mAs) e il chilovoltaggio di picco (kVp). C'è anche bisogno di una protezione appropriata. Il radiologo possiede molti metodi per ridurre i parametri in modo che il bambino effettui l'imaging diagnostico senza una irradiazione eccessiva. Il dimezzamento della dose di radiazioni, anche negli adulti sottoposti a TC, non altera l'efficacia diagnostica e la capacità del radiologo di confermare la diagnosi appropriata.

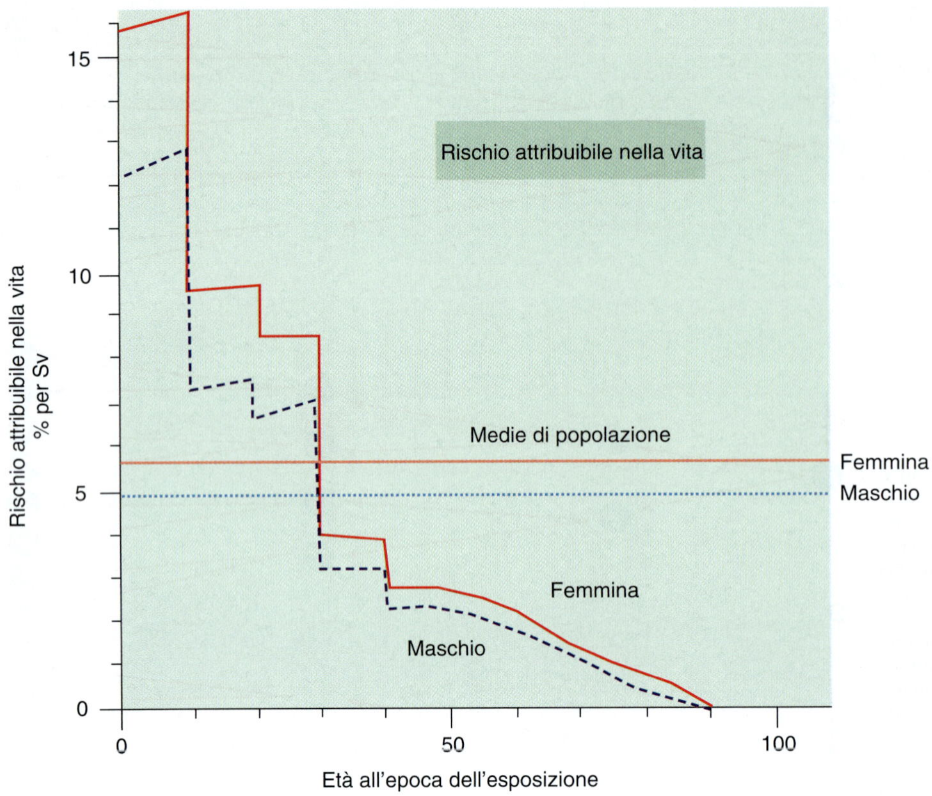

Figura 706-2. Rischio in vita di tumore in eccesso per sievert (Sv) in funzione dell'età al momento dell'esposizione. Dati ottenuti dai sopravvissuti alla bomba atomica. Il rischio medio per una popolazione è circa del 5% per sievert, ma varia significativamente con l'età: i bambini sono molto più sensibili rispetto agli adulti. In età precoci, le femmine sono più sensibili dei maschi. (Da Hall EJ: Introduction to session I: Helical CT and cancer risk. *Pediatr Radiol* 2002;32:225-227, figura 1. Per gentile concessione di Springer Science and Business Media.)

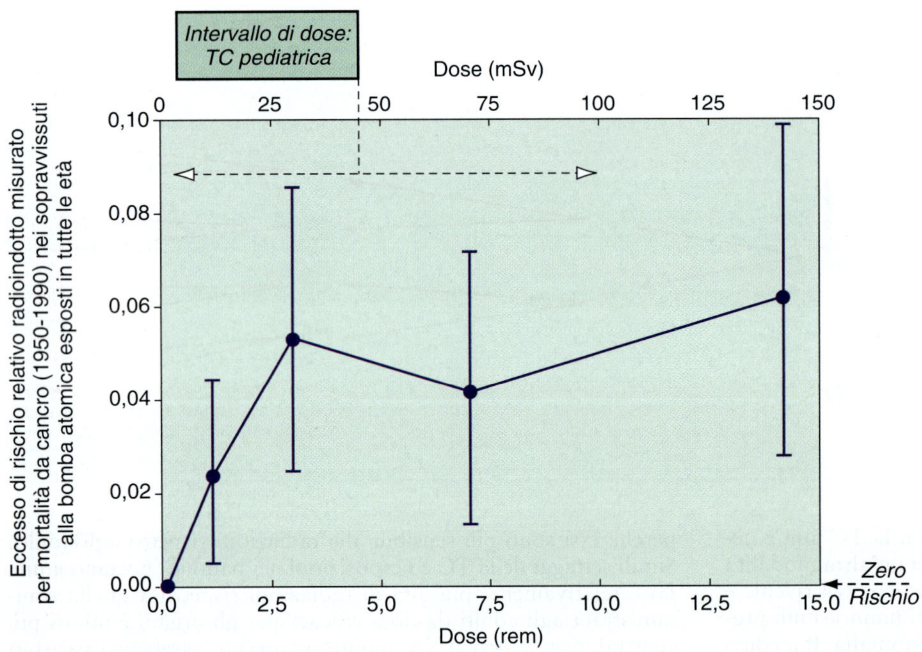

Figura 706-3. Intervallo di dose valido per la TC pediatrica: 6-100 mSv (0,006 = 0,1 Sv). "Vi sono segni diretti, statisticamente significativi di rischio nell'intervallo di dose compreso tra 0 e 0,1 Sv". Da Brenner DJ: Estimating cancer risks from pediatric CT: going from the qualitative to the quantitative. *Pediatr Radiol* 2002;32:228-231.

IRRADIAZIONE CORPOREA TOTALE

MANIFESTAZIONI CLINICHE. La Tabella 706-6 presenta le relazioni dose-effetto per le radiazioni acute penetranti di tutto il corpo. Un'ampia esposizione singola a radiazioni penetranti può portare alla **sindrome da irradiazione acuta**, i cui segni e sintomi risultano secondari al danno dei principali sistemi organici, che presentano differenti livelli di radiosensibilità modulati dalla velocità con cui si è verificata l'esposizione. Per esempio, 100 rad somministrati in 1 minuto sarebbero sintomatici, ma 1 rad/die per 100 giorni non lo sarebbe.

La **sindrome ematopoietica** è dovuta a dosi acute sull'intero corpo superiori a 200 rad. Una fase prodromica è caratterizzata da nausea e vomito entro le prime 12 ore, con sintomi che di solito durano fino a 48 ore. Segue un periodo di latenza di 2-3 settimane, durante il quale i pazienti possono sentirsi piuttosto bene. Anche se i pazienti sono asintomatici, si è verificata la compromissione del midollo osseo. Il reperto di laboratorio più evidente è la depressione dei linfociti (Tab. 706-7). La massima depressione del midollo osseo ha luogo dopo circa 30 giorni dall'esposizione, quando l'emorragia e l'infezione possono essere i disturbi maggiori. Se il midollo osseo non è stato completamente eradicato, segue poi una fase di ripresa. Tale effetto da radiazioni è simile a quello che avviene quando l'irradiazione sull'intero corpo (somministrata in 1200 rad per due trattamenti) viene usata per obliterare il midollo osseo nei bambini con leucemia prima del trapianto dello stesso.

TABELLA 706-6. Relazioni dose-effetto dopo irradiazione corporea totale da raggi γ o raggi X

DOSE ASSORBITA DAL CORPO, RAD (Gy)	REPERTI
5 (0,05)	Asintomatico
15 (0,15)	Asintomatico (ma possono essere presenti aberrazioni cromosomiche in linfociti periferici in coltura)
50 (0,5)	Asintomatico (depressione minima dei globuli rossi e delle piastrine in alcuni soggetti)
100 (1,0)	Nausea e vomito in circa il 10% dei pazienti entro 2 giorni dall'esposizione
200 (2,0)	Nausea e vomito nella maggior parte dei soggetti esposti, con franca depressione ematologica
400 (4,0)	Nausea, vomito e diarrea entro 48 ore; mortalità del 50% senza trattamento medico
600 (6,0)	Mortalità del 100% entro 30 giorni per insufficienza del midollo osseo senza trattamento medico
5000 (50,0)	Collasso cardiovascolare e danno del sistema nervoso centrale, con decesso in 24-72 ore

TABELLA 706-7. Esiti attesi in base alla conta linfocitaria assoluta dopo irradiazione acuta penetrante corporea totale

CONTA LINFOCITARIA MINIMA ENTRO 48 ORE DALL'ESPOSIZIONE	PROGNOSI
1000-3000 intervallo normale	Nessun danno significativo
1000-1500	Danno significativo ma probabilmente non letale, prognosi buona
500-1000	Danno grave, prognosi discreta
100-500	Danno molto grave, prognosi sfavorevole
<100	Letale in assenza di donatore compatibile di midollo osseo

La **sindrome gastrointestinale** è dovuta a una dose di irradiazioni del corpo intero superiore a 800 rad. La nausea, il vomito e la diarrea compaiono precocemente. Vi è un periodo di latenza di circa 1 settimana, seguito dalla recidiva dei sintomi gastrointestinali, dalla sepsi e da squilibri elettrolitici, che possono condurre alla morte.

Per dosi superiori a 3000 rad, predomina la **sindrome cardiovascolare/del sistema nervoso centrale**. Nausea, vomito, prostrazione, ipotensione, atassia e convulsioni sono pressoché immediati. Di solito il decesso si verifica rapidamente.

TRATTAMENTO. Per le sindromi ematopoietica e gastrointestinale la terapia è di supporto, con trasfusioni, liquidi, antibiotici e agenti antivirali.

IRRADIAZIONE LOCALIZZATA

MANIFESTAZIONI CLINICHE. Dal momento che l'irradiazione localizzata interessa una piccola quantità di tessuto, le manifestazioni sistemiche possono essere meno gravi e i pazienti possono sopravvivere anche se le dosi locali assorbite sono molto elevate. La mano è la sede più comune per le lesioni localizzate da irradiazione, dovute di solito al raccogliere o giocare con sorgenti radioattive smarrite. La seconda sede accidentale più comune è rappresentata dalle cosce e dalle natiche, prevalentemente per il fatto di mettere in tasca sorgenti altamente radioattive insospettate.

Gli effetti di un'ustione termica compaiono quasi immediatamente e i pazienti conoscono sempre l'origine dell'ustione. Le radiazioni dovrebbero essere sospettate anche quando i pazienti si presentano con sintomi simili a ustioni ma senza alcuna causa nota.

La penetrabilità delle radiazioni è un importante fattore negli esiti del danno locale. Nei casi d'irradiazione a bassa energia, la guarigione e l'innesto cutaneo sono possibili, anche in caso di elevate dosi cutanee assorbite. I raggi γ e i raggi X penetrano a livelli significativi e causano un'endoarterite obliterante progressiva che può portare a necrosi e gangrena. I sintomi si verificano nelle prime 12 ore sono pochi, a meno che la dose non sia estremamente elevata. I pazienti possono lamentare ipersensibilità, formicolio o dolore. L'eritema è simile a quello osservato in caso di ustione di primo grado; se compare nelle prime 48 ore, probabilmente si verificherà un'ulcerazione. Esso può presentarsi, scomparire e ritornare dopo 13 settimane. Il danno transepidermico è simile a una ustione termica di secondo grado. La formazione di bolle può avvenire a 1-2 settimane per dosi dell'ordine di 10000 rad.

Alcuni tessuti che possono subire una esposizione localizzata sono relativamente radiosensibili. La **formazione di cataratta** può avere luogo in caso di singole esposizioni a raggi γ dell'ordine di 200-500 rad. Di solito il suo sviluppo richiede da 2 mesi a diversi anni. Per il realizzarsi dell'**oligospermia** possono essere necessari fino a 2 mesi. L'infertilità transitoria nei maschi può essere secondaria a dosi anche di 15 rad, mentre la sterilità permanente può verificarsi in essi a dosi comprese fra 300 e 600 rad.

TRATTAMENTO. La terapia cutanea è diretta alla prevenzione delle infezioni. Il trattamento delle lesioni localizzate di solito comporta la chirurgia plastica e gli innesti, se l'esposizione non è stata molto penetrante (vedi Capitolo 74). La natura della chirurgia dipende dalla dose a varie profondità nel tessuto e dalla localizzazione della lesione. La piena espressione del danno da radiazioni spesso non è evidente prima di 1-2 anni, a causa del lento restringimento arteriolare che determina una necrosi ritardata. Dopo un'irradiazione relativamente penetrante, può essere necessaria l'amputazione, a causa delle alterazioni obliteranti dei piccoli vasi.

RADIOTERAPIA

La radioterapia utilizza alte dosi per uccidere le cellule maligne, ma la loro sensibilità è piuttosto simile a quella delle cellule normali, sicché per ottenere significativi tassi terapeutici il radio-oncologo deve accettare una certa percentuale di complicanze gravi (5-10%). I protocolli di radioterapia sono ragionevolmente standardizzati. Nella maggior parte degli schemi si utilizzano circa 50 Gy (5000 rad) somministrati pressappoco in 25 frazioni in 5 settimane. Uno schema di trattamento che si avvale di dosi di molto superiori al 10% di questo valore o che adopera tale dose in un numero di frazioni significativamente minore determina un'elevata incidenza di complicanze gravi.

Ogni anno i tumori infantili colpiscono 70-160 bambini su un milione di età compresa tra 0 e 14 anni. A causa della maggiore precocità della diagnosi e del miglioramento della terapia, oltre il 70% di essi sopravvive a lungo termine. Attualmente si stanno cercando metodi più opportuni per prevenire o ottimizzare l'assistenza per gli effetti tardivi della terapia per i tumori (vedi Tab. 706-9). È molto difficile a volte separare i risultati della chemioterapia, della radioterapia o della chemioterapia associata a radioterapia. Il tipo di effetti dipende dall'età al momento dell'irradiazione (livello di sviluppo rimanente, stato puberale). Le seconde neoplasie possono costituire il 6-10% di tutti i tumori nei bambini o negli adulti. Nei bambini sopravvissuti, il rischio di un secondo tumore è aumentato di 3-6 volte.

Dal 3 al 12% dei bambini trattati per una neoplasia svilupperà un secondo tumore maligno entro i 25 anni di vita (Tab. 706-8). Circa il 70% di questi è localizzato nel campo dell'irradiazione originale, dato che la radioterapia ne aumenta il rischio in modo dose-dipendente per le neoplasie non genetiche.

Le complicanze specifiche dipendono dalla localizzazione del campo di trattamento. Nei bambini, a causa della collocazione di molti tumori infantili, il sistema nervoso centrale (SNC) si trova comunemente nel campo di trattamento e subisce le complicanze. L'irradiazione standard del cervello nei bambini porta a un'atrofia corticale in oltre la metà di quelli che avevano ricevuto 2000-6000 rad; il 26% presenta alterazioni della sostanza bianca (leucoencefalopatia) e l'8% calcificazioni (Fig. 706-4). Più giovane è il bambino al momento dell'irradiazione, maggiore è l'atrofia. Alcuni pazienti sviluppano anche una microangiopatia mineralizzante (Fig. 706-5). Le alterazioni cerebrali radioindotte

TABELLA 706-8. Seconde neoplasie e loro relazione con neoplasie primarie*

SECONDE NEOPLASIE	NEOPLASIE PRIMARIE	LATENZA (MEDIANA IN ANNI)	FATTORI DI RISCHIO
Tumori cerebrali	ALL; tumori cerebrali; HD	9-10	Radiazioni; età più giovane
MDS/AML	ALL; HD; tumori ossei	3-5	Inibitori della topoisomerasi II; agenti alchilanti
Tumore della mammella	HD; tumori ossei; sarcomi dei tessuti molli; ALL; tumori cerebrali; tumori di Wilms; NHL	15-20	Radiazioni; sesso femminile
Tumore della tiroide	ALL; HD, neuroblastoma; sarcomi dei tessuti molli tumori ossei; NH:L	13-15	Radiazioni; età più giovane; sesso femminile
Tumori ossei	Retinoblastoma (ereditario); altri tumori ossei; sarcoma di Ewing; sarcomi dei tessuti molli; ALL	9-10	Radiazioni; agenti alchilanti; splenectomia
Sarcomi dei tessuti molli	Retinoblastoma (ereditario); sarcomi dei tessuti molli; HD; tumore di Wilms; tumori ossei; ALL	10-11	Radiazioni; età più giovane; antracicline

*Da Bhatia S, Sklar S. Second cancers in survivors of childhood cancer. *N Rev Cancer* 2002;2:124-132, per gentile concessione.

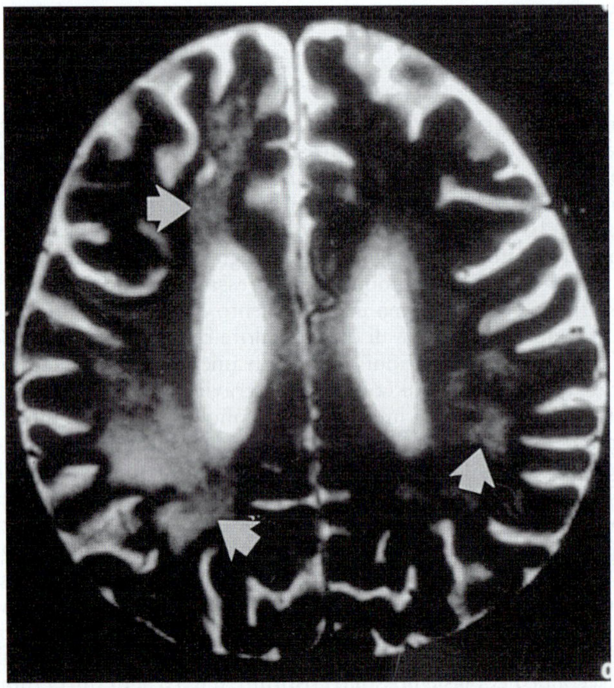

Figura 706-4. La scansione RM T2-pesata di un bambino dopo radioterapia mostra alterazioni della sostanza bianca (*frecce*).

sono potenziate dal metotrexato somministrato prima, durante o dopo la radioterapia.

La **necrosi cerebrale** è una grave complicanza della vasculopatia indotta dalle radiazioni. Di solito viene diagnosticata dopo 1-5 anni dall'irradiazione ma può comparire fino a 10 anni di distanza. Si verifica con moderata probabilità quando gli schemi di radioterapia superano i 4000 rad in 10 frazioni, 5000 rad in 20 frazioni o 6000 rad in 30 frazioni o quando le singole frazioni sono superiori a 300 rad. Si può manifestare con cefalea, aumento della pressione endocranica, convulsioni, deficit sensitivi e alterazioni psicotiche.

L'irradiazione del midollo spinale può portare a una **mielite da radiazioni**, transitoria o permanente. La mielite transitoria acuta spesso compare a distanza di 2-4 mesi dall'irradiazione. I pazienti di solito presentano il **segno di Lhermitte**, una sensazione di piccole scariche elettriche nelle braccia e nelle gambe che compaiono con la flessione del collo o con altri movimenti che stirano il midollo spinale. La regressione della mielopatia transitoria in genere avviene dopo 8-40 settimane e non progredisce necessariamente a una necrosi tardiva.

La **mielopatia tardiva** compare dopo un periodo di latenza medio di 20 mesi, ma anche più precocemente se la dose totale o per frazione è elevata. Di solito si manifesta con peggioramento intermittente ed è irreversibile. Nelle regioni cervicale e toracica si sviluppa una dissociazione sensoriale seguita dalla paresi spastica e flaccida. Nel midollo lombare la paresi flaccida è dominante. La mortalità per le lesioni toraciche alte e cervicali raggiunge il 70%, con decessi dovuti a polmonite e infezioni delle vie urinarie.

L'irradiazione provoca anche altri effetti specifici nei bambini (Tab. 706-9). L'**effetto sulla crescita** è più pronunciato quando essi sono di età inferiore a 6 anni o durante lo scatto di crescita nell'adolescenza. Scoliosi e ipoplasia delle ossa possono comparire se gli schemi di trattamento frazionati superano i 4000 rad. Dosi frazionate >2500 rad possono portare all'epifisiolisi della testa femorale. È stata riportata anche un'aumentata incidenza di osteocondromi benigni. L'irradiazione della parete toracica nelle femmine con 1500-2000 rad in 1 settimana compromette lo sviluppo mammario, mentre dosi frazionate di 3000-4000 rad causano fibrosi e atrofia del tessuto mammario.

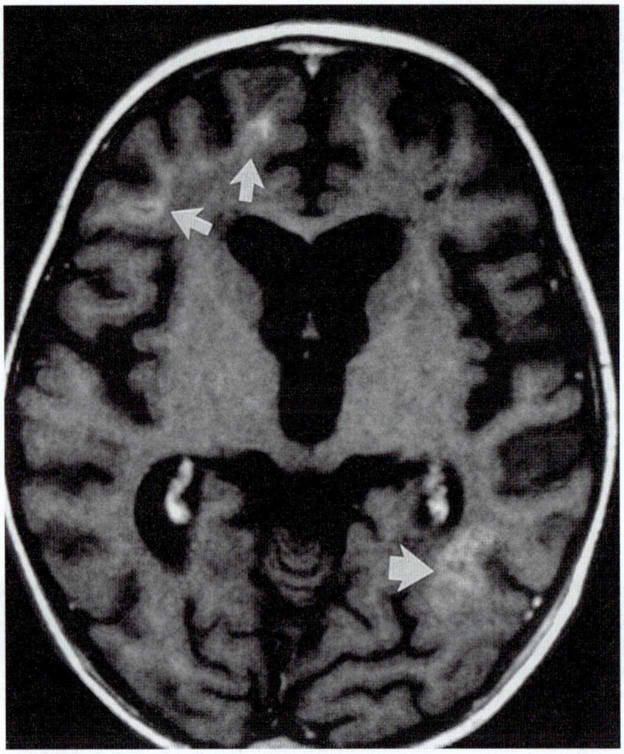

Figura 706-5. Alterazioni cerebrali generalizzate dopo radioterapia. La scansione RM T1-pesata di un bambino mostra atrofia centrale e corticale così come aree iperintense (*frecce*) dovute a microangiopatia mineralizzante.

CONTAMINAZIONE INTERNA

EPIDEMIOLOGIA. Gli episodi che comportano una contaminazione interna sono rari e di solito secondari a un'errata somministrazione in ambito ospedaliero o a una ingestione volontaria di materiali radioattivi contaminati insospettati. Altre possibili cause nei bambini comprendono l'ingestione di latte materno da madri che sono state sottoposte a scintigrafia diagnostica e l'esposizione alle radiazioni nei casi in cui un genitore o un fratello riceva una dose terapeutica di iodio 131.

TABELLA 706-9. Effetti tardivi della radioterapia nei bambini trattati per neoplasia

APPARATO	DOSE
Muscoloscheletrico	
Ipoplasia muscolare	>20 Gy
Scoliosi, cifosi, lordosi	10-20 Gy
Esostosi osteocartilaginea	?
Neuroendocrino (cranico o craniospinale)	
Compromissione dell'ormone della crescita	>18 Gy
Deficit di ACTH	>40 Gy
Deficit di TRH	>40 Gy
Pubertà precoce (prevalentemente nel sesso femminile)	>20 Gy
Deficit di gonadotropine	>40 Gy
Insufficienza gonadica	
Insufficienza ovarica	4-12 Gy
Insufficienza testicolare	>3 Gy
Disfunzione del sistema nervoso centrale*	
Alterazioni strutturali	>18 Gy
Alterazioni cognitive	?
Altro	
Fibrosi polmonare	
Nefropatia	
Insufficienza epatica	
Arterite	
Compromissione oculare	
Compromissione dell'orecchio	
Disfunzione del midollo osseo	
Compromissione cardiaca	

*Con chemioterapia intratecale (MTX).
Tratta da Halperin EC, Constine LS, Tarbell NJ, Kun LE (editors): *Pediatric Radiation Oncology*, 3th ed, Philadelphia, Lippincott Williams & Wilkins, capitoli 19-20, 1999.

TABELLA 706-10. Terapia specifica per la contaminazione interna

RADIONUCLIDE	APPROCCIO TERAPEUTICO
Trizio	Diluizione (forzare i liquidi)
Iodio 125 o Iodio 131	Blocco (SSKI o ioduro di potassio), mobilizzazione (farmaci antitiroidei)
Cesio 134 o Cesio 137	Riduzione dell'assorbimento gastrointestinale (blu di Prussia)
Stronzio 89 o Stronzio 90	Riduzione dell'assorbimento (gel antiacidi di fosfato di alluminio), blocco (lattato di stronzio), spostamento (fosfato per os), mobilizzazione (ammonio cloruro o estratto di paratiroide)
Plutonio e altri elementi transuranici	Chelazione con zinco o acido dietilentriamino pentacetico di calcio
Sconosciuto	Riduzione dell'assorbimento (emetici, lavaggio, carbone vegetale o lassativi) in caso di ingestione

SSKI, soluzione satura di ioduro di potassio (*saturated solution of potassium iodide*).
Da Mettler FA, Voelz GL: Major radiation exposureóWhat to expect and how to respond. *N Engl J Med* 2002; 346:1554.

MANIFESTAZIONI CLINICHE. I rischi da contaminazione interna dipendono dalla natura del radionuclide (in particolare relativamente alla sua solubilità in acqua, all'emivita e all'emissione radioattiva) e del composto chimico.

TRATTAMENTO. Per il trattamento più efficace, è necessario conoscere il radionuclide e la forma chimica che va istituito immediatamente (Tab. 706-10). Il **trattamento di rimozione** comporta la pulizia di una ferita contaminata e la lavanda gastrica o la somministrazione di catartici in caso d'ingestione. Anche gli antiacidi contenenti alginato risultano utili per la rimozione, in quanto riducono l'assorbimento nel tratto gastrointestinale. Un esempio di **terapia bloccante** è dato dalla somministrazione di ioduro di potassio o di altri composti stabili contenenti iodio a pazienti con una contaminazione interna nota da iodio radioattivo. Lo iodio stabile blocca opportunamente la tiroide, sebbene la sua validità si riduca in modo rapido con il trascorrere del tempo dalla contaminazione. La dose raccomandata di ioduro di potassio è di 16 mg per i neonati, 32 mg all'età di 3 anni e 65 mg dai 3 ai 18 anni. Ogni dose protegge soltanto per un giorno. La **terapia di diluizione** viene utilizzata nei casi di contaminazione da trizio (idrogeno radioattivo come acqua). Forzare i liquidi favorisce l'escrezione. Nei casi di contaminazione interna con elementi transuranici (americio e plutonio) può essere necessaria la **terapia chelante** con l'acido dietilentriamino pentacetico di calcio.

CONTAMINAZIONE ESTERNA

La presenza della contaminazione radioattiva esterna sulla cute del paziente non è un'emergenza medica immediata. Il trattamento comporta la rimozione e il controllo della diffusione dei materiali radioattivi. Se in un paziente si sospetta una contaminazione superficiale e non vi sono lesioni fisiche, la decontaminazione può essere effettuata in modo relativamente facile. Quando un trauma fisico significativo o altre lesioni minacciose per la vita sono associate a una contaminazione esterna, la decontaminazione dovrebbe procedere solo dopo che il paziente è stato stabilizzato fisiologicamente. In molti incidenti la terapia medica essenziale viene ritardata in modo inappropriato dal personale di emergenza ospedaliero per paura delle radiazioni o della diffusione della contaminazione nell'ospedale. Dopo l'episodio di irradiazione, il triage dei pazienti è critico e si basa sull'esposizione e sui sintomi (Fig. 706-6).

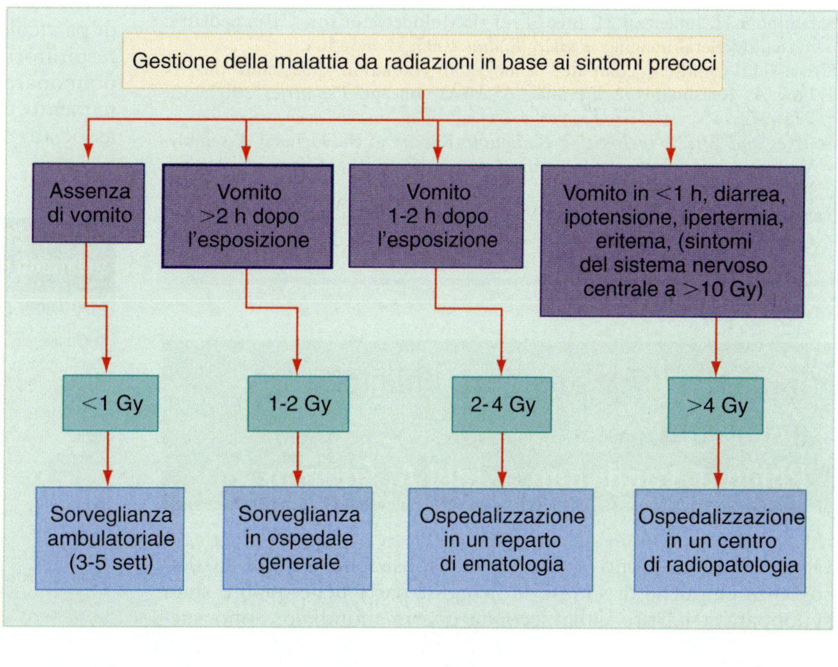

Figura 706-6. Trattamento della malattia da radiazioni a differenti livelli di assistenza medica, a seconda dell'aspetto dei sintomi precoci e della dose stimata di radiazioni per l'intero organismo. (Da Turai I, Veress K, Günalp B, Souchkevitch: Medical response to radiation incidents and radionuclear threats. *BMJ* 2204;328:568-572.)

American College of Radiology: *Practice Guidelines and Technical Standards.* Reston, VA: American College of Radiology, 2003.
Bernal B, Altman NR: Evidence-based medicine: Neuroimaging of seizures. *Neuroimag Clin North Am* 2003;13:211–224.
Berrington de Gonzalez A, Darby S: Risk of cancer from diagnostic X-rays: Estimates for the UK and 14 other countries. *Lancet* 2004;363:345–351.
Bhatia S, Sklar S: Second cancers in survivors of childhood cancer. *N Rev Cancer* 2002;2:124–132.
Brenner DJ, Elliston CD, Hall EJ, et al: Estimated risks of radiation-induced fatal cancer from pediatric CT. *AJR* 2001;176:289–296.
Cuthbertson DJ, Davidson J: What to tell patients about radioiodine therapy. *BMJ* 2006;333:271–272.
Doll R, Wakeford R: Risk of childhood cancer from fetal irradiation. *Br J Radiol* 1997;70:130–139.
Frush DP, Donnelly LF, Rosen NS: Computed tomography and radiation risks: What pediatric health care providers should know. *Pediatrics* 2003;112:951–957.
Gangopadhyay KK, Sundram F, De P: Triggering radiation alarms after radioiodine treatment. *BMJ* 2006;333:293–294.
Huda W, Atherton JV, Ware DE, et al: An approach for the estimation of effective radiation dose at CT in pediatric patients. *Radiology* 1997;203: 417–422.
Huda W: Effective dose to adult and pediatric patients. *Pediatr Radiol* 2002;32:272–279.
Imaizumi M, Usa T, Tominaga T, et al: Radiation dose-response relationships for thyroid nodules and autoimmune thyroid diseases in Hiroshima and Nagasaki atomic bomb survivors 55–58 years after radiation exposure. *JAMA* 2006;295:1011–1022.
Kal HB, Struikmans H: Radiotherapy during pregnancy: Fact and fiction. *Lancet Oncol* 2005;6:328 333.
Kasatkinan EP, Shilin DE, Rosenbloom AL, et al: Effects of low level radiation from the Chernobyl accident in a population with iodine deficiency. *Eur J Pediatr* 1997;156:916.
Koenig TR, Wolff D, Mettler FA, et al: Skin injuries from fluoroscopically guided procedures: Part I, characteristics of radiation injury. *AJR* 2001;177:3–11.
Martin D, Semelka RC: Health effects of ionizing radiation from diagnostic CT. *Lancet* 2006;367:1712–1714.
McLean D: Computed tomography doses in children. *Lancet* 2004;363: 1178.
Mettler FA, Voelz GL: Major radiation exposure–What to expect and how to respond. *N Engl J Med* 2002;346:1554–1561.
Oeffinger KC, Mertens AC, Sklar CA, et al: Chronic health conditions in adult survivors of childhood cancer. *N Engl J Med* 2006;355:1572–1582.
Pierce DA, Preston DL: Radiation-related cancer risks at low doses among atomic bomb survivors. *Radiat Res* 2000;154:178–186.
Pierce DA, Shimizu Y, Preston DL, et al: Studies of the mortality of atomic bomb survivors. Report 12, part 1. Cancer: 1950–1990. *Radiat Res* 1996;146:1–27.
Preston DL, Ron E, Yonehara S, et al: Tumors of the nervous system and pituitary gland associated with atomic bomb radiation exposure. *J Natl Cancer Inst* 2002;94:1555–1563.
Salamipour H, Jimenez RM, Bree SL, et al: Multidetector row CT in pediatric musculoskeletal imaging. *Pediatr Radiol* 2005;35:555–564.
Slovis TL: Children, computed tomography radiation dose, and the As Low As Reasonably Achievable (ALARA) concept. *Pediatrics* 2003;112: 971–972.
Sources and Effects of Ionizing Radiation. Report to the General Assembly. Vienna: United Nations Scientific Committee on the Effects of Atomic Radiation, 2000.
Turai I, Veress K, Günalp B, et al: Medical response to radiation incidents and radionuclear threats. *BMJ* 2004;328:568–572.

Capitolo 707 ■ Sostanze chimiche inquinanti

Philip J. Landrigan e Joel A. Forman

Oggi i bambini sono a rischio di esposizione a oltre 80 000 sostanze chimiche di sintesi, la maggior parte delle quali è stata sviluppata a partire dalla seconda guerra mondiale. Sono specialmente esposti a 2863 sostanze chimiche prodotte in elevate quantità, di cui vengono realizzate 500 000 tonnellate o più all'anno e che risultano le più ampiamente diffuse nell'ambiente. I dati di biomonitoraggio estrapolati dal *Third National Report on Human Esposition to Enviromental Chemicals* dei Center for Disease Control mette in evidenza che i bambini possono venire in contatto con un'ampia gamma di sostanze chimiche di sintesi e in alcuni casi presentano maggiori conseguenze corporee rispetto agli adulti. Questo tipo di dati documenta l'esposizione dei bambini, ma non affronta gli effetti sulla salute. In meno della metà delle sostanze chimiche prodotte in elevate quantità sono stati valutati i possibili rischi per la salute dell'uomo e in meno del 10% è stata determinata la tossicità pediatrica o dello sviluppo. Si è sempre più consapevoli del rischio per i bambini, ma c'è una conoscenza molto limitata dell'impatto delle esposizioni sulla salute.

I bambini sono vulnerabili in maniera particolare alle sostanze chimiche inquinanti per diversi motivi.

1. **Essi hanno un numero proporzionalmente maggiore di contatti con molte sostanze inquinanti ambientali rispetto agli adulti. Dato che bevono più acqua, mangiano più cibo e respirano più aria per kg di peso corporeo, si trovano molto maggiormente in relazione con le sostanze inquinanti dell'acqua, del cibo e dell'aria. Le loro esposizioni sono ulteriormente aumentate per il fatto di portare le mani alla bocca e di giocare a contatto con il suolo.**
2. **Le vie metaboliche dei bambini, specialmente nei primi mesi di vita, sono immature. Sebbene in alcuni casi essi siano più capaci degli adulti di fare fronte alle sostanze tossiche ambientali, in quanto non sono in grado di metabolizzarle alla loro forma attiva, tuttavia spesso sono meno abili nel detossificare ed eliminare le sostanze chimiche inquinanti.**
3. **I lattanti e i bambini sono in fase di crescita e sviluppo e i loro processi evolutivi risultano particolarmente sensibili alla distruzione da parte di sostanze chimiche inquinanti. L'invalidità secondaria alle esposizioni a sostanze chimiche durante i periodi di vulnerabilità precoce può essere grave e permanente (Tab. 707-1).**
4. **Dal momento che i bambini hanno molti anni di vita davanti, possiedono il tempo di sviluppare malattie croniche multistadio che possono essere scatenate da esposizioni precoci.**

SOSTANZE CHIMICHE INQUINANTI PIÙ PERICOLOSE

SOSTANZE INQUINANTI NELL'ARIA. Le sostanze inquinanti che destano maggiore preoccupazione nell'aria ambientale sono gli ossidanti fotochimici (specialmente l'ozono), gli ossidi di azoto (NO_x), i particolati sottili, gli ossidi di zolfo e il monossido di carbonio. Queste sostanze sono prodotte principalmente dalla combustione di combustibili fossili. Le emissioni degli autoveicoli sono la principale fonte d'inquinamento dell'aria in tutto il mondo, seguite dalle fonti immobili come le industrie per la produzione di energia.

Gli elevati livelli di sostanze inquinanti nell'aria, specialmente di particolati sottili, di ozono e di NO_x, sono associati a disturbi respiratori nei bambini quali la riduzione del flusso espiratorio polmonare, il wheezing e le riacutizzazioni dell'asma. L'inquinamento dell'aria da particolato sottile, anche a bassi livelli, è associato a lievi incrementi della mortalità cardiopolmonare e a

TABELLA 707-1. Effetti di sostanze chimiche inquinanti selezionate su lattanti e bambini

ESPOSIZIONE CHIMICA	EFFETTO
Dietilstibestrolo	Adenocarcinoma della vagina dopo esposizione intrauterina
Talidomide	Focomelia dopo esposizione intrauterina
Tricloroetilene	Elevato rischio di leucemia dopo esposizione intrauterina
Alcol	Sindrome fetoalcolica dopo esposizione intrauterina
Piombo	Tossicità neurocomportamentale da esposizione a basse dosi
Nitrosamina, vinilcloruro, radiazioni ionizzanti	Aumentato rischio di tumore dopo esposizione intrauterina
Insetticidi organofosforici	Neurotossicità evolutiva
Fumo di tabacco ambientale	Aumentato rischio di sindrome della morte improvvisa del lattante e di asma

un aumentato tasso di decesso per sindrome della morte improvvisa del lattante (vedi Capitolo 372). Uno studio prospettico di coorte in California sull'inquinamento dell'aria e lo sviluppo dei polmoni dimostra una ridotta crescita polmonare tra i 10 e i 18 anni, che porta a una diminuzione clinicamente significativa della funzione polmonare che persiste nella vita adulta.

Anche l'aria degli ambienti interni può essere un'importante fonte d'irritazione respiratoria, in quanto molti bambini trascorrono l'80-90% del loro tempo al chiuso. Questo tipo d'inquinamento è diventato specialmente importante negli Stati Uniti a partire dalle crisi energetiche degli anni '70, che portarono alla costruzione di case maggiormente a tenuta, più energeticamente efficienti. Gli allergeni nell'aria possono contribuire ai problemi respiratori e comprendono quelli di scarafaggi, acari, muffa, gatti e cani. Alcune muffe degli ambienti chiusi producono tossine chimiche denominate micotossine. Il fumo di tabacco è un altro dei principali fattori che contribuiscono alle riacutizzazione dell'asma infantile.

PIOMBO. L'esposizione al piombo si verifica in tutto il mondo (vedi Capitolo 709), ma è particolarmente comune nei Paesi che permettono ancora la benzina con il piombo. Negli Stati Uniti i livelli ematici pediatrici di piombo sono diminuiti di oltre il 90% negli ultimi 20 anni, principalmente in seguito alla rimozione del piombo dalla benzina. Ciononostante, i Center for Disease Control and Prevention stimano che oltre 310 000 bambini di età tra 1 e 5 anni abbiano ancora livelli ematici di piombo di 10 μg/dL e più. La diffusione è particolarmente elevata nei bambini delle minoranze povere nei centri urbani. Livelli di 5 μg/dL sono stati associati a tutta una serie di deficit neurocognitivi, tra cui la diminuzione dell'intelligenza, la riduzione della durata dell'attenzione e l'aumentato rischio di comportamento asociale. Sebbene l'estensione del danno sia direttamente proporzionale alla dose di piombo, le conseguenze relative sull'intelligenza sembrano maggiori per livelli ematici inferiori a 10 μg/dL. Le vernici a base di piombo sono la principale fonte di esposizione negli Stati Uniti. Dal momento che le superfici intatte verniciate con piombo si deteriorano immancabilmente producendo polvere di piombo, gli sforzi per ridurre ulteriormente il numero dei bambini intossicati da piombo negli Stati Uniti devono focalizzarsi sull'identificazione e sulla rimozione permanente di tutta la vernice a base di piombo, intatta o meno, dalle abitazioni. La benzina con piombo, le sostanze inquinanti industriali e le attività industriali basate su lavoro artigianale a domicilio rimangono le principali fonti di inquinamento da piombo in molti Paesi in via di sviluppo.

MERCURIO. I bambini possono essere esposti a mercurio inorganico o organico (vedi Capitolo 708). Il mercurio inorganico produce dermatite, gengivite, stomatite, tremore e acrodinia, mentre quello organico, o metilmercurio, è liposolubile, penetra facilmente nel sistema nervoso centrale (SNC) ed è neurotossico. L'esposizione a mercurio organico avviene principalmente con il consumo di pesce, che ha accumulato il mercurio depositato in laghi e oceani come ricaduta atmosferica dalla combustione del carbone, che normalmente ne contiene piccole quantità. È stato dimostrato che anche un'esposizione a basse dosi di mercurio organico è pericolosa per lo sviluppo del cervello fetale e quindi si raccomanda alle donne gravide di ridurre il consumo di pesce che contiene mercurio, come tonno e pesce spada. Sebbene effetti neurologici indesiderati non siano stati correlati all'esposizione al conservante comunemente usato nella preparazione dei vaccini e contenente etilmercurio o metilmercurio, tale sostanza, come misura precauzionale, è stata eliminata dai vaccini di routine dell'infanzia e dal vaccino materno Rh.

ASBESTO. Tra il 1947 e il 1973 l'asbesto fu utilizzato come materiale isolante sulle pareti delle aule e dei soffitti in circa 10 000 scuole negli Stati Uniti. Il suo successivo deterioramento ha rilasciato nell'aria fibre di asbesto inalabili, che rappresentano un rischio per i bambini. L'asbesto è infatti una sostanza cancerogena per l'uomo e i due principali tumori causati da esso sono il carcinoma del polmone e il mesotelioma. La legge federale degli Stati Uniti stabilisce che tutte le scuole siano ispezionate periodicamente per l'asbesto e che i risultati vengano resi pubblici. La rimozione è necessaria soltanto quando l'asbesto è visibilmente in fase di deterioramento o si trova alla portata dei bambini. Nella maggior parte dei casi, il posizionamento di barriere (muro a secco o soffitti a pannelli) offre una protezione appropriata.

FUMO DI TABACCO NELL'AMBIENTE. Il fumo durante la gravidanza è un rischio per il feto (vedi Capitolo 96). I neonati di madri fumatrici sono, in media, più piccoli del 10% rispetto ai neonati di madri non fumatrici e quelli di genitori che fumano hanno un più elevato rischio di sindrome della morte improvvisa neonatale. La nicotina del fumo di tabacco sembra essere una neurotossina che influisce sullo sviluppo.

Anche il fumo passivo è un rischio per i bambini. Negli Stati Uniti, il 43% dei bambini di età inferiore a 12 anni vive in un'abitazione con almeno un fumatore. I bambini esposti al fumo di tabacco nell'ambiente presentano un numero maggiore di malattie delle vie respiratorie inferiori, di versamenti dell'orecchio medio e di malattie respiratorie virali rispetto ai bambini non esposti.

PESTICIDI. I pesticidi sono un gruppo eterogeneo di sostanze chimiche utilizzate per controllare gli insetti, le erbe selvatiche, i funghi e i roditori. Circa 600 pesticidi sono registrati presso la U.S. Enviromental Protection Agency.

L'alimentazione è una delle principali vie di esposizione ai pesticidi nei bambini, a causa del contatto con residui di numerosi di essi sulla frutta e sulla verdura. I bambini possono anche essere esposti a casa o a scuola, nei prati o nei giardini e nelle aree agricole dove sono stati spruzzati. Negli Stati Uniti, i bambini che lavorano nei campi o che vivono negli accampamenti di lavoratori stagionali agricoli sono a rischio di contatto con molti pesticidi.

I pesticidi possono causare tutta una serie di effetti tossici cronici: polineuropatia e disfunzione del SNC (organofosfati); compromissione ormonale e riproduttiva (DDT, chepone, dibromocloropropano); neoplasie (aldrin, dieldrin, clorofenossi erbicidi [2,4,5-T]); fibrosi polmonare (paraquat). I bambini possono essere tenuti lontani dai pesticidi riducendo al minimo le applicazioni di questi a prati, giardini, scuole, parchi gioco e nelle derrate alimentari, nonché adottando tecniche di trattamento integrato degli insetti nocivi.

I bambini possono essere iperesposti acutamente a pesticidi (vedi Capitolo 58). Gli organofosfati e i carbamati, che causano entrambi neurotossicità attraverso l'inibizione dell'aceticolinesterasi, determinano il più ampio numero di casi d'intossicazione acuta. Tra i sintomi sono compresi miosi (sebbene non in tutti i casi), ipersalivazione, crampi addominali, vomito, diarrea e fascicolazione muscolare. Nei casi gravi il bambino può andare incontro a perdita di coscienza, aritmie cardiache e morte per arresto respiratorio. Il gas sarin usato a scopo bellico è un organofosfato. (Vedi Capitolo 58 per il trattamento dell'intossicazione da farmaci, da sostanze chimiche e da piante.)

PCB, DDT, DIOSSINE E ALTRI IDROCARBURI CLORATI. Gli idrocarburi clorati sono usati come insetticidi (DDT), plastiche (polivinilcloruro [PVC]), isolanti elettrici (bifenili policlorati [PCB, *PolyChlorinated Biphenyls*]) e solventi (tricloroetilene). Diossine e furani altamente tossici si possono formare durante la sintesi di erbicidi clorati o come prodotti di degradazione della combustione della plastica. Tutti questi materiali sono ampiamente diffusi nell'ambiente. Il DDT, i PCB e le diossine sono inoltre molto persistenti.

L'embrione, il feto e il bambino piccolo sono a rischio particolarmente elevato di danno da PCB, DDT e diossine. Tutti questi composti sono liposolubili, attraversano facilmente la placenta e si accumulano nel latte mammario. L'esposizione intrauterina ai PCB è stata ripetutamente collegata alla disfunzione neurocomportamentale persistente nei bambini.

Il pesce proveniente da acque contaminate è una delle principali fonti di esposizione ai PCB nei bambini, che possono venirne a contatto in utero o attraverso il latte mammario. Negli Stati Uniti, per proteggere bambini e donne gravide nei confronti dei PCB nel pesce le agenzie governative hanno emesso raccomandazioni per il consumo per alcuni laghi e fiumi. La combustione dei rifiuti medici contenenti PVC e l'uso di cloro per lo sbiancamento dei prodotti di carta sono le principali fonti prevenibili di diossina ambientale e dovrebbero essere disincentivati.

SOSTANZE CHE ALTERANO IL SISTEMA ENDOCRINO (ENDOCRINE DISRUPTORS). È stato dimostrato che numerose sostanze chimiche, tra cui il dietilstilbestrolo (DES), il DDT, i PCB e le diossine, influiscono in modo negativo sui sistemi endocrini degli animali e dell'uomo. Si sospetta che anche altre sostanze chimiche possiedano effetti negativi sul sistema endocrino, inclusi ulteriori pesticidi e ftalati (plasticizzanti). Gli effetti sulla flora e sulla fauna comprendono l'assottigliamento del guscio delle uova negli uccelli, la sterilità nelle foche, la femminilizzazione e il criptorchidismo nelle pantere, ridotti tassi di schiusura delle uova negli alligatori e molti altri. Nell'uomo la compromissione del sistema endocrino è stata implicata nelle osservazioni epidemiologiche della tendenza verso un telarca e un menarca più precoci nelle femmine, di crescenti tassi di tumori testicolari e ipospadia e della diminuzione della conta degli spermatozoi. Tra gli effetti più chiaramente riportati vi sono l'adenocarcinoma della vagina nelle donne e il criptorchidismo nei maschi le cui madri assunsero DES. L'esistenza di elevati livelli plasmatici di esteri ftalati è stata messa in relazione al telarca precoce nelle ragazze portoricane. Alcune sostanze che alterano il sistema endocrino possono avere effetti negativi anche sullo sviluppo cerebrale. La ricerca continua in quest'area è di particolare importanza, a causa dell'esposizione assai diffusa dell'uomo e della biopersistenza a lungo termine di molte di queste sostanze chimiche.

CANCEROGENI AMBIENTALI. I bambini possono essere esposti a sostanze inquinanti cancerogene in utero o dopo la nascita. Essi appaiono più sensibili rispetto agli adulti ad alcuni cancerogeni chimici e anche alle radiazioni (vedi Capitolo 706). Il rischio della cancerogenesi in utero fu riconosciuto per la prima volta con la scoperta che l'adenocarcinoma a cellule chiare della vagina poteva svilupparsi nelle donne dopo l'esposizione intrauterina al DES.

La cancerogenesi può anche essere associata a esposizioni domestiche e nella comunità. È stato riscontrato che i figli di lavoratori dell'asbesto e i bambini che sono cresciuti nelle vicinanze di industrie hanno un'incidenza più elevata di mesotelioma rispetto alle popolazione non esposte. I bambini cresciuti in fattorie presentano elevati tassi di leucemia; si sospetta che i pesticidi svolgano un ruolo eziologico. L'esposizione intrauterina al tricloroetilene attraverso acqua potabile contaminata è stata messa in relazione con l'aumentata incidenza di leucemia nelle ragazze che vivono in prossimità di una struttura industriale e di un sito di smaltimento industriale.

Il National Cancer Institute degli Stati Uniti riporta che la diffusione della leucemia e del glioma cerebrale, le due forme più comuni di tumore maligno dell'infanzia, è aumentata nelle ultime tre decadi, nonostante i grandi miglioramenti della terapia e la diminuzione dei tassi di decesso. L'aumento cumulativo dell'incidenza per glioma è attualmente di circa il 30%. Simili incrementi dei tumori infantili sono stati osservati nel Regno Unito. Sono in corso ricerche per stabilire se le sostanze chimiche inquinanti nell'ambiente abbiano contribuito a tali aumenti.

VIE DI ESPOSIZIONE

TRANSPLACENTARE. I metalli pesanti e le sostanze liposolubili come i PCB e i DDT attraversano facilmente la placenta e possono produrre effetti tossici gravi e irreversibili sugli organi nervosi, endocrini e riproduttivi in via di sviluppo, anche a livelli molto bassi.

ACQUA. Circa 200 sostanze chimiche sono state trovate in varia quantità nei rifornimenti idrici. Il piombo è particolarmente comune. Negli Stati Uniti, in alcuni quartieri più vecchi il piombo nell'acqua deriva da quello dei tubi, ma più comunemente viene disciolto (filtrato) dalla saldatura da parte dell'acqua poco dura e acida. I livelli più elevati di piombo si osservano nell'acqua che è rimasta nei tubi durante la notte; si consiglia pertanto di fare scorrere l'acqua per 2-3 minuti ogni mattina prima di preparare il latte artificiale per il bambino. Solventi e componenti della benzina come il metil terziario-butil etere (MTBE) e il benzene sono comunemente riscontrati nell'acqua del suolo.

ARIA. Le emissioni dei veicoli sono la principale fonte di inquinamento urbano dell'aria. Il gas di scarico dei motori diesel è cancerogeno per l'uomo. Nelle aree rurali, il fumo del legno può contribuire all'inquinamento aereo. I bambini che vivono vicino a fonderie e industrie chimiche possono essere esposti a emissioni tossiche industriali come piombo, benzene e 1,3-butadiene.

CIBO. Molte sostanze chimiche sono intenzionalmente aggiunte per migliorarne l'aspetto, il sapore, la consistenza o la conservazione, ma la possibile tossicità di molte di queste sostanze è stata poco valutata. Residui di molti pesticidi vengono riscontrati in cibi crudi ed elaborati. I livelli dei pesticidi risultano minori nei prodotti biologici piuttosto che nella frutta e nella verdura coltivate nella maniera convenzionale.

INDUMENTI DA LAVORO. Talvolta le malattie nei bambini possono essere fatte risalire a polveri contaminate provenienti dagli indumenti da lavoro dei genitori; si è verificata tossicità da piombo, berillio, diossina, pesticidi organofosfati e asbesto. Tale esposizione (denominata "fouling the nest", letteralmente "contaminazione del nido") può essere prevenuta fornendo attrezzature sul lavoro per cambiarsi e farsi la doccia.

SCUOLE. I bambini possono essere esposti nelle scuole, negli asili e nei nidi a vernici di piombo, muffe, asbesto, fumo di tabacco, pesticidi e materiali pericolosi di arti e mestieri. Esistono significative possibilità di prevenzione nell'ambiente scolastico e negli Stati Uniti spesso i pediatri vengono interpellati per un parere.

LAVORO MINORILE. Da 4 a 5 milioni di bambini e adolescenti negli Stati Uniti hanno un lavoro salariato e il lavoro minorile è ampiamente diffuso in tutto il mondo. I bambini che lavorano sono ad alto rischio di traumi e danni fisici. Essi possono anche essere esposti a un'ampia serie di sostanze chimiche tossiche, tra cui i pesticidi nei lavori agricoli e di giardinaggio, l'asbesto nella costruzione e nella demolizione di edifici e il benzene nei distributori di benzina.

IL RUOLO DEL MEDICO

I pediatri dovrebbero sempre essere attenti alla possibilità che un inquinante chimico abbia causato malattia in un bambino. Nel considerare le origini di una malattia non infettiva, essi dovrebbero porre domande sull'ambiente domestico, sull'occupazione professionale, su esposizioni insolite, sugli stabilimenti vicini. Una causa ambientale è particolarmente probabile quando diversi casi insoliti di malattia o gruppi di reperti compaiono insieme. Ogni adolescente con una lesione traumatica può essersela procurata sul lavoro.

L'anamnesi è l'unico e più importante strumento per ottenere informazioni sulle esposizioni ambientali. Bisognerebbe sempre avere informazioni sulle esposizioni attuali e pregresse (includendo domande su viaggi o residenze in Paesi in via di sviluppo) mediante poche semplici domande di screening. Modificazioni nelle modalità di esposizione o nuove esposizioni possono essere particolarmente importanti. Se si rilevano informazioni sospette, occorrerebbe svolgere un follow-up più dettagliato. Può essere indicato l'invio a una unità specialistica d'igiene ambientale pediatrica (www.ADEC.org). La diagnosi accurata di una origine ambientale di malattia può portare a una migliore assistenza per i bambini affetti e alla prevenzione della malattia in altri bambini.

American Academy of Pediatrics: *Handbook of Pediatric Environmental Health*, 2nd ed. Elk Grove Village, Il, American Academy of Pediatrics, 2003.

Centers for Disease Control and Prevention: *Third National Report on Human Exposure to Environmental Chemicals*. Atlanta, GA, Centers for Disease Control and Prevention, 2005.

Colón I, Caro D, Bourdony CJ, et al: Identification of phthalate esters in the serum of young Puerto Rican girls with premature breast development. *Environ Health Perspect* 2000;108:895–900.

Environmental Defense Fund: *Toxic Ignorance: The Continuing Absence of Basic Health Testing for Top-Selling Toxic Chemicals in the United States*. Washington, DC, Environmental Defense Fund, 1997.

Etzel RA, Balk SJ (editors): *Handbook of Environmental Health for Children*, 2nd ed.. Elk Grove Village, IL, American Academy of Pediatrics, 2003.

Frumkin H (editor): *Environmental Health: From Global to Local*. San Francisco, John Wiley & Sons, 2005.

Gauderman WJ, Avol E, Gilliland F, et al: The effect of air pollution on lung development from 10 to 18 years of age. *N Engl J Med* 2005;352:1276.

Gilliland FD, Gerhane K, Rappaport EB, et al: The effects of ambient air pollution on school absenteeism due to respiratory illnesses. *Epidemiology* 2001;12:43–54.

Jacobson JL, Jacobson SW: Intellectual impairment in children exposed to polychlorinated biphenyls in utero. *N Engl J Med* 1996;335:783–789.

Landrigan PJ, Trasande L, Thorpe LE, et al: The National Children's Study: A 21-year prospective study of 100,000 American children. *Pediatrics* 2006;118:2175–2186.

Landrigan PJ, Woolf AD, Gitterman B, et al: The Ambulatory Pediatric Association Fellowship in Pediatric Environmental Health: A five-year assessment. *Pediatrics* 2007 (in press).

Lanphear BP: Cognitive deficits associated with blood lead concentrations <10 μg/dL in US children and adolescents. *Public Health Rep* 2000;115:521–529.

Longnecker MP, Rogan WJ, Lucier G: The human health effects of DDT (dichlorodiphenyltrichloroethane) and PCBs (polychlorinated biphenyls) and an overview of organochlorines in public health. *Annu Rev Public Health* 1997;18:211–244.

Magnani C, Dalmasso P, Biggeri A, et al: Increased risk of malignant mesothelioma of the pleura after residential or domestic exposure to asbestos: A case-control study in Casale Monferrato, Italy. *Environ Health Perspect* 2001;109:915–919.

Paulson JA (editor): Children's Environmental Health. *Pediatr Clin North Am* 2001;48:xv–1337.

Tellez-Rojo MM, Bellinger DC, Arroyo-Quiroz C, et al: Longitudinal associations between lead concentrations lower than 10 microg/dL and neurobehavioral development in environmentally exposed children in Mexico City. *Pediatrics* 2006;118:323–330.

Capitolo 708 ■ Intossicazione da metalli pesanti Prashant V. Mahajan

Le principali minacce per l'uomo dovute ai metalli pesanti sono associate all'esposizione a piombo, cadmio, mercurio e arsenico. La causa più comune di tossicità è il piombo, che viene discusso separatamente nel Capitolo 709; nel presente Capitolo vengono invece trattati il mercurio e l'arsenico. La popolazione generale è esposta al mercurio principalmente attraverso il cibo; il pesce è una delle principali fonti per il metilmercurio. Il contatto con l'arsenico può da parte sua avvenire per contaminazione del cibo o dell'acqua. L'intossicazione da metallo pesante porta a diverse tossicità multiorgano attraverso la distruzione diffusa delle funzioni cellulari vitali. Le manifestazioni proteiformi dell'intossicazione acuta o cronica possono facilmente sfuggire alla diagnosi, a meno che non si ottenga una scrupolosa anamnesi dell'esposizione ambientale.

ARSENICO

EPIDEMIOLOGIA. L'arsenico è un metalloide che esiste in quattro forme: arsenico elementare, gas arsina, sali inorganici di arsenico (forma di arsenato pentavalente o forma di arsenato trivalente) e composti di arsenico organico. Le manifestazioni tossiche sono più elevate nei composti maggiormente solubili e a valenza più alta. Il *gas arsina* è la forma più tossica. Intossicazioni di massa dovute a esposizione all'arsenico si sono sempre verificate nella storia, tra cui una nel 1998 a Wakayama, in Giappone, in cui furono coinvolte 70 persone. I bambini possono avvelenarsi dopo il contatto con l'arsenico inorganico presente in pesticidi, erbicidi, tinture, medicinali omeopatici e determinati rimedi popolari contaminati in modo intenzionale o accidentale provenienti da Cina, India e Sudest asiatico (vedi Capitolo 59). I depositi del suolo possono contaminare i pozzi artesiani e quindi l'acqua, un problema comune nei Paesi in via di sviluppo. I prodotti alimentari (per es. il riso) cotti in acqua contaminata possono di fatto assorbire l'arsenico, concentrandolo così nell'alimento. L'Organizzazione Mondiale della Sanità (OMS) ha stabilito il limite inferiore di sicurezza a 10 ppb. L'esposizione professionale può verificarsi in industrie come quelle di fabbricazione del vetro, di ceramiche, di componenti elettronici, di semiconduttori, di laser, nell'industria mineraria, di fusione e raffinatura. Composti di arsenico organico possono essere riscontrati nei frutti di mare, nei pesticidi e in alcuni farmaci veterinari, anche se, a differenza del mercurio, le forme nei frutti di mare non sono tossiche.

FARMACOCINETICA. L'arsenico elementare è insolubile in acqua e nei liquidi corporei e, pertanto, non viene significativamente assorbito e non è tossico. Il gas arsina inalato viene invece rapidamente assorbito dai polmoni. I sali inorganici di arsenico sono ben assorbiti dal tratto gastrointestinale, dai polmoni e dalla cute; i composti di arsenico organico dal tratto gastrointestinale. Dopo un'esposizione acuta, inizialmente l'arsenico è legato alla porzione proteica dell'emoglobina nei globuli rossi e viene rapidamente distribuito a tutti i tessuti. L'arsenico inorganico è metilato e viene eliminato prevalentemente dai reni, essendo escreto per il 95% nelle urine e per il 5% nella bile. La maggior parte viene espulsa nei primissimi giorni, mentre la parte rimanente viene escreta lentamente nell'arco di diverse settimane. L'arsenico si concentra nei capelli, nelle unghie e nella cute. La misurazione della distanza delle **linee di Mees** (strie bianche trasverse sull'unghia) dal letto ungueale può fornire una stima del tempo di esposizione (le unghie crescono a una velocità di 0,4 mm al giorno).

FISIOPATOLOGIA. Dopo esposizione al gas arsina, quello assorbito entra nei globuli rossi e viene ossidato ad arsenico diidruro e arsenico elementare. La complessazione di questi derivati con i gruppi sulfidrilici del globulo rosso determina l'instabilità di membrana e una emolisi massiva. I sali inorganici di arsenico intossicano i processi enzimatici vitali per il metabolismo cellulare. L'arsenico trivalente si lega ai gruppi sulfidrilici, con una conseguente diminuzione della produzione di adenosina trifosfato attraverso l'inibizione di sistemi enzimatici come la piruvato deidrogenasi e i complessi α-chetoglutarato. L'arsenico pentavalente può essere biotrasformato in arsenico trivalente o sostituito con il fosfato nella via glicolitica, con un conseguente disaccoppiamento della fosforilazione ossidativa.

MANIFESTAZIONI CLINICHE. Il gas arsina è incolore, inodore, non irritante e altamente tossico. L'inalazione non provoca sintomi immediati. Dopo un periodo di latenza di 2-24 ore compare un'emolisi massiva assieme a malessere, cefalea, debolezza, dispnea, nausea, vomito, dolore addominale, epatomegalia, pallore, ittero, emoglobinuria e insufficienza renale (Tab. 708-1). L'ingestione acuta di arsenico produce tossicità gastrointestinale entro minuti o ore e si manifesta con nausea, vomito, dolore addominale e diarrea. La gastroenterite emorragica con ampia perdita di liquidi e accumulo nel terzo spazio può portare a uno shock ipovolemico. La tossicità cardiovascolare comprende l'allungamento dell'intervallo QT, la tachicardia ventricolare po-

TABELLA 708-1. Effetti dell'arsenico sui sistemi d'organo

APPARATO	EFFETTI DELL'ARSENICO
Sistema gastrointestinale	Vescicole sottomucose, diarrea acquosa o ematica, grave ematemesi
Sistema cardiovascolare	Ridotta contrattilità miocardica, intervalli Q-T prolungati, tachiaritmie
	Vasodilatazione, ipotensione
Reni	Ematuria, proteinuria, necrosi tubulare acuta
Sistema nervoso	Encefalopatia tossica con convulsioni, edema cerebrale e coma
	Esposizione cronica: neuropatia sensitivomotoria periferica dolorosa
Sistema ematologico e linfatico	Anemia e trombocitopenia; emolisi acuta con gas arsina
Fegato	Degenerazione adiposa con necrosi centrale
Cute	Desquamazione, alopecia, ipercheratosi, alterazioni ungueali
	Esposizione cronica: ipercheratosi, iperpigmentazione
Teratogenicità	Difetti del tubo neurale nel feto

limorfa, la cardiomiopatia congestizia, l'edema polmonare e lo shock cardiogeno. La tossicità neurologica acuta include delirio, convulsioni, edema cerebrale, encefalopatia e coma. Le dosi letali di arsenati sono di 5-50 mg/kg; quelle di arseniti di <5 mg/kg.

Le **sequele tardive** sono costituite da ematuria, proteinuria e necrosi tubulare acuta. Una neuropatia sensitivomotoria ritardata può comparire a distanza di giorni o settimane dall'esposizione acuta, secondariamente alla degenerazione assonale. La neuropatia si manifesta con disestesie dolorose seguite da una diminuzione della sensibilità vibratoria, dolorifica, tattile e termica, dalla riduzione dei riflessi tendinei profondi e, nei casi più gravi, da una paralisi ascendente con insufficienza respiratoria che simula la sindrome di Guillain-Barré (vedi Capitolo 615).

La **tossicità subacuta** è caratterizzata da affaticamento protratto, malessere, calo ponderale, cefalea, encefalopatia cronica, neuropatia sensitivomotoria periferica, leucopenia, anemia, trombocitopenia, tosse cronica e gastroenterite. Le linee di Mees nelle unghie diventano evidenti dopo 1-2 mesi dall'esposizione in circa il 5% dei pazienti. I reperti dermatologici comprendono alopecia, ulcerazione orale, edema periferico, rash maculare pruriginoso e desquamazione.

L'**esposizione cronica** a bassi livelli di arsenico di solito è dovuta a fonti ambientali o occupazionali. Nel corso degli anni si sviluppano lesioni dermatologiche, tra cui iperpigmentazione, ipopigmentazione, ipercheratosi (specialmente sui palmi delle mani e sulle piante dei piedi), carcinoma squamocellulare e basocellulare e **malattia di Bowen** (carcinoma cutaneo squamocellulare *in situ*). Possono essere presenti encefalopatia e neuropatia periferica e compaiono epatomegalia, ipersplenismo, fibrosi portale non cirrotica e ipertensione portale. La **malattia di Blackfoot** è un'arteriopatia obliterante degli arti inferiori associata a un contatto cronico con l'arsenico che è stata descritta a Taiwan. La cancerogenicità di tale contatto è rispecchiata dagli aumentati tassi di neoplasie della cute, dei polmoni, del fegato, della vescica e dei reni e di angiosarcomi.

REPERTI DI LABORATORIO. La diagnosi d'intossicazione da arsenico si basa sui reperti clinici caratteristici, un'anamnesi di contatto ed elevati livelli urinari di arsenico, che confermano l'esposizione. Un test estemporaneo per l'arsenico urinario dovrebbe essere effettuato nei pazienti sintomatici prima della chelazione, sebbene inizialmente il risultato possa essere negativo. Dal momento che l'escrezione urinaria di arsenico è intermittente, la diagnosi definitiva dipende dalla raccolta delle urine nelle 24 ore, considerando che concentrazioni maggiori di 50 μg/L sono compatibili con l'intossicazione (Tab. 708-2). I campioni devono essere deposti in contenitori privi di metallo. L'ingestione di frutti di mare contenenti arsenobetaina e arsenocolina non tossiche possono causare elevati livelli urinari di arsenico. I suoi livelli ematici raramente risultano utili, a motivo della loro elevata variabilità e della rapida clearance dell'arsenico dal sangue nelle intossicazioni acute. Elevati livelli nei capelli o nelle unghie vanno interpretati con cautela, per la possibilità di contaminazione esterna. Le radiografie addominali possono indicare la presenza di arsenico radiopaco ingerito.

TABELLA 708-2. Livelli normali e tossici di arsenico e mercurio

	ARSENICO	MERCURIO
Peso molecolare	74,9 d	200,59 d
Livello ematico normale	<5 μg/L (<0,665 nmol/L)	<10 μg/L (<50 nmol/L)
Livello urinario normale	<50 μg/L (<6,65 nmol/L) campione di urine delle 24 h	<20 μg/L (<100 nmol/L)
Intervenire a livelli ematici		>35 μg/L (>175 nmol/L)
Intervenire a livelli urinari	>100 μg/L (>13,3 nmol/L) campione di urine delle 24 h	>150 μg/L (>750 nmol/L)

Successivamente nel decorso della malattia, l'emocromo può mostrare anemia, trombocitopenia e leucocitosi seguite da leucopenia, carioressi e punteggiamento basofilo dei globuli rossi. I livelli sierici di creatinina, bilirubina e transaminasi possono apparire elevati; l'esame delle urine può segnalare proteinuria, piuria ed ematuria; l'esame del liquido cerebrospinale può indicare elevati livelli di proteine.

MERCURIO

EPIDEMIOLOGIA. Il mercurio esiste in tre forme: mercurio elementare, sali inorganici di mercurio e mercurio organico (Tab. 708-3). Il **mercurio elementare** è presente nei termometri, negli sfigmomanometri, nei barometri, nelle batterie e in alcune vernici in lattice prodotte prima del 1991. I lavoratori nelle industrie che fabbricano questi prodotti possono esporre i loro figli alla tossina quando il mercurio viene portato a casa sugli indumenti contaminati. La pulizia con aspirapolvere di tappeti contaminati da mercurio e la rottura di lampadine fluorescenti a mercurio possono portare all'esposizione al vapore di mercurio elementare. Gravi intossicazioni da inalazione si sono verificate in seguito a tentativi di separare l'oro dall'oro minerale grezzo o riscaldando il mercurio e formando un amalgama di oro-mercurio. Il mercurio elementare è stato utilizzato in rimedi popolari dalle popolazioni asiatica e messicana per il dolore cronico dello stomaco e dai latinoamericani e dai caraibici in pratiche occulte. Gli amalgami dentari contenenti mercurio elementare rilasciano tracce che non pongono un rischio significativo per la salute; ciò è stato confermato da un gruppo di esperti del National Institutes of Health, che ha concluso che non sarebbe necessario sostituire gli amalgami dentari per ridurre l'esposizione al mercurio.

I **sali inorganici di mercurio** vengono riscontrati in pesticidi, disinfettanti, antisettici, pigmenti, batterie a secco ed esplosivi e come conservanti in alcuni preparati medicinali. Il **mercurio organico** nella dieta, specialmente il pesce che contiene metilmercurio,

TABELLA 708-3. Caratteristiche differenziali dell'esposizione al mercurio

	ELEMENTARE	INORGANICO (SALE)	ORGANICO (ALCHILE)
Via primaria di esposizione	Inalazione	Orale	Orale
Tessuto primario di distribuzione	SNC, rene	Rene	SNC, rene, fegato
Clearance	Renale, GI	Renale, GI	Metile: GI Arile: renale, GI
Effetti clinici			
SNC	Tremore	Tremore	Parestesie, atassia, tremore, visione tubulare, disartria
Polmonare	+++	−	−
Gastrointestinale	+	+++ (caustici)	+
Renale	+	+++ (ATN)	+
Acrodinia	+	++	−
Terapia	BAL, DMSA	BAL, DMSA	DMSA (precocemente)

+, lieve; ++, moderata; +++, grave.

ATN, necrosi tubulare acuta (*Acute Tubular Necrosis*); BAL, British anti-Lewisite; SNC, sistema nervoso centrale; DMSA, acido 2,3-dimercaptosuccinico (*DiMercaptoSuccinic Acid*); GI, gastrointestinale.

Da Sue MJ: Mercury (heavy metals). In: Goldfrank LR, Flomenbaum NE, Lewin NA, et al (editors): *Goldfrank's Toxicologic Emergencies*, 7th ed. McGraw-Hill, 2002. Disponibile su http://www.knovel.com/knovel2/Toc.jsp?BookID=957. Per gentile concessione di The McGraw Hill Companies, Inc.

è una delle vie principali con cui la popolazione generale viene a contatto con il mercurio. Tra le industrie che possono produrre scarichi che comprendono il mercurio vi sono quelle per la produzione di cloro e soda caustica, l'industria mineraria e metallurgica, la placcatura galvanica, l'industria chimica e tessile, la produzione di carta e farmaci e la concia delle pelli. I composti di mercurio nell'ambiente sono metilati a metilmercurio dai microrganismi del suolo e dell'acqua. Il metilmercurio nell'acqua si accumula rapidamente nel pesce (pesce spada, sgombro, tonno fresco, pesce tegola, squalo) e in altri organismi acquatici, che a loro volta sono consumati dall'uomo. Tra le grandi epidemie ben note d'intossicazione da metilmercurio si possono ricordare gli incidenti in Giappone negli anni '50 (**malattia di Minamata,** da consumo di frutti di mare contaminati) e in Iraq nel 1971 (da consumo di cereali trattati con un fungicida contenente metilmercurio).

Il **thimerosal** è un conservante contenente mercurio usato in alcuni vaccini. Nel suo peso, esso ha il 49,6% di mercurio ed è metabolizzato a etilmercurio e tiosalicilato. Durante una revisione continua dei prodotti biologici in risposta al Modernization Act del 1997 della Food and Drug Administration (FDA), la FDA stessa ha stabilito che i bambini che avevano ricevuto vaccini contenenti thimerosal in più visite potevano avere assunto una quantità di mercurio superiore a quella raccomandata dalle linee guida federali. Come misura precauzionale, l'American Academy of Pediatrics, l'American Academy of Family Physicians, l'Advisory Committee on Immunization Practices e lo U.S. Public Health Service hanno emanato una raccomandazione congiunta nel 1999 per rimuovere il thimerosal dai vaccini il più presto possibile. Negli Stati Uniti questo conservante è stato tolto da tutti i vaccini del programma di vaccinazioni raccomandate nell'infanzia. Nei lattanti e nei bambini che hanno ricevuto vaccini con il thimerosal non è tuttavia necessario effettuare alcun test sul sangue, sulle urine o sul capello, in quanto le concentrazioni di mercurio sarebbero piuttosto basse e non richiederebbero un trattamento. I benefici e i rischi dei vaccini con il thimerosal dovrebbero essere discussi con i genitori (come del resto di tutti i vaccini). I maggiori rischi della mancata vaccinazione superano di gran lunga ogni rischio noto di esposizione ai vaccini con il thimerosal. Gli studi non hanno dimostrato un legame tra questi ultimi e le malattie dello spettro autistico (vedi Capitolo 29) e non vi sono prove che suggeriscano di modificare lo standard pratico relativamente alla loro somministrazione nelle aree del mondo dove vengono utilizzati. Un aumento dei livelli ematici di mercurio in seguito a una singola dose di vaccino antiepatite fu osservato in neonati pretermine, ma l'importanza clinica è sconosciuta. L'American Academy of Pediatrics raccomanda che l'inizio della serie di vaccini per l'epatite sia rinviato ai 2-6 mesi di vita nei bambini che sono nati da madri negative per l'antigene di superficie dell'epatite B.

FARMACOCINETICA. Il vapore di mercurio elementare inalato viene assorbito per l'80% dai polmoni e si distribuisce rapidamente al sistema nervoso centrale (SNC) a causa della sua elevata liposolubilità. Il mercurio elementare viene ossidato dalla catalasi a ioni di mercurio, la forma reattiva che provoca tossicità cellulare. Il mercurio elementare liquido viene scarsamente assorbito dal tratto gastrointestinale, essendolo per meno dello 0,1%. La sua emivita nei tessuti è di circa 60 giorni e la maggior parte di esso viene escreta con le urine.

I sali di mercurio inorganico sono assorbiti per il 10% circa dal tratto gastrointestinale e attraversano la barriera ematoencefalica in misura minore rispetto al mercurio elementare. I sali mercurici sono più solubili dei sali mercurosi e pertanto producono maggiore tossicità. L'eliminazione avviene prevalentemente nelle urine, con un'emivita di circa 40 giorni.

Tra i composti di mercurio organico, il **metilmercurio** è quello assorbito più avidamente, dal momento che lo è per circa il 90% dal tratto gastrointestinale. La struttura lipofila e alchilica a catena breve del metilmercurio gli consente di distribuirsi rapidamente attraverso la barriera ematoencefalica e la placenta. Esso viene poi eliminato per il 90% circa nella bile, mentre la parte rimanente viene escreta nelle urine. L'emivita è di 70 giorni.

FISIOPATOLOGIA. Dopo l'assorbimento, il mercurio si distribuisce a tutti i tessuti, in particolare al SNC e ai reni. Reagisce con i gruppi sulfidrilici, fosforilici, carbossilici e amidici, con la conseguente alterazione degli enzimi, dei meccanismi di trasporto, delle membrane e delle proteine strutturali. La disfunzione o la necrosi cellulari diffuse determinano la caratteristica tossicità multiorgano dell'intossicazione da mercurio.

MANIFESTAZIONI CLINICHE. La presentazione clinica dell'intossicazione da mercurio è descritta da cinque sindromi. L'**inalazione acuta del vapore di mercurio elementare** porta al rapido esordio di tosse, dispnea, dolore toracico, febbre, brividi, cefalea e disturbi visivi. I reperti gastrointestinali comprendono sapore metallico, salivazione, nausea, vomito e diarrea. A seconda della gravità dell'esposizione, la malattia può essere autolimitata o può progredire a bronchiolite necrotizzante, polmonite interstiziale, edema polmonare e morte per insufficienza respiratoria. I bambini più piccoli sono maggiormente suscettibili alla tossicità polmonare. I sopravvissuti possono sviluppare pneumopatia restrittiva. In fase subacuta possono comparire disfunzione renale e disturbi neurologici (atassia, debolezza persistente, labilità emotiva). È stato riscontrato che l'esposizione cronica al mercurio elementare volatilizzato negli amalgami dentari non ha alcuna rilevanza clinica.

L'**ingestione acuta di sali inorganici di mercurio** (tipicamente secondaria all'ingestione di una batteria a pastiglia) può presentarsi entro poche ore con una gastroenterite corrosiva che si manifesta con sapore metallico, bruciori orofaringei, nausea, ematemesi, dolore addominale grave, ematochezia, necrosi tubulare acuta, collasso cardiovascolare e morte.

L'**intossicazione cronica da mercurio inorganico** produce la **triade classica** di tremore, disturbi neuropsichiatrici e gengivostomatite. La sindrome può essere dovuta a un'esposizione cronica a mercurio elementare, sali inorganici di mercurio o determinati composti di mercurio organico, tutti i quali possono essere metabolizzati a ioni mercurici. Il tremore inizia come un fremito intenzionale fine delle dita delle mani che s'interrompe durante il sonno, ma successivamente può interessare il volto e progredire alla coreoatetosi e al ballismo spasmodico. Possono esservi anche neuropatia sensitivomotoria mista e disturbi visivi. I disturbi neuropsichiatrici comprendono labilità emotiva, delirio, cefalea, perdita della memoria, insonnia, anoressia e affaticamento. La disfunzione renale va da una proteinuria asintomatica a una sindrome nefrosica.

L'**acrodinia**, o **malattia rosa**, è una rara reazione idiosincrasica da ipersensibilità al mercurio che compare prevalentemente nei bambini esposti a polveri mercurose. Il complesso sintomatologico prevede un dolore generalizzato, parestesie e rash acrale (mani, piedi) che può diffondersi e interessare il volto. Esso è tipicamente rosso-rosa, papulare, pruriginoso e dolente; può progredire alla desquamazione e all'ulcerazione. Sono state descritte varianti morbilliformi, vescicolari ed emorragiche. Altre importanti caratteristiche comprendono l'anoressia, l'apatia, la fotofobia e l'ipotonia, specialmente del cingolo scapolare e del cingolo pelvico. Possono subentrare irritabilità, tremori, diaforesi, insonnia, ipertensione e tachicardia. Alcuni casi inizialmente furono diagnosticati come feocromocitomi. La prognosi è buona, dopo la rimozione della fonte dell'esposizione al mercurio.

L'**intossicazione da metilmercurio** è nota anche come **malattia di Minamata**, dopo l'intossicazione diffusa da mercurio verificatasi a Minamata Bay in Giappone in soggetti che avevano ingerito pesce contaminato. Si presenta come una neurotossicità ritardata dopo un periodo di latenza di settimane o mesi ed è caratterizzata da atassia, disartria, parestesie, tremori, disturbi del movimento, compromissione della vista, dell'udito, dell'olfatto e del gusto, perdita della memoria, demenza progressiva e morte. I bambini esposti in utero sono affetti più gravemente, con basso peso alla nascita, microcefalia, grave ritardo di sviluppo, paralisi cerebrale, sordità, cecità e convulsioni. Sebbene vi sia una significativa morbilità residua da neurotossicità da metilmercurio, le osservazioni nel follow-up a lungo termine dei bambini esposti in

Iraq rivelano una risoluzione completa o parziale nella maggior parte dei casi.

REPERTI DI LABORATORIO. La diagnosi di intossicazione da mercurio si basa su reperti clinici caratteristici, un'anamnesi di esposizione e l'aumento dei livelli di mercurio nel sangue intero o nelle urine, che confermano l'esposizione. Si possono utilizzare tecniche su strato sottile e gascromatografiche per distinguere tra mercurio organico e inorganico. Il sangue dovrebbe essere raccolto in apposite provette per elementi in traccia da laboratori che sono in grado di effettuare tali test. Livelli $<$10 μg/L nel sangue intero e $<$20 μg/L nelle urine raccolte nelle 24 ore sono considerati normali (vedi Tab. 708-2). Sebbene i livelli ematici di mercurio possano riflettere l'esposizione acuta, essi si riducono quando il mercurio si ridistribuisce nei tessuti. I livelli urinari risultano più utili per identificare le esposizioni croniche, tranne che nel caso del metilmercurio, perché esso viene eliminato in misura minima con le urine. I livelli urinari di mercurio sono utilizzati per monitorare l'efficacia della terapia chelante, mentre i livelli ematici si usano prevalentemente per il monitoraggio delle intossicazioni da mercurio organico. L'analisi del capello non è affidabile, in quanto i capelli rispecchiano l'esposizione endogena ed esogena al mercurio (i capelli legano avidamente il mercurio dall'ambiente). Le radiografie addominali possono mostrare mercurio radiopaco ingerito.

Tra i marker urinari di nefrotossicità precoce vi sono la microalbuminuria, la retinol-binding protein, la β_2-microglobulina e l'*N*-acetyl-β-D-glucosaminidasi. La neurotossicità precoce può essere identificata mediante test neuropsichiatrici e studi di conduzione nervosa, mentre la tossicità grave del SNC è evidente alla TC o alla RM.

TRATTAMENTO DELL'INTOSSICAZIONE DA ARSENICO E DA MERCURIO

I principi del trattamento dell'intossicazione da arsenico e da mercurio comprendono la tempestiva eliminazione della sorgente d'intossicazione, la stabilizzazione e la terapia di supporto aggressive, la decontaminazione e la terapia chelante quando appropriato. Se si sospetta la diagnosi, si dovrebbe contattare il servizio locale di controllo delle intossicazioni (o il centro antiveleni, *N.d.C.*) e si dovrebbero coordinare le terapie con medici che hanno familiarità con il trattamento dell'intossicazione da metallo pesante.

La terapia di supporto per i pazienti esposti a gas arsina richiede uno stretto monitoraggio dei segni di emolisi, compresi la valutazione dello striscio di sangue periferico e l'esame delle urine. Può essere necessaria la trasfusione di globuli rossi concentrati, così come la somministrazione per via endovenosa di liquidi, bicarbonato di sodio e mannitolo per prevenire l'insufficienza renale secondaria al deposito di emoglobina nei reni. In seguito all'inalazione di vapore di mercurio elementare, i pazienti vanno sottoposti a uno stretto monitoraggio dello stato respiratorio, che può comprendere la pulsossimetria, l'emogasanalisi arteriosa e la radiografia del torace. La terapia di supporto prevede la somministrazione di ossigeno supplementare e, nei casi gravi, l'intubazione e la ventilazione meccanica.

L'ingestione acuta di sali inorganici di arsenico e mercurio porta alla gastroenterite emorragica, al collasso cardiovascolare e alla disfunzione multiorgano. La rianimazione con fluidi, gli agenti pressori e la trasfusione di prodotti del sangue possono essere necessari per il trattamento dell'instabilità cardiovascolare. Un distress respiratorio grave, il coma con perdita dei riflessi delle vie aeree, convulsioni intrattabili e una paralisi respiratoria sono indicazioni all'intubazione e alla ventilazione meccanica. La funzionalità renale deve essere monitorata con attenzione e nel caso di segni d'insufficienza subentra la necessità dell'emodialisi.

La decontaminazione gastrointestinale dopo l'ingestione dei sali di arsenico e mercurio inorganico non è stata ben studiata. A causa degli effetti corrosivi di questi composti, l'induzione del vomito non è raccomandata e l'endoscopia può essere presa in considerazione prima della lavanda gastrica. L'arsenico e il mercurio non sono ben adsorbiti dal carbone attivo, ma il suo utilizzo può risultare utile se si sospettano ingestioni concomitanti. L'irrigazione intestinale in toto viene utilizzata per eliminare eventuale materiale radiopaco che rimane nel tratto gastrointestinale.

La **chelazione** per l'intossicazione acuta da arsenico e da mercurio è più efficace quando viene somministrata il più presto possibile dopo l'esposizione. Dovrebbe essere continuata fino a quando i livelli urinari delle 24 ore di arsenico o mercurio ritornano nella norma ($<$50 μg/L per l'arsenico e $<$20 μg /L per il mercurio), il paziente diventa asintomatico o si ritiene che gli effetti tossici residui siano irreversibili. L'efficacia della chelazione nelle esposizioni croniche è ridotta, perché il metallo pesante nel compartimento tissutale è relativamente non scambiabile e si è già verificato un certo grado di tossicità irreversibile.

Il **dimercaprolo**, noto anche come 2,3-dimercaptopropanolo o British anti-Lewisite (BAL), è il chelante di scelta se il paziente non può tollerare la terapia per os, come spesso avviene nei soggetti critici e dopo l'ingestione dei sali corrosivi di arsenico e di mercurio inorganico. Negli Stati Uniti il BAL è disponibile in sospensione in olio di arachidi e benzil benzoato in fiale da 3 mL a una concentrazione di 100 mg/mL per l'iniezione intramuscolare (im) profonda. Per l'**intossicazione da arsenico**, lo schema raccomandato di BAL è 2,5 mg/kg im ogni 6 h per i primi 2 giorni, 2,5 mg/kg im ogni 12 h il terzo giorno, quindi 2,5 mg/kg/die im per 10 giorni. Per l'intossicazione grave da arsenico, la dose di BAL viene aumentata a 3 mg/kg im ogni 4 h per 2 giorni, 3 mg/kg im ogni 6 h il terzo giorno, quindi 3 mg/kg im ogni 12 h per 10 giorni. La dose per l'**intossicazione da mercurio inorganico** è di 5 mg/kg im il primo giorno, quindi 2,5 mg/kg im ogni 12-24 h per 10 giorni. Il complesso BAL-metallo pesante viene escreto nelle urine e nella bile. Si raccomanda un periodo di 5 giorni tra i cicli di chelazione. Tra gli effetti avversi si possono citare il dolore nel punto d'iniezione, l'ipertensione, la tachicardia, la diaforesi, la nausea, il vomito, il dolore addominale, una sensazione urente nell'orofaringe e una sensazione di costrizione toracica. Il BAL può anche provocare emolisi nei soggetti con deficit della glucosio-fosfato deidrogenasi (G6PD). È importante notare che esso è controindicato per la chelazione del metilmercurio, perché lo ridistribuisce al cervello da altre sedi tissutali, con un conseguente aumento della neurotossicità.

La **D-penicillamina** è un chelante somministrato per os che può essere preso in considerazione per l'intossicazione meno grave da mercurio o in aggiunta alla terapia con il BAL nell'intossicazione da arsenico, ma il suo utilizzo è stato ampiamente limitato a causa del rischio di leucopenia, trombocitopenia e proteinuria significative. Un analogo studiato più recentemente, la *N*-acetyl-d,l-penicillamina, è stato adoperato con successo variabile nell'intossicazione da mercurio.

Gli agenti chelanti per os vengono usati in sostituzione delle iniezioni dolorose del BAL quando il paziente è sufficientemente stabile da tollerare la terapia orale e la chelazione prolungata si rende necessaria. Il **succimero**, noto anche come acido 2,3-dimercaptosuccinico (DMSA), è un derivato idrosolubile del BAL somministrato per os. Negli Stati Uniti è disponibile in capsule da 100 mg. Il regime terapeutico raccomandato è di 1050 mg/m^2/24 h (o 30 mg/kg/24 h) per os suddivisi in tre dosi per 5 giorni, quindi 700 mg/m^2/24 h (o 20 mg/kg/24 h) per os suddivisi in due dosi per 14 giorni. Il complesso DMSA-metallo pesante viene escreto nelle urine e nella bile. Si raccomanda un periodo di 2 settimane tra i cicli di chelazione. Tra gli effetti avversi lievi compaiono nausea, vomito, diarrea, inappetenza e transitori aumenti dei livelli degli enzimi epatici. Il DMSA può anche causare emolisi nei pazienti con un deficit di G6PD. Nei soggetti che hanno ingerito mercurio elementare non è necessario alcun follow-up, tranne che in presenza di una malattia sottostante che riduca il tempo di transito gastrointestinale. Sono raccomandate radiografie addominali seriali per documentare la progressione del metallo. In caso d'inalazione acuta di fumi di mercurio e d'ingestione di mercurio inorganico è necessaria l'ospedalizzazione per monitorare rispettivamente le condizioni respiratorie e gastrointestinali.

L'aborto terapeutico può essere preso in considerazione nelle pazienti gravide, a causa dell'effetto teratogeno del mercurio.

American Academy of Pediatrics, Committee on Environmental Health: Technical report: Mercury in the environment. Implications for pediatricians. *Pediatrics* 2001;108:197–204.

Bae M, Wantanabe C, Inaoka T, et al: Arsenic in cooked rice in Bangladesh. *Lancet* 2002;360:1839–1840.

Baum CR: Treatment of mercury intoxication. *Curr Opin Pediatr* 1999;11:265–268.

Bolger PM, Schwetz BA: Mercury and health. *N Engl J Med* 2002;347:1735–1736.

Centers for Disease Control and Prevention: Summary of the joint statement on thimerosal in vaccines. American Academy of Family Physicians, American Academy of Pediatricians, Advisory Committee on Immunization Practices, Public Health Service. *MMWR* 2000;49:622–631.

Centers for Disease Control and Prevention: Mercury exposure–Kentucky, 2004. *MMWR* 2005;54:797–798.

Clarkson TW, Magos L, Myers GJ: The toxicology of mercury–Current exposures and clinical manifestations. *N Engl J Med* 2003;349:1731–1736.

Cullen NM, Wolf LR, St Clair D: Pediatric arsenic ingestion. *Am J Emerg Med* 1995;13:432–435.

Ford M: Arsenic (heavy metals). In: Goldfrank LR, Flomenbaum NE, Lewin NA, et al (editors): *Goldfrank's Toxicologic Emergencies,* 7th ed. McGraw-Hill, 2002. Available at http://www.knovel.com/knovel2/Toc.jsp?BookID=957.

Heron J, Golding J; ALSPAC Study Team: Thimerosal exposure in infants and developmental disorders: A prospective cohort study in the United Kingdom does not support a causal association. *Pediatrics* 2004;114:577–583.

Horowitz Y, Greenberg D, Ling G, et al: Acrodynia: A case report of two siblings. *Arch Dis Child* 2002;86:453–455.

Innis SM, Palaty J, Vaghri Z, et al: Increased levels of mercury associated with high fish intakes among children from Vancouver, Canada. *J Pediatr* 2006;148:759–763.

Jacobson JL, Jacobson SW: Risks to child health from methylmercury exposure in immigrant populations. *J Pediatr* 2006;148:716–718.

Kondo K: Congenital Minamata disease: Warnings from Japan's experience. *J Child Neurol* 2000;15:458–464.

Lai MW, Boyer EW, Kleinman ME, et al: Acute arsenic poisoning in two siblings. *Pediatrics* 2005;116:249–257.

McLellan F: Arsenic contamination affects millions in Bangladesh. *Lancet* 2002;359:1127.

Mitchell RJ, Osborne PB, Haubenreich JE: Dental amalgam restorations: Daily mercury dose and biocompatibility. *J Long Term Eff Med Implants* 2005;15:709–721.

Parker SK, Schwartz B, Todd J, et al: Thimerosal-containing vaccines and autistic spectrum disorder: A critical review of published original data. *Pediatrics* 2004;114:793–804.

Pichichero ME, Cernichiari E, Lopreiato J, et al: Mercury concentrations and metabolism in infants receiving vaccines containing thiomersal: A descriptive study. *Lancet* 2002;360:1737–1740.

Schober SE, Sinks TH, Jones RL, et al: Blood mercury levels in US children and women of childbearing age, 1999–2000. *JAMA* 2003;289:1667–1674.

Stajich GV, Lopez GP, Harry SW, et al: Iatrogenic exposure to mercury after hepatitis B vaccination in preterm infants. *J Pediatr* 2000;136:679–681.

Sue YJ: Mercury (heavy metals). In: Goldfrank LR, Flomenbaum NE, Lewin NA, et al (editors): *Goldfrank's Toxicologic Emergencies,* 7th ed. McGraw-Hill, 2002. Available at http://www.knovel.com/knovel2/Toc.jsp?BookID=957.

Capitolo 709 ■ Intossicazione da piombo

Morri Markowitz

EPIDEMIOLOGIA

Il piombo è un metallo esistente in quattro forme isotopiche. Dal punto vista chimico, il suo basso livello di fusione e la capacità di formare composti stabili ha fatto sì che sia utilizzato nella manifattura di centinaia di prodotti. Dal punto di vista clinico è però una sostanza tossica; nessun organismo ha funzioni essenziali piombo-dipendenti. La sua attrattiva commerciale ha comunque determinato la lavorazione di milioni di tonnellate di minerale di piombo, portando a una sua grande diffusione nell'ambiente.

Il livello soglia a cui il piombo causa alterazioni biochimiche e disturbi subclinici o clinici è stato ridefinito molte volte negli ultimi 50 anni. Il livello di sangue nel piombo (BLL, *Blood Lead Level*) è il gold standard per determinare gli effetti sulla salute. I Centers for Disease Control and Prevention (CDC), l'American Academy of Pediatrics (AAP) e diverse altre organizzazioni nazionali e internazionali (per es. Global Lead Network – Alliance to End Childhood Lead Poisoning e The National Referral Centre for Lead Poisoning, in India) hanno stabilito che un BLL di 10 μg/dL o maggiore indica la necessità di intervenire per trattare il rischio. Tuttavia, effetti tossici da piombo sono stati osservati in bambini con un BLL inferiore a questa soglia, sicché il CDC sta attualmente considerando se abbassarlo.

CENNI STORICI DI SANITÀ PUBBLICA

Tra il 1976 e il 1980, oltre l'85% dei bambini americani in età prescolare aveva un BLL >10 μg/dL e tra essi il 98% era afroamericano. Nei successivi 15 anni, le disposizione governative hanno determinato una riduzione significativa dei tre principali fattori che determinano la produzione di piombo, mediante: (1) l'eliminazione dell'uso della benzina con piombo tetraetile; (2) la proibizione dell'uso di leghe-saldature contenenti piombo per sigillare i contenitori di alimenti e bevande; (3) l'applicazione di un regolamento federale che ha limitato la quantità di piombo consentita nelle vernici destinate alle abitazioni a meno dello 0,07% del loro peso. La sorveglianza da parte dei CDC ha evidenziato che la prevalenza di BLL elevati è diminuita in modo marcato e dal 2000 meno del 3% di tutti i bambini in età prescolare aveva livelli elevati. Dei bambini colpiti, circa il 10% avrà un BLL maggiore di quello clinicamente significativo, cioè 25 μg/dL. I bambini con livelli sufficientemente elevati da risultare a rischio di vita sono rari, ma i decessi continuano a verificarsi. Si stima che mezzo milione di bambini americani ha ancora livelli significativi di BLL. I fattori che indicano un aumento del rischio d'intossicazione da piombo, oltre all'età prescolare, comprendono un basso livello socioeconomico, vivere in case vecchie costruite prima del 1960, la permanenza in città, l'appartenenza alla razza afroamericana. Altri gruppi a rischio elevato includono gli immigrati recenti, inclusi gli adottati, provenienti da Paesi che usano ancora benzina con il piombo o ceramiche smaltate con vernici contenenti piombo.

Anche a livello mondiale sono comunque stati fatti progressi. Dal 1999, 29 Paesi hanno completamente eliminato il piombo dalla benzina e anche alcuni Paesi in via di sviluppo/in transizione di Asia, America Latina, Europa dell'Est, Nord Africa hanno sviluppato piani di rimozione. A Malta, dopo il divieto d'importazione di vernice contenente piombo rosso e il divieto di usare legno trattato con il piombo come combustibile nei forni, i livelli medi di piombo delle donne incinte e dei neonati si sono ridotti del 45%. In Messico l'introduzione di benzina senza piombo nel 1990 è stata associata a una riduzione della piombemia tra gli studenti di prima elementare dai 17 μg/dL di quell'anno a 6,2 μg/dL nel 1997. Dopo che è stato documentato che in Nicaragua i bambini che vivevano nelle vicinanze di un'industria di batterie avevano livelli medi di piombemia di 17,2 μg/dL, mentre quelli della comunità di controllo erano di 7,4 μg/dL, la fabbrica è stata chiusa. Tuttavia, malgrado i progressi si stima che a livello mondiale il 40% di tutti i bambini ha una piombemia maggiore di 5 μg/dL e il 20% di essi possiede livelli superiori a 10 μg/dL; il 90% di questi bambini vive nei Paesi in via di sviluppo, dove in alcune regioni i livelli di piombo sono 10-20 volte più alti rispetto a quelli dei Paesi sviluppati.

FONTI DI ESPOSIZIONE

L'intossicazione da piombo può avvenire in utero, dal momento che il piombo del sangue materno attraversa rapidamente la placenta. Lo spettro degli effetti tossici è simile a quello che riguarda i bambini dopo la nascita. La fonte del contenuto di piombo nel sangue materno dipende sia dalla ridistribuzione dalle riserve endogene (per es. lo scheletro della madre) sia dal piombo appena acquisito per un'esposizione ambientale in atto.

Diverse centinaia di prodotti contengono piombo, comprese le batterie, il rivestimento dei cavi, i cosmetici, i supplementi minerali, le plastiche e i giocattoli (Tab. 709-1). Le fonti principali di esposizione variano tra i vari Paesi e anche all'interno degli stessi; negli Stati Uniti le vecchie vernici contenenti piombo restano la fonte principale. Circa 25 milioni di famiglie vivono in case costruite prima del 1950, un periodo che ha visto il massimo uso di queste vernici. Quando si deteriorano, esse si sfaldano e producono polvere. Il lavoro di restauro-rinnovo effettuato in maniera non corretta delle superfici verniciate con questi prodotti (per es. sabbiatura, levigatura, carteggiatura) può produrre in casa polvere contenente piombo. Questa può ricoprire tutte le superfici, comprese le mani dei bambini. Tutte queste forme di piombo possono inoltre essere ingerite. Se viene usato il calore per eliminare la vernice, la concentrazione di vapori di piombo nella stanza può raggiungere livelli sufficienti a causare un'intossicazione attraverso l'inalazione.

METABOLISMO

L'abitudine dei bambini di portare le mani alla bocca rappresenta la via principale d'ingresso del piombo nell'organismo. In quasi tutti i casi il piombo viene ingerito, come polvere leccata dalle superfici o deglutita dai frammenti di vernice, attraverso l'acqua contaminata nel passaggio per tubature di piombo o per rubinetti di ottone, o con cibi e bevande contaminate per il contatto con contenitori di ceramica smaltata. La contaminazione cutanea con composti inorganici del piombo, come quelli dei pigmenti, non determina un assorbimento significativo. I composti organici come il piombo tetraetile possono penetrare attraverso la pelle.

La percentuale di piombo assorbita dall'intestino dipende da diversi fattori: dimensione delle particelle, pH, presenza di altri materiali nell'intestino stesso e stato nutrizionale degli elementi essenziali. I frammenti di vernice grandi sono difficili da digerire e per gran parte vengono escreti. La polvere sottile si può dissolvere più facilmente, soprattutto in un mezzo acido. Il piombo ingerito a digiuno viene assorbito meglio rispetto a quello assunto insieme a un pasto. La presenza di calcio e ferro può ridurre l'assorbimento del piombo mediante la competizione diretta con i siti di legame; il deficit di ferro (e probabilmente quello di calcio) determina invece un aumento dell'assorbimento di piombo, la sua ritenzione e la tossicità.

Dopo l'assorbimento, il piombo si distribuisce in tutto l'organismo, circolando legato agli eritrociti: circa il 97% si trova sulla loro superficie o dentro i globuli rossi. La frazione nel plasma è troppo piccola per essere misurata con le tecniche convenzionali; presumibilmente si tratta della porzione che entra nelle cellule e induce tossicità. Il piombo esercita diversi effetti nelle cellule. Si lega agli enzimi, soprattutto a quelli che hanno gruppi sulfidrilici disponibili, alterandone la struttura e riducendone l'attività.

La via sintetica dell'eme, presente in tutte le cellule, ha tre enzimi sensibili agli effetti inibitori esercitati dal piombo. L'ultimo enzima di questa via, la ferrochetalasi, permette alla protoporfirina di chelare il ferro, formando l'eme. La protoporfirina è facilmente misurabile nei globuli rossi. Livelli >di 35 μg/dL non sono considerati normali e sono indicativi di un'intossicazione da piombo, di carenza di ferro o di malattia flogistica recente. La scarsità di eme colpisce diverse vie metaboliche. L'accumulo di quantità eccessive di protoporfirine e di altri precursori dell'eme è comunque tossica, sicché la misurazione dei livelli di **protoporfirina eritrocitaria** (**EP**, *Erythrocyte Protoporphyrin*) rappresenta uno strumento utile per monitorare gli effetti biochimici dell'intossicazione da piombo. Questi livelli aumentano alcune settimane dopo che il BLL ha raggiunto 20 μg/dL in una porzione suscettibile della popolazione e saranno elevati in quasi tutti i bambini con un BLL >50 μg/dL. La caduta dei livelli dell'EP segue la riduzione del BLL di diverse settimane, sia per la cessazione da parte del midollo osseo di iperprodurre precursori dei globuli rossi sia per il turn-over cellulare.

Un secondo meccanismo di tossicità del piombo si attua attraverso la sua competizione con il calcio. Molte proteine leganti il calcio hanno un'affinità per il piombo maggiore rispetto a quella per il calcio stesso. il piombo legato a queste proteine può alterarne la funzione, determinando una falsificazione nel segnale intra- e intercellulare. Il rilascio dei neurotrasmettitori è un processo calciodipendente che viene in parte modificato dal piombo.

Sebbene questi due meccanismi tossici siano reversibili, ve ne è un terzo che previene lo sviluppo della struttura cerebrale terziaria normale. Nei mammiferi immaturi, il processo normale di riduzione che determina l'eliminazione delle connessioni multiple intercellulari cerebrali viene inibito dal piombo. L'incapacità di costruire una struttura cerebrale terziaria appropriata durante i primi anni di vita può provocare un'anomalia permanente. Si sta cercando di estrapolare da questi reperti anatomici i correlati clinici del disturbo da deficit dell'attenzione/iperattività osservato nei bambini intossicati con il piombo.

EFFETTI CLINICI

Il BLL è l'indicatore più studiato dell'accumulo di piombo nei bambini. Sebbene le caratteristiche cliniche e subcliniche si correlino al BLL nella popolazione, esiste una variabilità interindividuale considerevole in questa connessione. L'encefalopatia da piombo è più probabile nei bambini con un BLL >100 μg/dL; tuttavia, un bambino con un BLL di 300 μg/dL può non presentare sintomi, mentre un altro con gli stessi valori potrà sviluppare un edema cerebrale. La diversa suscettibilità può essere collegata al polimorfismo dei geni che codificano per le proteine leganti il piombo, come l'acido delta-aminolevulinico deidratasi, un enzima della via sintetica dell'eme.

Diversi **effetti subclinici** del piombo sono stati evidenziati da studi epidemiologici trasversali. Nei bambini l'**udito** e l'**altezza** sono inversamente correlati al BLL; tuttavia, in nessun caso l'effetto del piombo raggiunge un livello tale da richiedere la consultazione medica. All'aumentare del BLL nella popolazione allo studio, è necessario un suono più elevato (a tutte le frequenze) per raggiungere la soglia dell'udito. I bambini con un BLL più alto sono leggermente più bassi di quelli con livelli inferiori; ogni 10 μg d'incremento del BLL, essi risultano più bassi di 1 cm. L'esposizione cronica al piombo può anche essere responsabile di una pubertà ritardata.

Vari studi longitudinali hanno seguito gruppi di bambini dalla nascita fino ai 20 anni di età ed esaminato la relazione tra il BLL e i **punteggi ai test cognitivi** nel tempo. In generale, c'è accordo che i BLL, espressi sia come reperto ottenuto a circa 2 anni sia come parametro che integra diversi BLL ricavati dal soggetto nel tempo, sono inversamente correlati ai punteggi nei test cognitivi.

TABELLA 709-1. Fonti di piombo

Frammenti di vernice
Polvere
Terreno
Esposizione legata al lavoro dei genitori
Ceramica smaltata
Medicine a base di erbe (per es. ayurvediche)
Rimedi casalinghi tra cui antitraspiranti, deodoranti (per es. litargirio)
Gioielleria (dei genitori o bigiotteria dei giochi)
Magazzini di rivestimenti di batterie (o vivere vicino a fonderie di batterie)
Benzina con piombo
Dolci messicani
Poligono di tiro
Spezie importate (swanuri marili, zafron, kozhambu)
Cosmetici contenenti piombo (kohl, surma)
Tubature (acqua)
Cibi importati in contenitori a base di piombo

In media, ogni μg/dL di aumento nel BLL corrisponde a circa 1/4 o 1/2 di punto in meno nei punteggi dei test cognitivi. Questi dati non si basano su valutazioni concomitanti di piombo e cognitività. I livelli del BLL della prima infanzia sono predittori dei risultati nei test cognitivi eseguiti anni dopo e ciò indica che gli effetti cognitivi sono permanenti.

L'effetto dell'esposizione al piombo in utero è controverso. Sono stati raccolti punteggi alla Bayley Scale of Mental Development in maniera ripetuta ogni 6 mesi nei primi due anni di vita in un gruppo di neonati appartenenti alla classe media. I risultati sono inversamente correlati al BLL del cordone ombelicale, ma non al BLL ottenuto contestualmente al momento della valutazione dello sviluppo. Inoltre, dopo i 2 anni di età e nei successivi 10 anni tutti gli altri test cognitivi eseguiti nel gruppo si correlavano con il BLL a 2 anni e non con quello del cordone ombelicale, indicando che gli effetti dell'esposizione al piombo nel periodo prenatale sulla funzione cerebrale sono stati sostituiti da eventi nella prima infanzia e successivamente dal BLL.

Uno studio d'intervento, in cui bambini con un'intossicazione da piombo moderata con un BLL iniziale di 20-55 μg/dL sono stati trattati in modo aggressivo per 6 mesi, ha indirizzato l'interesse degli effetti del trattamento sullo sviluppo. La terapia ha compreso l'educazione sulle fonti del piombo e la sua eliminazione, un supporto nutrizionale, visite multiple a domicilio e in clinica e per un sottogruppo anche una terapia chelante. Il BLL medio diminuiva e i punteggi cognitivi erano inversamente correlati ai suoi cambiamenti. Per ogni μg/dL di riduzione del BLL, i punteggi ai test cognitivi erano più alti di 1/4 di punto.

Anche il **comportamento** è influenzato in modo grave dall'esposizione al piombo. In bambini piccoli in età scolare con un'anamnesi d'intossicazione da piombo o con un concomitante aumento del BLL è stata riscontrata iperattività. I bambini più grandi con un'elevata quantità di piombo nelle ossa risultano con maggiore probabilità più aggressivi e presentano comportamenti predittivi di una successiva delinquenza giovanile. Attraverso un unico piccolo studio si è valutato se gli effetti del piombo sul comportamento siano reversibili. Bambini iperattivi di 7 anni con un BLL di 20 sono stati sottoposti in modo randomizzato alla somministrazione o di un agente chelante (penicillamina), o di metilfenidato o di un placebo. Le valutazioni dell'insegnante e dei genitori rispetto al loro comportamento erano migliori nei primi due gruppi, ma non in quello che aveva ricevuto il placebo. Il BLL diminuiva solo nel gruppo che aveva ricevuto la terapia chelante.

SINTOMI CLINICI

SISTEMA GASTROINTESTINALE E SISTEMA NERVOSO CENTRALE. I **sintomi gastrointestinali** comprendono anoressia, dolore addominale, vomito e stipsi, che frequentemente si presentano o ricorrono dopo settimane. I bambini con un BLL >20 μg/dL hanno una probabilità doppia di avere disturbi gastrointestinali rispetto a quelli con un BLL più basso. I **sintomi a carico del SNC** sono correlati all'edema cerebrale e a un aumento della pressione endocranica. Cefalea, alterazione dell'attività mentale, letargia, papilledema, convulsioni e coma che porta al decesso sono rari con livelli <100 μg/dL, ma sono stati riportati anche in bambini con livelli bassi, di 70 μg/dL. L'ultimo decesso direttamente attribuibile alla tossicità da piombo negli Stati Uniti è avvenuto nel 2006, in un bambino con un BLL di 180 μg/dL. Non esiste un cut-off definito dei livelli ematici di piombo per la comparsa d'iperattività, ma questa si osserva con maggiore probabilità in bambini con livelli >20 μg/dL.

Possono venire colpiti anche altri organi dagli effetti tossici del piombo, ma i sintomi di solito non si evidenziano nei bambini. A livelli elevati (>100 μg/dL) si osserva una **disfunzione tubulare renale**. Il piombo può inoltre provocare la sindrome di Fanconi reversibile (vedi Capitolo 529). Quando il BLL risulta elevato, la **sopravvivenza dei globuli rossi** è minore e può portare ad anemia emolitica, sebbene la maggior parte dei casi di anemia nei bambini con intossicazione da piombo sia dovuta ad altri fattori, come la carenza di ferro e le emoglobinopatie. I pazienti più grandi possono sviluppare una neuropatia periferica.

DIAGNOSI

SCREENING. Si valuta che circa il 99% dei bambini intossicati dal piombo vengano identificati mediante procedure di screening piuttosto che tramite il riconoscimento clinico dei sintomi dell'intossicazione. Fino al 1997 lo screening con valutazione della piombemia in tutti i bambini di 12 e 24 mesi era lo standard negli Stati Uniti. Data la riduzione a livello nazionale della diffusione dell'intossicazione da piombo, si è poi raccomandato di eseguire questa valutazione nella popolazione a rischio. Il grado di rischio è direttamente correlato alla probabilità di esposizione. I Departments of Health sono responsabili della determinazione della diffusione a livello locale dell'intossicazione da piombo e della percentuale di abitazioni costruite prima del 1950, periodo di massimo uso di vernici contenenti piombo. Una volta che si sono ottenuti questi dati, si possono stabilire linee guida informative per lo screening per i medici di base. Per esempio, nello Stato di New York, dove una grande percentuale di case è stata costruita prima del 1950, il Department of Health ha stabilito che **tutti i bambini** devono essere esaminati per un'eventuale intossicazione mediante esami del sangue. In assenza di queste informazioni, i medici di base devono continuare a valutare tutti i bambini a 12 e a 24 mesi. In aree in cui la diffusione dell'intossicazione è bassa e le abitazioni vecchie sono poche, si effettua una valutazione del rischio per decidere chi sottoporre allo screening. Il questionario è formato da tre domande di base (Tab. 709-2), cui possono essere aggiunte notizie utili dal punto di vista locale o individuale. È indicato effettuare l'esame del sangue, se il bambino risiede nelle vicinanze di un complesso industriale che utilizza piombo, se è immigrato recentemente da zone in cui viene ancora consentito l'uso della benzina con il piombo, se presenta pica o ritardo dello sviluppo. Devono essere sottoposti a screening tutti i bambini assistibili da Medicaid. Il sangue venoso si preferisce a quello capillare, perché la possibilità di falsi positivi e negativi è minore.

INTERPRETAZIONE DEI LIVELLI EMATICI DI PIOMBO. Il livello soglia perché si verifichino gli effetti del piombo e il livello di attenzione che conduce al trattamento del rischio non sono gli stessi. Quest'ultimo, per i CDC e per l'AAP, attualmente è di 10 μg/dL; un valore di screening pari o maggiore indica la necessità di ripetere il test per confermare la diagnosi e definire l'intervento. Il momento in cui eseguire nuovamente la valutazione dipende dal valore iniziale (Tab. 709-3). Se il secondo test diagnostico

TABELLA 709-2. Questionario di rischio personale minimo

1. Il bambino vive o frequenta regolarmente abitazioni costruite prima del 1950? (Compresi asili, abitazione della baby-sitter o dei parenti)
2. Il bambino vive in, o frequenta regolarmente, abitazioni costruite prima del 1978 con recenti restauri o ristrutturazioni (negli ultimi 6 mesi)?
3. Il bambino ha fratelli o compagni di gioco che hanno o hanno avuto intossicazione da piombo?

Da *Screening Young Children for Lead Poisoning: Guidance for State and Local Public Health Officials*. Atlanta, GA, Centers for Disease Control and Prevention, 1997.

TABELLA 709-3. Follow-up del test di screening della piombemia

SE LO SCREENING DEL LIVELLO DI PIOMBEMIA (μg/dL) È:	*CDC* RIPETERE LA PIOMBEMIA SU SANGUE VENOSO IN:	*AAP* RIPETERE LA PIOMBEMIA SU SANGUE VENOSO IN:
10-19	3 mesi	1 mese
20-44	1 settimana-1 mese (prima se la piombemia è più alta)	1 settimana
45-59	48 ore	48 ore
60-69	24 ore	48 ore
≥70	immediatamente	immediatamente

AAP, American Academy of Pediatrics; CDC, Centers for Disease Control and Prevention.
Adattata da *Screening Young Children for Lead Poisoning: Guidance for State and Local Public Health Officials*. Atlanta, GA, Centers for Disease Control and Prevention, 1997; e American Academy of Pediatrics, Committee on Environmental Health: Screening for elevated blood lead levels. *Pediatrics* 1998;101:1072-1078.

conferma che il BLL è elevato, è necessario un ulteriore esame come da raccomandazioni (Tab. 709-4). **La conferma che il BLL nel sangue venoso è ≥45 μg/dL indica la necessità di una pronta terapia chelante.**

ALTRI STRUMENTI PER LA VALUTAZIONE. La determinazione della piombemia resta il gold standard per valutare i bambini. Sono disponibili tecniche per misurare il piombo in altri tessuti e liquidi corporei. Sperimentalmente, il metodo della fluorescenza a raggi X (XRF, *X-Ray Fluorescence*) permette una valutazione diretta e non invasiva dei depositi ossei del piombo. La tecnica XRF è stata usata per esaminare una popolazione che aveva avuto un'esposizione al piombo a lungo termine a causa dell'inquinamento originato da un impianto di riciclaggio delle batterie. Lo studio ha evidenziato che i bambini in età scolare presentavano nelle ossa livelli elevati di piombo, ma che non avevano alti BLL, ciò che risulta significativo, dal momento che è noto un turn over lento del piombo a livello dell'osso, valutabile negli anni, in contrasto con quello del sangue, dov'è rilevabile in settimane. Questo studio indica anche che i bambini possono avere piombo in quantità significative nel proprio corpo senza che esso venga rilevato dagli esami del sangue di routine per la piombemia. Questi depositi di piombo possono venire rilasciati e raggiungere livelli tossici, se il tasso di riassorbimento osseo aumenta in modo improvviso, come nel caso di una immobilizzazione che si prolunghi per oltre una settimana o durante la gravidanza. Quindi i bambini con un'anamnesi di BLL elevati sono potenzialmente a rischio di recrudescenza di tossicità da piombo molto dopo che il contatto è cessato e possono trasferire questo piombo alle generazioni successive. Il piombo può inoltre essere misurato nelle urine. L'escrezione spontanea, anche in bambini con BLL alti, di solito è bassa, ma può essere stimolata dalla terapia con agenti chelanti; la proprietà di questi farmaci costituisce anzi il motivo del loro impiego come parte della terapia dell'intossicazione da piombo ed è stata usata anche per sviluppare un test che contraddistingue i bambini con accumulo di piombo che rispondono alla terapia chelante: il **Test di Mobilizzazione del Piombo.**

In una sua versione, si usa un protocollo standardizzato che include una dose fissa di farmaco (500 mg/m^2 di calcio-disodio-edetato [$CaNa_2EDTA$] in una dose per via intramuscolare combinata con un 1% di procaina in rapporto di 1:1 per volume), seguita da una raccolta delle urine di 6-8 ore analizzate per il contenuto di piombo. I criteri applicati (Pb nelle urine/dose di calcio-disodio-edetato >0,6 o Pb nelle urine >200 μg/volume) portano alla selezione dei bambini che con maggiore probabilità rispondono all'intero ciclo terapeutico con un'aumentata escrezione del piombo. Interrogativi di tipo pratico (per es. raccogliere le urine del neonato per 6-8 ore in ambulatorio) e teorico (per es. avviene una ridistribuzione del piombo dopo una dose singola di agente chelante che può causare un aumento transitorio del piombo nel cervello? Esistono evidenze che dimostrino l'efficacia a lungo termine nei bambini chelati su questa base?) hanno limitato l'utilizzo di questo test diagnostico a pochi esperimenti nei centri medici.

Anche il piombo nei capelli si può determinare, ma ciò presenta problemi di contaminazione e d'interpretabilità. È necessaria una ricerca più approfondita, prima di definire indicazioni per l'esame dei capelli. Vengono pertanto utilizzati altri test per la valutazione indiretta dell'esposizione e dell'accumulo del piombo. Le radiografie delle ossa lunghe possono evidenziare bande dense a livello delle metafisi che possono risultare difficili da distinguere dalle linee di arresto della crescita, ma, quando causate dal piombo, sono indicative di un periodo di esposizione da mesi ad anni. Per i bambini con sintomi acuti, quando il BLL non è immediatamente disponibile, un KUB può rivelare macchie radiopache a livello intestinale, segno significativo d'ingestione recente d'intonaco o di frammenti di vernice contenenti piombo. Tuttavia, l'assenza di reperti radiografici non esclude la possibilità di un'intossicazione.

Dato che il BLL riflette l'ingestione recente o la ridistribuzione da altri tessuti, ma non è necessariamente correlato con l'accumulo di piombo nell'organismo o con la sua tossicità in un singolo bambino, possono essere utili test sugli effetti del piombo. Dopo alcune settimane di accumulo del piombo e un BLL >20 μg/dL, si può avere un incremento dei livelli di protoporfirina eritrocitaria (EP) >35 μg/dL. Un livello elevato di EP che non può essere attribuito a una carenza di ferro o a una malattia infiammatoria recente costituisce sia un indicatore dell'effetto del piombo sia un test utile per stabilire il successo del trattamento; i livelli inizieranno a diminuire poche settimane dopo il successo terapeutico, che riduce l'ingestione di piombo e ne aumenta l'escrezione. Dal momento che l'EP è sensibile alla luce, l'intero campione di sangue deve essere coperto da un foglio di alluminio (o equivalente) fino a che non viene analizzato.

TABELLA 709-4. Riepilogo delle raccomandazioni per bambini con concentrazioni elevate di piombemia confermata (nel sangue venoso)

PIOMBEMIA	RACCOMANDAZIONI

10-14 μg/dL	Educazione sull'esposizione al piombo
	  Nutrizionale
	  Ambientale
	Follow-up della piombemia con monitoraggio a 1-3 mesi

15-19 μg/dL	Educazione sull'esposizione al piombo
	  Nutrizionale
	  Ambientale
	Follow-up piombemia e monitoraggio a 1-2 mesi
	Procedere in accordo con quanto previsto per 20-24 μg/dL se al follow-up la concentrazione della piombemia è in questo range almeno 3 mesi dopo il test venoso iniziale o se la piombemia è aumentata

20-44 μg/dL	Educazione sull'esposizione al piombo
	  Nutrizionale
	  Ambientale
	Follow-up piombemia e monitoraggio a 1 settimana-1 mese (prima se più alto)
	Anamnesi completa ed esame obiettivo
	Esami di laboratorio
	  Emoglobina o ematocrito
	  Stato del ferro
	Investigazione ambientale
	Riduzione del rischio da piombo
	Monitoraggio dello sviluppo neurologico
	Radiografia addominale (se si sospetta l'ingestione di una particella di piombo) con decontaminazione dell'intestino se indicato

45-69 μg/dL	Educazione sull'esposizione al piombo
	  Nutrizionale
	  Ambientale
	Follow-up piombemia e monitoraggio
	Esami di laboratorio
	  Emoglobina o ematocrito
	  Stato del ferro
	  EP libera o ZPP
	Valutazione ambientale
	Riduzione del rischio di esposizione al piombo
	Monitoraggio dello sviluppo neurologico
	RX addome con decontaminazione dell'intestino se indicato
	Terapia chelante

≥70 μg/dL	Ricovero e inizio terapia chelante Procedere in accordo a quanto indicato per 45-69 μg/dL

NON RACCOMANDATO PER QUALSIASI CONCENTRAZIONE DI PIOMBEMIA

Ricerca delle linee gengivali causate dal piombo
Valutazione della funzionalità renale (eccetto durante terapia chelante con $CaNa_2EDTA$)
Valutazione capelli, denti, unghie delle mani per la presenza di piombo
RX ossa lunghe
Fluorescenza a raggi X delle ossa lunghe

EDTA, acido etilendiamminicotetracetico (*EthyleneDiamineTetraacetic Acid*); EP, protoporfirina eritrocitaria; ZPP, zinco protoporfirina.

Da American Academy of Pediatrics: Lead exposure in children: Prevention, defection, and management. *Pediatrics* 2005;116:1036-1046.

TRATTAMENTO

Una volta che il piombo è nell'osso, viene rilasciato lentamente ed è difficile rimuoverlo anche con l'uso di agenti chelanti. Dato che gli effetti cognitivi/comportamentali del piombo possono essere irreversibili, lo sforzo maggiore nel trattare l'intossicazione va fatto nel **prevenire** che accada ed **evitare** l'ulteriore ingestione da parte del bambino già intossicato. Gli elementi principali per impedire l'intossicazione sono universalmente applicabili a tutti i bambini (e agli adulti): (1) identificazione ed eliminazione delle fonti ambientali di esposizione al piombo; (2) modificazione dell'abitudine di portare le mani alla bocca; (3) counseling nutrizionale per assicurare un apporto adeguato di elementi essenziali quali calcio e ferro. Per una minor parte di bambini con un'intossicazione grave è disponibile il trattamento farmacologico per aumentare l'escrezione del piombo.

Durante le visite di controllo viene garantita una valutazione del rischio che include domande pertinenti alle fonti di esposizione più frequenti: lo stato delle vernici vecchie; l'esposizione occupazionale secondaria per un adulto che vive in casa; la vicinanza a una fonte industriale d'inquinamento. Se una di queste fonti viene identificata, la sua eliminazione solitamente necessiterà dell'assistenza da parte della sanità pubblica e delle agenzie abitative, così come di educazione per i genitori. La famiglia deve lasciare l'abitazione contaminata dal piombo fino a che non saranno completate le riparazioni, durante le quali sarà necessario lavare ripetutamente le superfici e usare un aspiratore dotato di un filtro ad alta efficienza per aria con particolato, che aiuterà nel ridurre il contatto con polveri contenenti piombo. È necessaria un'attenta selezione della ditta che svolgerà i lavori, la quale deve essere certificata nell'esecuzione dell'eliminazione del piombo. Un lavoro non accurato può generare la disseminazione di polvere e frammenti contenenti piombo nella casa o nell'edificio, determinando un ulteriore aumento del BLL nel bambino. Una volta che il lavoro sarà completato, vanno raccolti campioni di polvere asciutta dal pavimento, dal davanzale o dalla tromba delle scale per assicurarsi che il rischio d'intossicazione sia stato eliminato.

Spesso si scopre un caso singolo d'intossicazione in un componente di una famiglia costituita da più membri, inclusi bambini piccoli, anche in famiglie con una fonte comune di esposizione come la rimozione di vernice a base di piombo. La semplice presenza di piombo in un ambiente non determina necessariamente un'intossicazione. Il tentativo dei genitori di **evitare** che il bambino colpito **porti le mani alla bocca** è necessario per ridurre il rischio d'ingestione. Lavare le mani rimuove il piombo, ma in un'abitazione con polvere contenente piombo, esso si accumula velocemente sulle mani del bambino dopo il lavaggio. Di conseguenza, questa azione diventa utile solo prima di mangiare portando le mani alla bocca.

Dato che vi è competizione tra il piombo e i minerali essenziali, è ragionevole favorire una dieta sana con un apporto adeguato di calcio e ferro. L'assunzione giornaliera raccomandata di questi nutrienti varia con l'età. In generale, per i bambini di un anno e oltre è sufficiente un apporto di calcio di circa 1 g/die (pressappoco il contenuto di un quarto di latte [~1200 mg/qt] o di un succo d'arancia fortificato con calcio). L'assorbimento del calcio è vitamina D-dipendente; il latte è fortificato con la vitamina D, ma altre fonti nutrizionali di calcio spesso non lo sono. Nei bambini che non assumono latte in quantità sufficienti o che hanno un'esposizione alle radiazioni solari inadeguata può venire prescritto un multivitaminico con vitamina D. Anche il fabbisogno di ferro varia con l'età, andando da 6 mg/die per i neonati a 12 mg/die per gli adolescenti. Nei bambini che risultano carenti di ferro dal punto di vista biochimico, diventa appropriata una terapia a base di ferro alla dose giornaliera di 5-6 mg/kg per 3 mesi. L'assorbimento del ferro viene potenziato dall'assunzione di acido ascorbico (succo di agrumi). La somministrazione di supplementazioni di calcio o ferro, al di sopra dell'assunzione raccomandata quotidiana, a bambini che possiedono minerali in quantità sufficiente non esplica effetti benefici dal punto di vista terapeutico nel trattamento dell'intossicazione da piombo.

Il **trattamento farmacologico** per eliminare il piombo è salvavita nei bambini con l'encefalopatia da piombo, mentre in quelli non encefalopatici previene la progressione dei sintomi e l'ulteriore tossicità. Le linee guida per la chelazione si basano sul BLL. Un bambino con il BLL nel sangue venoso ≥4 μg/dL deve essere sottoposto a terapia. Negli Stati Uniti sono disponibili 4 farmaci: acido 2,3 dimercaptosuccinico (DMSA [succimero]), $CaNa_2EDTA$ (versenato), British anti-Lewisite (BAL [dimercaprolo]) e penicillamina. Il DMSA e la penicillamina vengono somministrati per via orale, mentre il $CaNa_2EDTA$ e il BAL solo per via parenterale. La scelta del farmaco dipende dalla gravità dell'intossicazione, dalla sua efficacia e dalla facilità di utilizzo (Tab. 709-5). I bambini con un BLL di 44-70 μg/dL possono essere trattati con un farmaco singolo, preferibilmente il DMSA; quelli con un BLL di 70 μg/dL o superiore necessitano di 2 farmaci: il $CaNa_2EDTA$ in combinazione con il DMSA o il BAL per chi risulta senza evidenze di encefalopatia o il $CaNa_2EDTA$ e il BAL per quelli con l'encefalopatia. Sono molto limitati i dati sul trattamento combinato del $CaNa_2EDTA$ e del DMSA nei bambini con un BLL >100 μg/dL.

Le tossicità correlate ai farmaci sono meno importanti e risultano reversibili. Gli effetti avversi comprendono distress gastrointestinale, aumento transitorio delle transaminasi, sedimento urinario attivo e neutropenia. Questi effetti sono minori per il $CaNa_2EDTA$ e il DMSA e più comuni per il BAL e la penicillamina. Tutti i farmaci sono efficaci nel ridurre il BLL se vengono somministrati alla dose sufficiente e per la durata prevista. Essi possono anche aumentare l'assorbimento del piombo da parte dell'intestino e vanno fatti assumere ai bambini in ambienti privi di piombo. Alcuni specialisti raccomandano, in aggiunta, la somministrazione di un lassativo immediatamente prima o in concomitanza con l'inizio della chelazione, per eliminare ogni traccia del piombo già presente nell'intestino.

Nessuno di questi agenti, in ogni caso, rimuove il piombo dall'intestino per intero. Entro giorni-settimane dalla fine del ciclo terapeutico, il BLL aumenta anche in assenza di una nuova ingestione di piombo. La causa di questo rebound si ritiene sia l'osso. Valutazioni in serie del contenuto di piombo dell'osso mediante XRF hanno evidenziato che la chelazione con $CaNa_2EDTA$ si associa a una riduzione dei suoi livelli ma la quota di piombo residuo a livello osseo resta evidente anche dopo cicli multipli di trattamento.

TABELLA 709-5. Terapia chelante

NOME	SINONIMO	DOSAGGIO	EFFETTI COLLATERALI
Succimero	Chemet, DMSA	350 mg/m^2/dose (**non 10 mg/kg**) ogni 8 ore, per os per 5 giorni, poi ogni 12 ore per 14 giorni	Disturbi gastrointestinali, rash, aumento test di funzionalità epatica, depressione leucocitaria
Edetato*	$CaNa_2EDTA$, versenato	1000-1500 mg/m^2/d; infusione ev: continua o intermittente; im suddivisi ogni 6 o ogni 12 ore. Per 5 giorni	Proteinuria, piuria, aumento BUN/creatinina: tutti rari. Ipercalcemia se troppo rapida come infusione Flogosi tissutale se infusione per infiltrazione
BAL	Dimercaprolo, British anti-Lewisite	300-500 mg/m^2/die; im solo suddivisi ogni 4 ore. Per 3-5 giorni. Solo per BLL ≥70	Disturbi gastrointestinali, alterazione attività mentali; aumento test di funzionalità epatica, emolisi se c'è deficit di G6PD; no terapia a base di ferro concomitante
D-Pen	Penicillamina	10 mg/kg/d per 2 sett aumentando a 25-40 mg/kg/d; orale, suddivisi ogni 12 ore. Per 12-20 settimane	Rash, febbre; discrasia ematica, aumento test di funzionalità epatica, proteinuria Reazione allergica cross-reattiva con la penicillina

***Somministrato sempre come sali di calcio; mai come sali di sodio senza calcio.**

BAL, British anti-Lewisite; BUN, azoto ureico (*Blood Urea Nitrogen*); $CaNa_2EDTA$, sodio calcio edetato; DMSA, acido 2,3-dimercaptosuccinico; G6PD, glucosio-6-fosfato deidrogenasi.

Da Markowitz ME: Lead poisoning. Pediatr Rev 2000;21:327-335.

La chelazione ripetuta è indicata se il rebound del BLL è ≥45 μg/dL. I bambini con un BLL iniziale >70 μg/dL probabilmente necessitano di più di un ciclo. Si raccomanda un intervallo di almeno 3 giorni tra i cicli di terapia, per prevenire gli effetti collaterali specialmente a livello renale.

L'indicazione per la terapia chelante per i bambini con un BLL <45 μg/dL è meno chiara. L'uso di questi farmaci in bambini con un BLL di 20-44 μg/dL determina una sua diminuzione transitoria e in alcuni ciò si accompagna all'annullamento dell'inibizione dell'enzima causata dal piombo. Tuttavia, in pochi soggetti l'escrezione di piombo durante la chelazione aumenterà in modo significativo e ciò solleva la questione se sia stato raggiunto un beneficio a lungo termine. In uno studio su bambini di 2 anni con un BLL di 20-44 μg/dL, ai quali venne somministrato random il DMSA o un placebo, si è visto che la riduzione del BLL era maggiore nei primi 6 mesi dopo l'arruolamento nel gruppo trattato con il DMSA, ma i livelli convergevano dopo 1 anno di follow-up. I punteggi ai test cognitivi a 4 e 7 anni non apparvero poi differenti in modo significativo nei due gruppi. La chelazione con il DMSA (e il $CaNa_2EDTA$) non è raccomandata in tutti quei bambini con un BLL di 20-44 μg/dL. Un altro gruppo da sottoporre alla terapia chelante comprende i bambini che rispondono alla dose test di un agente chelante con un aumento della escrezione urinaria di piombo (un'indicazione che il farmaco è efficace nel rimuovere il piombo in modo permanente dall'organismo). Questi bambini possono essere identificati mediante il test di mobilizzazione del piombo. Non sono disponibili dati per nessuno dei due casi, che dimostrino miglioramenti nei risultati cognitivi per chi è stato chelato su queste basi. Allo stesso modo resta da dimostrare che vi siano altri agenti chelanti, negli Stati Uniti o altrove, efficaci nel ridurre i depositi corporei (ossei) di piombo o nell'eliminare i deficit cognitivi attribuibili al piombo.

Con un intervento efficace, il BLL diminuisce e la riduzione più importante si ha nei primi 2 mesi dall'inizio della terapia. Successivamente la velocità di variazione del BLL cala lentamente, così che 6-12 mesi dopo l'identificazione il BLL del bambino medio con una intossicazione moderata (BLL >20 μg/dL) sarà inferiore (più basso) del 50%. I bambini con un BLL marcatamente elevato possono impiegare anni per raggiungere la soglia accettabile di 10 μg/dL, anche se tutte le fonti di esposizione al piombo sono state eliminate, il comportamento è stato modificato e la nutrizione implementata. Lo screening precoce resta il modo migliore di evitare e quindi di prevenire il bisogno del trattamento per l'intossicazione da piombo.

American Academy of Pediatrics: Lead exposure in children: prevention, detection, and management. *Pediatrics* 2005;116:1036–1046.

Berkowitz S, Tarrago R: Acute brain herniation from lead toxicity. *Pediatrics* 2006;118:2548–2551.

Canfield RL, Henderson CR Jr, Cory-Slechta DA, et al: Intellectual impairment in children with blood lead concentrations below 10 microg per deciliter. *N Engl J Med* 2003;348:1517–1526.

Centers for Disease Control and Prevention: Death of a child after ingestion of a metallic charm–Minnesota, 2006. *MMWR* 2006;55:340–341.

Centers for Disease Control and Prevention: Deaths associated with hypocalcemia from chelation therapy–Texas, Pennsylvania and Oregon, 2003–2005. *MMWR* 2006;55:204–206.

Centers for Disease Control and Prevention: Lead exposure from indoor firing ranges among students on shooting teams–Alaska, 2002–2004. *MMWR* 2005;54:577–579.

Centers for Disease Control and Prevention: Lead poisoning associated with use of litargirio–Rhode Island, 2003. *MMWR* 2005;54:227–229.

Centers for Disease Control and Prevention: Lead poisoning associated with Ayurvedic medications–Five states, 2000–2003. *MMWR* 2004;53: 582–586.

Centers for Disease Control and Prevention: Surveillance for elevated blood lead levels among children–United States, 1997–2001. *MMWR* 2003;52: 1–21.

Centers for Disease Control and Prevention: Childhood lead poisoning associated with Tamarind county and folk remedies. *MMWR* 2002;51:684–686.

Centers for Disease Control and Prevention: Fatal pediatric lead poisoning–New Hampshire, 2000. *MMWR* 2001;50:457–459.

Committee on Drugs, American Academy of Pediatrics: Treatment guidelines for lead exposure in children. *Pediatrics* 1995;96:155–160.

Committee on Environmental Health, American Academy of Pediatrics. Screening for elevated blood lead levels. *Pediatrics* 1998;101:1072–1078.

Dietrich KN, Ware JH, Salganik M, et al: Effect of chelation therapy on the neuropsychological and behavioral development of lead-exposed children after school entry. *Pediatrics* 2004;114:19–26.

Florin TA, Brent RL, Weitzman M: The need for vigilance: the persistence of lead poisoning in children. *Pediatrics* 2005;115:1767–1768.

Global Lead Network: Alliance to End Childhood Lead Poisoning. Website at http://www.globalleadnet.org.

Kemper AR, Cohn LM, Fant KE, et al: Follow-up testing among children with elevated screening blood lead levels. *JAMA* 2005;293:2232–2237.

Lanphear BP: Childhood lead poisoning prevention. *JAMA* 2005;293: 2274–2276.

Laraque D, Trasande L: Lead poisoning: successes and 21st century challenges. *Pediatr Rev* 2005;26:435–443.

Meyer PA, Pivetz T, Dignam TA, et al: Surveillance for elevated blood lead levels among children–United States, 1997–2001. *MMWR Surveill Summ* 2003;52(10):1–21.

Selevan SG, Rice DC, Hogan KA, et al: Blood lead concentration and delayed puberty in girls. *N Engl J Med* 2003;348:1527–1536.

Tellez-Rojo MM, Bellinger DC, Arroyo-Quiroz C, et al: Longitudinal associations between blood lead concentrations lower than 10 microg/dL and neurobehavioral development in environmentally exposed children in Mexico City. *Pediatrics* 2006;118:323–330.

Woolf AD, Woolf NT: Childhood lead poisoning in 2 families associated with spices used in food preparation. *Pediatrics* 2005;116:e314–e318.

Wright NJ, Thacher TD, Pfitzner MA, et al: Causes of lead toxicity in a Nigerian city. *Arch Dis Child* 2004;90:262–266.

Capitolo 710 ■ Intossicazione alimentare non batterica

Denise A. Salerno e Stephen C. Aronoff

710.1 • AVVELENAMENTO DA FUNGHI

La raccolta e il consumo di funghi selvatici, un'abitudine diffusa in Europa, sta diventando sempre più frequente negli Stati Uniti, dove ha comportato un aumento di avvelenamenti gravi e letali da funghi.

Le sindromi cliniche causate dall'avvelenamento da funghi si classificano in base alla rapidità d'insorgenza dei sintomi e al sistema principalmente coinvolto. I sintomi sono dovuti alla tossina presente nei funghi ingeriti. Le otto tossine principali prodotte dai funghi si dividono nelle seguenti categorie: ciclopeptidi, monometilidrazina, muscarina, indoli allucinogeni, isossazoli, coprini (reazione simile al disulfiran), orellanina, irritanti GI (gastrointestinali)-specifici. Inoltre, la parte edibile del *Tricholoma equestre* è stata associata alla rabdomiolisi ritardata, mentre si è visto che il *Clytocybe amoenolens* e il *Clitocybe acromelalgia* sono responsabili di eritromelalgia, ma sono sconosciute le tossine che generano questi effetti.

SISTEMA GASTROINTESTINALE: INSORGENZA RITARDATA

AVVELENAMENTO DA AMANITA. L'avvelenamento da specie *Amanita* e *Galerina* rende conto del 95% dei decessi dovuti a una intossicazione da funghi; il tasso di mortalità in questo gruppo è del 5-10%. La maggior parte delle specie produce due classi di tossine ciclopeptidiche: (1) fallotossine, che sono eptapeptidi ritenuti responsabili dei sintomi precoci dell'avvelenamento da *Amanita,* e (2) amanitotossina, un octapeptide che inibisce la

RNA polimerasi e la conseguente produzione di RNA messaggero. Le cellule a rapido turn-over, come quelle della mucosa gastrointestinale, dei reni e del fegato, sono le più gravemente colpite.

L'avvelenamento da *Amanita* determina una necrosi cellulare che può verificarsi in tutto il tratto gastrointestinale, il sistema maggiormente esposto. L'atrofia giallo-acuta del fegato e la necrosi dei tubuli renali prossimali si riscontrano nei casi letali.

Il **decorso clinico** legato all'avvelenamento da *Amanita* o da *Galerina* è bifasico, dopo un periodo asintomatico iniziale di latenza di 6-24 ore. Trascorso tale lasso di tempo dall'ingestione, si hanno nausea, vomito e dolore addominale severo; quindi segue una diarrea acquosa profusa che può durare 12-24 ore. In questa fase possono essere persi sino a 9 litri di liquidi. Da 24 a 48 ore dall'avvelenamento subentrano ittero, aumento delle transaminasi (con picco a 72-96 ore), insufficienza renale e coma. La morte avviene dopo 4-7 giorni. Un tempo di protrombina inferiore al 10% di quello di controllo rappresenta un fattore prognostico non favorevole.

Trattamento. Il trattamento dell'avvelenamento da *Amanita* è sia di supporto sia specifico. La perdita di liquidi legata alla diarrea severa nelle fasi iniziali è cospicua, necessitando di una terapia aggressiva per la sua correzione. Nella fase tardiva occorre trattare l'insufficienza renale ed epatica.

La terapia specifica mira a rimuovere rapidamente la tossina e a bloccare il legame al suo sito bersaglio. Il carbone attivo e il lattulosio per via orale combinati con la somministrazione di liquidi ed elettroliti sono raccomandati come parte del trattamento iniziale nei bambini. Dovrebbe essere evitata la diuresi forzata, in quanto aumenta l'esposizione del rene. La penicillina G endovena (400 000 U/kg/die) in infusione continua combinata con la silibinina, la forma idrosolubile del flavolignone silimarina (20-50 mg/kg/die ev), agisce in modo sinergico inibendo il legame delle tossine e interrompendo la circolazione enteroepatica dell'amanitotossina. Anche l'emodialisi e l'emoperfusione sono consigliate come parte del trattamento iniziale. Il trapianto ortotopico del fegato si raccomanda in bambini in cui si è sviluppata una grave insufficienza epatica (vedi Capitolo 365).

INTOSSICAZIONE DA MONOMETILIDRAZINA. La specie *Gyromitra* contiene monometilidrazina (CH_3NHNH_2), che inibisce la produzione enzimatica di acido γ-aminobutirrico nel sistema nervoso centrale (SNC). La monometilidrazina ossida inoltre il ferro dell'emoglobina con la formazione di metaemoglobina. I bambini con avvelenamento da *Gyromitra* sviluppano vomito, diarrea, ematochezia e dolore addominale entro 6-24 ore dall'ingestione della tossina. I sintomi della depressione del sistema nervoso centrale e le convulsioni si sviluppano in una fase successiva del decorso clinico. L'emolisi e la metaemoglobinemia rappresentano complicanze potenzialmente fatali. La **metaemoglobinemia** severa può richiedere la dialisi.

Trattamento. L'ipovolemia da perdita di liquidi gastrointestinali e le convulsioni richiedono una terapia di supporto. Il piridossalfosfato, il coenzima che catalizza la produzione di acido γ-aminobutirrico, può fare regredire gli effetti della monometilidrazina, se viene somministrato ad alto dosaggio. La **piridossina idrocloruro** (**25 mg/kg**) è inoculata endovena con una frequenza che dipende dal miglioramento clinico. La somministrazione per via parenterale di blu di metilene è indicata se la concentrazione di metaemoglobina supera il 30%. In caso di emolisi grave possono essere necessarie trasfusioni di sangue.

SISTEMA RENALE: INSORGENZA RITARDATA

AVVELENAMENTO DA ORELLANINA. La specie *Cortinarius* possiede la tossina termo-stabile orellanina bipiridina, responsabile di un danno renale non glomerulare severo caratterizzato da fibrosi interstiziale e necrosi tubulare acuta. Il meccanismo esatto del danno è sconosciuto. L'avvelenamento da *Cortinarius* è caratterizzato da nausea, vomito e diarrea, che insorgono 36-48 ore dopo l'ingestione. Sebbene i sintomi iniziali possano essere di scarsa rilevanza, dopo diversi giorni si può presentare una tossicità renale più grave. L'insufficienza renale acuta subentra nel 30-50% dei soggetti colpiti; inizia con una poliuria ed evolve verso l'insufficienza.

Trattamento. Il **trattamento** dell'avvelenamento da orellanina è di supporto. I sintomi iniziali, dopo 4-6 ore dall'ingestione, possono venire trattati con carbone attivo e lavanda gastrica. Nei pazienti con insufficienza renale può essere necessaria l'emodialisi. La maggior parte dei pazienti guarisce in un mese, ma dal 30 al 50% sviluppa una insufficienza renale cronica.

SISTEMA NERVOSO AUTONOMO: INSORGENZA RAPIDA

AVVELENAMENTO DA MUSCARINA. I funghi dei generi *Inocybe* e, in grado minore, *Clytocibe* contengono la muscarina o composti correlati a essa. Questi derivati dell'ammonio quaternario si legano ai recettori postsinaptici, provocando una risposta colinergica abnorme.

Le **manifestazioni cliniche** sono caratterizzate da una risposta colinergica con insorgenza rapida dei sintomi (30 minuti-2 ore dall'ingestione) e consistente in sudorazione intensa, lacrimazione eccessiva, scialorrea, miosi, incontinenza urinaria e fecale e vomito. La complicanza più grave è il distress respiratorio causato dal broncospasmo e dall'aumento delle secrezioni broncopolmonari. I sintomi regrediscono spontaneamente in 6-24 ore.

Trattamento. L'atropina solfato, l'antidoto specifico, è somministrata per via endovenosa (0,01 mg/kg; max 2 mg). Questo trattamento va ripetuto finché non si risolvono i sintomi respiratori o se il paziente diventa estremamente tachicardico.

INGESTIONE DI COPRINO. Il *Coprinus atramentarius* e il *Clytocibe clavipes* contengono il coprino. Come il disulfiram (antabuse), il coprino inibisce il metabolismo dell'acetaldeide in seguito all'ingestione di etanolo. La sintomatologia deriva dall'accumulo di acetaldeide.

L'intossicazione da coprino diviene evidente dopo l'ingestione di etanolo e può presentarsi fino a 5 giorni dopo il consumo dei funghi. L'iperemia del volto e del tronco, un formicolio alle mani, un sapore metallico, la tachicardia e il vomito sono sintomi che si manifestano in modo acuto. L'ipotensione può essere una conseguenza dell'intensa vasodilatazione periferica.

La sindrome generalmente si autolimita e dura solo alcune ore. Non è disponibile un antidoto specifico. Se l'ipotensione è grave, può essere necessaria la riespansione vascolare con soluzioni isotoniche. Sono state suggerite anche piccole dosi di propranololo per via orale.

SISTEMA NERVOSO CENTRALE: INSORGENZA RAPIDA

INTOSSICAZIONE DA ISOSSAZOLO. Sebbene l'*Amanita muscaria* e l'*Amanita panterina* possano contenere la muscarina, le tossine responsabili di sintomi a carico del SNC dopo l'ingestione di questi funghi sono il muscimolo e l'acido ibotenico, derivati termostabili degli isossazoli. Il muscimolo, un allucinogeno e l'acido ibotenico, un insetticida, hanno effetti colinergici. Da 30 minuti a 3 ore dopo, compaiono i sintomi a carico del SNC: ottundimento, alternanza di letargia e agitazione, occasionalmente convulsioni. Sono poco frequenti la nausea e il vomito. Se i funghi contengono quantità elevate di muscarina si possono avere sintomi di crisi colinergica.

La **terapia** specifica deve essere selezionata con attenzione. Se si osserva una risposta colinergica esagerata va utilizzata l'atropina. Dato che l'ingestione dell'*Amanita muscaria* è spesso associata a sintomi colinergici, viene usata la fisostigmina, inibitrice dell'acetilcolinesterasi, per fare regredire il delirio e il coma. Le convulsioni vengono controllate con il diazepam. Nella maggior parte dei casi, comunque, il trattamento in fase iniziale con l'ipecacuana (se il paziente è cosciente) e un'attenta osservazione sono tutto ciò che occorre.

INTOSSICAZIONE DA INDOLO. I funghi che appartengono al genere *Psylocibe* ("funghi magici") contengono psilocibina e psilocina, composti psicotropi. Entro 30 minuti dall'ingestione, i pazienti manifestano euforia e allucinazioni, spesso accompagnate da tachicardia e midriasi. Si sono osservate anche febbre e convulsioni nei bambini con avvelenamento da psilocibina. Questi sintomi sono di breve durata: in genere persistono per 6 ore dopo il consumo dei funghi. I pazienti con una forte agitazione possono essere trattati con il diazepam.

SISTEMA GASTROINTESTINALE: INSORGENZA RAPIDA

Molti funghi di vari generi provocano sintomi gastrointestinali. Le tossine responsabili sono diverse e in gran parte sconosciute. Entro 1 ora dall'ingestione, i pazienti presentano un dolore addominale acuto, nausea, vomito e diarrea. I sintomi possono durare ore o giorni, in base alla specie del fungo.

Il **trattamento** è prevalentemente di supporto. I bambini con una perdita cospicua di liquidi necessitano di una terapia reidratante parenterale. Risulta fondamentale differenziare l'ingestione di funghi appartenenti a questa classe dall'ingestione di specie di *Amanita* e *Galerina* che contengono tossine della classe dei ciclopeptidi.

Bedry R, Baudrimont I, Deffieux G, et al: Brief report: Wild mushroom intoxication as a cause of rhabdomyolysis. *N Engl J Med* 2001;345:798-804.

Berger KJ, Guss DA: Mycotoxins revisited: Part I. *J Emerg Med* 2005;28: 53-62.

Berger KJ, Guss DA: Mycotoxins revisited: Part II. *J Emerg Med* 2005;28: 175-183.

Diaz JH: Evolving global epidemiology, syndromic classification, general management, and prevention of unknown mushroom poisonings. *Crit Care Med* 2005;33:419-426.

Diaz JH: Syndromic diagnosis and management of confirmed mushroom poisonings. *Crit Care Med* 2005;33:427-436.

Klein AS, Hart J, Brems JJ, et al: *Amanita* poisoning: Treatment and the role of liver transplantation. *Am J Med* 1989;86:187-193.

McDonald A: Mushrooms and madness: Hallucinogenic mushrooms and some psychopharmacological implications. *Can J Psychiatry* 1980;25:586-594.

Sabeel AI, Kurkus J, Lindholm T: Intensive hemodialysis and hemoperfusion treatment of *Amanita* mushroom poisoning. *Mycopathologia* 1995;131:107-114.

710.2 • INTOSSICAZIONE DA SOLANINA

La solanina è una miscela di diverse tossine correlate che si trovano nelle patate verdi e germogliate. Le patate esposte alla luce e lasciate germogliare producono diversi glucosidi alcaloidi contenenti solanidina, un derivato del colesterolo. Due di questi glucosidi, l'α-solanina e l'α-caconina, si trovano in alte concentrazioni nelle bucce delle patate verdi e nei germogli. Gli alcaloidi della solanina si legano alla colinesterasi sierica, suggerendo un possibile meccanismo fisiopatologico.

Le **manifestazioni cliniche** dell'intossicazione da solanina si presentano entro 7-19 ore dall'ingestione. I sintomi più frequenti sono il vomito e la diarrea; nei casi più gravi si hanno febbre, dolore addominale generalizzato, coma e shock ipovolemico.

Il **trattamento** è in gran parte di supporto. Nei casi più gravi i sintomi si risolvono entro 11 giorni. Non è stato valutato il trattamento con l'atropina.

Korpan YI, Nazarenko EA, Skryshevskaya IV, et al: Potato glycoalkaloids: True safety or false sense of security? Trends Biotechnol 2004;22:147-151.

McMillan M, Thompson JC: An outbreak of suspected solanine poisoning in school boys: Examination of criteria of solanine poisoning. Q J Med 1979;48:227-243.

710.3 • INTOSSICAZIONE DA ALIMENTI MARINI

INTOSSICAZIONE DA PESCE CON CIGUATERA

Le principali epidemie d'intossicazione da pesce con ciguatera si sono verificate in Florida, Hawaii, Carabi, Sud Pacifico, Isole Vergini. Con i mezzi di trasporto attuali, la malattia si presenta ora in tutto il mondo. La cernia è la fonte principale in cui è stata identificata la tossina, seguita da pesce ballerino, pesce re, seriola, delfino, anguilla e barracuda. L'intossicazione è stata anche associata al salmone da allevamento.

La fonte di questo avvelenamento è il dinoflagellato *Gambierdiscus toxicus*, un microrganismo unicellulare riscontrato lungo i banchi corallini che produce concentrazioni elevate di ciguatossina e maitotossina. Le tossine vengono passate lungo la catena alimentare dai piccoli pesci erbivori che consumano i dinoflagellati dei banchi corallini ai pesci predatori più grandi e quindi all'uomo. Queste tossine sono innocue per i pesci, ma producono chiari sintomi clinici nell'uomo.

La ciguatossina-1, un lipide dal peso molecolare di 1,1 kd circa, è inodore, incolore e insapore e non viene distrutta dalla cottura e dal congelamento. Essa aumenta la permeabilità al sodio delle membrane eccitabili, un'azione inibita dal calcio e dalla tetrodotossina.

L'insorgenza delle **manifestazioni cliniche** dell'intossicazione da ciguatossina di solito si presenta entro 2-30 ore dall'ingestione di pesce contaminato. La patologia è spesso bifasica. I primissimi sintomi sono diarrea, vomito e dolore addominale; la seconda fase comprende prurito intenso, rash ai palmi delle mani e alle piante dei piedi, mialgie, disestesia periorale o degli arti. La disestesia è caratterizzata dall'inversione delle sensazioni di caldo e di freddo. Tachicardia, bradicardia e ipotensione appaiono poco frequenti. L'intossicazione da pesce con ciguatera si basa sul quadro clinico e la diagnosi viene confermata dimostrando la presenza della tossina nel pesce ingerito.

TRATTAMENTO. Il **trattamento** dell'intossicazione da pesce con ciguatera è di supporto. Si raccomanda la lavanda gastrica per rimuovere ogni residuo di tossina. I liquidi per via endovenosa sono necessari nel caso di una diarrea severa e ci si può avvalere della somministrazione parenterale di calcio per trattare l'ipotensione. In alcuni pazienti con coma o sintomatologia prolungata, l'assunzione di mannitolo entro 24 ore dall'insorgenza dei sintomi è efficace verso i sintomi neurologici dell'intossicazione. Tuttavia occorrono ulteriori studi perché il mannitolo possa essere raccomandato. Il gabapentin, per la stessa occorrenza, si è rivelato efficace in pochi pazienti. La maggior parte dei casi è autolimitante; i sintomi neurologici possono durare mesi. La morte si ha in meno del 10% dei casi.

INTOSSICAZIONE (PSEUDOALLERGIA) DA SCOMBROIDI

Le epidemie sono state associate all'ingestione di componenti della famiglia Scombresocidae o Scombridae, in particolare l'albacora, lo sgombro, il tonno, la bonita e il pesce re. Ma anche i pesci non scombroidei e i mammiferi marini come il mahi-mahi (delfino) e il pesce azzurro sono stati correlati a epidemie d'intossicazione.

La scombrotossina, che sia l'istamina o il prodotto dell'azione della tossina nella polpa del pesce, è responsabile della sindrome clinica. L'istidina è stata trovata in alta concentrazione nella carne dello sgombro e l'azione della decarbossilasi batterica durante la putrefazione la converte in istamina. Un pesce che contiene ≥20 mg di istamina per 100 g di polpa è tossico. Nei pazienti trattati con isoniazide, un potente bloccante dell'istaminasi, l'ingestione di polpa di pesce con una concentrazione anche bassa di istamina può risultare tossica.

L'insorgenza delle **manifestazioni cliniche** è acuta e avviene entro 10 minuti-2 ore dall'ingestione. I sintomi e i segni più comuni comprendono diarrea, arrossamento, sudorazione, orticaria, nausea e cefalea. Possono aversi anche dolore addominale, tachicardia, bruciore del cavo orale, vertigini, distress respiratorio ed edema al volto. La malattia solitamente si autolimita e termina in 8-10 ore.

TRATTAMENTO. Il **trattamento** è soprattutto di supporto. La lavanda gastrica riduce l'assorbimento continuo d'istamina. Nel caso di diarrea severa può rendersi necessaria la reidratazione. Gli antistaminici hanno dimostrato un'efficacia variabile. Quattro pazienti con tossicità grave trattati con cimetidina (un antistaminico) hanno risposto in modo rapido. Dal momento che gli studi sono pochi, occorre riservare la cimetidina o la ranitidina ai casi più gravi.

INTOSSICAZIONE PARALITICA DA MOLLUSCHI

I molluschi con alimentazione a filtro, come la cozza nera e le capesante, possono contaminarsi durante le fioriture dei dinoflagellati o durante le "maree rosse". Lo *Ptychodiscus brevis*, un dinoflagellato, è frequentemente responsabile di queste maree rosse e contiene diverse potenti neurotossine. L'intossicazione paralitica da molluschi è una malattia neurologica distinta causata da 20 tossine strettamente correlate, termostabili, di cui la saxitossina è quella più potente. Questa tossina impedisce la conduzione nervosa inibendo la pompa sodio-potassio. Altre tossine possono essere trasformate in composti meno tossici. Il consumo di bivalvi, come cozze, capesante e vongole, è la via abituale dell'intossicazione, sebbene siano stati chiamati in causa anche crostacei e pesci.

L'insorgenza delle **manifestazioni cliniche** avviene rapidamente, a 30 minuti-2 ore dall'ingestione. Sono frequenti dolore addominale e nausea, come anche le parestesie in area periorale, con distribuzione a guanto e a calza, o entrambe. Sono meno comuni l'intorpidimento periorale, il formicolio, la diplopia, l'atassia, la disartria e la sensazione di fluttuazione. Non è rara l'inversione delle sensazioni di caldo e di freddo. In casi gravi si può avere un'insufficienza respiratoria da paralisi diaframmatica.

TRATTAMENTO. Non è conosciuto un antidoto per l'intossicazione acuta da molluschi. Può essere necessaria una terapia di supporto che comprenda la ventilazione meccanica. Sebbene i sintomi di solito si autolimitino e siano di breve durata, debolezza e malessere possono persistere per settimane dopo l'ingestione.

INTOSSICAZIONE DIARROICA DA MOLLUSCHI

Diverse epidemie di intossicazione diarroica da molluschi sono state registrate in Europa dopo il consumo di cozze, telline e altri molluschi. I dinoflagellati *Dinophysis* e *Prorocentrum* producono l'acido ocadaico e i suoi derivati, dinophysistossine. Questi composti inibiscono le fosfatasi proteiche. L'accumulo intracellulare di proteine fosforilate causa un aumento della secrezione di liquidi dalle cellule intestinali attraverso l'afflusso di calcio, mediato dall'adenosin monofosfato ciclico e dalle prostaglandine.

I pazienti sviluppano una diarrea severa. La terapia è di supporto e volta alla reidratazione. La malattia si autolimita e la guarigione avviene in 3-4 giorni; pochi pazienti necessitano di ospedalizzazione.

INTOSSICAZIONE AMNESICA DA MOLLUSCHI

L'intossicazione amnesica da molluschi è stata individuata per la prima volta in Canada nel 1987, dopo che un gruppo di persone aveva sviluppato una gastroenterite severa e sintomi neurologici, inclusa la perdita di memoria, in seguito all'ingestione di cozze dell'Isola di Prince Edward. I casi successivi legati all'alimentazione con molluschi si sono avuti negli Stati Uniti, in Spagna e nel Regno Unito. La tossina responsabile, l'acido domoico, deriva da una diatomea, la *Pseudo-nitzschia multiseries,* ed è un potente agonista del glutammato, alterando la trasmissione neurochimica a livello cerebrale. Essa si lega anche ai recettori per il glutammato che aumentano l'afflusso di calcio, producendo un edema e la morte neuronale a livello dell'ippocampo.

Le **manifestazioni cliniche** iniziali sono di tipo gastrointestinale. La perdita della memoria è strettamente correlata all'età avanzata. I pazienti di età inferiore ai 40 anni probabilmente accuseranno solo diarrea, mentre quelli di età superiore ai 50 anni soffrono di perdita di memoria a breve termine della durata di mesi o anni.

INTOSSICAZIONE DA AZASPIRACIDE

Le azaspiracidi sono tossine delle alghe. L'intossicazione da azaspiracide deriva dall'ingestione di molluschi contaminati, soprattutto cozze. Le tossine sono distribuite nei tessuti muscolari dei molluschi. I sintomi iniziano 8-18 ore dall'ingestione e comprendono nausea, vomito, crampi gastrici severi e diarrea, che spesso persistono oltre 5 giorni.

Intossicazione da pesce con ciguatera

Caplan CE: Ciguatera fish poisoning. *CMAJ* 1998;159:1394.
CDC: Ciguatera fish poisoningóTexas 1997. *JAMA* 1998;280:1394-1395.
DiNubile MJ, Hokama Y: The ciguatera poisoning syndrome from farm-raised salmon. *Ann Intern Med* 1995;122:113-114.
Lange WR: Ciguatera fish poisoning. *Am Fam Physician* 1994;50:579-584.
Palafox NA, Jain LG, Pinano AZ, et al: Successful treatment of ciguatera fish poisoning with intravenous mannitol. *JAMA* 1988;259:2740-2742.
Perez CM, Vasquez PA, Perret CF: Treatment of ciguatera poisoning with gabapentin. *N Engl J Med* 2001;344:692-693.

Intossicazione da scombroidi

Gilbert RJ, Hobbs G, Murray CK, et al: Scombrotoxic fish poisoning: Features of the first 50 incidents to be reported in Britain (1976-9). *BMJ* 1980;281:71-72.
Hughes JM, Potter ME: Scombroid fish poisoning: From pathogenesis to prevention. *N Engl J Med* 1991;324:766-768.
Wu SF, Chen W: An outbreak of scombroid fish poisoning in a kindergarten. *Acta Paediatr Taiwan* 2003;44:297-299

Intossicazione paralitica da molluschi

Gessner BD, Middaugh JP: Paralytic shellfish poisoning in Alaska: A 20-year retrospective analysis. *Am J Epidemiol* 1995;141:766-770
Isbister GK, Kiernan MC: Neurotoxic marine poisoning. *Lancet Neurol* 2005;4:219-228.
Morris PD, Campbell DS, Taylor TJ, et al: Clinical and epidemiological features of neurotoxic shellfish poisoning in North Carolina. *Am J Public Health* 1991;81:471-474.
Shimizu Y, Yoshioka M: Transformation of paralytic shellfish toxins as demonstrated in scallop homogenates. *Science* 1981;212:547-549.
Whittle K, Gallacher S: Marine toxins. *BMJ* 2000;56:236-253.

Intossicazione da pesci

Bret MM: Food poisoning associated with biotoxins in fish and shellfish. *Curr Opin Infect Dis* 2003;16:461-465.

Capitolo 711 ■ Terrorismo biologico e chimico

Theodore J. Cieslak e Fred M. Henretig

Gli attacchi al World Trade Center e al Pentagono dell'11 settembre 2001, la successiva ondata di casi di antrace dovuti all'esposizione a lettere contaminate e gli attacchi terroristici ai mezzi di trasporto pubblici in Gran Bretagna e in India dimostrano che i terroristi fanno uso di "armi di distruzione di massa" biologiche o chimiche. L'attacco a una scuola di Beslan in Russia nel settembre del 2004, così come il tentativo fallito di rilasciare gas cloro a Disneyland, indicano che alcuni terroristi hanno intenzione di colpire i bambini. I pediatri devono avere familiarità con le manifestazioni cliniche delle malattie indotte da agenti biologici e chimici, molte delle quali possono essere trattate con successo se la diagnosi viene posta precocemente, se la terapia viene iniziata tempestivamente e se le misure preventive vengono messe in atto.

EZIOLOGIA

Centinaia di agenti biologici e chimici possono essere adattati dai terroristi per essere utilizzati a scopi funesti. I tentativi di accertare gli agenti che hanno la maggiore probabilità di essere utilizzati sono pieni di difficoltà. Questa analisi spesso dipende da un'accurata intelligence, che può risultare problematica. Gli attentatori possono scegliere di utilizzare **armi occasionali**, agenti che per qualche motivo sono facilmente disponibili a qualche membro del gruppo terroristico. Le intenzioni dei terroristi sono spesso oscure e difficili da prevedere. Per questo motivo, un gruppo di lavoro convocato dai Centers for Disease Control and Prevention (CDC) ha deciso di concentrare gli sforzi di risposta non tanto su quegli agenti che hanno la maggiore probabilità di venire utilizzati, quanto su quelli che, se adoperati, costituirebbero le minacce potenzialmente più gravi per la salute e la sicurezza pubbliche.

Nel caso degli agenti biologici, il gruppo di lavoro dei CDC ha suddiviso i patogeni e le tossine in tre categorie, delle quali la **categoria A** comprende le malattie generate dai sei agenti che rappresentano la minaccia più grave: antrace, peste, tularemia, vaiolo, botulismo e febbri emorragiche virali.

I terroristi potrebbero rilasciare un'ampia serie di sostanze chimiche potenzialmente dannose. Camion pieni di gas e liquidi industriali infiammabili, acidi e basi industriali corrosivi, composti velenosi come cianuri e nitriti, pesticidi, diossine ed esplosivi attraversano le nostre ferrovie e le nostre strade quotidianamente. Quattro classi di sostanze chimiche di "categoria militare", con una storia di utilizzo nella guerra o fabbricate in modo specifico per essere impegate come armi, comprendono gli **agenti nervini a base di organofosfati**, le **sostanze vescicanti**, "agenti ematici"(**cianuri**) e alcuni **irritanti polmonari** o "agenti soffocanti".

EPIDEMIOLOGIA E RISCHI SPECIFICI PER L'INFANZIA

Gli attacchi su ampia scala su obiettivi civili comportano probabilmente vittime pediatriche e i bambini possono essere più sensibili degli adulti agli effetti di determinati agenti biologici e chimici. La maggiore sottigliezza della cute rende le sostanze chimiche dermatologicamente attive, come la mostarda azotata, più rischiose per i bambini che per gli adulti. La maggiore area di superficie per unità di volume aumenta ulteriormente il problema. Un volume ematico relativo piccolo rende i bambini più suscettibili alle perdite di volume associate a infezioni enteriche quali il colera e a intossicazioni gastrointestinali come si potrebbero osservare in caso di esposizione alle enterotossine stafilococciche. La ventilazione per minuto, relativamente elevata nei bambini rispetto agli adulti, accresce la minaccia degli agenti somministrati per via inalatoria. Il fatto che i bambini vivano "più vicini al suolo" aggrava questo effetto quando sono implicate sostanze chimiche più pesanti della pioggia. L'immaturità della barriera ematoencefalica può alzare il rischio di tossicità da agenti nervini per il sistema nervoso centrale. Infine, fattori legati allo sviluppo riducono la probabilità che un bambino abbandoni rapidamente un'area di pericolo, aumentando così l'esposizione a vari effetti avversi (vedi Capitolo 707).

Sembra che i bambini abbiano una sensibilità particolare nei confronti di determinati agenti potenziali di cui si potrebbero avvalere i terroristi. Sebbene in genere gli adulti, per esempio, sperimentino soltanto una breve malattia invalidante autolimitata dopo un'infezione da parte del virus dell'encefalite equina venezuelana, i bambini piccoli hanno una maggiore probabilità di andare incontro a convulsioni, sequele neurologiche permanenti e morte. In caso di vaiolo, la diminuzione dell'immunità di gregge (*herd immunity*) può fare sì che i bambini restino colpiti in modo sproporzionato. L'immunità al vaiolo indotta dal vaccino probabilmente si riduce in modo significativo dopo 3-10 anni. Sebbene la maggior parte degli adulti sia considerata sensibile al vaiolo, quelli più grandi possono avere una certa protezione residua nei confronti della morte, se non dallo sviluppo della malattia, dal momento che fino ai primi anni '70 vigeva la vaccinazione pubblica di routine. Oggi i bambini sono tra i primi a crescere senza alcuna immunità individuale o di gregge nei confronti del vaiolo.

I bambini possono anche sperimentare manifestazioni di malattia peculiari non osservate negli adulti. In uno studio su casi di melioidosi infantile in Thailandia, fu osservata una parotite suppurativa come presentazione caratteristica; questa malattia in genere non viene riscontrata negli adulti con un'infezione da *Burkholderia pseudomallei*.

I pediatri hanno la possibilità di venire a contatto con problemi unici nel trattamento dei bambini che sono rimasti vittime di un attacco biologico o chimico. Molti dei farmaci utili nel trattamento di questi soggetti sono poco familiari ai pediatri, oppure presentano controindicazioni relative nell'infanzia. I fluorochinoloni e le tetracicline vengono comunemente citate come agenti di scelta nel trattamento e nella profilassi dell'antrace, della peste, della tularemia, della brucellosi e della febbre Q. Ma entrambe queste classi di farmaci sono spesso evitate nei bambini, sebbene il rischio di morbilità e mortalità dovute alle malattie indotte dagli agenti di bioterrorismo sia di gran lunga superiore ai rischi minori associati all'impiego di tali agenti a breve termine. La ciprofloxacina ha ricevuto, come sua prima indicazione pediatrica autorizzata, l'approvazione della U.S. Food and Drug Administration (FDA) per venire adoperata nella profilassi dell'antrace da esposizione inalatoria (terrorismo). La doxiciclina è attualmente autorizzata in modo specifico nei bambini per la stessa indicazione. Le vaccinazioni potenzialmente utili nella prevenzione delle malattie indotte da agenti biologici spesso non sono approvate per i pazienti pediatrici. Il vaccino contro l'antrace attualmente disponibile è permesso soltanto ai soggetti di età compresa fra 18 e 65 anni. Il vaccino contro la peste, attualmente non più prodotto e probabilmente inefficace contro le esposizioni inalatorie, è stato consentito solo per le persone di 18-61 anni. Quello per il vaiolo, un vaccino vivo che utilizza il virus attenuato, può causare vaccinia e morte fetale quando somministrato alle donne gravide.

Molti agenti farmacologici altrimenti utili non sono disponibili in regimi di dosaggio pediatrici. Negli Stati Uniti, l'esercito distribuisce kit di antidoto per il gas nervino che consistono in autoiniettori preriempiti finalizzati all'inoculazione rapida di atropina e pralidossima. Le dosi degli agenti contenuti nel kit sono calcolate per i militari e quindi risultano di molto superiori a quelle appropriate per i bambini piccoli, sebbene autoiniettori di atropina specificamente formulati per essi siano stati approvati dalla FDA e ci si aspetta che a ciò segua l'autorizzazione agli autoiniettori di pralidossima. Sebbene la protezione fisica non sarebbe probabilmente utile in un contesto civile, è degno di nota che negli Stati Uniti i dispositivi in commercio come le maschere a gas in genere non sono disponibili nelle taglie pediatriche.

Negli Stati Uniti, il numero di letti ospedalieri pediatrici potrebbe non essere sufficiente. Nel caso di un attacco terroristico su vasta scala, come avviene in ogni grande disastro, la capacità di letti aggiuntivi potrebbe potenzialmente essere fornita dagli ospedali civili e in quelli del Department of Veterans Affairs sotto gli auspici del National Disaster Medical System, ma questo sistema non fornisce specificamente letti pediatrici.

MANIFESTAZIONI CLINICHE

In caso di attacco terroristico, ai medici può essere richiesto di porre diagnosi tempestive e fornire rapidi trattamenti salvavita prima che i risultati dei test diagnostici di conferma siano disponibili. Sebbene ogni potenziale agente usato da attentatori produca proprie manifestazioni cliniche specifiche, appare utile circoscrivere i loro effetti in un limitato numero di sindromi cliniche distinte. Ciò aiuterà i medici a prendere decisioni tempestive e razionali riguardanti la terapia empirica. In generale, le vittime di un attacco svilupperanno sintomi immediati al momento dell'esposizione a una sostanza (o entro le prime ore) oppure nell'arco di giorni o settimane. Nel primo caso, la natura maligna dell'evento spesso risulta evidente ed è più probabile che l'eziologia sia convenzionale o chimica. Le sostanze biologiche differiscono dalle armi convenzionali, chimiche e nucleari (vedi Capitoli 706 e 707) per il fatto che possiedono periodi di incubazione intrinseci e quindi diviene probabile che i pazienti siano allontanati in tempo dal luogo di un'esposizione imprevista e inosservata a un agente biologico. Mentre il personale di emergenza (first responder) tradizionale, come pompieri e paramedici, può essere in prima linea in una risposta a un attacco convenzionale o chimico, il medico di assistenza primaria può costituire la prima linea di difesa di un agente biologico.

Le vittime possono presentarsi immediatamente o in un secondo momento. In entrambi i casi, possono essere ulteriormente classificate a seconda che abbiano manifestazioni prevalentemente respiratorie, neuromuscolari o dermatologiche (Tab. 711-1). Un limitato numero di agenti può causare ogni sindrome particolare, permettendo l'istituzione della terapia empirica rivolta a un elenco breve di possibili eziologie. Le febbri emorragiche virali possono presentarsi con febbre e diatesi emorragica; questi agenti vengono presi in considerazione separatamente nel Capitolo 268. Nella maggior parte dei casi, la terapia di supporto è il cardine del trattamento della febbre emorragica.

SINDROME NEUROMUSCOLARE A ESORDIO IMPROVVISO: AGENTI NERVINI. La comparsa molto rapida di sintomi neuromuscolari dopo un'esposizione dovrebbe indurre il medico a prendere in considerazione l'intossicazione da agente nervino. Gli agenti nervini (*tabun*, *sarin*, *soman* e *VX*) sono **organofosfati** analoghi ai comuni pesticidi che agiscono come potenti inibitori dell'enzima acetilcolinesterasi; sono nocivi per ingestione, inalazione o assorbimento cutaneo (vedi Capitolo 58).

L'inibizione della colinesterasi da parte di queste sostanze porta all'accumulo di acetilcolina in corrispondenza delle giunzioni neuromuscolari, provocando un'eccessiva stimolazione. La sindrome colinergica conseguente comporta effetti centrali, nicotinici e muscarinici. Gli effetti centrali comprendono alterazioni dello stato mentale, che progrediscono rapidamente a letargia e coma, così come atassia, convulsioni e depressione respiratoria. Gli effetti nicotinici includono fascicolazioni e spasmi muscolari, seguiti da una debolezza che può progredire a paralisi flaccida con affaticamento muscolare. Gli effetti muscarinici riguardano miosi, offuscamento del visus, lacrimazione profusa e rinorrea acquosa. Il broncospasmo e l'aumento delle secrezioni bronchiali portano a tosse, respiro affannoso, dispnea e cianosi. Le manifestazioni cardiovascolari comprendono bradicardia, ipotensione e blocco atrioventricolare. Si osservano anche flushing, sudorazione, salivazione, nausea, vomito, diarrea, crampi addominali e incontinenza urinaria. In assenza di un intervento tempestivo, la morte può sopraggiungere rapidamente, per la combinazione tra effetti centrali e paralisi dei muscoli respiratori.

TABELLA 711-1. Malattie causate da agenti del terrorismo chimico e biologico, classificate per sindrome

	SINTOMI NEUROMUSCOLARI PROMINENTI	SINTOMI RESPIRATORI PROMINENTI	REPERTI DERMATOLOGICI PROMINENTI
ESORDIO IMPROVVISO	Agenti nervini	Cloro Fosgene Cianuro	Mostarda azotata Lewisite
ESORDIO RITARDATO	Botulismo	Antrace Peste Tularemia	Vaiolo

SINDROME NEUROMUSCOLARE A ESORDIO TARDIVO: BOTULISMO. La comparsa tardiva (ore o giorni dopo l'esposizione) di sintomi neuromuscolari è caratteristica del botulismo. Il botulismo si verifica dopo il contatto con una delle sette neurotossine prodotte da alcuni ceppi di *Clostridium botulinum*, un bacillo Gram-positivo sporigeno strettamente anaerobio riscontrato nel suolo. Il botulismo contratto in modo naturale (vedi Capitolo 207) di solito fa seguito all'ingestione della tossina preformata (intossicazione alimentare) o deriva dalla produzione intestinale della tossina (forma infantile). Ciononostante, un'esposizione aerosolica potrebbe portare a un quadro di botulismo clinico indistinguibile da quello causato dalle esposizioni naturali.

In seguito al contatto con la tossina botulinica, le manifestazioni cliniche esordiscono tipicamente con paralisi bulbare, che portano alla comparsa di ptosi, fotofobia e offuscamento del visus secondario a difficoltà dell'accomodazione. I sintomi possono progredire fino a comprendere disartria e disfagia e, infine, una paralisi discendente simmetrica. La sensibilità e il sensorio sono tipicamente risparmiati. In assenza d'intervento, spesso sopraggiunge il decesso per insufficienza muscolare respiratoria.

SINDROME RESPIRATORIA A ESORDIO IMPROVVISO: CLORO, FOSGENE E CIANURO. L'esordio acuto di sintomi respiratori poco dopo un'esposizione dovrebbe portare il medico a prendere in considerazione tutta una serie di possibili agenti chimici. Gli agenti nervini possono colpire la respirazione, ma questi effetti sono di solito secondari alla paresi dei muscoli respiratori piuttosto che alla patologia polmonare di per sé. Tale distinzione dovrebbe essere facilmente evidente dal punto di vista clinico, perché la vittima da agente nervino presenterà un interessamento muscolare generalizzato. Al contrario, le sostanze tossiche inalatorie come il cloro e il fosgene determinano un distress respiratorio senza interessamento muscolare.

Il **cloro** è un gas denso, acre, giallo-verde, più pesante dell'aria. Dopo un'esposizione lieve o moderata compare un'irritazione oculare e nasale seguita da tosse, sensazione di soffocamento, broncospasmo e senso di oppressione retrosternale. L'edema polmonare, mediato dall'acido cloridrico e dalla produzione di radicali liberi dell'ossigeno, subentra in seguito a esposizioni da moderate a gravi entro 30 minuti o diverse ore. L'ipossiemia e l'ipovolemia secondarie all'edema polmonare sono responsabili del decesso nei casi fatali.

Il **fosgene**, come il cloro, è un comune composto industriale che fu utilizzato nei campi di battaglia della prima guerra mondiale. Il suo odore è stato descritto come quello di "fieno appena falciato". Similmente al cloro, si ritiene che anche esso porti alla produzione di acido cloridrico, contribuendo in particolare all'irritazione delle vie respiratorie, del naso e della congiuntiva. Le reazioni di acilazione causate dai suoi effetti sulla membrana alveolo-capillare conducono a un edema polmonare. Il danno polmonare può in parte essere mediato anche da una reazione infiammatoria associata alla produzione di leucotriene. I pazienti con contatti lievi o moderati con il fosgene possono risultare asintomatici, con il rischio che rimangano nell'area contaminata. L'edema polmonare compare a distanza di 4-24 h dall'esposizione ed è dose-dipendente, nel senso che esposizioni più intense determinano sintomi più precoci. La dispnea può precedere i reperti radiologici. Nelle esposizioni gravi, l'edema polmonare può essere così marcato da portare a ipovolemia e ipotensione. Come nel caso del cloro, la morte è dovuta a ipossiemia e asfissia.

Il **cianuro** è un veleno cellulare, con manifestazioni cliniche variabili. All'inizio la tossicità si presenta più probabilmente con tachipnea e iperpnea, progredendo rapidamente ad apnea nei casi di contatto significativo (vedi Capitolo 58). L'efficacia del cianuro come agente chimico terroristico è limitata dalla sua volatilità nell'aria libera e dalla sua letalità relativamente bassa rispetto agli agenti nervini. Tuttavia, rilasciato in una stanza chiusa, esso potrebbe avere effetti devastanti, come evidenziato dal suo utilizzo nelle camere a gas dei nazisti durante la seconda guerra mondiale. Il cianuro inibisce il citocromo a_3, interferendo con il normale metabolismo mitocondriale ossidativo e portando all'anossia cellulare e all'acidosi lattica. Oltre al distress respiratorio, i reperti precoci includono tachicardia, flushing, vertigini, cefalea, diaforesi, nausea e vomito. A esposizioni maggiori possono fare seguito entro pochi minuti convulsioni, coma, apnea e arresto cardiaco. Tipicamente si ha un'acidosi metabolica con gap anionico elevato, mentre la diminuzione dell'uso periferico di ossigeno porta a un elevato valore di saturazione dell'ossigeno venoso misto.

SINDROME RESPIRATORIA A ESORDIO TARDIVO: ANTRACE, PESTE E TULAREMIA. Un esordio ritardato (giorni dopo l'esposizione) di sintomi respiratori è caratteristico di diverse malattie infettive che possono essere modificate dai terroristi per scopi malvagi. Tra queste vi sono l'antrace, la peste e la tularemia.

L'**antrace** è causato dall'infezione da parte di *Bacillus antraci*, un bacillo sporigeno Gram-positivo la cui capacità di formare spore gli consente di sopravvivere per lunghi periodi nell'ambiente e aumenta il suo potenziale come arma.

La massima parte dei casi di antrace che si verifica in modo naturale è cutanea, acquisita per contatto ravvicinato con pelli, lana, osso e altri sottoprodotti di bovini, pecore e capre infetti. I casi cutanei possono anche risultare secondari all'impiego intenzionale di fomiti contaminati da antrace. L'antrace cutaneo può essere trattato con tutta una serie di antibiotici e viene facilmente riconosciuto dai medici esperti nelle aree endemiche; pertanto, raramente è fatale. Sebbene sia comune in alcune parti dell'Asia e dell'Africa subsahariana, soltanto due casi si sono verificati negli Stati Uniti nei 9 anni che precedettero gli 11 episodi osservati nel 2001. L'antrace gastrointestinale, che non è mai stato descritto negli Stati Uniti, può insorgere dopo l'ingestione di carne contaminata. In passato, l'antrace inalatorio, o **malattia dei cardatori di lana**, era un rischio professionale per coloro che lavoravano nei macelli o nell'industria tessile e attualmente rimane la minaccia più grande negli Stati Uniti, che hanno altrimenti eliminato la malattia contratta in modo naturale. In seguito alle emissioni accidentali nel 1979 da parte di una fabbrica di armi biologiche a Sverdlovsk, nella ex Unione Sovietica, morirono 66 adulti su 77 che erano stati vittime di antrace inalatorio. Negli Stati Uniti, 6 pazienti su 11 con antrace inalatorio sono sopravvissuti agli attacchi di bioterrorismo con le lettere contaminate. Non è ancora chiaro se il miglioramento di questo tasso di mortalità sia dovuto alle modalità della terapia intensiva, alle modifiche della terapia antibiotica o al riconoscimento più precoce.

L'antrace inalatorio sintomatico tipicamente inizia 1-6 giorni dopo l'esposizione, sebbene siano stati riportati periodi d'incubazione di diverse settimane. L'esordio è quello di una malattia simil-influenzale, caratterizzata da febbre, mialgia, cefalea e tosse. Spesso intercorre un breve periodo di miglioramento, ma in seguito si ha un rapido aggravamento; questa seconda fase è contraddistinta da febbre alta, dispnea, cianosi e shock. Fino nel 50% dei casi si verifica una meningite emorragica. Le radiografie del torace ottenute successivamente nel corso della malattia possono evidenziare l'ingrandimento del mediastino o una linfoadenopatia mediastinica prominente; si possono osservare anche versamenti pleurici. In questa fase, la colorazione di Gram del sangue periferico può evidenziare il microrganismo. Il trattamento precoce è imperativo; la morte sopraggiunge fino nel 95% dei casi di antrace inalatorio se esso viene invece ritardato per oltre 48 ore dalla comparsa dei sintomi.

Mentre l'antrace inalatorio è una malattia che riguarda in maniera prevalente il tessuto linfatico mediastinico, l'esposizione ai bacilli aerosolizzati della peste porta tipicamente a una polmonite primaria. La **peste** endemica viene di solito trasmessa attraverso il morso di pulci ed è discussa nel Capitolo 200.3. Il microrganismo scatenante di tutte le forme di peste umana, *Yersinia pestis*, è un bacillo intracellulare facoltativo Gram-negativo a colorazione bipolare. La capacità di sopravvivere all'interno del macrofago favorisce la sua disseminazione in sedi distanti dopo l'inoculazione o l'inalazione. Il segno caratteristico della peste bubbonica sono appunto i "bubboni", linfonodi regionali ingrossati, dolenti lungo la distribuzione di un morso. Febbre e malessere si riscontrano usualmente e spesso si sviluppa la setticemia quando i batteri raggiungono la circolazione. Comunemente compaiono petecchie, porpora e coagulopatia intravascolare disseminata imponente e l'80% delle vittime alla fine avrà emocolture positive. La peste è estremamente infettiva e letale, come illustrato dal fatto che la "Morte Nera" eliminò un terzo della popolazione europea durante il Medioevo. Anche allora ci si rese conto del suo possibile uso come arma, come evidenziato dal suo impiego intenzionale nel 1346 da parte dei Tartari invasori contro il presidio di Kaffa in Ucraina.

La disseminazione aerosolica intenzionale di *Y. pestis* potrebbe portare a una preponderanza di casi di peste polmonare. Questa può comparire anche in seguito alla disseminazione ai polmoni nei pazienti setticemici. I sintomi comprendono febbre, brividi, malessere, cefalea e tosse. Le radiografie del torace possono evidenziare un addensamento irregolare, mentre il classico reperto clinico è l'escreato striato di sangue. Coagulopatia intravascolare disseminata e sepsi fulminante si sviluppano tipicamente con la progressione della malattia. La peste polmonare non trattata ha un tasso di fatalità che si avvicina al 100%.

La **tularemia** è una malattia altamente infettiva causata da *Francisella tularensis*, un coccobacillo Gram-negativo. Quella che si contrae naturalmente viene discussa nel Capitolo 203. L'elevato grado di infettività di *F. tularensis* (si ritiene siano necessari <10 microrganismi per produrre un'infezione per via inalatoria), così come la capacità di sopravvivere nell'ambiente, contribuisce alla sua inclusione nell'elenco degli agenti a rischio. Sono note diverse forme cliniche di tularemia endemica, ma l'esposizione inalatoria in un attacco terroristico condurrebbe probabilmente a una polmonite primaria simile a quella della peste oppure alla tularemia tifoide, che si manifesta con tutta una serie di sintomi aspecifici tra cui febbre, malessere e dolore addominale.

SINDROME DERMATOLOGICA A ESORDIO IMPROVVISO: MOSTARDA AZOTATA E LEWISITE. La comparsa di lesioni cutanee poco dopo l'esposizione è una conseguenza caratteristica dei vescicanti chimici. Questi composti, spesso noti come "blistering agents" (letteralmente, "agenti vescicanti"), sono veleni cellulari e comprendono la mostarda azotata (agente alchilante) e la lewisite (arsenico organico). Il danno ai tessuti con cellule in rapida replicazione inizia entro minuti dal contatto. Nel caso della mostarda, gli effetti clinici in genere diventano evidenti diverse ore dopo l'esposizione, mentre i pazienti esposti alla lewisite avvertono un dolore immediato. Oltre alla formazione di vescicole cutanee, anche gli occhi e il tratto respiratorio vengono colpiti. Inoltre, l'esposizione alla mostarda può portare a una soppressione midollare e sia essa sia la lewisite possono provocare significativi sintomi gastrointestinali.

SINDROME DERMATOLOGICA A ESORDIO TARDIVO: VAIOLO. La comparsa di un esantema giorni o settimane dopo l'esposizione è probabilmente una caratteristica che contraddistingue la manifestazione del vaiolo. Il vaiolo, causato dal virus del vaiolo, un membro della famiglia degli ortopoxvirus, ha un periodo di incubazione di 7-17 giorni. Ciò potrebbe permettere l'ampia dispersione delle persone asintomatiche contagiate, contribuendo così alla diffusione di una epidemia. Durante il periodo di incubazione, il virus si replica nel tratto respiratorio superiore. Segue una viremia primaria, durante la quale si ha il passaggio del virus al fegato e alla milza. Si sviluppa quindi una seconda viremia, con l'estensione alla cute e la comparsa del classico esantema.

I sintomi appaiono improvvisamente durante la fase della viremia secondaria e includono febbre, brividi, vomito, cefalea, lombalgia e intenso malessere. Entro 2-4 giorni si osservano macule sul volto e agli arti, che successivamente progrediscono in modo sincrono in papule, pustole e infine croste, con la caduta delle quali nei sopravvissuti spesso rimangono cicatrici depigmentate deturpanti. La natura sincrona dell'eruzione e la sua distribuzione centrifuga distinguono il vaiolo dalla varicella, che ha invece una distribuzione centripeta. Dal punto di vista storico, il vaiolo ha un tasso di mortalità del 30%, con il decesso in genere dovuto all'interessamento di organi viscerali.

DIAGNOSI

In alcuni casi, la natura terroristica di un'aggressione chimica o biologica può essere evidente, per esempio quando si ha un attacco in cui le vittime soccombono in vicinanza temporale e geografica a un dispositivo di dispersione o quando i terroristi annunciano la loro offensiva. In altri casi il medico può avere bisogno di basarsi su dati epidemiologici per sospettare un'emissione intenzionale di agenti chimici o biologici. La presenza di un elevato numero di vittime ravvicinate nel tempo e nello spazio dovrebbe aumentare il livello di sospetto, così come i casi di morte imprevista o di malattia grave inspiegata. Analogamente, malattie insolite in un determinato ambiente, in un preciso gruppo di età o durante una stagione specifica dovrebbero giustificare ulteriori indagini. Anche epidemie simultanee di una malattia in aree non contigue dovrebbero indurre a prendere in considerazione emissioni intenzionali, così come epidemie di malattie multiple nella stessa area. Un singolo caso di una malattia rara come l'antrace o come alcune febbri emorragiche virali sarebbe già sospetto, allo stesso modo di un'occorrenza singola di vaiolo, che bisognerebbe quasi certamente far risalire a un'emissione intenzionale. Un numero elevato di decessi negli animali potrebbe essere il segno di un'emissione aerosolica non naturale, così come la presenza di un tasso di contaminazione significativamente diverso tra gli animali che notoriamente vivono in casa e quelli che vivono all'esterno in un determinato lasso temporale.

In caso di un attacco di massa, le diagnosi possono essere confermate in gran parte su elementi clinici. La diagnosi di intossicazione da agenti nervini si basa principalmente sul riconoscimento clinico e sulla risposta alla terapia con l'antidoto. Diversi dispositivi di rilevazione semplici e rapidi sviluppati per l'uso militare possono identificare gli agenti nervini. Alcuni di questi sono disponibili in commercio negli Stati Uniti e sono depositati in alcuni dipartimenti di emergenza e in veicoli di sicurezza pubblica. I test su carta M8 ed M9 segnalano la presenza di agenti nervini mediante una semplice variazione del colore. Il dosaggio dell'acetilcolinesterasi nel plasma o negli eritrociti delle vittime di questi agenti può essere utile per stabilire la prognosi a lungo termine, ma la correlazione tra i livelli di colinesterasi e gli effetti clinici è spesso scarsa e il test è raramente disponibile in emergenza.

Il **botulismo** dovrebbe essere sospettato clinicamente nei pazienti che si presentano con una paralisi flaccida, discendente, simmetrica. Sebbene la diagnosi differenziale del botulismo comprenda altre malattie neurologiche rare, come la miastenia grave e la sindrome di Guillain-Barré, molteplici vittime con sintomi simili dovrebbero consentire di stabilire l'esistenza di un'epidemia di botulismo.

Inizialmente, anche la diagnosi di **intossicazione da cianuro** può essere confermata in base a elementi clinici, di fronte alla sindrome tossica. Un'acidosi metabolica con gap anionico insolitamente elevato e una concentrazione di ossigeno nel sangue venoso maggiore del previsto vengono a supporto della diagnosi clinica. Elevate concentrazioni ematiche di cianuro possono confermare tale sospetto.

L'**antrace** andrebbe sospettato in base al rincontro di bacilli Gram-positivi nel materiale della biopsia cutanea (in caso di malattia cutanea), negli strisci ematici, nel liquido pleurico o nel liquido spinale. Anche le radiografie del torace che dimostrino un allargamento del mediastino nel contesto di una febbre e di segni costituzionali e in assenza di un'altra spiegazione (come per es. un trauma contusivo o un'infezione postchirurgica) dovrebbero indurre a prendere in considerazione la diagnosi. La conferma può essere ottenuta mediante l'emocoltura. I laboratori sanitari statali e le strutture federali presso i CDC e lo U.S. Army Medical Research Institute of Infectious Diseases possono confermare la diagnosi di antrace mediante la reazione a catena polimerasica e i saggi immunoistochimici.

La diagnosi di **peste** può venire sospettata in base al riscontro di bacilli con colorazione bipolare "a spilla da balia" nelle colorazioni di Gram o Wayson dell'escreato o nel materiale linfonodale aspirato; la conferma viene ottenuta coltivando *Y. pestis* dal sangue, dall'escreato o dall'aspirato linfonodale. Il microrganismo cresce su sangue standard o su agar MacConkey TRA®, ma spesso non viene identificato dai sistemi automatizzati. *F. tularensis* cresce invece poco nei terreni standard; la sua crescita aumenta nei terreni contenenti cisteina. A causa dell'elevata infettività di tale microrganismo, tuttavia, molti laboratori preferiscono determinare la diagnosi mediante la reazione a catena polimerasica oppure sierologicamente utilizzando un test di immunoassorbimento enzimatico (ELISA) o un test di agglutinazione del siero.

Il **vaiolo** dovrebbe essere sospettato clinicamente e potrebbe essere confermato dalla coltura o dall'esame delle croste o del liquido vescicolare al microscopio elettronico, sebbene la manipolazione del materiale clinico dalle vittime con sospetto vaiolo andrebbe tentata soltanto nei laboratori sanitari pubblici in grado di impiegare le massime precauzioni di biocontenimento (BSL-4). Occorrerebbe adottare una simile attenzione nel caso dei campioni prelevati da pazienti con varie febbri emorragiche virali.

PREVENZIONE

Le misure preventive possono essere prese in considerazione in un contesto pre- e postesposizione. La **protezione pre-esposizione** nei confronti di un attacco chimico o biologico può consistere in misure fisiche, chimiche o immunologiche. La **protezione fisica** nei riguardi dell'attacco primario spesso comporta maschere a gas e tute protettive; questo equipaggiamento è utilizzato dall'esercito e da alcuni gruppi d'intervento per materiali pericolosi, ma è poco probabile che sia disponibile ai civili nel preciso momento dell'emissione. Il personale medico deve conoscere i principi di protezione fisica e la loro applicazione per il controllo dell'infezione e della diffusione della contaminazione.

La peste polmonare si diffonde attraverso le goccioline respiratorie. Le precauzioni nei confronti delle goccioline, che comprendono l'uso di maschere chirurgiche semplici, sono quindi giustificate nell'assistenza dei pazienti con la peste. Il vaiolo viene trasmesso attraverso i nuclei delle goccioline, per cui sono giustificate le precauzioni contro i microrganismi trasmessi per via aerea, tra le quali (idealmente) una maschera con filtro HEPA (*High-Efficiency Particulate Air*). Analogamente, i pazienti con febbre emorragica virale dovrebbero, in generale, essere trattati utilizzando le cautele da contatto. La maggior parte delle altre vittime da agenti biologici può essere assistita temporaneamente in modo sicuro utilizzando le precauzioni standard. Nel caso degli agenti chimici, la mostarda residua o l'agente nervino sulla cute o sugli indumenti delle vittime potrebbero costituire un pericolo per il personale medico. I vestiti andrebbero dunque tolti a queste vittime, quando possibile, e bisognerebbe decontaminarle utilizzando abbondanti quantità di acqua prima di fornire l'assistenza medica completa. La maggior parte delle altre sostanze chimiche è sufficientemente volatile da rendere improbabile la diffusione dell'agente tra i pazienti o dal paziente all'assistente.

La **profilassi chimica pre-esposizione** potrebbe essere utilizzata sulla base di credibili rapporti dell'intelligence. Per esempio, qualora i funzionari ritenessero che la minaccia di emissione di un agente biologico specifico sia imminente, si potrebbe effettuare la distribuzione preventiva di antibiotici alla popolazione. Tuttavia le occasioni di utilizzo di questa strategia sono probabilmente piuttosto limitate.

Sebbene esistano vaccini autorizzati (**misure immunologiche pre-esposizione**) contro l'antrace e il vaiolo, l'uso esteso di entrambi i vaccini è probabilmente problematico, specialmente nei bambini. Il vaccino per l'antrace negli Stati Uniti è autorizzato soltanto per gli individui di età uguale o superiore a 18 anni; viene somministrato come ciclo da 6 dosi in 18 mesi e richiede richiami annuali. Questa situazione, associata a una fornitura limitata, rendono improbabile il suo impiego su larga scala; peraltro, negli Stati Uniti un nuovo vaccino ricombinante per l'antrace si trova nelle ultime fasi di sviluppo ed è allo studio come cicli da 3 dosi.

Significativi ostacoli esistono anche per l'uso ampio del vaccino contro il vaiolo, sebbene i responsabili dell'igiene pubblica abbiano contemplato la ripresa di una campagna vaccinale. Mentre in passato questo vaccino (preparato dal virus vaccinico, un ortopoxvirus correlato al vaiolo) era usato in modo sicuro e con successo nei bambini piccoli, esso comporta un tasso relativamente elevato di complicanze grave in alcuni pazienti. La *vaccinia fetale* e la morte possono subentrare quando vengono vaccinate le donne gravide; la *vaccinia gangrenosa*, una complicanza spesso fatale, può verificarsi nella vaccinazione di soggetti immunocompromessi; l'*eczema vaccinatum* colpisce i soggetti con dermatosi pre-esistenti (dermatite atopica). Una grave encefalite correlata al vaccino era ben nota già durante il periodo della vaccinazione diffusa; dal momento che questa si verifica soltanto nei vaccini primari, colpirebbe in modo sproporzionato i pazienti pediatrici. L'autoinoculazione può verificarsi quando il virus presente in corrispondenza del sito della vaccinazione viene trasferito manualmente ad altre aree della cute o all'occhio. I bambini piccoli sarebbero presumibilmente a maggiore rischio di tale trasmissione involontaria.

Per il trattamento di queste complicanze, dovrebbero essere disponibili immunoglobuline anti virus vaccinico (VIG, *Vaccinia Immune Globulin*), quando si intraprende una campagna vaccinale. Le VIG (0,6 mg/kg im) possono essere somministrate a coloro che ricevono il vaccino e che sperimentano gravi complicanze oppure a individui significativamente immunodepressi esposti al vaiolo, in cui la vaccinazione sarebbe pericolosa. Negli Stati Uniti, le provviste attuali di vaccino e di VIG sono controllate dai CDC e la produzione di un nuovo vaccino e la preparazione di VIG è in corso. Oltre a un ruolo potenziale nella profilassi pre-esposizione, la vaccinazione può essere efficace nella profilassi postesposizione se somministrata entro i primi 4 giorni circa.

Il vaccino contro l'antrace potrebbe essere impiegato in un contesto postesposizione. Negli Stati Uniti, alcuni enti raccomandano tre dosi di questo vaccino in aggiunta alla chemioprofilassi postesposizione dopo un contatto documentato con spore di antrace aerosolizzate. Ciononostante, l'assunzione postesposizione di antibiotici orali costituisce il cardine del trattamento delle vittime asintomatiche che si ritiene siano state esposte all'antrace, così come ad altri agenti come la peste e la tularemia. La Tabella 711-2 illustra gli appropriati regimi profilattici per le varie esposizioni biologiche.

TRATTAMENTO

Le Tabelle 711-2 e 711-3 mostrano le terapie raccomandate per le malattie conclamate causate da agenti chimici e biologici. Tuttavia, è piuttosto probabile che il medico che assiste le vittime avrà bisogno di prendere decisioni terapeutiche prima che i risultati dei test diagnostici di conferma siano disponibili e in situazioni in cui la diagnosi non è nota con certezza. In tali casi, è utile notare che molte malattie e molti sintomi causati da agenti chimici e biologici si risolveranno spontaneamente, con necessità soltanto della terapia di supporto. Le esposizioni al cloro e al fosgene possono quindi venire trattate con successo prestando una meticolosa attenzione all'ossigenazione e al bilancio dei liquidi. Le vittime della mostarda possono richiedere un intenso supporto multisistemico, ma nessun antidoto o terapia specifici sono disponibili.

TABELLA 711-2. Agenti biologici critici del terrorismo

MALATTIA	REPERTI CLINICI	PERIODO DI INCUBAZIONE	PRECAUZIONI DI ISOLAMENTO	TRATTAMENTO INIZIALE	PROFILASSI
Antrace (inalatorio)[*] I pazienti che sono clinicamente stabili dopo 14 giorni possono passare a un singolo farmaco per os (ciprofloxacina o doxiciclina) per completare un ciclo di 60 giorni[†]	Prodromi febbrili con rapida progressione a linfoadenite mediastinica e mediastinite, sepsi, shock e meningite	1-5 gg	Standard	Ciprofloxacina[‡] 10-15 mg/kg ev ogni 12 h O Doxiciclina 2,2 mg/kg ev ogni 12 h E Clindamicina[§] 10-15 mg/kg ev ogni 8 h E Penicillina G[‖] 400-600 k U/kg/d ev ÷ ogni 4 h	Ciprofloxacina 10-15 mg/kg per os ogni 12 h O Doxiciclina 2,2 mg/kg per os ogni 12 h
Peste (polmonare)	Prodromi febbrili con rapida progressione a polmonite fulminante, emottisi, sepsi, CID	2-3 gg	Goccioline di saliva (per i primi 3 gg di terapia)	Gentamicina 2,5 mg/kg ev ogni 8 h O Doxiciclina 2,2 mg/kg ev ogni 12 h O Ciprofloxacina 15 mg/kg ev ogni 12 h	Doxiciclina 2,2 mg/kg per os ogni 12 h O Ciprofloxacina 20 mg/kg per os ogni 12 h
Tularemia	Polmonare: esordio improvviso di febbre con polmonite fulminante Tifoidea: febbre, malessere, dolore addominale	2-10 gg	Standard	Come per la peste	Come per la peste
Vaiolo	Prodromi febbrili con esantema, sincrono, centrifugo, vescicolopustuloso	7-17 gg	Per via aerea (+ contatto)	Terapia di supporto	La vaccinazione può essere efficace se somministrata entro i primi giorni dall'esposizione
Botulismo	Paralisi flaccida simmetrica discendente afebbrile con paralisi dei nervi cranici	1-5 gg	Standard	Terapia di supporto; l'antitossina (vedi testo) può arrestare la progressione dei sintomi ma è improbabile che li faccia regredire	Nessuna
Febbri emorragiche virali	Prodromi febbrili con rapida progressione a shock, porpora e diatesi emorragica	4-21 gg	Contatto (prendere in considerazione la trasmissione aerea in caso di emorragia massiva)	Terapia di supporto; la ribavirina può essere vantaggiosa in casi selezionati	Nessuna

[*] In caso di attacco di massa, in cui le risorse sono gravemente limitate, può essere necessario sostituire la terapia per os con l'opzione parenterale preferita.
[†] Assumendo che il microrganismo sia sensibile, i bambini possono passare ad amoxicillina per os (80 mg/kg/d ÷ ogni 8 h) per completare un ciclo di 60 giorni. Gli Autori raccomandano che i primi 14 giorni di terapia o di profilassi postesposizione, tuttavia, includano ciprofloxacina e/o doxiciclina indipendentemente dall'età.
[‡] Levofloxacina o ofloxacina possono essere alternative accettabili alla ciprofloxacina.
[§] Rifampicina o claritromicina possono essere alternative accettabili alla clindamicina, in quanto farmaci diretti alla sintesi proteica batterica. Se si sceglie la ciprofloxacina o un altro chinolone, la doxiciclina può essere usata come secondo farmaco, perché anch'essa è diretta alla sintesi proteica.
[‖] Ampicillina, imipenem, meropenem o cloramfenicolo possono essere alternative accettabili alla penicillina, in quanto sono farmaci con una buona penetrazione nel sistema nervoso centrale.
CID, coagulazione intravascolare disseminata.

TABELLA 711-3. Agenti chimici critici del terrorismo

AGENTE	TOSSICITÀ	REPERTI CLINICI	ESORDIO	DECONTAMINAZIONE*	TRATTAMENTO
AGENTI NERVINI					
Tabun, Sarin, Soman, VX	Anticolinesterasi: effetti muscarinici, nicotinici, sul SNC	Vapore: miosi, rinorrea, dispnea	Secondi: vapore	Vapore: aria aperta, togliere gli indumenti, lavare i capelli	ABC Atropina: 0,05 mg/kg ev[†] im[‡] (minimo 0,1 mg, max 5 mg), ripetere ogni 2-5 minuti a.b. in caso di secrezioni marcate, broncospasmo
		Liquidi: diaforesi, vomito	Minuti-ore: liquidi	Liquidi: togliere gli indumenti, lavare la cute, i capelli con abbondanti acqua e sapone, irrigazione oculare	Pralidossima: 25 mg/kg ev, im[§] (max 1 g ev; 2 g im), si può ripetere entro 30-60 min a.b., quindi ancora ogni ora per una o due dosi a.b. per perdita di forza persistente, elevata necessità di atropina
		Entrambi: coma, paralisi, convulsioni, apnea			Diazepam: 0,3 mg/kg (max 10 mg) ev; lorazepam: 0,1 mg/kg ev, im (max 4 mg); midazolam: 0,2 mg/kg (max 10 mg) im a.b. per convulsioni o grave esposizione
VESCICANTI					
Mostarda	Alchilazione	Cute: eritema, vescicole Occhio: infiammazione	Ore	Cute: sapone e acqua Occhi: acqua (efficace solo se effettuato entro minuti dall'esposizione)	Terapia sintomatica
		Vie respiratorie: infiammazione			
Lewisite	Arsenicale		Dolore immediato		Possibilmente BAL 3 mg/kg im ogni 4-6 h per gli effetti della lewisite nei casi gravi
AGENTI POLMONARI					
Cloro, fosgene	HCl libero, alchilazione	Occhi, naso, irritazione alla gola (specialmente cloro)	Minuti: occhi, naso, irritazione alla gola, broncospasmo;	Aria fresca	Terapia sintomatica
		Respiratori: broncospasmo, edema polmonare (specialmente fosgene)	Ore: edema polmonare	Cute: acqua	
CIANURO					
	Inibizione della citocromo ossidasi: anossia cellulare, acidosi lattica	Tachipnea, coma, convulsioni, apnea	Secondi	Aria fresca	ABC, ossigeno 100%
				Cute: sapone e acqua	Na bicarbonato a.b. acidosi metabolica Na nitrito (3%): dose (mL/kg) — Hb stimata (g/dL) 0,27 — 10 0,33 — 12 (stimata per il bambino medio) 0,39 — 14 (max 10 mL) Na tiosolfato (25%): 1,65 mL/kg (max 50 mL)

*Decontaminazione, specialmente per i pazienti con significativa esposizione ad agente nervino o vescicante; dovrebbe essere effettuata da personale sanitario che indossi un adeguato equipaggiamento protettivo personale. Per lo staff del pronto soccorso questo consiste in tute chimicamente resistenti, non incapsulate, stivali e guanti con maschera/cappuccio di purificazione dell'aria che ricoprono tutto il volto.

†La via intraossea è probabilmente equivalente a quella endovenosa.

‡L'atropina può avere qualche beneficio attraverso il tubo endotracheale o per inalazione, così come l'ipratropio aerosolizzato.

§Il pralidossima viene ricostituito a 50 mg/mL (1 g in 20 mL di acqua) per la somministrazione ev e la dose totale viene infusa in 30 min o mediante infusione continua (dose da carico 25 mg/kg in 30 min, quindi 10 mg/kg/h). Per l'uso im può essere diluito a una concentrazione di 300 mg/mL (1 g aggiunto a 3 mL di acqua, per analogia con la concentrazione dell'autoiniettore dell'U.S. Army's Mark 1®), per realizzare un volume adeguato per l'iniezione. Ogni kit di Mark 1 contiene due autoiniettori, uno di atropina 2 mg (0,7 mL) e uno di pralidossima 600 mg (2 mL); sebbene non approvati per l'uso pediatrico, essi possono essere presi in considerazione come trattamento iniziale in circostanze molto gravi (specialmente preospedaliere) per i bambini con tossicità grave e potenzialmente fatale da agente nervino che non siano dotati di accesso endovenoso e per i quali un dosaggio mg/kg im più preciso sarebbe logisticamente impossibile. Sono presentate le linee guida suggerite per il dosaggio; occorre notare il potenziale eccesso della dose di atropina e pralidossima iniziali per età/peso, sebbene entro le linee guida generali per il totale raccomandato nei primi 60-90 minuti di terapia delle esposizioni gravi:

Età approssimativa	Peso approssimativo	Numero di autoiniettori (ogni tipo)	Intervallo della dose di atropina (mg/kg)	Intervallo della dose di pralidossima (mg/kg)
3-7 anni	13-25 kg	1	0,08-0,13	24-46
8-14 anni	26-50 kg	2	0,08-0,13	24-46
>14 anni	>51 kg	3	≤0,11	≤35

ABC, supporto delle vie aeree, della respirazione e della circolazione (*Airway, Breathing and Circulatory support*); BAL, British anti-Lewisite; SNC, sistema nervoso centrale; HCl, acido cloridrico; Hb, concentrazione di emoglobina; max, massimo; a.b., al bisogno.
Adattata da Henretig FH, Cieslak TJ, Eitzen EM: Biological and chemical terrorism. *J Pediatr* 2002; 141:311-326. Per gentile concessione.

Molte malattie virali, come il vaiolo, la maggior parte delle febbri emorragiche virali e le encefaliti equine, sono trattate con una terapia di supporto.

Oltre a garantire adeguate ossigenazione, ventilazione e idratazione, il medico può avere bisogno di fornire terapie empiriche specifiche in modo urgente. I pazienti che soffrono di gravi sintomi neuromuscolari a esordio acuto possono avere subito un'intossicazione da agente nervino e andrebbero trattati tempestivamente con l'atropina (0,05 mg/kg) per i suoi effetti antimuscarinici. Sebbene l'atropina allievi il broncospasmo e la bradicardia, riduca le secrezioni e migliori gli effetti gastrointestinali della nausea, del vomito e della diarrea, tuttavia non migliora la paralisi del muscolo scheletrico. La pralidossima (nota anche come 2-PAM) cliva la parte di organofosfato dalla colinesterasi e rigenera l'enzima intatto se l'"invecchiamento" dell'enzima non si è verificato. L'effetto è più evidente in corrispondenza della giunzione neuromuscolare e porta al miglioramento della forza muscolare. Il suo tempestivo utilizzo (a una dose di 25 mg/kg) in aggiunta all'atropina è raccomandato in tutti i casi gravi.

Idealmente, si dovrebbero somministrare atropina e pralidossima in questi casi gravi, sebbene anche la via intraossea possa risultare accettabile. Alcuni esperti raccomandando di inoculare l'atropina per via intramuscolare in presenza di ipossia, al fine di evitare le aritmie associate all'assunzione endovenosa. Negli Stati Uniti, molti sistemi EMS forniscono kit di autoiniettori militari costituiti da atropina e 2-PAM per l'iniezione intramuscolare. Gli autoiniettori di atropina pediatrici ora risultano autorizzati, sebbene anche i kit militari (con 2 mg di atropina e 600 mg di pralidossima) possano venire usati nei bambini con più di 2-3 anni di età. Gli studi sugli animali depongono a favore dell'impiego profilattico di routine di dosi anticonvulsivanti di benzodiazepine, anche in assenza di un'attività convulsiva osservabile.

Sintomi neuromuscolari tardivi nell'ambito di azioni terroristiche possono essere dovuti al botulismo. La terapia di supporto, con una meticolosa attenzione a quello ventilatorio, è il cardine del suo trattamento. Tale supporto può essere necessario per diversi mesi, rendendo il trattamento di un'epidemia su larga scala particolarmente problematico in termini di risorse mediche. Un'antitossina botulinica bivalente autorizzata (tipi A e B) e un'antitossina botulinica equina in corso di studio di tipo E sono disponibili negli Stati Uniti tramite i CDC (1-404-639-3670). È improbabile che la somministrazione di queste antitossine faccia regredire la malattia nei pazienti sintomatici, ma può comunque prevenire l'ulteriore progressione. Una dose test andrebbe somministrata prima della terapia e bisognerebbe desensibilizzare i pazienti che reagiscono a questo test. Un'antitossina in corso di studio eptavalente desensibilizzata (Fab_2), prodotta anche nei cavalli, è disponibile tramite lo U.S. Army Medical Research Institute of Infectious Diseases in un protocollo d'uso straordinario. Inoltre, un prodotto (autorizzato per il trattamento del botulismo di tipo A e B) pentavalente (tipi A-E), Botulism Immune Globulin Intravenous (Human), BabyBIG®, è disponibile tramite il California Department of Health Services (1-510-231-7600).

La **rapida comparsa di sintomi respiratori** può segnalare un'esposizione a cloro, fosgene, cianuro o a tutta una serie di altre sostanze chimiche tossiche industriali. Sebbene il cardine della terapia in quasi tutte queste occorrenze consista nel trasporto all'aria fresca e nella terapia intensiva di supporto, l'intossicazione da cianuro spesso richiede l'utilizzo di antidoti specifici, somministrati in due stadi. Un agente formante metaemoglobina come il sodio nitrito viene fatto assumere per primo, perché la metaemoglobina ha elevata affinità per il cianuro e ne causa la dissociazione dalla citocromo ossidasi. Il dosaggio dei nitriti nei bambini dovrebbe essere basato sul peso corporeo, per evitare l'eccessiva formazione di metaemoglobina e l'ipotensione indotta dai nitriti. Per gli stessi motivi, i nitriti andrebbero infusi lentamente in 5-10 minuti. Successivamente si somministra un donatore di zolfo, come il sodio tiosolfato, un composto che viene impiegato come substrato dall'enzima epatico rhodanese, che converte il cianuro in tiocianato, meno tossico ed escreto nelle urine. Il trattamento con il tiosolfato è efficace e relativamente benigno e, pertanto, può essere istituito da solo per i casi lievi e moderati. Il sodio nitrito e il sodio tiosolfato negli Stati Uniti sono confezionati insieme in kit di antidoto standard, con l'aggiunta anche di amilnitrito, un sostituto del sodio nitrito che può essere inalato in contesti preospedalieri in cui l'accesso endovenoso non è disponibile.

Nei casi in cui i **sintomi respiratori a esordio tardivo** possano essere dovuti a un attacco terroristico, bisognerebbe prendere in considerazione la somministrazione empirica di un antibiotico efficace contro l'antrace, la peste e la tularemia. La ciprofloxacina (10-15 mg/kg ev ogni 12 h) o la doxiciclina (2,2 mg/kg ev ogni 12 h) appaiono opzioni ragionevoli. Sebbene i ceppi di *B. anthracis* che si verificano naturalmente siano piuttosto sensibili alla penicillina G, i suddetti agenti vengono scelti a causa dell'esistenza di ceppi penicillino-resistenti. Inoltre, la ciprofloxacina e la doxiciclina risultano efficaci contro tutti i ceppi noti di *Y. pestis* e *F. tularensis*. Le preoccupazioni nei confronti delle β-lattamasi inducibili in *B. anthracis* hanno portato alcuni esperti a raccomandare uno o due antibiotici aggiuntivi nei pazienti con un antrace inalatorio. Rifampicina, vancomicina, penicillina o ampicillina, clindamicina, imipenem e claritromicina costituiscono opzioni ragionevoli basate sui dati di sensibilità in vitro. Dato che la virulenza di *B. anthracis* si basa sulla produzione di due tossine proteiche, la tossina dell'edema e la tossina letale, i farmaci che agiscono a livello ribosomiale per distruggere la sintesi proteica (per es. la clindamicina e i macrolidi) risultano teoricamente vantaggiosi. Il frequente coinvolgimento meningeo nelle vittime di antrace inalatorio rende desiderabili agenti con una penetrazione superiore nel sistema nervoso centrale. Una combinazione di ciprofloxacina più clindamicina e penicillina G è una buona terapia empirica iniziale per una presunta inalazione di antrace. La ciprofloxacina o la doxiciclina in monoterapia è probabilmente adeguata nei casi di antrace cutaneo, sebbene i pazienti con una malattia cutanea secondaria a un attacco terroristico inizialmente dovrebbero ricevere una terapia multifarmacologica, a causa della possibilità di un'esposizione inalatoria concomitante.

Nei pazienti in cui viene posta la diagnosi di peste o di tularemia, la streptomicina (15 mg/kg im ogni 12 h) è storicamente stata considerata come il farmaco di scelta. Dal momento che attualmente questo farmaco è in genere indisponibile, molti esperti considerano la gentamicina (2,5 mg/kg ev/im ogni 8 h) l'opzione preferita. Oltre alla doxiciclina e alla ciprofloxacina, il cloramfenicolo (25 mg/kg ev ogni 6 h) è un'accettabile alternativa. Quest'ultimo dovrebbe essere impiegato nel 6% dei casi di peste polmonare, con meningite concomitante. Per essere efficace, la terapia per la peste polmonare va intrapresa entro 24 h dalla comparsa dei sintomi.

Il trattamento del **danno indotto da vescicanti** è simile a quello per le vittime delle ustioni ed è in gran parte sintomatico (vedi Capitolo 74). Le vittime da mostarda trarranno beneficio dall'applicazione di lozioni cutanee allevianti, come la calamina e dalla somministrazione di analgesici. L'intubazione precoce dei pazienti gravemente esposti è giustificata per evitare la compromissione edematosa delle vie aeree. Possono essere necessari ossigeno e ventilazione meccanica, mentre la scrupolosa attenzione all'idratazione è d'importanza capitale. Le vittime da lewisite possono essere trattate all'incirca allo stesso modo di quelle da mostarda. Inoltre, il dimercaprolo (British antilewisite [BAL]) in olio per via intramuscolare può aiutare a migliorare gli effetti sistemici della lewisite.

Anche il trattamento delle vittime del vaiolo sintomatico è in gran parte di supporto e l'attenzione al controllo del dolore, allo stato d'idratazione e alla sufficienza respiratoria è sempre di primaria importanza. Il composto antivirale parenterale cidofovir, autorizzato per il trattamento della retinite da Cytomegalovirus nei pazienti con infezione da HIV, è efficace *in vitro* contro il vaiolo e altri ortopoxvirus, ma la sua utilità nel trattamento delle vittime non è stata valutata. Inoltre, di fronte a una vasta epidemia, l'uso parenterale su larga scala di questo farmaco sarebbe problematico.

Cieslak TJ, Henretig FM: Bioterrorism. *Pediatr Ann* 2003;32:154–165.

Cieslak TJ, Henretig FM: Ring-a-ring-a-roses: Bioterrorism and its peculiar relevance to pediatrics. *Curr Op Pediatr* 2003;15:107–111.

Franz DR, Jahrling PB, McClain DJ, et al: Clinical recognition and management of patients exposed to biological warfare agents. *Clin Lab Med* 2001;21:435–473.

Henretig FH, Cieslak TJ, Eitzen EM: Biological and chemical terrorism. *J Pediatr* 2002;141:311–326.

Markenson D, Redlener I: Pediatric terrorism preparedness national guidelines and recommendations: Findings of an evidence-based consensus process. *Biosecur Bioterror* 2004;2:301–319.

Markenson D, Reynolds S, American Academy of Pediatrics Committee on Pediatric Emergency Medicine, Task Force on Terrorism: The pediatrician and disaster preparedness. *Pediatrics* 2006;117:340–362.

Patt HA, Feigin RD: Diagnosis and management of suspected cases of bioterrorism: A pediatric perspective. *Pediatrics* 2002;109:685–692.

White SR, Henretig F, Dukes RG: Medical management of vulnerable populations and co-morbid conditions of victims of bioterrorism. *Emerg Med Clin North Am* 2002;20:365–392.

Capitolo 712 ■ Morsi di animali e morsi umani

Charles M. Ginsburg

I cani e i gatti negli Stati Uniti sono circa 100 milioni e questo dato comporta una media di 3,5-4,7 milioni di soggetti morsi ogni anno. Tra essi, oltre 400 000 l'anno si rivolgono al Pronto Soccorso e a centri per l'emergenza autonomi. Si stima che i soggetti che sono stati morsi ricorrono con maggiore frequenza agli ambulatori medici e alle cliniche di medicina generale piuttosto che alle strutture per l'emergenza.

EPIDEMIOLOGIA. Negli Stati Uniti, nelle ultime 3 decadi, ci sono stati circa 20 decessi all'anno per lesioni causate da cani; il 65% di queste si sono avute in bambini di età inferiore agli 11 anni. Sono varie le razze di cani che attaccano i bambini; la Tabella 712-1 descrive l'indice di rischio in base alla razza ricavato da uno studio su 342 morsi. I rottweiler, i pitt-bull e i pastori tedeschi sono responsabili di oltre il 50% delle ferite mortali correlate ai morsi. I cani maschi non castrati costituiscono la causa di circa il 75% degli attacchi; le femmine che allattano possono attaccare l'uomo quando i bambini cercano di toccare uno dei loro cuccioli.

La maggior parte degli **attacchi da parte dei cani** si ha in bambini tra i 6 e gli 11 anni di età. I bambini vengono morsi più frequentemente delle bambine (1,5:1). Circa 2/3 di questi eventi si hanno nei pressi di casa, il 75% degli animali che mordono è conosciuto dai bambini e quasi il 50% degli attacchi viene riportato come "non provocato". Il Canada contempla statistiche simili, con il 70% dei morsi che si verifica in bambini tra i 2 e i 14 anni; il 65% dei cani coinvolti che faceva parte della famiglia e che ha compiuto il proprio attacco in casa.

Sono stati riportati circa 450 000 **morsi di gatti** all'anno negli Stati Uniti, quasi tutti causati da animali domestici conosciuti. Dal momento che i morsi di ratti e gerbilli (un tipo di roditore) non sono condizioni riferibili, poco si sa circa l'epidemiologia di queste lesioni e l'incidenza delle infezioni dopo i morsi o i graffi dei roditori.

Esistono pochi dati sulla diffusione e sugli aspetti demografici delle lesioni da **morso umano** nei pazienti pediatrici; comunque l'età prescolare e i primi anni di scuola sembrano essere quelli a rischio maggiore. Negli Stati Uniti i morsi umani costituiscono una causa frequente di ferita negli asili, sebbene in alcuni gruppi la percentuale sia maggiore in età adolescenziale. Negli adolescenti le lesioni da pugni alla bocca (denti) sono associate alle risse.

MANIFESTAZIONI CLINICHE. Le lesioni da morso di cane si dividono in tre categorie simili: abrasione, perforazione, ferita e lacerazione con o senza associazione dell'avulsione del tessuto. I morsi possono determinare anche schiacciamento. Il tipo più frequente di lesione causata da gatti e ratti è la ferita perforante. I morsi dei gatti spesso penetrano profondamente nel tessuto. Le lesioni da morso umano sono di due tipi: una di specie occlusiva, che si ha quando i denti superiori e inferiori mordono insieme una parte del corpo e una lesione al pugno della mano, nei bambini più grandi e nei giovani adulti, quando viene sferrato un pugno, di solito della mano dominante, contro i denti di un altro soggetto.

TABELLA 712-1. Rischio di morsi da cani negli Stati Uniti tra i bambini in base alla razza dei cani

RAZZA CANINA	N° DI MORSI (%)	POPOLAZIONE CANINA (%)	INDICE DI RISCHIO
Pastore tedesco	105 (34)	12	2,83
Doberman	8 (3)	1,1	2,71
Spitz	5 (2)	1,1	1,81
Pechinese	10 (3)	1,9	1,56
Bassotto	22 (7)	5,2	1,35
Schnauzer	5 (2)	1,5	1,33
Collie	10 (3)	2,3	1,30
Basset-hound	15 (5)	3,9	1,29
Barboncino	10 (3)	3,1	0,98
Rottweiler	3 (1)	1,1	0,92
Beagle	3 (1)	1,2	0,80
Terrier	15 (5)	8,1	0,61
Bernese	3 (1)	1,7	0,58
Labrador-retriever	11 (4)	8,2	0,49
Meticcio	39 (13)	28	0,46
Spaniel	5 (2)	6,5	0,31
Shi-tzu	1 (0,3)	1,2	0,26
Maltese	0 (0,0)	1,1	0,00

*I dati sulla distribuzione della popolazione canina sono stati ricavati dall'anagrafe canina della comunità locale. L'indice di rischio è stato calcolato dividendo la proporzione delle razze tra il totale della popolazione canina per la proporzione di questa razza tra tutti i morsi di cani valutati.

Da Schalamon J, Ainoedhofer H, Singer G, et al: Analysis of dog bites in children who are younger than 17 years. *Pediatrics* 2006;117:e374-e379.

DIAGNOSI. Il trattamento delle vittime di morsi deve iniziare con l'anamnesi e l'esame obiettivo. Occorre porre attenzione alle variabili che caratterizzano il morso (per es. il tipo di animale, domestico o selvatico, provocato o non provocato; la sede del morso); all'anamnesi di allergia ai farmaci; allo stato immunitario del bambino (tetano) e dell'animale (rabbia). Durante l'esame obiettivo occorre rilevare attentamente tipo, sede e profondità della lesione; la presenza di materiali estranei nella ferita; lo stato delle strutture sottostanti; l'estensione del movimento dell'area affetta se il morso riguarda un arto. Occorre riportare nella cartella clinica del paziente uno schema della lesione o delle lesioni. Serve una radiografia della parte affetta, se c'è la possibilità che l'osso o l'articolazione possano essere stati penetrati o fratturati o se è presente materiale estraneo. L'ipotesi di una frattura o di una lesione penetrante del cranio va presa in considerazione nei soggetti, soprattutto neonati, che hanno una ferita da morso di cane al viso o al capo.

COMPLICANZE. La complicanza più frequente delle lesioni da morso è l'**infezione**, indipendentemente dalla specie di animale che ha portato l'attacco. La decisione di effettuare un esame colturale con il materiale presente nella ferita dipende dalla specie di animale, dal tempo trascorso dalla lesione, dalla profondità della ferita, dalla presenza di materiale estraneo che contamina la ferita e da un'eventuale evidenza di infezione. Sebbene siano stati isolati batteri potenzialmente patogeni dall'80% delle ferite da morso di cane che sono state sottoposte a una consultazione medica entro 8 ore dal morso, l'incidenza dell'infezione dalle ferite che ricevono terapie mediche prima delle 8 ore è minore (2,5-2,0%).

Di conseguenza, a meno che non sia profonda ed estesa, che non sussistano segni di contaminazione o di infezione, che il paziente non sia immunocompromesso, la ferita presente da meno di 8 ore non necessita di un esame colturale. Alcune specie di *Capnocytophaga canimorsus*, un patogeno non comune delle lesioni da morsi, sono stati isolate da quasi il 5% delle ferite infette nei pazienti immunocompromessi. La diffusione dell'infezione da ferite da **morso di gatto** che ricevono terapie mediche precocemente è almeno del 50%, per cui appare prudente ottenere materiale per coltura da tutte le ferite causate da un gatto, tranne da quelle lievi, e da tutte le altre ferite da morso di animale che non vengono portate alla consultazione medica entro 8 ore, indipendentemente dalla specie di animale.

Non è nota l'incidenza dell'infezione dopo una lesione da **morso di roditore**. La maggior parte della flora orale dei ratti è simile a quella di altri mammiferi; a ogni modo, circa rispettivamente il 50% e il 25% delle specie di *Streptobacillus moniliformis* e di *Spirillum minus* si trovano ospitate dalla flora della cavità orale dei ratti. Ognuno di questi agenti può causare potenzialmente infezione (vedi Capitolo 712.1).

Tutti i **morsi umani**, indipendentemente dal meccanismo della lesione, vanno considerati a elevato rischio di infezione e devono essere sottoposti all'esame colturale. A causa della grande incidenza di infezioni anaerobiche in seguito a una ferita da morsi occorre prelevare materiale per la coltura di anaerobi e aerobi.

Le cause più comuni di infezione batterica dei tessuti molli in seguito a morsi di cani, gatti ed esseri umani sono riportate nella Tabella 712-2. I morsi a elevato rischio di infezione riguardano le mani, i piedi, i genitali, la penetrazione ossea o tendinea; comprendono inoltre morsi umani o di gatti, ritardo del trattamento

TABELLA 712-2. Microrganismi associati a infezioni da ferite da morso di mammiferi

FREQUENTI	NON FREQUENTI
CANI	
Infezioni miste	*Acinetobacter* spp.
Pasteurella multocida	*Aeromonas hydrophila*
Staphylococcus aureus	Streptococco α, β, γ-emolitico
Staphylococcus epidermidis	*Staphylococcus epidermidis*
	Bacteroides spp.
	Brucella canis
	Capnocytophaga canimorsus (o DF-2)
	Enterobacter cloacae
	Enterococcus spp.
	Escherichia coli
	Klebsiella spp.
	Moraxella spp.
	Peptococcus spp.
	Peptostreptococcus spp.
	Pseudomonas spp.
GATTI	
P. multocida	*Acinetobacter* spp.
S. aureus	*Bacteroides* spp.
	Corynebacterium spp.
	E. cloacae
	Fusobacterium spp.
	Streptococcus spp.
	S. epidermidis
UOMO	
Streptococco α, β, γ-emolitico	*Enterococcus* spp.
Bacteroides spp.	*Eubacterium* spp.
Corynebacterium spp.	*Klebsiella pneumoniae*
Eikenella corrodens	*Neisseria* spp.
Fusobacterium spp.	*Peptococcus* spp.
Infezioni miste	*Pseudomonas* spp.
Peptostreptococcus spp.	*Veillonella* spp.
S. aureus	

TABELLA 712-3. Trattamento profilattico per la prevenzione delle infezioni delle ferite da morso o animale

TIPO DI TRATTAMENTO	TRATTAMENTO
Detersione	Detergere la ferita dallo sporco visibile usando una grande quantità di soluzione salina sterile mediante irrigazione con siringa ad alta pressione* Non irrigare le ferite penetranti. Utilizzare le precauzioni standard
Coltura della ferita	Non per la ferita fresca senza segni di infezione Sì per ferite di oltre 8-12 ore e per ferite che sembrano infette†
Radiografia	Indicata per ferite che penetrano nell'osso o nelle articolazioni sottostanti, nel sospetto di fratture o per valutare l'inoculazione di corpi estranei
Sbrigliamento	Rimuovere i tessuti devitalizzati
Sbrigliamento ed esplorazione chirurgici	Sì se c'è uno dei fattori seguenti: • Ferita estesa (tessuto devitalizzato) • Coinvolgimento dell'articolazione matacarpofalangea (ferita da pugno) • Ferita al cranio da animale di grossa taglia
Sutura della ferita	Sì per ferite non penetranti da morso recenti (vedi testo)
Valutare la copertura immunitaria verso tetano	Sì
Valutare il rischio di contrarre la rabbia mediante il morso dell'animale	Sì
Valutare il rischio di infezione da virus dell'epatite B per morso umano	Sì
Valutare il rischio di infezione da virus dell'immunodeficienza umana dopo morso umano	Sì
Iniziare la terapia antibiotica	Sì, per: • Ferite da morso moderate o severe, specialmente se ci sono edema e schiacciamento • Ferite penetranti, specialmente se c'è penetrazione ossea, dei tendini o delle articolazioni • Morso al viso • Morsi a mani e piedi • Morsi nell'area genitale • Ferite in soggetti compromessi o con asplenia • Ferite con segni di infezione
Follow-up	Monitorare la ferita per eventuali segni di infezione per 48 ore

*Usare un ago 18 gauge con una siringa che contenga un grande volume. Le soluzioni antibiotiche o antinfettive non danno vantaggi e possono aumentare l'irritazione tissutale.
†Eseguire coltura sia per gli aerobi sia per gli anaerobi.
Da American Academy of Pediatrics. Bite wounds. In: Pickering LK, Baker CJ, Long SS, McMillan JA, eds. *Red Book: 2006 Report of the Committee on Infectious Disease*. 27th ed. ElK Grove Village, IL, AAP, 2006: pp 191-195.

di oltre 24 ore, presenza di materiale estraneo, immunosoppressione (asplenia) e schiacciamento o ferita perforante profonda.

TRATTAMENTO (TAB. 712-3). Dopo che si è ottenuto il materiale necessario e adeguato per l'esame colturale, la ferita deve essere anestetizzata, pulita e irrigata con abbondante soluzione salina. L'irrigazione con soluzioni contenenti antibiotici non dà vantaggi rispetto a quella con la sola soluzione salina e può causare irritazione locale dei tessuti. La ferita perforante va pulita accuratamente e irrigata con delicatezza, con un catetere o con aghi a punta smussa; non bisogna eseguire un'irrigazione ad alta pressione. Occorre rimuovere i tessuti avulsi o devitalizzati ed eventuali aree fluttuanti devono essere incise e drenate.

Esistono pochi dati e molte controversie sulla questione se la ferita da morso debba venire sottoposta a una chiusura primaria o a una chiusura primaria ritardata (3-5 giorni) oppure debba essere lasciata guarire per seconda intenzione. I fattori da considerare sono il tipo, la dimensione e la profondità della ferita; la sede anatomica; la presenza di un'infezione; il tempo che è passato dalla lesione; la possibilità di un danno estetico. Appare necessario richiedere una consulenza chirurgica in tutti i casi in cui la ferita sia profonda o estesa; se coinvolge il viso, le ossa e le articolazioni; se la ferita infetta necessiti di drenaggio aperto. Sebbene vi sia accordo generale sul fatto che le ferite infette e quelle che sono presenti da oltre 24 ore non devono essere suturate, sussiste disaccordo e vi sono esperienze cliniche differenti circa l'efficacia e la sicurezza di chiudere una ferita che sia stata procurata da meno di 8 ore e senza evidenza di infezione. Dal momento che tutte le **ferite alle mani** hanno un elevato rischio di infezione, soprattutto se c'è stata una lesione dei tendini o una penetrazione ossea, la chiusura primaria ritardata è raccomandata per tutte le lesioni eccetto quelle lievi alle mani. Le **lacerazioni del volto** hanno basso rischio di infezione secondaria, a causa dell'elevata vascolarizzazione di questa regione. Molti chirurghi plastici consigliano la chiusura primaria delle ferite da morso al viso che siano state portate alla consultazione medica entro 6 ore e siano state irrigate completamente con la rimozione del tessuto infetto o danneggiato.

Esistono pochi studi che dimostrino in modo inequivocabile l'efficacia degli antibiotici per la **profilassi** delle lesioni da morsi. Vi è un consenso generale sul fatto che debbano essere somministrati gli antibiotici a tutti i soggetti che abbiano subito morsi umani e tutti i morsi, tranne quelli lievi, di cani, gatti e ratti, indipendentemente dalla presenza di infezione. La specie batteriologica delle infezioni delle ferite da morso deriva principalmente della flora del cavo orale dell'animale che ha morso e in secondo luogo è un riflesso della flora cutanea del ferito (vedi Tab. 712-2). Dal momento che ogni specie batterica aerobica e anaerobica che colonizza la cavità orale dell'animale che morde ha la potenzialità d'invadere i tessuti locali, moltiplicarsi e causare una distruzione tissutale, la maggior parte delle infezioni da morsi è polimicrobica. Le evidenze indicano che non meno di 5 differenti specie possono essere isolate da una ferita infetta determinata da un morso di cane.

Malgrado l'elevato grado di somiglianza della flora batterica della cavità orale dell'uomo, del cane e del gatto, esistono importanti differenze tra le specie che mordono e ciò si riflette nel tipo di infezione delle ferite. Le specie batteriche predominanti isolate dalla ferita infetta da morso di cane sono *Staphylococcus aureus* (20-30%), *Pasteurella multocida* (20-30%), *Staphylococcus intermedius* (25%) e *C. canimorsus*; circa la metà delle infezioni da morso di cane contiene anaerobi misti. Specie simili vengono isolate dalle ferite infette da morso di gatto; *P. multocida* è comunque la prevalente, trovandosi in almeno il 50% di esse. Almeno il 50% dei ratti ospita ceppi di *Streptobacillus moniliformis* nell'orofaringe e circa il 25% ospita *S. minor*, un microrganismo anaerobio Gram-negativo. Nelle ferite da morso umano le specie prevalenti sono costituite da ceppi non tipizzabili di *Haemophilus influenzae*, *Eikenella corrodens*, *S. aureus*, streptococco α-emolitico e aerobi produttori di β-lattamasi (circa il 50%). Le lesioni da pugno sono particolarmente suscettibili alle infezioni da *Eikenella* spp. (25%) e batteri anaerobi (50%).

La scelta tra un antibiotico per via orale oppure parenterale si basa sulla gravità della ferita, sulla presenza e sul grado di una infezione palese, sui segni di tossicità sistemica e sullo stato immunitario del paziente. L'amoxicillina-clavulanato costituisce un'ottima scelta per la terapia empirica per via orale nel caso di ferite da morso umano e animale, a motivo del suo ampio spettro d'azione verso la maggior parte dei batteri che sono stati isolati dalle ferite infette. Similmente, la ticarcillina-clavulanato o l'ampicillina e il sulbactam sono preferibili nei pazienti che necessitano di una terapia empirica per via parenterale. La procaina penicillina resta il farmaco d'elezione per la profilassi e il trattamento delle lesioni da ratto. Le cefalosporine di prima generazione hanno un'efficacia limitata verso *P. multocida* ed *E. corrodens*, per cui non vanno usate per la profilassi o la terapia empirica iniziale delle infezioni della ferita da morso. Altre scelte terapeutiche per i pazienti allergici alla penicillina sono limitate, perché i farmaci alternativi tradizionali generalmente non sono efficaci contro uno o più dei patogeni multipli responsabili delle infezioni. Sebbene l'eritromicina sia frequentemente raccomandata come agente alternativo nei pazienti allergici alla penicillina che hanno subito morsi di cani e gatti, essa possiede una non completa validità verso ceppi di *P. multocida* e *S. moniliformis* e non è efficace contro *E. corrodens*. Similmente, la clindamicina e la combinazione trimetoprim-sulfametoxazolo hanno un'attività limitata verso, rispettivamente, i ceppi della *P. multocida* e batteri anaerobi. Si può considerare l'impiego dell'azitromicina e di chetolidi, a causa della loro azione verso i batteri aerobi e anaerobi presenti sulla ferita da morso infetta. La tetraciclina è il farmaco di scelta per i pazienti allergici alla penicillina con una lesione da morso di ratto.

Sebbene il **tetano** venga contratto raramente dopo una lesione da morso umano o animale, è importante disporre di un'accurata anamnesi dello stato immunitario del soggetto e somministrare un tossoide tetanico a tutti quei pazienti che risultano immunizzati in modo incompleto o a quelli per cui sono trascorsi 10 anni dall'ultima dose di vaccino antitetanico. La necessità di una vaccinazione antirabbica postesposizione nelle persone morse da cani e gatti dipende dalla conoscenza sulla vaccinazione dell'animale colpevole e soprattutto dall'esperienza con gli animali rabbiosi nella comunità locale (vedi Capitolo 271). Occorre consultare il dipartimento di sanità locale per avere consigli in tutti i casi in cui non si conoscano le vaccinazioni dell'animale che ha morso e se la rabbia sia endemica nella comunità. La profilassi postesposizione per l'epatite B va considerata nel caso raro in cui un soggetto abbia ricevuto un morso da un individuo a rischio elevato di epatite B (vedi Capitolo 355).

Tutte le ferite, tranne quelle lievi, da morso alla mano vanno immobilizzate in posizione funzionale per 3-5 giorni e i pazienti con ferite da morsi a un arto devono tenere l'arto colpito sollevato per 24-36 ore, fino a che l'edema non si sia risolto. Tutti i pazienti vanno rivalutati entro 24-36 ore dalla lesione.

PREVENZIONE. È possibile ridurre il rischio di lesione mediante una educazione preventiva. I genitori devono ricevere di routine, durante le visite prenatali e le visite di controllo, un counseling sul rischio che comporta tenere animali domestici che possono mordere in famiglia. Tutti i pazienti vanno messi in guardia verso la custodia di animali esotici. Inoltre, occorre informare i genitori sulla propensione di alcune razze di cani ad attaccare e sull'istinto protettivo della femmina che accudisce i cuccioli. Tutti i bambini piccoli vanno attentamente sorvegliati, soprattutto quando si trovano in presenza di un animale e fino da un'età molto precoce va insegnato loro a rispettare gli animali e vanno informati sulla loro possibilità potenziale di provocare lesioni (Tabb. 712-4 e 712-5).

La riduzione delle lesioni da morso umano, soprattutto negli asili e nelle scuole, si può ottenere mediante una buona sorveglianza dei bambini e un adeguato rapporto tra numero di addetti e numero di bambini.

TABELLA 712-4. Regole di comportamento quando si ha a che fare con un cane

CANI	UMANI
Il cane annusa per comunicare	Prima di accarezzare un cane, lasciarsi annusare
Il cane segue gli oggetti in movimento	Non passare di corsa davanti a un cane
Il cane corre più velocemente degli umani	Non cercare di sorpassare un cane
Urlare può stimolare il comportamento da predatore	Restare tranquilli se si avvicina un cane
L'ordine di precedenza deve essere rispettato	Non abbracciare o baciare un cane
Il contatto oculare diretto può essere interpretato come aggressione	Evitare il contatto oculare diretto
I cani tendono ad attaccare gli arti, il viso e il collo	Se attaccati, restare calmi (piedi uniti) e proteggere collo e viso con braccia e mani
Distendersi a terra provoca l'attacco	Stare in piedi. Se attaccati mentre ci si distende, mettere il viso in basso e coprire le orecchie con le mani. Restare fermi
I cani che lottano mordono qualsiasi cosa sia vicina	Non cercare di separare due cani che lottano

Da Schalamon J, Ainoedhofer H, Singer G, et al: Analysis of dog bites in children who are younger than 17 years. *Pediatrics* 2006; 117: e374-e379.

TABELLA 712-5. Come prevenire i morsi dei cani

- Valutare in modo realistico l'ambiente e lo stile di vita e consultare un professionista (per es. un veterinario, un comportamentalista animale o un allevatore) per valutare quali razze di cani considerare.
- Cani con episodi di aggressioni precedenti non sono adatti a famiglie con bambini.
- Stare attenti ai segnali di paura e apprensione del bambino verso il cane e se ci sono ritardarne l'acquisto.
- Dedicare un tempo adeguato prima di comprare o accogliere un cane. Usare cautela nel portare un cane o un cucciolo in casa di un neonato o di un lattante.
- Castrare tutti i cani (questo solitamente riduce le tendenze aggressive).
- Non lasciare un neonato o un bambino piccolo solo con un cane.
- Socializzare e addestrare adeguatamente ogni cane che entri in famiglia. Insegnare al cane a obbedire (per es. mettersi a pancia in su, lasciare il cibo senza ringhiare).
- Chiedere immediatamente la consulenza di un professionista (per es. veterinario, comportamentalista animale, allevatore) se il cane sviluppa comportamenti aggressivi o indesiderati.
- Non fare giochi violenti con il proprio cane (per es. la lotta).
- Insegnare ai bambini le regole di sicurezza di base nel relazionarsi con il cane e riesaminarle regolarmente:
  – non avvicinare un cane che non si conosce;
  – non scappare mai urlando;
  – restare immobili quando si viene avvicinati da un cane con cui non si ha familiarità (per es. "fermo come un albero");
  – se buttati a terra da un cane, "accoccolarsi" e restare fermi (per es. "fermo come un tronco");
  – non giocare con un cane senza il controllo da parte di un adulto;
  – riferire immediatamente a un adulto se c'è un cane randagio in giro o se un cane mostra un comportamento insolito;
  – evitare il contatto oculare diretto con un cane;
  – non disturbare un cane mentre dorme, mangia o accudisce i cuccioli;
  – non accarezzare un cane senza avergli permesso di annusarci;
  – se morsi, riferirlo immediatamente a un adulto.

Da Centers for Disease Control and Prevention: Dog bite – related fatalities – United States, 1995-1996. *MMWR* 1997; 46:463-467.

Benson L, Edwards S, Schiff A, et al: Dog and cat bites to the hand: Treatment and cost assessment. *J Hand Surg* 2006;31:468–473.
Broder J, Jerrard D, Olshaker J, Witting M: Low risk of infection in selected human bites treated without antibiotics. *Am J Emer Med* 2004;22:10–12.

Centers for Disease Control and Prevention: Nonfatal dog bite-related injuries treated in hospital emergency departments–United States, 2001. *MMWR* 2003;52:605.
Centers for Disease Control and Prevention: Dog-bite–related fatalities–United States, 1995–1996. *MMWR* 1997;46:463–467.
Chapman S, Righetti J, Sung L: Preventing dog bites in children: Randomised controlled trial of an educational intervention. *BMJ* 2000;320:1512.
Chen E, Hornig S, Shepherd SM, Hollander JE: Primary closure of mammalian bites. *Acad Emer Med* 2000;7:157–161.
Cummings P: Antibiotics to prevent infection in patients with dog bite wounds: A meta-analysis of randomized trials. *Ann Emerg Med* 1994; 23:535.
Merchant RC, Fuerch J, Becker BM, Mayer KH: Comparison of the epidemiology of human bites evaluated at three US pediatric emergency departments. *Pediatr Emerg Care* 2005;21:833–838.
Schalamon J, Ainoedhofer H, Singer G, et al: Analysis of dog bites in children who are younger than 17 years. *Pediatrics* 2006;117:e374–e379.
Stefanopoulos PK, Tarantzopoulou: Facial bite wounds: management update. *Int J Oral Maxillofoc Surg* 2005;34:464–472.
Talan DA, Abrahamian M, Moran GJ, et al: Clinical presentation and bacteriologic analysis of infected human bites in patients presenting to emergency departments. *Clin Infect Dis* 2003;37:1481–1489.
Talan DA, Citron DM, Abrahamian FM, et al: Bacteriologic analysis of infected dog and cat bites. *N Engl J Med* 1999;340:85.

712.1 • FEBBRE DA MORSO DI RATTO

EZIOLOGIA. "Febbre da morso di ratto" è un termine generico che è stato applicato ad almeno due sindromi cliniche distinte, causate da microrganismi diversi.

Negli Stati Uniti, la forma più frequente di febbre da morso di ratto è determinata da *Streptobacillus moniliformis*, un microrganismo Gram-negativo presente nella flora dell'orofaringe di circa il 50% dei ratti sani. Solitamente l'infezione si contrae in seguito al morso di un ratto, ma si può presentare anche in soggetti che hanno subito un graffio o che hanno toccato ratti morti e in quelli che hanno consumato latte contaminato da *Streptobacillus moniliformis* (**febbre di Haverhill**).

La forma meno comune di febbre da morso di ratto (**sodoku**) è causata da *Spirillum minus*, un piccolo microrganismo spirillare, Gram-negativo aerobico. Il periodo d'incubazione è più lungo (14-21 giorni) rispetto alla forma della malattia causata da streptobacilli e le mialgie e l'artrite sono meno frequenti.

DECORSO CLINICO. Il periodo d'incubazione per la forma di febbre da morso di ratto causata da streptobacilli è variabile ed è compreso fra 3 e 10 giorni. La malattia è caratterizzata dall'insorgenza improvvisa di febbre, cefalea severa pulsante, mialgie intense, brividi e vomito. Virtualmente, in tutti i casi la lesione nella sede d'inoculazione guarisce nel momento in cui appaiono i primi segni di tipo sistemico. Subito dopo l'insorgenza della febbre, si ha un rash polimorfo in oltre il 75% dei pazienti, nella maggior parte dei quali il rash consiste in lesioni maculopapulari rosse a chiazze che spesso presentano una componente petecchiale; la distribuzione del rash è variabile, ma generalmente è più concentrata agli arti (Fig. 712-1). Circa la metà dei pazienti svilupperà un'artrite, i cui primi segni compaiono verso la fine della prima settimana di malattia; in fase iniziale l'artrite può essere migrante. Se non trattati, febbre, rash e artrite durano 14-21 giorni; spesso la febbre e l'artrite hanno un andamento bifasico. Un'ampia gamma di complicanze è stata riscontrata nei pazienti con febbre da morso di ratto, le più frequenti delle quali sono la polmonite, l'artrite persistente, gli ascessi cerebrali e dei tessuti molli e meno frequentemente la miocardite e l'endocardite.

Il segno patognomonico della malattia da *Spirillum* è una lesione che non guarisce, indurata e spesso suppurativa nella sede del morso. Sono sempre presenti una linfoadenite e una linfoadenopatia nei linfonodi regionali che drenano la sede d'inoculazione e molti pazienti sviluppano un rash maculare generalizzato che diventa più evidente con la febbre. Nei pazienti non trattati il sodoku ha un andamento recidivante; dopo 5-7 giorni di brividi e febbre la sintomatologia si attenua, ma si ripresenta trascorsi 7-10 giorni. Possono esserci più cicli se la malattia non viene riconosciuta e trattata.

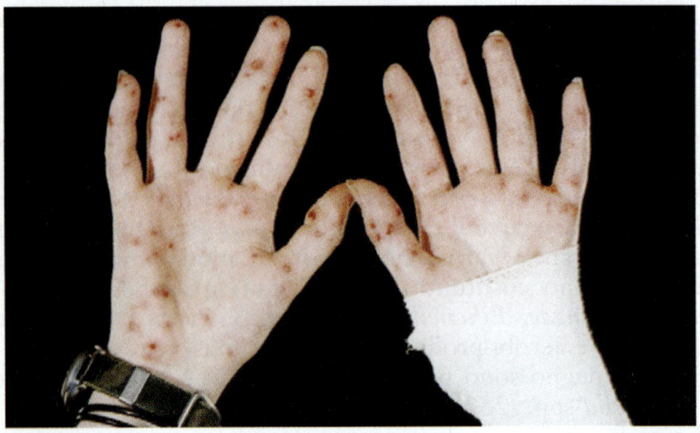

Figura 712-1. Rash maculopapulare con piccole eruzioni rosso scuro sulla mano di un soggetto con febbre da morso di ratto. (Da Van Nood E, Peters SH: Rat-bite fever. *Neth J Med* 2005;63:319-321.)

DIAGNOSI. La diagnosi di febbre da morso di ratto da streptobacilli è difficoltosa, dal momento che la malattia non è usuale e viene spesso confusa con la febbre maculosa delle Montagne Rocciose (vedi Capitolo 225) o meno di frequente con la meningococcemia (vedi Capitolo 190). Inoltre *Streptobacillus moniliformis* è difficilmente isolabile e identificabile mediante le abituali tecniche batteriologiche. Il microrganismo è "esigente", dato che necessita di terreni arricchiti per crescere ed è inibito dal sodio polianetosulfonato, un additivo presente nella maggior parte dei flaconi per emocoltura che si trovano in commercio. Si effettua una diagnosi definitiva quando si riscontra il microrganismo nel sangue o nel liquido articolare o si identifica in campioni umani mediante la tecnologia molecolare.

La diagnosi di sodoku è clinica, dato che non esistono test sierologici e che lo *Spirillum minus* non cresce su terreni artificiali. Raramente il microrganismo viene identificato mediante striscio colorato con colorazione di Gram ottenuto dal pus presente nella sede d'inoculazione infetta.

TRATTAMENTO. Il farmaco d'elezione è la penicillina per ambedue le forme di febbre da morso di ratto. Deve essere somministrata penicillina G endovena per 7-10 giorni, seguita da penicillina V per via orale per altri 7 giorni. Se il paziente risponde velocemente e migliora in 5-7 giorni senza segni di endocardite, si può effettuare in quel momento il passaggio alla penicillina per os. Alternative efficaci, in caso di allergia alla penicillina, sono rappresentate dalla tetraciclina e dall'eritromicina.

Berger C, Altwegg M, Meyer A, et al: Broad range polymerase chain reaction for diagnosis of rat-bite fever caused by *Streptobacillus moniliformis*. *Pediatr Infect Dis J* 2001;20:1181-1182.
Ojukwu IC, Christy C: Rat-bite fever in children: Case report and review. *Scand J Infect Dis* 2002;34:474-477.
Stehle P, Dubuis O, So A, et al: Rat bite fever without fever. *Ann Rheum Dis* 2003;62:894-897.
van Nood E, Peters SH: Rat-bite fever. *Neth J Med* 2005;63:319-321.

712.2 • VAIOLO DELLA SCIMMIA

EZIOLOGIA. Il vaiolo della scimmia è una rara malatia virale causata dal virus del vaiolo della scimmia, appartenente agli *Orthopoxvi-*

rus. La malattia è stata riscontrata per la prima volta nell'uomo in Africa occidentale e centrale. Le scimmie sono l'ospite principale per il virus, che tuttavia è stato anche ritrovato negli scoiattoli africani, nei ratti e nei topi; ne è stata osservata la presenza e la trasmissione anche nei cani della prateria degli Stati Uniti.

La trasmissione primaria della malattia dall'animale infetto all'uomo avviene attraverso il morso o tramite il contatto dell'uomo con sangue infetto dell'animale, ferite infette o liquidi corporei. La trasmissione interumana dell'infezione non è frequente, ma si ritiene essere stata una fonte importante per l'insorgenza di nuovi casi durante il picco epidemico della malattia che si è avuto negli Stati Uniti nel 2003.

DECORSO CLINICO. I segni clinici, i sintomi e il decorso del vaiolo della scimmia sono simili a quelli del vaiolo, anche se più lievi. Dopo un periodo di incubazione di 10-14 giorni, durante il quale il virus si moltiplica nei tessuti linfatici, gli esseri umani manifestano un malessere improvviso, febbre, mialgie, cefalea e mal di schiena severo. Possono presentarsi una tosse non produttiva, nausea, vomito e dolore addominale. La linfoadenopatia generalizzata, di raro riscontro nel vaiolo, è sempre presente nello stadio acuto. Dopo un periodo prodromico di 2-4 giorni, si ha un esantema che procede in senso cefalo-caudale. Al progredire del rash inizia la diminuzione del picco febbrile. Inizialmente il rash compare al viso sotto forma di macule eritematose, ma dopo poche ore dalla comparsa le macule si mutano in papule dure che rapidamente, in 2-3 giorni, si trasformano in vescicole e pustole. A differenza del vaiolo e similmente alla varicella, le lesioni del vaiolo della scimmia appaiono in gruppi. Successivamente, nella seconda settimana di malattia, la lesione si secca, forma la crosta e cade.

Si deve sospettare il vaiolo della scimmia in tutti i bambini che hanno i prodromi caratteristici associati a una forma atipica di varicella e un'anamnesi di contatto con cani della prateria o mammiferi esotici come i ratti del Gambia e gli scoiattoli africani. Ognuno dei seguenti criteri conferma la diagnosi in modo definitivo:

1. **isolamento del virus del vaiolo della scimmia nella coltura;**
2. **dimostrazione del DNA del vaiolo della scimmia mediante PCR di un campione clinico;**
3. **dimostrazione di un virus morfologicamente compatibile con un *Orthopoxvirus* mediante microscopia elettronica in assenza di esposizione a un altro *Orthopoxvirus*;**
4. **dimostrazione della presenza dell'*Orthopoxvirus* nel tessuto tramite metodi di valutazione immunoistochimici in assenza di esposizione a un altro *Orthopoxvirus*.**

TRATTAMENTO. Non esiste una terapia di provata efficacia per il vaiolo della scimmia. Sebbene vi sia evidenza che il vaccino per il vaiolo è efficace nel prevenire o attenuare la malattia nell'85% dei casi, la sua rarità non giustifica una vaccinazione di massa. In caso di esposizione nota o di epidemie, può sopravvenire l'indicazione a somministrare il vaccino. Occorre considerare se vaccinare i familiari stretti dei contatti e gli operatori sanitari che curano i soggetti infetti. Il vaccino sembra possedere un'azione preventiva se somministrato entro 2 ore dall'esposizione. I soggetti immunocompromessi e coloro che sono allergici in modo grave al lattice o al vaccino contro il vaiolo o ad alcuni dei suoi componenti (polimixina B, streptomicina, clortetraciclina, neomicina) non devono essere vaccinati.

Occorre porre attenzione all'igiene della cute, al mantenimento di un'alimentazione e di un'idratazione adeguate, a una rapida implementazione di una terapia locale o sistemica per una infezione batterica secondaria che può verificarsi. Per prevenire la diffusione interumana della malattia occorre implementare le linee guida dei Centers for Disease Control and Prevention per il controllo delle infezioni trasmesse attraverso le goccioline e per via aerea.

Cho CT, Wenner HA: Monkeypox virus. *Bacteriol Rev* 1973;37:1.
Earl PL, Americo JL, Wyatt LS, et al: Immunogenicity of a highly attenuated MVA smallpox vaccine and protection against monkeypox. *Nature* 2004;428:182.
Ligon BL: Monkeypox: A review of the history and emergence in the Western hemisphere. *Sem Pediatr Infect Dis* 2004:15:280.
Maskalyk J: Monkeypox outbreak among pet owners. *CMAJ* 2003;169:44.
Sejvar JJ, Chowdary Y, Schomogyi M, et al: Human monkeypox infection: A family cluster in the midwestern United States. *J Infect Dis* 2004:190:1833.

Capitolo 713 ■ Avvelenamenti

Steve Holve

La maggior parte dei morsi e delle punture da parte di ragni, serpenti, scorpioni e altri animali velenosi provoca dolore poco più che locale e non richiede un'attenzione medica. I bambini, tuttavia, sono a maggiore rischio di reazioni gravi, per il fatto che nel loro caso una determinata quantità di veleno ha un minore volume di distribuzione.

I sintomi di avvelenamento possono essere IgE-mediati, come l'anafilassi in risposta alle punture di Imenotteri, oppure mediati dal veleno, come nel caso dei morsi di ragni o di serpenti velenosi o della puntura di scorpioni. Le reazioni di ipersensibilità immediata vengono trattate in urgenza, come descritto nel Capitolo 148 a proposito dell'anafilassi. L'antidoto specie-specifico migliora i sintomi e previene la morte per gravi reazioni mediate dal veleno, ma il suo utilizzo comporta rischi significativi. L'appropriata valutazione del rapporto rischio:beneficio nell'uso dell'antidoto è importante nel trattamento dei morsi e delle punture.

ANTIDOTI

I **veleni** sono miscele specie-specifiche di polipeptidi, enzimi proteolitici, glicoproteine e sostanze vasoattive. Tutti gli **antidoti** sono costituiti da immunoglobuline derivate da animali che si legano alle proteine nel veleno neutralizzandole. L'origine animale di questi prodotti espone i pazienti a elevate quantità di proteine estranee, che causano reazioni di ipersensibilità immediata e ritardata.

Negli Stati Uniti, solo 4 antidoti sono autorizzati per il commercio dalla U.S. Food and Drug Administration (FDA). Per i morsi di crotalidi sono disponibili l'antiveleno (crotalidi) polivalente (ACP) derivato dal siero del cavallo e il Crotalidae Polyvalent Immune Fab (Crofab), derivato dalla pecora. Inoltre, si può trovare un antidoto prodotto dal siero di cavallo per i morsi del serpente corallo (*Micrurus fulvius*) e della vedova nera (*Latrodectus mactans*). Altri antidoti per specie più rare di serpenti o scorpioni possono essere reperibili presso l'American Zoo and Aquarium Association (1-301-562-0777) e l'Arizona Poison Control Center (1-800-222-1222).

Le reazioni da ipersensibilità immediata (vedi Capitolo 148) agli antidoti possono essere fatali, sebbene il rischio differisca enormemente a seconda del prodotto. L'incidenza di tali reazioni dopo la somministrazione di Crotalid equino può arrivare al 25-40%. L'antidoto ovino Crofab ha invece un tasso di reazione acuta molto minore (15%) e la maggior parte degli eventi è lieve. Le reazioni di ipersensibilità all'antidoto per la vedova nera e per il serpente corallo si verificano a un tasso dell'1% circa. In considerazione del rischio di anafilassi, l'antidoto andrebbe somministrato soltanto in una situazione in cui sono disponibili attrezzature complete di rianimazione, tra cui ossigeno, intubazione endotracheale, possibilità di somministrazione di liquidi endovenosi e adrenalina.

Bisognerebbe interrogare i pazienti circa eventuali allergie a farmaci e passate esposizioni ad antidoti. Se risulta necessario adoperare prodotti di derivazione equina si può effettuare un test cutaneo, ma questa pratica rimane controversa. Il test cutaneo ritarda il trattamento e di per sé ha scatenato anafilassi e malattia da siero. Il test cutaneo presenta anche elevati tassi di falsi positivi e di falsi negativi, fino al 30%. Il test cutaneo viene eseguito utilizzando 0,02 mL di un antidoto diluito a 1:10. Un risultato positivo non preclude l'uso dell'antidoto, ma avverte il medico che sussiste un aumentato rischio di anafilassi. In questi casi risulta necessario il pretrattamento con somministrazione endovenosa di difenidramina 1 mg/kg e metilprednisolone 1-2 mg/kg. Alcuni tossicologi raccomandano il pretrattamento in tutti i pazienti che ricevano l'antidoto.

Se si sviluppano segni di ipersensibilità immediata durante la somministrazione dell'antidoto, l'infusione dovrebbe essere interrotta finché il paziente non si sia stabilizzato. Se la gravità dell'avvelenamento giustifica l'infusione continua dell'antidoto, essa può riprendere a una velocità più lenta o simultaneamente alla somministrazione di adrenalina. In tali casi è raccomandabile la consulenza con il tossicologo più vicino in un centro antiveleni.

L'ipersensibilità ritardata, o malattia da siero (vedi Capitolo 149), si sviluppa fino nel 65% dei pazienti che ricevono l'antidoto equino-derivato e fino nel 15% di quelli trattati con i prodotti ovino-derivati. Di solito la malattia si sviluppa 5-21 giorni dopo l'esposizione e può durare per settimane. Si manifesta più comunemente con orticaria, prurito, artralgia e malessere generale, ma raramente può presentarsi con glomerulonefrite da immunocomplessi, neurite o miocardite. È stato dimostrato che i test cutanei intradermici non predicono il rischio di malattia da siero in modo accurato. L'uso profilattico di antistaminici e corticosteroidi può ridurre questo rischio ed essere sicuramente vantaggioso se i sintomi si sviluppano.

MORSO DI SERPENTE

Delle >3000 specie note di serpenti, solo 200 sono velenose per l'uomo. Il 90% dei serpenti velenosi fa parte di una di queste tre famiglie: Idrofidi, o serpenti d'acqua velenosi; Elapidi, che comprendono i cobra, i mamba e i serpenti corallo; Viperidi, o vipere vere (Tab. 713-1).

Negli Stati Uniti, il 95% dei morsi velenosi è inflitto dai Crotalidi, o vipere delle fossette, una sottofamiglia delle vipere vere. I Crotalidi possono essere identificati in base alla loro testa triangolare, agli occhi ellittici e alla fossetta identificabile tra gli occhi e il naso (Fig. 713-1). I membri di questa famiglia, negli Stati Uniti, comprendono il serpente a sonagli, il mocassino acquatico e la testa di rame. I serpenti corallo, gli altri serpenti velenosi nativi degli Stati Uniti, si trovano in Texas e nel sud-est e fanno parte della famiglia degli Elapidi. Sono piccoli, con testa piccola e rotondeggiante e bande rosse e nere brillanti separate da bande gialle più ristrette. Il detto "red on yellow, kill a fellow; red on black, venom lack" (Letteralmente "rosso e giallo, uccide una persona; rosso e nero senza veleno". Variante italiana: "Rosso e nero, sicuro è il sentiero; rosso e giallo è proprio un corallo", *N.d.C.*) serve per differenziare il serpente corallo dal *Lampropeltis triangulum elapsoides*, di aspetto simile ma non velenoso. I

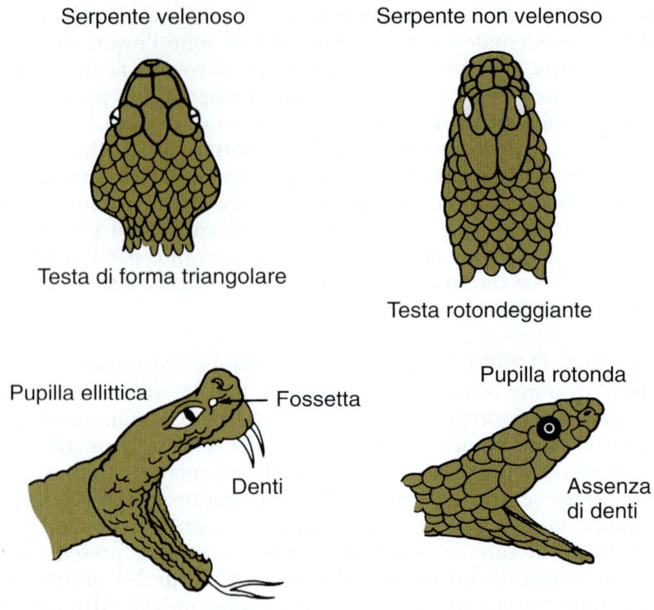

Figura 713-1. Identificazione dei serpenti velenosi. (Modificata da Rosen P et al [editors]: *Emergency Medicine*, 3th ed. St. Louis, CV Mosby, 1992.)

cobra e i bungari sono comuni in alcune parti dell'Asia, mentre le vipere, i cobra e i marassi (*Vipera berus*) sono comuni in alcune parti dell'Africa.

EPIDEMIOLOGIA. Negli Stati Uniti ogni anno vengono riportati circa 45 000 morsi di serpenti, solo 8000 dei quali sono inflitti da serpenti velenosi. L'incidenza è significativamente maggiore in Africa (stimata a 5 morsi per 1000 persone in Nigeria; 23 000 morti da morso di serpente per anno in Africa Occidentale), in Australia (da 0,6 a 5 morsi per 1000 persone), in Asia e in Sudamerica. Negli Stati Uniti la maggior parte si verifica in maschi giovani e vede implicata l'intossicazione da alcol; spesso la vittima ha provato a catturare o a giocare con il serpente. In Africa e in Asia la maggior parte dei morsi interessa gli arti inferiori, si verifica di notte ed è provocata dall'avere calpestato un serpente. Negli Stati Uniti si verificano solo 12-15 decessi ogni anno, mentre tassi di mortalità fino al 15% sono riportati nelle vittime di morso di serpente ospedalizzate in alcune parti dell'Africa e dell'Asia, in cui la terapia intensiva e l'accesso all'antidoto sono limitati. I bambini, a causa della loro minore massa corporea per la distribuzione del veleno, hanno una probabilità molto maggiore di presentare una reazione sistemica grave all'avvelenamento e costituiscono oltre la metà dei decessi.

PATOGENESI. Il veleno del serpente è una miscela specie-specifica di polipeptidi, enzimi proteolitici e tossine. Il veleno degli Ela-

TABELLA 713-1. Principali serpenti velenosi nel mondo

FAMIGLIA	SOTTOFAMIGLIA	DISTRIBUZIONE ED ESEMPI	COMMENTI
Viperidae	Crotalidae (crotali)	Nord America: specie crotalus e sistrurus (serpente a sonagli), specie agkistrodon (mocassino acquatico, testa di rame) America Centrale e Sudamerica: specie crotalus (serpente a sonagli), specie agkistrodon (testa di rame), specie bothrops (ferro-di-lancia), *Lachesis muta* (terrore dei boschi)	Fossetta termo-sensitiva tra ciascun occhio e la narice; pupille ellittiche; zanne canalizzate e retrattili
Viperidae	Viperinae (vipere vere)	Africa, Europa, Medio Oriente: *Bitis arietans* (puff adder), *B. gabonica* (vipera del Gabon), *B. nasicornis* (vipera cornuta-rinoceronte), specie echis (vipera rostrata-squamata), specie cerastes (vipere cornute o del deserto), specie vipera (vipere) Subcontinente indiano e Sudest asiatico: *Daboia russelli* (vipera di Russell)	Assenza di fossette sensitive
Elapidae		Zone tropicali e caldo-temperate: specie naja (cobra), specie dendroaspis (mamba), specie bungarus (bungari), specie micrurus, calliophis e maticora (serpenti corallo) e la maggior parte dei serpenti velenosi dell'Australia	Zanne corte, fisse; veleno iniettato da una successione di movimenti di masticazione
Hydrophidae	Hydrophinae (serpenti d'acqua veri)	Regione indopacifica: *Pelamis platurus* (serpente pelagico del mare)	Zanne simili a quelle degli Elapidae; veleno estremamente neurotossico; raramente morde l'uomo

Da Gold BS, Dart RC, Barish RA: Bites of venomous snakes. *N Engl J Med* 2002;347:347-356.

pidi e degli Idrofidi è prevalentemente neurotossico e possiede un effetto simil-curarico, per il blocco della neurotrasmissione in corrispondenza della giunzione neuromuscolare. La morte è secondaria alla depressione respiratoria. Il veleno dei Crotalidi è citolitico, provocando necrosi tissutale, stravaso vascolare e coagulopatie. La morte da morso di crotali è secondaria allo shock emorragico, a sindrome da distress respiratorio dell'adulto e a insufficienza renale.

Manifestazioni cliniche. I morsi dei Crotalidi di solito interessano gli arti; entro minuti compaiono dolore ed edema in corrispondenza del sito (Tab. 713-2). Via via che il veleno si sposta prossimalmente, l'edema e l'ecchimosi progrediscono; nei casi gravi fanno seguito la formazione di bolle e la necrosi tissutale (Fig. 713-2). I sintomi sistemici comprendono nausea, vomito, diaforesi, perdita di forza, formicolio al volto e alle fascicolazioni muscolari. Raramente i pazienti possono presentarsi con shock, con un edema generalizzato o aritmie cardiache. Spesso compaiono anomalie complesse della coagulazione.

I morsi della maggior parte degli Elapidi, tra cui i serpenti corallo, sono minimamente dolorosi, in quanto il veleno non possiede citotossine. Tuttavia, la mancanza di sintomi immediati non dovrebbe essere scambiata per l'assenza di un avvelenamento grave. Il veleno del serpente corallo è prevalentemente neurotossico e i sintomi possono progredire rapidamente in poche ore da una lieve sonnolenza alla paralisi dei nervi cranici, debolezza e morte per insufficienza respiratoria.

Trattamento. Il primo obiettivo è determinare se il morso è stato inflitto da un serpente velenoso e se si è verificato l'avvelenamento. Se il serpente è stato ucciso, esso dovrebbe essere portato al pronto soccorso per l'identificazione. Oltre l'80% dei morsi negli Stati Uniti viene inflitto da serpenti non velenosi; questi morsi provocano un dolore minimo senza la comparsa di un edema e richiedono soltanto la terapia locale della ferita.

Se si stabilisce invece che il morso è stato inflitto da un serpente velenoso, la terapia immediata consiste nell'immobilizzare l'arto interessato e trasportare rapidamente il paziente all'ospedale più vicino. Alcuni raccomandano un laccio emostatico prossimale sufficientemente lasso da consentire il passaggio di due dita e permettere il flusso ematico arterioso. Molti esperti attualmente evitano di applicare fasce di costrizione per il rischio di un'ischemia, che aggrava il danno tissutale locale. Si ritiene che il ghiaccio sul sito del morso o l'escissione o la suzione causino più danni che benefici tissutali e dovrebbero essere evitati. L'esperienza con i morsi da serpente a sonagli mostra che i trattamenti sul campo hanno aumentato il danno tissutale e triplicato la necessità di un intervento chirurgico successivo.

All'arrivo del paziente al pronto soccorso occorre inserire una linea endovenosa di grosso calibro e si devono effettuare esami del sangue basali. È necessario che gli esami del sangue iniziali comprendano la tipizzazione e le prove incrociate, in quanto una coagulopatia progressiva può successivamente rendere impossibile la tipizzazione. Gli altri test includono l'emocromo completo con conta delle piastrine; tempi di protrombina e di tromboplastina parziale; fibrinogeno e prodotti di degradazione della fibrina; azotemia, creatinina e creatinina fosfochinasi. Questi esami vanno ripetuti periodicamente, a seconda della gravità dell'avvelenamento. Occorre misurare i parametri vitali basali e la circonferenza dell'arto morsicato, contrassegnando l'ecchimosi e l'edema in modo da potere monitorare la progressione. La ferita

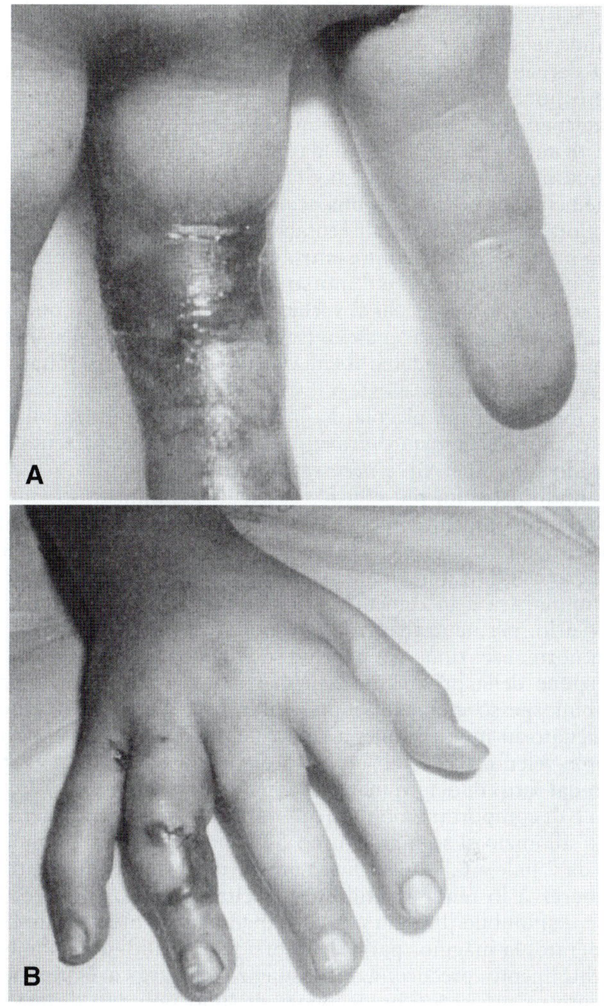

Figura 713-2. *A*, Avvelenamento da crotalidi; fotografia scattata 60 minuti dopo il morso. Sono evidenti l'edema marcato e l'ecchimosi. I segni dei denti sono appena visibili. *B*, Nello stesso paziente, il dorso della mano mostra un edema esteso. (Da Wolf MD: Evenomation. In Halbrook PR [ed]: *Textbook of Pediatric Critical Care*. Philadelphia, WB Saunders, 1993, p 1028.)

TABELLA 713-2. Linee guida per la valutazione della gravità degli avvelenamenti da Crotalidi del Nord America*

TIPO DI SEGNI O SINTOMI	GRAVITÀ DELL'AVVELENAMENTO		
	MINIMA	**MODERATA**	**GRAVE**
Locali	Edema, eritema o ecchimosi circoscritti al sito del morso	Progressione dell'edema, dell'eritema o dell'ecchimosi oltre il sito del morso	Edema, eritema o ecchimosi che coinvolgono rapidamente l'intera parte del corpo
Sistemici	Assenza di segni o sintomi sistemici	Assenza di segni e sintomi potenzialmente fatali (nausea, vomito, parestesie periorali, miochimia e lieve ipotensione)	Segni e sintomi marcatamente gravi (ipotensione [pressione arteriosa sistolica <80 mmHg], alterazione del sensorio, tachicardia, tachipnea e distress respiratorio)
Coagulazione	Assenza di anomalie della coagulazione o di altre importanti anomalie di laboratorio	Profilo della coagulazione lievemente anormale senza emorragie clinicamente significative; lievi anomalie di altri test di laboratorio	Profilo della coagulazione significativamente anormale con segni di emorragia o minaccia di emorragia spontanea (INR, APTT e fibrinogeno indosabili; grave trombocitopenia con conta piastrinica $<20\,000$ per mm^3); i risultati di altri test di laboratorio possono essere gravemente anormali

*Il grado di gravità definitivo di ogni avvelenamento viene determinato sulla base del segno, del sintomo o dell'anomalia di laboratorio più grave (per es. una pressione arteriosa sistolica <70 mmHg in assenza di edema locale dovrebbe essere classificata come un avvelenamento grave).

APTT, tempo di tromboplastina parziale attivata (*Activated Partial Thromboplastin Time*); INR, rapporto internazionale normalizzato (*International Normalized Ratio*).

Da Gold BS, Dart RC, Barish RA: Bites of venomous snakes. *N Engl J Med* 2002;347:347-356.

deve essere detersa e, se appropriato, si deve somministrare il tossoide tetanico.

La decisione di usare l'antidoto dipende dalla gravità e dalla progressione dei sintomi. In generale, esso risulta necessario per l'avvelenamento da serpente a sonagli, ma non per i morsi da testa di rame, mentre i morsi da mocassino acquatico ricadono tra questi due estremi. La gravità dell'avvelenamento viene comunemente classificata su una scala di 4 punti (Tab. 713-3). La maggior parte dei morsi di crotalide dà origine a sintomi entro pochi minuti e quasi sempre entro 6 h; se questi non si presentano, si può presumere che il morso sia "secco" e l'avvelenamento di grado 0. I morsi secchi si verificano fino nel 25% di quelli da crotali e non è necessario alcun trattamento. Per l'avvelenamento di grado 1 con un edema localizzato sono necessari soltanto il controllo del dolore e l'osservazione attenta. I bambini, a causa della loro taglia più piccola, hanno una maggiore probabilità di subire un avvelenamento grave; il 75% di essi ne presenta uno di grado 2 o 3, per cui è necessario l'antidoto.

L'**antidoto** risulta più efficace se viene somministrato entro 4 ore dal morso, mentre appare di scarsa utilità se è ritardato oltre 12 ore; comporta un piccolo ma significativo rischio di reazione da ipersensibilità immediata. L'antiveleno (crotalidi) polivalente si somministra a incrementi di 5 fiale e si ripete ogni 2 ore, se necessario, per neutralizzare il veleno circolante, come misurato dalla normalizzazione dei parametri della coagulazione e dall'interruzione della progressione dell'edema dell'arto interessato. I bambini spesso richiedono più antidoto rispetto a un adulto avvelenato in modo simile, a causa del loro più basso rapporto volume-veleno. Il Crofab derivato dagli ovini appare avvantaggiato dal fatto di determinare raramente un'ipersensibilità immediata e di comportare molto meno rischio di malattia da siero. Di solito all'inizio si somministrano 5-10 fiale di Crofab, con altre dosi da 2 fiale a 6, 12 e 18 h se necessario. Il suo migliore profilo di sicurezza lo rende l'**antidoto di scelta** per i morsi da crotalidi, se disponibile. In ogni caso, indipendentemente dall'antidoto adoperato, la maggior parte dei morsi da crotalidi risponde bene al trattamento precoce. La consulenza chirurgica è necessaria soltanto se sussistono preoccupazioni sullo sviluppo di una sindrome compartimentale.

A tutti i soggetti morsi da un serpente corallo si dovrebbero somministrare preventivamente 3-5 fiale di antidoto (*M. fulvius*). Questi soggetti possono essere asintomatici, prima di presentare paralisi e insufficienza respiratoria. L'antidoto è efficace solo se somministrato prima dello sviluppo dei sintomi, mentre è inutile per farli regredire dopo che sono comparsi.

PROGNOSI. Nonostante il rischio di mortalità e di grave morbilità in caso di morso di serpenti velenosi, questo può essere ridotto al minimo dall'uso tempestivo e assennato dell'antidoto. Anche gli arti con una marcata necrosi tissutale dovuta a morsi da serpente a sonagli ritorneranno alla loro funzione con la risoluzione dell'edema.

AVVELENAMENTO DA ARACNIDI

Gli aracnidi comprendono il numero più ampio di specie velenose note. Sono stati identificati oltre 20 000 ragni velenosi, ma la maggior parte non è pericolosa per l'uomo, perché sono privi di veleno potente o di zanne capaci di penetrare la cute umana. Negli Stati Uniti l'unica significativa morbilità è causata da ragni di due generi, il *Lactrodectus* (vedova nera) e il *Loxosceles* (ragno violino o *Loxosceles reclusa*).

MORSI DA VEDOVA NERA. La vedova nera si trova in tutti gli Stati Uniti, ma più comunemente nel sud. Appare di colore nero lucido e presenta segni rosso chiaro o arancione sulla superficie ventrale dell'addome; i classici marchi a clessidra sono osservati solo nella specie *L. mactans* (Fig. 713-3). Le femmine hanno un corpo lungo 1,5 cm con zampe di 4-5 cm; i maschi risultano di dimensioni quasi dimezzate rispetto a esse e non comportano alcuna minaccia per l'uomo, perché le loro zanne sono troppo corte per penetrare la cute. La vedova nera s'incontra comunemente in luoghi protetti come sotto i sassi o nelle cataste di legna, i gabinetti esterni e le stalle.

Patogenesi. Il veleno della vedova nera contiene una potente neurotossina, l'α-latrotossina, che si lega alle membrane nervose presinaptiche causando un enorme rilascio di acetilcolina e noradrenalina in corrispondenza della giunzione neuromuscolare. L'emissione di questi neurotrasmettitori determina un'eccessiva depolarizzazione muscolare e iperattività autonomica.

Manifestazioni cliniche. Il morso provoca effetti locali e sistemici. Una sensazione di puntura di spillo di solito viene percepita immediatamente in corrispondenza del sito del morso, che si trasforma in un'area pallida di 2-3 mm con un bordo rosso. Entro 1 h si avverte un dolore sordo, crampiforme attorno al sito, che gradualmente si estende a tutto il corpo. In passato si sosteneva che i morsi all'arto superiore si presentavano con un senso di oppressione toracica e grugniti respiratori, mentre i morsi all'arto inferiore con un dolore addominale e rigidità di tipo ligneo; tuttavia, entrambi questi segni possono comparire indipendentemente dalla localizzazione del morso. Oltre ai gravi crampi muscolari, la maggior parte dei bambini ha nausea, vomito e diaforesi, assieme ad agitazione e ipertensione. In casi estremamente rari i sintomi possono progredire fino all'arresto respiratorio e alla morte.

A causa della sua manifestazione con addome doloroso e rigido, un morso da vedova nera può simulare un'appendicite acuta o una peritonite. Un punto chiave nella **diagnosi differenziale** è che la maggior parte dei pazienti con morsi da vedova nera è ipertesa, agitata e tende a muoversi cercando una posizione confortevole, mentre i soggetti con peritonite da addome chirurgico spesso sono ipotesi e cercano di stare sdraiati e di evitare il movimento. Molti casi riportati in passato di decessi dovuti a morsi di vedova nera erano correlati al fatto che i pazienti furono erroneamente sottoposti a un intervento chirurgico per un presunto addome acuto. Pertanto, ottenere un'anamnesi accurata e porre la diagnosi corretta sono le fasi più importanti nel trattamento.

Trattamento. I crampi muscolari e l'agitazione sono le principali cause di disagio e di solito possono essere ben controllati

TABELLA 713-3. Classificazione della gravità dell'avvelenamento

Grado 0	Avvelenamento assente
Grado 1	Avvelenamento minimo (edema locale e dolore senza progressione)
Grado 2	Avvelenamento moderato (edema, dolore o ecchimosi che progrediscono oltre il sito della lesione; manifestazioni sistemiche o di laboratorio lievi)
Grado 3	Avvelenamento grave (marcata risposta locale, segni e sintomi sistemici gravi e significativa alterazione dei reperti di laboratorio)

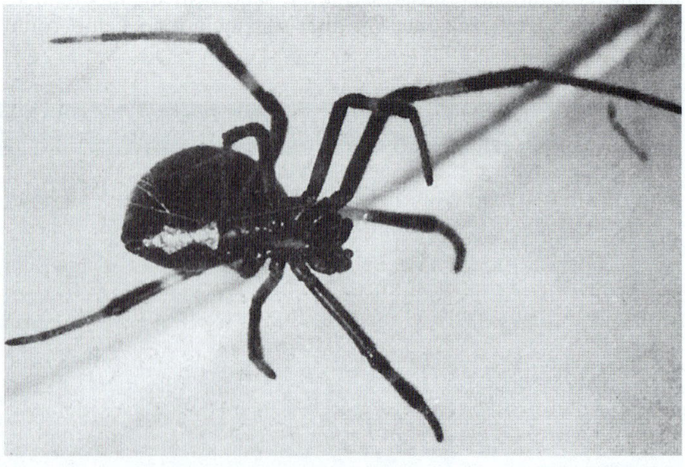

Figura 713-3. Il ragno vedova nera femmina presenta un corpo globulare, nero, lucido, con un segno rosso a forma di clessidra sull'addome. (Da Patan BC: Bites – Human, dog, spider, and snake. *Surg Clin North Am* 1963;43:537.)

con oppioidi endovenosi per il dolore e benzodiazepine per il rilassamento muscolare. In passato venivano adoperate infusioni di calcio e dantrolene per i crampi muscolari, che tuttavia non risultano efficaci e non sono più raccomandati.

L'uso dell'antidoto invece che del trattamento sintomatico è determinato dalla consapevolezza che senza trattamento tutti i sintomi si risolverebbero in 24-48 h, ma possono essere atroci. Le misure conservative dovrebbero essere tentate per prime. Se il controllo del dolore non viene ottenuto o sussiste un'instabilità autonomica, andrebbe preso in considerazione l'antidoto. Un albero decisionale per il trattamento è illustrato nella Figura 713-4.

L'antidoto è derivato dal siero equino. Se viene utilizzato, si può somministrare una dose test intradermica e si dovrebbero seguire tutte le precauzioni elencate nella precedente discussione sull'antidoto equino. Il rischio di anafilassi (<1%) è molto inferiore a quello associato all'antidoto equino contro i crotalidi. Una fiala di solito è sufficiente e i sintomi di avvelenamento diminuiscono rapidamente entro 1-3 h. Come con altri antidoti equini, si può sviluppare malattia da siero in 5-21 giorni.

MORSI DA LOXOSCELES. Sebbene il morso di numerosi ragni possa portare a lievi reazioni tissutali, soltanto le specie del genere *Loxosceles* possono causare una significativa necrosi cutanea. I membri di questo genere, negli Stati Uniti, sono comunemente noti come "brown recluse spider" (letteralmente "ragno marrone recluso", o "ragno bruno solitario", *N.d.C.*) a causa della loro predilezione a vivere in luoghi bui e indisturbati come cataste di legna e seminterrati; un'altra specie di *Loxosceles* è il *Loxosceles rufescens*, conosciuto come "ragno violino" a causa del segno marrone a forma di violino sul torace (Fig. 713-5).

Epidemiologia. Tutte le specie sono di colore opaco e presentano un corpo piccolo che misura 1 cm e zampe che arrivano fino a 5 cm. La specie con il morso più potente, la *Loxosceles reclusa*, è riscontrata più comunemente nella regione dei fiumi degli Stati Uniti medio-occidentali ma si trova anche nel Sud. Altri *Loxosceles* spp. meno potenti sono presenti in tutti gli Stati Uniti, ma il loro numero diminuisce alle latitudini più settentrionali.

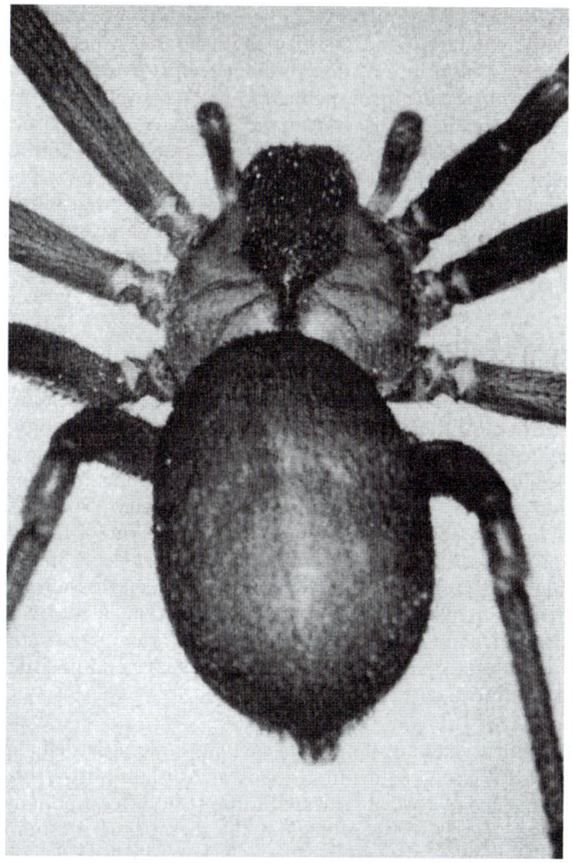

Figura 713-5. Il *Loxosceles reclusa* è lungo 10-15 mm, di colore da marrone chiaro a marrone scuro e con una banda dorsale specie-specifica, scura, a forma di violino. (Da Dillaha CJ, Jansen GT, Honeycutt WM, et al: North American loxoscelism. Necrotic bite of the brown recluse spider. *JAMA* 1964;188:33.)

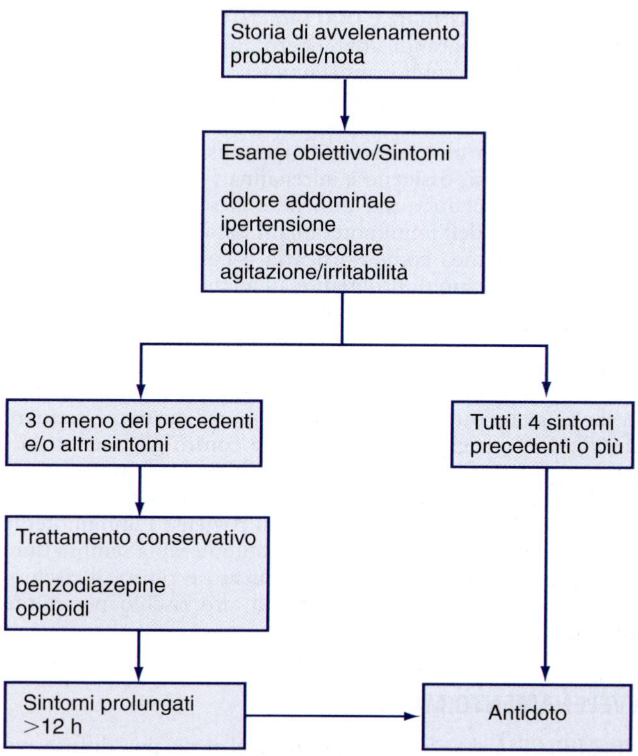

Figura 713-4. Processo decisionale per il trattamento pediatrico dell'avvelenamento da vedova nera. (Per gentile concessione di Robin Woestman, Loma Linda Children's Hospital, Loma Linda, CA.)

Manifestazioni cliniche. Il veleno del *Loxosceles reclusa* contiene la ialuronidasi, o fattore di diffusione e la sfingomielinasi D, una proteina che lisa le pareti cellulari. Il morso spesso non viene notato o è percepito soltanto come una puntura di spillo. Tipicamente si verifica quando un ragno è inavvertitamente intrappolato sulla cute mentre la vittima indossa gli indumenti, per cui spesso è localizzato all'arto superiore, al torace laterale, alla coscia mediale o, raramente, sulle mani e al volto. Entro 2 h, una macula di colore blu scuro, dolorosa, con un alone di infiammazione compare in corrispondenza del sito del morso, seguita da sintomi sistemici che comprendono febbre, brividi, nausea e vomito. In una minor parte di casi, ma più comunemente nei bambini piccoli, si può verificare emolisi, che si presume secondaria all'azione della tossina, in quanto i risultati del test di Coombs risultano negativi e il sistema della coagulazione non si è attivato secondo quanto rilevato dalla conta delle piastrine, dai prodotti di degradazione della fibrina e dal tempo di protrombina. Raramente può avvenire un'emolisi massiva, che può portare a una coagulazione intravascolare disseminata o a un'insufficienza renale emoglobinurica.

Oltre ai sintomi sistemici del morso, entro 1-2 giorni si forma una **vescicola emorragica**, che quando si rompe lascia l'ulcera necrotica caratteristica dei morsi di questo ragno. La maggior parte delle ulcere rimane di 1-2 cm, ma può ingrandirsi fino a 15 cm di diametro e interessare la cute a tutto spessore e in parte il tessuto sottostante.

Trattamento e prognosi. La prognosi nei morsi da *Loxosceles reclusa* è eccellente e la maggior parte si risolve solo con la terapia di supporto. I pazienti con sintomi sistemici o con una emolisi significativa dovrebbero essere ricoverati per il controllo del dolore e il monitoraggio. L'idratazione e il mantenimento della diuresi sono essenziali in presenza di un'emoglobinuria significativa. Anche il trattamento delle lesioni cutanee ulcerative è di supporto, con terapia locale della ferita. Il dolore di solito diminuisce in pochi giorni, sebbene per la completa guarigione della cute siano necessarie settimane. L'ossigeno iperbarico, che favorisce il risanamento della ferita, il dapsone per l'inibizione dei leucociti e la ciproeptadina, un inibitore dell'aggregazione piastrinica, sono stati consigliati per prevenire l'ingrandimento delle ulcere cutanee; tuttavia, nessuno di questi si è dimostrato vantaggioso. In rari casi, ampie ulcere necrotiche necessitano di innesti cutanei tardivi.

MORSI DI SCORPIONE

EPIDEMIOLOGIA. Nel mondo si trovano oltre 1000 specie di scorpioni, tutte in grado di liberare veleno attraverso un pungiglione localizzato all'estremità di una coda a 6 segmenti. Solo le poche specie della famiglia *Butidae* rivestono un'importanza medica, per il fatto che producono un veleno neurotossico. Tra queste, vi sono il *Leiurus* spp. dell'India e del medio Oriente e i *Centuroides* spp. in Messico e nel deserto del sud-ovest degli Stati Uniti. La maggior parte delle punture, anche da specie tossiche, causa soltanto una reazione dolorosa locale. Tuttavia, a motivo della loro taglia, i bambini piccoli e giovani che sono punti corrono il rischio di una disfunzione autonomica grave, un'insufficienza d'organo multisistemica e la morte.

PATOGENESI. I veleni di scorpione variano a seconda della specie, ma tutti possiedono ialuronidasi, sostanze rilascianti serotonina e istamina e neurotossine; queste ultime sono la componente più importante, perché possono legarsi alle membrane presinaptiche causando il rilascio di acetilcolina e la stimolazione del sistema nervoso simpatico e parasimpatico.

MANIFESTAZIONI CLINICHE. L'unica specie di scorpione significativa dal punto di vista medico negli Stati Uniti è la *Centuroides exilicauda*, che si trova nel sud-ovest. La maggior parte delle punture causa una reazione locale immediata, che può variare da bruciore lieve a dolore severo. L'avvelenamento grave provoca disfunzione autonomica entro 1 h dalla puntura (Tab. 713-4). I sintomi comprendono agitazione, irritabilità, salivazione, offuscamento del visus e tremore, con segni d'ipertensione, tachicardia, tachipnea e nistagmo. Rare volte nei bambini piccoli o nei neonati possono comparire l'insufficienza respiratoria, le convulsioni o il coma. In questi casi, se non si ottiene un'anamnesi di puntura, si può prendere in considerazione una diagnosi di encefalite e la diagnosi corretta di avvelenamento da scorpione risulta oscurata dal fatto che i bambini con un avvelenamento grave da *Centuroides* possono presentare una lieve pleiocitosi del liquido cerebrospinale.

L'avvelenamento da parte di altre specie di scorpioni può avere caratteristiche specifiche. Le punture da *Leiurus* spp. in India e in Medio Oriente possono causare una grave ipertensione, una miocardite tossica diretta e una ischemia miocardica potenzialmente fatale.

TABELLA 713-4. Avvelenamento da scorpione

Grado 1	Dolore e parestesia locale
Grado 2	Dolore e parestesia si estendono all'arto
Grado 3	Ipercinesia motoria Disfunzione dei nervi cranici Disfagia Instabilità oculare Parestesia facciale Irrequietezza
Grado 4	Disfunzione dei nervi cranici Iperscialorrea, movimenti incontrollabili degli occhi Fascicolazioni, muscoli facciali e distali Iperattività neuromuscolare Opistotono Convulsioni Respiro affannoso Ipertermia Cianosi

Da Wolf MD: Evenomation. In Holbrook PR (editor): *Textbook of Pediatric Critical Care*. Philadelphia, WB Saunders, 1993, p 1024.

TRATTAMENTO. Il dolore localizzato può venire trattato con l'applicazione di ghiaccio e analgesici e di solito diminuisce significativamente entro 24 h. Per le punture da *Centuroides exilicauda*, l'avvelenamento grave con instabilità autonomica richiede il ricovero ospedaliero per la sedazione e l'osservazione. I sintomi di solito si risolvono entro 24-48 h. In caso di compromissione cardiopolmonare, si dovrebbe prendere in considerazione la somministrazione dell'antidoto. Quello specifico per i *Centuroides* non è approvato dalla FDA, ma è disponibile contattando l'Arizona Poison Control Center (1-800-222-1222). Il suo impiego, se giustificato, determina la completa risoluzione dei sintomi entro 1 h. L'antidoto per le altre specie di scorpioni è disponibile nei Paesi in cui si trovano queste specie o attraverso le società di zoologia.

PUNTURE DI IMENOTTERI

Nella classe degli Imenotteri sono comprese le formiche, le api e le vespe, che sono caratterizzate dalla presenza di un pungiglione all'estremità dell'addome attraverso il quale viene iniettato il veleno. Essi sono presenti in tutto il mondo.

EPIDEMIOLOGIA. Il veleno degli Imenotteri, una miscela di proteine e sostanze vasoattive, non è molto potente; la maggior parte delle punture determina solo reazioni locali che possono essere trattate con l'applicazione di compresse di garza fredde e analgesici. Tuttavia, l'1-4% della popolazione è sensibilizzata al veleno degli Imenotteri e risulta a rischio di reazioni da ipersensibilità immediata. Ogni anno, 50-150 persone negli Stati Uniti muoiono di anafilassi causata da punture di Imenotteri (vedi Capitolo 145).

MANIFESTAZIONI CLINICHE E TRATTAMENTO. I bambini con reazioni locali piccole o grandi dovrebbero applicare impacchi freddi e ricevere corticosteroidi e antistaminici. Tutte le persone con un avvelenamento da Imenotteri che manifestano orticaria, angioedema, respiro affannoso o ipotensione andrebbero trattate aggressivamente per una reazione da ipersensibilità immediata con liquidi endovenosi, ossigeno e adrenalina (vedi Capitolo 148).

Il quesito terapeutico più difficile è la scelta dei pazienti che necessiterebbero dell'immunoterapia. I bambini che hanno avuto un'anafilassi cutanea come l'orticaria o l'angioedema sembrano essere a basso rischio di progredire ad anafilassi sistemica in caso di punture future. Quelli che hanno avuto reazioni sistemiche con respiro affannoso, ma non anafilassi, non hanno bisogno dell'immunoterapia, eppure dovrebbero portare con sé un kit di emergenza con adrenalina. I pazienti che hanno subito un'anafilassi con ipotensione o ostruzione delle vie aeree devono effettuare il test delle IgE per gli anticorpi specifici contro gli Imenotteri. Se queste sono negative, il soggetto può essere rassicurato sul fatto che gravi reazioni future sono improbabili. Al contrario, se il test per le IgE è positivo, occorre offrire al paziente l'immunoterapia specie-specifica. La protezione dell'immunoterapia sembra durare tutta la vita dopo 3-5 anni di trattamento e riduce il rischio di un'anafilassi sistemica nei soggetti ad alto rischio per punture future dal 30% a $<5\%$.

AVVELENAMENTO MARINO

EPIDEMIOLOGIA. Le creature marine velenose più diffuse comprendono le meduse (*Cnidaria*), le Dasiatidi (*Chondricthyes*) e membri della famiglia *Scorpaenidae*: il pesce zebra, il pesce scorpione, il pesce sasso.

PATOGENESI. Tutte le meduse possiedono cellule urticanti peculiari denominate nematocisti. Queste cellule contengono un tubulo altamente ripiegato che si apre all'esterno al contatto e inietta il veleno. Il veleno è antigenico e può essere dermatonecrotico, emolitico, cardiotossico o neuropatico, a seconda della specie. I nematocisti possono pungere anche dopo che il tentacolo si è separato dal corpo e dopo la morte della medusa. Le Dasiatidi hanno un aculeo alla base della coda che contiene una ghiandola di veleno, con proprietà vasocostrittive che possono predisporre a una necrosi tissutale e alla scarsa guarigione della ferita. Inoltre, gli aculei delle Dasiatidi sono retro-serrati e quindi causano comunemente una lacerazione dentellata, assieme all'avvelenamento. Le *Scorpaenidae* possiedono aculei velenosi che diventano eretti durante la stimolazione.

MANIFESTAZIONI CLINICHE. È noto che la medusa del Pacifico (*Chironex fleckeri*) causa una puntura fatale per il suo veleno cardiotossico, ma questo membro della famiglia *Cnidaria* si trova solo in Australia. Sebbene un'anafilassi fatale alle punture di medusa sia stata riportata nelle acque costiere degli Stati Uniti, questi eventi sono estremamente rari. Per i medici nelle Americhe, la principale preoccupazione riguardo alle punture di medusa è il dolore localizzato, che può essere associato a parestesie o prurito. Raramente le vittime possono avere sintomi sistemici di nausea, vomito, cefalea e brividi. Gli avvelenamenti da Dasiatidi sono degni di nota per il dolore immediato e intenso in corrispondenza del sito di lesione che dura 24-48 h. Alcuni pazienti possono anche avere nausea, vomito, crampi muscolari e, raramente, ipotensione o convulsioni. L'avvelenamento da parte di un membro delle *Scorpaenidae* genera un dolore immediato che può persistere per ore o giorni. Le vittime possono sperimentare un'intensa distruzione tissutale locale, in cui le sovrainfezioni appaiono comuni. I sintomi sistemici comprendono vomito, dolore addominale, cefalea, delirio, convulsioni e insufficienza respiratoria.

TRATTAMENTO. Il trattamento delle punture da medusa inizia nell'oceano; le ferite dovrebbero essere irrigate nell'acqua di mare, perché l'acqua dolce può lisare le nematocisti, portando a ulteriore avvelenamento. L'irrigazione del sito della puntura con aceto o alcol appare utile, in quanto inibisce il rilascio della nematocisti. I frammenti visibili dei tentacoli dovrebbero essere rimossi con le pinze, mentre i frammenti microscopici possono essere asportati depilando con delicatezza l'area interessata. Rimedi popolari come lo sfregamento della puntura con sabbia o l'applicazione di urine non sono utili e causano un'irritazione maggiore. Gli emollienti locali, un trattamento popolare lungamente utilizzato, non sono efficaci. Gli antistaminici e i corticosteroidi sono indicati per l'edema e l'orticaria. Gli antibiotici non sono necessari. Tutti i pazienti guariscono senza problemi.

Il trattamento delle punture da Dasiatidi e *Scorpaenidae* è simile, iniziando con un'accurata detersione della ferita e, se necessario, un richiamo antitetanico. Gli aculei delle Dasiatidi sono radiopachi e andrebbero rimossi dalla ferita, se presenti. Se la lacerazione è ampia, bisognerebbe consentire la chiusura tardiva. Le tossine sono termolabili e l'immersione in acqua calda (42 °C) per 30-60 minuti denatura gli elementi proteici del veleno e riduce significativamente il dolore. Un'ulteriore analgesia dovrebbe essere fornita secondo necessità. La sovrainfezione da parte di microrganismi aerobi e anaerobi è rara e la profilassi antibiotica non appare necessaria.

ERUZIONE DEL BAGNANTE

EPIDEMIOLOGIA E PATOGENESI. L'eruzione del bagnante è determinata dall'esposizione alle larve di due specie del phylum *Cnidaria*, l'anemone di mare, *Edwardsiella lineata*, che si trova al largo della costa degli Stati Uniti nordorientali e la medusa ditale, *Linuche unguiculata*, riscontrata nei Caraibi e nel Golfo del Messico. Sono stati riportati casi anche in Brasile. Epidemie di eruzione del bagnante si verificano in estate quando vi sono elevate quantità di larve nell'acqua.

MANIFESTAZIONI CLINICHE E TRATTAMENTO. Un'eruzione vescicolare o maculopapulare intensamente pruriginosa inizia entro 4-24 dall'esposizione e può persistere per giorni o settimane. I sintomi associati possono comprendere febbre, brividi, cefalea, malessere generale, congiuntivite e uretrite. La maggior parte di questi risponde agli antistaminici, sebbene i corticosteroidi topici o sistemici possano essere vantaggiosi nei casi gravi.

Morso di serpente

Boyer L, Seifert S, Cain J: Recurrence phenomena after immunoglobulin therapy for snake envenomations: Guidelines for clinical management with crotaline Fab antivenom. *Ann Emerg Med* 2001;37:196–201.

Gold BS, Dart RC, Barish RA: Bites of venomous snakes. *N Engl J Med* 2002;347:347–356.

Habib AG, Gebi UI, Onyemelukwe GC: Snake bite in Nigeria. *Afr J Med Sci* 2001;30:171–178.

Juckett G, Hancox J: Venomous snakebites in the United States: Management review and update. *Am Fam Phys* 2002;65:1367–1374.

Junghanss T, Bodio M: Medically important venomous animals: biology prevention, first aid and clinical management. *Clin Inf Dis* 2006;43: 1309–1317.

McKinney P: Out of hospital and interhospital management of crotaline snakebite. *Ann Emerg Med* 2001;37:168–174.

Tokish JT, Benjamin J, Walter F: Crotalid envenomation: The southern Arizona experience. *J Ortho Trauma* 2001;15:5–9.

Avvelenamento da aracnidi

Gomez HF, Krywko DM, Stoecker WV: A new assay for the detection of *Loxosceles* species (brown recluse) spider venom. *Ann Emerg Med* 202;39: 469–474.

Ibister G: Necrotic arachnidism: The mythology of a modern plague. *Lancet* 2004;364:549–553.

Ibister G, Gray MR: A prospective study of 750 definite spider bites, with expert spider identification. *Q J Med* 2002;95:723–731.

Ibister G, Graudins A, White J, et al: Antivenom treatment in arachnidism. *Clin Toxicol* 2003;41:291–300.

LoVecchio F, McBride C: Scorpion envenomation in young children in central Arizona. *J Toxicol Clin Toxicol* 2003;41:937–940.

Pauli I, Puka J, Gubert IC, Minozzo JC: The efficacy of antivenom in loxoscelism treatment. *Toxicon* 2006;48:123–137. Epub 2006, Jun 30.

Avvelenamento da insetti

Muller U: New developments in the diagnosis and treatment of Hymenoptera venom allergy. *Int Arch Allergy Immunol* 2001;124:447–453.

Freeman T: Hypersensitivity to hymenoptera stings. *N Engl J Med* 2004;351:1978–1984.

Avvelenamento marino

Perkins RA, Morgan S: Poisoning, envenomation and trauma from marine creatures. *Am Fam Phys* 2004;69:885–890.

Williams GC: Stinging seas. *Calif Wild* 2000;53(4):12–17.

Parte XXXIII ▪ Medicina di laboratorio

Capitolo 714 ▪ Test di laboratorio nei bambini Michael A. Pesce

A causa dell'eterogeneità genetica, della variabilità biologica e ambientale e della disomogeneità dello stato di salute subclinico, i valori normali di molti test di laboratorio non mostrano una curva di distribuzione gaussiana a campana. Di conseguenza, la media della popolazione e la deviazione standard (DS) sono frequentemente meno utili rispetto all'intervallo di riferimento dei valori normali, in genere indicato come il range di normalità del 95%, oppure come il range di valori ottenuto nel testare una popolazione normale meno il 2,5% inferiore e il 2,5% superiore. La concentrazione sierica di sodio nei bambini, che è controllata in modo rigoroso a livello fisiologico, presenta una distribuzione essenzialmente gaussiana; il valore medio ±2 DS fornisce un range che è molto vicino a quello effettivamente osservato nel 95% dei bambini (Tab. 714-1). In alternativa, il livello di creatina chinasi, soggetto a diverse influenze e non attivamente controllato, non mostra una distribuzione gaussiana, come evidenziato dalla mancanza di concordanza tra il range effettivamente osservato e quello predetto dal valore medio ±2 DS.

Un perfezionamento nella refertazione che viene sempre più utilizzato consiste nel riportare il valore ottenuto con il percentile dei valori normali entro cui cade il valore ottenuto. Questo metodo è utile nella valutazione dei fattori di rischio, come la determinazione del colesterolo sierico. Un'ulteriore modificazione che risulta necessaria per molti test effettuati nei lattanti e nei bambini consiste nel calcolare l'aggiustamento del range normale in relazione all'età. Questo aggiustamento e l'uso dei percentili vengono illustrati nei valori normali per il colesterolo sierico. Un'ultima modificazione necessaria per riportare i range normali consiste nel riferire lo stadio di Tanner della maturazione sessuale, che appare più utile nella valutazione della funzione ipofisaria e delle gonadi.

ACCURATEZZA E PRECISIONE DEI TEST DI LABORATORIO. L'accuratezza tecnica è un importante elemento da considerare nell'interpretazione dei risultati di un test di laboratorio. Grazie ai miglioramenti nei metodi di analisi e all'eliminazione dell'interferenza analitica, l'accuratezza della maggior parte dei test è limitata principalmente dalla loro precisione. L'**accuratezza** è la misura della vicinanza del risultato di un test al valore effettivo, mentre la **precisione** è la misura della riproducibilità di un risultato. Nessun test può essere più accurato che preciso. L'analisi della precisione mediante misurazioni ripetitive di un singolo campione dà origine a una distribuzione gaussiana con una media e una DS. La stima della precisione è il coefficiente di variazione (CV):

$$CV = \frac{DS}{Media} \times 100$$

Il CV non è probabilmente costante lungo tutto il range di valori ottenuti nei test clinici, ma è circa del 5% nel range normale. In genere il CV non viene riportato, ma è sempre noto al laboratorio. Esso è particolarmente importante nel valutare il significato delle alterazioni dei test di laboratorio. Per esempio, una situazione comune è la necessità di determinare l'epatotossicità contratta in seguito alla somministrazione di un farmaco terapeutico e riflessa nel valore dell'alanina aminotransferasi (ALT) sierica. Se il valore della ALT sierica aumenta da 25 U/L a 40 U/L, la variazione è significativa? Il CV per l'ALT è 7%. Utilizzando il valore ottenuto ±2 × CV per esprimere gli estremi dell'imprecisione, si può osservare che appare improbabile che un valore di 25 U/L rifletta una concentrazione effettiva >29 U/L e che un valore di 40 U/L rifletta una concentrazione effettiva <34 U/L. Pertanto, risulta invece probabile che la variazione del valore ottenuto dal test rifletta una reale modificazione nei livelli dell'ALT circolante. È indicato il monitoraggio continuo dell'ALT sierica, anche se entrambi i valori di ALT rientrano nei limiti della norma. *Verosimilmente* in questo caso è soltanto una probabilità. La variabilità biologica intrinseca è tale che i risultati di due test successivi possono suggerire una tendenza che scomparirà nei test seguenti.

La precisione di un test può anche essere indicata fornendo i limiti di confidenza per un determinato risultato. Normalmente si utilizzano intervalli di confidenza del 95%, che indicano una certezza del 95% che il valore ottenuto si trovi tra i due limiti riportati. I limiti di confidenza vengono calcolati utilizzando la media e la DS delle determinazioni ripetute:

$$\text{limiti di confidenza 95\%} = \text{media} \pm t \times DS$$

in cui t è una costante derivata dal numero di ripetizioni. Nella maggior parte dei casi, $t = 2$.

SENSIBILITÀ, ACCURATEZZA E TEST ANALITICI. In alcune circostanze, la sensibilità e l'accuratezza di un'analisi sono ridotte o aumentate in funzione dello scopo clinico. Per esempio, la cromatografia a scambio ionico degli aminoacidi plasmatici per la diagnosi degli errori congeniti del metabolismo viene di solito effettuata a una sensibilità analitica che consente la misurazione di tutti gli aminoacidi con un singolo set di standard. L'intervallo di riferimento è circa di 20-800 μmol/L, mentre l'accuratezza è scarsa per valori ≤20 μmol/L. L'identificazione dell'omocisteina in questo tipo di analisi suggerisce un errore congenito del metabolismo della metionina. Se l'analisi viene aggiustata per ottenere una maggiore sensibilità analitica, è possibile misurare accuratamente l'omocisteina nel plasma normale (3-12 μmol/L). Questo test più sensibile viene utilizzato per determinare lo stato della cobalamina e analizzare i fattori di rischio di malattia cardiovascolare aterosclerotica.

VALORE PREDITTIVO DEI TEST DI LABORATORIO. La teoria del valore predittivo (VP) si occupa dell'utilità dei test secondo quanto definito dalla loro sensibilità (capacità di identificare una malattia) e specificità (capacità di definire l'assenza di malattia) cliniche.

$$\text{Sensibilità} = \frac{\text{Numero di test positivi}}{\text{Numero totale di positivi}} \times 100$$

$$\text{Specificità} = \frac{\text{Numero di test negativi}}{\text{Numero totale senza malattia}} \times 100$$

$$\text{VP del test positivo} = \frac{\text{Risultati veri positivi}}{\text{Risultati positivi totali}} \times 100$$

$$\text{VP del test negativo} = \frac{\text{Risultati veri negativi}}{\text{Risultati negativi totali}} \times 100$$

I problemi cui è rivolta la teoria del VP sono i falsi negativi e i falsi positivi. Entrambi rappresentano gli elementi principali da prendere in considerazione nell'interpretazione dei risultati dei test di screening in generale e dei test di screening neonatali in particolare.

TABELLA 714-1. Valori di laboratorio gaussiani e non gaussiani in 458 bambini normali, scolari di 7-14 anni

	SODIO SIERICO (mmol/L)	CREATINA CHINASI SIERICA (U/L)
Media	141	68
DS	1,7	34
Media ±2 DS	138-144	0-136
Intervallo 95% effettivo	137-144	24-162

DS = deviazione standard.

I test per la sieroreattività dell'HIV illustrano alcune di queste considerazioni. Se si assume che circa 1 100 000 abitanti su 284 000 000 negli Stati Uniti siano infettati dall'HIV (prevalenza = 0,39%) e che il 90% di quelli infettati mostrino anticorpi contro l'HIV, è possibile prendere in considerazione l'utilità di un test semplice con una sensibilità del 99% e una specificità del 99,5%. Se l'intera popolazione degli USA fosse sottoposta a screening, sarebbe possibile identificare la maggior parte dei soggetti infettati da HIV.

$$1\,100\,000 \times 0{,}9 \times 0{,}99 = 980\,100\ (89{,}1\%)$$

Tuttavia, ci saranno 119 900 test falsi negativi. Anche con una specificità del 99,5%, il numero di falsi positivi del test sarebbe superiore al numero dei veri positivi:

$$284\,000\,000 \times 0{,}005 = 1\,420\,000$$

Inoltre, ci sarebbero 281 480 000 veri negativi.

$$\text{VP del test positivo} = \frac{980\,100}{(980\,100 + 1\,420\,000)} \times 100 = 41\%$$

$$\text{VP del test negativo} = \frac{281\,480\,000}{(281\,480\,000 + 119\,900)} \times 100 = 99{,}96\%$$

Considerati gli elevati costi associati al follow-up e l'angoscia provocata da un risultato falso positivo, è semplice osservare perché lo screening universale per la sieropositività da HIV abbia ricevuto una bassa priorità subito dopo l'introduzione dei test per l'infezione da HIV.

Per converso, si può prendere in considerazione lo screening di 100 000 individui di gruppi ad aumentato rischio di HIV in cui la prevalenza globale della malattia sia del 10%, mentre tutte le altre considerazioni rimangono invariate.

$$\text{Risultati veri positivi} = 0{,}9 \times 0{,}99 \times 10\,000 = 8910$$

$$\text{Risultati falsi positivi} = 0{,}005 \times 90\,000 = 450$$

$$\text{Risultati falsi negativi} = 10\,000 - 8910 = 1090$$

$$\text{VP del test positivo} = \frac{8910}{8910 + 450} \times 100 = 95\%$$

$$\text{VP del test negativo} = \frac{89\,500}{89\,550 + 1090} \times 100 = 99\%$$

Queste due strategie ipotetiche mostrano che l'efficienza diagnostica dei test dipende grandemente dalla diffusione della malattia che viene testata, anche con un test superiore, come quello per gli anticorpi anti-HIV. Dal momento che il trattamento delle donne gravide infettate da HIV risulta efficace nel prevenire la trasmissione verticale dell'infezione, lo screening è stato allargato a tutte loro. L'efficacia provata della terapia attuale nella prevenzione dell'infezione neonatale ha intensificato lo screening precoce per l'HIV nella gravidanza.

Tuttavia, a causa del lungo tempo necessario per testare gli anticorpi anti-HIV, era difficile sottoporre a screening le donne durante il travaglio e fornire la terapia necessaria. Recentemente sono state approvate le procedure di un test rapido per gli anticorpi anti-HIV in cui si utilizza un prelievo digitale o la puntura venosa per ottenere sangue, plasma o siero e test in cui si impiegano i liquidi orali (Tab. 714-2). Di solito i risultati del test HIV vengono ottenuti in <20 minuti. La raccolta di campioni di liquidi orali fornisce un'alternativa per i soggetti che evitano il test HIV a causa della loro antipatia per gli aghi. Il test HIV che utilizza sangue intero o liquidi orali è classificato come test waived secondo i **Clinical Laboratory Improvement Amendments del 1988 (CLIA)** e questi test sono consentiti in un contesto point-of-care. I test waived sono semplici procedure di laboratorio che utilizzano metodologie così semplici e accurate da rendere trascurabile la probabilità di un risultato erroneo da parte dell'utente. Un test rapido positivo per l'HIV viene successivamente confermato mediante l'analisi con Western blot o con l'immunofluorescenza.

Secondo gli U.S. Centers for Disease Control and Prevention, negli Stati Uniti tra 280 e 370 bambini sono nati con l'HIV nel 2000. Il test rapido per l'HIV durante il travaglio consente l'attuazione della terapia antiretrovirale per le donne infette che non sono state sottoposte al test o sono ignare del loro stato HIV. L'inizio della terapia al momento del travaglio o entro le prime 12 ore dalla nascita del bambino riduce significativamente il rischio di trasmissione dalla madre al bambino. Nel rapido intervento madre-bambino nello studio del parto è stato mostrato che la sensibilità e la specificità di un test rapido su sangue intero per l'HIV durante il travaglio erano rispettivamente del 100% e del 99,9%, con un VP positivo del 90%. Il tempo mediano di ritorno dei risultati dalla raccolta del sangue alla notifica al paziente era di soli 66 minuti. Il rendimento del test ematico rapido era migliore rispetto a quello del saggio immunoenzimatico standard per l'HIV, che aveva una sensibilità e una specificità rispettivamente del 100% e del 99,8%, con un VP positivo del 76%. Inoltre, il tempo mediano di ritorno dei risultati era di 28 ore. Di conseguenza, attualmente il test rapido per l'HIV su sangue intero è lo standard dell'assistenza per le donne in travaglio con stato HIV non documentato.

I test rapidi per l'HIV possono anche essere utilizzati nei Paesi in via di sviluppo. In condizioni di scarsi mezzi, a causa della mancanza di laboratori adeguatamente attrezzati, di tecnici esperti e di risorse di base come l'elettricità e l'acqua, questi test riservati, di point-of-care per l'HIV sono molto attraenti. In aree dell'Asia e dell'Africa in cui l'HIV è epidemico, lo screening delle donne gravide con questi test e l'offerta della terapia antiretrovirale possono ridurre significativamente la trasmissione dell'HIV a centinaia di migliaia di bambini.

TEST DI SCREENING NEONATALE. Quasi tutte le malattie identificate nei programmi di screening neonatale hanno una prevalenza molto bassa e per la maggior parte i test sono quantitativi piuttosto che qualitativi. In generale, la strategia consiste nell'utilizzare il test di screening iniziale per distinguere un gruppo di pazienti con elevato sospetto dai bambini normali (ossia per aumentare la prevalenza) e quindi seguire il gruppo sospetto in modo aggressivo. Tale strategia è illustrata da un programma usato nello screening dei neonati per l'ipotiroidismo congenito la cui prevalenza è di 25/100 000 bambini nati vivi. Il test che si esegue all'inizio è per

TABELLA 714-2. Test anticorpali rapidi per l'HIV e stato HIV secondo i Clinical Laboratory Improvement Amendments del 1988 (CLIA)

TEST RAPIDO PER HIV	TIPO DI CAMPIONE	CATEGORIA CLIA*	TEMPO PER EFFETTUARE IL TEST	TEMPO DI ATTESA PER LEGGERE I RISULTATI	PRODUTTORE
OraQuick ADVANCE Rapid Test anticorpale HIV-1/2 Antibody	Liquidi orali	Waived	<5 min	20-40 min	OraSure Technologies, Inc. www.orasure.com
	Sangue intero (prelievo digitale o puntura venosa)	Waived			
	Plasma	Complessità moderata			
Uni-Gold Recombigen HIV-1	Sangue intero (prelievo digitale o puntura venosa)	Waived	<5 min	10-12 min	Trinity Biotech www.unigoldhiv.com
	Siero e plasma	Complessità moderata			
Reveal G-2 Rapid HIV-1 Test anticorpale	Siero e plasma	Complessità moderata	<5 min	Leggere il risultato immediatamente	MedMira, Inc. www.medmira.com
MultiSpot HIV-1/HIV-2 Test rapido	Siero e plasma	Complessità moderata	10-15 min	Il risultato può essere letto immediatamente o fino a 4 ore dopo	BioRad Laboratories www.biorad.com

*Clinical Laboratory Improvement Amendment.

la tiroxina nel sangue intero e i bambini con il 10% più basso di risultati sono considerati sospetti. Se tutti i bambini con ipotiroidismo fossero inclusi in questo gruppo, la prevalenza della malattia in esso sarebbe di 250/100 000. I campioni originali ottenuti dal gruppo sospetto vengono sottoposti nuovamente al test per la tiroxina e per l'ormone tireostimolante. Questa seconda serie di test porta a un gruppo con un sospetto ancora più elevato, composto dallo 0,1% dei bambini sottoposti allo screening e con una prevalenza di ipotiroidismo di 25 000/100 000 soggetti. Questo gruppo finale viene seguito in modo aggressivo per ulteriori test e per il trattamento. Anche con un aumento di 1000 volte della prevalenza, il 75% della popolazione sottoposta a un test aggressivo è eutiroidea. Le giustificazioni avanzate per il programma sono che il trattamento è semplice ed efficace e che l'alternativa, se l'ipotiroidismo congenito non viene identificato e trattato (terapia di sorveglianza a lungo termine), è insoddisfacente e costosa.

Agli inizi, lo screening neonatale era guidato dalla selezione di malattie genetiche le cui manifestazioni cliniche si sviluppavano nel periodo postnatale, come la fenilchetonuria, la galattosemia e l'omocistinuria. Le malattie potrebbero venire trattate efficacemente con metodi semplici cominciati poco dopo la nascita. I test di screening classici sono saggi microbiologici specifici per malattia.

Anche malattie più comuni sono diventate oggetto dei programmi di screening neonatale. L'ipotiroidismo congenito fu selezionato a causa della sua frequenza e della sua semplicità di trattamento. La malattia a cellule falciformi, anch'essa facilmente identificata, può venire trattata più opportunamente se diagnosticata prima della comparsa dei segni clinici. Inoltre, i risultati dello screening neonatale per la fibrosi cistica (FC) mostrano che vi sono evidenti vantaggi correlati alla diagnosi preclinica, ma anche alcune difficoltà intrinseche associate allo screening genetico per malattie autosomiche recessive complesse che sono comuni e causate da un numero piuttosto ampio di mutazioni di un singolo gene. Il test diagnostico definitivo per la FC consiste nella misurazione delle concentrazioni di sodio e di cloro nel sudore, un test che non è pratico durante la prima settimana di vita. I neonati con FC in genere presentano un aumento del tripsinogeno nel sangue intero. Questo test consente di identificare un gruppo di neonati a rischio per la FC. La realizzazione dell'analisi del DNA per comuni mutazioni che causano questa malattia riduce le dimensioni del gruppo di sospetto e identifica i neonati con una più elevata probabilità di averla contratta. Questa strategia identifica un numero gestibile di neonati in cui effettuare i test del sudore. Tra i problemi sono inclusi: (1) le mutazioni rare non vengono comprese nel quadro dello screening (pertanto, casi di FC determinati da tali mutazioni possono sfuggire); (2) comuni mutazioni che danno origine ad aumenti clinicamente innocui del tripsinogeno nel sangue intero di neonati eterozigoti causano reperti falsi positivi potenzialmente allarmanti; (3) la FC nei pazienti con un risultato normale del test al sudore è rara, ma è probabile che non venga identificata. L'iperplasia surrenalica congenita, un'altra malattia comune, viene attualmente inclusa nei programmi di screening neonatale.

La **spettrometria di tandem massa (MS/MS)** è un metodo tecnicamente avanzato in cui molti composti vengono inizialmente separati in base al peso molecolare. Ogni composto subisce quindi una frammentazione per consentirne l'identificazione. Il processo richiede circa 2 min/campione e può riconoscere 20 o più errori congeniti del metabolismo. Gli effetti della prematurità, le malattie neonatali e la terapia intensiva neonatale sui metaboliti nel sangue complicano l'interpretazione dei risultati. Il VP di un test di screening positivo è probabilmente $<10\%$; in altre parole, il 90% dei risultati positivi non è indicativo di una malattia genetica del metabolismo. Ciononostante, la MS/MS permette di confermare una diagnosi prima dello sviluppo della malattia clinica. La MS/MS non è rivolta a malattie definite come trattabili, ma a tutte quelle malattie rare che la tecnica è in grado di identificare (Tab. 714-3).

La spettrometria di tandem massa a elettrospray permette l'identificazione di rari errori congeniti del metabolismo ed è stata introdotta come strumento di screening neonatale in Australia.

TABELLA 714-3. Screening neonatale mediante spettrometria di tandem massa

MALATTIE DEL METABOLISMO DEGLI ACIDI ORGANICI E DELL'OSSIDAZIONE DEGLI ACIDI GRASSI
Deficit di idrossimetilglutaril CoA liasi
Aciduria glutarica di tipo 1
Deficit di isobutiril CoA deidrogenasi
Acidemia isovalerica
Deficit di 2-metilbutiril CoA deidrogenasi
Deficit di 2,4-dienoil CoA reduttasi
Deficit di 3-metilcrotonil CoA carbossilasi
Deficit di 3-metilglutaconil CoA idratasi
Acidemia metilmalonica
Deficit di 3-chetotiolasi
Deficit multiplo di CoA carbossilasi
Acidemia propionica
Deficit di traslocatore carnitina/acilcarnitina
Deficit di acil CoA deidrogenasi a catena intermedia
Deficit di chetoacil CoA tiolasi a catena intermedia
Aciduria glutarica di tipo 2
Deficit di carnitina palmitoil transferasi
Deficit di acil CoA deidrogenasi a catena corta
Deficit di idrossi acil CoA deidrogenasi a catena corta
Deficit di proteina trifunzionale
Deficit di 3-idrossi acil CoA deidrogenasi a catena lunga
Deficit di acil CoA deidrogenasi a catena molto lunga
MALATTIE DEL METABOLISMO DEGLI AMINOACIDI
Aciduria argininosuccinica
Citrullinemia
Citrullinemia tipo II
Omocistinuria
Iperfenilalaninemia
Malattia delle urine a sciroppo d'acero
Fenilchetonuria
Tirosinemia

CoA, coenzima A.

Nei 4 anni trascorsi da quando la spettrometria fu introdotta, il tasso di identificazione ogni 100 000 nati è diventato di 15,7, significativamente più elevato rispetto a quello di 8,6-9,5 dei 6 anni precedenti. Le malattie dell'ossidazione degli acidi grassi, in particolare il deficit di acil coenzima A deidrogenasi a catena intermedia, hanno rappresentato la maggior parte delle diagnosi aumentate.

I programmi di screening neonatale allargati che utilizzano la MS/MS accrescono l'identificazione delle malattia metaboliche ereditarie. Dal 2006, 34 Stati degli Stati Uniti hanno usato la MS/MS nei loro programmi di screening neonatale. Tuttavia, le condizioni metaboliche sottoposte a questo screening variano nei diversi Stati, andando da <3 a >20.

Nel tentativo di standardizzare i programmi di screening neonatale, l'American College of Medical Genetics raccomanda che ogni bambino nato negli Stati Uniti venga sottoposto a screening per un pannello uniforme di 29 malattie. Anche la March of Dimes e l'American Academy of Pediatrics approvano questa raccomandazione. Tuttavia, l'allargamento della lista di test di screening solleva diversi problemi. Per esempio, il costo di realizzazione può essere significativo, in quanto molti Stati avranno bisogno di sistemi di MS/MS multipli. Inoltre, provvedere il laboratorio di personale tecnico qualificato per fare funzionare il sistema MS/MS e di scienziati clinici qualificati per interpretare i profili può essere difficoltoso. Con questi test di screening neonatale si otterrà anche un certo numero di risultati falsi positivi, molti dei quali saranno dovuti alla nutrizione parenterale, alla variazione biologica o al trattamento e non saranno secondari a un errore congenito del metabolismo. Pertanto, diventerà necessario personale qualificato per assicurarsi che i pazienti con risultati anormali vengano contattati e sottoposti a test e consulenza di follow-up, se necessario. Nonostante queste preoccupazioni, il rapporto dell'American College of Medical Genetics rappresenta un passo nella giusta direzione verso linee guida standardizzanti per i programmi di screening neonatale.

TEST NELL'AFFINAMENTO DI UNA DIAGNOSI DIFFERENZIALE. L'uso dei test di laboratorio nell'affinamento di una diagnosi differenziale soddisfa la teoria del VP, in quanto una diagnosi differenziale corretta dovrebbe portare a una prevalenza relativamente elevata della malattia che viene presa in considerazione. Un esempio di test per l'affinamento di una diagnosi differenziale è la misurazione dell'acido vanilmandelico urinario (VMA, *VanillylMandelic Acid*) per la diagnosi di neuroblastoma. Un semplice test spot per il VMA non è utile in generale nei programmi di screening, a causa della bassa prevalenza del neuroblastoma (3 casi/100 000) e la bassa sensibilità del test (69%). Anche se la specificità del VMA urinario è del 99,6%, la realizzazione del test su 100 000 bambini produrrebbe 2 veri positivi, 400 falsi positivi e 1 falso negativo. Il VP di un test positivo in questa situazione è dello 0,5% e quello di un test negativo è del 99,99%, non molto diverso dall'ipotesi che il neuroblastoma non sia presente. Tuttavia, la realizzazione di questo test in un bambino di 3 anni con una massa addominale dà un risultato utile, perché la prevalenza del neuroblastoma è almeno del 50% in questi casi. Se 100 di tali bambini venissero sottoposti al test e si assumesse che la prevalenza del neuroblastoma nel gruppo sia del 50%, si otterrebbe un VP soddisfacente.

$$\text{VP del test positivo} = \frac{0{,}69 \times 50}{0{,}69 \times 50 + (0{,}004 \times 50)} \times 100 = 99\%$$

$$\text{VP del test negativo} = \frac{0{,}996 \times 50}{0{,}996 \times 50 + (0{,}31 \times 50)} \times 100 = 76\%$$

Quindi, in questa situazione, un test di bassa sensibilità è potente nell'affinamento della diagnosi differenziale, perché il VP di un test positivo è quasi del 100% in caso di prevalenza elevata.

Test sierologici. L'utilizzo dei test di laboratorio per l'affinamento di una diagnosi differenziale pone problemi, come esemplificato dal test sierologico per la borreliosi di Lyme, che è un'infezione da parte della *Borrelia burgdorferi* trasmessa dal morso di zecca e che ha varie manifestazioni nelle fasi iniziali e tardive (vedi Capitolo 219). La dimostrazione diretta del microrganismo è difficile e i risultati del test sierologico per la borreliosi di Lyme non sono attendibilmente positivi nei pazienti giovani che si presentano precocemente con un eritema cronico migrante. Questi risultati diventano positivi dopo poche settimane dall'infezione e rimangono tali per un certo numero di anni. In una popolazione più anziana che venisse valutata per la borreliosi di Lyme in stadio tardivo, alcuni soggetti saranno guariti dalla forma clinica o subclinica, altri presenteranno una borreliosi di Lyme attiva ed entrambi i gruppi avranno risultati veri positivi al test sierologico. Tra gli individui senza borreliosi di Lyme, alcuni presenteranno risultati veri negativi al test sierologico, ma una significativa percentuale avrà anticorpi diretti contro altri microrganismi che possiedono una reazione incrociata con gli antigeni della *B. burgdorferi*.

Questa serie di circostanze solleva un certo numero di problemi. Innanzitutto, la natura proteiforme della borreliosi di Lyme rende difficile assicurare un'elevata prevalenza di malattia nei soggetti da sottoporre al test. In secondo luogo, gli anticorpi più appropriati da identificare sono mal definiti, portando a un'ampia varietà di test con variabili tassi di falsi positivi e falsi negativi. In terzo luogo, l'anamnesi naturale della risposta anticorpale all'infezione e la difficoltà di mostrare il microrganismo causale si combinano direttamente, rendendo difficile la diagnosi iniziale di borreliosi di Lyme. Infine, nella diagnosi di borreliosi di Lyme in stadio tardivo nei soggetti più anziani, quella di laboratorio è influenzata da risultati positivi ingannevoli (falsi positivi o veri positivi, ma clinicamente irrilevanti), tipicamente un *enzyme-linked immunosorbent assay* che utilizza microrganismi interi della *B. burgdorferi*. In una revisione su 788 pazienti inviati a una clinica specialistica con diagnosi di borreliosi di Lyme, la diagnosi era corretta in 180 pazienti, 156 pazienti presentavano una vera sieropositività senza borreliosi attiva e 452 non avevano mai avuto questa malattia, anche se nel 45% di essi fu riscontrata la sieropositività da almeno un test prima dell'invio.

TABELLA 714-4. Profilo di laboratorio come esame di sistemi

TEST DI LABORATORIO	VALUTAZIONE FACILITATA DAI TEST
Emocromo completo e piastrine	Nutrizione, stato degli elementi formati
Esame delle urine completo	Funzionalità renale/infiammazione delle vie genitourinarie
Albumina e colesterolo	Nutrizione
ALT, bilirubina, GGT	Funzionalità epatica
Azotemia, creatinina	Funzionalità renale, nutrizione
Sodio, potassio, cloro, bicarbonato	Omeostasi degli elettroliti
Calcio e fosforo	Omeostasi del calcio

ALT, alanina aminotransferasi; GGT, γ-glutamiltransferasi.

Si utilizza comunemente un approccio a due stadi, simile a quello adoperato nel test dell'HIV: un test di screening che ha una sensibilità elevata (per es. l'*enzyme-linked immunosorbent assay*) e un eccellente VP negativo, seguito da un test di conferma molto specifico per la verifica dei risultati positivi del test di screening (per es. Western blot per identificare gli anticorpi diretti contro antigeni batterici selettivi). Risultati negativi del test di screening e del test di verifica sono riferiti come negativi. Risultati positivi al test di verifica sono riferiti come positivi. Tuttavia, la standardizzazione delle procedure dei test è difficile in Nord America, dove si riscontra soltanto un ceppo patogeno della *B. burgdorferi* ed è inoltre più difficoltoso anche altrove nell'emisfero settentrionale, in cui sono presenti fino a tre ceppi patogeni. L'identificazione del DNA microbico nei liquidi corporei mediante la polymerase chain reaction è definitiva, ma invasiva.

Esami di laboratorio di screening. I profili di screening (Tab. 714-4) vengono usati nell'ambito di un esame completo degli apparati, per stabilire un valore basale o per facilitare la terapia del paziente in circostanze specifiche, come: (1) quando il paziente ha evidentemente una malattia, ma una diagnosi specifica non è ancora stata posta; (2) quando un paziente necessita di terapie intensive; (3) per la sorveglianza postmarketing e la valutazione di un nuovo farmaco; (4) quando si utilizza un farmaco che notoriamente possiede effetti collaterali sistemici. Gli esami di laboratorio di screening dovrebbero essere utilizzati in modo mirato, a integrazione, non in sostituzione, di un'anamnesi e di un esame obiettivo completi.

American Academy of Pediatrics and American Thyroid Association: Newborn screening for congenital hypothyroidism. *Pediatrics* 1987;80: 745–749.

Bulterys M, Jamieson DJ, O'Sullivan MJ, et al: Rapid HIV-1 testing during labor: A multicenter study. *JAMA* 2004;292:219–223.

Clayton EW: Issues in state newborn screening programs. *Pediatrics* 1992; 90:641–646.

Farrell PM, Kosrok MR, Rock MJ, et al: Early diagnosis of cystic fibrosis through neonatal screening prevents severe malnutrition and improves long-term growth. *Pediatrics* 2001;107:1–13.

Galen RS, Gambino SR: *Beyond Normality.* New York, Academic Press, 1975.

Hu LT, Klempner MS: Update on the prevention, diagnosis, and treatment of Lyme disease. *Adv Intern Med* 2001;46:247–275.

National Newborn Screening and Genetics Resource Center (website *http://genes-r-us.uthscsa.edu*).

Rinaldo P, Tortorelli S, Matern D: Recent developments and new applications of tandem mass spectrometry in newborn screening. *Curr Opin Pediatr* 2004;16:427–433.

Steere AC, Taylor E, McHugh GL, et al: The overdiagnosis of Lyme disease. *JAMA* 1993;269:1812–1826.

Wilcken B, Wiley V, Hammond J, et al: Screening newborns for inborn errors of metabolism by tandem mass spectrometry. *N Engl J Med* 2003;348: 2304–2312.

Zytkovicz TH, Fitzgerald EF, Marsden D, et al: Tandem mass spectrometric analysis for amino, organic, and fatty acid disorders in newborn dried blood spots: A two-year summary from the New England Newborn Screening Program. *Clin Chem* 2001;47:1945–1955.

Capitolo 715 ■ Valori di riferimento per esami e procedure di laboratorio

Michael A. Pesce

Nelle Tabelle da 715-1 a 715-6, gli intervalli di riferimento sono validi per i bambini piccoli, i bambini grandi e gli adolescenti, quando possibile. Per molte analisi, tuttavia, valori di riferimento separati per gli adolescenti e per i bambini non sono ben delineati. Nell'interpretare il risultato di un test, si dovrebbe usare sempre l'intervallo di riferimento fornito dal laboratorio che effettua il test. Vedi le Figure 715-1 e 715-2 per le stime relative ai dosaggi.

TABELLA 715-1. Prefissi indicanti fattori decimali

PREFISSO	SIMBOLO	FATTORE
Mega-	M	10^{6}
Chilo-	k	10^{3}
Etto-	h	10^{2}
Deca-	da	10^{1}
Deci-	d	10^{-1}
Centi-	c	10^{-2}
Milli-	m	10^{-3}
Micro-	μ	10^{-6}
Nano-	n	10^{-9}
Pico-	p	10^{-12}
Femto-	f	10^{-15}

TABELLA 715-2. Abbreviazioni

Ab	Assorbanza
BB	Isoenzima cerebrale della creatina chinasi
cap	Capillare
CH_{50}	Diluizione necessaria per lisare il 50% dei globuli rossi indice; indica l'attività del complemento
Cr	Creatinina
F	Femmina
g	Grammo
Hb	Emoglobina
HbCO	Carbossiemoglobina
hpf	*High-power field* (campo focale a elevato ingrandimento)
it	Intratecale
L	Litro
LCS	Liquido cerebrospinale
M	Maschio
MB	Isoenzima cardiaco della creatina chinasi
mEq/L	Milliequivalenti litro
min	Minuto, minuti
mm^3	Millimetro cubo, microlitro (μL)
mmHg	Millimetri di mercurio
mol	Moli
mmol	Millimoli
mOsm	Milliosmoli
MW	Peso molecolare relativo
ND	Non identificato
nm	Nanometro (lunghezza d'onda)
OMS	Organizzazione Mondiale della Sanità
Pa	Pascal
pc	Postprandiale
RBC	Globuli rossi, eritrociti
RT	Temperatura ambientale
s	Secondo, secondi
SD	Deviazione standard
sett	Settimana, settimane
Tr	Tracce
U	Unità Internazionale di attività enzimatica
UA	Unità arbitraria
UI	Unità Internazionale dell'attività ormonale
V	Volume
WBC	Globuli bianchi

TABELLA 715-3. Simboli

>	Maggiore di	≤	Minore o uguale a
≥	Maggiore o uguale a	±	Più o meno
<	Minore di	≈	Approssimativamente uguale a

TABELLA 715-4. Abbreviazioni per i campioni

S	Siero
P	Plasma
(H)	Eparina
(LiH)	Litio eparina
(E)	Acido etilendiaminotetracetico (EDTA)
(C)	Citrato
(O)	Ossalato
W	Sangue intero
U	Urina
F	Feci
LCS	Liquido cerebrospinale
AF	Liquido amniotico
(NaC)	Citrato di sodio
(NH_4H)	Ammonio eparinato

TABELLA 715-5. Legenda ai commenti

30 °C, 37 °C	Temperatura dell'analisi enzimatica (Celsius)
a	I valori ottenuti sono significativamente dipendenti dal metodo
b	I valori nei maschi più anziani sono più alti di quelli ottenuti nelle femmine più anziane
c	I valori nelle femmine più anziane sono più alti di quelli ottenuti nei maschi più anziani
d	Assorbimento atomico
e	Cromatografia di affinità al borato
f	Cromatografia a scambio di cationi
g	Vitros, sistema analitico di proprietà della Ortho Clinical Diagnostics, Inc.
i	Elettroforesi
j	Analisi enzimatica
k	*Enzyme-amplified immunoassay*
l	Metodo fluorometrico
m	Citometria a flusso (*Fluorescence-Activated Cell Sorting*, FACS)
n	Polarizzazione della fluorescenza
o	Gas cromatografia
p	Cromatografia liquida a elevata efficienza (*High-Performance Liquid Chromatography*, HPLC)
q	Analisi con anticorpi a fluorescenza indiretta (*Indirect Fluorescence Antibody* [IFA] *assay*)
r	Elettrodo ione-selettivo
s	Nefelometria
t	Densità ottica
u	Immunodiffusione radiale (*Radial ImmunoDiffusion*, RID)
v	Radioimmunoanalisi (*RadioImmunoAssay*, RIA)
w	Spettrofotometria

TABELLA 715-6. Valori di riferimento[*,†]

ANALITA O PROCEDURA	CAMPIONE	VALORI DI RIFERIMENTO (USA)		FATTORE DI CONVERSIONE	VALORI DI RIFERIMENTO (SI)	COMMENTI
Esame emocromocitometrico completo						
Acido urico	S		mg/dL		μmol/L	j (Meites, 1989)
		1-5 anni	1,7-5,8	×59,48	100-350	
		6-11 anni	2,2-6,6		130-390	
		M 12-19 anni	3,0-7,7		180-460	
		F 12-19 anni	2,7-5,7		160-340	
Alanina aminotransferasi (ALT, SGPT)	S	0-5 giorni	6-50 U/L	×1	6-50 U/L	37°bw (Lockitch, Halstead e Albersheim, 1988)
		1-19 anni	5-45		5-45	
Albumina	P	Prematuro 1 giorno	1,8-3,0 g/dL	×10	18-30 g/dL	g (Meites, 1989)
		A termine <6 giorni	2,5-3,4		25-34	
		<5 anni	3,9-5,0		39-50	
		5-19 anni	4,0-5,3		40-53	
Amilasi	S,P	1-19 anni	30-100 U/L	×1	30-100 U/L	(Lockitch, Halstead e Albersheim et al., 1988; Gillard et al., 1983)
			% frazione pancreatica		% frazione pancreatica	
Amilasi, isoenzimi	S,P(H)	Cordone-8 mesi	0-34%	×0,01	0-0,34%	
		9 mesi-4 anni	5-56%		0,05-0,56%	
		5-19 anni	23-59%		0,23-0,59%	
Ammoniaca	W	<30 giorni	21-95 μmol/L	×1	21-95 μmol/L	(Diaz et al., 1995)
		1-12 mesi	18-74		18-74	
		1-14 anni	17-68		17-68	
		>14 anni	19-71		19-71	
Anidride carbonica, pressione parziale (PCO_2)	W(H)		mmHg		kPa	
		Neonato	27-40	×0,1333	3,6-5,3	
		Bambino piccolo	27-41		3,6-5,5	
		Oltre M	35-48		4,7-6,4	
		F	32-45		4,3-6,0	
Aspartato aminotransferasi (AST, SGOT)	S		U/L		U/L	
		0-5 giorni	35-140	×1	35-140	37°b (Lockitch, Halstead, e Quigley et al., 1988)
		1-9 anni	15-55		15-55	
		10-19 anni	5-45		5-45	
Azotemia	S,P		mg/dL		mmol urea/L	
		Sangue cordonale	21-40	×0,357	7,5-14,3	
		Prematuro (1 sett)	3-25		1,1-9,0	
		Neonato	3-12		1,1-4,3	
		Bambino piccolo o grande	5-18		1,8-6,4	
		Oltre	7-18		2,5-6,4	
Bicarbonato	S,P		mmol/L	×1	mmol/L	
		Arterioso	21-28		21-28	
		Venoso	22-29		22-29	
Calcio, ionizzato (Ca)	S,P(H), W(H)		mg/dL		mmol/L	
		Sangue cordonale	5,0-6,0	×0,25	1,25-1,50	
		Neonato, 3-24 ore	4,3-5,1		1,07-1,27	
		24-48 ore	4,0-4,7		1,00-1,17	
		Oltre	4,8-4,92		1,12-1,23	
		oppure	2,24-2,46 Eq/L	×0,5	1,12-1,23	
Calcio, totale	S		mg/dL		mmol/L	
		Sangue cordonale	9,0-11,5	×0,25	2,25-2,88	
		Neonato, 3-24 ore	9,0-10,6		2,3-2,65	
		24-48 ore	7,0-12,0		1,75-3,00	
		4-7 giorni	9,0-10,9		2,25-2,73	
		Bambino	8,8-10,8		2,20-2,70	
		Oltre	8,4-10,2		2,10-2,55	
Captazione tiroidea di iodio radioattivo	Attività sulla ghiandola tiroidea	2 ore	<6%	×0,01	2 ore <0,06	
		6 ore	3-20%		6 ore 0,03-0,20	
		24 ore	8-30%		24 ore 0,08-0,30	
Captazione tiroidea di tecnezio 99 m	Attività sulla ghiandola tiroidea	Dopo 24 ore	0,4-3,0%	×0,01	Captazione frazionale 0,004-0,030	

TABELLA 715-6. Valori di riferimento*† – *continua*

ANALITA O PROCEDURA	CAMPIONE	VALORI DI RIFERIMENTO (USA)	FATTORE DI CONVERSIONE	VALORI DI RIFERIMENTO (SI)	COMMENTI
Clearance della creatinina (endogena)	S,P,U	Neonato 40-65 mL/min/1,73 m²			
		<40 anni, M 97-137			
		F 88-128			
		Diminuisce <6,5 mL/min/decade			
Cloro	S,P(H)	Sangue cordonale 96-104 mmol/L	×1	96-104 mmol/L	
		Neonato 97-110		97-110	
		Oltre 98-106		98-106	
Concentrazione emoglobinica corpuscolare media (MCHC)	W(E)	% Hb/cell o g Hb/dL RBC		mmol Hb/L RBC	
		Nascita 30-36	×0,155	4,65-5,58	
		1-3 giorni (cap) 29-37		4,50-5,74	
		1-2 sett 28-38		4,34-5,89	
		1-2 mesi 29-37		4,50-5,74	
		3 mesi-2 anni 30-36		4,65-5,58	
		2-18 anni 31-37		4,81-5,74	
		>18 anni 31-37		4,81-5,74	
Conta leucocitaria (conta WBC)	W(E)	×1000 cellule/mm³ (μL)		×10⁹ cellule/L	
		Parto 9,0-30,0	×1	9,0-30,0	
		24 ore 9,4-34,0		9,4-34,0	
		1 mese 5,0-19,5		5,0-19,5	
		1-3 anni 6,0-17,5		6,0-17,5	
		4-7 anni 5,5-15,5		5,5-15,5	
		8-13 anni 4,5-13,5		4,5-13,5	
		Adulto 4,5-11,0		4,5-11,0	
Conta piastrinica (conta dei trombociti)	W(E)	×10³/mm³ (μL)		×10⁹/L	
		Neonato 84-478 (dopo 1 sett, idem per l'adulto)	×10⁶	84-478	(Buck, 1996)
		Adulto 150-400		150-400	
Conta reticolocitaria	W(E,H,O)	Adulti 0,5-1,5% di eritrociti	×0,01	0,005-0,015 (numero della frazione)	
		o 25 000-75 000/mm³ (μL)	×10⁶	o 25 000-75 000 ×10⁶/L	
		%		Numero della frazione	
	W(cap)	1 giorno 0,4-6,0	×0,01	0,004-0,060	
		7 giorni <0,1-1,3		<0,001-0,013	
		1-4 sett <1,0-1,2		<0,001-0,012	
		5-6 sett <0,1-2,4		<0,001-0,024	
		7-8 sett 0,1-2,9		0,001-0,029	
		9-10 sett <0,1-2,6		<0,001-0,026	
		11-12 sett 0,1-1,3		0,001-0,013	
Cortisolo	S,P(H)	μg/dL		nmol/L	
		Neonato 1-24	×27,59	28-662	
		Adulti, 8.00 5-23		138-635	
		16.00 3-15		82-413	
		20.00 <50% delle 8.00	×0,01	Frazione delle 8.00 ≤0,50	
Creatina chinasi	S	Sangue cordonale 70-380 U/L	×1	70-380 U/L	30°b (Jedeikin et al., 1982)
		5-8 ore 214-1,175		214-1,175	
		24-33 ore 130-1,200		130-1200	
		72-100 ore 87-725		87-725	
		Adulto 5-130		5-130	
Creatinchinasi, isoenzimi	S	% MB	% BB		
		Sangue cordonale 0,3-3,1	0,3-10,5		
		5-8 ore 1,7-7,9	3,6-13,4		
		24-33 ore 1,8-5,0	2,3-8,6		
		72-100 ore 1,4-5,4	5,1-13,3		
		Adulto 0-2	0		
Creatinina					
Jaffe, cinetica, o enzimatica	S,P	mg/dL		μmol/L	
		Sangue cordonale 0,6-1,2	×88,4	53-106	
		Neonato 0,3-1,0		27-88	
		Bambino piccolo 0,2-0,4		18-35	
		Bambino grande 0,3-0,7		27-62	
		Adolescente 0,5-1,0		44-88	
		Adulto M 0,6-1,2		53-106	
		F 0,5-1,1		44-97	

TABELLA 715-6. Valori di riferimento*† – *continua*

ANALITA O PROCEDURA	CAMPIONE	VALORI DI RIFERIMENTO (USA)		FATTORE DI CONVERSIONE	VALORI DI RIFERIMENTO (SI)	COMMENTI
Eccesso di basi	W(H)		mmol/L		mmol/L	
		Neonato	(−10)–(−2)	×1	(−10)–(−2)	
		Bambino piccolo	(−7)–(−1)		(−7)–(−1)	
		Bambino grande	(−4)–(−2)		(−4)–(+2)	
		Oltre	(−3)–(−3)		(−3)–(−3)	
Ematocrito (HCT, Hct)	W(E)		% globuli rossi concentrati			
Calcolato dal volume corpuscolare medio			(V globuli rossi/V sangue intero)		Frazione di volume	
(MCV) e dalla conta dei RBC (dislocazione			cellule × 100		(V globuli rossi/V sangue intero)	
elettronica o laser)		1 giorno (cap)	48-69%	×0,01	0,48-0,69	
		2 giorni	48-75%		0,48-0,75	
		3 giorni	44-72%		0,44-0,72	
		2 mesi	28-42%		0,28-0,42	
		6-12 anni	35-45%		0,35-0,45	
		12-18 anni M	37-49%		0,37-0,49	
		F	36-46%		0,36-0,46	
		18-49 anni M	41-53%		0,41-0,53	
		F	36-46%		0,36-0,46	
Emoglobina (Hb)	W(E)		g/dL		mmol/L	
		1-3 giorni (cap)	14,5-22,5	×0,155	2,25-3,49	MW Hb = 64 500
		2 mesi	9,0-14,0		1,40-2,17	
		6-12 anni	11,5-15,5		1,78-2,40	
		12-18 anni M	13,0-16,0		2,02-2,48	
		F	12,0-16,0		1,86-2,48	
		18-49 anni M	13,5-17,5		2,09-2,27	
		F	12,0-16,0		1,86-2,48	
	P(H)	Vedi *Elementi chimici*				
Indici eritrocitari (indici RBC)						
Emoglobina corpuscolare media (MCH)	W(E)		pg/cell		fmol/cell	
		Parto	31-37	×0,0155	0,48-0,57	
		1-3 giorni (cap)	31-37		0,48-0,57	
		1 sett-1 mese	28-40		0,43-0,62	
		2 mesi	26-34		0,40-0,53	
		3-6 mesi	25-35		0,39-0,54	
		0,5-2 anni	23-31		0,36-0,48	
		2-6 anni	24-30		0,37-0,47	
		6-12 anni	25-33		0,39-0,51	
		12-18 anni	25-35		0,39-0,54	
		18-49 anni	26-34		0,40-0,53	
Ferritina	S		ng/mL		μg/L	
		Neonato	25-200	×1	25-200	
		1 mese	200-600		200-600	
		2-5 mesi	50-200		50-200	
		6 mesi-15 anni	7-140		7-140	
		Adulto M	15-200		15-200	
		F	12-150		12-150	
Ferro	S	Tutte le età	22-184 μg/dL	×0,1791	4-33 μmol/L	(Lockitch, Halstead e Wadsworth et al., 1988)
Ferro, capacità totale di legame (*Total Iron-Binding Capacity*, TIBC)	S	Bambino piccolo	100-400 μg/dL	×0,179	17,90-71,60 μmol/L	
		Oltre	250-400		44,75-71,60	
Folato	S	Neonato 7,0-32 ng/mL		×2,265	15,9-72,4 nmol/L	
		Oltre 1,8-9,0			4,1-20,4	
	W(E)	150-450 ng/mL RBC			340-1,020 nmol/L cellule	
Formula leucocitaria	W(E)	%			Numero della frazione	
Mielociti		0%		×0,01	0	
Neutrofili ("iposegmentati")		3-5%			0,03-0,05	
Neutrofili ("ipersegmentati")		54-62%			0,54-0,62	
Linfociti		25-33%			0,25-0,33	
Monociti		3-7%			0,03-0,07	
Eosinofili		1-3%			0,01-0,03	
Basofili		0-0,75%			0-0,0075	
		Cellule/mm³ (μL)			×10⁶ cellule/L	
Mielociti		0		×1	0	
Neutrofili ("iposegmentati")		150-400			150-400	
Neutrofili ("ipersegmentati")		3000-5800			3000-5800	
Linfociti		1500-3000			1500-3000	
Monociti		285-500			285-500	
Eosinofili		50-250			50-250	
Basofili		15-50			15-50	

TABELLA 715-6. Valori di riferimento*† – *continua*

ANALITA O PROCEDURA	CAMPIONE	VALORI DI RIFERIMENTO (USA)			FATTORE DI CONVERSIONE	VALORI DI RIFERIMENTO (SI)		COMMENTI
Fosfatasi, alcalina	S		U/L			U/L		
		1-9 anni	145-420		×1	145-420		37°C aw (Lockitch, Halstead, Albersheim et al., 1988)
		10-11 anni	130-560			130-560		
			M	F		M	F	
		12-13 anni	200-495	105-420		200-495	105-420	
		14-15 anni	130-525	70-230		130-525	70-230	
		16-19 anni	65-260	50-130		65-260	50-130	
Fosforo, inorganico	S,P(H)		mg/dL			mmol/L		
		0-5 giorni	4,8-8,2		×0,3229	1,55-2,65		w (Meites, 1989)
		1-3 anni	3,8-6,5			1,25-2,10		
		4-11 anni	3,7-5,6			1,20-1,80		
		12-15 anni	2,9-5,4			0,95-1,75		
		16-19 anni	2,7-4,7			0,90-1,50		
γ-glutamil transpeptidasi (GGT, GGTP)	S		U/L			U/L		
		Sangue del cordone ombelicale	37-193		×1	37-193		37°b (Knight e Haymond, 1981)
		0-1 mese	13-147			13-147		
		1-2 mesi	12-123			12-123		
		2-4 mesi	8-90			8-90		
		4 mesi-10 anni	5-32			5-32		
		10-15 anni	5-24			5-24		
Gap anionico (sodio − [cloro + bicarbonato])	P(H)	7-16 mEq/L			×1	7-16 mEq/L		
Glucosio	S		mg/dL			mmol/L		
		Sangue del cordone ombelicale	45-96		×0,0555	2,5-5,3		
		Prematuro	20-60			1,1-3,3		
		Neonato	30-60			1,7-3,3		
		Neonato						
		1 giorno	40-60			2,2-3,3		
		>1 giorno	50-90			2,8-5,0		
		Bambino	60-100			3,3-5,5		
		Adulto	70-105			3,9-5,8		
	W(H)	Adulto	65-95			3,6-5,3		
Glucosio, 2 ore post	S	<120 mg/dL				<6,7 mmol/L		
Glucosio-6-fosfato deidrogenasi (G6PD) negli eritrociti		W(E,H,C)						Bishop, modificata
		Adulto				Adulto		
		3,4-8,0 U/gHb			×0,0645	0,22-0,52 mU/molHb		
		98,6-232 U/10^{12} RBC			$\times 10^{-3}$	0,10-0,23 nU/10^{6} RBC		
		1,16-2,72 U/mL RBC			×1	1,16-2,72 kU/L RBC		
		Neonato: 50% più alto				Neonato: 50% più alto		
Immunoglobulina A (IgA)	S		mg/dL		×10	mg/L		
		Sangue del cordone ombelicale	1,4-3,6			14-36		s (Meites, 1989)
		1-3 mesi	1,3-53			13-530		
		4-6 mesi	4,4-84			44-840		
		7 mesi-1 anno	11-106			110-1060		
		2-5 anni	14-159			140-1590		
		6-10 anni	33-236			330-2360		
		Adulto	70-312			700-3120		
Immunoglobulina D (IgD)	S	Neonato: non rilevata				Non rilevata		
		Oltre: 0-8 mg/dL			×10	0-80 mg/L		
Immunoglobulina E (IgE)	S	M 0-230 UI/mL			×1	0-230 kUI/L		
		F 0-170				0-170		
Immunoglobulina G (IgG)	S		mg/dL			g/L		
		Sangue del cordone ombelicale	636-1606		×0,01	6,36-16,06		s (Meites, 1989)
		1 mese	251-906			2,51-9,06		
		2-4 mesi	176-601			1,76-6,01		
		5-12 mesi	172-1069			1,72-10,69		
		1-5 anni	345-1236			3,45-12,36		
		6-10 anni	608-1572			6,08-15,72		
		Adulto	639-1349			6,39-13,49		
Immunoglobulina M (IgM)	S		mg/dL			mg/L		
		Sangue del cordone ombelicale	6,3-25		×10	63-250		s (Meites, 1989)
		1-4 mesi	17-105			170-1050		
		5-9 mesi	33-126			330-1260		
		10 mesi-1 anno	41-173			410-1730		
		2-8 anni	43-207			430-2070		
		9-10 anni	52-242			520-2420		
		Adulto	56-352			560-3520		

TABELLA 715-6. Valori di riferimento*† – *continua*

ANALITA O PROCEDURA	CAMPIONE	VALORI DI RIFERIMENTO (USA)		FATTORE DI CONVERSIONE	VALORI DI RIFERIMENTO (SI)	COMMENTI
Isoenzimi	S		% di attività totale			
			1-6 anni 7-19 anni			
		LD1	20-38 20-35			
		LD2	27-38 31-38			
		LD3	16-26 19-28			
		LD4	5-16 7-13			
		LD5	3-13 5-12			
D-lattato	P(H)	6 mesi-3 anni	0,0-0,3	×1	0,0-0,3	j (Rosenthal e Pesce, 1985)
L+lattato	W		mmol/L		mmol/L	(Bonnefont et al., 1990)
		1-12 mesi	1,1-2,3	×1	1,1-2,3	
		1-7 anni	0,8-1,5		0,8-1,5	
		7-15 anni	0,6-0,9		0,6-0,9	
Lattato deidrogenasi	S		U/L		U/L	
		<1 anno	170-580	×1	170-580	37° a (Meites, 1989)
		1-9 anni	150-500		150-500	
		10-19 anni	120-330		120-330	
Lipasi	P,S	1-18 anni	145-216 U/L	×1	145-216 U/L	(Ghoshal e Soldin, 2003)
Magnesio	P(H)		mg/dL		mmol/L	
		0-6 giorni	1,2-2,6	×0,411	0,48-1,05	w (Meites, 1989)
		7 giorni-2 anni	1,6-2,6		0,65-1,05	
		2-14 anni	1,5-2,3		0,60-0,95	
Metaemoglobina (MetHb)	W(E,H,C)	0,06-0,24 g/dL o		×155	9,3-37,2 μmol/L	
		0,78 ± 0,37% dell'Hb totale		×0,01	0,0078 ± 0,0037 (frazione della massa)	
Monossido di carbonio (carbossiemoglobina)	W(E)	Non fumatore	<2% HbCO	×0,01	Frazione di HbCO <0,02	
		Fumatore	<10%		<0,10	
		Letale	>50%		>0,5	
Ormone antidiuretico (hADH), vasopressina	P(E)	Osmolarità plasmatica (mOsmL/kg)	ADH plasmatico (pg/mL)		ADH plasmatico ng/L	
		270-280	<1,5	×1	<1,5	
		280-285	<2,5		<2,5	
		285-290	1-5		1-5	
		290-295	2-7		2-7	
		295-300	4-12		4-12	
Ormone rilasciante la tireotropina (hTRH)	P	5-60 pg/mL		×2,759	14-165 pmol/L	
Ormone tireostimolante	S	Prematuro (28-36 sett)	mUI/L		mUI/L	
		Prima sett di vita	0,7-27,0	×1	0,7-27,0	(Nichols Institute Diagnostics)
		Neonati a termine				
		Sangue cordonale	2,3-13,2		2,3-13,2	
		1-2 giorni	3,2-34,6		3,2-34,6	
		3-4 giorni	0,7-15,4		0,7-15,4	
		2-20 sett	1,7-9,1		1,7-9,1	
		21 sett-20 anni	0,7-6,4		0,7-6,4	
Osmolalità	S	Bambino, adulto 275-295 mOsmol/kgH_2O				
Piombo	W(H)		μg/dL		mmol/L	
		Bambino	<10	×0,0483	<0,48	
		Tossico	≥70		≥3,38	
Piruvato	W	7-17 anni	0,076 ± 0,026 mmol/L	×1	0,076 ± 0,026 mmol/L	(Pianosi et al., 1995)
Potassio	S		mmol/L		mmol/L	
		<2 mesi	3,0-7,0	×1	3,0-7,0	r (Meites, 1989)
		2-12 mesi	3,5-6,0		3,5-6,0	Aumentato dall'emolisi; valori serici sistematicamente più alti dei valori plasmatici
		>12 mesi	3,5-5,0		3,5-5,0	
	P(H)	3,5-4,5 mmol/L			3,5-4,5 mmol/L	
Prealbumina (transtiretina)	P		mg/L		mg/L	
		2-6 mesi	142-330	×1	142-330	s (Sherry et al., 1988)
		6-12 mesi	120-274		120-274	
		1-3 anni	108-259		108-259	

TABELLA 715-6. Valori di riferimento*† – *continua*

ANALITA O PROCEDURA	CAMPIONE	VALORI DI RIFERIMENTO (USA)	FATTORE DI CONVERSIONE	VALORI DI RIFERIMENTO (SI)	COMMENTI
Proteina-C reattiva (alta sensibilità)	S				(Soldin et al., 2004)
		M (mg/dL) F (mg/dL)		M (mg/L) F (mg/L)	
		0-90 giorni 0,08-1,58 0,09-1,58	×10	0,8-15,8 0,9-15,8	
		91 giorni-12 mesi 0,08-1,12 0,05-0,79		0,8-11,2 0,5-7,9	
		13 mesi-3 anni 0,08-1,12 0,08-0,79		0,8-11,2 0,8-7,9	
		4-10 anni 0,06-0,79 0,5-1,0		0,6-7,9 0,5-10,0	
		11-14 anni 0,08-0,76 0,06-0,81		0,8-7,6 0,6-8,1	
		15-18 anni 0,04-0,79 0,06-0,79		0,4-7,9 0,6-7,9	
Proteine totali	S	g/dL		g/L	(Meites, 1989)
		Prematuro 4,3-7,6	×10	43-76	
		Neonato 4,6-7,4		46-74	
		1-7 anni 6,1-7,9		61-79	
		8-12 anni 6,4-8,1		64-81	
		13-19 anni 6,6-8,2		66-82	
Sodio	S,P (LiH,NH_4H)	mmol/L		mmol/L	
		Neonato 134-146	×1	134-146	
		Bambino piccolo 139-146		139-146	
		Bambino 138-145		138-146	
		Oltre 136-146		136-146	
Test di captazione della triiodotironina su resina (T_3RU)	S			Captazione frazionale	
		Neonato 26-36%	×0,01	0,26-0,36	
		Oltre 26-35%		0,26-0,35	
Test di tolleranza al glucosio (GTT)	S	mg/dL		mmol/L	
Dose orale Adulto: 75 g		Normale Diabetico		Normale Diabetico	
Bambino: 1,75 g/kg del peso ideale, fino a un massimo di 75 g		Digiuno 70-105 ≥126	×0,0555	3,9-5,8 ≥7,0	(American Diabetes Association, 1977)
		60 min 120-170 ≥200		6,7-9,4 ≥11	
		90 min 100-140 ≥200		5,6-7,8 ≥11	
		120 min 70-120 ≥200		3,9-6,7 ≥11	
Thyroxine-binding globulin (TBG)	S	mg/dL		mg/L	
		Sangue cordonale 1,4-9,4	×10	14-94	
		1-4 sett 1,0-9,0		10-90	
		1-12 mesi 2,0-7,6		20-76	
		1-5 anni 2,9-5,4		29-54	
		5-10 anni 2,5-5,0		25-50	
		10-15 anni 2,1-4,6		21-46	
		Adulto 1,5-3,4		15-34	
Tiroxina, libera	S	Neonati ng/dL	×12,9	Neonati a termine pmol/L	(Esoterix Endocrinology)
		3 giorni 2,0-4,9		3 giorni 26-63	
		Infanti 0,9-2,6		Bambini piccoli 12-33	
		Bambini in prepubertà 0,8-2,2		Bambini in prepubertà 10-28	
		Bambini in pubertà e adulti 0,8-2,3		Bambini in pubertà e adulti 10-30	
Tiroxina, totale	S	Neonati a termine	×12,9	Neonati a termine	(Esoterix Endocrinology)
		μg/dL		nmol/L	
		1-3 giorni 8,2-19,9		1-3 giorni 106-256	
		1 sett 6,0-15,9		1 sett 77-205	
		1-12 mesi 6,1-14,9		1-12 mesi 79-192	
		Bambini in prepubertà		Bambini in prepubertà	
		1-3 anni 6,8-13,5		1-3 anni 88-174	
		3-10 anni 5,5-12,8		3-10 anni 71-165	
		Bambini in pubertà e adulti 4,2-13,0		Bambini in pubertà e adulti 54-167	
	W	Screening neonatale (carta da filtro) 6,2-22,0 μg/dL	×12,9	80-283 nmol/L	
Titolo anti-desossiribonucleasi B (titolo anti-DNasi B)	S	Età Limite superiore della norma		Limite superiore della norma	
		4-6 anni 240-480 U	×1	240-480 U	(Kaplan et al., 1998)
		7-12 anni 480-800 U		480-800 U	
Titolo antistreptolisina-O (titolo ASO)	S	Età Limite superiore della norma		Limite superiore della norma	(Kaplan et al., 1998)
		2-5 anni 120-160 unità Todd	×1	120-160 unità Todd	
		6-9 anni 240 unità Todd		240 unità Todd	
		10-12 anni 320 unità Todd		320 unità Todd	

TABELLA 715-6. Valori di riferimento*† – *continua*

ANALITA O PROCEDURA	CAMPIONE	VALORI DI RIFERIMENTO (USA)		FATTORE DI CONVERSIONE	VALORI DI RIFERIMENTO (SI)	COMMENTI
Triiodotironina, libera	S		pg/dL		pmol/L	
		Sangue cordonale	20-240	×0,01536	0,3-3,7	
		1-3 giorni	200-610		3,1-9,4	
		6 sett	240-560		3,7-8,6	
		Adulti (20-50 anni)	230-660		3,5-10,0	
Triiodotironina, totale	S		ng/dL		nmol/L	
		Sangue cordonale	30-70	×0,0154	0,46-1,08	
		Neonato	75-260		1,16-4,00	
		1-5 anni	100-260		1,54-4,00	
		5-10 anni	90-240		1,39-3,70	
		10-15 anni	80-210		1,23-3,23	
		Oltre	115-190		1,77-2,93	
Volume corpuscolare medio (MCV)	W(E)		μm^3		fL	
		1-3 giorni (cap)	95-121	×1	95-121	
		0,5-2 anni	70-86		70-86	
		6-12 anni	77-95		77-95	
		12-18 anni M	78-98		78-98	
		F	78-102		78-102	
		18-49 anni M	80-100		80-100	
		F	80-100		80-100	

***Un elenco più esauriente dei valori di riferimento si può trovare online sul sito: *www.nelsonpediatrics.com*.**

†Nel preparare le liste dei valori di riferimento, sono stati utilizzati abbreviazioni, simboli e codici (vedi Tab. 715-2).

American Diabetes Association: Report of the Expert Committee on the Diagnosis and Classification of Diabetes Mellitus. *Diabetes Care* 1997;20:1183–1197.

Bonnefont JP, Specola NB, Vassault A, et al: The fasting test in children: Application to the diagnosis of pathological hypo- and hyperketotic states. *Eur J Pediatr* 1990;150:80–85.

Buck ML: Anticoagulation with warfarin in infants and children. *Ann Pharmacother* 1996;30:1316–1322.

Diaz J, Tornel PL, Martinez P: Reference intervals for blood ammonia in healthy subjects, determined by microdiffusion. *Clin Chem* 1995;41:1048.

Esoterix Endocrinology, Calabasas Hills, CA 91301.

Ghoshal A, Soldin S: Evaluation of the Dade Behring dimension R × L: Integrated chemistry system-pediatric reference ranges. *Clin Chim Acta* 2003;331:135–146.

Gillard BK, Simbala JA, Goodglick L: Reference intervals for amylase isoenzymes in serum and plasma of infants and children. *Clin Chem* 1983;29:1119–1123.

Jedeikin R, Makela SK, Shennan AT, et al: Creatine kinase isoenzymes in serum from cord blood and the blood of healthy full-term infants during the first three postnatal days. *Clin Chem* 1982;28:317–322.

Kaplan EL, Rothermel CD, Johnson DR: Antistreptolysin O and anti-deoxyribonuclease B titers: Normal values for children ages 2 to 12 in the United States. *Pediatrics* 1998;101:86–88.

Knight JA, Haymond RE: -Glutamyltransferase and alkaline phosphatase activities compared in serum of normal children and children with liver disease. *Clin Chem* 1981;27:48–51.

Lockitch G, Halstead AC, Wadsworth L, et al: Age-and sex-specific pediatric reference intervals and correlations for zinc, copper, selenium, iron, vitamins A and E, and related proteins. *Clin Chem* 1988;34:1625–1628.

Meites S (editor): *Pediatric Clinical Chemistry, Reference (Normal) Values*, 3rd ed. Washington, DC, American Association for Clinical Chemistry, 1989.

Muntau A, Streiter M, Kappler M, et al: Age-related reference values for serum selenium concentrations in infants and children. *Clin Chem* 2002;48:555–560.

Nichols Institute Diagnostics, San Juan Capistrano, CA 92675.

Nir A, Bar-Oz B, Perles Z, et al: N-terminal pro-B-type natriuretic peptide: Reference plasma levels from birth to adolescence. Elevated levels at birth and in infants and children with heart diseases. *Acta Paediatr* 2004;93:603–607.

Pianosi P, Seargeant L, Haworth JC: Blood lactate and pyruvate concentrations, and their ratio during exercise in healthy children: Developmental perspective. *Eur J Appl Physiol Occup Physiol* 1995;71:518–522.

Rosenthal P, Pesce MA: Long-term monitoring of D-lactic acidosis in a child. *J Pediatr Gastroenterol Nutr* 1985;4:674–676.

Sherry B, Jack RM, Weber A, et al: Reference interval for prealbumin for children 2 to 36 months old. *Clin Chem* 1988;34:1878–1880.

Soldin O, Bierbower L, Choi J, et al: Serum iron, ferritin, transferrin, total iron binding capacity, hs-CRP, LDL cholesterol and magnesium in children. New reference intervals using the Dade Dimension Clinical Chemistry System. *Clin Chim Acta* 2004;342:211–217.

Soldin SJ, Hicks JM, Bailey J, et al: Pediatric reference ranges for 25 hydroxy vitamin D during the summer and winter. *Clin Chem* 1997;43:S200.

TABELLA 715-7. Composizione delle soluzioni orali e parenterali comunemente usate negli Stati Uniti (Raymond Adelman e Michael Solhaug) [vedi le relative Tabelle di conversione da 715-8 a 715-10]

LIQUIDI	CARBOIDRATI (g/dL)	PROTEINE*	CALORIE/L	Na (mEq/L)	K (mEq/L)	Cl (mEq/L)	HCO_3† (mEq/L)	Ca (mEq/L)	P‡ (mEq/L)	Mg (mEq/L)	Osm§‖ ($mOsm/kgH_2O$)
ORALI											
Coca-Cola®	10,9	0	435	4,3	0,1	0	13,4	0	0	0	656
Gatorade®	5,9	0	250	21	2,5	17	0	0	6,8	0	377
Ginger®	9,0	0	360	3,5	0,1	0	3,6	0	0	0	565
Hydralyte®	2,5	0	100	84	10	59	15	<1	<1	0	300
Latte	4,9	3,5	670	22	36	28	30	60	54	0	260
Lytren®	7,0	0	280	30	25	25	36	4	5	4	267§‖
Pedialyte®	5,0	0	200	30	20	30	28	4	0	4	387
Pepsi-Cola®	12	0	480	6,5	0,8	0	7,3	0	0	0	0
Resol Solution®	2,0	0	83	50	20	50	34	4	5	4	269
Rhydrate®	2,5	0	100	75	25	65	30	0	0	0	305
Ricelyte Oral Solution® (solidi dello sciroppo di riso)	3,0	0	140	50	25	45	34	0	0	0	200
Root beer®	0	0	0	3,5	3,9	0	0	0	0	0	588
7Up®	8,0	0	320	7,5	0,2	0	0	0,3	0	0	564
Succo d'arancia	10,4	0,7	444	0,2	49	0	50	0	0	0	654
Succo d'ananas (in scatola)	13,5	0,4	556	0,2	38	0	0	7,5	9	0	783
Succo di mela¶	11,9	0,1	480	0	0,4	26	0	3	4,5	0	700
Succo di pomodoro (in scatola, salato)	4,3	0	172	100	59	150	10	3	18	0	592
Succo di pompelmo (in scatola, con zucchero)	17,8	0,6	736	0,2	35	0	0	6,5	0	0	591
Succo di prugne	19	0,4	776	0,9	60	0	0	7	20	0	0
Succo d'uva	16,6	0,2	672	0,4	30	0	32	0	0	0	1027
PARENTERALI											
Bicarbonato di sodio 5%	0	0	0	595	0	0	595	0	0	0	0
Butler 1 (a)	5	0	200	25	20	22	23	0	3	3	360
Butler 2 modificata (b)	5-10	0	200-400	56	25	49	26	0	12	5	423-719
Carboidrati# in H_2O	5-10	0	200-400	0	0	0	0	0	0	0	266-532
Destrano 6% (alto peso molecolare) [g]	5-10	0	200-400	0	0	0	0	0	0	0	0
Destrano 6% in fisiologica (h)	0	0	0	154	0	154	0	0	0	0	0
Destrano 10% (basso peso molecolare) [e]	5	0	200	0	0	0	0	0	0	0	0
Destrano 10% in fisiologica (f)	0	0	0	154	0	154	0	0	0	0	0
Fisiologica 3% (M/2)	0	0	0	513	0	513	513	0	0	0	969
Fisiologica 5%	0	0	0	855	0	855	855	0	0	0	1616
Fisiologica isotonica	0-5	0	0-200	154	0	154	0	0	0	0	292-558
1/2 fisiologica isotonica	2,5-5	0	100-200	77	0	77	0	0	0	0	280-415
Frazione delle proteine plasmatiche umane (d)	0	5	0	130	2	50	50	0	0	0	0
Lattato di sodio M/6	0	0	0	167	0	0	167	0	0	0	0
Mannitolo 20%**	0	0	0	0	0	0	0	0	0	0	0
Sangue	0	3	0	95	4	50	40	0	2	1-2	0
Soluzione Ringer lattato	0-5-10	0	0-20	130	4	109	28	3	0	0	261-531-801
			0-40	0	0	0	0	0	0	0	0
			0	0	0	0	0	0	0	0	0
Talbot (c)	5	0	200	40	35	40	20	0	15	0	409

ADDITIVI DISPONIBILI	
Acetato di potassio	2 e 4 mEq/mL
Acetato di sodio	2 e 4 mEq/mL
Bicarbonato di sodio	0,5 (4,2%) mEq/mL e 0,9 (7,5%) mEq/mL
Calcio gluconato 10%	9,3 mg (0,465 mEq/mL) calcio elementare
Cloruro di ammonio	5 mEq/mL
Cloruro di calcio 10%	27,3 mg (1,4 mEq/mL) calcio elementare
Cloruro di potassio	2 e 3 mEq/mL
Cloruro di sodio	2,5 e 5 mEq/mL
Fosfato di potassio	4,4 mEq/mL di potassio e 3 mM/mL di fosfato
Glucosio 50%	0,5 g/mL
Lattato di sodio	5 mEq/mL
Magnesio solfato	0,8 mEq/mL, 1 mEq/mL e 4 mEq/mL disponibile in soluzioni al 10%, 12,5% e 50%

PREPARAZIONI COMMERCIALI SELEZIONATE NEGLI STATI UNITI (SONO POSSIBILI PICCOLE VARIAZIONI NELLA COMPOSIZIONE RISPETTO AI VALORI NELLA TABELLA)	
(a)	Ionosol MB® in D_5W, Isolyte P con destrosio 5%
(b)	Ionosol B® in D_5W, Electrolyte #2® con zucchero invertito 10%, 10% Travert in electrolyte #2®
(c)	Ionosol T® in D_5W, Isolyte M®
(d)	Plasmatein®, Plasmanate®
(e) (f)	LMD® 10%, destrano 40, Rheomacrodex®, Gentran 40®
(g) (h)	Destrano 70, Macrodex®, Gentran® 75 in 10% Travert®

*Proteina o aminoacido equivalente.
†Bicarbonato reale o potenziale, come acetato, lattato o citrato.
‡Calcolato secondo una valenza di 1,8.
§Osmolalità, tranne per i valori mostrati (‖), che sono osmolarità (in mOsm/L).
¶La composizione varia leggermente, a seconda della fonte.
#Contenuto di globuli rossi non incluso nei calcoli.
**Disponibile anche: mannitolo 5%, 10%, 15% e 20%.
††Glucosio (destrosio, fruttosio o zucchero invertito).

Fonti: Pennington JAT (editor): *Bowes & Church's Food Values of Portions Commonly Used*, 17ª ed. Philadelphia, Lippincott Williams & Wilkins, 1997; Olin BR (editor): *Facts e Comparisons*. Philadelphia, JB Lippincott, 1993; Murray BN, Peterson LJ: Unpublished observations. Additional values in Wendland BE, Arbus GS: Oral fluid therapy: Sodium e potassium content e osmolality of some commercial soups, juices e beverages. *Can Med Assoc* J 1979;121:564.

TABELLA 715-8. Metodo per la conversione da milligrammi in milliequivalenti litro (o in millimoli litro)

mg = milligrammi mL = millilitro

g = grammi 1 mL = 1,000027 cc

dL = decilitro = 100 mL

$$\text{mEq/L (milliequivalenti litro)} = \frac{\text{mg/L}}{\text{Peso equivalente}}$$

$$\text{Peso equivalente} = \frac{\text{Peso atomico}}{\text{Valenza dell'elemento}}$$

Esempio: Un campione di sangue contiene 10 mg di Ca in 1 dL (100 mL).
La valenza del Ca è 2 e il peso atomico è 40. Il peso equivalente del Ca è perciò 40 ÷ 2, o 20.
I milliequivalenti di Ca per litro sono 10 (mg/dL) × 10 (dL/L) ÷ 20, o 5 milliequivalenti per litro.

$$\text{mmol/L (millimoli litro)} = \frac{\text{mg/L}}{\text{Peso molecolare}}$$

TABELLA 715-9. Fattori di conversione delle concentrazioni espresse in milliequivalenti litro a milligrammi decilitro (100 mL) e viceversa, per i comuni ioni che sono presenti nelle soluzioni fisiologiche

ELEMENTO O RADICALE		da mEq/L a mg/dL		da mg/dL a mEq/L
Bicarbonato (HCO_3^-)	1	6,1	1	0,1639
Calcio	1	2,005	1	0,4988
Cloro	1	3,55	1	0,2817
Magnesio	1	1,215	1	0,8230
Potassio	1	3,91	1	0,2558
Sodio	1	2,30	1	0,4348
Valenza del fosforo 1	1	3,10	1	0,3226
Valenza del fosforo 1,8	1	1,72	1	0,5814
Valenza dello Zolfo 2	1	1,60	1	0,625

Esempio: Per convertire i milliequivalenti di magnesio litro in milligrammi decilitro (100 mL), moltiplicare per il fattore 1,215; per convertire i milligrammi di potassio decilitro (100 mL) in milliequivalenti litro, moltiplicare per il fattore 0,2558.

TABELLA 715-10. Milliequivalenti e milligrammi di cationi e anioni presenti in 1 millimole di sali comunemente usati nelle soluzioni fisiologiche

SALE	SALE (mg/mmol)	CATIONE	SALE (mEq/mmol)	SALE (mg/mmol)	ANIONE	SALE (mEq/mmol)	SALE (mg/mmol)
Bicarbonato di sodio ($NaHCO_3$)	84,0	Na^+	1	23,0	HCO_3^-	1	61,0
Cloruro di ammonio (NH_4Cl)	53,5	NH^{4+}	1	18,0	Cl^-	1	35,5
Cloruro di calcio, anidroso ($CaCl_2$)	111,0	Ca^{2+}	2	40,0	Cl_2^{2-}	2	71,0
Cloruro di calcio diidrato ($CaCl_2{\cdot}2H_2O$)	147,0	Ca^{2+}	2	40,0	Cl_2^{2-}	2	71,0
Cloruro di magnesio, anidroso ($MgCl_2$)	95,2	Mg^{2+}	2	24,3	Cl_2^{2-}	2	71,0
Cloruro di magnesio esaidrato ($MgCl_2{\cdot}6H_2O$)	203,3	Mg^{2+}	2	24,3	Cl_2^{2-}	2	71,0
Cloruro di potassio (KCl)	74,6	K^+	1	39,1	Cl^-	1	35,5
Cloruro di sodio (NaCl)	58,5	Na^+	1	23,0	Cl^-	1	35,5
Fosfato di potassio monobasico (K_2HPO_4)	174,2	K^+	1	78,2	HPO_4^{2-}	2	96,0
Fosfato di potassio dibasico (KH_2PO_4)	136,1	K^+	1	39,1	$H_2PO_4^-$	1	97,0
Lattato di sodio ($CH_3CHOHCOONa$)	112,0	Na^+	1	23,0	$CH_3CHOHCOO^-$	1	89,0

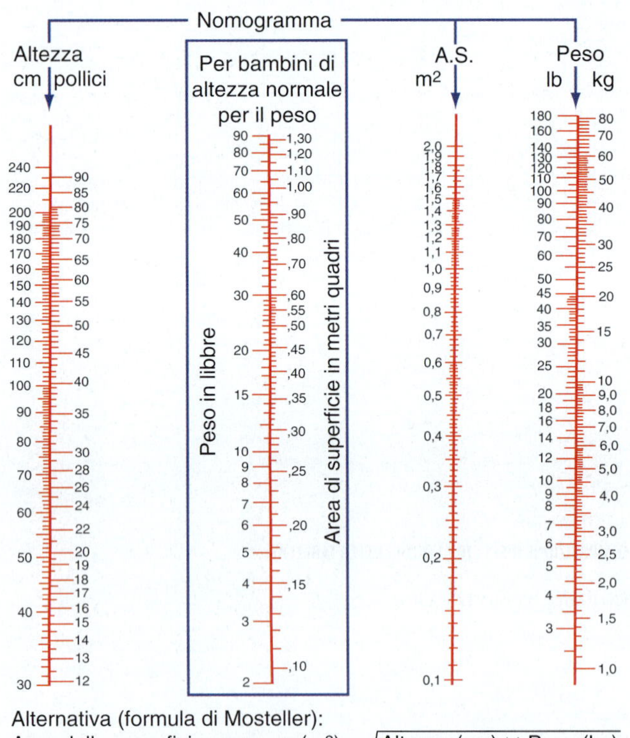

Alternativa (formula di Mosteller):

$$\text{Area della superficie corporea (m}^2\text{)} = \sqrt{\frac{\text{Altezza (cm)} \times \text{Peso (kg)}}{3600}}$$

Figura 715-1. Nomogramma per la valutazione della superficie corporea. L'area della superficie corporea è individuata nel punto in cui una linea retta che collega il livello del peso e quello dell'altezza interseca la colonna dell'area della superficie corporea, oppure se il paziente è approssimativamente di taglia media, dal peso da solo (*zona racchiusa nella cornice blu*). (Nomogramma modificato dai dati di E. Boyd da C. D. West. Vedi anche Briars GL, Bailey BJ: Surface area estimation: pocket calculator v nomogram. *Arch Dis Child* 1994;70:246-247.)

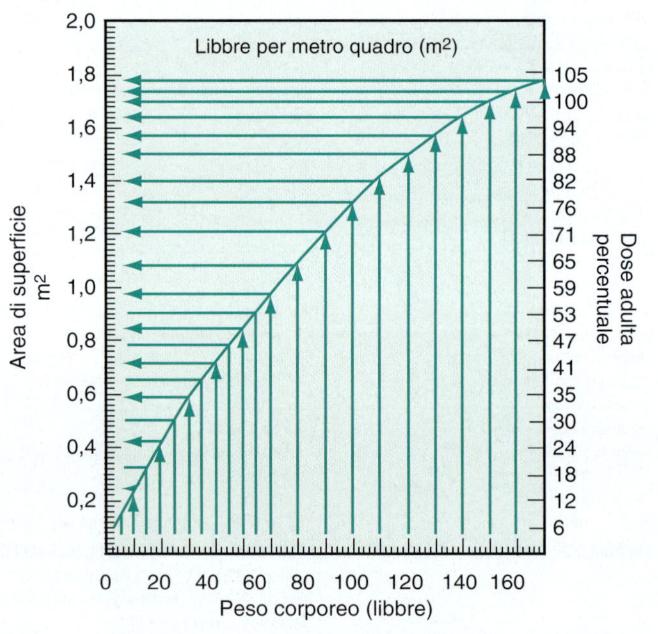

Figura 715-2. Relazioni tra peso corporeo (lb), superficie corporea e dosaggio nell'adulto. I valori della superficie corporea corrispondono a quelli indicati da Crawford JD, Terry ME, Rourke GM: Simplification of drug dosage calculation by application of the surface area principle. *Pediatrics* 1950;5:783-790. Si noti che il 100% della dose adulta è per un paziente che pesa approssimativamente 140 lb e che ha una superficie corporea di circa 1,7 m². (Tratta da Talbot NB, Richie RH, Crawford JH: *Metabolic Homeostasis: A Syllabus for Those Concerned with the Care of Patients*. Cambridge, Harvard University Press, 1959.)

TABELLA 715-11. Composizione del cibo per il metodo breve di analisi della dieta (Lewis A. Barness e John S. Curran)*

CIBO E PORZIONE APPROSSIMATIVA	PESO (g)	ENERGIA DEL CIBO (kcal)	PROTEINE (g)	GRASSI (g)	CARBOIDRATI (g)	CALCIO (mg)	FERRO (mg)	VITAMINA A (UI)	TIAMINA (mg)	RIBOFLAVINA (mg)	NIACINA (mg)	ACIDO ASCORBICO (mg)
LATTE, FORMAGGIO, PANNA; PRODOTTI CORRELATI												
Besciamella, media (1/2 c)	130	215	5	16	12	150	0,2	610	0,06	0,22	0,3	Tracce
Bevande al latte (1 c): cacao, bevanda al cioccolato prodotta con latte scremato; per latte al malto, aggiungere 4 cucchiai da cucina metà e metà (270 g)	245	210	8	8	26	280	0,6	300	0,09	0,43	0,3	Tracce
Dolci al latte, crema pasticcera (1 c), 248 g, gelato (240 mL circa), 142 g		290	8	17	29	210	0,4	785	0,07	0,34	0,1	1
Formaggio: tipo gorgonzola, cheddar, 17 g, cheddar process (30 g);	30	105	6	9	1	165	0,2	345	0,01	0,12	Tracce	0
cottage svizzero (30 g) (fiocchi di latte) con panna (1/2 c)	115	120	16	5	3	105	0,4	190	0,04	0,28	0,1	0
Latte: intero (3,5% di grassi) [1 c] liquido;	245	160	9	9	12	285	0,1	350	0,08	0,42	0,1	2
non grasso (scremato) e latticini (da latte cagliato)	245	90	9	Tracce	13	300	Tracce	0	0,10	0,44	0,2	2
Panna: metà e metà (panna e latte) [2 cucchiai da cucina]; per montatura leggera, aggiungere 1 panetto di burro	30	40	1	4	2	30	Tracce	145	0,01	0,04	Tracce	Tracce
Pudding all'amido di granoturco (248 g), gelato al latte (1 c) 187 g		280	9	10	40	290	0,1	390	0,08	0,41	0,3	2
Uovo: 1 grosso	50	80	6	6	Tracce	25	1,2	590	0,06	0,15	Tracce	0
CARNE, POLLAME, PESCE, CROSTACEI, PRODOTTI CORRELATI												
Bastoncini di pesce, impanati, cotti (3-4)	75	130	13	7	5	10	0,3	0	0,03	0,05	1,2	0
Carni a pranzo: mortadella (2 fette), salsiccia di maiale, cotto (60 g), würstel (1), pancetta, alla griglia o fritta croccante (3 fette)		185	9	16	0	5	1,3	0	0,21	0,12	1,7	0
Fegato: manzo, fritto (60 g)	55	130	15	6	3	5	5,0	30 280	0,15	2,37	9,4	15
Maiale: magro e grasso, cotto (90 g) [tutti i tagli]	85	325	20	24	0	10	2,6	0	0,62	0,20	4,2	
Solo magro, cotto (più di 60 g) [tutti i tagli]	60	150	18	8	0	5	2,2	0	0,57	0,19	3,2	
prosciutto, poco affumicato, magro e grasso, arrosto (90 g)	85	245	18	19	0	10	2,2	0	0,40	0,16	3,1	
Manzo, agnello, vitello: magro e grasso, cotto, incluso manzo salato (circa 90 g) [tutti i tagli]	85	245	22	16	0	10	2,9	25	0,06	0,19	4,2	0
solo magro, cotto; carne secca (più di 60 g) [tutti i tagli]	65	140	20	5	0	10	2,4	10	0,05	0,16	3,4	0
Manzo, relativamente grasso, come bistecca e costina, cotto (60 g)	85	350	18	30	0	10	2,4	60	0,05	0,14	3,5	0
Molluschi, in scatola; polpa di granchio, in scatola; aragosta; ostrica, cruda; capasanta; gamberetto, in scatola	85	75	14	1	2	65	2,5	65	0,10	0,08	1,5	0
Pesce azzurro, merluzzo, aringhe, pesce persico, alosa, cotti (tonno in scatola all'olio, 20 g)	85	160	19	8	2	20	1,0	60	0,06	0,11	4,4	0
Pollo: solo la carne, alla griglia (90 g);	85	115	20	3	0	10	1,4	80	0,05	0,16	7,4	0
fritto (più di 60 g)	75	170	24	6	1	10	1,6	85	0,05	0,23	8,3	0
Salmone, in scatola (90 g)	85	130	17	5	0	165	0,7	60	0,03	0,16	6,8	0
Sgombro, halibut, cotti	85	175	19	10	0	10	0,8	515	0,08	0,15	6,8	0
Tacchino, chiaro e scuro, arrosto (90 g)	85	160	27	5	0	0	1,5	0	0,03	0,15	6,5	0
FAGIOLI E PISELLI SECCHI MATURI, NOCI, ARACHIDI, PRODOTTI CORRELATI												
Fagioli: bianchi con maiale e pomodoro, in scatola (1 c)	260	320	16	7	50	140	4,7	340	0,20	0,08	1,5	5
Rossi (128 g), fagioli di Lima (96 g), fagioli dall'occhio (125 g), cotti (1/2 c)		125	8	0	25	35	2,5	5	0,13	0,06	0,7	0
Noci: mandorle (12), anacardi (8), arachidi (1 cucchiaio da cucina), burro d'arachidi (1 cucchiaio da cucina), noci americane (12), noci inglesi (2 cucchiai da cucina), noci di cocco (1/4 c)	15	95	3	8	4	15	0,5	5	0,05	0,9	0	
VEGETALI E PRODOTTI VEGETALI												
Asparago, cotto, punte tagliate (2/3 c)	115	25	3	Tracce	4	25	0,7	1055	0,19	0,20	1,6	30
Broccoli: cime, cotti (2/3 c)	100	25	3	Tracce	4	90	0,8	2500	0,09	0,20	0,8	90
Cavolini di Bruxelles, cotti (2/3 c)	85	30	3	Tracce	5	30	1,0	450	0,07	0,12	0,7	75
Cavolo (110 g); cavolfiore, cotto (80 g); crauti, in scatola (150 mg) [ridurre il valore di acido ascorbico di 1/3 per i crauti] [2/3 c]		20	1	Tracce	4	35	0,5	80	0,05	0,05	0,3	37
Carote, cotte (2/3 c)	95	30	1	Tracce	7	30	0,6	10 145	0,05	0,05	0,5	6
Fagioli: verdi (1/2 c), cotti, 60 g; in scatola, 120 g;		15	1	Tracce	3	30	0,4	340	0,04	0,06	0,3	8
di Lima, acerbi, cotti (1/2 c)	80	90	6	1	16	40	2,0	225	0,14	0,08	1,0	14
Grano, 1 spiga, cotta (140 g); in scatola (130 g) [1/2 c]		75	2	Tracce	18	5	0,4	315	0,06	0,06	1,1	6
Ketchup (2 cucchiai)	35	30	1	Tracce	8	10	0,2	480	0,04	0,02	0,6	6

TABELLA 715-11. Composizione del cibo per il metodo breve di analisi della dieta (Lewis A. Barness e John S. Curran)* – *continua*

CIBO E PORZIONE APPROSSIMATIVA	PESO (g)	ENERGIA DEL CIBO (kcal)	PROTEINE (g)	GRASSI (g)	CARBOIDRATI (g)	CALCIO (mg)	FERRO (mg)	VITAMINA A (UI)	TIAMINA (mg)	RIBOFLAVINA (mg)	NIACINA (mg)	ACIDO ASCORBICO (mg)
Patate: al forno, bollite (100 g), 10 pezzi;		85	3	Tracce	30	10	0,7	Tracce	0,08	0,04	1,5	16
dolci, in scatola (1/2 c);	110	120	2	0	27	25	0,8	8500	0,05	0,05	0,7	15
fritte (55 g) [per la frittura, aggiungi 1 cucchiaio di olio da cucina]												
Piselli, verdi (1/2 c)	80	60	4	1	10	20	1,4	430	0,22	0,09	1,8	16
Pomodoro, 1 fresco, 2/3 c in scatola, 2/3 c succo	150	35	2	Tracce	7	14	0,8	1350	0,10	0,06	1,0	29
Zucca, in scatola (1/2 c)	115	40	1	1	9	30	0,5	7295	0,03	0,06	0,6	6
Zucca, inverno, in scatola (1/2 c)	100	65	2	1	16	30	0,8	4305	0,05	0,14	0,7	14
Altro, comunemente consumato crudo: cavolo		10	Tracce	Tracce	2	15	0,3	100	0,03	0,03	0,2	20
(1/2 c, 50 g), sedano (3 gambi piccoli, 40 g),	25	10	Tracce	Tracce	2	10	0,2	2750	0,02	0,02	0,2	2
cocomero (1/4, 30 g), ravanelli (5, 40 g) (di media grandezza, 50 g), carote al pepe verde (1/2), 1/2 carota cruda, foglie di lattuga (2 grosse)	50	10	1	Tracce	2	34	0,7	950	0,03	0,04	0,2	9
Altro, cotto (barbabietole, funghi, cipolle, rape) [1/2 c]	95	25	1	0	5	20	0,5	15	0,02	0,10	0,7	7
FRUTTA E PRODOTTI DELLA FRUTTA												
Agrumi e fragole: arancia (1), pompelmo (1/2, 1/2 c di succo), fragole (1/2 c), limone (1), mandarino (1)		50	1	0	13	25	0,4	165	0,08	0,03	0,3	55
Gialla, fresca: albicocche (3), pesca (2 medie); frutta e succo in scatola (1/2 c) oppure secca, cotta, non zuccherata: albicocca, pesche (1/2 c)		85	0	0	22	10	1,1	1,005	0,01	0,05	1,0	5
Melone (1/2 medio)	385	60	1	Tracce	14	25	0,8	6540	0,08	0,06	1,2	63
Altro, mela fresca (1), banana (1), fichi (3), pera (1)		80	0	0	21	15	0,5	140	0,04	0,03	0,2	6
Altro, secca: datteri, frutta con nocciolo (4), fichi (2), uva passa (1/4 c)	40	120	1	0	31	35	1,4	20	0,04	0,04	0,5	0
PRODOTTI DEL GRANO												
Biscotti, normali (1)	25	120	1	5	18	10	0,2	20	0,01	0,01	0,01	0
Crostata, crostata senza copertura di pastafrolla (1/7 del totale)	20	95	1	6	8	3	0,3	0	0,04	0,03	0,3	0
Farina, bianca e arricchita (1 cucchiaio)	7	25	1	Tracce	5	1	0,2	0	0,03	0,02	0,2	0
Grano intero e arricchito: pane (1 fetta, 23 g), biscotti (1/2), cereali cotti (1/2 c), cereali preparati (30 g), cracker Graham (2 grossi), maccheroni, tagliatelle, spaghetti (1/2 c, cotti), frittella (1, 27 g), panino (1/2), cialda (1/2, 38 g)		65	2	1	16	20	0,6	10	0,09	0,05	0,7	0
Pane non arricchito (1 fetta, 23 g), cereali cotti (1/2 c), maccheroni, tagliatelle, spaghetti (1/2 c), pop-corn (1/2 c), pretzel, pretzel piccoli (15), panino (1/2)		65	2	1	16	10	0,3	5	0,02	0,02	0,3	0
Torta, liscia (1 pezzo), ciambella (1); per torta gelato o ciambella, aggiungere le calorie per lo zucchero (1 cucchiaio); per la torta al cioccolato, aggiungere il cioccolato (30 g)	45	145	2	5	24	30	0,4	65	0,02	0,05	0,2	0
GRASSI E OLI												
Burro, margarina (1 panetto, 1/2 cucchiaio)	7	50	Tracce	6	Tracce	1	0	230	0	0	0	0
Condimento per insalata, tipo maionese (1 cucchiaio)	15	80	Tracce	9	1	2	0,1	45	Tracce	Tracce	Tracce	0
Grassi e oli, cucinati (1 cucchiaio), vinaigrette (2 cucchiai)	14	125	0	14	0	0	0	0	0	0	0	0
ZUCCHERO, DOLCI												
Caramella, normale (15 g), marmellata e gelatina (1 cucchiaio), sciroppo (1 cucchiaio), dessert alla gelatina, normale (1/2 c), bevande, gassate (1 c)		60	0	0	14	3	0,1	Tracce	Tracce	Tracce	Tracce	Tracce
Cioccolato fondente (30 g), sciroppo di cioccolato (3 cucchiai)		125	1	2	30	15	0,6	10	Tracce	0,02	0,1	Tracce
Melassa (1 cucchiaio), caramello (15 g)		40	Tracce	Tracce	8	20	0,3	Tracce	Tracce	Tracce	Tracce	Tracce
Zucchero (1 cucchiaio)	12	45	0	0	12	0	Tracce	0	0	0	0	0
VARIE												
Cioccolato, amaro (30 g)	30	145	3	15	8	20	1,9	20	0,01	0,07	0,4	0
Sorbetto (1/2 c)	96	130	1	1	30	15	Tracce	55	0,01	0,03	Tracce	2
ZUPPE												
Fagioli, piselli (verdi) [1 c]		150	7	4	22	50	1,6	495	0,09	0,06	1,0	4
Noodle, manzo, pollo (1 c)		65	4	2	7	10	0,7	50	0,03	0,04	0,9	Tracce
Zuppa di mare, minestrone, pomodoro, verdure (1 c)		90	3	2	14	25	0,9	1880	0,05	0,04	1,1	3

C = tazza (*Cup*) = 110 g circa.
*Vedi le relative tabelle di conversione (Tabb. da 715-8 a 715-10).
Tratta da Wilson ED, Fisher KH, Fuqua ME: *Principles of Nutrition*, 2ª ed. New York, John Wiley & Sons, 1965, pp. 528-533.

TABELLA 715-12. Valori nutritivi dei cibi per bambini (per porzione)*

CIBO	PORZIONE (g)	ENERGIA (kcal)	PROTEINE (g)	GRASSI (g)	CARBOIDRATI (g)	SODIO (mg)	CALCIO (mg)	FERRO (mg)	VITAMINA A (UI)	TIAMINA (mg)	RIBOFLAVINA (mg)	NIACINA (mg)	ACIDO ASCORBICO (mg)
CARNI, POLLAME													
Agnello	99	111	15,0	5,2	2,5	73	7	1,6	30	0,02	0,20	3,2	2
Manzo	99	105	14,3	4,9	0	65	8	1,6	100	0,01	0,16	3,3	2
Pollo	99	148	14,6	9,5	0	50	54	1,0	200	0,01	0,16	3,4	2
Prosciutto	99	123	14,9	6,6	0	66	5	1,0	30	0,14	0,19	2,8	2
Tacchino	99	128	15,2	7,0	0	72	28	1,3	600	0,02	0,25	3,4	2
CEREALI													
Farina d'avena	2,4	10	0,3	0,2	1,7	1	18	1,8		0,07	0,06	0,9	0
Misti	2,4	9	0,3	0,1	1,8	1	18	1,5		0,06	0,07	0,8	0
Orzo	2,4	9	0,3	0,1	1,8	1	19	1,1		0,07	0,07	0,9	0
Proteine nobili	2,4	9	0,9	0,1	1,1	1	17	1,8		0,06	0,07	0,8	0
Riso	2,4	9	0,2	0,1	1,9	1	20	1,8		0,06	0,05	0,8	0
FRUTTA													
Banane, tapioca (vasetto)	220	147	0,8	0,4	39,1	21	17	0,7	100	0,03	0,04	0,5	57
Composta di mele (vasetto)	213	79	0,1	0,0	21,9	5	10	0,4	20	0,03	0,06	0,1	81
Composta di mele, albicocche (vasetto)	220	104	0,5	0,5	27,3	6	13	0,6	745	0,03	0,07	0,3	39
Pere	213	93	0,6	0,2	24,7	4	18	0,5	70	0,03	0,06	0,4	47
Pesche	220	157	1,3	0,4	41,6	10	11	0,6	400	0,03	0,07	1,4	42
PASTI, VASETTO													
Maccheroni e prosciutto	213	127	6,8	2,9	18,0	101	159	0,8	1100	0,12	0,21	1,7	5
Manzo e tagliatelle all'uovo	213	122	5,4	4,0	15,7	37	18	0,9	1400	0,06	0,08	1,2	3
Pollo e tagliatelle	213	109	4,1	3,0	16,1	36	36	0,8	1900	0,06	0,07	1,1	3
Spaghetti, pomodoro, manzo	213	135	5,4	2,7	21,6	42	39	1,1	1500	0,14	0,15	2,3	5
Tacchino e riso	213	104	3,8	2,9	15,3	33	50	0,6	2200	0,02	0,06	0,6	3
TUORLI D'UOVO	94	191	9,4	16,3	0,9	37	72	2,6	1200	0,07	0,25	1,45	1
VERDURE													
Barbabietole	128	43	1,7	0,1	9,8	106	18	0,4	40	0,01	0,06	0,2	4
Carote	213	67	1,7	0,4	15,4	104	49	0,8	25 000	0,05	0,09	1,1	12
Fagioli	206	51	2,5	0,3	11,8	3	133	2,2	900	0,04	0,21	0,7	17
Miste	213	88	3,1	0,8	17,4	77	24	0,9	9000	0,06	0,07	1,4	5
Patate dolci	220	113	2,4	0,3	30,7	49	35	0,8	15 000	0,06	0,08	0,8	21
Piselli	213	113	7,0	1,1	19,0	15	34	1,9	700	0,15	0,13	2,0	9
Zucca	213	51	1,8	0,4	12,0	3	50	0,7	4000	0,02	0,14	0,8	17

* Vedi le relative tabelle di conversione da 715-8 a 715-10. Tratta da Pennington JAT (editor): *Bowes e Church's Food Values of Portions Commonly Used*, 17th ed. Philadelphia, Lippincott Williams & Wilkins, 1997.

TABELLA 715-13. Valori equivalenti della temperatura (Celsius [C] e Fahrenheit [F])

C	F	C	F	C	F	C	F
0	32,0	37,2	99,0	39,2	102,6	41,2	106,2
20	68,0	37,4	99,3	39,4	102,9	41,4	106,5
30	86,0	37,6	99,7	39,6	103,3	41,6	106,9
31	87,8	37,8	100,1	39,8	103,7	41,8	107,2
32	89,6	38,0	100,4	40,0	104,0	42,0	107,6
33	91,7	38,2	100,8	40,2	104,4	43,0	109,4
34	93,2	38,4	101,2	40,4	104,7	44,0	111,2
35	95,0	38,6	101,5	40,6	105,1	100,0	212,0
36	96,8	38,8	101,8	40,8	105,4		
37	98,6	39,0	102,2	41,0	105,8		

*Per convertire i gradi Celsius (centigradi) in Fahrenheit, moltiplicare per 1,8 e aggiungere 32. Per convertire i gradi Fahrenheit in Celsius, sottrarre 32 e dividere per 1,8.

Capitolo 716 ■ Farmaci

Peter Gal e Michael D. Reed

TABELLA 716-1. Farmaci generali

FARMACO (PRINCIPIO ATTIVO, FORMULAZIONI)	INDICAZIONI (MECCANISMO D'AZIONE E DOSAGGIO)	COMMENTI (CAUTELE, EFFETTI INDESIDERATI, MONITORAGGIO)
Abciximab Soluzione endovenosa: 2 mg/mL in fiale da 5 mL.	**Inibisce l'aggregazione piastrinica attraverso l'inibizione della via del recettore della glicoproteina IIb/IIIa. Usato in associazione a immunoglobuline ev e acido acetilsalicilico per accelerare la regressione degli aneurismi coronarici nella malattia di Kawasaki. Negli adulti, usato per prevenire l'aggregazione piastrinica in varie procedure e nelle sindromi coronariche acute.** *Bambini e adulti:* dose da carico di 0,25 mg/kg, seguita da infusione di 0,125 µg/kg/min per 12 h.	*Effetti indesiderati:* sanguinamento.
Acarbosio Compresse: 25, 50, 100 mg.	**Trattamento del diabete mellito di tipo 2; trattamento dell'ipoglicemia postprandiale in bambini dopo fundoplicatio di Nissen.** *Bambini:* 12,5-50 mg a ogni pasto. *Adulti:* dose iniziale di 25 mg tid all'inizio di ogni pasto; titolare alla risposta (massimo: 100 mg tid).	*Effetti indesiderati:* flatulenza, dolore addominale, diarrea.
Acetato di alluminio Prodotto cutaneo topico. Polvere, per preparare la soluzione topica: 2 bustine/litro d'acqua = 1:40 soluzione. Soluzione, auricolare: acetato di alluminio 1:10 con acido acetico 2% (60 mL). Compresse: 2 compresse/L = diluizione 1:40.	**Preparazione umida astringente per la cura degli stati infiammatori della cute; profilassi dell'orecchio del nuotatore.** *Bambini e adulti:* Auricolare: instillare 4-6 gocce ogni 2-3 h inizialmente, poi ogni 4-6 h fino alla risoluzione del prurito o dell'arrossamento. Topico: impregnare l'area con soluzione per 15-30 min 2-4 volte al giorno.	*Effetti indesiderati:* irritazione locale.
Acetazolamide Diuretico, inibitore dell'anidrasi carbonica. Capsule, rilascio prolungato: 500 mg. Iniezione: 500 mg/5 mL. Compresse: 125, 250 mg.	**Idrocefalo dovuto a emorragia intraventricolare comunicante.** *Neonati:* 25 mg/kg/24 h per iniziare, e incrementare a bid, tid e qid nel giro di 4-7 giorni. **Glaucoma** (l'inibizione dell'anidrasi carbonica riduce la formazione di umore acqueo). *Bambini:* 8-30 mg/kg/24 h per os suddivisi ogni 6-8 h o 20-40 mg/kg/24 h ev suddivisi ogni 6 h. **Epilessia, in aggiunta ad altri farmaci nelle crisi refrattarie** (meccanismo non certo). *Bambini e adulti:* 8-30 mg/kg/24 h suddivisi in 1-4 dosi (massimo: 1 g/24 h). **Edema** (diuretico). *Bambini:* 5 mg/kg/24 h ev o per os. *Adulti:* 250-375 mg/24 h ev o per os.	*Cautela:* usato in combinazione con furosemide per idrocefalo. (l'inibizione dell'anidrasi carbonica riduce la produzione di liquido cerebrospinale). Ridurre la dose ed allungare l'intervallo di dosaggio se la funzionalità renale è compromessa. Evitare se il paziente è allergico allo zolfo. Somministrazione im molto dolorosa a causa del pH alcalino del farmaco. *Effetti indesiderati:* acidosi metabolica, ipocloremia, ipopotassiemia, nausea, anoressia, sonnolenza, affaticamento, debolezza muscolare, calcoli renali.
Acetilcisteina Antidoto, paracetamolo; agente mucolitico. Soluzione, con sodio: 10% (100 mg/mL) (4, 10, 30 mL); 20% (200 mg/mL) (4, 10, 30, 100 mL).	**Mucolitico** (il gruppo sulfidrilico libero apre i legami disulfidi nelle mucoproteine, riducendo la viscosità). Dose basata su 10% di soluzione o soluzione diluita al 20% (1:1) per inalazione. *Bambini piccoli:* 2-4 mL tid-qid. *Bambini grandi:* 6-10 mL tid-qid. *Adolescenti:* 10 mL tid-qid. Overdose acuta da paracetamolo (fornisce una via metabolica alternativa per la coniugazione dei metaboliti tossici, ripristinando i normali livelli di glutatione). *Bambini e adulti:* dose da carico di 140 mg/kg, seguita da 70 mg/kg ogni 4 h per 17 dosi. Ripetere la dose se si verifica emesi entro 1 ora dalla somministrazione.	*Cautela:* somministrare un broncodilatore 10-15 min prima del Mucomyst nebulizzato per evitare il broncospasmo. Seguire il trattamento con percussione toracica e aspirazione per il trattamento delle secrezioni aumentate. Diluire le dosi nebulizzate con acqua salina o sterile e soluzioni orali con bevande leggere o succo d'arancia. Preparare inalato come 1:1 e per os come soluzioni 1:3. *Effetti indesiderati:* stomatite nausea, vomito, orticaria. *Monitoraggio:* controllare la concentrazione di paracetamolo non prima di 4 h dopo l'overdose. Somministrare un ciclo completo di acetilcisteina, senza considerare le concentrazioni di paracetamolo.
Acido acetilsalicilico Analgesico, non-narcotico; agente anti-infiammatorio; agente antipiastrinico, antipiretico; agente anti-infiammatorio non steroideo, orale; salicilato. Supposta, rettale: 60, 120, 125, 130, 195, 200, 300, 325, 600, 650, 1200 mg. Compresse: 325, 500, 650 mg Compresse, tamponate: 325 mg con idrossido di alluminio 75 mg e idrossido di magnesio 75 mg; 325 mg con idrossido di alluminio 150 mg e idrossido di magnesio 150 mg; 500 mg con idrossido di alluminio 33 mg e idrossido di magnesio 150 mg. Masticabili: 75, 81 mg. Chewing gum: 227 mg. Compresse a rilascio controllato: 800 mg. Compresse gastroprotette (a rilascio ritardato): 80, 165, 325, 500, 650, 975 mg. Compresse a rilascio prolungato: 650 mg. Compresse, con caffeina: 400 mg e caffeina 32 mg; 500 mg e caffeina 32 mg.	**Dolore, infiammazione, febbre (inibizione della sintesi delle prostaglandine).** *Bambini:* 10-15 mg/kg/dose ogni 4-6 h. *Adulti:* 650-1000 mg/dose ogni 4-6 h (massimo: 4 g/24 h). **Malattia di Kawasaki (fase acuta).** *Bambini:* 80-100 mg/kg/24 h suddivisi ogni 6 h. ulcere gastriche, broncospasmo negli asmatici, perdita dell'udito, tinnito. **Febbre reumatica.** 60-100 mg/kg/24 h suddivisi ogni 6 h.	*Cautela:* controindicato nei bambini <16 anni con varicella o sintomi simil-influenzali per il rischio di sindrome di Reye. Sospendere se si verifica perdita dell'udito o tinnito. *Effetti indesiderati:* sanguinamento gengivale o del tratto gastrointestinale, *Monitoraggio:* controllare la concentrazione sierica 2 h dopo una dose per la malattia di Kawasaki (target 150-300 µg/mL) o per la febbre reumatica (target 250-400 µg/mL).

TABELLA 716-1. Farmaci generali – *continua*

FARMACO (PRINCIPIO ATTIVO, FORMULAZIONI)	INDICAZIONI (MECCANISMO D'AZIONE E DOSAGGIO)	COMMENTI (CAUTELE, EFFETTI INDESIDERATI, MONITORAGGIO)
Acido aminocaproico Agente emostatico. Iniezione: 250 mg/mL (20, 96, 100 mL). Sciroppo (gusto al lampone): 250 (480 mL). Compresse: 500 mg.	**Trattamento del sanguinamento eccessivo causato da iperfibrinolisi sistemica (inibisce l'attivazione del plasminogeno).** *Bambini:* per os, ev: dose da carico di 100-200 mg/kg, dose di mantenimento di 100 mg/kg ogni 6 h o 33,3 mg/kg/h infusione continua. Ifema traumatico: 100 mg/kg ogni 4 h (massimo: 30 g/24 h). *Adulti:* dose da carico di 5 g per 1 ora, poi 1-1,25 g/h fino all'arresto del sanguinamento (massimo: 30 g/24 h).	*Cautela:* evitare la coagulazione intravascolare disseminata e l'ematuria delle vie urinarie superiori. Contiene benzil alcol, quindi evitare nei neonati <1500 g. *Effetti indesiderati:* ipotensione, bradicardia, aritmie, vertigini, cefalea, congestione nasale. *Monitoraggio:* D-dimero o prodotti della degradazione della fibrina, tempo di coagulazione attivato (target 180-200 s), potassio sierico (specialmente in caso di ridotta funzione renale).
Acido ascorbico Supplemento nutrizionale; agente acidificante le urine; vitamina, idrosolubile. Capsule, a rilascio prolungato; 500 mg. Cristalli: 4 g/cucchiaio (1000 g). Iniezione: 25 mg/mL (2, 30 mL), 500 mg/mL (1, 2, 50 mL). Pastiglie: 60 mg. Polvere: 4 g/cucchiaio (1000 g). Soluzione, orale: 35 mg/0,6 mL (50 mL), 100 mg/mL (50 mL). Sciroppo: 500 mg/5 mL (5, 10, 120, 480 mL). Compresse: 25, 50, 100, 250, 500, 1000 mg. Compresse, masticabili: 100, 250, 500, 1000 mg. Compresse, a rilascio prolungato: 500, 1000, 500 mg.	**Scorbuto.** *Bambini:* 100-300 mg/24 h. *Adulti:* 100-250 mg bid. **Acidificazione urinaria.** *Bambini:* 500 mg ogni 6 h. *Adulti:* 4-12 g/24 h suddivisi in 3-4 dosi.	*Effetti indesiderati:* gastrite, calcoli renali.
Acido etacrinico Compresse: 25, 50 mg. Iniezione.	**Diuretico (agisce a livello del tratto ascendente dell'ansa di Henle).** *Bambini:* per os: 1-3 mg/kg/24 h. ev: 0,5-1 mg/kg/dose ogni 8-24 h. *Adulti:* per os: 25-400 mg/24 h. ev: 0,5-1 mg/kg/dose ogni 8-24 h.	*Effetti indesiderati:* ipotensione, deplezione di fluidi e deplezione di elettroliti, iperuricemia, ototossicità, tinnito.
Acido folico Iniezione. Compresse: 0,4, 0,8, 1 mg. Possono essere preparate formulazioni estemporanee.	**Trattamento dell'anemia da deficit di folati (cioè, megaloblastica, macrocitica) (cofattore per normale eritropoiesi).** *Neonati-6 mesi:* per os: 25-35 μg/24 h. *6 mesi-3 anni:* 50 μg/24 h. *4-6 anni:* 75 μg/24 h. *7-10 anni:* 100 μg/24 h. *11-14 anni:* 150 μg/24 h. *>15 anni e adulti:* 200 μg/24 h. Deficit di folati: 1 mg/24 h.	*Cautela:* dosi massive di folati possono mascherare gli effetti ematologici del deficit di vitamina B_{12} mentre permettono l'insorgenza di conseguenze neurologiche.
Acido tranexamico Iniezione: 100 mg/mL. Compresse: 500 mg.	**Usato nell'emofilia durante e dopo estrazioni dentali per ridurre o prevenire l'emorragia (inibisce in modo competitivo l'attivazione del plasminogeno).** *Bambini e adulti:* ev: 10 mg/kg subito prima dell'intervento chirurgico, poi 25 mg/kg/dose per os tid-qid per 2-8 giorni.	*Effetti indesiderati:* ipotensione, complicazioni tromboemboliche (incluso il SNC), trombocitopenia, nausea, vomito, diarrea. *Commento:* diminuire la dose nell'insufficienza renale (CrCl 50-80 mL/min: somministrare il 50% della dose; CrCl 10-50 mL/min; somministrare il 25% della dose; CrCl <10 mL/min: somministrare il 10% della dose).
Acido valproico e derivati Ccompresse rilascio ritardato, capsule sprinkle: 125, 250, 500 mg. Capsule: 250 mg. Sciroppo: 250 mg/5 mL. Iniezione.	**Trattamento delle convulsioni semplici e complesse generalizzate e parziali (blocca sodio e rallenta i canali T).** *Neonati:* Convulsioni refrattarie: per os: dose da carico di 20 mg/kg, poi 10 mg/kg/dose ogni 12 h. *Bambini e adulti:* Convulsioni: ev o per os. 10-15 mg/kg/24 h in 2-3 dosi; aumentare di 5-10 mg/kg/24 h alla sett fino all'effetto; possono essere necessari fino a 100 mg/kg/giorno in 3-4 dosi suddivise, specialmente se usato con induttori enzimatici concomitanti (per es. fenitoina, carbamazepina).	*Cautela:* sono stati riportati casi di insufficienza epatica fatale, specialmente per pazienti di età <2 anni o che ricevono altri anticonvulsivanti. Se usato nei neonati, monitorare l'ammonemia. *Effetti indesiderati:* sonnolenza, irritabilità, confusione, malessere, cefalea, tremore, sordità neurosensoriale, iperammoniemia, epatotossicità, nausea, vomito, diarrea, pancreatite, trombocitopenia, aumento di appetito, aumento di peso. *Monitoraggio:* concentrazioni di valproato: terapeutiche 50-100 μg/mL; tossiche >150 μg/mL.
Adenosina Agente antiaritmico, miscellanea. Iniezione, senza conservanti: 3 mg/mL (2 mL).	**Trattamento della tachicardia parossistica sopraventricolare** (rallenta il tempo di conduzione attraverso il nodo AV). *Neonati e bambini:* bolo di 0,05 mg/kg ev, poi aumentare le dosi del bolo di 0,05 mg/kg ogni 2 min fino a quando si verifica una risposta clinica o viene raggiunta la dose massima di 0,25 mg/kg o di 12 mg. *Adulti:* bolo di 6 mg ev; se non c'è risposta, bolo di 12 mg ev. Si può ripetere un bolo di 12 mg ev se necessario.	*Cautela:* usare una sede periferica ev. Può causare broncocostrizione negli asmatici. Le metilxantine (per es. teofillina o caffeina) antagonizzano gli effetti dell'adenosina, per cui sono necessarie dosi più alte di adenosina. Controindicato nel blocco AV di 2° o 3° grado o nella sindrome del seno malato. *Effetti indesiderati:* arresto cardiaco, flushing, palpitazioni al torace, bradicardia, ipotensione, dispnea, cefalea, vertigini, nausea. *Monitoraggio:* ECG continuo, pressione arteriosa, respirazioni.

TABELLA 716-1. Farmaci generali – *continua*

FARMACO (PRINCIPIO ATTIVO, FORMULAZIONI)	INDICAZIONI (MECCANISMO D'AZIONE E DOSAGGIO)	COMMENTI (CAUTELE, EFFETTI INDESIDERATI, MONITORAGGIO)
Adrenalina Iniezione: 0,01, 0,1, 1 mg/mL. Sospensione: 5 mg/mL. Aerosol inalatore a dosaggio controllato, soluzione inalatoria, soluzione oftalmica, soluzione topica.	**Trattamento dell'arresto cardiaco, broncospasmo, reazioni anafilattiche, glaucoma ad angolo aperto (stimola i recettori α, β_1, β_2).** *Neonati:* ev, intratracheale (it): 0,01-0,03 mg/kg (0,1-0,3 mL/kg di 1:10 000 soluzione) ogni 3-5 min. *Bambini piccoli e grandi:* sc: 0,01 mg/kg (0,01 mL/kg/dose di 1:1000 soluzione, o 0,005 mL/kg/dose di sospensione). ev: 0,01 mg/kg (0,1 mL/kg di soluzione 1:10 000) (massimo: 1 mg). it: 0,1 mg/kg/dose (0,1 mL/kg di soluzione 1:1000) (massimo: 0,2 mL/kg). Infusione continua: 0,1-1 μg/kg/min fino alla risposta. Nebulizzazione: 0,25-0,5 mL del 2,25% adrenalina racemica diluita in 3 mL di soluzione fisiologica normale. Oftalmica: instillare 1-2 gocce per occhio 1-2 volte al giorno. *Adulti:* ev: 1-5 mg ogni 3-5 min. it: 1 mg inizialmente (massimo: 12,5 mg/dose). im, sc: 0,1-0,5 mg ogni 10-15 min. Infusione continua: 1-10 μg/min. Oftalmica: Instillare 1-2 gocce per occhio 1-2 volte al giorno.	*Effetti indesiderati:* tachicardia, ipertensione, nervosismo, irritabilità, irritabilità, cefalea, tremore, debolezza, nausea, vomito, ritenzione urinaria acuta.
Albumina, umana Derivato dei prodotti del sangue; espansore del volume plasmatico. Iniezione: 5%. (50 mg/mL) (50, 250, 500, 1000); 25% (250 mg/mL) (10, 20, 50, 100 mL).	**Espansione del volume plasmatico e trattamento dell'ipovolemia** (aumenta la pressione oncotica intravascolare e mobilizza i fluidi dall'interstizio allo spazio intravascolare). *Neonati:* 0,5-1 g/kg/dose (massimo: 1g/kg/24 h). *Bambini piccoli e grandi:* 0,5-1 g/kg/dose (massimo: 6 g/kg/24 h). *Adulti:* 25 g/dose (massimo: 250 g/24 h).	*Cautela:* l'albumina al 25% può aumentare il rischio di emorragia intraventricolare nei neonati pretermine, quindi in questi casi è preferita la forma al 5%. Infondere per almeno 2 h nei neonati. L'infusione può essere per più di 30-60 min per l'ipovolemia. *Effetti indesiderati:* precipitazione dello scompenso cardiaco, edema polmonare, ipertensione, tachicardia dovuta a sovraccarico di volume. Reazioni immuni (per es. febbre, brividi, rash). Aumento della mortalità nei pazienti con malattie critiche. *Monitoraggio:* segni vitali.
Albuterolo Agente agonista adrenergico; agente agonista β_2 adrenergico; Broncodilatatore; simpaticomimetico. Aerosol, orale: 90 μg/spruzzo (200 inalazioni) (17 g). Capsule, microfini, per inalazione, come solfato: 200 μg. Soluzione, inalazione, come solfato: 0,083% Sciroppo, come solfato (gusto fragola): 2 mg/5 mL (480 mL). Compresse, come solfato: 2, 4 mg. Compresse, rilascio prolungato: 4 mg.	**Broncodilatatore** (β_2 agonista). **Dose da inalazione:** *Neonati, bambini piccoli, bambini grandi e adulti:* **Inalatore predosato:** 1-2 puff a.b. o 5 min prima dell'esercizio o tid-qid. **Rotahaler:** 1-2 capsule a.b., o ogni 4-6 h, o prima dell'esercizio. **Soluzione nebulizzata:** *Neonati:* 0,1-0,5 mg/kg/dose a.b. o ogni 2-6 h. *Bambini:* 1,25-2,5 mg a.b. o ogni 4-6 h. *Adulti:* 1,25-5 mg a.b. o ogni 4-6 h **per os:** *Neonati:* 0,1-0,3 mg/kg/dose ogni 6-8 h. *Bambini:* *<6 anni:* 0,1-0,2 mg/kg/dose tid. *6-12 anni:* 2 mg/dose tid-qid *>12 anni:* 2-4 mg tid-qid.	*Cautela:* l'aumento dell'uso e la mancanza di effetto possono indicare la perdita del controllo dell'asma, che richiede attenzione medica. Meglio usare a.b. o prima dell'esercizio fisico. *Effetti indesiderati:* iperglicemia, ipopotassiemia, tachicardia, palpitazioni, nervosismo, stimolazione SNC, insonnia, tremore.
Alfentanil idrocloruro Analgesico, narcotico; anestetico generale. Iniezione, senza conservanti: 500 μg/mL (2, 5, 10, 20 mL).	**Analgesia, anestesia** (analgesico narcotico). *Neonati, bambini piccoli, e bambini <12 anni:* 5-15 g/kg ev iniettata over 3-5 min o 0,5-3 μg/kg/min in infusione continua (limitata esperienza e dosi poco stabilite). *Adulti:* infusione continua ev 0,5-1,5 μg/kg/min.	*Cautela:* dose bolo di 9-15 μg/kg causa rigidità toracica in 9 neonati su 20, compromettendo la respirazione in 4 pazienti. Usare un rilassante del muscolo scheletrico in concomitanza. Evitare nei pazienti con pressione endocranica aumentata o depressione respiratoria grave. *Effetti indesiderati:* bradicardia, ipotensione, aumentata pressione endocranica, rilascio di ormone antidiuretico. *Commento:* dose basata sul peso magro per pazienti obesi
Alglucerasi Enzima, glucocerebrosidasi. Iniezione: 10 U/mL (5 mL); 80 U/mL (5 mL).	**Terapia di sostituzione enzimatica per la malattia di Gaucher di tipo I** (sostituisce la β-glucosidasi mancante necessaria per la degradazione e quindi per evitare l'accumulo di macrofagi pieni di glicosil ceramide nell'osso, nel fegato e nella milza nella malattia di Gaucher di tipo 1). 20-60 U/kg ev infuso per 1-2 h. In genere ripetuto ogni 2 sett, ma varia da ogni 2 giorni a ogni 4 sett, a seconda della risposta.	*Effetti indesiderati:* febbre, brividi, dolenzia addominale, nausea, vomito, arrossamento del sito locale ev o edema. *Monitoraggio:* risoluzione dell'anemia, trombocitopenia, tendenza al sanguinamento ed epatosplenomegalia (entro 6 mesi). Migliorata mineralizzazione ossea (di solito osservata a 80-104 sett di terapia).
Allopurinolo Agente antigottoso; agente che riduce l'acido urico. Compresse: 100, 300 mg.	**Previene gli attacchi di artrite gottosa e la nefropatia gottosa.** **Previene l'iperuricemia indotta dalla chemioterapia tumorale** (inibisce la xantino ossidasi, impedendo così la conversione dell'ipoxantina in acido urico). *Bambini* ≤10 anni: 10 mg/kg/24 h suddivisi in 2-3 dosi. *Bambini >10 anni e adulti:* 200-600 mg/24 h in 2-3 dosi suddivise. **Gotta, iperuricemia indotta da chemioterapia.** 600-800 mg/24 h in 2-3 dosi suddivise iniziando 1-2 giorni prima della chemioterapia e continuando per 3 giorni. **Insufficienza renale:** CrCl 10-50: ridurre la dose al 50%. CrCl <10: ridurre la dose al 30% di quanto suggerito.	*Cautela:* sospendere ai primi segni di rash. *Effetti indesiderati:* rash, inclusi eritema multiforme, insufficienza renale, epatite, neuropatia periferica, vasculite. *Monitoraggio:* i livelli di acido urico diminuiscono in 1-2 giorni, con il massimo effetto osservato in 1-3 sett.
Aloperidolo Concentrato orale: 2 mg/mL. Compresse: 0,5, 1, 2, 5, 10, 20 mg. Iniezione.	**Trattamento dei disturbi del comportamento gravi, incluse psicosi e sindrome di Tourette (bloccante competitivo dei recettori della dopamina).** *Bambini 3-12 anni:* per os: iniziare 0,25-0,5 mg/24 h in 2-3 dosi suddivise, poi aumenta alla sett di 0,25-0,5 mg al giorno in base alla risposta (massimo: 0,15 mg/kg/24 h). *6-12 anni:* im: 1-3 mg/dose ogni 4-8 h (massimo: 0,15 mg/kg/24 h). *Adulti:* pigmentazione retinica, epatopatiacolestatica, agranulocitosi, leucopenia. per os: 0,5-5 mg bid-tid al giorno. im: 2-5 mg ogni 4-8 h.	*Effetti indesiderati:* sonnolenza, irritabilità, ansia, sintomi extrapiramidali, distonia, acatisia, pseudoparkinsonismo, discinesia tardiva, sindrome neurolettica maligna, convulsioni, stipsi, aumento di peso, rigonfiamento delle mammelle, ipotensione, tachicardia, aritmie, ritenzione urinaria, visione offuscata, *Monitoraggio:* concentrazioni plasmatiche (terapeutiche 5-15 ng/mL, tossiche >42 ng/mL).

TABELLA 716-1. Farmaci generali – *continua*

FARMACO (PRINCIPIO ATTIVO, FORMULAZIONI)	INDICAZIONI (MECCANISMO D'AZIONE E DOSAGGIO)	COMMENTI (CAUTELE, EFFETTI INDESIDERATI, MONITORAGGIO)
Alprazolam Agente antiansia. Benzodiazepina. Compresse: 0,25, 0,5, 1, 2 mg.	**Trattamento dell'ansia o degli attacchi di panico** (non certo, ma può essere mediato dall'acido γ-aminobutirrico). *Bambini:* 0,005-0,02 mg/kg/dose tid. *Adulti:* 0,25-0,5 mg bid-tid (massimo: 4 mg/24 h) (ansia) (massimo: 10 mg/24 h) (panico).	*Cautela:* la sospensione improvvisa determina reazioni da sospensione, incluse convulsioni. La sicurezza non è stata stabilita nei bambini <18 anni. Fattore di rischio D per la gravidanza. *Effetti indesiderati:* sonnolenza, confusione, sedazione.
Alprostadil Prostaglandina. Iniezione: 500 μg/mL (1 mL).	**Mantiene la pervietà del dotto arterioso nelle cardiopatie cianogene.** Vasodilatazione diretta del muscolo liscio del dotto. *Neonati e bambini piccoli:* 0,05-0,1 μg/kg/min come infusione continua ev può gradualmente aumentare al massimo di 0,4 μg/kg/min o svezzare lentamente a 0,005 μg/kg/min, a seconda della risposta.	*Effetti indesiderati:* apnea, bradicardia, ipotensione, tachicardia, flushing, Attività simil-convulsiva, iperostosi corticale (con utilizzo >6 mesi), diarrea, ostruzione del tratto di efflusso gastrico (uso ≥5 giorni). *Monitoraggio:* la risposta terapeutica include aumento della pressione sanguigna sistemica, migliorata saturazione dell'ossigeno o Po_2, e minore acidosi al pH plasmatico. Sospendere immediatamente in caso di grave apnea o bradicardia.
Aminofillina (equivalenti della teofillina elencati tra parentesi.) Broncodilatatore; stimolante respiratorio; derivato della teofillina. Iniezione, ev : 25 mg/mL (19,7 mg/mL) (10, 20 mL). Liquida, orale: 105 mg/5 mL (90 mg/5 mL) (240 mL). Supposta, rettale: 250 mg (197,5 mg), 500 mg (395 mg). Compresse: 100 mg (79 mg), 200 mg (158 mg). Compresse, rilascio controllato (12 h) 225 mg (178 mg). Compresse, gastroprotetta: 100 mg (79 mg), 200 mg (158 mg). Vedi *Teofillina* per il dosaggio orale	**Apnea della prematurità, svezzamento dal respiratore nei neonati, broncodilatatore, deboli effetti anti-infiammatori polmonari.** Aumenta la contrattilità e riduce l'affaticamento del diaframma e dei muscoli respiratori; debole broncodilatatore, stimola il SNC; riduce la risposta delle vie aeree agli stimoli. I meccanismi esatti per questi effetti rimangono controversi. *Neonati* (per apnea della prematurità, svezzamento dal respiratore o broncospasmo): dose da carico: 6 mg/kg ev o per os; dose di mantenimento: 2,5-3 mg/kg/dose ogni 12 h ev o per os. **Terapia dell'asma cronico (vedi teofillina).** L'uso nella terapia acuta è di dubbia utilità. Se usato in infusione continua ev: *Bambini:* *6 sett-6 mesi:* 0,5 mg/kg/h. *6 mesi-1 anno:* 0,7 mg/kg/h. *1-9 anni:* 1 mg/kg/h. *9-12 anni:* 0,9 mg/kg/h. *12 anni-adulto:* 0,7 mg/kg/h.	*Cautela:* può causare o peggiorare aritmie, convulsioni o reflusso gastroesofageo. La clearance della teofillina è modificata da numerose patologie e farmaci, che richiedono aggiustamenti della posologia in base dalle concentrazioni seriche di teofillina. La clearance è ridotta da malattie virali, febbre >40 °C per >24 h, cor polmonare e farmaci che inibiscono gli enzimi del P450 (cimetidina, verapamil, macrolidi, chinolonici); ridurre la dose del 50%. *Effetti indesiderati:* intolleranza nutrizionale nei neonati, disagio gastrointestinale nei bambini e negli adulti, nausea, vomito, irritabilità del SNC, agitazione, tachicardia, tachiaritmie. *Monitoraggio:* i livelli plasmatici di teofillina sono correlati agli effetti clinici e alla tossicità. I livelli target sono talvolta controversi. *Neonati:* 6-15 mg/L (65% dei neonati non avrà apnea eliminato fino a che i livelli superano 10 mg/L se viene eseguito il monitoraggio elettronico continuo. Livelli >10 mg/L sono necessari per lo svezzamento dal respiratore. Livelli di 5-15 mg/L sono sufficienti per la broncodilatazione). *Bambini:* la teofillina da sola è inefficace per l'asma acuto. Nell'asma cronico livelli di teofillina di 5-15 mg/L sono efficaci, ma i livelli dovrebbero essere superiori a 10 mg/L per la prevenzione del broncospasmo indotto dall'esercizio.
Amiodarone idrocloruro Agente antiaritmico, classe III. Compresse: 200 mg. Iniezione: 50 mg/mL (3 mL).. Iniezione, privo di benzil alcol e polisorbati: 15 mg/mL (10 mL).	**Trattamento delle aritmie ventricolari resistenti, minacciose per la vita o della tachicardia parossistica sopraventricolare (TPSV) che non risponde ad agenti meno tossici** (agente antiaritmico di classe III; prolunga il potenziale d'azione e il periodo refrattario nel tessuto miocardico). **Dose orale:** *Bambini piccoli e grandi:* *<1 anno:* 600-800 mg/1,73 m^2/24 h in 2 dosi suddivise. *>1 anno:* 10-20 mg/kg/24 h suddivisi in 2 dosi per 10 giorni, poi 5-10 mg/kg/24 h. *Adulti:* 800 mg/24 h in 2 dosi suddivise. Dimezzare tutte le dosi (cioè, 1 dose/giorno) dopo 1-4 sett di trattamento o quando le aritmie sono controllate. **Dose ev:** *bambini piccoli e grandi:* dose da carico di 5 mg/kg per 1 ora, poi infusione continua di 5-15 μg/kg/min. *Adulti:* 150 mg per 10 min, poi 0,5 mg/min.	*Cautela:* usare il prodotto senza benzil alcol nei neonati. Minimizza il rischio di torsioni di punta correggendo le alterazioni del potassio e del magnesio. Inibisce gli enzimi del citocromo P450, così che molti farmaci che sono metabolizzati avranno livelli ed effetti marcatamente aumentati, tra cui teofillina, fenitoina, warfarin, altri antiaritmici, metotrexato e ciclosporina. *Effetti indesiderati:* proaritmie (possono essere bradiaritmie, tachiaritmie o arresto cardiaco), affaticamento, malessere, incubi, disturbi dell'umore, ipotiroidismo, iperglicemia, aumento dei trigliceridi, alterazioni del colore della cute (blu ardesia), fotosensibilità, rash, tossicità epatica (può essere fatale o solo con aumento degli enzimi epatici), tossicità polmonare (potenzialmente fatale) inclusa la fibrosi polmonare, polmonite interstiziale, polmonite da ipersensibilità (tosse, febbre, dispnea, alterazioni radiografiche del torace), fotofobia, trombocitopenia. *Monitoraggio:* test di funzionalità polmonare, epatica e tiroidea; radiografia del torace, ECG, esame dell'occhio; segni clinici e sintomi di tossicità. Concentrazione di Amiodarone: 2-4 μmol/L.
Amitriptilina idrocloruro Antidepressivo, triciclico; agente antiemicranico. Iniezione: 10 mg/mL (10 mL). Compresse: 10, 25, 50, 75, 100, 150 mg.	**Depressione (aumenta la concentrazione di serotonina e noradrenalina nel SNC inibendo il reuptake).** *Bambini:* 1-1,5 mg/kg/24 h suddivisi tid. *Adolescenti:* 30-100 mg prima di andare a dormire o suddivisi bid (massimo: 200 mg/24 h). *Adulti:* 30-100 mg ogni 24 h (massimo: 300 mg/24 h). **Analgesico per il dolore neuropatico o cronico o profilassi dell'emicrania.** *Bambini:* 0,1 mg/kg prima di andare a letto e attendere 2-3 sett per l'effetto (massimo: 2 mg/kg prima di andare a letto). *Adolescenti:* 25 mg suddivisi bid e aumentare la dose fino a ottenere l'effetto (massimo: 200 mg/24 h). *Adulti:* 25 mg prima di andare a letto e aumentare la dose fino a ottenere l'effetto (massimo: 300 mg/24 h).	*Cautela:* possono verificarsi disturbi della conduzione cardiaca, monitorare con ECG. Non sospendere improvvisamente perché può verificarsi sindrome da astinenza. *Effetti indesiderati:* secchezza delle fauci, stipsi, aumento ponderale, ipotensione posturale, sonnolenza, confusione, cefalea, disturbi della vista. *Monitoraggio:* concentrazioni terapeutiche di amitriptilina 100-250 ng/mL; concentrazioni di nortriptilina: terapeutiche 50-150 ng/mL.
Ammonio cloruro Alcalosi metabolica, agente di trattamento; agente acidificante urinario. Iniezione: 26,75% (5 mEq/mL) (20 mL). Compresse: 500 mg. Compresse, gastroprotette: 500 mg.	**Acidificazione sistemica o urinaria (dissociazione di ammonio e cloruro e sostituzione degli ioni bicarbonato con ioni cloruro).** *Bambini:* 75 mg/kg/24 h ev suddivisi ogni 6 h (massimo: 6 g al giorno). *Adulti:* 1,5 g/dose ev ogni 6 h.	*Effetti indesiderati:* ipercloremia, iperammoniemia, iperpotassemia.
Amrinone lattato Agente agonista adrenergico. Iniezione: 5 mg/mL (20 mL).	**Trattamento degli stati di bassa gittata cardiaca (aumenta i livelli cellulari di adenosina monofosfato).** *Neonati:* 0,75 mg/kg ev in bolo per 2-3 min, poi 3-5 μg/kg/min in infusione ev continua. *Bambini piccoli e grandi:* 0,75 mg/kg ev in bolo per 2-3 min, poi 5-10 μg/kg/min infusione continua. *Adulti:* bolo di 0,75 mg/kg ev per 2-3 min, poi 5-10 μg/kg/min.	*Cautela:* l'aumentata gittata cardiaca può causare diuresi eccessiva se le dosi di diuretico non sono modificate. Si può ripetere una dose bolo se la risposta clinica è inadeguata. *Effetti indesiderati:* ipotensione, aritmie, trombocitopenia.

TABELLA 716-1. Farmaci generali – *continua*

FARMACO (PRINCIPIO ATTIVO, FORMULAZIONI)	INDICAZIONI (MECCANISMO D'AZIONE E DOSAGGIO)	COMMENTI (CAUTELE, EFFETTI INDESIDERATI, MONITORAGGIO)
Antipirina e benzocaina Agente otologico, analgesico; agente otologico, ceruminolitico. Otologico: antipirina 5,4% e benzocaina 1,4% (10, 15 mL).	**Sollievo temporaneo per il dolore e l'infiammazione all'orecchio (anestetico e anti-infiammatorio topico).** *Tutti pazienti:* riempire il canale dell'orecchio malato e inumidire un tampone di cotone e posizionarlo nel meato. Si può ripetere ogni 1-2 h fino a risoluzione del dolore. Limitare l'uso a circa 3 giorni.	*Effetti indesiderati:* bruciore, metaemoglobinemia.
Antitossina tetanica Iniezione.	**Prevenzione o trattamento del tetano quando non è disponibile l'immunoglobulina tetanica.** *Bambini e adulti:* sc, im: Profilassi: <30 kg 1500 unità; >30 kg 3000-5000 unità. Trattamento: iniettare 10 000-40 000 unità nella ferita e 40 000-100 000 unità ev.	*Effetti indesiderati:* malattia da siero, orticaria, eruzioni cutanee, reazioni allergiche.
Antitrombina III **Thrombate III**	**Deficit di antitrombina III (ATIII) causato da coagulazione intravascolare disseminata o shock e complicanze chirurgiche. Trattamento della trombosi nel deficit di ATIII.** *Tutti i pazienti:* dose (UI) = (120 − ATIII del paziente) × peso (kg).	*Monitoraggio:* controllare i livelli di ATIII: mantenere all'80-120%.
Antiveleno (crotalidi) polivalente Antivenom. Iniezione: siero liofilizzato, diluente (10 mL); 1 fiala vacuum fino ad arrivare a 10 mL di antiveleno.	**Antiveleno per il morso di crotalidi del Nord e Sud America (cioè, crotalo, testa di rame, mocassino acquatico, mocassino, tropicale, terrore dei boschi).** Dose basata sulla gravità del morso: lieve, 1 fiala; moderato, 10 fiale; grave, >15 fiale.	*Cautela:* reazioni da ipersensibilità, inclusa anafilassi (trattare con adrenalina e antistaminico e breve tenuta della dose).
Arginina idrocloruro Agente diagnostico, funzionalità ormone delle crescita; alcalosi metabolica, agente terapeutico. Iniezione: 10% (0,475 mEq cloride/mL) (500 mL).	**Test di funzionalità dell'ipofisi (stimola l'ipofisi, rilascio dell'ormone della crescita e della prolattina).** *Bambini:* 500 mg/kg per 30 min. *Adulti:* 300 mL per 30 min.	*Effetti indesiderati:* flushing, cefalea, iperglicemia. iperpotassemia, acidosi metabolica. *Monitoraggio:* concentrazioni plasmatiche dell'ormone della crescita.
Asparaginasi Agente antineoplastico, miscellanea. Iniezione: 10 000 U/fiala.	**Chemioterapia tumorale (inibisce la sintesi delle proteine nelle cellule cancerogene prive di asparagina).** *Bambini e adulti:* le dosi possono variare a seconda del protocollo specifico utilizzato; 6000 unità/m^2 im, 3 × sett per 3 sett nell'ambito della terapia combinata. Terapia im ad alte dosi: 25 000 unità/m^2/dose ogni sett × 9 dosi. Terapia ev: 1000 unità/kg/24 h per 10 giorni; o 200 unità/kg/24 h per circa 28 giorni.	*Cautela:* sospendere il farmaco al minimo segno di insufficienza renale o pancreatite. Essere pronti a trattare l'anafilassi a ogni dose. *Effetti indesiderati:* mielosoppressione (leucociti e piastrine; lieve e rara) inizio, 7 giorni; nadir, 14 giorni; remissione, 21 giorni. Epatotossicità, pancreatite, distrubri gastrointestinali, uremia, iperglicemia, coagulopatia.
Astemizolo Antistaminico. Compresse: 10 mg	**Allergia e rinite (bloccante competitivo dei recettori H1).** *Bambini:* *<6 anni:* 0,2 mg/kg una volta al giorno. *6-12 anni:* 5 mg una volta al giorno. *>12 anni e adulti:* 10-30 mg/24 h	*Cautela:* episodi sincopali possono segnalare aritmie, tra cui il prolungamento dell'intervallo Q-T, che causa aritmie fatali. Sospendere se l'ECG mostra prolungamento del Q-T, in caso di episodio sincopale o se si aggiungono farmaci che alterano il metabolismo epatico (per es. eritromicina, ketoconazolo) .
Atenololo Agente antianginoso; antipertensivo; bloccante β-adrenergico. Iniezione: 0,5 mg/mL (10 mL). Compresse: 25, 50, 100 mg.	**Ipertensione, aritmie (bloccante competitivo β_1).** *Bambini:* 0,8-1,5 mg/kg/24 h (massimo: 2 mg/kg/24 h). *Adulti:* 25-200 mg/24 h per os, 5 mg ev per 5 min.	*Cautela:* Evitare la sospensione improvvisa; misurare per 1-2 sett. *Effetti indesiderati:* bradicardia, letargia, cefalea, stipsi, respiro affannoso, dispnea.
Atorvastatina calcio Compresse: 10, 20, 40 mg.	**Ipercolesterolemia, inclusa l'ipercolesterolemia familiare omozigote (inibisce l'HMG-CoA reduttasi).** *Bambini >6 anni:* 10-80 mg/24 h. *Adulti:* 10-80 mg/24 h.	*Effetti indesiderati:* dispepsia, flatulenza, pancreatite, epatite, mialgia, artralgia. *Monitoraggio:* quadro lipidico plasmatico.
Atracurio besilato Agente bloccante neuromuscolare; rilassante non depolarizzante del muscolo scheletrico; paralitico. Iniezione: 10 mg/mL (5, 10 mL).	**Bloccante neuromuscolare per la paralisi muscolare; si lega ai siti recettoriali colinergici per bloccare la trasmissione nervosa).** *Bambini:* *<2 anni:* 0,3-0,4 mg/kg se necessario. *>2 anni-adulti:* 0,4-0,5 mg/kg, poi 1 mg/kg 20-45 min dopo ogni blocco iniziale per mantenere l'effetto. Infusione continua ev: 0,4-0,8 mg/kg/h.	*Cautela:* assicurarsi che la via aerea e il supporto respiratorio siano secure prima dell'uso. Contiene benzil alcol; l'uso neonatale dovrebbe essere limitato. Non ha proprietà analgesiche o sedative, quindi dovrebbe essere prevista l'aggiunta di sedativo o analgesico. *Monitoraggio:* mioclonia riflessa in risposta allo stimolatore del nervo periferico.
Atropina solfato Agente anticolinergico; antidoto; oftalmico, avvelenamento da organofosfati; antispasmodico agente, gastrointestinale; broncodilatatore; oftalmico, agente midriatico. Iniezione oftalmica: 0,05 mg/mL; (5 mL); 0,1 mg/mL (5, 10 mL); 0,3 mg/mL (1, 30 mL); 0,4 mg/mL (1, 20, 30 mL); 0,5 mg/mL (1, 5, 30 mL); 0,8 mg/mL (0,5, 1 mL); 1 mg/mL (1, 10 mL). Pomata, oftalmica: 0,5% (3,5 g); 1% (3,5 g). Soluzione, oftalmica: 0,5% (1, 5 mL); 1% (1, 2, 5, 15 mL); 2% (1, 2 mL). Compresse: 0,4 mg. Compresse, solubili: 0,4, 0,6 mg.	**Medicazione preoperatoria per inibire le secrezioni e la salivazione (blocca l'azione dell'acetilcolina e antagonizza l'istamina e la serotonina).** *Neonati e bambini:* *<5 kg:* 0,2 mg/kg 30 min preoperatorio, poi ogni 4-6 h. *>5 kg:* 0,1-0,2 mg/kg/dose (massimo: 0,4 mg/dose). *Adulti:* 0,4-0,6 mg ev o sc 30 min prima dell'intervento. **Trattamento della bradicardia sinusale.** *Neonati e bambini:* 0,02 mg/kg (minimo: 0,1 mg); ev o intratracheale (massimo: 0,5 mg); si può ripetere 5 min più tardi, 1× *Adulti:* 0,5-1 mg ogni 5 min (dose massima totale: 2 mg). **Antidoto per l'avvelenamento da organofosfati.** 0,02-0,05 mg/kg ogni 10-20 min fino all'effetto dell'atropina (tachicardia, midriasi, febbre), poi ogni 1-4 h per almeno 24 h.	*Cautela:* evitare nel glaucoma ad angolo chiuso, nell'ostruzione gastrointestinale, nella tireotossicosi e nella tachicardia. *Effetti indesiderati:* tachicardia; palpitazioni; delirio; atassia; cute calda e secca; tremore; compromissione della vista.
Attapulgite Antidiarroico. Capsule: 750 mg. Liquida: 600 mg attapulgite attivata/15 mL (180, 240, 360, 480 mL); 750 mg attapulgite attivata/15 mL (120 mL). Sospensione: 600 mg/15 mL. Compresse, masticabili: 300, 600, 750 mg.	**Diarrea non complicata (azione assorbente).** *Bambini:* *3-6 anni:* 300-750 mg/dose (massimo: 7 dosi). *6-12 anni:* 600-1500 mg/dose (massimo: 7 dosi).	*Cautela:* non usare in caso di diarrea dovuta a dissenteria, enterocolite o batteri tossigeni.

TABELLA 716-1. Farmaci generali – *continua*

FARMACO (PRINCIPIO ATTIVO, FORMULAZIONI)	INDICAZIONI (MECCANISMO D'AZIONE E DOSAGGIO)	COMMENTI (CAUTELE, EFFETTI INDESIDERATI, MONITORAGGIO)
Attivatore tissutale del plasminogeno Iniezione.	**Terapia trombolitica (favorisce la conversione del plasminogeno in plasmina).** *Neonati:* 0,1-0,5 mg/kg/h per 3-10 h. *Bambini:* 0,1-0,6 mg/kg/h per 6 h. *Adulti:* 100 mg infusi come 60 mg nella prima ora, 20 mg alla seconda ora, 20 mg alla terza ora. *Monitoraggio:* D-dimero, fibrinogeno, tempo di sanguinamento.	*Cautela:* iniziare eparina concomitante per evitare trombosi ed emboli trombotici. *Effetti indesiderati:* sanguinamento, aritmie (correlate alla riperfusione post-primo infarto miocardico).
Auranofin Sale d'oro. Capsule: 3 mg (oro 29%).	**Trattamento dell'artrite reumatoide o psoriasica in fase attiva (effetto immunomodulante).** *Bambini:* dose iniziale: 0,1 mg/kg/24 h; dose di mantenimento abituale: 0,15 mg/kg/24 h in 1-2 dosi (massimo: 0,2 mg/kg/24 h). *Adulti:* 6 mg/24 h in 1-2 dosi (massimo: 9 mg/24 h in 1-3 dosi).	*Effetti indesiderati:* prurito, rash cutaneo, stomatite, congiuntivite, proteinuria, anemia, agranulocitosi, eosinofilia, neuropatia periferica, alopecia, glossite, leucopenia, trombocitopenia, ematuria, polmonite interstiziale, angioedema, epatotossicità. *Monitoraggio:* sospendere se leucociti $<4000/mm^3$, granulociti $<1500/mm^3$, piastrine $<100\,000/mm^3$.
Aurotioglucosio Sale d'oro. Sospensione, sterile: 50 mg/mL (oro al 50%) (10 mL).	**Trattamento immunomodulante dell'artrite reumatoide o psoriasica.** *Bambini:* 0,25 mg/kg/dose nella sett 1, aumentato di 0,25 mg/kg/dose ogni sett fino alla dose di mantenimento di 0,75-1,0 mg/kg alla sett (massimo: 25 mg/dose, totale 20 dosi). *Adulti:* 10 mg nella sett 1, poi 25 mg alla sett 2 e 3, poi 50 mg/sett fino alla dose cumulativa o alla somministrazione di 1 g.	*Cautela:* somministrato mediante iniezione im profonda. *Effetti indesiderati:* gli stessi di auranofin.
Azatadina maleato Antistaminico. Compresse: 1 mg	**Trattamento di allergia, rinite allergica e orticaria (antistaminico, anticolinergico).** *Bambini <12 anni:* non raccomandato. *Bambini >12 anni e adulti:* 1-2 mg due volte al giorno.	*Effetti indesiderati:* sedazione, secchezza delle fauci, ispessimento delle secrezioni bronchiali.
Azatioprina Agente immunosoppressivo. Iniezione, come sodio: 100 mg (10 mL). Compresse: 50 mg.	**Previene il rigetto del trapianto.** *Bambini e adulti:* dose iniziale di 2-5 mg/kg/24 h ev o per os, con una dose di mantenimento di 1-3 mg/kg/24 h. **Trattamento di malattie autoimmuni (per es. lupus, artrite, sindrome nefrosica).** Inibisce la sintesi di DNA, RNA, e proteine. Antagonizza il metabolismo della purina. *Adulti:* 1 mg/kg/24 h × 6-8 sett.	*Cautela:* l'utilizzo cronico causa aumentato rischio di linfoma e tumori cutanei. Può causare soppressione midollare irreversibile. Ridurre la dose al 25% del normale se usato in concomitanza con allopurinolo. *Effetti indesiderati:* febbre, brividi, nausea, vomito, diarrea, trombocitopenia, leucopenia, epatotossicità, rash.
Baclofene Rilassante del muscolo scheletrico; non paralitico. Iniezione, it: 0,5 mg/mL (20 mL); 2 mg/mL (5 mL). Compresse: 10, 20 mg.	**Spasticità associata a sclerosi multipla o a lesioni della colonna vertebrale.** **Nevralgia del trigemino (inibisce la trasmissione dei riflessi monosinaptici e polisinaptici a livello della colonna vertebrale).** *Bambini: 2-7 anni:* 10-15 mg/24 h suddivisi ogni 8 h e titolare fino a ogni 3 giorni (massimo: 40 mg/24 h per os). Intratecale 25-50 µg. *Adulti:* 5 mg ogni 8 h e aumentare gradualmente di 5 mg ogni 3 giorni (massimo: 80 mg/24 h per os). Intratecale 50 µg fino al massimo di 100 µg.	*Cautela:* evitare la sospensione improvvisa; scalare lentamente per la sospensione. *Effetti indesiderati:* sonnolenza, vertigini, reazioni psichiatriche, atassia, ipotonia.
Beclometasone Corticosteroide surrenalico; agente anti-infiammatorio; corticosteroide, inalatorio (orale); corticosteroide, nasale; glucocorticoide. Inalazione: Nasale: 42 µg/inalazione (200 dosi misurate) (16,8 g). Orale: 42 µg/inalazione (200 dosi misurate) (16,8 g). Spruzzo, acquoso, nasale: 42 µg /inalazione (200 dosi misurate) (25 g).	**Asma (inalazione orale), rinite (aerosol nasale) (anti-infiammatorio, immunomodulante).** *Adulti e bambini (inalato):* 1-2 puff bid-qid (massimo bambini: 10 puff al giorno; adulti: 20 puff al giorno). *Adulti e bambini (spruzzo nasale):* 1 spruzzo in ogni narice bid-qid.	*Effetti indesiderati:* candida orale, arrossamento e irritazione della mucosa nasale, tosse, raucedine, cefalea. *Monitoraggio:* i corticosteroidi inalatori dovrebbero essere somministrati utilizzando un distanziatore per migliorare la penetrazione nei polmoni e ridurre la tossicità locale.
Benzilpenicilloil-polilisina Agente diagnostico, test cutaneo dell'allergia alla penicillina. Iniezione: 0,25 mL.	**Valutazione del rischio di ipersensibilità alla penicillina (scatena reazioni di tipo 1, reazioni orticarioidi mediante reazione IgE-mediata).** *Bambini e adulti:* nella tecnica dello scratch si utilizza un ago da 20-gauge per realizzare un graffio di 3-5 mm sul derma; si applica quindi alla zona graffiata una piccola goccia di soluzione e la si sfrega delicatamente con un applicatore. Iniezione intradermica di 0,1-0,2 mL dell'agente e soluzione fisiologica 0,9% in 2 siti fra loro lontani.	*Monitoraggio:* lo scratch test è positivo se compare un pomfo pallido ≥5-15 mm entro 10 min. Il test intradermico è positivo in 5-15 min. Sospendere antistaminici prima di fare i tests (idrossizina e difenidramina per almeno 4 giorni, astemizolo per 6-8 sett).
Benzocaina Anestetico locale, orale; anestetico locale, topico. Aerosol: 5% (97,5, 105 mL) 20% (20, 60, 120 g). Crema: 5% (30, 454 g); 6% (28,4 g). Gel 15% (7 g). Liquido, con benzil benzoato e sapone leggero: 30 mL. Lozione: 8% (90 mL). Pomata: 5% (3,5, 30 g).	**Riduzione temporanea del dolore associato a traumi minori della cute (anestetico locale).** *Bambini e adulti:* applicare all'area interessata come necessario.	*Effetti indesiderati:* irritazione locale o sensibilizzazione.
Benzoil perossido Prodotti per l'acne, prodotto topico per la cute. Sapone detergente: 5% (120 g); 10% (120 g). Lozione detergente: 5% (120, 150, 240 mL); 10% (120, 150 mL). Crema: 5% (30 g); 10% (30, 45 g). Maschera facciale: 5%. Gel: 2,5% (45, 60, 90 g); 5% (45, 60, 90, 120 g); 10% (45, 60, 90, 120 g). Lozione: 5% (30, 42,5, 60 mL); 5,5% (25 mL); 10% (30, 42,5, 60 mL). Stick: 10%.	**Trattamento dell'acne (effetto cheratolitico e comedolitico e uccisione dei batteri anaerobi).** *Bambini e adulti:* applicare con parsimonia tid per 15 min. Si possono aumentare la forza e la durata dell'esposizione se tollerato.	*Effetti indesiderati:* dermatite da contatto, irritazione locale, bruciore, eritema.
Benzonatato Anestetico topico.	**Rimedio per la tosse non produttiva (azione come anestetico topico).** *Bambini <10 anni:* non indicato. *Bambini >10 anni e adulti:* 100 mg tid o ogni 4 h (massimo: 600 mg/24 h).	*Effetti indesiderati:* sedazione, parestesie, vertigini, cefalea.

TABELLA 716-1. Farmaci generali – *continua*

FARMACO (PRINCIPIO ATTIVO, FORMULAZIONI)	INDICAZIONI (MECCANISMO D'AZIONE E DOSAGGIO)	COMMENTI (CAUTELE, EFFETTI INDESIDERATI, MONITORAGGIO)
Benzotropina mesilato Agente anticolinergico: antidoto, reazioni distoniche indotte da farmaci; agente anti-parkinsoniano. Iniezione: 1 mg/mL (2 mL). Compresse: 0,5, 1, 2 mg.	**Parkinsonismo, reazione extrapiramidale indotta da farmaci (blocco dei recettori colinergici striatali).** *Bambini >3 anni:* 0,02-0,05 mg/kg/dose 1-2 × giorno. *Adulti:* 1-4 mg/dose 1-2 × giorno.	*Effetti indesiderati:* tachicardia, sonnolenza, nervosismo, allucinazioni, secchezza delle fauci, visione offuscata, midriasi.
Beractant Surfattante polmonare. Sospensione: 200 mg (8 mL).	**Profilassi e trattamento della sindrome da distress respiratorio nei bambini piccoli prematuri (recupera il deficit di surfattante endogeno).** *Neonati:* 4 mL/kg mediante tubo endotracheale. Si può ripetere ogni 6 h fino a un totale di 4 dosi. Ruotare il bambino a destra, poi a sinistra, e somministrare 1/2 dose su ogni lato per 2-3 s.	*Effetti indesiderati:* bradicardia, ipotensione, desaturazione dell'ossigeno, perdite di aria polmonare, ostruzione delle vie aeree, emorragia polmonare, ipocarbia. *Monitoraggio:* frequenza cardiaca, saturazione dell'ossigeno ed emogasanalisi arteriose frequenti. Regolare il ventilatore per ridurre al minimo gli episodi di iperossia e ipocarbia.
Betametasone Corticosteroide surrenalico; agente anti-infiammatorio; corticosteroide, sistemico; corticosteroide, topico; glucocorticoide. Base: Sciroppo: 0,6 mg/5 mL. Compresse: 0,6 mg. Benzoato: Crema, base emolliente: 0,025% (60 g). Gel, topico: 0,025% (15, 60 g). Lozione: 0,025% (60 mL). Dipropionato: Aerosol, topico: 0,1% (85 g). Crema: 0,05% (15, 45 g). Lozione: 0,05% (20, 30, 60 mL). Pomata, topica: 0,05% (15, 45 g). Diproprionato: Crema: 0,05% (15, 45 g). Dipropionato, augmented: Crema, base emolliente: 0,05% (15, 45 g). Gel, topico: 0,05% (15, 45 g). Lozione: 0,05% (30, 60 mL). Pomata, topica: 0,05% (15, 45 g). Valerato: Crema: 0,01% (15, 60 g); 0,1% (15, 45, 110, 430 g). Lozione: 0,1% (20, 60 mL). Pomata, topica: 0,1% (15, 45 g). Polvere per miscela: 5, 10 g. Fosfato di sodio: Iniezione: equivalente a 3 g/mL (5 mL). Fosfato e acetato di sodio: Iniezione, sospensione: 6 mg/mL (3 mg betametasone e betametasone sodio fosfato e 3 mg mbetametasone acetato/mL) (5 mL).	**Uso sistemico per stimolare la maturazione dei polmoni fetali nel parto pretermine. Uso topico per trattare le dermatosi infiammatorie.** *Bambini e adulti:* applicazione topica di un sottile film sull'area interessata bid-qid al giorno. *Donne in gravidanza:* 12 mg im ogni 24 h per 2 dosi.	*Effetti indesiderati:* edema polmonare materno e ipertensione, cefalea.
Betanecolo Agente colinergico. Iniezione: 5 mg/mL (1 mL). Compresse: 5, 10, 25, 50 mg.	**Trattamento della ritenzione urinaria non ostruttiva o del reflusso gastroesofageo (stimola i recettori colinergici nel muscolo liscio nelle vie urinarie e nel tratto gastrointestinale).** *Bambini:* 0,3-0,6 mg/kg/24 h suddivisi in 3-4 dosi. *Adulti:* 10-50 mg bid-qid.	*Effetti indesiderati:* ipotensione, crampi addominali, diarrea, vomito, scialorrea, pollachiuria, broncocostrizione, sudorazione.
Biotina Deficit di biotinidasi, agente terapeutico; vitamina, idrosolubile. Compresse: 300, 400, 600, 800 μg; 2,5, 3, 5, 10 mg.	**Trattamento del deficit primario di biotinidasi o del deficit alimentare di biotina, componente del complesso della vitamina B (necessaria per varie funzioni metaboliche).** *Bambini e adulti:* deficit di biotina: 5-20 mg al giorno. Deficit di biotinidasi: 5-10 mg al giorno.	
Bisacodil Lassativo, stimolante. Clistere: 10 mg/30 mL. Polvere: 1,5 mg con acido tannico 2,5 g/busta (25, 50). Supposta, rettale: 5, 10 mg. Compresse, gastroprotette: 5 mg.	**Trattamento della stipsi (irritazione diretta del muscolo liscio per stimolare la peristalsi gastrointestinale).** *Bambini:* *<2 anni:* 5 mg supposta rettale. *>2 anni:* 10 mg supposta rettale. *>6 anni:* 5-10 mg per os prima di andare a letto o prima di colazione. *Adulti:* 5-30 mg per os, 10 mg supposta rettale.	*Effetti indesiderati:* squilibrio idroelettrolitico, crampi addominali.
Bleomicina Agente antineoplastico, tipo antibiotico. Polvere per iniezione: 15 U.	**Trattamento palliativo di molti tumori e agente sclerosante per versamenti maligni (inibisce la sintesi di DNA).** *Bambini e adulti:* 10-20 U/m^2/dose ev, im, sc (0,25-0,5 U/kg) 1-2 × sett in regimi di combinazione.	*Cautela:* ridurre la dose in caso di disfunzione renale. *Effetti indesiderati:* polmonite interstiziale, fibrosi polmonare, tosse non produttiva, flebite, leucopenia, trombocitopenia, desquamazione, fenomeno di Raynaud; evitare l'uso di ossigeno. stomatite, vomito, alopecia, ipercheratosi delle mani e delle unghie,
Blu di metilene Iniezione: 10 mg/mL. Compresse: 65 mg	**Antidoto per l'avvelenamento da cianuro e metaemoglobinemia farmaco-indotte (promuove la conversione della metemoglobina a emoglobina; si combina con il cianuro per formare cian-metemoglobina).** *Bambini e adulti:* Metaemoglobinemia: ev: 1-2 mg/kg; si può ripetere dopo 1 ora se necessario. Deficit di NADP-metemoglobina reduttasi: per os: 1-1,5 mg/kg/24 h (somministrato con 5-8 mg/kg/24 h di acido ascorbico).	*Cautela:* evitare nel deficit di glucosio-6-fosfato deidrogenasi e nell'insufficienza renale. *Effetti indesiderati:* urine e feci virano al blu-verde; anemia.

TABELLA 716-1. Farmaci generali – *continua*

FARMACO (PRINCIPIO ATTIVO, FORMULAZIONI)	INDICAZIONI (MECCANISMO D'AZIONE E DOSAGGIO)	COMMENTI (CAUTELE, EFFETTI INDESIDERATI, MONITORAGGIO)
Bretilio Agente antiaritmico, classe III. Iniezione: 50 mg/mL (10, 20 mL); 100 mg/mL. Iniezione, premiscelato in D5W: 1 mg/mL (500 mL); 2 mg/mL (250 mL); 4 mg/mL (250, 500 mL).	**Trattamento delle aritmie gravi minacciose per la vita (inibisce il rilascio di noradrenalina in corrispondenza delle terminazioni nervose postgangliari).** *Bambini:* 2-5 mg/kg ev o im, si può ripetere ogni 10-20 min (massimo: 30 mg/kg). *Adulti:* dose iniziale o 5 mg/kg, poi 10 mg/kg ogni 15-30 min (massimo: 35 mg/kg). *Nota:* la cardioversione/defibrillazione deve essere tentata prima e dopo ogni dose di bretilio	*Effetti indesiderati:* ipotensione, aumento delle contrazioni ventricolari premature, bradicardia, congestione nasale, sudorazione, singhiozzo. *Monitoraggio:* ECG, pressione arteriosa.
Bromfeniramina Antistaminico. Compresse. Elisir: 2 mg/5 mL con alcol 3% (120, 480, 4000 mL). Iniezione: 10 mg/mL (10 mL). Compresse: 4, 8, 12 mg. Compresse, rilascio prolungato: 8, 12 mg.	**Trattamento dei sintomi allergici (per es. rinite, orticaria) (compete con l'istamina per i siti dei recettori H_1).** *Bambini:* *<6 anni:* 0,125 mg/kg/dose ogni 6 h (massimo: 8 mg/24 h) per os. *6-12 anni:* 2-4 mg/dose ogni 6-8 h (massimo: 16 mg/24 h) per os. *Adulti:* 4-8 mg/dose ogni 4-6 h (massimo: 24 mg/24 h) per os. ev, im, sc: *<12 anni:* 0,5 mg/kg/24 h suddivisi ogni 6 h. *>12 anni:* 10 mg/dose suddivisi ogni 6-12 h (massimo: 40 mg/24 h).	*Effetti indesiderati:* sedazione, secchezza delle fauci.
Budesonide Corticosteroide surrenalico; agente anti-infiammatorio; corticosteroide, nasale; glucocorticoide. Aerosol: rilasciato 50 µg/attuazione dell'erogazione ≈32 µg mediante adattatore nasale (200 dosi misurate) (7 g). Polvere inalatoria: 200 µg/inalazione.	**Trattamento della rinite o dell'asma cronico (sopprime l'infiammazione).** *Bambini >6 anni e adulti:* Rhinocort spruzzo nasale 2 puff in ogni narice bid o 4 puff in ogni narice una volta al giorno. *Bambini >6 anni:* Pulmicort Turbohaler 1-2 inalazioni bid. *Adulti:* 1-4 inalazioni bid.	*Effetti indesiderati:* stomatite aftosa orale, disfonia (minimizzata sciacquando la bocca dopo l'assunzione).
Bumetanide Antipertensivo: diuretico, dell'ansa. Iniezione: 0,25 mg/mL (2, 4, 10 mL). Compresse: 0,5, 1, 2 mg.	**Trattamento dell'edema o degli stati di sovraccarico di volume (impedisce il riassorbimento di sodio e cloro nell'ansa ascendente di Henle e nel tubulo prossimale).** per os, ev, im: *Neonati:* 0,01-0,05 mg/kg/dose ogni 24-48 h. *Bambini piccoli e grandi :* 0,015-0,1 mg/kg/dose ogni 6-24 h (massimo: 10 mg/24 h). *Adulti:* 0,5-2 mg/dose (massimo: 10 mg/24 h).	*Effetti indesiderati:* deplezione di elettroliti, disidratazione.
Bupivacaina Anestetico locale, iniettabile. Iniezione; senza conservanti: 0,25% (2,5 mg/mL); 0,5% (5 mg/mL); 0,75% (7,5 mg/mL). Con conservanti: 0,25% (2,5 mg/mL); 0,5% (5 mg/mL). Bupivacaine e adrenalina (2 : 2 milioni) iniezione, senza conservanti: 0,25% (2,5 mg/mL); 0,5% (5 mg/mL); 0,75% (7,5 mg/mL). Con conservanti: 0,25% (2,5 mg/mL); 0,5% (5 mg/mL). Bupivacaina in destrosio: 8,25%. Iniezione (spinale), senza conservante: 0,75% (7,5 mg/mL).	**Anestetico locale (blocca l'avvio e la conduzione degli impulsi nervosi diminuendo la permeabilità dei neuroni agli ioni sodio).** Blocco caudale: *Bambini:* 1-3,7 mg/kg. *Adulti:* 15-30 mL di 0,25% o 0,5%. Blocco epidurale: *Bambini:* 1,25 mg/kg/dose. *Adulti:* 10-20 mL di 0,25% o 0,5%. Blocco nervo periferico: 5 mL dose di 0,25% (12,5 mg) o 0,5% (25 mg) (massimo: 400 mg/24 h). Blocco nervoso simpatico: 20-50 mL di 0,25% (senza adrenalina).	*Cautela:* dosi eccessive possono portare a convulsioni, bradiaritmie, acidosi metabolica, apnea e metaemoglobinemia. Evitare l'adrenalina per il blocco nervoso in prossimità della terminazione arteriosa a causa del rischio di necrosi.
Bupropione Antidepressivo. Compresse: 75, 100 mg.	**Depressione, disturbo da deficit dell'attenzione, cessazione del fumo (blocca l'attività della serotonina e il reuptake della noradrenalina)** *Bambini:* l'esperienza aneddotica ha mostrato benefici a 75-100 mg 2-3 volte/24 h. *Adulti:* iniziare con 100 mg bid e si può gradualmente aumentare (massimo: 450 mg/24 h).	*Effetti indesiderati:* agitazione, insonnia, cefalea, psicosi, confusione, ansia, convulsioni, acatisia, febbre, brividi, secchezza delle fauci, stipsi, nausea, vomito.
Busulfano Agente antineoplastico; agente alchilante. Compresse: 2 mg.	**Trattamento della leucemia mieloide cronica (LM) o nell'ambito dell'ablazione midollare di condizionamento prima del trapianto di midollo (interferisce con l'alchilazione del DNA).** *Bambini:* (per la remissione della LM) 0,06-0,12 mg/kg/24 h; titolare la dose per mantenere la conta leucocitaria >40 000/mm^3; (per il condizionamento da trapianto del midollo) 1 mg/kg/dose ogni 6 h per 16 dosi. *Adulti:* (per la remissione della LM) 0,06 mg/kg/24 h.	*Effetti indesiderati:* grave pancitopenia, leucopenia, trombocitopenia, soppressione midollare (inizio, 7-10 giorni; nadir, 14-21 giorni; remissione, 28 giorni). *Monitoraggio:* emocromo completo con formula leucocitaria e conta delle piastrine (sospendere se leucociti <20 000/mm^3). Emoglobina, test di funzionalità epatica.
Caffeina, citrato Stimolante nel sistema nervoso centrale, non anfetaminico; stimolante respiratorio. Compresse: 65 mg (caffeina anidra 32,5 mg), citrati di caffeina, caffeina benzoato.	**Trattamento dell'apnea della prematurità (stimola l'impulso inspiratorio centrale e la sensibilità al diossido di carbonio).** *Neonati:* per os o ev (citrato o benzoato). Agisce come la caffeina base: dose da carico di 10 mg/kg. Dose di mantenimento di 5-10 mg/kg/24 h come 1 o 2 dosi/24 h.	*Cautela:* il benzoato di sodio sposta la bilirubina dal legame e dovrebbe essere evitato nei neonati con bilirubina indiretta elevata. *Effetti indesiderati:* tachicardia, agitazione, irritabilità, irritazione gastrica. *Monitoraggio:* concentrazioni di caffeina: terapeutiche >10 µg/mL; tossiche >50 µg/mL.
Calcifediolo 25-idrossicolecalciferolo; 25-idrossivitamina D_3; analogo della vitamina D. Capsule: 20, 50 µg.	**Trattamento della malattia metabolica dell'osso associata a insufficienza renale cronica (regola l'omeostasi del calcio sierico come analogo della vitamina D).** *Bambini piccoli:* 5-7 µg/kg/24 h. *Bambini e adulti:* 20-100 µg/kg al giorno titolato per ottenere normali livelli di calcio e fosfato serici.	*Cautela:* evitare in caso di ipercalcemia, ipervitaminosi D, stati di malassorbimento. Garantire un'adeguata assunzione di calcio durante l'uso. *Effetti indesiderati:* ipercalcemia, intolleranza gastrointestinale.

TABELLA 716-1. Farmaci generali – *continua*

FARMACO (PRINCIPIO ATTIVO, FORMULAZIONI)	INDICAZIONI (MECCANISMO D'AZIONE E DOSAGGIO)	COMMENTI (CAUTELE, EFFETTI INDESIDERATI, MONITORAGGIO)
Calcio, sali di (per os ed ev) Calcio carbonato. (Calcio elementare indicato tra parentesi.) Antacido; sale di calcio; supplemento elettrolitico. Capsule: 1500 mg (600 mg). Liquido: 1000 mg/5 mL (360 mL). Arresto cardiaco Pastiglia: 600 mg (240 mg). Polvere: 6,5 g/bustina. Sospensione, orale: 1250 mg/5 mL (500 mg). Compresse: 650 mg (260 mg); 1500 mg (600 mg). Compresse, masticabili.	**Tetania ipocalcemica e disturbi cardiaci da iperpotassemia (moderata performance nervosa e muscolare).** Tetania ipocalcemica. *Neonati:* 2,4 mEq/kg/24 h in dosi suddivise (se dovuta a trasfusione di sangue citrato, somministrare 0,45 mEq/dL di sangue trasfuso). *Bambini piccoli e grandi:* 10 mg/kg per 5-10 min (si può ripetere a 6-8 h), seguita da infusione con massimo 200 mg/kg/24 h. *Adulti:* 4,5-16 mEq ripetuti fino alla risposta. *Bambini piccoli e bambini:* 20 mg/kg ev e si può ripetere dopo 10 min. *Adulti:* 2-4 mg/kg ripetuti a 10 min se necessario. Calcio glucoeptato	*Cautela:* assicurarsi del sito di accesso ev per evitare gravi ustioni ev; bradicardia. *Effetti indesiderati:* stipsi, ipercalcemia, sindrome milk-alkali. *Monitoraggio:* ECG continuo; livelli serici di calcio, potassio e magnesio.
Calcio cloruro Sale di calcio; supplemento elettrolitico, parenterale. Cal Plus. (Calcio elementare indicato tra parentesi.) Iniezione: 10% = 100 mg/mL (27,2 mg/mL) (10 mL) (1,4 mEq calcio/mL).	**Prevenzione della deplezione di calcio e risoluzione dell'indigestione acida (fonte di calcio e neutralizza l'acido).** *Bambini:* *<6 mesi:* 400 mg/24 h. *6-12 mesi:* 600 mg/24 h. *1-5 anni:* 800 mg/24 h. *6-10 anni:* 800-1200 mg/24 h. *>10 anni e adulti:* 1000-1500 mg/24 h.	
Calcio edetato disodico Iniezione: 200 mg/mL.	**Antidoto per l'avvelenamento acuto e cronico da piombo (agente chelante).** *Bambini e adulti:* 500 mg/m²/dose una volta al giorno.	*Cautela:* controindicato nell'insufficienza renale grave e nei pazienti con tubercolosi attiva o lesioni tubercolari calcificate cicatrizzate. *Effetti indesiderati:* aritmie, ipotensione, convulsioni, cefalea, brividi, eruzioni cutanee, ipomagnesiemia, ipopotassemia, ipocalcemia, iperuricemia, vomito, diarrea, crampi addominali, dolore alla schiena, crampi muscolari, parestesia, tetano, nefrotossicità, arresto respiratorio. *Monitoraggio:* 24 h raccolta delle urine dopo la prima dose per il rapporto di escrezione di piombo/mg di calcio EDTA (test positivo >0,5-0,6); livello ematico di piombo.
Calcio glubionato Sale di calcio; Supplemento elettrolitico, orale. Sciroppo: 1,8 g/5 mL (115 mg/5 mL) (480 mL) (1,2 mEq calcio/mL).		
Calcitriolo Analogo della vitamina D; 1,25-diidrossicolecalciferolo, vitamina, liposolubile. Capsule: 0,25, 0,5 μg. Iniezione: 1 μg/mL (1 mL); 2 μg/mL (1 mL).	**Trattamento dell'ipocalcemia e della malattia metabolica dell'osso; riduce i livelli ormonali paratiroidei elevati e diminuisce la gravità delle lesioni psoriasiche nella psoriasi volgare (regola l'omeostasi del calcio sierico e aumenta l'assorbimento del calcio).** *Bambini piccoli prematuri* (ipocalcemia): 0,05 μg/kg/24 h ev o 1 μg/24 h per os. *Bambini:* 0,01-0,08 μg/kg/24 h. *Adulti:* 0,25-1 μg/24 h.	*Effetti indesiderati:* Ipercalcemia, tossicità da vitamina D.
Calfactant Sospensione intratracheale di surfattante polmonare di vitello (35 mg fosfolipidi, 0,65 mg proteine, 0,26 mg SP-B/mL).	**Profilassi o trattamento della sindrome da distress respiratorio e trattamento dell'ipertensione polmonare persistente.** *Neonati:* 3 mL/kg/dose 1-4 volte ogni 12 h. *Bambini e adulti:* non indicato.	*Cautela:* monitorare strettamente lo stato del ventilatore; può essere necessario uno svezzamento rapido entro min dalla dose. *Effetti indesiderati:* bradicardia, ostruzione delle vie aeree, cianosi.
Caolino e pectina Sospensione orale.	**Trattamento della diarrea non complicata (azione assorbente).** *Bambini:* *3-6 anni:* 15-30 mL/dose. *6-12 anni:* 30-60 mL/dose. *>12 anni:* 60-120 mL/dose.	*Cautela:* alcuni prodotti contengono subsalicilato bismuto e possono causare disordini del sanguinamento. Evitare nella dissenteria e nelle diarree tossigene.
Capsaicina Analgesico, topico; prodotto cutaneo topico. Crema: 0,025% (45, 90 g); 0,075% (30, 60 g). Gel: 0,025% (15, 30 mL).	**Trattamento topico del dolore associato a nevralgia posterpetica, artrite reumatoide, osteoartrite, neuropatia diabetica e dolore postchirurgico (induce il rilascio di sostanza P, con deplezione dei nervi periferici e impedendone il riaccumulo).** *Bambini >2 anni e adulti:* applicare sull'area interessata almeno tid-qid.	*Effetti indesiderati:* prurito locale, bruciore, arrossamento, eritema.
Captopril Inibitore dell'enzima di conversione dell'angiotensina (ACE); antipertensivo. Compresse: 12,5, 25, 50, 100 mg.	**Trattamento dell'ipertensione e dello scompenso.** *Neonati prematuri:* 0,01 mg/kg ogni 8-12 h. *Neonati:* dose iniziale di 0,05-0,1 mg/kg/dose ogni 8-24 h, titolata fino alla risposta (massimo: 0,5 mg/kg/dose ogni 6-24 h). *Bambini piccoli:* dose iniziale di 0,15-0,3 mg/kg/dose, titolata (massimo: 6 mg/kg/24 h in 1-4 dosi suddivise). *Bambini:* dose iniziale di 0,3-0,5 mg/kg/dose, titolata (massimo: 6 mg/kg/24 h suddivisi in 2-4 dosi). *Bambini più grandi :* dose iniziale di 6,25-12,5 mg/kg/dose ogni 12-24 h, titolata (massimo: 6 mg/kg/24 h in 2-4 dosi). *Adolescenti e adulti:* dose iniziale di 12,5-25 mg/dose, titolata (massimo: 450 mg/24 h).	*Cautela:* usare con cautela nella stenosi dell'arteria renale o nei pazienti con deplezione di volume. *Effetti indesiderati:* tosse, angioedema, oliguria, iperpotassemia.

Contenuto di sali di calcio

Sale	mg di calcio/g di sale (elementare)	mEq Ca^{2+}/g di sale
Carbonato di calcio	400	20
Cloruro di calcio	270	13,5
Calcio glubionato	64	3,2
Calcio glucoeptato	82	4,1
Calcio gluconato	90	4,5
Calcio lattato	130	6,5
Calcio fosfato	390	19,3

TABELLA 716-1. Farmaci generali – continua

FARMACO (PRINCIPIO ATTIVO, FORMULAZIONI)	INDICAZIONI (MECCANISMO D'AZIONE E DOSAGGIO)	COMMENTI (CAUTELE, EFFETTI INDESIDERATI, MONITORAGGIO)
Carbamazepina Anticonvulsivante, miscellanea. Sospensione, orale (gusto limone-vaniglia): 100 mg/5 mL (450 mL). Compresse: 200 mg. Compresse, masticabili: 100 mg. Compresse a rilascio prolungato: 100, 200, 400 mg.	**Trattamento delle convulsioni generalizzate tonico-cloniche e parziali, riduzione del dolore nella nevralgia del trigemino e nella neuropatia diabetica e trattamento del disturbo bipolare (limita l'afflusso di ioni sodio attraverso le membrane cellulari o mediante altri meccanismi sconosciuti).** *Bambini:* *<6 anni:* dose iniziale di 5 mg/kg/24 h in 2-4 dosi suddivise; si può aumentare ogni 5-7 giorni di 5 mg/kg, in base all'effetto o alla tossicità e alla concentrazione sierica. *6-12 anni:* dose iniziale di10 mg/kg/24 h in 2-4 dosi suddivise; aumentare di 100 mg o 5 mg/kg/24 h a intervalli settimanali fino al raggiungimento dei livelli terapeutici (dose usuale: 800-1200 mg/24 h). *Adulti:* dose iniziale di 200 mg bid; aumentare di 200 mg a intervalli settimanali fino terapeutiche al raggiungimento dei livelli (dose usuale: 1,6-2,4 g/24 h in 3-4 dosi suddivise).	*Cautela:* evitare nei pazienti con depressione del midollo osseo; può presentare reazione incrociata nei pazienti con ipersensibilità agli antidepressivi triciclici. *Effetti indesiderati:* sedazione, vertigini, affaticamento, atassia, confusione, nausea, vomito, offuscamento del visus, nistagmo, depressione del midollo osseo, leucopenia, neutropenia, trombocitopenia, pancitopenia, anemia aplastica, epatite, reazioni da ipersensibilità. *Monitoraggio:* concentrazioni seriche correlate alla risposta clinica (6-12 μg/mL), e tossicità neurologica e visiva (>8 μg/mL, ma particolarmente >12 μg/mL). La necessità di dosare il farmaco aumenteranno per le prime 4 sett a causa dell'induzione dell'enzima epatico da parte della carbamazepina. Monitorare le concentrazioni seriche per aumentare appropriatamente le dosi.
Carbamide perossido Agente otologico, ceruminolitico. Gel, orale: 11% (36 g). Soluzione, orale: 10% in glicerina (15, 22,5, 30, 60 mL). Otologico: 6,5% in glicerina (15, 30 mL).	**Riduzione dell'infiammazione lieve della mucosa orale, incluse gengive e labbra, e rimozione del cerume dall'orecchio (rilascio di perossido di idrogeno, che inibisce i batteri e ammorbidisce il cerume dell'orecchio).** *Bambini e adulti:* Gel: massaggiare delicatamente sull'area interessata qid. Soluzione orale: applicare diverse gocce sull'area interessata qid per un massimo di 7 giorni. (espettorare 2-3 min dopo ogni uso). Soluzione otologica: inclinare la testa da un lato e instillare 5-10 gocce bid fino a 4 giorni. Tenere le gocce nel canale uditivo per diversi min inclinando la testa e introducendo del cotone nell'orecchio.	*Effetti indesiderati:* irritazione locale.
Carbinoxamina e pseudoefedrina Antistaminico/associazione di decongestionanti. Gocce: carbinoxamina maleato 2 mg e pseudoefedrina idrocloruro 25 mg/mL (30 mL con contagocce). Sciroppo: carbinoxamina maleato 4 mg e pseudoefedrina idrocloruro 60 mg/5 mL (120, 480 mL). Compresse, rivestite da film: carbinoxamina maleato 4 mg e pseudoefedrina idrocloruro 60 mg. Compresse a rilascio prolungato: carbinoxamina maleato 8 mg e pseudoefedrina idrocloruro 120 mg.	**Riduzione temporanea di congestione nasale, rinorrea, starnuti e sintomi da allergia (antistaminico come bloccante H_1, e decongestionante come stimolante dei recettori α e β).** *Bambini:* somministrare qid: *1-3 mesi:* 1/4 contagocce (0,25 mL). *3-6 mesi:* 1/2 contagocce (0,5 mL). *6-9 mesi:* 3/4 contagocce (0,75 mL). *9-18 mesi:* 1 contagocce (1,0 mL). *18 mesi-6 anni:* 2,5 mL sciroppo. *6-12 anni:* 5 mL sciroppo o 1 compresse. *Bambini >12 anni e adulti:* 1 compressa qid o 1 compressa a rilascio prolungato bid.	*Cautela:* evitare in caso di glaucoma ad angolo stretto, cardiopatia coronarica, ostruzione gastrointestinale o genitourinaria o terapia con inibitori delle monoamino ossidasi. *Effetti indesiderati:* ipertensione, tachicardia, sonnolenza, sedazione, ispessimento delle secrezioni bronchiali.
Carbone vegetale Assorbente, antidoto.	**Trattamento di emergenza dell'avvelenamento dovuto a certi farmaci e sostanze chimiche; dialisi gastrointestinale per favorire l'eliminazione di determinati farmaci e tossine; trattamento della diarrea (assorbe le sostanze tossiche; interferisce con il ricircolo enteroepatico di certi farmaci).** *Bambini e adulti:* 1-2 g/kg o 5-10 × il peso della sostanza nociva ingerita (limitare il sorbitolo a 1-2 × giorno); le dosi si possono ripetere ogni 2-6 h.	*Effetti indesiderati:* stipsi, feci nere.
Carboplatino Agente antineoplastico; agente alchilante. Polvere per iniezione, liofilizzato: 50, 150, 450 mg.	**Trattamento di vari tumori, tra cui i tumori cerebrali pediatricio e il neuroblastoma (la platinazione del DNA interferisce con la funzione del DNA).** *Bambini:* Tumore solido: 300-600 mg/m² ev 1 × ogni 4 sett. Tumore cerebrale: 175 mg/m² ev 1 × sett per 4 sett (periodo di 2 sett di remissione tra i trattamenti). *Adulti:* 360 mg/m² ev 1 × ogni 4 sett.	*Effetti indesiderati:* neutropenia, leucopenia, trombocitopenia, neuropatia periferica, ototossicità, alterazioni della funzionalità epatica e renale, alopecia, nausea, vomito. *Monitoraggio:* la conta dei neutrofili e delle piastrine condiziona la scelta della dose come segue: piastrine <50 000/mm³ o neutrofili <500/mm³: somministrare il 75% della dose raccomandata (nadir: 14-21 giorni post dose).
Carmustina Agente antineoplastico; agente alchilante (nitrosourea). Polvere per iniezione: 100 mg/fiala confezionate con 3 mL di alcol assoluto da usare come diluente sterile.	**Trattamento dei tumori, tumore cerebrale, malattia di Hodgkin, linfoma non-Hodgkin e mieloma multiplo (inibisce le reazioni enzimatiche chiave coinvolte nella sintesi del DNA).** *Bambini:* 200-250 mg/m² ev ogni 4-6 sett in monosomministrazione. *Adulti:* 150-200 mg/m² ev ogni 6 sett in monosomministrazione.	*Effetti indesiderati:* nausea, vomito, mielosoppressione (nadir 4-6 sett post dose), alopecia, stomatite, anoressia, diarrea, vertigini, atassia, fibrosi polmonare, insufficienza renale ed epatica, retinite, neurite ottica.
Carnitina Supplemento alimentare. Capsule: 250 mg. Iniezione: 1 g/5 mL (5 mL). Liquido (gusto ciliegia): 100 mg/mL (10 mL). Compresse: 330 mg.	**Trattamento del deficit di carnitina; migliora l'uso delle emulsioni grasse ev nei neonati prematuri (facilita l'ingresso degli acidi grassi a catena lunga nei mitocondri e necessari nel metabolismo energetico).** *Neonati prematuri:* 8-16 mg/kg/24 h infusione ev. *Bambini:* 50-100 mg/kg/24 h in 2-3 dosi suddivise per os, 50 mg/kg/dose ogni 4-6 h ev (massimo: 300 mg/kg/24 h). *Adulti:* 0,33-1 g/dose bid-tid, per os, 50 mg/kg/dose ogni 4-6 h (massimo: 300 mg/kg/24 h).	*Effetti indesiderati:* nausea, vomito, crampi addominali, odore corporeo sgradevole.
Carvedilolo Compresse: 3,125, 6,25, 12,5, 25 mg.	**Bloccante dei recettori β con attività vasodilatante, usato per trattare lo scompenso cardiaco o l'ipertensione.** *Bambini:* dose iniziale di 0,08 mg/kg, aumentati gradualmente per 2-3 m, in base alla risposta (massimo: 0,5 mg/kg/24 h suddivisi ogni 12 h).	*Cautela:* può causare blocco AV, aritmie, bradicardia, o peggiorare l'asma o lo scompenso. *Interazioni farmacologiche:* può causare ipotensione eccessiva quando usato con altri antipertensivi.
Cascara sagrada Lassativo; stimolante. Liquido, estratto fluido aromatico: 5, 120 mL. Compresse: 325 mg.	**Risoluzione temporanea della stipsi (irritazione chimica diretta della mucosa gastrointestinale).** *Bambini piccoli:* 1,25 mL una volta al giorno. *Bambini 2-11 anni:* 2,5 mL una volta al giorno. *>12 anni e adulti:* 5 mL una volta al giorno.	*Cautela:* impattamento fecale, ostruzione gastrointestinale, sanguinamento gastrointestinale. Inizio dell'effetto 6-10 h, quindi somministrare all'ora di andare a letto. *Effetti indesiderati:* crampi gastrointestinali, urine di colore rosso o marrone.

TABELLA 716-1. Farmaci generali – *continua*

FARMACO (PRINCIPIO ATTIVO, FORMULAZIONI)	INDICAZIONI (MECCANISMO D'AZIONE E DOSAGGIO)	COMMENTI (CAUTELE, EFFETTI INDESIDERATI, MONITORAGGIO)
Cianocobalamina, vitamina B_{12} Supplemento nutrizionale. Iniezione: 100, 1000 μg/mL. Compresse: 25, 50,100, 250, 500, 1000 μg.	**Anemia perniciosa, deficit di vitamina B_{12} (coenzima per varie funzioni metaboliche).** Anemia perniciosa: *Bambini:* 30-50 μg/24 h fino alla dose totale di 1000-5000 μg, e poi proseguire con 100 μg/mese. *Adulti:* 100 μg/24 h per 6-7 giorni, poi 100 μg/mese. Deficit di vitamina B_{12}: *Bambini:* 100 μg/24 h per 10-15 giorni, poi 1-2×/sett per diversi mesi. *Adulti:* 30 μg/24 h per 5-10 giorni poi 100-200 μg/mese.	*Monitoraggio:* livelli serici di B_{12} (normali: 150-750 pg/mL). Sono stati riportati alcuni casi di problemi neuropsichiatrici per livelli <300 pg/mL.
Ciclizina Antinausea. Iniezione: 50 mg/mL. Compresse: 50 mg.	**Previene e tratta la nausea, il vomito e la vertigine da movimento; controlla la nausea e il vomito postoperatori (meccanismo sconosciuto).** *Bambini 6-12 anni:* per os: 25 mg/dose fino a 3×/24 h se necessario. *Adulti:* per os: 50 mg fino a ogni 4-6 h (30 min prima del viaggio) (massimo: 200 mg/24 h); im 50 mg ogni 4-6 h se necessario.	*Effetti indesiderati:* sonnolenza, secchezza delle fauci, cefalea, diplopia, ritenzione urinaria.
Ciclofosfamide Agente alchilante antineoplastico. Polvere per iniezione: 0,1, 0,2, 0,5, 1,0, 2,0 g. Compresse: 25, 50 mg.	**Trattamento di vari tumori, tra cui malattia di Hodgkin, linfomi maligni e leucemie; sindrome nefrosica; lupus eritematoso sistemico; artrite reumatoide; vasculite reumatoide (interferisce con la normale funzione del DNA mediante alchilazione).** *Bambini e adulti con problemi non ematologici:* Induzione: ev: 40-50 mg/kg (1,5-1,8 g/m²) in dosi suddivise per 2-5 giorni. per os: 1-5 mg/kg/24 h. Mantenimento: ev: 10-15 mg/kg (350-550 mg/m²) ogni 7-10 giorni o 3-5 mg/kg 2×/sett. per os: *Bambini:* 2-5 mg/kg 2×/sett. *Adulti:* 1-5 mg/kg/24 h. *Bambini:* LES: 500-750 mg/m²/mese. AR giovanile/vasculite: ev 10 mg/kg ogni 2 sett. Condizionamento per trapianto del midollo osseo: ev 50 mg/kg/24 h per 3-4 giorni. Sindrome nefrosica: per os: 2-3 mg/kg/24 h (quando gli steroidi falliscono, usare fino a 12 sett). Aggiustare le dosi per: Funzione renale: CrCl 25-50 mL/min: diminuire del 50%. CrCl <25 mL/min: evitare l'uso. Diminuita funzionalità del midollo osseo: ridurre la dose del 33-50%.	*Cautela:* mantenere un'elevata assunzione di liquidi per evitare la cistite emorragica, e prendere in considerazione la somministrazione di mesna. *Effetti indesiderati:* cardiotossicità ad alte dosi, versamento pericardico, scompenso cardiaco congestizio, alopecia, nausea, vomito, disgeusia, stomatite, anoressia, cistite emorragica, leucopenia (inizio: 7 giorni; nadir: 8-15 giorni; remissione: 21 giorni), trombocitopenia, epatotossicità, ittero, tossicità renale, neoplasia secondaria.
Ciclopentolato Midriatico. Soluzione oftalmica: 0,5%, 1%, 2%.	**Procedure diagnostiche che richiedono midriasi e cicloplegia (impedisce che i muscoli del corpo ciliare e dell'ride rispondano agli stimoli colinergici).** *Bambini piccoli:* 1 goccia 0,5% in ogni occhio 5-10 min prima dell'esame. *Bambini e adulti:* 1 goccia 0,5% o 1% nell'occhio 40-50 min prima della procedura (si può ripetere 1 goccia dopo 5 min se necessario); si può usare al 2% se l'iride è molto pigmentata.	*Cautela:* evitare in caso di glaucoma ad angolo stretto. *Effetti indesiderati:* tachicardia, stimolazione del SNC, psicosi, agitazione, arrossamento locale. *Monitoraggio:* cicloplegia e midriasi iniziano entro 15-60 min e durano fino a 24 h (ridurre a 3-6 h con pilocarpina).
Cimetidina Antagonista dell'istamina₂. Compresse: 200, 300, 400, 800 mg. Liquido: 300 mg/5 mL. Iniezione: 150 mg/mL.	**Trattamento a breve termine e profilassi a lungo termine del reflusso gastroesofageo, dell'ulcera gastrointestinale e dell'iperacidità (inibizione competitiva dell'istamina a livello dei recettori H_2).** *Neonati:* per os, ev, im: 5-10 mg/kg/24 h suddivisi ogni 8-12 h. *Bambini:* per os, ev, im: 20-40 mg/kg/24 h suddivisi ogni 6 h. *Adulti:* 300 mg ogni 6 h (aumentare l'intervallo delle dosi se clearance della creatinina è <40 mL/min).	*Cautela:* potente inibitore enzimatico che può causare accumulo tossico di farmaci che sono metabolizzati (per es. antidepressivi, anticonvulsivanti, teofillina, warfarin, cisapride). *Effetti indesiderati:* vertigini, sonnolenza, bradicardia. *Monitoraggio:* pH gastrico target ≥5.
Ciproeptadina idrocloruro Antistaminico. Sciroppo: 2 mg/5 mL. Compresse: 4 mg.	**Trattamento di sintomi allergici (antagonista dei recettori H_1 e della serotonina).** *Bambini:* *2-6 anni:* 2 mg/dose ogni 8-12 h (massimo: 12 mg/24h). *>7 anni-adulti:* 4 mg/dose ogni 8-12 h (massimo: 0,5 mg/kg/24 h).	*Effetti indesiderati:* sonnolenza, sedazione, ispessimento delle secrezioni bronchiali, broncospasmo, stimolazione dell'appetito, fotosensibilità.
Cisapride Agente gastrointestinale procinetico. Compresse: 10 mg.	**Trattamento del reflusso gastroesofageo, della gastroparesi e della stipsi refrattaria (aumenta il rilascio di acetilcolina a livello del plesso mioenterico).** *Neonati-bambini:* 0,15-0,3 mg/kg/dose tid-qid. *Adulti:* 10-20 mg qid. Somministrare la dose 15-30 min prima dei pasti.	*Cautela:* alte dosi o l'associazione con inibitori enzimatici (per es. eritromicina, cimetidina) può causare prolungamento del tratto Q-T, predisponendo a torsioni di punta. *Effetti indesiderati:* tachicardia, allungamento dell'intervallo Q-T, cefalea, ansia, insonnia, crampi gastrointestinali, flatulenza, diarrea. *Monitoraggio:* ECG basale e trattamento precoce.
Cisplatino Agente antineoplastico; agente alchilante. Iniezione, acqueo: 1 mg/mL. Polvere per iniezione: 10, 50 mg.	**Trattamento di vari tipi di tumore (inibisce la sintesi di DNA).** *Bambini e adulti:* 37-75 mg/m² una volta ogni 2-3 sett o 50-120 mg/m² una volta ogni 21-28 giorni (somministrare in 4-6 h). Modificare la dose nell'insufficienza renale: CrCl 10-50 mL/min = 75% della dose; CrCl <10 mL/min = 50% della dose.	*Effetti indesiderati:* nausea, vomito dura fino a 1settimana post dose), mielosoppressione (inizio, 10 giorni; nadir, 14-23 giorni; remissione, 21-39 giorni), insufficienza renale acuta, nefropatia cronica (perdita di sodio, magnesio e acqua; iperuricemia), neuropatia periferica (irreversibile), ototossicità (alta frequenza di perdita dell'udito), lesioni da stravaso, aumento degli enzimi epatici, alopecia, neurite ottica, aritmie.

TABELLA 716-1. Farmaci generali – *continua*

FARMACO (PRINCIPIO ATTIVO, FORMULAZIONI)	INDICAZIONI (MECCANISMO D'AZIONE E DOSAGGIO)	COMMENTI (CAUTELE, EFFETTI INDESIDERATI, MONITORAGGIO)
Cisteina Supplemento nutrizionale. Iniezione: 50 mg/mL.	**Supplemento alle soluzioni cristalline di aminoacidi per soddisfare le richieste nutrizionali di aminoacidi durante la nutrizione parenterale (corregge il deficit; aumenta anche la solubilità di calcio e fosfato nelle soluzioni parenterali totali nutritive).** *Neonati e bambini piccoli:* aggiungere 40 mg di cisteina a 1 g di aminoacidi (in genere porta a 20-100 mg/kg/24 h di cisteina).	*Effetti indesiderati:* acidosi metabolica, uremia, iperazotemia, nausea.
Citarabina HCl, Ara-C Antineoplastico; antimetabolita. Polvere per iniezione: 0,1, 0,5, 1, 2 g. Iniezione: 20 mg/mL.	**Utilizzata nella terapia di combinazione per trattare leucemie e linfomi (inibisce la DNA polimerasi a inibire la sintesi di DNA lavora nella S-fase della divisione cellulare).** *Bambini e adulti:* le dosi dipendono dai protocolli individuali. Dose tipica: Induzione: ev: 100-200 mg/m²/24 h per 5-10 giorni o fino alla remissione. Mantenimento: ev: 70-200 mg/m²/24 h per 2-5 giorni a intervalli mensili. im, sc: 1-1,5 mg/kg monodose a intervalli di 1-4 sett. it 5-75 mg/m² ogni 2-7 giorni fino a che i reperti del SNC si normalizzano (la concentrazione non dovrebbe eccedere i 100 mg/mL).	*Effetti indesiderati:* febbre, rash, ulcerazioni orali/anali, nausea, vomito, diarrea, mucosite, disfunzione epatica, sanguinamento, mielosoppressione (inizio, 4-7 giorni; nadir, 14-18 giorni; remissione 21-28 giorni), alopecia, congiuntivite (somministrare gocce oculari di corticosteroide per 24 ore prima, durante e dopo Ara-C ad alte dosi), vertigini, cefalea, neurite (previene tossicità SNC con piridossina somministrazione nei giorni Ara-C ad alte dosi).
Citrato, soluzioni Agente alcalinizzante. Citrato di sodio 500 mg e acido citrico 334 mg/5 mL = 1 mEq sodio + 1 mEq bicarbonato equivalente/mL. Citrato di sodio 500 mg e acido citrico 334 mg e citrato di potassio 550 mg/5 mL = 1 mEq sodio + 1 mEq potassio + 2 mEq bicarbonato equivalente/mL.	**Trattamento dell'acidosi metabolica cronica (i sali di citrato vengono ossidati nell'organismo per formare bicarbonato).** *Neonati, bambini piccoli e grandi:* 2-3 mEq/kg/24 h in 3-4 dosi suddivise con acqua dopo i pasti. *Adulti:* 15-30 mL con acqua dopo pasti e prima di andare a letto.	*Effetti indesiderati:* ipernatremia, iperpotassemia, alcalosi metabolica.
Clomipramina Antidepressivo. Capsule: 25, 50, 75 mg.	**Trattamento del disturbo ossessivo-compulsivo e degli attacchi di panico (agisce sull'uptake di serotonina e di noradrenalina).** *Bambini:* dose iniziale di 25 mg/24 h, gradualmente aumentata alla risposta (massimo: 200 mg/24 h). *Adulti:* dose iniziale di 25 mg/24 h, aumentata fino alla risposta (massimo: 250 mg/24 h).	*Effetti indesiderati:* vertigini, sonnolenza, secchezza delle fauci, stipsi, nausea, aumento del peso, nervosismo, ansia, convulsioni, ipotensione, aritmie, sindrome parkinsoniana, insonnia.
Clonazepam Benzodiazepina. Compresse: 0,5, 1, 2 mg.	**Profilassi di alcuni tipi di convulsioni: assenza, Lennox-Gastaut acinetica, mioclonica (deprime la trasmissione nervosa nella corteccia motoria).** *Bambini:* 0,01-0,3 mg/kg/24 h in 2-3 dosi suddivise, aumentati di 0,5 mg/24 h ogni 3-5 giorni alla risposta (massimo: 0,3 mg/kg/24 h). *Adulti:* dose iniziale di 0,1 mg bid; poi 0,2-2,4 mg/24 h in 2-4 dosi suddivise.	*Effetti indesiderati:* tachicardia, dolore toracico, sonnolenza, affaticamento, alterata memoria e coordinazione, depressione, visione offuscata, nausea, vomito, secchezza delle fauci, ipersalivazione, anoressia, ipersecrezione bronchiale, depressione respiratoria, dipendenza fisica e psicologica. *Monitoraggio:* concentrazioni di clonazepam: terapeutiche 20-80 ng/mL; tossiche >80 ng/mL; perdita di efficacia con l'uso prolungato (tachifilassi).
Clonidina Agonista α-adrenergico. Compresse: 0,1, 0,2, 0,3 mg. Cerotto transdermico: 0,1, 0,2, 0,3 mg/24 h.	**Trattamento dell'ipertensione, del disturbo da deficit dell'attenzione (ADD) e dell'astinenza da narcotici; aiuta nella diagnosi di feocromocitoma e di deficit dell'ormone della crescita (stimola gli adrenorecettori α_2 nel tronco cerebrale).** *Neonati:* astinenza da narcotici: 1 µg/kg ogni 6-8 h per iniziare e si può titolare fino allo score di astinenza calcolato (massimo: 2 µg/kg/dose ogni 4 h). *Bambini:* ADD: dose iniziale di 0,05 mg/24 h, aumentata ogni 3-7 giorni di 0,05 mg/24 h somministrati in 3-4 dosi suddivise alla risposta (massimo: 0,4 mg/24 h). Ipertensione: 5-10 µg/kg/24 h in 2-4 dosi suddivise (massimo: 0,9 mg/24 h). Test di tolleranza alla clonidina per il rilascio di ormone della crescita: 4 µg/kg × 1 dose. *Adulti:* Ipertensione: per os: 0,2-2,4 mg/24 h in 2-4 dosi titolate alla risposta. Transdermico: 0,1-0,3 mg/24 h titolato all'effetto.	*Cautela:* titolare le dosi gradualmente per evitare i sintomi dell'iperattività simpatica. *Effetti indesiderati:* sonnolenza, vertigini, secchezza delle fauci, stipsi, ipotensione.
Clorazepato Benzodiazepina. Compresse: 3,75, 7,5, 15 mg.	**Ansia e disturbo da panico; come aggiunta nel trattamento delle convulsioni parziali (facilita la trasmissione del neurotrasmettitore inibitorio, acido γ-aminobutirrico).** *Bambini:* *9-12 anni:* 3,75-7,5 mg/dose bid (massimo: 60 mg/24 h). *>12 anni e adulti:* 7,5 mg/dose bid-tid (massimo: 90 mg/24 h). *Adulti:* 7,5-15 mg/dose bid-qid.	*Effetti indesiderati:* sonnolenza, confusione, depressione, visione offuscata.
Cloralio idrato Ipnotico; sedativo. Capsule: 250, 500 mg. Sciroppo: 250, 500 mg/5 mL. Supposte: 324, 500, 648 mg.	**Sedativo-ipnotico a breve termine (meccanismo sconosciuto).** *Neonati:* 25 mg/kg/dose. *Bambini piccoli e bambini:* 25-100 mg/kg/dose. *Adulti:* 250-1000 mg/dose. La dose può essere ripetuta ogni 6-8 h. Dosi all'estremo inferiore causano sedazione; dosi all'estremo superiore causano ipnosi.	*Cautela:* la ripetizione delle dosi nei neonati può causare accumulo del metabolita attivo tricloroetanolo, che può causare tossicità epatica e spostamento della bilirubina.
Clorambucil Agente alchilante antineoplastico. Compresse: 2 mg.	**Trattamento di vari tumori, tra cui malattia di Hodgkin, linfoma non-Hodgkin e leucemia linfocitica cronica, e della sindrome nefrosica (interferisce con l'alchilazione della replicazione del DNA e la trascrizione dell'RNA).** *Bambini e adulti:* 0,1-0,2 mg/kg/24 h per 3-6 sett. Dosi di trattamento più lunghe sono calcolate in base all'emocromo.	*Effetti indesiderati:* soppressione del midollo osseo (inizio, 7 giorni; nadir, 10-14 giorni; remissione, 28 giorni); rash, iperuricemia, nausea, vomito, diarrea, ulcerazione orale, fibrosi polmonare, necrosi epatica, neuropatia periferica.

TABELLA 716-1. Farmaci generali – *continua*

FARMACO (PRINCIPIO ATTIVO, FORMULAZIONI)	INDICAZIONI (MECCANISMO D'AZIONE E DOSAGGIO)	COMMENTI (CAUTELE, EFFETTI INDESIDERATI, MONITORAGGIO)
Clorfeniramina maleato Antistaminico. Capsule: 12 mg. Capsule, a rilascio prolungato: 6, 8, 12 mg. Sciroppo: 2 mg/5 mL. Compresse: 4, 8, 12 mg. Compresse; masticabili: 2 mg. Compresse; a rilascio prolungato: 8, 12 mg.	**Trattamento dei sintomi allergici (compete con l'istamina per i siti recettoriali H_1).** *Bambini:* *2-6 anni:* 1 mg ogni 4-6 h. *6-12 anni:* 2 mg ogni 2-6 h, o formulazione a rilascio prolungato, 8 mg prima di andare a letto. *>12 anni e adulti:* 4 mg ogni 4-6 h, o formulazione a rilascio prolungato, 12 mg prima di andare a letto.	*Effetti indesiderati:* sonnolenza, eccitazione o iperattività (nei bambini), secchezza delle fauci, visione offuscata.
Clorpromazina Fenotiazina. Capsule: 30, 75, 150, 200, 300 mg. Concentrato orale: 30, 100 mg/mL. Supposte : 25, 100 mg. Sciroppo: 10 mg/5 mL. Compresse: 10, 25, 50, 100, 200 mg. Iniezione: 25 mg/mL.	**Trattamento di psicosi, mania, sindrome di Tourette, problemi comportamentali, nausea e vomito (blocca i recettori postsinaptici mesolimbici dopaminergici nel cervello, potente effetto bloccante α-adrenergico).** *Bambini >6 mesi:* per os: 0,5-1 mg/kg/dose ogni 4-6 h. rettale: 1 mg/kg/dose ogni 6-8 h. im o ev: 0,5-1 mg/kg/dose ogni 6-8 h. *Adulti:* Psicosi: per os: 30-800 mg/24 h in 1-4 dosi suddivise (partire a basse dosi e titolare fino all'effetto). ev o im: 25 mg dose iniziale, titolata fino all'effetto (massimo: 400 mg/dose ogni 4-6 h). Nausea o vomito: per os: 10-25 mg ogni 4-6 h. im o ev: 25-50 mg ogni 4-6 h. rettale: 50-100 mg ogni 6-8 h.	*Effetti indesiderati:* ipotensione, tachicardia, aritmie, pseudoparkinsonismo, discinesia tardiva, acatisia, distonie, stipsi, congestione nasale, secchezza delle fauci, iperpiressia maligna. *Monitoraggio:* concentrazioni di clorpromazina: terapeutiche 50-300 ng/mL; tossico >750 ng/mL.
Clorpropamide Sulfonilurea. Compresse: 100, 250 mg.	**Controllo della glicemia nel diabete mellito non-insulino-dipendente (tipo II)** (stimola il rilascio di insulina dalle cellule delle isole pancreatiche). *Adulti:* dose iniziale 250 mg una volta al giorno, si può aumentare alla risposta di 125 mg ogni 3-5 giorni alla risposta (massimo: 750 mg/24 h).	*Effetti indesiderati:* problemi gastrointestinali, fotosensibilità, epatotossicità, iponatremia, sindrome da inappropriata secrezione di ormone antidiuretico.
Clortalidone Diuretico tiazidico. Compresse: 20, 25, 100 mg.	**Trattamento del sovraccarico di volume e dell'ipertensione lieve (inibisce il riassorbimento di sodio e di cloro nel segmento corticale diluente dell'ansa ascendente di Henle).** *Bambini:* 1-2 mg/kg una volta al giorno. *Adulti:* 25-100 mg una volta al giorno.	*Effetti indesiderati:* fotosensibilità, alterazione dell'equilibrio idroelettrolitico, ipopotassemia.
Clortiazide Diuretico. Compresse: 250, 500 mg. Sospensione: 250 mg/5 mL. Polvere per iniezione: 500 mg.	**Trattamento degli stati di sovraccarico di volume e dell' ipertensione (inibisce il riassorbimento di sodio nel tubulo distale).** *Neonati e bambini piccoli <6 mesi:* per os: 20-40 mg/kg/24 h suddivisi ogni 12 h; ev: 2-8 mg/kg/24 h suddivisi ogni 12 h. *Bambini piccoli >6 mesi e bambini:* per os: 20 mg/kg/24 h in 2 dosi suddivise; ev: 4 mg/kg/24 h. *Adulti:* per os: 500 mg-2 g/24 h in 1-2 dosi; ev: 500-1,000 mg/24 h.	*Effetti indesiderati:* ipopotassemia, alcalosi ipocloremica, iperglicemia, iperlipidemia, ipercalcemia, iperuricemia, leucopenia, uremia prerenale.
Clorzoxazone Rilassante del muscolo scheletrico. Compresse: 250, 500 mg.	**Riduzione sintomatica dello spasmo muscolare e del dolore (deprime i riflessi polisinaptici nel midollo spinale e ai livelli subcorticali).** *Bambini:* 20 mg/kg/24 h in 3-4 dosi suddivise. *Adulti:* 250-500 mg tid-qid.	*Effetti indesiderati:* sonnolenza.
Clozapina Compresse: 25, 100 mg.	**Antipsicotico atipico, gruppo chimico dibenzepino.** *Bambini:* dose iniziale di 6,25 mg bid, aumentata a 6,25 mg/24 h alla sett se necessario. Dose tipica: 50-300 mg/24 h. *Adulti:* dose iniziale di 25 mg ogni 24 h, titolata fino a 25-50 mg/24 h fino a 450-500 mg/24 h suddivisi tid a 2 sett. Ulteriori aumenti di dose non dovrebbero superare i 100 mg/sett (massimo: 900 mg/24 h).	*Cautela:* agranulocitosi, talvolta fatale, è stata riportata nell'1,3% dei pazienti. Perciò, si deve effettuare la conta basale dei leucociti che deve essere ripetuta ogni sett per i primi 6 mesi di trattamento, poi ogni due sett. La conta dei leucociti deve essere controllata ogni altra sett dopo. Se la clozapina viene sospesa, controllare i leucociti settimanalmente per le successive 4 sett. *Effetti indesiderati:* convulsioni, ipotensione ortostatica, sintomi extrapiramidali (meno spesso degli antipsicotici tipici), iperglicemia, vertigini, sonnolenza, cefalea, tremore, salivazione eccessiva (specialmente durante il sonno). *Interazioni farmacologiche:* i livelli di clozapina possono aumentare con l'uso concomitante di inibitori enzimatici. La clozapina ha un elevato legame con le proteine e può spiazzare altri farmaci ad alto legame alle proteine (per es. warfarin).
Codeina Analgesico narcotico. Prodotti di combinazione. Iniezione. Compresse.	**Trattamento del dolore lieve moderato e della tosse (inibizione delle vie dolorifiche ascendenti; azione centrale nel midollo per sopprimere la tosse).** *Bambini:* Dolore: 0,5-1 mg/kg/dose ogni 4-6 h (massimo: 60 mg/dose). Tosse: 1-1,5 mg/kg/24 h suddivisi ogni 4-6 h. *Adulti:* Dolore: 15-60 mg/dose ogni 4-6 h se necessario. Tosse: 10-20 mg/dose ogni 4-6 h (massimo: 120 mg/24 h).	*Effetti indesiderati:* sonnolenza, stipsi, nausea, anoressia, vomito, sedazione, vertigini.

TABELLA 716-1. Farmaci generali – *continua*

FARMACO (PRINCIPIO ATTIVO, FORMULAZIONI)	INDICAZIONI (MECCANISMO D'AZIONE E DOSAGGIO)	COMMENTI (CAUTELE, EFFETTI INDESIDERATI, MONITORAGGIO)
Colchicina Agente anti-infiammatorio/antigottoso. Iniezione: 0,5 mg/mL. Compresse: 0,5, 0,6 mg.	**Trattamento della febbre mediterranea familiare e dell'artrite gottosa acuta e cronica (diminuisce la motilità dei leucociti e la fagocitosi nelle articolazioni).** *Bambini:* Profilassi della febbre mediterranea familiare: *<5 anni:* 0,5 mg/24 h *>5 anni:* 1-1,5 mg/24 h in 2-3 dosi suddivise. *Adulti:* Artrite gottosa: per os: 0,5-0,6 mg ogni 2 h fino al sollievo dei sintomi o in caso di tossicità gastrointestinale (massimo: 8 mg/24 h). ev: dose da carico di 1-3 mg, poi 0,5 mg/dose ogni 6 h fino alla risposta (massimo: 4 mg/24 h).	*Cautela:* ridurre la dose del 50% se CrCl <10 mL/min. *Effetti indesiderati:* nausea, vomito, diarrea, dolore addominale.
Colestiramina resina Agente antilipidemico. Polvere: 4 g resina/9 g polvere.	**Trattamento dell'ipercolesterolemia (forma complessi non assorbibili con i sali biliari e il colesterolo LDL).** *Bambini:* 240 mg/kg/24 h in 3 dosi suddivise. *Adulti:* 4 g/dose 1-6 × al giorno.	*Effetti indesiderati:* acidosi ipercloremica, stipsi, nausea, vomito, dolore e distensione addominale, malassorbimento delle vitamine liposolubili.
Colfosceril palmitato Surfattante polmonare. Sospensione intratracheale: 108 mg/10 mL.	**Sindrome neonatale da distress respiratorio (RDS) (sostituisce il surfattante deficitario, riduce la tensione superficiale in corrispondenza dell'interfaccia aria-liquido negli alveoli).** *Neonati:* 5 mL/kg/dose come profilassi o terapia rescue per la RDS (massimo: 4 dosi, sebbene non vi sia un benefico provato per >2 dosi).	*Cautela:* somministrare attraverso la porta laterale usando uno speciale adattatore del tubo endotracheale, 1/2 dose con la testa e il tronco piegati a sinistra e 1/2 dose con testa e tronco piegati a destra; somministrare ogni 1/2 in 1-2 min. *Effetti indesiderati:* emorragia polmonare, iperventilazione (che causa iperossia e ipocarbia), pervietà del dotto arterioso.
Colina magnesio trisalicilato Agente anti-infiammatorio non steroideo. Liquido: 500 mg salicilato/5 mL. Compresse: 500, 750, 1000 mg.	**Trattamento delle malattie artritiche (inibisce la sintesi di prostaglandine).** *Bambini:* 30-60 mg/kg/24 h in 3-4 dosi suddivise. *Adulti:* 500-1500 mg/dose 1-3 × al giorno.	*Cautela:* evitare nei pazienti con sospetta influenza o varicella a causa del rischio di sindrome di Reye; evitare nei soggetti con asma e in quelli a rischio di reazioni da ipersensibilità gravi. *Effetti indesiderati:* intolleranza gastrointestinale, tinnito, epatotossicità, edema polmonare. *Monitoraggio:* concentrazioni di salicilato: anti-infiammatorio 150-300 μg/mL; effetto analgesico o antipiretico 30-50 μg/mL.
Corticotropina, ACTH Corticosteroide surrenalico. Iniezione, repository: 40, 80 U/mL. Compresse: 5, 10, 25 mg.	**Spasmi infantili, agente diagnostico nell'insufficienza corticosurrenalica, riacutizzazioni della sclerosi multipla, grave debolezza muscolare nella miastenia gravis (stimola la corteccia surrenalica a rilasciare steroidi surrenalici, sostanze androgene e una piccola quantità di aldosterone).** *Bambini:* Infiammazione o immunosoppressione: ev, im, sc (acquosa): 1,6 U/kg/24 h o 50 U/m^2 suddivise ogni 6-8 h. im (gel): 0,8 U/kg/24 h o 25 U/m^2 giorno suddivise ogni 12-24 h. Spasmi infantili: 5-160 U/kg/24 h sono stati usati per 1 settimana-12 mesi come gel im (prednisone 2 mg/kg/24 h ha uguale efficacia). *Adulti:* Esacerbazioni acute della MS: 80-120 U/24 h per 2-3 sett.	*Cautela:* può mascherare i segni di infezione; non somministrare vaccini vivi; può esacerbare lo scompenso cardiaco o l'ipertensione. *Effetti indesiderati:* insonnia, nervosismo, aumento dell'appetito, indigestione, diabete mellito, dolori articolari, epistassi, sbalzi dell'umore, pancreatite, esofagite, perdita della massa muscolare, soppressione della crescita ossea, infezioni opportunistiche.
Cortisone acetato Corticosteroide surrenalico. Iniezione: 50 mg/mL. Compresse: 5, 10, 25 mg.	**Terapia dell'insufficienza corticosurrenalica (sostitutiva).** *Bambini:* per os: 0,5-0,75 mg/kg/24 h suddivisi ogni 8 h. im: 0,25-0,35 mg/kg/24 h. *Adulti:* per os, im: 20-300 mg/24 h in 1-2 dosi.	*Cautela:* evitare nell'infezione fungina attiva e in molte altre infezioni gravi a eccezione dello shock o della meningite. *Effetti indesiderati:* insonnia, nervosismo, pseudotumore cerebrale, cefalea, aumento dell'appetito, ulcera peptica, diabete mellito, edema, ipertensione, cataratta, glaucoma, ipopotassemia. *Commento:* vedi il confronto tra i corticosteroidi alla voce *Idrocortisone.*
Cosintropina Corticosteroide surrenalico. Polvere per iniezione: 0,25 mg.	**Diagnosi del deficit corticosurrenalico primario vs secondario (stimola la corteccia surrenalica a rilasciare steroidi surrenalici).** *Neonati:* 0,015 mg/kg/dose. *Bambini <2 anni:* 0,125 mg. *Bambini >2 anni e adulti:* 0,25 mg. Somministrare la dose al mattino presto.	*Effetti indesiderati:* flushing, lieve febbre, prurito, pancreatite. *Monitoraggio:* misurare il cortisolo plasmatico prima ed esattamente 30 min dopo la dose. La risposta normale consiste nell'aumento del cortisolo sierico >7 μg/dL (>193 nmol/L) o nell'aumento del picco di risposta >18 μg/dL (497 nmol/L).
Crotamiton Crema: 10%. Lozione: 10%.	**Trattamento della scabbia (meccanismo sconosciuto).** *Bambini piccoli, bambini grandi e adulti:* lavare completamente l'area, asciugare con un asciugamano asciutto, applicare uno strato sottile e massaggiare il farmaco sulla cute. Ripetere l'applicazione dopo 24 h. Effettuare un bagno detergente 48 h dopo l'applicazione finale. Si può ripetere dopo 7 giorni se necessario.	*Effetti indesiderati:* irritazione locale.
Dacarbazina Agente antineoplastico. Iniezione: 100, 200, 500 mg.	**Trattamento di vari tumori (agente alchilante e probabilmente una certa attività antimetabolita).** *Bambini:* Tumori solidi: 200-470 mg/m^2/24 h per 5 giorni ogni 21-28 giorni. Neuroblastoma: 800-900 mg/m^2 al giorno 1 della terapia di combinazione ogni 3-4 sett. Malattia di Hodgkin: 375 mg/m^2 ai giorni 1 e 15 della terapia di combinazione; ripetere ogni 28 giorni. *Adulti:* Malattia di Hodgkin: 150 mg/m^2/24 h per 5 giorni; ripetere ogni 4 sett.	*Effetti indesiderati:* dolore e arrossamento nel sito di infusione, nausea e vomito, leucopenia (inizio: 7 giorni; nadir: 10-14 giorni; remissione: 21-28 giorni), debolezza, polineuropatia, parestesie, aumento degli enzimi epatici, congestione sinusale, alopecia, sapore metallico.

TABELLA 716-1. Farmaci generali – *continua*

FARMACO (PRINCIPIO ATTIVO, FORMULAZIONI)	INDICAZIONI (MECCANISMO D'AZIONE E DOSAGGIO)	COMMENTI (CAUTELE, EFFETTI INDESIDERATI, MONITORAGGIO)
Dactinomicina Agente antineoplastico. Polvere per iniezione: 0,5 mg.	**Trattamento di vari tipi di tumore (si lega alla porzione guanina del DNA, bloccando la replicazione e la trascrizione dello stampo di DNA).** *Bambini >6 mesi e adulti:* 15 μg/kg/24 h o 400-600 μg/m^2/24 h per 5 giorni; si può ripetere ogni 3-6 sett.	*Effetti indesiderati:* mielosoppressione (inizio: 7 giorni; nadir: 14-21 giorni; remissione: 21-28 giorni), affaticamento, malessere, febbre, alopecia, eruzioni cutanee, acne, nausea e vomito gravi, diarrea, mucosite, stomatite, ipocalcemia, iperuricemia.
Danaparoid Agente antitrombotico. Iniezione: 750 unità anti-Xa in 0,6 mL.	**Agisce inibendo gli effetti anti-Xa e anti-IIa (attività anti Xa/anti-IIa >22). Eparinoide a basso peso molecolare, costituito principalmente da eparan solfato. Utilizzare per la trombocitopenia eparino-indotta (la cross-reattività con anticorpi anti-eparina è <10%, rispetto al >90% per l'eparina a basso peso molecolare).** *Bambini:* Dose da carico: 30 U/kg. Dose di mantenimento: 1,2-2,0 U/kg/h. *Adulti:* Trattamento: Dose da carico: <50 kg: 1500 U; 50-90 kg: 2250 U; >90 kg: 3000 U. Fare seguire la dose da carico con 400 U/h per 4 h, poi 300 U/h per 4 h, quindi dose di mantenimento di 150-200 U/h. Profilassi: <50 kg: 750 U ogni 12 h; 50-90 kg: 1500 U ogni 8 h; >90 kg: 1500 U ogni 12 h.	*Monitoraggio:* controllare i livelli plasmatici anti-Xa; target 0,5-0,8 U/mL per il trattamento; target 0,2-0,4 U/mL per la profilassi. Il monitoraggio dei test coagulativi tradizionali (per es. tempo di protrombina, tempo parziale di tromboplastina attivata, tempo di coagulazione attivato) non è vantaggioso; non si è osservato alcun effetto. *Effetti indesiderati:* sanguinamento (il rischio è minore che con l'eparina non frazionata).
Dantrolene sodico Rilassante muscolo-scheletrico. Capsule: 25, 50, 100 mg. Polvere per iniezione: 20 mg.	**Trattamento della spasticità associata a disordini del neurone motorio superiore come trauma al midollo spinale, ictus, paralisi cerebrale o sclerosi multipla; anche usato per il trattamento dell'ipertermia maligna (interferisce con il rilascio di ione calcio dal reticolo sarcoplasmatico).** Spasticità: *Bambini:* 0,5 mg/kg/dose bid; aumentare frequenza ogni 4-7 giorni a tid-qid; poi aumentare la dose di 0,5 mg/kg (massimo: 3 mg/kg/dose bid-qid). *Adulti:* dose iniziale di 25 mg/24 h, aumentando di 25 mg o la frequenza ogni 4-7 giorni (massimo. 100 mg bid-qid). Ipertermia: *Bambini e adulti:* per os: 4-8 mg/kg/24 h in 4 dosi suddivise somministrate 1-2 giorni prima dell'intervento (profilassi), o per 1-3 giorni dopo l'intervento (follow-up post-crisi). ev: 2,5 mg/kg iniziando 1,5 h prima dell'intervento e continuare per 1 ora (profilassi) o 1 mg/kg/dose ripetuta se necessario (crisi) (massimo: 10 mg/kg).	*Cautela:* non dovrebbe essere usato nei casi in cui la spasticità è usata per mantenere la postura o l'equilibrio; evitare nei pazienti con epatopatia attiva. *Effetti indesiderati:* sonnolenza, affaticamento, vertigini, confusione, visione offuscata, convulsioni, diarrea, crampi allo stomaco, nausea, vomito, versamento pleurico con pericardite, epatite.
Daunorubicina idrocloruro Antineoplastico. Polvere per iniezione: 20 mg.	**Trattamento della leucemia non linfocitica acuta (LNLA) e della leucemia mieloblastica (inibizione della sintesi di DNA e RNA).** *Bambini:* induzione della remissione per la leucemia linfocitica acuta (terapia di combinazione): 25-45 mg/m^2 al giorno 1 alla sett per 4 cicli (massimo: totale, 300 mg/m^2). *Adulti:* 30-60 mg/m^2/24 h per 3-5 giorni; ripetere la dose a 3-4 sett; la dose totale cumulative non dovrebbe essere maggiore di 400-600 mg/m^2 (estremo inferiore in caso di storia di cardiotossicità da farmaci o irradiazione del torace).	*Cautela:* evitare nei pazienti con scompenso cardiaco o aritmie. Si può verificare cardiotossicità irreversibile se l'esposizione alla dose totale è maggiore di 550 mg/m^2 negli adulti, 400 mg/m^2 in caso di irradiazione del torace, 300 mg/m^2 nei bambini >2 anni, 10 mg/kg nei bambini <2 anni. *Effetti indesiderati:* alopecia, urine colorate di rosso, nausea, vomito, diarrea, ulcerazione gastrointestinale, stomatite, mielosoppressione (inizio, 7 giorni; nadir, 14 giorni; remissione, 21-28 giorni), ulcerazioni e necrosi tessutali correlate a stravaso, scompenso cardiaco congestizio, iperuricemia, epatotossicità. *Monitoraggio:* bilirubina sierica e aspartato aminotransferasi (AST) (per adeguare le dosi in caso di compromissione epatica): bilirubina 1,2-3 mg/dL o AST 60-180 UI: ridurre dose al 75%; bilirubina 3,1-5 mg/dL o AST >180 UI: ridurre la dose del 50%; bilirubina >5 mg/dL: evitare l'uso.
Deferoxamina mesilato Agente chelante. Polvere per iniezione: 500 mg.	**Trattamento dell'intossicazione acuta da ferro o del sovraccarico secondario cronico da ferro (forma complessi con il ferro per formare ferrioxamina, che viene eliminata dai reni).** *Bambini:* Intossicazione acuta da ferro: im: 90 mg/kg/dose ogni 8 h. ev: 15 mg/kg/h (massimo: 6 g/24 h). Sovraccarico cronico di ferro: ev: 15 mg/kg/h (massimo: 12 g/24 h). sc: 20-40 mg/kg/24 h per 8-12 h attraverso dispositivo di infusione portatile. *Adulti:* Intossicazione acuta da ferro: im: 1 g STAT, poi 0,5 g ogni 4 h (massimo: 6 g/24 h). ev: 15 mg/kg/h (massimo: 6 g/24 h). Sovraccarico cronico di ferro: im: 0,5-1 g/24 h. sc: infondere 1-2 g/24 h per 8-24 h.	*Cautela:* Controindicato nei pazienti con emocromatosi primaria. *Effetti indesiderati:* dolore e indurimento locale, flushing, ipotensione, tachicardia, febbre, perdita dell'udito, visione offuscata, cataratta. *Monitoraggio:* ferritina sierica, ferro, total iron binding capacity. audiometrie ed esame oculistico in caso di utilizzo cronico.

TABELLA 716-1. Farmaci generali – *continua*

FARMACO (PRINCIPIO ATTIVO, FORMULAZIONI)	INDICAZIONI (MECCANISMO D'AZIONE E DOSAGGIO)	COMMENTI (CAUTELE, EFFETTI INDESIDERATI, MONITORAGGIO)
Desametasone Corticosteroide surrenalico. Aerosol: orale 84 μg/attivazione, nasale 84 μg/spruzzo. Crema: 0,1%, 0,04%. Iniezione: 4, 8, 10, 16, 20, 24 mg/mL. Pomata oftalmica: 0,05%. Sospensione oftalmica: 0,1, 0,5%. Soluzione orale: 0,5 mg/5 mL. Compresse: 0,25, 0,5, 0,75, 1, 1,5, 2, 4, 6 mg. Elisir: 0,5 mg/5 mL.	**Per via sistemica e locale per l'infiammazione acuta e cronica; malattie allergiche, neoplastiche e autoimmuni, edema cerebrale, shock settico, meningite da *Haemophilus influenzae*; agente diagnostico (diminuisce l'infiammazione e sopprime la normale risposta immune).** *Neonati:* edema delle vie aeree o estubazione: ev: 0,25 mg/kg ogni 12 h per 3-4 dosi (iniziare $>$4 h prima dell'estubazione programmata). Displasia broncopolmonare: ev, per os: 0,25 mg/kg/dose ogni 12 h per 6 dosi, poi misurare per 1-6 sett (i regimi possono iniziare già al giorno 1). *Bambini:* edema delle vie aeree o estubazione: per os, im, ev: 0,5-2 mg/kg/24 h suddivisi ogni 6 h (iniziare 24 h prima dell'estubazione e continuare per 4-6 dosi post estubazione). Antiemetico (chemioterapia-indotta): ev: 10 mg/m^2 prima dose, poi 5 mg/m^2/dose ogni 6 h se necessario (iniziare prima la chemioterapia). Anti-infiammatorio: per os, im, ev: 0,08-0,3 mg/kg/24 h suddivisi ogni 6-12 h. Meningite batterica: ev: 0,6 mg/kg/24 h suddivisi ogni 6 h per giorni 1-4 di antibiotici. Edema cerebrale: per os, im, ev: dose da carico di 1-2 mg/kg, poi 1-1,5 mg/kg/24 h suddivisi ogni 4-6 h, ridotti in 1-6 sett. Inalazione: 2 puff tid-qid. Spruzzo nasale: 1-2 spruzzi per narice bid. Sostituzione fisiologica: per os, im, ev: 0,03-0,15 mg/kg/24 h suddivisi ogni 6-12 h. *Adulti:* Anti-infiammatorio: per os, im, ev: 0,5-9 mg/24 h suddivisi ogni 6-12 h. Antiemetico: come per i bambini. Edema cerebrale: ev: 10 mg STAT, poi 4 mg ogni 6 h. Sindrome di Cushing: 1 mg alle 23.00; valutare il cortisolo plasmatico alle 8.00 del giorno seguente. Shock: ev: 1-6 mg/kg (massimo: 40 mg; si può ripetere ogni 2-6 h. *Bambini e adulti:* Oftalmico: Pomata: applicare un film sottile ogni 3-4 h nel sacco congiuntivale. Sospensione: instillare 2 gocce nel sacco congiuntivale ogni h durante il giorno e ogni due h di notte. Ridurre gradualmente le dosi a mano a mano che l'infiammazione si risolve. Topico: applicare 1-4 × al giorno.	*Cautela:* l'uso di desametasone nei neonati con displasia broncopolmonare, è stato associato associato ad aumentata incidenza di paralisi cerebrale, e questo rischio dovrebbe essere soppesato con i potenziali benefici. *Effetti indesiderati:* insonnia, nervosismo, aumento dell'appetito ipertensione, iperglicemia, iperacidità gastrointestinale (rischio di ulcera da stress), cataratta, soppressione adrenale, crescita ridotta. *Commento:* vedi il confronto di corticosteroidi alla voce *Idrocortisone*.
Desipramina idrocloruro Antidepressivo, triciclico. Compresse: 10, 25, 50, 75, 100, 150 mg. Capsule: 25, 50 mg.	**Trattamento della depressione, disturbo da deficit dell'attenzione, dolore neuropatico (aumenta le concentrazioni sinaptiche o la serotonina e la noradrenalina inibendone il reuptake).** *Bambini 6-12 anni:* 1-3 mg/kg/24 h (massimo: 5 mg/kg/24 h). *Adolescenti:* dose iniziale o 25-50 mg/24 h, aumentata gradualmente (massimo: 150 mg/24 h). *Adulti:* dose iniziale di 75 mg/24 h, aumentata gradualmente (massimo: 300 mg/24 h).	*Cautela:* la sospensione improvvisa può portare a sintomi da astinenza; le compresse contengono tartrazina (può essere un problema per gli asmatici), controindicata nel glaucoma ad angolo stretto.. *Effetti indesiderati:* vertigini, sonnolenza, cefalea, visione offuscata, bocca secca, stipsi, aumento dell'appetito, aritmie cardiache, ipotensione. *Monitoraggio:* concentrazioni di desipramina: terapeutiche 100-300 ng/mL, tossiche $>$300 ng/mL; controllare l'ECG.
Desmopressina acetato Analogo della vasopressina. Iniezione: 4 μg/mL. Soluzione nasale: 0,1 mg/mL.	**Trattamento del diabete insipido, controllo del sanguinamento in certi tipi di emofilia, enuresi primaria notturna (aumenta il riassorbimento di acqua nei reni, aumento dose-dipendente del fattore VIII e dell'attivatore del plasminogeno).** *Bambini:* Diabete insipido: *3 mesi-12 anni:* per os: 0,05 mg inizialmente, poi titolare fino alla risposta. ev: 5 μg/24 h in 1-2 dosi. Emofilia: *$>$3 mesi:* ev: 0,3 μg/kg, si può ripetere la dose se necessario, usare 30 min prima della procedura. Enuresi notturna: *$>$6 anni:* 20 μg prima di andare a letto. *Bambini $>$12 anni e adulti:* Diabete insipido: per os: 0,05 mg bid, poi titolare fino alla risposta. ev, sc: 2-4 μg/24 h. Intranasale: 5-40 μg/24 h in 1-3 dosi. Emofilia: ev: 0,3 μg/kg. Intranasale: $<$50 kg: 150 μg, $>$50 kg: 300 μg. Enuresi: per os: 0,2-0,4 mg prima di andare a letto.	*Cautela:* evitare l'uso nei pazienti con malattia di von Willebrand di tipo IIB o platelet-type, emofilia A con livelli di fattore VII $<$5% o emofilia B. *Effetti indesiderati:* flushing al volto, cefalea, vertigini, aumento della pressione arteriosa, iponatremia, intossicazione da acqua. *Monitoraggio:* elettroliti serici, osmolalità plasmatica e urinaria, diuresi, livelli dell'antigene del fattore VIII, tempo di tromboplastina parziale attivata, livello di attività del fattore VIII.

TABELLA 716-1. Farmaci generali – *continua*

FARMACO (PRINCIPIO ATTIVO, FORMULAZIONI)	INDICAZIONI (MECCANISMO D'AZIONE E DOSAGGIO)	COMMENTI (CAUTELE, EFFETTI INDESIDERATI, MONITORAGGIO)
Destrano Espansore del volume plasmatico. Destrano 40 (basso peso molecolare) Destrano 70 (alto peso molecolare).	**Espansore di volume plasmatico nello shock o nello shock imminente (simile all'albumina).** *Bambini:* fino a 20 mL/kg al giorno 1, poi 10 mL/kg/24 h per non più di 5 giorni. *Adulti:* 500-1000 mL a una velocità di 20-40 mL/min (massimo: 10 mL/kg/24 h per 5 giorni).	*Effetti indesiderati:* prevalentemente associati a dosi eccessive – edema polmonare, sanguinamento causato da alterata funzione piastrinica.
Destroamfetamina Stimolante del SNC. Compresse: 5, 10 mg. Capsule, rilascio prolungato: 5, 10, 15 mg.	**Trattamento del disturbo da deficit dell'attenzione, della narcolessia e dell'obesità esogena (blocca il reuptake della dopamina e della noradrenalina da parte delle sinapsi).** *Bambini 6-12 anni:* narcolessia e disturbo da deficit dell'attenzione: dose iniziale di 5 mg/24 h; si può aumentare di 5 mg/24 h a intervalli settimanali fino alla risposta (massimo: 60 mg/24 h). *>12 anni e adulti:* Dose iniziale di 20 mg/24 h; si può aumentare di incrementi di 10 mg alla sett (massimo: 60 mg/24 h).	*Cautela:* evitare l'uso concomitante di inibitori delle monoamino ossidasi. *Effetti indesiderati:* ipertensione, tachicardia, palpitazioni, aritmie, insonnia, agitazione, irritabilità, nervosismo, cefalea, depressione, tremore, esacerbazione di tic e disordini del movimento, midriasi, dipendenze fisica e psicologica, anoressia, nausea, diarrea, crampi addominali, soppressione della crescita. *Monitoraggio:* pressione arteriosa, crescita, attività del SNC.
Destrometorfano Antitussivo. Liquido: 7,5 mg/5 mL. Pastiglie: 5 mg.	**Rimedio sintomatico della tosse, meglio quando la tosse non è produttiva (deprime il centro midollare della tosse).** *Bambini 2-6 anni:* 2,5-7,5 mg ogni 4-8 h o rilascio-prolungato, 15 mg ogni 12 h (massimo: 30 mg/24 h). *6-12 anni:* 10-15 mg ogni 4-8 h, o rilascio-prolungato, 30 mg bid (massimo: 60 mg/24 h). *>12 anni e adulti:* 10-30 mg ogni 4-8 h, o rilascio-prolungato, 60 mg bid (massimo: 120 mg/24 h).	*Effetti indesiderati:* prevalentemente in caso di overdoseósonnolenza, vertigini, depressione respiratoria, visione offuscata, nausea, disturbi gastrointestinali, stipsi.
Diazepam Benzodiazepina. Compresse: 2, 5, 10 mg. Soluzione orale: 5 mg/mL. Iniezione: 5 mg/mL.	**Trattamento di ansia, attacchi di panico, stato epilettico, astinenza da alcol; fornisce sedazione; rilassante del muscolo scheletrico (si pensa aumenti l'azione neuroinibitoria dell'acido γ-aminobutirrico).** *Bambini piccoli e bambini:* Stato epilettico: ev: 0,05-0,3 mg/kg/dose somministrato per 2-3 min; si può ripetere ogni 30 min fino alla dose totale massima di 5-10 mg. Rettale: 0,5 mg/kg, poi 0,25 mg/kg in 10 min se necessario. Sedazione: per os: 0,2-0,3 mg/kg (massimo: 10 mg). im, ev: 0,04-0,3 mg/kg (massimo: 0,6 mg/kg/8 h). *Adulti:* Stato epilettico: ev: 5-10 mg ogni 30 min (massimo: 30 mg/8 h). Ansia, sedazione, miorilassante: per os, im, ev: 2-10 mg bid-qid.	*Effetti indesiderati:* ipotensione, bradicardia, arresto cardiaco (con dose ev), sonnolenza, atassia, affaticamento, confusione, alterata coordinazione, eccitazione paradossa, amnesia, visione offuscata, diplopia, sudorazione, secchezza delle fauci, stipsi o diarrea, aumento o diminuzione dell'appetito, singhiozzo, dipendenza fisica e psicologica. *Monitoraggio:* si dovrebbero monitorare gli end-point clinici desiderati e quelli tossici, le dosi per raggiungere gli effetti variano considerevolmente tra i pazienti.
Diazossido Antipertensivo. Iniezione: 15 mg/mL. Sospensione orale: 50 mg/mL. Capsule: 50 mg.	**Riduzione della pressione arteriosa in urgenza, trattamento dell'ipoglicemia iperinsulinemica correlata a tumori delle cellule insulari o a nesidioblastosi (rilassamento del muscolo liscio, inibisce il rilascio di insulina dal pancreas).** Ipertensione: *Bambini e adulti:* 1-3 mg/kg; si può ripetere dopo 5-15 min; dose ogni 4-24 h. Ipoglicemia iperinsulinemica: *Neonati e bambini piccoli:* per os: 8-15 mg/kg/24 h suddivisi ogni 8-12 h (iniziare con l'estremo inferiore). *Bambini e adulti:* per os: 3-8 mg/kg/24 h suddivisi ogni 8-12 h (iniziare con l'estremo inferiore).	*Effetti indesiderati:* ipotensione, vertigini, debolezza, nausea, vomito.
Dibucaina Anestetico locale. Crema: 0,5%. Pomata: 1%.	**Riduzione temporanea del dolore e del prurito causato da emorroidi e da lesioni o irritazione cutanee minori (blocca l'avvio e la conduzione degli impulsi nervosi).** *Bambini e adulti:* Topico: applicare con delicatezza sull'area interessata (bambini, 7,5 g/24 h; adulti, 30 g/24 h). Rettale: inserire con l'applicatore rettale la mattina, di sera e dopo ogni evacuazione intestinale.	*Effetti indesiderati:* irritazione locale, dermatite da contatto.
Diciclomina Agente anticolinergico. Capsule: 10, 20 mg. Compresse: 20 mg. Sciroppo: 10 mg/5 mL. Iniezione: 10 mg/mL.	**Trattamento dei disturbi funzionali della motilità gastrointestinale (per es. sindrome dell'intestino irritabile) (blocca l'azione dell'acetilcolina).** *Bambini piccoli >6 mesi:* per os: 5 mg/dose tid-qid. *Bambini:* 10 mg tid-qid. *Adulti:* 40 mg qid (iniziare con 1/2 dose e aumentare gradualmente). im: *Adulti:* 20 mg qid.	*Cautela:* evitare in caso di glaucoma ad angolo stretto, ostruzione gastrointestinale, ostruzione delle vie urinarie e miastenia grave. *Effetti indesiderati:* tachicardia, palpitazioni, nervosismo, irritabilità, confusione, ipotonia muscolare, visione offuscata, fotofobia, ritenzione urinaria, nausea, vomito, stipsi, secchezza delle fauci, orticaria, prurito.
Diclofenac sodico Agente anti-infiammatorio non steroideo. Compresse: 25, 50, 75 mg. Soluzione oftalmica: 0,1%.	**Trattamento del dolore acuto o cronico da lieve a moderato; infiammazione postoperatoria dopo estrazione di cataratta (inibisce la sintesi di prostaglandine).** per os: *Bambini:* 2-3 mg/kg/24 h in 2-4 dosi suddivise. *Adulti:* 100-200 mg/24 h in 2-4 dosi suddivise. Oftalmico: 1 goccia nell'occhio interessato qid per 2 sett, iniziare 24 h dopo l'intervento chirurgico per cataratta.	*Effetti indesiderati:* vertigini, cefalea, ritenzione idrica, indigestione, dolore addominale, ulcera peptica, sanguinamento gastrointestinale, insufficienza renale.
Difenidramina Capsule o compresse: 25, 50 mg. Iniezione: 10, 50 mg/mL. Sciroppo o elisir: 12,5 mg/5 mL. Crema o lozione: 1%	**Antistaminico (inibitore competitivo del recettore H_{1pe}).** *Bambini:* im, ev, per os: 5 mg/kg/24 h suddivisi ogni 6 h se necessario (massimo: 300 mg/24 h). *Adulti:* 10-50 mg/dose ogni 4 h se necessario (massimo: 400 mg/24 h). *Topico:* applicare tid-qid al giorno.	*Effetti indesiderati:* ipotensione, tachicardia, sonnolenza, eccitamento paradosso, secrezioni bronchiali ispessite, secchezza delle fauci.

TABELLA 716-1. Farmaci generali – *continua*

FARMACO (PRINCIPIO ATTIVO, FORMULAZIONI)	INDICAZIONI (MECCANISMO D'AZIONE E DOSAGGIO)	COMMENTI (CAUTELE, EFFETTI INDESIDERATI, MONITORAGGIO)
Difenossilato e atropina Compresse, soluzione orale.	**Antidiarroico (il difenossilato inibisce l'eccessiva motilità gastrointestinale; l'atropina è usata per prevenire l'abuso).** *Bambini:* *2-5 anni:* 4 mL (2 mg difenossilato) tid. *5-8 anni:* 4 mL qid. *8-12 anni:* 4 mL 5 × al giorno. *Adulti:* 15-20 mg/24 h in 3-4 dosi suddivise.	*Effetti indesiderati:* nervosismo, vertigini, sonnolenza, cefalea, bocca secca, ritenzione urinaria, visione offuscata, ileo paralitico.
Digossina Glicoside cardiaco. Capsule: 50, 100, 200 μg. Elisir: 50 μg/mL. Compresse: 125, 250, 500 μg. Iniezione: 100, 250 μg/mL.	**Trattamento dello scompenso cardiaco sistolico e tachiaritmie sopraventricolari (aumenta calcio intracellulare attraverso inibizione della pompa sodio/potassio adenosina trifosfatasi; soppressione della conduzione al nodo AV).** *Neonato:* dose da carico di 10-30 μg/kg ev, poi 5-10 μg/kg/24 h dose di mantenimento. *1 mese-2 anni:* dose da carico di 30 μg/kg, poi 10-15 μg/kg/24 h dose di mantenimento. *2-10 anni:* dose da carico di 30 μg/kg, poi 5-10 μg/kg/24 h dose di mantenimento. *Bambino >10 anni:* dose da carico di 10 μg/kg, poi 2-5 μg/kg/24 h dose di mantenimento. *Adulto:* dose da carico di 10-15 μg/kg, poi 0,1-0,5 mg/24 h dose di mantenimento. Aggiustare le dosi in caso di ridotta funzione renale: CrCl 10-15 mL/min: ridurre la dose al 25-75% del normale. CrCl <10 mL/min: ridurre la dose al 10-25% del normale.	*Cautela:* controindicato nel blocco AV, nella stenosi subaortica idiopatica ipertrofica o nella pericardite costrittiva. *Effetti indesiderati:* anoressia, nausea, vomito, diarrea, intolleranza alimentare, bradicardia, aritmie, letargia, depressione, vertigini, visione offuscata, diplopia, fotofobia, visione gialla o verde. *Monitoraggio:* l'efficacia e la tossicità sono strettamente correlate alle concentrazioni seriche e il dosaggio dovrebbe essere guidato misurando le concentrazioni di digossina nel siero: terapeutiche: 0,8-2 ng/mL; tossiche: >2-2,5 ng/mL. Sostanze immuni simili alla digossina (DLIS) possono aumentare falsamente i livelli di digossina nei neonati e nei bambini, pertanto si possono ottenere i livelli di digossina pretrattamento e sottrarli dai livelli di trattamento oppure si possono prelevare campioni attraverso un filtro free-level per rimuovere le DLIS prima dell'esame. Controllare i livelli post distribuzione (calcolati almeno 6-8 h dopo la dose) allo stato stazionario (2-4 sett) o in presenza di segni di tossicità all'ECG o clinici. Controllare ECG, elettroliti serici, calcio e magnesio. Controllare la frequenza cardiaca.
Digossina Immune Fab Antidoto della digossina. Polvere per iniezione: 38 mg.	**Trattamento dell'intossicazione digitalica da digossina o digitossina (si lega alle molecole non legate della digossina o della digitossina ed è escreta per via renale).** *Bambini piccoli, bambini grandi e adulti:* dose basata sulla quantità di digossina o digitossina ingerita o stimata in base al carico corporeo totale (TBL) calcolato sulla concentrazione sierica post distribuzione: TBL digossina = concentrazione (ng/mL) × 5,6 × peso (kg)/1000. TBL digossina = mg ingerita × 0,8, TBL digitossina = concentrazione (ng/mL) × 0,56 × peso (kg)/1000. TBL digitossina = mg ingeriti. Dose di digossina immune Fab (mg) = TBL digossina × 76, Dose di digossina immune Fab (n. di fiale) = TBL/0,5.	*Effetti indesiderati:* peggioramento dello scompenso cardiaco o della fibrillazione atriale, ipopotassemia, edema facciale, arrossamento. *Monitoraggio:* ECG; le concentrazioni seriche di digossina aumenteranno molto con la digossina immune Fab e non riflettono i depositi corporei o la correlata con la tossicità clinica.
Diidrotachisterolo Analogo della vitamina D. Capsule: 0,125 mg. Compresse: 0,125 mg. Soluzione: 0,2 mg/mL, 0,2 mg/5 mL.	**Trattamento dell'ipocalcemia associata a ipoparatiroidismo e a osteodistrofia renale (stimola l'assorbimento intestinale di calcio e fosfato).** *Neonati:* 0,05-0,1 mg/24 h. *Bambini piccoli e bambini giovani:* 1-5 mg/24 h per 4 giorni, poi 0,5-1,5 mg/24 h. *Bambini più grandi e adulti:* 0,75-2,5 mg/24 h per 4 giorni, poi 0,2-1 mg/24 h (massimo: 1,5 mg/24 h). Osteodistrofia renale: 0,1-0,6 mg/24 h.	*Effetti indesiderati:* ipercalcemia, ipercalciuria, elevata creatinina sierica.
Diltiazem Calcio antagonista. Compresse: 30, 60, 90, 120 mg. Capsule, rilascio prolungato: 60, 90, 120, 180, 240, 300 mg. Iniezione: 5 mg/mL.	**Trattamento dell'ipertensione e delle tachiaritmie atriali (inibisce l'ingresso di ioni calcio nei "canali-lenti" durante la depolarizzazione).** *Bambini:* per os: 1,5-2 mg/kg/24 h in 3-4 dosi suddivise. *Adolescenti e adulti:* per os: 90-480 mg/24 h in 3-4 dosi suddivise in compresse o 1-2 dosi a rilascio prolungato capsule. ev: dose da carico di 0,25 mg/kg, poi 5-15 mg/h infusione continua.	*Cautela:* il diltiazem è un inibitore dell'enzima epatico e può causare accumulo e tossicità dei farmaci usati in concomitanza che sono metabolizzati. *Effetti indesiderati:* ipotensione, bradicardia, edema, blocco AV, vertigini, nausea, vomito.
Dimenidrinato Antistaminico. Capsule: 50 mg. Iniezione: 50 mg/mL. Compresse: 50 mg. Liquido: 12,5 mg/4 mL.	**Trattamento di nausea, vomito e vertigini associati a cinetosi (compete con l'istamina per il recettore H_1).** *Bambini:* *2-5 anni:* 12,5-25 mg ogni 6-8 h (massimo: 75 mg/24 h). *6-12 anni:* 25-50 mg ogni 6-8 h (massimo: 150 mg/24 h). *Adulti:* 50-100 mg ogni 4-6 h (massimo: 400 mg/24 h).	*Effetti indesiderati:* sonnolenza, vertigini, ipotensione, tachicardia.
Dimercaprolo Iniezione: 100 mg/mL.	**Antidoto per l'avvelenamento da oro, arsenico e da mercurio e aggiunto a calcio edetato disodico nell'avvelenamento da piombo (chela i metalli pesanti per formare composti stabili non tossici).** *Bambini e adulti:* Lieve avvelenamento da arsenico e oro: 2,5 mg/kg/dose im ogni 6 h per 2 giorni, poi ogni 12 h al giorno 3, poi ogni 24 h per 10 giorni. Grave avvelenamento da arsenico e oro: 3 mg/kg/dose ogni 4 h per 2 giorni, poi ogni 6 h al giorno 3, poi ogni 12 h per 10 giorni. Avvelenamento da mercurio: dose da carico di 5 mg/kg, poi 2,5 mg/kg/dose 1-2 × giorno per 10 giorni. Avvelenamento da piombo: Lieve: dose da carico di 4 mg/kg, poi 3 mg/kg/dose ogni 4 h per 2-7 giorni. Grave: dose da carico di 4 mg/kg/dose ogni 4 h per 2-7 giorni.	*Effetti indesiderati:* ipertensione, tachicardia, convulsioni, nausea, vomito, febbre, cefalea, nervosismo, blefarospasmo, nefrotossicità. *Monitoraggio:* livelli specifici dei metalli pesanti; il pH urinario dovrebbe essere mantenuto alcalino.

TABELLA 716-1. Farmaci generali – *continua*

FARMACO (PRINCIPIO ATTIVO, FORMULAZIONI)	INDICAZIONI (MECCANISMO D'AZIONE E DOSAGGIO)	COMMENTI (CAUTELE, EFFETTI INDESIDERATI, MONITORAGGIO)
Disopiramide Capsule: 100, 150 mg.	**Trattamento delle aritmie ventricolari e tachiaritmie ventricolari (antiaritmico classe 1a, diminuisce l'eccitabilità e la velocità di conduzione miocardica).** *Bambini:* *<1 anno:* 10-30 mg/kg/24 h suddivisi ogni 6 h. *1-4 anni:* 10-20 mg/kg/24 h suddivisi ogni 6 h. *4-12 anni:* 10-15 mg/kg/24 h suddivisi ogni 6 h. *12-18 anni:* 6-15 mg/kg/24 h suddivisi ogni 6 h. *Adulti:* 100-200 mg ogni 6 h.	*Cautela:* evitare nel blocco AV 2- o 3-grado; peggiora lo scompenso, ritenzione urinaria, glaucoma e alcune aritmie. *Effetti indesiderati:* ritenzione o esitazione urinaria, secchezza delle fauci, affaticamento, malessere, stipsi, colestasi, enzimi epatici elevati. *Monitoraggio:* clearance della creatinina (diminuire la dose a ogni 8 h se 30-40 mL/min, ogni 12-h se 15-30 mL/min, ogni 24 h se <15 mL/min), ECG, pressione arteriosa, segni di scompenso cardiaco, livelli ematici (range terapeutico: aritmie atriali 2,8-3,2 μg/mL, aritmie ventricolari 3,3-7,5 μg/mL).
Dobutamina Iniezione.	**Trattamento dell'ipotensione (stimola recettori β_1-adrenergici).** *Neonati:* 2-20 μg/kg/min. *Bambini e adulti:* 2,5-40 μg/kg/min infusione costante.	*Cautela:* evitare nei pazienti con cardiomiopatia ipertrofica, fibrillazione o flutter atriale o sensibilità ai solfiti. *Effetti indesiderati:* tachicardia, battiti ectopici, angina, palpitazioni, tachiaritmie, sensazione di formicolio, parestesie, crampi alle gambe.
Docusato Capsule, liquido, sciroppo (può essere combinato con casantrolo).	**Emolliente delle feci, lassativo (riduce la tensione superficiale dell'interfaccia olio-acqua delle feci).** *<3 anni:* 10-40 mg/24 h in 1-4 dosi. *3-6 anni:* 20-60 mg/24 h in 1-4 dosi. *6-12 anni:* 40-150 mg/24 h. *>12 anni e adulti:* 50-400 mg/24 h.	*Effetti indesiderati:* diarrea, crampi addominali.
Dolasetron mesilato Compresse: 50, 100 mg. Iniezione.	**Prevenzione e trattamento del vomito e della nausea da chemioterapia e postoperatori (antagonista recettori 5-HT_3).** *Bambini >2 anni e adulti:* ev, per os: 1,8 mg/kg (massimo: 100 mg) in monosomministrazione 30 min prima della chemioterapia; 0,35 mg/kg (massimo: 12,5 mg) somministrato 15 min prima di interrompere l'anestesia per la nausea postoperatoria.	*Effetti indesiderati:* ipotensione, cefalea, tachicardia, vertigini.
Dopamina Iniezione.	**Trattamento dell'ipotensione e dello shock (stimola i recettori dopaminergici e i recettori adrenergici).** *Neonati, bambini grandi e adulti:* 1-20 μg/kg/min ev velocità d'infusione (mL/h) = 6 × peso (kg) × dose desiderata (μg/kg/min)/mg farmaco/100 mL di fluido ev.	*Cautela:* contiene solfiti. *Effetti indesiderati:* tachicardia, battiti ectopici, aritmie ventricolari, necrosi tissutale con stravaso, vasocostrizione, gangrena delle estremità, diuresi eccessiva (dosi <5 μg/kg/min), oliguria (dosi >10 μg/kg/min).
Dornase alfa Soluzione inalante: 1 mg/mL.	**Trattamento della fibrosi cistica per migliorare la funzionalità polmonare (enzima del DNA che riduce la viscosità del muco).** *Neonati, bambini e adulti:* 2,5 mL 1-2 volte al giorno, nebulizzato con compressore Pulmo-Aide o Pari-Proneb.	*Effetti indesiderati:* faringite, alterazione della voce, tosse, rinite, emottisi.
Doxacurio Iniezione: 1 mg/mL.	**Paralisi muscolo-scheletrica (fornisce blocco neuromuscolare competendo con l'acetilcolina per il recettore neuromuscolare).** *Bambini 2-12 anni:* dose iniziale di 30-50 μg/kg, poi 5-10 μg/kg/dose ogni 1-2 h. *Adulti:* dose iniziale di 50 μg/kg, poi 5-10 μg/kg/dose ogni 1-2 h.	*Effetti indesiderati:* debolezza muscoloscheletrica, ipotensione. *Monitoraggio:* stimolazione del nervo periferico.
Doxapram Iniezione: 20 mg/mL.	**Trattamento dell'apnea da prematurità refrattaria alle metilxantine (stimolante respiratorio e del SNC).** *Neonati:* dose iniziale di 2,5-3 mg/kg seguita da infusione di 1 mg/kg/h (massimo: 2,5 mg/kg/h).	*Cautela:* contiene benzil alcol (dose raccomandata da rilasciare 5,4-27 mg/kg/24 h). *Effetti indesiderati:* ipertensione, tachicardia, aritmie, stimolazione del SNC, irritabilità, convulsioni, iperpiressia , vomito, aumento del residuoi gastrico, iperglicemia.
Doxepina Antidepressivo triciclico. Capsule: 10, 25, 50, 75, 100, 150 mg. Concentrato orale: 10 mg/mL. Crema: 5%.	**Trattamento della depressione; analgesico per il dolore neuropatico (aumenta le concentrazioni sinaptiche di serotonina e noradrenalina).** *Bambini:* 1-3 mg/kg/24 h. *Adolescente:* dose iniziale di 25-50 mg/24 h (massimo: 100 mg/24 h). *Adulti:* dose iniziale di 30-150 mg/24 h (massimo: 300 mg/24 h; dose singola massimo: 150 mg).	*Cautela:* controindicato nel glaucoma ad angolo stretto. *Effetti indesiderati:* sedazione, sonnolenza, vertigini, cefalea, secchezza delle fauci, stipsi, appetito aumentato, aumento di peso, ritenzione urinaria, diuresi difficile, visione offuscata, ipotensione, aritmie. *Monitoraggio:* ECG, concentrazioni di doxepin: terapeutiche 30-150 ng/mL, tossiche >500 ng/mL.
Doxorubicina idrocloruro Polvere per iniezione. Iniezione: 2 mg/mL.	**Antineoplastico usato per vari tipi di tumore (inibisce la sintesi di DNA e RNA).** *Bambini:* 35-75 mg/m^2/dose, ripetuta ogni 21 giorni, o 20-30 mg/m^2, ripetuta ogni/sett, o 60-90 mg/m^2 somministrati in infusione continua per 96 h ogni 3-4 sett. *Adulti:* 60-75 mg/m^2/dose ogni 21 giorni. Epatopatia: ridurre la dose: bilirubina 1,2-3 (ridurre del 50%), bilirubina >3 (ridurre del 75%).	*Cautela:* controindicato se il paziente ha scompenso cardiaco congestizio, miocardiopatia o ha ricevuto una dose totale di 550 mg/m^2 (400 mg/m^2 in caso di precedente o concomitante daunorubicina, idarubicina, mitoxantrone, ciclofosfamide, irradiazione all'area cardiaca). *Effetti indesiderati:* cardiotossicità, alopecia, iperpigmentazione dei letti ungueali , iperuricemia, stomatite, esofagite, mucosite, nausea, vomito, trombocitopenia (inizio, 7 giorni; nadir, 10-14 giorni; remissione, 21-28 giorni), lacrimazione, necrosi tissutale da stravaso, flebite.
Dronabinol, tetraidrocannabinolo Capsule: 2,5, 5, 10 mg.	**Antiemetico per la chemioterapia tumorale (inibisce il centro del vomito).** *Bambini e adulti:* 5 mg/m^2/dose ogni 2-4 h iniziando 1-3 h prima della chemioterapia (massimo: 15 mg/m^2/dose).	*Effetti indesiderati:* sonnolenza, difficoltà di concentrazione, sbalzi di umore, allucinazioni. *Monitoraggio:* monitorare per l'abuso.
Droperidolo Iniezione: 2,5 mg/mL.	**Antiemetico, antipsicotico (altera l'azione della dopamina nel SNC e ha un blocco α-adrenergico).** *Bambini 2-12 anni:* ev, im: 0,05-0,06 mg/kg/dose ogni 4-6 h se necessario per la nausea. *Adulti:* ev, im: 2,5-5 mg/dose ogni 3-4 h se necessario.	*Effetti indesiderati:* ipotensione, tachicardia, reazioni extrapiramidali, confusione, perdita della memoria.
D-xilosio Polvere per soluzione orale.	**Agente diagnostico usato per valutare i disordini intestinali dovuti a malattia o trauma (meccanismo non noto).** *Bambini:* 500 mg/kg come soluzione al 5-10% (massimo: 25 g). *Adulti:* 5-25 g come soluzione al 10%, seguita da 200-400 mL di acqua.	*Effetti indesiderati:* nausea, vomito, crampi, gonfiore intestinale. *Monitoraggio:* concentrazioni ematiche e urinarie di D-xilosio.

TABELLA 716-1. Farmaci generali – *continua*

FARMACO (PRINCIPIO ATTIVO, FORMULAZIONI)	INDICAZIONI (MECCANISMO D'AZIONE E DOSAGGIO)	COMMENTI (CAUTELE, EFFETTI INDESIDERATI, MONITORAGGIO)
Edetato disodico Iniezione: 150 mg/mL.	**Trattamento di emergenza dell'ipercalcemia e delle aritmie ventricolari indotte dalla digitale (agente chelante).** *Bambini:* 40-70 mg/kg/24 h infusione lenta per 3-4 h; somministrare per 5 giorni, poi 5 giorni senza farmaco. *Adulti:* 50 mg/kg/dose per 5 giorni, poi 2 giorni senza, poi reiniziare per un totale di 15 dosi. aritmie da digitale (bambini e adulti): 15 mg/kg/h infusione continua (massimo: 60 mg/kg/24 h).	*Cautela:* controindicato in insufficienza renale grave e tubercolosi. *Effetti indesiderati:* aritmie, ipotensione, convulsioni, cefalea, brividi, ipopotassemia, ipocalcemia, ipomagnesiemia, iperuricemia, vomito, diarrea, crampi addominali, disuria, dolore alla schiena, nefrotossicità.
Edrofonio cloruro Iniezione: 10 mg/mL.	**Diagnosi di miastenia grave, differenziazione delle crisi colinergiche dalle crisi miasteniche, inversione dei bloccanti neuromuscolari non depolarizzanti, trattamento della tachicardia atriale parossistica (inibisce la degradazione dell'acetilcolina da parte dell'acetilcolinasterasi).** *Bambini piccoli:* im: 0,5-1 mg. ev: 0,1 mg, seguita da 0,4 mg (in assenza di risposta). *Bambini:* Diagnosi (iniziale): im: <34 kg: 1 mg; >34 kg: 5 mg. ev: 0,04 mg/kg per 1 min, seguita da 0,16 mg/kg data entro 45 s (in assenza di risposta) (massimo: 10 mg totali). Titolazione orale della terapia anticolinesterasica: ev 0,04 mg/kg somministrata 1 ora dopo la somministrazione orale del trattamento farmacologico; se la forza migliora, aumentare la dose di neostigmina o piridostigmina. *Adulti:* Diagnosi: im: inizialmente, 10 mg; se si verifica una reazione colinergica, somministrare 2 mg in 30 min per evidenziare una reazione falsa negativa. ev: 2 mg somministrata in 15 s, 8 mg dati 45 s più tardi (se non risposta). Titolazione della terapia orale anticolinesterasica: ev 1-2 mg data 1 ora dopo una dose orale. Aumentare la dose orale se la forza migliora.	*Effetti indesiderati:* aritmie, ipotensione, nausea, vomito, diarrea, crampi allo stomaco, sudorazione eccessiva, frequenza urinaria, lacrimazione, diplopia, miosi, laringospasmo, broncospasmo, paralisi respiratoria.
Emulsione lipidica Iniezione: 10%, 20%.	**Fonte di acidi grassi essenziali e calorie (supplemento nutrizionale con la nutrizione parenterale).** *Bambini prematuri:* iniziare con 0,5 g/kg/24 h e aumentare di 0,5 g/kg/24 h secondo quanto tollerato (massimo: 3g/kg/24 h). *Bambini piccoli e grandi:* iniziare con 0,5-1 g/kg/24 h e aumentare di 0,5 g/kg/24 h secondo quanto tollerato (massimo: 3-4 g/kg/24 h). *Adolescenti e adulti:* 1 g/kg/24 h e aumentare secondo quanto tollerato (massimo: 2,5 g/kg/24 h).	*Cautela:* le calorie provenienti dai grassi non dovrebbero superare il 60% delle calorie totali giornaliere. Controindicato nei pazienti con grave allergia all'uovo o alla soia. *Effetti indesiderati:* iperlipidemia, epatomegalia, dispnea e ipossiemia possono verificarsi se viene infusa troppo velocemente o in caso di dose eccessiva. *Monitoraggio:* trigliceridemia.
Enalapril/Enalaprilat Orale (enalapril): 2,5, 5, 10, 20 mg. Iniezione (enalaprilat): 1,25 mg/mL. Formulazione estemporanea.	**Trattamento dell'ipertensione e dello scompenso cardiaco congestizio (inibizione dell'enzima di conversione dell'angiotensina).** *Neonato:* per os: 0,1 mg/kg/24 h in 1-2 dosi (può essere aumentato a 0,4 mg/kg/24 h per lo scompenso cardiaco o adeguata risposta dell'ipertensione). ev: 5-10 µg/kg/dose ogni 8-24 h. *Bambini piccoli e grandi:* per os: 0,1-0,5 mg/kg/24 h in 1-2 dosi. ev: 5-10 µg/kg/dose ogni 8-24 h. *Adolescenti e adulti:* per os: 2,5-5 mg/24 h e titolare (massimo: 40 mg/24 h in 2 dosi). ev: 0,625-1,25 mg/dose ogni 6 h (massimo: 20 mg/24 h).	*Cautela:* evitare o aggiustare la dose nei pazienti con compromissione renale (CrCl 10-50 mL/min, somministrare il 75% della dose; CrCl <10 mL/min, somministrare il 50% della dose). *Effetti indesiderati:* ipotensione, tachicardia, sincope, affaticamento, vertigini, cefalea, tosse, iperpotassemia, ipoglicemia. *Commento:* ridurre le dosi in presenza di diuretici concomitanti o ridotta funzione renale; l'indometacina concomitante può mascherare la risposta.
Enoxaparina sodica Iniezione: 30 mg/0,3 mL.	**Profilassi e trattamento del tromboembolismo venoso (eparina a basso peso molecolare con attività contro i fattori IIa e Xa).** *Neonati e bambini:* sc: 1 g/kg ogni 8-12 h. *Adulti:* sc: 30 mg bid o 1 mg/kg bid (dipende dall'indicazione).	*Effetti indesiderati:* trombocitopenia ed emorragia (<eparina non frazionata). *Monitoraggio:* dose a livello plasmatico dell'eparina (test anti-fattore Xa) intervallo medio 0,5-1,0 U/mL, o attraverso 0,3-0,7 U/mL.
Eparina (non frazionata) Iniezione.	**Profilassi e trattamento del tromboembolismo (potenzia le azioni dell'antitrombina III).** *Neonati, bambini piccoli e grandi:* Trombosi e ossigenazione della membrana extracorporea: dose da carico bolo ev di 50 U/kg V, dose di mantenimento di 15-35 U/kg/h in infusione ev continua (aggiustare secondo il target tempo parziale di tromboplastina attivata (APTT) target o i livelli di eparina). Pervietà del catetere: 0,5-1 U/mL. *Adulti:* ev: dose da carico di 70-100 U/kg bolo ev, 15-25 U/kg/h infusione continua (APTT target o livelli di eparina). sc: 5000 unità ogni 8-12 h per profilassi.	*Cautela:* evitare se trombocitopenia grave, emorragia endocranica, endocardite batterica. *Effetti indesiderati:* sanguinamento da vari siti (per es. urine, gengive, naso); ecchimosi, trombocitopenia, trombosi. *Monitoraggio:* APTT (terapeutico, 1,5-2,5 × basale; tossico >2,5 × basale); concentrazione eparina plasmatica (test anti-fattore X: terapeutico 0,3-0,7 U/mL).
Epoetina alfa, eritropoietina, EPO Iniezione, fiala senza conservanti: 2000, 3000, 4000, 10 000 U/mL. Con conservanti: 10 000 U/mL.	**Anemia associata alla prematurità; nefropatia in stadio finale; pazienti con infezione da HIV trattati con zidovudina; pazienti neoplastici sottoposti a chemioterapia (induce eritropoiesi).** Somministrare ev, sc. *Neonati:* 100-500 U/kg/dose ogni 1-2 giorni per 10-21 giorni. *Bambini e adulti:* Pazienti tumorali: 150 U/kg/dose 3×/sett (si può aumentare a 300 U/kg/dose). Pazienti in emodialisi: 50-100 u 3×/sett. Pazienti trattati con zidovudina: 100 U/dose 3×/sett.	*Cautela:* ipertensione non controllata, la neutropenia nei neonati deve avere adeguati depositi di ferro e può richiedere supplemento di ferro orale o ev. *Effetti indesiderati:* ipertensione, edema, cefalea, febbre, rash, artralgie, ipersensibilità. *Monitoraggio:* ferro sierico, conta reticolocitaria, ematocrito (ridurre la dose o sospendere l'EPO se l'ematocrito >40), pressione arteriosa.

TABELLA 716-1. Farmaci generali – *continua*

FARMACO (PRINCIPIO ATTIVO, FORMULAZIONI)	INDICAZIONI (MECCANISMO D'AZIONE E DOSAGGIO)	COMMENTI (CAUTELE, EFFETTI INDESIDERATI, MONITORAGGIO)
Ergocalciferolo Compresse, capsule: 50 000 unità. Liquido: 8000 U/mL. Iniezione: 500 000 U/mL (1 μg = 4 u).	**Trattamento del rachitismo refrattario, ipofosfatemia, ipoparatiroidismo (analogo della vitamina D, stimola l'assorbimento di calcio e fosfato).** *Bambini piccoli prematuri:* 10-20 μg/24 h. Insufficienza renale: *Bambini:* 100-1000 μg/24 h. *Adulti:* 500 μg/24 h. Ipoparatiroidismo: *Bambini:* 1,25-5 mg/24 h. *Adulti:* 0,625-5 mg/24 h. Rachitismo: *Bambini:* 75-125 μg/24 h. *Adulti:* 0,25-1,5 mg/24 h.	*Effetti indesiderati:* ipercalcemia, debolezza, letargia, ipertensione, aritmie, lieve acidosi, ipercolesterolemia, nausea, vomito, stipsi, nefrocalcinosi, fotofobia. *Monitoraggio:* calcio e fosforo sierico, fosfatasi alcalina, radiografia ossea.
Ergotamina Compresse: 1, 2 mg. Aerosol: 9 mg/mL. Supposte: 2 mg.	**Previene o risolve le cefalee vascolari (per es. emicrania o cefalea a grappolo) (alcaloide dell'ergot bloccante α-adrenergico).** *Bambini più grandi e adolescenti:* 1 mg sublinguale o per os all'inizio dell'attacco e ogni 30 min fino al sollievo (massimo: 3 mg/attacco). *Adulti:* 1-2 mg per via sublinguale o per os, si può ripetere ogni 30 min fino al massimo di 6 mg (dose/massima sett: 10 mg).	*Cautela:* ridurre la dose del 50% se il paziente assume cronicamente metisergide. *Effetti indesiderati:* tachipnea, vasospasmo, nausea, vomito, diarrea, crampi alle gambe, debolezza muscolare, parestesie.
Esmololo Iniezione: 10 mg/mL.	**Antiaritmico, antipertensivo (β bloccante, antiaritmico classe II).** *Bambini:* 100-500 μg/kg per 1 min, poi infusione continua di 200-1000 μg/kg/min. *Adulti:* 500 μg/kg per 1min, poi 50-200 μg/kg/min.	*Cautela:* controindicato in bradicardia sinusale, blocco cardiaco, scompenso cardiaco. *Effetti indesiderati:* ipotensione, bradicardia, fenomeno di Raynaud, vertigini, confusione, letargia, broncocostrizione.
Etoposide, VP-16 Capsule: 50 mg. Iniezione: 20 mg/mL.	**Antineoplastico per il trattamento di vari tumori (inibisce l'attività mitotica).** *Bambini:* ev: 150 mg/m^2/24 h per 3 giorni per 2-3 cicli per la remissione della leucemia mielocitica acuta o tumore cerebrale; 160 mg/m^2/24 h per 4 giorni per il condizionamento del trapianto del midollo osseo. *Adulti:* ev: 50-100 mg/m^2/24 h per 3-5 giorni/ciclo. per os: ev dose ×2 fino a raggiungere i 50 mg.	*Effetti indesiderati:* ipotensione, tachicardia, febbre, cefalea, brividi, alopecia, rash, orticaria, nausea, vomito, diarrea, mucosite, mielosoppressione, anemia (nadir, 7-14 giorni), trombocitopenia (nadir, 9-16 giorni), neuropatia periferica, broncospasmo.
Etosuccimide Capsule: 250 mg. Sciroppo: 250 mg/5 mL.	**Anticonvulsante per il trattamento dell'epilessia assenza, mioclonica e acinetica (aumenta la soglia delle convulsioni).** *Bambini:* *<6 anni:* iniziare con 15 mg/kg/24 h in 2 dosi; aumentare ogni 4-7 giorni fino ai livelli terapeutici, di solito 15-40 mg/kg/24 h in 2 dosi (massimo: 1,5 g/24 h). *>6 anni e adulti:* iniziare con 250 mg bid; aumentare di 250 mg/24 h ogni 4-7 giorni fino ai livelli terapeutici o a 1,5 g/24 h.	*Effetti indesiderati:* sedazione, letargia, nausea, vomito, anoressia, dolore addominale, leucopenia, trombocitopenia, anemia aplastica. *Monitoraggio:* concentrazioni di etosuccimide: terapeutiche 40-100 μg/mL; tossiche 150 μg/mL.
Famotidina Compresse: 20, 40 mg. Iniezione.	**Trattamento dell'ulcera gastrica e duodenale e controllo del pH gastrico nei pazienti con malattia critica (blocca i recettori H_2).** *Bambini piccoli e grandi:* per os, ev: 1-12 mg/kg/24 h in 1-2 dosi (massimo: 40 mg/24 h). *Adulti:* per os: 40 mg/24 h prima di andare a letto. ev: 20 mg ogni 12 h.	*Cautela:* ridurre la dose in base alla funzione renale: CrCl 30-50 mL/min: somministrare il 50%, della dose; CrCl <30 mL/min: somministrare il 25% della dose. *Effetti indesiderati:* disturbi gastrointestinali, trombocitopenia, aumento edegli nzimi epatici.
Fattore IX complesso (umano) Iniezione.	**Agente antiemofilico per controllare il sanguinamento nei pazienti con deficit di fattore IX (cioè, emofilia B o malattia di Christmas), o con inibitori per il fattore VIII (cioè, emofilia A) (sostituzione del fattore deficitario).** *Bambini e adulti:* 20-25 U/kg/dose fino a ogni 24 h; deficit di fattore VIII: 75-100 U/kg/dose fino a ogni 6 h.	*Effetti indesiderati:* flushing, febbre, cefalea, brividi, orticaria, trombosi ad alte dosi), formicolio, rigidità al capo e al collo.
Fattore antiemofilico, umano Agente antiemofilico; derivato del prodotto del sangue. Iniezione (attività approssimativa fattore VIII/fiala): 200, 250, 500, 750, 1000, 1250, 1500 unità; potenza esatta indicata sull'etichetta di ogni fiala.	**Deficit di fattore VIII nell'emofilia (fornisce fattore VIII).** *Tutti i pazienti:* unità necessarie = peso (kg) × 0,5 × aumento desiderato di fattore VIII (% della norma).	*Effetti indesiderati:* tachicardia, allergia, infezioni virali ematogene. *Monitoraggio:* livelli plasmatici di fattore antiemofilico.
Felbamato Compresse: 400, 600 mg. Sospensione orale: 600 mg/5 mL.	**Terapia aggiuntiva usata prevalentemente per le convulsioni generalizzate e parziali refrattarie associate alla sindrome di Lennox-Gastaut (anticonvulsante con meccanismo d'azione sconosciuto).** *Bambini: 2-14 anni:* iniziare con 15 mg/kg/24 h in 3-4 dosi; aumentare ogni settimana di 15 mg/kg/24 h (massimo: 45 mg/kg/24 h o 3600 mg, a seconda di quale sia minore). *>14 anni:* iniziare con 1200 mg/24 h in 3-4 dosi; aumentare settimanalmente di 1200 mg/24 h (massimo: 3600 mg/24 h).	*Cautela:* sono stati riportati oltre 30 casi di insufficienza epatica e 30 di anemia aplastica con diversi decessi. *Effetti indesiderati:* cefalea, insonnia, sonnolenza, affaticamento, modificazioni dell'umore, depressione, atassia, anoressia, nausea, vomito, diarrea, trombocitopenia, granulocitopenia, leucopenia, agranulocitosi, anemia aplastica, epatite, insufficienza epatica acuta. *Monitoraggio:* interagisce con fenitoina, carbamazepina e valproato; monitorare i livelli di tali farmaci se si aggiunge felbamato.
Fenazopiridina Anestetico urinario. Compresse: 100, 200 mg.	**Possibile sollievo sintomatico del bruciore e del prurito urinari associati alle procedure urologiche o alle infezioni delle vie urinarie.** *Bambini:* per os: 12 mg/kg/24 h ogni 8 h. *Adulti:* per os: 100-200 mg ogni 6-8 h.	*Cautela:* discolora le urine ad arancio o rosso. *Effetti indesiderati:* cefalea, rash, metaemoglobinemia. Somministrare ai pasti per diminuire gli effetti indesiderati gastrointestinali.

TABELLA 716-1. Farmaci generali – *continua*

FARMACO (PRINCIPIO ATTIVO, FORMULAZIONI)	INDICAZIONI (MECCANISMO D'AZIONE E DOSAGGIO)	COMMENTI (CAUTELE, EFFETTI INDESIDERATI, MONITORAGGIO)
Fenilepinefrina idrocloruro Agonista del recettore α-adrenergico; vasocostrittore periferico. Iniezione: 10 mg/mL. Gocce nasali, spray: 0,16-1%. Gocce per occhio.	**Trattamento dell'ipotensione nello shock e usata in molti decongestionanti nasali.** Decongestionante nasale: *Bambini piccoli:* 1-2 gocce per narice ogni 3-4 h; soluzione 0,16%. *Bambini 1-6 anni:* 1-2 gocce o spruzzi per narice ogni 3-4 h; soluzione 0,125%. *6-12 anni:* 1-2 gocce o spruzzi ogni 3-4 h; soluzione 0,25%. *>12 anni e adulti:* 1-2 gocce o spruzzi per narice ogni 3-4 h; soluzione 0,25-0,5%. Ipotensione e shock: *Bambini:* ev: 5-20 μg/dose ogni 10-15 min. Si può somministrare per infusione continua ev e 0,1-0,5 μg/kg/min, titolato all'effetto desiderato (per es. pressione arteriosa). *Adulti:* ev 0,1-0,5 mg/dose ogni 10-15 min per infusione continua 100-180 μg/min, titolata all'effetto desiderato. Tachicardia parossistica sopraventricolare: *Bambini:* ev: 5-10 μg/kg per 20-30sec. *Adulti:* ev: 0,25-0,5 mg per 20-30sec.	*Cautela:* pazienti con ipertensione. Iniezione contiene solfiti. Rigidità nasale da rimbalzo con prolungato uso/abuso nasale. *Effetti indesiderati:* ipertensione, angina, bradicardia, irritabilità, necrosi se infiltrati ev. *Interazioni farmacologiche:* simpaticomimetici, antagonisti del recettore α, inibitori delle monoamino ossidasi.
Fenitoina Anticonvulsante e antiaritmico. Capsule, a rilascio lento-(lungo-): 30, 100 mg. Capsule, a pronto rilascio: 30, 100 mg. Sospensione: 125 mg/5 mL. Iniezione: 50 mg/mL.	**Stato epilettico**: *Bambini e adulti:* ev: 15-18 mg/kg (massimo: 1-3 mg/kg/min). Dose da carico: *Neonato:* ev: 15-20 mg/kg (massimo: 0,5 mg/kg/min). Dose di mantenimento: per os, ev: *Neonato:* 5 mg/kg/24 h ogni 12-24 h. *Bambini 0,5-0,6 anni:* 8-10 mg/kg/24 h. *7-9 anni:* 6-8 mg/kg/24 h ogni 12-24 h. *10-16 anni:* 6-7 mg/kg/24 h ogni 12-24 h. *Adulti:* 300-600 mg/24 h ogni 12-24 h.	*Cautela:* infondere lentamente ev; biodisponibilità orale variabile; compresse masticabili più consistente. Bisogna agitare la sospensione orale molto bene prima dell'uso. Seguire la farmacocinetica di saturazione (Michaelis-Menten). Alcuni stati patologici (insufficienza renale, trauma cranico acuto) possono portare a squilibrio tra farmaco libero e legato alle proteine. *Effetti indesiderati:* letargia, vertigini, nistagmo, ipotensione, irsutismo, iperplasia gengivale, rash, sindrome di Stevens-Johnson, epatite, tromboflebite. *Interazioni farmacologiche:* può aumentare il metabolismo di certi farmaci eliminati per via epatica; contraccettivi orali, griseofulvina, corticosteroidi, ciclosporina; è altamente legata alle proteine e può causare interazione da spiazzamento. *Monitoraggio:* concentrazioni di fenitoina: terapeutiche 8-20 μg/mL. Se necessario, misurare la concentrazione di farmaco libero: terapeutica 1-2 μg/mL.
Fenobarbital Barbiturico depressivo del SNC. Elisir: 15 mg/5 mL; 20 mg/5 mL. Compresse: 8, 15, 30, 60, 100 mg Iniezione: 30, 60, 130 mg/mL.	**Sedativo ipnotico anticonvulsante e anestetico.** Anticonvulsante: **Dose da carico:** *Bambini e adulti:* per os, ev: 15-20 mg/kg. Dose di mantenimento: *Neonati:* per os, ev: 3-4 mg/kg/24 h, ogni 12-24 h. *Bambini:* per os, ev: 5-6 mg/kg/24 h, ogni 12-24 h. Certi farmaci possono interagire con il metabolismo del fenobarbital: *Adulti:* per os, ev: 1-3 mg/kg/24 h ogni 12-24 h. Sedazione: *Bambini:* 2 mg/kg/dose. >60 μg/mL. Iperbilirubinemia: Sedazione: *Bambini:* per os, ev: 3-8 mg/kg/24 h ogni 12-24 h. *Adulti:* per os, ev: 90-180 mg/24 h ogni 12-24 h.	*Cautela:* dose titolata all'effetto desiderato. Somministrare ev ≤30 mg/min in bambini piccoli e grandi e ≤60 mg/min in adulti. *Effetti indesiderati:* ipotensione, sonnolenza, depressione respiratoria, iperattività paradossa. *Interazioni farmacologiche:* può aumentare il metabolismo di molti farmaci eliminati per via epatica; contraccettivi orali, griseofulvina, corticosteroidi. acido valproico, cloramfenicolo, felbamato. *Target concentrazioni sieriche:* 15-40 μg/mL; coma (acuto) *Monitoraggio:* concentrazioni di fenobarbital: sedazione 15-40 μg/mL; coma >60 μg/mL.
Fenossibenzamina Antagonista del recettore α-adrenergico Capsule: 10 mg.	**Trattamento sintomatico del feocromocitoma.** *Bambini:* per os: 0,2-2 mg/kg/24 h ogni 24 h. Titolare la dose all'effetto desiderato (per es. pressione arteriosa). *Adulti:* per os: 10 mg/dose ogni 12 h. Titolare la dose fino all'effetto.	*Cautela:* antagonista a lunga durata d'azione del recettore α. *Effetti indesiderati:* ipotensione posturale, sincope, vertigini. *Interazioni farmacologiche:* simpaticomimetici.
Fentanil citrato Iniezione, transdermico, pastiglia orale.	**Antidolorifico, sedativo, medicazione preoperatoria, narcotico analgesico (aggiunto all'anestesia, si lega ai recettori oppioidi).** *Neonati e bambini piccoli:* ev: 1-4 μg/kg/dose; si può ripetere ogni 2-4 h o infusione continua di 0,5-5 μg/kg/h. *Bambini 1-2 anni:* dolore: im, ev: 1-3 μg/kg/dose, si può ripetere ogni 30-60 min; infusione continua di 1-5 μg/kg/h. *Bambini >12 anni e adulti:* Dolore: ev, im: 0,5-1 μg/kg/dose; si può ripetere dopo 30-60 min. Transdermico: 25-100 μg/h secondo quanto necessario per il sollievo. Per os: 5 μg/kg o 400 μg, a seconda di quale è minore. Anestesia: ev, im: 2-50 μg/kg.	*Cautela:* l´infusione ev rapida può portare a rigidità muscoloscheletrica e della gabbia toracica, con alterata ventilazione e distress respiratorio; si può verificare dipendenza fisica in 3-5 giorni. *Effetti indesiderati:* ipotensione, bradicardia, depressione SNC, stipsi, spasmo del tratto biliare, nausea, vomito, spasmo delle vie urinarie, depressione respiratoria.

TABELLA 716-1. Farmaci generali – *continua*

FARMACO (PRINCIPIO ATTIVO, FORMULAZIONI)	INDICAZIONI (MECCANISMO D'AZIONE E DOSAGGIO)	COMMENTI (CAUTELE, EFFETTI INDESIDERATI, MONITORAGGIO)
Fentolamina Antagonista α-adrenergico. Iniezione: 5 mg/mL.	**Diagnosi e trattamento del feocromocitoma e stravaso dei farmaci con effetti α-adrenergici (per es. dopamina, dobutamina, adrenalina, noradrenalina, fenilepinefrina).** Feocromocitoma: Diagnosi: *Bambini:* ev 0,05-0,1 mg/kg/dose (massimo: 5 mg). *Adulti:* ev 5 mg/dose. Prima dell'intervento: *Bambini:* ev 0,05-0,1 mg/kg/dose ogni 1-2 h titolando fino all'effetto e alla durata necessaria. (massimo: 5 mg). Stravaso: 5-10 mg in 10 mL soluzione fisiologica normale. Infiltrare l'area con poco volume usando un ago da 27-30 gauge (massimo: 0,1 mg/kg).	*Cautela:* antagonista del recettore α a breve durata d'azione. *Effetti indesiderati:* ipotensione, vertigini, gastrite. *Interazioni farmacologiche:* simpaticomimetici.
Ferro Complesso ferro destrano (iniezione). Solfato ferroso, gluconato ecc. Orale.	**Trattamento del deficit di ferro, anemia ipocromica o microcitica (terapia sostitutiva).** Iniezione: im, ev: dose test di 0,25-0,5 mL 1 ora prima iniziando la terapia con ferro destrano. Dose (mL/kg) = Hgb (normale – attuale) × 0,0476 + 1 mL/5kg (massimo: <5 kg = 25 mg; 5-10 kg = 50 mg; >10 kg = 100 mg). per os (mg ferro): *Bambini:* Profilassi: 1-2 mg/kg/24 h. Deficit: 3-6 mg/kg/24 h in 1-3 dosi suddivise. *Adulti:* Profilassi: 60 mg/24 h. Deficit: 60 mg bid-qid.	*Effetti indesiderati:* (orale) irritazione gastrointestinale, nausea, stipsi, feci scure: (ev, im) ipotensione, flushing, vertigini, febbre, cefalea, gusto metallico, artralgia, anafilassi. *Monitoraggio:* emoglobina (normale <15 kg = 12 mg/dL, >15 kg = 14,8 mg/dL), conta reticolocitaria, ferritina sierica.
Fexofenadina Capsule: 60 mg. Compresse: 30, 60, 180 mg.	**Antistaminico con attività selettiva per i recettori H_1 periferici. Trattamento della rinite allergica stagionale e dell'orticaria cronica idiopatica.** *Bambini <12 anni:* 30 mg bid. *Bambini >12 anni e adulti:* 60 mg bid o 180 mg ogni 24 h.	*Effetti indesiderati:* profilo di sicurezza molto buono; la tossicità è rara, anche in caso di overdose (principalmente vertigini, sonnolenza e secchezza delle fauci).
Filgrastim Granulocyte colony-stimulating factor. Iniezione: 300 μg/mL	**Riduce la durata della neutropenia (stimola la produzione, la maturazione e l'attivazione dei neutrofili).** *Neonati:* 5 μg/kg/dose al giorno per 3-6 dosi. *Bambini e adulti:* 5-10 μg/kg/dose al giorno fino a 14 giorni; si può sospendere se la conta assoluta dei neutrofili rimane >1000/mm³ per 3 giorni consecutivi.	*Cautela:* tumori maligni con caratteristiche mieloidi. *Effetti indesiderati:* ipotensione, vasculite, febbre, riacutizzazione di malattie cutanee pre-esistenti, aumentato acido urico, trombocitopenia, dolore midollare (correlato alla dose e principalmente localizzato alla regione lombare, alla cresta iliaca e allo sterno), ematuria, proteinuria.
Fisostigmina Antagonista competitivo dell'acetilcolina. Iniezione, soluzione oftalmica, pomata.	**A differenza della neostigmina, attraversa la barriera ematoencefalica con effetti centrali. usato con estrema cautela nell'antagonizzare gli effetti anticolinergici.** im, ev, sc: *Bambini:* 0,001-0,03 mg/kg/dose ogni 15-20 min fino all'effetto desiderato (massimo: 2 mg). *Adulti:* 0,5-2 mg ogni 15-20 min all'effetto desiderato.	*Cautela:* pazienti con bradicardia, aritmie cardiache, asma, ulcera. Dovrebbe essere usato come antidoto solo in situazioni minacciose per la vita da persone esperte. *Effetti indesiderati:* palpitazioni, irritabilità, salivazione eccessiva, secrezioni, fascicolazioni muscolari, broncospasmo.
Fitonadione AquaMEPHYTON; Mephyton. Compresse: 5 mg. Iniezione.	**Vitamina K_1 per l'integrazione alimentare e per il trattamento della malattia emorragica del neonato o della tossicità da sostanze anticoagulanti warfarin-simili.** *Bambini:* im, ev, sc: 1-2 mg/dose dosato fino all'effetto; per os: la dose si può aumentare a 2,5-5 mg. *Adulti:* im, ev, sc: 10 mg/24 h; per os: 5-25 mg/24 h. Dosi più alte possono essere necessarie per antagonizzare la tossicità anticoagulante warfarin-simile.	*Cautela:* infondere lentamente ev (per 15-30 min) per evitare flushing. Possono essere necessarie dosi multiple per periodi prolungati, a seconda del tipo di anticoagulante cumarinico. *Effetti indesiderati:* flushing, ipotensione.
Flecainide Compresse: 50, 100, 150 mg. Possono essere preparate formulazioni estemporanee.	**Trattamento della tachicardia sopraventricolare e delle aritmie ventricolari (antiaritmico di classe 1c; rallenta la conduzione nel tessuto cardiaco).** *Bambini:* inizialmente, 1-3 mg/kg/24 h in 3 dosi suddivise; si può aumentare fino a 12 mg/kg/24 h. *Adulti:* inizialmente 100 mg ogni 12 h; si può aumentare di 100 mg/24 h ogni 4 giorni (massimo: 400 mg/24 h).	*Cautela:* diminuire la dose del 25-50% nell'insufficienza renale; evitare nel blocco cardiaco di 2° o 3° grado. *Effetti indesiderati:* bradicardia, blocco cardiaco, peggioramento di aritmie, scompenso cardiaco congestizio, vertigini, disturbi della vista, cefalea, affaticamento, astenia, nausea, stipsi, dolore addominale, aumento degli enzimi epatici, parestesie, tremore. *Monitoraggio:* attraverso le concentrazioni seriche (terapeutiche 0,2-1 μg/mL).
Fludarabina antineoplastica Antimetabolita. Iniezione polvere.	**Trattamento della leucemia linfocitica cronica a cellule B e della leucemia linfocitica acuta non responsiva alla precedente terapia.** *Bambini:* 10 mg/m² per 15 min, seguita da 30,5 mg/m²/24 h di infusione continua per 5 giorni. *Adulti:* 20-25 mg/m² per 30 min per 5 giorni.	*Effetti indesiderati:* neurotossicità (encefalopatia demielinizzante primariamente progressiva con deterioramento dello stato mentale), sonnolenza, debolezza, convulsioni, acidosi metabolica, iperuricemia, iperfosfatemia, iperpotassemia, ipocalcemia, nausea, vomito, diarrea, stomatite, gusto metallico, mielosoppressione (leucociti nadir, 8 giorni; piastrine nadir, 16 giorni; remissione, 5-7 sett), polmonite, dispnea, tosse non produttiva, polmonite interstiziale, perdita di udito, epatotossicità reversibile.
Fludrocortisone acetato Compresse: 0,1 mg.	**Terapia sostitutiva parziale per l'insufficienza adrenale (mineralcorticoide con attività glucocorticoide).** *Bambini piccoli e bambini:* 0,05-0,1 mg/24 h. *Adulti:* 0,05-0,2 mg/24 h.	*Effetti indesiderati:* ipertensione, edema, scompenso cardiaco congestizio, convulsioni, cefalea, acne, rash, contusioni, ipopotassemia, soppressione asse HPA (surrenalica), ulcera peptica, debolezza muscolare.

TABELLA 716-1. Farmaci generali – *continua*

FARMACO (PRINCIPIO ATTIVO, FORMULAZIONI)	INDICAZIONI (MECCANISMO D'AZIONE E DOSAGGIO)	COMMENTI (CAUTELE, EFFETTI INDESIDERATI, MONITORAGGIO)
Flumazenil Iniezione.	**Antagonista delle benzodiazepine per annullare gli effetti sedativi (antagonizza gli effetti delle benzodiazepine sul complesso recettoriale acido γ-aminobutirrico/ benzodiazepina).** *Bambini:* dose da carico di 0,005-0,01 mg/kg, poi infusione continua di 0,005-0,01 mg/kg/h (dose cumulativa massima: 1 mg).	*Cautela:* evitare se le benzodiazepine sono usate per trattare condizioni potenzialmente letali (per es. stato epilettico, aumentatapressione endocranica). *Effetti indesiderati:* aritmie, ipotensione o ipertensione, convulsioni, sintomi acuti da sospensione (se il paziente è dipendente da benzodiazepine o antidepressivo triciclico).
Flunisolide Steroide inalatorio; anti-infiammatorio. Inalatore a dosaggio controllato: 250 μg/puff. Spruzzo nasale: 25 μg/spruzzo.	**Trattamento di asma e rinite.** *Bambini e adulti:* Inalazione orale: 2-4 puff bid. Spruzzo nasale: 1-2 spruzzi per narice bid-tid.	*Effetti indesiderati:* infezioni da Candida di naso e gola, disfonia, mal di gola, sapore amaro, irritazione nasale, cefalea, vertigini, ritardo di crescita a breve termine.
Fluocinolone acetonide Corticosteroide surrenalico topico; anti-infiammatorio. Crema topica, pomata, shampoo, soluzione, olio: 0,01-0,025%	**Infiammazione e dermatosi che rispondono ai corticosteroidi.** *Bambini e adulti:* applicare uno strato sottile bid-qid.	*Effetti indesiderati:* acne, ipopigmentazione, dermatite allergica, atrofia cutanea, follicolite, infezione secondaria, soppressione asse HPA, ritardo di crescita.
Fluocinonide Corticosteroide surrenalico; anti-infiammatorio. Crema, gel, pomata, soluzione: 0,05%	**Infiammazione e dermatosi che rispondono ai corticosteroidi.** *Bambini e adulti:* applicare uno strato sottile bid-qid.	*Effetti indesiderati:* acne, ipopigmentazione, dermatite allergica, atrofia cutanea, follicolite, infezione secondaria, soppressione asse HPA, ritardo nella crescita.
Fluoro Gocce orali, gel topico, pastiglie, compresse, collutorio, soluzione orale.	**Prevenzione della carie dentale (promuove la remineralizzazione, aumenta la resistenza alla dissoluzione dovuta all'acido).** Collutorio o gel dentale: *Bambini:* 5-10 mL dopo lo spazzolamento. *Adulti:* 10 mL dopo lo spazzolamento.	*Effetti indesiderati:* gastrite se deglutito; il fluoro stannoso può colorare i denti.
Fluorometolone Glucocorticoide oftalmico; anti-infiammatorio. Pomata oftalmica: 0,1%. Sospensione oftalmica: 0,1%, 0,25%	**Condizioni infiammatorie dell'occhio.** *Bambini >2 anni e adulti:* Pomata: applicare tid nei casi lievi-moderati e ogni 4 h nei casi gravi. Gocce: instillare 1-2 gocce nel sacco congiuntivale ogni ora durante la veglia e ogni 2 h di notte fino alla risposta, poi ogni 4-8 h.	*Effetti indesiderati:* bruciore locale, aumentata pressione intraoculare.
Fluorouracile Iniezione, soluzione topica, crema.	**Chemioterapia tumorale (antimetabolita antineoplastico che inibisce la sintesi di timidilato, causando deplezione di timidina).** *Bambini e adulti:* ev: 12 mg/kg/24 h (massimo: 800 mg/24 h) per 4-5 giorni, poi 6 mg/kg a giorni alterni per 4 dosi. Ripetere a 4 sett. Crema o soluzione 5%: applicare sull'intera area interessata bid.	*Effetti indesiderati:* aritmie, ipotensione, scompenso cardiaco, atassia cerebellare, fotosensibilità, eritrodisestesia di mani e piedi, perdita delle unghie, iperpigmentazione del letto ungueale, nausea, vomito, diarrea, sonnolenza, alopecia, pigmentazione cutanea, rash maculo papulare pruriginoso, emorragia gastrointestinale, esofagite, stomatite, epatotossicità, congiuntivite, mielosoppressione (leucociti e piastrine: inizio, 7-10 giorni; nadir, 9-14 giorni; remissione, 21 giorni).
Fluoxetina idrocloruro Capsule: 10, 20 mg. Liquido: 20 mg/5 mL.	**Trattamento della depressione e del disturbo ossessivo-compulsivo (antidepressivo, inibisce l'uptake della serotonina nel SNC).** *Bambini 5-18 anni:* inizialmente, 5-10 mg/24 h, poi titolare lentamente fino all'effetto (massimo: 20 mg/24 h). *Adulti:* inizialmente, 20 mg/24 h, poi lentamente aumenta dose giornaliera di 20 mg fino all'effetto.	*Cautela:* evitare nei pazienti che assumono inibitori delle monoamino ossidasi. *Effetti indesiderati:* cefalea, nervosismo, insonnia, ansia, mania, idee suicidarie, tremore, nausea, anoressia, diarrea, stipsi, secchezza delle fauci, perdita di peso. *Monitoraggio:* concentrazioni seriche di fluoxetina (terapeutiche: 100-800 ng/mL), norfluoxetina (terapeutiche: 100-600 ng/mL).
Fluticasone Corticosteroide inalato. Soluzione nasale: 50 μg/spruzzo. Rotadisk: 50, 100, 250 μg/dose.	**Trattamento della rinite allergica e dell'asma cronico.** *Bambini e adulti:* Spruzzo nasale: 1-2 spruzzi in ogni narice una volta al giorno. MDI: 88-880 μg bid (a seconda della gravità dell'asma e bisogno di corticosteroidi Inalatore a dosaggio controllato (MDI): 44, 110, 220 μg/spruzzo. Rotadisk: 50-1000 μg bid (a seconda della gravità dell'asma e della necessità di corticosteroidi sistemici).	*Effetti indesiderati:* disfonia, stomatite aftosa orale, soppressione adrenale, arresto della crescita, cataratta.
Fluvoxamina Compresse: 25, 50, 100 mg.	**Inibitore del reuptake della serotonina; trattamento della depressione, del disturbo ossessivo-compulsivo.** *Bambini <12 anni:* iniziare con 25 mg/h, aumentare di 25 mg/24 h ogni 4-7 giorni fino all'effetto (massimo:200 mg/24 h). Dividere in 2 dosi al giorno se sono necessari >50 mg/24 h. *Bambini >12 anni:* iniziare con 25 mg/24 h; aumentare di 25 mg/24 h ogni 4-7 giorni fino all'effetto (massimo: 300 mg/24 h). Dividere in 2 dosi al giorno se sono necessari >50 mg/24 h. *Adulti:* iniziare con 50 mg/24 h; aumentare di 50 mg/24 h ogni 4-7 giorni fino all'effetto (massimo:300 mg/24 h). Se sono necessari >100 mg/24 h, dividere in 2 dosi/24 h.	*Cautela:* non sospendere improvvisamente la somministrazione o può verificarsi sindrome da astinenza per molti giorni. Ridurre la dose di 25-50 mg/24 h ogni 5-7 giorni. *Effetti indesiderati:* sonnolenza, cefalea, secchezza delle fauci, nausea, stipsi. *Interazioni farmacologiche:* inibisce gli enzimi epatici del citocromo 2D6; farmaci come il metadone e le fenotiazine possono avere livelli aumentati quando sono usati in concomitanza.
Fosfenitoina Iniezione: le fiale da 10 mL contengono 750 mg di fosfenitoina (500 mg fenitoina); le fiale da 2 mL ne contengono 150 mg.	**Trattamento delle convulsioni acute (può sostituire la fenitoina ev).** *Bambini e adulti:* dose da carico di 15-20 mg/kg dosi equivalenti di fenitoina (massimo: 150 mg/min). Può sostituire le dosi di mantenimento ev o im di fenitoina. Ogni 1,5 mg fosfenitoina = 1 mg dose equivalente di fenitoina.	*Cautela:* come per fenitoina. *Interazioni farmacologiche:* come per fenitoina.
Furosemide Iniezione: 10 mg/mL. Soluzione orale: 10 mg/mL, 40 mg/mL. Compresse: 20, 40, 80 mg.	**Diuretico (inibisce il riassorbimento di sodio e cloro nel tratto ascendente dell'ansa di Henle e nel tubulo distale).** *Bambini piccoli prematuri:* 0,5-2 mg/kg ev o 1-4 mg/kg per os ogni 12-48 h (dose fino alla risposta). *Bambini piccoli e bambini:* 1-2 mg/kg ev o 1-4 mg/kg per os ogni 6-24 h o infusione continua (iniziare con 0,05 mg/kg/h e aggiustare la dose fino alla risposta). *Adulti:* 10-600 mg/24 h in 1-4 dosi suddivise, o infusione continua o 0,05 mg/kg/h.	*Effetti indesiderati:* disidratazione, perdita di elettroliti, iperuricemia, fotosensibilità, epatite ischemica, ipercalciuria, calcoli renali, ototossicità (velocità di infusione ev >4 mL/min), intolleranza gastrointestinale.

TABELLA 716-1. Farmaci generali – *continua*

FARMACO (PRINCIPIO ATTIVO, FORMULAZIONI)	INDICAZIONI (MECCANISMO D'AZIONE E DOSAGGIO)	COMMENTI (CAUTELE, EFFETTI INDESIDERATI, MONITORAGGIO)
Gabapentin Capsule: 100, 300, 400 mg.	**Aggiunta al trattamento delle convulsioni generalizzate parziali e secondarie; trattamento del dolore neuropatico (meccanismo non certo).** *Bambini 2-12 anni:* 15-35 mg/kg/24 h in 3 dosi suddivise (massimo: 50 mg/kg/24 h). *Bambini >12 anni e adulti:* iniziare 300 mg al giorno, poi aumentare di 300 mg al giorno fino a 900-3600 mg/24 h in 3 dosi suddivise.	*Effetti indesiderati:* sonnolenza, vertigini, affaticamento, depressione, iperattività, aggressione, dispepsia, stipsi, nausea, aumento di peso, diplopia.
Gamma globulina Vedi Immunoglobulina, endovenosa.		
Glicopirrolato Iniezione: 0,2 mg/mL. Compresse: 1 mg.	**Inibisce la salivazione e le secrezioni eccessive del tratto respiratorio; broncodilatatore; aggiunta al trattamento dell'ulcera peptica; inverte gli effetti muscarinici sugli agenti colinergici (anticolinergico).** *Bambini:* Controllo delle secrezioni: per os: 40-100 μg/kg/dose tid-qid. im, ev: 4-10 μg/kg/dose ogni 3-4 h. Preoperatorio im: 4,4-8,8 μg/kg/dose 30-60 min prima della procedura.	*Effetti indesiderati:* tachicardia, nervosismo, cefalea, insonnia, sonnolenza, secchezza delle fauci, stipsi, nausea, ritenzione urinaria, visione offuscata.
Glucagone Polvere per iniezione.	**Trattamento dell'ipoglicemia (stimola la glicolisi e la gluconeogenesi epatica).** *Neonati:* ev, im, sc: 0,3 mg/kg/dose (massimo: 1 mg). *Bambini:* 0,025-0,1 mg/kg/dose (massimo: 1 mg); si può ripetere dopo 20 min sc, im, ev. *Adulti:* 0,5-1 mg; si può ripetere dopo 20 min se necessario, sc, im, ev.	*Effetti indesiderati:* nausea, vomito, reazioni da ipersensibilità.
Gonadorelina Iniezione.	**Valutazione della regolazione della gonadotropina nella pubertà precoce o ritardata; trattamento dell'amenorrea ipotalamica primaria (stimola il rilascio di ormone luteinizzante).** *Bambini:* ev (sale di HCl) 100 μg. *Bambini >12 anni e adulti:* ev, sc: 100 μg durante i giorni 1-7 del ciclo mestruale.	*Effetti indesiderati:* flushing, sventatezza, cefalea, fastidio addominale. *Monitoraggio:* ormone luteinizzante plasmatico e ormone follicolo-stimolante.
Gonadotropina corionica Gonadotropina; stimolante l'ovulazione. Polvere per iniezione: 200, 500, 1000, 2000 U/mL (10 mL).	**Trattamento dell'ipogonadismo ipogonadotropo e del criptorchidismo; induce l'ovulazione (stimola la produzione di ormoni steroidei gonadotropi; si sostituisce all'ormone luteinizzante per stimolare l'ovulazione).** *Bambini:* Criptorchidismo prepuberale: 1000-2000 unità/m^2/dose 3 ×/sett per 3 sett o 500 unità 3 ×/sett per 4-6 sett. Ipogonadismo ipogonadotropo: 500-1000 U/dose 3 ×/sett per 3 sett; o 4000 U 3 ×/sett per 6-9 mesi, poi ridurre a 2000 unità 3 ×/sett per 3 mesi. *Adulti* (dose di menotropina): 5000 unità 3 ×/sett per 4-6 mesi.	*Effetti indesiderati:* depressione mentale, stanchezza, pubertà precoce, chiusura prematura delle epifisi.
Granisetron Iniezione: 1 mg/mL. Compresse: 1 mg.	**Antiemetico (antagonista selettivo 5-HT$_3$).** *Bambini >2 anni e adulti:* agitazione, ansia, aumento degli enzimi epatici. ev 10-20 μg/kg 15-30 min prima della chemioterapia; si possono ripetere 2-3 dosi in 24 h. per os: 1 mg bid iniziando 1 ora prima della chemioterapia.	*Effetti indesiderati:* aritmie, bradicardia, alterazioni transitorie della pressione arteriosa,
Guaifenesin, glicerile guaiacolato espettorante Con o senza codeina, destrometorfano, fenilpropanolamina o fenilepinefrina. Sciroppo, compresse, capsula, liquido.	**Controllo temporaneo della tosse.** *Bambini <2 anni:* 12 mg/kg/24 h suddivisi in 6 dosi. *2-5 anni:* 50-100 mg ogni 4 h (massimo: 600 mg/24 h). *6-11 anni:* 100-200 mg ogni 4 h (massimo: 1200 mg/24 h). *>12 anni e adulti:* 200-400 mg ogni 4 h (massimo: 2,4 g/24 h).	*Cautela:* monitorare le dosi e le tossicità di altri farmaci nei prodotti in combinazione.
Guanetidina Compresse: 10, 25 mg.	**Trattamento dell'ipertensione moderata-grave (agisce come un falso neurotrasmettitore).** *Bambini:* 0,2 mg/kg/24 h; si può aumentare di 0,2 mg/kg/24 h ogni sett (massimo: 3 mg/kg/24 h). *Adulti:* iniziale 10 mg/24 h; aumentare ogni sett (massimo: 25-50 mg/24 h).	*Effetti indesiderati:* palpitazioni, dolore toracico, edema periferico, affaticamento, cefalea, sonnolenza, confusione, stipsi, anoressia, pollachiuria, nicturia, parestesie, disturbi della vista, ipotensione ortostatica.
Guanfacina HCL Compresse: 1 mg.	**Trattamento dell'ipertensione e del disturbo da deficit dell'attenzione (ADD) (stimola i recettori α-2 nel tronco cerebrale).** *Bambini:* ADD: 1 mg/24 h. *Adulti:* 1 mg/24 h; si può aumentare ogni 4 sett (massimo: 3 mg/24 h).	*Effetti indesiderati:* sonnolenza, vertigini, secchezza delle fauci, stipsi, gastrite.
Ialuronidasi Iniezione: 150 U/mL.	**Trattamento dello stravaso; aumenta l'assorbimento dei liquidi somministrati per ipodermoclisi (idrolisi dell'acido ialuronico per modificare la permeabilità del tessuto connettivo).** *Neonati, bambini piccoli e grandi:* iniettare usando un ago da 25-26 g (totale 1 mL, 150 U), sc, o intradermico in 5 siti (0,2 mL in ciascuno) in corrispondenza del margine principale dello stravaso.	*Effetti indesiderati:* tachicardia, ipotensione, eritema.
Ibuprofene Agente anti-infiammatorio non steroideo. Sospensione: 100 mg/5 mL. Compresse: 200, 300, 400, 600, 800 mg.	**Trattamento del dolore, della febbre, dell'artrite reumatoide (inibisce la sintesi delle prostaglandine).** *Bambini:* Dolore, febbre: 5-10 mg/kg/dose ogni 6-8 h. Artrite reumatoide giovanile: 30-50 mg/kg/24 h in 4 dosi suddivise. *Adulti:* 400-800 mg/dose tid-qid (massimo: 3,2 g/24 h).	*Effetti indesiderati:* crampi addominali, pirosi gastrica, nausea, sanguinamento e perforazione gastrointestinale, ritenzione idrica, edema, ipertensione, tachicardia, insufficienza renale acuta.

TABELLA 716-1. Farmaci generali – *continua*

FARMACO (PRINCIPIO ATTIVO, FORMULAZIONI)	INDICAZIONI (MECCANISMO D'AZIONE E DOSAGGIO)	COMMENTI (CAUTELE, EFFETTI INDESIDERATI, MONITORAGGIO)
Idralazina Iniezione: 20 mg/mL. Compresse. Possono essere preparate formulazioni estemporanee.	**Trattamento dell'ipertensione; in aggiunta al trattamento dello scompenso cardiaco congestizio con nitrati (vasodilatazione diretta delle arteriole).** *Neonati:* ev: 0,1-0,5 mg/kg/dose ogni 6-8 h. per os: 0,25-1 mg/kg/dose ogni 6-8 h. *Bambini piccoli e grandi:* im, ev: iniziare con 0,1-0,2 mg/kg/dose ogni 4-6 h e titolare fino all'effetto (massimo: 3,5 mg/kg/24 h). per os: 0,75-1 mg/kg/24 h in 2-4 dosi suddivise (massimo: 7,5 mg/kg/24 h). *Adulti:* im, ev: 10-20 mg/dose ogni 4-6 h (massimo: 40 mg/dose). per os: 10-25 mg/dose qid, e titolare fino all'effetto (massimo: 300 mg/24 h).	*Effetti indesiderati:* palpitazioni, flushing, tachicardia, cefalea, nausea, vomito, anoressia, diarrea, sindrome simil-lupus, artralgie, neuropatia periferica (correlata al deficit di piridossina).
Idroclortiazide Soluzione orale: 50 mg/5 mL. Compresse: 25, 50, 100 mg Prodotti di combinazione (per es. con spironolattone).	**Trattamento dell'ipertensione e degli stati di sovraccarico di volume (edema) (per es. displasia broncopolmonare, scompenso cardiaco congestizio, prevenzione dei calcoli renali di calcio recidivanti) (diuretico, inibisce il riassorbimento di sodio nel tubulo distale).** *Neonati e bambini piccoli:* 2-4 mg/kg/24 h in dosi suddivise. *Bambini piccoli >6 mesi e bambini grandi:* 2 mg/kg/24 h in 2 dosi suddivise. *Adulti:* 12,5-100 mg/24 h.	*Effetti indesiderati:* ipopotassemia, ipocloremia, ipomagnesiemia, iperglicemia, iperuricemia, iperlipidemia, pancreatite, leucopenia, trombocitopenia, anemia aplastica, epatite, colestasi intraepatica, uremia prerenale.
Idrocortisone Crema, pomata, gel, lozione, iniezione, sospensione orale, schiuma rettale.	**Trattamento dell'insufficienza surrenalica, dell'iperplasia surrenalica congenita, shock, delle dermatosi responsive ai corticosteroidi, trattamento aggiuntivo della colite ulcerosa (anti-infiammatorio, glucocorticoide).** *Neonati, bambini piccoli e bambini giovani :* Insufficienza surrenalica: 1-2 mg/kg ev bolo, poi 25-150 mg/24 h suddivisi ogni 6 h. Iperplasia surrenalica congenita: ev: iniziare 0,5-0,7mg/kg/24 h, poi 0,3-0,4 mg/kg/24 h terapia di mantenimento; somministrare dosi 1/4 al mattino, 1/4 a mezzogiorno e 1/2 alla sera. Shock: ev: 35-50 mg/kg, poi 50-150 mg/kg/24 h suddivisi ogni 6 h per 48-72 h. *Bambini piccoli e bambini più grandi :* Insufficienza surrenalica: 1-2 mg/kg bolo ev, poi 150-250 mg/24 h suddivisi ogni 6-8 h. Anti-infiammatorio: ev, im: 1-5 mg/kg/24 h in 1-2 dosi. per os: 2,5-10 mg/kg/24 h suddivisi ogni 6-8 h. Shock: ev: 50 mg/kg/dose ogni 4 h. Stato asmatico: ev: 1-2 mg/kg/dose ogni 6 h. *Adulti:* Anti-infiammatorio: ev, im, per os: 15-240 mg/dose ogni 12 h. Shock: ev: 0,5-2 g ogni 2-6 h. Rettale: applicare 1-2 volte/24 h per 2-3sett. Topico: applicare 3-4 volte/24 h.	*Cautela:* la sospensione improvvisa può causare insufficienza surrenalica acuta. *Effetti indesiderati:* ipertensione, iperglicemia, ipopotassemia, euforia, insonnia, cefalea, sindrome di Cushing, ulcera peptica, cataratta, immunosoppressione, atrofia cutanea e muscolare, acne, edema.

Potenza relativa dei corticosteroidi

Farmaco	Effetto antinfiammatorio (mg)	Effetto sodio ritentivo (mg)
Idrocortisone	100	100
Cortisone	80	80
Prednisolone	20	100
Prednisone	20	100
Metilprednisolone	16	0
Triamcinolone	16	0
Desametasone	2	0
Desossicorticosterone	0	2

FARMACO (PRINCIPIO ATTIVO, FORMULAZIONI)	INDICAZIONI (MECCANISMO D'AZIONE E DOSAGGIO)	COMMENTI (CAUTELE, EFFETTI INDESIDERATI, MONITORAGGIO)
Idromorfone Iniezione. Compresse: 2, 4 mg. Sciroppo: 1 mg/5 mL. Supposta : 3 mg.	**Analgesico, antitussivo (narcotico).** *Bambini 6-12 anni:* Tosse: per os: 0,5 mg ogni 3-4 h se necessario. Dolore: per os: 0,03-0,08 mg/kg/dose ogni 4-6 h se necessario. ev: 0,015 mg/kg/dose ogni 4-6 h se necessario. *Bambini >12 anni e adulti:* Tosse: per os: 1 mg ogni 3-4 h se necessario. Dolore: per os, ev, im, sc: 1-4 mg/dose ogni 4-6 h se necessario. *Commento:* idromorfone ev, im 1,5 mg = morfina 10 mg; orale idromorfone 7,5 mg = morfina 30 mg (acuta) o 60 mg (cronica).	*Cautela:* le compresse e lo sciroppo contengono tartrazina, che può riacutizzare l'asma; non sospendere improvvisamente dopo l'uso continuo. *Effetti indesiderati:* sedazione, sonnolenza, confusione, irritabilità, cefalea, tachicardia, ipotensione, assuefazione fisica e psicologica, nausea, vomito, stipsi, crampi allo stomaco, riduzione della diuresi, spasmo ureterale, depressione respiratoria, respiro affannoso, miosi, rilascio di ormone antidiuretico, reazioni da sensibilità (dovute al rilascio di istamina).
Idrossicobalamina, vitamina B_{12} Iniezione.	**Trattamento dell'anemia perniciosa, del deficit di vitamina B_{12}, aumentate richieste di vitamina B_{12} (terapia sostitutiva).** *Bambini:* 100 μg/24 h im fino a 1 mg totale per 2 sett, poi 30-50 μg/mese. *Adulti:* 30 μg/24 h per 5-10 giorni, poi 100-200 μg/mese.	*Commento:* può essere necessaria la co-somministrazione di folati.
Idrossiclorochina Compresse: 200 mg. Possono essere preparate formulazioni estemporanee.	**Soppressione o chemoprofilassi della malaria; trattamento del lupus eritematoso e dell'artrite reumatoide (interferisce con la funzione del vacuolo digestivo nei parassiti della malaria sensibili, altera le reazioni antigene-anticorpo complemento dipendenti).** *Bambini:* Chemioprofilassi della malaria: 5 mg/kg 1×/sett (iniziare 1-2 sett prima dell'esposizione e continuare per 4 sett dopo avere lasciato l'area a rischio). Attacco acuto di malaria: 10 mg/kg dose iniziale seguita da 5 mg/kg in 6-8 h al giorno 1400 mg una volta ai giorni 2 e 3. *Adulti:* Profilassi della malaria: 400 mg 1×/sett (timing come nei bambini). Attacco acuto di malaria: giorno 1: 800 mg, poi 400 mg in 6-8 h; giorni 2 e 3: 400 mg una volta. Artrite reumatoide e lupus eritematoso: 400 mg una volta al giorno, si può aumentare di 200 mg se la risposta è inadeguata in 4-12 sett, ridurre a 200- 400 mg/24 h dopo avere ottenuto la risposta ed è necessario un mantenimento a lungo termine.	*Cautela:* evitare nella porfiria o nella psoriasi. *Effetti indesiderati:* cefalea, confusione, agitazione, insonnia, incubi, psicosi, difetti del campo visivo, retinite, cecità, soppressione midollare, trombocitopenia, insufficienza epatica, anoressia, nausea, vomito, diarrea, dermatite lichenoide, sbiancamento dei capelli, prurito, ototossicità. *Monitoraggio:* esami oftalmologici per le alterazioni del campo visivo.

TABELLA 716-1. Farmaci generali – *continua*

FARMACO (PRINCIPIO ATTIVO, FORMULAZIONI)	INDICAZIONI (MECCANISMO D'AZIONE E DOSAGGIO)	COMMENTI (CAUTELE, EFFETTI INDESIDERATI, MONITORAGGIO)
Idrossiurea Compresse: 1000 mg. Capsule: 500 mg.	**Chemioterapia tumorale, anemia a cellule falciformi (interferisce con la sintesi di DNA durante la fase S della divisione cellulare).** *Bambini:* 1500-3000 mg/m² ogni 4-6 sett. *Adulti:* Chemioterapia tumorale: 80 mg/kg ogni 3 giorni, o 20-30 mg/kg/24 h. Anemia a cellule falciformi: 10-20 mg/kg/24 h.	*Effetti indesiderati:* sonnolenza, cefalea, allucinazioni, convulsioni, nausea, vomito, mucosite, stomatite, mielosoppressione (inizio, giorno 7; nadir, giorno 10; remissione, giorno 21), alopecia, rash maculopapulare, cute secca, eritema del volto e delle mani, epatite, aumento di azotemia e creatinina, iperuricemia.
Idrossizina Iniezione, sciroppo, compresse, capsule.	**Trattamento dell'allergia, prurito, ansia, nausea e come aggiunta per il trattamento del dolore cronico (bloccante del recettore H_1).** per os, im: *Bambini:* 0,6 mg/kg/dose ogni 6 h. *Adulti:* 10-100 mg/dose tid-qid.	*Cautela:* può peggiorare il glaucoma ad angolo stretto, l'ipertrofia prostatica, l'ostruzione del collo vescicale, l'asma e la pneumopatia cronica ostruttiva. *Effetti indesiderati:* ipotensione, sonnolenza, vertigini, cefalea, bocca secca, ritenzione urinaria, dolore nel sito di iniezione.
Idarubicina Iniezione.	**Chemioterapia di combinazione per la leucemia mielocitica e linfocitica acute (LMA e LLA) (inibisce la sintesi di DNA e RNA).** *Bambini:* LLA: 10-12 mg/m² ev una volta al giorno per un ciclo di 3 giorni/trattamento. *Adulti:* LMA: 8-12 mg/m² ev al giorno per un ciclo di 3 giorni/trattamento.	*Effetti indesiderati:* cefalea, infezione, emorragia, mucosite, stomatite, alopecia, rash, orticaria, nausea, vomito, diarrea, leucopenia (nadir, 8-19 giorni), trombocitopenia (nadir, 10-15 giorni), tossicità miocardica (aritmie, cardiomiopatia, scompenso cardiaco, modificazioni ECG). *Monitoraggio:* dose massima per tutta la vita = 137,5 mg/m², Abbassare la dose del 25% se è presente una mucosite grave o la creatinina sierica è >2 mg/dL; del 50% se la bilirubina è >2,5 mg/dL; non somministrare la dose se la bilirubina è >5 mg/dL.
Ifosfamide Agente alchilante. Iniezione.	**Chemioterapia tumorale.** *Bambini:* ev: 1200-1800 mg/m² 24 h per 5 giorni ogni 21-28 giorni, o 5 g/m² come infusione ev singola. *Adulti:* 700-2000 mg/m² 24 h per 5 giorni ogni 21-28 giorni, o 5 g/m² come infusione ev singola.	*Effetti indesiderati:* alopecia, nausea, vomito, stomatite, cistite emorragica (somministrare mesna per l'uroprotezione), ematuria, polineuropatia, psicosi depressiva, aumento degli enzimi epatici, danno renale, sonnolenza, confusione, allucinazioni, coma, mielosoppressione (inizio, giorno 7; nadir, 10-14 giorni), fibrosi polmonare, congestione nasale, cardiotossicità.
Imipramina Iniezione, capsule, compresse.	**Trattamento della depressione, dell'enuresi, del dolore (antidepressivo triciclico, aumenta le concentrazioni sinaptiche di noradrenalina e serotonina).** *Bambini:* Depressione: iniziare con 1,5 mg/kg/24 h; si può aumentare di 1 mg/kg/24 h ogni 3-4 giorni (massimo: 5 mg/kg/24 h). Enuresi: >6 anni: 10-25 mg prima di andare a letto. Dolore tumorale: 0,2-0,4 mg/kg prima di andare a letto; si può aumentare la dose del 50% ogni 3-4 giorni (massimo: 3 mg/kg). *Adolescenti:* per os: iniziare con 25-50 mg/24 h; si può gradualmente aumentare (massimo: 200 mg/24 h). *Adulti:* per os: 25 mg tid-qid; si può aumentare la dose gradualmente (massimo: 300 mg/24 h). im: inizialmente, somministrare fino a 100 mg in dosi suddivise.	*Effetti indesiderati:* aritmie, ipotensione posturale, sonnolenza, sedazione, confusione, cefalea, secchezza delle fauci, stipsi, ritenzione urinaria, aumento degli enzimi epatici, convulsioni, ritenzione urinaria. *Monitoraggio:* concentrazioni di imipramina (terapeutiche: imipramina e desipramina 150-250 ng/mL, tossiche >1000 ng/mL).
Immunoglobulina, endovenosa Iniezione.	**Sindrome da immunodeficienza, porpora trombotica trombocitopenica, infezioni batteriche o virali acute nei pazienti immunocompromessi o neutropenici, malattia di Kawasaki, sindrome di Guillain-Barré, polineuropatia demielinizzante (terapia sostitutiva o interferenza con i recettori Fc nel sistema reticolo endoteliale per le malattie autoimmuni).** *Neonati:* 500-750 mg/kg una volta. *Bambini e adulti:* Sindrome da immunodeficienza: 100-400 mg/kg/dose ogni 2-4 sett. Leucemia linfocitica cronica: 400 mg/kg/dose ogni 3 sett. Porpora trombotica trombocitopenica: 1000 mg/kg/dose per 2-5 giorni consecutivi, poi ogni 3-6 sett. Malattia di Kawasaki: 2 g/kg in dose singola. Infezione da Cytomegalovirus: 500 mg/kg/dose e ogni giorno per 7 dosi. Infezione sistemica grave: 500-1000 mg/kg/sett. Polineuropatia: 1 g/kg/24 h per 2 giorni consecutivi ogni mese.	*Cautela:* le dosi dovrebbero basarsi sul peso corporeo ideale (non sul peso corporeo totale). *Effetti indesiderati:* flushing, tachicardia, brividi, nausea, dispnea, febbre, reazioni da ipersensibilità, cefalea, meningite asettica.
Immunoglobulina tetanica Iniezione.	**Profilassi e trattamento del tetano.** Profilassi: *Bambini:* im 4 U/kg. *Adulti:* im: 250 unità. Trattamento: *Bambini:* im 500-3000 unità. *Adulti:* im 3000-6000 unità (infiltrare parte della dose attorno alla ferita).	*Effetti indesiderati:* reazioni allergiche.
Indometacina Capsule: 25, 50 mg. Sospensione: 25 mg/5 mL. Iniezione.	**Chiusura del dotto arterioso pervio nei neonati, trattamento dei disordini reumatoidi, artrite gottosa acuta, dolore (farmaco anti-infiammatorio non steroideo, inibizione delle prostaglandine), tubulopatie renali ereditarie ipopotassiemiche sale-disperdenti.** *Neonati:* ev: 0,10-0,25 mg/kg/dose ogni 12 h per 3-6 dosi. Disordini infiammatori reumatoidi: *Bambini:* 1-2 mg/kg/24 h in 2-4 dosi (massimo: 4 mg/kg/24 h). piastrinica, oliguria, insufficienza renale, ipertensione, edema. *Adulti:* 25-50 mg/dose bid-tid (massimo: 200 mg/24 h).	*Cautela:* evitare nei neonati prematuri con enterocolite necrotizzante, funzione renale ridotta, o sanguinamento attivo, e tutti i pazienti con sanguinamento gastrointestinale attivo. *Effetti indesiderati:* confusione, vertigini, cefalea, nausea, vomito, perforazione gastrointestinale, soppressione del midollo osseo, alterata aggregazione dolore addominale, sanguinamento gastrointestinale, ulcere, iperpotassemia. *Monitoraggio:* indometacina (concentrazioni nella chiusura del dotto arterioso pervio): terapeutiche 1-3 μg/mL.

TABELLA 716-1. Farmaci generali – *continua*

FARMACO (PRINCIPIO ATTIVO, FORMULAZIONI)	INDICAZIONI (MECCANISMO D'AZIONE E DOSAGGIO)	COMMENTI (CAUTELE, EFFETTI INDESIDERATI, MONITORAGGIO)
Insulina **Azione rapida**. **Azione-intermedia**. **Long-acting:** **Prodotti di combinazione**. Insulina umana (forma preferita); insulina di manzo, insulina di maiale. Iniezione.	**Trattamento del diabete mellito insulino-dipendente e non-insulino-dipendente non adeguatamente controllato dagli agenti ipoglicemizzanti orali (terapia sostitutiva).** *Neonati:* insulina regolare 0,01-0,1 U/kg/h in infusione continua, o sc 0,1-0,2 U/kg 6-12 h. *Bambini e adulti:* 0,5-1 U/kg/24 h. Aggiustare le dosi in base alla glicemia plasmatica e all'emoglobina A_{1C} *Adolescenti (durante lo scatto di crescita):* 0,8-1,2 U/kg/24 h. Chetoacidosi diabetica: Infusione continua ev: 0,1 U/kg/h aggiustare in base alla glicemia. Iperpotassemia: somministrare calcio gluconato e $NaHCO_3$ per primi, poi destrosio 50% 0,5-1 mL/kg e insulina regolare 1 U/4-5 g destroso.	*Cautela:* controllare gli aumenti o le diminuzioni dell'insulina correlati al farmaco. Non cambiare i tipi di insulina o le marche una volta che il paziente è regolato poiché i fabbisogni di dosaggio si modificheranno; nei nuovi pazienti iniziare con insulina umana se possibile. *Effetti indesiderati:* ipoglicemia (e sintomi associati vertigini, debolezza, parestesie, parestesia della bocca, affaticamento, confusione mentale, fame, nausea, problemi visivi), ipopotassemia. *Monitoraggio:* glicemia (insegnare al paziente a monitorare a casa e ad apportare le correzioni del dosaggio in base ai risultati), emoglobina A_{1C}, glicosuria e acetone.
Interferone α-2a Iniezione.	**Nei bambini, trattamento degli emangiomi dell'infanzia e polmonari (inibisce la crescita cellulare, altera la differenziazione cellulare).** *Bambini piccoli e bambini:* sc: 1-3 milioni U/m²/dose. *Adulti:* 3-20 milioni U/m²/dose/dose alla 3×/sett, a seconda dell'indicazione.	*Effetti indesiderati:* tachicardia, aritmie, ipotensione, edema, depressione del SNC, confusione, affaticamento, vertigini e sintomi simil-influenzali (iniziare 2-6 h dopo la dose e continuare fino a 24 h).
Iosciamina (con atropina, scopolamina e fenobarbital) Capsule, elisir, compresse.	**Trattamento dell'intestino irritabile, del colon spastico, della vescica spastica e della colica renale (anticolinergico).** *Bambini:* 0,1 mL/kg/dose ogni 4 h (massimo: 5 mL) *Adulti:* 1-2 compresse (o 5-10 mL) tid-qid.	*Cautela:* controindicato nel glaucoma ad angolo stretto, nella miastenia gravis e nell'ostruzione gastrointestinale e genitourinaria. *Effetti indesiderati:* tachicardia, palpitazioni, cefalea, sonnolenza, nervosismo, secchezza delle fauci, stipsi, disfagia, ileo paralitico, visione offuscata, congestione nasale.
Ipecacuana sciroppo Sciroppo: 70 mg/mL.	**Induce vomito per il trattamento dell'ingestione di alcune sostanze tossiche (stimola la zona trigger del chemorecettore midollare).** *Bambini:* si può ripetere dose in 20 min 1×. *6-12 mesi:* 5-10 mL, seguita da 20 mL/kg di acqua. *1-12 anni:* 15 mL, seguita da 20 mL/kg di acqua. *>12 anni e adulti:* 30 mL, seguita da 300 mL di acqua.	*Cautela:* non usare se il paziente non è cosciente, ha assenza del riflesso del vomito, o ha convulsioni, o dopo ingestione di basi o acidi forti o di oli volatili. Non confondere con ipecacuana estratto fluido, che è 14 volte più potente. *Effetti indesiderati:* letargia, vomito persistente, diarrea.
Ipratropio Anticolinergico. Soluzione da nebulizzare: 0,02%. Inalatore a dosaggio controllato (MDI): 18 μg/puff. Spruzzo nasale: 0,3%, 0,6%.	**Broncodilatatore, trattamento della rinite).** *Neonati:* nebulizzato 100 μg/dose o MDI 1-2 puff tid-qid. *Bambini piccoli e bambini:* nebulizzato 125-250 μg o MDI 1-2 puff 3-6 volte/24 h. *Adulti:* nebulizzato 500 μg o MDI 2 puff tid-qid. Spray nasale per la rinite: 1-2 spruzzi in ogni narice bid-tid.	*Effetti indesiderati:* secchezza delle fauci, nervosismo, vertigini, cefalea, visione offuscata, ritenzione urinaria.
Isoetarina Inalatore a dosaggio controllato (MDI), soluzione inalante.	**Broncodilatatore (stimolazione β-agonista).** *Bambini:* nebulizzare 0,01 mL/kg di soluzione 1%. *Adulti:* nebulizzare 0,5-1 mL di soluzione 0,5-1%; MDI 1-2 puff ogni 4 h se necessario.	*Effetti indesiderati:* tachicardia, cefalea, tremore, eccitamento, irritabilità, nausea.
Isoproterenolo Iniezione, compresse sublinguali, soluzione nebulizzata, inalatore a dosaggio controllato (MDI).	**Asma o broncopneumopatia cronica ostruttiva, aritmie ventricolari causate da blocco del nodo AV, stati di shock da bassa gittata (stimola i recettori β_1 e β_2)** *Neonati, bambini piccoli e grandi:* ev: infondere 0,05-2 μg/kg/min. *Bambini:* MDI: 1-2 puff e ogni 4 h se necessario; nebulizzare 0,01 mL di soluzione 1%; compresse sublinguali: 5-10 mg e ogni 3-4 h (massimo: 30 mg/24 h). *Adulti:* MDI: 1-2 puff 4-6 volte/24 h; nebulizzare 0,25-0,5 mL di soluzione 1%; compresse sublinguali: 10-20 mg ogni 3-4 h (massimo: 60 mg/24 h); ev infusione2-20 μg/min.	*Effetti indesiderati:* tachicardia, palpitazioni, dolore toracico, nervosismo, irritabilità, ansia, cefalea, insonnia, tremore, disturbi gastrointestinali, nausea, broncospasmo paradosso.
Istrelina Analogo del gonadotropin-releasing hormone. Iniezione.	**Pubertà precoce idiopatica centrale.** *Bambini:* sc: 10 μg/kg una volta al giorno. *Femmina adulta:* 100 μg/24 h per l'endometriosi.	*Effetti indesiderati:* ansia, depressione, irritabilità, insonnia, cefalee.
Ketamina Iniezione: 10, 100 mg/mL.	**Anestesia per procedure brevi (azione diretta su corteccia e sistema limbico per produrre un'anestesia dissociativa).** *Bambini:* somministrare 30 min prima della procedura. per os: 6-10 mg/kg. im: 3-7 mg/kg. ev: 0,5-2 mg/kg. *Adulti:* 3-8 mg/kg ev. ev: 1-4,5 mg/kg (dosi supplementari 1/3 della dose iniziale).	*Effetti indesiderati:* ipertensione, tachicardia, ipotensione, bradicardia, aumentato del flusso ematico cerebrale e della pressione endocranica, allucinazioni, delirio, movimenti tonico-clonici, aumento della velocità metabolica, ipersalivazione, nausea, vomito, depressione respiratoria, apnea, aumentate resistenze delle vie aeree, tosse, reazioni di emergenza.
Ketorolac Farmaco anti-infiammatorio non steroideo. Oftalmico. Toradol. Compresse, iniezione.	**Trattamento del dolore; del prurito oculare con congiuntivite (inibisce le prostaglandine).** *Bambini 2-16 anni:* im, ev: 0,4-1 mg/kg/dose. per os: 1 mg/kg/dose ogni 6 h se necessario. *Adulti:* im: 60 mg. ev: 30 mg fino a ogni 6 h se necessario. Oftalmico: 1 goccia in occhio qid fino a 7 giorni.	*Effetti indesiderati:* edema, sonnolenza, vertigini, cefalea, dispepsia, nausea, diarrea, dolore gastrointestinale, sanguinamento gastrointestinale, ulcera peptica, alterata aggregazione piastrinica, oliguria, insufficienza renale acuta, dispnea, respiro affannoso, dolore nel sito di iniezione.

TABELLA 716-1. Farmaci generali – *continua*

FARMACO (PRINCIPIO ATTIVO, FORMULAZIONI)	INDICAZIONI (MECCANISMO D'AZIONE E DOSAGGIO)	COMMENTI (CAUTELE, EFFETTI INDESIDERATI, MONITORAGGIO)
Labetalolo Iniezione: 5 mg/mL. Compresse: 100, 200, 300 mg.	**Trattamento dell'ipertensione da lieve a grave (blocca i recettori α e β adrenergici).** *Bambini:* per os: iniziare con 4 mg/kg/24 h in 2 dosi, poi aumentare gradualmente (massimo: 40 mg/kg/24 h). ev: iniziare 0,2-1 mg/kg/dose (massimo: 20 mg/dose), infusione ev continua di 0,4-1 mg/kg/h (massimo: 3 mg/kg/h). *Adulti:* per os: 100 mg bid; si può aumentare ogni 2-3 giorni (massimo: 2,4 g/24 h). ev: iniziare 20 mg; ripetere boli 40 mg ogni 10 min (massimo: dose totale 300 mg), infusione continua ev di 2 mg/min e titolare fino alla risposta.	*Effetti indesiderati:* ipotensione ortostatica, scompenso cardiaco congestizio, disturbi di conduzione, bradicardia, sonnolenza, affaticamento, cefalea, secchezza delle fauci, congestione nasale, broncospasmo.
Lamotrigina Compresse: 25, 100, 150, 200 mg. Compresse, masticabili, dispersibili: 2, 5, 25 mg.	**Trattamento delle convulsioni parziali (blocca i canali del sodio e inibisce il rilascio presinaptico di glutammato e aspartato).** *Bambini 2-12 anni:* 0,6 mg/kg/24 h in 1-2 dosi per 2 sett, poi 1,2 mg/kg/24 h in 2 dosi per 2 sett, poi 5-15 mg/kg/24 h in 2 dosi per la risposta (massimo: 400 mg/24 h). Pazienti che assumono valproato: 0,15 mg/kg/24 h in 1-2 dosi per 2 sett, poi 0,3 mg/kg/24 h in 2 dosi per 2 sett, poi 1-5 mg/kg/24 h in 2 dosi (massimo: 200 mg/24 h). *Adulti:* iniziare 50 mg/24 h per 2 sett, poi 100 mg/24 h, poi aumentare di 100 mg/24 h a intervalli settimanali fino alla risposta (massimo: 500 mg/24 h). Pazienti che assumono valproato: 25 mg ogni giorno per 2 sett, poi 25 mg/24 h per 2 sett, poi aumentare di 25 mg/24 h ogni sett fino alla risposta (massimo: 150 mg/24 h).	*Cautela:* si possono verificare rash seri (potenzialmente fatali) e sono particolarmente comuni nei bambini, specialmente se le dosi sono aumentate troppo velocemente. Un lento aumento del dosaggio è importante specialmente per i i pazienti che assumono acido valproico. *Effetti indesiderati:* vertigini, sedazione, cefalea, agitazione, esacerbazione delle convulsioni, rash (maculopapulare o eruzioni eritematose), angioedema, fotosensibilità, nistagmo, ambliopia, nausea, vomito.
Lansoprazolo Inibitore pompa-protonica. Capsule: 15, 30 mg. Bustine: polvere per sospensione orale 5 mg, 30 mg.	**Trattamento dell'ulcera gastrica o duodenale.** *Bambini:* 15-30 mg/24 h. *Adulti:* 15-30 mg/24 h.	
Lattulosio Sciroppo: 10 g/15 mL.	**Trattamento della stipsi, dell'encefalopatia epatica (effetto osmotico sulle feci nel colon; l'acidificazione delle feci promuove l'eliminazione di $NH4^+$).** *Bambini piccoli:* 2,5-10 mL/24 h in 3-4 dosi. *Bambini:* 40-90 mL/24 h in 3-4 dosi. *Adulti:* 30-45 mL/dose 3-4 volte/24 h.	*Effetti indesiderati:* flatulenza, fastidio addominale, diarrea, nausea, vomito. *Monitoraggio:* target 2-3 feci molli/giorno; ammoniemia.
Leucovorin Compresse: 5, 15 mg. Iniezione.	**Antidoto per gli antagonisti dell'acido folico (per es. metotrexato), trattamento delle anemie megaloblastiche da deficit di folati dell'infanzia, deficit nutrizionale di folati quando non si possono usare i folati orali (forma ridotta dell'acido folico, per cui non è necessaria la conversione, terapia sostitutiva).** *Bambini e adulti:* Metotrexato rescue: ev: 10 mg/m^2 per iniziare, poi 10 mg/m^2 per os ogni 6 h per 72 h; aumentare la dose a 100 mg/m^2 ogni 3 h se 24 h dopo la dose di metotrexato, la creatinina sierica è aumentata del >50%, o il livello sierico di metotrexato è $>5 \times 10^{-6}$M (continuare fino e quando il livello è $<1 \times 10^{-8}$M). Metotrexato rescue ad alte dosi: ev: 100-1000 mg/m^2 dose. Metotrexato intretecale: ev: 12 mg/m^2 in monosomministrazione. Anemia megaloblastica dell'infanzia: im 3-6 mg/24 h.	*Effetti indesiderati:* rash, prurito eritema. *Monitoraggio:* livelli plasmatici di metotrexato; è disponibile un nomogramma per il dosaggio di leucovorin e si basa sui livelli di metotrexato a vari tempi dopo la dose.
Leuprolide Iniezione.	**Trattamento della pubertà precoce, cancro alla prostata (diminuisce i livelli di ormone luteinizzante e follicolo-stimolante).** 0,15-0,3 mg/kg/dose ogni 28 giorni (minimo: 7,5 mg) im. sc: 20-45 μg/kg/24 h. *Adulti:* cancro alla prostata: im: 7,5 mg/dose/mese. sc: 1 mg/24 h.	*Effetti indesiderati:* aumento di peso, vampate, depressione, nausea, vomito, sanguinamento gastrointestinale, mialgia, dolore osseo, debolezza, visione offuscata, effetti estrogenici.
Levotiroxina Iniezione, compresse.	**Terapia tiroidea sostitutiva.** per os: *0-6 mesi:* 8-10 μg/kg/24 h. *6-12 mesi:* 6-8 μg/kg/24 h. *1-5 anni:* 5-6 μg/kg/24 h. *6-12 anni:* 4-5 μg/kg/24 h. *>12 anni:* 2-3 μg/kg/24 h. *Adulti:* 12,5-50 μg/24 h (massimo: 200 μg/24 h). ev, im: 50-75% di dose per os. Coma da mixedema: 200-500 μg per 1 dose. Terapia soppressiva tiroidea: 2-6 μg/kg/24 h per 7-10 giorni.	*Effetti indesiderati:* tachicardia, aritmie cardiache, ipertensione, nervosismo, cefalea, insonnia, perdita di capelli, appetito aumentato, perdita di peso, tremore, sudorazione.
Lidocaina Iniezione. Topico (solo o in combinazione con prilocaina [EMLA]).	**Trattamento delle aritmie ventricolari, anestetico locale (antiaritmico di classe 1B, blocca l'inizio e la conduzione degli impulsi).** *Bambini e adulti:* topico: applicare sull'area interessata (massimo: 3 mg/kg/dose) almeno 2 h dopo. Iniezione di anestetico locale: dosi secondo quanto necessario (massimo: 4,5 mg/kg), a distanza di 2 h l'una dall'altra. Aritmie: *Bambini:* dose da carico di 1 mg/kg (si può ripetere ogni 5-10 min (massimo: 3 mg/kg). ev: infusione continua: 20-50 μg/kg/min (1/2 dose per epatopatia o ridotta gittata cardiaca). *Adulti:* dose da carico di 1-1,5 mg/kg, ripetibile (massimo: 3 mg/kg). ev: infusione continua: 2-4 mg/min (1/2 dose per epatopatia o scompenso cardiaco). Via endotracheale: 2-2,5 × ev dose. Post-infarto miocardico preospedaliero: 300 mg im.	*Cautela:* evitare lidocaina con le preparazioni di adrenalina per le aritmie. *Effetti indesiderati:* aritmie, blocco cardiaco, letargia, coma, convulsioni, nausea, vomito, parestesie, visione offuscata, diplopia, irritazione cutanea locale o rash. *Monitoraggio:* livelli sierici di lidocaina (terapeutiche 1-5 μg/mL tossiche >6 μg/mL).

TABELLA 716-1. Farmaci generali – *continua*

FARMACO (PRINCIPIO ATTIVO, FORMULAZIONI)	INDICAZIONI (MECCANISMO D'AZIONE E DOSAGGIO)	COMMENTI (CAUTELE, EFFETTI INDESIDERATI, MONITORAGGIO)
Liotironina Orale. Iniezione.	**Terapia sostitutiva nell'ipotiroidismo.** *Neonati, bambini piccoli e bambini <3 anni:* ipotiroidismo congenito (cretinismo): per os: 5 µg/24 h inizialmente, poi si può aumentare 5 µg ogni 3 giorni (massimo: 20 µg/24 h (50 µg/24 h per bambini di età 1-3 anni)). Ipotiroidismo: *Bambini:* 5 µg/24 h; aumentare di 5 µg ogni 1-2 sett (di solito, 15-20 µg/24 h). *Adulti:* iniziare 5 µg/24 h; aumentare di 5 µg/24 h ogni 1-2 sett fino a 25 µg, poi di 12,5-25 µg ogni 1-2 sett (massimo: 100 µg/24 h).	*Effetti indesiderati:* palpitazioni, tachicardia, ipertensione, nervosismo, insonnia, cefalea, perdita di capelli, diarrea, crampi addominali, tremore, sudorazione. *Monitoraggio:* funzionalità tiroidea, T_3, ormone tireostimolante.
Litio Sciroppo: 300 mg/5 mL. Compresse: 300 mg. Capsule: 150, 300, 600 mg.	**Trattamento della mania acuta, del disordine bipolare e della depressione (altera lo scambio di cationi attraverso le membrane cellulari).** *Bambini:* 15-60 mg/kg/24 h in 3-4 dosi (iniziare con dosi basse e aumentare a intervalli settimanali). *Adolescenti:* 600-1800 mg/24 h in 3-4 dosi a intervalli regolari. *Adulti:* 300 mg tid-qid per iniziare; si può gradualmente aumentare per livelli plasmatici (massimo: 2,4 g/24 h). **Si può usare il dosaggio di due volte il giorno se viene usato il prodotto a rilascio prolungato.** *Insufficienza renale:* CrCl 10-50 mL/min: 50-70% della dose normale; CrCl 0,6-1,2 mEq/L; protezione contro futuri episodi <10 mL/min: 25-50% della dose normale.	*Effetti indesiderati:* polidipsia, nausea, diarrea, gusto alterato, sensazione di gonfiore, aumento di peso, tremore, mioclonia riflessa, debolezza, affaticamento, diabete insipido, atrofia dei nefroni aspecifica, acidosi tubulare renale, leucocitosi, problemi della vista, ipotiroidismo, gozzo, eruzioni cutanee, acne. *Monitoraggio:* le concentrazioni seriche di litio sono essenziali per un corretto utilizzo del litio, il prelievo deve essere effettuato 8-12 h dopo una dose (terapeutico: mania acuta 0,6-1mEq/L; tossiche >1,5 mEq/L; convulsioni >2,5 mEq/L). Fare attenzione all'accumulo durante la perdita di sale e gli stati di disidratazione.
Lomustina, CCNU Agente alchilante. Capsule: 10, 40, 100 mg.	**Trattamento di vari tumori (inibisce la sintesi di DNA e RNA).** *Bambini:* 75-100 mg/m^2 in monosomministrazione ogni 6 sett. *Adulti:* 100-130 mg/m^2 in monosomministrazione ogni 6 sett.	*Effetti indesiderati:* nausea, vomito, mielosoppressione (inizio, 14 giorni; nadir, 4-5sett; remissione, 6 sett), neurotossicità, stomatite, diarrea, anemia, alopecia, epatotossicità, insufficienza renale, fibrosi polmonare (con dosi cumulative >600 mg). *Monitoraggio:* ridurre la dose se CrCl <50 mL/min o conta piastrinica e leucociti rimangono bassi oltre le 6 sett.
Loperamide Liquido: 1 mg/5 mL. Compresse: 2 mg. Capsule: 2 mg.	**Trattamento della diarrea acuta e cronica (inibisce direttamente la peristalsi intestinale).** *Bambini:* *2-5 anni:* 1 mg tid. *6-8 anni:* 2 mg bid. *8-12 anni:* 2 mg tid. *Adulti:* 4 mg inizialmente, poi 2 mg dopo ogni scarica diarroica (massimo: 16 mg/24 h).	*Effetti indesiderati:* sedazione, affaticamento, vertigini, nausea, vomito, stipsi.
Loratadina Sciroppo: 1 mg/mL. Compresse: 10 mg.	**Trattamento dei sintomi allergici (antistaminico, antagonista dei recettori H_1).** *Bambini >3 anni:* <30 kg; 5 mg/24 h; >30 kg: 10 mg/24 h. *Adulti:* 10 mg/24 h.	*Cautela:* si può verificare un allungamento del tratto Q-T quando associata a farmaci che inibiscono gli enzimi epatici; attenzione alle interazioni farmacologiche. *Effetti indesiderati:* snnolenza, affaticamento, ansia, depressione, cefalea.
Lorazepam Iniezione. Compresse: 0,5, 1, 2 mg. Soluzione orale: 2 mg/mL.	**Trattamento dell'ansia, sedazione e convulsioni; aggiunta alla terapia antiemetica (benzodiazepina,aumenta l'azione dell'acido γ-amminobutirrico).** Terapia antiemetica: *Bambini:* ev: 0,04-0,08 mg/kg/dose ogni 6 h se necessario. Ansia/sedazione: *Neonati:* ev: 0,1-0,4 mg/kg/dose ogni 4-6 h se necessario. *Bambini piccoli e grandi:* ev: 0,05-0,1 mg/kg/dose ogni 4-8 h. *Adulti:* per os: 1-10 mg/24 h in 2-3 dosi suddivise. Insonnia: *Adulti:* 2-4 mg prima di andare a letto. Stato epilettico: *Neonati:* ev: 0,05-0,2 mg/kg/dose per 2-5 min; si può ripetere in 10-15 min. *Bambini piccoli e grandi:* ev: dose da carico di 0,1 mg/kg per 2-5 min; si può somministrare bolo addizionale di 0,05 mg/kg a 10-15 min. *Adolescenti:* ev: 0,07 mg/kg/dose in 2-5 min; si può ripetere a 10-15 min. *Adulti:* ev: 4 mg/dose in 2-5 min; si può ripetere a 10 min.	*Cautela:* non sospendere improvvisamente dopo un utilizzo a lungo termine per evitare i sintomi da possibile astinenza. *Effetti indesiderati:* sono stati riportati molti casi di mioclonia nei neonati; tachicardia, sonnolenza, depressione, confusione, eccitamento paradosso, visione offuscata, diplopia.
Magnesio citrato, citrato di magnesia Soluzione: 300 mL.	**Evacuazione dell'intestino (ritenzione osmotica di liquidi e aumentata peristalsi).** *Bambini <6 anni:* 2-4 mL/kg. *Bambini 6-12 anni:* 100-150 mL. *>12 anni e adulti:* 150-300 mL.	*Effetti indesiderati:* ipermagnesiemia, ipotensione, crampi addominali, debolezza muscolare, depressione SNC. *Monitoraggio:* tossicità correlata ai livelli serici di magnesio (>3 mg/dL, SNC depresso; >5 mg/dL, sonnolenza e riflessi tendinei profondi depressi; >12 mg/dL, paralisi respiratoria e arresto cardiaco).
Magnesio gluconato Compresse: 500 mg.	**Terapia sostitutiva del magnesio.** *Bambini:* 10-20 mg/kg/dose elementare di magnesio qid. *Adulti:* 300 mg magnesio elementare qid.	*Effetti indesiderati:* ipermagnesiemia (vedi *Magnesio citrato, citrato di magnesio*). *Monitoraggio:* concentrazione sierica di magnesio (normale: bambini, 1,5-1,9 mg/dL; adulti, 2,2-2,8 mg/dL).
Magnesio idrossido, latte di magnesio Liquido, compresse.	**Trattamento a breve termine della stipsi (la ritenzione osmotica di liquidi promuove la peristalsi).** *Bambini:* *<2 anni:* 0,5 mL/kg/dose. *2-5 anni:* 5-15 mL una volta al giorno. *6-12 anni:* 15-30 mL una volta al giorno. *>12 anni e adulti:* 30-60 mL una volta al giorno.	*Effetti indesiderati:* (vedi *Magnesio citrato, citrato di magnesio*).

TABELLA 716-1. Farmaci generali – *continua*

FARMACO (PRINCIPIO ATTIVO, FORMULAZIONI)	INDICAZIONI (MECCANISMO D'AZIONE E DOSAGGIO)	COMMENTI (CAUTELE, EFFETTI INDESIDERATI, MONITORAGGIO)
Magnesio, ossido di Compresse: 400, 420, 500 mg. Capsule: 140 mg.		
Magnesio solfato Granuli: 40 mEq/5 g. Iniezione: soluzione 50%.	**Trattamento dell'ipomagnesiemia e delle convulsioni associate a nefrite acuta nei bambini; usato anche come catartico (cofattore per molti enzimi dell'organismo e importante nell'omeostasi di calcio e potassio).** Ipomagnesiemia: *Neonati:* ev: 25-50 mg/kg/dose ogni 8 h per 2-3 dosi. *Bambini:* per os: 100-200 mg/kg/dose qid. im, ev: 25-50 mg/kg/dose ogni 6 h per 3-4 dosi. *Adulti:* per os: 3 g ogni 6 h per 4 dosi. im, ev: 1 g ogni 6 h per 4 dosi. Mantenimento giornaliero di magnesio: *Neonati, bambini piccoli e grandi:* ev: 30-60 mg/kg/24 h. *Adolescenti:* ev: 42-54 mg/kg/24 h. *Adulti:* ev: 0,5-3 g/24 h. Infondere dosi ev per 2-4 h (massimo: 125 mg/kg/h). Trattamento delle convulsioni e ipertensione: *Bambini:* im, ev: 20-100 mg/kg/dose ogni 4-6 h se necessario. Catartico: *Bambini:* per os: 0,25 g/kg/dose. *Adulti:* per os: 10-30 g.	*Cautela:* il magnesio si può accumulare a livelli tossici nell'insufficienza renale. *Effetti indesiderati:* (vedi *Magnesio citrato, citrato di magnesio*).
Manganese Iniezione: 0,1 mg/mL.	**Tracce di elemento aggiunte alla nutrizione parenterale (cofattore in molti sistemi enzimatici).** *Bambini piccoli:* 2-10 μg/kg/24 h in soluzioni parenterali totali nutritive. *Adulti:* 150-180 μg/24 h in soluzioni parenterali totali nutritive.	*Monitoraggio:* il livello plasmatico di riferimento del manganese è 4-14 μg/L.
Mannitolo Iniezione.	**Promozione della diuresi, riduzione dell'ipertensione endocranica.** *Bambini e adulti:* ev: 200 mg/kg dose test; iniziale, 0,5-1 g/kg; mantenimento, 0,25-0,5 g/kg ogni 4-6 h.	*Effetti indesiderati:* sovraccarico circolatorio, scompenso cardiaco congestizio, cefalea, brividi, convulsioni, alterazioni dell'equilibrio idroelettrolitico. *Monitoraggio:* dopo dose test, valutare diuresi di almeno 1 mL/kg/h (bambini) o 30-50 mL/h (adulti) per 2-3 h; per ipertensione endocranica, mantenere l'osmolarità sierica a 310-320 mOsm/kg.
Meclizina Compresse, capsule.	**Prevenzione e trattamento della cinetosi e trattamento della vertigine (effetti anticolinergici e depressivi sul SNC).** *Bambini e adulti:* per os: 25-50 mg 1 ora prima del viaggio per la cinetosi; 25-100 mg/ 24 h in dosi suddivise per la vertigine.	*Effetti indesiderati:* sonnolenza, cefalea, affaticamento, secchezza delle fauci, aumento dell'appetito, aumento di peso.
Mecloretamina, mostarda azotata Agente alchilante. Idrocloruro. Iniezione.	**Chemioterapia tumorale (inibisce la sintesi di DNA e RNA).** *Bambini:* ev: come parte del regime MOPP, 6 mg/m^2 ai giorni 1 e 8 del regime di 28 giorni. *Adulti:* ev: 0,4 mg/kg (12-16 mg/m^2) come singola dose mensile.	*Cautela:* lo stravaso dovrebbe essere trattato prontamente con sodio sterile tiosolfato (1/6 M) e applicando compresse fredde per 6-12 h. *Effetti indesiderati:* nausea, vomito, diarrea, mielosoppressione grave (inizio, 4-7 giorni; nadir, 14 giorni; remissione, 21 giorni), ototossicità, precipitazione dell'herpes zoster, alopecia, iperuricemia.
Medrisone Soluzione oftalmica.	**Trattamento della congiuntivite (inibisce la risposta infiammatoria).** *Bambini e adulti:* oftalmica: instillare 1 goccia nel sacco congiuntivale bid-qid (si può usare ogni 1-2 h per 1-2 giorni).	*Effetti indesiderati:* puntura locale e arrossamento, aumentata pressione intraoculare, cataratta.
Melfalan Agente alchilante. Iniezione. Compresse: 2 mg.	**Chemioterapia tumorale (inibisce la sintesi di DNA e RNA).** *Bambini:* ev: 10-35 mg/m^2 dose ogni 21-28 giorni; alta dose: 140-220 mg/m^2 prima del trapianto di midollo. per os: 4-20 mg/m^2/24 h per 1-21 giorni. *Adulti:* ev: 16 mg/m^2 dose ogni 2 sett per 4 dosi al mese. per os: 0,15 mg/kg/24 h per 7 giorni o 0,25 mg/kg/24 h per 4 giorni; ripetere ogni 4-6 sett.	*Effetti indesiderati:* mielosoppressione (inizio, 7 giorni; nadir, 8-10 giorni e 27-32 giorni; remissione, 42-50 giorni), tumore maligno secondario, alopecia, vescicolazione della cute, sindrome da inappropriata secrezione di ormone antidiuretico, nausea, vomito, diarrea, stomatite, cistite emorragica, fibrosi polmonare, polmonite interstiziale, vasculite.
Meperidina Iniezione, sciroppo: 50 mg/5 mL. Compresse: 50, 100 mg.	**Analgesico narcotico, aggiunta all'anestesia (si lega ai recettori oppiacei nel SNC).** *Bambini:* im, ev, sc: 1-1,5 ogni 3-4 h. *Adulti:* im, ev, sc: 50-100 mg/dose ogni 3-4 h se necessario (la dose equipotente orale è 3× dose ev).	*Cautela:* l'uso programmato può portare ad accumulo di metaboliti e diminuita funzionalità renale, che può condurre a stimolazione del SNC o a convulsioni. *Effetti indesiderati:* ipotensione, debolezza, stanchezza, cefalea, anoressia, crampi allo stomaco, allucinazioni, eccitazione paradossa, convulsioni, dipendenza fisica e psicologica. *Commento:* la dose equianalgesica a morfina 10 mg ev è meperidina 100 mg ev o im, o 300 mg per os.
Mefenitoina Compresse: 100 mg.	**Trattamento delle convulsioni tonico-cloniche e parziali (diminuisce l'afflusso di ioni sodio attraverso le membrane cellulari).** *Bambini:* 3-15 mg/kg/24 h in 3 dosi suddivise. *Adulti:* iniziare 50-100 mg/24 h; poi aumentare di 50-100 mg alla sett (massimo: 800 mg/24 h).	*Effetti indesiderati:* sonnolenza, eloquio farfugliato, problemi psichiatrici, confusione, nausea, vomito, stipsi, leucopenia, epatite, visione offuscata, nistagmo, fotofobia, linfoadenopatia. *Monitoraggio:* livello totale di mefenitoina (25-40 μg/mL).

TABELLA 716-1. Farmaci generali – *continua*

FARMACO (PRINCIPIO ATTIVO, FORMULAZIONI)	INDICAZIONI (MECCANISMO D'AZIONE E DOSAGGIO)	COMMENTI (CAUTELE, EFFETTI INDESIDERATI, MONITORAGGIO)
Mefenobarbital Compresse: 32, 50, 100 mg.	**Sedativo, trattamento dell'epilessia (aumenta la soglia delle convulsioni).** *Bambini:* 4-10 mg/kg/24 h in 2-4 dosi. *Adulti:* 200-600 mg/24 h in 2-4 dosi.	*Effetti indesiderati:* sonnolenza, letargia, confusione, depressione mentale, eccitamento paradosso, dipendenza fisica e psicologica, stipsi, nausea, vomito. *Monitoraggio:* concentrazioni di fenobarbital (terapeutiche 10-40 μg/mL).
Mercaptopurina Iniezione, compresse. Si possono preparare formulazioni estemporanee.	**Trattamento delle leucemie e del linfoma non-Hodgkin (antimetabolita, blocca la sintesi di purina).** *Bambini:* per os: induzione: 2,5-5 mg/kg una volta al giorno; mantenimento: 1,5-2,5 mg/kg/24 h. ev: infusione continua: 50 mg/m^2/h per 24-48 h. *Adulti:* per os: induzione: 2,5-5 mg/kg una volta al giorno; mantenimento: 1,5-2,5 mg/kg/24 h. Funzione renale: Crcl <50 mL/min: dose ogni 48 h.	*Effetti indesiderati:* epatotossicità (colestasi e necrosi), nausea, anoressia, vomito, diarrea, dolore allo stomaco, stomatite, mucosite, rash, iperpigmentazione, mielosoppressione (inizio, 7-10 giorni; nadir, 14 giorni; remissione, 21 giorni), tossicità renale, iperuricemia, eosinofilia, febbre da farmaci.
Mesna Iniezione: 100 mg/mL.	**Protegge dalla cistite emorragica da terapia con lifosamide e ciclofosfamide (si lega e detossifica i metaboliti urotossici attraverso il gruppo sulfidrilico attivo).** *Bambini e adulti:* ev: iniziare con 20% w/w di dose di lifosfamide o ciclofosfamide e 15 min prima della dose di agente alchilante. Ripetere la dose di mesna 3, 6, 9, e 12 h dopo la dose di agente alchilante. per os: 40% w/w di agente alchilante in 3 dosi 4 h dopo.	*Effetti indesiderati:* ipotensione, cefalea, nausea vomito, cattivo sapore in bocca, dolore agli arti. *Monitoraggio:* esame delle urine.
Metadone Iniezione: 10 mg/mL. Compresse: 5, 10 mg. Soluzione orale: 5 mg/mL.	**Trattamento del dolore grave, detossificazione da narcotici (si lega ai recettori oppiacei nel SNC).** *Neonati (sindrome da astinenza):* 0,05-0,2 mg/kg/dose ogni 12 h; poi aggiustare o ridurre in base agli score dell'astinenza. *Bambini:* analgesia: ev, im, per os: 0,1 mg/kg/dose ogni 4 h per 2-3 dosi, poi ogni 6-12 h. *Astinenza da narcotici:* iniziare con 0,05-0,1 mg/kg/dose ogni 6 h e ridurre in base agli score per astinenza. *Adulti:* ev, im, sc, per os. Analgesia: 2,5-20 mg ogni 6-8 h. Detossificazione: 15-40 mg/24 h.	*Effetti indesiderati:* debolezza, sonnolenza, vertigini, nausea, vomito, stipsi, ileo. *Monitoraggio:* il metadone si accumula in caso di dosi ripetute e come necessario. nei pazienti si dovrebbe monitorare l'eccessiva depressione del SNC.
Metaproterenolo, orciprenalina Inalatore a dosaggio controllato (MDI). Soluzione inalatoria. Compresse: 10, 20 mg. Sciroppo: 10 mg/5 mL.	**Broncodilatatore (stimola i recettori β_2).** *Bambini:* per os: *<2 anni:* 0,4 mg/kg/dose tid-qid. *2-6 anni:* 1,3-2,6 mg/kg/24 h suddivisi ogni 6 h. *6-9 anni:* 10 mg/dose qid. *>9 anni e adulti:* 20 mg/dose tid-qid. MDI: 2-3 puff ogni 4 h. Nebulizzatore: *Bambini piccoli e bambini:* 0,01-0,02 mL/kg di soluzione 5% ogni 4-6 h. *Adolescenti e adulti:* 0,3 mL di soluzione 5% ogni 4-6 h.	*Cautela:* alcune soluzioni generiche nebulizzate contengono solfiti che possono esacerbare l'asma. *Effetti indesiderati:* tremore, nervosismo, iperattività, tachicardia, ipotensione, cefalea. *Commento:* diluire la soluzione nebulizzata in 2,5 mL di soluzione fisiologica normale.
Metformina Compresse: 500, 850, 1000 mg.	**Trattamento del diabete di tipo 2; aumenta la sensibilità all'insulina e migliora la tolleranza al glucosio; effetto ipoglicemico.** *Bambini 10-16 anni:* iniziare con 500 mg bid con i pasti; aumentare con incrementi di 500 mg alla sett fino alla risposta (massimo: 2000 mg/24 h). *Adulti:* iniziare con 850 mg ogni 24 h o 500 mg bid; titolare di 500 mg una volta 1×/sett o 850 mg ogni 2 sett fino alla risposta (massimo: 2550 mg/24 h).	*Cautela:* evitare l'uso se clearance della creatinina <60 mL/min, creatinina serica >1,5 mg/dL (maschi) o >1,4 mg/dL (femmine). Monitorare l'acidosi lattica. Sospendere in caso di ogni processo che può predisporre all'acidosi metabolica o alla disfunzione renale fino a che la situazione è risolta. Evitare l'alcol. *Effetti indesiderati:* nausea, vomito, diarrea, indigestione, flatulenza.
Metildopa Iniezione: 50 mg/mL. Compresse: 125, 250, 500 mg. Sospensione orale: 250 mg/5 mL.	**Trattamento dell'ipertensione (metabolita falso neurotrasmettitore α stimola i recettori α-adrenergici inibitori).** *Bambini:* per os: iniziare con 10 mg/kg in 2-4 dosi; si può aumentare ogni 2 giorni (massimo: 65 mg/kg/24 h o 3 g/24 h). ev: iniziare 2-4 mg/kg/dose; si può aumentare a 5-10 mg/kg/dose per la risposta (massimo: 65 mg/kg/24 h). *Adulti:* per os: iniziare 250 mg tid; si può aumentare (massimo 3 g/24 h). ev: 0,25-1 g ogni 6 h (massimo: 4 g/24 h).	*Cautela:* tolleranza fino all'effetto, quindi per l'utilizzo cronico è necessario un diuretico concomitante. *Effetti indesiderati:* sonnolenza, depressione mentale, cefalea, secchezza delle fauci, febbre, brividi, vertigine, ritenzione idrica, edema, danno epatocellulare, diarrea, anemia emolitica, test di Coombs positivo, leucopenia, epatopatia colestatica, cirrosi, pancreatite, nausea, vomito, trombocitopenia, parestesie, debolezza, ipotensione, bradicardia. *Monitoraggio:* pressione arteriosa, enzimi epatici, test di Coombs diretto.
Metilfenidato Compresse: 5, 10, 20 mg. Compresse, rilascio prolungato: 20 mg.	**Disturbo da deficit dell'attenzione (ADD), narcolessia, aggiunta per il trattamento del dolore (stimolante del SNC).** *Bambini >5 anni:* 0,3-0,6 mg/kg/dose (massimo: 2 mg/kg/24 h). *Adulti:* 10 mg bid-tid (massimo: 60 mg/24 h).	*Cautela:* evitare nei pazienti con tic motori, sindrome di Tourette o marcata agitazione o psicosi. Può somministrare dipendenza se usato ad alte dosi a intervalli frequenti. *Effetti indesiderati:* nervosismo, insonnia, agitazione, anoressia, perdita di peso, tachicardia, disordini del movimento, tic, ritardo di crescita (controverso e minimo, se reale), dipendenza (non nel caso del dosaggio tipico per l´ADD).

TABELLA 716-1. Farmaci generali – *continua*

FARMACO (PRINCIPIO ATTIVO, FORMULAZIONI)	INDICAZIONI (MECCANISMO D'AZIONE E DOSAGGIO)	COMMENTI (CAUTELE, EFFETTI INDESIDERATI, MONITORAGGIO)
Metilprednisolone Glucocorticoide anti-infiammatorio e immunosoppressore. Iniezione. Compresse. Pomata topica.	**Usato nei disordini allergici, infiammatori e neoplastici e nel trauma della colonna vertebrale acuto.** *Bambini:* Anti-infiammatorio e immunosoppressivo: per os, im, ev: 0,5-2 mg/kg/24 h suddivisi ogni 6-12 h. Nefrite da lupus: ev: 30 mg/kg a giorni alterni per 6 dosi. Trauma acuto alla colonna vertebrale: 30 mg/kg per 15 min, seguito in 45 min da infusione continua di 5,4 mg/kg/h per 23 h. per os: 2-60 mg/24 h in 1-4 dosi. ev: 40-250 mg ogni 4-6 h. im: 10-80 mg/24 h.	*Cautela:* evitare se viene somministrato vaccino con virus vivo o in caso di tubercolosi o di infezione fungina. *Effetti indesiderati:* ipertensione, edema, nervosismo, agitazione, psicosi, pseudomotor cerebri, cefalea, sbalzi dell'umore, delirio, euforia, iperglicemia, ipopotassemia, alcalosi, soppressione dell'asse HPA-(surrene), sindrome di Cushing, atrofia cutanea, contusioni, iperpigmentazione, ulcera peptica, debolezza muscolare, osteoporosi, dolore articolare, ritardo di crescita, cataratta, glaucoma, immunosoppressione. *Commento:* vedi il confronto tra i corticosteroidi alla voce *Idrocortisone.*
Metimazolo Compresse: 5, 10 mg.	**Trattamento dell'ipertiroidismo (blocca la sintesi di iodio nella ghiandola tiroidea, inibisce la sintesi di ormone tiroideo).** *Bambini:* iniziare con 0,4 mg/kg/24 h, poi mantenimento con 0,2 mg/kg/24 h. *Adulti:* iniziare con 5 mg/kg ogni 8 h; dose di mantenimento: 5-15 mg/24 h (massimo: 60 mg/24 h).	*Effetti indesiderati:* febbre, rash, leucopenia, agranulocitosi, sindrome da lupus sistemico simil-eritematoso, nausea, vomito, dolore allo stomaco, ageusia, ittero colestatico, stipsi, aumento di peso. *Monitoraggio:* test di funzionalità tiroidea per ipotiroidismo o ipertiroidismo.
Metocarbamolo Iniezione: 100 mg/mL. Compresse: 500, 750 mg.	**Trattamento dello spasmo muscolare (rilassante muscoloscheletrico attraverso effetti depressivi sul SNC).** *Bambini:* trattamento del tetano: ev: 15 mg/kg/dose ogni 6 h per 3 giorni soltanto. *Adulti:* ev: 1-2 g ogni 6 h. per os: 1,5 g tid-qid per 2-3 giorni, quindi diminuire a 4-4,5 g/24 h.	*Effetti indesiderati:* sincope, bradicardia, ipotensione, sonnolenza, vertigini, cefalea, nausea, gusto metallico.
Metoclopramide Iniezione: 5 mg/mL. Compresse: 5, 10 mg. Soluzione orale: 10 mg/mL. Sciroppo: 5 mg/5 mL.	**Trattamento della gastroparesi diabetica, del reflusso gastro esofageo e della nausea associata a chemioterapia e chirurgia (blocca i recettori della dopamina nella zona trigger del chemorecettore, aumenta la motilità gastrointestinale e il tono dello sfintere gastroduodenale).** *Neonati, bambini piccoli e grandi:* reflusso gastroesofageo: ev, per os: 0,033-0,1 mg/kg/dose ogni 8 h. *Bambini:* Antiemetico postoperatorio: ev: 0,1-0,2 mg/kg/dose ogni 6-8 h se necessario. Antiemetico in chemioterapia: per os, ev: 1-2 mg/kg/dose ogni 2-4 h (pretrattare con difenidramina per evitare reazioni extrapiramidali). *Adulti:* Antiemetico: per os, ev: 1-2 mg/kg/dose ogni 2-4 h. Reflusso gastroesofageo: per os: 10-15 mg qid. Disfunzione renale: diminuire la dose.	*Cautela:* può precipitate le convulsioni, causare reazioni distoniche acute e peggiorare l'asma (se la formulazione contiene solfiti). Nell'anziano, l'uso cronico è associato ad aumentato rischio e inizio precoce di malattia di Parkinson (mancano studi pediatrici). *Effetti indesiderati:* debolezza, sonnolenza, diarrea, stimolazione della prolattina, dolenzia mammaria, reazione extrapiramidale, somministrazione ev associata a intenso senso di ansia e irritabilità, seguita da sonnolenza. *Commento:* somministrare dosi orali 30 min prima dei pasti e prima di andare a letto. *Monitoraggio:* clearance della creatinina: CrCl 40-50 mL/min: somministrare il 75% della dose raccomandata; CrCl <40 mL/min: somministrare il 50% della dose raccomandata; CrCl <10 mL/min: somministrare il 25% della dose raccomandata.
Metoexital Iniezione.	**Induzione e mantenimento dell'anestesia generale (barbiturato a durata d'azione ultrabreve).** *Bambini:* im: preoperatorio: 5-10 mg/kg/dose. ev: dose di induzione di 1-2 mg/kg/dose. Rettale: 20-35 mg/kg/dose. *Adulti:* ev: dose di induzione di 50-120 mg, poi 20-40 mg ogni 4-7 min.	*Effetti indesiderati:* apnea, depressione respiratoria, singhiozzo, laringospasmo, ipotensione, stiramento e rigidità del muscolo scheletrico, tremore, convulsioni, cefalea, nausea, vomito.
Metolazone Compresse.	**Trattamento degli stati da sovraccarico di volume (diuresi; inibisce il riassorbimento di sodio nei tubuli distali).** *Bambini:* 0,2-0,4 mg/kg/24 h in 1-2 dosi. *Adulti:* 2,5-20 mg/24 h.	*Effetti indesiderati:* alterazione dell'equilibrio idroelettrolitico, iperglicemia, ipocalcemia, ipomagnesiemia, nausea, vomito, discrasie plasmatiche.
Metoprololo Iniezione: 1 mg/mL. Compresse: 50, 100 mg.	**Trattamento dell'ipertensione, tachiaritmie, stenosi subaortica idiopatica ipertrofica, profilassi dell'emicrania (bloccante selettivo dei recettori β_1).** *Bambini:* per os: 1-5 mg/kg/24 h. *Adulti:* per os: 100-450 mg/24 h in 2-3 dosi. ev: 5 mg ogni 2 min per 3 dosi.	*Effetti indesiderati:* depressione mentale, stanchezza, debolezza, bradicardia, ridotta circolazione periferica; insonnia, incubi, peggiora il diabete mellito; peggiora l'asma.
Metosuccimide Capsule: 150, 300 mg.	**Controllo delle crisi da assenza e aggiunta nel trattamento delle convulsioni parziali complesse (aumenta la soglia delle convulsioni, sopprime la trasmissione nervosa).** *Bambini:* 10-15 mg/kg/14 h suddivisi in 3-4 dosi; si può aumentare a intervalli settimanali (massimo: 30 mg/kg/24 h). *Adulti:* iniziare 300 mg/24 h; si può aumentare di 300 mg/24 h a intervalli settimanali (massimo:1200 mg/24 h).	*Effetti indesiderati:* vertigini, sonnolenza, letargia, cefalea, atassia, aggressività, depressione, anoressia, nausea, vomito, singhiozzo, agranulocitosi, anemia aplastica, leucopenia, trombocitopenia. *Monitoraggio:* concentrazioni di metosuccimide (terapeutiche 10-40 μg/mL, tossiche >4 μg/mL).

TABELLA 716-1. Farmaci generali – *continua*

FARMACO (PRINCIPIO ATTIVO, FORMULAZIONI)	INDICAZIONI (MECCANISMO D'AZIONE E DOSAGGIO)	COMMENTI (CAUTELE, EFFETTI INDESIDERATI, MONITORAGGIO)
Metotrexato Iniezione. Compresse: 2,5 mg.	**Trattamento di neoplasie, psoriasi, artrite reumatoide (antimetabolita, inibizione del DNA e della sintesi di purina).** *Bambini:* Artrite reumatoide giovanile: per os, im: 5-15 mg/m^2/sett in monosomministrazione. Antineoplastico: per os, im: 7,5-30 mg/m^2 ogni 1-2 sett. ev: 10-33g/m^2 dose in bolo o infuso per 6-42 h. *Adulti:* Artrite reumatoide: per os: 7,5 mg 1×sett. Psoriasi: per os, im: 10-25 mg/dose 1×/sett. Antineoplastico: per os, im, ev: 25-50 mg/m^2/sett. Diminuita funzione renale: CrCl 61-80 mL/min: ridurre la dose del 25%. CrCl 51-60 mL/min: ridurre la dose del 33%. CrCl 10-50 mL/min: ridurre la dose del 50-70%.	*Cautela:* evitare nei pazienti con disfunzione epatica o renale grave. *Effetti indesiderati:* epatotossicità, nefropatia, vasculite, malessere, affaticamento, encefalopatia, cefalea, convulsioni, brividi, febbre, cistite, stomatite, enterite, nausea, vomito, diarrea, alopecia, fotosensibilità, aumenta o diminuisce la pigmentazione cutanea, orticaria, artralgia, iperuricemia mielosoppressione (inizio, 7 giorni; nadir, 10 giorni; remissione, 21 giorni). *Monitoraggio:* concentrazioni di metotrexato (tossiche se $>1 \times 10^{-7}$mol/L per >40 ore), assicurare un'adeguata idratazione e alcalinizzazione urinaria.
Mexiletina Capsule: 150, 200, 250 mg. Possono essere preparate formulazioni estemporanee.	**Trattamento delle aritmie ventricolari, del dolore neuropatico (antiaritmico classe 1B).** *Bambini:* 1,4-5 g/kg/dose ogni 8 h. *Adulti:* 200 mg ogni 8 h (massimo: 1,200 mg/24 h). Disfunzione renale: CrCl <10 mL/min: somministrare il 50% della dose.	*Effetti indesiderati:* aritmie atriali e ventricolari, bradicardia, ipotensione, confusione, vertigini, nervosismo, tremore, atassia, parestesie delle dita delle mani o dei piedi, debolezza, visione offuscata, tinnito, aumento degli enzimi epatici, fastidio gastrointestinale. *Monitoraggio:* concentrazioni di mexiletina: terapeutiche 0,5-2 μg/mL, tossiche >2 μg/mL.
Micofenolato mofetil Capsule: 250 mg.	**Previene il rigetto di trapianti allograft, usato in associazione con altri farmaci (metabolita attivo MPA inibisce la proliferazione delle cellule T- e B-, la generazione di cellule T e la secrezione di anticorpi).** *Bambini:* 660 mg/m^2/dose bid. *Adulti:* 1000 mg/dose bid.	*Effetti indesiderati:* ipertensione, insonnia, vertigini, febbre, cefalea, soppressione del midollo osseo, tremore, dolore alla schiena, mialgia, dispnea, tosse, faringite, ematuria, necrosi tubulare renale, malattia linfoproliferativa.
Midazolam Iniezione: 1, 5 mg/mL. Possono essere preparate formulazioni estemporanee.	**Sedazione, anticonvulsivante (benzodiazepina, aumenta l'acido γ-aminobutirrico).** *Neonati:* ev: infusione continua 0,15-0,5 μg/kg/min per sedazione; bolo ev 0,05-0,15 mg/kg ogni 2-4 h. *Bambini piccoli e grandi:* Stato epilettico: ev: dose da carico di 0,15 mg/kg seguita da infusione continua di 1 μg/kg/min. Sedazione: ev: dose da carico di 0,05-0,2 mg/kg, poi stessa dose ogni 1-2 h oppure infusione continua di 1-2 μg/kg/min. Intranasale: 2,5 mg (0,5 mL) per narice (totale, 5 mg) con fiala da 5 mg/mL. *>12 anni:* 0,5 mg ogni 3-4 min fino all'effetto. *Adulti:* 0,5-2 mg ogni 2 min fino all'effetto (di solito 2-5 mg).	*Effetti indesiderati:* molti casi di mioclono e disordini del movimento prolungati sono stati riportati nei neonati trattati con midazolam. Può insorgere una reazione da astinenza in caso di interruzione improvvisa. Sedazione, amnesia, eccitazione paradossa, visione offuscata, diplopia, arrossamento nasale, apnea, depressione respiratoria.
Mitomicina Agente alchilante. Iniezione.	**Chemioterapia tumorale (agente alchilante tipo-antibiotico inibisce la sintesi di DNA e RNA).** *Bambini e adulti:* dipende dal protocollo; tipicamente ev 3 mg/m^2/24 h per 5 giorni ogni 4-6 sett; fino a 40-50 mg/m^2 in dose singola per il trapianto del midollo osseo.	*Effetti indesiderati:* nausea, vomito, mielosoppressione (inizio, 21 giorni; nadir, 36 giorni; remissione, 42-56 giorni), formicolio agli arti, parestesie, alopecia, scoloramento delle unghie della mani, ulcere buccali, insufficienza cardiaca (dosi >30 mg), polmonite interstiziale, fibrosi polmonare.
Mitoxantrone, DHAD Iniezione.	**Chemioterapia tumorale (analogo dell'antraciclina, inibisce la sintesi di DNA e RNA attraverso l'intero ciclo cellulare).** Leucemie acute non linfocitiche: *Bambini <2 anni:* 0,4 mg/kg/24 h per 3-5 giorni. *>2 anni e adulti:* 8-12 mg/m^2/24 h per 5 giorni. Tumori solidi: *Bambini:* 18-20 mg/m^2 ogni 3-4 sett o 5-8 mg/m^2 alla sett. *Adulti:* 12-14 mg/m^2 ogni 3-4 sett (massimo: totale 80-120 mg/m^2).	*Effetti indesiderati:* cardiotossicità (minore che con altre antracicline), convulsioni, cefalea, febbre, enzimi epatici elevati, insufficienza renale, congiuntivite, mielosoppressione (inizio, 7-10 giorni; nadir, 14 giorni; remissione, 21 giorni).
Molindone idrocloruro Compresse: 5, 10, 25, 100 mg. Concentrato orale: 20 mg/mL.	**Trattamento del disordine psicotico (azioni simili alla clorpromazina, ma con effetti extrapiramidali e minore sedazione).** *Bambini:* *3-5 anni:* 1-2,5 mg/kg/24 anni in 4 dosi. *5-12 anni:* 0,5-1 mg/kg/24 h in 4 dosi. *Adulti:* 50-225 mg/24 h.	*Effetti indesiderati:* effetti extrapiramidali, acatisia, discinesie, stipsi, visione offuscata, ipotensione ortostatica, convulsioni, sindrome neurolettica maligna, secchezza delle fauci, aumento di peso, galattorrea, ritenzione urinaria, agranulocitosi, leucopenia, pigmentazione retinica.
Montelukast Bloccante il recettore del leucotriene. Compresse: 10 mg. Compresse masticabiie: 4,5 mg.	**Profilassi e trattamento cronico dell'asma (bloccante il recettore del leucotriene per LTD4).** *Bambini 2-5 anni:* 4 mg una volta al giorno di sera. *Bambini: 6-14 anni:* 5 mg una volta al giorno di sera. *>15 anni e adulti:* 10 mg una volta al giorno di sera.	*Effetti indesiderati:* cefalea, vertigini, dispepsia, affaticamento, aumento degli enzimi epatici.
Morfina Analgesico narcotico. Iniezione, soluzione orale, supposte. Compresse. Compresse, rilascio prolungato. Compresse, rilascio controllato.	**Sollievo del dolore moderato-grave.** *Neonati:* ev, im, sc: analgesia: 0,05-0,2 mg/kg/dose ogni 2-4 h; infusione continua di 0,025-0,05 mg/kg/h. *Bambini piccoli e grandi:* ev, im, sc: 0,1-0,2 mg/kg/dose ogni 2-4 h; per os: 0,2-0,5 mg/kg/dose ogni 4-6 h. *Adolescenti >12 anni:* ev: 3-4 mg; si può ripetere a 5 min se necessario. *Adulti:* per os: 10-30 mg ogni 4 h o compresse a rilascio controllato 15-30 mg ogni 8-12 h. ev, im, sc: 2,5-20 mg/dose ogni 2-6 h se necessario o infusione continua di 0,8-10 mg/h.	*Cautela:* si può sviluppare dipendenza fisica dopo >5-7 giorni di uso continuo; in questo caso, ridurre la dose. Alcune preparazioni contengono solfiti. *Effetti indesiderati:* ipotensione, bradicardia, nausea, vomito, stipsi, sedazione, confusione, diminuzione della diuresi, depressione respiratoria.

TABELLA 716-1. Farmaci generali – *continua*

FARMACO (PRINCIPIO ATTIVO, FORMULAZIONI)	INDICAZIONI (MECCANISMO D'AZIONE E DOSAGGIO)	COMMENTI (CAUTELE, EFFETTI INDESIDERATI, MONITORAGGIO)
Mupirocina Pomata: 2%.	**Trattamento topico dell'impetigine e di altre infezioni cutanee Gram-positive (inibisce la la sintesi di RNA e di proteina batterica).** *Bambini e adulti:* Applicare all'area interessata 4-5 volte al giorno. Intranasale (eliminare trasporto nasale di *Staphylococcus aureus*): applicare piccola quantità bid-qid per 5-14 giorni.	*Effetti indesiderati:* bruciore e irritazione nel sito di applicazione.
Muromonab-CD3, OKT3 Iniezione: 5 mg/5 mL.	**Trattamento del rigetto acuto di allograft nel trapianto renale (riveste i linfociti T circolanti, facilitando la loro opsonizzazione dal sistema reticolo endoteliale e promuove la rimozione di tutte le molecole CD3 dal complesso linfocita-T antigene recettore).** *Bambini <12 anni:* 0,1 mg/kg/24 h per 10-14 giorni, o se <30 kg, somministrare 2,5 mg/24 h per 10-14 giorni. *>12 anni e adulti:* 5 mg/24 h per 10-14 giorni.	*Cautela:* si possono verificare gravi reazioni da prima dose; somministrare metilprednisolone 1 mg/kg ev 2-6 h prima della dose di OKT3 e idrocortisone 100 mg ev 30 min dopo ogni dose di OKT3 e se necessario. *Effetti indesiderati:* respiro affannoso, edema polmonare, febbre, brividi, tremore, nausea, vomito, diarrea, cefalea, rigidità del collo, fotofobia, sintomi simil-influenzali. *Monitoraggio:* livelli serici di OKT3 (se mantenuto vicino a 1 μg/mL, la conta CD3 rimane bassa).
Nadololo Antagonista non selettivo del recettore β-adrenergico. Compresse: 20, 40, 80, 120, 160 mg.	**Antiaritmico, antipertensivo e profilassi dell'emicrania.** *Bambini:* per os: 0,5-2,5 mg/kg al giorno per tachicardia sopraventricolare. *Adulti:* 40 mg al giorno; titolare fino all'effetto desiderato (dose usuale: 40-80 mg/24 h fino a 640 mg/24 h).	*Cautela:* non usare nei pazienti con asma, broncocostrizione o scompenso cardiaco non controllato. Aggiustare la dose in caso di disfunzione renale (CrCl <50 mL/min). *Effetti indesiderati:* bradicardia, scompenso cardiaco, broncospasmo. *Interazioni farmacologiche:* altri farmaci ipotensivi, diuretici. Antagonizza i farmaci β-simpaticomimetici (per es. albuterolo).
Nalbufina Iniezione. im, ev, sc: 10 mg/mL.	**Analgesico (agonista oppiaceo con parziale attività antagonista oppiacea per il trattamento del dolore moderato-grave).** *Bambini ≥1anni:* ev, im, sc: 0,1-0,2 mg/kg ogni 3-4 h. Dose singola massima: 20 mg; dose massima giornaliera: 160 mg.	*Cautela:* come molti analgesici oppiacei, può stimolare il rilascio di istamina e causare depressione respiratoria e del SNC. Usare con cautela nell'epatopatia con altri depressivi respiratori. Potenziale dipendenza. *Effetti indesiderati:* ipotensione, sedazione, depressione respiratoria. Il naloxone ne annulla gli effetti.
Naloxone Antagonista oppiaceo. Iniezione: 0,4 mg/mL. Iniezione, neonate: 0,02 mg/mL.	**Antagonizza tutti i recettori oppiacei; usato nel trattamento dell'eccesso di oppiacei (overdose, avvelenamento).** *Neonati e bambini:* ev: 0,1 mg/kg (massimo: 2 mg). Se nessuna risposta, ripetere ogni 2-3 min fino all'effetto desiderato. Si può somministrare per infusione continua ev.	*Cautela:* può precipitare astinenza acuta da oppiacei. La durata dell'effetto di molti oppiacei può essere più lunga di questa o del naloxone, richiedendo un dosaggio di naloxone personalizzato. Somministrare bolo ev.
Naproxene Farmaco anti-infiammatorio non steroideo. Compresse: 220, 250, 275, 375, 550 mg. Sospensione: 125 mg/5 mL.	**Trattamento di dolore da lieve a moderato, infiammazione, febbre (inibisce la sintesi di prostaglandine).** *Neonati:* non usare a causa dei probabili effetti negativi sulla funzione renale. *Bambini:* per os: 5-7mg/kg ogni 8-12 h. *Adulti:* per os: 250-375 mg ogni 8-12 h (massimo: 1250 mg/24 h).	*Cautela:* disturbi o irritazione gastrointestinali, interferenza dell'aggregazione piastrinica reversibile. Non somministrare a bambini piccoli di età <3 mesi. *Effetti indesiderati:* vertigini, irritazione gastrointestinale, rash, diminuita funzione renale correlata all'età.
Nedocromil Stabilizzatore delle mastcellule. Aerosol: 1,75 mg/sessione.	**Trattamento cronico dell'asma e dei disordini allergici. Stabilizza le altre cellule al rilascio dei mediatori: neutrofili, eosinofili, piastrine; non steroideo.** *Bambini e adulti:* 1-2 puff bid-qid. Titolare la dose alla risposta clinica.	*Cautela:* efficace solo come terapia cronica. Non produce broncodilazione. *Effetti indesiderati:* disfonia, irritazione del torace e dolore.
Neostigmina Compresse: 15 mg (come bromide). Iniezione: 0,25, 0,5, 1 mg/mL (come metilsolfato).	**Trattamento della miastenia grave, antagonizza gli agenti bloccanti non depolarizzanti neuromuscolari (NDNM). Inibisce in modo competitivo l'acetilcolina esterasi aumentando gli effetti dell'acetilcolina endogena.** *Bambini:* ev, im, sc: 0,01-0,04 mg/kg ogni 2-4 h; titolare la dose all'effetto desiderato. Per invertire NDNM, 0,025-1 mg/kg/dose (dose massima nell'adulto: 5 mg).	*Cautela:* pazienti con asma o broncospasmo, bradicardia. Non antagonizza la succinilcolina. *Effetti indesiderati:* bradicardia, crampi addominali, pollachiuria.
Niacina Compresse: 25, 50, 100, 250, 500 mg. Compresse, a rilascio prolungato: 150, 250, 500, 750 mg. Capsule, a rilascio prolungato: 125, 250, 300, 400, 500 mg. Elisir: 50 mg/5 mL. Iniezione: 100 mg/mL.	**Supplemento vitaminico (vitamina B_3), iperlipidemia, vasodilatatore.** *Bambini:* ev, im, sc, per os: titolare all'effetto desiderato (massimo: 10 mg/kg/24 h).	*Cautela:* titolare la dose e somministrare ev lentamente per evitare o minimizzare il flushing. *Effetti indesiderati:* flushing, tachicardia, vertigini, iperuricemia. *Interazioni farmacologiche:* aumenta gli effetti ipotensivi degli antipertensivi.
Nifedipina Capsula (piena di liquido): 10, 20 mg. Capsule, a rilascio prolungato: 30, 60, 90 mg. Compresse, a rilascio prolungato: 30, 60, 90 mg.	**Antipertensivo, antiaritmico calcio-antagonista.** *Bambini piccoli e grandi:* Emergenza ipertensiva per os/sublinguale 0,25-0,5 mg/kg/dose ogni 4-6 h (massimo: 10 mg). Cardiomiopatia ipertrofica: per os: 0,2-0,3 mg/kg ogni 8 h. *Adulti:* 10 mg/dose titolare fino all'effetto (massimo: 120-180 mg/24 h).	*Cautela:* non rompere o tagliare le compresse a rilascio prolungato. *Effetti indesiderati:* ipotensione profonda, acuta, flushing, vertigini. Effetto più rapido se il farmaco viene somministrato senza cibo. Il succo di pompelmo concomitante può aumentare la biodisponibilità e gli effetti. *Interazioni farmacologiche:* cimetidina, ciclosporina, fenitoina e probabilmente digossina. *Commento:* la via di somministrazione preferita è quella orale, non sublinguale. Effetti clinici dovuti alla deglutizione. Contenuto nella capsula approssimativamente 10 mg in 0,34 mL e 20 mg in 0,45 mL.
Nitroprussiato Iniezione: 10, 25 mg/mL.	**Antipertensivo, scompenso cardiaco congestizio: controllo della pressione arteriosa controllata, titolabile.** *Bambini e adulti:* ev 0,3-0,5 μg/kg/min; titolare la dose all'effetto desiderato; raramente richiede >6 μg/kg/min (probabile massimo: 8 μg/kg/min).	*Cautela:* metabolizzato a tiocianato/cianuro, che si accumula con disfunzione renale. *Effetti indesiderati:* ipotensione profonda, tachicardia, soppressione tiroidea, acidosi, convulsioni. tossicità da cianuro-acidosi metabolica, cute rosa, metaemoglobinemia. Somministrare in infusione continua ev. Proteggere la soluzione dalla luce diretta. La cosomministrazione di tiosolfato previene la tossicità (10 mg di tiosolfato per ogni 1 mg nitroprussiato.

TABELLA 716-1. Farmaci generali – *continua*

FARMACO (PRINCIPIO ATTIVO, FORMULAZIONI)	INDICAZIONI (MECCANISMO D'AZIONE E DOSAGGIO)	COMMENTI (CAUTELE, EFFETTI INDESIDERATI, MONITORAGGIO)
Noradrenalina bitartrato Agonista simpaticomimetico/adrenergico. Iniezione: 1 mg/mL base.	**Ipotensione e shock.** *Bambini:* 0,05-0,1 μg/kg/min; titolare la dose all'effetto desiderato (massimo: 2 μg/kg/min).	*Cautela:* lo stravaso può causare grave necrosi tissutale. Somministrare in una grossa vena mediante infusione continua ev . Assicurarsi dello stato dei liquidi del paziente. Può causare vasocostrizione profonda. *Effetti indesiderati:* ipertensione, aritmie cardiache, cefalea. Dose di farmaco basata sulla base di noradrenalina.
Nortriptilina Antidepressivo triciclico; inibitore della serotonina noradrenalinica centrale sinaptica. Capsule: 10, 25, 50, 75 mg Soluzione: 10 mg/5 mL.	**Trattamento dell'enuresi notturna, depressione.** *Bambini:* Enuresi notturna: per os: 10-20 mg/24 h; titolare (massimo: 40 mg/24 h). Depressione: per os: 1-3 mg/kg/24 h (alla sera) titolare fino all'effetto. Si può somministrare in dosi suddivise ogni 6 h (massimo usuale: 150 mg/24 h).	*Cautela:* evitare nei pazienti con disturbi di conduzione cardiaca, malattia cardiaca. Lento aggiustamento della dose nei pazienti con disfunzione epatica. *Effetti indesiderati:* effetti anticolinergici (secchezza delle fauci, tachicardia, visione offuscata, ritenzione urinaria), sedazione. *Interazioni farmacologiche:* clonidina, inibitori della monoamino ossidasi.
Octreotide Iniezione: 0,05, 0,1, 0,2, 0,5, 1 mg/mL	**Analogo antisecretorio della somatostatina.** *Bambini:* diarrea secretoria: ev, sc: 1-10 μg/kg ogni 12 h; titolare la dose fino all'effetto. Si può somministrare per infusione continua ev. *Adulti:* trattamento dei tumori secernenti peptide intestinale vasoattivo: ev, sc: 100-150 μg ogni 12 h.	*Cautela:* l'uso continuo a lungo termine (mesi) può causare colelitiasi, ipotiroidismo. *Effetti indesiderati:* flushing, vertigini, ipo/iperglicemia. Infondere ev per 20-30 min, bolo ev per 3 min.
Olanzapina Compresse: 2,5, 5, 7,5, 10, 15, 20 mg.	**Antipsicotico atipico, antagonista monaminergico con elevata affinità per serotonina, dopamina, istamina, recettori muscarinici e α_1-adrenergici. Reale meccanismo d'azione sconosciuto.** *Bambini:* iniziare 2,5-5 mg ogni 24 h; titolare settimanalmente da 2,5-5 mg a 15-20 mg/24 h come ogni dosaggio giornaliero. *Adulti:* iniziare 5-10 mg/24 h; aumentare di 5 mg alla sett fino alla risposta (massimo: 20 mg/24 h).	*Effetti indesiderati:* ipotensione posturale, sonnolenza, tremore, vertigini, acatisia, astenia, secchezza delle fauci, stipsi, dispepsia, appetito aumentato, aumento di peso, iperglicemia, amenorrea, vaginite nelle femmine.
Olio di ricino Lassativo; stimolante. Emulsione, orale; liquido, orale: 100% (60, 120, 480 mL).	**Evacuazione dell'intestino o del retto per la chirurgia (stimola la peristalsi).** *Bambini piccoli <2 anni:* 1-5 mL dose singola. *Bambini 2-11anni:* 5-15 mL. *Bambini >12 anni e adulti:* 15-60 mL.	*Effetti indesiderati:* alterazioni dell'equilibrio elettrolitico, crampi addominali.
Olsalazina Anti-infiammatorio farmaco; derivato dell'acido 5-aminosalicilico. Capsule: 10, 20, 250 mg.	**Trattamento della malattia infiammatoria intestinale.** *Adulti:* 500 mg ogni 12 h.	*Cautela:* somministrare con cibo. *Effetti indesiderati:* cefalea, crampi, diarrea, vertigini, rash, colestasi.
Omatropina idrobromuro Anticolinergico. Soluzione oftalmica: 2%, 5%.	**Produce cicloplegia e midriasi per rifrazione; trattamento dell'uveite.** *Bambini:* Per midriasi: 1 goccia di soluzione 2% prima della procedura; si può ripetere ogni 10 min se necessario. Uveite: 1 goccia di soluzione 2% bid-tid. *Adulti:* Midriasi: 1-2 gocce di soluzione al 2% o 5% prima della procedura; si può ripetere ogni 10 min. Uveite: 1-2 gocce di soluzione al 2% o 5% bid-tid.	*Effetti indesiderati:* visione offuscata, fotofobia, puntura locale, congestione respiratoria.
Omeprazolo Inibitore della pompa protonica della secrezione di ioni idrogeno delle cellule parietali. Capsule: 10, 20 mg.	**Trattamento dell'ipersecrazione/ulcera gastrica.** *Bambini:* per os: 0,6-0,7mg/kg ogni 24 h. Dose titolata al pH gastrico desiderato. *Adulti:* per os: 20-40 mg/24 h.	*Cautela:* i granuli di farmaco in capsule devono essere ingeriti interi; non masticare. *Interazioni farmacologiche:* può diminuire la clearance di diazepam e fenitoina. Può ridurre l'assorbimento di itraconazolo e digossina.
Ondansetron Antiemetico, antagonista selettivo del recettore della serotonina-3. Compresse: 4, 8 mg. Iniezione: 2 mg/mL.	**Trattamento della nausea e del vomito associati a chemioterapia tumorale o chirurgia e altre cause (tossicità farmacologica).** *Bambini piccoli e grandi:* 0,15 mg/kg ev ogni 8 h; si può somministrare in infusione ev continua e 0,45 mg/kg/24 h (massimo: 24-32 mg/24 h). *Bambini:* nausea/vomito lievi-moderati: per os: 4-8 mg ogni 8-12 h.	*Effetti indesiderati:* cefalea, dolore toracico. Non causa distonia/sedazione. *Commento:* biodisponibilità orale ≈50%. Dosi somministrate ≈30 min prima di iniziare la chemioterapia.
Ormone della crescita umano Iniezione.	**Trattamento del ritardo di crescita causato da inadeguata secrezione di ormone della crescita (terapia sostitutiva).** *Bambini:* 0,06 mg/kg (0,15 UI/kg) 3×/sett. 0,043 mg/kg/24 h. 0,1 mg/kg (0,26 UI/kg) 3×/sett.	*Effetti indesiderati:* lipoatrofia locale, ipotiroidismo, dolore all'anca o al ginocchio.
Oxcarbazepina Compresse, rivestite da film: 150, 300, 600 mg. Sospensione: 300 mg/5 mL.	**Trattamento delle convulsioni (eccetto assenza).** *Bambini 3-17 anni:* iniziare 8-10 mg/kg/24 h suddivisi bid (massimo: 600 mg/24 h); aumenta per 2 sett a 30-45 mg/kg/24 h suddivisi bid per la risposta. *Adulti:* iniziare con 600 mg/24 h suddivisi bid, poi aumentare gradualmente per 2-4 sett fino a 1200 mg/24 h suddivisi bid (massimo: 2400 mg/24 h).	*Cautela:* dimezzare la dose se la clearance della creatinina è <30 mL/min. Tossicità principalmente del SNC (cefalea, sonnolenza, vertigini ecc.), diplopia, gastrointestinale (nausea, vomito, diarrea) e iponatriemia.
Oxibutinina Antispasmodico urinario. Compresse: 5 mg. Sciroppo: 5 mg/5 mL.	**Rilassa il muscolo liscio antagonizzando l'acetilcolina.** *Bambini:* per os: 0,2 mg/kg ogni 6-12 h (massimo: 5 mg per os ogni 8 h). *Adulti:* 5 mg/dose fino a 4× al giorno.	*Cautela:* pazienti con epatopatiae/o renale. *Effetti indesiderati:* tachicardia, sonnolenza, sedazione, secchezza delle fauci, visione offuscata. *Interazioni farmacologiche:* effetti anticolinergici additivi/depressione del SNC (per es. antistaminici).

TABELLA 716-1. Farmaci generali – *continua*

FARMACO (PRINCIPIO ATTIVO, FORMULAZIONI)	INDICAZIONI (MECCANISMO D'AZIONE E DOSAGGIO)	COMMENTI (CAUTELE, EFFETTI INDESIDERATI, MONITORAGGIO)
Oxicodone Analgesico oppiaceo. Compresse: 5 mg.	**Trattamento del dolore moderato-grave.** *Bambini:* per os: 0,05-0,15 mg/kg ogni 4-6 h (massimo: 5 mg). *Adulti:* per os: 5 mg/dose ogni 4-6 h (massimo: 5 mg).	*Cautela:* come molti analgesici oppiacei, può stimolare il rilascio di istamina e può causare depressione respiratoria e del SNC. Usare con cautela nell'epatopatia o con altri depressivi respiratori. Potenziale dipendenza. *Effetti indesiderati:* ipotensione, sedazione, depressione respiratoria. Il naloxone annulla gli effetti.
Pamidronato disodio Derivato dei bifosfonati. Iniezione: 30, 60, 90 mg.	**Trattamento dell'ipercalcemia, malattia di Paget, osteogenesi imperfetta, osteopenia. Si lega all'osso, inibendo il riassorbimento di calcio mediato dagli osteoclasti. Dose basata sulla concentrazione di calcio sierico.** *Bambini:* 1 mg/kg/24 h per giorni consecutivi ogni 3 mesi; 10-40 mg/m^2 per 5-8 h ogni mese. *Adulti:* Calcio sierico 12-13,5 mg/dL 60-90 mg; calcio sierico >13,5 mg/dL: 90 mg. Attendere 7 giorni per valutare l'effetto pieno della dose prima del ritrattamento. Malattia di Paget: 30 mg/24 h per 3 giorni consecutivi.	*Cautela:* leucopenia, tromboflebite. Farmaco incompatibile con soluzioni contenenti calcio ev. *Effetti indesiderati:* ipertensione, sincope, ipocalcemia, ipofosfatemia, ipotiroidismo, dolore osseo.
Pancreatina Capsule, compresse, capsule a rilascio prolungato, polvere.	**Sostituzione di enzima pancreatico. I prodotti individuali contengono differenti quantità di lipasi, amilasi e proteasi.** *Bambini e adulti:* dose titolata alla desiderata frequenza e consistenza delle feci.	*Cautela:* un dosaggio eccessivo può portare a impattamento; un dosaggio inadeguato può portare a steatorrea. Gli enzimi pancreatici esogeni sono inattivati dall'acido gastrico; usare forme microincapsulate quando possibile. *Interazioni farmacologiche:* riduzione dell'acido gastrico (per es. recettore-H_2 antagonisti/omeprazolo/antacidi) possono aumentare l'efficacia. *Effetti indesiderati:* rash, addominali sintomi, stipsi, iperuricemia, allergia.
Pancuronio Iniezione: 1, 2 mg/mL.	**Anestetico e rilassante del muscolo scheletrico. Antagonista non depolarizzante neuromuscolare.** *Bambini e adulti:* ev: 0,04-0,1 mg/kg ogni 20-30 min. Dose titolata all'effetto desiderato.	*Cautela:* durante il blocco neuromuscolare la ventilazione deve essere supportata. Aggiustamento della dose in caso di disfunzione renale. *Effetti indesiderati:* tachicardia, ipertensione, debolezza muscolare prolungata. *Interazioni farmacologiche:* possibile aumento della debolezza muscolare con aminoglicosidi, anestetici e colistina.
Papaverina idrocloruro Vasodilatatore; antiemicranico; rilassante generalizzato del muscolo liscio. Capsule: 150 mg. Compresse, a rilascio prolungato. Iniezione.	**Uso comune pediatrico per la preservazione dei cateteri arteriosi in modo da prolungarne il funzionamento.** *Bambini:* 30 mg papaverina più 250 U eparina/250 mL soluzione ev (0,45-0,9% NaCl) infuso.	*Cautela:* evitare nei neonati poiché può causare vasodilatazione cerebrale, predisponendo ad emorragia del SNC. *Effetti indesiderati:* flushing, tachicardia, ipotensione, vertigini. *Interazioni farmacologiche:* effetto ipotensivo additivo.
Paracetamolo Analgesico, non-narcotico; antipiretico. Capsule: 160, 325, 500 mg. Capsule: 325, 500 mg. Gocce: 100 mg/mL (15 mL); 120 mg/2,5 mL (35 mL). Granuli, packs predosati: 30 mg. Supposte: 120, 325 mg. Tra i prodotti con paracetamolo in combinazione vi sono preparati per tosse e raffreddore e quelli con codeina.	**Dolore da lieve a moderato** (inibisce la sintesi delle prostaglandine nel SNC e la generazione acuta dell'impulso periferico). **Febbre** (inibisce il centro di regolazione termica ipotalamico). *Bambini <12 anni:* 10-15 mg/kg/dose ogni 4-6 h. *Bambini >12 anni e adulti:* 325-650 mg ogni 4-6 h o 1000 mg 3-4 × die. Massimo: 5 dosi/24 h (bambini) o 4 g/24 h (adulti) somministrati per os o per via rettale.	*Cautela:* l'overdose può causare necrosi epatica fatale. Trattare le overdosi acute con acetilcisteina. L'utilizzo cronico concomitante di inibitori enzimatici, specialmente di alcol, può causare necrosi epatica. Evitare prodotti contenenti aspartame nei pazienti con fenilchetonuria (per es. compresse masticabili).
Paraldeide Anticonvulsante; sedativo; depressivo generalizzato del SNC. Liquido: 1 g/mL.	**Usato come aggiunta nel trattamento dello stato epilettico refrattario, sospensione di alcol.** *Bambini:* per os, rettale: 0,15 mL/kg/dose. Si può ripetere una volta dopo 4-6 h. Formulazione im non disponibile negli Stati Uniti. *Adulti:* 5-10 mL/dose.	*Cautela:* si può somministrare im, ma iniettare lontano dai nervi a causa del rischio di lesioni. Usare siringhe/provette di vetro poiché il farmaco reagisce con la plastica. Via rettale preferita alla via im. Soluzione mista rettale 2:1 in olio (per es. olio d'oliva) *Effetti indesiderati:* sedazione, irritazione gastrica, tromboflebite.
Paregoric Antidiarroico, analgesico. Liquido: 2 mg di morfina equivalente/5 mL.	**Tintura canforata di oppio.** *Bambini:* per os: 0,25-0,5 mL/kg ogni 6-12 h. *Adulti:* per os: 5-10 mL ogni 6-12 h. Sindrome da astinenza neonatale: dose titolata all'effetto desiderato.	*Commenti:* 5 mL di paregoric contengono 2 mg di morfina equivalente, 20 mg di canfora, 20 mg di acido benzoico. Contenuto finale di alcol 45%.
Paroxetina Inibitore del reuptake della serotonina. Compresse: 10, 20, 40 mg. Sospensione orale: 10 mg/5 mL.	**Trattamento della depressione, disturbo ossessivo-compulsivo, attacchi di panico e disturbo di ansia sociale.** *Bambini:* iniziare con 10 mg ogni al giorno; aumentare a intervalli settimanali di 10 mg/giorno (massimo: 60 mg/24 h). *Adulti:* iniziare con 20 mg al giorno aumentare di 10 mg al giorno a intervalli settimanali fino alla risposta (massimo: 60 mg/24 h).	*Cautela:* non sospendere improvvisamente o può insorgere la sindrome da sospensione. Misurare di 10 mg/24 h ogni 5-7 giorni per evitare problemi. Evitare l'uso con gli inibitori della monamino ossidasi eccetto in situazioni. estreme. *Effetti indesiderati:* sonnolenza, vertigini, insonnia, tremore, nervosismo, diminuzione dell'appetito, astenia, nausea, stipsi. *Interazioni farmacologiche:* la paroxetina inibisce l'isoenzima del citocromo 2D6 e può interagire con fenotiazine e antiaritmici tipo 1C. L'uso concomitante di tioridazina può aumentare i livelli di tioridazina, causando allungamento del tratto QTc e predisporre a torsioni di punta.
Pegaspargasi Agente antineoplastico. Iniezione.	**Usato in combinazione per l'induzione della leucemia linfoblastica acuta. Chiamato anche PEG-l-asparaginasi.** *Bambini e adulti:* im, ev: 2500 U/m^2 ogni 14 giorni. Dose di solito dettata dal protocollo specifico.	*Cautela:* reazioni epatotossiche, allergiche. Controindicato nei pazienti con pancreatite, eventi significativamente emorragici associati a L-asparaginasi. *Interazioni farmacologiche:* possibili interazioni con metotrexato, vincristina, corticosteroidi.

TABELLA 716-1. Farmaci generali – *continua*

FARMACO (PRINCIPIO ATTIVO, FORMULAZIONI)	INDICAZIONI (MECCANISMO D'AZIONE E DOSAGGIO)	COMMENTI (CAUTELE, EFFETTI INDESIDERATI, MONITORAGGIO)
Pemolina Stimolante del SNC. Compresse: 18,75, 37,5, 75 mg. Compresse: masticabile: 37,5 mg.	**Trattamento del disturbo da deficit dell'attenzione. Strutturalmente distinto dal metilfenidato.** *Bambini:* per os: 1 mg/kg/24 h in monosomministrazione ogni mattino. Titolare fino all'effetto 0,5 mg/kg/ 24 h ogni 1-2 sett. (massimo: 3 mg/kg/24 h; ≈112,5 mg/24 h).	*Cautela:* insonnia, anoressia, perdita di peso. *Effetti indesiderati:* stimolazione del SNC, convulsioni, ipertensione, aumentata funzione epatica, epatite, disordini del movimento. *Interazioni farmacologiche:* possibili con altri stimolanti del SNC, simpaticomimetici.
Penicillamina Agente chelante. Capsule: 12, 250 mg. Compresse: 250 mg.	**Agente chelante metallico con affinità per il rame (malattia di Wilson) e il piombo. Usato anche come aggiunta al trattamento dell'artrite reumatoide grave.** Malattia di Wilson: Dose titolata fino a mantenere >1 mg/24 h di escrezione urinaria di rame. *Bambini piccoli e grandi:* per os: 20 mg/kg/24 h ogni 6-12 h (massimo: 1 g/24 h). *Adulti:* per os: 1 g/24 h ogni 6-12 h (massimo: 2 g). Intossicazione da piombo: *Bambini piccoli e grandi:* per os: 30-40 mg/kg/24 h ogni 8-12 h (massimo: 1,5 g/24 h). *Adulti:* per os: 1-1,5 g/24 h ogni 8-12 h. Artrite reumatoide: *Bambini:* per os: 3 mg/kg/24 h ogni 12 h, incrementando di 3 mg/kg/24 h ogni 2-3 mesi (massimo: 10 mg/kg/24 h).	*Cautela:* cross-allergene nei pazienti allergici alla penicillina. Non somministrare con cibo o composti ferro/zinco. *Effetti indesiderati:* rash, prurito, nausea, vomito, anemia, soppressione del midollo, sindrome nefrosica, sindrome simil-lupus eritematoso sistemico. *Interazioni farmacologiche:* altri metalli, ferro, oro, mercurio, antimalarici.
Pentazocina Compresse: 50 mg con 50 mg naloxone (deterrente parenterale). Iniezione: 30 mg/mL.	**Analgesico oppiaceo del tipo benzorfano per il trattamento del dolore moderato- grave.** *Bambini >14 anni di età e adulti:* per os: 50 mg ogni 3-4 h, titolare fino all'effetto alla dose di 100 mg, non superare i 600 mg/24 h. Si può somministrare im o ev, riducendo la dose orale di 1/3,	*Cautela:* depressivo generalizzato del SNC possiede debole azione antagonista e può precipitare l'astinenza da oppiacei. *Effetti indesiderati:* depressione SNC, nausea, vomito, depressione respiratoria, rilascio di istamina.
Pentobarbital Barbiturici a breve durata d'azione. Capsule: 50, 100 mg. Elisir: 18,2 mg/5 mL. Supposta: 30, 60, 120, 200 mg. Iniezione.	**Usato come un anticonvulsivante, sedativo/ipnotico e anestetico.** Sedazione: *Bambini:* per os, im: 2-6 mg/kg/24 h ogni 6 h. Si può somministrare per via rettale dosato in base al peso corporeo: 4,5-10 kg: 30 mg 10-18 kg: 30-60 mg; 18-36 kg: 60 mg; 36-50 kg: 60-120 mg. Coma da pentobarbital: *Bambini:* ev: dose da carico di 10-15 mg/kg lentamente per 1-2 h, monitoraggio della pressione arteriosa e frequenza cardiaca. Infusione di mantenimento di 1 mg/kg/ora, aumentando fino a 5 mg/kg/h per mantenere la soppressione dei burst all'elettroencefalogramma.	*Cautela:* ipotensione nei pazienti ipovolemici; iniettabile contiene glicol propilene. *Effetti indesiderati:* aritmie bradicardia, ipotensione, depressione respiratoria, laringospasmo, dipendenza. *Interazioni con altri farmaci:* può aumentare il metabolismo di molti farmaci eliminati per via epatica, contraccettivi orali, griseofulvina, corticosteroidi. *Monitoraggio:* concentrazioni di pentobarbital: sedazione 1-5 μg/mL; coma 20-40 μg/mL.
Pentossifillina Compresse, a rilascio prolungato: 400 mg.	**Usata nel trattamento della vasculopatia periferica (sindrome di Raynaud) e sperimentalmente per ridurre il fattore di necrosi tumorale, l'adesione dei neutrofili e l'aggregazione piastrinica.** *Bambini:* effetto antipiastrinico nella malattia di Kawasaki: per os: 20 mg/kg/24 h ogni 8 h. *Adulti:* per os: 400 mg tid.	*Cautela:* somministrare con i pasti per ridurre la gastrite. *Effetti indesiderati:* ipotensione, tachicardia, vertigini, nausea, vomito. *Interazioni farmacologiche:* cimetidina, possibile aumento con il warfarin, effetti dell'eparina.
Piroxicam Agente anti-infiammatorio non steroideo. Capsule: 10, 20 mg.	**Analgesico e trattamento dei disordini reumatici.** per os: *Bambini:* 0,2-0,3 mg/kg ogni 24 h (massimo: 15 mg/kg/24 h). *Adulti:* 10-20 mg ogni 24 h.	*Cautela:* dati limitati nei bambini piccoli e grandi; possono essere necessari dosaggi giornalieri più frequenti nei bambini. Somministrare con il cibo o il latte per diminuire gli effetti indesiderati gastrointestinali. Non usare nei bambini piccoli. *Effetti indesiderati:* vertigini, gastrite, nausea/vomito, ulcera, epatite, diminuita funzione renale.
Polietilene glicole, soluzione elettrolitica Soluzione per lavaggio intestinale. Polvere da ricostituire.	**Usato prima di esami radiologici dell'intestino o negli avvelenamenti.** *Bambini:* 25-40 mL/kg/h fino a 1,5-2 L/h fino a che l'evacuazione rettale è chiara; la dose massima abituale di 4 L per radiografia può essere più elevata per gli avvelenamenti (per es. ferro). *Adulti:* 2400 mg ogni 10-20 min fino a consumare 4 L. Può essere più elevata per gli avvelenamenti.	*Cautela:* pazienti con malattia o ostruzione dell'intestino (colite). *Effetti indesiderati:* nausea, crampi, gonfiore.
Poractant alfa Sospensione intratracheale degli estratti suini di polmone, surfattante (80 mg fosfolipidi, 1 mg proteine, 0,3 mg SP-B/mL).	**Profilassi o trattamento della sindrome da distress respiratorio, trattamento dell'ipertensione polmonare persistente.** *Neonati:* 2,5 mL/kg (200 mg/kg) per la dose 1, si può ripetere la dose di 1,25 mL/kg (100 mg/kg) 2 × ogni 12 h. *Bambini e adulti:* non indicato.	*Cautela:* monitorare strettamente lo stato del ventilatore; può essere necessario uno svezzamento rapido entro min dalla dose. *Effetti indesiderati:* bradicardia, ostruzione delle vie aeree, cianosi.
Pralidossima Riattivazione dell'acetilcolinasterasi. Compresse: 500 mg. Iniettabile.	**Trattamento dell'avvelenamento da organofosfati; possibile trattamento della tossicità da farmaci colinergici.** im, ev: *Bambini:* 20-50 mg/kg/dose ripetuta in 1-2 h se non è stata rilevata debolezza muscolare; quando è ottenuto l'effetto desiderato, dose ogni 12 h. *Adulti:* 1-2 g ogni 5-6 h; dose basata sulla risposta clinica.	*Cautela:* come antidoto per l'avvelenamento da organofosfati; usare in combinazione con atropina. Il dosaggio eccessivo può causare effetti colinergici. Una somministrazione ev troppo rapida è associata a tachicardia, laringospasmo. Infondere ev per 15-30 min. *Effetti indesiderati:* ipertensione, vertigini, nausea, debolezza muscolare o rigidità.
Prazosin Capsule: 1, 2, 5 mg.	**Antagonista competitivo dei recettori postsinaptici α-adrenergici usato nel trattamento dell'ipertensione o dello scompenso cardiaco.** per os: *Bambini:* 0,1 mg/kg/24 h ogni 6 h, titolando la dose alla pressione arteriosa desiderata (massimo: 0,4 mg/kg/24 h o 15 mg dose totale). Considerare combinazioni aggiuntive/sinergiche con i diuretici. *Adulti:* 3 mg/24 h ogni 8-12 ore, titolando la dose alla pressione arteriosa desiderata. Range dose usuale: 3-15 mg/24 h.	*Cautela:* può verificarsi ipotensione grave dopo la prima dose (dose "fenomeno della prima dose"); più comune nei pazienti con deplezione di liquidi e/o sali. *Effetti indesiderati:* sincope, palpitazioni, vertigini, ritenzione idrica. *Interazioni farmacologiche:* altri farmaci per l'ipertensione (diuretici, β-bloccanti).

TABELLA 716-1. Farmaci generali – *continua*

FARMACO (PRINCIPIO ATTIVO, FORMULAZIONI)	INDICAZIONI (MECCANISMO D'AZIONE E DOSAGGIO)	COMMENTI (CAUTELE, EFFETTI INDESIDERATI, MONITORAGGIO)
Prednisolone Glucocorticoide. Compresse: 5 mg. Sospensione. Iniezione.	**Trattamento dei disordini infiammatori, inclusi allergici, respiratori, reumatici, endocrini e neoplastici.** Asma: per os, ev: *Bambini:* 0,5-4 mg/kg/24 h ogni 6-12 h. *Adulti:* 5-60 mg/24 h. Anti-infiammatorio: per os, ev: *Bambini:* 0,1-2 mg/kg/24 h ogni 6 h-al giorno.	*Cautela:* dose titolata all'effetto desiderato; usare il ciclo di trattamento più breve per evitare effetti indesiderati. Può rallentare la crescita, aumenta la ritenzione di sali. *Effetti indesiderati:* edema. ipertensione, psicosi, sindrome di Cushing, soppressione asse HPA (adrenale), ulcera peptica. *Interazioni farmacologiche:* barbiturici, fenitoina, rifampicina. *Commento:* vedi confronto tra i corticosteroidi alla voce *Idrocortisone*.
Prednisone Glucocorticosteroide. Compresse: 1, 2,5, 5, 10, 20, 50 mg. Sciroppo: 5 mg/5 mL. Iniezione.	**Trattamento delle malattie infiammatori, tra cui quelli allergici, respiratori, reumatici, endocrini e neoplastici.** Asma: per os: *Bambini:* 0,5-4 mg/kg/24 h ogni 6-12 h. *Adulti:* 5-60 mg/24 h. Anti-infiammatorio: per os, ev: *Bambini:* 0,1-2 mg/kg/24 h ogni 6-24 h.	*Cautela:* dose titolata all'effetto desiderato; usare il ciclo più breve di trattamento per evitare effetti indesiderati. Può rallentare la crescita, aumenta la ritenzione di sali. *Effetti indesiderati:* edema, ipertensione, psicosi, sindrome di Cushing, soppressione asse HPA (surrenalica), ulcera peptica. *Interazioni farmacologiche:* barbiturici, fenitoina, rifampicina. *Commento:* vedi confronto tra i corticosteroidi alla voce *Idrocortisone*.
Primidone Anticonvulsante. Compresse: 50, 250 mg. Sospensione: 250 mg/5 mL.	**Trattamento delle convulsioni generalizzate tonico-cloniche, complesse parziali, e focali.** per os: *Neonati:* 12-20 mg/kg/24 h ogni 8-12 h. *Bambini:* 10-25 mg/kg/24 h. ogni 8-12 h. *Bambini >8 anni e adulti:* 125-1500 mg/24 h ogni 8-12 h (massimo: 2 g/24 h).	*Effetti indesiderati:* sedazione, atassia, rash. *Interazioni farmacologiche:* valproato, griseofulvina, fenitoina. *Monitoraggio:* concentrazioni di PEMA: terapeutiche 5-12 µg/mL. *Cautela:* parzialmente metabolizzato a fenobarbital e PEMA.
Procainamide Antiaritmico di classe 1a. Compresse e capsule: 250, 375, 500 mg. Compresse, rilascio prolungato: 250, 500, 750, 1,000 mg. Iniezione.	**Trattamento della tachicardia ventricolare, contrazioni ventricolari premature, tachicardia atriale parossistica, fibrillazione atriale.** Dose da carico: *Bambini:* ev: 3-6 mg/kg/dose per 5 min, non superare i 100 mg/dose; ripetere ogni 5-10 min se necessario (massimo: 15 mg/kg dose totale). Non superare i 500 mg in 30 min. Dose di mantenimento: per os: *Bambini:* 15-50 mg/kg/24 h, ogni 3-6 h; 20-30 mg/kg/24 h, non superare i 4 g/ 24 h; infusione continua ev e di 20-80 µg/kg/min (massimo: 2 g/24 h). *Adulti:* 250-500 mg/dose ogni 3-6 h (massimo: 2-4 g/24 h).	*Cautela:* causa reazione positiva degli anticorpi antinucleo, cardiodepressivo generale. Metabolizzato a NAPA attivo. *Effetti indesiderati:* ipotensione, aritmie, blocco AV, confusione, agranulocitosi, sindrome simil lupus eritematoso sistemico, febbre, rash. *Interazioni farmacologiche:* cimetidina, β-bloccanti, anticolinergici. *Monitoraggio:* concentrazioni di procainamide: terapeutiche 4-10 µg/mL. Somma di procainamide e NAPA: terapeutiche 10-30 µg/mL.
Procarbazina Agente antineoplastico. Capsule: 50 mg.	**Trattamento della malattia di Hodgkin, del carcinoma broncogeno.** Malattia di Hodgkin: *Bambini:* per os: 1,5-3 mg/kg/24 h (50-100 mg/m^2) ogni 24 h per ciclo di 10-14/28 giorni. Preparazione per il trapianto del midollo osseo: 12,5 mg/kg/dose. Neuroblastoma e medulloblastoma: *Bambini:* 100-200 mg/m^2 dose per protocollo.	*Cautela:* dose calcolata sul protocollo della malattia e sui farmaci concomitanti. Evitare alcol (causa reazioni disulfiram-simili). Possiede una certa attività inibitoria della monoaminossidasi. *Effetti indesiderati:* depressione del SNC, confusione, atassia, soppressione midollare, alopecia, sindrome simil-influenzale. *Interazioni farmacologiche:* alcol, antidepressivi triciclici, fenotiazine, cibi simpaticomimetici contenenti tiramina.
Proclorperazina Compresse: 5, 10, 25 mg. Capsule, rilascio prolungato: 10, 15, 30 mg. Iniezione. Supposte : 2,5, 2, 25 mg. Sciroppo: 5 mg/5 mL.	**Antiemetico fenotiazinico piperazina-simile. L'uso nei bambini dovrebbe essere evitato.** *Bambini:* per os, rettale: 0,4 mg/kg/24 h ogni 6-8 h. im: 0,1-0,15 mg/kg/24 h ogni 8-12 h. *Adulti:* per os: 5-10 mg/dose tid-qid.	*Effetti indesiderati:* sedazione, reazioni extrapiramidali, fotosensibilità, ittero colestatico. *Interazioni farmacologiche:* effetti additivi sul SNC, antagonisti del recettore α. *Cautela:* reazione distonica acuta comune nei bambini.
Prometazina Compresse: 12,5, 25, 50 mg. Sciroppo. Supposta . Iniezione.	**Fenotiazina con attività antistaminica primaria usata nel trattamento di nausea, vomito, cinetosi, allergia.** Cinetosi: *Bambini:* per os: 0,5 mg/kg 30-60 min come inizio; poi ogni 8-12 h se necessario. Sedativo antiemetico: *Bambini:* im, ev, rettale: 0,25-1 mg/kg/dose ogni 4-6 h se necessario.	*Cautela:* potenzia gli effetti anticolinergici. *Effetti indesiderati:* sedazione, ipotensione, reazioni extrapiramidali, visione offuscata. *Interazioni farmacologiche:* effetti sedativi aggiuntivi.
Propafenone Agente antiaritmico di classe 1c. Compresse: 150, 225, 300 mg.	**Efficace contro la tachicardia pediatrica sopraventricolare.** *Bambini:* per os: 200-600 mg/m^2/24 h suddivisi. Causa anche vertigini, affaticamento, nausea, vomito e stipsi. *Adulti:* 150 mg ogni 8 h (450 mg/24 h). Si può titolare da intervalli di 3-5 giorni a 300 mg ogni 8 h (massimo: 900 mg/24 h).	*Cautela:* può peggiorare o causare aritmie, scompenso cardiaco o angina. *Interazioni farmacologiche:* aumenta i livelli di digossina (dose-correlati), ciclosporina e teofillina.
Propantelina bromuro Compresse: 7,5, 15 mg.	**Anticolinergico antispasticomodico sintetico usato come terapia aggiuntiva per spasmo gastrointestinale o vescicale, intestino irritabile.** *Bambini:* per os: 1,5-3 mg/kg/24 h ogni 4-8 h. Dose fino all'effetto desiderato.	*Cautela:* evitare nei pazienti con diminuita motilità intestinale. *Effetti indesiderati:* sedazione, tachicardia, secchezza delle fauci, visione offuscata, midriasi.
Propofol Iniezione.	**Sedativo non barbiturico, ipnotico, anestetico generale.** Sedazione: *Bambini:* ev: 1,5-3 mg/kg/dose per 1-2 min. Sedazione continua (ventilazione meccanica): *Bambini:* ev: 5,5 mg/kg per 30 min, aumentare a 6 mg/kg per 30 min, aumentare a 8 mg/kg per 1 ora, aumentare a 10 mg/kg per 1 ora, aumentare alla velocità di infusione finale di 12,5 mg/kg/h.	*Cautela:* regime di titolazione della dose per permettere un'adeguata sedazione che si adegui alla complessa farmacocinetica del farmaco. Fiale monouso in emulsione lipidica. *Effetti indesiderati:* ipotensione, bradicardia, iperlipidemia, dubbia acidosi metabolica.

TABELLA 716-1. Farmaci generali – *continua*

FARMACO (PRINCIPIO ATTIVO, FORMULAZIONI)	INDICAZIONI (MECCANISMO D'AZIONE E DOSAGGIO)	COMMENTI (CAUTELE, EFFETTI INDESIDERATI, MONITORAGGIO)
Propoxifene Capsule. Compresse.	**Analgesico per il dolore lieve moderato. Si lega ai recettori oppiacei. Minore suscettibilità alla dipendenza rispetto alla codeina.** per os: *Bambini:* 2-3 mg/kg/24 h ogni 4-6 h. Titolare la dose fino all'effetto desiderato. *Adulti:* idrocloruro 65 mg/dose ogni 4-6 h (massimo: 390 mg); sale napsilato 100 mg ogni 4-6 h (massimo: 600 mg).	*Cautela:* debole agonista oppiaceo con limitata possibilità di abuso. *Effetti indesiderati:* sedazione, vertigini, nausea, vomito, stipsi, dipendenza.
Propranololo Compresse: 10, 20, 40, 60, 80 mg. Soluzione: 4, 8, e concentrato 80 mg/mL. Iniezione: 1 mg/mL. Capsule, rilascio prolungato: 60, 80, 120, 160 mg.	**Antagonista non selettivo dei recettori β-adrenergici (β_1 e β_2)** *Neonati:* per os: 0,25 mg/kg/dose ogni 6-8 h; titolare fino alla risposta desiderata, aumentando lentamente (massimo: 5 mg/kg/24 h). ev: 0,01 mg/kg per 10-15 min; titolare all'effetto desiderato (massimo: 1 mg/kg/24 h). Aritmie/ipertensione: *Bambini:* per os: 0,5-1 mg/kg/24 h ogni 6-8 h titolare fino a 2-5 mg/kg/24 h, per 3-5 giorni. ev: 0,01-0,1 mg/kg/dose infusi in 10-15 min se necessario (massimo: 1 mg nei bambini piccoli; 3 mg bambini grandi). *Adulti:* per os: 40-80 mg/24 h, titolando fino al range di risposta: 40-320 mg/24 h ogni 6-8 h. Tireotossicosi: *Neonati:* per os: 2 mg/kg/24 h ogni 6-8 h; titolare fino alla risposta. *Bambini:* per os: 2-4 mg/kg/24 h ogni 6-8 h; titolare fino alla risposta. Profilassi dell'emicrania: *Bambini:* per os: 0,6-2 mg/kg/24 h ogni 6-8 h (massimo: 4 mg/kg/24 h).	*Cautela:* il farmaco va incontro a un significativo metabolismo di primo passaggio, giustificando la grossa differenza tra dosi ev e per os. Usare con cautela ev e nei pazienti con scompenso cardiaco congestizio, asma, pneumopatia cronica ostruttiva. Monitorare la frequenza cardiaca per l'effetto del farmaco. *Effetti indesiderati:* diminuita contrattilità cardiaca, ipotensione, bradicardia, ipoglicemia, broncospasmo.
Propiltiouracile (PTU) Compresse: 50 mg.	**Antitiroideo che inibisce la sintesi di ormone tiroideo interferendo con l'accumulo di iodio.** per os: *Neonati:* 5-10 mg/kg/24 h ogni 8 h; titolare fino all'effetto. *Bambini:* 5-7mg/kg/24 h ogni 8 h; titolare fino all'effetto. *Adulti:* 300-450 mg/24 h ogni 8 h; aumentando a 600-1200 mg/24 h.	*Cautela:* per un marcato effetto del farmaco di solito sono necessarie 24-36 h. *Effetti indesiderati:* vertigini, rash, discrasie ematiche, epatite, artralgia, polmonite interstiziale.
Protamina solfato Iniezione: 10 mg/mL.	**Antidoto dell'eparina, neutralizza il suo effetto anticoagulante.** 1 mg protamina neutralizza 90 unità USP di eparina derivata dai polmoni e 115 USP unità di di eparina derivata dall'intestino. La dose di protamina va calcolata considerando la durata di tempo dall'ultima dose di eparina usando l'emivita dell'eparina (h) per determinare una stima dei depositi di eparina.	*Cautela:* calcolare la dose con attenzione; l'eccesso di protamina può causare anticoagulazione. Monitorare il tempo di tromboplastina parziale durante l'uso. *Effetti indesiderati:* ipotensione, dispnea, ipersensibilità.
Pseudoefedrina Compresse: 30, 60 mg. Compresse, a rilascio prolungato: 12 mg. Capsule: 60 mg. Capsule, a rilascio prolungato: 120 mg. Sciroppo: 15 mg/mL.	**Simpaticomimetico ad azione indiretta usato come decongestionante nasale per trattare i sintomi del raffreddore comune.** per os: *Bambini piccoli e grandi:* 4 mg/kg/24 h ogni 6-12 h. *Adulti:* 6 mg/dose ogni 6-8 h (massimo: 240 mg/24 h).	*Cautela:* pazienti con ipertensione, cardiopatia. *Effetti indesiderati:* tachicardia, cefalea, nervosismo, tremore. *Interazioni farmacologiche:* inibitori di monoamino ossidasi, propranololo, pressori.
Piridostigmina Compresse: 60 mg. Compresse, rilascio prolungato 180 mg. Sciroppo: 60 mg/5 mL. Iniezione: 5 mg/mL.	**Inibitore della colinesterasi usato per trattare la miastenia gravis; inversione degli agenti bloccanti neuromuscolari.** Miastenia grave: *Bambini:* im, ev: 0,05-0,15 mg/kg/dose (massimo: 10 mg); titolare all'effetto desiderato. per os: 7 mg/kg/24 h in 5-6 dosi suddivise. *Adulti:* im, ev: 2 mg ogni 2-3 h. per os: 60 mg/dose ogni 8 h; titolare fino all'effetto desiderato. Inversione degli agenti bloccanti neuromuscolari: *Bambini:* im, ev: 01-0,25 mg/kg/dose; titolare fino all'effetto; può essere necessario co-somministrare atropina/glicopirrolato. *Adulti:* 10-20 mg/dose con atropina/glicopirrolato.	*Cautela:* pazienti con asma, disfunzione cardiaca o aritmie, ulcera peptica. *Effetti indesiderati:* bradicardia, blocco AV, convulsioni, cefalea, diarrea, crampi addominali, salivazione, pollachiuria, debolezza muscolare, miosi, lacrimazione, aumento delle secrezioni bronchiali.
Piridossina Compresse: 25, 50, 100 mg; Compresse, rilascio prolungato: 100 mg. Iniezione: 100 mg/mL.	**Vitamina B_6 usata per i deficit alimentari o farmaco-indotti (per es. isoniazide, idralazina) e le convulsioni B_6-dipendenti.** Convulsioni piridossina-dipendenti: *Bambini:* per os, im, ev: 50-100 mg; dose di mantenimento 50-100 mg/24 h. Deficit dietetico: *Bambini:* 5-15 mg/24 h per 3-4 sett, poi 2,5-5 mg/24 h. *Adulti:* 10-20 mg/24 h per 3-4 sett. Neurite farmaco-indotta: per os, im, ev: *Bambini:* 1 mg/kg/24 h al giorno. *Adulti:* 100-200 mg/24 h al giorno.	*Cautela:* può diminuire le concentrazioni sieriche di fenobarbital e fenitoina. Dosi ev elevate possono precipitate le convulsioni. *Effetti indesiderati:* nausea, diminuzione dell'acido folico, test di funzionalità epatica.
Quetiapina Antipsicotico atipico. Compresse: 25, 100, 200, 300 mg.	**Antagonista di serotonina, dopamina e dei recettori adrenergici $\alpha 1$ e $\alpha 2$,** *Bambini:* per os: iniziare con 12,5 mg bid, poi aumentare con incrementi di 25-50 mg fino a 300-400 mg/24 h suddivisi in 2-3 dosi. *Adulti:* per os: iniziare con 25 mg bid, poi aumentare con incrementi da 25-50 mg ogni 2-3 giorni fino alla risposta, a 300-400 mg/24 h suddivisi in 2-3 dosi (massimo: 800 mg/24 h).	*Effetti indesiderati:* sonnolenza, vertigini, cefalea, stipsi, bocca secca, dispepsia, ipotensione posturale, tachicardia.

TABELLA 716-1. Farmaci generali – *continua*

FARMACO (PRINCIPIO ATTIVO, FORMULAZIONI)	INDICAZIONI (MECCANISMO D'AZIONE E DOSAGGIO)	COMMENTI (CAUTELE, EFFETTI INDESIDERATI, MONITORAGGIO)
Quinidina Compresse (solfato): 200, 300 mg. Compresse a rilascio prolungato (solfato): 300 mg. Compresse, rilascio prolungato (gluconato): 324 mg. Iniezione (gluconato): 80 mg/mL.	**Depressivo miocardico usato nel trattamento delle aritmie: tachicardia sopraventricolare, tachicardia parossistica ventricolare, contrazioni atrio/ventricolari premature.** *Bambini:* per os, im, ev: 2 mg/kg Dose test per escludere l'idiosincrasia: 20-50 mg/kg/24 h sale solfato ogni 4 h per os; gluconato sale 2-10 mg/kg/dose ogni 3-6 h ev. *Adulti:* 199-600 mg/dose di sale solfato ogni 4-6 h per os; 324-972 mg/dose di gluconato ogni 8-12 h; 200-400 mg/dose di solfato ev; titolare fino all'effetto.	*Cautela:* sincope da prima dose; 267 mg di quinidina gluconato = 200 mg quinidina solfato. Infondere ev lentamente <10 mg/min. *Effetti indesiderati:* sincope, ipotensione, blocco cardiaco, febbre, dolore addominale, soppressione del midollo osseo, trombocitopenia, porpora trombotica trombocitopenica, cinconismo. *Interazioni farmacologiche:* verapamil, cimetidina, fenitoina, fenobarbital, rifampicina, digossina.
Ranitidina Compresse/capsule: 150, 300 mg. Sciroppo: 15 mg/mL. Iniezione: 25 mg/mL. Granuli effervescenti e compresse: 150 mg.	**Antagonista dei recettori H_2 inibisce in modo competitivo la secrezione acida gastrica nella malattia gastrica o nell'ulcera peptica e nella profilassi dell'ulcera da stress; reflusso gastroesofageo.** *Neonati:* per os, ev: 1,5-2 mg/kg/24 h ogni 12 h; infusione continua 24 h ev 0,04 mg/kg/h (massimo: 1 mg/kg/24 h). *Bambini:* per os, im, ev: 1-5 mg/kg/24 h ogni 6-8 h; infusione continua ev 24 h 2-5 mg/kg/24 h. *Adulti:* per os: 150 mg/dose ogni 12 h o 300 mg per os prima di andare a letto. im, ev: 50-100 mg/dose ogni 6-8 h.	*Cautela:* la dose può essere titolata al pH gastrico desiderato dall'aspirato gastrico. *Effetti indesiderati:* cefalea, confusione mentale, dolore al punto di iniezione. *Commento:* rare o assenti interazioni farmacologiche clinicamente importanti.
Risperidone Compresse: 0,25, 0,5, 1, 2, 3, 4 mg. Soluzione per os: 1 mg/mL.	**Antipsicotico atipico.** *Bambini:* iniziare 0,25 mg bid; aumentare per la risposta fino a 3 mg bid. *Adolescenti e adulti:* iniziare con 1 mg bid; aumentare fino a 3 mg bid o fino alla risposta.	*Cautela:* può causare prolungamento del tratto Q-T e aumenta il rischio di morte cardiaca improvvisa; monitorare l'ECG ed evitare l'uso concomitante con altri farmaci che prolungano l'intervallo QT. *Effetti indesiderati:* vertigini, sonnolenza, agitazione, cefalea, tachicardia, stipsi, secchezza delle fauci, ipotensione ortostatica, aumento di peso.
Riboflavina Compresse: 25, 50, 100 mg.	**Vitamina usata come supplemento e negli stati di deficit.** Deficit: *Bambini:* per os: 2,5-10 mg/24 h ogni 8-12 h. *Adulti:* per os: 5-30 mg/24 h ogni 8-12 h.	*Effetti indesiderati:* estremamente rari. *Interazioni farmacologiche:* probenecid.
Rocuronio Iniezione: 10 mg/mL.	**Anestetico/rilassante del muscolo scheletrico agente bloccante neuromuscolare non depolarizzante.** *Bambini e adulti:* dose iniziale: 0,6-12 mg/kg; dosi seguenti somministrate al bisogno a 0,2 mg/kg ogni 20-30 min. Infusione continua ev e o 10-12 μg/kg/min.	*Cautela:* durante il blocco neuromuscolare si deve utilizzata la ventilazione, aggiustamento della dose in caso di disfunzione epatica. *Effetti indesiderati:* tachicardia, ipotensione, debolezza muscolare prolungata, broncospasmo. *Interazioni farmacologiche:* possibile aumentata debolezza muscolare con aminoglicosidi, anestetici, colistina.
Salmeterolo Bomboletta di aerosol.	**Agonista β_2-adrenergico a lunga durata d'azione (≈8-12+ h); broncodilatatore usato per trattare una malattia reversibile delle vie aeree. Eccellente nei pazienti con asma notturno.** *Bambini e adulti:* 1-2 puff (21 μg), aerosol ogni 12 h; titolare fino all'effetto desiderato.	*Cautela:* non usare nell'attacco acuto di asma. *Effetti indesiderati:* tachicardia, palpitazioni, cefalea, nervosismo, tremore muscolare, tosse, irritazione delle vie aeree.
Sargramostim Iniezione: 250, 500 μg.	**Fattore stimolante le colonie di granulociti-macrofagi (GM-CSF) per l'accelerazione della remissione mieloide da chemioterapia o danno midollare.**	*Cautela:* monitorare la conta dei globuli bianchi per definire la durata della terapia. *Effetti indesiderati:* tachicardia, ipotensione, flushing, ritenzione idrica, febbre, malessere, dolore osseo, mialgia, rigidità, dispnea.
Scopolamina Patch transdermico.	**Agente anticolinergico usato per controllare le secrezioni; antiemetico postoperatorio; trattamento della cinetosi.** Emesi postoperatoria: *Bambini:* im, ev, sc: 6 μg/kg/dose ogni 6-8 h. *Adulti:* 0,3-0,65 mg/dose ogni 6-8 h. Cinetosi: *Bambini e adulti:* 1 patch dietro l'orecchio almeno 4 h prima del movimento.	*Cautela:* glaucoma ad angolo stretto, ileo. Usare il patch con attenzione nei bambini <12 anni. *Effetti indesiderati:* tachicardia, disorientamento, sedazione, psicosi, secchezza delle fauci, stipsi, ritenzione urinaria, visione offuscata. *Interazioni farmacologiche:* altri composti anticolinergici; può interferire con l'assorbimento gastrointestinale di certi farmaci.
Senna Sciroppo: 218 mg/5 mL. Compresse: 187, 217, 600 mg. Granuli: 326 mg/cucchiaio.	**Stimolante catartico per il trattamento a breve termine della stipsi; preparazione intestinale preliminare a esami radiologici.** *Bambini:* per os: 10-20 mg/kg/dose, ogni 12-24 h.	*Cautela:* evitare uso prolungato (>1 settimana); dipendenza. *Effetti indesiderati:* crampi addominali, diarrea, alterazioni dell'equilibrio idroelettrolitico.
Sertralina Antidepressivo; inibitore del reuptake della serotonina. Compresse: 25, 50, 100 mg. Soluzione orale (concentrate): 20 mg/mL.	**Trattamento di depressione, disturbo ossessivo-compulsivo, attacchi di panico, disturbo post-traumatico da stress, disturbo da deficit dell'attenzione.** *Bambini 6-12 anni:* iniziare con 25 mg ogni 24 h; aumentare di 25 mg alla sett fino alla risposta, dose ogni 24 h (massimo: 200 mg/24 h). *Bambini >12 anni e adulti:* iniziare con 50 mg ogni 24 h, aumentare di 25-50 mg alla sett fino alla risposta; dose ogni 24 h (massimo: 200 mg/24 h).	*Cautela:* non sospendere improvvisamente o sintomi da astinenza (sindrome da astinenza dell'inibitore selettivo del reuptake della serotonina) al verificarsi. Ridurre al massimo o 50 mg/24 h ogni 5-7 giorni. *Effetti indesiderati:* insonnia, sonnolenza, cefalea, secchezza delle fauci, nausea, diarrea.
Simeticone Compresse, masticabile: 40, 80, 125 mg. Capsule: 125 mg. Gocce: 40 mg/0,6mL.	**Antiflatulenza per il sollievo sintomatico della colica, del gas eccessivo.** *Bambini <2 anni:* per os: 20 mg/dose ogni 4-6 h. *Bambini 2-12 anni:* per os: 40 mg/dose ogni 6 h. *Bambini >12 anni e adulti:* per os: 40-120 mg ogni 6 h; dose titolata fino all'effetto.	*Commenti:* farmaco molto sicuro con rari effetti indesiderati. La dose può essere titolata fino all'effetto desiderato aumentando la dose o la frequenza di dosi/giorno. Evitare cibi formanti gas e irritanti gastrointestinali.

TABELLA 716-1. Farmaci generali – *continua*

FARMACO (PRINCIPIO ATTIVO, FORMULAZIONI)	INDICAZIONI (MECCANISMO D'AZIONE E DOSAGGIO)	COMMENTI (CAUTELE, EFFETTI INDESIDERATI, MONITORAGGIO)
Sodio cromoglicato Stabilizzatore delle mastcellule. Soluzione oftalmica. Capsule (orali): 100 mg. Inalazione: 20 mg. Inalatore a dosaggio controllato(MDI): 800 µg/spruzzo. Soluzione nebulizzata: 10 mg/mL (2 mL). Soluzione nasale: 40 mg/mL. Soluzione oftalmica: 4%.	**Prevenzione dei sintomi cronici di asma, riniti, congiuntivite, mastocitosi sistemica, allergia alimentare e malattia infiammatoria dell'intestino (previene il rilascio di istamina e leucotrieni da parte delle mastcellule).** *Bambini e adulti:* Asma: 1-2 puff (MDI) o 2 mL (soluzione nebulizzata) 3-4 tid-qid. Riniti: 1 spruzzo ogni narice tid-qid. Congiuntivite: 1-2 gocce 4-6 volte al giorno. Mastocitosi, allergia al cibo: *Bambini:* 100 mg/dose qid (massimo: 40 mg/kg/24 h). *Adulti:* 200 mg/dose qid (massimo: 400 mg/dose qid).	*Effetti indesiderati:* raucedine e tosse (principalmente con la polvere inalatoria), arrossamento e puntura al sito di somministrazione.
Sodio polistirene sulfonato Polvere per sospensione.	**Resina a scambio ionico che rimuove il potassio in cambio del sodio per il trattamento dell'iperpotassemia.** *Bambini:* per os: 4 g/kg/24 h, ogni 4-8 h; rettale: 4-12 g/kg/24 h ogni 2-6 h. *Adulti:* per os: 15 g/dose, ogni 6-12 h.	*Cautela:* monitorare strettamente il potassio sierico. Non miscelare con liquidi contenenti potassio (per es. succo d'arancia). *Effetti indesiderati:* crampi addominali, senso di sazietà, ipopotassemia.
Sodio tiosolfato Iniezione: 100, 250 mg/mL.	**Antidoto per il cianuro (nitroprussiato) e il cisplatino. Fornisce uno zolfo extra all'enzima rodanese per migliorare la detossificazione del cianuro.** Nitroprussiato: *Bambini e adulti:* ev: 1 g di sodio tiosolfato ogni 100 mg di nitroprussiato somministrati. Si può infondere nella stessa via ev. Cisplatino: *Adulti:* ev: 12 g infusi per 6 h prima o durante l'infusione di cisplatino. Alternato: bolo da 9 g/m^2 ev seguito da 1,2 g/m^2/h per 6 h prima o durante l'infusione di cisplatino.	*Cautela:* l'infusione rapida ev può causare ipotensione. *Effetti indesiderati:* molto rari. Ipotensione, irritazione locale nel sito di infusione.
Sotalolo Antiaritmico di classe III. Compresse: 80, 120, 160 mg.	**Trattamento delle aritmie sopraventricolari e ventricolari.** *Bambini:* per os: 2-8 mg/kg/24 h suddivisi ogni 8-12 h. *Adulti:* per os: iniziare con 80 mg ogni 12 h e titolare ogni 3-4 giorni fino alla risposta (massimo: 640 mg/24 h)	*Cautela:* effetto proaritmico che peggiora lo scompenso cardiaco congestizio o il diabete. Ridurre la dose in caso di diminuzione della funzione renale (1/2 dose. per CrCl <60 mL/min, 1/3 dose per CrCl <30 mL/min). Aumentare l'intervallo per diminuire la dose.
Spironolattone Compresse: 25, 50, 100 mg.	**Antagonista competitivo dell'aldosterone usato come lieve antipertensivo, diuretico risparmiatore di potassio, nell'epatopatia cronica.** *Neonati:* per os: 1-3 mg/kg/24 h suddivisi ogni 12-24 h. *Bambini:* per os: 1,5-3,3 mg/kg/24 h suddivisi ogni 8-24 h. *Adulti:* per os: 25-200 mg/dose ogni12-24 h.	*Cautela:* attento monitoraggio del potassio sierico/introito di potassio. La sospensione può essere realizzata frantumando le compresse in acqua/glicerina. *Effetti indesiderati:* letargia, iperpotassemia, ginecomastia, nausea, rash.
Streptochinasi Iniezione.	**Agente trombolitico usato per il trattamento di trombosi venosa profonda e ictus e per la pervietà del catetere.** Trombosi: ev: 3500-4000 unità infuse ev in 30 min seguita da 1000-1500 unità in infusione continua. Coagulo nel catetere: ev: 10 000-25 000 unità in soluzione fisiologica normale del volume del catetere instillate nel catetere per ~1 ora, poi rimosse (aspirate).	*Cautela:* un'infezione recente da streptococco può ridurne l'efficacia. *Effetti indesiderati:* sanguinamento, broncospasmo, flushing, rash. *Interazioni farmacologiche:* anticoagulanti, farmaci antipiastrinici.
Subsalicilato di bismuto Antidiarroico; agente gastrointestinale; trattamento dell'ulcera gastrica o duodenale. Liquido: 262 mg/15 mL (120, 240, 360, 480 mL); 524 mg/15 mL (120, 240, 360 mL). Compresse, masticabile: 262 mg.	**Trattamento della diarrea o dell'ulcera gastrointestinale (assorbe l'acqua in eccesso e le tossine nell'intestino crasso e uccide i batteri patogeni).** *Bambini o adulti:* fino a 8 dosi/24 h. *3-6 anni:* 1/3 compressa o 5 mL. *6-9 anni:* 2/3 compressa o 10 mL. *9-12 anni:* 1 compressa o 15 mL. *Adulti:* 2 compresse o 30 mL.	*Cautela:* evitare nei pazienti con influenza o varicella a causa del contenuto di salicilato. *Effetti indesiderati:* depigmentazione della lingua, feci grigiastre-nere.
Succimero Capsule: 100 mg.	**Chelante metallico che forma sali solubili in acqua con piombo, mercurio e arsenico.** *Bambini e adulti:* per os: 10 mg/kg/dose ogni 8 h per 5 giorni, poi 10 mg/kg/dose ogni 12 h per 14 giorni.	*Cautela:* mantenere un'adeguata idratazione. Le capsule possono essere aperte spargendo i granuli in cibi molli. *Effetti indesiderati:* cefalea, vertigini, nausea, crampi addominali, sintomi simil-influenzali.
Succinilcolina Iniezione.	**Agente bloccante neuromuscolare.** *Bambini:* ev: 1-2 mg dose iniziale; dose di mantenimento di 0,3-0,6 mg/kg ogni 5-10 min, titolata fino al livello del rilassamento del muscolo scheletrico. *Adulti:* ev: 0,6 mg/kg fino a 150 mg dose iniziale; dose di mantenimento di 0,04- 0,07 mg/kg ogni 5-10 min titolato fino all'effetto.	*Cautela:* pazienti con iperpotassemia, trauma grave, aumentata pressione endocranica o intraoculare. *Effetti indesiderati:* bradicardia, ipotensione, ipertermia maligna, iperpotassemia, broncospasmo. *Interazioni farmacologiche:* depressivi o rilassanti muscolari.
Sucralfato Compresse: 1 g. Sospensione: 1 g/10 mL.	**Sale di alluminio di saccarosio solfato che in presenza di acido forma una sorta simile di impasto che aderisce alla mucosa danneggiata.** *Bambini:* per os: 40-80 mg/kg/24 h suddivisi ogni 6-8 h. Stomatite: per os: 5-10 mL sciacquare e sputare o deglutire ogni 6 h. *Adulti:* per os: 1 g/dose ogni 4-6 h.	*Cautela:* si può usare per via topica per la stomatite. *Effetti indesiderati:* cefalea, stipsi, crampi addominali, rash. *Interazioni farmacologiche:* diminuisce l'assorbimento di fenitoina, tetraciclina, ketoconazolo, teofillina, digossina, cimetidina.
Sufentanil Iniezione.	**Analgesico oppioide usato in anestesia e per il trattamento del dolore.** *Bambini:* ev: 10-25 µg/kg dose iniziale, titolato all'effetto desiderato con 25-50 µg/kg. *Adulti:* ev: 0,5-8 µg/kg dose iniziale con dose di mantenimento di 10-50 µg/kg.	*Cautela:* nei pazienti con trauma cranico o concomitanti inibitori delle monoamino ossidasi, i profili degli effetti indesiderati di tutti gli oppiacei sono potenziati. *Effetti indesiderati:* bradicardia, vasodilatazione, nausea, vomito, visione offuscata, depressione respiratoria, possibile dipendenza. *Interazioni farmacologiche:* depressivi del SNC e respiratori.

TABELLA 716-1. Farmaci generali – *continua*

FARMACO (PRINCIPIO ATTIVO, FORMULAZIONI)	INDICAZIONI (MECCANISMO D'AZIONE E DOSAGGIO)	COMMENTI (CAUTELE, EFFETTI INDESIDERATI, MONITORAGGIO)
Sulfasalazina Compresse: 500 mg.	**Anti-infiammatorio derivato dell'acido 5-aminosalicilico combinato con sulfonamide usato nel trattamento della malattia infiammatoria intestinale.** *Bambini:* per os: inizialmente, 40-75 mg/kg/24 h suddivisi ogni 4-6 h (massimo: 6 g/24 h); dose di mantenimento di 30-50 mg/kg/24 h suddivisi ogni 6-8 h. *Adulti:* per os: 1 g/dose ogni 6-8 h (massimo: 6 g/24 h).	*Cautela:* ipersensibilità ai farmaci zolfo. *Effetti indesiderati:* rash, vertigini, cefalea, nausea, soppressione midollare. *Interazioni farmacologiche:* diminuisce l'assorbimento di folati e digossina.
Tacrolimus Immunosoppressore. Iniezione. Capsule: 1,5 mg. Possono essere preparate preparazioni estemporanee.	**Previene la graft versus host disease nel trapianto d'organo.** *Bambini:* per os: 0,15 mg/kg ogni 12 h; ev: infusione continua di 0,05-0,1 mg/kg/24 h. *Adulti:* per os: 0,075-0,15 mg/kg ogni 12 h; ev: infusione continua di 0,05-0,1 mg/kg/24 h.	*Effetti indesiderati:* ipertensione, cefalea, insonnia, dolore addominale e alla schiena, febbre, astenia, prurito, ipo/iperpotassemia, ipomagnesiemia, iperglicemia, nausea, vomito, diarrea, anemia, leucocitosi, danno epatico, nefrotossicità, dispnea, versamento pleurico, edema periferico. *Monitoraggio:* concentrazioni: di tacrolimus: terapeutiche 9,8-19,4 ng/mL usando test ELISA sul sangue intero; 0,5-1,5 ng/mL mediante cromatografia liquida ad alta pressione del siero.
Teniposide, VM-26 Iniezione: 10 mg/mL.	**Trattamento della leucemia linfocitica acuta (LLA) e del tumore polmonare (inibisce che le cellule entrino in mitosi).** *Bambini:* ev: iniziare 130 mg/m^2/sett, aumentare dopo 3 sett fino a 150 mg/m^2, e dopo 6 sett fino a 180 mg/m^2, *Adulti:* LLA: 250 mg/m^2 sett per 4-8 sett.	*Cautela:* aumenta l'accumulo intracellulare e quindi la tossicità del metotrexato. *Effetti indesiderati:* nausea, vomito, diarrea, mucosite, mielosoppressione, alopecia, rash, febbre, emorragia, neuropatia periferica. *Commento:* i pazienti con sindrome di Down dovrebbero iniziare con 1/2 della dose usuale.
Teofillina Sciroppo, soluzione, elisir, capsule, compresse (anche a rilascio prolungato). (vedi *Aminofillina* per il dosaggio ev).	**Trattamento dell'apnea della prematurità, sintomi di malattia reversibile delle vie aeree (influisce sul trasporto intracellulare di calcio, inibitore della fosfodiesterasi, debole agente anti-infiammatorio).** *Neonati:* Apnea, broncodilatazione: dose da carico o 6-10 mg/kg; dose di mantenimento o 2-4 mg/kg/ dose ogni 12 h. *Bambini piccoli e grandi:* *6 sett-6 mesi:* 10 mg/kg/24 h. *6 mesi-1 anno:* 12-18 mg/kg/24 h. *1-9 anni:* 20-24 mg/kg/24 h. *9-12 anni:* 16 mg/kg/24 h. *12-16 anni:* 13 mg/kg/24 h. *Adulti:* 10 mg/kg/24 h. Il dosaggio può essere aumentato per i fumatori e per i farmaci induttori enzimatici; diminuire la dose nei pazienti con inibitori enzimatici, malattia epatica, scompenso cardiaco o ipotiroidismo.	*Cautela:* può causare o peggiorare aritmie, convulsioni o reflusso gastroesofageo. La clearance della teofillina è modificata da numerose patologie e farmaci richiedendo aggiustamenti della dose guidata dalle concentrazioni seriche di teofillina. La clearance è ridotta da malattie virali, febbre >41 °C per >24 h, cor polmonare e farmaci che inibiscono gli enzimi del P450 (cimetidina, verapamil, macrolidi, chinoloni); ridurre la dose del 50%. *Effetti indesiderati:* tachicardia, nervosismo, iperattività, difficoltà di concentrazione, irritabilità, agitazione, cefalea, nausea, vomito, dolore addominale, intolleranza al cibo, diuresi frequente, convulsioni e aritmie a livelli tossici. *Monitoraggio:* concentrazioni di teofillina: terapeutiche: apnea neonatale: 6-15 μg/mL; previene l'intubazione o promuove l'estubazione: 10-20 μg/mL; broncodilatazione: 5-20 μg/mL; tossiche >20 μg/mL.
Terbutalina solfato Iniezione. Compresse: 2,5, 5 mg. Inalatore a dosaggio controllato (MDI).	**Broncodilatatore (agonista del recettore β_2).** *Bambini <12 anni:* per os: 0,05 mg/kg/dose ogni 8 h (massimo: 5 mg). sc: 0,005-0,01 mg/kg/dose; si può ripetere dopo 15-20 min (massimo: 0,4 mg). *Bambini ≥12 anni e adulti:* per os: 2,5-5 mg/dose ogni 6-8 h. sc: 0,25 mg/dose; si può ripetere dopo 15 min. *Bambini e adulti:* MDI: 1-2 puff ogni 6-8 h se necessario.	*Effetti indesiderati:* tachicardia, aritmie, flushing, cefalea, nervosismo, tremore, ipopotassemia, crampi muscolari, broncospasmo paradosso.
Terfenadina Compresse: 60 mg.	**Trattamento dei sintomi allergici (antistaminico).** *Bambini:* *3-6 anni:* 15 mg bid. *6-12 anni:* 30 mg bid. *>12 anni e adulti:* 60 mg bid.	*Cautela:* possono verificarsi allungamento del tratto Q-T e aritmie fatali se combinato con farmaci che inibiscono gli enzimi epatici. *Effetti indesiderati:* sonnolenza, affaticamento. *Interazioni farmacologiche:* antifungini azolici, macrolidi e cimetidina può allungare l'intervallo Q-T e causare aritmie.
Testosterone Iniezione.	**Sostituzione androgenica nell'ipogonadismo maschile e nella pubertà ritardata (terapia sostitutiva).** *Bambini:* im Ipogonadismo maschile: Inizio della crescita prepuberale e pubertà ritardata: 40-50 mg/m^2/dose mensile; Fase della crescita terminale: 100 mg/m^2/dose 2× mensile. *Adulti:* Ipogonadismo: im: 50-400 mg ogni 2-4 sett.	*Cautela:* può accelerare la maturazione ossea senza produrre un guadagno compensatorio della crescita lineare. *Effetti indesiderati:* acne, irritabilità della vescica, comportamento aggressivo, depressione, insonnia, cefalea, irsutismo, disfunzione epatica.
Tiagabina Compresse: 2, 4, 12 16, 20 mg.	**Trattamento delle convulsioni parziali. Usato come aggiuntivo, terapia add-on. Inibitore del reuptake dell'acido γ-aminobutirrico.** *Adolescenti e adulti:* per os: iniziare con 4 mg al giorno; aumentare di 4-8 mg ogni sett fino alla risposta (massimo: 56 mg/24 h).	*Cautela:* problemi del SNC, tra cui vertigini, sonnolenza, atassia, tremore e debolezza muscolare; può anche causare stato epilettico non convulsivo.

TABELLA 716-1. Farmaci generali – *continua*

FARMACO (PRINCIPIO ATTIVO, FORMULAZIONI)	INDICAZIONI (MECCANISMO D'AZIONE E DOSAGGIO)	COMMENTI (CAUTELE, EFFETTI INDESIDERATI, MONITORAGGIO)
Tiamina Iniezione. Compresse: 50, 100, 250, 500 mg.	**Supplemento nutrizionale, trattamento del beri-beri e dell'encefalopatia di Wernicke (coenzima essenziale nel metabolismo dei carboidrati).** Beri-beri: *Bambini:* im, ev: 10-25 mg/24 h. per os: 10-50 mg/24 h per 2 sett, poi 5-10 mg/24 h per 1 mese. *Adulti:* im, ev: 5-30 mg tid per 2 sett, poi 15-30 mg/24 h per os per 1 mese. Encefalopatia di Wernicke: im, ev: 100 mg/24 h fino al consumo di una dieta bilanciata.	*Effetti indesiderati:* collasso cardiovascolare con dosi ev ripetute, angioedema, rash, formicolio.
Timololo Soluzione oftalmica, gel oftalmico, compresse.	**Trattamento dell'ipertensione intraoculare (blocca i recettori β_1 e β_2 e diminuisce la produzione di umore acqueo).** *Bambini:* (solo uso oftalmico) instillare una soluzione allo 0,25% 1 goccia due volte al giorno; si può aumentare a una soluzione allo 0,5% se la risposta è inadeguata; si può diminuire a una volta al giorno se controllato. *Adulti:* stessa dose oftalmica dei bambini.	*Effetti indesiderati:* broncospasmo, bradicardia, ipotensione, disturbi alla vista, congiuntivite, cheratiti.
Tioguanina Compresse: 40 mg.	**Trattamento delle leucemie (analogo della purina inibisce la sintesi e l'uso di nucleotidi purinici).** *Bambini <3 anni:* leucemia non linfocitica acuta: per os: 3,3 mg/kg/24 h in 2 dosi per 4 giorni. *Bambini >3 anni e adulti:* per os: 2-3 mg/kg al giorno (fino a circa 20 mg) fino alla remissione.	*Effetti indesiderati:* mielosoppressione (inizio, 7-10 giorni; nadir, 14 giorni; remissione, 21 giorni), nausea, vomito, diarrea, anoressia, stomatite, iperuricemia, andatura instabile.
Tiomalato di oro e sodio Iniezione: 25 mg/mL.	**Trattamento dell'artrite reumatoide (meccanismo sconosciuto).** *Bambini:* dose test: 10 mg im, seguita da 1 mg/kg im ogni sett per 20 sett, poi 1 mg/kg/dose ogni 2-4 sett (massimo: 50 mg/dose). *Adulti:* Dose test: 10 mg im, poi 25-50 mg/sett, poi 25-50 mg im ogni 2-4 sett dopo avere notato la risposta.	*Cautela:* il paziente dovrebbe stare seduto o sdraiato per 10 min dopo la dose; evitare nei pazienti con lupus eritematoso sistemico o discrasie ematiche. *Effetti indesiderati:* cefalea, flushing, convulsioni, dermatite esfoliativa, eritema nodoso, orticaria, alopecia, perdita di unghie, stomatite, gengivite, glossite, congiuntivite, eosinofilia, leucopenia, trombocitopenia, ematuria, proteinuria, sindrome nefrosica, fibrosi polmonare e polmonite interstiziale, epatotossicità, neuropatia periferica. *Monitoraggio:* concentrazioni seriche di oro (terapeutiche 1-3 μg/mL).
Tiopentale Barbiturato a ultra breve durata d'azione. Iniezione.	**Induzione dell'anestesia e mantenimento, convulsioni intrattabili, aumento della pressione endocranica.** *Neonati:* ev: anestesia: 3-4 mg/kg. Convulsioni: 2-3 mg/kg; ripetere dosi da 1 mg/kg se necessario. *Bambini piccoli e grandi:* ev: Anestesia: 5-8 mg/kg. Convulsioni: 2-3 mg/kg. Aumento della pressione endocranica: 1,5-5 mg/kg, ripetuta se necessario. *Adulti:* ev: 25-250 mg se necessario per l'effetto. Sedazione: Rettale: *Bambini:* 5-10 mg/kg/dose. *Adulti:* 3-4 g/dose.	*Effetti indesiderati:* crampi, diarrea, sanguinamento rettale, ipotensione, depressione miocardica, sonnolenza e risveglio prolungati, delirio acuto, depressione respiratoria, tosse, broncospasmo, laringospasmo, singhiozzo, starnuti. *Monitoraggio:* concentrazioni di tiopentale: terapeutiche: ipnosi: 1-5 μg/mL; anestesia: 7-130 μg/mL; coma: 30-100 μg/mL.
Tioridazina Concentrato orale: 30, 100 mg/mL. Sospensione orale: 25 mg/5 mL, 100 mg/5 mL. Compresse: 10, 15, 25, 50, 100, 150, 200 mg.	**Trattamento di psicosi, nevrosi e gravi alterazioni comportamentali nei bambini (fenotiazina; blocca i recettori dopaminergici nel cervello).** *Bambini >2 anni:* 0,5-3 mg/kg/24 h in 2-3 dosi per os. *Bambini >12 anni e adulti:* 25-800 mg/24 h in 2-4 dosi per os.	*Effetti indesiderati:* pseudoparkinsonismo, discinesia tardiva, acatisia, distonie, vertigini, sindrome neurolettica maligna, alterata regolazione della temperatura, ipotensione ortostatica, retinopatia pigmentosa, ittero colestatico, leucopenia, agranulocitosi, ritenzione urinaria, stipsi, secchezza delle fauci, gastrite, iperpigmentazione, fotosensibilità.
Tiotepa Agente alchilante. Iniezione.	**Chemioterapia tumorale (inibisce la sintesi di DNA, RNA e proteine).** *Bambini:* ev (dipende dal protocollo): dose regolare: 25-65 mg/m^2 ogni 3-4 sett; alte dosi: 300 mg/m^2/24 h per 3 dosi. *Adulti:* ev: infusione continua di 15-35 mg/m^2 per 48 h.	*Effetti indesiderati:* mielosoppressione (inizio, 7-10 giorni; nadir, 14 giorni; remissione, 28 giorni), vertigini, febbre, cefalea, anoressia, nausea, vomito, alopecia, rash, prurito, iperuricemia, ematuria, cistite emorragica, stomatite.
Tiotixene Iniezione. Capsule: 1, 2, 5, 10, 20 mg. Concentrato orale: 5 mg/mL.	**Trattamento della psicosi (fenotiazina; blocca i recettori dopaminergici del SNC).** *Bambini <12 anni:* 0,25 mg/kg/24 h in dosi suddivise. *Bambini >12 anni e adulti:* per os: 6-60 mg/24 h in 3 dosi. im: 4 mg bid-qid (massimo: 30 mg/24 h).	*Effetti indesiderati:* ipotensione ortostatica, pseudoparkinsonismo, discinesia tardiva, acatisia, distonia, stipsi, ritenzione urinaria, bocca secca, dolore allo stomaco, congestione nasale, retinopatia pigmentaria, agranulocitosi, leucopenia, sindrome neurolettica maligna, alterata regolazione della temperatura, tremore delle dita, ittero colestatico.
Tolazolina Iniezione: 25 mg/mL.	**Trattamento dell'ipertensione polmonare persistente (bloccante α-adrenergico e rilascio di istamina).** *Neonati:* ev: dose da carico di 1-2 mg/kg, poi 1-2 mg/kg/h in infusione continua.	*Effetti indesiderati:* ipotensione, flushing, tachicardia, aumento delle secrezioni dal tratto respiratorio e gastrointestinale; sanguinamento e perforazione gastrointestinale; oliguria; emorragia polmonare; trombocitopenia. *Monitoraggio:* saturazione dell'ossigeno preduttale e postduttale, emogasanalisi arteriosa.

TABELLA 716-1. Farmaci generali – *continua*

FARMACO (PRINCIPIO ATTIVO, FORMULAZIONI)	INDICAZIONI (MECCANISMO D'AZIONE E DOSAGGIO)	COMMENTI (CAUTELE, EFFETTI INDESIDERATI, MONITORAGGIO)
Tolmetin sodio Agente antinfiammatorio non steroideo; inibitore delle prostaglandine. Compresse: 200, 600 mg. Capsule: 400 mg.	**Trattamento dell'artrite reumatoide, inclusa l'artrite reumatoide giovanile.** *Bambini >2 anni:* per os: 15-30 mg/kg/24 h in 3-4 dosi. Analgesia: 5-7 mg/kg/dose. *Adulti:* 400-600 mg tid (massimo: 2 g/24 h).	*Effetti indesiderati:* gastrite, ulcera peptica, ipertensione, edema, vertigini, cefalea, insufficienza renale acuta, tinnito.
Topiramato Capsule: 15, 25 mg. Compresse: 25, 100, 200 mg.	**Trattamento delle convulsioni. Ampio spettro di tipologie di convulsioni coperte e meccanismi multipli proposti.** *Bambini 2-16 anni:* per os: iniziare con 1-3 mg/kg/24 h prima di andare a letto per 1 sett; titolare l'aumento della dose ogni 1-2 sett di 1-3 mg/kg/24 h dosato bid; dose tipica 5-10 mg/kg/24 h suddivisi ogni 12 h. La capsula può essere frantumata nel cibo per la somministrazione. *Adulti:* per os: iniziare con 25-50 mg ogni 24 h; aumentare di 25-50 mg/24 h ogni sett (massimo: 1600 mg/24 h). Ridurre la dose del 50% se CrCl <60 mL/min.	*Cautela:* se usato con altri inibitori dell'anidrasi carbonica, gli effetti additivi possono predisporre a calcoli renali.
Trazodone Compresse: 50, 100, 150, 300 mg.	**Antidepressivo (inibisce il reuptake della serotonina, bloccante α-adrenergico).** *Bambini 6-18 anni:* iniziare con 1,5-2 mg/kg/24 h in 3 dosi; si può aumentare ogni 3-4 giorni (massimo: 6 mg/kg/24 h). *Adolescenti:* iniziare 25-50 mg/24 h; si può aumentare gradualmente (massimo: 150 mg) in 2-3 dosi. *Adulti:* iniziare con 50 mg tid; si può aumentare di 50 mg.	*Effetti indesiderati:* cefalea, confusione, vertigini, secchezza delle fauci, nausea, cattivo sapore in bocca, stipsi, visione offuscata, tremori muscolari, ipotensione, tachicardia. *Interazioni farmacologiche:* la fluoxetina può aumentare i livelli. *Monitoraggio:* concentrazioni di trazodone (limitata correlazione con l'efficacia clinica): terapeutiche 0,5-2,5 μg/mL; tossiche >4 μg/mL.
Tretinoina Crema: 0,025%, 0,05%, 0,1%. Gel topico: 0,01%, 0,025%. Liquido topico: 0,05%.	**Trattamento dell'acne vulgaris, della cute foto-danneggata e di alcuni tumori cutanei (inibisce la formazione di micro comedoni ed elimina le lesioni).** *Bambini >12 anni:* applicare la formulazione più debole una volta al giorno prima di andare a letto. Aumentare se necessario.	*Effetti indesiderati:* eccessiva secchezza cutanea, eritema, desquamazione, bruciore e arrossamento locali; fotosensibilità (usare creme protettive per il sole), acne in fase eruttiva.
Triamcinolone Corticosteroide. Generico. Iniezione. Orale. Topico Inalatore a dosaggio controllato. Spruzzo nasale.	**Trattamento delle condizioni infiammatorie e allergiche.** *Bambini 6-12 anni:* im: 0,03-0,2 mg/kg ogni 1-7 giorni. MDI: 2 puff bid-qid. Intranasale: 1 spruzzo in ogni narice 1-2 volte/24 h. Iniezione: intra-articolare, intraborsale o nella guaina tendinea: 2,5-15 mg (ripetere se necessario). *Bambini >12 anni* e adulti: MDI: 2-4 puff bid-qid. Intranasale: 2 spruzzi in ogni narice al giorno (massimo: 4 spruzzi/24 h). Intra-articolare, intrasinoviale: 2,5-40 mg. per os: 40-100 mg/24 h in 1-4 dosi. Topico: applicare un film sottile bid-tid.	*Effetti indesiderati:* atrofia del tessuto in corrispondenza del sito di applicazione locale, affaticamento, cataratta, osteoporosi, candidiasi orale (con MDI), crescita ridotta. *Commento:* vedi il confronto tra i corticosteroidi alla voce *Idrocortisone*.
Triamterene Capsule: 50, 100 mg (farmaci in combinazione, per es. con idroclorotiazide).	**Diuretico per trattare l'edema o l'ipertensione (compete con l'aldosterone per i siti recettoriali nei tubuli renali distali).** *Bambini:* per os: 2-4 mg/kg/24 h in 1-2 dosi (massimo: 6 mg/kg/24 h). *Adulti:* 100-300 mg/24 h in 1-2 dosi.	*Cautela:* non usare nei pazienti con insufficienza renale; evitare concomitanti supplementi di potassio per evitare l'iperpotassemia. *Effetti indesiderati:* stipsi, nausea, cefalea, affaticamento, iperpotassemia, iponatriemia, acidosi metabolica ipercloremica.
Trientina Agente chelante. Capsule: 250 mg.	**Trattamento della malattia di Wilson nei pazienti che non possono tollerare la penicillamina.** *Bambini <12 anni:* 500-1500 mg/24 h in 2-4 dosi. *Bambini >12 anni e adulti:* 750-2000 mg/24 h in 2-4 dosi.	*Commento:* assumere 1 ora prima o 2 h dopo i pasti. Non rompere le capsule in alcun modo e assumere con un bicchiere pieno d'acqua. Se la capsula si rompe, irrigare in modo esauriente con acqua l'area di cute venuta a contatto con il contenuto. *Effetti indesiderati:* deficit di ferro anemia, malessere, dolore epigastrico, ispessimento e fissurazione della cute, crampi muscolari, lupus eritematoso sistemico.
Trifluorperazina Concentrato orale: 10 mg/mL. Compresse: 1, 2, 5, 10 mg. Iniezione.	**Trattamento della psicosi (fenotiazina; blocca la dopamina nel SNC).** *Bambini 6-12 anni:* per os: 1 mg 1-2 volte/24 h, gradualmente aumenta fino all'effetto (massimo: 15 mg/24 h). im: 1 mg bid. *>12 anni e adulti:* per os: 1-2 mg bid. im: 1-2 mg ogni 4-6 h se necessario (massimo: 10 mg/24 h).	*Effetti indesiderati:* ipotensione, tachicardia, aritmie, pseudoparkinsonismo, discinesia tardiva, acatisia, distonie stipsi, congestione nasale, secchezza delle fauci, ipertensione maligna.
Trigliceridi a catena media Olio: 14 g/15 mL.	**Supplemento dietetico per i soggetti che non possono digerire grassi a catena lunga, dieta chetogenica per i disordini convulsivanti (supplemento nutrizionale).** *Bambini piccoli:* 0,5 mL a pasti alterni; si può passare a 0,5 mL ogni 2-3 giorni se tollerato. *Bambini:* Dieta chetogenica per convulsioni: 50-70% delle calorie totali (di solito circa 40 mL a ogni pasto). Fibrosi cistica: 1 cpr tid. *Adulti:* 15 mL tid-qid.	*Effetti indesiderati:* nausea, vomito, dolore addominale, chetosi.
Trimetafan camsilato Bloccante adrenergico e colinergico. Iniezione.	**Trattamento delle emergenze ipertensive.** *Bambini:* 50-150 μg/kg/min. *Adulti:* 0,5-2 mg/min.	*Effetti indesiderati:* anoressia, nausea, secchezza delle fauci, ileo, ritenzione urinaria, cicloplegia, prurito, orticaria, apnea, ipotensione.

TABELLA 716-1. Farmaci generali – *continua*

FARMACO (PRINCIPIO ATTIVO, FORMULAZIONI)	INDICAZIONI (MECCANISMO D'AZIONE E DOSAGGIO)	COMMENTI (CAUTELE, EFFETTI INDESIDERATI, MONITORAGGIO)
Trimetobenzamide Capsule: 100, 250 mg. Supposta rettale: 100, 200 mg. Iniezione: 100 mg/mL.	**Controllo della nausea e vomito (inibisce la stimolazione SNC della zona trigger del chemorecettore).** *Bambini:* per os, rettale: 15-20 mg/kg/24 h in 3-4 dosi. *Adulti:* per os: 250 mg tid-qid. im, rettale: 200 mg tid-qid.	*Effetti indesiderati:* sonnolenza, vertigini, cefalea, diarrea, crampi muscolari.
Trombina, topico Polvere.	**Emostasi per sanguinamento minore dai capillari e delle venule (catalizza la conversione di fibrinogeno in fibrina).** *Bambini e adulti:* applicare come soluzione topica 1000-2000 U/mL direttamente sul sito.	*Effetti indesiderati:* allergia.
Trometamina Iniezione: 0,3M (1 mEq THAM = 3,3 mL).	**Correzione dell'acidosi metabolica (si combina con gli ioni idrogeno a formare bicarbonato e tampone).** *Neonati, bambini piccoli e grandi e adulti:* dose (mL di 0,3M soluzione) = peso (kg) × deficit di basi o 1-2 mEq/kg/dose.	*Effetti indesiderati:* apnea, ipoglicemia, iperpotassemia, irritazione tissutale o necrosi in caso di contatto diretto.
Tropicamide Soluzione oftalmica: 0,5%, 1%.	**Agente midriatico a breve durata d'azione (blocca il muscolo sfintere dell'iride e il corpo ciliare impedendo la risposta alla stimolazione colinergica).** *Bambini e adulti:* Cicloplegia: Instillare 1-2 gocce di soluzione all'1%; si può ripetere in 5 min. Midriasi: Instillare 1-2 gocce di soluzione allo 0,5% 15-20 min prima dell'esame.	*Effetti indesiderati:* tachicardia, sonnolenza, cefalea, secchezza delle fauci, visione offuscata, fotofobia.
Tubocurarina Iniezione.	**Bloccante neuromuscolare usato in anestesia (blocca i recettori dell'acetilcolina).** *Neonati:* iniziare 0,3 mg/kg; dose di mantenimento di 0,1 mg/kg/dose. *Bambini:* iniziare 0,2-0,5 mg/kg, poi dose di mantenimento di 0,04-0,1 mg/kg/dose. *Adulti:* iniziare 6-9 mg, poi dose di mantenimento di 3-4,5 mg.	*Effetti indesiderati:* ipotensione, depressione respiratoria prolungata.
Urochinasi Iniezione.	**Agente trombolitico per il trattamento della trombosi di inizio recente (attiva la conversione del plasminogeno in plasmina).** *Neonati, bambini piccoli e grandi e adulti:* ev: dose da carico di 4400 U/kg; dose di mantenimento o 4000-10 000 U/kg/h. Catetere ev occluso: Riempire l'intero volume del catetere con urochinasi 5000 U/mL e lasciare nel lume per 1-4 h.	*Effetti indesiderati:* sanguinamento, ematoma, reazioni allergiche, broncospasmo. *Monitoraggio:* D-dimero, prodotti di degradazione della fibrina, tempo di coagulazione attivato.
Ursodiolo, acido ursodesossicolico Capsule: 300 mg. Può essere costituito da formulazioni estemporanee.	**Dissoluzione del calcolo della colecisti, contrasta la colestasi indotta dalla nutrizione parenterale totale nei neonati (diminuisce il contenuto di colesterolo della bile).** *Neonati:* per os: 10-18 mg/kg/24 h suddivisi in 1-3 dosi giorno. *Bambini piccoli:* 30 mg/kg/24 h suddivisi ogni 8-12 h. *Adulti:* 300 mg prima di andare a letto per 6-12 mesi.	*Effetti indesiderati:* diarrea, dispepsia, dolore biliare, rinite, prurito, cefalea.
Vasopressina Analogo dell'ormone antidiuretico. Iniezione: 20 pressor U/mL.	**Trattamento del diabete insipido; prevenzione e trattamento della distensione addominale postoperatoria; trattamento dell'emorragia gastrointestinale acuta.** *Bambini:* Diabete insipido: im, sc: 2,5-10 U/dose bid-qid. Emorragia gastrointestinale: ev: infusione continua di 0,002-0,01 U/kg/min. *Adulti:* Diabete insipido: im, sc: 5-10 U/dose bid-qid. Emorragia gastrointestinale. ev: infusione continua di 0,2-0,4 U/min.	*Effetti indesiderati:* aumento della pressione arteriosa, bradicardia, aritmie, febbre, flatulenza, crampi addominali, nausea, vomito, tremore, sudorazione, pallore periorale, intossicazione da acqua.
Vecuronio Iniezione.	**Aggiunta all'anestesia, bloccante neuromuscolare (impedisce il legame dell'acetilcolina con le placche motrici terminali).** *Neonati:* 0,03-0,15 mg/kg/dose ogni 1-2 h se necessario. *Bambini piccoli >7 sett-12 mesi:* 0,05-0,1 mg/kg ogni h se necessario. *Bambini 1 anno-adulti:* 0,05-0,1 mg/kg ogni ora se necessario.	*Effetti indesiderati:* tachicardia, ipotensione, flushing, bradicardia, collasso circolatorio, reazioni da ipersensibilità.
Venlafaxina Inibitore del reuptake della serotonina e della noradrenalina. Compresse: 25, 37,5, 50, 75, 100 mg.	**Trattamento di depressione, disturbo ossessivo-compulsivo, distrubo da deficit dell'attenzione** *Bambini:* 25-200 mg/24 h; iniziare a basse dosi e titolare fino all'effetto ogni 4-7 giorni. *Adulti:* iniziare 75 mg/24 h; titolare ogni 4-7 giorni fino all'effetto (massimo: 375 mg/24 h).	*Cautela:* ridurre lentamente (massimo: 25 mg/24 h ogni 5-7 giorni) se si interrompe il farmaco per evitare la sindrome da astinenza. *Effetti indesiderati:* cefalea, sonnolenza, vertigini, insonnia, nervosismo, nausea, secchezza delle fauci, stipsi, visione offuscata.
Verapamil Capsule, rilascio prolungato: 120, 180, 240, 360 mg. Compresse: 40, 80, 120 mg. Compresse, rilascio prolungato: 120, 180, 240 mg. Iniezione.	**Calcioantagonista usato per trattare l'ipertensione e le aritmie sopraventricolari.** Dosi nei bambini piccoli e giovani non ben stabilite. *Bambini piccoli:* ev: 0,1-0,2 mg/kg dose ripetuta fino all'effetto desiderato. *Bambini:* ev: 0,1-0,3 mg/kg dose ripetuta fino all'effetto desiderato. *Bambini:* per os: 4-8 mg/kg/24 h ogni 6-8 h; dose abituale 5 mg/kg/24 h. *Adulti:* per os: 240-480 mg/24 h suddivisi ogni 6-8 h; ogni 12 h con prodotti a rilascio-prolungato. Si può rompere il contenuto della capsula nel cibo molle senza che ciò alteri l'assorbimento del farmaco.	*Cautela:* aggiustare la dose nella malattia renale. Evitare l'uso ev nei neonati e nei bambini piccoli giovani o in quelli con scompenso cardiaco. *Effetti indesiderati:* ipotensione, bradicardia, blocco cardiaco, vertigini, convulsioni, dolore addominale. Evitare nei neonati perché molti casi fatali riportati in seguito a blocco cardiaco. *Interazioni farmacologiche:* può aumentare le concentrazioni di caffeina, digossina, carbamazepina, ciclosporina; diminuite concentrazioni con rifampicina, fenobarbital.
Vigabatrin Bustina di polvere secca. Compresse: 500 mg.	**Efficace contro gli spasmi infantili, le convulsioni parziali e altri tipi di convulsioni. Inibitore dell'acido γ-aminobutirrico transaminasi.** *Bambini:* 40-150 mg/kg/24 h in 1-2 dosi.	*Cautela:* può causare deficit bilaterale del campo visivo; eseguire un esame basale dell'occhio e poi ogni 6 mesi. Depressione del SNC, possono verificarsi reazioni psichiatriche, problemi comportamentali e intolleranza gastrointestinale.

TABELLA 716-1. Farmaci generali – *continua*

FARMACO (PRINCIPIO ATTIVO, FORMULAZIONI)	INDICAZIONI (MECCANISMO D'AZIONE E DOSAGGIO)	COMMENTI (CAUTELE, EFFETTI INDESIDERATI, MONITORAGGIO)
Vinblastina solfato Iniezione.	**Terapia di molti tumori (si lega al fuso mitotico per inibire la metafase).** *Bambini:* Malattia di Hodgkin: ev: 2,5-6 mg/m²/24 h ogni 1-2 sett per 3-6 sett (massimo: 12,5 mg/m²/sett). *Adulti:* 3,7-18,5 mg/m²/24 h ogni 7-10 giorni.	*Effetti indesiderati:* alopecia, nausea, vomito, crampi addominali, stipsi, diarrea, stomatite, mielosoppressione (inizio, 4-7 giorni; nadir, 4-10 giorni; remissione, 17 giorni), tachicardia, ipotensione ortostatica, dermatite, fotosensibilità, dolore muscolare, parestesie, ritenzione urinaria, iperuricemia, neuropatia periferica (perdita dei riflessi tendinei profondi, cefalea, debolezza).
Vincristina Iniezione.	**Trattamento di vari tumori (si lega al fuso mitotico per inibire la metafase).** *Bambini:* *<10 kg o area di superficie corporea <1 m²:* 0,05 mg/kg ogni/sett. *>10 kg o area di superficie corporea >1 m²:* 1-2 mg/m² ogni/sett. *Adulti:* 0,4-1,4 mg/m² ogni/sett.	*Effetti indesiderati:* stipsi, ileo paralitico, depressione, confusione, insonnia, cefalea, dolore mandibolare, atrofia ottica, cecità, perdita dei riflessi tendinei profondi delle gambe, parestesia, formicolio, dolore, bruciore e parestesie a calza e a guanto, piede cadente, polso cadente, sindrome da inappropriata secrezione di ormone antidiuretico, fotofobia, iperuricemia, stomatite, flebite, mielosoppressione (inizio, 7 giorni; nadir, 10 giorni; remissione, 21 giorni).
Violetto di genziana Soluzione topica: 1%, 2%.	**Trattamento delle infezioni cutanee e mucocutanee (uccide la Candida, le specie di stafilococco e alcuni batteri gram-positivi vegetativi).** *Bambini piccoli:* applicare 3-4 gocce di soluzione 0,5% sublinguale o sulla lesione dopo i pasti. *Bambini e adulti:* applicare 0,5-2% con cotone alla lesione bid-tid per 3 giorni.	*Cautela:* non deglutire. *Effetti indesiderati:* bruciore, irritazione locale o reazioni da sensibilità.
Vitamina A Iniezione. Gocce orali. Capsule.	**Trattamento o prevenzione del deficit; supplementazione nei pazienti con morbillo (cofattore per molti processi biochimici); migliora la crescita nei bambini con HIV o malaria. Prevenzione della displasia broncopolmonare nei neonati.** *Neonati:* im: 4000 UI 3× sett, o 2000 UI im a giorni alterni. Deficit di vitamina A con xeroftalmia: *Bambini 1-8 anni:* per os: 5000 U/24 h per 5 giorni; im: 5000-15 000 U/24 h per 10 giorni. *Bambini >8 anni e adulti:* per os: 500 000 U/24 h per 3 giorni, poi 50 000 U/24 h per 14 giorni, poi 20 000 U/24 h per 2 mesi. Deficit di vitamina A senza alterazioni corneali: *Bambini <1 anno:* im: 100 000 unità ogni 4-6 mesi. *>1 anno:* im: 200 000 unità ogni 4-6 mesi. *>8 anni e adulti:* im: 100 000 U/24 h per 3 giorni, poi 50,000 U/24 h per 14 giorni. Profilassi nei pazienti a rischio e supplementazione nel morbillo: Dose per os ogni 4-6 mesi. *Bambini <1 anno:* 100 000 unità. *>1 anni:* 200 000 unità Miglioramento della crescita nei bambini con HIV, malaria, o diarrea: *Bambini piccoli <1 anno:* 100 000 U/24 h per 2 dosi, poi 100 000 unità (1 dose) a 4 e 8 mesi. *Bambini >1 anno:* 200 000 U/24 h per 2 dosi, poi 200 000 unità (1 dose) a 4 e 8 mesi	*Effetti indesiderati:* irritabilità, vertigine, letargia, febbre, cefalea, ipercalcemia.
Vitamina E Capsule, gocce orali, compresse, crema, pomata.	**Supplemento nutrizionale (antiossidante).** *Neonati, bambini piccoli prematuri:* per os 25-50 U/24 h. *Bambini:* per os 1 U/kg/24 h. Anemia a cellule falciformi: per os 450 U/24 h. Fibrosi cistica: per os 100-400 U/24 h. β-talassemia: per os 750 U/24 h. *Adulti:* per os 60-75 U/24 h.	*Effetti indesiderati:* rari.
Warfarin Compresse: 1, 2, 2,5, 4, 5, 7,5, 10 mg.	**Anticoagulante che antagonizza la sintesi epatica di vitamina K, riducendo i fattori II, VII, IX e X vitamina K-dipendenti.** *Bambini:* per os: dose iniziale di 0,2 mg/kg, poi dose usuale intorno a 0,1 mg/kg/24 h. Dose titolata in base ai target desiderati di tempo di protrombina e INR (*International Normalized Ratio*). Evitare dosi da carico elevate perché un completo effetto anticoagulante dipende dall'emivita di eliminazione dei fattori di coagulazione target. Gli effetti completi possono non essere osservati prima di 2-3 giorni dopo un aggiustamento della dose di warfarin, annullando rapidi cambiamenti della dose.	*Cautela:* nei bambini piccoli più giovani sono necessarie dosi più alte (dose tipica media: 0,3 mg/kg/24 h). Evitare cibi con alto contenuto di vitamina K (vegetali a foglie verdi). *Effetti indesiderati:* sanguinamento, necrosi cutanea, emottisi. *Interazioni farmacologiche:* acido acetilsalicilico, barbiturici, carbamazepina, cimetidina, omeprazolo, fenitoina, rifampicina, vitamina K, ritonavir, delavirdina.
Xilometazolina Soluzione nasale: 0,05%, 0,1%.	**Sollievo sintomatico della congestione nasale (stimola i recettori α-adrenergici a produrre vasocostrizione).** *Bambini 2-12 anni:* instillare 2-3 gocce di soluzione 0,05% in ogni narice ogni 8-10 ore. *Bambini >12 anni e adulti:* instillare 2-3 gocce di soluzione 0,1% in ogni narice ogni 8-10 ore.	*Cautela:* non usare per più di 4 giorni consecutivi e non superare il dosaggio raccomandato perché può causare congestione da rebound e polmonite chimica e creare dipendenza. *Effetti indesiderati:* palpitazioni, cefalea, vertigini, sonnolenza, sudorazione, visione offuscata.
Zafirlukast Compresse: 20 mg.	**Antagonista del leukotriene D4 e E4, inibisce l'effetto delle sostanze a lenta reazione dell'anafilassi sulla muscolatura liscia bronchiale. Non efficace nel trattare la broncocostrizione acuta, sebbene la terapia possa essere continuata negli attacchi acuti.** *Bambini 7-11anni:* per os: 20 mg/24 h suddivisi ogni 12 h. *Adolescenti e adulti:* per os: 40 mg/24 h suddivisi ogni 12 h. Somministrare 1 ora prima o 2 h dopo i pasti.	*Cautela:* in base al meccanismo d'azione, questo farmaco è efficace per la profilassi e non antagonizza la broncocostrizione. *Effetti indesiderati:* cefalea, nausea, dispepsia, aumento dei test di funzionalità epatica. *Interazioni farmacologiche:* blocca gli isoenzimi epatici CYP2C9 e 3A4; macrolidi, teofillina, carbamazepina, terfenadina, astemizolo.

TABELLA 716-1. Farmaci generali – *continua*

FARMACO (PRINCIPIO ATTIVO, FORMULAZIONI)	INDICAZIONI (MECCANISMO D'AZIONE E DOSAGGIO)	COMMENTI (CAUTELE, EFFETTI INDESIDERATI, MONITORAGGIO)
Zileuton Compresse: 600 mg.	**Inibitore della 5-lipossigenasi inibendo la formazione dei leucotrieni LTB1, LTC1, LTD_1, e LTE_1, Non efficace nel trattare la broncocostrizione acuta, sebbene la terapia possa essere continuata negli attacchi acuti.** *Adolescenti e adulti:* per os: 2400 mg/24 h suddivisi ogni 6 h.	*Cautela:* in base al meccanismo d'azione, questo farmaco è efficace per la profilassi e non antagonizza la broncocostrizione. *Effetti indesiderati:* dolore toracico, cefalea, nausea, dispepsia, aumento dei test di funzionalità epatica. *Interazioni farmacologiche:* macrolidi, teofillina, propranololo, warfarin, terfenadina, astemizolo.
Zinco, supplementi dello Iniezione, liquido, compresse.	**Prevenzione e trattamento del deficit di zinco (terapia sostitutiva).** Deficit di zinco: per os: *Bambini piccoli e grandi:* 0,5-1 mg/kg/24 h in 1-3 dosi. *Adulti:* 25-50 mg/dose tid. Supplemento TPN: *Bambini piccoli pretermine:* 400 μg/kg/24 h. *Bambini piccoli <3 mesi:* 250 μg/kg/24 h. *Bambini piccoli >3 mesi:* 100 μg/kg/24 h. *Bambini grandi:* 50 μg/kg/24 h.	*Effetti indesiderati:* rari, ma se sono usate dosi eccessive, può causare deficit di rame.
Ziprasidone Capsule: 20, 40, 60, 80 mg.	**Antipsicotico atipico.** *Bambini:* iniziare 5 mg/24 h; aumentare ogni 48 h fino alla risposta. Dose bid. *Adulti:* iniziare 20 mg bid; aumentare ogni 48 h fino alla risposta (massimo: 80 mg bid).	*Cautela:* può prolungare l'intervallo OTc e predisporre ad aritmie (specialmente torsioni di punta); evitare uso concomitante di altri farmaci che possono prolungare l'intervallo QTc. *Effetti indesiderati:* agitazione, ansia, vertigini, sonnolenza, cefalea, insonnia, tachicardia, stipsi, secchezza delle fauci, ipotensione ortostatica, aumento di peso. *Interazioni farmacologiche:* gli inibitori del CYP3A4 diminuiranno la clearance e predisporranno alla tossicità. Gli induttori enzimatici aumenteranno la clearance e potranno aumentare le dosi necessarie.
Zonisamide Capsule (gelatina): 100 mg.	**Trattamento dei disordini convulsivi. Meccanismo incerto.** *Bambini:* iniziare 2-4 mg/kg/24 h; poi aumentare di 2-5 mg/kg/24 h ogni 2-4 giorni fino alla risposta, di solito 4-20 mg/kg/24 h. *Adulti:* iniziare con 100 mg/24 h; si può aumentare di 100 mg/24 h ogni 2 sett (massimo: 600 mg/24 h).	*Cautela:* i bambini sono predisposti a ipoidrosi e ipertermia con questo farmaco. Effetti indesiderati molto comuni sono sonnolenza, rash e calcoli renali.

Indice analitico

I numeri di pagina seguiti dalla f indicano le figure, quelli seguiti dalla t indicano le tabelle.

C

O